P9-DTK-403

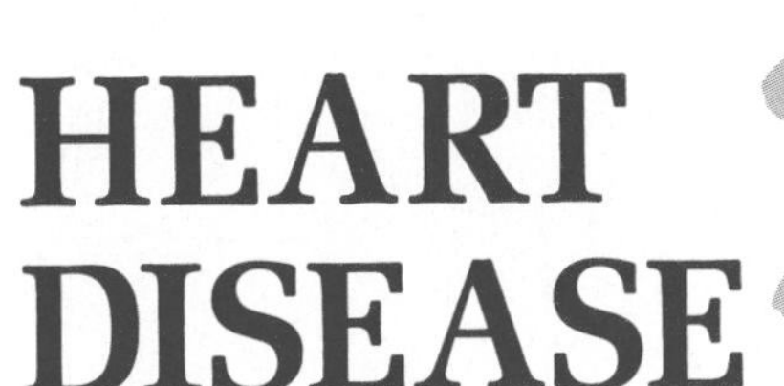

A Textbook of
Cardiovascular Medicine

Fourth Edition

HEART DISEASE

A Textbook of Cardiovascular Medicine

Edited by

EUGENE BRAUNWALD,
A.B., M.D., M.A. (hon.), M.D. (hon.), Sc.D. (hon.), F.R.C.P.

Hersey Professor of the Theory and Practice of Medicine,
Harvard Medical School;
Chairman, Department of Medicine,
Brigham and Women's Hospital, Boston

W. B. SAUNDERS COMPANY

Harcourt Brace Jovanovich, Inc.

Philadelphia, London, Toronto, Montreal, Sydney, Tokyo

W. B. SAUNDERS COMPANY
Harcourt Brace Jovanovich, Inc.

The Curtis Center
Independence Square West
Philadelphia, PA 19106

Library of Congress Cataloging-in-Publication Data

Heart disease : a textbook of cardiovascular medicine / edited by
Eugene Braunwald. — 4th ed.
p. cm.
Includes bibliographical references and index.
ISBN 0-7216-3097-9 (single volume). — ISBN
0-7216-3096-0 (set]. — ISBN 0-7216-2943-1 (v. 1). — ISBN
0-7216-3094-4 (v. 2)
1. Heart— Diseases. 2. Cardiovascular system—Diseases.
I. Braunwald, Eugene
[DNLM: 1. Heart Diseases. WG 200 H4364]
RC681.H362 1992
616.1′2—dc20
DNLM/DLC 91-27954

Manuscript Editor: Edna Dick
Production Manager: Frank Polizzano
Illustration Coordinator: Joan Sinclair
Indexer: Mark Coyle

ISBN Single Volume 0-7216-3097-9
ISBN Set 0-7216-3096-0
ISBN Volume 1 0-7216-2943-1
ISBN Volume 2 0-7216-3094-4

HEART DISEASE

Printed in the United States of America.

Last digit is the print number: 9 8 7 6 5 4 3 2

Dedicated to
NINA
KAREN, ALLISON, JILL
and
DANA

CONTRIBUTORS

ELLIOTT M. ANTMAN, M.D.

Associate Professor of Medicine, Harvard Medical School. Director, Samuel A. Levine Cardiac Unit, Cardiovascular Division, Department of Medicine, Brigham and Women's Hospital, Boston, Massachusetts

Medical Management of the Patient Undergoing Cardiac Surgery

DONALD S. BAIM, M.D.

Associate Professor of Medicine, Harvard Medical School. Director of Invasive Cardiology, Beth Israel Hospital, Boston, Massachusetts

Interventional Catheterization Techniques: Percutaneous Transluminal Balloon Angioplasty, Valvuloplasty, and Related Procedures

S. SERGE BAROLD, M.D.

Professor of Medicine, University of Rochester School of Medicine and Dentistry. Chief, Cardiology Division, Department of Medicine, The Genesee Hospital, Rochester, New York

Cardiac Pacemakers and Antiarrhythmic Devices

WILLIAM H. BARRY, M.D.

Nora Eccles Harrison Professor of Cardiology, University of Utah School of Medicine. Attending Physician, University of Utah Medical Center, Salt Lake City, Utah

Cardiac Catheterization

EUGENE BRAUNWALD, A.B., M.D., M.A.(hon.), M.D.(hon.), Sc.D.(hon.), F.R.C.P.

Hersey Professor of the Theory and Practice of Medicine, Harvard Medical School. Chairman, Department of Medicine, Brigham and Women's Hospital, Boston, Massachusetts.

The History; The Physical Examination; Mechanisms of Cardiac Contraction and Relaxation; Pathophysiology of Heart Failure; Assessment of Cardiac Function; Clinical Aspects of Heart Failure; The Management of Heart Failure; Pulmonary Edema: Cardiogenic and Noncardiogenic; Pulmonary Hypertension; Valvular Heart Disease; Coronary Blood Flow and Myocardial Ischemia; Acute Myocardial Infarction; Chronic Ischemic Heart Disease; The Cardiomyopathies and Myocarditides: Toxic, Chemical, and Physical Damage to the Heart; Primary Tumors of the Heart; Pericardial Disease; Traumatic Heart Disease; Pulmonary Embolism; Cor Pulmonale; General Anesthesia and Noncardiac Surgery in Patients with Heart Disease; Hematological-Oncological Disorders and Heart Disease; Endocrine and Nutritional Disorders and Heart Disease; Renal Disorders and Heart Disease

AGUSTIN CASTELLANOS, M.D.

Professor of Medicine, University of Miami School of Medicine. Director, Clinical Electrophysiology, Jackson Memorial Medical Center, Miami, Florida

Cardiac Arrest and Sudden Cardiac Death

BERNARD R. CHAITMAN, M.D.

Professor of Medicine, St. Louis University School of Medicine. Director, Division of Cardiology, St. Louis University Medical Center, St. Louis, Missouri

Exercise Stress Testing

PETER F. COHN, M.D.

Professor of Medicine and Chief, Cardiology Division, State University of New York Health Sciences Center, Stony Brook, New York

Traumatic Heart Disease

WILSON S. COLUCCI, M.D.

Associate Professor of Medicine, Harvard Medical School. Associate Physician, Cardiovascular Division, Brigham and Women's Hospital, Boston, Massachusetts

Primary Tumors of the Heart

CHARLES A. DENNIS, M.D.

Director, Comprehensive Cardiac Therapy, Scripps Clinic and Research Foundation, La Jolla, California

Rehabilitation of Patients with Coronary Artery Disease

ROMAN W. DeSANCTIS, M.D.

Professor of Medicine, Harvard Medical School. Physician, Director of Clinical Cardiology, Massachusetts General Hospital, Boston, Massachusetts

Diseases of the Aorta

KIM A. EAGLE, M.D.

Assistant Professor of Medicine, Harvard Medical School. Assistant Chief of Medicine-Residency Training, and Co-Director of Cardiology Fellowship Training, Massachusetts General Hospital, Boston, Massachusetts

Diseases of The Aorta

URI ELKAYAM, M.D.

Professor of Medicine, University of Southern California School of Medicine. Chief of Cardiology, USC University Hospital, Los Angeles, California

Pregnancy and Cardiovascular Disease

JOHN A. FARMER, M.D.

Associate Professor, Department of Medicine, Baylor College of Medicine. Associate Physician, Internal Medicine and Cardiology Service, The Methodist Hospital; Associate Physician, Ben Taub General Hospital, Houston, Texas

Risk Factors for Coronary Artery Disease

HARVEY FEIGENBAUM, M.D.

Distinguished Professor of Medicine, and Director, Hemodynamic Laboratory, Indiana University School of Medicine. Senior Research Associate, Krannert Institute of Cardiology, Indianapolis, Indiana

Echocardiography

CHARLES FISCH, M.D.

Distinguished Professor of Medicine, Indiana University School of Medicine, Indianapolis, Indiana

Electrocardiography and Vectorcardiography

WILLIAM F. FRIEDMAN, M.D.

J. H. Nicholson Professor of Pediatrics and Executive Chairman, Department of Pediatrics, University of California, Los Angeles, School of Medicine. Pediatrician-in-Chief, University of California at Los Angeles Medical Center, Los Angeles, California

Congenital Heart Disease in Infancy and Childhood; Acquired Heart Disease in Infancy and Childhood

GEOFFREY A. GARDINER, Jr., M.D.

Associate Professor of Radiology, Jefferson Medical College of Thomas Jefferson University. Director of Cardiovascular and Interventional Radiology, Thomas Jefferson University Hospital, Philadelphia, Pennsylvania

Coronary Arteriography

GARY GERSTENBLITH, M.D.

Associate Professor of Medicine, Johns Hopkins Hospital and Francis Scott Key Medical Center, Baltimore, Maryland

Aging and The Heart

SAMUEL Z. GOLDHABER, M.D.

Associate Professor of Medicine, Harvard Medical School. Associate Physician, Brigham and Women's Hospital, Boston, Massachusetts

Pulmonary Embolism

LEE GOLDMAN, M.D.

Professor of Medicine, Harvard Medical School. Vice-Chairman, Department of Medicine, Brigham and Women's Hospital, and Chief, Division of Clinical Epidemiology, Brigham and Women's Hospital and Beth Israel Hospital, Boston, Massachusetts

Cost-Effective Strategies in Cardiology; General Anesthesia and Noncardiac Surgery in Patients with Heart Disease

ANTONIO M. GOTTO, JR., M.D., D.Phil.

Professor of Medicine, and Chairman, Department of Medicine, Baylor College of Medicine. Chief, Internal Medicine Service, The Methodist Hospital, Houston, Texas

Risk Factors for Coronary Artery Disease

WILLIAM GROSSMAN, M.D.

Herman Dana Professor of Medicine, Harvard Medical School. Chief, Cardiovascular Division, Beth Israel Hospital, Boston, Massachusetts

Cardiac Catheterization; Clinical Aspects of Heart Failure; Pulmonary Hypertension

ROBERT I. HANDIN, M.D.

Associate Professor of Medicine, Harvard Medical School. Chief, Hematology Division, Brigham and Women's Hospital, Boston, Massachusetts

Hemostasis, Thrombosis, Fibrinolysis, and Cardiovascular Disease

CHARLES B. HIGGINS, M.D.

Professor of Radiology, University of California at San Francisco School of Medicine. Chief, Magnetic Resonance Imaging, University of California at San Francisco Medical Center, San Francisco, California

Newer Cardiac Imaging Techniques (CT, MRI)

ROLAND H. INGRAM, JR., M.D.

Professor and Vice Chairman of Medicine, University of Minnesota Medical School. Chief of Internal Medicine, Hennepin County Medical Center, Minneapolis, Minnesota

Pulmonary Edema: Cardiogenic and Noncardiogenic

NORMAN M. KAPLAN, M.D.

Professor of Internal Medicine, University of Texas Southwestern Medical School, Dallas, Texas

Systemic Hypertension: Mechanisms and Diagnosis; Systemic Hypertension: Therapy

WISHWA N. KAPOOR, M.D.

Professor of Medicine, University of Pittsburgh. Attending Physician, Presbyterian-University Hospital, Pittsburgh, Pennsylvania

Hypotension and Syncope

DONALD KAYE, M.D.

Professor and Chairman, Department of Medicine, Medical College of Pennsylvania. Chief of Medicine, Hospital of Medical College of Pennsylvania; Consultant, Philadelphia Veterans Administration Medical Center, Philadelphia, Pennsylvania

Infective Endocarditis

RALPH A. KELLY, M.D.

Assistant Professor of Medicine, Harvard Medical School. Associate Physician, Division of Cardiology, Department of Medicine, Brigham and Women's Hospital, Boston, Massachusetts

The Management of Heart Failure

OKSANA M. KORZENIOWSKI, M.D.

Associate Professor, Medical College of Pennsylvania, Philadelphia, Pennsylvania

Infective Endocarditis

EDWARD G. LAKATTA, M.D.

Professor of Medicine, Johns Hopkins University School of Medicine, and Professor of Physiology, University of Maryland School of Medicine. Visiting Physician, Francis Scott Key Medical Center, Baltimore, Maryland

Aging and The Heart

DAVID C. LEVIN, M.D.

Professor of Radiology, Jefferson Medical College of Thomas Jefferson University. Chairman, Department of Radiology, Thomas Jefferson University Hospital, Philadelphia, Pennsylvania

Radiology of the Heart; Coronary Arteriography

BEVERLY H. LORELL, M.D.

Associate Professor of Medicine, Harvard Medical School. Co-Director, Hemodynamic Research Laboratory, Beth Israel Hospital, Boston, Massachusetts

Pericardial Disease

JOSEPH LOSCALZO, M.D., PH.D.

Associate Professor of Medicine, Harvard Medical School. Director, Center for Research in Thrombolysis, Brigham and Women's Hospital; Chief, Cardiology Section, Brockton/West Roxbury Veteran's Administration Medical Center, Boston, Massachusetts

Hemostasis, Thrombosis, Fibrinolysis, and Cardiovascular Disease

VIJAK MAHDAVI, PH.D.

Associate Professor, Department of Pediatrics (Genetics), Harvard Medical School. Associate in Cardiology, Children's Hospital, Boston, Massachusetts

General Principles of Cardiovascular Cellular and Molecular Biology

MELVIN L. MARCUS, M.D. (Deceased)

Professor, Department of Internal Medicine, College of Medicine, The University of Iowa. Director, Coronary Physiology Laboratory, and Director, Specialized Center of Research in Ischemic Heart Disease, The University of Iowa College of Medicine; Consultant Physician, Department of Veterans Affairs Medical Center, Iowa City, Iowa

Relative Merits of Imaging Techniques

E. REGIS MCFADDEN, JR., M.D.

Argyle J. Beams Professor of Medicine, Case Western Reserve University School of Medicine. Director, Airway Disease Center, University Hospitals of Cleveland, Cleveland, Ohio

Cor Pulmonale

ROBERT J. MYERBURG, M.D.

Professor of Medicine and Physiology, and Director of the Division of Cardiology, University of Miami School of Medicine. Chief of Cardiology Services, Jackson Memorial Hospital, Miami, Florida

Cardiac Arrest and Sudden Cardiac Death

BERNARDO NADAL-GINARD, M.D., PH.D.

Alexander S. Nadas Professor of Pediatrics and Cellular and Molecular Physiology, Harvard Medical School. Chairman, Department of Cardiology, Children's Hospital, Boston, Massachusetts

General Principles of Cardiovascular Cellular and Molecular Biology

STEPHEN O. PASTAN, M.D.

Assistant Professor of Medicine, Indiana University School of Medicine. Attending Physician, Indiana University Hospitals, Indianapolis, Indiana

Renal Disorders and Heart Disease

RICHARD C. PASTERNAK, M.D.

Assistant Professor of Medicine, Harvard Medical School. Director, Coronary Care Unit, Beth Israel Hospital, Boston, Massachusetts

Acute Myocardial Infarction

D. GLENN PENNINGTON, M.D.

Professor of Surgery, and Director of Heart Replacement Services, St. Louis University Medical Center. Director of Cardiac Surgery, Cardinal Glennon Children's Hospital, St. Louis, Missouri

Assisted Circulation and the Mechanical Heart

JOSEPH K. PERLOFF, M.D.

Streisand/American Heart Association Professor of Medicine and Pediatrics, University of California, Los Angeles, School of Medicine. Division of Cardiology, Departments of Medicine and Pediatrics, UCLA Center for the Health Sciences, Los Angeles, California

Heart Sounds and Murmurs; Congenital Heart Disease in Adults; Neurological Disorders and Heart Disease

REED E. PYERITZ, M.D., PH.D.

Professor of Medicine and Pediatrics, Johns Hopkins University School of Medicine. Clinical Director, Center for Medical Genetics, Johns Hopkins Hospital, Baltimore, Maryland

Genetics and Cardiovascular Disease

ERIC C. RACKOW, M.D.

Professor and Chairman, Department of Medicine, St. Vincent's Hospital and Medical Center of New York Medical College, New York, New York

Acute Circulatory Failure

BRUCE A. REITZ, M.D.

Professor of Surgery, Johns Hopkins University School of Medicine. Cardiac Surgeon-in-Charge of New York Medical College, Johns Hopkins Hospital; Attending Cardiac Surgeon, Sinai Hospital, Baltimore, Maryland

Heart and Heart-Lung Transplantation

DAVID S. ROSENTHAL, M.D.

Associate Professor of Medicine, Harvard Medical School; Henry K. Oliver Professor of Hygiene, Harvard University. Physician and Hematologist, Brigham and Women's Hospital; Director and Physician, University Health Services, Harvard University, Boston, Massachusetts

Hematological-Oncological Disorders and Heart Disease

JOHN ROSS, JR., M.D.

Professor of Medicine, and Co-Director, Scientific Affairs, Department of Medicine, Division of Cardiology, University of California at San Diego. Attending Physician, University of California at San Diego Medical Center, San Diego, California; Editor-in-Chief, *Circulation*

Mechanisms of Cardiac Contraction and Relaxation

RUSSELL ROSS, PH.D., D.D.S.
Professor and Chairman of Pathology, University of Washington, Seattle, Washington
The Pathogenesis of Atherosclerosis

JOHN D. RUTHERFORD, M.B., Ch.B., F.R.A.C.P.
Assistant Professor of Medicine, Harvard Medical School. Co-Director, Clinical Cardiology Service, Brigham and Women's Hospital, Boston, Massachusetts
Chronic Ischemic Heart Disease

HEINRICH R. SCHELBERT, M.D.
Professor of Radiological Sciences, Division of Nuclear Medicine and Biophysics, Department of Radiological Sciences, University of California at Los Angeles School of Medicine. Principal Investigator, The Laboratory of Nuclear Medicine and The Laboratory of Biomedical and Environmental Sciences, University of California at Los Angeles, Los Angeles, California
Relative Merits of Imaging Techniques

DAVID J. SKORTON, M.D.
Professor and Associate Chair for Clinical Programs, Department of Internal Medicine, College of Medicine, and Professor, Department of Electrical and Computer Engineering, College of Engineering, University of Iowa. Consultant Physician, Department of Veterans Affairs Medical Center, Iowa City, Iowa
Relative Merits of Imaging Techniques

THOMAS W. SMITH, A.B., M.D.
Professor of Medicine, Harvard Medical School. Chief, Cardiovascular Division, and Senior Physician, Brigham and Women's Hospital, Boston, Massachusetts
The Management of Heart Failure

BURTON E. SOBEL, M.D.
Lewin Professor of Medicine, and Director, Cardiovascular Division, Washington University School of Medicine; Cardiologist-in-Chief, Barnes Hospital, St. Louis, Missouri
Coronary Blood Flow and Myocardial Ischemia; Acute Myocardial Infarction

EDMUND H. SONNENBLICK, M.D.
Olson Professor of Medicine, The Albert Einstein College of Medicine. Chief, Division of Cardiology, Hospital of The Albert Einstein College of Medicine and The Bronx Municipal Hospital Center, Bronx, New York
Mechanisms of Cardiac Contraction and Relaxation

ROBERT SOUFER, M.D.
Associate Professor of Diagnostic Radiology and Medicine (Cardiovascular Medicine), and Director, Positron Emission Tomography Center, Yale University. Attending Physician, Internal Medicine, Yale–New Haven Hospital; Director, Nuclear Medicine Service, West Haven VA Hospital, West Haven, Connecticut
Nuclear Cardiology

ROBERT M. STEINER, M.D.
Professor of Radiology and Associate Professor of Medicine, Jefferson Medical College of Thomas Jefferson University. Chief, Section of Thoracic Radiology and Director, Division of General Diagnostic Radiology, Thomas Jefferson University Hospital, Philadelphia, Pennsylvania
Radiology of the Heart

GENE H. STOLLERMAN, M.D.
Professor of Medicine, Boston University School of Medicine. VA Distinguished Physician, Edith Nourse Rogers Memorial Veterans Hospital, Bedford, Massachusetts
Rheumatic Fever and Other Rheumatic Diseases of the Heart

MARC T. SWARTZ
Director of Circulatory Support, St. Louis University Medical Center, St. Louis, Missouri
Assisted Circulation and the Mechanical Heart

MARTIN VON PLANTA, M.D.
Chief Resident, Department of Medicine, University Hospital Basle, Basle, Switzerland
Acute Circulatory Failure

FRANS J. TH. WACKERS, M.D.
Professor of Diagnostic Radiology and Medicine, and Director, Cardiovascular Nuclear Imaging and Exercise Laboratories, Yale University School of Medicine and Yale–New Haven Hospital, New Haven, Connecticut
Nuclear Cardiology

MYRON L. WEISFELDT, M.D.
Professor of Medicine, Johns Hopkins University School of Medicine and Francis Scott Key Medical Center, Baltimore, Maryland
Aging and the Heart

MAX HARRY WEIL, M.D., PH.D.
Distinguished Professor and Chairman, Department of Medicine, The Chicago Medical School, North Chicago, Illinois
Acute Circulatory Failure

GORDON H. WILLIAMS, M.D.
Professor of Medicine, Harvard Medical School. Chief, Endocrine-Hypertension Division, Department of Medicine, Brigham and Women's Hospital, Boston, Massachusetts
Endocrine and Nutritional Disorders and Heart Disease

GERALD L. WOLF, PH.D., M.D.
Professor of Radiology, Harvard Medical School. Director, Center for Imaging and Pharmaceutical Research, Massachusetts General Hospital, Boston, Massachusetts
Relative Merits of Imaging Techniques

JOSHUA WYNNE, M.D.
Professor of Medicine, Wayne State University. Chief of Cardiology, Harper Hospital, Detroit, Michigan
The Cardiomyopathies and Myocarditides: Toxic, Chemical, and Physical Damage to the Heart

BARRY L. ZARET, M.D.
Robert W. Berliner Professor of Medicine, Professor of Diagnostic Radiology, and Chief, Section of Cardiovascular Medicine, Yale University School of Medicine. Chief of Cardiology, Yale–New Haven Medical Center, New Haven, Connecticut
Nuclear Cardiology

DOUGLAS P. ZIPES, M.D.
Professor of Medicine, Indiana University School of Medicine. Attending Physician, University Hospital, Wishard Memorial Hospital, and Roudebush Veterans Administration Hospital, Indianapolis, Indiana
Genesis of Cardiac Arrhythmias: Electrophysiological Considerations; Management of Cardiac Arrhythmias: Pharmacological, Electrical, and Surgical Techniques; Specific Arrhythmias: Diagnosis and Treatment; Cardiac Pacemakers and Antiarrhythmic Devices

PREFACE to the Fourth Edition

The rates at which the various branches of medicine progress are by no means uniform. To even the most casual observer of the medical scene, it is evident that cardiology has been moving ahead at an unprecedented pace and more rapidly than most other medical subspecialties. As I complete my quadrennial task of preparing a new edition of *Heart Disease*, I am awed by the continued growth and progress in cardiovascular medicine. During my professional lifetime, I have been privileged to observe the field's advance to a point at which the safe and accurate diagnosis and the effective treatment of most forms of heart disease is now feasible, although many patients still receive far from optimal cardiac care. While the overall population is aging and the total prevalence of heart disease may therefore be rising, the age-adjusted mortality rate for cardiovascular disease has declined by approximately 1 per cent per year for the last 40 years, and this decline appears to be continuing. Five influences, I believe, have been especially important to this transformation of cardiology,[1] which is reflected in this textbook.

1. The rich heritage of basic cardiovascular science, particularly cardiovascular physiology, dating back to William Harvey, provided a framework for the understanding of cardiovascular diseases and for the development and perfection of a number of important clinical investigative techniques in cardiology, such as electrocardiography and cardiac catheterization. The early differentiation of the clinical subspecialty of cardiology provided a cadre of capable clinical cardiovascular investigators by mid-century.

2. The acceleration of technical and engineering developments during World War II led to instruments, devices, and techniques that improved enormously the diagnosis and treatment of the cardiac patient. The development or perfection during World War II of the cathode-ray oscilloscope, ultrasonography, radioisotopes, and computers and the successful surgical treatment of cardiac trauma — to name just a few — was of immense importance to the subsequent flowering of cardiovascular medicine, radiology, and surgery.

3. Spectacular clinical successes early in the post-World War II era — such as the prophylaxis of rheumatic fever, the development of orally effective diuretics for the management of hypertension and heart failure, and the development of open-heart surgery — caused excitement about our ability to control heart disease which built its own momentum. This momentum, in turn, has enhanced cardiology's ability to attract the most creative, talented, vigorous, and devoted new investigators and clinicians.

4. The federal commitment to cardiovascular research (expressed principally in the programs of the National Heart, Lung and Blood Institute) has fueled investigation — especially basic investigation — into cardiovascular function and disease and has supported the training of talented persons who have become the leaders in research, teaching, and clinical care of cardiovascular disease.

5. In the United States, voluntary organizations such as the American Heart Association, professional groups such as the American College of Cardiology, and analogous groups in other nations have set standards for and disseminated new information on cardiac care, and some have provided much-needed support for research and training. Industry also has recognized the enormous potential for improving cardiovascular health and has made substantial investments in research in this field.

---

[1] Braunwald, E.: The golden age of cardiology. *In* Knoebel, S.B., and Dack, S. An Era of Cardiovascular Medicine. New York, Elsevier Science Publishing Co., 1991, pp. 1–4.

The enormous advances in the field in just 4 years have required the most extensive changes yet made in any revision of this text. Therefore, the preparation of this edition proved to be more challenging and at the same time more intellectually invigorating than I had anticipated. However, the basic format of the fourth edition of *Heart Disease* remains the same as that of the previous editions. The book is divided into 5 parts: Part I deals with the examination of the patient in the broadest sense, including clinical findings and the theory and application of modern noninvasive and invasive techniques to elicit information about the heart and circulation. Part II is concerned with the pathophysiology, diagnosis, and treatment of the principal abnormalities of circulatory function, including heart failure, shock, arrhythmias, and abnormalities of arterial pressure. Part III, the longest in the book, consists of descriptions of the principal congenital and acquired diseases affecting the heart, pericardium, aorta, and pulmonary vascular bed in adults and children. Part IV deals with the interfaces between cardiology and broad fields such as genetics, aging, management of the postoperative cardiac patient, and the economics of cardiac care. Part V details the manner in which diseases of other organ systems affect the circulation and vice versa.

Fifteen new chapters have been added or substituted: Heart Sounds and Murmurs: Physiological Mechanisms by Joseph K. Perloff; Exercise Stress Testing by Bernard Chaitman; Radiology of the Heart by Robert M. Steiner and David C. Levin; Nuclear Cardiology by Barry Zaret, Frans J. Th. Wackers, and Robert Soufer; Relative Merits of Imaging Techniques by David J. Skorton, Heinrich R. Schelbert, Gerald L. Wolf, and Melvin L. Marcus; Heart and Heart-Lung Transplantation by Bruce A. Reitz; Assisted Circulation and Mechanical Hearts by D. Glenn Pennington and Marc T. Swartz; Hypotension and Syncope by Wishwa Kapoor; Congenital Heart Disease in Adults by Joseph K. Perloff; Infective Endocarditis by Oksana H. Korzeniowski and Donald Kaye; Rehabilitation of Patients with Coronary Artery Disease by Charles Dennis; General Principles of Cardiovascular Cellular and Molecular Biology by Bernardo Nadal-Ginard and Vijak Mahdavi; Genetics and Cardiovascular Disease by Reed Pyeritz; Medical Management of the Patient Undergoing Cardiac Surgery by Elliott M. Antman; and Pregnancy and Cardiovascular Disease by Uri Elkayam.

Many other important new areas are covered in detail. These include Doppler echocardiography; CT scanning and MR imaging of the heart; thrombolytic therapy of acute myocardial infarction and pulmonary embolism; newer concepts regarding the pathogenesis, treatment, and prevention of hypertension, atherosclerosis, cardiac arrhythmias, and congestive heart failure; percutaneous transluminal angioplasty and balloon valvuloplasty; atrial natriuretic peptide; normal and abnormal functions of vascular endothelium; and the role of electrical and surgical techniques in the treatment of tachyarrhythmias, to mention only a few. The fourth edition of *Heart Disease* is approximately 15 per cent longer than the third. This has been accomplished with no increase in the number of pages or bulk of the book through a more efficient page layout, the use of somewhat smaller illustrations, and the more liberal use of a special type face. It is hoped that the reader will find the two-color illustrations to be helpful.

The intelligent contemporary practice of cardiology involves much more than the use of advanced technology in patients with heart disease. It requires the careful integration of findings obtained on the clinical examination as well as the exercise of judgment and discretion in selection among the growing number of diagnostic and therapeutic modalities now available. Accordingly, the chapter on Physical Examination has been expanded and thoroughly revised, and a new chapter on Heart Sounds and Murmurs by Perloff has been included. In an effort to avoid costly, redundant information testing in clinical practice, the new chapter on the Relative Merits of Imaging Techniques by Skorton and colleagues provides a rational approach to the intelligent selection of the appropriate technique among the several now available to image the heart. The relative advantages and disadvantages of various diagnostic and therapeutic options are discussed throughout the book. The chapter on Cost-Effective Strategies in Cardiology by Goldman explains how cost-conscious practice need not impair the quality of care.

Normal cardiovascular function is affected profoundly by a large number of processes that are being understood increasingly at the molecular level. These processes involve membrane receptors, transmembrane ion channels, the production and utilization of high energy phosphate stores, the production of and response to growth factors, and the synthesis of a variety of proteins—such as the apoproteins involved in the transport of lipids and the contractile proteins—of both heart and vascular smooth muscle. It is becoming clear that abnormalities of these processes may be the basis of many cardiovascular diseases and that genetic influences can play critical roles in the development of these abnormalities. Therefore, I believe that the contemporary cardiologist should have some basic understanding of the impact of cell and molecular biology and of genetics on cardiovascular disease. The former is provided in the new chapter on this subject by Nadal-Ginard and Mahdavi, while the latter is summarized in the new chapter by Pyeritz. The important role played by genetics in cardiovascular disease is underscored by Figure 51–1, on pages 1624 and 1625, specially prepared for this book by Pyeritz, which shows the chromosomal location of 76 human genes whose mutations have been shown to produce deleterious effects on the cardiovascular system. This field is moving very swiftly indeed; undoubtedly many other genes will be identified and their chromosomal locations determined by the time the fifth edition of *Heart Disease* is readied. In addition, the chromosomal map in Figure 51–1 lists only monogenic disorders. Many forms of hyperlipoproteinemia and essential hypertension are not shown because they represent polygenic disorders. The important impact of "the new biology" is reflected not only in these two new chapters but throughout the book, especially in the chapters on the Mechanisms of Cardiac Contraction and Relaxation, on the Pathophysiology of Heart Failure, on the Genesis of Cardiac Arrhythmias, on the Pathogenesis of Atherosclerosis, on Risk Factors for Coronary Artery Disease, and on Coronary Blood Flow and Myocardial Ischemia.

An important responsibility of an editor is to establish the boundaries of a book. In approaching this task, I have deliberately taken a broad approach—in line with this book's subtitle "*A Textbook of Cardiovascular Medicine.*" I believe that the modern cardiologist will best serve his/her patients by being first a broadly based physician and second an accomplished technical specialist. The cardiologist must remain the master—not become the slave—of the powerful new diagnostic and therapeutic tools now available and must also understand the enormous impact that heart disease can exert on the function of other organ systems, as well as the equally important effect that disordered function of other organ systems can have on the circulation. The cardiologist should be able to function ably as a consultant to generalists, surgeons, and other specialists. For these reasons, ample space in *Heart Disease* is devoted to what might be considered to be the "boundaries" of cardiology. The chapters on Pulmonary Edema, Acute Circulatory Failure, Hypertension, Pulmonary Embolism, and Cor Pulmonale, and all of Part V (Heart Disease and Disorders of Other Organ Systems), explore the important interfaces between cardiology and other branches of medicine. The new chapter by Antman on the medical management of the patient undergoing cardiac surgery should be helpful to the cardiologist and internist in what is a steadily growing responsibility of both of these specialists.

Considerable revisions have been made in both galley proofs and page proofs to include information about the most recent advances in the field. Particular emphasis has been placed on ensuring a comprehensive and up-to-date bibliography, which includes 15,000 pertinent references. Hundreds of references to publications that appeared in 1991 are included. Many of the 1500 figures and 396 tables are new to this edition.

Despite these efforts, the rapid pace at which cardiology continues to advance makes it ever more difficult to provide a timely picture of this field in a traditional textbook. Therefore, we are publishing *Updates to Heart Disease*, a quarterly publication begun 4 years ago. The *Updates* complement *Heart Disease* and describe new developments in the field that have occurred since the preparation of the last edition. In addition, a *Question and Answer Self-Assessment and Review Book* will again accompany this edition of *Heart Disease*. It consists of 600 questions based on material discussed in the textbook and provides the answers as well as detailed explanations. In 1991 W. B. Saunders published *Cardiac Imaging: A Companion to Braunwald's Heart Disease* edited by Skorton, Schelbert, Wolf and Marcus, which consists of an elegant analysis of the most important cardiovascular diagnostic imaging techniques available. This book is especially useful given the profound advances in cardiovasular diagnosis made possible by modern imaging techniques. This multipronged educational effort—*Heart Disease*, the *Updates*, the *Self-Assessment and Review* book, and *Cardiac Imaging Companion*, as well as some other projects now under consideration—is designed to assist the reader with the awesome task of learning and remaining current in this dynamic field.

It is hoped that this textbook will prove useful to those who wish to broaden their knowledge of cardiovascular medicine. To the extent that it achieves this goal and thereby aids in the care of patients afflicted with heart disease, credit must be given to the many talented and dedicated persons involved in its preparation. My deepest appreciation goes to my fellow contributors for their professional expertise, knowledge, and devoted scholarship, which are at the very "heart" of this book. It has been a personal pleasure for me to deal with the W. B. Saunders Company. Its President and my editor, Mr. Lewis Reines, and Ms. Lorraine Kilmer, Manager of the Editorial/Design/Production Team, have been particularly helpful, as have been the effective members of this team—especially Mr. Frank Polizzano and Ms. Edna Dick. Ms. Kathryn Saxon in my office rendered most capable editorial and secretarial services. Dr. David Beier served as a valued consultant.

Without question, this edition could not have become a reality were it not for the skillful and dedicated efforts of several individuals. My responsibilities to the Harvard Medical School and the Brigham and Women's Hospital during the leave of absence that I required for much of my own writing were shouldered most effectively by my respected colleague and good friend, Dr. Marshall Wolf, who provided the Department of Medicine with exemplary leadership. My administrative assistant, Ms. Diane Rioux, was enormously helpful in maintaining the orderly flow of activity essential to a busy Department of Medicine. I am especially indebted to Dr. Daniel C. Tosteson, Dean of the Harvard Medical School, and to Dr. H. Richard Nesson, President of the Brigham and Women's Hospital, for graciously allowing me the freedom to devote myself to this task. On a personal note, my wife, Dr. Nina S. Braunwald, and my children, Karen Gail, Denise Allison, and Adrienne Jill, provided the personal support, encouragement, and understanding so essential for one who adds a task of this magnitude to an already full professional life.

EUGENE BRAUNWALD

Adapted from the PREFACE to the First Edition

Cardiovascular disease is the greatest scourge afflicting the population of the industrialized nations. As with previous scourges — bubonic plague, yellow fever, and smallpox — cardiovascular disease not only strikes down a significant fraction of the population without warning but causes prolonged suffering and disability in an even larger number. In the United States alone, despite recent encouraging declines, cardiovascular disease is still responsible for almost one million fatalities each year and more than one half of all deaths; almost 5 million persons afflicted with cardiovascular disease are hospitalized each year. The cost of this disease in terms of human suffering and of material resources is almost incalculable.

Fortunately, research focusing on the causes, diagnosis, treatment, and prevention of heart disease is moving ahead rapidly. In the last 25 years in particular we have witnessed an explosive expansion of our understanding of the structure and function of the cardiovascular system — both normal and abnormal — and of our ability to evaluate it in the living patient, sometimes by means of techniques that require pentration of the skin but also, with increasing accuracy, by noninvasive methods. Simultaneously, remarkable progress has been made in preventing and treating cardiovascular disease by medical and surgical means. Indeed, in the United States, the aforementioned steady reduction in mortality from cardiovascular disease during the past decade suggests that the effective application of this increased knowledge is beginning to prolong the human life span — the most valued resource on earth.

An attempt to summarize our present understanding of heart disease in a comprehensive textbook for the serious student of this subject is a formidable undertaking. Following the untimely death of Dr. Charles K. Friedberg, whose masterful text served as a bible to me and to a whole generation of cardiologists during the 1950's and 1960's, the W. B. Saunders Company invited me to accept this responsibility. Younger colleagues, particularly cardiology fellows and medical residents at the Brigham, convinced me of the need for such a book.

In order to provide a comprehensive, authoritative text in a field that has become as broad and deep as cardiovascular medicine, I chose to enlist the aid of a number of able colleagues. However, I hoped that my personal involvement in the writing of about half of the book would make it possible to minimize the fragmentation, gaps, inconsistencies, organizational difficulties, and impersonal tone that sometimes plague multiauthored texts. I also sought a compromise between a book that is too long as a result of excessive repetition and one in which all duplication is eliminated, resulting in fragmented coverage of certain subjects. To help achieve this objective, extensive cross references have been provided within the text.

Since the early part of this century, clinical cardiology has had a particularly strong foundation in the basic sciences of physiology and pharmacology. More recently, the disciplines of molecular biology, genetics, developmental biology, biophysics, biochemistry, experimental pathology, and bioengineering have also begun to provide critically important information about cardiac function and malfunction. Although *Heart Disease: A Textbook of Cardiovascular Medicine* is primarily a clinical treatise and not a textbook of fundamental cardiovascular science, an effort has been made to explain, in some detail, the scientific basis of cardiovascular diseases.

EUGENE BRAUNWALD, 1980

CONTENTS

PART I
EXAMINATION OF THE PATIENT

PART II

NORMAL AND ABNORMAL CIRCULATORY FUNCTION

PART III

DISEASES OF THE HEART, PERICARDIUM, AORTA, AND PULMONARY VASCULAR BED

PART IV

BROADER PERSPECTIVES ON HEART DISEASE AND CARDIOLOGIC PRACTICE

PART V

HEART DISEASE AND DISORDERS OF OTHER ORGAN SYSTEMS

PART I

EXAMINATION OF THE PATIENT

1

The History

by EUGENE BRAUNWALD, M.D.

IMPORTANCE OF THE HISTORY

Specialized examinations of the cardiovascular system, presented in Chapters 3 to 12, provide a large portion of the data base required to establish a specific anatomical diagnosis of cardiac disease and to determine the extent of functional impairment of the heart. The development of these methods represents one of the triumphs of modern medicine. However, their appropriate use is to *supplement but not to supplant* a careful clinical examination, which remains the cornerstone of the assessment of the patient with known or suspected cardiovascular disease. There is a temptation in cardiology, as in many other areas of medicine, to carry out expensive, uncomfortable, and occasionally even hazardous procedures to establish a diagnosis when a detailed and thoughtful history and physical examination may be sufficient. Obviously, it is undesirable to subject patients to the unnecessary risks and expenses inherent in many specialized tests when a diagnosis can be made on the basis of an adequate clinical examination or when management will not be altered significantly as a result of these tests.[1] Intelligent selection of investigative procedures from the ever-increasing array of tests now available requires far more sophisticated decision-making than was necessary when the choices were limited to the electrocardiogram and chest roentgenogram (Chaps. 12, 54). The history and physical examination provide the critical information necessary for these decisions.

THE ROLE OF THE HISTORY. The overreliance on laboratory tests has increased as physicians attempt to utilize their time more efficiently by delegating responsibility for taking the history to a physician's assistant or nurse or even by limiting the history to a questionnaire—an approach that I consider to be an undesirable trend insofar as the patient with known or suspected heart disease is concerned.[2] First, it must be appreciated that the history remains the richest source of information concerning the patient's illness,[3,4] and any practice that might diminish the quality of information provided by the history is likely ultimately to impair the quality of care. Second, the physician's attentive and thoughtful taking of a history establishes a bond with the patient that may be valuable later in securing the patient's compliance in following a complex treatment plan, undergoing hospitalization for an intensive diagnostic work-up or a hazardous operation, and, in some instances, accepting that heart disease is not present at all. It is largely through the direct contact established between the patient and the physician during the clinical examination that this confidence can best be established.

Taking a h[illegible]ry also permits the physician to evaluate the results of diagnostic tests that have strong subjective components, such as the determination of exercise capacity (Chap.

6). Perhaps most importantly, a careful history allows the physician to evaluate the impact of the disease, or the fear of the disease, on the patient's total life and to assess the patient's personality, emotion, and stability; often it provides a glimpse of the patient's responsibility, fears, aspirations, and threshold for discomfort as well as the likelihood of compliance with one or another therapeutic regimen. Whenever possible, the physician should question not only the patient but also relatives or close friends in order to obtain a clearer understanding of the extent of the patient's disability and a broader perspective concerning the impact of the disease on both the patient and the family. (For example, the patient's spouse is much more likely than the patient to provide a history of Cheyne-Stokes [periodic] respiration.)

In interpreting the history obtained from a patient with known or suspected heart disease, it must be appreciated that the combination of the widespread fear of cardiovascular disorders and the deep-seated emotional, symbolic, and sometimes even religious connotations concerning this organ's function may, on the one hand, provoke symptoms that mimic those of organic heart disease in persons with normal cardiovascular systems and, on the other, cause so much fear that serious symptoms are repressed or denied by patients with organic heart disease. Functional complaints referable to the cardiovascular system may also develop in patients with organic heart disease.

TECHNIQUE. Several approaches can be employed successfully in obtaining a medical history. I believe that patients should first be given the opportunity to relate their experiences and complaints in their own way. Although time-consuming and likely to include much seemingly irrelevant information, this technique has the advantage of providing considerable information concerning the patient's intelligence, emotional make-up, and attitude to his or her complaints, as well as providing the patient with the satisfaction that he or she has been "heard out" by the physician, rather than merely having had a few questions thrown at him or her and then been exposed to a series of laboratory examinations based on "high technology." After the patient has given an account of the illness, the physician should obtain information concerning the onset and chronology of symptoms; their location, quality, and intensity; the precipitating, aggravating, and alleviating factors, the setting in which the symptoms occur, and any associated symptoms; and the response to therapy.

Of course, a detailed general medical history including the personal past history, occupational history, nutritional history, and review of systems must be obtained. Concern should focus on a past history of rheumatic fever, chorea, venereal disease or exposure to it, thyroid disease, recent dental extractions or manipulations, catheterization of the bladder, and earlier examinations that showed abnormalities of the cardiovascular system as reflected in restriction from physical activity at school and in rejection for life insurance, employment, or military service. Personal habits such as exercise, cigarette smoking, alcohol intake, and parenteral use of drugs—illicit and otherwise—should be ascertained, and the exact nature of the patient's work should be assessed. The increasing appreciation of the importance of genetic influences in many forms of heart disease (Chap. 51) underscores the importance of the family history.

A wide variety of disorders including, but not limited to, neurological (Chap. 60), endocrine (Chap. 61), and rheumatological (Chap. 56) may have important effects on the cardiovascular system; it is vital to ascertain the presence of these and other conditions which are not *primarily* cardiological. A history of the risk factors for ischemic heart disease—the personal and family history, cigarette smoking, hypertension, hypercholesterolemia, diabetes mellitus, artificial or early menopause, and long-term contraceptive pill ingestion (Chap. 37)—should always be sought.

A cardinal principle of cardiovascular evaluation is that myocardial or coronary function that may be adequate at rest may be inadequate during exertion; therefore, specific attention should be directed to the influence of activity on the patient's symptoms. Thus, a history of chest pain or discomfort and/or undue shortness of breath that appears only during activity is characteristic of heart disease, whereas the opposite pattern, i.e., the appearance of symptoms at rest and their remission during exertion, is observed only rarely in patients with heart disease but is more characteristic of functional disorders. In attempting to assess the severity of functional impairment, both the *extent* of activity and the *rate* at which it is performed before symptoms develop should be determined and related to a detailed consideration of the therapeutic regimen. For example, the complaint of exertional dyspnea after walking slowly up a flight of stairs in a patient on maximal treatment for heart failure denotes far more severe functional disability than does a similar symptom occurring in an untreated patient who has run up a flight of stairs.

As the patient relates the history, important nonverbal clues are often provided. The physician should observe the patient's attitude, reactions, and gestures while being questioned, as well as his or her choice of words or emphasis. Tumulty has aptly likened obtaining a meaningful clinical history to playing a game of chess:[5] "The patient makes a statement and based upon its content, and mode of expression, the physician asks a counter-question. One answer stimulates yet another question until the clinician is convinced that he understands precisely all of the circumstances of the patient's illness."

CARDINAL SYMPTOMS OF HEART DISEASE

The cardinal symptoms of heart disease include dyspnea, chest pain or discomfort, syncope, collapse, palpitation, edema, cough, hemoptysis, and excess fatigue. Cyanosis is more often a sign rather than a symptom, but it may be a key feature of the history, particularly in patients with congenital heart disease. Without doubt, history-taking is the most valuable technique available for determining whether or not these symptoms are caused by heart disease. Examples of the manner in which these symptoms may serve as a guide to diagnosis are given in the following pages, and reference is made to other portions of the book that contain more detailed information.

DYSPNEA

(See also pp. 449 and 556)

Dyspnea is defined as an abnormally uncomfortable awareness of breathing; it is one of the principal symptoms of cardiac and pulmonary disease.[6] Since dyspnea is regularly caused by strenuous exertion in healthy, well-conditioned subjects and by only moderate exertion in those who are normal but unaccustomed to exercise, it should be regarded as abnormal only when it occurs at rest or at a level of physical activity not expected to cause this symptom. Dyspnea is associated with a wide variety of diseases of the heart and lungs, chest wall, and respiratory muscles as well as with anxiety[7,8]; the history is the most valuable means of establishing the etiology. Table 1–1 provides a list of the various syndromes which may cause dyspnea and the primary pathophysiological mechanisms that are responsible.[9] Borg and Noble have developed a scale which is useful in quantitating the severity of dyspnea.[10]

The *sudden* development of dyspnea suggests pulmonary embolism, pneumothorax, acute pulmonary edema, pneumonia, or airway obstruction. In contrast, in most forms of *chronic* heart failure, dyspnea progresses slowly over weeks or months. Such a protracted course may also occur in a variety of unrelated conditions, including obesity, pregnancy, and bilateral pleural effusion. *Inspiratory dyspnea* suggests obstruction of the upper airways, whereas *expiratory dyspnea* characterizes obstruction of the lower airways. Exertional dyspnea suggests the presence of organic diseases, such as left

TABLE 1-1 DISORDERS CAUSING DYSPNEA AND LIMITING EXERCISE PERFORMANCE, PATHOPHYSIOLOGY, AND DISCRIMINATING MEASUREMENTS*

DISORDERS	PATHOPHYSIOLOGY	MEASUREMENTS THAT DEVIATE FROM NORMAL
Pulmonary		
Airflow limitation	Mechanical limitation to ventilation, mismatching of $\dot{V}A/\dot{Q}$, hypoxic stimulation to breathing	$\dot{V}E$ max/MVV, expiratory flow pattern, VD, VT; $\dot{V}O_2$ max, $\dot{V}E/\dot{V}O_2$, $\dot{V}E$ response to hyperoxia, $(A - a)PO_2$
Restrictive	Mismatching $\dot{V}A/\dot{Q}$, hypoxic stimulation to breathing	
Chest wall	Mechanical limitation to ventilation	$\dot{V}E$ max/MVV, $PACO_2$, $\dot{V}O_2$ max
Pulmonary circulation	Rise in physiological dead space as fraction of VT, exercise hypoxemia	VD/VT, work-rate–related hypoxemia, $\dot{V}O_2$ max, $\dot{V}E/\dot{V}O_2$, $(a - ET)PCO_2$, O_2-pulse
Cardiac		
Coronary	Coronary insufficiency	ECG, $\dot{V}O_2$ max, anaerobic threshold $\dot{V}O_2$, $\dot{V}E/\dot{V}O_2$, O_2-pulse, BP (systolic, diastolic, pulse)
Valvular	Cardiac output limitation (decreased effective stroke volume)	
Myocardial	Cardiac output limitation (decreased ejection fraction and stroke volume)	
Anemia	Reduced O_2 carrying capacity	O_2-pulse, anaerobic threshold $\dot{V}O_2$, $\dot{V}O_2$ max, $\dot{V}E/\dot{V}O_2$
Peripheral circulation	Inadequate O_2 flow to metabolically active muscle	Anaerobic threshold $\dot{V}O_2$, $\dot{V}O_2$ max
Obesity	Increased work to move body; if severe, respiratory restriction and pulmonary insufficiency	$\dot{V}O_2$-work-rate relationship, PAO_2, $PACO_2$, $\dot{V}O_2$ max
Psychogenic	Hyperventilation with precisely regular respiratory rate	Breathing pattern, PCO_2
Malingering	Hyperventilation and hypoventilation with irregular respiratory rate	Breathing pattern, PCO_2
Deconditioning	Inactivity or prolonged bed rest; loss of capability for effective redistribution of systemic blood flow	O_2-pulse, anaerobic threshold $\dot{V}O_2$, $\dot{V}O_2$ max

* $\dot{V}A$ indicates alveolar ventilation; $\dot{Q}$, pulmonary blood flow; $\dot{V}E$, minute ventilation; MVV, maximum voluntary ventilation; VD/VT, physiological dead space/tidal volume ratio; O_2, oxygen; $\dot{V}O_2$, O_2 consumption; $(A - a)PO_2$, alveolar-arterial PO_2 difference; and $(a - ET)PCO_2$, arterial-end tidal PCO_2 difference.
Modified from Wasserman, D: Dyspnea on exertion: Is it the heart or the lungs? JAMA *248*:2042, 1982.

ventricular failure (Chap. 16) or chronic obstructive lung disease (Chap. 49), whereas dyspnea developing at rest may occur in pneumothorax, pulmonary embolism (Chap. 48), or pulmonary edema, or may be functional. Dyspnea that occurs *only* at rest and is absent on exertion is almost invariably functional. A functional origin is suggested when dyspnea, or simply a heightened awareness of breathing, is accompanied by brief stabbing pain in the region of the cardiac apex or by prolonged (more than 2 hours) dull chest pain, and is associated with difficulty in getting enough air into the lungs, claustrophobia, or sighing respirations that are relieved by exertion, by taking a few deep breaths, or by sedation. A history of relief of dyspnea by bronchodilators and corticosteroids suggests asthma as the etiology, whereas relief of dyspnea by rest, diuretics, and digitalis suggests left heart failure.

In patients with *heart failure,* dyspnea is a clinical expression of pulmonary venous and capillary hypertension (p. 452). It occurs either during exertion or, in resting patients, in the recumbent position and is relieved promptly by sitting upright or standing (orthopnea). In patients with heart failure, dyspnea may be accompanied by edema (p. 556), upper abdominal pain (due to congestive hepatomegaly), and nocturia. The *sudden* occurrence of dyspnea in a patient with a history of mitral valve stenosis suggests the development of atrial fibrillation, rupture of chordae tendineae, or pulmonary embolism.

Paroxysmal nocturnal dyspnea is due to interstitial pulmonary edema and sometimes intraalveolar edema most commonly secondary to left ventricular failure (p. 449). This condition, beginning usually 2 to 5 hours after the onset of sleep and often associated with sweating and wheezing, is frightening to the patient. Paroxysmal nocturnal dyspnea is often relieved by the patient's sitting on the side of the bed or getting out of bed. Although paroxysmal nocturnal dyspnea secondary to left ventricular failure is usually accompanied by coughing, a careful history often discloses that the dyspnea *precedes* the cough, not vice versa. In contrast, patients with *chronic pulmonary disease* may also awaken at night, but cough and expectoration often precede the dyspnea. These patients also often have a long history of smoking and a chronic cough with sputum production and wheezing and may be able to breathe more easily while leaning forward. Nocturnal dyspnea in patients with pulmonary disease is usually relieved after the patient rids himself or herself of secretions rather than specifically by sitting up. Details of the value and limitations of the history of dyspnea in differentiating between primary diseases of the heart and lungs[11,12] are presented on page 450.

Patients with *pulmonary embolism* usually experience sudden dyspnea that may be associated with apprehension, palpitation, hemoptysis, or pleuritic chest pain (Chap. 48). The development or intensification of dyspnea, sometimes associated with a feeling of faintness, may be the only complaint of the patient with pulmonary emboli. Dyspnea accompanying thoracic pain occurs in *acute myocardial infarction.* Occasionally dyspnea is an *"anginal equivalent"* (p. 1293), i.e., a symptom secondary to myocardial ischemia that occurs in place of typical anginal discomfort[12]. This form of dyspnea may be closely associated with a sensation of tightness in the chest, is present on exertion or emotional stress, is relieved by rest (more often in the sitting than in the recumbent position), has a duration similar to angina (i.e., 2 to 10 minutes), and is usually responsive to nitroglycerin but not to digitalis. The sudden development of severe dyspnea in the sitting rather than in the lying position, or whenever a particular position is assumed, suggests the possibility of a *myxoma* (p. 1454) or *ball-valve thrombus* in the left atrium. When dyspnea is relieved by squatting, it is caused most commonly by tetralogy of Fallot or a variant thereof (p. 935).

CHEST PAIN OR DISCOMFORT

(See also p. 1293)

Elucidation of the cause of chest pain is one of the key tasks of physicians and this symptom is responsible for many cardiac consultations. The history remains the most important technique for distinguishing among the many causes of chest discomfort. Although chest pain or discomfort is one of the cardinal manifestations of cardiac disease, it is critical to recognize that is may originate not only in the heart but also in (1) a variety of noncardiac intrathoracic structures, such as the aorta, pulmonary artery, bronchopulmonary tree, pleura, mediastinum, esophagus, and diaphragm; (2) the tissues of the neck or thoracic wall, including the skin, thoracic muscles, cervicodorsal spine, costochondral junctions, breasts, sensory nerves, and spinal cord; and (3) subdiaphragmatic organs such as the stomach, duodenum, pancreas, and gallbladder (Tables 1–2 and 1–3). Factitious pain or pain of functional origin may also occur in the chest. Although a wide variety of laboratory tests is available to aid in the differential diagnosis of chest pain, the history is without question the most valuable mode of examination. In obtaining the history of a patient with chest pain it is helpful to have a mental checklist and to ask the patient to describe the location, radiation, and character of the pain; what causes and relieves the pain; time relationships, including the duration, frequency, and pattern of recurrence of the pain; the setting in which it occurs; and associated symptoms. It is also particularly useful to observe the patient's gestures. Clenching the fist in front of the chest while describing the sensation (Levine's sign) is a strong indication of an ischemic origin for the pain.

QUALITY. *Angina pectoris* may be defined as a discomfort in the chest or adjacent area associated with myocardial ischemia but without myocardial necrosis.[17] It is important to recognize that angina means *choking*, not pain. Thus, the discomfort of angina often is described not as pain at all but rather as an unpleasant sensation; "pressing," "squeezing," "strangling," "constricting," "bursting," and "burning" are some of the adjectives commonly used to describe this sensation (Table 1–4). "A band across the chest" and "a weight in the center of the chest" are other frequent descriptions. Often with severe attacks the discomfort may radiate from the chest to the shoulders, upper extremities (particularly the ulnar aspect of the left arm), neck, jaws, and teeth. It is characteristic of angina that the intensity of effort required to incite it seems to vary from day to day and throughout the day in the same patient, but often a careful history will uncover explanations for this, such as meals ingested, weather, emotions, and the like. The anginal threshold is lower in the morning than at any other time of day; thus patients note frequently that activities that may cause angina in the morning or when first undertaken do not do so later in the day. When the threshold for angina is quite variable, defies any pattern, and is prominent at rest, the possibility that myocardial ischemia is caused by coronary spasm should be considered (p. 1207). Thus, a careful history may indicate not only the cause of the pain (i.e., myocardial ischemia) but can also provide a clue to the mechanism of the ischemia (spasm vs. organic obstruction).

TABLE 1–2 DIFFERENTIAL DIAGNOSIS OF EPISODIC CHEST PAIN RESEMBLING ANGINA PECTORIS

	DURATION	QUALITY	PROVOCATION	RELIEF	LOCATION	COMMENT
Effort angina	5–15 minutes	Visceral (pressure)	During effort or emotion	Rest, nitroglycerin	Substernal, radiates	First episode vivid
Rest angina	5–15 minutes	Visceral (pressure)	Spontaneous (? with exercise)	Nitroglycerin	Substernal, radiates	Often nocturnal
Mitral prolapse	Minutes to hours	Superficial (rarely visceral)	Spontaneous (no pattern)	Time	Left anterior	No pattern, variable character
Esophageal reflux	10 minutes to 1 hour	Visceral	Recumbency, lack of food	Food, antacid	Substernal, epigastric	Rarely radiates
Esophageal spasm	5–60 minutes	Visceral	Spontaneous, cold liquids, exercise	Nitroglycerin	Substernal, radiates	Mimics angina
Peptic ulcer	Hours	Visceral, burning	Lack of food, "acid" foods	Foods, antacids	Epigastric, substernal	
Biliary disease	Hours	Visceral (waxes and wanes)	Spontaneous, food	Time, analgesia	Epigastric, ? radiates	Colic
Cervical disc	Variable (gradually subsides)	Superficial	Head and neck movement, palpation	Time, analgesia	Arm, neck	Not relieved by rest
Hyperventilation	2–3 minutes	Visceral	Emotion, tachypnea	Stimulus removal	Substernal	Facial paresthesia
Musculoskeletal	Variable	Superficial	Movement, palpation	Time, analgesia	Multiple	Tenderness
Pulmonary	30 minutes +	Visceral (pressure)	Often spontaneous	Rest, time, bronchodilator	Substernal	Dyspneic

Reproduced with permission from Christie, L. G., Jr., and Conti, C. R.: Systematic approach to the evaluation of angina-like chest pain. Am. Heart J. *102*:897, 1981.

TABLE 1-3 MAIN DISTINCTIONS BETWEEN ANGINA AND LEFT BREAST (NONCARDIAC) PAIN

	ANGINA PECTORIS	LEFT BREAST PAIN (DA COSTA'S SYNDROME, NEUROCIRCULATORY ASTHENIA)
Site	Central; behind the sternum; across the chest	Left breast
Radiation	Both arms; jaws; back	Left arm
Quality	Constricting; crushing	Prolonged ache; sharp stabs
Duration	2–5 minutes	Seconds or hours
Provocation	During effort; emotion	After effort; fatigue; in bed
Additional symptoms	None	Breathlessness; exhaustion; palpitation; dizziness
ST depression with exercise	Invariable; unaffected by beta-blockade	Sometimes; abolished by beta-blockade
Coronary arteriogram	Abnormal (with rare exceptions)	Normal

From Somerville, W: Chest pain. *In* Weatherall, D. J., Ledingham, J. G. G., Warrell, D. A. (eds.): Oxford Textbook of Medicine. 2nd ed. Oxford, Oxford University Press, copyright 1987, by permission of the Oxford University Press.

A history of prolonged, severe anginal chest discomfort accompanied by profound fatigue often signifies acute myocardial infarction.[19] There is some relationship between location of the chest pain and the site of coronary artery occlusion[20]; patients with ischemic heart disease who complain of substernal or left chest pain with radiation to the left arm usually have heart disease involving the left coronary artery, while those with epigastric pain radiating to the neck or jaw usually do *not* have disease of the left anterior descending coronary artery.

When dyspnea is an "anginal equivalent," the patient may describe the midchest as the site of the shortness of breath, whereas true dyspnea is usually not as well localized. Other anginal equivalents are discomfort limited to areas that are ordinarily sites of secondary radiation, such as the ulnar aspect of the left arm and forearm, lower jaw, teeth, neck, or shoulders, and the development of gas and belching, nausea, "indigestion," dizziness, and diaphoresis. Anginal equivalents above the mandible or below the umbilicus are quite uncommon. In patients with either typical or atypical angina, it is useful to determine whether the patient has symptoms or complications caused by atherosclerosis of other vascular beds, e.g., intermittent claudication, transient ischemic attacks, and stroke. In patients with suspected angina, a history of one of these manifestations of extracardiac atherosclerosis lends weight to the diagnosis of myocardial ischemia.

TABLE 1-4 SOME FEATURES DIFFERENTIATING CARDIAC FROM NONCARDIAC CHEST PAIN

FAVORING ISCHEMIC ORIGIN	AGAINST ISCHEMIC ORIGIN
1. Character of Pain	
Constricting	dull ache
Squeezing	"knife-like," sharp, stabbing
Burning	"jabs" aggravated by respiration
"Heaviness," "heavy feeling"	
2. Location of Pain	
Substernal	in the left submammary area
Across mid-thorax, anteriorly	in the left hemithorax
In both arms, shoulders	
In the neck, cheeks, teeth	
In the forearms, fingers	
In the interscapular region	
3. Factors Provoking Pain	
Exercise	pain *after* completion of exercise
Excitement	provoked by a specific body motion
Other forms of stress	
Cold weather	
After meals	

From Selzer, A.: Principles and Practice of Clinical Cardiology. 2nd ed. Philadelphia, W. B. Saunders Company, 1983, p. 17.

The chest discomfort of *pulmonary hypertension* (p. 806) may be identical to that of typical angina; it is caused by dilation of the pulmonary arteries, most commonly acute pulmonary embolism, and/or by right ventricular ischemia. The chest discomfort of *unstable angina* and *acute myocardial infarction* (p. 1215) is similar in quality to that of angina pectoris in location and character; however, it usually radiates more widely than does angina and is more severe and therefore is generally referred to as true *pain* rather than *discomfort* by the patient. This pain generally develops unrelated to unusual effort or emotional stress, often with the patient at rest or even sleeping. Usually nitroglycerin does not provide complete or lasting relief.

Acute pericarditis (p. 1469) is frequently preceded by a history of a viral upper respiratory infection. The inflammation causes pain that is sharper than is anginal discomfort, is more left-sided than central, and is often referred to the neck. The pain of pericarditis lasts for hours and is little affected by effort but often aggravated by breathing, turning in bed, swallowing, or twisting the body; unlike angina, the pain of acute pericarditis may lessen when the patient sits up and leans forward.

Aortic dissection (p. 1535) is suggested by persistent, severe pain with radiation to the back and into the lumbar region in an individual with a history of hypertension. An expanding *thoracic aortic aneurysm* may erode the vertebral bodies and cause localized, severe, boring pain that may be worse at night. An aneurysmally enlarged left atrium in patients with mitral valve disease rarely causes chest pain; instead, patients commonly complain of discomfort in the back or right side of the chest that intensifies on exertion.

Chest-wall pain due to *costochondritis* or *myositis* is common in patients who present with fear of heart disease.[21] It is associated with both local costochondral and muscle tenderness, which may be aggravated by moving or coughing. Chest-wall pain may also accompany or follow herpes zoster, chest injury, or *Tietze syndrome* (i.e., discomfort localized in swelling of the costochondral and costosternal joints, which are painful on palpation). When *herpes zoster* affects the left chest it may mimic myocardial infarction. However, its persistence, its localization to a dermatome, and the appearance of the characteristic vesicles allow recognition of this condition.

Functional or *psychogenic chest pain* may be one feature of an anxiety state, also called Da Costa syndrome or neurocirculatory asthenia[22-24] (Table 1-3). It is localized typically to the area of the cardiac apex and consists of a dull, persistent ache that lasts for hours and is often accentuated by or alternates with attacks of sharp, lancinating stabs of inframammary pain of 1 or 2 seconds' duration. The condition may occur with emotional strain and fatigue, bears little relation to exertion, and may be accompanied by precordial tenderness. Attacks are usually associated with palpitation, hyperventilation, numbness and tingling in the extremities, sighing, dizziness,[25] dyspnea, generalized weakness, and a history of panic attacks and other signs of emotional instability or depression. The pain may not be completely relieved by any medication other than analgesics, but it is partially attenuated by many types of interventions, including rest, exertion, tranquilizers, and placebos. Therefore, in contrast to ischemic discomfort, functional pain is more likely to show variable responses to interventions on different occasions. Since functional chest pain is often preceded by hyperventilation, which in turn may cause increased muscle tension and be responsible for diffuse chest tightness, some instances of so-called functional chest pain may, in fact, have an organic basis. Chest pain is common in patients with *prolapse of the mitral valve* (p. 1029). The pain varies considerably among patients with this condition; it may be similar to that of classic angina pectoris or may resemble the chest pain of neurocirculatory asthenia described above.

LOCATION. Embryologically the heart is a midline viscus; thus, cardiac ischemia produces anginal symptoms that are characteristically felt across both sides of the chest or chiefly substernally (Fig. 1–1). Some patients complain of discomfort only to the left or less commonly to the right of the midline. If the pain or discomfort can be localized to the skin or superficial structures, and can be reproduced by localized pressure, it generally arises from the chest wall. Thus, if the patient can point directly to the site of discomfort, it is usually not angina pectoris, which, like other symptoms arising in deeper structures, tends to be diffuse and eludes precise localization. Pain that is localized to the region of or under the left nipple or that radiates to the right lower chest[26] is usually noncardiac in origin and may be functional or due to osteoarthritis, gaseous distention of the stomach, or the splenic flexure syndrome. Although pain due to myocardial ischemia often radiates to the left arm or left shoulder, such radiation also occurs in pericarditis and disorders of the cervical spine. Chest pain that radiates to the neck and jaw occurs in pericarditis as well as in myocardial ischemia. Dissection of the aorta or enlargement of an aortic aneurysm produces pain in the *back* rather than in the front of the chest.

DURATION. The duration of the pain is important in determining its etiology.[27] Angina pectoris is relatively short, usually lasting from 2 to 10 minutes. However, if the pain is very brief, i.e., a momentary, lancinating, sharp pain, "stitch," or other discomfort that lasts less than 20 seconds, angina can usually be excluded; such a short duration points instead to musculoskeletal pain, pain due to hiatal hernia, or functional pain. Chest pain lasting for hours may be seen with acute myocardial infarction, pericarditis, aortic dissection, musculoskeletal disease, herpes zoster, and anxiety.

PRECIPITATING AND AGGRAVATING FACTORS. Angina pectoris occurs characteristically on exertion, particularly when hurrying or walking on an upgrade. Thus, the development of chest discomfort or pain when walking, typically in the cold and against a wind, and after a heavy meal, is characteristic of angina pectoris. An exception is *Prinzmetal's (variant) angina*, which characteristically occurs at rest (p. 1342), and may or may not be affected by exertion; however, it must be remembered that classic (nonvariant) angina, although most often precipitated by effort, not uncommonly may be experienced at rest, as in unstable angina (p. 1334); in these patients exertion intensifies the discomfort. Emotional stress also may precipitate angina.

DIFFERENTIAL DIAGNOSIS. Chest pain that occurs after protracted vomiting may be due to the *Mallory-Weiss syndrome*, i.e., a tear in the lower portion of the esophagus. Pain that occurs while bending over is often radicular and may be associated with *osteoarthritis* of the cervical or upper thoracic spine. Chest pain occurring when moving the neck may be due to a *herniated intervertebral disk*.

Esophageal Pain. Substernal and epigastric discomfort during swallowing may be due to *esophageal spasm or esophagitis*, often with acid reflux, with or without a hiatal hernia. These conditions may also be associated with substernal or epigastric burning pain that is brought on by eating or lying

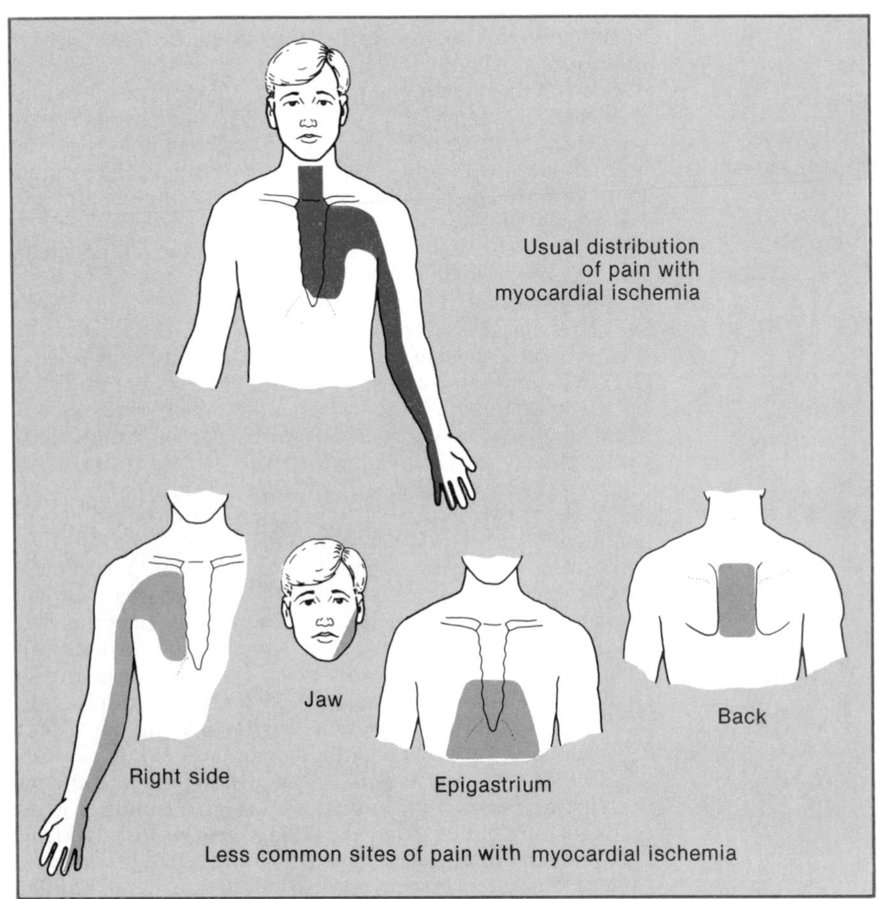

FIGURE 1–1. Pain patterns with myocardial ischemia. The usual distribution is referral to all or part of the sternal region, the left side of the chest, the neck, and down the ulnar side of the left forearm and hand. With severe ischemic pain, the right chest and right arm are often involved as well, although isolated involvement of these areas is rare. Other sites sometimes involved, either alone or together with other sites, are the jaw, epigastrium, and back. (From Horwitz, L. D.: Chest pain. *In* Horwitz, L. D., and Groves, B. M. [eds.]: Signs and Symptoms in Cardiology. Philadelphia, J. B. Lippincott, 1985, p. 9.)

down after meals and that may be relieved with antacids. Pain due to esophageal spasm has many of the features of and may be difficult to differentiate from angina pectoris.[26] Indeed, it is a common cause of chest pain considered atypical of angina pectoris.[17] The presence of acid reflux into the mouth (water brash) and/or dysphagia[29] may be a useful diagnostic clue pointing to esophageal disease.[30] The chest discomfort secondary to esophageal reflux is most common after meals and occurs in the supine position or on bending. The difficulty in distinguishing angina from esophageal disease is compounded by the frequent coexistence of these two common conditions, and by the observation that esophageal reflux lowers the threshold for the development of angina[31] and that esophageal spasm may be precipitated by ergonovine and relieved by nitroglycerin. Esophageal pain radiates to the back more frequently than does angina pectoris.[16]

The discomfort produced by *peptic ulcer disease* may also resemble angina pectoris, but its characteristic relationship to food ingestion and its relief by antacids are important differentiating features. While *acute pancreatitis* may mimic acute myocardial infarction, with the former there is usually a history of alcoholism or biliary tract disease. The pain of pancreatitis, like that of myocardial infarction, may be predominant in the epigastrium. However, unlike the pain of myocardial infarction, it is usually transmitted to the back, is position-sensitive, and may be relieved in part by leaning forward.[26] Chest pain aggravated by swallowing may also be due to acute pericarditis, whereas pain intensified by coughing may be due to pericarditis, bronchitis, or pleurisy or may be of radicular origin. *Congenital absence of the pericardium* (p. 1506) produces chest pain that is relieved by changing position in bed, is brought on by lying on the left side, and lasts a few seconds. Pain due to the *scalenus anticus (thoracic outlet) syndrome* may be confused with angina because it is often associated with paresthesias along the ulnar distribution of the arm and forearm. However, in contrast to angina, not only is it typically precipitated by abduction of the arm, lifting a weight, or working with the hands above the shoulders, but it is not brought on by walking.

RELIEF OF PAIN. Rest and nitroglycerin characteristically relieve the discomfort of angina in approximately 1 to 5 minutes. If more than 10 minutes transpire before relief, the diagnosis of chronic stable angina becomes questionable and instead may be unstable angina, acute myocardial infarction, or pain not caused by myocardial ischemia at all. Although nitroglycerin commonly relieves the pain of angina pectoris, the discomfort of esophageal spasm and esophagitis may also be relieved by this drug. Angina pectoris is alleviated by quiet standing or sitting; sometimes the recumbent position does not relieve angina. Chest pain secondary to *acute pericarditis* is characteristically relieved by leaning forward, whereas pain that is relieved by food or antacids may be due to *peptic ulcer disease* or esophagitis. Pain that is alleviated by holding the breath in deep expiration is commonly due to pleurisy. Some patients with upper gastrointestinal disease or anxiety report relief of symptoms after belching.

ACCOMPANYING SYMPTOMS. The physician should always be respectful of the patient who reports the presence of chest pain and profuse sweating. This combination of symptoms frequently signals a serious disorder, often acute myocardial infarction. Severe chest pain accompanied by nausea and vomiting is also often due to myocardial infarction. The latter diagnosis, as well as pneumothorax or pulmonary embolism, is suggested when pain is associated with shortness of breath. Chest pain accompanied by palpitation may be due to the acute myocardial ischemia that results from a tachyarrhythmia-induced increase in myocardial oxygen consumption in the presence of coronary artery disease. Chest pain accompanied by hemoptysis suggests pulmonary embolism with infarction or lung tumor, whereas pain accompanied by fever occurs in pneumonia, pleurisy, and pericarditis. Functional pain is commonly accompanied by frequent sighing, anxiety, or depression.

CYANOSIS

(See also pp. 895 and 901)

Cyanosis, both a symptom and a physical sign, is a bluish discoloration of the skin and mucous membranes resulting from an increased quantity of reduced hemoglobin or of abnormal hemoglobin pigments in the blood perfusing these areas.[32] There are two principal forms of cyanosis: (1) *central cyanosis*, characterized by decreased arterial oxygen saturation due to right-to-left shunting of blood or impaired pulmonary function, and (2) *peripheral cyanosis*, most commonly secondary to cutaneous vasoconstriction due to a low cardiac output or exposure to cold air or water; if peripheral cyanosis is confined to an extremity, localized arterial or venous obstruction should be suspected. A history of cyanosis localized to the hands suggests *Raynaud's phenomenon*. Central cyanosis due to congenital heart disease or pulmonary disease characteristically worsens during exertion, whereas the resting peripheral cyanosis of congestive heart failure may be accentuated only slightly, if at all, during exertion.

Central cyanosis usually becomes apparent at a mean capillary concentration of 4 gm/dl reduced hemoglobin (or 0.5 gm/dl methemoglobin). In general, a history of cyanosis in Caucasians is rarely elicited unless arterial saturation is 85 per cent or less; in pigmented races arterial saturation has to drop far lower before cyanosis is perceptible. Cyanosis generally occurs in patients with *congenital heart disease* when the volume of a right-to-left shunt exceeds 25 per cent of the left ventricular output. Since it is the *absolute* quantity of reduced hemoglobin in the blood that is responsible for cyanosis, the higher the total hemoglobin content, the greater the tendency toward cyanosis; thus, patients with marked polycythemia become cyanotic at higher levels of arterial oxygen saturation than do patients with normal hematocrit values, and cyanosis may be absent in patients with severe anemia despite marked arterial desaturation. Patients with congenital heart disease often have a history of cyanosis which is intensified during exertion because of the lower saturation of blood returning to the right side of the heart and the augmented right-to-left shunt.

Although a history of cyanosis beginning in infancy suggests a congenital cardiac malformation with a right-to-left shunt, *hereditary methemoglobinemia* is another, albeit rare, cause of congenital cyanosis; the diagnosis of this condition is supported by a family history of cyanosis in the absence of heart disease.

A history of cyanosis limited to the neonatal period suggests the diagnosis of atrial septal defect with transient right-to-left shunting or, more commonly, pulmonary parenchymal disease or central nervous system depression. Cyanosis beginning at age 1 to 3 months may be reported when spontaneous closure of a patent ductus arteriosus causes a reduction of pulmonary blood flow in the presence of right-sided obstructive cardiac anomalies (p. 914). If cyanosis appears at age 6 months or later in childhood, it may be due to the development or progression of obstruction to right ventricular outflow in patients with ventricular septal defect. A history of the development of cyanosis between ages 5 and 20 years in a patient with congenital heart disease suggests an Eisenmenger's reaction with right-to-left shunting as a consequence of a progressive increase in pulmonary vascular resistance (p. 911).

SYNCOPE

(See also Chap. 30)

Syncope, which may be defined as a loss of consciousness, results most commonly from reduced perfusion of the brain. The history is extremely valuable in the differential diagnosis of syncope (Table 1–5). Several daily attacks of loss of consciousness suggest (1) Stokes-Adams attacks, i.e., transient asystole or ventricular fibrillation in the presence of atrioventricular block; (2) other cardiac arrhythmias; or (3) a seizure disorder, i.e., petit mal epilepsy. These diagnoses are suggested when the

TABLE 1-5 CLUES FROM THE HISTORY IN ELUCIDATING THE CAUSE OF SYNCOPE

PRECEDING EVENTS	
Drugs:	Orthostatic hypotension (antihypertensives), hypoglycemia (insulin)
Severe pain, emotional stress:	Vasovagal syncope, hyperventilation
Movement of head and neck:	Carotid sinus hypersensitivity
Exertion:	Any form of obstruction to left ventricular outflow, Takayasu's arteritis
Upper extremity exertion:	Subclavian "steal"
TYPE OF ONSET	
Sudden:	Neurological (seizure disorder); arrhythmia (ventricular tachycardia or fibrillation, Stokes-Adams)
Rapid with premonition:	Vasovagal, neurological (aura)
Gradual:	Hyperventilation, hypoglycemia
POSITION AT ONSET	
Arising:	Orthostatic hypotension
Prolonged standing:	Vasovagal
Any position:	Arrhythmias, neurological, hypoglycemia, hyperventilation
POST SYNCOPAL CLEARING OF SENSORIUM	
Slow:	Neurological
Rapid:	All others
ASSOCIATED EVENTS	
Incontinence, tongue biting, injury:	Neurological

Modified from Lindenfeld, J. A.: Syncope. *In* Horwitz, L. D., and Groves, B. M. (eds.): Signs and Symptoms in Cardiology. Philadelphia, J. B. Lippincott, 1985, 506 pp.

loss of consciousness is abrupt and occurs over 1 or 2 seconds; a more gradual onset suggests vasodepressor syncope (i.e., the common faint) or syncope due to hyperventilation or, much less commonly, hypoglycemia.

Cardiac syncope is usually of rapid onset without aura, and is usually *not* associated with convulsive movements, urinary incontinence, and a postictal confusional state. Syncope in aortic stenosis is usually precipitated by effort.[33] Patients with epilepsy often have a prodromal aura preceding the seizure. Injury from falling is common, as are urinary incontinence and a postictal confusional state, associated with headache and drowsiness. Unconsciousness developing gradually and lasting for a few seconds suggests vasodepressor syncope or syncope secondary to postural hypotension, whereas a longer period suggests aortic stenosis or hyperventilation. *Hysterical fainting* is usually not accompanied by any untoward display of anxiety or change in pulse, blood pressure, or skin color, and there may be a question about whether any true loss of consciousness occurred. It is often associated with paresthesias of the hands or face, hyperventilation, dyspnea, chest pain, and feelings of acute anxiety.

Syncope independent of body position suggests Stokes-Adams attacks, hyperventilation, or epilepsy, whereas syncope of other etiologies usually occurs in the upright position. Syncope occurring upon bending, leaning, or assuming a particular body position should raise the possibility of a left atrial myxoma (p. 1454) or a ball-valve thrombus. Since syncope is an unusual feature of mitral stenosis, when it does occur in a patient thought to have this condition, the possibility of left atrial *myxoma* or *ball-valve thrombus* should be considered. Syncope occurring during or immediately following exertion suggests *aortic stenosis, hypertrophic obstructive cardiomyopathy,* or *primary pulmonary hypertension.* Syncope is rare in patients with angina pectoris unless the latter is secondary to one of the aforementioned conditions. Syncope following insulin administration suggests a hypoglycemic etiology; syncope several hours after eating is characteristic of reactive hypoglycemia. Loss of consciousness following an emotional stress suggests that it is vasodepressor syncope or secondary to hyperventilation.

Patients with *vasodepressor syncope* often have a long history of fainting, commonly associated with emotional or painful stimuli. This, the most common form of syncope, may be precipitated by the sight or loss of blood or by physical or emotional stress; it can be averted by promptly lying down, and it is characteristically preceded by symptoms of autonomic hyperactivity such as dim vision, giddiness, yawning, sweating, and nausea (p. 875). Syncope secondary to *cerebrovascular disturbance* is often preceded by aphasia, unilateral weakness, or confusion. A history of fainting following sudden movements of the head, shaving the neck, or wearing a tight collar suggests carotid sinus syncope (p. 878). Syncope associated with chest pain may be secondary to massive acute myocardial infarction or infarction associated with arrhythmias; occasionally, following recovery of consciousness, the associated chest pain may be forgotten, and the infarction may be recognized only by means of characteristic changes in serum enzymes and on the electrocardiogram.

REGAINING CONSCIOUSNESS. Consciousness is usually regained quite promptly in syncope of cardiovascular origin but more slowly with epilepsy. When consciousness is regained after vasodepressor syncope, the patient is often pale and diaphoretic with a slow heart rate, whereas after a Stokes-Adams attack, the face is often flushed and there may be cardiac acceleration. Patients who sustain an injury when falling during a fainting spell usually have epilepsy or occasionally syncope of cardiac origin, but patients who have unconsciousness related to emotional disturbance rarely sustain physical trauma.

DIFFERENTIAL DIAGNOSIS. A *family history of syncope* or near syncope can often be elicited in patients with hypertrophic obstructive cardiomyopathy (p. 1407) or ventricular tachyarrhythmias associated with Q-T prolongation (p. 879). A family history of epilepsy is positive in approximately 4 per cent of patients with convulsive disorders. Syncope associated with progressive intensification of cyanosis in an infant or child with cyanotic congenital heart disease is likely to be due to cerebral anoxia as a consequence of an increase in the right-to-left shunt, secondary to an increase in the obstruction to right ventricular outflow or a reduction in systemic vascular resistance (p. 898). A history of *syncope during childhood* suggests the possibility of a cardiovascular anomaly obstructing left ventricular outflow—valvular, supravalvular, or subvalvular aortic stenosis. In patients with hypertrophic obstructive cardiomyopathy, syncope may be post-tussive and occurs characteristically in the erect position, when arising suddenly, after standing erect for long periods, and during or immediately after cessation of exertion.

Patients with syncope secondary to *orthostatic hypotension* may have a history of drug therapy for hypertension or of abnormalities of autonomic function, such as impotence, disturbances of sphincter function, peripheral neuropathy, and anhidrosis (p. 876). When syncope is secondary to hypovolemia, there is often a history of melena, anemia, menorrhagia, or treatment with anticoagulants. Syncope due to *cerebrovascular insufficiency* is frequently associated with a history of unilateral blindness, weakness, paresthesias, or memory defects.

PALPITATION

This common symptom is defined as an unpleasant awareness of the forceful or rapid beating of the heart. It may be brought about by a variety of disorders involving changes in cardiac rhythm or rate, including all forms of tachycardia, ectopic beats, compensatory pauses, augmented stroke volume due to valvular regurgitation, hyperkinetic (high cardiac output) states, and the sudden onset of bradycardia. In the case of premature contractions the patient is more commonly aware of the postextrasystolic beat than of the premature beat itself, and it appears that it is the increased motion of the heart within the chest that is perceived rather than the increase in cardiac contractility. This explains why palpitation is not a characteristic feature of aortic or pulmonic stenosis or of severe systemic or pulmonary hypertension, conditions characterized by an increased force of cardiac contraction.

When episodes of palpitation last for an instant, they are described as "skipped beats" or a "flopping sensation" in the chest and most commonly are due to extrasystoles. On the other hand, the sensation that the heart has "stopped beating" often correlates with the compensatory pause following a premature contraction.

DIFFERENTIAL DIAGNOSIS. Palpitation characterized by a slow heart rate may be due to atrioventricular block or sinus node disease. When palpitation begins and ends abruptly, it is often due to a paroxysmal tachycardia such as paroxysmal atrial or junctional tachycardia, atrial flutter, or atrial fibrillation, whereas a gradual onset and cessation of the attack suggest sinus tachycardia and/or an anxiety state. A history of chaotic, rapid heart action suggests the diagnosis of atrial fibrillation; fleeting and repetitive palpitation suggests multiple ectopic beats. A history of multiple paroxysms of tachycardia followed by palpitation that occurs only with effort or excitement suggests paroxysmal atrial fibrillation that has become permanent—the palpitation being experienced only when the ventricular rate rises. Some patients have taken their pulse during palpitation or have asked a companion to do so. A regular rate between 100 and 140 beats/min suggests *sinus tachycardia,* a regular rate of approximately 150 beats/min suggests *atrial flutter,* and a regular rate exceeding 160 beats/min suggests *paroxysmal supraventricular tachycardia.* As an adjunct to the history, it may be possible to ascertain the rhythm responsible for the palpitation by tapping the finger on the patient's chest in a variety of rhythms and asking the patient to identify the pattern which most closely resembles the abnormal feeling.

A history of palpitation during strenuous physical activity is normal, whereas palpitation during mild exertion suggests the presence of heart failure, atrial fibrillation, anemia, or thyrotoxicosis, or that the individual is severely "out of condition." A feeling of forceful heart action accompanied by throbbing in the neck suggests aortic regurgitation. When palpitation can be relieved suddenly by stooping, breath-holding, or induced gagging or vomiting, i.e., by vagal maneuvers, the diagnosis of paroxysmal supraventricular tachycardia is suggested. A history of syncope following an episode of palpitation suggests either asystole or severe bradycardia following the termination of a tachyarrhythmia or a Stokes-Adams attack. A history of palpitation associated with anxiety, a lump in the throat, dizziness, and tingling in the hands and face suggests sinus tachycardia accompanying an anxiety state with hyperventilation. Palpitation followed by angina suggests that myocardial ischemia has been precipitated by increased oxygen demands induced by the rapid heart rate.

In many individuals no obvious cause for palpitation emerges despite careful work-up, including a correlation between episodes of palpitation with a simultaneously recorded ambulatory electrocardiogram (p. 615) or an electrocardiogram recorded by transtelephonic transmission. Anxiety is responsible for the symptom in many such patients, some of whom have known heart disease and may be receiving a vasodilator for the treatment of hypertension or nifedipine for the treatment of myocardial ischemia. In these patients palpitation may be due to postural hypotension resulting in reflex cardiac acceleration.

EDEMA

(See also Ch. 20)

LOCALIZATION. This is helpful in elucidating the etiology of edema.[34] Thus a history of edema of the legs that is most pronounced in the evening is characteristic of heart failure or bilateral chronic venous insufficiency. Inability to fit the feet into shoes is a common early complaint. In most patients any visible edema of both lower extremities is preceded by a weight gain of at least 7 to 10 lbs. Cardiac edema is generally symmetrical. As it progresses, it usually ascends to involve the legs, thighs, genitalia, and abdominal wall. In patients with heart failure who remain chiefly in bed, the edema localizes particularly in the sacral area. Edema located in both the abdomen and the legs is observed in heart failure and hepatic cirrhosis. Edema may be generalized (anasarca) in the nephrotic syndrome, severe heart failure, and hepatic cirrhosis. A history of edema around the eyes and face is characteristic of the nephrotic syndrome, acute glomerulonephritis, angioneurotic edema, hypoproteinemia, and myxedema. A history of edema limited to the face, neck, and upper arms may be associated with obstruction of the superior vena cava, most commonly by carcinoma of the lung, lymphoma, or aneurysm of the aortic arch. A history of edema restricted to one extremity is usually due to venous thrombosis or lymphatic blockage of that extremity.

ACCOMPANYING SYMPTOMS. A history of dyspnea associated with edema is most frequently due to heart failure but may also be observed in patients with large bilateral pleural effusions, elevation of the diaphragms due to ascites, angioneurotic edema with laryngeal involvement, and pulmonary embolism. When dyspnea precedes edema, the underlying disorder is usually left ventricular dysfunction, mitral stenosis, or chronic lung disease with cor pulmonale. A history of jaundice suggests that edema may be of hepatic origin, whereas edema associated with a history of ulceration and pigmentation of the skin of the legs is most commonly due to chronic venous insufficiency or postphlebitic syndrome. When cardiac edema is *not* associated with orthopnea, it may be due to tricuspid stenosis or regurgitation or constrictive pericarditis; in these conditions edema is not always most prominent in the lower extremities but may be generalized and may even involve the face.

A history of ascites *preceding* edema suggests cirrhosis, whereas a history of ascites *following* edema suggests cardiac or renal disease. *Angioneurotic edema* occurs intermittently, particularly after emotional stress or eating certain foods. *Idiopathic cyclic edema* is associated with menstruation. A history of edema on prolonged standing is observed in patients with chronic venous insufficiency.

COUGH

Cough, one of the most frequent of all cardiorespiratory symptoms, may be defined as an explosive expiration which provides a means of clearing the tracheobronchial tree of secretions and foreign bodies. It can be caused by a variety of infectious, neoplastic, or allergic disorders of the lungs and tracheobronchial tree. Cardiovascular disorders most frequently responsible for cough include those that lead to pulmonary venous hypertension, interstitial and alveolar pulmonary edema, pulmonary infarction, and compression of the tracheobronchial tree (aortic aneurysm). Cough due to pulmonary venous hypertension secondary to left ventricular failure or mitral stenosis tends to be dry, irritating, spasmodic, and nocturnal. When cough accompanies exertional dyspnea, it suggests either chronic obstructive lung disease or heart failure, whereas in a patient with a history of allergy and/or wheezing, cough is often a concomitant of bronchial asthma. A history of cough associated with expectoration for months or years occurs in chronic obstructive lung disease and/or chronic bronchitis.

The *character* of the sputum may be helpful in the differential diagnosis. Thus, a cough producing frothy, pink-tinged sputum occurs in pulmonary edema; clear, white, mucoid sputum suggests viral infection or longstanding bronchial irritation; thick, yellowish sputum suggests an infectious cause; rusty sputum suggests pneumococcal pneumonia; blood-streaked sputum suggests tuberculosis, bronchiectasis, carcinoma of the lung, or pulmonary infarction.

A history of a combination of cough with *hoarseness* without upper respiratory disease may be due to pressure of a greatly enlarged left atrium on an enlarged pulmonary artery compressing the recurrent laryngeal nerve.

HEMOPTYSIS

The expectoration of blood or of sputum, either streaked or grossly contaminated with blood, may be due to (1) escape of red cells into the alveoli from congested vessels in the lungs (acute pulmonary edema); (2) rupture of dilated endobronchial vessels that form collateral channels between the pulmonary and bronchial venous systems (mitral stenosis); (3) necrosis and hemorrhage into the alveoli (pulmonary infarction); (4) ulceration of the bronchial mucosa or the slough of a caseous lesion (tuberculosis); minor damage to the tracheobronchial mucosa, produced by excessive coughing of any cause, can result in mild hemoptysis; (5) vascular invasion (carcinoma of the lung); or (6) necrosis of the mucosa with rupture of pulmonary-bronchial venous connections (bronchiectasis).

The history is often decisive in pinpointing the etiology of hemoptysis.[35] Recurrent episodes of minor bleeding are observed in patients with chronic bronchitis, bronchiectasis, tuberculosis, and mitral stenosis. Rarely, these conditions result in the expectoration of large quantities of blood, i.e., more than one-half cup. Massive hemoptysis may also be due to rupture of a pulmonary arteriovenous fistula; exsanguinating hemoptysis may occur with rupture of an aortic aneurysm into the bronchopulmonary tree. Hemoptysis associated with a history of expectoration of clear, gray sputum suggests chronic obstructive lung disease and of yellowish-green sputum, pulmonary infection. Hemoptysis associated with shortness of breath suggests mitral stenosis; in this condition the hemoptysis is often precipitated by sudden elevations in left atrial pressure during effort or pregnancy and is attributable to rupture of small pulmonary or bronchopulmonary anastomosing veins. Blood-tinged sputum in patients with mitral stenosis may also be due to transient pulmonary edema; in these circumstances it is usually associated with severe dyspnea.

A history of hemoptysis associated with acute pleuritic chest pain suggests pulmonary embolism with infarction. Recurrent hemoptysis in a young, otherwise asymptomatic woman favors the diagnosis of bronchial adenoma. Hemoptysis associated with congenital heart disease and cyanosis suggests Eisenmenger syndrome (p. 978). A history of recurrent hemoptysis with chronic excessive sputum production suggests the diagnosis of bronchiectasis. Hemoptysis associated with the production of putrid sputum occurs in lung abscess, whereas hemoptysis associated with weight loss and anorexia in a male smoker suggests carcinoma of the lung. When blunt trauma to the chest is followed by hemoptysis, lung contusion is the probable cause.

A history of drug ingestion may be helpful in elucidating the etiology of hemoptysis; e.g., anticoagulants and immunosuppressive drugs can cause bleeding. A history of ingestion of contraceptive pills may be a risk factor for the development of deep vein thrombosis and subsequent pulmonary embolism and infarction.

OTHER SYMPTOMS

Cardiovascular disorders can cause symptoms emanating from every organ system. Several of these are mentioned here primarily to point out how detailed the history should be in providing a comprehensive evaluation of a patient suspected of having cardiovascular disease; fuller discussions are found elsewhere in this text.

FATIGUE. This is among the most common symptoms in patients with impaired cardiovascular function. However, it is also one of the most nonspecific of all symptoms in clinical medicine; in patients with an impaired systemic circulation as a consequence of a depressed cardiac output, it may be associated with muscular weakness. In other patients with heart disease, fatigue may be caused by drugs, such as beta-adrenoceptor blocking agents, or by excessive blood pressure reduction in patients treated too vigorously for hypertension or heart failure. In patients with heart failure, fatigue may also be caused by excessive diuresis and by diuretic-induced hypokalemia.

Extreme fatigue sometimes precedes or accompanies acute myocardial infarction.[19] *Nocturia* is a common early complaint in patients with congestive heart failure. *Anorexia,* abdominal fullness, right upper quadrant discomfort, weight loss, and cachexia are symptoms of advanced heart failure (p. 451). Anorexia, *nausea, vomiting,* and *visual changes* are important signs of digitalis intoxication (p. 490). Nausea and vomiting occur frequently in patients with acute myocardial infarction. *Hoarseness* may be caused by compression of the recurrent laryngeal nerve by an aortic aneurysm, a dilated pulmonary artery, or a greatly enlarged left atrium. A history of *fever* and *chills* is common in patients with infective endocarditis (p. 1085).

The aforementioned symptoms are examples of the wide variety not obviously associated with abnormalities of the cardiovascular system that can be of critical importance in differential diagnosis when they are elicited in patients known to have or suspected of having heart disease. They serve to reemphasize that the physician whose responsibility it is to care for patients with heart disease must be first and foremost a broadly based clinician.

THE HISTORY IN SPECIFIC FORMS OF HEART DISEASE

Just as the history is of central importance in determining whether or not a specific symptom is caused by heart disease, it is equally valuable in elucidating the *etiology* of recognized heart disease. A few examples are given below; considerably greater detail is provided in later chapters that deal with each specific disease entity.

HEART DISEASE IN INFANCY AND CHILDHOOD

The history is particularly helpful in establishing a diagnosis of *congenital heart disease.* In view of the familial incidence of certain congenital malformations (Chs. 31 and 51), a history of congenital heart disease, cyanosis, or heart murmur in the family should be ascertained. Rubella in the first 2 months of pregnancy is associated with a number of congenital cardiac malformations (patent ductus arteriosus, atrial and ventricular septal defect, tetralogy of Fallot, and supravalvular aortic stenosis). A maternal viral illness in the last trimester of pregnancy may be responsible for neonatal myocarditis. Syncope on exertion in a child with congenital heart disease suggests a lesion in which the cardiac output is fixed, such as aortic or pulmonic stenosis. Exertional angina in a child suggests severe aortic stenosis, pulmonary stenosis, primary pulmonary hypertension, or anomalous origin of the left coronary artery. A history of syncope or faintness with straining and associated with cyanosis suggests tetralogy of Fallot.

In infants or children with cardiac murmurs, it is important to ascertain as precisely as possible when the murmur was first heard. Murmurs due to either aortic or pulmonic stenosis are usually audible within the first 48 hours of life, whereas those produced by a ventricular septal defect are usually apparent a few days or weeks later. On the other hand, the murmur produced by an atrial septal defect often is not heard until age 2 to 3 months.

Frequent episodes of pneumonia early in infancy suggest a large left-to-right shunt, and excessive diaphoresis occurs in left ventricular failure, most commonly due to ventricular septal defect in this age group. A history of squatting is most frequently associated with tetralogy of Fallot or tricuspid atresia (p. 895). Dysphagia suggests the presence of an aortic arch anomaly such as double aortic arch or an anomalous origin of the right subclavian artery passing behind the esophagus. A history of headaches, weakness of the legs, and intermittent claudication is compatible with the diagnosis of coarctation of the aorta (p. 975). Weakness or lack of coordination in a child with heart disease suggests cardiomyopathy associated with Friedreich's ataxia or muscular dystrophy (p. 1816). Recurrent bleeding from the nose, lips, or mouth, associated with dizziness and visual disturbances, and a family history of bleeding in a cyanotic child suggest hereditary hemorrhagic telangiectasia (Osler-Weber-Rendu disease) with pulmonary arteriovenous fistula(s). A cerebrovascular accident in a cyanotic patient may be due to cerebral thrombosis or abscess or paradoxical embolization (p. 895).

MYOCARDITIS AND CARDIOMYOPATHY

Rheumatic fever (p. 1721) is suggested by a history of sore throat followed by symptoms including rash and chorea (St. Vitus dance), and manifested as a period of twitching or clumsiness for a few months in childhood, as well as by frequent epistaxes and growing pains, i.e., nocturnal pains in the legs. In patients suspected of having myocarditis or cardiomyopathy, a history of Raynaud's phenomenon, dysphagia, or tight skin suggests scleroderma (p. 1746), a history of dyspnea following an influenza-like illness with myalgia suggests acute myocarditis. Pain in the hip or lower back that awakens the patient in the morning and is followed by morning back stiffness suggests rheumatoid spondylitis, which is often associated with aortic valve disease (p. 1741). *Carcinoid heart disease* is associated with a history of diarrhea, bronchospasm, and flushing of the upper chest and head (p. 1424). A history of diabetes, particularly if resistant to insulin and associated with bronzing of the skin, suggests *hemochromatosis* (p. 1747), which may be associated with heart failure due to cardiac infiltration. *Amyloid heart disease* (p. 1416) is often associated with a history of postural hypotension and peripheral neuropathy. *Hypertrophic cardiomyopathy* (p. 1404) is often associated with a family history of this condition and sometimes with a family history of sudden death. The characteristic symptoms are angina, dyspnea, and syncope, which are often intensified paradoxically by digitalis and which occur during or immediately after exercise.

HIGH-OUTPUT HEART FAILURE AND CORPULMONALE

Patients with symptoms of heart failure (breathlessness and excess fluid accumulation) with warm extremities often have *high-output heart failure* (p. 458). They should be questioned about a history of anemia and of its common causes and accompaniments, such as menorrhagia, melena, peptic ulcer, hemorrhoids, sickle cell disease, and the neurological manifestations of vitamin B_{12} deficiency. Also, in such patients an attempt should be made to elicit a history of thyrotoxicosis (p. 1831) (weight loss, polyphagia, diarrhea, diaphoresis, heat intolerance, nervousness, breathlessness, muscle weakness, and goiter). Patients with beriberi heart disease responsible for high-output heart failure often present with a history characteristic of peripheral neuritis, alcoholism, poor eating habits, fad diets, or upper gastrointestinal surgery.

Patients with chronic *cor pulmonale* (see Chap. 49) frequently have a history of smoking, chronic cough and sputum production, dyspnea, and wheezing relieved by bronchodilators. Alternatively, they may present with a history of pulmonary emboli, phlebitis, and the sudden development of dyspnea at rest with palpitations, pleuritic chest pain, and, in the case of massive infarction, syncope.

PERICARDITIS AND ENDOCARDITIS

In patients in whom *pericarditis* or *cardiac tamponade* is suspected (Chap. 45), an attempt should be made to elicit a history of chest trauma, a recent viral infection, recent cardiac surgery, neoplastic disease of the chest with or without extensive radiation therapy, myxedema, scleroderma, tuberculosis, or contact with tuberculous patients. The *sequence of development* of abdominal swelling, ankle edema, and dyspnea should be determined since, in patients with chronic constrictive pericarditis, ascites often precedes edema, which in turn usually precedes exertional dyspnea. A history of joint symptoms with a face rash suggest the possibility of systemic lupus erythematosus (SLE), an important cause of pericarditis, and it should be recalled that procainamide, hydralazine, and isoniazid can produce an SLE-like syndrome (p. 638).

The diagnosis of *infective endocarditis* is suggested by a history of fever, severe night sweats, anorexia and weight loss, and embolic phenomena expressed as hematuria, back pain, petechiae, tender finger pads, and a cerebrovascular accident (p. 1085).

DRUG-INDUCED HEART DISEASE

The increasing appreciation that a wide variety of cardiac abnormalities can be induced by drugs makes a meticulous history of drug intake of great importance. Catecholamines, whether administered exogenously or when secreted by a pheochromocytoma (p. 1839), may produce a myocarditis and arrhythmias. Digitalis glycosides can be responsible for a variety of tachy- and bradyarrhythmias as well as gastrointestinal, visual, and central nervous system disturbances (p. 490). Quinidine may cause Q-T prolongation, ventricular tachycardia of the torsades de pointes variety, syncope, and sudden death, presumably due to ventricular fibrillation (p. 635). Paradoxically, the administration of antiarrhythmic drugs is one of the major causes of serious cardiac arrhythmias (p. 633).

Disopyramide (p. 630), beta-adrenoceptor blockers (p. 864), and the calcium channel antagonists, diltiazem and verapamil (p. 648), may depress ventricular performance, and in patients with ventricular dysfunction these drugs may intensify heart failure. Alcohol is also a potent myocardial depressant and may be responsible for the development of cardiomyopathy (p. 1402), arrhythmias, and sudden death. Tricyclic antidepressants may cause orthostatic hypotension and arrhythmias. Lithium, also used in the treatment of psychiatric disorders, can aggravate preexisting cardiac arrhythmias, particularly in patients with heart failure in whom the renal clearance of this ion is impaired. Cocaine can cause coronary spasm with resultant myocardial ischemia, myocardial infarction, and sudden death.[36,37]

The anthracycline compounds doxorubicin (Adriamycin) and daunorubicin, which are widely used because of their

TABLE 1-6 A COMPARISON OF THREE METHODS OF ASSESSING CARDIOVASCULAR DISABILITY

CLASS	NEW YORK HEART ASSOCIATION FUNCTIONAL CLASSIFICATION	CANADIAN CARDIOVASCULAR SOCIETY FUNCTIONAL CLASSIFICATION	SPECIFIC ACTIVITY SCALE
I	Patients with cardiac disease but without resulting limitations of physical activity. Ordinary physical activity does not cause undue fatigue, palpitation, dyspnea, or anginal pain.	Ordinary physical activity, such as walking and climbing stairs, does not cause angina. Angina with strenuous or rapid or prolonged exertion at work or recreation.	Patients can perform to completion any activity requiring ≥ 7 metabolic equivalents, e.g., can carry 24 lb up eight steps; carry objects that weigh 80 lb; do outdoor work (shovel snow, spade soil); do recreational activities (skiing, basketball, squash, handball, jog/walk 5 mph).
II	Patients with cardiac disease resulting in slight limitation of physical activity. They are comfortable at rest. Ordinary physical activity results in fatigue, palpitation, dyspnea, or anginal pain.	Slight limitation of ordinary activity. Walking or climbing stairs rapidly, walking uphill, walking or stair climbing after meals, in cold, in wind, or when under emotional stress, or only during the few hours after awakening. Walking more than two blocks on the level and climbing more than one flight of ordinary stairs at a normal pace and in normal conditions.	Patients can perform to completion any activity requiring ≥ 5 metabolic equivalents but cannot and do not perform to completion activities requiring ≥ 7 metabolic equivalents, e.g., have sexual intercourse without stopping, garden, rake, weed, roller skate, dance fox trot, walk at 4 mph on level ground.
III	Patients with cardiac disease resulting in marked limitation of physical activity. They are comfortable at rest. Less than ordinary physical activity causes fatigue, palpitation, dyspnea, or anginal pain.	Marked limitation of ordinary physical activity. Walking one to two blocks on the level and climbing more than one flight in normal conditions.	Patients can perform to completion any activity requiring ≥ 2 metabolic equivalents but cannot and do not perform to completion any activities requiring ≥ 5 metabolic equivalents, e.g., shower without stopping, strip and make bed, clean windows, walk 2.5 mph, bowl, play golf, dress without stopping.
IV	Patient with cardiac disease resulting in inability to carry on any physical activity without discomfort. Symptoms of cardiac insufficiency or of the anginal syndrome may be present even at rest. If any physical activity is undertaken, discomfort is increased.	Inability to carry on any physical activity without discomfort—anginal syndrome *may be* present at rest.	Patients cannot or do not perform to completion activities requiring ≥ 2 metabolic equivalents. *Cannot* carry out activities listed above (Specific Activity Scale, Class III).

From Goldman L., et al.: Comparative reproducibility and validity of systems for assessing cardiovascular functional class: Advantages of a new specific activity scale. Circulation 64:1227, 1981, by permission of the American Heart Association, Inc.

broad spectrum of activity against various tumors, may cause or intensify left ventricular failure, arrhythmias, myocarditis, and pericarditis (p. 1756). Cyclophosphamide, an antineoplastic alkylating agent, may also cause left ventricular dysfunction (p. 1769). Radiation therapy to the chest may cause acute and chronic pericarditis (p. 1765), a pancarditis, or coronary artery disease; further, it may enhance the aforementioned cardiotoxic effects of the anthracyclines.

ASSESSING CARDIOVASCULAR DISABILITY

(Table 1–6)

One of the greatest values of the history is in categorizing the *degree* of cardiovascular disability, so that a patient's status can be followed over time, the effects of a therapeutic intervention assessed, and patients compared with one another. The Criteria Committee of the New York Heart Association has provided a widely used classification that relates symptoms to "ordinary" activity.[38] The term "ordinary," of course, is subject to varying interpretation, as are terms such as "undue fatigue" that are used in this classification, and this has limited its accuracy and reproducibility. Somewhat more detailed and specific criteria were provided by the Canadian Cardiovascular Society,[39] but this classification and grading are limited to patients with angina pectoris. Goldman et al.[40] developed a specific activity scale in which classification is based on the estimated metabolic cost of various activities. This scale appears to be more reproducible and to be a better predictor of exercise tolerance than either the New York Heart Association Classification or the Canadian Cardiovascular Society Criteria.

A key element of the history is to determine whether the patient's disability is stable or progressive. A useful way to accomplish this is to inquire whether a specific task which now causes symptoms, e.g., dyspnea after climbing two flights of stairs, did so 3, 6, and 12 months previously. Precise questioning on this point is important since a gradual reduction of ordinary activity as heart disease progresses may lead to an underestimation of the apparent degree of disability.[41]

REFERENCES

1. Sandler, G.: The importance of the history in the medical clinic and the cost of unnecessary tests. Am. Heart J. *100*:928, 1980.
2. Hickman, D. H., Soc, H. C., Jr., and Soc, C. H.: Systematic bias in recording the history in patients with chest pain. J. Chronic Dis. 38:91, 1985.
3. Sapira, J. D.: The history. *In* The Art and Science of Bedside Diagnosis. Baltimore, Urban Schwartzenberg, 1990, pp. 9–45.
4. Hampton, J. R., Harrison, M. J. G., Mitchell, J. R. A., et al.: Relative contributions of history-taking, physical examination, and laboratory investigation to diagnosis and management of medical outpatients. Br. Med. J. 2:486, 1975.
5. Tumulty, P. A.: Obtaining the history. *In* The Effective Clinician. Philadelphia, W. B. Saunders Company, 1973, pp. 17–28.
6. Fishman, A. P.: The first approach to the patient with respiratory signs and symptoms. *In* Fishman, A. P. (ed.): Pulmonary Diseases and Disorders. New York, McGraw-Hill Book Co., 1980, pp. 3–28.
7. Weber, K. T., and Szidon, J. P.: Exertional dyspnea. *In* Weber, K. T., and Janick, J. S. (eds.): Cardiopulmonary Exercise Testing. Philadelphia, W. B. Saunders Company, 1986, pp. 290–301.
8. Cherniack, N. S.: Dyspnea. *In* Murray, J. F., and Nadel, J. A. (eds.): Textbook of Respiratory Medicine. Philadelphia, W. B. Saunders Company, 1988, pp. 389–96.
9. Wasserman, K.: Dyspnea on exertion. Is it the heart or the lungs? JAMA *248*:2039, 1982.
10. Borg, G., and Noble, B.: Perceived exertion. *In* Wilmore, J. H. (ed.): Exercise and Sports. Science Reviews. New York, Academic Press, 1974, pp. 131–153.
11. Loke, J.: Distinguishing cardiac versus pulmonary limitation in exercise performance. Chest *83*:441, 1983.
12. Schmitt, B. P., Kushner, M. S., and Weiner, S. L.: The diagnostic usefulness of the history of the patient with dyspnea. J. Gen. Intern. Med. *1*:386, 1986.
13. Christie, L. G., and Conti, C. R.: Systematic approach to the evaluation of angina-like chest pain. Am. Heart J. *102*:897, 1981.
14. Constant, J.: The clinical diagnosis of nonanginal chest pain: The differentiation of angina from nonanginal chest pain by history. Clin. Cardiol. 6:11, 1983.
15. Levine, H. J.: Difficult problems in the diagnosis of chest pain. Am. Heart J. *100*:108, 1980.
16. Schofield, P. M., Whorwell, P. J., Jones, P. E., et al.: Differentiation of "esophageal" and "cardiac" chest pain. Am. J. Cardiol. *62*:315, 1988.
17. Conte, M. R., Orzan, F., Magnacca, M., et al.: Atypical chest pain: Coronary or esophageal disease? Int. J. Cardiol. *13*:135, 1986.
18. Matthews, M. B., and Julian, D. G.: Angina pectoris: Definition and description. *In* Julian, D. G. (ed.): Angina Pectoris. New York, Churchill Livingstone, 1985, p. 2.
19. Appels, A., and Mulder, P.: Excess fatigue as a precursor of myocardial infarction. Eur. Heart J. *9*:758, 1988.
20. Lichstein, E., Breitbart, S., Shani, J., et al.: Relationship between location of chest pain and site of coronary artery occlusion. Am. Heart J. *115*:564, 1988.
21. Cook, D. G., and Shaper, A. G.: Breathlessness, angina pectoris and coronary artery disease. Am. J. Cardiol. *63*:921, 1989.
22. Bass, C., Chambers, J. B., Kiff, P., et al.: Panic anxiety and hyperventilation in patients with chest pain: A controlled study. Q. J. Med. *69*:260:949–959, 1988.
23. Beitman, B. D., Basha, I., Flaker, G. et al.: Atypical or nonanginal chest pain: Panic disorder or coronary artery disease? Arch. Intern. Med. *147*:1548, 1987.
24. Kane, F. J., Jr., Harper, R. G., and Wittels, E.: Angina as a symptom of a psychiatric illness. South. Med. J. *81*:1412, 1988.
25. Selzer, A.: History. *In* Principles and Practice of Clinical Cardiology. 2nd ed. Philadelphia, W. B. Saunders Company, 1983, pp. 14–22.
26. Horwitz, L. D., and Groves, B. M. (eds.): Signs and Symptoms in Cardiology. Philadelphia, J. B. Lippincott, 1985, 506 pp.
27. Sutton, G. C.: Symptoms of heart disease. *In* Julian, D. G. (ed.): Diseases of the Heart. London, Balliere Tindall, 1989, pp. 89–99.
28. Mellow, M. H.: A gastroenterologist's view of chest pain. Curr. Probl. Cardiol. *7*:36, 1983.
29. Patterson, D. R.: Diffuse esophageal spasm in patients with undiagnosed chest pain. J. Clin. Gastroenterol. *4*:415, 1982.
30. DeMeester, T. R., O'Sullivan, G. C., Bermudez, G. et al.: Esophageal function in patients with angina-type chest pain and normal coronary angiograms. Ann. Surg. *196*:488, 1982.
31. Davies, H. A., Rush, E. M., Lewis, M. J., et al.: Oesophageal stimulation lowers exertional angina threshold. Lancet *1*:1011, 1985.
32. Braunwald, E.: Cyanosis. *In* Wilson, J., Braunwald, E., et al. (eds.): Harrison's Principles of Internal Medicine. 12th ed. New York, McGraw-Hill, 1991, pp. 226–228.
33. Forssell, G., Jonasson, R., and Orinius, E.: Identifying severe aortic valvular stenosis by bedside examination. Acta Med. Scand. *218*:397, 1985.
34. Braunwald, E.: Edema. In Wilson, J., Braunwald, E., et al. (eds.): Harrison's Principles of Internal Medicine. 12th ed. New York, McGraw-Hill, 1991, pp. 228–232.
35. Bristow, M. R. (ed.): Drug-Induced Heart Disease. Amsterdam, Elsevier, 1980, 476 pp.
36. Virmani, R., Robinowitz, M., Smialek, J. E., and Smyth, D. F.: Cardiovascular effect of cocaine: An autopsy study of 40 patients. Am. Heart J. *115*:1068, 1988.
37. Isner, J. M., and Chokshi, S. K.: Cocaine and vasospasm. N. Engl. J. Med. 321:1604, 1989.
38. The Criteria Committee of the New York Heart Association: Diseases of the Heart and Blood Vessels; Nomenclature and Criteria for Diagnosis. 6th ed. Boston, Little, Brown and Co., 1964
39. Campeau, L.: Grading of angina pectoris. Circulation *54*:522, 1975.
40. Goldman, L., Hashimoto, B., Cook, E. F., and Loscalzo, A.: Comparative reproducibility and validity of systems for assessing cardiovascular functional class: Advantages of a new specific activity scale. Circulation *64*:1227, 1981.
41. Goldman, L., Cook, E. F., Mitchell, N., et al.: Pitfalls in the serial assessment of cardiac functional status. How a reduction in "ordinary" activity may reduce the apparent degree of cardiac compromise and give a misleading impression of improvement. J. Chronic Dis. *35*:763, 1982.

GENERAL REFERENCES

Braunwald, E.: Alterations in circulatory and respiratory function. *In* Wilson, J., Braunwald, E., et al. (eds.): Harrison's Principles of Internal Medicine. 12th ed. New York, McGraw-Hill Book Co., 1991, pp. 217–241.

Constant, J.: The evolving check list in history-taking. *In* Bedside Cardiology. 3rd ed. Boston, Little, Brown and Co., 1985, pp. 1–22.

Dressler, W.: Clinical Aids in Cardiac Diagnosis. New York, Grune and Stratton, 1970.

Fowler, N. O.: The history in cardiac diagnosis. *In* Fowler, N. O. (ed.): Cardiac Diagnosis and Treatment. 3rd ed. Hagerstown, Md., Harper and Row, 1980, pp. 23–29.

Kraytman, J.: Cardiorespiratory system. *In* The Complete Patient History. New York, McGraw-Hill Book Co., 1979, pp. 11–112.

Oram, S.: Clinical examination. *In* Clinical Heart Disease. 2nd ed. London, William Heinemann, 1981, pp. 45–60.

Parkinson, J.: Cardiac symptoms. Ann. Intern. Med. *35*:499, 1951.

White, P. D.: Clues in the Diagnosis and Treatment of Heart Disease. Springfield, Ill., Charles C Thomas, 1955.

Wood, P.: The chief symptoms of heart failure. *In* Diseases of the Heart and Circulation. 3rd ed. Philadelphia, J. B. Lippincott, 1968, pp. 1–25.

The Physical Examination

by EUGENE BRAUNWALD, M.D.

Two of the most common pitfalls in cardiovascular medicine are the failure by the cardiologist to recognize the effects of systemic illnesses on the cardiovascular system and the failure by the noncardiologist to recognize the cardiac manifestations of systemic illnesses that have major effects on other organ systems. In order to avoid these pitfalls, patients known to have or suspected of having heart disease require not only a detailed examination of the cardiovascular system but a meticulous general physical examination as well. For example, the condition of patients with previously stable rheumatic valvular or coronary artery disease may suddenly deteriorate, not because of the progression of the underlying cardiac condition, but rather because of the development of an unrelated disease—such as a painless bleeding peptic ulcer or a malignant neoplasm—and a change in the patient's cardiac condition, such as the intensification of angina or dyspnea, may result from an anemia caused by the other disorder.

The presence of cardiac disease should prompt a careful search for frequent noncardiac concomitants such as atherosclerosis of the carotid arteries and of the arteries of the lower extremities and aorta in patients with ischemic heart disease. Conversely, the very high incidence (approximately 50 per cent) of coronary artery disease in patients with cerebrovascular disorders must be considered in dealing with patients who have these disorders. In some patients an underlying cardiovascular abnormality may be responsible for the involvement of other organ systems; for example, retarded physical development and failure to thrive in infants may be secondary to congenital heart disease, and embolic strokes are important complications of rheumatic mitral stenosis and atrial fibrillation, of mitral valve prolapse, and of infective endocarditis.

Examples of disorders which have effects principally on other organs but which often also affect the heart include the following:[1]

1. *Muscular dystrophies* (Chap. 60) causing cardiomyopathies.
2. *Metabolic disorders,* such as hemochromatosis (p. 1747), glycogen storage disease (p. 1645), Gaucher's disease (p. 1419), and Fabry's disease (p. 1646) (myocardial infiltration, heart failure, and conduction defects).
3. *Chromosomal disorders,* such as the Turner syndrome (p. 1629) associated with a variety of congenital cardiac defects, particularly coarctation of the aorta.
4. *Endocrine disorders,* such as acromegaly (p. 1827) associated with accelerated coronary atherosclerosis and myocardial hypertrophy; hyperthyroidism (p. 1833) associated with heart failure and atrial fibrillation, and myxedema associated with pericardial effusion.
5. *Congenital deafness* (p. 889) associated with Q-T interval prolongation and serious cardiac arrhythmias.
6. *Raynaud's disease* associated with primary pulmonary hypertension (p. 804), coronary spasm, and sclerodermatous involvement of the heart (p. 1736).
7. *Inherited connective tissue disorders* (Chap. 51), such as Marfan syndrome, osteogenesis imperfecta, Ehlers-Danlos syndrome, pseudoxanthoma elasticum, associated with aortic dilatation, dissection and regurgitation, mitral valve prolapse, coronary artery disease, and pericarditis; Hurler syndrome and related disorders of mucopolysaccharide metabolism (p. 1646) associated with arrhythmias, valvular disease, and heart failure.
8. *Collagen vascular diseases* (Chap. 56): systemic lupus erythematosus (valvulitis, myocarditis, coronary arteritis, and pericarditis), ankylosing spondylitis (diseases of the aorta and aortic valve), rheumatoid arthritis (pericarditis and valve disease), vasculitis (coronary arteritis and myocarditis), polymyositis (arrhythmias, pericarditis, and myocarditis).
9. *Sarcoidosis* (p. 763) associated with restrictive cardiomyopathy and arrhythmias.
10. *Chronic hemolytic anemia* (p. 1743) causing cardiac dilatation and myocarditis secondary to transfusional hemosiderosis.

In patients in whom these and related systemic disorders are present or suspected, the physical examination should be conducted so as to allow recognition of the systemic disorder and evaluation of the presence and severity of cardiovascular involvement.

THE GENERAL PHYSICAL EXAMINATION

Although a variety of techniques may be employed in carrying out the physical examination I favor commencing with an assessment of the general appearance of the patient and then utilizing the regional approach, starting with the head and ending with the lower extremities. It is desirable, whenever possible, to examine the patient on an examining table or

Editor's Note: Examination of the cardiovascular system includes inspection and palpation of the arterial and venous pulses and of the chest as well as auscultation of the heart. The findings elicited on physical examination can be aided enormously by graphic recordings. The details of carrying out the cardiovascular examination and the interpretation of the findings are presented in this chapter and in Chapter 3. These two chapters should be considered as a unit, since the subjects covered are similar and the material does not lend itself well to a rigid separation between physical and graphic modes of examination; some degree of overlap in content among these chapters is therefore unavoidable.

bed whose head section may be raised. Examination in a quiet room at a comfortable temperature and in daylight is optimal.

GENERAL APPEARANCE

An assessment of the patient's general appearance is usually begun with a detailed inspection at the time when the history is being obtained.[1-3] The general build and appearance of the patient, the skin color, and the presence of pallor or cyanosis should be noted, as well as the presence of shortness of breath, orthopnea, periodic (Cheyne-Stokes) respiration (p. 454), and distention of the neck veins. If the patient is in pain, is he or she sitting quietly (typical of angina pectoris); moving about, trying to find a more comfortable position (characteristic of acute myocardial infarction); or most comfortable sitting upright (heart failure) or leaning forward (pericarditis)? Simple inspection will also reveal whether the patient's whole body shakes with each heartbeat and whether Corrigan's pulses (bounding arterial pulsations, as occur with the large stroke volume of severe aortic regurgitation, arteriovenous fistula, or complete atrioventricular block) are present in the head, neck, and upper extremities. Marked weight loss, malnutrition, and cachexia, which occur in severe chronic heart failure (p. 454), may also be readily evident on inspection. The cold, sweaty palms and frequent sighing respirations typical of *neurocirculatory asthenia* may be detected, as well as the marked obesity, somnolence, and cyanosis suggestive of the *Pickwickian syndrome* (p. 801). Abdominally located obesity (diameter of waist/diameter of hips > 0.85; normal $= 0.7$) is associated with adult onset diabetes and coronary artery disease and should also be looked for.

The distinctive general appearance of the *Marfan syndrome* (p. 1641) is often apparent, i.e., long extremities with an arm span that exceeds the height; a longer lower segment (pubis to foot) than upper segment (head to pubis); arachnodactyly (spider fingers); and a variety of thoracic deformities, including kyphoscoliosis, pectus carinatum, and pectus excavatum. Patients with *muscular dystrophy*—a cause of cardiomyopathy (Chap. 60)—may have difficulty rising from a chair or walking. The diagnosis of *hyperthyroidism*, which frequently causes cardiac disease (p. 1832), can often be suspected from simple inspection (exophthalmos, lid lag, perspiration, a fine tremor). In *Cushing's syndrome*, a cause of secondary hypertension (p. 1837), there is truncal obesity and rounding of the face, with disproportionately thin extremities.

Many congenital somatic abnormalities such as cleft palate or harelip are frequently apparent on simple inspection and are observed in 25 per cent of infants with congenital heart disease; their presence should prompt a search for a cardiac malformation. In the *Ellis–van Creveld syndrome*, dwarfism, polydactyly, and ectodermal dysplasia frequently accompany congenital heart disease.[4] In patients with *coarctation of the aorta*, the lower extremities may be poorly developed, whereas the upper extremities are normal. Although heart failure may be associated with slight elevation of temperature (p. 454), if the latter exceeds 38°C, it should not be attributed to heart failure alone; it is possible that a complication such as a respiratory or urinary tract infection, endocarditis, or pulmonary embolus is responsible.

HEAD AND FACE

Examination of the face often aids in the recognition of many disorders that can affect the cardiovascular system. *Myxedema* (p. 1834) is characterized by a dull, expressionless face; periorbital puffiness; loss of the lateral eyebrows; a large tongue; and dry, sparse hair. An *earlobe crease* occurs more frequently in patients with coronary artery disease than in those without this condition.[5,6] The presence of an earlobe crease in a relatively young person (i.e., under 45 years), in particular, should alert the examiner to the possibility of premature coronary artery disease.

Patients with *rheumatic heart disease* and severe mitral stenosis may exhibit a characteristic facies—a malar flush, cyanotic lips, and slight jaundice due to hepatic congestion. Bobbing of the head coincident with each heartbeat (de Musset's sign) is characteristic of severe aortic regurgitation. Facial edema may be present in patients with *tricuspid valve disease* and *constrictive pericarditis. Infective endocarditis* may result in a "café au lait" complexion. Anemia, cyanosis, and polycythemia may all be suspected from examination of the conjunctivae and oral mucosa. Telangiectasia of the lips and tongue may be associated with pulmonary arteriovenous fistula.

In *Down syndrome* (mongolism, trisomy 21), which is often associated with congenital heart disease, especially endocardial cushion defects and pulmonary hypertension (p. 1628), there is mental deficiency, a prominent medial epicanthus, and a large, often protruding tongue, low-set ears, a poorly formed nasal bridge, and hypoplastic mandible. In *Hurler syndrome*, a form of mucopolysaccharidosis,[7] the facial features are grotesque (hence the name "gargoylism"); mitral and/or aortic valve disease (stenosis and/or regurgitation) and coronary artery narrowing may be present. Adenoma sebaceum of the face may be accompanied by a cardiac *rhabdomyoma* (p. 1456). Approximately 5 per cent of infants with congenital heart disease (most commonly ventricular septal defect) have the so-called cardiofacial syndrome, characterized by unilateral partial lower facial weakness, which may become apparent only when the patient cries. In the so-called *velocardiofacial syndrome*,[8] a cleft of the secondary palate, a long vertical face, and deep overbite with retruded mandible accompany congenital heart disease, most commonly a ventricular septal defect.

Hypertelorism (widely set eyes) is observed in patients with *Noonan syndrome*,[9] who often have pulmonic stenosis; *Turner syndrome,* often accompanied by coarctation of the aorta (p. 1629); the *multiple lentigines syndrome* (also termed LEOPARD syndrome), often associated with pulmonic stenosis and hypertrophic cardiomyopathy[10]; and *Hurler syndrome* (arrhythmias and valvular regurgitation). The facies of one group of patients with a nonfamilial type of *supravalvular aortic stenosis* and mental retardation is quite characteristic (Fig. 31–35, p. 927) and includes hypertelorism; a broad, high forehead; strabismus and epicanthal folds; low-set ears; upturned nose; a long upper lip and wide mouth; and hypoplasia of the mandible, with a pointed chin, small teeth, and dental deformities.[11] Patients with *stenosis of the pulmonary artery* and/or its branches often have an unusual facial appearance characterized by a large mouth, a blunt upturned nose, wide-set eyes, internal strabismus, and malformed teeth.[2,4]

Scleroderma, which can cause several forms of heart disease (p.1736), can often be recognized in the face, where skin becomes firm, thickened, and leathery in texture and is tightly bound to the underlying subcutaneous tissues. In the late stages of this disease the skin is atrophic, and there is immobility, particularly around the mouth. Patients with *systemic lupus erythematosus* (which may cause pericarditis, myocarditis, and endocarditis) (p. 1734) may present with a butterfly rash on the face. *Acromegaly,* which may cause cardiomyopathy (p. 1827), is associated with enlargement of the head, coarse facial features, prognathism, and macroglossia. *Cushing's syndrome*, in which hypertension is often present, is characterized by moon facies, hirsutism, and acne. *Paget's disease* of bone, which may be associated with a high cardiac output state (p. 462), is characterized by enlargement of the skull. Episodic facial flushing occurs in patients with *carcinoid tumors* and *pheochromocytoma* (p. 1839). A high, arched palate, prominent ears, and shimmering irides are characteristic of the *Marfan syndrome* (p. 1641).

The *muscular dystrophies*, the cardiac manifestations of which are described in Chapter 60, may also affect facial appearance profoundly. Patients with *myotonic dystrophy* exhibit a dull, expressionless face, with ptosis due to weakness of the levator muscles; the forehead is furrowed, and the temporalis and sternocleidomastoid muscles are atrophied. In the *facioscapulohumeral type* of *muscular dystrophy* (Landouzy-Déjerine) (p. 1813), nearly all the facial muscles are weak, particularly the orbicularis oris, preventing the patients from puckering the mouth and whistling; weakness of the orbicularis oculi, diffuse fattening of the face, and facial asymmetry (particularly around the mouth) are also characteristic.

In patients with *Werner syndrome*, who are at high risk of developing premature coronary and arterial atherosclerosis, there is premature graying of the hair, frontal baldness, beaking of the nose, cataract formation, and proptosis. Myotonic muscular dystrophy (p. 1815) may also cause premature graying of the hair, frontal thinning or baldness, and early cataracts.

EYES

External ophthalmoplegia and ptosis due to muscular dystrophy of the extraocular muscles occur in the *Kearns-Sayre syndrome*, which may be associated with complete heart block and myocardial failure[12] (Fig. 60–15, p. 1818).

Exophthalmos and stare occur not only in hyperthyroidism, which can cause high-output cardiac failure (p. 458), but also in advanced congestive heart failure, in which there is severe pulmonary venous hypertension and weight loss (p.454).[13] The stare is probably due to lid retraction caused by the increased adrenergic tone that accompanies heart failure. Severe tricuspid regurgitation and a carotid artery–cavernous sinus fistula can also cause pulsation of the eyeballs[14,15] (pulsatile exophthalmos), as well as of the earlobes.

Attention should be directed to the *iris* to look for an arcus, a circumferential light ring around the iris. When this ring begins inferiorly, leaving a rim peripherally, and occurs in a young person, it is frequently associated with hypercholesterolemia,[16] xanthelasma (small yellowish deposits of cholesterol on the eyelids), and premature atherosclerosis. (In blacks, an arcus often does not reflect hypercholesterolemia.) Iridodonesis (tremulous iris), in which the iris is not properly supported by the lens because of dislocation or weakness of the suspensory free ligament, occurs in Marfan syndrome. Gray-white spots (Brushfield's spots) (Fig. 2–1C) in the iris occur in Down syndrome. Iridocyclitis and enlargement of the lacrimal glands are seen in sarcoidosis, which may be associated with cardiomyopathy (p. 1420).

Blue sclerae may be seen in patients with Marfan syndrome, Ehlers-Danlos syndrome, and osteogenesis imperfecta[17]—disorders that may be associated with aortic dilatation, regurgitation, and dissection and with prolapse of the mitral valve (Chaps. 51 and 56). *Argyll Robertson pupils* (small, irregular, unequal pupils that do not dilate properly on administration of mydriatic drugs and that fail to react to light but constrict on accommodation) are diagnostic of central nervous system syphilis; this may be associated with cardiovascular syphilis, characterized by aneurysm of the ascending aorta, coronary ostial stenosis, and aortic regurgitation (p. 1043). The *cornea* may be clouded in the Hurler syndrome.[7] *Cataracts* are associated with the so-called rubella syndrome, in which a variety of congenital cardiac malformations occur (p. 888); premature cataracts also occur in Refsum's disease and in myotonic muscular dystrophy, both of which may be associated with cardiomyopathy; *vitreous opacities* are frequent in patients with familial amyloidosis, in whom a restrictive cardiomyopathy may be present (p. 1415).

FUNDI. Examination of the *fundi* allows classification of arteriolar disease in patients with hypertension (Fig. 2–2*A*) and may be helpful in the recognition of arteriosclerosis. Beading of the retinal artery may be present in patients with hypercholesterolemia (Fig. 2–2*B*), and wreathlike arteriovenous anastomoses around the disc are characteristic of Takayasu's disease (p. 802) (Fig. 2–2*C*). Hemorrhages near the discs with white spots in the center (Roth's spots) occur in infective endocarditis (p. 1078) (Fig. 2–2*D*). Embolic retinal occlusions may occur in patients with rheumatic heart disease, left atrial myxoma, and atherosclerosis of the aorta or arch vessels. Papilledema may be present not only in patients with malignant hypertension (Chap. 28) but also in cor pulmonale with severe hypoxia. In coarctation of the aorta, the retinal arteries are particularly tortuous and often display "U turns" but may not show other changes characteristic of hypertensive retinopathy.[18] In patients with cyanosis and polycythemia, the retinal veins are particularly dilated and edema and retinal papilledema are occasionally present. *Angioid streaks* are reddish-brown lines which are wider than retinal vessels and which radiate from the optic discs; they occur in *pseudoxanthoma elasticum* (p. 1644) as well as in *Paget's disease* of bone (p. 462).

SKIN AND MUCOUS MEMBRANES

Central cyanosis (due to intracardiac or intrapulmonary right-to-left shunting) involves the entire body, including warm, well-perfused sites such as the conjunctivae and the mucous membranes of the oral cavity, while peripheral cyanosis (due to reduction of peripheral blood flow, such as occurs in heart failure and peripheral vascular disease) is characteristically most prominent in cool, exposed areas that may not be well-perfused, such as the extremities, particularly the nailbeds and nose. Polycythemia can often be suspected from inspection of the conjunctivae, lips, and tongue, which in anemia are pale and in polycythemia are darkly

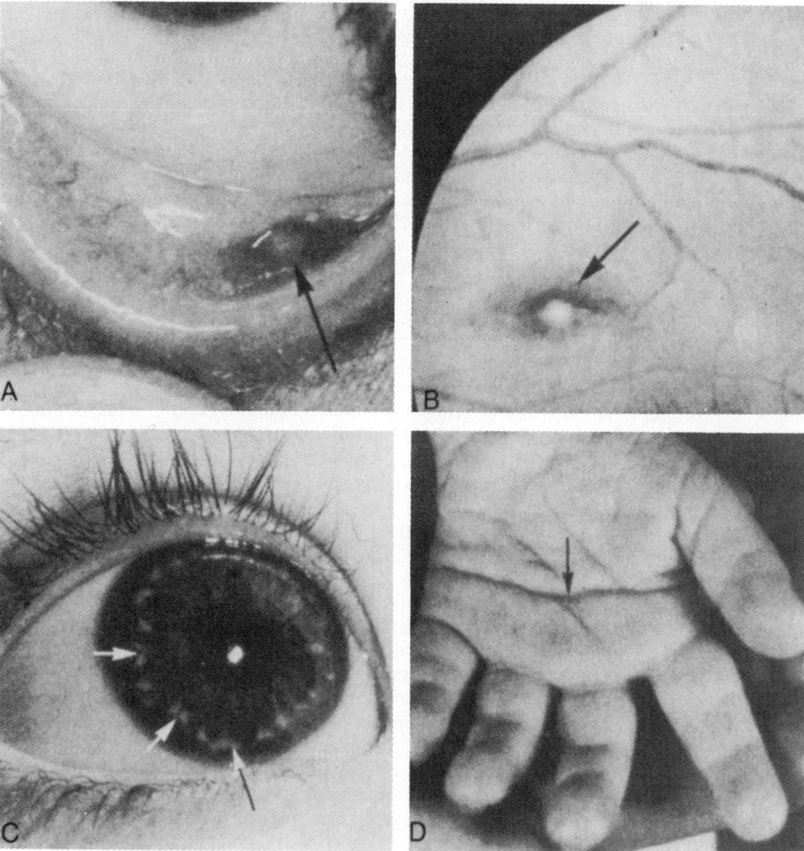

FIGURE 2–1. ***A,*** **Typical lower lid white-centered conjunctival petechia (arrow) in a young man with infective endocarditis of the aortic valve.** ***B,*** **Retinal Roth spot (white center) (arrow) surrounded by hemorrhage in a young woman with mitral valve infective endocarditis.** ***C,*** **Typical Brushfield spots (circle of depigmented dots along the outer circumference of the iris, arrows) and sparse, thin eyelashes in a child with Down syndrome and a partial endocardial cushion defect.** ***D,*** **The hand of a 6-month-old child with Down syndrome and complete endocardial cushion defect. A simian crease (arrow) traverses the palm. (From Perloff, J. K.: Physical Examination of the Heart and Circulation. 2nd ed. Philadelphia, W. B. Saunders Company, 1990.)**

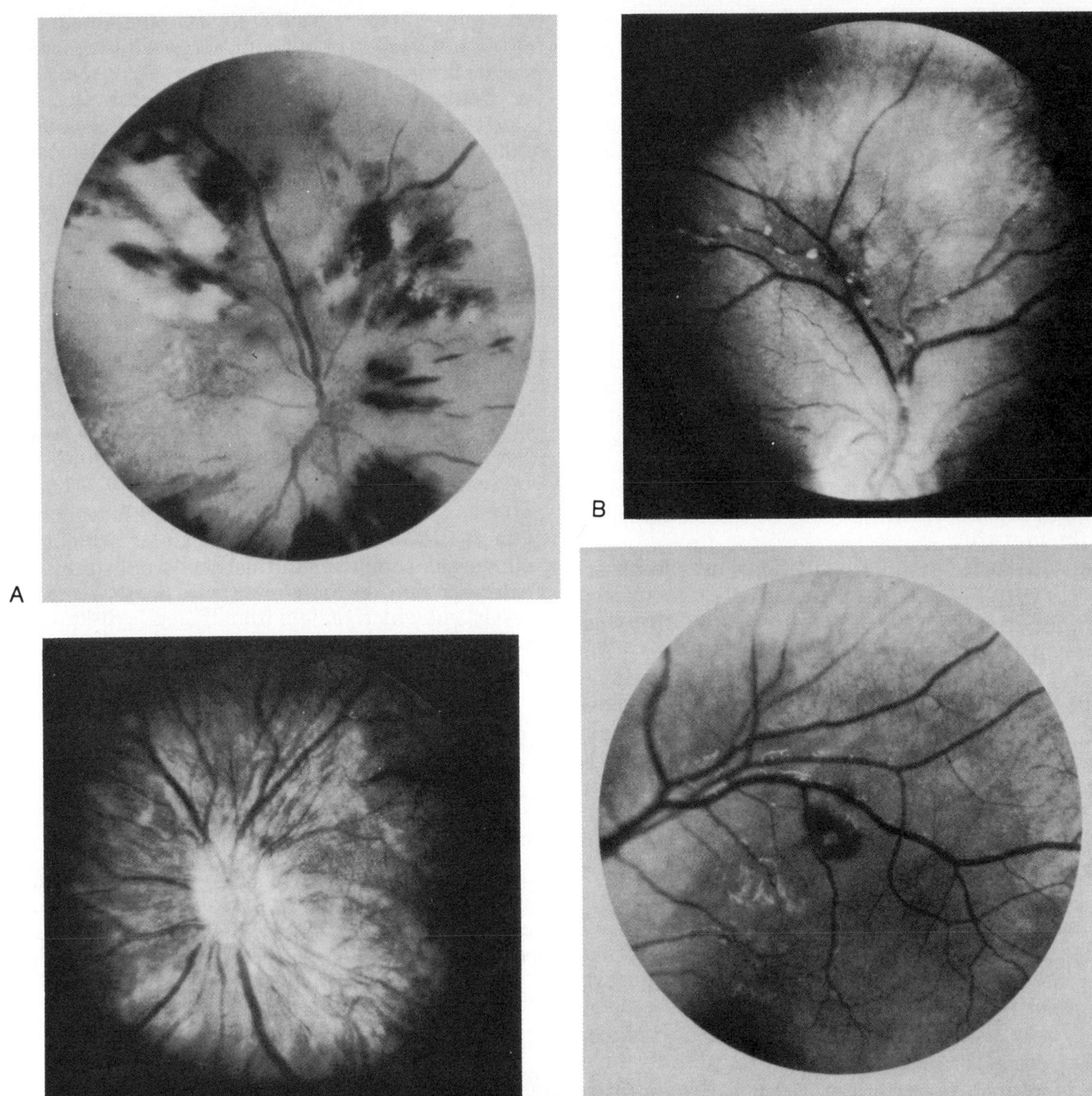

FIGURE 2–2. ***A,*** **Severe hypertensive retinopathy. The patient was a 43-year-old man with the symptoms of malignant hypertension. He subsequently died of massive cerebral hemorrhage.** ***B,*** **Beading of the retinal artery in a patient with hypercholesterolemia. The patient was a 37-year-old man with a serum cholesterol level of 400 mg per 100 ml.** ***C,*** **Proliferative retinopathy of Takayasu-Ohnishi disease. The patient was a 27-year-old Oriental woman with postural amaurosis and hemiplegia. Brachial pulses unobtainable.** ***D,*** **Roth spots (hemorrhage with white center) in a patient with subacute bacterial endocarditis. (From Cogan, D. G.: Ophthalmic Manifestations of Systemic Vascular Disease. Philadelphia, W. B. Saunders Company, 1974, p. 52.)**

congested. A blotchy cyanotic tinge to the skin associated with episodic flushing, particularly of the face, occurs in patients with *carcinoid tumors,* which may be associated with valvular heart disease (p. 1424).

Bronze pigmentation of the skin and loss of axillary and pubic hair occur in *hemochromatosis* (which may result in cardiomyopathy owing to iron deposits in the heart, p. 1419). Jaundice may be observed in patients following pulmonary infarction as well as in patients with congestive hepatomegaly or cardiac cirrhosis. *Lentigines,* i.e., small brown macular lesions on the neck and trunk that begin at about age 6 and do not increase in number with sunlight, are observed in patients with pulmonic stenosis and hypertrophic cardiomyopathy.[10]

The skin is ruddy in patients with polycythemia and Cushing's syndrome; sallow and yellowish in myxedema and in uremia; café au lait in late stages of infective endocarditis[19]; fine and silky in thyrotoxicosis; coarse and dry in myxedema and acromegaly; thickened and yellow (particularly in the neck and antecubital region) in pseudoxanthoma elasticum; smooth and glossy in longstanding Raynaud's syndrome; and warm and moist in anemia, beriberi, and other high-output states (Chap. 16). Increased sweating, most commonly a cold sweat in the palms, is observed in patients with neurocirculatory asthenia. *Erythema marginatum* (evanescent lesions confined primarily to the trunk) and *subcutaneous nodules* (which occur on the extensor surface of the elbows or over bony prominences such as the spine or skull) may be present in acute rheumatic fever (p. 1727). *Petechiae* occur in infective endocarditis; café-au-lait spots, freckles, and cutaneous neurofibromas occur in patients with pheochromocytoma (p. 1839), whereas *symmetric vitiligo* of the extremities is seen in patients with hyperthyroidism. Bluish pigmentation of the ear and nose cartilage is characteristic of *ochronosis,* which can produce serious valvular deformities (Chap. 34). Large areas of *psoriasis* or *exfoliative dermatitis* may be responsible for high-output heart failure.

Several types of xanthomas, i.e., cholesterol-filled nodules, are found either subcutaneously or over tendons in patients with hyperlipoproteinemia (Chap. 37). Premature atherosclerosis frequently develops in these individuals. *Tuberoeruptive xanthomas*, present subcutaneously or on the extensor surfaces of the extremities, and *xanthoma striatum palmare*, which produces yellowish, orange, or pink discoloration of the palmar and digital creases, occur most commonly in patients with type III hyperlipoproteinemia (Fig. 37–11, p. 1139). Patients with *xanthoma tendinosum* (Fig. 2–3), i.e., nodular swellings of the tendons, especially of the elbows, extensor surfaces of the hands, and Achilles' tendons, usually have type II hyperlipoproteinemia (p. 1138). *Xanthelasma* also occurs in this condition but is less specific. *Eruptive xanthomas* are tiny yellowish nodules, 1 to 2 mm in diameter on an erythematous base, which may occur anywhere on the body and are associated with hyperchylomicronemia and are therefore often found in patients with type I and type V hyperlipoproteinemia (pp. 1137 and 1139).

Hereditary telangiectasias are multiple capillary hemangiomas occurring in the skin, lips (Fig. 2–4), nasal mucosa, and upper respiratory and gastrointestinal tracts that resemble the spider nevi seen in patients with liver disease. When present in the lung, they are associated with pulmo-

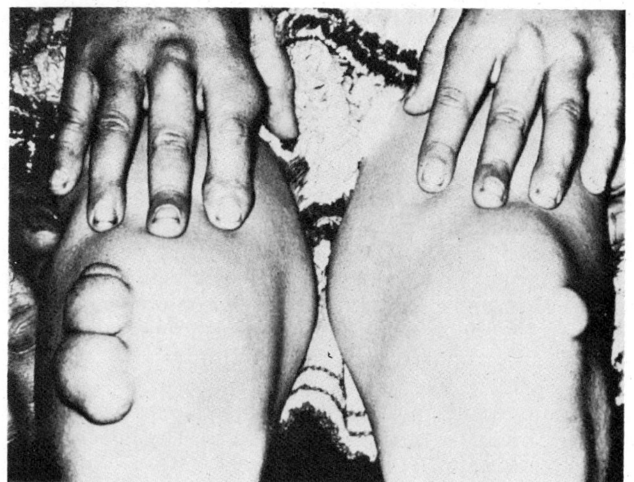

FIGURE 2-3. Tendinous xanthomas of the knees in a patient with familial hypercholesterolemia. The patient was a 10-year-old girl with a serum cholesterol level of 665 mg/100 ml. Several other members of the family had a similar syndrome. (From Cogan, D. G.: Ophthalmic Manifestations of Systemic Vascular Disease. Philadelphia, W. B. Saunders Company, 1974, pp. 14 and 15.)

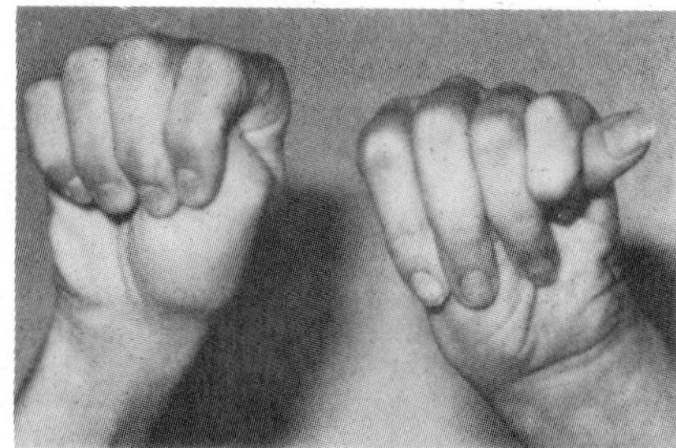

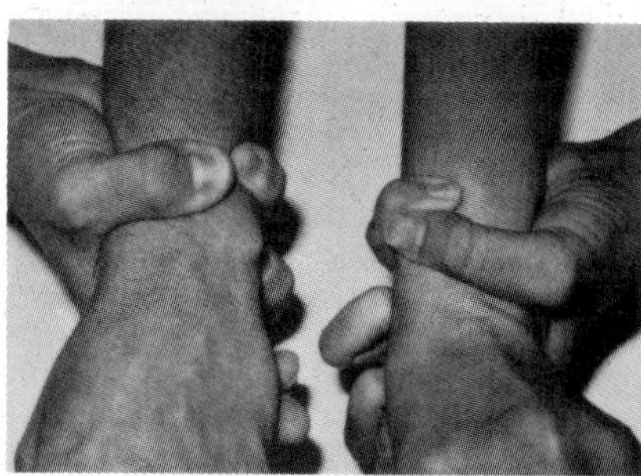

FIGURE 2-5. *A*, At left is the hand of a normal subject, who is unable to protrude his thumb beyond his clenched fingers, as can the patient with Marfan syndrome at right, who can do this because of a long thumb and lax joints. *B*, The normal patient at left cannot overlap his thumb and little finger around his wrist because, unlike the patient with Marfan syndrome at right, his fingers are not long relative to his wrist. (From Constant, J.: Bedside Cardiology. 3rd ed. Boston, Little, Brown & Co., 1985, pp. 30 and 31.)

nary arteriovenous fistulas and cause central cyanosis. Spider nevi on the face occur in patients with *chronic liver disease*, which may be associated with a high cardiac output state. Nicotine staining of the fingers suggests excessive cigarette smoking, an important risk factor for the development of coronary artery and peripheral vascular disease (p. 1146).

EXTREMITIES

A variety of congenital and acquired cardiac malformations are associated with characteristic changes in the extremities. Among the congenital lesions, short stature, cubitus valgus, and medial deviation of the extended forearm are characteristic of *Turner syndrome* (p. 1629). Patients with the *Holt-Oram syndrome* (Table 51-7, p. 1632), i.e., atrial septal defect with skeletal deformities, often have a thumb with an extra phalanx, a so-called "fingerized thumb," which lies in the same plane as the fingers, making it difficult to appose the thumb and fingers. In addition, they may exhibit deformities of the radius and ulna, causing difficulty in supination and pronation. There is often asymmetry of skeletal involvement, with the left side more severely affected. Polydactyly and hypoplastic fingernails are part of the *Ellis-van Creveld syndrome* (chondroectodermal dysplasia), a disorder frequently associated with atrial or ventricular septal defect (p. 1633). Arachnodactyly is characteristic of *Marfan syndrome* (p. 1641). Normally, when a fist is made over a clenched thumb, the latter does not extend beyond the ulnar side of the hand, but it usually does so in Marfan syndrome (Fig. 2-5*A*). When the wrist is encircled by the thumb and little finger of the opposite hand, the little finger will overlap the thumb by at least 1 cm in more than three-fourths of patients with Marfan syndrome but will rarely do so in individuals without this syndrome[20] (Fig. 2-5*B*). In *osteogenesis imperfecta*, hyperextensibility of the joints is common, but arachnodactyly is not.[18] In patients with *homocystinuria*, the extremities may be elongated and other skeletal abnormalities, such as kyphoscoliosis and pectus carinatum, may be present. Ulnar deviation of the fourth and fifth fingers and flexion at the metacarpophalangeal joints occur in *Jaccoud's arthritis*, a rare concomitant of rheumatic heart disease. In *Down syndrome*, there is a simian palm crease (Fig. 2-1*D*) and sometimes increased space between the fourth and fifth fingers, and a short fifth finger that is curved inward, whereas in Turner syndrome the fingers tend to be short.

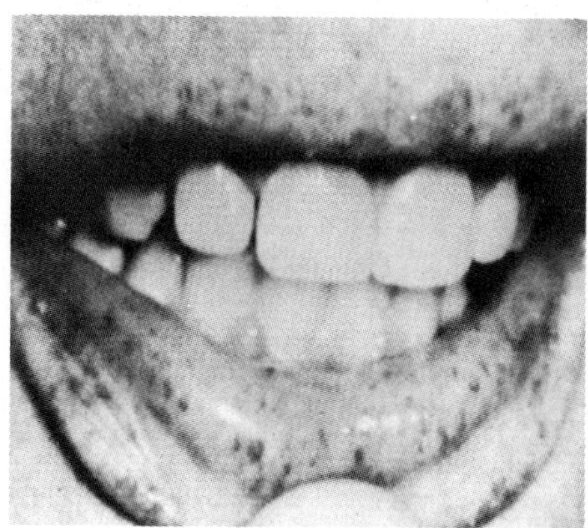

FIGURE 2-4. Hemorrhagic telangiectasia on the lips of a 25-year-old woman with pulmonary arteriovenous fistulas. (From Perloff, J. K.: The Clinical Recognition of Congenital Heart Disease. Philadelphia, W. B. Saunders Company, 1987, p. 645.)

SKIN. *Raynaud's phenomenon*, which sometimes occurs in association with primary pulmonary hypertension (p. 804), scleroderma (p. 1736), and coronary spasm (p. 262), is characterized by intermittent pallor and/or cyanosis of the extremities precipitated by exposure to cold. With the passage of time, the skin overlying the fingers and under the nails becomes atrophic. Cold, pale, or blue hands accompanied by collapse of the forearm veins signify peripheral vasoconstriction, which may be a normal response to cold, anxiety, or a low cardiac output. In patients with peripheral vascular disease, the ischemic foot typically exhibits paleness on elevation and rubor on dependency.

High cardiac output states (Chap. 16) produce warm, pink hands associated with distention of the forearm veins (signs of vasodilatation). Redness of the palmar eminences may be a sign of severe liver disease, whereas a fine tremor of the outstretched hands suggests thyrotoxicosis. Peripheral *arteriovenous fistula* or *Paget's disease* of bone may cause local warmth and excessive growth of the affected limb. Systolic flushing of the nailbeds, which can be readily detected by pressing a flashlight against the terminal digits (Quincke's sign), is a sign of aortic regurgitation and of other conditions characterized by a greatly widened pulse pressure. *Differential cyanosis*, in which the hands and fingers (especially on the right side) are pink and the feet and toes are cyanotic, is indicative of patent ductus arteriosus with reversed shunt due to pulmonary hypertension (p. 913); this finding can often be brought out by exercise. On the other hand, *reversed differential cyanosis*, in which cyanosis of the fingers exceeds that of the toes, suggests transposition of the great arteries, pulmonary hypertension, preductal narrowing of the aorta, and reversed flow through a patent ductus arteriosus.[21]

CLUBBING OF THE FINGERS AND TOES[22] (Fig. 2-6). Clubbing of the digits is characteristic of central cyanosis (cyanotic congenital heart disease or pulmonary disease with hypoxia). It may also appear within a few weeks of the development of infective endocarditis but usually develops after 2 or 3 years of central cyanosis. Clubbing is also observed in a variety of suppurative pulmonary lesions and carcinoma of the lung as well as in gastrointestinal disorders, including biliary cirrhosis and regional enteritis; occasionally, it is a harmless familial condition. The earliest forms

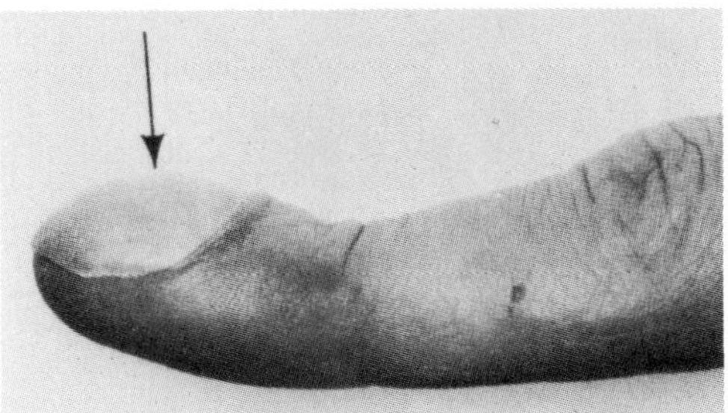

FIGURE 2-6. Typical cyanosis and clubbing, close-up, profile. (From Perloff, J. K.: The Clinical Recognition of Congenital Heart Disease. 3rd ed. Philadelphia, W. B. Saunders Company, 1987, p. 6.)

of clubbing are characterized by increased glossiness and cyanosis of the skin at the root of the nail.[23] Following obliteration of the normal angle between the base of the nail and the skin, the soft tissue of the pulp becomes hypertrophied, the nail root floats freely, and its loose proximal end can be palpated. In the more severe forms of clubbing, bony changes occur, i.e., *hypertrophic pulmonary osteoarthropathy;* these changes involve the terminal digits and in rare instances even the wrists, ankles, elbows, and knees. *Unilateral clubbing* of the fingers is rare but can occur when an aortic aneurysm interferes with the arterial supply to one arm. Not to be confused with clubbing are the subungual fibromas of the fingers that occur in tuberous sclerosis, a condition often associated with cardiac rhabdomyoma (p. 1457).

Osler's nodes are small, tender, purplish erythematous skin lesions due to infected microemboli and occurring most frequently in the pads of the fingers or toes and in the palms of the hands or soles of the feet,[24] whereas *Janeway lesions* are slightly raised, nontender hemorrhagic lesions in the palms of hands and soles of the feet; both these lesions as well as petechiae occur in infective endocarditis (p. 1086). When the latter occur under the nailbeds, they are termed *splinter hemorrhages*. The terminal digits may also show, early in endocarditis, a mottled pink followed by a bluish discoloration which darkens as necrosis occurs; it is probably due to arteriolar embolism.[20]

Edema of the extremities is a common finding in congestive heart failure; however, if it is present in only one leg, it is more likely due to obstructive venous or lymphatic disease than to heart failure. Firm pressure on the pretibial region for 10 to 20 seconds may be necessary for the detection of edema in ambulatory patients. In patients confined to bed, edema appears first in the sacral region. Edema may involve the face in children with heart failure of any etiology and in adults with heart failure associated with marked elevation of systemic venous pressure (e.g., constrictive pericarditis and tricuspid valve disease).

CHEST AND ABDOMEN

Examination of the thorax should begin with observations of the respiratory rate, effort, and regularity. The shape of the chest is important as well; thus, a barrel-shaped chest with low diaphragms suggests emphysema, bronchitis, and possibly cor pulmonale. In chronic obstructive pulmonary disease, accessory muscles are used during inspiration, while expiration is prolonged and often accompanied by wheezing.

Inspection of the chest may reveal a bulging to the right of the upper sternum caused by an aortic aneurysm. This can also produce a venous collateral pattern caused by obstruction of the superior vena cava. *Kyphoscoliosis* of any etiology can cause cor pulmonale; this skeletal abnormality as well as pectus excavatum (funnel chest) and pectus carinatum (pigeon breast) is often present in Marfan syndrome, with mitral prolapse or atrial septal defect. It is also seen in the *Noonan syndrome*, in which it is often associated with pulmonic stenosis. Percussion of the chest will reveal dullness at the bases, most commonly the right base in heart failure.

Pericardial effusion often causes dullness at the angle of the left scapula (Ewart's sign).[25] Left ventricular failure and other causes of elevation of pulmonary venous pressure may cause pulmonary rales; wheezing is sometimes audible in pulmonary edema (cardiac asthma).

Painful enlargement of the *liver* may be due to venous congestion; the tenderness disappears in longstanding heart failure. Hepatic systolic expansile pulsations occur in patients with severe tricuspid regurgitation (Fig. 16-3, p. 453), and presystolic pulsations can be felt in patients with pure tricuspid stenosis and sinus rhythm. Patients with constrictive pericarditis also often have pulsatile hepatomegaly, the contour of the pulsations resembling those of the jugular venous pulse in this condition.[26,27] Transmitted (as opposed to intrinsic) pulsations of the liver occur in patients with right ventricular enlargement, aneurysmal dilatation of the upper abdominal aorta, and a widened pulse pressure. When firm pressure over the abdomen (see Fig. 2-19F) causes cervical venous distention, i.e., when there is *abdominojugular reflux*, right heart failure is usually present.[28] *Ascites* is also characteristic of heart failure, but is especially characteristic of tricuspid valve disease and chronic constrictive pericarditis.

Splenomegaly may occur in the presence of severe congestive hepatomegaly, most frequently in patients with constrictive pericarditis or tricuspid valve disease. The spleen may be enlarged and painful in infective endocarditis as well as following splenic embolization. Splenic infarction is frequently accompanied by an audible friction rub.

Both *kidneys* may be palpably enlarged in patients with hypertension secondary to polycystic disease. Auscultation of the abdomen should be carried out in all patients with hypertension; a systolic bruit secondary to renal artery stenosis may be audible near the umbilicus or in the flank (Table 28-9, p. 835).

Atherosclerotic aneurysms of the abdominal aorta are usually readily detected on palpation (p. 1530), except in markedly obese patients. In patients with *coarctation of the aorta*, no abdominal pulsations are palpable despite the presence of prominent arterial pulses in the neck and upper extremities; arterial pulses in the lower extremities are reduced or absent.

THE JUGULAR VENOUS PULSE

Important information concerning the dynamics of the right side of the heart can be obtained by inspection of the jugular venous pulse.[29,30] The *internal* jugular vein is ordinarily employed in the examination; the venous pulse can usually be analyzed more readily on the right than on the left side of the neck, because the right innominate and jugular veins extend in an almost straight line cephalad to the superior vena cava, thus favoring transmission of hemodynamic changes from the right atrium, while the left innominate vein may be kinked or compressed by a variety of normal structures, by a dilated aorta, or by an aneurysm.

The patient should be lying comfortably during the examination; clothing should be removed from the neck and upper thorax, and although the head should rest on a pillow, it must not be elevated at a sharp angle from the trunk. The jugular venous pulse may be examined effectively by shining a light tangentially across the neck. Most patients with heart disease are examined most effectively in the 45-degree position, but in patients in whom venous pressure is high, a greater inclination (60 or even 90 degrees) is required to obtain visible pulsations, while in those in whom jugular venous pressure is low, a lesser inclination (30 degrees) is desirable. In order to amplify the pulsations of the jugular veins, it may be helpful to place the patient in the supine position and try to increase venous return by elevating the patient's legs.

The internal jugular vein is located deep within the neck, where it is covered by the sternocleidomastoid muscle and is therefore not usually visible as a discrete structure, except in the presence of severe venous hypertension. However, its pulsations are transmitted to the skin of the neck, where they are usually easily visible. Sometimes considerable difficulty may be experienced in differentiating between the carotid and jugular venous pulses in the neck, particularly when the latter exhibits prominent *v* waves, as occurs in patients with tricuspid regurgitation, in whom the valves in the internal jugular veins may be incompetent. However, there are several helpful clues[31]: (1) The arterial pulse is a sharply localized rapid movement that may not be readily visible but that strikes the palpating fingers with considerable force; in contrast, the venous pulse, while more readily visible, often disappears when the palpating finger is placed lightly on or below the pulsating area. (2) The arterial pulse usually exhibits a single upstroke while the venous pulse has two peaks and two troughs per cardiac cycle. (3) The arterial pulsations do not change when the patient is in the upright position or during respiration, whereas venous pulsations usually disappear or diminish greatly in the upright position and during inspiration, unless the venous pressure is greatly elevated. (4) Compression of the root of the neck does not affect the arterial pulse but usually abolishes venous pulsations, except in the presence of extreme venous hypertension.

Two principal observations can usually be made from examination of the neck veins: the level of venous pressure and the type of venous wave pattern. In order to estimate jugular venous pressure, the height of the oscillating top of the distended proximal portion of the internal jugular vein, which reflects right atrial pressure, should be determined. The upper limit of normal is 4 cm above the sternal angle, which corresponds to a central venous pressure of approximately 9 cm H_2O, since the right atrium is approximately 5 cm below the sternal angle. When the veins in the neck collapse in a subject breathing normally in the horizontal position, it is likely that the central venous pressure is subnormal. When obstruction of veins in the lower extremities is responsible for edema, pressure in the neck veins is not elevated and the abdominal-jugular reflux is negative.

ABDOMINAL-JUGULAR REFLUX.[28] This can be tested by applying firm pressure to the periumbilical region for 10 to 30 seconds with the patient breathing quietly while the jugular veins are observed (Fig. 2–19*F*); increased respiratory excursions or strain should be avoided. In normal subjects jugular venous pressure rises less than 3 cm H_2O and only transiently, while pressure is continued, whereas in right or left ventricular failure and/or tricuspid regurgitation the jugular venous pressure remains elevated. In the absence of these conditions a positive abdominal-jugular reflux suggests an elevated pulmonary artery wedge[29] or central venous pressure.[31]

PATTERN OF THE VENOUS PULSE. The events of the cardiac cycle, shown in Figure 13–32, p. 374, provide an explanation for the details of the jugular venous pulse pattern (Fig. 2–7). The *a* wave in the venous pulse results from venous distention due to right atrial systole, while the x descent is due to atrial relaxation. The *c* wave, which occurs simultaneously with the carotid arterial pulse, is an inconstant wave in the jugular venous pulse and/or interruption of the descent following the peak of the *a* wave. The x descent may be due in part to forceful closure of the tricuspid valve; sometimes it is an artifact produced by the adjacent carotid arterial pulse. It is followed by the x′ descent or trough, caused by the pulling down of the floor of the atrium (descent of the base) by ventricular contraction. (Many investigators refer to this wave as the x descent.) The *v* wave results from the rise in right atrial pressure when blood flows into the right atrium during ventricular systole when the tricuspid valve is shut, and the *y* descent, i.e., the downslope of the *v* wave, is related to the decline in right atrial pressure when the tricuspid valve reopens. Following the bottom of the *y* descent (the *y* trough) and beginning of the *a* wave is a period of relatively slow filling of the atrium or ventricle, the diastasis period, a wave termed the *H* wave.

While all or most of these events can usually be recorded, they may not be distinguishable readily on inspection. The descents or downward collapsing movements of the jugular veins are more rapid, produce larger excursions, and are therefore more prominent to the eye than are the ascents (Fig. 2–7). The normal dominant jugular venous descent, the x′ descent, occurs just prior to the second heart sound, while the *y* descent ends after the second heart sound. With an increase in central venous pressure, the *v* wave becomes higher and the *y* collapse becomes more prominent. The *a* wave can be recognized when it is abnormally prominent; it occurs just before the first sound or carotid pulse and has a sharp rise and fall. The *v* wave occurs just after the arterial pulse and has a slower, undulating pattern.

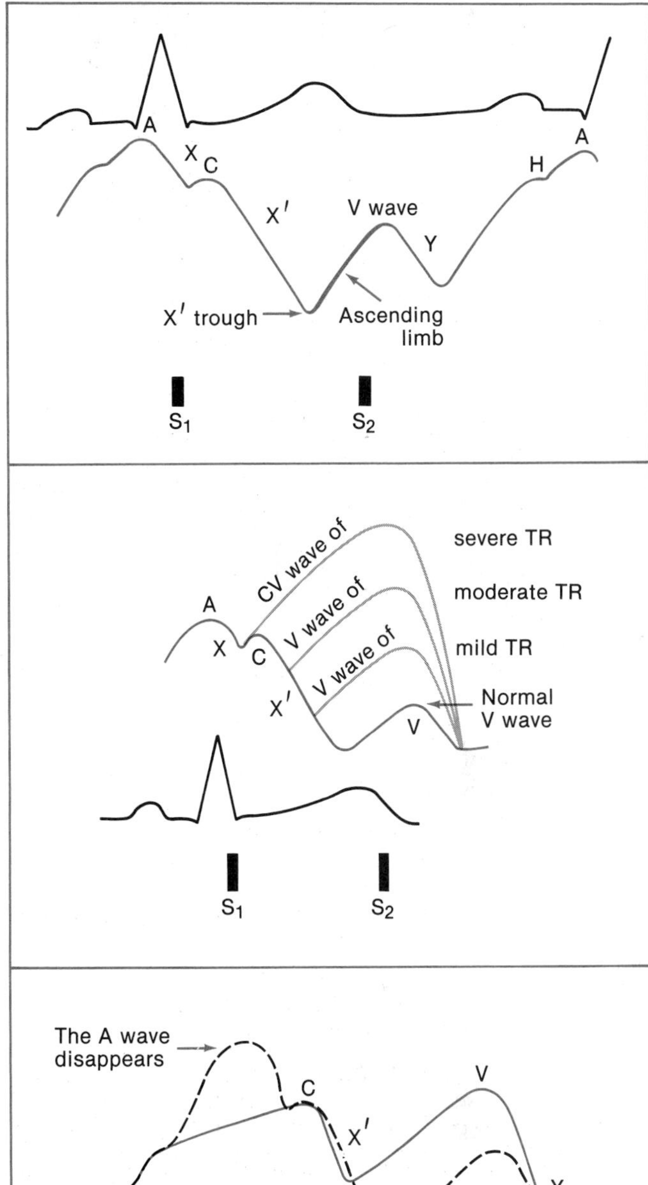

FIGURE 2–7. ***Top,*** **Normal jugular venous pulse: the jugular *v* wave is built up during systole, and its height reflects the rate of filling and the elasticity of the right atrium. Between the bottom of the *y* descent (*y* trough) and beginning of the *a* wave is the period of relatively slow filling of the "atrioventricle" or diastasis period. The wave built up during diastasis is the *H* wave. The *H* wave height also reflects the stiffness of the right atrium. S_1 and S_2 refer to the first and second heart sounds, respectively. *Center,* As the degree of tricuspid regurgitation (TR) increases, the *x′* descent is increasingly encroached upon. With severe TR, no *x′* descent is seen, and the jugular pulse wave is said to be "ventricularized." *Bottom,* Black broken line = normal jugular venous pulse and sinus rhythm; red continuous line = following development of atrial fibrillation. The dominant descent in atrial fibrillation is almost always the *y* descent, i.e., it has the superficial appearance of the pulse wave of TR. (From Constant, J.: Bedside Cardiology. 3rd ed. Boston, Little, Brown & Co., 1985, pp. 95, 105, and 108.)**

ALTERATIONS IN DISEASE. Elevation of jugular venous pressure reflects an increase in right atrial pressure and occurs in heart failure, reduced compliance of the right ventricle, pericardial disease, hypervolemia, and obstruction of the superior vena cava. During inspiration, the jugular venous pressure normally declines but the *amplitude* of the pulsations increases. *Kussmaul's sign* is a paradoxical rise in the height of the jugular venous pressure during inspiration, which occurs frequently in patients with chronic constrictive pericarditis and sometimes in congestive heart failure and tricuspid stenosis.

The *a* wave is particularly prominent in conditions in which the resistance to right atrial emptying is increased, such as right ventricular hypertrophy and pulmonary hypertension (Fig. 2–8*A*). The *a* wave may also be tall in left ventricular hypertrophy when the thickened ventricular septum interferes with right ventricular filling. Tall *a* waves are present in patients with sinus rhythm and tricuspid stenosis or atresia, right atrial myxoma, or reduced compliance and/or marked hypertrophy of the right ventricle. Cannon (giant) *a* waves are noted in patients with atrioventricular dissociation when the right atrium contracts against a closed tricuspid valve. In atrial fibrillation, the *a* wave and x descent disappear, and the x′ descent becomes more prominent. In right ventricular failure and sinus rhythm, there may be increases in prominence of both the *a* and *v* waves. A steeply rising *H* wave is observed (or recorded) in restrictive cardiomyopathy, constrictive pericarditis, and right ventricular infarction. The *a* wave is absent in atrial fibrillation, accompanied by a diminished x′ descent and a prominent *v* wave (Fig. 2–7 *Bottom*). The x descent may be prominent in patients with enlarged *a* waves, as well as in patients with right ventricular volume overload (atrial septal defect). Constrictive pericarditis (Fig. 2–8*B*) is characterized by a rapid and deep *y* descent followed by a rapid rise to a diastolic plateau (*H* wave) without a prominent *a* wave; occasionally, the x′ descent is prominent in this condition as well, causing a "W"-shaped jugular venous pulse. However, it is in cardiac tamponade that the x descent is most prominent (Fig. 45–12, p. 1479). A prominent *v* wave or *c-v* wave, i.e., fusion of the *c* and *v* waves in the absence or attenuation of an x′ descent, occurs in tricuspid regurgitation, sometimes causing a systolic movement of the earlobe (Figs. 2–7 *Center* and 3–23, p. 54 and Fig. 34–43, p. 1058). A prominent *v* wave and *y* descent are also seen in atrial septal defect; the *y* descent is gradual when right atrial emptying is impeded, as in tricuspid stenosis and rapid when it is unimpeded, as in tricuspid regurgitation. A steep *y* descent is seen in any condition in which there is myocardial dysfunction, ventricular dilatation, and an elevated central venous pressure.

INDIRECT MEASUREMENT OF ARTERIAL PRESSURE

Systolic arterial pressure can be *estimated* without a sphygmomanometer cuff by gradually compressing the brachial artery while palpating the radial artery; the force required to obliterate the radial pulse represents the systolic blood pressure, and with practice, one can often estimate this level within 20 mm Hg. Ordinarily, however, a sphygmomanometer is used to obtain an indirect measurement of blood pressure. The cuff should fit snugly around the arm, with its lower edge at least 1 inch above the antecubital space, and the diaphragm of the stethoscope should be placed close to or under the edge of the sphygmomanometer cuff. The width of the cuff selected should be at least 40 per cent of the circumference of the limb to be used. The standard size, with a 5-inch-wide cuff, is designed for adults with an arm of average size. When this cuff is applied to a large upper arm or a normal adult thigh, arterial pressure will be overestimated, leading to spurious hypertension in the obese (arm circumference > 35 cm)[3,32,33]; when it is applied to a small arm, the pressure will be underestimated. The cuff width should be approximately 1½ inches in infants and small children, 3 inches in young children (2 to 5 years), and 8 inches in obese adults. The bag should be long enough to extend at least halfway around the limb (10 inches in adults). In patients with rigid, sclerotic vessels the systolic pressure may also be overestimated, by as much as 30 mm Hg. Mercury manometers are, in general, more accurate and reliable than the aneroid type; the latter should be calibrated at least once yearly.

BLOOD PRESSURE IN THE UPPER EXTREMITIES. In order to measure arterial pressure in the upper extremity,[34] the patient should be seated or lying comfortably and relaxed, the arm should be slightly flexed and at heart level, and the arm muscles should be relaxed. The cuff should be inflated rapidly to approximately 30 mm Hg above the anticipated systolic pressure.[35] These maneuvers, which diminish the volume of blood in the venous bed, decrease the tissue pressure distal to the cuff and thereby increase the flow into the occluded brachial artery. The cuff is then deflated slowly, no faster than 3 mm Hg/sec; the pressure at which the brachial pulse can be palpated is close to the systolic pressure.

The cuff should be deflated rapidly after the diastolic pressure is noted and a full minute allowed to elapse before pressure is remeasured in the same limb. Although excessive pressure on the stethoscope head does

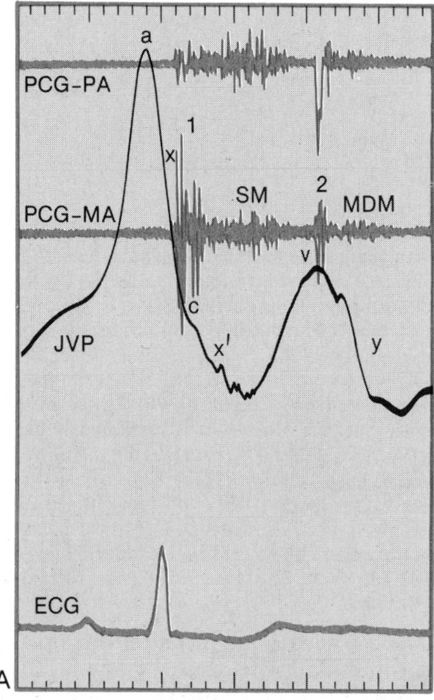

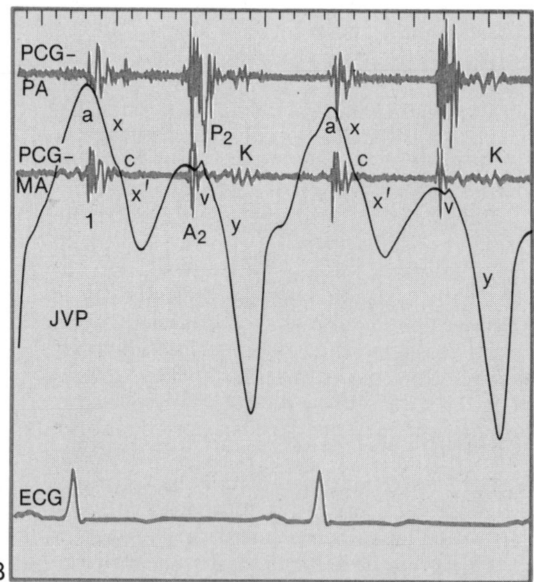

FIGURE 2–8. ***A,*** **Jugular venous pressure (JVP) in mitral stenosis with pulmonary hypertension. The JVP is dominated by a very large *a* wave resulting from diminished compliance of the right ventricle associated with pulmonary hypertension. The peaked *a* wave represents a brief period of retrograde flow from right atrium to great veins. *B,* Jugular venous pressure (JVP) in constrictive pericarditis. In this severe and longstanding case, the *x′* descent has become very shallow and the *y* descent is the principal feature, indicating that antegrade flow from the venous system to the right heart is now limited to early diastole.[124] A pericardial knock (K) is seen at approximately the nadir of the *y* descent. (From Craige, E., and Smith, P.: Heart sounds. *In* Braunwald, E. [ed.]: Heart Disease: A Textbook of Cardiovascular Medicine. 3rd ed. Philadelphia, W. B. Saunders Company, 1988, pp. 61 and 62.)**

not affect systolic pressure, it does erroneously lower diastolic readings.[36] In one study, the anxiety associated with blood pressure measurement was shown to elevate arterial pressure by an average of 27/17 mm Hg:[37] ("white coat hypertension"). It is desirable for the patient to reduce anxiety and bladder distention and to avoid exercise, caffeine, eating, and smoking for a half hour preceding the screening.

BLOOD PRESSURE IN THE LOWER EXTREMITIES. To measure pressure in the legs, the patient should lie on his or her abdomen, an 8-inch-wide cuff should be applied with the compression bag over the posterior aspect of the midthigh and should be rolled diagonally around the thigh to keep the edges snug against the skin, and auscultation should be carried out in the popliteal fossa. In order to measure pressure in the lower leg, an arm cuff is placed over the calf, and auscultation is carried out over the posterior tibial artery. Regardless of where the cuff is applied, care must be taken to avoid letting the rubber part of the balloon of the cuff extend beyond its covering and to avoid placing the cuff on so loosely that central ballooning occurs.

KOROTKOFF SOUNDS. There are five phases of Korotkoff sounds, i.e., sounds produced by the flow of blood as the constricting blood pressure cuff is gradually released. The first appearance of clear, tapping sound (phase I) represents the systolic pressure. These sounds are replaced by soft murmurs during phase II and by louder murmurs during phase III, as the volume of blood flowing through the constricted artery increases. The sounds suddenly become muffled in phase IV, when constriction of the brachial artery diminishes as arterial diastolic pressure is approached. Korotkoff sounds disappear in phase V, which is usually within 10 mm Hg of phase IV. Diastolic pressure measured directly through an intraarterial needle and external manometer corresponds closely to phase V.[30] In severe aortic regurgitation, however, when the disappearance point is extremely low, sometimes 0 mm Hg, the sound of muffling (phase IV) is much closer to the intraarterial diastolic pressure than is the disappearance point (phase V). When there is a sizable difference between phases IV and V of the Korotkoff sounds (>10 mm Hg), both pressures should be recorded (e.g., 142/54/10 mm Hg). Korotkoff sounds may be difficult to hear and arterial pressure difficult to measure when arterial pressure rises at a slow rate (as in aortic stenosis), when the vessels are markedly constricted (as in shock), and when the stroke volume is reduced (as in severe heart failure). Very soft or inaudible Korotkoff sounds can often be accentuated by dilating the blood vessels of the upper extremities simply by opening and closing the fist repeatedly. Sometimes in states of shock, the indirect method of measuring blood pressure is unreliable, and arterial pressure should be measured through an intraarterial needle.

The Auscultatory Gap. This is a silence that sometimes separates the first appearance of the Korotkoff sounds from their second appearance at a lower pressure. The phenomenon tends to occur when there is venous distention or reduced velocity of arterial flow into the arm. If the first muffling of sounds is considered to be the diastolic pressure, it will be overestimated. If the second appearance is taken as the systolic pressure, it will be underestimated. On the other hand, sounds transmitted through the arterial tree from prosthetic aortic valves may be responsible for falsely high readings.

BLOOD PRESSURE IN THE BASAL CONDITION. In order to determine arterial pressure in the basal condition, the patient should have rested in a quiet room for 15 minutes. It is desirable to record the arterial pressure in both arms at the time of the initial examination; differences in systolic pressure exceeding 10 mm Hg between the two arms when measurements are made simultaneously or in rapid sequence[39] suggest obstructive lesions involving the aorta or the origin of the innominate and subclavian arteries, or supravalvular aortic stenosis (in which pressure in the right arm exceeds that in the left). In patients with vertebral-basal artery insufficiency, a difference in pressure between the arms may signify that a subclavian "steal" is responsible for the cerebrovascular symptoms. In order to determine whether orthostatic hypotension is present, arterial pressure should be determined with the patient in both the supine and the erect positions. However, regardless of the patient's posture, the brachial artery should be at the level of the heart to avoid superimposition of the effects of gravity on the recorded pressure.

Normally, the systolic pressure in the legs is up to 20 mm Hg higher than in the arms, but the diastolic pressures are usually virtually identical. The recording of a higher diastolic pressure in the legs than in the arms suggests that the thigh cuff is too small. When systolic pressure in the popliteal artery exceeds that in the brachial artery by more than 20 mm Hg (Hill's sign), aortic regurgitation is usually present.[40] Blood pressure should be measured in the lower extremities in patients with hypertension to detect coarctation of the aorta or when obstructive disease of the aorta or its immediate branches is suspected.

To be *certain* from physical examination that the systolic pressure is different in the two arms or in the upper and lower extremities, two examiners should measure the pressures simultaneously, then switch extremities.[3]

The volume and contour of the arterial pulse are determined by a combination of factors, including the left ventricular stroke volume, the ejection velocity, the relative compliance and capacity of the arterial system, and the pressure waves that result from the antegrade flow of blood and reflections of the arterial pressure pulse returning from the peripheral circulation.[41] Bilateral palpation of the carotid, radial, brachial, femoral, popliteal, dorsalis pedis, and posterior tibial pulses should be part of the examination of all cardiac patients. The frequency, regularity, and shape of the pulse wave and the character of the arterial wall should be determined.[42] The carotid pulse (Figs. 2–9*C,D*) provides the most accurate representation of the central aortic pulse.[43] For palpation of the left carotid artery, the observer applies the right thumb to the patient's left carotid artery in the lower third of the neck[2] (Fig. 2–9*C*). The left femoral artery should be palpated with the right thumb. The patient should be lying supine with the head and chest at a 45-degree angle. The brachial artery is the vessel ordinarily most suitable for appreciating the rate of rise of the pulse and the contour, volume, and consistency of the peripheral vessels. This artery is located at the medial aspect of the elbow, and it may be helpful to flex the arm in order to palpate it; palpation of the artery should be carried out with the thumb exerting pressure on the artery until its maximal movement is detected (Fig. 2–9*A* and *B*). A normal rate of rise of the arterial pulse suggests that there is no obstruction to left ventricular outflow, whereas a pulse wave of small amplitude with normal configuration suggests a reduced stroke volume.

THE NORMAL PULSE (Fig. 2–10). The pulse in the ascending aorta normally rises rapidly to a rounded dome; this initial rise reflects the peak velocity of blood ejected from the left ventricle. A slight anacrotic notch or pause is frequently

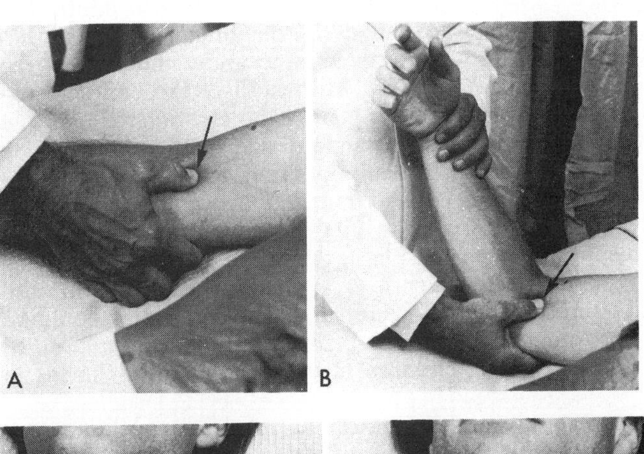

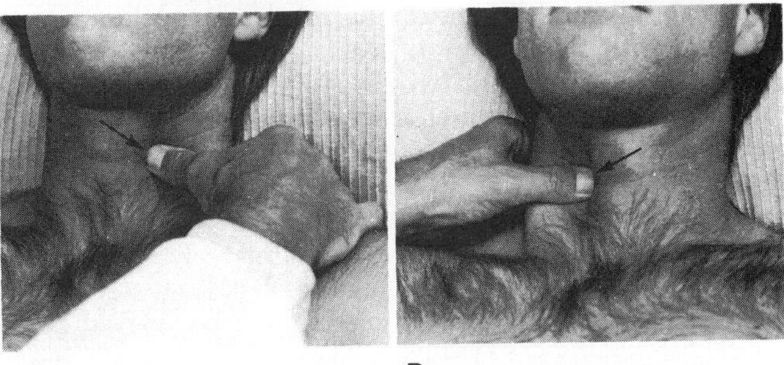

FIGURE 2–9. *A*, **Palpation of the right brachial pulse with the thumb while the patient's arm lies at the side with the palm up.** *B*, **Palpation of the right brachial pulse with the patient's elbow resting in the palm of the examiner's hand. The thumb explores the antecubital fossa (arrow), while the patient's forearm is passively raised and lowered to achieve maximum relaxation of muscles around the elbow.** *C* **and** *D*, **Palpation of the carotid pulse. The examiner places the right thumb (arrow) on the patient's left carotid artery (*C*). The left thumb (arrow) is then applied separately to the right carotid (*D*). (From Perloff, J. K.: Physical Examination of the Heart and Circulation. Philadelphia, W. B. Saunders Company, 1982, pp. 58 and 60.)**

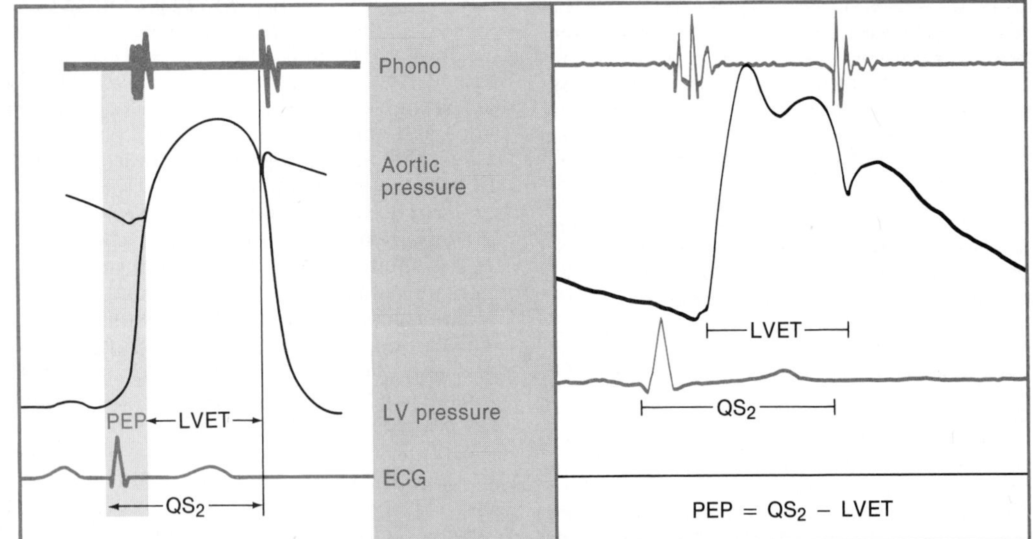

FIGURE 2–10. Recording of a normal phonocardiogram, external carotid pulse, and electrocardiogram. (From Lewis, R. P., et al.: A critical review of the systolic time intervals. Circulation *56:*146, 1977, by permission of the American Heart Association, Inc.)

recorded, but only occasionally felt, on the ascending limb of the pulse. The descending limb of the central aortic pulse is less steep than is the ascending limb, and it is interrupted by the incisura, a sharp downward deflection related to closure of the aortic valve. Immediately thereafter, the pulse wave rises slightly and then declines gradually throughout diastole. As the pulse wave is transmitted to the periphery, its upstroke becomes steeper, the systolic peak becomes higher, the anacrotic shoulder disappears, and the sharp incisura is replaced by a smoother, later dicrotic notch followed by a dicrotic wave.[44] Normally, the height of this dicrotic wave diminishes with age, hypertension, and arteriosclerosis. In the central arterial pulse (central aorta and innominate and carotid arteries), the rapidly transmitted shock of left ventricular ejection results in a peak in early systole, referred to as the *percussion wave*; a second, smaller peak, the *tidal wave*, presumed to represent a reflected wave from the periphery, can often be recorded but is not normally palpable. However, in older subjects, particularly those with increased peripheral resistance, as well as in patients with arteriosclerosis and diabetes, the tidal wave may be somewhat higher than the percussion wave; i.e., the pulse reaches a peak in late systole. In peripheral arteries, the pulse wave normally has a single sharp peak.

ABNORMAL PULSES. When vascular resistance and arterial stiffness are increased, as in hypertension or with the increased arterial stiffness that accompanies normal aging, there is an elevation in pulse wave velocity, and the pulse contour has a more rapid upstroke and greater amplitude. Reduced or unequal carotid arterial pulsations occur in patients with carotid atherosclerosis and with diseases of the aortic arch, including aortic dissection, aneurysm, and Takayasu's disease (p. 1545). In *supravalvular aortic stenosis* there is a streaming of the jet toward the innominate artery, and the carotid and brachial arterial pulses are stronger and rise more rapidly on the right than on the left side, and pressures are higher in the right than in the left arm (p. 926). The pulses of the upper extremity may be reduced or unequal in a variety of other conditions, including arterial embolus or thrombosis, anomalous origin or aberrant path of the major vessels, and cervical rib or scalenus anticus syndrome. Asymmetry of right and left popliteal pulses is characteristic of iliofemoral obstruction. Weakness or absence of radial, posterior

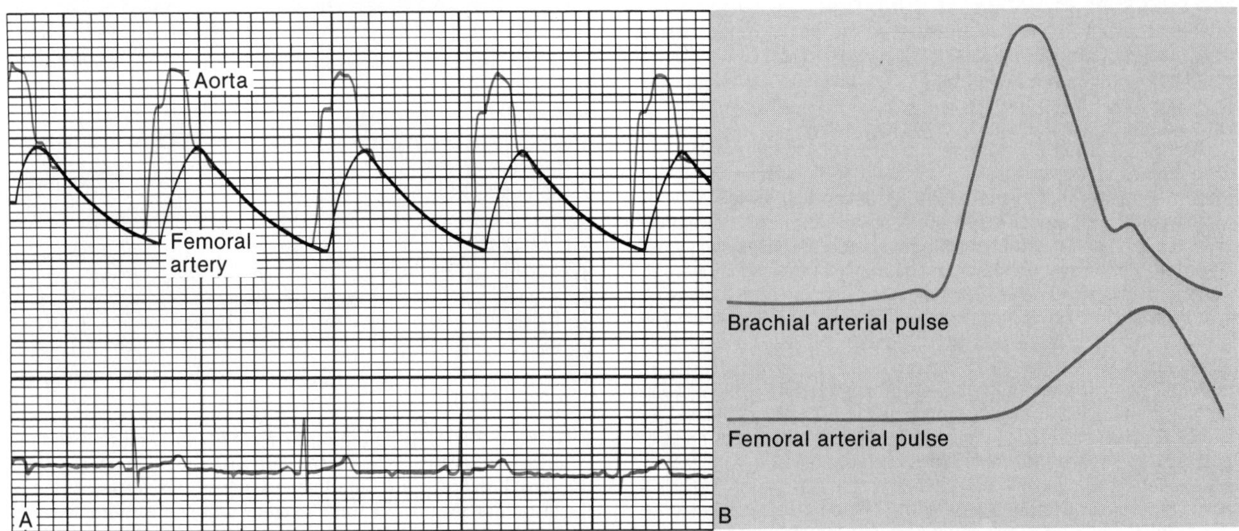

FIGURE 2–11. *A*, Pulses recorded in the aorta proximal to a coarctation (red) and in the femoral artery (black) together with the electrocardiogram. The systolic pressure difference is seen as well as the delay in onset of the upstroke of the femoral pulse. *B*, Diagrammatic representation of simultaneous brachial and femoral arterial pulses in a patient with coarctation. The onset of the upstroke in the femoral pulse is delayed relative to the onset of the upstroke in the brachial pulse. (From Sutton, G. C.: Examination of the cardiovascular system. *In* Julian, D. G., Camm, A. J., Fox, K. M., et al. [eds.]: Diseases of the Heart. London, Balliere Tindall, 1989.)

tibial, or dorsalis pedis pulses on one side suggests arterial insufficiency. In *coarctation of the aorta* the carotid and brachial pulses are bounding, rise rapidly, and have large volumes, while in the lower extremities, the systolic and pulse pressures are reduced, their rate of rise is slow, and there is a late peak (Fig. 2–11). This delay in the femoral arterial pulses can usually be readily detected by simultaneous palpation of the femoral and radial arterial pulses.

In patients with fixed obstruction to left ventricular outflow (valvular aortic stenosis, and congenital fibrous subaortic stenosis), the carotid pulse rises slowly (*pulsus tardus*) (Fig. –12); the upstroke is frequently characterized by a thrill (the *carotid shudder*); and the peak is reduced, occurs late in systole, and is sustained. There is a notch on the upstroke of the carotid pulse (anacrotic notch) that is so distinct that two separate waves can be palpated in what is termed an *anacrotic pulse. Pulsus parvus* is a pulse of small amplitude, usually because of a reduction of stroke volume. *Pulsus parvus et tardus* refers to a small pulse with a delayed systolic peak, which is characteristic of severe aortic stenosis. This type of pulse is more readily appreciated by palpating the carotid rather than a more peripheral artery. Patients with severe aortic stenosis and heart failure usually exhibit simply a reduced pulse amplitude, i.e., *pulsus parvus*, and the delay in the upstroke is not readily apparent. However, this delay is readily recorded. In elderly patients with inelastic peripheral arteries, the pulse may rise normally despite the presence of aortic stenosis.

The carotid arterial pulse may be prominent or exaggerated in any condition in which pulse pressure is increased, including anxiety, the hyperkinetic heart syndrome, anemia, fever, pregnancy, or other high cardiac output states (Chap. 16), as well as in bradycardia, and peripheral arteriosclerosis with loss of arterial distensibility. In patients with *mitral regurgitation* or *ventricular septal defect*, the forward stroke volume (from the left ventricle into the aorta) is usually normal, but the fraction ejected during early systole is greater than normal; hence, the arterial pulse is of normal volume (the pulse pressure is normal), but the pulse may rise abnormally rapidly.[45] Exaggerated or bounding arterial pulses may be observed in patients with an elevated stroke volume, with sympathetic hyperactivity, and in patients with a rigid, sclerotic aorta. In *aortic regurgitation*, there is a very brisk rate of rise with an increased pulse pressure. The *Corrigan* or *water-hammer pulse* of aortic regurgitation consists of an abrupt upstroke (percussion wave) followed by rapid collapse later in systole, but no dicrotic notch. Corrigan's pulse reflects a low resistance in the reservoir into which the left ventricle rapidly discharges an abnormally elevated stroke volume, and it can be exaggerated by raising the patient's arm. In *acute* aortic regurgitation, the left ventricle may not be greatly dilated, and premature closure of the mitral valve may occur and limit the volume of aortic reflux; therefore, the aortic diastolic pressure may *not* be very low, the arterial pulse *not* bounding, and the pulse pressure *not* widened despite a serious abnormality of valve function (p. 1047). Signs characteristic of severe chronic aortic regurgitation include "pistol-shot" sounds heard over the femoral artery when the stethoscope is placed on it (*Traube's sign*); a systolic murmur heard over the femoral artery when it is gradually compressed proximally; a diastolic murmur when the artery is compressed distally (*Duroziez's sign*[40,46]) and Quincke's sign. Of these, Duroziez's sign is the most predictive. Bounding arterial pulses are also present in patients with patent ductus arteriosus or large arteriovenous fistulas; in hyperkinetic states such as thyrotoxicosis, pregnancy, fever, and anemia; in severe bradycardia; and in vessels proximal to a coarctation of the aorta. *Hill's sign* of aortic regurgitation (or any condition leading to an increased stroke volume, or the hyperkinetic circulatory state) the indirectly recorded systolic pressure in the lower extremities exceeds that in the arms by more than 20 mm Hg. Other signs of increased pulse pressure include *Becker's sign* (visible pulsations of the retinal arterioles) and *Mueller's sign* (pulsating uvula).

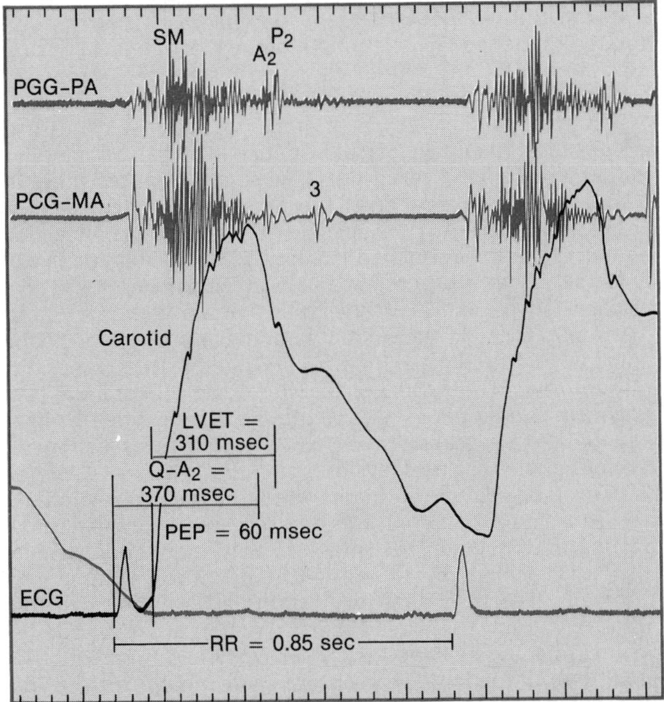

FIGURE 2–12. Valvular aortic stenosis in an 11-year-old boy with moderately severe obstruction (gradient = 50 to 60 mm Hg across the aortic valve). A loud midsystolic murmur is seen in all valve areas. The carotid upstroke is delayed and shattered by coarse vibrations. A_2 is well preserved. A third sound (3) is present, probably a normal finding in this youthful subject. (From Craige, E., and Smith, D.: Heart sounds. *In* Braunwald, E. [ed.]: Heart Disease: A Textbook of Cardiovascular Medicine. 3rd ed. Philadelphia, W. B. Saunders Company, 1988, p. 56.)

In the presence of atrioventricular dissociation, when atrial activity is irregularly transmitted to the ventricles, the strength of the peripheral arterial pulse depends on the time interval between atrial and ventricular contractions. In a patient with rapid heart action, the presence of such variations is suggestive of ventricular tachycardia; with an equally rapid rate, an absence of variation of pulse strength suggests a supraventricular mechanism.

BISFERIENS PULSE (Fig. 2–13). A bisferiens pulse is characterized by *two systolic peaks*, the percussion and tidal waves, separated by a distinct midsystolic dip; the peaks may be equal or either may be larger. This type of pulse may be detected most readily by palpation of the carotid and less commonly of the radial arteries. It occurs in conditions in which a large stroke volume is ejected rapidly from the left ventricle[47] and is observed most commonly in patients with pure aortic regurgitation or with a combination of aortic regurgitation and stenosis; it may disappear as heart failure supervenes.

A bisferiens pulse is also noted in patients with *hypertrophic obstructive cardiomyopathy*,[48,49] but the bifid nature may only be recorded, not palpated; on palpation there may merely be a rapid upstroke. In these patients the initial prominent percussion wave is associated with rapid ejection of blood into the aorta during early systole, followed by a rapid decline as obstruction becomes manifest in midsystole and by a tidal (reflected) wave. In some patients with hypertrophic cardiomyopathy with no or little obstruction to left ventricular outflow, the arterial pulse is normal or simply hyperkinetic in the basal state, but obstruction and a bisferiens pulse can be elicited by means of the Valsalva maneuver or inhalation of amyl nitrite. Occasionally, a bisferiens pulse is observed in hyperkinetic circulatory states, and very rarely it occurs in normal individuals.

DICROTIC PULSE (Fig. 2–14). Not to be confused with a bisferiens pulse, in which both peaks occur in systole, is a dicrotic pulse in which the second peak is in diastole immediately after the second heart sound.[42,44] The normally small wave that follows aortic valve closure (i.e., the dicrotic notch)

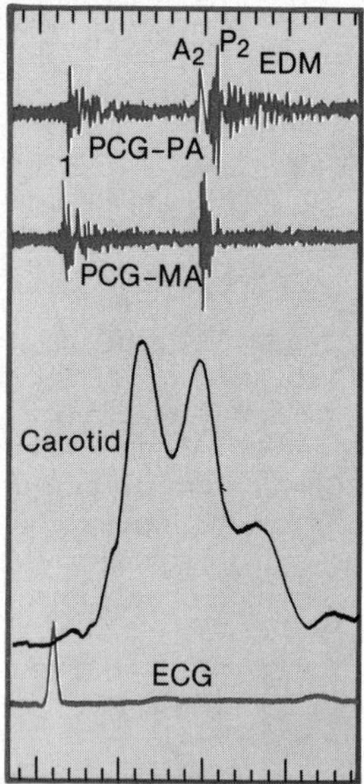

FIGURE 2-13. Bisferiens pulse in aortic regurgitation. The carotid pulse is bifid, and there is a large excursion reflecting the wide pulse pressure. The phonocardiogram establishes that both humps of the carotid pulse are systolic in time (i.e., prior to A_2), thus separating the bisferiens pulse from a large dicrotic wave (Fig. 2-14), with which it may be confused at the bedside. There is no incisura, owing to aortic incompetence. EDM = early diastolic murmur. (From Craige, E., and Smith, D.: Heart sounds. *In* Braunwald, E. [ed.]: Heart Disease: A Textbook of Cardiovascular Medicine. 3rd ed. Philadelphia, W. B. Saunders Company, 1988, p. 56.)

is exaggerated and measures more than 50 per cent of the pulse pressure on direct pressure recordings and in which the dicrotic notch is low (i.e., near the diastolic pressure). It may be present in normal hypotensive subjects with reduced peripheral resistance, as occurs in fever, and it may be elicited or exaggerated by inspiration or the inhalation of amyl nitrite. Rarely, a dicrotic pulse may be noted in healthy adolescents or young adults, but it usually occurs in conditions such as cardiac tamponade, severe heart failure, and hypovolemic shock, in which a low stroke volume is ejected into a soft elastic

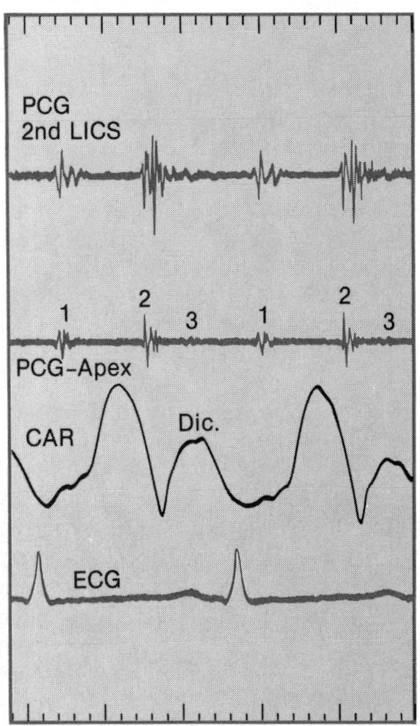

FIGURE 2-14. Dicrotic pulse in cardiomyopathy. Note two pulsations, the second of which is diastolic—the dicrotic wave (Dic.). Note also the prominent incisural notch. (From Craige, E., and Smith, D.: Heart sounds. *In* Braunwald, E. [ed.]: Heart Disease: A Textbook of Cardiovascular Medicine. 3rd ed. Philadelphia, W. B. Saunders Company, 1988, p. 56.)

aorta. In these conditions the dicrotic pulse is due to a shrinkage of the systolic wave with preservation of the incisura. A dicrotic pulse is rarely present when systolic pressure exceeds 130 mm Hg.

PULSUS ALTERNANS (alternating strong and weak pulses) (Fig. 2-15). Mechanical alternans is a sign of severe depression of myocardial function (p. 380). Although more readily recognized on sphygmomanometry, when the systolic pressure alternates by more than 20 mm Hg it can be detected by palpation of a peripheral (femoral or radial) pulse more frequently than a more central pulse or by the recording of an indirect carotid pulse tracing. Palpation should be carried out with light pressure and with the patient's breath held in mid-expiration to avoid the superimposition of respiratory variation on the amplitude of the pulse. Pulsus alternans is generally accompanied by alternation in the intensity of the Korotkoff sounds and occasionally by alternation in intensity of the heart sounds. Rarely, pulsus alternans is so marked that the weak beat is not perceived at all. Aortic regurgitation, systemic hypertension, and reducing venous return by tilting the patient into the upright position or nitroglycerin all exaggerate pulsus alternans and assist in its detection. Pulsus alternans, which is frequently precipitated by a premature ventricular contraction, is characterized by a regular rhythm and must be distinguished from pulsus bigeminus (see below), which is usually irregular.

PULSUS BIGEMINUS. A bigeminal rhythm is caused by the occurrence of premature contractions, usually ventricular, after every other beat and results in alternation of the strength of the pulse, which can be confused with pulsus alternans. However, in contrast to the latter, in which the rhythm is regular, in pulsus bigeminus the weak beat always follows the shorter interval. In normal persons or in patients with fixed obstruction to left ventricular outflow, the compensatory pause following a premature beat is followed by a stronger-than-normal pulse. However, in patients with hypertrophic obstructive cardiomyopathy, the postpremature ventricular contraction beat is weaker than normal because of increased obstruction to left ventricular outflow[50] (p. 1410).

PULSUS PARADOXUS (see also p. 1476). This is an exaggerated reduction in the strength of the arterial pulse during normal inspiration or an exaggerated inspiratory fall in systolic pressure (more than 10 mm Hg during quiet breathing). When marked, i.e., an inspiratory reduction of pressure greater than 20 mm Hg, it can be detected by palpation of the radial or brachial arterial pulse; in some instances there is inspiratory disappearance of the pulse. Milder degrees of a paradoxical pulse can be readily detected on sphygmomanometry: the cuff is inflated to suprasystolic levels and is deflated slowly at a rate of about 2 mm Hg per heartbeat; the peak systolic pressure during expiration is noted. The cuff is then deflated even more slowly, and the pressure is again noted when Korotkoff sounds become audible throughout the respiratory cycle. Normally, the difference between the two pressures should not exceed 10 mm Hg during quiet respiration. (Pulsus alternans can also be detected by this maneuver by noting whether peak systolic pressure or the intensity of the Korotkoff sounds alternates when the breath is held.)

Pulsus paradoxus represents an exaggeration of the normal decline in systolic arterial pressure with inspiration, which results from the reduced left ventricular stroke volume and the transmission of negative intrathoracic pressure to the aorta. It is a frequent, indeed characteristic, finding in patients with cardiac tamponade (p. 1473), occurs less frequently (in about half) in patients with chronic constrictive pericarditis (p. 1482), and is also observed in patients with emphysema and bronchial asthma (who have wide respiratory swings of intrapleural pressure),[51] as well as in hypovolemic shock, pulmonary embolus, pregnancy, and extreme obesity. Aortic regurgitation tends to prevent the development of pulsus paradoxus despite the presence of cardiac tamponade. *Reversed* pulsus paradoxus (an inspiratory rise in arterial pressure) may occur in hypertrophic obstructive cardiomyopathy.[52]

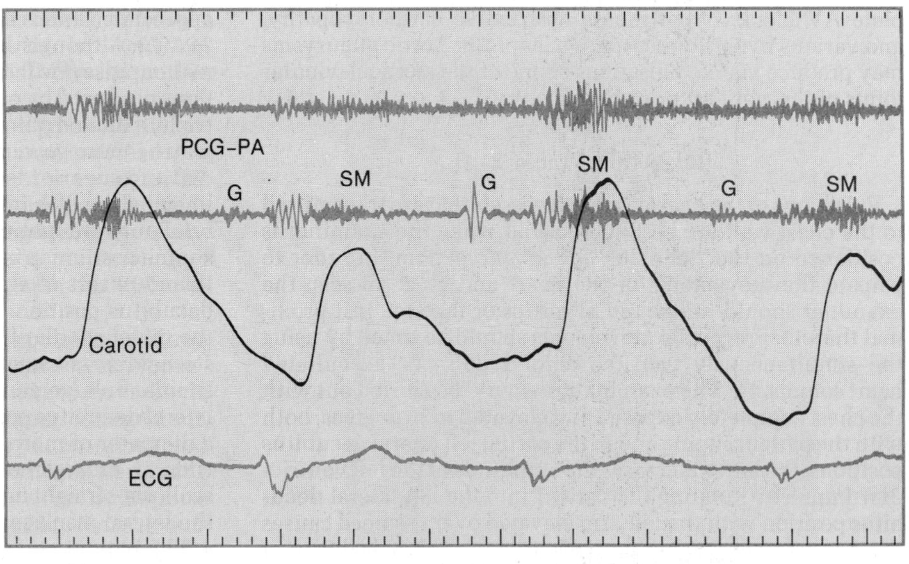

FIGURE 2–15. Pulsus alternans in a man with aortic stenosis and left ventricular failure. The first and third beats are of greater amplitude than are the second and fourth beats. The stronger beats are also marked by a louder murmur (SM) and less abnormality of STI. The diastolic sound (G) is louder after the second (weak) beat. It is a summation sound caused by merging of S_3 and S_4, resulting from the combined effect of a rapid heart rate and a prolonged P-R interval. (From Craige, E., and Smith, D.: Heart sounds. *In* Braunwald, E. [ed.]: Heart Disease: A Textbook of Cardiovascular Medicine. 3rd ed. Philadelphia, W. B. Saunders Company, 1988, p. 57.)

THE ARTERIAL PULSE IN VASCULAR DISEASE. Examination of the arterial pulses is of critical importance in the diagnosis of extracardiac obstructive arterial disease. Systematic bilateral palpation of the common carotid, brachial, radial, femoral, popliteal, dorsalis pedis, and posterior tibial vessels, as well as palpation of the abdominal aorta, should be part of every examination in patients suspected of having ischemic heart disease.[53] To diminish cold-induced vasoconstriction, peripheral pulses should be palpated after the patient has been in a warm room for at least 20 minutes.[54] Absent or weak peripheral pulses usually signify obstruction. However, the dorsalis pedis and posterior tibial arteries may be absent in approximately 2 per cent of normal persons because they pursue an abnormal course. Arterial bruits should be searched for by examination of specific anatomical sites. When the lumen diameter is reduced by approximately 50 per cent, a soft early systolic bruit is heard; as the obstruction becomes more severe, the bruit becomes high-pitched, louder, and longer. With approximately 80 per cent diameter reduction it spills into early diastole, but it disappears with very severe stenosis or complete occlusion. Arterial bruits are augmented by elevations of cardiac output (e.g., as occurs in anemia), by poor development of collaterals, and augmented arterial outflow (as occurs in regional exercise).

Auscultation of the interscapular region in patients with coarctation of the aorta may reveal a systolic or continuous murmur, and a systolic murmur may be heard over the lower abdomen in patients with aortic or iliofemoral obstructions.

EXAMINATION OF THE HEART

INSPECTION

The cardiac examination proper should commence with inspection of the chest, which can best be accomplished with the examiner standing at the foot of the bed or examining table. Respirations—their frequency, regularity, and depth—as well as the relative effort required during inspiration and expiration, should be noted (p. 37). Simultaneously, one should search for cutaneous abnormalities, such as spider nevi (seen in hepatic cirrhosis and Osler-Weber-Rendu disease). Dilation of veins on the anterior chest wall with caudal flow suggests obstruction of the superior vena cava, whereas cranial flow occurs in patients with obstruction of the inferior vena cava. Precordial prominence is most striking if cardiac enlargement developed before puberty, but it may also be present, although to a lesser extent, in patients in whom cardiomegaly developed in adult life, after the period of thoracic growth.[55,56]

A heavy muscular thorax, contrasting with less developed lower extremities, may occur in coarctation of the aorta, in which visible collateral arteries may be present in the axillae and along the lateral chest wall. The upper portion of the thorax exhibits symmetrical bulging in children with stiff lungs in whom the inspiratory effort is increased. An anterior bulge in the area of the manubrium in a child suggests pulmonary hypertension. A "shield chest" is a broad chest in which the angle between the manubrium and the body of the sternum is greater than normal and is associated with widely separated nipples; it is frequently observed in the Turner and Noonan syndromes. Careful note should be made of other deformities of the thoracic cage, such as *kyphoscoliosis*, which may be responsible for cor pulmonale (Ch. 49); *ankylosing spondylitis*, sometimes associated with aortic regurgitation (p. 1731); and *pectus carinatum* (pigeon chest), which may be associated with Marfan syndrome but does not directly affect cardiovascular function.

Pectus excavatum, a condition in which the sternum is displaced posteriorly, is commonly observed in Marfan syndrome, homocystinuria, Ehlers-Danlos syndrome, Hunter-Hurler syndrome (Chap. 51), and a small fraction of patients with mitral valve prolapse (p. 1029). This thoracic deformity rarely compresses the heart or elevates the systemic and pulmonary venous pressures, and the signs of heart disease are more often apparent rather than real. Displacement of the heart into the left thorax, prominence of the pulmonary artery, and a parasternal midsystolic murmur all may falsely suggest the presence of organic heart disease. It may be associated with palpitation, tachycardia, fatigue, mild dyspnea, and some impairment of cardiac function.[57] Lack of normal thoracic kyphosis, i.e., the *straight back* syndrome,[1] is often associated with expiratory splitting of the second heart sound, a parasternal midsystolic murmur, and enlargement of the pulmonary artery on x-ray; therefore, it may be confused with atrial septal defect. It is frequently associated with mitral valve prolapse and/or a bicuspid aortic valve.[58]

Cardiovascular pulsations should be looked for on the entire chest but specifically in the regions of the cardiac apex, the left parasternal region, and the third left and second right intercostal spaces. Prominent pulsations in these areas suggest enlargement of the left ventricle, right ventricle, pulmonary artery, and aorta, respectively. A thrusting apex exceeding 2 cm in diameter suggests left ventricular enlargement; systolic retraction of the apex may be visible in constrictive pericarditis. Normally, cardiac pulsations are not visible lateral to the midclavicular line; when present there, they signify cardiac enlargement unless there is thoracic deformity or congenital absence of the pericardium. Shaking of the entire precordium with each heartbeat may occur in patients with severe valvular regurgitation, large left-to-right shunts, com-

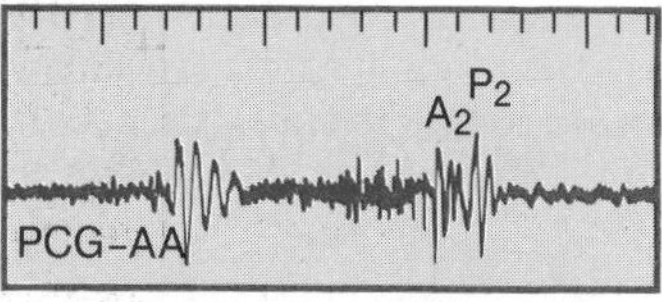

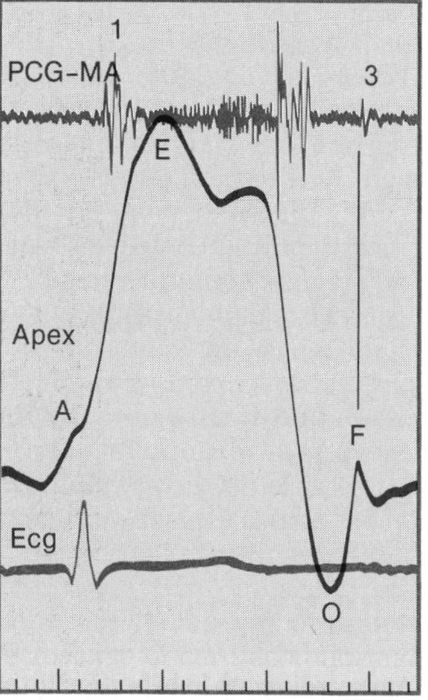

FIGURE 2-18. Hyperdynamic apexcardiogram in mitral regurgitation. The configuration of the tracing in systole is qualitatively similar to a normal curve, although the amplitude was clearly exaggerated by palpation. The rapid filling wave (F) is higher than normal and terminates in a sharp point coincident with its audible counterpart, the third heart sound (3). (From Craige, E., and Smith, D.: Heart sounds. *In* Braunwald, E. [ed.]: Heart Disease: A Textbook of Cardiovascular Medicine. 3rd ed. Philadelphia, W. B. Saunders Company, 1988, p. 58.)

mented, as occurs in patients with reduced left ventricular compliance associated with concentric left ventricular hypertrophy, myocardial ischemia, and myocardial fibrosis, a presystolic pulsation (usually accompanying a fourth heart sound) is palpable, resulting in a double outward movement of the left ventricular impulse. This presystolic expansion is most readily discernible during expiration, when the patient is in the left lateral decubitus position, and it can be confirmed by detecting the motion of the stethoscope placed over the left ventricular impulse or by observing the motion of the tip of a pencil or tongue depressor when the proximal portion is placed near the left ventricular impulse. It can be enhanced by sustained handgrip. Presystolic expansion of the left ventricle is usually associated with marked elevation of left ventricular end-diastolic (rather than early diastolic) pressure. In contrast to prominence of early diastolic filling, in patients without ischemic heart disease presystolic expansion is usually associated with normal or almost normal left ventricular function.[59] In patients with ischemic heart disease presystolic pulsation is usually associated with left ventricular dysfunction.[63] Presystolic expansion of the right ventricle occurs in right ventricular hypertrophy and pulmonary hypertension. It may be appreciated by subxiphoid palpation of the right ventricle during inspiration.

THE RIGHT VENTRICLE. Normally, this chamber, or its motion, is not palpable. A palpable anterior systolic movement (replacing systolic retraction) in the left parasternal region (Fig. 2-19*A*), best felt by the proximal palm or fingertips, and with the patient supine, usually represents *right ventricular enlargement*. In the absence of associated left ventricular enlargement, this may be accompanied by reciprocal systolic retraction of the apex. In patients with pulmonary emphysema even an enlarged right ventricle is not readily palpable at the left sternal edge but better appreciated in the subxiphoid region. Exaggerated motion of the entire parasternal area, i.e., a hyperdynamic impulse with normal contour, usually reflects increased right ventricular recoil due to augmented stroke volume, as occurs in patients with atrial septal defect or tricuspid regurgitation, while a sustained left parasternal outward thrust reflects right ventricular hypertrophy due to pressure overload, as occurs in pulmonary hypertension or pulmonic stenosis. With marked right ventricular enlargement, this chamber occupies the apex and the left ventricle is displaced posteriorly.

When both ventricles are enlarged, both the left parasternal and the apical areas may rise with systole, but an area of systolic retraction between them can sometimes be appreciated. In patients with emphysema or obesity, an enlarged right ventricle is sometimes detected most readily in the subxiphoid region by palpating the epigastrium and pointing the fingers upward (Fig. 2-19*B*). With marked isolated right ventricular enlargement, the heart may rotate in a clockwise manner, and the right ventricle may form the cardiac apex, producing findings that may be confused with those of left or biventricular enlargement. When acute myocardial ischemia or myocardial infarction causes dyskinetic movement of the ventricular septum, there may be a transient left parasternal impulse not caused by right ventricular enlargement.

PULMONARY ARTERY. *Pulmonary hypertension* and/or increased pulmonary blood flow frequently produces a prominent systolic pulsation of the pulmonary artery in the second intercostal space just to the left of the sternum. This pulsation is often associated with a prominent left parasternal impulse, reflecting right ventricular enlargement, and a palpable shock synchronous with the second heart sound, reflecting forceful closure of the pulmonic valve.

LEFT ATRIUM. An enlarged left atrium or a large posterior left ventricular aneurysm can make right ventricular pulsations more prominent by displacing the right ventricle anteriorly against the left parasternal area, and in severe mitral regurgitation an expanding left atrium may be responsible for marked left parasternal movement, even in the absence of right ventricular hypertrophy. The systolic bulging of the left atrium, which is transmitted through the right ventricle, commences and terminates *after* the left ventricular thrust. It can be appreciated by placing the index finger of one hand at the left ventricular apex and the index finger of the other in the left parasternal region in the third intercostal space; the movement of the latter finger begins and ends slightly later than that of the former. While this difference in timing may be difficult to appreciate on palpation, particularly when the heart rate is rapid, recordings of chest wall motion in severe chronic mitral regurgitation demonstrate a delayed fall in the left lower precordium compared to the cardiac apex. Outward movement of the chest wall that is more marked to the right than to the left of the sternum is usually due to aneurysm of the aorta or to marked enlargement of the right atrium. Occasionally, a giant left atrium is palpable in the right hemithorax. The left atrial appendage is sometimes palpable in the third left intercostal space.

AORTA. Enlargement or aneurysm of the ascending aorta or aortic arch may cause visible or palpable systolic pulsations of the right or left sternoclavicular joint; it may also cause a systolic impulse in the suprasternal notch or the first or second right intercostal space.[1]

PALPABLE SOUNDS. Valve closure, if abnormally forceful or if normal in a patient with a thin chest wall, can be appreciated as a tapping sensation. It occurs most prominently in the second left intercostal space in patients with pulmonary hypertension (pulmonic valve closure), in the second right intercostal space in patients with systemic hypertension (aortic valve closure), and at the cardiac apex in patients with mitral stenosis (mitral valve closure). Occasionally, in congenital aortic stenosis, aortic ejection sounds can be palpated at the cardiac apex; ejection sounds originating in a dilated aorta or pulmonary artery can sometimes be felt at the base of the heart.[64] Prominent third and fourth heart sounds are often palpable as diastolic movements at the cardiac apex. In patients with mitral stenosis an opening snap may be palpated at the apex.

THRILLS. The flat of the hand or the fingertips usually best appreciate thrills, vibratory sensations which are palpable manifestations of loud, harsh murmurs *having low-fre-*

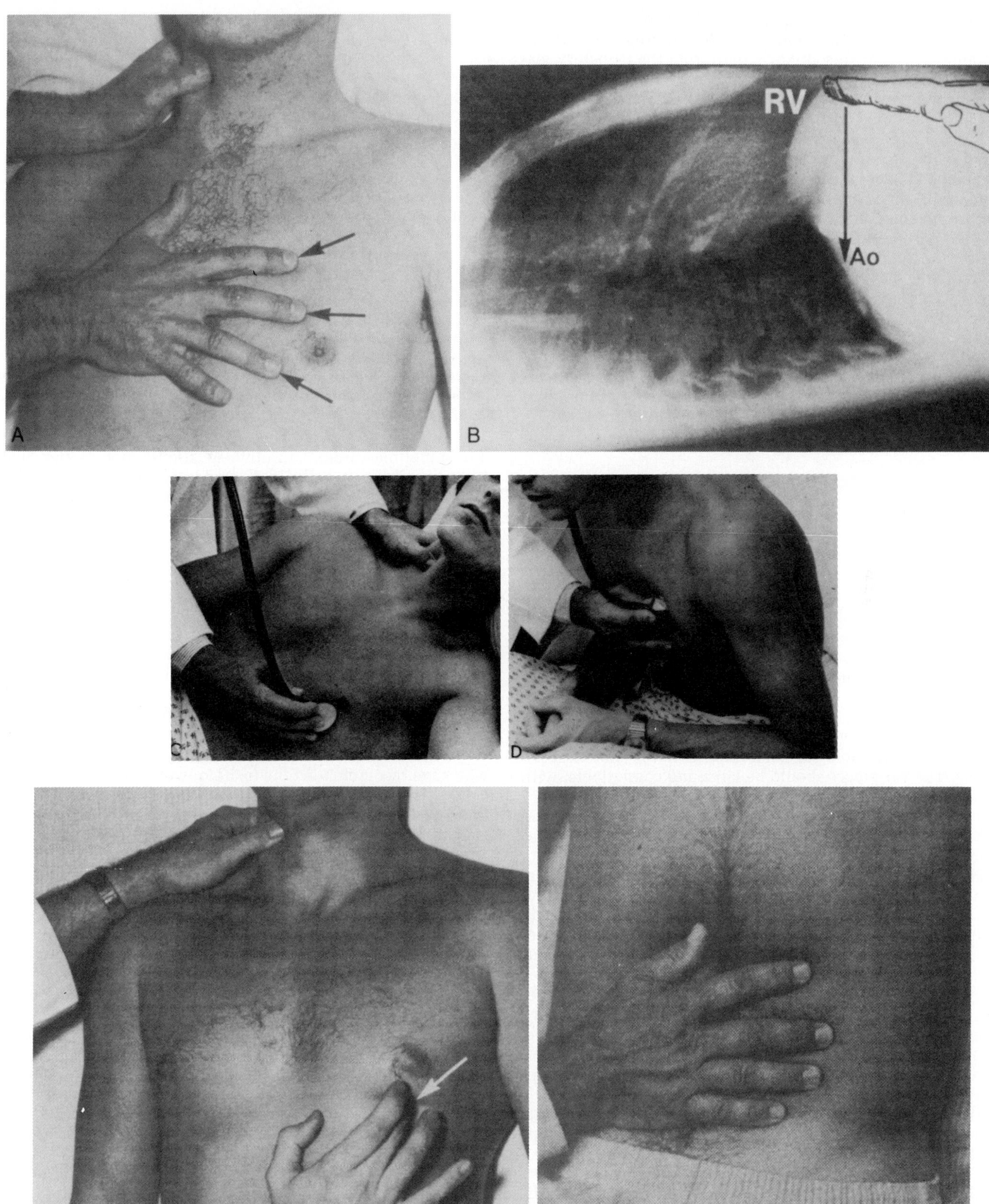

FIGURE 2–19. *A*, Palpation of the anterior wall of the right ventricle by applying the tips of three fingers in the third, fourth, and fifth interspaces, left sternal edge (arrows), during full held exhalation. Patient is supine with the trunk elevated 30 degrees. *B*, Subxiphoid palpation of the inferior wall of the right ventricle (RV) with the relative position of the abdominal aorta (Ao) shown by the arrow. *C*, The stethoscope is applied to the cardiac apex while the patient lies in a partial left lateral decubitus position. The examiner's free left hand is used to palpate the carotid artery for timing purposes. *D*, The soft–high frequency early diastolic murmur of either aortic regurgitation or pulmonary hypertensive regurgitation is best elicited by applying the stethoscopic diaphragm very firmly to the mid-left sternal edge. The patient leans forward with breath held in full exhalation. *E*, Palpation of the left ventricular impulse with a fingertip (arrow). The patient's trunk is 30 degrees above the horizontal. The examiner's right thumb palpates the carotid pulse for timing purposes. *F*, Testing for abdominojugular reflux is performed with the palm of the hand gently but firmly applied to the center of the abdomen. (From Perloff, J. K.: Physical Examination of the Heart and Circulation. 2nd ed. Philadelphia, W. B. Saunders Company, 1990.)

quency components.[65] Since the vibrations must be quite intense before they are felt, far more information can be obtained from the auscultatory than from the palpatory features of heart murmurs. High-pitched murmurs such as those produced by valvular regurgitation, even when loud, are not usually associated with thrills.

PERCUSSION. Palpation is far more helpful than is percussion in determining cardiac size. However, in the absence of an apical beat, as occurs in patients with pericardial effusion, or in some patients with dilated cardiomyopathy, heart failure, and marked displacement of a hypokinetic apical beat, the left border of the heart can be outlined by means of percussion. Also, percussion of dullness in the right lower parasternal area may, in some instances, aid in the detection of a greatly enlarged right atrium. Percussion aids in determining visceral situs, i.e., in ascertaining the side on which the heart, stomach, and liver are located. When the heart is in the right chest, but the abdominal viscera are located normally, congenital heart disease is usually present. When both the heart and abdominal viscera are in the opposite side of the chest (situs inversus), congenital heart disease is uncommon.

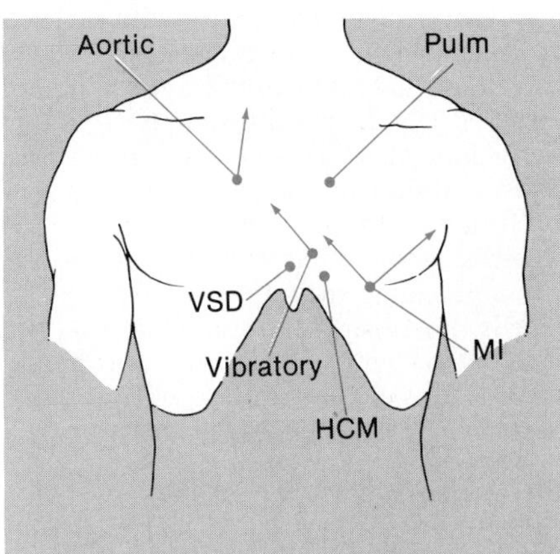

FIGURE 2-20. Maximal intensity and radiation of six isolated systolic murmurs. HCM = hypertrophic cardiomyopathy; MI = mitral incompetence; Pulm = pulmonary; VSD = ventricular septal defect. (From Barlow, J. B.: Perspectives on the Mitral Valve. Philadelphia, F. A. Davis, 1987, p. 140.)

CARDIAC AUSCULTATION

GENERAL PRINCIPLES. Vibrations on the surface of the chest set into motion a column of air that is collected and conducted to the ear by the stethoscope.[66-68] Since the transmission of high frequencies are dampened by a large volume of air between the chest and the ear, the most effective stethoscopes are made of plastic tubing 10 to 12 inches in length with an internal diameter of ⅛ inch; the thicker and shorter the tubing, the more room noise is eliminated. The stethoscope should have two chest pieces, a shallow bell and a stiff diaphragm. Since their ability to collect sound is proportional to their diameter, they should be as large as is practical, without impairing contact with the chest wall. A small bell and diaphragm are desirable for examining children and thin patients. The ear pieces should be large and comfortable, with their axes parallel to the long axes of the external auditory canals. Air leaks—anywhere between the patient's chest and the examiner's auditory canal—are the greatest source of auscultatory difficulties, and must be avoided.

High-frequency sounds, such as the first and second heart sounds, and systolic clicks and high-pitched murmurs, such as those of valvular regurgitation, are best appreciated by using the diaphragm, which has a relatively high natural frequency and damps out low frequencies (<300 Hz), particularly when firm pressure is applied to the stethoscope. In order to detect low frequency vibrations (30 to 150 Hz), the bell of the stethoscope should be applied to the chest with slight pressure, just enough to prevent detection of room noise. When the bell is applied too tightly, the skin under the bell forms a diaphragm, defeating the purpose of the bell by damping out low-frequency sounds. Third and fourth heart sounds and diastolic murmurs originating from the mitral and tricuspid valves, which are usually low pitched, are best heard through the bell.

Cardiac auscultation should be carried out in a quiet room with the patient comfortable and the chest exposed.[69] Ordinarily the examiner should be on the patient's right side, and the patient should be examined routinely in three positions: supine, sitting, and left lateral decubitus (Fig. 2-19C and *D*). A simultaneously palpated carotid pulse (or apex impulse) is helpful in timing the auscultatory events. Occasionally, the effects of squatting, standing, or the prone position (p. 39) and other physiological and pharmacological interventions are studied (p. 40). Although the principal areas of cardiac auscultation (Fig. 2-20) are the second right interspace ("aortic" area), the second left interspace ("pulmonic" area), the fourth interspace adjacent to the left sternal border ("tricuspid" area), and the cardiac apex ("mitral" area), auscultation should not be limited to these sites, since important findings are sometimes present in other locations, such as the right parasternal region, axilla, neck, and interscapular regions. For example, auscultation just above the sternoclavicular joints is best for detecting a venous hum. Murmurs produced by pulmonary arteriovenous fistula, bronchial collateral vessels, and systemic arterial collaterals in patients with coarctation of the aorta as well as murmurs of pulmonary branch stenosis may be heard over the posterior chest. In some patients with pulmonary emphysema, heart sounds are best heard in the epigastrium.

A logical sequence for auscultation is to begin at the apex, where the first heart sound is usually prominent, then to proceed along the left sternal border to the upper right sternal edge and then the carotid arteries. When the heart rate is rapid, it may be difficult to identify the phase of the cardiac cycle and the resultant auscultatory events. Levine and Harvey have recommended the technique of first listening at the apex, where the first heart sound is normally the loudest sound audible and can usually be readily identified because it occurs just before the carotid arterial upstroke, and then "inching up" the chest along the left sternal border, using the diaphragm and bell alternately.[70] This allows correct identification of systole and diastole at other precordial sites. Auscultation should be carried out during normal quiet respiration, during normal held expiration, and during forced expiration; the effects of variations in respiration and posture on auscultatory findings should be determined.

A systematic plan should be employed for cardiac auscultation, listening to only one part of the cardiac cycle at a time and in sequence. It is desirable to listen selectively to the first heart sound (S_1), and then the second heart sound (S_2), the systolic interval, and then the diastolic interval. An attempt should be made to listen to each component separately. The intensity, quality, and splitting of each of the sounds should be determined and the effects of respiration on the splitting of S_2 ascertained.[69-75] The systolic and diastolic intervals should then be listened to separately for extra sounds and murmurs.

Heart Sounds (See also pp. 43 to 50)

FIRST AND SECOND HEART SOUNDS (Fig. 3-1, p. 44). S_1 occurs just *before* the palpable arterial upstroke of the carotid pulse and can be distinguished from S_2, which occurs immediately *after* the peak of the carotid pulse. S_1 is heard best with the diaphragm of the stethoscope, usually medial to the apex at the lower sternal border. The mitral component of S_1 is usually loudest at the apex, whereas the tricuspid component is often loudest at the lower left sternal edge. The intensity of S_1 is increased in mitral stenosis, left atrial myxoma,[76] mitral valve prolapse, short P-R interval, and any condition that causes tachycardia or unusually vigorous ventricular contraction. S_1 is diminished or absent with P-R prolongation, fibrosis or calcification of the mitral valve, severe left ventricular failure, left bundle branch block, and mitral regurgitation (not due to prolapse). Narrow splitting of S_1 frequently is heard at the lower left sternal border in normal subjects. Wide splitting of S_1 with an audible delayed tricuspid component is best heard in inspiration and at the lower left sternal border; it may occur in tricuspid stenosis, Ebstein's anomaly, right bundle branch block, and pacing from the left ventricle.

S_2 is ordinarily most readily audible in the second right and left intercostal spaces along the sternal borders. S_2 is higher pitched than S_1 and is also heard best with the diaphragm of the stethoscope. It is normally split into two components,[77] the aortic (A_2) and pulmonic (P_2) closure sounds, because of asynchronous closure of these two valves (see below). P_2 is normally softer than A_2 and is less widely transmitted. Splitting of S_2 is most readily assessed with the patient supine, first during normal respiration and then during slow, deep respiration (Figs. 2–21 to 2–23 and Table 2–2). A single S_2 may result from inaudibility of either component or their fusion, as in Eisenmenger's complex.

The intensity of A_2 depends on the anatomical relationship between the aorta and the anterior chest wall as well as on the level of the aortic pressure. It is loud in systemic hypertension, with a "tambour" quality, and in congenital malformations such as transposition of the great arteries, in which the aorta arises anteriorly. The intensity of P_2 varies directly with the level of pulmonary artery pressure and the degree of dilatation of the pulmonary artery. P_2 is not normally audible at the apex; when it is audible, pulmonary hypertension is usually present. Stenosis of the aortic and pulmonic valves causes decreased intensity of A_2 and P_2, respectively. P_2 may not be audible in emphysematous subjects.

TABLE 2–2 CAUSES OF SPLITTING OF THE SECOND HEART SOUND

NORMAL SPLITTING

DELAYED PULMONIC CLOSURE
- Delayed electrical activation of the right ventricle
  - Complete RBBB (proximal type)
  - Left ventricular paced beats
  - Left ventricular ectopic beats
- Prolonged right ventricular mechanical systole
  - Acute massive pulmonary embolus
  - Pulmonary hypertension with right heart failure
  - Pulmonic stenosis with intact septum (moderate to severe)
- Decreased impedance of the pulmonary vascular bed (increased hang-out)
  - Normotensive atrial septal defect
  - Idiopathic dilatation of the pulmonary artery
  - Pulmonic stenosis (mild)
  - Atrial septal defect, postoperative (70%)

EARLY AORTIC CLOSURE
- Shortened left ventricular mechanical systole (LVET)
  - Mitral regurgitation
  - Ventricular septal defect

REVERSED SPLITTING

DELAYED AORTIC CLOSURE
- Delayed electrical activation of the left ventricle
  - Complete LBBB (proximal type)
  - Right ventricular paced beats
  - Right ventricular ectopic beats
- Prolonged left ventricular mechanical systole
  - Complete LBBB (peripheral type)
  - Left ventricular outflow tract obstruction
  - Hypertensive cardiovascular disease
  - Arteriosclerotic heart disease
    - Chronic ischemic heart disease
    - Angina pectoris
- Decreased impedance of the systemic vascular bed (increased hang-out)
- Poststenotic dilatation of the aorta secondary to aortic stenosis or insufficiency
- Patent ductus arteriosus

EARLY PULMONIC CLOSURE
- Early electrical activation of the right ventricle
  - Wolff-Parkinson-White syndrome, type B

RBBB = right bundle-branch block; LVET = left ventricular ejection time; LBBB = left bundle-branch block.

Modified from Shaver, J. A., O'Toole, J. D.: The second heart sound: Newer concepts. Parts 1 and 2. Mod. Concepts Cardiovasc. Dis. *46*:7 and 13, 1977.

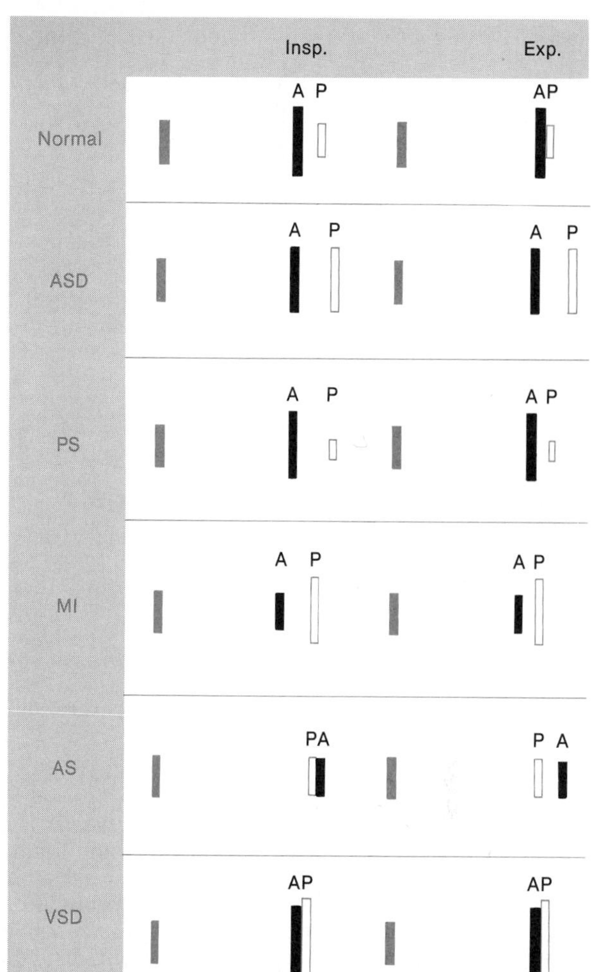

FIGURE 2–21. Diagrammatic representation of normal and abnormal patterns in the respiratory variation of the second heart sound. The heights of the bars are proportional to the sound intensity. A = aortic component; P = pulmonary component; ASD = atrial septal defect; PS = pulmonary stenosis; MI = mitral incompetence; AS = aortic stenosis; VSD = ventricular septal defect. (From Barlow, J. B.: Perspectives on the Mitral Valve. Philadelphia, F. A. Davis, 1987, p. 23.)

EJECTION SOUNDS (Fig. 3–5, p. 45). These systolic sounds usually coincide with the full opening of the semilunar valves, are high-pitched and clicking, and are heard best with the diaphragm of the stethoscope. They are not heard in normal persons but are caused by opening of the stenotic semilunar valves or from the ejection of blood into a dilated aorta or pulmonary artery. Pulmonary ejection sounds are heard in patients with valvular pulmonic stenosis (as long as the cusps retain some mobility) (Fig. 3–3, p. 45), in pulmonary hypertension, and in idiopathic dilatation of the pulmonary artery. Aortic ejection sounds are heard best in the second right interspace and at the apex and are not notably affected by respiration, while pulmonic ejection sounds are heard best in the second left interspace and often increase in intensity during expiration. Aortic ejection sounds are heard most frequently in aortic stenosis (congenital or acquired) as long as the valve is mobile. They are also heard in systemic hypertension and aortic dilatation.

If more than two heart sounds are heard during each cardiac cycle, it must be determined whether the extra sound occurs in systole or diastole, whether it is early or late, and whether it is high-pitched (such as a systolic click) or low-pitched (such

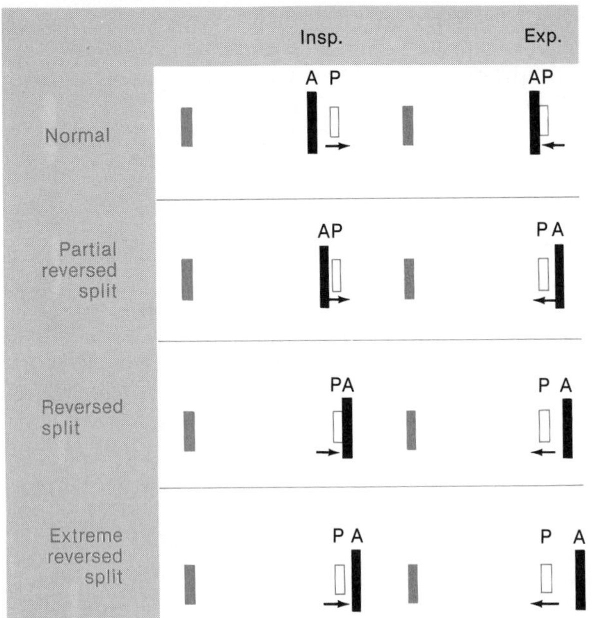

FIGURE 2–22. Reversed and partially reversed splitting of the second heart sound. Arrows indicate the direction of the movement of P during inspiration and expiration. (From Barlow, J. B.: Perspectives on the Mitral Valve. Philadelphia, F. A. Davis, 1987, p. 24.)

as a third or fourth heart sound). When two heart sounds are heard at the time of S_1, it is often difficult to differentiate between a split S_1, a combination of S_4 and S_1, and a combination of S_1 and an ejection click.[73] The S_4 is usually audible only at the apex and often in the left lateral decubitus position; it is low-pitched, associated with palpable presystolic distention of the left ventricle, and attenuated by increased pressure on the bell of the stethoscope. It is rarely heard at the lower left sternal border, where splitting of S_1 is most easily detected. The ejection click is usually louder than the second (tricuspid) component of a split S_1 and is often audible at the base of the heart, whereas splitting of S_1 is rarely heard in this area.

MID-SYSTOLIC CLICKS (Fig. 3–7, p. 46). These sounds are associated most frequently with mitral (or rarely tricuspid) valve prolapse (p. 1029). They are high-pitched, heard best with the diaphragm of the stethoscope, variable in timing (p. 000) and intensity, and are sometimes multiple. Midsystolic clicks occur at the time of the maximum excursion of the prolapsed leaflets and elongated chordae. These clicks are sometimes audible in severe aortic regurgitation.[78]

OPENING SNAPS. These diastolic sounds usually occur with mitral or tricuspid valves that are stenotic but mobile and are analogous to the systolic ejection sounds produced by opening of stenotic semilunar valves. Opening snaps are high-pitched and heard best through the diaphragm. It may be difficult to differentiate an opening snap from P_2 by clinical examination. However, the former radiates more widely and is often heard both at the apex and in the second right intercostal space; P_2 also usually changes its relationship to A_2 during respiration, whereas an opening snap does not. Finally, the A_2-opening snap interval is usually longer (>40 msec) than the A_2-P_2 interval. Opening snaps precede third heart sounds (Table 2–3) and are higher pitched (Fig. 3–11*B*, p. 48). Opening snaps originating from the tricuspid valve are usually heard best at the lower left sternal edge, commonly signify rheumatic tricuspid stenosis and frequently increase in intensity during inspiration.

THIRD AND FOURTH HEART SOUNDS (Fig. 3–1*A*, p. 44). The diastolic sound during passive filling which occurs during the *y* descent of the atrial pressure pulse is termed the *third heart sound* (S_3), while the sound which occurs during ventricular filling caused by atrial contraction is called the *fourth heart sound* (S_4).[79–88] When S_3 and S_4 are abnormal, they are referred to as third or fourth sound *gallops*. Third and fourth heart sounds are low-pitched sounds that are heard best with the bell of the stethoscope and are intensified by the recumbent position and by exercise, such as a few sit-ups or sustained handgrip. Inspiration enhances third or fourth heart sounds originating from the right ventricle but has little de-

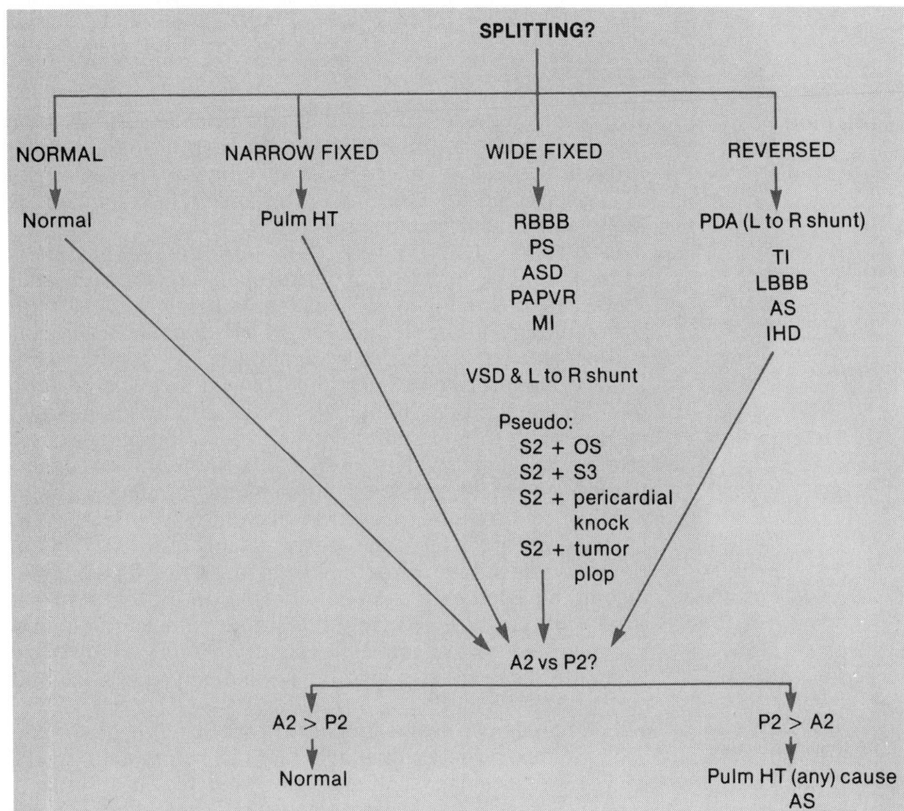

FIGURE 2–23. Branching logic tree for S_2 splitting. Pulm HT, pulmonary hypertension; RBBB, right bundle branch block; PS, pulmonic stenosis; ASD, atrial septal defect; PAPVR, partial anomalous pulmonary venous return; MI, mitral insufficiency; VSD, ventricular septal defect; L to R, left-to-right shunt; OS, opening snap; PDA, patent ductus arteriosus; TI, tricuspid insufficiency; LBBB, left bundle branch block; AS, aortic stenosis; IHD, ischemic heart disease; HT, hypertension. (From Sapira, J. D.: The Art and Science of Bedside Diagnosis. Baltimore, Urban & Schwartzenberg, 1990.)

TABLE 2-3 EARLY DIASTOLIC INTERVALS

A2-P2 (normal expiration)	<0.03 sec
A2-P2 (inspiration, young persons)	0.04–0.05 sec
A2-P2 (right bundle branch block)	0.06–0.08 sec
A2-Opening snap	0.03–0.15 sec
A2-Pericardial knock	0.10–0.12 sec
AS-S3 (adults with heart disease)	0.14–0.16 sec
A2-S3 (normal children)	0.12–0.20 sec

Adapted from Sapira, J. D.: The Art and Science of Bedside Diagnosis. Baltimore, Urban and Schwartzenberg, 1990.

tectable effect on such sounds originating from the left ventricle. At heart rates above 100 beats/min, when both S_3 and S_4 gallops are present they may fuse, producing a loud sound, a so-called *summation gallop.* Third and fourth heart sounds originate in the ventricle and require unimpeded filling for their generation.

S_3 occurs as active ventricular relaxation (reflected in the decline in ventricular pressure) ends and passive filling (reflected in a diastolic rise in ventricular pressure) commences.[74,79,86] It appears to be caused by an early diastolic impact of the ventricle on the chest wall; it is intensified by rapid early diastolic filling, by an elevated atrial pressure, and by increased or abnormal diastolic distensibility of the ventricle. S_3 is often heard in hyperkinetic states, such as hyperthyroidism and with severe mitral regurgitation. Left-sided S_3 sounds are heard best at the apex, whereas those originating from the right ventricle are heard best along the left sternal border and are accentuated by inspiration. Third heart sounds may be audible in normal children and young adults. However, when they are heard in men over the age of 40 and women over 50, they are generally abnormal. The disappearance of a normal S_3 with age appears to result from a decrease in the rate of early ventricular filling and resulting deceleration.[80,84] S_3 is usually maximally audible at the apex, with the patient in the left lateral recumbent position and during expiration. An S_4 originating from the right ventricle, due to tricuspid regurgitation or right ventricular failure, is heard best along the lower left sternal border.

Conditions causing ventricular diastolic overload with atrial hypertension are often responsible for an S_3 which is audible in states of increased cardiac output,[81] such as during the third trimester of pregnancy, after exertion, and in anxiety-related tachycardia (Table 2–4). It also occurs with impaired left ventricular function of any cause.[82] In the presence of ischemic heart disease, an S_3 strongly suggests left ventricular dyskinesia or aneurysm. In patients with aortic regurgitation, a third heart sound usually signifies a reduced ejection fraction and elevated end-systolic volume.[83] In patients with reduced cardiac reserve it correlates well with the response to digitalis.[88]

Healthy older adults rarely may have an S_4, but when heard in the young, this sound is usually abnormal. S_4 is probably caused by vibrations of the ventricular wall during the rapid influx of blood during atrial contraction and is best heard with the patient in the left lateral recumbent position and with the bell of the stethoscope gently applied to the chest; it is generally associated with an elevated ventricular end-diastolic pressure and a high ratio of left ventricular wall thickness-to-cavity diameter. As left ventricular compliance decreases, atrial systole becomes responsible for more than 25 per cent of ventricular filling, and an S_4 may become prominent. Vigorous atrial contraction is necessary to produce an audible S_4, which can be recorded phonocardiographically in about 50 per cent of normal adults, but it is extremely low in intensity and usually not audible. It is not present in atrial fibrillation, nor when atrial systole is weak, as following cardioversion. A distinctly audible, palpable S_4 is usually abnormal (Table 2–4). The common denominators with which it is associated are left ventricular hypertrophy, increased left ventricular end-diastolic pressure, some restriction to diastolic filling, and a high ratio of left ventricular wall thickness-to-cavity diameter. An S_4 is characteristic of aortic stenosis with a significant left ventricular-aortic pressure gradient, systemic hypertension, hypertrophic cardiomyopathy, ischemic heart disease, and *acute* mitral regurgitation. Reduced left ventricular compliance following myocardial infarction often results in an audible S_4. A right ventricular S_4 is common in pulmonary hypertension and pulmonary stenosis.

Murmurs and Other Adventitious Sounds

The etiology of various murmurs is presented in Tables 2–5 and 2–6, and Figures 2–24 and 2–25 illustrate a variety of murmurs and sounds. A discussion of the most important heart murmurs is presented in Chapter 3.

Murmurs and adventitious sounds are caused, at least in part, by turbulence of blood flow, which in turn results from a

TABLE 2-4 PHYSIOLOGICAL AND PATHOLOGICAL STATES WITH A THIRD AND FOURTH HEART SOUND

THIRD HEART SOUND
- Physiological
  - Children and young adults (<40 yr)
- Pathological
  - Hyperdynamic states
    - High output
    - Anemia
    - Thyrotoxicosis
    - Arteriovenous fistula
  - Hypertrophic cardiomyopathy
  - Regurgitant atrioventricular valve lesions
    - Mitral regurgitation
    - Tricuspid regurgitation
  - Increase in end-systolic volume
    - Ventricular dysfunction
    - Left ventricle:
      - Congenital heart disease
      - Valvular disease
      - Systemic hypertension
      - Ischemic heart disease
      - Cardiomyopathy
    - Right ventricle:
      - Congenital heart disease
      - Valvular disease
      - Pulmonary hypertension
      - Right ventricular infarct
      - Cardiomyopathy
  - Constrictive pericarditis

FOURTH HEART SOUND
- Physiological
  - Recordable but not audible
- Pathological
  - Left ventricular hypertrophy
    - Left ventricular outflow tract obstruction
    - Systemic hypertrophic cardiomyopathy
  - Right ventricular hypertrophy
    - Right ventricular outflow tract obstruction
    - Pulmonic hypertension
    - Idiopathic hypertrophic cardiomyopathy (rarely)
  - Ischemic heart disease
    - Angina
    - Acute myocardial infarction
    - Left ventricular dysfunction
  - Hyperkinetic states
    - Anemia
    - Thyrotoxicosis
    - Arteriovenous fistula
  - Acute valvular regurgitation
    - Acute mitral regurgitation
    - Acute aortic regurgitation
    - Acute tricuspid regurgitation
  - Arrhythmia
    - Heart block
    - Atrial flutter

From Reddy, P. S., Salerni, R., and Shaver, J. A.: Normal and abnormal heart sounds in cardiac diagnosis. Part II. Diastolic sounds. Cur. Probl. Cardiol. *10*(4):26 and 44, 1985.

TABLE 2–5 PRINCIPAL CAUSES OF HEART MURMURS

A. ORGANIC SYSTOLIC MURMURS
1. Midsystolic (Ejection)
   a. Aortic
      (1) Obstructive
         (a) Supravalvular—supraaortic stenosis, coarctation of the aorta
         (b) Valvular—AS and sclerosis
         (c) Infravalvular—HOCM
      (2) Increased flow, hyperkinetic states, AR, complete heart block
      (3) Dilatation of ascending aorta, atheroma, aortitis, aneurysm of aorta
   b. Pulmonary
      (1) Obstructive
         (a) Supravalvular—pulmonary arterial stenosis
         (b) Valvular—pulmonic valve stenosis
         (c) Infravalvular—infundibular stenosis
      (2) Increased flow, hyperkinetic states, left-to-right shunt (e.g., ASD, VSD)
      (3) Dilatation of pulmonary artery
2. Pansystolic (Regurgitant)
   a. Atrioventricular valve regurgitation (MR, TR)
   b. Left-to-right shunt to ventricular level

B. EARLY DIASTOLIC MURMURS
1. Aortic regurgitation
   a. Valvular; rheumatic deformity; perforation post-endocarditis, post-traumatic, post-valvulotomy
   b. Dilatation of valve ring: aorta dissection, annuloectasia, cystic medial necrosis, hypertension
   c. Widening of commissures: syphilis
   d. Congenital: bicuspid valve, with ventricular septal defect
2. Pulmonic regurgitation
   a. Valvular: post-valvulotomy, endocarditis, rheumatic fever, carcinoid
   b. Dilatation of valve ring: pulmonary hypertension; Marfan syndrome
   c. Congenital: isolated or associated with tetralogy of Fallot, VSD, pulmonic stenosis

C. MID-DIASTOLIC MURMURS
1. Mitral stenosis
2. Carey-Coombs murmur (mid-diastolic apical murmur in acute rheumatic fever)
3. Increased flow across nonstenotic mitral valve (e.g., MR, VSD, PDA, high-output states, and complete heart block)
4. Tricuspid stenosis
5. Increased flow across nonstenotic tricuspid valve (e.g., TR, ASD, and anomalous pulmonary venous return)
6. Left and right atrial tumors

D. CONTINUOUS MURMURS
1. Patent ductus arteriosus
2. Coronary AV fistula
3. Ruptured aneurysm of sinus of Valsalva
4. Aortic septal defect
5. Cervical venous hum
6. Anomalous left coronary artery
7. Proximal coronary artery stenosis
8. Mammary souffle
9. Pulmonary artery branch stenosis
10. Bronchial collateral circulation
11. Small (restrictive) ASD with MS
12. Intercostal AV fistula

AR = aortic regurgitation; AS = aortic stenosis; ASD = atrial septal defect; AV = arteriovenous; HOCM = hypertrophic obstructive cardiomyopathy; MR = mitral regurgitation; MS = mitral stenosis; PDA = patent ductus arteriosus; TR = tricuspid regurgitation; VSD = ventricular septal defect. (*A* and *C* modified from Oram, S. [ed.]: Clinical Heart Disease. London, William Heinemann Medical Books, Ltd., 1981; *D* modified from Fowler, N. O. [ed.]: Cardiac Diagnosis and Treatment. Hagerstown, MD, Harper and Row, 1980.)

disproportion between the velocity of blood flow and the dimensions of the orifice through which it flows. The turbulence is most prominent in the structure *beyond* the obstruction. There are eight characteristics of heart murmurs which should be considered. These are: (1) timing, (2) shape, (3) location, (4) radiation, (5) pitch (tone), (6) timbre (purity of pitch), (7) intensity, and (8) effects of special maneuvers, including changes in patient position, respiration, and sometimes drugs.

Cardiac murmurs should be timed, and their length in the cardiac cycle and their shape, i.e., their intensity (or loudness) as a function of time, should be determined. Murmurs are classified as systolic (between S_1 and S_2) or diastolic (between S_2 and S_1) and continuous (enveloping S_2). Each of these major categories is then subclassified as early, mid, late or pan (systolic or diastolic). Their shape is characterized as crescendo, decrescendo, or crescendo-decrescendo. The *intensity* of a murmur is determined by the quantity and velocity of blood flow across the sound-producing area, by its distance from the stethoscope, and by the transmission qualities of the tissue between the origin of the murmur and the stethoscope. Murmurs are accentuated in thin persons and diminished in patients who are obese, with emphysema, and in the presence of pleural or pericardial fluid.[66] They are accentuated in hyperdynamic and reduced in hypodynamic states. Murmurs radiate in the direction of the blood flow responsible for the murmur.

It is helpful to grade the intensity of murmurs; six grades, as described by Freeman and Levine, are commonly distinguished.[89] A *Grade 1/6* murmur is the faintest that can be detected, often only after close concentration and adjustment of the stethoscope. A *Grade 2/6* murmur is a faint murmur but can be detected immediately by an experienced observer. A *Grade 3/6* murmur is moderately loud, and a *Grade 4/6* murmur is loud. A *Grade 5/6* murmur is a very loud murmur but requires placement of the stethoscope on the chest to be audible. A *Grade 6/6* murmur is so loud that it can be heard even without placing the stethoscope on the chest. The *duration* of a murmur depends upon the duration of the event, such as the pressure gradient, which is responsible for it, while the *radiation* of a murmur is determined by its site of origin, its intensity, the direction of the blood flow responsible for the mur-

TABLE 2–6 DIFFERENTIAL DIAGNOSIS OF CONTINUOUS THORACIC MURMURS (IN ORDER OF DECREASING FREQUENCY)

DIAGNOSIS	KEY FINDINGS
Cervical venous hum	Disappears on compression of the jugular vein
Hepatic venous hum	Often disappears with epigastric pressure
Mammary souffle	Disappears upon pressing hard with stethoscope
Patent ductus arteriosus	Loudest at 2nd left intercostal space
Coronary arteriovenous fistula	Loudest at lower sternal borders
Ruptured aneurysm of sinus of Valsalva	Loudest at upper right sternal border, sudden onset
Bronchial collaterals	Associated signs of congenital heart disease
High-grade coarctation	Brachial-pedal arterial pressure gradient
Anomalous left coronary artery arising from pulmonary artery	Electrocardiographic changes of myocardial infarction
Truncus arteriosus	
Pulmonary artery branch stenosis	Heard outside the area of cardiac dullness
Pulmonary AV fistula	Same as above
Atrial septal defect with mitral stenosis or atresia	Altered by the Valsalva maneuver
Aortic-atrial fistulas	

Adapted from Sapira, J. D.: The Art and Science of Bedside Diagnosis. Baltimore, Urban & Schwartzenberg, 1990.

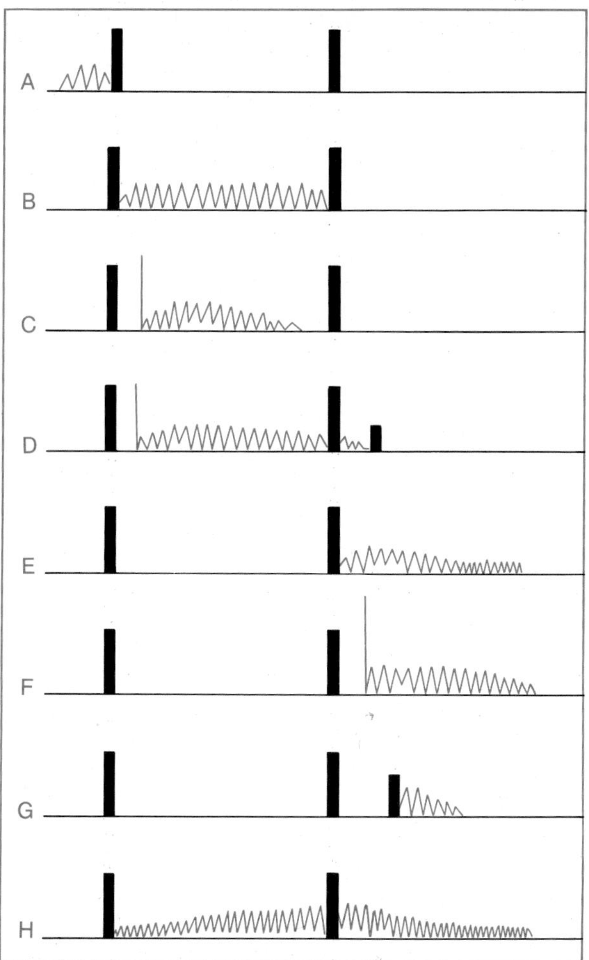

FIGURE 2-24. Diagram depicting principal heart murmurs:
A, Presystolic murmur of mitral or tricuspid stenosis.
B, Pansystolic murmur of mitral or tricuspid incompetence or of ventricular septal defect.
C, Aortic ejection murmur beginning with an ejection click and fading before the second heart sound.
D, Systolic murmur in pulmonic stenosis spilling through the aortic second sound, pulmonic valve closure being delayed.
E, Aortic pulmonary diastolic murmur.
F, Long diastolic murmur of mitral stenosis following the opening snap.
G, Short mid-diastolic inflow murmur following a third heart sound.
H, Continuous murmur of patent ductus arteriosus. (From Wood, P.: Diseases of the Heart and Circulation. Philadelphia, J. B. Lippincott, 1968, p. 75.)

mur (Fig. 2-20), and the physical characteristics of the chest. The *quality* of murmurs should be described using adjectives such as blowing, harsh, rumbling, scratchy, musical, and high- or low-pitched. Murmurs with mixed high and medium frequencies sound harsh or rasping, while those with a narrow frequency range, often owing to vibration of an intracardiac structure such as a valve leaflet, are musical or honking in quality (Fig. 3-17, p. 51).[90]

The interpretation of heart murmurs is based equally on their characteristics (timing, shape, intensity, duration, location, quality, and pitch) and the accompanying auscultatory features, such as the character of the splitting of S_2 as well as the presence of ejection sounds and of S_3 and S_4.

Mid-Systolic Murmurs (Fig. 3-16, p. 51). These commence after S_1 and terminate before S_2, and may be caused, as Perloff has pointed out, by at least five conditions[2] operating individually or in combination: (1) obstruction to outflow from either ventricle; (2) dilatation of the aorta and/or pulmonary trunk, (3) hyperkinetic ejection and accelerated flow into these two major trunks, (4) innocent (flow) murmurs, (5) *some* forms of mitral regurgitation. The intensity of outflow murmurs (Nos. 1 to 4 above) often vary proportionately with the duration of the preceding diastole, while the murmurs of atrioventricular valve regurgitation (No. 5) do not (or less so). *Innocent murmurs* (No. 4) usually originate from the pulmonary valve in children or young adults and result from the transmission of normal vibrations—presumably of the pulmonary valve—through a thin chest wall; they are often heard in patients with the "straight back syndrome."

begin with the first heart sound and end with the second sound on its side of origin and result from flow (usually abnormal) from a chamber or vessel whose pressure is higher than that of the recipient throughout systole. The prototypes are mitral and tricuspid regurgitation and ventricular septal defect (although the lesions frequently cause shorter murmurs as well). The holosystolic murmur of mitral regurgitation is usually directed posterolaterally into the left atrium and radi-

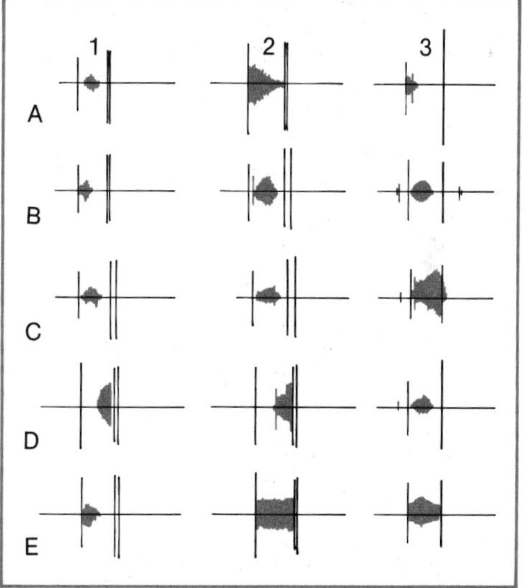

FIGURE 2-25. Sketches of various murmurs and heart sounds.
A-1, Short, midsystolic murmur, with normal aortic and pulmonic components of S_2-findings consistent with an innocent murmur.
A-2, Holosystolic murmur that decreases in the latter part of systole-a configuration observed in acute mitral regurgitation.
A-3, An ejection sound and a short early systolic murmur, plus accentuated, closely split S_2-consistent with pulmonary hypertension, as with Eisenmenger's ventricular septal defect.
B-1, Early to midsystolic murmur with vibratory component-typical of an innocent murmur.
B-2, An ejection sound followed by a diamond-shaped murmur and wide splitting of S_2 that may be present with atrial septal defect or mild pulmonic stenosis; an ejection sound is more likely with valvular pulmonic stenosis.
B-3, Crescendo-decrescendo systolic murmur, not holosystolic; S_3 and S_4 are present-findings consistent with mitral systolic murmur heard in congestive cardiomyopathy or coronary artery disease with papillary muscle dysfunction and cardiac decompensation.
C-1, Longer, somewhat vibratory crescendo-decrescendo systolic murmur with wide splitting of S_2 sound. If S_2 becomes fused with expiration, atrial septal defect is less likely; if the remainder of the cardiovascular evaluation is normal, this finding is consistent with an innocent murmur.
C-2, Midsystolic murmur and wide splitting of S_2 that was "fixed"-findings typical of atrial septal defect.
C-3, Prolonged diamond-shaped systolic murmur masking A_2 with delayed P_2, S_4, and ejection sound-findings typical of valvular pulmonic stenosis of moderate severity.
D-1, Late apical systolic murmur of prolapsing mitral valve leaflet.
D-2, Systolic click-late apical systolic murmur of prolapsing mitral leaflet syndrome.
D-3, S_4 and midsystolic murmur consistent with mitral systolic murmur of cardiomyopathy or ischemic heart disease.
E-1, Early crescendo-decrescendo systolic murmur ending in midsystole consistent with innocent murmur and small ventricular septal defect.
E-2 and *E-3*, Holosystolic murmurs consistent with mitral or tricuspid regurgitation and ventricular septal defect. (From Harvey, W. P.: Innocent vs. significant murmurs. Curr. Probl. Cardiol. Vol. 1, No. 8, 1976.)

ates into the axilla. Occasionally, when the murmur is transmitted anteromedially, it radiates to the base of the heart and may be confused with the murmur of semilunar valve stenosis. The murmur of tricuspid regurgitation is usually holosystolic, is heard best along the left sternal edge, and increases in intensity with inspiration. In some patients with mitral or tricuspid regurgitation and ventricular septal defect in whom the pressure difference between the two chambers diminishes and disappears at the end of systole, the murmur may be early rather than holosystolic. This occurs characteristically in acute mitral regurgitation with very tall left atrial *v* wave or in patients with muscular ventricular septal defects which may close in midsystole.

Late Systolic Murmurs (Fig. 3–8, p. 46). These are most commonly due to mitral (and occasionally tricuspid) valve prolapse and are often ushered in by a mid-systolic click. They can usually be recognized by physiological or pharmacological maneuvers (see pp. 39 and 40).

Early Diastolic Murmurs (Figs. 3–6, p. 46; 3–26, p. 56; 3–27, p. 56). When caused by aortic regurgitation, these begin with A_2 (or in the case of pulmonary regurgitation with P_2), are high-pitched, decrescendo, blowing in quality, and heard best with the diaphragm of the stethoscope. Regurgitant diastolic murmurs originating from the aortic valve are usually heard best along the left sternal border, whereas those in which a dilated aorta is primarily responsible tend to be most readily audible along the right sternal border. The diastolic murmur is shorter and rougher in acute severe aortic regurgitation. The early diastolic murmur of pulmonary regurgitation (the Graham Steell murmur) resembles that of aortic regurgitation, and is also commonly heard best along the left sternal edge; it usually follows an accentuated P_2, is usually shorter than the murmur of aortic regurgitation, and is *not* accompanied by a wide pulse pressure or physical findings thereof (p. 56).

Mid-Diastolic Murmurs (Fig. 3–28, p. 57). These murmurs are usually low-pitched and heard best with the bell of the stethoscope. They follow a pause after S_2 and are due to turbulence in the ventricle secondary to a disproportion between the atrioventricular valve orifice and the flow rate across it. Thus mid-diastolic murmurs can be present when normal (or even reduced) blood flow traverses a stenotic atrioventricular valve or when there is increased blood flow across a normal orifice; the latter may occur in the left side in mitral regurgitation or ventricular septal defect and in the right side in tricuspid regurgitation or atrial septal defect. In atrioventricular valve stenosis the duration of the murmur correlates roughly with the severity of the obstruction. The mid-diastolic murmur of tricuspid stenosis is accentuated by inspiration and is heard best along the left sternal edge, whereas that produced by mitral stenosis is not greatly affected by respiration and is usually heard best at the apex.

Mid-diastolic flow murmurs across nonobstructed atrioventricular valves are usually short, medium-pitched and usually follow an S_3.

Presystolic (Late Diastolic) Murmurs (Fig. 3–33, p. 59; Fig. 3–34, p. 59). These murmurs usually are caused by turbulent flow across a stenotic atrioventricular valve, are low-pitched, and therefore are most readily appreciated with the bell of the stethoscope. They require an appropriately timed atrial contraction and are not present in atrial fibrillation. When originating from the mitral valve they are heard best at the apex and when originating from the tricuspid valve they are heard best along the left sternal edge. The presystolic murmur of tricuspid stenosis is accentuated by inspiration.

Continuous Murmurs (Fig. 3–35, p. 60). These commence during systole and continue through (envelop) S_2 into diastole. They may be, but often are *not*, continuous through the entire cardiac cycle. Continuous murmurs usually originate from connections between high and low pressure chambers or vessels that persist throughout the cardiac cycle and are high pitched and best heard with the diaphragm of the stethoscope. They may occur with flow across constricted arteries as in constriction of the peripheral pulmonary arteries or with excessive flow through nonconstricted vessels, as in the mammary souffle. The *venous hum* is an example of a continuous venous murmur.

Cervical Venous Hum (Fig. 3–37, p. 60). This is a continuous murmur heard best with the stethoscopic bell placed lightly on the lateral portion of the right supraclavicular fossa with the patient sitting or standing, with the patient's head turned to the left. It can be confused with the murmur produced by a patent ductus arteriosus.[91] It is due to the rapid downward flow of blood through a jugular vein that becomes artificially stenosed when the patient is in the upright position, and it disappears when the jugular vein is compressed above, with the stethoscope, or when the patient assumes the recumbent position. A venous hum can be intensified by tilting the chin upward and can be abolished by pressure over the upper part of the jugular vein. It is common in normal children and in conditions in which the circulation is hyperkinetic, such as anemia, thyrotoxicosis, or pregnancy.

Mammary Souffle. This is a systolic or continuous murmur sometimes heard over the breasts of pregnant or lactating women[92] that can be confused with continuous murmurs produced by pulmonary arteriovenous fistula, patent ductus arteriosus, and other forms of congenital heart disease (Table 2–5*D*). It is presumably caused by the increased flow of blood through the engorged breast, generally commences just after the first heart sound, is best heard with the patient supine and may disappear in the upright position or with pressure from the stethoscope.

Pericardial Friction Rubs. These are not murmurs but are the sounds made by two inflamed layers of the pericardium sliding over one another, but they may be present even when there is considerable pericardial effusion (p. 1472). Friction rubs are generally described as scratching, grating, crunching, and creaking; they seem close to the ear and may vary in distribution from a site that is sharply localized to a small area of the precordium to the entire left hemithorax.[93] Usually they are most readily audible along the left sternal edge in the third and fourth intercostal spaces using the diaphragm with firm pressure and are often better heard during deep inspiration and with the patient leaning forward or in the prone position and propped up by the elbows.[94] They often exhibit nonrespiratory variations in intensity from beat to beat.[95] The sounds are commonly "to and fro" and have a systolic and either one or two diastolic components. In some patients, however, only a systolic component is audible. Friction rubs may be confused with the to-and-fro murmurs of combined aortic stenosis and regurgitation. Pleural-pericardial friction rubs are caused by the inflamed pleura against the parietal pericardium and are usually heard only during inspiration.

Acute Mediastinal Emphysema. This condition produces loud, bizarre, crunching sounds (again not murmurs) over the precordium, mainly during systole, that are audible most prominently near the apex and sometimes only with the patient in the left lateral recumbent position.[70] *Diaphragmatic flutter* produces regular sounds that are independent of the pulse and are audible over the entire thorax, even in the right axilla, far removed from the heart.[70]

Cardiorespiratory murmurs are systolic (rarely continuous) murmurs heard on inspiration but not when the breath is held or during expiration, and they may result from the movement of air in the bronchial tree during systole and inspiration.[93]

DYNAMIC AUSCULTATION

This is the technique of altering circulatory dynamics by means of respiration and a variety of physiological and pharmacological maneuvers and determining their effects on heart sounds and murmurs.[96–99] As outlined in Figures 2–21, 2–22, 2–26, 2–27, and 3–8, p. 46, and Tables 2–7 and 2–8, an appreciation of the effects of these interventions can be of great value in the interpretation of a variety of auscultatory findings. The interventions most commonly employed in dynamic auscultation include respiration, postural changes, the Valsalva maneuver, premature ventricular contractions, isometric exercise, and one of the vasoactive agents—amyl nitrite, methoxamine, or phenylephrine.

RESPIRATION

SPLITTING OF S_2 (see also pp. 47 and 48). The splitting of S_2 is best audible along the left sternal border and can usually be appreciated when A_2 and P_2 are separated by more than 0.02 sec. During inspiration A_2 ordinarily becomes softer in part because of the increased volume of lung that becomes interposed between the heart and chest wall; P_2 becomes louder because of increased flow into the pulmonary artery. A_2 normally occurs less than 0.02 sec after the pressure in the left ventricle falls below that in the aorta, whereas P_2 occurs 0.03 to 0.09 sec after the decline of pressure in the right ventricle below that in the central pulmonary artery; these intervals have been termed the "hang-out" intervals[100] and their durations are inversely proportional to the impedance to blood flow in the aortic and pulmonic circuits. The higher capacitance and lower resistance of the systemic compared to the pulmonary circulation result in a longer hang-out interval in the pulmonary artery than in the aorta and this difference contributes to the normal delay in P_2 compared to A_2 and therefore to the splitting of S_2. As the impedance to pulmonary flow increases with progressive pulmonary hypertension, the hang-out interval in the pulmonary artery shortens, and there is a reduction in the width of splitting of S_2, so that in severe pulmonary hypertension S_2 may become fused. Several factors play a role in the normal widening of the separation between A_2 and P_2 during inspiration.

During inspiration, venous return to the right side of the heart is augmented, resulting in an increased right ventricular stroke volume and lengthening of the duration of right ventricular ejection. When the respiratory rate is normal, these changes are accompanied by a reduced return of blood to the left side of the heart and a lower left ventricular stroke volume and shorter ejection time. In part, the difference in the effects of respiration on the stroke volumes of the two ventricles is due to the delay in transmission of the augmented right ventricular stroke volume through the pulmonary vascular bed, so that it reaches the left ventricle three or four cardiac cycles later, i.e., during the following respiration.[101] The greater delay in P_2, which accounts for about three-fourths of the widening of the splitting,[72] results from the increased right ventricular stroke volume and ejection time and an inspiratory decline in pulmonary vascular impedance, with further prolongation of the hang-out interval. The pooling of blood in the lungs during inspiration, with decreased venous return to the left heart, is responsible for shortening of left ventricular systole; earlier occurrence of A_2 accounts for about one-fourth of the inspiratory augmentation of the width of splitting of S_2.

Splitting of S_2 with 0.03 sec between components is usually detected readily by auscultation, while intervals <0.02 sec are not. In normal adults, A_2 and P_2 are separated by 0.04 to 0.05 sec during inspiration, with a single S_2 heard during expiration (split ≤ 0.02 sec). Occasionally there may be residual audible splitting in expiration (0.03 to 0.04 sec) in the supine position, but in normal adults auditory expiratory splitting disappears in the sitting or standing position. Expiratory splitting heard in both the supine and upright positions is uncommon in normal subjects of any age. Expiratory splitting of ≥ 0.03 sec, with an increase of ≤ 0.015 sec in the width of splitting, is perceived to be "fixed" splitting.

There are four types of abnormal splitting of S_2: (1) Absent splitting (single S_2), (2) splitting that is persistent during expiration, (3) fixed splitting, and (4) paradoxical splitting. A "branching logic tree" for analyzing the splitting of S_2 is given in Figure 2–23. Further discussion of this subject can be found beginning on p. 46.

S_3, S_4, AND EJECTION SOUNDS. When third and fourth sounds originate from the right ventricle, they are characteristically diminished during expiration and augmented during inspiration, whereas they exhibit the opposite response when they originate from the left side of the heart. Like other left-sided events, the opening snap of the mitral valve may become softer during inspiration and louder during expiration owing to respiratory alterations in venous return, whereas the opening snap of the tricuspid valve behaves in the opposite fashion. Inspiration also diminishes the intensity of valvular pulmonic ejection sounds, since the elevation of right ventricular diastolic pressure causes partial presystolic opening of the pulmonic valve and therefore less upward motion of the valve during systole. On the other hand, respiration does not affect the intensity of nonvalvular pulmonic ejection sounds or of aortic ejection sounds.

MURMURS. Respiration exerts more pronounced and consistent alterations on murmurs originating from the right than from the left side of the heart. During inspiration, the

TABLE 2–7 PHYSIOLOGICAL AND PHARMACOLOGICAL MANEUVERS USEFUL IN DIFFERENTIAL DIAGNOSIS OF SIMILAR AUSCULTATORY FINDINGS

AUSCULTATORY PROBLEMS	HELPFUL MANEUVERS*
Systolic murmur of valvular aortic stenosis vs. hypertrophic subaortic stenosis	Sudden squatting, Valsalva maneuver
Systolic murmur of valvular aortic stenosis vs. mid- to late systolic mitral valve dysfunction	Sudden standing, amyl nitrite
Systolic murmur of valvular aortic stenosis vs. mitral regurgitation	Amyl nitrite, phenylephrine, variation in cycle length
Diastolic rumble of mitral stenosis vs. Austin Flint murmur	Amyl nitrite
Diastolic murmur of mitral stenosis vs. tricuspid stenosis	Respiration
Systolic murmur of mitral regurgitation vs. tricuspid regurgitation	Respiration
Supraclavicular bruit vs. aortic stenosis	Extension of shoulder, compression of subclavian artery
Ejection sound in pulmonic stenosis vs. aortic stenosis	Respiration
Small ventricular septal defect vs. pulmonic stenosis	Amyl nitrite, phenylephrine
Large ventricular septal defect with fixed vs. hyperkinetic pulmonary hypertension	Amyl nitrite
Systolic murmur of pulmonic stenosis vs. tetralogy of Fallot	Amyl nitrite
Continuous murmur of patent ductus arteriosus vs. cervical venous hum	Compression of neck veins
Fourth sound plus first sound vs. separation of two components of first heart sound	Respiration, sudden standing, lying with passive leg-raising
Second sound plus opening snap vs. wide separation of second heart sound components	Respiration, phenylephrine, sudden standing

* See Table 2–8 for typical response. (From Criscitiello, M. G.: Physiologic and pharmacologic aids in cardiac auscultation. *In* Fowler, N. O. [ed.]: Cardiac Diagnosis and Treatment, Hagerstown, MD, Harper and Row, 1980, p. 89.)

TABLE 2-8 RESPONSE OF MURMURS AND HEART SOUNDS TO PHYSIOLOGICAL AND PHARMACOLOGICAL INTERVENTIONS

CLINICAL DISORDER	INTERVENTION AND RESPONSE
SYSTOLIC MURMURS	
Aortic outflow obstruction	
Valvular aortic stenosis	Louder with passive leg-raising, with sudden squatting, with Valsalva release (after five to six beats), following a pause induced by a premature beat, or after amyl nitrite; fades during Valsalva strain and with isometric handgrip
Hypertrophic obstructive cardiomyopathy	Louder with standing, during Valsalva strain, or with amyl nitrite; fades with sudden squatting, recumbency, or isometric handgrip
Pulmonic stenosis	Midsystolic murmur increases with amyl nitrite except with marked right ventricular hypertrophy; also increases during first few beats after Valsalva release
Mitral regurgitation	
Rheumatic	Murmur louder with sudden squatting, isometric handgrip, or phenylephrine; softens with amyl nitrite
Mitral valve prolapse	Midsystolic click moves toward S_1 and late systolic murmur starts earlier with standing, Valsalva strain, and amyl nitrite; click may occur earlier on inspiration; murmur starts later and click moves toward S_2 during squatting, with recumbency, and often after pause induced by a premature beat
Papillary muscle dysfunction	Late systolic murmur generally softer after a pause induced by a premature beat; response to amyl nitrite variable, depending on acute or chronic nature of this disorder
Tricuspid regurgitation	Murmur increases during inspiration, with passive leg-raising, and with amyl nitrite
Ventricular septal defect	
Small defect with pulmonary hypertension	Fades with amyl nitrite; increases with isometric handgrip or phenylephrine
Large defect with hyperkinetic pulmonary hypertension	Louder with amyl nitrite; fades with phenylephrine
Large defect with severe pulmonary vascular disease	Little change with any of above interventions
Tetralogy of Fallot	Murmur softens with amyl nitrite
Supraclavicular bruit	Altered by compression of subclavian artery; may be eliminated by extension of ipsilateral shoulder
DIASTOLIC MURMURS	
Aortic regurgitation	
Blowing diastolic murmur	Increases with sudden squatting, isometric handgrip, or phenylephrine
Austin Flint murmur	Fades with amyl nitrite
Pulmonary regurgitation	
Congenital	Early or mid-diastolic rumble increases on inspiration and with amyl nitrite
Pulmonary hypertension	High-frequency blowing murmur not altered by above interventions
Mitral stenosis	Mid-diastolic and presystolic murmurs louder with exercise, left lateral position, coughing, isometric handgrip, or amyl nitrite; phenylephrine widens A_2-OS interval; inspiration produces sequence of A_2-P_2-OS
Tricuspid stenosis	Mid-diastolic and presystolic murmurs increase during inspiration, with passive leg-raising, and with amyl nitrite
CONTINUOUS MURMURS	
Patent ductus arteriosus	Diastolic phase amplified with isometric handgrip or phenylephrine; diastolic phase fades with amyl nitrite
Cervical venous hum	Obliterated by direct compression of jugular veins or by Valsalva strain
ADDED HEART SOUNDS	
Gallop rhythm	
Ventricular gallop (S_3) and atrial gallop (S_4)	Accentuated by lying flat with passive leg-raising; decreased by standing or during Valsalva; right-sided gallop sounds usually increase during inspiration; left-sided during expiration
Summation gallop	Separates into ventricular gallop (S_3) and atrial gallop (S_4) sounds when heart rate slowed by carotid sinus massage
Ejection sounds	Ejection sound in pulmonary stenosis fades and occurs closer to the first sound during inspiration

OS = opening snap of mitral value
From Criscitiello, M. G.: Physiologic and pharmacologic aids in cardiac auscultation. *In* Fowler, N. O. (ed.): Cardiac Diagnosis and Treatment. Hagerstown, MD, Harper and Row, 1980.

diastolic murmurs of tricuspid stenosis (Fig. 3–34, p. 59) and pulmonic regurgitation, the systolic murmurs of tricuspid regurgitation[102] (Carvallo's sign) and of mild or moderate pulmonic stenosis, the diastolic murmur of pulmonary regurgitation, and the presystolic murmur of Ebstein's anomaly may all be accentuated. During expiration, the increased venous return to the left side of the heart may result in mild accentuation of the diastolic murmur of mitral stenosis and the systolic murmurs of mitral regurgitation, ventricular septal defect, and valvular aortic stenosis. The inspiratory reduction in left ventricular size in patients with mitral valve prolapse increases the redundancy of the mitral valve and therefore the degree of valvular prolapse; consequently, the midsystolic click and the systolic murmurs occur earlier during systole and frequently become accentuated.[103] The effects of inspiration on auscultatory findings may be accentuated by the use of the Müller maneuver, i.e., forced inspiration against a closed glottis. Deep, maintained expiration tends to accentuate soft, early diastolic murmurs of aortic or pulmonic regurgitation.

POSTURAL CHANGES

Sudden assumption of the *lying* from the standing or sitting position or sudden passive elevation of both legs results in an increase in venous return, which augments first right ventricular and, several cardiac cycles later, left ventricular stroke volume. The principal auscultatory changes include widening of the splitting of S_2 in all phases of respiration and augmentations of right-sided S_3 and S_4 and, several cardiac cycles later, left-sided S_3 and S_4. The systolic murmurs of valvular pulmonic and aortic stenosis, the systolic murmurs of mitral and tricuspid regurgitation and ventricular septal defect, and most functional systolic murmurs are augmented. On the other hand, since left ventricular end-diastolic volume is increased, the systolic murmur of hypertrophic obstructive cardiomyopathy is diminished, and the midsystolic click and systolic murmur associated with mitral valve prolapse are delayed and sometimes attenuated (p. 1032) (Fig 3–8, p. 46).

Rapid standing or sitting up from a lying position or rapid standing from a squatting posture has the opposite effect; in patients in whom there is relatively wide splitting of S_2 during expiration—a finding that may be confused with fixed splitting—the width of the splitting is reduced, so that a normal pattern emerges during the respiratory cycle. No change in splitting occurs in patients with true fixed splitting. The decrease in venous return reduces stroke volume and innocent pulmonary flow murmurs as well as the murmurs of semilunar valve stenosis and of atrioventricular valve regurgitation. The auscultatory changes in hypertrophic cardiomyopathy and mitral valve prolapse are opposite to those on assumption of the lying posture described above.

SQUATTING (Fig. 2–27). A sudden change from standing to squatting increases venous return and systemic resistance simultaneously. Stroke volume and arterial pressure rise, and the latter may induce a transient reflex bradycardia. The auscultatory features include augmentation of S_3 and S_4 (from both ventricles) and as a consequence of an increase in stroke volume, the systolic murmurs of pulmonic and aortic stenosis and the diastolic murmurs of tricuspid and mitral stenosis become louder, with right-sided events preceding left-sided events. Squatting may make audible a previously inaudible murmur of aortic regurgitation and a pericardial knock. The elevation of arterial pressure increases blood flow through the right ventricular outflow tract of patients with tetralogy of Fallot and increases the volume of mitral regurgitation and of the left-to-right shunt through a ventricular septal defect, thereby increasing the intensity of the systolic murmur in these conditions. Also, the diastolic murmur of aortic regurgitation is augmented consequent to an increase in aortic reflux. The combination of elevated arterial pressure and increased venous return increases left ventricular size, which reduces the obstruction to outflow and therefore the intensity of the systolic murmur of hypertrophic obstructive cardiomyopathy[1]; the midsystolic click of mitral valve prolapse and the systolic murmur are delayed.

Assumption of the left lateral recumbent position accentuates the intensity of S_1, S_3, and S_4 originating from the left side of the heart; the opening snap and the murmurs associated with mitral stenosis and regurgitation; the midsystolic click and late systolic murmur of mitral valve prolapse; and the Austin Flint murmur associated with aortic regurgitation. *Sitting up and leaning forward* make the diastolic murmurs of aortic and pulmonic regurgitation more readily audible. Assuming the *prone* position and then rising onto hands and knees accentuates pericardial friction rubs.

THE VALSALVA MANEUVER (Fig. 2–26). This consists of a forced exhalation against a closed glottis or blowing into a manometer to maintain a level of 40 mm Hg for 10 sec. It may briefly reduce coronary blood flow and therefore should not be utilized in patients with acute myocardial ischemic syndromes. During the initial phase of the Valsalva maneuver, phase I, intrathoracic pressure rises, producing a transient increase in left ventricular output. During the straining phase, phase II, systemic venous return declines; filling of the right and then of the left side of the heart is reduced; and the stroke volume and mean arterial and pulse pressures fall and heart rate increases. As a consequence, S_3 and S_4 become attenuated and the A_2-P_2 interval normally narrows.[72] As stroke volume and arterial pressure fall, the systolic murmurs of aortic and pulmonic stenosis and of mitral and tricuspid regurgitation, and the diastolic murmurs of aortic and pulmonic regurgitation and of tricuspid and mitral stenosis all diminish. However, as left ventricular volume is reduced, the systolic murmur of hypertrophic obstructive cardiomyopathy becomes louder,[104,105] and the systolic click and murmur of mitral valve prolapse commence earlier. With the cessation of straining, phase III, there is an abrupt decline in arterial pressure, and the aortic and pulmonic components of S_2 normally become more widely separated.[72,106] During the first two cycles following release of the Valsalva maneuver, murmurs and filling sounds (S_3 and S_4) originating from the right side of the heart return to normal and may be transiently accentuated. Filling sounds and murmurs originating from the left side of the heart also return to pre-Valsalva levels after six to eight beats and then may be transiently augmented during phase IV, the so-called overshoot phase, in which systemic arterial pressure normally rises and reflex bradycardia occurs.

An abnormal "square-wave" response to the Valsalva maneuver (see Fig. 16–4, p. 456) occurs in patients with atrial septal defect, mitral stenosis, and heart failure of any etiology. With such a response, the aforementioned changes in hemodynamics and therefore in the auscultatory findings do *not* occur.

POSTPREMATURE VENTRICULAR CONTRACTIONS. When a premature contraction is followed by a significant pause, both an increase in ventricular filling and an augmentation of cardiac contractility occur. Consequently, during the postpremature beat, the systolic murmurs of aortic and pul-

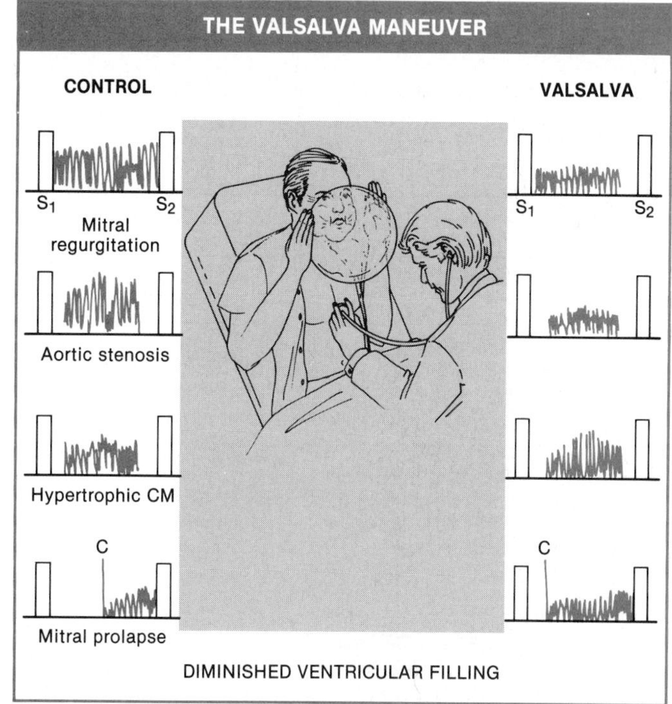

FIGURE 2–26. Changes in four left-sided systolic murmurs during the strain phase of the Valsalva maneuver. (From Grewe, K., Crawford, M. H., and O'Rourke, R. A.: Differentiation of cardiac murmurs by auscultation. Curr. Probl. Cardiol. *13*(10):669, 1988.)

monic stenosis and of hypertrophic obstructive cardiomyopathy are augmented,[50] while the systolic murmurs of rheumatic mitral regurgitation and of ventricular septal defect are not altered significantly (Fig. 3–18, p. 52). The diastolic murmur of aortic regurgitation becomes louder consequent to increased right ventricular filling and an elevated arterial pressure. The increase in left ventricular size delays the systolic click and the systolic murmur of mitral valve prolapse. Similar auscultatory changes follow prolonged diastolic pauses in atrial fibrillation and sinus arrhythmia.

ISOMETRIC EXERCISE. This can be carried out simply and reproducibly using a calibrated handgrip device or tennis ball. (It is useful to carry out isometric exercise bilaterally simultaneously.) Isometric exercise should be avoided in patients with ventricular arrhythmias and myocardial ischemia, both of which can be intensified by this activity. Handgrip should be sustained for 20 to 30 seconds, but a Valsalva maneuver during the handgrip must be avoided. Isometric exercise results in transient but significant increases in systemic vascular resistance, arterial pressure, heart rate, cardiac output, left ventricular filling pressure, and heart size. As a consequence, (1) S_3 and S_4 originating from the left side of the heart become accentuated, (2) the systolic murmur of aortic stenosis is diminished as a result of reduction of the pressure gradient across the aortic valve,[107,108] (3) the diastolic murmur of aortic regurgitation and the systolic murmurs of rheumatic mitral regurgitation and ventricular septal defect increase, (4) the diastolic murmur of mitral stenosis becomes louder consequent to the increase in cardiac output, and (5) the systolic murmur of hypertrophic obstructive cardiomyopathy diminishes and the systolic click and murmur secondary to mitral valve prolapse is delayed because of the increased left ventricular volume.

PHARMACOLOGICAL AGENTS (Fig. 2–27)

Inhalation of *amyl nitrite* is carried out by placing an ampule in gauze near the supine patient's nose and then crushing the ampule. The patient is asked to take three or four deep breaths over 10 to 15 seconds, after which the amyl nitrite is removed. It produces marked vasodilatation, resulting in the first 30 seconds in a reduction of systemic arterial pressure, and 30 to 60 seconds later in a reflex tachycardia, followed in turn by a reflex *increase* in cardiac output, velocity of blood flow, and heart rate.[2,95–99] The major auscultatory changes occur in the first 30 seconds following inhalation. S_1 is augmented and A_2 is diminished. The opening snaps of the mitral and tricuspid valves become louder, and as arterial pressure falls, the A_2-opening snap interval shortens. An S_3 originating in either ventricle is augmented, owing to greater rapidity of ventricular filling, but since mitral regurgitation is reduced, the S_3 associated with this lesion is diminished. The systolic murmurs of valvular aortic stenosis, pulmonic stenosis, hypertrophic obstructive cardiomyopathy, tricuspid regurgitation, and functional systolic mumurs are all accentuated. The reduction of arterial pressure increases the right-to-left shunt and decreases the blood flow from the right ventricle to the pulmonary artery and diminishes the systolic ejection murmur in patients with tetralogy of Fallot. The increase in cardiac output augments the diastolic murmurs of mitral and tricuspid stenosis and of pulmonary regurgitation and the systolic murmur of tricuspid regurgitation. However, as a result of the fall in systemic arterial pressure, the systolic murmurs of mitral regurgitation and ventricular septal defect, the diastolic murmurs of aortic regurgitation (Fig. 3–31, p. 58), and the Austin Flint murmur as well as the continuous murmurs of patent ductus arteriosus and of systemic arteriovenous fistula are all diminished.[107] The reduction of cardiac size results in an earlier appearance of the midsystolic click and systolic murmur of mitral valve prolapse; the intensity of the systolic murmur exhibits a variable response.

The response to amyl nitrite is useful in distinguishing (1) the systolic murmur of aortic stenosis (which is augmented) from that of mitral regurgitation (which is diminished),[109] (2) the systolic murmur of tricuspid regurgitation (augmented) from that of mitral regurgitation (diminished), (3) the systolic murmur of isolated pulmonic stenosis (augmented) from that of tetralogy of Fallot (diminished), (4) the systolic murmur of isolated pulmonic stenosis (increased) from that of ventricular septal defect (diminished), (5) the diastolic rumbling murmur of mitral stenosis (augmented) from the Austin Flint murmur of aortic regurgitation (diminished), and (6) the early blowing

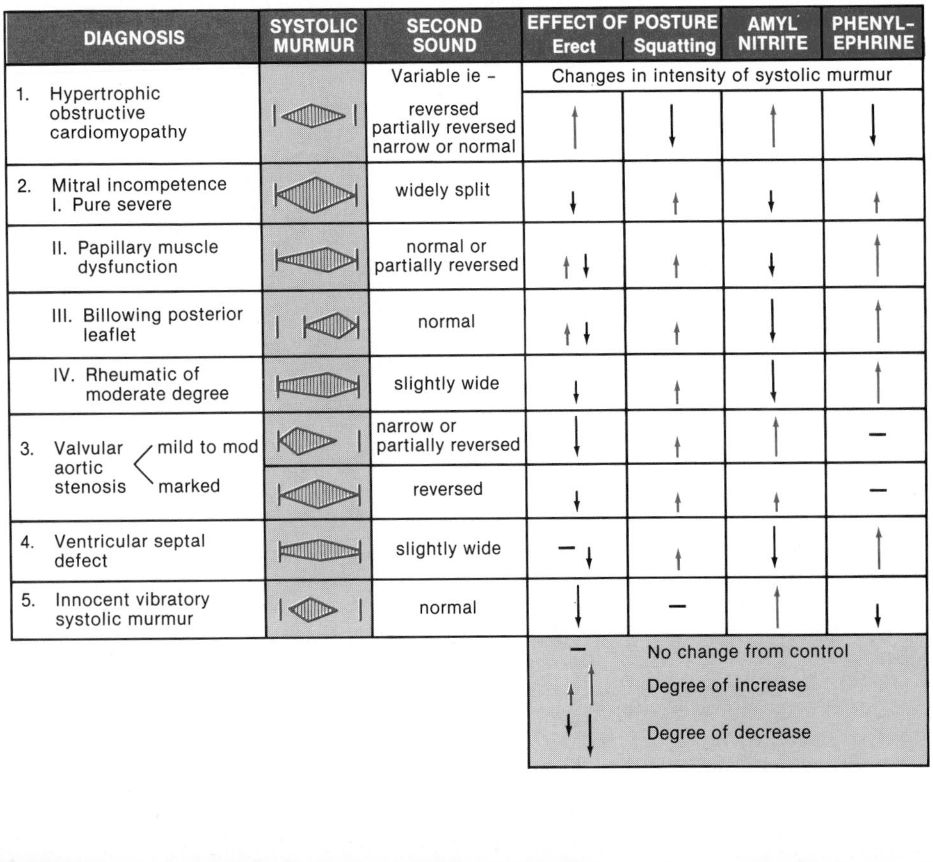

DIAGNOSIS	SYSTOLIC MURMUR	SECOND SOUND	EFFECT OF POSTURE Erect	EFFECT OF POSTURE Squatting	AMYL NITRITE	PHENYLEPHRINE
			Changes in intensity of systolic murmur			
1. Hypertrophic obstructive cardiomyopathy		Variable ie – reversed partially reversed narrow or normal	↑	↓	↑	↓
2. Mitral incompetence I. Pure severe		widely split	↓	↑	↓	↑
II. Papillary muscle dysfunction		normal or partially reversed	↑ ↓	↑	↓	↑
III. Billowing posterior leaflet		normal	↑ ↓	↑	↓	↑
IV. Rheumatic of moderate degree		slightly wide	↓	↑	↓	↑
3. Valvular aortic stenosis — mild to mod		narrow or partially reversed	↓	↑	↑	—
3. Valvular aortic stenosis — marked		reversed	↓	↑	↑	—
4. Ventricular septal defect		slightly wide	— ↓	↑	↓	↑
5. Innocent vibratory systolic murmur		normal	↓	—	↑	↓

— No change from control
↑ Degree of increase
↓ Degree of decrease

FIGURE 2–27. Diagrammatic representation of the character of the systolic murmur and of the second heart sound in five conditions. The effects of posture, amyl nitrite inhalation, and phenylephrine injection on the intensity of the murmur are shown. (From Barlow, J. B.: Perspectives on the Mitral Valve. Philadelphia, F. A. Davis, 1987, p. 138.)

diastolic murmur of pulmonic regurgitation (augmented) from that of aortic regurgitation (diminished).

Methoxamine and *phenylephrine* increase systemic arterial pressure and exert an effect opposite to amyl nitrite. In general, methoxamine, 3 to 5 mg intravenously, elevates arterial pressure by 20 to 40 mm Hg for 10 to 20 minutes, but phenylephrine is preferred because of its shorter duration of action; 0.3 to 0.5 mg of phenylephrine administered intravenously elevates systolic pressure by approximately 30 mm Hg for only 3 to 5 minutes. Both drugs cause a reflex bradycardia and decreased contractility and cardiac output. They should not be used in the presence of congestive heart failure and essential hypertension.

After administration the intensity of S_1 and A_2 is usually reduced, and the A_2-mitral opening snap interval becomes prolonged. The responses of S_3 and S_4 are variable. As a result of the increased arterial pressure, the diastolic murmur of aortic regurgitation; the systolic murmurs of mitral regurgitation (Fig. 3–29, p. 57), ventricular septal defect, and tetralogy of Fallot; and the continuous murmurs of patent ductus arteriosus and systemic arteriovenous fistula all become louder.[107] On the other hand, as a consequence of the increase in left ventricular size, the systolic murmur of hypertrophic obstructive cardiomyopathy becomes softer, and the click and murmur of mitral valve prolapse syndrome are delayed. The reduction in cardiac output diminishes the systolic murmur of valvular aortic stenosis, functional systolic murmurs, and the diastolic murmur of mitral stenosis. On the other hand, the rumbling diastolic murmurs of mitral regurgitation and the Austin Flint murmur diminish.

REFERENCES

THE GENERAL PHYSICAL EXAMINATION

1. Abrams, J.: Essentials of Cardiac Physical Diagnosis. Philadelphia, Lea and Febiger, 1987.
2. Perloff, J. K.: Physical Examination of the Heart and Circulation. 2nd ed. Philadelphia, W. B. Saunders Company, 1990.
3. Sapira, J. D.: The Art and Science of Bedside Diagnosis. Baltimore, Urban & Schwartzenberg, 1990.
4. Greenwood, R. D., Rosenthal, A., Parisi, L., et al.: Extracardiac abnormalities in infants with congenital heart disease. Pediatrics 55:485, 1975.
5. Brady, P. M., Zive, M. A., Goldberg, R. J., et al.: A new wrinkle to the earlobe crease. Arch. Intern. Med. *147*:65, 1987.
6. Kirkham, N., Murrels, T., Melcher, S. H., and Morrison, E. A.: Diagonal ear lobe creases and fatal cardiovascular disease: A necropsy study. Br. Heart J. *61*:361, 1989.
7. Renteria, V. G., Ferrans, V. J., and Roberts, W. C.: The heart in the Hurler syndrome: Gross, histologic and ultrastructural observations in five necropsy cases. Am. J. Cardiol. *38*:487, 1976.
8. Young, D., Shprintzen, R. J., and Goldberg, R. B.: Cardiac malformations in the velocardiofacial syndrome. Am. J. Cardiol. *46*:643, 1980.
9. Noonan, J. A.: Hypertelorism with Turner phenotype. Am. J. Dis. Child. *116*:373, 1968.
10. St. John Sutton, M. G., Tajik, A. J., Giuliani, E. R., et al.: Hypertrophic obstructive cardiomyopathy and lentiginosis: A little known neural ectodermal syndrome. Am. J. Cardiol. *47*:214, 1981.
11. Beuren, A. J., Schultze, C., Eberle, P., et al.: The syndrome of supravalvular aortic stenosis, peripheral pulmonary stenosis, mental retardation and similar facial appearance. Am. J. Cardiol., *13*:471, 1964.
12. Roberts, N. K., Perloff, J. K., Kark, R. A. P.: Cardiac conduction in the Kearns-Sayre syndrome (a neuromuscular disorder associated with progressive external ophthalmoplegia and pigmentary retinopathy). Am. J. Cardiol. *44*:1396, 1979.
13. Cogan, D. G.: Ophthalmic Manifestations of Systemic Vascular Disease. Philadelphia, W. B. Saunders Company, 1974.
14. Allen, S. J., and Naylor, D.: Pulsation of the eyeballs in tricuspid regurgitation. Can. Med. Assoc. J. *133*:119, 1985.
15. Byrd M. D.: Lateral systolic pulsation of the earlobe: A sign of tricuspid regurgitation. Am. J. Cardiol *54*:244, 1984.
16. Walker, G. L., and Stanfield, T. F.: Retinal changes associated with coarctation of the aorta. Trans. Am. Ophthalmol. Soc. *50*:407, 1952.
17. Criscitiello, M. G., Ronan, J. A., Besterman, E. M., and Schoenwetter, W.: Cardiovascular abnormalities in osteogenesis imperfecta. Circulation *31*:255, 1965.
18. Winder, A. F.: Relationship between corneal arcus and hyperlipidemia is clarified by studies in familial hypercholesterolaemia. Br. J. Ophthalmol. *67*:789, 1983.
19. Proudfit, W. L.: Skin signs of infective endocarditis. Am. Heart J. *106*:1451, 1983.
20. Walker, B. A., and Murdoch, J. L.: The wrist sign. Arch. Intern. Med. *126*:276, 1970.
21. Buckley, M. J., Mason, D. T., Ross, J., Jr., and Braunwald, E.: Reversed differential cyanosis with equal desaturation of the upper limbs. Syndrome of complete transposition of the great vessels with complete interruption of the aortic arch. Am. J. Cardiol. *15*:111, 1965.
22. Finger clubbing. Lancet *1*:1285, 1975.
23. Lanken, P. N., and Fishman, A. P.: Clubbing and hypertrophic osteoarthropathy. *In* Fishman, A. P. (ed.): Pulmonary Diseases and Disorders. New York, McGraw-Hill Book Co., 1980, pp. 84–91.
24. Yee, J., McAllister, C. K.: The utility of Osler's nodes in the diagnosis of infective endocarditis. Chest *92*:751, 1987.
25. Parrino, T. A.: The art and science of percussion. Hospital Practice, September 1987, pp 25–36.
26. Manga, P., Vythilingum, S., and Mitha, A. S.: Pulsatile hepatomegaly in constrictive pericarditis. Br. Heart J. *52*:465, 1984.
27. Coralli, R. J., and Crawley, I. S.: Hepatic pulsations in constrictive pericarditis. Am. J. Cardiol. *58*:370, 1986.
28. Ewy, G. A.: The abdominojugular test: Technique and hemodynamic correlates. Ann. Intern. Med. *109*:456, 1988.
29. Swartz, M. H.: Jugular venous pressure pulse: Its value in cardiac diagnosis. Primary Cardiol. *8*:197, 1982.
30. Constant, J.: Bedside Cardiology. 3rd ed. Boston, Little, Brown & Co., 1985.
31. Ducas, J., Magder, S., and McGregor, M.: Validity of the hepatojugular reflux as a clinical test for congestive heart failure. Am. J. Cardiol. *52*:1299–1303, 1983.
32. Linfors, E. W., Feussner, J. R., Blessing, C. L., et al.: Spurious hypertension in the obese patient. Effect of sphygmomanometer cuff size on prevalence of hypertension. Arch. Intern. Med. *144*:1482, 1984.
33. Manning, D. M., Kuchirka, C., and Kaminski, J.: Miscuffing: Inappropriate blood pressure cuff application. Circulation *68*:763, 1983.
34. Nelson, W. P., and Egbert, A. M.: How to measure blood pressure—accurately. Prim. Cardiol. *10*:14, 1984.
35. Kirkendall, W. M., Burton, A. C., Epstein, F. H., and Freis, E. D.: Recommendations for human blood pressure determination by sphygmomanometers. Circulation *36*:980, 1967.
36. Londe, S., and Klitzner, T. S.: Auscultatory blood pressure measurement —Effect of pressure on the head of the stethoscope. West. J. Med. *141*:193, 1984.
37. Mancia, G., Grassi, G., Pomidossi, G., et al.: Effects of blood-pressure measurement by the doctor on patient's blood pressure and heart rate. Lancet *2*:695, 1983.
38. Finnie, K. J. C., Watts, D. G., and Armstrong, P. W.: Biases in the measurement of arterial pressure. Crit. Care Med. *12*:965, 1984.
39. Gould, B. A., Hornung, R. S., Kieso, H. A., et al.: Is the blood pressure the same in both arms? Clin. Cardiol. *8*:423, 1985.
40. Sapira, J. D.: Quincke, de Musset, Duroziez, and Hill: Some aortic regurgitations. South. Med. J. *74*:459, 1981.
41. Abrams, J.: The arterial pulse. Prim. Cardiol. *8*:138, 1982.
42. Schlant, R. C., and Feiner, J. M.: The arterial pulse—clinical manifestations. Curr. Probl. Cardiol. Vol. 1, No. 5, 1976, 50 pp.
43. Perloff, J. K.: The physiologic mechanisms of cardiac and vascular physical signs. J. Am. Coll. Cardiol. *1*:184, 1983.
44. Smith, D., and Craige, E.: Mechanism of the dicrotic pulse. Br. Heart J. *56*:531, 1986.
45. Elkins, R. C., Morrow, A. G., Vasko, J. S., and Braunwald, E.: The effects of mitral regurgitation on the pattern of instantaneous aortic blood flow. Clinical and experimental observations. Circulation *36*:45, 1967.
46. Rowe, G. G., Afonso, S., Castillo, C. A., and McKenna, D. H.: The mechanism of the production of Duroziez's murmur. N. Engl. J. Med. *272*:1207, 1965.
47. Fleming, P. R.: The mechanism of the pulsus bisferiens. Br. Heart J. *19*:519, 1957.
48. Braunwald, E., Lambrew, C. T., Rockoff, S. D., et al.: Idiopathic hypertrophic subaortic stenosis. I. A description of the disease based upon an analysis of 64 patients. Circulation *30*(Suppl. 4):3, 1964.
49. Bartall, M., Auber, S., Desser, K. B., and Benchimol, A.: Normalization of the external carotid pulse tracing of hypertrophic subaortic stenosis during Müller's maneuver. Chest *74*:77, 1978.
50. Brockenbrough, E. C., Braunwald, E., and Morrow, A. G.: A hemodynamic technic for the detection of hypertrophic subaortic stenosis. Circulation *23*:189, 1961.
51. Rebuck, A. S., and Pengelly, L. D.: Development of pulsus paradoxus in the presence of airways obstruction. N. Engl. J. Med. *288*:66, 1973.
52. Massumi, R. A., Mason, D. T., Zakauddin, V., et al.: Reversed pulsus paradoxus. N. Engl. J. Med. *289*:1272, 1973.
53. Kurtz, K. J.: Dynamic vascular auscultation. Am. J. Med. *76*:1066, 1984.
54. Linhart, J.: Bedside examination of peripheral vascular disease. Eur. Heart J. *4*:137, 1983.

EXAMINATION OF THE HEART

55. Davies, H.: Chest deformities in congenital heart disease. Br. J. Dis. Chest *53*:151, 1959.
56. Perloff, J. K.: Diagnostic inferences drawn from observation and palpation of the precordium with special reference to congenital heart disease. Adv. Cardiopulm. Dis. *4*:13, 1969.
57. Beiser, G. D., Epstein, S. E., Stampfer, M., et al.: Impairment of cardiac function in patients with pectus excavatum. N. Engl. J. Med. *287*:267, 1972.
58. Ansari, A.: The "straight back" syndrome. Clin. Cardiol. *8*:290, 1985.
59. Abrams, J.: Precordial palpation. *In* Horwitz, L. D., and Groves, B. M. (eds): Signs and Symptoms in Cardiology. Philadelphia, J. B. Lippincott, 1985, pp. 156–177.

60. O'Neill, T. W., Smith, M., Barry, M., and Graham, I. M.: Diagnostic value of the apex beat. Lancet *1*(8635):410, 1989.
61. Eilen, S. D., Crawford, M. H., and O'Rourke, R. A.: Accuracy of precordial palpation for detecting increased left ventricular volume. Ann. Intern. Med. *99*:628, 1983.
62. Bancroft, W. H., Jr., Eddleman, E. E., Jr., and Larkin, L. N.: Methods and physical characteristics of the kineto-cardiographic and apex cardiographic systems for recording low-frequency precordial motion. Am. Heart J. *73*:756, 1967.
63. Ranganathan, Juma, Z., and Sivaciyan, V.: The apical impulse in coronary heart disease. Clin. Cardiol. *8*:20, 1985.
64. Dressler, W.: Clinical Aids in Cardiac Diagnosis. New York, Grune and Stratton, 1970, 246 pp.
65. Counihan, T. B., Rappaport, M. B., and Sprague, H. B.: Physiologic and physical factors that govern the clinical appreciation of cardiac thrills. Circulation *4*:716, 1951.
66. Rappaport, M. B., and Sprague, H. B.: Physiologic and physical laws that govern auscultation, and their clinical application: The acoustic stethoscope and the electrical amplifying stethoscope and stethograph. Am. Heart J. *21*:257, 1941.
67. Stein, P. D.: A Physical and Physiological Basis for the Interpretation of Cardiac Auscultation. Mt. Kisco, N. Y., Futura Publishing Co., 1981, 288 pp.
68. Kindig, J. R., Beeson, T. P., Campbell, R. W., et al.: Acoustical performance of the stethoscope: A comparative analysis. Am. Heart J. *104*:269, 1982.
69. Leatham, A.: Auscultation of the Heart and Phonocardiography. Edinburgh, Churchill Livingstone, 1975, p. 181.
70. Levine, S. A., and Harvey, W. P.: Clinical Auscultation of the Heart. 2nd ed. Phildelphia, W. B. Saunders Company, 1959, 657 pp.
71. Luisada, A. A., and Portaluppi, F.: The Heart Sounds. New York, Praeger Publishers, 1982, 246 pp.
72. Aygen, M. M., and Braunwald, E.: The splitting of the second heart sound in normal subjects and in patients with congenital heart disease. Circulation *25*:328, 1962.
73. Abrams, J.: The first heart sound. Prim. Cardiol. *8*:15, 1982.
74. Shaver, J. A., Salerni, R., and Reddy, P. S.: Normal and abnormal heart sounds in cardiac diagnosis. Part I. Systolic sounds. Cur. Probl. Cardiol. *10*(3):1, 1985.
75. Reddy, P. S., Salerni, R., and Shaver, J. A.: Normal and abnormal heart sounds in cardiac diagnosis. Part II. Diastolic sounds. Cur. Probl. Cardiol. *10*(4):1, 1985.
76. Gershlick, A. H., Leech, G., Mills, P. G., and Leatham, A.: The loud first heart sound in left atrial myxoma. Br. Heart J. *52*:403, 1984.
77. Stein, P. D., and Sabbah, H.: Second heart sound: Mechanism and clinical utility of auscultatory changes. Am. J. Noninvas. Cardiol. *1*:68, 1987.
78. Robertson, W. S., and Tavel, M. E.: Mid-systolic sound associated with aortic insufficiency and bisferiens pulse. Chest *83*:141, 1983.
79. Van de Werf, F., Minten, J., Carmeliet, P., et al.: The genesis of the third and fourth heart sounds. A pressure-flow study in dogs. J. Clin. Invest. *73*:1400, 1984.
80. Van de Werf, F., Geboers, J., Kesteloot, H., et al.: The mechanism of disappearance of the physiologic third heart sound with age. Circulation *73*:877, 1986.
81. Van de Werf, F., Boel, A. N., Geboers, J., et al.: Diastolic properties of the left ventricle in normal adults and in patients with third heart sounds. Circulation *69*:1070, 1984.
82. Reddy, P. S.: The third heart sound. Int. J. Cardiol. *7*:213, 1985.
83. Abdulla, A. M., Frank, M. J., Erdin, R. A., Jr., and Canedo, M. I.: Clinical significance and hemodynamic correlates of the third heart sound gallop in aortic regurgitation: A guide to optimal timing of cardiac catheterization. Circulation *64*:463, 1981.
84. Wilken, M. K., Meyers, D. G., Laski, P. A., et al: Mechanism of disappearance of S_3 with maturation. Am. J. Cardiol. *64*:1394, 1989.
85. Ishmail, A. A., Wing, S., Ferguson, J., et al: Interobserver agreement by auscultation in the presence of a third heart sound in patients with congestive heart failure. Chest *91*:870, 1987.
86. Vancheri, F., and Gibson, D.: Relation of third and fourth heart sounds to blood velocity during left ventricular filling. Br. Heart J. *61*:144, 1989.
87. Jordon, M. D., Taylor, C. R., Nyhuis, A. W., and Tavel, M. E.: Audibility of the fourth heart sound: Relationship to presence of disease and examiner experience. Arch. Intern. Med. *147*:721, 1987.
88. Lee, D. C-S., Johnson, R. A., Bingham, J. B., et al.: Heart failure in outpatients: A randomized trial of digoxin versus placebo. N. Engl. J. Med. *306*:699, 1982.
89. Freeman, A. R., and Levine, S. A.: The clinical significance of the systolic murmur. A study of 1000 consecutive "noncardiac" cases. Ann. Intern. Med. *6*:1371, 1933.
90. Sheikh, M. U., Lee, W. R., Mills, R. J., and Dais, K.: Musical murmurs: Clinical implications, long-term prognosis, and echo-phonocardiographic features. Am. Heart J. *108*:377, 1984.
91. Fowler, N. O., and Gause, R.: The cervical venous hum. Am. Heart J. *67*:135, 1964.
92. Tabatznik, R., Randall, T. W., and Hersch, C.: The mammary souffle of pregnancy and lactation. Circulation *22*:1069, 1960.
93. Harvey, W. P.: Auscultatory findings in diseases of the pericardium. Am. J. Cardiol. *7*:15, 1961.
94. Dressler, W.: Effect of respiration on the pericardial friction rub. Am. J. Cardiol. *7*:130, 1961.

DYNAMIC AUSCULTATION

95. Tavel, M. E.: Clinical Phonocardiography and External Pulse Recording. Chicago, Year Book Medical Publishers, 1985.
96. Grewe, K., Crawford, M. H., and O'Rourke, R. A.: Differentiation of cardiac murmurs by dynamic auscultation. Curr. Probl. Cardiol. *13*:671, 1988.
97. Lembro, N. J., Dell'Italia, L. J., Crawford, M. H., and O'Rourke, R. A.: Bedside diagnosis of systolic murmurs. N. Engl. J. Med. *318*:1572, 1988.
98. Baragan, J., Fernandez, F., and Thiron, J. M.: Dynamic Auscultation and Phonocardiography. Tavel, M. E. and Tavel, M. E. (eds.). Maryland, Charles Press, 1979.
99. Rothman, A., and Goldberger, A. L.: Aids to cardiac auscultation. Ann. Intern. Med. *99*:346, 1983.
100. Shaver, J. A.: Clinical implications of the hangout interval. Int. J. Cardiol. *5*:391, 1984.
101. Goldblatt, A., Harrison, D. C., Glick, G., and Braunwald, E.: Studies on cardiac dimensions in intact, unanesthetized man. II. Effects of respiration. Circ. Res. *13*:455, 1963.
102. Cha, S. D., and Gooch, A. S.: Diagnosis of tricuspid regurgitation. Arch. Intern. Med. *143*:1763, 1983.
103. Barlow, J. B.: Perspectives on the Mitral Valve. Philadelphia, F. A. Davis, 1987.
104. Braunwald, E., Oldham, H. N., Jr., Ross, J., Jr., et al: The circulatory response of patients with idiopathic hypertrophic subaortic stenosis to nitroglycerin and to the Valsalva maneuver. Circulation *29*:422, 1964.
105. Nishimura, R. A., and Tajik, A. J.: The Valsalva maneuver and response revisited. Mayo Clin. Proc. *61*:211, 1986.
106. van der Hauwaert, L. G.: The effect of the Valsalva maneuver on the splitting of the second sound. Acta Cardiol. *19*:518, 1964.
107. Criscitiello, M.: Physiologic and pharmacologic aids in cardiac auscultation. *In* Fowler, N. O. (ed.): Cardiac Diagnosis and Treatment. 3rd ed. Hagerstown, Harper and Row, 1980, pp. 77–90.
108. McCraw, D. B., Siegel, W., Stonecipher, H. K., et al: Response of the heart murmur intensity to isometric (handgrip) exercise. Br. Heart J. *34*:605, 1972.
109. Barlow, J., and Shillingford, J.: The use of amyl nitrite in differentiating mitral and aortic systolic murmurs. Br. Heart J. *20*:162, 1958.

Heart Sounds and Murmurs: Physiological Mechanisms

by JOSEPH K. PERLOFF, M.D.

HISTORICAL CONSIDERATIONS

Immediate auscultation, performed by applying the ear directly to the chest, was an established diagnostic technique in ancient medicine, practiced by Hippocrates, circa 400 B.C.[1] However, there is no recorded account of precordial auscultation until William Harvey (1616) referred to the heartbeat as "two clacks of a water-bellows," and later wrote (1628) that" . . . with each motion of the heart when there is the delivery of a quantity of blood from the veins to the arteries . . . a pulse takes place and can be heard within the chest."[2] Not only was Robert Hooke familiar with heart sounds, but he also foresaw the value of clinical auscultation, stating in his Cutlerian Lectures published posthumously in 1705, "I have been able to hear very plainly the beating of a man's heart . . . "[3] The modern era of cardiac auscultation began in 1816 with René Théophile Hyacinthe Laënnec, who initiated what McKusick called "the Golden Century of Stethoscopy."[4,5] The development of graphic methods for the registration of heart sounds—phonocardiography—was a major step that set the stage for analyses of the timing of auscultatory events. The first phonocardiograms in anything approaching the modern sense were made by Willem Einthoven of Leyden in 1894 using Lippman's capillary electrometer, with which the first electrocardiogram had also been made.[6] Subsequent developments by Otto Frank in Munich, Carl J. Wiggers in Cleveland, and Orias and Braun-Menendez in Argentina anticipated Weiss' 1909 monograph, in which auscultatory signs were graphically displayed and the term "phonocardiogram" was first used.[5]

Simultaneous recordings of high-fidelity phonocardiograms with reference tracings initiated investigations of the physiological mechanisms of heart sounds and murmurs,[7] an area of inquiry fostered in the 1950's by Paul Wood and in the 1980's by Aubrey Leatham at the National Heart Hospital, London.[8,9] It is to Wood and Leatham that I owe my greatest debt for the background of this chapter. The electrocardiogram as a reference tracing was followed by simultaneous recordings of phonocardiograms with the carotid and jugular venous pulses, the apex cardiogram, intracardiac pressure pulses, intracardiac phonocardiograms, cineangiographic frames, and, most recently, echocardiograms.[10,11] These modalities have permitted considerable elucidation of the *mechanisms of auscultatory signs,* which is the central concern of this chapter. Chapter 2 deals with bedside elicitation (physical examination) of heart sounds and murmurs.

In 1825, William Stokes argued eloquently that the stethoscope was indispensable.[12] Is a defense still necessary? Apparently so, according to Ernest Craige, who recently asked (rhetorically perhaps) whether auscultation should be rehabilitated.[13] "Should it be reserved for the occupational therapy of a dwindling coterie of antiquarians or should it be promoted more vigorously as a viable part of our diagnostic armamentarium?" Auscultation *should* be rehabilitated, not as a symbolic gesture to a distinguished past, but "to decipher the auscultatory language of diseases of the heart, . . . an affair requiring labor and use and docility."[14]

THE HEART SOUNDS

(See also pp. 30 to 33)

Heart sounds are relatively brief, discrete auditory vibrations of varying intensity (loudness), frequency (pitch), and quality (timbre). The first heart sound identifies the onset of ventricular systole and the second heart sound identifies the onset of diastole. These two auscultatory events establish a framework within which other heart sounds and murmurs can be placed and timed.[1]

The basic heart sounds are the first, second, third, and fourth sounds (Fig. 3–1*A*). Each of these sounds can be normal or abnormal. Other heart sounds are, with few exceptions, abnormal, either intrinsically so or iatrogenically (e.g., prosthetic valve sounds, pacemaker sounds). A heart sound should first be assigned simple descriptive terms that identify where in the cardiac cycle it occurs. Accordingly, heart sounds within the framework established by the first and second sounds are designated as "early systolic, midsystolic, late systolic," and "early diastolic, mid-diastolic, late diastolic (presystolic)" (Fig. 3–1*B*).[1] The next step is to draw conclusions regarding what a sound so identified might represent. An *early systolic* sound might be an ejection sound (aortic or pulmonic) or an aortic prosthetic sound. Mid- and late systolic sounds are typified by the click(s) of mitral valve prolapse but occasionally are "remnants" of pericardial rubs. *Early diastolic* sounds are represented by opening snaps (usually mitral), early third heart sounds (constrictive pericarditis, less commonly mitral regurgitation), the opening of a mechanical mitral prosthesis, or the abrupt seating of a pedunculated mobile atrial myxoma (tumor "plop"). *Mid-diastolic* sounds are generally third heart sounds or occasionally summation sounds (synchronous occurrence of third and fourth heart sounds). *Late diastolic* or *presystolic* sounds are almost always fourth heart sounds, rarely pacemaker sounds.

THE FIRST HEART SOUND

The first heart sound consists of two major components (Fig. 3–1*C*). The initial component is most prominent at the cardiac apex when the apex is occupied by the left ventricle.[15] The second component, if present, is normally confined to the

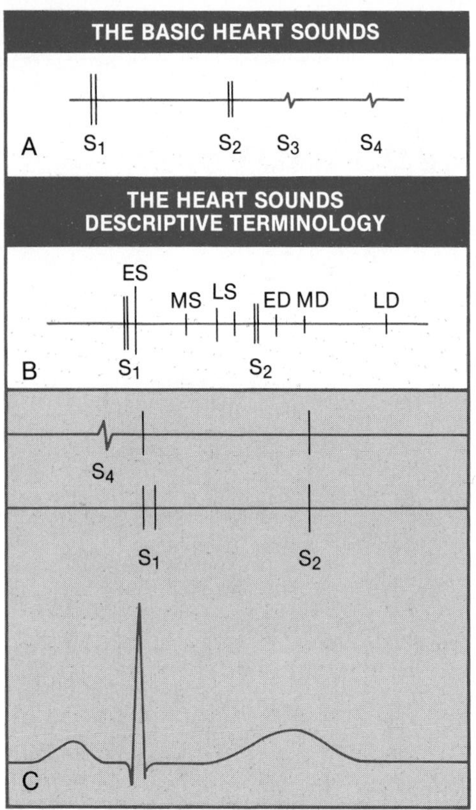

FIGURE 3–1. ***A,*** **The basic heart sounds consist of the first heart sound (S_1), the second heart sound (S_2), the third heart sound (S_3), and the fourth heart sound (S_4).** ***B,*** **Heart sounds within the auscultatory framework established by the first heart sound (S_1) and the second heart sound (S_2). The additional heart sounds are designated descriptively as early systolic (ES), midsystolic (MS), late systolic (LS); early diastolic (ED), mid-diastolic (MD), and late diastolic (LD), or presystolic.** ***C,*** **Upper tracing illustrates a low-frequency fourth heart sound (S_4) preceding a single first sound, and the lower tracing illustrates a split first heart sound (S_1), the two components of which are of the same quality.**

lower left sternal edge, and is less commonly heard at the apex and seldom at the base. The first major component is associated with closure of the mitral valve and coincides with abrupt arrest of leaflet motion when the cusps—especially the larger and more mobile anterior mitral cusp—reach their fully closed positions (maximal systolic excursion into the left atrium). While the origin of the second major component of the first heart sound has been debated, it is assigned to closure of the tricuspid valve on the basis of an analogous line of reasoning.[16] Opening of the semilunar valves and ejection of blood into the great arteries (aortic root or pulmonary trunk) usually produce no audible sound in the normal heart, although phonocardiograms sometimes record a low-amplitude sound following the mitral and tricuspid components and coinciding with the maximal opening excursion of the aortic cusps.[1] In complete right bundle branch block, the first heart sound is widely split owing to delay in the tricuspid component.[17] In complete left bundle branch block, the first heart sound is single because of delay in the mitral component.[18]

Because the two major audible components of the first heart sound are believed to originate in the closing movements of the atrioventricular valves, the quality of the two components is similar. When the first heart sound is split, its first component is the louder and is the only component normally heard at the base. The intensity of the first heart sound, particularly its first major audible component, depends chiefly on the position of the bellies of the mitral leaflets, particularly the anterior leaflet, at the time the left ventricle begins to contract and depends less on the rate of left ventricular contraction.[19] The first heart sound—especially its first component—is therefore loudest when the beginning of left ventricular systole finds the mitral leaflets maximally recessed into the left ventricular cavity as in the presence of a rapid heart rate, a short P-R interval[20] (Fig. 3–2), short cycle lengths in atrial fibrillation, or mitral stenosis with a mobile anterior leaflet. In Ebstein's anomaly of the tricuspid valve the first heart sound is widely split (delayed right ventricular activation) and loud (large mobile anterior tricuspid leaflet).[22]

EARLY SYSTOLIC SOUNDS

Aortic or pulmonic ejection sounds are the most common early systolic sounds.[21] The term "ejection sound" is preferred to the term "click." The latter designation is best reserved for the mid- to late systolic clicks of mitral origin (see later). The ejection sound coincides with the fully opened position of the relevant semilunar valve, as in congenital aortic valve stenosis (Fig. 3–3), bicuspid aortic valve, or dilated aortic root in the left side of the heart, or pulmonary valve stenosis (Fig. 3–4), or a dilated pulmonary trunk in the right side of the heart.[22,23] Ejection sounds are relatively high in frequency, and, depending on intensity, have a pitch similar to that of the two major components of the first heart sound. An ejection sound that originates in the aortic valve (congenital aortic stenosis or bicuspid aortic valve) indicates that the valve is mobile, because the ejection sound is caused by abrupt cephalad doming (Fig. 3–3).[23] Less certain is the origin of an ejection sound within a dilated arterial trunk that is guarded by a normal or near-normal semilunar valve. Origin of the sound is either valvular (opening movement of the leaflets resonating in the dilated arterial trunk) or in the wall of the dilated great artery per se. Aortic ejection sounds do not vary with respiration except those that originate in the large biventricular aorta of truncus arteriosus or Fallot's tetralogy with pulmonary atresia

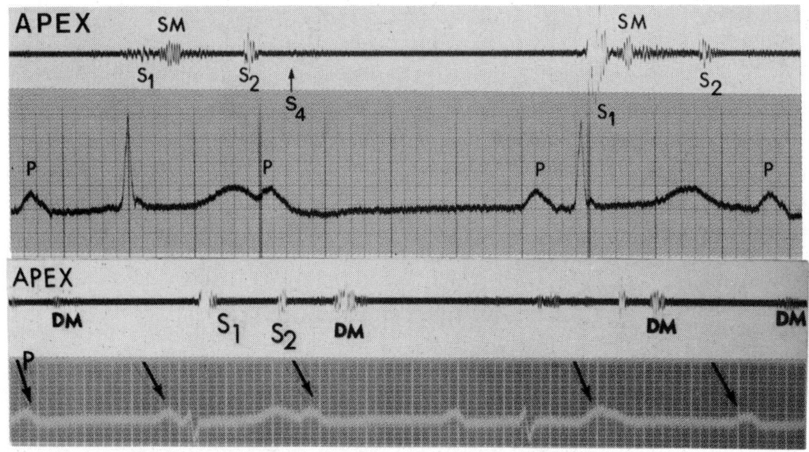

FIGURE 3–2. ***Upper tracing,*** **Phonocardiogram and electrocardiogram (lead 2) from a 12-year-old girl with congenital complete heart block. The first heart sound (S_1) varies from soft (long P-R interval) to loud (short P-R interval). There is a grade 2/6 vibratory midsystolic murmur (SM). A soft fourth heart sound (arrow) follows the second P wave.** ***Lower tracing,*** **Phonocardiogram and electrocardiogram from a 15-year-old boy with congenital complete heart block. Arrows point to independent P waves. The first heart sound (S_1) varies from loud to soft. The short diastolic murmurs (DM) are especially prominent when atrial contraction (P wave) coincides with the rapid filling phase (shortly after the T wave).**

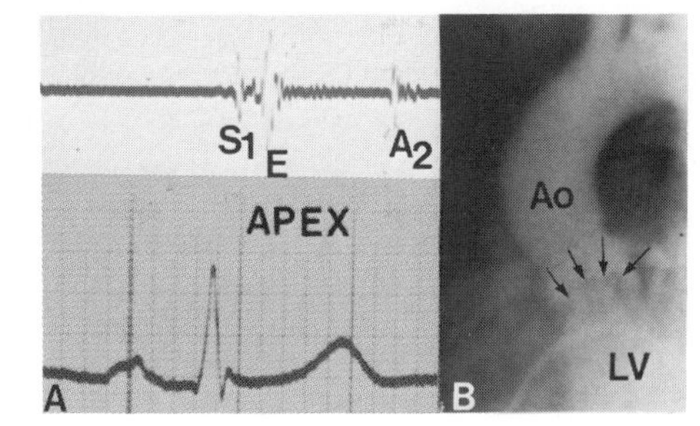

FIGURE 3-3. **Phonocardiogram over the left ventricular impulse in a patient with mild congenital aortic valve stenosis. The aortic ejection sound (E) is louder than the first heart sound (S_1). A_2 = aortic component of the second heart sound. *B,* Left ventriculogram (LV) in another patient with congenital aortic valve stenosis. The cephalad systolic doming of the stenotic valve (arrows) produces the ejection sound.**

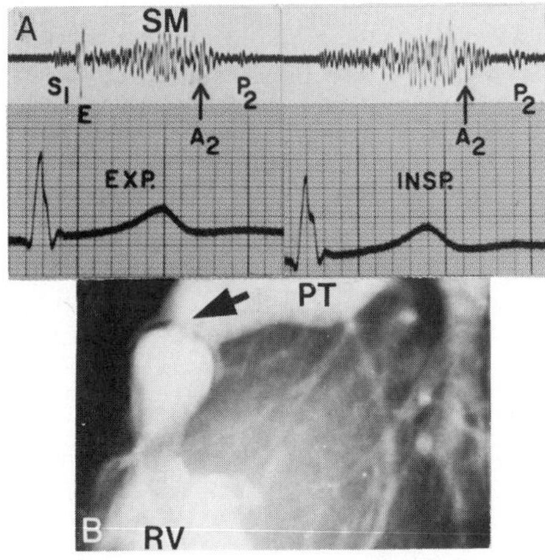

FIGURE 3-4. ***A,* Phonocardiogram in the second left intercostal space of a patient with congenital pulmonary valve stenosis. The ejection sound (E) is obvious during expiration (EXP) but disappears entirely during casual inspiration (INSP). The pulmonic component of the second heart sound (P_2) is delayed and soft. SM = systolic murmur; S_1 = first heart sound. *B,* Right ventriculogram (RV) in another patient with pulmonic valve stenosis. The cephalad systolic doming of the stenotic valve (arrow) produces the pulmonic ejection sound. There is poststenotic dilatation of the pulmonary trunk (PT).**

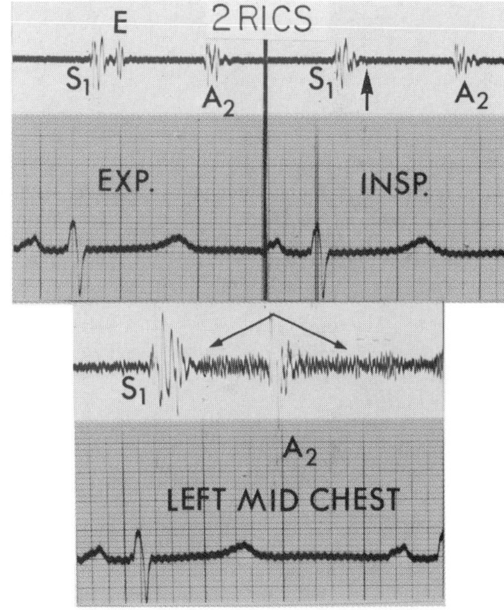

FIGURE 3-5. **Phonocardiograms from an 11-year-girl with Fallot's tetralogy, pulmonary atresia, and a right aortic arch. The upper tracing from the second right intercostal space (2RICS) shows an aortic ejection sound (E) that is prominent during expiration (EXP) but absent during inspiration (INSP). The lower tracing from the left midchest shows a continuous murmur of aortopulmonary collaterals. S_1 = first heart sound; A_2 = second heart sound.**

(Fig. 3-5).[22] The mechanism responsible for the respiratory variation in this setting is unclear.

PULMONIC EJECTION SOUNDS. These are associated with abrupt cephalad doming of a mobile stenotic pulmonic valve (Fig. 3-4) or dilatation of the pulmonary trunk guarded by a normal or near-normal semilunar valve. The mechanisms are analogous if not identical to those just described for the aortic ejection sound.[23] Pulmonic ejection sounds often selectively and distinctively decrease in intensity during normal inspiration (Fig. 3-4*A*) in contrast to aortic ejection sounds, which seldom vary with respiration except as already noted. The mechanism responsible for respiratory variation of a pulmonic ejection sound is most convincing in the setting of typical pulmonary valve stenosis.[24] An inspiratory increase in right atrial contractile force is transmitted into the right ventricle and to the ventricular surface of the mobile stenotic valve, moving its cusps upward *before* the onset of ventricular contraction. The result is diminished cephalad excursion of the valve during inspiration, accounting for the inspiratory decrease in intensity of the pulmonic ejection sound. This mechanism would not apply to the respiratory variation of a pulmonic ejection sound associated with a dilated hypertensive pulmonary trunk (Fig. 3-6).[22]

Early systolic sounds accompany ball-in-cage mechanical prostheses in the aortic location (especially the Starr-Edwards valve), less so with a tilting disc valve (such as the Björk-Shiley valve). Early systolic sounds do not accompany bioprosthetic valves (tissue valves) in either the aortic or pulmonic location.

MID- TO LATE SYSTOLIC SOUNDS

Far and away the most common mid- to late systolic sound(s) are associated with mitral valve prolapse[25] (p. 1029). The term "click" is appropriate because these mid- to late systolic sounds are of relatively high frequency and often, but not invariably, "clicking." Mid- to late systolic clicks associated with mitral valve prolapse coincide with the maximal systolic excursion of the leaflet(s) into the left atrium and are ascribed to sudden tensing of the redundant leaflet(s) and elongated chordae tendineae (Fig. 3-7). Variability epitomizes mitral systolic clicks, which from time to time may be replaced by a cluster of discrete late systolic "crackles." Physical or pharmacological interventions that *reduce* left ventricular volume, such as the Valsalva maneuver or a change in position from squatting to standing (Fig. 3-8), cause the click(s) to occur earlier in systole.[25-27] Conversely, physical or

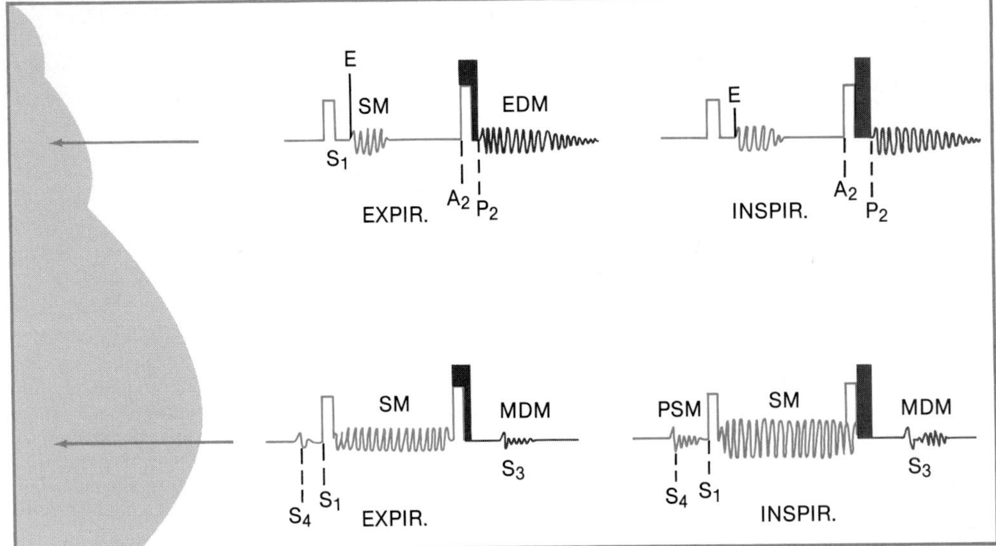

FIGURE 3–6. Composite of the principal auscultatory and phonocardiographic manifestations of pulmonary hypertension. (From Perloff, J. K.: Auscultatory and phonocardiographic manifestations of pulmonary hypertension. Prog. Cardiovasc. Dis. *9*:303, 1967.)

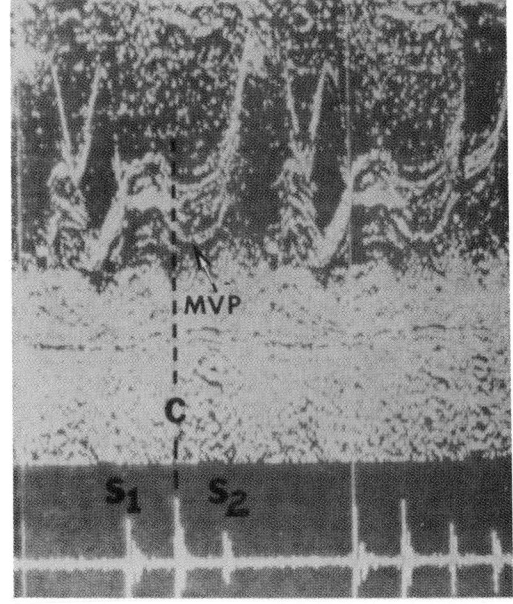

FIGURE 3–7. One of the earliest echophonocardiographic recordings that timed the systolic click (C) of mitral valve prolapse (MVP). The click coincides with the onset of superior systolic displacement of the anterior mitral leaflet as illustrated on the simultaneously recorded M-mode echocardiogram. (From Devereux, R., Perloff, J. K., Reichek, N., and Josephson, M.: Mitral valve prolapse. Circulation *54*:3, 1976, by permission of the American Heart Association, Inc.)

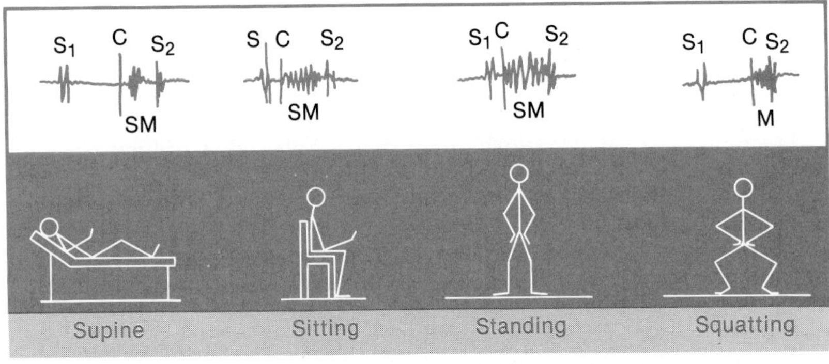

FIGURE 3–8. Postural maneuvers that affect the click(s) and late systolic murmur (SM) of mitral valve prolapse. A change from supine to sitting or standing causes the click to become earlier and the murmur longer although softer. Conversely, squatting delays the timing of the click, and the murmur gets shorter but louder. (From Devereux, R., Perloff, J. K., Reichek, N., and Josephson, M.: Mitral valve prolapse. Circulation *54*:3, 1976, by permission of the American Heart Association, Inc.)

pharmacological interventions that *increase* left ventricular volume such as squatting (Fig. 3–8) or sustained handgrip delay the timing of the click(s). Multiple clicks are thought to arise from asynchronous tensing of different portions of redundant mitral leaflets, especially the triscalloped posterior leaflet.

On rare occasions, a pericardial friction rub leaves in its wake mid- to late systolic sounds—remnants of rubs—that persist for varying periods of time after disappearance of the systolic phase of the rub. Carl Potain, in 1894, described "small, short clicking sounds, well localized and such that one can scarcely attribute them to anything except the tensing of a pericardial adhesion."[28]

THE SECOND HEART SOUND

(See also Figs. 2–21, p. 30; 2–22, p. 32; and 2–23, p. 32, and Table 2–2, p. 31)

Respiratory splitting of the second heart sound was described by Potain in 1866,[29] and Leatham called the second heart sound the "key to auscultation of the heart."[30] The first

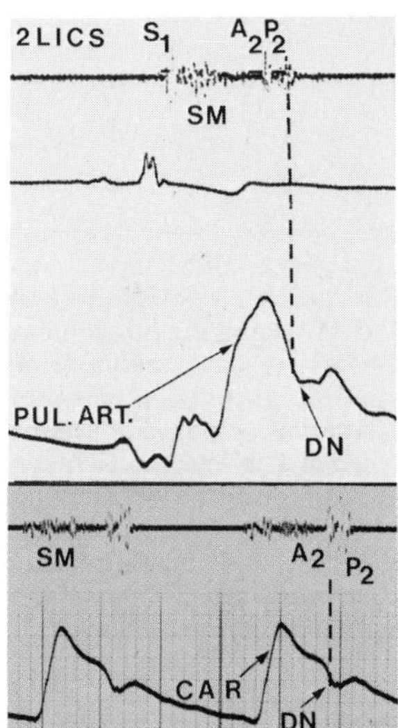

FIGURE 3-9. **Tracings from a 28-year-old woman with an uncomplicated ostium secundum atrial septal defect. In the second left interspace (2LICS) the pulmonic component (P_2) of a widely split second heart sound is synchronous with the dicrotic notch (DN) of the pulmonary arterial pressure pulse. (S_1 = first heart sound; SM = systolic murmur.) In the lower tracing, the aortic component (A_2) of the widely split second heart sound is synchronous with the dicrotic notch of the carotid arterial pulse (CAR).**

component of the second heart sound is designated "aortic" and the second "pulmonic."[31,32] Each component coincides with the dicrotic incisura of its great arterial pressure pulse (Fig. 3-9).[15] Inspiratory splitting of the second heart sound is due chiefly to a delay in the pulmonic component, less to earlier timing of the aortic component.[33] During inspiration, the pulmonary arterial dicrotic incisura moves away from the descending limb of the right ventricular pressure pulse because of an inspiratory increase in capacitance of the pulmonary vascular bed, delaying the pulmonic component of the second heart sound.[34] Expiration has the opposite effect. The earlier inspiratory timing of the aortic component of the second heart sound is attributed to a transient reduction in left ventricular volume coupled with unchanged impedance (capacitance) in the systemic vascular bed. Accordingly, normal respiratory variations in the timing of the second heart sound are ascribed principally to the variations in impedance characteristics (capacitance) of the pulmonary vascular bed, not to an inspiratory increase in right ventricular volume as originally believed. When an increase in capacitance of the pulmonary bed is lost because of a rise in pulmonary vascular resistance, inspiratory splitting of the second heart sound narrows and, if present at all, reflects an increase in right ventricular ejection time and/or earlier timing of the aortic component.

The frequency compositions of the aortic and pulmonic components of the second heart sound are similar, but their normal amplitudes differ appreciably, reflecting the differences in systemic (aortic) and pulmonic arterial closing pressures. Accordingly, splitting of the second heart sound is most readily identified in the second left intercostal space, because the softer pulmonic component is normally confined to that site, whereas the louder aortic component is heard at the base, sternal edge, and apex.[1]

ABNORMAL SPLITTING OF THE SECOND HEART SOUND. Three general categories are recognized: (1) persistently single, (2) persistently split (fixed or nonfixed), and 3) paradoxically split (reversed). When the second heart sound remains single throughout the respiratory cycle, either one component is absent or the two components remain synchronous. The most common cause of the single second heart sound is inaudibility of the *pulmonic* component in older adults with increased anteroposterior chest dimensions. In the setting of congenital heart disease, a single second heart sound due to absence of the pulmonic component is a feature of pulmonary atresia (Fig. 3-5), severe pulmonary valve stenosis, or complete transposition of the great arteries (pulmonic component inaudible because of the posterior position of the pulmonary trunk).[22] Conversely, a single second heart sound due to inaudibility of the *aortic* component occurs when the aortic valve is immobile (severe calcific aortic stenosis) or atretic (aortic atresia). A single second heart sound due to synchronous occurrence of its two components is a feature of Eisenmenger's complex, in which the aortic and pulmonary arterial dicrotic incisurae are virtually identical in timing.[22]

Both components of the second heart sound are sometimes inaudible at *all* precordial sites. This is likely to be so in older adults in whom fibrocalcific changes limit mobility of the aortic valve and the pulmonic component is inaudible because of a large anteroposterior chest dimension (see above).

A single semilunar valve does not necessarily generate what is perceived on auscultation as a single second heart sound but instead this may be due to asynchronous closure of the quadricuspid valve of truncus arteriosus.[22] In systemic or pulmonary hypertension, a single loud second heart sound may be sufficiently prolonged and slurred (reduplicated) to encourage the mistaken impression of splitting.

Persistent Splitting of the Second Heart Sound. This term means that the two components remain audible (or recordable) during both inspiration and expiration. Persistent splitting may be due to a delay in the pulmonic component, as in simple complete right bundle branch block (Fig. 3-10*A*),[15] or to early timing of the aortic component as occasionally occurs in mitral regurgitation.[35] Normal inspiratory and expiratory directional changes in the interval of the split (greater with inspiration, less with expiration) indicate that the split is *persistent* but not *fixed* (Fig. 3-10*A*).

Fixed Splitting of the Second Heart Sound. This term means that the interval between the aortic and pulmonic components is not only wide and persistent but also remains unchanged during the respiratory cycle.[15] Fixed splitting is an auscultatory hallmark of uncomplicated ostium secundum atrial septal defect (Fig. 3-10*B*). The aortic and pulmonic components are widely separated during expiration and exhibit little or no change in the degree of splitting during inspiration or with the Valsalva maneuver. The *wide* splitting is caused by a delay in the pulmonic component because a marked increase in pulmonary vascular capacitance delays the interval between the descending limbs of the pulmonary arterial and right ventricular pressure pulses ("hangout"), and accordingly delays the pulmonic incisura and the pulmonic component of the second heart sound (Fig. 3-9). Because the capacitance (impedance) of the pulmonary bed is appreciably increased, there is little or no additional increase during inspiration and little or no inspiratory delay in the pulmonic component of the second sound. Phasic changes in systemic venous return during respiration in atrial septal defect are associated with reciprocal changes in the volume of the left-to-right shunt, minimizing respiratory variations in right ventricular filling. The net effect is wide fixed splitting of the two components of the second heart sound.

Paradoxical Splitting of the Second Heart Sound. This term refers to a reversed sequence of semilunar valve closure, the pulmonic component (P_2) preceding the aortic component (A_2).[15] Common causes of paradoxical splitting are complete left bundle branch block or a right ventricular pacemaker, both of which are associated with initial activation of the right side of the ventricular septum, resulting in delayed activation of the left ventricle because of transseptal (right-to-left) depolarization.[36] When the second heart sound splits paradoxically, its two components separate during *expiration* and become single (synchronous) during *inspiration*. Inspiratory synchrony is achieved as the two components fuse owing primarily to a delay in the pulmonic component and less to earlier timing of the aortic component.

Abnormal Loudness (Intensity) of the Two Components of the Second Heart Sound. Assessment requires comparison of both components when assessed simultaneously at the same

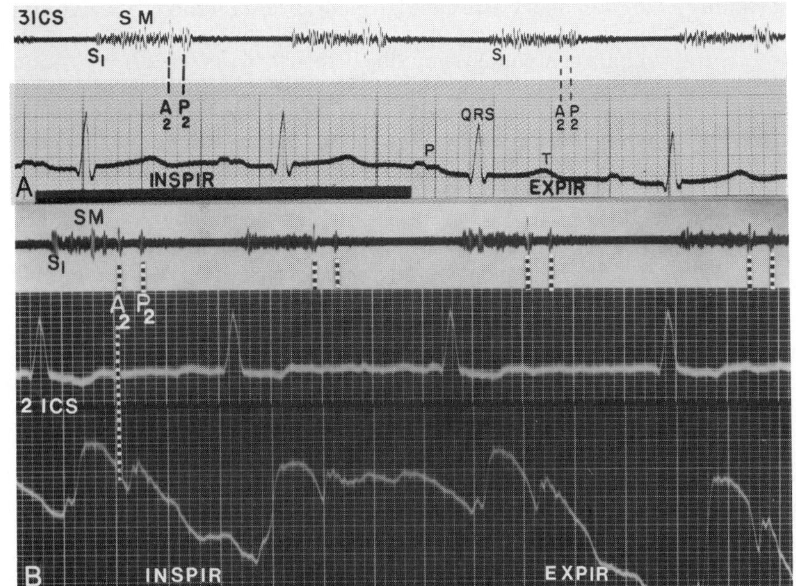

FIGURE 3–10. *A,* Phonocardiogram from the third left intercostal space (3ICS) and electrocardiogram of a patient with complete right bundle branch block. The aortic component (A_2) and the pulmonic component (P_2) of the second heart are persistently split. The interval increases during inspiration and decreases during expiration. (S_1 = first heart sound; SM = systolic murmur.) *B,* Phonocardiogram (second left intercostal space [2ICS]), electrocardiogram, and carotid pulse from a patient with an uncomplicated ostium secundum atrial septal defect. The aortic component (A_2) and pulmonic component (P_2) of the second heart sound are widely split, but the split remains fixed during inspiration and expiration.

site. The relative softness of the normal pulmonic component is responsible for its localization in the second left intercostal space (see earlier), whereas the relative loudness of the normal aortic component accounts for its audibility at all precordial sites.[1] An increase in intensity of the *aortic* component of the second heart sound commonly occurs in systemic hypertension. The aortic component also increases in loudness when the aorta is closer to the anterior chest wall due to aortic root dilatation or transposition of the great arteries, or when an anterior pulmonary trunk is small or absent, as in pulmonary atresia (Fig. 3–5).[22]

A loud *pulmonic* component of the second heart sound is a feature of pulmonary hypertension (Fig. 3–6).[37] The intensity is further amplified by dilatation of the hypertensive pulmonary trunk. Graham Steell, in describing the auscultatory signs of pulmonary hypertension, remarked that "Extreme accentuation of the pulmonary second sound is always present, the closure of the pulmonary semilunar valve being generally perceptible to the hand placed over the pulmonary area, as a sharp thud."[38] When very loud, the accentuated pulmonic component of the second sound is transmitted throughout the precordium from base to lower left sternal edge to apex (Fig. 3–11*A*).

An alternative mechanism responsible for an increase in the intensity of the pulmonic component of the second heart sound in patients with normal pulmonary arterial pressure was alluded to earlier. A moderate increase in intensity sometimes occurs when the pulmonary trunk is dilated, as in idiopathic dilatation or ostium secundum atrial septal defect,[22] or when there is a decrease in anteroposterior chest dimension (loss of thoracic kyphosis) that serves to place the pulmonary trunk closer to the anterior chest wall.[39]

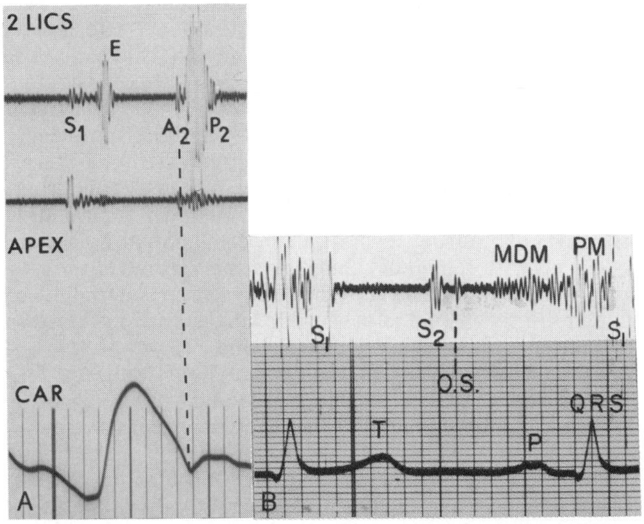

FIGURE 3–11. *A,* Tracings from a 32-year-old woman with an ostium secundum atrial septal defect, pulmonary hypertension, and a small right-to-left shunt. In the second left intercostal space (2LICS), the first heart sound is followed by a prominent pulmonic ejection sound (E). The second sound remains split. The pulmonic component (P_2) is very loud and is transmitted to the apex. (CAR = carotid pulse.) *B,* Phonocardiogram recorded in the left lateral decubitus position over the left ventricular impulse in a patient with pure rheumatic mitral stenosis. The first heart sound (S_1) is loud. The second heart sound (S_2) is followed by an opening snap (OS). There is a mid-diastolic murmur (MDM) and a prominent presystolic murmur (PM) that go up to the subsequent loud first heart sound.

EARLY DIASTOLIC SOUNDS

(See also Table 2–3, p. 23)

The best known early diastolic sound is the opening snap of rheumatic mitral stenosis (Fig. 3–11*B*). The term was introduced in 1908 by W. S. Thayer as the English equivalent to the "claquement d' ouverture" of Rouchès.[40] The diagnostic value of the presence, quality, loudness, and timing of the opening snap in the assessment of rheumatic mitral stenosis was clarified by Wood in his classic monograph *An Appreciation of Mitral Stenosis*.[41] An audible opening snap indicates that the mitral valve is mobile, at least that its longer anterior leaflet is.[42] The snap is generated when superior systolic bowing of the anterior mitral leaflet is rapidly reversed toward the left ventricle in early diastole by the high left atrial pressure. The mechanism of the opening snap is therefore a corollary to the loud first heart sound (Fig. 3–11*B*), which is generated by abrupt superior systolic displacement of an anterior mitral leaflet that was recessed into the left ventricle by high left atrial pressure until the onset of left ventricular isovolumetric contraction (see earlier). The designation "snap" is appropriate for the relatively high frequency of the sound. The timing of the opening snap (OS) relative to the aortic component of the second heart sound (A_2) has important physiological meaning in rheumatic mitral stenosis. A short A_2-OS interval generally reflects the high left atrial pressure of *severe* mitral stenosis. However, in older subjects with systolic hypertension, mitral stenosis of appreciable severity can occur with a relatively long A_2-OS interval because the elevated left ventricular systolic pressure takes longer to fall below the left atrial pressure. When atrial fibrillation occurs with mitral stenosis, the A_2-OS interval varies inversely with cycle length, because (all else being equal) the higher the left atrial pressure (short cycle length), the earlier the stenotic valve opens and vice versa.

Early diastolic sounds are not confined to the opening snap of rheumatic mitral stenosis. In 1842, Dominic Corrigan, in a presentation before the Pathological Society of Dublin, described a "very loud bruit de frappement" in a patient with chronic constrictive pericarditis.[43] In French, *frapper* means "to knock," implying that the "bruit de frappement" was what has come to be known as the pericardial "knock" of chronic constrictive pericarditis.[44] The knock has also been applied to an early diastolic sound in pure severe mitral regurgitation with reduced left ventricular compliance. Both Corrigan's "pericardial knock" and the "knock" of mitral regurgitation are rapid filling sounds that are early *and* loud because a high-pressure atrium decompresses rapidly across an unobstructed atrioventricular valve into a recipient ventricle whose compliance is impaired.

Early diastolic sounds are sometimes caused by atrial myxomas (see also p. 1454). The requirement for the generation of such a sound, called a tumor "plop," is a mobile myxoma attached to the atrial septum by a long stalk. The "plop" is believed to result from abrupt diastolic seating of the tumor within the right or left atrioventricular orifice.[45]

An early diastolic sound is generated by the opening movement of a mechanical prosthesis in the mitral location. The opening sound is especially prominent with a ball-in-cage prosthesis (Starr-Edwards), less prominent with a tilting-disc prosthesis (Björk-Shiley).

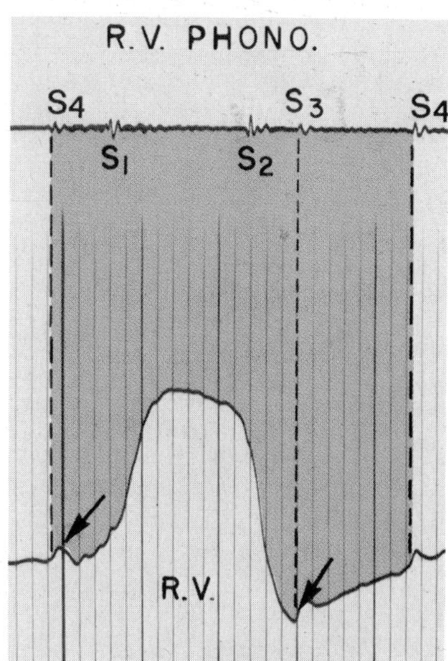

FIGURE 3–13. Right ventricular (RV) phonocardiogram with simultaneous RV pressure pulse in a normal subject. The third heart sound (S_3) coincides with the onset of a low-frequency diastolic wave generated by rapid filling (arrow). The fourth heart sound (S_4) coincides with the onset of a low-frequency wave generated by the atrial contribution to right ventricular filling (arrow).

MID-DIASTOLIC AND LATE DIASTOLIC (PRESYSTOLIC) SOUNDS

Mid-diastolic sounds are, for all practical purposes, either normal or abnormal third heart sounds, and most if not all late diastolic or presystolic sounds are fourth heart sounds (Fig. 3–1*A*). Each sound coincides with its relevant diastolic filling phase.[46] In sinus rhythm, the ventricles receive blood during two filling phases (Fig. 3–12). The first phase occurs when ventricular pressure drops sufficiently to allow its atrioventricular valve to open; blood then flows from atrium into ventricle. Flow coincides with the *y* descent of the atrial pressure pulse (Fig. 3–12) and is designated the "rapid filling phase" of ventricular diastole, accounting for about 80 per cent of normal filling. This phase is not a passive event in which in-flow merely expands the recipient ventricle; rather, ventricular relaxation is an active, complex, energy-dependent process. The sound generated during the rapid filling phase is called the third heart sound (Fig. 3–12).[47] The second filling phase—diastasis—is variable in duration, usually accounting for less than 5 per cent of ventricular filling. The third phase of diastolic filling is in response to atrial contraction, which accounts for about 15 per cent of normal ventricular filling. The sound generated during the atrial filling phase is called the fourth heart sound (Fig. 3–12). Importantly, both third and fourth heart sounds occur *within* the recipient ventricle as that chamber receives blood (Fig. 3–13). Potain in 1876 attributed the third heart sound to sudden cessation of distention of the ventricle in early diastole, and he attributed the fourth heart sound to " . . . the abruptness with which the dilatation of the ventricle takes place during the presystolic period, a period which corresponds to the contraction of the auricle."[48] He was not far from the mark.

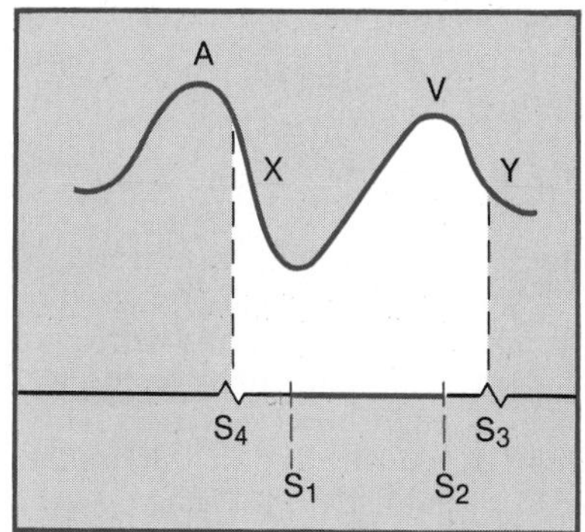

FIGURE 3–12. Atrial pressure pulse showing the *a* wave and *x* descent, and the *v* wave and *y* descent. The fourth heart sound (S_4) coincides with the phase of ventricular filling following atrial contraction. The third heart sound (S_3) coincides with the *y* descent (the phase of rapid ventricular filling). S_1 = first heart sound; S_2 = second heart sound.

The addition of either a third or a fourth heart sound to the cardiac cycle produces a *triple* rhythm. If both third *and* fourth heart sounds are present, a *quadruple* rhythm is produced. When diastole is short or the P-R interval long, third and fourth heart sounds may fuse to form a summation sound.[1]

Children and young adults often have normal (physiological) *third* heart sounds but do not have normal fourth heart sounds. Normal third heart sounds sometimes persist beyond age 40 years, especially in women.[49] However, after that age, especially in men, the third heart sound is likely to be abnormal. Fourth heart sounds are sometimes heard in healthy older adults without clinical evidence of heart disease, particularly after an exercise stress test.[50] Such observations have led to the conclusion, still debated, that these fourth heart sounds are normal in older adults.

Third and fourth heart sounds may originate in either the left or right ventricle. Because a fourth heart sound requires active atrial contribution to ventricular filling, the sound disappears when coordinated atrial contraction ceases, as in atrial fibrillation. When the atria and ventricles contract independently as in complete heart block (Fig. 3–2), fourth heart sounds or summation sounds occur randomly in diastole because the relationship between the P wave and the QRS of the electrocardiogram is random. Because third and fourth heart sounds are events of ventricular filling, obstruction of an atrioventricular valve, by impeding ventricular in-flow, removes one of the prime preconditions for the generation of these sounds. Accordingly, the presence of a third or fourth heart sound implies an unobstructed (or relatively unobstructed) atrioventricular orifice in the side of the heart in which the sound originates. It is intuitive that third and fourth heart sounds originating within the *left* ventricular cavity are best heard over the left ventricular impulse, and *right* ventricular third and fourth heart sounds are best heard over the *right* ventricular impulse. *Right ventricular* third or fourth heart sounds often respond selectively and distinctively to respiration by becoming more audible during inspiration.[1] The inspiratory increase in right atrial flow is converted into an inspiratory augmentation of both mid-diastolic and presystolic flow.

Third and fourth heart sounds, either normal or abnormal, are relatively low-frequency events that vary considerably in intensity (loudness). An understanding of this simple physical principle sets the stage for bedside detection. The same physical principles can be used to advantage to distinguish a fourth heart sound preceding a single first heart sound from splitting of the two components of the first heart sound (Fig. 3-1C). As described earlier, the two components of the first heart sound are similar in frequency (pitch) although not in intensity (loudness) but differ in pitch from a preceding fourth heart sound.

Audibility of third heart sounds is improved by isotonic exercise that serves to augment venous return and mid-diastolic atrioventricular flow. A few situps may suffice to produce the desired increase in venous return and acceleration in heart rate that increase the rate and volume of atrioventricular flow. Venous return can also be increased by simple passive raising of both legs with the patient supine. The heart rate is transiently increased by vigorous coughing. Left ventricular *fourth heart sounds*, especially in patients with ischemic heart disease, can be induced or augmented by increasing the resistance to left ventricular discharge in response to sustained handgrip (isometric exercise, see later).

In the presence of sinus tachycardia, atrial contraction may coincide with the rapid filling phase, making it impossible to determine whether a given filling sound is a third heart sound, a fourth heart sound, or a summation sound. Carotid sinus massage transiently slows the heart rate, so the diastolic sound or sounds can be assigned proper timing in the cardiac cycle.[1]

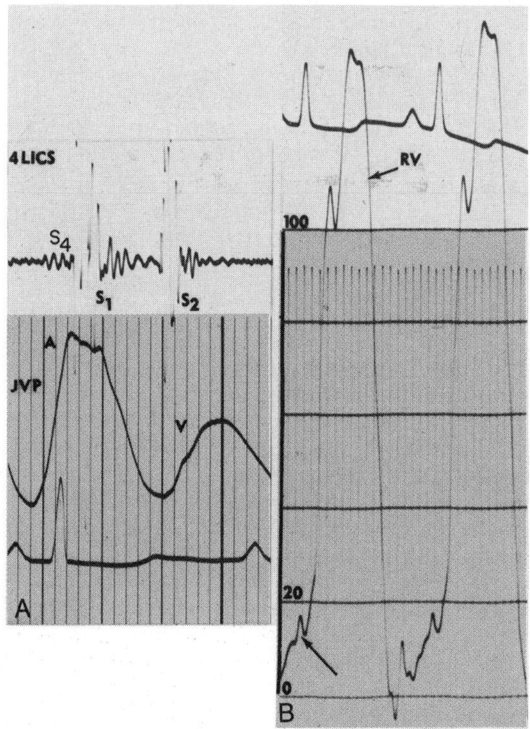

FIGURE 3–14. Tracings from an 18-year-old man with primary pulmonary hypertension. *A,* The phonocardiogram from the fourth left intercostal space (4LICS) shows a fourth heart sound (S_4). The jugular venous pulse (JVP) exhibits a prominent *a* wave. (S_1 = first heart sound; S_2 = second heart sound.) *B,* The increased force of right atrial contraction, reflected in the large *a* wave, results in presystolic distention (arrow) of the right ventricle (RV).

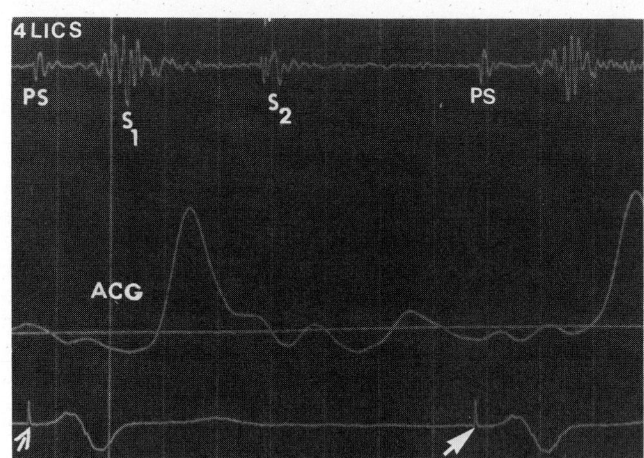

FIGURE 3–15. Phonocardiogram in the fourth left intercostal (4LICS) space with simultaneous apex cardiogram (ACG) and electrocardiogram in a patient with a right ventricular pacemaker. The pacemaker sound (PS) is synchronous with the pacemaker stimulus (arrows) shown in the electrocardiogram.

CAUSES OF THIRD AND FOURTH SOUNDS (see also Table 2–4, p. 33). The normal *third* heart sound is believed to be caused by sudden intrinsic limitation of longitudinal expansion of the left ventricular wall during early diastolic filling.[51,52] The majority of abnormal third heart sounds are generated by altered physical properties of the recipient ventricle and/or an increase in the rate and volume of atrioventricular flow during the rapid filling phase of the cardiac cycle.[53] Abnormal *fourth* heart sounds occur when augmented atrial contraction is required to generate presystolic distention of a ventricle (an increase in end-diastolic segment length) so that the chamber can contract with greater force.[37,54] Typical examples are the left ventricular hypertrophy of aortic stenosis or systemic hypertension in the left side of the heart,[55] or the right ventricular hypertrophy of pulmonic stenosis or pulmonary hypertension in the right side of the heart (Fig. 3–14).[37] Fourth heart sounds are also common in ischemic heart disease and are almost universal during angina pectoris or acute myocardial infarction, because the atrial "booster pump" is needed to assist the relatively stiff ischemic ventricle in maintaining adequate contractile force.

A variation on the theme of presystolic sounds is the *pacemaker sound* (Fig. 3–15).[56] A pacemaker electrode in the apex of the right ventricle may produce a presystolic sound that is relatively high-pitched and clicking and therefore different in pitch from a fourth heart sound. The consensus is that the pacemaker sound is extracardiac, resulting from contraction of chest wall muscle following spread of the electrical impulse from the pacemaker site.[56,57]

MURMURS

(See also pp. 33 to 36 and Table 2–5, p. 34)

According to O. H. Perry Pepper, *murmur* is a Latin word with probable onomatopoeic origins.[58] A cardiovascular murmur is a series of auditory vibrations more prolonged than a sound and characterized according to intensity (loudness), frequency (pitch), configuration (shape), quality, duration, direction of radiation, and timing in the cardiac cycle. Once these features are established, the stage is set for diagnostic conclusions that can be drawn from a murmur of a given description.

The intensity or loudness of a murmur is graded from one to six, based on the original recommendations of Samuel A. Levine and A. R. Freeman in 1933.[59] The frequency or pitch of a murmur varies from high to low. The configuration or shape of a systolic murmur is best characterized as crescendo, decrescendo, crescendo-decrescendo (diamond-shaped), plateau (even), or variable (uneven). The duration of a murmur varies from short to long with all gradations in between. A loud murmur radiates from its site of maximal intensity, and the direction of radiation sometimes provides useful diagnostic information. The timing of a murmur within the cardiac cycle is the basis for its classification.

There are three basic categories of murmurs: systolic, diastolic, and continuous. A *systolic* murmur begins with or after the first heart sound and ends at or before the second heart sound on its site of origin. A *diastolic* murmur begins with or after the second heart sound and ends before the first heart sound. A *continuous* murmur begins in systole and continues without interruption through the timing of the second heart sound into all or part of diastole. The following descriptive classification of murmurs is based on their timing relative to the first and second heart sounds.

SYSTOLIC MURMURS

(See also Figs. 2–24, p. 35, and 2–25, p. 35)

Systolic murmurs are best classified according to their time of onset and termination as midsystolic, holosystolic, early systolic, or late systolic. A midsystolic murmur begins after the first heart sound and ends perceptibly before the second sound. The termination of the murmur must be related to the relevant component of the second heart sound. Accordingly, midsystolic murmurs originating in the *left* side of the heart end before the *aortic* component of the second heart sound; midsystolic murmurs originating in the *right* side of the heart end before the *pulmonic* component of the second sound. A *holosystolic* murmur begins with the first heart sound, occupies all of systole, and ends with the second heart sound on its side of origin. Holosystolic murmurs originating in the *left* side of the heart end with the *aortic* component of the second heart sound, and holosystolic murmurs originating in the *right* side of the heart end with the *pulmonic* component of the second sound.

The term "regurgitant systolic murmur," originally applied to murmurs that occupied all of systole,[13] has fallen into disuse because "regurgitation" can be accompanied by holosystolic, midsystolic, early systolic, or late systolic murmurs. Similarly, the term "ejection systolic murmur," originally applied to midsystolic murmurs, should be discarded, because midsystolic murmurs are not necessarily due to "ejection."[1]

MIDSYSTOLIC MURMURS. Midsystolic murmurs occur in five settings: (1) obstruction to ventricular outflow, (2) dilatation of the aortic root or pulmonary trunk, (3) accelerated systolic flow into the aorta or pulmonary trunk, (4) innocent midsystolic murmurs, including those due to morphological changes of functionally normal semilunar valves (generally aortic), and (5) some forms of mitral regurgitation. The physiological mechanism of *outflow* midsystolic murmurs reflects the pattern of phasic flow across the left or right ventricular outflow tract as originally described by Leatham (Fig. 3–16).[15] Following isovolumetric contraction and generation of the first heart sound, ventricular pressure rises and the semilunar valves open. Ejection commences, and the murmur begins. As ejection proceeds, the murmur increases in crescendo; as ejection decreases, the murmur decreases in decrescendo. The murmur ends before ventricular pressure drops below the central great arterial pressure, at which time the aortic and pulmonic valves close with generation of the aortic and pulmonic components of the second heart sound.

A prototypical midsystolic murmur originating in the left side of the heart is caused by stenosis of the aortic valve. The

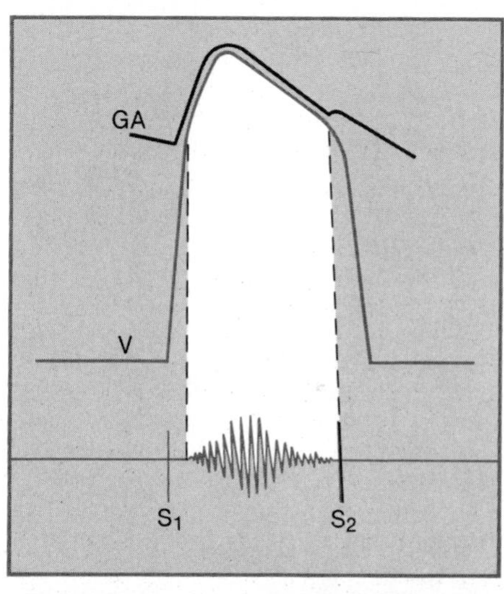

FIGURE 3–16. Illustration of the physiological mechanism of an outflow midsystolic murmur generated by phasic flow into the aortic root or pulmonary trunk. Ventricular (V) and great arterial (GA) pressure pulses are shown with phonocardiogram. The murmur begins after the first heart sound (S_1). The murmur rises in crescendo to a peak as flow proceeds and then declines in decrescendo as flow diminishes, ending just before the second heart sound (S_2) as ventricular pressure falls below the pressure in the great artery.

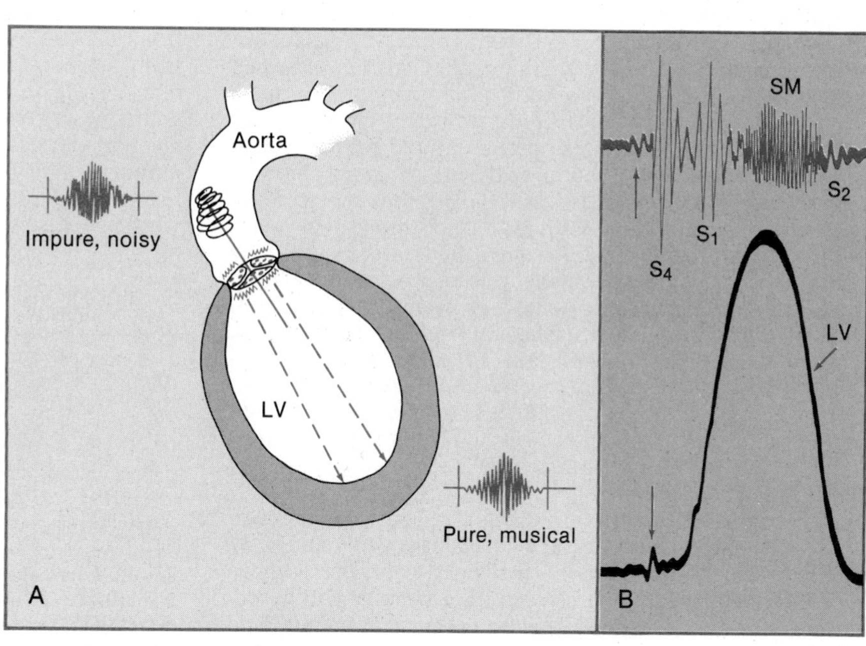

FIGURE 3–17. *A,* Illustration of "Gallavardin dissociation" of the murmurs associated with a fibrocalcific stenotic trileaflet aortic valve in older adults. The impure, noisy midsystolic murmur at the right base originates within the aortic root because of turbulence caused by the high-velocity jet. The pure, musical midsystolic murmur at the apex results from periodic high-frequency vibrations originating in the fibrocalcific but mobile aortic cusps and radiates selectively into the left ventricular cavity (LV). *B,* Left ventricular intracardiac phonocardiogram of an older adult with calcific aortic stenosis on a previously normal trileaflet valve. The pure, musical midsystolic murmur (SM) is recorded at the apex of the left ventricle (LV). A prominent fourth heart sound (S_4) coincides with presystolic distention of the left ventricle (lower vertical arrow). Upper vertical arrow identifies inaudible low-frequency vibrations preceding the fourth heart sound. S_1 = first heart sound; S_2 = second heart sound.

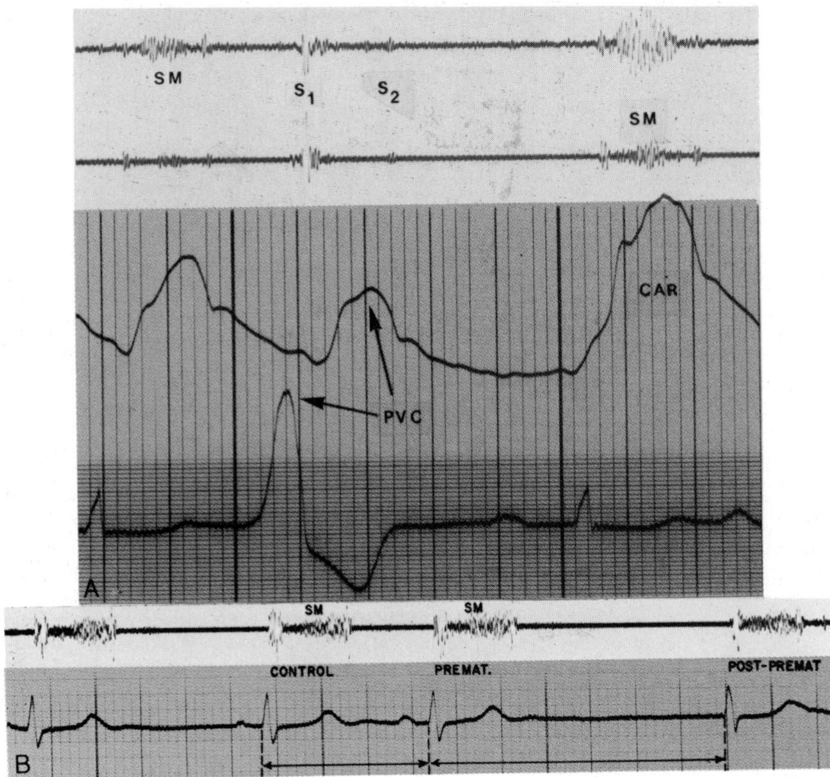

FIGURE 3-18. *A,* Phonocardiograms from the second right interspace and apex of a patient with an aortic sclerotic midsystolic murmur (SM). After the compensatory pause initiated by a premature ventricular contraction (PVC), the midsystolic murmur appreciably increased in intensity. CAR = carotid pulse. *B,* The effect of changes of cycle length on the holosystolic murmur (SM) of mitral regurgitation. The intensity of the murmur changes little if at all when the control beat is compared with the postpremature beat.

direction of the high-velocity jet within the aortic root results in radiation of the murmur upward, to the right (second right intercostal space) and into the neck. An interesting and important variation on the theme occurs in older adults with previously normal trileaflet aortic valves rendered sclerotic or stenotic by fibrocalcific changes.[60] The accompanying murmur in the second right intercostal space is harsh, noisy, and impure, whereas the murmur over the left ventricular impulse is pure and often musical (Fig. 3-17*A*). These two distinctive midsystolic murmurs—the noisy right basal and the musical apical—were described by Gallavardin in 1925,[61] and the designation "Gallavardin dissociation" is still used. The impure right basal component of the murmur originates within the aortic root because of turbulence caused by the high-velocity jet. The pure musical component of the murmur heard over the left ventricular impulse is ascribed to periodic high-frequency vibrations of the fibrocalcific aortic cusps without commissural fusion. The musical apical midsystolic murmur is sometimes dramatically loud. William Stokes (1855) reported that such a murmur was heard at a distance of 3 feet from the chest, and that "this gentleman once observed to me that his entire body was one humming top."[62]

The high-frequency apical midsystolic murmur of aortic sclerosis or stenosis requires differentiation from the apical murmur of mitral regurgitation, a difference that may be difficult or impossible to establish, especially if the aortic component of the second heart sound is soft or absent. However, when premature ventricular contractions are followed by pauses longer than the dominant cycle length, the apical midsystolic murmur of aortic stenosis or sclerosis increases in intensity in the beat following the premature contraction (Fig. 3-18*A*),[55] whereas the murmur of mitral regurgitation (whether midsystolic or holosystolic) remains relatively unchanged in intensity (Fig. 3-18*B*). The same patterns hold following longer cycle lengths in atrial fibrillation. The validity of these observations assumes that aortic and mitral murmurs do not coexist at the apex, which is often the case.

Prototypical of midsystolic murmurs originating in the *right* side of the heart is the murmur of pulmonary valve stenosis.[22] The murmur begins after the first heart sound or with an ejection sound, rises in crescendo to a peak, and then decreases in decrescendo to end before a delayed pulmonic component of the second heart sound (midsystolic, right-sided) (Fig. 3-4*A*). The length and configuration of the murmur are useful signs of the degree of obstruction.[22] The relative durations of right and left ventricular ejection can be compared by relating the end of the pulmonic stenotic murmur (right-sided event) to the timing of the *aortic* component of the second heart sound (left-sided event) (Fig. 3-4*A*).

Short, soft midsystolic murmurs can originate within a dilated aortic root or dilated pulmonary trunk. Midsystolic murmurs are also generated by rapid ejection into a *normal* aortic root or pulmonary trunk, as is often the case during pregnancy, fever, thyrotoxicosis, or anemia. The pulmonic midsystolic murmur of ostium secundum atrial septal defect results from a combination of *rapid* ejection into a *dilated* pulmonary trunk (Fig. 3-9). *Normal* (innocent) systolic murmurs are, with the exception of the systolic mammary souffle, all midsystolic.[22] The normal vibratory midsystolic murmur described by George Still (1909)[63] is short, buzzing, pure, and medium-frequency (Fig. 3-19), and is believed to originate from low-frequency periodic vibrations of normal pulmonic leaflets at their attachments. A second type of innocent pulmonic midsystolic murmur occurs in children, adolescents, and young adults and represents an exaggeration of normal ejection vibrations within the pulmonary trunk. This normal pulmonic midsystolic murmur is relatively impure and is best heard in the second left intercostal space, in contrast to the vibratory midsystolic murmur of Still, which is typically

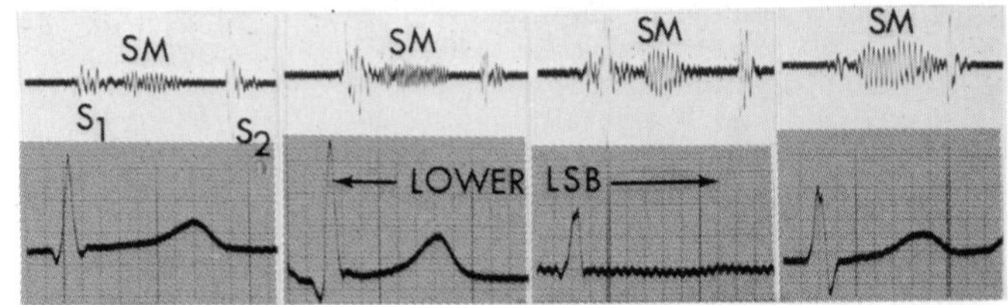

FIGURE 3-19. Four vibratory midsystolic murmurs (SM) from healthy children. These murmurs, designated "Still's murmur," are pure, medium frequency, relatively brief in duration, and maximal along the lower left sternal border (LSB). The last of the four murmurs was from a 5-year-old girl who was febrile. Following defervescence, the murmur decreased in loudness and duration.

heard between the lower left sternal edge and apex. Normal pulmonic midsystolic murmurs are also heard in thin patients with diminished anteroposterior chest dimensions (loss of thoracic kyphosis, for example).[39]

The most common form of "innocent" midsystolic murmur in older adults is designated the "*aortic sclerotic*" murmur (see above). The cause of this functionally benign murmur is fibrous or fibrocalcific thickening of the bases of otherwise normal aortic cusps as they insert into the sinuses of Valsalva.[22] As long as the fibrosis or fibrocalcific thickening is confined to the *base* of the leaflets, the free edges move well and there is no obstruction. Commissural fusion is absent and therefore does not contribute to restricted leaflet motion. The Gallavardin dissociation phenomenon was described earlier.

Some forms of *mitral regurgitation* generate midsystolic murmurs.[35,64] The clinical setting is usually ischemic heart disease associated with left ventricular regional wall motion abnormalities. The physiological mechanism responsible for the midsystolic murmur of mitral regurgitation in this setting relates to early systolic competence of the valve, midsystolic incompetence, followed by late systolic decrease in regurgitant flow. In any event, these midsystolic murmurs have nothing to do with "ejection."

HOLOSYSTOLIC MURMURS. Just as the term "midsystolic" is preferable to "ejection systolic," the term "holosystolic" is preferable to "regurgitant" because murmurs in the latter category are not necessarily due to regurgitant flow. A holosystolic murmur begins with the first heart sound and occupies all of systole (Gr. *holos* = entire) up to the second sound on its side of origin.[15] Such murmurs are generated by flow from a chamber or vessel whose pressure or resistance throughout systole is higher than the pressure or resistance in the chamber or vessel receiving the flow. Holosystolic murmurs occur in the left side of the heart with mitral regurgitation, in the right side of the heart with tricuspid regurgitation, between the ventricles with restrictive ventricular septal defects, and between the great arteries through an aortopulmonary window or patent ductus arteriosus when pulmonary vascular resistance eliminates diastolic flow and the diastolic component of the murmur (see below).

The timing of holosystolic murmurs within the framework established by the first and second heart sounds reflects the physiological and anatomical mechanisms responsible for their genesis. Figure 3–20 illustrates the mechanism of the holosystolic murmur of mitral regurgitation or high-pressure tricuspid regurgitation. Because ventricular pressure exceeds atrial pressure at the very onset of systole (isovolumetric contraction), regurgitant flow begins with the first heart sound.

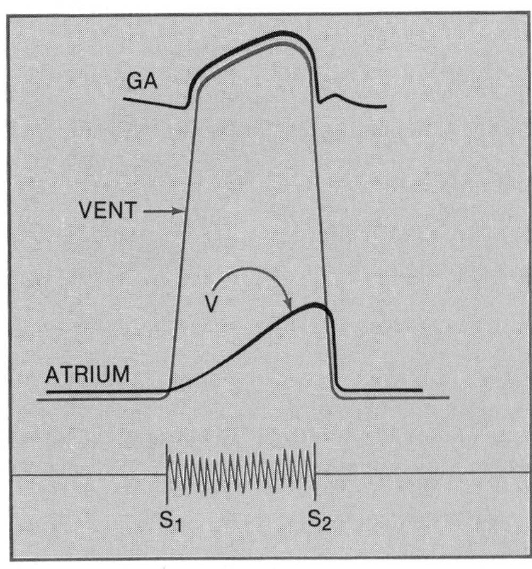

FIGURE 3–20. Illustration of great arterial (GA), ventricular (VENT), and atrial pressure pulses with phonocardiogram showing the physiological mechanism of holosystolic murmurs in some forms of mitral regurgitation and tricuspid regurgitation. Ventricular pressure exceeds atrial pressure from the onset of systole, so regurgitant flow and murmur commence with the first heart sound (S_1). The murmur persists up to or slightly beyond the second heart sound (S_2), because regurgitation persists to the end of systole (ventricular pressure still exceeds atrial pressure). V = atrial *v* wave.

The murmur persists up to or slightly beyond the relevant component of the second heart sound, provided that the ventricular pressure at end systole exceeds the atrial pressure and provided that the atrioventricular valve remains incompetent.

Direction of radiation of the intraatrial jet of mitral regurgitation may be reflected in the chest wall distribution of the murmur.[35,65] When the direction of the intraatrial jet is forward and medial against the atrial septum near the base of the aorta, the murmur radiates to the left sternal edge, to the base, and even into the neck (Fig. 3–21*A*). When the flow generating the murmur of mitral regurgitation is directed posterolaterally within the left atrial cavity, the murmur radiates into the axilla, to the angle of the left scapula, and occasionally to the vertebral column with bone conduction from the cervical to the lumbar spine (Fig. 3–21*B*).

The murmur of *tricuspid regurgitation* is holosystolic when there is a substantial elevation of right ventricular systolic pressure, as schematically illustrated in Figure 3–20. A dis-

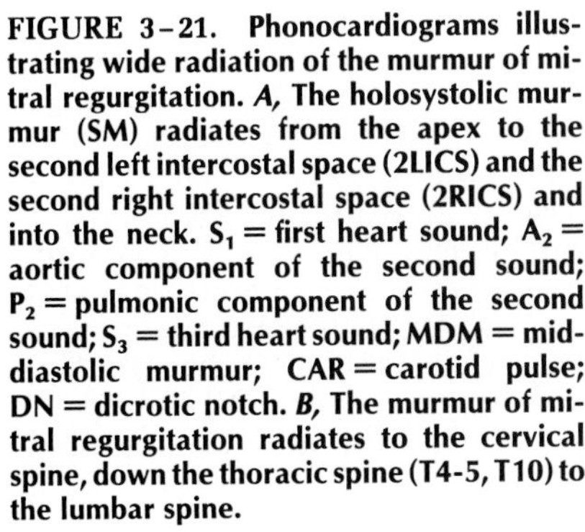

FIGURE 3–21. Phonocardiograms illustrating wide radiation of the murmur of mitral regurgitation. *A*, The holosystolic murmur (SM) radiates from the apex to the second left intercostal space (2LICS) and the second right intercostal space (2RICS) and into the neck. S_1 = first heart sound; A_2 = aortic component of the second sound; P_2 = pulmonic component of the second sound; S_3 = third heart sound; MDM = mid-diastolic murmur; CAR = carotid pulse; DN = dicrotic notch. *B*, The murmur of mitral regurgitation radiates to the cervical spine, down the thoracic spine (T4-5, T10) to the lumbar spine.

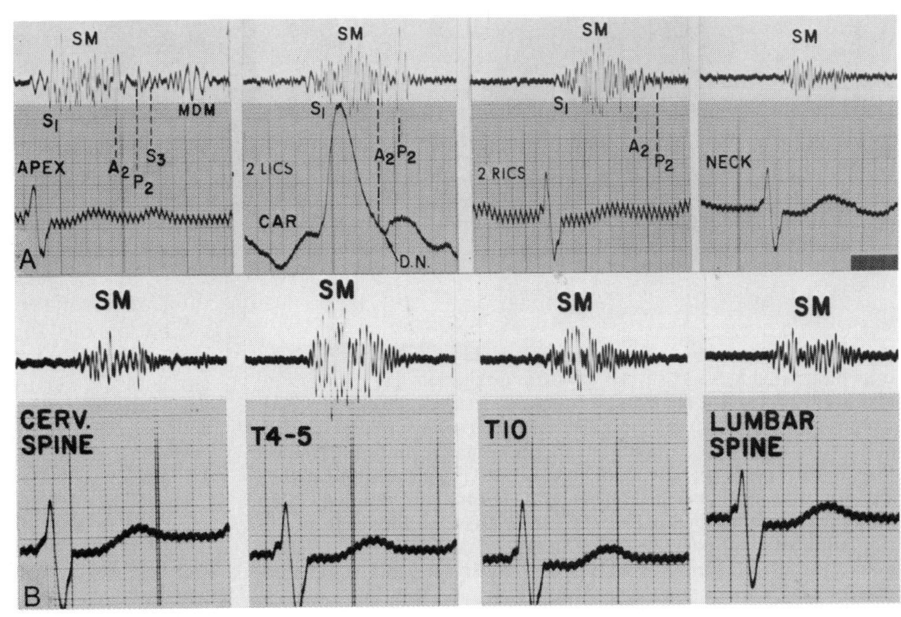

tinctive and diagnostically important feature of the murmur is a selective inspiratory increase in loudness—Carvallo's sign.[66,67] The tricuspid murmur is occasionally audible only during inspiration. The increase in intensity occurs because the inspiratory augmentation in right ventricular volume is converted into an increase in stroke volume and in the velocity of regurgitant flow.[54] When the right ventricle fails, this capacity is lost, so Carvallo's sign vanishes.

The murmur of an uncomplicated restrictive *ventricular septal defect* is holosystolic because the left ventricular systolic pressure and systemic resistance exceed right ventricular systolic pressure and pulmonary resistance from the onset to the end of systole. Holosystolic murmurs are perceived as such in patients with large aortopulmonary connections (aortopulmonary window, patent ductus arteriosus) when a rise in pulmonary vascular resistance abolishes the diastolic portion of the continuous murmur, leaving a murmur that is holosystolic or nearly so.[22]

EARLY SYSTOLIC MURMURS. Early systolic murmurs begin with the first heart sound, diminish in decrescendo, and end well before the second heart sound, generally at or before midsystole. Certain types of mitral regurgitation, tricuspid regurgitation, or ventricular septal defects are examples.

Acute severe mitral regurgitation is accompanied by an early systolic murmur, or a holosystolic murmur that is decrescendo, diminishing if not ending before the second heart sound (Fig. 3–22).[68–70] The physiological mechanism responsible for this early systolic decrescendo murmur is regurgitation into a relatively normal-sized left atrium of limited distensibility. A steep rise in left atrial V wave approaches the left ventricular pressure at end diastole; a late systolic decline in left ventricular pressure favors this tendency (Figs. 3–22 and 2–23). The stage is set for regurgitant flow that is maximal in early systole and minimal in late systole. The systolic murmur parallels this pattern, declining or vanishing before the second heart sound (Figs. 3–22 and 3–23).

An early systolic murmur is a feature of "low-pressure" tricuspid regurgitation, that is, tricuspid regurgitation with *normal* right ventricular systolic pressure.[71] An example is the regurgitation accompanying tricuspid valve infective en-

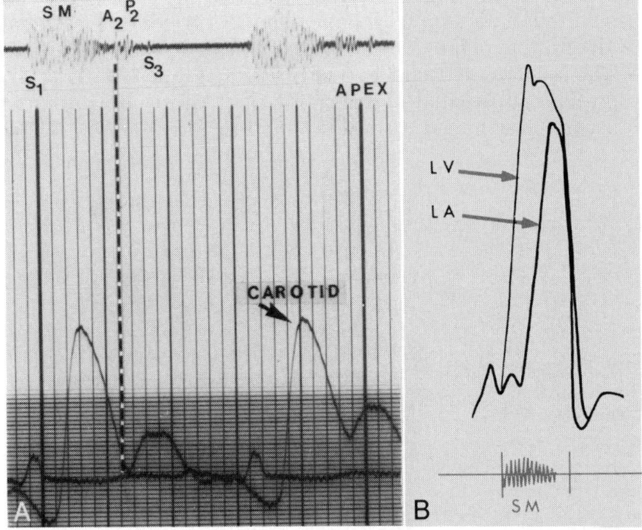

FIGURE 3–22. ***A,*** **Phonocardiogram recorded from the cardiac apex of a patient with acute severe mitral regurgitation due to ruptured chordae tendineae. There is an early systolic decrescendo murmur (SM) diminishing if not ending before the aortic component (A_2) of the second heart sound. P_2 = pulmonic component of the second heart sound; S_1 = first heart sound; S_3 = third heart sound.** ***B,*** **Left ventricular (LV) and left atrial (LA) pressure pulses with schematic illustration of the phonocardiogram showing the relationship between the decrescendo configuration of the early systolic murmur and late systolic approximation of the tall left atrial *v* wave and left ventricular end-systolic pressure.**

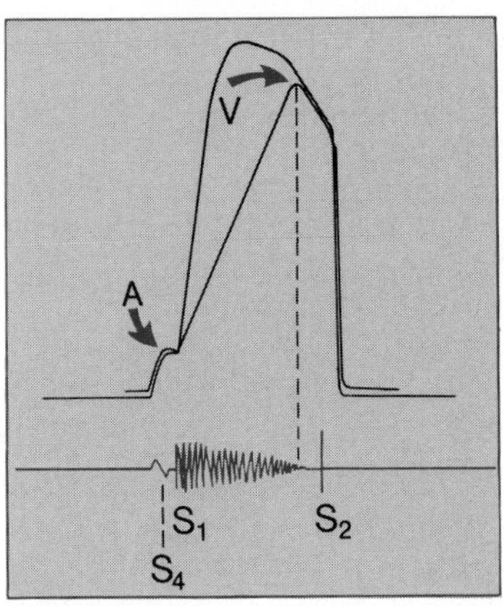

FIGURE 3–23. **Ventricular and atrial pressure pulses with phonocardiogram illustrating the mechanism of the *early* systolic murmur of acute severe mitral regurgitation or low-pressure tricuspid regurgitation. The *v* wave reaches ventricular pressure at end systole (upper curved arrow) so regurgitant flow diminishes or ceases. The murmur is therefore early systolic and decrescendo, paralleling the hemodynamic pattern of regurgitation. (S_4 = fourth heart sound.)**

docarditis in drug abusers. The mechanisms responsible for the timing and configuration of the early systolic murmur of low-pressure tricuspid regurgitation are analogous to those described in the preceding paragraph (and illustrated in Figure 3–23). The tall right atrial *v* wave reaches the level of normal right ventricular pressure in latter systole; therefore, the regurgitation and murmur are chiefly, if not exclusively, *early* systolic. These murmurs are of medium or low frequency, because normal right ventricular systolic pressure generates a comparatively low velocity of regurgitant flow in contrast to the high-frequency *holosystolic* murmur of tricuspid regurgitation generated by *elevated* right ventricular systolic pressure (see earlier).

Early systolic murmurs also occur in the presence of ventricular septal defects but under two widely divergent anatomical and physiological circumstances. A soft, pure, high-frequency, early systolic murmur localized to the mid- or lower left sternal edge is typical of a very small ventricular septal defect in which the shunt is confined to early systole.[22] A murmur of similar timing and configuration occurs through a nonrestrictive ventricular septal defect when an elevation in pulmonary vascular resistance decreases or abolishes late systolic shunting.[22]

LATE SYSTOLIC MURMURS. The term "late systolic" applies when a murmur begins in mid- to late systole and proceeds up to the aortic component of the second heart sound. The late systolic murmur of mitral valve prolapse is prototypical.[25,72] One or more mid- to late systolic clicks often introduce the murmur. The responses of the late systolic murmur and clicks to postural maneuvers (see earlier discussion) are illustrated in Figure 3–8. A *diminution* in left ventricular volume, best achieved by prompt standing after squatting,[27] but also achieved by the Valsalva maneuver, causes the late systolic murmur to become longer although softer. An *increase* in left ventricular volume associated with squatting or sustained handgrip causes the murmur to become shorter but louder. Pharmacological interventions that variably alter left ventricular volume, especially amyl nitrite (Fig. 3–24), produce analogous results but are less practical at the bedside.

The late systolic murmur of mitral valve prolapse is occasionally converted into an intermittent, striking, and sometimes disconcerting systolic whoop or honk, either spontaneously or in response to physical maneuvers.[25] The whoop is high-frequency, musical, widely transmitted and occasionally loud enough to be disquieting to the patient and sometimes to the physician.[73] The musical whoop is thought to arise from mitral leaflets and chordae tendineae set into high-frequency periodic vibration.

SYSTOLIC ARTERIAL MURMURS. Systolic arterial murmurs originate in anatomically normal arteries in the

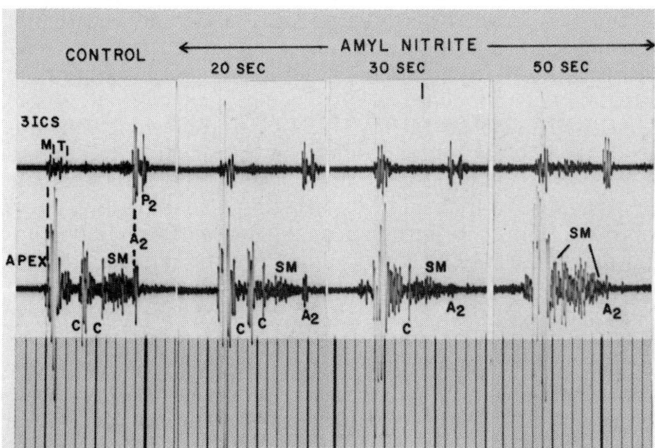

FIGURE 3–24. Phonocardiograms illustrating the response of the systolic clicks (C) and late systolic murmur (SM) of mitral valve prolapse to amyl nitrite inhalation. At 20 to 30 seconds, the clicks become earlier and the systolic murmur becomes longer but softer. At 50 seconds, the murmur is holosystolic and louder. M_1 = mitral component of the first heart sound; T_1 = tricuspid component of the first heart sound; A_2 = aortic component of the second heart sound; P_2 = pulmonic component of the second sound.

presence of normal or increased flow, or in abnormal arteries because of tortuosity or luminal narrowing. Detection of systolic arterial murmurs requires auscultation at nonprecordial sites. Timing with the first and second heart sounds is necessarily imprecise because the murmurs begin at variable distances from the heart. Nevertheless, the arterial murmurs dealt with here are essentially systolic, and tend to have a crescendo-decrescendo configuration that reflects a rise and fall of pulsatile arterial flow.[1]

The "supraclavicular systolic murmur" (Fig. 3–25*A*), a normal systolic arterial murmur that is often heard in children and adolescents, is believed to originate at the aortic origins of normal major brachiocephalic arteries.[22,74] The configuration of these murmurs is crescendo-decrescendo, the onset is abrupt, the duration brief, and the intensity at times is surprisingly loud, with radiation below the clavicles. Normal supraclavicular systolic murmurs decrease or vanish in response to hyperextension of the shoulders, which is achieved by bringing the elbows back until the shoulder girdle muscles are taut (Fig. 3–25*B*).[74]

In older adults, the most common cause of a systolic arterial murmur is atherosclerotic disease that results in narrowing of a carotid, subclavian, or iliofemoral artery. A variation on this theme is the "compression artifact" of free aortic regurgitation in which a systolic arterial murmur is generated when a femoral artery is moderately compressed by the examiner's stethoscopic bell. Further compression serves to make the systolic murmur continue into diastole, a sign described in 1861 by Duroziez.[22] The eponym is still in use.

A systolic "mammary souffle" is sometimes heard over the breasts because of increased flow through normal arteries during late pregnancy but especially in the postpartum period in lactating women.[22,75] The murmur begins well after the first heart sound because of the interval between left ventricular ejection and arrival of flow at the artery of origin.

Still another type of systolic arterial murmur can be present in the back between the scapulae over the site of coarctation of the aortic isthmus.[22] Transient systolic arterial murmurs in the pulmonary artery and its branches are heard occasionally in normal neonates because the angulation and disparity in size between the pulmonary trunk and its branches set the stage for turbulent systolic flow. These normal or innocent pulmonary arterial systolic murmurs disappear with maturation of the pulmonary bed, generally within the first few weeks or months of life.[22,76] Similar if not identical pulmonary arterial systolic murmurs are generated across zones of congenital stenosis of the pulmonary artery and its branches. Rarely, a pulmonary arterial systolic murmur is caused by luminal narrowing following a pulmonary embolus.[37]

DIASTOLIC MURMURS

(See also Table 2–5, p. 34)

Diastolic murmurs are descriptively classified according to their time of *onset* as early diastolic, mid-diastolic, or late diastolic (presystolic) (Fig. 3–26). An *early* diastolic murmur begins with the aortic or pulmonic component of the second heart sound, depending on its side of origin. A mid-diastolic murmur begins at a clear interval *after* the second heart sound. A late diastolic or presystolic murmur begins immediately before the first heart sound.

EARLY DIASTOLIC MURMURS. An early diastolic murmur originating in the left side of the heart is represented by aortic regurgitation. The murmur begins with the aortic component of the second heart sound (Fig. 3–27*A*), i.e., as soon as left ventricular pressure crosses (falls below) the aortic incisura. The murmur tends to be decrescendo, reflecting a progressive decline in volume and rate of regurgitant flow during the course of diastole. In moderate chronic aortic regurgita-

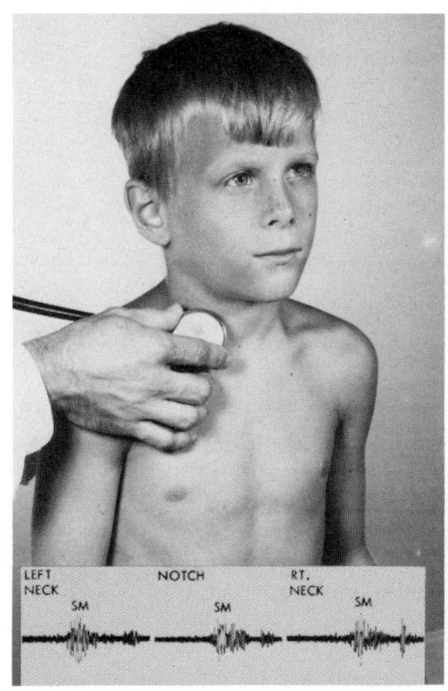

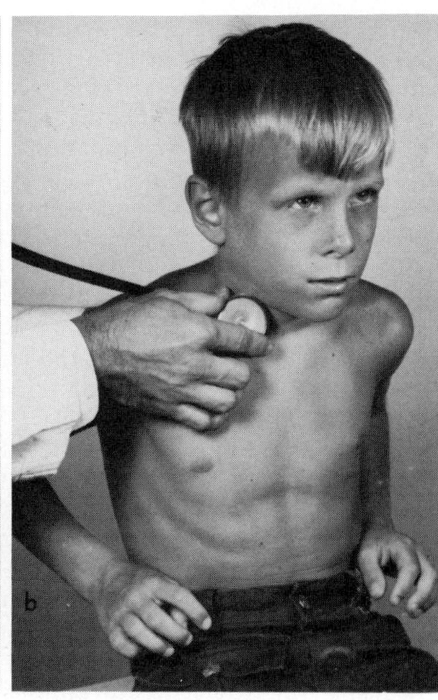

FIGURE 3–25. *A,* Phonocardiogram showing a normal supraclavicular systolic arterial murmur maximal above the clavicles (left neck, right neck) and in the suprasternal notch. Auscultation is initially carried out while the patient sits with shoulders relaxed and arms resting in the lap. *B,* When the elbows are brought well behind the back (hyperextension of the shoulders), the murmur markedly diminishes or disappears.

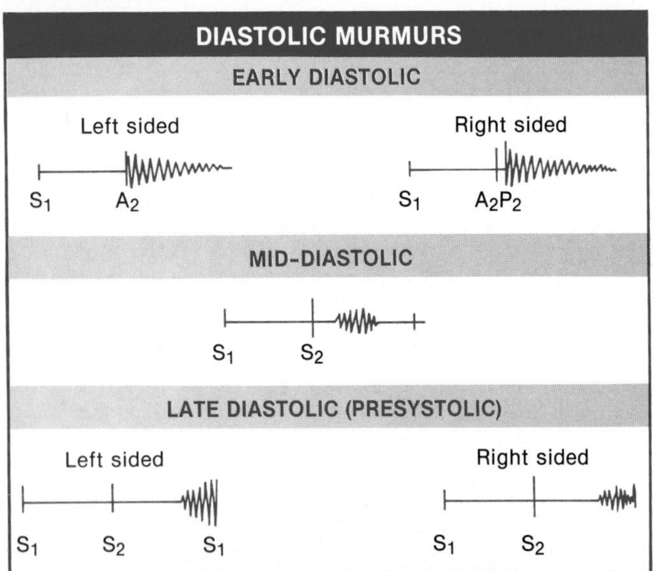

FIGURE 3-26. Diastolic murmurs are descriptively classified according to their time of *onset* as early diastolic, mid-diastolic, or late diastolic (presystolic). Diastolic murmurs originate in either the left or the right side of the heart.

tion, the aortic diastolic pressure consistently and appreciably exceeds left ventricular diastolic pressure so the decrescendo is less obvious, and the murmur is well heard throughout diastole. In chronic *severe* aortic regurgitation, the decrescendo is more obvious, paralleling the dramatic decline in aortic root diastolic pressure. Selective radiation of the murmur of aortic regurgitation to the *right* sternal edge implies aortic root dilatation, as in the Marfan syndrome. When an inverted cusp is set into high-frequency periodic vibration by aortic regurgitation, the accompanying murmur is musical, early diastolic, and decrescendo (Fig. 3-27*B*).

The early diastolic murmur of *acute severe* aortic regurgitation differs importantly from the murmur of chronic severe aortic regurgitation as just described.[77] When regurgitant flow is both sudden *and* severe (bicuspid aortic valve infective endocarditis, aortic dissection), the diastolic murmur is relatively short because of early equilibration of aortic diastolic pressure with the steeply rising diastolic pressure in the poorly compliant left ventricle. The pitch of the murmur is likely to be medium rather than high because the velocity of regurgitant flow is less rapid than in chronic severe aortic regurgitation. The short, medium-frequency diastolic murmur of sudden severe aortic regurgitation may be disarmingly soft. These auscultatory features are in contrast to the long, pure, high-frequency blowing early diastolic murmur of chronic severe aortic regurgitation (Fig. 3-27*A*).

Early diastolic murmurs in the *right* side of the heart are represented by the Graham Steell murmur of pulmonary hypertensive pulmonary regurgitation described in 1888. "I wish to plead for the admission among the recognized auscultatory signs of disease of a murmur due to . . . long-continuing excess blood pressure in the pulmonary artery. . . . When the second sound is reduplicated, the murmur proceeds from its latter part. That such a murmur as I have described does exist, there can, I think, be no doubt."[38]

The Graham Steell murmur begins with a loud *pulmonic* component of the second heart sound as Steell originally described (Fig. 3-6), because the elevated pressure exerted on the incompetent pulmonic valve begins at the moment that the right ventricular pressure crosses (drops below) the pulmonary arterial incisura.[37] The high diastolic pressure generates a high velocity of regurgitant flow and results in a high-frequency blowing murmur that may last throughout diastole. Because of the persistent and appreciable difference between pulmonary arterial diastolic pressure and right ventricular diastolic pressure, the amplitude of the murmur may be relatively uniform through most if not all of diastole rather than distinctly decrescendo.

MID-DIASTOLIC MURMURS. A mid-diastolic murmur begins at a clear interval following the second heart sound (Fig. 3-26). The majority of mid-diastolic murmurs originate across mitral or tricuspid valves during the rapid filling phase of the cardiac cycle (atrioventricular valve obstruction or abnormal patterns of atrioventricular flow) or across an incompetent pulmonic valve, provided the pulmonary arterial pressure is not elevated.[78]

The mid-diastolic murmur of rheumatic mitral stenosis is an example.[79] The murmur characteristically follows the mitral opening snap (Fig. 3-11*B*). Because the murmur originates within the left ventricular cavity, transmission to the chest wall is maximal at the site where the left ventricular impulse is palpated. In atrial fibrillation, the *duration* of the mid-diastolic murmur is a useful sign of the degree of obstruction at the mitral orifice. A murmur that lasts up to the first heart sound even after long cycle lengths implies a persistent gradient at the end of long diastoles (Fig. 3-28).

The mid-diastolic murmur of *tricuspid* stenosis occurs in the presence of atrial fibrillation. The tricuspid mid-diastolic murmur differs from the *mitral* mid-diastolic murmur in two important respects: (1) the tricuspid murmur selectively and

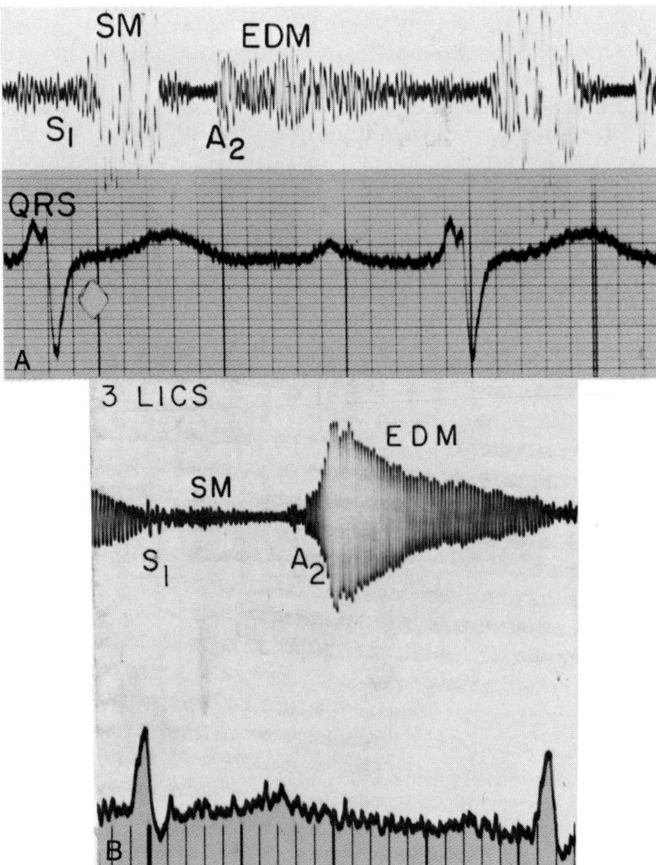

FIGURE 3-27. *A*, Phonocardiogram recorded from the mid-left sternal edge of a patient with chronic pure severe aortic regurgitation. An early diastolic murmur (EDM) proceeds immediately from the aortic component (A_2) of the second heart sound. The murmur has an early crescendo followed by a late long decrescendo. There is a prominent midsystolic flow murmur (SM) across an unobstructed aortic valve. S_1 = first heart sound. *B*, Phonocardiogram in the third left intercostal space (3LICS) records a high-frequency, musical, decrescendo early diastolic murmur (EDM) caused by eversion of an aortic cusp. S_1 = first heart sound; SM = midsystolic murmur; A_2 = aortic component of the second sound.

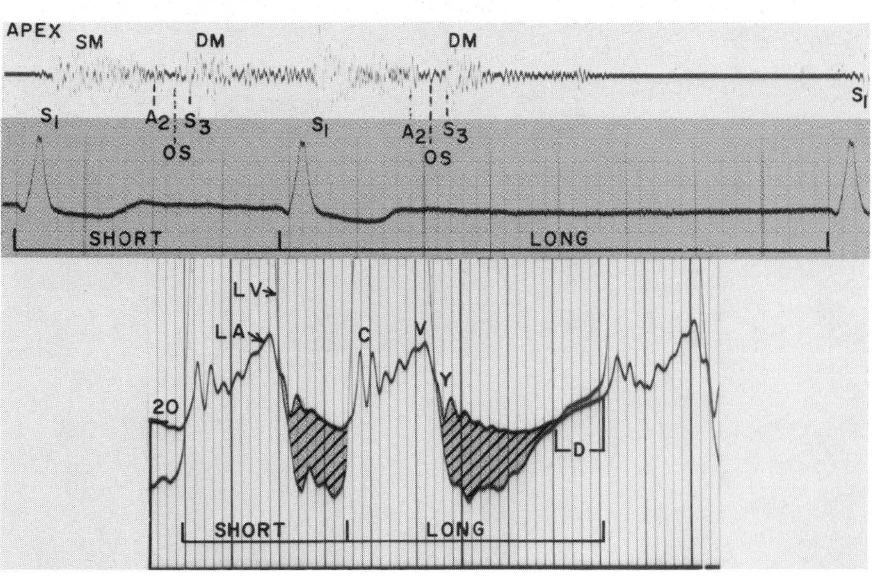

FIGURE 3–28. Tracings from a patient with rheumatic mitral stenosis, appreciable mitral regurgitation, and atrial fibrillation. The first heart sound (S_1) varies in intensity with cycle length. The aortic component of the second heart sound (A_2) is followed by a soft opening snap (OS) and a prominent third heart sound that introduces an early diastolic murmur (DM). With a short cycle length, the diastolic murmur proceeds throughout diastole because (as seen in nonsimultaneously recorded pressure tracings at the bottom), there is an end-diastolic gradient between left atrium (LA) and left ventricle (LV). In the second cycle (long), the diastolic murmur ends, and the remainder of diastole is murmur-free, paralleling the equilibration of left atrial and left ventricular diastolic pressures. D = diastasis; C = *c* wave; V = *v* wave; Y = *y* descent.

distinctively increases in loudness during inspiration; and (2) the tricuspid murmur is confined to a relatively localized area along the left lower sternal edge. The inspiratory increase in loudness occurs because inspiration is accompanied by an augmentation in right ventricular volume, by a fall in right ventricular diastolic pressure, and by an increase in the gradient and flow rate across the stenotic tricuspid valve.[80] The murmur is localized to the left lower sternal edge because it originates within the in-flow portion of the right ventricle and is transmitted to the overlying chest wall.

Mid-diastolic murmurs across *unobstructed* atrioventricular valves occur in the presence of augmented volume and velocity of flow. Examples in the left side of the heart are the mid-diastolic flow murmur of pure mitral regurgitation (Fig. 3–29) and the mid-diastolic mitral flow murmur that accompanies a large left-to-right shunt through a ventricular septal defect (Fig. 3–30). Mid-diastolic murmurs due to augmented flow across unobstructed *tricuspid* valves are generated in the presence of severe triscuspid regurgitation or in the presence of a left-to-right shunt through an ostium secundum atrial septal defect (Fig. 3–30*B*). These mid-diastolic murmurs occur with appreciable atrioventricular valve incompetence or large left-to-right shunts and are often preceded by third heart sounds, especially in the presence of mitral or tricuspid regurgitation.

Short, mid-diastolic atrioventricular flow murmurs occur intermittently in *complete heart block* when atrial contraction coincides with the phase of rapid diastolic filling (Fig. 3–2). These murmurs are believed to result from antegrade flow across atrioventricular valves that are closing rapidly during filling of the recipient ventricle.[78] A similar mechanism is believed to be responsible for the Austin Flint murmur (Fig. 3–31), as Flint originally described (see below).[81,82]

A mid-diastolic murmur is a feature of *pulmonary valve regurgitation* provided that the pulmonary arterial pressure is normal or low (Fig. 3–32*A*). The diastolic murmur typically begins at a perceptible interval after the pulmonic component of the second heart sound, and is crescendo-decrescendo, ending well before the subsequent second heart sound.[22] The physiological mechanism responsible for the timing of the murmur of low-pressure pulmonary regurgitation is shown in Figure 3–32*B*. The diastolic pressure exerted on the incompe-

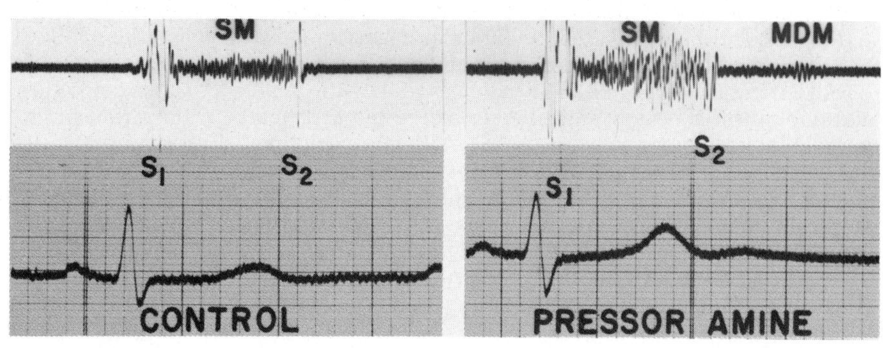

FIGURE 3–29. Phonocardiogram recorded over the left ventricular impulse of a patient with pure mitral regurgitation. When regurgitant flow is augmented in response to a pressor amine, the holosystolic crescendo murmur (SM) becomes more prominent and a mid-diastolic flow murmur (MDM) appears.

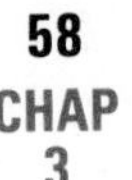

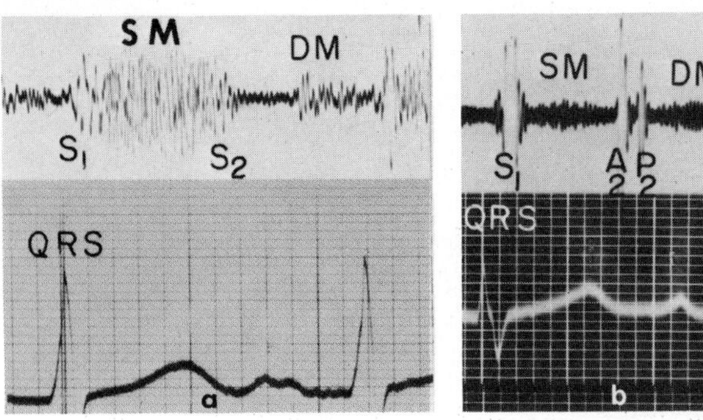

FIGURE 3–30. *A,* Phonocardiogram recorded at the apex of a patient with a moderately restrictive ventricular septal defect and increased pulmonary arterial blood flow. The mid-diastolic murmur (DM) results from augmented flow across the mitral valve. SM = holosystolic murmur; S_1 = first heart sound; S_2 = second heart sound. *B,* Phonocardiogram at the lower left sternal edge of a patient with an ostium secundum atrial septal defect and increased pulmonary arterial blood flow. A mid-diastolic murmur (DM) resulted from augmented flow across the tricuspid valve. SM = midsystolic murmur; A_2 and P_2 = aortic and pulmonic components of a conspicuously split second heart sound.

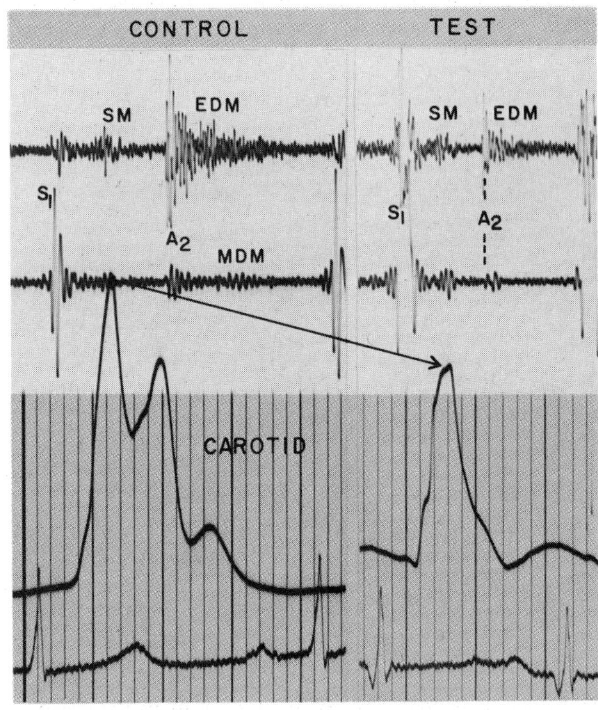

FIGURE 3–31. Phonocardiograms and simultaneous carotid pulse from a patient with chronic pure severe aortic regurgitation. Following amyl nitrite inhalation (test), the prominent early diastolic murmur (EDM) decreases, a mid-diastolic (MDM) Austin-Flint murmur disappears, and the bisferiens carotid pulse becomes single-peaked.

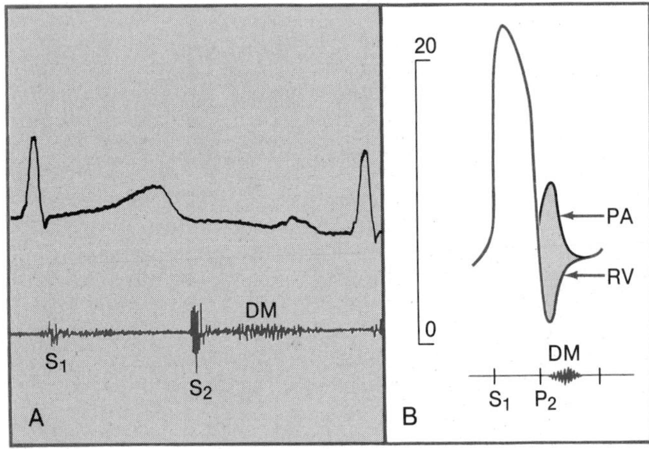

FIGURE 3–32. *A,* Phonocardiogram illustrating the mid-diastolic murmur (DM) of low-pressure pulmonary regurgitation in a heroin addict who had pulmonary valve infective endocarditis. The murmur begins well after the second heart sound (S_2), is medium-frequency and mid-diastolic, and ends well before the subsequent first heart sound (S_1). *B,* Pressure pulses and phonocardiogram illustrate the physiological mechanism of the mid-diastolic murmur of low-pressure pulmonary regurgitation. Because the pressure exerted against the incompetent pulmonic valve is low, the murmur does not begin until well after the right ventricular (RV) and pulmonary arterial (PA) pressure pulses diverge. The murmur is maximal when the diastolic gradient (shaded area) is greatest. Following an early diastolic dip in the RV pressure pulse, there is equilibration of the pulmonary arterial and right ventricular pressure in later diastole, so the regurgitant gradient disappears and the murmur disappears.

tent pulmonic valve is negligible at the inscription of the pulmonic component of the second sound, so regurgitant flow is minimal at that time. Regurgitation accelerates as right ventricular pressure dips below the diastolic pressure in the pulmonary trunk; at that point the murmur reaches its maximum (Fig. 3–32*B*). Late diastolic equilibration of pulmonary arterial and right ventricular pressures eliminates regurgitant flow and abolishes the murmur prior to the next first heart sound.

LATE DIASTOLIC OR PRESYSTOLIC MURMURS. A late diastolic murmur occurs immediately before the first heart sound, that is, in *presystole* (Fig. 3–26). With few exceptions, the late diastolic timing of the murmur coincides with the phase of ventricular filling that follows atrial systole and implies coordinated atrial contraction, generally sinus rhythm. Late diastolic or presystolic murmurs originate at the mitral or tricuspid orifice, usually because of obstruction, but occasionally because of abnormal patterns of presystolic atrioventricular flow.

The best known presystolic murmur accompanies rheumatic mitral stenosis in sinus rhythm as atrioventricular flow is augmented by an increase in the force of left atrial contraction (Figs. 3–11*B* and 3–33).[41] "Presystolic" accentuation of a mid-diastolic murmur is occasionally heard in mitral stenosis with atrial fibrillation, especially during short cycle lengths,[83,84] but the timing is actually early systolic, and the mechanism is different from the true presystolic murmur as shown in Figure 3–11*B*.

In *tricuspid stenosis* with sinus rhythm, a late diastolic or presystolic murmur typically occurs in the absence of a perceptible mid-diastolic murmur (Fig. 3–33*B*). This is so because the timing of tricuspid diastolic murmurs coincides with the maximal acceleration of flow and gradient, which is usually negligible until the powerful right atrium contracts.[80] The presystolic murmur of tricuspid stenosis is crescendo-decrescendo in shape and relatively discrete, fading in decrescendo before the first heart sound (Fig. 3–33*B*). This is in contrast to

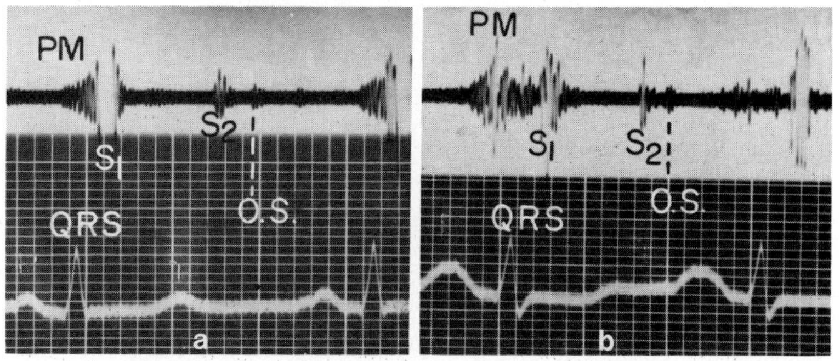

FIGURE 3-33. *A,* Phonocardiogram from the cardiac apex of a patient with pure rheumatic mitral stenosis. A presystolic murmur (PM) rises in crescendo to a loud first heart sound (S_1). S_2 = second heart sound; OS = mitral opening snap. *B,* Phonocardiogram from the lower left sternal edge of a patient with rheumatic tricuspid stenosis. The first cycle is during inspiration and is accompanied by a prominent presystolic murmur (PM) that is crescendo-decrescendo, decreasing before the first heart sound (S_1). During expiration (second cycle) the presystolic murmur all but vanishes.

the presystolic murmur of mitral stenosis, which tends to rise in crescendo to the first heart sound (Fig. 3-33*A*). The most valuable auscultatory sign of tricuspid stenosis in sinus rhythm is the effect of respiration on the intensity of the presystolic murmur. Inspiration increases right atrial volume, provoking an increase in right atrial contractile force in the face of a fall in right ventricular end-diastolic pressure. The result is an increase in the tricuspid gradient, the velocity of tricuspid flow, and the intensity of the tricuspid stenotic presystolic murmur (Fig. 3-33*B* and 3-34).

Short, crescendo-decrescendo presystolic murmurs are occasionally heard in *complete heart block* when atrial contraction fortuitously falls in late diastole. However, the diastolic murmur in complete heart block is usually mid-diastolic as already described, occurring when atrial contraction coincides with and reinforces the rapid filling phase of the cardiac cycle (Fig. 3-2).

In 1862, Austin Flint described a presystolic murmur in patients with aortic regurgitation and proposed a mechanism that was astonishingly perceptive.[81,82,85,86] "Now in cases of considerable aortic insufficiency, the left ventricle is rapidly filled with blood flowing back from the aorta as well as from the auricle, before the auricular contraction takes place. The distention of the ventricle is such that the mitral curtains are brought into coaptation, and when the auricular contraction takes place, the mitral direct current passing between the curtains throws them into vibration and gives rise to the characteristic blubbering murmur."[81]

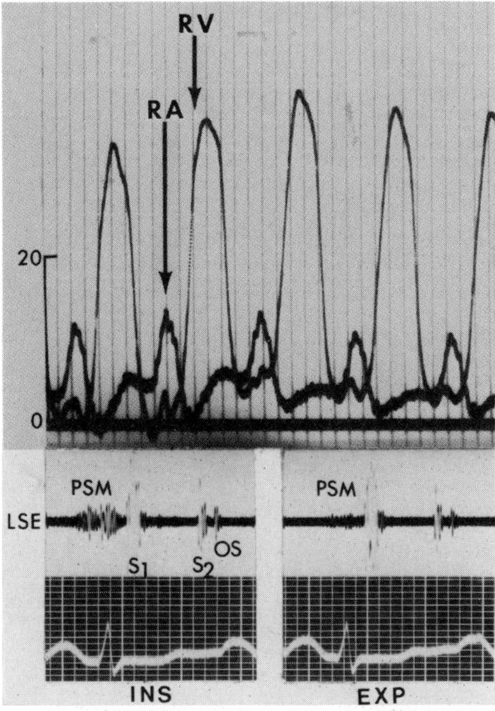

FIGURE 3-34. Pressure pulses and phonocardiogram illustrating the physiological mechanism of the respiratory variation in the presystolic murmur of tricuspid stenosis. During inspiration, a fall in intrathoracic pressure and a rise in systemic venous return result in an increase in the right atrial (RA) *a* wave and a decline in right ventricular (RV) end-diastolic pressure, so the presystolic murmur (PSM) increases in loudness. During expiration, the right atrial *a* wave declines, the right ventricular diastolic pressure increases, the tricuspid gradient is at its minimum, and the presystolic murmur all but vanishes.

CONTINUOUS MURMURS

(See also Table 2-6, p. 34)

The term "continuous" appropriately applies to murmurs that begin in systole and *continue* without interruption through the timing of the second heart sound into all or part of diastole (Fig. 3-35). The presence of murmurs throughout both phases of the cardiac cycle (holosystolic followed by holodiastolic) (Fig. 3-35) is not a requirement. Conversely, a murmur that fades completely before the subsequent first heart sound is continuous provided that the systolic murmur proceeds without interruption through the second heart sound (Fig. 3-35).

Continuous murmurs are generated by flow from a zone of higher resistance into a zone of lower resistance without phasic interruption between systole and diastole. Such murmurs are usually due to: (1) aortopulmonary connections, (2) arteriovenous connections, (3) disturbances of flow patterns in arteries, and (4) disturbances of flow patterns in veins (Fig. 3-35).

The best known continuous murmur is associated with the aortopulmonary connection of patent ductus arteriosus (Fig. 3-36). The murmur characteristically peaks just before and after the second heart sound, decreases appreciably in late diastole, and may be soft or even absent before the subsequent first heart sound.[22] In 1847, the *London Medical Gazette* published the description of "a murmur accompanying the first heart sound . . . prolonged into the second sound so that there is no cessation of the murmur before the second sound had already commenced."[87] The author correctly assigned the cause of the murmur to patent ductus arteriosus and established the proper meaning of "continuous" as "no cessation of the murmur before the second sound had already commenced." George Gibson's description in 1900 was even more precise.[88] "It persists through the second sound and dies away gradually during the long pause. The murmur is rough and thrilling. It begins softly and increases in intensity so as to reach its acme just about at, or immediately after, the incidence of the second sound, and from that point gradually wanes until its termination" (Fig. 3-36).

Arteriovenous continuous murmurs can be congenital or acquired and are represented in part by the murmurs of arteriovenous fistulas, coronary arterial fistulas, anomalous origin of the left coronary artery from the pulmonary trunk, and sinus of Valsalva-to-right heart communications.[22] The configuration, location, and intensity of arteriovenous continuous murmurs vary considerably among these different lesions. *Acquired* systemic arteriovenous fistulas occur after surgically created forearm connections created for chronic hemodialysis. A *congenital* arteriovenous continuous murmur occurs in the setting of a coronary arterial fistula that

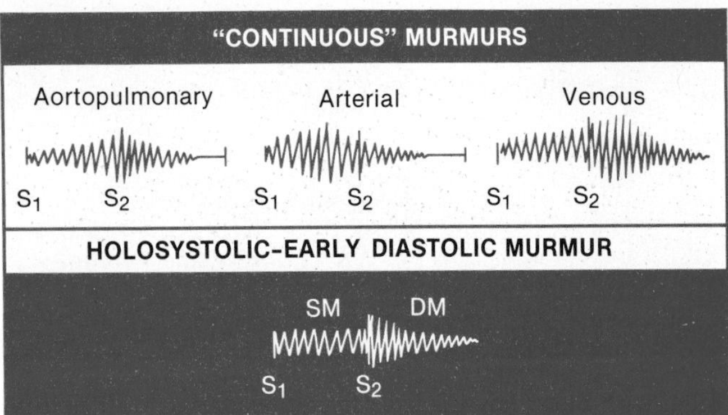

FIGURE 3-35. Continuous murmurs begin in systole and *continue* without interruption through the timing of the second heart sound (S_2) into all or part of diastole. The continuous murmurs shown here are aortopulmonary, systemic arterial, and venous. A holosystolic murmur (SM) followed by a holodiastolic murmur (DM) represents two separate murmurs, not one continuous murmur.

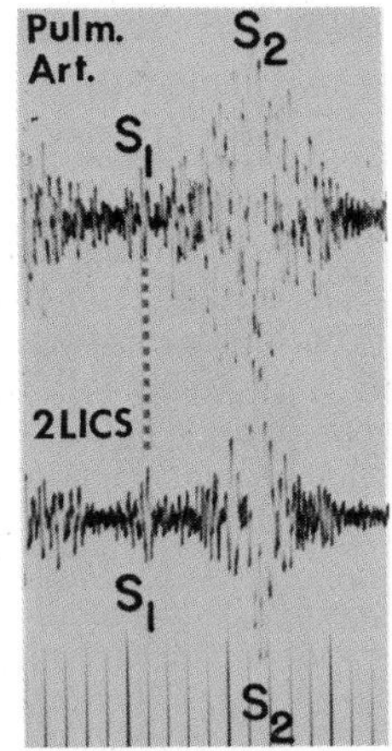

FIGURE 3-36. The classic continuous murmur of patent ductus arteriosus recorded from within the main pulmonary artery (*upper tracing*) and simultaneously at the second left intercostal space (2LICS). The murmur "begins softly and increases in intensity so as to reach its acme just about at, or immediately after the incidence of the second sound, and from that point gradually wanes until its termination," as originally described by Gibson in 1900.[88]

enters the pulmonary trunk, right atrium, or right ventricle. At the latter site, the continuous murmur can be either softer or louder in systole, depending on the degree of compression exerted on the fistulous coronary artery by right ventricular contraction.[22] Rupture of a congenital aortic sinus aneurysm into the right heart results in a continuous murmur that does not peak before and after the second sound but instead tends to be louder in either systole or diastole, sometimes creating a to-and-fro impression.

Arterial continuous murmurs originate in *constricted* or *nonconstricted* arteries. A common example of a continuous murmur arising in a constricted artery is atherosclerotic carotid or femoral arterial obstruction. Not surprisingly, these arterial continuous murmurs are characteristically louder in systole (Fig. 3-35) and more often than not are purely systolic rather than continuous.

Disturbances of flow patterns in *normal, nonconstricted* arteries sometimes produce continuous murmurs. The "mammary souffle" described earlier,[75] which is an innocent murmur heard during late pregnancy and the puerperium, is an arterial murmur that is sometimes continuous but typically louder in systole and maximal over either lactating breast. A distinct gap separates the first heart sound from the onset of the mammary souffle because of the interval that elapses before blood ejected from the left ventricle arrives at the artery of origin.[22] Light pressure with the stethoscope tends to augment the murmur and bring out its continuous features, whereas firm pressure with the stethoscope or by digital compression adjacent to the site of auscultation often abolishes the murmur.

Continuous murmurs originating in nonconstricted arteries can originate in the large systemic-to-pulmonary arterial collaterals in certain types of cyanotic congenital heart disease, typically Fallot's tetralogy with pulmonary atresia (Fig. 3-5). These continuous murmurs are randomly located throughout the thorax because of the random location of the aortopulmonary collaterals.[22]

Continuous venous murmurs are well-represented by the innocent cervical venous hum (Fig. 3-37) described by Potain in 1867[89] (Fig. 3-35, p. 60). The hum is far and away the most common type of normal continuous murmur, almost universal in healthy children and frequently present in healthy young adults, especially in women during pregnancy. Thyrotoxicosis and anemia, by augmenting cervical venous flow, initiate or reinforce the venous hum. The term "hum" does not necessarily characterize the quality of these cervical venous murmurs, which may be rough and noisy and are occasionally accompanied by a high-pitched whine.[22] The hum is truly continuous, although typically louder in diastole, as is the case with venous continuous murmurs in general (Fig. 3-35). The mechanism of the venous hum is unsettled. Silent laminar flow in the internal jugular vein may be disturbed by deformation of the vessel at the level of the transverse process of the atlas during head rotation designed to elicit the hum.[90]

PERICARDIAL RUBS

(See also Chap. 45)

In sinus rhythm, the classic pericardial rub is triple-phased, that is, midsystolic, mid-diastolic, and presystolic.[91] Recognition is simplest when all three phases are present, and when

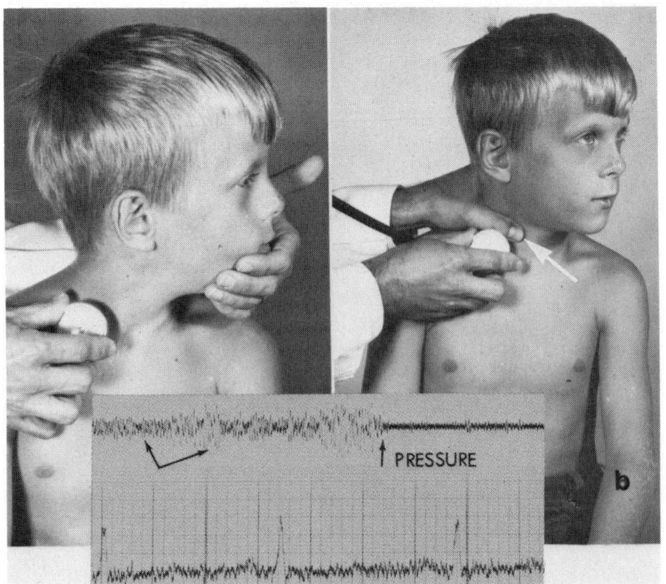

FIGURE 3-37. The phonocardiogram shows the continuous murmur of a normal venous hum. The *diastolic* component is louder (paired arrows). Digital pressure over the right internal jugular vein (vertical arrow) abolishes the murmur. The accompanying photographs show maneuvers used to elicit or abolish the venous hum. *Left,* The bell of the stethoscope is applied to the medial aspect of the right supraclavicular fossa as the examiner's left hand grasps the patient's chin from behind and pulls it tautly to the left and upward, stretching the neck. *Right,* The patient's head has returned to a more neutral position, and digital compression of the right internal jugular vein (arrow) abolishes the hum.

the typical superficial scratchy, leathery quality is evident. The term "rub" is appropriate because the auscultatory sign is generated by abnormal visceral and parietal surfaces "rubbing" against each other. In the supine position, firm pressure with the stethoscopic diaphragm during full held expiration serves to reinforce visceral and parietal pericardial contact and to accentuate the rub. Apposition of visceral and parietal pericardium can be even better achieved by examination while the patient rests on elbows and knees.

Of the three phases of the pericardial rub, the systolic phase is the most consistent, followed by the presystolic phase. In atrial fibrillation, the presystolic component necessarily disappears. A corollary is that the diagnosis of a pericardial rub is least secure (and often impossible) when only one phase remains, typically the midsystolic. The most common clinical setting in which pericardial rubs are heard is following open heart surgery. However, auscultation may detect instead a "crunch" synchronous with the heartbeat and heard over the cardiac apex, especially in the left lateral decubitus position. This is not a pericardial rub but rather *Hamman's sign* caused by air in the mediastinum.[92]

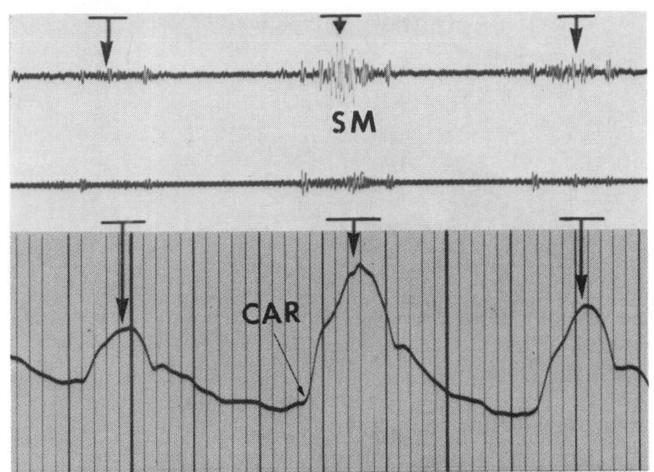

FIGURE 3-38. Phonocardiogram from the right base and apex of a 58-year-old man with an aortic sclerotic midsystolic murmur (SM). The intensity of the murmur varies with the pulsus alternans of a simultaneously recorded carotid arterial pulse (CAR).

PHYSICAL MANEUVERS

(See also pp. 36 to 41 and Figs. 2-26, p. 39; 2-27, p. 40; Tables 2-7, p. 37, and 2-8, p. 38)

A number of physical maneuvers that influence heart sounds and murmurs have already been discussed and will now be brought into focus.[26,27] Pharmacological interventions, except for amyl nitrite inhalation, will not be dealt with because they are less practical at the bedside. They are discussed on p. 40.

Changes in position that are useful in assessing heart sounds and murmurs are listed in Table 3-1. A partial *left lateral decubitus position* assists in identifying the left ventricular impulse, which is an important auscultatory site. During the act of turning, the heart rate sometimes transiently increases sufficiently to improve audibility of mid-diastolic and presystolic murmurs of mitral stenosis. The left lateral decubitus position occasionally results in premature ventricular beats that may assist in distinguishing an aortic midsystolic murmur heard at the apex from the apical murmur of mitral regurgitation (Fig. 3-18) and may initiate pulsus alternans with alternation of the murmur (Fig. 3-38).

Sitting and leaning forward in full expiration assists in detecting soft, high-frequency early diastolic murmurs of aortic regurgitation or high-pressure pulmonary regurgitation (Graham Steell). *Standing, squatting, and prompt standing* are maneuvers that influence both systemic vascular resistance and left ventricular volume, and are useful in assessing the murmurs of aortic and mitral regurgitation, mitral valve prolapse (Fig. 3-8), and hypertrophic obstructive cardiomyopathy.[27]

Hyperextension of the shoulders is an important positional maneuver in assessing supraclavicular systolic murmurs (Fig.3-25).[74] The mechanism responsible for diminution of supraclavicular systolic murmurs with hyperextension of the shoulders apparently relates to the effect of the maneuver on the site of origin of the murmurs in the proximal brachiocephalic arteries as they leave the aortic arch.

TABLE 3-1 CHANGES IN POSITION DURING AUSCULTATION

Left lateral decubitus
Sitting, leaning forward
Sitting with legs dangling
Standing to squatting and vice versa
Hyperextension of the shoulders
"Stretching" of the neck
Passive elevation of the legs
Elevation of precordium on elbows and knees

Passive elevation of both legs with the patient supine transiently increases venous return and augments third heart sounds. Pericardial rubs may be more readily detected when the patient is examined on the *elbows and knees*, a physical maneuver designed to increase the contact of visceral and parietal pericardium (see earlier).

Physical maneuvers other than positional changes include respiration, the Valsalva and Müller maneuvers, and isometric exercise (sustained handgrip).[27] Respiration is routinely employed in the form of normal inspiration and expiration. *Exaggerated respiratory excursions* are useful for analysis of splitting of the second heart sound, right-sided third and fourth heart sounds, tricuspid systolic and diastolic murmurs, and pulmonic ejection sounds. *Full held expiration* is employed when searching for the soft, early diastolic murmur of aortic regurgitation or pulmonary hypertensive pulmonary regurgitation while the patient sits and leans forward. A subtle pericardial friction rub may be more audible during held exhalation while the patient is supine. Innocent pulmonic midsystolic murmurs associated with a decreased anteroposterior chest dimension (loss of thoracic kyphosis) may appreciably amplify when the diaphragm of the stethoscope is pressed firmly in the second left intercostal space during full held expiration, a maneuver designed to bring the pulmonary trunk close to the chest wall.

THE VALSALVA MANEUVER. This procedure was described in 1704 as a method for expelling pus from the middle ear by straining with the mouth and nose closed.[22] The normal Valsalva response consists of four phases. *Phase I* is associated with a transient rise in systemic blood pressure as straining commences. This phase cannot, as a rule, be identified at the bedside. *Phase II* is accompanied by a perceptible decrease in blood pressure and pulse pressure (small pulse) and readily detectible reflex tachycardia. *Phase III* begins with cessation of straining and is associated with an abrupt, transient decrease in blood pressure. Phase III is generally not perceived at the bedside and is followed promptly by *phase IV*, which is characterized by an overshoot of systemic arterial pressure and relatively obvious reflex bradycardia.

THE MÜLLER MANEUVER. This maneuver is the converse of the Valsalva maneuver but is less frequently employed because it is not as useful.[26] The maneuver is continued for about 10 seconds as the patient forcibly *inspires* while the nose is held closed and the mouth firmly sealed. The Müller manuever exaggerates the inspiratory effort and occa-

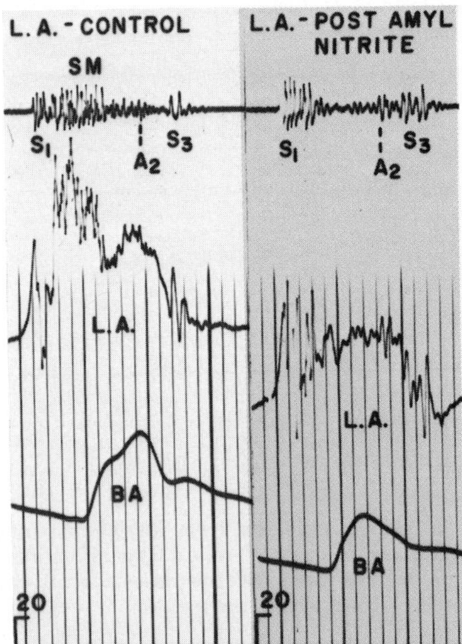

FIGURE 3-39. Phonocardiogram recorded from within the left atrium (LA, *top tracing*) with simultaneous left atrial and brachial arterial (BA) pressure pulses in a patient with mitral regurgitation. After amyl nitrite inhalation, the holosystolic decrescendo murmur (SM) in the control tracing vanishes as the left atrial and brachial arterial pressures decline. S_1 = first heart sound; S_3 = third heart sound.

sionally augments the murmur of tricuspid regurgitation or stenosis.

ISOMETRIC EXERCISE. This is best generated by sustained handgrip and is a useful, simple, safe maneuver readily performed at the bedside. The physiological response to sustained handgrip is an increase in systolic blood pressure, an increase in left ventricular systolic pressure and end-diastolic pressure, and an increase in heart rate and cardiac index, with prompt return to control values on cessation of the maneuver. The duration of handgrip depends in part on when and whether a positive auscultatory response is elicited. As a rule, 20 seconds of maximum isometric exercise more than suffices. The physiological response to sustained handgrip reinforces left ventricular fourth heart sounds; the murmurs of mitral and aortic regurgitation get louder. The click(s) of mitral valve prolapse occur later in systole, and the late systolic murmur shortens but increases in intensity. The systolic murmur of hypertrophic obstructive cardiomyopathy decreases in response to the isometric exercise of sustained handgrip.

AMYL NITRITE INHALATION. Of the many pharmacological interventions, *amyl nitrite inhalation* occasionally has a place in analyses of heart sounds and murmurs. The drug results in a prompt fall in systemic vascular resistance and blood pressure and an increase in heart rate, cardiac output, and ejection velocity.[93] The auscultatory effects of amyl nitrite inhalation mirror these hemodynamic effects. An increase in cardiac output and ejection velocity is accompanied by an increase in loudness of the systolic murmur of aortic stenosis or of isolated pulmonary stenosis. A decrease in systemic vascular resistance is accompanied by a decrease in the systolic murmur of mitral regurgitation (Fig. 3-39) and in the diastolic murmur of aortic regurgitation (Fig. 3-31). The mid- to late systolic clicks and the late systolic murmur of mitral valve prolapse occur earlier (reduction in left ventricular volume), and the murmur becomes softer (decreased resistance to left ventricular discharge) (Fig. 3-24). In hypertrophic obstructive cardiomyopathy, the systolic murmur intensifies because amyl nitrite causes a decrease in left ventricular volume and an increase in ejection velocity.

REFERENCES

HISTORICAL CONSIDERATIONS

1. Perloff, J. K.: Physical Examination of the Heart and Circulation. 2nd ed. Philadelphia, W. B. Saunders Company, 1990.
2. Harvey, W.: An Anatomical Disquisition on the Motion of the Heart and Blood in Animals. London, 1628 (translated from the Latin by Robert Willis, Barnes, Surrey, England, 1847). *In* Williams, F. A., and Keys, T. E. (eds.): Classics of Cardiology. Vol. 1. Malabar, FL., Robert E. Krieger Publishing Co., 1983.
3. Hooke, R.: The Posthumous Works of Robert Hooke, containing his Cutlerian Lectures and Other Discourses Read at the Meeting of the Illustrious Royal Society. *In* McKusick, V. A.: Cardiovascular Sound. Baltimore, William and Wilkins Co., 1958.
4. Laënnec, R.T.H.: A Treatise on the Diseases of the Chest (translated by John Forbes). Philadelphia, James Webster, 1823.
5. McKusick, V. A.: Cardiovascular Sound in Health and Disease. Baltimore, Williams and Wilkins, 1958.
6. Einthoven, W., and Geluk, M.A.J.: Die regostroerimg der herztone. Pflugers Arch. ges. Physiol. *57*:617, 1894.
7. Rappaport, M. B., and Sprague, H. B.: The graphic registration of the normal heart sounds. Am. Heart J. *23*:591, 1942.
8. Wood, P.: Diseases of the Heart and Circulation. Philadelphia, J. B. Lippincott Co., 1956.
9. Leatham, A.: Auscultation and phonocardiography: a personal view of the past 40 years. Br. Heart J. *57*:397, 1987.
10. Mills, P. G., and Craige, E.: Echophonocardiography. Prog. Cardiovasc. Dis. *20*:337, 1978.
11. Craige, E.: On the genesis of heart sounds: Contribution made by echocardiographic studies. Circulation *53*:207, 1976.
12. Stokes, W.: An Introduction to the Use of the Stethoscope. Edinburgh, Maclachlan and Stewart, 1825.
13. Craige, E.: Should auscultation be rehabilitated? N. Engl. J. Med. *318*:1611, 1988.
14. Latham, P. M.: Lectures on Subjects Connected with Clinical Medicine Comprising Diseases of the Heart. Philadelphia, Barrington and Hoswell, 1847.

THE HEART SOUNDS

15. Leatham, A.: Auscultation of the heart. Lancet *II*:703, 1958.
16. O'Toole, J. D., Reddy, P. S., Curtiss, E. L., et al.: The contribution of tricuspid valve closure to the first heart sound. An intracardiac micromanometer study. Circulation *53*:752, 1976.
17. Brooks, N., Leech, G., and Leatham, A.: Complete right bundle branch block: Echophonocardiographic study of the first heart sound and right ventricular contraction times. Br. Heart J. *41*:637, 1979.
18. Burggraf, G. W.: The first heart sound in left bundle branch block: An echophonocardiographic study. Circulation *63*:429, 1981.
19. Burggraf, G. W., and Craige E.: The first heart sound in complete heart block. Circulation *50*:17, 1974.
20. Leech, G., Brooks, N., Green-Wilkinson, A., and Leatham, A.: Mechanism of influence of PR interval on loudness of first heart sound. Br. Heart J. *43*:138, 1980.
21. Waider, W., and Craige, E.: The first heart sound and ejection sounds: Echophonocardiographic correlation wih valvular events. Am. J. Cardiol. *35*:346, 1975.
22. Perloff, J. K.: The Clinical Recognition of Congenital Heart Disease. Philadelphia, W. B. Saunders Company, 1987.
23. Mills, P. G., Brodie, B., McLaurin, L., et al.: Echocardiographic and hemodynamic relationships of ejection sounds. Circulation *56*:430, 1977.
24. Hultgren, H. N., Reeve, R., Cohn, K., and McLeod, R.: The ejection click of valvular pulmonic stenosis. Circulation *40*:631, 1969.
25. Devereux, R., Perloff, J. K., Derchek, N., and Josephson, M.: Mitral valve prolapse. Circulation *54*:3, 1976.
26. Rothman, A., and Goldberger, A. L.: Aids to cardiac auscultation. Ann. Intern. Med. *99*:346, 1983.
27. Lembo, N. J., Dell'Italia, J. L., Crawford, M. H., and O'Rourke, R. A.: Bedside diagnosis of systolic murmurs. N. Engl. J. Med. *318*:1572, 1988.
28. Potain, P. C.: Clinique médicale de la Charité. Paris, Masson, 1894. *In* McKusick, V. A.: Cardiovascular Sound in Health and Disease. Baltimore, Williams and Wilkins, 1958.
29. Potain, P. C.: Note sur les dédoublements normaux des bruits du coeur. Bull. Mem. Soc. Med. Hop. Paris. *3*:138, 1866.
30. Leatham, A.: The second heart sound. Key to auscultation of the heart. Acta Cardiol. *19*:395, 1964.
31. Leatham, A.: Splitting of the first and second heart sounds. Lancet *II*:607, 1954.
32. Kupari, M.: Aortic valve closure and cardiac vibrations in the genesis of the second heart sound. Am. J. Cardiol. *52*:152, 1983.
33. Curtiss, E. I., Matthews, D. G., and Shaver, J. A.: Mechanism of normal splitting of the second heart sound. Circulation *51*:157, 1975.
34. Shaver, J. A., Nadolny, R. A., O'Toole, J. D., et al.: Sound-pressure correlates of the second heart sound. Circulation *49*:316, 1974.
35. Perloff, J. K, and Harvey, W. P.: Auscultatory and phonocardiographic manifestations of pure mitral regurgitation. Prog. Cardiovasc. Dis. *5*:172, 1962.
36. Hultgren, H. N., Craige, E., Nakamura, T., and Bilisoly, J.: Left bundle

branch block and mechanical events of the cardiac cycle. Am. J. Cardiol. 52:755, 1985.

37. Perloff, J. K.: Auscultatory and phonocardiographic manifestations of pulmonary hypertension. Prog. Cardiovasc. Dis. 9:303, 1967.
38. Steell, G.: The murmur of high pressure in the pulmonary artery. Med. Chron. (Manchester) 9:182, 1888–1889.
39. de Leon, A. C., Perloff, J. K., Twigg, H., and Moyd, M.: The straight back syndrome. Circulation 32:193, 1965.
40. Thayer, W. S.: On the early diastolic sound (the so-called third heart sound). Boston Med. Surg. J. 158:713, 1908.
41. Wood, P.: An appreciation of mitral stenosis. I. Clinical features. Br. Med. J. 1:1051, 1954; II. Investigations and results. 1:1113, 1954.
42. Joyner, C. R., Jr., and Dear, W. E.: The motion of the normal and abnormal mitral valve. A study of the opening snap. J. Clin. Invest. 45:1029, 1966.
43. Connolly, D. C., and Mann, R. J.: Dominic J. Corrigan (1802–1880) and his description of the pericardial knock. Mayo Clin. Proc. 55:771, 1980.
44. Tyberg, T. I, Goodyer, A. V. N., and Langou, R. A.: Genesis of the pericardial knock in constrictive pericarditis. Am. J. Cardiol. 46:570, 1980.
45. Bass, N. M., and Sharatt, G. J. P.: Left atrial myxoma diagnosed by echocardiography with observations on tumor movement. Br. Heart J. 35:1332, 1973.
46. Van de Werf, F., Minten, J., Carmeliet, P., et al.: Genesis of the third and fourth heart sounds. J. Clin. Invest. 73:1400, 1984.
47. Van de Werf, F., Boel, A., Geboers, J., et al.: Diastolic properties of the left ventricle in normal adults and in patients with third heart sounds. Circulation 69:1070, 1984.
48. Potain, P. C.: Concerning the cardiac rhythm called gallop rhythm. Bull. Men. Soc. Med. Hop. (Paris) 12:137, 1876.
49. Van de Werf, F., Geboers, J., Math, L., et al.: The mechanism of disappearance of the physiologic third heart sound with age. Circulation 73:877, 1986.
50. Aronow, W. S., Papageorge's, N. P., Uyeyama, R. R., and Cassidy, J.: Maximal treadmill stress test correlated with postexercise phonocardiogram in normal subjects. Circulation 43:884, 1971.
51. Ozawa, Y., Smith D., and Craige, E.: Origin of the third heart sound. I. Studies in dogs. Circulation 67:393, 1983.
52. Ozawa, Y., Smith, D., and Craige, E.: Origin of the third heart sound. II. Studies in human subjects. Circulation 67:399, 1983.
53. Ishimitsu, T., Smith, D., Berko, B., and Craige, E.: Origin of the third heart sound: comparison of ventricular wall dynamics in hyperdynamic and hypodynamic types. J. Am. Coll. Cardiol. 5:268, 1985.
54. Gibson, T. C., Madry, R., Grossman, W., et al.: The A wave of the apex cardiogram and left ventricular diastolic stiffness. Circulation 49:441, 1974.
55. Perloff, J. K.: Clinical recognition of aortic stenosis. Progr. Cardiovasc. Dis. 10:323, 1964.
56. Cheng, T. O., Ertem, G., and Vera, Z.: Heart sounds in patients with cardiac pacemakers. Chest 62:66, 1972.
57. Harris, A.: Pacemaker "heart sound." Br. Heart. J. 29:608, 1967.

MURMURS

58. Pepper, O.H.P.: Medical Etymology. Philadelphia, W. B. Saunders Company, 1949.
59. Freeman, A. R., and Levin, S. A.: The clinical significance of the systolic murmur. A study of 1000 consecutive "non-cardiac" cases Ann. Intern. Med. 6:1371, 1933.
60. Roberts, W. C., Perloff, J. K., and Costantino, T.: Severe valvular aortic stenosis in patients over 65 years of age. Am. J. Cardiol. 27:497, 1971.
61. Gallavardin, L., and Pauper-Ravault: Le souffle du rétré cissement aortique peut changer de timbre et devenir musical dans se propagation apexienne. Lyon Med. 1925, p. 523.
62. Stokes, W.: Diseases of the Heart in Aorta. Philadelphia, Lindsay and Blakiston, 1855.
63. Still, G. F.: Common Disorders and Diseases of Childhood. London, Henry Frowde, 1909.
64. Burch, G. E., DePasquale, N. P., and Phillips, J. H.: The syndrome of papillary muscle dysfunction. Am. Heart J. 75:399, 1968.
65. Perloff, J. K., and Roberts, W. C.: The mitral appartus: functional anatomy of mitral regurgitation. Circulation 46:227, 1972.
66. Rivero-Carvallo, J. M.: Sitno para el diagnostico de las insuficiencias tricuspideas. Arch. Inst. Cardiol. Mexico 16:531, 1946.
67. Leon, D. F., Leonard, J. J., Lancaster, J. F., et al.: Effect of respiration on pansystolic regurgitant murmurs as studied by biatrial intracardiac phonocardiography. Am. J. Med. 39:429, 1965.
68. Sanders, C. A., Scannell, J. G., Harthorne, J. W., and Austen, W. G.: Severe mitral regurgitation secondary to ruptured chordae tendineae. Circulation 31:506, 1965.
69. Sutton, G. C., and Craige, E.: Clinical signs of acute severe mitral regurgitation. Am. J. Cardiol. 20:141, 1967.
70. Ronan, J. A., Steelman, R. B., DeLeon, A. C., et al.: The clinical diagnosis of acute severe mitral insufficiency. Am. J. Cardiol. 27:284, 1971.
71. Rios, J. C., Massumi, R. A., Breesman, W. T., and Sarin, R. K.: Auscultatory features of acute tricuspid regurgitation. Am. J. Cardiol. 23:4, 1969.
72. Ronan, J. A., Perloff, J. K., and Harvey, W. P.: Systolic clicks and the late systolic murmur—intracardiac phonocardiographic evidence of their mitral valve origin. Am. Heart J. 70:319, 1965.
73. Osler, W.: On a remarkable heart murmur, heard at a distance from the chest wall. Med. Times Gaz. Lond. 2:432, 1980.
74. Nelson, W. P., and Hall, R. J.: The innocent supraclavicular arterial bruit—utility of shoulder maneuvers in its recognition. N. Engl. J. Med. 278:778, 1968.
75. Grant, R. P.: A precordial systolic murmur of extracardiac origin during pregnancy. Am. Heart J. 52:944, 1965.
76. Danilowicz, D. A., Rudolph, A. M., Hoffman, J.I.E., and Heyman, M.: Physiologic pressure differences between the main and branch pulmonary arteries in infants. Circulation 45:410, 1972.
77. Morganroth, J., Perloff, J. K., Zeldis, S. M., and Dunkman, W. B.: Acute severe aortic regurgitation: pathophysiology, clinical recognition and management. Ann. Intern. Med. 87:223, 1977.
78. Fortuin, N. J., and Craige, E.: Echocardiographic studies of genesis of mitral diastolic murmurs. Br. Heart J. 35:75, 1973.
79. Ross, R. S., and Criley, J. M.: Cineangiocardiographic studies of the origin of cardiovascular physical signs. Circulation 30:255, 1964.
80. Perloff, J. K., and Harvey, W. P.: Clinical recognition of tricuspid stenosis. Circulation 22:346, 1960.
81. Flint, A.: On cardiac murmurs. Am. J. Med. Sci. 44:23, 1862.
82. Fortuin, N. J., and Craige, E.: On the mechanisms of the Austin Flint murmur. Circulation 45:558, 1972.
83. Criley, J. M., and Hermer, H. A.: Crescendo pre-systolic murmur of mitral stenosis with atrial fibrillation. N. Engl. J. Med. 285:1284, 1971.
84. Criley, J. M., Feldman, J. M., and Meredith, T.: Mitral valve closure and the crescendo presystolic murmur. Am. J. Med. 51:456, 1971.
85. Reddy, P. S., Curtiss, E. L., and Salerni, R.: Sound-pressure correlates of the Austin Flint murmur: An intracardiac sound study. Circulation 53:210, 1976.
86. Berman, P.: Austin Flint—America's Laënnec revisited. Arch. Intern. Med. 148:2053, 1988.
87. Williams, X.: Comment in discussion of case of patent ductus arteriosus with aortic valve disease, coarctation of aorta and infective endocarditis reported by Babington. London Med. Gazette 4:822, 1847.
88. Gibson, G. A.: Persistence of the arterial duct and its diagnosis. Edinb. Med. J. 8:1, 1900.
89. Potain, P. C.: Des movements et de bruits qui se passent dans les veines jugulaires. Bull. Mem. Soc. Med. Hop. Paris 4:3, 1867.
90. Cutforth, R., Wideman, J., and Sutherland, R. D.: The genesis of the cervical venous hum. Am. Heart J. 80:488, 1970.
91. McGuire, J., Kotte, J. H., and Helm, R. A.: Acute pericarditis. Circulation 9:425, 1954.
92. Hamman, L.: Mediastinal emphysema. J. A. M. A. 128:1, 1945.
93. Perloff, J. K., Calvin, J., de Leon, A. C., and Bowen, P.: Systemic hemodynamic effects of amyl nitrite in normal man. Am. Heart J. 66:460, 1963.

4

Echocardiography

by HARVEY FEIGENBAUM, M.D.

PRINCIPLES OF ECHOCARDIOGRAPHY

CREATION OF IMAGES USING PULSED REFLECTED ULTRASOUND

The term *echocardiography* refers to a group of tests that utilize ultrasound to examine the heart and record information in the form of echoes, i.e., reflected sonic waves.[1-3] The upper limit for audible sound is 20,000 cycles/second, or 20 kiloHertz (kHz = 1000 cycles/second).[1] The sonic frequency used for echocardiography ranges from 1 to 10 million cycles/second, or 1 to 10 megaHertz (MHz).[2] In adults the frequencies commonly employed are 2.0 to 5.0 MHz, while in children they are usually higher, ranging from 3.5 to 10.0 MHz. The *resolution* of the recording, which is the ability to distinguish two objects that are spatially close together, varies directly with the frequency and inversely with the wave length. High-frequency (short wave length) ultrasound can identify separate objects that are less than 1 mm apart. Beams having lower frequencies and longer wave lengths have poorer resolution. However, the degree of *penetration,* which is the ability to transmit sufficient ultrasonic energy into the chest to provide a satisfactory recording, is inversely proportional to the frequency of the signal. Since a high-frequency ultrasonic beam (i.e., 5 or 10 MHz) is unable to penetrate a thick chest wall, lower frequency ultrasonic beams are used in adults. While this permits penetration through the chest wall, it partially sacrifices resolution; however, even with a transducer producing a beam of 2.50 MHz, which is commonly used in adult echocardiography, it is still possible to resolve objects that are 1 to 2 mm apart.

PRINCIPLES OF ULTRASOUND IMAGING. The principles by which ultrasound creates an image are depicted in Figure 4–1. The transducer at the side of the beaker of water has a piezoelectric element that vibrates very rapidly and produces ultrasound when activated by an electrical field.[3] If a burst of electrical energy is imparted to the transducer, it will emit a burst of ultrasound, which travels through the beaker. As long as the medium through which the sound travels is homogeneous, the ultrasonic waves will travel in a straight line. When the ultrasound strikes an interface between two media that have different acoustical properties, the sound behaves according to the laws of reflection and refraction,[1,2] analogous to light. Whether or not ultrasound is reflected by an interface depends upon the difference in the acoustical impedances of the two media. Although acoustical impedance is the product of the density of the object and the velocity of sound through that object, for all practical purposes one can consider the acoustical impedance to be a function of density. Thus, if the interface is between a liquid and a solid, the ultrasonic wave will generally be reflected. If the interface is between two solids of different densities, the quantity of reflected ultrasound is usually less. Thus, the quantity of energy reflected is directly proportional to the difference in the acoustical impedances (or densities) of the object and its surrounding media.

The left panel of Figure 4–1 shows diagrammatically an ultrasonic beam, which consists of individual bursts of ultrasound that leave the transducer, travel through the fluid, strike the far side of the beaker, are reflected by this interface, retrace their original path, and again strike the transducer. The piezoelectric element in the transducer not only converts electrical energy into ultrasonic impulses but also converts ultrasound back to electrical energy. Thus, when the reflected ultrasound (echo) strikes the piezoelectric element in the transducer, an electrical signal is produced. If the time it takes for (a) the ultrasound to leave the transducer

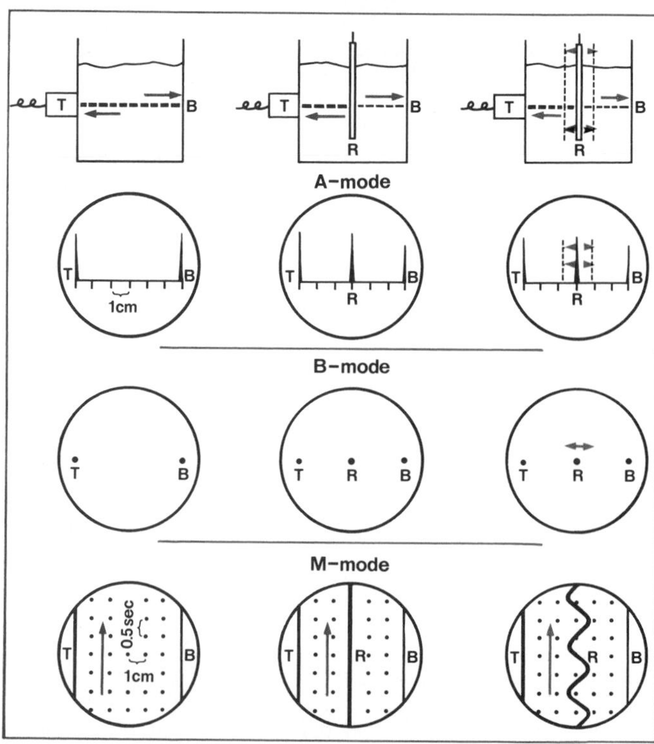

FIGURE 4–1. Diagrams illustrating the principles of acoustic imaging using pulsed reflected ultrasound (see text for details). T = transducer, B = beaker, R = rod. (Modified from Feigenbaum, H., and Zaky, A.: Use of diagnostic ultrasound in clinical cardiology. J. Indiana State Med. Assoc. *59*:140, 1966.)

and return and (b) the velocity of sound through the medium are both known, the distance between the transducer and the reflected interface can be calculated. By calibration of the echograph for a velocity of sound in the medium under examination, the time that it takes for the ultrasound to leave and return as an echo can be automatically converted to distance. Thus, the far wall of the beaker is depicted on the oscilloscope as being 6 cm from the transducer.

If a rod is placed in the water so that it transects the ultrasonic beam, part of the energy will strike and be reflected by the rod before the beam strikes the far side of the beaker. Thus, the returning ultrasonic energy or echo from the rod will strike the transducer sooner than that returning from the far side of the beaker, and the corresponding electrical signal produced by the echo from the rod will be closer to the transducer than will that from the beaker. Also, since some of the ultrasonic energy is reflected by the rod, less energy will remain to strike the far wall of the beaker, and the magnitude of the echo (Fig. 4–1, center panel) will be reduced. If the interface is a very strong reflector of sound, no energy may traverse the object and no images are obtained behind the object, i.e., acoustic shadowing. There are adjustments in ultrasonic instrumentation which provide depth compensation and thereby correct for the usually gradual loss of ultrasonic energy from distant or far objects. From examination of the A-mode echo ("A" refers to amplitude) in Figure 4–1 (center panel), one could deduce that the far wall of the beaker is 6 cm from the transducer and that an echo-reflecting object is present in the center of the beaker, 3 cm from the transducer.

IMAGING A MOVING OBJECT. If the rod were moving back and forth as in the right panel of Figure 4–1, the ultrasonic examination would differ. The transducer functions as a transmitter of ultrasound for a very short period of time, just over 1 μsec in commercial echocardiographs. During the remaining time the transducer functions as a receiver, waiting for echoes to be converted into electrical signals. The rapidity or the repetition rate with which the transducer fires the 1 μsec impulses varies depending upon the design of the instrument. In most situations the transducer functions as a receiver for over 90 per cent of the time.

A-MODE, B-MODE, AND M-MODE PRESENTATIONS. In the left and center panels of Figure 4–1, the wall of the beaker and the rod are not moving. All the ultrasonic impulses firing at a rate of 1000/sec take the same time to leave the transducer and return as echoes. Therefore, the signals or echoes seen on the oscilloscope are static. In the right panel, the object moves constantly and therefore the time required for the ultrasound to leave the transducer and return as an echo varies correspondingly and the echo signal on the oscilloscope moves. In the A-mode presentation the echo from the rod moves back and forth within the center of the beaker. To record the motion of the rod, one converts the amplitude of the echo to brightness, which changes the display from the A-mode to the B-mode (the "B" refers to brightness), in which the returning echoes are displayed on the oscilloscope as dots rather than as spikes. Stronger signals are therefore taller on the A-mode and brighter on the B-mode presentation. On the M-mode presentation ("M" refers to motion) displayed in Figure 4–1, the oscilloscope sweeps from bottom to top. In the left and center panels the structures are fixed, and therefore the M-mode presentation shows simply a series of parallel lines. In the right panel the rod moves back and forth in a regular manner, its echo inscribing a sinusoidal curve on the M-mode oscilloscope.

Thus, the M-mode presentation permits recording of amplitude and of the rate of motion of moving objects with great accuracy; the sampling rate is essentially 1000 pulses/second, the repetition rate of the transducer. Since electrocardiograms and other cardiac parameters are conventionally displayed on the oscilloscope together with the echocardiographs, the oscilloscope usually sweeps from left to right rather than from bottom to top; therefore, the transducer is generally displayed at the top of the oscilloscopic image rather than on the left side, as depicted in Figure 4–1.

M-MODE ECHOCARDIOGRAPHY

TECHNIQUE. The ultrasonic transducer is ordinarily placed on the surface of the chest, usually along the left sternal border, and the ultrasonic beam is directed toward the part of the heart to be examined. In Figure 4–2 the ultrasound is depicted as passing through a small portion of the right ventricle, the interventricular septum, and the cavity and posterior wall of the left ventricle. Structures such as the chest wall which do not move with cardiac activity are depicted as horizontal lines. Cardiac walls and valves that move with cardiac action inscribe wavy signals, while the blood-filled cavities are relatively echo-free.

THE M-MODE TRACING. An M-mode recording is sometimes called a one-dimensional or an "ice-pick" view of the heart. However, since time is the second dimension on M-mode tracings, this display is not truly one-dimensional. The information provided by an isolated M-mode views of the heart, such as in Figure 4–2, can be augmented by changing the direction of the ultrasonic beam, as in an arc or sector. With the transducer placed along the left sternal border in approximately the third or fourth intercostal space, the ultrasonic beam can be swept in a sector between the apex and the base of the heart. When the transducer is pointed toward the apex of the heart, the ultrasonic beam traverses the left ventricular cavity at the level of the papillary muscles and passes through a small portion of the right ventricular cavity (Fig. 4–3, position 1). Tilting the transducer superiorly and medially causes the ultrasonic beam to traverse the left ventricular cavity at the level of the edges of the mitral valve leaflets or the chordae (position 2). The beam again passes through a small portion of the right ventricle. By directing the transducer more superiorly and medially (position 3), more of the anterior leaflet of the mitral valve can be recorded and the beam may traverse part of the left atrial cavity. Further tilting of the transducer superiorly and medially (position 4) directs the beam through the root of the aorta, the leaflets of the aortic valve, and the body of the left atrium.

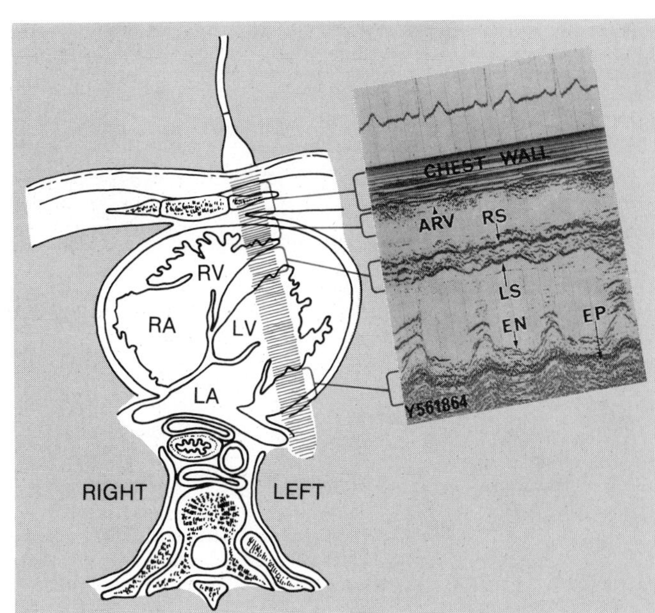

FIGURE 4–2. Diagrammatic cross-section of the heart and corresponding echocardiogram showing the cardiac structures transected by an ultrasonic beam directed toward the left ventricle. The ultrasound passes through the chest wall, the anterior right ventricular wall (ARV), a small portion of the right ventricular cavity, the interventricular septum, the cavity of the left ventricle, and the posterior left ventricular wall. RS = right side of interventricular septum, LS = left side of interventricular septum, EN = posterior left ventricular endocardium, EP = posterior left ventricular epicardium. (Modified from Popp, R. L., et al.: Estimation of right and left ventricular size by ultrasound. A study of the echoes from the interventricular septum. Am. J. Cardiol. *24*:523, 1969.)

Figure 4–4 shows echoes from the aorta and aortic valve; by tilting the transducer medially from the aortic valve, it is possible to record the anterior leaflet of the tricuspid valve, which is similar in appearance to the recording from the anterior leaflet of the mitral valve. When the transducer is directed superiorly and laterally from the aortic valve, a posterior leaflet of the pulmonary valve can be recorded (Fig. 4–4).

TWO-DIMENSIONAL ECHOCARDIOGRAPHY

The principle of two-dimensional (2-D) echocardiography is depicted in Figure 4–5. The ultrasonic beam now moves in a sector so that a pie-shaped slice of the heart is interrogated.

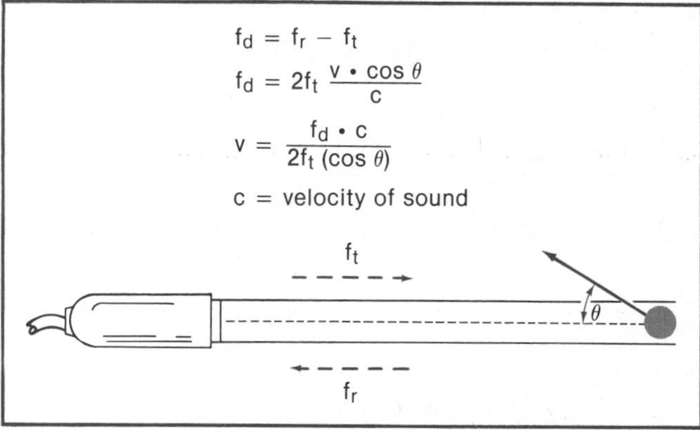

$f_d = f_r - f_t$
$f_d = 2f_t \frac{v \cdot \cos\theta}{c}$
$v = \frac{f_d \cdot c}{2f_t (\cos\theta)}$
c = velocity of sound
f_t
θ
f_r

FIGURE 4–8. Doppler equations relating Doppler frequencies (f_d), received frequency (f_r), transmitted frequency (f_t), and the angle (θ) between the direction of the moving target and the path of the ultrasonic beam. (From Feigenbaum, H.: Echocardiography. 4th ed. Philadelphia, Lea and Febiger, 1986.)

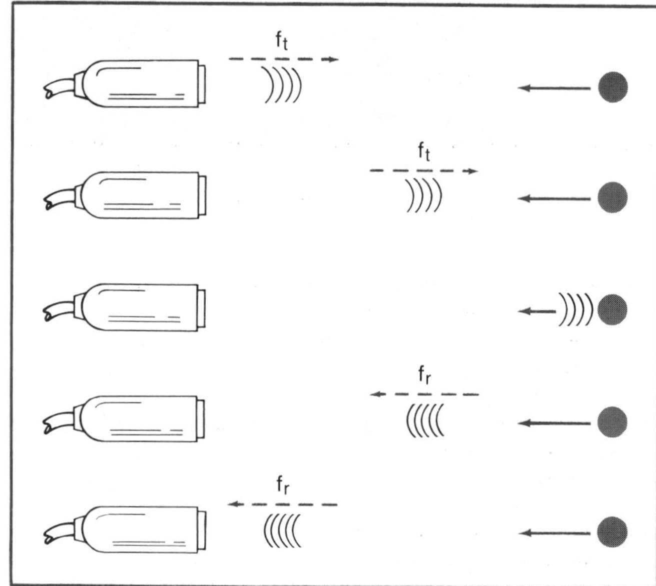

FIGURE 4–9. Drawings demonstrating the principle of pulsed Doppler echocardiography. If the object reflecting the pulses with ultrasound is moving toward the transducer, the frequency of the received pulse (f_r) is greater than the transmitted frequency (f_t). (From Feigenbaum, H.: Echocardiography. 4th ed. Philadelphia, Lea and Febiger, 1986.)

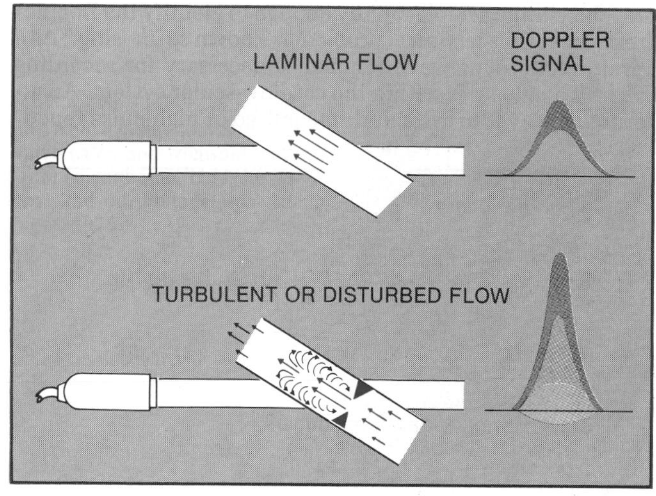

FIGURE 4–10. Doppler signals recorded from laminar flow and turbulent or disturbed flow. With laminar flow, all the velocities are similar. The Doppler signal produces a relatively thin wave form with minimal spectral broadening. When blood flows across an area with a significant change in the caliber of the vessel, flow with multiple velocities in different directions is produced. Such disturbed flow produces a Doppler signal with multiple frequencies and marked spectral broadening. (From Feigenbaum, H.: Echocardiography. 4th ed. Philadelphia, Lea and Febiger, 1986.)

tion frequency (high PRF) Doppler system. High PRF allows simultaneous imaging and recording of high flow rates; however, it is technically more difficult. The continuous wave approach is the more commonly used technique for recording high-frequency flows.[10]

The diagram in Figure 4–10 illustrates two types of flow that can be recorded using Doppler echocardiography. Laminar flow produces a Doppler signal consisting of fairly uniform frequencies all moving in the same direction. If blood flow is turbulent or disturbed, multiple frequencies will be recorded, some of which may be moving in opposite directions as depicted by signals below the baseline. The Doppler recording is a spectral display using fast Fourier analysis of the audible Doppler signal. The recording is usually on strip chart paper or videotape. The audio signal is helpful in interpreting the various types of flow and represents an important aspect of the Doppler examination.

COLOR DOPPLER. Doppler information from the cardiovascular system can also be recorded in a spatially correct format superimposed on an M-mode or 2-D echocardiogram.[11] Doppler flow imaging is created by multiple Doppler gates that are spatially correct and display the moving blood within the 2-D or M-mode recording.[12–14] The direction of the blood is displayed in *color* as in Figure 4–11. With this particular instrument blood moving toward the transducer is depicted in shades of yellow and red, whereas blood moving away from the transducer is in shades of blue. Figure 4–12 shows an M-mode color Doppler or M/Q study of a patient with valvular disease. The tracing shows how turbulent flow can be displayed as green or as a mosaic of colors.[15]

Figure 4–11. See color plate 1.

Figure 4–12. See color plate 1.

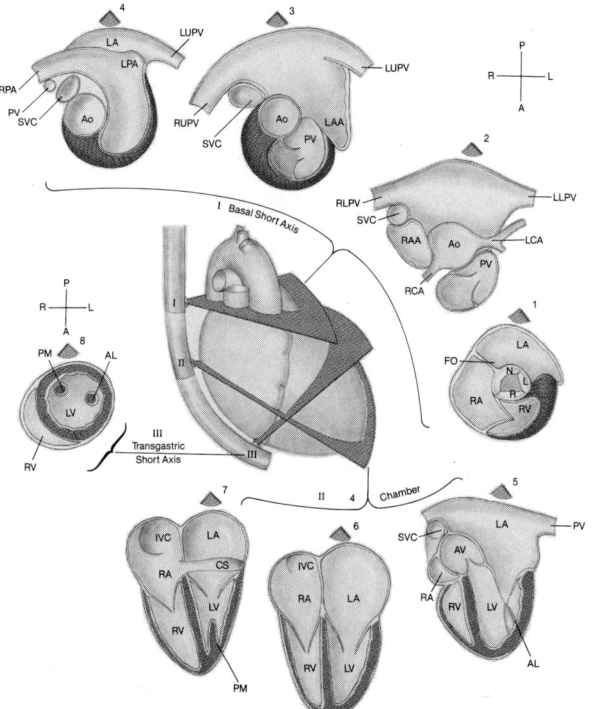

FIGURE 4–13. **Diagram demonstrating the various views of the heart that can be obtained using transesophageal echocardiography. With the transducer in position I the base of the heart can be visualized. With the transducer in position II and tilted in a retroflex manner, apical four and five chamber views may be obtained. Advancing the transducer into the stomach (position III) and anteflexing the transducer gives a short-axis view of the left ventricle. (From Seward, J. B., Khandheria, B. K., Oh, J. K., et al.: Transesophageal echocardiography: Technique, anatomic correlations, implementation, and clinical applications. Mayo Clin. Proc. *63*:649, 1988.)**

TRANSESOPHAGEAL ECHOCARDIOGRAPHY

Although echocardiography is one of the most common noninvasive examinations, this ultrasonic examination need not be limited to merely placing the transducer on the surface of the chest. Transesophageal echocardiography has been available for many years. With the technical advances in placing a 2-D transducer at the end of a flexible endoscope it is now possible to obtain high-quality 2-D images via the esophagus[19,20] (Fig. 4–13). It is also possible to obtain Doppler information with this approach. Figure 4–14 demonstrates a transesophageal echocardiogram in a patient with mitral regurgitation. The regurgitant jet is multicolored instead of green.

Transesophageal echocardiography is useful in patients in whom examination from the usual position is impossible technically. As noted, this approach is particularly helpful in assessing prosthetic valves, vegetations, and aortic dissections. The other major application for esophageal echocardiography is in the patient undergoing cardiac surgery.[21] The esophageal ultrasonic probe can be used to monitor cardiac left ventricular function throughout the surgical procedure and into the postoperative state. Transesophageal echocardiography is also being used in the operating room during open heart surgery.[21,22] Cardiac surgeons are finding echocardiography to be helpful in assessing cardiac morphology and function before and after surgical repair of valvular or congenital conditions.[23–26]

Echocardiography can also be used in conjunction with other invasive procedures[27,28] such as pericardiocentesis.[29] A similar type of monitoring has been useful to follow an endomyocardial biopsy,[30] especially from the right ventricle.[31] Therapeutic catheter techniques using balloon valvuloplasty or septostomy are also monitored effectively using echocardiography.[32] The ultrasonic transducer can be placed in a small

Figure 4–14. See color plate 1.

catheter so that a vessel can be imaged via the lumen to provide an intravascular echocardiogram, a technique known as intravascular ultrasound. Several intravascular ultrasonic devices are currently under development.[33–36] The techniques utilize a rotating transducer, rotating ultrasonic mirror, or phased array multielement systems. These devices are generating considerable interest, especially for the ability to evaluate atherosclerotic arteries.

CONTRAST ECHOCARDIOGRAPHY

Ultrasound is an extremely sensitive detector of intravascular bubbles. The injection of almost any liquid into the intravascular spaces will introduce many microbubbles that appear as a cloud of echoes on the echocardiogram. Figure 4–15 demonstrates an M-mode echocardiogram of a patient with a right-to-left shunt at the ventricular level. The contrast can be seen initially in the right ventricle. It then traverses the intraventricular septum and appears in the left ventricle. This technique is obviously a sensitive method of detecting right-to-left shunts. The contrast agents that have been used include the patient's blood, saline, indocyanine green dye, agitated or sonicated angiographic contrast agents, and sonicated albumen. In all cases the contrast effect originates from suspended microbubbles in the fluid. Commercially manufactured microbubbles that traverse the pulmonary capillaries will be available soon.[16–18] The potential clinical uses for contrast echocardiography are numerous. There is much ongoing research in this area.

FETAL ECHOCARDIOGRAPHY

Examination of the fetal heart in utero has become an important subspecialty of echocardiography. The examination is extremely demanding and requires great technical skill as well as an excellent understanding of fetal anatomy, physiology, and potential pathology.[37] The field is primarily in the hands of a few pediatric echocardiographers. Because of the highly specialized nature of this work it is beyond the scope of this particular discussion of echocardiography.

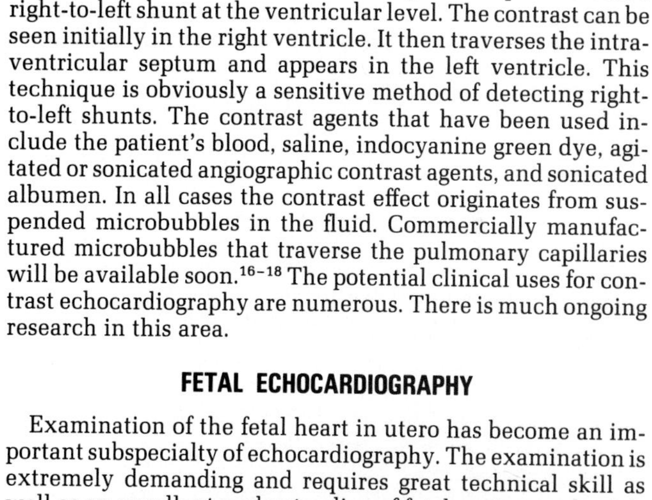

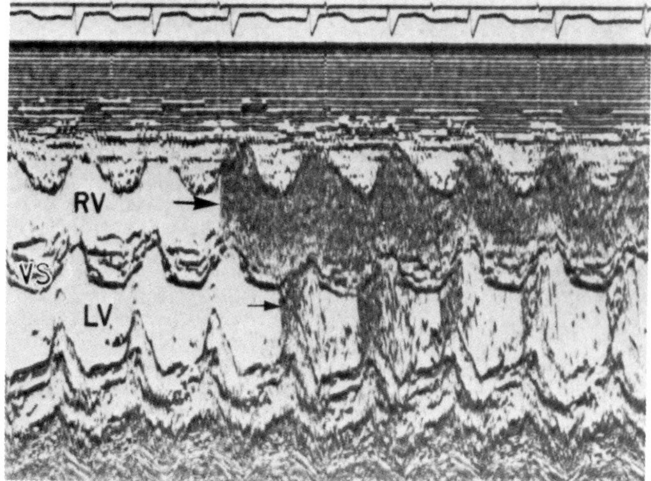

FIGURE 4–15. **A contrast M-mode echocardiogram in a patient with a right-to-left shunt at the ventricular level. The dark mass of echoes from the injected contrast (large arrow) is initially seen in the right ventricular cavity (RV) and next is seen (small arrow) in the left ventricle (LV) above the mitral valve. Normally the contrast should not appear on the left side of the heart at all. If the shunt were at the atrial level, contrast would appear in the left and right ventricles simultaneously and would be seen posterior to the mitral valve. VS = ventricular septum. (From Seward, J. B., et al.: Echocardiographic contrast studies: Initial experience. Mayo Clin. Proc. *50*:163, 1975.)**

ADVANTAGES AND LIMITATIONS OF ECHOCARDIOGRAPHY

The advantages of echocardiography are numerous. The examination is painless, as best as can be determined it is virtually harmless,[38] and it is less costly than other sophisticated imaging techniques. However, some technical difficulties exist which require expertise on the part of the examiner and interpreter of the echocardiographic recordings. The principal problem is posed by the poor transmission of ultrasound through bony structures or air-containing lungs. The examiner must thus try to avoid these structures. A variety of techniques have been developed to circumvent this problem. The patient is commonly placed in the left recumbent position to move the heart from beneath the sternum. The subxiphoid or subcostal transducer position is frequently used in patients with hyperinflated lungs and a low diaphragm. The apical examination with 2-D echocardiography has greatly increased the success rate in difficult examinations. Transesopheal echocardiography is available for the patient in whom examination is extremely difficult. The suprasternal notch approach offers yet another useful echocardiographic window especially for Doppler studies. Thus many examining techniques have been developed to minimize the technical difficulties in performing an echocardiographic examination.

EXAMINATION OF THE NORMAL HEART

M-MODE ECHOCARDIOGRAM

Figure 4–16 shows an M-mode scan that encompasses the full length of the *mitral valve apparatus*. The echoes from this structure are striking and are readily identified. The anterior leaflet of the mitral valve shows a downward motion in mid-diastole, and the characteristic "M" pattern is recorded. The posterior mitral leaflet is essentially a mirror image of the anterior leaflet, except the amplitude of its motion is less.

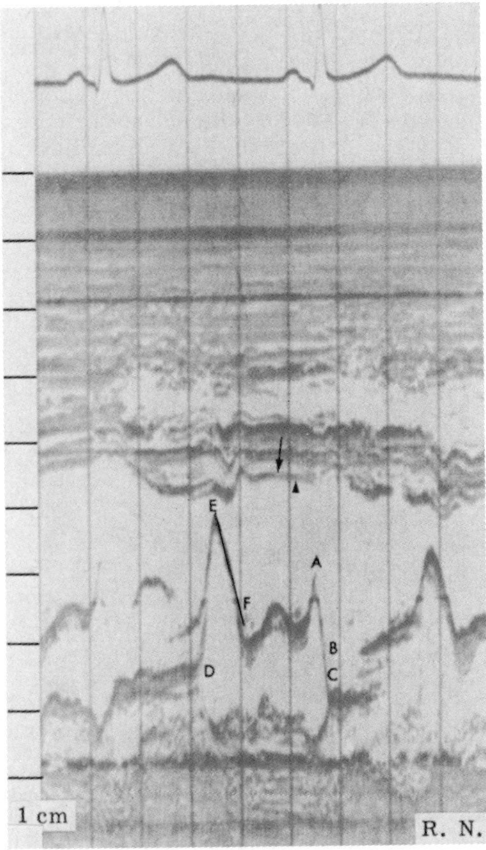

FIGURE 4–16. M-mode echocardiogram of a normal mitral valve. The letters A through F denote various portions of the anterior leaflet motion. The arrow indicates the leading edge of the echo from the left side of the interventricular septum; the arrowhead denotes the trailing edge of that echo. (From Feigenbaum, H.: Echocardiography. 2nd ed. Philadelphia, Lea and Febiger, 1976.)

Figure 4–16 is an M-mode examination of a normal mitral valve. The end of systole, just prior to the opening of the valve, is designated "D." The maximum excursion of the anterior leaflets is designated "E" and the nadir of the initial diastolic closing wave "F." The diastolic closing rate, or the "E to F slope," is indicated by the line drawn on Figure 4–16. This slope is frequently curved rather than straight. With atrial systole, blood is propelled through the mitral orifice and the leaflets reopen. The peak of this reopening of the mitral valve is designated "A"; with atrial relaxation, the valve begins to close again. Ventricular systole begins during the downward slope of the mitral leaflet and may produce a slight interruption of the closure wave, at point "B." (This is not always evident and is not so in Figure 4–16.) Complete closure occurs following the onset of ventricular systole at "C."

The *left ventricular cavity* is bordered by the interventricular septum anteriorly and the posterior left ventricular wall posteriorly (Fig. 4–3). Both walls move toward each other during systole, so that the diameter of the cavity decreases with systole. Both walls are approximately 1 cm thick in diastole, and the thickness increases during systole. A small portion of the right ventricular cavity lies anterior to the interventricular septum, and the anterior wall of the right ventricle is shown at the top of the tracing; the latter structure cannot always be imaged, especially in adults.

As the ultrasonic beam is swept superiorly and medially toward the base of the heart, the posterior leaflet of the mitral valve drops out and the posterior left atrial wall is seen to lie behind the anterior leaflet of the mitral valve. At the junction between the left atrium and ventricle the ultrasonic beam traverses both chambers during a given cardiac cycle. Because the atrioventricular junction moves in a superoinferior direction during each cycle, the stationary ultrasonic beam may record the left atrial wall during systole and the left ventricular wall during diastole. As the beam is directed more superiorly into the body of the left atrium, the relatively stationary posterior wall of the left atrium is imaged. The aorta, represented by two parallel echoes that move anteriorly during systole and posteriorly during diastole, lies anterior to the left atrium. The anterior wall of the aorta is in continuity with the echoes from the interventricular septum, and the posterior wall of the aorta is in continuity with the echoes of the anterior leaflet of the mitral valve. The aortic valve leaflets lie within the root of the aorta; only the anterior aorta valve leaflet is recorded in Figure 4–3. Two of the leaflets, probably the right coronary leaflet and the noncoronary leaflet, make up the boxlike configuration observed during systole as the aortic valve opens (Fig. 4–4). As the leaflets come together in diastole a *single* echo is commonly recorded.

M-MODE ECHOCARDIOGRAPHIC MEASUREMENTS

Numerous measurements have been suggested for M-mode echocardiography. Figure 4–17 demonstrates some of the measurements that can be obtained from an M-mode echocardiogram. Most of these measurements involve the left ventricle, the aortic root, and the left atrium. The American Society of Echocardiography has standardized the common measurements used in M-mode echocardiography.[39] A key consideration in these measurements is that the leading edge of an echo, i.e., that portion of the echo closest to the transducer, is more readily identified and precisely measured than is the trailing edge. The left ventricular dimension should be taken just beyond the mitral valve or at the chordae tendineae. In infants and young children, left ventricular dimensions are probably best recorded at the level of the mitral valve. The end-diastolic dimension is taken at the onset of the QRS complex, while end-systolic measurement is obtained at the instant of maximum posterior (downward) position of the interventricular septum, which usually precedes the peak anterior (upward) position of the posterior left ventricular wall. When septal motion is abnormal, the instant of peak upward position of the posterior ventricular endocardium may be taken at end-systole. A true right ventricular dimen-

PLATE 1

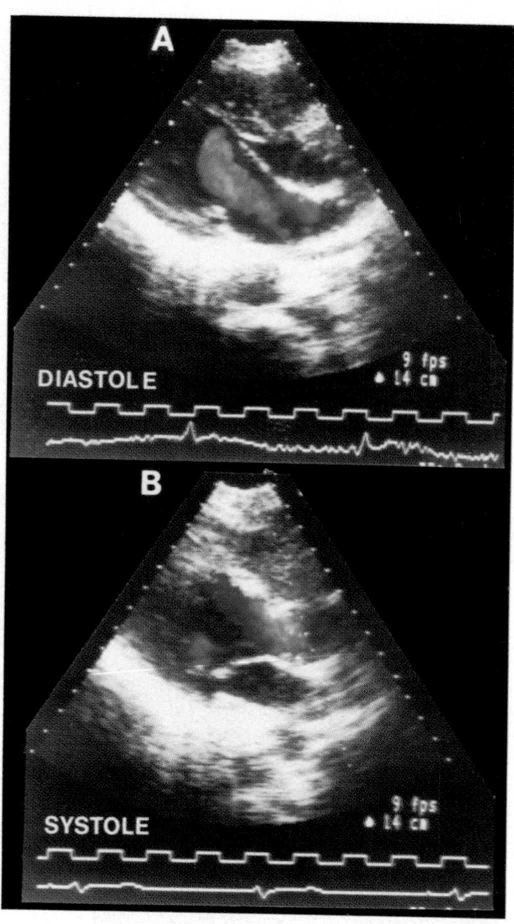

FIGURE 4–11 (See page 68)

Two-dimensional color flow Doppler image of the left ventricular inflow (A) and outflow (B) in the parasternal long-axis view. The blood passing through the mitral valve during diastole (A) is moving toward the transducer and is encoded in red. During systole (B) the blood passes through the left ventricular outflow tract and is encoded in blue. As the velocity increases toward the aortic root, the intensity or brightness of the color increases. (From Feigenbaum, H.: Doppler Color Flow Imaging. *In* Braunwald, E. (ed.): Heart Disease: A Textbook of Cardiovascular Medicine, 3rd ed. Update No. 2, pp. 35–48. Philadelphia, W. B. Saunders Co., 1988.)

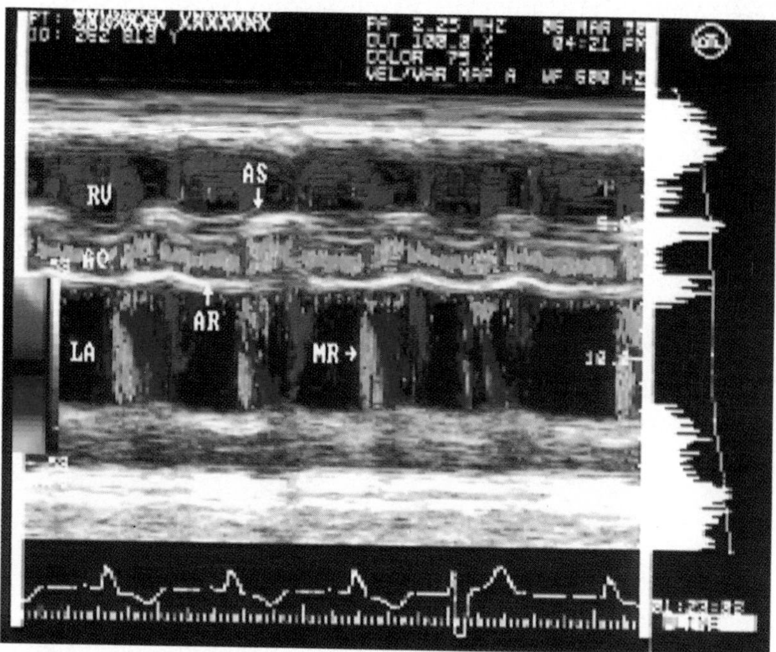

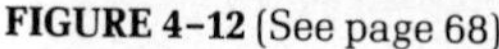

FIGURE 4–12 (See page 68)

Color-encoded Doppler flow superimposed on an M-mode tracing in a patient with valvular heart disease. The high-velocity turbulent blood is encoded in green. Both the systolic aortic stenosis flow (AS) and the diastolic aortic regurgitation flow (AR) can be seen within the aorta (AO). The high velocity mitral regurgitation jet (MR) is detected within the left atrium (LA) in systole. RV = right ventricle.

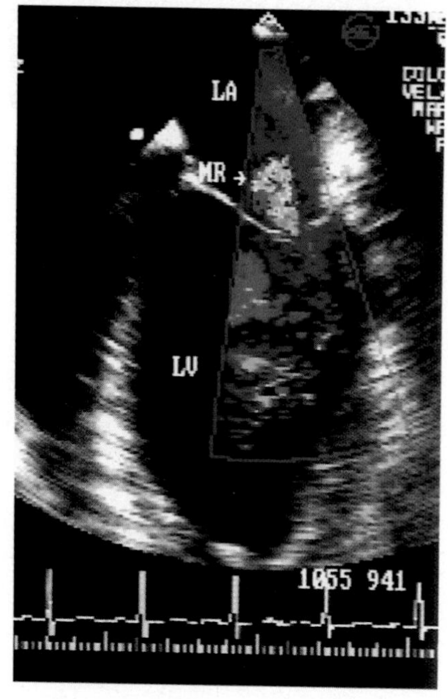

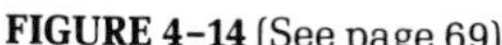

FIGURE 4–14 (See page 69)

Transesophageal echocardiographic examination demonstrating mitral regurgitation (MR) utilizing color flow Doppler. LA = left atrium, LV = left ventricle.

PLATE 2

FIGURE 4–48 (See page 83)

Color flow Doppler of a patient with mitral regurgitation (MR) as viewed from the four-chamber (A) and two-chamber (B) views. There is acceleration of flow on the left ventricular side of the regurgitant mitral orifice (AC). LV = left ventricle, LA = left atrium, RV = right ventricle, RA = right atrium.

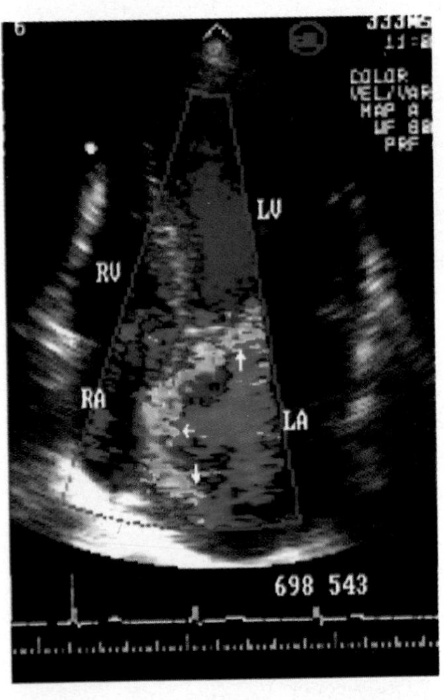

FIGURE 4–49 (See page 83)

Color flow Doppler study of a patient with mitral regurgitation in whom the regurgitant jet (arrows) is eccentric and directed toward the interatrial septum. RV = right ventricle, LV = left ventricle, RA = right atrium, LA = left atrium.

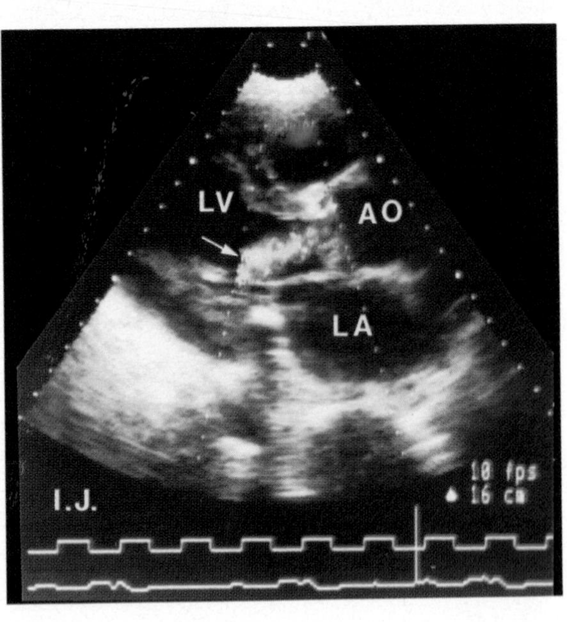

FIGURE 4–57 (See page 87)

Color flow mapping of a patient with aortic regurgitation. The brightly colored, high velocity jet can be seen passing from the aorta (AO) to the left ventricle (LV). The center of the jet is white and the edges are shades of blue. Even though the velocity is extremely high, most of the jet is blue because the flow is almost perpendicular to the ultrasonic beam, and the velocities are registered as being lower than they actually are. (From Feigenbaum, H.: Dopper Color Flow Imaging. *In* Braunwald E. (ed.): Heart Disease: A Textbook of Cardiovascular Medicine, 3rd ed. Update No. 2, pp. 35–48. Philadelphia, W. B. Saunders Co., 1988.)

PLATE 3

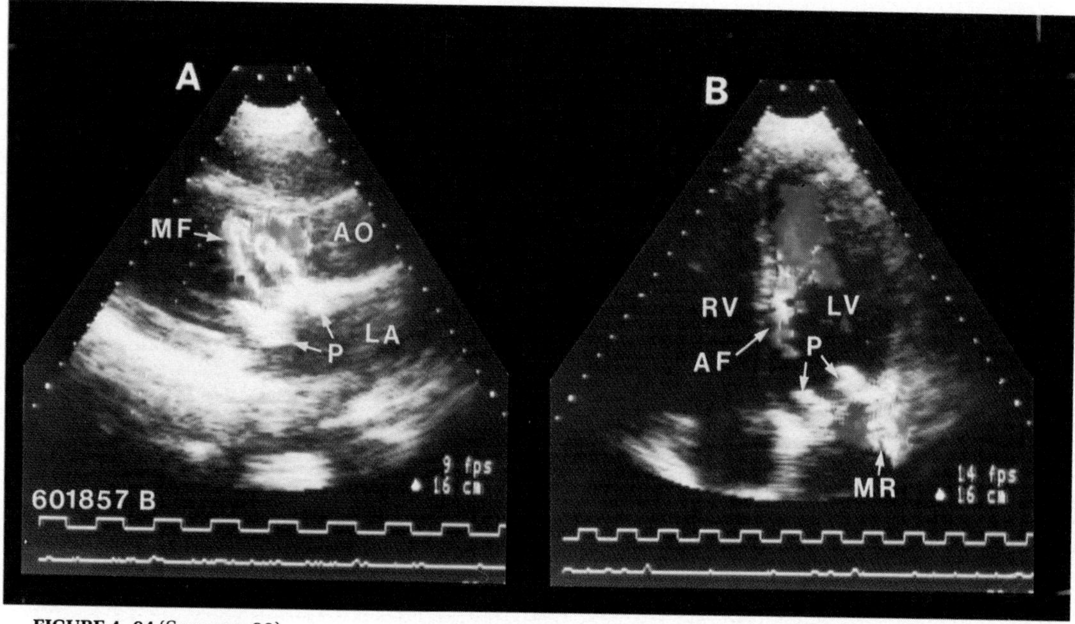

FIGURE 4-64 (See page 89)

Color Doppler images in the left parasternal projection diastole *(A)* and the four chamber view systole *(B)* of a patient with a prosthetic mitral valve (P). During diastole *(A)*, turbulent multidirectional antegrade mitral flow (MF) is present. During systole *(B)*, a regurgitant jet (MR) is present within the left atrium along the lateral border of the prosthetic valve (P). Aortic flow (AF) exhibits aliasing in this patient, who also had left ventricular outflow obstruction. The apical half of the left ventricular outflow tract is blue and the portion near the aorta is red. AO = aorta, LA = left atrium, RV = right ventricle, LV = left ventricle. (From Feigenbaum, H.: Doppler Color Flow Imaging. *In* Braunwald, E. (ed.): Heart Disease: A Textbook of Cardiovascular Medicine, 3rd ed. Update No. 2, pp. 35–48. W. B. Saunders Co., 1988.)

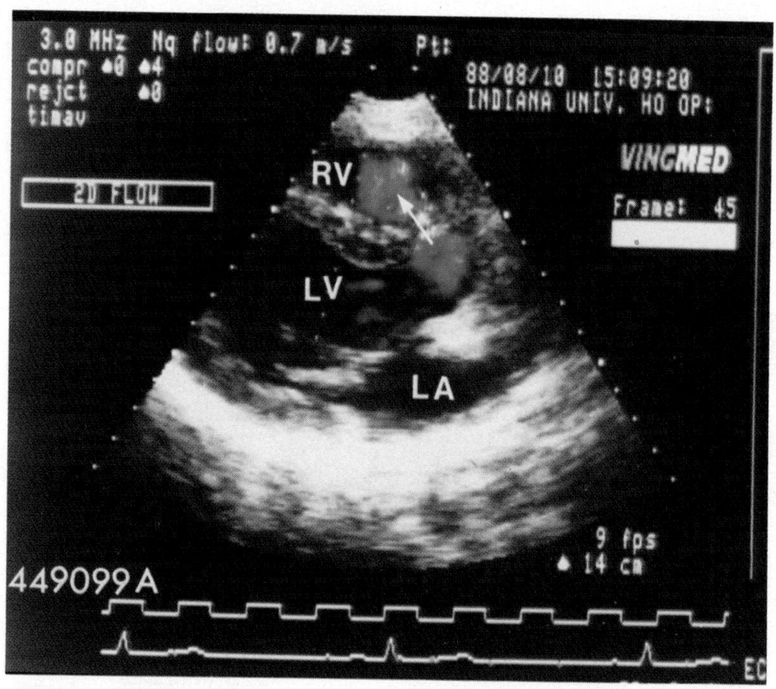

FIGURE 4-73 (See page 92)

Color flow Doppler study in the parasternal view of a patient with a membranous ventricular septal defect. The blood can be seen flowing toward the transducer and the right ventricle (R), and is encoded in red (arrow). At the site of the defect the width of the jet is narrowed and the velocity is increased as noted by the multicolor nature of the flow map. LV = left ventricle, LA = left atrium.

PLATE 4

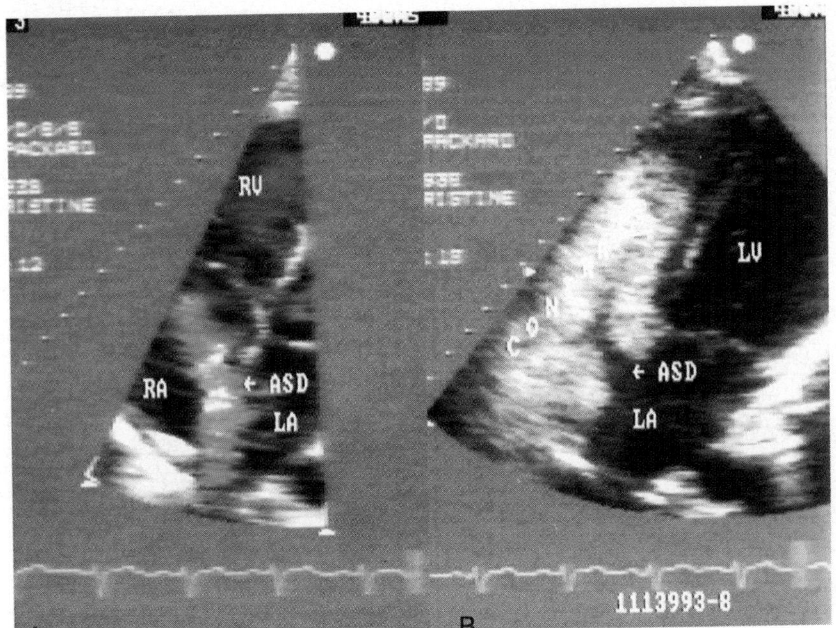

FIGURE 4–79 (See page 94)

Color flow Doppler (left) and contrast echocardiogram (right) of a patient with a secundum atrial septal defect. The defect (ASD) is noted by red-encoded blood passing through the atrial septum on the color study and as a negative contrast with the contrast echocardiogram. RV = right ventricle, RA = right atrium, LA = left atrium, LV = left ventricle.

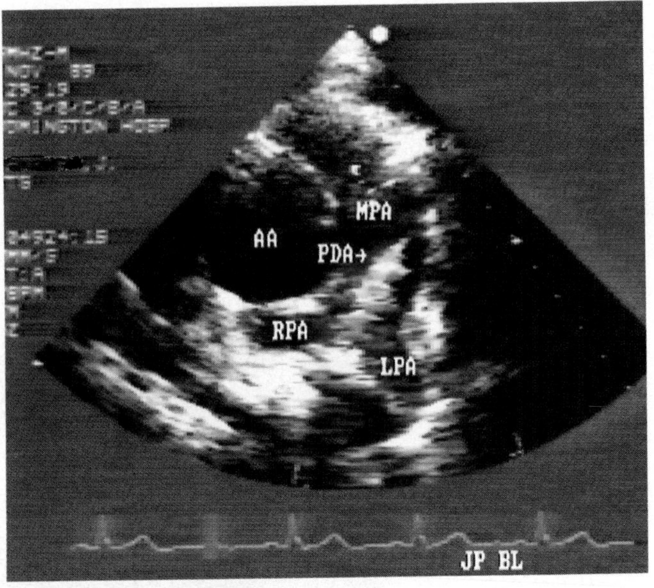

FIGURE 4–81 (See page 94)

Doppler image of a patient with patent ductus arteriosus. The shunt flow passing from the aorta into the pulmonary artery can be seen as a blue jet (PDA) within the main pulmonary artery (MPA). RPA = right pulmonary artery, LPA = left pulmonary artery, AA = aorta.

FIGURE 4–110 (See page 107)

Dissection of the aorta. A 2-D echocardiogram *(A)* shows the dilated circular arch of the aorta with an intimal flap (IF). The Doppler flow study *(B)* records blood flow in the true lumen (T) and virtually no flow in the false lumen (F). (From Feigenbaum, H.: Doppler Color Flow Imaging. *In* Braunwald, E. (ed.): Heart Disease: A Textbook of Cardiovascular Medicine, 3rd ed. Update No. 2, pp. 35–48. Philadelphia, W. B. Saunders Co., 1988.)

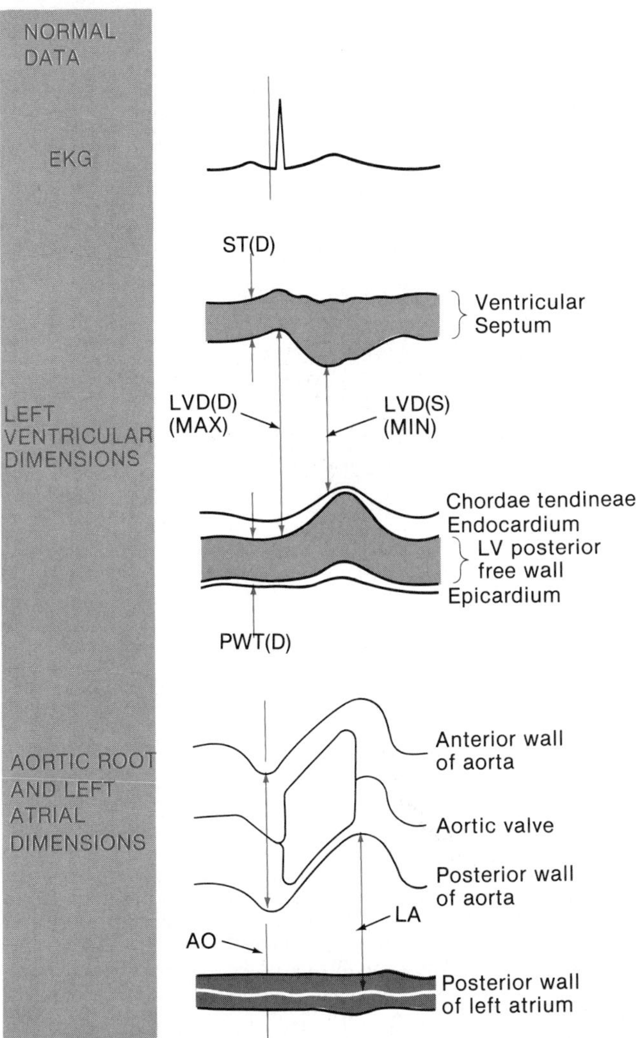

FIGURE 4-17. Methods for obtaining M-mode echocardiographic measurements. ST(D) = diastolic septal thickness; LVD(D) and LVD(S) = diastolic and systolic left ventricular diameter; PWT(D) = diastolic posterior wall thickness; AO = aorta; LA = left atrium. (From Henry, W. L., Gardin, J. M., and Ware, J. H.: Echocardiographic measurements in normal subjects from infancy to old age. Circulation 62:1054, 1980, by permission of the American Heart Association, Inc.)

sion can be obtained only when the anterior right ventricular wall is well delineated; otherwise, only an estimate of this dimension can be made.

Wall thickness is also measured from leading edge to leading edge. The width of the interventricular septum is the distance from the anterior surface of the right to the anterior surface of the left septal echo. The thickness of the posterior left ventricular wall is measured from the anterior surface of the posterior left ventricular endocardial echo to that from the anterior surface of the posterior left ventricular epicardium.

Table 4-1 provides normal values for commonly used M-mode echocardiographic measurements. These data represent approximations and do not conform in all instances to the criteria developed by the American Society of Echocardiography. Nor do they take into account that some changes in measurements occur during aging.[40] Normal values for children can be quite complex. The reader is encouraged to refer to some of the references, since more exhaustive normal values have been obtained.[2]

Although M-mode measurements have been made since the development of echocardiography in the 1950's, the role played by these measurements is decreasing. The closing velocity or E to F slope of the mitral valve is nonspecific and has relatively little diagnostic value. Even the left ventricular dimensions have significant limitations, especially in patients with regional wall motion abnormalities, such as with coronary artery disease or left bundle branch block. Thus, although M-mode measurements are still clinically helpful and are being used in many laboratories, they are gradually being replaced by quantitative 2-D and Doppler measurements.

An infinite number of slices of the heart can theoretically be obtained using 2-D echocardiography. The American Society of Echocardiography has attempted to standardize and simplify the many 2-D examinations.[41] The Society thought that all views could be categorized into three orthogonal planes, as illustrated in Figure 4-18. These planes are the long-axis, short-axis, and four-chamber. The long-axis plane is the imaging plane that transects the heart perpendicular to the dorsal and ventral surfaces of the body and parallel to the long axis of the heart. The plane transecting the heart perpendicular to the dorsal and ventral surfaces of the body, but perpendicular to the long axis of the heart, is defined as the short-axis plane. The plane that transects the heart approximately parallel to the dorsal and ventral surfaces of the body is referred to as the four-chamber plane. It should be emphasized that these views or planes are with reference to the heart and not to the thorax or body.

TRANSDUCER LOCATIONS. These ultrasonic planes or views can be obtained from more than one transducer location. Figure 4-19*A* demonstrates that the long-axis view can be obtained with the transducer in the apical position, in the parasternal position (left sternal border), or in the suprasternal notch. A short-axis view (Fig. 4-19*B*) cuts across the heart so that the left ventricle resembles a circle. The right ventricle can be seen curving around the left ventricle. Such an examination can be obtained with the transducer in the parasternal position or in the subcostal (subxiphoid) position. The four-chamber view is depicted in Figure 4-19*C*. Such a view permits the examination of all four cardiac chambers simultaneously. This type of examination can be obtained with the transducer over the cardiac apex or with the transducer in the subcostal position.

Table 4-2 lists the various 2-D echocardiographic examinations categorized according to the location of the transducer, the plane of the examination, and the cardiac structure being examined.

The right ventricle, right atrium, and tricuspid valve can be recorded with the transducer in the parasternal position (Fig. 4-20). The plane of the transducer does not exactly fit either the long axis or the short axis. However, the plane is closer to that of the long axis than that of the short axis and thus is categorized as a long-axis study. Figure 4-21 shows the right ventricular inflow tract and right atrium by way of such a parasternal examination.

TABLE 4-1 NORMAL VALUES OF ECHOCARDIOGRAPHIC MEASUREMENTS IN ADULTS

	RANGE (CM)	MEAN (CM)	NUMBER OF SUBJECTS
Age (years)	13 to 54	26	134
Body surface area (M^2)	1.45 to 2.22	1.8	130
RVD-flat	0.7 to 2.3	1.5	84
RVD-left lateral	0.9 to 2.6	1.7	83
LVID-flat	3.7 to 5.6	4.7	82
LVID-left lateral	3.5 to 5.7	4.7	81
Posterior LV wall thickness	0.6 to 1.1	0.9	137
Posterior LV wall amplitude	0.9 to 1.4	1.2	48
IVS wall thickness	0.6 to 1.1	0.9	137
Mid IVS amplitude	0.3 to 0.8	0.5	10
Apical IVS amplitude	0.5 to 1.2	0.7	38
Left atrial dimension	1.9 to 4.0	2.9	133
Aortic root dimension	2.0 to 3.7	2.7	121
Aortic cusps' separation	1.5 to 2.6	2.9	93
Percentage of fractional shortening*	34% to 44%	36%	20%
Mean rate of circumferential shortening (Vcf),† or mean normalized shortening velocity	1.02 to 1.94 circ/sec	1.3 circ/sec	38

$*\ \frac{\text{LVIDd} - \text{LVIDs}}{\text{LVIDd}}$

$\dagger\ \frac{\text{LVIDd} - \text{LVIDs}}{\text{LVIDd} \times \text{Ejection time}}$

RVD = Right ventricular dimension
LVID = Left ventricular internal dimension; d = end diastole; s = end systole
LV = Left ventricle
IVS = Interventricular septum

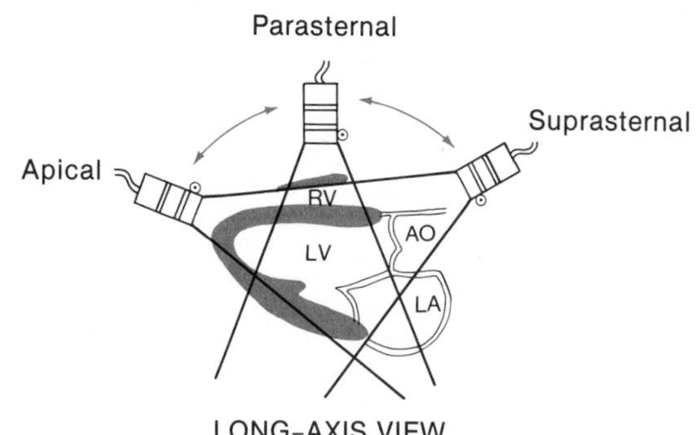

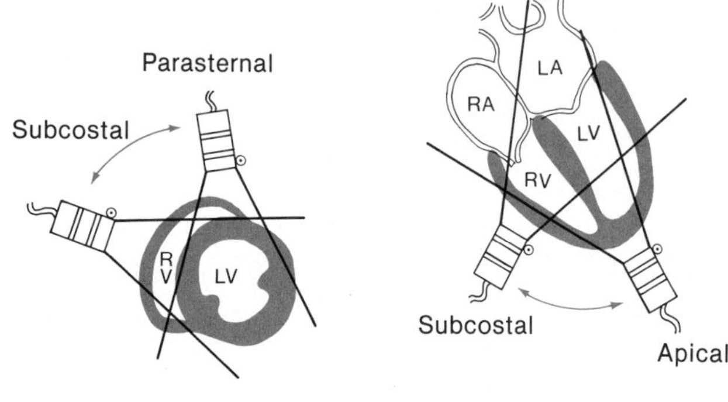

FIGURE 4-18. Diagram demonstrating the three orthogonal planes for 2-D echocardiographic imaging. AO = aorta; PA = pulmonary artery; LA = left atrium; RA = right atrium; RV = right ventricle; LV = left ventricle. (From Henry, W. L. et al.: Report of the American Society of Echocardiography Nomenclature and Standards in Two-dimensional Echocardiography. Circulation *62*:212, 1980, by permission of the American Heart Association, Inc.)

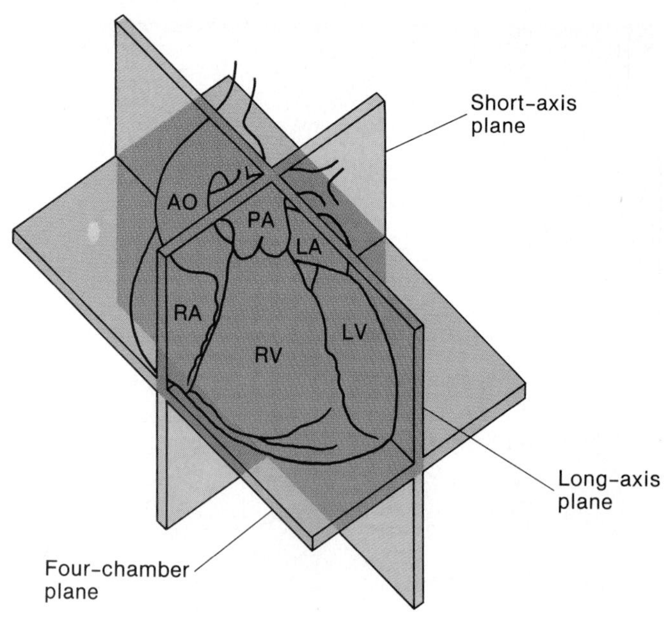

FIGURE 4-19. Diagrams demonstrating how one can obtain the various orthogonal planes from different transducer positions. (From Henry, W. L, et al.: Report of the American Society of Echocardiography Nomenclature and Standards in Two-dimensional Echocardiography. Circulation *62*:212, 1980, by permission of the American Heart Association, Inc.)

TABLE 4-2 TWO-DIMENSIONAL ECHOCARDIOGRAPHIC EXAMINATION

Parasternal Approach
- Long-axis plane
  - Root of aorta-aortic valve, left atrium, left ventricular outflow tract
  - Body of left ventricle-mitral valve
  - Left ventricular apex
  - Right ventricular inflow tract-tricuspid valve
- Short-axis plane
  - Root of the aorta-aortic valve, pulmonary valve, tricuspid valve, right ventricular outflow tract, left atrium, pulmonary artery, coronary arteries
  - Left ventricle-mitral valve
  - Left ventricle-papillary muscles
  - Left ventricle-apex

Apical Approach
- Four-chamber plane
  - Four chamber
  - Four chamber with aorta
- Long-axis plane
  - Two chamber-left ventricle, left atrium
  - Two chamber with aorta

Subcostal Approach
- Four-chamber plane-all four chambers and both septae
- Short-axis plane
  - Left ventricle
  - Right ventricle
  - Inferior vena cava

Suprasternal Approach
- Four-chamber plane
  - Arch of aorta-descending aorta
- Long-axis plane
  - Arch of aorta-pulmonary artery, left atrium

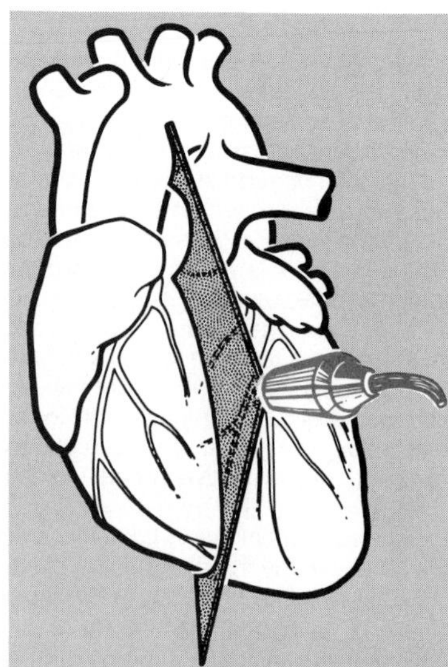

FIGURE 4-20. Transducer position for long-axis parasternal examination of the tricuspid valve, right atrium, and right ventricular inflow tract. (From Feigenbaum, H.: Echocardiography. 4th ed. Philadelphia, Lea and Febiger, 1986.)

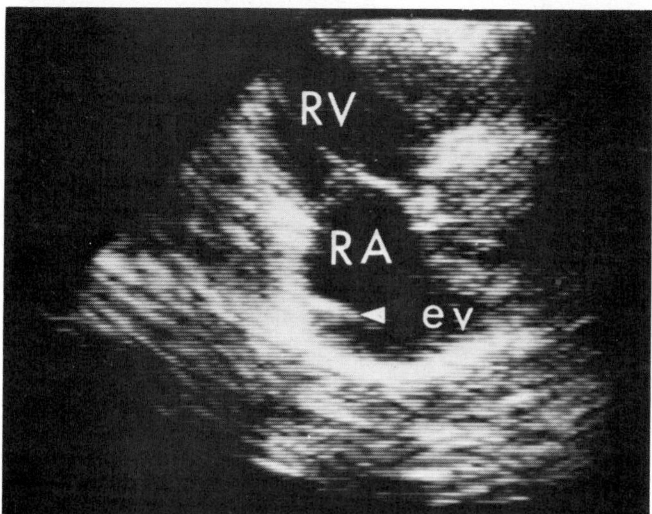

FIGURE 4–21. Two-dimensional echocardiogram of the right atrium (RA) and right ventricular inflow tract (RV). ev = eustachian valve. (From Feigenbaum, H.: Echocardiography. 4th ed. Philadelphia, Lea and Febiger, 1986.)

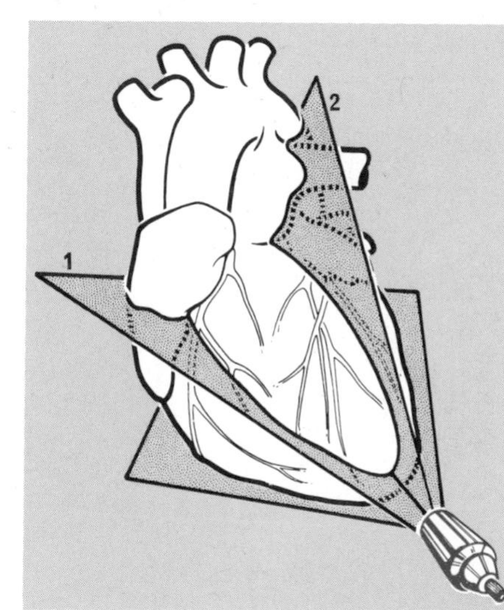

FIGURE 4–23. Transducer position and examining planes for apical 2-D echocardiograms. Plane 1 passes through the four chamber plane of the heart. Plane 2 represents the path of the ultrasonic beam for the two-chamber apical examination. (From Feigenbaum, H.: Echocardiography. 4th ed. Philadelphia, Lea and Febiger, 1986.)

Various *short-axis examinations* are diagrammatically illustrated in Figure 4–22. The short-axis views are commonly obtained at the level of the apex, the papillary muscles, the mitral valve, and the base of the heart. With slight variation in angulation the short-axis examination of the base of the heart can also record the pulmonary valve and the pulmonary artery with its bifurcation. It is also possible to use this examination to record the origins of the coronary arteries and the left atrial appendage.

Figure 4–23 diagrammatically illustrates the two commonly used 2-D echocardiographic views with the transducer placed at the *cardiac apex.* Plane 1 demonstrates the apical four-chamber view of the heart. Figure 4–24*A* shows an example of a four-chamber apical echocardiogram. It is possible to obtain an apical view of the long axis of the heart similar to that seen from the parasternal view. Such an examination would include portions of the right ventricle and the aorta. A more common examination is a so-called apical two-chamber view (Fig. 4–23, plane 2). This examination requires slight clockwise rotation of the transducer to avoid the right ventricle and the aorta completely. Thus one records only the left ventricle and the left atrium (Fig. 4–24*B*). This view is similar to the right anterior oblique ventriculogram commonly obtained at cardiac catheterization.

The *subcostal transducer location* produces examinations roughly in

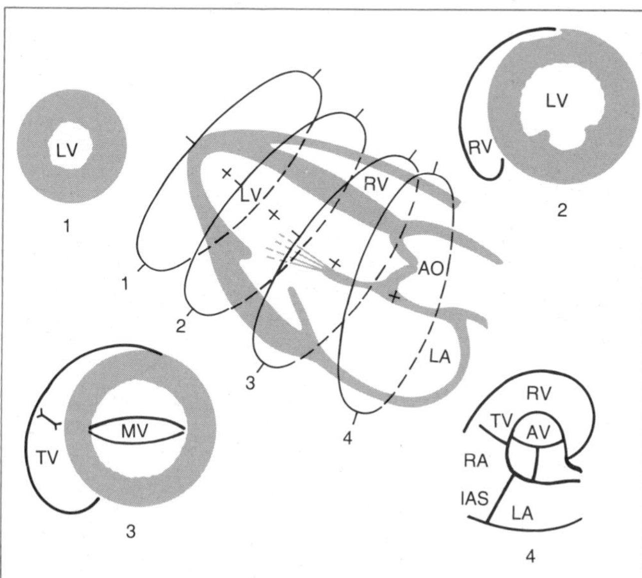

FIGURE 4–22. Diagrams showing how short-axis echocardiographic cross-sectional images of the heart, which are perpendicular to the long axis of the left ventricle, are obtained. Diagram 1 shows a short-axis left ventricular echocardiogram near the cardiac apex. Diagram 2 demonstrates part of the right ventricle (RV) and the circular left ventricular cavity (LV) at the level of the papillary muscles, which can be seen to bulge into the LV cavity. Diagram 3 is closer to the base of the heart and shows the left ventricle at the level of the mitral valve (MV). Diagram 4 shows a short-axis cross-section of the base of the heart with the aorta, aortic valve (AV), left atrium (LA), interatrial septum (IAS), right atrium (RA), tricuspid valve (TV), and right ventricular outflow tract (RV). (From Feigenbaum, H.: Echocardiography. 4th ed. Philadelphia, Lea and Febiger, 1986.)

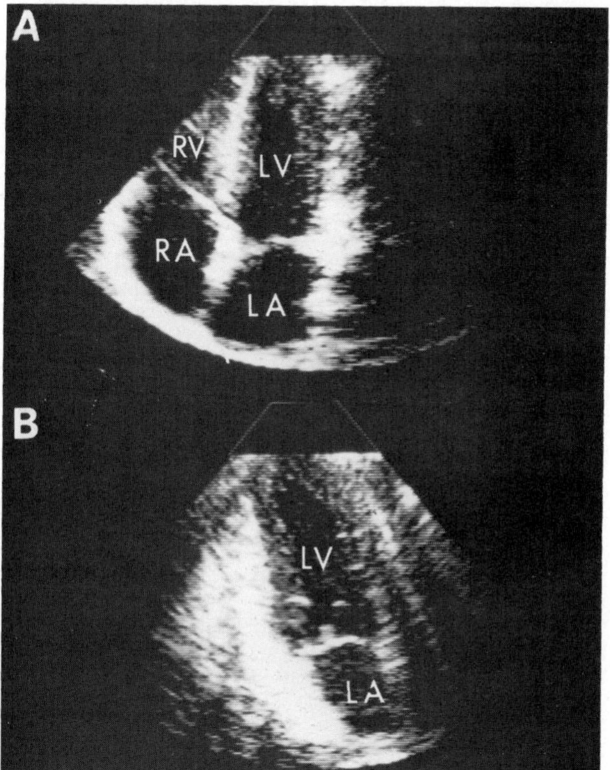

FIGURE 4–24. Four-chamber *(A)* and two-chamber *(B)* apical 2-D echocardiograms. RV = right ventricle; LV = left ventricle; RA = right atrium; and LA = left atrium. (From Feigenbaum, H.: Echocardiography. 4th ed. Philadelphia, Lea and Febiger, 1986.)

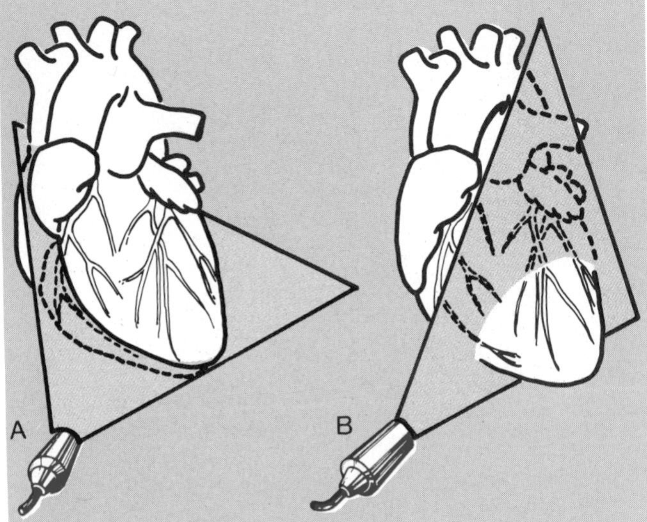

FIGURE 4–25. Diagrams showing the transducer position and examining planes for a subcostal four-chamber examination *(A)* and a subcostal short-axis examination *(B)*. (From Feigenbaum, H.: Echocardiography. 4th ed. Philadelphia, Lea and Febiger, 1986.)

the four-chamber and short-axis planes. The ultrasonic plane indicated in Figure 4–25*A* is similar to examining plane 1 in Figure 4–23. The resultant subcostal four-chamber echocardiogram appears in Figure 4–26*A*. Figures 4–25*B* and 4–26*B* show how the transducer can be rotated 90 degrees to provide a subcostal short-axis examination of the heart. The subcostal four-chamber view is particularly helpful in examining the interatrial and interventricular septa. By directing the transducer in a slightly modified short-axis examination, one can obtain an excellent view of the right side of the heart. The subcostal location also permits an opportunity to direct the ultrasonic beam through the inferior vena cava and hepatic veins (Figs. 4–27*B* and 4–28).

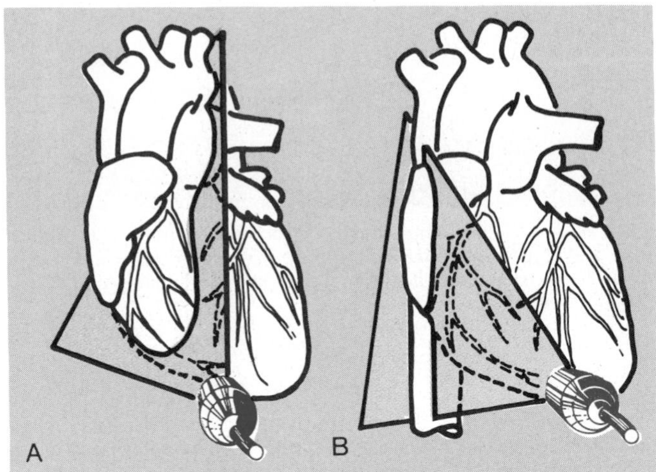

FIGURE 4–27. Diagrams demonstrating the examining planes and transducer positions for the subcostal examination for the right side of the heart *(A)* and the inferior vena cava *(B)*. (From Feigenbaum, H.: Echocardiography. 4th ed. Philadelphia, Lea and Febiger, 1986.)

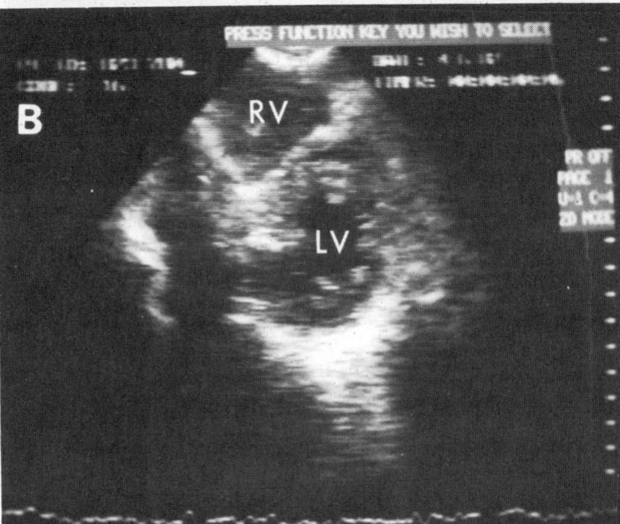

FIGURE 4–26. Two-dimensional echocardiograms obtained with the transducer in the subcostal position. Echocardiogram *A* represents a four-chamber view and *B* is a short-axis examination. RV = right ventricle; RA = right atrium; LA = left atrium; LV = left ventricle.

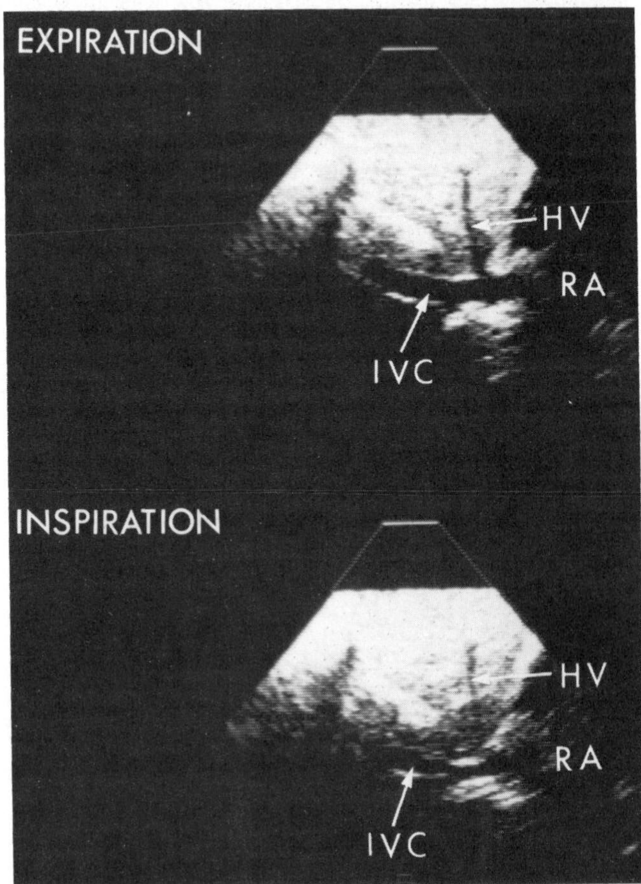

FIGURE 4–28. Subcostal 2-D echocardiograms of the inferior vena cava (IVC) and hepatic veins (HV). The inferior vena cava decreases in size with inspiration. RA = right atrium. (From Feigenbaum, H.: Echocardiography. 4th ed. Philadelphia, Lea and Febiger, 1986.)

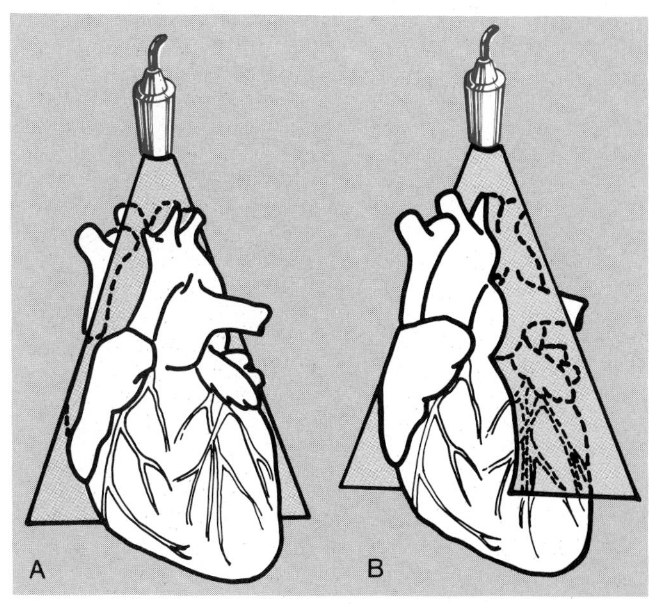

FIGURE 4-29. Transducer position in examining planes for the suprasternal examination parallel to the arch of the aorta *(A)* and perpendicular to the arch of the aorta *(B)*. (From Feigenbaum, H.: Echocardiography. 4th ed. Philadelphia, Lea and Febiger, 1986.)

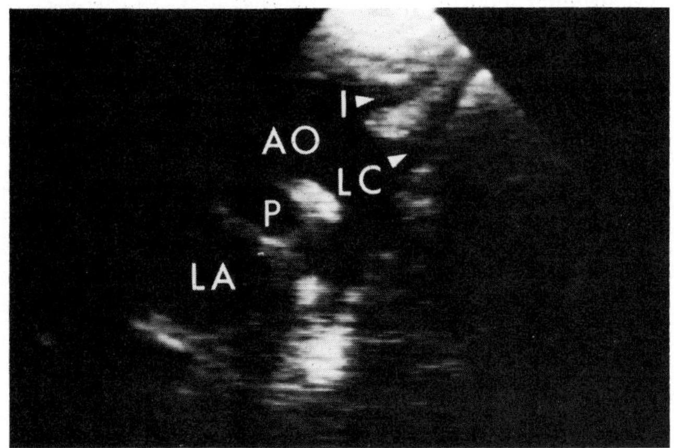

FIGURE 4-30. Suprasternal echocardiographic examination of the arch of the aorta (AO), pulmonary artery (P), and left atrium (LA). I = innominate artery; LC = left common carotid artery.

The two examining planes with the transducer in the suprasternal notch are depicted in Figure 4-29. The ultrasonic view in Figure 4-29*A* is roughly equivalent to that of a four-chamber plane, and the view in Figure 4-29*B* is somewhat comparable to that of the long-axis plane. However, it is probably best to orient the ultrasonic beam with regard to the arch of the aorta rather than to the heart, since one does not record much of the heart with the transducer in this position, especially in the adult. In addition, the planes are different from those with the transducer at the apex or subcostal region. Thus, better terminology with regard to the examining plane from the suprasternal location would be parallel or perpendicular to the arch of the aorta. Figure 4-30 shows a suprasternal examination parallel to the arch of the aorta.

DOPPLER ECHOCARDIOGRAPHY

Doppler echocardiographic recordings of the normal heart consist primarily of two types of flow patterns. The two types of blood flow are ventricular outflow and ventricular inflow. Figure 4-31 shows Doppler recordings of left ventricular outflow in the ascending aorta, the descending aorta, and the left ventricular outflow tract. The only difference in the recordings is whether the flow is toward or away from the transducer. With the transducer in the suprasternal notch the normal systolic flow in the ascending aorta is toward the transducer. In the descending aorta systolic flow is away from the transducer and the Doppler signal is below the baseline. With the transducer at the cardiac apex and the Doppler

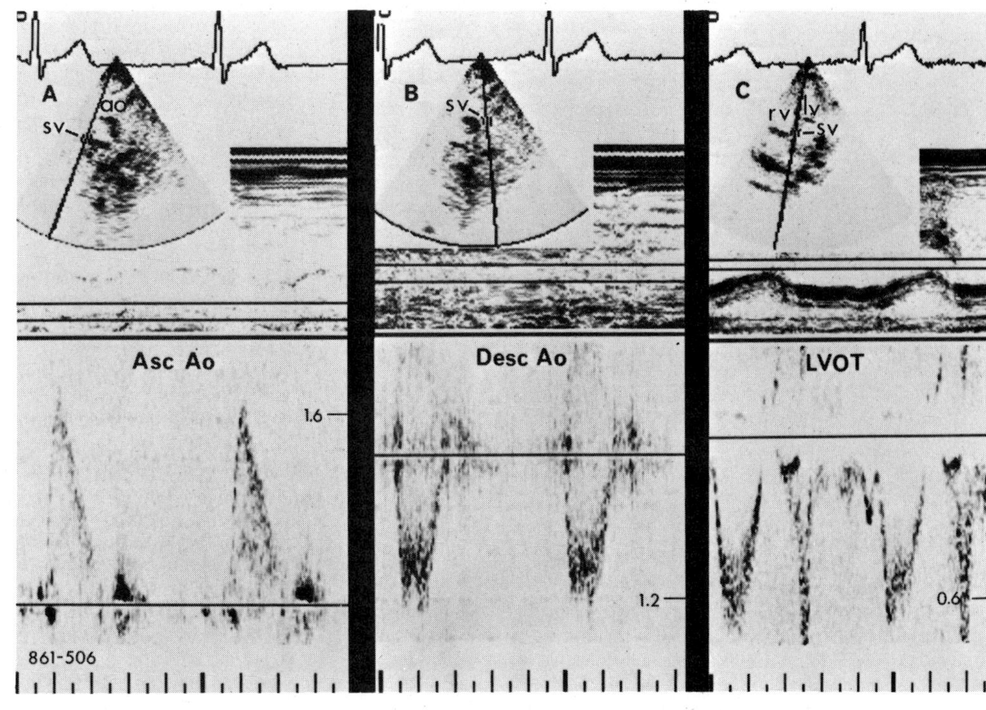

FIGURE 4-31. Pulsed Doppler echocardiogram of flow in the ascending aorta (Asc Ao) with the transducer in the suprasternal notch *(A)*, flow in the descending aorta (Desc Ao) with the transducer in the suprasternal notch *(B)*, and Doppler flow in the left ventricular outflow tract (LVOT) with the transducer at the apex *(C)*. sv = sample volume; lv = left ventricle; ao = aortic root; rv = right ventricle. (From Feigenbaum, H.: Echocardiography. 4th ed. Philadelphia, Lea and Febiger, 1986.)

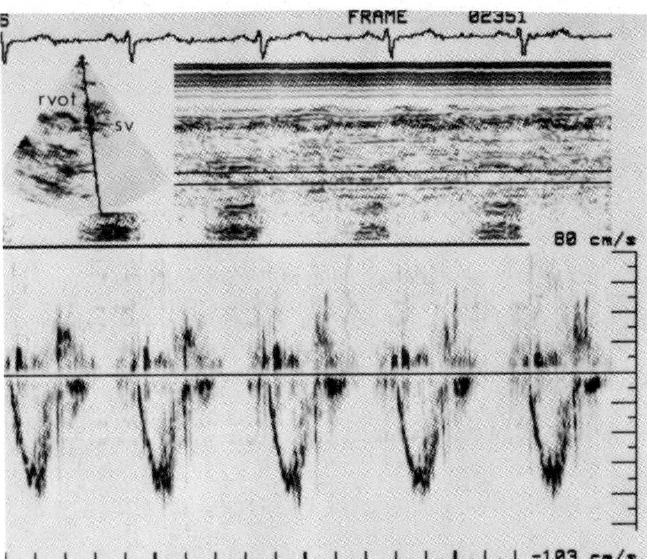

FIGURE 4–32. Pulsed Doppler recording of pulmonary artery flow. The 2-D scan is a parasternal short-axis examination through the base of the heart. rvot = right ventricular outflow tract; sv = sample volume. (From Feigenbaum, H.: Echocardiography. 4th ed. Philadelphia, Lea and Febiger, 1986.)

sample in the left ventricular outflow tract, blood flow is again away from the transducer. A similar flow pattern is noted in the right ventricular outflow tract (Fig. 4–32). The peak velocity and acceleration are greater in the aorta than in the pulmonary artery.

Figure 4–33 illustrates the Doppler flow pattern in the left ventricular inflow tract just beyond the mitral valve. The Doppler recording superficially resembles an M-mode tracing of the anterior mitral leaflet. There is rapid inflow in early diastole, decreasing flow in mid-diastole, and a subsequent increase in flow with atrial systole. Doppler tricuspid flow is almost identical to that of mitral flow except that the peak velocity is somewhat lower.

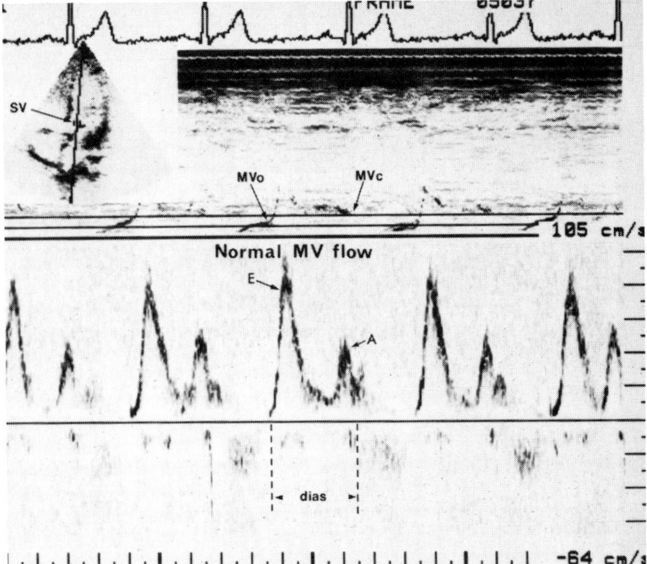

FIGURE 4–33. Normal mitral valve (MV) flow with the transducer at the apex and the sample volume (SV) in the left ventricle. MVo = mitral valve opening; MVc = mitral valve closure. (From Feigenbaum, H.: Echocardiography. 4th ed. Philadelphia, Lea and Febiger, 1986.)

EVALUATION OF CARDIAC PERFORMANCE

(See Chap. 15)

M-MODE ECHOCARDIOGRAPHY

The ability to evaluate the function of the left ventricle by means of echocardiography has been one of the principal factors in the increasing application of this technique. The standard M-mode technique may be used to record a dimension of the left ventricle between the left side of the interventricular septum and the endocardial surface of the posterior left ventricular wall (Fig. 4–17).[42] This dimension may be measured in end-diastole and end-systole. Although these dimensions can be used to estimate ventricular volume, many errors can occur in such calculations,[43,44] since many assumptions that are not always valid are required to obtain the volume of a three-dimensional object from measurement of a single dimension. Irrespective of whether or not M-mode echocardiography can calculate true left ventricular volumes, simple dimensions of the left ventricle can provide an estimate of the overall size and performance of the left ventricle in many patients.[45] *Fractional shortening*, i.e., the difference between the end-diastolic and end-systolic dimensions divided by the end-diastolic dimension,[45] provides information about left ventricular systolic function. The quotient of fractional shortening and ejection time provides the mean fractional or circumferential shortening.[46] While these measurements are useful in judging left ventricular performance (Table 4–1), it must be appreciated that the ventricle must be contracting uniformly for them to reflect global function. These echocardiographic measurements assess the status of only the basal portion of the chamber and must be interpreted with caution in patients with segmentally diseased left ventricles,[47] with left bundle branch block, with a dilated right ventricle, or with a low echocardiographic window so that the M-mode measurement is closer to the major axis rather than the minor axis.

Another useful M-mode echocardiographic technique for assessing left ventricular size is to measure the distance between the E point of the mitral valve and the left side of the interventricular septum.[48,49] Normally, the mitral E point and the left side of the septum are within a few millimeters of each other. The upper limits of normal of the mitral E point–septal separation (EPSS) is approximately 8 mm. As the left ventricular ejection fraction decreases, the EPSS increases. As the left ventricle dilates, the septum moves anteriorly. The opening of the mitral valve is largely dependent upon the volume of blood passing through that orifice. As the mitral valve flow or left ventricular stroke volume decreases, the amplitude of the E point is decreased. Thus, with a decreased stroke volume and/or left ventricular dilatation, the septum and anterior mitral leaflet would move in opposite directions. Naturally, if there is intrinsic valvular disease, such as mitral stenosis, then the excursion of the mitral valve is not a reliable indicator of flow through that orifice. In patients with aortic regurgitation, mitral valve flow is not an indicator of total left ventricular stroke volume, and one would not be able to provide an assessment of ejection fraction.

TWO-DIMENSIONAL ECHOCARDIOGRAPHY

The limited number of sampling sites for the M-mode dimensions and the lack of spatial orientation limits the clinical usefulness of these measurements. Thus, it is not surprising that there has been interest in using 2-D echocardiography for assessing the cardiac chambers. Hesitancy to use the 2-D approach has been caused by the inconvenience associated with analyzing a recording made on videotape. With the advent of newer videotape and video disc systems, electronic calipers, bit pads, light pens, and computers, it is becoming more convenient to make the necessary measurements from the 2-D examination.

There have been numerous attempts to use 2-D echocardiography to calculate left ventricular volumes.[50–54] Several geometric formulas have been suggested. These include the *area-length technique* commonly used for angiographic volumes. The *Simpson's rule* formula is attractive because it minimizes the effect of geometric shape for calculating volumes.[55] An intriguing formula is that which describes the left ventricle as a bullet, which consists of a cylinder and half of a prolate ellipse. The formula for calculating left ventricular volume using the *bullet formula* is volume equals five-sixths the area of the left ventricle times the length of the left ventricle

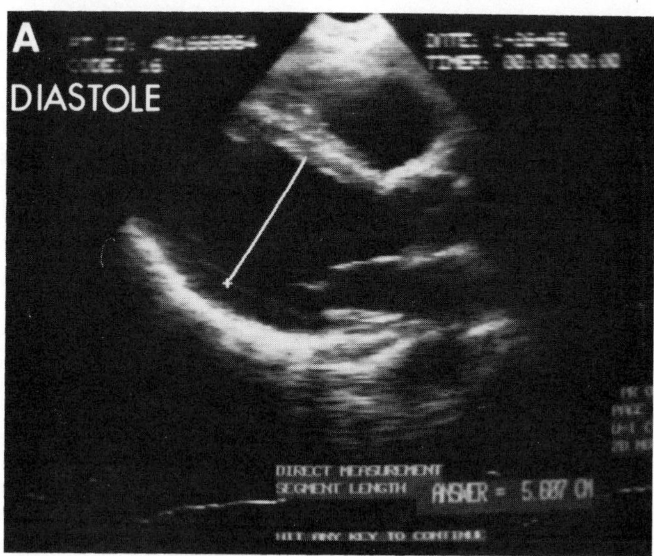

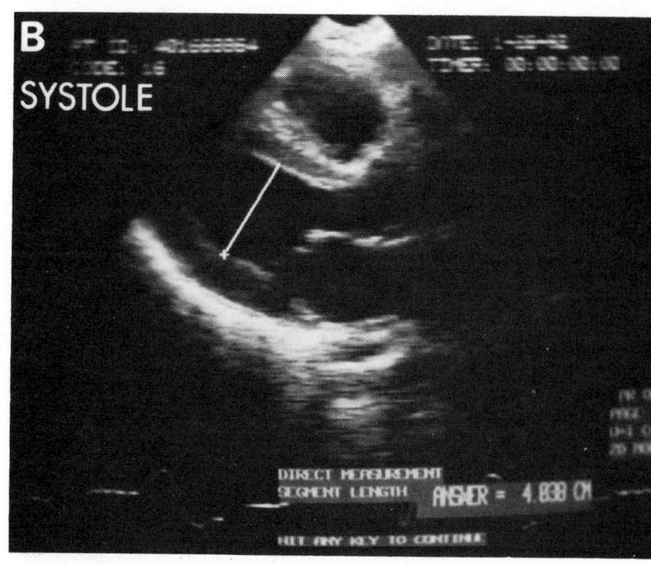

FIGURE 4–34. Parasternal long-axis examinations demonstrating how a minor dimension of the left ventricle can be measured in diastole and systole.

(V = 5/6 AL). This formula is attractive because of its simplicity and because the area of the left ventricle and the length of the left ventricle can be easily obtained with 2-D echocardiography.

Another simplified approach to assessing the left ventricle with 2-D echocardiography is merely to obtain minor axis measurements using the parasternal long-axis and short-axis views.[2,55] It is possible to obtain a true minor dimension using the parasternal long-axis examination. One can also obtain a short-axis area at the level of the papillary muscles. Derived indices, such as fractional shortening or fractional area change, can be obtained with this approach. Figures 4–34 and 4–35 illustrate how one can obtain the minor dimension from the parasternal long-axis examination (Fig. 4–34) and how the short-axis area can be measured at the level of the papillary muscles (Fig. 4–35).

DOPPLER ECHOCARDIOGRAPHY

This technique can be used to evaluate left ventricular systolic function with a recording of flow in the ascending aorta. Acceleration time, from the onset of flow to the time of peak acceleration (Fig. 4–36), and peak acceleration have been shown to be related to global left ventricular systolic function.[56–58]

DIASTOLIC FUNCTION

Echocardiography has been used to evaluate left ventricular diastolic function. M-mode techniques have been used to record the rate of relaxation of the left ventricular cavity. This technique utilizes digitization of the borders of the left ventricular cavity, with the rapidity with which the left ventricular dimension increases in early diastole being noted.[59] Doppler echocardiography is the primary technique used for evaluating left ventricular diastolic function.[60,61] Early diastolic flow is reduced and the velocity following atrial contraction is increased in certain disease states.[62–67]

FIGURE 4–35. ***A, B,*** **Short-axis 2-D echocardiograms demonstrating how the area of the left ventricle at the papillary muscle level can be measured in diastole (A) and systole (B). (From Feigenbaum, H.: Echocardiography. 4th ed. Philadelphia, Lea and Febiger, 1986.)**

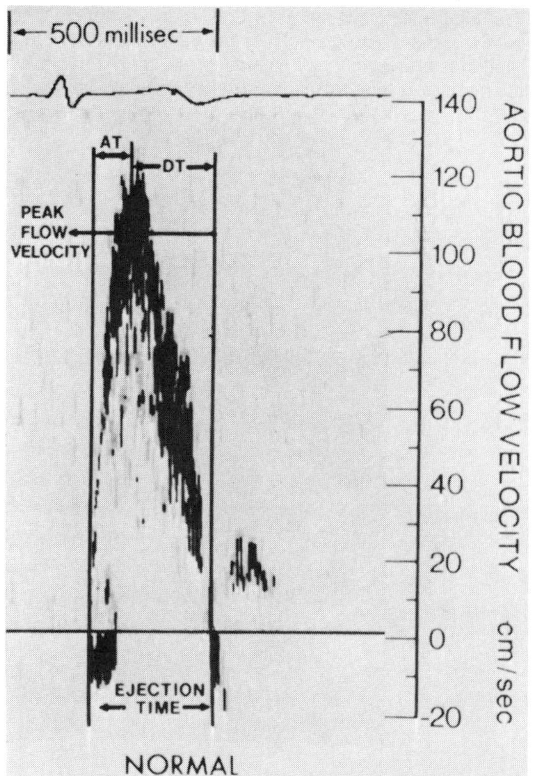

FIGURE 4–36. Pulsed Doppler recording of aortic blood flow velocity demonstrating how ejection time, peak flow velocity, acceleration time (AT), and deceleration time (DT) are measured. (From Gardin, J. M., et al.: Evaluation of blood flow velocity in the ascending aorta and main pulmonary artery of normal subjects by Doppler echocardiography. Am. Heart J. ***107*****:310, 1984.)**

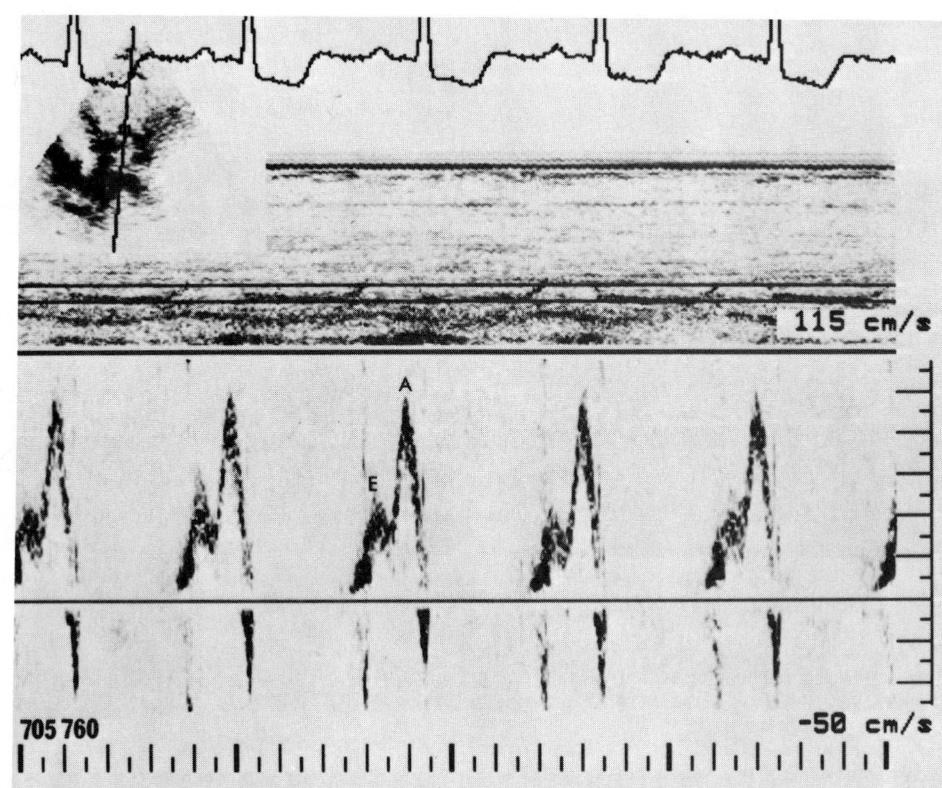

FIGURE 4–37. Mitral valve flow pattern in a patient with reduced early left ventricular filling. Early diastolic velocity (E) is reduced, and late velocity following atrial contraction (A) is increased. (From Feigenbaum, H.: Echocardiography. 4th ed. Philadelphia, Lea and Febiger, 1986.)

This phenomenon has been quantitated in several ways. The simple technique is to take a ratio of the peak velocity with early filling or E point and the peak velocity with atrial filling or A point. Normally the velocity at the E point is significantly higher than at the A point (Fig. 4–33). With reduced early left ventricular filling this ratio is reversed (Fig. 4–37). With restrictive ventricular filling the diastolic velocities may again reverse with a tall E wave and reduced A wave; thus "pseudonormalization" can occur.[68] To complicate matters further, the diastolic velocities vary with normal aging (p. 1662).[69–71]

EXERCISE ECHOCARDIOGRAPHY

Although echocardiography has been used primarily for evaluating the cardiac chambers at rest, there is increasing interest in performing the ultrasonic examination during or immediately after some form of stress. These studies have utilized supine[72] or upright bicycle exercise,[73,74] immediate post-treadmill exercise, pharmacological stress, and atrial pacing.[75] Many of the technical difficulties involved in recording an echocardiogram while the patient is hyperventilating following exercise have been overcome by using digital techniques which record a single cardiac cycle in a continuous loop display.[76] This digital approach eliminates respiratory artifacts and permits the resting and exercise studies to be presented side by side for ease of interpretation. This type of examination is being done primarily for detecting exercise-induced regional wall motion abnormalities in patients with coronary artery disease. Exercise studies using Doppler measurements of ascending aortic flow have also been used to assess global changes in left ventricular function during exercise[77] and hemodynamic changes in patients with valvular heart disease.

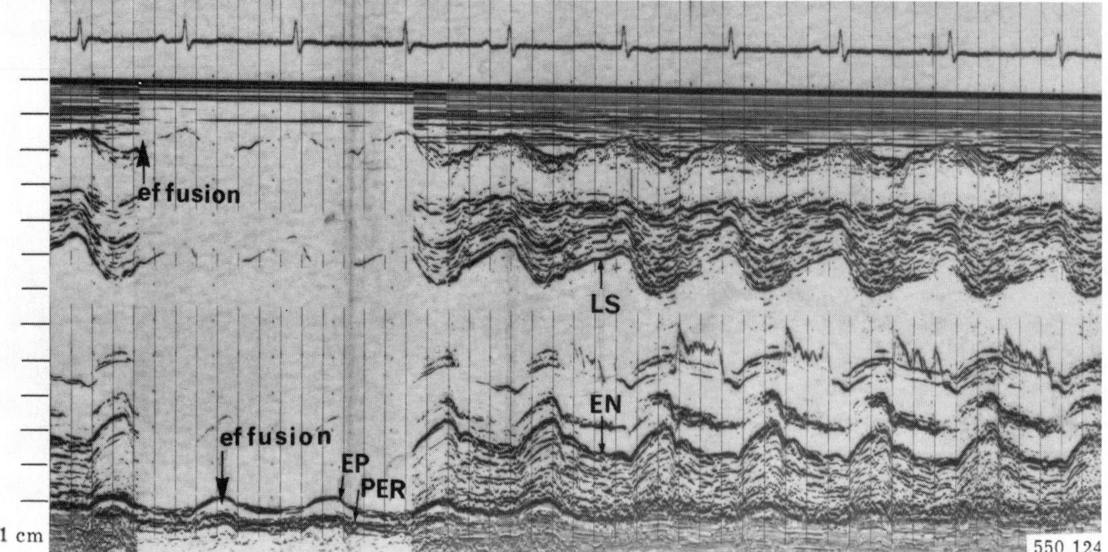

FIGURE 4–38. Left ventricular echocardiogram from a patient with left ventricular hypertrophy and a small pericardial effusion. The thickness of the interventricular septum and posterior left ventricular wall is markedly increased. LS = left septum, EN = posterior left ventricular endocardium, EP = posterior left ventricular epicardium, PER = posterior pericardium. (From Chang, S.: M-Mode Echocardiographic Techniques and Pattern Recognition. Philadelphia, Lea and Febiger, 1976.)

WALL THICKNESS

Echocardiography may also be employed to measure the thickness of the walls of the ventricle.[78] The absolute thickness of the ventricle is important in determining the presence of left ventricular hypertrophy (Fig. 4–38), in estimating left ventricular mass,[79–83] and in calculating left ventricular end-systolic stress.[84,85] Echocardiography also permits measurement of changes in left ventricular thickness during the cardiac cycle.[86] Normally, the left ventricular wall thickens during systole, but in pathological conditions this thickening decreases and actual systolic thinning has been noted in acute ischemia or myocardial infarction.[87]

OTHER CHAMBERS

LEFT ATRIUM. Echocardiography offers the opportunity to evaluate all four cardiac chambers and not just the left ventricle. Left atrial dilatation is readily recognized on the M-mode[88] or 2-D echocardiogram.[89,90] A variety of quantitative measurements have been introduced. A simple anteroposterior dimension of the chamber is usually sufficient for identifying patients with dilated left atria. Such measurements can be done with either the M-mode or parasternal long-axis 2-D view. In patients in whom the left atrium does not uniformly expand or if there is distortion by a dilated aorta,[91] other views including the suprasternal M-mode and the apical 2-D views can be used to assess the size of the left atrium.[92,93]

RIGHT VENTRICLE AND ATRIUM. The right ventricle is more difficult to evaluate quantitatively because of its unusual shape.[94,95] However, gross dilatation is easily assessed with M-mode[96] or 2-D examinations. Probably the most common technique is to use the relative size of the right and left ventricles in the apical four-chamber view. The thickness of the right ventricular walls can also be detected using either M-mode or 2-D echocardiography.[97] With right ventricular dilatation there is frequently distortion of the shape of the interventricular septum.[98] Whether this distortion occurs primarily during diastole or systole will indicate whether or not there is primarily a pressure or volume overload of the right ventricle.[99] With a diastolic overload the septum is flat in diastole and assumes a more normal curvature in systole. With a pressure overload the flattened interventricular septum can be seen with systole.

The right atrium can also be evaluated with 2-D echocardiography using the apical four-chamber view.

HEMODYNAMIC INFORMATION

DOPPLER ECHOCARDIOGRAPHY. This is now the principal ultrasonic technique for obtaining hemodynamic information. By recording the velocity of intracardiac blood flow, one can obtain quantitative data concerning both blood flow and intracardiac pressures. The principle is illustrated in Figure 4–39. To calculate flow the mean velocity passing through an orifice or vessel and the cross-sectional area of the orifice or vessel must be known. The mean velocity is acquired by measuring the velocity time integral of the Doppler signal which is the area under the recording. The cross-sectional area of the orifice through which the blood is flowing can be obtained directly with 2-D echocardiography; alternatively, the diameter can be measured with either 2-D[100] or M-mode[101] echocardiography and then the area can be calculated. Such flow determinations are feasible through any orifice or vessel.[102]

Blood flow in the ascending aorta is commonly used for cardiac output calculations.[103] The integrated velocity from the ascending aorta is combined with the calculated cross-sectional area determined at any of three locations: the aortic annulus, the separation of the aortic valve leaflets, or just past the sinus of Valsalva. All three approaches have been used with reasonable success. In a similar manner pulmonary blood flow can be measured by taking Doppler pulmonary artery velocity and multiplying it by the cross-sectional area of the pulmonary artery. Flow through the mitral[104,105] and tricuspid[106] valves has also been calculated. Atrioventricular valve flow is somewhat more complicated because the flow is phasic and early and late diastolic flow must be allowed for.[107] Although the measurements are more complex, they have been reasonably accurate.

The effectiveness of Doppler echocardiography for measuring flow has been validated.[108] There are many technical details in making such calculations. The biggest limitation is the calculation of the orifice or vessel area. It is difficult to obtain an accurate cross-sectional area of the various orifices. Because the measured diameter must be squared in the calculation of blood flow, any error would also be squared. For example, in many adult patients it is difficult to obtain an accurate orifice measurement of the main pulmonary artery.

Although the Doppler technique for measuring blood flow is not routinely done in many laboratories, the potential clinical utility is readily apparent. It can be used to measure cardiac output or stroke volume.[103,109] The technique is particularly useful for following *directional changes* in these variables in a given patient.[110] By calculating flow through different orifices, regurgitant fractions[111] and shunt ratios can be quantified.[112] For example, pulmonary to systemic flow ratios can be obtained by measuring aortic and pulmonary artery flows. Mitral regurgitant fraction can be calculated by measuring aortic flow and mitral valve flow. With the increasing availability of computer analysis, the difficulties of making these determinations have been resolved. However, some limitations still exist.[113,114]

DOPPLER MEASUREMENT OF PRESSURE GRADIENTS. Possibly the most important development in Doppler echocardiography has been the utilization of a modified version of the Bernoulli equation to calculate the pressure drop or gradient across a narrowed part of the cardiovascular system[5]; the principle is shown in Figure 4–40. Although the Bernoulli equation is fairly complex and involves convective acceleration, flow acceleration, and viscous friction, the equation can be limited to convective acceleration alone because flow acceleration and viscous friction are probably not relevant in the clinical setting. Essentially the equation relates the difference in pressure across a stenosis with the differences in velocities. As blood flows through a narrowed orifice, the velocity increases proportionally. With a few assumptions which seem to be clinically appropriate, a fairly complicated equation can be condensed to the difference in pressure (ΔP) equals 4 times the square of the velocity distal to the obstruction. The accuracy and validity of this approach has been confirmed in numerous laboratories.[116–118] This observation is now the basis for many clinical applications of Doppler echocardiography.

CLINICAL APPLICATIONS: THE ESTIMATION OF INTRACARDIAC PRESSURES. An early application of Doppler echocardiography was calculating a pressure gradient across a stenotic mitral valve.[116] The approach was then

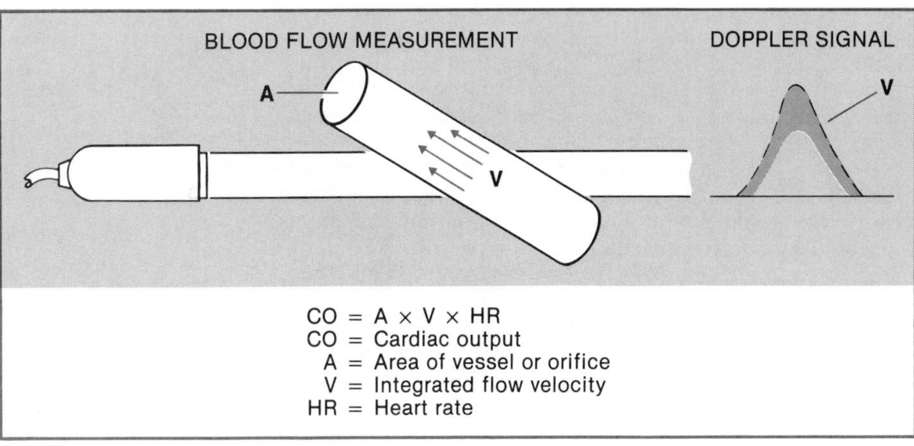

FIGURE 4–39. Principles of using Doppler echocardiography to measure blood flow. (From Feigenbaum, H.: Echocardiography. 4th ed. Philadelphia, Lea and Febiger, 1986.)

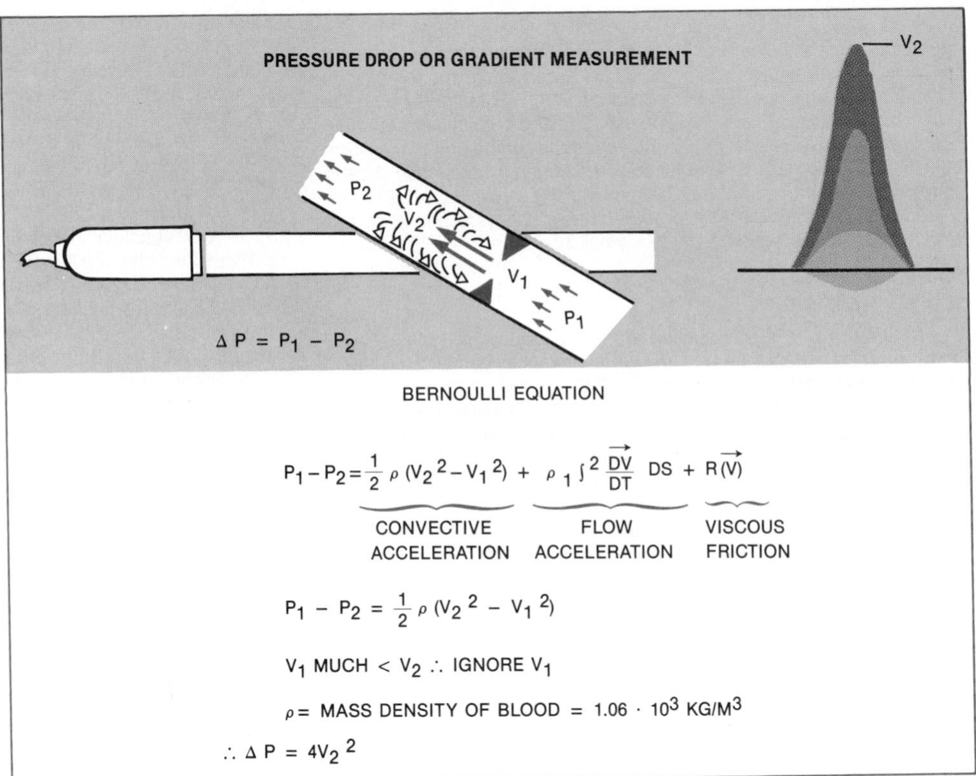

$$P_1 - P_2 = \frac{1}{2}\rho(V_2^2 - V_1^2) + \rho \int_1^2 \frac{\vec{DV}}{DT} DS + R(\vec{V})$$

$$P_1 - P_2 = \frac{1}{2}\rho(V_2^2 - V_1^2)$$

$$\therefore \Delta P = 4V_2^2$$

FIGURE 4-40. Principles of using Doppler echocardiography to measure a pressure drop or gradient across an obstruction. P_2 = pressure distal to an obstruction, V_2 = blood velocity distal to an obstruction, V_1 = velocity proximal to an obstruction, P_1 = pressure proximal to an obstruction. (From Feigenbaum, H.: Echocardiography. 4th ed. Philadelphia, Lea and Febiger, 1986.)

used with stenotic semilunar valves.[117] This same technique can be used to assess the difference in pressure across a regurgitant valve as well as a stenotic valve. For example, in the presence of tricuspid regurgitation the difference in pressure between the right ventricle and the right atrium in systole can be assessed by noting the peak velocity of the regurgitant jet.[119,120] By knowing the pressure differential between the right ventricle and right atrium and adding an estimate of the right atrial pressure, one can calculate right ventricular systolic pressure. If there is no obstruction to right ventricular outflow, the pulmonary artery systolic pressure is also known. If the velocity of blood flow across a ventricular septal defect is measured, the difference in pressure between the left and right ventricles can also be calculated. By knowing the left ventricular systolic pressure and the gradient between this chamber and the right ventricle, one can calculate right ventricular systolic pressure.[121,122] A similar approach is possible with aortic-pulmonary shunts.[123] With the help of the modified Bernoulli equation Doppler echocardiography is playing an increasing role in estimating intracardiac pressures.

The timing of the Doppler flow velocities can also provide hemodynamic information. For example, the flow pattern within the pulmonary artery can give clues to the presence of pulmonary hypertension.[124,125] However, these techniques have been replaced by measurement of right ventricular systolic pressure. There have been many studies correlating echocardiographic *mitral valve* motion with hemodynamics. In the setting of aortic regurgitation, premature closure of the mitral valve is a sign of a high left ventricular diastolic pressure.[126] This finding may be particularly helpful in the recognition of this hemodynamic abnormality in patients with acute aortic regurgitation secondary to infective endocarditis[127] (Ch. 35). The mitral valve M-mode echogram becomes distorted in patients who have tall and prominent *a* waves reflected in the left ventricular diastolic pressure.[128] Following atrial systole, closure of the valve is interrupted, and there is a plateau or notch between the A and C points just before the onset of ventricular systole.[129]

DOPPLER MEASUREMENT OF VALVE AREA. Combining the Doppler principles for measuring blood flow and pressure gradient permits one to calculate a valve area utilizing the "continuity equation." Figure 4-41 shows the principle of how the area of a stenotic orifice can be calculated using a combination of Doppler and imaging ultrasound. From the blood flow calculations (Fig. 4-39) stroke volume is a function of the product of the integrated velocity with the area. The *continuity equation* states that the blood flow proximal to an area of obstruction must equal the blood flow passing through the area of obstruction. Thus, if the volume of blood flow proximal to an obstruction and the velocity of blood through the obstruction are known, the area of the stenotic orifice can be calculated (Fig. 4-41). In the case of aortic stenosis the velocity and the area of the left ventricular outflow tract must be measured in order to calculate the blood flow proximal to a stenotic valve. Then by measuring the velocity of flow across the valve the aortic valve area can be calculated.

AORTIC VALVE ECHOCARDIOGRAMS. Analysis of *aortic valve* motion also provides useful hemodynamic information. In patients with hypertrophic obstructive cardiomyopathy, closure of the aortic valve occurs during midsystole as the subaortic obstruction suddenly becomes mani-

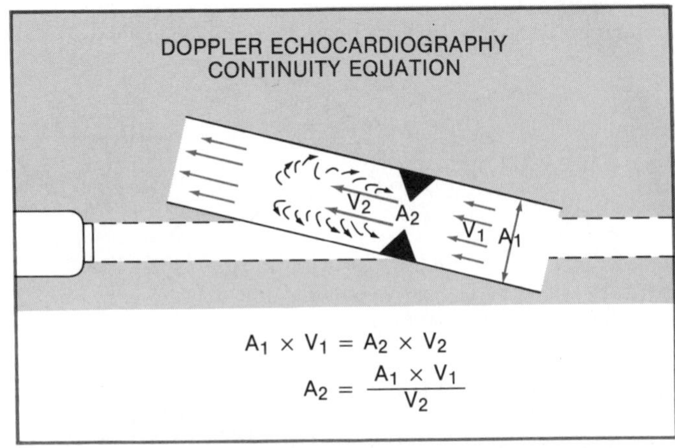

$$A_1 \times V_1 = A_2 \times V_2$$

$$A_2 = \frac{A_1 \times V_1}{V_2}$$

FIGURE 4-41. Diagram illustrating the principles of using Doppler echocardiography and the continuity equation for calculating the area of a stenotic orifice. A_1 = area proximal to the stenosis, A_2 = area of the stenosis, V_1 = velocity proximal to the stenosis, V_2 = velocity through the stenosis.

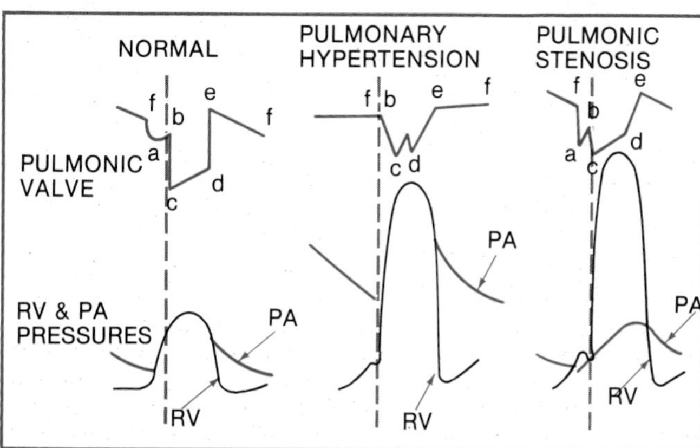

FIGURE 4–42. Diagrams demonstrating the relationship of the pulmonic valve echocardiogram and right-heart pressure in the normal state, with pulmonary hypertension, and with pulmonic stenosis. PA = pulmonary artery pressure, RV = right ventricular pressure. (See text for details.) (From Feigenbaum, H.: Echocardiography. 2nd ed. Philadelphia, Lea and Febiger, 1976.)

fested (Fig. 4–95C, p. 100).[130] Patients with mitral regurgitation exhibit a gradual premature closure of the aortic valve late during systole as blood regurgitates into the left atrium and forward flow into the aorta diminishes.[2] This gradual late systolic closure of the aortic valve may also be seen in low cardiac output states in which the left ventricle may not be capable of sustaining a continuous flow of blood across the aortic valve. In patients with severe aortic regurgitation and markedly elevated left ventricular diastolic pressure the aortic valve may open before ventricular systole.[131]

PULMONARY VALVE ECHOCARDIOGRAMS. M-mode echocardiograms of the *pulmonary valve* have proved to be useful in reflecting hemodynamic events as well. Although the pulmonary valve echocardiogram is probably influenced in part by the movement of structures to which it is attached,[132] the pressure relationship between the right ventricle and the pulmonary artery also influences the motion of the pulmonary valve (Fig. 4–42). Normally, atrial systole produces a slight downward motion of the pulmonary valve.[133] In pulmonic stenosis, the right ventricular systolic and end-diastolic pressures rise without any similar elevation in pulmonary artery pressure, and the atrial contribution to right ventricular pressure is exaggerated and usually sufficient to open the pulmonary valve prior to ventricular systole (Fig. 4–42).[134] In patients with elevated right ventricular diastolic pressure due to right ventricular failure, tricuspid regurgitation, constrictive pericarditis, or a communication between the aorta and right ventricle, the elevated pressure in the right ventricle in early diastole may cause opening of the pulmonic valve even before the onset of atrial systole.[135]

An increase in pulmonary artery pressure has been shown to influence pulmonary valve motion in several ways (Fig. 4–42).[136,137] One of the most consistent changes is the elimination of atrial systolic motion, and the absence or marked reduction of the pulmonary valve *a* wave is one of the echocardiographic signs of pulmonary hypertension. As might be expected, when right ventricular failure occurs in pulmonary hypertension, right ventricular diastolic pressure may rise sufficiently so that a small *a* wave may again be recorded.[2] Another sign of pulmonary hypertension is midsystolic closure of the pulmonary valve.[136] Although this finding has not been explained, it is probably related to elevated pulmonary vascular resistance.[138]

The pulmonary valve echogram has been used to calculate systolic time intervals of the right side of the heart,[139] and these intervals, in turn, have been used to estimate pulmonary artery pressure and right ventricular performance.[140] Most of these measurements have now been replaced by calculations from Doppler echocardiography[141,142] (p. 67).

With the 2-D echocardiographic examination of the inferior vena cava and hepatic vein, more information concerning right-sided hemodynamics may be obtained (Fig. 4–43).[143,144] This particular examination can be helpful in assessing the central venous pressure by noting the size of the veins[115] and the lack of the normal respiratory variation in the size of the inferior vena cava.

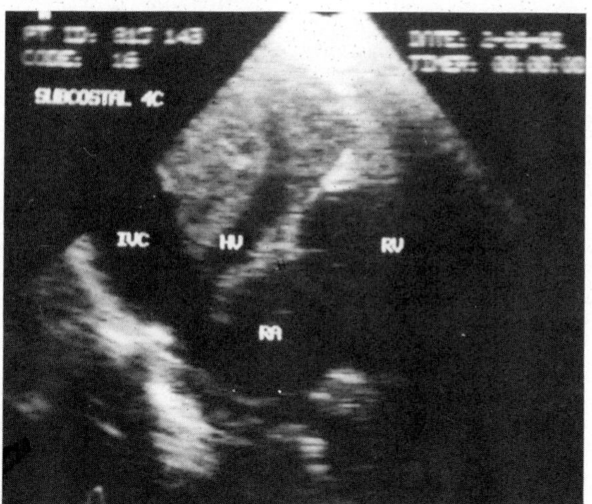

FIGURE 4–43. Subcostal 2-D echocardiogram of the right atrium (RA) and right ventricle (RV) in a patient with elevated right atrial pressure and a markedly dilated inferior vena cava (IVC) and hepatic vein (HV).

ACQUIRED VALVULAR HEART DISEASE

(See also Chap. 34)

MITRAL STENOSIS

The detection of mitral stenosis (MS) was the first clinical application of echocardiography.[145] It remains an important technique in the evaluation of patients with suspected mitral valve disease because echocardiography can allow visualization of the mitral valve in a manner not possible with any other procedure. The M-mode examination provides a sensitive assessment of the motion and thickness of the valve leaflets, while the 2-D technique provides a spatial image of the valve and allows direct measurement of the valve orifice.[146] Doppler echocardiography provides a hemodynamic assessment of the stenotic orifice.

Figure 4–44 shows an M-mode echocardiogram of a patient with calcific MS. The motion of the mitral valve is considerably altered from the normal pattern seen in Figures 4–3 and 4–16; the normal "M"-shaped configuration during diastole is no longer present, since the presence of a holodiastolic atrioventricular pressure gradient (diastasis) prevents rapid closure of the valve in mid-diastole. Although sinus rhythm was present, there was no reopening of the valve with atrial contraction and no *a* wave. Thus, the M-mode echocardiographic hallmark of MS is the absence of valve closure in mid-diastole and of reopening in late diastole. Although this decreased (flat) diastolic (E-F) slope is characteristic of MS, it is not specific. Other conditions such as decreased left ventricular compliance or a low cardiac output may also reduce the diastolic slope of mitral valve motion.[147]

In addition to the change in motion of the valve, the number of echoes originating from the valve is increased when it is fibrotic or calcified, and another echocardiographic sign of MS is increased thickness of the valve leaflets. (Note that the quantity of echoes originating from the mitral valve in Figure 4–44 is considerably greater than in Figure 4–16). Inadequate separation of the anterior and posterior leaflets of the valve occurs during diastole.[147] Normally, the two leaflets move in opposite directions during diastole, but when fused, as in MS, they do not separate widely and may actually appear to move in the same direction (Fig. 4–44). The echocardiographic findings of reduced diastolic slope, increased thickness, and decreased separation of the valve leaflets provide a sensitive and accurate method for detection of MS. The diagnosis of MS by 2-D echocardiography is made by noting thickening, doming, and restricted motion of the leaflets (Fig. 4–45A).

Doming of *any* valve on 2-D echocardiography is a characteristic sign of stenosis. This distortion in shape with opening of the valve indicates that the tips of the leaflets are restricted in their ability to open, whereas the bodies of the leaflets still wish to accommodate more blood flow; thus, the leaflets are curved, or domed. The presence of doming distinguishes a

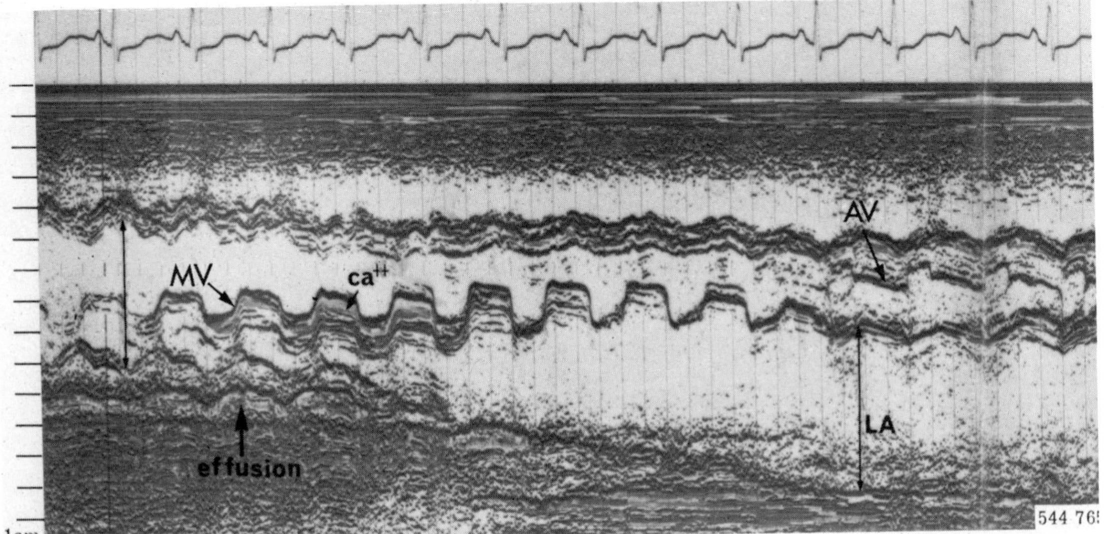

FIGURE 4–44. M-mode scan from a patient with mitral stenosis. The valve is calcified (Ca^{++}) and immobile. The left atrium (LA) is dilated and there is moderate posterior pericardial effusion. AV = aortic valve. (From Chang, S.: M-Mode Echocardiographic Techniques and Pattern Recognition. Philadelphia, Lea and Febiger, 1976.)

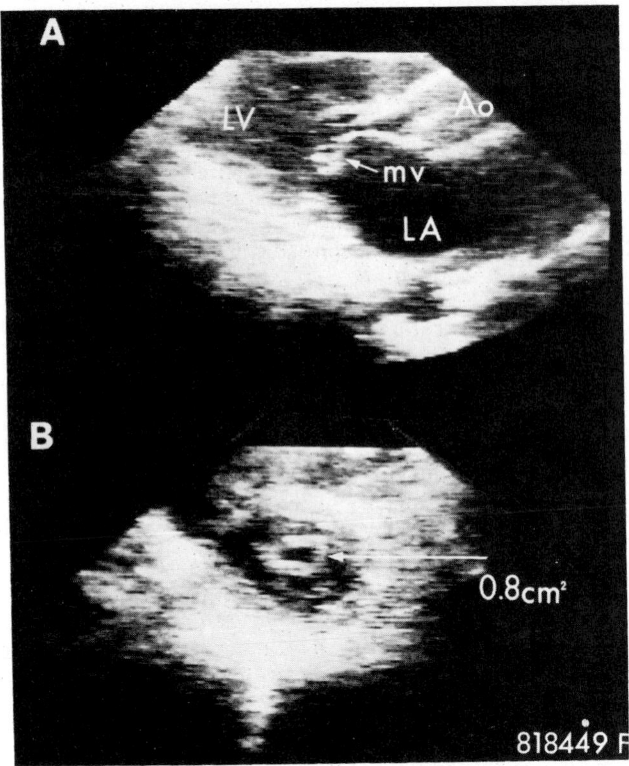

FIGURE 4–45. Two-dimensional echocardiograms of a patient with mitral stenosis. The domed mitral valve (mv) can be seen in the long-axis examination *(A)*. The short-axis examination *(B)* demonstrates the orifice of the stenotic valve and provides the opportunity for determining the degree of stenosis.

valve that is truly stenotic from one that opens poorly because of low flow. Two-dimensional echocardiography provides an opportunity to visualize and measure the flow-restricting orifice of the stenotic mitral valve directly (Fig. 4–45*B*).[148]

Doppler echocardiography provides another means of quantitating the degree of MS.[149] Figure 4–46 shows a pulsed Doppler recording of a patient with MS and atrial fibrillation; there is no atrial contraction. The peak velocities are increased and the fall in velocity in early diastole is decreased. The technique for quantitating the degree of MS depends on the rate of velocity decrease in early diastole. The time interval required for the peak velocity to reach half of its initial level is related directly to the severity of the obstruction of the mitral orifice.[150] This pressure half-time correlates reasonably well with the mitral valve area; however, there are some limitations to this technique.[151–153] The modified Bernoulli equation can also be used to calculate the mean gradient transmitral valve pressure gradient. Mitral valve area can then be calculated using the Gorlin formula and a Doppler measurement for mitral blood flow.[154]

Echocardiography can help determine whether or not a stenotic valve is suitable for valvotomy by estimating its pliability and degree of calcification.[155] This ability is particularly valuable in evaluating patients for balloon valvuloplasty.[156–157] Two-dimensional echocardiography is the procedure of choice for assessing the fibrosis and pliability of the mitral valve apparatus, especially when subvalvular adhesions are present.[158] Secondary effects of mitral stenosis, such as left atrial dilatation and pulmonary hypertension, can be detected with various echocardiographic examinations.

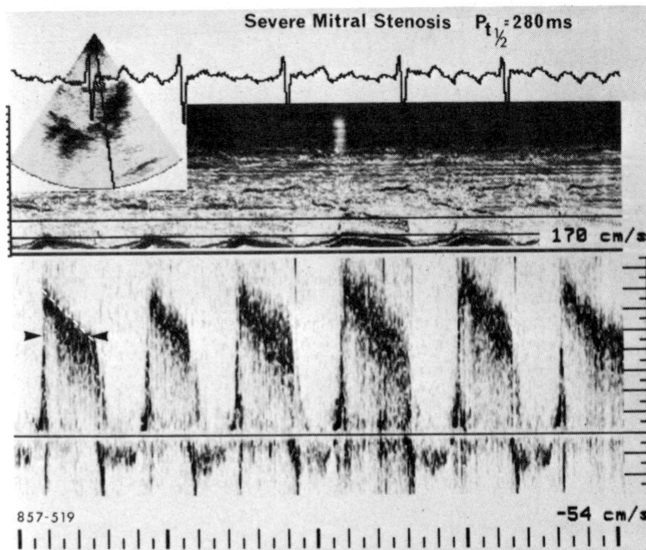

FIGURE 4–46. Pulsed Doppler echocardiogram of mitral flow in a patient with mitral stenosis. This echocardiogram demonstrates how the pressure half-time ($P_{t_{1/2}}$) (arrowheads) is measured. (From Feigenbaum, H.: Echocardiography. 4th ed. Philadelphia, Lea and Febiger, 1986.)

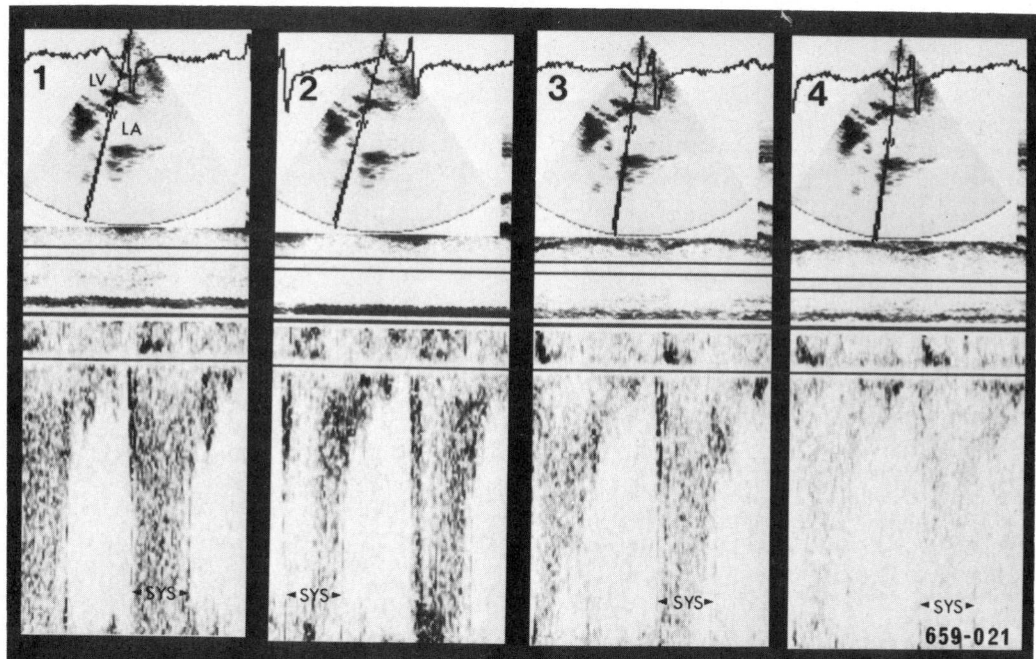

FIGURE 4–47. Serial Doppler examinations showing mapping from mitral regurgitation with the transducer in the parasternal long-axis position. SYS = systole. The regurgitant signal becomes progressively fainter as the sampling site is moved progressively from the mitral valve. (From Feigenbaum, H.: Echocardiography. 4th ed. Philadelphia, Lea and Febiger, 1986.)

MITRAL REGURGITATION

DOPPLER ECHOCARDIOGRAPHY. This is the ultrasonic procedure of choice for the detection of any valvular regurgitation.[159,160] Figure 4–47 shows a pulsed Doppler recording with the Doppler sample in the left atrium. With this type of examination a high-velocity recording during ventricular systole in the left atrium is visualized. The severity of the mitral regurgitation (MR) is generally assessed by the distance from the valve orifice that the regurgitant jet can still be detected on the Doppler recording. For example, in Figure 4–47 the Doppler sample is in the mid portion of the left atrium and regurgitation is still detected. This finding would generally be interpreted as indicating a moderate degree of MR. If the jet were present only near the orifice, as in Figure 4–47, then a mild degree of MR would be present. Detecting high-velocity systolic flow with the sample volume near the back of the left atrial wall indicates a more severe form of MR.

COLOR FLOW DOPPLER. This is another technique for assessing the presence of MR[14,160] (Fig. 4–48). The regurgitant blood flows into the left atrium during ventricular systole. The velocity is very high and a mosaic, multicolored pattern is recorded because of aliasing. The location, direction, and size of the MR flow are readily depicted by the color flow system. There is a rough relationship between the size of the regurgitant jet and the extent of regurgitation,[161,162] but this relationship is influenced by many factors, such as the direction of the regurgitant jet (Fig. 4–49). In Figure 4–48 the jet enters the center of the left atrium and fills much of the left atrium. However, in Figure 4–49 the jet is directed towards the interatrial septum and the flow curves around the atrial septum (arrows). A useful sign when using color flow Doppler for valvular regurgitation is to look at the acceleration of flow proximal to the regurgitant orifice (AC) (Fig. 4–48). This acceleration is due to blood velocity increasing as it approaches the small regurgitant orifice.[163] This finding is usually indicative of significant blood flow or regurgitant flow.

Unfortunately, all flow mapping techniques either with color mapping or standard pulsed Doppler have only a limited relationship to the degree of MR.[164–166] Thus the quantitation of valvular regurgitation using Doppler flow mapping is at best semiquantitative. An alternative Doppler technique for quantifying MR is to calculate stroke volumes through two different orifices, one which reflects flow ejected from the left ventricle to the aorta and one measuring flow passing from the left atrium to the left ventricle.[167,168] The difference is the regurgitant volume, and regurgitant fraction can be calculated. This approach requires accurate stroke volume measurements and may not be possible in all patients.

Echocardiography is also helpful in assessing the hemodynamic consequences of the MR. The left atrium is invariably dilated and left ventricular stroke volume increases with frequent left ventricular dilatation.[169] All of these findings are detectable on the echocardiogram. Possibly one of the most important uses of echocardiography is in identifying the *etiology* of the MR. Rheumatic MR almost always produces some thickening of the mitral valve and at least minimal echocardiographic evidence of MS. There are numerous other causes for MR, and echocardiography plays an important role in identifying these.

Figure 4–48. See color plate 2.

Figure 4–49. See color plate 2.

Nonrheumatic Mitral Regurgitation

MITRAL VALVE PROLAPSE (see p. 1029). Echocardiography is particularly useful in the diagnosis of this condition. Figure 4–50 demonstrates the principal M-mode—a fairly abrupt posterior (downward) motion of the mitral valve apparatus in mid- or late systole.[170] This motion often commences simultaneously with the mid- or late systolic click (Fig. 4–50), a typical auscultatory and phonocardiographic finding in this condition (p. 54). Although this mid- or late systolic posterior motion of the mitral valve is a reasonably *specific* sign of mitral valve prolapse, it is not a very *sensitive* sign. Many patients with this lesion fail to show it, while in others the prolapse is a holosystolic event, i.e., there is posterior displacement of the valve throughout systole (Fig. 34–23, p. 1034).[171] Minor degrees of posterior displacement of the mitral valve can occur normally, and there is a troublesome "gray zone" in which it is difficult to determine whether the prolapse is normal or not.[172] Late or holosystolic prolapse, as in Figure 4–50, in which the leaflets move posteriorly by at least 5 mm, is generally accepted as abnormal. However, when the holosystolic "hammocking" is less than 5 mm,[173] the diagnosis is not clear-cut.

Several findings on 2-D echocardiography have been suggested for the diagnosis of mitral valve prolapse,[174,175] including the recording of buckling of one or both mitral leaflets into the left atrium during systole. Figure 4–51 (and also 4–59) demonstrates a parasternal long-axis on a four-chamber examination of a patient with mitral valve prolapse. The posterior or mitral leaflet can be seen buckling or herniating into the left atrium in late systole. Unfortunately, the amount of systolic prolapse noted on the 2-D echocardiograms also exhibits a continuum from normal to abnormal, and there may still be a problem in differentiating between prolapse and a normal variant with this technique.[176,177] The parasternal long-axis view is probably more specific for the diagnosis of prolapse.[178]

Other echocardiographic findings in patients with mitral valve prolapse include excessive amplitude of motion of the valve during diastole which can be appreciated in both M-mode and 2-D examinations. Thickening of the leaflets is

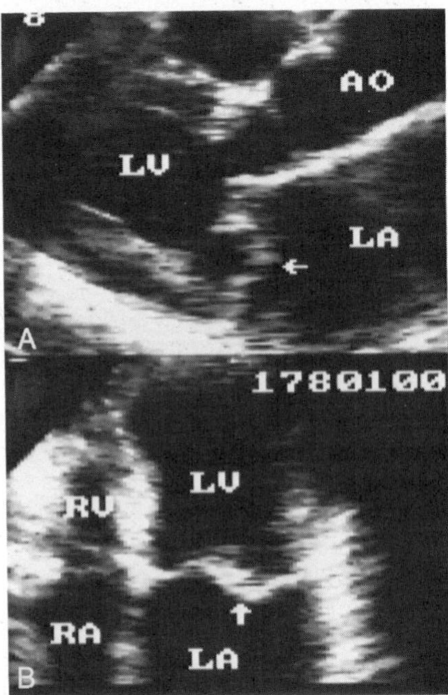

FIGURE 4–51. Two-dimensional echocardiogram in the parasternal long-axis (A) and apical four-chamber (B) views of a patient with mitral valve prolapse (arrows). LV = left ventricle, AO = aorta, LA = left atrium, RV = right ventricle, RA = right atrium.

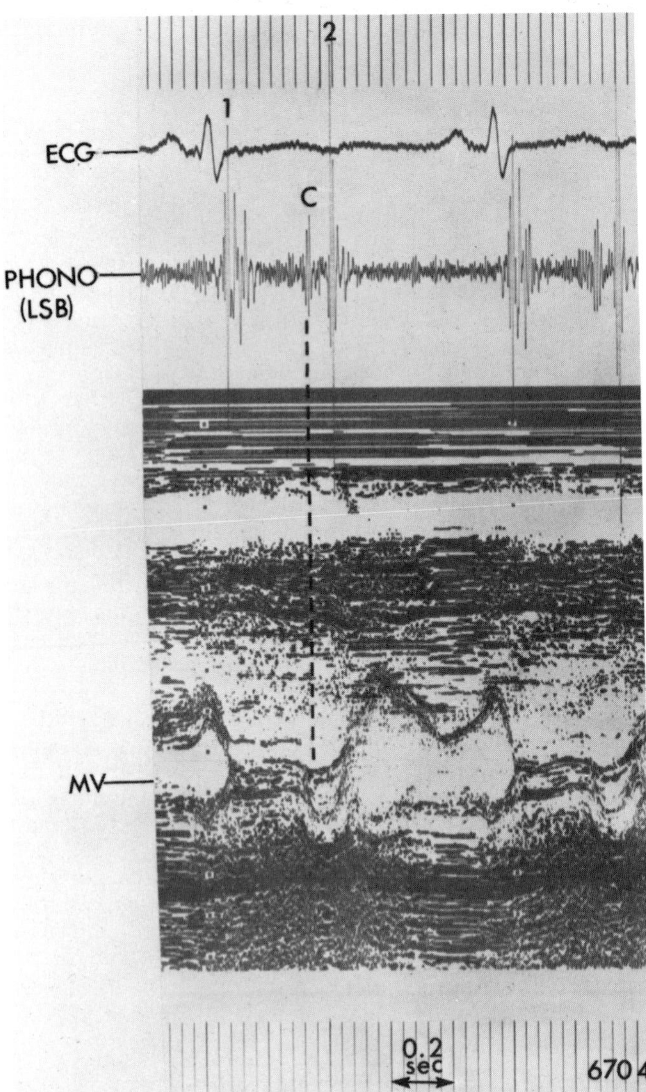

FIGURE 4–50. Phonocardiogram and M-mode echocardiogram from a patient with mitral valve prolapse. The late systolic click (C) on the phonocardiogram corresponds to late systolic posterior displacement of the mitral valve (MV). (From Tavel, M. E.: Clinical Phonocardiography and External Pulse Recordings. 3rd ed. Chicago, Year Book Medical Publishers, 1978.)

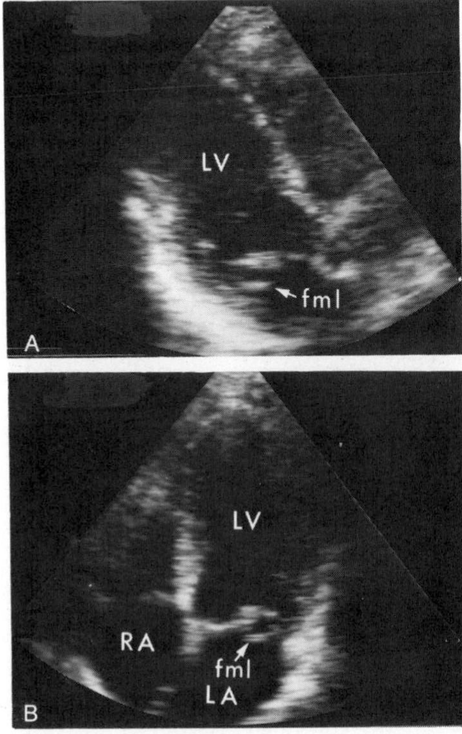

FIGURE 4–52. *A*, Apical two-chamber and *B*, four-chamber views of a patient with a flail mitral leaflet. The flail leaflet (fml) can be seen protruding into the left atrium (LA) during ventricular systole. LV = left ventricle; RA = right atrium. (From Feigenbaum, H.: Echocardiography. 4th ed. Philadelphia, Lea and Febiger, 1986.)

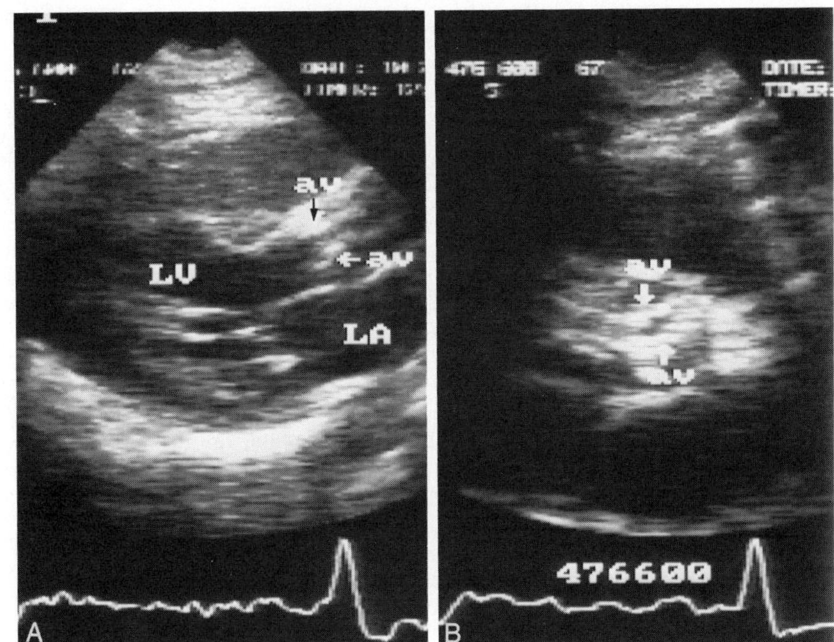

FIGURE 4–53. Long-axis *(A)* and short-axis *(B)* 2-D echocardiograms of a patient with a thickened stenotic aortic valve (av). LV = left ventricle, LA = left atrium.

common and is presumably due to myxomatous degeneration.[179] The leaflets may also be redundant and seem to fold on themselves in diastole. When there is redundancy and thickening of the leaflets, the diagnosis of mitral valve prolapse is more secure than when the leaflets are seen to move into the left atrium in systole.[180] It must be emphasized that although echocardiography can frequently be used to make a positive diagnosis of mitral valve prolapse, it is also difficult to distinguish minor degrees of prolapse from a normal variant.

Two-dimensional echocardiography is the examination of choice for establishing the presence of a flail mitral leaflet.[181] With this abnormality the leaflets are seen to protrude into the left atrium (Fig. 4–52).[182] The differentiation between a flail mitral leaflet and mitral valve prolapse depends on whether the tips of the leaflet point toward the left atrium (flail valve) or curve back and point toward the left ventricle (prolapse).[183]

PAPILLARY MUSCLE DYSFUNCTION. Two-dimensional echocardiography provides an opportunity to detect incomplete closure of the mitral valve because of left ventricular dilatation or scarring of the papillary muscles. In this condition the leaflets in the four-chamber view fail to reach the level of the mitral annulus (Fig. 4–53).[184]

AORTIC STENOSIS

Doppler echocardiography has revolutionized the role of echocardiography and indeed the management of patients with AS. M-mode and 2-D echocardiography have always provided an excellent qualitative diagnosis of AS. Doppler echocardiography now provides an opportunity for the quantitative diagnosis. The 2-D echocardiographic diagnosis of valvular aortic stenosis is doming, thickening, and restricted motion of the leaflets (Fig. 4–53).[185,186] The valve may be heavily calcified and immobile, in which case only distorted, echo-producing, immobile valve leaflets are apparent.[187] It is possible to make a semiquantitative assessment of AS with 2-D echocardiography by judging the mobility of the leaflets, especially in the short-axis view (Fig. 4–53).

The best ultrasonic technique for quantifying AS utilizes continuous wave Doppler.[117,188–190] Using the modified Bernoulli equation (Fig. 4–40) it is possible to measure the pressure gradient across the aortic valve. Figure 4–54 shows a composite of simultaneous Doppler recordings and intracardiac pressure measurements in four patients with AS; an increase in the Doppler velocity occurs as the gradient increases.

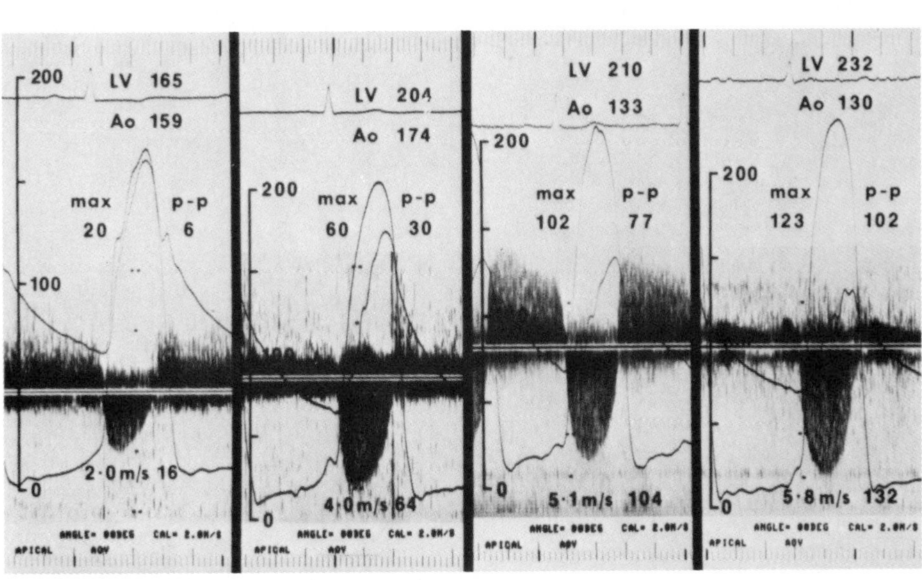

FIGURE 4–54. Simultaneous continuous wave Doppler and hemodynamic measurements in four different patients with valvular aortic stenosis. The peak velocity increases as the gradient between the left ventricular and aortic pressures increases. (From Currie, P. J., et al.: Continuous wave Doppler echocardiographic assessment of severity of calcific aortic stenosis: A simultaneous Doppler-catheter correlative study in 100 adult patients. Circulation *71*:1162, 1985, by permission of the American Heart Association, Inc.)

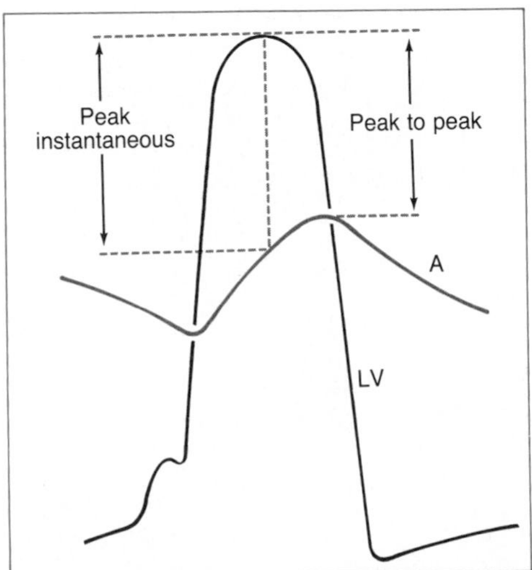

FIGURE 4-55. Diagram of left ventricular (LV) and aortic (A) pressures in aortic stenosis. The peak instantaneous pressure difference or gradient is greater than the peak-to-peak gradient because the peak aortic pressure occurs later than the peak left ventricular pressure. (From Feigenbaum, H.: Echocardiography. 4th ed. Philadelphia, Lea and Febiger, 1986.)

There is an excellent relationship between the instantaneous gradient across the stenotic valve as measured by both catheterization and Doppler techniques.[188]

In the cardiac catheterization laboratory it is customary to measure the aortic valve gradient difference between the peak left ventricular pressure and the peak aortic pressure (the *"peak to peak" gradient*) (Fig. 4-55). This gradient actually does not exist at any instant in time because the peak aortic pressure occurs later than the peak left ventricular pressure. The *peak instantaneous pressure gradient* measured by the Doppler technique is invariably larger. If one measures the more accurate *mean gradients* both in the catheterization laboratory and with the Doppler examination, then the measurements are quite similar.

The Doppler technique thus gives a good estimate of the gradient across the aortic valve. Obviously the gradient is dependent on both the aortic valve area and the flow across the valve. With a reduced cardiac output one can have a small gradient in a patient with severe AS. Cardiac output could be measured with a right heart catheter and thermodilution techniques[191] or by use of one of the Doppler stroke volume measurements through an orifice that does not have a diseased valve. Another Doppler approach for calculating aortic valve area uses the "continuity equation"[192] (Fig. 4-41). This technique has been used with reasonable accuracy to calculate the aortic valve orifice in patients with valvular AS. A modification of the continuity equation uses blood flow through the mitral orifice rather than the left ventricular outflow tract.[193]

The theoretical basis for using Doppler echocardiography for calculating valve gradient is well established. However, there are technical details which must be recognized.[194,195] It is crucial that the maximal velocity be recorded and that the ultrasonic beam be parallel to the aortic stenotic jet. This requirement can make the examination fairly lengthy. Various ultrasonic windows must be tried to make certain that the optimal jet is identified.

From a practical point of view, if a high-velocity jet (in excess of 4 m/sec) is identified, the probability of critical AS is extremely high and the patient's condition can be managed accordingly. On the other hand, if the velocity is within normal limits or mildly elevated, the possibility of significant AS can be excluded. When the velocity is in an intermediate zone, which would indicate a pressure gradient between 25 and 50 mm Hg, additional hemodynamic information may be necessary for proper management.[196]

There are secondary signs of AS which can be noted on the echocardiogram. Both M-mode and 2-D echocardiography can detect left ventricular hypertrophy with increased thickness of the left ventricular walls. Although the degree of left ventricular hypertrophy has been used to assess the severity of AS,[197] this technique is not nearly as reliable as use of Doppler for valve gradients and valve area.

AORTIC REGURGITATION

As with all valvular regurgitation, Doppler echocardiography is the examination of choice for detecting the presence of aortic regurgitation (AR).[198,199] Figure 4-56 shows a Doppler sample in the left ventricular outflow tract and the recording of high-velocity flow during diastole. This type of examination is both sensitive and specific for the presence of AR. Color-flow Doppler provides a 2-D display of the AR jet (Fig. 4-57). The accuracy of Doppler flow mapping for quantitating AR is at best semiquantitative.[200] The same limitations pertain to AR as were discussed with MR (p. 83). Some investigators are using the width of the aortic jet at the valve orifice as judged by color flow Doppler to judge the severity of AR.[13,201-203] The validity of this observation has yet to be confirmed. The rate of decrease in velocity of the regurgitant blood as recorded in the left ventricle using continuous-wave

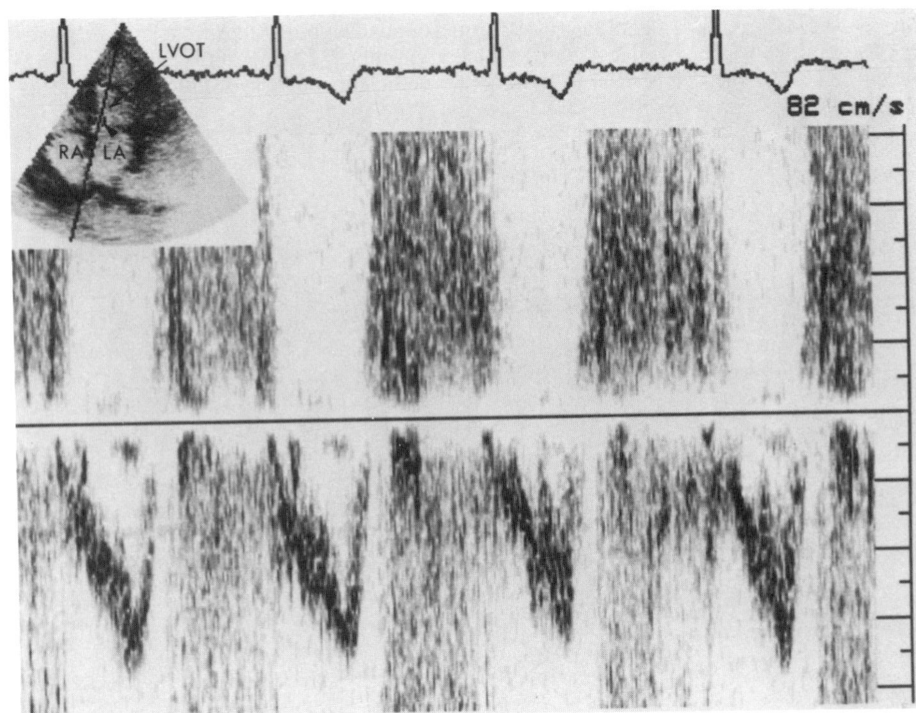

FIGURE 4-56. Pulsed Doppler echocardiogram with the sample volume (arrow) in the left ventricular outflow tract (LVOT) in a patient with aortic regurgitation. RA = right atrium; LA = left atrium. (From Feigenbaum, H.: Echocardiography. 4th ed. Philadelphia, Lea and Febiger, 1986.)

Figure 4–57. See color plate 2.

Doppler has been used as a reflection of severity of the AR (Fig. 4–58). Severe AR produces a faster fall in velocity as the pressure difference between the aorta and left ventricle falls rapidly.[204] AR can also be judged by the difference between aortic flow and pulmonary artery flow or mitral flow.[205]

There are several indirect echocardiographic signs of AR which have become obsolete with the advent of Doppler techniques. Fluttering of the mitral valve on the M-mode echocardiogram was the principal indication for the qualitative diagnosis of AR. The sign is not nearly as sensitive or specific for AR as is Doppler. The regurgitant jet will also influence the Doppler mitral inflow.[206,207]

One M-mode sign of AR which remains very useful is the premature closure of the mitral valve in the presence of severe, usually acute, AR[126,127] (p. 1051). With an elevated left ventricular diastolic pressure there may even be early opening of the aortic valve on the M-mode recording.[131] Both of these signs represent severe AR and markedly elevated left ventricular diastolic pressures. The secondary effects of AR on the left ventricle can be detected with both M-mode and 2-D echocardiographic examinations. Serial measurements of left ventricular size and systolic function are important in following patients with chronic AR or judging the efficacy of surgery.[208,209] Deterioration in left ventricular systolic function is one criterion for valve replacement[210] (p. 1052).

TRICUSPID STENOSIS. The echocardiographic findings of tricuspid stenosis and regurgitation are very similar to those for MS and MR. Two-dimensional and Doppler echocardiography are the procedures of choice for detecting tricuspid stenosis. Doming of the tricuspid valve on 2-D echocardiography is the hallmark of MS.[211,212] The Doppler findings of tricuspid stenosis are similar to those with mitral stenosis. The velocities passing through the orifice are increased and the rate of diastolic decline in velocity is reduced. The pressure half-time can also be used to calculate the severity of the valvular obstruction.

TRICUSPID REGURGITATION. This abnormality is also best determined by pulsed, continuous wave, or color flow Doppler echocardiography.[213,214] As noted previously the Doppler recording of tricuspid regurgitation can be used to estimate the pressure gradient across the tricuspid valve. This measurement provides an opportunity for estimating right ventricular systolic pressure by adding an estimate of right atrial pressure. Contrast echocardiography can be used for detecting tricuspid regurgitation but is being replaced by the Doppler approach.[213,215]

Two-dimensional echocardiography can help determine the etiology of tricuspid regurgitation. *Rheumatic tricuspid regurgitation* usually has an element of tricuspid stenosis and invariably exhibits MS. Pulmonary hypertension can be detected by estimating the right ventricular systolic pressure.

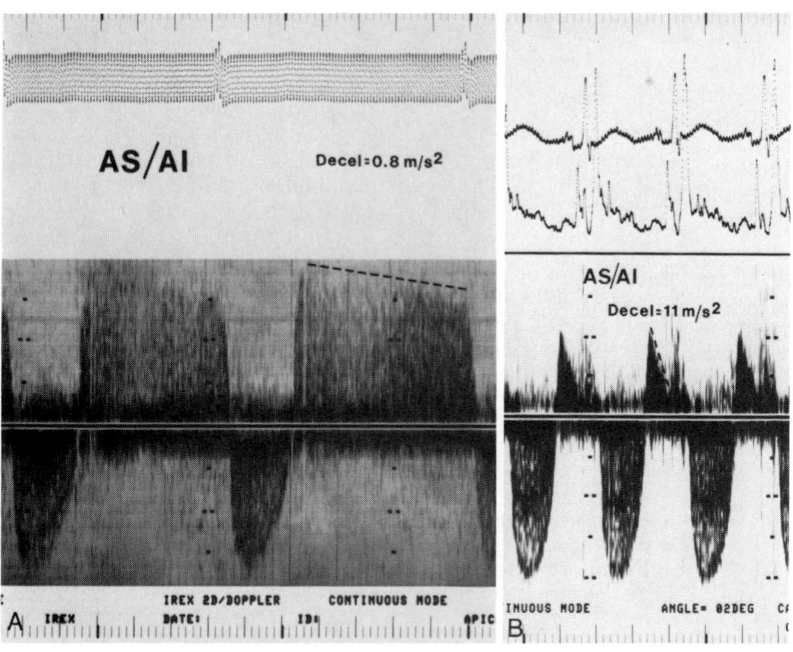

FIGURE 4–58. Continuous wave Doppler recordings of two patients with aortic regurgitation. The diastolic deceleration rate is less rapid with mild aortic regurgitation *(A)* than with more severe regurgitation *(B)*.

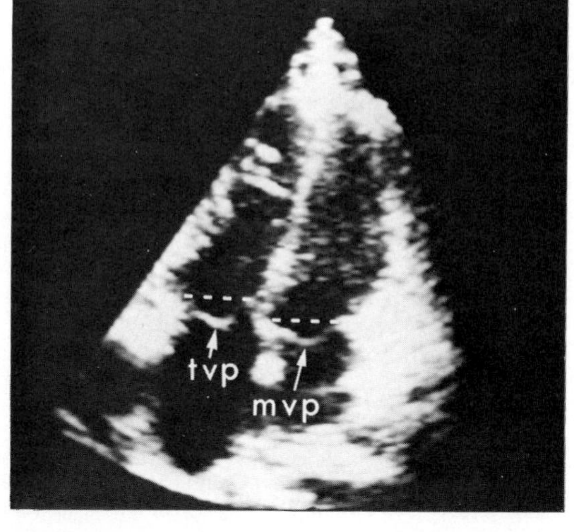

FIGURE 4–59. Apical four-chamber 2-D echocardiogram of a patient with tricuspid valve prolapse (tvp) and mitral valve prolapse (mvp). (From Feigenbaum, H.: Echocardiography. 4th ed. Philadelphia, Lea and Febiger, 1986.)

Tricuspid valve prolapse gives an appearance similar to that of mitral valve prolapse (Fig. 4–59).[216] A *flail* tricuspid valve is indicated by the finding of parts of the tricuspid valve protruding into the right atrium in ventricular systole.[217] *Carcinoid valve disease* (p. 1056) produces stiff immobile tricuspid leaflets that are continuously open.[218] Tricuspid valvular *vegetations* and *Ebstein's anomaly* are discussed on pp. 1083 and 940, respectively.

Secondary effects of tricuspid regurgitation can be noted on both M-mode and 2-D studies. Right ventricular and right atrial dilatation are invariably present. Abnormal motion of the interventricular septum indicates that a right ventricular volume overload may be present.

INFECTIVE ENDOCARDITIS

(See Chap. 35)

Echocardiography provides a means for visualizing the vegetations of infective valvular endocarditis, which appear as echo-producing masses attached to the infected valve (Fig. 35–2, p. 1085).[219,220] Vegetations must be approximately 3 to 4 mm in diameter before they can be appreciated on a transthoracic echocardiogram[221] (Fig. 4–60). They are usually asymmetrical, commonly involving one leaflet more than another, but may be present on more than one valve. If the vegetation is associated with destruction of the valve or if it is on a long "stalk," it can be readily imaged; its excessive motion can be appreciated on both M-mode[222,223] and 2-D echocardiography.[223] Transesophageal echocardiography is proving to be much more sensitive than transthoracic echocardiography in detecting valvular vegetations.[224] Fig. 4–61 shows a small vegetation on the aortic valve. This lesion was not seen on the routine transthoracic echocardiogram. The greater sensitivity of transesophageal echocardiography for the detection of valvular vegetations may change our understanding as to why echocardiographic vegetations are frequently seen in patients with endocarditis and whether or not this ultrasonic technique can exclude the diagnosis.[225]

Vegetations visualized echocardiographically need not be bacterial[226–231] or even infected. Infected vegetations may be difficult to distinguish from myxomatous degeneration of the valve,[223] although this differentiation is usually readily accomplished clinically.

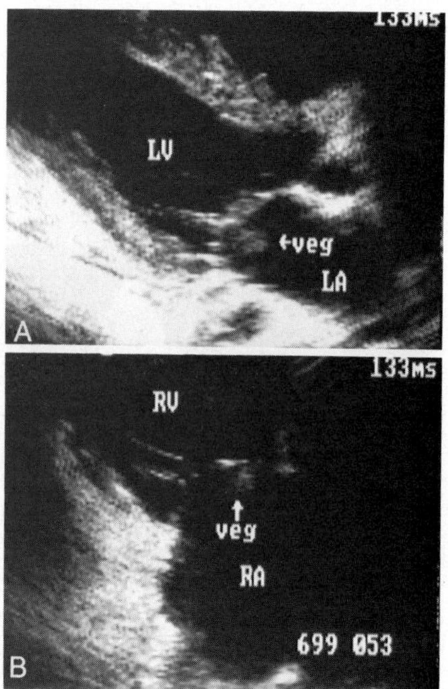

FIGURE 4–60. **Two-dimensional echocardiograms of a patient with vegetation (veg) on the mitral *(A)* and tricuspid valves *(B)*. LV = left ventricle, LA = left atrium, RV = right ventricle, RA = right atrium.**

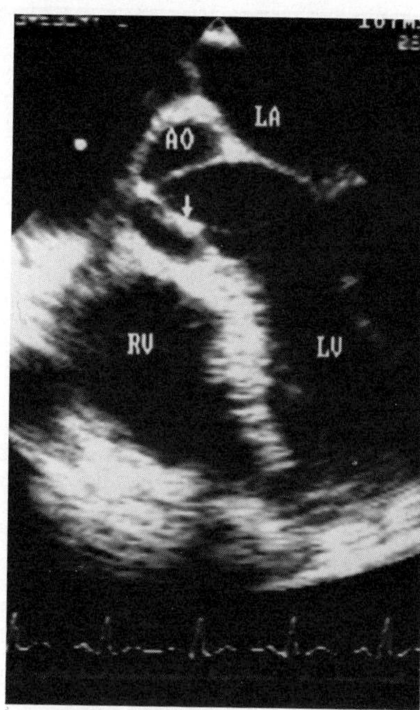

FIGURE 4–61. **Transesophageal echocardiogram of a patient with a small vegetation (arrows) on the aortic valve. AO = aorta, LA = left atrium, RV = right ventricle, LV = left ventricle.**

One of the major applications of echocardiography in patients with endocarditis is in the identification of complications. When the valve is damaged to the point that it is grossly incompetent, echocardiography can both detect and assess the hemodynamic importance of the valvular regurgitation. When the aortic valve is involved, premature closure of the mitral valve because of the very high left ventricular diastolic pressure may be evident. Another serious complication of aortic valve endocarditis is the development of an aortic abscess (Fig. 4–62).[232,233] This problem is seen as a relatively echo-free space adjacent to the aortic root. Mitral valve diverticulum can be detected by means of esophageal echocardiography.[234]

PROSTHETIC VALVES

There is a variety of echocardiographic signs of prosthetic valve malfunction. Most published reports of prosthetic valve malfunction represent isolated case studies.[235–237] Abnormal motion of a ball or disc usually results from a thrombus[238] or from ball variance.[239] A useful sign of a malfunctioning Björk-Shiley valve in the mitral position is a rounding of the E point on the M-mode echocardiogram.[240] An abnormal rocking motion of a prosthetic valve resulting from the sutures pulling loose from the annulus has been reported.[241] The significance of the *fine* intracavitary echoes

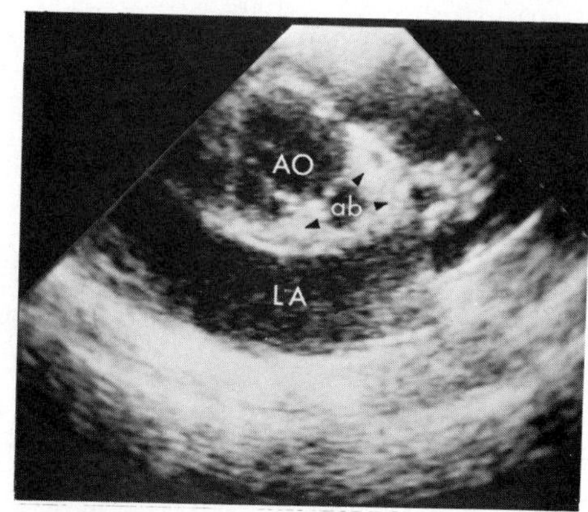

FIGURE 4–62. **Short-axis 2-D echocardiogram through the root of the aorta in a patient with an abscess (ab) involving the aortic root (AO). LA = left atrium.**

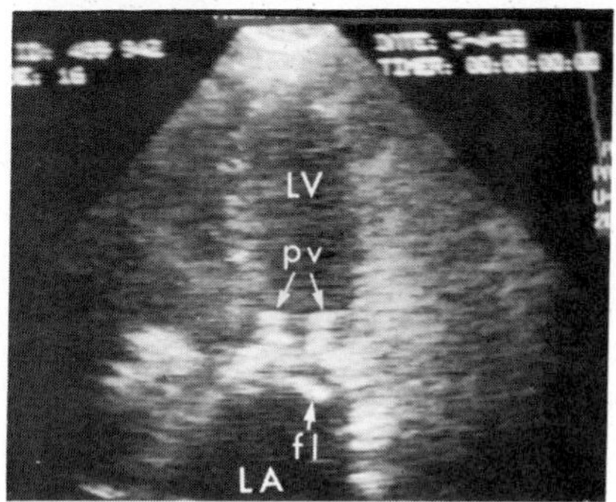

FIGURE 4-63. Apical four-chamber view of a patient with a degenerated flail porcine mitral prosthesis (pv). The flail leaflet (fl) can be seen protruding into the left atrium (LA) in systole. LV = left ventricle. (From Feigenbaum, H.: Echocardiography. 4th ed. Philadelphia, Lea and Febiger, 1986.)

originating from prosthetic valves in the mitral position is unclear.[242] Thickening of the porcine valve leaflets is useful in judging deterioration of this valve.[243] A flail porcine valve, especially in the mitral position, can be easily identified with 2-D echocardiography (Fig. 4-63).[244]

DOPPLER ECHOCARDIOGRAPHY. This technique is very helpful in evaluating prosthetic valves.[245-247] Valvular regurgitation is detected readily with the Doppler technique. Color Doppler has the advantage of locating some of these unusually located valvular regurgitations (Fig. 4-64).[248,249] Doppler echocardiography can also assist in judging stenotic prosthetic valves. The technique is most effective with valves which have a central orifice, such as a tissue valve[250,251] or St. Jude mechanical valve.[252] Ball valves or tilting disc valves present more difficulties in judging the flow characteristics through the valve.

Figure 4-64. See color plate 3.

TRANSESOPHAGEAL ECHOCARDIOGRAPHY. This technique has made a major contribution to the detection of malfunctioning prosthetic valves,[253,254] particularly of prosthetic mitral valves.[255] Acoustic shadowing frequently prohibits the detection of mitral regurgitation involving a prosthetic valve when the examination is done through the chest.[22] When the ultrasonic examination is performed via the esophagus and the left atrium, the regurgitant jet is unobstructed and easily detected (Fig. 4-15).[256] In addition, the high resolution inherent in the higher frequency transducer provides better visualization of the prosthetic valve, especially for the detection of minor abnormalities such as small thrombi or vegetations.

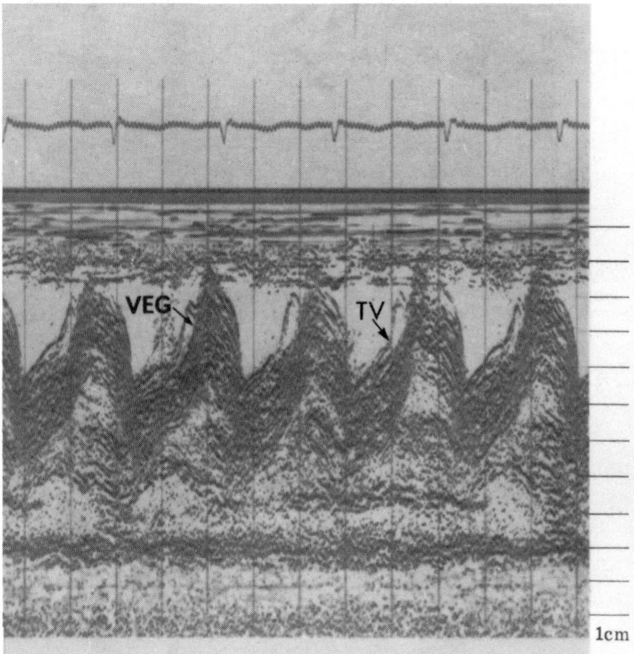

FIGURE 4-65. M-mode echocardiogram demonstrating a large bacterial vegetation (veg) on the tricuspid valve (tv). (From Feigenbaum, H.: Echocardiography. 4th ed. Philadelphia, Lea and Febiger, 1986.)

CALCIFIED MITRAL ANNULUS (see p. 1018)

Calcification of a mitral annulus can be readily demonstrated by echocardiography.[257-258] The principal finding is a band of dense echoes between the mitral valve and the posterior left ventricular wall (Fig. 4-65). Calcification can be extensive and involve the posterior mitral leaflet and much of the base of the heart.

CONGENITAL HEART DISEASE

(See also Chaps. 31 and 32)

DEDUCTIVE ECHOCARDIOGRAPHY

With the advent of 2-D echocardiography and Doppler techniques, echocardiography is rapidly becoming a definitive study for many patients with congenital heart disease.[259,260] This type of study is providing critical morphological and functional information in the management of these patients. Even the most complex anomalies have been recognized with echocardiography. The question is now being raised as to how often these patients require cardiac catheterization following an adequate echocardiographic examination.[261,262]

There are many ways in which echocardiography can be used to decipher the riddle of a congenitally malformed heart. The term *deductive echocardiography* refers to a technique by which an attempt is made to deduce the anatomy of the heart by identifying systematically the atria, atrioventricular valves, ventricles, semilunar valves, and great vessels.[263] Initially this type of examination was done by combining the chest roentgenogram with the M-mode echocardiogram. Two-dimensional echocardiography alone can now recognize almost all of the cardiovascular components.[264,265] Locating the vena cava identifies the right atrium. The pulmonary veins can be imaged in the apical four-chamber view and signify the location of the left atrium. The pulmonary artery bifurcation distinguishes this vessel from the aorta and its arch branches. The tricuspid valve is identified by the fact that it inserts into the interventricular septum closer to the apex than does the mitral valve.[266] Distinguishing between the mitral and tricuspid valves helps to identify the ventricles since they always accompany the appropriate atrioventricular valve. The semilunar valves are always a part of the appropriate great vessel. Thus these valves are identified once the aorta and pulmonary artery are recognized. This deductive approach can frequently unravel the mystery of even the most complex malformation.

CONGENITAL VALVULAR DISEASE

VALVULAR STENOSIS. A *bicuspid aortic valve* (p. 967) is probably the most common congenital cardiac anomaly. The best echocardiographic criterion for making this diagnosis utilizes 2-D echocardiography. With this technique two cusps rather than the normal three cusps can be identified (Fig. 4-66). The diagnosis can be confusing since occasionally a fused commissure may resemble a third leaflet echocardiographically. In addition, if the commissure is in an anterior-posterior direction, it is sometimes difficult to record echocardiographically.[267] The M-mode technique of identifying eccentric closure of the aortic valve within the aorta[268] is less reliable.

In *aortic stenosis* (p. 1035) most echocardiographic findings are similar whether the valve is deformed on a congenital (p. 922) or acquired basis. In the adult the valve is frequently heavily calcified and the etiology is difficult to determine. The qualitative diagnosis is made by finding doming and/or restricted motion of the valve during systole. The quantitative

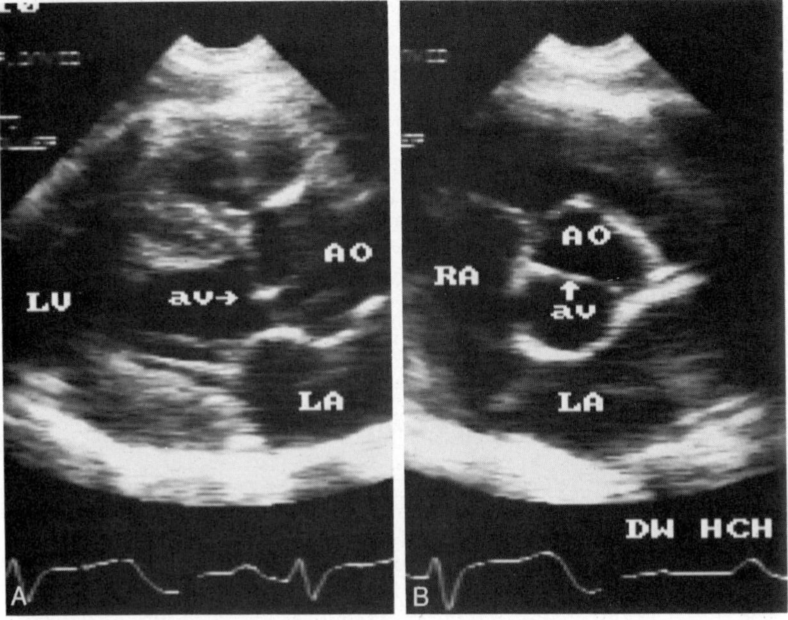

FIGURE 4-66. Long-axis (A) and short-axis (B) 2-D echocardiograms of a patient with a bicuspid aortic valve (av). LV = left ventricle, AO = aorta, LA = left atrium, RA = right atrium.

diagnosis is now best obtained using continuous wave Doppler (p. 67).

A host of types of congenitally deformed mitral valves can be detected echocardiographically.[269] *Congenital mitral stenosis* is rare but has been recognized by echocardiography. A *parachute mitral valve* has also a fairly characteristic echocardiographic appearance. Two-dimensional echocardiography can identify a *double orifice mitral valve*.[270] The domed *stenotic pulmonary valve* resembles the congenitally stenotic aortic valve on 2-D echocardiography.[271] Normally, the open leaflets are parallel to the wall of the pulmonary artery during systole, but when the valve is domed and stenotic, they curve away from the wall (Fig. 4-67). Though only a single leaflet of the pulmonary valve is ordinarily imaged, its domed appearance is sufficient to establish the diagnosis. The *severity* of congenital pulmonic stenosis may also be assessed by Doppler

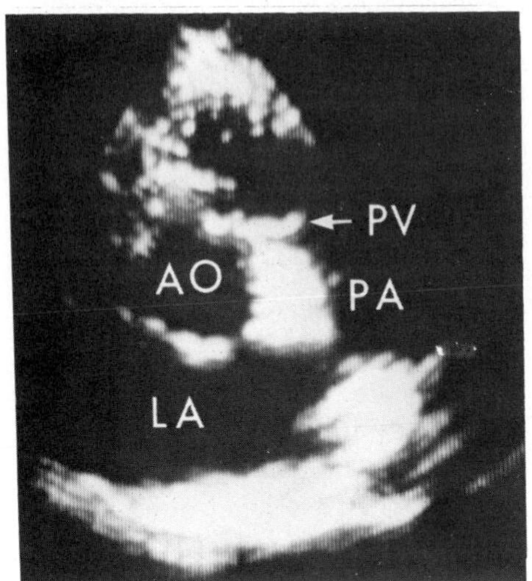

FIGURE 4-67. Two-dimensional echocardiogram of a patient with pulmonic stenosis. The domed, stenotic pulmonary valve (PV) curves into the pulmonary artery (PA) in the systolic frame. AO = aorta, LA = left atrium. (From Feigenbaum, H.: Echocardiography. 4th ed. Philadelphia, Lea and Febiger, 1986.)

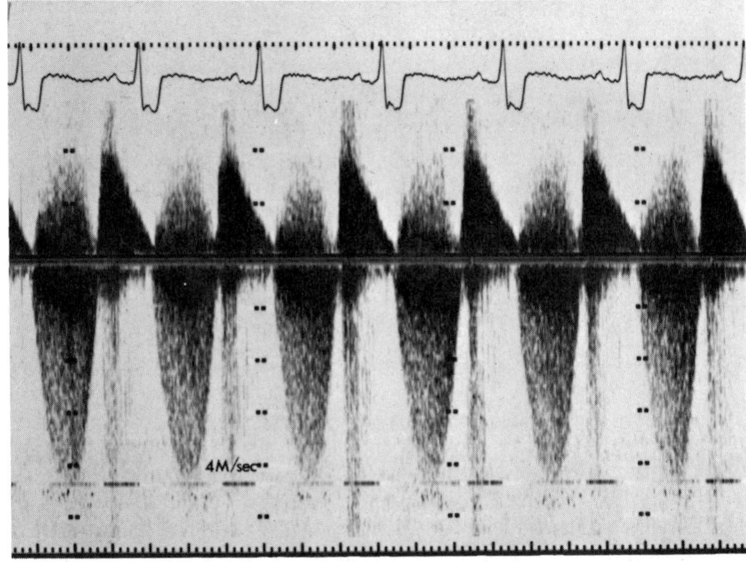

FIGURE 4-68. Continuous wave Doppler recording of a patient with pulmonic stenosis and pulmonary regurgitation. In systole (downward deflection) the velocity is very high and exceeds 4 m/sec. The diastolic reverse flow signifies the presence of pulmonic regurgitation.

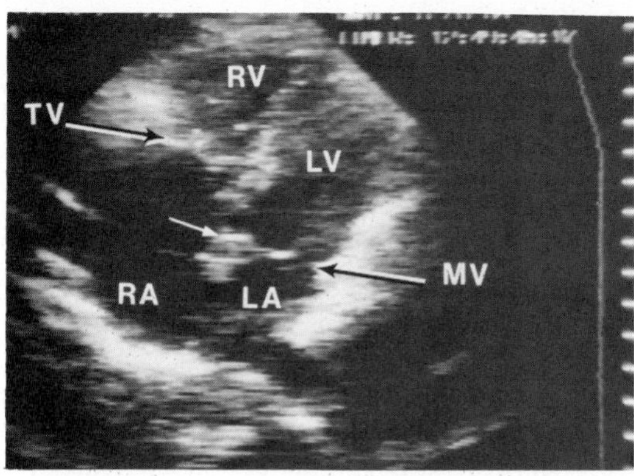

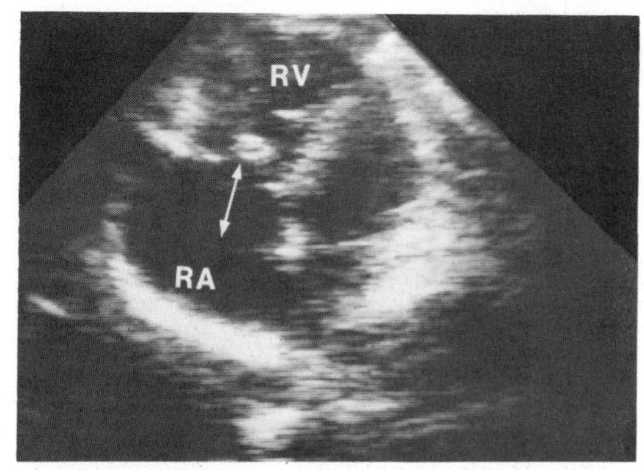

FIGURE 4-69. Apical four-chamber view in a patient with Ebstein's anomaly. The tricuspid valve (TV) is displaced from the tricuspid annulus (arrow). The effective right ventricular volume (RV) is decreased and the volume of the right atrium (RA) is increased. LV = left ventricle, LA = left atrium, MV = mitral valve. (From Feigenbaum, H.: Echocardiography. 4th ed. Philadelphia, Lea and Febiger, 1986.)

echocardiography.[272,273] Utilizing continuous wave Doppler echocardiography and criteria similar to those for aortic stenosis (p. 86), the gradient across the stenotic pulmonary valve can be estimated (Fig. 4-68). A common abnormality associated with congenital pulmonic stenosis is pulmonic regurgitation. This abnormality is noted using Doppler recordings which reveal diastolic flow into the right ventricle.

EBSTEIN'S ANOMALY. (See p. 940). The echocardiographic diagnosis of Ebstein's anomaly is based on the displacement of the tricuspid valve leaflets within the body of the right ventricle on the 2-D echocardiogram (Fig. 4-69).[274,275] Normally the tricuspid valve inserts on the interventricular septum slightly above the insertion of the mitral valve. However, with Ebstein's anomaly this displacement is marked and much of the tricuspid valve lies within the body of the right ventricle. On M-mode echocardiography the diagnosis of Ebstein's anomaly is based on delayed closure of the tricuspid valve.[276] The 2-D echocardiogram is more specific and reliable for this diagnosis.

VALVULAR ATRESIA. Atresia of cardiac valves is generally associated with hypoplasia of the ipsilateral ventricle (Chap. 31). Thus, aortic or mitral atresia is associated with a hypoplastic left ventricle,[277] while tricuspid or pulmonary atresia is associated with hypoplasia of the right ventricle.[278] Diminutive ventricles and the atretic valves have been imaged with both M-mode[277] and 2-D techniques (Fig. 4-70).[279,280]

SUBVALVULAR OBSTRUCTIONS. A variety of congenital subvalvular obstructions have been detected echocardiographically. Early systolic closure of the aortic valve has been observed in patients with both *discrete* (Fig. 4-71)[281] and *hypertrophic obstructive cardiomyopathy* (Fig. 43-11, p. 1406).[130] In addition, systolic fluttering of the aortic valve is often exaggerated, although some degree of aortic valve fluttering may be seen normally. Although midsystolic closure and fluttering of the aortic valve are not specific findings for subaortic stenosis, they can be very helpful in differentiating valvular from subvalvular obstruction, since they do not occur in the former condition.

Examination of the outflow tract is accomplished with 2-D echocardiography, and the subvalvular obstruction can be identified directly by this technique (Fig. 4-72).[282,283] The 2-D technique also permits the classification of discrete obstruction into the discrete membranous and the diffuse types.[284] Distinguishing between them may be of considerable clinical importance, since their management may differ. The membranous form is frequently situated just below the aortic valve and may therefore be difficult to recognize at catheterization, since the short subvalvular chamber can be missed on a pull-out pressure recording. Indeed, the thin membrane can even be missed on the angiogram, so that its recognition by 2-D echocardiography can be very helpful. Doppler echocardiography can be used to assess the severity of subvalvular as well as valvular stenosis.[285]

In *subpulmonic obstruction* the M-mode tracing exhibits coarse fluttering of the pulmonary valve.[286] The actual subpulmonic obstruction can be detected and its severity quantified in patients with tetralogy of Fallot by means of 2-D examination of the right ventricular outflow tract and subpulmonic area.[287]

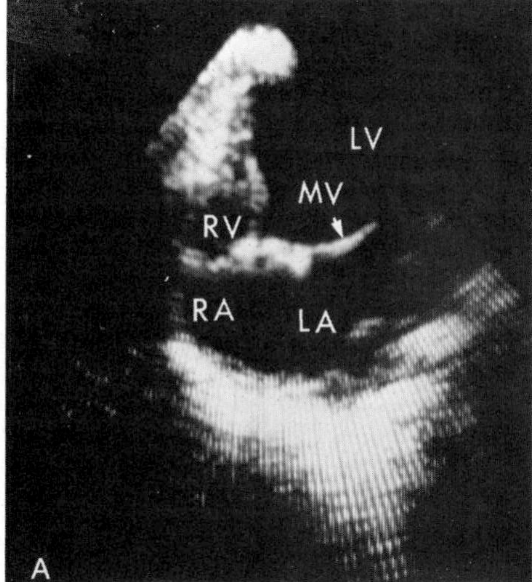

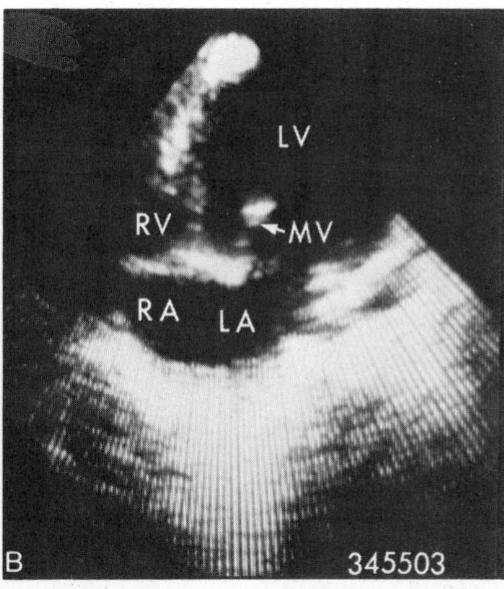

FIGURE 4-70. Apical four-chamber 2-D echocardiograms of a patient with tricuspid atresia. The mitral valve (MV) can be seen opening into a large left ventricular chamber (LV). The right ventricle (RV) is small and is separated from the right atrium (RA) by a dense band of linear echoes. No valvular structure could be identified in the region of the tricuspid valve. LA = left atrium. (From Feigenbaum, H.: Echocardiography. 3rd ed. Philadelphia, Lea and Febiger, 1981.)

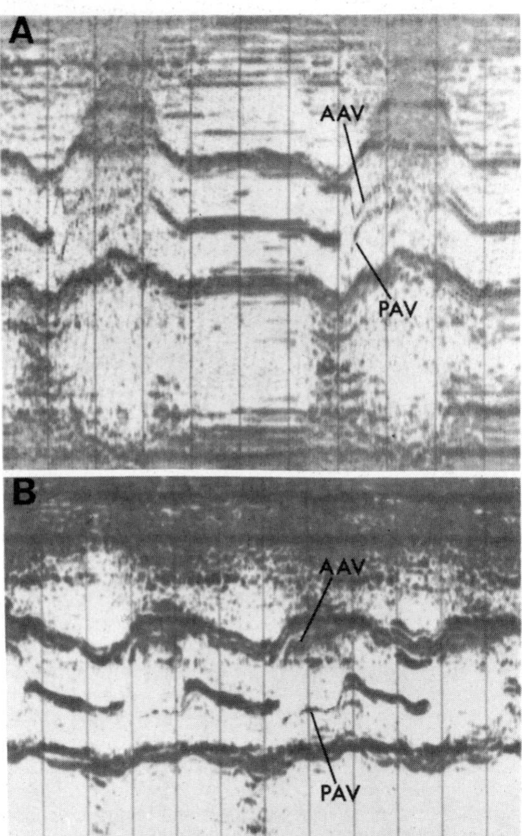

FIGURE 4–71. Aortic valve echocardiograms from a patient with discrete subaortic stenosis before *(A)* and *(B)* surgery for the subaortic obstruction. Prior to surgery the aortic valve anterior (AAV) and posterior (PAV) leaflets come together shortly after the onset of ventricular ejection and remain essentially closed throughout systole. This systolic closure of the valve leaflets is no longer present following surgery. (From Davis, R. H., et al.: Echocardiographic manifestation of discrete subaortic stenosis. Am. J. Cardiol. *33*:277, 1974.)

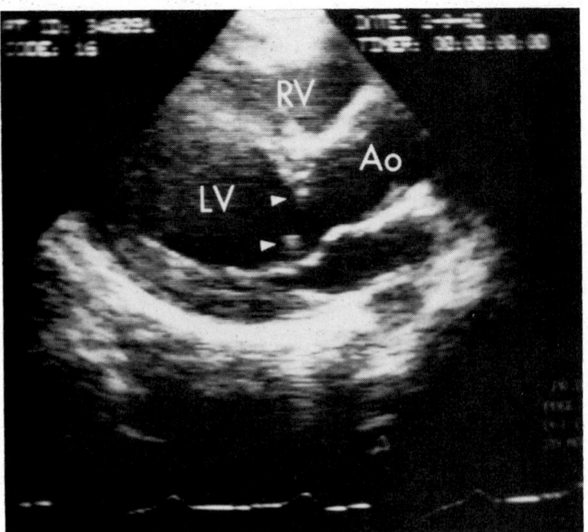

FIGURE 4–72. Parasternal, long-axis 2-D echocardiogram of a patient with a membranous discrete subaortic stenosis. The echoes from the subvalvular membrane (arrowheads) can be seen between the left ventricle (LV) and the aorta (AO). RV = right ventricle.

CARDIAC SHUNTS

Echocardiography can be helpful in the diagnosis of cardiac shunts by detecting the actual defect between the two sides of the heart, by evaluating the hemodynamic consequences of the shunt, and by recording the shunted blood using color flow Doppler or contrast methods.

VENTRICULAR SEPTAL DEFECT. Pulsed Doppler is useful for detecting ventricular septal defects,[288] but color flow Doppler has become the technique of choice for visualizing these abnormalities[289] (Fig. 4–73). The examination is particularly helpful when multiple defects exist.[290] The defects can also be seen with 2-D echocardiography.[291] Figure 4–74 demonstrates a small membranous ventricular septal defect using 2-D echocardiography and contrast. Figure 4–75 demonstrates an apical four-chamber view in a patient with total absence of a ventricular septum or a single ventricle.[292] The Doppler velocity across the ventricular septal defect can reflect the pressure difference between the left and right ventricles during systole.[293] Subtracting the pressure gradient from the left ventricular systolic pressure provides an estimate of the right ventricular systolic pressure.

ATRIAL SEPTAL DEFECT. The 2-D echocardiographic examination, especially from the subcostal position, provides an opportunity for direct examination of the interatrial septum (Fig. 4–26*A*, p. 74).[294] Figure 4–76 demonstrates findings in a patient with an ostium secundum atrial septal defect. A remnant of the interatrial septum can be seen attached to the ventricular septum. In contrast, Figure 4–77 demonstrates an atrial septal defect in a patient with an ostium primum defect. There is no residual septum attached to the ventricular septum. Thus, the 2-D technique not only helps to identify the presence of an atrial septal defect, but it is also an excellent means of differentiating a secundum from a primum type abnormality. One can also identify more severe forms of endocardial cushion defect with a coexistent ventricular septal defect (Fig. 4–78). A sinus venosus type atrial septal defect is the most difficult type of atrial septal defect to detect with 2-D echocardiography.[294a]

Color flow Doppler and contrast echocardiogram can both be used to demonstrate atrial septal defects. Figure 4–79 shows a color flow Doppler and a contrast echocardiogram in a patient with a secundum type atrial septal defect.[295] With the Doppler study one can see the red encoded blood passing from the left atrium to the right atrium through the defect. With the contrast examination one sees an echo-filled right atrium and right ventricle. The left atrium and left ventricle are echo-free. As the noncontrast containing left atrial blood passes through the atrial septal defect, a negative contrast effect within the right atrium (ASD) is apparent.[296,297] If there were a right-to-left shunt then contrast would be seen within the left atrium and left ventricle with such an injection.[241]

In *total anomalous pulmonary venous return* all four pulmonary veins empty into a common pulmonary venous chamber behind the left atrium which produces additional echoes posterior to the left atrium (Fig. 31–67, p. 980).[298] From an echocardiographic viewpoint the recording is similar to that in *cor triatriatum*, in which the additional echoes are imaged in the left atrium.[299]

Besides septal defects one can also record septal aneurysms frequently associated with septal defects. The aneurysm involving the membranous portion of the interventricular septum can be imaged on the right side of the septum.[300] Atrial septal aneurysms can also be detected by 2-D echocardiography.[301,302] These aneurysm are frequently quite mobile and may be seen moving between the two atria throughout the cardiac cycle.

Figure 4–73. See color plate 3.

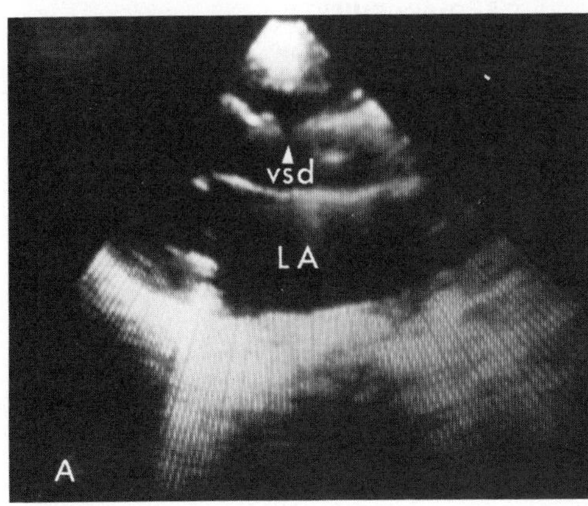

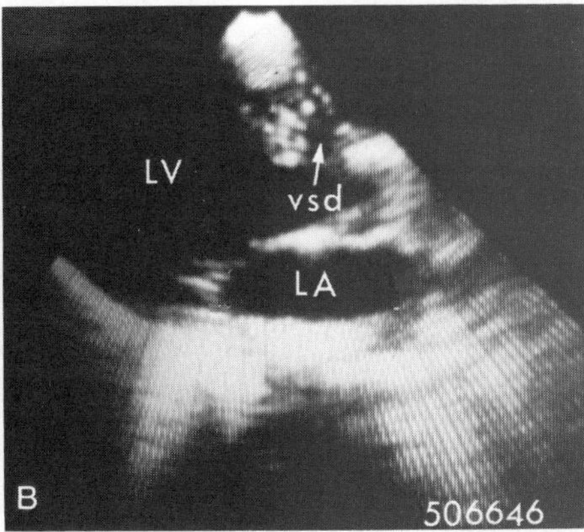

FIGURE 4-74. Two-dimensional long-axis echocardiograms of a patient with a membranous ventricular septal defect. *A*, The discontinuity of echoes from the ventricular septal defect (vsd) can be seen. *B*, A peripheral contrast injection fills the right ventricle, but an echo-free jet, i.e., negative contrast, can be seen anterior to the ventricular septal defect. LV = left ventricle; LA = left atrium. (From Feigenbaum, H.: Echocardiography. 4th ed. Philadelphia, Lea and Febiger, 1986.)

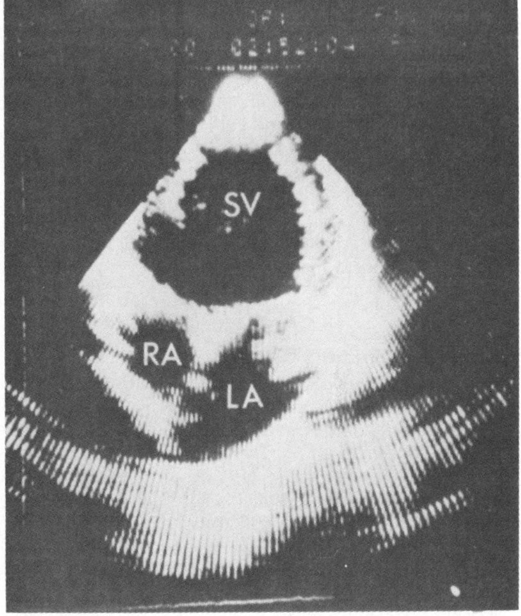

FIGURE 4-75. Cross-sectional echocardiogram of a patient with a single ventricle (SV). The ultrasonic probe is placed at the apex of the heart, and the plane of the scan transects the interatrial septum so that all chambers can be seen simultaneously. This view is particularly helpful in demonstrating the absence of the interventricular septum. RA = right atrium, LA = left atrium.

FIGURE 4-76. Subcostal 2-D echocardiogram of a patient with an ostium secundum atrial septal defect. Remnants of the interatrial septum are visible on both sides of the defect (ASD). RA = right atrium; LA = left atrium; LV = left ventricle. (From Feigenbaum, H.: Echocardiography. 3rd ed. Philadelphia, Lea and Febiger, 1981.)

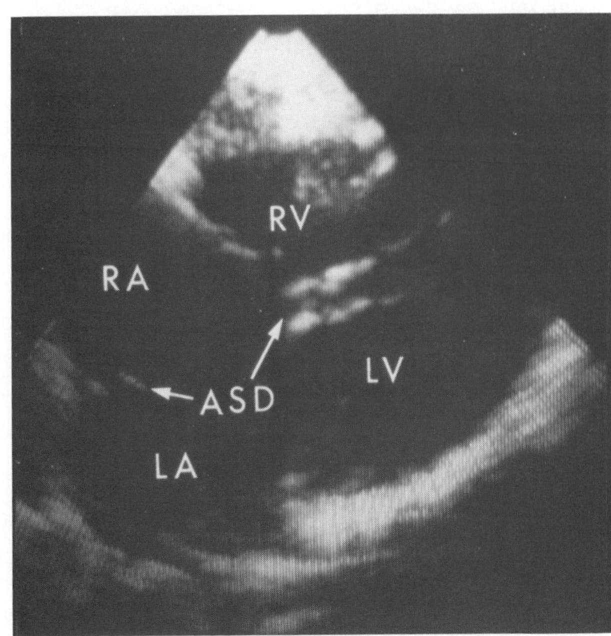

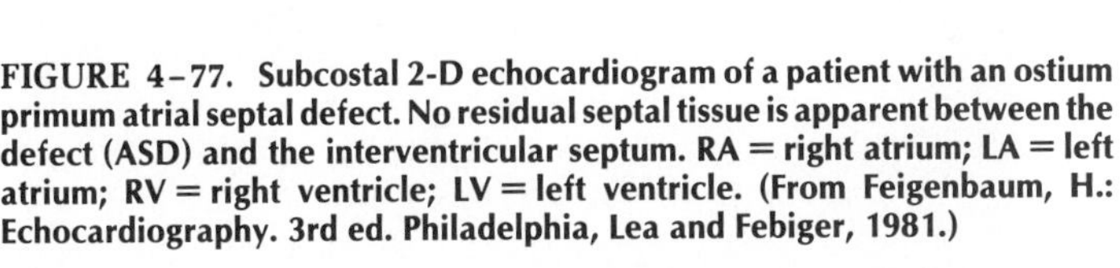

FIGURE 4-77. Subcostal 2-D echocardiogram of a patient with an ostium primum atrial septal defect. No residual septal tissue is apparent between the defect (ASD) and the interventricular septum. RA = right atrium; LA = left atrium; RV = right ventricle; LV = left ventricle. (From Feigenbaum, H.: Echocardiography. 3rd ed. Philadelphia, Lea and Febiger, 1981.)

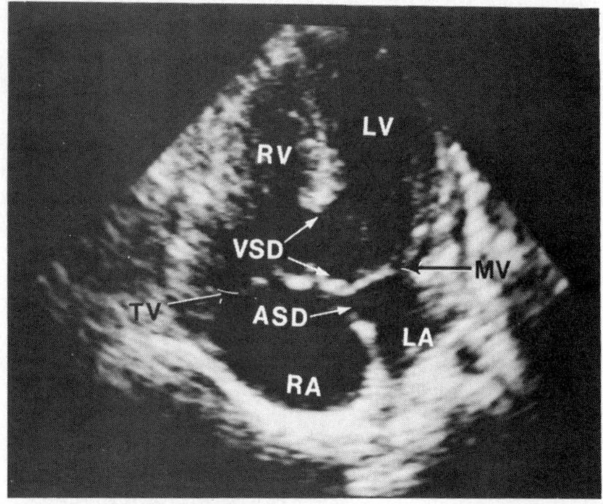

FIGURE 4-78. Apical four-chamber view of a patient with an endocardial cushion defect showing the perimembranous ventricular septal defect (VSD) and primum atrial septal defect (ASD). RA = right atrium; LA = left atrium; RV = right ventricle; LV = left ventricle; MV = mitral valve; TV = tricuspid valve. (From Feigenbaum, H.: Echocardiography. 4th ed. Philadelphia, Lea and Febiger, 1986.)

Figure 4-79. See color plate 4.

ASSOCIATED LESIONS. Intracardiac shunts are frequently associated with other anomalies of the heart that can be recognized echocardiographically. For example, in patients with defects of the atrioventricular canal, anomalies of the mitral and/or tricuspid valves can be appreciated on the echocardiogram.[303] The mitral valve appears to be closer than normal to the interventricular septum, a finding consistent with the abnormal insertion of the mitral leaflet in this anomaly. Also, the tricuspid valve echo appears to traverse the interventricular septum as a result of its abnormal position. The cleft in the mitral valve commonly present with ostium primum atrial septal defect may be detected using 2-D echocardiography.[304]

Another valvular anomaly that may be associated with an intracardiac shunt is a tricuspid valve that overrides the ventricular septum, which can pose major problems in the repair of a ventricular septal defect and which is therefore important to recognize preoperatively. The echocardiographic findings in this condition resemble those in atrioventricular canal defects in that the tricuspid valve is recorded to the left of the interventricular septum.[305,306]

PATENT DUCTUS ARTERIOSUS. Although 2-D echocardiography can occasionally visualize the patent ductus between the aorta and pulmonary artery, Doppler is more sensitive and reliable in detecting the abnormal communication.[307] Although continuous flow within the ductus itself has been detected, since the ductus is frequently perpendicular to the sample volume the Doppler signal can be somewhat difficult to record. It is actually easier to make the diagnosis by obtaining Doppler recordings from the aorta and pulmonary artery. By placing the sampling volume in the pulmonary artery, flow into the pulmonary artery can be noted in both systole and diastole as the shunted blood comes from the aorta (Fig. 4-80). Figure 4-81 shows a color flow Doppler study of a patient with a patent ductus arteriosus. The abnormal flow within the pulmonary artery can be readily detected.[308]

Figure 4-81. See color plate 4.

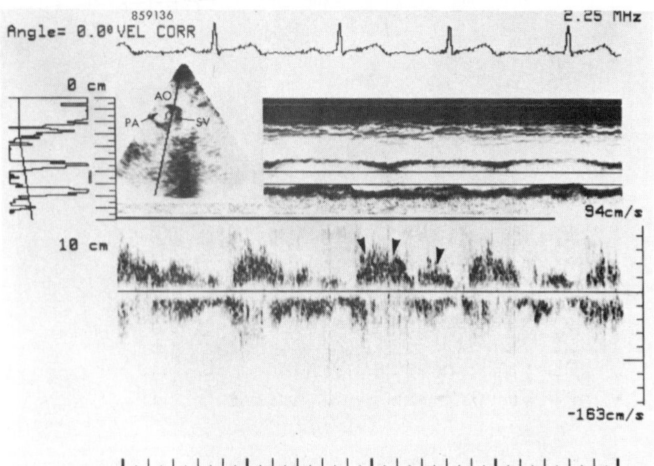

FIGURE 4-80. Pulsed Doppler examination with the sample volume (SV) placed in the wall of the pulmonary artery (PA) in the region of the presumed patent ductus. Note the presence of continuous flow in the region of the ductus (arrowheads). Ao = aorta. (From Feigenbaum, H.: Echocardiography. 4th ed. Philadelphia, Lea and Febiger, 1986.)

ABNORMALITIES OF THE GREAT ARTERIES

Supravalvular aortic stenosis can be detected using 2-D echocardiography.[279,309,310] The method of examination is similar to that used for the detection of valvular aortic stenosis, except that the scanning is carried out superior to the aortic valve.

Coarctation of the aorta (Fig. 32-2, p. 968) is detected with 2-D echocardiography by placing the probe in the suprasternal notch,[311] which allows imaging of both the narrowed segment of the aorta and the poststenotic dilation and detection of the excessive pulsation of the aorta proximal to the coarctation. Doppler echocardiography can be used to assess the hemodynamic obstruction across the coarctation.[312-319] Color flow Doppler is improving the ability to assess the severity of a coarctation.[315]

Tetralogy of Fallot is detected echocardiographically by noting a membranous ventricular septal defect and a dilated aorta that overrides the interventricular septum (Fig. 4-82 and Fig. 31-47, p. 935). The short-axis view also demonstrates a narrowing of the right ventricular outflow tract, usually at the subpulmonic level.[287] *Double-outlet right ventricle* (p. 948) is clinically similar to tetralogy of Fallot but can be differentiated echocardiographically from the more common anomaly when a mass of tissue can be noted between the anterior mitral leaflet and the aorta.[316] This tissue indicates that the aorta is communicating directly with the right ventricle and cannot be repaired surgically as is possible in tetralogy of Fallot. For the diagnosis of *truncus arteriosus* (p. 915), 2-D echocardiography helps establish the position of the vessel leaving the heart.[317] The definitive diagnosis is made by identifying the branch from the truncus that supplies the lungs.

Two-dimensional echocardiography has greatly improved the ultrasonic detection of *anomalies of the great arteries*.[317,318] In the diagnosis of *truncus arteriosus*, 2-D echocardiography helps to establish the number of great arteries leaving the heart.[319] Normally, with a short-axis view of the

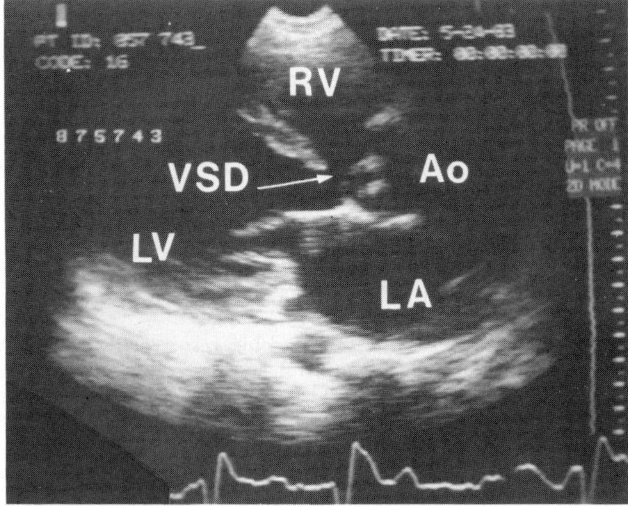

FIGURE 4-82. Parasternal long-axis examination of an adult with uncorrected tetralogy of Fallot. The ventricular septal defect (VSD) in the area of a membranous septum and overriding of the aorta (Ao) are apparent. LA = left atrium, LV = left ventricle, RV = right ventricle. (From Feigenbaum, H.: Echocardiography. 4th ed. Philadelphia, Lea and Febiger, 1986.)

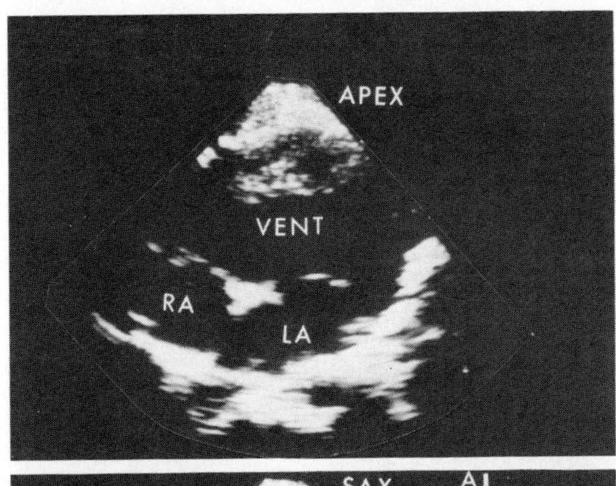

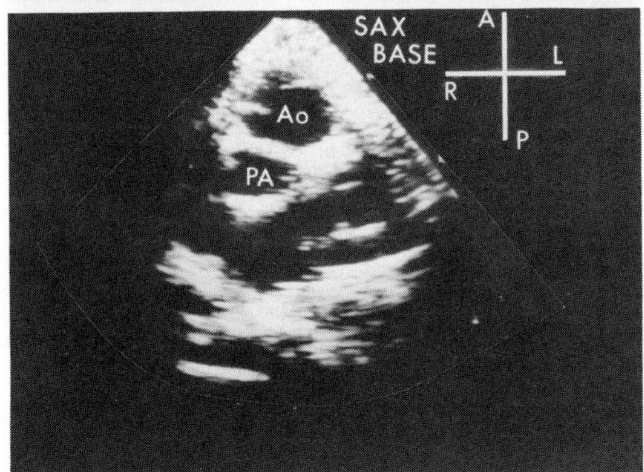

FIGURE 4-83. Apical four-chamber view (top) and short-axis (SAX) view (bottom) of the great vessels in a patient with a single ventricle and transposition of the great arteries. A single ventricular chamber (VENT) can be seen which receives blood from both the right and left atria (RA, LA). In the short-axis view two great vessels oriented in a parallel direction can be seen. The aorta (Ao) is anterior and to the left of the pulmonary artery (PA). (From Feigenbaum, H.: Echocardiography. 4th ed. Philadelphia, Lea and Febiger, 1986.)

great vessels, a circular aorta surrounded by a curved, tubular right ventricular outflow tract and pulmonary artery is recorded (Fig. 4-22, diagram 4); in truncus arteriosus only a single large circular vessel can be visualized. In addition, a new technique has been devised by actual recording of the branch of the truncus that supplies the lungs in an effort to establish definitely the diagnosis of truncus arteriosus.

The 2-D technique for the detection of *transposition of the great arteries* (p. 941) is based on determining the relationship between the two great arteries[287,320]; normally the pulmonary artery twists around the aorta as the latter passes posteriorly. With transposition of the great arteries, on the other hand, the two arteries run parallel to each other, and with a 2-D view parallel to the arteries it is possible to appreciate how the transposed arteries do not twist around each other.[321] A perpendicular or short-axis view of the great vessels demonstrates two circular structures (Fig. 4-83) rather than the pulmonary artery normally wrapping around the circular aorta. Doppler examination together with 2-D echocardiography helps in the recognition of corrected transposition.[322]

ISCHEMIC HEART DISEASE

DETECTION OF MYOCARDIAL ISCHEMIA

Echocardiography can detect ischemic myocardium by allowing appreciation of the motion, thickening, and thickness of various segments of the heart.[323-326] Figure 4-84 shows long-axis and short-axis 2-D echocardiograms of a patient with an acute anterior myocardial infarction. The posterior left ventricular wall moves and thickens normally in systole (arrowheads). The anterior and septal walls fail to move or thicken from diastole to systole. This finding is characteristic of acute ischemia. The four-chamber view in Figure 4-85 shows the findings with chronic ischemia. The basal half of the left ventricle contracts normally (inward-pointing arrowheads, Fig. 4-85). The normal muscle moves toward the left ventricular cavity and increases in thickness during systole. The apical half of the septum and the apex is much thinner than the basal half and fails to move with systole. The loss of myocardial tissue is indicative of scar formation (outward pointing arrowheads).[327] When the myocardium decreases in total thickness, the muscle is irreversibly damaged. As long as the myocardium retains normal thickness (Fig. 4-84), the damage is potentially reversible.

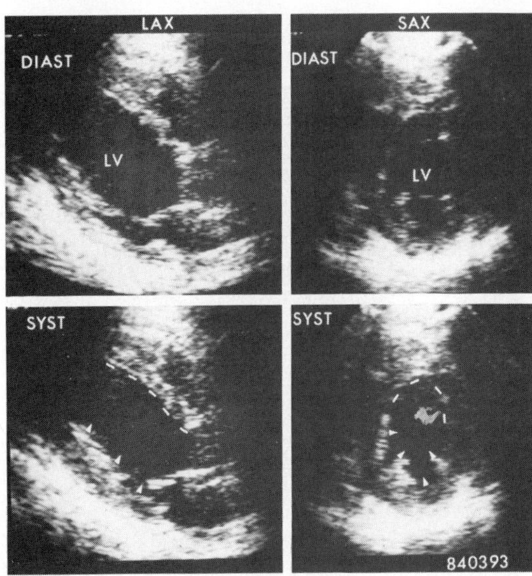

FIGURE 4-84. Long-axis (LAX) and short-axis (SAX) 2-D echocardiograms of a patient with an acute anterior myocardial infarction with an akinetic anterior interventricular septum and left ventricular free wall. In systole the nonischemic walls move normally (arrowheads). The ischemic muscle fails to contract (dashed line). LV = left ventricle. (From Feigenbaum, H.: Echocardiography. 4th ed. Philadelphia, Lea and Febiger, 1986.)

Figure 4-86 shows an M-mode recording of a patient with reversible ischemia.[328] The control recording shows normal septal and posterior ventricular wall motion. With handgrip,

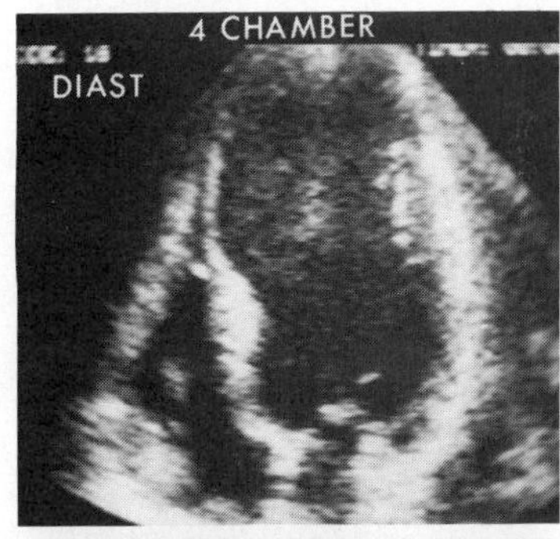

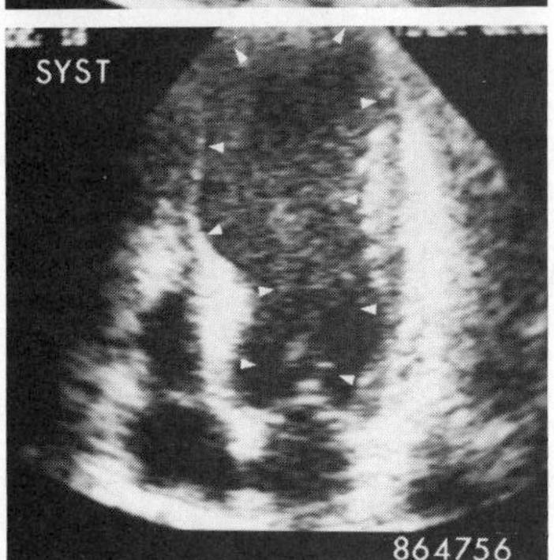

FIGURE 4-85. Apical four-chamber view of a patient with a scarred, dilated, aneurysmal apex and distal interventricular septum. The proximal half of the septum has normal thickness and contracts normally with systole. (From Feigenbaum, H.: Echocardiography. 4th ed. Philadelphia, Lea and Febiger, 1986.)

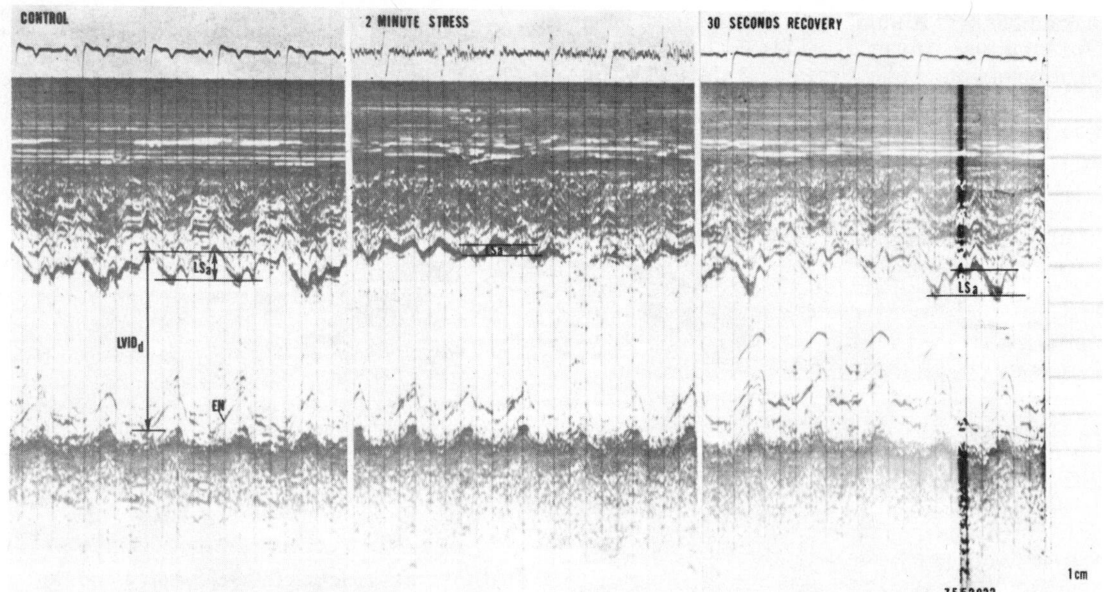

FIGURE 4–86. Serial M-mode echocardiograms from a patient with spasm of the left anterior descending coronary artery. At rest, the left septal echo amplitude (LS_a) is normal. During handgrip stress, the patient develops angina, and the amplitude of septal motion is markedly reduced. Following cessation of handgrip and the disappearance of pain, septal motion returns to normal. (From Widlansky, S., et al.: Coronary angiography, echocardiographic, and electrocardiographic studies on a patient with variant angina due to coronary artery spasm. Am. Heart J. *90*:631, 1975.)

ischemia is produced and septal motion and thickening are abolished. Total wall thickness remains normal. The posterior ventricular wall motion is unchanged. Following recovery from ischemia, septal motion and thickening return to normal. Because wall motion and thickening are excellent indicators of ischemia, echocardiography using exercise, pacing, or pharmacological agents is becoming increasingly popular.[329–332] Many of the technical difficulties involved in performing echocardiograms during or immediately after exercise have been resolved with the use of computer technology and the construction of continuous loop 2-D echocardiograms.[76] With these digital techniques the resting and exercise continuous loops can be placed side by side on a split screen or a four-screen format. Thus, subtle changes in wall motion as a result of exercise-induced ischemia can be detected.[333,335] Figure 4–87 shows a long-axis echocardiogram before and immediately after treadmill exercise. At rest, systolic motion of the interventricular septum is normal; however, with exercise the distal half of the septum becomes ischemic and akinetic (reverse arrows). Considerable investigation is under way to detect ischemic myocardium by ultrasonic tissue identification. The technique depends upon evaluation of integrated backscatter.[338,339]

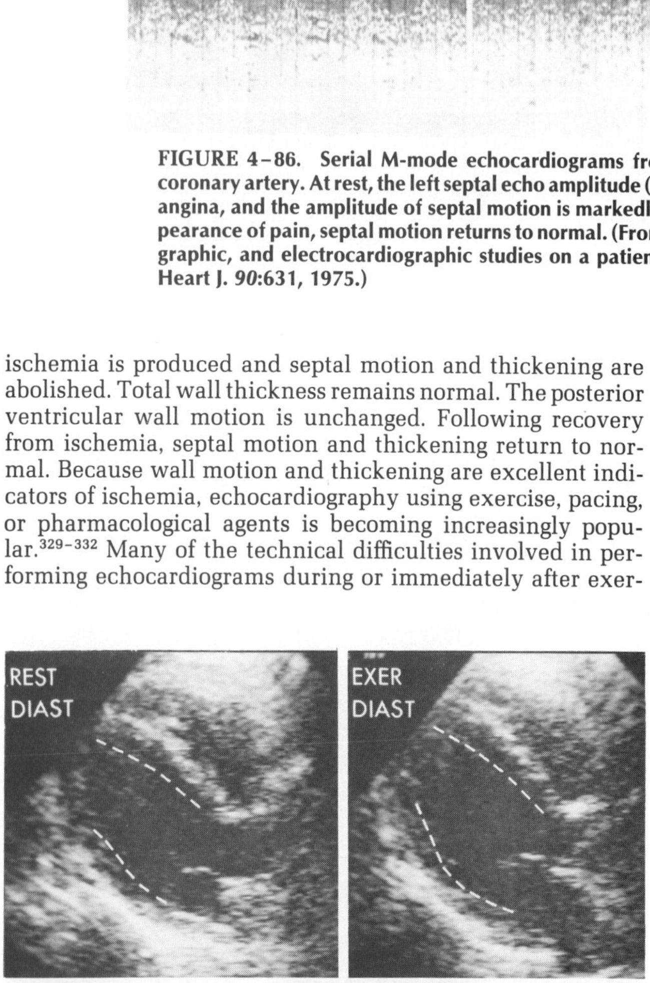

FIGURE 4–87. Resting and immediate postexercise echocardiograms of a patient with an obstruction in the left anterior descending coronary artery. At rest the septal motion is normal (arrow) (REST, SYST). Immediately following exercise the septum becomes dyskinetic (reverse arrows) (EXER, SYST). (From Feigenbaum, H.: Echocardiography. 4th ed. Philadelphia, Lea and Febiger, 1986.)

ASSESSMENT OF LEFT VENTRICULAR PERFORMANCE

There are many echocardiographic techniques available for assessing left ventricular performance in patients with ischemic heart disease. Although the M-mode left ventricular dimensions are of limited value in patients with regional heart disease, measurements such as mitral valve E point septal separation and abnormal closure of the mitral valve can give a reasonable assessment of altered left ventricular function in patients with ischemic heart disease. The E point–septal separation increases when left ventricular ejection fraction decreases and abnormal closure of the mitral valve occurs in patients with elevated atrial components of the left ventricular diastolic pressure. Doppler echocardiography can also be used to evaluate global left ventricular function. Acceleration and peak velocity are reduced as global left ventricular function deteriorates. Instantaneous mitral valve flow can reflect altered left ventricular filling.[340] With ischemia the early diastolic flow or E point is reduced and the velocity of flow with atrial systole (A point) is increased. As a result, the E/A ratio changes from a normal positive value to a negative one.[341]

The best echocardiographic technique for evaluating regional left ventricular performance utilizes 2-D echocardiography and the assessment of regional wall motion.[342,343] The left ventricle is divided into a number of segments. Determining the motion of each segment provides a *wall motion score* for the entire chamber.[55,344] A number of schemes have been suggested in the literature. Any or all of these techniques provide a reasonable assessment of both regional and global left ventricular function. Standard ejection fractions can also be calculated from the apical two-chamber or four-chamber views in patients with ischemic heart disease.[345,346] Because of the frequently distorted shape of the ventricle in these patients, Simpson's rule technique is preferred.[55] Minor axis measurements using parasternal long-axis or short-axis views can also be very helpful in patients with coronary artery disease by providing regional systolic function. Frequently the status of the base of the left ventricle is a better predictor of prognosis than is global ejection fraction, especially in patients who have apical aneurysms.[347,348]

MYOCARDIAL INFARCTION

COMPLICATIONS. All of the common complications of acute myocardial infarction (AMI) may be detected with echocardiographic techniques. A common problem is the development of a *left ventricular aneurysm*.[348,349] Figure 4–85 shows the echocardiographic findings characteristic of aneurysm. There is a loss of myocardial thickness, scar formation, localized dilatation, and frequently dyskinesis. A *pseudoaneurysm* (p. 1258) is a serious complication of MI, which represents rupture of the free wall. The blood leaving the cavity of the left ventricle is trapped in the pericardium, clot forms within the pericardial sac, and an aneurysmal wall consisting of clot and pericardium keeps the patient from exsanguinating. The echocardiographic appearance of this complication is fairly characteristic, with the neck of the aneurysm being smaller than the body (Fig. 4–88).[350] Doppler flow patterns, especially color flow Doppler, within the aneurysm can help differentiate between a true and a false aneurysm.[351,352] Indications for surgery are more urgent with a pseudoaneurysm; therefore, the diagnosis is crucial.

Aneurysmal dilatation and subsequent *perforation of the ventricular septum* (p. 1258) is another complication of MI.

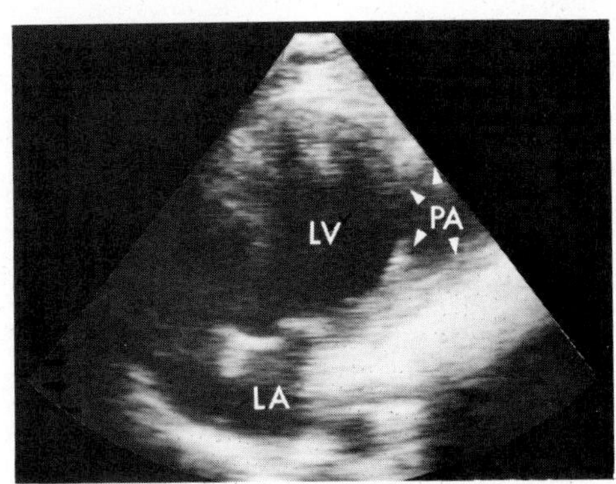

FIGURE 4–88. Four-chamber 2-D echocardiogram of a patient with a pseudoaneurysm (PA) adjacent to the posterior lateral free wall of the left ventricle (LV). LA = left atrium. (From Feigenbaum, H.: Echocardiography. 4th ed. Philadelphia, Lea and Febiger, 1986.)

The septal aneurysm may be seen on the 2-D echocardiogram.[353] On rare occasions the actual perforation can be visualized.[354] The echocardiographic diagnosis, however, is best made with Doppler echocardiography.[355] When the sample volume is put on the right ventricular side of the interventricular septum, the high-velocity systolic flow going from the left ventricle to the right ventricle through the ruptured septum can be recorded (Fig. 4–89). Color flow Doppler recording of such a defect is probably the procedure of choice.[356,357]

Right ventricular infarction (p. 1255) is an increasingly recognized complication of MI and can have important clinical implications for management. Figure 4–90 shows the common echocardiographic findings with right ventricular infarction.[358–360] These patients usually have evidence of an inferior infarction. The inferior-posterior wall of the left ventricle is akinetic in systole (dashes) as noted in the short-axis view. The evidence for right ventricular infarction is right ventricular dilatation and right ventricular free wall motion akinesis (dashes) (Fig. 4–90). Premature pulmonary valve opening may

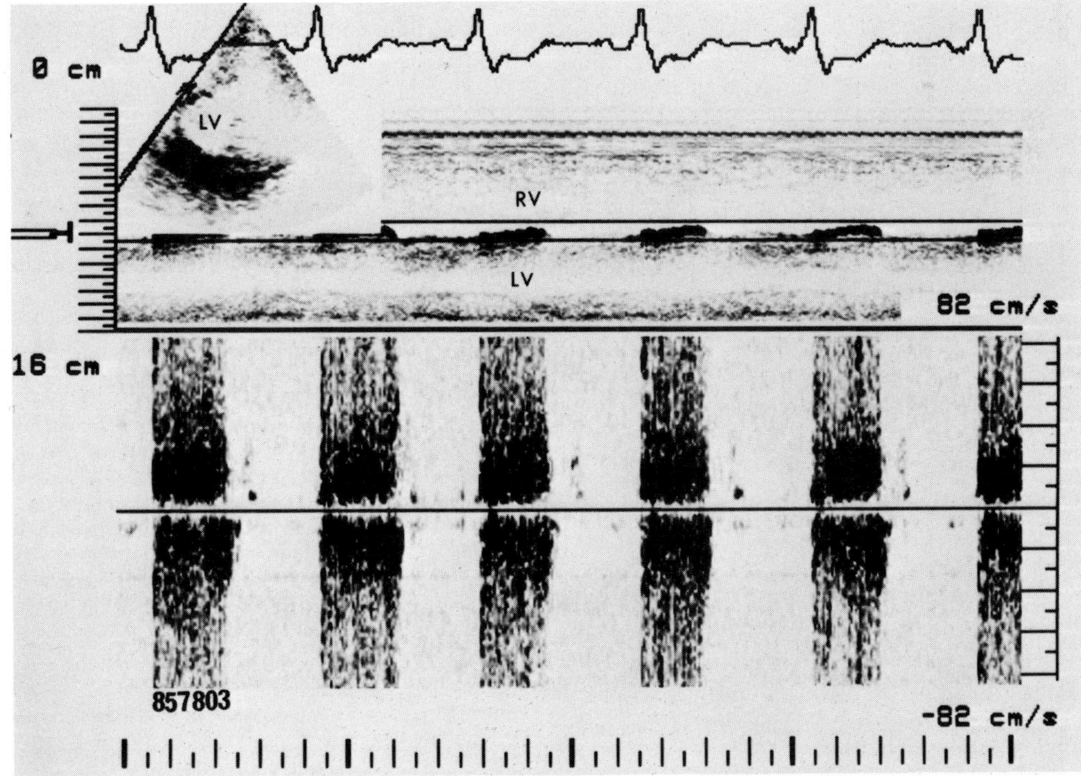

FIGURE 4–89. Pulsed Doppler echocardiogram of a patient with a ruptured ventricular septum following an acute myocardial infarction. With the sample volume to the right of the interventricular septum one records a high velocity systolic flow from the left-to-right shunt. RV = right ventricle, LV = left ventricle.

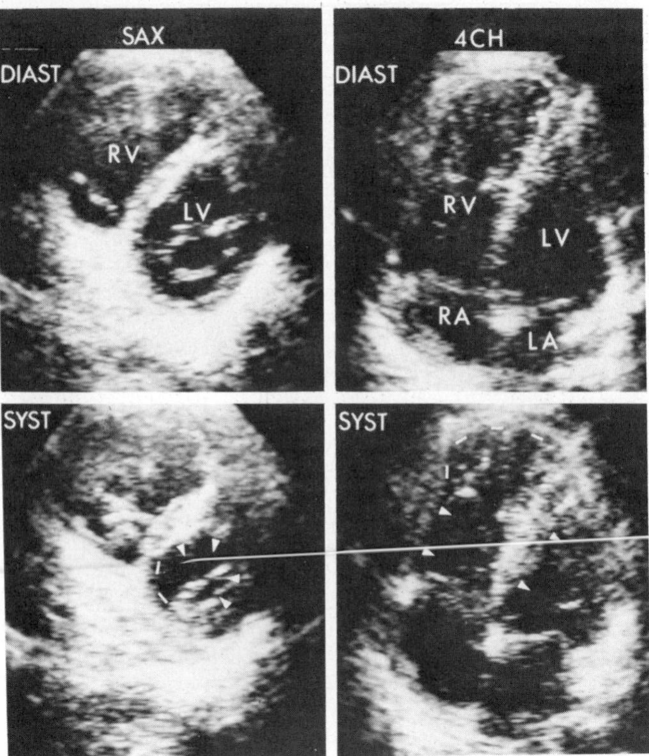

FIGURE 4-90. Short-axis (SAX) and four-chamber (4CH) 2-D echocardiograms of a patient with an inferior myocardial infarction complicated by right ventricular infarction. The posterior-inferior wall is akinetic (dashed line, SAX SYST). In addition, the apical half of the right ventricular free wall is akinetic (arrowheads, 4CH SYST). The right ventricle (RV) is also dilated. RA = right atrium; LV = left ventricle; LA = left atrium. (From Feigenbaum, H.: Echocardiography. 4th ed. Philadelphia, Lea and Febiger, 1986.)

occur with right ventricular infarction.[361] There may also be distortion of the interatrial septum so that it bulges toward the left atrium.[362]

Mural thrombus (p. 1261) represents another common complication of AMI that can be detected with echocardiography.[363,364] These clots occur most often with aneurysms, especially those involving the anterior wall and apex. Figure 4-91 shows two patients with left ventricular clots. The thrombi may have a variety of configurations; those which protrude into the cavity and may be mobile, such as in Figure 4-91*B* and *C*, are easier to detect echocardiographically and may have a greater likelihood of producing systemic emboli.[365-367] Other thrombi are layered along the wall and may not be as likely to break loose (Fig. 4-91*A*). Certain left ventricular echocardiographic flow patterns may be precursors of thrombi.[368]

Other complications of AMI, such as mitral regurgitation[369,370] and pericardial effusion,[371] are easily detected echocardiographically.

NATURAL HISTORY AND PROGNOSIS. Echocardiography is ideal for serial studies in patients with MI. Two-dimensional echocardiography carried out early in the course of an infarction is helpful in establishing the diagnosis[372,373] and provides prognostic information as well.[374-376] This examination is useful in the assessment of the status of the myocardium not involved in the current infarction[377] because an unsuspected previous MI may be discovered. An early echocardiographic study also can serve as a baseline for detecting future ischemic events such as MI expansion[378,379] or complications. The initial examination may even help identify the patients who are at high risk of experiencing complications.[380,381] A resting[382] or stress[383] 2-D echocardiogram before discharge can also provide long-term prognostic information.

Possibly one of the most important uses of echocardiography in patients with acute MI is the efficacy of reperfusion therapy.[384-388] Figure 4-92 shows serial studies on a patient who underwent angioplasty for an occluded left anterior descending coronary artery. During the acute infarction and before angioplasty the anterior septum was dyskinetic (reverse arrows). After successful reopening of the artery and recovery of the stunned myocardium, the septal motion returned to normal (arrows LX post, SX post).

EXAMINATION OF THE CORONARY ARTERIES

Two-dimensional echocardiography can provide an indirect evaluation of myocardial perfusion and therefore can be helpful in predicting obstruction in specific coronary arteries because of the predictable relationship between certain myocardial segments and specific coronary arteries.[389] For example, the anterior interventricular septum and apex are usually perfused by the left anterior descending coronary artery while the posterior septum and inferior wall are supplied by the posterior descending coronary artery, which usually arises

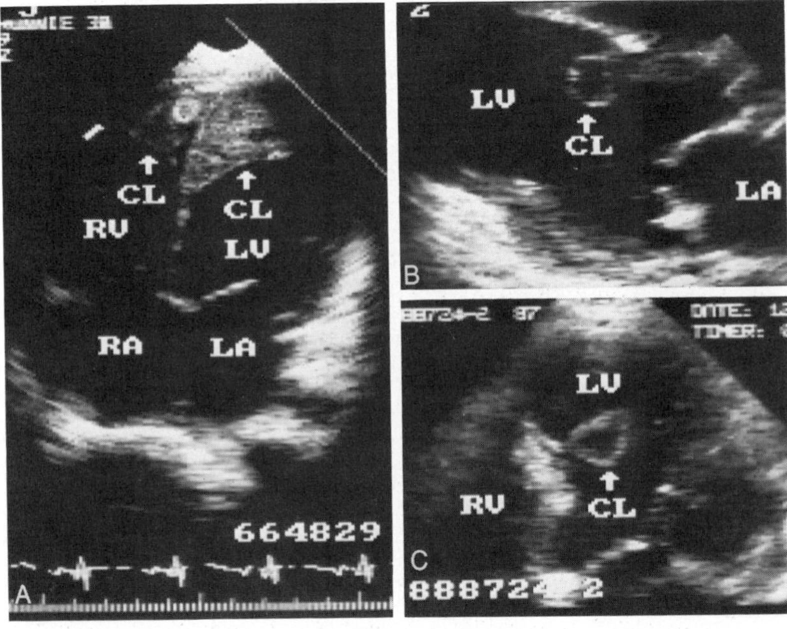

FIGURE 4-91. Two patients with mural thrombi. In *A* the clots (CL) can be seen both in the right ventricle and the right atrium. The left ventricular clot is smooth and layered against the ventricular wall. In *B* and *C* the clot is pedunculated and mobile within the cavity of the left ventricle (LV). RV = right ventricle, RA = right atrium, LA = left atrium.

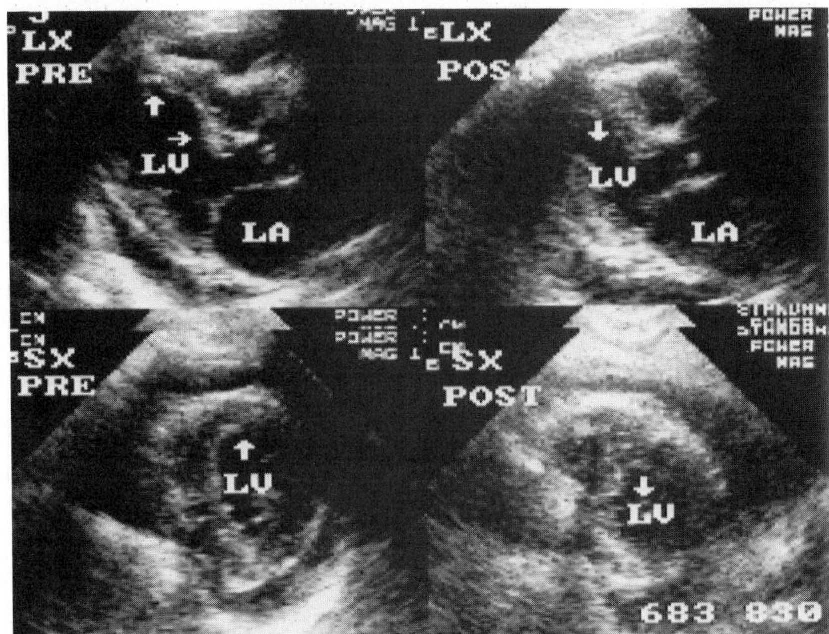

FIGURE 4-92. Long-axis (LX) and short-axis (SX) echocardiograms of a patient with an acute anterior myocardial infarction before (PRE) and after (POST) angioplasty of the left anterior descending coronary artery. Before PTCA the anterior septum is dyskinetic (upward arrows). After successful PTCD the motion of the septum is normal (downward arrows).

from the right coronary artery. Thus one can usually predict the vessel with severe obstruction from a 2-D echocardiogram showing impaired regional myocardial contraction.

Direct visualization of the proximal coronary arteries is also feasible.[390,391] With improved technology, especially the development of annular array and transesophageal 2-D echocardiographic systems, the resolution required for visualizing the coronary arteries has been improved dramatically.[392-394] Figure 4-93 shows an annular array study of the left proximal coronary artery system in which it is possible to identify the left main, proximal circumflex, left anterior descending, and diagonal arteries. The ultimate value of examining the coronary arteries echocardiographically has yet to be determined. Investigators have noted the ability of transesophageal echocardiography to detect atherosclerotic obstructions in proximal coronary arteries.[395]

Congenital anomalies of the coronary arteries (pp. 918 and 969) can be detected by 2-D, Doppler, and Doppler color echocardiography.[396-398] The value of 2-D echocardiography in visualizing coronary artery aneurysms in Kawasaki disease has been well demonstrated (Fig. 33-5, p. 998).[399] Coronary arteriovenous fistulas can also be detected echocardiographically.[400,401]

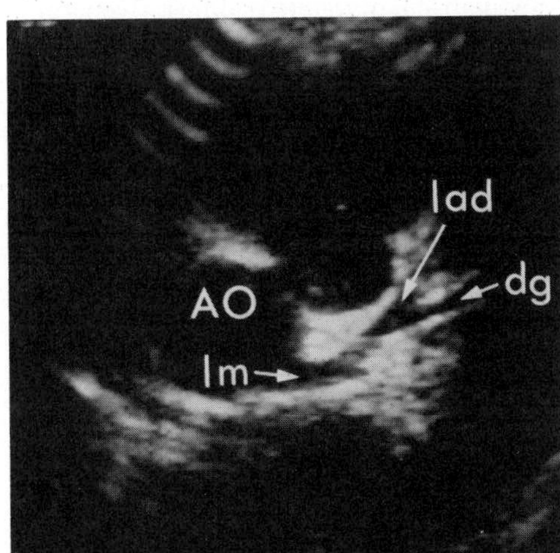

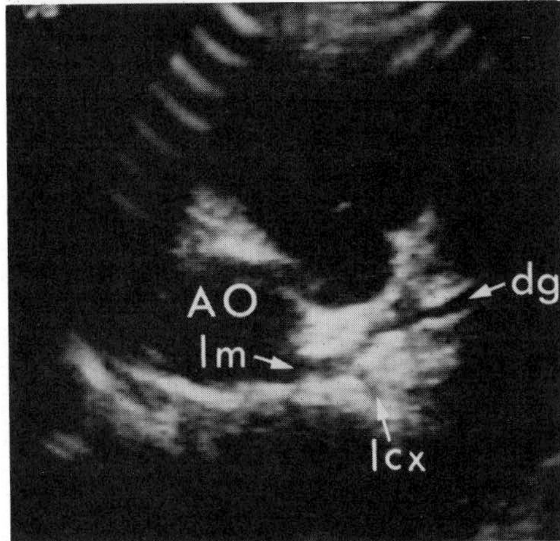

FIGURE 4-93. Short-axis 2-D echocardiogram of the left coronary artery using an annular phased array system. AO = aorta; lm = left main coronary artery; lcx = left circumflex; dg = diagonal; lad = left anterior descending.

MYOCARDIAL PERFUSION USING CONTRAST ECHOCARDIOGRAPHY. Contrast echocardiography may also be employed to study myocardial perfusion.[402-405] If a fluid containing microbubbles is injected into the root of the aorta or directly into the coronary arteries, the echogenicity of the myocardium will be increased (Fig. 4-94),

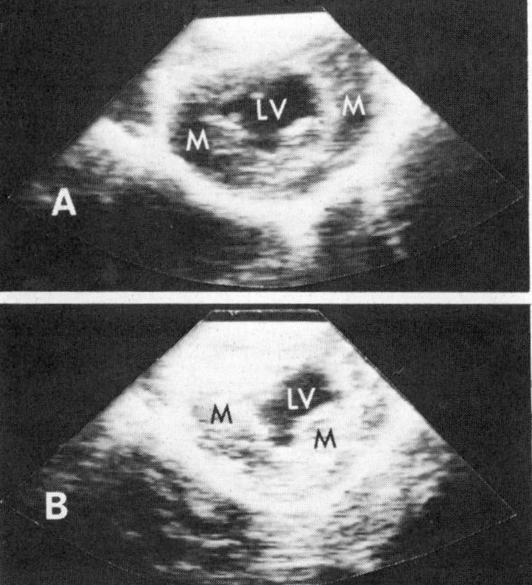

FIGURE 4-94. Short-axis 2-D echocardiogram of a dog before and after injection of contrast in the root of the aorta. Before contrast (A) the myocardium (M) is relatively echo-free. Following the injection of fluid containing tiny microbubbles (B) the myocardium becomes uniformly echogenic.

provided that the blood supply is intact. When blood flow is impeded, the increase in echogenicity in that segment is reduced or absent. Such studies have been done extensively in animal models. One can determine infarct size and myocardial perfusion rather precisely with this technique. There is only limited experience in patients thus far. The examination is obviously invasive and requires injections into the aortic root or coronary artery; the clinical role for this procedure has yet to be determined.

CARDIOMYOPATHIES

(See also Chap. 43)

HYPERTROPHIC CARDIOMYOPATHY (HCM)

(See also p. 1404)

Echocardiography is an important diagnostic tool in patients with HCM and has enriched our understanding of this abnormality. An early echocardiographic abnormality to be noted was systolic anterior motion of the mitral valve (termed "SAM") (Fig. 4-95*B*, p. 1406),[406] which appeared to be related to and was correlated with the presence of obstruction to left ventricular outflow.[407] The shorter the distance between the septum and the leaflet and the longer the duration of apposition between these two structures, the more severe the obstruction.[408] This echocardiographic finding also demonstrated the critical importance of involvement of the mitral valve apparatus in the obstruction in this condition.[409] More recently SAM has been noted in a variety of other patients, some of whom had no evidence of left ventricular hypertrophy.[410,411] It has been observed in patients with anemia and hypovolemia as well as in patients with a hyperdynamic left ventricle.[410] It is possible that SAM is a nonspecific sign that occurs whenever the left ventricular systolic volume is reduced, either because of hypertrophy, as in HCM, or in the presence of a hyperdynamic state.[412,413]

A second echocardiographic finding in patients with obstructive HCM is midsystolic closure of the aortic valve (Fig. 4-95C). However, as noted earlier, this sign is not specific for HCM and is also present in patients with discrete subaortic stenosis. While this finding is not sensitive, when present, it usually indicates a significant amount of obstruction.

Hypertrophy of the septum with abnormal organization of myocardial cells may be one of the basic abnormalities of HCM[414] (p. 1405), and key echocardiographic findings are disproportionate hypertrophy of the septum in relation to the posterior wall of the left ventricle, so that the ratio of thickness of the septum to the free wall exceeds 1.3/1.0 (Fig. 4-95*A*),[415] and the motion of the hypertrophied septum is reduced.[416] It has also been shown that asymmetrical septal hypertrophy (ASH) is frequently transmitted as an autosomal dominant trait and that there are patients with asymmetrical septal hypertrophy who do not show SAM and therefore do not have obstruction to left ventricular outflow.[415,417] These patients may be considered to have HCM without obstruction. While the concept of recognizing ASH with or without obstruction to left ventricular outflow by echocardiography is an important one, there are limitations to echocardiographic diagnosis. First, the thickness of the septum may be difficult to measure precisely echocardiographically. (In Figure 4-95 the left side of the septum is clearly identified, but the right side is not as distinct.) Second, it must be appreciated that ASH is not pathognomonic for HCM and related myopathies and can occur in a variety of other disease states, including right ventricular hypertrophy. In addition, some patients with HCM may have concentric rather than asymmetrical hypertrophy, in which the septal and posterior left ventricular walls are equal in thickness (p. 1404).

Two-dimensional echocardiography provides additional information by indicating the shape and location of the hypertrophied septum in patients with known or suspected HCM.[418] A variety of hypertrophied septal segments has been recorded by this technique. Figure 4-96 shows a hypertrophied septum limited to the basal two-thirds of the septum, while the apex is virtually free of muscular hypertrophy. Other patients exhibit an apical form of hypertrophy with the proximal septum being relatively thin.[419] Concentric hypertrophy is also a fairly common form of hypertrophic myopathy (Fig. 4-97). Cavity obliteration with ventricular systole is almost always present with this type of disease. Two-dimensional echocardiography is useful in assessing the effectiveness of myotomy and myectomy. An intriguing observation is that the echoes from the diseased septum in HCM are more reflective or "speckled" than those from the free posterior wall.

Doppler echocardiography may also be helpful in evaluating patients with hypertrophic cardiomyopathy.[420,421] The Doppler recording of the left ventricular outflow may show an abnormal pattern with the abnormally high velocity occurring in late systole (Fig. 4-95*D*). The systolic gradient can be

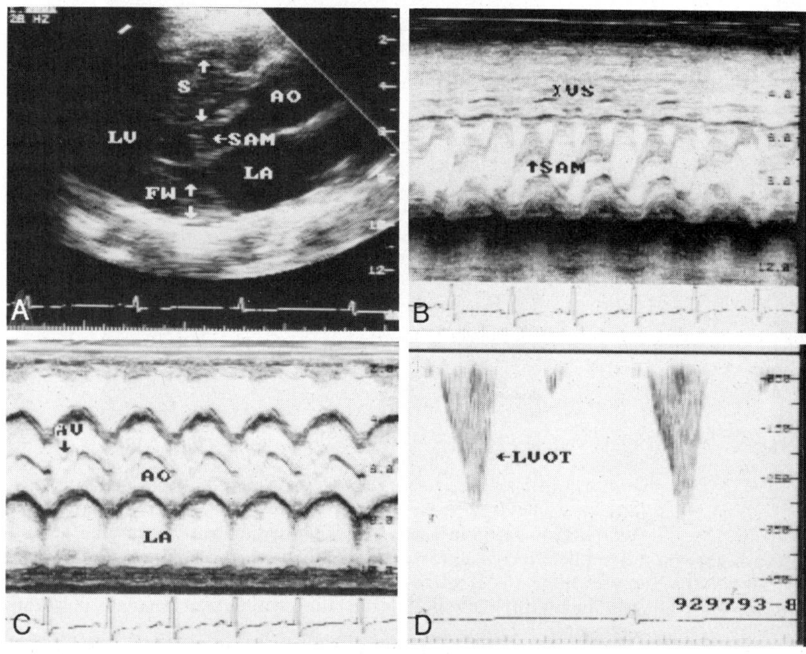

FIGURE 4-95. Two-dimensional, M-mode, and Doppler studies of a patient with hypertrophic obstructive cardiomyopathy. The 2-D long-axis study shows the thickened interventricular septum (S) and the systolic anterior motion of the mitral valve (SAM). The abnormal mitral motion and the thickened septum are also seen on the M-mode recording (B). The M-mode recording of the aortic valve shows mid systolic closure (AV). The Doppler recording of the left ventricular outflow tract shows how the velocity within the outflow tract increases in the latter half of systole. LV = left ventricle, AO = aorta, FW = left ventricular free wall, LA = left atrium, IVS = interventricular septum, LVOT = left ventricular outflow tract.

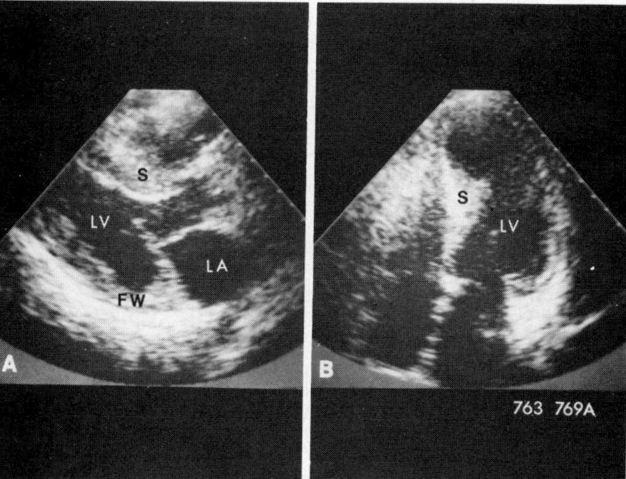

FIGURE 4-96. Long-axis *(A)* and apical four-chamber *(B)* echocardiograms of a patient with hypertrophic cardiomyopathy whose hypertrophy primarily involves the proximal two-thirds of the interventricular septum (S). The apex is spared from the hypertrophic process. LV = left ventricle, FW = left ventricular free wall, LA = left atrium. (From Feigenbaum, H.: Echocardiography. 4th ed. Philadelphia, Lea and Febiger, 1986.)

estimated using the Doppler technique.[422] The left ventricular hypertrophy and reduced left ventricular compliance alters the Doppler recording of mitral valve flow. The early diastolic velocity or E point is reduced and the late velocity with atrial systole is increased.[423] Color Doppler provides a spatial visualization of the altered blood flow in patients with obstructive HCM.[424]

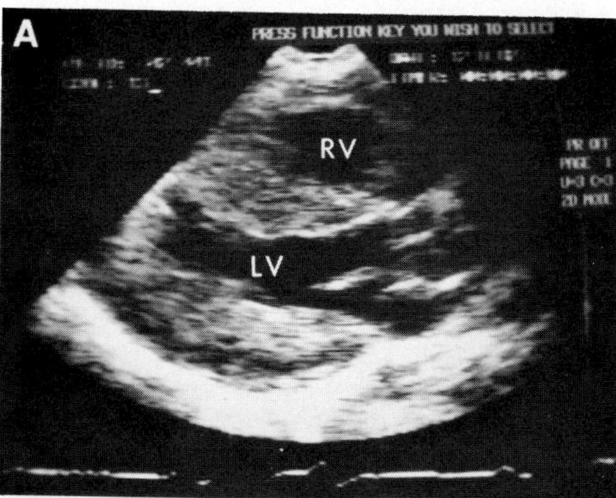

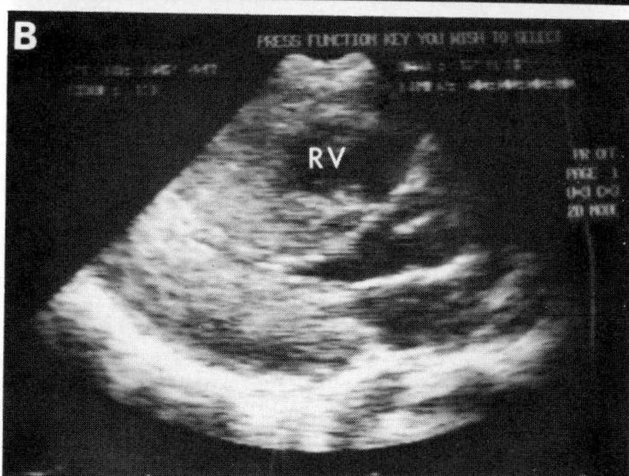

FIGURE 4-97. Long-axis 2-D echocardiogram of a patient with hypertrophic cardiomyopathy who exhibits uniform hypertrophy of the entire left ventricle (LV). RV = right ventricle, A = diastole, B = systole. (From Feigenbaum, H.: Echocardiography. 4th ed. Philadelphia, Lea and Febiger, 1986.)

CONGESTIVE (DILATED) CARDIOMYOPATHY

(See also p. 1398)

The echocardiogram characteristically reveals a dilated, poorly contracting left ventricle in patients with congestive cardiomyopathy.[425,426] Signs of reduced cardiac output include a poorly moving aorta, reduced opening of the mitral valve, and slow closure of the aortic valve. The left atrium is dilated, and the abnormal closure of the mitral valve indicative of elevated left diastolic pressure is frequently noted. The rate of left ventricular filling on the digitized M-mode and Doppler echograms is reduced.[427] It must be appreciated that these findings are nonspecific and may also occur in patients with ischemic heart disease. However, at least one portion of the left ventricle, usually the posterior wall, continues to exhibit normal motion in most, although not all, patients with severe coronary artery disease.[425] In patients with cardiomyopathy the impairment of left ventricular wall motion is diffuse and includes the posterior wall. If mitral regurgitation develops in patients with cardiomyopathy, septal motion may increase slightly in keeping with the left ventricular volume overload, although this increase in septal motion is certainly not as striking as that which occurs in primary mitral valve disease with secondary myocardial failure.

RESTRICTIVE (INFILTRATIVE) CARDIOMYOPATHY

(See also p. 1415)

The principal echocardiographic findings in patients with infiltrative cardiomyopathy are reduced wall motion and thickening of the left ventricular wall without dilatation[428-430]; these changes are usually uniform throughout the

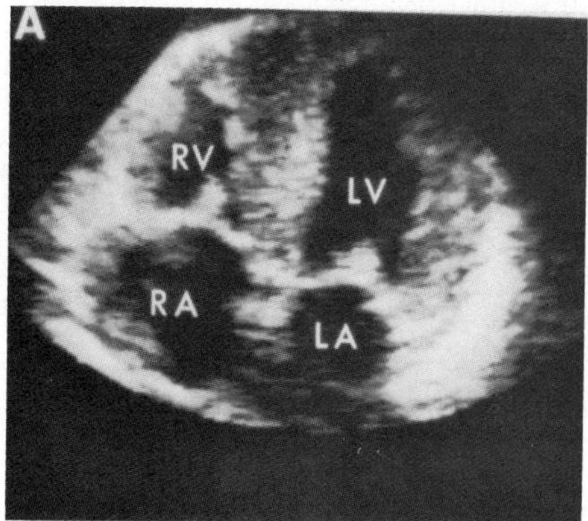

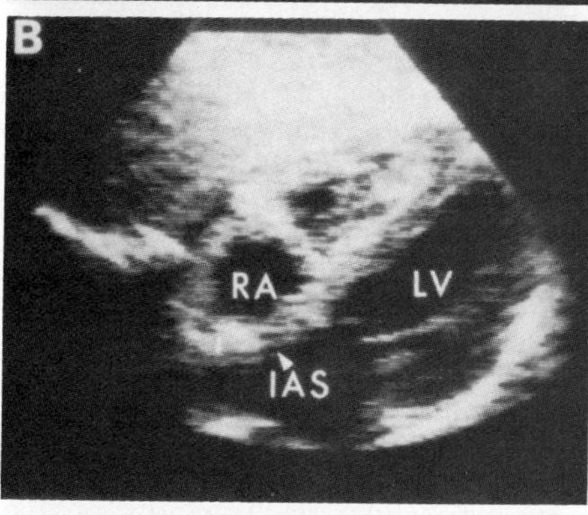

FIGURE 4-98. Four-chamber *(A)* and subcostal *(B)* 2-D echocardiograms of a patient with hereditary amyloidosis. The four-chamber view demonstrates markedly hypertrophied cardiac walls, especially the interventricular septum and free wall of the right ventricle. The tricuspid and mitral valve leaflets are also thickened. The left ventricle (LV) and right ventricle (RV) cavities are small. The subcostal examination demonstrates a thickened interatrial septum (IAS). RA = right atrium, LA = left atrium (From Feigenbaum, H.: Echocardiography. 4th ed. Philadelphia, Lea and Febiger, 1986.)

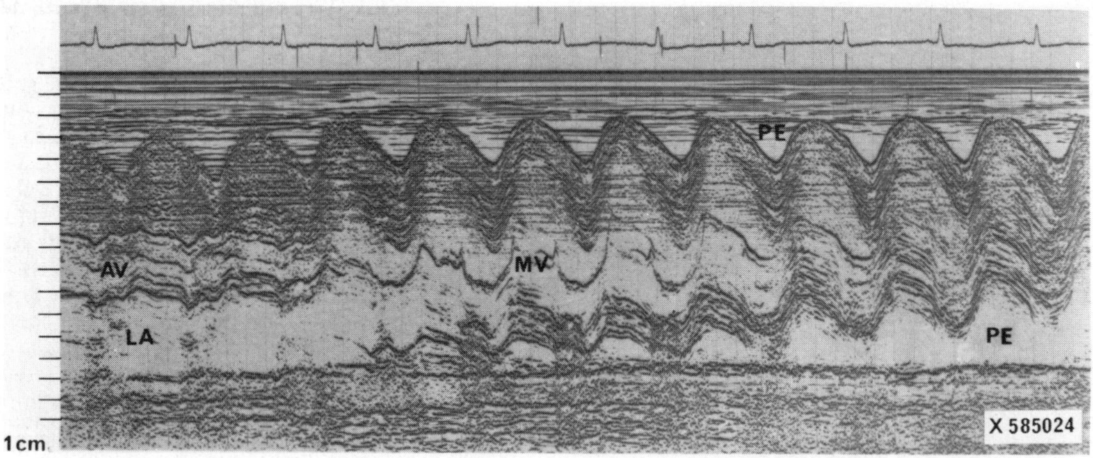

FIGURE 4-99. M-mode echocardiographic scan of a patient with a large pericardial effusion. Fluid (PE) can be seen both anteriorly and posteriorly. The entire heart is moving posteriorly during ventricular systole, producing distortion of all the echoes, including those from the mitral valve (MV). AV = aortic valve, LA = left atrium. (From Bonner, A. J., et al.: An unusual precordial pulse and sound associated with large pericardial effusion. Chest *68*:829, 1975.)

ventricle. Obviously, these findings are not specific for infiltrative cardiomyopathy and, like those obtained by means of electrocardiography, chest roentgenography, hemodynamics, and angiocardiography, they must be interpreted in terms of the total clinical setting. In patients with amyloid heart disease (Fig. 4-98)[431-432] the echocardiographic findings are usually nonspecific and show left ventricular hypertrophy. There are also frequently more specific findings in that the valves may be uniformly thickened in addition to the hypertrophy of the ventricular walls. The interatrial septum may also be unusually thick, and a peculiar speckled appearance of the myocardium may be noted, reflecting localized variations in echo density.[433] Diastolic relaxation as judged by digitized M-mode recordings is impaired.[434] In the beginning course of amyloid heart disease early left ventricular filling is reduced. The Doppler mitral E wave is decreased and the A wave is increased. Later, filling becomes more restrictive and the E and A waves are reversed "pseudonormalization."[68]

PERICARDIAL DISEASE

(See Chap. 45)

PERICARDIAL EFFUSION

(See also p. 1472)

The theory underlying the use of ultrasound in the recognition of pericardial effusion is relatively simple; since the acoustical properties of fluid differ significantly from those of cardiac muscle, the effusion surrounding the heart is less echogenic than is the myocardium. Accordingly, the detection of effusion was one of the first and has remained one of the most useful applications of echocardiography.[435,436] Figure 4-38 shows the echocardiographic appearance of a relatively small pericardial effusion in a patient with left ventricular hypertrophy. There is a clear space between the posterior left ventricular epicardial echo and the surrounding pericardium and between the anterior wall of the right ventricle and the chest wall. This figure demonstrates the sensitivity of echocardiography in detecting a small quantity (as little as 20 ml) of pericardial fluid,[437] which would easily be missed by other techniques.

Figures 4-99 and 45-10 (p. 1478) are echocardiograms from patients with large pericardial effusions; although there is a potential space behind the left atrium, it rarely fills with pericardial fluid. When it does,[438] the quantity is considerably less than that behind the posterior wall of the left ventricle. There is a large echo-free space anteriorly, and during much of the cardiac cycle, the anterior and posterior cardiac walls move in the same direction rather than in opposite directions, and the amplitude of motion of the anterior wall of the right ventricle is excessive. This type of cardiac motion has been referred to as a "swinging heart."[439,440] As would be expected, the motion of all the cardiac structures is distorted by this excessive cardiac displacement, and any diagnosis based on

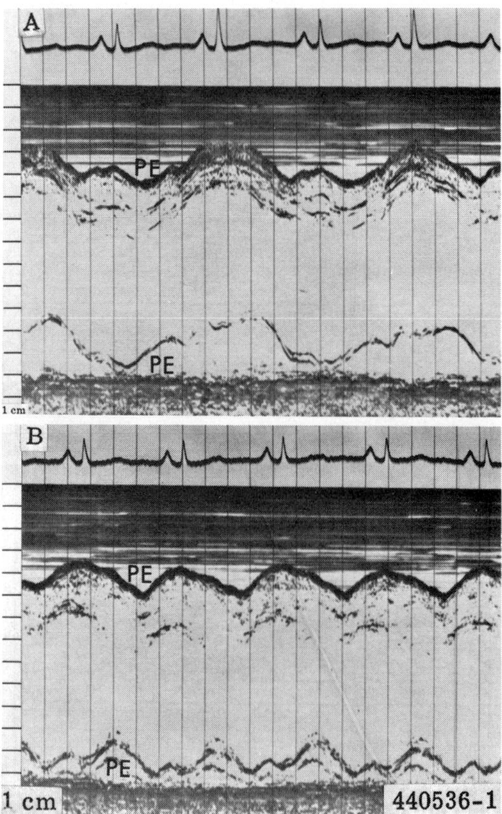

FIGURE 4-100. Echocardiograms from a patient with massive pericardial effusion (PE). *A*, Anterior right ventricular echo (ARV) and posterior left ventricular epicardial echoes move essentially in similar directions. The position of the heart differs slightly with each cardiac cycle. The corresponding electrocardiogram shows electrical alternation. Upon removal of some of the pericardial fluid *(B)*, cardiac excursions are synchronous with each electrical depolarization, and electrical alternation is no longer present. (From Feigenbaum, H.: Echocardiography. 2nd ed. Philadelphia, Lea and Febiger, 1976.)

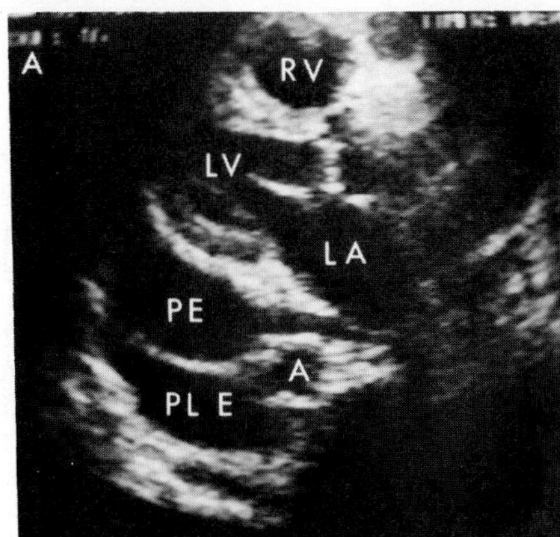

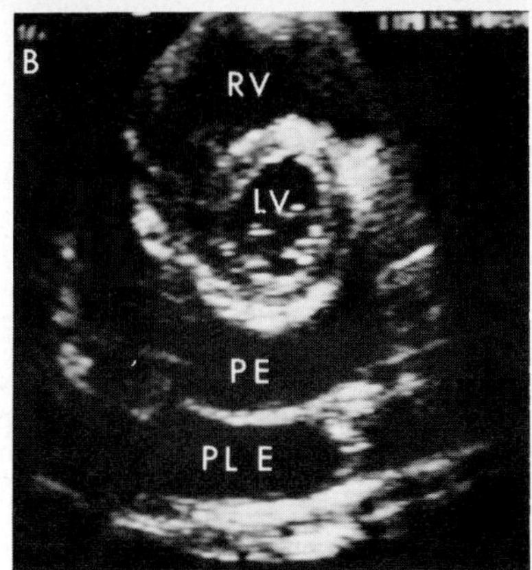

FIGURE 4-101. Long-axis *(A)* and short-axis *(B)* 2-D echocardiograms of a patient with pericardial effusion (PE) and pleural effusion (PL E). In the long-axis view the aorta (A) lies between the two bodies of fluid. RV = right ventricle, LV = left ventricle, LA = left atrium. (From Feigenbaum, H.: Echocardiography. 4th ed. Philadelphia, Lea and Febiger, 1986.)

this pattern of motion can be misleading. False-positive findings of prolapse of the mitral valve, of systolic anterior motion of the mitral valve, and of abnormal septal motion have all been reported in such patients.[441]

When the motion of the heart within the pericardial effusion is increased markedly and, in particular, when this is accompanied by tachycardia, the heart may not have returned to its previous position by the time the next cardiac cycle commences. Figure 4-100*A* demonstrates an echocardiogram in such a patient; with each depolarization the heart is in a slightly different position, and the electrocardiographic QRS complex also varies[439] with alternating heights of R waves on the electrocardiogram, i.e., electrical alternans (p. 149). When the cardiac motion becomes regular in such a patient, as reflected in the echogram in Figure 4-100*B*, electrical alternation ceases.

Although M-mode echocardiography can make the qualitative diagnosis of pericardial effusion, there are many situations in which the fluid collects in a nonuniform fashion around the heart, and 2-D echocardiography is more reliable in identifying the location and amount of fluid.[442] Figure 4-101 demonstrates long-axis *(A)* and short-axis *(B)* views of a patient with both pericardial and pleural effusions. The pleural effusion can be identified since it is separated from the heart by the descending aorta.[443] Pericardial effusion, on the other hand, is between the aorta and the heart.

CARDIAC TAMPONADE (p. 1473). Once the diagnosis of pericardial effusion has been established, a number of echocardiographic findings which are characteristic of cardiac tamponade should be sought.[444,445] A reliable echocardiographic finding with tamponade is compression of the right ventricular free wall in early diastole. This finding is noted by posterior displacement of the anterior free wall on the M-mode echocardiogram (Fig. 4-102).[439] The free wall then moves anteriorly following atrial systole. This observation has been confirmed with 2-D echocardiography by noting a diastolic collapse of the right ventricular free wall (Fig. 4-103).[445,446] Rarely, the left ventricle[447] or left atrium may collapse. Another finding is a diastolic indentation (collapse) of the right atrial free wall on the 2-D four-chamber view (Fig. 4-104).[448] Both of these signs (diastolic collapse of the right atrium and right ventricle) are very sensitive for detecting hemodynamic impairment secondary to tamponade and may precede the clinical signs of tamponade. Exaggerated respiratory variation of transvalvular Doppler flow and altered hepatic venous flow are also characteristic of tamponade.[450-452] The other echocardiographic signs of tamponade, such as reduction of the size of the right ventricular cavity, flat diastolic motion of the left ventricular wall, and variations in the E to F slope of the mitral valve,[444] have not proven reliable.

CONSTRICTIVE PERICARDITIS (p. 1482). Echocardiography is of some, albeit limited, value in the diagnosis of a thickened pericardium with constrictive pericarditis.[449,453-455] Although a thickened pericardium can be detected in many patients,[2,455] particularly those who also have pericardial fluid, this finding by itself does not imply the presence of constriction. The echocardiographic signs of constriction include lack of diastolic motion, i.e., a flat diastolic slope of the posterior left ventricular wall,[2,456,457] abnormal motion of the interventricular septum,[457] a very short and steep E to F slope of the mitral valve,[2] and a dilated inferior vena cava that does not get smaller with inspiration. Doppler studies of the pulmonary and systemic veins provide alternative approaches to the diagnosis of constrictive pericarditis.[458-461] The echocardiographic signs of constriction are not very sensitive and are certainly not specific; at best they raise the suspicion of this condition.

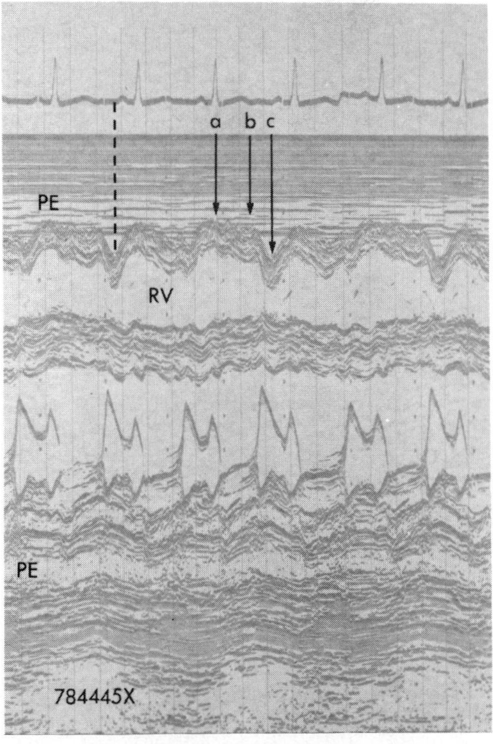

FIGURE 4-102. M-mode echocardiogram of a patient with pericardial effusion and clinical evidence of tamponade. The right ventricular free wall moves gradually posteriorly during systole (from a to b). In early diastole there is an abrupt downward or posterior motion of the right ventricular free wall (c and dashed line). PE = pericardial effusion, RV = right ventricle. (From Feigenbaum, H.: Echocardiography. 4th ed. Philadelphia, Lea and Febiger, 1986.)

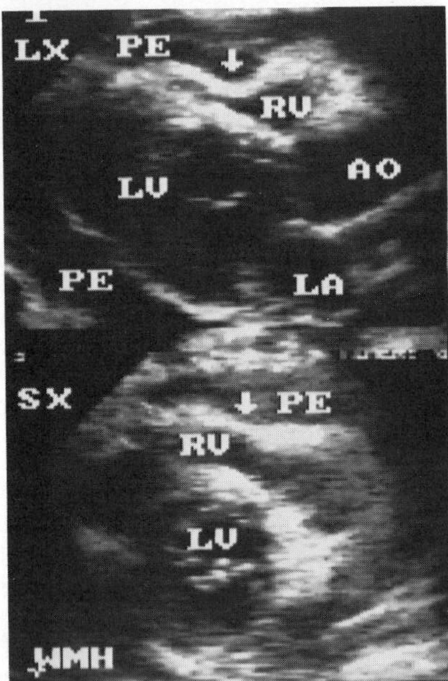

FIGURE 4–103. Long-axis (LX) and short-axis (SX) 2-D echocardiograms of a patient with pericardial effusion and collapse of the right ventricular free wall (arrows). PE = pericardial effusion, RV = right ventricle, LV = left ventricle, AO = aorta, LA = left atrium.

CONGENITALLY ABSENT PERICARDIUM (p. 952). On the M-mode echocardiogram, the right ventricle is usually dilated and there is paradoxical septal motion similar to a right ventricular volume overload. Two-dimensional echocardiography reveals bulging or displacement of part of the left ventricle or left atrium in a distorted manner that suggests an absent pericardium.[462,463]

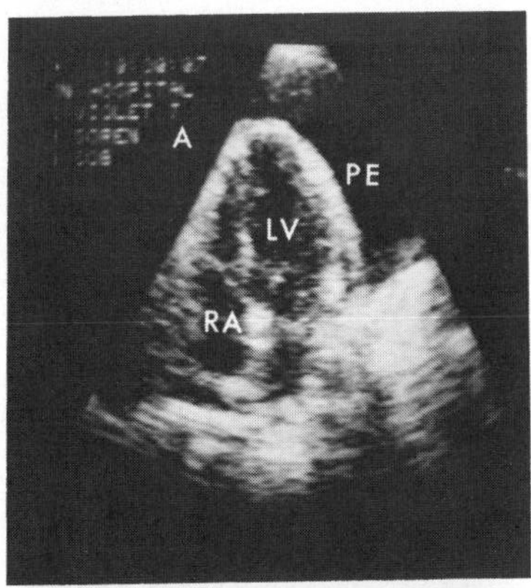

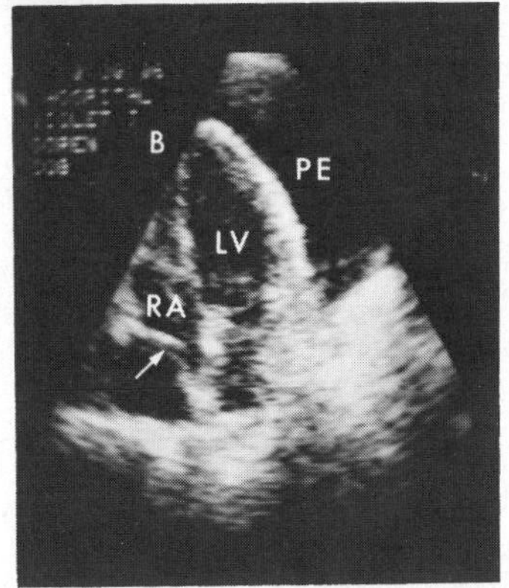

FIGURE 4–104. Apical four-chamber 2-D echocardiograms of a patient with a large pericardial effusion (PE) during systole *(A)*. Collapse (arrow) of the right atrial (RA) free wall during diastole *(B)*. LV = left ventricle. (From Feigenbaum, H.: Echocardiography. 4th ed. Philadelphia, Lea and Febiger, 1986.)

CARDIAC TUMORS AND THROMBI

(See Chap. 44)

ATRIAL TUMORS. Left atrial myxoma (p. 1452) is by far the most common cardiac tumor, and echocardiography has proved to be an extremely important diagnostic technique for its recognition.[464–468] Figure 4–105 demonstrates a 2-D echocardiogram of a patient with left atrial myxoma. The spatial orientation inherent in this examination provides additional useful information, and the size and shape of the mass are apparent. In addition, the site of attachment of the mass to the cardiac structure can frequently be detected. Transesophageal echocardiography provides an outstanding view of the left atrium.[469] Even further definition of left atrial masses can be seen with this unobstructive view. Figure 4–106 shows four images of a small left atrial mass which is attached to the atrial septum (IAS). Although this tumor was seen on a transthoracic 2-D echocardiogram, the clarity and detail were far greater with the transesophageal examination.

LEFT ATRIAL THROMBI. Other space-occupying structures—atrial thrombi—have been identified in the left atrium by means of echocardiography (Fig. 4–107).[2,470,471] However, since most of them are located in or near the left atrial appendage, transesophageal echocardiography is superior to conventional echocardiography in visualizing left atrial thrombi.[472]

RIGHT ATRIAL MYXOMA (p. 1453). These tumors are not as common as the left atrial variety. They can also be detected echocardiographically.[467,473] Such tumors appear as extraneous echoes behind the *tricuspid* valve in the right atrium during systole and within the right ventricle during diastole. As on the left side of the heart, a large vegetation involving the tricuspid valve can simulate a right atrial myxoma. Bilateral atrial myxomas have also been detected echocardiographically.[474,475]

OTHER INTRACARDIAC ECHOGENIC STRUCTURES. *Right atrial thrombi* that have the potential of producing massive pulmonary emboli have been detected with 2-D echocardiography.[476,477] However, it should be kept in mind that not all echogenic structures in the right atrium are pathologic. It is possible to detect various structures in the right atrium which are possibly normal variants. The so-called *Chiari network* may produce mobile echoes within the right atrium which may not be pathologic.[478] In addition, the eustachian valve may be prominent and simulate a pathologic mass.[473,479]

There are nonpathologic echo-producing structures on the left side of the heart as well.[480] Left ventricular bands or false tendons straddling the left ventricular chamber can frequently be imaged.[481–483]

Moderator bands are routinely seen in the right ventricle. Iatrogenic masses, such as various catheters, are also easily detected on the 2-D echocardiogram. Frequently this examination can help detect an incorrectly placed catheter or pacemaker catheter which may have perforated one of the cardiac walls.[484]

VENTRICULAR TUMORS. Myxomas can occur in the ventricles as well as in the atria[485,486] (p. 1453) and have been imaged in both ventricles. When the tumors are mobile, they can produce very dramatic echograms on both M-mode and 2-D examinations; they may move above the mitral valve into the left ventricular outflow tract during systole.[487] Pedunculated right ventricular masses can prolapse into the pulmonary artery[488] or simulate pulmonic stenosis.[489] Rhabdomyomas[490] and fibromas[491] can also involve the ventricles; these two types of lesion have been imaged successfully.[492]

VALVULAR TUMORS. Neoplasms may involve the cardiac valves. Cardiac papillary fibroelastoma represent small tumors on the edges of the valve leaflets, primarily the mitral valve[493] and rarely the tricuspid valve.[494] Systemic emboli and stroke occur in patients with these neoplasms.[495] Other neoplasms, such as a rhabdomyosarcoma, may also involve the mitral valve and can be detected echocardiographically.[496] Primary myxoma can also be attached to the mitral valve.[497]

INVASION AND METASTASIS TO THE HEART (p. 1752). Invasion of the walls of the heart[498] and compression of the heart[499,500] by neoplasms arising elsewhere have been imaged echocardiographically. Seeding of the pericardium with metastases and the production of pericardial effusion (p. 1473) probably represent the most common types of cardiac involvement with malignant disease. Occasionally, a massively thickened pericardium is produced.[2] On echocardiography the position and configuration of the heart may be distorted by a large tumor mass in the mediastinum. Echocardiography has also been shown to be helpful in distinguishing between cystic and solid tumors involving the heart.[501,502]

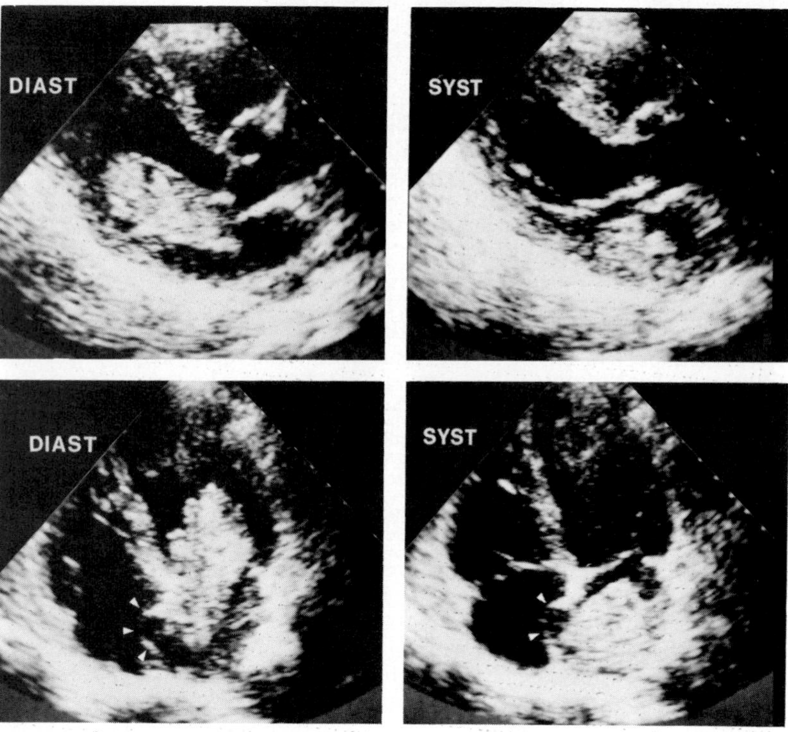

FIGURE 4-105. Long-axis (top) and apical four-chamber (bottom) 2-D echocardiograms in diastole and systole in a patient with a left atrial myxoma and an atrial septal aneurysm. The septal aneurysm (arrowheads) can be seen bulging towards the right atrium in both diastole and systole in the four-chamber view. (From Feigenbaum, H.: Echocardiography. 4th ed. Philadelphia, Lea and Febiger, 1986.)

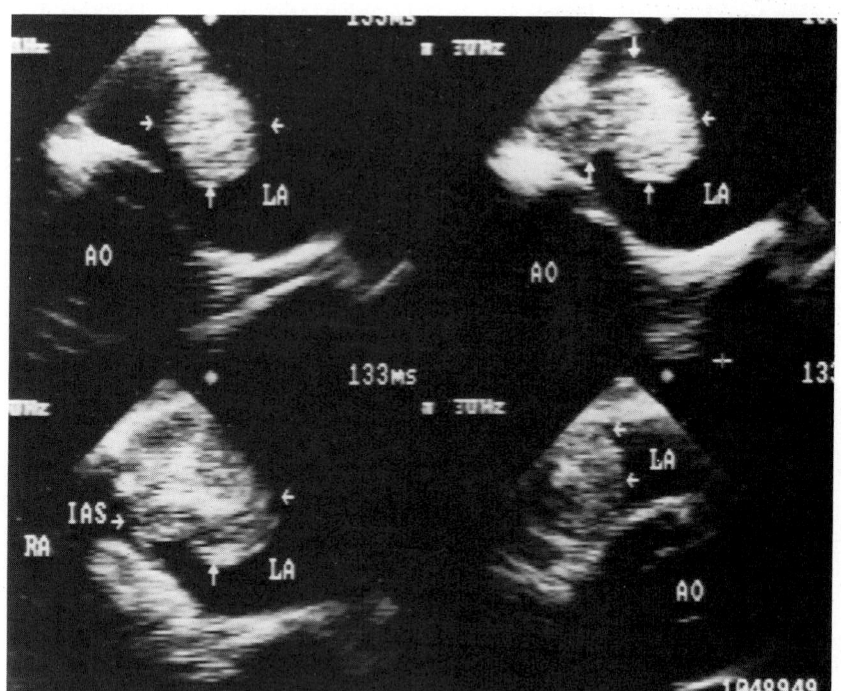

FIGURE 4-106. Transesophageal echocardiogram of a patient with a left atrial tumor (arrows). The tumor is attached to the interatrial septum (IAS). RA = right atrium, LA = left atrium, AO = aorta.

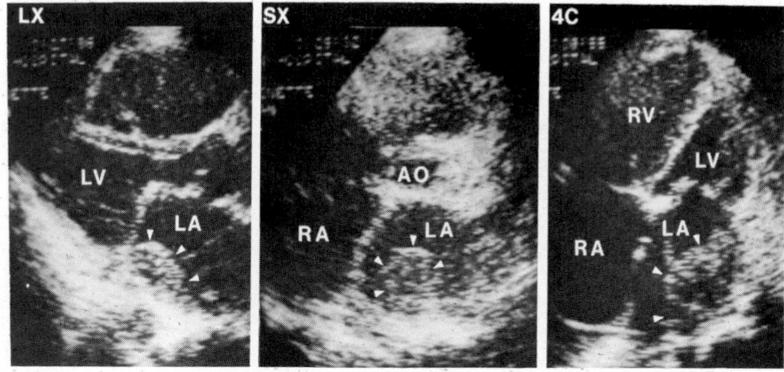

FIGURE 4-107. Long-axis (LX), short-axis (SX), and four-chamber (4C) 2-D echocardiograms of a patient with a large clot (arrowheads) in the left atrium (LA). LV = left ventricle, AO = aorta, RA = right atrium. (From Feigenbaum, H.: Echocardiography. 4th ed. Philadelphia, Lea and Febiger, 1986.)

DISEASES OF THE AORTA

(See also Chap. 47)

DILATATION AND ANEURYSM (p. 1530). It is possible to examine almost the entire aorta using echocardiography. The root of the aorta and proximal portion of the ascending aorta may be recorded with both M-mode and 2-D echocardiography. The 2-D technique utilizing the parasternal long-axis examination permits recording of the descending aorta posterior to the left atrium and left ventricle.[503] The suprasternal approach provides visualization of the arch of the aorta and the proximal portion of the descending aorta. The abdominal aorta can then be imaged with the transducer in the subcostal position or over the abdomen itself. Transesophageal echocardiography provides the most spectacular images of the aorta. Aside from a small section of the arch of the aorta all of the aorta can be imaged very accurately with the transesophageal approach.

Supravalvular aortic stenosis (p. 926) can be detected echocardiographically using either 2-D or Doppler echocardiography. As might be expected, dilatation of the aorta, such as occurs in the Marfan syndrome and cystic medial necrosis, is imaged relatively easily (Fig. 4-108).[504] The echocardiographic detection of coarctation of the aorta has already been discussed (p. 94). Aneurysms of the abdominal aorta are routinely examined quite successfully by 2-D echocardiography (Fig. 47-1, p. 1529).

AORTIC DISSECTION (p. 1535). Two-dimensional echocardiography has been used extensively for the detection of aortic dissection (Fig. 4-109).[505-507] In addition to the usual transducer position, the right parasternal position may be useful in detecting dissection with its true and false lumina and indicating systolic fluttering of the intimal flap.[508] Transesophageal echocardiography is becoming the procedure of choice in the diagnosis of aortic dissection.[509-511] Doppler echocardiography has also been useful in the diagnosis of aortic dissection.[512, 513] The flow characteristics in the false channel are distinctly different from those in the true channel. Color flow Doppler helps in establishing the correct diagnosis by indicating the difference between the false and true lumina (Fig. 4-110) and helps to identify the entry point of the dissection.[514-516]

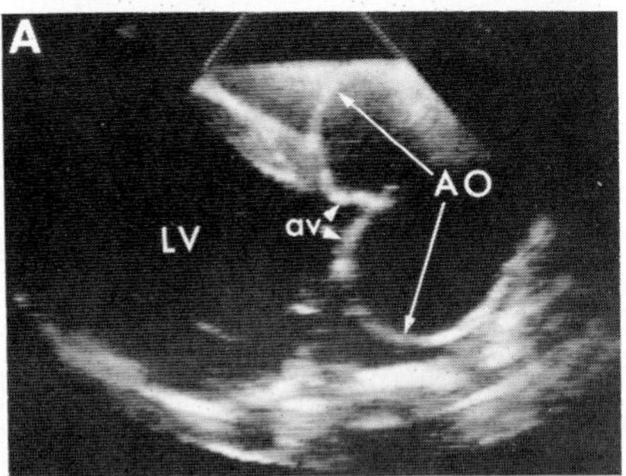

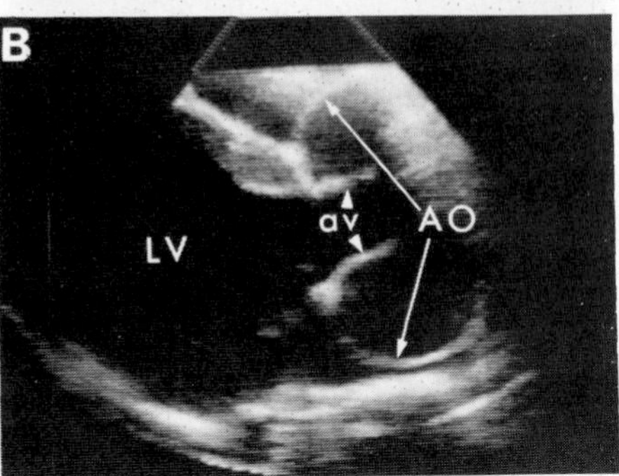

FIGURE 4-108. Diastolic *(A)* and systolic *(B)* long-axis, parasternal 2-D echocardiograms of a patient with Marfan syndrome. The aorta (AO) is markedly dilated. Note the marked discrepancy between the aortic valve (av) opening and the size of the aorta. LV = left ventricle. (From Feigenbaum, H.: Echocardiography. 3rd ed. Philadelphia, Lea and Febiger, 1981.)

ANEURYSM OF THE SINUS OF VALSALVA. Because examination of the root of the aorta is possible, 2-D and transesophageal echocardiography have been used to image the sinuses of Valsalva, allowing detection of aneurysms of these sinuses.[517] Bulging of the sinus, usually the anterior or right coronary sinus, into the right ventricular outflow tract[518] or interventricular septum[519-521] has been recorded. With rupture there is discontinuity of the anterior wall of the sinus and

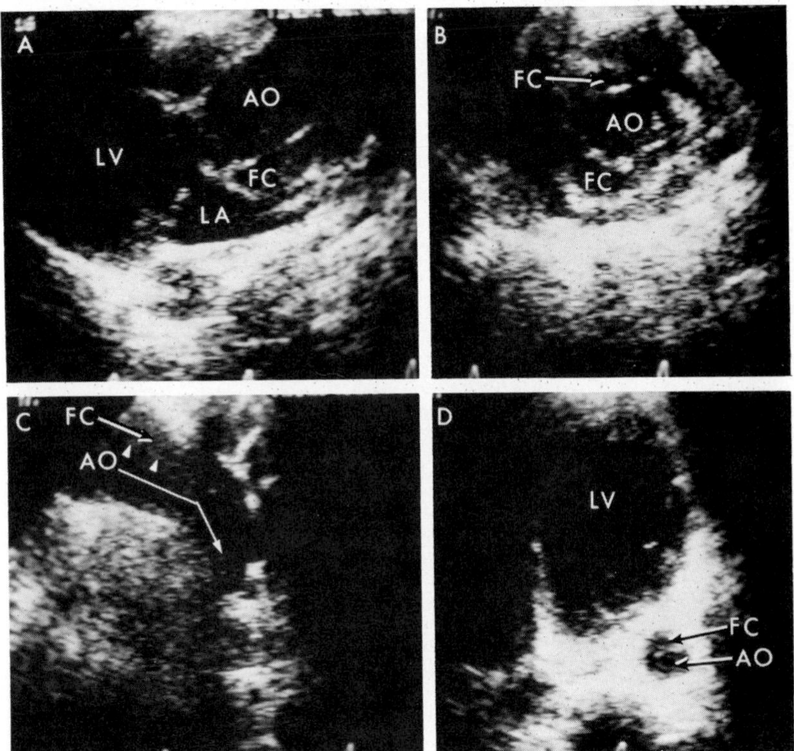

FIGURE 4-109. Parasternal long-axis *(A)*, short-axis *(B)*, suprasternal *(C)*, and apical *(D)* views of a patient with aortic dissection. The false channel (FC) can be seen in every view. The intimal flap (arrowheads) is only faintly seen in the suprasternal examination *(C)*. AO = true aortic lumen, LV = left ventricle, LA = left atrium. (From Feigenbaum, H.: Echocardiography. 4th ed. Philadelphia, Lea and Febiger, 1986.)

Figure 4–110. See color plate 4.

mid-systolic closure and coarse fluttering of the right coronary cusp of the aortic valve.[522] With rupture of the sinus of Valsalva into the right side of the heart, fluttering of the tricuspid valve as well as premature opening of the pulmonary valve has been reported.[136] Doppler echocardiography, especially color flow, is very helpful[523] in the diagnosis of sinus of Valsalva aneurysms. The abnormal jets of blood can be readily identified.

REFERENCES

PRINCIPLES OF ECHOCARDIOGRAPHY

1. Carlsen, E. N.: Ultrasound physics for the physician: A brief review. J. Clin. Ultrasound *3*:69, 1975.
2. Feigenbaum, H.: Echocardiography. 4th ed. Philadelphia, Lea and Febiger, 1986.
3. Wells, P. N. T.: Ultrasonics in Clinical Diagnosis. 2nd ed. New York, Churchill Livingstone, 1977.
4. Von Ramm, O. T., and Thurstone, F. L.: Cardiac imaging using a phased array ultrasound system. Circulation *53*:258, 1976.
5. Hatle, L., and Angelsen, B.: Doppler ultrasound in cardiology: Physical principles and clinical applications. 2nd ed. Philadelphia, Lea and Febiger, 1984.
6. Goldberg, S. J., Allen, H. D., Marx, G. R., and Flinn, C. J.: Doppler Echocardiography. Philadelphia, Lea and Febiger, 1985.
7. Baker, D. W., Rubenstein, S. A., and Lorch, G. S.: Pulsed Doppler echocardiography: Principles and applications. Am. J. Med. *63*:69, 1977.
8. Burns, P. N.: The physical principles of Doppler and spectral analysis. J. Clin. Ultrasound *15*:567, 1987.
9. Bom, K., deBoo, J., and Rijsterborgh, H.: On the aliasing problem in pulsed Doppler cardiac studies. J. Clin. Ultrasound *12*:559, 1984.
10. Steward, W. J., Galvin, K. A., Gillam, L. D., et al.: Comparison of high pulse repetition frequency and continuous wave Doppler echocardiography in the assessment of high flow velocity in patients with valvular stenosis and regurgitation. J. Am. Coll. Cardiol. *6*:565, 1985.
11. Sahn, D. J.: Instrumentation and physical factors related to visualization of stenotic and regurgitant jets by Doppler color flow mapping. J. Am. Coll. Cardiol. *12*:1354, 1988.
12. Omoto, R.: Color Atlas of Real-time Two-dimensional Doppler Echocardiography. 2nd ed. Tokyo, Shindan-to-Chiryo Co. Ltd., 1987.
13. Nanda, N. C.: Textbook of Color Doppler Echocardiography. Philadelphia, Lea and Febiger, 1989.
14. Stevenson, J. G.: Appearance and recognition of basic concepts in color flow imaging. Echocardiography *6*:451, 1989.
15. Ritter, S. B.: Red, green and blue: The flag of color flow mapping. 1989. Echocardiography *6*:369, 1989.
16. Keller, M. W., Glasheen, W., and Kaul, S.: Albunex: A safe and effective commercially produced agent for myocardial contrast echocardiography. J. Am. Soc. Echo. *2*:48, 1989.
17. Meltzer, R. S., Klig, V., and Teichholz, L. E.: Generating precision microbubbles for use as an echocardiographic contrast agent. J. Am. Coll. Cardiol. *5*:978, 1985.
18. Smith, M. D., Elion, J. L., McClure, R. R., et al.: Left heart opacification with peripheral venous injection of a new saccharide echo contrast agent in dogs. J. Am. Coll. Cardiol. *13*:1622, 1989.
19. Daniel, W. G., Erbel, R., Kasper, W., et al.: Safety of transesophageal echocardiography: A multicenter survey of 10,419 examinations. Circulation *83*:817, 1991.
20. Seward, J. B., Khandheria, B. K., Oh, J. K., et al.: Transesophageal echocardiography: Technique, anatomic correlations, implementation, and clinical applications. Mayo Clin. Proc. *63*:649, 1988.
21. Smith, J. S., Cahalan, M. K., Benefiel, D. J., et al.: Intraoperative detection of myocardial ischemia in high-risk patients: Electrocardiography versus two-dimensional transesophageal echocardiography. Circulation *72*:1015, 1985.
22. Mindich, B. P., Goldman, M. E., Fuster, V., et al.: Improved intraoperative evaluation of mitral valve operations utilizing two-dimensional contrast echocardiography. J. Thorac. Cardiovasc. Surg. 90:112, 1985.
23. Ren, J. F., Panidis, I. P., Kotler, M. N., et al.: Effect of coronary bypass surgery and valve replacement on left ventricular function: Assessment by intraoperative two-dimensional echocardiography. Am Heart J. *109*:281, 1985.
24. Sutherland, G. R., Balaji, S., and Monro, J. L.: Potential value of intraoperative Doppler colour flow mapping in operations for complex intracardiac shunting. Br. Heart J. *62*:467, 1989.
25. Sheikh, K. H., DeBruijn, N. P., Rankin, J. S., et al.: The utility of transesophageal echocardiography and Doppler color flow imaging in patients undergoing cardiac valve surgery. J. Am. Coll. Cardiol. *15*:363, 1990.
26. Stewart, W. J., Currie, P. J., Salcedo, E. E., et al.: Intraoperative Doppler color flow mapping for decision making in valve repair for mitral regurgitation. Circulation 81:556, 1990.
27. Perry, L. W., Galioto, F. M., Jr., Blair, T., et al.: Two-dimensional echocardiography for catheter location and placement in infants and children. Pediatrics *67*:541, 1981.
28. Kronzon, I., Glassman, E., Cohen, M., and Winer, H.: Use of two-dimensional echocardiography during transeptal cardiac catheterization. J. Am. Coll. Cardiol. *4*:425, 1984.
29. Callahan, J. A., Seward, J. B., Nishimura, R. A., et al.: Two-dimensional echocardiographically guided pericardiocentesis: Experience in 117 consecutive patients. Am. J. Cardiol. *55*:476, 1985.
30. Mortensen, M.: Endomyocardial biopsy guided by cross-sectional echocardiography. Br. Heart J. *50*:246, 1983.
31. Strachovsky, G., Zeldis, S. M., Katz, S., and McNulty-Mackey, M.: Two-dimensional echocardiographic monitoring during percutaneous endomyocardial biopsy. J. Am. Coll. Cardiol. *6*:609, 1985.
32. Lin, A. E., DiSessa, T. G., Williams, R. G., et al.: Balloon and blade atrial septostomy facilitated by two-dimensional echocardiography. Am. J. Cardiol. *57*:273, 1986.
33. Leon, M., Keren, G., Pichard, A., et al.: Intravascular ultrasound assessment of plaque responses to PTCA helps to explain angiographic findings. J. Am. Coll. Cardiol. (abstr) *17*:47a, 1991.
34. Tobis, J. M., Mallery, J. A., Gessert, J., et al.: Intravascular ultrasound cross-sectional arterial imaging before and after balloon angioplasty in vitro. Circulation *80*:873, 1989.
35. Gussenhoven, E. J., Essed, C. E., Lancee, C. T., et al.: Arterial wall characteristics determined by intravascular ultrasound imaging. An in vitro study. J. Am. Coll. Cardiol. *14*:947, 1989.
36. Pandian, N. G.: Intravascular and intracardiac ultrasound imaging. Circulation *80*:1091, 1989.
37. Martin, G. R., and Ruckman, R. N.: Fetal echocardiography: A large clinical experience and follow-up. J. Am. Soc. Echo. *3*:4, 1990.
38. Stewart, H. D., Stewart, H. F., Moore, R. M., and Garry, J.: Compilation of reported biological effects data and ultrasound exposure levels. J. Clin. Ultrasound *13*:167, 1985.

EXAMINATION OF THE NORMAL HEART

39. Sahn, D. J., DeMaria, A., Kisslo, J., and Weyman, A.: Recommendations regarding quantitation in M-mode echocardiography: Results of a survey of echocardiographic measurements. Circulation *58*:1072, 1978.
40. Henry, W. L., Gardin, J. M., and Ware, J. H.: Echocardiographic measurements in normal subjects from infancy to old age. Circulation *62*:1054, 1980.
41. Henry, W. L., DeMaria, A., Gramiak, R., et al.: Report of the American Society of Echocardiography Nomenclature and Standards in Two-dimensional Echocardiography. Circulation *62*:212, 1980.

EVALUATION OF CARDIAC PERFORMANCE

42. Feigenbaum, H., Popp, R. L., Wolfe, S. B., et al.: Ultrasound measurements of the left ventricle: A correlative study with angiography. Arch. Intern. Med. *129*:461, 1972.
43. Teichholz, L. E., Kreulen, T., Herman, M. V., and Gorlin, R.: Problems in echocardiographic volume determinations: Echocardiographic-angiographic correlations in the presence or absence of asynergy. Am. J. Cardiol. *37*:7, 1976.
44. Rasmussen, S., Corya, B. C., Phillips, J. F., and Black, M. J.: Unreliability of M-mode left ventricular dimensions for calculating stroke volume and cardiac output in patients without heart disease. Chest *81*:614, 1982.
45. McDonald, I. G., Feigenbaum, H., and Chang, S.: Analysis of left ventricular wall motion by reflected ultrasound: application to assessment of myocardial function. Circulation *46*:14, 1972.
46. Quinones, M. A., Gaasch, W. H., and Alexander, J. K.: Echocardiographic assessment of left ventricular function: With special reference to normalized velocities. Circulation *50*:42, 1974.
47. Feigenbaum, H.: Echocardiographic examination of the left ventricle. Circulation *51*:1, 1975.
48. Rosoff, M. H., and Cohen, M. V.: Significance of E point-septal separation by M-mode echocardiography in patients with aortic regurgitation. Am. J. Cardiol. *56*:809, 1985.
49. Ahmadpour, H., Shah, A. A., Allen, J. W., et al.: Mitral E point septal separation: A reliable index of left ventricular performance in coronary artery disease. Am. Heart J. *106*:21, 1983.
50. Schiller, N. B., Acquatella, H., Ports, T. A., et al: Left ventricular volume from paired biplane two-dimensional echocardiography. Circulation *60*:547, 1979.
51. Himelman, R. B., Cassidy, M. M., Landzberg, J. S., and Schiller, N. B.: Reproducibility of quantitative two-dimensional echocardiography. Am. Heart J. *115*:425, 1988.
52. Starling, M. R., Crawford, M. H., Sorensen, S. G., et al.: Comparative accuracy of apical biplane cross-sectional echocardiography and gated equilibrium radionuclide angiography for estimating left ventricular size and performance. Circulation *63*:1075, 1981.
53. Rokey, R., Kuo, L. C., Zoghbi, W. A., et al.: Determination of parameters of left ventricular diastolic filling with pulsed Doppler echocardiography: Comparison with cineangiography. Circulation *71*:543, 1985.
54. Erbel, R., Schweizer, P., Lambertz, H., et al.: Echoventriculography—A

simultaneous analysis of two-dimensional echocardiography and Cineventriculography. Circulation 67:205, 1983.
55. Schiller, N. B., Shah, P. M., Crawford, M., et al.: Recommendations for quantitation of the left ventricle by two-dimensional echocardiography. J. Am. Soc. Echo. 1:3A, 1989.
56. Gardin, J. M.: Doppler measurements of aortic blood flow velocity and acceleration: Load-independent indexes of left ventricular performance? Am. J. Cardiol. 64:935, 1989.
57. Isaaz, K., Ethevenot, G., Admant, P., et al.: A new Doppler method of assessing left ventricular ejection force in chronic congestive heart failure. A. J. Cardiol. 64:81, 1989.
58. Harrison, M. R., Clifton, G. D., Berk, M. R., and DeMaria, A. N.: Effect of blood pressure and afterload on Doppler echocardiographic measurements of left ventricular systolic function in normal subjects. Am. J. Cardiol. 64:905, 1989.
59. St. John Sutton, M. G., Reichck, N., Kastor, J. A., and Giuliani, E. R.: Computerized M-mode echocardiographic analysis of left ventricular dysfunction in cardiac amyloid. Circulation 66:790, 1982.
60. Smith, S. A., Stoner, J. E., Russell, A. E., et al.: Transmitral velocities measured by pulsed Doppler in healthy volunteers: Effects of acute changes in blood pressure and heart rate. Br. Heart J. 61:344, 1989.
61. Strok, T. V., Myller, R. M., Piske, G. J., et al.: Noninvasive measurement of left ventricular filling pressures by means of transmitral pulsed Doppler ultrasound. Am. J. Cardiol. 64:655, 1989.
62. Nishimura, R. A., Housmans, P. R., Hatle, L. K., and Tajik, A. J.: Assessment of diastolic function of the heart: Background and current applications of Doppler echocardiography. Part I. Physiologic and pathophysiologic features. Mayo Clin. Proc. 64:71, 1989.
63. Nishimura, R. A., Hatle, L. K., Abel, M. D., and Tajik, A. J.: Assessment of diastolic function of the heart: Background and current applications of Doppler echocardiography. Part II. Clinical studies. Mayo Clin. Proc. 64:181, 1989.
64. Sheikh, K. H., Bashore, T. M., Kitzman, D. W., et al.: Doppler left ventricular diastolic filling abnormalities in aortic stenosis and their relation to hemodynamic parameters. Am. J. Cardiol. 63:1360, 1989.
65. Stoddard, M. F., Pearson, A. C., Kern, M. J., et al.: Left ventricular diastolic function: Comparison of pulsed Doppler echocardiographic and hemodynamic indexes in subjects with and without coronary artery disease. J. Am. Coll. Cardiol. 13:327, 1989.
66. Douglas, P. S., Berko, B., Lesh, M., and Reichek, N.: Alterations in diastolic function in response to progressive left ventricular hypertrophy. J. Am. Coll. Cardiol., 13:461, 1989.
67. Wisenbaugh, T., Harlamert, E., and DeMaria, A. N.: Relation of left ventricular filling dynamics to alterations in load and compliance in patients with and without pressure-overload hypertrophy. Circulation 81:101, 1990.
68. Klein, A. L., Hatle, L, K., Burstwo, D. J., et al.: Doppler characterization of left ventricular diastolic function in cardiac amyloidosis. J. Am. Coll. Cardiol. 13:1017, 1989.
69. Miyatake, K., Okamoto, M., Kinoshita, N., et al.: Augmentation of atrial contribution to the left ventricular inflow with aging as assessed by intracardiac Doppler flowmeter. Am. J. Cardiol. 53:586, 1984.
70. Spirito, P., and Maron, B. J.: Influence of aging on Doppler echocardiographic indices of left ventricular diastolic function. Br. Heart J. 59:672, 1988.
71. Kuecherer, H., Ruffmann, K., and Kuebler, W.: Effect of aging on Doppler echocardiographic filling parameters in normal subjects and in patients with coronary artery disease. Clin. Cardiol. 11:303, 1988.
72. Maeda, M., Yokota, M., Iwase, M., et al.: Accuracy of cardiac output measured by continuous wave Doppler echocardiography during dynamic exercise testing in the supine position in patients with coronary artery disease. J. Am. Coll. Cardiol. 13:76, 1989.
73. Ginzton, L. E., Conant, R., Brizendine, M., et al.: Quantitative analysis of segmental wall motion during maximal upright dynamic exercise: Variability in normal adults. Circulation 73:268, 1986.
74. Presti, C. F., Armstrong, W. F., and Feigenbaum, H.: Comparison of echocardiography at peak exercise and after bicycle exercise in evaluation of patients with known or suspected coronary artery disease. J. Am. Soc. Echo. 1:119, 1988.
75. Iliceto, S., Sorino, M., D'Ambrosio, G., et al.: Detection of coronary artery disease by two-dimensional echocardiography and transesophageal atrial pacing. J. Am. Coll. Cardiol. 5:1188, 1985.
76. Feigenbaum, H.: Digital recording, display, and storage of echocardiograms. J. Am. Soc. Echo. 1:378, 1988.
77. Gardin, J. M., Kozlowski, J., Dabestani, A., et al.: Studies of Doppler aortic flow velocity during supine bicycle exercise. Am. J. Cardiol. 57:327, 1986.
78. Feigenbaum, H., Popp, R. L., Chip, J. N., and Haine, C. L.: Left ventricular wall thickness measured by ultrasound. Arch. Intern. Med. 121:391, 1969.
79. Devereux, R. B., Alonso, D. R., Lutas, E. M., et al.: Echocardiographic assessment of left ventricular hypertrophy: Comparison to necropsy findings. Am. J. Cardiol. 57:450, 1986.
80. Collins, H. W., Kronenberg, M. W., and Byrd, B. F.: Reproducibility of left ventricular mass measurements by two-dimensional and M-mode echocardiography. J. Am. Coll. Cardiol. 14:672, 1989.
81. Reichek, N., Helak, J., Plappert, T. A., et al.: Anatomic validation of left ventricular mass estimates from clinical two-dimensional echocardiography: Initial results. Circulation 67:348, 1983.
82. Daniels, S. R., Meyer, R. A., Liang, Y., and Bove, K. E.: Echocardiographically determined left ventricular mass index in normal children, adolescents and young adults. J. Am. Coll. Cardiol. 12:703, 1988.
83. Byrd, B. F., Finkbeiner, W., Bouchard, A., et al.: Accuracy and reproducibility of clinically acquired two-dimensional echocardiographic mass measurements. Am. Heart J. 118:133, 1989.
84. Roman, M. J., Devereux, R. B., and Cody, R. J.: Ability of left ventricular stress-shortening relations, end-systolic stress/volume ratio and indirect indexes to detect severe contractile failure in ischemic or idiopathic dilated cardiomyopathy. Am. J. Cardiol. 64:1338, 1989.
85. Heng, M. K., Bai, J. X., and Marin, J.: Changes in left ventricular wall stress during isometric and isotonic exercise in healthy men. Am. J. Cardiol. 62:794, 1988.
86. Goldberg, S. J.: Analysis and interpretation of thickening and thinning phases of left ventricular wall dynamics. Ultrasound Med. Biol. 10:797, 1984.
87. Corya, B. C., Rasmussen, S., Feigenbaum, H., et al.: Systolic thickening and thinning of the septum and posterior wall in patients with coronary artery disease, congestive cardiomyopathy, and atrial septal defect. Circulation 55:109, 1977.
88. Feigenbaum, H.: Estimation of left atrial size using ultrasound. Am. Heart J. 78:43, 1969.
89. Schabelman, S., Schiller, N. B., Silverman, N. H., and Ports, T. A.: Left atrial volume and estimation by two-dimensional echocardiography. Cathet. Cardiovasc. Diagn. 7:165, 1981.
90. Hoglund, C., and Rosenhamer, G.: Echocardiographic left atrial dimension as a predictor of maintaining sinus rhythm after conversion of atrial fibrillation. Acta Med. Scand. 217:411, 1985.
91. Lemire, F., Tajik, A. J., and Hagler, D. J.: Asymmetric left atrial enlargement: An echocardiographic observation. Chest 59:779, 1976.
92. Gehl, L. G., Mintz, G. S., Kotler, M. N., and Segal, B. L.: Left atrial volume overload in mitral regurgitation: A two-dimensional echocardiographic study. Am. J. Cardiol. 49:33, 1982.
93. Hiraishi, S., DiSessa, T. G., Jarmakani, J. M., et al.: Two-dimensional echocardiographic assessment of left atrial size in children. Am. J. Cardiol. 52:1249, 1983.
94. Gibson, T. C., Miller, S. W., Aretz, T., et al.: Method for estimating right ventricular volume by planes applicable to cross-sectional echocardiography: Correlation with angiographic formulas. Am. J. Cardiol. 55:1584, 1985.
95. Silverman, N. H., and Hudson, S.: Evaluation of right ventricular volume and ejection fraction in children by two-dimensional echocardiography. Pediatr. Cardol. 4:197, 1983.
96. Popp, R. L., Wolfe, S. B., Hirata, T., and Feigenbaum, H.: Estimation of right and left ventricular size by ultrasound. A study of the echoes from the interventricular septum. Am. J. Cardiol. 24:523, 1969.
97. Baker, B. J., Scovil, J. A., Kane, J. J., and Murphy, M. L.: Echocardiographic detection of right ventricular hypertrophy. Am. Heart J. 105:611, 1983.
98. King, M. E., Braun, H., Goldblatt, A., et al.: Interventricular septal configuration as a predictor of right ventricular systolic hypertension in children: A cross-sectional echocardiographic study. Circulation 68:68, 1983.
99. Ryan, T., Petrovic, O., Dillon, J. C., et al.: An echocardiographic index for separation of right ventricular volume and pressure overload. J. Am. Coll. Cardiol. 5:918, 1985.
100. Robson, S. C., Murray, A., Peart, I., et al.: Reproducibility of cardiac output measurement by cross-sectional and Doppler echocardiography. Br. Heart J. 59:680, 1988.
101. Bouchard, A., Blumlein, S., Schiller, N. B., et al.: Measurement of left ventricular stroke volume using continuous wave Doppler echocardiography of the ascending aorta and M-mode echocardiography of the aortic valve. J. Am. Coll. Cardiol. 9:75, 1987.
102. Sahn, D. J.: Determination of cardiac output by echocardiographic Doppler methods: Relative accuracy of various sites for measurement. J. Am. Coll. Cardiol. 6:663, 1985.
103. Ihlen, H., Amlie, J. P., Dale, J., et al.: Determination of cardiac output by Doppler echocardiography. Br. Heart J. 51:54, 1984.
104. Zhang, Y., Nitter-Hauge, N., Ihlen, H., and Myhre, E.: Doppler echocardiographic measurement of cardiac output using the mitral orifice method. Br. Heart J. 53:130, 1985.
105. Ascah, K. J., Stewart, W. J., Gillam, L. D., et al.: Calculation of transmitral flow by Doppler echocardiography: A comparison of methods in a canine model. Am. Heart J. 117:402, 1989.
106. Meijboom, E. J., Horowitz, S., Valdes-Cruz, L. M., et al.: A Doppler echocardiographic method for calculating volume flow across the tricuspid valve: Correlative laboratory and clinical studies. Circulation 71:551, 1985.
107. Valdes-Cruz, L. M., Horowitz, S., Goldberg, S. J., and Allen, H. D.: The mitral valve orifice method for noninvasive two-dimensional echo Doppler determinations of cardiac output. Circulation 67:872, 1983.
108. Alverson, D. C., Eldridge, M., Dillon, T., et al.: Noninvasive pulsed Doppler determination of cardiac output in neonates and children. J. Pediatr. 101:46, 1982.
109. Nishimura, R. A., Callahan, M. J., Schaff, H. V., et al.: Non-invasive measurement of cardiac output by continuous-wave Doppler echocardiography: Initial experience and review of the literature. Mayo Clin. Proc. 59:484, 1984.
110. Ihlen, H., Myhre, E., Amlie, J. P., et al.: Changes in left ventricular stroke volume measured by Doppler echocardiography. Br. Heart J. 54:378, 1985.
111. Goldberg, S. J., and Allen, H. D.: Quantitative assessment by Doppler echocardiography of pulmonary or aortic regurgitation. Am. J. Cardiol. 56:131, 1985.
112. Jenni, R., Ritter, M., Vieli, A., et al.: Determination of the ratio of pulmo-

nary blood flow to systemic blood flow by derivation of amplitude weighted mean velocity from continuous wave Doppler spectra. Br. Heart J. *61*:167, 1989.

113. Meijboom, E. J., Rijsterborgh, H., Bot, H., et al.: Limits of reproducibility of blood flow measurements by Doppler echocardiography. Am. J. Cardiol. *59*:133, 1987.
114. Dittmann, H., Voelker, W., Karsch, K-R., and Seipel, L.: Influence of sampling site and flow area on cardiac output measurements by Doppler echocardiography. J. Am. Coll. Cardiol. *10*:818, 1987.
115. Nicolosi, G. L., Pungercic, E., Cervesato, E., et al.: Feasibility and variability of six methods for the echocardiographic and Doppler determination of cardiac output. Br. Heart J. *59*:299, 1988.
116. Hatle, L., Brubakk, A., Tromsdal, A., and Angelsen, B.: Noninvasive assessment of pressure drop in mitral stenosis by Doppler ultrasound. Br. Heart J. *40*:131, 1978.
117. Stamm, R. B., and Martin, R. P.: Quantification of pressure gradients across stenotic valves by Doppler ultrasound. J. Am. Coll. Cardiol. *2*:707, 1983.
118. Teirstein, P. S., Yock, P. G., and Popp, R. L.: The accuracy of Doppler ultrasound measurement of pressure gradients across irregular, duel, and tunnellike obstructions to blood flow. Circulation *72*:577, 1985.
119. Yock, P. G., and Popp, R. L.: Non-invasive estimation of right ventricular systolic pressure by Doppler ultrasound in patients with tricuspid regurgitation. Circulation *70*:657, 1984.
120. Chan, K-L., Currie, P. J., Seward, J. B., et al.: Comparison of three Doppler ultrasound methods in the prediction of pulmonary artery disease. J. Am. Coll. Cardiol. *9*:549, 1987.
121. Marx, G. R., Allen, H. D., and Goldberg, S. J.: Doppler echocardiographic estimation of systolic pulmonary artery pressure in pediatric patients with interventricular communications. J. Am. Coll. Cardiol. *6*:1132, 1985.
122. Silbert, D. R., Brunson, S. C., Schiff, R., and Diamant, S.: Determination of right ventricular pressure in the presence of a ventricular septal defect using continuous wave Doppler ultrasound. J. Am. Coll. Cardiol. *8*:379, 1986.
123. Marx, G. R., Allen, H. D., and Goldberg, S. J.: Doppler echocardiographic estimation of systolic pulmonary artery pressure in patients with aortic-pulmonary shunts. J. Am. Coll. Cardiol. *7*:880, 1986.
124. Kosturakis, D., Goldberg, S. J., Allen, H. D., and Loeber, C.: Doppler echocardiographic prediction of pulmonary arterial hypertension in congenital heart disease. Am. J. Cardiol. *53*:1110, 1984.
125. Isobe, M., Yazaki, Y., Takaku, F., et al.: Prediction of pulmonary arterial pressure in adults by pulsed Doppler echocardiography. Am. J. Cardiol. *57*:316, 1986.
126. Pridie, R. B., Beham, R., and Oakley, C. M.: Echocardiography of the mitral valve in aortic valve disease. Br. Heart J. *33*:296, 1971.
127. Botvinick, E. H., Schiller, N. B., Wickramasekaran, R., et al.: Echocardiographic demonstration of early mitral valve closure in severe aortic insufficiency. Its clinical implications. Circulation *51*:836, 1975.
128. Konecke, L. L., Feigenbaum, H., Chang, S., et al.: Abnormal mitral valve motion in patients with elevated left ventricular diastolic pressures. Circulation *47*:989, 1973.
129. Lewis, J. R., Parker, J. O., and Burggraf, G. W.: Mitral valve motion and changes in left ventricular end-diastolic pressures: A correlative study of the PR-AC interval. Am. J. Cardiol. *42*:383, 1978.
130. Sabbah, H. N., and Stein, P. D.: Mechanism of early systolic closure of the aortic valve in discrete membranous subaortic stenosis. Circulation *65*:399, 1982.
131. Nathan, M. P. R., Arora, R., and Rubenstein, H.: Mid-diastolic aorta valve opening in bacterial endocarditis of aortic valve. Clin. Cardiol. *5*:294, 1982.
132. Green, S. E., and Popp, R. L.: The relationship of pulmonary valve motion to the motion of surrounding cardiac structures: a two-dimensional and dual M-mode echocardiographic study. Circulation *64*:107, 1981.
133. Gramiak, R., Nanda, N. C., and Shah, P. M.: Echocardiographic detection of pulmonary valve. Radiology *102*:153, 1972.
134. Weyman, A. E., Dillon, J. C., Feigenbaum, H., and Chang, S.: Echocardiographic patterns of pulmonic valve motion in pulmonic stenosis. Am. J. Cardiol. *34*:644, 1974.
135. Wann, L. S., Weyman, A. E., Dillon, J. C., and Feigenbaum, H.: Premature pulmonary valve opening. Circulation *55*:128, 1977.
136. Weyman, A. E., Dillon, J. C., Feigenbaum, H., and Chang, S.: Echocardiographic patterns of pulmonary valve motion with pulmonary hypertension. Circulation *50*:905, 1974.
137. Turkevich, D., Groves, B. M., Micco, A., et al.: Early partial systolic closure of the pulmonic valve relates to severity of pulmonary hypertension. Am. Heart J. *115*:409, 1988.
138. Tahara, M., Tanaka, H., Nakao, S., et al.: Hemodynamic determinants of pulmonary valve motion during systole in experimental pulmonary hypertension. Circulation *64*:1249, 1981.
139. Hirschfeld, S., Meyer, R., Schwartz, D. C., et al.: Measurement of right and left ventricular systolic time intervals by echocardiography. Circulation *51*:304, 1975.
140. Hirschfeld, S., Meyer, R., Schwartz, D. C., et al.: The echocardiographic assessment of pulmonary artery pressure and pulmonary vascular resistance. Circulation *52*:642, 1975.
141. Stevenson, J. G.: Comparison of several noninvasive methods for estimation of pulmonary artery pressure. J Am. Soc. Echo. *2*:157, 1989.
142. Chang, K. L., Currie, P. J., Seward, J. B., et al.: Comparison of three Doppler ultrasound methods in the prediction of pulmonary artery pressure. J. Am. Coll. Cardiol. *9*:549, 1987.
143. Moreno, F. L. L., Hagan, A. D., Holman, J. R., et al.: Evaluation of size and dynamics of the inferior vena cava as an index of right-sided cardiac function. Am. J. Cardiol. *53*:579, 1984.
144. Reeves, W. C., Leaman, D. M., Bounocore, E., et al.: Detection of tricuspid regurgitation and estimation of central venous pressure by two-dimensional contrast echocardiography of the right superior hepatic vein. Am. Heart J. *102*:374, 1981.

ACQUIRED VALVULAR HEART DISEASE

145. Edler, I.: Ultrasound cardiogram in mitral valve disease. Acta Chir. Scand. *111*:230, 1956.
146. Wann, L. S., Weyman, A. E., Dillon, J. C., and Feigenbaum, H.: Determination of mitral valve area by cross-sectional echocardiography. Ann. Intern. Med. *88*:337, 1978.
147. Duchak, J. M., Jr., Chang, S., and Feigenbaum, H.: The posterior mitral valve echo and the echocardiographic diagnosis of mitral stenosis. Am. J. Cardiol. *29*:628, 1972.
148. Motro, M., Schneeweiss, A., Lehrer, E., et al.: Correlation between cardiac catheterization and echocardiography in assessing the severity of mitral stenosis. Int. J. Cardiol. *1*:25, 1981.
149. Diebold, B., Theroux, P., Bourassa, M. G., et al.: Non-invasive pulsed Doppler study of mitral stenosis and mitral regurgitation: Preliminary study. Br. Heart J. *42*:168, 1979.
150. Smith, M. D., Handshoe, R., Handshoe, S., et al.: Comparative accuracy of two-dimensional echocardiography and Doppler pressure half-time methods in assessing severity of mitral stenosis in patients with and without prior commissurotomy. Circulation *73*:100, 1986.
151. Loyd, D., Ask, P., and Wranne, B.: Pressure half-time does not always predict mitral valve area correctly. J. Am. Soc. Echo. *1*:313, 1988.
152. Chen, C., Wang, Y., Guo, B., and Lin, Y.: Reliability of the Doppler pressure half-time method for assessing effects of percutaneous mitral balloon valvuloplasty. J. Am. Coll. Cardiol. *13*:1309, 1989.
153. Thomas, J. D., Wilkins, G. T., Choong, C. Y. P., et al.: Inaccuracy of mitral pressure half-time immediately after percutaneous mitral valvotomy. Circulation *78*:980, 1988.
154. Fredman, C. S., Pearson, A. C., Labovitz, A. J., and Kern, M. J.: Comparison of hemodynamic pressure half-time method and Gorlin formula with Doppler and echocardiographic determination of mitral valve area in patients with combined mitral stenosis and regurgitation. Am. Heart J. *119*:121, 1990.
155. Zanolla, L., Marino, P. Nicolosi, G. L., et al.: Two-dimensional echocardiographic evaluation of mitral valve calcification. Sensitivity and specificity. Chest *82*:154, 1982.
156. Reid, C. L., Chandraratna, A. N., Kawanishi, D. T., et al.: Influence of mitral valve morphology on double-balloon catheter balloon valvuloplasty in patients with mitral stenosis. Circulation *80*:515, 1989.
157. Chen, C., Wang, X., Wang, Y., and Lan, Y.: Value of two-dimensional echocardiography in selecting patients and balloon sizes for percutaneous balloon mitral valvuloplasty. J. Am. Coll. Cardiol. *14*:1651, 1989.
158. Zaretskii, V. V., Kuznetsoa, L. M., Bobkov, V. V., and Aksiuk, M. A.: Diagnosis of subvalvular adhesions in mitral stenosis by 2-dimensional echocardiography. Kardiologiia *25*:68, 1985.
159. Patel, A. K., Rowe, G. G., Thomsen, J. H., et al.: Detection and estimation of rheumatic mitral regurgitation in the presence of mitral stenosis by pulsed Doppler echocardiography. Am. J. Cardiol. *51*:986, 1983.
160. Miyatake, K., Izumi, S., Okamoto, M., et al.: Semiquantitative grading of severity of mitral regurgitation by real-time two-dimensional Doppler flow imaging technique. J. Am. Coll. Cardiol. *7*:82, 1986.
161. Nanda, N. C., Cooper, J. W., Philpot, E. F., and Fan, P: Evaluation of valvular regurgitation by color Doppler. J. Am. Soc. Echo. *2*:56, 1989.
162. Spain, M. G., Smith, M. D., Grayburn, P. A., et al.: Quantitative assessment of mitral regurgitation by Doppler color flow imaging: Angiographic and hemodynamic correlations. J. Am. Coll. Cardiol. *13*:585, 1989.
163. Appleton, C. P., Hatle, L. K., Nellesen, U., et al.: Flow velocity acceleration in the left ventricle: A useful Doppler echocardiographic sign of hemodynamically significant mitral regurgitation. J. Am. Soc. Echo. *3*:35, 1990.
164. Simpson, I. A., and Sahn, D. J.: Hydrodynamic investigation of a hemodynamic problem: A review of the in vitro evaluation of mitral insufficiency by color Doppler flow mapping. J. Am. Soc. Echo. *2*:67, 1989.
165. Hoit, B. D., Jones, M., Eidbo, E. E., et al.: Sources of variability for Doppler color flow mapping of regurgitant jets in an animal model of mitral regurgitation. J. Am. Coll. Cardiol. *13*:1631, 1989.
166. Smith, M. D., Grayburn, P. A., Spain, M. G., et al.: Observer variability in the quantitation of Doppler color flow jet areas for mitral and aortic regurgitation. J. Am. Coll. Cardiol. *11*:579, 1988.
167. Zhang, Y., Ihlen, H., Myhre, E., et al.: Measurement of mitral regurgitation by Doppler echocardiography. Br. Heart J. *54*:384, 1985.
168. Ascah, K. J., Stewart, W. J., Jiang, L., et al.: A Doppler two-dimensional echocardiographic method for quantitation of mitral regurgitation. Circulation *72*:377, 1985.
169. Zile, M. R., Gaasch, W. H., Carroll, J. D., and Levine, H. J.: Chronic mitral regurgitation: Predictive value of preoperative echocardiographic indexes of left ventricular function and wall stress. J. Am. Coll. Cardiol. *3*:235, 1984.
170. Dillon, J. C., Haine, C. L., Chang, S., and Feigenbaum, H.: Use of echocardiography in patients with prolapsed mitral valve. Am. J. Cardiol. *43*:503, 1971.
171. DeMaria, A. N., King, J. F., Bogren, H. G., et al.: The variable spectrum of echocardiographic manifestations of the mitral valve prolapse syndrome. Circulation *50*:33, 1974.

172. Sahn, D. J., Wood, J., Allen, H. D., et al.: Echocardiographic spectrum of mitral valve motion in children with and without mitral valve prolapse: The nature of false positive diagnosis. Am. J. Cardiol. *39*:422, 1977.
173. Markiewicz, W., Stoner, J., London, E., et al.: Mitral valve prolapse in one hundred presumably healthy young females. Circulation *53*:464, 1976.
174. Sahn, D. J., Allen, H. D., Goldberg, S. J., and Friedman, W. F.: Mitral valve prolapse in children. A problem defined by real-time cross-sectional echocardiography. Circulation *53*:651, 1976.
175. Morganroth, J., Jones, R. H., Chen, C. C., and Naito, M.: Two-dimensional echocardiography in mitral aortic and tricuspid valve prolapse. The clinical problem, cardiac nuclear imaging considerations and a proposed standard for diagnosis. Am. J. Cardiol. *46*:1164, 1980.
176. Wann, L. S., Gross, C. M., Wakefield, R. J., and Kalbfleisch, J. H.: Diagnostic precision of echocardiography in mitral valve prolapse. Am. Heart J. *109*:803, 1985.
177. Krivokapich, J., Child, J. S., Dadourian, B. J., and Perloff, J. K.: Reassessment of echocardiographic criteria for diagnosis of mitral valve prolapse. Am. J. Cardiol. *61*:131, 1988.
178. Levine, R. A., Stathogiannis, E., Newell, J. B., et al.: Reconsideration of echocardiographic standards for mitral valve prolapse: Lack of association between leaflet displacement isolated to the apical four chamber view and independent echocardiographic evidence of abnormality. J. Am. Coll. Cardiol. *11*:1010, 1988.
179. Chun, P, K. C., and Sheehan, M. W.: Myxomatous degeneration of mitral valve M-mode and two-dimensional echocardiographic findings. Br. Heart J. *47*:404, 1982.
180. Ballester, M., Presbitero, P., Foale, R., et al.: Prolapse of the mitral valve in secundum atrial septal defect: A functional mechanism. Eur. Heart J., *4*:472, 1983.
181. Avgeropoulou, C. C., Rahko, P. S., and Patel, A. K.: Reliability of M-mode, two-dimensional, and Doppler echocardiography in diagnosing a flail mitral valve leaflet. J. Am. Soc. Echo. *2*:433, 1988.
182. Ballester, M., Foale, R., Presbitero, P., et al.: Cross-sectional echocardiographic features of ruptured chordae tendineae. Eur. Heart J. *4*:795, 1983.
183. Himelman, R. B., Kusumoto, F., Oken, K., et al.: The flail mitral valve: Echocardiographic findings by precordial and transesophageal imaging and Doppler color flow mapping. J. Am. Coll. Cardiol. *17*:272, 1991.
184. Godley, R. W., Wann, L. S., Rogers, E. W., et al.: Incomplete mitral leaflet closure in patients with papillary muscle dysfunction. Circulation *63*:565, 1981.
185. Gramiak, R., and Shah, P.M.: Echocardiography of the normal and diseased aortic valve. Radiology *96*:1, 1970.
186. Weyman, A. E., Feigenbaum, H., Dillon, J. C., and Chang, S.: Cross-sectional echocardiography in assessing the severity of valvular aortic stenosis. Circulation *52*:828, 1975.
187. Godley, R. W., Green, D., Dillon, J. C., et al.: Reliability of two-dimensional echocardiography in assessing the severity of valvular aortic stenosis. Chest *79*:657, 1981.
188. Currie, P. J., Seward, J. B., Reeder, G. S., et al.: Continuous-wave Doppler echocardiographic assessment of severity of calcific aortic stenosis: A simultaneous Doppler-catheter correlative study in 100 adult patients. Circulation *71*:1162, 1985.
189. Hegrenaes, L., and Hatle, L.: Aortic stenosis in adults. Non-invasive estimation of pressure differences by continuous wave Doppler echocardiography. Br. Heart J. *54*:396, 1985.
190. Teien, D., and Ericksson, P.: Quantification of transvalvular pressure differences in aortic stenosis by Doppler ultrasound. Int. J. Cardiol. *7*:121, 1985.
191. Warth, D. C., Stewart, W. J., Block, P. C., and Weyman, A. E.: A new method to calculate aortic valve area without left heart catheterization. Circulation *70*:978, 1984.
192. Zoghbi, W. A., Farmer, K. L., Soto, J. G., et al.: Accurate noninvasive quantification of stenotic aortic valve area by Doppler echocardiography. Circulation *73*:452, 1986.
193. Richards, K. L., Cannon, S. R., Miller, J. F., and Crawford, M. H.: Calculation of aortic valve area by Doppler echocardiography: A direct application of the continuity equation. Circulation *73*:964, 1986.
194. Danielsen, R., Nordrehaug, J. E., and Vik-Mo, H.: Factors affecting Doppler echocardiographic valve area assessment in aortic stenosis. Am. J. Cardiol. *63*:1107, 1989.
195. Danielsen, R., Nordrehaug, J. E., Strangeland, L., Vik-Mo, H.: Limitations in assessing the severity of aortic stenosis by Doppler gradients. Br. Heart J. *59*:551, 1988.
196. Yeager, M., Yock, P. G., and Popp, R. L.: Comparison of Doppler-derived pressure gradient to that determined at cardiac catheterization in adults with aortic valve stenosis: Implications for management. Am. J. Cardiol. *57*:644, 1986.
197. Reichek, N., and Devereux, R. B.: Reliable estimation of peak left ventricular systolic pressure by M-mode echographic-determined end-diastolic relative wall thickness: Identification of severe valvular aortic stenosis in adult patients. Am. Heart J. *103*:202, 1982.
198. Ciobanu, M., Abbasi, A. S., Allen, M., et al.: Pulsed Doppler echocardiography in the diagnosis and estimation of severity of aortic insufficiency. Am. J. Cardiol. *49*:339, 1982.
199. Grayburn, P. A., Smith, M. D., Handshoe, R., et al.: Detection of aortic insufficiency by standard echocardiography, pulsed Doppler echocardiography, and auscultation. Ann. Intern. Med. *104*:599, 1986.
200. Bouchard, A., Yock, P., Schiller, N. B., et al.: Value of color Doppler estimation of regurgitant volume in patients with chronic aortic insufficiency. Am. Heart J. *117*:1099, 1989.
201. Byard, C. E., Perry, G. J., Roitman, D. I., and Nanda, N. C.: Quantitative assessment of aortic regurgitation by color Doppler. Circulation *72*(suppl. III):146, (abstract) 1986.
202. Perry, G. J., Helmcke, F., Nanda, N. C., et al.: Evaluation of aortic insufficiency by Doppler color flow mapping. J. Am. Coll. Cardiol. *9*:952, 1987.
203. Masuyama, T., Kodama, K., Kitabatake, A., et al.: Noninvasive evaluation of aortic regurgitation by continuous-wave Doppler echocardiography. Circulation *73*:460, 1986.
204. Samstad, S. O., Hegrenaes, L., Skjaerpe, T., and Hatle, L.: Half-time of the diastolic aortoventricular pressure difference by continuous wave Doppler ultrasound: A measure of the severity of aortic regurgitation? Br. Heart J. *61*:336–343, 1989.
205. Zhang, Y., Nitter-Hauge, S., Ihlen, H., et al.: Measurement of aortic regurgitation by Doppler echocardiography. Br. Heart J. *55*:32, 1986.
206. Robertson, W. S., Stewart, J., Armstrong, W. F., et al.: Reverse doming of the anterior mitral leaflet with severe aortic regurgitation. J. Am. Coll. Cardiol. *3*:431, 1984.
207. Oh, J. K., Hatle, L. K., Sinak, L. J., and Tajik, A. J.: Characteristic Doppler echocardiographic pattern of mitral inflow velocity in severe aortic regurgitation. J. Am. Coll. Cardiol. *14*:1712, 1989.
208. Fioretti, P., Roelandt, J., Sclavo, M., et al.: Postoperative regression of left ventricular dimensions in aortic insufficiency: A long-term echocardiographic study. J. Am. Coll. Cardiol. *5*:856, 1985.
209. Henry, W. L., Bonow, R. O., Borer, J. S., et al.: Observations on the optimum time for operative intervention for aortic regurgitation. I. Evaluation of the results of aortic valve replacement in symptomatic patients. Circulation *61*:741, 1980.
210. Bonow, R. O., Rosing, D. R., Kent, K. M., and Epstein, S. E.: Timing of operation for chronic aortic regurgitation. Am. J. Cardiol. *50*:325, 1982.
211. Guyer, D. E., Gillam, L. D., Foale, R. A., et al.: Comparison of the echocardiographic and hemodynamic diagnosis of rheumatic tricuspid stenosis. J. Am. Coll. Cardiol. *3*:1135, 1984.
212. Parris, T. M., Panidis, I. P., Ross, J., and Mintz, G. S.: Doppler echocardiographic findings in rheumatic tricuspid stenosis. Am. J. Cardiol. *60*:1414, 1987.
213. Skjaerpe T., and Hatle, L.: Diagnosis of tricuspid regurgitation. Sensitivity of Doppler ultrasound compared with contrast echocardiography. Eur. Heart J. *6*:429, 1985.
214. Missri, J., Agnarsson, U., and Sverrisson, J.: The clinical spectrum of tricuspid regurgitation detected by pulsed Doppler echocardiography. Angiology *36*:746, 1985.
215. Curtius, M. M., Thyssen, M., Breuer, H. W. M., and Loogen, F.: Doppler versus contrast echocardiography for diagnosis of tricuspid regurgitation. Am. J. Cardiol. *56*:333, 1985.
216. Ogawa, S., Hayashi, J., Sasaki, H., et al.: Evaluation of combined valvular prolapse syndrome by two-dimensional echocardiography. Circulation *65*:174, 1982.
217. Eckfeldt, J. H., Weir, E. K., and Chesler, E.: Echocardiographic findings in ruptured chordae tendineae of the tricuspid valve. Am. Heart J. *105*:1033, 1983.
218. Forman, M. B., Byrd, B. F., Oates, J. A., and Robertson, R. M.: Two-dimensional echocardiography in the diagnosis of carcinoid heart disease. Am. Heart J. *107*:492, 1984.
219. Sheikh, M. U., Covarrubias, E. A., Ali, N., et al.: M-mode echocardiographic observations in active bacterial endocarditis limited to the aortic valve. Am. Heart J. *102*:66, 1981.
220. Berger, M., Gallerstein, P. E., Benhuri, P., et al.: Evaluation of aortic valve endocarditis by two-dimensional echocardiography. Chest *80*:61, 1981.
221. Dillon, J. C., Feigenbaum, H., Konecke, L. L., et al.: Echocardiographic manifestations of valvular vegetations. Am. Heart J. *86*:698, 1973.
222. Roy, P., Tajik, A. J., Giuliani, E. R., et al.: Spectrum of echocardiographic findings in bacterial endocarditis. Circulation *53*:474, 1976.
223. Gallis, H. A., Johnson, M. L., and Kisslo, J. A.: Two-dimensional echocardiographic assessment of vegetative endocarditis. Circulation *55*:346, 1977.
224. Klodas, E., Edwards, W. D., and Khandheria, B. K.: Use of transesophageal echocardiography for improving detection of valvular vegetations in subacute bacterial endocarditis. J. Am. Soc. Echo. *2*:386, 1989.
225. Mugge, A., Daniel, W. G., Frank, G., and Lichtlen, P. R.: Echocardiography in infective endocarditis: Reassessment of prognostic implications of vegetation size determined by the transthoracic and the transesophageal approach. J. Am. Coll. Cardiol. *14*:631, 1989.
226. Zee-Cheng, C-S., Gibbs, H. R., Johnson, K. P., and Smith, J. C.: Giant vegetation due to *Staphylococcus aureus* endocarditis simulating left atrial myxoma. Am. Heart J. *111*:414, 1986.
227. Berger, M., Delfin, L. A., Jelveh, M., and Goldberg, E.: Two-dimensional echocardiographic findings in right-sided infective endocarditis. Circulation *61*:855, 1980.
228. Pruett, T. L., Rotstein, O. D., Anderson, R. W., and Simmons, R. L.: Tricuspid valve candida endocarditis. Am. J. Med. *80*:116, 1986.
229. Wann, L. S., Dillon, J. C., Weyman, A. E., and Feigenbaum, H.: Echocardiography in bacterial endocarditis. N. Engl. J. Med. *295*:135, 1976.
230. Rakowski, H., and Popp, R. L.: Clinical utility of two-dimensional echocardiography in infective endocarditis. Am. J. Cardiol. *46*:379, 180.
231. Gomes, J. A., Calderon, J., Lajam, F., et al.: Echocardiographic detection of fungal vegetations in Candida parasilopsis endocarditis. Am. J. Med. *61*:273, 1976.
232. Pollak, S. J., and Felner, J. M.: Echocardiographic identification of an aortic valve ring abscess. J. Am. Coll. Cardiol. *7*:1167, 1986.
233. Saner, H. E., Asinger, R. W., Homans, D. C., et al.: Two-dimensional echocardiographic identification of complicated aortic root endocarditis: Implications for surgery. J. Am. Coll. Cardiol. *10*:859, 1987.
234. Teskey, R. J., Chan, K-L., and Beanlands, D. S.: Diverticulum of the mitral

valve complicating bacterial endocarditis: Diagnosis by transesophageal echocardiography. Am. Heart J. *118*:1063, 1989.
235. Bloch, W. N., Jr., Felner, J. M., Wickliffe, C., and Symbas, P. N.: Echocardiographic diagnosis of thrombus on a heterograft aortic valve in the mitral position. Chest *70*:399, 1976.
236. Bernal-Ramirez, J. A., and Philips, J. H.: Echocardiographic study of malfunction of the Björk-Shiley prosthetic heart valve in the mitral position. Am. J. Cardiol. *40*:449, 1977.
237. Wann, L. S., Pyhel, H. J., Judson, W. E., et al.: Ball variance in a Harken mitral prosthesis. Echocardiographic and phonocardiographic features. Chest *72*:785, 1977.
238. Pfeifer, J., Goldschlager, N., Sweatman, T., et al.: Malfunction of mitral ball valve prosthesis due to thrombus. Am. J. Cardiol. *29*:95, 1972.
239. Wann, L. S., Pyhel, H. J., Judson, W. E., et al.: Ball variance in a Harken mitral prosthesis. Echocardiographic and phonocardiographic features. Chest *72*:785, 1977.
240. Clements, S. D., and Perkins, J. V.: Malfunction of a Björk-Shiley prosthetic heart valve in the mitral position producing an abnormal echocardiographic pattern. J. Clin. Ultrasound *6*:334, 1978.
241. Mehta, A., Kessler, K. M., Tamer, D., et al.: Two-dimensional echographic observations in major detachment of a prosthetic aortic valve. Am. Heart J. *101*:231, 1981.
242. Schuchman, H., Feigenbaum, H., Dillon, J. C., and Chang, S.: Intracavitary echoes in patients with mitral prosthetic valves. J. Clin. Ultrasound *3*:111, 1975
243. Alam, M., Goldstein, S., and Lakier, J. B.: Echocardiographic changes in the thickness of porcine valves with time. Chest *79*:663, 1981.
244. Bansal, R. C., Morrison, D. L., and Jacobsen, J. G.: Echocardiography of porcine aortic prostheses with flail leaflets due to degeneration and calcification. Am. Heart J. *107*:591, 1984.
245. Burstwo, D. J., Nishimura, R. A., Bailey, K. R., et al.: Continuous wave Doppler echocardiographic measurement of prosthetic valve gradients. Circulation *80*:504, 1989.
246. Ryan, T., Armstrong, W. F., Dillon, J. C., and Feigenbaum, H.: Doppler echocardiographic evaluation of patients with porcine mitral valves. Am. Heart J. *111*:237, 1986.
247. Ferrara, R. P., Labovitz, A. J., Wiens, R. D., et al.: Prosthetic mitral regurgitation detected by Doppler echocardiography. Am. J. Cardiol. *55*:229, 1985.
248. Alam, M., Rosman, H. S., McBroom, D., et al.: Color flow Doppler evaluation of St. Jude medical prosthetic valves. Am. J. Cardiol. *64*:1387, 1989.
249. Chambers, J., Monaghan, M., and Jackson, G.: Colour Doppler mapping in the assessment of prosthetic valve regurgitation. Br. Heart J. *62*:1, 1989.
250. Gross, C. M., and Wann, L. S.: Doppler echocardiographic diagnosis of porcine bioprosthetic cardiac valve malfunction. Am. J. Cardiol. *53*:1203, 1984.
251. Rothbart, R. M., Castriz, J. L., Harding, L. V., et al.: Determination of aortic valve area by two-dimensional and Doppler echocardiography in patients with normal and stenotic bioprosthetic valves. J. Am. Coll. Cardiol. *15*:817, 1990.
252. Weinstein, I. R., Marbarger, J. P., and Perez, J. E.: Ultrasonic assessment of the St. Jude prosthetic valve: M-mode, two-dimensional and Doppler echocardiography. Circulation *68*:897, 1983.
253. Gindea, A. J., Schwinger, M., Freedberg, R. S., et al.: Dehiscence of a Carpentier mitral ring: Diagnosis by transesophageal echocardiography. Am. Heart J. *118*:841, 1989.
254. Nellessen, U., Schnittger, I., Appleton, C. P., et al.: Transesophageal two-dimensional echocardiography and color Doppler flow velocity mapping in the evaluation of cardiac valve prostheses. Circulation *78*:848, 1988.
255. van den Brink, R. B. A., Visser, C. A., Basart, D. C. G., et al.: Comparison of transthoracic and transesophageal color Doppler flow imaging in patients with mechanical prostheses in the mitral valve position. Am. J. Cardiol. *63*:1471, 1989.
256. Taams, M. A., Gussenhoven, E. J., Cahalan, M. K., et al.: Transesophageal Doppler color flow imaging in the detection of native and Björk-Shiley mitral valve regurgitation. J. Am. Coll. Cardiol. *13*:95, 1989.
257. Nair, C. K., Aronow, W. S., Sketch, M. H., et al.: Clinical and echocardiographic characteristics of patients with mitral annular calcification. Am. J. Cardiol. *51*:992, 1983.
258. Nair, C. K., Thomson, W., Ryschon, K., et al.: Long-term follow-up of patients with echocardiographically detected mitral anular calcium and comparison with age- and sex-matched control subjects. Am. J. Cardiol. *63*:465, 1989.
259. Reeder, G. S., Currie, P. J., Hagler, D. J., et al.: Use of Doppler techniques (continuous-wave, pulsed-wave, and color flow imaging) in the noninvasive hemodynamic assessment of congenital heart disease. Mayo Clin. Proc. *61*:725, 1986.
260. Dickinson, D. F., Goldberg, S. J., and Wilson, N.: A comparison of information obtained by ultrasound examination and cardiac catheterization in paediatric patients with congenital heart disease. Int. J. Cardiol. *9*:275, 1985.
261. Lipshultz, S. E., Sanders, S. P., Mayer, J. E., et al.: Are routine preoperative cardiac catheterization and angiography necessary before repair of ostium primum atrial septal defect? J. Am. Coll. Cardiol. *11*:373, 1988.
262. Huhta, J. C., Glasow, P., Murphy, D. J., et al.: Surgery without catheterization for congenital heart defects: Management of 100 patients. J. Am. Coll. Cardiol. *9*:823, 1987.
263. Pasquini, L., Sanders, S. P., Parness, I., et al.: Echocardiographic and anatomic findings in atrioventricular discordance with ventriculoarterial concordance. Am. J. Cardiol. *62*:1256, 1988.
264. Foale, R., Stefanini, L., Rickards, A., and Somerville, J.: Left, and right ventricular morphology in complex congenital heart disease defined by two dimensional echocardiography. Am. J. Cardiol. *49*:93, 1982.
265. Silverman, N. H.: An ultrasonic approach to the diagnosis of cardiac situs, connections, and malpositions. Cardiol. Clin. *1*:473, 1983.
266. Hagler, D. J., Tajik, A. J., Seward, J. B., et al.: Atrioventricular and ventriculoarterial discordance (corrected transposition of the great arteries). Wide-angle two-dimensional echocardiographic assessment of ventricular morphology. Mayo Clin. Proc. *56*:591, 1981.
267. Lesbre, J. P., Scheuble, C., Kalisa, A., et al.: Echocardiography in the diagnosis of severe aortic valve stenosis in adults. Arch. Mal. Coeur *76*:1, 1983.
268. Brandenburg, R. O., Jr., Tajik, A. J., Edwards, W. D., et al.: Accuracy of two-dimensional echocardiographic diagnosis of congenitally bicuspid aortic valve: Echocardiographic-anatomic 115 patients. Am. J. Cardiol. *51*:1469, 1983.
269. Smallhorn, J., Tommasini, G., Deanfield, J., et al.: Congenital mitral stenosis. Anatomical and functional assessment by echocardiography. Br. Heart J. *45*:527, 1981.
270. Trowitzsch, E., Bano-Rodrigo, A., Burger, B. M., et al.: Two-dimensional echocardiographic findings in double orifice mitral valve. J. Am. Coll. Cardiol. *6*:383, 1985.
271. Weyman, A. E., Hurwitz, R. A., Girod, D. A., et al.: Cross-sectional echocardiographic visualization of the stenotic pulmonary valve. Circulation *56*:769, 1977.
272. Johnson, G. L., Kwan, O. L., Handshoe, S., et al.: Accuracy of combined two-dimensional echocardiography and continuous wave Doppler recordings in the estimation of pressure gradient in right ventricular outlet obstruction. J. Am. Coll. Cardiol. *3*:1013, 1984.
273. Hagler, D. J., Tajik, A. J., Seward, J. B., and Ritter, D. G.: Noninvasive assessment of pulmonary valve stenosis, aortic valve stenosis, and coarctation of the aorta in critically ill neonates. Am. J. Cardiol. *57*:369, 1986.
274. Shiina, A., Seward, J. B., Edwards, W. D., et al.: Two-dimensional echocardiographic spectrum of Ebstein's anomaly: Detailed anatomic assessment. J. Am. Coll. Cardiol. *3*:356, 1984.
275. Radford, D. J., Graff, R. F., and Neilson, G. H.: Diagnosis and natural history of Ebstein's anomaly. Br. Heart J. *54*:517, 1985.
276. Milner, S., Meyer, R. A., Venables, A. W., et al.: Mitral and tricuspid valve closure in congenital heart disease. Circulation *53*:513, 1976.
277. Lundstrom, N. R.: Ultrasound cardiographic studies of the mitral valve region in young infants with mitral atresia, mitral stenosis, hypoplasia of the left ventricle and cor triatriatum. Circulation *45*:324, 1972.
278. Meyer, R. A., and Kaplan, S.: Echocardiography in the diagnosis of hypoplasia of the left or right ventricle in the neonate. Circulation *46*:55, 1972.
279. Weyman, A. E., Caldwell, R. L., Hurwitz, R. A., et al.: Cross-sectional echocardiographic characterization of aortic obstruction. I. Supravalvular aortic stenosis and aortic hypoplasia. Circulation *57*:491, 1978.
280. Cabrera, A., Pastor, E., and Lekuona, I.: Congenital aortic atresia with intact ventricular septum and normal left ventricle. Diagnosis by cross-sectional echocardiography. Int. J. Cardiol. *8*:339, 1985.
281. Davis, R. A., Feigenbaum, H., Chang, S., et al.: Echocardiographic manifestations of discrete subaortic stenosis. Am. J. Cardiol. *33*:277, 1974.
282. DiSessa, T. G., Hagan, A. D., Isabel-Jones, J. B., et al.: Two-dimensional echocardiographic evaluation of discrete subaortic stenosis from the apical long axis view. Am. Heart J. *101*:774, 1981.
283. Isaaz, K., Cloez, J. L., Canchin, N., et al.: Assessment of right ventricular outflow tract in children by two-dimensional echocardiography using a new subcostal view. Am. J. Cardiol. *56*:539, 1985.
284. Motro, M., Schneeweiss, A., Shem-Tov, A., et al.: Two-dimensional echocardiography in discrete subaortic stenosis. Am. J. Cardiol. *53*:896, 1984.
285. Valdes-Cruz, L. M., Jones, M., Scagnelli, S., et al.: Prediction of gradients in fibrous subaortic stenosis by continuous wave two-dimensional Doppler echocardiography: Animal studies. J. Am. Coll. Cardiol. *5*:1363, 1985.
286. Weyman, A. E., Dillon, J. C., Feigenbaum, H., and Chang, S.: Echocardiographic differentiation of infundibular from valvular pulmonary stenosis. Am. J. Cardiol. *36*:21, 1975.
287. Caldwell, R. L., Weyman, A. G., Hurwitz, R. A., et al.: Right ventricular outflow tract assessment by cross-sectional echocardiography in tetralogy of Fallot. Circulation *59*:395, 1979.
288. Magherini, A., Azzolina, G., Weichmann, V., and Fantini, F.: Pulsed Doppler echocardiography for diagnosis of ventricular septal defects. Br. Heart J. *43*:143, 1980.
289. Helmcke, F., deSouza, A., Nanda, N. C., et al.: Two-dimensional and color Doppler assessment of ventricular septal defect of congenital origin. Am. J. Cardiol. *63*:1112, 1989.
290. Sutherland, G. S., Smyllie, J. H., Ogilvie, B. C., and Keeton, B. R.: Colour flow imaging in the diagnosis of multiple ventricular septal defects. Br. Heart J. *62*:43, 1989.
291. Sharif, D. S., Huhta, J. C., Maranttz, P., et al.: Two-dimensional echocardiographic determination of ventricular septal defect size: Correlation with autopsy. Am. Heart J. *117*:1333, 1989.
292. Rigby, M. L., Anderson, R. H., Gibson, D., et al.: Two dimensional echocardiographic categorisation of the univentricular heart. Br. Heart J. *46*:603, 1981.
293. Houston, A. B., Lim, M. K., Doig, W. B., et al.: Doppler assessment of the interventricular pressure drop in patients with ventricular septal defects. Br. Heart J. *60*:50, 1988.

294. Shub, C., Dimopoulos, I. N., Seward, J. B., et al.: Sensitivity of two-dimensional echocardiography in the direct visualization of atrial septal defect utilizing the subcostal approach: Experience with 154 patients. J. Am. Coll. Cardiol. *2*:127, 1983.
294a. Nasser, F. N., Tajik, A. J., Stewart, J. B., and Hagler, D. J.: Diagnosis of sinus venosus atrial septal defect by two-dimensional echocardiography. Mayo Clin. Proc. *56*:568, 1981.
295. Pollick, C., Sullivan H., Cujec B., and Wilansky, S.: Doppler color-flow imaging assessment of shunt size in atrial septal defect. Circulation *78*:522, 1988.
296. Weyman, A. E., Wann, L. S., Caldwell, R. L., et al.: Negative contrast echocardiography: A new method for detecting left-to-right shunts. Circulation *59*:498, 1979.
297. VanHare, G. G., and Silverman, N. H.: Contrast two-dimensional echocardiography in congenital heart disease: Techniques, indications and clinical utility. J. Am. Coll. Cardiol. *13*:673, 1989.
298. Chin, A. J., Sanders, S. P., Sherman, F., et al.: Accuracy of subcostal two-dimensional echocardiography in prospective diagnosis of total anomalous pulmonary venous connection. Am. Heart J. *113*:1153, 1987.
299. Lengyel, M., Arvay, A., and Biro, V.: Two-dimensional echocardiographic diagnosis of cor triatriatum. *59*:484, 1987.
300. Barron, J. V., Sahn, D. J., Valdes-Cruz, L. M., et al.: Two-dimensional echocardiographic features of ventricular septal aneurysm paradoxically bulging into the left ventricular outflow tract. Am. Heart J. *104*:156, 1982.
301. Wolf, W. J., Casta, A., and Sapire, D. W.: Atrial septal aneurysms in infants and children. Am. Heart J. *113*:1149, 1987.
302. Belkin, R. N., Waugh, R. A., and Kisslo, J.: Interatrial shunting in atrial septal aneurysm. Am. J. Cardiol. *57*:310, 1986.
303. Beppu, S., Nimura, Y., Nagata, S., et al.: Diagnosis of endocardial cushion defect with cross-sectional and M-mode scanning of echocardiography. Differentiation from secundum atrial septal defect. Br. Heart J. *38*:911, 1976.
304. Beppu, S., Nimura, Y., Sakakibara, H., et al.: Mitral cleft in ostium primum atrial septal defect assessed by cross-sectional echocardiography. Circulation *62*:1099, 1980.
305. Rice, M. J., Seward, J. B., Edwards, W. D., et al.: Straddling atrioventricular valve: Two-dimensional echocardiographic diagnosis, classification and surgical implications. Am. J. Cardiol. *55*:505, 1985.
306. Smallhorn, J. F., Tommasini, G., and Macartney, F. J.: Detection and assessment of straddling and overriding atrioventricular valves by two-dimensional echocardiography. Br. Heart J. *46*:254, 1981.
307. Milne, M. J., Sung, R. Y. T., Fok, T. F., Crozier, I. G.: Doppler echocardiographic assessment of shunting via the ductus arteriosus in newborn infants. Am. J. Cardiol. *64*:102, 1989.
308. Liao, P-K., Su, W-J., and Hung, J-S.: Doppler echocardiographic flow characteristics of isolated patent ductus arteriosus: Better delineation by Doppler color flow mapping. J. Am. Coll. Cardiol. *12*:1285, 1988.
309. Weyman, A. E., Feigenbaum, H., Dillon, J. C., et al.: Localization of left ventricular outflow obstruction by cross-sectional echocardiography. Am. J. Med. *60*:33, 1976.
310. Vogt, J., Rupprath, G., Grimm, T., and Beuren, A. J.: Qualitative and quantitative evaluation of supravalvular aortic stenosis by cross-sectional echocardiography. Pediatr. Cardiol. *3*:13, 1982.
311. Snider, A. R., and Silverman, N. H.: Suprasternal notch echocardiography: A two-dimensional technique for evaluating congenital heart disease. Circulation *63*:165, 1981.
312. Shaddy, R. E., Snider, A. R., Silverman, N. H., and Lutin, W.: Pulsed Doppler findings in patients with coarctation of the aorta. Circulation *73*:82, 1986.
313. Rao, P. S., and Carey, P.: Doppler ultrasound in the prediction of pressure gradients across aortic coarctation. Am. Heart. J. *118*:299, 1989.
314. VanSon, J. A. M., Skotnicki, S. H., VanAsten, W. N., et al.: Quantitative assessment of coarctation in infancy by Doppler spectral analysis. Am. J. Cardiol. *63*:1282, 1989.
315. Simpson, I. A., Sahn, D. J., Valdes-Cruz, L. M., et al.: Color Doppler flow mapping in patients with coarctation of the aorta: New observations and improved evaluation with color flow diameter and proximal acceleration as predictors of severity. Circulation *77*:736, 1988.
316. Hagler, D. J., Tajik, A. J., Seward, J. B., et al.: Double-outlet right ventricle: Wide-angle two dimensional echocardiographic observations. Circulation *63*:419, 1980.
317. Hagler, D. J., Tajik, A. J., Seward, J. B., et al.: Wide-angle two-dimensional echocardiographic profiles of conotruncal abnormalities. Mayo Clin. Proc. 55:73, 1980.
318. Daskalopoulos, D. A., Edwards, W. D., Driscoll, D. J., et al.: Correlation of two-dimensional echocardiographic and autopsy findings in complete transposition of the great arteries. J. Am. Coll. Cardiol. *2*:1151, 1983.
319. Marin-Garcia, J., and Tonkin, I. L. D.: Two-dimensional echocardiographic evaluation of persistent truncus arteriosus. Am. J. Cardiol. *50*:1376, 1982.
320. Marino, B., DeSimone, G., Pasquini, L., et al.: Complete transposition of the great arteries: Visualization of left and right outflow tract obstruction by oblique subcostal two-dimensional echocardiography. Am. J. Cardiol. 55:1140, 1985.
321. Sahn, D. J., Terry, R., O'Rourke, R., et al.: Multiple crystal cross-sectional echocardiography in the diagnosis of cyanotic congenital heart disease. Circulation *50*:230, 1974.
322. Meissner, M. D., Panidis, I. P., Eshaghpour, E., et al.: Corrected transposition of the great arteries: Evaluation by two-dimensional and Doppler echocardiography. Am. Heart J. *111*:599, 1986.

ISCHEMIC HEART DISEASE

323. Jacobs, J. J., Feigenbaum, H., Corya, B. C., and Phillips, J. F.: Detection of left ventricular asynergy by echocardiography. Circulation *48*:263, 1973.
324. Lima, J. A., Becker, L. C., Melin, J. A., et al.: Impaired thickening of nonischemic myocardium during acute regional ischemia in the dog. Circulation *71*:1048, 1985.
325. Buda, A. J., Zotz, R. J., Pace, D. P., and Krause, L. C.: Comparison of two-dimensional echocardiographic wall motion and wall thickening abnormalities in relation to the myocardium at risk. Am. Heart J. *111*:587, 1986.
326. Heger, J. J., Weyman, A. E., Wann, L. S., et al.: Cross-sectional echocardiographic analysis of the extent of left ventricular asynergy in acute myocardial infarction. Circulation *61*:1113, 1980.
327. Rasmussen, S., Corya, B. C., Feigenbaum, H., and Knoebel, S. B.: Detection of myocardial scar tissue by M-mode echocardiography. Circulation *57*:230, 1978.
328. Distante, A., Picano, E., Moscarelli, E., et al.: Echocardiographic versus hemodynamic monitoring during attacks of variant angina pectoris. Am. J. Cardiol. *55*:1319, 1985.
329. Berthe, C., Pierard, L. A., Hiernaux, M., et al.: Predicting the extent and location of coronary artery disease in acute myocardial infarction by echocardiography during dobutamine infusion. Am. J. Cardiol. *58*:1167, 1986.
330. Jaarsma, W., Visser, C. A., Kupper, A. J. F., et al.: Usefulness of two-dimensional exercise echocardiography shortly after myocardial infarction. Am. J. Cardiol. *57*:86, 1986.
331. Iliceto, S., D'Ambrosio, G., Sorino, M., et al.: Comparison of postexercise and transesophageal atrial pacing two-dimensional echocardiography for detection of coronary artery disease. Am. J. Cardiol. *57*:547, 1986.
332. Picano, E., Severi, S., Michelassi, C., et al.: Prognostic importance of dipyridamole-echocardiography test in coronary artery disease. Circulation *80*:450, 1989.
333. Armstrong, W. F., O'Donnell, J., Ryan, T., and Feigenbaum, H.: Effect of prior myocardial infarction and extent and location of coronary disease on accuracy of exercise echocardiography. J. Am. Coll. Cardiol. *10*:531, 1987.
334. Oberman, A., Fan, P-H., Nanda, N. C., et al.: Reproducibility of two-dimensional exercise echocardiography. J. Am. Coll. Cardiol. *14*:923, 1989.
335. Sawada, S. G., Ryan, T., Fineberg, N. S., et al.: Exercise echocardiographic detection of coronary artery disease in women. J. Am. Coll. Cardiol. *14*:1440, 1989.
336. Labovitz, A. J., Lewen, M., Kern, M. J., et al.: The effects of successful PTCA on left ventricular function: Assessment by exercise echocardiography. Am. Heart J. *117*:1003, 1989.
337. Segar, D. S., Sawada, S. G., Brown, S. E., et al.: Dobutamine stress echocardiography: Correlation of dose responsiveness and quantitative angiography. J. Am. Coll. Cardiol. *15*:234A, 1990. (Abstract)
338. Milunski, M. R., Mohr, G. A., Perez, J. E., et al.: Ultrasonic tissue characterization with integrated backscatter. Circulation *80*:491, 1989.
339. Vered, Z., Mohr, G. A., Barzilai, B., et al.: Ultrasound integrated backscatter tissue characterization of remote myocardial infarction in human subjects. J. Am. Coll. Cardiol. *13*:84, 1989.
340. Stoddard, M. F., Pearson, A. C., Kern, M. J., et al.: Left ventricular diastolic function: Comparison of pulsed Doppler echocardiographic and hemodynamic indexes in subjects with and without coronary artery disease. J. Am. Coll. Cardiol. *13*:327, 1989.
341. Fujii, J., Yazaki, Y., Sawada, H., et al.: Noninvasive assessment of left and right ventricular filling in myocardial infarction with a two-dimensional Doppler echocardiographic method. J. Am. Coll. Cardiol. *5*:1155, 1985.
342. Erbel, R., Schweizer, P., Meyer, J., et al.: Sensitivity of cross-sectional echocardiography in detection of impaired global and regional left ventricular function: Prospective study. Int. J. Cardiol. *7*:375, 1985.
343. Ren, J-F., Kotler, M. N., Hakki, A-H., et al.: Quantitation of regional left ventricular function by two-dimensional echocardiography in normals and patients with coronary artery disease. Am. Heart J. *110*:552, 1985.
344. Shiina, A., Tajik, A. J., Smith, H. C., et al.: Prognostic significance of regional wall motion abnormality in patients with prior myocardial infarction: A prospective correlative study of two-dimensional echocardiography and angiography. Mayo Clin. Proc. *61*:254, 1986.
345. Van Reet, R. E., Quinones, M. A., Poliner, L. R., et al.: Comparison of two-dimensional echocardiography with gated radionuclide ventriculography in the evaluation of global and regional left ventricular function in acute myocardial infarction. J. Am. Coll. Cardiol. *3*:243, 1984.
346. Illiceto, S., Ricci, A., Sorino, M., et al.: Evaluation of the ejection fraction using two simplified echocardiographic methods in patients with ischemic heart disease and left ventricular asynergy. G. Ital. Cardiol. *15*:142, 1985.
347. Ryan, T., Petrovic, O., Armstrong, W. F., et al.: Quantitative two-dimensional echocardiographic assessment of patients undergoing left ventricular aneurysmectomy. Am. Heart J. *111*:714, 1986.
348. Visser, C. A., Kan, G., Meltzer, R. S., et al.: Assessment of left ventricular aneurysm resectability by two-dimensional echocardiography. Am. J. Cardiol. *56*:857, 1985.
349. Matsumoto, M., Watanabe, F., Gotto, A., et al.: Left ventricular aneurysm and the prediction of left ventricular enlargement studied by two-dimensional echocardiography: Quantitative assessment of aneurysm size in relation to clinical course. Circulation *72*:280, 1985.

350. Hamilton, K., Ellenbogen, K., Lowe, J. E., and Kisslo, J.: Ultrasound diagnosis of pseudoaneurysm and contiguous ventricular septal defect complicating inferior myocardial infarction. J. Am. Coll. Cardiol. 6:1160, 1985.
351. Bach, M., Berger, M., Hecht, S. R., and Strain, J. E.: Diagnosis of left ventricular pseudoaneurysm using contrast and Doppler echocardiography. Am. Heart J. 118:854, 1989.
352. Sutherland, G. R., Smyllie, J. H., and Croelandt, J. R. T.: Advantages of colour flow imaging in the diagnosis of left ventricular pseudoaneurysm. Br. Heart J. 61:59, 1989.
353. Stephens, J. D., Giles, M. R., and Banim, S. O.: Ruptured postinfarction ventricular septal aneurysm causing chronic congestive cardiac failure. Detection by two-dimensional echocardiography. Br. Heart J. 46:216, 1981.
354. Smith, G., Endresen, K., Sivertssen, E., and Semb, G.: Ventricular septal rupture diagnosed by simultaneous cross-sectional echocardiography and Doppler ultrasound. Eur. Heart J. 6:631, 1985.
355. Panidis, I. P., Mintz, G. S., Goel, I., et al.: Acquired ventricular septal defect after myocardial infarction: Detection by combined two-dimensional and Doppler echocardiography. Am. Heart J. 111:427, 1986.
356. Harrison, M. R., MacPhail, B., Gurley, J. C., et al.: Usefulness of color Doppler flow imaging to distinguish ventricular septal defect from acute mitral regurgitation complicating acute myocardial infarction. Am. J. Cardiol. 64:697, 1989.
357. Fortin, D. F., Sheikh, K. H., and Kisslo, J.: The utility of echocardiography in the diagnostic strategy of postinfarction ventricular septal rupture: A comparison of two-dimensional echocardiography versus Doppler color flow imaging. Am. Heart J. 121:25, 1991.
358. Sharkey, S. W., Shelley, W., Carlyle, P. F., et al.: M-mode and two-dimensional echocardiographic analysis of the septum in experimental right ventricular infarction: Correlation with hemodynamic alterations. Am. Heart J. 110:1210, 1985.
359. Bellamy, G. R., Rasmussen, H. H., Nasser, F. N., et al.: Value of two-dimensional echocardiography, electrocardiography, and clinical signs in detecting right ventricular infarction. Am. Heart J. 112:304, 1986.
360. Jugdutt, B. I., Sussex, B. A., Sivaram, C. A., and Rossall, R. E.: Right ventricular infarction: Two-dimensional echocardiographic evaluation. Am. Heart J. 107:505, 1984.
361. Doyle, T., Troup, P. J., and Wann, L. S.: Mid-diastolic opening of the pulmonary valve after right ventricular infarction. J. Am. Coll. Cardiol. 5:366, 1985.
362. Lopez-Sendon, J., DeSa, E. L., Roldan, I., et al.: Inversion of the normal interatrial septum convexity in acute myocardial infarction: Incidence, clinical relevance and prognostic significance. J. Am. Coll. Cardiol. 15:801, 1990.
363. Asinger, R. W., Mikell, F. L., Elsperger, J., and Hodges, M.: Incidence of left-ventricular thrombosis after acute transmural myocardial infarction. Serial evaluation by two-dimensional echocardiography. N. Engl. J. Med. 305:297, 1981.
364. Sharma, B., Carvalho, A., Wyeth, R., and Franciosa, J. A.: Left ventricular thrombi diagnosed by echocardiography in patients with acute myocardial infarction treated with intracoronary streptokinase followed by intravenous heparin. Am. J. Cardiol. 56:422, 1985.
365. Keren, A., Goldberg, S., Gottlieb, S., et al.: Natural history of left ventricular thrombi: Their appearance and resolution in the posthospitalization period of acute myocardial infarction. J. Am. Coll. Cardiol. 15:790, 1990.
366. Weintraub, W. S., and Ba'albaki, H. A.: Decision analysis concerning the application of echocardiography to the diagnosis and treatment of mural thrombi after anterior wall acute myocardial infarction. Am. J. Cardiol. 64:708, 1989.
367. Jugdutt, B. I., Sivaram, C. A., Wortman, C., et al.: Prospective two-dimensional echocardiographic evaluation of left ventricular thrombus and embolism after acute myocardial infarction. J. Am. Coll. Cardiol. 13:554, 1989.
368. Delemarre, B. J., Visser, C. A., Bot, H., et al.: Prediction of apical thrombus formation in acute myocardial infarction based on left ventricular spatial flow pattern. J. Am. Coll. Cardiol. 15:355, 1990.
369. Barzilai, B., Gessler, C., Perez, J. E., et al.: Significance of Doppler-detected mitral regurgitation in acute myocardial infarction. Am. J. Cardiol. 61:220, 1988.
370. Patel, A. M., Miller, F. A., Jr., Khandheria, B. K., et al.: Role of transesophageal echocardiography in the diagnosis of papillary muscle rupture secondary to myocardial infarction. Am. Heart J. 118:1330, 1989.
371. Pierard, L. A., Albert, A., Henrard, L., et al.: Incidence and significance of pericardial effusion in acute myocardial infarction as determined by two-dimensional echocardiography. J. Am. Coll. Cardiol. 8:517, 1986.
372. Horowitz, R. S., Morganroth, J., Parrotto, C., et al.: Immediate diagnosis of acute myocardial infarction by two dimensional echocardiography. Circulation 65:323, 1982.
373. Oh, J. K., Miller, F. A., Shub, C., et al.: Evaluation of acute chest pain syndromes by two-dimensional echocardiography: Its potential application in the selection of patients for acute reperfusion therapy. Mayo Clin. Proc. 62:59, 1987.
374. Stamm, R. B., Gibson, R. S., Bishop, H. L., et al.: Echocardiographic detection of infarction: Correlation with the extent of angiographic coronary disease. Circulation 67:233, 1983.
375. Kan, G., Visser, C. A., Koolen, J. J., and Dunning, A. J.: Short and long term predictive value of admission wall motion score in acute myocardial infarction. Br. Heart J. 56:422, 1986.
376. Erlebacher, J. A., Weiss, J. L., Weisfeldt, M. L., and Bulkley, B. H.: Early dilation of the infarcted segment in acute transmural myocardial infarction: role of infarct expansion in acute left ventricular enlargement. J. Am. Coll. Cardiol. 4:201, 1984.
377. Ginzton, L. E., Conant, R., Rodrigues, D. M., and Laks, M. M.: Functional significance of hypertrophy of the noninfarcted myocardium after myocardial infarction in humans. Circulation 80:816, 1989.
378. Jugdutt, B. I., and Michorowski, B. L.: Role of infarct expansion in rupture of the ventricular septum after acute myocardial infarction: A two-dimensional echocardiographic study. Clin. Cardiol. 10:641, 1987.
379. Isaacsohn, J. L., Earle, M. G., Kemper, A. J., and Parisi, A. F.: Postmyocardial infarction pain and infarct extension in the coronary care unit: Role of two-dimensional echocardiography. J. Am. Coll. Cardiol. 11:246, 1988.
380. Nishimura, R. A., Tajik, A. J., Shib, C., et al.: Role of two-dimensional echocardiography in the prediction of in-hospital complications after acute myocardial infarction. J. Am. Coll. Cardiol. 4:1080, 1984.
381. Abrams, D. S., Starling, M. R., Crawford, M. H., and O'Rourke, R. A.: Value of noninvasive techniques for predicting early complications in patients with clinical class II acute myocardial infarction. J. Am. Coll. Cardiol. 2:818, 1983.
382. Bhatnagar, S. K., and Al-Yusuf, A. R.: The role of prehospital discharge two-dimensional echocardiography in determining the prognosis of survivors of first myocardial infarction. Am. Heart J. 109:472, 1985.
383. Ryan, T., Armstrong, W. F., O'Donnell, J. A., and Feigenbaum, H.: Risk stratification after acute myocardial infarction by means of exercise two-dimensional echocardiography. Am. Heart J. 114:1305, 1987.
384. Force, T., Kemper, A., Leavitt, M., and Parisi, A. F.: Acute reduction in functional infarct expansion with late coronary reperfusion: Assessment with quantitative two-dimensional echocardiography. J. Am. Coll. Cardiol. 11:192, 1988.
385. Bourdillon, P. D. V., Broderick, T. M., Williams, E. S., et al.: Early recovery of regional left ventricular function after reperfusion in acute myocardial infarction assessed by serial two-dimensional echocardiography. Am. J. Cardiol. 63:641, 1989.
386. Otto, C. M., Stratton, J. R., Maynard, C., et al.: Echocardiographic evaluation of segmental wall motion early and late after thrombolytic therapy in acute myocardial infarction: The Western Washington tissue plasminogen activator emergency room trial. Am. J. Cardiol. 65:132, 1990.
387. Marino, P., Zanolla, L., and Zardini, P.: Effect of streptokinase on left ventricular modeling and function after myocardial infarction: The GISSI (Gruppo Italiano per lo Studio della Streptochinasi nell'Infarto Miocardico) Trial. J. Am. Coll. Cardiol. 14:1149, 1989.
388. Presti, C. F., Gentile, R., Armstrong, W. F., et al.: Improvement in regional wall motion after percutaneous transluminal coronary angioplasty during acute myocardial infarction: Utility of two-dimensional echocardiography. Am. Heart J. 115:1149, 1988.
389. Stamm, R. B., Gibson, R. S., Bishop, H. L., et al.: Echocardiographic detection of infarction: Correlation with the extent of angiographic coronary disease. Circulation 67:233, 1983.
390. Ross, J. J., Jr., Mintz, G. S., and Chandrasekaran, K.: Transthoracic two-dimensional high frequency (7.5 MHz) ultrasonic visualization of the distal left anterior descending coronary artery. J. Am. Coll. Cardiol. 15:373, 1990.
391. Rink, L. D., Feigenbaum, H., Godley, R. W., et al.: Echocardiographic detection of left main coronary artery obstruction. Circulation 65:719, 1982.
392. Presti, C. F., Feigenbaum, H., Armstrong, W. F., et al.: Digital two-dimensional echocardiographic imaging of the proximal left anterior descending coronary artery. Am. J. Cardiol. 60:1254, 1987.
393. Zwicky, P., Daniel, W. G., Mugge, A., and Lichtlen, P. R.: Imaging of coronary arteries by color-coded transesophageal Doppler echocardiography. Am. J. Cardiol. 62:639, 1988.
394. Douglas, P. S., Fiolkoski, J., Berko, B., and Reichek, N.: Echocardiographic visualization of coronary artery anatomy in the adult. J. Am. Coll. Cardiol. 11:565, 1988.
395. Samdarshi, T. E., Chang, L. K., Ballal, R. S., et al.: Transesophageal color Doppler echocardiography in assessing proximal coronary artery stenosis. J. Am. Coll. Cardiol. 15:93A, 1990. (Abstract)
396. Sanders, S. P., Parness, I. A., and Colan, S. D.: Recognition of abnormal connections of coronary arteries with the use of Doppler color flow mapping. J. Am. Coll. Cardiol. 13:922, 1989.
397. Shah, R. M., Nanda, N. C., Hsiung, M. C., et al.: Identification of anomalous origin of the right coronary artery from pulmonary trunk by Doppler color flow mapping. Am. J. Cardiol. 57:366, 1986.
398. Vaksmann, G., Mauran, P., Rey, C., et al.: Visualization of anomalous origin of the left main coronary artery from the pulmonary trunk by pulsed and color Doppler echocardiography. Am. Heart J. 116:181, 1988.
399. Capannari, T. E., Daniels, S. R., Meyer, R. A., et al.: Sensitivity, specificity, and predictive value of two-dimensional echocardiography in detecting coronary artery aneurysms in patients with Kawasaki disease. J. Am. Coll. Cardiol. 7:355, 1986.
400. Valvis, H., Schmidt, K. G., Silverman, N. H., and Turley, K.: Diagnosis of coronary artery fistula by two-dimensional echocardiography, pulsed Doppler ultrasound and color flow imaging. J. Am. Coll. Cardiol. 14:968, 1989.
401. Kimball, T. R., Daniels, S. R., Meyer, R. A., et al.: Color flow mapping in the diagnosis of coronary artery fistula in the neonate: Benefits and limitation. Am. Heart J. 117:968, 1989.
402. Armstrong, W. F., Mueller, T. M., Kinney, E. L., et al.: Assessment of myocardial perfusion abnormalities with contrast-enhanced two-dimensional echocardiography. Circulation 66:166, 1982.

403. Kemper, A. J., Force, T., Kloner, R., et al.: Contrast echocardiographic estimation of regional myocardial blood flow after acute coronary occlusion. Circulation *72*:1115, 1985.
404. Reisner, S. A., Ong, L. S., Lichtenberg, G. S., et al.: Myocardial perfusion imaging by contrast echocardiography with use of intracoronary sonicated albumin in humans. J. Am. Coll. Cardiol. *14*:660, 1989.
405. Feinstein, S. B., Lang, R. M., Dick, C., et al.:Contrast echocardiography during coronary arteriography in humans: Perfusion and anatomic studies. J. Am. Coll. Cardiol. *11*:59, 1988.

CARDIOMYOPATHIES

406. Shah, P. M., Taylor, R. D., and Wong, M.: Abnormal mitral valve coaptation in hypertrophic obstructive cardiomyopathy: Proposed role in systolic anterior motion of mitral valve. Am. J. Cardiol. *48*:258, 1981.
407. Henry, W. L., Clark, C. E., Glancy, D. L., and Epstein, S. E.: Echocardiographic measurement of the left ventricular outflow gradient in idiopathic hypertrophic subaortic stenosis. N. Engl. J. Med. *288*:989, 1973.
408. Pollick, C., Rakowski, H., and Wigle, E. D.: Muscular subaortic stenosis: The quantitative relationship between systolic anterior motion and the pressure gradient. Circulation *69*:43, 1984.
409. Henry, W. L., Clark, C. E., Griffith, J. M., and Epstein, S. E.: Mechanism of left ventricular outflow obstruction in patients with obstructive asymmetric septal hypertrophy (idiopathic hypertrophic subaortic stenosis). Am. J. Cardiol. *35*:337, 1975.
410. Mintz, G. S., Kotler, M. N., Segal, B. L., and Parry, W. R.: Systolic anterior motion of the mitral valve in the absence of asymmetric septal hypertrophy. Circulation *57*:256, 1978.
411. Maron, B. J., Epstein, S. E., Bonow, R. O., et al.: Obstructive hypertrophic cardiomyopathy associated with minimal left ventricular hypertrophy. Am. J. Cardiol. *53*:377, 1984.
412. Maron, B. J., Gottdiener, J. S., and Perry, L. W.: Specificity of systolic anterior motion of anterior mitral leaflet for hypertrophic cardiomyopathy. Br. Heart J. *45*:206, 1981.
413. Jiang, L., Levine, R. A., King, M. E., and Weyman, A. E.: An integrated mechanism for systolic anterior motion of the mitral valve in hypertrophic cardiomyopathy based on echocardiographic observations. Am. Heart J. *113*:633, 1987.
414. Henry, W. L., Clark, C. E., Roberts, W. C., et al.: Difference in distributions of myocardial abnormalities in patients with obstructive and non-obstructive asymmetric septal hypertrophy (ASH): Echocardiographic and gross anatomic findings. Circulation *50*:447, 1974.
415. Henry, W. L., Clark, C. E., and Epstein, S. E.: Asymmetric septal hypertrophy (ASH). Echocardiographic identification of the pathognomonic anatomic abnormality of IHSS. Circulation *47*:225, 1973.
416. TenCate, F. J., Hugenholtz, P. G., and Roelandt, J.: Ultrasound study of dynamic behaviour of left ventricle in genetic asymmetric septal hypertrophy. Br. Heart J. *39*:627, 1977.
417. Clark, C. E., Henry, W. L., and Epstein, S. E.: Familial prevalence and genetic transmission of idiopathic hypertrophic subaortic stenosis. N. Engl. J. Med. *289*:709, 1973.
418. Maron, B. J., Gottdiener, J. S., and Epstein, S. E.: Patterns and significance of distribution of left ventricular hypertrophy in hypertrophic cardiomyopathy. A wide angle, two-dimensional echocardiographic study of 125 patients. Am. J. Cardiol. *48*:418, 1981.
419. Webb, J. G., Sasson, Z., Rakowski, H., et al.: Apical hypertrophic cardiomyopathy: Clinical follow-up and diagnostic correlates. J. Am. Coll. Cardiol. *15*:83, 1990.
420. Maron, B. J., Gottdiener, J. S., Arce, J., et al.: Dynamic subaortic obstruction in hypertrophic cardiomyopathy: Pulsed Doppler echocardiography. J. Am. Coll. Cardiol. *6*:1, 1985.
421. Zoghbi, W. A., Haichin, R. N., and Quinones, M. A.: Mid-cavity obstruction in apical hypertrophy: Doppler evidence of diastolic intraventricular gradient with higher apical pressure. Am. Heart J. *116*:1469, 1988.
422. Sasson, Z., Yock, P. G., Hatle, L. K., et al.: Doppler echocardiographic determination of the pressure gradient in hypertrophic cardiomyopathy. J. Am. Coll. Cardiol. *11*:752, 1988.
423. Spirito, P., and Maron, B. J.: Relation between extent of left ventricular hypertrophy and diastolic filling abnormalities in hypertrophic cardiomyopathy. J. Am. Coll. Cardiol. *15*:808, 1990.
424. Hoit, B. D., Penonen, E., Dalton, N., and Sahn, D. J.: Doppler color flow mapping studies of jet formation and spatial orientation in obstructive hypertrophic cardiomyopathy. Am. Heart J. *117*:1119, 1989.
425. Douglas, P. S., Morrow, R., Ioli, A., and Reichek, N.: Left ventricular shape, afterload and survival in idiopathic dilated cardiomyopathy. J. Am. Coll. Cardiol. *13*:311, 1989.
426. Goldberg, S. J., Valdes-Cruz, L. M., Sahn, D. J., and Allen, H. D.: Two dimensional echocardiographic evaluation of dilated cardiomyopathy in children. Am. J. Cardiol. *52*:1244, 1983.
427. Lavine, S. J., and Arends, D.: Importance of the left ventricular filling pressure on diastolic filling in idiopathic dilated cardiomyopathy. Am. J. Cardiol. *64*:61, 1989.
428. Borer, J. S., Henry, W. L., and Epstein, S. E.: Echocardiographic observations in patients with systemic infiltrative disease involving the heart. Am. J. Cardiol. *39*:184, 1977.
429. Siegel, R. J., Shah, P. K., and Fishbein, M. C.: Idiopathic restrictive cardiomyopathy. Circulation *70*:165, 1984.
430. Gross, D. M., Williams, J. C., Caprioli, C., et al.: Echocardiographic abnormalities in the mucopolysaccharide storage diseases. Am. J. Cardiol. *61*:170, 1988.
431. Cueto-Garcia, L., Reeder, G. S., Kyle, R. A., et al.: Echocardiographic findings in systemic amyloidosis: Spectrum of cardiac involvement and relation to survival. J. Am. Coll. Cardiol. *6*:737, 1985.
432. Hongo, M., and Ikeda, S-I.: Echocardiographic assessment of the evolution of amyloid heart disease: A study with familial amyloid polyneuropathy. Circulation *73*:249, 1986.
433. Chandrasekaran, K., Aylward, P. E., Fleagle, S. R., et al.: Feasibility of identifying amyloid and hypertrophic cardiomyopathy with the use of computerized quantitative texture analysis of clinical echocardiographic data. J. Am. Coll. Cardiol. *13*:832, 1989.
434. Morgan, J. M., Raposo, L., Clague, J. C., et al.: Restrictive cardiomyopathy and constrictive pericarditis: Non-invasive distinction by digitised M mode echocardiography. Br. Heart J. *59*:629, 1988.

PERICARDIAL DISEASE

435. Edler, I.: Diagnostic use of ultrasound in heart disease. Acta Med. Scand. *308*:32, 1955.
436. Feigenbaum, H., Waldhausen, J. A., and Hyde, L. P.: Ultrasound diagnosis of pericardial effusion. J.A.M.A. *191*:107, 1965.
437. Horowitz, M. S., Schultz, C. S., Stinson, E. B., et al.: Sensitivity and specificity of echocardiographic diagnosis of pericardial effusion. Circulation *50*:239, 1974.
438. Nanda, N. C., Reeves, W., and Gramiak, R.: Echocardiographic demonstration of pericardial effusion behind the left atrium. Clin. Res. *24*:232A, 1976.
439. Feigenbaum, H., Zaky, A., and Grabhorn, L.: Cardiac motion in patients with pericardial effusion: A study using ultrasound cardiography. Circulation *34*:611, 1966.
440. Kreuger, S. K., Zucker, R. P., Dzindzio, B. S., and Forker, A. D.: Swinging heart syndrome with predominant anterior pericardial effusion. J. Clin. Ultrasound *4*:113, 1976.
441. Nanda, N. C., Gramiak, R., and Gross, C. M.: Echocardiography of cardiac valves in pericardial effusion. Circulation *54*:500, 1976.
442. Houppe, J. P., Villemot, J. P., Houppe-Nousse, M. P., et al.: Compressive peridardial effusion after heart surgery in the adult. Contribution of bidimensional echocardiographic findings. Presse Med. *14*:1591, 1985.
443. Haaz, W. S., Mintz, G. S., Kotler, M. N., et al.: Two dimensional echocardiographic recognition of the descending thoracic aorta: Value in differentiating pericardial from pleural effusions. Am. J. Cardiol. *46*:739, 1980.
444. Schiller, N. B., and Botvinick, E. H.: Right ventricular compression as a sign of cardiac tamponade. An analysis of echocardiographic ventricular dimensions and their clinical implications. Circulation *56*:774, 1977.
445. Armstrong, W. F., Schilt, B. F., Helper, D. J., et al.: Diastolic collapse of the right ventricle with cardiac tamponade: An echocardiographic study. Circulation *65*:1491, 1982.
446. Singh, S., Wann, L. S., Klopfenstein, H. S., et al.: Usefulness of right ventricular diastolic collapse in diagnosing cardiac tamponade and comparison to pulsus paradoxus. Am. J. Cardiol. *57*:652, 1986.
447. Conrad, S. A., and Byrnes, T. J.: Diastolic collapse of the left and right ventricles in cardiac tamponade. Am. Heart J. *115*:475, 1988.
448. Gillam, L. D., Guyer, D. E., Gibson, T. C., et al.: Hydrodynamic compression of the right atrium: A new echocardiographic sign of cardiac tamponade. Circulation *68*:294, 1983.
449. Brodyn, N. E., Rose, M. R., Prior, F. P., and Haft, J. I.: Left atrial diastolic compression in a patient with a large pericardial effusion and pulmonary hypertension. Am. J. Med. *88*:1, 1990.
450. Burstow, D. J., Oh, J. K., Bailey, K. R., et al.: Cardiac tamponade: Characteristic Doppler observations. Mayo Clin. Proc. *64*:312, 1989.
451. Leeman, D. E., Levine, M. J., and Come, P. C.: Doppler echocardiography in cardiac tamponade: Exaggerated respiratory variation in transvalvular blood flow velocity integrals. J. Am. Coll. Cardiol. *11*:572, 1988.
452. Appleton, C. P., Hatle, L. K., and Popp, R. L.: Cardiac tamponade and pericardial effusion: Respiratory variation in transvalvular flow velocities studied by Doppler echocardiography. J. Am. Coll. Cardiol. *11*:1020, 1988.
453. Lewis, B. S.: Real time two dimensional echocardiography in constrictive pericarditis. Am. J. Cardiol. *49*:1789, 1982.
454. Engel, P. J., Fowler, N. O., Tei, C., et al.: M-mode echocardiography in constrictive pericarditis. J. Am. Coll. Cardiol. *6*:471, 1985.
455. Schnittger, I., Bowden, E. E., Abrams, J., and Popp, R. L.: Echocardiography: Pericardial thickening and constrictive pericarditis. Am. J. Cardiol. *42*:388, 1978.
456. Morgan, J. M., Raposo, L., Clague, J. C., et al.: Restrictive cardiomyopathy and constrictive pericarditis: Non-invasive distinction by digitised M mode echocardiography. Br. Heart J. *61*:29, 1989.
457. Voelkel, A. G., Pietro, D. A., Folland, E. D., et al.: Echocardiographic features of constrictive pericarditis. Circulation *58*:871, 1978.
458. Schiavone, W. A., Calafiore, P. A., Currie, P. J., and Lytle, B. W.: Doppler echocardiographic demonstration of pulmonary venous flow velocity in three patients with constrictive pericarditis before and after pericardiectomy. Am. J. Cardiol. *63*:145, 1989.
459. von Bibra, H., Schober, K., Jenni, R., et al.: Diagnosis of constrictive pericarditis by pulsed Doppler echocardiography of the hepatic vein. Am. J. Cardiol. *63*:483, 1989.
460. Hatle, L. K., Appleton, C. P., and Popp, R. L.: Differentiation of constrictive pericarditis and restrictive cardiomyopathy by Doppler echocardiography. Circulation *79*:357, 1989.
461. Schiavone, W. A., Calafiore, P. A., and Salcedo, E. E.: Transesophageal

Doppler echocardiographic demonstration of pulmonary venous flow velocity in restrictive cardiomyopathy and constrictive pericarditis. Am. J. Cardiol. 63:1286, 1989.
462. Ruys, F., Paulus, W., Stevens, C., and Brutsaert, D.: Expansion of the left atrial appendage is a distinctive cross-sectional echocardiographic feature of congenital defect of the pericardium. Eur. Heart J. 4:738, 1983.
463. Kansal, S., Roitman, D., and Sheffield, L. T.: Two-dimensional echocardiography of congenital absence of pericardium. Am. Heart J., 109:912, 1985.

CARDIAC TUMORS AND THROMBI

464. Charuzi, Y., Bolger, A., Beeder, C., and Lew, A. S.: A new echocardiographic classification of left atrial myxoma. Am. J. Cardiol. 55:614, 1985.
465. Markel, M. L., Armstrong, W. F., Waller, B. F., and Mahomed, Y.: Left atrial myxoma with multicentric recurrence and evidence of metastases. Am. Heart J. 111:409, 1986.
466. Wolfe, S. B., Popp, R. L., and Feigenbaum, H.: Diagnosis of atrial tumors by ultrasound. Circulation 39:615, 1969.
467. Perry, L. S., King, J. F., Zeft, H. J., et al.: Two-dimensional echocardiography in the diagnosis of left atrial myxoma. Br. Heart J. 45:667, 1981.
468. Obeid, A. I., Marvasti, M., Parker, F., and Rosenberg, J.: Comparison of transthoracic and transesophageal echocardiography in diagnosis of left atrial myxoma. Am. J. Cardiol. 63:1006, 1989.
469. Tway, K. P., Shah, A. A., and Rahimtoola, S. H.: Multiple bilateral myxomas demonstrated by two-dimensional echocardiography. Am. J. Med. 71:896, 1981.
470. Bansal, R. C., Heywood, J. T., Applegate, P. M., and Jutzy, K. R.: Detection of left atrial thrombi by two-dimensional echocardiography and surgical correlation in 148 patients with mitral valve disease. Am. J. Cardiol. 64:243, 1989.
471. Hsu, T. L., Chen, C. C., Chen, C. Y., et al.: Two-dimensional echocardiographic features of floating left atrial thrombus. Am. J. Cardiol. 57:701, 1986.
472. Aschenberg, W., Schluter, M., Kremer, P., et al.: Transesophageal two-dimensional echocardiography for the detection of left atrial appendage thrombus. J. Am. Coll. Cardiol. 7:163, 1986.
473. Riggs, T., Paul, M. H., DeLeon, S., and Ilbawi, M.: Two dimensional echocardiography in evaluation of right atrial masses: Five cases in pediatric patients. Am. J. Cardiol. 48:961, 1981.
474. Gustafson, A. G., Edler, I. G., and Dahlback, O. K.: Bilateral atrial myxomas diagnosed by echocardiography. Acta Med. Scand. 201:391, 1977.
475. Dittmann, H., Voelker, W., Karsch, K. R., and Seipel, L.: Bilateral atrial myxomas detected by transesophageal two-dimensional echocardiography. Am. Heart J. 118:172, 1989.
476. Cameron, J., Pohlner, P. G., Stafford, E. G., et al.: Right heart thrombus: Recognition and management. J. Am. Coll. Cardiol. 5:1239, 1985.
477. Sans, P., Provansal, D., Balansard, P., and Gerard, R.: Large right intracardiac thrombus cause of recurrent pulmonary embolism. Arch. Mal. Coeur 78:650, 1985.
478. Cloez, J. L., Neimann, J. L., Chivoret, G., et al.: Echocardiographic rediscovery of an anatomical structure: The Chiari network. Apropos of 16 cases. Arch. Mal. Coeur. 76:1284, 1983.
479. Limacher, M. C., Gutgesell, H. P., Vick, G. W., et al.: Echocardiographic anatomy of the eustachian valve. Am. J. Cardiol. 57:363, 1986.
480. Keren, A., Billingham, M. E., and Popp, R. L.: Echocardiographic recognition and implications of ventricular hypertrophic trabeculations and aberrant bands. Circulation 70:836, 1984.
481. Glover, M. U., Bloor, C., and Vieweg, W. V. R.: Anomalous left ventricular band diagnosed by two-dimensional echocardiography. Am. Heart J. 111:805, 1986.
482. Casta, A., and Wolf, W. J.: Left ventricular bands (false tendons): Echocardiographic and angiocardiographic delineation in children. Am. Heart J. 111:321, 1986.
483. Malouf, J., Charzuddine, W., and Kutayli, F.: A reappraisal of the prevalence and clinical importance of left ventricular false tendons in children and adults. Br. Heart J. 55:587, 1986.
484. Chazal, R. A., and Feigenbaum, H.: Two-dimensional echocardiographic identification of epicardial pacemaker wire perforation. Am. Heart J. 107:165, 1984.
485. Meller, J., Teichholz, L. E., Pichard, A. O., et al.: Left ventricular myxoma. Echocardiographic diagnosis and review of the literature. Am. J. Med. 63:816, 1977.
486. Roelandt, J., Bletter, W. B., Leuftink, E. W., et al.: Ultrasonic demonstration of right ventricular myxoma. J. Clin. Ultrasound 5:191, 1977.
487. Levisman, J. A., MacAlpin, R. N., Abbasi, A. S., et al.: Echocardiographic diagnosis of a mobile, pedunculated tumor in the left ventricular cavity. Am. J. Cardiol. 36:957, 1975.
488. Nanda, N. C., Barold, S. S., Gramiak, R., et al.: Echocardiographic features of right ventricular outflow tumor prolapsing into the pulmonary artery. Am. J. Cardiol. 40:272, 1977.
489. Grantham, N.: Echocardiographic, angiocardiographic, and surgical correlations in right ventricular myxoma simulating valvar pulmonic stenosis. Circulation 55:619, 1977.
490. Bass, J. L., Breningstall, G. N., and Swaiman, K. F.: Echocardiographic incidence of cardiac rhabdomyoma in tuberous sclerosis. Am. J. Cardiol. 55:1379, 1985.
491. Yabek, S. M., Isabel-Jones, J., Gyepes, M. T., and Jarmakani, J. M.: Cardiac fibroma in a neonate present with severe congestive heart failure. J. Pediatr. 91:310, 1977.
492. Ports, T. A., Schiller, N. B., and Strunk, B. L.: Echocardiography of right ventricular tumors. Circulation 56:439, 1977.
493. Topol, E. J., Biern, R. O., and Reitz, B. A.: Cardiac papillary fibroelastoma and stroke. Am. J. Med. 80:129, 1986.
494. Schwinger, M. E., Katz, E., Rotterda, H., et al.: Right atrial papillary fibroelastoma: Diagnosis by transthoracic and transesophageal echocardiography and percutaneous transvenous biopsy. Am. Heart J. 118:1047, 1989.
495. Fowles, R. E., Miller, D. C., Egbert, B. M., et al.: Systemic embolization from mitral valve papillary endocardial fibroma detected by two dimensional echocardiography. Am. Heart J. 102:128, 1981.
496. Hajar, R., Roberts, W. C., and Folger, G. M.: Embryonal botryoid rhabdomyosarcoma of the mitral valve. Am. J. Cardiol. 57:376, 1986.
497. Grosse, P., Herpin, D., Roudaut, R., et al.: Myxoma of the mitral valve diagnosed by echocardiography. Am. Heart J. 111:803, 1986.
498. Weg, I. L., Mehra, S., Azueta, V., and Rosner, F.: Cardiac metastasis from adenocarcinoma of the lung. Am. J. Med. 80:108, 1986.
499. Canedo, M. I., Otken, L., and Stefadouros, M. A.: Echocardiographic features of cardiac compression by a thymoma simulating cardiac tamponade and obstruction of the superior vena cava. Br. Heart J. 39:1038, 1977.
500. Cueto-Garcia, L., Shub, C., Sheps, S. G., and Puga, F. J.: Two-dimensional echocardiographic detection of mediastinal pheochromocytoma. Chest 87:834, 1985.
501. Farooki, Z. Q., Adelman, S., and Green, E. W.: Echocardiographic differentiation of a cystic and solid tumor of the heart. Am. J. Cardiol. 39:107, 1977.
502. Kruger, S. R., Michaud, J., and Cannon, D. S.: Spontaneous resolution of a pericardial cyst. Am. Heart J. 109:1390, 1985.

DISEASES OF THE AORTA

503. Come, P. C., Sacks, B., Vine, H., et al.: Ultrasonic visualization of the posterior thoracic aorta in long axis: Diagnosis of a saccular mycotic aneurysm. Chest 79:470, 1981.
504. Come, P. C., Fortuin, N. J., White, R. I., Jr., and McKusick, V. A.: Echocardiographic assessment of cardiovascular abnormalities in the Marfan syndrome. Am. J. Med. 74:465, 1983.
505. Victor, M. F., Mintz, G. S., Kotler, M. N., et al.: Two-dimensional echocardiographic diagnosis of aortic dissection. Am. J. Cardiol. 48:1155, 1981.
506. Diehl, J. T., Kaiser, L. R., Howard, R. J., and Salerno, T. A.: Two-dimensional echocardiography for diagnostic acute ascending aortic dissection. Can. J. Surg. 28:345, 1985.
507. Granato, J. E., Dee, P., and Gibson, R. S.: Utility of two-dimensional echocardiography in suspected ascending aortic dissection. Am. J. Cardiol. 56:123, 1985.
508. D'Cruz, I. A., Jain, M., Campbell, C., and Goldberg, A. N.: Ultrasound visualization of aortic dissection by right parasternal scanning, including systolic flutter of the intimal flap. Chest 80:239, 1981.
509. Erbel, R., Borner, N., Steller, D., et al.: Detection of aortic dissection by transesophageal echocardiography. Br. Heart J. 58:45, 1987.
510. Mohr-Kahaly, S., Erbel, R. Rennollet, H., et al.: Ambulatory follow-up of aortic dissection by transesophageal two-dimensional and color-coded Doppler echocardiography. Circulation 80:24, 1989.
511. Erbel, R., Borner, N., Steller, D., et al.: Detection of aortic dissection by transesophageal echocardiography. Br. Heart J. 58:45, 1987.
512. Mohri, M., Nagata, Y., Hisano, R., et al.: Detection of different blood flow patterns in the true and false lumen with aortic root dissection by pulsed Doppler echocardiography. Clin. Cardiol. 8:225, 1985.
513. Hashimoto, S., Kumada, T., Osakada, G., et al.: Assessment of transesophageal Doppler echography in dissecting aortic aneurysm. J. Am. Coll. Cardiol. 14:1252, 1989.
514. Dagli, S. V., Nanda, N. C., Roitman, D., et al.: Evaluation of aortic dissection by Doppler color flow mapping. Am. J. Cardiol. 56:497, 1985.
515. Iliceto, S., Nanda, N. C., Rizzon, P., et al.: Color Doppler evaluation of aortic dissection. Circulation 75:748, 1987.
516. Chia, B. L., Yan, P. C., Ee, B. K., et al.: Two-dimensional echocardiography and Doppler color flow abnormalities in aortic root dissection. Am. Heart J. 116:192, 1988.
517. Lewis, B. S.: Echocardiographic diagnosis of unruptured sinus of Valsalva aneurysm. Am. Heart J. 107:1025, 1984.
518. Kiefaber, R. W., Tabakin, B. S., Coffin, L. H., and Gibson, T. C.: Unruptured sinus of Valsalva aneurysm with right ventricular outflow obstruction diagnosed by two-dimensional and Doppler echocardiography. J. Am. Coll. Cardiol. 7:438, 1986.
519. Hands, M. E., Lloyd, B. L., and Hung, J.: Cross-sectional echocardiographic diagnosis of unruptured right sinus of Valsalva aneurysm dissecting into the interventricular septum. Int. J. Cardiol. 9:380, 1985.
520. Chen, W. W. C., and Tai, Y. T.: Dissection of interventricular septum by aneurysm of sinus of Valsalva. Br. Heart J. 50:293, 1983.
521. Chamsi-Pasha, H., Musgrove, C., and Morton, R.: Echocardiographic diagnosis of multiple congenital aneurysms of the sinus of Valsalva. Br. Heart J. 59:724, 1988.
522. Terdjman, N., Bourdarias, J. P., Farcot, J. C., et al.: Aneurysms of sinus of Valsalva: two dimensional echocardiographic diagnosis and recognition of rupture into the right heart cavities. J. Am. Coll. Cardiol. 3:1227, 1984.
523. Chia, B. L., Ee, B. K., Choo, M. H., and Yan, P. C.: Ruptured aneurysm of sinus of Valsalva: Recognition by Doppler color flow mapping. Am. Heart J. 115:686, 1988.

5

Electrocardiography and Vectorcardiography

by CHARLES FISCH, M.D.

The clinical electrocardiogram (ECG) records the changing potentials of the electrical field imparted by the heart. The ECG *does not record directly the electrical activity of the source itself.* Such activity is registered only when an electrode is in immediate contact with the tissue generating the current and at the moment when the electrode senses the edge of the wave of activation or recovery. In all other circumstances only potential differences in an electrical field are registered. It is important to appreciate that the ECG, while recording the changes of an electrical field, often provides only an *approximation of the actual* voltage generated by the heart. Efforts to predict surface potentials from the knowledge of behavior of the cardiac generator—the so-called electrocardiographic *forward problem*—or to predict the electrical behavior of the cardiac generator from the body surface potentials—the so-called electrocardiographic *inverse problem*—have to date been unsuccessful.[1]

Despite this basic limitation, the ECG has evolved into an extremely useful clinical laboratory tool and is the only practical means of recording the electrical behavior of the heart. Its usefulness as a diagnostic method is the result of careful, often purely deductive analysis of innumerable patient records and of studies correlating the ECG with basic electrophysiological properties of the heart; with clinical and laboratory findings; and with anatomical, pathological, and experimental observations.[2] The result has been that electrocardiography can be used, within limits, to identify anatomical, metabolic, ionic, and hemodynamic changes. It is often an independent marker of cardiac disease and occasionally the only indicator of a pathological process.[3-15]

Electrocardiography serves as a gold standard for the diagnosis of arrhythmias, which are discussed in detail in Chapters 22 to 25. Although arrhythmias have been studied by a variety of methods for centuries, none has approached the levels of sensitivity and specificity offered by the ECG. Free of the assumptions required for interpreting the electrocardiographic waveforms, arrhythmias recorded from the surface of the body, with rare exceptions, accurately reflect intracardiac events. However, while most arrhythmias are due to disordered impulse formation or conduction (or both) of the specialized tissue, the ECG reflects the electrical behavior of the myocardium and not of the specialized tissue. This limitation, once appreciated as inherent in the ECG, rarely interferes with proper analysis of even the most complex arrhythmias.[14]

As with any other laboratory procedure, the sensitivity and specificity of the ECG and of its individual components are critical determinants of its clinical usefulness. This is far more complex for the ECG than for other laboratory techniques developed for any single purpose, since its multiple waveforms may be identically or differentially influenced by a wide spectrum of physiological, pathophysiological, or anatomical changes. Thus, it may be difficult—if not impossible—to identify a single cause for any given ECG abnormality.

THE NORMAL ELECTROCARDIOGRAM AND VECTORCARDIOGRAM

THEORETICAL CONSIDERATIONS

Essential to an understanding of the derivation and interpretation of the clinical ECG is information about (1) the physical and electrophysiological events responsible for the electrical potential recorded as the transmembrane action potential, and the spread of excitation; (2) the role of the volume conductor; and (3) the theoretical basis of the lead systems.

Electrical Bases and Theory

At any instant, the cardiac generator can be viewed as a dipole consisting of a positive and a negative charge separated by a small distance. Since the dipole generates a force that has magnitude and direction, it can be expressed as a vector. By convention the arrowhead of the vector indicates the positive pole. When such a dipole is immersed in a volume conductor, an electrical field is generated.[16,17] In a homogeneous volume conductor, the field is symmetrically distributed. The lines of the electrical field are symmetrical in relation to a line that is perpendicular to and transects the dipole at its midpoint.

At any instant, the magnitude of the potential at a given point (P) in the volume conductor can be estimated using the solid-angle concept, or the concept relating the potential to an angle formed by a line drawn from P to the midpoint of the dipole axis and the dipole axis itself (Fig. 5–1).

The electrical surface with its boundary projected to P results in a cone and defines the solid angle subtended by the area in question. The seg-

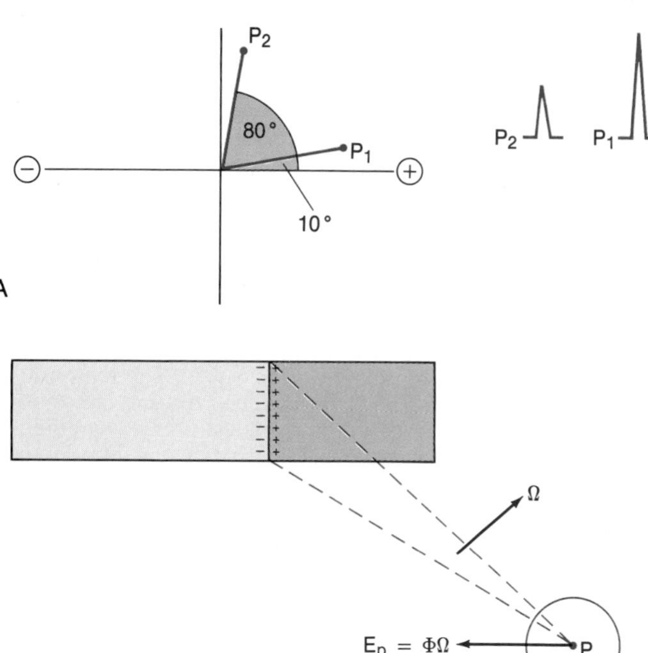

FIGURE 5-1. ***A,*** **The potentials at points P_1 and P_2 are inversely proportional to the square of the distance from the source and proportional to the cosine of angle formed by a line drawn from point P to the midpoint of the dipole axis and the axis itself.** ***B,*** **The potential E is proportional to the solid angle Ω and the strength of the charged surface. (Modified from Wolff, L: Electrocardiography: Fundamentals and Clinical Application. 3rd ed. Philadelphia, W. B. Saunders Company, 1962, p. 15.)**

ment of a sphere inscribed by a radius of unity drawn about point P, with P as the center of the sphere, and its border delineated by the cone, is proportional to the area of electrical activity. With variables such as tissue resistance and geometry being constant, the voltage at P can be expressed as $Ep = \phi \cdot \Omega$, where ϕ is voltage per unit of the solid angle and Ω is the solid angle. An alternative and perhaps clinically more applicable approach to estimating Ep considers the distance (r) of P from the source, the strength of the source (m), and the cosine of the angle formed by a line drawn from P to the midpoint of the dipole axis and the dipole axis (Θ), with the magnitude of the angle estimated in reference to the positive pole of the dipole. This relationship can be expressed as

$$Ep = \frac{m \cos \Theta}{r^2}$$

According to this formula, when the angle is 90°, the line drawn from P is perpendicular to the dipole axis and the Ep is zero. In the ECG the inscription would be isoelectric or equiphasic. On the other hand, with the angle becoming smaller, the P is closer to the positive pole of the dipole and the voltage becomes greater.

Assuming that the volume conductor is homogeneous and infinite and has a uniform boundary and that the generator is located in the center of the volume conductor, both approaches for estimation of Ep at P are correct. Such assumptions, however, are not entirely valid in humans (see below).

The influence of polarity of the dipole, the distance of the electrode from the dipole, and the strength of the electrical field on waveform are important in analysis of the ECG. These relationships can be studied using a hypothetical dipole or tissue immersed in a homogeneous volume conductor. An electrode, located outside the electrical field, when moved into the negative field records a gradually increasing negativity. Halfway between the two poles, a sharp reversal of polarity is registered (intrinsic deflection) and the electrode enters the positive field. As the electrode is moved, positive voltage declines gradually until a potential difference is no longer registered. A similar sequence of events is registered with the electrode stationary and the electrical field moving relative to the electrode. When the positive field moves toward the electrode, a positive potential is recorded; when the electrode finds itself in the negative field, a negative potential is recorded.

Transmembrane ionic fluxes are responsible for voltage differences between activated and resting tissue. These ionic fluxes are reflected as the transmembrane action potential, the cellular counterpart of the clinical ECG. The ECG counterparts of the phases 0, 1, 2, 3, and 4 of the transmembrane action potential are the QRS complex, the ST segment, the T wave, and the isoelectric baseline, respectively (Chap. 22).

DEPOLARIZATION AND REPOLARIZATION. To progress logically toward an understanding of the ECG, we will review the effect of a muscle strip immersed in a homogenous volume conductor on the electrical field generated by the muscle strip and on the electrode immersed in the field. A muscle strip, when uniformly positive on the outside, is in a resting or polarized state. Because it exhibits no difference of potential and fails to impart an electrical field, an electrode immersed in the volume conductor registers an isoelectric line. Stimulation of the muscle strip at any given point increases membrane permeability, and positive ions, largely sodium, enter the cell. The result is depolarized muscle whose external field is relatively negative in apposition to polarized muscle whose external field is relatively positive, with a potential difference across a boundary. In the surrounding medium the current flows from the positively (source) to the negatively (sink) charged muscle. The moving boundary between the polarized (positive) and the depolarized (negative) muscle can be represented by a dipole or vector. This dipole or vector moves along the muscle fiber from the point of excitation, leaving in its wake tissue that is electrically negative (depolarized) in relation to the still polarized (resting) muscle. When the wave of depolarization reaches the end of the muscle strip, the surface becomes uniformly negative and the strip is now completely depolarized. Since a difference of potential no longer exists, an isoelectric baseline is inscribed. The most intense difference of potential exists at the boundary between depolarized and resting tissue, and the recorded voltage changes reflect the events taking place at this boundary.[16,17]

Restitution of membrane polarity, *repolarization,* can be viewed as a "wave" of positivity sweeping across the cells or tissue. As a result, the outside of the cell is again uniformly positive. Since the boundary moves in the direction of the depolarized, negative muscle, an electrode located at the point of origin of repolarization records a positive potential, while an electrode placed at the opposite end records a negative potential. In a preparation of *isolated myocardial tissue* (not the intact heart), the direction of repolarization is the same as that of depolarization but is preceded by the negative pole of the dipole. The repolarization inscribes an area equal to that inscribed by depolarization but of opposite polarity.

EFFECT OF THE BOUNDARY OF DEPOLARIZATION ON THE POLARITY OF THE RECORDED POTENTIAL. Three electrodes placed on a muscle strip will illustrate the effect of a boundary potential, which can be represented as a dipole or vector, on the recording electrode (Fig. 5-2). Electrode A is located at the point of excitation, electrode B at the midpoint of the muscle strip, and electrode C at the opposite end of the muscle strip. Immediately after excitation, electrode A is in the most intensively negative field. As the dipole moves away, the potential becomes less negative, and at the end of depolarization the inscription returns to the baseline. Thus, the electrode at point A inscribes a negative deflection. At the moment of excitation, electrode B is located in the positive field of the dipole and, as the dipole moves toward the recording electrode, the latter registers a gradually increasing positivity and records an upright deflection. When the dipole passes the electrode, there is a sudden reversal of polarity, termed the *intrinsic deflection,* and the electrode finds itself in a strongly negative field. A downward, negative deflection is recorded. With the dipole moving away, the electrode at point B registers a less negative potential, and finally, when the strip is completely depolarized, an isoelectric baseline is recorded. Thus, the electrode at point B registers a positive-negative deflection. Electrode C is located in the positive field throughout the entire process of depolarization. As the dipole approaches the electrode, the field becomes more intensively positive, with the most intense positivity occurring at the mo-

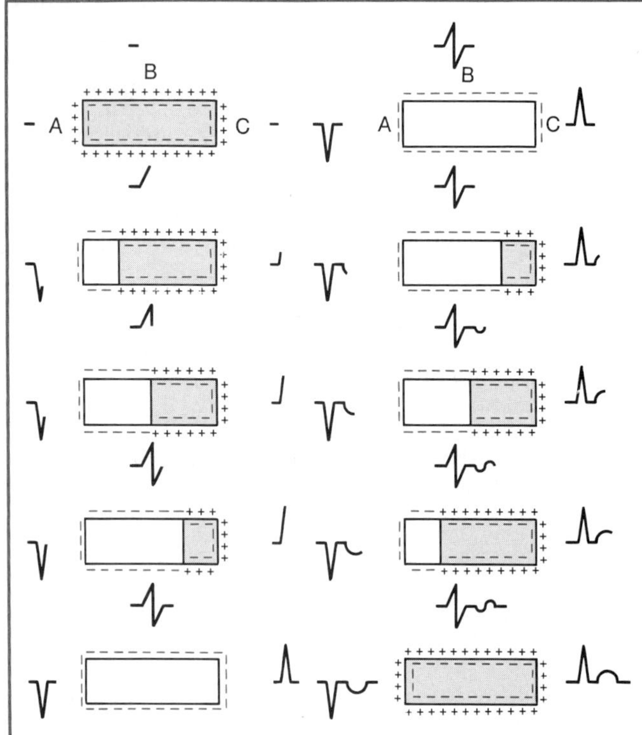

FIGURE 5-2. Potential generated during depolarization (left vertical sequence of panels) and repolarization (right vertical sequence of panels) recorded with an exploring electrode located at the endocardium (A), epicardium (C), and midway between the two (B). (Modified from Barker, J. M.: The Unipolar Electrocardiogram: A Clinical Interpretation. New York, Appleton-Century-Crofts, Inc., 1952.)

ment immediately before completion of depolarization. Thus, the electrode at point C records an upright deflection.

SEQUENCE OF CARDIAC ACTIVATION. The sequence of cardiac activation has been studied in animals, primarily in the dog, and in the isolated perfused human heart.[18] The normal impulse originates in the sinoatrial (SA) node and traverses the atria in a wavelike front with a velocity of approximately 1000 mm/sec. The wave of atrial activation resembles a wavefront seen when a pebble is thrown into water. The sinoatrial node is located in the right atrium and initially activates the right atrium in a right and anterior direction, followed by excitation of the left atrium in a left and posterior direction. It has been suggested that preferential internodal pathways connect the SA node and the atrioventricular (AV) junctional tissue and that these specialized internodal pathways are capable of conducting an impulse in the presence of a quiescent atrium.[19]

The impulse arrives at the AV node, where it is delayed, most probably because of decremental conduction (p. 607). Study of the sequence of ventricular activation in the dog reveals an early (0 to 5 msec) and almost simultaneous activation of the central left side of the septum and the high anterior and apical posterior paraseptal areas of the left ventricle. At 5 to 10 msec after the onset of ventricular activation, the wave of activation envelops left and right ventricular walls and the remainder of the septum; the latter is completely activated at 12 msec. The earliest epicardial breakthrough occurs at the anterior right epicardial surface near the apex, followed by anterior and posterior paraseptal areas of the left ventricle. At 18 msec, activation of the central portion of the two ventricles is complete. Excitation continues along the lateral and basal aspects of the left ventricle, with the basal portion of the septum the last to become depolarized.

Studies of perfused human heart indicate that its path of activation closely follows that of the canine heart (Fig. 5-3).[18] The results obtained from the resuscitated human heart were validated by comparison of the process of activation with that of a perfused and in situ dog heart. The only difference was that the activation proceeded more rapidly in the perfused dog preparation. Intracardiac mapping during surgery indicates that initial epicardial breakthrough occurs in the right ventricle followed by activation of the anterior and inferior left ventricle.

Human studies indicate that atrial repolarization follows approximately the same path as atrial depolarization, with the polarity of repolarization opposite to that of depolarization. Ventricular repolarization proceeds in a direction *opposite* to that of depolarization, and its polarity is therefore the *same* as that of depolarization. The process of repolarization in the intact ventricle begins at the epicardium—a sequence opposite to that observed in isolated muscle strip. The reason for the reversal in vivo of the order of repolarization is not entirely clear. The presence of a transmural pressure gradient may be an important factor, since it prolongs the duration of the excited state of the endocardium and, consequently, recovery begins at the epicardium.

VENTRICULAR GRADIENT. The ventricular gradient (G), introduced by Wilson, describes the relationships between depolarization (QRS) and repolarization (T).[20] In an isolated muscle strip depolarization and repolarization are equal in duration and follow the same path. The net areas of the QRS complex (AQRS) and the T wave (AT) are equal but of opposite polarity, so that their sum is zero and there is no gradient. In the intact heart, on the other hand, repolarization proceeds from the epicardium to endocardium, in a direction *opposite* to that of depolarization; the algebraic sum of their respective areas is no longer zero; and a gradient is said to exist. AQRS, AT, and G can be expressed as a vectorial quantity from any two of the three bipolar limb leads of the ECG. AQRS and AT are expressed in the form of vectors and are plotted using the Einthoven triangle or Bayley triaxial reference system. A parallelogram of the AQRS and the AT is constructed, with the resultant diagonal vector being the manifest AQRST vector or gradient (G). The G vector and the mean QRS vector are located in about the same plane. The G forms an angle of approximately 30° with the mean spatial QRS vector.

THEORETICAL BASES OF SURFACE LEADS. At any instant the surface leads reflect projection of the electrical field of the equivalent or "net" dipole expressed as the mean instantaneous spatial vector. Orientation of a lead axis is defined as one that records a maximal voltage when its axis is parallel to that of the axis or vector of the equivalent dipole. The voltage registered in any lead, having magnitude and direction, can be expressed as a vector (lead vector), with the amplitude of deflection in any lead paralleling the magnitude of the vector. Since more than one dipole may exist at any instant, the net potential and consequently the resultant lead vector reflect the contribution of all such dipoles. Furthermore, because dipole vectors may vary in magnitude and direction, the equivalent or "net" dipole is an approximation of these forces and consequently its expression on a lead axis is also an approximation.

LEADS. *Bipolar limb leads*, introduced by Einthoven, register the direction, magnitude, and duration of voltage changes in the frontal plane. The three bipolar leads—I, II, and III—record the differences in potential between left arm

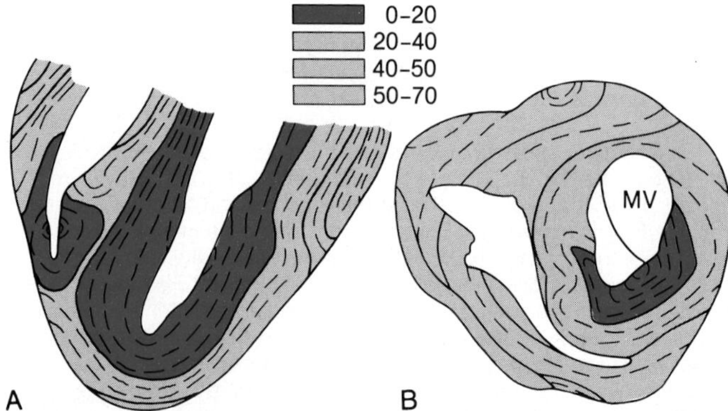

FIGURE 5-3. Sequence of ventricular activation of an isolated human heart. *A* and *B* represent sagittal and coronal sections, respectively. The dotted lines denote 5-msec sequences, while changes in pattern represent 20-msec intervals. (Durrer, D., et al.: Total excitation of the isolated human heart. Circulation *41*:899, 1970, by permission of the American Heart Association, Inc.)

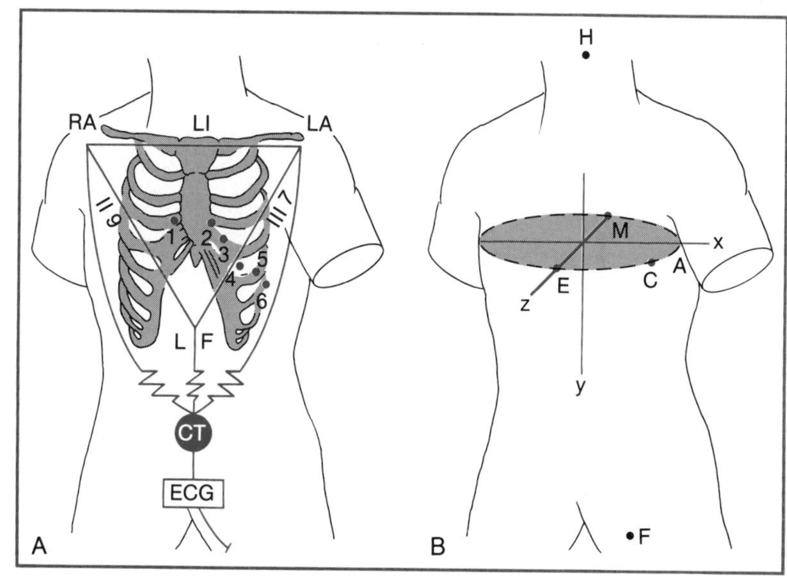

FIGURE 5-4. *A*, ECG lead system. Leads I, II, and III are formed by connecting RA-LA, RA-LF, and LA-LF, respectively. The indifferent electrode of the unipolar system is obtained by connecting RA, LA, and LF through 50,000-ohm resistance into a central terminal (CT). (For details about positioning of the exploring unipolar electrode, see discussion under Leads.) *B*, Frank electrode system. Five horizontal electrodes are placed at the level where the fifth intercostal space intersects the sternal line. Specific locations include fifth intercostal space and sternum (E), the midaxillary line (A,I) and the vertebral column (M). Electrode C is located halfway between points E and A, while electrodes H and F are on the back of the neck and left lower extremity, respectively.

(LA) and right arm (RA), left leg (LF) and RA, and LF and LA, respectively.

Unipolar limb leads are constructed by connecting all three extremities to a "central terminal" (Fig. 5-4*A*). Although in reality the central terminal registers a small voltage, for practical purposes it is considered to have a zero potential and serves as the *indifferent* or *reference electrode*. The potential differences recorded by the positive terminal, the *exploring electrode*, are dominated by local electrical events. When placed on the right arm, left arm, or left foot, the exploring electrode registers the potential from the respective limb. The letter *V* identifies a unipolar lead and the letters *r*, *l*, and *f* the respective extremities. If one disconnects the central terminal from the extremity from which the potential is being recorded, the amplitude registered by the respective unipolar limb lead is augmented, and the leads are designated as aV_r, aV_l, and aV_f.

Locations of the exploring electrode for the *precordial leads* are as follows: V_1—fourth interspace to the right of the sternum; V_2—fourth interspace to the left of the sternum; V_3—midway between leads V_2 and V_4; V_4—fifth interspace at the midclavicular line; V_5—anterior axillary line at the level of lead V_4; and V_6—midaxillary line at the level of lead V_4 (Fig. 5-4*A*).[21]

Of the six precordial leads, it is assumed that in the absence of major thoracic deformity or cardiac malposition, three pairs of precordial leads, i.e., leads V_1 and V_2, V_3 and V_4, and V_5 and V_6, face the right side of the septum, the septum itself, and the left side of the septum, respectively, and are referred to as right ventricular, septal or transitional, and left ventricular leads, respectively. Right precordial leads are of increasing interest because of their importance in the diagnosis of right ventricular infarction. The leads are recorded from the following positions on the right chest: V_3R—between V_1 and V_4R; V_4R—right midclavicular line in the fifth intercostal space; V_5R—right anterior axillary line in the same horizontal plane as V_4R; V_6R—right midaxillary line in the same horizontal plane as V_4R. Normally, an rS configuration is present in 98 per cent of V_3R leads. Secondary R wave (r′) increases in frequency and amplitude in the right lateral leads (for details see ref. 22).

THE NORMAL ELECTROCARDIOGRAM

The P Wave

The cardiac impulse originating in the SA node activates the right and left atria in the general direction from right to left, inferiorly and posteriorly. Initial activation of the right atrium, an anterior chamber, is directed anteriorly and inferi-

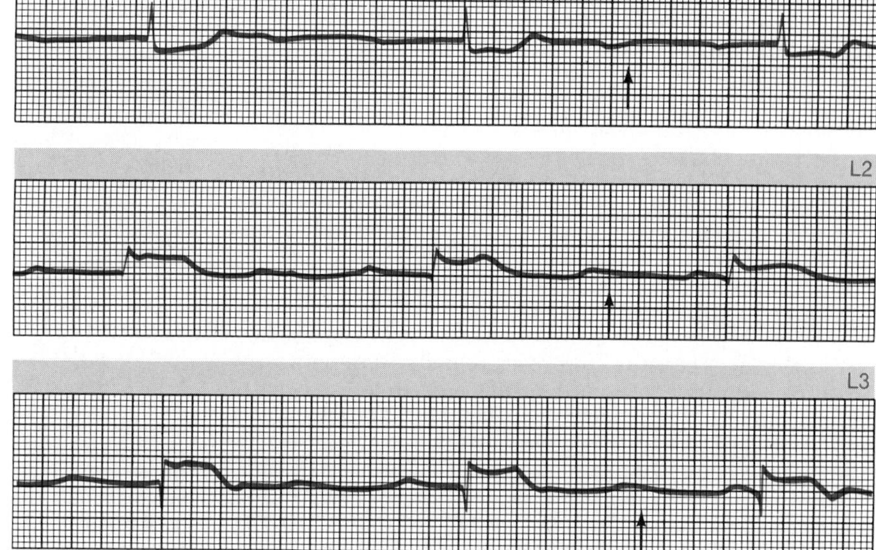

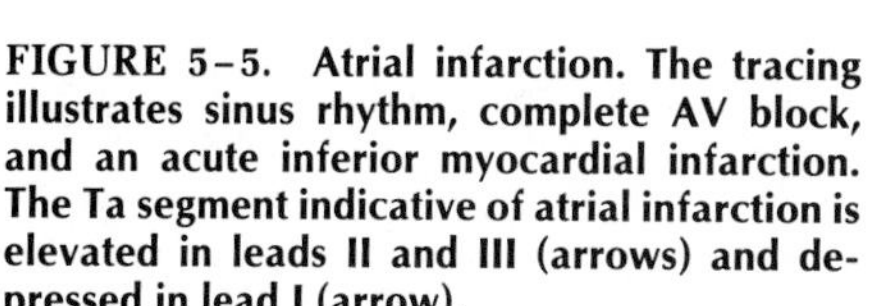
FIGURE 5-5. Atrial infarction. The tracing illustrates sinus rhythm, complete AV block, and an acute inferior myocardial infarction. The Ta segment indicative of atrial infarction is elevated in leads II and III (arrows) and depressed in lead I (arrow).

TABLE 5-1 P WAVE: AMPLITUDE AND DURATION IN NORMAL ADULTS

	LEAD I	LEAD II	LEAD III	LEAD V_1*
P Amplitude (mv)				
Mean	0.049	0.103	0.069	0.040
Range	0.02 to 0.10	0.03 to 0.20	0 to 0.20	0.005 to 0.080
P Duration (sec)				
Mean	0.08	0.09	0.16	0.05
Range	0.05 to 0.12	0.05 to 0.12	0.12 to 0.20	0 to 0.08
P-R Interval (sec)				
Mean	0.16	0.16		
Range	0.12 to 0.20	0.12 to 0.20		

AMPLITUDE OF Q, R, S, AND T WAVES IN SCALAR ELECTROCARDIOGRAM OF 100 NORMAL ADULTS†

	I	II	III	aV_r	aV_l	aV_f	V_1	V_5	V_6
Patients with Q Wave	38%	41%	50%	—	38%	40%	0%	60%	75%
Q Amplitude									
Mean	0.4	0.6	0.09	—	0.04	0.07	0	0.03	0.03
Range	0 to 0.1	0 to 0.16	0 to 0.23		0 to 0.11	0 to 0.17	0	0 to 0.18	0 to 0.18
R Amplitude									
Mean	0.56	0.89	0.45	0.13	0.34	0.6	0.19	1.2	1.0
Range	0.1 to 1.0	0.2 to 1.6	0.1 to 1.2	0 to 0.29	0 to 0.82	0 to 1.38	0.1 to 0.6	0.7 to 2.1	0.5 to 1.8
S Amplitude									
Mean	0.2	0.2	0.24	0.7	0.26	—	0.8	0.25	0.13
Range	0 to 0.5	0 to 0.37	0 to 0.64	0.22 to 1.18	0 to 0.58	—	0.3 to 1.3	0 to 0.5	0 to 0.2
T Amplitude									
Mean	0.19	0.23	0.1	—	0.03	0.17	0.1	0.33	0.1
Range	0.1 to 0.3	0.1 to 0.2	−0.2 to 0.2	—	−0.1 to 0.2	0 to 0.4	−0.2 to 0.2	0.2 to 0.7	0.1 to 0.4

* Twenty-five per cent of the series had a small terminal negative deflection of the P wave in lead V_1.
† Amplitude values are in millivolts (0.1 mV = 1 mm).
From Cooksey, J. D., et al.: Clinical Vectorcardiography and Electrocardiography. 2nd ed. Chicago, Year Book Medical Publishers, 1977.

orly and is followed by activation of the left or posterior atrium, directed to the left, posteriorly, and inferiorly.

The P wave is rounded with a notch corresponding to the separation between right and left atrial activation. Amplitude of the P wave is normally less than 0.20 mV (2.0 mm) with a duration less than 0.12 sec (Table 5-1). The P wave and the *Ta segment*, or atrial repolarization, define atrial electrical systole. The P vector varies from −50° to +60°. In the precordial leads the P wave is positive except in lead V_1, where the P wave may be upright, biphasic, or negative.

The Ta segment is inscribed during the QRS complex and the early part of the ST segment. It is best seen in the presence of AV block (Fig. 5-5). Duration of the Ta segment varies from 0.15 to 0.45 sec, and its amplitude is low, reaching 0.08 mV. The magnitude of the Ta is directionally related to the area of the P wave. The orientation of the Ta segment is opposite to that of the P wave. The P wave and Ta areas are equal and opposite in direction, and the resultant gradient is zero. In the presence of atrial enlargement, the Ta segment may result in displacement of the ST segment.

P-R INTERVAL. The P-R interval includes the time for intraatrial, AV nodal, and His-Purkinje conduction, and its duration varies from 0.12 to 0.20 or 0.22 sec (Table 5-1; Chap. 22).

The QRS Complex

Ventricular activation proceeds chiefly symmetrically about the septum and from the endocardium to the epicardium. Consequently, much of its voltage is canceled; in fact, only 10 to 15 per cent of the potential generated by the heart is ultimately recorded on the surface ECG.

The normal QRS complex can be described by four vectors (Fig. 5-6): (1) initial septal activation from left to right, anteriorly, inferiorly, or superiorly, followed by further septal activation from left to right (0.01 sec); (2) an overlapping wave of excitation involving both ventricles, with the vector directed inferiorly and slightly to the left (0.02 sec); (3) unopposed activation of the apical and central portions of the left ventricle, the thin right ventricular wall having been depolarized, with a resultant vector directed posteriorly, inferiorly, and to the left (0.04 sec); and, finally, (4) activation of the posterior basal portion of the left ventricle and septum, with a vector directed superiorly and posteriorly (0.06 sec).

Septal activation from left to right and anteriorly results, normally, in an initial Q wave in leads I, II, III, aV_l, V_5, and V_6

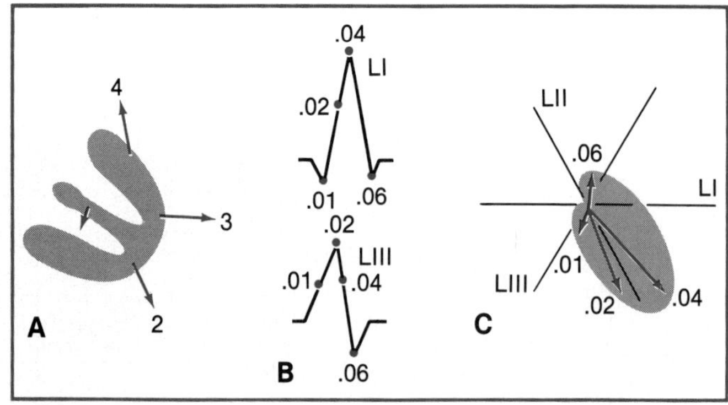

FIGURE 5-6. Correlation between the order of ventricular activation *(A)*, scalar ECG *(B)*, and vectorcardiogram *(C)*. *A*, The sequence of ventricular activation is represented by four instantaneous frontal plane vectors. *B*, The four vectors plotted on leads I and III at the appropriate time during inscription of the QRS. *C*, Using the method of construction of vectors described in Figure 5-7, one can derive each of the four vectors in the frontal plane. A line joining the ends of the vectors results in a frontal plane QRS loop. The same method can be used to derive the orthogonal X, Y, and Z leads from the frontal, transverse, or sagittal planes. (Times given are in seconds.)

and an R wave in the right precordial and septal leads V_1 to V_4. Lead aV_f registers an R or Q wave depending on whether the septal vector is directed superiorly or inferiorly. The ventricular vector directed inferiorly and to the left is reflected by an R wave in leads II and III and in the transitional or septal leads V_3 and V_4. The third vector, that of the unopposed force directed to the left, posteriorly, and somewhat inferiorly, gives rise to an R wave in leads I, II, III, aV_l, aV_f, V_5, V_6, and occasionally V_4, with an S wave in leads aV_r, V_1, V_2, V_3, and at times V_4. The terminal force directed superiorly and posteriorly and perhaps to the right may result in a terminal S wave in leads I, V_5, and V_6. A lead positioned in the right fourth interspace in the midclavicular line (V_{4r}) may record a terminal R wave (R′), which may also occasionally be recorded in lead V_1.[21]

The magnitude of the Q, R, and S waves is given in Table 5–1.

THE QRS AXIS, POSITION, AND ROTATION. The electrical position of the heart can be described by the QRS axis and the rotation of the heart on the anteroposterior and longitudinal (apex-to-base) axes. As the *order* of activation can be viewed as a sequence of instantaneous dipoles or vectors, *total* cardiac activation can be presented as a mean QRS vector. When such a vector is placed within the triangle formed by leads I, II, and III, which define the frontal plane, and assuming that this triangle is equilateral, that the heart is located in its center, and that the thorax is a homogeneous volume conductor with a uniform boundary, projection of the vector on the respective leads permits an estimate of the magnitude of voltage recorded in each lead. Similarly, if the voltage in each of the leads is known, the mean QRS vector can be reconstructed and the axis of the QRS complex can be estimated (Fig. 5–7).

The preceding assumptions—the Einthoven postulates—are applicable in the experimental setting. In the human, however, the heart is a large organ; it is not a point generator

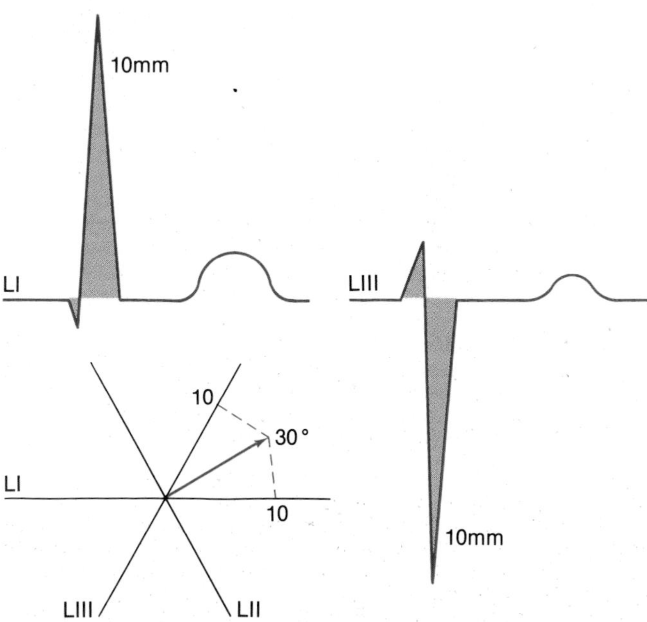

FIGURE 5–7. Electrical axis plotted in leads I and II of the Einthoven triangle. Peak amplitudes of the R wave in lead I and of the S wave in lead III—in this instance each measuring 10 mm—are plotted on their respective leads. Perpendicular lines are dropped and the point at which these cross is identified. A line drawn from the point where leads I, II, and III cross to the point where the two "perpendicular" lines intersect identifies the electrical axis of the QRS (30°). The same approach is used for plotting the P and T axes.

When the P, QRS, or T wave area is plotted on the respective lead, the mean P, QRS, or T vector is identified. The latter represents the mean magnitude, direction, and polarity of the entire period of depolarization. This is a more accurate but impractical method of estimating the electrical axis. Although the direction of the QRS axis and of the mean QRS vector differ, as a rule both lie in the same quadrant.

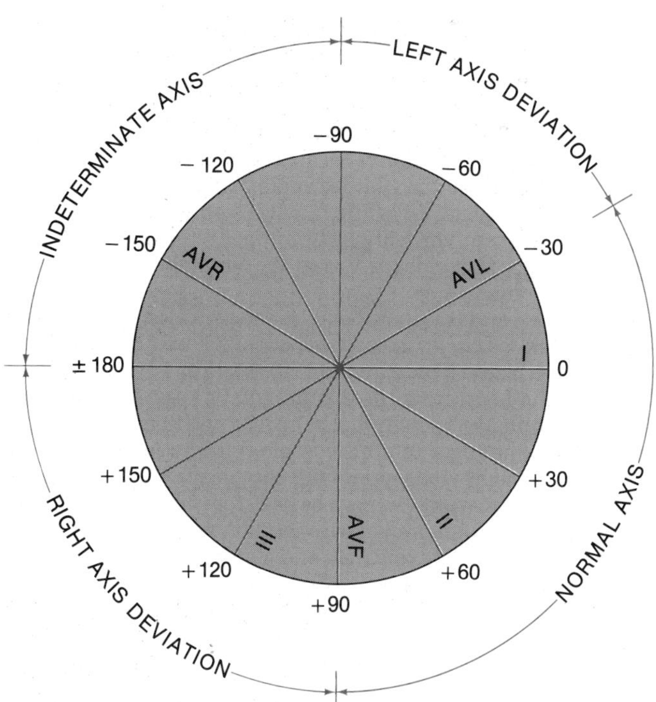

FIGURE 5–8. The frontal plane hexaxial reference system and the respective ranges of axis deviation.

nor is it centrally located, and the thorax is not a homogeneous conductor within a uniform boundary. Burger, using a model of a human torso, with nonhomogeneous conduction to reflect the nature of human organs and an eccentrically located generator, found that the triangle formed by the axes of leads I, II, and III is not equilateral but is scalene, with lead I being shortest and lead III longest.[23] The scalene triangle configuration is more consistent with clinical electrocardiography.

The most accurate method for determining the QRS axis is based on estimation of the QRS area in each of the limb leads and a plot of these as vectors on the respective lead axis of a triaxial reference system. From the positive end of the vector, lines perpendicular to the lead axis are dropped. A vector is drawn from the center of the triaxial reference system to the point where the perpendicular lines cross. This vector defines the direction and magnitude of the mean QRS vector. The same method is used to estimate the T vector. Normally, the angle between the QRS and T vectors does not exceed 30°. For practical purposes, however, the assumption that the magnitude of the force projected on a given lead axis is directionally related to the cosine of the angle subtended by the lead vector and lead axis allows a rapid and reasonably accurate estimate of the QRS axis. Thus, if the mean QRS vector is perpendicular to a given lead axis, the angle between the two is 90°, the cosine of the angle is zero, and the QRS will be isoelectric, very small, or equiphasic. On the other hand, when the mean QRS vector is parallel to a lead axis, the angle between the two is zero, the cosine of the angle is one, and the amplitude of the QRS will be greatest in that lead.

Plotted on a hexaxial reference system, axes of −30° to +90°, −30° to −90°, +90° to 180°, and −90° to 180° are normal, left, right, and indeterminate, respectively (Fig. 5–8).[24]

An *anteroposterior axis* allows the apex to face either the left arm or the left foot or to assume a position between the two. Thus, when a QRS complex in aV_l resembles that in leads V_5 and V_6, the electrical position is said to be horizontal. On the other hand, when the QRS complex in aV_f reflects that in leads V_5 and V_6, the position is said to be vertical. Similarly, in the horizontal position the QRS complex in aV_f and in the vertical position the QRS complex in aV_r resemble the QRS

patterns can be recognized in the transverse plane. Patterns with a superior or inferior orientation require frontal projection for analysis. Of these, the most commonly encountered abnormalities include block of the divisions of the left bundle and inferior myocardial infarction.

Like the P loop, analysis of the T loop also ordinarily requires that the loop be magnified. In the frontal plane, its inscription is variable, with a maximal orientation similar to that of the QRS loop. In the transverse plane, the inscription is counterclockwise and the maximal T vector is located in the left anterior quadrant. In the right sagittal plane, the loop is inscribed clockwise and its maximal vector is located in the anterior and inferior quadrants.

The loops illustrated in this chapter are interrupted every 2.5 msec, each dot representing a 2.5-msec interval. The dot or line is comma shaped, with the thin end indicating the direction of the loop. The spacing of the dots reflects the speed of conduction, i.e., the closer the dots, the slower the conduction.

Normal values for the VCG are given in Tables 5–2 to 5–4.

BODY SURFACE POTENTIAL MAPPING

Body surface potential mapping may contribute information not available from the 12-lead ECG or the VCG, i.e., it provides regional electrophysiological information that cannot be extracted using these methods.[34] Analysis of surface potentials has been applied to the diagnosis of old inferior myocardial infarction, localization of the bypass pathway in the Wolff-Parkinson-White syndrome,[35] recognition of ventricular hypertrophy, estimation of the size of a myocardial infarction, and the effects of different interventions designed to reduce infarct size.[36] The limiting factor at present is the complexity of the recording and analysis, which requires 100 or more electrodes, sophisticated instrumentation, and dedicated personnel. Initial efforts toward reducing the number of electrodes without loss of pertinent information are promising. Once the technical obstacles are overcome, large numbers of patients can be studied and the ultimate utility of this procedure can be evaluated.

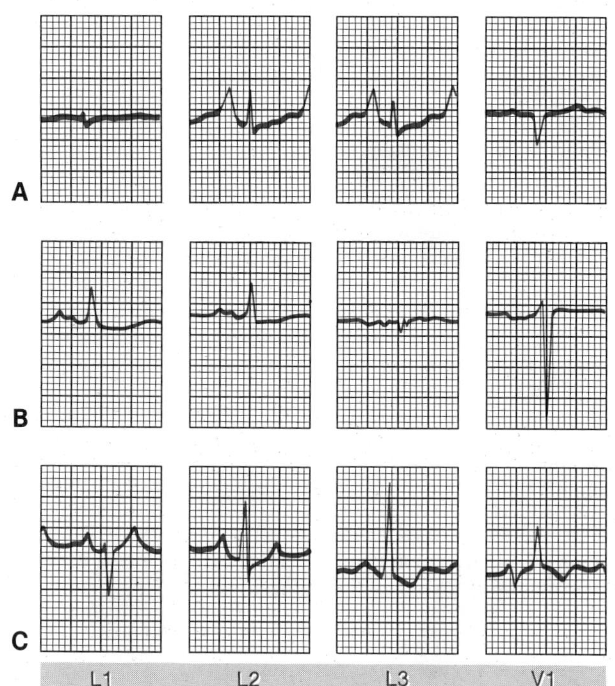

FIGURE 5–10. Atrial hypertrophy. *A*, Recording from a patient with chronic obstructive lung disease showing right atrial enlargement manifested by right-axis deviation of the P wave and a tall, peaked P wave in leads II and III. *B*, Recording from a patient with mitral stenosis showing left atrial enlargement characterized by prolonged duration and notching of the P wave, left-axis deviation of the P wave, and a negative orientation in lead V_1. A common feature not clearly visible in this tracing is loss of the P-R segment. *C*, Recording from a patient with mitral stenosis showing biatrial enlargement manifested by a tall P wave in lead II, a notched P wave in lead III, and a large biphasic P wave in lead V_1.

THE ABNORMAL ELECTROCARDIOGRAM AND VECTORCARDIOGRAM

ABNORMAL P WAVE AND THE Ta SEGMENT

Although an atrial abnormality often implies atrial enlargement or hypertrophy, P-wave changes may reflect altered intraatrial pressure, volume, or conduction. Furthermore, shift of the site of origin of the P wave with an intraatrial conduction disturbance may simulate a pathological state. *Right atrial enlargement* or preponderance is manifested by an atrial vector that is increased in magnitude and shifted to the right. The P wave is normal in duration, low or isoelectric in lead I, and tall—but more importantly, peaked or pointed—in leads II, III, and aV_f (Fig. 5–10*A*). P waves in leads V_{4r}, V_1, and V_2 may be upright and increased in amplitude. A P-wave axis of +90° or greater, with an isoelectric P wave in lead I, is rarely, if ever, a normal finding (Fig. 5–10*A*). In the adult the most common cause of right atrial abnormality is chronic obstructive lung disease (p. 144). The predictive value of P-wave amplitude for detecting right atrial enlargement diagnosed with two-dimensional echocardiography is low. P pulmonale pattern in the absence of right atrial enlargement, termed "pseudo–P pulmonale," has been found in association with a variety of disorders of the left heart, including coronary artery disease with angina pectoris, and less often in the absence of heart disease. It has been suggested that in the presence of left heart disease, "pseudo–P pulmonale" reflects an increase of the left atrial component of the P waves.[37] This suggestion is supported by a recent observation that damage to the left atrium increases the right atrial vector and damage to the right atrium simulates left atrial enlargement.[38]

Left atrial enlargement is manifested by prolongation of the P wave, shortening or absence of the P-R segment, and a shift of the P vector to the left and posteriorly (Fig. 5–10*B*). The duration of the P wave is 0.12 sec or longer, the prolongation is at the expense of the P-R segment, the P wave is notched, and its axis is shifted to the left. Because the vector is increased in magnitude and oriented posteriorly, lead V_1 registers a prominent negative P wave. A negative P wave in lead V_1, 0.04 sec in duration and 0.1 mV in depth, is consistent with left atrial preponderance, the so-called P mitrale. In a study relating the terminal force of P in V_1 to echocardiographically determined left atrial enlargement, the product of the duration of the terminal portion of the P wave in lead V_1 in seconds and the negative deflection in millimeters of 0.03 to 0.08 mm sec was associated with 80 per cent correct diagnosis of left atrial enlargements.[39] In another study of 57 patients with echocardiographically confirmed left atrial enlargement, the sensitivity of the various ECG criteria for left atrial enlargements varied from as low as 15 per cent for notched P wave with interpeak duration more than 0.04 sec, to as high as 83 for negative P wave of more than 0.04 sec in lead V_1. The specificity varied from 64 per cent for a foreshortened P-R segment to nearly 100 per cent for notched P wave with interpeak more than 0.04 sec.[40] Although P mitrale is common in mitral valve disease, the most frequent cause is left ventricular disease, with the increased left ventricular end-diastolic pressure reflected in the atrium.

In *biatrial* enlargement, both anterior and posterior forces are increased. The abnormality includes a prominent initial part of the P wave coupled with the left axis of the terminal portion of the P wave and a biphasic P wave in leads V_1 and occasionally in V_2 (Fig. 5–10*C*).

In the presence of atrial fibrillation, atrial disease can occasionally be suspected from an analysis of the QRS complex. With severe tricuspid regurgitation, right atrial enlargement displaces the tricuspid valve down and to the left. As a result, lead V_1 (and sometimes V_2), normally subtended by the right ventricle, now reflects the intracavitary (qR) right atrial potential as indicated by QR, qR, or qrS complexes in leads V_1 or V_1 and V_2 followed by a normal progression of R-wave amplitude from leads V_2 or V_3 to V_6. Atrial enlargement can also be suspected when coarse, relatively large fibrillatory waves are present, especially in lead V_1. This is in contrast to atrial fibrillation complicating arteriosclerotic and hypertensive heart disease, in which the fibrillatory waves are fine and frequently unidentifiable.

In the VCG, the P loop parallels the changing direction of the maximal P vector. There is a significant increase of the spatial vector and of the loop. In the transverse plane, *right atrial enlargement* is recognized when a major portion of the loop is displaced anteriorly. The inscription is counterclockwise. In the right sagittal plane, the loop is inscribed counterclockwise and is displaced anteriorly and inferiorly; the posteriorly located component remains unaltered. In the frontal plane, the loop is narrow and has a vertical orientation.

In the transverse plane, *left atrial enlargement* is inscribed in a counterclockwise direction or in the form of a figure-of-eight. Both the spatial vector and magnitude of the loop are increased. The increase is not as marked as in right atrial enlargement. With the exception of an initial component located anteriorly, the loop is shifted posteriorly and to the left. In the right sagittal plane, the loop is located more superiorly than normal and the major portion of the loop is located posteriorly; the inscription is clockwise. In the frontal plane, the loop is shifted to the left of normal; this is especially true for the left atrial component of the P wave.

In *biatrial enlargement,* the horizontal plane loop inscribes both the increased early anterior and the late posterior components of the loop. The size of the loop increases with large anterior and posterior components.

Intraatrial conduction abnormalities can result in enlargement of the loop in the absence of dilatation or hypertrophy. The loop displays localized conduction and anatomical abnormalities, the latter in the form of "notches" and "bites."[41]

Alteration of atrial repolarization (Ta), recognized by deviation from the T-P segment, can be either secondary or primary. Secondary changes appear in response to and are obligatory to atrial depolarization (Fig. 5–10*A*), while primary Ta changes are independent of atrial depolarization and indicate nonuniformity of atrial repolarization (Fig. 5–5). The usual pathological causes of secondary Ta-segment depression, which may exceed 1 mm (0.1 mV), include atrial dilation, hypertrophy, and intraatrial block. In chronic obstructive lung disease, for example, depression of the Ta segment may be exaggerated and mistaken for ST-segment displacement.

The usual causes of *primary* Ta-segment changes are pericarditis, atrial infarction, and atrial injury due to penetrating wounds.[42] *Pericarditis* exaggerates the normally negative Ta segment, and Ta-segment depression is recorded in all leads except aVR, in which it is elevated. Occasionally, a Ta-segment abnormality may be the only convincing evidence of acute pericarditis.

The incidence of *atrial infarction* in myocardial infarction (p. 1201) is difficult to estimate and the reported numbers vary widely.[42] Isolated atrial infarction in the absence of ventricular infarction is a most unlikely event. The manifestations of infarction may include elevation of the Ta segment in leads I, II, III, V_5, or V_6 or a depression that may exceed 0.15 mV in precordial leads and 0.1 mV in leads I, II, and III. Displacement of Ta segment in an opposite direction, a reciprocal change, may be recorded in "distal" leads, i.e., those facing noninfarcted areas of the atrium (Fig. 5–5). Attempts to localize the site of atrial infarction by ECG have been unsuccessful. Supraventricular arrhythmias frequently accompany atrial infarction.

Penetrating injury of the atria due to gunshot wounds (p. 1521) or perforation in the course of cardiac catheterization may be associated with diagnostic Ta-segment depression. Ta-segment displacement is also frequently observed following open heart surgery, and whether or not the displacement reflects mechanical injury, associated pericarditis, hemopericardium, or a combination of these factors is still unclear.

VENTRICULAR HYPERTROPHY

Left Ventricular Hypertrophy (LVH)

ECG manifestations of LVH include an increase in voltage; shift of the mean QRS axis posteriorly, superiorly, and to the left; prolongation of depolarization (delayed intrinsicoid deflection); and gradual shift of the ST segment and T wave in a direction opposite to that of the QRS complex. The exact mechanism of the voltage increase is not clear.[43] In addition to the muscle mass, other factors may play a role, such as intracavitary blood volume,[44] proximity to the chest wall, conducting properties of intrathoracic organs, location of the heart within the thorax, intraventricular and transmural pressures, and perhaps unopposed inscription of a portion of the QRS complex due to delayed activation.

The left superior and posterior orientation of the mean QRS vector in LVH is most likely related to hypertrophy of the basal portion of the left ventricle with delayed, and at times unopposed, activation. Variables that may be responsible for delayed depolarization include increased muscle mass, increased Purkinje activation, and localized intraventricular conduction delays. Marked superior orientation is noted in association with left anterior divisional block.

Prolongation of the excited state through the myocardium and prolongation of activation result in a change in the order of repolarization, which proceeds from endocardium to epicardium, resulting in a reversal of T-wave polarity. Of the mechanisms responsible for this reversal of repolarization, increased muscle mass without a concomitant increase in the capillary bed—so-called relative coronary insufficiency—may be an important factor. It is also possible that as the muscle mass outgrows the Purkinje fiber mass, more of the activation proceeds through the myocardium, and this can contribute to a change in the T-wave vector. ST-segment depression may be due to the onset of repolarization before the completion of depolarization.

The mean QRS vector, increased in magnitude and oriented toward the left, posteriorly and superiorly, results in a positive deflection in leads I, II, aV_1, V_5, and V_6 and a positive or negative deflection in leads III and aV_f. The precordial transitional zone is shifted to the left. Leads V_1 and V_2 record an rS pattern, but in some instances the initial R wave may be absent for reasons that may remain obscure. Lack of the initial R wave may be erroneously interpreted as an anteroseptal myocardial infarction.

QRS voltage criteria for LVH include $R_I + S_{III} \geq 2.5$ mV, R in $aV_1 > 1.2$ mV, R in $aV_f > 2.0$ mV, S in $V_1 \geq 2.4$ mV, R in V_5 or $V_6 > 2.6$ mV, R in V_5 or V_6 + S in $V_1 > 3.5$ mV.[45] The following point system for diagnosing LVH has been suggested.[46] Amplitude of R or S wave in limb leads ≥ 2.0 mV *or* S in V_1 or $V_2 \geq 3.0$ mV *or* R wave in V_5 or $V_6 \geq 3.0$ mV = 3 points. ST-segment changes with or without digitalis = 1 or 2 points, respectively. Left atrial enlargement = 3 points. Left-axis deviation of $-30°$ or more = 2 points. QRS duration ≥ 0.09 sec and intrinsicoid deflection in V_5 and $V_6 \geq 0.05$ sec = 1 point each. Left ventricular hypertrophy is considered to be likely if the points total 4 and to be present if the total is 5 or more. The diagnosis of LVH is strengthened by a delayed intrinsicoid deflection in lead V_5 or V_6, measuring more than 0.05 sec in the adult. The *intrinsicoid deflection,* based on the concept of intrinsic deflection (p. 117) and applied to the indirect surface leads, is theoretically related to muscle mass. In the clinical ECG the time from the onset of the QRS to the peak of the R wave is an estimate of the intrinsicoid deflection. In the right (namely, V_1, V_2) and left (namely, V_5, V_6) precordial leads, the time from onset of the QRS to appearance of the intrinsicoid deflection is 0.035 and 0.055 sec or less, respectively. For practical purposes in the study of conduction delays, the term "R peak time" is preferred.[24]

The direction of the ST segment and T wave is opposite to that of the QRS complex in LVH. Characteristically, the T wave is negative and asymmetrical, its ascending limb being steeper with an occasional terminal positive inscription. The J point and the ST segment are depressed in leads I, aV_1, V_5, and V_6. The T-wave inversion is greater in lead V_6 than in V_4. In the presence of a vertical position, these changes are recorded in leads II, III, and aV_f. It has been suggested that depression of the J point, asymmetry of the T wave with a more rapid return to the baseline, terminal positivity of the T wave ("overshoot"), T-wave inversion in lead V_6 greater than 3 mm, and T-wave change greater in lead V_6 than V_4 support the diagnosis of LVH and help to distinguish LVH from coronary artery disease in the absence of voltage criteria for LVH.[47] Left atrial preponderance is common with LVH.

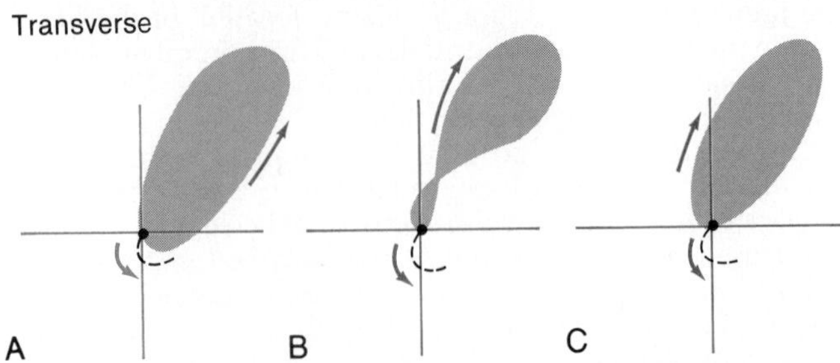

FIGURE 5-11. VCG loops in the transverse plane in left ventricular hypertrophy. The loops illustrate the occasional loss of the initial rightward force *(A)* and rightward and anterior forces *(B, C)* as a result of LVH. Such changes are reflected in the precordial ECG by diminution or loss of the initial R wave in right precordial leads, which could mistakenly suggest myocardial infarction. The dashed lines represent the initial normal forces.

The limitations of the sensitivity of the ECG criteria for LVH are recognized. This is true for both the voltage criteria and the point system. Anatomical and echocardiographic studies suggest a sensitivity of about 25 per cent for Sokolow-Lyons voltage criteria and approximately 50 per cent for Romhilt-Estes point score.[46] The specificity is approximately 95 per cent for both.[48] In a study of 421 hearts, the ECG signs of LVH were correlated with postmortem findings, and the following ECG criteria showed high reliability with a sensitivity, specificity, and predictive value for LVH: SV1 + RV5 > 4.0 mV with strain type ST-T changes, 35.4, 93.3, and 67.3 per cent, respectively; SV1 + RV5 > 4.0 mV with strain type ST-T change, 29.3, 94.9, and 69.0 per cent, respectively; and a right anteriorly directed T vector, 39.4, 89.4, and 59.1 per cent, respectively.[49] Sensitivity of the criteria for LVH varies depending on the etiology of the underlying heart disease, with the sensitivity lowest in the presence of coronary artery disease.[50,51]

In a population with a true prevalence of LVH of less than 10 per cent, there are more false-positive than true-positive diagnoses.[48] Similarly, autopsy data indicate that voltage changes consistent with LVH can be present in the absence of LVH.

The concept of *diastolic overload* may be useful clinically.[52] It may point to such lesions as patent ductus arteriosus, ventricular septal defect, or aortic or mitral valve regurgitation, in which there is volume overload. The ECG pattern is one of LVH but with a prominent Q wave in the leads facing the left side of the septum, namely, I, aV_1, V_5, and V_6, and a reciprocal, prominent R wave in the leads facing the right side of the septum, namely, V_1 and V_2. As a rule, the Q wave is narrow, measuring 0.025 sec or less, and its depth is 0.2 mV or greater. Systolic or "pressure" overload is characterized by high-amplitude R waves and ST-segment and T-wave changes in the left ventricular leads and may be present in disorders with an increased resistance to left ventricular outflow. However, the accuracy of the pattern of LVH is not high in predicting the hemodynamic abnormality.

VECTORCARDIOGRAM. The VCG changes in LVH are due to an increase in and rotation of the forces farther to the left and posteriorly. These events are best reflected in the transverse plane. The VCG loop is increased in magnitude, elongated, inscribed counterclockwise as a rule, and shifted posteriorly. The occasional posterior orientation of the initial part of the loop simulates anteroseptal myocardial infarction (Fig. 5-11). The termination of the loop is anterior, to the right, and superior to the origin of the loop. The loop is therefore open, and this displacement is reflected in the ECG by the ST-segment shift. *Secondary T-wave* changes, the result of alteration of timing and sequence, or both, of depolarization (p. 117), shift the T loop in a direction opposite to that of the QRS loop, namely, anteriorly, to the right, and superiorly.

Right Ventricular Hypertrophy (RVH)

In contrast to LVH, RVH is not simply an exaggeration of the norm. For RVH to become manifest, the right ventricular mass must be sufficiently large to overcome the left ventricular forces. For this reason, the specificity of the ECG pattern of RVH is much greater but the sensitivity is relatively low, varying from 25 to 40 per cent depending on the criteria used.[43] While the ECG changes of RVH result largely from the chamber's anatomical dominance, the cause of the heart disease and associated hemodynamic alterations often contribute to the abnormal ECG pattern. At times, the origin of the cardiac disorder and the severity of right ventricular pressure can be estimated from an analysis of the ECG.

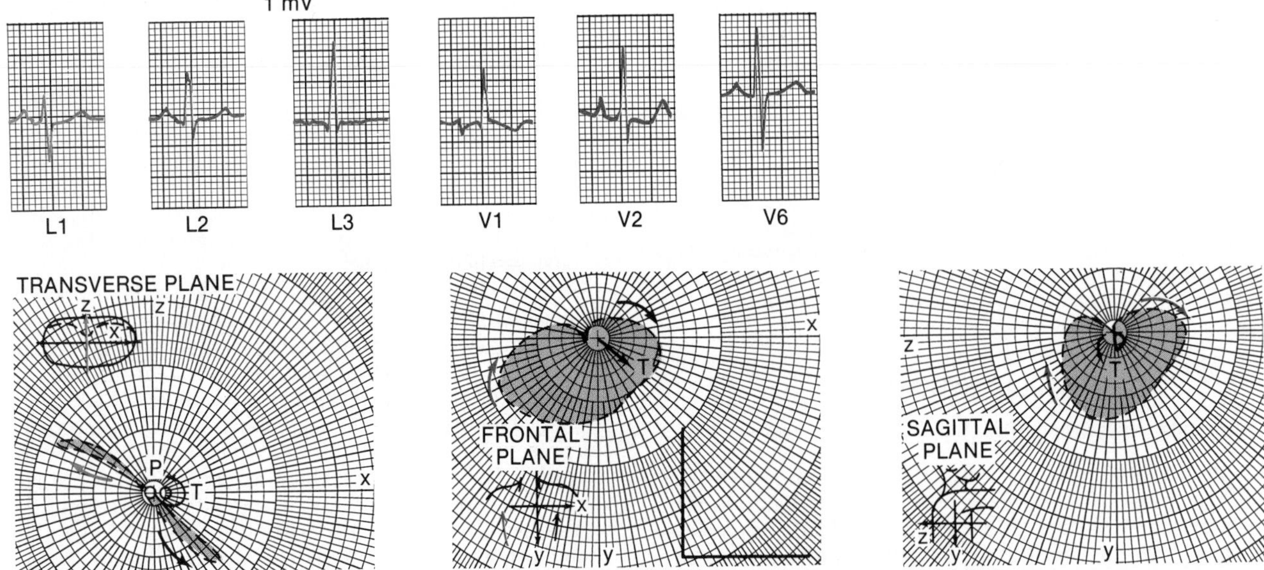

FIGURE 5-12. Right ventricular hypertrophy (RVH), Type A variant. In the transverse plane of the VCG there is anterior and rightward displacement of the mid and late portions of the QRS loop with a figure-of-eight inscription. In the frontal plane, the QRS loop is inscribed clockwise and displaced to the right. In the sagittal plane the loop is inscribed clockwise and displaced anteriorly. The T-wave loop is inscribed counterclockwise. The ECG illustrates the classic pattern of moderately severe to severe RVH (see text).

In RVH the axis shifts to the right, the degree of axis deviation varying with the clinical disorder, and this is accompanied by vertical position and clockwise rotation. Based on the QRS pattern in lead V_1, RVH can generally be separated into three groups, namely, a dominant R wave (qR, rR, rsR′) (Fig. 5–12), RS (Rs, Rsr′), and rS or rsr′complex. The different QRS patterns may provide a clue to the degree of elevation in right ventricular pressure. In general a qR complex, a prominent R wave with a slur on the upstroke, or an rsR′ complex (incomplete RBBB) suggests that right ventricular pressure exceeds (qR), is equal to (R or rR), or is lower than (rsR′) left ventricular pressure, respectively. Examples include severe pulmonary stenosis or primary pulmonary hypertension (qR), tetralogy of Fallot or Eisenmenger complex (R or rR), and atrial septal defect (rsR′), respectively. In the latter, hypertrophy of the outflow tract of the right ventricle is responsible for the r′ wave.

In the presence of RVH the delay of ventricular activation results in earlier recovery of the endocardium, and, as in LVH, repolarization proceeds from endocardium to epicardium. The ST segment is thereby depressed and the T wave inverted in lead V_1 and occasionally in V_2. Significant ST-segment depression and T-wave inversion are, as a rule, indicative of moderate or severe right ventricular hypertension.

In the adult with acquired RVH the most commonly encountered ECG changes include right-axis deviation and an R/S ratio equal to or greater than 1 in V_1, with an R wave 0.5 mV or greater. Isolated right-axis deviation of +100° to −90° is considered by some to be indicative of RVH, but this criterion alone is less sensitive. An R/S ratio greater than 1 in lead V_1 alone is not diagnostic of RVH, since it may be recorded in patients with a posterior infarction or occasionally in the absence of heart disease.

ACUTE PULMONARY EMBOLISM (ACUTE COR PULMONALE) (see Chap. 48). The most characteristic ECG feature of this disorder is probably the transient nature of the changes and for this reason serial tracings are most helpful. In the Urokinase–Pulmonary Embolism Trial,[53] the ECG was normal in 6 to 23 per cent of the patients depending on the severity of the embolism. The most common abnormalities were nonspecific T-wave changes and nonspecific ST-segment elevation or depression, the incidence being 42 and 41 per cent, respectively. The more classical changes—the S_1-Q_3T_3 pattern described by McGinn and White[54] (Fig. 5–13), RBBB, right axis deviation, and P pulmonale—were recorded in only 26 per cent of the patients. Other abnormalities included $S_1S_2S_3$ pattern, RVH, and right-axis deviation with clockwise rotation.[55] The ECG changes are most likely related to acute pulmonary hypertension with right atrial and ventricular dilation, hypoxia, and perhaps myocardial ischemia. Acute atrial dilation coupled with myocardial ischemia is probably responsible for the frequent atrial arrhythmias. Despite the high incidence of abnormal tracings the diagnosis is difficult because of the nonspecific nature of the ECG changes. While a single ECG is rarely helpful, a comparison with a tracing obtained before the acute episode and serial tracings after the episode increase significantly the sensitivity of the ECG.

CHRONIC OBSTRUCTIVE LUNG DISEASE (COLD) AND COR PULMONALE (see Chap. 49). The ECG pattern of COLD and COLD with pulmonary hypertension (cor pulmonale) can be ascribed to a combination of positional changes, increased lung volume, and RVH. ECG changes include right-axis deviation of the P wave, increased amplitude and "peaked" appearance of the P wave in the limb leads, and "peaked" and biphasic morphology wave in lead V_1 (Figs. 5–10*A* and 5–14). A P-wave axis of +90° is highly suggestive of COLD. The shift of the P-wave axis is most likely due to overinflation of the

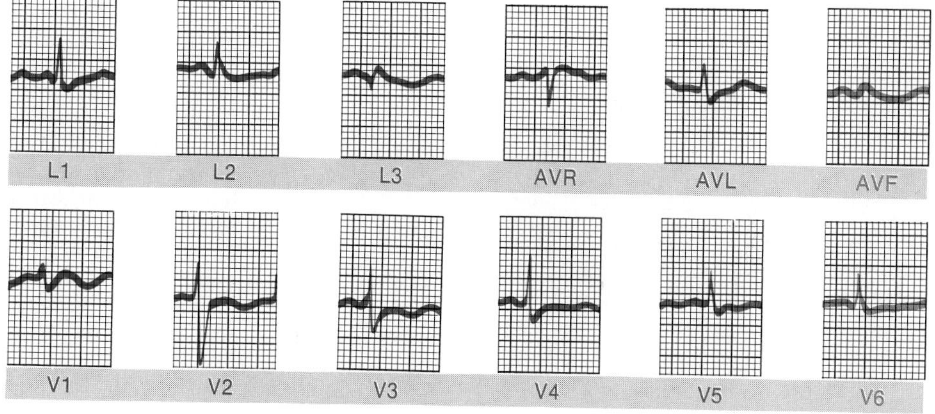

FIGURE 5–13. S_1Q_3 pattern of acute pulmonary embolism. In addition, some of the more common features of acute pulmonary embolism including inversion of T waves in leads V_1, V_2, and V_3, clockwise rotation, intraventricular conduction defect, and probable incomplete RBBB are also present.

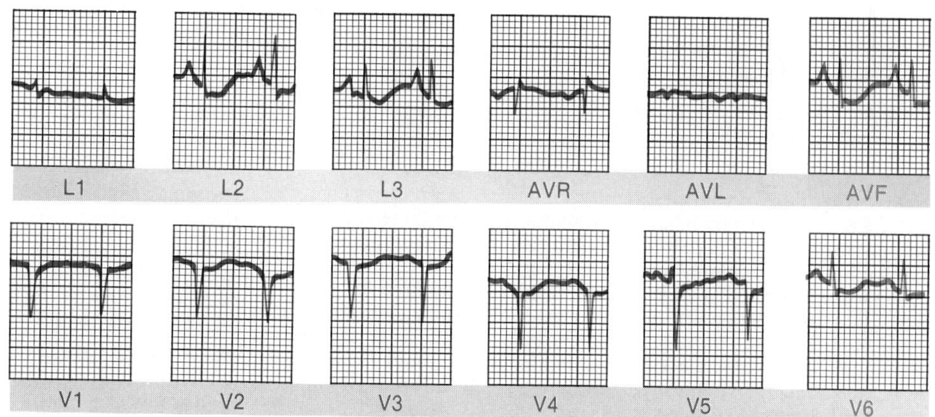

FIGURE 5–14. Chronic obstructive lung disease (COLD) simulating an anteroseptal myocardial infarction. The characteristic features of COLD include "pointed" tall P waves in leads II, III, AV_f with right-axis deviation (+90°), tendency to right axis of the QRS, clockwise rotation, and "pseudo" ST-segment depression. The latter reflects atrial repolarization. The clockwise rotation simulates anteroseptal myocardial infarction.

lungs. It is not seen with interstitial fibrosis.[56] Because of the large P-wave area, the Ta segment is exaggerated and occasionally interpreted as ST-segment depression. Right-axis deviation and clockwise rotation are characteristic findings. Occasionally, an $S_1S_2S_3$ pattern may be present.[56a] Amplitude of the precordial R wave is reduced in leads V_5 and V_6, often measuring less than 0.7 mV. When the clockwise rotation is marked, absence of the R wave in precordial leads simulates an anterior myocardial infarction. With progression to pulmonary hypertension and RVH, prominent R waves may appear in leads V_1 and V_2. These changes are probably due to unopposed late activation of the crista terminalis and right ventricular free wall. Right atrial dilatation is probably responsible for the QR pattern in V_1, with the Q wave reflecting right atrial intracavitary potential (as occurs also in tricuspid regurgitation.) As indicated, the sensitivity of the ECG for cor pulmonale is relatively low, the test being diagnostic in about 25 to 40 per cent of patients with confirmed RVH.

In *biventricular hypertrophy,* the LV forces are dominant and often obscure the RVH.

VECTORCARDIOGRAM. In RVH, the characteristic VCG changes of the QRS loop are recorded in the transverse plane, and these fall into three general types (Fig. 5–15). In type A, the configuration varies considerably. It may be oval, narrow, or figure-of-eight (Fig. 5–12). The major segment of the loops is located anteriorly and to the right. The loop is inscribed clockwise or, as in the case of the figure-of-eight loop, initially counterclockwise with the latter component recorded clockwise (Fig. 5–12). An oval loop is illustrated in Figure 5–15. In type B, the loop is inscribed clockwise, or counterclockwise, is often figure-of-eight, and is located primarily in the left anterior and to a lesser extent in the left and right posterior quadrants. In type C, the loop is inscribed counterclockwise, with 50 per cent of the loop located in posterior left and right quadrants. Of the three, type A usually reflects severe RVH, while type B is most often encountered in patients with atrial septal defect and mitral stenosis. Type C can be recorded with chronic obstructive lung disease.

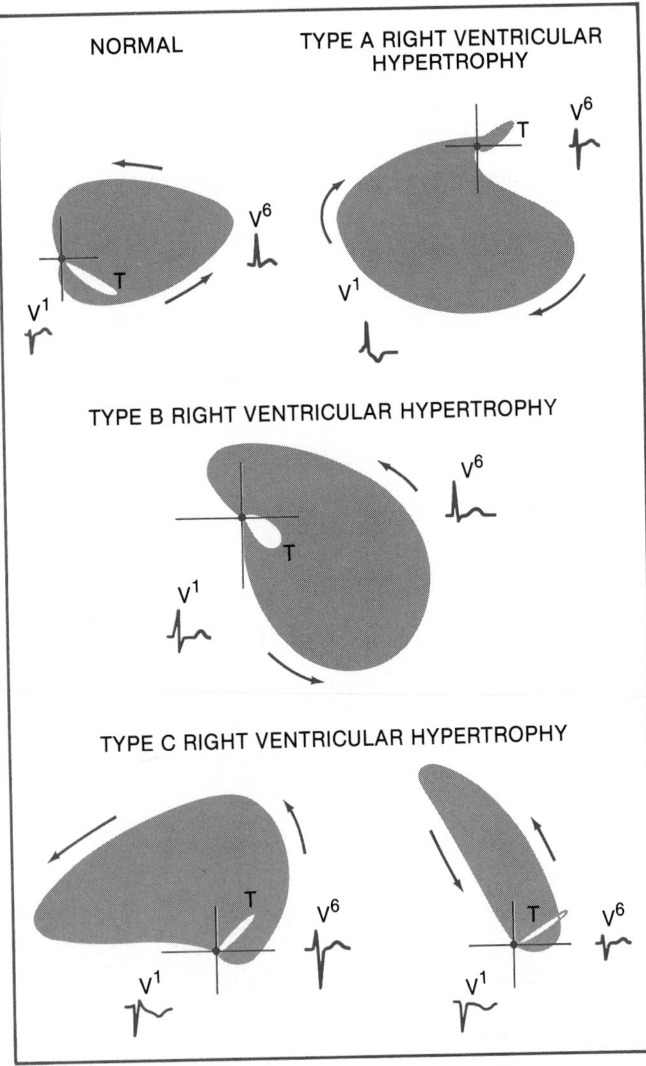

FIGURE 5–15. Diagrammatic representation of the three common, but not exclusive, VCG patterns of right ventricular hypertrophy recorded in the horizontal plane. When compared with the normal, the QRS loops are located in the right and left anterior quadrants in Type A and in the left anterior and to a lesser extent left and right posterior quadrants in Type B; a major portion of the loop is located in the left and right posterior quadrants in Type C. (Modified from Chou, T. C., Helm, R. A., and Kaplan, S.: Clinical Vectorcardiography. 2nd ed. New York, Grune and Stratton, 1974, pp. 87, 99, and 102.)

Ventricular Hypertrophy in the Presence of Conduction Defects

The diagnosis of ventricular hypertrophy in the presence of BBB is difficult, if not impossible, owing in part to the fact that a portion of cardiac activation may be unopposed for a period of time, resulting in misleading voltage changes. It has been suggested that in the presence of RBBB, an R′ greater than 1.0 to 1.5 mV indicates associated RVH. However, it is not unusual to record preoperatively a normal QRS complex in lead V_1, only to register postoperatively an RBBB with an R′ wave greater than 1.0 or 1.5 mV, indicating that this criterion of RVH may not be valid in the presence of RBBB. LBBB makes a diagnosis of RVH and LVH essentially impossible. In the presence of RBBB, LVH may be suspected when the S wave in lead V_1 and the R wave in lead V_6 satisfy voltage criteria for LVH. However, such an interpretation is subject to the limitations imposed by the relatively low sensitivity and specificity of the voltage criteria.[57] It has also been suggested that the QRS is significantly longer in LBBB with LVH than with isolated LBBB.[58]

In a study of 50 patients with left anterior fascicular block, the sum of S in lead III and the maximal R + S in any precordial lead equal to or exceeding 3 mV (30 mm) showed a specificity of 87 per cent, a sensitivity of 96 per cent, a positive predictive value of 89 per cent, and a negative predictive value of 95 per cent for left ventricular hypertrophy.[59]

INTRAVENTRICULAR CONDUCTION DEFECTS

The bundle of His bifurcates into right and left bundles (see Fig. 22–5, p. 590). The ribbon-like right bundle descends subendocardially on the right side of the septum. At the base of the right ventricular anterior papillary muscle, it divides and supplies fibers to the free right ventricular wall and the right side of the septum. The left bundle divides into an anterior division (LAD) and posterior division (LPD), which supply the left ventricular wall and left side of the septum. Discrete anatomical lesions, asynchrony of conduction in the bundles or its branches, nonuniformity of refractoriness, changes in membrane responsiveness, and a decrease in the magnitude of phase 4 of the transmembrane action potential (p. 117) may, singly or in combination, cause block of conduction in the bundle branches (BBB) and the divisions of the left bundle. However, most commonly BBB is due to an anatomical lesion. In transient BBB, the specific underlying electrophysiological mechanism may be difficult to define.

A study of 522 patients with BBB confirmed that LBBB, but not RBBB, is a strong and independent predictor of cardiovascular mortality.[60]

Left Bundle Branch Block

Interruption of the left bundle branch results in early activation of the right side of the septum and of the right ventricular myocardium. Transseptal activation from right to left is transmyocardial and thus slow, and probably a major cause of the prolonged ventricular activation. Initial activation of the ventricles proceeds from right to left, inferiorly, and more often anteriorly than posteriorly. This is followed by continued activation of the septum and of the adjacent free left ventricular wall, with the activation proceeding to the left, posteriorly, and inferiorly. This phase of activation is rapid, presumably because the impulse enters the Purkinje system below the site of the BBB. Last to be activated are the lateral

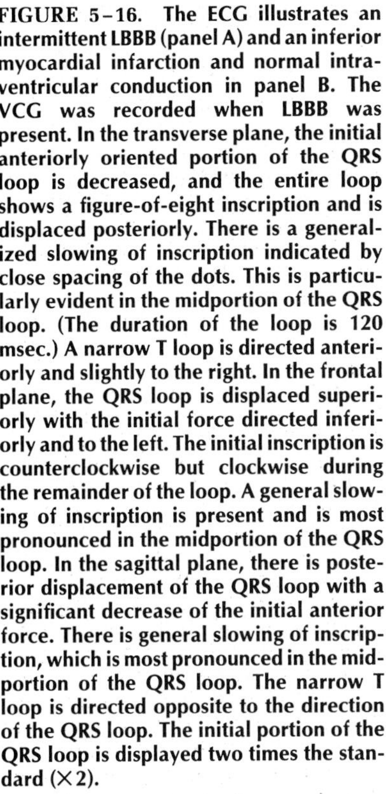

FIGURE 5-16. The ECG illustrates an intermittent LBBB (panel A) and an inferior myocardial infarction and normal intraventricular conduction in panel B. The VCG was recorded when LBBB was present. In the transverse plane, the initial anteriorly oriented portion of the QRS loop is decreased, and the entire loop shows a figure-of-eight inscription and is displaced posteriorly. There is a generalized slowing of inscription indicated by close spacing of the dots. This is particularly evident in the midportion of the QRS loop. (The duration of the loop is 120 msec.) A narrow T loop is directed anteriorly and slightly to the right. In the frontal plane, the QRS loop is displaced superiorly with the initial force directed inferiorly and to the left. The initial inscription is counterclockwise but clockwise during the remainder of the loop. A general slowing of inscription is present and is most pronounced in the midportion of the QRS loop. In the sagittal plane, there is posterior displacement of the QRS loop with a significant decrease of the initial anterior force. There is general slowing of inscription, which is most pronounced in the midportion of the QRS loop. The narrow T loop is directed opposite to the direction of the QRS loop. The initial portion of the QRS loop is displayed two times the standard (×2).

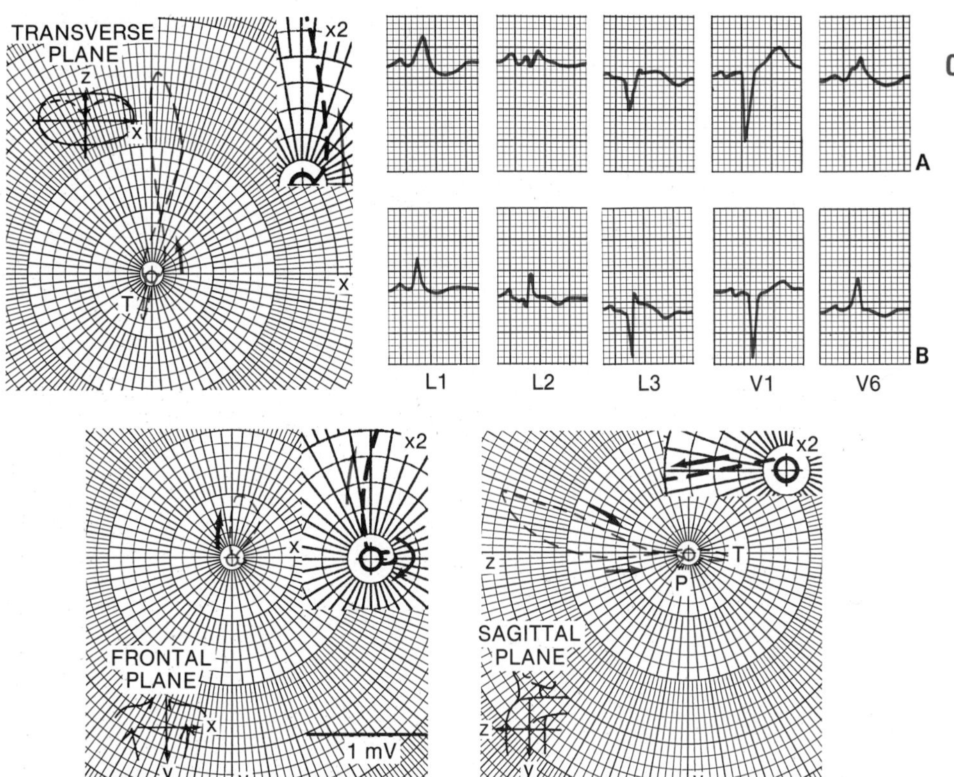

wall and basal aspect of the left ventricle, with a vector oriented posteriorly, superiorly, and, less frequently, inferiorly.

In complete LBBB, the QRS complex is prolonged, measuring 0.12 to 0.18 sec (Fig. 5-16).[61] An upright notched or slurred R wave reflecting the right-to-left myocardial activation is recorded in leads I and V_6. A small R wave followed by an S wave is present in aV_f; the R wave and the S wave reflect, respectively, the initial septal activation directed inferiorly and the superior orientation of the final vector. An rS or a QS complex, depending on whether the initial activation is oriented anteriorly or posteriorly, is recorded in lead V_1, with the S wave reflecting activation of the left ventricle from right to left. An initial R wave in lead V_1 is present in about 45 per cent of cases of LBBB. The precordial leads V_1 to V_4 may exhibit a small R wave, with the R waves in the midprecordial leads occasionally lower in amplitude than those in the right precordial leads. One clinically important feature of LBBB is an absence of a septal Q, owing to the initial right-to-left septal activation. Similarly, a Q wave fails to register when either myocardial infarction complicates preexisting LBBB or when LBBB complicates an acute myocardial infarction (p. 136). The frontal axis in LBBB may be either normal or directed to the left (−30° to −90°), the prevalence of the two being about equal. Although it has been accepted that an abnormal left axis in excess of −45° is nearly always due to a left anterior divisional block, LBBB per se may also result in pronounced left-axis deviation.

In LBBB, the direction of the ST-segment and T-wave vectors is opposite to that of the QRS vector. In the presence of an upright QRS complex in leads I, aV_1, and V_6 the ST segment is depressed and the T waves are inverted. The opposite is true in leads V_1, V_2, and V_3, in which a predominantly negative QRS complex is recorded. The ST-segment and T-wave changes are secondary to the conduction disturbance, and the magnitude of the change parallels the magnitude of the QRS aberration. Occasionally LBBB is associated with an isoelectric ST segment and a T-wave vector concordant with the QRS vector. Such primary T-wave changes suggest a myocardial abnormality independent of the LBBB, which may be due, for example, to accompanying myocardial ischemia. However, this is not always a reliable sign of a primary myocardial disorder.

Incomplete LBBB implies a greater delay of conduction in the left than in the right bundle, with initial right-to-left septal activation and loss of the septal Q wave. In contrast to complete LBBB, the left bundle ultimately contributes to activation of the septum and left ventricular wall. ECG criteria for incomplete LBBB include a QRS complex of 0.10 to 0.12 sec, loss of the initial septal Q wave, slurring or notching (Fig. 5-17), and often high voltage of the QRS complex.

In the transverse plane of the VCG, the QRS loop of LBBB is oriented to the left and posteriorly. The initial portion of the loop reflects septal activation and is inscribed slowly from right to left and anteriorly. The remainder of the loop is inscribed clockwise with slow inscription of the midportion, most likely reflecting slow intramyocardial conduction through the left ventricular wall. The T loop points in a direction opposite to that of the QRS (Fig. 5-16).

Right Bundle Branch Block

In RBBB the septum is activated normally, from left to right. While the left ventricle is activated normally, right ventricular depolarization is delayed, the right ventricle being last to be activated, and this terminal activation is unopposed. Prolongation of the QRS complex is largely due to delayed activation of the septum and right ventricular wall. The initial dominant septal force is directed from left to right, anteriorly and superiorly, followed by a vector dominated by the left ventricle, oriented to the left, inferiorly, and either somewhat anteriorly or posteriorly. The final vector representing activation of the right ventricle is directed to the right, anteriorly, and either superiorly, inferiorly, or horizontally.

The characteristic ECG changes of RBBB are recorded in lead V_1. The initial normal septal activation inscribes an R wave, followed by an S wave reflecting left ventricular activation and a final R′ wave due to depolarization of the right ventricle from left to right and anteriorly. The depth of the S wave in lead V_1 varies depending on whether the left ventricular activation generates a more posteriorly or anteriorly oriented vector. In the former, a prominent S wave separates the R wave from the R′ wave, while in the latter, the S wave may be shallow or a slur or, indeed, may be absent. Leads facing the left side of the septum, namely, I, aV_1, V_5, and V_6, record an

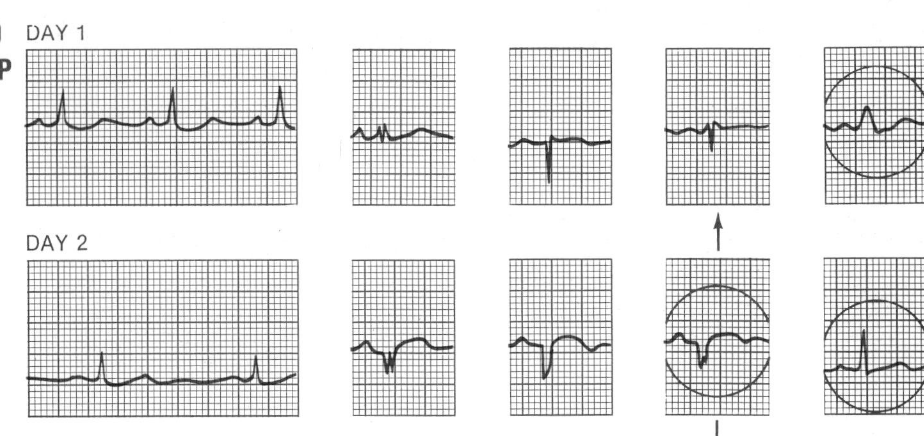

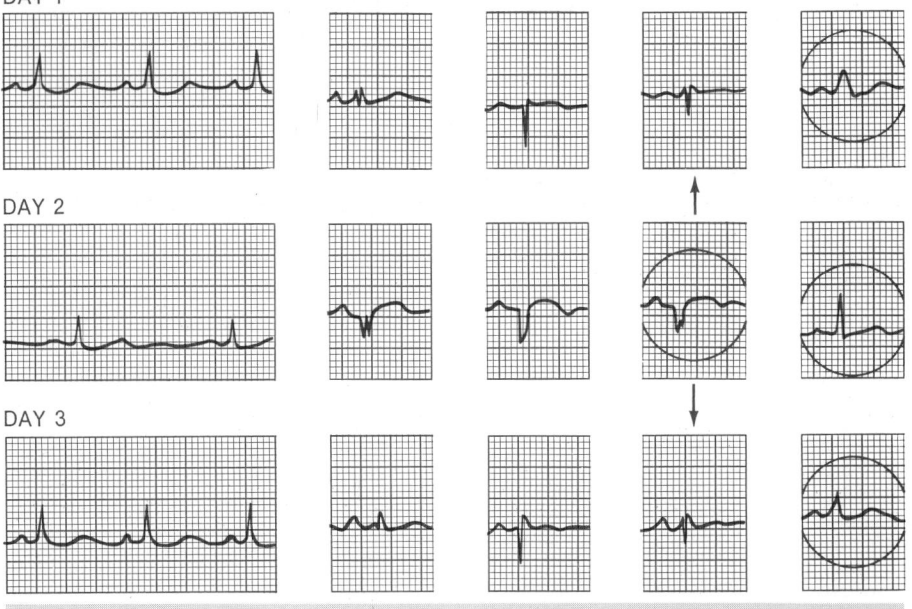

FIGURE 5-17. Inferior myocardial infarction obscured by incomplete LBBB due to acceleration of the heart rate. On day 1, the heart rate was 83 beats/min with incomplete LBBB as reflected by loss of the septal Q wave in lead V_6 and prolongation of the QRS complex (circle). On day 2, the heart rate slowed to 60 beats/min and incomplete LBBB is no longer evident (circle). Features of inferior myocardial infarction are now recorded in leads II, III, and aV_f (circle). On day 3, the heart rate accelerated to 88 beats/min, and incomplete LBBB recurred, masking the inferior myocardial infarction (arrows).

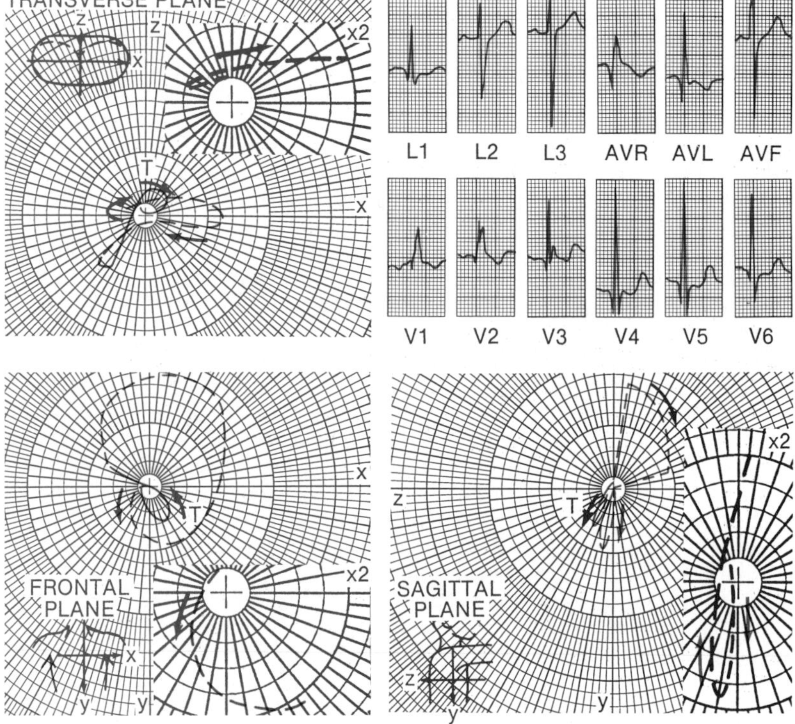

FIGURE 5-18. The ECG illustrates an anterior myocardial infarction, RBBB, and left anterior divisional block (LADB). In the transverse plane, the VCG displays an initial QRS force directed to the right and slightly anteriorly with a clockwise inscription. The decrease in the anteriorly directed initial QRS force is due to the infarction. A delayed terminal QRS loop exhibiting a figure-of-eight inscription is displaced anteriorly. The terminal, anteriorly directed, slowly inscribed part of the loop is due to RBBB. The clockwise-inscribed T-wave loop is oriented in a direction opposite to that of the main QRS force. In the frontal plane, the initial QRS is directed to the right and inferiorly. The loop is inscribed counterclockwise and is displaced superiorly and to the left. The superior and leftward displacement of the loop is due to LADB. The delayed terminal QRS forces are shifted superiorly and to the right. In the sagittal plane, the initial QRS loop is directed inferiorly and slightly anteriorly, with a decrease of the initial anteriorly directed QRS force. The delayed terminal loop is displaced anteriorly and superiorly. The initial portion of the QRS loop is displayed at two times the standard (×2).

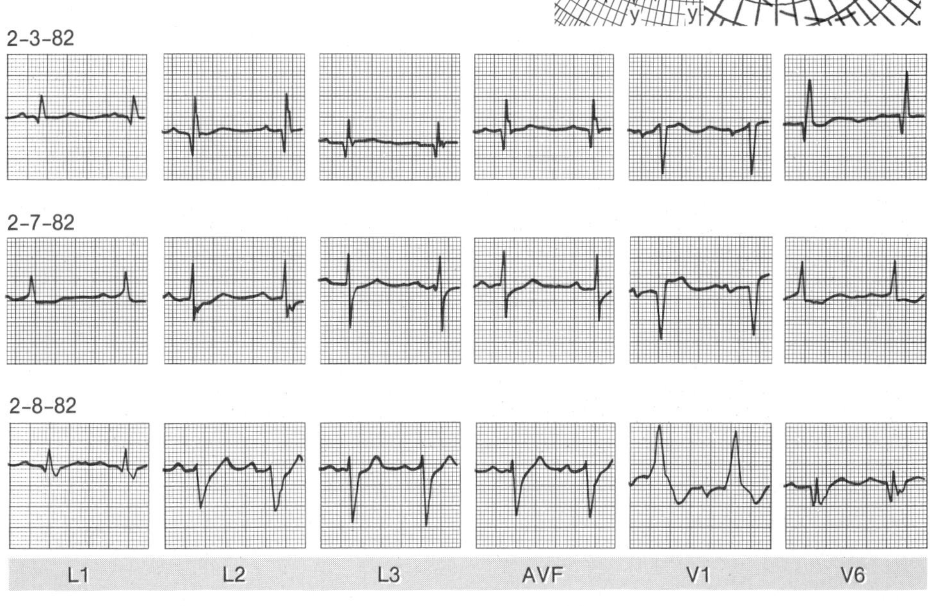

FIGURE 5-19. Masking of myocardial infarction Q waves by intraventricular conduction defects. Top trace (2-3-82) illustrates an inferolateral infarction manifest by Q waves in leads II, III, aV_f, and V_6. Incomplete LBBB and LADB in the middle trace (2-7-82) mask the inferior and lateral infarction. In the bottom trace (2-8-82), the LAFB masks the inferior infarction. The RBBB, in contrast to the incomplete LBBB in the middle trace, does not obscure the lateral infarction. (From Fisch, C.: Evolution of the clinical electrocardiogram. Reprinted with permission of the American College of Cardiology. J. Am. Coll. Cardiol. *14*:1127, 1989.)

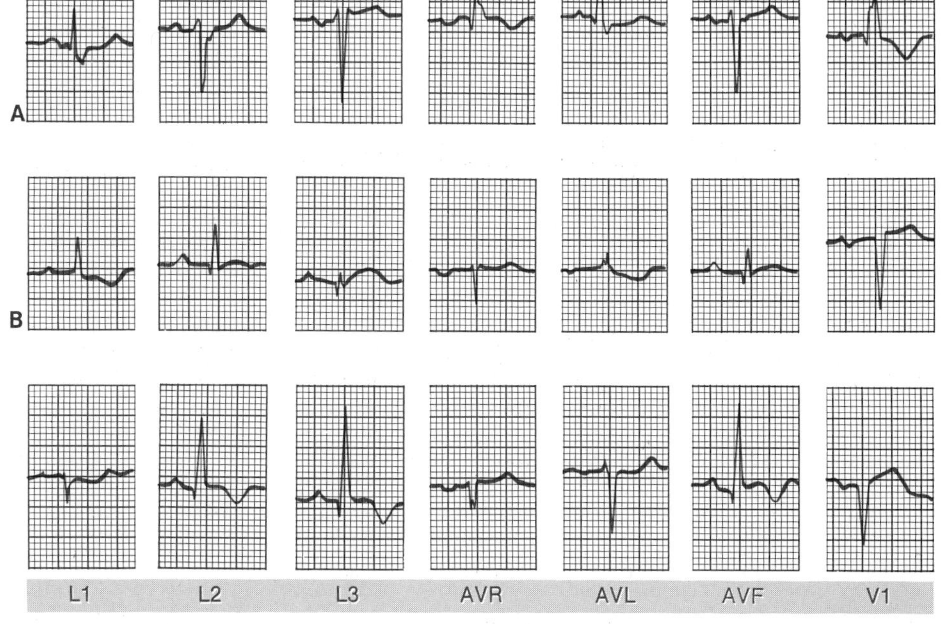

FIGURE 5-20. ***A,*** **Right bundle branch block with left anterior divisional block.** ***B,*** **Upper trace, the control trace, illustrates an inferior myocardial infarction with a normal QRS axis. The bottom trace demonstrates left posterior divisional block (LPDB). Because the latter may be due to causes other than LPDB a diagnosis of LPDB requires evidence of normal conduction prior to appearance of LPDB such as illustrated in upper trace of panel B.**

initial Q wave followed by an R wave of normal duration and a prolonged, relatively shallow S wave. The latter reflects delayed activation of the right ventricle (Figs. 5-18 to 5-20). Because the initial septal activation is normal, namely, left to right, RBBB, in contrast to LBBB, does not obscure myocardial infarction.

The T wave is usually inverted in lead V_1 and occasionally in V_2, while it is upright in the remaining precordial and limb leads, a direction opposite to the *terminal* portion of the QRS complex.

The characteristic VCG feature is evident in the transverse plane and consists of a slowly inscribed terminal appendage directed to the right and anteriorly. The initial septal and left ventricular portion of the loop is normal (Fig. 5-18).

Divisional (Fascicular) Blocks

The ventricular conduction system, including the right bundle branch and the two divisions of the left bundle, can be considered for purposes of clinical electrocardiography to consist of three divisions (fascicles) (Fig. 5-21). Divisional blocks are, with rare exception, acquired. Although the evidence for the existence of anatomically discrete divisions of the left bundle branch is not convincing, experimental data support a functional divisional conduction system.[62-64]

Furthermore, nearly simultaneous early endocardial activation at three sites—the middle anterior and posterior paraseptal areas—is consistent with the concept of functional divisions of the left bundle. This concept is also supported by distinctive and predictable ECG patterns. Thus, from the ECG standpoint, the concept of divisions of the left bundle is a useful one.[65]

BLOCK OF ANTERIOR DIVISION OF THE LEFT BUNDLE BRANCH (ANTERIOR FASCICULAR BLOCK). In the presence of left anterior divisional block, the initial septal activation proceeds inferiorly, anteriorly, to the right, and occasionally to the left. This is followed by activation of inferior and apical areas with the vector oriented inferiorly, to the left, and anteriorly. Final activation is that of the anterolateral and posterobasal left ventricular wall, the vector oriented superiorly, posteriorly, and to the left.

The resultant ECG pattern is characteristic (Figs. 5-20 and

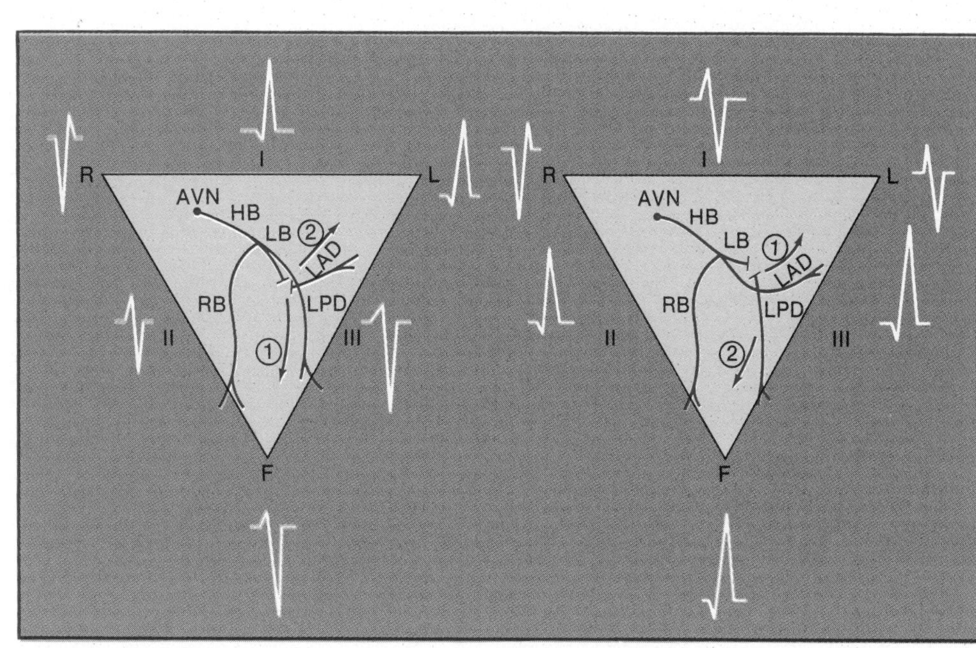

FIGURE 5-21. Diagrammatic representation of the conduction system. Interruption of the LAD ***(left)*** **results in an initial inferior** ***(1)*** **followed by a dominant superior** ***(2)*** **direction of activation; interruption of the LPD** ***(right)*** **results in an initial superior** ***(1)*** **followed by a dominant inferior** ***(2)*** **direction of activation. AVN = atrioventricular node; HB = His bundle; LB = left bundle; RB = right bundle; LAD = left anterior division; LPD = left posterior division.**

5–21). Lead I records a dominant R wave, with or without an initial Q wave. The criterion of a small Q wave in leads I and aV_l is the subject of continued controversy.[24] The presence or absence of a Q wave depends on whether the initial septal activation is directed to the right or to the left. Since the initial activation is directed inferiorly, leads II, III, and aV_f inscribe an R wave followed by a deep S wave reflecting activation of the anterolateral and posterobasal segments of the left ventricle. The QRS axis varies from −45° to −90°. The duration of the QRS is less than 0.12 sec[24] (Figs. 5–18 and 5–20).

The precordial transitional zone is frequently displaced to the left. The amplitude of the R wave is diminished, with a prominent S wave in V_5 and V_6 reflecting the superior orientation of the mean left ventricular vector. The S wave is exaggerated when the final order of activation is directed to the right. Because of the inferior orientation of the initial vector, the right and midprecordial leads may register an initial Q wave. Such patterns could be mistaken for anteroseptal myocardial infarction were it not for the fact that an R wave is recorded when the leads are placed an interspace lower. The T waves are normally upright except in lead aV_r and occasionally in leads aV_1 and V_1.

The frontal plane is the most useful for visualization of left anterior divisional block (Fig. 5–22). The inscription of the loop is counterclockwise, initially directed to the right and inferiorly, with the remaining major portion of the loop displaced superiorly. The superior orientation reflects activation of the anterior and lateral left ventricular wall. Left anterior divisional block is nearly always an acquired abnormality and thus a marker of organic disease. Often, however, it is present without clinical evidence of heart disease. The prognosis depends on the underlying disease.

BLOCK OF POSTERIOR DIVISION OF THE LEFT BUNDLE BRANCH (POSTERIOR FASCICULAR BLOCK). Left posterior divisional block is a rare finding and its pattern is nonspecific. It can be recorded in asthenic individuals and patients with emphysema, RVH, and extensive lateral infarction.[65] Diagnosis is secure only if a normal ECG is recorded before appearance of the block.

In the presence of left posterior divisional block, activation begins in the midseptal and paraseptal areas, with the vector directed to the left, anteriorly, and superiorly. This is followed by activation of the left ventricular anterior and anterolateral walls, with the vector directed to the left and anteriorly. Final activation is of the inferior and posterior walls with the vector directed inferiorly, posteriorly, and to the right. The QRS duration is less than 0.12 sec.[24] In the limb leads, the initial superior and left orientation of septal vectors is reflected as R waves in leads I and aV_1 and a narrow, 0.025-msec Q wave in leads II, III, I, and aV_f. The R waves in leads I and aV_1 are small and followed by deep S waves reflecting the inferior, posterior, and right orientation of the wave of activation (Figs. 5–20 and 5–21). The initial superior force and final inferior force result in a QR complex in leads II, III, and aV_f. The amplitude of the R wave in lead III exceeds the R wave in lead II. The frontal axis varies from about +90° to +120°, or perhaps +80° to +140°. The T wave is usually normal.

In the frontal plane of the VCG, the inscription is clockwise, initially superior and to the left, but with the major portion of the loop located in the right inferior quadrant.

RIGHT BUNDLE BRANCH BLOCK AND DIVISIONAL BLOCKS. RBBB with left anterior divisional block is the most common combination. The activation during the first 0.08 sec determines the axis and identifies the left anterior divisional block. The delay of polarization due to RBBB results in a final activation of the right ventricle to the right and anteriorly (Fig. 5–20).

RBBB with left posterior divisional block is a rare combination. The initial 0.08 sec defines the axis and divisional block while the final delayed activation, oriented to the right and anteriorly, reflects RBBB.

Block of the right bundle and both divisions of the left bundle (trifascicular block) can occur in the presence of RBBB with alternating left anterior and posterior divisional blocks. Such patterns are usually associated with Mobitz (type II) AV block. It has been suggested that RBBB with either hemiblock and a prolonged P-R interval may be a manifestation of trifascicular block. Although the prolonged P-R interval may be due to delayed conduction in the remaining division, the delay may also reflect AV nodal delay.[66]

VECTORCARDIOGRAM. The VCG records the characteristic terminal portion of the RBBB loop in the transverse plane, while the left anterior divisional block and left posterior hemiblock are best visualized in the frontal plane. The characteristic features of RBBB and left anterior divisional block with and without RBBB are shown in Figures 5–18 and 5–22. An initial inferior with rapid upward displacement of the loop or an initial

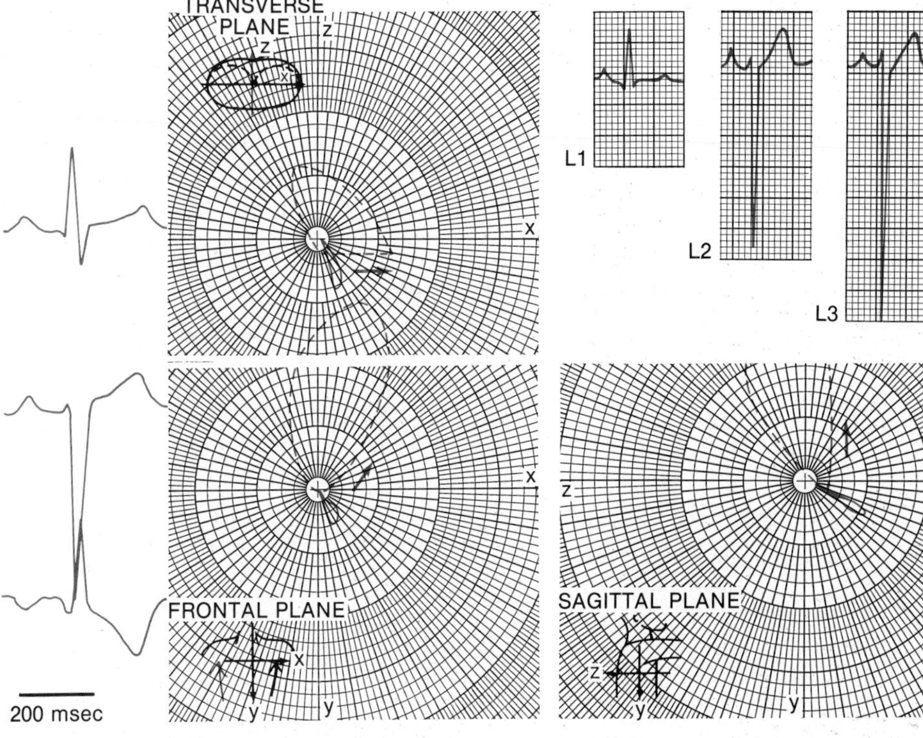

FIGURE 5–22. Left anterior divisional block and left ventricular hypertrophy (LVH). The ECG pattern of qR in lead I and rS in leads II and III indicates presence of left anterior divisional block. The diagnostic VCG features of left anterior divisional block are an initial small inferior deflection with rapid superior and counterclockwise displacement of the loop in the frontal plane, and the major area of the loop located in the left upper quadrant. LVH is suggested on ECG by the ST-T changes in lead I and the QRS voltage in leads II and III. On the VCG, LVH is indicated by posterior displacement of the loop in the transverse plane.

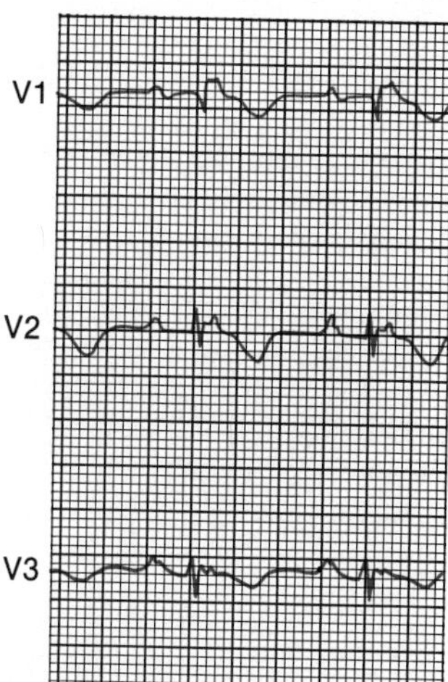

FIGURE 5-23. Epsilon potential of right ventricular dysplasia. Right intraventricular conduction defect manifested by a sharp deflection inscribed within the ST segment, the epsilon potential.

superior with rapid inferior displacement in the frontal plane is recorded with left anterior or left posterior divisional block, respectively. A terminal and delayed activation to the right and anteriorly in the transverse plane is the characteristic finding in RBBB.

NONSPECIFIC INTRAVENTRICULAR CONDUCTION DEFECT (IVCD). The QRS complex may be abnormally prolonged but without the characteristic pattern of either RBBB or LBBB. Such conduction delays are referred to as "nonspecific" IVCD. These often resemble LBBB or LBBB with an abnormal left-axis deviation, a combination suggesting left anterior hemiblock with peripheral conduction delay. Presence of a normal Q wave supports peripheral delay as the cause of QRS prolongation. Although such a nonspecific prolongation may be due to drugs or electrolyte abnormalities, it is most often due to organic heart disease. An interesting form of right ventricular conduction delay has been described in patients with arrhythmogenic ventricular dysplasia. The delayed activation is inscribed in the form of a sharp deflection after termination of the QRS, during the ST segment or upstroke of the T wave (Fig. 5-23).[67,68]

BILATERAL BUNDLE BRANCH BLOCK. This diagnosis can be considered when alternating RBBB and LBBB are present. Any other combination of conduction delays cannot be differentiated from block in the AV junction. For example, simultaneous block in both bundles results in complete AV block. Similarly, intermittent delay or block in one bundle and complete block of conduction in the contralateral bundle will manifest either as bundle branch block with a prolonged P-R interval or intermittent AV block. In the presence of BBB, a superimposed AV block due to failure of conduction in the contralateral bundle branch cannot be differentiated from block in the AV junction.

Aberration

Intraventricular aberration describes a supraventricular impulse with abnormal, bizarre intraventricular conduction (Fig. 5-24).[69] It refers to intraventricular conduction abnormalities related to changing heart rate or other functional alterations in electrophysiological properties, anomalous AV conduction, metabolic and electrolyte abnormalities, and toxic effects of drugs. The term aberration, as used currently, does not include fixed organic conduction defects.

The mechanisms responsible for, or contributory to, aberration with changing cycle length include: (1) excitation prior to completion of repolarization (i.e., in the presence of a reduced transmembrane potential), (2) unequal refractoriness of conducting tissue resulting in local delay or block of conduction, (3) prolongation of the action potential due to prolongation of the preceding cycle length, (4) failure of restitution of transmembrane electrolyte concentration during diastole, (5) failure of the refractory period to shorten in response to acceleration of the heart rate, (6) a reduced take-off potential secondary to diastole depolarization, (7) concealed transseptal conduction with delay or block of bundle branch conduction, and (8) diffuse depression of intraventricular conduction including that of specialized as well as myocardial tissue.

Aberration may result when any of these mechanisms alter conduction in the bundle branches or the divisions of the left bundle branch (or a combination of the two), the Purkinje fibers, or the myocardium. RBBB is the most common form of aberrancy and is frequently associated with left anterior divisional block. Aberrancy due to LBBB is much less common and in our experience often due to heart disease, although the heart disease may not be clinically evident. An abnormality of intraventricular conduction due to diffuse depression of conduction in the Purkinje system and in the myocardium should be suspected when both the initial and terminal portions of the QRS complex are abnormal.

Of the mechanisms and manifestations of aberration, seven will be considered in further detail: (1) premature excitation, (2) the Ashman phenomenon, (3) acceleration-dependent aberrancy, (4) deceleration-dependent aberrancy, (5) concealed conduction, (6) diffuse myocardial depression of conduction, and (7) postextrasystolic aberrancy.

PREMATURE EXCITATION. Conduction will fail or be delayed if the stimulus falls during the effective or the relative refractory period of recovery. When the impulse falls during the relative refractory period of a single bundle branch, the unilateral delay results in a bundle branch block. The duration of the refractory period may equal that of the transmembrane action potential, so-called voltage-dependent refractoriness, or it may exceed it, so-called time-dependent refractoriness. Duration of the refractory period depends to a great extent on the basic heart rate and on the duration of the immediately preceding cycle(s). Normally, the refractory period shortens with acceleration of the heart rate and lengthens with slowing of the heart rate.[70] With all variables affecting conduction being constant, the degree of aberration is usually a function of prematurity of excitation.

The site of conduction depression and thus the morphology of the aberrant QRS complex is determined by the length of the refractory period of the AV node, the bundle of His, and the bundle system itself. Normally, at slow heart rates, the right bundle branch has the longest refractory period, with the left bundle and the AV node somewhat shorter and the bundle of His the shortest. Only at very rapid rates may the duration of the refractory period of the left bundle exceed that of the right bundle.

EFFECT OF CHANGING CYCLE LENGTH ON REFRACTORINESS (ASHMAN PHENOMENON). This form of aberrancy, also a function of premature excitation, differs from that due to early excitation just described in that the abnormal conduction is a function of an altered duration

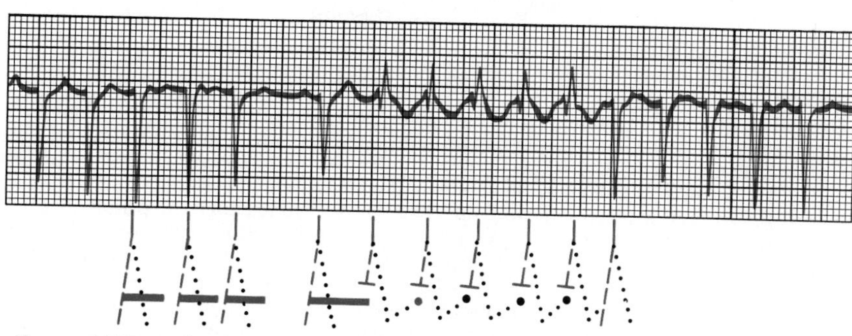

FIGURE 5-24. Atrial tachycardia with Wenckebach (type I) AV block, ventricular aberration due to the Ashman phenomenon, and probably concealed transseptal conduction. The long pause of the atrial tachycardia is followed by five QRS complexes with RBBB morphology. The RBBB of the first QRS reflects the Ashman phenomenon. The aberration is perpetuated by concealed transseptal activation from the left bundle into the right bundle with block of the anterograde conduction of the subsequent sinus impulse in the right bundle. Foreshortening of the R-R cycle, a manifestation of the Wenckebach structure, disturbs the relationship between transseptal and anterograde sinus conduction, and RBB conduction is normalized. In the ladder diagram below the tracing, the solid lines represent the His bundle, the dashes the RBB and the dots the LBB, while the solid horizontal bars denote the refractory period. Neither the P waves nor the AV node is identified in the diagram.

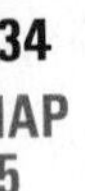

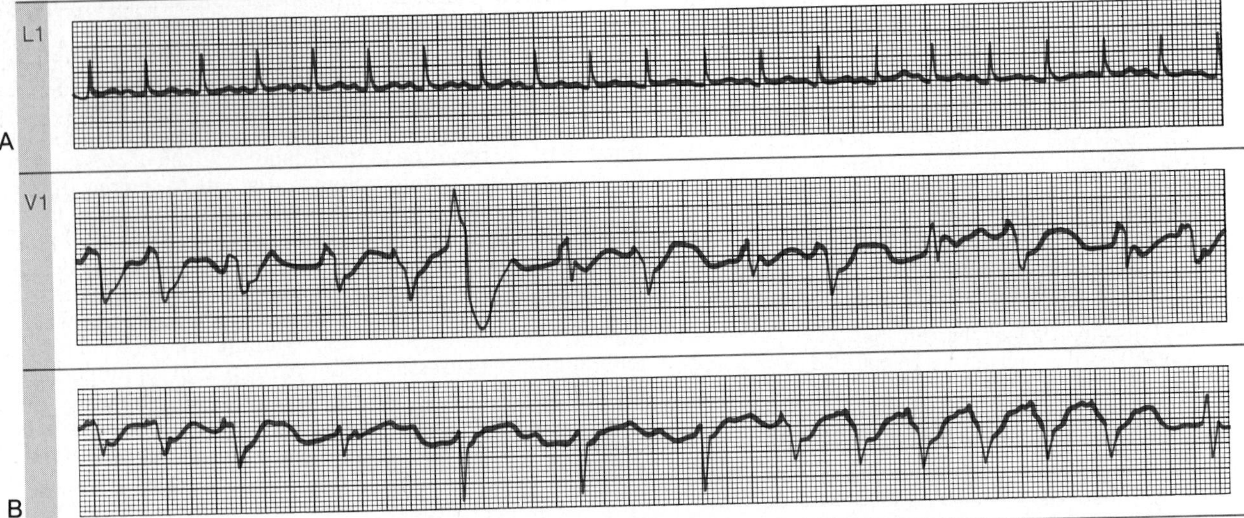

FIGURE 5–25. Intraventricular aberration due to quinidine and acceleration of the heart rate. In panel *A*, control tracing, the ECG is normal with a sinus rate of 130 beats/min. After administration of quinidine (panel *B*), the heart rate is 120 beats/min and the QRS widened to 0.20 sec with a 3:2 Wenckebach (type I) AV block interrupted by one VPC. P-wave duration is prolonged and the P-R interval is increased to 0.28 sec. The QRS complex which follows the longer pauses are narrower, probably owing to a longer period of recovery. In the bottom trace 1:1 AV conduction is interrupted by 2:1 AV conduction. P waves measure 0.20 sec in duration, the P-R interval is 0.40 sec, and the QRS complexes at onset of 2:1 AV block are foreshortened to 0.16 sec. The QRS prolongation to 0.16 sec is due to quinidine, while further widening of the QRS complexes to 0.20 sec in presence of 1:1 A-V conduction reflects both the effect of quinidine and the accelerated heart rate.

of the refractory period rather than of changing prematurity of stimulation. Since the duration of the refractory period is a function of the immediately preceding cycle length, the longer the preceding cycle, the longer the refractory period that follows. Consequently, with a relatively constant heart rate, sudden prolongation of the immediately preceding cycle length may result in aberration. This relationship of aberrancy to changes in the preceding cycle length is known as the Ashman phenomenon.[70] Aberrancy so initiated may persist for a number of cycles (Fig. 5–24), usually exhibits RBBB morphology, and may be associated with left anterior or rarely with left posterior divisional block.

In the presence of irregular supraventricular rhythms, such as atrial fibrillation, repetitive atrial tachycardia, or atrial tachycardia with Wenckebach (type 1) AV block (Fig. 5–24), aberration due to the Ashman phenomenon is suggested by the following: (1) a relatively long cycle immediately preceding the cycle terminated by the aberrant QRS complex, (2) RBBB aberrancy with normal orientation of the initial QRS vector, (3) irregular coupling of the aberrant QRS complex, and (4) lack of a compensatory pause following the aberrant QRS complex.

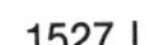

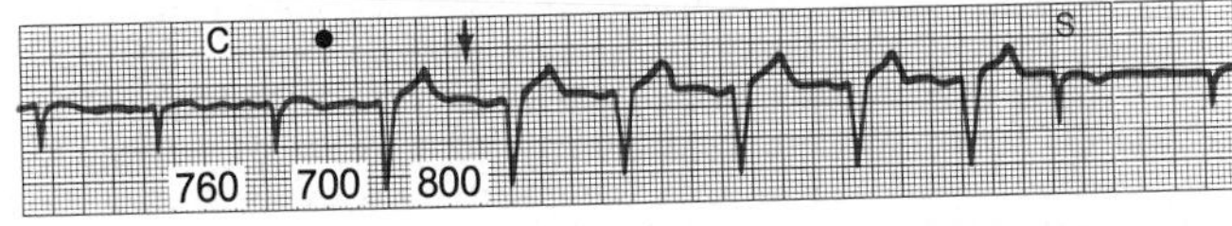

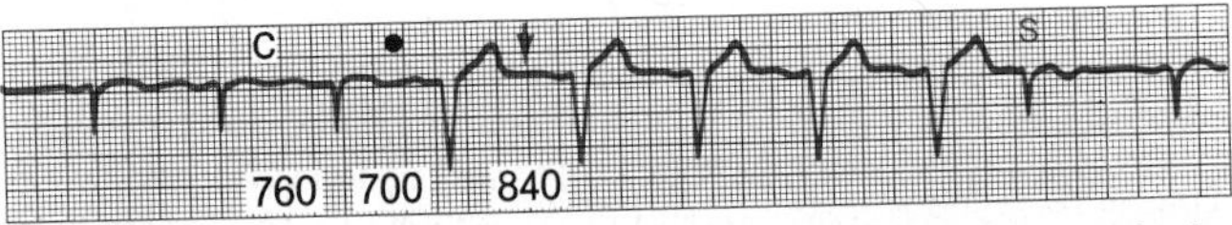

FIGURE 5–26. Acceleration-dependent QRS aberration with the paradox of persistence at a longer cycle and normalization at a shorter cycle than that which initiated the aberration. The duration of the basic cycle (C) is 760 msec. LBBB appears at a cycle length of 700 msec (•) and is perpetuated at cycle lengths of 800 (↓) and 840 (↓) msec; conduction normalizes after a cycle length of 600 msec (S). Perpetuation of LBBB at a cycle length of 800 and 840 (↓) msec is probably due to transseptal concealment, similar to that described in Figure 5–24. Unexpected normalization of the QRS (S) following the atrial premature contraction is probably due to equalization of conduction in the two bundles; however, supernormal conduction in the left bundle cannot be excluded. (From Fisch, C., et al.: Rate dependent aberrancy. Circulation *48*:714, 1973, by permission of the American Heart Association, Inc.)

ACCELERATION-DEPENDENT ABERRANCY (TACHYCARDIA-DEPENDENT ABERRANCY, PHASE 3 ABERRANCY). This form of aberration has been recognized since 1913.[71] At certain critical heart rates, impaired intraventricular conduction results in aberrancy (Figs. 5–25 and 5–26). This phenomenon has been described as tachycardia-dependent aberrancy or phase 3 aberrancy; however, the term *acceleration-dependent aberrancy* appears most appropriate. Aberration often appears at relatively slow rates, frequently below 75 beats/min; similarly, because of the slow rate at which the conduction fails, one would have to postulate an extremely long transmembrane action potential in order to accept excitation during phase 3 as the cause of the impaired conduction. Finally, conduction will also fail with excitation during phase 2 of the action potential.

The appearance and disappearance of aberration often depends on very small changes in cycle length, a change frequently difficult if not impossible to detect in the ECG. Assuming that a reasonably long recording is available, a comparison of the earliest available cycle length terminated by a normal QRS complex with the cycle length terminated by the first aberrant QRS complex will aid in the diagnosis of acceleration-dependent aberrancy. The difference in the duration of two such cycles is often less than 0.04 sec.

Acceleration-dependent aberrancy differs in a number of respects from the physiological aberrancy observed in a normal heart. Differences include (1) appearance of aberrancy at relatively slow heart rates, (2) predominance of LBBB morphology, (3) independence from the immediately preceding cycle length, (4) occasional appearance without or with only a slight change in cycle length, and (5) association with heart disease.

QRS aberrancy may persist at an R-R interval considerably longer than the interval that initiated the aberrancy (Fig. 5–26). Three mechanisms have been suggested to explain this paradox: (1) concealed transseptal activation blocking conduction in the contralateral bundles; (2) "fatigue" of the bundle; and (3) concealed transseptal conduction coupled with suppression of conduction due to the increased heart rate, somewhat analogous to suppression of pacemakers by an ectopic tachycardia.[72] A discrepancy of as much as 210 msec between the cycles initiating and terminating the aberration suggests that concealed transseptal conduction may not be the sole factor responsible for the unexpected persistence of aberrancy at the longer cycle lengths. The difference cannot be explained solely on the basis of time consumed by conduction along the contralateral bundle and across the septum. Normal transseptal activation in the human heart is about 40 to 45 msec;[18] in the diseased heart, it may be prolonged to 115 msec.[73] It is likely, therefore, that a combination of mechanisms is operative.

One mechanism that would explain the unexpected delay in normalization of intraventricular conduction is "fatigue," a descriptive term that may reflect failure of restitution of transmembrane ionic gradients and lowering of the transmembrane resting potential and/or a shift of the membrane

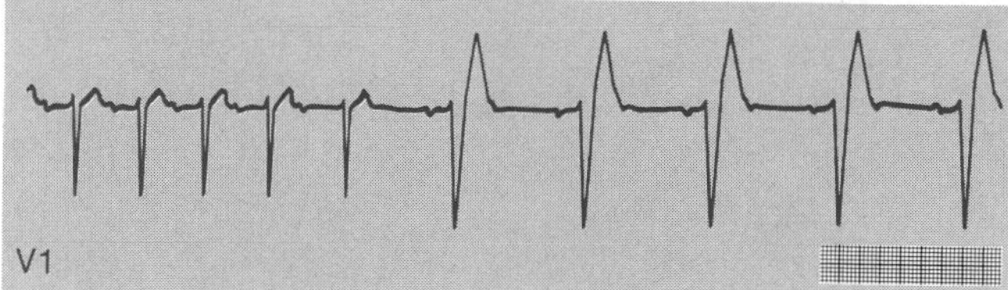

FIGURE 5-27. Deceleration-dependent aberration. The basic rhythm is sinus with Wenckebach (type I) AV block. With 1:1 AV conduction, the QRS complexes are normal in duration; with 2:1 AV block or after the longer pause of a Wenckebach sequence, LBBB appears. Slow diastolic depolarization (phase 4) of the transmembrane action potential during the prolonged cycle is implicated as the cause of the LBBB.

responsiveness to the right. The latter denotes a decrease in upstroke velocity of phase 0 for any given magnitude of transmembrane resting potential. A different mechanism, namely, concealed conduction, may explain the delayed normalization of bundle branch conduction in patients with atrial fibrillation. Concealed conduction of atrial fibrillatory impulses into the blocked bundle may result in a true bundle-to-bundle interval that is consistently shorter than the manifest QRS interval.

Occasionally, paradoxical normalization of the QRS complex without a change in heart rate—or, in fact, with acceleration of the heart rate—has been documented (Fig. 5-26). Mechanisms that may explain this phenomenon include physiological shortening of the refractory period in response to acceleration of the heart rate, equalization of conduction in the two bundles and conduction during the supernormal period, and the gap phenomenon.

DECELERATION-DEPENDENT ABERRANCY (BRADYCARDIA-DEPENDENT ABERRANCY, PHASE 4 ABERRANCY). A prolonged cycle may be terminated by an aberrant QRS and foreshortening of the cycle may normalize the QRS (Fig. 5-27).[74] It has been suggested that this form of aberrancy is due to a gradual loss of transmembrane resting potential during a prolonged diastole with excitation from a less negative take-off potential.[75] Because a small change in resting potential may have a pronounced effect on the rate of rise of phase 0 of the action potential, deceleration aberrancy may be seen with a relatively small prolongation of the cycle length.

CONCEALED CONDUCTION. Conduction in the bundle branches may be impaired by concealed penetration of a supraventricular impulse or by transseptal activation from the contralateral bundle (Fig. 5-24). In atrial fibrillation, concealed conduction into a bundle branch can be considered when acceleration-dependent aberrancy persists at a QRS cycle that is longer than a cycle terminated by a normal QRS. Transseptal concealed conduction into a bundle branch from the contralateral bundle should be suspected if aberrancy, once initiated, persists at rates slower than the rate that initiated the aberrancy (Fig. 5-26).

MYOCARDIAL DEPRESSION. Drugs and metabolic and electrolyte disorders are frequent causes of QRS aberrancy (Fig. 5-25). The severity of depression of conduction varies, and the QRS may exhibit RBBB or LBBB, divisional block, or the two combined. As indicated previously, aberrancy can be differentiated from ordinary BBB by the presence of distortion in the initial and terminal components of the QRS complex. The appearance of aberration is often rate related (Fig. 5-25).

POSTEXTRASYSTOLIC ABERRATION. Aberrant intraventricular conduction of a sinus impulse terminating a compensatory pause is rare and must be differentiated from an aberrant escape complex. The exact mechanism of the postpausal aberrancy is not clear. It may be due to slow diastolic depolarization, unequal recovery of conducting or myocardial tissue, or increased diastolic volume.

Wolff-Parkinson-White (WPW) Syndrome

(See pp. 611 and 693)

WPW, or preexcitation,[76] is an electrocardiographic syndrome characterized by a short P-R ($\leq$ 0.12 sec) interval, prolonged QRS ($\geq$ 0.12 sec) complex, a slur on the upstroke of the QRS (delta wave), and (as a rule) a normal P-J interval (Figs. 5-28 and 5-29). Secondary ST-segment and T-wave changes are nearly always present. Paroxysmal supraventricular tachycardia is recorded in about 50 per cent of patients with WPW. The characteristic pattern of WPW can be altered by abnormalities of AV and intraventricular conduction. The prevalence of WPW in the general population is approximately 3 per thousand; the fact that this figure is identical for both the young and the aged supports a congenital origin for WPW.[5]

Although Wilson is credited with the initial report of WPW,[77] it was Cohn who brought the electrocardiograph to America and first described an ECG pattern to become known as WPW. His patient, described in 1913, exhibited the WPW pattern and supraventricular tachycardia.[78] In 1930, this pattern was recognized as a discrete ECG syndrome.[76] Shortly thereafter the bypass concept of WPW was proposed, and this concept has stood the test of time.[79]

In WPW the QRS complex is a fusion between the impulse traversing the bypass and the normal AV junction. The bypass component of the QRS complex, or *delta wave*, varies depending on the size of the ventricular muscle mass activated through the bypass. In some instances, especially in the presence of AV conduction delay, the entire ventricular mass may be activated by the impulse propagated through the bypass, and the entire QRS complex becomes essentially a delta wave.

Traditionally, WPW has been classified into types A and B. *Type A* is characterized by a prominent positive initial QRS deflection in leads V_1 and V_2 (Fig. 5-29) and *type B* by a predominantly negative deflection in leads V_1 and V_2 (Fig. 5-28).[80] In type A, the initial inscription of the QRS complex, the delta wave, reflects early activation of the posterior left ventricle and, in type B, early activation of the anterior superior right ventricle. *Type C WPW*, characterized by a negative delta wave in the left lateral leads, has also been described. Studies using surface potential mapping, epicardial mapping during surgery, and electrophysiological studies have identified a number of preexcitation sites.[35,81,82] Presence of more than one QRS pattern in an individual patient suggests the possibility of multiple bypass tracts. A short P-R interval with a normal QRS complex accompanied by paroxysmal supraventricular tachycardia has been suggested as a variant of WPW (p. 693).

First-, second-, and third-degree AV block have been reported with WPW, as have right and left BBB. In the presence of a BBB, an ipsilateral bypass, by preexciting the ventricle normally activated by the blocked bundle branch, will obscure the BBB. Both supernormal and concealed conduction have been invoked to explain unexpected patterns of behavior of bypass conduction.

WPW often complicates ECG interpretation because it may obscure or simulate a variety of patterns. It may mask (Fig. 5-29) or simulate myocardial infarction.[82a] When the QRS vector is directed toward the left ventricular cavity, the cavity becomes initially positive and a Q wave will not be recorded. A diagnosis of ventricular hypertrophy in the presence of WPW (as in BBB) may be difficult if not impossible. WPW has been mistaken for RBBB, LBBB, and RVH.[35] Supraventricular arrhythmias with aberration, resulting from conduction through the bypass, have been mistaken for ventricular tachycardia. Aberration due to WPW should be suspected when the ventricular rate is rapid, often approaching 300 beats/min, or when the QRS morphology of the bizarre complexes is upright in leads V_1 and V_2 as well as in V_5 and V_6.

VECTORCARDIOGRAM. The characteristic VCG feature of WPW syndrome is a slowly inscribed initial portion of the loop, the delta wave of the ECG, which is best seen in the transverse plane. The delta is defined as that portion of the loop which begins at point E, the resting or isoelectric point of the electronic beam, and ends with resumption of normal conduction speed. The direction of this initial portion of the loop classifies the WPW into type A, B, or C. Normally, the duration of the slow inscription varies from 0.02 to 0.08 sec, depending on how much of the ventricle is activated through the anomalous pathway.

In *type A WPW*, the slow portion of the loop is directed to the left or slightly to the right and anteriorly. The remainder of the QRS loop, usually inscribed counterclockwise, maintains the same direction as the delta wave and is located in the left anterior quadrant. In about 20 per cent of cases, the maximal vector of the loop points in the direction of the left posterior quadrant. In the ECG these changes are manifested by an upright QRS complex in leads V_1 and V_6.

Type B WPW is characterized by an initial slow inscription oriented to the left and posteriorly or slightly anteriorly. The major portion of the loop is

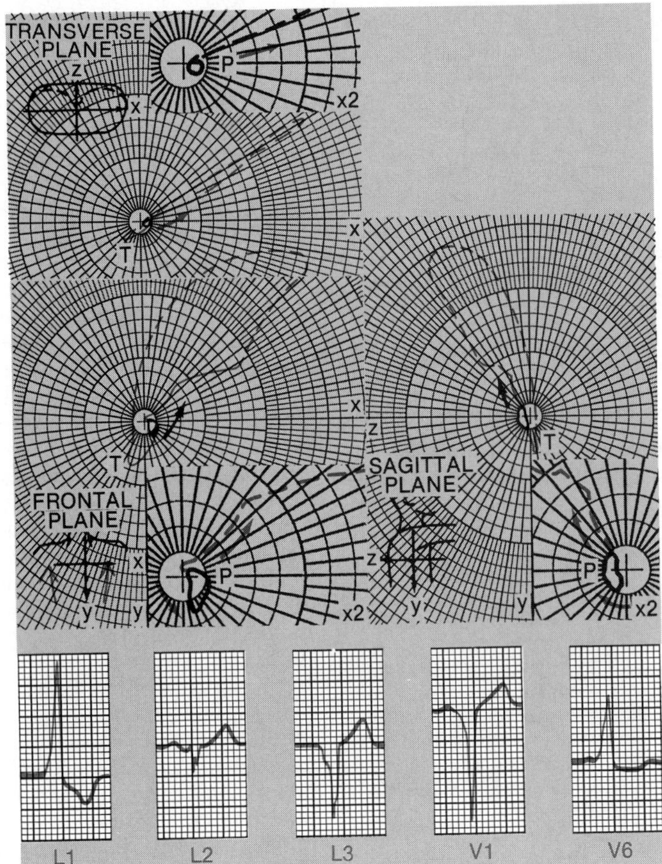

FIGURE 5-28. The ECG illustrates type B Wolff-Parkinson-White syndrome and simulates an inferior myocardial infarction. The VCG displays a delayed initial QRS force, indicated by close spacing of the dots. This initial force is directed to the left, posteriorly, and superiorly. The T-wave loop is oriented in a direction opposite to that of the initial QRS force. The initial portion of the QRS loop is also recorded at twice the standard (×2).

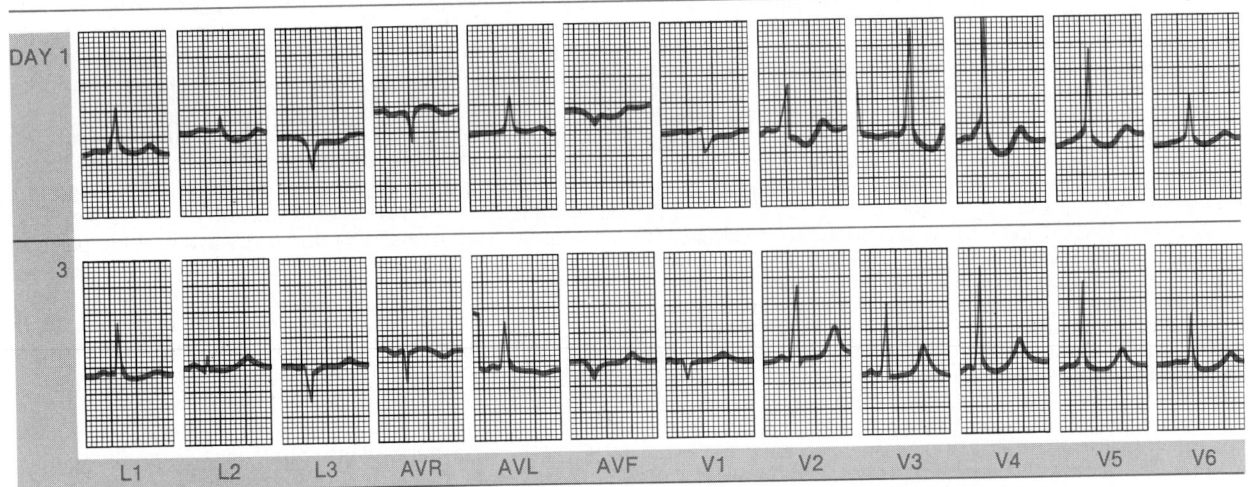

FIGURE 5-29. Acute myocardial infarction obscured by W-P-W. On day 1 of the infarction, the current of injury is manifested by sagging ST segments in leads II, III, aV_f, V_2 to V_6. On day 3, the ST segments are essentially isoelectric and the T wave of greater amplitude than on day 1. Early ventricular activation through the accessory results in an initial positivity of the left ventricular cavity precluding inscription of a Q wave. The mechanism by which the Q wave is obscured is similar to that noted with LBBB.

located in the left posterior quadrant. In the ECG these are reflected as a QS complex in leads V_1 and V_2 and an R wave in leads V_5 and V_6 (Fig. 5-28).

Type C WPW is a rarely encountered variant characterized by a Q wave in leads V_5 and V_6. The slowly inscribed initial portion of the loop is directed anteriorly to the right, with the remainder of the loop inscribed normally.

MYOCARDIAL INFARCTION

(See Chap. 39)

The ECG changes of myocardial infarction, first described in man in 1920 by Pardee,[83] are those of ischemia, injury, and cellular death and are, within limits, reflected by T-wave changes, ST-segment displacement, and the appearance of Q waves, respectively. Such a clear-cut differentiation, although clinically useful, may be overly simplistic and artificial. For example, T-wave changes may be due to ischemia, injury, or death of muscle. Similarly, a Q wave may be due to impairment of transmembrane ionic fluxes and not necessarily cellular death. However, for the purpose of this discussion, T-wave changes, ST-segment displacement, and appearance of a Q wave are assumed to reflect ischemia, injury, and cell death, respectively.

ISCHEMIA. In the dog, the earliest change following ligation of a coronary artery is the almost immediate appearance of a primary, as a rule negative, T wave. After 60 or 90 seconds, there is a maximal shift of the ST segment. The T wave becomes positive and peaked, and the change is as a rule a primary change. The amplitude of the R wave decreases during the first 30 seconds after experimental occlusion. This is followed by an increase in the amplitude which peaks 20 to 30 seconds after the maximal increase of the left ventricular volume.[84] In humans, unless an ECG is recorded at the moment of occlusion, the initial T-wave change is usually missed. Occasionally, a giant R wave is recorded early during the ischemic episode. Such changes in the QRS could contribute to the T-wave abnormality, and the abnormal T wave would reflect both primary and secondary changes of repolarization.

Normally the process of repolarization proceeds from the epicardium to the endocardium, and an upright T wave is recorded. Ischemia prolongs the regional duration of recovery, with the ischemic area being last to repolarize. If the ischemia is subendocardial, the direction of repolarization remains unchanged and the polarity of the T wave remains upright. In the presence of subepicardial ischemia, the duration of the excited state is longer in the epicardium; the normal order of repolarization is reversed, proceeding from endocardium to epicardium; and an inverted T wave is inscribed. Because of local prolongation of recovery, the late phase of repolarization may be unopposed, and a large and prolonged T wave may be registered.

INJURY. Two concepts based on systolic and diastolic phenomena have been suggested to explain the ST-segment displacement. One postulates local reduction or loss of resting potential, resulting in a *diastolic current of injury*. The second concept assumes an unopposed current flowing from the injured area during the isoelectric ST segment, resulting in a *systolic current of injury*. These systolic and diastolic phenomena cannot be differentiated with the ordinary clinical alternating-current (AC) electrocardiograph but can be recorded experimentally with direct-current (DC) equipment (Fig. 5–30).

The concept of the *diastolic current* of injury proposes that localized injury is associated with a flow of current from the uninjured to the injured area. As a result, the T-Q segment is displaced downward but is automatically shifted to control level by the capacitor-coupled amplifier of the ECG. When the entire heart (including the injured area) is depolarized, the ST segment is elevated with respect to the depressed but rectified (isoelectric) diastolic T-Q segment (Fig. 5–31).

The concept of the *systolic current* of injury proposes that during the ST segment, the normal heart is depolarized but the injured area undergoes early repolarization. The result is a current flow from the more positive injured area to a more negative or uninjured area. The result is true elevation of the ST segment. Similarly, if, rather than repolarizing early, the injured area fails to depolarize with the normal myocardium, a current of injury would exist and an elevated ST segment would be recorded (Fig. 5–31).

Earlier experimental studies indicate that during injury both systolic and diastolic currents are present,[85] and at times the systolic precedes the diastolic current of injury. A more recent study suggests that the diastolic current predominates while the systolic current plays a lesser role and that the magnitude of the current is modified by the heart rate[86] (Fig. 5–30). As indicated, the clinical ECG does not differentiate between systolic and diastolic currents of injury. Furthermore, unless the onset of the injury is recorded, even a DC coupled ECG would not identify the mechanism of the ST-segment shift.

An electrode facing subendocardial injury registers an elevated ST segment, while an epicardial electrode subtended by the normal myocardium registers ST-segment depression. Similarly, an electrode facing epicardial injury registers elevation of the ST segment, while the endocardial electrode inscribes ST-segment depression.

INFARCTION. The diagnostic feature of infarction (myocardial necrosis) is the *Q wave*. Two concepts have been invoked to explain the appearance of the Q wave. The theory of proximity, the "window" theory, suggests that the electrically inert myocardium allows an electrode to record the intracavitary negativity.[87] There is ample evidence, however, to suggest that a Q wave can be recorded in the absence of a transmural infarction. Heterogeneity of electrophysiological changes associated with the dynamic events of ischemia and subsequent healing, with intermingling of fibrous and viable tissue, has been suggested as an explanation.[87–89]

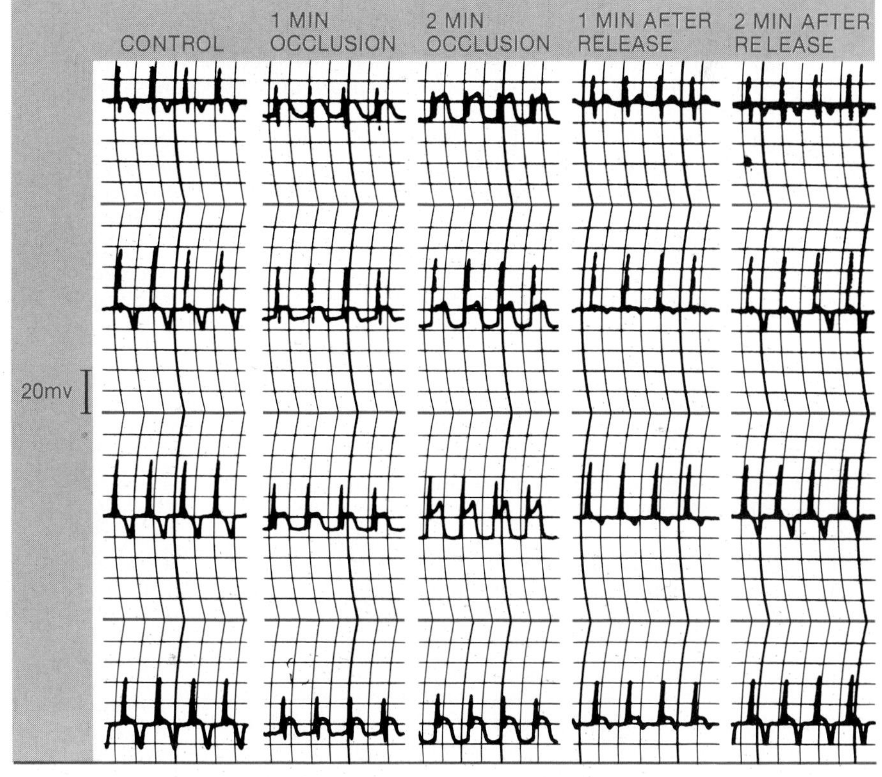

FIGURE 5–30. Simultaneous epicardial electrograms recorded from four sites. The electrodes were distributed randomly in the ischemic area, with some closer to the center of the ischemic area than others. After one minute of occlusion, TQ-segment depression is apparent in all recordings. After two minutes of occlusion, TQ-segment depression has increased. The ST-segment takeoff is slightly elevated or isoelectric in all recordings. The polarity of the T wave is changed from negative during the control period to positive. These recordings emphasize that major changes in action potential downstroke, shape, and timing can occur without significant alteration of phase 2 and of the action potential. Similarly, T-wave changes can occur without a significant shift of the true ST segment. True TQ-segment depression appears to be the major cause of ST-segment displacement and the true ST-segment shift of lesser magnitude and variable. T waveform is markedly altered with occlusion. (From Vincent, G. M., et al.: Mechanisms of ischemic ST-segment displacement. Circulation *56*: 559, 1977, by permission of the American Heart Association, Inc.)

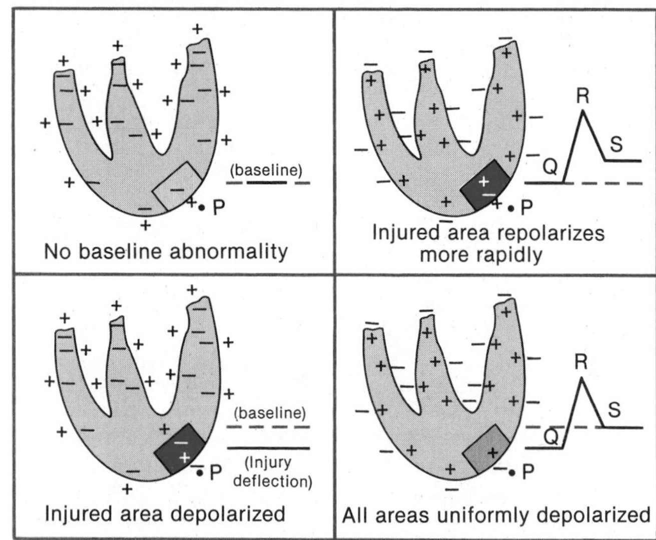

FIGURE 5-31. Systolic *(upper row)* and diastolic *(lower row)* currents of injury. *Upper row,* The ischemic area (pink) is electrically identical to the nonischemic heart at rest, and there is no shift of the baseline potential. During repolarization, however, the ischemic area (red) has repolarized early and is positive relative to the depolarized heart, the baseline is shifted upward (positive), and the ECG records an elevated ST segment. Similarly, if the ischemic area fails to depolarize with the remainder of the heart, it would be positive relative to the remainder of the heart and a positive ST segment would be recorded. This latter mechanism may also be operative.

Lower row, The ischemic area (red) is depolarized at rest, thus negative relative to the remainder of the heart, and the baseline is shifted down (negative). This shift is not recognizable on ECG. However, with completion of depolarization the injured area is also depolarized; its potential becomes identical to that of the rest of the heart; and the ST segment, although isoelectric, is elevated relative to the depressed baseline; so that an elevated ST segment is registered.

These two mechanisms cannot be differentiated with the ECG, and although both contribute to the current of injury, the systolic is thought to dominate (Fig. 5-30). (From Scher, A. M.: Electrocardiogram. *In* Ruch, I. C., and Patton, H. D. [eds.]: Physiology and Biophysics. Philadelphia, W. B. Saunders Company, 1974, p. 94.)

According to the vectorial concept, the electrically inert myocardium fails to contribute to the normal electrical forces and the result is a vector that points away from the area of infarction, reflected by a Q wave. Theoretically, the infarction vector represents the force that alters the normal vector. It is equal to but opposite in direction from the vector generated by the infarcted myocardium before infarction. If the net vector is directed normally but is reduced in magnitude, a Q wave will not be recorded, but the amplitude of the QRS complex will be reduced, indicating loss of myocardium. However, the specificity of such a change for infarction is low.

Diagnosis

One of the most valuable contributions of the ECG is in the diagnosis of myocardial infarction.[90] Usually it is the first laboratory test performed; the technique is reliable and reproducible, can be applied serially, and when properly interpreted is the cornerstone of the laboratory diagnosis of myocardial infarction.

THE INITIAL ECG. The initial ECG is "diagnostic" of acute infarction in approximately 60 per cent of the patients, abnormal but not diagnostic in approximately 25 per cent, and normal in about 15 per cent. Serial tracings increase the sensitivity to near 95 per cent. A single ECG may never be "diagnostic." However, a pattern of ST-segment displacement, especially with associated Q-wave and T-wave changes, and a clinical history suggestive of ischemic heart disease is highly suggestive—if not diagnostic—of acute myocardial infarction.

CLASSIC PATTERN AND EVOLUTION OF INFARCTION. As in the experimental animal, if the ECG is inscribed at the onset of myocardial infarction, the characteristic early change—namely, an abnormal T wave—is often recorded. The T wave may be prolonged, increased in magnitude, and either upright or inverted. This is followed by ST-segment elevation in leads facing the area of injury, with reciprocal depression in the "remote" opposite leads. The upright T wave may exhibit terminal inversion at a time when the ST segment is still elevated. A Q wave may be present in the first ECG or may not appear for hours or sometimes days. The amplitude of the QRS complex may diminish and may be replaced by a QS pattern. As the ST segment returns to the baseline, symmetrically inverted T waves evolve.[83] The time of appearance and the magnitude of the changes vary among patients (Fig. 5-32).

The classic evolution of acute myocardial infarction is documented in approximately one-half to two-thirds of the patients (Fig. 5-33), while in those remaining the infarct is manifested by ST-segment, T-wave, and non-Q QRS changes (Fig. 5-34).

SUBTLE, ATYPICAL, NONSPECIFIC PATTERNS OF INFARCTION. Atypical features and characteristics of early infarction seen in about 40 to 50 per cent of the first ECG's include a normal ECG; subtle ST-segment and T-wave changes; isolated T-wave abnormality; transient normalization of the ST segment, T wave, or QRS complex; involvement of electrically "silent" areas (Fig. 5-35); or the masking effect of conduction defects (Figs. 5-17, 5-19, and 5-29). Awareness and recognition of the early, nondiagnostic, "atypical" or subtle abnormalities will improve the diagnostic sensitivity of the ECG.

Although ECG changes can be documented within seconds after experimental coronary occlusion and in humans during angioplasty,[91] such changes may be delayed. A normal initial ECG in a patient with evolving clinical acute myocardial infarction may be due to absence of ischemia at the time of the initial tracing, a delay in evolution of the characteristic pattern, an initially small infarct that produces diagnostic ECG changes only after extension, transient normalization of the ECG in the course of evolution of acute myocardial infarction, or infarction of an electrocardiographically silent area of the myocardium (Fig. 5-35).

Early changes of myocardial infarction may alter the terminal part of the QRS (Fig. 5-34). With an inferior infarction these may be manifested by an increase of the R wave amplitude in lead III and appearance of an S wave in AVL. There may also be an associated increase in S wave amplitude in leads V_2 and V_3.[92] These changes are most likely due to conduction delays in the ischemic and injured areas, in some way similar to periinfarction block[92] (p. 1241).

Evolution of the characteristic ST-segment and T-wave changes coupled with appearance of Q waves is highly specific for acute myocardial infarction. In the first ECG, the sensitiv-

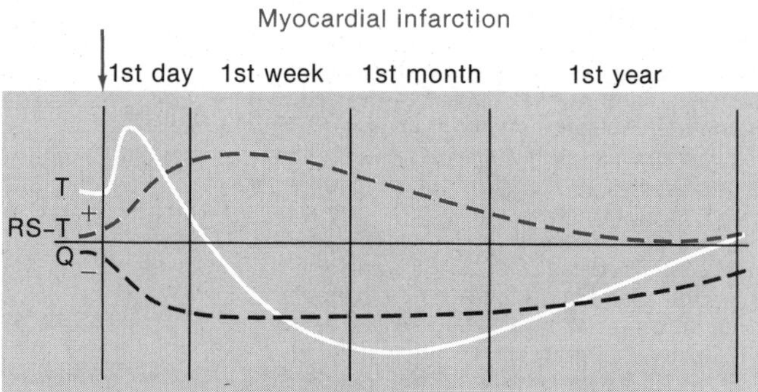

FIGURE 5-32. Evolution of the T wave, ST segment, and Q wave after myocardial infarction. (From Lepeschkin, E.: Modern Electrocardiography. Baltimore, Williams and Wilkins Co., 1951.)

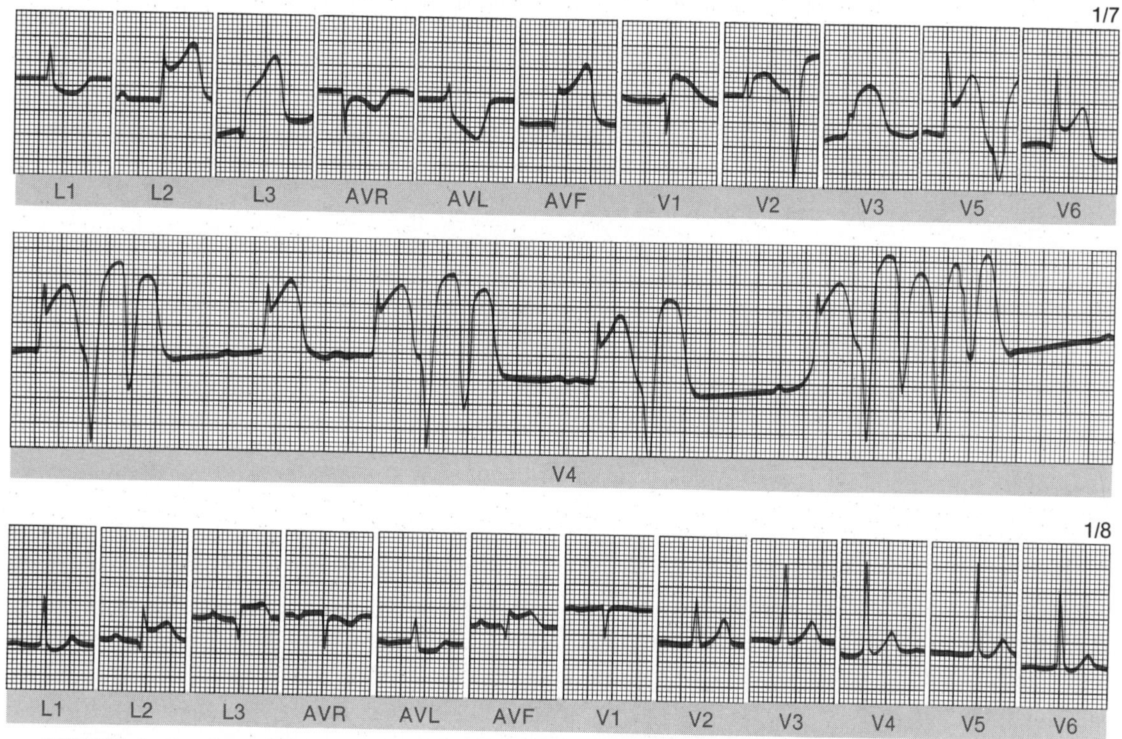

FIGURE 5-33. Acute inferior myocardial infarction and transient extensive anterior injury. Tracing made on 1/7 shows elevation of the ST segment in leads II, III, and aV_f, V_1 through V_6 with reciprocal depression of the ST segment in leads I and aV_1. In the second row the acute injury is accompanied by ventricular premature complexes (isolated and couplets) and a short run of ventricular tachycardia. In the tracing of 1/8, the anterior current of injury is no longer present, and the residual pattern is that of an acute inferior myocardial infarction manifest by a Q wave and ST-segment elevation in leads II, III, and aV_f. The tall R in lead V_2 and upright right precordial R waves suggest an associated posterior infarction.

ity and specificity of the ST-segment change alone, especially when marked, is high. With the passage of 4 to 12 hours, however, *evolving* changes in the ST segment need to be demonstrated, since conditions such as pericarditis, early repolarization, and ventricular aneurysm may also manifest ST-segment elevation but it is usually persistent. Transient hyperkalemia and Prinzmetal's angina, like acute myocardial infarction, can also cause transient ST-segment elevations. Although subtle, minor ST-segment elevation can be easily overlooked, and it is a relatively common, isolated early finding.

ST-segment depression may reflect subendocardial ischemia, infarction, or reciprocal changes secondary to infarction at a "remote" (opposite) site.[93,93a,93b] It has also been suggested

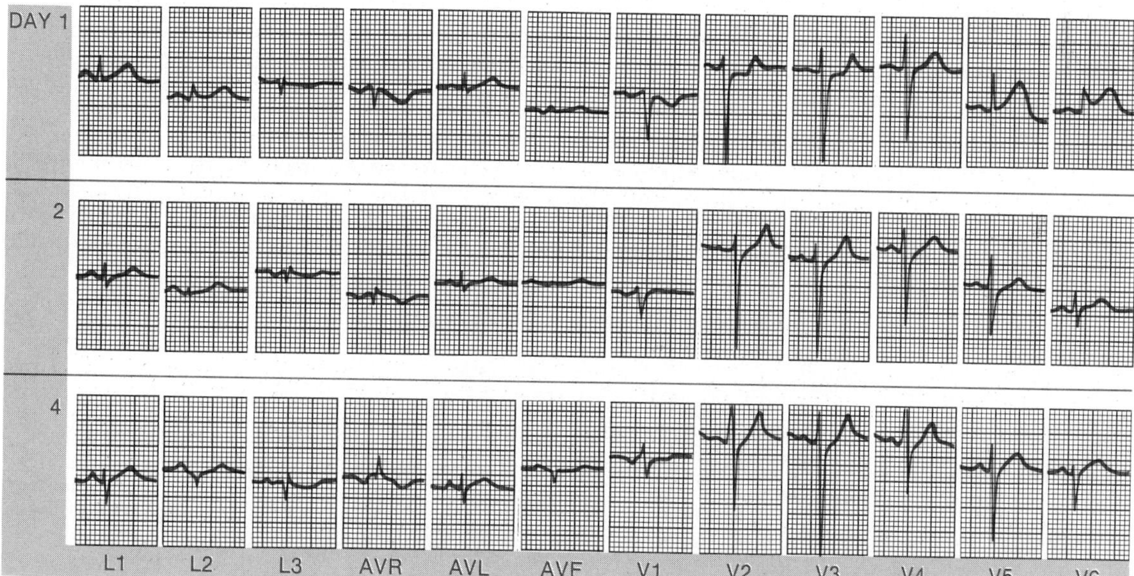

FIGURE 5-34. Acute myocardial infarction manifested by an altered sequence of ventricular activation. Tracing recorded on day 1 suggests a lateral infarction with reciprocal ST segment depression in leads V_1 to V_3. A shift of axis to right with prominent S waves in leads V_5 and V_6 is noted in the middle trace. The Q waves in leads II, III, and aV_f with R waves of higher amplitude in leads V_1 and V_2 suggest that the infarct is inferior and probably posterior. The marked right-axis duration and the prominent S waves in leads V_5 and V_6 indicate an inferior and posterior periinfarction block with the terminal ventricular excitation directed toward the infarction.

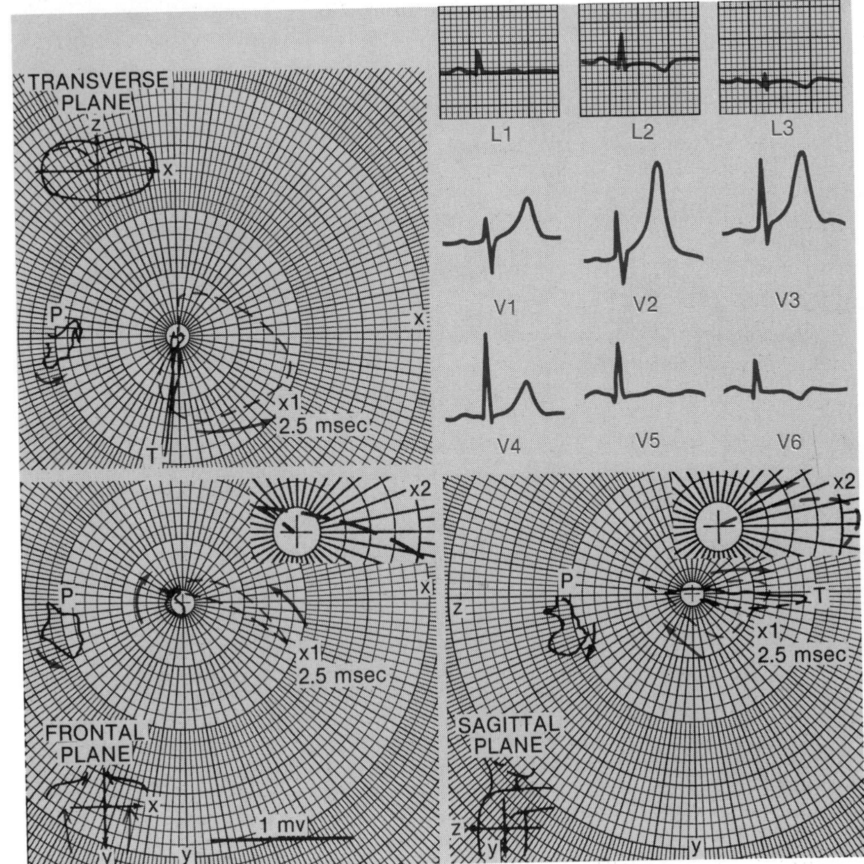

FIGURE 5–35. The ECG illustrates an inferior and posterior infarction. In the transverse plane, the VCG displays anterior displacement of the QRS loop with the anteriorly displaced area about 70 per cent of the entire loop owing to the posterior infarction. The large but narrow T loop is directed anteriorly and to the right and is inscribed counterclockwise at a uniform rate. In the frontal plane, the initial QRS force is directed superiorly and is inscribed clockwise with an inscription of 20 msec located superiorly. The initial leftward QRS magnitude, along the 0 to 180° axis, is 0.25 mV. In the sagittal plane, the initial QRS force is directed superiorly and anteriorly and is inscribed clockwise with a portion displaced superiorly. The entire QRS loop is also shifted anteriorly consistent with a posterior infarction. The large but narrow T-wave loop is directed anteriorly and is inscribed clockwise at an almost uniform rate. The initial QRS force in the frontal and sagittal planes is displayed at two times the standard (×2), while the P-wave loop is displayed at four times the standard in each of the three planes. The Q waves in leads II, III, and V_6 and T-wave changes in leads I, II, III, V_5, and V_6 indicate an inferior apical infarction, while the tall R waves in leads V_1, V_2, and V_3 reflect the posterior infarction. The tall T waves in leads V_1, V_2, and V_3 may be due to the inferior or posterior infarction or both.

that depression of the ST segment in leads V_1 to V_4 in the presence of an inferior infarction may indicate ischemia secondary to significant obstruction of the left anterior descending coronary artery. However, evidence indicates that the ST-segment depression is reciprocal to the inferior or posterolateral infarction[94–98] and that the severity of the anterior wall ST-segment depression is related to the severity and extent of the inferior ischemia rather than to anterior wall ischemia.[99–101] There is evidence that inferior ST-segment depression noted with anterior ischemia is also a reciprocal phenomenon and does not reflect inferior ischemia.[102]

Minor, subtle ST-segment depression is a common early finding of acute myocardial infarction, especially non-Q wave infarction. However, since ST-segment depression is often a nonspecific change it should be evaluated in light of other clinical and laboratory findings.

Tall, peaked T waves seen in experimental coronary occlusion are occasionally recorded in man and are thought to reflect subendocardial ischemia. More often, initially the T waves are isoelectric, negative, or biphasic. While subtle T-wave changes are often the earliest recorded signs of infarction, their value is limited because of nonspecificity. In about 20 to 30 per cent of patients with myocardial infarction, a T-wave abnormality is the only sign of acute infarction.

An *abnormal U wave* is a frequent marker of ischemic heart disease. Negative or biphasic U waves have been reported in up to 30 per cent of patients with chronic angina pectoris, either as a persistent finding or as a transient manifestation during an episode of angina. It is most often recorded in leads I, II, and V_4 to V_6. Appearance of a negative U wave during exercise-induced ischemia has been appreciated for some time and is highly specific for disease of the left anterior descending coronary artery.[103,103a] A negative U wave is seen in 10 to 60 per cent of patients with anterior infarction and in up to 30 per cent of patients with inferior infarction. Appearance of a negative U wave may precede other ECG changes of infarction by several hours (Fig. 5–36).

An abnormal QRS complex, ST segment, and T wave may normalize transiently in the course of evolution of acute myocardial infarction. This may be due to reversible ischemia or injury or conduction defects but it is also frequently observed in the normal evolution of acute myocardial infarction.[104] A

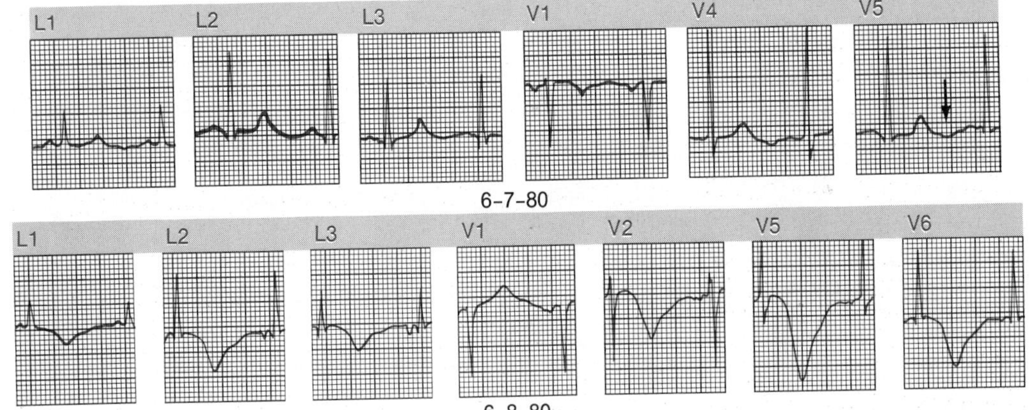

FIGURE 5–36. Negative U wave as the only marker of an acute ischemic episode. On 6/7/80 a negative U wave (↓) was recorded in leads I, II, III, V_4 and V_5, and an upright reciprocal U wave was present in lead V_1. In the tracing of 6/8/80 a prolonged Q-T interval and deeply inverted T waves are present in all the leads—evolutionary changes consistent with an acute myocardial infarction. At necropsy a subendocardial infarction was found.

premature ventricular complex with a qR or QR morphology even in the absence of ECG findings of infarction suggests the presence of myocardial infarction. This finding may prove particularly useful when the myocardial infarction is masked, for example, by LBBB or WPW. A recent study, however, questions the value of this finding in the absence of other ECG findings of myocardial infarction.[105]

OLD INFARCTION. ECG diagnosis of old myocardial infarction is often difficult and frequently impossible without the availability of tracings documenting the acute episode. A definitive diagnosis of old infarction depends on the presence of a pathological Q wave. Only rarely can it be based on T-wave changes alone. While abnormal Q waves may be absent in transmural infarction[87,89] and present in nontransmural infarction, the sensitivity and specificity of the ECG for diagnosis of an old myocardial infarction still depend on such Q waves. The specificity of abnormal Q waves for myocardial infarction is relatively high; however, the sensitivity is quite low. Within 6 to 12 months after an acute myocardial infarction, about 30 per cent of the tracings, although abnormal, are no longer diagnostic of infarction, because the Q wave(s) are absent. Similarly, by the end of 10 years, or sooner, some 6 to 10 per cent of the cardiograms revert to normal. There is evidence to suggest that loss of Q waves following anterior myocardial infarction is associated with smaller areas of infarction.[106]

In a series of 1184 tracings correlating myocardial infarction with postmortem findings, the specificity and sensitivity of the Q wave were 89 and 61 per cent, respectively, and varied with location of the infarction. Anteriorly located Q waves (leads V_1 to V_4) and inferiorly located Q waves (leads II, III, and aV_f) were falsely positive in 46 per cent. Q waves longer than 0.03 sec in lateral leads (V_5 and V_6) or Q waves in more than one "electrocardiographic zone," i.e., inferior and lateral, were false positive in only 4 per cent. The sensitivity of the Q wave was lowest for infarction located in the lateral basal portion of the left ventricle.[107] This anatomical area is usually reflected in leads I and aV_l.

MYOCARDIAL INFARCTION AND CONDUCTION DELAYS. Conduction defects may not interfere with, may mask, or may falsely suggest the diagnosis of myocardial infarction. In RBBB, the initial order of activation is normal and thus the pattern of infarction is unaltered (Figs. 5–18 and 5–19). Rarely, the development of RBBB will unmask an anteroseptal infarction.[108] In LBBB the sequence of early activation is altered, with the initial septal vector directed from right to left. As a result the earliest left ventricular intracavitary potential is positive. In keeping with the "window" concept of infarction, a Q wave cannot be registered except when there is extensive septal infarction. Restated in terms of the dipole or vector concept, since the free wall infarct is inscribed during the latter part of the QRS complex after the septal activation is complete, the direction of initial activation expressed as a dipole or vector is unaltered by the infarction, and the infarct is masked (Figs. 5–16, 5–17, and 5–19).

LEFT BUNDLE BRANCH BLOCK. Numerous attempts at defining diagnostic criteria for myocardial infarction in the presence of LBBB have proven unsuccessful. The proposed criteria rarely correlate with autopsy findings. In a study of 52 patients with LBBB and autopsy findings of myocardial infarction, the following ECG findings were thought to correlate with myocardial infarction: (1) a Q wave 0.04 sec or greater in leads I, aV_l, V_5, or V_6; (2) rapid serial ST-segment and T-wave changes; (3) acute ST-segment elevation disproportionate to the area of the QRS complex; and (4) a Q wave of any size in lead V_6. Others suggest that a deep S wave in leads V_5 and V_6, a qRs complex with a slurred S wave in leads V_5 and V_6, loss of the R wave in the precordial leads, or a Q wave in leads II, III, and aV_f is consistent with myocardial infarction complicating LBBB. However, in another study of patients with LBBB, the significance of Q waves, broad R waves, notched mid and left precordial S waves, rsR′ complexes, ST-segment elevation, and T-wave changes was addressed and found to lack significant correlation with myocardial infarction.[109] In patients with LBBB, ischemia, and infarction, the following criteria were found highly specific and predictive for myocardial infarction in a range of 90 to 100 per cent: Q wave in at least two leads, leads I, aV_l, V_5 or V_6; R-wave regression from V_1 to V_4; notching on the upstroke of the S wave in at least two leads (leads V_3, V_4, or V_5), and primary ST-T changes in two or more adjacent leads.[110] A somewhat better correlation was noted between an ECG suggestive of acute inferior myocardial infarction and postmortem findings. Observations made during angioplasty indicate that in the presence of LBBB with acute transmural ischemia, the ST segment becomes elevated over the area of the acute ischemia; this is a change similar to that observed with normal intraventricular conduction.[111]

Studies of patients with intermittent LBBB and myocardial infarction provide additional evidence that LBBB masks myocardial infarction (Fig. 5–17). It should be noted, however, that occasionally when acute infarction is evident during normal intraventricular conduction, acute changes are also recognizable in the presence of LBBB.

Block of divisions of the LBBB may simulate[112] or obscure myocardial infarction (Fig. 5–19).[65] In addition, in WPW as in LBBB, the initial vector may be directed from right to left, precluding the appearance of a Q wave (Fig. 5–29). The ECG pattern of infarction masked by WPW is recognizable during normalization of intraventricular conduction and during preexcitation is suggested by ST-segment and T-wave changes.

PERIINFARCTION BLOCK. As originally defined, periinfarction block is a specific conduction abnormality due to myocardial infarction.[113,113a] The ECG changes include a Q wave of 0.04 sec and a QRS complex in the limb leads of 0.10 sec, with a slurred prolonged terminal component facing the site of infarction. Periinfarction block is not synonymous with left anterior divisional block. Periinfarction block may be of help in the diagnosis of old inferior infarction when the characteristic changes are no longer evident. Presence of terminal, somewhat delayed activation facing leads II, III, or aV_f and a terminal negative wave in leads I, V_5, and V_6—signs of periinfarction block—strengthen the diagnosis of inferior myocardial infarction (Fig. 5–37).

THE ECG AND SITE OF CORONARY ARTERY OBSTRUCTION. The correlation of ECG pattern and site of obstruction early in the course of myocardial infarction was investigated arteriographically in 152 patients. The sensitivity, specificity, and predictive value for (1) ECG indicative of anterior infarction and occlusion of the left anterior descending coronary was 90, 95, and 96 per cent, respectively; (2) ECG indicative of inferior infarction and occlusion of the right coronary artery was 56, 97, and 80 per cent, respectively; (3) ECG indicative of posterior or lateral infarction and obstruction of the left circumflex coronary was 24, 98, and 75 per cent, respectively; (4) ECG indicative of inferior infarction and obstruction of the right or left circumflex coronary was 53, 98, and 94 per cent, respectively; and (5) ECG indicative of posterior or lateral infarction and obstruction of the right or left circumflex coronary was 53, 98, and 94 per cent, respectively.[114]

In acute inferior myocardial infarction, changes in the lateral leads (aV_l, V_5, and V_6) with an isoelectric or elevated ST in lead I identified obstruction of the circumflex coronary artery with a sensitivity, specificity, and predictive value of 83, 96, and 93, respectively. Changes in the lateral leads are rare, with inferior infarction resulting from obstruction of the right coronary artery.[115]

Two hundred four consecutive patients with unstable angina manifesting abnormal ST-segment and terminal T-wave inversion in leads V_2 and V_3 without abnormal Q waves were found to have more than 50 per cent narrowing of proximal left anterior descending artery. Of this group, 33 had complete obstruction and 75 had collateral circulation to the affected vessel.[116] Others have made similar observations.[117]

Presence of ST-segment elevation equal to or greater than 1 mm in lead V_4R has a sensitivity of 100 per cent and specificity of 87 per cent and a predictive accuracy of 92 per cent for occlusion of right coronary above the first right ventricular branch. The absence of ST-segment elevation of 1 mm excludes such lesions. Similarly, presence of ST-segment elevation in V_4R excluded isolated obstruction of left circumflex artery.[118]

THE ECG AND LOCATION OF INFARCTION. A precise anatomical location of anterior myocardial infarction based on ECG is not always possible. Accuracy of such localization is influenced, for example, by distance of the electrode from the heart, which varies considerably among individuals. The area subtending a given precordial electrode varies with the anteroposterior (AP) diameter of the chest and is greater in individuals with an increased diameter. Consequently, the same size anterior infarct would be recorded in more leads than in an individual with a normal AP diameter.

The diagnosis of transmural and nontransmural infarction when based on presence or absence of a Q wave shows a poor correlation with autopsy findings.[119] Experimental[120] and autopsy findings indicate that while nontransmural lesions may be accompanied by a Q wave, the Q wave may be absent in transmural infarction.[121] It has been suggested that as many as

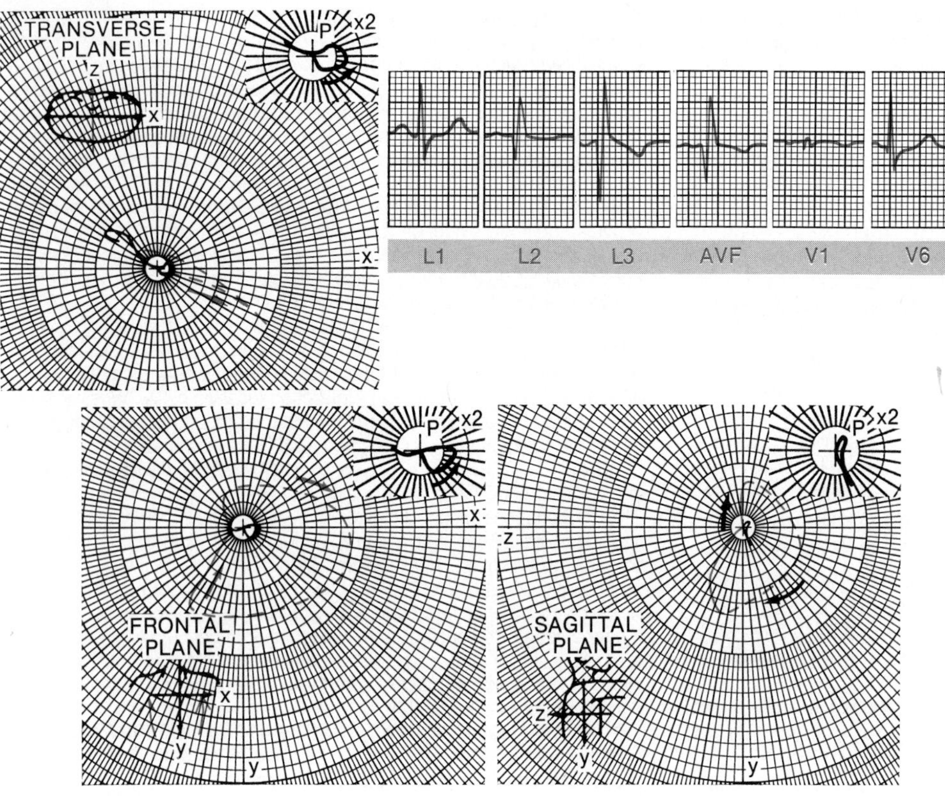

FIGURE 5-37. Inferior myocardial infarction and periinfarction block. Q waves in leads II, III and aV_f coupled with T-wave changes are indicative of inferior myocardial infarction. QRS duration is 0.10 sec. S waves in leads I and V_6 and terminal positivity of QRS in leads II, III, and aV_f suggest inferior periinfarction block.

In the VCG, superior displacement of the initial forces with clockwise rotation indicates an inferior myocardial infarction. In the sagittal plane, the superior displacement and clockwise rotation of the increased initial forces are consistent with inferior myocardial infarction. In the frontal plane terminal delay of the forces located inferiorly and to the right of the E point is indicated by close spacing of the dots and identifies periinfarction block. Total duration of the QRS is 10 msec. Slowing of conduction is also recorded in the transverse and sagittal planes.

50 per cent of nontransmural myocardial infarctions manifest Q waves, making differentiation of nontransmural and transmural infarction based on the Q wave highly tenuous.[119] It appears, therefore, that the terms Q and non-Q wave infarction (Fig. 5-36) may be preferable to transmural and nontransmural,[119,121] unless necropsy findings are available.[122] Early elevation of the ST segment is a poor predictor of subsequent Q-wave evolution.[123]

On the basis of the presence of Q waves, an infarct is considered septal when a Q wave is present in leads V_1 and V_2[124]; anterior when they are present in leads V_3 and V_4 (Fig. 5-18); anteroseptal if present in V_1 to V_4; lateral when present in leads I, aV_l, and V_6; anterolateral when present in leads I, aV_l, and V_3 to V_6; extensive anterior when present in leads I, aV_l, and V_1 to V_6, high lateral when present in leads I and aV_l, inferior when present in leads II, III, and aV_f (Figs. 5-5, 5-16,

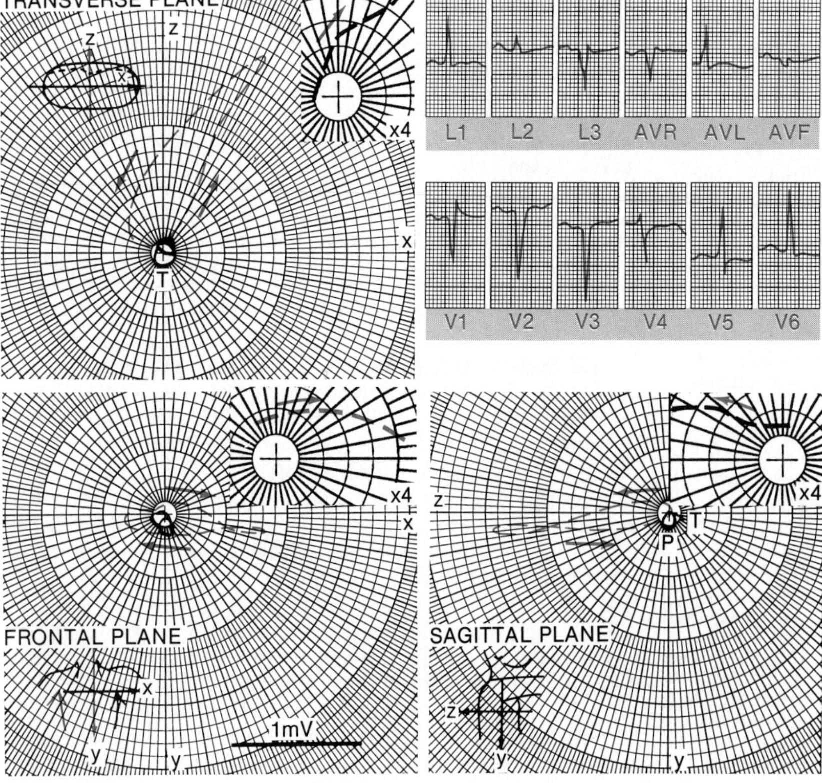

FIGURE 5-38. The ECG illustrates an anteroseptal and inferior myocardial infarction. On VCG, the transverse plane displays an initial QRS force directed to the left and posteriorly, with the entire QRS loop displaced posteriorly. The small oval T loop is situated anteriorly and to the right. In the frontal plane, the initial QRS force is directed to the right and superiorly and is inscribed clockwise. The duration of the superiorly displaced initial force is 22.5 msec and the amplitude of the superiorly displaced and leftward directed force along the 0 to 180° axis is 0.3 mV. In the sagittal plane, the initial QRS force is directed posteriorly and superiorly, with posterior displacement of the QRS loop. The small T-wave loop is located anteriorly. The initial QRS force is displayed four times the standard (×4).

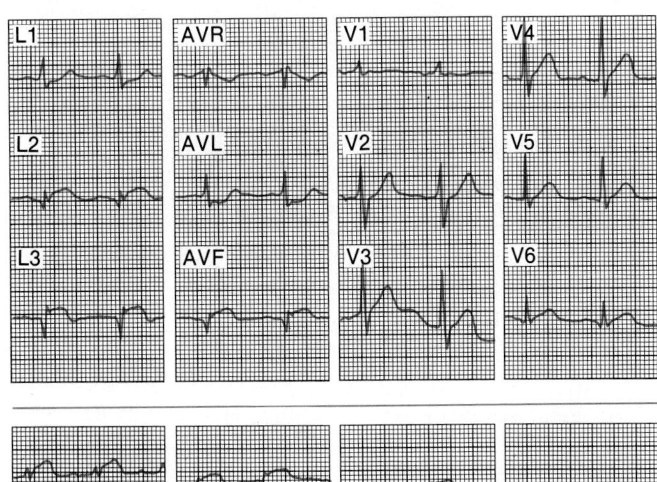

FIGURE 5-39. Inferior, right ventricular, and posterior myocardial infarction. The inferior infarct is manifested by Q waves and elevated ST segments in leads II, III, and aV_f, the posterior by the prominent R waves in leads V_1 and V_2, and the right ventricular by ST segment elevation in leads V_3R to V_6R.

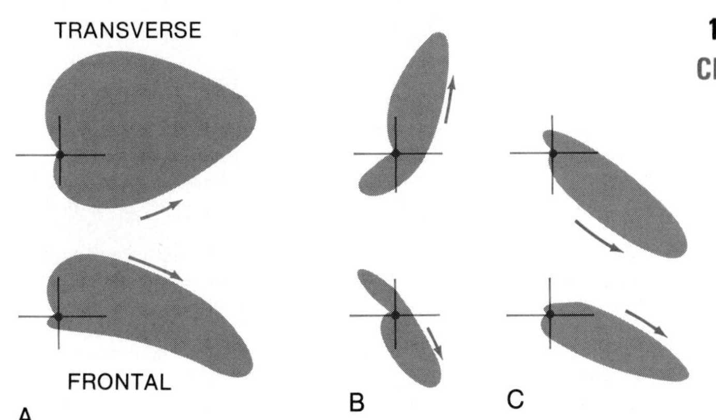

FIGURE 5-41. Vectorcardiogram of inferior and posterior myocardial infarction. *A*, Inferior; *B*, inferolateral; *C*, true posterior. (Modified from Chou, T. C., et al.: Clinical Vectorcardiography, 2nd ed. New York, Grune and Stratton, 1974, pp. 208, 220, 226.)

5-17, 5-33, 5-34); and anteroinferior, or apical, when present in leads II, III, aV_1, and in one or more of the V_1 to V_4 leads (Fig. 5-38). A posterior infarct is recognized by prominent R waves in lead V_1 or V_2 (Fig. 5-35).

A right ventricular infarction is likely when an elevated ST segment in lead V_1 or V_2 complicates a Q-wave inferior left ventricular septal infarction (Fig. 5-39).[125] Although Q waves and ST elevation may appear in leads V_1 through V_3, their specificity is too low to be useful in the diagnosis of right ventricular infarction.[126] Right ventricular infarction is therefore more likely when the changes are recorded in right precordial leads, especially V_4R.[127-129] The sensitivity and specificity of ST-segment elevation in lead V_4R alone has been estimated between 82 to 100 and 68 to 77 per cent, respectively. ST-segment elevation equal to or greater than 1 mm in one or more leads V_4R to V_6R has been shown to have a sensitivity and specificity for infarction of the right ventricle of 90 and 91 per cent, respectively. It has been suggested that ST-segment elevation when greater in lead V_4R than in V_1, V_2, and V_3 reaches a specificity of 100 per cent but its sensitivity is somewhat lower (78 per cent) than that of an elevated ST segment in V_4R alone.[130] Right ventricular conduction delay is a frequent finding in patients with right ventricular ischemia with an elevated ST segment.[131]

Infarction isolated to the posterior left ventricular wall is rarely detected. This area of the left ventricle, the last to be depolarized, is inscribed during the terminal 0.04 to 0.06 sec of the QRS complex. Theoretically, therefore, it cannot be expressed as an initial positive wave in leads V_1 and V_2. In keeping with the dipole concept, however, the S wave may become smaller, a sign that lacks any degree of specificity. In a small number of patients, posterior myocardial infarction may be suspected when there is ST-segment depression in lead V_1 or V_2 or both, an R wave in lead V_1 of 0.04 sec, and an R/S ratio greater than 1. The exact mechanism of the change in the initial QRS forces in leads V_1 and V_2 is not clear. Some have suggested that posterior myocardial infarction is not manifested in the ECG but that the findings in lead V_1 or V_2 or both reflect an associated lateral infarction. In patients with an inferior or lateral myocardial infarction, an R wave of increased amplitude 0.04 sec in duration in leads V_1 and V_2, and an upright T wave in lead V_1, suggest concomitant posterior wall involvement (Fig. 5-36). On occasion, ST-segment depression in leads V_2 and V_3 may be the early evidence of an evolving posterolateral myocardial infarction.[132,133]

In an effort to estimate the size of infarction a QRS scoring system based on duration of the Q and R waves and loss of R-wave amplitude expressed in amplitude ratio of R/Q or R/S has been proposed.[134]

THE VCG IN MYOCARDIAL INFARCTION

The appearance of the vector loop in myocardial infarction depends on the site and size of the infarction. Deviation from normal reflects loss of forces normally generated by the infarcted area and resultant dominance of the noninfarcted myocardium. Anterior myocardial infarction is best visualized in the transverse plane, while inferior infarction is best displayed in the frontal or sagittal planes (Fig. 5-40 and 5-41).

Anteroseptal myocardial infarction is recognized in the transverse plane by loss of the first 10- to 20-msec forces, with the initial position of the loop oriented posteriorly and to the left. The entire loop is displaced posteriorly with loss of the anterior convexity. In the vast majority of cases, the loop is inscribed in a counterclockwise direction. The initial posterior and leftward orientation of the loop is reflected in the ECG as a QS complex in leads V_1 to V_4 (Figs. 5-38 and 5-40).

In *localized anterior infarction*, the transverse loop is similar in appearance to that present in anteroseptal myocardial infarction except for a normally inscribed initial force in a left and anterior direction. This initial inscription is displayed in the ECG as an R wave in lead V_1 and at times in V_2 (Figs. 5-18 and 5-40). In *extensive anterior infarction*, the transverse loop reflects loss of both the septal and free left ventricular walls. The initial normal anteriorly inscribed portion of the loop is lost, and the loop is shifted

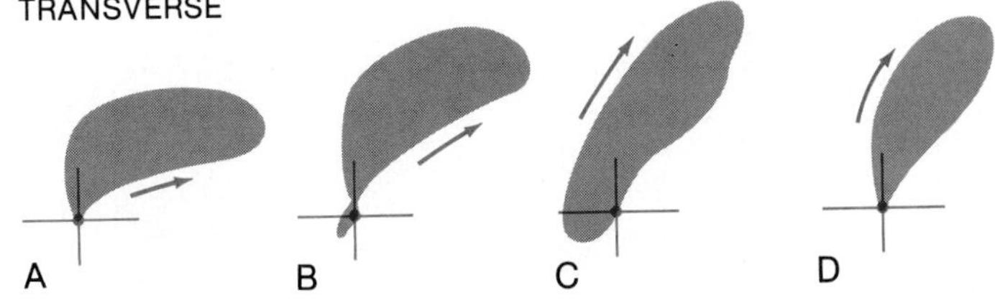

FIGURE 5-40. Vectorcardiogram (diagram) of anterior myocardial infarction. *A*, Anteroseptal; *B*, localized anterior; *C*, anterolateral; *D*, extensive anterior. (Modified from Chou, T. C., et al.: Clinical Vectorcardiography, 2nd ed. New York, Grune and Stratton, 1974, pp. 191, 196, 199.)

posteriorly and inscribed clockwise. The ECG shows a loss of R wave, at times, in all precordial leads.

Anterolateral infarction is inscribed clockwise or as a figure-of-eight in the transverse plane. The initial normal part of the loop is followed by posterior and somewhat rightward displacement, reflecting the more extensive loss of left ventricular wall. Loss of the lateral wall may result in an increase in magnitude of the initial left-to-right portion of the loop, reflected in the ECG as a tall R wave inscribed in the right precordial leads (Fig. 5–40).

Inferior myocardial infarction is best displayed in the frontal and sagittal planes (Figs. 5–35 and 5–41). In the frontal plane, the loop is most often inscribed in a clockwise direction. The initial portion is directed superiorly, the superior displacement exceeding 25 to 30 msec. The loop crosses the X axis to the left of the point of origin. It has been suggested that when the above diagnostic findings are absent, a shift to the left of the QRS loop combined with clockwise rotation is strongly indicative of an inferior infarction. Occasionally, when the inferior septum is spared, the initial loop may have a normal orientation, that is, to the right and inferiorly. This is followed by clockwise inscription and superior displacement of the remainder of the loop. In such instances the ECG will record small initial R waves in leads II, III, and aV_f.

In *posterior myocardial infarction* the initial forces are normal in the transverse plane, but more than half the loop is ultimately displaced anteriorly. In the majority of cases, inscription of the loop is counterclockwise. The anterior displacement of the loop is reflected in the ECG by a prominent R wave in lead V_1 or V_2 that may exceed 0.04 sec in duration (Figs. 5–35 and 5–41).

A summary of VCG criteria for myocardial infarction is presented in Table 5–5 and Figures 5–40 and 5–41.

TABLE 5–5 SUMMARY OF VECTORCARDIOGRAPHIC CRITERIA FOR DIAGNOSIS OF MYOCARDIAL INFARCTION (MI)

Anteroseptal MI (1 and 2)*
1. Initial anterior QRS forces absent
2. 0.02-sec QRS vector directed posteriorly

Localized Anterior MI (1, 2, and 3)
1. Initial anterior septal forces present
2. 0.02-sec QRS vector directed posteriorly
3. Voltage criteria for left ventricular hypertrophy absent

Anterolateral MI (1, 2, and 3)
1. Initial anterior septal forces normal
2. Initial rightward QRS forces > 0.022 sec
3. Efferent limb of transverse plane QRS loop inscribed clockwise
4. Initial rightward QRS forces > 0.16 mV
5. Maximum frontal plane QRS vector > 40°, QRS loop inscribed counterclockwise

Extensive Anterior MI (1 and 2)
1. Initial anterior QRS forces absent
2. Transverse plane QRS loop inscribed clockwise

Inferior MI (1 or more)
1. Initial superior QRS forces > 0.025 sec
2. Initial superior QRS forces ≥ 0.020 sec, maximum left superior force ≥ 0.25 mV
3. Maximum frontal plane QRS vector < 10°, efferent limb of frontal QRS loop inscribed clockwise
4. Bites in afferent limb of frontal QRS loop

Inferolateral MI (1 and 2)
1. Initial rightward QRS forces > 0.022 sec
2. Initial superior QRS forces > 0.025 sec

* Numbers in parentheses after each type of infarction indicate the minimum requirements for the diagnosis.

From Chou, T.-C., et al.: Clinical Vectorcardiography. 2nd ed. New York, Grune and Stratton, 1974, p. 229.

NONINFARCTION Q WAVES

While the vast majority of abnormal Q waves are due to myocardial infarction, a significant number are due to other causes.

Noninfarction Q waves may be transient or permanent. Transient Q waves have been produced experimentally in animals and observed in patients during ischemic episodes.[135,136] Such Q waves have been explained by a transient loss of electrophysiological function, but without irreversible cellular damage, a phenomenon referred to by some as "myocardial concussion."[137–140] Q waves have been recorded with severe metabolic disturbances accompanying shock or pancreatitis. Similarly, transient Q waves have been noted during cardiac surgery and ascribed variously to transient ischemia and hypoxia, coronary spasm, localized metabolic and electrolyte disturbances, and possible hypothermia. Rarely a transient Q wave may result from tachycardia.

The largest group of noninfarction Q waves is due to myocardial disease, including myocarditis, cardiac amyloidosis, neuromuscular disorders such as progressive muscular dystrophy, myotonia atrophica, Friedreich's ataxia, scleroderma, postpartum myopathy, myocardial replacement by tumor (Fig. 5–42), sarcoidosis, idiopathic cardiomyopathy, anomalous coronary artery, and coronary embolism.

Noninfarction Q waves are common in hypertrophic cardiomyopathy[140a,140b,140c] and may simulate anterior or inferior myocardial infarction (Fig. 5–43). Although the exact mechanism of the abnormal Q waves in this condition is unclear, increased septal mass or abnormal depolarization because of anomalous architecture of the septal myocardium, or both, have been proposed as the cause.

Abnormal Q waves can be associated with chronic obstructive lung disease (COLD) with or without cor pulmonale, pulmonary embolism, and pneumothorax. In COLD, findings in the precordial leads frequently simulate anterior myocardial infarction. The mechanism responsible for the QS complex is clockwise rotation and downward displacement of the diaphragm and of the heart. As a result, the electrodes are located superior to the initial vector; when this vector is directed inferiorly, a QS pattern results. By placing the electrode one interspace lower, it is often possible to record an R wave and thus provide strong evidence against myocardial infarction. Occasionally in COLD the Q wave may simulate inferior myocardial infarction. The positional origin of the anterior or inferior Q waves may be suspected when the Q wave is accompanied

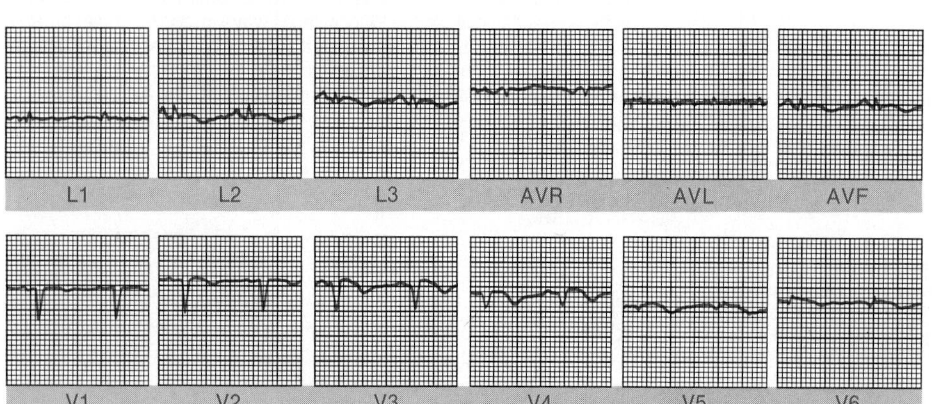

FIGURE 5–42. Extensive anterior and inferior myocardial infarction simulated by extensive myocardial metastasis of carcinoma of the breast.

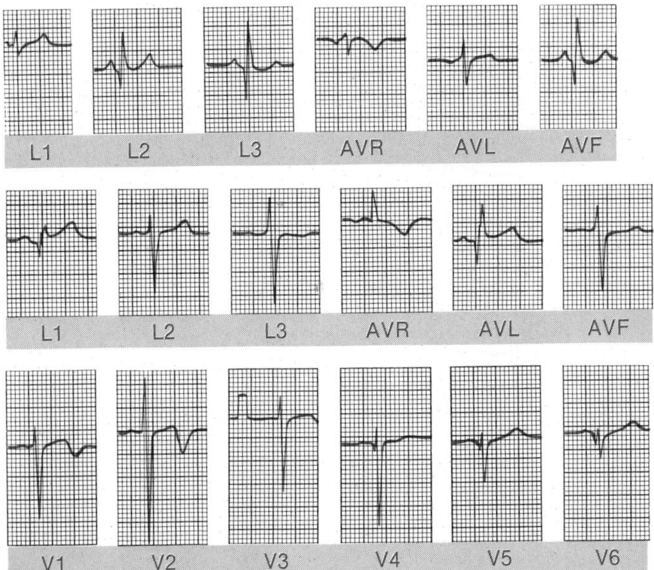

FIGURE 5–43. Hypertrophic cardiomyopathy simulating an inferior, high lateral (precordial leads, not shown, are normal) and anterolateral myocardial infarction in the upper, middle, and lower trace, respectively. (From Fisch, C.: Evolution of the clinical electrocardiogram. Reprinted by permission of the American College of Cardiology. J. Am. Coll. Cardiol. *14*:1127, 1989.)

by other ECG findings of COLD (p. 1590). However, since both COLD and myocardial infarction frequently coexist, differential diagnosis may at times be difficult or impossible (Fig. 5–14).

Abnormal Q waves, especially in lead III and rarely in lead aV_f, with an S wave in lead I, can be recorded in acute cor pulmonale due to *pulmonary embolism* (see Fig. 5–13, p. 127). Clockwise rotation with superior orientation of the initial vector is most likely responsible for the Q waves in lead III. A Q wave in lead II is rarely recorded. Occasionally acute pulmonary embolus may simulate anterior myocardial infarction.

Spontaneous pneumothorax, particularly on the left, may result in a pattern simulating anterior myocardial infarction with occasional absence of the R wave in all the precordial leads.

In LBBB the initial forces are directed from right to left and either superiorly or inferiorly. When the inferiorly directed forces dominate, a QS complex may be recorded in the precordial leads, simulating an anterior myocardial infarction. If the initial vector is oriented to the left and superiorly, a QS complex may be registered in the inferior leads, suggesting inferior myocardial infarction.

With left anterior divisional block, the transitional zone is shifted to the left, and an initial Q wave may appear in the right precordial leads. Loss of the forces normally contributed by the left anterior division results in a vector directed inferiorly, posteriorly, and to the right. Consequently, right precordial leads may register a qrS complex suggestive of an anteroseptal infarction. By placement of the electrodes one interspace lower, an rS complex can be recorded attesting to the positional nature of the Q wave.[65]

Noninfarction Q waves are frequent in WPW (p. 693). WPW type B, with the initial forces directed from right to left, registers a QS complex in the right precordial leads and may be mistaken for anteroseptal or anterior myocardial infarction. Rarely, preexcitation of the left lateral wall, with the vector oriented anteriorly and to the right, simulates lateral infarction. Most often, however, WPW simulates inferior infarction (Fig. 5–28). The Q waves recorded in leads II, III, and aV_f are due to superior orientation of the initial vector and may be seen with either type A or type B WPW.

In LVH, failure to record an R wave in leads V_1 to V_4 may suggest an anteroseptal myocardial infarction (Fig. 5–11). Similarly, reciprocal elevation of the ST segments in these leads may contribute to an erroneous diagnosis of myocardial infarction. The exact mechanism of the initial negative deflection of the QRS is not clear, but it may be related to posterior rotation or inferior orientation of the initial vector.

ST-SEGMENT AND T-WAVE CHANGES

ST-SEGMENT ELEVATION. In addition to the three most common organic causes of ST-segment elevations—acute myocardial infarction, pericarditis, and Prinzmetal's angina (Fig. 5–44)—ST-segment elevation is occasionally observed in acute cor pulmonale, hyperkalemia, cerebrovascular accidents, LVH, LBBB, hypertrophic cardiomyopathy, invasion of the heart by neoplastic tissue, and hypothermia. Elevation of the ST segment may also be an artifact caused by excessive inertia of the stylus of the electrocardiograph. In the normal heart the most common cause of ST-segment elevation is so-called *early repolarization*, a normal variant (Fig. 5–45).

T-WAVE ABNORMALITIES. A *primary T-wave change* indicates a regional alteration in the duration of the depolarized state. Some common clinical conditions associated with primary T-wave changes include myocardial ischemia, electrolyte abnormalities (Fig. 5–46), drugs, and a variety of primary myocardial and extracardiac disorders such as myocarditis and subarachnoid hemorrhage. A clinically important sequence of T-wave changes is one of abnormal baseline with normalization of the T wave during ischemia and return to the abnormal baseline after ischemia subsides. Unavailability of a control tracing could lead to an erroneous conclusion of non-Q wave infarction (Fig. 5–47).

Giant negative or, at times, upright T waves, usually associated with a prolonged Q-T interval, have been described in subarachnoid hemorrhage, complete heart block with marked bradycardia, myocardial ischemia (Fig. 5–36), hypertrophic cardiomyopathy,[140d,140e] and following cardiac resuscitation.

Secondary T-wave changes result from alterations of the timing or sequencing of depolarization or both, with an obligatory change of the order of repolarization. For example, in LBBB, left ventricular epicardial activation is delayed because of slow conduction through the ventricular myocardium. As a result, repolarization begins in the subendocardium and an inverted T wave is recorded in precordial leads. The change in the area of the QRS complex and T waves is identical but opposite in direction. Occasionally LBBB is associated with an upright T wave in the left ventricular leads, suggesting that in addition to altered activation due to LBBB, regional abnormalities of repolarization contribute to the T-wave morphology.

RATE-RELATED T-WAVE CHANGES. Postextrasystolic T-wave change was first described in 1915.[141] Since then, a number of mechanisms have been proposed to explain this observation, including an abnormal pathway of repolarization, prolonged diastolic filling time, and an abrupt change in the cycle length. Minor T-wave changes following an abrupt cycle change or after an interpolated ventricular premature complex may be recorded in normal tissue, while more pronounced T-wave alterations suggest an underlying myocardial disorder.

T-wave inversion is occasionally noted following supraventricular or ventricular tachycardia. The magnitude of the T-wave inversion varies, and when extreme, it may resemble the T-wave changes seen with cerebrovascular accidents or myocardial ischemia. The exact mechanism of the posttachycardia T wave is obscure.

T-WAVE ALTERNANS. Isolated T-wave alternans, i.e., without a change in either the QRS complex or the P wave, was first noted in the cat papillary muscle.[142] It is relatively rare and its mechanism not clear. Alternans of phases 2 and 3 of the action potential of the T wave has been recorded without any demonstrable change in phase 0, supporting the concept that isolated alternation of repolarization reflected in the T wave is possible. T-wave alternans of the type already mentioned is most often present during tachycardia or during a sudden change in cycle length. Isolated T-wave alternans, independent of tachycardia or premature systole, is nearly always associated with advanced heart disease or severe electrolyte disturbance (Fig. 5–48) or may follow cardiac resuscitation.

NOTCHED, BIFID T WAVES. Notched, bifid T waves are relatively common in the absence of heart disease, especially in children.[143] These waves may also be present in congenital organic heart disease, the pro-

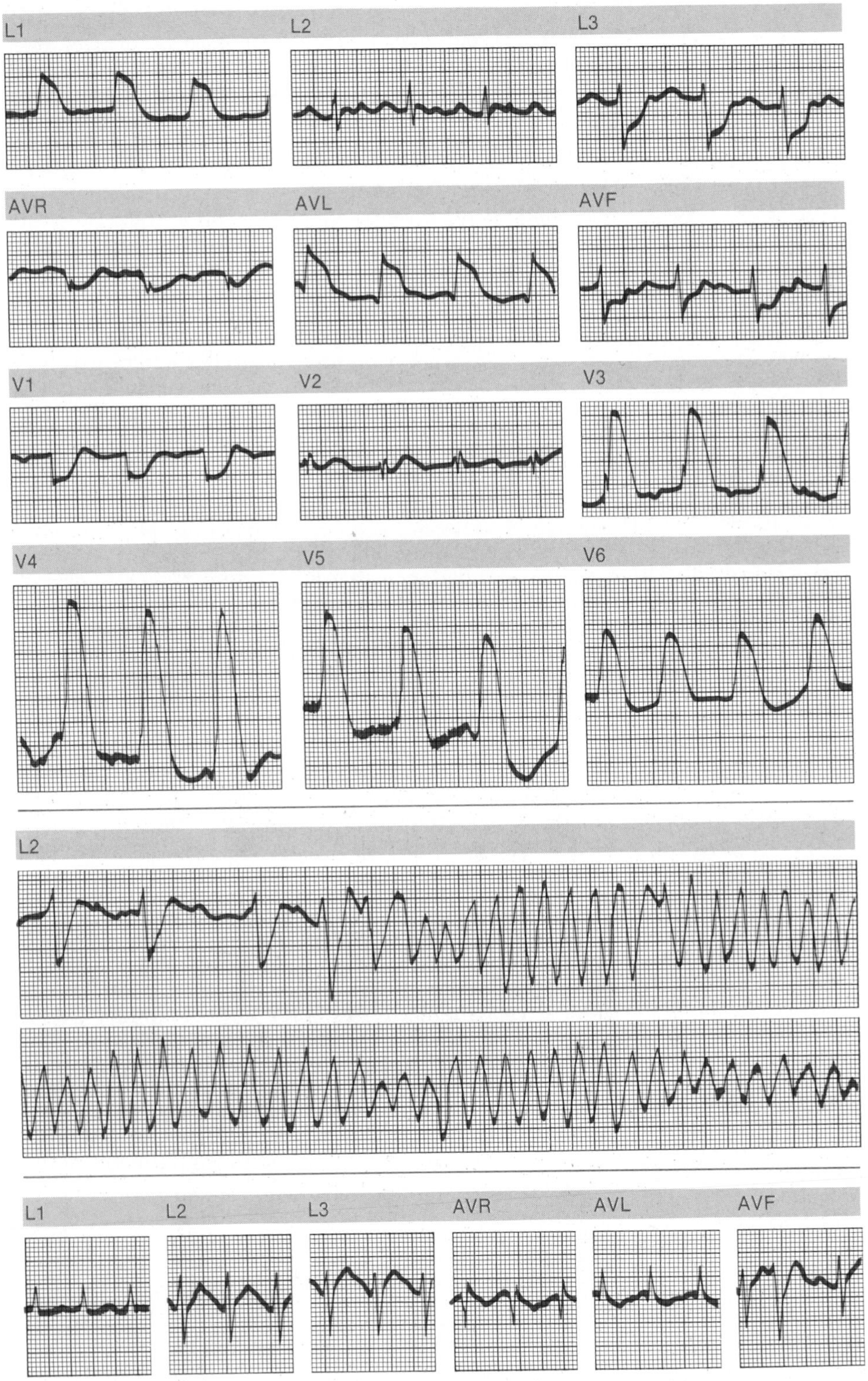

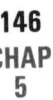

FIGURE 5-44. **Prinzmetal's angina. Current of injury resembling a monophasic action potential manifest by elevated ST segment over the anterior wall and reciprocal depression over the inferior wall is illustrated in top panel. Delayed A-V and intraventricular conduction, progressing to ventricular flutter and possibly ventricular fibrillation, is recorded in the middle trace. Sinus tachycardia with LAFB but otherwise normal tracing is present in the bottom trace.**

longed Q-T syndrome (Fig. 5-49), central nervous system disorders, alcoholic cardiomyopathy, and following the administration of drugs, especially the phenothiazines. The mechanism of bifid or notched T waves is unclear. It has been suggested that in some instances they are caused by nonuniform repolarization secondary to differential innervation of the anterior and posterior ventricular walls. It has also been proposed that in patients with left ventricular disease they may reflect regional delay of repolarization of the left ventricle.[143]

NONSPECIFIC ST-SEGMENT AND T-WAVE CHANGES. Although the ST segment and T wave represent different electrophysiological events and their respective changes may have different clinical connotations, the widespread practice among electrocardiographers is to refer to either one or both as *ST-T changes.* While it is more appropriate to discuss the two separately, it should be recognized that abnormalities of the ST segment and T wave frequently coexist.

Nondiagnostic ST-segment and T-wave changes are the most common ECG abnormality and account for about 50 per cent of the abnormal tracings recorded in a general hospital and in 2.4 per cent of all cardiograms.[144] An abnormal T wave is extremely common because the wave is highly sensitive to physiological, pharmacological, and organic changes and therefore is least likely to suggest a specific diagnosis.[145,146] This fact has been recognized since 1923, when Wilson first recorded inversion of the T wave following the ingestion of cold water.[147]

Although an abnormal T wave suggests the presence of an abnormal or, more appropriately, an altered state, it is recorded with relative frequency in the absence of any disorder

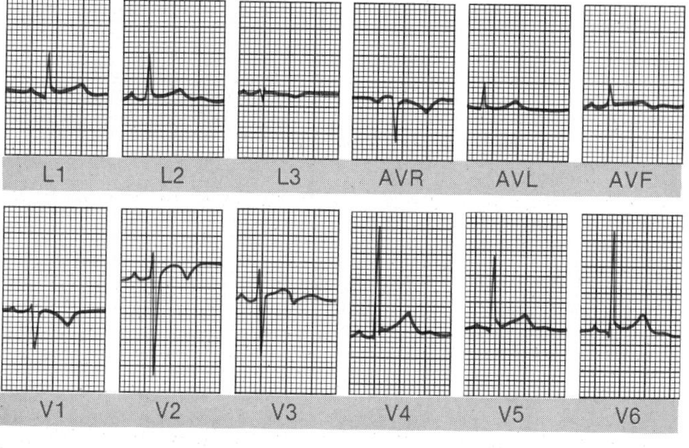

FIGURE 5-45. Normal tracing with juvenile T-wave inversion in leads V_1, V_2, and V_3 and early repolarization manifest by ST segment elevation in leads I, II, aV_f, V_4, V_5, and V_6.

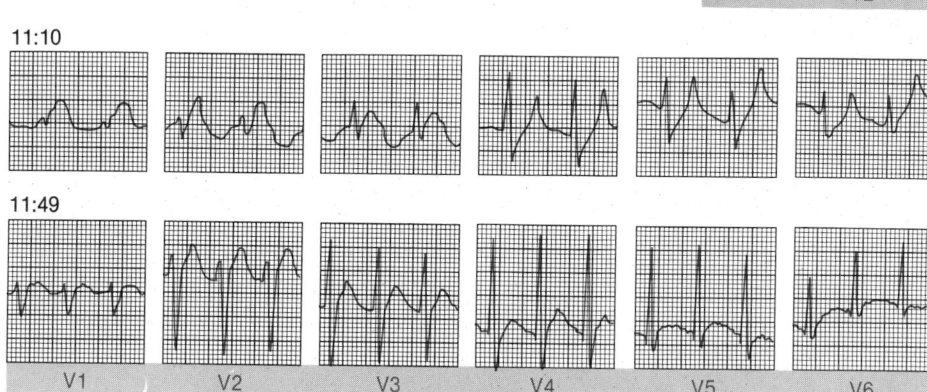

FIGURE 5-46. "Dialyzable" current of injury due to hyperkalemia manifested by ST segment elevation in leads V_1, V_2, V_3 is recorded at 11:10. At 11:49, following therapy, the ECG signs of hyperkalemia are no longer present.

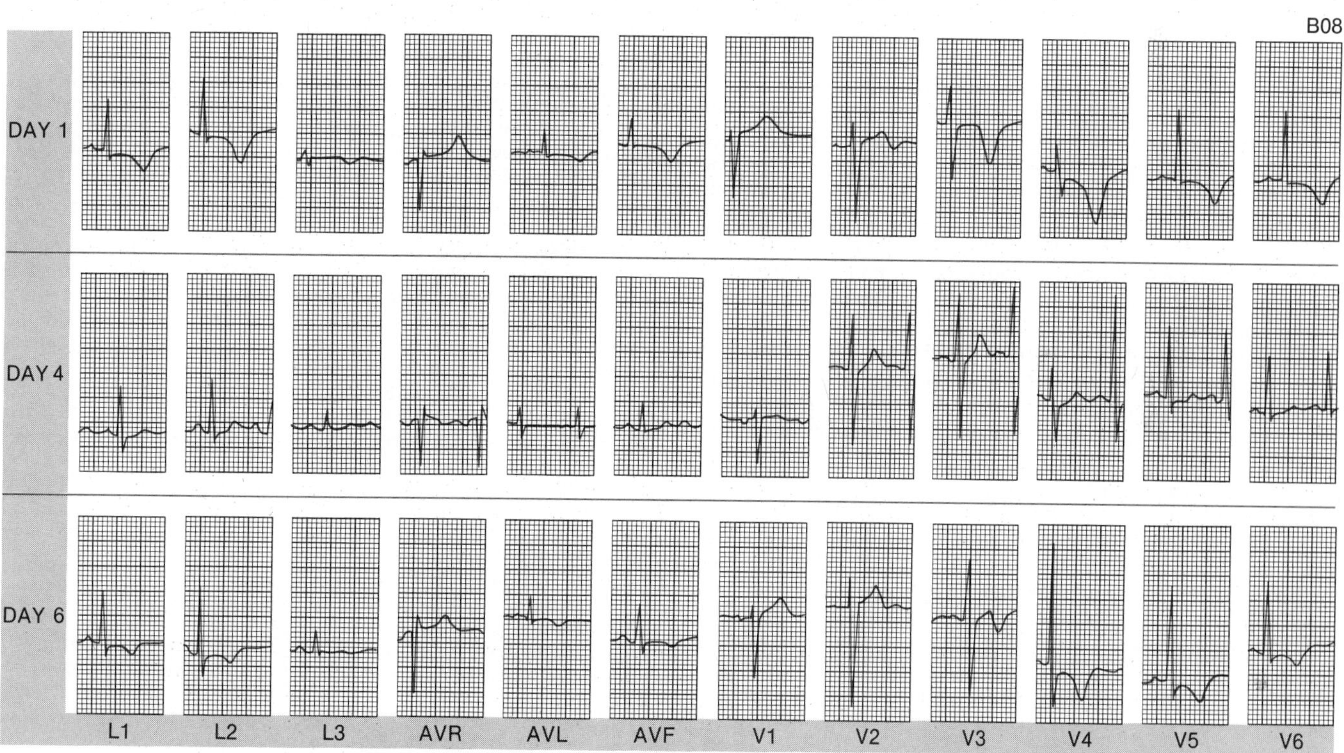

FIGURE 5-47. The top, control, trace recorded when the patient was asymptomatic illustrates symmetrical T-wave inversion consistent with ischemic heart disease. During pain, on day 4, the T waves normalized, only to return to control after the pain subsided. If the top trace had been unavailable, the sequence of changes noted in the middle and lower traces coupled with the history could have been mistaken for a new non-Q-wave infarction.

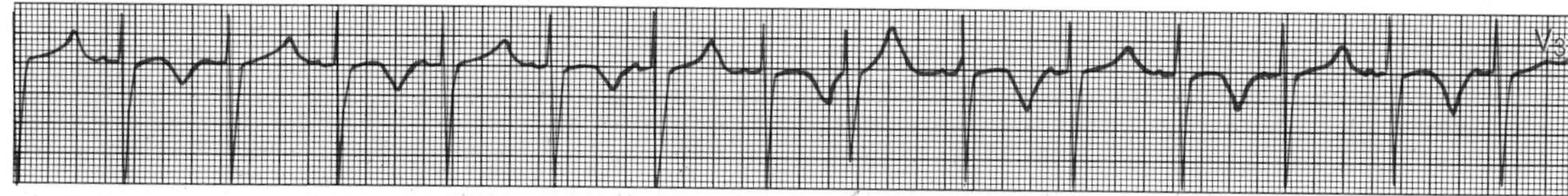

FIGURE 5-48. Isolated alternation of the T wave. The rhythm is sinus with occasional supraventricular premature complexes, probably atrial in origin. The QRS is normal in duration, with alternation of polarity of the T wave.

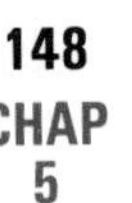

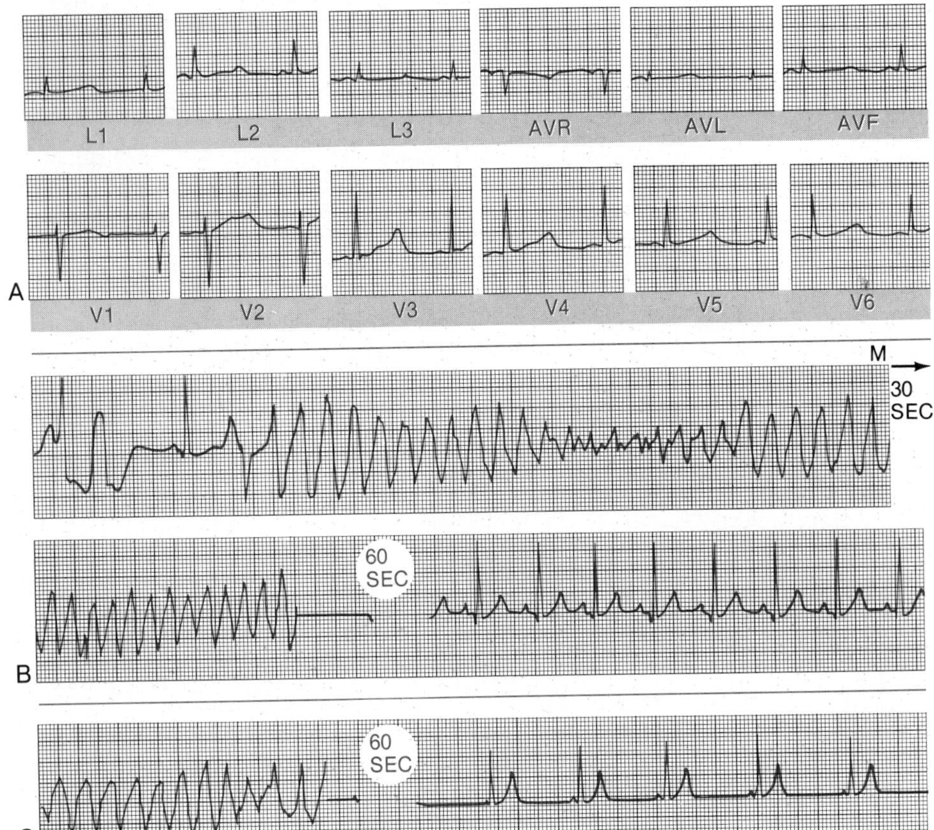

FIGURE 5-49. Congenital prolongation of the Q-T interval with spontaneous onset and termination of ventricular tachycardia and fibrillation. ***A,*** **The rhythm is sinus with a rate of 55 beats/min, the Q-T interval measures approximately 0.56 sec, and the T wave is notched, particularly in leads V_2 to V_4.** ***B,*** **The tracing is continuous and illustrates spontaneous onset and termination of a ventricular tachycardia and (?) fibrillation lasting about 90 sec.** ***C,*** **Spontaneous termination of an episode of ventricular tachycardia and fibrillation lasting about 90 sec. Both the Q-T interval and the T-wave morphology normalize after termination of ventricular arrhythmia. In addition to normalization of the Q-T interval and the T wave, the P-R interval is foreshortened. A possible mechanism that could explain the normalization of repolarization and shortening of the P-R interval is an increase in the level of catecholamines in response to the ventricular arrhythmia. The morphology of the T waves in C also suggests hyperkalemia.**

(Fig. 5–45), as a reflection of physiological influences, e.g., in highly trained athletes,[148,149] or during paroxysmal supraventricular tachycardia.[150] For these reasons, an isolated T-wave change must be interpreted with caution and must *always* be correlated with all available clinical and laboratory information. Misinterpretation of the significance of a T-wave abnormality is the most common cause of "atrogenic ECG heart disease." Attempts to identify the etiology of an abnormal ST segment, T wave, or ST-T segment in isolation from clinical and other laboratory findings often fail.

The specificity of the purported "classic" ST-T changes, such as those seen with LVH, digitalis administration, and ischemic heart disease, is relatively low. For example, a negative T wave reflecting persistence of a juvenile pattern cannot be differentiated from the symmetrically inverted T wave due to myocardial ischemia. The "classic" ST-T change of LVH may also be due to ischemic heart disease or digitalis, while the marked ST-segment depression due to ischemia or subendocardial infarction may be simulated by the administration of digitalis in the presence of moderate or severe disease. However, when correlated with clinical and other laboratory data, ST-T changes assume a greater predictive value. In a series of 410 abnormal tracings analyzed without regard to clinical data, 70 per cent could be interpreted only as "nonspecific ST-T change." This number was reduced to 10 per cent when such changes were correlated with available clinical information.[144]

The nonspecific and labile nature of the ST segment and the T wave, especially the latter, is expected. Repolarization is a much more diverse process than depolarization. Depolarization is rapid, with a reasonably uniform potential difference across the boundary of activation, and is reflected in the rate of rise of phase 0 and the amplitude of the action potential (p. 358). Repolarization, displayed as the ST segment and T wave, reflects phases 2 and 3 of the action potential, is considerably longer, and is nonuniform, with many simultaneous boundaries and with differing potentials across various boundaries. It has been shown that shortening of the monophasic action potential by as little as 12 to 18 msec will alter the morphology of the T wave, and importantly, the change can be seen with involvement of 10 per cent or less of the myocardial mass.[151] The magnitude of the T-wave changes, unlike that of the QRS complex, is not related to the mass of the myocardium. This condition has been ascribed to cancellation of repolarization voltages and to uneven contributions from the different regions of repolarization to the genesis of the T wave. Such experimental findings explain, at least partially, the nonspecific character of ST-segment and T-wave changes.

A number of the clinical conditions which may alter the ST segment and T waves are listed in Table 5–6.

U-WAVE ABNORMALITIES. An abnormal U wave may be increased in amplitude, inverted, or prolonged. A negative U wave is documented in about 1 per cent of cardiograms recorded in a general hospital. An exaggerated upright U wave may be due to hypokalemia, a variety of drugs (particularly digitalis), and some of the antiarrhythmic agents (e.g., amiodarone).

The most common causes of a *negative U wave* are hypertension, aortic and mitral valve disease, RVH, and myocardial ischemia (Fig. 5–36).[103a,152] A negative U wave can occasionally be found in other metabolic

TABLE 5-6 CAUSES OF ST-SEGMENT AND T-WAVE CHANGES (SELECTED)

Physiological:
Position, temperature, hyperventilation, anxiety, food (glucose), tachycardia, neurogenic influences, physical training
Pharmacological:
Digitalis, antiarrhythmic and psychotrophic drugs (phenothiazines, tricyclics, lithium)
Extracardiac Disorders:
Electrolyte abnormalities, cerebrovascular accidents, shock, anemia, allergic reactions, infections, endocrine disorders, acute abdominal disorders, pulmonary embolism
Primary Myocardial Disease:
Congestive, hypertrophic, postpartum cardiomyopathy, myocarditis
Secondary Myocardial Disease:
Amyloidosis, hemochromatosis, neoplasm, sarcoidosis, connective tissue, neuromuscular disorders
Ischemic Heart Disease:
Myocardial infarction

or organic diseases. In hypertension, a negative U wave may be the earliest sign of myocardial involvement, appearing long before any change in the T wave, and has been reported in about 16 per cent of ECG's with an upright T wave and 45 per cent with negative T waves. It may revert to normal with control of the hypertension.[153] The majority of patients with aortic regurgitation and about 10 per cent of patients with aortic stenosis manifest negative U waves. Approximately 5 and 80 per cent of patients with systolic and diastolic overload of the right ventricle, respectively, manifest negative U waves in leads II, III, V_1, and V_2. In essence, a negative U wave, even as an isolated finding in an otherwise normal ECG, is strongly suggestive of a pathophysiological state.

Q-T INTERVAL ABNORMALITY (see also p. 122). *Shortening of the Q-T interval* may be recorded with hyperkalemia, digitalis, hypercalcemia, and acidosis. *Prolongation of the Q-T interval* may be primary and independent of the QRS, or it may reflect secondary changes of repolarization due to abnormal depolarization, or a combination of the two. Prolongation of the Q-T interval, independent of QRS duration, can be congenital (Fig. 5–49) or acquired.[154,155] Acquired disorders include ischemic heart disease, hypothermia, cardiomyopathy, mitral valve prolapse, complete heart block, the condition following cardiac resuscitation, electrolyte changes, and administration of drugs.[156–158] Q-T interval prolongation is a relatively frequent complication of acquired cerebral lesions, especially subarachnoid hemorrhage, and can also be present during and following neurosurgical procedures.

ELECTRICAL ALTERNANS. Alternation of amplitude and direction of the QRS complex was noted in the experimental animal and humans as early as 1909 and 1910, respectively,[159,160] followed by documentation of alternation of the P wave, ST segment, and T wave (Fig. 5–48). Isolated *alternation of the P wave* is seen frequently in the experimental setting but is rare in humans. Most often it accompanies alternation of the QRS complex and occasionally the QRS complex and the T wave. The latter is referred to as *total alternans* and suggests pericardial effusion, usually due to malignancy and frequently associated with tamponade or impending tamponade.

Although pericardial effusion is the most common cause of alternation of the QRS complex (p. 120), *QRS alternans* is also seen with myocardial ischemia and myocardial disease due to other causes. Two mechanisms of QRS alternans have been proposed: positional oscillation and aberrancy of intraventricular conduction. The early suggestion that oscillation or alternation of position is the mechanism of alternans of the QRS complex[161] was proven by means of echocardiography.[162] The concept of oscillation also explains the fact that P-wave alternans is seen predominantly with massive pericardial effusion.

ST segment alternans has been described in dogs after ligation of the coronary artery, in severely ill infants with congenital heart disease, and in patients with Prinzmetal's angina. *T-wave alternans* is discussed on page 145. *U-wave alternans* is least common and very difficult to recognize.

The mechanism of alternans in severe myocardial disorders but in the absence of pericardial effusion is obscure. It has been ascribed to uneven duration of the excited state or to two alternating foci of impulse formation. However, the fact that alternation of depolarization, activation, and repolarization can be recorded in a single cell suggests that the mechanism is probably related to transmembrane ionic fluxes. Alternans of a human atrial monophasic action potential adds further credence to the primary role of transmembrane ionic events.

THE OSBORNE WAVE. An Osborne wave, seen in hypothermia, is a deflection inscribed between the QRS complex and the beginning of the ST segment (Fig. 5–50).[163] It has been variously suggested that this wave reflects delay of depolarization, a current of injury, or early repolarization. In the left ventricular leads the polarity of the wave is positive and its amplitude is inversely related to body temperature. The electrophysiological mechanism of the Osborne wave remains unclear.

ABNORMAL ECG IN ABSENCE OF CLINICAL HEART DISEASE

Abnormal ECG's may be recorded in patients with clinically normal hearts.[164,164a] The abnormalities may be those of the QRS, ST segment, or T wave. Common abnormalities of the QRS include QS complexes in lead aV_l, or QS or QR complexes in leads III and aV_f, a QS complex in leads V_1 and V_2, a tall R wave in leads V_1 and V_2,[165,166] and high voltage of the R wave over the left ventricle. A frequent "normal" alteration of the ST segment is an elevation, the so-called early repolarization, which may be recorded in the inferior, left precordial, and rarely right precordial leads. Abnormal T waves include persistence of juvenile T-wave inversion over the right precordium (p. 122), isolated midprecordial T-wave inversion (Fig. 5–45), and terminal T-wave inversion associated with ST-segment elevation due to early repolarization and right precordial T-wave inversion in middle-aged women. A variety of physiological influences alter the T wave of a normal heart (Table 5–6).

An abnormal ECG in the absence of clinical evidence of heart disease in the young should be evaluated carefully, because the prevalence of true heart disease in this setting is low and the chances are high that the tracing is false positive for disease.[167]

THE ECG AND ELECTROLYTE ABNORMALITIES

Potassium (K)

HYPERKALEMIA. There is a good correlation between plasma K and the surface ECG in experimental hyperkalemia. The earliest ECG change, at a plasma level of about 5.7 mEq/

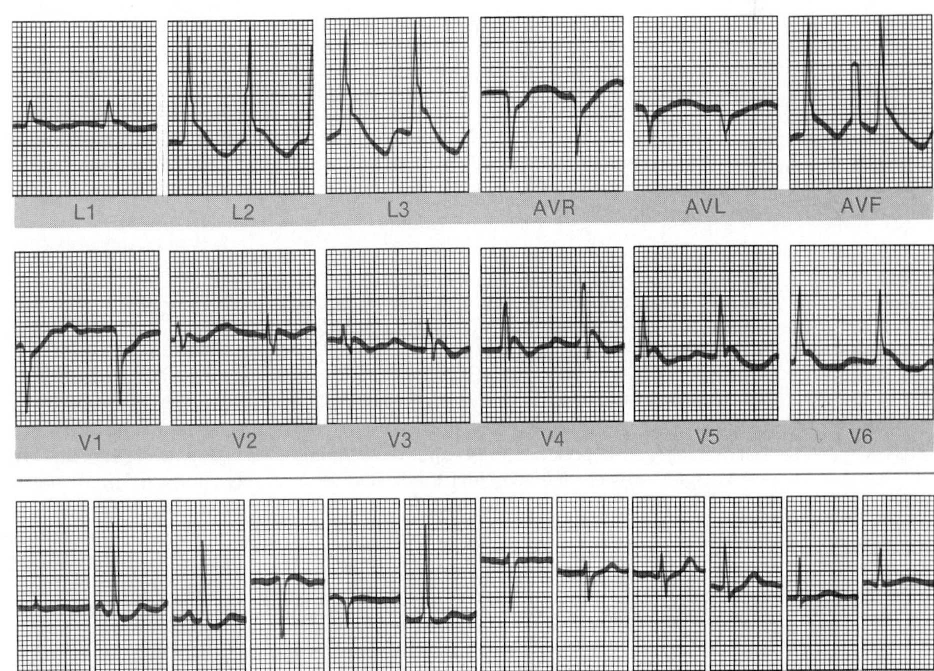

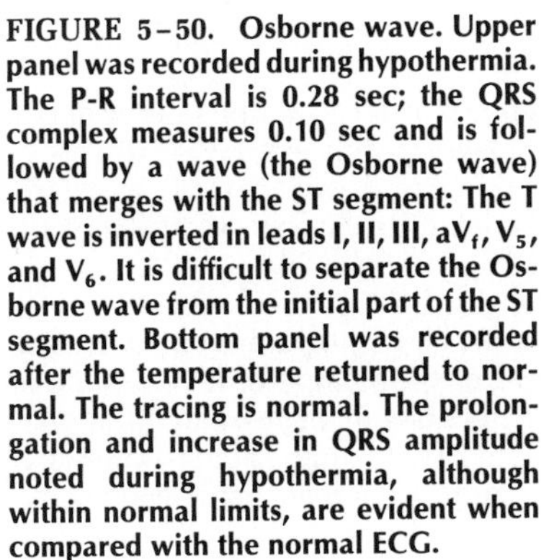
FIGURE 5–50. Osborne wave. Upper panel was recorded during hypothermia. The P-R interval is 0.28 sec; the QRS complex measures 0.10 sec and is followed by a wave (the Osborne wave) that merges with the ST segment: The T wave is inverted in leads I, II, III, aV_f, V_5, and V_6. It is difficult to separate the Osborne wave from the initial part of the ST segment. Bottom panel was recorded after the temperature returned to normal. The tracing is normal. The prolongation and increase in QRS amplitude noted during hypothermia, although within normal limits, are evident when compared with the normal ECG.

liter, is a tall, peaked, most often symmetrical T wave with a narrow base and a normal or decreased Q-Tc interval. The QRS complex widens uniformly at a level of 9 to 11 mEq/liter and an occasional acute current of injury resembling myocardial infarction may be present. Reduction in P-wave amplitude, intraatrial conduction delay, and P-R interval prolongation are recorded at a plasma level of about 7.0 mEq/liter. At plasma K levels of about 8.4 mEq/liter or higher, the P wave is no longer recognizable. When the plasma concentration exceeds 12 mEq/liter, either ventricular fibrillation or arrest follows. SA node fibers, being more resistant to the depressive action of K than is atrial myocardium, continue to generate impulses that are now delayed in their exit or may fail to propagate because of depressed intraatrial conduction. The result may be Wenckebach (type I) or Mobitz (type II) sinoatrial (SA) block (p. 710). Junctional escape and junctional rhythm are relatively common in experimental hyperkalemia.

In clinical hyperkalemia, abnormalities of impulse information and conduction appear at K levels lower than those observed in the experimental animal, and the correlation between plasma K and the ECG is less reliable. A tall, peaked, symmetrical T wave with a narrow base, the so-called "tented" T wave, is the earliest ECG abnormality, usually best seen in leads II, III, V_2, V_3, and V_4. The pointed, symmetrical appearance and narrow base of the T wave help to differentiate the effect of hyperkalemia from other causes of tall T waves, including normal variants. The tented appearance and the narrow base are probably more characteristic of hyperkalemia than is the amplitude of the T wave. A decrease in amplitude of the R wave, appearance of a prominent S wave, widening of the QRS complex, depression of the ST segment, and an occasional elevation of the ST segment evolve as plasma K continues to rise and approaches 8 to 9 mEq/liter (Fig. 5-51). A decrease in amplitude and prolongation of the P wave and lengthening of the P-R interval followed by disappearance of the P wave often makes recognition of arrhythmias in hyperkalemia difficult, if not impossible. At times hyperkalemia induces a current of injury called *dialyzable current of injury*, which may be mistaken for acute ischemia (Fig. 5-46).

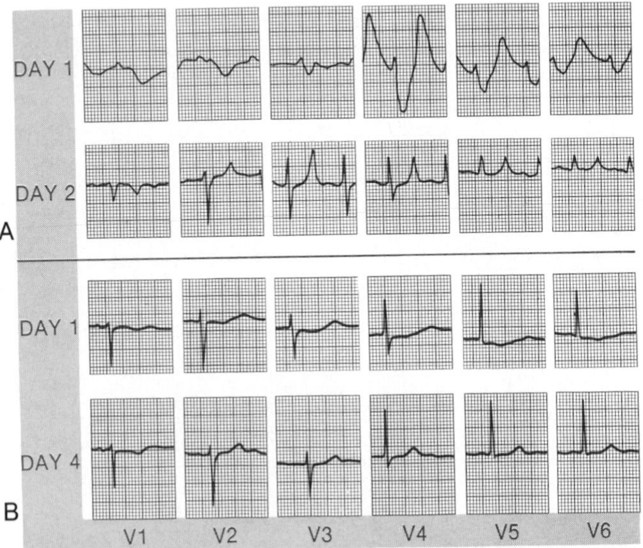

FIGURE 5-51. ECG changes in hyperkalemia *(A)* and hypokalemia *(B)*. Panel *A*, On day 1, at a K^+ level of 8.6 mEq/liter the P wave is no longer recognizable and the QRS complex is diffusely prolonged. Initial and terminal QRS delay is characteristic of K^+-induced intraventricular conduction and is best illustrated in leads V_2 and V_6. On day 2, at a K^+ level of 5.8 mEq/liter, the P wave is recognizable with a P-R interval of 0.24 sec, the duration of the QRS complex is approximately 0.10 sec, and the T waves are characteristically "tented." Panel *B*, On day 1, at a K^+ level of 1.5 mEq/liter the T and U waves are merged. The U wave is prominent and the Q-U interval prolonged. On day 4, at a K^+ level of 3.7 mEq/liter the tracing is normal.

With hyperkalemia, depression of intraventricular conduction is characteristically diffuse and fairly uniform and results in prolongation of both the initial and terminal parts of the QRS complex. The resulting pattern may resemble RBBB, LBBB, left anterior or posterior divisional block, or a combination of the four. When the ECG resembles RBBB, the initial phase of the QRS complex is prolonged, in contrast to the conventional RBBB, in which only the terminal portion of the QRS complex is delayed. Similarly, when the ECG simulates LBBB, an S wave indicates slowing of the terminal portion of the QRS (Fig. 5-51). In conventional LBBB, on the other hand, prolongation involves only the initial component of the QRS complex.

In humans, as in animals, SA block (p. 710), either Wenckebach (type I) or Mobitz (type II), passive or accelerated junctional or ventricular escape rhythms may be present. Potassium may normalize physiologically or functionally inverted T waves, but as a rule it has no effect on T-wave inversion due to organic disorders or drugs.

HYPOKALEMIA. The ECG in *hypokalemia* is characterized by gradual depression of the ST segment, decrease of T-wave amplitude, occasionally inversion of the T wave, and a prominent U wave but without a significant change in the Q-T interval (Fig. 5-51). In advanced hypokalemia the ST segment gradually fuses with the U wave, the latter greater in amplitude than the T wave. An increase in amplitude of the QRS complex may be present. There is reasonable correlation between ECG changes and K concentrations below 2.3 or 3.0 mEq/liter. Prominent U waves with ST-segment and T-wave changes are not specific for hypokalemia, however. Such abnormalities can be the result of administration of digitalis and other drugs, ventricular hypertrophy, and bradycardia.

Calcium (Ca)

The effects of Ca on the ECG were recognized in 1922.[168] In general, the ECG changes due to alteration in Ca concentrations correlate with the effect of Ca ions on the transmembrane action potential. Changes in duration of phase 2 parallel the altered duration of the ST segment and the Q-T interval.

Hypocalcemia prolongs phase 2, reflected by prolongation of the ST segment and Q-T interval (Fig. 5-51). The Q-aT (Q to the apex of the T wave) and the Q-T intervals are prolonged, but the Q-Tc interval rarely exceeds 140 per cent of the normal. If longer, the U wave is likely to be included in the measurement. Hypocalcemia does not affect phase 3 of the action potential or the T wave. Hypocalcemia with hyperkalemia, most often seen in patients with chronic renal disease, results in a prolonged ST segment and a "tented" T wave (Fig. 5-52). Hypocalcemia and hypokalemia exhibit a prolonged ST segment and a prominent terminal wave that includes both T and U waves.

Hypercalcemia shortens phase 2 of the action potential and the ST segment. The Q-T interval is shortened (Fig. 5-52), the ST segment occasionally depressed, and the T wave inverted.[169] A prominent J wave similar to that of hypothermia has been observed.[170]

The correlation between the Q-T interval and serum Ca concentration is unpredictable, largely because the Q-T duration is affected by factors other than calcium levels, such as age, sex, heart rate, myocardial disease, drugs, and other electrolytes. It has been suggested that when factors known to alter the Q-T interval are eliminated, a reasonably good correlation is found between the ECG and calcium levels. This assumption is supported by the fact that Ca levels in pure hypocalcemia induced by EDTA show a reasonably good correlation with the Q-T interval. Of the three intervals—Q-T, Q-oT (Q to the onset of the T wave), and Q-aT (Q to the apex of the T wave)—the Q-aT interval can be measured with greatest accuracy and correlates best with the Ca level.

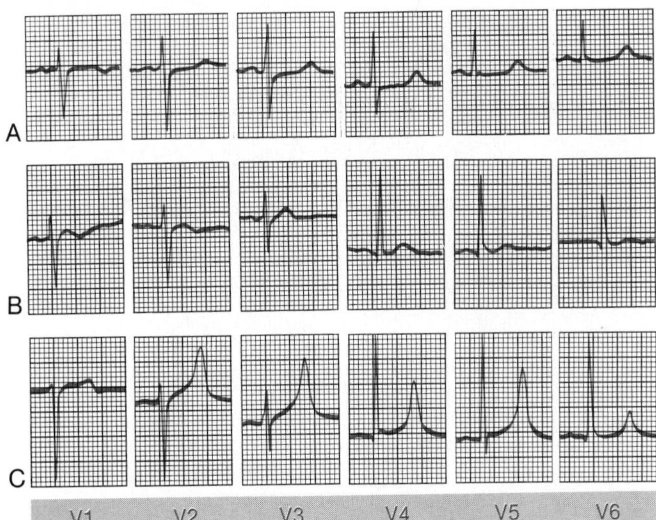

FIGURE 5-52. ECG changes of hypocalcemia, hypercalcemia, and hypocalcemia with hyperkalemia. ***A,*** **At a Ca^{++} level of 5.7 mg/dl the QT interval is prolonged, characteristic of hypocalcemia.** ***B,*** **Tracing recorded at a Ca^{++} level of 16.0 mg/dl shows the short ST segment of hypercalcemia.** ***C,*** **Tracing recorded at a K^+ level of 6.0 mEq/liter, Ca^{++} of 5.5 mg/dl, and phosphorus of 12.0 mg/dl. The prolonged Q-T interval and the tented T wave reflect hypocalcemia and hyperkalemia often present in chronic renal disease.**

Magnesium

Administration of magnesium may result in shortening of the Q-T interval, prolongation of the P-R interval, QRS complex, and intraatrial conduction. As a rule, however, abnormalities of the ST segment due to hypermagnesemia cannot be identified on the ECG because the changes are dominated by calcium. Hypomagnesemia cannot be recognized on the ECG.[171]

EFFECTS OF DRUGS ON THE ECG

The effect of antiarrhythmic drugs on the ECG is considered in Chapter 24.

Digitalis

(See p. 691)

Alterations of the ST segment and the T wave are the earliest recognizable changes due to the digitalis glycosides. The T-wave amplitude is lowered, and the ST segment is depressed and shortened, with occasional appearance of a prominent U wave.[172] While the "characteristic" digitalis-induced ST segment is described as sagging, it is often difficult if not impossible to differentiate it from ST-segment depression of other causes. When the ST segment is also shortened, digitalis is the likely cause of the depression. ST-segment displacement due to digitalis may be greatly exaggerated by myocardial disease, tachycardia, and high-amplitude QRS complexes. Rarely, digitalis causes symmetrical inversion of the T wave similar to that in pericarditis and ischemia, but there is usually associated shortening of the Q-T interval. A peaked, "tented" T wave, probably due to concomitant hyperkalemia, can also be present. Digitalis has no significant effect on depolarization of the atrium or ventricle. Consequently, prolongation of intraatrial and intraventricular conduction is rare.

DIGITALIS-INDUCED ARRHYTHMIAS. Digitalis has been known to induce nearly every known arrhythmia.[173,174]

1. Ectopic rhythms due to enhanced automaticity, reentry, or delayed diastolic afterdepolarizations (Fig. 5-53): atrial tachycardia with block (Fig. 24-13, p. 684), atrial fibrillation and flutter, nonparoxysmal junctional tachycardia (Fig. 24-17, p. 687), ventricular premature contractions, ventricular tachycardia (Fig. 5-53), ventricular flutter and fibrillation, multiple ectopic rhythms, bidirectional ventricular tachycardia (Fig. 5-54), or accelerated escape.
2. Depression of pacemaker: SA node arrest.
3. Depression of conduction: SA block, AV block, exit block, or reciprocation.
4. AV dissociation: Suppression of the dominant pacemaker with passive escape of the lower junctional focus or inappropriate acceleration of a subsidiary pacemaker, or, rarely, dissociation within the AV junction (double junctional tachycardia).

Arrhythmias identical to those due to digitalis toxicity can also be caused by heart disease, drugs other than digitalis, and a variety of extracardiac factors.

THERAPEUTIC AND TOXIC EFFECTS. Appearance of ectopic rhythms in the course of digitalis administration is nearly always a sign of toxicity. On the other hand, depression of AV conduction may at times be a desirable therapeutic endpoint. Acknowledging that some degree of overlap is unavoidable and that the clinical significance of an arrhythmia may differ depending on the setting, the effects of digitalis on the ECG can be divided into three general groups—therapeutic, excessive and/or toxic, and unequivocally toxic.

The wide spectrum of arrhythmias induced by digitalis and the coexistence of a number of different arrhythmias in the same tracing can be explained by the interplay between digitalis and myocardial and extracardiac factors on the electrophysiological properties of cardiac tissues. The drug may have different effects on the same specialized tissue, i.e., it may depress conduction or enhance automaticity, or both. Also, digitalis may act directly on the specialized tissue or its action may be mediated through the sympathetic or parasympathetic system or both.[175] In addition, the sensitivity of the tissues to digitalis may be altered by factors such as a changing acid-base balance, plasma and intracellular electrolyte levels, oxygen tension, and mechanical stretch.

Selected arrhythmias due to digitalis have been chosen for the following discussion here because of their frequency and relatively high specificity for digitalis toxicity.

ATRIAL TACHYCARDIA WITH BLOCK (see p. 684). The cause of this arrhythmia can be ascribed almost equally to severe heart disease and to digitalis toxicity. The diagnosis of atrial tachycardia with block may occasionally be difficult. At rapid rates it resembles atrial flutter. The amplitude of the atrial deflections may be low, and only careful attention to lead V_1 may disclose the true nature of the arrhythmia.

NONPAROXYSMAL JUNCTIONAL TACHYCARDIA (see also p. 687). In the proper setting, this arrhythmia is highly specific for digitalis excess or toxicity.[176] Other less common causes of nonparoxysmal junctional tachycardia—acute myocardial infarction, open heart surgery, myocarditis, and general anesthesia—must be ruled out. Nonparoxysmal junctional tachycardia differs from paroxysmal junctional or supraventricular tachycardia. It appears and disappears gradually and, when repetitive, the coupling, or relation of the first ectopic complex to the dominant impulse, varies. The rate is 70 to 130 beats/min. AV dissociation resulting from acceleration of the AV junctional pacemaker is recorded in 85 per cent of patients. The ectopic junctional focus activates both atria and ventricles in the remaining 15 per cent. Rarely, two junctional foci coexist, one controlling the atria and the other the ventricles, resulting in a double junctional tachycardia.

In the absence of exit block, the rhythm in nonparoxysmal junctional tachycardia is generally perfectly regular and the diagnosis usually simple. Recognition becomes more difficult in the presence of exit block. A high degree of exit block may suggest a slow junctional rhythm or AV block. If the exit block is Mobitz (type II) (p. 710) with 3:2 exit block, a bigeminal rhythm appears, with longer cycles exact multiples of shorter cycles. If the exit block is Wenckebach (type I), the gradually shortening R-R interval and lack of the expected relationship of the long pause to the shorter cycles (i.e., the pause is not a

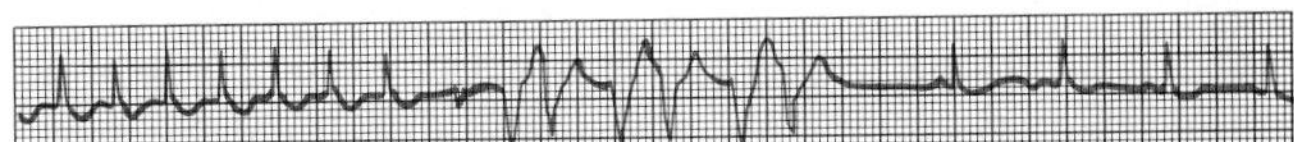

FIGURE 5-53. Supraventricular tachycardia treated with large doses of digitalis terminating with ventricular tachycardia with a 3:2 Wenckebach (type 1) exit block. Atrial tachycardia at a rate of 230 beats/min is followed by a bigeminal rhythm, with ventricular complexes all of similar morphology. The longer cycles are less than twice the shorter cycle, suggesting a ventricular tachycardia with a 3:2 Wenckebach exit block. The interectopic ventricular cycle length is 0.22 sec. One possible mechanism of the ventricular tachycardia is delayed afterdepolarization, or "triggered" automaticity.

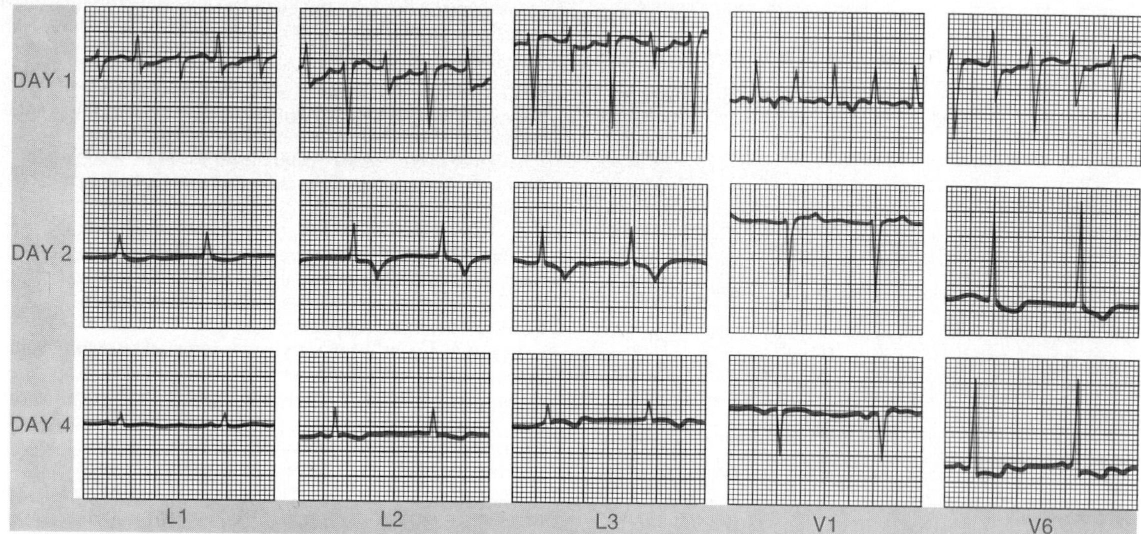

FIGURE 5-54. Bidirectional ventricular tachycardia and junctional tachycardia due to digitalis. On day 1, the ECG shows bidirectional ventricular tachycardia with alternation of the axis and RBBB. The divisions of the left bundle are the site of the tachycardia. On day 2, after discontinuation of digitalis, the rhythm is junctional at a rate of 83 beats/min, with retrograde P waves in leads II and III and an R-P interval of about 0.20 sec. On day 4, normal sinus rhythm is accompanied by nonspecific T-wave changes in leads II, III, and V_6.

multiple of the shorter cycle), atrial fibrillation may be suggested. Only a careful search for the Wenckebach structure will reveal the true nature of the arrhythmia. Nonparoxysmal junctional tachycardia with an irregular ventricular response without conforming to the Wenckebach (type I) or Mobitz (type II) structure precludes the diagnosis, and nonparoxysmal junctional tachycardia cannot be differentiated from atrial fibrillation. Occasionally, this arrhythmia is masked and becomes evident with slowing of the dominant rhythm; it may appear as nonparoxysmal junctional tachycardia or as a single accelerated escape impulse.

VENTRICULAR ARRHYTHMIAS. Ventricular premature contractions (VPC) are the most common manifestation of digitalis toxicity but, at the same time, are the least specific as a sign of glycoside toxicity. None of the morphological features of the QRS complex helps to differentiate VPC due to digitalis from those of other causes. The exception is ventricular bigeminy, with accurate coupling but varying morphology —a criterion that is suggestive of digitalis toxicity.

The problems of recognition associated with digitalis-induced VPC are also applicable to ventricular tachycardia. Ventricular tachycardia with exit block (Fig. 5-52) and bidirectional ventricular tachycardia (Fig. 5-54) strongly suggest digitalis intoxication. When the ventricular tachycardia originates in the divisions of the left bundle branch, the QRS complex may be normal in duration, and the diagnosis rests on the presence of ventricular capture and fusion complexes. Studies in animals and man confirm that narrow QRS complex tachycardias may be ventricular in origin.

In rare instances, ventricular parasystole (p. 717) is due to digitalis. This is quite likely when parasystole is accompanied by other arrhythmias known to be due to digitalis intoxication.

Digitalis-induced ventricular fibrillation is rarely, if ever, the initial manifestation of digitalis toxicity but is usually preceded by other digitalis-induced arrhythmias. It is seldom recorded in humans.

AV DISSOCIATION (see also p. 715). AV dissociation appearing in the course of digitalis administration is strongly indicative of digitalis intoxication.

AV CONDUCTION DELAY. Depression of AV conduction may be due to a vagal effect of the glycoside and can be reversed with atropine or catecholamines released during normal activities or during exercise. Such depression may also be due to a "direct" extravagal effect of the drug on the cell.[175]

In contrast to ectopy, which is a sign of digitalis toxicity, depression of conduction may be either a desirable therapeutic effect or a manifestation of toxicity. The differentiation of the two is a clinical decision. For example, in atrial fibrillation and atrial flutter depression of AV conduction is desirable. In the presence of sinus rhythm, however, AV delay, other than simple prolongation of the P-R interval, is, with rare exception, evidence of digitalis overdose. Although AV block in the presence of sinus rhythm is a frequently mentioned sign of digitalis intoxication, third-degree AV block is a relatively rare manifestation of glycoside toxicity.

ACCELERATED JUNCTIONAL ESCAPE. This arrhythmia is seen in the same clinical conditions as is nonparoxysmal junctional tachycardia and its clinical significance is probably the same. Accelerated junctional escape follows the rules set for cardiac arrhythmias induced by delayed afterdepolarization[177] and may be the clinical counterpart of the arrhythmias induced in the Purkinje fiber and the intact animal.

REFERENCES

THE NORMAL ELECTROCARDIOGRAM AND VECTORCARDIOGRAM

1. Macfarlane, P. W., and Lawrie, V.T.D.: Comprehensive Electrocardiology, Vol. I. New York, Pergamon Press, 1989.
2. Horan, L. G.: Manifest orientation: The theoretical link between the anatomy of the heart and the clinical electrocardiogram. J. Am. Coll. Cardiol. 9:1049, 1987.
3. Burch, G. E., and DePasquale, N. P.: A History of Electrocardiography. Chicago, Year Book Medical Publishers, 1964.
4. Krikler, D. M.: Historical aspects of electrocardiography. Cardiol. Clin. 5:349, 1987.
5. Fisch, C.: Evolution of the clinical electrocardiogram. J. Am. Coll. Cardiol. *14*:1127, 1989.
6. Waller, A. D.: A demonstration on man of electromotive changes accompanying the heart's beat. J. Physiol. *8*:229, 1887.
7. Burchell, H. B.: A centennial note on Waller and the first human electrocardiogram. Am. J. Cardiol. *59*:979, 1987.
8. Einthoven, W.: Selected Papers on Electrocardiography. *In* Snellen, A. (ed.): Leiden, the Netherlands, University Press, 1977.
9. Lewis, T.: The Mechanism and Graphic Registration of the Heart Beat. London, Shaw and Sons, Ltd., 1920, p. 228.
10. Wilson, F. N.: Selected Papers, Johnston. Edited by F.D.E. Lepeschkin. Ann Arbor, MI, Edward Brothers, Inc., 1954.
11. Chou, T. C.: Electrocardiography in clinical practice. 2nd ed. Orlando, Grune and Stratton, 1986.
12. Durrer, D.: Selected Papers. Edited by F. L. Meijler and H. B. Burchell. Amsterdam, North Holland Publishing Co., 1986.
13. Dunn, M. I., and Lipman, B. S.: Lipman-Massie Clinical Electrocardiography. Chicago, Year Book Medical Publishers, Inc., 1989.
14. Fisch, C.: Electrocardiography of Arrhythmias. Philadelphia, Lea and Febiger, 1989.

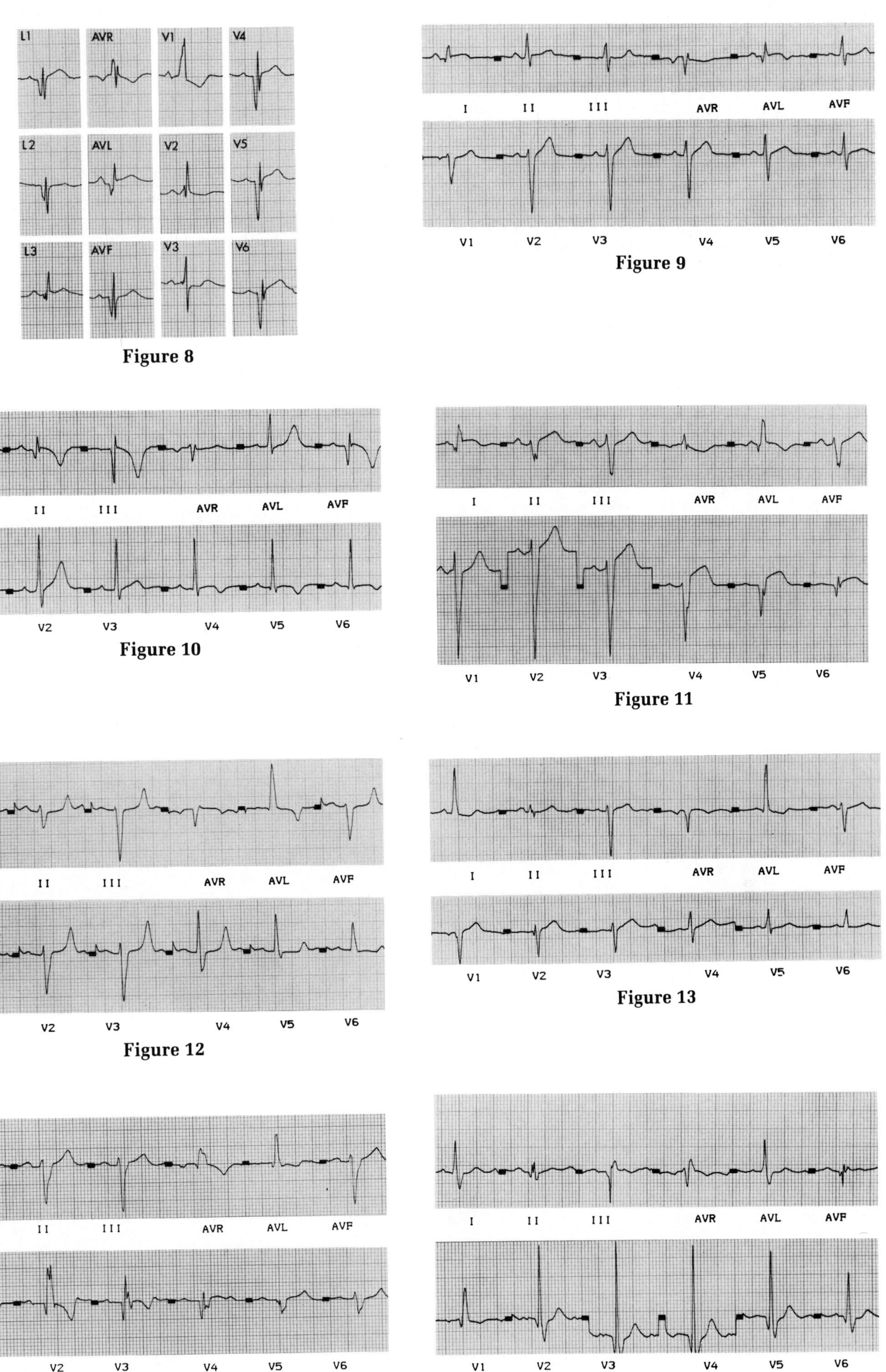

Figure 8

Figure 9

Figure 10

Figure 11

Figure 12

Figure 13

Figure 14

Figure 15

Figure 16

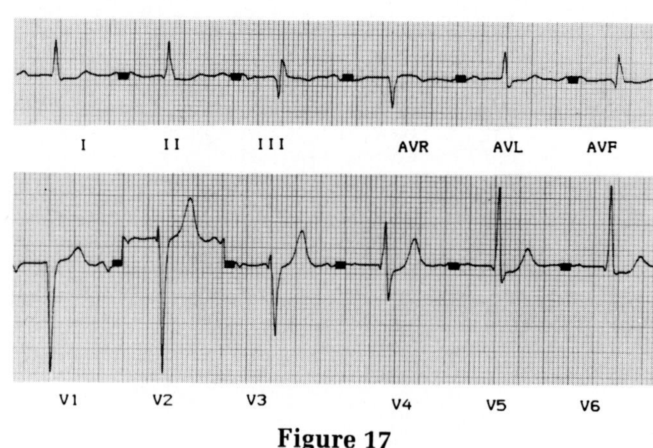

Figure 17

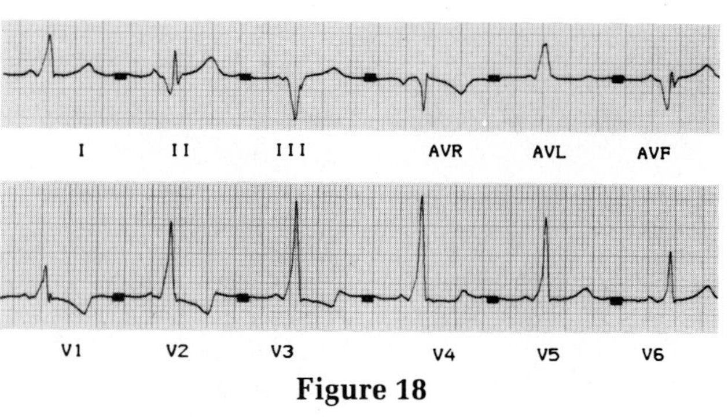

Figure 18

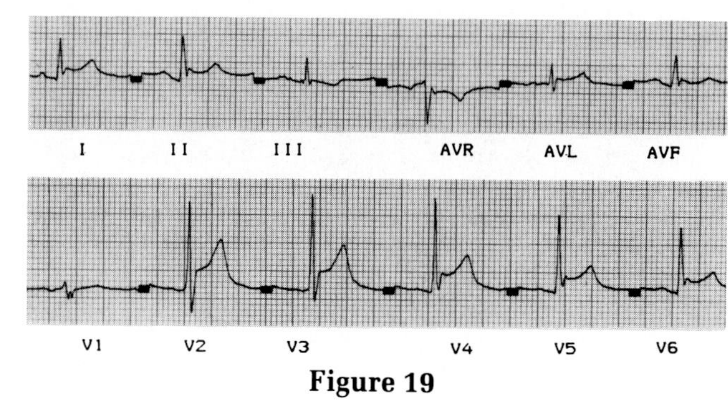

Figure 19

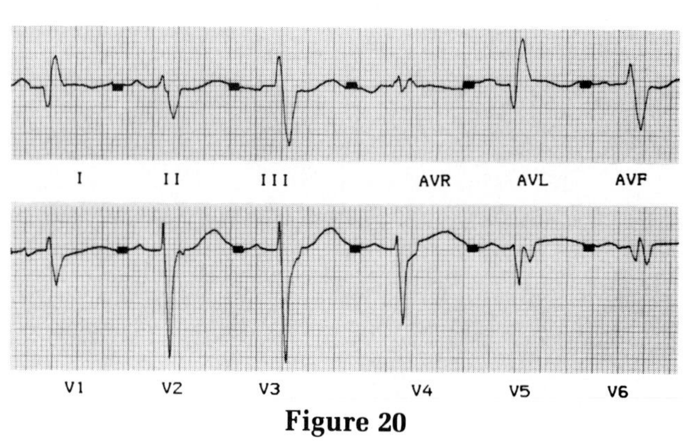

Figure 20

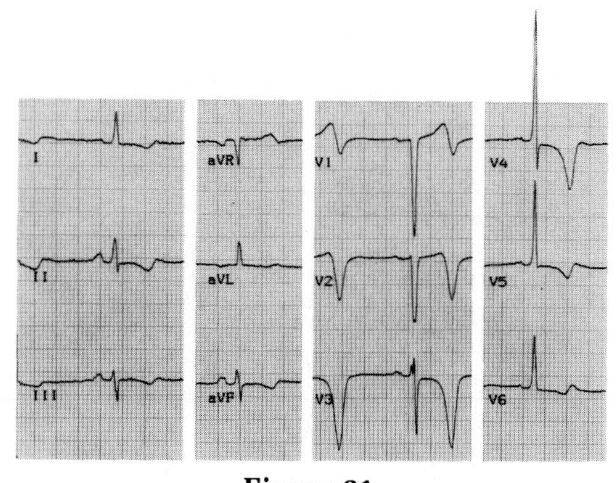

Figure 21

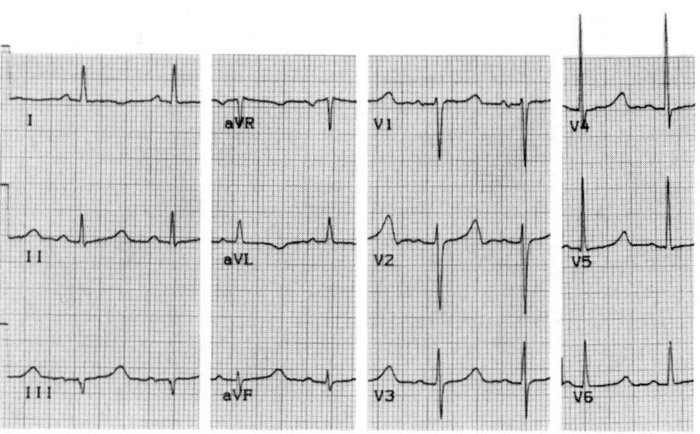

Figure 22

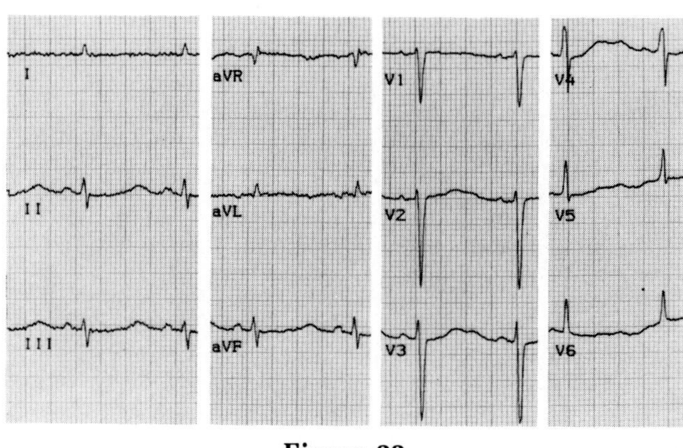

Figure 23

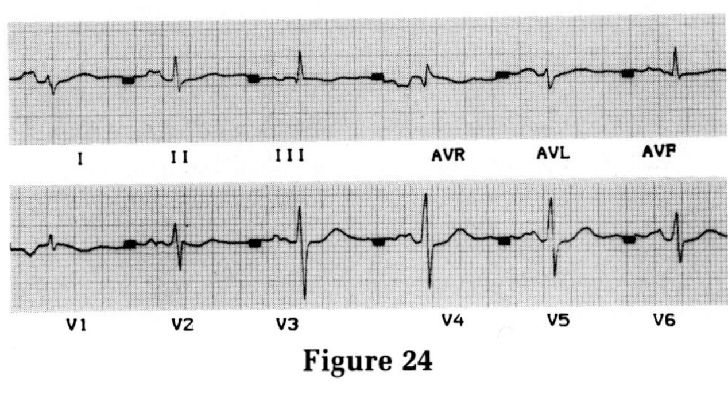

Figure 24

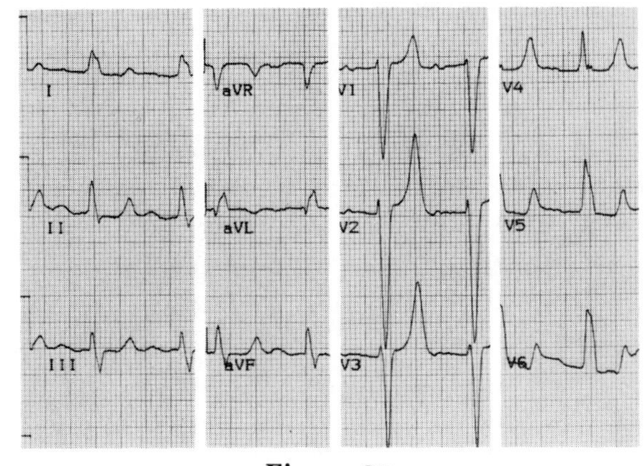

Figure 25

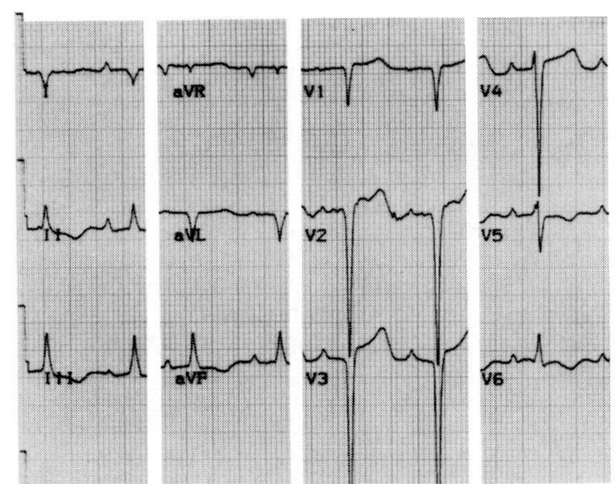

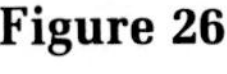

Figure 26

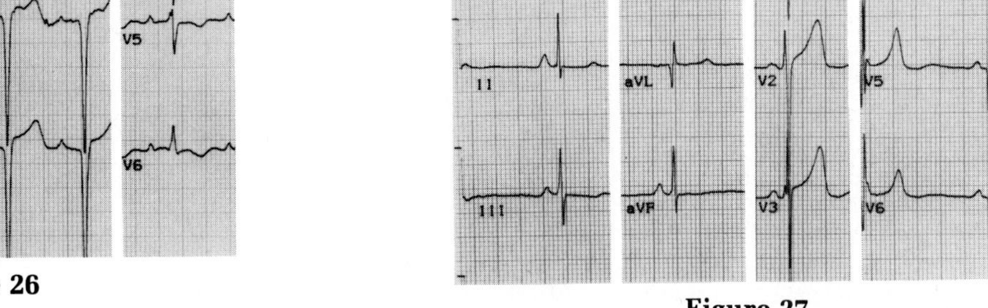

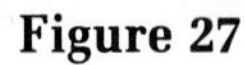

Figure 27

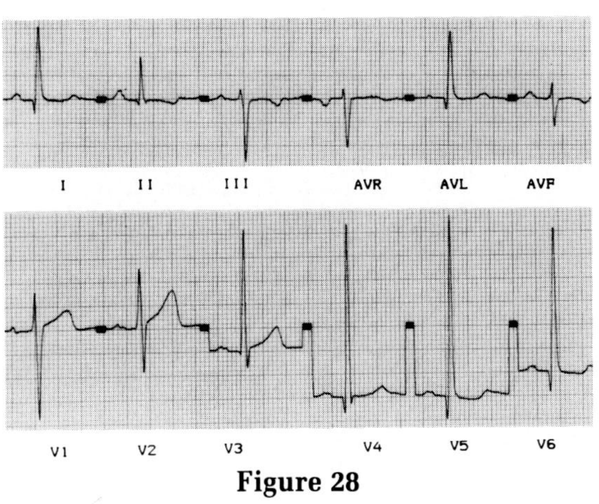

Figure 28

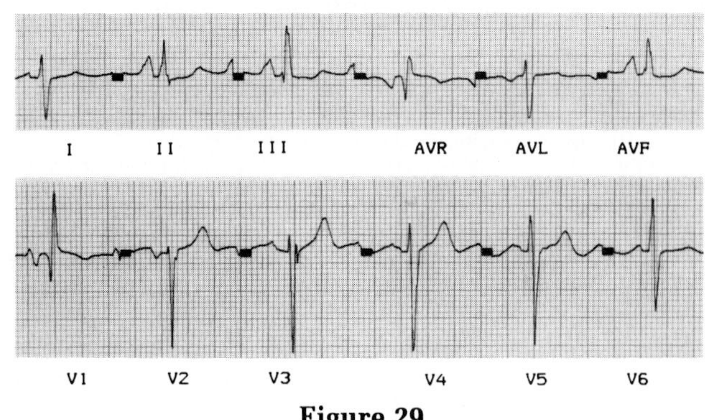

Figure 29

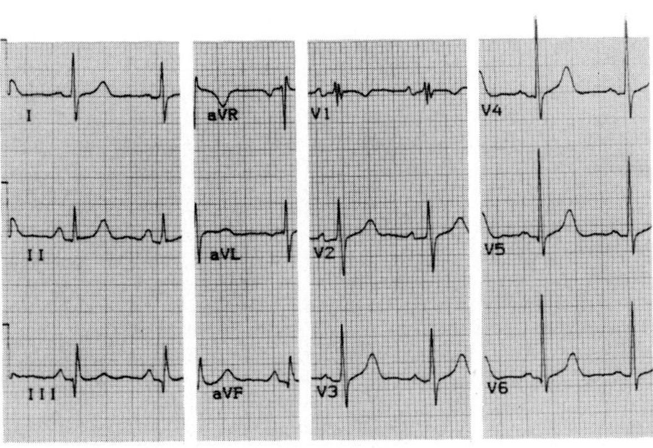

Figure 30

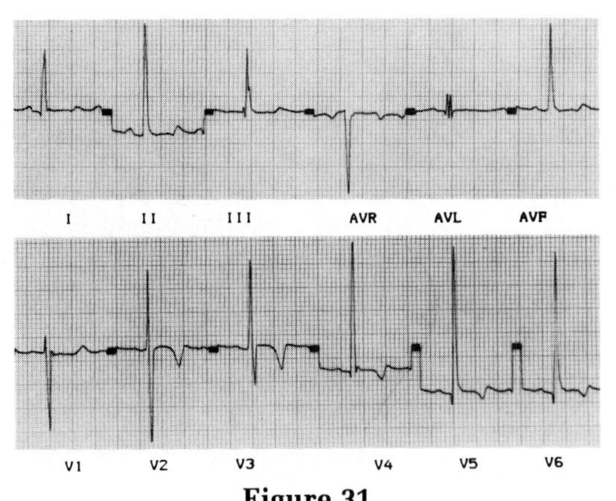

Figure 31

ABBREVIATIONS

AF = atrial fibrillation
c/w = consistent with
HCM = hypertrophic cardiomyopathy
IVCD = intraventricular conduction defect
LBBB = left bundle branch block
LDEA = left deviation of the electrical axis
LVH = left ventricular hypertrophy
non-QWMI = non Q wave myocardial infarction
RBBB = right bundle branch block
RDEA = right deviation of the electrical axis
RVH = right ventricular hypertrophy
SR = sinus rhythm
Tw = T wave
1° AV block = first degree atrioventricular block

Figure 1
SR
Nonspecific IVCD
Inferior MI of indeterminate age
Poor R-wave progression, V1–V3, c/w lead reversal or old anteroseptal MI
(coronary artery disease)

Figure 2
AF, well-controlled ventricular response
RDEA and prominent R wave, V1, c/w RVH
Low voltage, limb leads
Anterior ST and Tw abnormalities c/w ischemia or RV "strain" (systolic overload) pattern
Lateral ST and Tw abnormalities c/w ischemia or digitalis effect
(rheumatic heart disease)

Figure 3
SR
Left atrial abnormality
LDEA, marked
QS pattern in anteroseptal leads with minimal R-wave progression across precordium
Nonspecific inferior ST and Tw abnormalities
(HCM, with pseudoinfarction pattern, age 26)

Figure 4
Atrial fibrillation, well-controlled ventricular response
Right-axis deviation and deep lateral S waves, c/w RVH
(mitral stenosis 2° rheumatic valvular disease)

Figure 5
SR
P-wave flattening
RBBB
Markedly peaked Tw with associated ST abnormalities
(marked hyperkalemia)

Figure 6
SR
LVH with "strain pattern"
Anterior J-point elevation c/w normal early repolarization
(aortic stenosis from rheumatic valvular disease)

Figure 7
SR
Right atrial enlargement, marked
RDEA, prominent R wave in V1, deep lateral S waves, anterior ST and Tw abnormalities all c/w RVH with systolic overload pattern
(pulmonic stenosis, congenital)

Figure 8
SR
RBBB
Marked Q waves, lateral and inferior leads
Diffuse ST and Tw abnormalities
(HCM with "pseudoinfarction" pattern)

Figure 9
SR
Q waves I,L, and associated ST elevation, Tw abnormality c/w high lateral MI
(coronary artery disease)

Figure 10
SR, 1° AV block
Inferoposterior MI of indeterminate age (large R and upright T wave in V2)
Lateral ST and Tw abnormalities c/w ischemia or non-Qw MI
(coronary artery disease)

Figure 11
SR, nonspecific IVCD
Left anterior fascicular block
Q waves in I,L,V5–6 and associated ST segment elevation c/w evolving anterolateral MI or persistent ST and Tw abnormality c/w aneurysm formation
(coronary artery disease, anterior aneurysm 9 mos. after MI)

Figure 12
SR with low P-wave amplitude, 1° AV block
Nonspecific IVCD
Peaked T waves V2–V4
(hyperkalemia in chronic renal disease)

Figure 13
SR
LDEA
Anteroseptal MI of indeterminate age
Lateral (I, AVL) ST and Tw abnormalities suggestive of ischemia
(coronary artery disease)

Figure 14
SR, 1° AV block, RBBB
Left anterior fascicular block
Anterior MI of indeterminate age
(coronary artery disease with associated conduction abnormalities)

Figure 15
SR
Nonspecific IVCD
Old inferior MI, old anterior MI
(coronary artery disease)

Figure 16
SR, RBBB, left anterior fascicular block
(conduction system disease, subclinical)

Figure 17
SR, 1° AV block
Inferior MI, indeterminate age
Anteroseptal MI, indeterminate age
(coronary artery disease)

Figure 18
Sinus atrial mechanism
Short PR interval, delta wave
Left-axis deviation and Q waves in inferior leads (due to superior direction of the delta wave)
(WPW, type A, from a "routine" preoperative tracing)

Figure 19
SR
P-R segment depression, leads I, II, V4–6
ST elevation, diffuse
(acute pericarditis)

Figure 20
SR
Left atrial abnormality, LDEA, IVCD
Lateral Q waves
Diffuse ST and Tw abnormalities
(congestive cardiomyopathy, normal coronary arteries)

Figure 21
SR
Anteroseptal MI, indeterminate age
Marked ST and Tw abnormalities, V2–V5, c/w ischemia or non-Q wave MI
(coronary artery disease, non-Q wave MI)

Figure 22
SR
Mild Q-T prolongation
Lateral (I,L) Tw inversion c/w ischemia or electrolyte disturbance
(hypocalcemia)

Figure 23
SR
Prominent V waves, V2–V4 (pseudo Q-T prolongation II,III,F due to Tw flattening and prominent U wave)
Diffuse Tw flattening
(hypokalemia)

Figure 24
SR
Biatrial abnormality
RDEA, R > S in V1, prominent lateral S waves, and anterior ST and Tw abnormalities all c/w RVH with "strain"
(mitral stenosis 2° rheumatic heart disease)

Figure 25
SR, 1° AV block with flattening of P waves
LBBB
Markedly peaked Tw with associated ST abnormalities
(hyperkalemia)

Figure 26
SR
RDEA
Anteroseptal Q waves with associated ST-segment elevation
Inferolateral ST and Tw abnormalities
(amyloid disease with normal coronary arteries)

Figure 27
SR
Mild P-R "slurring" into tall R waves (e.g. III, V2)
Tall R waves, V1, V2 with tallest precordial R waves in mid-precordial leads
Prominent anterior T waves
Deep, narrow Q waves in lateral leads
Nonspecific St and Tw abnormalities, inferior leads
(HCM, with pseudoinfarction pattern, age 29)

Figure 28
SR
LVH with lateral "strain pattern"
(aortic regurgitation 2° rheumatic valvular disease)

Figure 29
SR
Biatrial abnormality
RDEA, prominent R wave in V1, deep lateral S waves all c/w RVH
(primary pulmonary hypertension with RVH)

Figure 30
SR
Right atrial abnormality
Incomplete RBBB
(atrial septal defect, secundum type)

Figure 31
SR
Prominent R waves in precordial leads, with large voltage, equiphasic complexes in mid-precordial leads, c/w biventricular hypertrophy (Katz-Wachtel phenomenon)
Tw inversions in precordial leads c/w biventricular "strain" (systolic overload)
(ventricular septal defect)

6

Exercise Stress Testing

by BERNARD CHAITMAN, M.D.

Exercise testing is an important diagnostic and prognostic procedure in the assessment of patients with ischemic heart disease. The diagnostic utility of the electrocardiogram was recognized by Feil and Siegel as early as 1928, when ST and T wave changes following exercise were reported in three of four patients with chronic stable angina.[1] Master and Oppenheimer developed a standardized exercise protocol to assess functional capacity and hemodynamic response in 1929.[2] Continued research into causal mechanisms of ST segment displacement, effect of lead position, refinement of exercise protocols, and determination of diagnostic and prognostic exercise variables in clinical patient subsets characterized the subsequent 30 years. Shortly after the advent of coronary angiography, the limitation of exercise-induced ST-segment depression as a diagnostic marker for obstructive coronary disease in patient populations with a low disease prevalence became apparent.[3] The test is now most frequently used to estimate prognosis and to determine functional capacity, likelihood and extent of coronary disease, and effects of therapy. Ancillary techniques such as metabolic gas analysis, radionuclide imaging, and echocardiography enhance the information content of exercise testing in selected patients.

EXERCISE PHYSIOLOGY

Anticipation of dynamic exercise results in an acceleration of ventricular rate due to vagal withdrawal, increase in alveolar ventilation, and increased venous return as a result of sympathetic vasoconstriction. In normal subjects, the net effect is to increase resting cardiac output before the start of exercise. The magnitude of hemodynamic response during exercise depends on the severity and amount of muscle mass involved. In the early phases of exercise in the upright position, cardiac output is increased by an augmentation in stroke volume mediated through the use of the Frank-Starling mechanism and heart rate; the increase in cardiac output in the latter phases of exercise is primarily due to an increase in ventricular rate[4] (see also p. 385). During strenuous exertion, sympathetic discharge is maximal and parasympathetic stimulation is withdrawn, resulting in vasoconstriction of most circulatory body systems, except for that in exercising muscle and in the cerebral and coronary circulations. Venous and arterial norepinephrine release from sympathetic postganglionic nerve endings is increased, and epinephrine levels are increased at peak exertion; this enhances ventricular contractility. As exercise progresses, skeletal muscle blood flow is increased, oxygen extraction increases by as much as threefold, total calculated peripheral resistance decreases, and systolic blood pressure, mean arterial pressure, and pulse pressure usually increase. Diastolic blood pressure is unchanged or may increase or decrease by approximately 10 mm Hg. The pulmonary vascular bed can accommodate as much as a sixfold increase in cardiac output with only modest increases in pulmonary artery pressure, pulmonary capillary wedge pressure, and right atrial pressure; in normal subjects, this is not a limiting determinant of peak exercise capacity.

Cardiac output increases by four- to sixfold above basal levels during strenuous exertion in the upright position, depending on genetic endowment and level of training.[5] The maximum heart rate and cardiac output are decreased in older individuals (see also p. 1662). Maximum heart rate can be calculated from the formula 220 − age (years) with a standard deviation of 10 to 12 beats per minute.[6] The age-predicted maximum heart rate is a useful measurement for safety reasons. However, the wide standard deviation seen in the various regression equations used and the impact of drug therapy limit the usefulness of this parameter in arbitrary selection of limits of age-predicted maximum heart rate to define the adequacy of cardiac reserve in individual patients.

In the postexercise phase, hemodynamics return to baseline within minutes of termination. Intense physical work, or important cardiorespiratory impairment, may interfere with achievement of a steady state, and an oxygen deficit occurs during exercise. The total oxygen uptake in excess of the resting oxygen uptake during the recovery period is the oxygen debt.

PATIENT POSITION. At rest, the cardiac output and stroke volume are higher in the supine than in the upright position. With exercise in normal supine subjects, the elevation of cardiac output results almost entirely from an increase in heart rate with little augmentation of stroke volume. In the upright posture, the increase in cardiac output in normal subjects results from a combination of elevations in stroke volume and heart rate. A change from supine to upright posture causes decreases in venous return, left ventricular end diastolic volume and pressure, stroke volume, and cardiac index. Renin and norepinephrine levels are increased. End-systolic volume and ejection fraction are not significantly changed. In normal individuals, end-systolic volume decreases and ejection fraction increases to a similar extent from rest to exercise in the supine and upright positions. The magnitude and direction of change in end-diastolic volume from rest to maximum exercise in both positions are small and may vary according to the patient population studied. The net effect on exercise performance is an approximate 10 per cent increase in exercise time, cardiac index, heart rate, and rate pressure product at peak exercise in the upright as compared with the supine position.[7]

Cardiopulmonary exercise testing involves measurements of respiratory oxygen uptake ($\dot{V}_{O_2}$), carbon dioxide production ($\dot{V}_{CO_2}$), and ventilatory parameters during a symptom-limited exercise test. During testing, the patient usually wears a nose clip and breathes through a nonrebreathing valve that separates expired air from room air. Important measurements of expired gas are O_2 tension, CO_2 tension, and air flow. A flow meter is used to determine air flow. Ventilatory measurements include respiratory rate, tidal volume, and minute ventilation (VE). O_2 and CO_2 tension are sampled breath-by-breath or by use of a mixing chamber. The $\dot{V}_{O_2}$ and $\dot{V}_{CO_2}$ can be computed on-line from ventilatory volumes and differences between inspired and expired gases.[8] Under steady-state(equilibrium) conditions, $\dot{V}_{O_2}$ and $\dot{V}_{CO_2}$ measured at the mouth are equivalent to total body oxygen consumption and CO_2 production. The relationship between work output, oxygen consumption, heart rate, and cardiac output during exercise is linear (Fig. 6–1). $\dot{V}_{O_2max}$ is the product of maximal arterial venous oxygen difference and cardiac output. In untrained persons, the arterial–mixed venous O_2 difference at peak exercise is relatively constant, and $\dot{V}_{O_2max}$ is an approximation of maximum cardiac output. Measured $\dot{V}_{O_2max}$ can be compared with predicted values from empirically derived formulas based on age, sex, weight, and height.[9,10] Peak exercise capacity is decreased when the ratio of measured to predicted $\dot{V}_{O_2max}$ is <85 to 90 per cent. Oximetry, determined noninvasively, can be used to monitor arterial oxygen saturation and normally does not decrease by more than 5 per cent during exercise.[10,11]

ANAEROBIC THRESHOLD. $\dot{V}_{O_2}$ increases rapidly in the initial stages of exercise, and in most subjects steady-state conditions are reached after 2 to 4 minutes[8–10] (Fig. 6–2). Lactic acid begins to accumulate when a healthy untrained subject reaches about 50 to 60 per cent of the maximal capacity for aerobic metabolism.[10] The increase in lactic acid becomes greater as exercise becomes more intense, resulting in metabolic acidosis. The gas exchange anaerobic threshold (AT_{ge}) is the point at which VE increases disproportionately relative to $\dot{V}_{O_2}$ and work; it occurs at 40 to 60 per cent of $\dot{V}_{O_2max}$ in normal untrained individuals.[10] There are several methods to determine AT_{ge}, which include (1) the point at which the $\dot{V}_{O_2}$ and $\dot{V}_{CO_2}$ slopes intersect and (2) the point at which the ratio of VE/$\dot{V}_{O_2}$ and end tidal O_2 tension begins to increase systematically without an immediate increase in the VE/$\dot{V}_{CO_2}$ (Figs. 6–1 and 6–2).[11,12] The AT_{ge} is a useful parameter because work below AT_{ge} encompasses most activities of daily living. Changes in anaerobic threshold with repeat testing can be used to assess disease progression, response to medical therapy, and improvement in cardiovascular fitness with training.

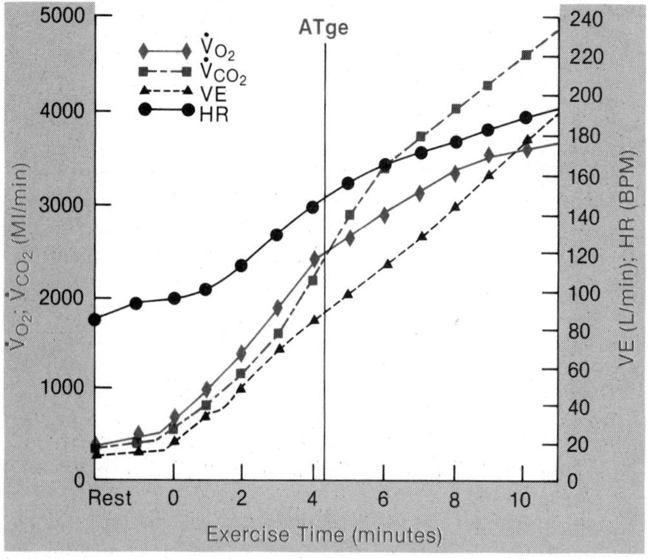

FIGURE 6–1. Cardiopulmonary exercise test in a 34-year-old healthy man using a ramp protocol. The relationship between work output, heart rate, and oxygen consumption ($\dot{V}_{O_2}$) is linear. The subject completed 10 minutes and 23 seconds of exercise, and peak $\dot{V}_{O_2}$ was 3.5 liters/min. The anaerobic threshold (AT_{ge}) occurred at 4 minutes and 15 seconds of exercise, at approximately 70 per cent of peak $\dot{V}_{O_2}$ and above the predicted value for a normal sedentary population. The AT_{ge} is determined at the point where the $\dot{V}_{O_2}$/$\dot{V}_{CO_2}$ curves intersect. Steady-state conditions are not reached using ramp protocols.

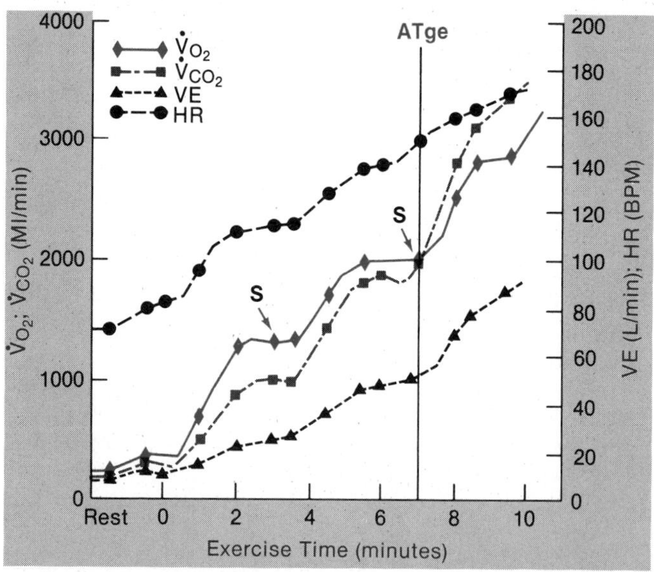

FIGURE 6–2. Cardiopulmonary exercise test in a 40-year-old man using the Bruce protocol. The patient reached steady-state conditions (S) after 2 min in Bruce stage I, and II. The anaerobic threshold (AT_{ge}) was reached at 7 min (vertical line).

METABOLIC EQUIVALENT. The current usage of the term MET refers to the resting $\dot{V}_{O_2}$ for a 70 kg, 40-year-old male, and 1 MET is equivalent to 3.5 ml/min/kg of body weight. Work activities can be calculated in multiples of METs; this measurement is useful to determine exercise prescriptions, assess disability, and standardize the reporting of submaximal and peak exercise workloads when different protocols are employed. However, estimating $\dot{V}_{O_2}$ from work rate or treadmill time in individual patients may lead to misinterpretation of data if exercise equipment is not correctly calibrated or if the patient fails to achieve steady-state, is obese, or has peripheral vascular disease, pulmonary vascular disease, or cardiac impairment. $\dot{V}_{O_2}$ does not increase linearly in some patients with cardiovascular or pulmonary disease as work rate is increased and may lead to overestimation of $\dot{V}_2$.[10] The measurements obtained with cardiopulmonary exercise testing are useful in understanding an individual patient's response to exercise and can be quite useful in the diagnostic evaluation of a patient with dyspnea.

PATHOPHYSIOLOGY OF THE MYOCARDIAL ISCHEMIC RESPONSE

(See also p. 1161)

Myocardial oxygen consumption ($M\dot{V}_{O_2}$) is determined by heart rate, systolic blood pressure, left ventricular end-diastolic volume, wall thickness, and contractility. The rate-pressure product (heart rate × systolic blood pressure) increases progressively with increasing work and is a reliable index of the myocardial perfusion requirement in normal subjects and in many patients with coronary artery disease. The heart is an aerobic organ with little capacity to generate energy through anaerobic metabolism. O_2 extraction in the coronary circulation is nearly maximal at rest. The only significant mechanism available to the heart to increase oxygen consumption is to increase perfusion, and there is a direct linear relationship between $M\dot{V}_{O_2}$ consumption and coronary blood flow in normal individuals. The principal mechanism for increasing coronary blood flow during exercise is to decrease resistance at the coronary arteriolar level. In patients with progressive atherosclerotic narrowing of the epicardial vessels, an ischemic threshold occurs beyond which exercise can produce abnormalities in diastolic and systolic ventricular function, electrocardiographic changes, and chest pain. The subendocardium is more susceptible to myocardial ischemia than the subepicardium because of increased wall tension, causing a relative increase in myocardial O_2 demand.

Dynamic changes in coronary artery tone at the site of an atherosclerotic plaque may result in diminished coronary flow during static or dynamic exercise; i.e., perfusion pressure distal to the stenotic plaque actually falls during exercise, resulting in reduced subendocardial blood flow[13] (see also p. 404). Thus, regional left ventricular myocardial ischemia may result not only from an increase in myocardial O_2 demand during exercise but also from a limitation of coronary flow as a result of coronary vasoconstriction near the site of an atherosclerotic plaque.

EXERCISE PROTOCOLS

The two main types of exercise are dynamic or isotonic exercise and static or isometric exercise. In daily living, a person frequently performs both types simultaneously. Dynamic protocols most frequently are used to assess cardiovascular reserve, and those suitable for clinical testing should include a low-intensity "warm-up" phase. In general, 6 to 10 minutes of continuous progressive exercise during which the myocardial O_2 demand is elevated to the patient's maximal level is optimal for diagnostic and prognostic purposes.[6,7] The protocol should include a suitable recovery or "cool-down" period. If the protocol is too strenuous for an individual patient, early test termination will result and will not allow an opportunity to observe clinically important responses. If the exercise protocol is too easy for an individual patient, the prolonged procedure will test endurance and not aerobic capacity. Thus, exercise protocols should be individualized to accommodate the patient's limitations. Protocols may be set up at a fixed duration of exercise for a certain intensity to meet minimal qualifications for certain industrial tasks or sports programs.

STATIC EXERCISE. This form of isometric exercise generates force with little muscle shortening and produces a greater pressor response than with dynamic exercise.[14] In a common form, the patient's maximal force on a hand dynamometer is recorded. The patient then sustains 25 to 33 per cent of maximal force for 3 to 5 minutes while ECG and blood pressures are recorded. The increase in myocardial V_{O_2} is often insufficient to initiate an ischemic response.

ARM ERGOMETRY. Arm crank ergometry protocols involve arm cranking at incremental workloads of 10 to 20 watts for 2 or 3 minute stages.[15] The heart rate and blood pressure responses to a given workload of arm exercise usually are greater than those for leg exercise. A bicycle ergometer with the axle placed at the level of the shoulders is used, and the subject sits or stands and cycles the peddles so that the arms are alternately fully extended. The most common frequency is 50 RPM's. In normal subjects, maximum $\dot{V}_{O_2}$ and VE for arm cycling approximates 50 to 70 per cent of leg cycling. Peak heart rate is approximately 70 per cent of that during leg testing.

BICYCLE ERGOMETRY. Bicycle protocols involve incremental workloads calibrated in watts or kilopond (KPD) meters/minute. One watt is equivalent to 6 KPD meters/min. In mechanically braked bicycles, work is determined by force and distance and requires a constant pedaling rate of 60 to 80 rpm, according to subject preference. Electronically braked bicycles provide a constant workload in spite of changes in pedaling rate and are less dependent on patient cooperation; although they are more costly than a mechanically braked bicycle, they are preferred for diagnostic and prognostic assessment. Most protocols begin at a workload of 25 watts and increase in 25 watt increments every 2 minutes. Younger subjects may start at 50 watts, with 50 watt increments every 2 minutes. A ramp protocol differs from the staged protocols in that the patient starts at 3 minutes of unloaded pedaling at a cycle speed of 60 rpm. Work rate is increased by a uniform amount each minute ranging from 5 to 30 watt increments depending on expected patient performance.[10] Exercise is terminated if the patient is unable to maintain a cycling frquency above 40 rpm. In the cardiac catheterization laboratory, hemodynamic measurements may be made during supine bicycle ergometry at rest and at one or two submaximal workloads.

In subjects unfamiliar with bicycle exercise, the muscles required for optimal performance are not as well developed as for treadmill exercise and early fatigue may be a limiting factor. The bicycle ergometer is associated with a lower maximum $\dot{V}_{O_2}$ and anaerobic threshold than the treadmill, although maximal heart rate, maximal VE, and maximal lactate values are often similar. The metabolic requirements of ergometric workloads are inversely related to body mass, whereas the requirements of treadmill exercise are relatively independent of body mass. The bicycle ergometer has the advantage of requiring less space than a treadmill, is quieter, and permits sensitive precordial measurements without much motion artifact. However, in North America, treadmill protocols are more widely used in the assessment of patients with coronary disease.

TREADMILL PROTOCOL. The treadmill protocol should be consistent with the patient's physical capacity and the purpose of the test. In healthy individuals, the standard Bruce protocol is popular, and a large diagnostic and prognostic data base has been published.[7,16] In older individuals, or those whose exercise capacity is limited by cardiac disease, the Bruce protocol can be modified by two 3-minute warm-up stages at 1.7 mph and 0 per cent grade, and 1.7 mph and 5 per cent grade. The Bruce multistage maximal treadmill protocol has 3-minute periods to allow achievement of a steady state before workload is increased (Fig. 6–2). A limitation of the Bruce protocol is the relatively large increase in $\dot{V}_{O_2}$ between stages and the additional energy cost of running as compared with walking at stages in excess of Bruce stage III. The Naughton, Weber, and Balke Ware protocols use 1- to 2-minute stages with 1 MET increments between stages; these protocols may be more suitable for patients with limited exercise tolerance such as patients with congestive heart failure (Fig. 6–3). The Cornell protocol is a modification of the Bruce protocol with smaller increments in 2-minute stages, permitting a more reliable estimate of ST/HR slope measurements, a parameter useful in diagnostic testing.[17]

Ramp protocols start the patient at a relatively slow treadmill speed, which is gradually increased until the patient has a good stride. The ramp angle of incline is progressively increased at fixed intervals (e.g., 10 to 60 seconds) starting at zero grade with the increase in grade calculated on the patient's estimated functional capacity such that the protocol will be complete at between 6 and 10 minutes.[18] In this type of protocol, the rate of work increase is continuous, steady-state conditions are not reached, cardiovascular fitness is assessed, and estimates of $\dot{V}_{O_2}$ appear to be more precise than staged exercise protocols. A limitation of ramp protocols is the requirement to estimate functional capacity from an activity scale; occasionally, under- or overestimation of functional capacity will result in an endurance test or premature cessation. One formula for estimating $\dot{V}_{O_2}$ from treadmill speed and grade is $\dot{V}_{O_2}(mlO_2/kg/min) = (MPH \times 2.68) + (1.8 \times 26.82 \times MPH \times grade \div 100) + 3.5$.[19]

It is important to encourage the patient not to grasp the handrails of the treadmill during exercise. Functional capac-

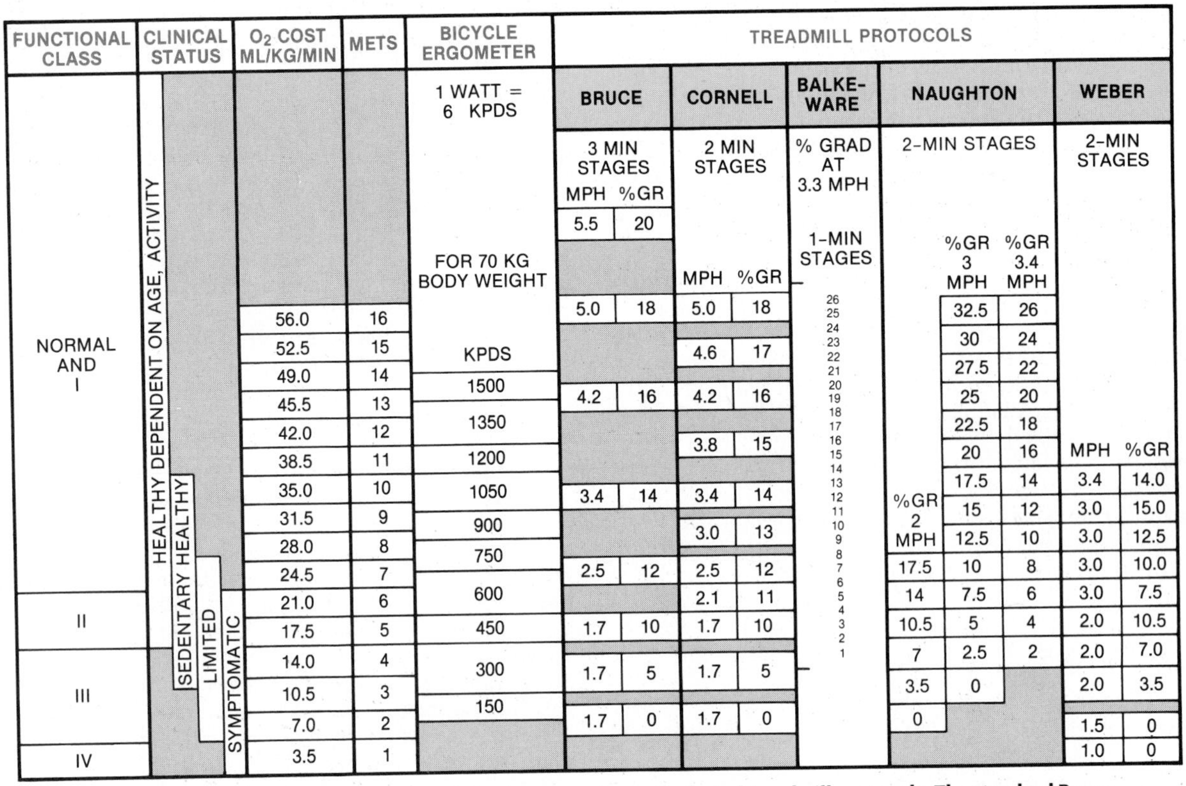

FUNCTIONAL CLASS	CLINICAL STATUS	O_2 COST ML/KG/MIN	METS	BICYCLE ERGOMETER (1 WATT = 6 KPDS; FOR 70 KG BODY WEIGHT) KPDS	TREADMILL PROTOCOLS: BRUCE (3 MIN STAGES) MPH	BRUCE %GR	CORNELL (2 MIN STAGES) MPH	CORNELL %GR	BALKE-WARE (% GRAD AT 3.3 MPH; 1-MIN STAGES)	NAUGHTON (2-MIN STAGES) %GR 2 MPH	NAUGHTON %GR 3 MPH	NAUGHTON %GR 3.4 MPH	WEBER (2-MIN STAGES) MPH	WEBER %GR
					5.5	20								
NORMAL AND I	HEALTHY DEPENDENT ON AGE, ACTIVITY	56.0	16		5.0	18	5.0	18	26 25 24		32.5	26		
		52.5	15				4.6	17	23 22		30	24		
		49.0	14	1500					21 20		27.5	22		
		45.5	13		4.2	16	4.2	16	19 18		25	20		
		42.0	12	1350					17 16		22.5	18		
		38.5	11	1200			3.8	15	15 14		20	16		
	SEDENTARY HEALTHY	35.0	10	1050	3.4	14	3.4	14	13 12		17.5	14	3.4	14.0
		31.5	9	900			3.0	13	11 10		15	12	3.0	15.0
	LIMITED	28.0	8	750					9 8		12.5	10	3.0	12.5
		24.5	7		2.5	12	2.5	12	7 6	17.5	10	8	3.0	10.0
II	SYMPTOMATIC	21.0	6	600			2.1	11	5 4	14	7.5	6	3.0	7.5
		17.5	5	450	1.7	10	1.7	10	3 2	10.5	5	4	2.0	10.5
III		14.0	4	300	1.7	5	1.7	5	1	7	2.5	2	2.0	7.0
		10.5	3	150						3.5	0		2.0	3.5
		7.0	2		1.7	0	1.7	0		0			1.5	0
IV		3.5	1										1.0	0

FIGURE 6–3. Estimated oxygen cost of bicycle ergometer and selected treadmill protocols. The standard Bruce protocol starts at 1.7 mph and 10 per cent grade (5 METS) with a larger increment between stages than protocols such as the Naughton, which starts at < 2 METS at 2 mph and increases by 1 MET every 2 minutes. The Bruce protocol can be modified by two 3 min warm-up stages at 1.7 mph, 0 per cent grade, and 1.7 mph, 5 per cent grade.

ity can be overestimated by as much as 20 per cent in tests in which handrail support is permitted, and V_{O_2} is decreased. Since the degree of handrail support is difficult to quantify from one test to another, more consistent results can be obtained during serial testing when handrail support is not permitted.

ELECTROCARDIOGRAPHIC MEASUREMENTS

Lead Systems

The Mason-Likar modification of the standard 12-lead electrocardiogram requires that the extremity electrodes be moved to the torso to reduce motion artifact. The arm electrodes should be located in the lateralmost aspects of the infraclavicular fossae and the leg electrodes in a stable position above the anterior iliac crest and below the rib cage (Fig. 6–4). The Mason-Likar modification results in a right axis shift and increased voltage in the inferior leads and may produce a loss of inferior Q waves and the development of new Q waves in lead aVl. The more cephalad the leg electrodes are placed, the greater the degree of change. Thus, the body torso limb lead positions cannot be used to interpret a diagnostic rest 12-lead ECG.[20]

Bipolar lead groups place the negative or reference electrode over the manubrium (CM5), right scapula (CB5), RV5 (CC5), or on the forehead (CH5), and the active electrode at V5 or proximate location to optimize R wave amplitude. In bipolar lead ML, which reflects inferior wall changes, the negative reference is at the manubrium and the active electrode in the left leg position. Bipolar lead groups may provide additional diagnostic information, and in some medical centers lead CM5 is substituted for lead aVr in the Mason-Likar modified lead system (Fig. 6–4). Bipolar leads are frequently used when only

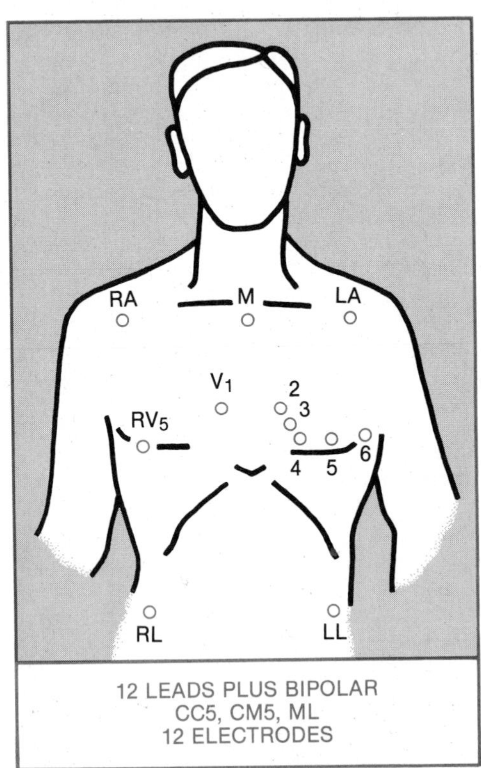

FIGURE 6–4. This lead group set reflects the Mason-Likar leads with the precordial electrodes in standard position and the arm and leg electrodes moved proximally to the subclavicular fossa and just above the anterior iliac crest. The position of the negative reference manubrial electrode and RV5 electrode illustrates the position required for lead CM5 and lead CC5. In lead ML, the active electrode is in the left leg position.

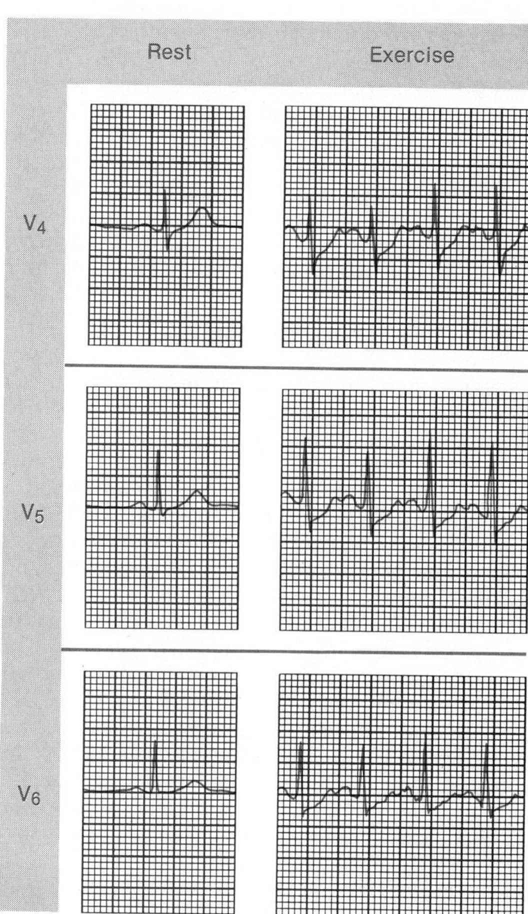

FIGURE 6–5. J point depression of 2 to 3 mm in leads V_{4-6} with rapid upsloping ST segments depressed approximately 1 mm 80 msec after the J point. The ST-segment slope in leads V_4, V_5 is ≥ 3.0 mV/second. This response should not be considered abnormal.

a limited ECG set is required (e.g., in cardiac rehabilitation programs). The use of more elaborate lead sets such as 87 lead body surface mapping provides the potential for insight into mechanisms of ST-segment displacement.[21]

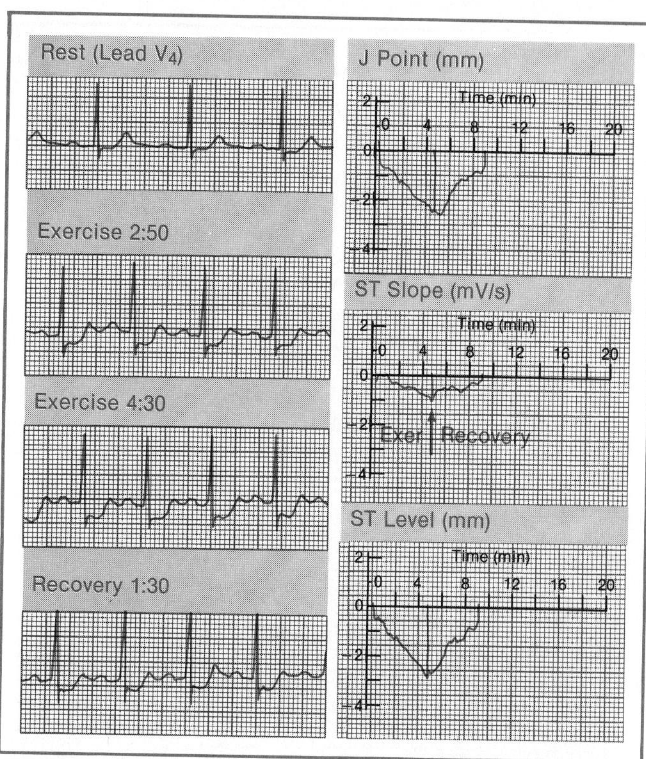

FIGURE 6–6. Bruce protocol. In lead V_4, the exercise ECG is abnormal early in the test, reaching 3 mm (0.3 mV) of horizontal ST-segment depression at the end of exercise. The ischemic changes persist for at least 1 min and 30 sec into the recovery phase. The right panel provides a continuous plot of the J point, ST slope, and ST-segment displacement at 80 msec after the J point (ST level) during exercise and in the recovery phase. Exercise ends at the vertical line at 4.5 min. The computer trends permit a more precise identification of initial onset and offset of ischemic ST-segment depression. This type of ECG pattern, with early onset of ischemic ST-segment depression, reaching > 3 mm of horizontal ST-segment displacement, and persisting several minutes into the recovery phase, is consistent with a severe ischemic response.

TYPES OF ST-SEGMENT DISPLACEMENT

In normal subjects, the P-R, QRS, and Q-T intervals shorten as heart rate increases. P amplitude increases and the P-R segment becomes progressively more downsloping in the inferior leads. J point, or junctional, depression is a normal finding during exercise (Fig. 6–5). However, in patients with myocardial ischemia, the ST segment usually becomes more horizontal (flattens) as the severity of the ischemic response worsens. With progressive exercise, the depth of ST-segment depression may increase, involving more ECG leads, and the patient may develop angina. In the immediate postrecovery phase, the ST-segment displacement may persist, with downsloping ST segments and T wave inversion, gradually returning to baseline after 5 to 10 minutes (Figs. 6–6 and 6–7). However, ischemic ST-segment displacement may be seen only during exercise, emphasizing the importance of adequate skin preparation and electrode placement to capture high-quality recordings during maximum exertion (Fig. 6–8). In about 10 per cent of patients, the ischemic response may appear only in the recovery phase.[22] The patient should not leave the exercise laboratory area until the postexercise ECG has returned to baseline.

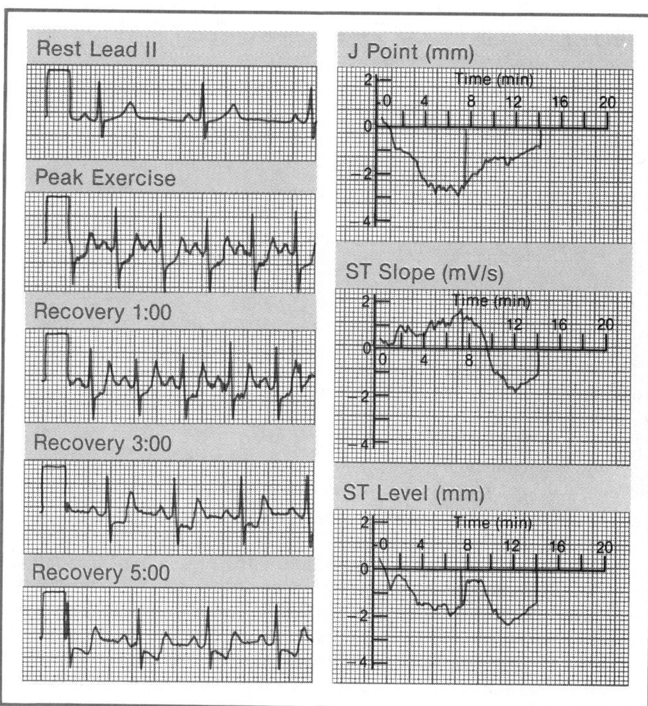

FIGURE 6–7. Bruce protocol. In this type of ischemic pattern, the J point at peak exertion is depressed 2.5 mm, the ST-segment slope is 1.5 mV/second, and the ST-segment level at 80 msec after the J point is depressed 1.6 mm. This "slow upsloping" ST segment at peak exercise indicates an ischemic pattern in patients with a high coronary disease prevalence pretest. A typical ischemic pattern is seen at 3 minutes of the recovery phase when the ST segment is horizontal and 5 minutes postexertion when the ST segment is downsloping. Exercise is discontinued at the vertical line in the right panels at 7.5 min.

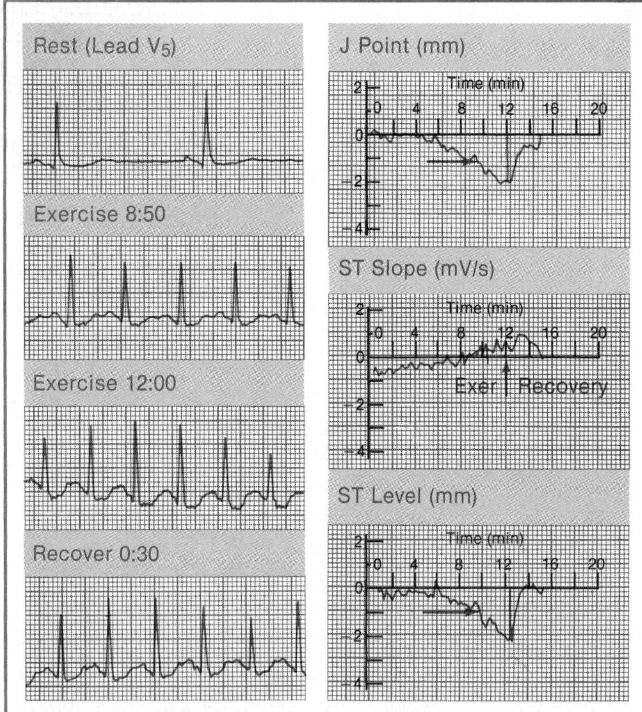

FIGURE 6–8. Bruce protocol. The exercise ECG becomes abnormal at 9:30 min of a 12 min exercise (horizontal panel, arrow *right*) and resolves in the immediate recovery phase. This ECG pattern in which the ST segment becomes abnormal only at high exercise workloads and returns to baseline in the immediate recovery phase may indicate a false-positive test in an asymptomatic subject without atherosclerotic risk factors. Exercise thallium scintigraphy would provide more diagnostic and prognostic information if this were an older person with several atherosclerotic risk factors.

MEASUREMENT OF ST-SEGMENT DISPLACEMENT. For purposes of interpretation, the PQ junction is usually chosen as the isoelectric point. The TP segment represents a true isoelectric point but is an impractical choice for most routine clinical measurements. The development of ≥ 0.10 mV (1mm) of J point depression measured from the PQ junction, with a relatively flat ST-segment slope (< 1 mV/sec), depressed ≥ 0.10 mV 60 to 80 msec after the J point in three consecutive beats with a stable baseline is considered to be an abnormal response. Occasionally, the ST segment at rest may be depressed. When this occurs, the J point and ST60 to ST80 measurements should be depressed an additional ≥ 0.10 mV to be considered abnormal. In patients with early repolarization and resting ST-segment elevation, return to the PQ junction is normal. Abnormal ST-segment depression in a patient with early repolarization should be measured from the PQ junction. A slow, upsloping ST segment is defined as J point depression with an upsloping ST segment (> 1 mV/sec), depressed ≥ 0.15 mV at 60 to 80 msec after the J point, in three consecutive beats (Fig. 6–7).

Exercise-induced ST-segment elevation may occur in Q wave or non-Q wave leads. The development of ≥ 0.10 mV (1 mm) of J point elevation, persistently elevated ≥ 0.10 mV at 60 to 80 msec after the J point in three consecutive beats, is considered an abnormal response (Fig. 6–9).

Exercise-induced ST-segment depression does *not* localize the site of myocardial ischemia, *nor* does it provide a clue as to which coronary artery is involved.[23] For example, it is not unusual for patients with isolated right coronary disease to exhibit exercise-induced ST-segment depression only in leads V_{4-6}, nor is it unusual for patients with disease of the left anterior descending coronary artery to exhibit exercise-induced ST-segment displacements in leads II, III, and aVf. The finding of exercise-induced ST-segment elevation is relatively specific for the territory of myocardial ischemia and the coronary artery involved (Fig. 6–10).

T-WAVE CHANGES. The morphology of the T wave is influenced by body position, respiration, and hyperventilation. Occasionally, a patient may be referred for exercise testing who has T-wave inversion on the resting 12-lead ECG Pseudonormalization of T waves (inverted at rest and becoming upright with exercise) is a nondiagnostic finding. Although in rare instances this finding may be a marker for myocardial ischemia in a patient with documented coronary disease, it would need to be substantiated by an ancillary technique, such as the concomitant finding of a reversible thallium defect.[24]

COMPUTER-ASSISTED ANALYSIS

The use of computers has facilitated the routine analysis and measurements required from exercise electrocardiography. When the raw ECG data are high quality, the computer can filter and average or select median complexes from which the degree of J point displacement, ST-segment slope, and ST displacement 60 to 80 msec after the J point (ST60 to 80) can be measured. The selection of ST60 or ST80 is dependent on the heart rate response. At ventricular rates ≥ 130 beats/min, the ST80 measurement may fall on the upslope of the T wave, and the ST60 measurement should be employed instead. In some computerized systems, the PQ junction or isoelectric interval is detected by scanning before the R wave for the 10 msec interval with the least slope. J point, ST slope, and ST levels are determined and the ST integral can be calculated from the area below the isoelectric line from the J point to ST60 to ST80. Computerized treatment of ECG complexes permits reduction of motion and myographic artifacts. However, the averaged or median beats occasionally may be erroneous because of ECG signal distortion caused by noise, baseline wander, or changes in conduction, and identification of the PQ junction and ST-segment onset may be imperfect. Therefore, it is critically important to ensure that the computer-determined averages or median complexes are reflective of the raw ECG data, and physicians should program the computer to print out raw data during exercise and inspect the raw data to ensure that the QRS template is accurately reproduced before accepting the automatic measurements.

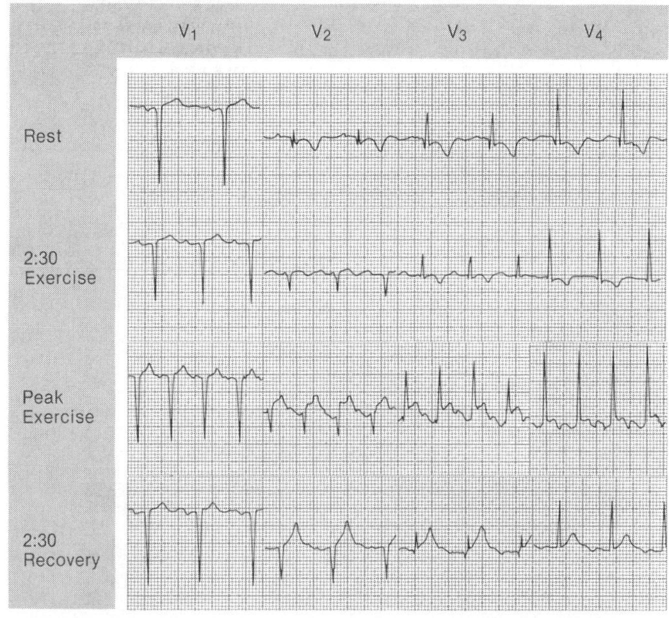

FIGURE 6–9. The rest tracing reveals a recent anterior wall myocardial infarction with persistent ischemic ST-T wave abnormalities. At peak exercise, 3 mm, 4 mm, and 2 mm of ST-segment elevations are noted in leads V_2, V_3, and V_4, respectively. The ST-segment elevation in lead V_3 persists 2 minutes and 30 seconds into the recovery phase. Exercise-induced ST-segment elevation is less frequent 6 weeks after infarction than on the predischarge test. In leads with abnormal Q waves or in the postinfarction setting, exercise-induced ST elevation is usually indicative of left ventricular regional wall motion abnormalities as opposed to myocardial ischemia.

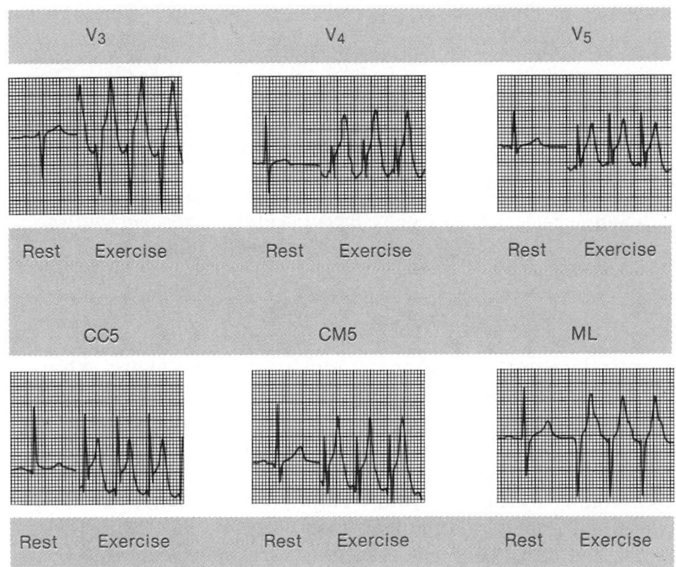

FIGURE 6-10. Marked ST-segment elevation in non-Q-wave leads V_3–V_5, and bipolar leads CC5 and CM5 is consistent with coronary vasospasm or a proximal high grade coronary narrowing causing epicardial ischemia. Bipolar lead ML (negative electrode at manubrium, positive electrode at left leg), an inferior lead, shows loss of R wave amplitude and 1 mm of J point elevation. This type of ECG pattern with ST-segment elevation usually warrants coronary angiography to clarify the cause of this response.

MECHANISM OF ST-SEGMENT DISPLACEMENT

The mechanism of exercise-induced ST-segment displacement is not completely understood (see also Fig. 5–30, p. 137). In normal persons, the action potential duration of the endocardial region is longer than that of the epicardial region, and ventricular repolarization is from epicardium to endocardium. The action potential duration is shortened in the presence of myocardial ischemia, and electrical gradients are created, resulting in ST-segment depression or elevation, depending on the surface ECG leads.[21] Increased myocardial oxygen demand associated with a failure to increase or an actual decrease in regional coronary blood flow will usually cause ST-segment depression; occasionally, ST-segment elevation may occur, depending on the severity of coronary flow reduction. ST-segment elevation in a non-Q wave lead is associated with a more severe degree of myocardial ischemia than is ST-segment depression.

EXERCISE TESTING

INDICATIONS. The most frequent indications for exercise testing are to aid in establishing the diagnosis of coronary artery disease in determining functional capacity, and in estimating prognosis. The indications continue to evolve, with some that are uniformly accepted and others that are more controversial. The AHA and ACC Exercise Task Force determined several categories of test indications drawn from a large body of published literature on exercise testing[25] (Table 6–1). The indications are classified according to conditions for which there is general agreement that exercise testing is justified, conditions for which the test may be indicated and conditions for which there is general agreement that the test is of marginal value.

TECHNIQUES. The patient should be instructed not to eat, drink caffeinated beverages or smoke for 3 hours prior to testing, and to wear comfortable shoes and loose-fitting clothes. Unusual physical exertion should be avoided prior to testing. A brief history and physical examination should be performed and the patient should be advised about the risks and benefits of the procedure. A written informed consent form is usually required. The indication for the test should be known. In many laboratories, the presence or absence of atherosclerotic risk factors is noted, and cardioactive medication recorded. A 12-lead ECG should be obtained with the electrodes at the distal extremities.

Following recording of the standard 12-lead ECG, a torso ECG should be obtained in the supine position and in the sitting or standing position. Postural changes can bring out labile ST-T wave abnormalities. Hyperventilation is not recommended before exercise. If a false-positive test is suspected, hyperventilation should be performed after the test, and the hyperventilation tracing compared with the maximum ST-segment abnormalities observed. The ECG and blood pressure should be recorded in both positions, and the patient should be instructed on how to perform the test.

Adequate skin preparation is essential for high-quality recordings, and the superficial layer of skin needs to be removed to augment signal-to-noise ratio. The areas of electrode application are rubbed with an alcohol-saturated pad to remove oil and rubbed with fine sandpaper or a rough material to reduce skin resistance to 5000 ohms or less. Silver chloride electrodes with a fluid column to avoid direct metal-to-skin contact produce high-quality tracings; these electrodes have the lowest offset voltage.

Cables connecting the electrodes and recorders should be light, flexible, and properly shielded. In a small minority of patients, a fishnet may be required over the electrodes and cables to reduce motion artifact. The electrode-skin interface can be verified by tapping on the electrode and examining the cathode-ray screen or by measuring skin impedance. Exces-

TABLE 6–1 INDICATIONS FOR EXERCISE TESTING

CLEAR INDICATION

Patients with Suspected or Proven Coronary Artery Disease:

1. Diagnosis: men with atypical symptoms
2. Prognostic assessment and functional capacity evaluation in patients with chronic stable angina or postmyocardial infarction
3. Symptomatic recurrent exercise-induced arrhythmias
4. Evaluation after revascularization procedure

TEST MAY BE INDICATED

1. Diagnosis: women with typical or atypical angina pectoris
2. Functional capacity evaluation to monitor cardiovascular therapy in patients with CAD or heart failure
3. Evaluation of patients with variant angina
4. Annual follow-up of patients with known CAD
5. Evaluation of asymptomatic men over 40; those who are in special occupations (pilots, firemen, police officers, bus or truck drivers, and railroad engineers) or who have two or more atherosclerotic risk factors or who plan to enter a vigorous exercise program

TEST PROBABLY NOT INDICATED

1. Evaluation of patients with isolated premature ventricular beats and no evidence of CAD
2. Multiple serial testing during the course of cardiac rehabilitation program
3. Diagnosis of CAD in patients who have preexcitation syndrome or complete left bundle branch block or are on digitalis therapy
4. Evaluation of young or middle-aged asymptomatic men or women; those who have no atherosclerotic risk factors or who have noncardiac chest discomfort

INDICATIONS FOR EXERCISE TESTING IN PATIENTS WITH VALVULAR HEART DISEASE OR HYPERTENSION

Test in Common Usage:

1. Evaluation of functional capacity in selected patients with valvular heart disease
2. Evaluation of blood pressure of hypertensive patients who wish to engage in vigorous dynamic or static exercise

CAD = coronary artery disease.

Adapted from Leff, A. R.: Cardiopulmonary Exercise Testing. Orlando, Grune and Stratton, 1986.

sive noise indicates that the electrode needs to be replaced; replacement before the test rather than during exercise can save time. The ECG signal can be digitized systematically at the patient end of the cable by some systems, reducing power-line artifact. Exercise equipment should be calibrated on a regular basis.

Treadmill walking should be demonstrated. The heart rate, blood pressure, and electrocardiograms should be recorded at the end of each stage of exercise, immediately before and immediately after stopping exercise, and for each minute for at least 5 to 10 minutes in the recovery phase. A minimum of three leads should be displayed continuously on the cathode-ray screen during the test. There is some controversy regarding optimal patient position in the recovery phase. In the sitting position, less space is required for a stretcher, and patients are more comfortable immediately after exertion. The supine position increases end-diastolic volume and has the potential to augment ST-segment changes.

DIAGNOSTIC USE OF EXERCISE TESTING

Appreciation of the exercise test literature requires an understanding of standard terminology such as sensitivity, specificity, and test accuracy (Table 6–2). The literature on the use of diagnostic exercise testing is extensive. The sensitivity of exercise ECG for single-vessel disease ranges from 25 to 71 per cent, with exercise-induced ST-segment displacement most frequent in patients with left anterior descending coronary artery disease, followed by those with right coronary artery disease, and is least frequent in patients with isolated left circumflex coronary disease. An obstruction in an isolated left circumflex coronary artery has the tendency to exaggerate the depth of ST-segment depression when the ECG is abnormal, most likely related to the fact that the ischemic territory underlies the lateral precordial leads. Approximately 75 to 80 per cent of the diagnostic information on exercise-induced ST-segment depression is contained in leads V_{4-6}. The ability to detect ECG changes in patients with right coronary disease can be augmented by recording lead V_5R.[26]

Gianrossi et al. performed an overview or meta analysis of 147 consecutive published reports involving 24,074 patients who underwent both coronary angiography and exercise testing.[27] The mean sensitivity was 68 (range 23 to 100) per cent and mean specificity was 77 (range 17 to 100) per cent. In patients with multivessel coronary disease, the mean sensitivity was 81 (range 40 to 100) per cent and mean specificity was 66 (range 17 to 100) per cent.[28] The weighted mean sensitivity was 86 ± 11 per cent and mean specificity was 53 ± 24 per cent for left main or three-vessel coronary disease. Decreased sensitivity was reported when nondiagnostic tests were classified as normal and when the exercise test was compared with a radionuclide test instead of a coronary arteriogram. The exercise ECG tends to be less sensitive in patients with extensive Q wave anterior wall myocardial infarction and when a limited-exercise ECG lead set is used. Increased sensitivity was noted when patients taking digitalis were excluded.

Selective referral of patients with a positive test for further study both decreases the rate of detection of true negative tests and increases the rate of detection of false-positive results, thus increasing sensitivity and decreasing specificity.[29] In Gianrossi's report, decreased specificity was more common when upsloping ST-segment depression was classified as abnormal, when patients with previous myocardial infarction were excluded, when preexercise hyperventilation was used, and when patients with left bundle branch block were included in the data analysis.[27] Adjustment for heart rate increased the specificity to predict left main or three-vessel coronary disease.[28,28a] There are other recognized noncoronary causes of ST-segment depression that may result in a false-positive test and decreased specificity, most notably digitalis use and left ventricular hypertrophy (Table 6–3).

SEVERITY OF ELECTROCARDIOGRAPHIC ISCHEMIC RESPONSE. The exercise ECG is more likely to be abnormal in patients with more severe coronary arterial obstruction, more extensive coronary disease, and after more strenuous levels of exercise. Early onset of ischemic ST-segment depression, profound ST-segment displacement, ischemic changes in five or more ECG leads, and persistence of the changes late in the recovery phase of exercise are associated with more severe myocardial ischemia and increase the probability of more extensive disease (Table 6–4).

CORRELATION OF EXERCISE TEST RESULTS WITH CORONARY ANGIOGRAPHY. The traditional reference standard against which the exercise ECG has been measured is a qualitative assessment of the coronary angiogram using 50

TABLE 6–2 TERMS USEFUL IN EVALUATION OF TEST RESULTS

True-positive (TP)	= abnormal test result in individual with disease
False-positive (FP)	= abnormal test result in individual without disease
True-negative (TN)	= normal test result in individual without disease
False-negative (FN)	= normal test result in individual with disease
Sensitivity:	percentage of patients with CAD who have an abnormal test = TP/(TP + FN)
Specificity:	percentage of patients without CAD who have a normal test = TN/(TN + FP)
Predictive value: of abnormal test	percentage of patients with abnormal test who have CAD = TP/(TP + FP)
Predictive value: of normal test	percentage of patients with normal test and without CAD = TN/(TN + FN)
Test accuracy:	percentage of true test results = (TP + TN)/total number tests performed
Likelihood ratio:	odds of a test result being true: of an abnormal test: sensitivity/(1-specificity); of a normal test: specificity/(1-sensitivity)
Relative risk:	$\frac{\text{disease rate in persons with a positive test result}}{\text{disease rate in persons with a negative test result}}$

TABLE 6–3 NONCORONARY CAUSES OF ST-SEGMENT DEPRESSION

Severe aortic stenosis	Glucose load
Severe hypertension	Left ventricular hypertrophy
Cardiomyopathy	Hyperventilation
Anemia	Mitral valve prolapse
Hypokalemia	Intraventricular conduction disturbance
Severe hypoxia	Preexcitation syndrome
Digitalis	Severe volume overload (aortic, mitral regurgitation)
Sudden excessive exercise	Supraventricular tachyarrhythmias

TABLE 6–4 EXERCISE PARAMETERS ASSOCIATED WITH AN ADVERSE PROGNOSIS AND MULTIVESSEL CORONARY ARTERY DISEASE

- Duration of symptom-limiting exercise (<6 METS)
- Failure to increase systolic blood pressure ≥120 mm Hg, or a sustained decrease ≥10 mm Hg, or below rest levels, during progressive exercise
- ST-segment depression ≥2 mm, downsloping ST segment, starting at <6 METS, involving ≥5 leads, persisting ≥5 minutes into recovery
- Exercise-induced ST-segment elevation (aVR excluded)
- Angina pectoris during exercise
- Reproducible sustained (>30 sec) or symptomatic ventricular tachycardia

to 70 per cent obstruction of the luminal diameter as the angiographic cutpoint. There are limitations of the angiographic classification of patients into one-, two-, and three-vessel coronary disease, and the length of the coronary artery narrowing and the impact of serial lesions are not accounted for in correlative studies comparing diagnostic exercise testing with coronary angiographic findings. Other approaches, including intracoronary Doppler flow studies and quantitative coronary angiography, have been proposed to assess coronary vascular reserve which may be more accurate than qualitative assessment of the angiogram.

BAYESIAN THEORY (see also p. 1697). The depth of exercise-induced ST-segment depression and the extent of the myocardial ischemic response can be thought of as continuous variables. Cutpoints such as 1 mm of horizontal or downsloping ST-segment depression as compared with baseline cannot completely discriminate patients with disease from those without disease, and the requirement of more severe degrees of ST-segment depression to improve specificity will decrease sensitivity. Sensitivity and specificity are inversely related, and false-negative and false-positive results are to be expected when ECG or angiographic cutpoints are selected to optimize the diagnostic accuracy of the test.[29]

The use of Bayesian theory incorporates the pretest risk of disease and the sensitivity and specificity of the test (likelihood ratio) to calculate the posttest probability of coronary disease (Fig. 6–11). The results of the patient's clinical information and exercise test results are used to make a final estimate of the probability of coronary disease. The diagnostic power of the exercise test is maximal when the pretest probability of coronary artery disease is intermediate (30 to 70 per cent). Exercise testing to diagnose coronary artery disease in young or middle-aged asymptomatic subjects without risk factors is not useful, since the pretest risk is very low and a normal or abnormal exercise ECG result does not alter significantly the posttest risk of coronary artery disease (Fig. 6–11).

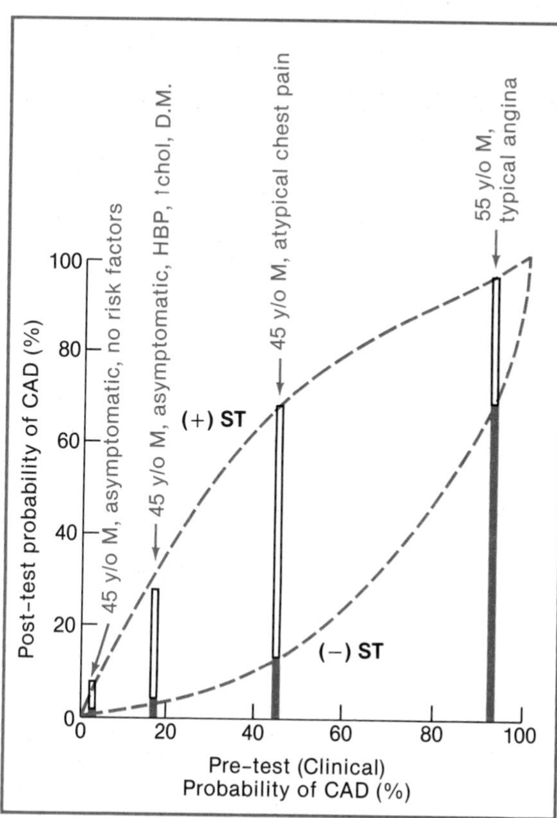

FIGURE 6–11. Use of Bayes theorem to calculate the probability of coronary artery disease (CAD). Four specific patient examples are shown by vertical bars where the height of the solid dark bar illustrates results for a negative exercise electrocardiogram (ECG)(−) ST, and a clear bar shows the results for a positive exercise ECG (+) ST. The posttest probability of coronary disease is optimal in patients with an intermediate coronary disease prevalence. (From Patterson, R. E., and Horowitz, S. F.: Importance of epidemiology and biostatistics in deciding clinical strategies for using diagnostic tests: A simplified approach using examples from coronary artery disease. Reprinted by permission of the American College of Cardiology. J. Am. Coll. Cardiol. *13:*1653, 1989.)

MULTIVARIATE ANALYSIS. Multivariate analysis of exercise test variables to estimate posttest risk can also provide important diagnostic information. There is some controversy concerning whether to use Bayesian theory or multivariate analysis to estimate final posttest risk. Multivariate analysis offers the potential advantage that it does not require that the tests be independent of each other or that sensitivity and specificity remain constant over a wide range of disease prevalence rates. However, the multivariate technique depends critically on how patients are selected to establish the reference data base. Both Bayesian and multivariate techniques are acceptable.[30]

UPSLOPING ST SEGMENTS. Junctional or J point depression is a normal finding during maximum exercise, and a rapid upsloping ST segment (>1 mV/sec) depressed <1.5 mm (0.15 mV) after the J point should be considered to be normal. Occasionally, however, the ST segment will be depressed ≥ 1.5 mm (0.15 mV) at 80 msec after the J point. This type of "slow upsloping" ST segment may be the only ECG finding in patients with well-defined obstructive coronary disease and may depend on the lead set employed (Fig. 6–7). In patient subsets with a high disease prevalence, a slow upsloping ST segment depressed ≥ 1.5 mm at 80 msec after the J point should be considered to be abnormal. The importance of this finding in asymptomatic subjects or those with a low coronary disease prevalence is less certain. Increasing the degree of ST-segment depression at 80 msec after the J point to ≥ 2.0 mm (0.20mV) in patients with a slow upsloping ST segment increases specificity but decreases sensitivity.[31]

ST-SEGMENT ELEVATION. Exercise-induced ST-segment elevation in a Q lead with an abnormal Q wave is a marker for poor left ventricular function and an adverse prognosis.[32] This finding occurs in approximately 30 per cent of patients with anterior myocardial infarctions and 15 per cent of those with inferior ones tested early (within 2 weeks) after the index event (Fig. 6–9) and decreases in frequency by 6 weeks. As a group, patients with exercise-induced ST-segment elevation have a lower ejection fraction than those without and greater severity of resting wall motion abnormalities. Exercise-induced ST-segment elevation in leads with abnormal Q waves is *not* a marker of more extensive coronary artery disease, nor does it indicate myocardial ischemia.[33] Occasionally, exercise-induced ST-segment elevation may occur in a patient who has regenerated R waves after an acute myocardial infarction; the clinical significance of this finding is similar to that observed when Q waves are present.

When ST-segment elevation develops during exercise in a non-Q wave lead in a patient without a previous myocardial infarction, the finding should be considered as likely evidence of transmural myocardial ischemia caused by coronary vasospasm or a high-grade coronary narrowing (Fig. 6–10). This finding is relatively uncommon, occurring in approximately 1 per cent of patients with obstructive coronary disease. The ECG site of ST-segment elevation is relatively specific for the coronary artery involved, and thallium scintigraphy will usually reveal a defect in the territory involved.

OTHER ELECTROCARDIOGRAPHIC MARKERS. Changes in R wave amplitude during exercise are relatively nonspecific and are related to the level of exercise performed. When the R wave amplitude meets voltage criteria for left ventricular hypertrophy the ST-segment response *cannot* be used reliably to diagnose coronary disease, even in the absence of a left ventricular strain pattern. Loss of R wave amplitude, commonly seen after myocardial infarction, reduces the sensitivity of the ST-segment response in that lead to diagnose obstructive coronary artery disease. In patients with a high clinical pretest risk of disease, an exercise-induced reduction in septal Q wave amplitude in bipolar CM5 and CC5 leads is suggestive of left anterior descending coronary stenosis.[34] Occasionally, U wave inversion may be seen in the precordial leads at heart rates < 120 beats/min. While this finding is relatively specific for disease of the left anterior descending coronary artery in the absence of left ventricular hypertrophy or cardiomyopathy, it is relatively insensitive, seen only in approximately 10 to 15 per cent of patients with disease of the left anterior descending coronary artery.

ST/HEART RATE SLOPE MEASUREMENTS. Heart rate adjustment of ST-segment depression appears to improve the sensitivity of the exercise test, particularly the prediction of multivessel coronary disease.[17,35] The ST/heart rate slope depends on the type of exercise performed, number and location of monitoring electrodes, method of measuring ST-segment depression, and clinical characteristics of the study population. Calculation of maximal ST/heart rate slope in mV/beats/min is performed by linear regression analysis relating the measured amount of ST-segment depression in individual leads to the heart rate at the end of each stage of exercise, starting at end exercise. The maximal ST/heart rate slope from all leads measured excluding lead aVR, aVl and V_1 is selected. An ST/heart rate slope ≥ 2.4 mV/beats/min is considered abnormal, and values ≥ 6 mV/beats/min are suggestive evidence of three-vessel coronary disease.[35] The use of this measurement requires modification of the exercise protocol such that increments in heart rate are gradual as in the Cornell protocol as opposed to more abrupt increases in heart rate between stages such as in the Bruce or Ellestad protocols, which limit the ability to calculate statistically valid ST-segment heart rate slopes.[17] The measurement is not accurate in the early postinfarction phase. A modification to the ST-segment/heart rate slope method is the Δ ST-segment/heart rate index calculation, which represents the average change of ST-segment depression with heart rate throughout the course of the exercise test. The Δ ST/heart rate index measurements are less than the ST/heart rate slope measurements and a Δ ST/heart rate index ≥ 1.6 is defined as abnormal. More research on ST-segment/heart rate slope measurements is required before the use of this measurement can be widely adopted.[36]

NONELECTROCARDIOGRAPHIC OBSERVATIONS

The ECG is only one part of the exercise response, and abnormal hemodynamics or functional capacity is just as important if not more so than ST-segment displacement.

BLOOD PRESSURE. The normal exercise response is to increase systolic blood pressure progressively with increasing workloads to a peak response ranging from 160 to 220 mm Hg, with the higher range of the scale seen in older patients with less compliant vascular systems.[6,7,16] As a group, black patients tend to have a higher systolic blood pressure response than do whites.[37] At high exercise workloads, it is sometimes difficult to obtain an accurate determination of systolic blood pressure.[38] In normal subjects the diastolic blood pressure does not change significantly, fluctuating ± 10 mm Hg as compared to that at rest. Failure to increase systolic blood pressure ≥ 120 mm Hg, or a sustained decrease ≥ 10 mm Hg repeatable within 15 seconds, or a fall in systolic blood pressure below standing rest values is abnormal and reflects either inadequate elevation of cardiac output because of left ventricular systolic pump dysfunction or an excessive reduction in systemic vascular resistance.[39,40] The prevalence of exertional hypotension ranges from 2.7 to 9.3 per cent and is higher in patients with three-vessel or left main coronary disease.[7,16] The finding of an abnormal systolic blood pressure response in patients with a high prevalence of coronary artery disease is associated with more extensive coronary disease and more extensive thallium defects. Conditions other than myocardial ischemia that have been associated with the failure to increase or an actual decrease in systolic blood pressure during progressive exercise are cardiomyopathy, cardiac arrhythmias, vasovagal reactions, left ventricular outflow tract obstruction, ingestion of antihypertensive drugs, hypovolemia, and prolonged vigorous exercise.

It is important to make the distinction between a decline in blood pressure in the *postexercise* phase and a decrease or failure to increase systolic blood pressure *during* progressive exercise. The incidence of postexertional hypotension in asymptomatic subjects was 1.9 per cent in 781 asymptomatic volunteers in the Baltimore Longitudinal Study on Aging, with a 3.1 per cent incidence noted in subjects younger than age 55 and 0.3 per cent incidence in patients older than age 55.[41] In this series, most hypotensive episodes were symptomatic, and only two patients had hypotension associated with bradycardia and vagal symptoms. Although ST-segment abnormalities suggestive of ischemia occurred in one-third of the patients with hypotension, none of the patients had a cardiac event during 4 years of follow-up. Occasionally, in young patients, vasovagal syncope can occur in the immediate postexercise phase, progressing through sinus bradycardia to several seconds of asystole and hypotension before reverting to sinus rhythm.

POSTEXERCISE SYSTOLIC BLOOD PRESSURE RATIOS. In the postexercise phase, there is a progressive decline in systolic and diastolic blood pressure. An abnormal postexercise systolic blood pressure response has been defined as a ratio of systolic blood pressure in the 3 minute recovery phase to the peak exercise systolic blood pressure reading. When the ratio is ≥ 0.9, some authors have reported a greater extent of exercise-induced myocardial ischemia, left ventricular dysfunction, and more extensive coronary disease. Other investigators have not found the ratio to improve diagnostic accuracy as compared with exercise ST-segment depression alone.[42]

MAXIMAL WORK CAPACITY. This variable is one of the most important prognostic measurements obtained from an exercise test.[43-45] Maximal work capacity in normal individuals is influenced by familiarization with the exercise test equipment, level of training, and environmental conditions at the time of testing. In patients with known or suspected coronary artery disease, a limited exercise capacity is associated with an increased risk of cardiac events, and, in general, the more severe the limitation, the worse the coronary disease extent and prognosis. In estimating functional capacity, the amount of work performed (or exercise stage achieved) should be the parameter measured and not the number of minutes of exercise, since peak workload is totally dependent on the protocol employed. Estimates of peak functional capacity for age and gender have been well established for most of the exercise protocols in common usage, subject to the limitations described in the section on cardiopulmonary testing.[10] Comparison of an individual's performance against normal standards provides an estimate of the degree of exercise impairment.

Serial comparison of functional capacity in individual patients to assess significant interval change requires a careful examination of the exercise protocol used during both tests, of drug therapy and time of ingestion, of systemic blood pressure, and of other conditions that might influence test performance. All of these variables need to be considered before attributing changes in functional capacity to progression of coronary artery disease or worsening of left ventricular function. Major reductions in exercise capacity usually indicate significant worsening of cardiovascular status; modest changes may not.

SUBMAXIMAL EXERCISE. The interpretation of an exercise test for diagnostic and prognostic purposes requires consideration of maximum work capacity. When a patient is unable to complete moderate levels of exercise or reach at least 85 to 90 per cent of age-predicted maximum, the level of exercise performed may be inadequate to test cardiac reserve. Thus, ischemic ECG, scintigraphic, or ventriculographic abnormalities may not be evoked and the test may be nondiagnostic.[46] Nondiagnostic tests are more common in patients with peripheral vascular disease, orthopedic limitation, or neurological impairment, and in patients with poor motivation.

HEART RATE RESPONSE. The sinus rate increases progressively with exercise, mediated in part through sympathetic and parasympathetic innervation of the sinoatrial node, and circulating catecholamines. In some patients who may be anxious about the exercise test, there may be an initial overreaction of heart rate and systolic blood pressure at the beginning of exercise with stabilization after approximately 30 to 60 seconds. Maximum heart rate during exercise is highest in childhood, decreases with age, and is slightly reduced in a trained athlete.

There are two types of abnormal heart rate responses to exercise. In patients with chronotropic incompetence, the heart rate increment per stage of exercise is less than normal and the heart rate may plateau at submaximal workloads.[47] This finding may indicate sinus node disease, may be present with drug therapy such as beta blockers, or may indicate a myocardial ischemic response. The second type of abnormal heart rate response is an inappropriate increase in heart rate at low exercise workloads. This response may occur in patients who are physically deconditioned, hypovolemic, or anemic or who have marginal left ventricular function and may persist for several minutes in the recovery phase.

RATE-PRESSURE PRODUCT. The heart rate–systolic blood pressure product, an indirect measure of myocardial oxygen demand (see also p. 1162), increases progressively with exercise, and the peak rate pressure product can be used to characterize cardiovascular performance. Most normal subjects develop a peak rate pressure product of 20 to 35 mm Hg $\times$ beats/min $\times 10^{-3}$. In many patients with significant ischemic heart disease, rate-pressure products exceeding 25 mm Hg $\times$ beats/min $\times 10^{-3}$ are unusual. However, the cutpoint of 25 mm Hg $\times$ beats/min $\times 10^{-3}$ is not a useful diagnostic parameter; significant overlap exists between patients with disease and those without disease. Furthermore, cardioactive drug therapy will significantly influence this measurement.

CHEST DISCOMFORT. Characterization of chest discomfort during exercise can be a useful diagnostic finding, particularly when the symptom complex is compatible with typical angina pectoris. In some patients, the exercise level during the test may exceed that which the patient exhibits in day-to-day activities. Exercise-induced chest discomfort usually occurs after the onset of ischemic ST-segment abnormalities and may be associated with diastolic hypertension.[48] However, in some patients, chest discomfort may be the only marker that obstructive coronary artery disease is present. In patients with chronic stable angina, exercise-induced chest discomfort occurs less frequently than ischemic ST-segment depression. The severity of myocardial ischemia in a patient with exercised-induced angina and a normal ECG can often be assessed using thallium scintigraphy. The new development of an S3, holosystolic apical murmur, or basilar rales in the early recovery phase of exercise will enhance the diagnostic accuracy of the test.

EXERCISE TESTING IN EVALUATING PROGNOSIS

ASYMPTOMATIC POPULATION. The prevalence of an abnormal exercise electrocardiogram in middle-aged asymptomatic men ranges from 5 to 12 per cent.[49–51] The risk of developing a cardiac event such as angina, myocardial infarction, or death in men is 9 times greater when the test is abnormal as when it is normal; however, over 5 years of follow-up, only one in four such men will suffer a cardiac event, and this will most commonly be the development of angina. The risk is slightly greater when the test is strongly positive. In the LRC Prevention Trial, a strongly positive test was defined as one in which the ST response was ≥ 2 mm (0.2 mV) or occurred during the first 6 minutes of exercise or at heart rate at or below $163 - 0.66 \times$ age. Of 3806 middle-aged asymptomatic men who had a total cholesterol ≥ 265 mg/dl at entry, 3 per cent had a strongly positive test; the event rate was 2 per cent per year over an average of 4 years of follow-up.[49] A positive test was *not* significantly associated with nonfatal myocardial infarction; this indicates the difficulty in identifying patients destined to develop abrupt changes in plaque morphology.

In the Seattle Heart Watch, Bruce noted that an abnormal ST response to exercise in asymptomatic men did *not* increase the likelihood of developing cardiac events within 6 years in the absence of conventional risk factors. However, the likelihood of developing a cardiac event was increased when the patient had any conventional atherosclerotic risk factor (see Chap. 37) and two or more abnormal responses to exercise, with an abnormal exercise response defined as chest discomfort during the test, exercise duration < 6 minutes or two stages, failure to achieve 90 per cent of age-predicted maximum heart rate, or ≥ 1 mm (0.1 mV) of horizontal or downsloping ST depression with exercise in early recovery. Only 1.1 per cent of the asymptomatic healthy men in this study were in a high-risk category.[51] The lead set and criteria for an abnormal ECG response were different in both studies. In the Baltimore Longitudinal Study on Aging, Fleg et al. performed maximal treadmill exercise electrocardiography and thallium scintigraphy in 407 asymptomatic volunteers whose mean age was 60 years. The only combination of test results predictive of subsequent cardiac events occurred in the 6 per cent of patients who had *both* an abnormal exercise ECG and thallium scan; 48 per cent had a cardiac event over an average 4-year follow-up[52] (Fig. 6–12).

In asymptomatic middle-aged or older men with several atherosclerotic risk factors, a markedly abnormal exercise response is associated with a significant increased risk of subsequent cardiac events, particularly when there is additional supporting evidence for underlying coronary artery disease (e.g., coronary calcification, abnormal thallium scan, and the like).[53] Serial change of a negative exercise ECG to a positive one in an asymptomatic subject carries the same prognostic importance as an initially abnormal test.[54] However, when an asymptomatic subject with an initially abnormal test has significant worsening of the ECG abnormalities at lower exercise workloads, this finding may indicate significant coronary artery disease progression and warrants a more aggressive diagnostic work-up.

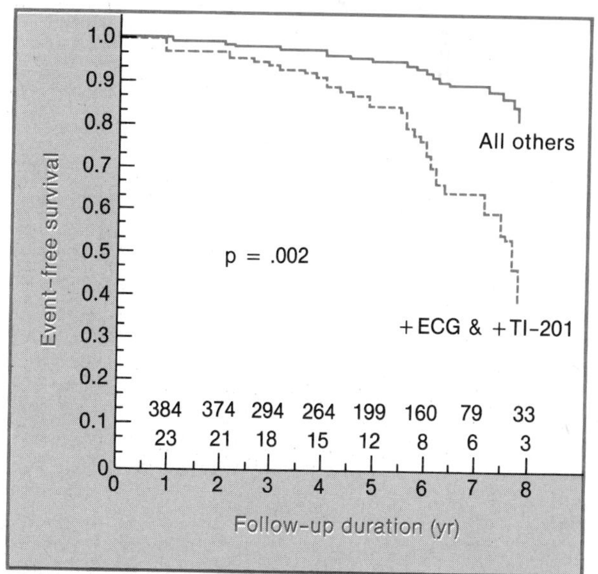

FIGURE 6–12. The incidence of cardiac events in 407 asymptomatic subjects with a mean age of 60 years was significantly greater in the 6 per cent of patients who had both an abnormal exercise electrocardiogram and abnormal thallium scan. (From Fleg, J. L., et al.: Prevalence and prognostic significance of exercise-induced silent myocardial ischemia detected by thallium scintigraphy and ECG in asymptomatic volunteers. Circulation *81:*428, 1990. Reprinted by permission of the American Heart Association, Inc.)

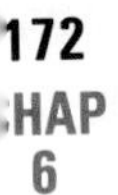

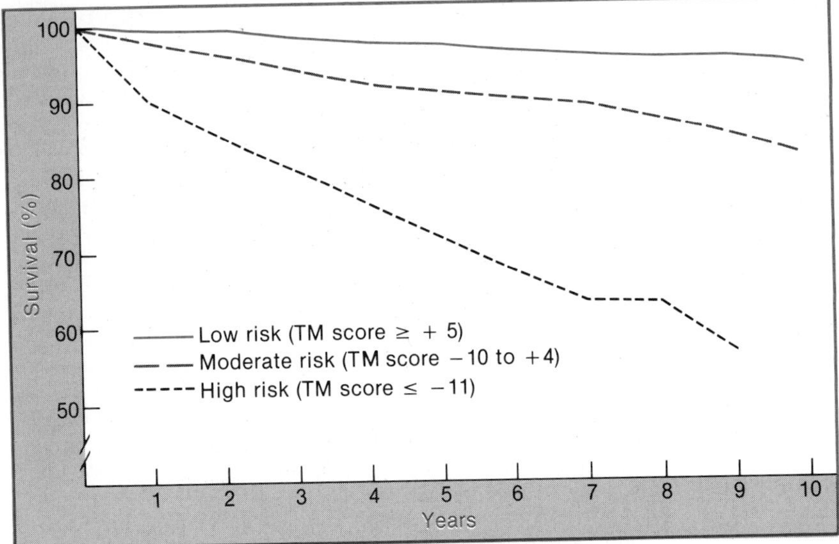

FIGURE 6–13. Exercise treadmill score based on exercise time, angina, and extent of ST deviation separates 2842 patients who underwent exercise testing and coronary angiography into low- and high-risk groups. The treadmill score (TM) is calculated as follows: exercise time − (5 × ST deviation) − (4 × treadmill angina index), when angina index is assigned a value of 0 if angina is absent, 1 if typical angina occurred during exercise, and 2 if angina was the reason for terminating the test. Exercise-induced ST deviation is defined as the largest net ST displacement in any lead. (From Mark, D. B., et al.: Exercise treadmill score for predicting prognosis in coronary artery disease. Ann. Intern. Med. *106*:793, 1987.)

The prevalence of an abnormal exercise ECG in middle-aged asymptomatic women ranges from 20 to 30 per cent.[7,16] In general, the prognostic value of an ST segment shift in women is less than in men. However, there are few prognostic data on asymptomatic women stratified by age and atherosclerotic risk factors, and additional research is required in this area.

SYMPTOMATIC PATIENTS. Exercise testing should be routinely performed (unless this is not feasible or unless there are contraindications) before coronary angiography in patients with chronic ischemic heart disease. Patients who have excellent exercise tolerance (e.g., > 10 METS) usually have an excellent prognosis regardless of the anatomical extent of coronary artery disease. The test provides an estimate of the functional significance of angiographically documented coronary artery stenoses. The impact of exercise testing in patients with documented coronary artery disease was studied by Weiner et al. in 4083 medically treated patients in the CASS study.[45] A high-risk patient subset was identified (12 per cent of the population) with an annual mortality ≥ 5 per cent a year when exercise workload was < Bruce stage I and the exercise ECG exhibited ≥ 1 mm (0.1 mV) ST-segment depression. A low-risk patient subset (34 per cent of the population) able to exercise into ≥ Bruce stage III who had a normal exercise ECG had an annual mortality < 1 per cent per year over 4 years of follow-up. Similar ECG and workload parameters were useful in risk stratifying patients with three-vessel coronary artery disease likely to benefit from coronary bypass grafting.[55]

Mark et al. developed a treadmill score based on 2842 consecutive patients in the Duke data bank with chest pain who had treadmill testing using the Bruce protocol and cardiac catheterization.[44] Patients with left bundle branch block or those with exercise-induced ST elevation in a Q wave lead were excluded. The treadmill score is calculated as follows: exercise time − (5 × ST deviation) − (4 × treadmill angina index). Angina index was assigned a value of 0 if angina was absent, 1 if typical angina occurred during exercise, and 2 if angina was the reason the patient stopped exercising. Exercise-induced ST deviation was defined as the largest net ST displacement in any lead. The 13 per cent of patients with a treadmill score ≤ − 11 had a 5-year survival of 72 per cent compared with 97 per cent in the 34 per cent of patients at low risk with a treadmill score ≥ +5. The score added independent prognostic information to that provided by clinical data, coronary anatomy, and left ventricular ejection fraction (Fig. 6–13).

SILENT MYOCARDIAL ISCHEMIA (see also p. 1347). In patients with documented coronary artery disease, the presence of exercise-induced ischemic ST-segment depression confers increased risk of subsequent cardiac events regardless of whether angina occurs during the test. The magnitude of the prognostic gradient in patients with an abnormal exercise ECG with or without angina varies considerably in the published literature, most likely a feature of patient selection. In the CASS data bank, 7-year survival in patients with silent or symptomatic exercise-induced myocardial ischemia was similar in patients stratified by coronary anatomy and left ventricular function[56,57] (Fig. 6–14). In the Duke data bank, patients with exercise-induced angina tended to have more severe coronary artery disease than patients with exercise-induced silent ST-segment changes, and 5-year survival was worse in patients with angina.[58] There are important patient selection differences between the two series; the prevalence of prior myocardial infarction was lower in the Duke series, and all patients had a prior history of angina in comparison with only 65 per cent of patients in the CASS series.

UNSTABLE ANGINA (see also p. 1334). The incidence of exercise-induced angina or ischemic ST-segment abnormalities in patients with unstable angina who undergo a predischarge low-level protocol ranges from 30 to 40 per cent. The finding of ischemic ST-segment changes or limiting chest pain is associated with a significantly increased risk of subsequent cardiac events. The *absence* of these findings identifies a low-risk patient subset, and in one patient series admitted to the CCU with rest angina and transient ST-T wave changes, 8-

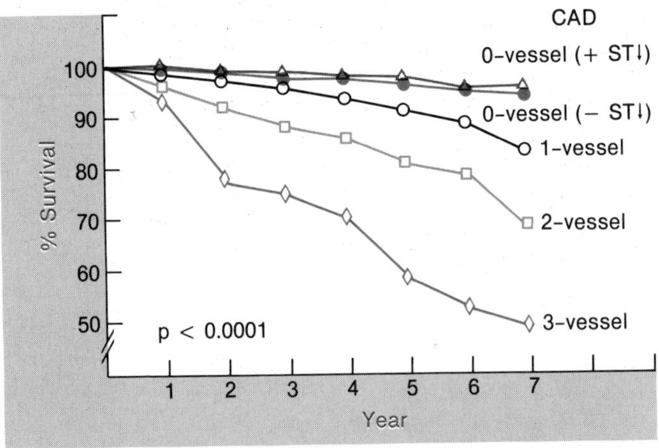

FIGURE 6–14. The 7-year survival in the 424 patients in the CASS Registry with silent exercise-induced myocardial ischemia is significantly worse according to extent of coronary disease. The prognosis of 424 patients enrolled in the CASS registry with silent exercise-induced ischemic ST depression is worse than in a separate group of 282 CASS patients without coronary disease who had abnormal ST-segment depression (+ST ↓) without angina, and a control group of 1117 without coronary disease and without ST-segment depression (−ST ↓) or angina during the test. (From Weiner, D. A. et al.: Significance of silent myocardial ischemia during exercise testing in patients with coronary artery disease. Am J. Cardiol. *59*:725, 1987.)

year survival was 100 per cent in the 54 patients who had a normal predischarge exercise test.[59]

MYOCARDIAL INFARCTION (see also Ch. 39). A low-level exercise test (achievement of 5 to 6 METS or 70 to 80 per cent of age-predicted maximum) is frequently performed before hospital discharge to establish the hemodynamic response and functional capacity for exercise prescriptions, to identify serious ventricular arrhythmia, and to identify patients at increased risk of cardiac events. The ability to complete 5 to 6 METS of exercise or 70 to 80 per cent of age-predicted maximum in the absence of abnormal ECG or blood pressure abnormalities is associated with a 1-year mortality of 1 to 2 per cent.[60] Approximately 30 per cent of postinfarction patients have predischarge exercise-induced ischemic ST-segment depression and 15 per cent have exertional hypotension. In the early postinfarction phase, exertional hypotension is not as specific a prognosis marker as in patients with chronic ischemic heart disease and occurs less frequently when patients are tested later (6 weeks). The prognostic importance of exercise-induced ST-segment changes is influenced by the fact that many patients who have an abnormal test undergo coronary angiography and revascularization, which may alter the natural history of the disease process. The performance of a predischarge maximum, symptom-limited test as opposed to a submaximal low-level test is gaining in popularity and is associated with an increased incidence of ischemic ST-segment depression and angina. However, the safety and incremental increase in prognostic information in this approach require further study.

Froelicher et al. performed an overview or meta analysis of the published literature on exercise testing postinfarction and identified several variables associated with an adverse outcome. The parameters associated with increased risk were inability to perform the low-level predischarge exercise test, an abnormal systolic blood pressure response, poor exercise capacity, and exercise-induced ST-segment depression in patients with inferior wall myocardial infarctions.[60] The clinical importance of painless ST-segment depression in patients able to complete a low-level predischarge exercise test is uncertain.[61,62]

The relative prognostic value of a 6-week postdischarge exercise test is minimal once clinical variables and the results of the low-level predischarge test are adjusted for.[63] However, the 6-week test is useful in clearing patients to return to work in occupations involving physical labor and to provide a better estimate of cardiovascular reserve at peak exercise performance. Exercise testing performed later after the acute infarction (e.g., ≥ 6 months) is useful in risk stratification.[64]

Left ventricular ejection fraction is one of the most important prognostic determinants of mortality following acute myocardial infarction (see also pp. 1251 and 1267). The additional value of exercise testing in patients with a left ventricular ejection fraction < 35 per cent by gated radionuclide scans 1 month after acute myocardial infarction was examined by Pilote et al.[65] Patients with an exercise capacity < 4 METS have a 3.5 fold greater risk of dying than patients with an exercise capacity ≥ 7 METS.

Approximately 20 to 30 per cent of patients with non-Q-wave infarct have exercise-induced ST-segment depression. This finding is associated with a significant increased risk of cardiac events, particularly in patients with complicated infarcts.[66-68]

Patients who receive thrombolytic therapy are in a different clinical subset than are patients studied in the prethrombolytic era and tend to have a better prognosis. In the TIMI II trial, patients who were able to perform a predischarge supine low-level exercise test had a 1-year mortality of only 1 per cent, and ST-segment depression during or after the test did *not* increase mortality.[68a] Prognostic variables that increase 1-year mortality in postinfarction patients treated with thrombolytic drugs include inability to take the test, inability to complete the protocol, and inability to increase systolic blood pressure ≥ 120 mm Hg.

CARDIAC ARRHYTHMIAS AND CONDUCTION DISTURBANCES

The genesis of cardiac arrhythmias includes reentry, delayed afterpotentials, and enhanced automaticity of ectopic foci (Chap. 22). Increased catecholamines during exercise accelerate impulse conduction velocity, shorten the myocardial refractory period, increase the amplitude of delayed afterpotentials, and increase the slope of phase 4 spontaneous depolarization of the action potential. Other potentiators of cardiac rhythm disturbance include metabolic acidosis and exercise-induced myocardial ischemia.[69,70] Ventricular premature beats occur frequently during exercise testing and increase with age[71] (Fig. 6-15). Repetitive forms occur in 0 to 5 per cent of asymptomatic subjects without suspected cardiac disease and are not associated with an increased risk of cardiac death. Exercise-induced ventricular ectopic activity is not a useful diagnostic marker of ischemic heart disease in the absence of ischemic ST-segment depression. Suppression of ventricular ectopic activity during exercise is a nonspecific finding and may occur in patients with coronary artery disease as well as in normal subjects. The prognostic importance of ventricular arrhythmias in patients with chronic ischemic heart disease after adjustment for baseline, clinical, and left ventricular function characteristics is small.[69] Approximately 20 per cent of patients with known heart disease and 50 to 75 per cent of sudden cardiac death survivors have repetitive ventricular beats induced by exercise. In patients with a recent myocardial infarction, the presence of exercise-induced repetitive forms is associated with an increased risk of subsequent cardiac events.

Exercise-induced ventricular arrhythmias tend to be more frequent in the recovery phase of exercise because peripheral plasma norepinephrine levels continue to increase for several minutes after cessation of exercise and vagal tone is high in the immediate recovery phase.[72] Beta-adrenergic blocking drugs may suppress exercise-induced ventricular arrhythmias. Continuous recording of the exercise test will enhance documentation of the cardiac arrhythmia.

EVALUATION OF VENTRICULAR ARRHYTHMIAS (see also Chap. 24). Exercise testing is useful in the assessment of patients with ventricular arrhythmias and has an important adjunctive role along with ambulatory monitoring and electrophysiological studies.[70] Exercise testing provokes repetitive ventricular premature beats in most patients with a his-

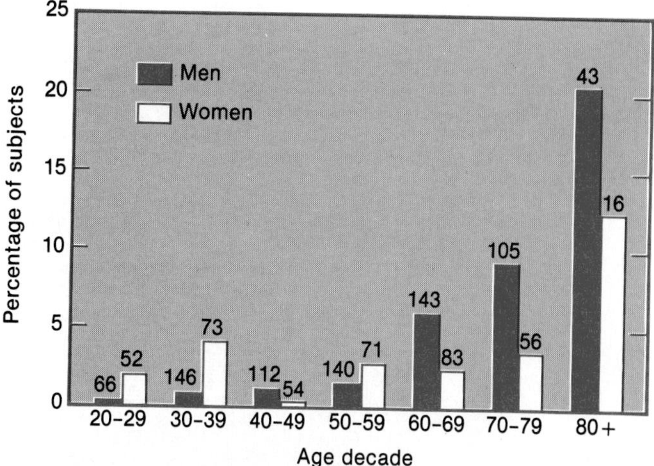

FIGURE 6-15. Prevalence of frequent or repetitive ventricular ectopic beats induced by maximal treadmill exercise as a function of age and gender in 1160 apparently healthy volunteers. The numbers above each bar indicate the number of subjects tested in each decade. (From Busby, M. J., et al.: Prevalence and long-term significance of exercise-induced frequent or repetitive ventricular ectopic beats in apparently healthy volunteers. Reprinted by permission of the American College of Cardiology. J. Am. Coll. Cardiol. *14:*1659, 1989.)

tory of sustained ventricular tachyarrhythmia, and, in approximately 10 to 15 per cent of such patients, spontaneously occurring arrhythmias are observed only during exercise testing. The test is useful in the evaluation of the effects of antiarrhythmic drugs, the detection of supraventricular arrhythmias, the management of patients with chronic atrial fibrillation, and exposing possible drug toxicity in patients placed on antiarrhythmic drugs. Approximately 50 per cent of patients with sustained ventricular tachyarrhythmias without pharmacological intervention will have reproducible findings on repeat testing within a reasonable time interval.[73] Paradoxical prolongation of the QT_C interval ≥ 10 msec with exercise identifies patients likely to develop a proarrhythmic effect on type 1A antiarrhythmic drugs.[74]

SUPRAVENTRICULAR ARRHYTHMIAS. Supraventricular premature beats induced by exercise are observed in 4 to 10 per cent of normal subjects and up to 40 per cent of patients with underlying heart disease. Sustained supraventricular tachyarrhythmias occur in only 1 to 2 per cent of patients, although the frequency may approach as much as 10 to 15 per cent in patients referred for management of episodic supraventricular arrhythmias. The presence of supraventricular arrhythmias is *not* diagnostic for ischemic heart disease.

ATRIAL FIBRILLATION (see also p. 682). Patients with chronic atrial fibrillation tend to have a rapid ventricular response in the initial stages of exercise and 60 to 70 per cent of the total change in heart rate usually occurs within the first few minutes of exercise. The effect of digitalis preparations and beta-adrenergic and calcium antagonists on attenuating this rapid increase in heart rate for individual patients can be measured using exercise testing. Pharmacological control of the ventricular rate does not necessarily result in a significant increase in exercise capacity, which in many patients is related to the underlying cardiac disease process and not adequacy of control of the ventricular rate.

SICK SINUS SYNDROME (see also p. 677). In general, patients with sick sinus syndrome have a lower heart rate at submaximal and maximal workloads compared with control subjects. However, as many as 40 to 50 per cent of patients will have a normal exercise heart rate response.

AV BLOCK. Exercise testing may help determine the need for AV sequential pacing in selected patients. In patients with congenital AV block, exercise-induced heart rates are low and some patients develop symptomatic rapid junctional rhythms which can be suppressed with DDD devices. In patients with acquired conduction disease, exercise can occasionally bring out advanced AV block.

LEFT BUNDLE BRANCH BLOCK (LBBB) (see also p. 128). Exercise-induced ST-segment depression is seen in most patients with LBBB and cannot be used as a diagnostic or prognostic indicator regardless of the degree of ST-segment abnormality. In patients referred to a tertiary center in whom exercise testing is carried out, the new development of exercise-induced transient left hemiblock is 0.3 per cent and left bundle branch block is 0.4 per cent, with a slightly greater incidence in older patients.[75] The development of ischemic ST-segment depression before the LBBB pattern appears or in the recovery phase after the LBBB has resolved does not attenuate the diagnostic yield of the ST-segment shift (Fig. 6–16). The ventricular rate at which the LBBB appears and disappears can be significantly different. In one series, permanent LBBB was reported in approximately half of the patients who developed transient LBBB during exercise and who were followed for an average 6.6 years. High-grade AV block did not develop in any of the patients in this 15-patient series.[76]

RIGHT BUNDLE BRANCH BLOCK (RBBB). The rest ECG in RBBB is frequently associated with T wave and ST-segment changes in the early anterior precordial leads (V_{1-3}). Exercise-induced ST depression in leads V_{1-4} is a common finding in patients with RBBB and is nondiagnostic. The new development of exercise-induced ST-segment depression in leads $V_{5,6}$ is useful in detecting patients with coronary artery disease who have a high clinical pretest risk of disease. The new development of exercise-induced RBBB is relatively uncommon, occurring in approximately 0.1 per cent of tests.[75]

PREEXCITATION SYNDROME (see also p. 693). The presence of WPW syndrome invalidates the use of ST-segment analysis as a diagnostic method for detecting coronary artery disease in preexcited as well as normally conducted beats; false-positive ischemic changes are frequently registered. In patients with persistent preexcitation, exercise may normalize the QRS complex with disappearance of the delta wave in 20 to 50 per cent of cases dependent on the series studied.[77-79] Abrupt disappearance of the delta wave is presumptive evidence of a longer anterograde effective refractory period of the accessory pathway. Progressive disappearance of the delta wave is less reassuring and occurs when the improvement in AV node conduction is greater than in the accessory pathway; this finding does not exclude a possible significant or even critical shortening of the anterograde effective refractory period in the accessory pathway under the influence of sympathetic stimulation.[77,78] Exercise-induced disappearance of the delta wave is more frequent with type A than type B WPW patterns.[79] Although tachyarrhythmias appearing during an

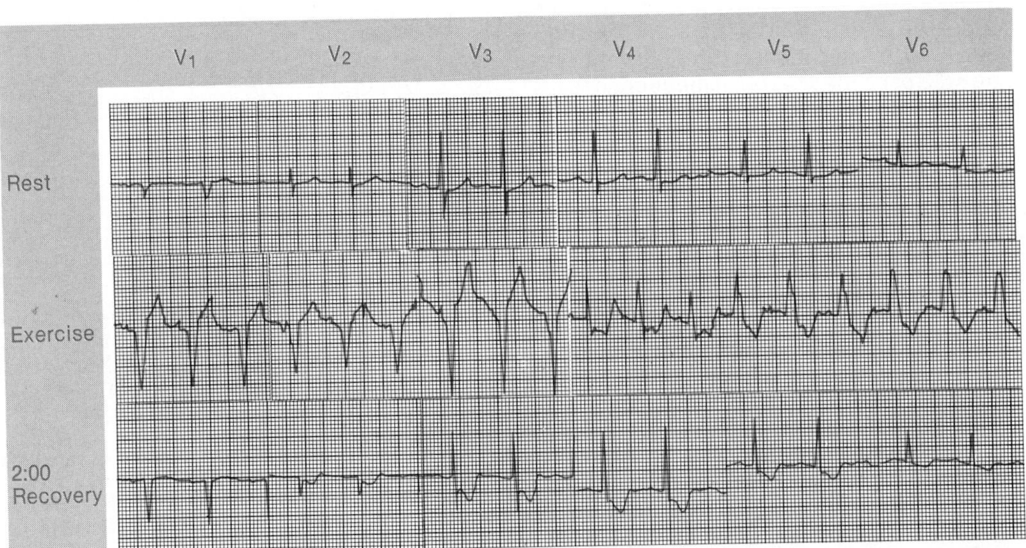

FIGURE 6–16. The rest, exercise, and recovery precordial lead set in a patient with exercise-induced left bundle branch block. In the absence of LBBB in the 2-minute recovery phase of exercise, the ST-segment changes can be used as a diagnostic marker for obstructive coronary disease.

exercise test in patients with WPW are rare, when they do occur, they provide an opportunity to evaluate AV conduction velocity. The presence of WPW does not cause a limitation of physical work capacity.

SPECIFIC CLINICAL APPLICATIONS

WOMEN. The specificity of exercise-induced ST-segment depression for obstructive coronary artery disease is less in women than in men. The decreased specificity results in part from a lower prevalence and extent of coronary artery disease in young and middle-aged women. Exercise-induced ST-segment depression is more likely to be a false-positive for coronary artery disease when the changes are seen only in the inferior leads appearing at moderate-to-high workloads.[80] Women tend to have a greater release of catecholamines during exercise, which could potentiate coronary vasoconstriction and augment the incidence of abnormal exercise ECGs, and false-positive tests have been reported to be more common during menses or preovulation.[81] Exercise myocardial scintigraphy (e.g., thallium-201) will improve the diagnostic yield of the test in patients with a suspected false-positive result.

HYPERTENSION. Exercise testing has been used in an attempt to identify patients with abnormal blood pressure response destined to subsequently develop hypertension.[82] The optimal exercise protocol, and consensus on what constitutes an abnormal exercise response, requires additional study.[83] Different criteria may be required for blacks and whites, men and women, and younger versus older patients.[37,83] Severe systemic hypertension may interfere with subendocardial perfusion and cause exercise-induced ST-segment depression in the absence of atherosclerosis, even when the rest ECG does not show significant ST or T wave changes. Beta and calcium channel blocking drugs decrease submaximal and peak systolic blood pressure in many hypertensive patients.

CONGESTIVE HEART FAILURE. Cardiac and peripheral compensatory mechanisms are activated in patients with chronic congestive heart failure to partly or fully restore impaired left ventricular performance. There is a wide range of exercise capacity in patients who have a markedly reduced ejection fraction, with some patients having near-normal peak exercise capacity.[6,7] Symptoms in patients with congestive heart failure are related to an excessive increase in blood lactate during low exercise levels, reduction in quantity of oxygen consumed at peak exertion, and disproportionate increase in ventilation at submaximal and peak workloads.[84] Fatigue may be related to altered skeletal muscle metabolism secondary to chronic physical deconditioning as well as impaired perfusion.[85] Dyspnea and fatigue are the usual reasons for exercise termination. Peak $\dot{V}_{O_2}$ measurements in patients with compensated congestive heart failure are useful in risk stratifying patients with congestive heart failure to determine subsequent incidence of cardiac events (Fig. 6–17).[84] The ability to achieve a peak $\dot{V}_{O_2}$ of > 20 ml/min/kg and AT_{ge} > 14 ml/min/kg is associated with a relatively good long-term prognosis and a maximum cardiac output > 8 l/min/m^2. Patients who are unable to achieve a peak $\dot{V}_{O_2}$ of 10 ml/min/kg and AT_{ge} of 8 ml/min/kg have a poor prognosis, and their maximum exercise cardiac output is usually < 4 l/min/m^2. A blunted heart rate response is not uncommon in patients with congestive heart failure caused by postsynaptic desensitization of beta-adrenergic receptors (see also p. 411).

DRUGS. Digitalis glycosides can produce exertional ST-segment depression even if the effect is not evident on the resting ECG (see p. 481). Absence of ST-segment deviation during an exercise test in a patient receiving a cardiac glycoside is considered a valid negative response. Antiischemic drug therapy with nitrates, beta-blocking drugs, or calcium channel blocking drugs will prolong the time to onset of ischemic ST-segment depression, increase exercise tolerance, and, in a small minority of patients, may normalize the exercise ECG response in patients with documented coronary artery disease.[6,7,16] The time and dose of drug ingestion may affect exercise performance. In some laboratories, cardioactive drug therapy is withheld for 3 to 5 half-lives and digitalis for 1 to 2 weeks before diagnostic testing. However, this is impractical in many cases. Heparin therapy may increase total exercise duration and ability to achieve a higher rate pressure product before the onset of angina, and at peak exertion.[86] The onset of ischemic ST-segment depression in patients with chronic ischemic heart disease occurs earlier in patients who are cold sensitive and who are exposed to low levels of carbon monoxide.[87,88] Amiodarone therapy increases the QRS duration during exercise by approximately 6 per cent in patients with a QRS duration < 110 msec compared to 15 per cent in patients with a QRS duration > 110 msec.[89]

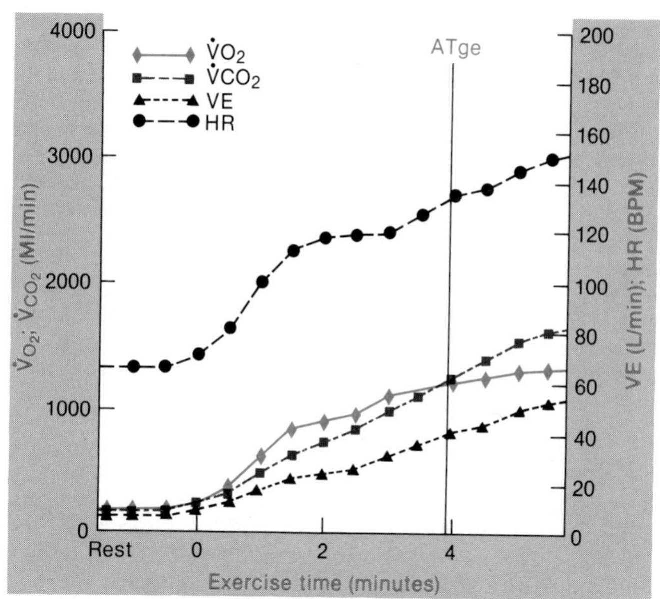

FIGURE 6–17. Cardiopulmonary exercise test in a patient with compensated congestive heart failure. The test reveals limited exercise capacity, with the AT_{ge} occurring at 3:50 minutes into exercise, and a peak $\dot{V}_{O_2}$ of only 1.3 liters/min, indicating that the patient is in a high-risk category.[84]

CORONARY REVASCULARIZATION PROCEDURES. The degree of improvement in exercise-induced myocardial ischemia and aerobic capacity after coronary bypass grafting depends in part on the degree of revascularization achieved and left ventricular function. Exercise-induced ischemic ST-segment depression may persist when incomplete revascularization is achieved, albeit at higher exercise workloads, and in approximately 5 per cent of patients in whom complete revascularization has been achieved. It usually takes at least 6 weeks of convalescence before maximum exercise can be performed. The natural history of saphenous vein grafts and internal mammary artery conduits is different, and serial conversion from an initially normal to abnormal exercise ECG will depend in part on the type of conduit used and coronary disease progression in nongrafted vessels. The diagnostic and prognostic utility of exercise testing late after coronary revascularization (e.g., 5 to 10 years) is much greater than early (< 1 year) testing, since a late abnormal exercise response is more likely to indicate graft occlusion, stenosis, or progression of coronary artery disease.[90]

After coronary angioplasty (PTCA), restenosis occurs in approximately 20 to 30 per cent of patients, usually within the first 6 months, and is more common in patients with proximal LAD disease, long coronary artery narrowings, diabetic patients, patients with multivessel or multilesion dilation, and those in whom post PTCA luminal obstruction is > 50 per cent. In the early post PTCA phase (< 1 month) an abnormal exercise ECG may be secondary to a suboptimal PTCA result, impaired coronary vascular reserve in a successfully dilated vessel, or incomplete revascularization.[91] The optimal time to perform an exercise test following PTCA depends in part on the success of the procedure, and the degree of revascularization obtained. Exercise testing early after PTCA (within days) can often be used to help determine the need for a staged procedure and to provide a reference baseline for subsequent follow-up. In an otherwise asymptomatic patient, a 6-month postprocedure test allows a sufficient amount of time to document restenosis should it occur and allows the dilated vessel an opportunity to heal. Serial conversion of an initially normal exercise test post PTCA to an abnormal test in the initial 6 months after the procedure, particularly when it occurs at a lower exercise workload, is usually associated with restenosis. The use of thallium scintigraphy in selected patients enhances greatly the diagnostic content of the test and can help localize the territory of myocardial ischemia and guide indications for repeat coronary angiography in patients who have undergone multivessel/multilesion PTCA.

CARDIAC TRANSPLANTATION (see also Chap. 18). Exercise performance in postransplant recipients is influenced by the fact that the donor heart is surgically denervated without efferent parasympathetic or sympathetic innervation and by the occurrence of rejection and scar formation, donor-recipient size mismatch, systemic and pulmonary vascular resistance, and development of coronary atherosclerosis in the graft.[92] Maximum oxygen uptake and work capacity are reduced after cardiac transplantation compared with age-matched controls but are usually markedly improved compared with preoperative findings. Abnormalities of the ventricular rate response include a resting tachycardia due to parasympathetic denervation, a slow heart rate response during mild-to-moderate exercise, a more rapid response during more strenuous exercise, and a more prolonged time for the ventricular rate to return to baseline during recovery.[93] The transplanted heart relies heavily on the Frank-Starling mechanism to increase cardiac output during mild-to-moderate exercise. Systemic vascular resistance may be increased because of cyclosporine therapy. The new development of an abnormal exercise ECG several years following cardiac transplantation may be secondary to accelerated coronary atherosclerosis.

VALVULAR HEART DISEASE (see also Chap. 34). The hemodynamics of exercise provide an excellent opportunity to measure gradients across stenotic valves, to assess ventricular function in patients with primary valvular regurgitation or mixed lesions, and to assess pulmonary and systemic vascular resistance. The use of echocardiographic Doppler techniques is particularly valuable in evaluating patients whose symptoms are out of proportion to the degree of valvular disease observed and in assessing the results of valvulotomy or valve replacement.[94] Clinical and exercise noninvasive assessment of patients with valvular heart disease can provide very useful information on the timing of operative intervention and help achieve a more precise estimate of a patient's degree of incapacitation than can assessment of symptoms alone.[95]

CARDIAC PACEMAKERS (see also Chap. 25). The exercise protocol used to assess chronotropic responsiveness in patients before and after cardiac pacemaker insertion should adjust for the fact that many such patients are older individuals and may not tolerate high exercise workloads or abrupt and relatively large increments in work between stages of exercise. An optimal physiological cardiac pacemaker should normalize the heart rate response to exercise in proportion to oxygen uptake and increase heart rate 2 to 4 beats/min for an increase in $\dot{V}_{O_2}$ of 1 ml/min/kg, with a slightly steeper slope for patients with severe left ventricular function impairment.[96]

ELDERLY PATIENTS (see also Chap. 52). The exercise protocol in elderly patients should be selected according to estimated aerobic capacity. In patients with limited exercise tolerance, the test should be started at the slowest speed with a 0 per cent grade and adjusted according to the patient's ability. Older patients may need to grasp the handrails for support. Limited exercise tolerance is to be expected in many persons ≥ 80 years old. There are few data on the prognostic value of exercise testing in older patients.

SAFETY AND RISKS OF EXERCISE TESTING

Exercise testing has an excellent safety record. The risk is determined by the clinical characteristics of the patient referred for the procedure. In nonselected patient populations, the mortality is < 0.01 per cent and morbidity < 0.05 per cent.[97] The risk is greater when the test is performed soon after an acute ischemic event. In a survey of 151,941 tests conducted within 4 weeks of an acute myocardial infarction, mortality was 0.03 per cent, and 0.09 per cent of patients had either a nonfatal reinfarction or were resuscitated from cardiac arrest.[98] The relative risk of a major complication is about twice as great when a symptom-limited protocol is used as compared with a low-level protocol. Nevertheless, in the early postinfarction phase, the risk of a fatal complication during symptom-limited testing is only 0.03 per cent. Exercise testing can be performed safely in patients with compensated congestive heart failure, with no major complications reported in 1286 tests in which a bicycle ergometer was used.[99] The risk of exercise testing in patients referred for life-threatening ventricular arrhythmias was examined by Young et al.[100] in a series of 263 patients who underwent 1377 tests; 2.2 per cent developed sustained ventricular tachyarrhythmias that required cardioversion, cardiopulmonary resuscitation, or antiarrhythmic drugs to restore sinus rhythm. The ventricular arrhythmias were more frequent in tests performed on antiarrhythmic drug therapy as compared with the baseline drug-free state.[100] In contrast to the high risk in the aforementioned patient subsets, the risk of complications in asymptomatic subjects is extremely low, with no fatalities reported in several series.[49,101]

The risk of incurring a major complication during exercise testing can be reduced by performing a careful history and physical examination before the test and observing the patient closely during exercise with monitoring of the electrocardiogram, arterial pressure, and symptoms. The standard 12-lead ECG should be verified before the test for any acute or recent change. There are well-defined contraindications to exercise testing (Table 6–5). After an episode of unstable angina, patients should be free of rest pain, of other evidence of ischemia, or of heart failure for at least 48 to 72 hours before testing. After an uncomplicated acute myocardial infarction, it is wise to wait at least 5 to 7 days before testing. Patients with critical obstruction to left ventricular outflow are at increased risk of cardiac events during exercise. In selected patients, low-level exercise can be quite useful in determining the severity of the left ventricular outflow tract gradient. The "cool-down" period should be prolonged to at least 2 minutes in patients with stenotic valves or those who have exertional hypotension, to avoid sudden pressure-volume shifts that occur in the immediate postexercise phase.

Uncontrolled systemic hypertension is a contraindication to exercise testing. Patients who present with systemic arterial pressure readings of ≥ 220/120 mm Hg should rest for 15 to 20 minutes and the blood pressure should be remeasured. If blood pressure remains at these levels, the test should be postponed until the hypertension is better controlled.

TABLE 6–5 CONTRAINDICATIONS TO EXERCISE TESTING

Unstable angina with recent rest pain
Untreated life-threatening cardiac arrhythmias
Uncompensated congestive heart failure
Advanced atrioventricular block
Acute myocarditis or pericarditis
Critical aortic stenosis
Severe hypertrophic obstructive cardiomyopathy
Uncontrolled hypertension
Acute systemic illness

TERMINATION OF EXERCISE

The use of standard test indications to terminate an exercise test will reduce risk (Table 6–6). Termination of exercise should be determined in part by the patient's recent activity level. The rate of perceived patient exertion can be estimated by the Borg scale (Table 42–1, p. 1385).[102] Borg readings of 14 to 16 approximate anaerobic threshold, and readings ≥ 18 approximate a patient's maximum exercise capacity. Ataxia may indicate cerebral hypoxia. It is helpful to grade exercise-induced chest discomfort on a 1 to 4 scale with 1 indicating the initial onset of chest discomfort and 4 the most severe chest pain the patient has ever experienced. The exercise technician should note the onset of grade 1 chest discomfort on the worksheet, and the test should be stopped when the patient reports grade 3 chest pain. In the absence of symptoms, it is prudent to stop exercise when a patient demonstrates ≥ 3 mm (0.3 mV) of ischemic ST-segment depression or ≥ 1 mm (0.1 mV) of ST-segment elevation in a lead without an abnormal Q wave. Significant worsening of ambient ventricular ectopy during exercise or the unsuspected appearance of ventricular tachycardia is an indication to terminate exercise. A progressive, reproducible decrease in systolic blood pressure ≥ 10 mm Hg may indicate transient left ventricular dysfunction or an inappropriate decrease in systemic vascular resistance and is an indication to terminate exercise. The test should be stopped if the systemic blood pressure is ≥ 250 to 270/120–130 mm Hg.

A resuscitory cart and defibrillator should be available in the room where the test procedure is carried out and appropriate cardioactive medication available to treat cardiac arrhythmias, atrioventricular block, hypotension, and persistent chest pain. An intravenous line should be started in high-risk patients such as those being tested for adequacy of control of life-threatening ventricular arrhythmias. The equipment and supplies in the cart should be checked on a regular basis. A previously specified routine for cardiac emergencies needs to be determined which includes patient transfer and admission to a coronary care unit if necessary.

Clinical judgment is required to determine which patients can be safely tested in an office as opposed to a hospital-based setting. High-risk patients, such as those with evident left ventricular dysfunction, severe angina pectoris, history of cardiac syncope, and signficant ambient ventricular ectopy on the pretest examination, should be tested in the hospital. Low-risk patients, such as asymptomatic subjects and those with a low pretest risk of disease, may be tested by specially trained nurses or physician assistants who have received ACLS certification, *with a physician in close proximity.*[101]

TABLE 6–6 INDICATIONS FOR TERMINATING EXERCISE TEST

Severe fatigue or dyspnea
Ataxia
Grade III/IV chest pain
Ischemic ST-segment depression ≥3.0 mm
Ischemic ST-segment elevation ≥1 mm in a non-Q wave lead
Unsuspected appearance of ventricular tachycardia
Ectopic supraventricular tachycardia
Progressive reproducible decrease in systolic blood pressure
Abnormal elevation of systolic blood pressure
Decreasing heart rate
Technical problems interfering with ECG or blood pressure interpretation

REFERENCES

EXERCISE TESTING FOR CARDIAC DISEASE

1. Feil, H., and Siegel, M. L.: Electrocardiographic changes during attacks of angina pectoris. A. J. Med. Sci. *175*:255, 1928.
2. Master, A. M., and Oppenheimer, E. T.: A simple exercise tolerance test for circulatory efficiency with standard tables for normal individuals. Am. J. Med. Sci. *177*:223, 1929.
3. Froelicher, V. F., Yanowitz, F. G., Major, A. J. T., and Lancaster, M. C.: The correlation of coronary angiography and the electrocardiographic response to maximal treadmill testing in 76 asymptomatic men. Circulation *48*:597, 1973.
4. Flamm, S. D., Taki, J., Moore, R., et al.: Redistribution of regional and organ blood volume and effect on cardiac function in relation to upright exercise intensity in healthy human subjects. Circulation *81*:1550, 1990.
5. Guyton, A. C.: Textbook of Medical Physiology. 7th ed. Philadelphia, W. B. Saunders Company, 1986.
6. Froelicher, V. F., and Marcondes, G. D.: Manual of Exercise Testing. Chicago, Year Book Medical Publishers, Inc., 1989.
7. Froelicher, V. F.: Exercise and the Heart. Clinical Concepts. 2nd ed. Chicago, Year Book Medical Publishers, Inc., 1987.

EXERCISE PHYSIOLOGY

8. McKelvie, R. S., and Jones, N. L.: Cardiopulmonary exercise testing. Clin. Chest Med. *10*:277, 1989.
9. Weber, K. T., and Janicki, J. S.: Cardiopulmonary Exercise Testing: Physiologic Principles and Clinical Applications. Philadelphia, W. B. Saunders Company., 1986.
10. Wasserman, K., Hansen, J. E, Sue, D. Y., and Whipp, B. J.: Principles of Exercise Testing and Interpretation. Philadelphia, Lea & Febiger, 1987.
11. Wasserman, K., Beaver, W. L., and Whipp, B. J.: Gas exchange theory and the lactic acidosis (anaerobic) threshold. Circulation *81*(Suppl. 11):14, 1990.
12. Sullivan, M. J., and Cobb, F. R.: The anaerobic threshold in chronic heart failure: relation to blood lactate, ventilatory basis, reproducibility, and response to exercise training. Circulation *81*(Suppl. 11):47, 1990.
13. Nabel, E. G., Selwyn, A. P., and Ganz, P.: Paradoxical narrowing of atherosclerotic coronary arteries induced by increases in heart rate. Circulation *81*:850, 1990.
14. Wilke, N. A., Sheldahl, L. M., Levandoski, S. G. et al.: Weight carrying versus handgrip exercise testing in men with coronary artery disease. Am. J. Cardiol. *64*:736, 1989.
15. Balady, G. J., Weiner, D. A., Rose, L., and Ryan, T. J.: Physiology responses to arm ergometry exercise relative to age and gender. J. Am. Coll. Cardiol. *16*:130, 1990.
16. Ellestad, M. H.: Stress Testing. Principles and Practice. 3rd ed. Philadelphia, F. A. Davis, 1986.
17. Okin, P. M., and Kligfield, P.: Effect of exercise protocol and lead selection on the accuracy of heart rate-adjusted indices of ST-segment depression for detection of three-vessel coronary artery disease. J. Electrocardiol. *22*:187, 1989.
18. Myers, J., Walsh, D., Buchanan, N., and Froelicher, V. F.: Can maximal cardiopulmonary capacity be recognized by a plateau in oxygen uptake? Chest *96*:1312, 1989.
19. Blair, S. N., Gibbons, L. W., Painter, P. et al.: Guidelines for Exercise Testing and Prescriptions. 3rd ed. Philadelphia, Lea & Febiger, 1986.
20. Sevilla, D. C., Dohrmann, M. L., Somelofski, C. A. et al: Invalidation of the resting electrocardiogram obtained via exercise electrode sites as a standard 12-lead recording. Am. J. Cardiol. *63*:35, 1989.
21. Kubota, I., Hanashima, K., Ideda, K. et al.: Detection of diseased coronary artery by exercise ST-T maps in patients with effort angina pectoris, single-vessel disease, and normal ST-T wave on electrocardiogram at rest. Circulation *80*:120, 1989.
22. Lachterman, B., Lehmann, K.G., Abrahamson, D., and Froelicher, V. F.: "Recovery only" ST-segment depression and the predictive accuracy of the exercise test. Ann. Intern. Med. *112*:11, 1990.

DIAGNOSTIC TESTING

23. Mark, D. B., Hlatky, M. A., Lee, K. L. et al.: Localizing coronary artery obstructions with the exercise treadmill test. Ann. Intern. Med. *106*:53, 1987.
24. Marin, J. J., Heng, M. K., Sevrin, R., and Udhoji, V. N.: Significance of T wave normalization in the electrocardiogram during exercise stress test. Am. Heart J. *114*:1342, 1987.
25. Schlant, R. C., Blonqvist, C. G.,Brandenburg, R. O., et al.: Guidelines for exercise testing: A report of the Joint American College of Cardiology-American Heart Association Task Force on Assessment of Cardiovascular Procedures (Subcommittee on Exercise Testing). Circulation *74*:(Suppl. III) 653A, 1986.
26. Couhan, L., Krone, R. J., Keller, A., and Eisenkramer, G.: Utility of lead V_4R in exercise testing for detection of coronary artery disease. Am. J. Cardiol. *64*:938, 1989.
27. Gianrossi, R., Detrano, R., Mulvihill, D., et al.: Exercise-induced ST depression in the diagnosis of coronary artery disease. A meta analysis. Circulation *80*:87, 1989.

7

Cardiac Catheterization*

by WILLIAM GROSSMAN, M.D.

HISTORICAL ASPECTS

THE EARLY PERIOD. According to André Cournand,[1] cardiac catheterization was first performed (and so named) in 1844 by Claude Bernard, who catheterized both the right and the left ventricles of a horse by means of a retrograde approach from the jugular vein and carotid artery. There followed an era of investigation of cardiovascular physiology in animals that resulted in the development of many important techniques and principles—including pressure manometry and the application of the Fick principle for measuring cardiac output—subsequently applied to the study of patients with heart disease.

Although others had previously passed catheters into the great veins, Werner Forssmann is generally credited as the first to pass a catheter into the heart of a living human being.[2] At age 25, as a surgical resident, he exposed a vein in his own left arm, introduced a ureteral catheter into the venous system, and advanced it under fluoroscopic control into the right atrium. He then walked to the Radiology Department, where the catheter position was documented by a chest x-ray. During the next 2 years, Forssmann continued to perform catheterization studies, including six attempts to catheterize himself.

The potential of Forssmann's technique was appreciated by other investigators. In 1930, Klein reported on catheterization of the right ventricle in 11 patients and measurement of cardiac output using the Fick principle.[3] Except for these and several other studies, application of cardiac catheterization to evaluate the circulation in normal and disease states was limited and fragmentary until the work of Cournand and Richards, who in 1941 began a remarkable series of investigations of right-heart physiology in humans.[4-6] In 1947, Dexter and his colleagues at the Peter Bent Brigham Hospital reported their studies of congenital heart disease and mentioned some observations on "the oxygen saturation and source of pulmonary capillary blood" obtained from a catheter in the pulmonary artery "wedge" position.[7] Subsequent work from Dexter's laboratory[8] showed that the pressure measured in the pulmonary artery "wedge" position was an accurate estimate of pulmonary venous and left atrial pressure. During this exciting early period, catheterization was used to investigate problems in cardiovascular physiology by McMichael in England,[9] Lenegre in Paris,[10] and Cournand, Dexter, Warren, Stead, Bing, Burchell, E. Wood, and their respective coworkers in this country.[11-14]

THE 1950'S AND BEYOND. Further developments came rapidly. Some of the highlights include the following: retrograde left-heart catheterization was first introduced by Zimmerman[15] and Limon Lason[16] and their respective coworkers in 1950. The percutaneous technique developed by Seldinger in 1953 was soon applied to cardiac catheterization of both the left and right heart chambers.[17] Transseptal left-heart catheterization was developed[18] and applied clinically by Ross, Braunwald, and Morrow.[19] Selective coronary arteriography was developed by Sones et al. in 1959[20] and was perfected in the ensuing years.[21] In 1970, a practical balloon-tipped flow-guided catheter technique was introduced by Swan, Ganz, and their collaborators, making possible the applicability of catheterization outside the conventional catheterization laboratory.[22] Many other landmark events could be mentioned and the contributions of many individuals could be recognized, but these have been detailed elsewhere.[23]

* This chapter is a revision of Chapter 9 in the third edition of *Heart Disease*, which was written by W. Grossman and W. H. Barry.

TECHNICAL ASPECTS OF CARDIAC CATHETERIZATION

THE CARDIAC CATHETERIZATION FACILITY

A modern cardiac catheterization laboratory should be housed in a room of 500 to 700 square feet. A report by the Intersociety Commission for Heart Disease Resources on Optimal Resources for Cardiac Catheterization Facilities[24] dealt with a number of critical issues concerning the cardiac catheterization facility. These included the location of a catheterization laboratory (within a hospital as opposed to freestanding); outpatient catheterization; administration, staff organization, and criteria for professional privileges; optimal annual caseload for physicians and for the laboratory; radiation safety and radiological techniques; and physiological measurements and patient safety.

Outpatient catheterization[25] has been demonstrated to be safe, practical, and cost-effective by a variety of groups. In properly selected cases, outpatient catheterization should be encouraged as part of an overall effort to use hospital facilities more efficiently and to contain costs of medical care.

The requirement for same-day admission for cardiac catheterization has been imposed increasingly by insurance carriers; this appears to be safe in most elective cases, although no randomized trials have been done to address this point. The issue of whether cardiac catheterization laboratories should be hospital-based, freestanding, or mobile has been addressed by a number of study groups, and much of the debate on this subject has been summarized by Conti.[25a] As he points out, there are many potential concerns about performance of cardiac catheterization in a freestanding facility, although the available data from such facilities are limited. Mobile cardiac catheterization laboratories may be either freestanding or hospital-based (as is the case for mobile MRI and other mobile diagnostic units), and it is important that the terms *mobile* unit and *freestanding* unit not be equated automatically. Careful prospective studies of the safety and cost-effectiveness of these innovative approaches to diagnostic cardiac catheterization need to be done before meaningful policies can be drafted.

An issue addressed in the Intersociety Report[24] concerns the proximity and availability of *cardiac surgical facilities*. Although this report states that "optimally, cardiovascular catheterization laboratories should be located only in institutions with well-organized and closely related programs of cardiovascular surgery," many community hospital-based catheterization laboratories have demonstrated that properly selected patients can safely undergo catheterization even in hospitals without on-site heart surgery programs. Procedures that are more likely to require urgent cardiac surgical support should not be done in such laboratories, and immediately

TABLE 7-1 GENERAL RECOMMENDATIONS FOR CASELOADS OF CATHETERIZATION LABORATORIES AND PHYSICIANS

Catheterization Laboratories	
1. Adults	≥300 cases/year
2. Pediatric	≥150 cases/year
Physician caseload	
1. Adult catheterizations	≥150 but ≤600
2. Pediatric catheterizations	≥50

Data from Friesinger, G. C., et al.: Optimal resources for evaluation of the heart and lungs: Cardiac catheterization and radiologic facilities. Circulation *68*:893A, 1983 reprinted with permission of the American Heart Association, Inc.

Note: The report indicates that physicians with extensive experience can perform fewer catheterizations to maintain their skill levels.

available cardiac surgical back-up is particularly critical for laboratories performing coronary artery interventions (angioplasty, atherectomy, stents, and laser therapies), endomyocardial biopsy, transseptal catheterization, and studies on patients suspected to have left main coronary artery disease, severe aortic stenosis, or other conditions that increase the risk of the catheterization procedure.

Utilization levels as well as optimal *physician caseload* are additional issues of importance in the operation of a cardiac catheterization facility, and current recommendations are given in Table 7-1.

RADIOGRAPHIC EQUIPMENT

Radiographic equipment must be capable of extremely high-quality image resolution, and it must include a system for permanent recording. The system usually consists of three components: an x-ray generating system, an image intensifier, and an image recording system consisting of a video camera, videotape recorder, and 35-mm cine camera. Many laboratories are now switching to all-electronic techniques for permanent recording, eliminating the need for the 35-mm cine camera.

Details concerning radiographic principles and practice are beyond the scope of this text, and the reader is referred elsewhere[23] for further information. The radiographic equipment must be mounted on an appropriate support stand to allow multiple complex angulation. Cardiac catheterization and angiography should only be carried out in a room where complex angulation (including cranial and caudal angulation as well as right and left anterior oblique angulation) can be accomplished. A strict quality assurance program must be implemented, with regular checks on performance of the apparatus.

RADIATION SAFETY

It is essential that details of radiation safety be considered in the operation of any facility. A radiation safety officer must be appointed, with the proper credentials to interpret and enforce existing laws and regulations. Units of x-ray exposure are the roentgen (R), rad, and rem. The roentgen unit is defined in terms of the amount of ionization created per unit volume of air. The rad (radiation absorbed dose) is a unit of absorbed dose defined as the amount of energy deposited per unit mass of a radiation material. The relation of radiation exposure expressed in R to the absorbed dose expressed in rad varies with the type of tissue exposed. An exposure of soft tissue to 1 R by either direct beam or scatter results in an absorbed dose of approximately 0.9 rad. Bone, which absorbs more, would receive a dose of 4 rad. Rem (roentgen equivalent, man) is the unit of dose used in state and federal radiation control regulations. The rem is intended to account for different types of radiation that produce varying damage for the same absorbed dose. For example, radiation caused by alpha particles and neutrons produces a different number of rems than the number of rad; however, for x-rays and gamma rays, rem and rad are practically identical.

RECOMMENDED RADIATION LIMITS. It is not known whether there exists a lower limit for radiation exposure, below which there is no risk of biological damage. For regulatory purposes, however, the recommended limits for the general population is 0.5 rem per person per year; for people involved in professions in which radiation exposure is necessary (e.g., radiology technicians, physicians in cardiac catheterization laboratories) the maximal permissible dose is 5.0 rem per year. Obviously, these limits cannot guarantee complete elimination of any hazard.

People who work in a cardiac catheterization facility must wear film badges, which monitor radiation exposure. No dose higher than 3 rem should be allowed within a 3-month period. Protection against radiation is achieved by wearing lead aprons and using lead neck wraps to protect the thyroid and wearing leaded eyeglasses to protect the lens. Most important, however, is to minimize the use of fluoroscopy and cineangiography during the procedure. The operator must avoid the temptation to fluoroscope continuously. Guidelines for radiation protection in the cardiac catheterization laboratory have been issued by the Society for Cardiac Angiography.[26]

TECHNIQUE OF CARDIAC CATHETERIZATION

The majority of catheterizations performed today utilize either of two approaches: catheterization by direct exposure of an artery and a vein (e.g., brachial vessels, umbilical vessels in neonates) and catheterization by the percutaneous approach (including transseptal catheterization). Each method has its advantages and disadvantages, and it is our belief that the physician performing cardiac catheterization should be well versed in both techniques. The methods used in the author's laboratory are described below.

BRACHIAL ARTERIAL APPROACH

This approach usually involves surgical exposure of the brachial artery and brachial or basilic vein in the antecubital fossa and insertion of the catheters directly after vessel incision. The percutaneous approach of Seldinger also may be used in adults by way of the brachial vessels if catheters of small size (No. 5 French) are used. The brachial approach has advantages in patients with obstructive and/or thrombotic arterial disease that involves the abdominal aorta, iliac artery, or femoral artery; suspected thrombosis of the femoral vein or inferior vena cava; defective hemostatic mechanisms (e.g., marked thrombocytopenia); or coarctation of the aorta. It also may be advantageous in obese patients, in whom the percutaneous femoral technique may be technically quite difficult and in whom bleeding may be hard to control after removal of the catheter.

PROCEDURE. After the brachial artery is localized by means of palpation in the right antecubital fossa, local anesthesia is induced with 5 to 15 ml of 1 to 2 per cent lidocaine, and a single transverse incision is made just proximal to the flexor crease. Tissues are separated by blunt dissection, and a medial vein is isolated and encircled proximally and distally with 3-0 or 4-0 silk. The brachial artery is isolated from adjacent nerves and fascia, and is encircled proximally and distally with moistened umbilical tape or silicone elastomer surgical tape.

Right-heart catheterization is accomplished by means of antegrade passage of an appropriate catheter (e.g., Cournand, Goodale-Lubin, or Swan-Ganz balloon-flotation) by way of the basilic or brachial vein to the right atrium, right ventricle, pulmonary artery, and pulmonary capillary "wedge" positions under fluoroscopic guidance. In the wedge position, the catheter occludes the distal pulmonary artery segment, and thus the catheter tip is exposed to only the pulmonary venous pressure. Pulmonary capillary wedge pressure provides an accurate estimate of left atrial pressure if appropriate attention is paid to pressure waveform, oximetric confirmation, and correction for time delay.[27] Left-heart catheterization is then accomplished by means of retrograde passage of an appropriate catheter (e.g., Sones, NIH) through a transverse brachial arteriotomy to the ascending aorta and left ventricle.

Systemic administration of heparin (5000 units) at the time of left-heart catheterization and coronary arteriography is indicated to prevent thrombotic complications. In case of difficulty in passing catheters from the brachial artery around the shoulder, an end-hole catheter with a flexible guidewire protruding beyond the tip should be used. As catheters with or without the aid of guidewires are advanced in the vascular system, their passage should be monitored fluoroscopically; if progress of the catheter is difficult, or if the patient complains of pain, caution should be exercised to avoid dissection or perforation of the vessel wall. Occasionally, spasm of the vessel around the catheter may occur, owing to the relatively small size of vessels in the upper extremities. In this case, administration of small amounts of morphine should promptly facilitate catheter manipulation; if not, a catheter of smaller diameter should be used.

Termination of the Procedure. After completion of hemodynamic and angiographic studies, the catheters are withdrawn, and the artery is repaired. In our laboratory, a Fogarty balloon catheter is routinely passed proximally and distally to remove any thrombi that may have formed within the arterial lumen during the catheterization. After flow is deemed adequate, 15 ml of heparinized solution (1500 units in 15 ml of 5 per cent dextrose in water) are infused into the artery through the Sones catheter. The artery is immediately occluded with vascular clamps proximal and distal to the arteriotomy site. A stay suture is placed at each end of the arteriotomy, which is then closed using a continuous stitch of 6-0 Tevdek. It is important not to raise an intimal flap or to penetrate the posterior intima with the needle. After suturing, first the distal and then the proximal clamp are removed. Minor leaks usually respond to gentle pressure applied directly with a finger over the site of the arteriotomy repair. The radial pulse should be palpable and as strong as it was before catheterization. If it is absent or markedly reduced, the artery should be reopened, a Fogarty balloon catheter passed again, and the vessel repaired. If this does not result in return of the pulse, an experienced vascular surgeon should be consulted. The vein may be tied off or repaired directly.

The wound is then flushed with sterile saline and a 1 per cent povidone-iodine solution, and the skin incision is closed. For skin closure, the author uses a subcuticular stitch with 4-0 Dexon, an absorbable polyglycolic acid suture material which makes a return visit for suture removal unnecessary. Antibiotic ointment (10 per cent povidone-iodine) is applied to the suture line, and the area should be covered with a dressing.

Postcatheterization orders should include the following:

1. Resume all previous medications.
2. Measure blood pressure and pulse and inspect dressing every 15 minutes for 1 hour, every hour for 4 hours, then every 4 hours for 12 hours.
3. Call a house officer or attending physician *and* a member of the catheterization laboratory staff in the event of bleeding, loss of pulse, hypotension, or chest pain.
4. Encourage oral fluid intake of 2 to 3 liters over 6 to 8 hours (if an angiographic contrast agent has been administered).
5. Administer analgesic medication, as needed.

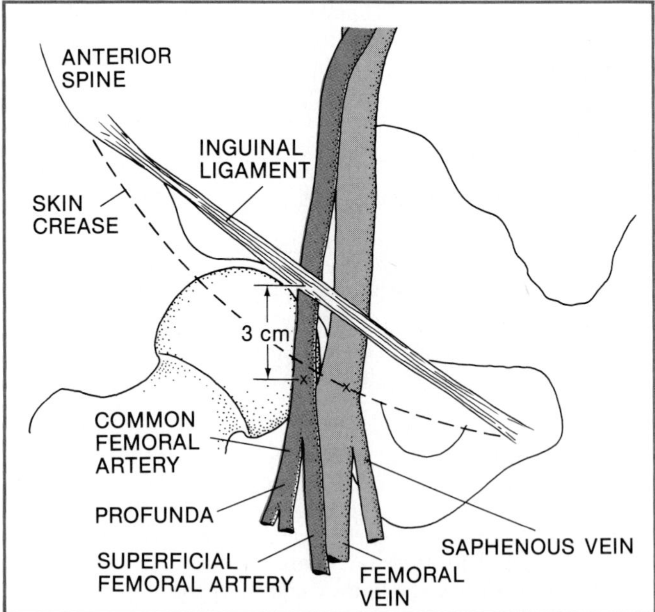

FIGURE 7–1. Anatomy relevant to percutaneous catheterization of femoral artery and vein: the right femoral artery and vein run underneath the inguinal ligament, which connects the anterior-superior iliac spine and pubic tubercle. The arterial skin nick (indicated by X) should be placed approximately 1½ to 2 fingerbreadths (3 cm) below the inguinal ligament and directly over the femoral artery pulsation. The venous skin nick should be placed at the same level, but approximately 1 fingerbreadth medial. (From Baim, D. S., and Grossman, W.: Percutaneous approach. *In* Grossman, W., and Baim, D. S. [eds.]: Cardiac Catheterization, Angiography, and Intervention. 4th ed. Philadelphia, Lea and Febiger, 1991.)

FEMORAL ARTERIAL APPROACH

Right- and left-heart catheterization by way of the femoral approach usually is performed from the right groin, although the left groin may be used, if necessary. The major landmarks of the femoral area are the anterior superior iliac spine, the pubic tubercle, and the inguinal ligament running between them. The femoral nerve, artery, and vein are located in the femoral triangle below the inguinal ligament. Proceeding from lateral to medial, the relationship of these structures may be remembered with the aid of the mnemonic NAVY (nerve, artery, vein, empty space).

PROCEDURE. The femoral artery is located by means of palpation at a point approximately 1½ to 2 fingerbreadths below the inguinal ligament (Fig. 7–1). The skin and subcutaneous tissue over the artery and vein are anesthetized with 10 to 15 ml of 1 per cent lidocaine. The anesthetic must be given carefully and must not be injected directly into a vessel. It is important that percutaneous puncture of the femoral vessels be a correct distance below the inguinal ligament; if it is too high, hemostasis may be impaired, owing to the posterior course of the vessels in the pelvic cavity; if it is too low, the vein may run behind the artery, and the artery may be entered after it bifurcates into the profunda and superficial femoral branches. Although the inguinal crease usually is just below the inguinal ligament, this relation is not constant, and the use of the inguinal ligament as the primary landmark is therefore advised.

Right-Heart Catheterization. When performing right- and left-heart catheterization by way of the femoral approach, the author prefers to enter the femoral vein first. This is accomplished using an 18-gauge Seldinger needle, which consists of a blunt, tapered external cannula with a sharp obturator. After a one-fourth-inch skin incision has been made at the correct distance below the inguinal ligament and medial to the arterial pulse, the needle and obturator are inserted with a smooth motion at a 45-degree angle (Fig. 7–2). If the patient has discomfort as the needle penetrates the deeper femoral tissues, additional lidocaine can be infiltrated through the needle, after the obturator is removed and it is confirmed that the needle is extravascular. A small syringe is then attached to the needle, which is slowly withdrawn while continuous gentle aspiration is performed. When the vein is entered, blood is easily aspirated. The syringe is removed without moving the needle, and a Teflon-coated guidewire (preferably a J tip) is inserted into the needle and advanced into the vein. The guidewire should pass easily, with its course checked fluoroscopically. The needle is then withdrawn over the guide, and a venous sheath of appropriate size with obturator is placed into the vein over the guidewire. The sheath should be inserted with a twisting, forward pressure. The obturator and guidewire are then removed, and the sheath is flushed by means of a stopcock. Right-heart catheterization is then performed using a balloon-flotation (Swan-Ganz), Cournand, or Goodale-Lubin catheter (Fig. 7–3). As the catheter is advanced through the sheath and into the inferior vena cava, its motion should be observed on fluoroscopy. The movement of the catheter should be gentle and the passage effortless; catheter advancement should never be forced. While the right-heart catheter is passed from the groin, it frequently enters the renal or hepatic veins. If this occurs, the catheter should be withdrawn and rotated before it is advanced farther. A guidewire may be used if a tortuous venous system makes catheter passage difficult.

The catheter is passed initially to the superior vena cava, where blood is sampled for measurement of oxygen saturation. The catheter is then withdrawn to the right atrium, where pressure is recorded. If a balloon-flotation catheter is used, the balloon is inflated with air (or carbon dioxide, if an intracardiac shunt is suspected) and advanced to the right ventricle, where pressure is recorded, and then to the pulmonary artery and immediately to the pulmonary wedge position. Pressure is again measured during balloon deflation so that pulmonary capillary wedge and pulmonary artery pressures can be recorded. A pulmonary artery blood sample is obtained for measurement of oxygen saturation, and if this value is greater than or equal to 7 per cent higher than superior vena caval oxygen saturation, a left-to-right shunt may be present.[28] In patients with left bundle branch block, a balloon-flotation catheter is preferred because of the reduced likelihood of trauma to the right bundle branch during right-heart catheterization with this type of catheter. Catheter-induced right bundle branch block in a patient with complete left bundle branch block results in complete heart block and can cause asystole. A right-heart pacing catheter also may be used in this situation to initiate emergency pacing, if necessary.

To re-obtain wedge pressure, the balloon is *slowly* inflated while catheter pressure is monitored until the pressure waveform changes to a wedge contour. Overinflation of the balloon, or inflation of the balloon in a

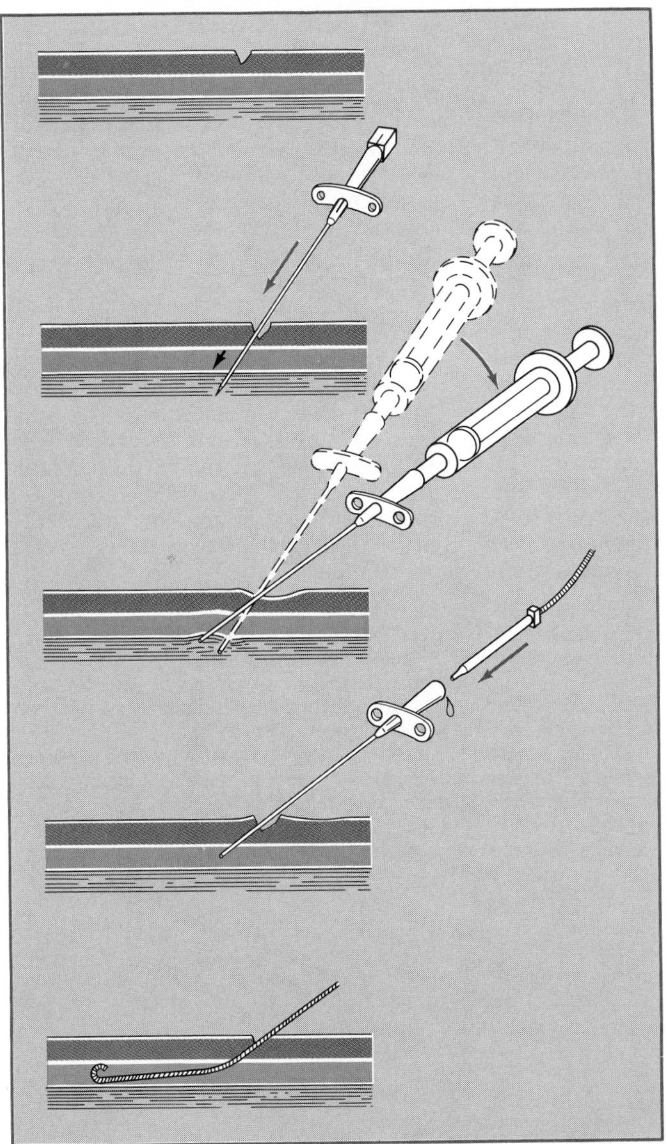

FIGURE 7-2. Seldinger technique for venous puncture and catheterization. In the top panel, a skin nick has been made overlying the desired vein, which is then transfixed through and through by Seldinger needle with obturator in place. The center panel shows the obturator removed and the needle cannula attached to a syringe. Lowering of the syringe toward the skin surface facilitates proper alignment of the needle tip at the moment that withdrawal brings the tip into the vessel lumen. Entry into the vesel lumen during withdrawal is recognized by sudden appearance of free-flowing blood in the syringe, which is held under gentle negative pressure. The syringe is then removed and a J guidewire (shown with plastic guide in place) is advanced into the vessel; after this, the needle cannula is removed and replaced with an intravascular sheath through which catheters may be advanced. A similar technique is used for arterial puncture, except that a syringe is unnecessary, since arterial pressure will cause blood to spurt backward through the needle once the needle tip is in the vessel lumen. (From Baim, D. S., and Grossman, W.: Percutaneous approach. *In* Grossman, W., and Baim, D. S. [eds.]: Cardiac Catheterization, Angiography, and Intervention. 4th ed. Philadelphia, Lea and Febiger, 1991.)

distal vessel, carries the risk of pulmonary artery rupture. Also, to reduce the likelihood of pulmonary infarction and/or pulmonary artery rupture, the balloon should not be left inflated for longer than the time required to record pressure (if needed) and to obtain a sample of blood to determine oxygen saturation. Positioning of the Cournand or balloon-tipped catheter during right-heart catheterization may be facilitated by the use of guidewires, but catheters should not be advanced into the wedge position with a guidewire protruding beyond the catheter tip.

Left-Heart Catheterization. After completion of right-heart catheterization, the femoral artery may be punctured at a 45-degree angle with the Seldinger needle, once a skin incision one-fourth-inch long and deep has been made directly over the arterial pulse. The obturator is removed, and the needle is slowly withdrawn until the tip enters the artery lumen and a pulsatile flow of arterial blood exits from the needle hub. In patients receiving heparin or other anticoagulants, an attempt should be made to puncture the front wall of the artery only, to prevent hematoma formation caused by bleeding from the posterior wall of the artery. A Teflon-coated J guidewire is inserted into the needle and advanced into the artery. The guidewire should advance easily, with its position observed on fluoroscopy as it passes into the abdominal aorta. The needle is then withdrawn over the guidewire, and the artery is compressed firmly at the puncture site. A No. 8 French arterial sheath with a proximal hemostasis valve and a side-port extension tube is inserted into the artery over the guidewire. The sheath obturator and guidewire are removed, and the sheath is flushed by means of the side-arm extension tube, which is connected to a pressure transducer for continuous monitoring of femoral arterial pressure. It is, of course, possible to insert an end-hole catheter into the artery directly over the guidewire without use of a sheath. This would be appropriate if only one arterial catheter were to be used. Use of the arterial sheath, however, greatly facilitates catheter changes, permits use of a greater variety of catheters, and allows continuous monitoring of femoral artery pressure during left-heart catheterization.[29]

When using a right femoral artery sheath, left-heart catheterization may be performed with a variety of catheters. In most laboratories, the most commonly used initial catheter for left-heart catheterization is the "pigtail" catheter, which has multiple side holes and an end hole and can be used for angiography as well as pressure measurement. After introduction of the left-heart catheter, 5000 units of heparin are administered intravenously for anticoagulation.

When preformed catheters are used (pigtail, Judkins, or Amplatz), a J-shaped guidewire is inserted into the catheter before introducing the catheter into the sheath. Then, when the catheter tip is within the sheath, the J guide is advanced beyond the tip and into the femoral artery for several centimeters. Under fluoroscopic observation, the catheter is then advanced into the aorta, with the guidewire tip preceding it. Again, the catheter passage should be effortless. When the catheter is in the abdominal aorta at the level of the diaphragm, the guidewire is removed, and the catheter and sheath are aspirated and then flushed with heparinized saline. The catheter and sheath should be flushed every 5 minutes after heparin administration and every 2 to 3 minutes if heparin is not used.

The catheter is advanced carefully around the aortic arch to avoid inadvertently entering the aortic arch vessels. The pressure just above the aortic valve is recorded, along with simultaneous femoral artery pressure, by means of the side arm of the sheath. As will be discussed later, the peak femoral artery pressure frequently is slightly higher than the peak central aortic pressure; however, mean systolic pressures usually are identical. The catheter is then passed across the aortic valve into the left ventricle (Fig. 7-4). If the aortic valve is abnormal, a guidewire may be required to

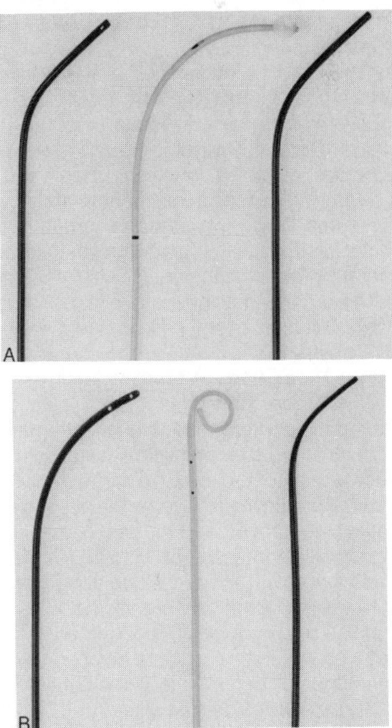

FIGURE 7-3. Various cardiac catheters. *A,* From left to right: Goodale-Lubin, balloon-flotation Swan-Ganz, and Cournand. *B,* From left to right: NIH, Nycore-pigtail, and Sones.

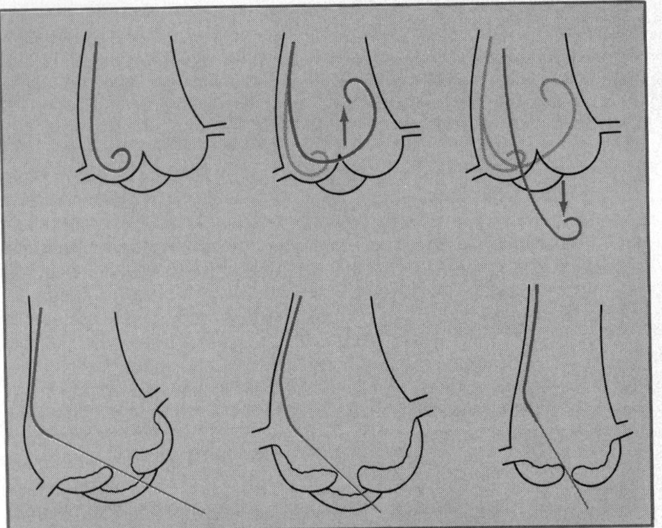

FIGURE 7-4. Technique for retrograde crossing of an aortic valve using a pigtail catheter. The upper three panels show the technique for crossing a normal aortic valve. In the bottom row, the use of a straight guidewire and pigtail catheter in combination is shown. Increasing the length of protruding guidewire straightens the catheter curve and causes the wire to point more toward the right coronary ostium; reducing the length of protruding wire restores the pigtail contour and deflects the guidewire tip toward the left coronary artery. Once the correct length of wire and the correct rotational orientation of the catheter have been found, repeated advancement and withdrawal of catheter and guidewire together will allow retrograde passage across the valve. In a dilated aortic root, the angled pigtail catheter is preferable. In a small aortic root (bottom row, right) a right coronary Judkins catheter may have advantages. (From Baim, D. S., and Grossman, W.: Percutaneous approach. *In* Grossman, W., and Baim, D. S. [eds.]: Cardiac Catheterization, Angiography, and Intervention. 4th ed. Philadelphia, Lea and Febiger, 1991.)

stiffen the catheter to permit crossing of the aortic valve. In aortic stenosis, the valve is best traversed with a straight-tip guidewire, and the catheter is then advanced over the wire into the ventricle for pressure measurement (Fig. 7-4). Other catheters, such as the Sones, right Judkins, and Gensini, may be preferable in selected patients. Not more than 15 minutes or so should be expended in attempting to cross an aortic valve with a single type of catheter before trying another.

When the catheter enters the left ventricle, the left ventricular and femoral artery pressures are recorded to evaluate aortic valve function, and the left ventricular and pulmonary artery wedge pressures are recorded to evaluate mitral valve function. Cardiac output is measured, and a right-heart pullback is performed to evaluate the pulmonic and tricuspid valves by recording, in close time sequence, pulmonary artery, right ventricular, and right atrial pressures. If left ventricular angiography is planned, and the aortic valve was not crossed with a pigtail or other catheter suitable for ventricular angiography, an exchange guidewire may be introduced into the left ventricle, the catheter may be removed over the guidewire, and a pigtail catheter then advanced over the exchange guidewire back into the left ventricle.

Termination of the Procedure. After completion of the hemodynamic and angiographic studies (coronary arteriography is discussed in Chap. 9), the catheters are removed. Preformed arterial catheters should be withdrawn from the artery into the sheath with several centimeters of guidewire protruding from the catheter tip to avoid trauma to the arterial intima. After administration of protamine to reverse the heparin effect, the arterial and venous sheaths are removed, and the vessels are compressed firmly by hand or a mechanical compressor for 15 to 20 minutes, with control of bleeding during this time. With this technique, significant hematoma formation occurs in fewer than 2 per cent of patients. In patients with hypertension, or wide pulse pressure (aortic regurgitation), longer groin compression times may be required to achieve hemostasis.

The patient should rest in bed and keep the right leg immobile after a right femoral catheterization. Most patients find it uncomfortable to be supine for several hours, and this is *not* necessary unless there is a problem with hypotension. Elevation of the head of the bed to 30 to 45 degrees does not increase the risk of femoral bleeding as long as the leg is kept immobile and Valsalva maneuver is avoided.

TRANSSEPTAL LEFT-HEART CATHETERIZATION

When the aortic valve cannot be crossed by the retrograde approach from either the brachial or the femoral artery, and it is essential that the left ventricular pressure be measured, transseptal catheterization of the left ventricle may be performed. In our experience, approximately 5 per cent of severely stenotic valves cannot be crossed in a retrograde manner within a reasonable period of time, and these patients, as well as those with tilting-disc prosthetic aortic valves, are candidates for this procedure. Patients with porcine heterograft valves and ball-cage prosthetic aortic valves can safely undergo retrograde left ventricular catheterization.[30] Transseptal left-heart catheterization also is indicated in patients with suspected mitral valve obstruction in whom a pulmonary artery wedge pressure cannot be measured. There has been a revival of interest in transseptal catheterization in recent years,[31] and newer techniques that involve the combination of an introducer and a sheath increase the safety and versatility of the procedure.[32] In addition, the transseptal technique is essential for some of the newer interventional techniques, such as balloon mitral valvuloplasty[33] (Chap. 41).

PROCEDURE. Transseptal catheterization is commonly performed using the Teflon 70-cm No. 8 French catheter developed by Brockenbrough and Braunwald.[34] Before insertion of the catheter into the right femoral vein, a Brockenbrough needle is inserted into the catheter, with a Bing stylet protruding 1 cm or so beyond the needle tip to prevent penetration of the catheter wall by the needle (Fig. 7-5).

With the patient positioned for a straight frontal projection, the Brockenbrough catheter is advanced to the junction of the right atrium and the superior vena cava by means of a guidewire. The guidewire is removed, the catheter is flushed, and right atrial pressure is recorded. The transseptal needle with its stylet is inserted and then gently advanced through the

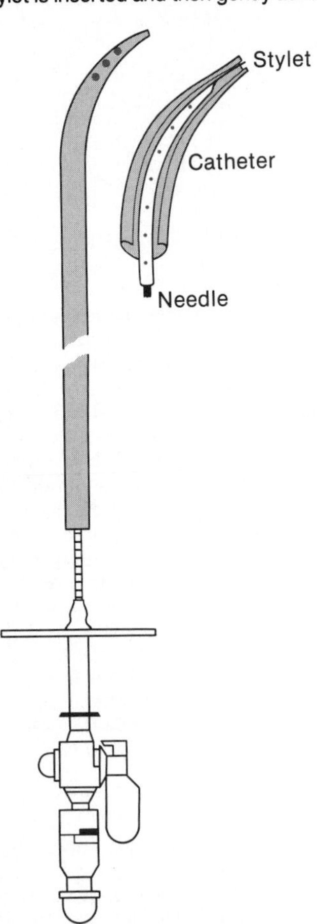

FIGURE 7-5. The Brockenbrough transseptal needle, catheter, and stylet. Use of the stylet prevents inadvertent puncture of the catheter by the needle tip during insertion of the needle into the catheter. The wide flange near the needle hub is pointed on one side to indicate the direction of the needle tip. (From Grossman, W., and Baim, D. S. [eds.]: Percutaneous approach. *In* Cardiac Catheterization, Angiography, and Intervention. 4th ed. Philadelphia, Lea and Febiger, 1991, p. 77.)

transseptal catheter under fluoroscopic observation. It is important to allow free rotation of the needle as it is advanced by holding the needle itself (not the direction indicator) between the fingertips. When the tip of the stylet is near the tip of the catheter, the stylet is removed and the needle is advanced until the needle tip is just within the catheter. The needle is firmly held in this position, with the direction indicator pointing up, to prevent inadvertent extension of the needle tip out of the catheter. The needle is flushed and connected to a pressure transducer, so that a phasic right atrial pressure and a mean pressure can be recorded through the needle. It is important not to use soft or excessively long lengths of connecting tubing for this purpose, since it is possible to overdamp the pressure recorded through the 21-gauge needle tip.

Puncture of Atrial Septum. After right atrial pressure has been recorded, the catheter and needle are slowly withdrawn as a unit while the direction indicator is rotated clockwise to point posteromedially at the 4 o'clock position with fluoroscopic and pressure monitoring. The catheter tip will move over the aortic root in a sudden leftward motion; further inferior pull usually will result in a second, smaller leftward motion, as the catheter tip enters the fossa ovalis. Right atrial phasic pressure should be monitored during this time. The catheter and needle (with the needle tip still within the catheter) are then advanced, and the catheter tip will move superiorly, sliding up the interatrial septum. It usually will "hang up" on the lip of the fossa ovalis, at the level of or slightly superior to the plane of the aortic valve. Occasionally, the catheter will pass easily into the left atrium through a patent foramen ovale, and this will be manifest as leftward motion of the catheter tip and by the appearance of a left atrial phasic waveform. If this occurs, the oxygen saturation of blood aspirated through the needle should be checked and the pressure recorded to document entry into the left atrium. The catheter is then gently advanced 1 or 2 cm over the needle, and the needle is removed. More commonly, the foramen ovale is not patent and must be punctured with the needle tip. This is done during pressure and fluoroscopic monitoring by advancing the needle 1 cm beyond the catheter tip, when the tip is firmly wedged in the fossa ovalis.

After the needle penetrates the interatrial septum, a left atrial pressure waveform (usually a higher mean pressure than in the right atrium) will be evident. Entry into the left atrium should be confirmed by measurement of oxygen saturation. The needle and catheter are then advanced slowly into the left atrium, with the needle position indicator maintained in the 4 o'clock position. Resistance usually is encountered as the catheter tip punctures the septum, and it is important to stabilize the catheter position by holding the catheter in the groin with the left hand while advancing the catheter and needle with the right hand. When the catheter traverses the septum and enters the left atrium (a 1- to 2-cm leftward motion), the needle is withdrawn, the catheter is flushed, left atrial pressure is recorded, and blood is withdrawn through the catheter for measurement of oxygen saturation. Passage of the catheter from the left atrium into the left ventricle is achieved by advancing the catheter tip through the mitral valve. The transseptal catheter may enter a pulmonary vein or left atrial appendage. In this case, the left ventricle may be entered by withdrawing the catheter slowly while rotating it counterclockwise and/or by inserting a coiled-tip occluder to increase the bend in the catheter tip. An improved technique more widely used today is to place a Mullins sheath in the left atrium at the time of the initial transseptal puncture, and advance a balloon-flotation catheter through this sheath into the left atrium and left ventricle.[32] It is important to emphasize that transseptal catheterization—indeed all cardiac catheterization procedures—should be done only by or under the supervision of physicians experienced in the technique. The transseptal needle may perforate the right atrial wall, enter the coronary sinus or the aorta, or perforate the left atrial wall. The small needle tip itself (21 gauge) is not likely to cause a major problem unless an atrial wall is torn; however, passage of the catheter through these structures may result in tamponade and death. Thus, the emphasis placed on pressure monitoring through the needle is important.

PEDIATRIC CARDIAC CATHETERIZATION[35]

The methods described above are broadly applicable to the cardiac catheterization of children, but *special considerations for the newborn* should be emphasized. In such patients, meticulous attention must be given to maintenance of body temperature by means of heating pads, an infrared lamp, or other devices designed for this purpose. In addition, precise attention must be paid to fluid balance, with care being taken to replace exactly the volume of fluid and blood removed, so as to cause neither hypovolemia and hypotension nor hypervolemia with pulmonary edema. In the newborn, the umbilical vein may be used for catheterization for about 72 hours after birth and the umbilical artery for up to 10 days of age. Of course, catheters should be of small diameters and lengths in procedures that involve neonates, infants, and children. The reader is referred to texts and reviews detailing special technical considerations in cardiac catheterization of newborns.[35]

CATHETER SIZES AND CONSTRUCTION

In addition to the above-mentioned considerations, it is important that individuals involved in cardiac catheterization understand the sizing of catheters, needles, and guidewires, and that they have a knowledge of different methods and materials used in their construction. Cardiac catheters differ in size, length, shape, and material of construction. The last factor determines the friction coefficient, hardness, curve retention, moisture absorption, and autoclavability. In addition, it is clear that different catheter materials have varying degrees of thrombogenicity. Cardiac catheters usually are constructed of woven Dacron, polyethylene, or polyurethane. Some catheter walls are reinforced with stainless steel braids to increase torque control and to enable the catheter to withstand high intraluminal pressures during the injection of angiographic contrast material. In addition, the walls of most cardiac catheters are impregnated with lead or barium salts to render them radiopaque.

The outside diameter (OD) of a catheter is indicated in French units: one French (F) unit = 0.33 mm (0.013 inches). Thus a No. 7 French (7F) catheter has an OD of 2.33 mm. The internal diameter (ID) of a catheter is always, of course, less than the OD, the exact relation between OD and ID depending on the thickness of the catheter wall. The ID of the catheter determines the thickness of the guidewire that can be passed through the catheter. The guidewire must in turn be small enough to fit through the lumen of the needle used for vessel puncture in percutaneous catheterization techniques. The diameter of the guidewire usually is expressed in inches (0.032, 0.035, 0.038, and so on), whereas needle size is expressed in "gauge," indicating the OD of the needle. An 18-gauge thin-walled needle has an OD of 0.086 inches. The cardiologist beginning to use these techniques must be familiar with these units. In addition, it is wise to check that catheter, guidewire, and needle are all compatible in size and length before the vessel is punctured.

HEMODYNAMIC MEASUREMENTS

MEASUREMENT OF INTRAVASCULAR AND INTRACARDIAC PRESSURES

THEORETICAL CONSIDERATIONS. Myocardial contractile force is transmitted through the fluid medium of blood as a pressure wave. An important objective of the cardiac catheterization procedure is to assess accurately the forces, and therefore the pressure waves, generated by various cardiac chambers. *A pressure wave may be considered a complex periodic fluctuation in force per unit area,* with one cycle consisting of the time interval from the onset of one wave to the onset of the next. The number of cycles within 1 second is termed the *fundamental frequency* of the waveform. Thus, for a left ventricular pressure waveform at a heart rate of 120 beats/min, the fundamental frequency would be 2 sec^{-1}, or 2 Hz.

Considered as a complex periodic waveform, the pressure wave may be subjected to a type of analysis developed by the French physicist Fourier, whereby any complex waveform may be considered to be the mathematical summation of a series of simple sine waves of differing frequencies and amplitudes. The practical consequence of this analysis is that to accurately record pressure, a system must respond in such a way that output amplitude is directly proportional to input throughout the range of frequencies contained within the pressure wave. If components in a given frequency range are either suppressed or exaggerated by the transducer system, the recorded signal will be a grossly distorted version of the original physiological waveform. For example, the incisura of the aortic pressure wave contains frequencies above 10 cycles/sec; if the pressure measurement system were unable to respond to these, the incisura would be slurred or absent.

The *frequency response* for a pressure measurement system may be defined as the ratio of output amplitude to input amplitude over a range of frequencies of the input or pressure wave. An ideal pressure measurement system would have an output-input ratio of one over an infinite range of input frequencies. In practice, this is never the case, and the frequency response characteristics reflect the interaction of the *natural frequency* of the system and the degree of *damping.* If the sensing membrane in a pressure measurement system were

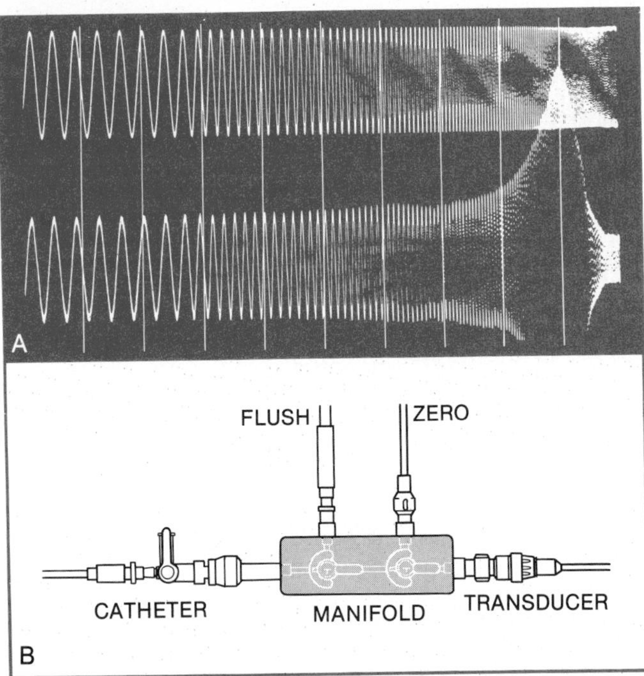

FIGURE 7-6. Recording of phasic pressures with a fluid-filled catheter system. *A,* The upper trace shows a "true" phasic pressure of 20 mm Hg (sine wave of increasing frequency) generated within a closed chamber. The lower trace shows the same pressure recorded with a fluid-filled 110-cm catheter-external transducer system. Note that the pressures are equal in amplitude up to a frequency of about 15 Hz. As the frequency of the pressure sine wave increases above this point, an increase in amplitude occurs owing to resonance in the catheter-transducer system. The "resonant frequency" is about 40 Hz, and above this frequency, the amplitude of the signal falls rapidly. In this case, because the resonant frequency is well above most frequencies contained in the intracardiac pressure waveforms, little distortion of intracardiac pressure by the catheter-transducer recording system will be present. (The vertical lines are 1 sec apart.) *B,* The system used to record the pressure in *A.* A small volume-displacement transducer is attached directly to the back end of a two-side-arm manifold. Fluid-filled tubings are attached to the side arms for "zero" pressure reference and catheter flushing, and the front end of the manifold is connected directly to the catheter. Care must be taken during filling of the transducer and manifold to remove all air bubbles, which can markedly lower the resonant frequency of the system.

shock-excited, in the absence of friction it would oscillate for an indefinite period of time in simple harmonic motion. The frequency of this motion would be the *natural frequency* of the system. The amplitude of the output signal tends to be augmented as the frequency of that signal approaches the natural frequency of the system (Fig. 7-6A). Optimal damping dissipates the energy of the oscillating system gradually, thereby maintaining the frequency response curve nearly flat (constant input-output ratio) as it approaches the region of the pressure measurement system's natural frequency. An extensive literature on the question of what frequency response is desirable and on the testing, construction, and evaluation of different pressure measurement systems is available.[23,36]

FLUID-FILLED CATHETER SYSTEMS. With fluid-filled catheters, an external pressure transducer is used to detect changes in pressure at the catheter tip that are transmitted to the transducer by the fluid column in the catheter. A pressure transducer consists basically of a diaphragm that is deformed in a linear manner by the application of pressure within the physiological range. Deformation of the diaphragm produces a proportional change in electrical resistance within the transducer. By use of a Wheatstone bridge type of circuit, this change in transducer resistance is converted into an electrical potential, which is then amplified and recorded as an analog signal that represents pressure applied to the transducer. Operation of the bridge requires an excitation voltage, usually supplied by the pressure amplifier. A variable resistance control by means of which the electrical potential can be adjusted to zero when no pressure is applied permits balancing of the transducer. Calibration of the system is performed by applying known pressures to the transducer by means of a mercury manometer and observing the analog voltage output. The sensitivity of the amplifiers used in pressure recording systems is adjustable, so that a given pressure may be made to correspond to a precise deflection of the recorder.

Because movement of the transducer diaphragm is necessary to produce a voltage output for a given pressure, a certain volume of fluid must move through the catheter-connector tubing system to the transducer to produce a pressure recording. This tends to cause low-frequency resonance in the system. The resonant frequency of a fluid-filled system should be above the frequencies contained in intracardiac pressure waveforms (see above). For usual clinical purposes, a system with frequency response that is flat to 10 or 12 Hz with a resonant frequency above this level is adequate. This can be achieved most easily by use of small volume-displacement transducers, with imposition of as few stopcocks and connecting tubings as possible between the catheter hub and the transducer. The system used in our cardiac catheterization laboratory is shown in Figure 7-6*B*.

With an aqueous fluid-filled catheter attached to a transducer, the transducer will indicate zero pressure when the catheter tip is at the same height as the transducer. If the catheter tip is elevated above the transducer, a positive pressure of 1 mm Hg will be indicated for every 1.36 cm of height difference; if the catheter tip is below the transducer level, a negative pressure of the same magnitude will be indicated. These effects are due simply to gravitational force acting on the fluid column in the catheter and the specific gravity of mercury of 13.6. The transducer is therefore positioned at a level approximately the same as that of the heart, usually the midchest. If the transducer is placed at a different height, attaching a second fluid-filled catheter to the transducer and positioning the tip of that catheter at the zero (midchest) level permit proper zeroing of the transducer relative to the catheter tip position within the heart (Fig. 7-6*B*). It is important to note that pressures measured inside the heart chambers do not necessarily equal the true transmural pressures because of the normal intrathoracic negative pressure, which ranges between 0 and −8 mm Hg during normal respiration.

Even when a pressure measurement system has a high degree of sensitivity, uniform frequency response, and optimal damping, and is properly zeroed and balanced, distortions and inaccuracies in the pressure waveform may occur. Motion of the catheter within the heart and great vessels accelerates the fluid contained within the catheter, and such *catheter whip* artifacts may produce superimposed waves of ±10 mm Hg. Catheter whip artifacts are particularly common in tracings from the pulmonary arteries and are difficult to avoid.

MANOMETER-TIPPED CATHETERS. To minimize artifacts associated with low resonant frequency systems, catheter whip, and excessive damping, some laboratories use micromanometer-tipped catheters, with which the pressure transducer is actually placed in the cardiac chamber in which pressure is being measured. As is evident in Figure 7-7, there may be a distinct difference in waveform between "true" left ventricular pressure (as recorded using an intracardiac micromanometer) and that recorded through a standard fluid-filled catheter system. Low resonant frequency and inadequate damping of the fluid-filled system in this example resulted in exaggeration of the high-frequency components in the left ventricular pressure rise and fall, with corresponding artifactual overshoot of the pressures in early diastole and early systole. More optimal damping and natural frequency characteristics of the fluid-filled system can minimize these artifacts but cannot eliminate them. In addition, a 30- to 40-msec delay in the pressure waveform occurs with fluid-filled catheter systems, necessitating the use of manometer-tipped catheters in situations in which recording of simultaneous pressure and angiographic volume, echocardiographic, phonocardiographic, or electrocardiographic data are required. The high-frequency response of manometer-tipped catheter transducers (resonant frequency = 25 to 40 kHz) permits their application for the detection and recording of intracardiac sounds.

Some manometer-tipped catheters do not have an end-hold and must therefore be inserted by means of arteriotomy or a vascular sheath. Millar* manufactures several No. 8 French end-hold manometer-tipped angiocatheters that can be used with a guidewire. Because the zero level of the manometer-tipped catheter may drift, it is most useful to have a fluid-filled lumen in the catheter by means of which a true zero pressure reference level can be established.

Representative Pressure Tracings

In evaluating pressure tracings, specific phasic and mean pressure values should be measured, the phasic pressure waveform contours noted, and pressures in different

* Millar Instruments, Inc., Houston, Texas.

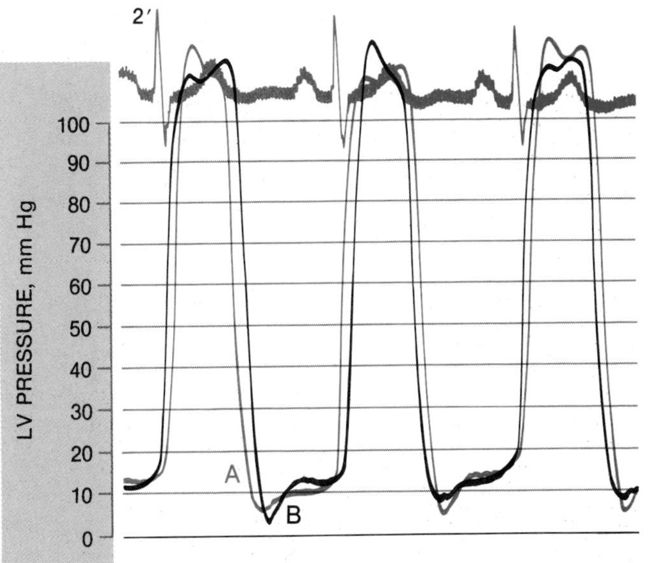

FIGURE 7–7. Left ventricular pressures recorded with a manometer-tipped catheter *(A)* and a fluid-filled catheter–extended transducer system with a low resonant frequency *(B)*. Note undershoot of pressure in early diastole, overshoot of pressure in early systole, and delay of fluid-filled catheter pressure relative to the "true" pressure. (From Grossman, W.: Pressure measurement. *In* Grossman, W., and Baim, D. S. [eds.]: Cardiac Catheterization, Angiography, and Intervention. 4th ed. Philadelphia, Lea and Febiger, 1991.)

chambers compared. Analysis of these data, interpreted in the light of cardiac output and angiographic measurement, permits detection and quantitation of valvular, myocardial, and pericardial abnormalities.

NORMAL PRESSURE WAVEFORMS. An understanding of pressure waveforms, both under normal conditions and in various disease states, is predicated on a thorough comprehension of the events of the cardiac cycle (Fig. 13–32, p. 374). Shown in Figure 7–8 are normal pressure waveforms obtained with fluid-filled catheters.

The *right atrial pressure waveform* consists of two major positive deflections—the *a* and *v* waves. The *a* wave is due to atrial systole and follows the P wave of the electrocardiogram. As the pressure declines from the peak of the *a* wave (the *x* descent), a small positive deflection, the *c* wave, occurs concomitant with tricuspid valve closure. After the "c" wave, right atrial pressure continues to fall (*x* descent) even though the atrium is filling with blood (the tricuspid valve is closed), owing to atrial relaxation. After full atrial relaxation occurs, at the nadir of the *x* descent, the pressure in the atrium starts to rise as atrial filling continues from peripheral venous return. This rise in the right atrial pressure during right ventricular systole is termed the *v* wave, and it reaches a peak just before the opening of the tricuspid valve. After opening of the tricuspid valve, the right atrium empties into the right ventricle, and pressure in the atrium falls, constituting the *y* descent. After the *y* descent, pressure in the atrium is equal to ventricular diastolic pressure and slowly increases as the ventricle fills. Peak *a* and *v* pressures are measured, and the mean pressure is obtained electronically. Normal values are shown in Table 7–2.

The *diastolic phase of the right ventricular pressure pulse* consists of an early rapid filling wave, during which approximately 60 per cent of ventricular filling occurs; a slow filling period, accounting for approximately 25 per cent of ventricular filling; and an atrial systolic wave (*a*), accounting for approximately 15 per cent of ventricular filling. During diastole, right atrial and right ventricular pressures are nearly equal because of the low resistance to flow across the tricuspid valve. Two pressures usually are measured: the peak systolic right ventricular pressure and the end-diastolic right ventricular pressure immediately after the *a* wave. The normal range of values for the pressures is shown in Table 7–2.

The *pulmonary artery pressure waveform* contains a systolic pressure owing to flow of blood into the pulmonary artery from the right ventricle. As right ventricular ejection ends,

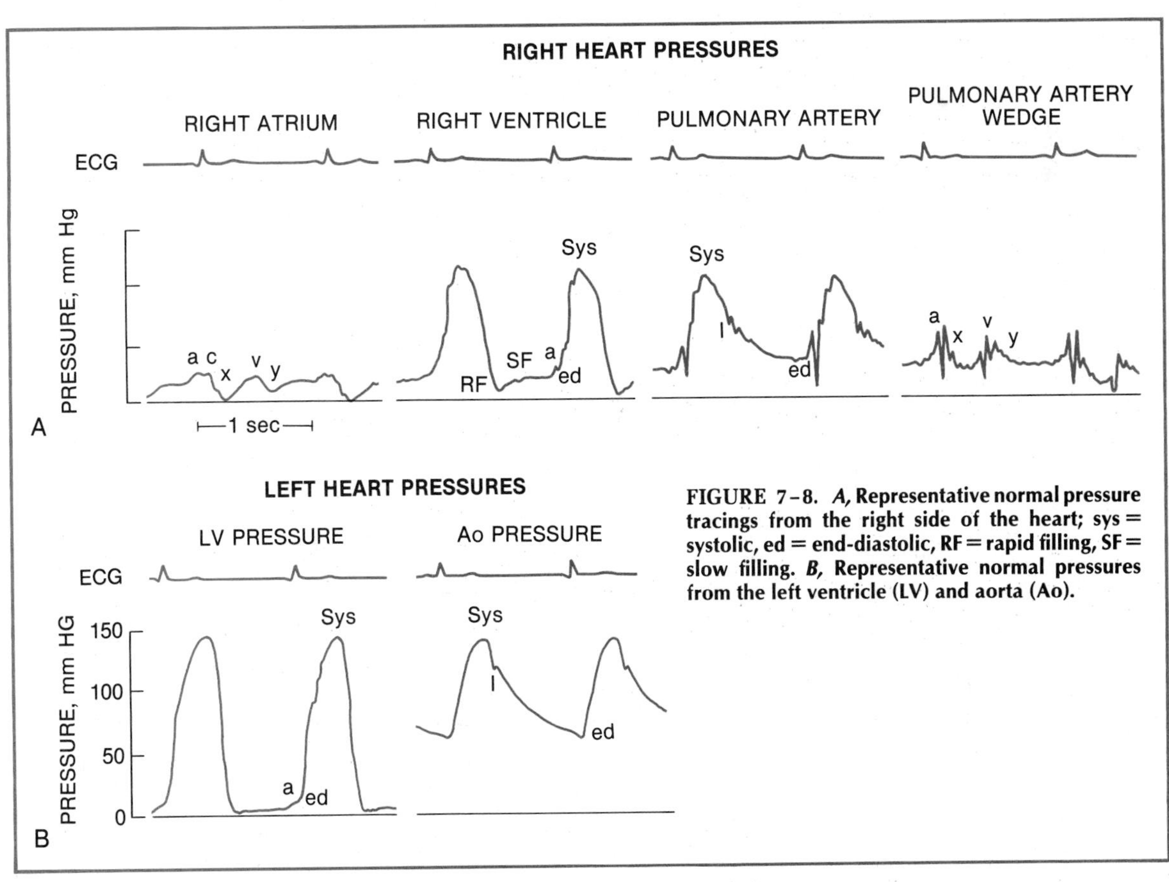

FIGURE 7–8. *A*, Representative normal pressure tracings from the right side of the heart; sys = systolic, ed = end-diastolic, RF = rapid filling, SF = slow filling. *B*, Representative normal pressures from the left ventricle (LV) and aorta (Ao).

TABLE 7–2 RANGE OF NORMAL RESTING HEMODYNAMIC VALUES

	a WAVE	v WAVE	MEAN	SYSTOLIC	END-DIASTOLIC	MEAN
Pressures						
Right atrium	2–10	2–10	0–8			
Right ventricle				15–30	0–8	
Pulmonary artery				15–30	3–12	9–16
Pulmonary artery wedge and left atrium	3–15	3–12	1–10			
Left ventricle				100–140	3–12	
Systemic arteries				100–140	60–90	70–105
Oxygen consumption index (ml/min/m²)		110–150				
Arteriovenous oxygen difference (ml/liter)		30–50				
Cardiac output index (liter/min/m²)		2.6–4.2				
Resistances (dynes-sec-cm⁻⁵)						
Pulmonary vascular		20–130				
Systemic vascular		700–1600				

pressure in the pulmonary artery falls, and when right ventricular pressure drops below the pulmonary pressure, the pulmonary valve closes, resulting in the incisura on the pressure waveform. Pressure in the pulmonary artery then falls gradually as blood flows through the pulmonary arteries and veins into the left atrium and ventricle. The nadir of this pressure in late diastole is termed the end-diastolic pulmonary artery pressure. This pressure and the peak systolic pressure and the mean pulmonary artery pressure are the parameters usually measured. It is not unusual to observe a small (≤5 mm Hg) gradient in peak systolic pressure between the right ventricle and the pulmonary artery.

The *pulmonary artery wedge pressure* (also termed *pulmonary capillary wedge pressure*) has a waveform similar to that of the left atrial pressure but is both damped and delayed by transmission through the capillary vessels.[27] A normal wedge pressure should show *a* and *v* waves, which reflect, respectively, left atrial systole and left atrial filling during left ventricular systole (see discussion of right atrial pressure above). However, *c* waves may not be apparent on the wedge pressure tracing. The x and y descents should be distinct in a wedge pressure tracing if it is not overdamped. The peak *a* and *v* wave pressures usually are measured, as is the mean wedge pressure. In a normal pulmonary circulation of low vascular resistance, the pulmonary artery flow is diminished at end diastole, so that end-diastolic pulmonary artery and mean pulmonary artery wedge pressures are approximately equal. Mean pulmonary artery pressure is always higher than mean wedge pressure (Table 7–2).

Normal left-heart pressure waveforms are shown in Figure 7–8. The *left atrial pressure waveform* was discussed in the description of the pulmonary artery wedge pressure. Unless a transseptal catheterization is performed, pulmonary artery wedge pressure is recorded as an acceptable substitute for the actual left atrial pressure. It is important to recognize that this can be a source of error, unless a properly damped wedge pressure is observed and confirmed by determination of oxygen saturation.

The components of the *left ventricular waveform* are similar to those already described for that of the right ventricle. The pressures in the left ventricle in diastole (as well as in systole) are normally higher than those in the right ventricle, owing in part to the greater wall thickness of the left ventricle, which results in greater chamber stiffness.

The *central aortic pressure tracing* consists of a systolic wave, followed by the incisura, which denotes closure of the aortic valve, and then a gradual fall in pressure as the blood flows from the aorta through the peripheral arterial, capillary, and venous vessels. Pressure normally is measured at peak systole and at end diastole, and the mean pressure is determined electronically.

The *peripheral arterial pressure*, commonly measured during cardiac catheterization in the radial or femoral artery, has a waveform similar to that described for the central aorta. However, because of reflected waves within the arterial system, the peripheral arterial pressure may show a wider pulse pressure with a higher peak systolic pressure than that seen in the central aorta. The mean pressure usually is identical to or up to 5 mm Hg lower than the central aortic pressure. Thus the peak systolic pressure gradients measured between the left ventricle and the systemic arterial system may vary, depending on whether the central aortic pressure or a peripheral arterial pressure is measured.

ABNORMAL PRESSURE TRACINGS. As discussed in greater detail in subsequent chapters, pressure tracings may be virtually diagnostic of certain conditions. In *valvular aortic stenosis* (p. 1035), there is a pressure gradient between the left ventricle and the aorta; however, in addition, the rise in aortic pressure is slow and delayed compared with that of the left ventricle (Fig. 7–9). In contrast, hypertrophic obstructive cardiomyopathy (p. 1404), also may result in a large systolic pressure gradient but will show near identity of the slopes and timing of the left ventricular and aortic pressure increases.

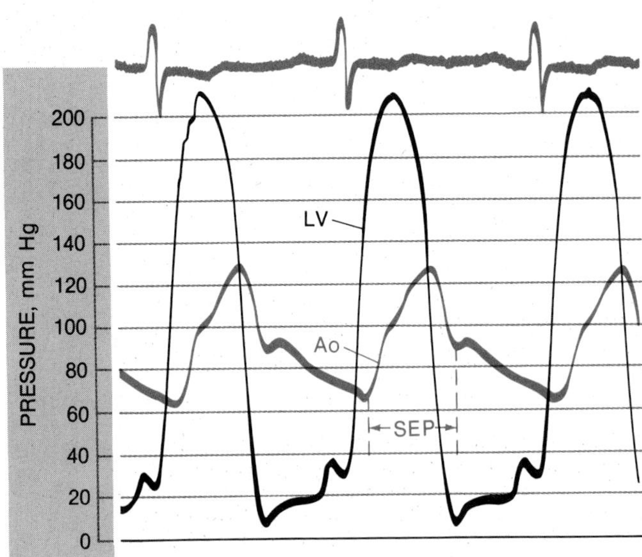

FIGURE 7–9. Left ventricular (LV) and aortic (Ao) pressure tracings in aortic stenosis. During systole, there is a large pressure gradient between LV and Ao, and the rate of rise of the aortic pressure is slow. The systolic ejection period (SEP) is the period of time in each cycle during which blood is being ejected from the left ventricle into the aorta. The vertical time lines are 1 sec apart. (From Grossman, W.: Profiles in valvular heart disease. *In* Grossman, W., and Baim, D. S. [eds.]: Cardiac Catheterization, Angiography, and Intervention. 4th ed. Philadelphia, Lea and Febiger, 1991.)

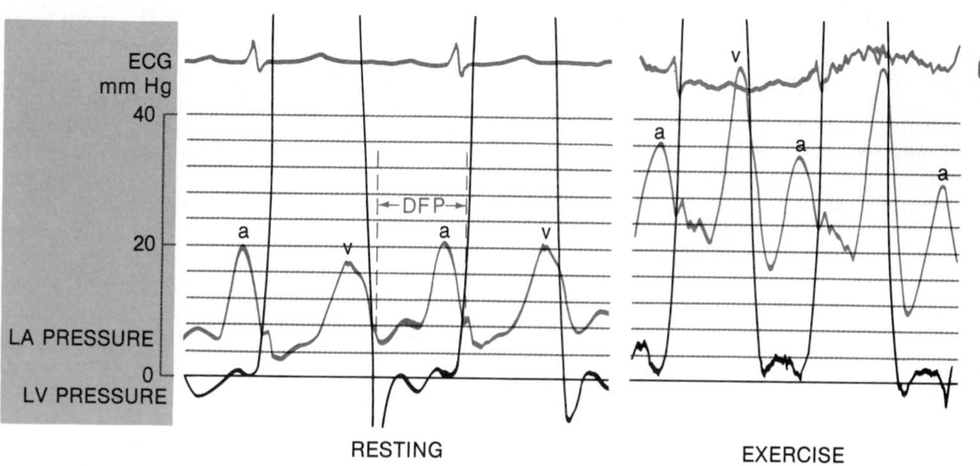

FIGURE 7-10. Left atrial (LA) and left ventricular (LV) pressures in a patient with mitral stenosis at rest *(left)* and during exercise *(right)*. During diastole, there is a pressure gradient between LA and LV. The diastolic filling period (DFP) is the period of time in each cycle when the mitral valve is open. The gradient is greater during exercise as flow across the stenotic valvular orifice increases. (From Lorell, B. H., and Grossman, W.: Dynamic and isometric exercise during cardiac catheterization. *In* Grossman, W., and Baim, D. S. [eds.]: Cardiac Catheterization, Angiography, and Intervention. 4th ed. Philadelphia, Lea and Febiger, 1991.)

Both conditions are associated with increased ventricular stiffness, and therefore may show prominent atrial systolic *a* waves transmitted into the left ventricular pressure tracing in late diastole.[37] *Aortic regurgitation* is characterized by near equalization of aortic and left ventricular pressures at end diastole, marked widening of the aortic pulse pressure, and slurring of the aortic incisura. *Mitral stenosis* is associated with a diastolic pressure gradient (pulmonary artery wedge or left atrium vs. left ventricle) across the mitral valve, which increases substantially with exercise (Fig. 7-10). If the patient is in sinus rhythm, there is a marked discrepancy between the large left atrial systolic wave (*a* wave) and the small or absent *a* wave in the left ventricular tracing.

A large *v* wave in the pulmonary artery wedge tracing may be present in patients with *mitral regurgitation* (p. 1018), and in severe mitral regurgitation the *v* wave may be transmitted back to the pulmonary arterial pressure tracing.[38] The amplitude of the *v* wave is increased because the left atrium is being filled during systole not only with blood entering from the pulmonary veins but also with blood leaking across the mitral valve. Accurate evaluation of mitral valve function by measuring simultaneous pulmonary artery wedge and left ventricular pressures is based on the assumption that the wedge pressure accurately reflects both phasic and mean left atrial pressure (Fig. 7-11). If the wedge pressure is overdamped, it is possible, because the *v* wave height is reduced and the decline of the *v* wave delayed, to overestimate the severity of mitral stenosis and underestimate the severity of mitral regurgitation.

Detection of *stenosis and regurgitation of the tricuspid* (p. 1053) and *pulmonic valves* (p. 1059) during right-heart catheterization usually is assessed by pullback of the catheter from the pulmonary artery to the right ventricle and then to the right atrium. More precise measurement of simultaneous pressures can be performed using a double-lumen right-heart catheter, in which the lumen openings are separated at the end of the catheter by a distance sufficient to permit monitoring pressures on opposite sides of the tricuspid valve or pulmonary outflow tract and valve.

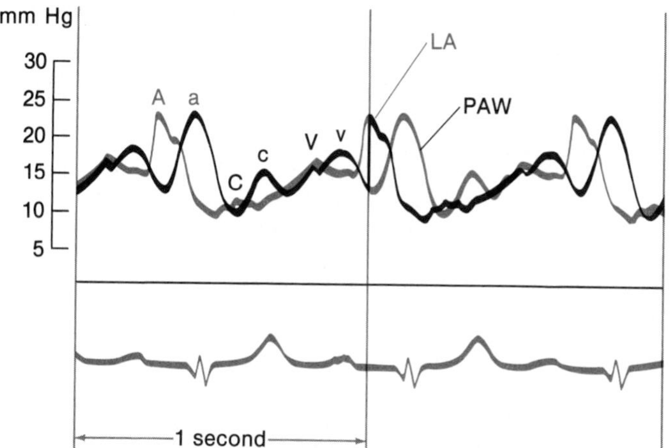

FIGURE 7-11. Simultaneous pulmonary artery wedge (PAW) and left atrial (LA) pressures. *a, c,* and *v* refer to the PAW and *A, C,* and *V* to the LA pressure pulses, respectively. The PAW pressure wave is delayed relative to the LA pressure because of the time required for retrograde propagation of the pressure wave through the pulmonary capillary bed. (From Kory, R. C., et al.: A Primer of Cardiac Catheterization. Springfield, Ill. Courtesy of Charles C Thomas, 1965.)

MEASUREMENT OF CARDIAC OUTPUT

FICK OXYGEN METHOD. Of the numerous techniques devised over the years to measure cardiac output,[39] two have won general acceptance in cardiac catheterization laboratories: the Fick oxygen method and the indicator-dilution technique. These methods resemble each other in that they are based on the theoretical principle enunciated by Adolph Fick in 1870.[40] The principle, which was never applied by Fick, states that total uptake or release of any substance by an organ is the product of blood flow to the organ and the arteriovenous concentration difference of the substance. For the lungs, the substance released to the blood is oxygen, and the pulmonary blood flow can be determined by measurement of the *arteriovenous difference of oxygen* across the lungs and the *oxygen consumption* per minute. If there is no intracardiac shunt, pulmonary blood flow is virtually equal to systemic blood flow, and this application of the Fick principle thus provides a measure of systemic blood flow.

Oxygen consumption is commonly estimated by measurement of oxygen extracted by the lungs over a given time period. A "steady state" is required in which oxygen consumption and cardiac output are constant over the time period of measurement.

Two methods are commonly used for measurement of oxygen consumption: the polarographic method and the Douglas bag method.

The polarographic method is easily utilized using an instrument such as the metabolic rate meter (MRM).* This instrument consists of a polarographic oxygen sensor cell, a hood or face mask, and a blower of variable speed connected with the oxygen sensor by a servocontrol loop (Fig. 7-12). This device is convenient and accurate and represents a significant advance over the older, standard procedure of collecting expired

* Waters Instruments, Rochester, Minnesota.

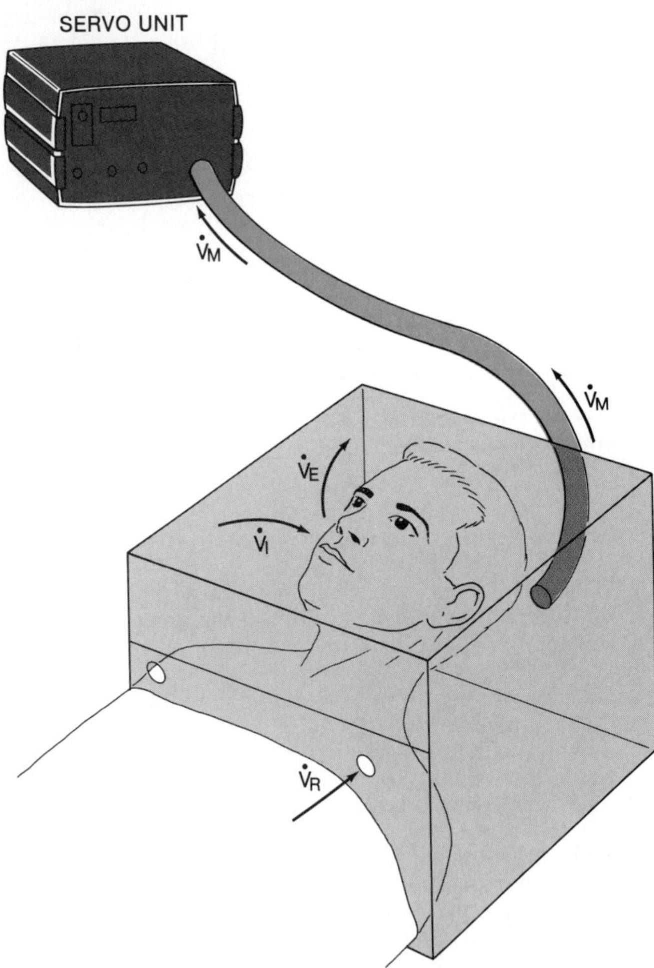

FIGURE 7–12. Measurement of oxygen consumption by a polarographic cell technique, using the metabolic rate meter (Waters instruments). A transparent hood fits snugly over the patient's head, resting on the pillow. Air enters the hood through holes in a plastic sheet at a flow rate, $\dot{V}_R$. Subtract the patient's inspiratory ($\dot{V}_I$) from the expiratory ($\dot{V}_E$) flow rates and add to $\dot{V}_R$ to yield $\dot{V}_M$, the flow rate leaving the hood and entering the servo-unit. A blower monitor in the servo-unit adjusts $\dot{V}_M$ to keep oxygen sensed by the polarographic cell constant. See text for details. (From Grossman, W.: Blood flow measurement: The cardiac output. *In* Grossman, W., and Baim, D. S. [eds.]: Cardiac Catheterization, Angiography, and Intervention. 4th ed. Philadelphia, Lea and Febiger, 1991, p. 111.)

air for 3 minutes in a Douglas bag and measuring volume (Tissot spirometer) and oxygen content. The principle of the polarographic method involves using a variable-speed blower to maintain a unidirectional flow of air from the room through the hood and by way of a connecting hose to the polarographic oxygen sensing cell. As shown in Figure 7–12, room air enters the hood at a rate, $\dot{V}_R$ (ml/min), which is determined by the blower's discharge rate $\dot{V}_M$ (ml/min) as well as the patient's ventilatory rate ($\dot{V}_I$, inhaled air in ml/min; $\dot{V}_E$, exhaled air). The blower's speed, $\dot{V}_M$, is controlled by a servo-loop designed to maintain the oxygen content of air flowing past the polarographic cell constant at a predetermined value. In a steady state, the patient's oxygen consumption, $\dot{V}_{O_2}$, can be calculated as follows:

$$\dot{V}_{O_2} = (F_RO_2 \cdot \dot{V}_R) - (F_MO_2 \cdot \dot{V}_M), \qquad (1)$$

where F_RO_2 and F_MO_2 are fractional contents of oxygen in room air and in the air flowing past the polarographic cell, respectively. As is apparent from Figure 7–12, $\dot{V}_M = \dot{V}_R - \dot{V}_I + \dot{V}_E$, which can be rewritten as $\dot{V}_R = \dot{V}_M + \dot{V}_I - \dot{V}_E$. Substituting this in equation 1 gives:

$$\dot{V}_{O_2} = \dot{V}_M(F_RO_2 - F_MO_2) + F_RO_2(\dot{V}_I - \dot{V}_E). \qquad (2)$$

Because the fractional content of oxygen in room air (F_{RO_2}) is 0.209, oxygen consumption is given by $\dot{V}_{O_2} = \dot{V}_M(0.209 - F_MO_2) + 0.209(\dot{V}_I - \dot{V}_E)$. Thus, in a steady state (where $\dot{V}_I - \dot{V}_E$ is constant), oxygen consumption can be determined by measurement of the volume rate of air moved by the blower motor ($\dot{V}_M$) and the fractional O_2 content of air moving past the polarographic sensor. For practical purposes, the respiratory quotient (RQ) is assumed to be 1.0; accordingly, $\dot{V}_I = \dot{V}_E$. If the RQ is actually 0.9 (i.e., the patient releases 0.9 liters of carbon dioxide for each liter of oxygen consumed), the error in $\dot{V}_{O_2}$ resulting from the assumption of an RQ of 1.0 is 1.6 per cent; if the RQ is 0.8, the error would be 3.2 per cent. Further details of this method, and the older Douglas bag method, are given elsewhere.[23]

The O_2 consumption in milliliters per minute usually is divided by body surface area to correct for differences in O_2 consumption rate, owing to differences in size among patients. The normal basal oxygen consumption index is between 110 and 150 ml O_2/min/m^2 body surface area.

The arteriovenous oxygen difference across the lungs is determined as the difference between the oxygen content of pulmonary arterial blood and that of left ventricular or systemic arterial blood, since pulmonary venous blood usually is not sampled. Actually, because of bronchial venous and thebesian venous drainage, the oxygen content of systemic arterial blood is commonly 2 to 5 ml/liter lower than that of pulmonary venous blood as it leaves the alveoli, and a small overestimation of cardiac output, of little clinical significance, results.

The pulmonary arterial blood is used for determination of mixed venous blood oxygen content and can be measured by a variety of methods. The most widely used methods measure the O_2 saturation of hemoglobin by reflectance oximetry. Oxygen content (ml O_2/liter blood) is then calculated by multiplying the fraction of O_2 saturation by the theoretical oxygen-carrying capacity ([hemoglobin, gm/100 ml] × 1.36 [ml O_2/gm Hb]) × 10. The arteriovenous oxygen content difference is then simply calculated as the arterial minus the venous blood O_2 content.

Cardiac output/m^2 (cardiac index) is calculated as:

$$\frac{O_2 \text{ consumption (ml/min/m}^2)}{\text{Arteriovenous } O_2 \text{ difference (ml/liter)}}$$

and is expressed in liters per minute per square meter.

The normal range is 2.6 to 4.2 liters/min/m^2. The average error in determining oxygen consumption is approximately 6 per cent. The error for arteriovenous oxygen difference determination is approximately 5 per cent, and the total error in measurement of cardiac output by this method is probably about 10 per cent.[39,41–44] The Fick oxygen method is most accurate in patients with low cardiac output, in whom the arteriovenous oxygen difference is wide.

INDICATOR-DILUTION METHOD. The Fick method is merely a specific application of the indicator-dilution method, in which O_2 being continuously infused by the lungs is the indicator and is diluted in the pulmonary blood flow. Stewart was the first to use a dye indicator-dilution method to measure cardiac output; he used the continuous infusion technique and reported his first studies in 1987.[45] Numerous indicators have since been used successfully.[46–49] Indocyanine green dye has been used extensively in clinical practice, although currently thermodilution (in which cold saline is the indicator) has become the most widely used indicator-dilution method.[50–52]

Thermodilution Method. A thermal indicator method for measuring cardiac output is widely used in clinical practice today.[51–53] In the initial report by Ganz et al.,[51] two thermistors were used—one in the superior cava at the site where the cold indicator was injected into the bloodstream and a second "downstream" thermistor located in the proximal pulmonary artery. This permitted accurate measurement of the temperature of the injectate as well as the temperature of blood downstream from the injectate. These parameters, together with knowledge of the specific heat of blood and injectate, permit calculation of cardiac output. Mathematical details of indicator-dilution theory, as well as calculation of cardiac output using thermodilution method, are given elsewhere.[23,51]

The thermodilution method for measuring cardiac output has several advantages over the indocyanine green dye method. These include the following: (1) it does not require withdrawal of blood; (2) it does not require an arterial puncture; (3) an inert and inexpensive indicator is used; and (4) there is virtually no recirculation, making computer analysis of the primary curves simple.

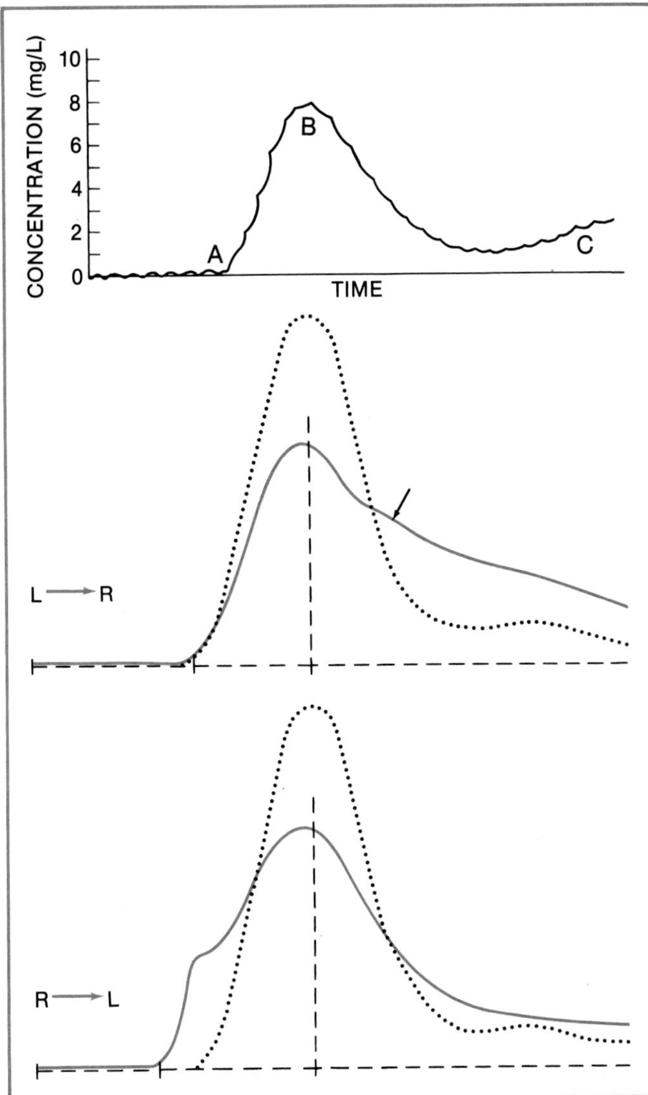

FIGURE 7–13. Time-concentration curves generated by injecting indocyanine green dye into the right heart and sampling in the brachial artery. *Top,* Normal curve showing appearance of the dye in arterial blood *(A)* and the peak concentration *(B),* followed by an exponential disappearance and then recirculation of the dye. *(C). Center,* The solid line is a schematic drawing of the time-concentration curve in a patient with left-to-right shunt. There is an early recirculation "bump" *(arrow)* on the downslope of the curve owing to the dye that is shunted from left to right and then reappears in the left circulation. The dotted line represents a normal dye concentration curve. *Bottom,* Time-concentration curve in the presence of a right-to-left shunt, showing early appearance of the dye in the brachial artery. The early-appearing dye passes through the shunt and thus does not traverse the pulmonary circulation. The dotted line represents a normal dye concentration curve. (Top panel from Grossman, W.: Measurement of cardiac output. *In* Grossman, W., and Baim, D. S. [eds.]: Cardiac Catheterization, Angiography, and Intervention. 4th ed. Philadelphia, Lea and Febiger, 1990. Center and lower panels from Kory, R. C., et al.: A Primer of Cardiac Catheterization. Springfield, Ill. Courtesy of Charles C Thomas, 1965.)

INDOCYANINE GREEN DYE METHOD. When indocyanine green dye is used, a bolus is injected rapidly into the pulmonary artery, and its appearance and concentration in arterial blood are recorded from a peripheral systemic artery (e.g., brachial, femoral, or radial). A time-concentration curve is thus recorded that exhibits a rapid rise to a peak and then a gradual decline in concentration that is interrupted by a secondary rise, owing to recirculation of the dye (Fig. 7–13, *top*). The problem of isolating those data that relate only to the first pass of the indicator has been approached by several investigators, but the method originally proposed by Kinsman, Moore, and Hamilton[54] is the one still used most widely today. Kinsman and coworkers showed mathematically that the true "first-pass" curve will be given by plotting the concentration decline on semilogarithmic paper and extrapolating the early linear part of the plot.

The cardiac output (CO) is then calculated as $CO = i/(\bar{c} \times t)$, where i is the quantity of indicator injected, $\bar{c}$ is the average concentration of the indicator during its first pass, and t is the total duration of the curve. The product of $\bar{c}$ and t is easily measured as the area under the first-pass curve, determined by planimetry. This may be simplified further by the use of any number of available computer methods in which the semilogarithmic replotting, area computation, and cardiac output calculation are all accomplished electronically. More precise methodological details, as well as a discussion of sources of error, can be found elsewhere.[23,39]

Most laboratories,[46,55–57] but not all,[49,53] have found that there is excellent agreement between the indicator-dilution methods (either thermodilution or green dye) and independent methods for measuring cardiac output, particularly when the cardiac output is normal or elevated. The error of the indicator-dilution method is greatest in patients with extremely low outputs,[53] severe mitral or aortic regurgitation, or intracardiac shunts. Therefore, it complements the Fick method of cardiac output determination, in which the accuracy is greatest in patients having low cardiac output with wide arteriovenous oxygen differences.

It is important to note that indocyanine green dye can cause interference when oxygen content is determined by spectrophotometric methods. Therefore, if cardiac output is to be determined by both Fick and the indocyanine green dye indicator-dilution methods *in the same patient,* the former measurement should be done first. Not only does the use of cold saline (thermodilution) as an indicator avoid this problem, but also this technique can be performed repeatedly without buildup of indicator or recirculation problems. For these reasons, the thermodilution method has become the most commonly used indicator-dilution technique for measuring cardiac output.

ANGIOGRAPHIC MEASUREMENT OF CARDIAC OUTPUT

Measurement of left ventricular end-diastolic and end-systolic volumes by quantitative left ventricular angiography, described on p. 422, permits calculation of left ventricular stroke volume. In the absence of atrial fibrillation or significant mitral or aortic regurgitation, systemic cardiac output may be estimated by multiplying the stroke volume by the heart rate during the angiogram. This method is a less accurate method of measuring cardiac output than either the indicator-dilution or the Fick method.

REGIONAL BLOOD FLOWS. The principles discussed above may be applied to measure regional blood flows. Three common examples are intracardiac shunt flow as measured by the Fick principle, coronary sinus flow by thermodilution, and regurgitant valve flow by a combination of angiographic and Fick measurements of cardiac output.

INTRACARDIAC SHUNTS

Detection, localization, and quantification of intracardiac shunts can be accomplished with precision at cardiac catheterization. Although intracardiac shunts usually are suspected before catheterization, this is not always the case. Therefore, the operator must be alert to the possibility of an intracardiac shunt and must search for one when unexpected arterial oxygen desaturation is detected or an inappropriately high pulmonary artery oxygen saturation is observed.

DETECTION AND LOCALIZATION OF SHUNTS. In a patient with a *left-to-right shunt* (e.g., atrial septal defect, ventricular septal defect, patient ductus arteriosus), pulmonary blood flow is higher than systemic blood flow, and the pulmonary artery oxygen saturation is greater than the true mixed venous blood saturation. The anatomical location of the shunt is determined by obtaining multiple samples for oxygen saturation. In the traditional "oximetry run,"[7,23,58] samples are drawn in rapid succession from the left, right, and main pulmonary arteries; the outflow tract, body, and inflow area of the right ventricle; the low, mid, and high right atrium; the low and high superior vena cava; and the inferior vena cava at the level of the diaphragm.

The technique of the oximetry run is based on the work of Dexter et al.,[7] who reported in 1947 that multiple samples drawn from the right atrium of normal subjects could vary in oxygen content by as much as 2 volumes per cent (20 ml O_2/liter), reflecting the fact that the right atrium receives its blood from three sources: the superior vena cava, the inferior vena cava, and the coronary sinus. Maximal normal variation within the right ventricle was found to be 10 ml O_2/liter, while maximal variation within the pulmonary artery was 5 ml O_2/liter. Using these criteria, a significant oxygen "step-up" is present at the atrial level when the highest oxygen content in blood samples drawn from the right atrium exceeds the highest content in the venae cavae by 20 ml O_2/liter. Similarly, a significant step-up at the ventricular level is present if the highest right ventricular sample is 10 ml O_2/liter higher than the highest right atrial sample, and a significant step-up at the level of the pulmonary artery requires a pulmonary artery oxygen content more than 5 ml O_2/liter greater than the highest right ventricular sample. Few laboratories currently measure oxygen content of blood directly, but rather measure blood oxygen saturation using reflectance oximetry.

The findings in a study[28] in which normal variation of both oxygen content and oxygen saturation of blood in the right-heart chambers in a large number of patients undergoing diagnostic cardiac catheterization were analyzed are summarized in Table 7–3. As can be seen, different criteria exist, depending on whether an average of oxygen saturation (or oxygen content) values obtained for multiple samples is used, or whether only the highest value for oxygen saturation or content in a particular chamber is used. Using averaged samples, an oxygen saturation step-up of greater than or equal to 7 per cent is necessary to diagnose a left-to-right shunt at the atrial level, whereas greater than or equal to 5 per cent suffices at the ventricular or great vessel level. Thus, for a patient in whom average right ventricular oxygen saturation (three samples) is 72 per cent and average pulmonary artery saturation (again, three samples) is 79 per cent, the diagnosis of left-to-right shunt at the pulmonary artery level is suggested. The anatomical defect causing the shunt could be a patent ductus arteriosus, an aortic-pulmonary window, or, rarely, aberrant coronary artery origin (e.g., left anterior descending artery originating from the pulmonary artery) with left-to-right shunt.

One limitation of the oxygen method of detecting intracardiac shunts is its low degree of sensitivity. Small shunts ($\dot{Q}_p/\dot{Q}_s \leq 1.3$) at the level of the pulmonary artery or right ventricle and shunts at the atrial level with $\dot{Q}_p/\dot{Q}_s < 1.5$ are not detected consistently by this technique alone because of the normal variability in O_2 saturation described above. A more sensitive technique for the detection of small left-to-right intracardiac shunts involves detection of the early appearance of hydrogen in the right heart after inhalation of hydrogen gas using a right-heart hydrogen-sensitive platinum-tipped electrode catheter to measure direct-current voltage changes. In addition, in the presence of a left-to-right shunt, injection of indocyanine green dye into the pulmonary artery with sampling from the femoral artery will demonstrate early recirculation on the downslope of the dye curve.[23,58,59] These techniques are easily performed and sometimes can detect left-to-right shunts too small to be detected by the oxygen step-up method (Fig. 7–13, *center*).

In patients with *right-to-left* shunts, arterial blood is unsaturated, and cyanosis commonly is present. Clinically, the site of entry of a right-to-left intracardiac shunt may be localized by noting which of the left-heart chambers is the first to show desaturation. It usually is difficult to enter the pulmonary veins and left atrium in the adult, as discussed previously. Small right-to-left shunts may be detected by injecting indocyanine dye into a vena cava and detecting the early appearance of the dye in arterial blood before the primary peak (Fig. 7–13, *bottom*). The origin of the shunt can then be localized by injecting dye at a more distal site in the right heart until its early appearance disappears.

It should be remembered that an abnormal catheter position also can be useful in detecting an abnormal communication. This is particularly true for atrial septal defects and for anomalous pulmonary veins that empty into the right atrium. In addition, angiographic methods may be used to detect and localize intracardiac shunts (Chap. 9).

SHUNT QUANTIFICATION. The usefulness of the oximetry run method of shunt detection is enhanced by the fact that the data obtained also are used in quantification of the shunt. When the shunt is unidirectional (e.g., left-to-right), its magnitude is calculated simply as the difference between the pulmonary and systemic blood flows. Pulmonary blood flow ($\dot{Q}_p$) in liters per minute is given as:

$$\dot{Q}_p = \frac{O_2 \text{ consumption (ml/min)}}{\underset{\text{(ml/liter)}}{\text{PV } O_2\text{content}} - \underset{\text{(ml/liter)}}{\text{PA } O_2\text{content}}},$$

where PV and PA refer to pulmonary venous and pulmonary arterial blood, respectively. If a pulmonary vein has not been entered, systemic arterial oxygen content may be used in lieu of PV O_2 content, as long as the systemic arterial oxygen saturation is 95 per cent or more. If systemic oxygen saturation is less than 95 per cent, one must determine whether a right-to-

TABLE 7–3 DETECTION OF LEFT-TO-RIGHT SHUNT BY OXIMETRY

	CRITERIA FOR SIGNIFICANT STEP-UP					
LEVEL OF SHUNT	Mean of Distal Chamber Samples	Mean of Proximal Chamber Samples	Highest Value in Distal Chamber	Highest Value in Proximal Chamber	APPROXIMATE MINIMAL Q_P/Q_S REQUIRED FOR DETECTION (ASSUMING SBFI = 3l/min/m²)	POSSIBLE CAUSES OF STEP-UP
	O_2% Sat	*O_2 Vol%*	*O_2% Sat*	*O_2 Vol%*		
Atrial (SVC/IVC to RA)	≥7	≥1.3	≥11	≥2.0	1.5–1.9	Atrial septal defect; partial anomalous pulmonary venous drainage; ruptured sinus of Valsalva; VSD with TR; coronary fistula to RA
Ventricular (RA to RV)	≥5	≥1.0	≥10	≥1.7	1.3–1.5	VSD; PDA with PR; primum ASD; coronary fistula to RV
Great vessel (RV to PA)	≥5	≥1.0	≥5	≥1.0	1.3	PDA; aorta-pulmonic window; aberrant coronary artery origin
Any level (SVC to PA)	≥7	≥1.3	≥8	≥1.5	1.5	All of the above

SVC and IVC, superior and inferior venae cavae; RA, right atrium; RV, right ventricle; PA, pulmonary artery; VSD, ventricular septal defect; TR, tricuspid regurgitation; PDA, patent ductus arteriosus; PR, pulmonic regurgitation; ASD, atrial septal defect; SBFI, systemic blood flow index; Q_P/Q_S, pulmonary to systemic flow ratio.

From Grossman, W., and Baim, D. S. (eds.): Cardiac Catheterization, Angiography, and Intervention. 4th ed. Philadelphia, Lea and Febiger, 1991.

left shunt is present. If such a shunt exists, then a value of PV O_2 content is calculated from the assumption that it is 98 per cent of blood oxygen-carrying capacity, and this is used in calculating $\dot{Q}_p$. If arterial desaturation is present but is not due to a right-to-left intracardiac shunt, the observed systemic arterial oxygen content is used to calculate $\dot{Q}_p$.

Systemic blood flow ($\dot{Q}_s$) in liters per minute is calculated as

$$\dot{Q}_s = \frac{O_2 \text{ consumption (ml/min)}}{\left[\begin{array}{c}\text{Systemic arterial}\\ O_2 \text{ content (ml/liter)}\end{array}\right] - \left[\begin{array}{c}\text{Mixed venous}\\ O_2 \text{ content (ml/liter)}\end{array}\right]}.$$

Mixed venous oxygen content is obtained as the average oxygen content of blood in the chamber immediately upstream in relation to the shunt, as defined by the level of the O_2 step-up in the oximetry run. The formula used to calculate mixed venous oxygen content when the shunt is at the level of the right atrium, as in atrial septal defect, was derived by Flamm and coworkers.[60] They found that $\dot{Q}_s$ calculated from mixed venous oxygen content derived as

$$\frac{3 \text{ SVC } O_2 \text{ content} + 1 \text{ IVC } O_2 \text{ content}}{4}$$

most closely approximated $\dot{Q}_s$ measured by left ventricular to brachial artery indicator-dilution curves in patients with atrial septal defect.

Calculation of the shunt flow itself is then given as $\dot{Q}_p - \dot{Q}_s$. If the shunt is wholly left to right, this value is positive, whereas a negative value is observed in patients with pure right-to-left shunts (e.g., tetralogy of Fallot). When there is *bidirectional shunting*, the more complicated formula below must be used.

$$L \rightarrow R = \frac{\dot{Q}_p \text{ (PA } O_2 \text{ content} - \text{MV } O_2 \text{ content)}}{\text{(PV* } O_2 \text{ content} - \text{MV } O_2 \text{ content)}}$$

$$R \rightarrow L = \frac{\dot{Q}_p \text{ (PV* } O_2 \text{ content} - \text{SA } O_2 \text{ content)} \cdot \text{(PV* } O_2 \text{ content} - \text{PA } O_2 \text{ content)}}{\text{(SA } O_2 \text{ content} - \text{MV } O_2 \text{ content)} \cdot \text{(PV* } O_2 \text{ content} - \text{MV } O_2 \text{ content)}},$$

where MV and SA are mixed venous and systemic arterial blood samples, respectively.

REGURGITANT FLOWS

In aortic or mitral valve regurgitation, left ventricular stroke volume measured angiographically is greater than the forward stroke volume (calculated by dividing the Fick cardiac output by the heart rate), and the difference is the volume of regurgitant blood that leaks across the abnormal valve(s) during each cardiac cycle. Calculation of this regurgitant flow from data obtained during cardiac catheterization can be helpful in evaluating the severity of regurgitant lesions. The regurgitant fraction (RF) is defined as

$$RF = \frac{\left[\begin{array}{c}\text{Angiographic}\\ \text{stroke volume}\end{array}\right] - \left[\begin{array}{c}\text{Fick stroke}\\ \text{volume}\end{array}\right]}{\text{Angiographic stroke volume}}$$

As a general rule, the correspondence of calculated regurgitant fraction to subjectively estimated severity of regurgitation from cineangiography is as follows: 1 + regurgitation corresponds to a RF of less than or equal to 20 per cent; 2 + regurgitation, RF 21 to 40 per cent; 3 + regurgitation, RF 41 to 60 per cent; 4 + regurgitation, RF greater than or equal to 60 per cent. Thus, regurgitant fractions exceeding 30 to 40 per cent are considered hemodynamically important. However, because of potential errors of measurement of both the angiographic and Fick stroke volume, this measurement must be interpreted in light of other hemodynamic, angiographic, and clinical data.

*If actual PV is not measured, assume 98 per cent blood O_2 capacity in a patient whose pulmonary function is normal or presumed to be so.

CORONARY BLOOD FLOW

Coronary sinus blood flow may be measured during cardiac catheterization by the thermodilution technique.[61-63] A thermodilution catheter is inserted into the coronary sinus by way of the right internal jugular vein or a left antecubital vein. Saline or 5 per cent dextrose solution at room temperature is infused continuously, and the temperature of the blood–saline mixture downstream in the coronary sinus is monitored by an external thermistor on the catheter. The temperature of the injected saline is monitored by an internal thermistor near the catheter injection orifice. The theoretical aspects of coronary venous thermodilution are summarized in Figure 7–14.

$$F_B = F_I \times 1.19 \times \left(\frac{T_M - T_I}{T_B - T_M}\right) \text{ ml/min}$$

where

F_B = coronary sinus blood flow
F_I = flow of room temperature saline injectate (ml/min)
T_B = body temperature (°C)
T_I = injectate temperature (°C)
T_M = temperature of blood–injectate mixture (°C)

Other techniques also may be used to estimate coronary blood flow.[23] For example, a small amount of the inert gas isotope xenon-133 may be injected selectively into a coronary artery, and the initial washout of radioactivity from the heart can be recorded with a scintillation camera (p. 276). The regional myocardial blood flow in the distribution of that coronary artery can be estimated from the rate constant (κ) derived from a semilogarithmic plot of the radioactivity washout curve, the partition coefficient of the tracer in myocardial tissue (λ), and the specific gravity of myocardial tissue (ρ). The formula used is

$$\text{Myocardial blood flow (cm}^3\text{/100 gm tissue} \times \text{min)} = \frac{\kappa \text{ (min}^{-1}) \; \lambda \; 100}{\rho \text{ (gm/cm}^3)}$$

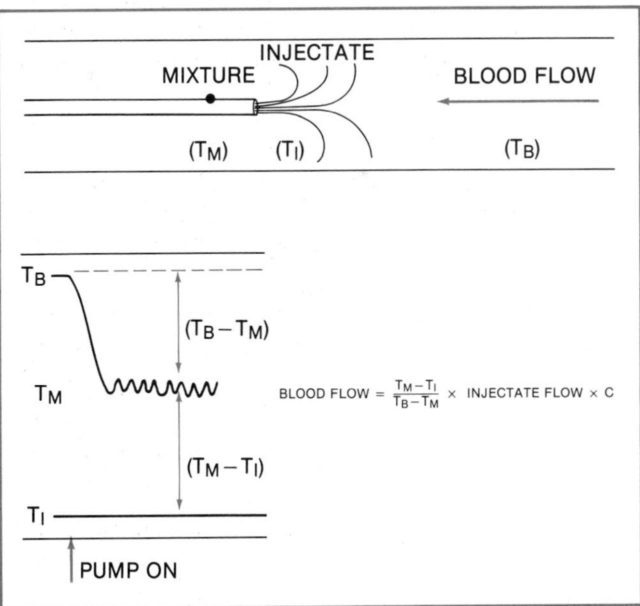

FIGURE 7–14. **Schematic illustration of coronary venous thermodilution. The thermal indicator (injectate) at temperature T_I is infused at a constant rate (e.g., 15 ml/min). Turbulence causes mixing of the injectate with coronary venous blood at temperature T_B, resulting in a blood–injectate mixture at temperature T_M. The catheter tip thermistor monitors T_B and T_M, while an internal thermistor monitors T_I, and these are recorded continuously on a uniform temperature scale *(lower left)*. Because heat loss by blood is gained by injectate, coronary venous flow is calculated using the measured temperatures, the rate of indicator injection, and the constant derived from the specific heats of blood and injectate. (From Bradley, A. B., and Baim, D. S.: Measurement of coronary blood flow in man. Methods and implications for clinical practice. Cardiovasc. Clin. *14*:67, 1984.)**

Inaccuracies in the measurement of coronary blood flow with this method may occur because of recirculation of the isotope, deposition of xenon in myocardial fat, and the local inhomogeneity of flow.

Adaptation of Doppler methodology to the measurement of coronary artery blood flow velocity has been developed to a point of practical applicability.[64] A piezoelectric crystal is mounted into the wall of a woven Dacron catheter and passed into the coronary arteries selectively through a No. 8 French coronary guiding catheter. Measurement of a Doppler coronary blood flow velocity signal can be obtained continuously, and the measured signal can be shown to reflect instantaneous changes in coronary blood flow. Striking increases in coronary blood flow velocity (e.g., fivefold increases) have been noted using the Doppler technique in normal coronary arteries after an infusion of intravenous dipyridamole. This technique seems well suited to the selective measurement of coronary vasodilator reserve in the catheterization laboratory.

DETERMINATION OF VASCULAR RESISTANCE

THEORETICAL CONSIDERATIONS. Hydraulic resistance (R) is defined by analogy to Ohm's law as the ratio of the mean pressure drop (ΔP) to flow (Q) between two points in a liquid flowing in a tube. The applicability of this simple equation to pulsatile flow in vascular beds is dubious. Nevertheless, vascular resistance calculated in this manner has become standard practice in hemodynamic laboratories, and the calculated resistances so obtained often yield important clinical information. Poiseuille's studies of laminar steady-state flow in rigid glass tubes showed that

$$Q = \frac{\pi(\Delta P)r^4}{8\,\eta l},$$

where r = radius of the tube, l = length of the tube, and η = viscosity of the fluid.[36] By rearrangement, it can be seen that resistance (R) is given by

$$R = \frac{\Delta P}{Q} = \frac{8\,\eta l}{\pi r^4}.$$

Thus, under the ideal conditions of laminar fluid flow in rigid tubes, resistance is directly proportional to the length of the tube and to the viscosity of the fluid and *inversely proportional to the fourth power of the tube's radius.* It is clear from this that reduction in the cross-sectional area of a vessel lumen is the most powerful determinant of resistance to flow. It was observed by Reynolds in 1883 that the pressure drop across a length of tubing exceeded that predicted by the Poiseuille equation at a critical flow rate, dependent on the diameter of the tube and the viscosity of the fluid. He defined the Reynold's number (R_e) as being equal to $\frac{\bar{V}D\rho}{\eta}$, where $\bar{V}$ = average velocity of flow, D = diameter of the tube, ρ = density of the fluid, and η = its viscosity.[36] When this number is exceeded, flow becomes turbulent, and the pressure drop exceeds that predicted by the Poiseuille equation, which assumes laminar flows. For blood, $R_e = 2000$, and it appears likely that during normal blood flow in arteries, R_e is not exceeded and that flow remains laminar. However, across severely stenotic valves or in areas of severe luminal arterial narrowing, this may not be the case. This will be considered further in the subsequent discussion of calculation of stenotic valve areas.

CALCULATIONS. Vascular resistance for the systemic and pulmonary vascular beds (SVR and PVR, respectively) usually is calculated as

$$SVR = \frac{80\,(AO_m - RA_m)}{\dot{Q}_s}$$

and

$$PVR = \frac{80\,(PA_m - LA_m)}{\dot{Q}_p},$$

where AO_m, RA_m, PA_m, and LA_m are the aortic, right atrial, pulmonary artery, and left atrial mean pressures in mm Hg; $\dot{Q}_s$ and $\dot{Q}_p$ are the systemic and pulmonary blood flows in liters per minute (which are equal to the cardiac output in the absence of a shunt); and 80 is the factor used to convert resistance from "hybrid" units (mm Hg/liter/min) to metric units (dynes-sec-cm^{-5}). (See also Chap. 27.) These values can be corrected for body size by multiplying (not dividing) them by body surface area—an important factor in evaluating vascular resistance in infants and adolescents.

Cardiac output, usually measured by the Fick or indicator-dilution method, is used in the calculation of systemic and pulmonary vascular resistances. It is important to appreciate that in the presence of an intracardiac shunt, in which pulmonary and systemic blood flows are not equal, the respective blood flows through each circuit must be measured and used in the calculation of resistance. The mean pulmonary artery wedge pressure often is used as an approximation of mean left atrial pressure, since there is ample evidence that these two measurements, when properly obtained, closely approximate each other.[27]

The normal value for systemic vascular resistance in the author's laboratory is 1170 ± 270 dynes-sec-cm^{-5} (mean ± standard deviation),[23] or 2130 ± 450 dynes-sec-cm^{-5} · m^2. Thus values for systemic vascular resistance less than 1700 dynes-sec-cm^{-5} are probably normal. The normal pulmonary vascular resistance in the author's laboratory is 67 ± 30 dynes-sec-cm^{-5}, or 123 ± 54 dynes-sec-cm^{-5} · m^2. Therefore, values of pulmonary vascular resistance less than 130 dynes-sec-cm^{-5} are probably normal.

Abnormal increases of systemic and pulmonary vascular resistance may be seen in a variety of conditions (Chaps. 27 and 28). It may be important to determine whether the increased resistance is fixed (i.e., owing to chronic anatomical and pathological changes) or functional (i.e., owing to increased tone in small muscular arteries and arterioles), since this finding can have important clinical implications. For example, major elevations in vascular resistance in the systemic bed may lead to a low cardiac output and left ventricular failure, particularly in the presence of mitral regurgitation. Lowering systemic resistance with specific agents (e.g., sodium nitroprusside) at the time of cardiac catheterization may yield important information about the potential therapeutic usefulness of such reduction of afterload in chronic therapy (Chap. 17). Marked fixed increases in pulmonary vascular resistance in patients with congenital heart disease and abnormal communication between the pulmonary and systemic circuits (e.g., ventricular septal defect, atrial septal defect, patent ductus arteriosus) may contraindicate corrective surgery. Therefore, a demonstration that the increased resistance is not fixed may be of considerable importance in the individual patient. In the catheterization laboratory, various agents and manipulations have been utilized to assess the reversibility of high pulmonary vascular resistance, including infusions of acetylcholine,[65,66] infusions of tolazoline hydrochloride,[67,68] oxygen inhalation (Chap. 27), and exercise.

Because blood flow is pulsatile, and the vascular beds have nonlinear elastic and capacitative properties, the concept of *vascular impedance* has been used. Resistance varies continuously with pressure, and blood flow is influenced by many factors, such as inertia, reflected waves, and the phase angle between pulse and flow velocities.[36,69] The impedance modulus is calculated to express the spectrum of impedance versus the frequency of a pressure wave.[36]

Stenotic Valves: Calculations of Orifice Area

The evaluation of valvular stenosis in the catheterization laboratory includes a calculation of orifice size based on measurement of the pressure gradient and flow across a valve. The equations used for the aortic and mitral valves were derived and validated by Gorlin.[23,70,71,71a]

The following equations are used when valvular gradients are measured directly:

$$\text{Aortic valve area (cm}^2\text{)} = \frac{F}{44.3\sqrt{\Delta P}}$$

and

$$\text{Mitral valve area (cm}^2\text{)} = \frac{F}{37.7\sqrt{\Delta P}},$$

where F = flow across the orifice in milliliters per second and ΔP = mean pressure gradient in millimeters of mercury across the orifice. A pressure drop across a stenotic valve occurs because of viscous resistance to flow (Poiseuille) and turbulent flow (Reynolds). The empirical constants 44.3 and 37.7 relate these factors to valve area and differ between aortic and mitral valves because of variations in flow pattern.

For specific application to cardiac valves, F is derived as:

$$\text{Flow (F) (ml/sec)} = \frac{\text{Cardiac output (ml/min)}}{\text{DFP (sec/min) or SEP (sec/min)}}.$$

The diastolic filling period (DFP) and systolic ejection period (SEP) are derived by measuring the diastolic filling time (mitral valve opening to closure, Fig. 7–10) or systolic ejection time (aortic valve opening to closure, Fig. 7–9) per beat and multiplying by the heart rate.

In a typical patient, cardiac output might be 4300 ml/min, mean transmitral diastolic pressure gradient = 14 mm Hg, diastolic filling time per beat directly measured from the pressure tracings = 0.42 sec/beat, and heart rate = 72 beats/min. Thus the mitral valve area will be

$$\frac{(4300\text{ ml/min}) \div (0.42\text{ sec/beat} \times 72\text{ beats/min})}{37.7\sqrt{14\text{ mm Hg}}} = 1.0\text{ cm}^2$$

It is important to remember that variations in flow patterns may alter the relation between orifice area and pressure gradient. In addition, stiff valve leaflets may be more widely opened at high flow velocities (and higher pressure gradients). Therefore, estimation of valve areas, particularly at low flow rates, may be in error and should be considered measurements of functional orifice size. In addition, the presence of valvular regurgitation will result in falsely low valve area calculation, since the actual valve flow per beat is greater than the flow calculated from the systemic cardiac output. Stenotic valve areas calculated in patients with regurgitation across the stenotic valve should therefore be considered to be the lower limits of the true valve area. In general, errors in estimation of valve flow cause greater inaccuracies in calculations of valve area than do errors in measurement of the pressure gradient across the valve. Nevertheless, hemodynamic measurement of valve area has proved very useful in the clinical management of patients.

There are many pitfalls in the calculation of valve areas. For calculation of mitral valve area, pulmonary capillary wedge pressure commonly is substituted for left atrial pressure under the assumption that a properly confirmed wedge pressure accurately reflects left atrial pressure. The weight of evidence and experience supports this assumption as correct,[27] except in some patients with pulmonary veno-occlusive disease or cor triatriatum. Failure to wedge the catheter properly, however, may cause inappropriate comparison of a damped pulmonary artery pressure to left ventricular pressure, yielding a falsely high gradient. To insure that the right-heart catheter is wedged properly, one should verify that (1) the mean wedge pressure is lower than the mean pulmonary artery pressure and (2) blood withdrawn from the wedged catheter is greater than or equal to 95 per cent saturated with oxygen, or at least equal in saturation to arterial blood. If these two criteria are not fulfilled, serious error may result from acceptance of pulmonary capillary wedge pressure as accurately reflective of left atrial pressure.

Failure to properly calibrate pressure transducers and to adjust them to the same zero reference point also may yield erroneous gradient measurements. A quick way to check the validity of an unexpected mitral or aortic pressure gradient is to switch catheters to opposite transducers, which, if calibrated equally and adjusted to the same zero reference, will yield the same gradient.

Inaccurate cardiac output determination may induce significant error in valve area calculation. Even in the absence of significant regurgitation across the valve whose area is being calculated, small errors in cardiac output measurement will substantially affect valve area determination. Cardiac output measurement should be carried out simultaneously with gradient determination.

Substitution of peripheral arterial pressure for central aortic pressure is done commonly during the measurement of gradients in patients with aortic stenosis. Because the peripheral arterial pressure is delayed temporally compared with central aortic pressure, appropriate realignment of pressure tracings is required before planimetry of gradients. In addition to distortion from temporal delay, peripheral arterial pressure waveforms are distorted by systolic amplification and spreading out of the pressure waveforms, and errors are introduced as a result of this substitution.[72] Specific techniques have been developed to correct for these errors, including the method of Krueger and coworkers which involves subtracting the planimetered mean peripheral arterial systolic pressure from the mean left ventricular systolic pressure.[73]

Certain modifications and simplifications of the Gorlin formula have been introduced.[73–75] The reader is referred elsewhere for details.[23]

HEMODYNAMICS DURING EXERCISE

In many patients with heart disease, hemodynamics may be normal or only slightly disturbed at rest, but they become markedly abnormal during the stress of exercise. Exercise of a patient during cardiac catheterization can therefore provide important information regarding the cause of symptoms that are exercise-related. Most commonly, bicycle ergometry in the supine position is used during catheterization; upright bicycle exercise, upper-extremity exercise, or straight leg raising also may be used, if appropriate.

For supine bicycle ergometry, the patient's feet are strapped to the pedals of a bicycle ergometer, which is attached to the catheterization table or suspended from the ceiling. The workload may be adjusted by varying the speed of and resistance to turning of the pedals. When the subject's feet are on the pedals, intracardiac pressures normally increase slightly (i.e., by 2 to 4 mm Hg), owing to increased venous return by gravity from the legs and elevation of the diaphragm. As the exercise load is increased, oxygen consumption is increased. Exercise level is frequently expressed as metabolic equivalents of resting O_2 consumption (METS), a level of 2 METS corresponding to a doubling of O_2 consumption and usually achieved at a workload of about 75 kg-meter/min. During exercise, increased O_2 consumption by skeletal muscles is supplied by increased cardiac output (C.O.) and a widened arteriovenous O_2 content difference. When exercise is carried out in the supine position, cardiac output normally is increased mainly by an increase in heart rate, with only slight increases in stroke volume. Patients with cardiac disease may be unable to increase cardiac output normally with exercise because of their inability to maintain stroke volume with increased heart rate, and thus will supply most of the increased O_2 required by exercising tissue through an increase in the arteriovenous O_2 difference. The "exercise factor," expressed as ΔC.O. during exercise (ml/min)/ΔO_2 consumption (ml/min), is a measure of this response. It normally is greater than or equal to 6.0, since cardiac output normally increases linearly with increasing O_2 consumption. If the exercise factor is less than 6.0, the increase in cardiac output in response to exercise is impaired.

Changes in intracardiac pressures during exercise also are important. The left ventricular end-diastolic pressure does not normally increase above 16 mm Hg during exercise, but in ischemic, myocardial, and valvular disease it may rise to considerably higher levels. In some patients, exercise may exacerbate mitral or tricuspid regurgitation and usually markedly increases the left atrial–left ventricular pressure gradient in mitral stenosis (Fig. 7–10). Thus an abnormal increase in pressures, an inadequate rise in the cardiac output, or both in response to the stress provided by mild to moderate exercise in the supine position can be an important finding at catheterization (p. 163). In practice, it is important to maintain a given exercise load for at least 3 to 4 minutes before measuring cardiac output and pressures to insure a steady state of O_2 consumption and cardiac output. Pressures and the electrocardiogram, as well as the patient's symptoms, should be carefully monitored during exercise to avoid complications.

Figure 7–15 shows the hemodynamic findings during exercise in a 55-year-old man with mitral regurgitation. Pressures are recorded on a scale chosen so that all pressures may be visualized simultaneously, with the same baseline and sensitivity. After a brief recording of all three pressures in phasic mode at a paper speed of 25 to 50 mm/sec, the paper speed is slowed to 5 to 10 mm/sec and systemic arterial and pulmonary capillary pressures are recorded as "mean" pressures.

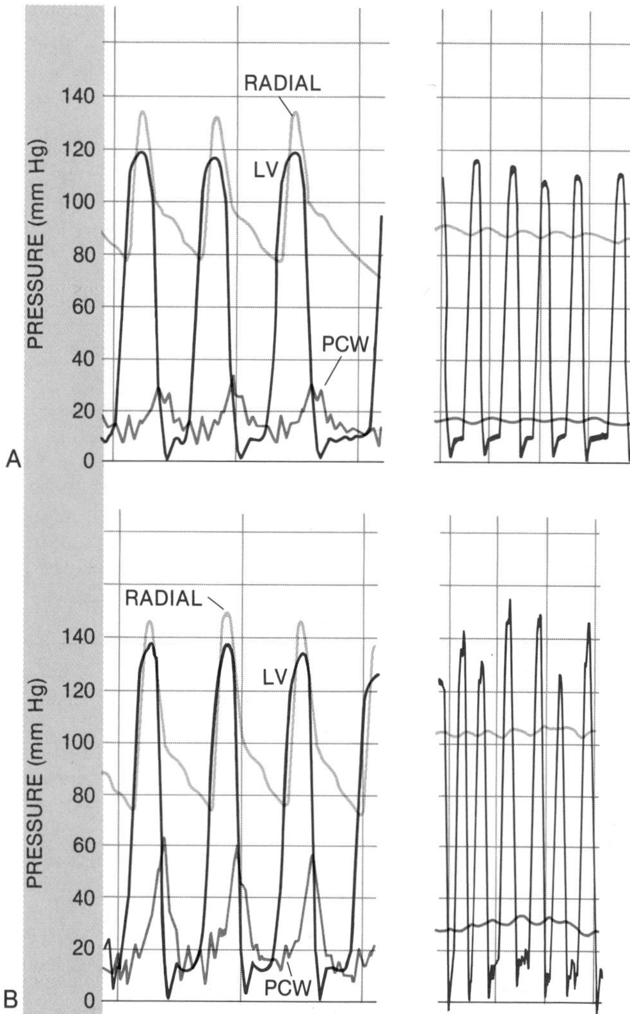

FIGURE 7–15. Hemodynamic findings during exercise in a 55-year-old man with mitral regurgitation. Left ventricular (LV), pulmonary capillary wedge (PCW), and radial artery pressure tracings are shown before *(A)* and during *(B)* the 6th minute of supine bicycle exercise. The peak systolic pressure normally is higher in the radial artery than in the left ventricle. (From Lorell, B. H., and Grossman, W.: Dynamic and isometric exercise during cardiac catheterization. *In* Grossman, W., and Baim, D. S. [eds.]: Cardiac Catheterization, Angiography, and Intervention. 4th ed. Philadelphia, Lea and Febiger, 1991.)

TABLE 7–4 RESPONSE TO SUPINE BICYCLE EXERCISE IN A 60-YEAR-OLD MAN WITH DILATED CARDIOMYOPATHY

	RESTING	EXERCISE (6 MINUTES)
O_2 consumption index (ml/min/m²)	128	469
AV O_2 difference (ml/liter)	40	96
Cardiac index (liter/min/m²)	3.2	4.9
Heart rate (beats/min)	90	141
Systemic arterial pressure (mm Hg), systolic/diastolic (mean)	91/62 (73)	107/67 (88)
Right atrial mean pressure (mm Hg)	5	20
Pulmonary capillary wedge mean pressure (mm Hg)	12	34
Left ventricular pressure (mm Hg)	91/16	107/34
Exercise factor	—	4.9

From Lorell, B. H., and Grossman, W.: Dynamic and isometric exercise during cardiac catheterization. *In* Grossman, W., and Baim, D. S., eds.: Cardiac Catheterization, Angiography, and Intervention. 4th ed. Philadelphia, Lea and Febiger, 1991.

The continuous observation and recording of pressures is quite important during exercise, since it permits accurate monitoring of any rise in filling pressure or fall in arterial pressure and insures that the catheters remain in correct position for the measurements during exercise. After the patient had achieved a steady-state level of exercise for 4 minutes, simultaneous left ventricular and systemic arterial, left ventricular and pulmonary capillary wedge pressure, and pulmonary capillary wedge pressure pull-back to pulmonary artery were recorded during minutes 4 through 6 of continued exercise. In the patient whose data are shown in Figure 7–15, during exercise, there was a substantial rise in pulmonary capillary mean pressure, as well as the development of tall *v* waves in the pulmonary capillary wedge tracing.

Dynamic bicycle exercise can be helpful in the evaluation of symptoms. Table 7–4 shows the response to supine exercise in a 60-year-old man with cardiomegaly, fatigue, and marked dyspnea with exertion. The right atrial mean pressure and cardiac index were normal at rest. Pulmonary capillary wedge pressure and left ventricular end-diastolic pressure were only minimally elevated. Interestingly, with exercise the patient failed to increase his forward cardiac output appropriately, and achieved an exercise factor of 4.9 (less than the normal of ≥ 6.0). Simultaneously, marked elevations occurred in both right- and left-heart filling pressures. Coronary angiography was normal, and a diagnosis of dilated cardiomyopathy was suggested.

APPLICATIONS OF CARDIAC CATHETERIZATION

INDICATIONS. As with any diagnostic procedure, the decision to perform cardiac catheterization must be based on a careful balance between the risk of the procedure and the anticipated value of the information obtained. Cardiac catheterization usually is recommended when there is a need to confirm the presence of a clinically suspected condition, define its anatomical and physiological severity, and determine the presence of associated conditions. This need most commonly arises when clinical assessment suggests that the patient may benefit from an interventional procedure (e.g., coronary angioplasty, balloon valvuloplasty) or heart surgery. Cardiac catheterization usually is coupled with angiographic examination and may yield information that will be crucial in defining the need for further intervention as well as the risks and anticipated benefit for a given patient.

Although few would disagree that consideration of heart surgery is an adequate reason for performance of catheterization, there are differences of opinion about whether *all* patients being considered for such procedures should undergo preoperative cardiac catheterization.[76-78] In this regard, it should be emphasized that the risks of catheterization are small compared with those of operation in patients in whom (1) an incorrect diagnosis was made, (2) the presence of an unsuspected additional condition prolongs and complicates the planned surgical approach, or (3) the hemodynamic assessment by clinical means was inaccurate. The operating room is not a good place for surprises; preoperative cardiac catheterization can provide the surgical team with a precise and complete road map of the course ahead and thereby permit a carefully reasoned and maximally efficient operative procedure. Furthermore, information obtained by cardiac catheterization may be invaluable in the assessment of the crucial determinants of prognosis, such as left ventricular function and patency of the coronary arteries. For these reasons, we recommend that cardiac catheterization be carried out on almost all adult patients for whom a cardiac operation is contemplated. Of course, it is possible that in time noninvasive techniques may be further perfected and shown to be acceptable substitutes for catheterization data.[78] After operation, catheterization may be necessary to evaluate the results of operation (graft patency, prosthetic valve function, and so forth).

A second broad indication for performing cardiac catheterization combined with coronary arteriography (Chap. 9) is to clarify the diagnosis in patients with *chest pain of uncertain cause,* in whom there is confusion regarding the presence of obstructive coronary disease. The data obtained will help to relieve the anxiety of patients and aid the physician in advising them concerning the appropriateness of their future personal or professional plans. Another example within this category might be the symptomatic patient with a suspected *cardiomyopathy.* Although some may be satisfied with a clinical diagnosis of this condition, the implications of such a diagnosis in terms of therapy and prognosis are so important that cardiac catheterization usually is recommended in such patients to rule out potentially correctable conditions (e.g., occult valvular or pericardial disease), even though the likelihood of their presence may appear remote on clinical grounds.

A third important indication for cardiac catheterization is the need to define the response of a patient to *specific pharmacological therapy.* This may be necessary during treatment of an unstable condition (e.g., after acute myocardial infarction) or in an intensive care unit setting, when monitoring of right and left atrial pressures, systemic pressures, and cardiac output is essential to patient management. In addition, the response of patients with chronic heart failure to afterload reduction or to changes in ventricular preload may be most precisely determined by cardiac catheterization. Pharmacological intervention with vasodilators in the treatment of pulmonary hypertension, or with anticoagulation in suspected acute pulmonary embolism (Chap. 48), might well be considered of sufficient potential risk to warrant cardiac catheterization and/or angiography.

CONTRAINDICATIONS. If it is important to consider the *indications* for cardiac catheterization in each patient, it is equally important to ascertain whether there are any *contraindications.* Over the past several years, our concept of contraindications has been modified because patients previously considered too ill for this procedure, with serious conditions such as acute myocardial infarction, intractable ventricular tachycardia, and cardiogenic shock, have tolerated catheterization and coronary arteriography surprisingly well. A long list of relative contraindications (Table 7–5) must be kept in mind, however, and these include all intercurrent conditions that can be corrected and whose correction would improve the safety of the procedure. Ventricular irritability may greatly increase the risk of left-heart catheterization and can interfere with the interpretation of ventriculography. Hypertension should be controlled before and during cardiac catheterization. Other conditions that should be corrected before elective cardiac catheterization, if possible, include febrile illness, decompensated left-heart failure, anemia, digitalis toxicity, and electrolyte disturbance. Infective endocarditis and pregnancy are relative, though not absolute, contraindications to cardiac catheterization.

TABLE 7–5 RELATIVE CONTRAINDICATIONS TO CARDIAC CATHETERIZATION AND ANGIOGRAPHY

1. **Uncontrolled ventricular irritability (increases the risk of ventricular tachycardia/fibrillation during catheterization)**
2. **Uncorrected hypokalemia or digitalis toxicity**
3. **Uncorrected hypertension (predisposes to myocardial ischemia and/or heart failure during angiography)**
4. **Intercurrent febrile illness**
5. **Decompensated heart failure (especially acute pulmonary edema, unless the catheterization can be done with patient sitting up)**
6. **Anticoagulated state (prothrombin time >18 seconds)**
7. **Severe allergy to radiographic contrast agent**
8. **Severe renal insufficiency and/or anuria (unless dialysis is planned to remove fluid and radiographic contrast fluid or if contrast radiography is not planned)**

From Grossman, W.: Cardiac Catheterization: Historical perspective and current practice. In Grossman, W., and Baim, D. S. (eds.): Cardiac Catheterization, Angiography, and Intervention. 4th ed. Philadelphia, Lea and Febiger, 1991.

Anticoagulant therapy may increase the risk of serious bleeding during or after cardiac catheterization. It is our policy to maintain the prothrombin time less than 18 seconds and to avoid heparin administration for 4 to 6 hours before the procedure. If anticoagulant therapy cannot be interrupted, we prefer heparin because it can be easily and immediately reversed by intravenous administration of protamine sulfate, if uncontrollable bleeding or cardiac perforation should occur in the course of catheterization. If transseptal catheterization is planned, it is mandatory that coagulation be normal.

DESIGN OF CATHETERIZATION PROTOCOL. Every cardiac catheterization should have a protocol, that is, a carefully reasoned sequential plan designed specifically for the individual patient being studied. Certain general principles should be considered in the design of a protocol. First, hemodynamic measurements should precede angiographic studies, whenever possible, so that the physiological state may be as basal as possible at the time of pressure and flow measurements. Second, pressure and blood oxygen saturation should be measured and recorded for each chamber immediately after entry and before passing on to the next chamber. If problems should develop during the later stages of a catheterization procedure (atrial fibrillation or other arrhythmia, pyrogen reaction, hypotension, or reaction to contrast material), the physician will wish that pressures and saturations had been measured initially rather than waiting until the catheter is being withdrawn. A third principle is that pressure and cardiac output measurements should be made simultaneously insofar as this is possible. Beyond these general guidelines, the protocol will reflect individual differences from patient to patient. With regard to angiography, it is important to give the contrast injections in sequence, so that the most important diagnostic study is performed first in a given patient.

PREPARATION AND PREMEDICATION OF THE PATIENT. The emotional as well as the "medical" preparation of the patient for cardiac catheterization is the responsibility of the operator. It is proper practice always to inform patients and their families that there are some risks involved, and to be specific as to what those risks are (e.g., death, heart attack, stroke). When appropriate, patients and their families may be reasonably reassured that special problems are unlikely. The discomfort and duration of the procedure should not be understated.

Patients scheduled for elective cardiac catheterization commonly are admitted to the hospital on the day of the pro-

TABLE 7-6 COMPLICATIONS OF CARDIAC CATHETERIZATION[82]

	DIAGNOSTIC CATHETERIZATION (n = 1609)	PTCA (n = 993)	BALLOON VALVULOPLASTY (n = 199)
Death	2 (0.12%)	3 (0.3%)	3 (1.5%)
Myocardial infarction	0	3 (0.3%)	1 (0.5%)
Neurological events			
Transient	2 (0.1%)	0	1
Persistent (stroke)	2 (0.1%)	1 (0.1%)	1 (0.5%)
Emergency CABG	0	12 (1.2%)	0
Cardiac perforation			
Observed, no intervention	1	0	0
Pericardiocentesis	0	0	1
Heart surgery	0	0	5 (2.5%)
Arrhythmias requiring countershock or temporary pacemaker	5 (0.3%)	6 (0.6%)	5 (2.5%)
Local vascular problem requiring repair	26 (1.6%)	15 (1.5%)	15 (7.5%)
Vasovagal reactions	33 (2.1%)	7 (0.7%)	4 (2.0%)
Allergic			
Hives	32	5	0
Hypotension/anaphylaxis	1	1	0

Of the diagnostic catheterizations, associated procedures included temporary pacemaker insertion (n = 193), intraaortic balloon counterpulsation (n = 38), and endomyocardial biopsy (n = 36). Sixty-one of the 199 balloon valvuloplasties involved transseptal catheterization. CABG = coronary artery bypass graft surgery. Mean patient age was 62 ± 13 years.

cedure and discharged the next morning. However, as mentioned earlier, some centers are now performing cardiac catheterization on an outpatient basis for selected patients whose conditions are stable.[25]

A wide variety of sedatives have been used for premedication. The authors routinely use diazepam (Valium), 5 to 10 mg orally, and diphenhydramine (Benadryl), 25 to 50 mg orally, one-half hour before starting the procedure. When coronary arteriography is to be part of the procedure, some operators favor the addition of 0.4 mg atropine subcutaneously to avoid excessive bradycardia. It is the author's practice to have the patient fasting (except for oral medications) after midnight. A light breakfast is allowed if the patient is not scheduled for catheterization until late in the morning or the afternoon.

Before catheterization, the skin overlying the vessels to be entered (femoral areas or antecubital fossa) should be prepared by shaving and thorough cleansing with iodine or Zephiran chloride solution. This procedure as well as careful sterile technique during the catheterization procedure minimize the incidence of infection.

COMPLICATIONS OF CARDIAC CATHETERIZATION

There is an extensive literature describing a wide array of complications associated with cardiac catheterization. Three large, multicenter studies[79-81] have been published, reporting the experience of the Society of Cardiac Angiography Registry[79,80] and the VA Cooperative Study on Valvular Heart Disease.[81] Major complications of cardiac catheterization and angiography in these reports included death (0.1 to 0.2 per cent), myocardial infarction (0.06–0.1 per cent), and cerebrovascular complications (0.07 to 0.10 per cent). None of these multicenter studies[79-81] included significant numbers of interventional procedures, such as percutaneous transluminal coronary angioplasty (PCTA) or balloon valvuloplasty. In this regard, a recent report[82] assessed complications in 2883 consecutive cardiac catheterization procedures performed during an 18-month period. Procedures performed during the study period included 1609 diagnostic catheterizations, 933 PTCAs, 199 percutaneous balloon valvuloplasties, and 142 other procedures performed by the catheterization team (intraaortic balloon placements, right ventricular endomyocardial biopsy, and pericardiocentesis). Complications in these patients are listed in Table 7–6.

These data indicate that the incidence of complications of cardiac catheterization as currently practiced is low, although careful attention to detail and meticulous technique are required to achieve this standard of performance.

RISK FACTORS. Characteristics of patients who have an increased risk of dying from cardiac catheterization are summarized in Table 7–7. Actual risks will vary among laboratories, depending on case mix. Laboratories where the percentage of normal or nearly normal studies is high might well be expected to have a lower rate of death and other major complications associated with cardiac catheterization and angiography. As indicated in Table 7–7, mortality in Class IV patients is more than 10 times greater than in Class I and Class II patients. Similarly, the mortality for patients with left main

TABLE 7-7 PATIENT CHARACTERISTICS ASSOCIATED WITH INCREASED MORTALITY FROM CARDIAC CATHETERIZATION

1. *Age:* Infants (<1 year old) and the elderly (>60 years old) are at increased risk of death during cardiac catheterization.
2. *Functional Class:* Mortality in Class IV patients is more than 10 times greater than in Class I or II patients.
3. *Severity of Coronary Obstruction:* Mortality for patients with left main disease is more than 10 times greater than for patients with single-vessel disease.
4. *Valvular Heart Disease:* When combined with coronary disease, valvular disease is associated with a higher risk of death at cardiac catheterization than coronary artery disease alone.
5. *Left Ventricular Dysfunction:* Mortality for patients with LV ejection <30% is more than 10 times greater than if ejection fraction is ≥50%.
6. *Severe Non-Cardiac Disease:* Patients with renal insufficiency, insulin-dependent diabetes, advanced cerebrovascular and/or peripheral vascular disease, and severe pulmonary insufficiency appear to have an increased incidence of death and other major complications from cardiac catheterization.

From Grossman, W., and Baim, D. S. (eds.): Cardiac Catheterization, Angiography, and Intervention. 4th ed. Philadelphia, Lea and Febiger, 1991.

coronary disease is more than 10 times greater than for patients with one- or two-vessel disease. Patients with substantial left ventricular dysfunction (left ventricular ejection fraction <30 per cent) also have a risk of dying during cardiac catheterization more than 10 times that in patients with normal ejection fractions. Thus the risk of a serious complication from cardiac catheterization and angiography, although small, is not insignificant, especially in patients who are seriously ill.

Prevention of a fatal outcome in patients with one or more of the risk factors listed in Table 7–7 requires attention to many issues. During the cardiac catheterization procedure itself, keeping the volume of radiographic contrast to a minimum (especially in patients known to have depressed left ventricular contractile function) is important. The use of the newer nonionic contrast agents may be appropriate in such patients. If physiological measurements (e.g., measurement of pulmonary capillary wedge pressure, cardiac output) routinely precede angiography, such high-risk patients will be identified more easily and can be pretreated with intravenous furosemide, oxygen, and a vasodilator (e.g., nitroglycerin, sodium nitroprusside) before angiographic studies. The author has found that a tilting cardiac catheterization table, which allows rapid transition to Trendelenburg position (for hypotension) or reverse Trendelenburg (for pulmonary congestion and edema), is valuable in helping very sick patients get through cardiac catheterization and angiography. Meticulous attention to the details of technique is important in preventing deaths in the cardiac catheterization laboratory, since even a minor complication, such as vasovagal reaction or arrhythmia, may be fatal in a patient with severely limited cardiac reserve. Despite all such measures, it seems likely that a certain irreducible mortality rate will be associated with cardiac catheterization in patients with the characteristics listed in Table 7–7.

Factors predisposing to *myocardial infarction* during or immediately after cardiac catheterization are unstable angina, recent subendocardial infarction, and insulin-dependent diabetes mellitus. Documentation of a small myocardial infarction may be difficult after cardiac catheterization, since intramuscular injections (e.g., lidocaine) and soft-tissue trauma of the catheterization procedure itself may lead to increases in serum enzymes (LDH, SGOT, total CPK) often used to assess the presence or absence of myocardial infarction. Such elevations of enzyme levels may be seen with either brachial or femoral approaches. An increase in serum CPK-MB activity is not to be expected after routine cardiac catheterization and angiography, and ordinarily indicates the presence of myocardial necrosis.[83]

CEREBROVASCULAR COMPLICATIONS. These are rare events during cardiac catheterization. Prevention of cerebral emboli can be accomplished by using systemic anticoagulation, paying meticulous attention to proper technique of catheter flushing, wiping guidewires free of blood or clot before insertion, and restricting time for the use of guidewires to 2 to 3 minutes at a time (after which the guidewire is removed and the catheter aspirated and flushed before reentry of the wire).

ARTERIAL THROMBOSIS. This problem deserves special attention. Brachial artery thrombosis can be avoided by use of heparin during catheterization and by appropriate attention to the details of arterial repair.[23] It is generally acknowledged that the incidence of thrombosis is related to the duration of the procedure, the number of catheters used, the presence of underlying arterial disease, and the technique of arterial repair. With regard to the percutaneous femoral approach, local complications include thrombosis, distal embolization, false aneurysm, and delayed hemorrhage.[84] Serious complications involving the femoral artery usually are related to the presence of preexisting iliofemoral disease, and in such patients, it is preferable to avoid a percutaneous femoral approach.

PERFORATION OF THE HEART OR INTRATHORACIC GREAT VESSELS. This complication can occur with any approach, but most commonly it involves the right ventricular outflow tract and apex. These areas are subject to perforation during right ventricular angiography or pacemaker placement. Perforations of the aorta, iliac artery, subclavian artery, or great veins have all been reported, and usually are associated with excessive catheter manipulation. In many such instances, catheter manipulation was continued despite resistance to passage or complaints by the patient of pain related to the catheter passage. Because transseptal left-heart catheterization entails controlled perforation of the interatrial septum, perforation of the heart is its main hazard. Unintentional perforation of the aorta, atrial wall, coronary sinus, or right atrial appendage may occur, leading to cardiac tamponade.

OTHER COMPLICATIONS. *Vagal reactions* are common and may be quite serious. They are frequently, but not always, incited by pain in a tense, anxious patient, and consist of nausea, hypotension, and bradycardia. In older patients, the entire picture of a vagal reaction may be present without bradycardia. If promptly recognized, vagal reactions usually respond dramatically to cessation of catheter manipulation, intravenous atropine (0.5 to 1.0 mg), and tilting of the patient or elevation of the legs to increase venous return. If the blood pressure does not increase promptly, pressor agents (particularly phenylephrine or metaraminol) should be administered intravenously. If the hypotension and bradycardia persist for any period of time, serious arrhythmias and/or irreversible shock may develop, particularly in patients with ischemic heart disease or aortic stenosis.

Electrical hazards have been reported in association with cardiac catheterization. Currents of only a few microamperes transmitted to a small area of myocardium by the wires of electrode catheters, catheters filled with saline, thermistor catheters, or manometer-tipped catheters may produce ventricular fibrillation. This occurrence is now rare because of the use of common grounding of all electrical equipment, transformer isolation of electrical equipment from the power line by means of current-limiting devices, and establishment of an equal potential environment.

Contamination of catheters or fluids administered during cardiac catheterization with sterile bacterial products or other foreign substances can result in a *pyrogen reaction*, characterized by rigors followed by temperature elevation. If this occurs during catheterization, catheters and fluids should be set aside for subsequent culture; the reaction itself usually responds to small amounts of morphine sulfate (2 mg) administered intravenously. Pyrogen reactions are best treated by prevention. Careful cleaning and sterilization of catheters are essential in this regard.

OTHER PROCEDURES INVOLVING CARDIAC CATHETERIZATION

Cardiac catheterization techniques are now being used in an increasing number of procedures for purposes other than hemodynamic or angiographic study. In many instances, the approaches and catheters used and the indications and complications for these procedures differ; they will therefore be discussed separately.

INTRACARDIAC ELECTROCARDIOGRAPHY AND PACING. Electrodes mounted on the tips of cardiac catheters can be used to record intracardiac electrical activity and to stimulate the heart at selected sites. This technique is of great value in elucidating the mechanism and treating a variety of arrhythmias, as discussed in Chaps. 22 to 24. Both temporary and permanent pacing also are carried out, most commonly through pacing catheters, as described in Chap. 25.

TRANSVENOUS ENDOMYOCARDIAL BIOPSY. Nonoperative cardiac biopsy was initially developed as a needle biopsy technique similar to needle biopsy of the kidney or liver. In 1962, Japanese workers reported a method for transvenous endomyocardial biopsy of the right ventricle[85]; this has subsequently been modified and applied to endomyocardial biopsy of both right and left ventricles by a number of

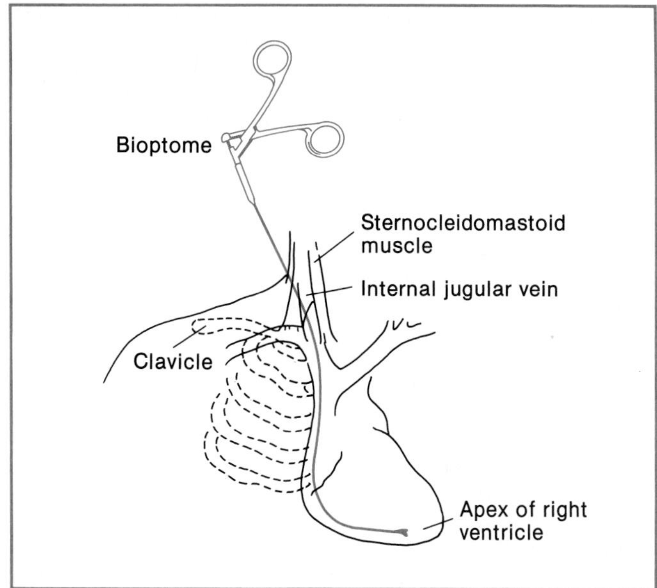

FIGURE 7-16. Endomyocardial biopsy. The bioptome is introduced by way of the right internal jugular vein and is passed across the tricuspid valve into the right ventricle. With the bioptome, a small segment of right ventricular endocardium is removed from the interventricular septum for microscopic examination. (From Mason, J. W., et al.: Myocardial biopsy. *In* Willerson, J. T., and Sanders, C. A. [eds.]: Clinical Cardiology. New York, Grune and Stratton, 1977.)

investigators.[86-90] This method is shown in Figure 7-16. A No. 9 French venous sheath is placed in the internal jugular vein by way of a percutaneous approach. The bioptome is inserted into the sheath and advanced to the right atrium and across the tricuspid valve. After positioning the end of the bioptome against the endocardium of the interventricular septum, using fluoroscopic guidance, the bioptome is opened, gently advanced against the endocardium, and then closed. On withdrawal of the bioptome, a small (1 to 2 mm in diameter) portion of right ventricular myocardium with attached endocardium is obtained. This maneuver is repeated three times, and specimens are processed for light and electron microscopic study. This technique is useful in the diagnoses of myocarditis,[91,92] hypertrophic and dilated cardiomyopathies (Chap. 43),[92,93] amyloid and other infiltrative cardiomyopathies (p. 1451),[94] and immunological rejection in cardiac transplant recipients (Ch. 18).[86,87,89] Serial endomyocardial biopsies have been used to evaluate cardiac toxicity in patients receiving high-dose systemic doxorubicin (Adriamycin) therapy for carcinoma (p. 1756).[95] A particularly promising application of this technique may be detection of inflammatory myocarditis. In a report of clinicopathological correlates in 100 consecutive patients undergoing right ventricular endomyocardial biopsy at the Mayo Clinic,[92] myocarditis was detected in 15 per cent of patients with unexplained congestive heart failure and in 15 per cent of patients with unexplained dysrhythmia or syncope. Similar clinical utility for endomyocardial biopsy was found by Parillo et al.[93] In their study, pathological information obtained was judged useful to the clinician in 54 of 100 consecutive patients undergoing biopsy (Table 7-8). In some cases, inflammatory myocarditis and associated congestive heart failure may respond to immunosuppressive drugs.[91] Complications include cardiac perforation and tamponade, pericarditis, coronary arteriovenous fistulas, and atrial and ventricular tachyarrhythmias.

PERCUTANEOUS INTRAAORTIC BALLOON PUMP INSERTION. Intraaortic balloon pump (IABP) counterpulsation provides mechanical circulatory assistance by lowering aortic pressure in systole and increasing aortic pressure in diastole. Cardiac output is increased and left ventricular filling pressure is decreased by the reduction in afterload; myocardial ischemia is alleviated by reduction in oxygen demand while oxygen supply is increased. Therefore, this technique can have a dramatic beneficial effect in patients with cardiogenic shock (p. 580) and severe, acute myocardial ischemia (p. 1340). It has become a well-accepted method of providing temporary circulatory support for critically ill patients, tiding them over during a stressful procedure, such as cardiac catheterization and angiography, and/or until cardiac surgery can be performed.[96] In the past, IABP catheters had been inserted by way of a direct surgical approach, requiring a cutdown on the femoral artery and surgical repair of the artery after the balloon pump had been removed. Currently, IABP placement is most commonly accomplished percutaneously, in the cardiac catheterization laboratory. There are several brands of IABP catheters that may be inserted percutaneously through a guiding sheath. All these catheters have a central lumen which allows insertion of a guidewire and provides the extra safety associated with guidewire-directed advancement of the catheter through potentially tortuous iliofemoral arterial systems. The central lumen also may be used for arterial pressure monitoring to adjust the timing of balloon counterpulsation. For details of the technique for balloon placement, the reader is referred elsewhere.[23] Once inserted, adjustment of balloon

TABLE 7-8 INDICATIONS AND FINDINGS OF ENDOMYOCARDIAL BIOPSY IN 100 PATIENTS

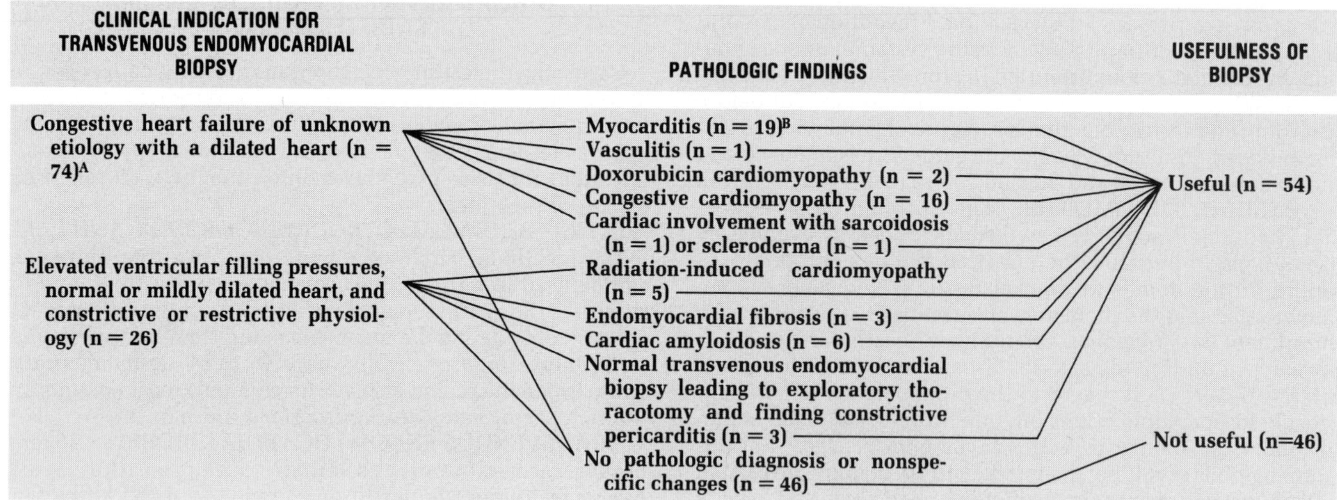

CLINICAL INDICATION FOR TRANSVENOUS ENDOMYOCARDIAL BIOPSY	PATHOLOGIC FINDINGS	USEFULNESS OF BIOPSY
Congestive heart failure of unknown etiology with a dilated heart (n = 74)[A]	Myocarditis (n = 19)[B]	Useful (n = 54)
	Vasculitis (n = 1)	Useful (n = 54)
	Doxorubicin cardiomyopathy (n = 2)	Useful (n = 54)
	Congestive cardiomyopathy (n = 16)	Useful (n = 54)
	Cardiac involvement with sarcoidosis (n = 1) or scleroderma (n = 1)	Useful (n = 54)
Elevated ventricular filling pressures, normal or mildly dilated heart, and constrictive or restrictive physiology (n = 26)	Radiation-induced cardiomyopathy (n = 5)	Useful (n = 54)
	Endomyocardial fibrosis (n = 3)	Useful (n = 54)
	Cardiac amyloidosis (n = 6)	Useful (n = 54)
	Normal transvenous endomyocardial biopsy leading to exploratory thoracotomy and finding constrictive pericarditis (n = 3)	Useful (n = 54)
	No pathologic diagnosis or nonspecific changes (n = 46)	Not useful (n=46)

[A]Numbers in parentheses refer to the number of patients. [B]Three patients had two diagnoses; one patient had amyloidosis and myocarditis, one patient had endomyocardial fibrosis with eosinophilic myocarditis, and one patient had vasculitis and myocarditis, so that the number of patients or indications totals 100 and the number of pathologic findings totals 103.

From Parillo, J. E., et al.: The results of intravenous endomyocardial biopsy frequently can be used to diagnose myocardial disease in patients with heart failure. Circulation 69:93. 1984, by permission of the American Heart Association, Inc.

timing is critical. Timing is adjusted with the balloon control console so that balloon inflation occurs with the central aortic dicrotic notch (aortic valve closure), while deflation occurs immediately before aortic valve opening.

An example of the effectiveness of IABP counterpulsation in a patient with cardiogenic shock caused by mitral regurgitation is shown in Figure 7–17. The patient was a 45-year-old woman who developed cardiogenic shock and pulmonary edema from acute ruptured chordae and massive mitral regurgitation. As seen in panel A, the patient's left ventricular systolic pressure is approximately 80 mm Hg with *v* waves in the pulmonary capillary wedge tracing of 50 to 60 mm Hg. Panel B shows that with IABP counterpulsation of the pulmonary capillary wedge, *v* waves are greatly reduced. Left ventricular systolic pressure, however, is lower than in panel A. Panel C shows the unusual tracing obtained when the left ventricular catheter was pulled back into the aorta. Close inspection demonstrates that the pressure waves to 100 mm Hg in the aorta are *diastolic* waves, resulting from expansion of the intraaortic balloon. The small systolic waves preceding each diastolic wave represent left ventricular systolic ejection. The patient's condition stabilized sufficiently to permit cardiac surgery and successful mitral valve replacement.

Successful percutaneous insertion of IABP catheters can be achieved in more than 90 per cent of patients. However, complications remain a significant problem. In a study of 103 patients undergoing percutaneous IABP placement at our hospital, Alderman et al.[97] found that detectable limb ischemia occurred in 40 per cent of patients, requiring balloon removal in nearly 30 per cent of all patients. Factors predisposing to limb ischemia included the presence of diabetes, peripheral vascular disease, and female gender. There was no correlation of ischemic leg complication and body surface area, age, No. 10.5 French versus No. 12 French balloon size, or adequacy of anticoagulation. The newer No. 9.5 French balloon and sheathless insertion techniques, currently gaining increasing acceptance, were not used during the duration of Alderman's study.[97] Advances in catheter design and insertion technique may reduce the complication rates.

CARDIOPULMONARY SUPPORT PUMPS. Percutaneous cardiopulmonary support systems analogous to the heart-lung machine have recently been introduced. In one system (Bard CPS), large venous and arterial cannulae (No. 20 French) are introduced percutaneously and positioned in the right atrium and aorta. Blood is pumped from the venous cannula to an external circuit, through a heat exchanger and a membrane oxygenator and then back into the aorta by way of the arterial cannula. In another system (Nimbus Hemopump), a single, large (No. 21 French) coaxial catheter is passed retrograde into the left ventricle after having been introduced into the femoral artery by direct surgical exposure. A smaller device which can be introduced percutaneously is under development. The Hemopump is connected to an external motor, and a rotating turbine within the catheter pumps blood from the left ventricle to the aorta at rates up to 3.5 liters/min. Both Bard CPS and Hemopump systems can support the circulation during cardiogenic shock and even for brief periods during cardiac arrest. These systems are being studied as adjuncts to high-risk angioplasty as well as therapy for cardiogenic shock.[98–100]

THERAPEUTIC PROCEDURES. Coronary angioplasty, intracoronary thrombolysis balloon valvuloplasty, and balloon dilatation of stenotic pulmonary and systemic arteries are described in Chap. 41.

Special "snare" catheters can *retrieve from within the heart catheter fragments* introduced iatrogenically.[101,102] These techniques can obviate thoracotomy and cardiotomy.

An exciting and rapidly growing technology involves the use of transcatheter interventions for treating patients with congenital heart disease[35] (Chap. 41). Among the first inter-

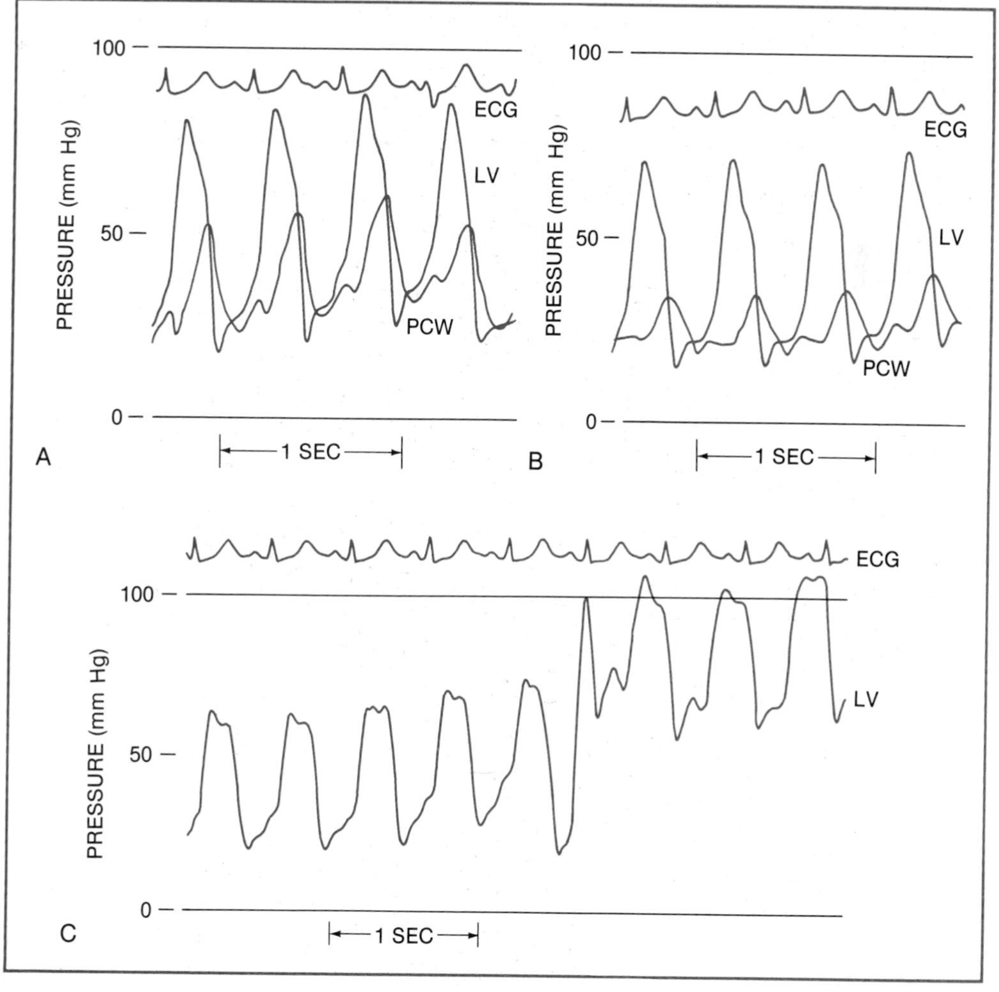

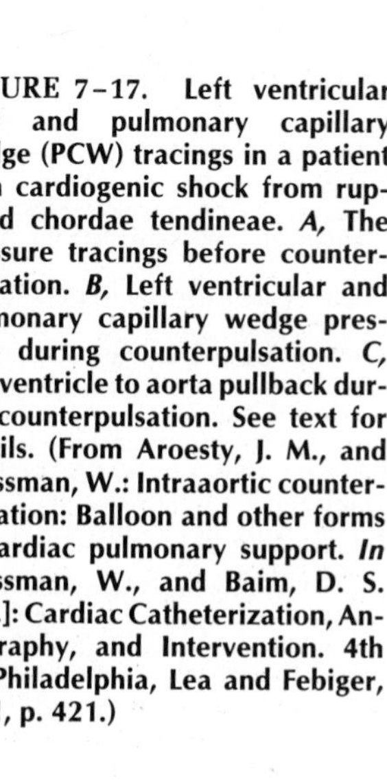
FIGURE 7–17. Left ventricular (LV) and pulmonary capillary wedge (PCW) tracings in a patient with cardiogenic shock from ruptured chordae tendineae. *A,* The pressure tracings before counterpulsation. *B,* Left ventricular and pulmonary capillary wedge pressure during counterpulsation. *C,* Left ventricle to aorta pullback during counterpulsation. See text for details. (From Aroesty, J. M., and Grossman, W.: Intraaortic counterpulsation: Balloon and other forms of cardiac pulmonary support. *In* Grossman, W., and Baim, D. S. [eds.]: Cardiac Catheterization, Angiography, and Intervention. 4th ed. Philadelphia, Lea and Febiger, 1991, p. 421.)

ventional procedures in this condition is the technique balloon atrial septostomy, developed by Rashkind, a therapeutic procedure to improve mixing between systemic and pulmonary circulations in neonates with transposition of the great arteries.[103] There has been extensive experience with nonoperative closure of patent ductus arteriosus.[103–106] Initially this was accomplished by insertion of a plug, mounted on the tip of a catheter, into the patent ductus.[103–105] Subsequently, a double-umbrella technique was developed by Rashkind.[103] This technique has been further modified by Lock and coworkers[105] and applied to a transcatheter technique for the closure of atrial septal defects. In addition, this technique has also been applied by Lock to the transcatheter closure of acquired and congenital ventricular septal defects.[104,105] Pediatric cardiologists use balloon dilatation as a treatment for congenital pulmonic stenosis.[107] Excellent results have led to the application of balloon dilatation techniques to a variety to other congenital lesions. Balloon dilatation is being used widely as a treatment for congenital aortic stenosis.[109] Similar techniques have also been applied to the nonoperative treatment of coarctation of the aorta, [109] as well as balloon dilatation of branch pulmonary artery stenosis.[110] Finally, a number of techniques have been applied by pediatric cardiologists, which involve therapeutic embolization of unwanted thoracic vessels with a variety of coils. These have included closure of aortopulmonary collaterals, Blalock-Taussig shunts, and coronary artery fistulas.[111]

This is by no means an exhaustive description or list of all the therapeutic uses of cardiac catheterization, but it should serve to illustrate how techniques originally developed to perform hemodynamic measurements have evolved into therapeutic procedures. Thus it is clear that cardiac catheterization can no longer be considered solely a diagnostic procedure.

REFERENCES

HISTORICAL ASPECTS

1. Cournand, A: Cardiac catheterization. Development of the technique, its contributions to experimental medicine, and its initial application in man. Acta Med. Scand. 579 (Suppl.):1, 1975.
2. Forssmann, W.: Die Sondierung des rechten Herzens. Klin. Wochenschr. 8:2085, 1929.
3. Klein, O.: Zur Bestimmung des zirkulatorischen Minutensvohumen nach dem Fickschen Prinzip. Münch. Med. 77:1311, 1930.
4. Cournand, A. F., and Ranges, H. S.: Catheterization of the right auricle in man. Proc. Soc. Exp. Biol. Med. 46:462, 1941.
5. Richards, D. W.: Cardiac output by the catheterization technique in various clinical conditions. Fed. Proc. 4:215, 1945.
6. Cournand, A. F., Riley, R. L., Breed, E. S., et al.: Measurement of cardiac output in man using the technique of catheterization of the right auricle. J. Clin. Invest. 24:106, 1945.
7. Dexter, L., Haynes, F. W., Burwell, C. S., et al.: Studies of congenital heart disease. II. The pressure and oxygen content of blood in the right auricle, right ventricle, and pulmonary artery in control patients, with observations on the oxygen saturation and source of pulmonary "capillary" blood. J. Clin. Invest. 26:554, 1947.
8. Hellems, H. K., Haynes, F. W., and Dexter, L.: Pulmonary "capillary" pressure in man. J. Appl. Physiol. 2:24, 1949.
9. McMichael, J., and Sharpey-Schafer, E. P.: The action of intravenous digoxin in man. Q. J. Med. 13:1123, 1944.
10. Lenegre, J., and Maurice, P.: Premiers recherches sur la pression ventriculaire droite. Bull. Mem. Soc. Med. Hop. Paris 80:239, 1944.
11. Stead, E. A., Jr., Warren, J. V., and Brannon, E. S.: Cardiac output in congestive heart failure: Analysis of reasons for lack of close correlation between symptoms of heart failure and resting cardiac output. Am. Heart J. 35:529, 1948.
12. Bing, R. J., Vandam, L. D., Gregoire, F., et al.: Measurement of coronary blood flow, oxygen consumption and efficiency of the left ventricle in man. Am. Heart J. 38:1, 1949.
13. Burchell, H. B.: Cardiac catheterization in diagnosis of various cardiac malformations and diseases. Proc. Mayo Clin. 23:481, 1948.
14. Wood, E. H., Geraci, J. E., Pollack, A. A., et al.: General and special techniques in cardiac catheterization. Proc. Mayo Clin. 23:494, 1948.
15. Zimmerman, H. A., Scott, R. W., and Becker, N. D.: Catheterization of the left side of the heart in man. Circulation 1:357, 1950.
16. Limon Lason, R., and Bouchard, A.: El cateterismo intracardico; cateterization de las cavidades izquierdas en el hombre. Registro simultaneo depression y electrocardiograma intracavetarios. Arch. Inst. Cardiol. Mexico 21:271, 1950.
17. Seldinger, S. I.: Catheter replacement of the needle in percutaneous arteriography: A new technique. Acta Radiol. 39:368, 1953.
18. Ross, J., Jr.: Transseptal left heart catheterization: A new method of left atrial puncture. Ann. Surg. 149:395, 1959.
19. Ross, J., Jr., Braunwald, E., and Morrow, A. G.: Transseptal left atrial puncture: A new method for the measurement of left atrial pressure in man. Am. J. Cardiol. 3:653, 1959.
20. Sones, F. M., Jr., Shirey, E. K., Proudfit, W. L., and Westcott, R. N.: Cine coronary arteriography. Circulation 20:773, 1959.
21. Sones, F. M., Jr., and Shirey, E. K.: Cine coronary arteriography. Mod. Concepts Cardiovasc. Dis. 31:735, 1962.
22. Swan, H. J. C., Ganz, W., Forrester, J., et al.: Catheterization of the heart in man with use of a flow directed balloon-tipped catheter. N. Engl. J. Med. 283:447, 1970.

TECHNICAL ASPECTS

23. Grossman, W., and Baim, D. S.: Cardiac Catheterization, Angiography, and Intervention. 4th ed. Philadelphia, Lea and Febiger, 1991.
24. Friesinger, G. C., Adams, D. F., Bourassa, M. G., et al.: Optimal resources for evaluation of the heart and lungs: Cardiac catheterization and radiographic facilities. Circulation 68:893A, 1983.
25. Block, P. C., Ockene, I., Goldberg, R. J., et al.: A prospective randomized trial of outpatient versus inpatient cardiac catheterization. N. Engl. J. Med. 319:1251, 1988.

25a. Conti, C. R.: Cardiac catheterization laboratories: Hospital-based, free-standing or mobile? J. Am. Coll. Cardiol. 15:748, 1990.

26. Guidelines for Radiation Protection in the Cardiac Catheterization Laboratory. Cathet. Cardiovasc. Diagn. 10:87, 1984.
27. Lange, R. A., Moore, D. M., Jr., Cigarroa, R. G., and Hillis, L. D.: Use of pulmonary capillary wedge pressure to assess severity of mitral stenosis. Is true left atrial pressure needed in this condition? J. Am. Coll. Cardiol. 13:825, 1989.
28. Antman, E. M., Marsh, J. D., Green, L. H., and Grossman, W.: Blood oxygen measurement in the assessment of intracardiac left to right shunts: A critical appraisal of methodology. Am. J. Cardiol. 46:265, 1980.
29. Barry, W. H., Levin, D. C., Green, L. H., et al.: Left heart catheterization and angiography via the percutaneous femoral approach using an arterial sheath. Cathet. Cardiovasc. Diagn. 5:401, 1979.
30. Karsh, D. L., Michaelson, S. P., Langon, R. A., et al.: Retrograde left ventricular catheterization in patients with an aortic valve prosthesis. Am. J. Cardiol. 41:893, 1978.
31. O'Keefe, J. H., Jr., Vliestra, R. E., Hanley, P. C., and Seward, J. C.: Revival of the transseptal approach for catheterization of the left atrium and ventricle. Mayo Clin. Proc. 60:790, 1985.
32. Mullins, C. E.: Transseptal left heart catheterization: Experience with a new technique in 520 pediatric and adult patients. Ped. Cardiol. 4:239, 1983.
33. Levine, M. J., Weinstein, J. S., Diver, D. J., et al.: Progressive improvement in pulmonary vascular resistance following percutaneous mitral valvuloplasty. Circulation 79:1061, 1989.
34. Brockenbrough, E. C., and Braunwald, E.: A new technique for left ventricular angiocardiography and transseptal left heart catheterization. Am. J. Cardiol. 6:1062, 1960.
35. Lock, J. E., Keane, J. F., and Fellows, K. E.: Diagnostic and Interventional Catheterization in Congenital Heart Disease. Boston, Martinus Nijhoff, 1987.
36. Milnor, W. R.: Hemodynamics. 2nd ed. Baltimore, Williams & Wilkins, 1989.
37. Grossman, W., McLaurin, L. P., and Stefadouros, M. A.: Left ventricular stiffness associated with chronic pressure and volume overloads in man. Circ. Res. 35:793, 1974.
38. Grose, R., Strain, J., and Cohen, M. W.: Pulmonary arterial V waves in mitral regurgitation: Clinical and experimental observations. Circulation 69:214, 1984.
39. Guyton, A. C., Jones, C. E., and Coleman, T. G.: Circulatory Physiology: Cardiac Output and Its Regulation. 2nd ed. Philadelphia, W. B. Saunders Company, 1973.
40. Fick, A.: Über die Messung des Blutquantums in den Herzventrikeln. Sitz der Physik. Med. Ges. Wurzburg 1870, p. 16.
41. Barratt-Boyes, B. G., and Wood, E. H.: The oxygen saturation of blood in the venae cavae, right heart chambers, and pulmonary vessels of healthy subjects. J. Lab. Clin. Med. 50:93, 1957.
42. Selzer, A., and Sudrann, R. B.: Reliability of the determination of cardiac output in man by means of the Fick principle. Circ. Res. 6:485, 1958.
43. Thomassen, B.: Cardiac output in normal subjects under standard conditions. The repeatability of measurements by the Fick method. Scand. J. Clin. Lab. Invest. 9:365, 1957.
44. Visscher, M. B., and Johnson, J. A.: The Fick principle: Analysis of potential errors and its conventional application. J. Appl. Physiol. 5:635, 1953.
45. Stewart, G. N.: Researches on the circulation time and on the influences which affect it. IV. The output of the heart. J. Physiol. 22:159, 1987.
46. Hamilton, W. F., Riley, R. L., Attyah, A. M., et al.: Comparison of Fick and dye injection methods of measuring cardiac output in man. Am. J. Physiol. 153:309, 1948.
47. Rahimtoola, S. H., and Swan, H. J. C.: Calculation of cardiac output from indicator dilution curves in the presence of mitral regurgitation. Circulation 31:711, 1965.
48. Shepherd, R. L., Higgs, L. M., and Glancy, D. L.: Comparison of left ventricular and pulmonary arterial injection sites in determination of cardiac output by the indicator dilution technique. Chest 62:175, 1972.
49. Reddy, P. S., Curtiss, E. I., Bell B., et al.: Determinants of variation between Fick and indicator dilution estimates of cardiac output during diagnostic catheterization. Fick vs. dye outputs. J. Lab. Clin. Med. 87:568, 1976.
50. Branthwaite, M. A., and Bradley, R. D.: Measurement of cardiac output by thermodilution in man. J. Appl. Physiol. 24:434, 1968.

51. Ganz, W., Donoso, R., Marcus, H. S., et al.: A new technique for measurements of cardiac output by thermodilution in man. Am. J. Cardiol. *27*:392, 1971.
52. Weisel, R. D., Berger, R. L., and Hechtman, H. B.: Measurement of cardiac output by thermodilution. N. Engl. J. Med. *292*:682, 1975.
53. Van Grondelle, A., Ditchey, R. V., Groves, B. M., et al.: Thermodilution method overestimates low cardiac output in humans. Am. J. Physiol. *245*:H690, 1983.
54. Kinsman, J. M., Moore, J. W., and Hamilton, W. F.: Studies on the circulation. I. Injection method. Physical and mathematical considerations. Am. J. Physiol. *89*:322, 1929.
55. Moore, J. W., Kinsman, J. M., Hamilton, W. G., and Spurling, R. G.: Studies on the circulation. II. Cardiac output determinations; comparison of the injection method with the direct Fick procedure. Am. J. Physiol. *89*:331, 1929.
56. Doyle, J. T., Wilson, J. S., Lepine, C., and Warren, J. V.: An evaluation of the measurement of the cardiac output and of the so-called pulmonary blood volume by the dye-dilution method. J. Lab. Clin. Med. *41*:29, 1953.
57. Eliasch, H., Lagerlof, H., Bucht, H., et al.: Comparison of the dye dilution and the direct Fick methods for the measurement of cardiac output in man. Scand. J. Lab. Clin. Invest. *7* (Suppl. 20):73, 1955.
58. Swan, H.J.C., and Wood, E. H.: Localization of cardiac defects by dye dilution curves recorded after injection of T-1824 at multiple sites in the heart and great vessels during cardiac catheterization. Proc. Staff Meet. Mayo Clin. *28*:95, 1953.
59. Castillo, C. A., Kyle, J. C., Gilson, W. E., and Rowe, G. G.: Simulated shunt curves. Am. J. Cardiol. *17*:691, 1966.
60. Flamm, M. D., Cohn, K. E., and Hancock, E. W.: Measurement of systemic cardiac output at rest and exercise in patients with atrial septal defect. Am. J. Cardiol. *23*:258, 1969.
61. Ganz, W., Tamura, K., Marcus, H. S., et al.: Measurement of coronary sinus blood flow by continuous thermodilution in man. Circulation *44*:181, 1971.
62. Baim, D. S., Rothman, M. T., and Harrison, D. C.: Improved catheter for regional coronary sinus blood flow and metabolic studies. Am. J. Cardiol. *46*:997, 1980.
63. Baim, D. S., Rothman, M. T., and Harrison, D. C.: Simultaneous measurement of coronary venous flow and oxygen saturation during transient alterations in myocardial oxygen supply and demand. Am. J. Cardiol. *49*:743, 1982.
64. Wilson, R. F., Laughlin, D. E., Ackell, P. H., et al.: Transluminal, subselective measurement of coronary artery blood flow velocity and vasodilator reserve in man. Circulation *72*:82, 1985.
65. Fritts, H. W., Harris, P., Clauss, R. H., et al.: The effect of acetylcholine on the human pulmonary circulation under normal and hypoxic conditions. J. Clin. Invest. *37*:99, 1958.
66. Wood, P., Besterman, E. M., Towers, M. K., and McIlroy, M. B.: The effect of acetylcholine on pulmonary vascular resistance and left atrial pressure in mitral stenosis. Br. Heart J. *19*:279, 1957.
67. Rudolph, A. M., Paul, M. H., Sommer, L. S., and Nadas, A. S.: Effects of tolazoline hydrochloride (Priscoline) on circulatory dynamics of patients with pulmonary hypertension. Am. Heart J. *55*:424, 1958.
68. Grover, R. F., Reeves, T. J., and Blount, S. G., Jr.: Tolazoline hydrochloride (Priscoline): An effective pulmonary vasodilator. Am. Heart J. *61*:5, 1961.
69. Nichols, W. W., Conti, C. R., Walker, W. E., and Milnor, W. R.: Input impedance of the systemic circulation in man. Circ. Res. *40*:421, 1977.
70. Gorlin, R., and Gorlin, G.: Hydraulic formula for calculation of area of stenotic mitral valve, other valves, and central circulatory shunts. Am. Heart J. *41*:1, 1951.
71. Cohen, M. V., and Gorlin, R.: Modified orifice equation for the calculation of mitral valve area. Am. Heart J. *84*:839, 1972.
71a. Gorlin, W. B., and Gorlin, R.: A generalized formulation of the Gorlin formula for calculating the area of the stenotic mitral valve and other stenotic cardiac valves. J. Am. Coll. Cardiol. *15*:246, 1990.
72. Folland, E. D., Parisi, A. F., and Carbone, C.: Is peripheral arterial pressure a satisfactory substitute for ascending aortic pressure when measuring aortic valve gradients? J. Am. Coll. Cardiol. *4*:1207, 1984.
73. Krueger, S. K., Orme, E. C., King, C. S., and Barry, W. H.: Accurate determination of the transaortic pressure gradient using simultaneous left ventricular and femoral artery pressures. Cathet. Cardiovasc. Diagn. *16*:202, 1989.
74. Hakki, A. H., Iskandrain, A. S., Bemis, C. E., et al.: A simplified formula for the calculation of stenotic cardiac valves. Circulation *63*:1050, 1981.
75. Cannon, S. R., Richards, K. L., and Crawford, M.: Hydraulic estimation of stenotic orifice area: A correction of the Gorlin formula. Circulation *71*:1170, 1985.

APPLICATIONS

76. St. John Sutton, M. G., St. John Sutton, M., Oldershaw, P., et al.: Valve replacement without preoperative cardiac catheterization. N. Engl. J. Med. *305*:1233, 1981.
77. Roberts, W. C.: Reasons for cardiac catheterization before cardiac valve replacement. N. Engl. J. Med. *306*:1291, 1982.
78. Alpert, J. S., Sloss, L. J., Cohn, P. F., and Grossman, W.: The diagnostic accuracy of combined clinical and noninvasive cardiac evaluation: Comparison with findings at cardiac catheterization. Cathet. Cardiovasc. Diagn. *6*:359, 1980.
79. Kennedy, J. W.: Complications associated with cardiac catheterization and angiography. Cathet. Cardiovasc. Diagn. *8*:5, 1982.
80. Johnson, L. W., Lozner, E. C., Johnson, S., et al.: Coronary angiography 1984–1987: A report of the Registry of the Society for Cardiac Angiography and Interventions. I. Results and complications. Cathet. Cardiovasc. Diagn. *17*:5, 1989.
81. Folland, E. D., Oprian, C., Giacomini, J., et al.: Complications of cardiac catheterization and angiography in patients with valvular heart disease. Cathet. Cardiovasc. Diagn. *17*:15, 1989.
82. Wyman, R. M., Safian, R. D., Portway, V., et al.: Current complications of diagnostic and therapeutic cardiac catheterization. J. Am. Coll. Cardiol. *12*:1400, 1988.
83. Roberts, R., Ludbrook, P. A., Weiss, E. S., and Sobel, B. E.: Serum CPK isoenzymes after cardiac catheterization. Br. Heart J. *37*:1144, 1975.
84. Skillman, J. J., Kim, D., and Baim, D. S.: Vascular complications of percutaneous femoral cardiac interventions. Arch. Surg. *123*:1207, 1988.
85. Sakakibara, S., and Konno, S.: Endomyocardial biopsy. Jpn. Heart J. *3*:537, 1962.
86. Caves, P., Billingham, M. B., Coltart, J., et al.: Transvenous endomyocardial biopsy—application of a method for diagnosing heart disease. Postgrad. Med. J. *51*:286, 1975.
87. Mason, J. W., and O'Connell, J. B.: Clinical merit of endomyocardial biopsy. Circulation *79*:971, 1989.
88. Popma, J. J., Cigarroa, R. G., Buja, M. B., and Hillis, L. D.: Diagnostic and prognostic utility of right sided catheterization and endomyocardial biopsy in idiopathic dilated cardiomyopathy. Am. J. Cardiol. *63*:955, 1989.
89. Mason, J. W.: Endomyocardial biopsy: Balance of success and failure. Circulation *71*:185, 1985.
90. Kawai, C., and Kitaura, Y.: New endomyocardial biopsy catheter for the left ventricle. Am. J. Cardiol. *40*:63, 1977.
91. Mason, J. W., Billingham, M. E., and Ricci, D. R.: Treatment of acute inflammatory myocarditis assisted by endomyocardial biopsy. Am. J. Cardiol. *45*:1037, 1980.
92. Nippoldt, T. B., Edwards, W. D., Holmes, D. R., et al.: Right ventricular endomyocardial biopsy. Clinicopathologic correlates in 100 consecutive patients. Mayo Clin. Proc. *57*:407, 1982.
93. Parillo, J. E., Aretz, H. T., Palacios, I., et al.: The results of transvenous endomyocardial biopsy frequently can be used to diagnose myocardial diseases in patients with heart failure. Circulation *69*:93, 1984.
94. Colucci, W. S., Lorell, B. H., Schoen, F. J., et al.: Hypertrophic obstruction due to Fabry's disease. N. Engl. J. Med. *307*:926, 1982.
95. Bristow, M. R., Mason J. W., Billingham, M. E., and Daniels, J. R.: Doxorubicin cardiomyopathy: Evaluation by phonocardiography, endomyocardial biopsy, and cardiac catheterization. Ann. Intern. Med. *88*:168, 1978.
96. Weintraub, R. M., Aroesty, J. M., Paulins, S., et al.: Medically refractory unstable angina pectoris. I. Long-term follow-up of patients undergoing intraaortic balloon counterpulsation and operation. Am. J. Cardiol. *43*:887, 1979.
97. Alderman, J. D., Gabliani, G. I., McCabe, C. H., et al.:Incidence and management of limb ischemia with percutaneous wire guided intraaortic balloon catheters. J. Am. Coll. Cardiol. *9*:524, 1987.
98. Shawl, F. A., Domanski, M. J., Punja, S., and Hernandez, T. J.: Emergency percutaneous cardiopulmonary (bypass) support in cardiogenic shock. J. Am. Coll. Cardiol. *13*:160A, 1989.
99. Vogel, R. A., Tommaso, C. L., and Gundry, S. R.: Initial experience with coronary angioplasty and aortic valvuloplasty using elective semipercutaneous cardiopulmonary support. Am. J. Cardiol. *62*:811, 1988.
100. Smalling R. W., Cassidy, D. B., Merhige, M., et al.: Improved hemodynamic and left ventricular unloading during acute ischemia using the Hemopump left ventricular assist device compared to intraaortic balloon counterpulsation. J. Am. Coll. Cardiol. *13*:160A, 1989.
101. Massumi, R. A., and Ross, A. M.: Atraumatic non-surgical techniques for removal of broken catheters from cardiac cavities. N. Engl. J. Med. *277*:195, 1967.
102. Bloomfield, A.: Techniques of non-surgical retrieval of iatrogenic foreign bodies from the heart. Am. J. Cardiol. *27*:538, 1971.
103. Rashkind, W. J., Mullins, C. E., Hellenbrand, W. E., and Tait, M. A.: Non-surgical closure of patent ductus arteriosus: Clinical application of the Rashkind PDA occluder system. Circulation *75*:583, 1987.
104. Lock, J. E., Rome, J. J., David, R., et al.: Transcatheter closure of atrial septal defects: Experimental studies. Circulation *(in press)*
105. Lock, J. E., Block, P. C., McKay, R. G., et al.: Transcatheter closure of ventricular septal defects. Circulation *78*:361, 1988.
106. Goldstein, S.A.N., Perry, S. B., Keane, J. F., et al.: Transcatheter closure of congenital ventricular septal defects. J. Am. Coll. Cardiol. *15*:240A, 1990.
107. Stranger, P., Cassidy, S. C., Girod, D. A., et al.: Balloon pulmonary valvuloplasty: Results of the Valvuloplasty and Angioplasty of Congenital Anomalies Registry. Am. J. Cardiol. *65*:775, 1990.
108. Rocchini, A. P., Beckman, R. H., Schachr, G. B., et al.: Balloon aortic valvuloplasty: Results of the Valvuloplasty and Angioplasty of Congenital Anomalies Registry. Am. J. Cardiol. *65*:784, 1990.
109. Tynan, M., Finley, J. P., Fontes, V., et al.: Balloon angioplasty for the treatment of native coarctation: Results of the Valvuloplasty and Angioplasty of Congenital Anomalies Registry. Am. J. Cardiol. *65*:790, 1990.
110. Rothman, A., Perry, S. B., Keane, J. F., and Lock, J. E.: Early results and follow-up of balloon angioplasty for branch pulmonary artery stenosis. J. Am. Coll. Cardiol. *15*:1109, 1990.
111. Perry, S. B., Radtke, W., Fellows, K. E., et al.: Coil embolization to occlude aortopulmonary collateral vessels and shunts in patients with congenital heart disease. J. Am. Coll. Cardiol. *13*:100, 1989.

8

Radiology of the Heart

by ROBERT M. STEINER, M.D., and DAVID C. LEVIN, M.D.

The chest roentgenogram provides unique and valuable information about the structure and function of the heart and thoracic blood vessels. As a survey examination that most patients undergo when entering a hospital or when examined in an office or clinic for a wide variety of cardiothoracic as well as other disorders, the chest film presents an opportunity to identify subtle or overlooked cardiac pathology including significant vascular and pericardial calcification, chamber enlargement, and evidence of pulmonary arterial or venous hypertension. Adult-onset congenital heart disease, often overlooked clinically, may also be identified by the plain film chest roentgenogram. It often helps to confirm a clinical impression of valvular heart disease, acute or chronic pericarditis, ischemic heart disease, left ventricular failure, and pulmonary edema.

For the diagnosis of cardiac disease the chest x-ray and particularly the four-view cardiac series with a barium esophagram and cardiac fluoroscopy have been largely supplanted by more sensitive and specific imaging modalities.[1,2] These include echocardiography (Chap. 4),[2-5] magnetic resonance imaging (MRI) (Chap. 11),[6-8,8a-c] radionuclide scanning (Chap. 10),[9] and computed tomography (CT) (Chap. 11).[6,10-13a] However, chest roentgenography remains a valuable examination that offers important insights into the cardiovascular status of the patient.[14-17] It has gained special importance in recent years in the evaluation of the patient with cardiac disease in the intensive care unit and in the postoperative cardiac patient.[18]

In this chapter we discuss the role of plain film chest roentgenography, emphasizing cardiovascular anatomy and alterations of that anatomy in a variety of pathological states. Correlation with cross-sectional imaging helps to clarify important anatomical problems.

NORMAL CARDIAC ANATOMY

ANALYSIS OF THE CHEST X-RAY

Because of the excellent contrast between the air-filled lung and soft tissue structures, the pulmonary arteries and veins and the interlobar fissures are visualized in great detail with chest roentgenography. For this reason, it remains the study of first choice for the evaluation of pulmonary parenchymal and vascular disease. On the other hand, the heart and other mediastinal structures appear as a featureless, opaque silhouette. Blood, myocardium, pericardium, coronary arteries and great vessels, valves, and mediastinal fat cannot be separated because they have similar attenuation characteristics and there is little or no contrast available to differentiate these structures. However, the cardiac borders are clearly outlined and deviation from the normal configuration suggests disease. Thus, knowledge of the appearance of the normal and pathological cardiac silhouette is essential for the evaluation of the cardiac patient.

FRONTAL VIEW. In a well-positioned posteroanterior (PA) or frontal chest x-ray, the contour of the normal cardiac structures is predictably outlined against the lung (Fig. 8–1). A series of indentations and bulges along the right and left mediastinal borders is associated with normal cardiac and vascular structures. Along the upper left mediastinal border above the aortic arch, the left subclavian artery is the border-forming structure. Although the left innominate vein actually lies lateral in position to the left subclavian artery, it is adjacent to the anterior chest wall so that there is no available contrast in the PA view to permit recognition of the left innominate vein as a distinct structure. The left subclavian artery usually forms a concave border with the lung, extending from the aortic arch to the clavicle. The left subclavian artery may bulge laterally when there is increased blood flow, as in postductal coarctation of the aorta or when the head and neck vessels are tortuous due to atherosclerosis. A straight or a convex left supraaortic border is found in patients with persistent left superior vena cava (Fig. 8–2).

The aortic arch or "knob" forms a sharply marginated convex border immediately below the left subclavian artery. It is usually small in the young patient, with a diameter of 2.0 cm ± 1 cm, and represents the posterior portion of the arch. The trachea at the level of the arch is displaced slightly to the right. When a right aortic arch is present, the trachea is displaced slightly to the left, a clear indication of that anomaly. A small bump or "nipple" representing the left superior intercostal vein measuring about 3 mm in diameter can be seen along the aortic arch in a small number of patients (4 to 10 per cent).[17,18] When enlarged, the left superior intercostal vein or "nipple" has the same significance as a dilated azygos vein, i.e., increased central venous pressure or increased blood flow resulting from diversion from other major venous structures as may occur in superior vena caval syndrome, inferior vena caval obstruction, or deep mediastinal venous blockage.

In older individuals with pronounced atherosclerosis, systemic hypertension, or aortic regurgitation, the aortic arch is prominent on the frontal view. It is wider and higher and may even reach the level of the clavicle. The ascending aorta protrudes further to the right side. The descending aorta assumes a tortuous or serpentine configuration (Fig. 8–3). The brachiocephalic vessels also dilate and become tortuous. At times, a dilated right brachiocephalic artery may mimic the appear-

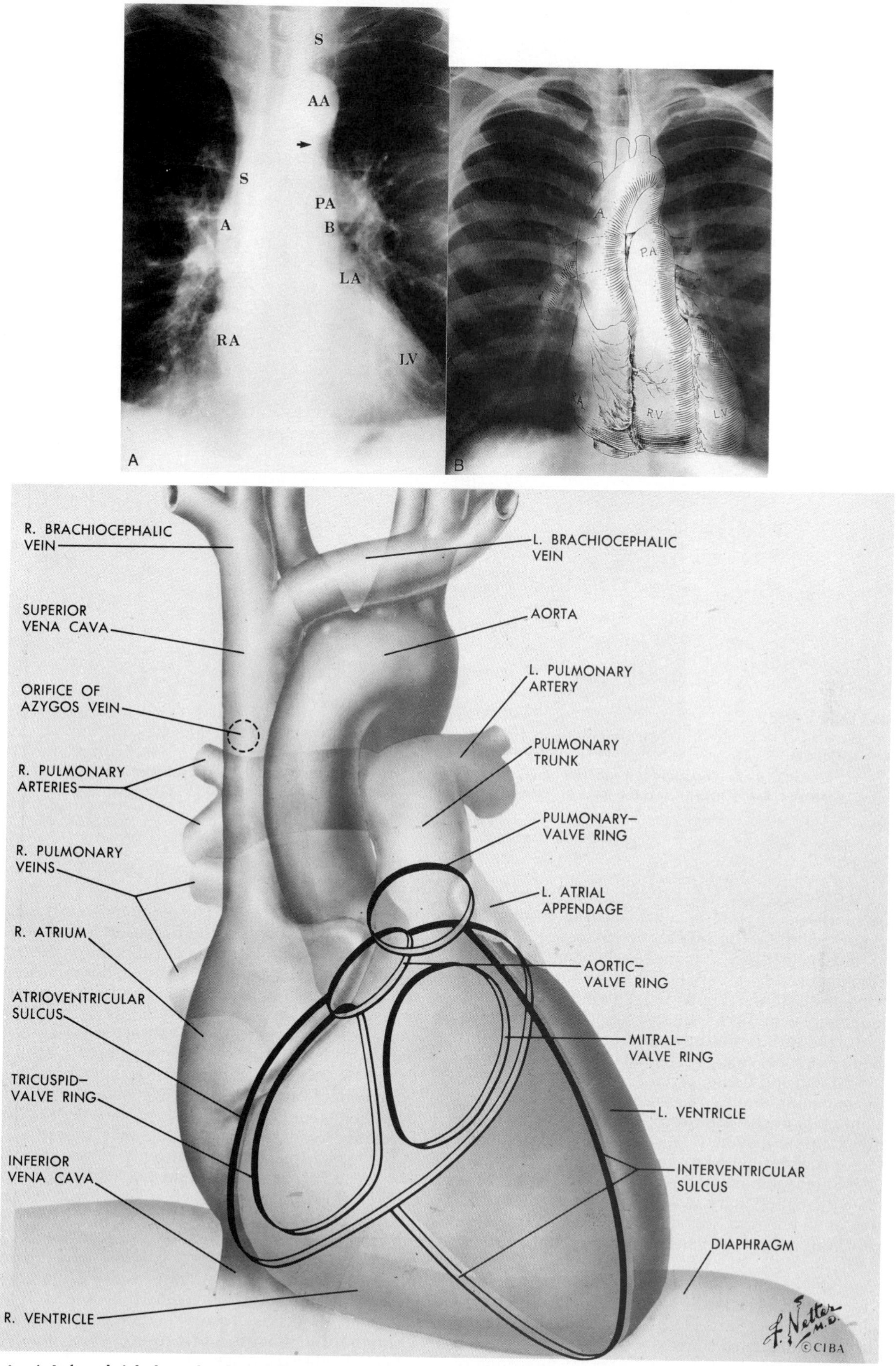

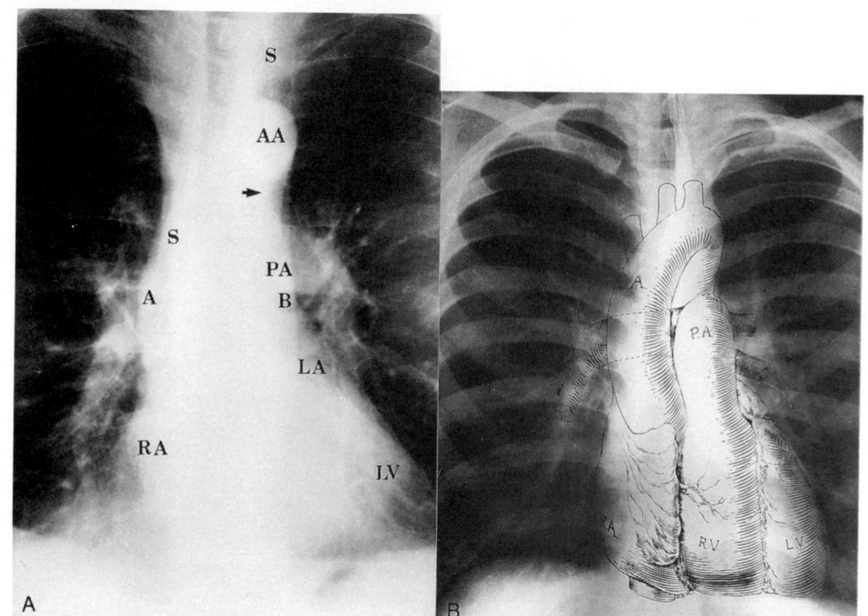

R. BRACHIOCEPHALIC VEIN
L. BRACHIOCEPHALIC VEIN
SUPERIOR VENA CAVA
AORTA
L. PULMONARY ARTERY
ORIFICE OF AZYGOS VEIN
PULMONARY TRUNK
R. PULMONARY ARTERIES
PULMONARY-VALVE RING
R. PULMONARY VEINS
L. ATRIAL APPENDAGE
R. ATRIUM
AORTIC-VALVE RING
ATRIOVENTRICULAR SULCUS
MITRAL-VALVE RING
TRICUSPID-VALVE RING
L. VENTRICLE
INFERIOR VENA CAVA
INTERVENTRICULAR SULCUS
DIAPHRAGM
R. VENTRICLE
F. Netter M.D.
© CIBA
C

FIGURE 8-1. *A,* Left and right heart borders in the frontal projection. SC = Left subclavian artery, A = Ascending aorta, LV = Left ventricle, B = Left bronchus, LA = Left atrial appendage, PA = Main pulmonary artery, RA = Right atrium, S = Superior vena cava, AA = Aortic arch, Arrow = Aortico-pulmonary window. *B,* Superimposed line drawing demonstrates the position of the heart and great vessels. PA = Pulmonary artery, RV = Right ventricle, A = Aorta, LV = Left ventricle, RA = Right atrium. (From van Houten, F. X. et al.: Radiology of valvular heart disease. *In* Sonnenblick, E., and Lesch, M. [eds.]: Valvular Heart Disease. New York, Grune and Stratton, 1974.) *C,* Line drawing in the frontal projection demonstrates the relationship of the cardiac valves, rings, and sulci to the cardiac silhouette. (Reproduced with permission from CIBA collection of medical illustrations by Frank H. Netter, M.D. Vol. 5, *The Heart,* edited by F. Y. Yonkman and Murray G. Baron, M.D. Copyright 1969, CIBA Pharmaceutical Co. All rights reserved.)

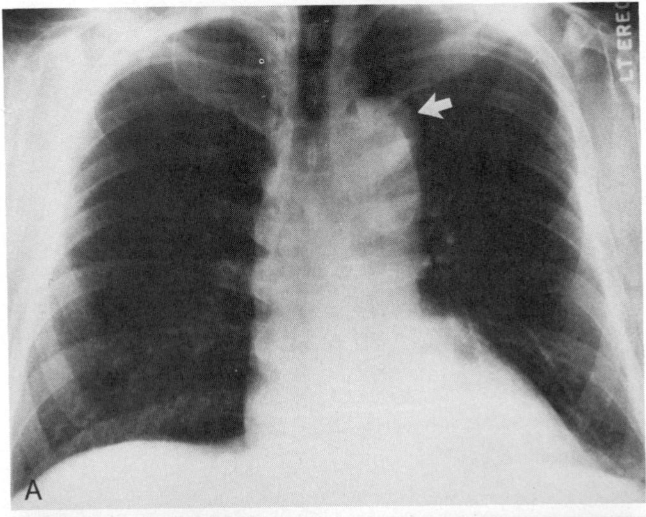

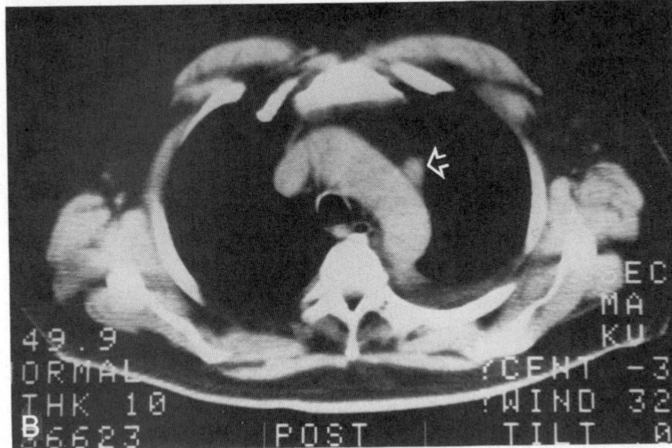

FIGURE 8–2. Persistent left superior vena cava (LSVC). *A,* There is a convex "mass" overlying the aortic knob (arrow). *B,* Enhanced CT at the level of the aortic arch shows the mass to conform with a LSVC (arrow).

ance of a substernal thyroid or other superior mediastinal mass and may require CT or MRI for diagnosis.

The left mediastinal border immediately below the aortic arch is characterized by a variable-sized indentation of the lung into the mediastinum (Fig. 8–1*A*). This indentation is the aorticopulmonary window. It is limited superiorly by the inferior margin of the aortic arch and inferiorly by the upper margin of the left pulmonary artery. This small space contains, in addition to fat and soft tissue, several important anatomical structures, including the left recurrent laryngeal nerve and the ligamentum or ductus arteriosus. Lymphadenopathy or a ductus diverticulum may cause a convex bulge in the normally concave mediastinal reflection of the aorticopulmonary window.[19,20] Encroachment on the recurrent laryngeal nerve within the aorticopulmonary window by a mass, ductus diverticulum, or an enlarged lymph node or extrinsic pressure from an aortic aneurysm can cause paralysis of the left vocal cord.

The origin of the left main pulmonary artery is border-forming, with the lung located immediately below the aorticopulmonary window. It is recognized as a small to moderate sized, smoothly marginated convexity at the level where the branch pulmonary arteries converge. Another indication of the location of the left main pulmonary artery is the position of the left mainstem bronchus (Fig. 8–1*A*). The left pulmonary artery arches over the left mainstem bronchus. When enlarged, the normally flat or slightly convex main pulmonary artery will form a prominent convex bulge; this is commonly found in pulmonary valvular stenosis, idiopathic pulmonary artery dilatation, pulmonary arterial hypertension, and a left-to-right shunt (Fig. 8–4). The pulmonary artery may be small or not seen in patients with transposition of the great arteries, truncus arteriosus, tetralogy of Fallot, or pulmonary atresia.

The left atrial appendage or auricle lies immediately below the left main stem bronchus in the frontal projection. Normally, the left atrial appendage forms a smooth and slightly concave border. When the left atrial border is straightened or bulges to the left, left atrial enlargement is suspected (Figs. 8–5, 8–6, and 8–7). Nonvascular pathology may simulate enlargement of vascular structures such as the left atrial appendage. For example, a pericardial fibroma or cyst, thymoma, or other mediastinal or pleural tumor may present as a convexity of the mediastinal border. Congenital absence of the pericardium also causes bulging of the left atrial appendage.

The left ventricular border blends with the left atrial border without a specific landmark to differentiate between the two chambers. The left ventricular border is mildly convex extending to the diaphragm. It may be rounded and the apex elevated because of hypertrophy resulting from aortic stenosis or hypertrophic cardiomyopathy (Fig. 8–8*A*). When the left ventricle is enlarged because of dilatation as may occur with chronic aortic stenosis, aortic regurgitation, or aneurysm, the apex is displaced downward and laterally. Much of the downward displacement may be obscured by the overlying left diaphragmatic dome (Fig. 8–8*B* and *C*).

With dilatation of the left ventricle due to volume overload as occurs in mitral regurgitation, the width of the chamber increases markedly and the heart assumes a globular appearance. The left ventricular border extends to the left and may even reach the rib convexities. As the left ventricle enlarges, it

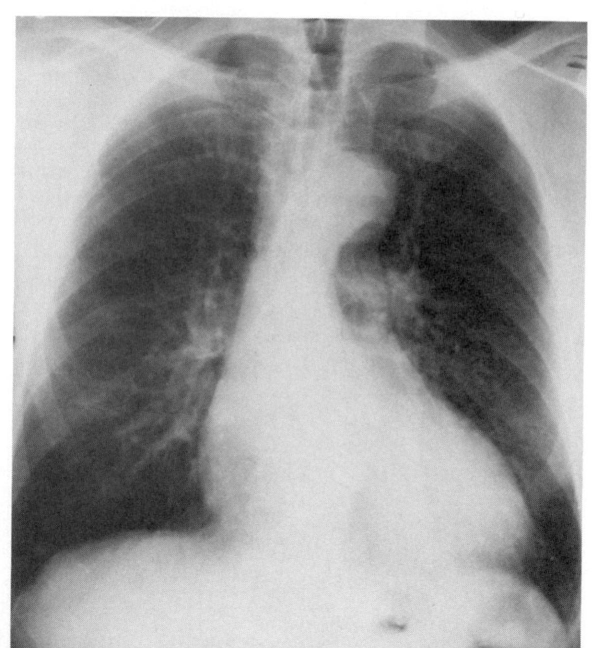

FIGURE 8–3. Aortic enlargement. A 63-year-old man with longstanding hypertension and aortic regurgitation. There is marked dilatation and uncoiling of the arch and descending aorta.

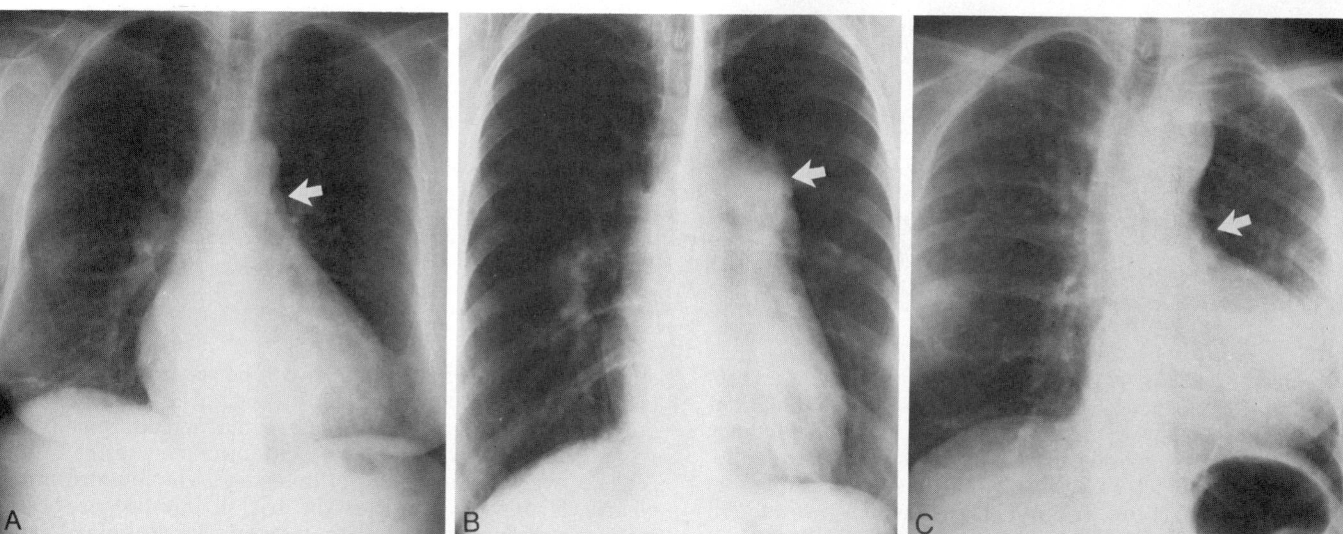

FIGURE 8–4. The pulmonary artery contour. *A,* Normal pulmonary artery segment in a 36-year-old woman with sickle cell anemia and moderate cardiomegaly (arrow). *B,* The main pulmonary artery is grossly enlarged in this patient with primary pulmonary hypertension (arrow). *C,* The pulmonary artery contour is small in this 16-year-old with tetralogy of Fallot and moderate pulmonary infundibular stenosis (arrow).

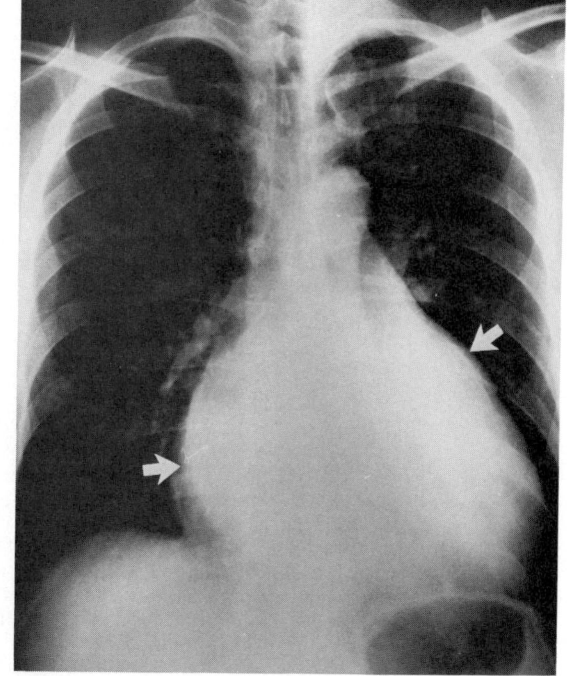

FIGURE 8–5. Prominent left atrial (LA) contour. The LA appendage bulges to the left in this patient with multivalvular rheumatic heart disease (arrow). The double convex contour of enlarged right and left atria is present along the right atrial border (arrow).

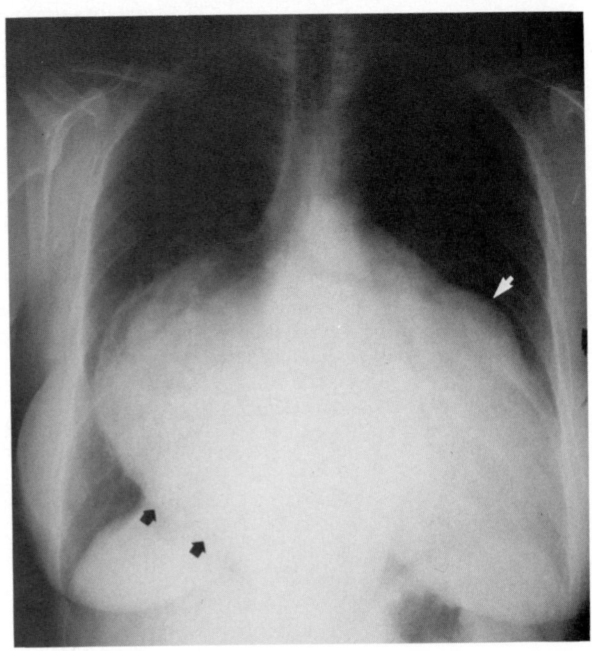

FIGURE 8–6. Left atrial (LA) enlargement. A large convex bulge is seen in the area of the LA appendage (white arrow). The LA is grossly enlarged and is border-forming on the right side after "overtaking" the smaller RA. The inferior border of the left atrium is visualized (black arrows) as it extends back toward the midline. If this were instead the RA border, it would have blended imperceptibly with the right hemidiaphragm.

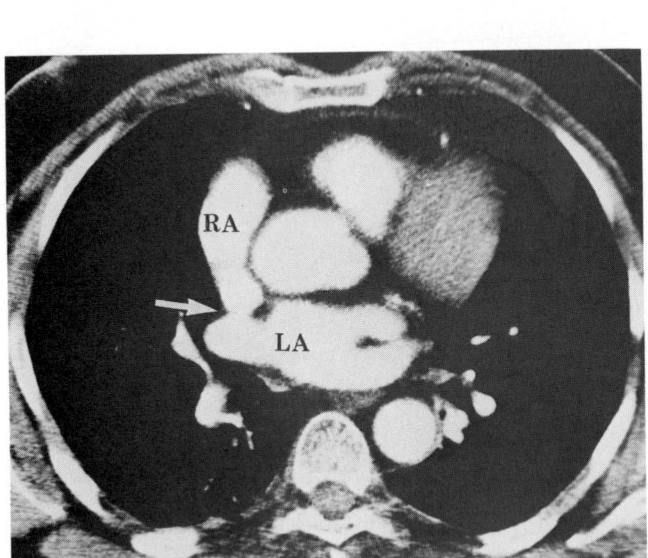

FIGURE 8–7. Enhanced CT demonstrates the anatomical relationship between the anterior RA and the posterior LA. The indentation of lung and fat between the atria (arrow) permits separation of the right-sided borders of both atria as seen in the PA chest radiograph.

obscures the left atrial border. The left anterior oblique projection will help to separate out the two chambers so that their relative sizes can be discerned. This assumes importance when the differential diagnosis lies between ischemic cardiomyopathy (in which case the left ventricle is larger than the left atrium) and mitral regurgitation (in which case the left atrium *can* be larger than the left ventricle).

In the frontal projection, the right atrial border forms a gentle convex interface against the adjacent right middle lobe. The caval border below the right atrium is usually straight, and in a good inspiratory film it can be separated from the convex right atrial border.[10] Deep to the right atrial border, the outline of the normal left atrium is seen as an additional convex density. The confluence of right pulmonary veins is directed toward the epicenter of this bulge. The left atrium is clearly visualized within the right atrial shadow because of an interface of lung between the posteriorly positioned left atrium and the more anteriorly positioned right atrium (Figs. 8–5, 8–6, 8–7, and 8–9). If the left atrium is markedly enlarged, the left atrial border will be lateral to the right atrium

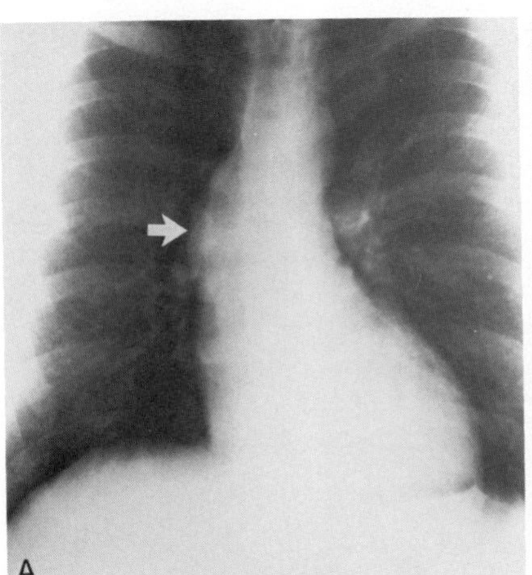

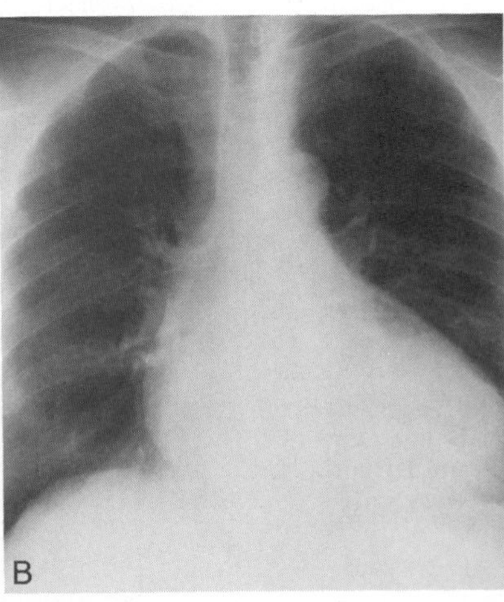

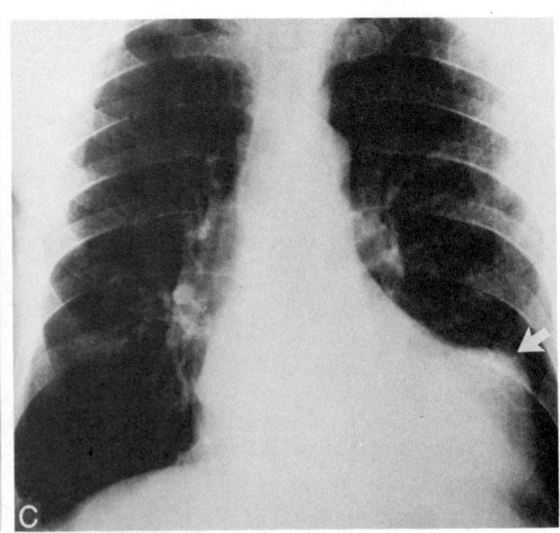

FIGURE 8–8. *A,* Aortic stenosis. The left ventricular border is rounded and prominent due to left ventricular hypertrophy. The proximal ascending aorta is prominent due to poststenotic dilatation (arrow). *B,* Aortic regurgitation. Prominent left ventricular (LV) border. The LV chamber is dilated due to aortic regurgitation and the ascending aorta is convex. The descending aorta is dilated. *C,* Left ventricular aneurysm. The prominent bulge of the LV apex (arrow) is separated from the pulmonary artery segment by the border of a relatively flat LA appendage.

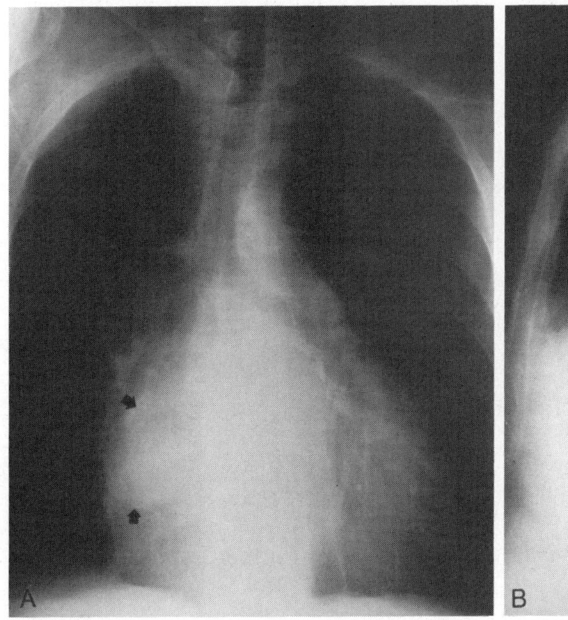

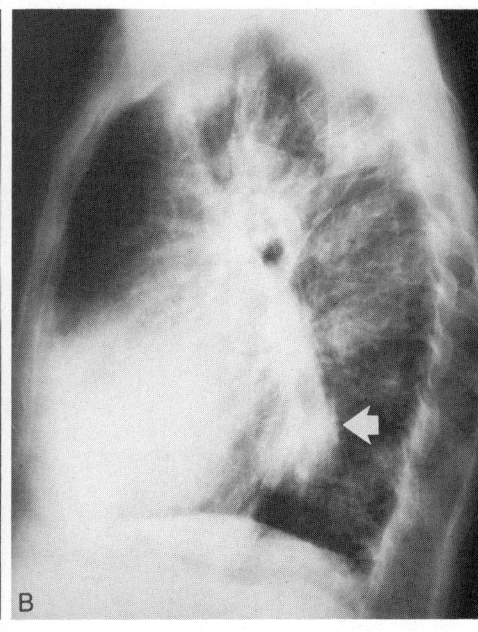

FIGURE 8–9. Prominent right atrial contour. *A,* The RA border is convex and the LA is seen deep (arrow) to the enlarged RA in this patient with mitral stenosis and regurgitation. *B,* In the lateral view, the pulmonary venous confluence bulges posteriorly because of LA enlargement (arrow).

(Fig. 8–6). The right and left atrium can be differentiated because the inferior border of the right atrium blends with the inferior vena cava while the left atrial density crosses toward the left side of the heart (Figs. 8–6, 8–7, and 8–9).

The right atrial border blends, superiorly with the superior vena cava, which forms a straight interface with the adjacent lung as it continues toward the neck. The normal right atrial border is considered enlarged when it bulges more than 5.5 cm to the right from the midline.[10] The right ventricle is not border-forming in the frontal projection and cannot be directly viewed (Fig. 8–1). As the right ventricle dilates, the left ventricle is displaced to the left and posteriorly, causing widening of the cardiac shadow. In selected cases such as in tetralogy of Fallot, the right ventricle forms a high round border on the left side of the heart and displaces the left ventricle[21] (Fig. 8–4*C*).

The ascending aorta is superimposed on the superior vena cava and forms a convex border above the right atrium. The azygos vein is an elliptical structure at the junction of the right distal tracheal air column and the right upper lobe bronchus. Normally measuring 0.7 to 1 cm in the erect position and 1 to 1.3 cm in the horizonal diameter in the supine anteroposterior (AP) position, it is a good indicator of changing cardiovascular dynamics (Fig. 8–10). It is enlarged in superior vena caval and inferior vena caval obstruction, in the absence of the inferior vena cava, and in both left- and right-sided cardiac failure.[22] A change in diameter of this vessel will parallel changes in pulmonary venous pressure, making the azygos vein a useful guide to the development of congestive heart failure on plain film x-rays. The cardiac valves, coronary arteries, and pericardium are not seen unless they are calcified, because they are as opaque as the remainder of the heart and mediastinum.

LATERAL VIEW. Proper positioning of the patient in the lateral projection is critical for accurate identification of cardiac structures[23] (Fig. 8–11). In the lateral view, the right atrial border of the heart is usually not seen. The right ventricle is border-forming in the subxyphoid area and generally extends superiorly about one-third of the distance between the diaphragm and the thoracic apex. As the right ventricle dilates, it encroaches upon the retrosternal space.[24] The relationship between the size of the right ventricle and the extent of substernal encroachment is affected by body habitus and lung volume. For example, in a patient with a small AP diameter or pectus excavatum deformity, the retrosternal space may be obliterated despite the absence of right ventricular enlargement. In the emphysematous patient, right ventricular enlargement may coexist with an expanded retrosternal space. CT and MRI as well as echocardiography portray relationships of the right ventricle to nearby structures with better accuracy and permit a clear analysis of right ventricular volume.[10,24]

The anterior margin of the pulmonary artery and the ascending aorta lie above the right ventricle; however, because of abundant mediastinal fat, neither structure is visualized distinctly in the normal patient. In patients with chronic obstructive pulmonary disease, the increased volume of lung permits the main pulmonary artery and the ascending aorta to be outlined clearly (Fig. 8–12*A*). The arch of the aorta usually is visualized except at the level where the superior vena cava crosses the aorta and where head and neck arteries enter the aorta. The inferior margin of the posterior aortic arch is often visible because of the indentation of the lung into the aorticopulmonary window. The semilunar lucency of the aorticopulmonary window outlines the superior margin of the left pulmonary artery, in addition to the inferior border of the aortic arch (Fig. 8–12*A*). The descending aorta is usually not clearly seen in the normal individual because it lies adjacent to the spine and the posterior mediastinal fat. However, in patients

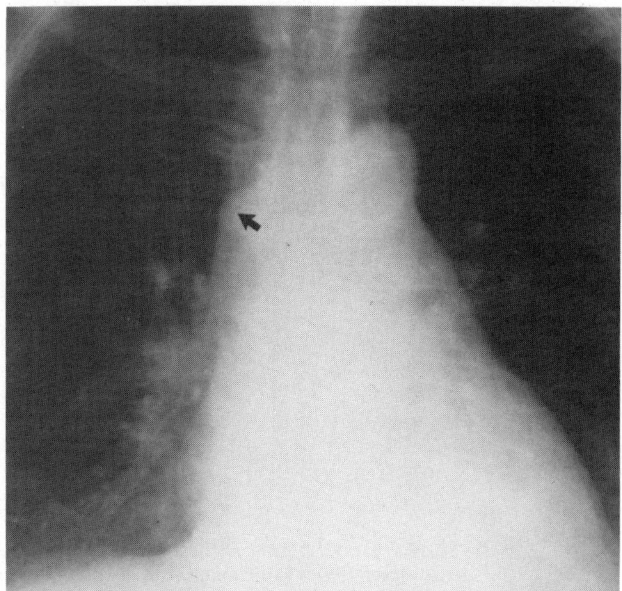

FIGURE 8–10. The azygos vein forms an elliptical opacity at the junction of the trachea and right mainstem bronchus. It is enlarged in this patient with a history of chronic congestive heart failure (arrow).

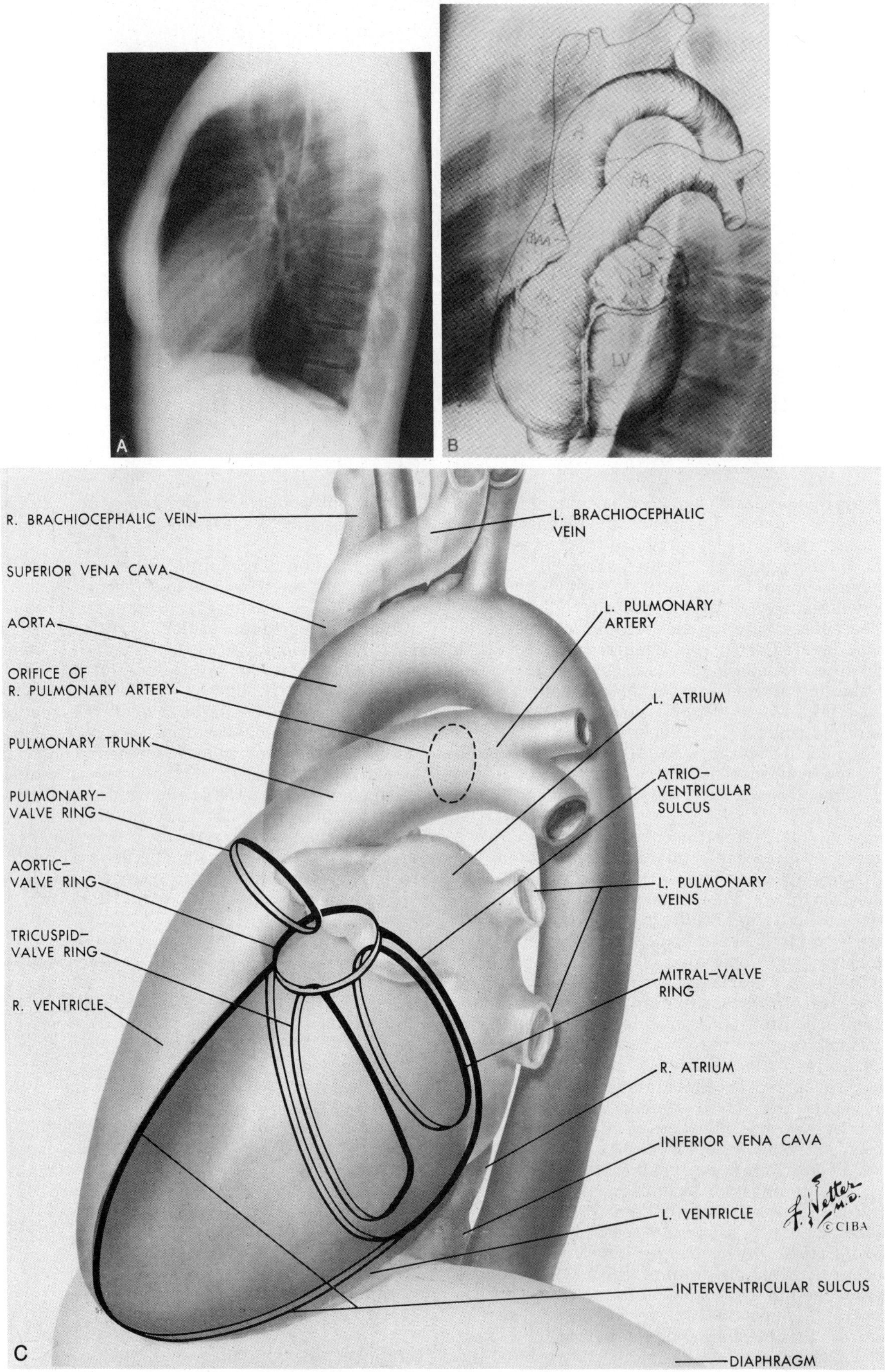

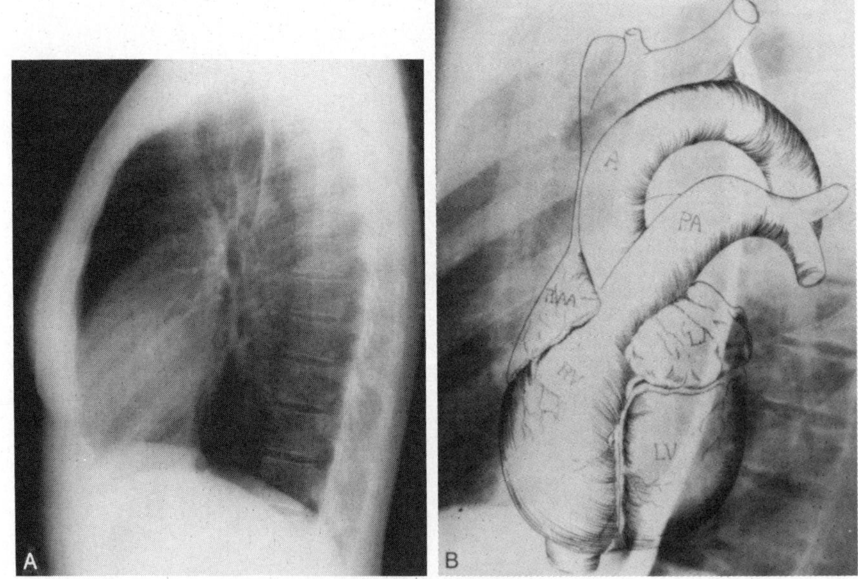

FIGURE 8-11. *A,* Lateral chest examination. *B,* Superimposed anatomical drawing of the cardiac chambers and great vessel. (From van Houten, F. X., et al: Radiology of valvular heart disease. *In* Sonnenblick, E., and Lesch, M. [eds.]: Valvular Heart Disease. New York, Grune and Stratton, 1974.) *C,* Lateral projection of the heart showing position of valve rings. (Reproduced with permission from CIBA collection of medical illustrations by Frank H. Netter, M.D. Vol. 5 *The Heart,* edited by F. Y. Yonkman and Murray G. Baron, M.D. Copyright 1969, CIBA Pharmaceutical Co. All rights reserved.)

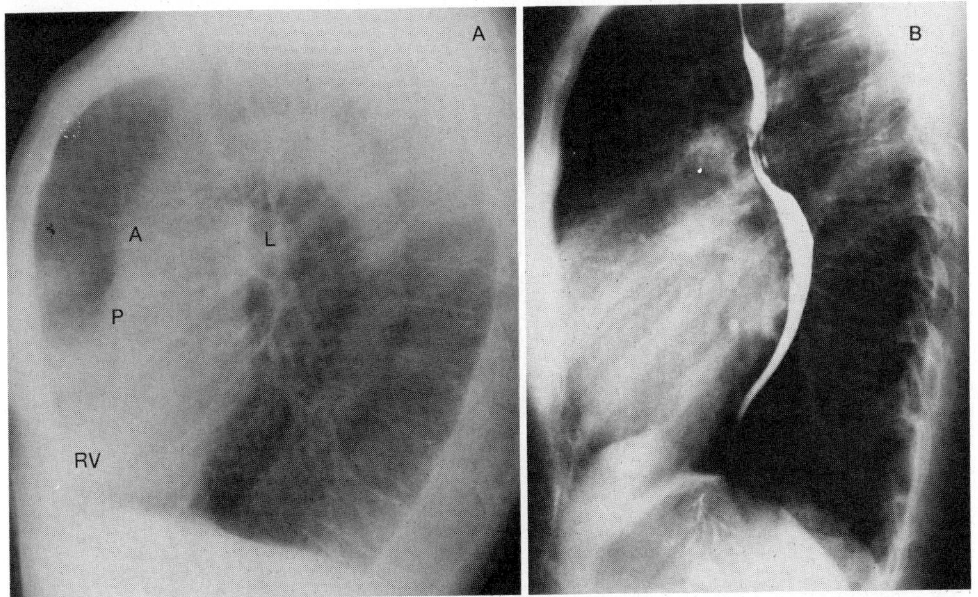

FIGURE 8–12. *A,* **In this patient with chronic obstructive lung disease, the hyperinflated lung permits improved visualization of the borders of the heart and great arteries. A = aorta, P = pulmonary artery, L = left pulmonary artery, RV = right ventricle.** *B,* **Discrete posterior displacement of the barium esophagram due to LA enlargement in a patient with mitral stenosis.**

with hyperaeration or those with a tortuous or calcified aorta due to atherosclerotic disease, the aorta is more distinct.

The left atrium forms a shallow convex bulge at the upper aspect of the posterior border of the heart on the lateral view. The normal left ventricle is a long convexity at the posterior-inferior heart border just above the diaphragm. Enlargement of the left ventricle is suggested by the use of the Hoffman-Rigler sign—a measurement determined by drawing a 2-cm line upward along the inferior vena cava from the point where the left ventricle and inferior vena cava cross in the lateral projection. At this point a second line is drawn parallel with the vertebral bodies. The distance between the left ventricle and the inferior vena cava should not exceed 1.8 cm. If it does, left ventricular enlargement is suggested. While this sign is helpful, it is far from accurate because obliquity of the chest or backward displacement of the left ventricle owing to right ventricular enlargement may influence this measurement.[25]

The esophagus lies immediately behind the left atrium and, when filled with contrast medium, can be used to locate the posterior border of the left atrium. Although normally the left atrium does not displace the esophagus, when the left atrium is enlarged, it causes posterior displacement of the esophagus from the area of the left mainstem bronchus to the level of the left ventricle (Fig. 8–12*B*). The normal left ventricle usually does not indent the esophagus but rather extends posterior and lateral to the esophagus. When both the left atrium and left ventricle are enlarged, the barium-filled esophagus may be pushed backward in one long curve.[21] Sometimes the left atrium enlarges without displacing the barium-filled esophagus because the esophagus may slide off the left atrium. When the aorta is tortuous and dilated, it carries the esophagus with it, and the esophagus cannot be used to evaluate left atrial size.

RIGHT ANTERIOR OBLIQUE PROJECTION (Figs. 8–13 and 8–14). This projection is performed with the patient in a 45-degree right anterior projection in relation to the film cassette (right shoulder toward the cassette). In this view there is elongation of the ventricles so that the long axes of the ventricles are in view and the atrioventricular groove is in profile. This permits clear visualization of a calcified mitral or tricuspid valve. The right anterior oblique view is helpful to the angiographer in determining the presence or absence of mitral and tricuspid regurgitation and stenosis. The aortic arch is foreshortened in this view, so that the arch and proximal descending aorta are often obscured. The anterior border of the heart consists of the sinus portion of the right ventricle inferiorly and the right ventricular outflow tract and the main pulmonary artery superiorly. The right-sided or posterior heart border consists of the right atrium superiorly and the left atrium inferiorly.[21,26]

LEFT ANTERIOR OBLIQUE PROJECTION. The left anterior oblique view is performed with the patient in the 60-degree oblique projection (Figs. 8–15 and 8–16). This is a useful angiographic view to diagnose the presence of left ventricular enlargement. In this projection the aortic and pulmonary valves are in profile, so that valve calcification can be clearly visualized and aortic stenosis and regurgitation can be assessed.[26–28] The aortic arch is also in profile so that abnormalities of the arch including dissection, contained rupture, aneurysm, and coarctation can be detected.[29] The anterior (right) heart border consists of the right atrium above and right ventricle below. Along the posterior (left) heart border, the left atrium is border-forming superiorly and the left ventricle inferiorly. The left anterior oblique projection is superior to other views in detecting right ventricular enlargement, indicated by a generalized increase in the convexity of the anterior border of the cardiac silhouette. Right atrial enlargement will cause bulging of the upper anterior border of the cardiac shadow, producing a shelf-like configuration.[29]

CARDIAC FLUOROSCOPY

Fluoroscopy is performed to study cardiac motion and to identify cardiac and other mediastinal calcifications.[26,30] Today, cardiac fluoroscopy is no longer performed routinely but is limited largely to solving specific clinical questions. Because fluoroscopy potentially causes significant radiation risk to the patient, it should be used selectively, with careful beam collimation. Exposure time should be kept to a minimum, preferably not more than 5 minutes. Perhaps the most important applications of fluoroscopy today are to detect coronary calcifications[11,31–34] and valvular and pericardial

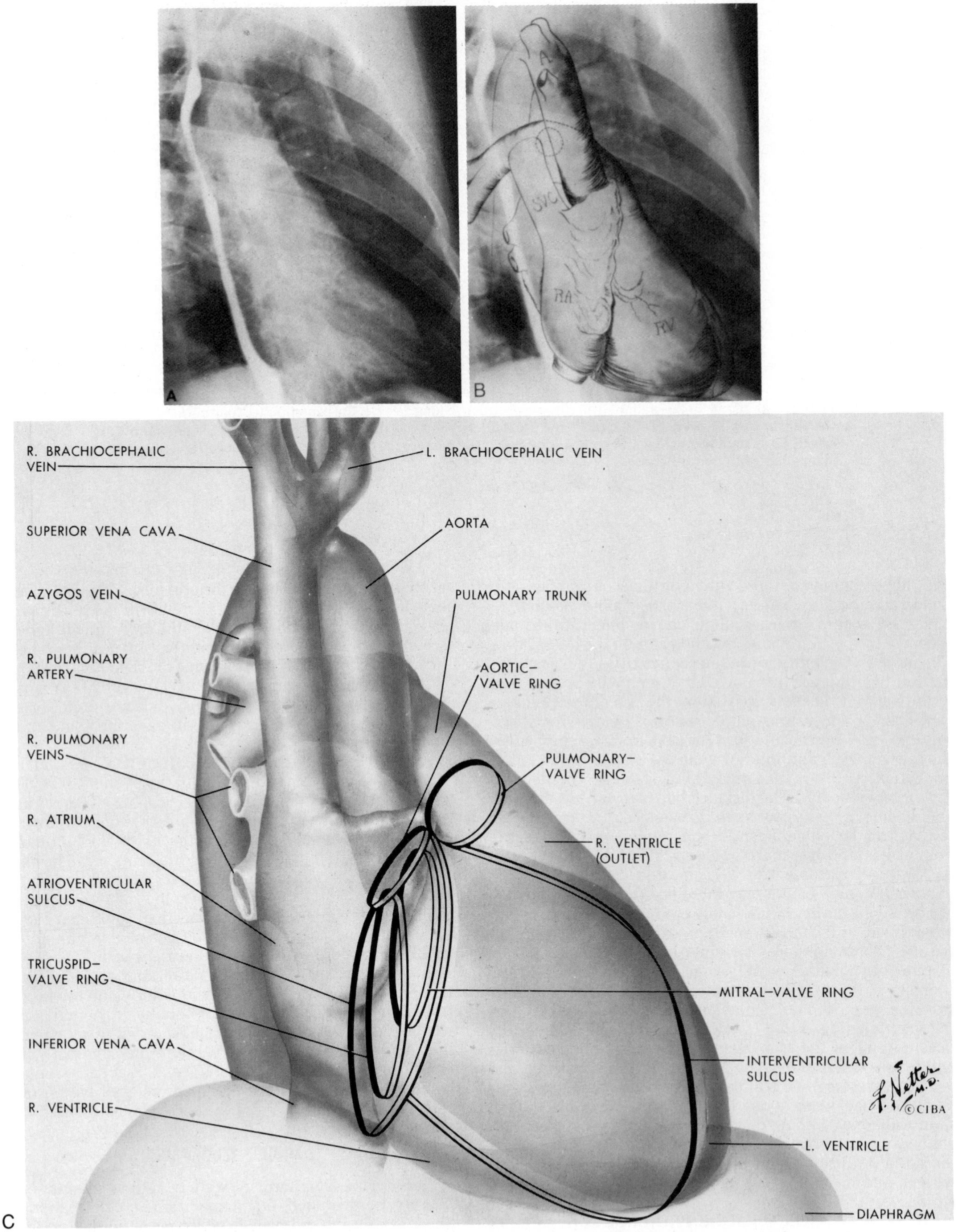

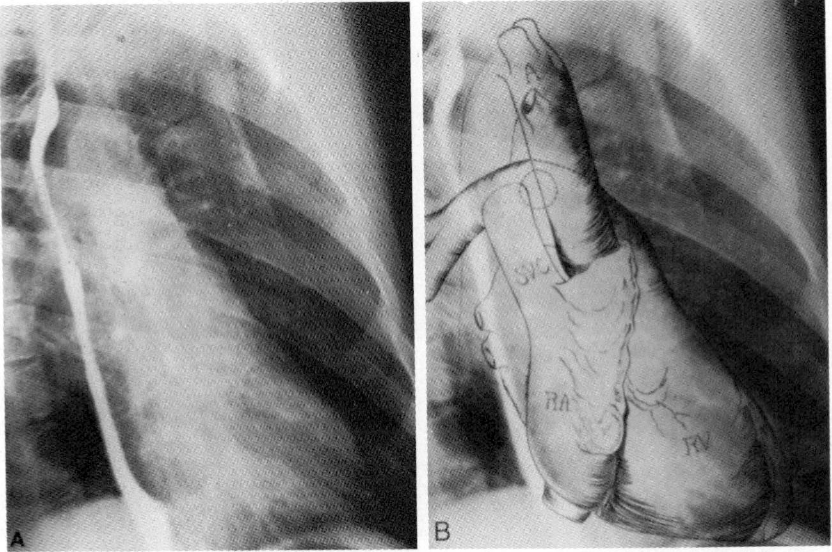

C

R. BRACHIOCEPHALIC VEIN
L. BRACHIOCEPHALIC VEIN
SUPERIOR VENA CAVA
AORTA
AZYGOS VEIN
PULMONARY TRUNK
R. PULMONARY ARTERY
AORTIC–VALVE RING
R. PULMONARY VEINS
PULMONARY–VALVE RING
R. ATRIUM
R. VENTRICLE (OUTLET)
ATRIOVENTRICULAR SULCUS
TRICUSPID–VALVE RING
MITRAL–VALVE RING
INFERIOR VENA CAVA
INTERVENTRICULAR SULCUS
R. VENTRICLE
L. VENTRICLE
DIAPHRAGM
F. Netter M.D.
©CIBA

FIGURE 8–13. Right anterior oblique (45-degree) projection. *A,* Chest radiograph with barium esophagram. *B,* Superimposed line drawing shows position of cardiac chambers. (From van Houten, F. X., et al: Radiology of valvular heart disease. *In* Sonnenblick, E., and Lesch, M. [eds.]: Valvular Heart Disease. New York, Grune and Stratton, 1974.) *C,* Drawing by Frank H. Netter, M.D., shows position of valve rings. (Reproduced with permission from CIBA collection of medical illustrations by Frank H. Netter, M.D. Vol. 5 *The Heart,* edited by F. Y. Yonkman 1969 and Murray G. Baron, M.D. Copyright 1969, CIBA Pharmaceutical Co. All rights reserved.)

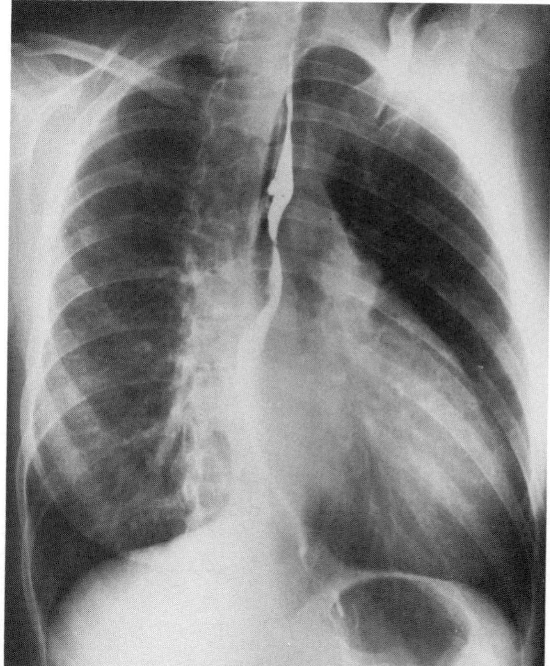

FIGURE 8–14. **Right anterior oblique view. There is posterior displacement of the barium column by an enlarged LA in this patient with mitral stenosis.**

calcifications,[35–38] and to evaluate prosthetic valve function.[39–41]

Fluoroscopy is usually performed with the patient in the upright position utilizing 68 to 75 kvp to enhance contrast and reduce mottle. The patient's position is determined by the structure to be studied. For example, if the presence or absence of aortic valve calcification is to be determined, a left anterior oblique or lateral position is optimal. If the function of a mitral valve prosthesis is in question, or if the presence of mitral calcification is suspected, then the right anterior oblique projection is most suitable. Coronary calcifications are best studied in the left and right oblique projections. In the 60-degree left anterior oblique projection, the right coronary artery, left circumflex, and left main coronary artery are seen to advantage. In the lateral and right anterior oblique projections, the left anterior descending artery is well seen[31] (Fig. 8–17).

Although large calcifications may be seen on the chest film, small calcifications are often obscured because of motion. On the other hand, motion is an advantage with fluoroscopy and coronary artery calcifications are seen clearly, because of their rhythmic movements, as opaque tracks moving perpendicular to their long axes in a "to and fro" motion. The right main and circumflex coronary arteries move more vigorously than the anterior and posterior descending arteries. Subepicardial fat represents an important landmark for the identification of vascular and valvular anatomy and is best seen with fluoroscopy. Fat surrounding the coronary arteries and within the atrioventricular grooves is well visualized so that the location of the mitral and tricuspid valves, the coronary sinus, and circumflex and right coronary arteries can be determined.

Fluoroscopy with videotape or spot film recording is useful in analyzing the integrity of the sewing ring and the mechanical components of prosthetic valves.[40–43] Excursion of the sewing ring exceeding 9 to 12 degrees between systole and diastole is associated with significant dehiscence (Fig. 8–18). Limitation of poppet or disc occluder motion suggests the presence of thrombus or vegetation. The results of fluoroscopic analysis of mechanical components compare favorably with echocardiography and phonocardiography but do not yield useful information about the degree of valvular regurgitation as do Doppler echocardiography and angiography.[39]

CARDIAC SIZE

Measurement of the heart with plain film radiology has been deemphasized because more accurate analysis of cardiac chamber dimensions and volume is available with echocardiography, radioisotope scanning, CT, and MRI. However, since an enlarged heart is abnormal, estimation of the cardiothoracic ratio remains a valuable yardstick to gain an impression of cardiac size. This may be done subjectively by estimating whether a heart is normal in size, enlarged, or grossly enlarged on the basis of an average cardiothoracic ratio of ≤ 0.5.[26] Using objective criteria, the cardiothoracic ratio may be expressed as the ratio between the maximum transverse diameter of the heart divided by the maximum width of the thorax. To obtain these diameters, a vertical line is drawn through the midpoint of the spine from the sternum to the diaphragm. The maximum transverse diameter of the heart is obtained by adding the widest distance of the heart border from the midline on the right and the left. This value is then divided by the maximum transverse diameter of the thorax[44–46] (Fig. 8–19). A normal range of cardiac transverse diameters of 10 cm in a small, thin individual to 16.5 cm in a heavy, tall person is described. A measurement 10 per cent beyond these values represents the upper limits of normal.[29] While the cardiothoracic ratio is helpful, it serves only as a guide. The normal heart may appear large in the frontal projection because of a small anterior-posterior (AP) diameter of the thorax caused by pectus excavatum deformity or straight back. The heart may appear smaller than it really is because of a downwardly displaced cardiac apex in patients with aortic regurgitation. In such patients the heart is actually enlarged but the cardiothoracic ratio remains within the normal range. Normal differences of transverse cardiac diameter in systole and diastole of 0.3 to 0.9 cm must be taken into account when analyzing cardiac size.[45] Cardiac volumes can be calculated from the PA and lateral radiographs using the following formula for the volume of an ellipsoid:

$$V = \frac{L \times S \times D \times K \times M}{A}$$

V = Heart volume in ml/square meter of body surface area;
L = Long-axis diameter from the junction of the right atrium and superior vena cava to the cardiac apex;
S = Short-axis or "broad" diameter from the right cardiophrenic angle to the base of the main pulmonary artery in the frontal projection (junction of left atrium and pulmonary arteries);
D = The greatest width or "depth" of the heart in the lateral view;
K = Constant for anode to film distance;
M = Magnification factor;
A = Body surface area in square meters.

The upper limits of normal have been calculated as 550 ml/m^2 body surface area for males and 500 ml/m^2 body surface area for females[26,29,44,47] (Fig. 8–20). This measurement correlates more closely with left heart size than does the cardiothoracic ratio, which does not take into account the AP dimension of the heart.

Because of magnification of the heart on AP films (including portable x-rays), a visual correction must be made in order to avoid overdiagnosis of cardiomegaly. A correction of 10 to 12.5 per cent depending on the anode-to-tube distance will correct this discrepancy.[48] High-kilovoltage PA airgap films are also magnified approximately 6.6 per cent when compared with low KV films in which airgap is not used.[49]

For the most part, calculated cardiothoracic ratios and volume measurements are of historical or research interest. In practice, these calculations are seldom performed because they are time consuming, and more accurate estimations of cardiac volume and size may be obtained with other imaging techniques.[7,8,12,14,15,50] However, knowledge of these guidelines is valuable when subjectively estimating cardiac size using chest x-rays.

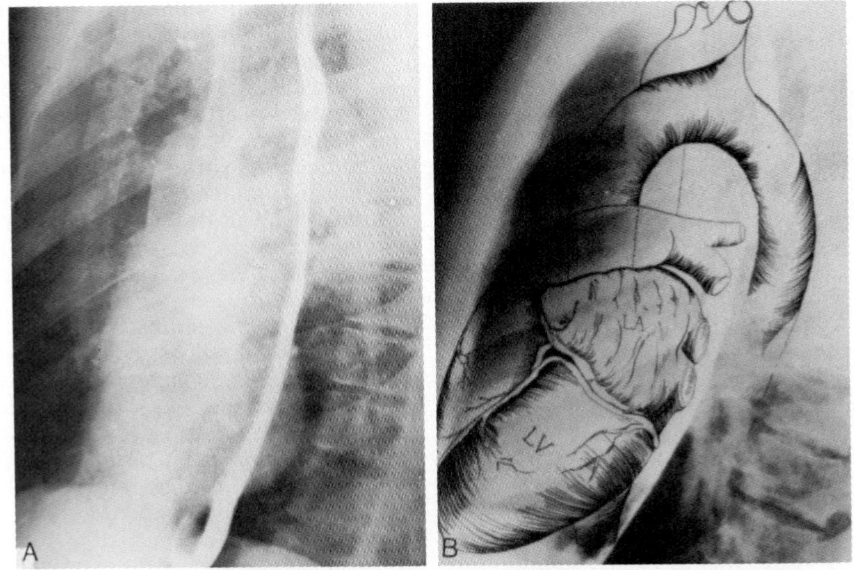

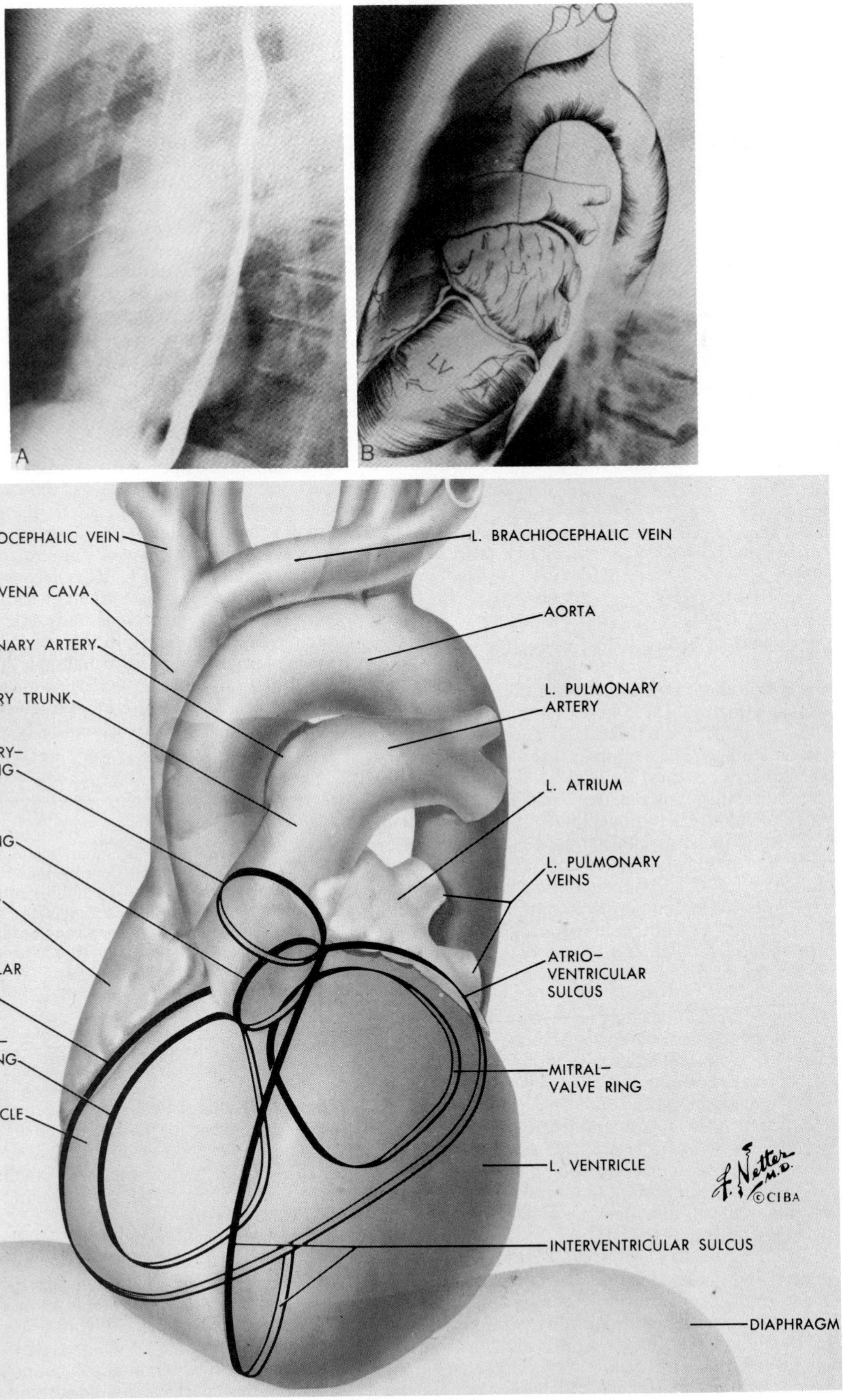

R. BRACHIOCEPHALIC VEIN
L. BRACHIOCEPHALIC VEIN
SUPERIOR VENA CAVA
AORTA
R. PULMONARY ARTERY
PULMONARY TRUNK
L. PULMONARY ARTERY
PULMONARY-VALVE RING
L. ATRIUM
AORTIC-VALVE RING
L. PULMONARY VEINS
R. ATRIUM
ATRIO-VENTRICULAR SULCUS
ATRIO-VENTRICULAR SULCUS
TRICUSPID-VALVE RING
MITRAL-VALVE RING
R. VENTRICLE
L. VENTRICLE
F. Netter M.D.
©CIBA
INTERVENTRICULAR SULCUS
DIAPHRAGM
C

FIGURE 8–15. Sixty-degree left anterior oblique projection. *A,* Chest x-ray with barium-filled esophagus. *B,* Superimposed line drawing in the same patient. (From van Houten, F. X. et al.: Radiology of valvular heart disease. *In* Sonnenblick, E., and Lesch, M. [eds.] Valvular Heart Disease, New York, Grune and Stratton, 1974.) *C,* Left anterior oblique projection. (Reproduced with permission from the CIBA collection of medical illustrations by Frank H. Netter, M.D. Vol. 5 *The Heart,* edited by F. Y. Yonkman 1969 and Murray G. Baron, M.D. Copyright 1969, CIBA Pharmaceutical Co. All rights reserved.)

FIGURE 8–16. Left atrial and ventricular enlargement, left anterior oblique view. There is a double bulge along the posterior border of the cardiac contour. Elevation of the left main stem bronchus is well visualized in this projection in a patient with aortic and mitral valve disease.

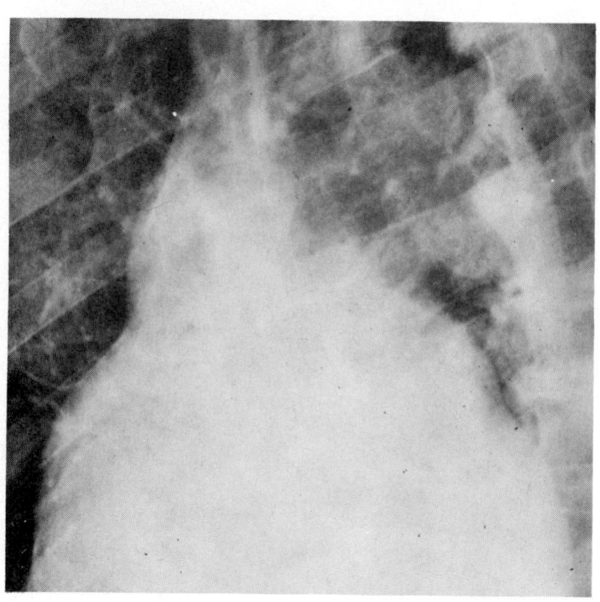

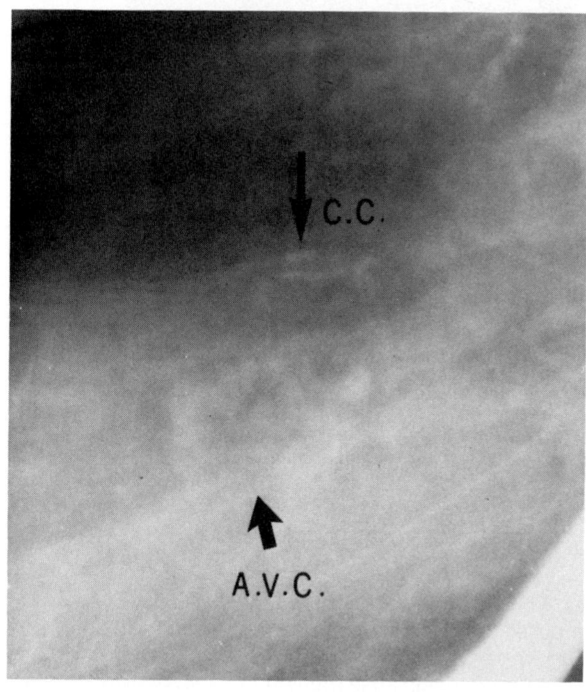

FIGURE 8–17. Coronary calcification. Coronary artery calcification may be clearly visualized with fluoroscopy or plain film radiography. In this patient, the left anterior descending coronary artery is calcified (CC), as is a bicuspid aortic valve (AVC) seen in the lateral projection.

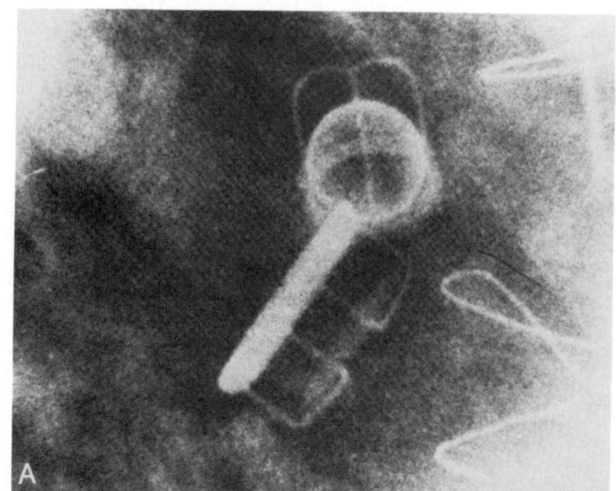

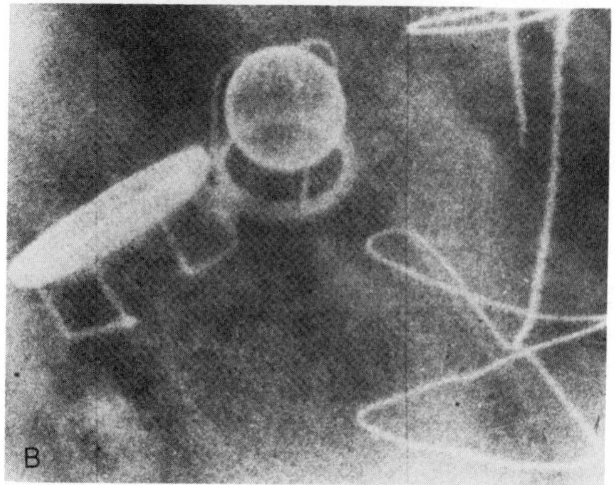

FIGURE 8–18. Abnormal excursion of a Beall mitral valve prosthesis due to partial dehiscence at the sewing ring. There was no abnormality of the aortic valve prosthesis. *A*, Diastole; *B*, Systole.

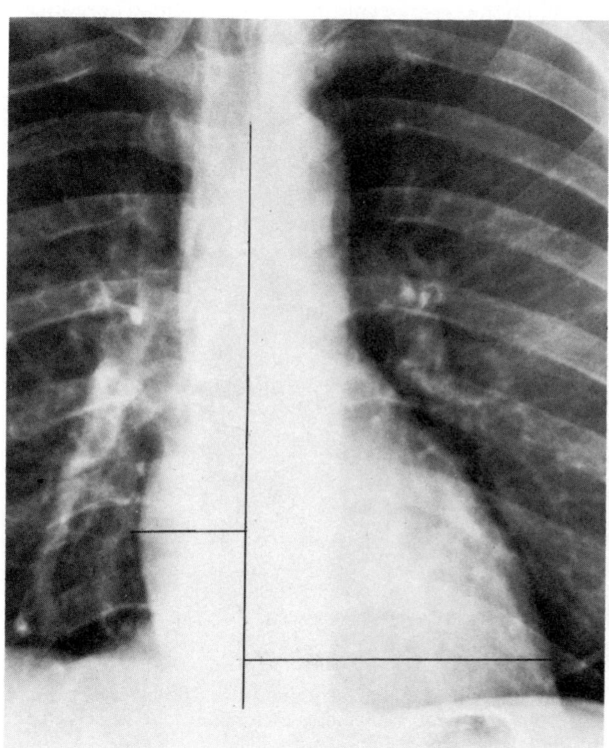

FIGURE 8–19. Measurement of the transverse cardiac diameter. A vertical reference line is drawn through the spinous process of the vertebrae. The greatest distance from this line to the right and left margins of the cardiac shadow are then measured. The sum is the transverse cardiac diameter.

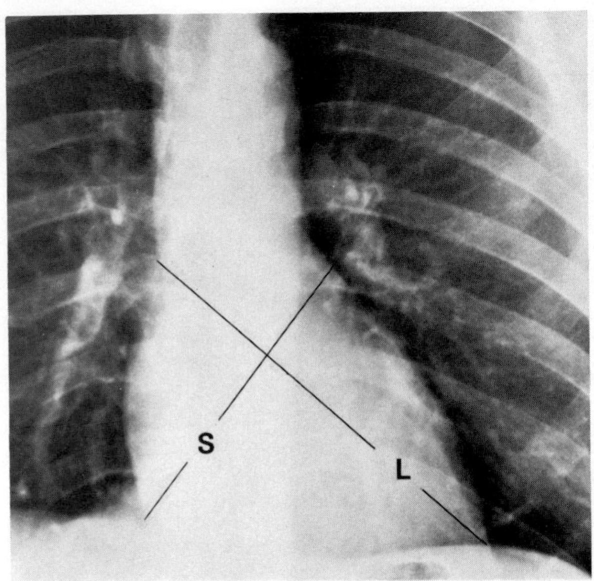

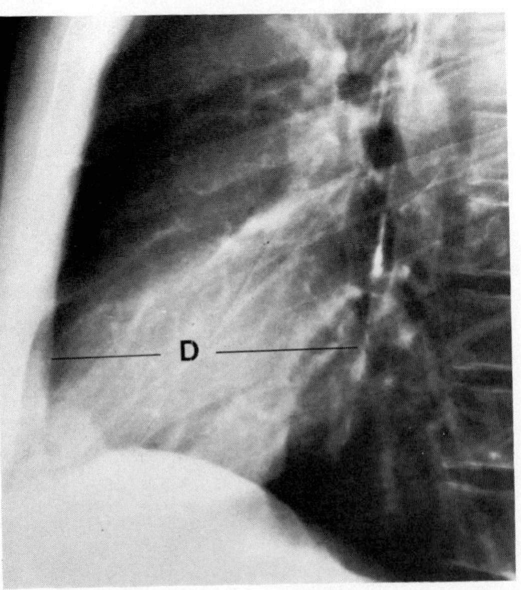

FIGURE 8-20. Measurement of relative cardiac volume: In the (*A*) frontal and (*B*) lateral views
V = Heart volume in ml/m² of body surface area
L or long axis is measured from the junction of the superior vena cava and right atrium to the cardiac apex.
S or short axis extends from the right cardiophrenic angle to the junction of the left atrium and pulmonary arteries.
D or depth is the widest cardiac dimension on the lateral view.

$$V = \frac{L \times S \times D \times K \text{ (constant for anode to film distance)} \times M \text{ (magnification factor)}}{A \text{ (body surface area in m}^2\text{)}}$$

THE PULMONARY VASCULATURE

NORMAL RADIOGRAPHIC ANATOMY

The pulmonary blood flow mirrors the pathophysiology of the heart. Since the pulmonary blood vessels are clearly visualized on the chest film, abnormal patterns of blood flow can be identified and increased, decreased, or redistributed flow can be appreciated and correlated with other indications of disease.

The main pulmonary artery bifurcates within the mediastinum. The left pulmonary artery courses to the left and posteriorly; its borders are visible just above the center of the left hilum. In the lateral view, the left pulmonary artery passes over the left main stem bronchus paralleling the aortic arch. The right pulmonary artery follows a horizontal course within the mediastinum, forming a circular or elliptical opacity on the lateral view anterior to the right main stem bronchus. It divides within the mediastinum proximal to the right hilum. The intrapulmonary branches parallel the bronchi, divide in an orderly manner, and gradually taper toward the periphery of the lung. The arteries and bronchi are approximately the same diameter at any particular level, with a ratio of 1.2 : 1.0. This relationship assumes importance when objective criteria are needed to support the impression of increased or redistributed blood flow.

In the erect position, blood flow is greater to the lower lobes than to the upper lobes (Fig. 20-8, p. 555), partly because of the effects of gravity (Fig. 8-21). Another contributing factor affecting the normal distribution of pulmonary blood flow is differential intraalveolar pressures as described by West.[51] In the supine and prone chest film, blood flow appears equal in both the upper and lower lung zones. Actually, flow will be greatest in the dependent or posterior third of each lung in the recumbent position; this is best appreciated with axial CT images. In normal individuals, the pulmonary arteries and veins in the outer third of the lung are too small to be seen clearly on chest x-rays. The central pulmonary veins usually can be distinguished from pulmonary arteries because they follow different pathways. Pulmonary veins course centrally in the interlobular septa, converging in the left atrium 2 to 3 cm below the hila. The pulmonary arteries radiate from the hila several centimeters above the pulmonary venous confluences. The veins of the upper lobes are usually lateral to or superimposed on their companion pulmonary arteries and, for the most part, the veins are larger and branch less than arteries. In practice, because the venous drainage and arterial supply to the upper lobes are so variable, it is often difficult to distinguish vein from artery.

ABNORMAL PULMONARY BLOOD FLOW

INCREASED PULMONARY FLOW. The size of the pulmonary arteries is proportional to the volume of pulmonary blood flow so that if there is an increase in right-sided cardiac output the vessels will enlarge as long as the reserve of the pulmonary vascular bed (8 times normal flow) is not exceeded. When the reserve volume is overwhelmed or reduced

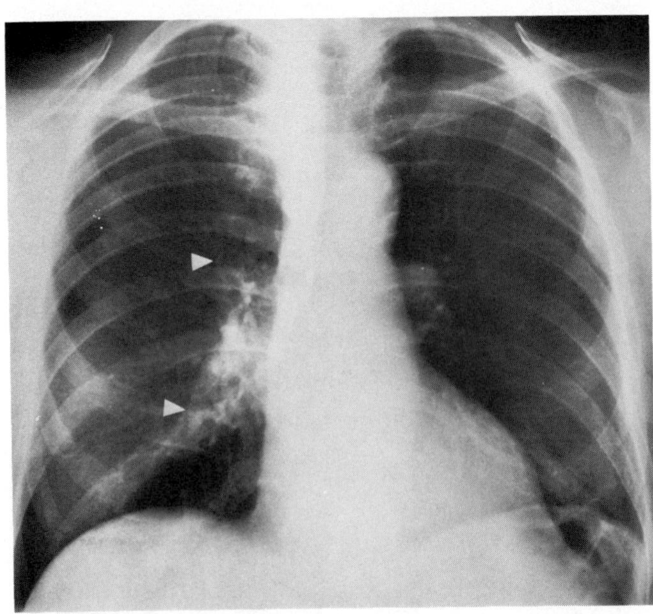

FIGURE 8-21. Normal pulmonary blood flow. The lower lobe vessels are 2 to 3 times greater in diameter than upper lobe vessels due to gravity and relative lung volumes (arrowheads).

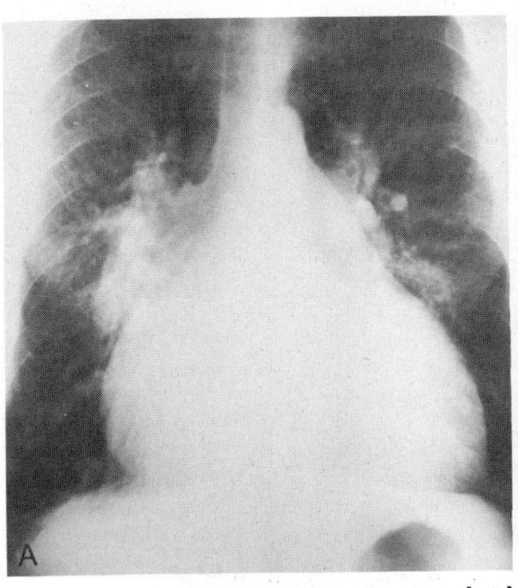

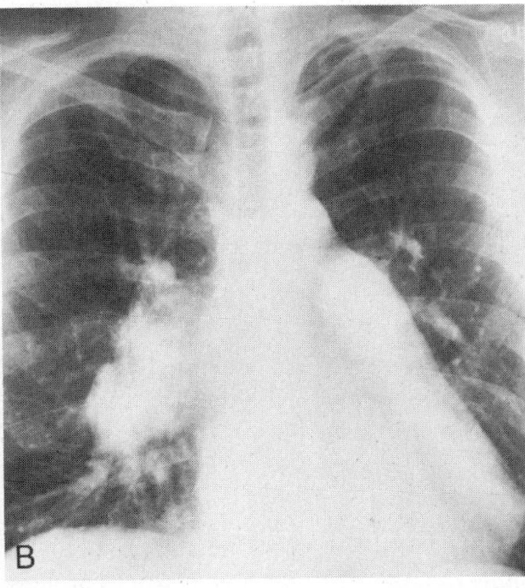

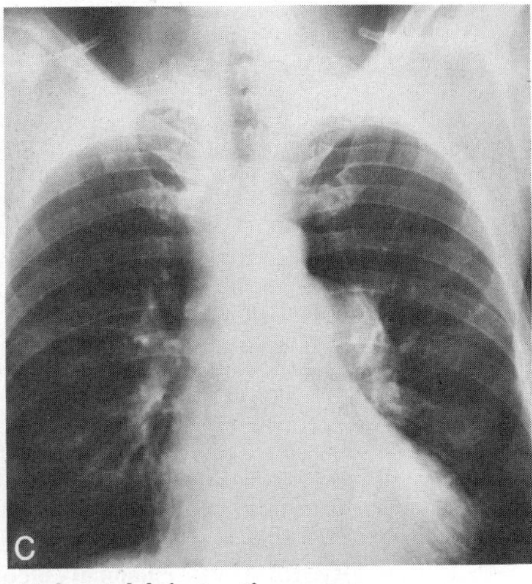

FIGURE 8–22. **Increased pulmonary blood flow. This 59-year-old man has an atrial septal defect, ostium secundum type with a pulmonary to systemic flow ratio of 4 : 1. There is secondary mitral regurgitation due to mitral valve prolapse. *A*,The right atrial border and the upper and lower lobe vessels are enlarged and their branches are visible in the outer third of both lungs. *B*, There is a disparity between large central and smaller peripheral vessels in this patient with ventricular septal defect and pulmonary arterial hypertension (Eisenmenger physiology). *C*, PA view in a 54-year-old man with marked disparity of central and peripheral vessels due to an atrial septal defect with longstanding pulmonary hypertension.**

because of vascular disease, the size of the vessels will be related to both blood flow and blood pressure or to pressure alone.[26] The pulmonary veins also enlarge as pulmonary arterial blood flow rises. Enlarged pulmonary vessels are found in a variety of conditions including left-to-right shunt, admixture lesions such as truncus arteriosus, severe anemia, hyperthyroidism, arteriovenous fistula, pregnancy, and other conditions that cause an increase in cardiac output (Fig. 8–22*A*) (see Chap. 14).

Roentgenographically, the blood vessels enlarge and are more clearly visible in the outer third of the lungs. With a small left-to-right shunt, the increase may appear confined to the lower lobes, but in larger shunts there is recruitment of the upper lobe vessels so that the differential flow between the upper and lower lobe vessels is lost. In occasional shunt cases, no pulmonary vascular abnormalities can be detected at all. The size of the pulmonary vessels can be measured objectively by determining the transverse diameter of the right descending pulmonary artery just above the origin of the right middle lobe branch. The normal transverse diameter of this vessel is 10 to 15 mm in males and 9 to 14 mm in females. A variation of +/− 1.0 mm beyond these limits is abnormal.[52]

PULMONARY ARTERIAL HYPERTENSION. As the pulmonary vascular reserve is fully recruited or the vascular reserve is reduced by pulmonary arteritis or chronic obstructive lung disease, pulmonary arterial pressure rises (see Chap. 27). The vascular engorgement that characterizes increased pressure is accompanied by vasospasm, peripheral vasoconstriction, and vessel wall thickening. Eventually, there is a decrease in peripheral blood flow and the outer one-third of the lungs appears more lucent radiographically. The central elastic vessels enlarge, including the main pulmonary artery, the right and left pulmonary arteries, and second-order branching vessels. Calcification of the main pulmonary artery and the proximal branches develops in chronic pulmonary arterial hypertension. Pulmonary arterial hypertension may be primary or result secondarily from pulmonary thromboembolic disease, a longstanding left-to-right shunt, or pulmonary venous hypertension[29,53] (Fig. 8–22*B*) (also see Chap. 27).

PULMONARY VENOUS HYPERTENSION. Left ventricular failure, mitral stenosis, and other causes of obstruction distal to the pulmonary arterial bed cause an increase in pulmonary venous pressure above the normal range of 8 to 12 mm Hg. As this pressure rises, pulmonary blood flow is redirected into the upper lobes (Fig. 20–8, p. 555) so that there is reversal of the normal difference in size between the small upper lobe and larger lower lobe vessels. With further elevation of pulmonary venous resistance above 25 mm Hg, pulmonary edema ensues. Radiographically, "cephalization" or redistribution of pulmonary venous and arterial flow to the upper lobes is the earliest sign of pulmonary venous hypertension. A clue to the recognition of pulmonary venous hypertension is the diameter of vessels in the first anterior interspace. Normally, they do not measure more than 3 mm in diameter. If they are larger, increased or redirected flow should be considered.

Although the exact mechanism of vascular redistribution is obscure, one possible explanation has been proposed by several authors.[21,26,54–56,56a] With an increase in pulmonary venous pressure, there is leakage of fluid from the pulmonary veins into the interlobular spaces, occurring first in the lower lobes because of gravitational effects. Fluid accumulation in the interlobular spaces decreases pulmonary compliance and increases interstitial pressure. These two phenomena restrict flow to the lower lobes. Arterial spasm may also be a factor. Since these processes first develop in the lower lobes, redistribution of blood flow to the upper lobes follows (Figs. 8–23 and 8–24).

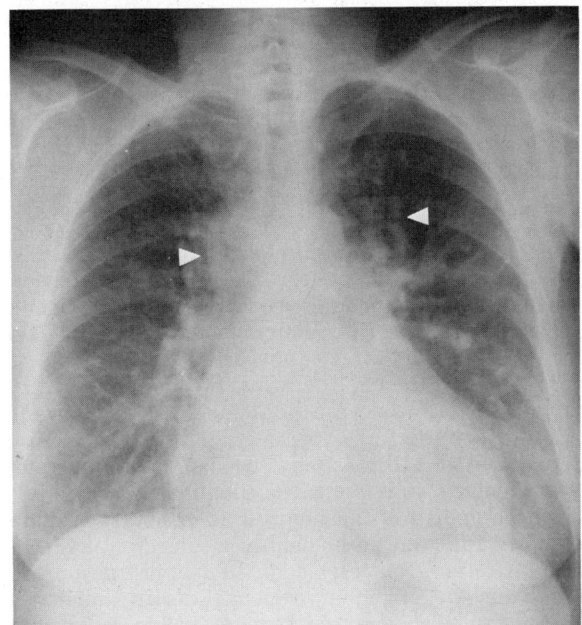

FIGURE 8–23. **Pulmonary vascular redistribution. This 60-year-old woman has a history of congestive heart failure. There is prominent vascular redistribution to the upper lobes due to elevated pulmonary venous pressure (arrowheads).**

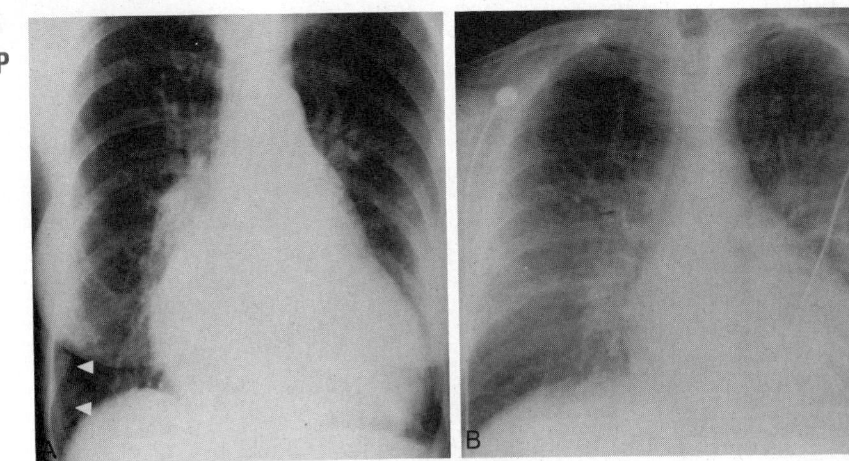

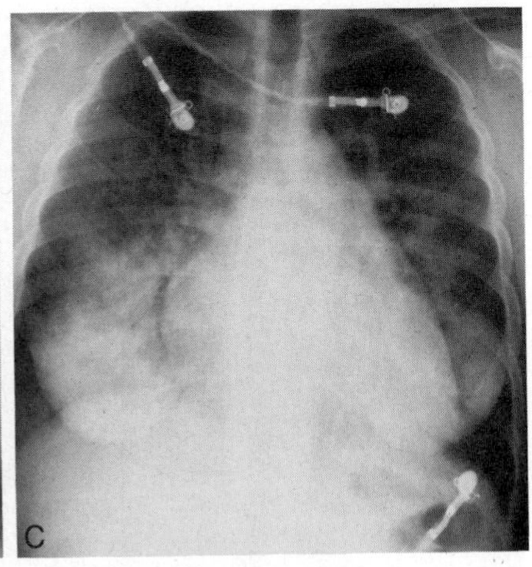

FIGURE 8-24. **Pulmonary blood flow redistribution. *A,* Enlargement of the upper lobe vessels in this patient with ischemic cardiomyopathy and elevated pulmonary venous pressure. Kerley B lines are present at the right base (arrowheads). *B,* Pulmonary interstitial edema: The vessels are indistinct and enlarged. There is peribronchial cuffing. *C,* Pulmonary alveolar edema in a patient with congestive cardiomyopathy. The central parahilar distribution or "batwing" edema is typical of cardiovascular or fluid overload (uremic) pulmonary alveolar edema.**

DECREASED PULMONARY VASCULATURE. When blood flow is reduced, usually because of pulmonary outflow tract obstruction or an intracardiac right-to-left shunt, the pulmonary arteries and veins are reduced in size. The central vessels narrow and the peripheral vessels are not visible. Reduced pulmonary blood flow may be generalized, as in tetralogy of Fallot, or may be regional as a result of pulmonary embolus, emphysema, and narrowing of vessels owing to tumor or to the reduced perfusion of arteritis. When pulmonary perfusion is reduced as in pulmonary atresia with ventricular septal defect, there is an increase in bronchial and other collateral arterial circulation. Radiographically, bronchial vessels are tortuous, small, and nontapered, and because they emanate from the aorta they do not radiate from the hilum. Normal but small pulmonary arteries and veins also contribute to pulmonary opacity in lungs with significant bronchial circulation because pulmonary arteries and bronchial arteries interconnect and preferential flow from the higher pressure systemic bronchial arteries to the lower pressure pulmonary arteries occurs.

ASYMMETRICAL PULMONARY BLOOD FLOW. Asymmetrical pulmonary blood flow is due to the presence of vessels in one lung that are smaller than in the other lung. As already indicated, these patterns of differential flow may be localized as in pulmonary embolism, chronic obstructive pulmonary disease, or arteritis. Unilateral decrease in pulmonary blood flow may occur also in patients with pulmonary artery branch atresia, hemitruncus, and tetralogy of Fallot with unilateral pulmonary atresia. In addition, asymmetrical increased flow may be found after creation of a Blalock-Taussig, Waterston, Potts, or Glenn shunt. Sometimes, the differences in blood flow in congenital heart disease are caused by orientation of the pulmonary outflow tract. For example, in pulmonary valvular stenosis, the flow of blood through the stenotic valve is occasionally directed toward the left pulmonary artery.[57] In patent ductus arteriosus, the preferential flow is often toward the left because the ductus is oriented toward the left pulmonary artery.

PULMONARY EDEMA (see also Chap. 20). In the normal subject, there is continuous transudation of fluid from the pulmonary veins into neighboring interlobular lymphatics that return the fluid to the central mediastinal veins. If the lymphatic reserve is overcome by increased transudate as a result of elevated pulmonary venous pressure, the interlobular septa are thickened and become visible radiologically. Blood flow redistribution, or "cephalization," will occur following reduction in compliance or vasoconstriction in the lower lobes roughly paralleling the increase in pulmonary venous pressure.[53,54,58-60] Interlobular septal lines, or Kerley B lines, are visible as thin horizontal lines present at both lung bases perpendicular to the lateral pleural surface on the frontal chest x-ray (Fig. 8-24*A*).[58] Increased interstitial opacities throughout the lung reflect additional thickened septal lines. If the cause of the pulmonary interstitial edema is cardiovascular in origin, the heart may be normal or enlarged depending upon the chronicity of cardiac failure. In addition to cardiac failure, prominent interstitial lines may occur in a wide variety of diseases including sarcoidosis, lymphatic spread of tumor, interstitial pneumonia and asbestosis. In pulmonary interstitial edema, the lungs may be clear to auscultation—a clue that the extravascular fluid is confined to the interstitium. With further increases in pulmonary venous pressure above 25 mm Hg, there is leakage of fluid into the airspaces, leading to alveolar edema (Fig. 8-24*C*). Radiographically, this pattern of pulmonary alveolar edema preferentially involves the inner two-thirds of the lung, giving a "butterfly" or "bat wing" appearance. An explanation for this pattern is that the outer third of the lung or cortex has better aeration and compliance as well as more efficient lymphatic drainage than the inner two-thirds, and for this reason fluid concentrates in the central portion of the lung[54,57,61] (Fig. 8-23).

Distinguishing pulmonary edema caused by congestive heart failure from that caused by increased capillary permeability or overhydration edema is often difficult. Recent studies have attempted to separate cardiovascular pulmonary edema from the other forms by specific characteristics such as heart size, the width of the pulmonary vascular pedicle, blood flow distribution, interstitial thickening, and regional distribution of pulmonary edema.[54,62,63] In these studies, cardiovascular pulmonary edema characteristically presents with a large heart, vascular redistribution, diffuse distribution of pulmonary edema fluid, a widened vascular pedicle and increased pulmonary blood volumes, septal lines, and pleural effusions. Overhydration pulmonary edema is characterized by a balanced blood flow and perihilar pulmonary edema. In capillary permeability pulmonary edema there is no cardiac enlargement, the vascular pedicle is normal or reduced in size, no septal lines are found, and the pulmonary edema presents with a more peripheral pattern.[62,63]

CARDIAC CALCIFICATION

PERICARDIAL CALCIFICATION (see also Chap. 45). Pericardial calcification occurs most often in association with previous inflammatory disease or trauma.[64] The most common causes are viral illness, especially Coxsackie or influenza A and B virus, granulomatous disease including that resulting from tuberculosis and histoplasmosis, hemopericardium following trauma, or autoimmune disease—particularly rheumatic heart disease. Occasionally, tumors (among them intrapericardial teratomas and cysts) will calcify.[36,65,66] Calcification is present in up to 50 per cent of patients with constrictive pericarditis (Fig. 45–16, p. 1485). On the other hand, extensive calcification may be present without the signs and symptoms of pericardial constriction. Pericardial and myocardial calcifications are frequently confused with each other. In general, pericardial calcifications can be distinguished from myocardial calcification by differences in their distribution. Pericardial calcifications are most abundant along the right atrial and ventricular borders and in the area of the atrioventricular groove (Fig. 8–25). The pericardium adjacent to the left ventricle usually is spared probably because of its vigorous pulsation, and calcification rarely occurs along the left atrial border because of the absence of pericardium behind the left atrium. Myocardial calcification is usually localized to the left ventricle and is very rare in the right heart chambers.

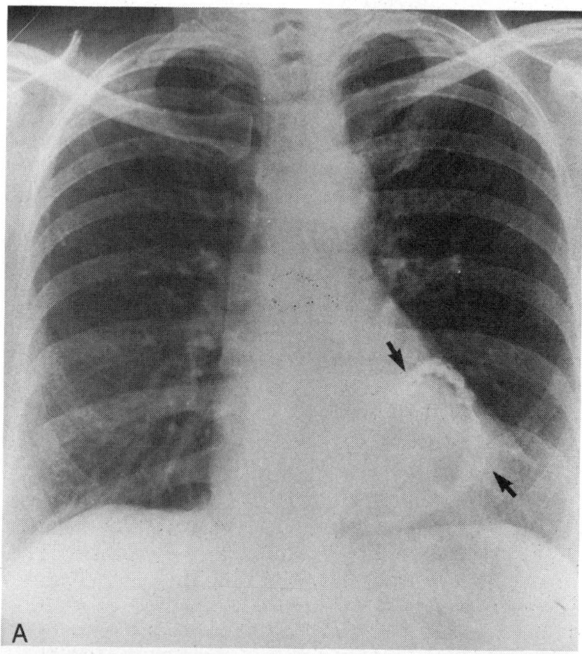

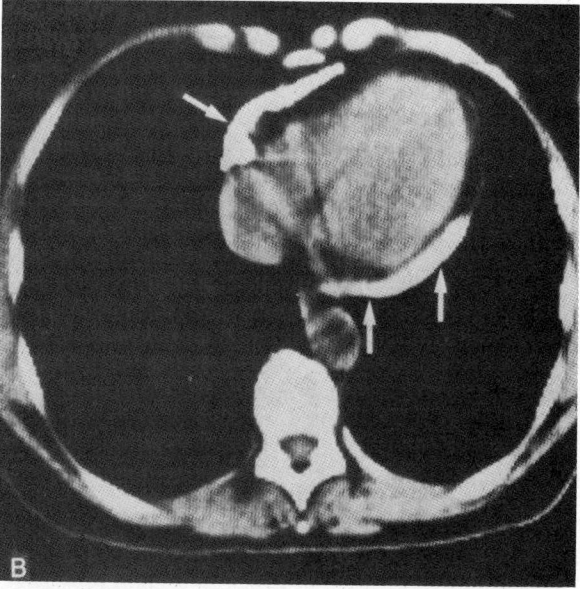

FIGURE 8–25. Pericardial calcification. *A,* Extensive calcification of the pericardium in the atrioventricular groove in a patient with a history of rheumatic heart disease (arrow). *B,* In another patient, CT demonstrates extensive calcification of the pericardium (arrows). (From Moncada, R., et al.: Multimodality approach to pericardial imaging. *In* Kotler, M. N., and Steiner, R. M. [eds.]: Cardiac Imaging: New Technologies and Clinical Applications, Philadelphia, F. A. Davis, 1986.)

MYOCARDIAL CALCIFICATION. Calicification of the myocardium is usually caused by a previous large myocardial infarction and has been reported to occur in 8 per cent of myocardial infarctions more than 6 years old.[26,38] Most frequently, myocardial calcification occurs in a ventricular aneurysm and in the apical and anterior lateral aspects of the left ventricular wall. The calcium deposits are usually curvilinear within the periphery of the infarct and occasionally may be homogenous when an entire infarcted area calcifies (Fig. 8–26). Calcification may also occur within the left atrium and left atrial appendage, particularly in patients with rheumatic heart disease, usually associated with mitral stenosis or mitral regurgitation. Left atrial calcification is most often found in the endo- or subendocardial layers and less often lies within an organized thrombus adherent to the chamber wall.[38] It is usually thin-walled and curvilinear, forming a shell around the circumference of the left atrial chamber or the left atrial appendage[26,38,67,68] (Fig. 8–27).

VALVULAR CALCIFICATION (see also Chap. 34). The radiological presence of calcification within a cardiac valve indicates the presence of either sclerosis or hemodynamically significant stenosis.[69] In the mitral valve, calcification is clump-like or linear, usually measuring about 2 to 4 cm in diameter, and is most often due to rheumatic heart disease. Aortic valve calcification in patients under age 40 generally signifies marked aortic stenosis. In patients over 65 years, calcification can be due to sclerosis with degeneration of normal valve leaflets or may be a manifestation of hemodynamically significant aortic stenosis. The radiological appearance of the calcification may help to determine the origin of the valvular deformity. A thickened irregular semilunar ring configuration with a central bar or knob is typical of stenotic bicuspid valve and is found in 65 per cent of patients with congenital aortic stenosis.[36,70] This pattern is due to calcification of the annulus and the dividing ridge or raphe of one of the two cusps (Fig. 8–28). The abundance of calcification is thought to be due to constant wear and tear from the abnormal tensions of movement of bicuspid valve leaflets. Calcification of the pulmonary valve occurs occasionally in pulmonary valve stenosis with gradients in excess of 80 mm Hg. Calcification of the tricuspid valve is usually caused by rheumatic disease and is also unusual.

Annular calcification is found in the valve rings or fibroskeleton of the heart. It is a degenerative process occurring with aging and is found most often in individuals above the age of 40 years, especially women.[71] Mitral annular calcification (p. 1018) presents radiographically as a crennated *O-*, *J-* or C-shaped opacity (Fig. 8–29). If extreme, it may involve the valve leaflets and cause limitation of valve motion leading to regurgitation.[37,71] Atrial fibrillation, conduction abnormalities, and mitral valve prolapse are associated findings. Aortic annular calcification is often associated with valve calcification and may extend into the ascending aorta and down into the interventricular septum.[29] Tricuspid annular calcification is rare, usually occurring in patients with longstanding pulmonary valvular stenosis and right ventricular hypertension.

Several methods have been suggested to identify the location of valvular calcification on plain films. Extending a line drawn on the lateral chest film from the junction of the anterior chest wall and the diaphragm through the hilum to the apex will separate anterior superior aortic calcifications from posterior inferior mitral calcifications (Fig. 8–30). Another approach is to divide the heart on the lateral view into six sections; this will also permit identification of the aortic valve in the upper row middle section and mitral calcification in the lower row posterior section.

CORONARY ARTERY CALCIFICATION. A number of studies have been performed to compare the efficacy of fluoroscopy with arteriography and exercise testing in identifying significant coronary artery disease.[11,31–34,72] As a result of these studies, a direct relationship between fluoroscopically identified coronary calcification and the frequency and severity of stenotic lesions is well established. In one study on 360 pa-

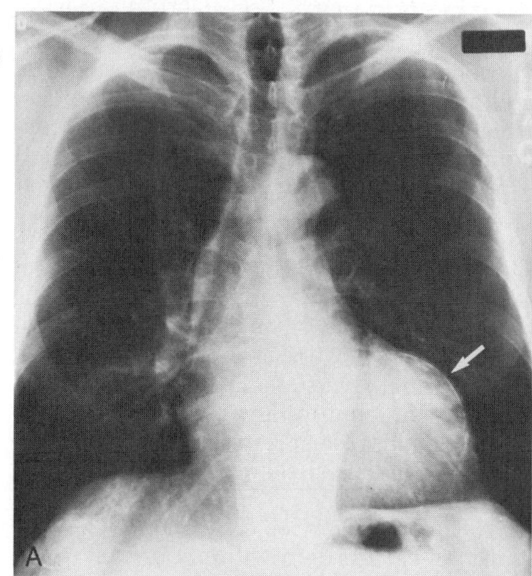

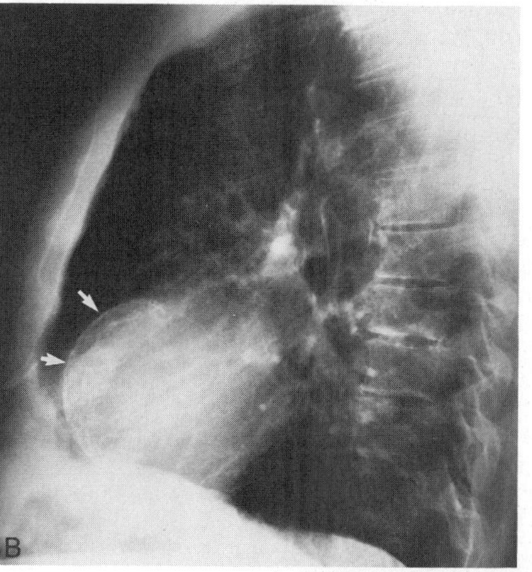

FIGURE 8–26. Myocardial calcification. A ring of calcification in the anterior left ventricular wall outlines a left ventricular aneurysm. *A,* PA and *B,* Lateral views (arrows). (Courtesy of Stephanie Flicker, M.D.)

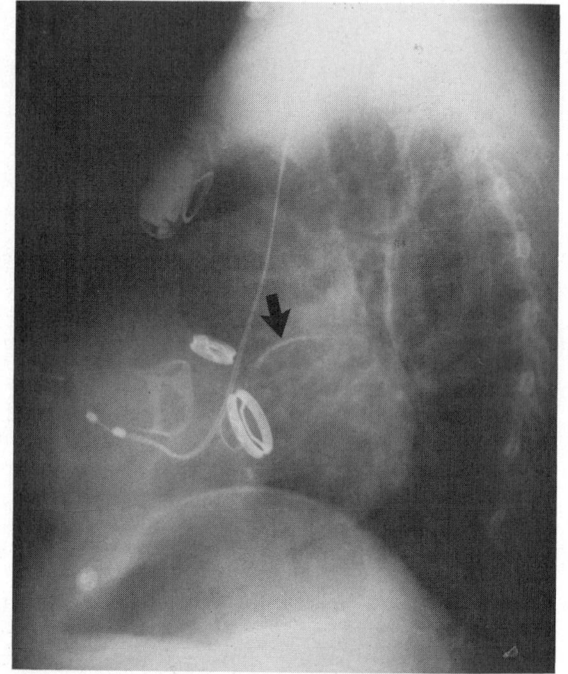

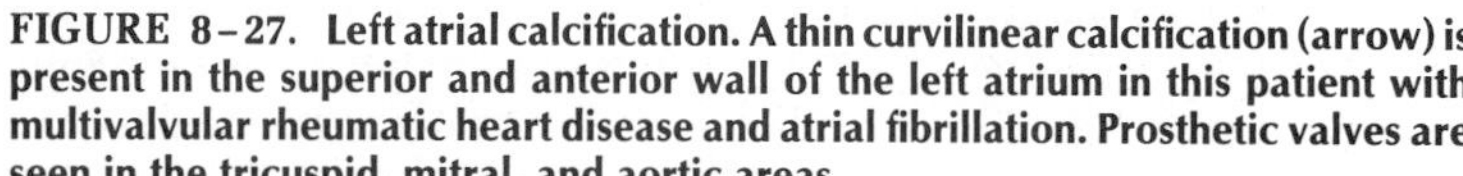
FIGURE 8–27. Left atrial calcification. A thin curvilinear calcification (arrow) is present in the superior and anterior wall of the left atrium in this patient with multivalvular rheumatic heart disease and atrial fibrillation. Prosthetic valves are seen in the tricuspid, mitral, and aortic areas.

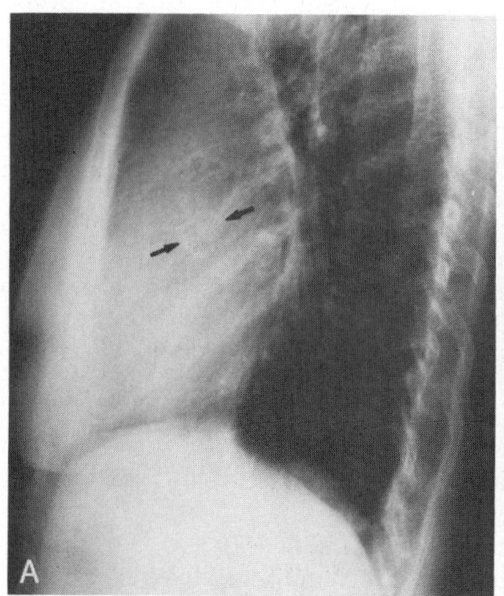

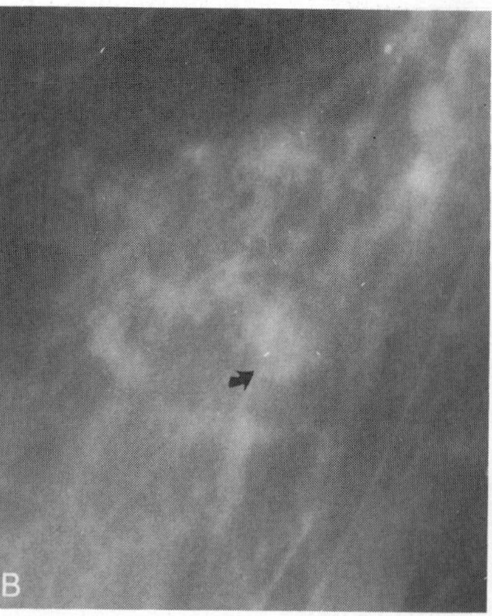

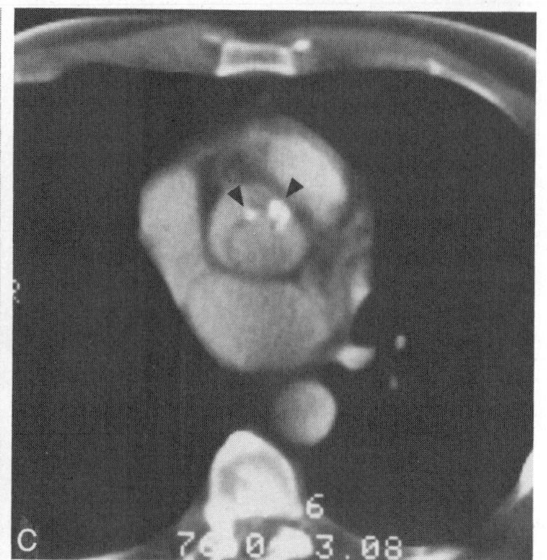

FIGURE 8–28. Aortic valve calcification. *A,* Lateral view shows the typical pattern of calcification of congenital bicuspid aortic valve in a 60-year-old woman with secondary aortic regurgitation (arrow). *B,* A fluoroscopic spot film shows the calcified valve to better advantage (curved arrow indicates calcified raphe). *C,* Cine CT demonstrates calcification of the aortic valve leaflets in a different patient with congenital bicuspid aortic valve (arrowheads). (Courtesy of Stephanie Flicker, M.D.)

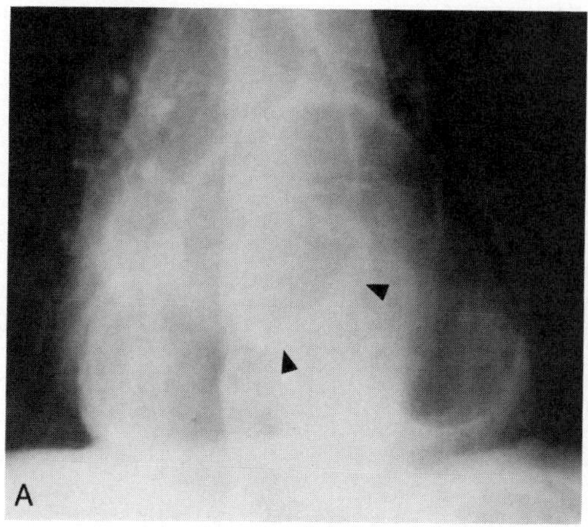

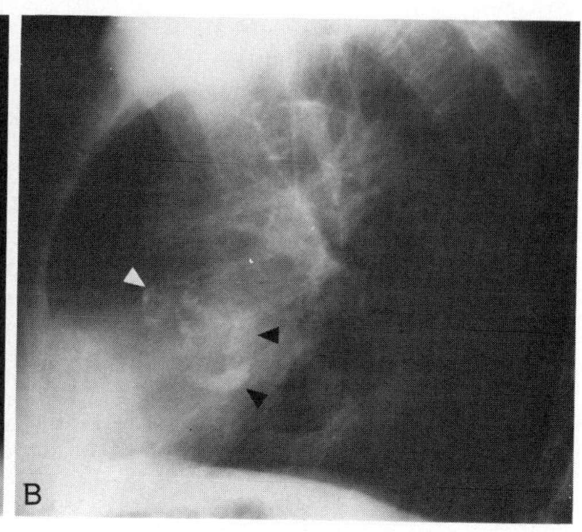

FIGURE 8–29. Calcified aortic and mitral annulus in an elderly woman. The air in a large hiatal hernia permits excellent visualization of the mitral annulus (arrows) in the PA view (*A*). In the lateral view (*B*), calcification can be seen in both the aortic (white arrowhead) and mitral (black arrowheads) annuli.

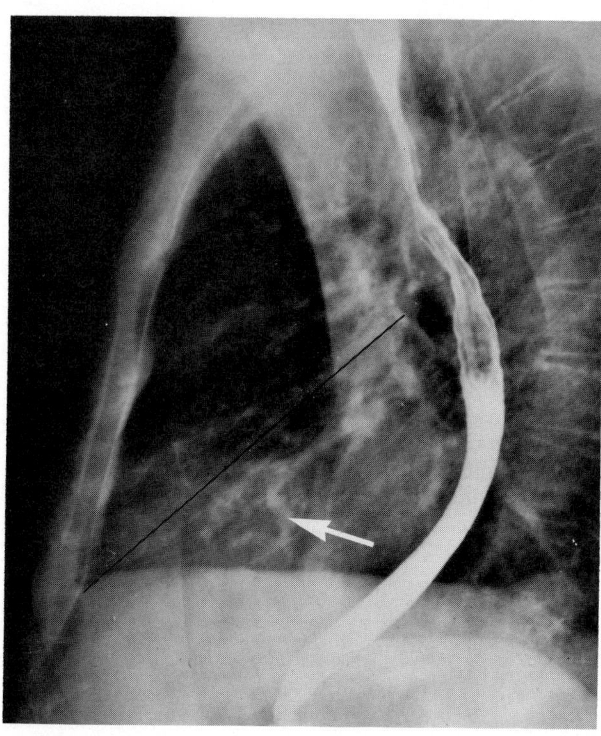

FIGURE 8–30. Mitral valve calcification in the lateral view. The valve calcification (arrow) lies below the line drawn from the left main bronchus to the anterior costophrenic sulcus localizing it to the mitral valve. The aortic valve in this view lies more anteriorly and above the line.

tients undergoing arteriography for coronary artery disease who also had cardiac fluoroscopy, 97 per cent of those with calcified coronary arteries on fluoroscopy had significant (≥70 per cent) coronary artery stenosis of at least one major vessel on arteriography. Of those with significant coronary disease on arteriography, 56 per cent had calcification on fluoroscopy.[34] Another study was performed in asymptomatic patients with Type II hyperlipidemia who were under the age of 55 years. Of those with both positive exercise tests and coronary calcification on fluoroscopy, 92 per cent had angiographically determined coronary artery disease. Fluoroscopy had an 82 per cent accuracy in the detection of significant (≥50 per cent) coronary artery disease.[72,73] In yet another study,[32] a randomly selected group of 108 asymptomatic men underwent cardiac fluoroscopy and exercise testing; 81 per cent with a positive exercise test had coronary calcifications; 35 per cent with calcified coronary arteries had a positive exercise test. Only 4 per cent of those without calcified coronary arteries had a positive exercise test. Finally, in this same series, 92 per cent had at least one critically stenosed (≥50 per cent) coronary artery diagnosed by angiography.[32]

Bartel el al. showed that approximately 90 per cent of patients with fluoroscopically detectable coronary calcifications had significant coronary disease.[34] Since exercise tests alone yield 10 to 20 per cent positive results in an asymptomatic middle-aged male population, fluoroscopy is an effective additional screening test for selection of patients with critical coronary artery disease. Fluoroscopy is most valuable when there is atypical chest pain or cardiomyopathy or for screening asymptomatic patients, particularly those at risk because of smoking, hyperlipidemia, and other prognostic indicators.

Coronary calcifications in the proximal left coronary artery may be identified in the frontal projection medial to the left atrial appendage. In the lateral view, calcification of the left anterior descending artery is often seen clearly as a double line of calcification extending along the anterior border of the cardiac silhouette. Circumflex and right coronary artery calcification may also be identified by means of chest radiography (Figs. 8–17 and 8–31).

CT is superior to fluoroscopy in the detection of coronary calcification[11,73] (Fig. 11–7, p. 316). Approximately twice as many patients will be found to have calcified coronary arteries with CT than with fluoroscopy.[74] There is a similar yield of critical coronary artery disease detection results when compared with those obtained by fluoroscopy. Although CT has been considered impractical as a screening test because of cost and availability, recent studies with cine CT have emphasized its value as a highly sensitive screening procedure in selected populations.[73,74] Since CT is performed routinely for other thoracic indications, it is important to make note of coronary calcifications and their distribution on CT to alert the clinician to their significance (Fig. 8–31).

CALCIFICATION OF THE GREAT VESSELS. The main pulmonary artery occasionally calcifies following surgery, particularly after infundibulectomy for total correction of tetralogy of Fallot. Calcification of the pulmonary artery is also found occasionally in severe longstanding pulmonary hypertension; calcified thrombi and emboli in the pulmonary artery may also occur. Aortic calcification, particularly in the region of the arch, is almost ubiquitous in individuals over the age of 50 years. It is usually noted on chest radiographs as a thin curvilinear opacity which may be more prominent when located deep to the aortic border in dissection (Fig. 8–32). Other causes of aortic calcification are syphilis (usually involving the ascending aorta), sinus of Valsalva aneurysm,[75] and Takayasu's arteritis.[76]

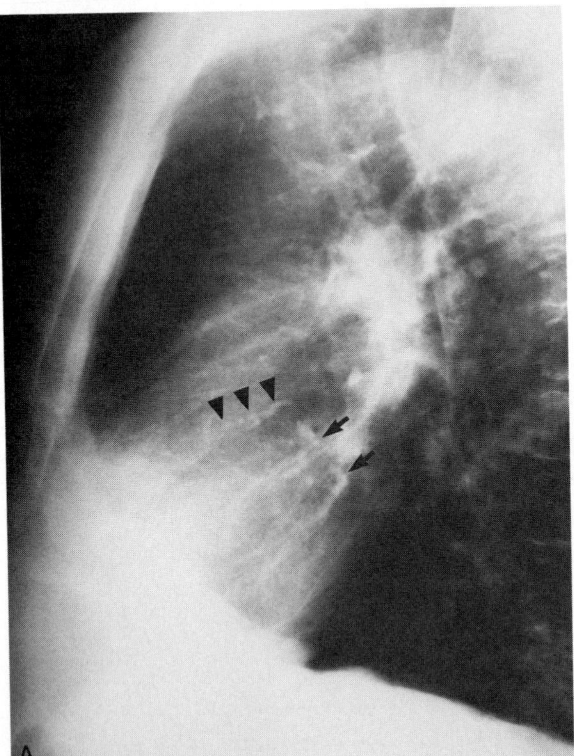

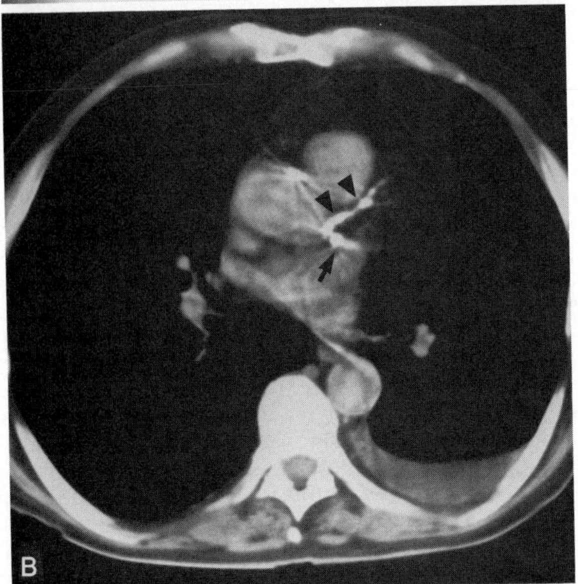

FIGURE 8–31. *A,* **Lateral view demonstrates the "tram track" pattern of coronary artery calcifications involving the left anterior descending (arrowheads) and circumflex coronary arteries (arrow).** *B,* **With cine CT calcifications of the left anterior descending (arrowhead) and circumflex arteries (arrow) are clearly identified.**

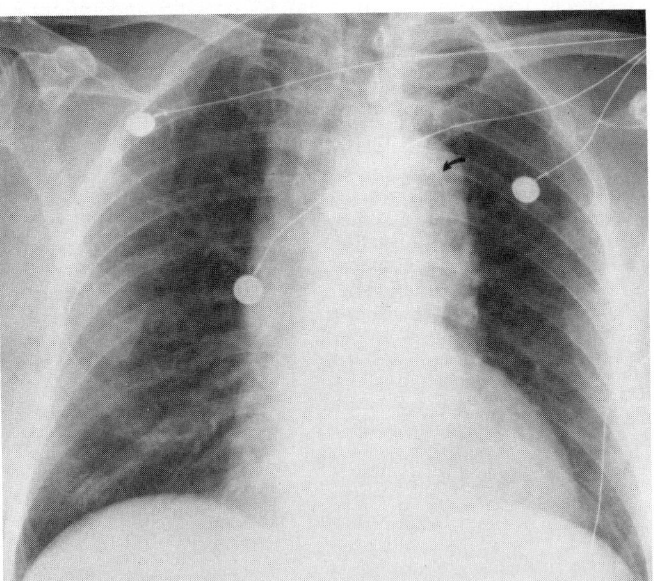

FIGURE 8–32. Calcified atherosclerotic plaque in the arch of the aorta deep to the outer surface of the vessel is demonstrated in this PA chest radiograph (arrow).

TUMOR CALCIFICATION (see also Chap. 44). The most common primary tumor of the heart is myxoma, most frequently occurring in the left atrium (p. 1454); 10 per cent will calcify sufficiently to be seen by x-ray.[77,77a] Occasionally, calcifications occurring in rhabdomyomas, fibromas,[78] osteosarcomas, and angiosarcomas are described. Calcifications in cardiac tumors vary from a speckled pattern to a large clump of calcium mimicking mitral valve calcification.[78a] Calcification may be visible on plain film or may be seen only with fluoroscopy or CT.[78b] With fluoroscopy, two-dimensional echocardiography, or cine CT, a calcified atrial tumor may be seen to prolapse through the atrioventricular valve during diastole.[3]

ACQUIRED HEART DISEASE

The diagnosis and assessment of the severity of acquired heart disease is assisted by a combination of imaging studies including plain films.[79,80] The chest x-ray is particularly useful to assess cardiac size and pulmonary vascularity and identify valvular, coronary artery, and myocardial calcification. It offers important clues to the enlargement of individual cardiac chambers, although cine angiography, echocardiography,[2,80a] and other cross-sectional imaging techniques are more reliable.[81,81a,81b] Nevertheless, the plain film remains a useful first examination in the work-up of the cardiac patient.[82]

VALVULAR HEART DISEASE

AORTIC STENOSIS (see also p. 1035). Aortic stenosis is due to reduction in the size of the aortic valve orifice from a normal cross-sectional area of 2.5 to 3.5 cm^2 to a cross-sectional area of less than 0.7 cm.^{2} With mild and moderate aortic stenosis, there is compensatory concentric hypertrophy of the left ventricle. With further increases in the severity of stenosis, cardiac output and left ventricular contractility decrease, resulting in left ventricular dilatation, elevated left ventricular end-diastolic pressure, and pulmonary venous pressure together with the signs and symptoms of congestive heart failure.

Typical roentgenographic changes of mild and moderate aortic stenosis include a normal-sized heart with rounding of the left ventricular border or a longer than normal heart with downward displacement of the cardiac apex due to left ventricular hypertrophy.[28,69] In most patients there is a discrete bulge on the right side of the ascending aorta due to poststenotic dilatation best visualized in the left anterior oblique or PA projection[26] (Fig. 8–8*A*). The aortic arch remains normal in size. Aortic valve calcification is frequent and increases with the severity of stenosis and the age of the patient so that by the age of 40 years, more than 90 per cent of patients with aortic stenosis have visible aortic calcification as demonstrated on the lateral chest x-ray.[26] Aortic valvular calcification has been associated with a peak systolic gradient of greater than 30 mm Hg in 97 per cent of another group of patients.[26] With cardiac decompensation, the left atrium and ventricle enlarge. The degree of enlargement of these chambers is correlated with increased severity of aortic stenosis and with mitral regurgitation due to left ventricular dilation or associated intrinsic mitral valve disease.

Congenital aortic stenosis (p. 922) may take two principal forms. One is a bicuspid valve with congenital commissural fusion and a central or eccentric orifice. The second form is an isolated bicuspid valve that is initially nonobstructive but undergoes commissural fusion with time. Recurrent trauma will cause irregular nodular scarring of both valve leaflets, which undergo gradual fusion and calcification[36] (Fig. 8–28). With time, these valves may also become regurgitant due to poor coaptation of the valve leaflets or because of infective endocarditis.

Degenerative and rheumatic aortic valvular stenoses are found in normally tricuspid valves. On the chest x-ray, thin or clumped calcifications are found in the area of the aortic valve leaflets and annulus. In patients with rheumatic aortic stenosis, mitral calcifications can also be seen.[28,79]

Both the obstructive and nonobstructive forms of hypertrophic cardiomyopathy and membranous subaortic stenosis are characterized radiographically by left ventricular enlargement.[4,80] Dilatation of the ascending aorta is absent or of mild degree. No calcification of the aortic valve is seen. Left atrial enlargement, when present, usually is associated with mitral regurgitation.[80]

AORTIC REGURGITATION (see also p. 1043). This lesion may result from a bicuspid valve that is stenotic and then develops regurgitation due to endocarditis or degeneration. Rheumatic fever and infective endocarditis are other important primary causes. A secondary cause of aortic regurgitation is dilatation of the aortic annulus (p. 1044) in diseases preferentially affecting the ascending aorta, such as ankylosing spondylitis, annuloaortic ectasia, Marfan syndrome (Fig. 8–33), Reiter's syndrome, psoriatic arthritis, and others.[82,83] The aortic regurgitation found in rheumatic heart disease is commonly associated with mitral regurgitation. Aortic regurgitation may also be caused by trauma or may accompany dissection of the ascending aorta.

In mild aortic regurgitation, the aorta is normal or mildly enlarged and the left ventricle is normal in size. With moderate or severe regurgitation, there is increased dilatation of the left ventricle, and the cardiothoracic ratio usually exceeds 0.5 (Figs. 8–3 and 8–8*B*). The aorta is diffusely dilated, unlike in aortic stenosis, in which only the ascending portion is involved. If the sinus portion of the ascending aorta is the only portion selectively dilated, Marfan syndrome (annuloaortic ectasia) is the most likely diagnosis (Fig. 8–33). If the ascending aorta is also calcified, syphilis is a likely diagnostic possibility. If the valve itself is calcified, aortic regurgitation secondary to a congenital bicuspid aortic valve should be considered.

MITRAL STENOSIS (see also p. 1007). Rheumatic carditis is the most common cause of mitral stenosis. Left atrial myxoma, and, rarely, congenital mitral stenosis are also causes of mitral valve obstruction. Early roentgenographic signs of mitral stenosis are often subtle and include mild left atrial enlargement and posterior displacement of the barium-filled esophagus on the lateral chest view. The left ventricle is of normal size and the pulmonary vessels are normal in appearance.

With more severe stenosis, the left atrium usually increases further in size; however, in any given patient, there is poor correlation between the severity of mitral stenosis and the size of the left atrial chamber.[84] The left atrial appendage is disproportionately enlarged except in those patients with thrombus, in whom the left atrial border may be flat[68,85,86] (Figs. 8–34 and 8–35). The right atrium is displaced to the right and there is evidence of vascular redistribution or "cephalization" of pulmonary blood flow to the upper lobes. The main pulmonary artery is enlarged and the left ventricle and aorta are usually small. Often, the mitral valve is calcified. In addition, calcification of the left atrial wall (often associated with atrial fibrillation) may be seen. Left atrial wall calcification is most common in the posterior portion of the left atrial chamber and the appendage in patients with rheumatic heart disease. There is evidence of pulmonary interstitial edema, characterized by Kerley B lines at the lung bases as pulmonary venous pressure rises above 25 mm Hg.[56,84] Interlobular effusions are also seen as Kerley C lines, a reticular pattern representing superimposed Kerley B lines. Kerley A lines are best seen in the lateral projection as long, opaque lines merging into the hila representing thickened perivascular connective tissue planes.[58-60] Hemosiderosis due to recurrent small hemorrhages because of chronically elevated capillary pressure is associated with chronic mitral stenosis. The radiological appearance of hemo-

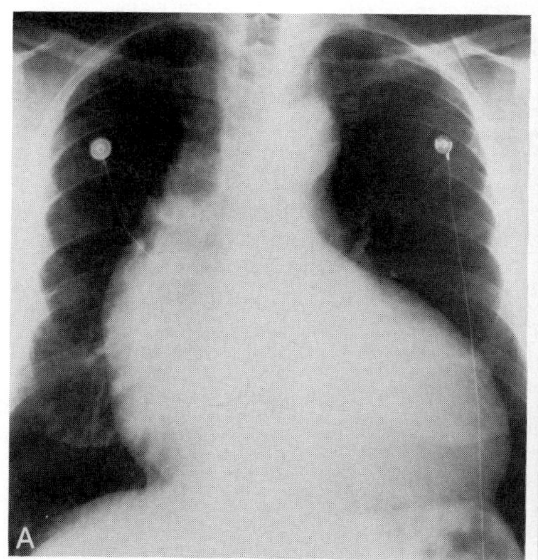

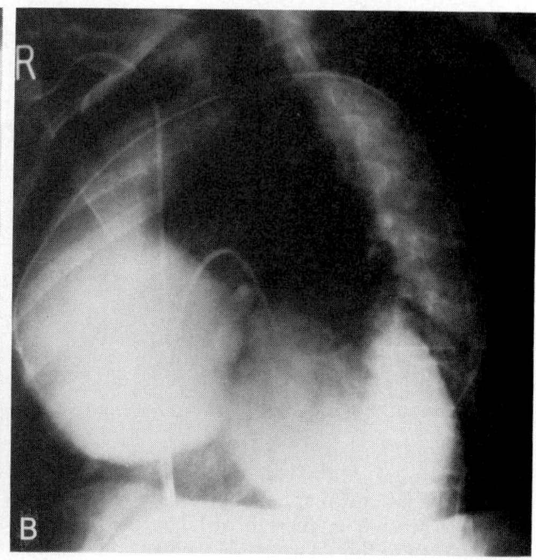

FIGURE 8–33. Aortic regurgitation in Marfan syndrome. *A*, There is marked left ventricular enlargement and aortic dilatation in this patient with aortic regurgitation. *B*, Aortography shows marked ascending aortic enlargement with regurgitation at the aortic valve.

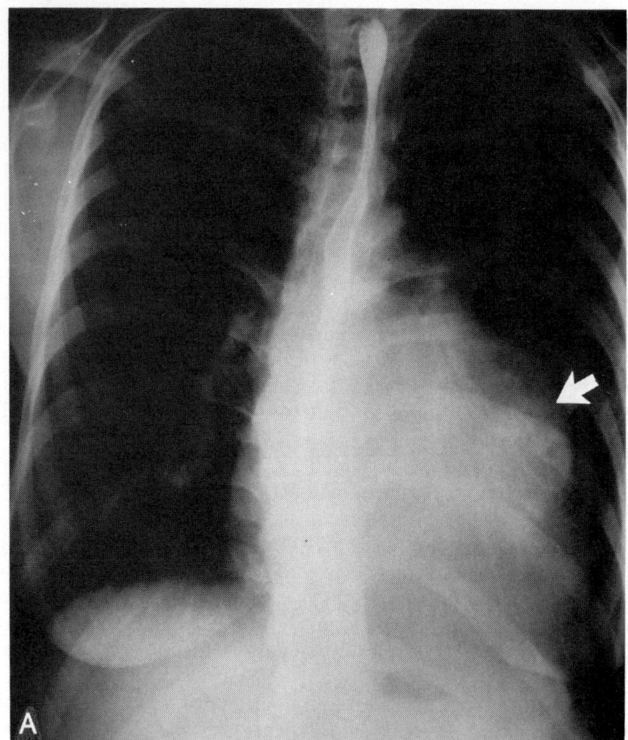

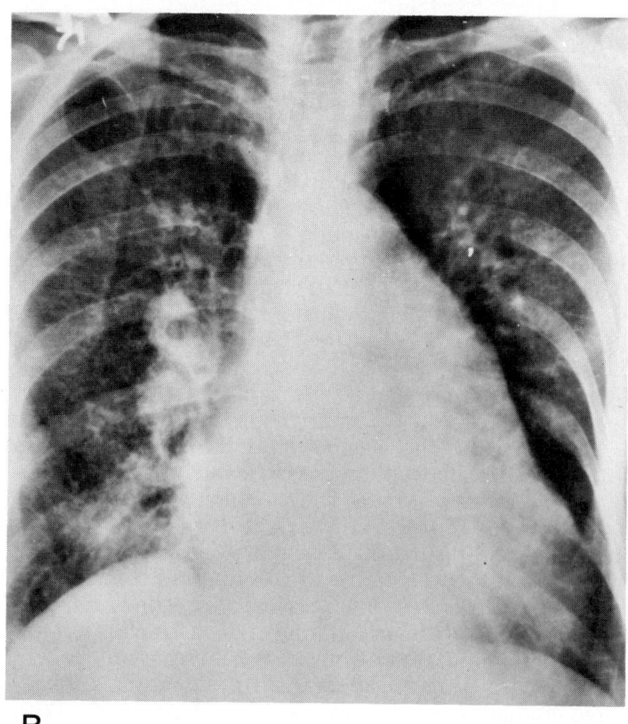

FIGURE 8–34. Mitral stenosis. *A,* The left atrial border is prominently convex. The aorta is small in this 19-year-old patient with mitral stenosis (arrow). *B,* In another patient, the lungs are studded with small nodules of moderate radiodensity due to hemosiderosis. The left atrium and left ventricle are enlarged. Kerley B lines are present in the lateral basal portions of the lungs.

siderosis is that of interstitial or miliary lung disease most prominent in the mid and lower lung zones[21] (Fig. 8–34*B*). With chronic pulmonary interstitial edema, pulmonary ossifications may be found as small islands of bone within the alveoli and visible as dense nodules on chest x-ray.

MITRAL REGURGITATION (see also p. 1018). Acute mitral regurgitation may be related to ruptured chordae tendinae, ischemic dysfunction or rupture of the papillary muscles, or infective endocarditis. In acute mitral regurgitation, while the heart may not be enlarged, severe pulmonary edema is frequently present as a result of left-sided cardiac failure.[87,88] Chronic mitral regurgitation may be secondary to rheumatic heart disease, mitral prolapse due to myxomatous degeneration, infective endocarditis, ischemic cardiomyopathy, hypertrophic cardiomyopathy, extensive mitral annulus calcification, Marfan syndrome, and congenital lesions such as parachute mitral valve. In chronic mitral regurgitation, the left atrium is enlarged and may be massive in size because of volume overload and increased pressure; the left ventricle is also enlarged. The enlarged left atrium may extend toward the right and may be seen as a double shadow along the right atrial border. In the left anterior oblique view it causes upward displacement of the left main stem bronchus. Coexistent pulmonary arterial hypertension or tricuspid regurgitation may cause dilatation of the right atrium and ventricle and enlargement of the pulmonary arteries.[10]

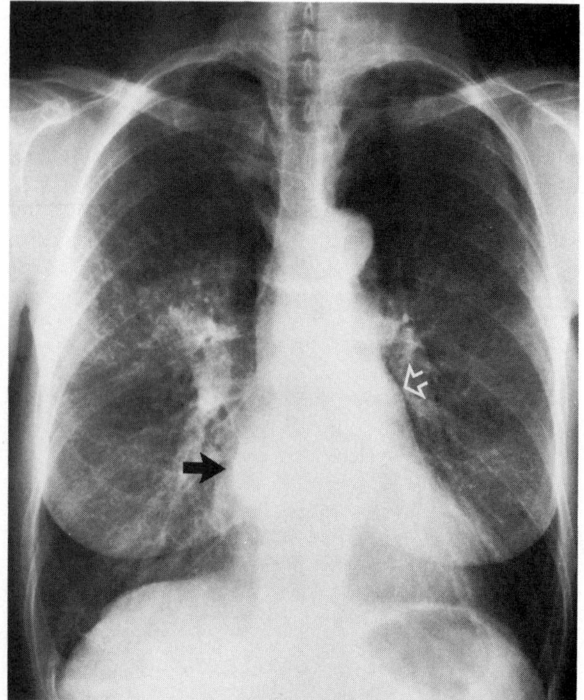

FIGURE 8–35. Mitral stenosis. There is a subtle convex bulge at the level of the left atrial appendage (white open arrow). A double atrial shadow is present on the right atrial border (black arrow). The heart is not enlarged in this 54-year-old woman with mitral stenosis.

ISCHEMIC HEART DISEASE

(See also Chaps. 39 and 40)

Many imaging modalities contribute to the diagnosis of ischemic heart disease, including coronary arteriography, radionuclide scintigraphy, echocardiography, CT, and MRI.[89,90] The chest roentgenogram can be entirely normal even in patients with advanced disease; however, left ventricular enlargement and/or aneurysm are often present. Plain film studies, fluoroscopy, and CT may demonstrate calcification of the coronary arteries.[11,32,33,34] Following myocardial infarction, pulmonary edema can occur, even in patients with a normal-sized heart. When congestive heart failure persists in spite of treatment, complications of myocardial infarction, including aneurysm, papillary muscle rupture, and interventricular septal defect, should be ruled out.[89,91]

Postmyocardial infarction interventricular septal defect occurs in 0.5 to 1.0 per cent of patients and can be characterized by cardiomegaly, pulmonary edema, and poor myocardial contractility. The typical shunt pattern may not be appreciated because of pulmonary edema but can emerge months

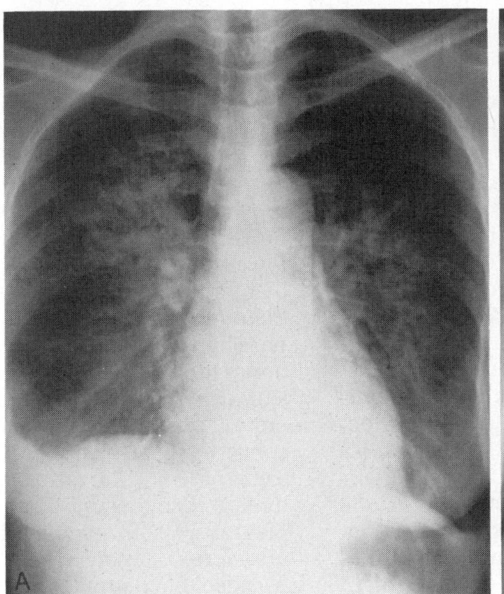

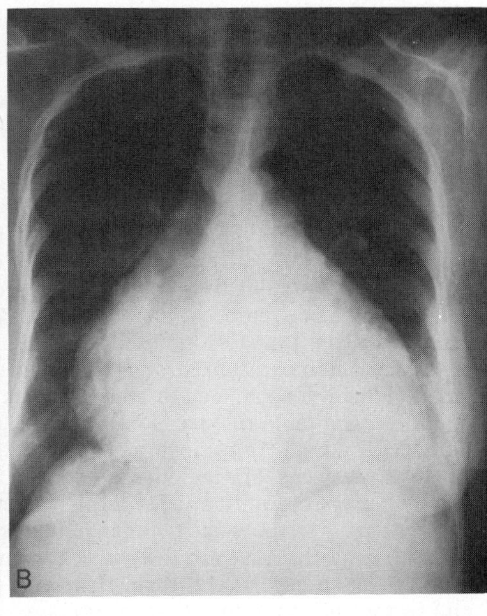

FIGURE 8-36. ***A,*** **Acute postmyocardial infarction papillary muscle dysfunction. Acute pulmonary interstitial edema is present but there is no cardiac enlargement.** ***B,*** **Dilated cardiomyopathy. There is diffuse dilatation of the heart in this woman with systemic lupus erythematosus.**

later if the patient survives. Such defects usually involve the muscular septum and occur within one week after myocardial infarction. Two-thirds of postmyocardial infarction ventricular septal defects occur in the anterior apical portion of the left ventricle and one-third occur in the posterior portion.[89,89a] The roentgenographic picture of postmyocardial infarction syndrome (Dressler syndrome)[92] is that of an enlarged heart due to pericardial effusion, pleural effusion, and lower lobe consolidation. It occurs weeks to months following the infarction and is analogous to the postpericardiotomy syndrome.

Aneurysm of the left ventricle is an abnormal bulge or outpouching of the myocardial wall that develops in 12 to 15 per cent of patients following myocardial infarction.[89] It occurs most commonly at the cardiac apex or the anterior wall. The chest film shows a localized bulge along the left ventricular wall near the apex with or without a thin rim of calcification (Figs. 8-8C and 8-26). Angiography, CT, MRI, and echocardiograms will also show the filling defect of a mural thrombus (if one is present) in the aneurysm. The differential diagnosis of aneurysm of the left ventricle includes pericardial cyst, mediastinal tumor, and thymoma. Cardiac rupture usually occurs in patients who have had acute transmural infarction.[93] Most die immediately, but in a minority of patients the rupture is contained and a pseudoaneurysm is formed. Radiographically, a paracardiac mass is present with sharply marginated edges free of calcification. The mass is usually posterior on the lateral view, unlike the more anterior position of a true aneurysm.[93] A firm diagnosis is made by echocardiography, MRI, or ventriculography. Coronary arteriography will show a complete absence of vessels in the region of the pseudoaneurysm wall, unlike a true aneurysm, which may have a rim of mural vessels.

The development of papillary muscle rupture following myocardial infarction occurs in approximately 1 per cent of patients. Plain radiographic findings vary from a normal chest examination to a marked increase in cardiac size with left ventricular and atrial enlargement as well as pulmonary edema (Fig. 8-36*A*). Left ventriculography or echocardiography will demonstrate the flail mitral valve leaflets and help in estimating the degree of mitral regurgitation.[89]

CARDIOMYOPATHY

(See also Chap. 43)

Cardiomyopathy describes a spectrum of myocardial disorders, including dilated or congestive, hypertrophic, restrictive, and ischemic cardiomyopathies.[21,26,94] In congestive, dilated, and ischemic cardiomyopathy, ventricular ejection fraction is reduced, often severely. Chest radiographs show diffuse nonspecific cardiac enlargement that may resemble a large pericardial effusion (Fig. 8-36*B*). Echocardiography will show decreased ventricular contraction and enlargement of the left atrium and ventricle. In time, the right atrium and ventricle will also enlarge. Doppler echocardiography may reveal mitral regurgitation caused by dilatation of the valve annulus. With time, left-sided and eventually biventricular failure will occur in most patients, an important predictive indicator of shortened survival.[94]

The pathophysiology of hypertrophic cardiomyopathy is discussed on p. 1404. Chest views demonstrate a normal heart or enlargement of the left ventricle, which can be focal or diffuse. If mitral regurgitation is present, the left atrium is enlarged. Unlike aortic valvular stenosis, no ascending aortic dilatation is present unless the patient has coincidental systemic hypertension or atherosclerotic uncoiling of the aorta.[2,80,95] The diagnosis is established by echocardiography. Cardiac catheterization and angiography are reserved for those cases in which noninvasive techniques are technically inadequate, coronary disease is suspected, or surgery is contemplated.[4] Angiography demonstrates, in systole, a narrow slit-like left ventricular chamber, marked wall thickening, and hyperdynamic contractions. CT and MRI are alternatives to angiography.[4,96,97,98]

Restrictive cardiomyopathy (p. 1415) is characterized by marked myocardial rigidity with poor left ventricular diastolic relaxation.[4,99] Radiographically, there are no consistent features of restrictive cardiomyopathy. The heart is normal in size or may be moderately or even markedly enlarged. The left atrium may also be enlarged when mitral regurgitation is present. Pulmonary congestion occurs in most patients, and calcification of the right or left ventricular wall may be seen. Contrast ventriculography demonstrates rapid relaxation during early diastole followed by "plateauing" and absence of an "atrial kick."

THE POSTOPERATIVE CHEST ROENTGENOGRAM

(See also Chap. 53)

With the great increase in coronary bypass graft surgery and the frequency of other cardiac surgical procedures, the postoperative chest roentgenogram has become one of the most frequently ordered studies. In the department of radiology at Thomas Jefferson University Hospital, over 50 per cent of inpatient chest x-rays are performed at the bedside, usually in the intensive care unit. About one-third of these studies are of postsurgical cardiac patients. In order to interpret adequately the postoperative chest x-ray, special attention must be given to optimization of technique.[100,101] Adequate equipment and careful positioning are needed to overcome the effects of low-capacity portable equipment and motion artifacts. Knowledge of the appearance of the preoperative film will often aid in clarifying abnormalities seen in the portable postoperative x-ray. When the pre- and postoperative films are compared, the differences in cardiac size between the preoperative erect PA and the postoperative supine AP films must be taken into account.[102,103]

Most cardiac surgery is performed through an extrapleural median sternotomy with the use of cardiopulmonary bypass. Except for specific problems related to the patient's preexisting cardiac disorder or to the specific surgical procedure, alterations in the postoperative chest film are common to all cardiac surgical procedures. Ideally, the lungs will appear normal with slight mediastinal widening due to intraoperative edema or hemorrhage. However, varying degrees of subsegmental lower lobe atelectasis are present in most patients, related to incomplete reexpansion of the lungs after cardiopulmonary bypass. A number of tubes and catheters are present in the postoperative chest. An endotracheal tube is virtually always present and should be positioned 5 to 7 cm above the carina to allow excursion in both flexion and extension of the neck.[104] A central venous pressure catheter is placed in the superior vena cava. However, its tip is often found in the right atrium, in which pressure measurements are accurate. There is, however, an increased risk of arrhythmia when this occurs.[18] A Swan-Ganz catheter is placed in the pulmonary artery (ideally with the tip lying in a dependent branch) (Fig. 8–37) to monitor pulmonary artery or pulmonary capillary wedge pressure and because of the need to obtain mixed venous blood samples.

Anterior mediastinal drainage catheters are located in the parasternal area, and posterior mediastinal drainage catheters usually lie on the left behind the heart. Epicardial pacing wires project over the heart and lungs.[105,106] When circulatory assistance is needed, an intraaortic counterpulsation balloon catheter may be positioned with its tip just below the level of the left subclavian artery within the proximal descending aorta.[107] Pacemaker leads,[18] prosthetic valves[40] (Fig. 8–18), and an implantable cardioverter-defibrillator[108] require careful observation for lead or component malposition or fracture. A nasogastric tube is also usually present.

THE EARLY POSTOPERATIVE FILM. The first postoperative chest film usually demonstrates varying degrees of lower lobe atelectasis, mediastinal widening, pulmonary edema, and pleural effusion. Bilateral and unilateral lower lobe atelectasis is the source of lower lobe opacities found in almost all cardiac surgery patients.[106] Elevation of the involved hemidiaphragm is also present.[107] The lower lobe opacities usually

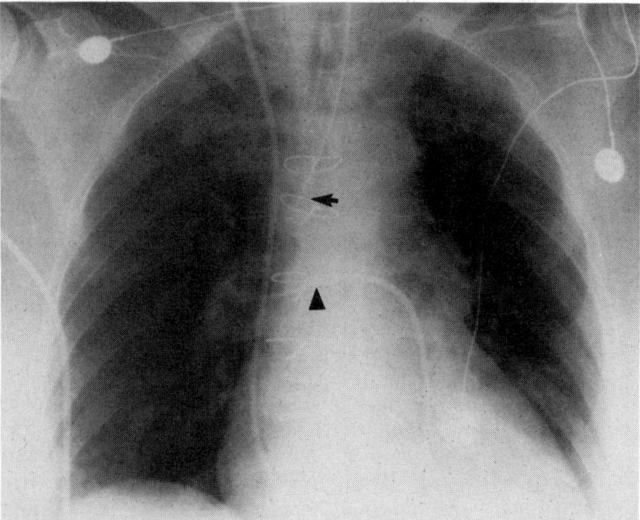

FIGURE 8–37. An early postoperative chest radiograph. There is a Swan-Ganz catheter in the right pulmonary artery (arrowhead). The endotracheal tube lies 2 cm above the carina (black arrow). It should be repositioned proximally to prevent selective bronchial placement.

appear within 8 hours after surgery and clear within 5 to 7 days. Although pneumonia can occur as a complication, it is unusual. These changes occur most commonly on the left side. The mechanisms for preferential left lower lobe atelectasis include paralysis of the phrenic nerve caused by cardioplegic solutions administered for myocardial preservation and retained secretions.[107] Decreased diaphragmatic motion may persist for many weeks after surgery but will usually resolve. Small pleural effusions are frequent and usually accompany lower lobe atelectasis. Radiographically, they are manifested by blunting of the costophrenic angle, loss of sharpness of the diaphragmatic contour, and increased opacity behind the diaphragmatic dome. These effusions are probably related to pericardial fluid that leaks into the pleural space through the surgically created pericardial window or to irritation of the pleura during surgery. Postpericardiotomy syndrome and congestive heart failure are the sources of pleural effusions in some patients. Larger or persistent pleural effusions may be due to hemomediastinum, with blood escaping into the pleural space through a pleural tear. Larger pleural effusions are more common in left internal mammary bypass surgery because the pleural space is entered in that procedure.

Patchy consolidation in both lungs is usually caused by some form of pulmonary edema. Capillary permeability pulmonary edema or adult respiratory distress syndrome is common after cardiac surgery, because of vasoactive substances released during cardiopulmonary bypass which affect capillary permeability.[106] Pulmonary edema usually occurs within 2 days of surgery and is reversible with supportive therapy including diuretics.[106] Postperfusion pulmonary edema occurs after cardiopulmonary bypass, which causes a marked increase in fluid in the extravascular space. The mechanism for postperfusion pulmonary edema is thought to be related to the contact of blood with foreign surfaces during bypass.[102] Congestive heart failure following cardiac surgery occurs in patients with poor cardiac output after bypass. Typically, vascular redistribution to the upper lobes, Kerley B lines, small bilateral effusions, and the patchy opacities due to pulmonary edema are present (Figs. 8–23 and 8–24).

Other early complications include fractures of the first three ribs, sternal dehiscence, pneumothorax, pneumomediastinum, pneumopericardium, and subcutaneous emphysema. Rib fractures occur in 2 to 4 per cent of patients and are usually identified by plain films, although additional fractures may be found with radionuclide scanning. Their importance lies in the possible misdiagnosis of chest pain of another cause including angina or dissection.

Pneumothorax is often difficult to identify in the supine patient. It is characterized as a poorly defined radiolucency overlying the lower lung fields. Decubitus views are helpful in clearly defining the presence of a pleural air collection. Pneumomediastinum may occur when the mediastinum is entered during surgery. In most cases the mediastinal air resolves spontaneously within several days. A radiolucency in the middle of the sternum following sternotomy is due to a small gap in the sternum and soft tissues at the surgical site; this occurs in approximately one-third of patients. There is no proven correlation between this thin radiolucency and sternal dehiscence.[108]

Mediastinal hemorrhage is common after cardiac surgery but seldom is serious enough to require reoperation (Fig. 8–38). In general, in these cases the mediastinum is widened by up to 35 per cent compared with preoperative PA chest films. Katzberg et al. found that if the mediastinum is widened more than 70 per cent compared with the baseline radiograph, surgery is usually required to remove the hematoma.[101] However, considerable bleeding may be present without visible mediastinal widening, especially if the patient is receiving PEEP therapy that compresses the mediastinum. Some patients may have a wide mediastinum but are hemodynamically stable, have no significant bloody drainage, and do not require reoperation. Enlargement of the cardiac silhouette occurring during the early postoperative period may be due to cardiac failure with or without myocardial infarction or to a mediastinal

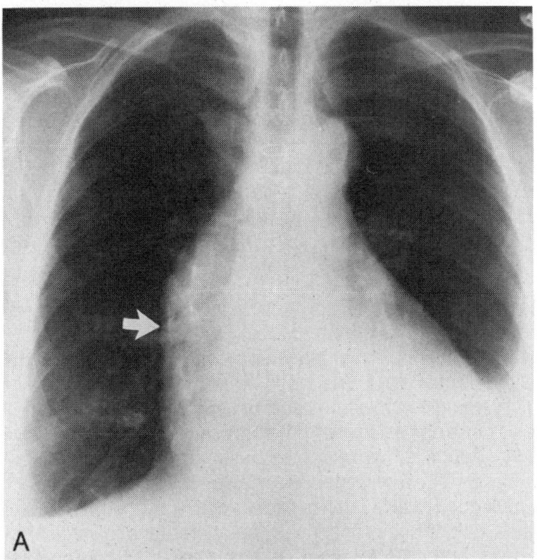

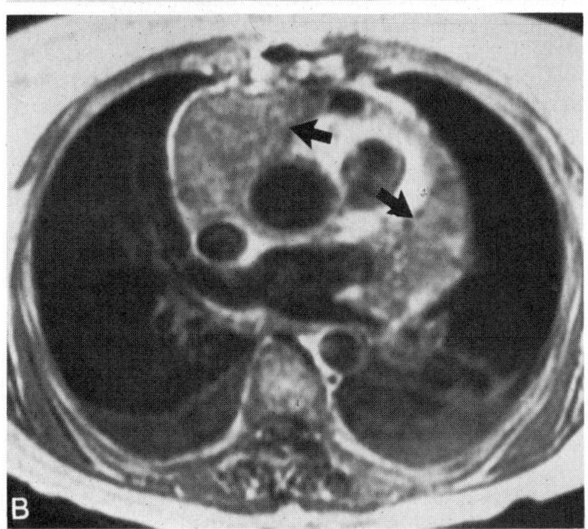

FIGURE 8–38. Mediastinal hemorrhage. ***A,*** **There is marked widening of the right side of the mediastinum in the area of the ascending aorta (arrow). A large left pleural effusion is also present three days after CABG surgery.** ***B,*** **MRI demonstrates a large mediastinal hematoma which was subsequently drained (arrows).**

or pericardial fluid collection. In some patients, pericardial tamponade occurs from bleeding of small arteries in the area of the sternal incision.[109] Equalization of diastolic pressures and elevation of the pulmonary capillary wedge pressure without pulmonary redistribution or edema, together with diffuse enlargement of the cardiac silhouette, suggests pericardial tamponade (p. 1473). Although x-ray is suggestive, CT or echocardiography will reveal the presence of pericardial fluid. CT is the procedure of choice to detect a mediastinal fluid collection.[109] Because of the sternotomy, echocardiography may be technically difficult as a result of the presence of mediastinal drains and pneumomediastinum.

LATE COMPLICATIONS OF CARDIAC SURGERY. The postpericardiotomy syndrome (p. 1503) is a common late complication of cardiac surgery characterized by pleuritis, pericarditis, and fever. It is thought to be the result of an immune response to the necrotic epicardium. It generally occurs several weeks after surgery and is self-limited. Occasionally, cardiac tamponade or constrictive pericarditis will occur as a complication of the postpericardiotomy syndrome. Radiographically, unilateral or bilateral pleural effusions, diffuse enlargement of the cardiac silhouette caused by pericardial effusion, and small basilar pulmonary opacities are found. Echocardiography or CT will identify the pleural or pericardial fluid collections.[110] Other late postoperative complications of cardiac surgery include sternal osteomyelitis, dehiscence, and mediastinitis. There is an increased risk of pseudoaneurysm of the thoracic aorta associated with sternal and mediastinal inflammation. Pseudoaneurysm is a rare but serious complication that can occur at the site of an aortic cannulation or vent, the aortic clamp line, or the saphenous graft–aortic anastomosis (Fig. 8–39). Cardiac pseudoaneurysms can occur at sites where full thickness cardiac incisions were made. Although plain-film radiographs will demonstrate a mass in the cardiac or aortic regions, CT or MRI is diagnostic and should be performed before reoperation.[111–113] Aortic dissection occurs very rarely in patients who have undergone surgery of the aorta and aortic valve replacement, but should be considered in the differential diagnosis of mediastinal widening or anterior mediastinal mass. A dissection may appear immediately after operation but more likely will occur weeks to months later. Although aortography is diagnostic, contrast enhanced CT will permit distinction between dissection on the one hand, and hematoma, abscess, tumor, or prominent mediastinal fat on the other.

PROSTHETIC VALVE SURGERY. The chest roentgenogram is helpful when following patients for the potential complications of valve implantation. Localization of the prosthetic valve is not as simple as with calcified native cardiac valves because only an AP film may be available during the early postoperative period and the prosthetic valves vary in position and often overlap.[114,115] If the patient fails to improve clinically after valve replacement or if there is pulmonary edema after a brief period of improvement, malfunction of the prosthetic valve may be the cause. Major malfunctions result from sewing ring dehiscence (Fig. 8–18), strut fracture, tissue encroachment into the ring orifice, disc or poppet thrombosis, and infective endocarditis.[39,40] Plain films may show enlargement of the involved cardiac chambers or pulmonary edema.[116] Calcification of a tissue valve may suggest degeneration and valve insufficiency.[115] Fracture and separation of mechanical components and their distal migration may be identified.[42,43]

Fluoroscopy documents valve motion, the integrity of the mechanical components, and the presence of calcification. If there is more than 12 degrees of rocking of the mitral or aortic sewing ring in systole and diastole, prosthesis dehiscence at the ring should be considered[41] (Fig. 8–18). Reduced excursion of the valve occluder, e.g., less than 60 degrees for the Björk-Shiley hinged disc valve, suggests thrombus or vegetation. Doppler echocardiography will document regurgitant blood flow proximal to the valve. Cine CT[12,117] is a complementary study for the diagnosis of valvular regurgitation. Pseudoaneurysm formation in the area of the aortic root can

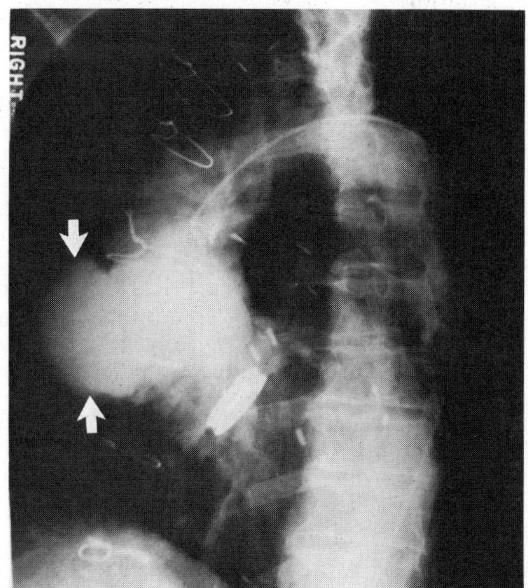

FIGURE 8–39. Pseudoaneurysm of the ascending aorta. This saccular pseudoaneurysm (arrows) developed five months after valve replacement at the aortotomy site in a 78-year-old man. (From Sullivan, K. L., et al.: Pseudoaneurysm of the ascending aorta following cardiac surgery. Chest ***93:*****138, 1988.)**

occur as a result of infection or weakened aortic wall secondary to the surgical procedure[113,118] (Fig. 8–39).

CORONARY ARTERY SURGERY. Early radiological findings after coronary bypass surgery are nonspecific and are similar to those of other cardiac surgical procedures. These include mediastinal widening, left pleural effusion, and pulmonary consolidation or atelectasis. The signs of pneumopericardium and pulmonary edema are less common abnormalities following coronary artery bypass graft surgery.[50] Radiological evaluation of coronary bypass grafts sometimes aids in distinguishing graft occlusion from other causes of postoperative chest pain. CT (particularly cine CT)[73,119] and MRI[120] have been used with success to determine graft patency (Fig. 11–6, p. 316). However, these noninvasive techniques do not exclude nonocclusive stenosis nor do they document progression of disease in native vessels. They do not eliminate the need to perform cardiac catheterization in patients in whom reoperation is contemplated. MRI has an accuracy of 91 per cent for determination of patency and 72 per cent for determination of occlusion.[120] This compares with CT, which exhibits 85 to 95 per cent accuracy in demonstrating occlusions and up to 100 per cent accuracy in demonstrating patency.[119]

CARDIAC TRANSPLANTATION (see also Chap. 18). Most transplant candidates have a history of end-stage cardiac failure caused by ischemic heart disease or cardiomyopathy. The heart is invariably enlarged and pulmonary vascular redistribution or edema is generally present. In orthotopic cardiac transplantation, the recipient heart is removed and the donor heart with an intact aorta and pulmonary arteries is attached to a cuff of native left atrium containing the pulmonary veins. Following transplant surgery, typical radiographic changes associated with median sternotomy are found, including a widened mediastinum, pleural effusion, left lower lobe consolidation, and atelectasis. Within 2 months, the heart becomes smaller and it reaches stability 6 months after transplant surgery. Persistent cardiomegaly most likely is caused by pericardial effusion, which may result from cyclosporin therapy or placement of a small donor heart in a large pericardial sac. The normal postoperative radiograph often has a double density in the vicinity of the right atrial border because of the overlapping donor and recipient atria. MRI and CT clearly depict postoperative transplantation anatomy as well as pericardial effusion and lymphadenopathy.[121]

When graft rejection occurs, the heart enlarges but pulmonary edema is usually not present. The diagnosis of rejection is made by endomyocardial biopsy showing increased lymphocytic infiltration and myocytic necrosis.[122] MRI can demonstrate alterations in signal intensity in moderate and severe rejection.[123] Accelerated coronary atherosclerosis can lead to myocardial infarction and left ventricular enlargement. Pulmonary infection due to immunosuppressive therapy is common; bacterial, viral, fungal, and protozoal infections can all occur.

Heart-lung transplantation is usually performed in patients with a history of primary pulmonary hypertension, end-stage chronic pulmonary disease with right ventricular decompensation, or Eisenmenger physiology. Early complications in the immunosuppressed patient include cytomegalovirus and bacterial pneumonia. Long-term sequelae include accelerated coronary atherosclerosis and bronchiolitis obliterans with or without organizing pneumonia. The parenchymal pattern of bronchiolitis obliterans is characterized by coarse, asymmetrical nodular or reticular-nodular densities throughout the lungs and relative sparing of the upper lobes.[124–126]

CONGENITAL HEART DISEASE IN THE ADULT

(See also Chap. 32)

Congenital cardiac disorders in adults fall into three different clinical groups: those whose cardiac disorder was recognized in childhood and surgically treated, those whose cardiac abnormalities were recognized but did not undergo surgery and were followed medically, and those patients who survived into adulthood with unrecognized or misdiagnosed congenital cardiac disease.[83]

The radiological findings in adult congenital heart disease can be classified in a number of ways based on the frequency of the disorder or a combination of the hallmarks of disease, including the state of the pulmonary vasculature, the position of the aortic arch, cardiac size and abdominal situs.[127–128c] Combining the radiological findings with a history of the presence or absence of cyanosis, the time of onset of cardiac murmur, and the clinical state of the patient should narrow the diagnostic choices.

CONGENITAL BICUSPID AORTIC VALVE

(See also p. 967)

Congenital bicuspid aortic valve is the most common congenital anomaly of the heart, occurring in up to 2 per cent of the population.[36,83] Aortic stenosis that presents first in the young adult is associated with bicuspid aortic valve in most cases. The aortic valve in this condition has a single or two partially fused commissures and an eccentric orifice. With time, valvular stenosis develops as a result of progressive fusion of the valve leaflets and calcific deposits, which often assume a ring-like or a ring-knob shape[36] (Fig. 8–28). Aortic stenosis may be followed years later by aortic regurgitation due to valve deformity or infective endocarditis. Radiographical findings include the presence of the characteristic valve calcification. The left heart border is rounded and the apex may be downwardly displaced due to left ventricular hypertrophy. The ascending aorta is dilated (Fig. 8–8*A*). The diagnosis is usually confirmed by echocardiography. Cine CT can demonstrate both the calcified aortic valve and left ventricular wall hypertrophy (Fig. 8–28*C*). MRI can demonstrate valvular regurgitation.

COARCTATION OF THE AORTA (See also p. 967)

Coarctation of the aorta is a common anomaly, accounting for 8 per cent of congenital heart defects in children and about 6 per cent of adult congenital heart disease.[83] In the adult patient, localized postductal narrowing of the aorta is most common. It represents a deformity in the aortic media that narrows the lumen by a curtain-like infolding of the vessel wall.[26] The clinical presentation is highly variable and ranges from left ventricular failure in infancy to hypertension in otherwise asymptomatic adult patients, depending on the site and severity of the coarctation and the presence of associated abnormalities. The most common associated anomaly is bicuspid aortic valve, which occurs in as many as 85 per cent of patients with coarctation of the aorta. Other associated congenital anomalies include ventricular septal defect, stenosis or atresia of the left subclavian artery, patent ductus arteriosus, Noonan syndrome, Turner syndrome, and malformations of the mitral valve.

The diagnosis of coarctation of the aorta can be established from the PA chest film alone in up to 92 per cent of patients.[129,129a] The most useful radiological sign is an abnormal contour of the aortic arch, which may appear as a double bulge above and below the usual site of the aortic knob. This pattern has been described as a figure "3" sign. The upper arc of the "3" is the dilated arch proximal to the coarctation and/or a dilated left subclavian artery. The lower arc or bulge is the poststenotic dilatation of the aorta immediately below the coarctation. The indentation between the two bulges is the coarctation itself. With a barium-filled esophagus, a reverse "3" or "E" sign is often seen, representing a mirror image of the areas of pre- and poststenotic dilatation (Fig. 8–40). The "3" sign is variable in that the upper arc may be small and the lower arc large or vice versa. Superior mediastinal widening due to large internal mammary collateral arteries is seen in some cases.[130] The aortic arch may also be obscured in the frontal view due to overlapping by an enlarged left subclavian artery.[131] Left ventricular enlargement usually occurs with coarctation, particularly when associated aortic stenosis is present.

Bilateral symmetrical rib notching, which is readily appreciated on the chest x-ray, is diagnostic of aortic coarctation. It is due to obstruction to blood flow at the narrowed aortic segment with collateral blood flow through the intercostal vessels. Rib notching is unusual in infancy but it becomes more prominent with increased age, and is present in 75 per cent of adults with coarctation.[132] Rib notching involves the inferior margin of the third to the eighth ribs due to pulsation of the dilated intercostal arteries. Typical pathways of collateral flow are (1) from the subclavian artery to internal mammary artery to intercostal arteries; (2) subclavian artery to the costovertebral trunk; and (3) transverse cervical and suprascapular arteries to the intercostal arteries. Dilatation of the internal mammary arteries acting as a collateral pathway may cause scallop-like retrosternal notching.[130,132]

Cardiac catheterization and angiography are diagnostic, demonstrating both the site of the coarctation and associated anomalies including aortic valvular disease (Fig. 32–2, p. 968). Cross-sectional imaging modalities yield important diagnostic information. Echocardiography (Fig. 4–66, p. 90), for example, demonstrates the presence or absence of bicuspid valve and mitral valve deformities. MRI is useful in demonstrating both the coarctation itself (Fig. 11–39, p. 331) and restenosis of the aorta following surgery or angioplasty.[6]

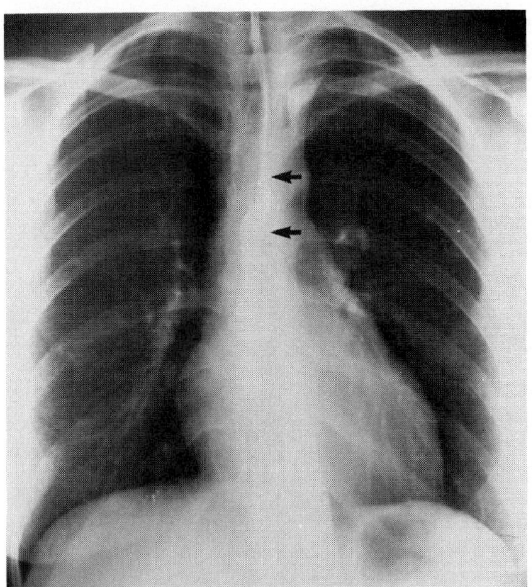

FIGURE 8–40. Coarctation of the aorta. There is displacement of the barium esophagram to the right above and below the coarctation (arrows).

LEFT-TO-RIGHT SHUNTS

Atrial Septal Defect (ASD) (see also p. 973). ASD is the most common left-to-right shunt diagnosed in adult life, accounting for over 40 per cent of adult congenital heart disease in some series.[133,134] Although the radiograph may be normal in a patient with a small shunt, typically the main pulmonary artery is enlarged, the peripheral vessels are uniformly enlarged (Fig. 8–22*A*) and the right atrial and right ventricular borders are prominent (Fig. 8–41*A*). Differentiation from other left to right shunts is often possible. There is usually less pulmonary artery dilatation in patent ductus arteriosus (PDA) than in ASD and both PDA and ventricular septal defect (VSD) are associated with enlarged left cardiac chambers. In the adult over the age of 50 years, the radiographical findings are often atypical and may include left atrial enlargement, evidence of pulmonary venous hypertension, and pulmonary edema. These changes are associated with smaller shunts and a higher prevalence of left ventricular dysfunction and pulmonary arterial hypertension.[135] Echocardiography is diagnostic in ASD; right ventricular chamber dilatation and paradoxical anterior systolic motion of the interventricular septum are seen. The size and location of the atrial septal defect can often be visualized, as well as associated abnormalities including mitral valve prolapse. Cine CT and MRI also demonstrate the defect of the atrial septum.[6]

Patent Ductus Arteriosus (PDA) (see also p. 969). PDA is an unusual diagnosis in adults. The size of the shunt and the degree of pulmonary hypertension determine the severity of symptoms; if the shunt is small, the chest x-ray is usually normal. When there is a large shunt, the main pulmonary artery and the right and left pulmonary artery branches are enlarged as a result of increased pulmonary blood flow (Fig. 8–41*B*). The ductus may sometimes calcify as a curvilinear or upside-down Y-shaped opacity, especially if a ductus aneurysm is present[19] (Fig. 32–5, p. 969). The left atrium, left ventricle, and ascending aorta are enlarged in high-flow PDA.

Ventricular Septal Defect (VSD) (see also p. 971). VSD accounts for 30 per cent of cardiac malformations in the newborn but comprises only 10 per cent of adult-onset congenital heart disease. The relatively smaller incidence in adults is due to spontaneous closure of the defect in childhood or surgical repair. If the VSD is small, the chest x-ray is normal. However, if there is a large left-to-right shunt or secondary pulmonary hypertension, the pulmonary arteries will be enlarged (Fig. 8–41*C*), as will both ventricles and the left atrium.[136] The ascending aorta will be normal in size or small, whereas it is enlarged in PDA. Cine CT, MRI, and echocardiography (Fig. 4–74, p. 93) often demonstrate the site of the defect.

PULMONARY VALVULAR STENOSIS (see also p. 972)

Pulmonary valvular stenosis in adults is usually an isolated anomaly.[35,137] Most patients are asymptomatic even with severe obstruction. There is mild to moderate enlargement of the main pulmonary artery (Fig. 8–42*A*). The enlargement represents poststenotic dilatation resulting from the jet effect of blood flow through the narrowed pulmonary valve orifice. Since the jet is directed toward the left, the left pulmonary artery is often preferentially enlarged. Calcification of the pulmonary valve is rare in this condition. The differential diagnosis of pulmonary valvular stenosis includes primary and secondary pulmonary hypertension and idiopathic pulmonary artery dilatation.

CONGENITAL CORRECTED TRANSPOSITION OF THE GREAT ARTERIES (see also p. 969)

In this condition, ventricular inversion and transposition of the pulmonary artery and aorta result from formation of a left (levo or l) rather than a right (dextro or d) bulboventricular loop. The systemic venous flow is transmitted to the lungs by way of a right-sided anatomic left ventricle and the transposed pulmonary artery. Pulmonary venous flow traverses a left-sided anatomic right ventricle to the aorta. The ascending aorta is positioned to the left, forming a long continuous prominence along the left cardiac border from the left ventricular apex to the aortic arch.[138] The main pulmonary artery lies behind and to the right of the aorta and is not border-forming with the lung in the PA view. Left-to-right shunts may or may not be present (Fig. 8–42*B*), and left atrioventricular valve regurgitation and conduction abnormalities leading to heart block are fairly common. The heart is normal to enlarged in size, depending on the degree of atrioventricular valve regurgitation. Cross-sectional imaging supports the plain film diagnosis, showing an anterior left-sided aorta and a pulmonary artery lying behind and medial to the aorta.[139]

CYANOTIC CONGENITAL HEART DISEASE

Tetralogy of Fallot (see also p. 971). Tetralogy of Fallot is the most common cyanotic congenital cardiac lesion in adults, although it is usually

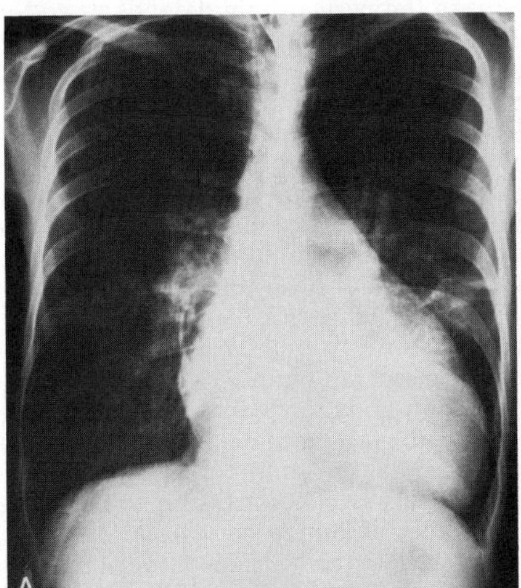

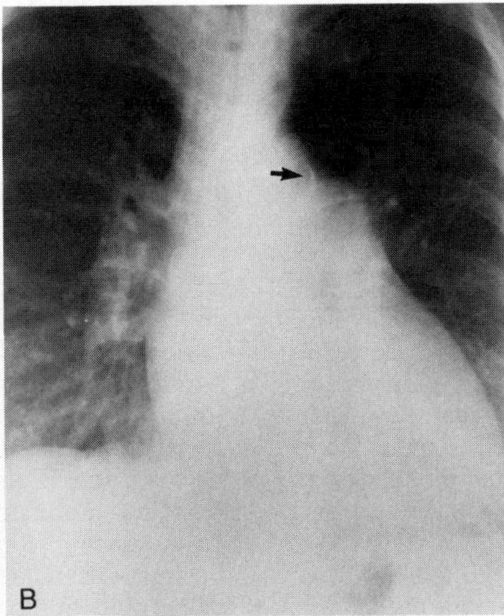

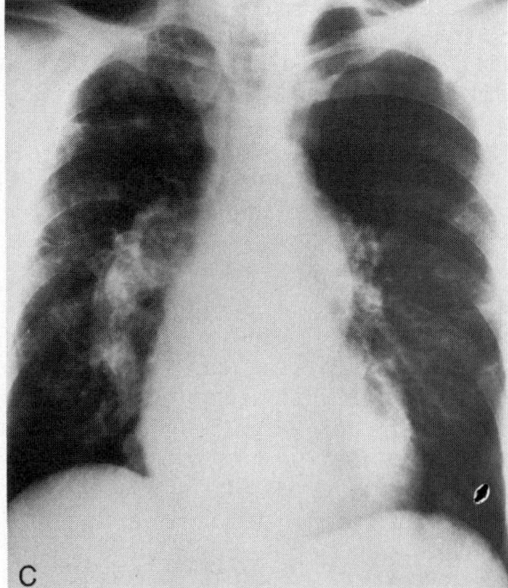

FIGURE 8–41. *A,* Atrial septal defect. A 45-year-old woman with an ostium secundum defect. The pulmonary artery is enlarged and there is prominence of the right atrial border. The enlargement of the right ventricle causes rounding of the left heart border. *B,* Patent ductus arteriosus. A curvilinear calcification is present above an enlarged pulmonary artery (arrow). C, Ventricular septal defect. There is an increase in the size of the central pulmonary arteries in this patient with VSD and Eisenmenger physiology.

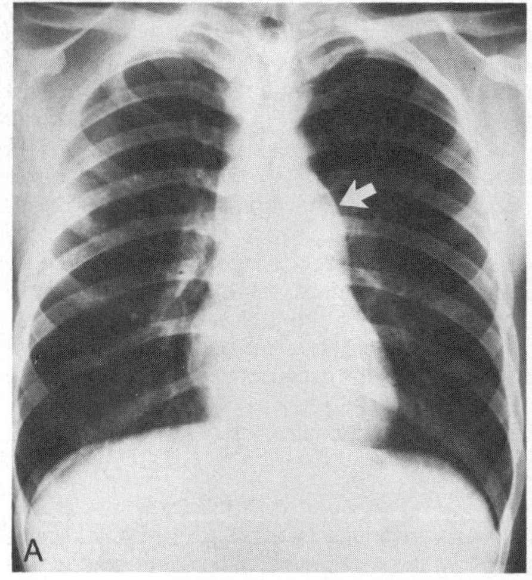

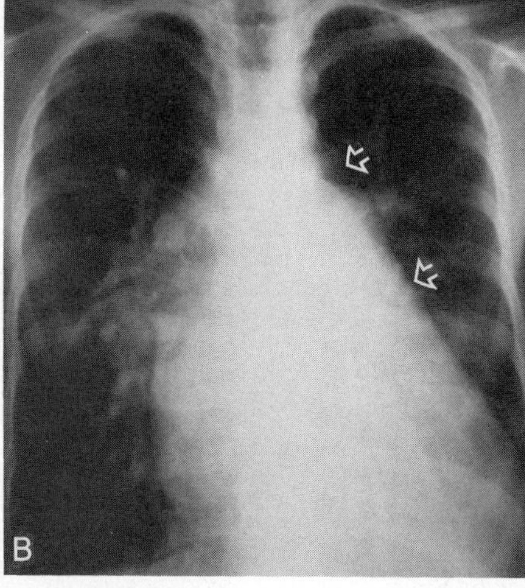

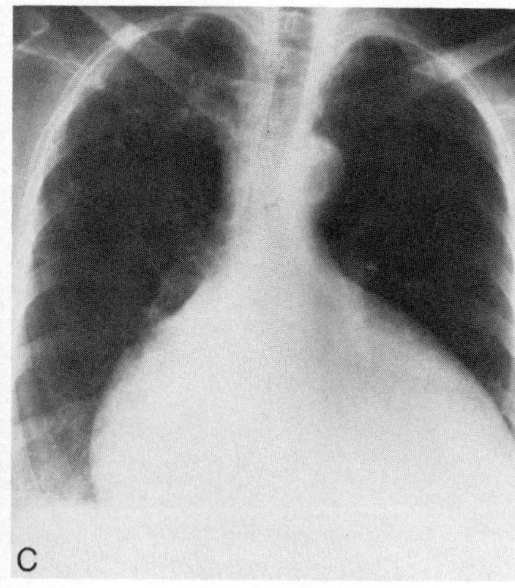

FIGURE 8-42. ***A,*** **Pulmonary valvular stenosis. Pulmonary blood flow and cardiac size are normal but the main pulmonary artery is enlarged (arrow) in this young woman with pulmonary valvular stenosis.** ***B,*** **Congenital corrected transposition of the great arteries. The left-sided ascending aorta (open arrows) confirms the diagnosis. There is increased pulmonary blood flow due to an atrial septal defect. Pulmonary valvular stenosis is also present.** ***C,*** **Ebstein's anomaly. There is globular cardiac enlargement due to severe tricuspid regurgitation and right heart enlargement. The pulmonary blood flow is reduced.**

diagnosed in childhood. Most adults with tetralogy of Fallot demonstrate mild to moderate pulmonary hypovascularity (Fig. 8-4*C*). Those with very mild infundibular pulmonary stenosis will have normal pulmonary blood flow. Small tortuous bronchial arteries are found in both lungs when severe pulmonary outflow tract stenosis or atresia is present. There is a right aortic arch in 25 per cent of patients. The combination of right aortic arch and cyanosis should suggest the diagnosis of tetralogy of Fallot, athough this combination can also be found in the rare examples of truncus arteriosus or double-outlet right ventricle in the adult patient. Echocardiography often demonstrates the high ventricular septal defect, overriding of the ventricular septum by the aorta, and right ventricular hypertrophy. Cine CT and MRI[140] can demonstrate the septal defect and the large ascending aorta, as well as evidence of a right aortic arch. Plain films show a boot-shaped heart in some adult patients, but this is less common than in children.

Ebstein's Anomaly (see also p. 972). In this abnormality, the tricuspid valve is malformed and partially fused to the walls of the right ventricle. This results in downward displacement of the orifice and tricuspid regurgitation.[141-144] There is a right-to-left shunt at the atrial level causing cyanosis. The right heart chambers are enlarged, often markedly, as a manifestation of the tricuspid regurgitation. The typical roentgenographic findings are those of a large rounded or triangular heart with a narrow vascular pedicle (Fig. 8-42*C*). The pulmonary vasculature is reduced, depending upon the degree of right to left shunting. The greater the shunt, the more diminished the vascularity. Echocardiography shows the abnormal position of the tricuspid valve with downward displacement of the septal and posterior leaflets. Tricuspid regurgitation can be evaluated by a combined two-dimensional and Doppler echocardiographic study. MR and CT also demonstrate the downward displacement of the valve and enlargement of the right atrium.

THE PERICARDIUM

(See also Chap. 45)

The pericardium is a double-layered sac composed of a parietal outer layer and an inner visceral layer (the epicardium) with a potential space containing 20-25 ml of lubricating lymphoid fluid. The serous lining of the parietal pericardium folds back on itself to cover the origins of the great vessels and lines a series of perivascular and retroaortic pericardial recesses.[145] Below the visceral pericardium lies the subepicardial fat. The subepicardial fat is localized around the coronary arteries, the atrioventricular grooves, the interventricular grooves, and along the posterior margin of the heart.

NORMAL PERICARDIUM. The normal pericardium is occasionally seen with plain film views in the lateral projection as a thin linear opacity separating the anterior subxiphoid mediastinal fat from the subepicardial fat.[146] The pericardium may also be visualized in the frontal projection paralleling the left heart border. With CT and MRI, the extent of the normal and abnormal pericardium is appreciated to better advantage because of the superior contrast resolution of both techniques.[146a] With both modalities, the anterior, lateral, and posterior pericardium are clearly separated from mediastinal fat. Subtle areas of pericardial thickening and loculated effusions are clearly seen. Echocardiography is probably the most sensitive technique for the diagnosis of small pericardial effusions (Fig. 4-101, p. 103). It usually is the imaging study of choice when pericardial effusion is suspected clinically or by x-ray.[5,146] With MRI or CT, the pericardial recesses are clearly defined but occasionally may mimic the appearance of aortic dissection or mediastinal lymphadenopathy (Fig. 11-8, p. 317).[145]

PERICARDIAL EFFUSION. The response of the pericardium to insult is limited to the development of pericardial effusion or cellular proliferation with development of calcification, adhesions, or constriction. Pericardial effusion, the initial manifestation of pericarditis, has many causes and may be a transudate or exudate, gaseous or chylous.[26,147] As fluid accumulates in the pericardial spaces, the cardiac silhouette develops a "globular" or "flask-like" configuration. The normal indentations and prominences along the heart border are effaced so that the shape of the cardiac silhouette is smooth and featureless. Because the pericardium extends up to the pulmonary bifurcation, the hilar structures are draped and obscured by the distended pericardial cavity. This may help distinguish a large pericardial effusion from massive cardiomegaly, which will not obscure the hilar vessels (Fig. 8-43*A*).

In the lateral view, in the patient with pericardial effusion, the retrosternal space is narrowed or obliterated by the expanding cardiac silhouette. Normally the low-radiographic-density epicardial fat merges imperceptibly with the mediastinal fat, since they are separated only by the potential space of the pericardium. However, with pericardial effusion, the epicardial fat is displaced posteriorly by the higher density fluid and may be visible as a distinct radiolucent stripe between the anterior border of the heart and the mediastinum. This positive epicardial fat pad sign, seen on the lateral projection, is highly specific for pericardial effusion[146,147] (Fig. 8-43*B*). If pericardial effusion is suspected, echocardiography is the primary method for detection of simple pericardial effusions, because it can be transported to the bedside to study critically ill patients and is sensitive and noninvasive. When the fluid volume is small, the fluid appears as an elliptical hypoechoic area localized behind the left ventricle. As fluid increases further, the hypoechoic area envelops the ventral aspect of the right atrium and ventricle. CT can be particularly helpful in detecting pericardial thickening, diffuse or loculated effusion,

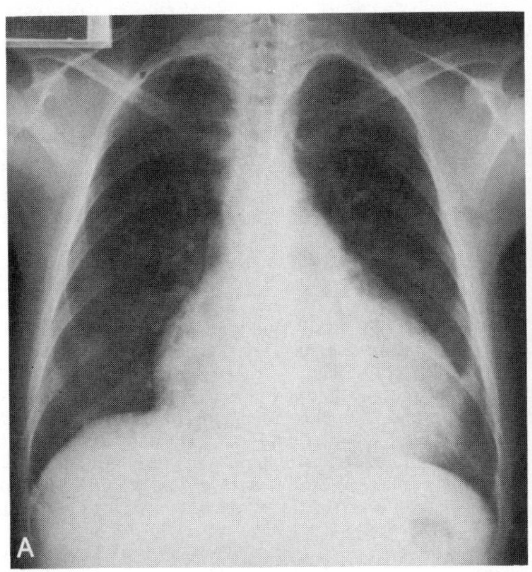

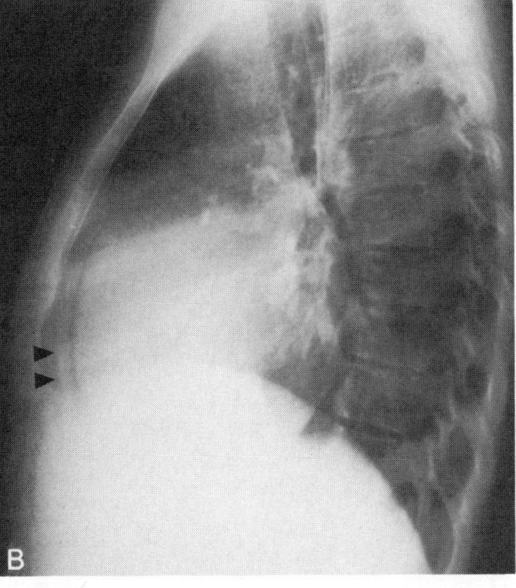

FIGURE 8-43. Pericardial effusion. ***A,*** **The heart assumes a globular rounded shape following development of a pericardial effusion. The normal indentations along the heart borders are effaced so that the cardiac silhouette is smooth and featureless.** ***B,*** **The subepicardial radiolucent fat stripe is separated from the subxiphoid fat by the higher density fluid of the pericardial effusion (arrowheads).**

calcification, adjacent mediastinal and pulmonary disease, and neoplasm (Fig. 11-10, p. 318).[109,148] The nature of the fluid may be suggested by analysis of CT density numbers. For example, there are higher CT density values in hemopericardium than in serous effusions. In chylous pericardial effusion the attenuation values may be lower.

MRI can clearly detect pericardial effusion as an area of signal void on T_1 weighted images, although artifacts sometimes accentuate this (Fig. 8-44). Intrapericardial masses, pericardial cysts, and thickening are also well demonstrated with MRI. In addition, MRI can clearly define pericardial recesses, mediastinal fat, and other anatomical landmarks that may present pitfalls for the echocardiographer.[148]

PERICARDIAL CONSTRICTION. Pericardial constriction may complicate viral or tuberculous pericarditis, hemopericardium, pericarditis associated with radiation, and postpericardiotomy syndrome.[65,66,149] Constriction may be acute or chronic. Acute intrapericardial pressure elevation secondary to tamponade will cause restriction of diastolic expansion of the heart with equalization of diastolic pressures in the cardiac chambers and reduction of venous inflow.[5] When unrecognized, acute pericardial constriction can lead to shock and even death. In chronic pericardial constriction, the overall heart size appears large when the left atrium is enlarged or when the pericardium is thickened to more than 2 cm; otherwise it will appear normal or small. The right atrial border is flattened and there may be pulmonary vascular redistribution. Pleural effusions are present in 60 per cent of patients and enlargement of the azygos vein and left atrium occurs in 20 per cent of patients. Pericardial calcification is present in 30 per cent of patients with chronic pericardial constriction and is usually best seen along the anterior and inferior cardiac border or in the atrioventricular grooves (Figs. 8-25 and 45-16, p. 1485). While the presence of pericardial calcification indicates chronic pericarditis, it does not in itself establish the diagnosis of pericardial constriction.[149]

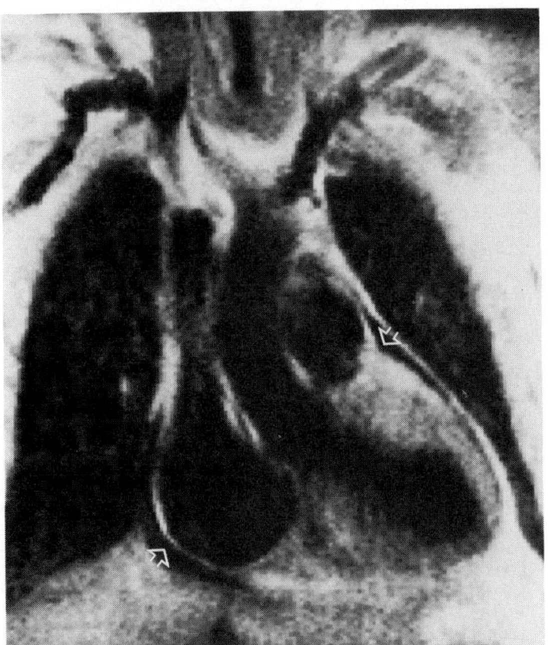

FIGURE 8-44. Pericardial effusion. Coronal T1W MRI at 0.5 T. The signal void fluid in the pericardial cavity indicates the presence of pericardial effusion (open arrows). (From Moncada, R., et al.: Multimodality approach to pericardial imaging. ***In*** **Kotler, M. N., and Steiner, R. M. [eds.]: Cardiac Imaging. Philadelphia, F. A. Davis, 1986.)**

PERICARDIAL NEOPLASM. Pericardial tumors are demonstrated best by CT, MRI, or echocardiography (Chaps. 11 and 45).[148,150] They generally do not cause a discrete bulge; however, there may be enlargement of the cardiac silhouette due to an associated pericardial effusion. CT can identify associated pleural and parenchymal disease including metastatic lesions in the pleural space. Metastatic neoplasm of the pericardium is far more common than primary neoplasm. The most common sources of pericardial metastases are the lung, the breast, lymphoma, leukemia, or melanoma. Benign tumors are unusual and include teratomas, lipomas, and fibromas.[65,148] The principal primary pericardial neoplasm is mesothelioma, a rare pericardial lesion generally associated with asbestosis. With extensive encasement, pericardial mesothelioma presents with a clinical picture of pericardial constriction.

CONGENITAL ANOMALIES. Congenital absence of the pericardium may be partial or complete (Fig. 8-45). Complete absence is more common and is usually left-sided. Partial absence occurs along the upper border of the pericardium on either side. Herniation of the left atrial appendage and pulmonary trunk through a left-sided defect radiographically can resemble pulmonary stenosis, mitral stenosis, or a mediastinal tumor (Fig. 8-45). When a partial right-sided defect is present, right atrial herniation may occur. In the absence of the left pericardium, with plain films the aortic knob remains in its usual position, but the rest of the cardiac silhouette shifts

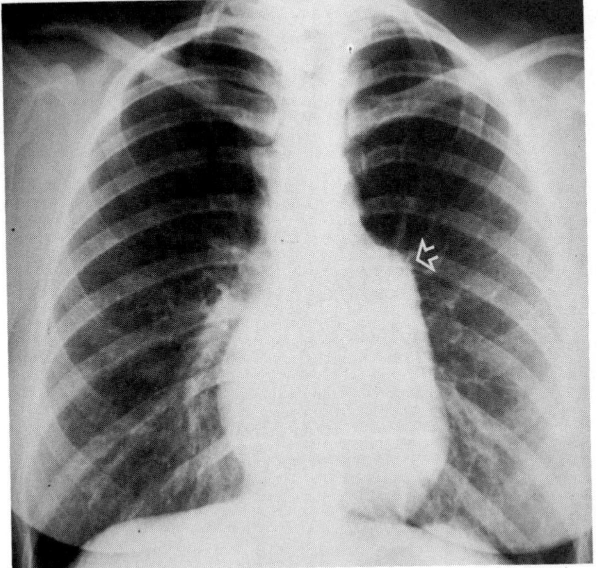

FIGURE 8-45. Partial absence of the pericardium: There is a convex bulge (open arrow) along the left atrial border due to herniation of the left atrial appendage through the pericardial defect.

to the left. The pulmonary artery and left atrial appendage are prominent. CT demonstrates absence of the left anterior pericardium and bulging of the heart toward the left side.

PERICARDIAL CYSTS. Most pericardial cysts are seen as smooth round convex bulges along the middle or lower right heart border, usually near the cardiophrenic sulcus. However, 20 per cent lie along the left heart border. Occasionally, cysts of pericardial recesses present as soft tissue masses along the aortic arch or in the area of the superior vena cava. Pericardial cysts are usually asymptomatic, although chest pain has been described in 20 per cent of patients.[151] They rarely calcify, seldom communicate with the pericardial space, and are best diagnosed by CT or MRI as smoothly marginated, fluid-filled structures adjacent to the right heart border.[148,150]

REFERENCES

NORMAL CARDIAC ANATOMY

1. Higgins, C. B.: New horizons in cardiac imaging. Radiology *156*:577, 1985.
2. Newell, J. D., Higgins, C. B., and Kelley, M. J.: Radiographic-echocardiographic approach to acquired heart disease: Diagnosis and assessment of severity. Radiol. Clin. N. Am. *18*:387, 1980.
3. Bogren, H. G., DeMaria, A. N., and Mason, D. T.: Imaging procedures in the detection of cardiac tumors with emphasis on echocardiography: A review. Cardiovasc. Intervent. Radiol. *3*:107, 1980.
4. Needleman L., Gardiner, G. A., Jr., and Levin, D. C.: Hypertrophic cardiomyopathy: Changing concepts over the last two decades. A.J.R. *150*:1219, 1988.
5. Gordon, S., and Butler, M.: Echocardiography in cardiac tamponade. J.C.U. *17*:428, 1989.
6. Bank, E. R., and Hernandez, R. J.: CT and MR of congenital heart disease. Radiol. Clin. N. Am. *26*:241, 1988.
7. Utz, J. A., Herfkens, R. J., Heinsimer, J. A., et al.: Cine MR determination of left ventricular ejection fraction. A.J.R. *148*:839, 1987.
8. Sechtem, U., Pflugfelder, P. W., Gould, R. G., et al.: Measurement of right and left ventricular volumes in healthy individuals with cine MR imaging. Radiology *163*:697, 1987.

8a. Cranney, G. B., Lotan, C. S., Dean, L., et al.: Left ventricular volume measurement using cardiac axis nuclear magnetic resonance imaging. Validation by calibrated ventricular angiography. Circulation *82*:154, 1990.

8b. Kersting-Sommerhoff, B. A., Diethelm, L., Stanger, P., et al.: Evaluation of complex congenital ventricular anomalies with magnetic resonance imaging. Am. Heart J. *120*:133, 1990.

8c. Mitchell, L., Jenklins, J.P.R., Watson, Y., et al.: Diagnosis and assessment of mitral and aortic valve disease by cine-flow magnetic resonance imaging. Magn. Res. Med. *12*:181, 1989.

9. Ahmad M., Johnson, R. F., Jr., Fawcett, H. D., et al.: Left ventricular aneurysm in short axis: A comparison of magnetic resonance, ultrasound and thallium-201 spect images. Mag. Reson. Imag. *5*:293, 1987.
10. Stanford, W., and Galvin, J. R.: The radiology of right heart dysfunction: Chest roentgenogram and computed tomography. J. Thorac. Imag. *4*:7, 1989.
11. Schultz, K. W., Thorsen, M. K., Gurney, J. W., et al.: Comparison of fluoroscopy, angiography and CT in coronary artery calcification. Applied Radiology *6*:38, 1989.
12. Lipton, M. J.: Quantitation of left ventricular anatomy and function by ultrafast cine CT. Cardiovasc. Intervent. Radiol. *10*:348, 1987.
13. Sinak, L. J., Hoffman, E. A., Schwartz, R. S., et al.: Three-dimensional cardiac anatomy and function in heart disease in adults: Initial results with the dynamic spatial reconstructor. Mayo Clin. Proc. *60*:383, 1985.

13a. Holt, W. W., Wong, E., and Lipton, M. J.: Conventional and ultra-fast cine-computed tomography in cardiac imaging. Curr. Opin. Radiol. *1*:159, 1989.

14. Chikos, P. M., Figley, M. M., and Fisher, L.: Correlation between chest film and angiographic assessment of left ventricular size. A.J.R. *128*:367, 1977.
15. Rose, C. P., and Stolberg, H. O.: The limited utility of the plain chest film in the assessment of left ventricular structure and function. Invest. Radiol. *17*:139, 1982.
16. Wachtel, T. J., and Fredericks, R.: Prediction of ventricular function from plain film chest roentgenogram. Rhode Island Med. J. *69*:589, 1986.
17. Ball, J. B., and Proto, A. V.: The variable appearance of the left superior intercostal vein. Radiology *144*:445, 1982.
18. Wechsler, R. J., Steiner, R. M., and Kinori, I.: Monitoring the monitors: The radiology of thoracic catheters, wires and tubes. Semin. Roentgen. *23*:61, 1988.
19. Danza, F. M., Fusco, A., Breda, M., et al.: Ductus arteriosus aneurysm in an adult. A.J.R. *143*:131, 1984.
20. Salomonowitz, E., Edwards, J. E., Hunter D. W., et al.: The three types of aortic diverticula. A.J.R. *142*:673, 1984.
21. Baron, M. G.: Radiological and angiographic examination of the heart. *In* Braunwald, E. (ed): Heart Disease: A Textbook of Cardiovascular Medicine. 3rd ed. Philadelphia, W. B. Saunders Company, 1988, p. 140.
22. Berdon, W. E., and Baker, D. H.: Plain film findings in azygos continuation of the inferior vena cava. A.J.R. *104*:452, 1968.
23. Amplatz, K., Formanek, A., Knight, L., et al.: Radiographic changes in the postoperative patient. Prog. Cardiovasc. Dis. *17*:403, 1985.
24. Murphy, M. L., Blue, L. R., Ferris, E. J., et al.: Sensitivity and specificity of chest roentgenogram criteria for right ventricular hypertrophy. Invest. Radiol. *23*:853, 1988.
25. Hoffman, R. B., and Rigler, L. G.: Evaluation of left ventricular enlargement in the lateral projection of the chest. Radiology *85*:93, 1965.
26. Chen, J.T.T.; Essentials of Cardiac Roentgenology. Boston, Little Brown, 1987.
27. Bachman, D. M., Ellis, K., and Austin, J.H.M.: The effect of minor degrees of obliquity on the lateral chest radiograph. Radiol. Clin. N. Am. *16*:465, 1978.
28. Van Houten, F. X., Adams, D. F., and Abrams, H. L. Radiology of valvular heart disease. *In* Sonnenblick, E., and Lesch, M. (eds.): Valvular Heart Disease. New York, Grune and Stratton, 1974.
29. Jefferson, K., and Rees, S.: Clinical Cardiac Radiology. 2nd ed. London, Butterworths, 1980.
30. Sos, T. A., Levin, D. C., Sniderman, K. W., et al.: Cinefluoroscopy in evaluating left ventricular contractility and aneurysms. Circulation *56* (Suppl. III):18, 1977.
31. Green, C. E., and Kelley, M. J.: A renewed role for fluoroscopy in the evaluation of cardiac disease. Radiol. Clin. N. Am. *18*:345,1980.
32. Kelley, M. J., Huang, E. K., and Langou, R. A.: Correlations of fluoroscopically detected coronary artery calcification with exercise stress testing in asymptomatic men. Radiology *729*:1, 1978.
33. Margolis, J. R., Chen, J.T.T., Kong, Y., et al.: The diagnostic and prognostic significance of coronary artery calcification. Radiology *137*:609, 1980.
34. Bartel, A. G., Chen, J.T.T., Peter, R. H., et al.: The significance of coronary calcification detected by fluoroscopy: A report of 360 patients. Circulation *49*:1247, 1974.
35. Covarrubias, E. A., Sheikh, M. U., Isner, J. M., et al.: Calcific pulmonic stenosis in adulthood. Chest *75*:399, 1979.
36. Spindola-Franco, H., Fish, B. G., Dachman, A., et al.: Recognition of bicuspid aortic valve by plain film calcification. A.J.R. *139*:867, 1982.
37. Fulkerson, P. K., Beaver, B. M., Auseon, J. C., et al.: Calcification of the mitral annulus: Etiology, clinical associations, complications, and therapy. Am. J. Med. *66*:967, 1979.
38. Freundlich, L. M., and Lind T. A.: Calcification of the heart and great vessels. C.R.C. Crit. Rev. Clin., Radiol. Nucl. Med. *6*:171, 1975.
39. Kotler, M. N., Mintz, G. S., Panidis, I., et al.: Noninvasive evaluation of normal and abnormal prosthetic valve function. J. Am. Coll. Cardiol. *2*:151, 1983.
40. Steiner, R. M., Mintz, G., Morse, D., et al.: Radiology of cardiac valve prosthesis. Radiographics *8*:277, 1988.
41. Sands, M. H., Jr., Lachman, A. S., O'Reilly, D. J., et al.: Diagnostic value of cinefluoroscopy in the evaluation of prosthetic heart valve dysfunction. Am. Heart J. *104*:622, 1982.
42. Gutierrez, F., McKnight, R., Clark, R., et al.: Chest film diagnosis of disc embolization in patients with Beall mitral valve prosthesis. J. Thorac. Cardiovasc. Surg. *81*:758, 1981.
43. Guit, G. L., Van Voorthuisen, A. E., and Steiner, R. M.: Outlet strut fracture of the Björk-Shiley mitral prosthesis. Radiology *154*:298, 1985.
44. Keats, T. E., and Enge, I. P.: Cardiac mensuration by the cardiac volume method. Radiology *85*:850, 1965.
45. Gammill, S. L., Krebs, C., Meyers, P., et al.: Cardiac measurements in systole and diastole. Radiology *94*:115, 1970.
46. Kabala, J. E., and Wilde, P.: Measurement of heart size in the anteroposterior chest radiograph. Br. J. Radiol. *60*:981, 1987.

47. Glover, L., Baxley, W. A., and Dodge, H. T.: A quantitative evaluation of heart size measurements from chest roentgenograms. Circulation *47*:1289, 1973.
48. Milne, E.N.C., Burnett, K., Aufrichtig, D., et al.: Assessment of cardiac size on portable chest films. J. Thorac. Imag. *3*:64, 1988.
49. Peerry, M. M., Irfan, A. Y., Simmons, S. P., et al.: Heart size in high-kilovoltage chest radiography. Clin. Radiol. *36*:335, 1985.
50. Righetti, A., Crawford, M. H., O'Rourke, R. A., et al.: Echocardiographic and roentgenographic determination of left ventricular size after coronary arterial bypass graft surgery. Chest *72*:455, 1977.

THE PULMONARY VASCULATURE

51. West, J. B.: Regional differences in gas exchange in the lung in erect man. J. Appl. Physiol. *17*:893, 1963.
52. Chang, C. H.: The normal roentgenographic measurement of the right descending artery in 1085 cases. A.J.R. *87*:929, 1962.
53. Harrison, M. O., Conte, P. J., and Heitzman, E. R.: Radiological detection of clinically occult cardiac failure following myocardial infarction. Br. J. Radiol. *44*:265, 1971.
54. Milne, E.N.C., Pistolesi, M., Miniati, M., et al.: The radiologic distinction of cardiogenic and noncardiogenic edema. A.J.R. *144*:879, 1985.
55. Friedman, W. F., and Braunwald, E.: Alterations of regional pulmonary blood flow in mitral valve disease studied by radioisotope scanning: A simple nontraumatic technique for estimation of left atrial pressure. Circulation *34*:363, 1966.
56. Chen, J.T.T., Behar, V. S., Morris, J. J., Jr., et al.: Correlation of Roentgen findings with hemodynamic data in pure mitral stenosis. A.J.R. *102*:280, 1968.
56a. Herman, P. C., Khan, A., Kallman, C. E., et al.: Limited correlation of left ventricular end-diastolic pressure with radiographic assessment of pulmonary hemodynamics. Radiology *174*:721, 1990.
57. Chen, J.T.T., Robinson, A. E., Goodrich, F. K., et al.: Uneven distribution of pulmonary blood flow between left and right lungs in isolated valvular pulmonary stenosis. A.J.R. *107*:343, 1969.
58. Grainger, R. G.: Interstitial pulmonary oedema and its radiological diagnosis. A sign of pulmonary venous and capillary hypertension. Br. J. Radiol. *31*:201, 1958.
59. Kerley, P. J.: Radiology in heart disease. Br. Med. J. *2*:594, 1933.
60. Fleischner, F. G., and Reiner, L.: Linear x-ray shadows in acquired pulmonary hemosiderosis and congestion. N. Engl. J. Med. *250*:900, 1954.
61. Fleischner, F. G.: The butterfly pattern of acute pulmonary edema. Am. J. Cardiol. *20*:39, 1967.
62. Milne, E.N.C., Pistolesi, M., Miniati, M., et al.: The vascular pedicle of the heart and the vena azygos. I: The normal subject. Radiology *152*:1, 1984.
63. Pistoles, M., Milne, E.N.C., Miniati, M., et al.: The vascular pedicle and the vena azygos. II: Acquired heart disease. Radiology *152*:9, 1984.

CARDIAC CALCIFICATION

64. Soulen, R. L., and Freeman, E.: Radiologic evaluation of traumatic heart disease. Radiol. Clin. N. Am. *9*:285, 1971.
65. Moncada, R., Baker, M., Salinas, M., et al.: Diagnostic role of computed tomography in pericardial heart disease: Congenital defects, thickenings, neoplasms and effusions. Am. Heart J. *103*:263, 1982.
66. Doppman, J. L., Rienmuller, R., Lissner, J., et al.: Computed tomography in constrictive pericardial disease. J. Comput. Assist. Tomogr. *5*:1, 1981.
67. Leonard, J. J., Katz, S., and Nelson, D.: Calcification of the left atrium: Its anatomic location, diagnostic significance, and roentgenologic demonstration. N. Engl. J. Med. *256*:629, 1957.
68. Matsuyama, S., Watabe, T., Kuribayashi, S., et al.: Plain film diagnosis of thrombosis of left atrial appendage in mitral valve disease. Radiology *146*:15, 1983.
69. Rodan, B. A., Chen, J.T.T., Halber, M. D., et al.: Chest roentgenographic evaluation of the severity of aortic stenosis. Invest. Radiol. *17*:453, 1982.
70. Spindola-Franco, H., and Fish, B. G.: Radiology of the Heart. New York, Springer-Verlag, 1985, p. 259.
71. Roberts, W. C., and Waller, B. F.: Mitral valve "anular" calcium forming a complete circle or "O" configuration. Clinical and necropsy observations. Am. Heart J. *101*:619, 1981.
72. Aldrich, R. F., Brensike, J. F., Battaglini, J. W., et al.: Coronary calcification in the detection of coronary artery disease and comparison with electrocardiographic exercise testing. Circulation *59*:113, 1979.
73. Stanford, W., Rooholamini, M., Rumberger, J., et al.: Evaluation of coronary bypass graft patency by ultrafast computed tomography. J. Thorac. Imag. 3(2):52, 1988.
74. Moore, E. H., Greenberg, R. W., Merrick, S. H., et al.: Coronary artery calcifications: Significance of incidental detection on CT scans. Radiology *172*:711, 1989.
75. Ominsky, S. H., and Kricun, M. E.: Roentgenology of sinus of Valsalva aneurysms. A.J.R. *125*:571, 1975.
76. Deutsch, V., Wexler, L., and Deutsch, H.: Takayasu's arteritis. A.J.R. *122*:13, 1974.
77. Davis, C. D., Kincaid, O. W., and Hallermann, F. J.: Roentgen aspects of cardiac tumors. Semin. Roentgenol. *4*:384, 1969.
77a. Nomeir, A. M., Watts, L. E., Seagle, R., et al.: Intracardiac myxomas: Twenty-year echocardiographic experience with review of the literature. J. Am. Soc. Echo. *2*:139, 1989.
78. Abrams, H. L., Adams, D. F., and Grant, H. A.: The radiology of tumors of the heart. L. Radiol. Clin. N. Am. *9*:299, 1971.
78a. Pucillo, A. L., Schechter, A. G., Kay, R. H., et al.: Identification of calcified intracardiac lesions using gradient echo MR imaging. J. Comput. Assist. Tomogr. *14*:743, 1990.
78b. Baumgartner, R. A., Das, S. K., Shea, M., et al.: The role of echocardiography and CT in the diagnosis of cardiac tumors. Int. J. Cardio. Imag. *3*:57, 1988.

ACQUIRED HEART DISEASE

79. Klatte, E. C., Yune, H., and Burney, B.: Radiographic manifestation of arteriostenosis and aortic valvular insufficiency. Semin. Roentgenol. *14*:122, 1979.
80. Braunwald, E., Morrow, A. G., Cornell, W. P., et al.: Idiopathic hypertrophic subaortic stenosis: Clinical, hemodynamic and angiographic manifestations. Am. J. Med. *29*:924, 1960.
80a. Gal, R. A., Shalev, Y., and Schmidt, D. H.: Mitral regurgitation: Parameters that affect the correlation between Doppler echocardiography and contrast venticulography. Int. J. Cardiol. *28*:87, 1990.
81. Lipton, M. J.: Quantitation of cardiac function by cine CT. Radiol. Clin. N. Am. *23*:613, 1985.
81a. de Roos, A., Reichek, N., Axel, L., et al.: Cine MR imaging in aortic stenosis. J. Comput. Assist. Tomogr. *13*:421, 1989.
81b. Utz, J. A., Herfkens, R. J., Heinsimer, J. A., et al.: Valvular regurgitation: Dynamic MR imaging. Radiology *168*:91, 1988.
82. Carlsson, E., Gross, R., and Holt, R. G.: The radiological diagnosis of cardiac valvular insufficiencies. Circulation *55*:921, 1977.
83. Roberts, W. C.: Congenital cardiovascular abnormalities usually silent until adulthood. *In* Roberts, W. C. (ed): Adult Congenital Heart Disease. Philadelphia, F. A. Davis, 1987.
84. Probst, P., Goldschlager, N., and Selzer, A.: Left atrial size and atrial fibrillation in mitral stenosis: Factors influencing their relationship. Circulation *48*:1282, 1973.
85. Kelley, M. J., Elliott, L. P., Shulman, S. T., et al.: The significance of the left atrial appendage in rheumatic heart disease. Circulation *54*:146, 1976.
86. Green, C. E., Kelley, M. J., and Higgins, C. B.: Etiologic significance of enlargement of the left atrial appendage in adults. Radiology *142*:21, 1982.
87. Raphael, M. J., Steiner, R. E., and Raftery, E. B.: Acute mitral incompetence. Clin. Radiol. *18*:126, 1967.
88. Gurney, J. W., and Goodman, L. R.: Pulmonary edema localized to the right upper lobe accompanying mitral regurgitation. Radiology *171*:397, 1989.
89. Higgins, C. B., and Lipton, M. J.: Radiography of acute myocardial infarction. Radiol. Clin. N. Am. *18*:359, 1980.
89a. Topaz, O., DiSciascio, G., and Vetrovec, G. W.: Acute ventricular septal rupture: Perspectives on the current role of ventriculography and coronary arteriography and their implication for surgical repair. Am. Heart J. *120*:412, 1990.
90. Revel, D., and Higgins, C. B.: Magnetic resonance imaging of ischemic heart disease. Radiol. Clin. N. Am. *23*:719, 1985.
91. Björk, L.: Radiology in diagnosis of mitral valve prolapse. Ann. Radiol. *245*:327, 1981.
92. Levin, J., and Byrk, D.: Dressler syndrome (postmyocardial infarction syndrome). A.J.R. *87*:731, 1966.
93. Higgins, C. B., Lipton, M. J., Johnson, A. D., et al.: False aneurysms of the left ventricle. Radiology *127*:21, 1978.
94. Johnson, R. A., and Palacios, I.: Dilated cardiomyopathies of the adult. N. Engl. J. Med. *307*:1051, 1119, 1982.
95. Maron, B. J., and Epstein, S. E.: Recent observations regarding the specificity of three hallmarks of the disease: Asymmetrical septal hypertrophy, septal disorganization, and systolic anterior motion of the anterior mitral leaflet. Am. J. Cardiol. *45*:141, 1980.
96. Higgins, C. B., Byrd, B. F. III, and Stark, D.: Magnetic resonance imaging in hypertrophic cardiomyopathy, Am. J. Cardiol. *55*:1121, 1985.
97. Wojtowicz, J., Pawlak, B., Lehman, Z., et al.: Cardiac chambers and their walls in cardiomyopathies as evaluated with CT. Europ. J. Radiol. *4*:93, 1984.
98. Bisset, G. S., III, and Meyer, R. A.: Obstructive left heart lesions. Semin. Roentgenol. *20*:244, 1985.
99. Chiles, C., Adams, G. W., and Ravin, C. E.: Radiographic manifestations of cardiac sarcoid. A.J.R. *145*:711, 1985.
100. Goodman, L. R.: Postoperative chest radiograph: II. Alterations after major intrathoracic surgery. A.J.R. *134*:803, 1980.
101. Katzberg, R. W., Whitehouse, G. H., and deWeese, J. A.: The early radiologic findings in the adult chest after cardiopulmonary bypass surgery. Cardiovasc. Radiol. *1*:205, 1978.
102. Henry, D. A., Jolles, H., Berberich, J. J., and Schmelzer, V.: The post-cardiac surgery chest radiograph: A clinically integrated approach. J. Thorac. Imag. *4*:20, 1989.
103. Harris, R. S.: The preoperative chest film in relation to post-operative management—some effects of different projection, posture and lung inflation. Br. J. Radiol. *53*:196, 1950.
104. Goodman, L. R., Conrardy, P. A., Laing, F., et al.: Radiologic evaluation of endotracheal tube position. A.J.R. *127*:433, 1976.
105. Steiner, R. M., Tegtmeyer, C. J., Morse, D., et al.: Radiology of cardiac pacemakers. Radiographics *6*:373, 1986.
106. Thorsen, M. K., and Goodman, L. R.: Extracardiac complications of cardiac surgery. Semin. Roentgenol. *23*:32, 1988.

107. Wheeler, W. E., Rubis, L. J., and Jones, C. W.: Etiology and prevention of topical cardiac hypothermia-induced phrenic nerve injury and left lower lobe atelectasis during cardiac surgery. Chest 88:680, 1985.
108. Escovitz, E. S., Okulski, T. A., and Lapayowker, M. S.: The midsternal stripe: A sign of dehiscence following median sternotomy. Radiology 121:521, 1976.
109. Moncada, R., Kotler, M. N., Churchill, R. J., et al.: Multimodality approach to pericardial imaging. In Kotler, M. N., and Steiner, R. M. (eds.): Cardiac Imaging: New Technologies and Clinical Applications. Philadelphia, F. A. Davis, 1986, p. 409.
110. Kaminsky, M. E., Rodan, B. A., Osborne, D. R., et al.: Postpericardiotomy syndrome. A.J.R. 138:503, 1982.
111. Goodwin, J. D.: Conventional CT of the aorta. J. Thorac. Imag. 5:18, 1990.
112. Thorsen, M. K., Goodman, L. R., Sagel, S. S., et al.: Ascending aorta complications of cardiac surgery: CT evaluation. J. Comput. Assist. Tomogr. 10:219, 1986.
113. Sullivan, K. L., Steiner, R. M., Smullens, S. N., et al.: Pseudoaneurysm of the ascending aorta following cardiac surgery. Chest 93:138, 1988.
114. Gross, B. H., Shirazi, K. K., and Slater, A. D.: Differentiation of aortic and mitral valve prosthesis based on postoperative frontal chest radiographs. Radiology 149:389, 1983.
115. Hipona, F. A., Lerona, P. T., and Paredes, S.: Radiologic diagnosis of late complications associated with cardiac valve surgery in acquired heart disease. Radiol. Clin. N. Am. 9:265, 1971.
116. Rubin, S. A., Hightower, C. W., and Flicker, S.: Giant right atrium after mitral valve replacement: Plain film findings in 15 patients. A.J.R. 149:257, 1987.
117. Diethelm, L., Simonson, J. S., Dery, R., et al.: Determination of left ventricular mass with ultrafast CT and two-dimensional echocardiography. Radiology 171:213, 1989.
118. Sherry, C. S., and Harms, S. E.: MR imaging of pseudoaneurysms in aorticocoronary bypass graft. J. Comput. Assist. Tomogr. 13(3):426, 1989.
119. Goodwin, J. D., Califf, R. M., Korobkin, M., et al.: Clinical value of coronary bypass graft evaluation with CT. A.J.R. 140:649, 1983.
120. White, R., Caputo, G., Mark, A., et al.: Coronary bypass graft patency: Noninvasive evaluation with MR imaging. Radiology 164:681, 1987.
121. Henry, D. A., Corcoran, H. L., Lewis, T. D., et al.: Orthotopic cardiac transplantation: Evaluation with CT. Radiology 170:343, 1988.
122. Florence, S. H., Hutton, L. C., McKenzie, F. N., et al.: Cardiac transplantation: Postoperative chest radiographs. J. Can. Assoc. Radiol. 39:115, 1989.
123. Aherne, T., Tscholakoff, D., FInkbeiner, W., et al.: Magnetic resonance imaging of cardiac transplants: The evaluation of rejection of cardiac allografts with and without immunosuppression. Circulation 74(1):145, 1986.
124. Griffith, J. P., Hardesty, R. L., Trento, A., et al.: Heart-lung transplantation: Lessons learned and future hopes. Ann. Thorac. Surg. 43:6, 1987.
125. Bonser, R. S., Fragomeni, L.S.U., and Jamieson, S. W.: Heart-lung transplantation. Invest. Radiol. 24:310, 1989.
126. Holland, S. A., Hutton, L. C., and McKenzie, F. N.: Radiologic findings in heart-lung transplantation: A preliminary experience. J. Can. Assoc. Radiol. 40:94, 1989.

CONGENITAL HEART DISEASE IN THE ADULT

127. Tonkin, I. L., Kelley, M. J., Bream, P. R., et al.: The frontal chest film as a method of suspecting transposition complexes. Circulation 53:1016, 1976.
128. Proto, A. V., Cuthbert, N. W., and Raider, L.: Abberant right subclavian artery: Further observations. A.J.R. 148:253, 1987.
128a. Grollman, J. H.: The aortic diverticulum: A remnant of the partially involuted dorsal aortic root. Cardiovasc. Intervent. Radiol. 12:14, 1989.
128b. van der Horst, R. L., Fischer, E. A., DuBrow, I. W., et al.: Right aortic arch, right patent ductus arteriosus, and mirror image branching of the brachiocephalic vessels. Cardiovasc. Radiol. 1:147, 1978.
128c. Gomes, A. S.: MR imaging of congenital anomalies of the thoracic aorta and pulmonary arteries. Radiol. Clin. N. Am. 27:1171, 1989.
129. Martin, E. C., Stratford, M. A., and Gersony, W. M.: Initial detection of coarctation of the aorta: An opportunity for the radiologist. A.J.R. 127:1015, 1981.
129a. Nyman, R., Hallberg, M., Sunnegardh, J., et al.: Magnetic resonance imaging and angiography for the assessment of coarctation of the aorta. Acta Radiol. 30:481, 1989.
130. Woodring, J. H., and Rhodes, R. A.: Posterior superior mediastinal widening in aortic coarctation. A.J.R. 144:23, 1985.
131. Chen, J.T.T., Khoury, M., and Kirks, D. R.: Obscured aortic arch on lateral radiographics in coarctation of aorta. Radiology 153:595, 1984.
132. Figley, M. M.: Accessory Roentgen signs of coarctation of the aorta. Radiology 62:671, 1954.
133. Green, C. E., Gottdiener, J. S., and Goldstein, H. A.: Atrial septal defect. Semin. Roentgenol. 20:214, 1985.
134. Hipona, F. A., Paredes, S., and Lerona, P. T.: Roentgenologic analysis of common postoperative problems in congenital heart disease. Radiol. Clin. N. Am. 9:229, 1971.
135. Sanders, C., Bittner, V., Nath, P. H., et al.: Atrial septal defects in older adults: Atypical radiographic appearances. Radiology 167:123, 1988.
136. Soto, B., Bergeron, L. M., Jr., and Dethlein, E.: Ventricular septal defect. Semin. Roentgenol. 20:200, 1985.
137. Hoeffel, J. C., Dally, P., Legras, B., et al.: Roentgen aspects of isolated pulmonary valvular stenosis. Radiology 26:248, 1986.
138. Guit, G. L., Kroon, H. M., Van Voorthuisen, A., et al.: Congenitally corrected transposition in adults with left atrioventricular valve incompetance. Radiology 155:567, 1985.
139. Takasugi, J. E., Godwin, J. D., and Chen, J.T.T.: CT in congenitally corrected transposition of the great vessels. Computerized Radiol. 11:215, 1987.
140. Soulen, R. L., Donner, R. M., and Capitanio, M.: Postoperative evaluation of complex congenital heart disease by magnetic resonance imaging. Radiographics 7:975, 1987.
141. Deutsch, V., Wexler, L., Blieden, L. C., et al.: Ebstein's anomaly of tricuspid valve: Critical review of roentgenological features and additional angiographic signs. A.J.R. 125:395, 1985.
142. Giuliani, E. R., Fuster, V., Brandenburg, R. O., and Mair, D. D.: Ebstein's anomaly. Mayo Clin. Proc. 54:163, 1979.
143. Cooley, D. A., Hallman, G. L., and Hammam, A. S.: Congenital cardiovas± anomalies in adults: Results of surgical treatment in 167 patients over age of 35. Am. J. Cardiol. 17:303, 1966.
144. Mu-sheng, T., Partridge, J., and Radford, D.: The plain film chest radiograph in uncomplicated Ebstein's disease. Clin. Radiol. 37:551, 1986.

THE PERICARDIUM

145. Levy-Ravetch, M., Auh, Y. H., Rubenstein, W. A., et al.: CT of the pericardial recesses. A.J.R. 144:707, 1985.
146. Carsky, E. W., Mauceri, R. A., and Azimi, R.: The epicardial fat pad sign. Radiology 137:303, 1980.
146a. Olson, M. C., Posniak, H. V., McDonald, V., et al.: Computed tomography and magnetic resonance imaging of the pericardium. Radiographics 9:633, 1989.
147. Baron, M. G.: Pericardial effusion. Circulation 44:294, 1977.
148. Brown, J. J., Barakos, J. A., and Higgins, C. B.: Magnetic resonance imaging of cardiac and paracardiac masses. J. Thorac. Imag. 4(2):58, 1989.
149. Ellis, K., and King, D. L.: Pericarditis and pericardial effusion. Radiol. Clin. N. Am. 11:393, 1973.
150. Sechtem, U., Tscholakoff, D., and Higgins, C. B.: MRI of the abnormal pericardium. A.J.R. 147:245, 1986.
151. Feigin, D. S., Fenoglio, J. J., McAllister, H. A., et al.: Pericardial cysts. A radiologic-pathologic correlation and review. Radiology 125:15, 1977.

9

Coronary Arteriography

by DAVID C. LEVIN, M.D., and GEOFFREY A. GARDINER, Jr., M.D.

Despite the numerous advances in imaging technology within recent years, coronary arteriography remains the definitive examination for establishing the presence, site, and severity of coronary artery disease in living patients. The era of modern coronary arteriography began in 1959 with the development by Sones of a technique for selectively catheterizing the coronary arteries by way of a brachial artery cutdown and recording the images by cineangiography.[1] A detailed and delightful account of the first (and inadvertent) selective coronary arteriogram has been recorded by Hurst in an interview with Sones.[2] Another major landmark in the field occurred in 1967 with the development by Judkins of preformed catheters for selectively cannulating the coronary arteries by way of a percutaneous femoral approach.[3] Sones and Judkins, both of whom died in 1985, will be linked together in medical history as the two major pioneers in this most important diagnostic technique. Because of its ease, rapidity, and somewhat lower complication rate, the Judkins technique has become the most widely used approach for coronary arteriography throughout the world. For this reason, it will be described in some detail.

Technique of Coronary Arteriography

JUDKINS TECHNIQUE

Equipment for Coronary Arteriography

Although a wide variety of guidewires is available, the standard wire for percutaneous transfemoral coronary arteriography is the 0.035-inch or 0.038-inch guidewire with a 3-mm J-shaped tip. The J configuration and flexible tip allow the wire to be passed safely through most iliac arteries, even those with considerable tortuosity and atherosclerotic irregularity.

The Judkins coronary catheters, shown in Figure 9–1*A*, are shaped specifically to facilitate entry into the coronary ostia. They contain a fine wire braid within the wall for stability and directional control, and are fabricated of either polyethylene or polyurethane. The catheters are available in different sizes; the appropriate size selected depends on the size of the aortic arch. In some cases, depending on the body habitus of the patient and the size of the aortic root, additional alterations may be necessary, such as reshaping of the catheter in a steam jet or cutting off the tip with a blade to shorten it.

In most laboratories, the coronary catheter is attached to a three-stopcock manifold (Fig. 9–1*B*), which enables the angiographer to switch rapidly between pressure monitoring, flushing the catheter with saline, and performing contrast injections, all in a closed system that allows for speed and maintenance of sterility. In addition to the three side ports, one end of the manifold has a rotating adapter for attachment to the catheter itself, while the other end has a Luer-Lok fitting to which a syringe is attached.

Some angiographers now use a side arm arterial sheath (Fig. 9–1*C*) for performing coronary arteriography. The sheath is inserted into the femoral artery percutaneously over a Teflon introducer which is then withdrawn, leaving only the sheath in place. It has a rubber check valve at its external end to maintain hemostasis and provide access for the catheter. It also has a side arm through which femoral artery pressure can be monitored. The inner diameter of the sheath is somewhat larger than the outer diameter of the angiographic catheter, and it is the column of blood between them which transmits pressure through the side arm to the transducer. Other advantages of the sheath are that it allows multiple catheter exchanges to be performed without compression of the groin, and that it lessens patient discomfort caused by catheter manipulation. Although the sheath has the potential disadvantage of creating a larger hole in the arterial wall than if a catheter alone is used, experience has shown that the use of this technique does not create an increased risk of local arterial complications.

Catheterization Technique

The groin area is palpated to ascertain the point of maximal impulse of the femoral artery. This usually is at or just below the level of the inguinal crease and always is several centimeters below the inguinal ligament. The skin area 1 to 2 cm below and slightly lateral to the point of maximal impulse is anesthetized locally. The artery is then punctured with a Seldinger type of needle using a relatively shallow approach (i.e., the needle direction is more parallel to the artery than perpen-

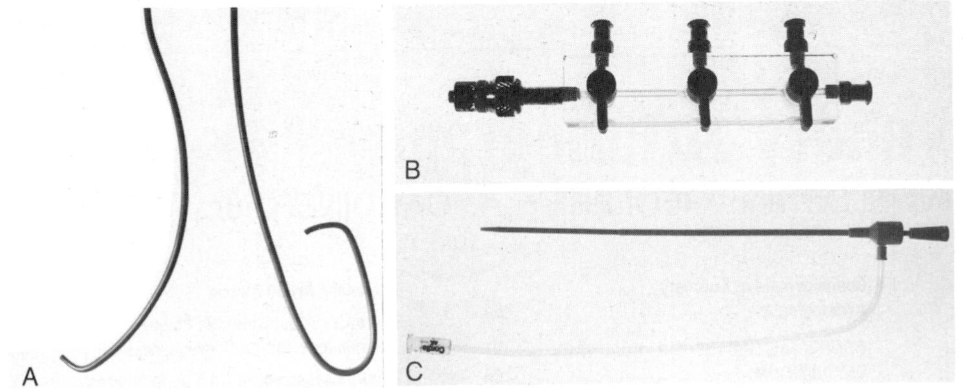

FIGURE 9–1. *A,* **Right and left Judkins coronary catheters. The right coronary catheter is on the left of the photograph.** *B,* **Three-stopcock manifold used in coronary arteriography.** *C,* **Side arm sheath used in transfemoral coronary arteriography. (From Abrams, H.L. [ed.]: Coronary Arteriography. A Practical Approach. Boston, Little, Brown, 1983, with permission.)**

dicular to it). The operator should be sure that the actual level of arterial entry is distal to the inguinal ligament. If the needle enters the femoral artery proximal to this ligament, it may be impossible to control bleeding by manual compression at the end of the procedure.

The guidewire is then passed through the needle into the aorta. The needle is removed over the guidewire, and the introducer–sheath combination is inserted over the wire. Once the sheath is positioned correctly in the artery, both the guidewire and the introducer are removed, leaving only the sheath in place. Careful flushing of the side arm of the sheath is performed to extract any small clots that may have formed during this maneuver, and the side arm is then connected to a pressure transducer for continuous monitoring of femoral artery pressure.

A pigtail catheter is loaded onto a 3-mm J-shaped guidewire, so that the flexible tip of the wire protrudes beyond the catheter tip. This combination is then inserted through the check valve of the sheath and into the aorta, using fluoroscopic control. The guidewire–catheter combination is passed up to the descending thoracic aorta, the wire is removed, and the catheter is connected to the rotating adapter of the three-stopcock manifold. The catheter is carefully flushed, and central aortic pressure is recorded through one of the side ports of the manifold, which has been connected to a second transducer. At this point, the operator should check both pressure tracings: one from the catheter tip (monitored through the manifold) and the other from the femoral artery (monitored through the side arm of the arterial sheath). If the pressure tracings are satisfactory, the catheter is advanced over the aortic arch and through the aortic valve into the left ventricle. Left ventricular pressure measurements, particularly left ventricular end-diastolic pressure (LVEDP), are recorded, and left ventriculography is performed as described on page 270.

After left ventriculography, LVEDP should again be measured. The contrast injection usually results in at least some degree of elevation of LVEDP. This is well tolerated, as long as it remains below 25 to 30 mm Hg. The pigtail catheter is then removed over a guidewire, and a selective coronary catheter is inserted in its place. To catheterize either coronary artery, the image intensifier should be positioned so that the angiographer views the patient's heart in the left anterior oblique (LAO) projection. When viewed in this projection, the left coronary artery (LCA) originates from the left side of the aorta, while the right coronary artery (RCA) originates from the right side of the aorta. (From a true anatomical point of view, the LCA originates from the left posterolateral aspect of the aorta, while the RCA originates from its anterior aspect.)

The technique for catheterizing the LCA is shown in Figure 9–2. In advancing the left Judkins catheter toward the left coronary ostium, the most important rules are to advance it slowly and to keep it positioned so that it remains in full profile (i.e., so that both curves of the catheter are clearly visible). If the catheter begins to turn out of profile, it should be gently rotated with the rotating adapter as it is advanced slowly. If the catheter is advanced too rapidly, it may snap forcefully into the left coronary ostium and cause dissection.

After the left coronary ostium is entered, the pressure at the catheter tip should be checked immediately to be sure that it still coincides with femoral artery pressure. If so, it can be safely assumed that the catheter tip is free within the lumen of the LCA, a fact which can be verified by a small test injection of contrast medium. If the pressure tracing shows significant damping or "ventricularization" (normal systolic pressure but a low diastolic pressure), this may indicate the presence of significant stenosis of the LCA. Although these pressure changes can occur merely from abutment of the catheter tip on the arterial wall, it should be assumed that left main coronary stenosis is present until proven otherwise. Whenever ventricularization or damping occurs, the catheter should be removed from the left coronary ostium and an attempt at repositioning should be made. If the pressure abnormality persists, it is wise to withdraw the catheter slightly and perform a nonselective injection of contrast material with the

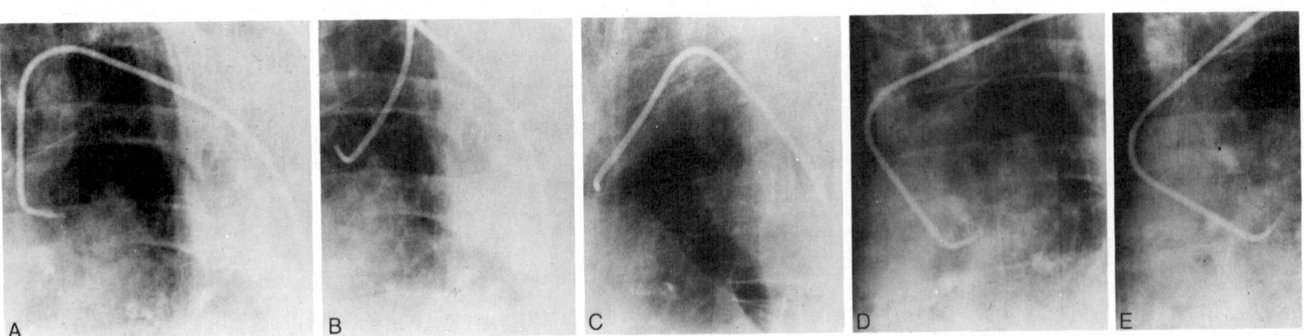

FIGURE 9–2. Technique for catheterizing the left coronary artery (LCA) while the patient is viewed in the left anterior oblique (LAO) projection. *A,* **The catheter is seen in full profile as it is advanced around the aortic arch. Note that both curves of the catheter are clearly seen.** *B,* **The catheter is rotated too far in one direction. The curves are distorted.** *C,* **The tip is now rotated too far in the other direction, resulting again in loss of visualization of the tip curve.** *D,* **After proper rotation of the catheter, both curves are again seen in profile as it is advanced toward the aortic root.** *E,* **The tip of the catheter has now passed into the left coronary ostium. (From Abrams, H.L. [ed.]: Coronary Arteriography. A Practical Approach. Boston, Little, Brown, 1983, with permission.)**

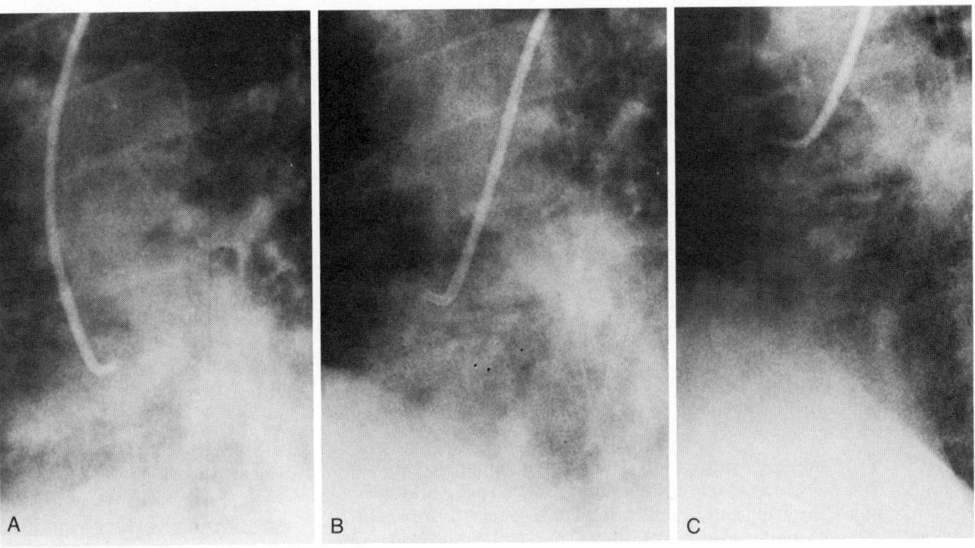

FIGURE 9–3. Catheterization of the right coronary artery (RCA) while viewing the patient in the LAO projection. *A*, The catheter tip is advanced to the root of the aorta with its tip directed to the left. *B*, The catheter is rotated in a clockwise direction as it is withdrawn. *C*, Further clockwise rotation and withdrawal result in passage of the tip into the right coronary ostium. (From Abrams, H.L. [ed.]: Coronary Arteriography. A Practical Approach. Boston, Little, Brown, 1983, with permission.)

catheter tip in the left aortic cusp just outside the ostium of the vessel. This often allows demonstration of left main coronary stenosis, if it is present.

If the catheter tip pressure is normal and a small test injection of contrast material shows that the main LCA is not stenotic, left coronary arteriography is then performed using multiple projections. A frontal or shallow right anterior oblique (RAO) view often is obtained first to visualize the ostium of the LCA and to make sure that there is no stenosis at that site. Other views that are most helpful include standard RAO, cranially angulated RAO, caudally angulated RAO, cranially angulated LAO, and direct lateral projections. If these fail to provide complete visualization of the left coronary system, a caudally angulated LAO view may be added, or the degrees of sagittal or transverse angulation may be varied. The advantages of cranial and caudal angulation are discussed on p. 245. A forceful hand injection of 6 to 9 ml of contrast material usually is required to fill the left coronary system; in some laboratories, these injections are performed with a power injector to provide complete opacification.

Catheterization of the RCA also is performed in the LAO position, but this requires different maneuvers than catheterization of the LCA. Whereas the left coronary catheter tends to seek out the left coronary ostium almost automatically, the right coronary catheter must be rotated by the angiographer to engage the vessel. This usually is accomplished by first passing the catheter to a point just above the aortic valve and then rotating it clockwise while slowly withdrawing it (Fig. 9–3). Entry into the RCA usually is signified by a sudden rightward movement of the catheter tip. Here again, the catheter tip pressure should be checked to be sure that damping or ventricularization has not occurred. If it has, this may signify ostial stenosis. These pressure changes also can result from a small RCA, inadvertent superselective entry of the catheter tip into the conus branch, presence of total obstruction shortly beyond the right coronary ostium, or spasm of the RCA.

Catheter-induced spasm of the RCA is relatively common, but it is extremely rare in the left coronary system, for reasons which are not entirely clear. Right coronary spasm can be alleviated by administration of sublingual nitroglycerin. If persistent damping or ventricularization of the pressure tracing is seen after use of nitroglycerin, a cusp injection should be performed to attempt to visualize a possible stenosis of the right coronary ostium. Alternatively, a very small injection of contrast medium into the RCA itself can be performed with immediate withdrawal of the catheter tip at the end of the injection (sometimes referred to as the "shoot-and-run" technique).

If the pressure tracing is normal on entry of the catheter tip, the RCA should be visualized in at least two projections. The standard LAO and RAO projections usually will suffice, but on occasion cranial angulation should be added. Hand injections of 3 to 6 ml of contrast material usually are enough to fill the right coronary system; the actual quantity should be judged by the angiographer, depending on the size of the vessel.

OTHER TECHNIQUES OF CORONARY ARTERIOGRAPHY

Sones Technique

The Sones catheter, shown in Figure 9–4, is constructed of either woven Dacron or polyurethane and has an end hole and four small side holes close to the catheter tip. The most commonly used catheter is the No. 7 or 8 French, with a tip that tapers to a No. 5 French. The brachial artery cutdown is performed by blunt dissection, and a small incision is made in the vessel.[4] A catheter is first introduced into the distal segment of the brachial artery, and heparinized saline is injected to prevent clotting during the remainder of the procedure when there is no blood flow. The Sones catheter is then advanced into the ascending aorta. The technique most commonly used to enter the left coronary ostium with this catheter is to form an open loop on the right aortic cusp so that the shaft of the catheter and its tip form a 45-degree angle pointed toward the left coronary cusp. Alternate advancement and withdrawal of the catheter then often results in entry of the tip into the left coronary ostium. Stable seating of the catheter tip can be accomplished in some patients by advancing the catheter, whereas in other cases slight retraction is necessary. To enter the right coronary ostium, a slightly smaller open loop is formed, once again pointing toward the left coronary cusp. The catheter is then slowly withdrawn during clockwise rotation. This maneuver often causes the tip to rotate and pass into the RCA.

AMPLATZ TECHNIQUE. During the same year the Judkins catheters were developed, Amplatz et al.[5] developed another set of catheters for percutaneous coronary arteriography by way of the femoral approach (Fig. 9–5). Although the Amplatz catheters are much less commonly used than those devised by Judkins, they are an excellent alternative in the occasional cases in which the Judkins catheters are not appropriately shaped to enter the coronary arteries. To catheterize the LCA, the broad secondary curve of the appropriately sized left Amplatz catheter is positioned so it rests on the right aortic cusp with its tip pointing toward the left aortic cusp. Alternating advancement and retraction of the catheter in a

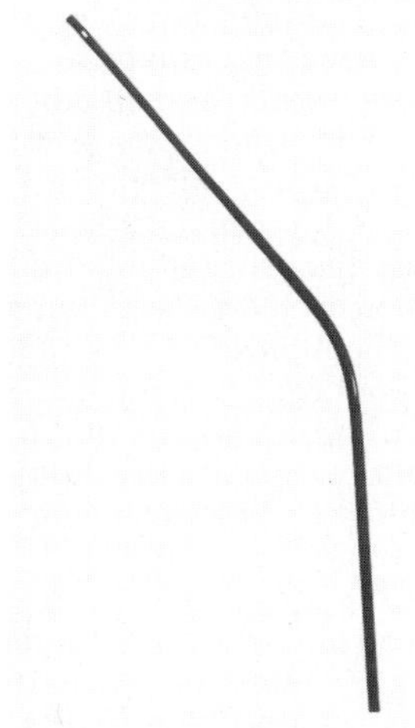

FIGURE 9–4. Sones coronary catheter.

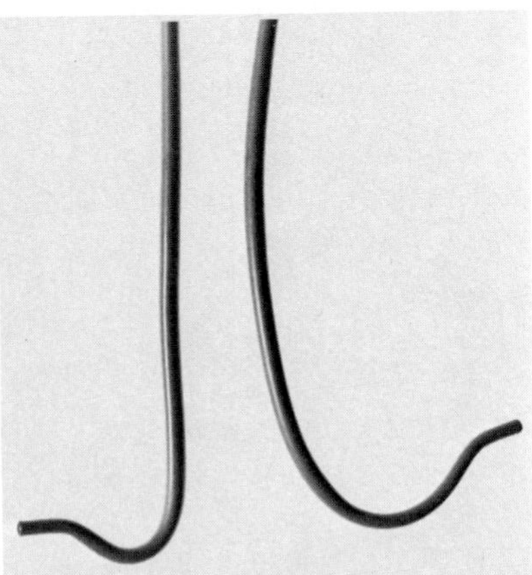

FIGURE 9-5. Amplatz right and left coronary catheters. The right coronary catheter is on the left of the photograph. (From Abrams, H.L. [ed.]: Coronary Arteriography. A Practical Approach. Boston, Little, Brown, 1983, with permission.)

slow and gentle manner usually produces entry of the tip into the left coronary ostium. Once the tip enters the ostium, the position of the catheter usually can be stabilized by slight retraction. Catheterizing the RCA with the right Amplatz catheter requires a technique similar to that used with the right Judkins catheter.

MULTIPURPOSE CATHETER TECHNIQUE. A single catheter which can be inserted percutaneously by way of the femoral approach and used to catheterize both the right and the left coronary arteries was originally described by Schoonmaker and King[6] and in greater detail by King and Douglas.[7] The catheter has a configuration similar to that of the Sones catheter, although the tip is shorter. The maneuvers used to seat the catheter also are similar to those used in the Sones technique.

TECHNICAL FEATURES

Cineangiographic Equipment

Cineangiographic equipment is expensive and complex.[8,9] In brief, the following types of equipment are needed: (1) A three-phase, 12-pulse, or constant-potential x-ray generator with cine pulsing, output of 100 or more kilowatts, and an automatic brightness control with very rapid response. (2) A high-heat-capacity x-ray tube capable of rotating at 10,000 rpm with a target angle of 10 degrees or less. Dual focal spots should be available, with a small focal spot size of approximately 0.6 mm and a large focal spot size of approximately 1.2 mm. (3) Carbon fiber grids and a grid ratio of 8:1 and approximately 100 lines per inch. (4) A dual- or triple-mode cesium iodide image intensifier with a resolution capability of approximately 5 line pairs per millimeter, a contrast ratio of greater than 15:1, and a conversion factor of greater than 50 for the small mode. The intensifier should have at least two modes, with the large mode approximating 9 inches to be able to image large ventricles, and a small mode (magnified mode) of 6 inches or less. Large-mode image intensifiers (14 or 16 inches) are commonly used in abdominal and peripheral angiography but are not recommended for cardiac catheterization laboratories because the considerable bulk of these units interferes with the need to obtain steep cranial and caudal angulation and to bring the intensifier face into close contact with the patient. (5) An optical system consisting of an objective lens, an image-distributing mirror, and a cine camera lens. The focal length of the camera lens should allow the proper degree of overframing. A diaphragm should be interposed in front of the cine camera lens, and ideally, the entire system should be set up so that the lens can operate at two f-stops above maximum aperture. (6) A cine camera capable of operating at either 30 or 60 frames per second with low vibration levels. (7) Cine film carefully chosen with a speed and average gradient appropriate for the system and a low level of "base + fog."[9] (8) A cine film processor which can maintain highly stable developer temperature and immersion time; it also must provide adequate replenishment of chemical solutions, proper agitation, and recirculation.

Drugs Used During Coronary Arteriography

Adequate premedication is important for efficient operation of the catheterization laboratory and the welfare of the patient. A variety of regimens are used in different laboratories. King and Douglas recommend diazepam in 2.5 to 5-mg increments and 0.6 mg atropine, both given intravenously.[7] Atropine is avoided in patients whose condition is unstable, those with a rapid heart rate, or those in whom ergonovine provocation is contemplated. In the cardiac catheterization laboratory at Thomas Jefferson University Hospital, diazepam, 5 to 10 mg, and diphenhydramine (Benadryl), 25 mg, are given orally 1 hour before the procedure.

Heparin (also see p. 1780) is used routinely in most laboratories. This is done despite the fact that it has not been clearly shown to exert a beneficial effect in the prevention of complications.[10] It is administered intravenously at a dose of 5000 units at the time the first arterial catheter is inserted.

Nitroglycerin has several effects on the cardiovascular system (p. 1304), but from the point of view of the angiographer, its principal effect is to diminish vascular tone in the epicardial coronary arteries. It is given shortly before the procedure, at a dose of 0.30 mg sublingually, to prevent catheter-induced spasm. This dose may not be sufficient to obviate spasm completely, so additional doses may well be necessary during the procedure. Nitroglycerin also can be administered intravenously or directly into a coronary artery. Most angiographers use this drug routinely except in patients with suspected variant angina. In these people, nitroglycerin might mask the demonstration of spasm.

The use of *atropine* is more controversial. Some laboratories avoid it in most cases. Atropine diminishes the likelihood of vasovagal reactions and the sinus bradycardia that frequently occurs after selective coronary injections. A drawback to its use is that it usually increases heart rate, which leads to increased myocardial oxygen demand and may make adequate opacification of the coronary arteries more difficult. When it is used, 0.6 mg should be given intravenously at the start of the procedure, provided the patient's heart rate is below 80 beats/min.

The monomeric ionic *contrast agents* that have been used in coronary arteriography for many years are high-osmolar methylglucamine and sodium salts of diatrizoic acid. These substances dissociate into cations and iodine-containing anions,[11,12] resulting in aqueous solutions with an osmolality of 1940 mOsm/kg. The osmolality of human plasma is 300 mOsm/kg. The hypertonicity of these compounds produces a number of adverse electrophysiologic and hemodynamic effects during coronary arteriography. These include sinus bradycardia, heart block, QT interval and QRS prolongation, ventricular tachycardia or fibrillation, ST depression, increased T wave amplitude, decreased left ventricular contractility, decreased systolic pressure, and increased LVEDP. Another contributing factor in the genesis of at least some of these effects is the presence of calcium-chelating agents like sodium citrate and EDTA (ethylenediaminetetraacetic acid) as preservatives in certain ionic contrast agents.

Nonionic agents such as iohexol and iopamidol also are available. Because they go into solution as single neutral molecules, their osmolality is substantially reduced (under 850 mOsm/kg). They also do not contain calcium-chelating agents. Another, similar new agent is the low-osmolality ionic dimer methylglucamine-sodium ioxaglate. Clinical trials of these agents have shown a lower incidence of the aforementioned adverse effects when compared with ionic contrast agents.[11,13-15] The major drawback to the low-osmolality agents is their substantially increased cost (10 to 15 times that of the standard agents). Another drawback is the fact that standard ionic contrast agents have an inhibitory effect on clot formation when mixed with blood, whereas nonionic agents exhibit less of this inhibitory effect.[16,17] Because contrast and blood are in direct contact in syringes and tubing for varying time intervals during arteriography, clots are more likely to form when nonionic agents are used. Serious thromboembolic complications have been anecdotally reported during coronary arteriography with nonionic contrast media.[16,17] This risk may be reduced with careful attention to catheter technique and maintenance of adequate systemic heparinization.

Although some laboratories routinely use low-osmolality agents, it appears that most have avoided doing so because of the associated high costs. A rational and cost-effective policy would seem to be that the standard ionic agents should be used for most elective procedures, but that the use of low-osmolality agents be considered for certain higher-risk patients, such as those with congestive heart failure, severely unstable angina, acute myocardial infarction, or a history of a previous adverse reaction to ionic contrast.

ELECTROCARDIOGRAPHIC AND HEMODYNAMIC CHANGES IN CORONARY ARTERIOGRAPHY. The selective injection of methylglucamine–sodium diatrizoate or other ionic contrast agents into coronary arteries characteristically results in a variety of electrocardiographic and hemodynamic changes. Right coronary arteriography often produces T-wave inversion in leads II, III, and aVF. Sinus bradycardia and systemic hypotension also occur frequently, and sometimes can be severe. Left coronary arteriography usually results in peaking of the T wave in leads II, III, and aVF. Sinus bradycardia and hypotension may occur, but usually are less pronounced than during right coronary arteriography. If the patient has total right coronary occlusion, a biphasic response can occur during left coronary arteriography. The left coronary injection first produces T-wave elevation, but as the contrast passes through collaterals to the distal right coronary tree, the characteristic T-wave inversion normally seen with right coronary arteriography occurs.

ANATOMY AND VARIATIONS OF THE CORONARY ARTERIES

Angiography visualizes only a small portion of the coronary circulation: the major epicardial branches and their second-, third-, and perhaps fourth-order branches. The myriad of small intramyocardial branches are not visualized because of their small size, cardiac motion, and limitations in resolution of cine imaging systems. Although these small "resistance" vessels play a major role in regulation of coronary blood flow, they are not thought to be important in human coronary artery disease (CAD).

In viewing the coronary arteries by cineangiography, the direct frontal and lateral views are less commonly used than the RAO and LAO views. This is because the heart is oriented obliquely in the thoracic cavity. Because the major coronary arteries traverse the atrioventricular and interventricular grooves, which in turn are aligned with the long and short axes of the heart, it follows that the best angiographic projections to visualize these vessels in profile are the oblique views. In the following discussion, most of the anatomical descriptions refer to the RAO and LAO projections.

The term "dominance" often is used to describe coronary artery anatomy. With this nomenclature, the dominant vessel is the one which supplies the posterior diaphragmatic portion of the interventricular septum and the diaphragmatic surface of the left ventricle. The RCA is dominant in about 85 per cent of humans. The use of the term "dominance" is somewhat misleading because it suggests that in this 85 per cent, the RCA is the more important vessel. Because human CAD is primarily the result of interruption of blood supply to the left ventricular myocardium, a nondominant LCA is almost always more important than the dominant RCA. With this understanding, the term "dominance" nevertheless is used because it is a commonly accepted anatomical concept.

Figure 9–6 is a diagram of the coronary anatomy in a typical patient with RCA dominance. The anatomy is demonstrated

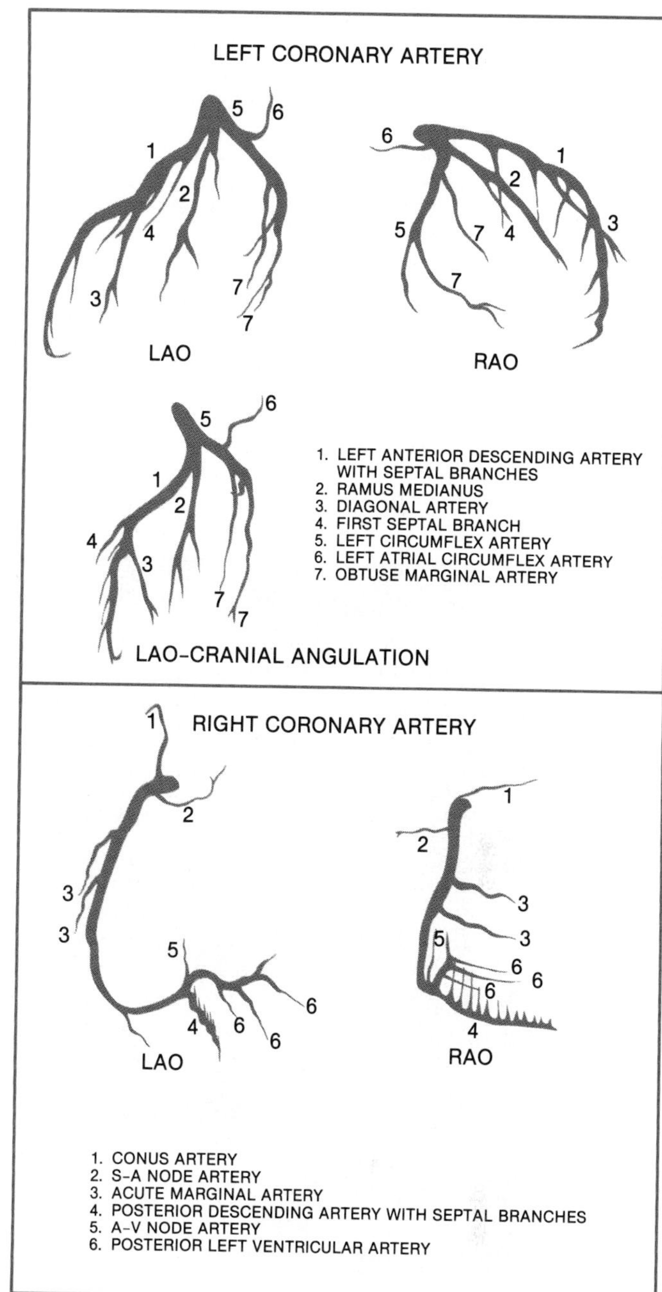

FIGURE 9–6. Anatomy of the coronary arteries. (From Grossman, W.G. [ed.]: Cardiac Catheterization and Angiography. Philadelphia, Lea and Febiger, 1991.)

in the standard LAO and RAO projections for both the right and the left coronary system. In addition, an LAO view of the left coronary system with cranial angulation is shown, since this is the most commonly used sagittal-angulation view.

LEFT CORONARY ARTERY

(Figs. 9–7*A* and *B* and 9–8*A* through *C*)

The main LCA arises from the upper portion of the left aortic sinus, just below the sinotubular ridge. It passes behind the right ventricular outflow tract and may extend for 0 to 10 mm. It then usually bifurcates into left anterior descending (LAD) and circumflex branches.

Left Anterior Descending Artery

The LAD passes down the anterior interventricular groove toward the cardiac apex. In the RAO projection, it extends toward the anterior aspect of the heart. In the LAO projection, it passes down the cardiac midline, between the right and left ventricles. Its major branches are the *septal* and *diagonal* branches.

The *septal* branches pass downward into the interventricular septum. They vary in size, number, and distribution. In some cases, there is a large first septal branch, which is vertically oriented and breaks up into a number of secondary branches that ramify throughout the septum. In other cases, a more horizontally oriented, large first septal branch is present, which passes parallel to and below the LAD itself. In still others, a number of septal arteries are roughly comparable in size. These septal branches interconnect with similar septal branches passing upward from the posterior descending branch of the RCA to produce a network of potential collateral channels. The interventricular septum is the most densely vascularized area of the heart, and the first septal branch is its most important potential collateral channel.

The *diagonal* branches of the LAD pass over the anterolateral aspect of the heart, and it usually is one of these branches which supplies the apex itself. Although virtually all patients have a single LAD in the anterior interventricular groove, there is wide variability in the number and size of diagonal branches. More than 90 per cent have one to three such branches.[18] Less than 1 per cent of patients have no diagonal branches. Thus, if none are seen, the angiographer should suspect the possibility that a diagonal branch might have originally been present but become totally occluded at its origin from the LAD. This is particularly true in cases in which there are unexplained contraction abnormalities of the anterior left ventricle.

In 37 per cent of patients, the LCA has a trifurcation instead of a bifurcation.[18] In these cases, a *ramus medianus* arises between the LAD and circumflex arteries; this vessel is analogous to a diagonal branch and usually supplies the free wall along the lateral aspect of the left ventricle.

In 78 per cent of patients, the LAD passes all the way around

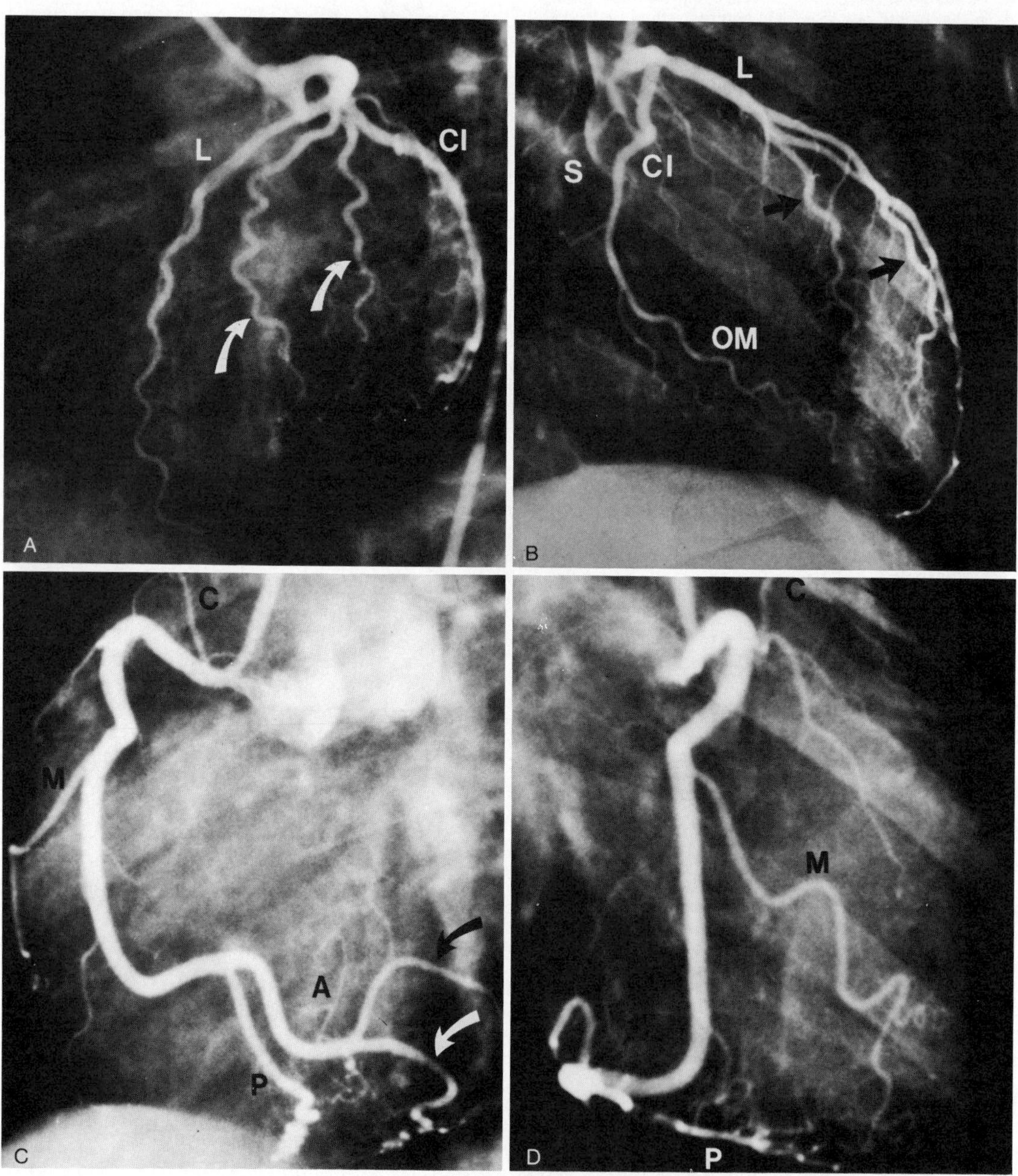

FIGURE 9–7. *A,* LCA in the LAO projection. *B,* LCA in the RAO projection. L = Left anterior descending artery (LAD); CI = Circumflex artery; OM = Obtuse marginal branch of the circumflex; S = Sinoatrial node artery; arrows point to two diagonal branches of the LAD. The small branches originating from the LAD and passing downward are the septal branches. *C,* RCA in the LAO projection. *D,* RCA in the right anterior oblique (RAO) projection. C = Conus branch; M = Acute marginal branch; P = Posterior descending artery; A = Atrioventricular node artery; arrows point to posterior left ventricular branches.

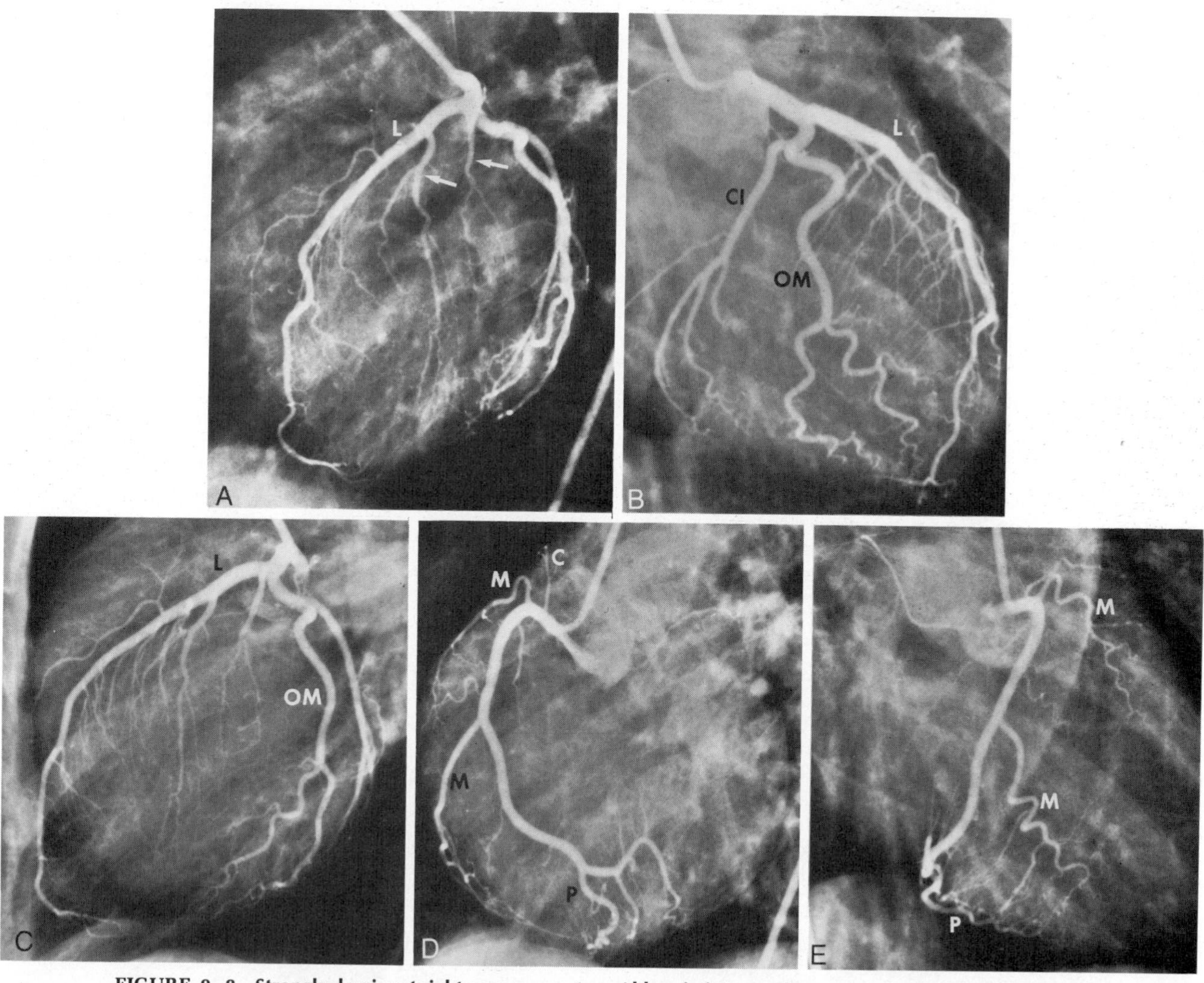

FIGURE 9–8. Strongly dominant right coronary system. Abbreviations are the same as in Figure 9–7. *A, B,* and *C,* LCA in the LAO, RAO, and left lateral projections. Arrows point to diagonal branches of the LAD. Note the large obtuse marginal branch of the left circumflex artery, which compensates for the small diagonal branches. *D* and *E,* RCA in the LAO and RAO projections.

the apex and terminates along the diaphragmatic aspect of the left ventricle. In 22 per cent of patients, however, the LAD fails to reach the diaphragmatic surface, terminating instead either at or even before the cardiac apex.[19] In these cases, the posterior descending branch of the RCA is larger and longer than usual, and supplies the apex. Correspondingly, because the LAD does not supply the cardiac apex in such cases, its distal segment is smaller and shorter than usual. Early attenuation and a narrow distal caliber do not necessarily signify LAD disease if some or all of the cardiac apex is supplied by the posterior descending artery.

Circumflex Artery

The left circumflex artery originates at the bifurcation (or trifurcation) of the main LCA and passes down the left atrioventricular groove. In about 85 per cent of human hearts, the left circumflex artery is the nondominant vessel and varies in size and length, depending on the actual degree of right coronary dominance. The left circumflex artery usually gives off one to three large *obtuse marginal branches* as it passes down the atrioventricular groove. These are the principal branches of the circumflex, since they supply the free wall of the left ventricle along its lateral aspect. Beyond the origins of these obtuse marginal branches, the distal left circumflex tends to be small. The actual position of the circumflex artery can best be determined on the late phase of a left coronary injection, when the coronary sinus becomes opacified with diluted contrast material. The position of the coronary sinus identifies the position of the left atrioventricular groove and the proper circumflex artery which runs in or near it. In the LAO projection, the obtuse marginal branches and the proper circumflex artery may be directly superimposed, or nearly so. Therefore, it is best to try and localize lesions of these vessels on either frontal or RAO projections.

The circumflex artery also may give rise to one or two *left atrial circumflex branches.* These branches supply the lateral and posterior aspects of the left atrium.

RIGHT CORONARY ARTERY

(Figs. 9–6, 9–7*C* and *D*, and 9–8*D* and *E*)

The RCA originates from the right aortic sinus at a point somewhat lower than the origin of the LCA from the left aortic sinus. It passes down the right atrioventricular groove toward the crux (a point on the diaphragmatic surface of the heart where the right atrioventricular groove, the left atrioventricular groove, and the posterior interventricular groove come together).

The first branch of the RCA is considered to be the *conus artery.* In about 50 per cent of hearts, this vessel arises at the right coronary ostium or within the first few millimeters of the RCA. It passes upward and anteriorly over the right ventricular outflow tract toward the LAD. Its primary importance is to serve as a source of collateral circulation in patients with LAD occlusion. In the other 50 per cent of hearts, the conus artery is not actually a branch of the RCA, but arises from a small, separate ostium in the right aortic sinus just above the right coronary ostium.[20] In this group of patients, selective right coronary arteriography may fail to opacify the conus artery unless sufficient reflux of contrast medium occurs to fill the separate ostium. In a series from the authors' laboratory, it was found that opacification of the right coronary artery failed to adequately visualize the conus artery in 20 per cent of cases.[20] Presumably this group came from the half of the population in which the conus artery has a separate origin.

The second branch of the RCA usually is the *sinoatrial node artery*. Kyriakidis et al. found that this vessel originated from the RCA in 59 per cent, from the left circumflex in 38 per cent, and had a dual supply in the remaining 3 per cent.[21] When it originates from the RCA, it passes obliquely backward through the upper portion of the atrial septum and the anteromedial wall of the right atrium. It sends branches to the sinus node, and usually also to the right atrium or both atria. When it originates from the left circumflex artery, it may pass backward in the atrial septum or around the posterolateral wall of the left atrium to reach the sinus node area.

The midportion of the RCA usually gives rise to one or several medium-sized *acute marginal* (or right ventricular) *branches*. These branches supply the anterior wall of the right ventricle and are relatively unimportant, except insofar as they also may serve as sources of collateral circulation in patients with LAD occlusion.

The next important branch of the RCA is the *posterior descending artery* (PDA). As indicated earlier, about 85 per cent of patients have a dominant RCA. The dominant artery is considered to be that vessel (either the RCA or the circumflex artery) which supplies the diaphragmatic aspect of the left ventricle and the lower portion of the interventricular septum. When the RCA is dominant, the PDA originates at or shortly before the crux and passes forward in the posterior interventricular groove. During its course along this groove, it gives rise to a number of small *inferior septal branches*, which pass upward to supply the lower portion of the interventricular septum and interdigitate with superior septal branches passing down from the LAD. After giving rise to the PDA, a dominant RCA continues beyond the crux and begins to pass upward along the distal portion of the left atrioventricular groove. Here it usually terminates by giving rise to one or several *posterior left ventricular* (PLV) *branches*, which supply the diaphragmatic surface of the left ventricle.

About 15 per cent do not have RCA dominance; about half of these have LCA dominance. With this anatomical pattern, the left circumflex artery is large and continues down to the diaphragmatic surface of the left ventricle, where it gives rise to the PLV branches and then reaches the crux and turns forward to become the PDA. In these cases, the RCA is very small and terminates before reaching the crux, and therefore does not supply any blood to left ventricular myocardium. The other half of patients without RCA dominance have a mixed or "balanced" circulation, wherein the RCA gives rise to the PDA, while the left circumflex artery gives rise to the PLV branches.

At or near the crux, the dominant artery gives rise to a small *atrioventricular node artery*, which passes upward to supply this node.

In about one-fourth of patients with right coronary dominance, there are significant anatomical variations in the origin of the PDA. These variations include partial supply of the PDA territory by acute marginal branches, double PDA, and early origin of the PDA proximal to the crux.

ARTERIOGRAPHIC EXAMPLES

Figures 9–7 through 9–9 are examples of three patients with dominant RCAs. The patient whose arteriogram is shown in Figure 9–7 has two diagonal branches of the LAD,

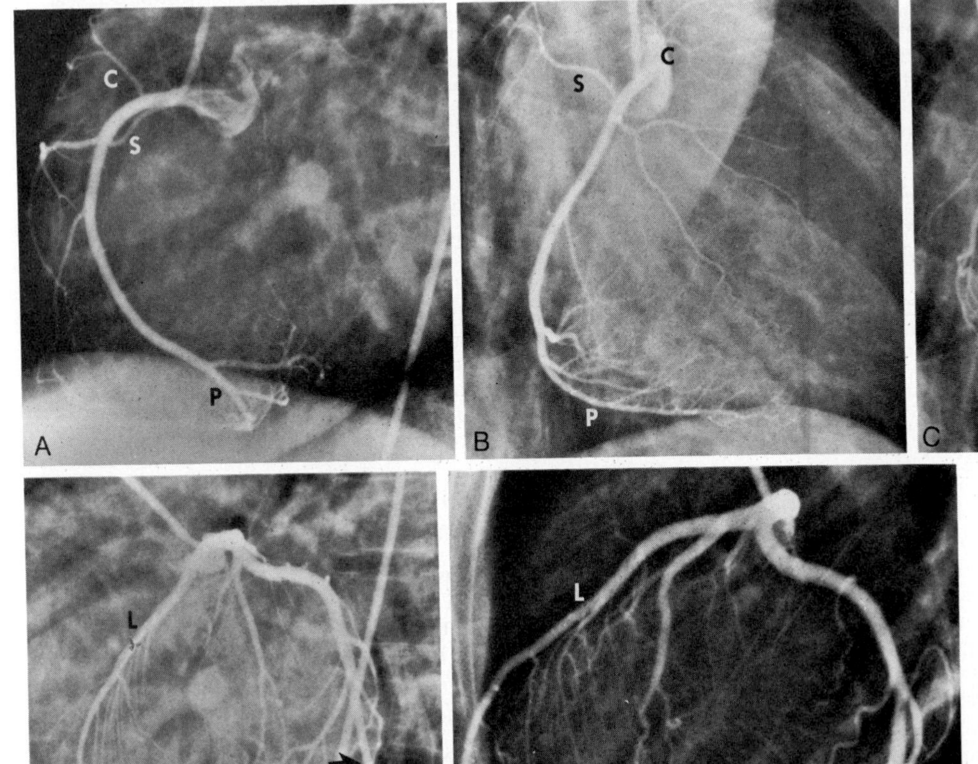

FIGURE 9–9. Weakly dominant right coronary system. *A* and *B*, LAO and RAO views of the RCA. Both the conus and the sinoatrial node artery arise from the RCA. The distal portion of the RCA beyond the origin of the posterior descending artery (P) is short and gives rise only to a single small posterior left ventricular branch. *C, D,* and *E,* LCA in the RAO, LAO, and left lateral projections. Note that the circumflex artery gives rise to four obtuse marginal branches, the most distal of which (arrow) supplies some of the diaphragmatic portion of the left ventricle. The LAD gives rise to two small and one medium-sized diagonal branches.

one of which closely parallels the LAD itself in the RAO projection. In this projection, it is still possible to differentiate the two because the LAD is the longer of the two vessels, passes all the way around the cardiac apex, and gives rise to septal branches. This patient's sinoatrial node artery arises from the left circumflex artery. In the patient whose arteriogram is shown in Figure 9–8, the sinoatrial node artery arises from the RCA. As is true in the preceding illustration, the arteriogram shown in Figure 9–8 exhibits relatively strong dominance of the RCA. In addition to the PDA, this patient's RCA gives rise to two relatively large PLV arteries. The patient also has two diagonal branches of the LAD, but both are relatively small. This is due to the presence of a very large first obtuse marginal branch of the left circumflex artery, which supplies much of the anterolateral free wall of the left ventricle. This area more commonly is supplied by diagonal branches. The numerous septal branches are clearly seen, and the LAD again passes all the way around the cardiac apex. The patient whose arteriogram is shown in Figure 9–9 has relatively weak dominance of the RCA. After the origin of the PDA, the terminal portion of the RCA gives rise to only a single, relatively small PLV branch. The left coronary arteriogram in this patient shows that four obtuse marginal branches arise from the left circumflex artery. The most distal of these is quite large, and supplies some of the diaphragmatic portion of the left ventricle, an area usually supplied by PLV branches. This patient has three diagonal branches of the LAD, two of which are quite small and one of which is medium-sized.

Figure 9–10 is an example of left coronary arterial dominance. The RCA is small and terminates well before reaching the crux of the heart. It does not supply any portion of left ventricular myocardium. On the other hand, the left circumflex artery in this patient is quite large and gives rise to three large PLV branches and the PDA. In addition, this circumflex artery gives rise to two large obtuse marginal branches.

The preceding arteriographic examples all show instances in which the LAD passes all the way around the cardiac apex. Figure 9–11 shows the coronary arteriogram of a patient with a short LAD that terminates before reaching the cardiac apex. Instead, the apex is supplied by the PDA branch of the RCA.

Figure 9–12*A* and *B* show an example of extremely strong dominance of the RCA. In this patient, the distal RCA passes

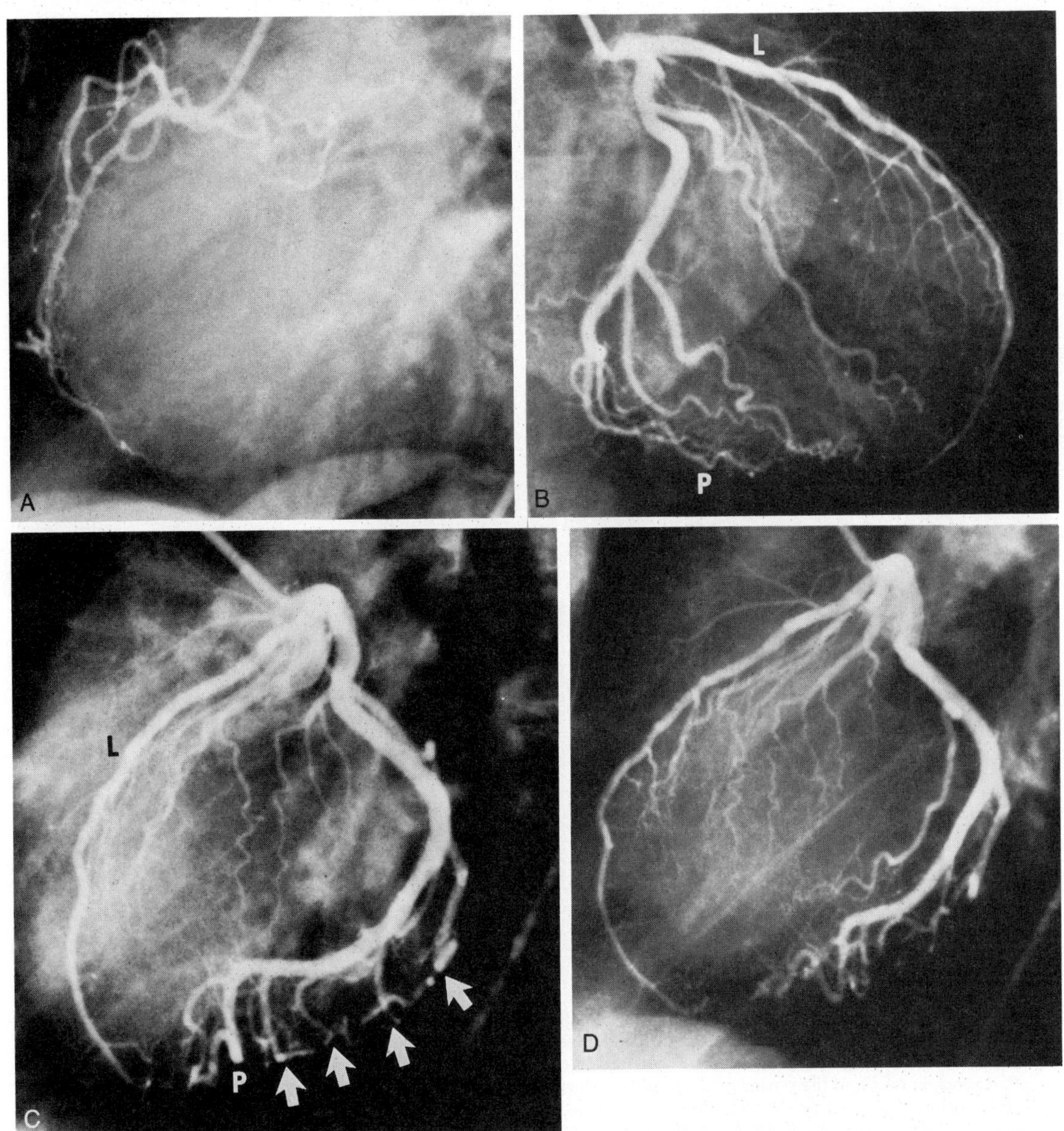

FIGURE 9–10. Dominant left coronary system. *A*, RCA in LAO projection. The RCA is small and terminates well before reaching the crux. *B*, *C*, and *D*, LCA in the RAO, LAO, and left lateral projections. The circumflex artery is large and gives rise to the posterior descending artery at the crux of the heart, and also to a number of large posterior left ventricular branches (arrows). Thus, the entire diaphragmatic surface of the left ventricle is supplied by left circumflex branches.

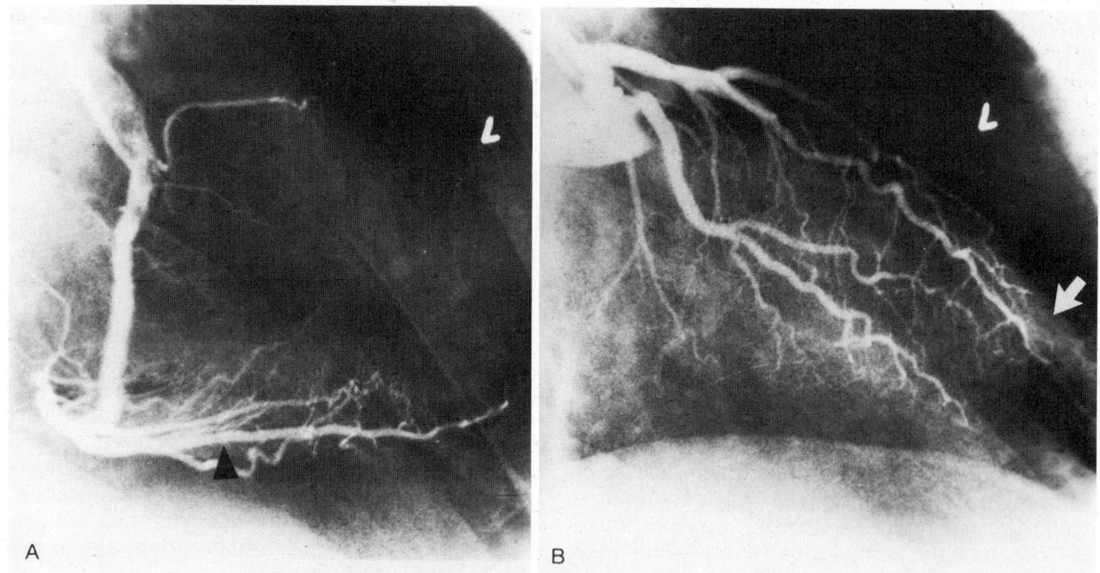

FIGURE 9–11. Short LAD. *A,* RAO right coronary arteriogram shows that the posterior descending branch (arrowhead) is longer than usual and supplies the apex. *B,* RAO left coronary arteriogram shows that the LAD terminates (arrow) before reaching the cardiac apex.

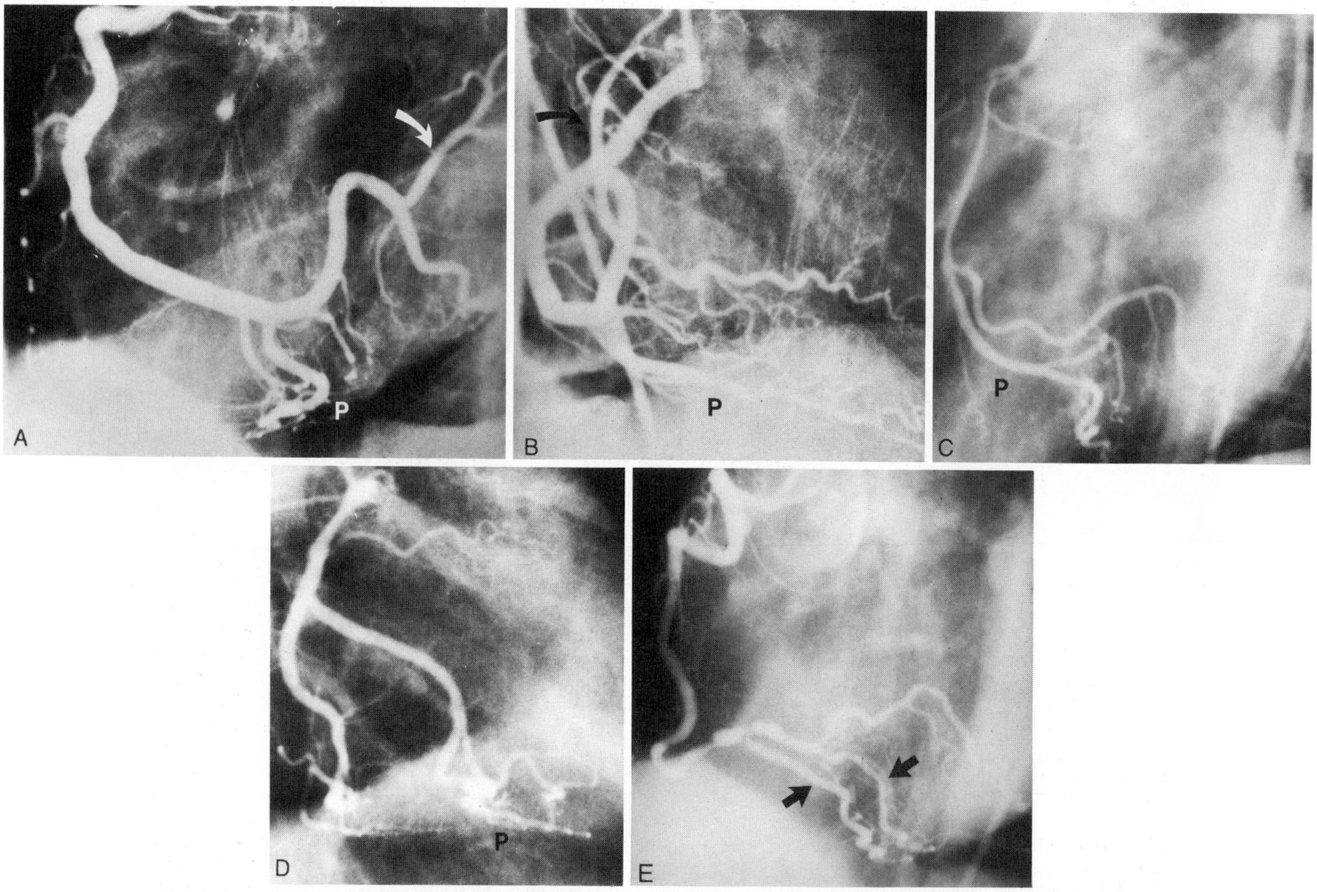

FIGURE 9–12. Unusually strong dominance of the RCA. *A* and *B,* LAO and RAO views of the RCA show that the distal segment of this vessel (arrows) extends all the way up the left atrioventricular groove. After giving rise to the posterior descending artery (P), it gives rise to multiple posterior left ventricular and obtuse marginal branches. *C,* Variations in origin of the posterior descending artery. LAO view of a dominant RCA. The posterior descending artery (P) originates early, then parallels the distal RCA before turning forward in the posterior interventricular groove. (From Levin, D.C., and Baltaxe, H.A.: Angiographic demonstration of important anatomic variations of the posterior descending coronary artery. A.J.R. *116*:41, 1972, with permission.) *D,* RAO right coronary arteriogram showing the posterior descending artery (P) arising from a right ventricular branch of the RCA. *E,* LAO right coronary arteriogram showing duplicated posterior descending arteries (arrows). (From Levin, D.C., and Baltaxe, H.A.: Angiographic demonstration of important anatomic variations of the posterior descending coronary artery. A.J.R. *116*:41, copyright 1972, American Roentgen Ray Society.)

almost all the way up the left atrioventricular groove and supplies most of the obtuse marginal branches. The left circumflex system consists only of a single, high obtuse marginal branch.

Figure 9–12*C* through *E* show three variations in origin of the PDA. Figure 9–12*C* is an instance of early origin of the PDA, which then closely parallels the distal RCA itself before turning forward in the posterior interventricular groove. Figure 9–12*D* is an example of origin of the PDA from a right ventricular branch of the RCA. Figure 9–12*E* is an example of a double PDA in a patient with multiple obstructive lesions in the RCA system.

ANGULATED VIEWS OF THE CORONARY ARTERIES

In the early 1970's, Bunnell et al. called attention to the fact that the routine RAO and LAO projections of the coronary arteries had serious shortcomings.[22,23] Foreshortening and superimposition of branches occurred in these projections, which frequently resulted in failure to detect significant lesions. In addition to rotation of the x-ray beam about the patient in the transverse plane, these investigators proposed rotation of the beam in the sagittal plane. Their studies revealed that lesions often missed on the standard LAO and RAO projections could be detected when a combination of both sagittal and transverse angulation of the x-ray beam was utilized. Sagittal angulation is most useful in evaluation of the left coronary system but also can aid in right coronary arteriography. Equipment has been developed which allows this kind of multiplanar angulation without moving the patient.

The terminology originally used to describe these views was somewhat confusing, in that a variety of terms were used by different authors. A simple nomenclature which is now generally accepted relates the cineangiographic projection to the relative positions of the image intensifier and the patient. In most modern cardiac catheterization laboratories, the x-ray tube is under the patient table, and the image intensifier, with its coupled video and cine cameras, is over the patient table. If this overtable image intensifier is tilted up toward the head of the patient, this is referred to as the "cranial" view. The resulting images appear as if the angiographer were looking down at the heart from the patient's head. Conversely, if the image intensifier is tilted down toward the feet of the patient, this is referred to as the "caudal" view, and provides images as if the angiographer were looking up at the heart from the patient's feet. Cranial and caudal angulations have become a standard part of coronary arteriography and are routinely used in most laboratories that have the necessary U or C arm mounting units for their cine systems.

Figure 9–13 shows a series of radiographs of a paraffin-embedded human heart specimen in which the coronary arteries are filled with a barium mixture. They demonstrate the advantages of the cranial and caudal views. In Figure 9–13*A*, the heart was filmed in a standard LAO projection. The left main coronary artery cannot be seen well because of overlap by the LAD. Also, the proximal portions of the LAD and its large diagonal branch are not well visualized because of foreshortening. In Figure 9–13*B*, the same degree of LAO rotation was used, but cranial angulation was added; this view clearly demonstrates the main LCA and its bifurcation, the proximal portion of the LAD, and the origin of its large diagonal branch. Figure 9–13*C* is an LAO caudal view which also demonstrates the main LCA and proximal LAD well, and is the best view for demonstrating the proximal portion of the left circumflex artery, which often is obscured in other views.

Figure 9–13*D* through *F* are three RAO views of the same specimen. Figure 9–13*D* shows a standard RAO projection in which there is considerable superimposition of the LAD and its diagonal branch. There also is foreshortening of the entire proximal portion of the left circumflex artery. The cranial angulation in Figure 9–13*E* displaces the LAD downward and the first diagonal branch upward, so that these two vessels are no longer superimposed. The LAD can be seen along its entire length without any overlap. However, this is not a good projection for the left circumflex artery. Figure 9–13*F* is an RAO caudal view which displaces the LAD upward and the diagonal branch downward, thereby providing another unobstructed view of both vessels. The origin of the diagonal branch is better demonstrated in this view than in the RAO cranial view. The RAO caudal view is also particularly helpful in demonstrating the entire length of the left circumflex artery, which is foreshortened in both the standard and the cranial RAO projections.

Figure 9–14*A* is an example of a standard RAO projection of a left coronary arteriogram, in which there is marked overlap of the LAD with its diagonal branches and the proximal left circumflex artery. Figure 9–14*B* is an RAO cranial view in the same case in which the overlap has been eliminated. The LAD can be seen along its entire length without superimposition of the other branches, and the latter are themselves well visualized. Figure 9–15 is an example of a patient who had severe stenoses of both the left main coronary artery and the LAD, neither of which could be properly appreciated on the standard RAO or LAO view or the RAO caudal view. The LAD lesion could be seen only on the LAO and RAO cranial views, and the left main coronary lesion could be seen only on the RAO cranial view. Figure 9–16 is an arteriogram in which a severe proximal LAD stenosis is clearly visualized in the standard RAO projections. A second, more distal LAD lesion was visualized only on the RAO cranial view, and not on the RAO caudal or LAO cranial projection.

It is difficult to predict which angulated views will be most useful in any given patient. This depends largely on body habitus, variations in the coronary anatomy, and location of lesions. For this reason, it is recommended that coronary angiographers routinely use cranial and caudal angulation views in both the LAO and RAO projections of the left coronary system. These views also can be helpful on occasion during examination of the right coronary system, though much less frequently.

PITFALLS OF CORONARY ARTERIOGRAPHY

Main Left Coronary Artery Stenosis

Stenosis of the main LCA is the most serious of all coronary lesions and is considered an indication for immediate bypass surgery (Chap. 40). The likelihood of angiographic complications is increased in this condition because the tip of the catheter may dissect the plaque on entry into the left coronary ostium or may occlude the already narrowed orifice. At times, ostial stenosis of the LCA may be unrecognized, particularly if careful attention is not paid to catheter and filming technique. On the standard LAO and RAO views, the LCA may be inadequately visualized because of superimposition by the LAD and circumflex branches, as demonstrated in Figure 9–15. The LCA usually is best visualized on a direct frontal projection or by use of the sagittal-angulation views. LCA stenosis also can escape detection if the catheter tip passes across it, so that the injected contrast material passes entirely in the antegrade direction and fails to opacify the narrowed orifice. In still other cases, a forceful injection can result in filling of the LCA to such a degree that an eccentric plaque is obscured by overlying contrast material, at least in some cine frames.

Figure 9–17 shows an angiogram of a patient with ostial stenosis of the LCA. Figure 9–17*A* shows a cine frame in which an intraluminal filling defect caused by an eccentric plaque is clearly visible adjacent to the catheter tip. Figure 9–17*B* is another frame from the same run in which rapidly injected contrast material obscures this lesion. These two images, taken less than 1 second apart, illustrate how a life-threatening lesion could be overlooked purely as a result of angiographic technique. Figure 9–18 is an example of another

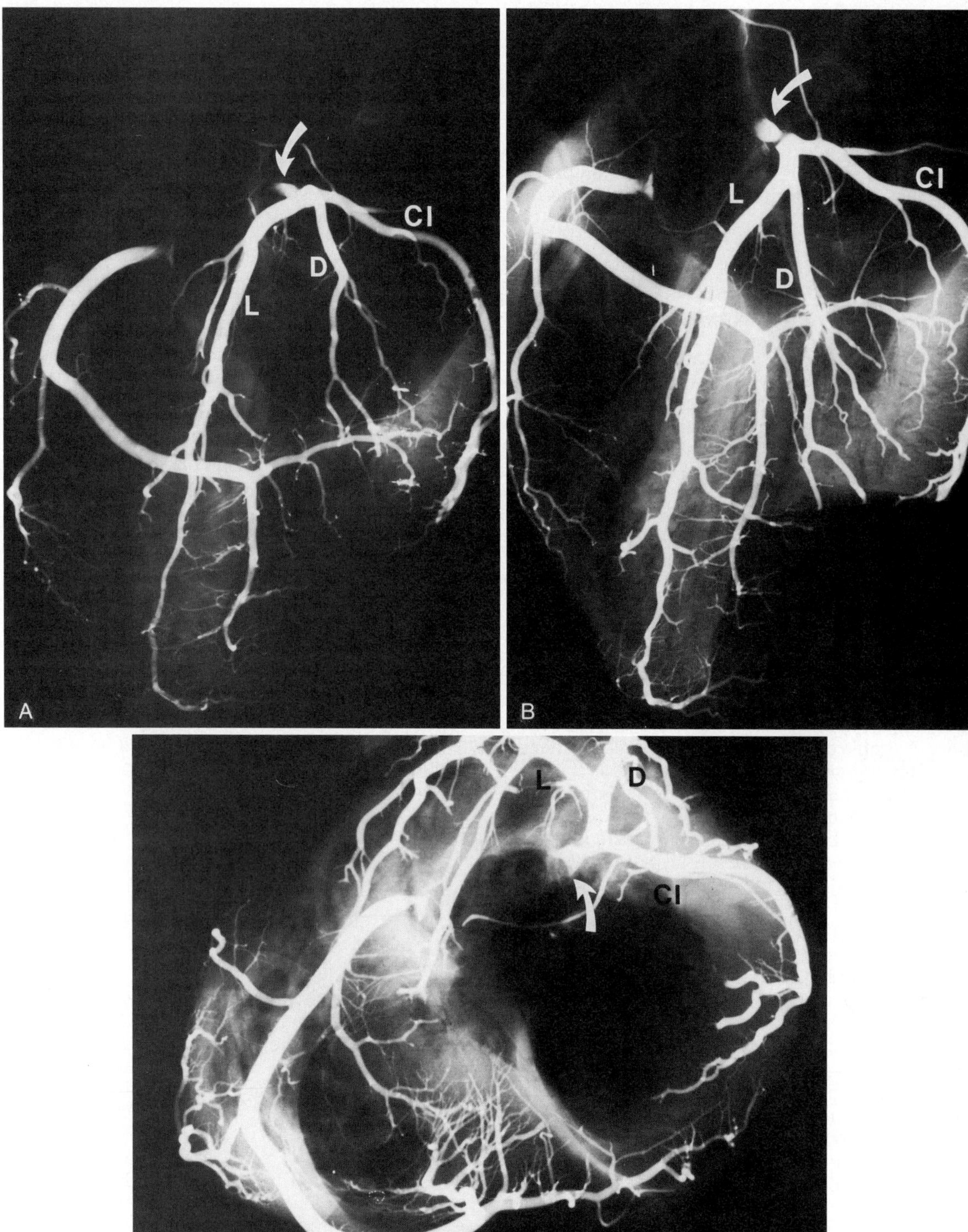

FIGURE 9–13. Views of an injected heart specimen in which a constricting ligature was placed around the main LCA to simulate an obstructing lesion. *A,* Standard LAO view. The main LCA (arrow) is not well seen. The proximal portions of both the LAD (L) and its diagonal branch (D) are not well seen because of foreshortening. The origin of the circumflex artery (CI) is obscured by the diagonal branch. *B,* LAO cranial view. The LCA is seen clearly and the bandlike narrowing created by the ligature can now be visualized. The proximal portions of the LAD and its diagonal branch are well seen. *C,* LAO caudal view. The main LCA is again well visualized, as is the origin of the LAD. This view is especially good for visualizing the origin of the circumflex artery. *D,* Standard RAO view. The LAD and its diagonal branch are almost completely superimposed. The circumflex artery is foreshortened. The arrow points to the first septal branch. *E,* RAO cranial view. The LAD is thrown downward and can now be seen along its entire length without superimposition. The diagonal and circumflex branches are thrown upward. *F,* RAO caudal view. The LAD is now thrown upward and its diagonal branch is thrown downward. Both vessels are well seen without superimposition. The circumflex artery is elongated in this view and is seen well along its entire length. (From Abrams, H.L. [ed.]: Coronary Arteriography. A Practical Approach. Boston, Little Brown, 1983, with permission.)

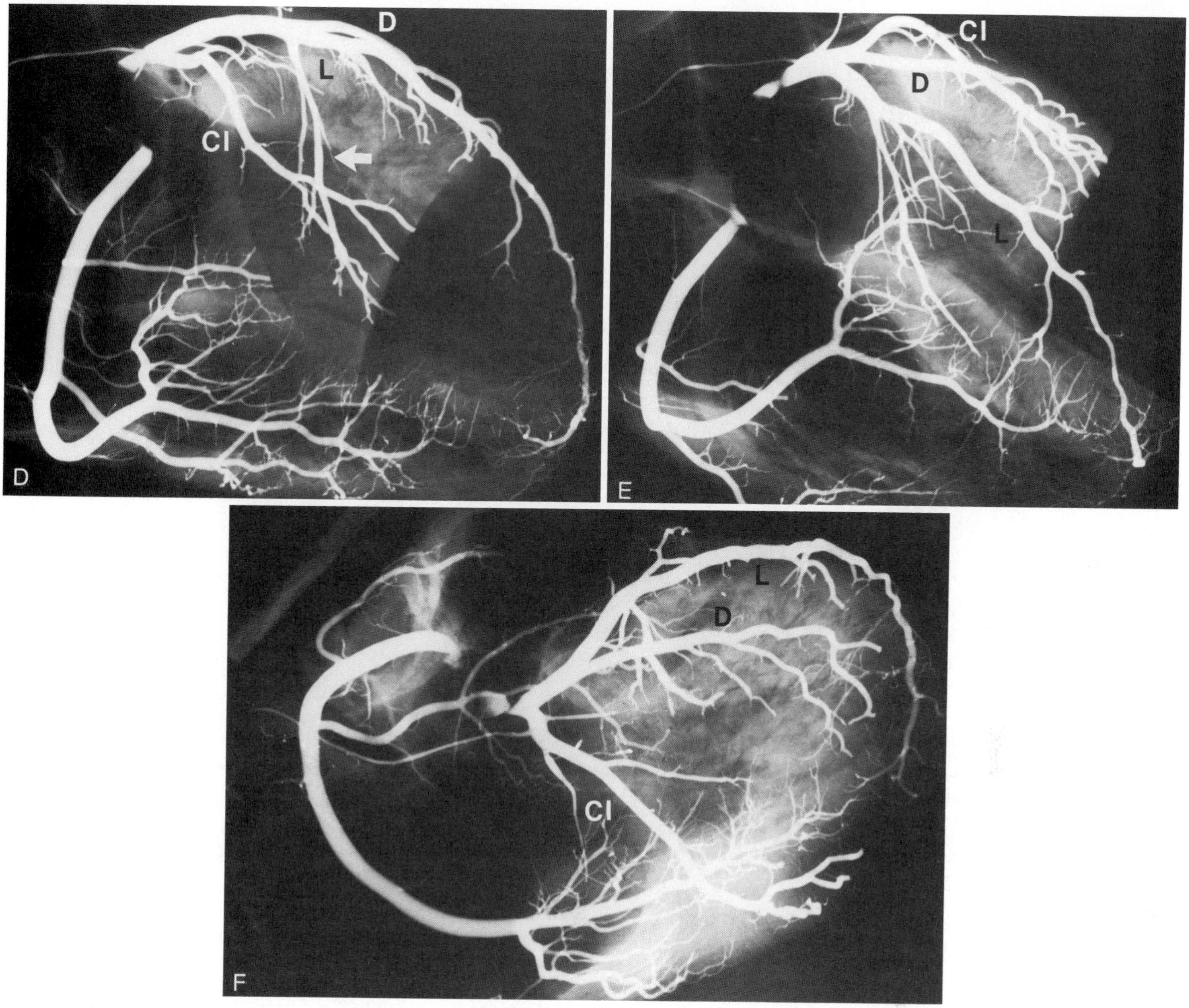

FIGURE 9–13 *Continued.*

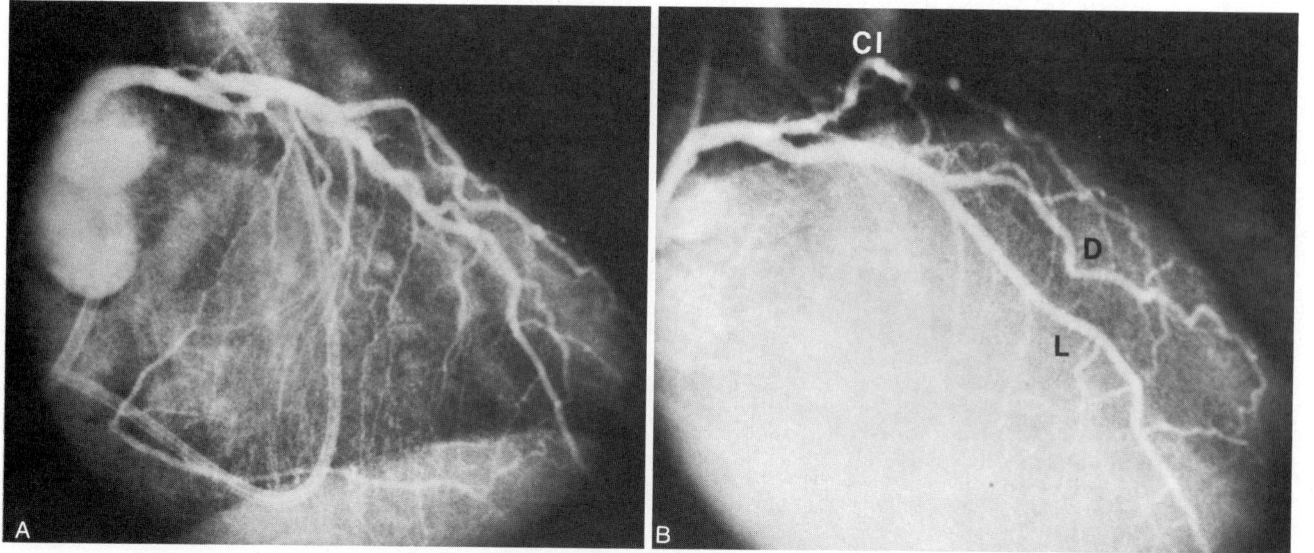

FIGURE 9–14. Standard RAO left coronary arteriogram, showing extensive superimposition of the circumflex and diagonal arteries upon the LAD. *B,* RAO cranial view throws the circumflex (CI) and diagonal (D) arteries upward and the LAD (L) downward. The LAD is now seen well along its entire length without superimposition.

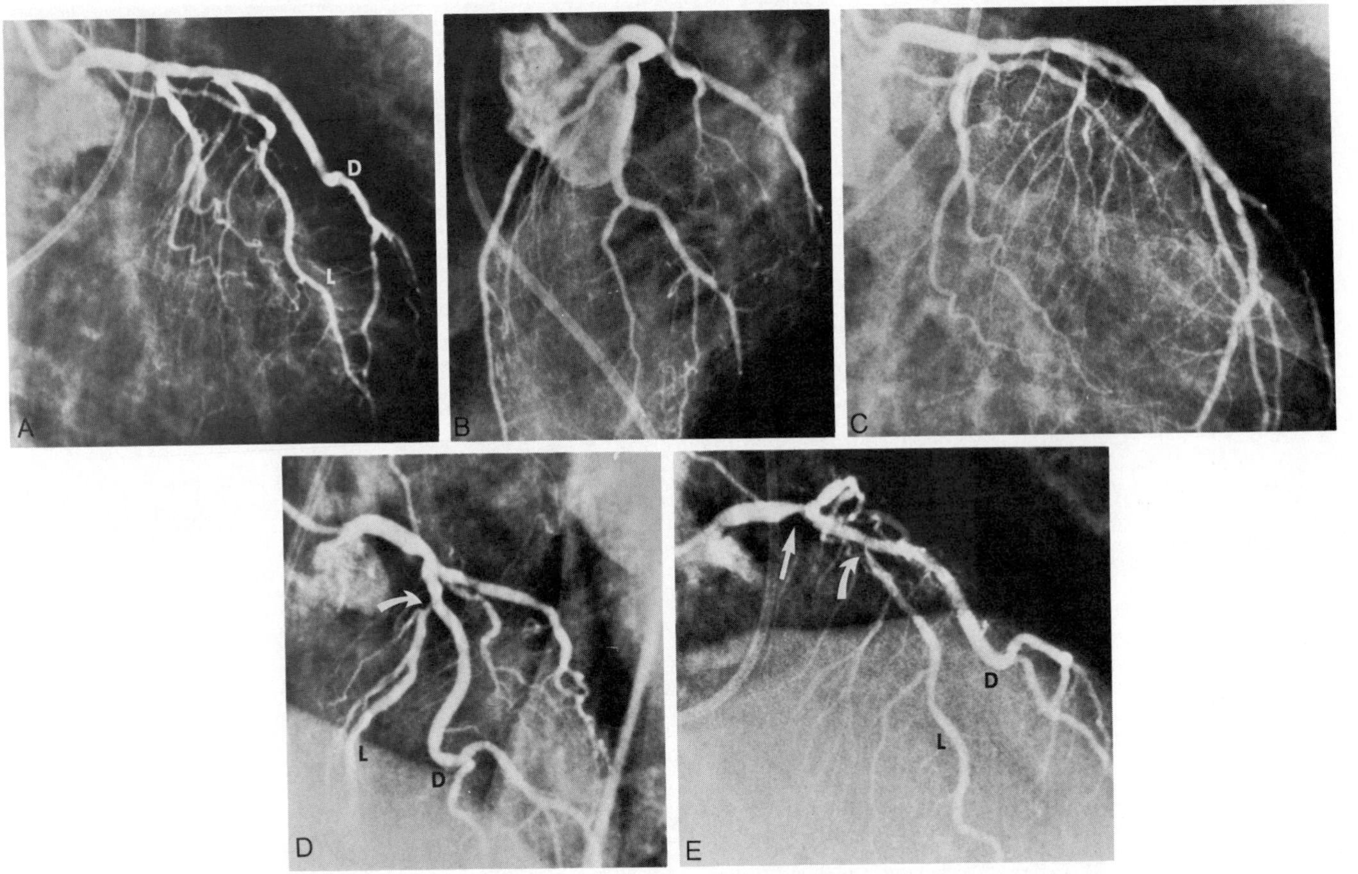

FIGURE 9–15. *A, B,* and *C,* left coronary arteriography in the standard RAO, LAO, and RAO caudal views fails to demonstrate significant stenoses of the main LCA or LAD. Note that in this patient, the diagonal branch (D) is larger than the LAD itself. *D,* LAO cranial view shows severe stenosis (curved arrow) of the LAD (L) just beyond the origin of its diagonal branch. *E,* RAO cranial view again shows the LAD stenosis (curved arrow) but also shows severe stenosis of the main LCA (straight arrow) at its bifurcation. This highly significant lesion could not be appreciated on other views.

patient with ostial stenosis of the LCA. In some projections and in some frames of certain cine runs, this severe lesion was difficult to appreciate. A right coronary arteriogram in this patient revealed collateral circulation from the PDA to the distal LAD, thereby proving that the ostial LCA narrowing was hemodynamically significant.

In most cases, a forceful injection of contrast into the LCA produces sufficient reflux back through the left coronary ostium to provide satisfactory visualization of the proximal portion of the LCA. If no reflux occurs, and the ostium is therefore not seen (as occurred in Fig. 9–18), this may signify a stenotic lesion which is just wide enough to admit the catheter tip. Another clue to the presence of main LCA stenosis is the demonstration of damping or ventricularization of catheter-tip

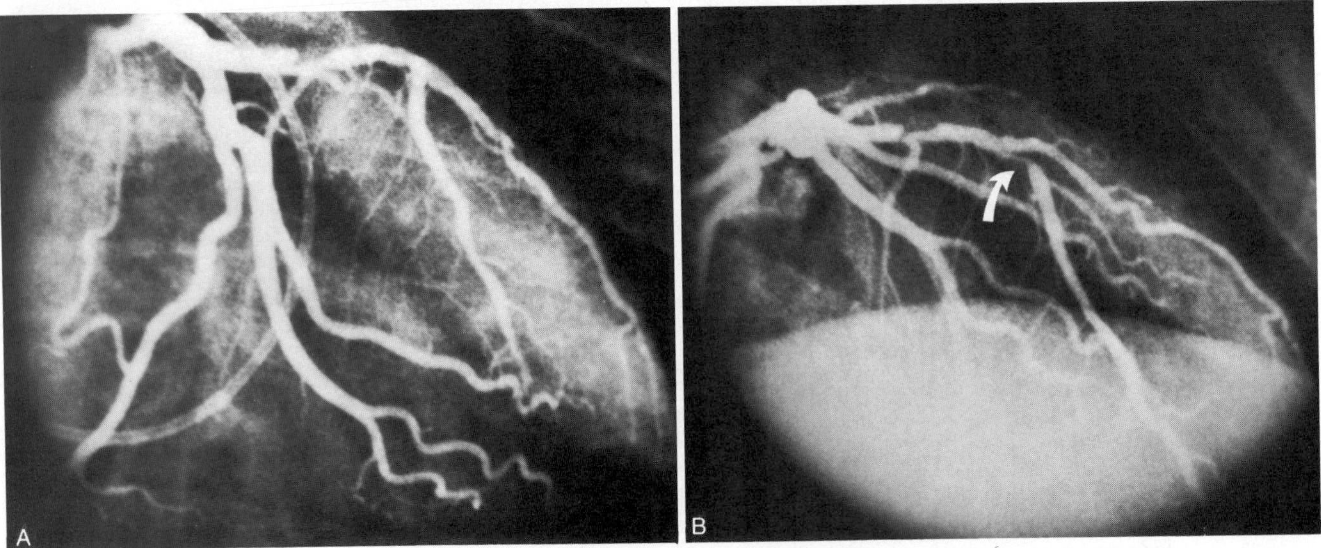

FIGURE 9–16. Left coronary arteriogram in a patient with a clearly visible proximal LAD stenosis. A second lesion is present 2 cm farther distally but cannot be seen in most views. *A,* Standard RAO projection. *B,* RAO cranial view. The latter was the only one of many views to show the second LAD lesion (arrow).

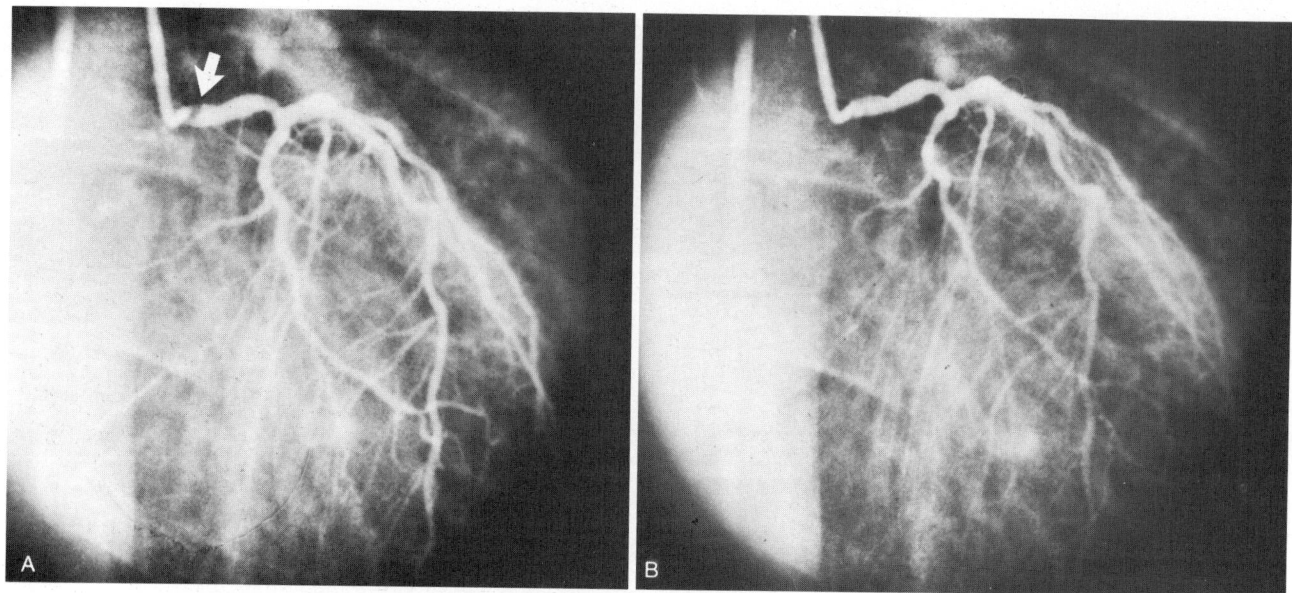

FIGURE 9–17. Obscuration of an ostial LCA stenosis by forcefully injected contrast material. ***A,*** **A filling defect caused by the ostial stenosis is clearly seen adjacent to the catheter tip (arrow).** ***B,*** **On another cine frame from the same injection, contrast material obscures the lesion.**

pressure when the catheter passes from the aorta into the left coronary ostium. Under either of these circumstances, the catheter should be withdrawn into a nonselective position in the left aortic sinus. Contrast injections with the catheter in this position may satisfactorily demonstrate ostial or proximal LCA stenosis.

EARLY BIFURCATION OF THE LEFT CORONARY ARTERY. In 1 to 2 per cent of human hearts, the LCA either is absent or bifurcates immediately beyond the ostium. If the LCA is completely absent, there are instead two separate ostia in the left aortic sinus, one for the LAD and the other adjacent to it for the left circumflex artery. Alternatively, there may be a single ostium with immediate bifurcation into the LAD and circumflex branches. In either case, catheterization of what is thought to be the LCA will invariably result in passage of the catheter tip into either the LAD or the circumflex branch. Subsequent contrast injection may demonstrate only that branch, thereby creating the erroneous impression that the other branch is totally occluded. In some cases, there may be enough reflux of contrast material back into the left aortic sinus to partially opacify the other vessel (Fig. 9–19). Whenever separate origin of the LAD and circumflex arteries is suspected, the catheter should be withdrawn to a nonselective position in the left aortic sinus and the arteriogram repeated, using forceful contrast injections. This often results in some degree of visualization of the second vessel. As seen in Figure 9–19, additional catheter manipulation or substitution of another catheter with a different shape or size usually allows selective entry into the second vessel.

CATHETER-INDUCED SPASM. Insertion of a catheter into the RCA can trigger pronounced spasm adjacent to the catheter tip. For reasons which are not entirely clear, this phenomenon is extremely rare in the LCA. Whenever right coronary arteriography reveals narrowing of the proximal portion of the RCA, the angiographer must rule out the possibility of catheter-induced spasm. The catheter should be removed, nitroglycerin administered sublingually or intravenously, and arteriography repeated shortly thereafter. Nitroglycerin reduces vasomotor tone in large coronary arteries,[24,25] and in most cases, it should be given prophylactically to prevent spasm from occurring during selective arteriography. The duration of action of this drug, however, is relatively short (20 to 30 minutes), and it may have a variable effect in different patients. Thus, even if it is given prophylactically at the start of the procedure, by the time right coronary arteriography is performed, its effect may have largely abated.

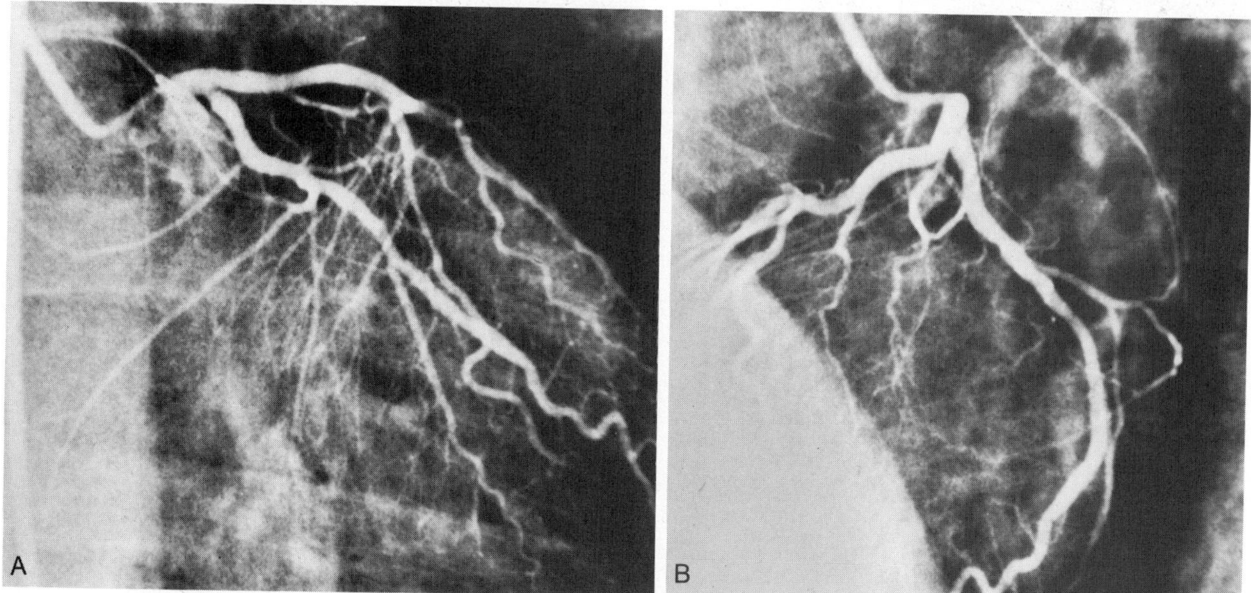

FIGURE 9–18. Example of the difficulty sometimes encountered in detecting ostial LCA stenoses. ***A,*** **Shallow RAO views of the LAD with the catheter not well seated in the vessel. The LAD ostium is not well visualized.** ***B,*** **LAO cranial view showing the catheter tip selectively positioned in the LCA and no reflux of contrast material around the catheter tip.**

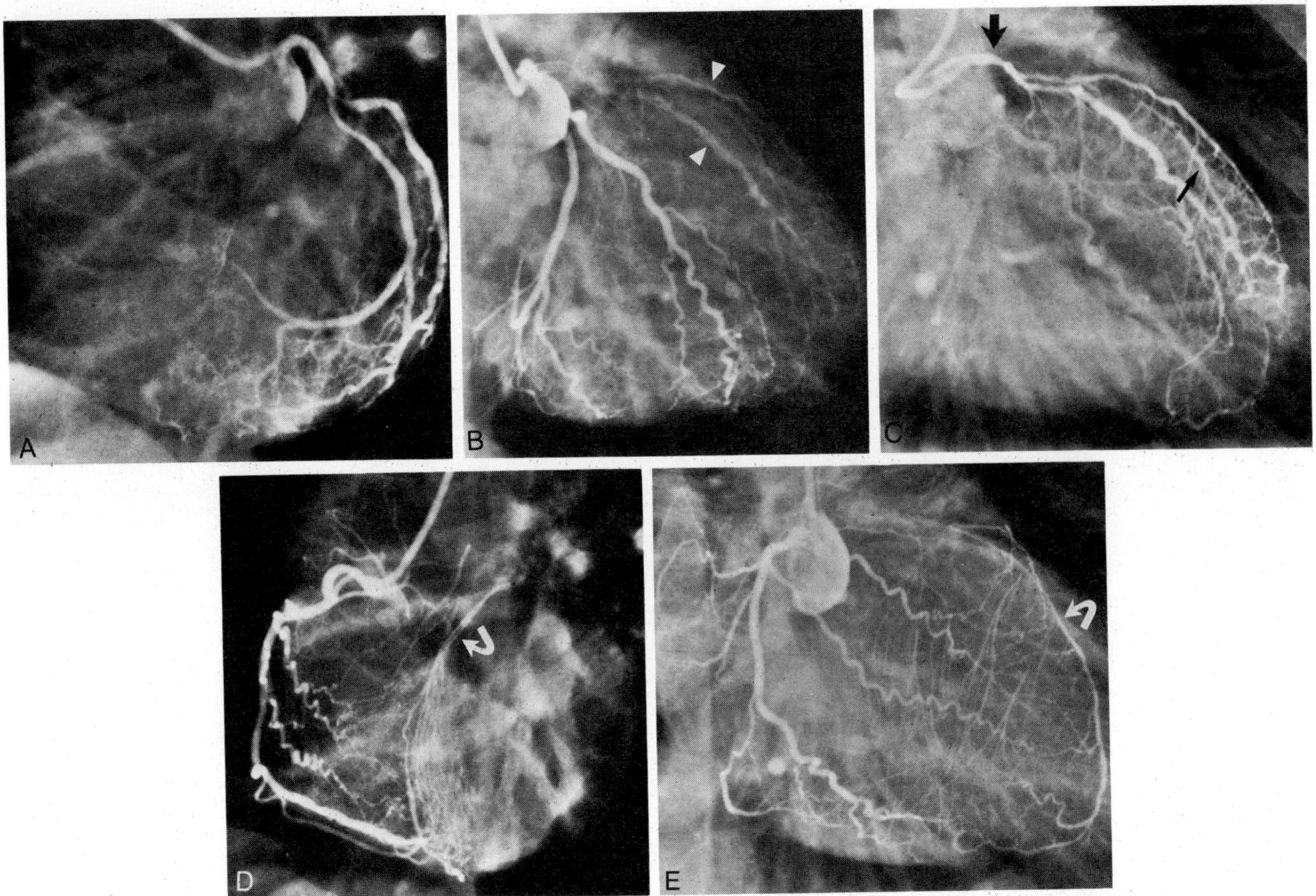

FIGURE 9–19. Separate origins of the LAD and circumflex arteries from the left aortic sinus. *A* and *B*, LAO and RAO views of a selective injection of what was thought to be the LCA. Only the left circumflex artery is visualized, although on the RAO projection there appears to be some faint spillover into LAD branches (arrowheads). *C*, RAO view (after repositioning the left Judkins catheter) of a selective injection of the LAD. The LAD is occluded proximally just beyond the origin of a large diagonal branch (large arrow). The distal portion of the LAD (small arrow) fills by means of collateral circulation from the diagonal branches. *D* and *E*, LAO and RAO projections of the right coronary arteriogram show distal filling of the obstructed LAD (curved arrows) by means of collaterals from the posterior descending branch up through the interventricular septum.

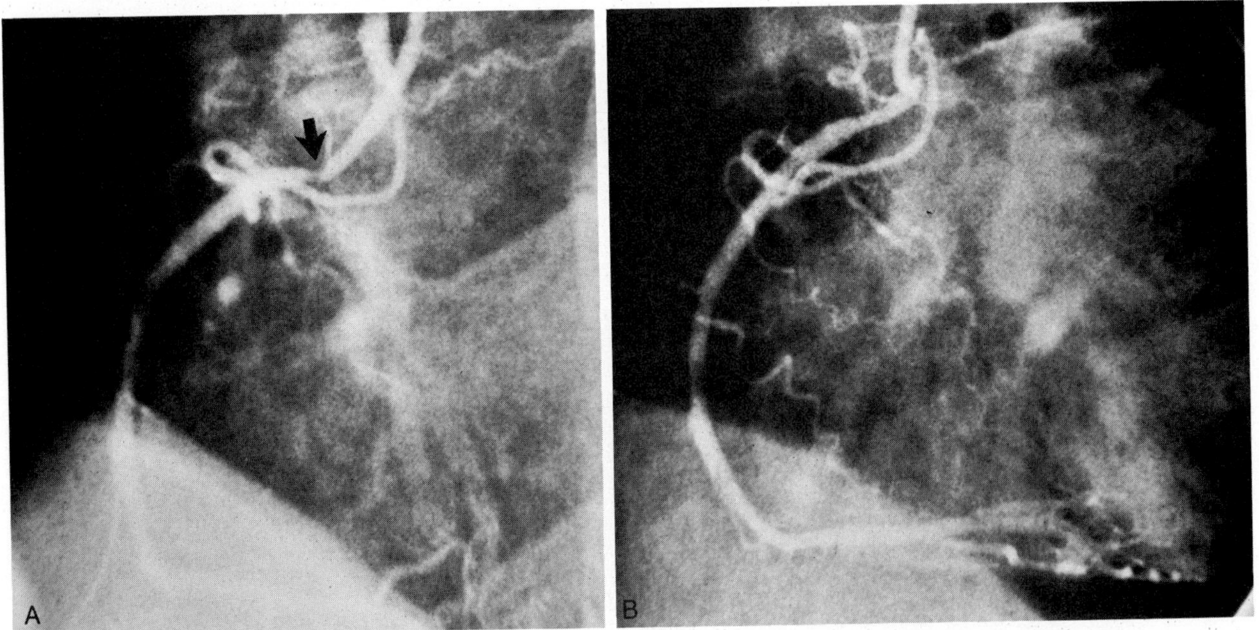

FIGURE 9–20. Catheter-induced spasm of the origin of the RCA. *A*, LAO view of a right coronary arteriogram. There is apparent severe narrowing of the origin of the RCA immediately adjacent to the catheter tip. *B*, After administration of sublingual nitroglycerin and repositioning of the catheter tip, the narrowing is much less pronounced.

Figure 9–20 shows catheter-induced spasm of the proximal RCA, relieved by sublingual nitroglycerin. A nonselective injection of contrast also helped to demonstrate this. Because of the rarity of catheter-induced spasm of the main LCA, angiographically demonstrated narrowing of this vessel is much more likely to represent organic disease.

FLOW ARTIFACTS DURING ARTERIOGRAPHY. It has been assumed that the pattern of flow of contrast material during arteriography accurately portrays blood flow under normal physiological circumstances. The assumption was that as long as the caliber of a catheter tip is somewhat smaller than the caliber of the artery into which it has been inserted, the force of the contrast injection would be dissipated out into the aorta. Therefore, the injection itself would not alter flow and pressure in the catheterized vessel. Experimental studies have shown that this assumption is incorrect. Injection of contrast material or other fluids through standard, nonoccluding catheters positioned selectively will raise significantly both flow and pressure in the vessel for the duration of the injection.[26] In effect, contrast is forced through the arterial tree, and artifactual flow patterns or accentuated filling of branch vessels and collateral circulation may result. The degree to which this occurs is largely related to the force of the injection itself, and to the relative sizes of the catheter tip and the artery into which it has been inserted. The smaller the size of the artery relative to that of the catheter tip, the greater the rise in flow and pressure during contrast injection. Thus, in a given patient, the speed and direction of flow seen on arteriography, the degree of opacification of distal branches, and the degree of filling of collateral vessels may not accurately reflect blood flow that occurs under physiological conditions.

Eccentric Stenoses

Eccentric or slitlike atherosclerotic narrowings of the coronary arteries commonly occur. If, in such cases, the x-ray beam passes through the lesion perpendicular to the long axis of the lumen, the vessel may appear to have a normal or near-normal caliber. Only if the beam passes parallel to the long axis of the stenotic lumen will the narrowing be visible. For this reason, *coronary arteries must be viewed in at least two projections 90 degrees apart.*

A related problem is that of the bandlike or membranous stenosis. Lesions such as this may be exceedingly difficult to detect. Figure 9–21 shows a severe bandlike lesion of the RCA which could be adequately seen only on the LAO view, whereas two other projections failed to demonstrate it. It is not clear whether these peculiar lesions represent pure atherosclerotic stenosis or are caused in some instances by congenital membranous bands.[27] Aside from the difficulty in detecting these lesions, it is difficult to ascertain their hemodynamic significance. Measurement of the pressure gradient across the lesion through a small inner catheter inserted through the angiographic catheter may be useful in this regard.

Unrecognized Occlusions

Occlusions of major coronary arteries often occur at branch points. Because of this, and the fact that there are anatomical variations in the number and distribution of branches, it is possible for occlusions at branch origins to go undetected. In some cases, occlusion of a branch can be recognized only by late filling of the distal segment of this branch by means of collateral circulation (Fig. 9–22).

Superimposition of Branches

Superimposition of major branches of the left coronary tree in the LAO and RAO projections can result in failure to detect stenoses or total obstructions of these branches. This problem is particularly applicable to branches of the LAD. As indicated earlier, the anatomy of diagonal branches of the LAD is variable. In some cases, a large diagonal branch is present, which closely parallels the LAD in both the LAO and RAO projections. If this diagonal branch or the LAD itself is totally occluded at its branch point, the obstruction could go undetected. Examples of this type of anatomy are shown in Figures 9–22 and 9–23. Because of overlapping of the LAD and diagonal branches in RAO projections, stenoses may be obscured. This problem often can be alleviated by the use of cranial or caudal angulation (p. 245). Septal branches can mimic the LAD in the LAO projection. In this projection, the LAD and the septal branches occupy the same plane. When the LAD is totally occluded beyond the origin of the first septal branch, this branch often becomes quite enlarged in an attempt to provide collateral circulation to the vascular bed of the distal LAD. In the case shown in Figure 9–24, the LAD is completely obstructed just beyond the origin of the first septal branch. The latter has become considerably enlarged and could be confused with the LAD itself on the LAO projection.

Myocardial Bridging

The major coronary arteries pass over the epicardial surface of the heart. In some cases, however, short segments descend into the myocardium for a variable distance. This occurs in 5 to 12 per cent of humans and is almost exclusively confined to the LAD.[28] Because a "bridge" of myocardial fibers passes over the involved segment of the LAD, each systolic contraction of these fibers can cause narrowing of the artery. Myocardial bridging has a characteristic appearance on cineangiography. The bridged segment is of normal caliber during diastole but

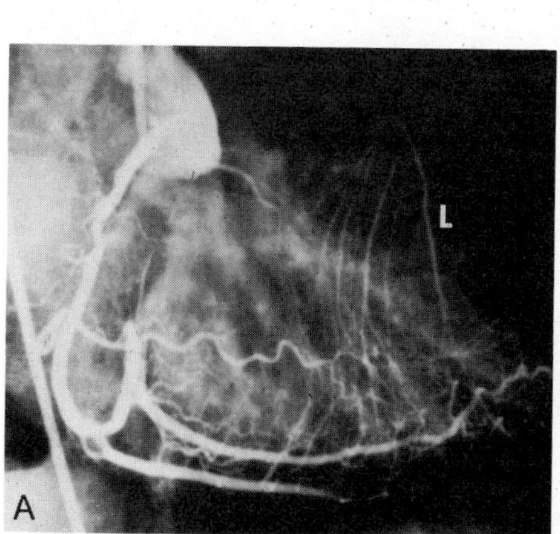

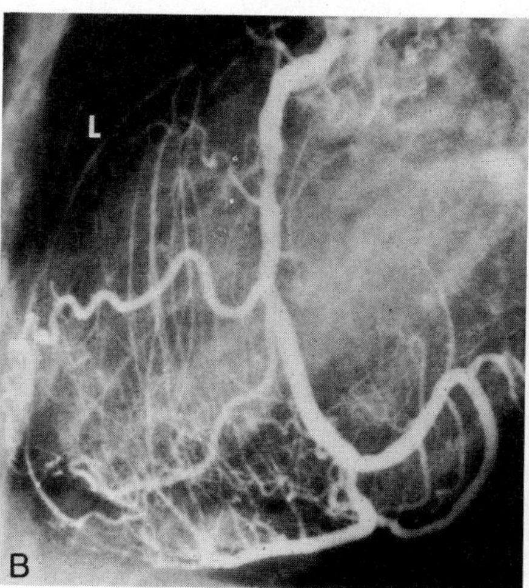

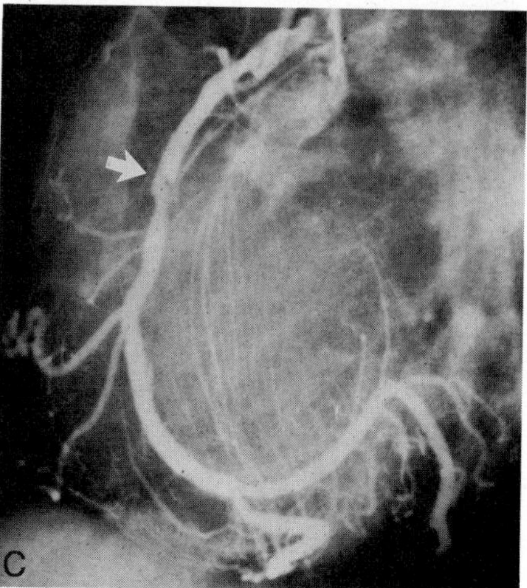

FIGURE 9–21. RAO *(A)* and left lateral *(B)* views of a right coronary arteriogram showing mild diffuse narrowing of the proximal RCA without severe localized obstruction. The LAD in this patient is totally occluded and can be seen filling by means of collateral circulation from the posterior descending artery. *C,* LAO view of the right coronary arteriogram. In this projection, but not in the others, a severe focal, bandlike narrowing is noted in a segment which otherwise has relatively normal caliber.

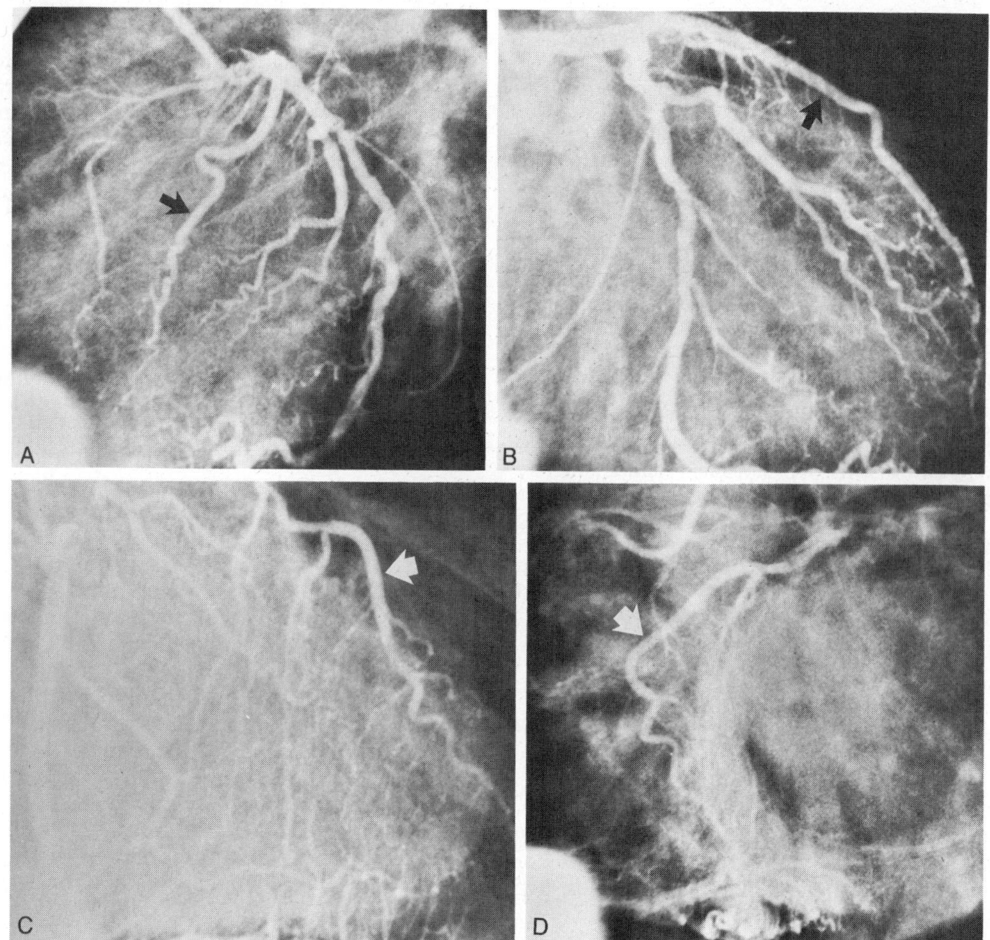

FIGURE 9–22. LAO *(A)* and RAO *(B)* views of a left coronary arteriogram. The LAD is totally occluded, although the point of occlusion is not visualized. There is a large diagonal branch (black arrows) which closely parallels the LAD in both projections and could be mistaken for the LAD. Late-phase frames from an RAO *(C)* and LAO (D) right coronary arteriogram. The distal segment of the obstructed LAD (white arrows) can be seen filling through septal collaterals.

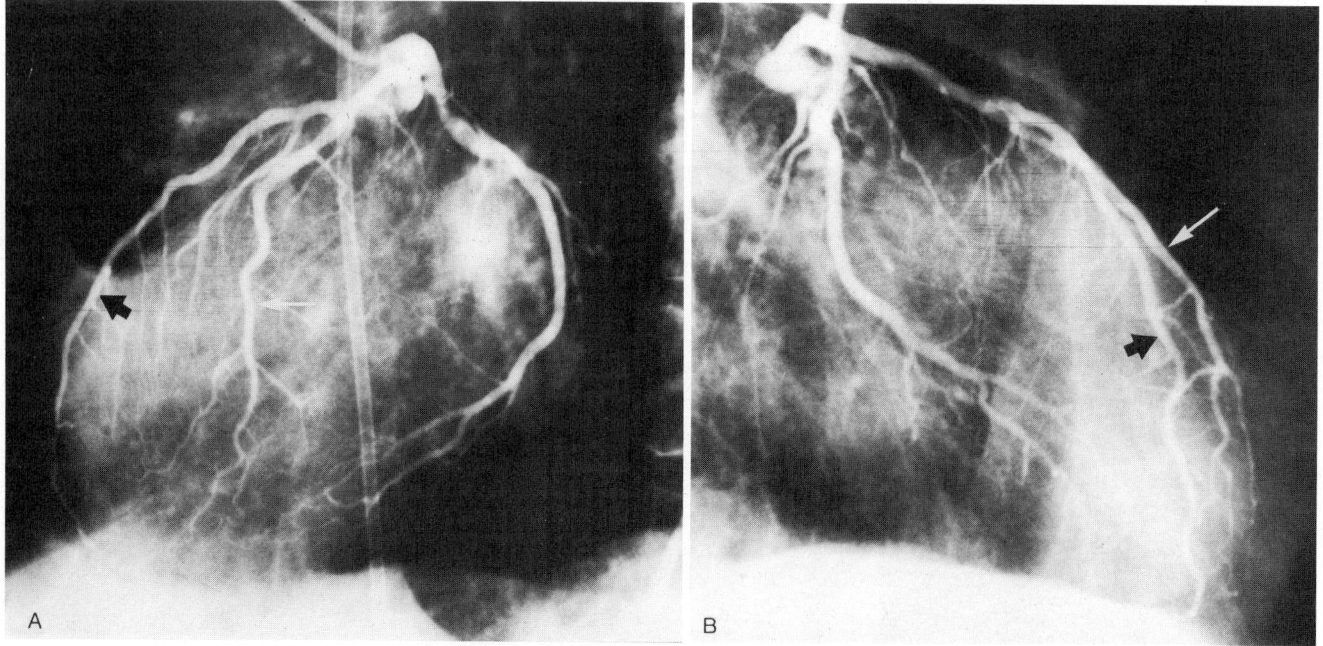

FIGURE 9–23. *A* and *B,* LAO and RAO views of a left coronary arteriogram. The LAD (black arrow) is normal in size and position. It has a large diagonal branch (white arrow) which closely parallels it. In either projection, if the LAD had become totally occluded at the origin of this diagonal branch, the latter might have then been mistaken for the LAD itself. (From Levin, D.C., Baltaxe, H.A., and Sos, T.A.: Potential sources of error in coronary arteriography. II. In interpretation of the study. A.J.R. *124*:386, copyright 1975, American Roentgen Ray Society.)

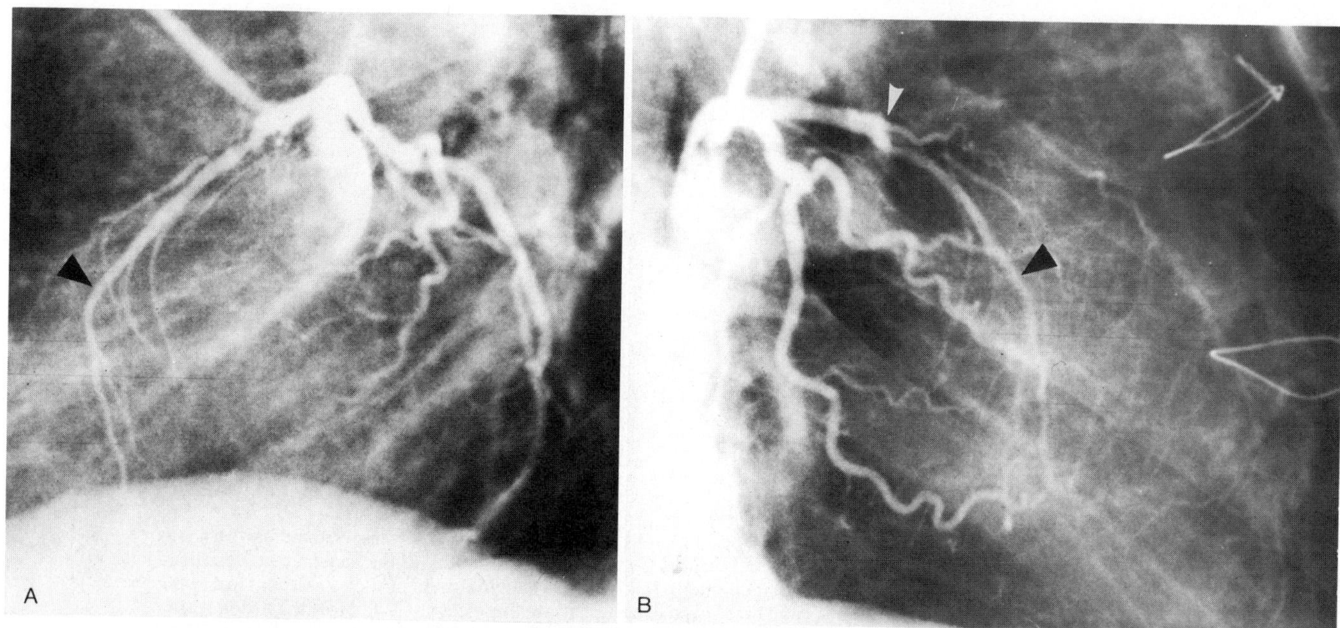

FIGURE 9–24. *A,* Septal branch mimicking the LAD, LAO left coronary arteriogram. The arrowhead points to an enlarged first septal branch which occupies the same course as the LAD and could be mistaken for the LAD. *B,* The RAO view shows that the LAD is totally obstructed (white arrowhead). The septal branch (black arrowhead) occupies a course roughly parallel to the normal position of the LAD but is below it and lies within the interventricular septum. (From Levin, D.C., Baltaxe, H.A., and Sos, T.A.: Potential sources of error in coronary arteriography. II. In interpretation of the study. A.J.R. *124*:386, copyright 1975, American Roentgen Ray Society.)

abruptly narrows with each systole. Systolic narrowing caused by myocardial bridging should not be confused with an atherosclerotic plaque. Although bridging is not thought to have any hemodynamic significance in *most* cases, some have suggested that when it produces severe systolic narrowing, or during tachycardia, myocardial ischemia can result.[29] An example of pronounced bridging is shown in Figure 9–25.

Recanalization

A narrowed segment of a coronary artery seen on arteriography usually is considered a "stenosis." Such lesions may actually be segments which once were totally occluded but have recanalized. Pathological studies have shown that as many as one-third of totally occluded coronary arteries ultimately recanalize.[30] The cineangiographic appearances of stenosis and recanalization may be indistinguishable. Figure 9–26 shows a *postmortem* injection specimen of a recanalized segment of an RCA, along with the corresponding histological section. Recanalization usually results in the development of multiple tortuous channels, which are quite small and close to one another, creating an impression on cineangiography of a single, slightly irregular channel. The fine detail of the postmortem angiogram in Figure 9–26 shows the multiple tortuous and irregular channels, but it is unlikely that the spatial resolution of cineangiography would be sufficient to demonstrate this degree of detail in living patients. Spontaneous or drug-induced lysis of thrombi also can account for reopening of previously occluded coronary arteries, particularly in the clinical setting of recent acute myocardial infarction.

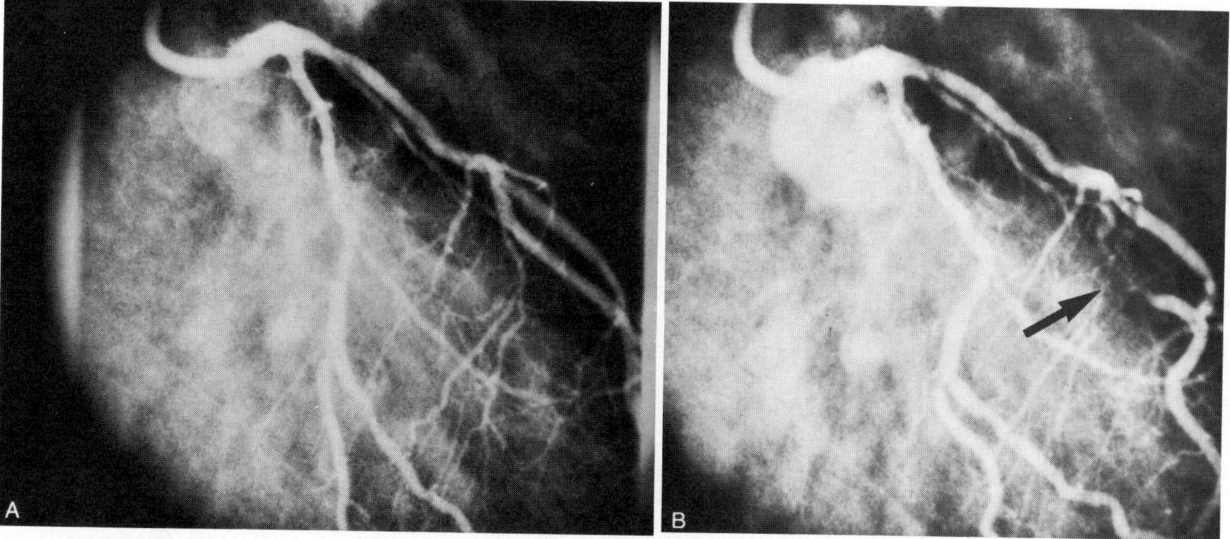

FIGURE 9–25. Myocardial bridging. *A,* RAO left coronary arteriogram, showing a normal LAD during diastole. *B,* During systole, there is pronounced narrowing of the LAD (arrow) at a point where it passes down into the myocardium.

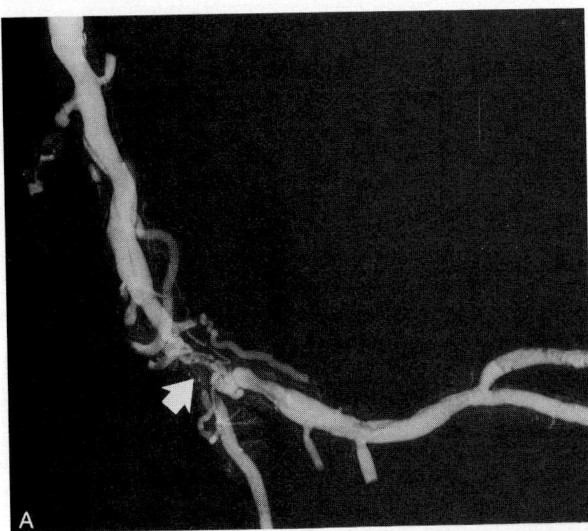

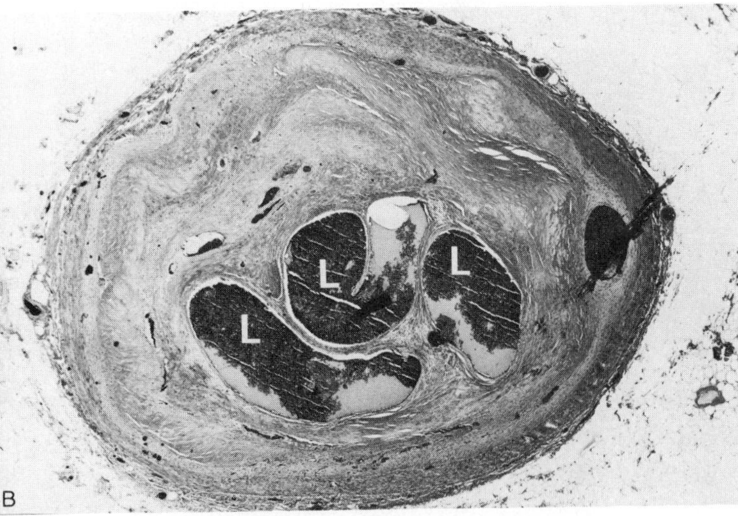

FIGURE 9–26. **Recanalized segment of a totally occluded RCA.** ***A,*** **Postmortem injection specimen. The RCA was injected with a barium-gelatin mixture and then dissected off the epicardial surface of the heart. The recanalized segment (arrow) demonstrates several irregular channels. It is likely that angiography of such a segment in a living patient would not have sufficiently high spatial resolution to demonstrate these channels and that the lesion would instead appear simply as a localized stenosis.** ***B,*** **Histologic section of the recanalized segment. L = Recanalized lumina filled with the barium-gelatin mixture.**

COMPLICATIONS OF CORONARY ARTERIOGRAPHY

Considerable data have now been accumulated from a variety of sources on the incidence of complications of coronary arteriography. In 1979, Davis et al. reported on the complications occurring in 7553 consecutive patients undergoing coronary arteriography at 13 institutions participating in the Coronary Artery Surgery Study (CASS) registry.[31] They compared the complications in 1087 patients studied by the brachial approach and 6328 patients studied by the percutaneous femoral approach. Death occurred in 0.51 per cent of patients in the brachial group and in 0.14 per cent of the femoral group. Ventricular fibrillation unrelated to myocardial infarction occurred in 0.63 per cent of the entire population. Cerebral ischemia occurred in 0.17 per cent of the brachial group compared with 0.08 per cent of the femoral group. Local vascular complications were considerably higher in the brachial group, with arterial thrombosis occurring in 1.85 per cent of this group, as opposed to 0.24 per cent in the femoral group.

In 1985, Klinke et al. discussed the complications occurring in 3071 outpatient coronary arteriograms, almost all of which were performed by the percutaneous femoral approach.[32] The mortality rate was 0.13 per cent, whereas nonfatal myocardial infarction occurred in 0.07 per cent and arrhythmias in 0.42 per cent. Central nervous system complications occurred in 0.14 per cent and local vascular complications in 0.35 per cent.

By far the most extensive analysis of complications of coronary arteriography is the report of the Registry of the Society for Cardiac Angiography and Interventions.[33] Among 222,553 patients entered into this registry between 1984 and 1987, death occurred in 0.10 per cent, myocardial infarction in 0.06 per cent, stroke in 0.07 per cent, serious arrhythmias in 0.47 per cent, vascular complications in 0.46 per cent, and unspecified contrast reactions in 0.23 per cent. Major complications (death, myocardial infarction, and stroke) occurred with similar frequencies using both the femoral and the brachial approaches, but vascular complications are four times as common with the latter. The incidence of death was much higher in patients with left main coronary disease (0.55 per cent), ejection fraction less than 30 per cent (0.30 per cent), and New York Heart Association functional class IV (0.29 per cent).

Abnormalities of the Coronary Circulation

CONGENITAL ANOMALIES OF THE CORONARY ARTERIES

(See also Chaps. 31 and 32)

Congenital anomalies of the coronary arteries can be divided into two broad categories: those that alter myocardial perfusion and those that do not.

ANOMALIES THAT ALTER MYOCARDIAL PERFUSION

Coronary Artery Fistulas (See p. 917)

A review of a large series of patients with congenital anomalies of the coronary arteries revealed that coronary artery fistula is by far the most common.[34] Although about half the patients with these lesions remain asymptomatic, the other half develop congestive heart failure, infective endocarditis, myocardial ischemia, or rupture of an aneurysmal fistula. About half of these fistulas arise from the RCA or its branches; slightly fewer than half arise from the LAD or circumflex arteries or their branches; and in the remaining cases there are multiple origins. Drainage occurs into the right ventricle in 41 per cent, the right atrium in 26 per cent, the pulmonary artery in 17 per cent, the left ventricle in 3 per cent, and the superior vena cava in 1 per cent.[34] Thus a left-to-right shunt exists in more than 90 per cent of cases. Selective coronary arteriography is the only way to demonstrate the origin of these fistulas. Figure 9–27 shows an example of a fistula arising from both the LAD and the circumflex arteries and draining into the left ventricle.

Origin of the Left Coronary Artery from the Pulmonary Artery

(See p. 918)

Most patients with origin of the LCA from the main pulmonary artery develop myocardial ischemia early in life. About 25 per cent survive to adolescence or adulthood but fre-

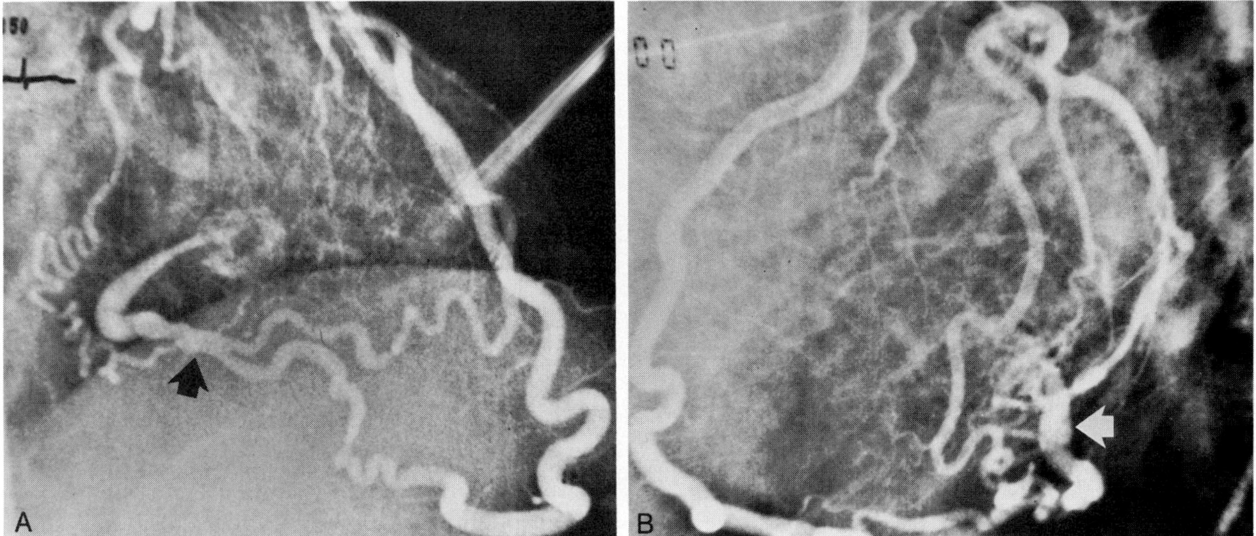

FIGURE 9–27. Congenital fistula arising from branches of both the LAD and circumflex arteries and draining into the left ventricle. *A*, RAO cranial view of the left coronary arteriogram. *B*, LAO view of the left coronary arteriogram. The arrows point to the fistula.

quently experience mitral regurgitation, angina, or congestive heart failure.[35] Aortography (Fig. 9–28) typically shows a large RCA with absence of a left coronary ostium in the left aortic sinus. During the late phase of the aortogram, the LAD and circumflex branches fill by means of collateral circulation from RCA branches. Still later in the filming sequence, retrograde flow from the LAD and circumflex opacifies the LCA and its origin from the main pulmonary artery. The clinical course of the patient tends to be more favorable if extensive collateral circulation exists. In rare instances, the RCA rather than the LCA may arise from the main pulmonary artery.

CONGENITAL CORONARY STENOSIS OR ATRESIA. Congenital stenosis or atresia of a coronary artery can occur as an isolated lesion or in association with other congenital diseases such as calcific coronary sclerosis, supravalvular aortic stenosis, homocystinuria, Friedreich's ataxia, Hurler's syndrome, progeria, and rubella syndrome.[34] In these cases, the atretic vessel usually fills by means of collateral circulation from the contralateral side.

ORIGIN OF EITHER CORONARY ARTERY FROM THE CONTRALATERAL SINUS WITH PASSAGE BETWEEN THE AORTA AND THE RIGHT VENTRICULAR OUTFLOW TRACT. Origin of the LCA from the proximal RCA or the right aortic sinus with subsequent passage between the aorta and the right ventricular outflow tract has been clearly shown to be a dangerous lesion, frequently associated with sudden death during or shortly after exercise in young people.[36–38] After its aberrant origin, the LCA takes an abrupt leftward turn and tunnels between the aorta and the right ventricular outflow tract (Fig. 9–29). Sudden death is thought to result from occlusion of the anomalous LCA. This may be caused by an increase in blood flow through the aorta and pulmonary artery that occurs during exercise and creates either a kink at the sharp leftward bend or a pinchcock mechanism in the tunnel. Origin of the RCA from the LCA or left aortic sinus with passage between the aorta and the right ventricular outflow tract is somewhat less dangerous. This anomaly, however, has also been associated with myocardial ischemia or sudden death, presumably through the same mechanism.[37–39] In rare cases of anomalous origin of the LCA from the right aortic sinus, myocardial ischemia may occur even if the LCA passes anterior to the right ventricular outflow tract or posterior to the aorta (i.e., not through a tunnel between the two great vessels).[40] The cause of the perfusion deficit is not clear in these cases.

CORONARY ANOMALIES NOT ALTERING MYOCARDIAL PERFUSION

In this category of anomalies, the coronary arteries originate from the aorta, but their origins are in unusual positions. Although myocardial perfusion is normal, the angiographer may have trouble locating them. These anomalies occur in about 0.5 to 1.0 per cent of adult patients undergoing coronary arteriography.[41,42]

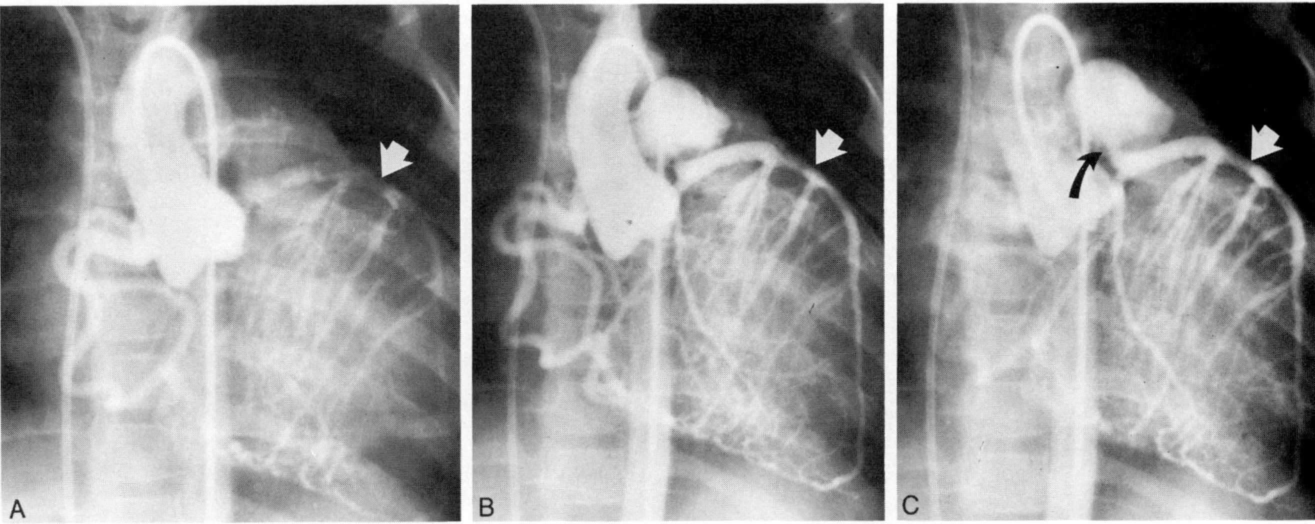

FIGURE 9–28. Anomalous origin of the LCA from the pulmonary artery. *A*, *B*, and *C*, Three frames from a thoracic aortogram demonstrating a large RCA and no antegrade filling of the LCA. The LCA fills primarily through extensive collaterals from the RCA to the LAD (white arrows). The anomalous origin of the LCA from the pulmonary artery is demonstrated (curved black arrow in C) in the late phases.

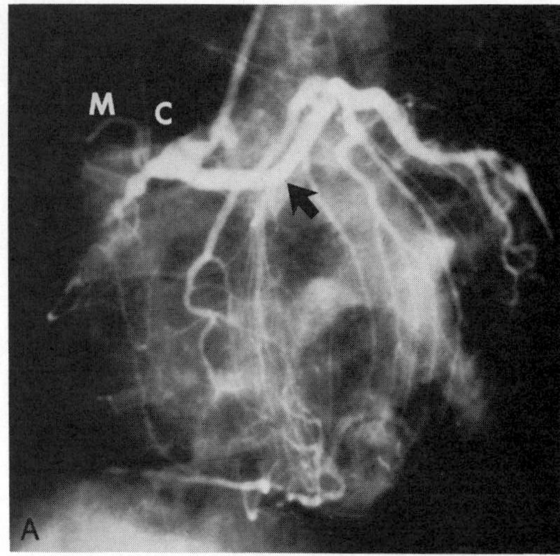

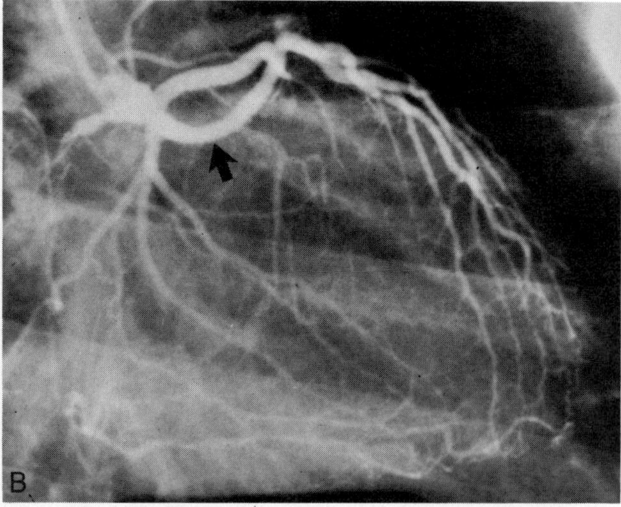

FIGURE 9-29. Origin of the LCA from the proximal portion of the RCA with subsequent passage of the LCA between the aorta and right ventricular outflow tract. *A,* LAO view of the right coronary arteriogram. The RCA is totally occluded. The black arrow points to the anomalous LCA, which passes behind the right ventricular outflow tract and then bifurcates into the usual LAD and circumflex branches. Small conus (C) and acute marginal (M) branches mark the position of the right ventricular outflow tract, clearly indicating that the aberrant LCA passes behind it. *B,* Standard RAO view of the right coronary arteriogram, again showing the course of the anomalous LCA as well as occlusion of the RCA.

ORIGIN OF THE CIRCUMFLEX ARTERY FROM THE RIGHT AORTIC SINUS. Anomalous origin of the circumflex artery from the right aortic sinus is by far the most common of these anomalies. In a series of almost 3000 patients, this anomaly was found in 0.67 per cent.[42] In these cases, the circumflex artery originates from the right aortic sinus by way of a common ostium with the RCA or a separate ostium of its own. It then passes posteriorly around the noncoronary aortic sinus toward the left atrioventricular groove (Fig. 9-30). Left coronary arteriography shows only the LAD arising from the left aortic sinus.

ORIGIN OF THE LEFT ANTERIOR DESCENDING ARTERY FROM THE RIGHT AORTIC SINUS. The LAD arises by means of a common ostium with the RCA or has a separate ostium in the right aortic sinus. It usually passes anterior to the right ventricular outflow tract on its way to the anterior interventricular groove.

When either the LCA or the LAD arise from the right aortic sinus, it may be difficult to determine angiographically whether the aberrant vessel passes in front of the right ventricular outflow tract or behind it in a tunnel between the outflow tract and the aorta. This can be an important consideration, in view of the potential for acute occlusion posed by the latter type of anomaly. In the authors' experience, the best way to determine this is to first pass a catheter into the main pulmonary artery and then perform an arteriogram of the aberrant coronary artery in the direct lateral projection. The catheter localizes the position of the pulmonary artery, and it is then usually possible to determine whether the course of the aberrant vessel is anterior or posterior to it.

SINGLE CORONARY ARTERY. There are numerous variations of this anomaly. Perhaps the best classification system is that of Lipton et al., which divided them into nine categories.[43] Some cases of this anomaly, however, do not fall into any of these categories. Single coronary artery can be hemodynamically significant when a major branch passes between the aorta and the right ventricular outflow tract, as described earlier.

ORIGIN OF ALL THREE CORONARY ARTERIES FROM EITHER RIGHT OR LEFT AORTIC SINUSES VIA MULTIPLE SEPARATE OSTIA. This rare anomaly is similar to single coronary artery. There is absence of a coronary ostium in either the left or right aortic sinus. The missing vessels arise in the contralateral aortic sinus, but instead of arising as a single coronary artery, they arise through two or even three separate ostia.

HIGH ORIGIN OF THE CORONARY ARTERIES. The right and left coronary arteries usually arise in the upper portion of the aortic sinuses, just below the sinotubular ridges. On occasion, one or both coronary arteries may originate farther up the ascending aorta above this ridge.

EFFECT OF STENOSIS ON CORONARY BLOOD FLOW

(See also Chap. 38)

Important concepts regarding the relation between arterial stenosis and blood flow (Fig. 9-31) have resulted from the studies of Shipley and Gregg and Gould et al.[44-46a] Under resting conditions, progressive narrowing of a major artery does not cause a corresponding reduction in flow. Instead,

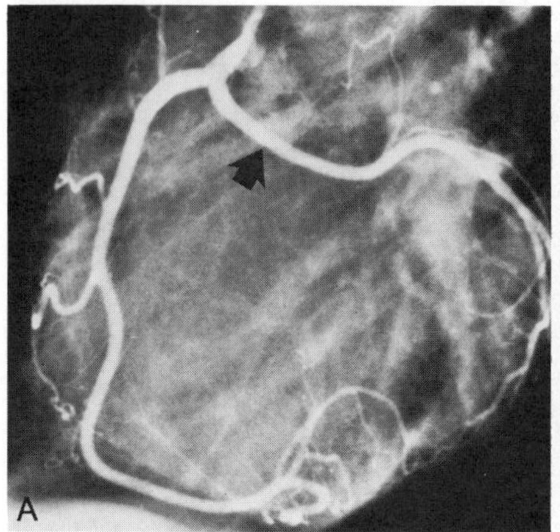

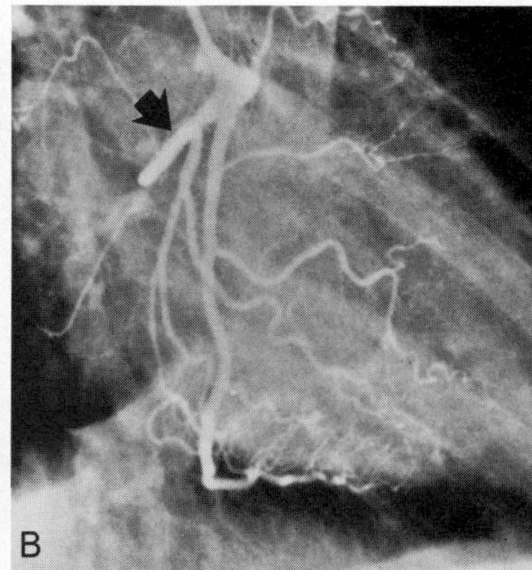

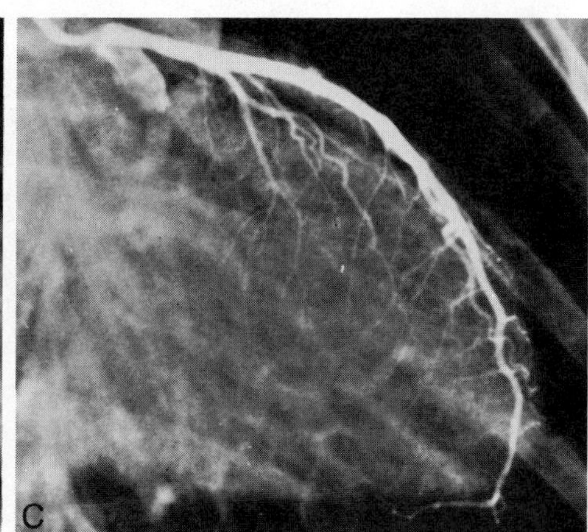

FIGURE 9-30. LAO *(A)* and RAO *(B)* views of a right coronary arteriogram. The patient has a dominant RCA and there is an anomalous left circumflex artery (arrows) which arises from the proximal portion of the RCA and passes behind the aortic root to the left atrioventricular groove. *C,* RAO view of the left coronary arteriogram shows only an LAD artery.

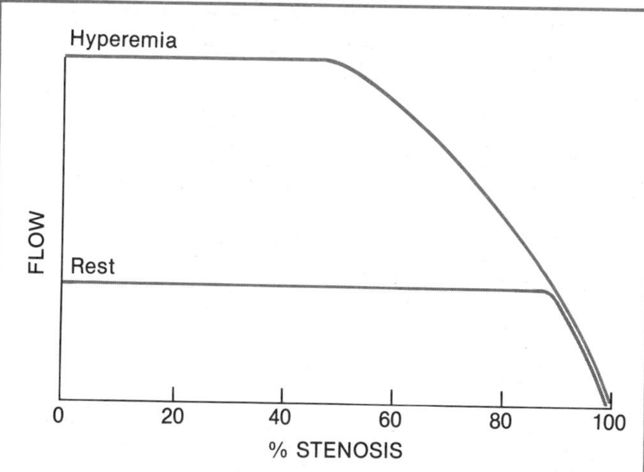

FIGURE 9–31. Relation between arterial stenosis and blood flow under resting and hyperemic conditions.

flow remains relatively constant until the luminal area has been markedly reduced, at which time an abrupt decrease occurs. Under hyperemic conditions in the same artery, a considerably milder degree of stenosis will reduce peak blood flow. In normal human coronary arteries, it has been noted that hyperemic or peak coronary blood flow (such as can occur during exercise) is about six times the normal resting blood flow.[47] The hyperemic state is mediated by dilatation of the distal arteriolar bed, which often is referred to as *coronary flow reserve*.[46] The point at which reduction in flow begins to occur can be called the *point of critical stenosis* (PCS). Expressed in different terms, Figure 9–31 shows that in a major artery, under resting conditions, the PCS is not reached until severe stenosis (about 90 per cent of the luminal diameter) exists. In the same artery under hyperemic conditions, the PCS occurs with much less severe stenosis (about 50 per cent).

Some authors have postulated that the maintenance of resting blood flow in the face of progressively severe proximal stenosis results from compensatory vasodilation of the arteriolar bed distal to the lesion.[47,48] Presumably, when the proximal arterial luminal area is about 90 per cent narrowed, the maximum vasodilatory capacity of the small arterioles is reached, and they cannot compensate any further. Additional narrowing of the major artery beyond this PCS then leads to the rapid falloff in flow. It is further assumed that during hyperemia, some of the coronary flow reserve has already been encroached on to maintain resting flow, so that the maximum vasodilatory capacity of the arteriolar bed is reached with lesser degrees of arterial stenosis. Therefore, according to this theory, the PCS during a hyperemic state is reduced to only 40 to 60 per cent stenosis.

Experiments in the authors' laboratory and in others[49,50] and the earlier study by Shipley and Gregg[44] have provided alternative explanations for the relationship shown in Figure 9–31. In these studies, measurements of arterial pressure distal to progressive stenoses failed to show a pressure drop as the degree of stenosis increased. Instead, both pressure and flow remained constant until the PCS was reached. This meant that peripheral resistance was being maintained as stenosis increased. It further suggested that compensatory peripheral arteriolar dilatation is not the explanation for the maintenance of resting blood flow.

A more likely explanation for this phenomenon has been discussed by Logan.[50] The rate of flow through a vessel equals the driving pressure divided by the total resistance in its vascular bed. Total resistance (R_t) is the sum of stenosis resistance (R_s) in the proximal artery and peripheral resistance in the arteriolar bed (R_p). Under resting conditions, when flow is relatively low and R_p is high, R_t is high but consists almost entirely of R_p. As major arterial stenosis increases, R_s begins to increase but is initially of very small magnitude compared with R_p, and therefore has little overall effect on the magnitude of R_t of the entire system. Only when proximal arterial stenosis becomes severe does R_s begin to approach R_p. At this point, further increase in R_s significantly elevates R_t, which in turn causes flow through the entire system to drop off rapidly. During hyperemic states induced by exercise or other vasodilator stimuli, R_p and therefore R_t are much lower to begin with. A given degree of arterial stenosis will create a level of R_s that is more significant relative to R_p. Any increase in the severity of that stenosis will begin to raise R_t by significant increments at an earlier stage, and the PCS accordingly also is reached at an earlier stage.

These concepts explain why resting blood flow may be entirely normal even when a significant proximal stenosis is present, and why ischemic symptoms develop during exercise when they are not present at rest. They also explain why a minor increase in degree of an already-existing stenosis can cause a profound decrease in blood flow and lead to the abrupt onset of severe ischemia.

Other important aspects of the flow-stenosis relationship relate to the effects of sequential arterial stenoses and length of the lesion. Gould and Lipscomb showed that the resistances of coronary stenoses in series are additive.[51] The effects of such sequential lesions are not determined solely by the most severe lesion. Feldman et al. showed that the hemodynamic effects of coronary stenoses increased significantly as their length increased.[52]

White et al. have called into question the reliability of coronary arteriography in predicting the hemodynamic significance of a coronary stenosis.[53] They compared the degree of coronary stenosis measured by arteriography with the reactive hyperemic response measured during coronary bypass surgery by a Doppler probe after 20 seconds of arterial occlusion. In each case, the ratio of peak to resting flow velocity (coronary flow reserve) was measured. It would be expected that if arteriography is an accurate way of assessing the hemodynamic significance of stenoses, the ratio of peak to resting flow would consistently be lower for severe stenoses than for minor stenoses. However, the study revealed lack of significant correlation between this ratio and the degree of stenosis as measured by arteriography. They suggested that the lack of correlation could be explained by a variety of factors, including interobserver and intraobserver variability, technical problems relating to radiographic magnification and distortion, and the diffuse nature of coronary atherosclerosis (which makes it difficult to establish an accurate denominator for the expression of percentage of stenosis). The nonphysiological circumstances of the measurements also could play a role. Their findings emphasize the importance of high-quality cineangiography with visualization of coronary lesions in multiple projections if any degree of accuracy is to be achieved.

The possible presence of diffuse coronary atherosclerosis is a particular drawback of using only percent diameter stenosis to angiographically assess the status of the coronary arteries in human patients. If diffuse symmetrical disease is present in a vessel, it may appear normal to the angiographer, who cannot see its outer wall and has no reference point other than the opacified lumen. A site of additional localized narrowing in such a vessel may appear to be only a mild stenosis angiographically, when in fact it actually severely compromises the original, *true* lumen of the vessel. Diffuse atherosclerosis is more likely to be present in patients with multivessel disease.[54] Studies utilizing intracoronary injections of acetylcholine in human patients with "normal" coronary arteries have demonstrated paradoxical constriction in some patients, suggesting the presence of angiographically undetected symmetrical atherosclerosis in these people.[55]

The accuracy of angiographic assessment of coronary lesions which appear to be of borderline significance can be enhanced by the measurement of pressure gradients across the stenoses at the time of diagnostic coronary arteriography.[56] This can be accomplished by first passing a small (No. 2 French) catheter coaxially through the diagnostic arteriographic catheter and through the stenosis and then recording pressure measurements during pullback both at rest and under hyperemic conditions induced by the injection of contrast material. Rest and exercise thallium myocardial scintigraphy also can help to evaluate such lesions.

CORONARY COLLATERAL CIRCULATION

(See also p. 1164)

In the normal human heart, a myriad of tiny anastomotic branches interconnect the major coronary arteries.[57] Most of these anastomotic vessels are less than 200 μm in diameter, and they are the precursors of the collateral circulation. In coronary arteriograms of patients with normal or mildly diseased coronary arteries, they cannot be visualized because they carry only minimal flow and their small caliber is well beyond the spatial resolution capabilities of cine imaging systems. If, however, obstruction of a major coronary artery occurs, a pressure gradient is created in the anastomotic vessels connecting the distal segment of the involved artery with either its proximal segment or the nearby segments of other vessels. With the creation of this gradient, an increased volume of blood is propelled through the anastomotic vessels, which progressively dilate and eventually become visible angiographically as collateral channels. The reason this process seems to occur effectively in some patients and ineffectively in others is not entirely clear, but it may well have to do with the rate at which the obstruction develops. The most favorable clinical circumstance is gradual development of the obstruction, thereby allowing collateral channels to enlarge and become functional before the native vessel becomes totally occluded.

Other factors that affect collateral development are patency of the feeding arteries and the size and vascular resistance of the postobstructive segment.[58] Some interesting observations on the temporal sequence of collateral development resulted from an angiographic study of patients who showed persistent occlusion of the infarct artery after acute myocardial infarction.[59] Among patients studied within 6 hours of infarction, about half demonstrated angiographically visible collaterals. Among those studied more than 24 hours after infarction, virtually all had visible collaterals. This suggests that collateral flow may develop more quickly than previously thought, perhaps within hours after total occlusion. In any event, collateral circulation does not represent the formation of new vessels, but rather the utilization of vessels which already exist but carry little blood flow until the need arises. Collaterals usually cannot be demonstrated at coronary arteriography unless the recipient vessel has developed at least 90 per cent diameter stenosis.[57,60]

A wide variety of collateral pathways exist in patients with severe coronary artery disease. These pathways are diagrammed in Figures 9–32 through 9–34. Figure 9–35 shows an example of early collateral circulation to a stenotic LAD seen on right coronary arteriography. Figure 9–36 shows a patient with LAD occlusion and collaterals from the RCA. Figure 9–37 shows an example of LAD occlusion and collaterals from both the RCA and a diagonal branch. The patient shown in Figure 9–38 has occlusions of both the RCA and the LAD, with a strikingly enlarged conus branch providing collaterals to both vessels. Figure 9–39 shows collaterals from the circumflex artery to the distal RCA. Figure 9–40 shows a patient with total occlusion of all three coronary arteries who is obviously surviving on collaterals. Figure 9–41 shows an example of collaterals from the proximal to distal circumflex artery.

The functional role of coronary collateral circulation has been debated for many years. An early study suggested that collateral circulation did not protect against development of regional left ventricular contraction abnormalities.[61] This study included patients both with and without total occlusions of coronary arteries, and some patients in the latter group undoubtedly had no demonstrable collaterals because their stenoses were not severe enough. A subsequent study of one of the authors (D.C.L.) addressed the same issue but included only patients in whom total occlusion of a coronary artery was present, thereby insuring that the degree of obstruction was absolutely identical in all cases.[57] This study revealed that regional left ventricular contraction was significantly better in segments supplied by adequate collateral circulation than in those segments supplied by inadequate or no collateral circulation.

Several recent studies have confirmed the protective effect which coronary collaterals confer on myocardial viability and function, both before and at the time of myocardial infarction.[62–64] In another important study, conducted before the era of thrombolytic therapy, patients with acute myocardial infarction undergoing emergency cardiac catheterization were divided into those with adequate collateral circulation to the infarct vessel and those with inadequate or no collateral circulation to the infarct vessel.[65] The group with adequate collaterals had significantly lower LVEDP, higher cardiac index, higher ejection fraction, and lower percentage of area dyssynergy. None of the patients with adequate collaterals died, whereas the majority with inadequate or no collaterals died. Patients with severe coronary obstruction without collateral circulation were found to have a significantly higher incidence of thallium-201 myocardial perfusion defects than those with collateral circulation.[66] This suggests that collaterals may improve myocardial perfusion in the ischemic zone. Frequent absence of thallium-201 perfusion defects also has been reported in noninfarcted, collaterized myocardial regions with totally occluded coronary arteries.[67]

The advent of percutaneous transluminal coronary angioplasty (PTCA) has provided interesting opportunities to study hemodynamic aspects and angiographic patterns of the coronary collateral circulation, since balloon inflation during PTCA simulates abrupt occlusion of a previously stenotic vessel. Using this model and a collateral grading system of 0 to 3 (0 = no distal filling, 1 = filling of side branches only, 2 = partial filling of the distal epicardial segment, 3 = complete filling of the distal epicardial segment), Cohen and Rentrop found that with balloon inflation during PTCA, patients

Text continued on p. 262

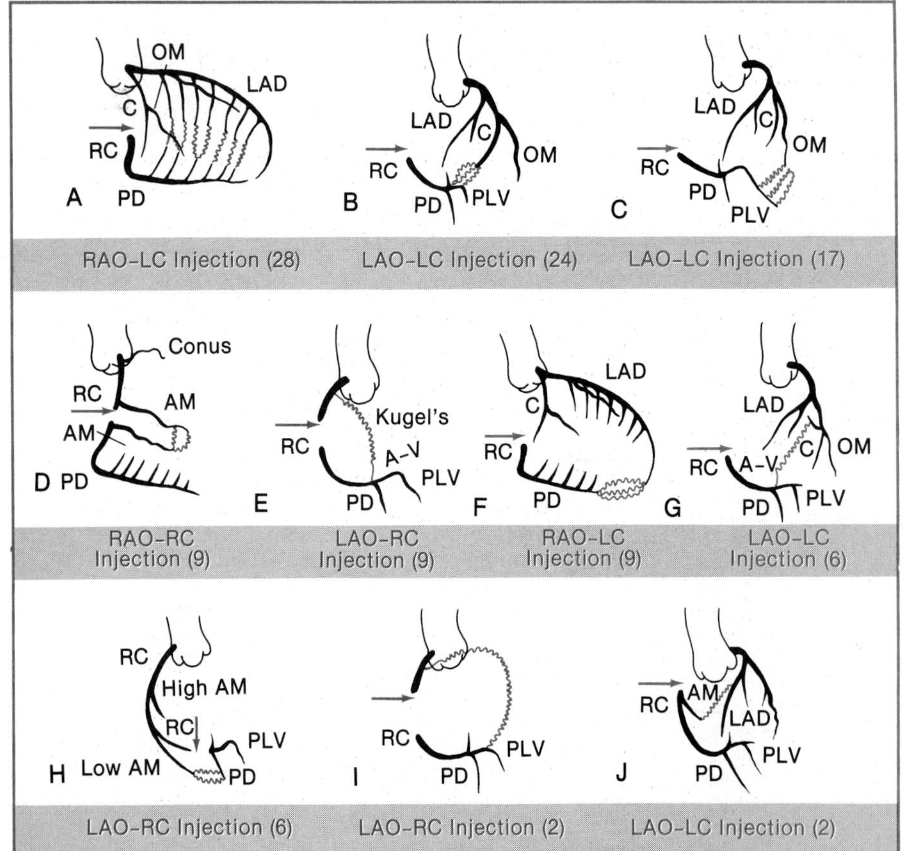

FIGURE 9–32. Common collateral pathways seen with RCA occlusion. The arrows point to the site of obstruction. The small tortuous channels represent the collateral connections. Numbers in parentheses refer to the frequency with which each pathway was visualized in a series of 200 patients with significant coronary disease. (From Levin, D.C.: Pathways and functional significance of the coronary collateral circulation. Circulation *50*:831, 1974, by permission of the American Heart Association, Inc.)

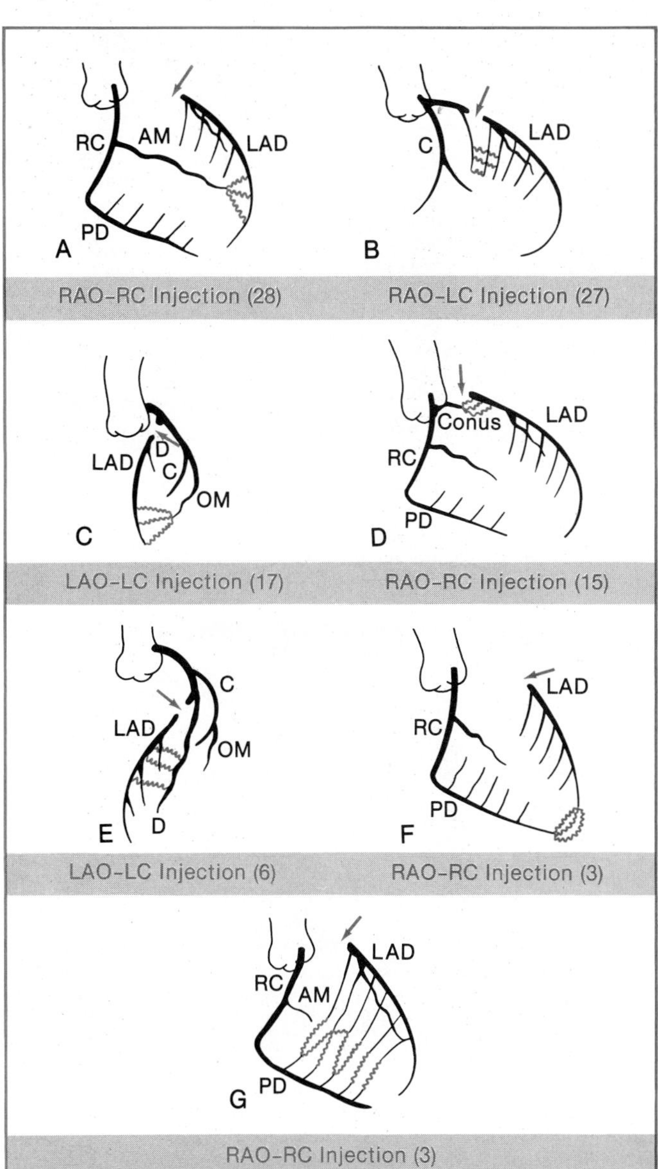

FIGURE 9-33. Common collateral pathways seen with LAD occlusion. (From Levin, D.C.: Pathways and functional significance of the coronary collateral circulation. Circulation *50*:831, 1974, by permission of the American Heart Association, Inc.)

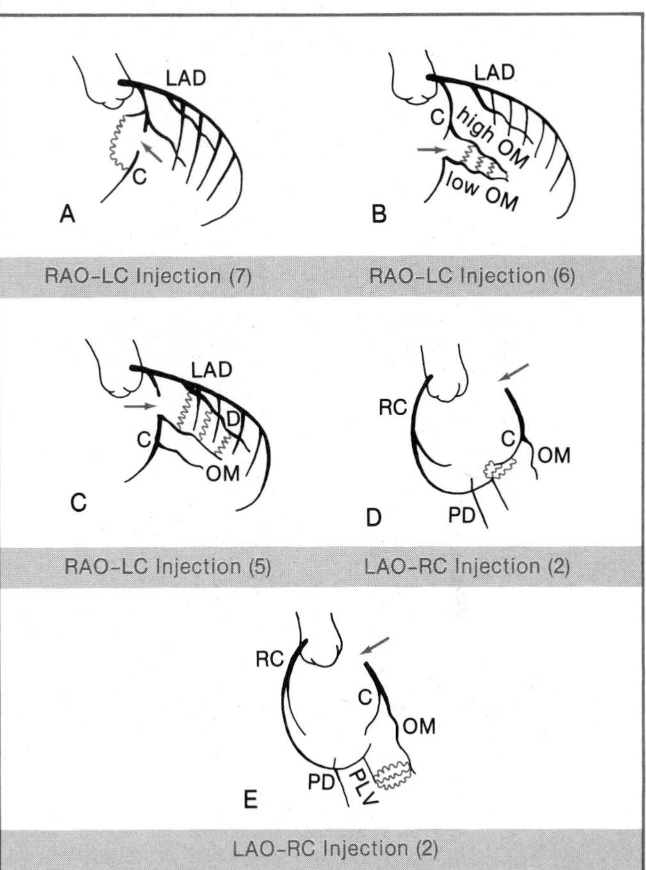

FIGURE 9-34. Common collateral pathways seen with left circumflex occlusion. (From Levin, D.C.: Pathways and functional significance of the coronary collateral circulation. Circulation *50*:831, 1974, by permission of the American Heart Association, Inc.)

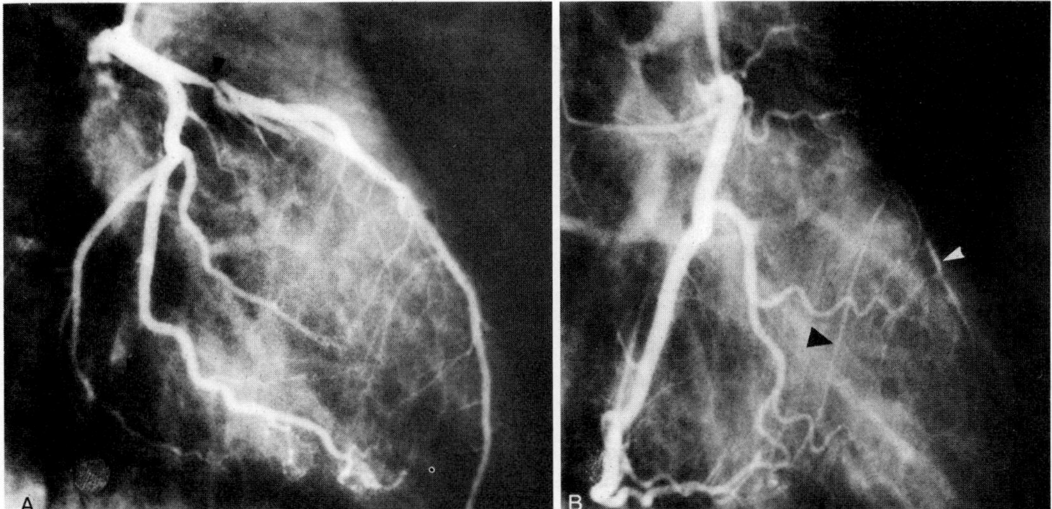

FIGURE 9-35. Early collateralization in a patient with severe LAD stenosis. *A*, RAO left coronary arteriogram, showing severe proximal LAD stenosis (arrowhead), *B*, RAO right coronary arteriogram. Early collateral circulation is seen extending from the posterior descending artery up through the interventricular septum (black arrowhead) and partially filling the distal LAD (white arrowhead).

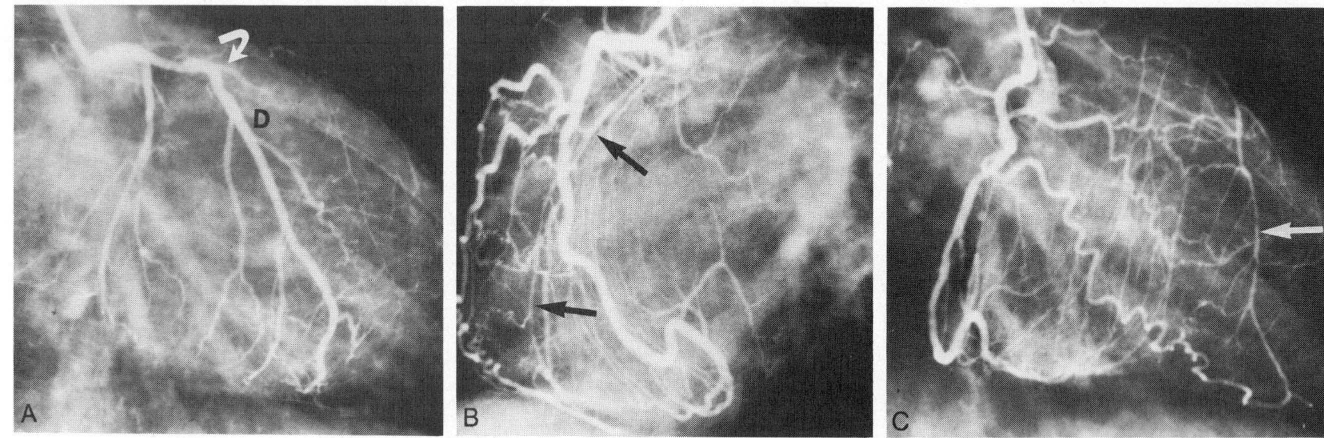

FIGURE 9-36. Total occlusion of the LAD with collateral filling from the RCA. *A,* RAO left coronary arteriogram showing total occlusion (curved arrow) of the LAD just beyond the origin of a large diagonal branch (D). LAO *(B)* and RAO *(C)* views of the right coronary arteriogram. The distal portion of the obstructed LAD (straight arrows) fills by means of extensive collateral circulation from the RCA. The primary collateral pathways are two large, acute marginal branches of the RCA and also septal branches from the posterior descending artery.

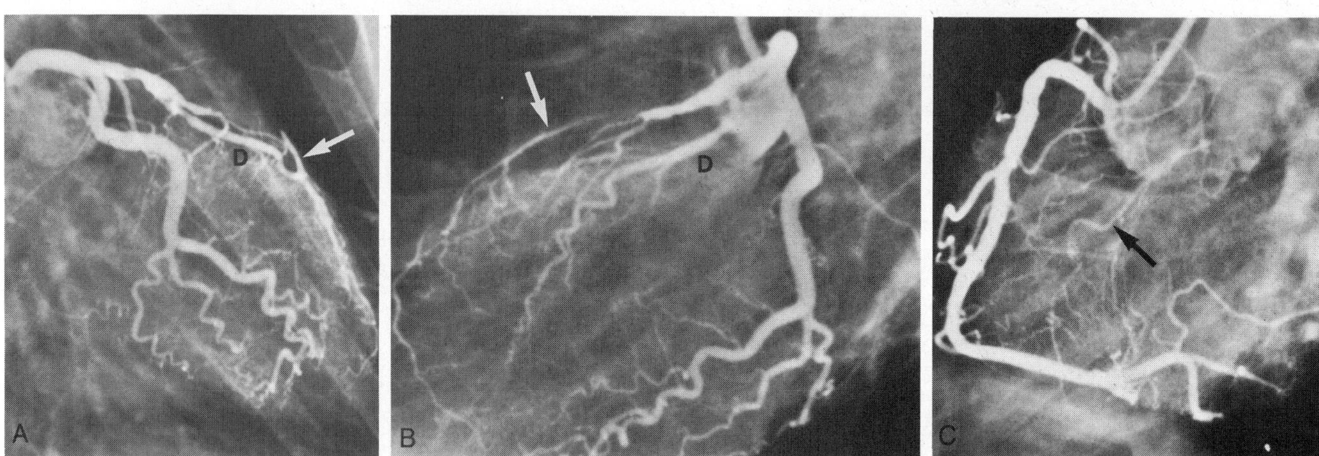

FIGURE 9-37. Total obstruction of the LAD with collateral circulation to the distal segment from both the right and left coronary systems. RAO *(A)* and left lateral *(B)* views of the left coronary arteriogram showing total occlusion of the LAD. Its distal segment (arrows) fills by means of collateral circulation from the diagonal branch (D) and also from obtuse marginal branches of the left circumflex artery. *C,* LAO view of the right coronary arteriogram. The patient has a strongly dominant RCA. Collateral filling of the distal segment of the LAD (arrow) is seen by means of the conus, acute marginal and posterior descending branches of the RCA.

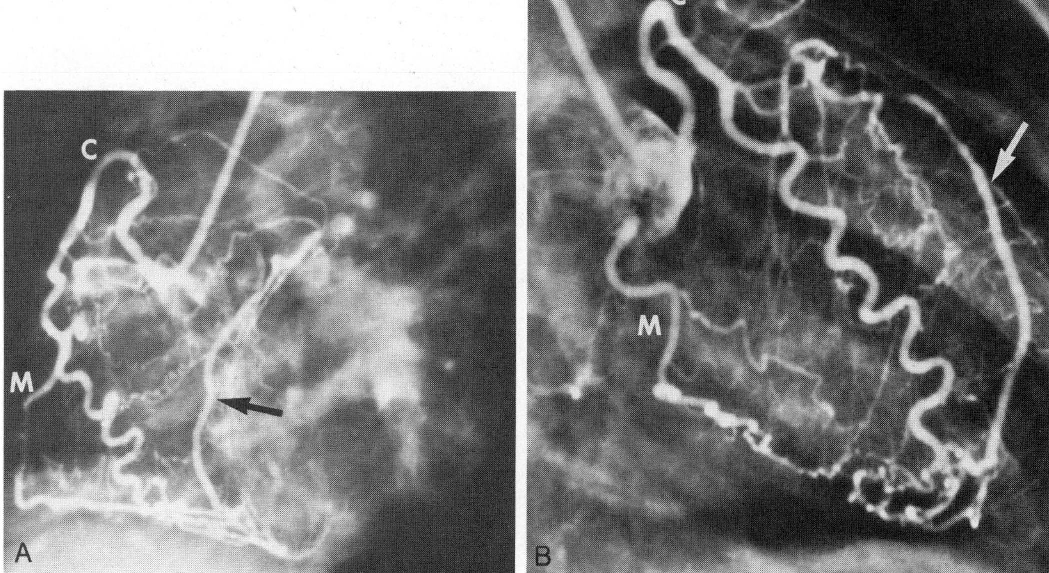

FIGURE 9-38. Total occlusion of both the LAD and RCA. LAO *(A)* and RAO *(B)* views of the right coronary arteriogram. The conus artery (C) arises proximal to the RCA occlusion and is massively enlarged. It supplies flow to both the distal segment of the obstructed LAD (arrows) and an acute marginal branch (M) of the RCA. Note the tortuosity of the collateral connections.

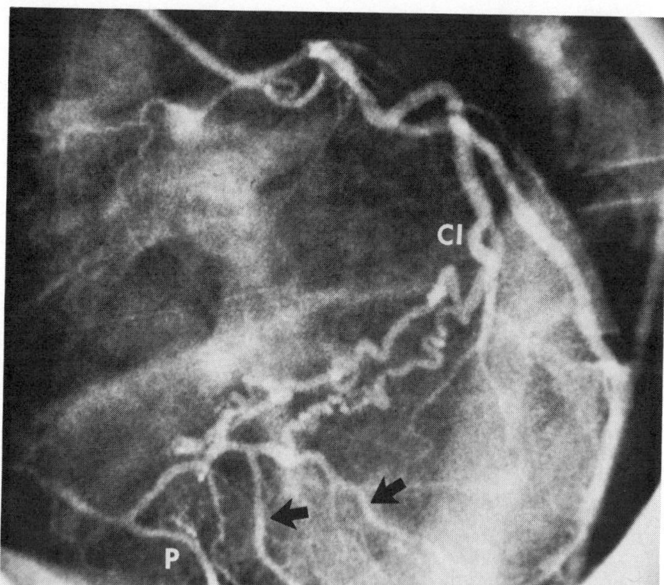

FIGURE 9-39. LAO view of a left coronary arteriogram in a patient with occlusions of both the LAD and RCA. The distal RCA and its posterior descending (P) and posterior left ventricular branches (arrows) also fill by means of collateral circulation from the left circumflex artery (CI). Note the tortuosity of the collateral connections.

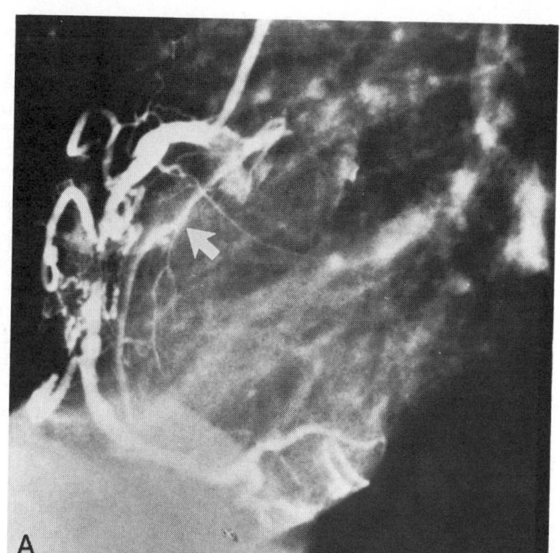

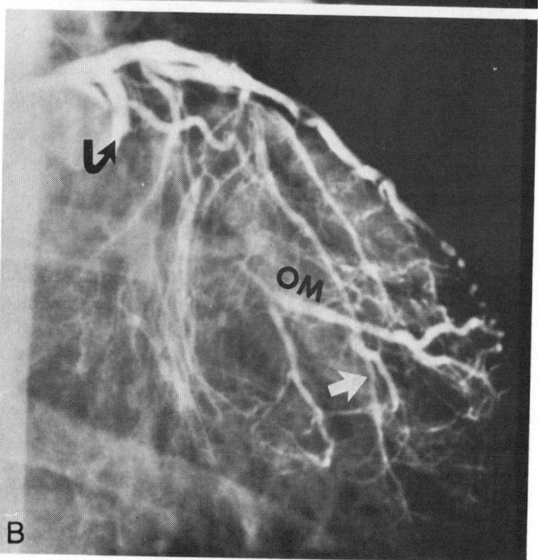

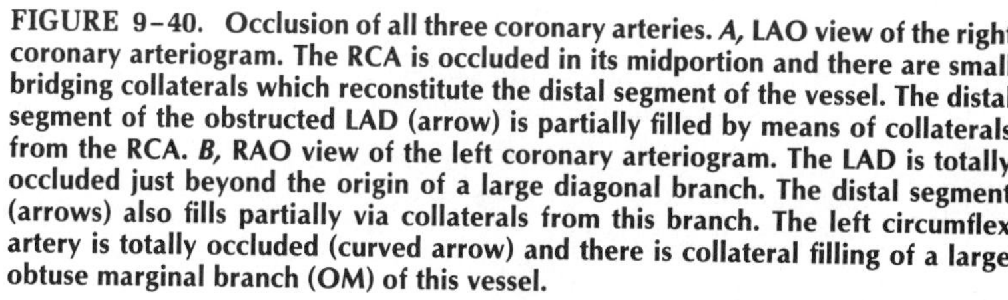

FIGURE 9-40. Occlusion of all three coronary arteries. *A,* LAO view of the right coronary arteriogram. The RCA is occluded in its midportion and there are small bridging collaterals which reconstitute the distal segment of the vessel. The distal segment of the obstructed LAD (arrow) is partially filled by means of collaterals from the RCA. *B,* RAO view of the left coronary arteriogram. The LAD is totally occluded just beyond the origin of a large diagonal branch. The distal segment (arrows) also fills partially via collaterals from this branch. The left circumflex artery is totally occluded (curved arrow) and there is collateral filling of a large obtuse marginal branch (OM) of this vessel.

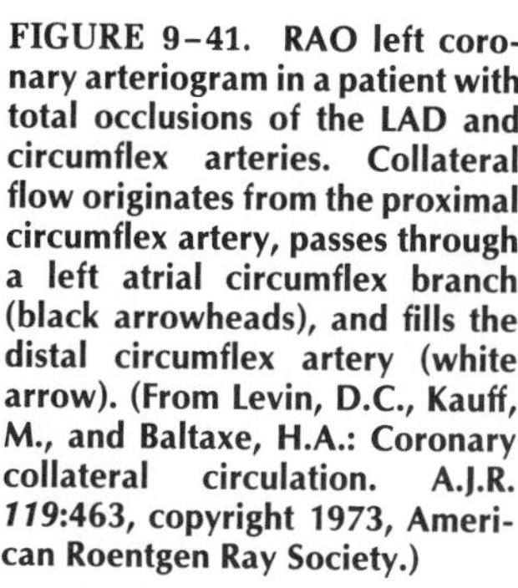

FIGURE 9-41. RAO left coronary arteriogram in a patient with total occlusions of the LAD and circumflex arteries. Collateral flow originates from the proximal circumflex artery, passes through a left atrial circumflex branch (black arrowheads), and fills the distal circumflex artery (white arrow). (From Levin, D.C., Kauff, M., and Baltaxe, H.A.: Coronary collateral circulation. A.J.R. *119*:463, copyright 1973, American Roentgen Ray Society.)

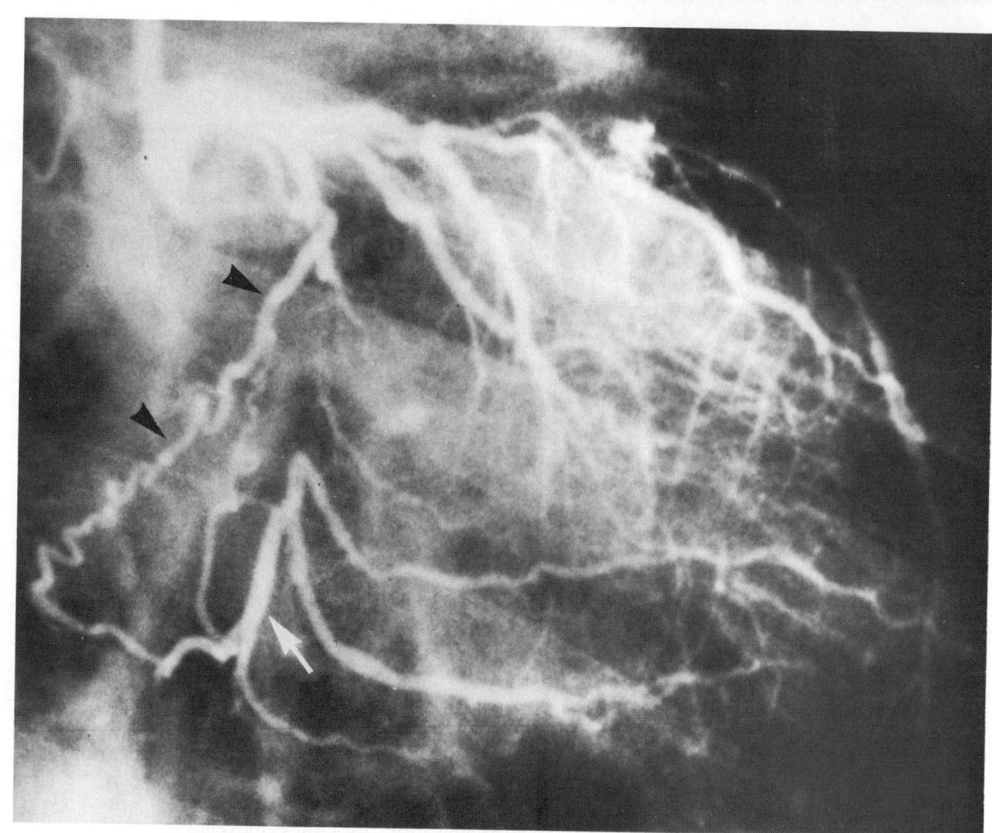

with well-developed collaterals experienced less pain, less left ventricular asynergy, and less summed ST segment elevation than those with poorly developed collaterals.[68] Other studies have revealed similar findings,[69] as well as the fact that distal coronary perfusion pressure during balloon inflation is higher in patients with well-developed collaterals than in those with poorly developed collaterals.[69-71]

CORONARY ARTERY SPASM (see also p. 1207)

Over three decades have elapsed since Prinzmetal et al. described an unusual or variant form of angina in which the onset of chest pain was not provoked by the usual factors, such as exercise, emotional upset, cold, and ingestion of a meal.[72] According to currently accepted theories, patients considered to have variant angina are those in whom chest pain commences at rest or both at rest and during exertion.[73] The pain often occurs in a cyclical pattern at the same time every day, generally in the morning, and usually is noted to be accompanied by ST-segment elevation if an electrocardiogram is recorded. Symptoms may occur many times daily, then cease for weeks or months, and then recur. Although the ST elevation often is striking, it rapidly reverts to normal when the pain disappears spontaneously or is terminated by the administration of nitroglycerin. Ischemic episodes may be accompanied by atrioventricular block, ventricular ectopic activity, ventricular tachycardia, or ventricular fibrillation. Although the original description of this syndrome emphasized its transient nature and its onset at rest, it has become apparent through further studies that coronary spasm also can play a role in exercise-induced angina, unstable angina, acute myocardial infarction, and sudden death.[73]

Coronary arteriography has played an important role in understanding the pathophysiology and clinical consequences of coronary artery spasm. In the early 1970's, several studies angiographically demonstrated spasm in patients with clinical variant angina.[74-76] These studies showed that although spasm usually was superimposed on areas of stenosis, in some cases it occurred in segments of coronary arteries that appeared normal. In the late 1970's, intravenous ergonovine maleate was used to provoke spasm in patients with suspected variant angina who were undergoing coronary arteriography.[77-79] These studies revealed that the vast majority of patients with this syndrome will demonstrate spasm on arteriograms performed immediately after the administration of ergonovine. Calcium channel blockers are effective in treating variant angina.

Ergonovine-induced provocation of coronary artery spasm entails intravenous administration of the drug in progressively increasing doses, usually starting with an initial dose of 0.05 mg. After each dose, the patient is observed for several minutes for the detection of ST-segment elevation or the onset of chest pain. If neither occurs, the next dose is administered and the cycle is repeated. Most laboratories terminate the study when a cumulative ergonovine dose of 0.5 mg has been reached. If no chest pain or ST-segment elevation occurs and the patient's systemic blood pressure rises by 10 per cent, it can be assumed that the ergonovine has had a physiological effect. When any of these endpoints is reached, repeat arteriography is performed to determine if coronary spasm has occurred. Although the ergonovine provocative test is widely used and usually safe, it should be borne in mind that serious complications, including irreversible occlusion, can occur on rare occasions.[80] Figure 9–42 shows an example of ergonovine-induced spasm in a vessel which appeared normal arteriographically.

Perhaps the most comprehensive angiographically oriented study of the frequency and role of coronary spasm is that of Bertrand et al.[81] They performed ergonovine provocation in 1089 consecutive patients undergoing coronary arteriography for a variety of clinical symptoms, excluding only those patients with main LCA disease, severe triple-vessel disease, New York Heart Association functional class III or IV, or spontaneously occurring spasm. One hundred thirty-four patients exhibited spasm after ergonovine; in 59 per cent of these patients spasm was superimposed on an organic stenosis, whereas in 41 per cent it occurred in an angiographically normal segment. Although ergonovine-induced spasm occurred rarely (less than 5 per cent) in patients with atypical chest pain and exertional angina, it occurred in 14 per cent of patients with symptoms of both exertional and resting angina. In patients with primarily resting angina who were observed to have episodes of ST-segment elevation during hospitalization, it was seen in 85 per cent. However, in resting angina patients without electrocardiographic abnormalities during hospitalization, spasm could only be provoked in 14 per cent. Finally, in patients with myocardial infarction within the previous 6 weeks, spasm was noted in 20 per cent.

The mechanisms of coronary vasospasm appear to be varied. Early attention focused on local, nonspecific arterial hypersensitivity to vasoconstrictor and alpha-adrenergic mechanisms.[82] More recently studies have been carried out on the function of coronary vascular endothelium and aggregating platelets in atherosclerotic vessels.[83-85] Normal endothe-

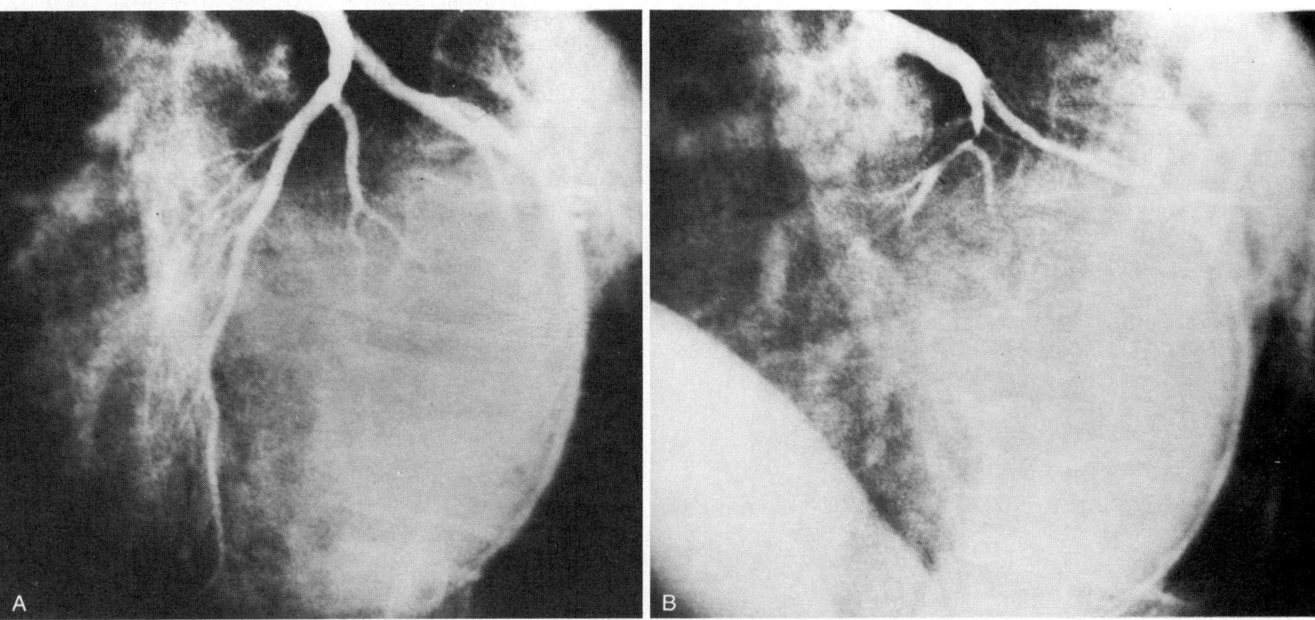

FIGURE 9–42. Ergonovine-induced spasm of the LAD. *A,* LAO left coronary arteriogram at the onset of intravenous ergonovine infusion. The LAD appears normal. *B,* After intravenous administration of 0.1 mg of ergonovine. Severe spasm has developed, causing nearly total occlusion of the LAD. The patient was experiencing mild chest pain and had pronounced ST-segment elevation. Spasm was quickly relieved with sublingual nitroglycerin.

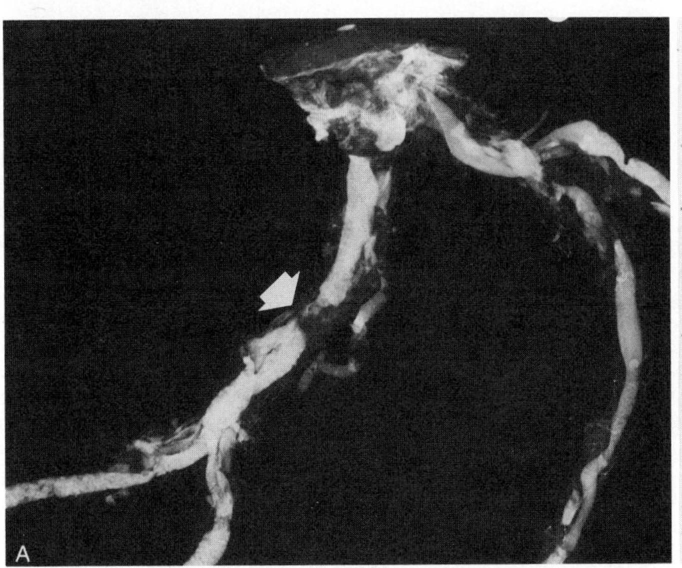

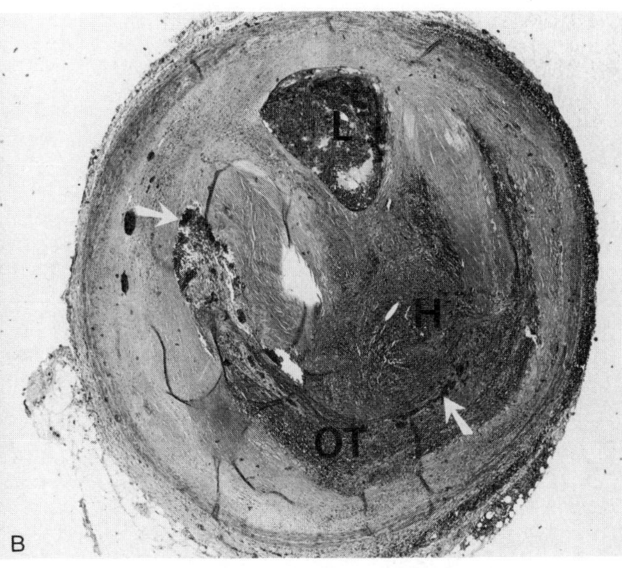

FIGURE 9–43. Complicated atherosclerotic plaque of the LAD. *A,* Postmortem injection specimen, in which the left coronary system has been dissected from the epicardial surface of the heart. A severe irregular stenosis of the proximal LAD is present (arrow). *B,* Corresponding histological section. L = residual lumen; H = large area of hemorrhage within the plaque; OT = organizing thrombus within the plaque; arrows point to small recanalized channels within the organizing thrombus.

lium produces substances like endothelium-derived relaxing factor (EDRF) and prostacyclin (PGI_2), which relax the underlying vascular smooth muscle and produce vasodilatation. It also produces endothelium-derived constricting factors (EDCF's) such as endothelin. Aggregating platelets release vasoconstricting substances like thromboxane A_2 and serotonin (5-HT). Atherosclerosis interferes with the synthesis and action of the vasoactive substances produced by endothelium, and this complex balance may be further altered by varying amounts of platelet aggregation. It is likely that these factors play an important role in the genesis of spasm.

Other factors affect this balance as well. For example, acetylcholine has been shown to dilate normal arteries by stimulating the release of EDRF from endothelium.[55,83] Ludmer et al. administered graded doses of intracoronary acetylcholine in human patients both with and without angiographically visible coronary disease.[85] In normal coronary arteries, dilatation occurred, but they noted a paradoxical vasoconstrictor response in diseased vessels—even those with mild disease. Some severely stenotic segments became totally occluded temporarily. They believed that this response resulted from direct action on the arterial wall and suggested that it represented a defect in endothelial vasodilator function, which might play a role in the pathogenesis of coronary vasospasm.

CORONARY ATHEROSCLEROTIC PLAQUE MORPHOLOGY AND ITS CONSEQUENCES

(See also p. 1112)

Postmortem studies have provided abundant evidence that acute thrombosis in stenotic coronary arteries occurs in association with plaques which have undergone rupture, ulceration, or subintimal hemorrhage (p. 1113). By contrast, it seems less likely to occur with uncomplicated fatty or fibrous plaques having intact luminal surfaces. Among 40 coronary artery segments containing occluding thrombi, the thrombus overlay a plaque rupture in 39.[86] Intraplaque hemorrhage was frequently noted, as was partial recanalization. Thrombi were found in 67 of 69 coronary arteries supplying zones of recently infarcted myocardium.[87] In 64 of these 67 vessels, ulcers or ruptures in the plaque surface underlay the thrombus. Horie et al. reported that 91 per cent of occlusive coronary artery thrombi formed at sites of rupture of atheromatous plaques.[88] In a pathological study of 51 recent coronary thrombi, 40 were associated with underlying ruptured atherosclerotic plaques and 2 others had rethrombosis of old recanalized occlusions.[89]

Willerson et al. have discussed the mechanism by which atherosclerotic plaque rupture can lead to acute thrombosis.[90] They postulate that at the site of coronary stenosis, there is decreased local prostacyclin concentration to begin with. Plaque fissuring and hemorrhage lead to platelet aggregation and the release of vasoactive substances and activators of further platelet aggregation, including thromboxane A_2, serotonin, histamine, and platelet-activating factor. As circulating platelets become activated and adhere to this nidus, a vicious cycle is initiated, leading rapidly to occlusive thrombosis.

An attempt was made in the laboratory of one of the authors (D.C.L.) to determine whether "complicated" or complex coronary atherosclerotic plaques (those characterized by plaque rupture, subintimal hemorrhage within the plaque, superimposed partially occluding thrombi, or recanalized thrombi) could be differentiated on postmortem angiography from "uncomplicated" fatty or fibrous plaques having intact luminal surfaces.[91] Postmortem coronary angiograms were studied and angiographic morphology was correlated with histological sections of 73 significant coronary stenoses to ascertain whether complicated and uncomplicated atherosclerotic lesions could be differentiated angiographically.

Lesions were angiographically divided into "smooth" and "irregular" categories; the former had smooth, tapered borders and no intraluminal lucencies, whereas the latter had irregular borders, intraluminal lucencies, or both. Only 4 of the 35 lesions (11 per cent) with smooth angiographic morphology were complex stenoses on histological examination. However, 30 of the 38 (79 per cent) lesions characterized by irregular angiographic morphology were complex stenoses histologically. Postmortem angiography had a sensitivity of 88 per cent and a specificity of 79 per cent in detecting complex coronary artery stenoses on the basis of the presence of irregular borders or intraluminal lucencies.

Figure 9–43 shows a postmortem coronary arteriogram of a complex LAD stenosis, along with its corresponding histological section. It was postulated that because it was possible to detect complex atherosclerotic plaques by postmortem angiography, it also might be possible (although undoubtedly more difficult) to detect such lesions in living patients by observing irregular borders or intraluminal lucencies on coronary angiograms. If present, they could create a greater danger to the patient because of their propensity to lead to acute thrombosis. Revascularization by means of angioplasty or bypass surgery might be more urgently needed in such cases.

A number of studies have suggested that angiographic plaque morphology can in fact be evaluated on coronary angiograms in living patients, and that it can be correlated with both the clinical status and the prognosis of the patient. In a study of 110 patients with stable or unstable angina, Ambrose et al. classified their lesions angiographically into four categories (Fig. 9–44).[92] The first category included those with concentric stenoses and smooth borders. The second category was referred to as type I eccentric stenoses—lesions which were eccentric but had smooth borders and a broad neck. The third category was designated type II eccentric stenoses–eccentric lesions usually in the form of a convex intraluminal obstruction with a narrow base or neck caused by overhanging edges, or borders that were irregularly scalloped. The fourth category included those lesions having multiple irregularities. The latter two categories (type II eccentric stenoses and lesions with multiple irregularities) probably correspond to le-

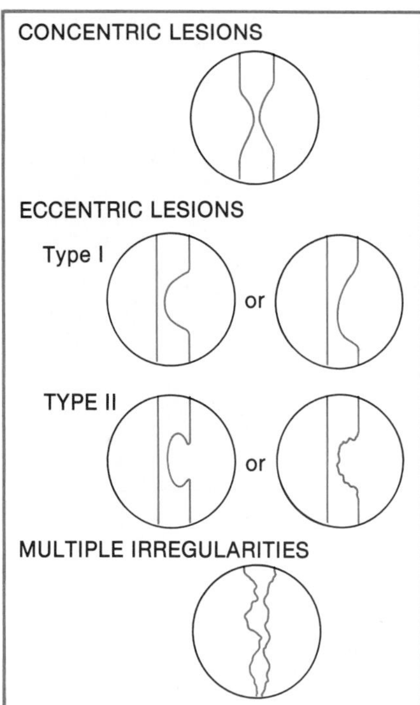

FIGURE 9–44. Method of Ambrose et al. of angiographically classifying coronary stenoses. (From Ambrose, J.A., Winters, S.L., Arpra, R.R., Haft, J.I., Goldstein, J., Rentrop, K.P., Gorlin, R., and Fuster, V.: Coronary angiographic morphology in myocardial infarction: A link between the pathogenesis of unstable angina and myocardial infarction. J. Am. Coll. Cardiol. 6:1233, 1985. Reprinted with permission of the American College of Cardiology.)

sions that would have been categorized as irregular (or complex) stenoses on the authors' postmortem angiograms. Among Ambrose's patients with stable angina, complex angiographic stenoses were present in 18 per cent of coronary arteries. Among the patients with unstable angina, 56 per cent had complex lesions. Ambrose further identified a group of patients in whom the "angina-producing" artery could be clearly identified by angiographic, electrocardiographic, or radionuclide techniques. In this subgroup, lesions that produced stable angina showed a 20 per cent incidence of complex angiographic morphology. By comparison, 71 per cent of the lesions that produced unstable angina were complex. These data show that in patients with unstable angina, lesions characterized by overhanging edges, scalloped borders, irregular borders, or multiple irregularities were more than three times as common as in patients with stable angina. They postulated that such complex lesions represent ruptured plaques or partially occlusive thrombi, or a combination of the two.

In a similar study, Rehr et al. compared the coronary angiographic findings in patients with stable angina and in those with prolonged rest angina.[93] Among the stable group, 17 per cent were noted to have intracoronary thrombi, 14 per cent had complex stenoses (defined as those having haziness, a smudged or inhomogeneous appearance, ill-defined or irregular margins, or ulceration), and 21 per cent had either or both. Among the patients with prolonged rest angina, 42 per cent were found to have intracoronary thrombi, 44 per cent had complex lesions, and 70 per cent had either or both. A study by the authors revealed that in patients with stable angina, 18 per cent of diseased coronary arteries had complex lesions and 2 per cent had thrombi; among patients with unstable angina, 55 per cent had complex lesions and 13 per cent had thrombi.[94] These and other studies clearly demonstrate a strong association between the presence of acute ischemic syndromes and coronary lesions having complex angiographic morphology.

Still other investigations have addressed the relation between lesion morphology and myocardial infarction. Ambrose et al. performed coronary angiography on 41 patients with recent myocardial infarction who were found to have subtotally occluded infarct-related vessels.[95] Twenty-seven of the 41 infarct vessels (66 per cent) were found to have complex stenoses. Among 18 other noninfarct-related lesions in this group of patients, only 2 (11 per cent) were complex. Another group of 23 patients were studied during acute myocardial infarction. All either had received intracoronary streptokinase infusion and had reperfused (17 cases), or had subtotal occlusion before the streptokinase infusion (6 cases). Fourteen of the 23 infarct vessels (61 per cent) contained a complex stenosis, whereas only 1 of 11 (9 per cent) diseased but noninfarct-related vessels had complex stenoses. The CASS investigators compared lesion morphology in comparable groups of patients with LAD stenosis and long-term medical management who subsequently either developed or did not develop anterior myocardial infarction.[96] The presence of a roughened or irregular stenosis at angiography increased the risk of future infarction more than fourfold. Lesion morphology ranked second only to percent stenosis as a predictor of risk of infarction.

Several groups of investigators have commented on the difficulties in assessing plaque morphology on coronary angiograms in living patients.[93,96] This is particularly true when lesion surface irregularities are subtle or when the spatial resolution of the cine imaging system is suboptimal. Figure 9–45 shows an LAD lesion which is difficult to characterize despite good image quality and optimal visualization of the lesion of profile. On the other hand, Figure 9–46 shows three patients who clearly have high-grade, complicated atherosclerotic plaques.

On the basis of our current knowledge, there seems to be general agreement on certain aspects of coronary lesion morphology. First, coronary thrombosis is almost always associated with complex or disrupted atheromatous lesions. Second, these lesions can be detected angiographically in living patients, although probably with relatively low sensitivity. Third, there is a high incidence of complex lesions in patients with unstable angina and acute myocardial infarction. Finally, the risk of myocardial infarction is probably greater in patients with complex lesions than in those with smooth lesions. A number of questions remain unanswered; principal among these is why atherosclerotic plaques which initially are smooth and intact undergo ulceration, rupture, or hemorrhage.

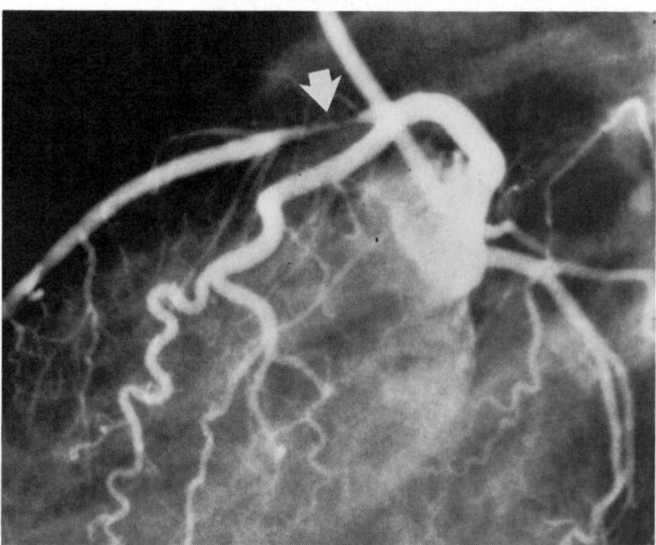

FIGURE 9–45. High-grade proximal LAD stenosis (arrow) as seen on a left lateral projection of a left coronary arteriogram. The lesion appears to have subtle irregularities, suggesting possible plaque ulceration. The case illustrates the difficulties that can be encountered in trying to differentiate complex from smooth stenoses angiographically.

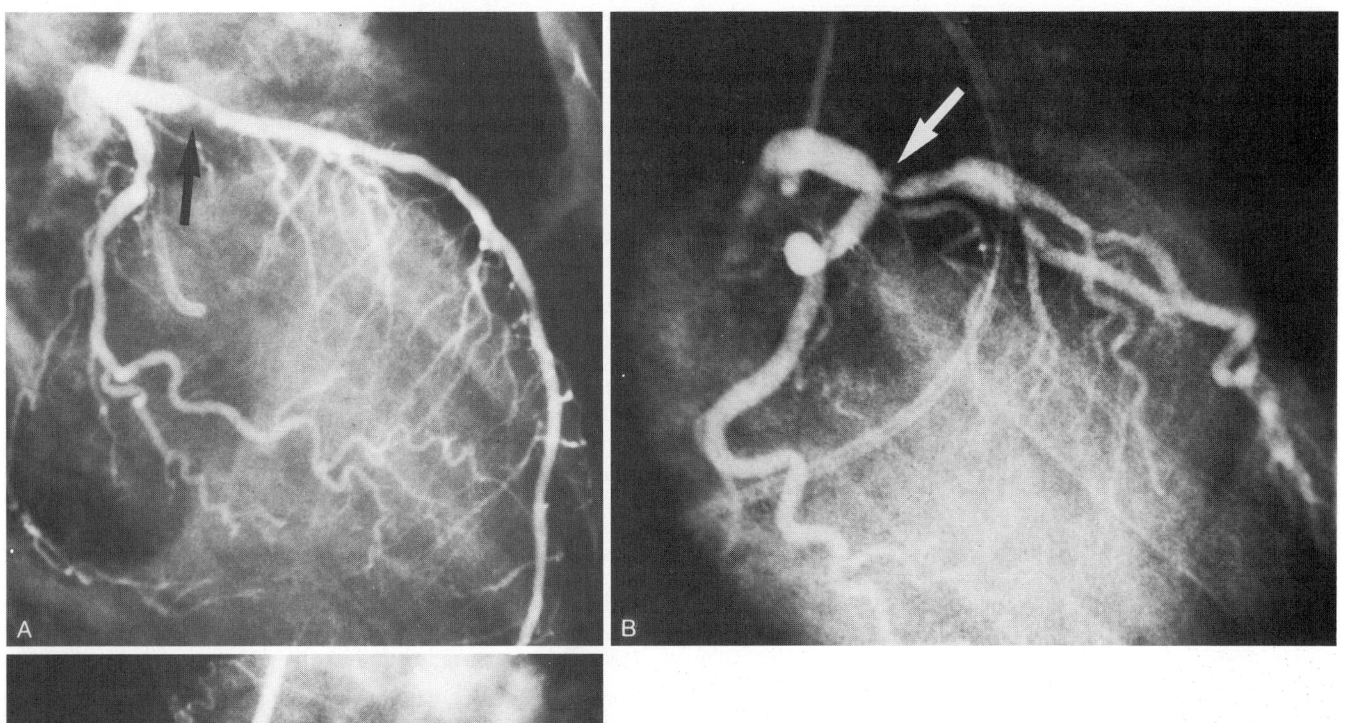

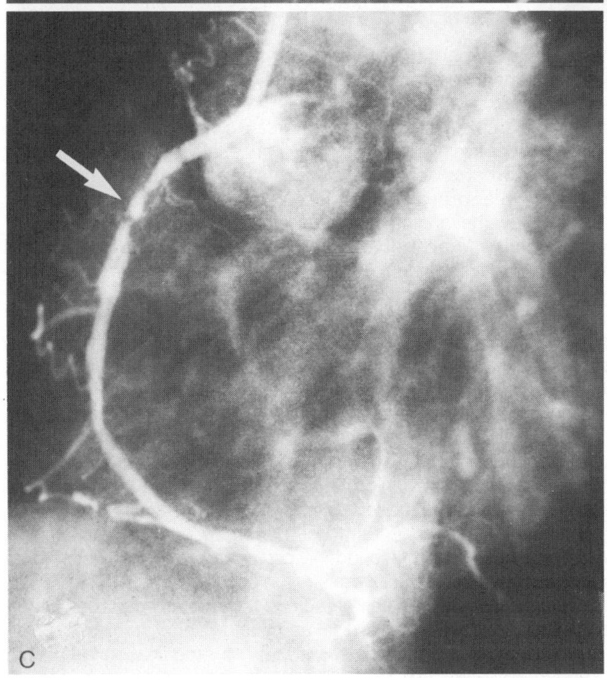

FIGURE 9–46. Examples of complicated plaques seen on coronary arteriography in three patients. *A,* Ulcerated stenosis in the proximal LAD (arrow). This patient died suddenly 3 days later. (From Levin, D.C., and Fallon, J.T.: Significance of the angiographic morphology of localized coronary stenoses: Histopathologic correlations. Circulation 66:316, 1982, by permission of the American Heart Association, Inc.) *B,* Ulcerated stenosis at the origin of the LAD (arrow). *C,* Diffusely irregular stenosis in the proximal portion of the RCA (arrow).

RISK ASSESSMENT IN CORONARY ARTERY DISEASE AS RELATED TO ARTERIOGRAPHIC FINDINGS

Numerous studies have directly and indirectly related the arteriographic findings to risk assessment in patients with mild and severe coronary disease. Because 15 to 20 per cent of coronary arteriograms in the average cardiac catheterization laboratory reveal normal or mildly diseased vessels despite the presenting symptom of chest pain, it is important to know the degree of risk facing these patients. A review of 4051 such cases in the CASS registry revealed a 7-year survival rate of 96 per cent among patients with normal coronary arteries and 92 per cent among patients with less than 50 per cent stenosis of one or more coronary segments.[97] Among 1977 patients followed in the Duke University Cardiovascular Disease Databank, those with normal vessels had an infarct-free 10-year survival rate of 98 per cent.[98] Patients with less than 75 per cent diameter stenosis of any coronary artery had an infarct-free 10-year survival rate of 90 per cent.

The CASS registry also has assessed risk in patients with more severe coronary disease, based on the number of diseased arteries and the ejection fraction.[99] This study analyzed 4-year survival of 20,088 patients enrolled between 1975 and 1979 and treated medically thereafter. The 4-year survival rate for patients with more than 70 per cent diameter reduction of one coronary artery was 92 per cent. For patients with two-vessel disease, survival was 84 per cent, and for three-vessel disease, it was 68 per cent. The CASS investigators found, however, that left ventricular ejection fraction (EF) was a more important predictor of survival. Thus patients with one-vessel disease and an EF of more than 50 per cent had 95 per cent 4-year survival. If EF ranged from 35 to 49 per cent, survival was 91 per cent, and if EF was less than 35 per cent, it dropped to 74 per cent. In patients with two-vessel disease, survival rates at 4 years were 93 per cent, 83 per cent, and 57 per cent, respectively, in these three EF categories. In patients with three-vessel disease, survival rates at 4 years were 82 per cent, 71 per cent, and 50 per cent, respectively.

Califf et al. have described a useful "jeopardy score" to assess the prognostic significance of the arteriographic findings in 462 consecutive nonsurgically treated patients with at least 75 per cent diameter stenosis

TABLE 9-1 FIVE-YEAR SURVIVAL BASED ON NUMBER OF DISEASED VESSELS AND JEOPARDY SCORE

	JEOPARDY SCORE					
	2	4	6	8	10	12
One-vessel disease	0.97	1.0	0.84			
Two-vessel disease		0.86	0.82	0.80	0.72	
Three-vessel disease			1.0	0.77	0.75	0.55
All patients	0.97	0.95	0.85	0.78	0.75	0.56

From Califf, R. M., et al.: Prognostic value of a coronary artery jeopardy score. J. Am. Coll. Cardiol. Reprinted by permission of the American College of Cardiology. 5:1055, 1985.

of at least one coronary artery.[100] Patients with main LCA stenosis were excluded. To determine the jeopardy score, the coronary circulation was considered as six arterial segments: the LAD, its major diagonal branch, its first major septal branch, the left circumflex artery, its major obtuse marginal branch, and the posterior descending branch of the RCA. Each segment with a 75 per cent or greater diameter reduction was given a score of 2 points. Thus, for example, a patient with 75 per cent stenosis of the LAD proximal to both the first septal and major diagonal branches would be assigned a score of 6:2 points for the LAD, 2 points for the septal branch, and 2 points for the diagonal branch. Thus, the maximal jeopardy score in any patient was 12. The results, according to both number of diseased vessels and jeopardy score, are shown in Table 9-1. By taking into account the quantity of myocardium at risk, the jeopardy score appears to provide a more reliable estimate of prognosis than does simply the number of diseased vessels.

Patients with significant stenosis of the main LCA are clearly in a higher-risk category. Conley et al. found that cumulative survival among a group of medically treated patients with more than 70 per cent diameter stenosis of the LCA was 72 per cent at 1 year and only 41 per cent at 3 years.[101] The prognosis in patients with LCA stenosis of between 50 and 70 per cent was somewhat more favorable (91 per cent survival at 1 year and 66 per cent survival at 3 years). Takaro et al. documented a cumulative survival at 42 months of 48 per cent in patients with at least 75 per cent main LCA stenosis on medical therapy, compared with 83 per cent survival in patients undergoing coronary bypass surgery.[102] As a result of these and other, similar studies, it is now widely accepted that the presence of main LCA stenosis is an indication for immediate bypass surgery.

THE POSTINFARCT PATIENT. Coronary arteriography and left ventriculography also help to identify risk in patients who have survived recent myocardial infarction. Sanz et al. studied 259 consecutive male survivors under age 60 who were catheterized a month after infarction and then followed for a mean of 34 months.[103] They found that in patients with a normal EF, survival was uniformly high (more than 95 per cent), regardless of the number of diseased vessels. It remained high in patients with EFs between 21 and 49 per cent who had one-vessel and two-vessel disease. In patients with three-vessel disease and an EF from 21 and 49 per cent, and in all patients with an EF of 20 per cent or less, 4-year survival was significantly reduced. DeFeyter et al. evaluated 179 patients in a similar manner.[104] During a mean follow-up period of 28 months, the mortality rate was 22 per cent in patients with an EF less than 30 per cent or three-vessel disease, but was only 1 per cent in patients with an EF greater than 30 per cent and either one or two diseased vessels.

SEVERITY OF OBSTRUCTION. For many years, the risk posed to the patient by a given coronary artery stenosis was intuitively equated with the severity of the lesion: the greater the degree of narrowing, the greater the presumed risk of subsequent occlusion and, possibly, myocardial infarction or death. Conversely, stenoses of moderate or mild degrees (less than 75 per cent or 50 per cent, respectively, of lumen diameter) were assumed to cause less risk. Investigations involving sequential coronary arteriograms have called both these assumptions into question. Danchin et al. noted that 12 of 13 patients with severely stenotic coronary arteries that totally occluded between diagnostic coronary arteriography and a subsequently scheduled PTCA had benign clinical courses.[105] Ambrose et al. compared the degree of baseline coronary stenoses in 38 patients who underwent two separate coronary arteriograms and had experienced either myocardial infarction or new total occlusion without infarction during the interval.[106] The median stenosis on the initial angiogram in the infarct group was only 48 per cent versus 74 per cent in the noninfarct group. In the infarct group, only 22 per cent of the culprit lesions were initially greater than 70 per cent, whereas in the noninfarct group, 61 per cent of lesions that subsequently progressed to total occlusion were initially greater than 70 per cent.

Another, similar study of patients undergoing sequential angiography while on medical therapy for coronary disease revealed that only 15 per cent of lesions that produced interval infarctions were of severe degree (greater than 75 per cent) on the initial angiogram.[107] Half were less than 50 per cent. Most patients who developed new total occlusions did not experience infarcts; 48 per cent of these stenoses were greater than 75 per cent on the initial study. In a study of 10 patients who underwent arteriography a mean of 21 months before myocardial infarction and then again more than 1 month post infarction, Hackett et al. noted that no culprit stenosis was greater than 60 per cent on the initial study, and most were less than 40 per cent.[108] Little et al. reviewed coronary arteriograms of 42 consecutive patients who had been studied both before and shortly after acute myocardial infarction; 29 of these patients had a new total occlusion on the second study.[109] Among the 29, 66 per cent of the culprit stenoses had been less than 50 per cent on the initial arteriogram and almost all of them had been less than 70 per cent.

One might question the significance of these angiographically based studies, since they represent retrospectively selected cohorts of patients whose clinical circumstances resulted in the performance of sequential coronary angiograms. However, they correlate closely with the results of a long-term prospective evaluation by McHenry et al. of 916 initially healthy men who underwent treadmill exercise tests and were then followed serially for 8 to 15 years (mean 12.7) to ascertain the incidence of significant new coronary events (angina, myocardial infarction, or sudden death).[110] Among 61 men who either had initially positive exercise tests or had converted to positive during follow-up, there were 21 subsequent coronary events. The vast majority of them (90 per cent) were onset of angina, rather than myocardial infarction or death. As expected, the incidence of coronary events was much lower in subjects with consistently negative exercise tests (44 events among 833 subjects), but when events did occur, the large majority (73 per cent) were infarction or death, rather than onset of angina. The authors hypothesized that subjects with positive exercise tests had a low incidence of catastrophic events (infarction or death) because their ischemia-producing lesions stimulated the development of collaterals, which then protected them against the consequences of subsequent occlusion. Those subjects with normal exercise tests who later experienced death or acute myocardial infarction probably had noncritical coronary stenoses that suddenly occluded without allowing for the protective development of collaterals.

Epstein and others have commented on the interesting paradoxes presented by the results of these clinical and angiographic studies and how they may undermine traditional ideas about risk stratification in patients with coronary disease.[111,112] On the one hand, patients experiencing subsequent myocardial infarction have been found to have lesser, rather than greater, degrees of coronary stenosis when they undergo angiography at some interval before the event. On the other hand, patients who experience coronary artery occlusion without infarction tend to have had higher-grade stenoses to begin with. It thus appears that patients with severe stenoses are at relatively low risk of myocardial infarction or sudden death. Presumably this is because the ischemia caused by the lesion has stimulated collateral development, which then provides protection. Patients with mild or moderate stenoses cannot be presumed to be at low risk because they may suffer a catastrophic event if spasm or plaque rupture or hemorrhage causes acute occlusion. This formulation helps to explain why some coronary disease patients survive for many years with chronic ischemia, while others initially experience infarction or death without any premonitory symptoms or signs. It greatly complicates the task of preventing catastrophic coronary events by screening asymptomatic subjects.[112]

CORONARY BYPASS ANGIOGRAPHY

Angiography after coronary bypass surgery commonly is performed to evaluate patients with recurrent angina. Because it is not possible to determine clinically whether symptoms are the result of compromise of the grafts or progression

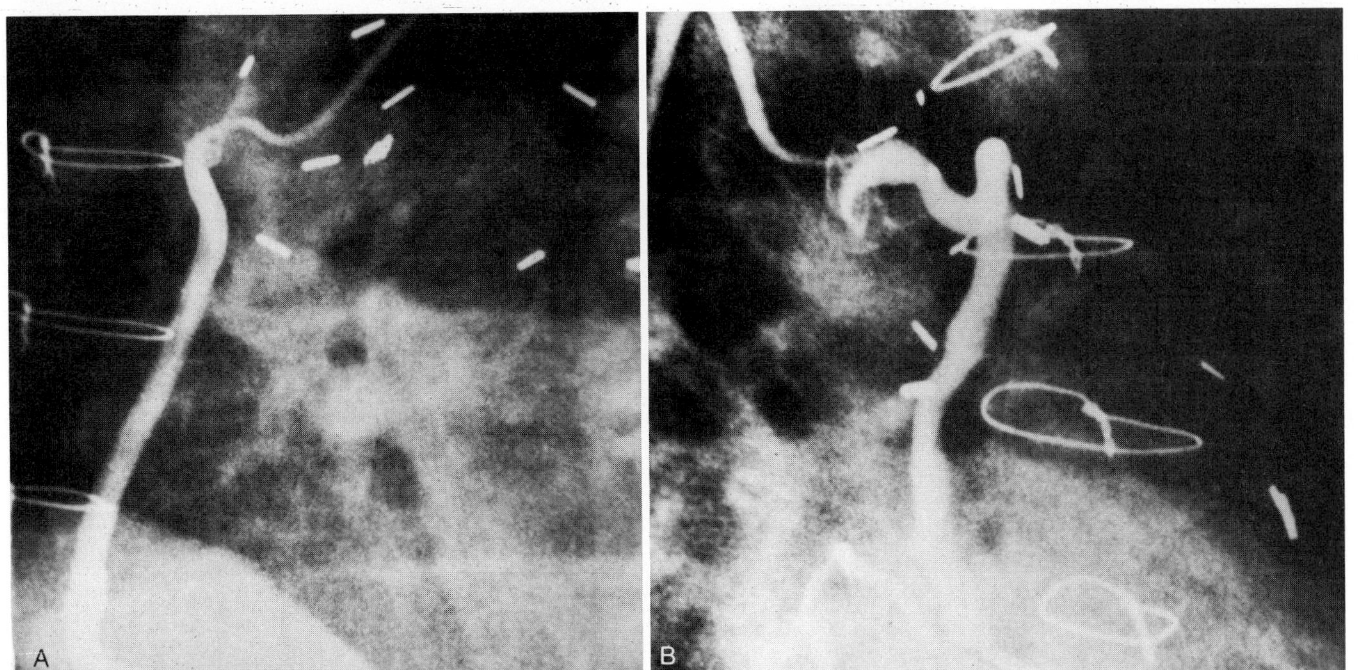

FIGURE 9–47. *A,* LAO angiogram of a saphenous vein bypass from the aorta to the distal RCA. *B,* RAO angiogram of a saphenous vein bypass from the aorta to the obtuse marginal branch of the circumflex artery. Both these angiograms utilized a No. 2 right Amplatz catheter.

of disease in the native coronary arteries, careful angiographic evaluation of both is necessary.

Technique of Coronary Bypass Angiography

Catheterization of coronary bypass grafts may be technically more difficult than catheterization of the native coronary arteries because the locations of graft ostia are not totally predictable unless they are marked with surgical clips. However, even if clips are not used, or if they migrate, the experienced angiographer usually can successfully locate the ostia.

Saphenous vein grafts (SVGs) from the aorta to the distal RCA usually are placed so they originate from the right anterolateral aspect of the aorta, whereas SVGs to the LAD and circumflex arteries usually are attached to the anterior aspect of the aorta. To catheterize SVGs, the authors recommend using No. 1 or 2 right Amplatz catheters by way of a percutaneous femoral approach. To enter right coronary SVGs, the patient is positioned in the LAO projection (Fig. 9–47*A*). To enter SVGs to either the LAD or circumflex arteries, the patient is positioned in the RAO projection (Fig. 9–47*B*). With the patient in the appropriate position, slow movement of the catheter tip up and down the aorta with varying degrees of rotation usually results in entry into the graft, which is signified by an abrupt outward movement of the tip. When this occurs, a small test injection of contrast material verifies that the catheter is in the SVG. Even if the graft is occluded, a small stump usually remains into which the catheter tip can pass. The stump can be demonstrated by injection of a small amount of contrast (Fig. 9–48) and invariably indicates total graft occlusion. If neither a patent graft nor a stump can be located, it may be necessary to perform an ascending aortogram (preferably using biplane cineangiography) in an attempt at visualization.

Internal mammary arteries (IMAs) are being used for coronary bypass with increasing frequency, as a result of evidence that they have significantly higher patency rates than SVGs.[113,114] To catheterize the IMA, a specially designed J-shaped catheter, usually referred to simply as the "femoral-internal mammary artery catheter" by the commercial manufacturers, is used by way of the percutaneous femoral approach. Rotation of the catheter tip in the aortic arch usually results in entry into the innominate artery or left subclavian artery. A guidewire is then passed through the catheter to a point in the subclavian artery distal to the expected origin of the IMA. The catheter is advanced to this point and then slowly withdrawn and rotated anteriorly until it enters the IMA. Figure 9–49 shows an angiogram of a left IMA-to-LAD

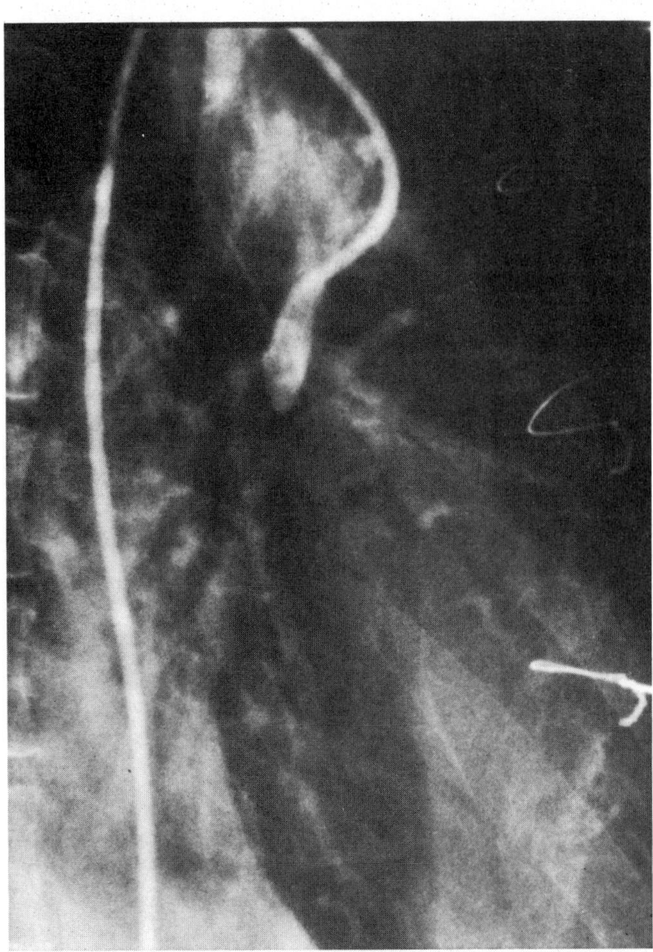

FIGURE 9–48. Stump of an occluded right coronary bypass.

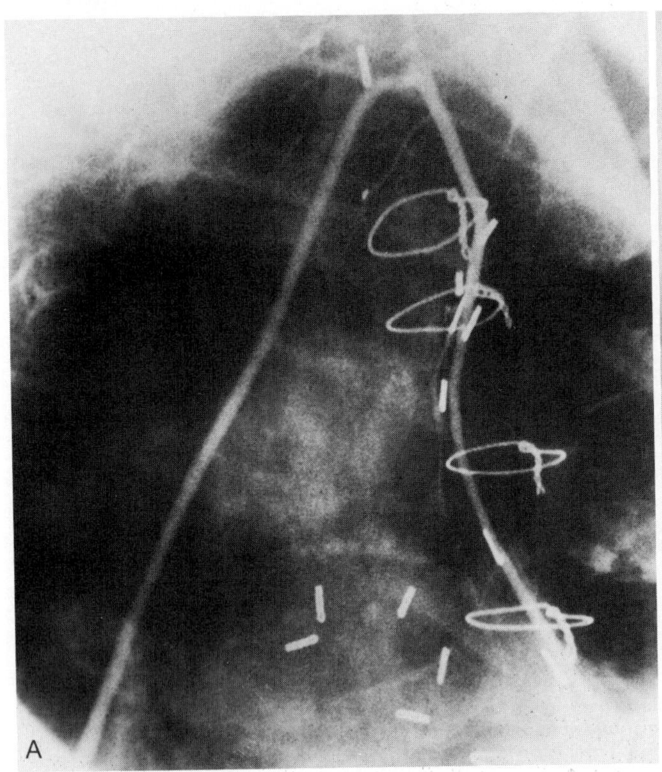

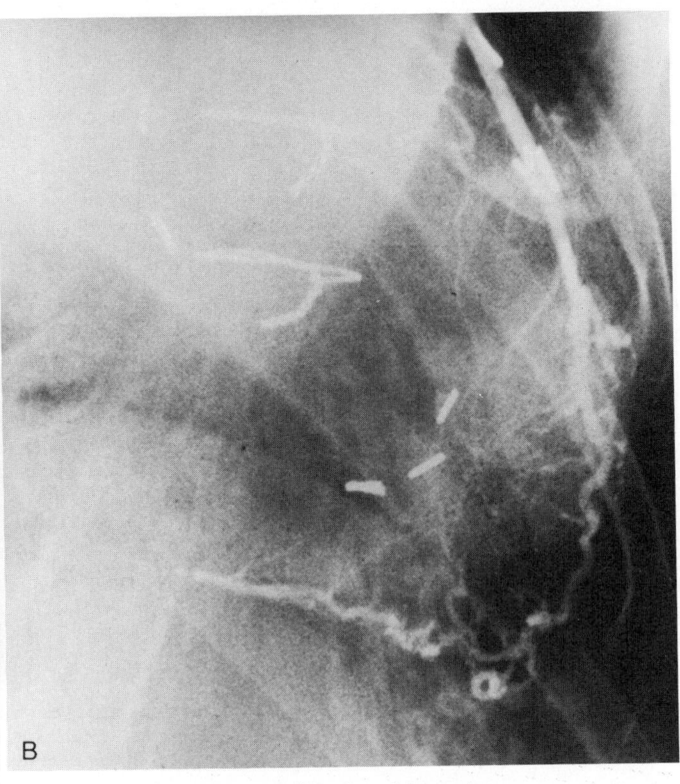

FIGURE 9–49. Angiogram of an internal mammary artery-to-LAD bypass. *A,* Proximal portion of the graft, seen in the RAO projection. *B,* Distal anastomosis of the internal mammary artery with the LAD.

graft. Internal mammary arteriograms can be quite painful because contrast enters branches leading to thoracic wall muscles, and the patient should be forewarned about this. Another vessel which is now being used for coronary bypass in some patients is the right gastroepiploic artery.[115] To adequately visualize this artery, a catheter must be advanced into the celiac axis and then superselectively into the hepatic and then the gastroduodenal branch. The right gastroepiploic artery can be used either as an in situ graft to the coronary arteries on the diaphragmatic aspect of the heart or as a free graft.

Angiographic studies of grafts must assess not only their patency, but also the status of the distal anastomoses. It has been shown that about 10 per cent of patent grafts are compromised by significant stenoses[116]; these stenoses are most likely to occur at the distal anastomosis (Fig. 9–50).

GRAFT PATENCY. Considerable data from several large clinical trials regarding the short- and long-term patency rates of SVGs have been reported. In the CASS trial, patency of SVGs was 90 per cent within 60 days after surgery; this decreased to 82 per cent at about 18 months after surgery and then appeared to remain stable over the next 3 years.[116] Similar results were obtained in the European Coronary Surgery Study, in which SVGs were noted to have a 77 per cent patency rate on studies performed from 9 to 18 months after surgery.[117] Among a larger series of patients at the Montreal Heart Institute, SVG patency at 1 year was about 80 per cent, and there was no further reduction in patency between 1 and 6 years after operation.[116] The most comprehensive longer-term experience comes from the same group. By the time 10 to 12 years had elapsed after surgery, the patency rate of SVGs had dropped to 63 per cent.[116] Moreover, almost half the grafts still patent showed significant atherosclerotic changes.

The Cleveland Clinic group compared patency rates of SVGs and IMA grafts.[113] After a mean follow-up period of 36 months, the patency rate for IMA grafts was 96 per cent. The patency rate for SVGs at a mean follow-up period of 39 months was 77 per cent. At 7 to 10 years after surgery, IMA graft patency has been shown to range from 85 to 95 per cent.[113,118] Furthermore, IMA grafts are only rarely involved by atherosclerosis. For these reasons, there is an increasing tendency among surgeons to choose the IMA for coronary bypass.[114]

SVG occlusion occurring within 1 month of surgery is almost invariably due to thrombosis.[116] Occlusions that occur between 1 month and 1 year after operation are primarily the result of intimal smooth muscle cell proliferation, which probably follows early platelet deposition on the walls of the graft. Figure 9–51 shows an example of fibrous initimal proliferation developing within 10 months after surgery. Chesebro et al. showed that this process can be favorably altered by the early and continued administration of dipyridamole and aspirin, with significant reduction in late SVG occlusion rates.[119] More recently, the Veterans Administration Cooperative Study showed that the SVG occlusion rate at 1 year was 13.2 per cent in patients taking aspirin, 325 mg daily, compared with 22.6 per cent in

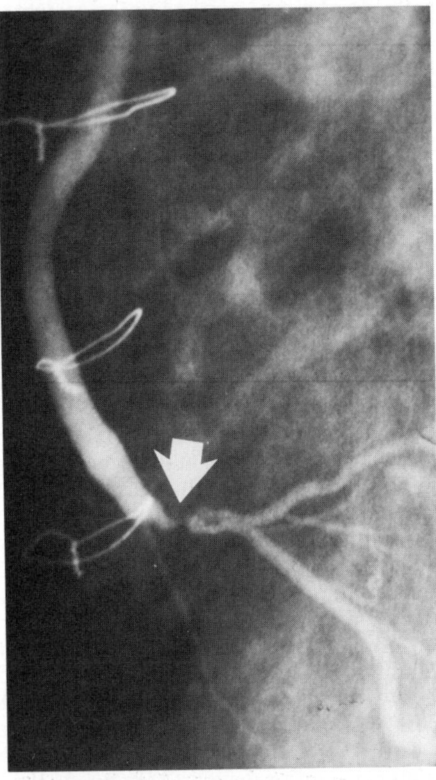

FIGURE 9–50. LAO view of a saphenous vein bypass graft to the distal RCA. Severe narrowing at the anastomosis is seen (arrow). (From Levin, D.C., Beckmann, C.F., Sos, T.A., and Sniderman, K.: Incomplete myocardial reperfusion despite a patent coronary bypass: A generally unrecognized shortcoming of the surgical approach to coronary artery disease. Radiology *142*:317, 1982, with permission.)

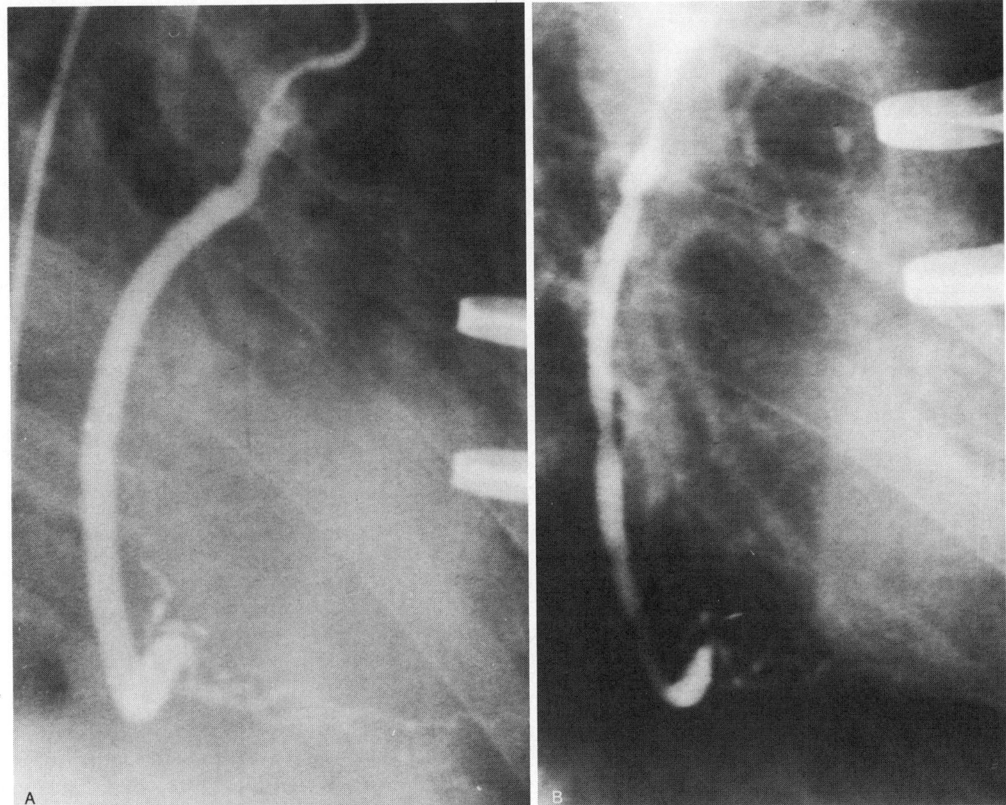

FIGURE 9–51. Fibrous intimal proliferation developing in a saphenous vein bypass graft to the RCA within 10 months after operation. *A,* Graft angiogram 4 weeks after operation. No significant narrowing is seen. *B,* Graft angiogram 10 months after surgery. Multiple areas of diffuse narrowing are seen along the course of the graft. (From Levin, D.C., Beckmann, C.F., Sos, T.A., and Sniderman, K.: Incomplete myocardial reperfusion despite a patent coronary bypass: A generally unrecognized shortcoming of the surgical approach to coronary artery disease. Radiology *142*:317, 1982, with permission.)

patients taking placebos.[120] Late graft occlusions more than 1 year after operation appear to be caused by atherosclerosis, which in turn probably results from lipid incorporation in areas of intimal proliferation. Graft atherosclerosis, therefore, seems to be a continuum from early platelet deposition to intimal smooth muscle cell proliferation to late incorporation of lipid into a fully developed atherosclerotic plaque.

DIGITAL AND QUANTITATIVE CORONARY ARTERIOGRAPHY

(See also p. 343)

Digital coronary arteriography is a video-based, computer-assisted method of imaging that was developed in the early 1980's. It was once thought that this technology might replace cine imaging, but this has not yet happened. To create images, digital systems usually use video cameras with "progressive" rather than "interlaced" scan readout capability, which permits higher resolution image acquisition. The analog video signal is passed through an analog-to-digital converter, and this digitized signal is stored in computer memory as optical density information for each of hundreds of thousands of tiny boxlike "pixels" that make up each frame of the image. The series of images is stored on tape or disk.

The most important advantage of digital coronary arteriography is that the images can be manipulated in various ways (Fig. 9–52), either to enhance visualization or for quantitative analysis. Subtraction techniques produce images without overlying densities such as bone and improve contrast resolution, allowing better visualization of poorly opacified structures. By subtracting a stored digital image from a fluoroscopic image, a "road map" can be obtained. This allows visualization of the arterial anatomy for accurate manipulation of wires or catheters under fluoroscopic control. Motion is a major problem when using digital subtraction techniques.

Parameters such as coronary flow reserve, myocardial perfusion, and degree of coronary stenosis can be measured using digital images. Quantification of arterial stenosis has so far proved to be the most widespread and useful quantitative application of digital coronary arteriography. Although lesion severity may not be the most important factor in predicting subsequent coronary artery occlusion, accurate assessment of the degree of coronary artery narrowing remains crucial in planning therapy and evaluating outcomes of various interventions.[109] Subjective analyses of coronary angiograms have demonstrated significant intraobserver and interobserver variability in grading the degree of coronary artery stenoses.[121-123] Therefore, several quantitative methods have been developed which allow automatic quantitation of arterial stenosis by computer.

Quantitative analysis of coronary artery stenosis requires a digital image, either obtained directly from a digital angiographic unit or created by digitizing a cine frame. Two fundamentally different techniques have been developed and are now commonly used: edge detection and densitometry. Both methods give an accurate estimation of the degree of coronary artery stenosis.[124]

QUANTITATIVE ANGIOGRAPHY. Using edge detection methods, a variety of algorithms have been created for detecting and tracing the vessel wall and calculating the percentage of stenosis by comparing the maximum or "normal" vessel diameter with the minimum diameter of a lesion (Fig. 9–53). Absolute measurements are possible with this method by using the known diameter of the angiographic catheter as a scaling device. For the most accurate calculations possible, the arterial segment of interest is magnified and the distortions related to image acquisition are corrected. Measurements of experimental and clinical stenoses using this method have been accurate and precise.[125-127] Such measurements are not completely operator-independent, however, and therefore may not be entirely objective. For instance, frame-to-frame variability in the measured vessel diameter can be demonstrated, apparently related to the degree of opacification and projection of the lesion in a rapidly moving artery.[128]

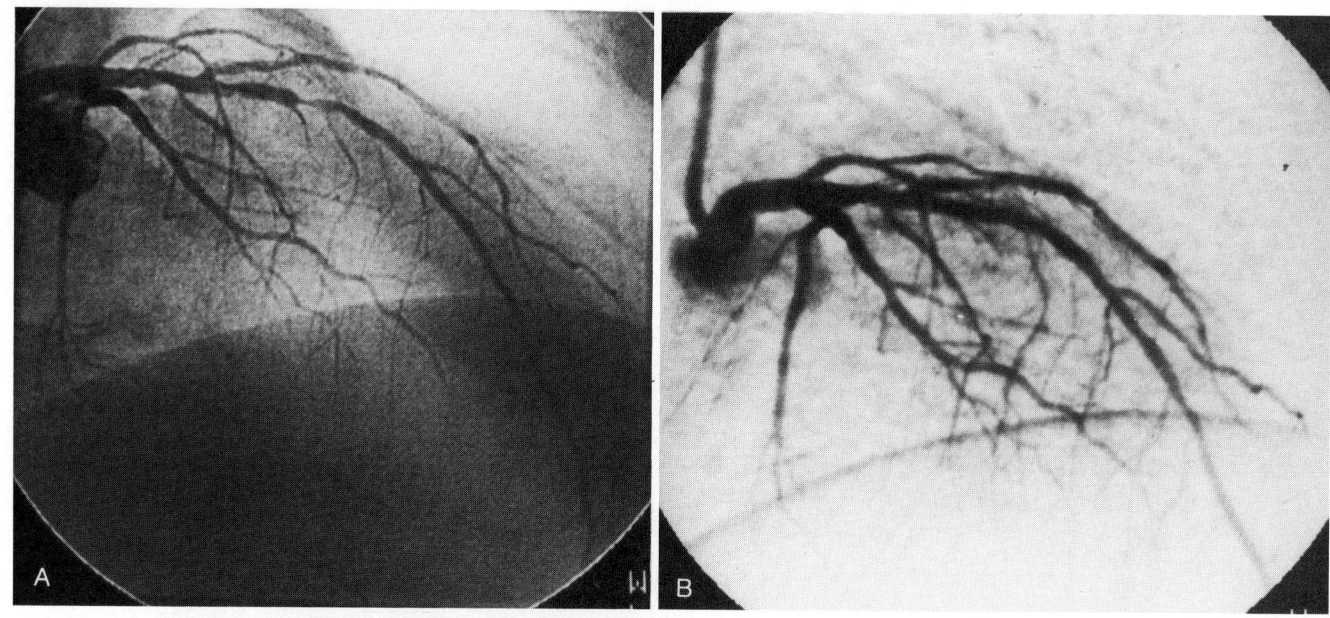

FIGURE 9-52. RAO cranial digital coronary arteriograms of the LCA. ***A,*** **Unsubtracted video image before LAD angioplasty.** ***B,*** **Subtracted image in the same projection, after LAD angioplasty.**

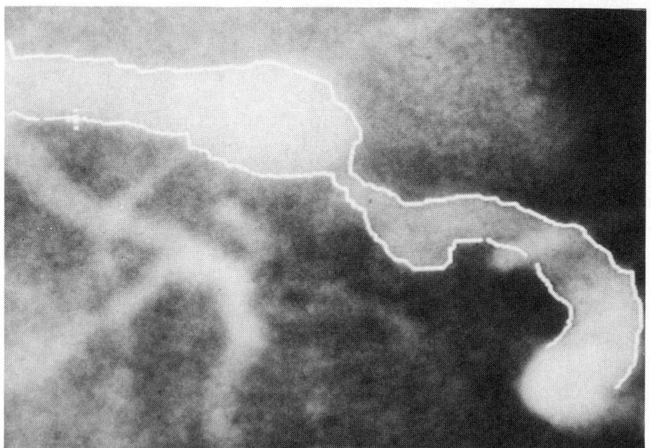

FIGURE 9-53. Coronary artery outline traced by an automatic edge-detecting program for quantitative arteriography.

Other pitfalls of this method include a normal biological variability in vessel diameter, crossing vessels or arterial branches, eccentric lesions, and diffusely diseased arteries.[126] The selection of the arterial segment considered normal by the operator or computer program significantly influences the calculated percentage of stenosis.

A second method of quantitative analysis is videodensitometry. This technique measures aggregate levels of brightness (opacification) across narrowed and normal arterial segments to calculate lesion severity. The precision of this technique also has been validated in multiple studies.[129-131] Although this method is better at calculating the percentage of stenosis of eccentric lesions than are edge-detecting methods, it also has many potential sources of inaccuracy. The most important of these is variation in background density overlying vessels or lesions of interest. Another is variability in vessel opacification owing to acceleration and deceleration of blood flow and injection rate. It should be emphasized that although both edge-detection techniques and densitometry can improve accuracy and consistency compared with subjective evaluation, neither is completely independent of operator judgement and both methods are susceptible to some degree of inaccuracy.

LEFT VENTRICULOGRAPHY AS AN ADJUNCT TO CORONARY ARTERIOGRAPHY

(See also Chap. 8)

Left ventriculography is an essential part of cardiac catheterization in most patients with known or suspected cardiac disease because it allows evaluation of segmental and global myocardial function, and also demonstrates anatomical details of the ventricular chamber and associated valves. In patients with CAD, ventriculography provides evidence of the effect of coronary obstruction on myocardial contractility, and it can reliably demonstrate complications resulting from myocardial infarction. In patients with cardiomyopathies and congenital or valvular heart disease, ventriculography often is helpful in establishing an accurate diagnosis and in properly classifying the disease.

Left ventriculography is performed from an arterial approach by passing a catheter across the aortic valve into the left ventricle. Ideally, it should be performed before coronary arteriography because of the depressant effect of radiographic contrast medium on myocardial function, which may last for up to an hour after injection.[132] The average injection rate for ventriculography is 12 to 15 ml/sec for a total volume of 40 to 50 ml; this may be increased or decreased, depending on the size of the left ventricle and the clinical status of the patient. The ventriculogram is imaged using the 9-inch mode of the image intensifier and 35-mm cine film at a rate of at least 30 frames/sec in the 30-degree RAO and 45- to 60-degree LAO projections. If only one view is possible, the RAO view is preferred. The LAO view may be angled 20 to 40 degrees cranially to profile optimally the ventricular cavity. This improves visualization of the septum and especially the ventricular outflow tract.

Ventricular injections of contrast medium adversely affect myocardial contractility and produce several hemodynamic changes.[133-135] In addition, there is rapid expansion of intravascular volume as water moves into the vascular system from the extravascular space owing to the hypertonicity of most contrast media.[136,137] These effects of contrast present some risk to patients with severely compromised myocardial function or with severe aortic stenosis. The hemodynamic effects of ventriculography can be minimized by using digital imaging with very small quantities of contrast material[138] or by using the newer low-osmolality agents (p. 238). Although injection of low-osmolality agents produces similar responses, the degree of hemodynamic change and myocardial toxicity is less severe compared with the standard hypertonic agents.[13,15]

Complications such as embolization from mural thrombus or valvular vegetations are possible, but a far more common cause of peripheral embolization is inadvertent injection of thrombus formed in or on the catheter. Routine heparinization may lower the incidence of this complication, especially if the procedure is prolonged, but careful technique is essential and is probably the most important factor in avoiding it.

Abnormalities of Ventricular Contour

The ventricular contour can be divided into segments for purposes of analyzing myocardial motion (Fig. 9–54). The left ventricular cavity normally is oval or ellipsoid. The septum is free of trabeculations, and usually is concave to the left ventricular cavity. The papillary muscles are best visualized during systole, and appear as elongated filling defects on the diaphragmatic and anterior ventricular borders in the RAO view.

Localized abnormalities of ventricular contour include filling defects, which usually represent thrombus. In most cases, ventricular thrombus is associated with severely hypokinetic, akinetic, or dyskinetic myocardial segments along the anterior wall or apex. At ventriculography, mural thrombus can range in appearance from a smooth defect following the contour of the left ventricle to an irregular polypoid mass extending into the left ventricular cavity. Thrombi which are pedunculated may be more prone to peripheral embolization.[139,140]

A well-demarcated bulge in the ventricular contour, contained by a smooth, thin wall and demonstrating paradoxical motion during systole are the classic findings of a *true ventricular aneurysm* at ventriculography. The wall of a true left ventricular aneurysm is composed of residual elements of the myocardial wall and fibrous tissue resulting from healing of the underlying myocardial infarction (p. 314). These aneurysms occur most often along the anterolateral and apical wall of the left ventricle after occlusion of the LAD or its branches. Poor collateral blood supply after coronary artery occlusion plays a major role in the formation of a ventricular aneurysm.[62,141]

The frequency of occurrence of true left ventricular aneurysms is uncertain because of variations in diagnostic criteria and definitions, but they have been demonstrated in 22 per cent of patients by echocardiography after an initial transmural myocardial infarction.[142] The presence of a ventricular aneurysm alone may not have significant prognostic implications, but can be clinically important because of associated rhythm disturbances, or hemodynamic and possibly thromboembolic consequences. Rupture of a true ventricular aneurysm, once scar formation occurs, is an extremely rare event.

False ventricular aneurysms are formed when complete rupture of the

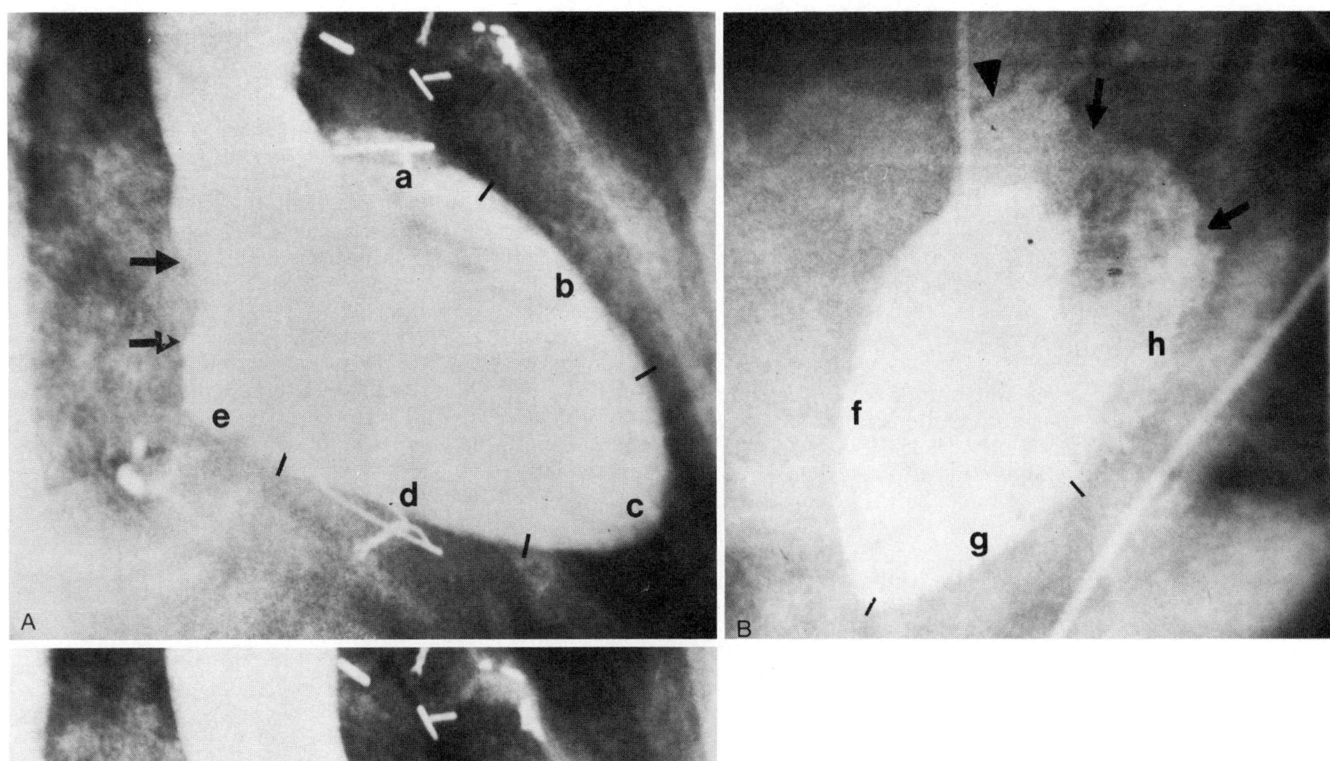

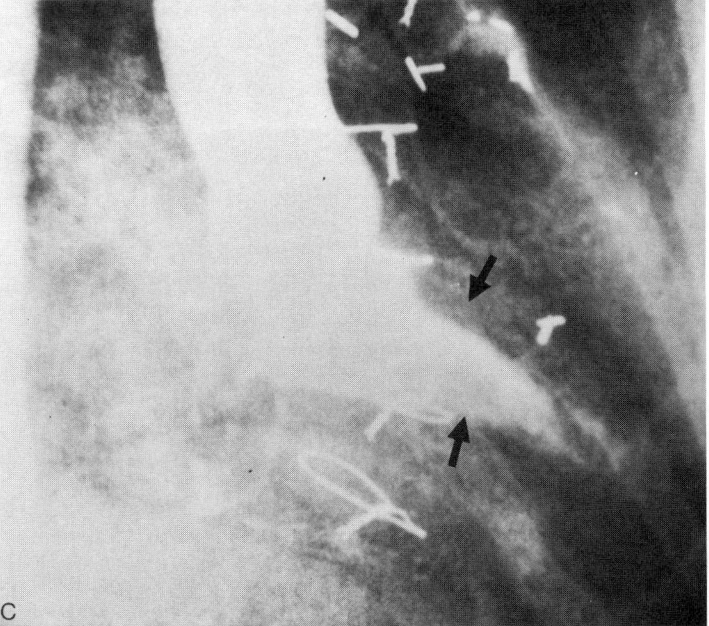

FIGURE 9–54. Normal ventricular function in a patient who had previously undergone LAD bypass surgery. *A,* End-diastole, 30-degree RAO projection provides the best view of mitral valve (arrows), and anterobasal (a), anterolateral (b), apical (c), diaphragmatic (d), and posterobasal (e) myocardial walls. *B,* End-diastole, 60-degree LAO–25-degree cranial projection shows the mitral valve en face (arrows), and provides good views of the septal (f), posterolateral (g), and superolateral (h) myocardial walls. *C,* End-systole, 30-degree RAO projection shows normal contraction of all myocardial segments. The papillary muscles are well demonstrated (arrows).

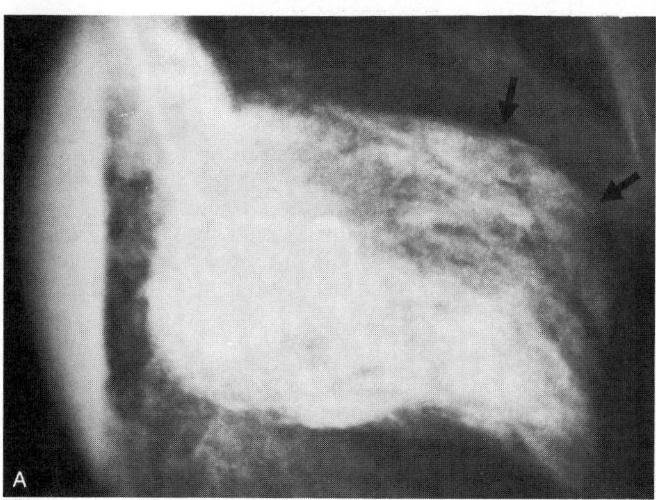

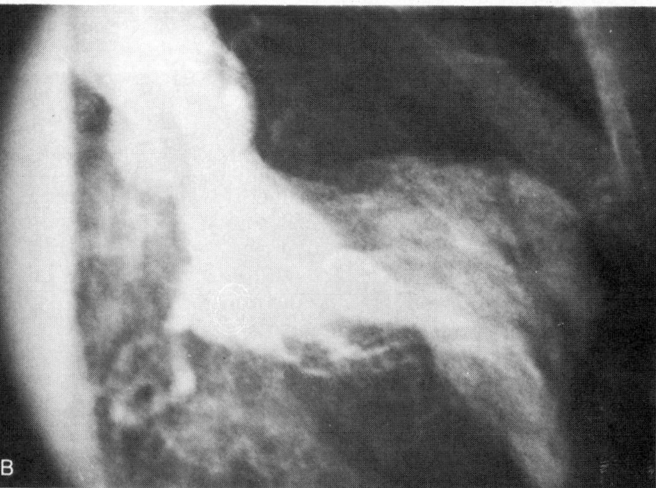

FIGURE 9-55. Akinesis in a patient with previous anterior myocardial infarct. *A,* RAO view, end-diastole, shows a prominent bulge of the anterolateral wall (arrows). *B,* RAO view, end-systole, shows no motion of the apex or anterolateral wall. The remaining myocardial segments contract normally.

left ventricular wall occurs, but is contained by adherent pericardium. Characteristically, false aneurysms form an outpouching or chamber which communicates with the left ventricular cavity by a relatively narrow neck. As with true aneurysms, false aneurysms are a complication of transmural myocardial infarction, but usually are found on the posterolateral and diaphragmatic segments, and therefore are most commonly associated with occlusions of the right or circumflex coronary arteries. Similar to true aneurysms, false aneurysms may contain thrombus, and may have significant hemodynamic consequences, but are most important because of their tendency to rupture. A key feature of false aneurysms on serial chest radiographs is their tendency to grow in size or change in configuration, a finding not associated with true ventricular aneurysms.

Other conditions that cause abnormalities of the left ventricular contour include myocardial diverticula, anomalous bands, and cardiomyopathies.

Abnormalities of Ventricular Function

(See also p. 823)

Considerable intraobserver and interobserver variability has been documented in the interpretation of segmental wall motion.[143-145] Several factors may be responsible for this variability, including cardiac rotation and positional changes during the cardiac cycle. Improved accuracy and consistency have been demonstrated when more objective methods are used.[144-146] Segmental wall motion, however, is not always an accurate predictor of coronary disease. Patients with severe CAD may have normal ventriculograms. On the other hand, segmental motion abnormalities occur in a wide variety of conditions in the presence of normal coronary arteries.[147-149]

Regional myocardial dysfunction (hypokinesia, akinesia, or dyskinesia) is the hallmark of CAD on ventriculography (Fig. 9-55). *Hypokinesia* is defined as reduced contractility during systole. *Akinesia* is defined as absence of contraction during systole. *Dyskinesia* means paradoxical outward bulging during systole, and usually is associated with ventricular aneurysm. Hypokinesis may occur in ischemia without infarction, as well as in myocardial infarction with varying degrees of myocardial fibrosis. Differentiation of these two conditions is an important factor in treatment and prognosis. Areas of dyskinesis are rarely, if ever, associated with significant amounts of viable myocardium.

Demonstration of the reversibility of wall motion abnormalities is an important way of differentiating underperfused but viable myocardium from myocardial scar. Methods such as nitroglycerin administration, postextrasystolic potentiation, and epinephrine infusion have been used successfully to determine the viability of myocardium in areas of compromised myocardial function.[150,151] There is good correlation between improvement in ventricular function using these methods and improvement after reperfusion by coronary bypass.[152,153] In some patients with normal myocardial contractility associated with CAD, myocardial dysfunction may be induced by ischemia resulting from tachycardia produced by atrial pacing. Segmental wall motion abnormalities produced by this method signify hemodynamically significant stenoses.[154]

Left ventricular volumes and global myocardial function are important aspects of ventriculography. There is close correlation between the overall effectiveness of myocardial contractility and prognosis, no matter what the therapy.[99,103,104,] Accurate calculation of ventricular volumes is essential for reliable calculation of stroke volume and ejection fraction. Ventricular volume calculations (Chap. 15) are based on the geometric formula for the volume of an ellipsoid,[155] with correction factors to compensate for magnification, and the use of a regression equation to compensate for consistent overestimation of the true volume.[156]

The sequelae of myocardial infarction may produce complications which are more serious than loss of myocardial function per se. These include ruptures of the ventricular septum, free wall, or papillary muscle (pp. 1256 to 1259). These may be life-threatening situations that require immediate surgical attention.

Acknowledgment

The authors express their deep gratitude and appreciation to Eileen Judkins, R.N., and the late Melvin Judkins, M.D., for allowing us to use their cases in Figures 9-8, 9-9, 9-10, 9-19, 9-21, 9-29, 9-30, 9-36, 9-37, 9-38, 9-40, and 9-41. During his career, Dr. Judkins amassed a huge library of serial film coronary arteriograms of outstanding quality, and this collection has been carefully maintained by Mrs. Judkins for use in teaching and research activities.

REFERENCES

TECHNIQUE OF CORONARY ARTERIOGRAPHY

1. Sones, F. M., and Shirey, E. K.: Cine coronary arteriography. Mod. Concepts Cardiovasc. Dis. *31*:735, 1962.
2. Hurst, J. W.: History of cardiac catheterization. *In* King, S. B., III, and Douglas, J. S., Jr. (eds.): Coronary Arteriography and Angioplasty. New York, McGraw-Hill Book Co., 1985, p. 1.
3. Judkins, M. P.: Selective coronary arteriography. I. A percutaneous transfemoral technique. Radiology *89*:815, 1967.
4. Gensini, G. G.: Coronary arteriography. *In* Braunwald, E. (ed.): Heart Disease. 2nd ed. Philadelphia, W. B. Saunders Company, 1984, p. 304.
5. Amplatz, K., Formanek, G., Stranger, P., and Wilson, W.: Mechanics of selective coronary artery catheterization via femoral approach. Radiology *89*:1040, 1967.
6. Schoonmaker, F. W., and King, S. B., III: Coronary arteriography by the single catheter percutaneous femoral technique. Circulation *50*:735, 1974.
7. King, S. B., III, and Douglas, J. S., Jr.: Coronary arteriography and left ventriculography: Multipurpose technique. *In* King, S. B., III, and Douglas, J. S., Jr. (eds.): Coronary Arteriography and Left Ventriculography. New York, McGraw-Hill Book Co., 1985, p. 239.

8. Friesinger, G. C., Adams, D. F., Bourassa, M. G., et al.: Report of the Inter-Society Commission for Heart Disease Resources: Optimal resources for examination of the heart and lungs: Cardiac catheterization and radiographic facilities. Circulation *68*:891A, 1983.
9. Levin, D. C., Dunham, L. R., and Stueve, R.: Causes of cine image quality deterioration in cardiac catheterization laboratories. Am. J. Cardiol. *52*:881, 1983.
10. Davis, K., Kennedy, J. W., Kemp, H. G., Jr., et al.: Complications of coronary arteriography. Circulation *59*:1105, 1979.
11. Benotti, J.: Comparative effects of ionic versus nonionic agents in cardiac catheterization. Invest. Radiol. *23* (Suppl 2):S 366, 1988.
12. Bettmann, M.: Radiographic contrast agents—a perspective. N. Engl. J. Med. *317*:891, 1987.
13. Bettmann, M. A., Bourdillon, P. D., Barry, W. H., et al.: Contrast agents for cardiac angiography: Effects of a nonionic agent vs. a standard ionic agent. Radiology *153*:583, 1984.
14. Missri, J., and Jeresaty, R. M.: Ventricular fibrillation during coronary angiography: Reduced incidence with nonionic contrast media. Cathet. Cardiovasc. Diagn. *19*:4, 1990.
15. Bettmann, M. A., and Higgins, C. B.: Comparisons of an ionic with a nonionic contrast agent for cardiac angiography: Results of a multicenter trial. Invest. Radiol. *20* (Suppl 1):S70, 1985.
16. Grollman, J. H., Liu, C. K., Astone, R. A., and Lurie, M. D.: Thomboembolic complications in coronary angiography associated with the use of nonionic contrast medium. Cathet. Cardiovasc. Diagn. *14*:159, 1988.
17. Hwang, M. H., Piao, Z. E., Murdock, D. K., et al.: Potential risk of thrombosis during coronary angiography using nonionic contrast media. Cathet. Cardiovasc. Diagn. *16*:209, 1989.
18. Levin, D. C., Harrington, D. P., Bettmann, M. A., et al.: Anatomic variations of the coronary arteries supplying the anterolateral aspect of the left ventricle. Possible explanation for the "unexplained" anterior aneurysm. Invest. Radiol. *17*:458, 1982.
19. Perlmutt, L. M., Jay, M. E., and Levin, D. C.: Variations in the blood supply of the left ventricular apex. Invest. Radiol. *18*:138, 1983.
20. Levin, D. C., Beckmann, C. F., Garnic, J. D., et al.: Frequency and clinical significance of failure to visualize the conus artery during coronary arteriography. Circulation *63*:833, 1981.
21. Kyriakidis, M. K., Kourouklis, C. B. Papaioannou, J. T., et al.: Sinus node coronary arteries studied with angiography. Am. J. Cardiol. *51*:749, 1983.
22. Bunnell, I. L., Greene, D. G., Tandon, R. N., and Arani, D. T.: The half axial projection. A new look at the proximal left coronary artery. Circulation *48*:151, 1973.
23. Arani, D. T., Bunnell, I. L., and Greene, D. G.: Lordotic right posterior oblique projection of the left coronary artery. A special view for special anatomy. Circulation *52*:504, 1975.
24. Feldman, R. L., Pepine, C. J., Curry, R. C., and Conti, C. R.: Coronary arterial responses to graded doses of nitroglycerin. Am. J. Cardiol. *43*:91, 1979.
25. Brown, B. G., Bolson, E., Peterson, R. B., et al.: The mechanisms of nitroglycerin action: Stenosis vasodilatation as a major component of the drug response. Circulation *64*:1089, 1981.
26. Levin, D. C., Phillips, D. A., Lee-Son, S., and Maroko, P. R.: Hemodynamic changes distal to selective arterial injection. Invest. Radiol. *12*:116, 1977.
27. Haraphongse, M., and Rossall, R. E.: Diaphragmatic coronary lesion mimics significant coronary stenosis: Report of 4 cases. Cathet. Cardiovasc. Diagn. *11*:173, 1985.
28. Kramer, J. R., Kitazume, H., Proudfit, W. L., and Sones, F. M., Jr.: Clinical significance of isolated coronary bridges: Benign and frequent condition involving the left anterior descending artery. Am. Heart J. *103*:283, 1982.
29. Faruqui, A.M.A., Maloy, W. C., Felner, J. M., et al.: Symptomatic myocardial bridging of coronary artery. Am. J. Cardiol. *41*:1305, 1978.
30. Friedman, M.: The coronary canalized thrombus: Provenance, structure, function and relationship to death due to coronary artery disease. Br. J. Exp. Pathol. *48*:556, 1967.
31. Davis, K., Kennedy, J. W., Kemp, H. G., Jr., et al.: Complications of coronary arteriography from the Collaborative Study of Coronary Artery Surgery (CASS). Circulation *59*:1105, 1979.
32. Klinke, W. P., Kubac, G., Talibi, T., and Lee, S.J.K.: Safety of outpatient catheterizations. Am. J. Cardiol. *56*:639, 1985.
33. Johnson, L. W., Lozner, E. C., Johnson, S., et al.: Coronary arteriography 1984–1987: A report of the Registry of the Society for Cardiac Angiography and Interventions. I. Results and Complications. Cathet. Cardiovasc. Diagn. 17:5, 1989.

ABNORMALITIES OF THE CORONARY CIRCULATION

34. Levin, D. C., Fellows, K. E., and Abrams, H. L.: Hemodynamically significant primary anomalies of the coronary arteries. Angiographic aspects. Circulation *58*:25, 1978.
35. Wilson, C. L., Dlabal, P. W., Holeyfield, R. W., et al.: Anomalous origin of left coronary artery from pulmonary artery. Case reports and review of literature concerning teenagers and adults. J. Thorac. Cardiovasc. Surg. *73*:887, 1977.
36. Cheitlin, M. D., De Castro, C. M., and McAllister, H. A.: Sudden death as a complication of anomalous left coronary origin from the anterior sinus of valsalva. A not-so-minor congenital anomaly. Circulation *50*:780, 1974.
37. Roberts, W. C.: Major anomalies of coronary artery origin seen in adulthood. Am. Heart J. *111*:941, 1986.
38. Kragel, A. H., and Roberts, W. C.: Anomalous origin of either the right or left main coronary artery from the aorta with subsequent coursing between aorta and pulmonary trunk: Analysis of 32 necropsy cases. Am. J. Cardiol. *62*:771, 1988.
39. Brandt, B., III, Martins, J. B., and Marcus, M. L.: Anomalous origin of the right coronary artery from the left sinus of Valsalva. N. Engl. J. Med. *309*:596, 1983.
40. Kimbiris, D., Iskandrian, A. S., Segal, B. L., and Bemis, C. E.: Anomalous aortic origin of coronary arteries. Circulation *58*:606, 1978.
41. Click, R. L., Holmes, D. R., Vlietstra, R. E., et al.: Anomalous coronary arteries: Location, degree of atherosclerosis and effect on survival—a report from the Coronary Artery Surgery Study. J. Am. Coll. Cardiol. *12*:531, 1989.
42. Page, H. L., Jr., Engel, H. J., Campbell, W. B., and Thomas, C. S., Jr.: Anomalous origin of the left circumflex coronary artery. Recognition, angiographic demonstration and clinical significance. Circulation *50*:768, 1974.
43. Lipton, M. J., Barry, W. H., Obrez, I., et al.: Isolated single coronary artery: Diagnosis, angiographic classification, and clinical significance. Radiology *130*:39, 1979.
44. Shipley, R. E., and Gregg, D. E.: The effect of external constriction of a blood vessel on blood flow. Am. J. Physiol. *141*:289, 1944.
45. Gould, K. L., Lipscomb, K., and Hamilton, G. W.: Physiologic basis for assessing critical coronary stenosis. Instantaneous flow response and regional distribution during coronary hyperemia as measures of coronary flow reserve. Am. J. Cardiol. *33*:87, 1974.
46. Gould, K. L., Kirkeeide, R. L., and Buchi, M.: Coronary flow reserve as a physiologic measure of stenosis severity. J. Am. Coll. Cardiol. *15*:459, 1990.
46a. White, C. W.: Physiologic assessment of coronary artery stenosis severity. Trends Cardiovasc. Med. *1*:70, 1991.
47. Klocke, F. J.: Measurements of coronary blood flow and degree of stenosis: Current clinical implications and continuing uncertainties. J. Am. Coll Cardiol. *1*:31,1983.
48. Nichols, A. B., Brown, C., Han, J., et al.: Effect of coronary stenotic lesions on regional myocardial blood flow at rest. Circulation *74*:746, 1986.
49. Levin, D. C., Beckmann, C. F., and Serur, J. R.: Vascular resistance changes distal to progressive arterial stenosis: A critical re-evaluation of the concept of vasodilator reserve. Invest. Radiol. *15*:120, 1980.
50. Logan, S. E.: On the fluid mechanics of human coronary artery stenosis. IEEE Trans. Biomed. Eng. *22*:327, 1975.
51. Gould, K. L., and Lipscomb, K.: Effects of coronary stenoses on coronary flow reserve and resistance. Am. J. Cardiol. *34*:48, 1974.
52. Feldman, R. L., Nichols, W. W., Pepine, C. J., and Conti, C. R.: Hemodynamic significance of the length of a coronary arterial narrowing. Am. J. Cardiol. *41*:865, 1978.
53. White, C. W., Wright, C. B., Doty, D. B., et al.: Does visual interpretation of the coronary arteriogram predict the physiologic importance of a coronary stenosis? N. Engl. J. Med. *310*:819, 1984.
54. Marcus, M. L., Skorton, D. J., Johnson, M. R., et al.: Visual estimates of percent diameter coronary stenosis: "A battered gold standard." J. Am. Coll. Cardiol. *11*:882, 1988.
55. Vita, J. A., Treasure, C. B., Nabel, E. G., et al.: Coronary vasomotor responses to acetylcholine relates to risk factors for coronary artery disease. Circulation *81*:491, 1990.
56. Ganz, P., Abben, R., Friedman, P. L., et al.: Usefulnesss of transstenotic coronary pressure gradient measurements during diagnostic catheterization. Am. J. Cardiol. *55*:910, 1985.
57. Levin, D. C.: Pathways and functional significance of the coronary collateral circulation. Circulation *50*:831, 1974.
58. Newman, P. E.: Coronary collateral circulation: Determinants and functional significance in ischemic heart disease. Am. Heart J. *102*:431, 1981.
59. Schwartz, H., Leiboff, R. H., Bren, G. B., et al.: Temporal evolution of the human coronary collateral circulation following acute myocardial infarction. J. Am. Coll. Cardiol. *4*:1088, 1984.
60. Freedman, S. B., Dunn, R. F., Bernstein, L., et al.: Influence of coronary collateral blood flow on the development of exertional ischemia and Q wave infarction in patients with severe single-vessel disease. Circulation *71*:681, 1985.
61. Helfant, R. H., Kemp, H. G., and Gorlin, R.: Coronary atherosclerosis, coronary collaterals and their relation to cardiac function. Ann. Intern. Med. *73*:189, 1970.
62. Forman, M. G., Collins, H. W. Kopelman, H. A., et al.: Determinants of left ventricular aneurysm formation: A clinical and angiographic study. J. Am. Coll. Cardiol. *8*:1256, 1986.
63. Sedlis, S. P., Cohen, K. H., Sequeira, J. M., and El-Sherif, N.: Preservation of left ventricular function in patients with total occlusion of the left anterior descending coronary artery and wide-caliber distal vessel filling by collateral vasculature. Cathet. Cardiovasc. Diagn. *15*:139, 1988.
64. Juilliere, Y., Danchen, N., Grentzinger, A., et al.: Role of previous angina pectoris and collateral flow to preserve left ventricular function in the presence or absence of myocardial infarction in isolated total occlusion of the left anterior descending coronary artery. Am. J. Cardiol. *65*:277, 1990.
65. Williams, D. O., Amsterdam, E. A., Miller, R. R., and Mason, D. T.: Functional significance of coronary collateral vessels in patients with acute myocardial infarction: Relation to pump performance, cardiogenic shock, and survival. Am. J. Cardiol. *37*:345, 1976.

66. Tubau, J. F. Chaitman, B. R., Bourassa, M. G., et al.: Importance of coronary collateral circulation in interpreting excercise test results. Am. J. Cardiol. *47*:27, 1981.
67. Eng, C., Patterson, R. E., Horowitz, S. F., et al.: Coronary collateral function during exercise. Circulation *66*:309, 1982.
68. Cohen, M., and Rentrop, K. P.: Limitation of myocardial ischemia by collateral circulation during sudden controlled coronary artery occlusion in human subjects: A prospective study. Circulation *74*:469, 1986.
69. Mizuno, K., Horiuchi, K., Matui, H., et al.: Role of coronary collateral vessels during transient coronary occlusion during angioplasty assessed by hemodynamic, electrocardiographic, and metabolic changes. J. Am. Coll. Cardiol. *12*:624, 1988.
70. Probst, P., Zangl, W., and Pachinger, O.: Relation of coronary arterial occlusion pressure during percutaneous transluminal coronary angioplasty to presence of collaterals. Am. J. Cardiol. *55*:1264, 1985.
71. Meier, B., Luethy, P., Fincy, L., et al.: Coronary wedge pressure in relation to spontaneously visible and recruitable collaterals. Circulation *75*:906, 1987.
72. Prinzmetal, M., Kennamer, R., Merliss, R., et al.: Angina pectoris. I. Variant form of angina pectoris. Am. J. Med. *27*:375, 1959.
73. Braunwald, E.: Coronary artery spasm. Mechanisms and clinical relevance. J.A.M.A. *256*:1957, 1981.
74. Dhurandhar, R. W., Watt, D. L., Silver, M. D., et al.: Prinzmetal's variant form of angina with arteriographic evidence of coronary arterial spasm. Am. J. Cardiol. *30*:902, 1972.
75. Cheng, T. O., Bashour, T., Kelser, G. A., et al.: Variant angina of Prinzmetal with normal coronary arteriogram: Variant of the variant. Circulation *47*:476, 1973.
76. Oliva, P. B., Potts, D. E., and Pluss, R. G.: Coronary arterial spasm in Prinzmetal angina. Documentation by coronary arteriography. N. Engl. J. Med. *288*:745, 1973.
77. Schroeder, J. S., Bolen, J. L., Quint, R. A., et al.: Provocation of coronary spasm with ergonovine maleate. New test with results in 57 patients undergoing coronary arteriography. Am. J. Cardiol. *40*:487, 1977.
78. Curry, R. C., Jr., Pepine, C. J., Varnell, J. H., et al.: Clinical usefulness and safety of the ergonovine test in patients with chest pain. Am. J. Cardiol. *41*:369, 1978.
79. Heupler, F. A., Jr., Proudfit, W. L., Razavi, M., et al.: Ergonovine maleate provocative test for coronary arterial spasm. Am. J. Cardiol. *41*:631, 1978.
80. Crevy, B. J., Owen, S. F., and Pitt, B.: Irreversible coronary occlusion related to administration of ergonovine. Circulation *64*:853, 1981.
81. Bertrand, M. E., LaBlanche, J. M., Tilmant, P. Y., et al.: Frequency of provoked coronary arterial spasm in 1089 consecutive patients undergoing coronary arteriography. Circulation *65*:1299, 1982.
82. Freedman, S. B., Richmond, D. R., and Kelly, D. T.: Clinical studies of patients with coronary spasm. Am. J. Cardiol. *52*:67A, 1983.
83. Furchgott, R. F.: Role of endothelium in responses of vascular smooth muscle. Circ. Res. *53*:557, 1983.
84. Vanhoutte, P. M., and Shimokawa, H.: Endothelium-derived relaxing factor and coronary vasospasm. Circulation *80*:1, 1989.
85. Ludmer, P. L., Selwyn, A. P., Shook, T. L., et al.: Paradoxical vasoconstriction induced by acetylcholine in atherosclerotic coronary arteries. N. Engl. J. Med. *315*:1046, 1986.
86. Friedman, M., and van den Bovenkamp, G. J.: Pathogenesis of coronary thrombus. Am. J. Pathol. *48*:19, 1966.
87. Ridolfi, R. L., and Hutchins, G. M.: Relationships between coronary artery lesions and myocardial infarcts: Ulceration of atherosclerotic plaques precipitating coronary artery thrombosis. Am. Heart J. *93*:468, 1977.
88. Horie, T., Sekiguchi, M., and Hirosawa, K.: Relation between myocardial infarction and preinfarction angina. A histopathological study of coronary arteries in two sudden death cases employing serial section. Am. Heart J. *95*:81, 1978.
89. Falk, E.: Plaque rupture with severe pre-existing stenosis precipitating coronary thrombosis: Characteristics of coronary atherosclerotic plaques underlying fatal occlusive thrombi. Br. Heart J. *50*:127, 1983.
90. Willerson, J. T., Campbell, W. B., Winniford, M. D., et al.: Conversion from chronic to acute coronary artery disease: Speculation regarding mechanisms. Am. J. Cardiol. *54*:1349, 1984.
91. Levin, D. C., and Fallon, J. T.: Significance of the angiographic morphology of localized coronary stenoses: Histopathologic correlation. Circulation *66*:316, 1982.
92. Ambrose, J. A., Winters, S. L., Stern A., et al.: Angiographic morphology and the pathogenesis of unstable angina pectoris. J. Am. Coll. Cardiol. *5*:609, 1985.
93. Rehr, R., Disciascio, G., Vetrovec, G., and Cowley, M.: Angiographic morphology of coronary artery stenoses in prolonged rest angina: Evidence of intracoronary thrombosis. J. Am. Coll. Cardiol. *14*:1429, 1989.
94. Levin, D. C., and Gardiner, G. A., Jr.: Complex and simple coronary artery stenoses: A new way to interpret coronary angiograms based upon lesion morphology. Radiology *164*:675, 1987.
95. Ambrose, J. A., Winters, S. L., Arora, R. R., et al.: Coronary angiographic morphology in myocardial infarction: A link between the pathogenesis of unstable angina and myocardial infarction. J. Am. Coll. Cardiol. *6*:1233, 1985.
96. Ellis, S., Alderman, E. L., Cain, K., et al.: Morphology of left anterior descending coronary territory lesions as a predictor of anterior myocardial infarction: A CASS registry study. J. Am. Coll. Cardiol. *13*:1481, 1989.
97. Kemp, H. G., Kronmal, R. A., Vlietstra, R. E., et al.: Seven year survival of patients with normal or near normal coronary arteriograms: A CASS registry study. J. Am. Coll. Cardiol. *7*:479, 1986.
98. Papanicolaou, M. N., Califf, R. M., Hlatky, M. A., et al.: Prognostic implications of angiographically normal and insignificantly narrowed coronary arteries. Am. J. Cardiol. *58*:1181, 1986.
99. Mock, M. B., Ringqvist, I., Fisher, L. D., et al.: Survival of medically treated patients in the Coronary Artery Surgery Study (CASS) registry. Circulation *66*:562, 1982.
100. Califf, R. M., Phillips, H. R., II, Hindman, M. C., et al.: Prognostic value of coronary artery jeopardy score. J. Am. Coll. Cardiol. *5*:1055, 1985.
101. Conley, M. J., Ely, R. L., Kisslo, J., et al.: The prognostic spectrum of left main stenosis. Circulation *57*:947, 1978.
102. Takaro, T., Peduzzi, P., Detre, K. M., et al.: Survival in subgroups of patients with left main coronary artery disease. Veterans Administration Cooperative Study of Surgery for Coronary Arterial Occlusive Disease. Circulation *66*:14, 1982.
103. Sanz, G., Castaner, A., Betriu, A., et al.: Determinants of prognosis in survivors of myocardial infarction. A prospective clinical angiographic study. N. Engl. J. Med. *306*:1065, 1982.
104. DeFeyter, P. J., van Eenige, M. J., Dighton, D. H., et al.: Prognostic value of exercise testing, coronary angiography and left ventriculography 6–8 weeks after myocardial infarction. Circulation *66*:527, 1982.
105. Danchin, N., Oswald, T., Voiriot, P., et al.:Significance of spontaneous obstruction of high degree coronary artery stenoses between diagnostic angiography and later percutaneous transluminal coronary angioplasty. Am. J. Cardiol. *63*:660, 1989.
106. Ambrose, J. A., Tannenbaum, M. A., Alexopoulos, D., et al.: Angiographic progression of coronary artery disease and the development of myocardial infarction. J. Am. Coll. Cardiol. *12*:56, 1988.
107. Webster, M. W., Chesebro, J. H., Smith, H. C., et al.: Myocardial infarction and coronary artery occlusion: A prospective 5-year angiographic study (abstr.). J. Am. Coll. Cardiol. *15*:218A, 1990.
108. Hackett, D., Verwilghen, J., Davies, G., and Maseri, A.: Coronary stenoses before and after acute myocardial infarction. Am. J. Cardiol. *63*:1517, 1989.
109. Little, W. C., Constantinescu, M., Applegate, R. J., et al.: Can coronary angiography predict the site of a subsequent myocardial infarction in patients with mild-to-moderate coronary artery disease? Circulation *78*:1157, 1988.
110. McHenry, P. L., O'Donnell, J., Morris, S. N., and Jordan, J. J.: Abnormal exercise electrocardiogram in apparently healthy men: A predictor of angina pectoris as an initial coronary event during long-term followup. Circulation *70*:547, 1984.
111. Epstein, S. E.: Influence of stenosis severity of coronary collateral development and importance of collaterals in maintaining left ventricular function during acute coronary occlusion. Am. J. Cardiol. *61*:866, 1988.
112. Epstein, S. E., Quyyumi, A. A., and Bonow, R. O.: Sudden cardiac death without warning. Possible mechanisms and implications for screening asymptomatic populations. N. Engl. J. Med. *321*:320, 1989.
113. Loop, F. D., Lytle, B. W., Cosgrove, D. M., et al.: Influence of the internal-mammary-artery graft on 10-year survival and other cardiac events. N. Engl. J. Med. *314*:1, 1986.
114. Spencer, F. C.: The internal mammary artery: The ideal coronary bypass graft? N. Engl. J. Med. *314*:50, 1986.
115. Lytle, B. W., Cosgrove, D. M., Ratliff, N. B., and Loop, F. D.: Coronary artery bypass grafting with the right gastroepiploic artery. J. Thorac. Cardiovasc. Surg. *97*:826, 1989.
116. Bourassa, M. G., Fisher, L. D., Campeau, L., et al.: Long-term fate of bypass grafts: The Coronary Artery Surgery Study (CASS) and the Montreal Heart Institute experiences. Circulation *72* (Suppl. V):V-71, 1985.
117. European Coronary Surgery Study Group: Long term results of prospective randomized study of coronary artery bypass surgery in stable angina pectoris. Lancet *2*:1173, 1982.
118. Tector, A. J., Schmahl, T. M., and Canino, V. R.: The internal mammary artery graft: The best choice for bypass of the diseased left anterior descending coronary artery. Circulation *68* (Suppl. II):II-214, 1983.
119. Chesebro, J. H., Clements, I. P., Fuster, V., et al.: Effect of dipyridamole and aspirin on late vein-graft patency after coronary bypass operations. N. Engl. J. Med. *310*:209, 1984.
120. Goldman, S., Copeland, J., Moritz, T., et al.: Saphenous vein graft patency 1 year after coronary artery bypass surgery and effects of antiplatelet therapy. Circulation *80*:1190, 1989.
121. Zir, L. M., Miller, S. W., Dinsmore, R. E., et al.: Interobserver variability in coronary angiography. Circulation *53*:627, 1976.
122. Detre, K. M., Wright, E., Murphy, M. L., and Takaro, T.: Observer agreement in evaluating coronary angiograms. Circulation *52*:979, 1975.
123. DeRouen, T. A., Murray, J. A., and Owen, W.: Variability in the analysis of coronary arteriograms. Circulation *55*:324, 1977.
124. Wijns, W., Serruys, P. W., Rieber, J.H.C., et al.: Quantitive angiography of the left anterior descending coronary artery: Correlations with pressure gradient and results of exercise thallium scintigraphy. Circulation *71*:273, 1985.
125. Brown, B. G., Bolson, E., Frimer, M., and Dodge, H. T.: Quantitative coronary arteriography: Estimation of dimensions, hemodynamic resistance, and atheroma mass of coronary artery lesions using the arteriogram and digital computation. Circulation *55*:329, 1977.
126. Reiber, J.H.C., Serruys, P.W., Kooijman, C. J., et al.: Assessment of short-, medium-, and long-term variations in arterial dimensions from computer-assisted quantitation of coronary cineangiograms. Circulation *71*:280, 1985.
127. Spears, J. R., Sandor, T., Als, A. V., et al.: Computerized image analysis for quantitative measurement of vessel diameter from cineangiograms. Circulation *68*:453, 1983.
128. Selzer, R. H., Hagerty, C., Azen, S. P., et al.: Precision and reproducibility

of quantitative coronary angiography with applications to controlled clinical trials. J. Clin. Invest. *83*:520, 1989.

129. Nichols, A. B., Gabrieli, C.F.O., Fenoglio, J. J., Jr., and Esser, P. D.: Quantification of relative coronary arterial stenosis by cinevideodensitometric analysis of coronary arteriograms. Circulation *69*:512, 1984.
130. Jaques, P., DiBianca, F., Pizer, S., et al.: Quantitative digital fluorography: Computer vs. human estimation of vascular stenoses. Invest. Radiol. *20*:45, 1985.
131. Johnson, M. R., McPherson, D. D., Fleagle, S. R., et al.: Videodensitometric analysis of human coronary stenoses: Validation in vivo by intraoperative high-frequency epicardial echocardiography. Circulation *77*:328, 1988.
132. Mattleman, S., Hakki, A-H., Iskandrian, A. S., and Kane, S. A.: Effects of angiographic contrast medium on left ventricular function: Evaluation by contrast angiography and radionuclide angiography. Cathet. Cardiovasc. Diagn. *10*:129, 1984.
133. Salem, D. N., Konstam, M. A., Isner, J. M., and Bonin, M. A.: Comparison of the electrocardiographic and hemodynamic responses to ionic and nonionic radiocontrast media during left ventriculography: A randomized double-blind study. Am. Heart J. *111*:533, 1986.
134. Gertz, E. W., Wisneski, J. A., Chiu, D., et al.: Clinical superiority of a new nonionic contrast agent (iopamidol) for cardiographic angiography. J. Am. Coll. Cardiol. *5*:250, 1985.
135. Tani, M., Handa, S., Norma, S., et al.: Changes in left ventricular diastolic function after left ventriculography: A comparison with iopamidol and urografin. Am. Heart J. *110*:617, 1985.
136. Bristow, J. D., Porter, G. A., Kloster, F. F., and Griswold, H. E.: Hemodynamic changes attending angiocardiography. Radiology *88*:939, 1976.
137. Morris, T. W., Harnish, P. P., Reece, K., and Katzberg, R. W.: Tissue fluid shifts during renal arteriography with conventional and low osmolality agents. Invest. Radiol. *18*:335, 1983.
138. Mancini, G.B.J., and Higgins, C. B.: Digital subtraction angiography: A review of cardiac applications. Prog. Cardiovasc. Dis. *17*:111, 1985.
139. Hartman, R. B., Harrison, E. E., Pupello, D. F., et al.: Characteristics of left ventricular thrombus resulting in perioperative embolism: A complication of coronary artery bypass grafting. J. Thorac. Cardiovasc. Surg. *86*:706, 1983.
140. Cabin, H. S., and Roberts, W. C.: Left ventricular aneurysm, intra-aneurysmal thrombus and systemic embolus in coronary heart disease. Chest *77*:586, 1980.
141. Hirai, T., Fujita, M., Nakajima, H., et al.: Importance of collateral circulation for prevention of left ventricular aneurysm formation in acute myocardial infarction. Circulation *79*:791, 1989.
142. Visser, C. E., Kan, G., Meltzer, R. S., et al.: Incidence, timing and prognostic value of left ventricular aneurysm formation after myocardial infarction: A prospective, serial echocardiographic study of 158 patients. Am. J. Cardiol. *57*:729, 1986.
143. Sheehan, F. H., Stewart, D. K., Dodge, H. T., et al.: Variability in the measurement of regional left ventricular wall motion from contrast angiograms. Circulation *68*:550, 1983.
144. Chaitman, B. R., DeMots, H., Bristow, D., et al.: Objective and subjective analysis of left ventricular angiograms. Circulation *52*:420, 1975.
145. Vas, R., Diamond, G. A., Forrester, J. S., et al.: Computer-enhanced digital angiography: Correlation of clinical assessment of left ventricular ejection fraction and regional wall motion. Am. Heart J. *104*:732, 1982.
146. Nissen, S. E., Booth, D., Waters, J., et al.: Evaluation of left ventricular contractile pattern by intravenous digital subtraction ventriculography: Comparison with cineangiography and assessment of interobserver variability. Am. J. Cardiol. *52*:1293, 1983.
147. Simon, A. L., Ross, J., Jr., and Gault, J. H.: Angiographic anatomy of the left ventricle and mitral valve in idiopathic hypertrophic subaortic stenosis. Circulation *36*:852, 1967.
148. Williams, R. S., Behar, V. S., and Peter, R. H.: Left bundle branch block: Angiographic segmental wall motion abnormalities. Am. J. Cardiol. *44*:1046, 1979.
149. Cohn, P. F., Herman, M. V., and Gorlin, R.: Ventricular dysfunction in coronary artery disease. Am. J. Cardiol. *33*:307, 1974.
150. Banka, V. S., Bodenheimer, M. M., Shah, R., and Helfant, R. H.: Intervention ventriculography: Comparative value of nitroglycerin, post-extrasystolic potentiation and nitroglycerin plus post-extrasystolic potentiation. Circulation *53*:632, 1976.
151. McAnulty, J. H., Hattenhauer, M. T., Rösch, J., et al.: Improvement in left ventricular wall motion following nitroglycerin. Circulation *51*:140, 1975.
152. Helfant, R. H., Pine, R., Meister, S. G., et al.: Nitroglycerin to unmask reversible asynergy: Correlation with post-coronary bypass ventriculography. Circulation *50*:108, 1974.
153. Popio, K. A., Gorlin, R., Bechtel, D., and Levine, J. A.: Postextrasystolic potentiation as a predictor of potential myocardial viability: Preoperative analyses compared with studies after coronary bypass surgery. Am. J. Cardiol. *39*:944, 1977.
154. Hood, W. P., Jr., Rackley, C. E., and Grossman, W.: Cardiac ventriculography. *In* Grossman, W. (ed.): Cardiac Catheterization and Angiography. 2nd ed. Philadelphia, Lea and Febiger, 1980, p. 170.
155. Dodge, H. T., Sandler, H., Ballew, D. W., and Lord, J. D., Jr.: Use of biplane angiocardiography for the measurement of left ventricular volume in man. Am. Heart J. *60*:762, 1960.
156. Wynne, J., Green, L. H., Mann, T., et al.: Estimation of left ventricular volumes in man from biplane cineangiograms filmed in oblique projections. Am. J. Cardiol. *41*:726, 1978.

10

Nuclear Cardiology

by BARRY L. ZARET, M.D., FRANS J. Th. WACKERS, M.D., and ROBERT SOUFER, M.D.

Nuclear cardiology developed as a new discipline in the 1970's. Since that time, new techniques have evolved progressively, while the clinical relevance of currently available procedures is being assessed on an ongoing basis. The discipline has moved from the diagnostic sphere to a broad emphasis on the functional characterization of patients with known disease. This has provided insights into patient risk stratification and prognosis. Major new methods of tomographic imaging and radiopharmaceutical techniques based upon biological activity of the tracers are being developed, and the role of technology in diagnosis and prognosis is being evaluated. In this chapter, following a brief introductory review of scintillation camera instrumentation, the major techniques of nuclear cardiology are discussed. In each section, relevant technical issues necessary for adequate test performance are presented together with the clinical and investigative impact of the derived data.

INSTRUMENTATION

THE SCINTILLATION (GAMMA) CAMERA

The acquisition and processing of imaging studies in cardiovascular nuclear medicine are performed with a scintillation camera interfaced to a computer. The visual display of radioactivity is a result of photons passing through the gamma camera. The gamma rays pass through three principal camera components, including a collimator, a large sodium iodide crystal of varying thickness (from 6 mm to 9 mm), and a hexagonal array of 37 to 91 photomultiplier tubes. The final positioning of the actual signal in relation to the image results from the interaction between the gamma ray and the crystal, which converts part of this energy into light. The photomultiplier tubes translate these scintillations into voltage pulses; these are measured as an electrical signal that defines the position at which gamma ray and crystal interact. This is accomplished by electronic circuits that compute the x and y coordinates of the crystal interaction, which is displayed in a two-dimensional matrix anatomically analogous to the site of occurrence within the patient. A multichannel analyzer defines the appropriate energy of the event. As a result, low-energy scatter events are not accepted.

COLLIMATION. This is an important concept in nuclear data acquisition. A collimator is composed of lead with channels designed in either a parallel or a diverging manner. Gamma rays must pass through a collimator before reaching the crystal. The purpose of the collimator is to approximate the origin of the photon emission within the patient to an analogous location within the crystal. Parallel-hole collimators are of either the high-resolution or high-sensitivity variety. The high-resolution collimation permits better spatial resolution (the ability of the detector source to discriminate between neighboring sources of activity and visually resolve various components within the field of view) but with a loss of count sensitivity (the number of counts the camera may acquire per unit time). Alternatively, a high-sensitivity collimator would result in maximizing the count rate at the expense of spatial resolution.

The compromise between the two is termed a low-energy all-purpose or general purpose collimator, which is intermediate with respect to sensitivity and resolution. The thickness of the crystal and the type of collimation will determine the sensitivity of a gamma camera. With this background, one may predict the type of collimation to be used for a particular study. Thus, a parallel-hole high-sensitivity collimator would be appropriate for rapidly acquired studies such as first-pass blood pool studies. Finally, a slant hole collimator in which the holes are angled with respect to the detector can be used when differentiation between the atria and ventricle is needed. This would be appropriate if one wanted to calculate right ventricular ejection fraction from the LAO image of a equilibrium radionuclide study in which separation of the right ventricle from the atrium is important.

Other important characteristics that influence the performance of the gamma camera are field uniformity, energy resolution, and count rate linearity. Most scintillation cameras have a spatial resolution of 4 mm with a count rate linearity of approximately 75,000 counts per second and a flood uniformity of ± 5 per cent.

COMPUTING. The computer is now a principal factor in nuclear imaging systems. These data processing systems are interfaced to the scintillation camera. Information is downloaded from the imaging device, where it is organized in a digital manner to be displayed quantitatively. The computers have software containing algorithms for quantification of both static images and dynamic events. In addition, software may be programmable to meet the specific needs of an individual laboratory. The principal hardware components of the computer include analog digital convertor, central processing unit, image memory, mass storage, an array processor, and a display monitor. The scintigraphic matrix is generally 256 × 256 pixels (picture elements). Capabilities for high temporal resolution (50 frames/second) are important. The computer must have special hardware and software requirements for tomographic (SPECT) imaging.

A more detailed discussion of instrumentation utilized in cardiovascular nuclear medicine is found elsewhere.[1,2]

Myocardial Perfusion Imaging

The regional distribution of myocardial blood flow can be visualized utilizing radiopharmaceuticals that accumulate proportional to regional myocardial perfusion. The first scintigraphic images of myocardial perfusion were acquired in 1964 by Carr et al.[3] using cesium-131. Exercise-induced myocardial ischemia was initially visualized with potassium-43 in 1973 by Zaret and colleagues.[4] Thallium-201 (^{201}Tl), a potassium analog, became available in 1974 and has since been employed successfully.[5-8,8a] More recently, new technetium-99m (^{99m}Tc)-labeled cationic compounds with better imaging characteristics and novel biological properties have been introduced for visualization of myocardial perfusion.[9] With these imaging agents, the *relative* distribution of myocardial blood flow can be visualized. *Absolute* quantification of myocardial blood flow is not feasible using single photon-emitting radioisotopes.

The most important clinical application of myocardial perfusion imaging is in conjunction with stress testing for evaluation of ischemic heart disease. Numerous investigators have shown the diagnostic usefulness of ^{201}Tl exercise imaging[8] (see also p. 1298). Although the experience with ^{99m}Tc-labeled imaging agents is still limited, it appears that its clinical usefulness is *at least comparable* to that of imaging with ^{201}Tl.[10,11] There is generally good agreement between the results of ^{201}Tl stress imaging and findings on contrast coronary angiography. More importantly, it has been demonstrated that abnormal findings on ^{201}Tl images reflect the hemodynamic and functional significance of coronary artery stenoses and thus provide important prognostic information.

RADIOPHARMACEUTICALS

THALLIUM-201. ^{201}Tl is cyclotron-produced and emits mercury x-rays at 69-83 keV (88 per cent) and gamma rays at 135, 165, and 167 keV (12 per cent). Its physical half-life is 74 hours; however, its biological half-life is approximately 58 hours. The estimated absorbed radiation dose to the whole body is 0.21 rad/mCi, to the kidney 0.24 rad/mCi, and to the large intestine 0.54 rad/mCi. Because of the relatively long half-life of ^{201}Tl, only a relatively small amount of radiation can be administered. For planar imaging, usually 2 to 2.5 mCi is administered, whereas for tomographic imaging 3.5 mCi is given. The first pass myocardial extraction fraction of ^{201}Tl of 85 per cent is relatively high.[12] The initial myocardial accumulation of ^{201}Tl is proportional to myocardial blood flow. Once ^{201}Tl has entered the myocyte, a continuous exchange of ^{201}Tl takes place across the cell membrane. This process involves the Na^+, K^+-ATPase pump. The intrinsic half-life of ^{201}Tl within the myocardial cell is approximately 85 minutes. However, because of continued cellular reaccumulation of ^{201}Tl, the effective half-life of ^{201}Tl from the heart is 7.5 hours. A unique aspect of ^{201}Tl studies is that images obtained early and late after injection provide different pathophysiological information:

1. Images immediately after injection reflect the flow-dependent initial distribution and thus regional myocardial blood flow.
2. Images taken after a delay of 2 to 24 hours reflect the distribution of the potassium pool and hence myocardial viability.

^{99m}Tc HEXAKIS 2-METHOXY-2-ISOBUTYL ISONITRILE (SestaMIBI). A number of compounds of the isonitrile family have been evaluated for myocardial imaging. The most promising compound is ^{99m}Tc-SestaMIBI, a lipophilic monovalent cation. The ^{99m}Tc label emits gamma rays at 140 keV and has a physical half-life of 6 hours. Because of the slow body clearance, the biological half-life of ^{99m}Tc-SestaMIBI is approximately the same. The whole-body absorbed radiation dose is 0.02 rad/mCi. The target organ is the upper large intestine, which receives 0.18 rad/mCi. Because of favorable dosimetry compared with ^{201}Tl, up to 30 mCi of ^{99m}Tc-SestaMIBI can be administered per day. The initial distribution of ^{99m}Tc-SestaMIBI is similar to that of ^{201}Tl and proportional to the distribution of myocardial blood flow. However, in contrast to ^{201}Tl, there is simultaneous rapid accumulation in the liver and subsequent clearance into the biliary tract.[10] Myocardial extraction fraction of ^{99m}Tc-SestaMIBI is substantially less efficient than that of ^{201}Tl: 65 per cent. The mechanism of myocardial uptake probably primarily involves passive diffusion. In contrast to ^{201}Tl, once the radiopharmaceutical has entered the myocardial cell, it is bound relatively stably to mitochondria. Because of intracellular retention and additional subsequent myocardial uptake during recirculation, the absolute net retention of ^{99m}Tc-SestaMIBI several minutes after administration is comparable with that of ^{201}Tl.[13] Because myocardial distribution of ^{99m}Tc-SestaMIBI remains relatively fixed and no significant redistribution occurs, the distribution of myocardial blood flow *at the time of injection* is "frozen" over time and can be imaged for several hours.

^{99m}Tc-TEBOROXIME. Another recently developed ^{99m}Tc-labeled myocardial perfusion imaging agent is teboroxime, a neutral cation. ^{99m}Tc-teboroxime is a boronic acid adduct of technetium oxime (BATO). In contrast with the other tracers, this imaging agent has both the rapid and efficient myocardial

TABLE 10-1 COMPARATIVE CHARACTERISTICS OF VARIOUS MYOCARDIAL PERFUSION IMAGING AGENTS

	^{201}Tl	^{99M}Tc-SestaMIBI	^{99M}Tc-TEBOROXIME
Energy emissions	69-83 (x-rays), 135,165,167 keV	140 keV	140 keV
Physical t ½	74 hrs	6 hrs	6 hrs
Biological t ½	58 hrs	6 hrs	?
Heart t ½	3-4 hrs	6-7 hrs	<10 min
Dose	2.5-3.5 mCi	30 mCi	30 mCi
Radiation dose:			
Whole body	0.21 rad/mCi	0.02 rad/mCi	0.02 rad/mCi
Intestines	0.54 rad/mCi	0.18 rad/mCi	0.11 rad/mCi
Myoc. exact. fraction	85%	65%	80-90%
% I.D. heart	4%	1.5%	?
Visualizes:			
Blood flow	+	+	+
Viability	+ (delayed image)	± ?	−
Redistribution	+	− or minimal	−
LVEF (first pass)	−	+	+
ECG gating	−	+	−
Imaging time/views			
Planar	10 min	5 min	1-2 min
Tomographic	21 min	11 min	?

Abbreviations: t ½ = half life; I.D. = injected dose

extraction (80 to 90 per cent myocardial extraction fraction) and subsequent rapid washout from the heart.[11] There is also intense early hepatic activity, which may hinder complete evaluation of myocardial uptake, particularly of the inferior wall. Myocardial washout of teboroxime is biexponential; 5 minutes after injection, only 25 per cent of its initial activity remains in the heart. The estimated whole-body absorbed radiation dose is 0.02 rad/mCi. The target organs are liver and large intestine, which receive 0.12 rad/mCi and 0.11 rad/mCi, respectively. This imaging agent requires rapid serial imaging during the first 5 minutes immediately after injection.

The principal characteristics of the three imaging agents are summarized in Table 10–1.

TECHNICAL CONSIDERATIONS IN MYOCARDIAL PERFUSION IMAGING

GAMMA CAMERA. For planar imaging, a camera with a 10-inch diameter detector and a $\frac{1}{4}$-inch thick crystal is preferred. Low-energy photons of ^{201}Tl do not adequately penetrate thicker crystals, resulting in images of inadequate count density. Tomographic cameras with large field of view (20-inch diameter) as a rule have a $\frac{3}{8}$-inch thick crystal and thus are not ideally suited for ^{201}Tl imaging.

COLLIMATION. For both planar and SPECT imaging with ^{201}Tl, a general all-purpose parallel-hole collimator is preferred to ensure adequate count density. Employing ^{99m}Tc-labeled imaging agents, the count rate is sufficiently high to allow use of a high-resolution parallel-hole collimator.

ENERGY WINDOW. For ^{201}Tl imaging, a dual window is preferred: a 25 per cent window over the 80 keV mercury x-ray peak and a 20 per cent window over the 167 gamma-ray peak. The latter window accounts for approximately 10 per cent additional counts. For ^{99m}Tc-labeled imaging agents, a 20 per cent window is placed over the 140 keV peak.

COMPUTER ACQUISITION. Images should be acquired on computer and stored on computer disc or magnetic tape for data processing. For planar myocardial perfusion imaging, acquisition in 128 × 128 matrix is preferred, whereas for tomographic imaging a 64 × 64 matrix is commonly used.

IMAGING PROTOCOL. For ^{201}Tl stress imaging, one single dose of ^{201}Tl is injected at peak exercise. Initial stress imaging should be started *within 5 minutes* of the injection. Delayed or redistribution imaging is performed *2 to 4 hours later.* (The timing of delayed imaging should be standardized.) For complete assessment of viable myocardium, a second injection of ^{201}Tl is administered in selected patients (see below).

With ^{99m}Tc-labeled perfusion imaging agents *two* injections are given: the first during exercise and a second at rest. Employing ^{99m}Tc-SestaMIBI, imaging is performed *30 to 60 minutes after injection.* With ^{99m}Tc-teboroxime the patient should be imaged rapidly, starting at *1 minute after injection.*

PATIENT IMAGING TECHNIQUES

PLANAR IMAGING. To acquire optimal myocardial perfusion images, some basic requirements should be met.[14,15] The most frequent reasons for poor quality images are (1) insufficient count density within the heart, (2) inconsistent *patient positioning and repositioning,* (3) use of *too large a zoom factor,* and (4) inadequate display of images.

ADEQUATE COUNT DENSITY. One should aim for at least 600,000 counts in the field of view. When extracardiac activity is present, e.g., in lungs or subdiaphragmatic organs, greater count density is needed. Because of the relatively low dose of ^{201}Tl, it is at times difficult to obtain adequate count density in the heart. Count density with ^{201}Tl can be optimized in several ways:

1. Administration of adequate dose, at least 2.5 mCi (92.5 MBq) of ^{201}Tl; in obese patients and for SPECT imaging a larger dose, not exceeding 3.5 mCi/kg, is administered.
2. Imaging on both energy peaks of ^{201}Tl.
3. The use of a general all-purpose collimator.
4. Imaging for a preset time rather than for counts, e.g., 10 minutes per view. This is of particular importance when substantial extracardiac activity is present, e.g., after dipyridamole infusion or in patients with increased pulmonary uptake (see below).

With ^{99m}Tc-labeled imaging agents, adequate count density is readily achieved, since 20 to 30 mCi is administered. With the latter agents, one should aim for 1.5 to 2 million counts/field of view.

PATIENT POSITIONING. Imaging is routinely performed in three projections. The *left anterior oblique* (LAO) view usually is obtained with the patient lying supine. This angulation should be used as a reference angle for the other views. The *anterior view* is obtained with the patient lying supine, 45 degrees to the right of the LAO view. For the *left lateral view,* the patient should be turned on to the *right side,* with the camera head in the same position as for the anterior view. The detector head should be angled in such a way that it is as close as possible to the patient's chest wall. On all views the heart should be in the *center* of the field of view. *Repositioning* of the patient at delayed imaging should be done with great care. The position of the heart on the exercise images should be reproduced as close as possible to those at rest.

ZOOM FACTOR. When a large field of view camera is used, the *zoom factor* (magnification) should not exceed 1.2 times. On an optimal image, the heart is approximately one-third to one-fourth of the diameter of the field of view.

PLANAR IMAGE DISPLAY

The *display* of myocardial perfusion images is important for reproducible and consistent interpretation. Color display of *planar* images is to be discouraged. "White on black" display using a linear gray scale is preferred (Fig. 10–1). On these images the heart is white (radioactivity). This display is preferred because cardiologists are accustomed to the heart shown in white on contrast angiograms. When interpretation is done from a computer screen, standardization of display is important. Arbitrary changing of contrast intensity and gray scales should be minimized. The linear gray scale should be normalized to the "hottest pixel" within the heart. In this manner the gray scale is utilized fully in the representation of the heart. This is particularly important for display of images acquired with ^{99m}Tc-labeled agents.

Exercise and rest/delayed images should be displayed side by side. Hard copies for documentation in the patient's chart can be obtained with photographic paper, exposed in a standard video imager. Because of the poor gray scale characteristics of Polaroid film, it should *not* be used for diagnostic purposes.

TOMOGRAPHIC IMAGING (SPECT)

Careful attention to technical details is even more important for SPECT imaging. For ^{201}Tl imaging, energy settings are the same as for planar imaging. Usually a general all-purpose collimator is employed. For imaging with ^{99m}Tc-labeled myocardial perfusion agents, high-resolution parallel-hole collimator is preferred because of higher count rate. During cardiac SPECT imaging, the gamma camera rotates through a 180-degree arc with 32 stops, each 40 seconds in duration. With ^{99m}Tc-SestaMIBI, the time for each stop can be shortened to 20 seconds.

TOMOGRAPHIC ARTIFACTS. Patient positioning and patient preparation are extremely important for optimal SPECT imaging. Most common artifacts on SPECT imaging are caused by motion and attenuation.[16] *Motion* may involve movement of the patient's upper body but also may result from a change in position of the heart within the chest. Immediately after exercise, because of deeper breathing, the heart may be in a vertical position. While the patient recovers from exercise, the heart may move into a horizontal position. This phenomenon of "upward creep" can cause artifactual inferior wall defects on reconstructed slices.[17] This can be avoided by delaying the start of SPECT imaging after termination of exercise for approximately 10 minutes. This allows for acquisition of one *planar* image immediately after exercise, which is useful for evaluation of increased lung uptake. Other common artifacts are caused by *attenuation.*

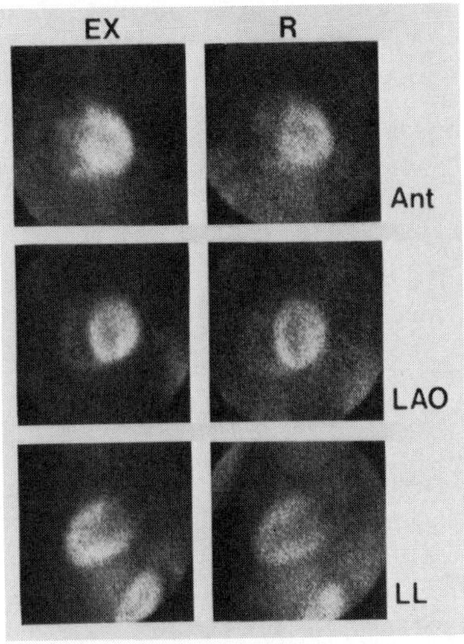

FIGURE 10–1. Normal planar exercise (EX) and redistribution (R) planar ^{201}Tl images. Ant = Anterior view, LAO = left anterior oblique view, LL = left lateral view.

The supine position of the patient may cause inferior wall defects by attenuation by the left hemidiaphragm. To avoid such artifacts, alternative patient positioning has been proposed. For instance, the image can be obtained with the patient prone (lying on the stomach)[18,19] or turned on the right side.[20] Attenuation by breast tissue can cause artifacts, which are difficult to recognize on reconstructed SPECT images. The authors have found that artifacts can be recognized best by means of breast markers used on regular planar images. For these reasons the authors routinely acquire "backup" planar images as an aid in interpretion of SPECT images.

ADEQUATE COUNT DENSITY. This is a frequently ignored aspect of tomographic perfusion imaging. As already mentioned, gamma camera for SPECT imaging has a three-fourths inch thick crystal, which is not optimal for ^{201}Tl imaging. Therefore, a relatively high dose of ^{201}Tl should be administered (3.5 mCi or 129.5 MBq).

SPECT ORBIT. Many cameras provide a choice of various acquisition orbits; the camera may rotate around the patient in a perfect *circle* or may follow the patient's *body contour.* A body contour orbit may cause artifacts because of varying gamma camera resolution with varying distance of the detector head from the target organ. These artifacts are typical and consist of small 180-degree diametrical defects on the short-axis slices.[21] A high-resolution collimator reduces the effect of varying spatial resolution and resulting artifacts.

TOMOGRAPHIC IMAGE DISPLAY. The display of reconstructed SPECT slices should be standardized in each laboratory. As a general rule, images should be displayed "white on black" using a linear gray scale (Fig. 10–2). It is recommended that three sets of slices be reconstructed: short-axis slices, horizontal long-axis slices, and vertical long-axis slices. The exercise and delayed (rest) images should be displayed side by side to facilitate comparison. Because of the multitude of images, it is useful to "condense" all information into one color-colded polar map or "bull's eye" image.

CHARACTERISTICS OF MYOCARDIAL PERFUSION IMAGES

In planar imaging, perfusion is visualized as the projection of myocardial radioactivity on a plane parallel to the crystal surface of the gamma camera. The "left ventricular cavity" as it appears on planar images is in part an optical illusion.[14] The familiar horseshoe appearance of the left ventricle on ^{201}Tl images is a result of (1) the attenuation of radiation from the distant myocardial wall by the ventricular blood pool and (2) the relatively greater myocardial mass of the walls perpendicular to the plane of view. The "facing" myocardial wall contains relatively less radiopharmaceutical. Because of overprojection of myocardial regions in one plane, it is necessary to obtain multiple planar images from different angles to visualize all segments of the left ventricular myocardium. The anatomy of the heart as projected on various planar views and the various coronary artery territories are shown in Figure 10–3.

NORMAL VARIATIONS OF THE THALLIUM-201 IMAGE

The interpretation of myocardial perfusion images at times may be difficult because of normal variations in the pattern of radiotracer uptake.[14]

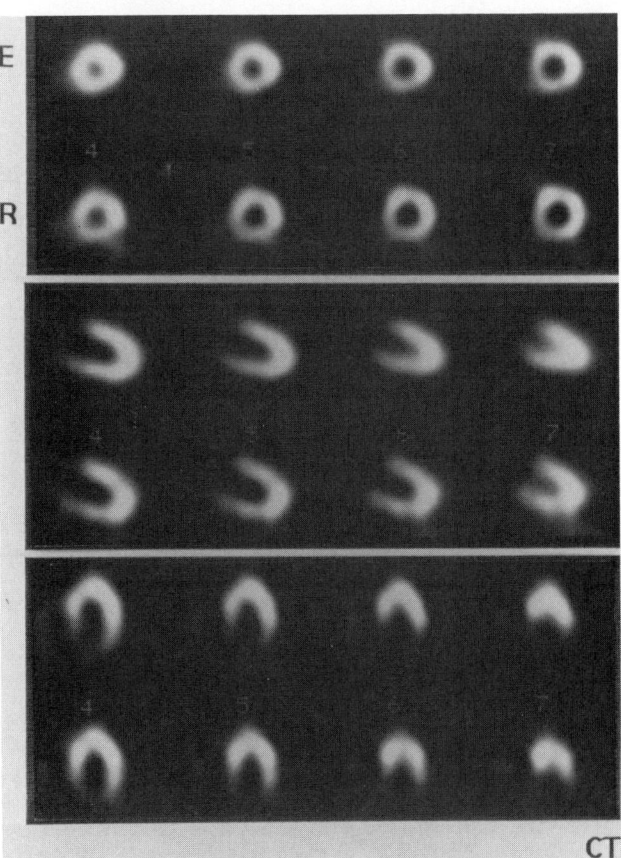

FIGURE 10–2. Normal exercise (E) and redistribution (R) ^{201}Tl SPECT images. Short-axis sections *(top),* vertical long-axis *(center),* and horizontal long-axis slices *(bottom)* are shown.

APEX. There is a well-recognized area of normally decreased tracer activity at the apex of the left ventricle. In a patient whose heart is in a vertical position, this may be a prominent feature. An apical variant appears as a narrow slit or cleft-like area, aligned with the long axis of the left ventricle. In patients with abnormally dilated left ventricles, this apical defect may be considerably larger and at times difficult to differentiate from apical infarction. However, an apical *infarct* frequently extends into either the anterior wall or inferior wall and therefore is not aligned with the long axis.

AORTIC VALVE PLANE. On the left anterior oblique view the membranous septum and aortic valve plane are projected at the open end of the horseshoe; at times they may cause an apparent high septal defect. This may be seen in patients with a horizontal position of the heart.

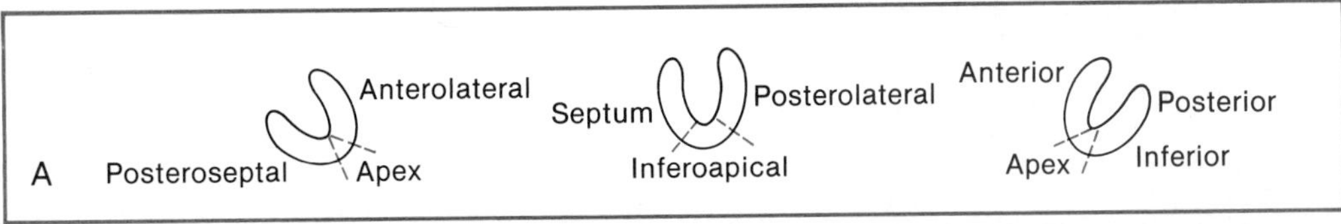

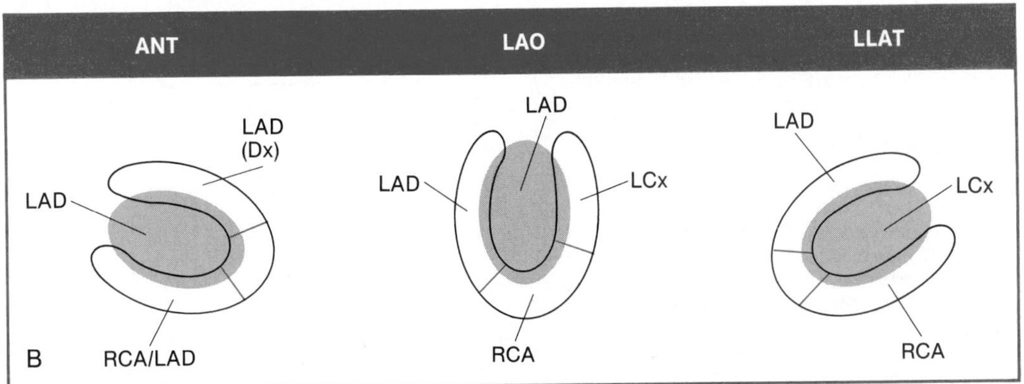

FIGURE 10–3. ***A,*** **Anatomy of the heart as projected on planar views.** ***B,*** **Coronary artery territories on three planar views. The shaded areas indicate the myocardium overlying the left ventricular cavity. LAD = Left anterior descending coronary artery, RCA = right coronary artery, Dx = diagonal artery, LCx = left circumflex artery, ANT = anteroposterior, LAO = left anterior oblique, LLAT = left lateral.**

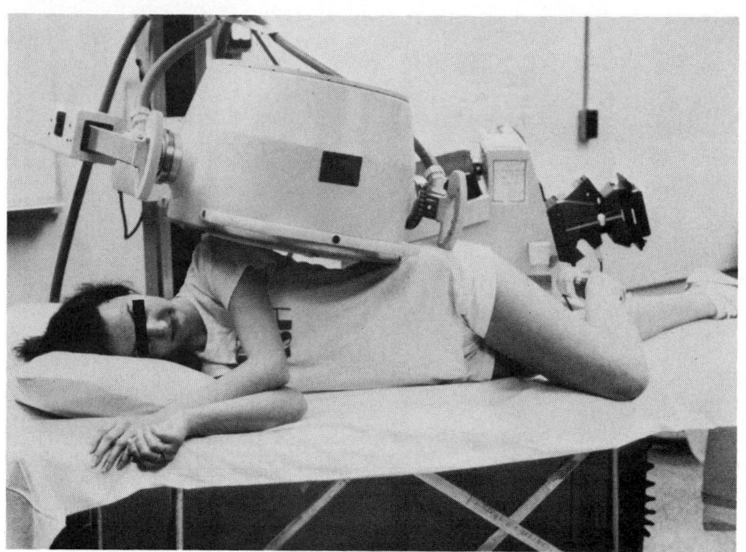

FIGURE 10–4. Correct positioning of a patient for obtaining the left lateral view. The patient should be lying on the right side, with the camera detector above the table. The camera detector should be placed as close as possible to the chest wall. (From Wackers, F.J.T.: Myocardial perfusion imaging. *In* Gottschalk, A., Hopper P. B., and Potchan, E. J. [eds.]: Diagnostic Nuclear Medicine. 2nd ed: Baltimore, Williams and Wilkins, 1988, p. 291.)

MITRAL VALVE PLANE. The mitral valve plane is seen as the open end of the horseshoe in all three views.

TYPICAL ARTIFACTS

ANTERIOR VIEW. In most normal subjects the intensity of uptake in the inferoseptal wall is approximately equal to that of the anterolateral wall. However, in a patient with enlargement of the right ventricle (e.g., in chronic obstructive pulmonary disease), the right ventricular blood pool may attenuate inferoseptal activity and produce an apparent defect. Such artifacts can be unmasked by imaging the patient in the upright position, thereby changing the position of the right ventricle in the chest.

LEFT ANTERIOR OBLIQUE VIEW. The appearance of the heart in the left anterior oblique view depends on both the position of the heart in the chest and the size of the heart. In patients with left ventricular dilatation, there may be clockwise rotation. In the latter situation a routine 45-degree left anterior oblique view may display an image similar to that usually seen in the anterior projection. The (normal) open end of the horseshoe could be misinterpreted as a septal defect. A steeper (e.g., 60-degree) angulation may project the left ventricle correctly along the long axis, thereby restoring the "typical" doughnut-shaped configuration.

LEFT LATERAL VIEW. Acquisition of a "steep" left anterior oblique or left lateral image with the patient *supine* may cause artifactual inferior wall defects (Fig. 10–4). This artifact is seen in approximately one-fourth of patients imaged in the supine position.[22] This artifact is caused by attenuation of the inferior wall activity by the left hemidiaphragm. Turning the patient on the right side causes the heart to shift into a vertical position. Moreover, in this position the left hemidiaphragm makes larger excursions. This results in less attenuation and improved projection of the inferoposterior wall.

OBESE PATIENTS/LARGE BREASTS. In extremely obese patients, or in females with large breasts, attenuation of radiation may cause apparent defects. These artifactual defects often appear as anterior defects on the anterior and left lateral views, whereas the location of artifacts is less predictable on the left anterior oblique view. The authors find it useful to employ radioactive string markers to outline the breasts and thus define the relationship between the breasts and any cardiac defects. Superimposition of breast tissue over the heart may also result in linear areas of relatively *increased* activity. This linear artifact is believed to be caused by a small-angle scatter from the breast tissue fold. Because breast artifacts are the most frequent cause of false-positive ^{201}Tl studies, the use of breast markers is an important aid in interpreting ^{201}Tl images.[14,15]

NORMAL ^{99m}Tc-SestaMIBI IMAGES

^{99m}Tc-SestaMIBI images are generally of better quality than ^{201}Tl images. Compared with ^{201}Tl, these images have substantially less low-radiation background scatter and are therefore clearer than ^{201}Tl images. The normal variants and artifacts already described can also be observed on ^{99m}Tc-SestaMIBI images. The most important difference, in comparison with ^{201}Tl, is the substantial amount of subdiaphragmatic uptake on ^{99m}Tc-SestaMIBI images. Images obtained immediately after injection show, in addition to uptake in the heart, accumulation in the liver and spleen. During the subsequent 30 to 60 minutes, most of the radiopharmaceutical in the liver is excreted in the biliary tract, improving heart-to-liver and spleen ratios.[10] Because of significant extracardiac activity, SestaMIBI images should be displayed with the gray scale normalized to the "hottest" pixel within the heart. Myocardial distribution of ^{99m}Tc-SestaMIBI does not change significantly for several hours after administration.

NORMAL ^{99m}Tc-TEBOROXIME IMAGES

^{99m}Tc-Teboroxime images are characterized by rapid initial accumulation of the radiotracer within the heart, subsequent fast clearance (within 2 to 3 minutes) from the heart, and intensive accumulation (within 2 to 3 minutes) in the liver.[11] Consequently, the heart can be imaged only for a few minutes after administration of this radiopharmaceutical. The appearance of the heart with this agent is very similar in quality to that with ^{201}Tl. The intense subdiaphragmatic activity also may interefere with analysis of the inferior wall.

NORMAL SPECT IMAGES

SHORT-AXIS SLICES. The short-axis slices should be analyzed in three groups: apical slices, mid-ventricular slices, and basal slices. To avoid artifacts by partial volume effect, only apical slices that clearly show the ventricular cavity should be analyzed. The SPECT anatomy and coronary territories are shown in Figure 10–5. Slightly less inferoseptal uptake can be noted in male patients as a normal variant, whereas radiotracer distribution is more or less homogeneous in females. The basal short-axis

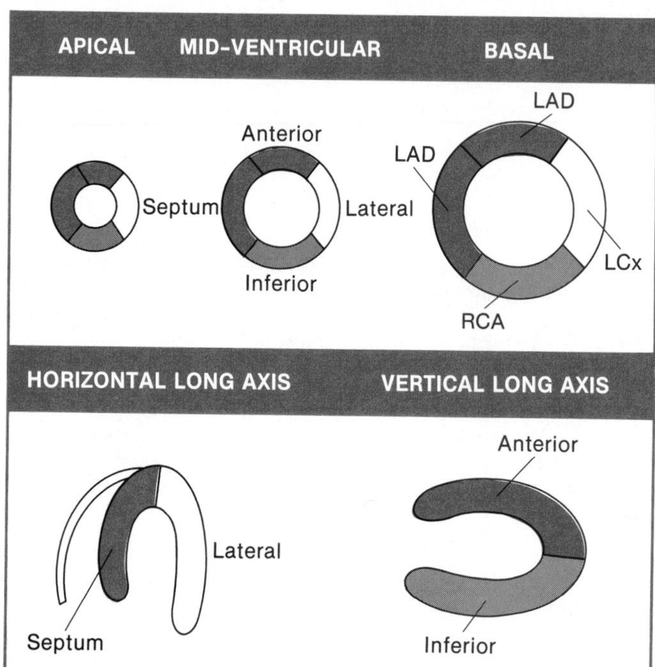

FIGURE 10–5. Left ventricular anatomy and coronary artery territories on SPECT slices.

slices usually show a septal defect, a normal finding that represents the membranous portion of the septum. A practical rule for interpreting a SPECT study is that a perfusion defect should be seen on at least three consecutive slices in order to be considered a true abnormality.

The *vertical long-axis slices* and the *horizontal long-axis* slices contain the same information shown on the short-axis slices. However, the apex and base of the heart can be analyzed without partial volume artifacts. Only slices that clearly show left ventricular cavity should be analyzed. On the horizontal long-axis slices the septum is usually shorter than the lateral wall; this normal variant is caused by the membranous septum.

POLAR MAPS. To simplify the interpretation of tomographic slices, the data are best consolidated as a *"polar map"* or *"bull's eye"* display. On this map all short-axis slices are displayed in a concentric manner, the apex in the center and the base of the heart at the periphery. It should be emphasized that tomographic studies should never be interpreted from the polar map alone but only after critical quality control of raw data and of reconstructed slices. Typical artifacts (and how to avoid them) have been discussed above.

QUALITY CONTROL. This should be performed systematically as a part of the interpretation of a SPECT study and should involve the following:

1. Inspection of cine display of 32 planar images to assess motion of the patient or of the heart. This display also allows the operator to observe whether the heart is in the center of rotation.
2. Aiming for a count density of *at least 100 counts* within the "hottest" pixel of the heart (anterior projection).
3. Assessment of attenuation of posterior wall by comparison of the left lateral "supine" view with a left lateral "right side down" view.
4. Assessment of breast artifacts on planar backup images.

Image Interpretation

Planar and tomographic images are interpreted qualitatively by visual analysis, often aided by computer quantification. Image interpretation can be described as follows:

NORMAL. Homogeneous uptake of the radiopharmaceutical throughout the myocardium.

DEFECT. A localized myocardial area with a relative decrease in radiotracer uptake. Defects may vary in intensity, from slightly reduced activity to almost total absence of activity.

REVERSIBLE DEFECT. A defect that is present on the initial stress images and no longer present, or present to a lesser degree, on the resting or delayed images. This pattern indicates myocardial ischemia. The change over time is called *redistribution*.

FIXED DEFECT. A defect that is unchanged and present on both exercise and rest (delayed) images. This pattern generally indicates infarction and scar tissue. However, in some patients with fixed ^{201}Tl defects at 2- to 4-hour delayed imaging, improved uptake can be noted on 24-hour redistribution imaging or after a new resting injection (see below).[23,24]

REVERSE REDISTRIBUTION. The initial images are either normal or show a defect, whereas the delayed or rest images show a (more severe) defect.[25] This pattern is frequently observed in patients who have undergone thrombolytic therapy or percutaneous coronary angioplasty. This phenomenon is thought to be caused by initial *excess* of tracer uptake in a reperfused area with a mixture of scar tissue and viable myocytes. Initial accumulation is thus followed by rapid clearance from scar tissue. Although the significance of this finding is controversial, it does *not* represent evidence of exercise-induced ischemia.

THALLIUM-201 LUNG UPTAKE. Normally no, or very little, ^{201}Tl is noted in the lung fields on postexercise images. Increased lung uptake can be quantitated as lung : heart ratio (normal < 0.5) or as lung washout (normal < 42 per cent). This abnormality indicates exercise-induced left ventricular dysfunction.[26]

TRANSIENT LEFT VENTRICULAR DILATION. Occasionally, the left ventricle is noted to be larger following exercise than on the rest or delayed image. This pattern indicates exercise-induced left ventricular dysfunction.[27]

Planar Image Quantification

THALLIUM-201 IMAGES. These images are difficult to interpret visually. Considerable intra- and interobserver variability exists, even among experienced readers.[28] Reproducibility of interpretation is related to a number of factors: (1) the overall quality of the raw data, (2) the quality of image display, (3) the degree of abnormality, (4) the degree of change between exercise and rest images, and (5) observer familiarity with normal variations. Important features of *quantitative analysis* are (1) comparison of the patient's myocardial distribution of radiopharmaceutical to a normal database, (2) quantitative comparison of defect size after exercise with that at delayed imaging, and (3) quantification of myocardial kinetics.

Myocardial Thallium-201 Kinetics

After injection at peak exercise, ^{201}Tl accumulates rapidly in myocardium supplied by normal coronary arteries and subsequently clears slowly from the myocardium (Fig. 10–6). The net myocardial half-life of ^{201}Tl after intravenous injection is 4 to 8 hours. In normal patients, washout at 2 hours after injection is approximately 30 per cent and at 4 hours 35 per cent. The rate of ^{201}Tl washout is related to peak exercise heart rate, exercise duration, and ^{201}Tl blood level. The kinetics of ^{201}Tl in *ischemic myocardium* is variable.[29] When a significant coronary artery stenosis is present, the initial uptake of ^{201}Tl during exercise is lower than in normal myocardium. Subsequently, the washout of ^{201}Tl from this ischemic tissue is lower compared to normal, and accumulation of ^{201}Tl may even occur over time. The initial uptake of ^{201}Tl in infarcted or scarred myocardium is considerably lower than in normal

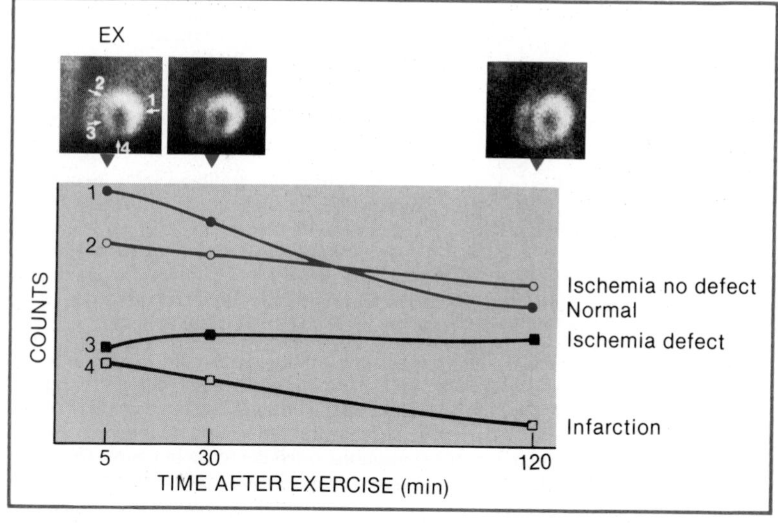

FIGURE 10–6. Thallium-201 time activity curves after exercise (EX) in normal myocardium (1), transiently ischemic myocardium without visual defect (2), transiently ischemic myocardium with a visible defect (3), and old myocardial infarction (4). Normal myocardium (1) shows a gradual decrease of ^{201}Tl activity over time. After transient ischemia, ^{201}Tl may clear more slowly than normally (2) or its concentration may actually increase (3) in the myocardium over time. An old infarct area (4) without exercise-induced myocardial ischemia shows gradual decrease in ^{201}Tl activity over time similar to normal myocardium. The images show an example of a septal defect that gradually fills in over time, except at the apex (4), where an old scar is present. (From Wackers, F.J.T., Myocardial perfusion imaging. *In* Gottschalk, A., Hopper P. B., and Potchan, E. J. [eds.]: Diagnostic Nuclear Medicine. 2nd ed. Baltimore, Williams and Wilkins, 1988, p. 291. Copyright 1988, The Williams and Wilkins Company, Baltimore.)

myocardium. On planar images ^{201}Tl clearance from the infarct parallels that of normal myocardium. This is probably explained by overlap of normal myocardium on planar images.

Computer Processing and Analysis

Whole body images acquired immediately after exercise and at delayed imaging show marked differences in total body distribution of ^{201}Tl.[14] Thus, cardiac background activity is different after exercise compared with that at rest. Because of this difference, normalization of images should be performed for quantitative comparison of initial and delayed cardiac ^{201}Tl activity. Most quantitative algorithms for ^{201}Tl imaging employ an interpolative background correction as described by Goris et al.[30] and later modified by Watson et al.[31] This computer algorithm creates a background image for the cardiac region on the basis of sampling and weighing background activities surrounding the heart. The various published algorithms and commercially available software for quantitative analysis of planar ^{201}Tl images are all similar in concept and differ only in details and data display. Watson et al. proposed use of transverse profile slices across each set of myocardial images (rest and delayed). In this algorithm the quantification of ^{201}Tl distribution and washout is based upon maximal ^{201}Tl activity in a transverse profile. Time activity curves are generated to assess ^{201}Tl kinetics.

Garcia et al.[32] and Wackers et al.[33] proposed circumferential profiles of relative ^{201}Tl distribution and ^{201}Tl washout. Garcia et al.[32] measured maximal ^{201}Tl activity along radii,

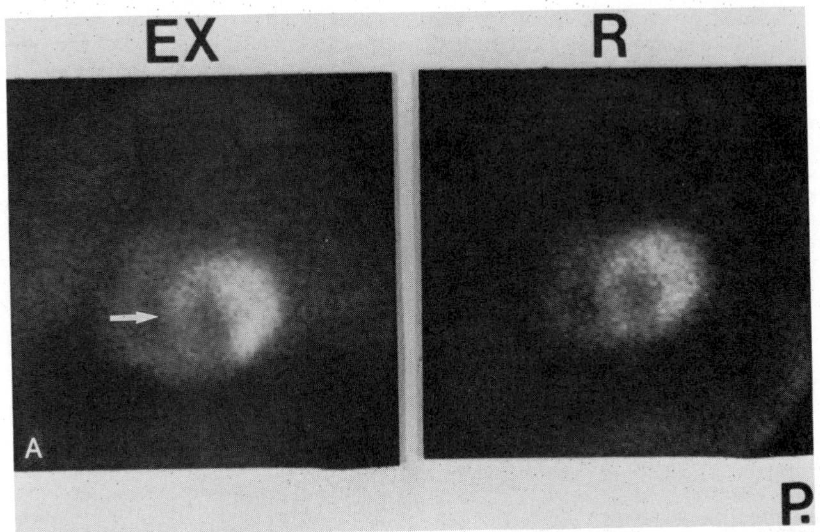

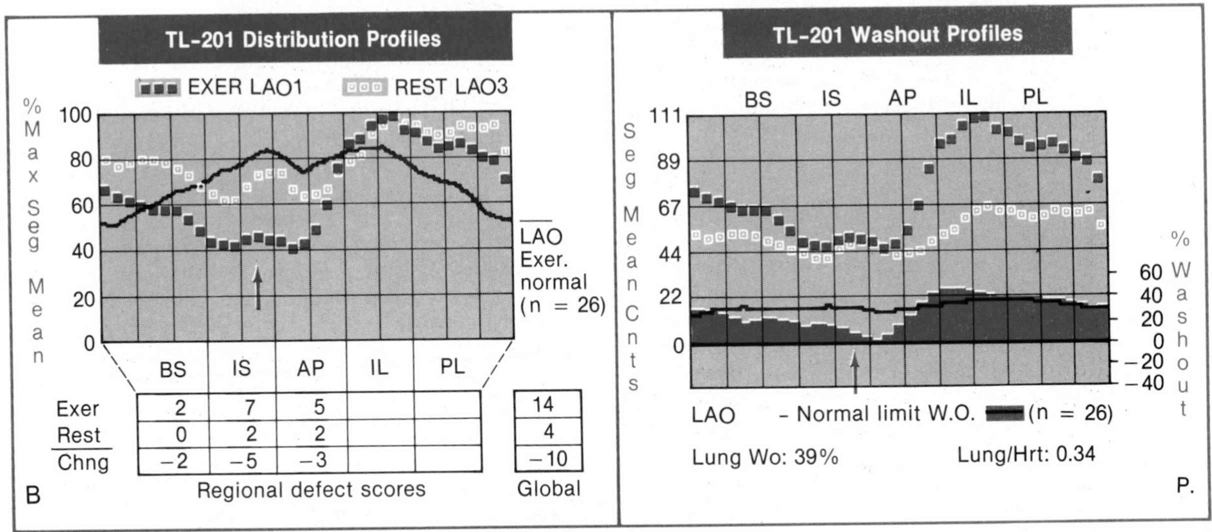

FIGURE 10–7. Left anterior oblique images after exercise (EX) and at redistribution (R) imaging, and circumferential count distribution and washout profiles generated from these images. *A*, The analog images show a reversible exercise-induced anteroseptal defect (arrow).

B, Left, Circumferential count distribution profiles display myocardial activity from basal septum (BS) to posterolateral (PL) wall. The continuous black line indicates the lower-limit-of-normal ^{201}Tl distribution (mean − 2 deviations). The exercise (black dots) and delayed (small dots) profiles are normalized to the area with maximal counts (i.e., PL wall). The exercise profile is below the lower limit of normal in the basal septal (BS), inferoseptal (IS), and apicoseptal (AP) segments. This exercise defect (arrow) is quantified as an integral of 14. The delayed profile shows the graphic representation of a reversible defect (closer to the lower limit of normal). The defect on the delayed images is 4. The change in defect size (reversibility) is 10.

Right, The washout profiles show thallium distribution as absolute counts. In the (normal) inferolateral and posterolateral area absolute counts decreased over time, with a measured washout of approximately 40 per cent. This is shown as the gray histogram on the bottom. The continuous black line indicates the lower limit of normal washout (W.O.). In the ischemic basal septal, inferoseptal, and apicalseptal area, there is no change in absolute counts (inferoseptal and apex) or only a small decrease in counts (basal septal). In these areas the washout is below the lower-limit-of-normal curve (arrow). The patient's lung washout is normal at 39 per cent, and the lung/heart ratio is normal at 0.34.

whereas Wackers[33] used the mean ^{201}Tl activity in 10-degree myocardial segments. Circumferential count distribution profiles are compared to a lower-limit-of-normal profile generated from a normal database consisting of patients in whom there is low probability of coronary artery disease. In a normal study, all circumferential count profile data points after exercise and at delayed imaging are above the lower limit of normal. In a patient with a myocardial perfusion defect, the profile displays data points below the normal limit (Fig. 10–7). This area below normal can be quantitated as an integral, reflecting the size and intensity of a myocardial perfusion defect.[34,43] By comparing the size of the defect after exercise with that at delayed imaging, defect reversibility can be quantified. The reproducibility of these methods has been established.[34]

Tomography Computer Processing and Analysis

The basic principle of SPECT reconstruction is to acquire multiple planar images around an object and reconstruct the three-dimensional object by "back projection." For cardiac tomography, since the heart is eccentrically located in the chest, usually only 180-degree image acquisition is employed.[35] The posterior 180-degree arch is not utilized because it contains poor data as a result of larger distance from the heart and substantial attenuation. After back projection, filtering techniques are used to deal with reconstruction artifacts and enhance the image quality. Tomographic slices are generated perpendicular to the anatomical axes of the heart rather than those of the body.

In most instances, tomographic slices are interpreted mainly by visual inspection. Similar to planar imaging, tomographic images are described qualitatively in terms of normal, fixed, or reversible perfusion defects. The bull's eye or polar map is analyzed either visually or quantitatively with respect to a gender-specific database (Fig. 10–8).[36] Areas that are more than 2 or 2.5 standard deviations below normal distribution are shown as "blackout" or abnormal areas. The comparison of the exercise and delayed polar maps is still subjective. True quantification of defect size and defect reversibility has only recently been developed.[37]

CLINICAL APPLICATIONS OF MYOCARDIAL PERFUSION IMAGING

MYOCARDIAL INFARCTION

DETECTION. Myocardial perfusion imaging with either ^{201}Tl or ^{99m}Tc-SestaMIBI is an extremely sensitive and reliable means of visualizing acute myocardial infarction (Fig. 10–9). The timing of imaging after the onset of acute chest pain is relevant for the results of imaging. Images obtained during the first 6 hours after the onset of myocardial infarction show perfusion abnormalities at the anatomical location of infarction almost without exception.[38] However, as the time interval after onset of chest pain increases, some patients may have normal perfusion images. Serial imaging in patients with acute myocardial infarction revealed that in some patients the size of the myocardial perfusion defect may decrease over time. These observations, initially made in 1974 with ^{201}Tl, are presently better understood. In approximately 20 per cent of patients with acute infarction, spontaneous thrombolysis

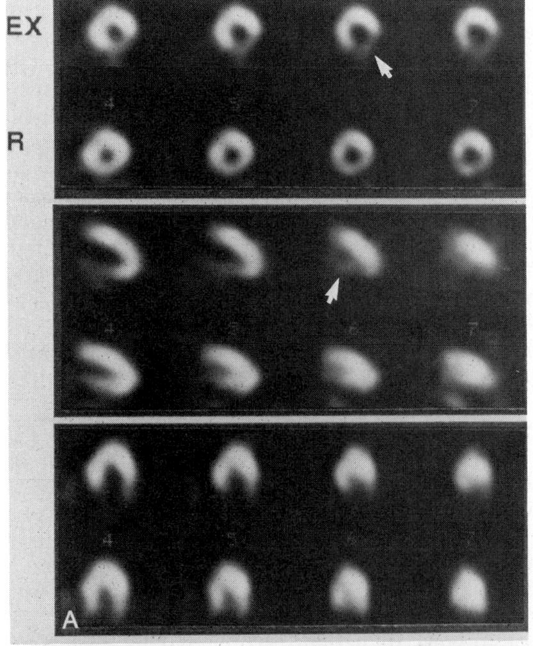

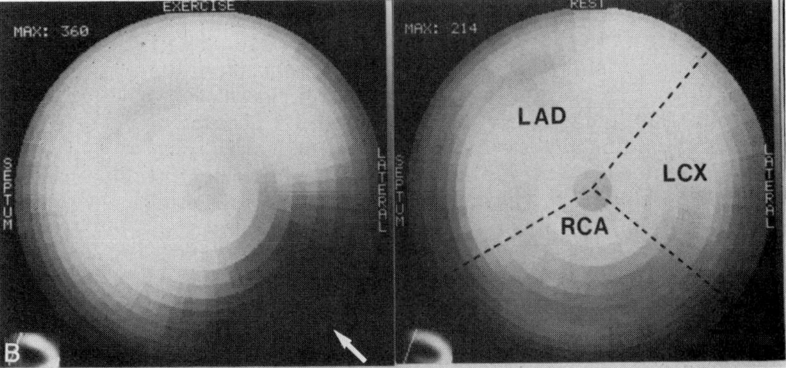

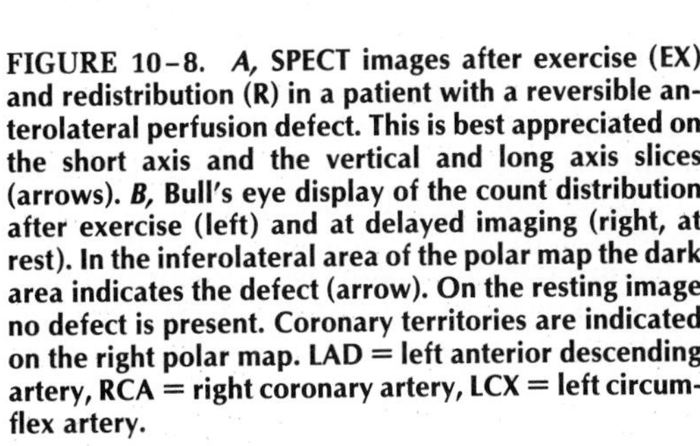

FIGURE 10–8. ***A,*** **SPECT images after exercise (EX) and redistribution (R) in a patient with a reversible anterolateral perfusion defect. This is best appreciated on the short axis and the vertical and long axis slices (arrows).** ***B,*** **Bull's eye display of the count distribution after exercise (left) and at delayed imaging (right, at rest). In the inferolateral area of the polar map the dark area indicates the defect (arrow). On the resting image no defect is present. Coronary territories are indicated on the right polar map. LAD = left anterior descending artery, RCA = right coronary artery, LCX = left circumflex artery.**

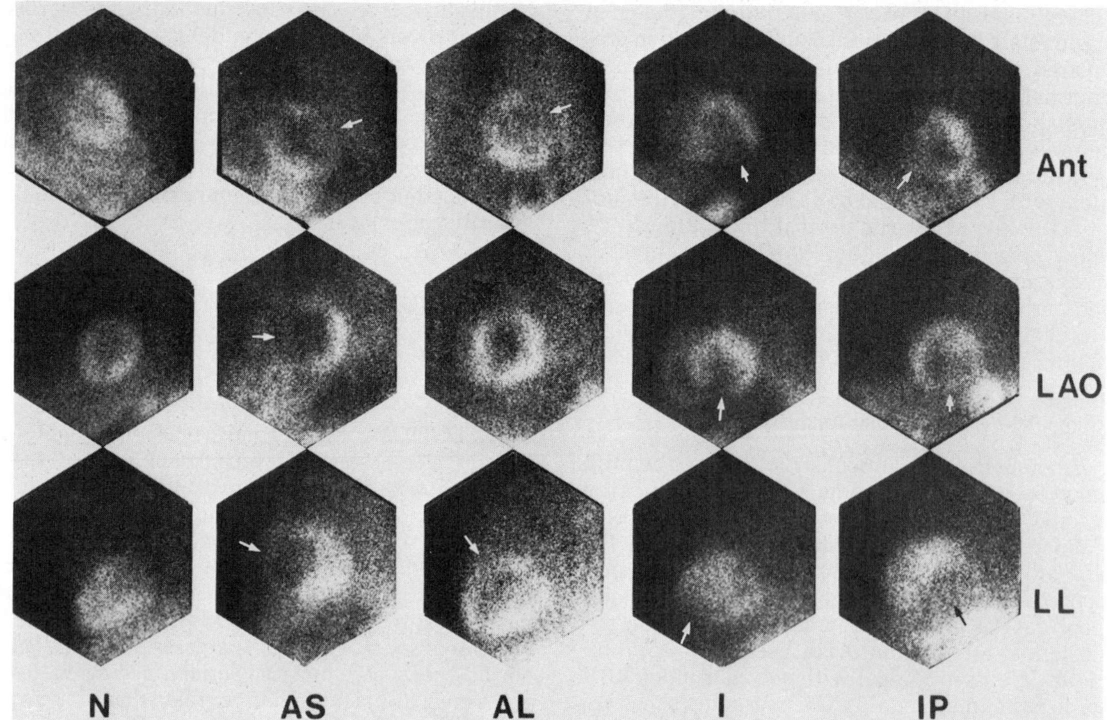

FIGURE 10–9. Thallium-201 images in AMI. Typical images of AMI in three projections. The first column shows normal ^{201}Tl images (N); the second to fourth show typical images of acute myocardial infarcts at anteroseptal (AS), anterolateral (AL), inferior (I), and inferoposterior (IP) locations. The defects are marked by arrows. (Reprinted by permission from Wackers, F.J.T., Busemann Sokole, E., Samson, G., et al.: Value and limitations of thallium-201 scintigraphy in the acute phase of myocardial infarction. N. Engl. J. Med. *295:*1, 1976.)

occurs, which could result in spontaneous improvement of myocardial perfusion images. The location and size of myocardial perfusion defects in acute myocardial infarction correlate well with findings at postmortem.[39]

MYOCARDIAL PERFUSION IMAGING FOR PATIENT TRIAGE. Since acute regional myocardial hypoperfusion can be visualized immediately with myocardial perfusion imaging, the potential use of this method as a means to triage patients in the emergency department has been evaluated. Among patients seen in an emergency department with atypical chest pain and nondiagnostic electrocardiogram but suspected of having acute coronary syndromes, more than 80 per cent who later were proven to have an acute ischemic syndrome (i.e., acute infarction or unstable angina) had abnormal ^{201}Tl perfusion images.[40] However, this clinical application has not found acceptance as a method to evaluate patients in the emergency department, probably because of the cost and limited availability of the ^{201}Tl as well as logistic problems of imaging in the emergency setting. It is possible that with the simpler logistics of imaging with ^{99m}Tc-labeled myocardial perfusion imaging agents, there may be renewed interest in this particular application.

THROMBOLYTIC THERAPY (see also p. 1230). During the early hours of acute myocardial infarction, evaluation of myocardial perfusion is of interest in patients who have thrombolytic therapy. Serial imaging with ^{201}Tl can demonstrate a decrease in the size of a myocardial perfusion defect over time in patients who had successful reperfusion of the infarct artery.[41] However, imaging with ^{201}Tl in the setting of thrombolytic therapy is not practical clinically. Because of ^{201}Tl redistribution, myocardial imaging has to be performed before initiation of therapy. This would cause a clinically unacceptable delay. A more practical approach is the use of ^{99m}Tc-SestaMIBI. Because of the lack of significant redistribution, this imaging agent can be injected *before* initiation of thrombolytic therapy, and imaging of myocardial perfusion can be performed later using either planar imaging at the patient's bedside or SPECT imaging in the nuclear cardiology laboratory.[42–44a] Successful thrombolysis of the infarct artery could be predicted by a decrease of the size of myocardial perfusion defects on serial ^{99m}Tc-SestaMIBI imaging (Fig. 10–10).

The noninvasive demonstration of successful myocardial reperfusion by thrombolysis could be useful in defining the management of individual patients.[44b] For example, patients who apparently have failure of thrombolytic therapy (i.e., no change in myocardial perfusion defect), may be candidates for a more aggressive and invasive approach. On the other hand, patients who apparently have successful reperfusion as demonstrated by improvement of myocardial perfusion may be more appropriate candidates for conservative management. With use of a "split dose" technique (i.e., a small dose initially followed by a larger dose later), it will be feasible to obtain the same information on risk area and salvage within a few hours after the patient's arrival in the emergency department.

PROGNOSIS. The size of myocardial perfusion defects in stable patients after acute myocardial infarction has been shown to be of prognostic significance. Silverman et al.[45] showed that patients with large resting myocardial perfusion defects had a significantly poorer prognosis and survival than patients with small myocardial perfusion defects. This was independent of other clinical parameters. Visualization of the right ventricle at rest[46] or increased ^{201}Tl uptake in the lung at rest in patients with recent infarction[47] has been reported as an additional indicator of a higher incidence of future adverse cardiac events.

UNSTABLE ANGINA (see also p. 1334). In patients with unstable angina and without prior myocardial infarction, myocardial perfusion defects have been demonstrated. These perfusion defects not only are demonstrable when the radiopharmaceutical is injected *during* chest pain but also for considerable time *after* the angina has subsided.[48–50] Initially, it was thought that impaired transmembrane transport of ^{201}Tl by depletion of ATP was responsible for such defects. However, it is now well recognized that ^{201}Tl uptake is primarily flow-dependent. ATP depletion in ischemia is not sufficient to explain perfusion defects in unstable angina. Resting ^{201}Tl defects in patients with unstable angina are invariably reversible, indicating viable myocardium. Similar observations have been reported in patients with unstable angina, using

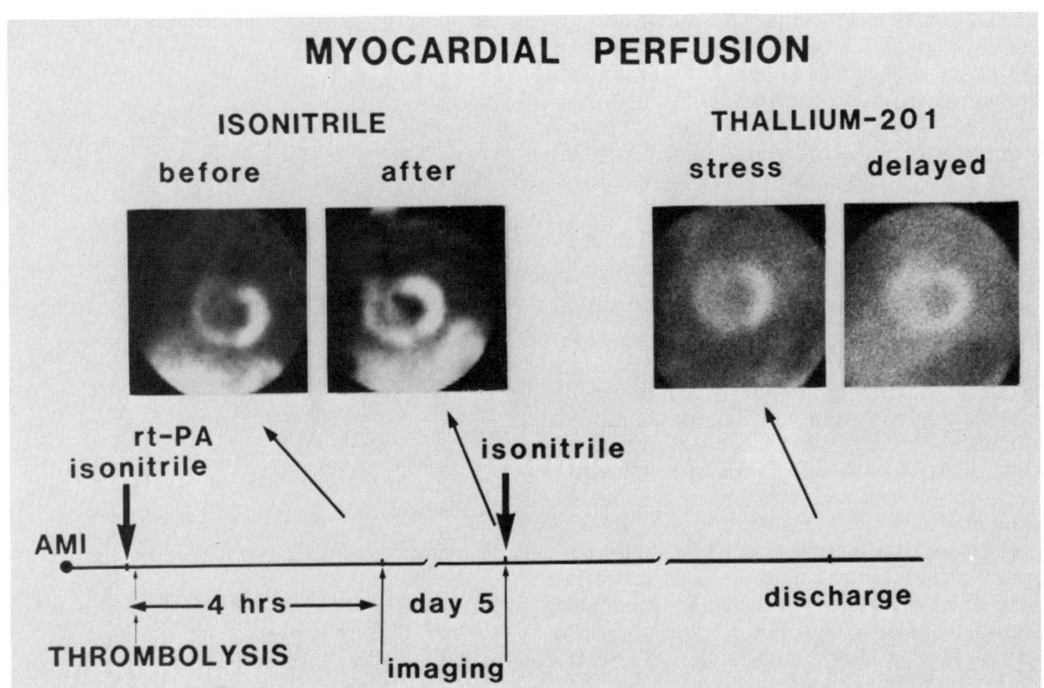

FIGURE 10-10. Serial ^{99m}Tc isonitrile images before and after thrombolysis and ^{201}Tl stress/delayed imaging at hospital discharge. The patient had an acute anteroseptal infarction. ^{99m}Tc SestaMIBI (isonitrile) was injected immediately before thrombolytic therapy with rtPA. Four hours later, when the patient was in the coronary care unit, an image was obtained of the risk area before thrombolysis that showed a septal defect. Imaging was repeated 5 days later. The septum was partially visualized, indicating reperfusion of the infarct artery. The patient had a further uncomplicated clinical course and had predischarge ^{201}Tl stress imaging. This showed a reversible exercise-induced septal defect. This imaging sequence demonstrates reperfusion by isonitrile imaging and residual jeopardized viable myocardium by ^{201}Tl stress imaging. (From Kayden, D. S., Mattera, J. A., Zaret, B. L., and Wackers, F.J.T.: Demonstration of reperfusion after thrombolysis with technetium-99m isonitrile myocardial imaging. J. Nucl. Med. *29*:1865, 1988.)

^{99m}Tc-SestaMIBI.[51] Patients with abnormal electrocardiographic findings during pain had larger myocardial perfusion defects than those who did not. These findings in patients with unstable angina indicate that in this condition impaired myocardial blood flow persists longer than can be judged from the patients' clinical status or electrocardiogram. Patients with reversible resting myocardial perfusion defects usually have severe multivessel coronary artery disease.

Resting imaging in patients with recurrent chest pain after infarction or with unstable angina is useful to demonstrate objectively the presence of transient myocardial hypoperfusion and viable myocardium. This information can be very helpful when myocardial revascularization is considered.

DETECTION OF OLD MYOCARDIAL INFARCTION. Myocardial perfusion imaging does not differentiate between acute myocardial infarction, acute ischemia, or old scar. A substantial number of patients with small or old myocardial infarction may have normal images. Frequently, prior myocardial infarction can be recognized only as "thinner" myocardial segments. In about one-half of patients with old infarction, ^{201}Tl images may become normal. This occurs particularly in patients with old inferior wall myocardial infarcts.

CHRONIC CORONARY ARTERY DISEASE

(See also p. 1293)

In patients with chronic stable coronary artery disease, myocardial perfusion imaging is used in conjunction with exercise testing. Physical exercise can be performed either on a treadmill, which is most popular in the United States, or on an upright bicycle, which is frequently employed in Europe. Physical exercise has the advantage of providing additional useful clinical and physiological parameters, such as duration of exercise, total workload capability, maximum heart rate, presence of exercise-induced symptoms and electrocardiographic changes, and blood pressure response. However, a substantial number of patients referred to a nuclear cardiology laboratory cannot exercise because of orthopedic, neurological, or peripheral vascular problems. In the latter group of patients, pharmacological vasodilatation with dipyridamole or adenosine provides a useful alternative approach.

PHYSICAL EXERCISE. Several standardized treadmill exercise protocols exist. The most widely used protocol was designed by Bruce (Fig. 6-2, p. 162). Nonimaging end points are reproduction of the patient's symptoms, exhaustion, hypotension or decrease in systolic blood pressure of 20 mm Hg or more, ventricular arrhythmias, and severe ST-segment depression on electrocardiography. An intravenous line should be in place in a large anticubital vein for injection of the radiopharmaceutical agent. When the end point of exercise is approached, the radiopharmaceutical is injected rapidly into the intravenous line and flushed with saline. The patient is then encouraged to exercise for another 1 to 2 minutes at the same level of exercise. This continuation of exercise after injection of the radiotracer is crucial for diagnostic stress imaging. It is important to maintain heart rate, and thus myocardial blood flow, at peak exercise level to allow accumulation of the radiotracer during a "steady ischemic state." If the patient is unable to continue exercising at the same level, the speed and grade of the treadmill can be reduced to a lower level. For bicycle exercise, a similar graded exercise protocol is used. Usually the patient starts at 25 kpm, and the resistance is increased every 3 minutes until an exercise end point is reached. The purpose of exercise is to increase cardiac metabolic demands and to test the ability of the coronary circulation to meet these demands by an appropriate increase of myocardial blood flow. Consequently, myocardial ischemia is frequently provoked with physical exercise.

PHARMACOLOGICAL VASODILATION. A substantial number of patients referred to the nuclear cardiology laboratory are incapable of exercising on a treadmill or bicycle. Patients with orthopedic, neurological, or peripheral vascular problems can be evaluated for the presence of significant coronary artery disease by use of pharmacological vasodilation in combination with ^{201}Tl imaging. Furthermore, patients on beta-blocking medication who are unable to increase their heart rate adequately by physical exercise have been studied successfully with pharmacological dilatation. The most extensive clinical experience exists with intravenous dipyridamole. Pharmacological vasodilation by dipyridamole infusion frequently does not provoke myocardial ischemia.[52] Intravenous infusion of dipyridamole blocks the cellular reabsorption of adenosine and thus increases the concentrations of adenosine, an endogenous vasodilator that activates specific receptors. Coronary blood flow is autoregulated by adenosine to meet myocardial metabolic demands (p. 1168).[52] In patients without coronary artery disease, dipyridamole infusion (and physical exercise) causes vasodilatation and increases coronary blood flow 3 to 5 times above baseline levels. In patients with significant coronary artery disease, the resistance vessels distal to the stenosis are already dilated, often maximally, in order to maintain normal resting flow. In these patients, infusion of dipyridamole does not cause further significant vasodilation in the diseased vascular bed. However, in the adjacent myocardium supplied by normal coronary arteries, a substantial increase in myocardial blood flow occurs. In this manner, *heterogeneity of myocardial blood flow is created:* territories supplied by diseased arteries are relatively hypoperfused compared with normal regions. This can be imaged with a gamma camera employing a radiotracer, such as ^{201}Tl, ^{99m}Tc-SestaMIBI, or ^{99m}Tc-teboroxime.

Dipyridamole Infusion Protocol. Dipyridamole is infused over a 4-minute period (0.568 mg/kg).[52] At approximately 4 minutes after completion of the infusion, maximal dilatory effect is achieved. This is usually associated with a modest increase in heart rate (10 beats per minute), and slight decrease (10 mm Hg) in systolic blood pressure. At this point in time the radiotracer is injected intravenously.[52a] In some laboratories dipyridamole infusion is combined with handgrip exercise. This appears to decrease the incidence of side effects that occur in about 50 per cent of the patients during infusion of dipyridamole.[53] Approximately 20 per cent may have electrocardiographical changes, and 10 per cent may experience angina, although most frequent complaints are of headache, flushing, and nausea. Chest discomfort is probably caused by "coronary steal." In this situation, the marked increase in blood flow in the *normal* myocardial zones "steals" blood away via collaterals from the vascular bed supplied by significantly diseased coronary arteries. This, and other undesirable side effects, can usually be reversed quickly by blocking adenosine receptor sites with intravenous aminophylline.

Adenosine Infusion. Initial clinical experience of direct intravenous infusion of adenosine (140 μg/kg/min) has been reported.[54a] It appears that the coronary vasodilatory effect of adenosine is more potent and more consistent than that of dipyridamole.[54b] Side effects, however, are also more common, occurring in about 75 per cent of the patients (Table 10–2). Approximately 50 per cent of the patients may experience chest discomfort and many have headache, nausea, and flushing. Atrioventricular conduction abnormalities have been reported occasionally in patients receiving adenosine infusion. This has been of some concern. However, because of

TABLE 10–2 REPORTED SIDE EFFECTS (% OF PATIENTS) OF INTRAVENOUS DIPYRIDAMOLE AND ADENOSINE THALLIUM 201 IMAGING

	DIPYRIDAMOLE Ranhosky et al.[53]	ADENOSINE Verani et al.[54]
CARDIAC		
Fatal MI	0.05	0
Nonfatal MI	0.05	0
Chest pain	19.7	57
ST-T changes on ECG	7.5	12
Ventricular ectopy	5.2	?
Tachycardia	3.2	?
Hypotension	4.6	?
Blood pressure liability	1.6	?
Hypertension	1.5	?
AV block	0	10
NONCARDIAC		
Headache	12.2	35
Dizziness	11.8	?
Nausea	4.6	?
Flushing	3.4	29
Pain (nonspecific)	2.6	?
Dyspnea	2.6	15
Paraesthesia	1.3	?
Fatigue	1.2	?
Dyspepsia	1.0	?
Acute bronchospasm	0.15	0

MI = myocardial infarction; ECG = electrocardiogram; AV = atrioventricular.
Patients with history of bronchospasm excluded.
? Not reported.

the short half-life of adenosine, side effects can be reversed almost instantaneously by terminating the infusion of adenosine. As of this writing, adenosine has not been approved by the Food and Drug Administration for use with myocardial perfusion imaging.

ASSESSMENT OF MYOCARDIAL VIABILITY. Myocardial viability occasionally may be underestimated in patients who appear to have a "scintigraphic scar," i.e., a fixed ^{201}Tl defect on 2- to 4-hour delayed imaging.[23,24] Some of these patients show normal ^{201}Tl uptake in the same area after coronary bypass surgery or coronary angioplasty. Depending on patient selection, approximately 30 to 50 per cent of patients with fixed ^{201}Tl stress defect on 2- to 3-hour delayed imaging may show "late filling-in" on either 24-hour redistribution imaging or after reinjection at rest (Fig. 10–11).[55–57] Since 24-hour redistribution images are generally of suboptimal quality, reinjection of ^{201}Tl at rest is preferred. This can be done either on the day following the stress test by administration of a new dose (2 mCi) of ^{201}Tl, or immediately after delayed imaging by administration of an additional 1 mCi of ^{201}Tl. The phenomenon of late filling-in cannot be predicted by clinical parameters such as the presence of prior infarction, the presence of angina, or electrocardiographic signs of ischemia. Late filling-in correlates in selected patients with improvement of wall motion after revascularization and metabolically viable

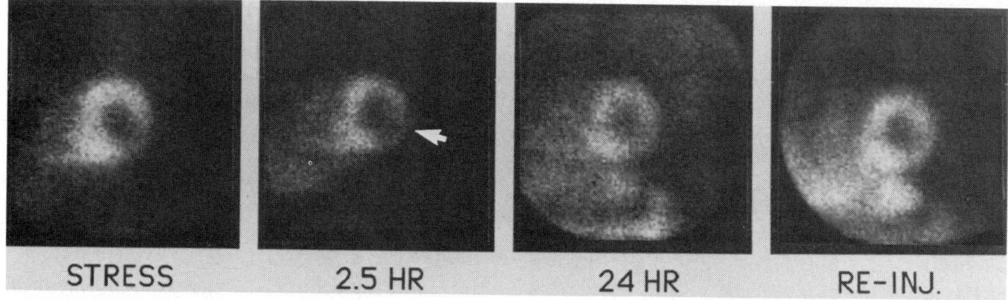

FIGURE 10–11. Thallium-201 images after exercise (stress), 2.5-hr delayed imaging, 24-hr delayed imaging, and after a reinjection of ^{201}Tl at rest. This patient had an apparently fixed defect (arrow) at 2.5-hr delayed imaging. However, at 24-hr redistribution imaging, filling in of the defect can be recognized. After reinjection of ^{201}Tl at rest, further normalization of the image can be seen.

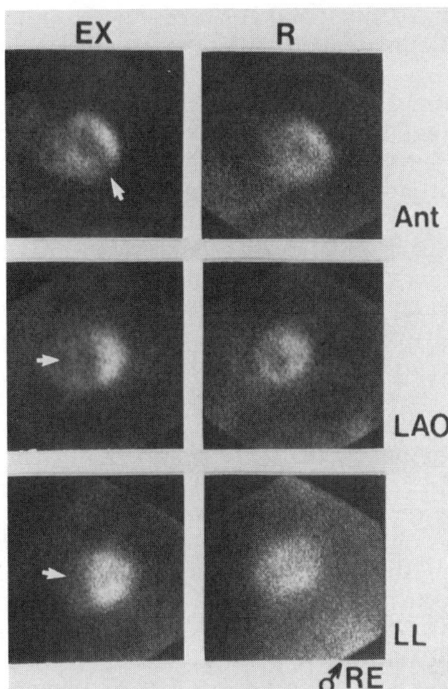

FIGURE 10–12. Thallium-201 stress imaging in a patient with a critical stenosis of the left anterior descending coronary artery. After exercise (EX), an anteroseptal myocardial perfusion defect is present (arrows). On redistribution (R) imaging, the defect has almost completely filled in.

myocardium seen on positron F-18-deoxyglucose imaging[58a] (p. 302).

Clinical Results of Exercise Testing and Myocardial Perfusion Imaging

Each year more than 1,000,000 patients undergo ^{201}Tl exercise testing in the United States (Fig. 10–12). Over the last 15 years the clinical usefulness of the tests has been established. A review of the literature in 1982 showed that the overall published sensitivity and specificity of ^{201}Tl exercise imaging by visual analysis of images was 83 and 90 per cent, respectively, for a total of 2084 patients.[59] This compares favorably with that of traditional exercise electrocardiography, which in the same review had a sensitivity of 58 per cent and a specificity of 82 per cent. The introduction of computer processing and quantification of ^{201}Tl images has improved the overall detection of coronary disease (Table 10–3). Several investigators have reported a sensitivity and specificity greater than 90 per cent.[33,60–62] Most false-negative results occurred in patients with single-vessel disease. Nevertheless, the detection of single-vessel disease improved from 55 per cent by visual analysis to 84 per cent by computer-assisted quantitative analysis. Almost all patients with double- or triple-vessel disease are detected by quantitative imaging. The ability to predict accurately the number of diseased vessels and to identify specific vessels by planar imaging is suboptimal and reflects an inherent limitation of planar technology. The improved detection of patients with significant coronary disease by quantitative analysis is achieved in a number of ways.[63,64] The graphic display of ^{201}Tl distribution and of ^{201}Tl washout (Figs. 10–6 and 10–7*B*) significantly increases the confidence with which images are categorized as either definitely normal or definitely abnormal. The assessment and quantification of ^{201}Tl washout is a major factor responsible for improved detection of extensive and multivessel coronary disease. However, washout analysis should be performed with caution, because many variables affect the reliability of quantification of myocardial clearance on planar imaging.

TABLE 10–3 SENSITIVITY AND SPECIFICITY FOR DETECTION OF CORONARY ARTERY DISEASE BY QUANTITATIVE PLANAR THALLIUM-201 SCINTIGRAPHY

AUTHOR		NO. PATIENTS	SENSITIVITY %	SPECIFICITY %
Berger[49]	1981	140	91	90
Maddahi[61]	1981	67	93	91
Wackers[33]	1985	150	89	95
Kaul[63]	1986	325	90	80
VanTrain[62]	1986	157	84	88

Pharmacological stress ^{201}Tl imaging with intravenous dipyridamole is widely used for detection of coronary artery disease in patients who cannot exercise (Fig. 10–13). The reported sensitivity and specificity are similar to those with physical exercise.[54,54a,65–67]

DETECTION OF HIGH-RISK CORONARY ARTERY DISEASE. The more severe the coronary artery disease which is present, the more likely it is that exercise ^{201}Tl images will be abnormal. Most patients (approximately 95 per cent) with left main coronary disease have abnormal ^{201}Tl stress images.[64] However, the expected typical left main pattern, i.e., defects in the anteroseptal and posterolateral walls, is found in only a minority (approximately 14 per cent) of patients with left main coronary artery disease.[64,68,69] The majority (approximately 75 per cent) of patients have multiple ^{201}Tl defects and frequently abnormally increased lung uptake of ^{201}Tl as well.[70] Although most patients with three-vessel disease have abnormal ^{201}Tl stress images, only approximately 60 per cent have multiple defects in two or more vascular regions. Most frequently, disease in the left circumflex coronary artery is not detected on ^{201}Tl planar images.

High-risk planar ^{201}Tl images (Fig. 10–14) can be characterized by (1) multiple reversible defects and/or washout of abnormalities in two or more coronary artery territories, (2) increased pulmonary ^{201}Tl uptake after exercise, and (3) transient dilatation of the left ventricle immediately after exercise. This high-risk pattern is highly specific (approximately 95 per cent) for multivessel coronary artery disease; however, the sensitivity is only about 70 per cent. Therefore, in absence of the aforementioned scintigraphic characteristics, the presence of multivessel disease cannot be ruled out.

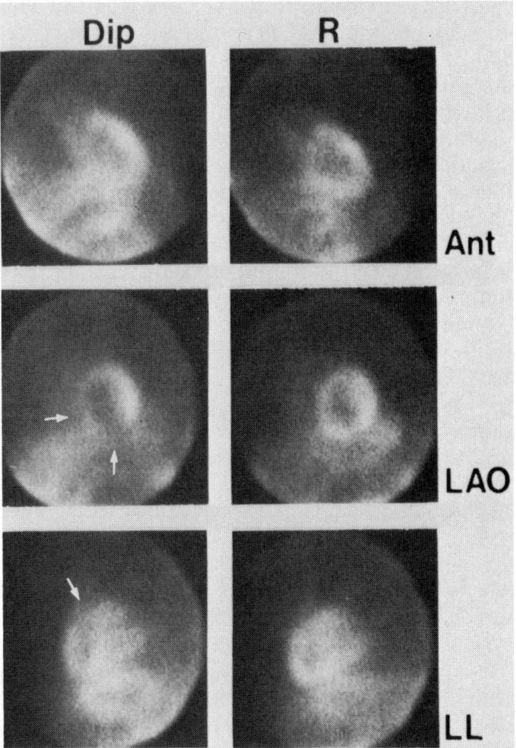

FIGURE 10–13. Thallium-201 imaging after pharmacological stress with dipyridamole (Dip). There is excellent visualization of the heart, but substantial uptake also has occurred in the subdiaphragmatic organs. A reversible anteroseptal and apical defect is present (arrows). R = redistribution image.

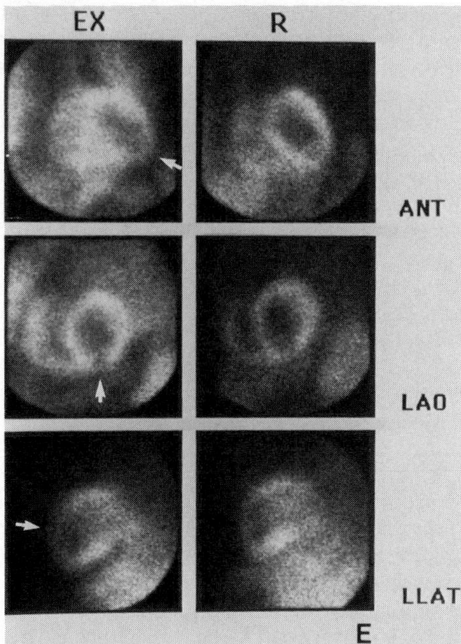

FIGURE 10–14. High-risk ^{201}Tl images. After exercise the heart is enlarged and there is increased lung uptake of ^{201}Tl. Furthermore, there is a partially reversible anteroapical myocardial perfusion defect (arrows).

SEVERITY OF THALLIUM-201 DEFECTS. ^{201}Tl defects vary in intensity. A defect can be very dense (severe), i.e., almost without any ^{201}Tl uptake. On the other hand, some residual activity may still be present within the defect. The severity of perfusion defects is often assessed using a semiquantitative scoring system: 0 = normal, 1 = mildly reduced or equivocal, 2 = moderately reduced, and 3 = severely reduced. Computer analysis of ^{201}Tl distribution circumferential profiles provides a means to quantify precisely the extent (the number of angles below the lower limit) and severity (area below the lower limit) of a perfusion defect. This measurement can be expressed as an integrated defect score.[34,71]

THALLIUM-201 STRESS IMAGING AND PROGNOSIS. The detection of coronary artery disease is only one aspect of the clinical value of ^{201}Tl stress imaging. An important additional feature is the ability to determine prognosis. The first critical finding on ^{201}Tl images is the presence or absence of a reversible defect and ^{201}Tl redistribution, i.e., ischemia.[63] Patients with evidence of transient ischemia have a higher incidence of future cardiac events than patients with fixed defects. In patients without prior myocardial infarction, semiquantitative assessment of the number of reversible ^{201}Tl defects or quantitative measurement of the extent, severity, and degree of reversibility of ^{201}Tl defects correlates with the occurrence of subsequent cardiac events (Fig. 10–15).[72–76] Gibson et al.[77] evaluated patients after uncomplicated myocardial infarction by quantitative ^{201}Tl stress imaging. Patients with a fixed single ^{201}Tl stress defect and without washout abnormalities (i.e., with normal clearance rate of ^{201}Tl from the heart) at hospital discharge had only a 6 per cent cardiac event rate (death, recurrent infarction, or unstable angina). Patients who had high-risk findings on predischarge ^{201}Tl stress images (multiple defects in more than one vascular region, abnormal washout, or increased lung uptake) had a 51 per cent cardiac event rate. Several other investigators have reported similar results on the prognostic value of ^{201}Tl stress imaging after myocardial infarction using either physical or pharmacological stress.[78–81] Transient postexercise dilatation of the left ventricle is another scintigraphic marker of poor prognosis. Brown et al.[82] reported that patients with recurrent chest pain *after myocardial infarction* frequently had ischemia *within* the infarct region (75 per cent of patients), whereas only 25 per cent of patients had ischemia at a distance. Patients with evidence of defect reversibility had a substantially poorer prognosis and higher incidence of revascularization procedures than did patients who did not have demonstrable reversibility.

On the other hand, the presence of *normal ^{201}Tl stress images* by quantitative analysis, even when coronary artery stenosis is angiographically documented, indicates favorable prognosis with low cardiac event rate.[83–86] A number of studies have shown a yearly nonfatal myocardial infarction rate of 0.6 per cent per year and a mortality rate of 0.5 per cent per year in patients with *normal quantitative* ^{201}Tl stress tests.

These data on abnormal and normal ^{201}Tl stress tests indicate that the extent of myocardial perfusion defects, or the lack thereof, provide significant functional or prognostic information that can surpass the anatomical information obtained from coronary angiograms. Optimally, both techniques are used together.

TOMOGRAPHIC THALLIUM-201 STRESS IMAGING. A major *limitation* of planar ^{201}Tl imaging is the overlap by projection of various coronary supply territories. SPECT allows separation of these territories by reconstruction of slices through the heart at different orientations and at different levels. In many laboratories SPECT imaging has replaced or is performed in addition to planar imaging (Fig. 10–16). However, it should be recognized that SPECT imaging with ^{201}Tl also has its limitations. The gamma cameras generally employed for tomography have $\frac{3}{4}$-inch thick crystals, which is not optimal for imaging with ^{201}Tl and frequently results in suboptimal count density. Although the separation of various vascular territories is improved over planar imaging, the spatial resolution of the SPECT slices is inferior compared with that of planar imaging (12 mm for planar imaging versus 19 mm for SPECT imaging). The SPECT slices are heavily processed and filtered. On reconstructed images it may be difficult to recog-

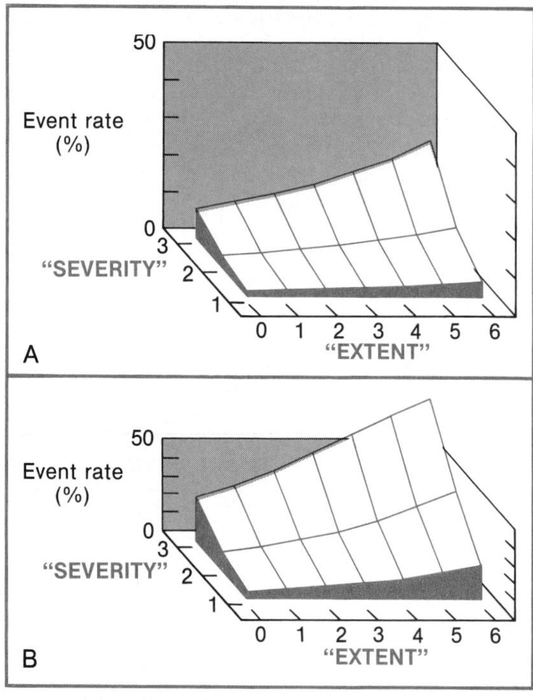

FIGURE 10–15. Extent and severity of ^{201}Tl myocardial hypoperfusion defects as predictors of prognosis in patients with coronary artery disease. The data are from 1114 patients who were able to exercise to at least 85 per cent of maximal heart rate (panel A) and 275 patients who were not able to achieve 85 per cent of maximal heart rate (panel B). In both groups, cardiac event rate (death, nonfatal myocardial infarction, and referral for coronary bypass surgery) rises as a curvilinear function of the extent and severity of ^{201}Tl defects. There is at least a threefold increase in event rate for group B in comparison with group A. (Note that the event rate axis for B is half of that for A.) (From Ladenheim, M. L., Pollock, B. H., Rozanski, A., et al.: Extent and severity of myocardial hypoperfusion as predictors of prognosis in patients with suspected coronary artery disease. Reprinted by permission of the American College of Cardiology. J. Am. Coll. Cardiol. *7*:464, 1986.)

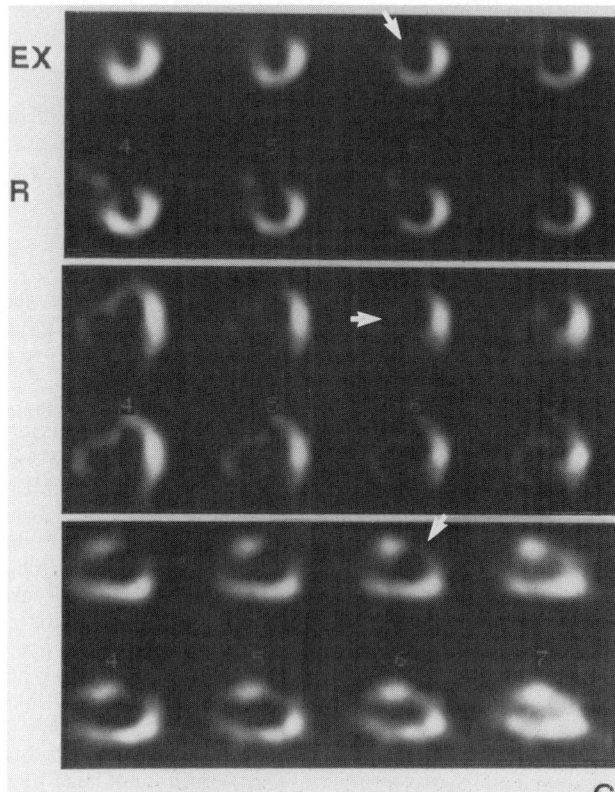

FIGURE 10–16. Thallium-201 SPECT images after exercise (EX) and at redistribution (R) in a patient with recent anteroseptal myocardial infarction. A fixed anteroseptal defect is present (arrows) on all reconstructed slices. No convincing evidence of reversibility is present.

nize suboptimal raw data, such as low count density, motion, and attenuation artifacts. The detection of coronary artery disease by SPECT imaging is very similar to that of planar imaging (Table 10–4).[87–93] However, the identification of disease in specific coronary artery distributions, in particular of the left circumflex artery, is improved by SPECT in comparison with planar imaging.

The *sensitivity* to detect coronary artery disease by SPECT has been reported to be over 90 per cent. However, many investigators report a rather low *specificity*, ranging from 60 to 70 per cent. This lack of specificity has been explained by "referral bias."[94] That is, ^{201}Tl stress imaging has become so well accepted in the clinical practice of cardiology that patients with normal ^{201}Tl stress tests are now rarely referred for cardiac catheterization; this has served to decrease the number of apparent false-negatives. On the other hand, the occasional patient who has normal coronary arteries on angiography almost always is referred for the latter examination because of abnormal ^{201}Tl stress test results. The true specificity of ^{201}Tl stress SPECT therefore can no longer be assessed in patients undergoing coronary angiography because of referral bias. However, specificity should be tested in patients with low probability of coronary artery disease. In these patients the "normalcy rate" is determined. The normalcy rate of planar imaging is generally over 95 per cent; with tomographic imaging this has been reported to be in the range of 85 per cent. This suggests that false-positive tests are frequently obtained with SPECT imaging. We believe that referral bias is only partially responsible for suboptimal specificity; technical aspects of imaging also play a significant role.

TABLE 10–4 SENSITIVITY AND SPECIFICITY FOR DETECTION OF CORONARY ARTERY DISEASE BY SINGLE PHOTON EMISSION TOMOGRAPHY (SPECT)

AUTHOR		NO. PATIENTS	SENSITIVITY %	SPECIFICITY %
Tamaki[87]	1984	104	Q 91	92
			V 80	93
De Pasquale[88]	1988	210	V 95	71
Borges-Neto[89]	1988	100 (dip.)	V 92	69
Maddahi[90]	1989	110	V 96	56
Fintel[91]	1989	112	V 91	90
Iskandrian[92]	1989	164	V 88	62
Mahmarian[93]	1990	360	Q 93	87
			V 95	76

Q = Quantitative analysis.
V = Visual analysis.
dip. = Dipyridamole.

Few investigators have compared planar ^{201}Tl imaging with SPECT ^{201}Tl imaging in the same patients. Fintel et al.[91] performed receiver operating curve analysis of planar and SPECT studies in the same patients and found a slight but definite superiority of tomographic imaging over planar imaging. Others found similar sensitivity and specificity for planar and SPECT imaging. However, most investigators report consistently improved detection of disease in specific coronary arteries. For this reason, SPECT imaging has been extensively used in the evaluation of patients before and after percutaneous transluminal coronary angioplasty. When the coronary anatomy is known, SPECT ^{201}Tl imaging can be extremely helpful in directing therapeutic and procedural decisions.

THALLIUM-201 IMAGING FOR PREOPERATIVE SCREENING. An important clinical application of ^{201}Tl imaging is in evaluating patients with coronary disease who are considered for major noncardiac surgery. In these patients it is of clinical importance to identify those at increased risk for perioperative coronary events. In patients with peripheral arterial disease, in whom the co-existence of coronary artery disease is very likely, dipyridamole-^{201}Tl imaging has been shown to be useful. Boucher et al.[95] showed that patients with reversible ^{201}Tl defects after dipyridamole infusion had a high incidence of perioperative cardiac events. Although other parameters for increased risk were identified (patient age, prior myocardial infarction, and clinical angina), the presence or absence of reversible ^{201}Tl defects was the single most important additional prognostic indicator. As expected, patients with extensive defect reversibility (greater ischemic burden), pulmonary ^{201}Tl uptake, and cavitary dilatation were at higher risk than those with only small abnormalities.[96,96a,96b]

^{99m}Tc-SestaMIBI STRESS IMAGING. Since the introduction of ^{99m}Tc-SestaMIBI in 1989, many thousands of patients have been evaluated with this myocardial perfusion agent (Fig. 10–17). Several comparative studies, both by planar and SPECT techniques, have shown that the detection of coronary artery disease with ^{99m}Tc-SestaMIBI is comparable to that with ^{201}Tl.[10,97,98] ^{99m}Tc-SestaMIBI can also be used in conjunction with dipyridamole pharmacological vasodilatation in patients who are not capable of physical exercise. Initial reports indicate diagnostic results similar to those with ^{201}Tl.

With respect to detection of ischemia and scar, a greater than 80 per cent agreement between the two imaging agents has been found consistently. Because of the absence of significant redistribution, exercise and rest tests with ^{99m}Tc-SestaMIBI imaging were performed initially on two separate days: one for injection during exercise, a second for injection at rest. Taillefer et al.[99] reported the feasibility of performing rest and exercise images on the same day by administering a smaller dose at rest and then a second larger dose during exercise. This sequence is preferred because, in some patients with large exercise defects, defect reversibility can be underestimated when the exercise study is performed first.

The relatively high dose of ^{99m}Tc-SestaMIBI that is permitted makes it possible to perform first-pass angiocardiography in combination with myocardial perfusion imaging.[100,101] The clinical importance of both resting and peak exercise left ventricular ejection fractions is discussed on p. 299. With ^{99m}Tc-SestaMIBI, it is feasible to obtain concomitant peak exercise left ventricular ejection fraction and perfusion data.

The high photon flux of ^{99m}Tc-SestaMIBI also makes it feasible to acquire ECG-gated myocardial perfusion images. The

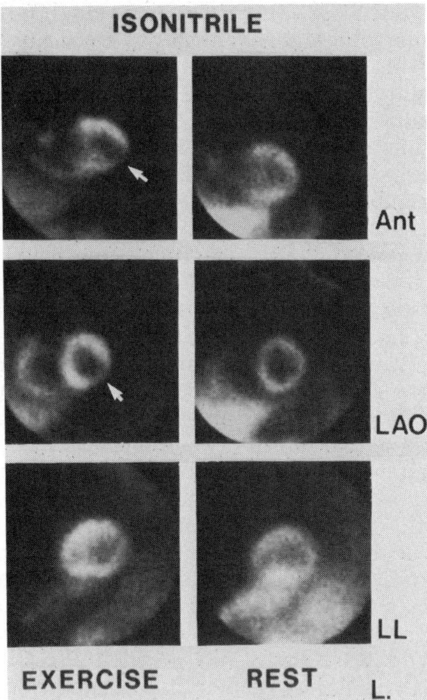

FIGURE 10–17. Technetium-99m SestaMIBI (isonitrile) images after exercise and at rest. Reversible inferolateral and inferoapical perfusion defect (arrows) is present. (From Wackers, F.J.T., Berman, D. S., Maddahi, J., et al.: Technetium-99m hexakis 2-methoxyisobutyl isonitrile: Human biodistribution, dosimetry, safety and preliminary comparison to thallium-201 for myocardial perfusion imaging. J. Nucl. Med. *30:*301,1989.)

ECG-gated myocardial perfusion imaging can be displayed as an endless loop movie, similar to the format commonly employed for ECG-gated blood pool imaging. The authors have developed a nongeometric count-based method to create functional images from ECG-gated ^{99m}Tc-SestaMIBI images.[102] Initial validation in an animal model has shown good correlation between a quantitative regional functional index of contraction and myocardial thickening as measured by sonomicrometer crystals. Using this method, it is feasible to obtain simultaneous information on myocardial perfusion and regional myocardial contraction.

The relative value of ^{99m}Tc-SestaMIBI in comparison with ^{201}Tl can be summarized as follows. Because of the relative high photon flux, ^{99m}Tc-SestaMIBI images are of consistently better quality. The interpretation of SestaMIBI images is consequently easier and more reproducible. ^{99m}Tc-SestaMIBI also is a superior agent for SPECT myocardial perfusion imaging. ^{99m}Tc-SestaMIBI allows for simultaneous assessment of left ventricular function and perfusion. Since the timing of imaging after injection is not critical, unique clinical applications and imaging protocols are feasible in acutely ill patients. Furthermore, this pharmaceutical provides great flexibility in patient scheduling as well as in the sequence of imaging. On the other hand, ^{201}Tl has a unique place as a marker of myocardial viability when imaging is performed at rest or after redistribution.

^{99m}Tc-TEBOROXIME STRESS IMAGING. The clinical experience with ^{99m}Tc-teboroxime is still limited to a relatively small number of patients (Fig. 10–18). The sensitivity of this agent to detect coronary artery disease appears comparable to that of ^{201}Tl.[11] This imaging agent is of particular interest because the relative short time it remains in the heart allows for multiple injections and repeat simultaneous assessment of left ventricular function by first-pass radionuclide angiocardiography and myocardial perfusion.

As already mentioned, ^{99m}Tc-teboroxime imaging requires a unique and rapid imaging protocol with multiple images obtained within 3 to 5 minutes after injection of the tracer.[102a,102b] This approach could enhance the efficiency of patient scheduling significantly. One could employ this methodology in clinical situations involving rapid changes in cardiac function and perfusion, such as during exercise, during administration of a short-acting vasodilator such as adenosine, or during mental stress. A potential limitation of this tracer is the suboptimal count density obtained in images acquired more than 3 minutes after injection.

PATIENT SELECTION FOR MYOCARDIAL PERFUSION STRESS IMAGING. Although the sensitivity and specificity of myocardial perfusion imaging for detection of coronary artery disease is better than that of electrocardiographical stress testing, the method is far from a perfect diagnostic test. False-negative and false-positive results occur. According to Bayes' theorem (Fig. 6–11, p. 169), the significance of test results relates not only to the sensitivity and specificity of a test but also to the prevalence of disease in the population under study.[103,104] With quantitative planar ^{201}Tl and ^{99m}Tc-SestaMIBI stress imaging, a sensitivity of approximately 90 per cent and a specificity of approximately 95 per cent have been reported. A positive result obtained in a population with a very low prevalence of coronary disease (e.g., less than 3 per cent) will have a predicted value of only 36 per cent, because, compared with expected true-positive results, a relatively large absolute number of false-positive results can be anticipated. However, in a patient population with a high prevalence of coronary disease, e.g., 90 per cent, a positive result has a predictive value of 99 per cent. In this setting, only a few false-positive results are obtained relative to the true positive results. On the other hand, in a population with a high prevalence of disease, a relatively large number of false-negative results are also obtained, and the predictive value of the negative test for absence of coronary disease is only 51 per cent.

Thus, in a population with a low prevalence of coronary disease (such as young asymptomatic subjects), a positive test

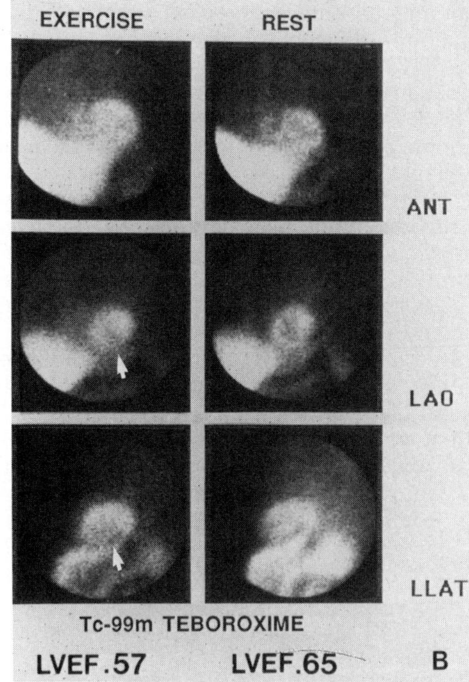

FIGURE 10–18. Technetium-99m teboroxime imaging at rest and during exercise. The patient had myocardial imaging as well as first-pass angiocardiography performed with ^{99m}Tc teboroxime. At peak exercise, 30 mCi of ^{99m}Tc teboroxime was injected. Left ventricular ejection fraction (LVEF) was 57 per cent. Immediately thereafter, planar images were obtained in the three standard views. An inferolateral myocardial perfusion defect (arrows) is present. First-past angiography measured a LVEF of 65 per cent at rest. This study shows reversibility of the defect and demonstrates the feasibility of assessing both left ventricular function and myocardial perfusion with a single injection of radiotracer. Note the intense subdiaphragmatic uptake in the liver, both after exercise and at rest.

is of little predictive value, while a negative test virtually excludes the diagnosis. In contrast, in a population with a high prevalence of coronary artery disease (50- to 60-year-old men with typical angina pectoris) a negative test is of little practical diagnostic value, while a positive test virtually assures the diagnosis. The difference between the pretest probability of disease (determined by the patient's age, symptoms, and a stress electrocardiogram) and the posttest probability (determined by the results of myocardial perfusion stress imaging) indicates the practical value of the test. ^{201}Tl scintigraphy has optimal discriminatory value in a patient population with a pretest probability of coronary artery disease ranging from about 40 to 70 per cent. This population includes patients with atypical chest pain, asymptomatic patients with major risk factors, and asymptomatic patients with a positive stress electrocardiogram.[105]

MYOCARDIAL PERFUSION IMAGING IN PATIENTS WITH LEFT BUNDLE BRANCH BLOCK. In patients with complete left bundle branch block, the conduction abnormality precludes the use of conventional electrocardiographical criteria for the diagnosis of infarction or exercise-induced ischemia. It was hoped that myocardial distribution of ^{201}Tl would be unaffected by the electrocardiographical abnormality.[106] Indeed, in patients with left bundle branch block without prior myocardial infarction, *resting* ^{201}Tl images are generally normal. However, the septum is frequently thin, and in older patients the left ventricle is often dilated.

A number of investigators have reported exercise-induced myocardial perfusion defects in anteroapical and anteroseptal areas in patients with complete left bundle branch block and angiographic normal coronary arteries.[107,108] In some patients, partial or complete reversibility of these defects has been observed. Hirzel et al.[109] proposed diminished septal myocardial blood flow as a result of the abnormal sequence of depolarization as an explanation for this finding. The authors found no difference in the quantitative distribution of ^{201}Tl injected during rapid pacing of the right atrium or injection during rapid pacing of the right ventricle (left bundle branch block).[109a] Thus, it seems unlikely that the altered sequence of ventricular depolarization *itself* is a cause for ^{201}Tl perfusion defects.

The authors have also found a relationship between the presence of exercise-induced ^{201}Tl defects in left bundle branch block and the degree of left ventricular dilatation. Altered geometry appears to be another plausible explanation for defects observed after exercise in patients with left bundle branch block, who often have clinically unexpected cardiomyopathy.

THALLIUM-201 STRESS IMAGING IN NONCORONARY ARTERY DISEASE. ^{201}Tl imaging has been employed in a number of clinical conditions that may be present with symptoms of chest pain but angiographically normal epicardial arteries.[110,111] In a number of these patients, abnormal and "false-positive" ^{201}Tl images have been observed. Legrand et al.[112] demonstrated that in patients with this "syndrome" (p. 1346), abnormal coronary reserve also could be demonstrated. Cannon et al.[113] found that these patients also had abnormal global and regional systolic and diastolic function. It would appear that at least some of the so-called "false-positive" ^{201}Tl images in patients with angiographic normal coronary arteries may in fact reveal true abnormalities in myocardial microcirculation. In patients with mitral valve prolapse and atypical chest pain, several investigators have demonstrated normal ^{201}Tl stress images.

Infarct Imaging

From the early days of nuclear cardiology, myocardial infarction was visualized either as a "cold spot" (perfusion defect) or as a "hot spot." Cold spot imaging has been extensively discussed above. When a radiopharmaceutical agent sequesters specifically in an area of recent infarction, the infarct is visualized as a "hot spot." The advantage of a hot spot imaging is that it is generally easier to image the presence of a tracer than its absence.

^{99m}Tc-Sn-Pyrophosphate

The first clinically useful hot spot imaging of acute infarction was performed using ^{99m}Tc-Sn-pyrophosphate (Fig. 10–19). This imaging agent is very sensitive for detecting acute myocardial infarction from 24 hours to 5 days after the onset of chest pain.[114] However, small and nontransmural infarcts are often not detected. Although scintigraphy is usually negative very early after infarction, some infarcts have been shown to be positive within a few hours after onset of chest pain. On the basis of present knowledge, it seems likely that spontaneous reperfusion occurred in these patients.[115] On the other hand, some very large acute infarcts remained scintigraphically negative, apparently because of absence of residual flow to the infarct region. The intensity and pattern of ^{99m}Tc-Sn-pyrophosphate uptake was found to be of prognostic significance. As of this writing ^{99m}Tc-Sn-pyrophosphate infarct imaging is mainly of historic interest and is performed infrequently in most laboratories. In occasional patients who are suspected of having sustained an acute infarction 2 to 3 days before hospital admission, ^{99m}Tc-Sn-pyrophosphate imaging may be useful in establishing the diagnosis at a time when plasma enzyme levels have returned to normal.

Indium-111 Leukocytes

Another approach to hot spot infarction imaging that has never had routine clinical application involves the use of

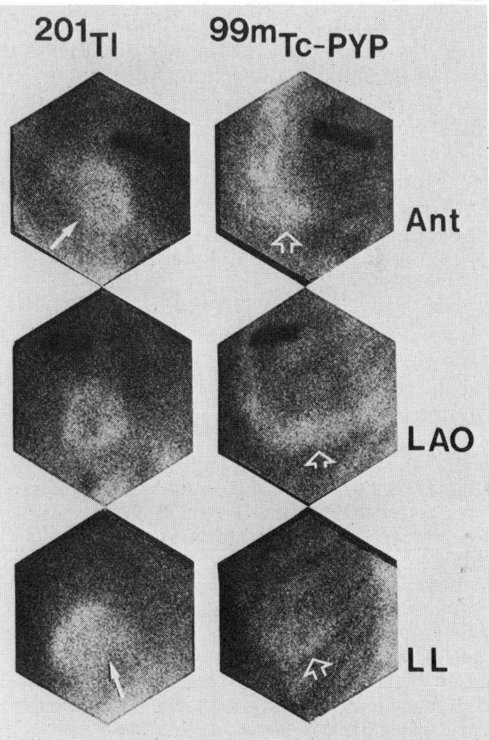

FIGURE 10–19. ***Left,*** **^{201}Tl images in a patient with acute inferior wall MI. An inferior ^{201}Tl myocardial perfusion defect can be seen (arrow).** ***Right,*** **Technetium-99m-Sn pyrophosphate (PYP) imaging in the same patient. Uptake of ^{99m}Tc pyrophosphate occurred in matching area (open arrow). On the LAO view, intense uptake of ^{99m}Tc pyrophosphate is present in the inferior wall, and extends into the right ventricle. This patient had, in addition to left ventricular infarction, right ventricular involvement.**

indium-111(^{111}In)-labeled leukocytes.[116] The patient's own white blood cells are labeled in vitro with ^{111}In and then reinjected. On the second or third day after acute infarction, migration of white cells occurs into the infarct area, which can be visualized by imaging with ^{111}In.

Indium-111 Antimyosin

More recently, imaging with a monoclonal antibody specific for intracellular myosin has shown promising clinical results. Indium-111 murine monoclonal antimyosin binds selectively to irreversibly damaged myocytes. Imaging is performed after administration of approximately 2 mCi of ^{111}In antimyosin. Planar or SPECT imaging is performed 24 hours after antibody injection. The gamma camera is peaked on both photopeaks (171 and 245 keV) of ^{111}In. A medium-energy collimator is used. The conventional three planar views, i.e., anterior, left anterior oblique, and left lateral view, are obtained, or 360 degree SPECT.

Typical ^{111}In antimyosin images of an acute infarct demonstrate discrete uptake in the myocardium. In addition, substantial liver and spleen uptake may be seen. Initial clinical studies have been encouraging. Indium-111-labeled antimyosin appears highly specific (100 per cent) and sensitive (92 per cent) for the detection of acute myocardial necrosis.[117] In addition to positive images in patients with acute myocardial infarction, uptake of ^{111}In antimyosin has been noted in patients with unstable angina. The intensity and extent of ^{111}In antimyosin accumulation appears to be of prognostic significance, both in patients with acute infarction and in those with unstable angina. Patients with extensive antimyosin uptake, i.e. greater than 50 per cent of the myocardium, had a 4 to 9 times increased risk for future cardiac events (cardiac death and nonfatal myocardial infarction) than patients with less or no uptake. The positive uptake seen in patients with unstable angina probably should be interpreted as the noninvasive demonstration of small, clinically undetectable focal areas of necrosis.

The clinical usefulness of ^{111}In antimyosin imaging still requires clear definition. In the majority of patients the diagnosis of acute myocardial infarction can be made readily on the basis of simple and inexpensive tests, such as electrocardiography and cardiac enzyme analysis. The potential prognostic significance of the extent of antimyosin uptake is important and has to be investigated in a larger number of patients. It has been proposed that simultaneous dual tracer imaging (^{201}Tl and ^{111}In antimyosin) may have a role for the assessment of myocardial salvage after thrombolytic therapy (Fig. 10-20).

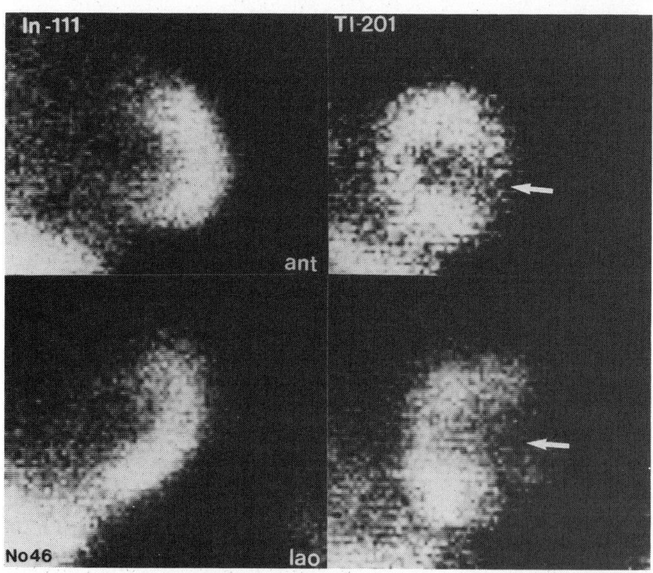

FIGURE 10-20. Indium-111 antimyosin (left) and ^{201}Tl imaging in a patient with acute anterolateral infarction. The ^{201}Tl defects (arrows) correspond with areas of ^{111}In antimyosin accumulation. (From Lahiri, A., and Jain, D.: New radionuclide imaging in cardiovascular disease. Curr. Opin. Cardiol. *2*:1070, 1987.)

In addition to imaging of acute myocardial infarction, ^{111}In antimyosin imaging may have a role in cardiac transplant patients having cardiac rejection.[118] Furthermore, in patients with active myocarditis, diffuse ^{111}In antimyosin uptake has been observed.[119] More patients (55 per cent) had abnormal ^{111}In antimyosin images than abnormal endomyocardial biopsies (22 per cent). Nearly all patients with abnormal myocardial biopsies had abnormal ^{111}In antimyosin images. More than half of the patients with positive antimyosin images showed improvement of left ventricular function over time, whereas only 18 per cent of patients with normal scans improved. This clinical course occurred irrespective of biopsy results. These observations suggest that imaging with ^{111}In antimyosine provides independent important clinical information in myocarditis. Further studies are needed to define the usefulness of ^{111}In antimyosin imaging in acute ischemic syndromes and other cardiac diseases associated with cellular necrosis.[120]

ASSESSMENT OF CARDIAC PERFORMANCE

Cardiac performance can be assessed with radionuclide techniques by either of two generic approaches. The first involves analysis of the first transit of a radionuclide bolus through the central circulation (first pass radionuclide angiocardiogram). The second, more widely applied method involves analysis following equilibrium intravascular labeling, which allows repeat imaging over several hours (equilibrium radionuclide angiocardiogram). There are variations of each technique that involve assessment of the right and left ventricles, diastolic as well as systolic function, regional or global performance, ventricular volumes, and adaptations for longer term or ambulatory monitoring. These specific approaches, their clinical implications, and applications are discussed below.

EQUILIBRIUM RADIONUCLIDE ANGIOCARDIOGRAPHY (ERNA)

The concept of utilizing a physiological signal such as the electrocardiogram to "gate," or physiologically control, the otherwise static imaging of the cardiac blood pool was initially proposed in 1971.[121,122] Since that time substantial technical and methodological advances have occurred and broad clinical application has been established.[123] The ERNA utilizes electrocardiographic events to define the temporal relationship between the acquisition of nuclear data and the volumetric components of the cardiac cycle. Sampling is performed repetitively over several hundred heartbeats with physiological segregation of nuclear data according to occurrence within the cardiac cycle (Fig. 10-21). Data are accumulated until radioactivity count density is sufficient for statistically meaningful analysis. The electrocardiogram provides a reasonably sensitive and easily defined physiological signal with which to link the static imaging technique. Currently, the technique involves major computer interactions, with automated or semiautomated analysis being the routine.[124] Data are quantified and displayed in an endless loop cine format for additional qualitative visual interpretation and analysis.

TECHNICAL CONSIDERATIONS. Because analysis involves the summation of several hundred cardiac cycles, a number of factors must be considered for the study to be deemed adequate. First, the patient must be able to remain relatively still beneath the detector during the period of data acquisition. In general, studies should be obtained in multiple views for interpretation to be complete. These include the standard anterior and left anterior oblique views, as well as the left lateral and/or left posterior oblique views (Figs. 10-22 to 10-25). The need for multiple views is inherent in this study because overlying radioactivity in multiple

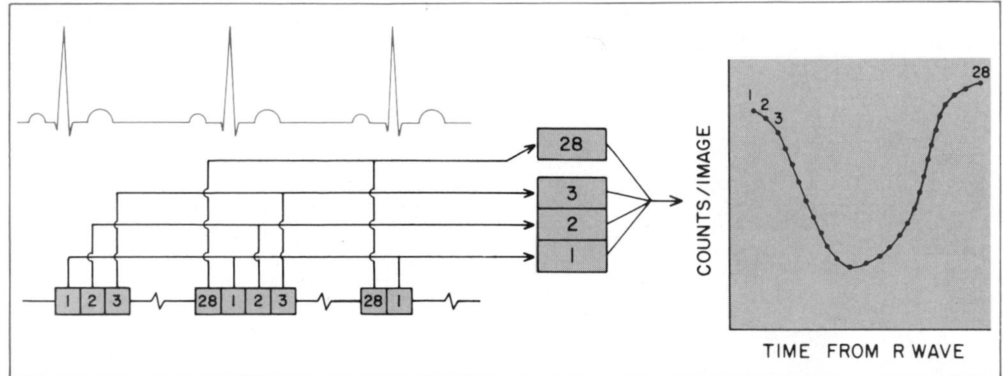

FIGURE 10-21. Diagrammatic representation of the technique for equilibrium radionuclide angiocardiography. Each cardiac cycle is divided into 28 equal segments. For each heartbeat, data are accumulated and then stored in separate file. To the right, these data for the 28 portions of the cycle are displayed as a single summed ventricular volume curve. The numbers 1-28 refer to the temporal sequence within the cardiac cycle. (From Zaret, B. L., and Berger, H. J.: Nuclear cardiology. *In* Hurst, J. W. (ed.): The Heart, Arteries and Veins. 7th ed. New York, McGraw-Hill, 1990, p. 1899.)

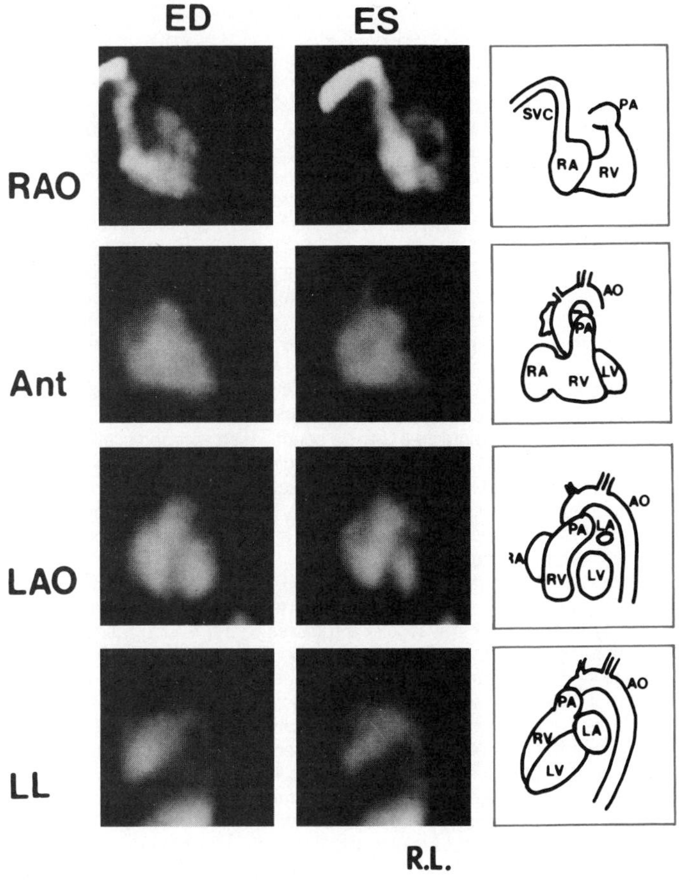

FIGURE 10-22. End-diastolic (ED) and end-systolic (ES) images obtained from a gated first-pass and equilibrium radionuclide angiocardiogram study. The anatomic configuration is shown diagrammatically to the right. In the upper panel, a gated first-pass study for evaluating the right ventricle is shown in the right anterior oblique (RAO) view. In the lower three panels (the equilibrium radionuclide angiocardiogram), images are shown for the anterior (Ant), left anterior oblique (LAO), and left lateral (LL) views. Note a normal contraction pattern in each view. (AO = aorta, LA = left atrium, LV = left ventricle, PA = pulmonary artery, RA = right atrium, RV = right ventricle, SVC = superior vena cava.)

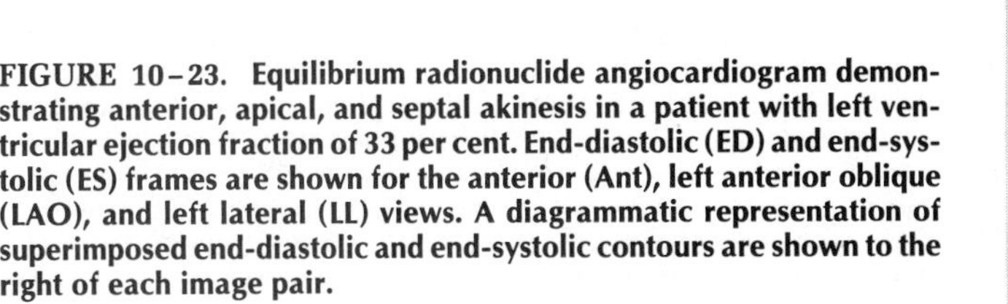

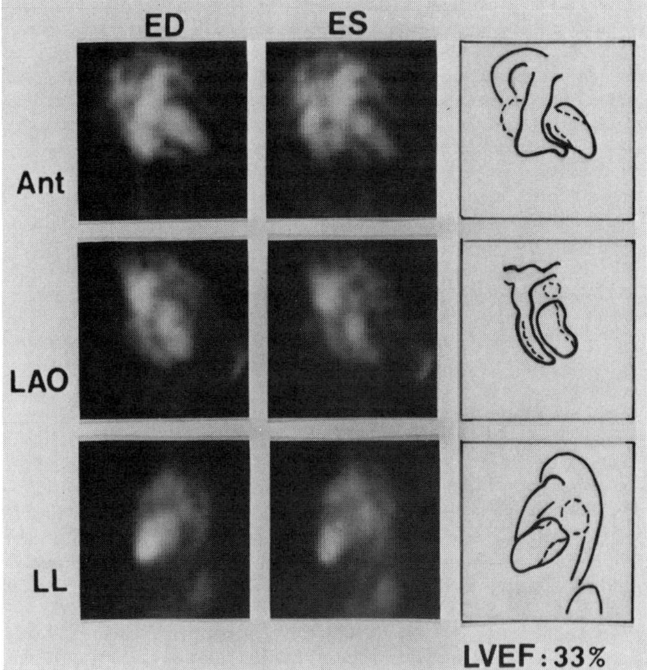

FIGURE 10-23. Equilibrium radionuclide angiocardiogram demonstrating anterior, apical, and septal akinesis in a patient with left ventricular ejection fraction of 33 per cent. End-diastolic (ED) and end-systolic (ES) frames are shown for the anterior (Ant), left anterior oblique (LAO), and left lateral (LL) views. A diagrammatic representation of superimposed end-diastolic and end-systolic contours are shown to the right of each image pair.

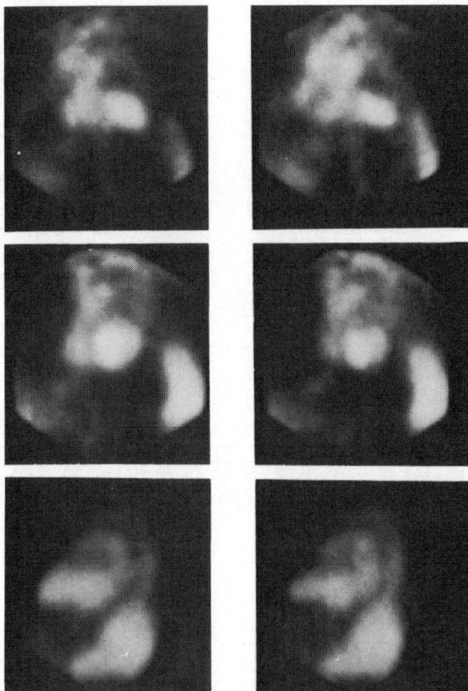

FIGURE 10-24. End-diastolic (left) and end-systolic (right) equilibrium radionuclide angiocardiogram images in a patient with a posterobasal left ventricular aneurysm. Anterior images are shown in the upper panel, left anterior oblique in the middle panel and left lateral images in the lower panel. Note the bulging posterobasal aneurysm in the left lateral images. This is the best view for defining this particular wall motion abnormality.

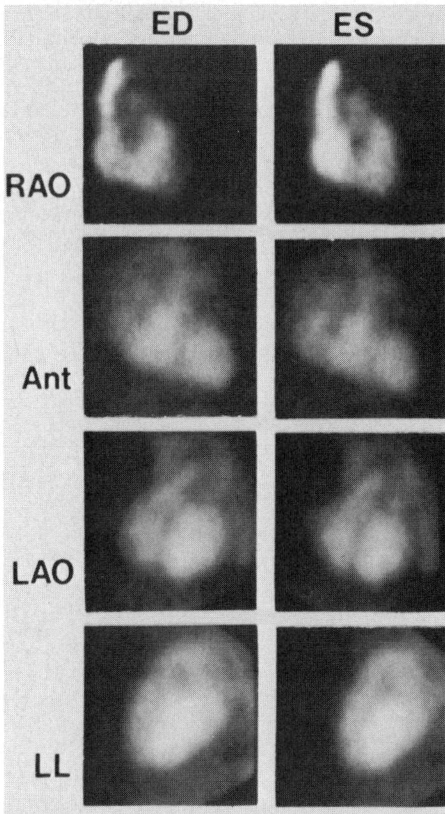

FIGURE 10-25. Equilibrium angiocardiogram in a patient with diffuse hypokinesis. End-diastolic (ED) images are shown at the left and end-systolic (ES) images are shown at the right. The gated first-pass radionuclide angiocardiogram in the right anterior oblique (RAO) view is shown at the top and the equilibrium studies in the anterior (ANT) left anterior oblique (LAO) and left lateral (LL) are shown in the three lower panels. In this patient with cardiomyopathy, there is readily apparent diffuse dysfunction of both right and left ventricles.

cardiac and noncardiac structures can obscure a given ventricular region in any one view.[125] In addition, specific abnormalities in regional left ventricular performance, such as ventricular aneurysms or akinesis of the posterobasal segment, may be appreciated only in lateral or posterior oblique views.[126] It is also assumed that cardiac performance remains relatively stable during the entire period of acquisition. This obviously will not be the case in the presence of substantial arrhythmia such as atrial fibrillation or frequent premature beats.

The presence of major arrhythmia must be accounted for in interpretation; otherwise, the potential exists for substantially underestimating ventricular performance. Some currently available programs routinely exclude premature beats. Finally, the radionuclide label also must remain stable during the period of analysis, and the interval of data acquisition (framing interval) must be sufficiently short to allow adequate temporal resolution for definition of both systolic and diastolic performance parameters.

PERFORMANCE

Equilibrium blood pool labeling is achieved using technetium-99m. The intravascular label is established with the patient's own red blood cells, using an in vitro or modified in vitro technique. Unlabeled stannous pyrophosphate is used to facilitate this reaction. The labeling techniques are now well standardized and quality control can be assured.[127] Following a single labeling procedure, serial studies can be readily obtained for periods ranging from 4 to 6 hours. If necessary, additional labeling can be achieved and the duration of observation extended.

Conventional Anger scintillation cameras are employed for these studies. Equipment is sufficiently portable to be brought to the bedside of acutely ill patients. As noted already, data are analyzed by computer, generally with some operator interaction. Analysis may be obtained in either the "frame" or "list" mode.[128] Radionuclide data are collected and segregated temporally. In the frame mode, which is employed most frequently, the R-R interval of electrocardiogram is divided into 20 to 50 msec portions, depending upon the patient's intrinsic heart rate and the conditions of the study, i.e., rest or exercise. If one is interested in defining diastolic filling events, a relatively short framing interval is required.[128] The process generally requires 3 to 10 minutes for completion of each view. Following data acquisition, the data from the several hundred individual beats are summed, processed, and displayed as a single "representative cardiac cycle."

Data from the left anterior oblique view also are utilized for qualitative analysis of global left ventricular function. In this view, there is minimal overlap of the two ventricles. Using a count based approach, left ventricular ejection fraction as well as other indices of filling and ejection are calculated from the left ventricular radioactivity present at various points throughout the cardiac cycle (Fig. 10-26). Measurements obtained in this manner correlate well with other defined standards, such as contrast left ventricular angiography.[128]

BACKGROUND ACTIVITY. Since radioactivity is present within the entire intravascular space, it is necessary to correct for contribution of activity in adjacent intravascular structures to the overall measured left ventricular radioactivity. Major contributions to this "backgound" come from lungs, left atrium, and, to a lesser extent, chest wall. Since in the left anterior oblique view the left atrium is posterior to the left ventricle, it will have its background contribution attenuated substantially by the more anterior left ventricular blood pool. Consequently, left atrial activity does not have a major impact on left ventricular measurements. Semiautomated methods are now routine for determining regions of interest as well as background zones. With the equilibrium technique, a variable region of interest is used for determining the left ventricular blood pool for each frame of the cardiac cycle. This is necessary because using a so-called "fixed" or single region of interest throughout the cardiac cycle will introduce error and result in an underestimation of ejection fraction.

INTERPRETATION

Interpretation of ERNA requires both visual and quantitative analysis. The approximate 45-degree left anterior oblique view provides data for the quantitative count based assessment of left ventricular function. In the equilibrium study, quantitative analysis of right ventricular function is difficult because of contamination from overlying anterior right atrial activity. For this reason, right ventricular function is best evaluated by first-pass techniques (p. 287). The degree of left anterior obliquity must be individualized based upon specific patient anatomy and cardiac orientation within the thorax. The degree of obliquity is determined in a manner providing optimal separation of right and left ventricles ("best septal view"). This is a relatively straightforward approach that can be used by the technologist without physician interaction. The left anterior oblique view also provides qualitative information concerning contraction of the septal, inferoapical, and lateral walls.[125] The anterior view provides data concern-

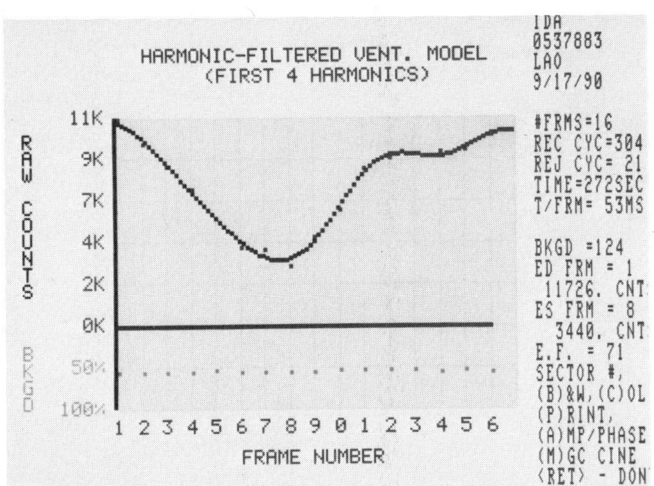

FIGURE 10-26. Ventricular volume curve derived from an equilibrium radionuclide angiocardiographic study. The raw data have been smoothed using a Fourier filter technique to four harmonics. Note the discrimination of the period of rapid diastolic filling as well as the atrial contribution to diastolic filling.

ing regional motion of the anterior and apical segments. The left lateral or left posterior oblique views provide optimal qualitative information concerning contraction of the inferior wall and posterobasal segment.[125,126]

Ventricular aneurysm can be assessed best in the lateral views as well. Analysis of only the anterior and left anterior oblique views may give the false impression of an enlarged diffusely hypokinetic ventricle, when in fact there are additional obscured zones of normally contracting myocardium. In addition to a purely visual assessment, a point scoring system can be utilized for assessing regional function. This is generally done with a 5-point score for each segment, with specific numerical grades assigned for dyskinesis, akinesis, mild and severe hypokinesis, and normal function.[129]

An advantage of labeling the entire intravascular blood pool involves visualization of all cardiac and vascular structures. Such a visual assessment can provide information concerning relative cardiac chamber sizes and the relative adequacy of contraction of each chamber. In addition, the size and orientation of the great vessels can be defined. The equilibrium study is helpful in detecting aneurysm formation of either the aorta or pulmonary artery. The relative thickness of the interventricular septum can be appreciated, as can the presence of filling defects representing intracardiac masses such as left atrial myxoma or intraventricular thrombus.[125]

The ERNA can easily be combined with additional physiological stress testing or provocation. This may either be in the form of physiological stress such as exercise, pharmacological stress with positive ionotropic agents such as dobutamine or isoproterenol, or psychological stress induced in the laboratory by tasks such as arithmetic problem solving or stressed speech.[130-131a] Since equilibrium labeling is stable for the short term, studies can be repeated, allowing for multiple stress measurements with interspersed adequate control and restabilization periods.

VENTRICULAR VOLUMES

Computer-based quantitative approaches to the ERNA are now well established.[124] Ventricular volume also can be determined by count-based methods.[132,133] This is now used most widely, rather than contrast angiography-derived area-length methods. Since radioactivity at equilibrium is directly proportional to volume, it is straightforward to establish a relationship between volume of a chamber and counts emanating from a region of interest representing that chamber in the two-dimensional display. The study also requires a blood sample to serve as a calibration standard. In addition, radiation attenuation must be accounted for.[134] Attenuation measurement represents the major source of error of the technique. However, volumes measured in this manner correlate well with other analyses. Since analysis is count-based, data are independent of the constraints and errors associated with fitting a deformed left ventricle to a geometrically ideal shape. Recently, a new count-based approach to measuring volume that does not involve attenuation correction has been described.[135] This innovative new approach may simplify substantially current volumetric analyses.

The ability to measure ventricular volumes is quite important, because volumetric changes may be critical for analysis of patients with heart failure and severely depressed systolic function. In such individuals, therapeutic benefit may be documented by a reduction in ventricular size while ejection fraction does not change.[136] Furthermore, linking volumetric analysis to concomitantly obtained pressure measurements can provide important insights into ventricular pressure-volume relations during both systole and diastole. This particular approach has been employed using both nonimaging nuclear probes and gamma camera equilibrium studies in the cardiac catheterization laboratory in which direct intracavitary pressure measurements are available.[137]

Marmor et al. have utilized equilibrium blood pool studies in conjunction with a noninvasive Doppler technique for accurately measuring central aortic systolic pressure from peripheral signals.[138] With this procedure, an assessment of systolic pressure-volume relationships as well as a measure of ventricular power can be obtained noninvasively. In preliminary studies, measures of power and the rate of change of power following exercise appear more sensitive to physiological manipulation than does ejection fraction.[138]

Concomitant assessment of the relative stroke volume of each cardiac chamber also can be obtained with the equilibrium technique. This provides a means of detecting and quantifying the presence and degree of valvular regurgitation.[139] However, it should be noted that significant error can be introduced with this measurement, particularly in the presence of ventricular enlargement and cardiac dysfunction.[140] Presently, the assessment of valvular regurgitation is best done by Doppler echocardiographic rather than radionuclide techniques (Chap. 12).

QUANTIFICATION OF REGIONAL FUNCTION

Recently, the equilibrium technique has been adapted for quantitative measurement of regional left ventricular function. In the left anterior oblique view, this is best done using a regional ejection fraction technique.[141] This technique is based upon the same principles utilized for measuring global ejection fraction. However, when regional function is assessed, the left ventricular blood pool is divided into several discrete regions with well-established anatomical correlates. The best approach involves division of the left ventricular blood pool into five regions of equal size (Fig. 10-27). These are upper and lower septal regions and inferoapical, inferolateral, and posterolateral regions. An upper zone involving the valve planes is excluded. This particular technique has been utilized in the TIMI multicenter trial and has provided meaningful insights into regional left ventricular function at rest and exercise following thrombolytic therapy.[141-142a]

THE CENTERLINE METHOD. An alternative regional approach is geometric in nature and is based upon modification of a technique developed for contrast left ventricular angiography, the "centerline" method[143] (Fig. 15-8, p. 426). The left lateral or left posterior oblique views are utilized since these represent mirror images of the contrast ventriculogram right anterior oblique view and provide an optimal view along the long axis of the left ventricle. This experimental approach employs new methods of edge detection based on principles of artificial intelligence.[144] Contours of the end-diastolic and end-systolic images are determined. A centerline midway between both contours is generated by computer. Cords are gener-

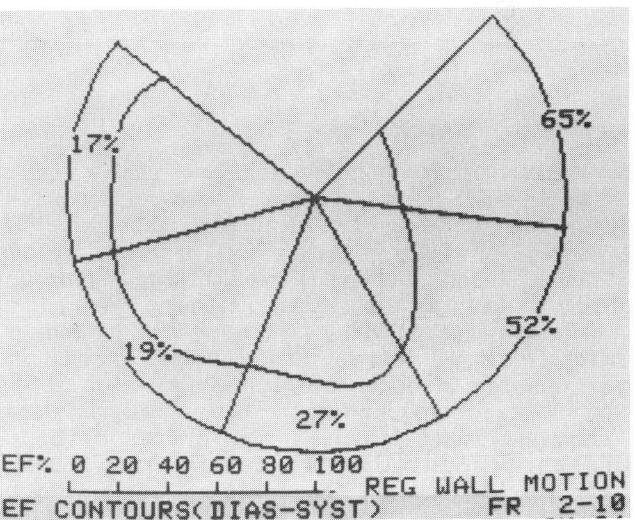

FIGURE 10-27. A typical regional ejection fraction display obtained from a left anterior oblique equilibrium study. The left ventricle is divided into five sectors. An upper sector involving the valve planes is excluded. These sectors, from upper left to upper right counterclockwise, involve upper septum, lower septum, apex, and inferolateral and posterolateral segments. In this particular study, there is a diminuition of regional ejection fraction in the upper and lower septum as well as the apex, with maintained contraction of the two lateral segments.

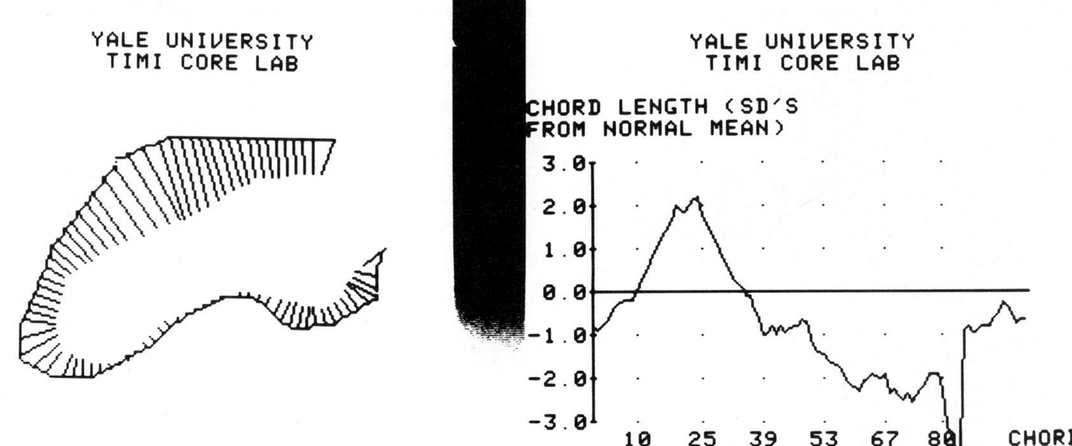

FIGURE 10-28. Centerline display in a patient with inferior and posterobasal akinesis and severe hypokinesis, and associated anterior wall hyperkinesis. A centerline display is shown at the left, and quantitative plot of the data in terms of standard deviation of each cord from normal is shown at the right. The image is obtained in the left lateral view. The length of the cords is a representation of effective contraction of each segment. There is akinesis of the inferior segment and severe hypokinesis of the posterobasal segment. The anterior wall appears hypercontractile. This is borne out from the quantitative standard deviation plot shown on the right. Segments 50 through 100 represent the inferior and posterobasal segments, while 0 through 50 represent the anterior and apical wall.

ated perpendicular to this centerline. The length of these cords defines the regional contraction within each particular zone (Fig. 10-28). Generally, 100 cords are generated per study. Data are related to a normal data base, and regional contraction is expressed both in absolute numbers and in relationship to deviation from normal. From the same contours, quantitative assessment also can be made of left ventricular shape. This involves the introduction of several additional mathematical analyses, one of which is based on the principle of "bending energy."[145] These approaches are limited by the spatial resolution of the nuclear technique, a problem not associated with the count-based, nongeometric methods.

PHASE ANALYSIS OF CONTRACTION

Regional function can also be assessed from phase analysis based upon the onset, timing, and extent of contraction.[146] The phase and amplitude images also can be used for specific localization of bypass tracts in Wolff-Parkinson-White syndrome, as well as for definition of the site of sustained ventricular ectopy or tachycardia.[147]

OTHER CIRCULATORY BEDS. With the same study in which an ERNA is obtained, it is also possible to gather quantitative data concerning circulatory beds other than the heart. Changes in pulmonary blood volume can be assessed under a variety of circumstances as well as changes in splanchnic and peripheral venous capacity.[148,149] Since counts are proportional to volume, relative change in counts provides important information concerning alterations in volume of various capacitance beds. This approach has been utilized to assess the effects of exercise and of drugs.[149,150]

Nonimaging Probe Studies

A variation of the equilibrium technique involves application of nonimaging probes for longer term (several hours) ventricular function monitoring. Nonimaging probes were first developed for first-pass (p. 297) studies. The technology then was modified and interfaced to a dedicated microprocessor suitable for equilibrium measurements. The probes employed initially were high sensitivity devices that provided beat-by-beat analysis as well as equilibrium analysis.[151] High temporal resolution also allowed relatively easy assessment of diastolic filling.[152] The nonimaging probe has been utilized in a number of clinical studies; one example involved evaluation of graded infusions of intravenous nitroglycerin in patients with unstable angina[153] (Fig. 10-29). The principle of monitoring ventricular function in unstable intensive care unit patients is appealing. The initial nonimaging probe called the "nuclear stethoscope" is no longer commercially available. However, a new miniaturized device involving a cadmium iodide detector has been developed recently. This device can be affixed easily to the patient's chest and allows for serial monitoring in the intensive care unit environment. Preliminary data indicate that ejection fraction measured in this manner correlates well with that measured with conventional gamma cameras.[154,154a] With this device, data also are available on-line for immediate analysis and input into patient care.

Ambulatory Monitoring

Further application of the technique of equilibrium angiocardiography relates to utilization of miniaturized equipment suitable for monitoring patients during routine activities. A

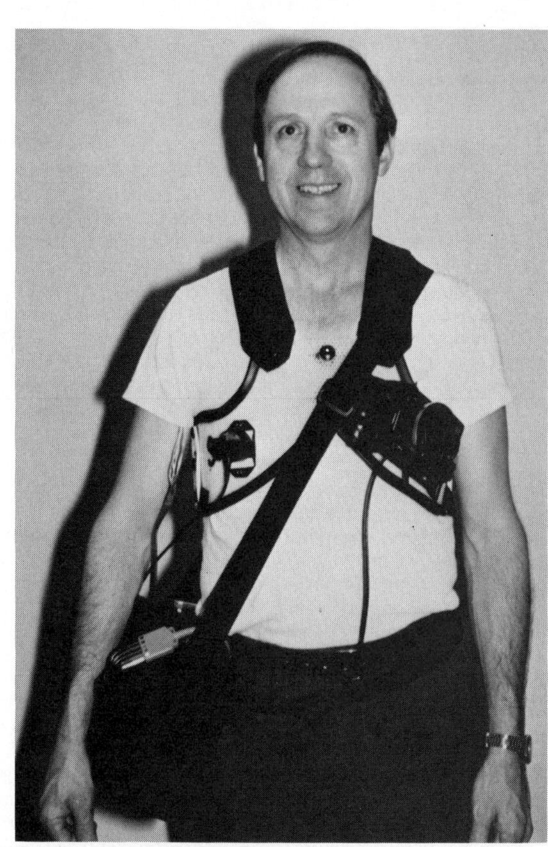

FIGURE 10-29. The ambulatory ventricular function monitor (VEST) seen in place as utilized for data accumulation. (From Zaret, B. L., and Kayden, D. S.: Ambulatory monitoring of left ventricular function: A new modality for assessing client myocardial ischemia. *In* Kellerman, J. J., and Braunwald, E. (eds.): Silent Myocardial Ischemia: A Critical Appraisal. Basel, Karger, 1990, p. 105.)

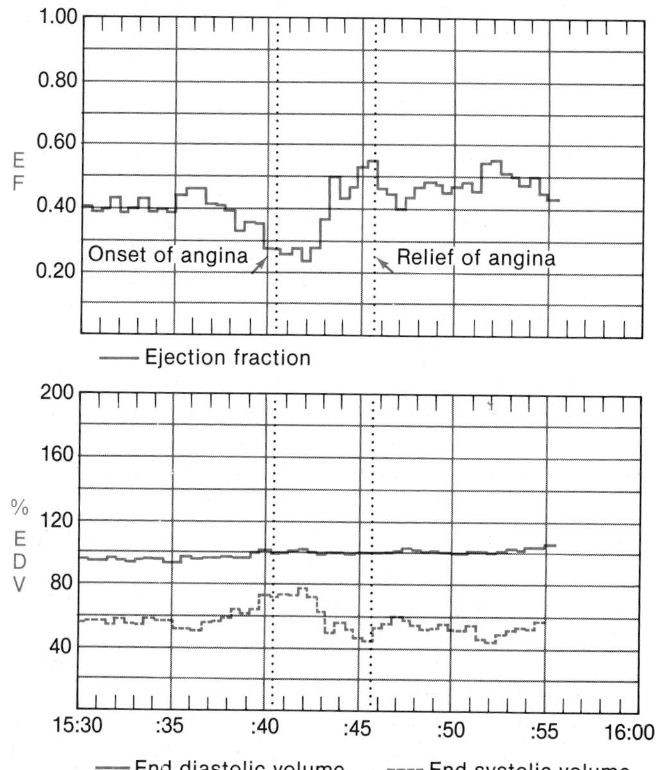

FIGURE 10–30. Trended data obtained with the VEST in a patient developing postmyocardial infarction ischemia. Data for ejection fraction are shown in the upper panel and data for relative end-diastolic volume and end-systolic volume are shown in the lower panel. Continuous data are shown for a 25-minute period. The times of onset and relief of angina are indicated. The fall in ejection fraction precedes the clinical occurrence of angina. This fall is associated predominantly with a rise in end-systolic volume, with minimal change in end-diastolic volume. (From Kayden, D. S., Wackers, F. J., and Zaret, B. L.: Silent left ventricular dysfunction during routine activity after thrombolytic therapy for acute myocardial infarction. Reprinted by permission of the American College of Cardiology. J. Am. Coll. Cardiol. *15*:1500, 1990.

newly developed instrument, called the VEST, allows for monitoring over several hours following blood pool labeling.[155] It again employs the basic principles of ERNA. The device is worn by patients so that they are fully ambulatory (Fig. 10–30). Radionuclide and electrocardiographic data are stored on tape in a manner comparable to that of the Holter monitor employed for arrhythmia detection. Offline analysis provides trended data concerning ventricular function (Fig. 10–31). This instrumentation has been validated and standardized in several laboratories and is ready for broader clinical application. Initial studies suggest a potential major role for this device in the assessment of silent myocardial ischemia.[156,157]

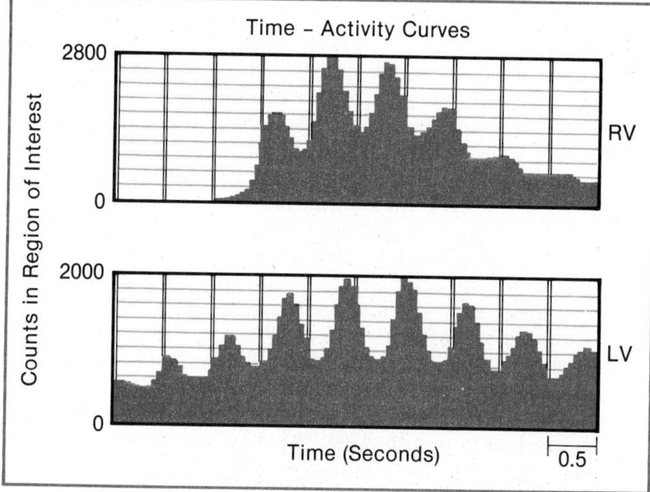

FIGURE 10–31. Radionuclide time activity curves obtained from a right ventricular (RV) and left ventricular (LV) region of interest during a first pass radionuclide angiocardiogram. Each peak and valley represents a single cardiac cycle. Data from this study are summed to provide right and left ventricular ejection fractions. (From Zaret, B. L., and Berger, H. J.: Nuclear Cardiology. *In* Hurst, J. W. (ed.): The Heart, Arteries and Veins. 7th ed. New York, McGraw-Hill, 1990, p. 1899.)

SPECT Studies

The equilibrium radionuclide technique may also be suitable for application to SPECT studies. As of this writing, work in this area is still relatively early and experimental.[158] However, it can be anticipated that appropriate software for ECG gating of SPECT equilibrium blood pool studies will soon be routinely available. Such studies could provide important information on a tomographic basis concerning regional ventricular wall thickening as well as regional contraction.

FIRST-PASS RADIONUCLIDE ANGIOCARDIOGRAPHY (FPRNA)

The first-pass radionuclide angiocardiogram was the first radionuclide technique applied to the study of cardiac physiology. The initial reports of Blumgart and Weiss occurred in 1927.[159] Prinzmetal described the gross characteristics of the first pass radionuclide angiocardiogram in the late 40's.[160] However, it was not until the early 70's that the clinical and investigative impact of the measurement was appreciated.[161] The first-pass approach remains a viable alternative to equilibrium studies. Presently, it is performed much less frequently than the equilibrium radionuclide angiocardiogram. However, with the availability of technetium-labeled myocardial perfusion agents (p. 277), the first-pass technique may take on new significance because ventricular function can be assessed by first-pass methods at the time of injection of the perfusion agent before subsequent static perfusion imaging.[100,101]

TECHNICAL CONSIDERATIONS

The first-pass radionuclide angiocardiographic technique involves sampling for only seconds during the initial transient of the bolus through the central circulation. The high-frequency components of this radioactive passage are recorded and analyzed quantitatively[125] (Fig. 10–32). It is assumed that there is sufficient mixing of the indicator with blood such that changes in count rates are proportional to volumetric changes. During the initial passage, there should be temporal and anatomical separation of radioactivity within each ventricle. Because of this, it is possible to analyze right and left ventricular function independently during this brief transit. Regional function also can be assessed from generated outlines of ventricular silhouettes.

THE SCINTILLATION CAMERA. In contrast to the equilibrium study, the choice of scintillation camera for the first-pass study is critical. Instrumentation must be utilized that provides high sensitivity with respect to count rate acquisition. If system linearity is lacking and there are major dead time losses, then data will be inaccurate. For this reason the multicrystal scintillation camera was initially developed.[125] This instrument has since been replaced by second- and third-generation digital cameras that are suitable for rapid acquisition of the high count rate data necessary for first-pass studies.

Several technical issues are relevant to performance of first-pass studies. First, the injection technique must be impeccable; it is necessary to have a compact radionuclide bolus without streaming. Injections can be made from either the jugular or the antecubital venous systems. Injections at more peripheral sites are not suitable. The presence of major arrhythmia during the evaluation will invalidate the data. Since analysis is based upon at most 8 to 10 cardiac cycles, the presence of rhythmic irregularity or premature beats will negate the validity of the study.

RADIOPHARMACEUTICALS. ^{99m}Tc radiopharmaceuticals are used for first-pass studies; for the most part, technetium pertechnetate or technetium complexed to either DTPA or sulfur colloid has been employed. Thus, based on the clearance of individual tracers, multiple injections can be made during a single study. Again, with the advent of technetium-labeled perfusion agents, it may be possible also to utilize these perfusion

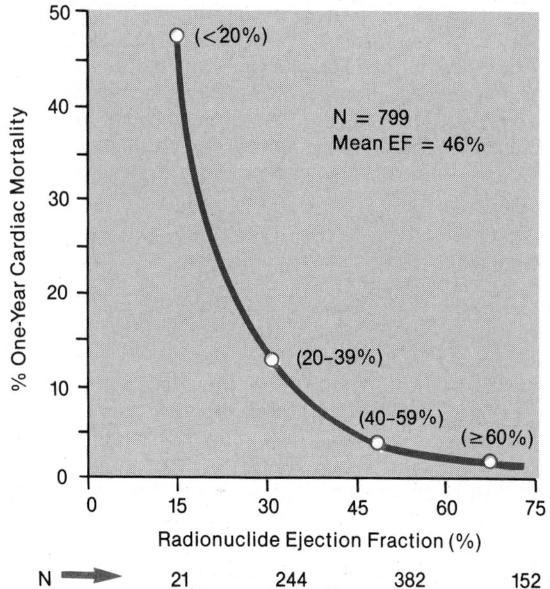

FIGURE 10-32. Relationship of ejection fraction at hospital discharge to cardiac mortality at one year in the multicenter postinfarction research study. As can be seen from the survival curve, there is a steep increase in mortality as ejection fraction falls below 30 per cent. (Reprinted with permission from The Multicenter Postinfarction Research Group: Risk stratification and survival after myocardial infarction. N. Engl. J. Med. *309*:331, 1983.)

agents for several purposes including first-pass functional evaluation.[100,101] In the past, attempts have been made to develop additional radiopharmaceuticals suitable for first-pass techniques. These have included generator-produced gold-195m, tantalum-178, and iridium-191m.[163,164] As of this writing, these short-lived generator systems have been purely investigational and have been employed for the most part only in individual laboratories with a specific research interest in their use.

PROCESSING OF FIRST-PASS STUDIES. The first-pass study is computer-processed in frame mode. Regions of interest are selected over either the right or left ventricle; generally, a fixed region of interest is used. Activity is analyzed only when the initial bolus passes through the specific chamber of interest. This temporal segregation of radioactivity compensates for the potential problem of overlapping regions of interest. Background corrections are necessary for which a variety of approaches have been described. The same approach utilized for the equilibrium study can be applied to the first-pass technique. In such a manner, global and regional left ventricular performance can be assessed. The first-pass technique is the modality of choice for assessing *right* ventricular function.[165] This can be carried out in concert with left ventricular analysis as part of a total first-pass evaluation.

GATED FIRST-PASS TECHNIQUE. Alternatively, a gated first-pass technique can be employed at the time of tracer injection for a subsequent equilibrium study. With this latter technique, first-pass data are acquired synchronously with the electrocardiogram. They are stored temporally and several beats are subsequently summed, forming a representative cardiac cycle obtained during the right heart phase. This particular approach provides higher count rate data than could be obtained with simple bolus injection and conventional Anger camera acquisition. The data from this study also can be viewed in endless loop cine format. Unlike the case for the left ventricle, poor contrast angiographic standards exist with which right ventricular radionuclide data can be compared. For this reason, normal values for right ventricular ejection fraction have been established independently and the technique standardized.[165] Right ventricular ejection fraction is a highly afterload-dependent measure. The finding of abnormal right ventricular ejection in the absence of intrinsic right ventricular disease is excellent evidence of acquired pulmonary hypertension.[166]

Shunt Studies

The first-pass study also can be used to detect and quantify intracardiac shunts.[167] With this particular approach, a region of interest is selected over the lung field. A pulmonary time-activity curve from the region is analyzed. Normally, there is a sharp rise and subsequent fall-off of radioactivity as it enters and leaves the pulmonary vasculature. A second, lower amplitude peak occurs as a result of normal recirculation of the bolus. In the presence of a significant left-to-right shunt, persistent activity remains in the lungs and there is relatively slow washout. Techniques have been developed for applying this approach to quantification of the degree of shunting.[168] By deconvolution of the pulmonary time-activity curve using a gamma-variate fit, the magnitude of shunting can be determined. This correlates extremely well with oximetry measures of left-to-right shunting. For right-to-left shunting, qualitative assessment demonstrating early appearance of activity in the aorta is often sufficient. Quantitative approaches also exist for defining the degree of right-to-left shunts.[167]

Comparison of First-Pass and Equilibrium Techniques

Both the equilibrium and first-pass radionuclide angiocardiographic techniques have advantages, limitations, and specific clinical indications. In addition, any one laboratory should perform that study with which it is most familiar and for which its equipment is optimal. The equilibrium technique (ERNA) has several distinct advantages: (1) multiple studies can be performed following a single radionuclide injection; (2) regional assessment can be done in as many views as are relevant for analysis; (3) sequential and serial data can be obtained during a variety of control, physiological, and/or pharmacological states; (4) the statistical reliability of high count rate equilibrium studies is superior to that of the first-pass technique; (5) the entire cardiovascular blood pool may be viewed at equilibrium; and (6) the equilibrium study is less prone to invalidation because of transient arrhythmia than is the first-pass study. On the other hand, additional activity from adjacent or overlying tissues can hinder optimal visualization of a specific ventricular segment in the ERNA. Evaluation of right ventricular performance, as well as shunt detection, is better achieved with the first-pass than the equilibrium technique. While equipment necessary for performing first-pass studies is more complex, as already stated, first-pass techniques may achieve resurgent popularity if combined with perfusion studies involving technetium-labeled agents.

Diastolic Function

Diastolic function of the ventricles (pp. 370, 402, and 438) can be evaluated from either the equilibrium or first-pass study, although the former has been more frequently used. A number of indices have been described for assessing diastolic function. The most widely employed are the peak filling rate and the time-to-peak filling rate.[169] Filling fraction also has been recently studied.[170] High temporal resolution is necessary for performing these studies. Equilibrium studies have often been obtained in list mode so that ectopic or irregular beats could be eliminated from analysis.[170] It is critical that there be high temporal resolution and reliability of the diastolic filling phase if accurate data are to be obtained. Fourier filtering techniques, in conjunction with polynomial mathematical algorithms, have been applied to volume curves obtained by frame mode equilibrium studies of lower temporal resolution in a manner that provides accurate data.[171] High temporal resolution nuclear probe studies also provide excellent analyses of diastole.[152]

Assessment of diastolic function has achieved increasing importance with clinical recognition of the entity of congestive heart failure associated with normal systolic and abnormal diastolic function (p. 402). This has been most commonly observed in left ventricular hypertrophy and coronary artery disease,[169,172] as well as in restrictive cardiomyopathies. Abnormal peak filling rates have been noted in a majority of patients with coronary disease, even in the presence of normal systolic function.[49] Improvement in filling parameters has been noted following successful coronary angioplasty or after the institution of antianginal therapy.[173,174] Abnormal diastolic function has been estimated to occur in as many as 30 to

40 per cent of patients hospitalized with congestive heart failure.[175]

A group of 54 such patients was described. The majority of patients with unequivocal heart failure and intact systolic performance had hypertensive or coronary disease, alone or in combination.[152] Follow-up of these patients over a 5-year period has indicated substantial cardiovascular morbidity and mortality that is not dissimilar to that of individuals manifesting systolic dysfunction alone.[176] Treatment with verapamil has been shown to improve objective and clinical parameters of heart failure as well as left ventricular filling in such patients.[177] Measurement of diastolic function offers a new dimension to the assessment of ventricular performance in patients with heart failure. However, it must be noted that parameters of diastolic filling are age-dependent. Abnormal filling is noted, proportional to age, in the absence of disease.[178,179]

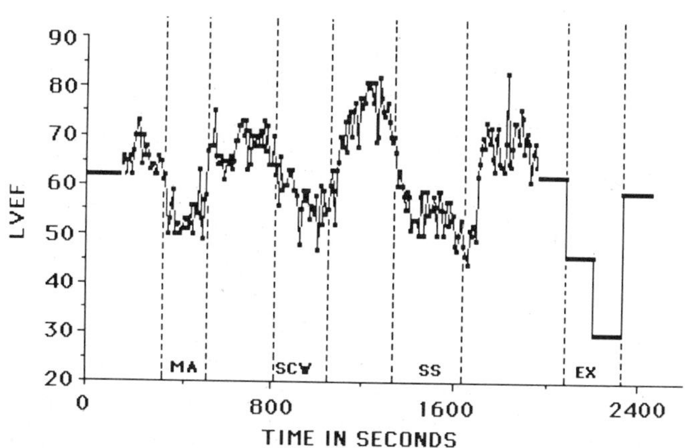

FIGURE 10–34. Serial ejection fraction measurements obtained with a nuclear probe in a patient with coronary artery disease undergoing a variety of mental stresses followed by exercise. The patient was studied with three types of mental stress: mental arithmetic (MA), the Stroop color word test (SCW), and stressed speech (SS). As is readily apparent in this study, with each mental stress the patient has a significant fall in ejection fraction. With supine bicycle exercise (EX) there is a further drop in ejection fraction. (From La Veau, P. J., Rozanski, A., Krantz, D. S., et al.: Cardiac dysfunction during mental stress. Am. Heart J. *118:*1, 1989.)

CLINICAL ASSESSMENT OF CARDIAC PERFORMANCE

RESTING VENTRICULAR PERFORMANCE. Measurement of right and left ventricular performance at rest is clearly of value in the evaluation of patients with congestive heart failure. In the simplest assessment, this particular study can be utilized to distinguish cardiac from pulmonary or other noncardiac causes of the symptom complex. Resting function is valuable in assessing preoperative surgical risk.[180,181] The cause of heart failure may be inferred from the involvement of the right and/or the left ventricles as well as the presence of diffuse left ventricular dysfunction as opposed to regional dysfunction.[125,128] Systolic versus diastolic heart failure may be differentiated by this study. Relative chamber size may also provide important insights concerning the occurrence of concomitant or primary valvular disease.[128]

Myocardial Infarction. Perhaps the widest clinical and investigative application of resting radionuclide ventricular function studies has been in the assessment of patients with myocardial infarction. Several reports have documented the importance of prognostic stratification on the basis of global ventricular function as measured by ejection fraction. Ejection fraction, certainly in the prethrombolytic era, has been a key factor in defining prognosis[182–184] (Fig. 10–33). In the thrombolytic era, ejection fraction still remains an important prognostic index; however, for any level of ejection fraction, mortality is substantially lower than noted in the prethrombolytic period.[185] The CASS trial has also indicated the importance of prognostic stratification based upon ejection fraction in patients with multivessel disease when survival was compared in patients assigned to surgical as opposed to medical therapy.[186] In patients who have survived out-of-hospital cardiac arrest, the single best prognostic factor also has been the degree of impairment in global function as measured by ejection fraction.[187]

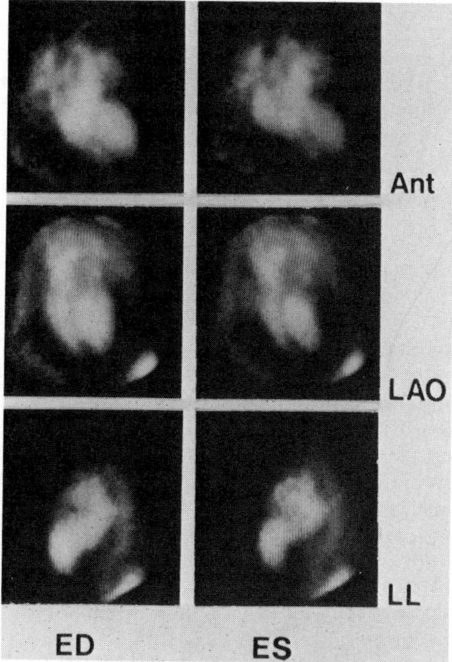

FIGURE 10–33. End-diastolic (ED) and end-systolic (ES) images in a patient with an anteroapical aneurysm. Anterior (Ant) images are shown in the upper panel, left anterior oblique (LAO), images in the middle panel and left lateral (LL) images in the lower panel. Note the marked regional wall motion abnormality that is readily apparent in the left lateral but not in the other views. The findings of diastolic deformity, regional akinesis or dyskinesis, and normally contractile myocardium are cardinal features of a left ventricular aneurysm.

In addition, the finding of a postinfarction functional left ventricular aneurysm carries further prognostic significance (Fig. 10–34). In one study involving patients with an anterior wall infarction, the finding of aneurysm formation, as defined by nuclear data, provided relevant prognostic information not available from the ejection fraction alone.[188] In the setting of acute infarction, radionuclide studies at rest also are of major value in distinguishing true from pseudoaneurysm and in distinguishing right from left ventricular infarction.[125]

EXERCISE STUDIES. Ventricular performance during exercise can be assessed with either equilibrium or first-pass techniques.[125] In general, exercise may be performed in the supine, semisupine, or nearly upright positions. A normal exercise response is generally defined by an increment of at least 5 per cent (in absolute terms) in global ejection fraction of both right and left ventricles. In patients with coronary artery disease, abnormal ventricular reserve is generally manifested by failure of such augmentation.[125,128] The finding of a major fall (>5 per cent) in ejection fraction from rest to exercise carries with it a poor prognosis.[189] Jones and colleagues have defined the prognostic impact of exercise ejection fraction data.[190,191] They have noted that the exercise ejection fraction itself as an absolute number provides the most relevant prognostic information. In addition, the exercise response is a major factor in predicting symptomatic outcome to surgical treatment in patients with coronary artery disease.[192]

A decrease in the specificity of exercise radionuclide ventricular function studies has been noted.[94] This change was attributed to differences in the selection of normal populations during the initial period of development of the technique. As a test is utilized more frequently, it is probably employed in patients with a higher pretest probability of disease, thereby leading to a decline in overall specificity (Fig. 6–11, p. 169). It also should be noted that some patients who contribute to the lower specificity have chest pain, angiographically normal coronary arteries, abnormal exercise radionuclide studies, and abnormal coronary vascular reserve despite epicardial coronary arteries that appear angiographically normal. These findings may indicate a new clinical entity characterized by inadequate coronary vasodilatation. (p. 1346).[112]

SILENT MYOCARDIAL ISCHEMIA (see also p. 1347). The prognosis associated with ischemia appears not to be affected by the presence or absence of a concomitant pain syndrome.[193] Since it is recognized that radionuclide exercise studies generally add to the sensitivity and specificity of the exercise ECG, it is not surprising that the study of left ventricular function during rest and exercise provides additional information concerning prognosis in silent ischemia.[194] The ability to detect silent myocardial ischemia during routine activities (as opposed to exercise in the laboratory) is of additional and perhaps greater importance. It is within this context that ambulatory ventricular function monitoring has achieved prominence (Figs. 10–30 and 10–31). Transient abnormalities in global left ventricular function during routine activity frequently occur silently.[157,195] Abnormal VEST responses have also been noted in the absence of symptoms during balloon occlusion at the time of coronary angioplasty, a situation producing transient transmural ischemia.[196]

Silent ventricular dysfunction also is relatively common under conditions of mental stress (Fig. 10–35). This phenomenon has been demonstrated in studies using the gamma camera or nuclear probe during several forms of induced mental stress.[130,131] Regional wall motion abnormalities were readily demonstrated during mental stress in patients with coronary artery disease, with or without an associated abnormal global ejection fraction response. These responses occurred in the absence of major increments in heart rate; this suggests that altered myocardial oxygen supply is the major mechanism.

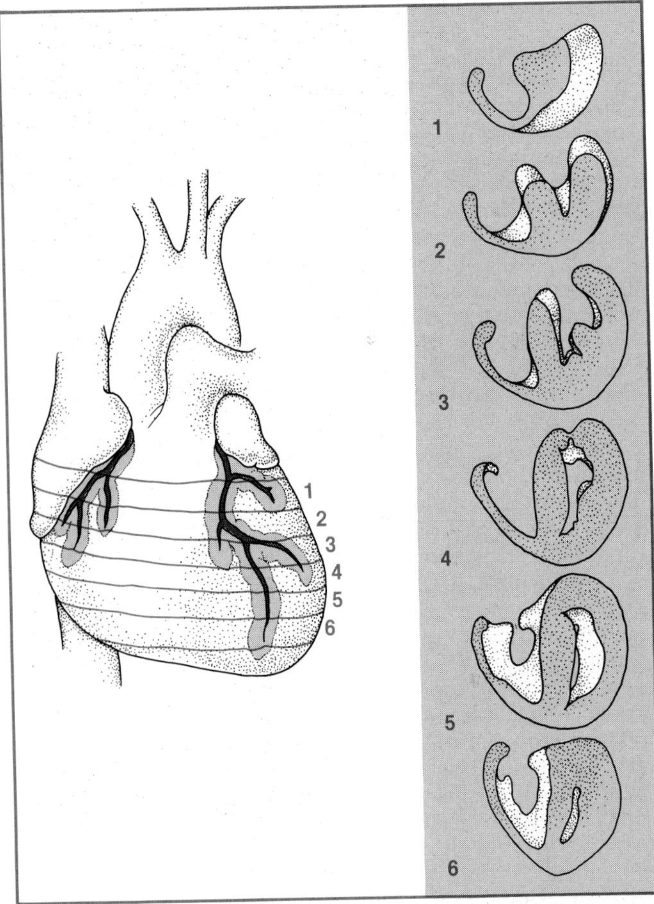

FIGURE 10–35. Schematic representation of the manner in which cross-sectional slices are obtained and acquired with PET imaging. Present technology is capable of imaging up to 21 slices simultaneously, although only six are shown in this example. It is from these initial slices that reconstruction occurs along a short axis, oblique sagittal and coronal axis similar to the reconstruction performed with single photon emission tomography. (From Brunken, R. C., and Schelbert, H. R.: Positron emission tomography in clinical cardiology. Cardiol. Clin. *7*:607, 1989.)

TABLE 10–5 GUIDELINES FOR MONITORING PATIENTS RECEIVING DOXORUBICIN

Perform baseline radionuclide angiocardiography at rest for LVEF prior to administration of 100 mg/m² doxorubicin. Subsequent studies at least 3 weeks after the indicated total cumulative doses have been given, but before next dose.

A. PATIENTS WITH NORMAL BASELINE LVEF (≥50%)
Perform the second study after 250 to 300 mg/m²
Repeat study after 400 mg/m² in patients with known heart disease, radiation exposure, abnormal electrocardiogram, or cyclophosphamide therapy; or after 450 mg/m² in the absence of any of these risk factors
Perform sequential studies thereafter before each dose
Discontinue doxorubicin if absolute decrease in LVEF ≥10% (EF units) with a decline to a level ≤50% (EF units)

B. PATIENTS WITH ABNORMAL BASELINE LVEF (<50%)
Doxorubicin therapy should not be initiated with baseline LVEF ≤30%
In patients with LVEF >30% and <50%, sequential studies should be obtained before each dose
Discontinue doxorubicin if absolute decrease in LVEF ≥10% (EF units) and/or final LVEF ≤30%

Modified from Schwartz, R. G., McKenzie, W. B., Alexander, J., et al.: Congestive heart failure and left ventricular dysfunction complicating doxorubicin therapy: Seven-year experience using serial radionuclide myocardiography. Am. J. Med. *82*:1109, 1987.

CONGESTIVE HEART FAILURE. Analysis of left ventricular function is cardinal for the assessment of patients with known or presumed congestive heart failure. Radionuclide studies provide systolic and diastolic data of relevance. The finding of diastolic dysfunction as the primary pathophysiological abnormality may necessitate use of a different therapeutic regimen (p. 507) from that used when systolic dysfunction alone is noted. The radionuclide study also can provide insight into the presence of valvular problems complicating or mimicking heart failure. Serial radionuclide studies provide a basis for monitoring the effects of therapy. In the presence of unexplained congestive heart failure, the demonstration of intact right ventricular function with abnormal left ventricular function speaks against primary cardiomyopathy disease as a cause. Generally, the most likely culprits in such a circumstance are coronary artery disease (ischemic cardiomyopathy), hypertensive heart disease, or aortic valvular disease. However, it should be noted that the converse is not necessarily true; patients with advanced left ventricular dysfunction may develop secondary pulmonary hypertension and, with this, secondary right ventricular dysfunction.[166]

DOXORUBICIN CARDIOTOXICITY (see also p. 1756). A major role for serial radionuclide left ventricular function studies involves the monitoring of patients with neoplastic disease for drug-induced cardiotoxicity. Doxorubicin, a commonly employed antineoplastic agent, may be associated with development of a severe cardiomyopathy that is often both irreversible and ultimately fatal. Radionuclide ventriculography has become established as a means of detecting presymptomatic cardiotoxicity.[197–199]

Guidelines for patient management with doxorubicin based upon resting ejection fraction data have been developed and are now currently employed (Table 10–5). Retrospective analysis noted marked differences in outcome between individuals who were managed with adherence to the radionuclide guidelines and those who were not.

It appears that resting ejection fraction provides an optimal means of assessing patients receiving cardiotoxic medication.

The addition of exercise stress does not appear to add significantly to this prognostic assessment.

VALVULAR HEART DISEASE (see also Chap. 34). Rest and exercise ventricular performance studies have been employed in the study of valvular heart disease. It has been suggested that exercise left ventricular responses are of value in patients with aortic regurgitation with respect to defining the indications for aortic valve replacement, even in the asymptomatic state.[200] At the present time, this general approach is not popular. Resting studies of ventricular performance clearly play a role in the assessment of patients with suspected or known valvular disease in whom surgery is being contemplated. In the context of the mitral regurgitation, such an evaluation may be particularly relevant clinically with respect to the definition of operability.

CONGENITAL HEART DISEASE. Radionuclide studies in patients with congenital heart disease initially focused on shunt detection. Within this context, valuable clinical data have been demonstrated both in adults and neonates.[168,201] In the future, far greater emphasis will be placed on the assessment of persons who have undergone either palliative or total repair for complex congenital abnormalities such as tetralogy of Fallot or transposition of the great arteries.[202]

CHRONIC OBSTRUCTIVE PULMONARY DISEASE. Patients with chronic obstructive pulmonary disease were studied intensively when radionuclide techniques for assessing the right ventricle were developed initially.[165] It is recognized that the right ventricle is an extremely afterload-dependent structure. The presence of abnormal right ventricular ejection fraction in such patients strongly suggests the presence of significant pulmonary hypertension.[170] Abnormalities in right ventricular performance also can be related to the degree of ventilatory and physiological impairment.[83] Right ventricular performance, as measured by ejection fraction, is responsive to agents that both augment inotropic performance as well as serve as pulmonary vasodilators.[165]

Recent work has evaluated the impact of positive end expiratory pressure (PEEP) upon right ventricular function.[204] Therapy involving PEEP is now routine in patients with severe respiratory insufficiency. Patients with normal baseline right ventricular function have no change in right ventricular volumetric status or contractile performance with PEEP. In contrast, those with depressed baseline right ventricular function manifest abnormal right ventricular hemodynamic responses to PEEP. On the basis of such data, a baseline evaluation of right ventricular performance before the institution of PEEP therapy would seem reasonable. In addition, the impact of right coronary flow upon right ventricular responses to PEEP has been studied. Abnormal right ventricular performance during PEEP frequently occurs under conditions of coronary stenosis or obstruction.[204] This also has been confirmed in experimental animal preparations.[205]

Special Imaging Techniques

IMAGING OF CARDIAC ADRENERGIC NERVES

MIBG (^{123}I metaiodobenzylguanidine) was initially developed as a radioactive imaging agent suitable for detection of pheochromocytoma.[206] MIBG behaves as an analog of the adrenergic neurotransmitter norepinephrine. Uptake of the analog occurs in preganglionic sympathetic nerves. In addition, there may be nonspecific extraneuronal uptake mechanisms.[207] In view of the rich cardiac sympathetic nerve supply, it is appropriate to consider this imaging technique for studying the pathophysiology of cardiac nerves. Two principal lines of investigation have been pursued with MIBG cardiac imaging. The first involves the demonstration of altered regional cardiac adrenergic innervation in the setting of acute myocardial ischemia and infarction. This has been studied in animal models of infarction as well in models designed to assess regional denervation (the removal of the stellate ganglion or topical administration of phenol).[208-210] Observations have now been extended to human myocardial infarction.[211,211a] The ultimate goal of these studies is to determine whether a relationship exists between regional neuronal integrity and either arrhythmogenesis or myocardial stunning.[211] MIBG studies of regional denervation generally involve reference imaging with thallium to assess concomitant perfusion defects. Regional denervation is inferred from a mismatch between the magnitude of the regional MIBG defect and the associated thallium defect, with the MIBG defect being larger.[210,211]

A second line of investigation involves the study of congestive heart failure. It has long been recognized that advanced congestive heart failure is associated with a relative decrement in cardiac catecholamine stores. With respect to MIBG imaging, a general correlation is seen between the magnitude of ventricular dysfunction and both a decrement in initial global left ventricular MIBG uptake and altered MIBG myocardial washout.[212,213]

THROMBUS IMAGING

PLATELET IMAGING. The major approach to imaging thrombus within the heart involves the use of indium-111–labeled platelets. This technique has been applied to experimental coronary thrombosis and to arterial, venous, intraventricular, and intraatrial thrombi in experimental animals and in humans.[214-218] This imaging technique appears to be as sensitive as echocardiography (Fig. 4–107, p. 105) for detecting left ventricular thrombus, particularly in the setting of anterior wall myocardial infarction.[215] A positive platelet study affects the prognosis with respect to subsequent embolic events[99] and supplements information obtained by echocardiography, suggesting that platelet imaging defines "activity" of the thrombus.

Additional platelet imaging approaches have been proposed recently that are based upon the use of monoclonal antibodies to specific platelet components such as glycoprotein IIb/IIIa.[220] With the use of antibody approaches, additional methods must be developed to allow for appropriate clearance of antibody from the intravascular blood pool so that imaging can be undertaken propitiously without excessive background present.

FIBRINOGEN/FIBRIN IMAGING. Radiolabeled fibrinogen and monoclonal antibody to fibrin also have been used to image thrombi.[221-223] To date, this technique has been utilized primarily to evaluate venous thrombosis. Its role in thrombus imaging in the arterial circulation remains unclear.

ATHEROSCLEROTIC PLAQUE IMAGING

Attempts are currently under way to develop new imaging techniques for identifying atherosclerosis as well as plaque activity with respect to the potential for instability. Preliminary studies have employed radioiodinated LDL cholesterol as an imaging agent.[224]

FATTY ACID ANALOG IMAGING

Substantial effort has been expended in developing planar imaging techniques involving radiolabeled fatty acids and their analogs. Initial studies with simple iodination of fatty acids proved to be inaccurate because of rapid elution of the iodinated label from the fatty acid.[225] Recently, a number of newer fatty acid analogs have been synthesized and employed in animal studies. Specific analogs may be trapped within the myocyte in a manner similar to the PET tracer fluorodeoxyglucose[226] (p. 302). The addition of a phenyl ring has provided stability for the iodinated label.[227] Studies have been performed in humans at rest and exercise stress with specific tracers.[228-230] Whether imaging with these agents provides metabolic data that is additive to that of their flow-related distribution remains unclear as of this writing. A number of positron emitting analogs currently are available and would appear to offer better metabolic insights than can be obtained from these single-photon fatty acids analogs alone (see below).

POSITRON-EMISSION TOMOGRAPHY

Positron-emission tomography (PET) is an imaging technique that has evolved over the past 20 years and is suitable for clinical application.[230a] The uniqueness of PET imaging lies in its ability to image and quantify metabolic processes, receptor occupancy, and blood flow. These unique properties depend on an ability to image biological phenomena by means of the availability of biologically active positron-emitting radiopharmaceuticals. Since there is no attenuation, as exists with single-photon imaging, with an appropriate kinetic model absolute quantitative measurements may be made noninvasively.

TECHNICAL CONSIDERATIONS

There are several limitations to conventional single-photon emitters such as ^{99m}Tc, ^{123}I, ^{201}Tl, and ^{111}In. These isotopes decay with emission of a single photon traveling in a random direction. The percentage of photons that reach the detector depends upon scatter attenuation and the distance between photon source and detector. These factors result in loss of relevant physiological information, which precludes accurate quantification of volumes, blood flow, and metabolism. Positron-emitting isotopes overcome these limitations. Positron-emitting radionuclides are characterized by excess protons. This unstable structure results in the conversion of an excess proton to a neutron; in the process, a positron (antielectron) is emitted. The positron travels a few millimeters in tissue; when it encounters an electron, an annihilation ensues. This results in the release of a photon pair with characteristic energy of 511 keV.

These photon gamma rays travel at 180 degrees from each other. Using detectors that are paired and aligned, the photons emitted from the positron annihilation can be detected. Images are obtained in a tomographic fashion similar to that in SPECT imaging. However, in SPECT studies a camera head (or heads) usually is used, which rotates on a gantry. PET imaging utilizes multiple stationary detector pairs arranged in a circular array. Present technology allows up to 21 simultaneous tomographic slices to be obtained, with reconstruction along various cardiac planes similar to those displayed in cardiac SPECT imaging.

PROCEDURES. Current PET imaging protocols depend on both the positron emitter and detector source. Briefly, the heart must be localized by either fluoroscopy or various transmission scan programs. The patient is positioned with arms above the head, so that the heart is within the 12-cm detector range. After the patient is made comfortable, a 10- to 30-minute attenuation scan (depending upon the ring souce) is acquired. This allows subtraction of activity in noncardiac structures from the overall field of view, thereby providing an isolated image of cardiac activity. The positron-emitting radionuclide is then injected. Allowance must be made for individual variation in the time needed for accumulation and subsequent acquisition of each radiopharmaceutical. For example, metabolic imaging with ^{18}FDG (fluorodeoxyglucose) requires injection of 5 to 10 millicuries. Then 30 to 40 minutes must elapse before FDG image acquisition is initiated for an additional 20 to 30 minutes. Data processing is generally performed off line after completion of acquisition.

RADIOPHARMACEUTICALS. Many positron emitters are unique because their naturally occurring counterparts (hydrogen, carbon, nitrogen, and oxygen) are predominant constituents of natural compounds. Positron-emitting isotopes of fluorine, carbon, nitrogen, and oxygen may replace their stable counterparts in the synthesis of metabolic substrate, receptor ligands, drugs, and other biologically active compounds without disrupting biochemical properties or activity. Fluorine-18 is a suitable substitute for naturally occurring hydrogen because of its strong carbon-fluorine bond and stearic effect similar to that of hydrogen. Positron-emitting tracers generally have shorter physical half-lives than most single photon emitters. This property allows for repeat injections as a means of observing rapidly changing events over time. Table 10–6 summarizes the isotopes, half-lives, and uses of the major positron emitters suitable for use in cardiovascular medicine.

ASSESSMENT OF MYOCARDIAL VIABILITY

An accurate assessment of the presence and extent of viable yet poorly contractile myocardium, and its discrimination from purely infarcted tissue, is of paramount clinical importance.[210a] This issue is particularly relevant to current cardiology practice because multiple pharmacological and mechanical interventions to establish reperfusion are now available. An assessment of viability is important with respect to establishing the appropriateness of these procedures as well as their ultimate efficacy. Available imaging techniques must be able to differentiate "stunned" or "hibernating"myocardium (p. 1176) from true infarcted tissue.

In the absence of capabilities for PET, myocardial viability is generally assessed with ^{201}Tl scintigraphy (p. 277). As already stated, delayed (18 to 72 hr) thallium imaging improves the detection of viable myocardium but still will not predict whether revascularization will result in improvement in myocardial function.[98] Clearly, a reduction in global left ventricular systolic performance in association with a fixed perfusion defect does *not* necessarily represent irreversible myocardial scar. Conventional assessment of left ventricular myocardial performance is not an adequate technique for the identification of patients who may improve after revascularization.[158] The assessment of myocardial viability with PET may provide insight into this area. Assessment of viability by PET involves comparison of perfusion and regional glucose utilization. Hypoperfused myocardial regions are visualized and/or quantified with flow tracers such as ^{82}Rb, ^{13}N ammonia, and ^{15}O water. Subsequently, these hypoperfused regions are then superimposed on and compared with the same regions visualized in a second study obtained with ^{18}F-fluorodeoxyglucose (FDG). Experimental studies have demonstrated that glucose utilization is *augmented* in segments that are hypoperfused and ischemic but nevertheless viable. During ischemia there is a shift of energy production from the oxidation of free fatty acids to that of glucose. Under normal conditions, glycolysis (glucose utilization) results predomi-

TABLE 10–6 POSITRON EMITTERS IN CARDIOVASCULAR IMAGING

ISOTOPE	HALF LIFE	LABELED COMPOUND	APPLICATION
^{18}F	109 min	^{18}F Fluoro-2-deoxyglucose (^{18}FDG)	Carbohydrate metabolism
		^{18}F Fluorodopamine	Adrenergic neuronal imaging
		^{18}F-6 Fluorometaraminol	Adrenergic neuronal imaging
^{13}N	10 min	^{13}N Ammonia	Perfusion
		^{13}N Amino acids (glutamate, alanine, leucine, aspartate)	Amino acid metabolism
^{11}C	20 min	^{11}C Amino acids (alanine, leucine, tryptophan)	Amino acid metabolism
		^{11}C Palmitate	Fatty acid metabolism
		^{11}C Acetate	Myocardial oxygen consumption
		^{11}C Butanol	Perfusion
		^{11}C Hydroxyephedrine	Adrenergic neuronal imaging
^{15}O	2 min	^{15}O Oxygen	Oxygen utilization
		^{15}O Water	Blood flow quantification
^{82}Rb	75 sec	^{82}Rb Chloride	Perfusion
^{68}Ga	68 min	^{68}Ga Platelets	Thrombus formation

nantly in CO_2 production with minimal lactate generation. However, during ischemia, lactate production is increased relative to CO_2 production; glucose may contribute up to 70 per cent of the total energy production in ischemia.[231-235]

Metabolism, as assessed with ^{18}F-FDG, traces exogenous glucose utilization. When FDG exchanges across the cellular membrane in proportion to glucose, it competes for hexokinase. The phosphorylated glucose analog FDG-6-phosphate, unlike its parent substance, is a poor substrate for glycolysis, glycogen synthesis, or the fructose-pentose shunt. It is also relatively impermeable to cell membranes because the enzyme that catalyzes the reverse reaction, glucose-6-phosphatase, is absent or present only in negligible quantities. Therefore, the tracer becomes trapped in the myocardium and its activity reflects regional rates of exogenous glucose utilization.[236] In myocardial segments with irreversible injury, tissue glucose utilization declines linearly with blood flow. Thus, in the presence of ischemic heart disease, PET imaging with ^{18}F deoxyglucose, a tracer of regional exogenous glucose utilization, has been useful in discriminating hypoperfused but viable tissue from regions with irreversible injury.[237-242]

Cross-sectional images are acquired 2 to 5 minutes following intravenous injection of a flow tracer. Then, 5 to 15 mCi of FDG is injected. However, 30 to 50 minutes must pass before images are obtained. These images are submitted to circumferential activity profile analysis similar to that employed with thallium image processing.[243] Three patterns of comparative blood flow and metabolism activity are demonstrable (Fig. 10–36). First, there may be a match between flow and metabolic uptake with homogeneous myocardial distribution of each tracer (normal). Second, blood flow is decreased but glucose utilization in the same area is increased relative to that in normally perfused myocardium or to the regions with reduced blood flow. This pattern of blood flow-metabolism mismatch is the PET scintigraphic marker of ischemia. Third, regional myocardial blood flow and glucose utilization are concordantly decreased. This pattern is the marker of myocardial scar and irreversible damage.

There have been two clinical investigations demonstrating that blood flow–metabolism mismatch on PET images is representative of ischemic but viable myocardium. Both have been based on the demonstration of improvement in regional wall motion after revascularization in regions demonstrating blood flow–metabolism mismatch (diminished flow, increased glucose uptake) preoperatively.[58,242] Both studies included patients with resting wall motion abnormalities as determined by equilibrium radionuclide ventriculography or contrast ventriculography.

Tillisch and colleagues evaluated 17 patients with a total of 73 regions with abnormal resting wall motion.[58] Those myocardial segments that showed preserved glucose uptake in regions of abnormal wall motion predicted reversibility of those wall motion abnormalities following bypass surgery. In contrast, abnormal motion in regions with depressed glucose uptake did not improve following revascularization. Abnormal contraction in 35 of 41 segments was correctly predicted to be reversible (85 per cent predictive accuracy). Abnormal contraction in 24 of 26 regions was correctly predicted to be irreversible (92 per cent predictive accuracy). In the 17 patients, left ventricular ejection fraction averaged 32 per cent $\pm$ 14 per cent before and 41 per cent $\pm$ 15 per cent after revascularization. This improvement was more marked in 11 patients with 2 or more regions that were either normal or revealed glucose activity in hypoperfused segments. Left ventricular ejection fraction increased in these patients from 30 per cent $\pm$ 11 per cent to 45 per cent $\pm$ 14 per cent ($P < 0.05$) as compared to no improvement in the remaining 6 patients with only 1 or no mismatched FDG/blood flow regions.

In a comparable study, Tamaki et al. performed PET perfusion and metabolic imaging before and 5 to 7 weeks after coronary artery bypass grafting in 22 patients.[242] Postoperative improvement in wall motion abnormalities was observed more often in the metabolically active segments (78 per cent) than in the metabolically inactive segments (22 per cent) ($P < 0.001$). Thus, the persistence of metabolic activity with FDG identifies dysfunctional myocardium that is viable.

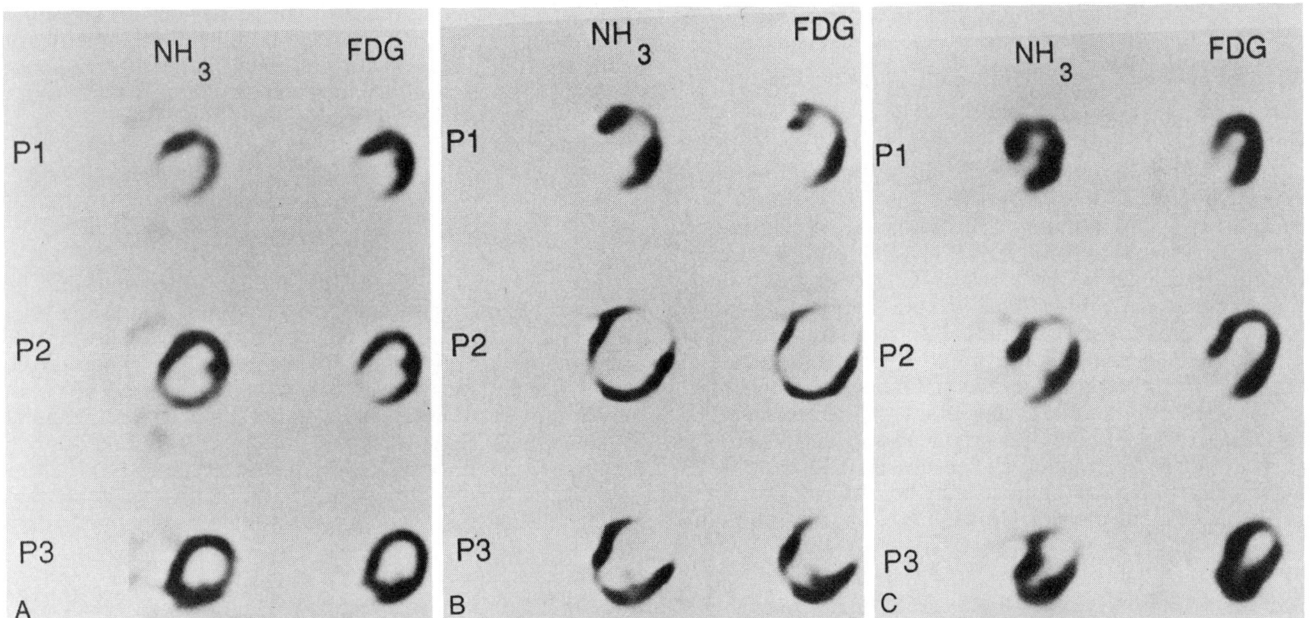

FIGURE 10–36. Three examples of paired PET images. Each example contains three cross-sectional images (p1 to 3 = planes 1 to 3) that are oriented with the anterior wall superiorly, the interventricular septum on the left and the free wall to the right. Panel A shows homogeneous uptake of perfusion images obtained with ^{13}N ammonia and of ^{18}F-FDG postprandially. This is an example of normal homogeneous perfusion and glucose (FDG) uptake. Panel B is an example of previous myocardial infarction in which there are concordant decreases in perfusion in the anterior wall on the ^{13}N ammonia image and the corresponding image obtained with ^{18}F-FDG. The images in panel C were obtained in a patient with critical obstruction of the left anterior descending coronary artery. Although there is decreased perfusion in the anterior wall on the ^{13}N ammonia study, there is significant uptake of FDG in that corresponding area. This mismatched defect is representative of intact metabolic activity in the presence of decreased perfusion. (From Chan, S. Y., Brunken, R. C., and Buxton, D. B.: Cardiac positron emission tomography: The foundations and clinical applications. J. Thorac. Imaging 5:9, 1990.)

COMPARISON OF PET WITH THALLIUM-201 REDISTRIBUTION SCINTIGRAPHY

Fixed defects on conventional thallium scintigraphy (comparison of stress and 3- to 4-hour redistribution images) have, until recently, been regarded as valid markers of myocardial scar without viability. However, repeat thallium imaging in patients after revascularization has shown improvement or normalization of thallium-201 uptake in up to 75 per cent of preinterventional fixed defects.[244,245] Repeat imaging in patients with fixed 4-hour defects as late as 72 hours after injection is considered a better predictor of postrevascularization functional improvement than is routine 3- to 4-hour redistribution alone.[98] However, 37 per cent of the segments that are fixed and irreversible at 48 hours of imaging still improve function after revascularization.

Studies directly comparing thallium scintigraphy and PET have been performed.[246–249a] A comparison of planar and SPECT thallium scintigraphy with tomographic images obtained by PET with FDG and ^{13}N ammonia showed that 58 per cent of the fixed planar thallium defects and 47 per cent of the fixed SPECT thallium defects were identified as viable on the basis of FDG uptake.[246,247] Comparative studies of SPECT thallium and PET imaging showed that 40 per cent of the regions with fixed (irreversible) thallium defects demonstrated FDG uptake and thus were viable by PET scintigraphic criteria.[248,249] These data, although based on small numbers of patients, indicate that metabolic imaging using PET may be superior to standard thallium scintigraphy in the delineation of viable myocardium. However, additional studies are needed in which PET imaging is compared to delayed thallium imaging with reinjection in large numbers of patients.[55,58a,250]

OTHER TECHNICAL CONSIDERATIONS

Several additional considerations require resolution. The dietary state of patients undergoing metabolic imaging should be standardized; some investigators study patients with FDG in the fasting state and others only after feeding and glucose loading. It is also not clear how accurate PET assessments of viability will be when tomography is performed early in the postinfarct period. Most studies to date have been performed late after the acute event. Other issues concern the accuracy of this technique in patients with diabetes and the lack of data concerning inter- and intraobserver variability.

There is agreement that the identification of viability is a recommended clinical indication for PET imaging. This has particular relevance in determining the need for percutaneous transluminal coronary angioplasty and coronary bypass surgery and in the assessment of congestive heart failure resulting from ischemic cardiomyopathy.

ASSESSMENT OF MYOCARDIAL BLOOD FLOW

The assessment of myocardial blood flow with PET is performed with rubidium-82 (^{82}Rb), ^{13}N ammonia, ^{15}O-labeled water, and copper pyruvaldehyde bis (N^4-methylthiosemicarbazonate) (PTSM). Rubidium-82 and ^{13}N ammonia are transiently trapped in the myocardium and in a distribution that is proportional to blood flow.[251–253] ^{15}O water is an inert diffusible tracer that accumulates and clears in the myocardium as a function of blood flow.[252] Rubidium is a potassium analog that in part requires the sodium potassium transport pump for uptake and thus utilizes energy for its myocardial trapping.[254,255] Its first-pass extraction fraction is 65 per cent.[253] Rubidium-82 is potentially a convenient radiopharmaceutical to use because it is generator-produced and not dependent upon a cyclotron for production. Because its half-life is only 76 seconds, repeated measurements may be performed to assess the effects of rapid physiological interventions.[253] Although the initial cost of a rubidium generator is less than a cyclotron, the monthly operating expenses may counterbalance this advantage.

Copper PTSM is another noncyclotron, generator-produced tracer with a high single pass extraction. It is not influenced by flow and may prove to be another alternative for use in measuring blood flow with PET.[256,256a] As of this writing, this agent is experimental and has been applied to human study in a limited manner.[256b] ^{13}N ammonia has a first-pass extraction fraction of 80 per cent and requires energy for myocardial trapping.[251] ^{13}N ammonia is converted to ^{13}N glutamine by the glutamine synthetase reaction.[243,256] For flows between 44 and 200 ml/min/100 gm myocardial blood flow measured with ^{13}N ammonia correlates linearly with that measured by means of radioactive microspheres. However, a plateau is reached at flows higher than 200 ml/min/100 gm, making flow measurement inaccurate in this range. Similarly, beta-probe experiments have confirmed that the net myocardium uptake of ^{82}Rb falls off as flows increase above 250 ml/min/100 gm.[254] Thus, at high flow rates, ^{82}Rb and $^{13}NH_3$ underestimate regional blood flow.

It has not been firmly established that flow measurements with either of these positron emitters are totally independent of metabolic conditions. Accumulation of these tracers is dependent upon some level of tissue viability following the ischemic insult.[240,260,261] Therefore, absolute quantification of blood flow with these two tracers may be limited by the nonlinear uptake at high flow rates and the extent to which metabolic factors affect the myocardial retention of these tracers. In contrast, water labeled with ^{15}O (half-life = 2.1 minutes) is a diffusible tracer of myocardial blood flow whose extraction fraction is independent of the metabolic state of the myocardium.[258] Accurate measurements of absolute myocardial blood flow may be performed across a wide spectrum of flow values.[262] Noninvasive calculation of absolute regional myocardial blood flow has been validated in experimental animals and has also been carried out in humans.[263]

The augmentation of myocardial perfusion reserve after coronary angioplasty has been quantified by PET H_2 ^{15}O studies.[264] Unfortunately, the high concentration of ^{15}O water in the intracavitary blood pool occurs concomitantly with myocardial activity. This results in suboptimal images and necessitates subtraction of the blood pool activity in order to obtain an accurate assessment of myocardial perfusion. This cumbersome process limits the wide clinical applicability of this technique.[265,266]

DIAGNOSIS OF CORONARY ARTERY DISEASE

The anatomical delineation of coronary artery luminal narrowing by coronary angiography may not accurately reflect the functional significance of coronary artery disease.[267] PET imaging with $^{13}NH_3$ and ^{82}Rb has identified abnormal flow reserve in patients with coronary artery disease.[210b] As of this writing, most studies involve relatively small patient numbers (Table 10–7). However, these studies do reinforce the view that perfusion imaging by PET (using either ^{82}Rb, ^{13}N ammonia, or ^{15}O-labeled water) can identify with acceptable sensitivity and specificity abnormal blood flow reserve in patients

TABLE 10–7 DIAGNOSTIC ASSESSMENT OF CORONARY ARTERY DISEASE WITH POSITRON EMISSION TOMOGRAPHY

STUDY	NO. PATIENTS	TRACER	STRESS	SENSITIVITY (PERCENTAGE)	SPECIFICITY (PERCENTAGE)
Schelbert[268]	45	$^{13}NH_3$	Dipyridamole	97	100
*Gould[269]	50	$^{82}Rb/^{13}NH_3$	Dipyridamole	95	100
Tamaki[270]	51	$^{13}NH_3$	Exercise-bicycle	88	90
*Demer[271]	193	$^{82}Rb/^{13}NH_3$	Dipyridamole	95	74
Stewart[273]	60	^{82}Rb	Dipyridamole	87	82
Total	399			92	89

* End-point coronary flow reserve vs. coronary artery luminal narrowing.

with obstructive coronary artery disease.[268–271] At the time of this writing only one large clinical study (193 patients) has been reported in which comparisons were made and a significant correlation found between the assessment of regional myocardial flow reserve by PET and coronary arteriography in all the subjects.

In another study, 50 patients were studied with either ^{82}Rb or ^{13}N ammonia after intravenous dipyridamole and isometric handgrip stress. Again, quantitative coronary arteriography was obtained to determine coronary flow reserve. Those patients with a coronary flow reserve of less than 3 were identified by PET imaging with a sensitivity of 95 and specificity of 100 per cent.[269]

Limited coronary artery perfusion reserve can also be delineated with ^{15}O-labeled water. Abnormalities in myocardial perfusion reserve have been reported in relative and absolute terms.[252,264,272] In one study, perfusion distal to a coronary stenosis after dipyridamole increased to only 64 per cent of that in normal anatomical areas. However, as quantified with PET, areas with successfully dilated arteries had post-dipyridamole perfusion similar to areas supplied by nonstenotic vessels.

COMPARISON WITH THALLIUM-201 SCINTIGRAPHY

The inherent cost and complexity of PET imaging mandates the need for a careful comparison between established, less costly modalities such as thallium scintigraphy. The higher energy photons released from positron-emitting tracers in conjunction with higher resolution images overcome the problems with photon attenuation commonly encountered with thallium studies. Little information is available directly comparing thallium-201 stress scintigraphy and PET perfusion studies in the same patient.[270,273]

Tamaki and colleagues studied 51 patients (48 with coronary artery disease) with exercise thallium SPECT and PET employing dipyridamole and ^{13}N ammonia. Both qualitative and semiquantitative image interpretation and qualitative analysis of the coronary arteriogram were employed. Of the 48 CAD patients, SPECT showed abnormal perfusion in 46 (96 per cent), while PET detected abnormalities in 47 (98 per cent). The sensitivity for detecting disease in individual coronary arteries (>50 per cent stenosis) was similar for SPECT (81 per cent) and PET (88 per cent).

Preliminary data in 60 patients who underwent ^{82}Rb PET and Tl-SPECT imaging within a 4-week interval recorded a higher specificity for PET.[273] However, at the time of this writing, it is not certain that PET has a clear advantage over conventional imaging techniques in the diagnosis of CAD. Further large scale comparisons are necessary. Current guidelines do not recommend PET perfusion imaging as a replacement for other nuclear diagnostic modalities.[275] However, it is possible that PET could become the perfusion study of choice in the future.

GATED PERFUSION STUDIES

Gated myocardial PET has also been performed, quantified, and compared with magnetic resonance imaging in normal subjects and with left ventriculography in patients with CAD.[274] In controls, percentage of wall thickening showed a good correlation with percentage of count increase. In CAD patients, count increase decreased significantly as wall motion worsened. This technique could eventually provide assessment of left ventricular regional function at the time of PET perfusion imaging.

OTHER PET MARKERS OF MYOCARDIAL METABOLISM

Flow/function relationships may not be the only reflection of regional myocardial ischemia. Metabolic perturbation may occur on a cellular level as a result of acute or chronic ischemia and not be detected by flow/function relationships. The ability to perform cardiac work depends on the availability of high-energy phosphate production. This is derived normally from the oxidation of long-chain fatty acids.[232] When fatty acid levels are low and glucose levels are high (as in the postprandial state), the heart utilizes glucose oxidation as a major source of energy.

^{11}C-palmitate is a position-emitting radiopharmaceutical that has been widely employed to characterize fatty acid metabolism experimentally and clinically.[276–283] The initial extraction fraction of ^{11}C-palmitate exceeds 50 per cent; therefore, its initial uptake reflects blood flow.[283] Oxidative fatty acid metabolism is reflected in the clearance of this tracer from the myocardium as $^{11}C\text{-}CO_2$ is produced. In this manner, PET imaging after injection allows the delineation of palmitate kinetics.[280–284] Alterations in myocardial substrate use and cardiac workload have been shown to alter cardiac ^{11}C fatty acid metabolism.[280] Impaired mitochondrial function, as a result of ischemia, is reflected by a slower ^{11}C clearance that presumably reflects decreased $^{11}C\text{-}CO_2$ production. Pacing-induced ischemia results in a slower ^{11}C clearance in the post-stenotic segment of the left ventricle. The same areas of slow ^{11}C clearance were noted to develop stress-related echocardiographic wall motion abnormalities in 50 per cent of the patients. The role that ^{11}C-palmitate studies will play in future diagnostic and functional characterization of cardiac patients is not clear.

Dynamic PET studies of ^{11}C-acetate kinetics provide a noninvasive measurement of regional myocardial oxygen consumption.[285] The clearance of ^{11}C-acetate from the myocardium is biexponential.[286] The decay constant of the initial component of the clearance curve is linearly related to myocardial oxygen consumption. Analysis of ^{11}C kinetics is thought to reflect accurately myocardial oxygen consumption and thus mitochondrial oxidative flux in human subjects.

NEUROCARDIOLOGIC POSITRON EMISSION TOMOGRAPHIC IMAGING

PET neurocardiac studies may develop into a new discipline focusing on sympathetic and parasympathetic interactions, neural regulation of the coronary circulation, adrenergic mechanisms in the genesis of arrhythmias, cardiac reflexes, and sympathetic innervation in the failing heart. Currently, PET may assess pre- and postganglionic neurochemistry, providing the opportunity to gain substantial insights in cardiovascular neurohormonal interactions. In one study, ^{18}F-fluorodopamine was used to visualize sympathetic innervation and function in vivo.[287] ^{18}F-fluorodopamine is converted to ^{18}F-fluoronorepinephrine in synaptic adrenergic vesicles. Imaging with this agent allows depiction of tissue sites of uptake, retention, and excretion for 3 hours after injection. The homogeneous uptake of the tracer occurs within 2 to 5 minutes after injection and is independent of blood flow because displacement with reserpine and desipramine inhibit uptake and retention of the tracer.

Visualization of the cardiac sympathetic nervous system has also been performed with ^{11}C hydroxyephedrine (^{11}C HED), an analog of norepinephrine.[288,288a] Comparative studies were performed between six normal volunteers and five cardiac transplant patients, the latter representing a model of global cardiac denervation. The normal volunteers showed homogeneous uptake of ^{11}C HED as well as the flow marker ^{82}Rb. However, the transplant patients, while demonstrating normal blood flow with ^{82}Rb, had a markedly reduced uptake of ^{11}C HED. Other cardiac neuronal agents such as [^{18}F] 6-fluorometaraminol are under investigation.[289] Furthermore, true postganglionic receptor imaging may be possible with the ongoing development of muscarinic and beta-receptor ligands.[290]

REFERENCES

INSTRUMENTATION

1. Budinger, T. F.: Single photon emission computed tomography. *In* Gottschalk, A., Hoffer, P. B., and Potchen, J. E., (eds.): Diagnostic Nuclear Medicine. Baltimore, Williams and Wilkins, 1988, p. 108.
2. Rullo, F., and Patton, J. A.: Instrumentation and information portrayal. *In* Freeman L. M., (eds.): Freeman and Johnson's Clinical Radionuclide Imaging. Orlando, Grune & Stratton, Inc., 1988, p. 203.

MYOCARDIAL PERFUSION IMAGING

3. Carr, E. A., Gleason, G., Shaw, J., et al.: The direct diagnosis of myocardial infarction by photoscanning after administration of cesium-131. Am. Heart J. *68*:627, 1964.
4. Zaret, B. L., Strauss, H. W., Martin, N. D., et al.: Noninvasive regional myocardial perfusion with radioactive potassium. N. Engl. J. Med. *288*:809, 1973.

5. Bradley-Moore, P. R., Lebowitz, E., Greene, M. W., et al.: Thallium-201 for medical use. II: Biologic behavior. J. Nucl. Med. *16*:156, 1975.
6. Strauss, H. W., Harrison, K., Langan, J.K., et al.: Thallium-201 for myocardial imaging. Relation of thallium-201 to regional myocardial perfusion. Circulation *51*:641, 1975.
7. Wackers, F.J.T., van der Schoot, J. B., Busemann Sokole, E., et al.: Noninvasive visualization of acute myocardial infarction in man with thallium-201, Br. Heart J. *37*:741, 1975.
8. Kaul, S.: A look at 15 years of planar thallium-201 imaging. Am. Heart J. *118*:581, 1989.
8a. Brown, K. A.: Prognostic value of thallium-201 myocardial perfusion imaging: A diagnostic tool comes of age. Circulation *83*:363, 1991.
9. Holman, B. L., Jones, A. G., Lister-James, J., et al.: A new Tc-99m-labeled myocardial imaging agent, hexakis(t-Butylisonitrile)-Technetium(I) [Tc-99m TBI]: Initial experience in the human. J. Nucl. Med. *25*:1350, 1984.
10. Wackers, F.J.T., Berman, D. S., Maddahi, J., et al.: Technetium-99m-hexakis 2-methoxyisobutyl isonitrile: Human biodistribution, dosimetry, safety and preliminary comparison to thallium-201 for myocardial perfusion imaging. J. Nucl. Med. *30*:301, 1989.
11. Seldin, D. W., Johnson, L. L., Blood, D., et al.: Myocardial perfusion imaging with technetium-99m SQ30217: Comparison with thallium-201 and coronary anatomy. J. Nucl. Med. *30*:312, 1989.
12. Weich, H. F., Strauss, H. W., and Pitt, B.: The extraction of thallium-201 by the myocardium. Circulation *56*:188, 1977.
13. Marshall, R. C., Leidholdt, E. M., Zhang, D. Y., et al.: Technetium-99m hexakis 2-methoxy-2-isobutyl isonitrile and thallium-201 extraction, washout, and retention at varying coronary flow rates in rabbit heart. Circulation *82*:998, 1990.
14. Wackers, F.J.T.: Myocardial perfusion imaging. *In* Gottschalk, A., Hoffer, P. B., and Potchen, E. J., (eds.): Diagnostic Nuclear Medicine. 2nd ed. Baltimore, Williams and Wilkins, 1988, p. 291.
15. Wackers, F.J.T., and Mattera, J.A.: Optimizing planar Tl-201 imaging: Computer quantification. Cardio *7*:103, 1990.
16. DePuey, E. G., and Garcia, E. V.: Optimal specificity of thallium-201 SPECT through recognition of imaging artifacts. J. Nucl. Med. *30*:441, 1989.
17. Friedman, J., Van Train, K., Maddahi, J., et al.: "Upward creep" of the heart: A frequent source of false-positive reversible defects during thallium-201 stress-distribution SPECT. J. Nucl. Med. *30*:1718, 1989.
18. Segal, G. M., and Davis, M. J.: Prone versus supine thallium myocardial SPECT: A method to decrease artifactual inferior wall defects. J. Nucl. Med. *30*:548, 1989.
19. Esquerre, J. P., Coca, F. J., Martinez, S. J., et al.: Prone decubitus: A solution to inferior wall attenuation in thallium-201 myocardial tomography. J. Nucl. Med. *30*:398, 1989.
20. Suzki, A., Muto, S., Oshima, M., et al.: A new scanning method for thallium-201 myocardial SPECT: Semi-decubital position method. Clin. Nuc. Med. *14*:736, 1989.
21. Maniawski, P. J., Morgan, H. T., and Wackers, F.J.T.: Orbit-related variation in spatial resolution as a source of artifactual defects in Tl201 SPECT. J. Nucl. Med. *(in press)*.
22. Johnstone, D. E., Wackers, F.J.T., Berger, H. J., et al.: Effect of patient positioning on left lateral thallium-201 myocardial images. J. Nucl. Med. *20*:183, 1979.
23. Cloninger, K. G., DePuey, E. G., Garcia, E. V., et al.: Incomplete redistribution of delayed thallium-201 single photon emission computed tomographic (SPECT) images: An overestimation of myocardial scarring. J. Am. Coll. Cardiol. *12*:955, 1988.
24. Kiat, H. K., Berman, D. S., Maddahi, J., et al.: Late reversibility of tomographic myocardial thallium-201 defects: An accurate marker of myocardial viability. J. Am. Coll. Cardiol. *12*:1456, 1988.
25. Weiss, A. T., Maddahi, J., Lew, A. S., et al.: Reverse redistribution of thallium-201. A sign of nontransmural myocardial infarction with patency of the infarct-related coronary artery. J. Am. Coll. Cardiol. *7*:61, 1986.
26. Boucher, C. A., Zir, L. M., Beller, G. A., et al.: Increased lung uptake of thallium-201 during exercise myocardial imaging: Clinical, hemodynamic and angiographic implications in patients with coronary artery disease. Am. J. Cardiol. *46*:189, 1980.
27. Weiss, A. T., Berman, D. S., Lew, A. S., et al.: Transient ischemic dilation of the left ventricle on stress thallium-201 scintigraphy: A marker of severe and extensive coronary artery disease. J. Am. Coll. Cardiol. *9*:752, 1987.
28. Trobaugh, G. B., Wackers, F.J.T., Busemann Sokole, E., et al.: Thallium-201 myocardial imaging: An interinstitutional study of observer variability. J. Nucl. Med. *19*:359, 1978.
29. Beller, G. A., Watson, D. D., and Pohost, G. M.: Kinetics of thallium distribution and redistribution: Clinical applications in sequential myocardial imaging. *In* Strauss, H. W., and Pitt, B., (eds.): Cardiovascular Nuclear Medicine, 2nd ed. St. Louis, C. V. Mosby Company, 1979.
30. Goris, M. L., Daspit, S. G., McLaughlin, P., et al.: Interpolative background subtraction. J. Nucl. Med. *17*:744, 1976.
31. Watson, D. D., Campbell, N. P., Read, E. K., et al.: Spatial and temporal quantitation of plane thallium myocardial images. J. Nucl. Med. *22*:577, 1981.
32. Garcia, E., Maddahi, J., Berman, D. S., et al.: Space/time quantitation of thallium-201 myocardial scintigraphy. J. Nucl. Med. *22*:309, 1981.
33. Wackers, F.J.T., Fetterman, R. C., Mattera, J. A., et al.: Quantitative planar thallium-201 stress scintigraphy: A critical evaluation of the method. Semin. Nucl. Med. *15*:46, 1985.
34. Sigal, S.L., Soufer, R., Fetterman, R.T., et al.: Reproducibility of quantitative planar thallium-201 scintigraphy: Quantitative criteria for reversibility of myocardial perfusion defects. J. Nucl. Med. *(in press)*.
35. Coleman, R. E., Jaszczak, and Cobb, F. R.: Comparison of 180° and 360° data collection in thallium-201 imaging using SPECT. J. Nucl. Med. *23*:655, 1982.
36. Eisner, R. I., Tamas, M. J., Colinger, K., et al.: Normal SPECT thallium-201 bull's eye display: Gender differences. J. Nucl. Med. *29*:1901, 1988.
37. Klein, J.L., Garcia, E. V., DePuey, G., et al.: Reversibility bulls-eye: A new polar bulls-eye may to quantify reversibility of stress-induced SPECT thallium-201 myocardial perfusion defects. J. Nucl. Med. *31*:1240, 1990.

CLINICAL APPLICATIONS OF MYOCARDIAL PERFUSION IMAGING

38. Wackers, F.J.T., Busemann Sokole, E., Samson, G., et al.: Value and limitations of thallium-201 scintigraphy in the acute phase of myocardial infarction. N. Engl. J. Med. *295*:1, 1976.
39. Wackers, F.J.T., Becker, A. E., Samson, G., et al.: Location and size of acute transmural myocardial infarction estimated from thallium-201 scintiscans. Circulation *56*:71, 1977.
40. Wacker, F.J.T., Lie, K. I., Liem, K. I., et al.: Potential value of thallium-201 scintigraphy as a means of selecting patients for the coronary care unit. Br. Heart J. *41*:111, 1979.
41. DeCoster, P. M., Melin, J. A., Detry, J. R., et al.: Coronary artery reperfusion in acute myocardial infarction: Assessment by pre-and post-intervention thallium-201 myocardial perfusion imaging. Am. J. Cardiol. *55*:889, 1985.
42. Gibbons, R. J., Verani, M. S., Behrenbeck, T., et al.: Feasibility of tomographic ^{99m}Tc-hexakis-2-methoxy-2-methylpropyl-isonitrile imaging for the assessment of myocardial area at risk and the effect of treatment in acute myocardial infarction. Circulation *80*:177, 1989.
43. Wackers, F.J.T., Gibbons, R. J., Verani, M. S., et al.: Serial quantitative planar technetium-99m-isonitrile imaging in acute myocardial infarction: Efficacy for noninvasive assessment of thrombolytic therapy. J. Am. Coll. Cardiol. *14*:861, 1989.
44. Santoro, G. M., Bisi, G., Sciagra, R., et al.: Single photon emission computed tomography with technetium-99m-hexakis 2-methoxy isobutyl isonitrile in acute myocardial infarction before and after thrombolytic treatment: Assessment of salvaged myocardium and prediction of late functional recovery. J. Am. Coll. Cardiol. *15*:301, 1990.
44a. De Coster, P.M., Wijns, W., Cauwe, F., et al.: Area-at-risk determination by technetium-99m-Hexakis-2-Methoxyisobutyl isonitrile in experimental reperfused myocardial infarction. Circulation *82*:2152, 1990.
44b. Wackers, F.J.Th.: Thrombolytic therapy for myocardial infarction: Assessment of efficacy by myocardial perfusion imaging with technetium-99m-sestaMIBI. Am. J. Cardiol. *66*:36E, 1990.
45. Silverman, K. J., Becker, L. C., Bulkley, B. H., et al.: Value of early thallium-201 scintigraphy for predicting mortality in patients with acute myocardial infarction. Circulation *61*:996, 1980.
46. Nestico, P. E., Hakki, A., Felsher, J., et al.: Implications of abnormal right ventricular thallium uptake in acute myocardial infarction. Am. J. Cardiol. *58*:230, 1986.
47. Jain, D., Lahiri, A., Raftery, E. B., et al.: Clinical and prognostic significance of lung thallium uptake on rest imaging in acute myocardial infarction. Am. J. Cardiol. *65*:154, 1990.
48. Wackers, F.J.T., Lie, K. I., Liem, K. L., et al.: Thallium-201 scintigraphy in unstable angina pectoris. Circulation *57*:738, 1978.
49. Berger, B. C., Watson, D. D., Burwell, L. R., et al.: Redistribution of thallium at rest in patients with stable and unstable angina and the effect of coronary artery bypass surgery. Circulation *60*:1114, 1979.
50. Maseri, A., Parodi, O., Severi, S., et al.: Transient transmural reduction of myocardial blood flow demonstrated by thallium-201 scintigraphy, as a cause of variant angina. Circulation *54*:280, 1976.
51. Gregoire, J., and Theroux, P: Detection and assessment of unstable angina using myocardial perfusion imaging: Comparison between technetium-99m Sesta-MIBI: SPECT and 12-lead electrocardiogram Am. J. Cardiol *66*:42E, 1990.
52. Gould, K. L.: Noninvasive assessment of coronary stenoses by myocardial perfusion imaging during pharmacologic coronary vasodilatation. I. Physiologic basis and experimental validation. Am. J. Cardiol. *41*:267, 1978.
52a. Zhu, Y. Y., Chung, W. S., Botvinick, E. H., et al.: Dipyridamole perfusion scintigraphy: The experience with its application in one hundred seventy patients with known or suspected unstable angina. Am. Heart J. *121*:33, 1991.
53. Ranhosky, A., Rawson, J., et al.: The safety of intravenous dipyridamole thallium myocardial perfusion imaging. Circulation *81*:1205, 1990.
54. Verani, M. S., Mahmarian, J. J., Hixson, J. B., et al.: Diagnosis of coronary artery disease by controlled coronary vasodilation with adenosine and thallium-201 scintigraphy in patients unable to exercise. Circulation *82*:80, 1990.
54a. Nguyen, T., Heo, J., Ogilby, J.D., and Iskandrian, A.S.: Single photon emission computed tomography with thallium-201 during adenosine-induced coronary hyperemia: Correlation with coronary arteriography, exercise thallium imaging and two-dimensional echocardiography. J. Am. Coll. Cardiol. *16*:1375, 1990.
54b. Wilson, R.F., Wyche, K., Christensen, B.V., et al.: Effects of adenosine on human coronary arterial circulation. Circulation *82*:1595, 1990.
55. Dilsizian, V., Rocco, T. P., Freedman, NMT., et al.: Enhanced detection of ischemic but viable myocardium by the reinjection of thallium after stress-redistribution imaging. N. Engl. J. Med. *323*:141, 1990.
56. Rocco, T. P., Dilsizian, V., McKusick, K. A., et al.: Comparison of thallium

redistribution with rest "reinjection" imaging for the detection of viable myocardium. Am. J. Cardiol. 66:158, 1990.
57. Kayden, D. S., Zaret, B. L., Wackers, F.J.T., et al.: Twenty-four-hour planar thallium-201 delayed imaging: Is reinjection necessary? (abstract). Circulation 80:376, 1989.
58. Tillisch, J., Brunken, R., Marshall, R., et al.: Reversibility of cardiac wall-motion abnormalities predicted by positron tomography. N. Engl. J. Med. 314:884, 1986.
58a. Bonow, R.O., Dilsizian, V., Cuocolo, A., and Bacharach, S.L.: Identification of viable myocardium in patients with chronic coronary artery disease and left ventricular dysfunction. Comparison of thallium scintigraphy with reinjection and PET imaging with ^{18}F-fluorodeoxyglucose. Circulation 83:26, 1991.
59. Gibson, R. S., and Beller, G. A.: Should exercise electrocardiographic testing be replaced by radioisotope methods? *In* Rahimtoola, S. H., and Brest, A. N., (eds.): Controversies in Coronary Artery Disease. Philadelphia, F. A. Davis Company, 1981, p. 1.
60. Berger, B. C., Watson, D. D., Taylor, G. J., et al.: Quantitative thallium-201 exercise scintigraphy for detection of coronary artery disease. J. Nucl. Med. 22:585, 1981.
61. Maddahi, J., Garcia, E. V., Berman, D. S., et al.: Improved noninvasive assessment of coronary artery disease by quantitative analysis of regional stress myocardial distribution and washout of thallium-201. Circulation 64:924, 1981.
62. van Train, K. F., Berman, D. S., Garcia, E. V., et al.: Quantitative analysis of stress thallium-201 myocardial scintigrams: A multicenter trial. J. Nucl. Med. 27:17, 1986.
63. Kaul, S., Boucher, C. A., Newell, J. B., et al.: Determination of the quantitative thallium imaging variables that optimize detection of coronary artery disease. J. Am. Coll. Cardiol. 7:527, 1986.
64. Maddahi, J., Abdulla, A., Garcia, E. V., et al.: Noninvasive identification of left main and triple vessel coronary artery disease: Improved accuracy using quantitative analysis of regional myocardial stress distribution and washout of thallium-201. J. Am. Coll. Cardiol. 7:53, 1986.
65. Albro, P. C., Gould, K. L., Westcott, R. J., et al.: Noninvasive assessment of coronary stenoses by myocardial imaging during pharmacologic coronary vasodilatation. III. Clinical trial. Am. J. Cardiol. 42:751, 1978.
66. Sochor, H., Pachinger, O., Ogris, E., et al.: Radionuclide imaging after coronary vasodilation: Myocardial scintigraphy with thallium-201 and radionuclide angiography after administration of dipyridamole. Eur. Heart J. 5:500, 1984.
67. Josephson, M. A., Brown, B. G., Hecht, H. S., et al.: Noninvasive detection and localization of coronary stenoses in patients: Comparison of resting dipyridamole and exercise thallium-201 myocardial perfusion imaging. Am. Heart J. 103:1008, 1982.
68. Rehn, T., Griffith, L.S.C., Achuff, S.C., et al.: Exercise thallium-201 myocardial imaging in left main coronary artery disease: Sensitive but not specific. Am. J. Cardiol. 48:217, 1981.
69. Nygaard, T. W., Gibson, R. S., Ryan, J. M., et al.: Prevalence of high-risk thallium-201 scintigraphic findings in left main coronary artery stenosis: Comparison with patients with multiple- and single-vessel coronary artery disease. Am. J. Cardiol. 53:462, 1984.
70. Kushner, F. G., Okada, R. D., Kirshenbaum, H. D., et al.: Lung thallium-201 uptake after stress testing in patients with coronary artery disease. Circulation 63:341, 1981.
71. Reisman, S., Maddahi, J., van Train, K., et al.: Quantitation of extent, depth, and severity of planar thallium defects in patients undergoing exercise thallium-201 scintigraphy. J. Nucl. Med. 27:1273, 1986.
72. Brown, K. A., Boucher, C. A., Okada, R. D., et al.: Prognostic value of exercise thallium-201 imaging in patients presenting for evaluation of chest pain. J. Am. Coll. Cardiol. 1:994, 1983.
73. Abraham, R. D., Freedman, S. B., Dunn, R. F., et al: Prediction of multivessel coronary artery disease and prognosis early after acute myocardial infarction by exercise electrocardiography and thallium-201 myocardial perfusion scanning. Am. J. Cardiol. 58:423, 1986.
74. Ladenheim, M. L., Pollock, B. H., Rozanski, A., et al.: Extent and severity of myocardial hypoperfusion as predictors of prognosis in patients with suspected coronary artery disease. J. Am. Coll. Cardiol. 7:464, 1986.
75. Kaul, S., Finkelstein, D. M., Homma, S., et al.: Superiority of quantitative exercise thallium-201 variables in determining long-term prognosis in ambulatory patients with chest pain: A comparison with cardiac catheterization. J. Am. Coll. Cardiol. 12:25, 1988.
76. Bairey, C. N., Rozanski, A., Maddahi, J., et al.: Exercise thallium-201 scintigraphy and prognosis in typical angina pectoris and negative exercise electrocardiography. Am. J. Cardiol. 64:282, 1989.
77. Gibson, R. S., Watson, D. D., Craddock, G. B., et al.: Prediction of cardiac events after uncomplicated myocardial infarction: A prospective study comparing predischarge exercise thallium-201 scintigraphy and coronary angiography. Cirlculation 68:321, 1983.
78. Leppo, J. A., O'Brien, J., Rothendler, J. A., et al.: Dipyridamole-thallium-201 scintigraphy in the prediction of future cardiac events after acute myocardial infarction. N. Engl. J. Med. 3101014, 1984.
79. Heller, L. I., Tresgallo, M., Sciacca, R. R., et al.: Prognostic significance of silent myocardial ischemia on a thallium stress test. Am. J. Cardiol. 65:718, 1990.
80. Koss, J. H., Kobren, S., Grunwald, A. W., et al.: Role of exercise thallium-201 myocardial perfusion scintigraphy in predicting prognosis in suspected coronary artery disease. Am. J. Cardiol. 59:531, 1987.
81. Gill, J. B., Ruddy, T. R., Newell, J. B., et al.: Prognostic importance of thallium uptake by the lungs during exercise in coronary artery disease. N. Engl. J. Med. 317:1485, 1987.
82. Brown, K. A., Weiss, R. M., Clements, J. P., et al.: Usefulness of residual ischemic myocardium within prior infarct zone for identifying patients at high risk late after acute myocardial infarction. Am. J. Cardiol. 60:15, 1987.
83. Wackers, F.J.T., Russo, D. J., Russo, D., et al.: Prognostic significance of normal quantitative planar thallium-201 stress scintigraphy in patients with chest pain. J. Am. Coll. Cardiol. 6:27, 1985.
84. Pamelia, F. X., Gibson, R. S., Watson, D.D., et al.: Prognosis with chest pain and normal thallium-201 exercise scintigrams. Am. J. Cardiol. 55:920, 1985.
85. Wahl, J., Hakki, A. H., and Iskandrian, A. S.: Prognostic implications of normal exercise thallium-201 images. Arch. Intern. Med. 145:253, 1985.
86. Staniloff, H. M., Forrester, J. S., Berman, D. S., et al.: Prediction of death, myocardial infarction, and worsening chest pain using thallium scintigraphy and exercise electrocardiography. J. Nucl. Med. 27:1842, 1986.
87. Tamaki, N., Yonekura, Y., Mukai, T., et al.: Stress thallium-201 transaxial emission computed tomography: Quantitative versus qualitative analysis for evaluation of coronary artery disease. J. Am. Coll. Cardiol. 4:1213, 1984.
88. DePasquale, E. E., Nody, A. C., DePuey, E.G., et al.: Quantitative rotational thallium-201 tomography for identifying and localizing coronary artery disease. Circulation 77:316, 1988.
89. Borges-Neto, S., Mahmarian, J. J., Jain, A., et al.: Quantitative thallium-201 single photon emission computed tomography after oral dipyridamole for assessing the presence, anatomic location and severity of coronary artery disease. J. Am. Coll. Cardiol. 11:962, 1988.
90. Maddahi, J., Van Train, K., Prigent, F., et al.: Quantitative single photon emission computed thallium-201 tomography for detection and localization of coronary artery disease: Optimization and prospective validation of a new technique. J. Am. Coll. Cardiol. 14:1689, 1989.
91. Fintel, D. J., Links, J. M., Brinker, J. A., et al.: Improved diagnostic performance of exercise thallium-201 single photon emission computer tomography over planar imaging in the diagnosis of coronary artery disease: A receiver operating characteristic analysis. J. Am. Coll. Cardiol. 13:600, 1989.
92. Iskandrian, S., Heo, J., Kong, B., et al.: Effect of exercise level on the ability of thallium-201 tomographic imaging in detecting coronary artery disease: Analysis of 461 patients. J. Am. Coll. Cardiol. 14:1477, 1989.
93. Mahmarian, J. J., Boyce, T. M., Goldberg, R. K., et al.: Quantitative exercise thallium-201 single photon emission computed tomography for the enhanced diagnosis of ischemic heart disease. J. Am. Coll. Cardiol. 15:318, 1990.
94. Rozanski, A., Diamond, G., Forrester, J. S., et al.: Declining specificity of exercise radionuclide ventriculography. N. Engl. J. Med. 309:518, 1983.
95. Boucher, C. A., Brewster, D. C., Darling, R. C., et al.: Determination of cardiac risk by dipyridamole-thallium imaging before peripheral vascular surgery. N. Engl. J. Med. 312:389, 1985.
96. Levinson, J. R., Boucher, C. A., Coley, G. M., et al.: Usefulness of semi-quantitative analysis of dipyridamole-thallium-201 redistribution for improving risk stratification before vascular surgery. Am. J. Cardiol. 66:406, 1990.
96a. Iskandrian, A.S., Heo, J., Nguyen, T., et al.: Left ventricular dilatation and pulmonary thallium uptake after single-photon emission computer tomography using thallium-201 during adenosine-induced coronary hyperemia. Am. J. Cardiol. 66:807, 1990.
96b. Lette, J., Lapointe, J., Waters, D., et al.: Transient left ventricular cavitary dilation during dipyridamole-thallium imaging as an indicator of severe coronary artery disease. Am. J. Cardiol. 66:1163, 1990.
97. Taillefer, R., DuPras, G., Sporn, V., et al.: Myocardial perfusion imaging with a new radiotracer, technetium-99m-hexamibi (methoxy isobutyl isonitrile): Comparison with thallium-201 imaging. Clinical Nuclear Medicine 14:89, 1989.
98. Kiat, H., Maddahi, J., Roy, L. T., et al.: Comparison of technetium 99m methoxy isobutyl isonitrile and thallium 201 for evaluation of coronary artery disease by planar and tomographic methods. Am. Heart J. 117:1, 1989.
99. Taillefer, R., Gagnon, A., Laflamme, L., et al.: Same-day injections of Tc-99m methoxy isobutyl isonitrile (hexamibi) for myocardi tomographic imaging. Comparison between rest-stress and stress-rest injection. Eur. J. Nucl. Med. 15:113, 1989.
100. Baillet, G., Mena, I. G., Kuperus, J. H., et al.: Simultaneous technetium-99m MIBI angiography and myocardial perfusion imaging. J. Nucl. Med. 30:38, 1989.
101. Iskandrian, A., Kong, H. J., and Lyons, E.: Use of technetium-99m isonitrile (RP-30A) in assessing left ventricular perfusion and function at rest and during exercise in coronary artery disease and comparison with coronary arteriography and exercise thallium-201 SPECT imaging. Am. J. Cardiol. 64:270, 1989.
102. Maniowski, P. J., Allam, A. H., Wackers, F.J.T., et al.: A new non-geometric technique for simultaneous evaluation of regional function and myocardial perfusion from gated planar isonitrile images (abstract). Circulation 80:544, 1989.
102a. Hendel, R.C., McSherry, B., Karimeddini, M., and Leppo, J.A.: Diagnostic value of a new myocardial perfusion agent, teboroxime (SQ 30,217), using a rapid planar imaging protocol: Preliminary results. J. Am. Coll. Cardiol. 16:855, 1990.
102b. Iskandrian, A. S., Heo, J., Nguyen, T., and Mercuro J.: Myocardial imaging with Tc-99m teboroxime: Technique and initial results. Am. Heart J. 121:889, 1991.
103. Diamond, G. A., and Forrester, J. S.: Analysis of probability as an aid in the clinical diagnosis of coronary artery disease. N. Engl. J. Med. 300:1350, 1979.
104. Epstein, S. E.: Implications of probability analysis on the strategy used for

noninvasive detection of coronary artery disease. Role of single or combined use of exercise electrocardiographic testing, radionuclide cineangiography and myocardial perfusion imaging. Am. J. Cardiol. *46*:491, 1980.

105. Hamilton, G. W., Trobaugh, G. B., Ritchie, J. C., et al.: Myocardial imaging with ^{201}Thallium: An analysis of clinical usefulness based on Bayes' Theorem. Semin. Nucl. Med. *8*:358, 1978.

106. Wackers, F.J.T.: Complete left bundle branch block: Is the diagnosis of myocardial infarction possible? Int. J. Cardiol. *2*:521, 1983.

107. McGowan, R. L., Welch, T. G., Zaret, B. L., et al.: Noninvasive myocardial imaging with potassium-43 and rubidium-81 in patients with left bundle branch block. Am. J. Cardiol. *38*:422, 1976.

108. DePuey, E. G., Guertler-Krawczynska, E., and Robbins, W. L.: Thallium-201 SPECT in coronary artery disease patients with left bundle branch block. J. Nucl. Med. *29*:1479, 1988.

109. Hirzel, H. O., Senn, M., Neusch, K., Buettner, C., et al.: Thallium-201 scintigraphy in complete left bundle branch block. Am. J. Cardiol. *53*:764, 1984.

109a. Shefcyk, D.L., Gingrich, S., Nino, A.F., et al.: Altered left ventricular depolarization sequence in left bundle branch block is not a cause for false-positive thallium-201. J. Am. Coll. Cardiol. (abstract), *(in press)*.

110. Berger, H. J., Sands, M. J., Davies, R. A., et al.: Exercise left ventricular performance in patients with chest pain, ischemic-appearing exercise electrocardiograms, and angiographically normal coronary arteries. Ann. Intern. Med. *94*:186, 1981.

111. Berger, B. C., Abramowitz, R., Park, C. H., et al.: Abnormal thallium-201 scans in patients with chest pain and angiographically normal coronary arteries. Am. J. Cardiol. *52*:365, 1983.

112. Legrand, V., Hodgson, J. M.., Bates, E. R., et al.: Abnormal coronary flow reserve and abnormal radionuclide exercise test results in patients with normal coronary angiograms. J. Am. Coll. Cardiol. *6*:1245, 1985.

113. Cannon, R. O., Bonow, R. O., Bacharach, S. L., et al.: Left ventricular dysfunction in patients with angina pectoris, normal epicardial coronary arteries and abnormal vasodilator reserve. Circulation *71*:218, 1985.

INFARCT IMAGING

114. Rude, R. E., Parkey, R. W., Bonte, F. J., et al.: Clinical implications of the technetium-99m stannous pyrophosphate myocardial scintigraphic "doughnut" pattern in patients with acute myocardial infarcts. Circulation *59*:721, 1979.

115. Schofer, J., Spielmann, R. P., Bromel, T. et al.: Thallium-201/technetium-99m pyrophosphate overlap in patients with acute myocardial infarction after thrombolysis: Prediction of depressed wall motion despite thallium uptake. Am. Heart J. *112*:291, 1986.

116. Davies, A. D., Thakur, M. L., Berger, H. J., et al.: Imaging the inflammatory response to acute myocardial infarction in man using indium-111–labeled autologous leukocytes. Circulation *63*:826, 1981.

117. Johnson, L. L., Seldin, D. W., Becker, L. C., et al.: Antimyosin imaging in acute transmural myocardial infarctions: Results of a multicenter clinical trial. J. Am. Coll. Cardiol. *13*:27, 1989.

118. Carrio, I., Bernia, L., Ballester, M., et al.: Indium-111 antimyosin scintigraphy to assess myocardial damage in patients with suspected myocarditis and cardiac rejection. J. Nucl. Med. *29*:1900, 1988.

119. Dec, G. W., Palacios, I. Yasuda, T., et al.: Antimyosin antibody cardiac imaging: Its role in the diagnosis of myocarditis. J. Am. Coll. Cardiol. *16*:97, 1990.

120. Lahiri, A., and Jain, D.: New radionuclide imaging in cardiovascular disease. Curr. Opin. Cardiol. *2*:1070, 1987.

ASSESSMENT OF CARDIAC PERFORMANCE

121. Zaret, B. L., Strauss, H. W., Hurley, P. J., et al.: A noninvasive scintiphotographic method for detecting regional ventricular dysfunction in man. N. Engl. J. Med. *284*:1165, 1971.

122. Strauss, H. W., Zaret, B. L., Hurley, P. J., et al.: A scintiphotographic method for measuring left ventricular ejection fraction in man without cardiac catheterization. Am. J. Cardiol. *28*:575, 1971.

123. Strauss, H. W., McKusick, K. A., Boucher, C. A., et al.: Of linens and laces: The eighth anniversary of the gated blood pool scan. Semin. Nucl. Med. *9*:296, 1979.

124. Rollo, F. D., and Patton, J. A.: Quantification of the radionuclide image: theoretical concepts and the role of the computer. *In* Freeman, L. M., (ed.): Freeman and Johnson's Clinical Radionuclide Imaging. 3rd ed. New York, Grune and Stratton, 1984, p. 261.

125. Berger, H. J., and Zaret, B. L.: Radionuclide assessment of cardiovascular performance. *In* Freeman, L. M., (ed.): Freeman and Johnson's Clinical Radionuclide Imaging. 3rd ed. New York, Grune and Stratton, 1984, p. 364.

126. Kelly, M. J., Giles, R. W., Simon, T. S., et al.: Multigated equilibrium radionuclide and angiocardiography: Improved detection of left ventricular wall motion abnormalities and aneurysms with the addition of the left lateral view. Radiology *139*:167, 1981.

127. Callahan, R. J., Froelich, J. W., McKusick, K. A., et al.: A modified method for the in vivo labeling of red blood cells with Tc-99m: Concise communication. J. Nucl. Med. *23*:315, 1982.

128. Zaret, B. L., and Berger, H. J.: Nuclear cardiology. *In* Hurst, J. W., (ed.): The Heart, Arteries and Veins. 7th ed. New York, McGraw-Hill, 1990, p. 1899.

129. Kimchi, A., Rozanski, A., Fletcher, C., et al.: Reversal of rest myocardial asynergy during exercise: A radionuclide scintigraphic study. J. Am. Coll. Cardiol. *6*:1004, 1985.

130. Rozanski, A., Bairey, C. N., and Krantz, D. S., et al.: Mental stress and the induction of silent myocardial ischemia in patients with coronary artery disease. N. Engl. J. Med. *318*:1005, 1988.

131. LaVeau, P. J., Rozanski, A., Krantz, D. S., et al.: Cardiac dysfunction during mental stress. Am. Heart J. *118*:1, 1989.

131a. Bairey, C.N., deYang, L., Berman, D.S., et al.: Comparison of physiologic ejection fraction to activities of daily life: Implications for clinical testing. J. Am. Coll. Cardiol. *16*:847, 1990.

132. Links, J. M., Becker, L. C., Shindledecker, J. G., et al.: Measurement of absolute left ventricular volume from gated blood pool studies. Circulation *65*:82, 1982.

133. Verani, M. S., Gaeta, J., LeBlanc, A. D., et al.: Validation of left ventricular volume measurements by radionuclide angiography. J. Nucl. Med. *26*:1394, 1985.

134. Fearnow, E. C., Stanfield, J. A., and Jaszczak, R. J., et al.: Factors affecting ventricular volume as determined by a count-based equilibrium method. J. Nucl. Med. *26*:1042, 1985.

135. Massardo, T., Gal, R. A., Grenier, R. P., et al.: Left ventricular volume calculation using a count-based ratio method applied to multigated radionuclide angiography. J. Nucl. Med. *31*:450, 1990.

136. Fritch, B. G., Dehmer, G. J., and Markham, R. V.: Assessment of vasodilator therapy in patients with severe congestive heart failure: Limitations of measurements of left ventricular ejection fraction and volume. Am. J. Cardiol. *50*:954, 1982.

137. Magorien, D. J., Shaffer, P., Bush, C. A., et al.: Assessment of left ventricular pressure-volume relations using gated radionuclide angiography, echocardiography and micromanometer pressure records. Circulation *67*:844, 1983.

138. Marmor, A., Sharir, T., and Ben Shlomo, I., et al.: Radionuclide ventriculography and central aortic pressure change in noninvasive assessment of myocardial performance. J. Nucl. Med. *30*:1657, 1989.

139. Rigo, P., Alderson, P. O., Robertson, R. M., et al.: Measurement of aortic and mitral regurgitation by gated cardiac blood pool scans. Circulation *60*:306, 1979.

140. Lam, W., Pavel, D., Byrom, E., et al.: Radionuclide regurgitant index: Value and limitations. Am. J. Cardiol. *47*:292, 1981.

141. Wackers, F. J., Terrin, M. L., Kayden, D. S., et al.: Quantitative radionuclide assessment of regional ventricular function after thrombolytic therapy for acute myocardial infarction: Results of phase I thrombolysis in myocardial infarction (TIMI) trial. J. Am. Coll. Cardiol. *13*:998, 1989.

142. Zaret, B. L., Wackers, F. J., Terrin, M. L., et al.: Exercise ventricular function following thrombolysis: Effect of invasive versus conservative strategies in the TIMI II trial. Circulation *80*(Suppl. II):608, 1989.

142a. Zaret, B.L., Wackers, F.J., Terrin, M.L., et al.: Assessment of global and regional left ventricular performance at rest and during exercise following thrombolytic therapy for acute myocardial infarction: Results of the thrombolysis in myocardial infarction (TIMI) II-B study. Submitted for publication.

143. Zaret, B. L., and Wackers, F. J.: Radionuclide methods for evaluating the results of thrombolytic therapy. Circulation *76*(Suppl. II):8, 1987.

144. Duncan, J. S., Fetterman, R., Greene, R., et al.: Quantification of left ventricular wall motion from multiple view equilibrium angiocardiography (ERNA). Automedica *10*:1, 1988.

145. Duncan, J., Smeulders, A., Lee, F., et al.: Measurement of end diastolic shape deformity using bending energy. IEEE Proceedings of Computers in Cardiology, 277, 1988.

146. Starling, M. R., Walsh, R. Z., Lasher, J. C., et al.: Quantification of left ventricular regional dyssynergy by radionuclide angiography. J. Nucl. Med. *28*:1725, 1987.

147. Botvinick, E. H., Dae, M. W., O'Connell, J. W., et al.: First harmonic Fourier (phase) analysis of blood pool scintigrams for the analysis of cardiac contraction and conduction. *In* Gerson, M. C., (ed.): Cardiac Nuclear Medicine. New York, McGraw-Hill, 1987, p. 109.

148. Okada, R. D., Pohost, G. M., Kirshenbaum, H. D., et al.: Radionuclide determined change in pulmonary blood volume with exercise: Improved sensitivity of multigated blood-pool scanning in detecting coronary artery disease. N. Engl. J. Med. *301*:569, 1979.

149. Robinson, V.J.B., Smiseth, O. A., Scott-Douglas, N. W., et al.: Assessment of splanchic vascular capacity and capacitance using quantitative equilibrium blood pool scintigraphy. J. Nucl. Med. *31*:154, 1990.

150. Flamm, S. D., Taki, J., and Moore, R., et al.: Redistribution of regional and organ blood volume and effect on cardiac function in relation to upright exercise intensity in healthy human subjects. Circulation *81*:1550, 1990.

151. Wagner, H. N., Wake, R., Nickoloff, E., et al.: The nuclear stethoscope: A simple device for generation of left ventricular volume curves. Am. J. Cardiol. *38*:747, 1976.

152. Soufer, R., Wohlgelernter, D., Vita, N. A., et al.: Intact systolic left ventricular function in clinical congestive heart failure. Am. J. Cardiol. *55*:1032, 1985.

153. Breisblatt, W. M., Vita, N. A., Armuchastegui, M., et al.: Usefulness of serial radionuclide monitoring during graded nitroglycerin infusion for unstable angina pectoris for determining left ventricular function and individualized therapeutic dose. Am. J. Cardiol. *61*:685, 1988.

154. Broadhurst, P., Cashman, P., Crawley, J., et al.: Clinical validation of a miniature nuclear probe system for continuous on-line monitoring of cardiac function and ST-segment. J. Nucl. Med. *32*:37, 1991.

154a. Jain, D., Allam, A. H., Wackers, F. J., et al.: Validation of a new nonimaging miniature probe for serial on-line left ventricular ejection fraction. Submitted for publication.

155. Tamaki, N., Yasuda, T., Moore, R., et al.: Continuous monitoring of left ventricular function by an ambulatory radionuclide detector in patients with coronary artery disease. J. Am. Coll. Cardiol. *12*:669, 1988.
156. Kayden, D. S., Wackers, F. J., and Zaret, B. L.: Silent left ventricular dysfunction during routine activity after thrombolytic therapy for acute myocardial infarction. J. Am. Coll. Cardiol. *15*:1500, 1990.
157. Zaret, B. L., and Kayden, D. S.: Ambulatory monitoring of left ventricular function: A new modality for assessing silent myocardial ischemia. *In* Kellerman, J. J., and Braunwald, E. (eds.): Silent Myocardial Ischemia: A Critical Appraisal. Basel, Karger, 1990, p. 105.
158. Faber, T. L., Stokely, E. M., Templeton, G. H., et al.: Quantification of three dimensional left ventricular segmental wall motion and volumes from gated tomographic radionuclide ventriculograms. J. Nucl. Med. *30*:638, 1989.

FIRST-PASS RADIONUCLIDE ANGIOCARDIOGRAPHY (FPRNA)

159. Blumgart, H. L., and Weiss, S.: Studies on the velocity of blood flow. VII. The pulmonary circulation time in normal resting individuals. J. Clin. Invest. *4*:399, 1927.
160. Prinzmetal, M., Corday, E., and Sprizler, R. J.: Radiocardiography and its clinical applications. J.A.M.A. *139*:617, 1949.
161. Van Dyke, D. C., Anger, H. O., Sullivan, R. W., et al.: Cardiac evaluation from radioisotope dynamics. J. Nucl. Med. *13*:585, 1972.
162. Gal, R., Grenier, R. P., Carpenter, J., et al.: High count rate first-pass radionuclide angiography using a digital gamma camera. J. Nucl. Med. *27*:198, 1986.
163. Wackers, F. J., Stein, R., Pytlik, L., et al.: Gold-195m for serial first pass radionuclide angiocardiography during upright exercise in patients with coronary artery disease. J. Am. Coll. Cardiol. *2*:497, 1983.
164. Cheng, C., Trevis, S., Samuel, A., et al.: A new osmium-191-iridium-191m generator. J. Nucl. Med. *21*:1169, 1980.
165. Zaret, B. L., and Wackers, F. J.: Measurement of right ventricular function. *In* Gerson, M. C. (ed.): Cardiac Nuclear Medicine. 2nd ed. New York, McGraw-Hill, (in press).
166. Brent, B. N., Mahler, D., Matthay, R. A., et al.: Noninvasive diagnosis of pulmonary hypertension in chronic obstructive pulmonary disease; Utility of resting right ventricular ejection fraction. Am. J. Cardiol. *53*:1349, 1984.
167. Gelfand, M. J., and Hannon, D. W.: Pediatric Nuclear Cardiology. *In* Gerson, M. C. (ed.): Cardiac Nuclear Medicine, 1st ed. New York, McGraw-Hill, p. 437, 1987.
168. Treves, S.: Detection and quantification of cardiovascular shunts with commonly available radionuclide. Semin. Nucl. Med. *10*:16, 1980.
169. Bonow, R. O., Bacharach, S. L., Green, M. V., et al.: Impaired left ventricular diastolic filling in patients with coronary artery disease: Assessment with radionuclide angiography. Circulation *64*:315, 1981.
170. Bashore, T. M., and Shaffer, P.: Diastolic function. *In* Gerson, M. C. (ed.): Cardiac Nuclear Medicine. New York, McGraw-Hill, 1987, p. 137.
171. Lee, F. A., Fetterman, R., Zaret, B. L., et al.: Rapid radionuclide-derived systolic and diastolic cardiac function using cycle-dependent background correction and fourier analysis. IEEE Computer Society, p. 443, 1983.
172. Fouad, F. M., Slominski, J. M., and Tarazi, R. C.: Left ventricular diastolic function in hypertension: Relation to left ventricular mass and function. J. Am. Coll. Cardiol. *3*:1500, 1984.
173. Bonow, R. O., Kent, K. M., Rosing, D. R., et al: Improved left ventricular diastolic filling in patients with coronary artery disease after percutaneous transluminal coronary angioplasty. Circulation *66*:1159, 1982.
174. Bonow, R. O., Leon, M. B., Rosing, D. R., et al.: Effects of verapamil and propranolol on left ventricular systolic function and diastolic filling in patients with coronary artery disease: Radionuclide angiographic studies at rest and during exercise. Circulation *65*:1337, 1981.
175. Cohn, J. N., Johnson, G., and the Veterans Administration Cooperative Study Group: Heart failure with normal ejection fraction. Circulation *81*(Suppl. III):4A, 1990.
176. Setaro, J. F., Remetz, M., Zaret, B. L., et al.: Prognosis of patients with congestive heart failure and intact systolic function: A seven-year followup. Circulation *80*(Suppl. II):275, 1989.
177. Setaro, J. F., Zaret, B. L., Schulman, D. S., et al.: Usefulness of verapamil for congestive heart failure, abnormal diastolic filling and normal left ventricular systolic performance. Am. J. Cardiol *66*:981, 1990.
178. Iskandrian, A. S., and Hakki, A.: Age-related changes in left ventricular diastolic performance. Am. Heart J. *112*:75, 1986.
179. Miller, T. R., Grossman, S. J., Schectman, K. B., et al: Left ventricular diastolic filling in its association with age. Am. J. Cardiol. *58*:531, 1986.

CLINICAL APPLICATIONS OF CARDIAC PERFORMANCE STUDIES

180. Kazmers, A., Cerqueira, M. D., and Zierler, R. E.: The role of preoperative radionuclide left ventricular ejection fraction for risk assessment in carotid surgery. Arch. Surg. *123*:416, 1988.
181. Kazmers, A., Cerqueira, M. D., and Zierler, R. E.: The role of preoperative radionuclide ejection fraction in direct abdominal aortic aneurysm repair. J. Vasc. Surg. *8*:128, 1988.
182. The Multicenter Postinfarction Research Group: Risk stratification and survival after myocardial infarction. N. Engl. J. Med. *309*:331, 1983.
183. Abraham, R. D., Harris, P. G., Rubin, G. S., et al.: Usefulness of ejection fraction response to exercise one month after acute myocardial infarction in predicting coronary anatomy and prognosis. Am. J. Cardiol. *60*:225, 1987.
184. Ahnve, S., Gilpin, E., Henning, H., et al.: Limitations and advantages of the ejection fraction for defining high risk after acute myocardial infarction. Am. J. Cardiol. *58*:872, 1986.
185. Zaret, B. L., Wackers, F. J., Terrin, M., et al.: Does left ventricular ejection fraction following thrombolytic therapy have the same prognostic impact described in the prethrombolytic era? Results of the TIMI II trial. J. Am. Coll. Cardiol. In press.
186. CASS Principal Investigators: Coronary artery surgery study (CASS): A randomized trial of coronary bypass surgery. Survival data. Circulation *68*:939 1983.
187. Ritchie, J. L., Hallstrom, A. P., Troubaugh, C. B., et al.: Out-of-hospital sudden coronary death: Rest and exercise left ventricular function in survivors. Am. J. Cardiol. *55*:645, 1985.
188. Meizlish, J., Berger, H. J., and Plankey, R. T., et al.: Functional left ventricular aneurysm formation following acute anterior transmural myocardial infarction: Incidence, natural history and prognostic implications. N. Engl. J. Med. *311*:101, 1984.
189. Bonow, R. O., Kent, K. M., Rosing, D. R., et al.: Exercise-induced ischemia in mildly symptomatic patients with coronary artery disease and preserved left ventricular function: Identification of subgroups at risk of death during medical therapy. N. Engl. J. Med. *311*:1339, 1984.
190. Pryor, D. D., Harrell, F. E., Lee, K. I., et al.: Prognostic indicators from radionuclide angiography in medically treated patients with coronary artery disease. Am. J. Cardiol. *53*:18, 1984.
191. Morris, K. G., Palmeri, S. T., Califf, R. M., et al.: Value of radionuclide angiography in predicting specific cardiac events after acute myocardial infarction. Am. J. Cardiol. *55*:318, 1985.
192. Jones, R. H., Floyd, R. D., Austin, E. H., et al.: The role of radionuclide angiocardiography in the preoperative prediction of pain relief and prolonged survival following coronary artery bypass grafting. Ann. Surg. *187*:743, 1983.
193. Schlant, R. C.: The prognosis of individuals with silent myocardial ischemia. *In* Kellerman, N.J.J., and Braunwald, E. (eds.): Silent Myocardial Ischemia: A Critical Appraisal. Vol. 37. Basel, Karger, 1990, p. 187.
194. Breitenbucher, A., Pfisterer, M., Hoffman, A., et al.: Long-term followup of patients with silent ischemia during exercise radionuclide angiography. J. Am. Coll. Cardiol. *15*:999, 1990.
195. Rocco, M. V., Nabel, E. G., Campbell, S., et al.: Prognostic significance of myocardial ischemia detected by ambulatory monitoring in patients with stable coronary artery disease. Circulation. *78*:877, 1988.
196. Kayden, D. S., Remetz, M. S., Cabin, H. S., et al.: Validation of continuous radionuclide ventricular monitoring during coronary angioplasty. Submitted for publication.
197. Alexander, J., Dainiak, N., Berger, H. J., et al.: Serial assessment of doxorubicin cardiotoxicity with quantitative radionuclide angiocardiography. N. Engl. J. Med. *300*:278, 1979.
198. Schwartz, R. G., McKenzie, W. B., Alexander, J., et al.: Congestive heart failure and left ventricular dysfunction complicating doxorubicin therapy: Seven-year experience using serial radionuclide angiocardiography. Am. J. Med. *82*:1109, 1987.
199. Palmeri, S. T., Bonow, R. O., Myers, C. E., et al.: Prospective evaluation of doxorubicin cardiotoxicity by rest and exercise radionuclide angiography. Am. J. Cardiol. *58*:607, 1986.
200. Borer, J. S., Bacharach, S. L., Green, M. V., et al.: Exercise-induced left ventricular dysfunction in symptomatic and asymptomatic patients with aortic regurgitation: Assessment by radionuclide cineangiography. Am. J. Cardiol. *42*:351, 1978.
201. Hurwitz, R. A., Caldwell, R. L., Mahony, L., et al.: The role of radionuclide shunt studies in management of infants and children. Clin. Nucl. Med. *11*:781, 1986.
202. Parrish, M. D., Graham, T. V., Bender, H. W., et al.: Radionuclide angiographic evaluation of right and left ventricular function during exercise after repair of transposition of the great arteries: Comparison with normal subjects and patients with congenitally corrected transposition. Circulation *67*:178, 1983.
203. Brent, B. N., Berger, H. J., Matthay, R. A., et al.: Physiologic correlates of right ventricular ejection fraction in chronic obstructive pulmonary disease: A combined radionuclide and hemodynamic study. Am. J. Cardiol. *50*:255, 1982.
204. Schulman, D. S., Biondi, J. W., Matthay, R. A., et al.: Differing responses in ventricular filling, loading and volumes during positive end exploratory pressure in man. Am. J. Cardiol. *64*:772, 1989.
205. Schulman, D. S., Biondi, J. W., Zohgbi, S., et al.: Coronary flow limits right ventricular performance during positive and exploratory pressure. Am. Rev. Respir. Dis. *141*:1531, 1990.

SPECIAL IMAGING TECHNIQUES

206. Von Moll, L., McEwan, A. J., Shapiro, B., et al.: Iodine-131 MIBG scintigraphy of neuroendocrine tumors other than pheochromocytoma and neuroblastoma. J. Nucl. Med. *28*:979, 1987.
207. Sisson, J. C., Wieland, D. M., Sherman, P., et al.: Metaiodobenzylguanidine as an index of the adrenergic nervous system integrity and function. J. Nucl. Med. *28*:1620, 1987.
208. Rabonivitch, M. A., Rose, C. P., Rouleau, J. L., et al.: Metaiodobenzylguanidine(^{131}I) scintigraphy detects impaired myocardial sympathetic neuronal transport function of canine mechanical-overload heart failure. Circ. Res. *61*:797, 1987.

209. Sisson, J. C., Lynch, J. J., Johnson, J., et al.: Scintigraphic detection of regional disruption of adrenergic neurons in the heart. Am. Heart J. *116*:67, 1988.
210. Dae, M. W., O'Connell, J. W., Botvinick, E. H., et al.: Scintigraphic assessment of regional cardiac adrenergic innervation. Circulation *79*:634, 1989.
210a. Mody, F. V., Brunken, R. C., Stevenson, L. W., et al.: Differentiating cardiomyopathy of coronary artery disease from nonischemic dilated cardiomyopathy utilizing positron emission tomography. J. Am. Coll. Cardiol. *17*:373, 1991.
211. Stanton, M. S., Tuli, M. M., Radtke, N. L., et al.: Regional sympathetic denervation after myocardial infarction in humans detected noninvasively using I-123-metaiodobenzylguanidine. J. Am. Coll. Cardiol. *14*:1519, 1989.
211a. McGhie, A. I., Corbett, J. R., Akers, M. S., et al.: Regional cardiac adrenergic function using I-123 meta-iodobenzylguanidine tomographic imaging after acute myocardial infarction. Am J. Cardiol. *67*:236, 1991.
212. Schofer, J., Spielman, N. R., Schuchert, A., et al.: Iodine-123 metaiodobenzylguanidine scintigraphy: A noninvasive method to demonstrate myocardial adrenergic nervous system disintegrity in patients with idiopathic dilated cardiomyopathy. J. Am. Coll. Cardiol. *12*:1252, 1988.
213. Henderson, E. B., Kahn, J. K., Corbett, J. R., et al.: Abnormal I-123 metaiodobenzylguanidine myocardial washout and distribution may reflect myocardial adrenergic derangement in patients with congestive cardiomyopathy. Circulation *78*:1192, 1988.
214. Riba, A. L., Thakur, M. L., Gottschalk, A., et al.: Imaging experimental coronary artery thrombosis with indium-111 platelets. Circulation *60*:767, 1979.
215. Ezekowitz, M. D., Wilson, D. A., Smith, E. O., et al.: Comparison of indium-111 platelet scintigraphy and two-dimensional echocardiography in diagnosis of left ventricular thrombi. N. Engl. J. Med. *306*:1509, 1982.
216. Pope, C. F., Ezekowitz, M. D., Smith, E. O., et al.: Detection of platelet deposition at the site of peripheral balloon angioplasty using indium-111 platelet scintigraphy. Am. J. Cardiol. *55*:495, 1985.
217. Seabold, J. E., Conrad, G. R., Ponto, J. A., et al.: Deep venous thrombophlebitis; detection with 4 hour vs. 24 hour platelet scintigraphy. Radiology *165*:355, 1987.
218. Vandenberg, B. F., Seabold, J. E., Conrad, G. R., et al.: 111-In–labeled platelet scintigraphy and two dimensional echocardiography for detection of left atrial appendage thrombi: Studies in a new canine model. Circulation *78*:1040, 1988.
219. Stratton, J. R., and Ritchie, J. L.: 111-In platelet imaging of left ventricular thrombi: Predictive value for systemic emboli. Circulation *81*:1182, 1990.
220. Oster, Z. H., Srivastava, S. C., Som, P., et al.: Thrombus radioimmunoscintigraphy: An approach using monoclonal antiplatelet antibody. Proc. Natl. Acad. Sci. *82*:3465, 1985.
221. Knight, I. C., Maurer, A. H., Mattis, J. A., et al.: Evaluation of In-111 labeled anti-fibrin antibody for imaging vascular thrombi. J. Nucl. Med. *27*:975, 1986.
222. Rosebrough, S. F., Kudryk, B., Grossman, Z. D., et al.: Radioimmunoimaging of venous thrombi using iodine-131 monoclonal antibody. Radiology *156*:515, 1985.
223. Vorne, M., Likes, S., Sakki, S., et al.: Radionuclide venography and uptake imaging using 99m Tc-fibrinogen in detection of venous thrombosis and its correlation with contrast venography. Nucl. Med. Commun. *8*:921, 1987.
224. Lees, A. M., Lees, R. S., Schoen, F. J., et al.: Imaging human atherosclerosis with 99m Tc labeled low density lipoproteins. Arteriosclerosis *8*:461, 1988.
225. Visser, F. C., van Eenige, M. J. van der Wall, E. E., et al.: The mechanism of the elimination of rate of ^{123}I-hepadecanoic acid from the myocardium. J. Am. Coll. Cardiol. *3*:476, 1984.
226. Livni, E., Elmaleh, D. R., Barlai-Kovach, M. M., et al.: Radioiodinated beta-methylphenyl fatty acids as potential tracers for myocardial imaging and end metabolism. Eur. Heart J. (Suppl. B)*6*:85, 1985.
227. Reske, S. N.:^{123}I-phenylpentadecanoic acid as a tracer of cardiac free fatty acid metabolism: Experimental and clinical results. Eur. Heart J. (Suppl. B) *6*:39, 1985.
228. Kennedy, P. L., Corbett, J. R., Kulkarni, P.V., et al.: Iodine-123-phenylpentadecanoic acid myocardial scintingraphy. Usefulness in the identification of myocardial ischemia. Circulation *74*:1007, 1986.
229. Hansen, C. L., Corbett, J. R., Pippin, J. J., et al.: Iodine-123-phenylpentadecanoic acid and single photon emission computed tomography in identifying left ventricular regional metabolic abnormalities in patients with coronary heart disease: Comparison with thallium-201 tomography. J. Am. Coll. Cardiol. *12*:78, 1988.
230. Kahn, J. K., Pippin, J. J., Akers, M. S., et al.: Estimation of jeopardized left ventricular myocardium in symptomatic and silent ischemia as determined by iodine-123-phenylpentadecanoic acid rotational tomography. Am. J. Cardiol. *63*:540, 1989.
230a. Rehr, R. B.: Cardiovascular nuclear magnetic resonance imaging and spectroscopy. Curr. Prob. Cardiol. Vol. xvi, 1991.

POSITRON EMISSION TOMOGRAPHY

231. Brachfeld, N., and Scheuer, J.: Metabolism of glucose by the ischemic dog heart. Am. J. Physiol. *212*:603, 1967.
232. Liedtke, A. J.: Alterations of carbohydrate and lipid metabolism in the acutely ischemic heart. Prog. Cardiovasc. Dis. *23*:321, 1981.
233. Marshall, R. C., Nash, W. W., Shine, K. L., et al.: Glucose metabolism during ischemia due to excessive oxygen demand or altered coronary flow in the isolated arterially perfused rabbit septum. Circ. Res. *49*:640, 1981.
234. Opie, L. H., Owen, P., and Riemersma, R. A.: Relative rates of oxidation of glucose and free fatty acids by ischemic and nonischemic myocardium after coronary artery ligation in the dog. Eur. J. Clin. Invest. *3*:419, 1973.
235. Myears, D. W., Sobel, B. E., and Bergmann, S. R.: Substrate use in ischemic and reperfused canine myocardium: Quantitative considerations. Am. J. Physiol. *253*:H107, 1987.
236. Chan, S. Y., Brunken, R. C., and Buxton, D. B.: Cardiac positron emission tomography: The foundations and clinical applications. J. Thorac, Imaging *5*:9, 1990.
237. Schelbert, H. R., Phelps, M. E., Hoffman, E., et al.: Regional myocardial blood flow, metabolism, and function assessed noninvasively with positron emission tomography. Am. J. Cardiol. *80*:1269, 1980.
238. Marshall, R. C., Tillisch, J. H., Phelps, M. E., et al.: Identification and differentiation of resting myocardial ischemia and infarction in man with positron computed tomography, ^{18}F-labeled fluorodeoxyglucose and N-13 ammonia. Circulation *67*:766, 1983.
239. Brunken, R., Tillisch, J., Schwaiger, M., et al.: Regional perfusion, glucose metabolism, and wall motion in patients with chronic electrocardiographic Q wave infarctions: Evidence for persistence of viable tissue in some infarct regions by positron emission tomography. Circulation *73*:951, 1986.
240. Schelbert, H. R., and Buxton, D.: Insights into coronary artery disease gained from metabolic imaging. Circulation *78*:496, 1988.
241. Fudo, T., Kambara, H., Hashimoto, T., et al.: F-18 deoxyglucose and stress N-13 ammonia positron emission tomography in anterior wall healed myocardial infarction. Am. J. Cardiol. *61*:1191, 1988.
242. Tamaki, N., Yonekura, Y., Yamashita, K., et al.: Positron emission tomography using fluorine-18 deoxyglucose in evaluation of coronary artery bypass grafting. Am. J. Cardiol. *64*:860, 1989.
243. Brunken, R. C., and Schelbert, H. R.: Positron emission tomography in clinical cardiology. Cardiol. Clin. *7*:607, 1989.
244. Liu, P., Kiess, M. C., Okada, R. D., et al.: The persistent defect on exercise thallium imaging and its fate after myocardial revascularization: Does it represent scar or ischemia: Am. Heart J. *110*:996, 1985.
245. Gibson, R. S., Watson, D. D., Taylor, G. J., et al.: Prospective assessment of regional myocardial perfusion before and after coronary revascularization surgery by quantitative thallium-201 scintigraphy. J. Am. Coll. Cardiol. *1*:804, 1983.
246. Brunken, R., Schwaiger, M., Grover-McKay, M., et al.: Positron emission tomography detects tissue metabolic activity in myocardial segments with persistent thallium perfusion defects. J. Am. Coll. Cardiol. *10*:557, 1987.
247. Brunken, R. C., Kottou, S., Nienabar, C. A.., et al.: PET detection of viable tissue in myocardial segments with persistent defects at Tl-201 SPECT. Radiology *172*:65, 1989.
248. Tamaki, N., Yonekura, Y., Yamashita, K., et al.: Relation of left ventricular perfusion and wall motion with metabolic activity in persistent defects on thallium-201 tomography in healed myocardial infarction. Am. J. Cardiol. *62*:202, 1988.
249. Tamaki, N., Yonekura, Y., Yamashita, K., et al.: SPECT thallium-201 tomography and positron tomography using N-13 ammonia and F-18 fluorodeoxyglucose in coronary artery disease. Am. J. Cardiac Imaging *3*:3, 1989.
249a. Go, R.T., Marwick, T.H., MacIntyre, W.J., et al.: A prospective comparison of rubidium-82 PET and thallium-201 SPECT myocardial perfusion imaging utilizing a single dipyridamole stress in the diagnosis of coronary artery disease. J. Nucl. Med. *31*:1899, 1990.
250. Bonow, R. O., Bacharach, S. L., Cuocolo, A., et al.: Myocardial viability in coronary artery disease and left ventricular dysfunction: Thallium-201 reinjection vs. fluorodeoxyglucose (abstract). Circulation *80*(Suppl. II):377, 1989.
251. Shah, A., Schelbert, H. R., Schwaiger, M., et al.: Measurement of regional myocardial blood flow with N-13 ammonia and positron emission tomography in intact dogs. J. Am. Coll. Cardiol. *5*:92, 1985.
252. Bergmann, S. R., Herrero, P., Markham, J., et al.: Noninvasive quantitation of myocardial blood flow in human subjects with oxygen-15-labeled with water and positron emission tomography. J. Am. Coll. Cardiol. *14*:639, 1989.
253. Kirkeeide, R. L., Gould, K. L., and Parsel, L.: Assessment of coronary stenoses of myocardial perfusion imaging during pharmacologic coronary vasodilation. VII. Validation of coronary flow reserve as a single integrated functional measure of stenosis severity reflecting all its geometric dimensions. J. Am. Coll. Cardiol. *7*:103, 1986.
254. Goldstein, R. A., Mullani, N. A., Marani, S. K., et al.: Myocardial perfusion with rubidium-82. II. Effects and pharmacologic intervention. J. Nucl. Med. *24*:907, 1983.
255. Mullani, N. A., Goldstein, R. A., Gould, K. L., et al.: Myocardial perfusion with rubidium-82. I. Measurement of extraction fraction and flow with external detectors. J. Nucl. Med. *24*:898, 1983.
256. Shelton, M. E., Green, M. A., Mathias, C. J., et al.: Kinetics of copper-PTSM in isolated hearts. A novel tracer for measuring blood flow with positron emission tomography. J. Nucl. Med. *30*:1843, 1989.
256a. Shelton, M.E., Green, M.A., Mathias, C.J., et al.: Assessment of regional myocardial and renal blood flow with copper-PTSM and positron emission tomography. Circulation *82*:990, 1990.
256b. Green, M.A., Mathias, C.J., Welch, M.J., et al.: Copper-62-labeled pyruvaldehyde bis(N^4-methylthiosemicarbazonato) copper(II): Synthesis

and evaluation as a positron emission tomography tracer for cerebral and myocardial perfusion. J. Nucl. Med. *31*:1989, 1990.
257. Schwaiger, M., Hutchins, G. D., and Guibourg, H.: Evaluation of myocardial blood flow and metabolism using positron emission tomography. Am. J. Cardiac Imaging *3*:266, 1989.
258. Bergmann, S. T., Hack, S., Tweson, T., et al.: Dependence of accumulation of $^{13}NH_3$ by myocardium on metabolic factors and its implications for the quantitative assessment of perfusion. Circulation *61*:34, 1980.
259. Hutchins, G. D., Schwaiger, M., Rosenspire, K. C., et al.: Noninvasive quantification of regional blood flow in the human heart using *N*-13 ammonia and dynamic positron emission tomographic imaging. J. Am. Coll. Cardiol. *10*:32, 1990.
260. Goldstein, R.A.: Kinetics of rubidium-82 after coronary occlusion and reperfusion: Assessment of patency and viability in open-chested dogs. J. Clin. Invest. *75*:1131, 1985.
261. Goldstein, R. A.: Rubidium-82 kinetics after coronary occlusion: Temporal relation of net myocardial accumulation and viability in open-chested dogs. J. Nucl. Med. *27*:1456, 1986.
262. Bergmann, S. R., Fox, K.A.A., Rand, A. L., et al.: Quantification of regional myocardial blood flow in vivo with $H_2{}^{15}O$. Circulation *70*:724, 1984.
263. Bergmann, S. R., Herrero, P., Markham, J., et al.: Noninvasive quantitation of myocardial blood flow in human subjects with oxygen-15-labeled water and positron emission tomography. J. Am. Coll. Cardiol. *14*:639, 1989.
264. Walsh, M. N., Geltman, E. M., Steele, R. L., et al.: Augmented myocardial perfusion reserve after coronary angioplasty quantified by positron emission tomography with $H_2{}^{15}O$. J. Am. Coll. Cardiol. *15*:119, 1990.
265. Soufer, R., and Zaret, B. L.: Positron emission tomography and the quantitative assessment of regional myocardial blood flow (editorial). J. Am. Coll. Cardiol. *15*:128, 1990.
266. Huang, S. C., Schwaiger, M., Carson, R. E., et al.: Quantitative measurement of myocardial blood flow with oxygen-15 water and positron computed tomography: An assessment of potential and problems. J. Nucl. Med. *26*:616, 1985.
267. Gould, K. L.: Percent coronary stenosis: Battered gold standard, pernicious relic or clinical practicality. J. Am. Coll. Cardiol. *11*:886, 1988.
268. Schelbert, H. R., Wisenberg, C., Phelps, M. E., et al.: Noninvasive assessment of coronary stenoses by myocardial imaging during pharmacologic coronary vasodilation. VI. Detection of coronary artery disease in human beings with intravenous N-13 ammonia and positron computed tomography. Am. J. Cardiol. *49*:1197, 1982.
269. Gould, K. L., Goldstein, R. A., Mullani, N. A., et al.: Noninvasive assessment of coronary stenoses by myocardial perfusion imaging during pharmacologic coronary vasodilation. VIII. Clinical feasibility of positron cardiac imaging without a cyclotron using generator-produced rubidium-82. J. Am. Coll. Cardiol. *7*:775, 1986.
270. Tamaki, N., Yonekura, Y., Senda, M., et al.: Value and limitation of stress thallium-201 single photon emission computed tomography: Comparison with nitrogen-13 positron tomography. J. Nucl. Med. *29*:1181, 1988.
271. Demer, L. L., Gould, K. L., Goldstein, R. A., et al.: Assessment of coronary artery disease severity by positron emission tomography: Comparison with quantitative arteriography in 193 patients. Circulation *79*:825, 1989.
272. Walsh, M. N., Bergmann, S. R., Steele, R. L., et al.: Delineation of impaired regional myocardial perfusion by positron emission tomography with $H_2{}^{15}O$. Circulation *78*:620, 1988.
273. Stewart, R., Kalus, M., Molina, E., et al.: Rubidium-82 PET versus thallium-201 SPECT for the diagnosis of regional coronary artery disease. Circulation *80*:209, 1989.
274. Yamashita, K., Tamaki, N., Yonekura, Y., et al.: Quantitative analysis of regional wall motion by gated myocardial positron emission tomography: Validation and comparison with left ventriculography. J. Nucl. Med. *30*:1775, 1989.
275. Cardiovascular Imaging Committee: Position Paper on Positron Emission Tomography. Cardiology (ACC Newsletter) 4, June 1990.
276. Goldstein, R. A., Klein, M. S., Welch, M. J., et al.: External assessment of myocardial metabolism with C-11 palmitate in vivo. J. Nucl. Med. *21*:342, 1980.
277. Kelin, M. S., Goldstein, R. A., Welch, M. J., et al.: External assessment of myocardial metabolism with ^{11}C-palmitate in rabbit hearts. Am. J. Physiol. *237*:H51, 1979.
278. Schon, H. R., Schelbert, H. R., Najafi, A., et al.: C-11 labeled palmitic acid for the noninvasive evaluation of regional myocardial fatty acid metabolism with positron computed tomography; I. Kinetics of C-11 palmitic acid in normal myocardium. Am. Heart J. *103*:532, 1982.
279. Schwaiger, M., Schelbert, H. R., Ellison, D., et al.: Sustained regional abnormalities in cardiac metabolism after transient ischemia in the chronic dog model. J. Am. Coll. Cardiol. *6*:336, 1985.
280. Schelbert, H. R., Henze, E., Schon, H. R., et al.: C-11 palmitate for the noninvasive evaluation of regional myocardial fatty acid metabolism with positron computed tomography. III. In vivo demonstration of the effects of substrate availability on myocardial metabolism. Am. Heart J. *105*:492, 1983.
281. Sobel, B. E., Geltman, E. M., Tiefenbrunn, A. J., et al.: Improvement of regional myocardial metabolism after coronary thrombolysis induced with tissue-type plasminogen activator or streptokinase. Circulation *69*:983, 1984.
282. Sobel, B. E., Weiss, E. S., Welch, M. J., et al.: Detection of remote myocardial infarction in patients with positron emission transaxial tomography and intravenous ^{11}C-palmitate. Circulation *55*:853, 1977.
283. Schwaiger, M., Schelbert, H. R., Keen, R., et al.: Retention and clearance of C-11 palmitic acid in ischemic and reperfused canine myocardium. J. Am. Coll. Cardiol. *6*:310, 1985.
284. Grover-McKay, M., Schelbert, H. R., Schwaiger, M., et al.: Identification of impaired metabolic reserve in patients with significant coronary artery stenosis by atrial pacing. Circulation *74*:281, 1986.
285. Armbrecht, J. J., Buxton, D. B., Brunken, R. C., et al.: Regional myocardial oxygen consumption determined noninvasively in humans with [1-^{11}C] acetate and dynamic positron tomography. Circulation *80*:863, 1989.
286. Buxton, D. B., Nienaber, C. A., Luxen, A., et al.: Noninvasive quantitation of regional myocardial oxygen consumption in vivo with [1-^{11}C]acetate and dynamic positron emission tomography. Circulation *79*:134, 1989.
287. Goldstein, D. S., Chang, P. C., Eisenhofer, G., et al.: Positron emission tomographic imaging of cardiac sympathetic innervation and function. Circulation *81*:1606, 1990.
288. Schwaiger, M., Kalff, V., Rosenspire, K., et al.: Noninvasive evaluation of sympathetic nervous system in human heart by positron emission tomography. Circulation *82*:457, 1990.
288a. Schwaiger, M., Kalff, V., Rosenspire, K., et al.: Noninvasive evaluation of sympathetic nervous system in human heart by positron emission tomography. Circulation *82*:457, 1990.
289. Rosenspire, K. C., Gildersleeve, D. L., Massin, C. C., et al.: Metabolic fate of the heart agent [18F]6-fluorometaraminol. Nucl. Med. Biol. *16*:735, 1989.
290. Syrota, A.: In vivo investigation of myocardial perfusion, metabolism and receptors by positron emission tomography. Int. J. Microcirc. Clin. Exp. *411*:22, 1989.

11

Newer Cardiac Imaging Techniques (Computed Tomography, Magnetic Resonance Imaging)

by CHARLES B. HIGGINS, M.D.

Computed Tomography

TECHNICAL ASPECTS

Computed tomographic (CT) scanning of the heart usually requires modification of the standard CT techniques used for investigating other parts of the body. For some purposes, such as evaluation of thoracic aortic disease, pericardial disease, paracardiac and intracardiac tumors, and patency of coronary arterial bypass grafts, newer standard CT scanners with exposure times of less than 2 secs are usually adequate.[1-4] However, assessment of cardiac function and precise definition of intracardiac anatomy necessitate either electrocardiographic (ECG) gating of standard CT scanners or, preferably, the use of millisecond CT scanners.[5,6]

GATED CT SCANNING. A method for overcoming the problem of cardiac motion is crucial in obtaining quantitative dimensional data and ejection fractions when standard CT scanners are employed. Two gating techniques have been used: retrospective and prospective gating.[4,7] With *retrospective gating* the CT scan data and the ECG are recorded simultaneously, but the ECG signal does not guide the acquisition of x-ray data in any manner. Subsequently, the image is reconstructed from data obtained within a selected time window (biological window), bracketing the desired portion of the ECG cycle, such as the QRS complex at end-diastole.

The *prospective gating system* allows preselection of a fraction of the R-R interval to be monitored. The biological window width sets the fraction of the cardiac cycle to be represented by each image. Prospective gating ensures the even distribution of R waves throughout the scanning circle in the minimal number of scans. This is accomplished by launching of the x-ray tube at the appropriate time relative to the R wave of the ECG input, so that one of the R waves falls into the largest gap in the already-acquired angular x-ray data.

Many of the limitations of the standard CT scanner in cardiac applications have been overcome by the successful construction of CT scanners specifically designed to evaluate central cardiovascular anatomy and function. The *ultrafast* (millisecond) *CT scanners*, developed by Boyd and colleagues[5] and Ritman and associates,[6] obtain scans at exposure times of 50 msec or less and can generate CT scans at multiple anatomical levels.

The ultrafast (cine) CT scanner employs a scanning focused x-ray beam, which provides complete cardiac imaging in real time without the need for ECG gating (Fig. 11-1). This CT scanner is not limited by the

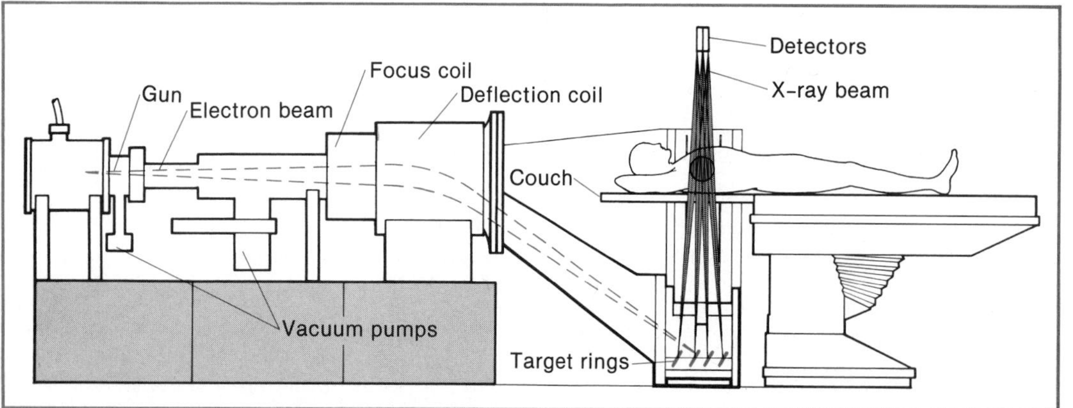

FIGURE 11-1. Diagram of cine CT scanner. Electron gun produces a stream of electrons that are magnetically focused and directed onto four tungsten target rings. Each target ring emits two fan beams of x-ray. Transmission of x-rays through the subject is registered by detectors arranged over a 180-degree arc.

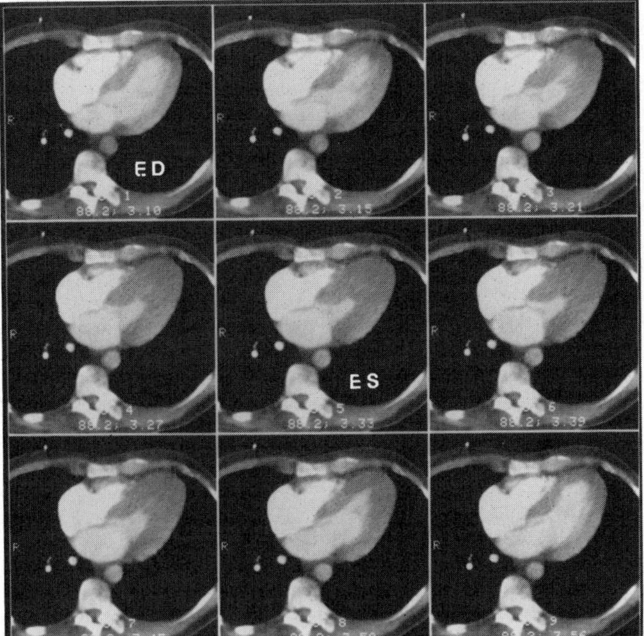

FIGURE 11–2. Series of CT scans of the same anatomical level acquired every 50 msec during a single cardiac cycle in a patient with hypertrophic cardiomyopathy. These are 9 of 17 scans acquired in approximately one cardiac cycle. Frame at upper left is near end diastole and middle frame is near end systole. Note the change in ventricular volumes during the cardiac cycle and wall thickening during systole. (Courtesy of J. Rumberger, Ph.D., M.D., Mayo Clinic.)

inertia associated with moving mechanical parts. It uses a focused electron beam that is successively swept across four cadmium tungstate target arcs at the speed of light. Each of the four targets generates a fan beam of photons that pass from beneath the patient to a bank of photon detectors arranged in a semicircle above the patient.

The cine CT scanner can be operated in three different modes. The *cine mode* is used to assess global and regional myocardial function. The scans are obtained at an exposure time of 50 msec and at a rate of 17 scans per sec (Fig. 11–2).[2] The *triggered mode,* used for flow analysis, employs a series of 20 to 40 successive scans in which each 50-msec exposure is triggered at a specific phase of the cardiac cycle of successive heartbeats or every other heartbeat. From such a series of scans, time-density curves can be constructed for specific regions of interest in the cardiac chamber or myocardium, providing an estimate of transit time, perfusion, or blood flow.[3] The *volume mode* provides eight scans by the use of all four targets arcs in an imaging period of approximately 200 msec. These eight transverse scans (1 cm thick) frequently can encompass the entire left ventricular chamber and thereby provide an estimate of left ventricular volume and mass. Usually 10 to 12 tomographic levels are needed to encompass the heart entirely.

Since multiple images can be acquired at multiple levels with only an 8 msec interscan delay, cine CT permits the acquisition of images at true end-diastole and end-systole, since both are approximately 60 msec in duration. Real-time sequential imaging is accomplished within a single heartbeat at multiple levels, and these images are then displayed in a closed-loop cine format (cine CT display).

Ten tomographic levels can be acquired during a single imaging sequence, using table incrementation. The maximum number of images that can be acquired in one sequence is 80. Consequently, if 8 tomographic levels are utilized, then only 10 images can be acquired at each level, or if 10 tomographic levels are employed, only 8 images can. The sequential images at each level are acquired during a single heartbeat, beginning immediately after the peak of the R-wave (end-diastole). When the entire heart is encompassed with tomographic levels, cine CT permits three-dimensional cardiac evaluation.

CONTRAST ENHANCEMENT. For nearly all purposes, intravenous injection of iodinated contrast medium is used to delineate the blood pool on CT scans. The contrast medium can be given as an intravenous bolus injection or a rapid infusion. For evaluation of the heart and great vessels, contrast medium is usually delivered in a bolus over several seconds and in a volume of approximately 30 to 60 ml. Scans are exposed at the estimated time of peak enhancement of the structure of interest. In order to identify the time of arrival of contrast medium in the left-sided cardiac chamber and aorta, a preliminary bolus injection of indocyanine dye is given to define circulation time. This time is then used to specify the time of acquisition of the series of cine CT scans. Scans are sometimes obtained without contrast medium in order to identify calcification of cardiac structures.

EVALUATION OF CARDIAC DIMENSIONS AND FUNCTION

CT scans have the capability of identifying not only the inner endocardial wall but also the epicardial surface. Wall thickness and myocardial mass have been estimated accurately both on ECG-gated CT scans[8–10] and with ultrafast CT[11] (Fig. 11–3). A close correlation has been found between CT measurements and postmortem anatomical measurements of wall thickness and mass[9–11] (Fig. 11–3). Ultrafast CT has been used to demonstrate regression of hypertrophy after relief of pressure overload lesions of the left ventricle.[12] It has also been employed to estimate right ventricular mass by measurement of the mass of the free wall.[13] Right ventricular mass was demonstrated to be substantially increased in patients with pulmonary arterial hypertension compared with measurements in normal subjects.[13]

CT scanning can be used in the assessment of the dynamics of regional myocardial wall thickening.[14–16] The method of (1) objective edge detection of the endocardium and epicardium and (2) realignment of end-diastolic and end-systolic images has been used with ultrafast CT scans to quantitate wall thickening dynamics during pharmacological intervention.[15] A series of tomograms in a short-axis plane acquired during multiple phases of the cardiac cycle provides the capability to measure area ejection fraction and wall thickening at various levels of the left ventricle, extending from the base to the apex. In normal human subjects, a variation in both regional ejection fraction and extent of wall thickening has been defined; there is a gradient in both area ejection fraction and extent of wall thickening increasing progressively from basal to apical layers.[17] Cine CT has been used also to demonstrate regional function in pathological states. In an animal model of regional ischemia, it has identified the region of ischemia by demonstrating loss of wall thickening during the cardiac cycle.[18]

Left ventricular volumes and ejection fraction can be estimated by contrast angiography (p. 422), echocardiography (p. 76), and gated blood pool nuclear images (p. 294). While the quantitation of ventricular volumes and ejection fraction by cine CT is not a unique capability, the accuracy of CT can potentially exceed that of the other techniques. Other cardiac

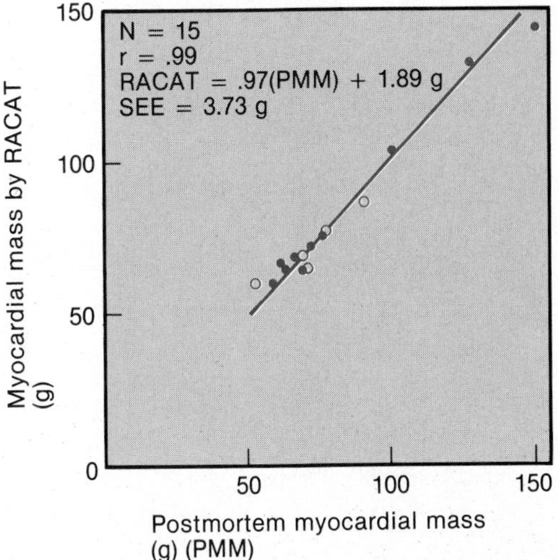

FIGURE 11–3. Graph plots mass determined by rapid-acquisition computer assisted tomography (RACAT) vs. postmortem measurement of left ventricular mass (PMM). RACAT is another denotation for cine CT. This study was done in anesthetized dogs. (From Feiring, A., et al.: Determination of left ventricular mass in dogs with rapid-acquisition cardiac CT scanning. Circulation *72*:1355, 1985, by permission of the American Heart Association, Inc.)

imaging techniques such as echocardiography and left ventricular angiography estimate left ventricular volume, making geometric assumptions and measurements in one or two planes. These assumptions lead to inaccuracies of volume measurement in the presence of left ventricular conformational abnormalities. Cine CT directly measures chamber volumes by planimetry of the cardiac blood pool on each tomogram, allowing precise volume determination. It has been demonstrated that left ventricular volume, ejection fraction, and stroke volume can be acquired by ultrafast (cine) CT with high accuracy and close reproducibility among observers and among studies on different occasions in the same subject.[19,20] In normal subjects, the stroke volumes of the right and left ventricle as measured by ultrafast CT were equal.

Ultrafast CT provides a measurement of total ventricular stroke volume. If an independent technique is used for the measurement of forward (effective) stroke volume, these measurements can be combined in order to estimate regurgitant volume; regurgitant volume is the difference between total stroke volume and forward stroke volume. Ultrafast CT also can be applied for the simultaneous quantification of the right and left ventricular stroke volumes.[21] The difference between the stroke volumes of the ventricles is equal to the total regurgitant volume of valves on one side of the heart. The method is not relevant for circumstances in which there is regurgitation of valves of both the right and left ventricle. Nearly identical stroke volumes for the right and left ventricles have been measured by cine CT in normal subjects.[20]

EVALUATION OF SPECIFIC CARDIAC DISEASES

ISCHEMIC HEART DISEASE

After myocardial infarction, CT can be used to demonstrate regional wall thinning[22-25] (Fig. 11–4) and complications of infarction, such as left ventricular aneurysm (Fig. 11–5) and mural thrombus. Gated CT or cine CT can also demonstrate left ventricular segmental dysfunction, such as reduced wall thickening and wall motion. In one large series in which ECG-gated CT was compared with left ventricular cineangiography, a sensitivity of 94 per cent and specificity of 87 per cent were shown for the detection of a regional wall abnormality.[22]

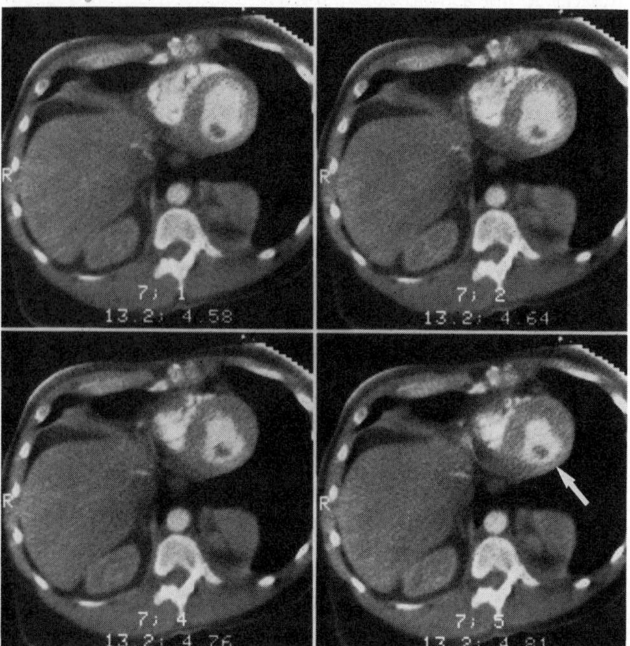

FIGURE 11–4. Diastolic (upper panels) and systolic (lower panels) images in a patient with prior posterior myocardial infarction. In diastole the posterior wall is thinner than at other regions and there is no thickening in systole (arrow).

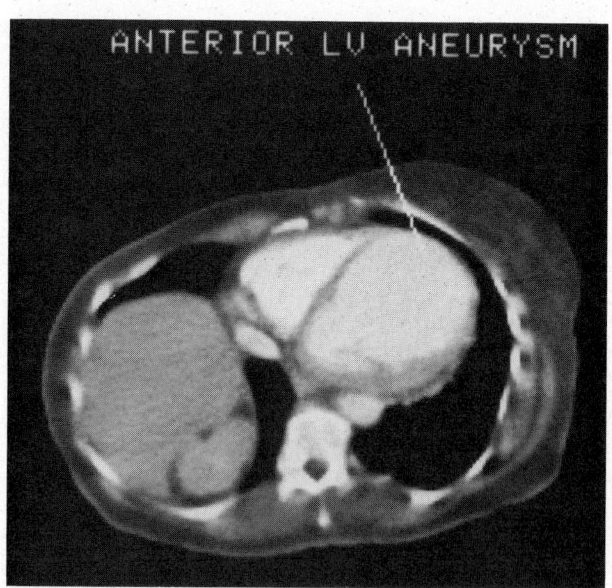

FIGURE 11–5. Anterior left ventricular aneurysm. There is severe thinning of the anteroseptal and anterior walls and bulging of the left ventricle anteriorly (Courtesy of W. Stanford, M.D., Iowa University Medical Center.)

The accuracy of detecting the anatomical and functional sequelae of infarction is substantially better for the anterior wall compared with the posterior and diaphragmatic walls of the left ventricle because of the orientation of the heart in relation to the fixed transverse imaging. In one study, all 13 anterior infarcts were detected as either wall thinning or decreased mural density on contrast-enhanced CT scans. However, the infarction site was not identified in three of six patients with inferior infarctions.[23] The ability of present-day methodology to acquire images in a plane approximating the cardiac short axis by elevation and tilting of the table should alleviate this problem.

CT provides unequivocal spatial separation between various regions of the left ventricle, enabling better localization and estimation of the extent of wall thinning after infarction compared with projectional techniques such as left ventriculography and most scintigraphic techniques. Likewise, the site and extent of anterior (Fig. 11–5) and posterior aneurysms of the left ventricle can be well demonstrated. The differentiation by CT between true aneurysm and pseudoaneurysm depends on the identification of the small ostium connecting the left ventricular cavity and the aneurysm. False aneurysms are usually substantially larger than true aneurysms and frequently arise from the posterior or inferior wall of the left ventricle.

REGIONAL WALL MOTION. Quantitation of systolic myocardial wall thickening appears to be a particularly useful technique for evaluating regional myocardial contractile function in patients with ischemic heart disease. Gated CT scans[7] and ultrafast CT[18] have been effective in identifying the region of ischemia by demonstrating loss of regional wall thickening during acute coronary occlusion in the canine model. With the combination of ultrafast CT scanning and contrast enhancement for demonstrating regional contraction abnormalities in patients with prior infarctions, a 91 per cent correlation with left ventriculography for identifying abnormal myocardial segments has been reported.[24] Regional wall thickening and inward motion were used as the parameters of regional function; they correlated well with wall motion abnormalities demonstrated on left ventriculography and critical coronary stenoses shown by coronary angiography.[25] Using the cine mode in which 17 frames per second are obtained, wall thickening was monitored during the course of a single cardiac cycle at the time of peak opacification of the left ventricle (Fig. 11–4).

MYOCARDIAL PERFUSION. Ultrafast CT may also be

able to provide an indication of *regional myocardial perfusion*.[26-28] Estimates of myocardial perfusion are obtained when regions of interest are drawn over various sites of the myocardium displayed on the transverse CT scans. The density of the myocardial regions is measured on sequential 50-msec scans acquired during an appropriate duration of the myocardial contrast enhancement phase. From these measurements, time-density curves are constructed; analyses of these curves in regard to contrast appearance and washout are used to estimate regional myocardial perfusion. Thus, ultrafast CT has the potential of providing both regional function and perfusion in a single study. Further study is needed to confirm that flow can be estimated reliably under variable physiological (vasodilatation) and pathological (stenosis) conditions and with equal accuracy at various myocardial sites. Studies in animals have shown the capability of the technique to measure blood flow at various regions in the LV and to monitor the increase in regional blood flow caused by injection of a vasodilator.[27] These measurements of regional flow in response to a vasodilator could be used to test coronary flow reserve in various regions and to identify a region served by an artery with a critical stenosis by failure of flow to rise in response to a vasodilator.

CT has been found to be at least as accurate as two-dimensional echocardiography for identifying left ventricular *mural thrombus*.[29,30] Indeed, comparative studies have shown greater accuracy of CT compared with two-dimensional echocardiography in demonstration of thrombus in the left atrium.[31]

MYOCARDIAL INFARCTION. Computed tomography with contrast enhancement provides direct visualization of the infarction because of differences between normal and infarcted myocardium in the distribution kinetics of iodinated contrast media.[32-34] After intravenous administration of contrast material, temporally distinct phases of enhancement of normal and ischemically damaged myocardium have been depicted on CT. During the perfusion phase, normal myocardium is maximally enhanced (maximum increase in x-ray attenuation value), whereas the area of damage is nonenhanced or minimally enhanced. Several minutes after administration of contrast material, enhancement of normal myocardium has declined and the damaged myocardium is nearly maximally enhanced. In the perfusion phase, the ischemically damaged area appears as a negative image within the myocardium, whereas in the later phase it appears as a positive image.

The delayed enhancement of the ischemic area after the intravenous administration of contrast material has been associated with a much higher concentration of iodine in infarcted compared with normal myocardium.[33,34] The concentration of iodinated contrast material in the center, periphery, and margin of the infarct and in normal myocardium demonstrated a close linear relationship to the distribution of technetium-99m-pyrophosphate (^{99m}Tc-PYP).[35] Both iodinated contrast material and ^{99m}Tc-PYP (p. 291) are markers of myocardial necrosis. Measurement of regional myocardial blood flow with indium-111–labeled microspheres indicated that both contrast material and ^{99m}Tc-PYP accumulated in the center of the infarct when residual blood flow was at least 5 per cent of normal.[35] These studies suggest that contrast enhancement of ischemically damaged tissue is a marker of myocardial necrosis, but its occurrence depends on the presence of a threshold level of residual myocardial perfusion. After intravenous administration, iodine-containing contrast material does not enter normal myocardial cells but does accumulate in ischemically damaged ones.[36]

In animal studies, quantitation of infarct volume or mass from a series of transverse CT scans encompassing the full extent of the left ventricle has been found to correlate closely with postmortem measurements.[10,37-39] In a canine model, sequential CT scans have been utilized to monitor the mass of the infarct and of the remaining normal myocardium during the initial month after coronary occlusion.[10] Infarct size was shown to increase beginning shortly after occlusion and continuing to 4 days after occlusion and then to decrease progressively. The noninfarcted myocardial mass in animals with infarcts was found to increase 27 per cent during the initial month after occlusion, presumably representing compensatory hypertrophy. CT scans have also been used to document the beneficial effects of reperfusion 2 hours after occlusion in the dog.[39]

CORONARY ARTERY BYPASS GRAFTS. The patency of coronary artery bypass grafts can be assessed by sequential CT scans during the transit of intravenously administered contrast medium through the arterial side of the circulation. An early study[1] showed a 93 per cent sensitivity and 95 per cent specificity for defining graft patency using coronary angiography as the standard of reference. Subsequent reports in larger numbers of patients have shown somewhat lower diagnostic accuracy of standard CT in defining graft patency.[2,3] While all reports show high diagnostic accuracy for evaluation of grafts to the left anterior descending coronary artery system, the accuracy for assessing grafts to the circumflex and right coronary arterial systems is poorer.[1-3] Another limitation of the technique is the inability to identify grafts with significant stenoses.[40] In recent years, several reports have appeared demonstrating a high accuracy of ultrafast CT for defining the patency of coronary artery bypass grafts.[41-44] The diagnostic accuracy of ultrafast CT for defining the patency of grafts and internal coronary bypasses has been shown to be greater than 95 per cent in a multicenter study.[41] High accuracy was shown for defining patency of grafts to the left anterior descending, circumflex, and right coronary arterial branches. It is possible that stenoses might be detected in grafts by time-density analysis or contrast transit time techniques applied to sequential scans of the same anatomical level acquired before and after pharmacological flow augmentation using the ultrafast CT scanner. The feasibility of such an approach using ultrafast CT has been shown.[44]

CT scanning has been used to assess graft patency within the first several days after bypass surgery with a view to reoperation in the event of documented early occlusion.[45,46] CT revealed a 70 per cent graft patency rate in patients with perioperative infarction compared with 95 per cent patency in those without infarction.[46]

The site of the bypass graft on contrast-enhanced CT scans can be related to a clock viewed from the feet looking upward. The grafts to the right coronary artery are situated between 9 and 11 o'clock; grafts to the left anterior descending artery system, at 12 to 2 o'clock, and the graft to the circumflex coronary artery system, at 2 to 4 o'clock (Fig. 11-6). Diagnostic confidence is enhanced by visualizing the graft at two adjacent anatomical levels and by showing contrast enhancement of the graft simultaneously with aortic opacification (Fig. 11-6). Dynamic CT scanning (multiple sequential CT scans at the same level) demonstrates opacification and washout of contrast from the grafts.

IDENTIFICATION OF CORONARY ARTERIAL CALCIFICATION. Calcification in the coronary arteries usually indicates the presence of atherosclerosis. While the early stages of atherosclerosis exist without calcification and calcification can exist in the coronary arteries in the absence of hemodynamically significant arterial obstruction, the detection of calcification increases the likelihood of significant coronary arterial obstructive disease. Several studies[47-49] have revealed that in patients being studied by coronary arteriography the *absence* of fluoroscopically detectable coronary arterial calcification is usually associated with no significant arterial stenoses and the presence of calcification with significant stenoses ($>$ 50 per cent reduction in luminal diameter). Since the population used in these studies contains a preponderance of patients with symptomatic disease, the role of detection of calcium as an indicator of occult disease is an unresolved question. Hamby et al.[47] demonstrated in a large group of patients that fluoroscopically detectable calcification increased the likelihood of significant coronary arterial disease several-

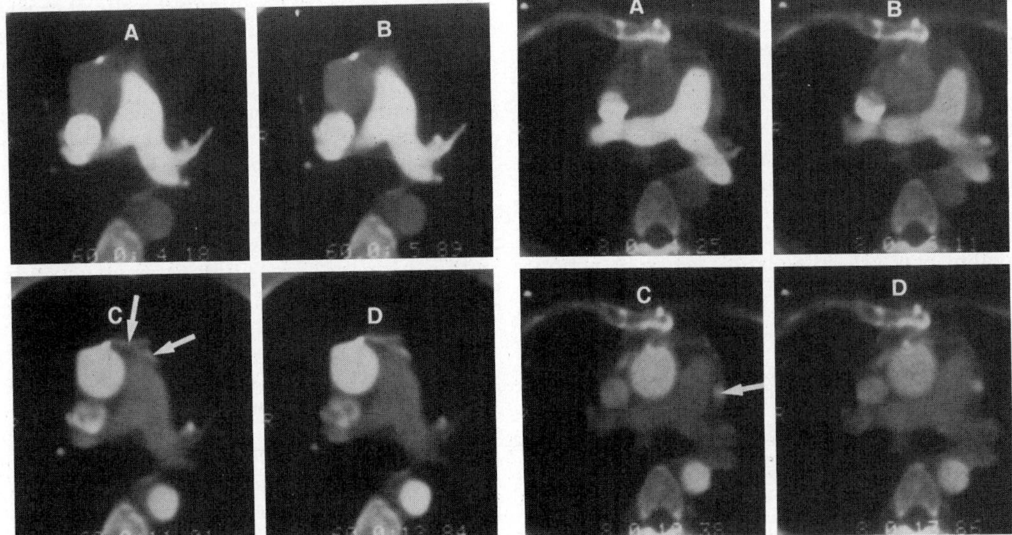

FIGURE 11–6. *Left,* Sequential cine CT scans show two patent bypass grafts (arrows) to the left anterior descending artery and acute diagonal. *Right,* Graft to the obtuse marginal branch of the circumflex artery (arrow). Note that the grafts opacify simultaneously with the ascending aorta. Each set of four images was obtained at the same anatomical level. The images were done with the passage of contrast medium through the central circulation. Early images (A,B) show contrast in the pulmonary artery and later images (C,D) show contrast in the aorta and bypass grafts.

fold in patients younger than 60 years. The positive predictive value was highest in younger subjects and in women. In comparison to exercise electrocardiography, fluoroscopic detection of calcification has been shown to be more sensitive for defining the presence of some degree of atherosclerotic disease but was less specific than exercise electrocardiography for identifying hemodynamically significant lesions.[49]

Ultrafast CT can be both sensitive and specific for predicting the presence of significant coronary obstructive disease in nonselected asymptomatic patients. Computed tomography is an extremely effective technique for detecting calcification in tissues; it is much more sensitive than fluoroscopy in this regard. The specificity of ultrafast CT is established by quantifying both the density and the extent of the calcification (coronary calcification score) in the regions of the three major coronary arteries on CT scans encompassing the entire heart.[50] Using the calcification quantification method (Fig. 11–7), ultrafast CT has been shown to be extremely sensitive and reasonably specific for predicting the presence of significant coronary obstructive disease (> 75 per cent reduction in luminal diameter). The coronary calcification score has been found to be higher for patients with multivessel than for those with single vessel involvement. These findings should stimulate a more extensive study in order to establish this technique as a screening test for coronary arterial disease in various patient populations at risk for the disease.

PERICARDIAL DISEASE

(See also Chap. 45)

Computed tomography provides distinct visualization of the pericardium in most patients (Fig. 11–8). Discrimination

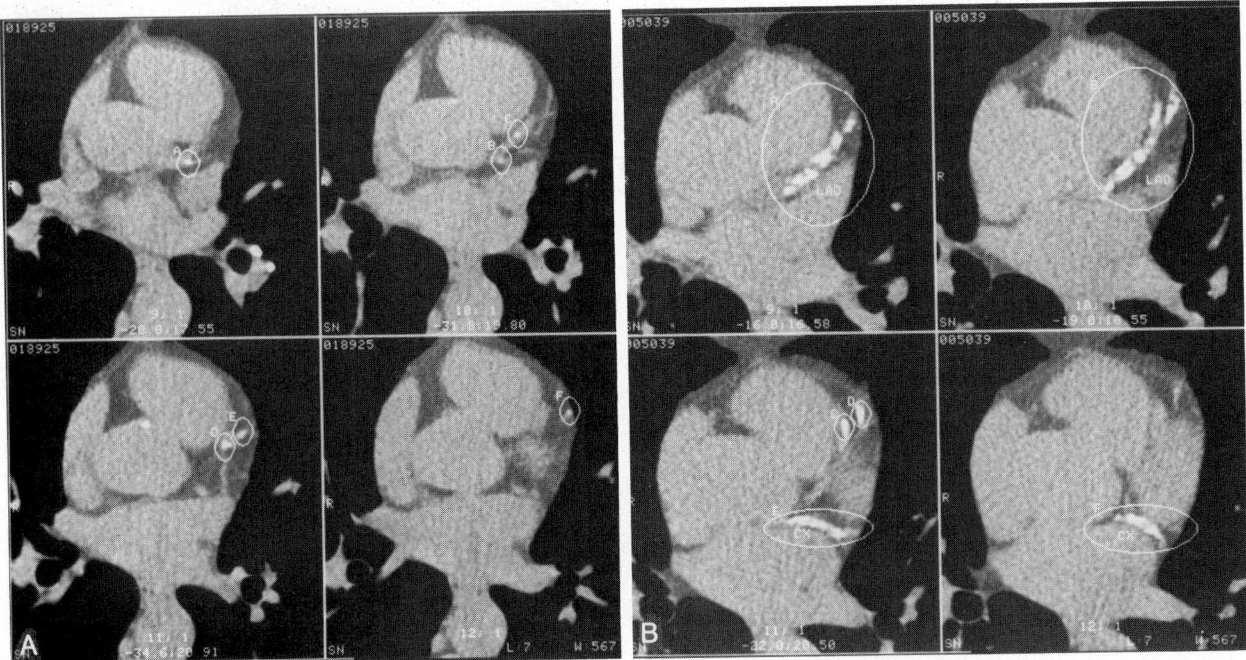

FIGURE 11–7. Cine CT scans obtained without contrast medium used to detect the presence, severity, and extent of coronary arterial calcification. *Left (A),* Mild calcification in a single vessel (left anterior descending). Sites of calcification are labeled *A* to *F. Right (B),* Severe calcification of multiple major coronary arterial branches (left anterior descending [LAD] and circumflex [Cx]). Sites of calcium are labeled *A* to *D.* (Courtesy of Imatron.)

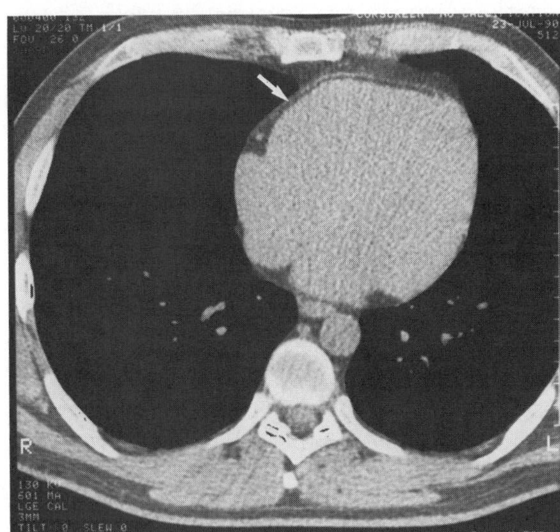

FIGURE 11-8. Nonenhanced cine CT image demonstrates the thin pericardium (arrow), which is readily visible anteriorly when it is outlined by epicardial and pericardial fat.

of the pericardial line from the myocardium depends on the presence of some epicardial and pericardial fat; it has been reported to be visible on CT scans of 95 per cent of normal subjects.[51] Although visible over the right atrium and ventricle in most subjects, it is frequently not detectable on the lateral and posterior wall of the left ventricle. The mean width of the line in normal subjects is 2.2 mm and is always less than 4 mm. Pericardial thickness is usually greatest near its diaphragmatic attachments. CT also frequently demonstrates the superior recesses of the pericardium extending over the ascending aorta and lateral to the main pulmonary artery. These recesses may be distended in the presence of a pericardial effusion.

Two-dimensional echocardiography is an extremely effective technique for the diagnosis of pericardial abnormalities and is the primary modality for evaluation of suspected pericardial disease (pp. 102 and 1473). Although it is extremely sensitive for the detection of pericardial effusion, it has some limitations in the defining of loculated effusions, hemorrhagic effusions, and especially pericardial thickening. CT is especially effective in depicting these entities.[52-54] Consequently, it is complementary to echocardiography in the diagnosis and assessment of pericardial disease.

CONGENITAL ABNORMALITIES AND CYSTS. Congenital abnormalities such as absence of the pericardium[55] and pericardial cyst[52,53,56,57] can be well demonstrated by CT; other techniques are usually not definitive for diagnosis of these abnormalities. Pericardial defect (usually partial or complete absence of left-sided pericardium) is recognized on CT by the discontinuity of the pericardial line over the left aspect of the heart, with shift of the heart leftward or bulging of the left atrial appendage through the defect. CT demonstrates direct continuity of the heart and the left lung without intervening pericardium or pericardial fat. A pericardial cyst appears as a paracardiac mass with a thin capsule, which is occasionally partially or completely calcified and which has a homogeneous internal density nearly equivalent to that of water. However, rarely the cyst contains mucoid material, causing the density to be higher than water; such a cyst usually cannot be reliably distinguished from a solid mass. *Thymic cysts*, which may be adjacent to the pericardium, also may show homogeneous water density on CT densitometry and may be indistinguishable from pericardial cysts.

PERICARDIAL FLUID. Fluid in the pericardial space may be reliably detected by CT.[52,58] This technique can also provide an accurate estimate of the volume of this fluid.[58] Although two-dimensional echocardiography is sufficient and, for economic and logistic reasons, more clinically efficacious for the primary evaluation of most pericardial effusions, CT is indicated in some special situations. Loculated effusions (especially anterior loculations), which may pose difficulty for echocardiography, are readily demonstrated on CT[53] because of the wide field of view provided and the potentially three-dimensional nature of the technique. CT can be effective not only for diagnosing loculated effusions but also for guiding pericardiocentesis.[59] CT density measurements provide some degree of characterization of pericardial fluid.[52-54,58] Density numbers (Hounsfield numbers) exceeding water density (water density = 0-12 units) are suggestive of hemopericardium, purulent exudate, or effusions associated with hypothyroidism. Low-density pericardial effusions have been reported in the presence of chylopericardium.[58]

CONSTRICTIVE PERICARDITIS. The establishment of the diagnosis of constrictive pericarditis can be substantially aided by CT. Since CT shows the pericardium, it can document pericardial thickening, defined as thickness greater than 4 mm. Focal plaques of thickening or the greater thickness of the pericardium near the diaphragm should not be confused with the more extensive pericardial thickening associated with constrictive pericarditis. However, the pericardial thickening may be limited to the right side of the heart, a form that appears to be more prevalent in patients who have undergone coronary arterial bypass surgery.

The documentation of pericardial thickening is the major discriminatory feature between constrictive pericarditis and restrictive cardiomyopathy (Fig. 11-9). However, thickened pericardium per se is not indicative of constrictive disease. Pericardial thickening without constriction frequently is observed in the early postoperative period and may persist for several months following operation in patients with the post-pericardiotomy syndrome.[52] Thickened pericardium without constriction has also been observed in association with inflammation of the pericardium caused by a variety of conditions including rheumatic heart disease, rheumatoid arthritis, sarcoidosis, and postmediastinal irradiation.[60] Pericardial thickening may also be caused by metastatic carcinoma, thymoma,[61] and lymphoma.[52,54] These conditions are usually associated with effusion.[54] Moreover, thickened pericardium is to be expected in all patients for several weeks after cardiac surgery. It may be present for a prolonged period in patients afflicted with the postpericardiotomy syndrome (Dressler's syndrome).

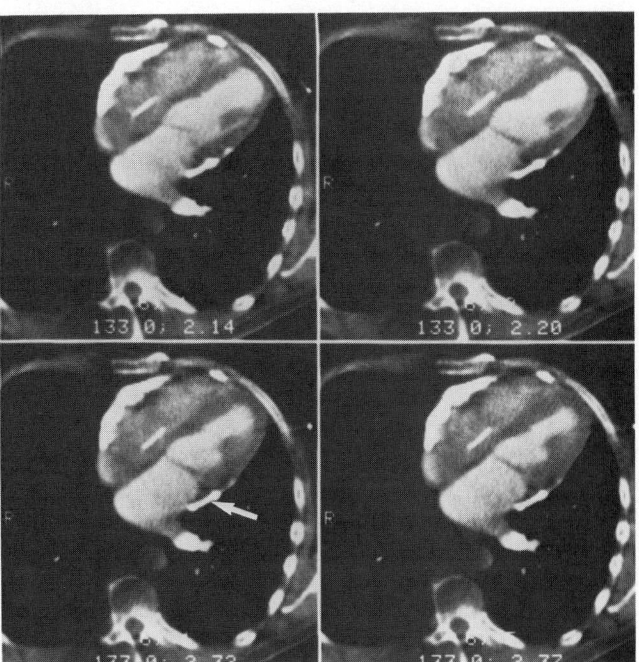

FIGURE 11-9. Calcific constrictive pericarditis. Four cine CT scans acquired during a single cardiac cycle. Images in diastole are shown above and during systole below. Note the heavy calcification located over the right ventricle and at the posterior atrioventricular groove.

EFFUSIVE-CONSTRICTIVE AND CONSTRICTIVE PERICARDITIS. This condition is demonstrated by an effusion in association with thickened pericardium; however, it may not always be possible to distinguish a small effusion from thickened pericardium.[52] Pericardial thickening alone usually measures between 5 to 20 mm, whereas greater thickening generally indicates associated effusion or effusion alone. Contrast enhancement of the thickened pericardium is indicative of pericardial inflammation[62] (Fig. 11-10). Additional CT findings in constrictive pericarditis often reflect the anatomical and physiological consequences of the thickened pericardium on the cardiac chambers.[63,64] CT shows substantial dilatation of the inferior vena cava and some enlargement of the atria, especially the right atrium (Fig. 11-9). The ventricles tend to have a small volume and a narrow tubular configuration.[63] In some cases, a sigmoid-shaped ventricular septum or prominent leftward convexity of the septum has been observed. Unusual contours, such as straightening or focal indentation of the free wall of either the right or left ventricle, have been noted on CT scans.[63]

The density resolution of CT makes it the most sensitive technique for identifying pericardial calcification (Fig. 11-9). Pericardial calcific deposits are usually residual of pericardial inflammation and are most commonly found in the visceral layer along the atrioventricular and interventricular grooves. Extensive calcification of the pericardium suggests but does not prove the presence of cardiac constriction.

PARACARDIAC AND CARDIAC MASSES

CT is useful for the evaluation of pericardial and paracardiac masses. CT and more recently magnetic resonance imaging (MRI) have emerged as the preferential techniques for defining the site and extent of such masses and in some cases even indicating their nature.[52,53,56,57,65,66] CT may show the water density of pericardial cysts; this is an especially useful finding when the cyst is located in an unusual mediastinal location[58] or when it protrudes inwardly, displacing the atrial wall.[67] In one series CT detected eight of eight intrapericardial masses compared with echocardiography, which identified only one.[66] CT and MRI currently are the best techniques for defining the extension of mediastinal neoplasms (including lymphoma) and of carcinoma of the lung into the pericardium. Metastatic involvement of the pericardium is suggested by the CT finding of effusion with an irregularly thickened pericardium or the actual demonstration of a mass involving the pericardium.[52,53,66] An effusion with high CT density (hemopericardium) along with pericardial thickening also suggests metastatic pericardial involvement.[53,58]

CT sometimes provides insight into the nature of the mass by demonstrating the shape, defining the density measurements, or showing multiple masses. The CT demonstration of multiple pericardial nodules suggests metastatic tumor or, rarely, multicentric mesothelioma. Pericardial cysts have water density, while lipomas have a very low density value (−55 or fewer Hounsfield units). Demonstration by CT of calcium or bone and fat in a paracardiac mass suggests teratoma.

Intracardiac masses can be detected quite well by echocardiography and angiography. However, CT not only can detect masses within the cardiac chambers but also can define fully their extent (Fig. 11-11). CT can demonstrate components of the mass within the myocardial wall and extending outside of the heart. The contrast resolution of CT may provide some insight into the composition of the mass, such as demonstrating the presence of fat or calcium. CT has detected simple intracardiac masses such as atrial myxoma[22,68,69] and complex masses involving the myocardial wall with extracardiac extension.[22] Finally, by defining clearly the myocardial wall, CT allows discrimination of the extracardiac location of tumors that produce compression and invagination of cardiac walls, simulating an intracardiac origin.[67]

INTRACARDIAC THROMBUS. The most frequent intracardiac mass is a thrombus. Intracardiac thrombi usually are located in the left atrium in patients with mitral valve disease or patients with atrial fibrillation from any cause and in the left ventricle in patients with recent myocardial infarction or patients with dilated (congestive) cardiomyopathy. While echocardiography is usually the initial study used to detect intracardiac thrombi or an intracardiac source of peripheral embolism, recent studies have revealed that CT is as sensitive but more specific for identifying ventricular thrombus[30] and more sensitive for defining left atrial thrombus[31] (Fig. 11-11). Thrombi in the left atrial appendage and lateral wall of the atrium are more readily detected with MRI and CT than with echocardiography. MRI and CT are the most effective techniques for the detection of intracardiac thrombus.

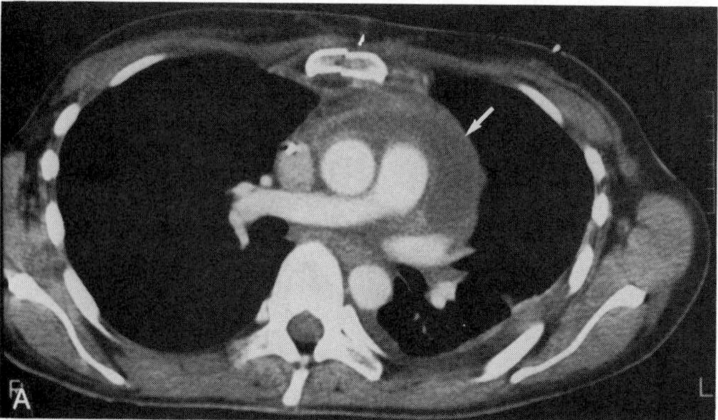

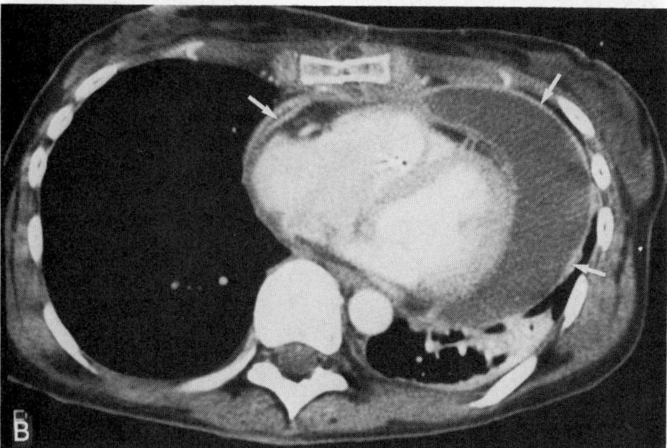

FIGURE 11-10. Cine CT scans at the levels of the right pulmonary artery (*A*) and at the ventricles (*B*) in a patient with a pericardial inflammation and large effusion (outlined by the arrows). The effusion extends over the pulmonary artery as well as the ventricles. There is contrast enhancement of the pericardium, suggesting pericardial inflammation. (Courtesy of Imatron.)

CONGENITAL HEART DISEASE

Standard CT, ultrafast CT (cine CT), and MRI are useful noninvasive techniques for the visualization of cardiovascular anatomy in patients with congenital heart disease. Ultrafast CT and MRI can also provide assessment of cardiovascular function in these patients. MRI appears to be the most suitable of these techniques for assessing congenital heart disease. The x-ray exposure, contrast media requirement, and inability to image in multiple plane are limitations of CT for the evaluation of congenital heart disease.

STANDARD CT. This technique has been found to be useful for evaluation of suspected *anomalies of the aortic arch*.[70-72] Contrast-enhanced CT is usually required to show the vascular tissue surrounding the trachea in the presence of double aortic arch and the retroesophageal vascular structure indicating anomalous origin of the subclavian artery. Double arch is also suggested by the presence of four paratracheal vessels arranged symmetrically.[70]

Although many cardiac anomalies such as septal defects,

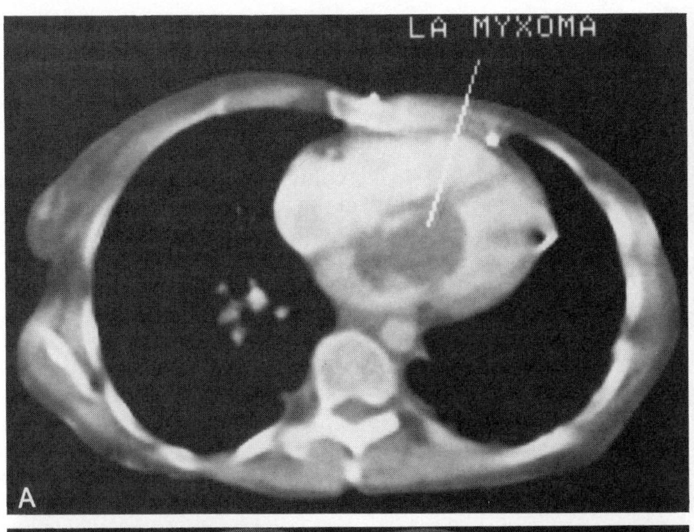

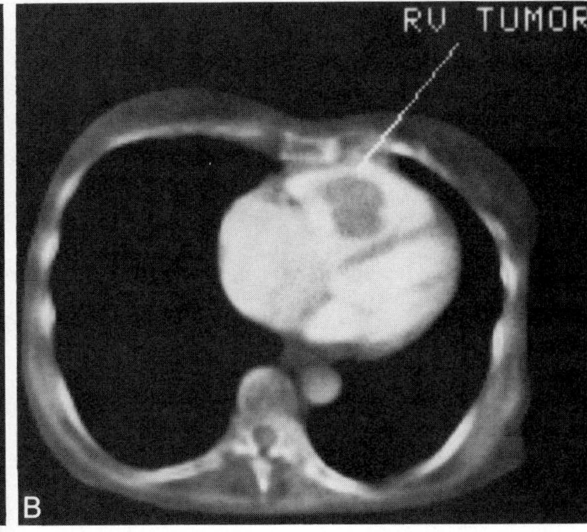

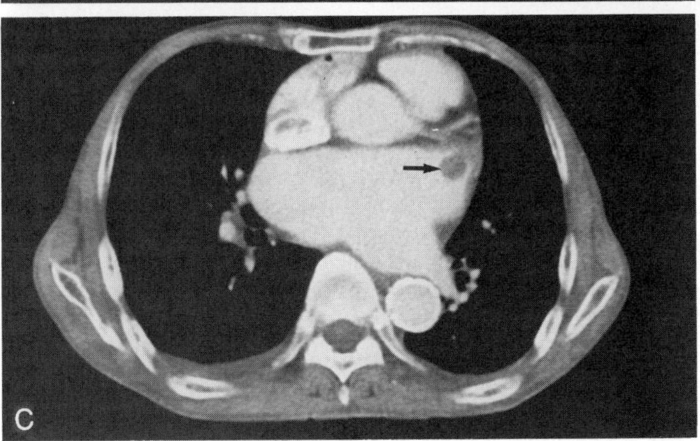

FIGURE 11-11. Cine CT scans of left atrial (LA) myxoma (*A*). The attachment of the myxoma to the atrial septum and prolapsing across the mitral valve are shown in the ultrafast CT scan. *B*, Right ventricular (RV) tumor that causes a filling defect in the opacified RV. *C*, A round filling defect in the dilated left atrial appendage (denoted by arrow) represents a left atrial thrombus. (Courtesy of W. Stanford, Iowa University Medical Center.)

tetralogy of Fallot, Ebstein's anomaly, abnormal arterioventricular connections, and others have been demonstrated by CT,[71,73] the technique has not found widespread use because of the ease and the usual diagnostic superiority of two-dimensional echocardiography and more recently MRI. An exception is the definitive demonstration of systemic veins, liver, and spleen possible with CT; this information is important for complete evaluation of the situs-splenic syndrome.[73]

ULTRAFAST CT. At a few centers ultrafast (cine) CT has also been employed in recent years for evaluation of congenital heart disease.[73,74] Cine CT has been found to be accurate in defining systemic and pulmonary venous connections. Likewise, it has demonstrated atrial (Fig. 11-12) and ventricular septal defects (Fig. 11-13). Transverse tomograms provide clear spatial separation of the inflow and outflow portions of the ventricular septum. This permits localization of defects and facilitates detection of multiple ventricular septal defects.[74] In addition, an assessment of the hemodynamic effects of septal defects (and of other lesions) can be made by evaluation of chamber dimension and wall thickness. Because of the absence of overlying structures defined on CT scans and the three-dimensional nature of cine CT, the size of the ventricles can be measured.

Normal and abnormal atrioventricular valves can be demonstrated by cine CT,[74] which can be used to diagnose both tricuspid and mitral atresia. It can also demonstrate the size of the atrium above the atretic valve. A common atrioventricular valve spanning both ventricles can be identified on the transverse image.

Cine CT has been effective for abnormal arterioventricular connections, including transposition complexes and double-outlet right ventricle[74] (Fig. 11-14). Abnormalities of the pulmonary arteries, such as congenital absence, peripheral coarctations, and hypoplasia have been demonstrated by this technique.[74] However, cine CT is not recommended for this purpose because multiplanar MRI has been shown recently to be the most effective technique for assessing pulmonary arterial anomalies.

Cine CT appears to be an excellent technique for the evaluation of both right and left ventricular function in surgically corrected congenital heart disease. Because ventricular volumes[17,19,20] and mass[9-11] can be measured accurately by CT, this technique can be used to evaluate the expected regression

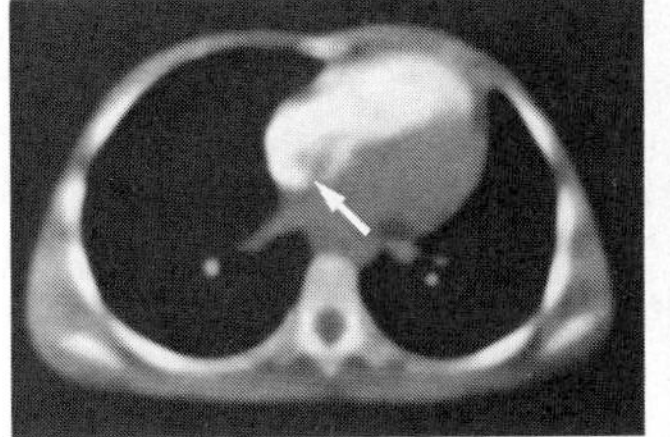

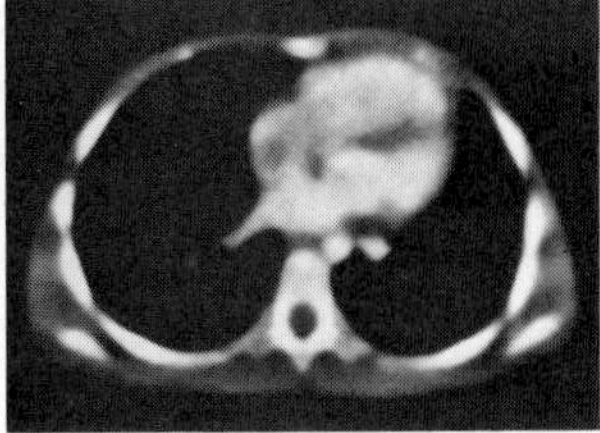

FIGURE 11-12. Cine CT scans of a patient with secundum atrial septal defect (ASD) after intravenous injection of contrast media. Sequential scans at same level obtained at time of the passage of contrast bolus through right heart *(left)* and left heart *(right)*. Unopacified blood crosses ASD into RA early (arrow) and on levophase, contrast-enhanced blood is observed crossing the ASD. (Courtesy of J. Eldridge, M.D., Deborah Heart Institute.)

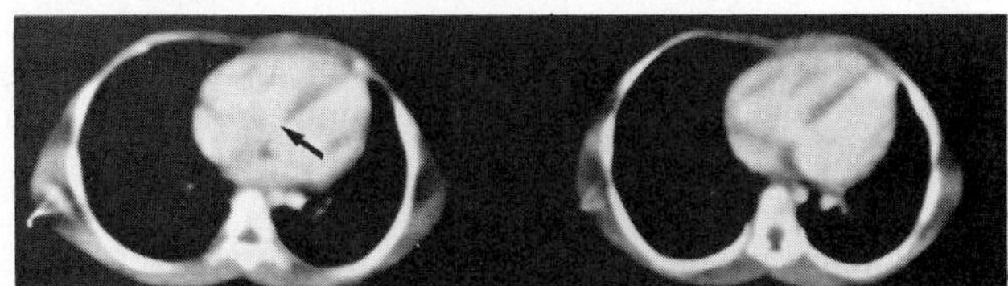

FIGURE 11-13. Cine CT scans of patient with ventricular septal defect. During the period of enhancement of both ventricles the ventricular septal defect is evident (arrow). (Courtesy of J. Eldridge, M.D., Deborah Heart Institute.)

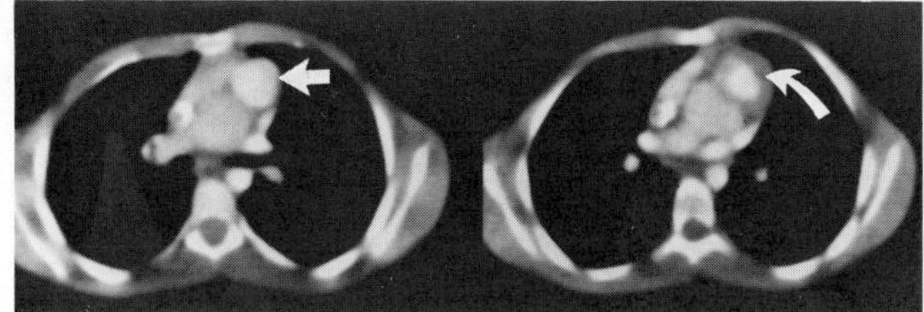

FIGURE 11–14. Cine CT scans of patient with levo-transposition. The aorta (arrow) is positioned anterior and to the left of the pulmonary artery. Scan at base of heart *(right)* shows that the aorta arises from the infundibulum (curved arrow). (Courtesy of J. Eldridge, M.D., Deborah Heart Institute.)

of ventricular dilatation and hypertrophy after corrective procedures.

EVALUATION OF CARDIAC FUNCTION (see also Chap. 15). This can be accomplished in patients with congenital heart disease by ultrafast CT, which, along with cine MRI, may be the best technique for quantitating right ventricular volumes and ejection fraction. In addition, cine CT can be used to estimate the volume of shunts; its accuracy has been documented in an experimental right-to-left shunt model in the dog.[75] This is done by measuring density of contrast medium within a cardiac chamber receiving shunt flow on sequential CT scans obtained during passage of contrast medium through the central circulation. A density-versus-time curve can be generated for such a region of interest. The normal curve is unimodal as contrast medium enters and leaves a cardiac chamber. A bimodal time-density curve may be generated from a region-of-interest cursor placed over any chamber involved in a shunt. With a gamma variate fit method, the areas under the primary and secondary portions of the curve can be measured in order to calculate pulmonary to systemic flow ratios. A close correlation has been found for the measurement of pulmonary-to-systemic flow ratio by cine CT and oximetry in experimental animals[75] and in patients.[74]

Another method for calculating the net shunt is to compare the difference in stroke volume between the two ventricles. For a left-to-right shunt at the ventricular level, the difference between the larger left ventricular stroke volume and right ventricular stroke volume indicates the net shunt value. Such an approach also can be used to calculate net volume and fraction of regurgitant lesions.

DISEASES OF THE THORACIC AORTA

(See also Chap. 47)

CT has been shown to be extremely accurate for the diagnosis of thoracic aortic aneurysm and dissection.[76–81]

AORTIC DISSECTION. In one prospective study in 26 patients with suspected aortic dissection, there were no false-negative or false-positive CT scans for this diagnosis.[80] In this study, CT correctly indicated the true extent of dissection in some patients in whom it was underestimated by angiography. In general, CT has an accuracy of approximately 90 per cent and is equivalent to angiography and MRI for the diagnosis of a variety of diseases of the thoracic aorta.[81] However, some instances of false-negative CT examination in aortic dissection have been reported.[74–81] Diagnosis of dissection requires the demonstration of the intimal flap, appearing as a lucency within the lumen of the contrast-enhanced aortic lumen on CT scans (Fig. 11–15). Intramural hematoma also has been reported recently as a feature of aortic dissection

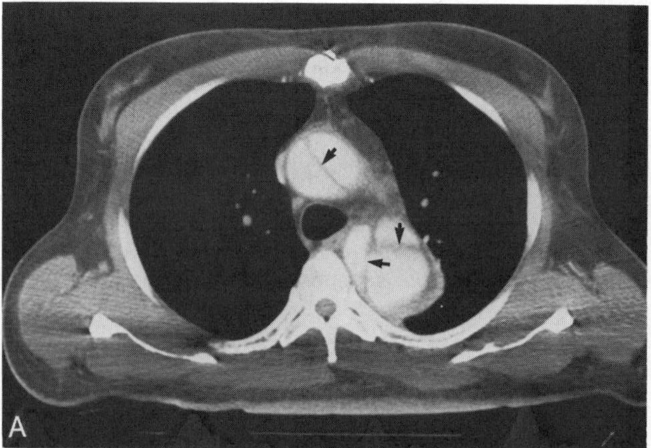

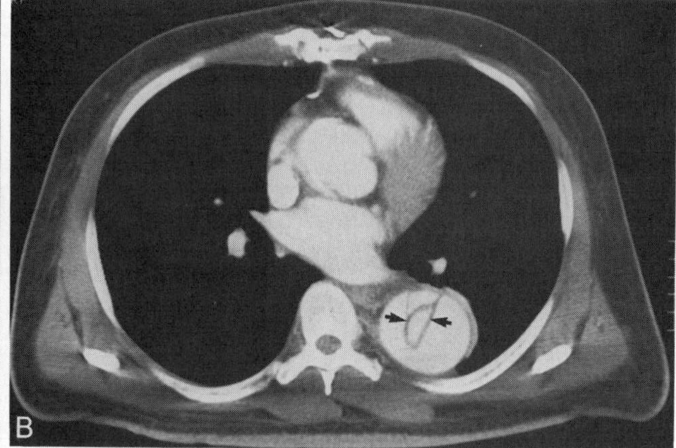

FIGURE 11–15. Cine CT scans just below aortic arch (*left, A*) and at level of the left atrium (*right, B*) show Type A aortic dissection. Intimal flaps (arrows) are visible in the descending aorta. (Courtesy of J. Eldridge, M.D., Deborah Heart Institute.)

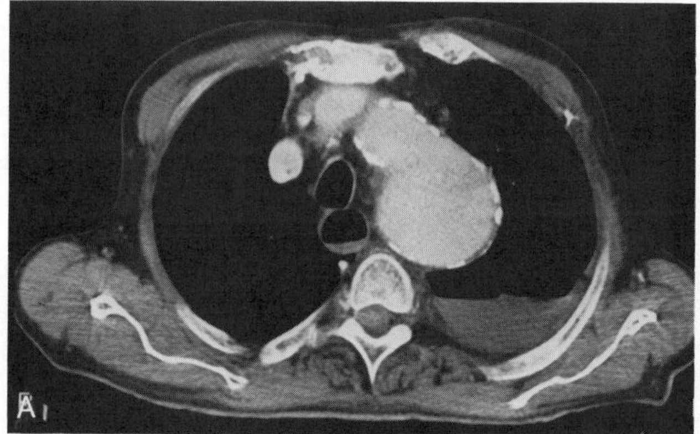

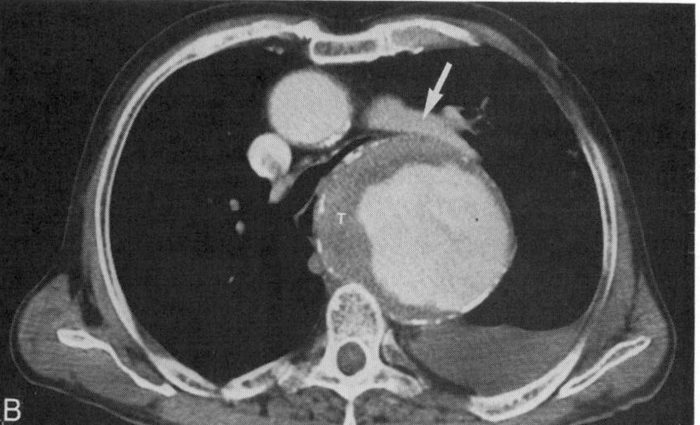

FIGURE 11–16. Cine CT scans at the level of the aortic arch (*A*) and descending aorta (*B*). The aneurysm involves the aortic arch. Thrombus partially fills the enormous aneurysm of the descending aorta and the aneurysm causes displacement and compression of the left pulmonary artery (arrow). There is heavy calcification of the ascending arch and the descending portions of the aorta. (Courtesy of Imatron.)

without entry into the lumen of the aorta.[82] While this has been reported in approximately 30 per cent of patients with dissection in a report from Japan, intramural hematoma is rarely encountered in the United States. Although it is possible that this is an early stage of an acute dissection, no evidence in this regard is extant. Supportive diagnostic findings are differential temporal enhancement of the true and false aortic channels and compression of the opacified true lumen by a thrombosed false channel. Inward displacement of calcium in the aortic wall is also a sign of aortic dissection. CT can distinguish between dissections that involve the ascending aorta and those that are limited to the descending aorta. In the former, the intimal flap can be demonstrated in the ascending aorta. It may be difficult to differentiate a dissection with thrombus of the false channel from an aortic aneurysm with mural thrombus (Fig. 11–16). A dissection is more likely when CT scans at multiple levels show the thrombus extending for more than 10 cm longitudinally. Also, dissection usually results in a compressed true aortic lumen, while aneurysm has a normal or increased lumen.

CT also may be used for following the course of thoracic aortic dissections after initial treatment.[79,83,84] After surgical placement of an ascending aortic graft, the false channel beyond the distal anastomosis of the graft frequently remains patent. Sequential CT studies have also revealed persistent patency of the false channel after medical as well as surgical therapy: eventual thrombosis of the false channel or even its disappearance is seen in some patients.[85,86] CT has also been used to follow the alterations in the false channel of untreated Type B dissections; in a minority of patients the aorta reverts to a normal appearance after months to years.[84]

AORTIC ANEURYSM. This is characterized by an increase in aortic diameter and by outward displacement of calcium of the aortic wall (Fig. 11–16). CT is an effective method for defining the maximum diameter of the aneurysm and monitoring it over time. A diameter of the thoracic aorta exceeding 5 cm is considered aneurysmal and one exceeding 6 cm is usually an indication for surgery of thoracic aortic aneurysm (Fig. 47–2, p. 1529).

Magnetic Resonance Imaging of the Heart

Brief descriptions of the MRI process, general imaging techniques, and specific imaging techniques for the heart are given below, and some useful terminology for MRI and spectroscopy is presented as a glossary. A more detailed description of the principles underlying MRI is available elsewhere.[87]

MAGNETIC RESONANCE IMAGING GLOSSARY

Echoplanar Imaging. A method for obtaining MR images in 30 to 50 msecs. Data for all points in the image matrix are obtained with a single pulse repetition (single TR). In echoplanar imaging, a very rapid series of spin echoes is generated by rapidly switching a strong phase-encoding gradient in the presence of a weaker read gradient.

Free Induction Decay. The signal produced by the release of energy absorbed by the nuclei from a previously applied radiofrequency pulse. The free induction decay is the signal analyzed in MRI and spectroscopy.

Gradient-Echo Imaging Sequence. A method by which images are acquired more rapidly than is possible with spin-echo imaging by substantially reducing the repetition time (TR). The technique uses a flip angle of less than 90 degrees and a short TR. This reduction is achieved by switching of the read gradient to focus the signal rather than by a time-consuming refocusing of the radiofrequency pulse. Contrast on these images is quite different from that of spin-echo images. A major difference is that blood flow produces strong signal and appears light.

Hydrogen Density (Spin Density, Proton Density). Density of protons at a site in a sample which are resonating as part of the magnetic resonance process. From the point of view of quantum mechanics, these are the protons making transitions from high-energy states to lower ones and vice versa, when energy that is just equal to the difference between these two states is applied.

Magnetic Moment. Intensity and direction of the net magnetic field of spinning nuclei. In a magnetic field, nuclei align to produce a net magnetic moment parallel to the field (Fig. 11–17).

Magnetic Resonance Imaging (MRI). Spatial two- or three-dimensional map of nuclei resonating at a characteristic frequency when placed in a magnetic field and subjected to intermittently applied radiofrequency pulses.

Magnetic Resonance Signal. During relaxation after cessation of a radiofrequency pulse, energy absorbed from this pulse is released and provides a radiofrequency signal.

Magnetic Resonance Spectroscopy. Spectrum of resonant frequencies of a specific nucleus contained within a sample. This spectrum results from the chemical shift of a nucleus caused by the influence of the local chemical environment. Consequently, the resonant frequency of phosphorus in the inorganic state is slightly different from its frequency in creatine phosphate. Magnetic resonance spectroscopy detects and maps these chemical shifts of a nucleus.

Multinuclear MRI. Imaging using nuclei other than hydrogen, such as sodium 23 and phosphorus 31.

Paramagnetic Substances. Substances that alter the natural relaxation times of nuclei undergoing the magnetic resonance process. These are

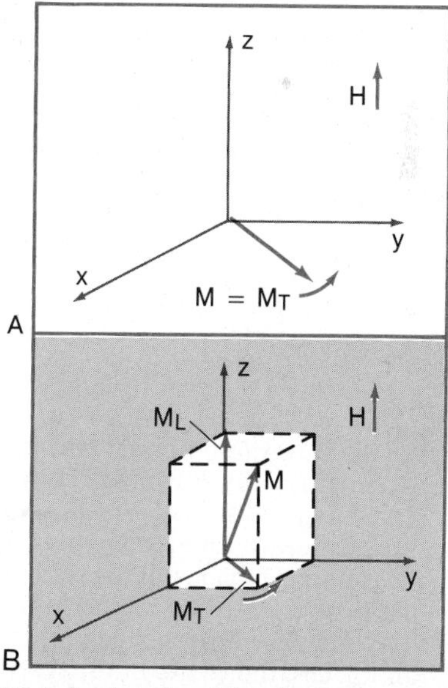

FIGURE 11–17. Behavior of nuclei undergoing magnetic resonance. Strong magnetic field (H) is present along the Z axis. After application of a 90-degree radiofrequency pulse the net magnetic moment of the nuclei is rotated into the transverse (XY) plane, causing the net magnetization to be equal to transverse magnetization (M_T). Subsequently, M_T decays as longitudinal magnetization (M_L) grows. The net magnetization vector (M) at any instant is the result of the instantaneous values of M_L and M_T. Since M_T decays more rapidly than M_L grows, the length of the vector changes as it returns to equilibrium. (From Margulis, A. R., et al.: Clinical Magnetic Resonance Imaging. San Francisco, Radiology Research and Education Foundation, 1983.)

usually molecules with unpaired electrons that reduce the relaxation times of resonating nuclei. These substances are being used and developed as contrast media for magnetic resonance imaging.

Proton MRI. Imaging dependent upon the concentration and relaxation time of hydrogen nuclei.

Proton Spectroscopy. Spectrum of resonant frequencies of hydrogen nuclei (protons) in relation to the chemical environment. Proton spectroscopy can define chemical peaks representative of substances such as fats, water, lactic acid, choline, and carnitine.

Relaxation. Return of nuclei to the original state of alignment with a magnetic field after having been tilted by a radiofrequency pulse.

Relaxation Times. Relaxation of nuclei undergoing the magnetic resonance process has two components called T1 and T2 relaxation times. These relaxation times are time-constants, measured as the magnetization vector precesses into alignment with the magnetic field after perturbation by a radiofrequency pulse.

Resonant Frequency. Each nucleus that is sensitive to the magnetic resonance process must be tilted in the magnetic field by a specific frequency (resonant frequency) in order to induce resonance. When this frequency is applied, the nucleus is rotated away from its equilibrium alignment with the magnetic field. When the radiofrequency pulse ceases, the nucleus realigns with the magnetic field through a process of magnetic relaxation.

Spin-Echo Imaging Sequence. Images are produced by sampling signal after an initial 90-degree radiofrequency pulse, followed by one or more 180-degree pulses. The 180-degree pulse refocuses spins and thereby enhances the signal from them. Signal is sampled some time after the 180-degree pulse.

Surface Coils. Radiofrequency receiver coils placed upon the surface of the subject or upon an organ of interest in order to detect the magnetic resonance signal. These coils increase the efficiency and signal strength for both MRI and spectroscopy.

T1 Relaxation Time. Also called spin-lattice or longitudinal relaxation time. T1 relaxation is a measure of the exponential rate of growth of the magnetization vector along the direction of the external magnetic field after the nuclei have been tilted (flipped) by a radiofrequency pulse (Fig. 11–18).

T1-Weighted Image. Image in which the intensity of image voxels is heavily dependent upon the T1 relaxation time of tissues. For the spin-echo technique, this is done with a short TR and TE.

T2 Relaxation Time. Also called spin-spin or transverse relaxation time. Immediately after cessation of a 90-degree radiofrequency pulse, the nuclei process in phase, resulting in a magnetization vector in the transverse plane (Fig. 11–19). There is gradual dephasing of nuclei, leading to cancellation of the magnetization vector in the transverse plane.

T2-Weighted Image. Image in which the intensity of image voxels is heavily dependent upon the T2 relaxation time of tissues. For the spin-echo technique, this is done with a long TR and TE.

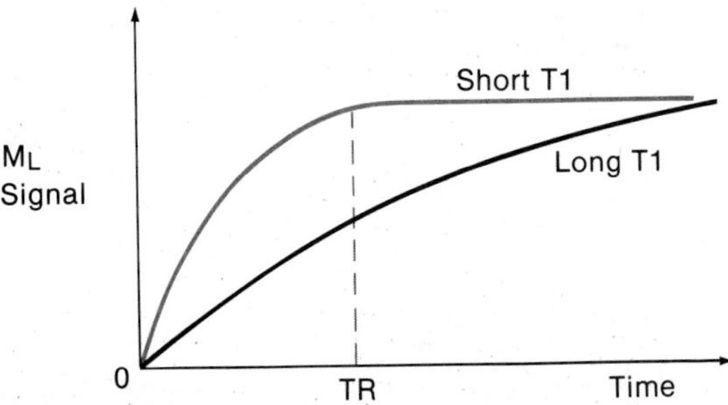

FIGURE 11–18. After perturbation of magnetic resonance–sensitive nuclei by a radiofrequency pulse, the magnetic resonance signal, owing to longitudinal magnetization (M_L), grows exponentially to the equilibrium value at a rate determined by T1. If the system is allowed a time TR to recover, contrast between tissues with different T1 values is produced. In general, there will be greater T1 contrast for shorter TR values and lower contrast for longer TR values. (From Margulis, A. R., et al.: Clinical Magnetic Resonance Imaging. San Francisco, Radiology Research and Education Foundation, 1983.)

TE. Echo delay time. Time between the initiation of a pulse sequence (90-degree pulse) and the sampling of the spin-echo signal. For the spin-echo sequence, this sampling is done after the 180-degree pulse. For example, the first spin-echo signal is sampled at a time that is twice the duration between the initial 90-degree pulse and the 180-degree refocusing pulse.

Tesla. Unit of the strength of the magnetic field.

Voxel. Volume element of the image matrix.

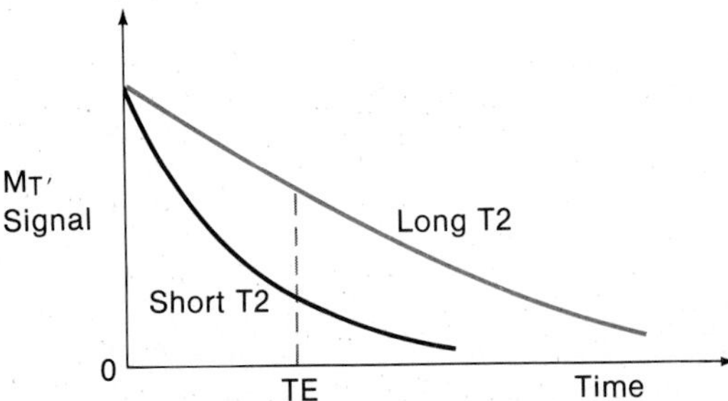

FIGURE 11–19. After perturbation of magnetic resonance–sensitive nuclei by a radiofrequency pulse, transverse magnetization (M_T) exponentially decays at a rate determined by T2. The TE determines contrast between two tissues with different values of T2. In general, there is greater T2 contrast for longer TE values up to a maximum point at which signal declines severely. (From Margulis, A. R., et al.: Clinical Magnetic Resonance Imaging. San Francisco, Radiology Research and Education Foundation, 1983.)

Magnetic resonance imaging has several important attributes that make it intrinsically advantageous for cardiovascular diagnosis. First, a high natural contrast exists between the blood pool and the cardiovascular structures because of the lack of signal from flowing blood with the spin-echo MRI technique or bright signal from blood with gradient-echo (cine MRI) technique. When the spin-echo technique is used, blood appears black on images; therefore, internal structures of the heart can be visualized within the signal void of the cardiac chambers (Fig. 11–20). Using the gradient-echo technique, the blood pool appears white and has substantially higher signal than the myocardium, again providing good edge definition of the endocardial margin (Fig. 11–21). Consequently, contrast medium is not required for discrimination of the blood pool, as MRI is an entirely noninvasive imaging technique. Second, a wide range of soft tissue contrast provides the potential for the characterization of myocardial tissue. This contrast among tissues is dependent upon proton (hydrogen nuclei) density and magnetic relaxation times of the protons. Third, imaging can be done in any plane, including those parallel and perpendicular to the major axis of the ventricles.

TECHNICAL ASPECTS

Atomic nuclei with a net charge have a magnetic moment. A net charge exists when a nucleus contains unpaired (an odd number of) protons, neutrons, or both. The hydrogen nucleus contains only a proton; it is positively charged and has a strong magnetic moment. The magnetic properties of nuclei are expressed when they are placed in an external magnetic field. When protons or other nuclei with magnetic moment lie within a magnetic field and are then exposed to electromagnetic radiation (radiofrequency waves), energy is absorbed and subsequently emitted. This absorption and release of energy causes resonance—nuclear magnetic resonance. The radiofrequency (RF) necessary to induce resonance has to be proportional to the local magnetic field (H_L) and a constant (magnetogyric ratio) related to the specific nucleus involved. The relationship between frequency (f) and magnetic field is expressed by the follow-

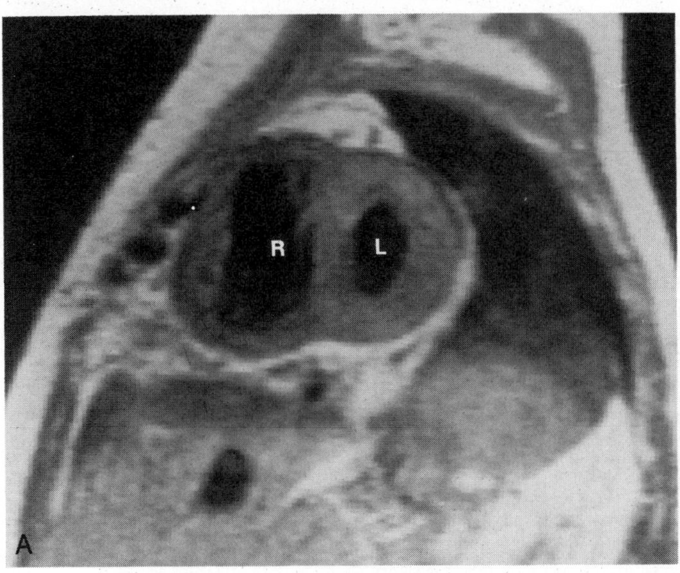

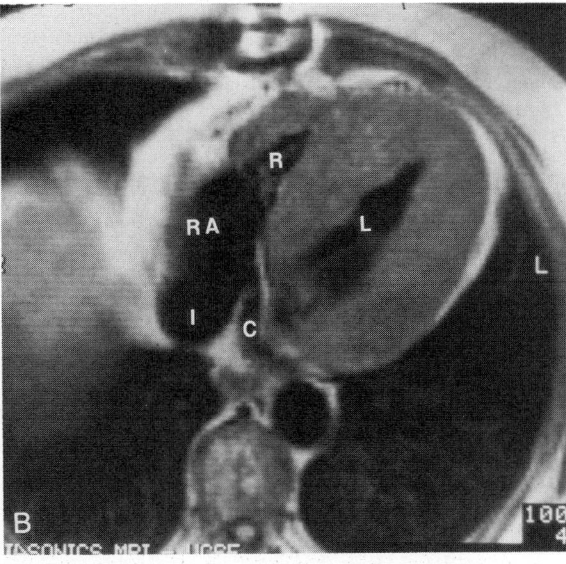

FIGURE 11–20. *A*, ECG-gated spin-echo MR image acquired in the short-axis plane through the middle of the ventricles. On this type of image the moving blood within the chambers of the heart produces little or no signal, resulting in high contrast between the blood pool and myocardial walls. The right ventricular wall is thickened in this patient. L = left ventricle; R = right ventricle. *B*, ECG-gated spin-echo image acquired in the transverse plane. The endocardial border is sharply demarcated due to the contrast between the blood pool and the myocardium. There is severe left ventricular hypertrophy. I = inferior vena cava; L = left ventricle; RA = right atrium; R = right ventricle; C = coronary sinus. Note that the cardiac short-axis image transects the heart perpendicular to the long axis of the heart while the transverse plane sections the ventricles obliquely.

ing equation:

$$f = \delta H_L/2\pi$$

When nuclei at equilibrium in a magnetic field are irradiated at the resonant frequency, they attain a higher energy state. When they return to equilibrium, they emit energy at the same frequency, if the magnetic field remains constant. If the magnetic field changes between the times of excitation and emission, then the emission occurs at a frequency corresponding to the new field strength as expressed by this equation.

LOCALIZATION OF MAGNETIC RESONANCE SIGNAL

MRI depends on the reception of the emitted radiofrequency (RF) signal from resonating nuclei and on the capability of locating these nuclei in space. Location of the resonating nuclei can be achieved by spatially varying the field strength in a known manner. Because resonance frequency of a nucleus at a specific site is related to local field strength, the emitted frequency will characterize the spatial location of the nucleus when a magnetic gradient exists in one or more planes.

Selection of a transverse section for imaging is done by applying a magnetic gradient along the Z axis (long axis of the body). In such a gradient each transverse plane (XY plane) has a specific and different resonant frequency. If the body is irradiated with a 90-degree RF pulse consisting of a narrow range of frequencies corresponding to the resonance frequency of a single plane, only the nuclei in this plane will resonate. By this means, called *selection irradiation,* the image plane is delineated.

Once a plane is excited by selective irradiation, spatial localization is attained in this plane by another gradient oriented parallel to this plane. After the selective 90-degree RF pulse is applied, a magnetic field gradient is produced in the X or Y direction. Nuclei at the stronger end of the field gradient will resonate at a higher frequency than those at the weaker end of the gradient. This provides spatial localization within the selected plane.

The magnetic signal from a sample undergoing MRI is detected by an RF receiver coil. The intensity of the signal at foci in the imaging plane depends on the concentration of resonating nuclei at the site and the magnetic relaxation times of the nuclei. The relaxation times are measures of the interaction of the resonating protons with the static magnetic field and the intermittently applied RF pulses.

The net magnetic moment of nuclei at any site can be expressed as a vector with length (intensity) and direction. At equilibrium, the vector points along the main static magnetic field. The vector can be tipped 90 degrees by application of an RF pulse. The component of the net magnetic moment that points along the main magnetic field is called *longitudinal magnetization.* The component at 90 degrees to the main field is the *transverse magnetization.* After completion and before attainment of full alignment with magnetic field (equilibrium), the vector varies continuously between longitudinal and transverse magnetization and gradually approaches full longitudinal magnetization.

MAGNETIC RELAXATION TIMES. After the application of a 90-degree RF pulse, net magnetization is rotated from the longitudinal direction (ZY plane) into the transverse direction (XY plane) (Fig. 11–17). At this instant, transverse magnetization is maximum and longitudinal magnetization is zero. Immediately after this, longitudinal magnetization gradually recovers toward its equilibrium value. This exponential growth has a time constant called *T1.* Likewise, after the 90-degree pulse, transverse magnetization exponentially decays and the time constant is called *T2.* In tissues, T2 is much shorter than T1. These relaxation times are related to several characteristics of tissues, including temperature. Tissues have different relaxation times, and these differences contribute to contrast among tissues during imaging. Contrast between two tissues can be accentuated by sampling signal at an instant when there is maximum difference between the relaxation times of the two tissues.

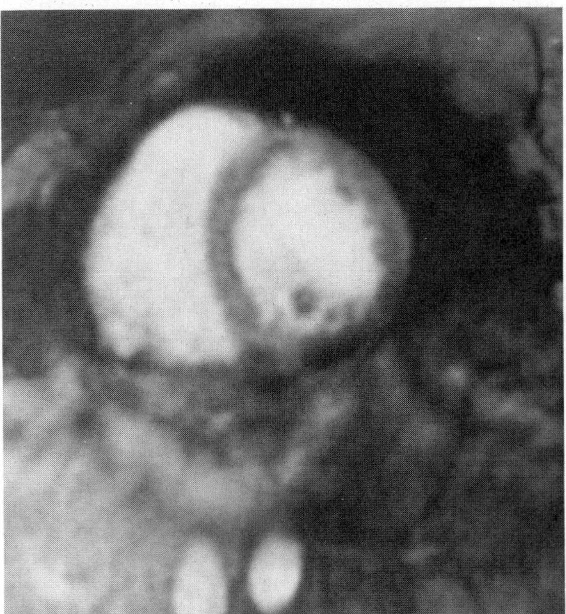

FIGURE 11–21. Cine MR image acquired in the short-axis plane through the middle of the ventricles. On this type of image the blood pool produces higher signal than the myocardium, resulting in substantial contrast between the two and sharp delineation of the endocardial margin.

IMAGING, REPETITION TIME, AND ECHO DELAY TIME. The MR image is produced by applying the sets of RF pulses many times over several minutes; generally, 256 to 512 pulse sequences are used. The time between application of sets of RF pulses is called the *repetition time* (TR). Depending on the technique employed for imaging, each set consists of one or more RF pulses. The time between the initial pulse in a sequence and the instant when signal is acquired from the sample is called the *echo delay time* (TE). It is possible to alter the pulse sequences in such a way that differences in T1 and T2 relaxation times among the tissues can be accentuated to produce contrast among these tissues. This is referred to as *T1* or *T2 weighting of the images.* With use of the spin-echo technique, T1-weighted images have short TR and TE intervals, while T2-weighted images have long TR and TE intervals when the spin-echo technique is used. T1 and T2 weighting for the fast gradient-echo imaging techniques are achieved to some extent by variations in the flip angles induced in the nuclei by the initial RF pulses.

Thus, as described above, MRI depends upon radiofrequency (RF radiowave) signals that result from the interaction of protons (hydrogen nuclei) with a strong magnetic field (0.15 to 2.0 tesla) and intermittent applied RF pulses. Although imaging possibly could be carried out for other atoms that have a magnetic moment, imaging is now carried out almost exclusively with hydrogen nuclei (protons). The combined effect of the magnetic field and the RF pulses causes protons to resonate at a characteristic frequency. Spatial identification of the resonating protons is achieved by an intermittently applied weak magnetic gradient. This causes slight variations in resonant frequency, depending on the site of the proton within the magnetic gradient, because of the proportionality between resonant frequency and magnetic field strength.

EFFECTS OF MOVING BLOOD. During an imaging sequence, the motion of nuclei through the region that is being imaged greatly influences signal intensity. Although the influence of blood flow on magnetic resonance images is complex, motion of the excited nuclei during the MRI sequence generally causes a loss of signal intensity. Consequently, moving blood in the lumina of vessels appears dark (no signal), providing considerable natural contrast for visualization of the internal surfaces of the blood vessels and walls of the cardiac chambers (Fig. 11–20). Because contrast medium is not required to mark the blood pool, MRI is a totally noninvasive technique for cardiovascular diagnosis. When blood velocity is such that protons move through the thickness of the tomogram (usually 5 to 10 mm) in the time between the 90- and 180-degree pulses of the spin-echo sequence, signal is lost from the blood. Using standard spin-echo sequences, this time (TE/2) is usually 15 msec for the first such image. On the other hand, with the fast imaging techniques recently introduced, signal is received from blood flowing at normal velocities in the cardiac chambers and all blood vessels. In this circumstance, blood appears substantially brighter (white) than the cardiac walls (Fig. 11–21). High-velocity jets produced by flow across stenotic or regurgitant valves can be recognized as a signal void within the signal-filled cardiac chambers.

Techniques for Magnetic Resonance Imaging of the Heart

Cardiac imaging requires some form of physiological gating of the imaging sequence. Acquisition of MR signals of the thorax without gating results in poor cardiac images owing to two factors. The first is the loss of the signal from moving structures while the second is the variable position of the cardiac structure relative to imaging pixels when data are acquired indiscriminately throughout the cardiac cycle.

GATING WITH MRI. This is associated with unique problems. Sensors, wire leads, and transducers are usually composed of ferromagnetic materials, which can generate noise or may grossly distort the images within the RF-shielded room containing the MRI device. Consequently, gating with MRI requires the use of a nonferromagnetic physiological signal-sensing circuit. An electronically isolated ECG electrode-lead circuit containing very little metal has been used for repetitive synchronization, i.e., ECG gating, of pulse sequences to fixed segments of the cardiac cycle. The uses and results of gating for the acquisition of MR images are described subsequently in this chapter.

MULTISLICE TECHNIQUES. Several imaging strategies have been employed depending upon the information desired. For anatomical diagnosis, the *ECG-gated multislice technique* is used. This technique is economical in time, requiring less than 10 minutes for the acquisition of tomograms (1 cm thickness) at 10 anatomical levels, which usually encompasses the entire heart and root of the great vessels. A difference of 50 to 100 msec exists between each adjacent level, so the images are obtained at different phases of the cardiac cycle. The reason why images can be obtained at multiple anatomical levels during a single imaging sequence is that the time required to complete a set of RF pulses and sample the emitted signal for each line on that image is usually 30 to 60 msec (T-E interval), while the time duration between the application of repetitive sets of pulses is approximately 500 to 1000 msec (T-R interval). Consequently, the inactive time for each cycle is long, frequently greater than 90 per cent of the cycle. Efficiency is improved by applying the set of spin-echo pulses at other levels during the magnetization recovery period. Therefore, upon completion of a 50-msec duty cycle at one level, the full set of pulses is selectively applied at the next adjacent tomographic level and then the next, and so forth. With this multislice technique, the total number of tomographic levels that can be imaged is approximately TR/TE. As indicated earlier, TR equals the length of the cardiac cycle (R-R interval) when ECG gating is used.

For imaging small anatomical structures such as the coronary arteries, thin slices (0.25 to 0.5 cm thickness) are acquired. Each anatomical level is also imaged at multiple phases of the cardiac cycle in order to minimize the effect of movement of the structures into and out of the imaging plane during the cardiac cycle. In this manner, each adjacent tomogram is acquired at the same phase of the cardiac cycle during both systole and diastole. The gating window for such images is less than 30 msec using the spin-echo technique: Thus the time is minimized for coronary motion during image acquisition.

The *multiphasic multislice technique* is also used for the evaluation of cardiac dimensions and function. With this technique, each anatomical section is imaged at five phases of the cardiac cycle. From end-diastolic and end (late)-systolic images of each anatomical level, measurement can be made of diastolic and systolic volumes, stroke volume, ejection fraction, myocardial mass, and extent of left ventricular regional wall thickening. With this technique, wall thickening dynamics have been measured for various regions of the left ventricle in normal subjects and patients with global and regional myocardial dysfunction and in patients with focal and generalized hypertrophy.

CINE MR IMAGING. This can be accomplished by ECG referencing of fast imaging sequences. This approach can produce approximately 30 images (20 to 30 msec in duration) during the cardiac cycle. The images are laced together in a cinematic display so that a wall motion of the ventricles, valve motion, and blood flow patterns in the heart and great vessels can be visualized.

Volume or three-dimensional data acquisition has also been achieved with an ECG-gated sequence. With this technique, images of any desired plane can be reconstructed later, and all reconstructed planes are in the same phase of the cardiac cycle (in contrast to the multislice technique). The time cost of volume imaging is considerable; the acquisition time for volume imaging of an equal portion of the heart is longer for this technique than for the multislice technique.

INTERPRETATION OF MAGNETIC RESONANCE IMAGES

Information on morphology, function, and tissue characteristics can be derived from MR images. Most abnormalities are evident from alterations in morphology, such as regional wall thinning in patients with ischemic heart disease. Occasionally, however, no morphological changes are evident but the disease process can be diagnosed because of abnormal tissue characteristics. Abnormal myocardial tissue may be manifested as a regional difference in myocardial intensity, such as the increased intensity of acutely infarcted myocardium compared with normal myocardium. Tissue characterization by MRI is achieved by measurements of relative signal intensity and relaxation times of tissue. It is still imprecise because motion-related artifactual variations occur in the magnetic relaxation times of myocardial tissue which are currently relied upon for such characterization. Signal intensity increases with increases in hydrogen density and T2 relaxation time and decreases with decreases in T1 relaxation time. The contrast in intensity between tissues can be augmented by variation of the technical factors used to acquire the MR images.

Decrease of the TR (repetition time) and TE (echo delay time) factors produces greater contrast related to differences in T1 magnetic relaxation times among tissues (T1-weighted images), and increase of TR and TE causes greater contrast primarily on the basis of difference in T2 relaxation times among tissues (T2-weighted image).

EVALUATION OF SPECIFIC CARDIAC DISEASES

The clinical use of MRI has been primarily for the demonstration of pathological anatomy. However, in the past few years cine MRI has been employed for the quantification of global and regional function of the right and left ventricles and for the estimation of valvular regurgitation. Precise demonstration of anatomical abnormalities has been useful for the evaluation of patients with ischemic heart disease, cardiomyopathies, pericardial disease, neoplastic disease, congenital heart disease, and thoracic aortic disease.

ISCHEMIC HEART DISEASE

MRI provides direct visualization of the myocardium with excellent delineation of the epicardial and endocardial interfaces. Consequently, it can define accurately segmental wall thinning that is indicative of previous myocardial infarction.[88-90] In some patients with a history of transmural infarction, residual myocardium can be demonstrated at the site of the infarction. In others, MRI shows virtually complete absence of remnant muscle. Direct visualization of the myocardium could be used to determine whether there is sufficient residual myocardium in the region jeopardized by a coronary arterial lesion to warrant a bypass graft (Fig. 11–22). Regional wall thickening can also be assessed.[91]

The recognition of decreased signal intensity of the myocardial wall at the site of old myocardial infarction suggests that MRI can identify the replacement of myocardium by fibrous scar.[89] Gated MRI has also demonstrated complications of myocardial infarctions, such as left ventricular thrombus and aneurysms[88,89] (Figs. 11–23 and 11–24). Transverse or short-axis tomograms facilitate the recognition of the small ostium connecting the LV chamber and the false aneurysm (see Fig. 11–30); this is a distinguishing feature for the false compared with the true LV aneurysm.

Acute myocardial infarction has been demonstrated by gated MRI. The region of ischemically damaged myocardium displays increased signal intensity compared with normal myocardium[92-96] (Fig. 11–25). Contrast between infarcted and normal myocardia increases on images with greater T2

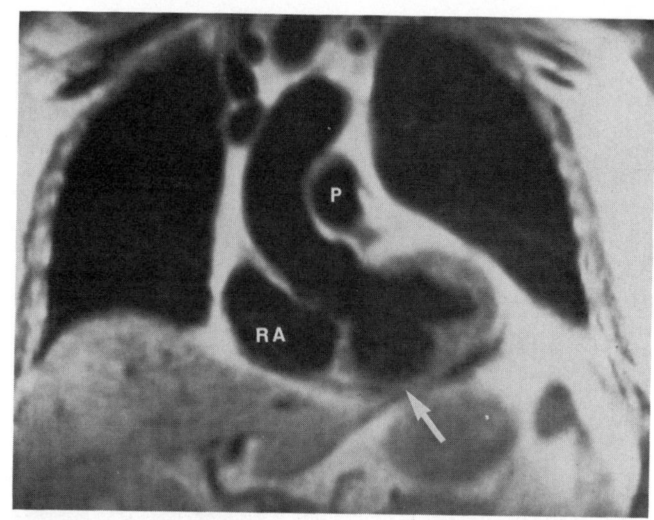

FIGURE 11–23. ECG-gated spin-echo image in the coronal plane displays a chronic transmural myocardial infarction (arrow) of the diaphragmatic wall of the left ventricle, which has caused severe wall thinning and aneurysmal bulging. P = pulmonary artery; RA = right atrium.

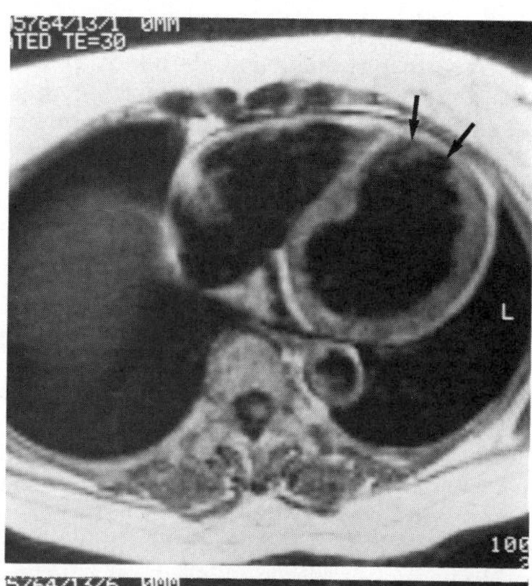

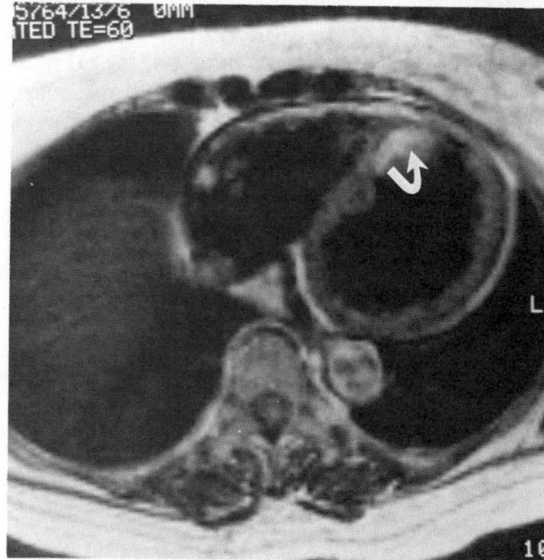

FIGURE 11–22. Chronic anterior myocardial infarction. First *(top)* and second *(bottom)* (spin-echo) images show absence of myocardium in the anterior wall of the LV (area between black arrows). Second echo image detects high signal from blood stasis (curved arrow) at the site of the old infarction, presumably due to segmental contractile dysfunction. (From Higgins, C. B.: MRI of the heart—1986. AJR *146*:907, copyright 1986, American Roentgen Ray Society.)

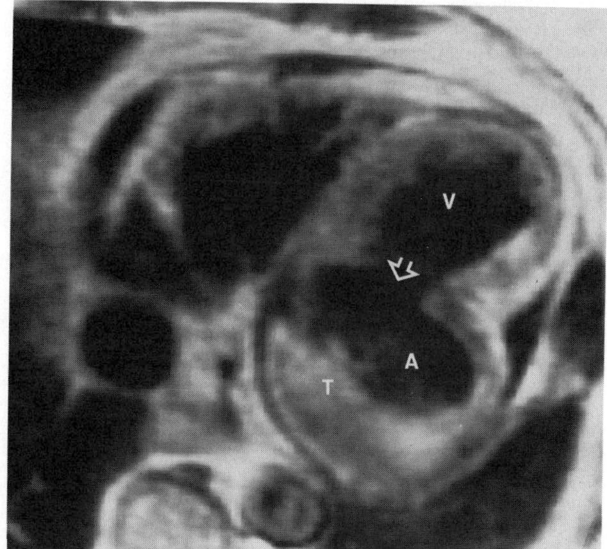

FIGURE 11–24. ECG-gated spin-echo image of a false aneurysm of the left ventricle. There is a narrow ostium (open arrow) connecting the large posterior aneurysm (A) to the ventricular (V) chamber. There is thrombus (T) in the aneurysm.

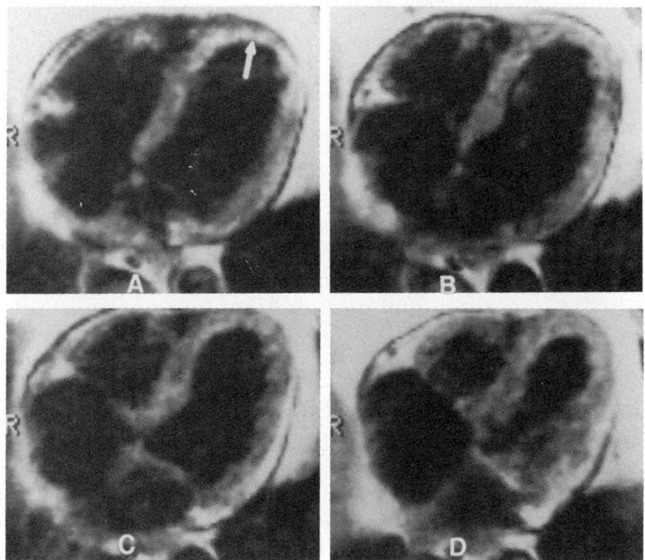

FIGURE 11-25. Anterior acute myocardial infarction. Images at four anatomical levels extending from cranial *(A)* to caudal *(D)* levels of the LV. Note the higher signal intensity (arrow) of the myocardium of the anterior wall of the LV at the site of the acute infarction. (From Higgins, C. B.: MRI of the heart — 1986. AJR *146*:907, copyright 1986, American Roentgen Ray Society.)

contribution to signal intensity. Since cardiac pulsations and respiration can cause high-intensity artifacts projected over the myocardial region, caution must be used in the interpretation of this finding.[97] Comparison of changes in contrast among images with increasing TE value and calculation of T2 relaxation times can alleviate this problem.[93]

The role of MRI in the evaluation of ischemic heart disease has been limited because it has not been capable of distinguishing ischemic noninfarcted myocardium from normal myocardium. Although studies in animal models indicate that this can be done using various MRI contrast media, little experience currently exists with patients in this regard. The potential role of MRI contrast media in ischemic heart disease is discussed later in this chapter.

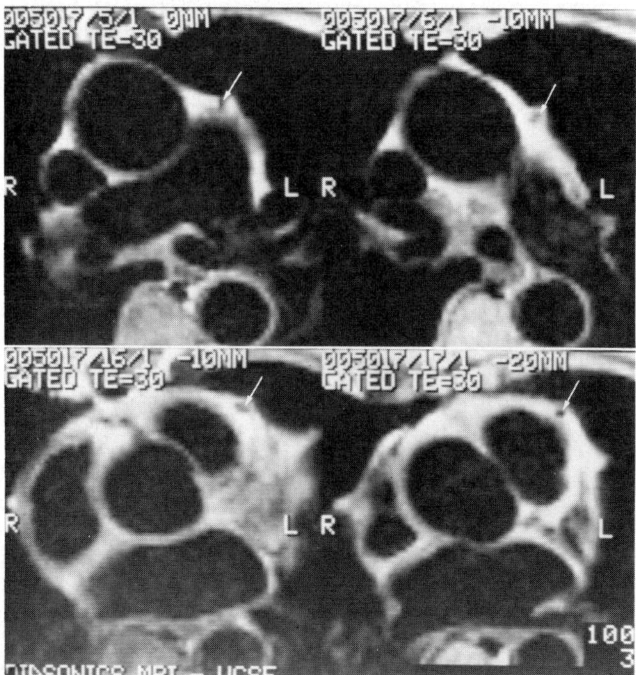

FIGURE 11-26. Multislice gated images extending from cranial *(upper left)* to caudal *(lower right)*. A graft to the left anterior descending coronary artery is visible at each level (arrow). Absence of luminal signal indicates patency of the graft.

CORONARY ARTERY BYPASS GRAFTS. Gated MRI has been used to evaluate the patency of bypass grafts. Since blood usually flows rapidly through the grafts, they appear as small circular structures with absence of a luminal signal (Fig. 11-26). For visualization of grafts, ECG-gated images are acquired in order to minimize the effect of motion of the grafts. Generally, images are acquired at each anatomical level during multiple phases of the cardiac cycle to ensure that an image is acquired at a phase when there is a rapid rate of flow through the graft. High flow rate in the graft produces a flow void in the lumen of the graft using spin-echo MRI and thus indicates patency of the graft. With the cine (gradient echo) MRI techniques, flowing blood causes bright signal intensity; therefore, bright signal rather than flow void would indicate graft patency with this technique. In order to achieve specificity in establishing patency, it is necessary to visualize absence of a luminal signal on at least two transverse images. MRI has an accuracy of 80 to 90 per cent for defining graft patency.[98-101]

CARDIOMYOPATHIES

(See also Chap. 43)

Gated MRI has been used to define the presence, distribution, and severity of hypertrophic cardiomyopathies.[102,103] Gated MRI has revealed the extent of septal involvement (Fig. 11-27) and has been particularly useful for identifying the unusual distribution of hypertrophy in the variant forms of hypertrophic cardiomyopathy. Quantification of left ventricular[104,105] and right ventricular[105,106] mass and wall thickness has been done using spin-echo and cine MRI. Substantial right ventricular hypertrophy has been shown by MRI measurements in patients with hypertrophic cardiomyopathy.[105,106] Cine MRI has also been used to assess right ventricular diastolic parameters by constructing volume-time curves during the cardiac cycle; reduced filling rate and time to peak filling have been demonstrated in patients with hypertrophic cardiomyopathy.[106]

DILATED CARDIOMYOPATHY (see p. 1398). MRI has depicted the morphological[107] and functional[108] alterations in congestive (dilated) cardiomyopathy. It has shown the degree of ventricular dilatation in patients with congestive cardiomyopathies.[102,107] Since MRI provides excellent discrimination of the edges of the myocardium, it can also be used to assess myocardial mass and wall thickness in patients with cardiomyopathies; recent studies have indicated the accuracy of MRI for quantifying myocardial mass in both normally and abnormally shaped left ventricles.[109,110] Cine MRI has also been found to be highly reproducible in measuring LV mass and volumes between two studies in the same subject.[109,110] The interstudy variability of mass measurements is less than 3 per cent. Cine MRI has demonstrated considerable increase in left ventricular mass and markedly elevated end-systolic wall

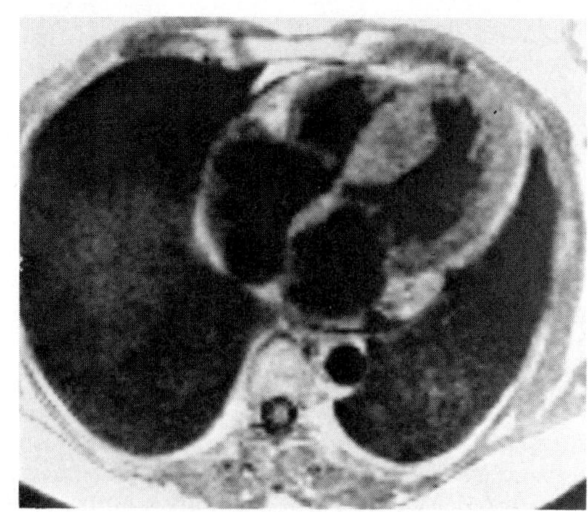

FIGURE 11-27. Hypertrophic cardiomyopathy. MRI displays severe hypertrophy of the entire septum and normal thickness of the lateral wall.

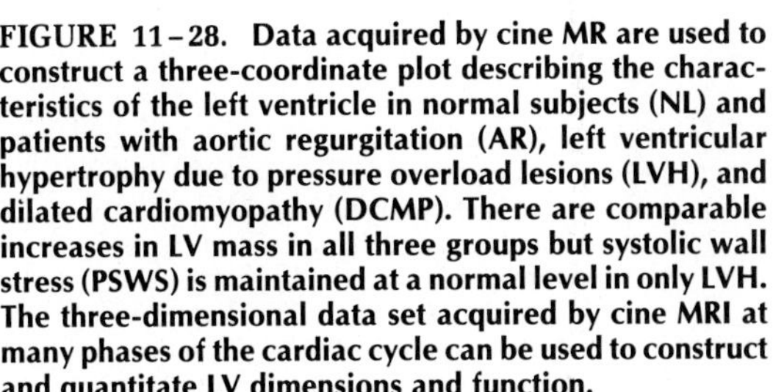

FIGURE 11-28. Data acquired by cine MR are used to construct a three-coordinate plot describing the characteristics of the left ventricle in normal subjects (NL) and patients with aortic regurgitation (AR), left ventricular hypertrophy due to pressure overload lesions (LVH), and dilated cardiomyopathy (DCMP). There are comparable increases in LV mass in all three groups but systolic wall stress (PSWS) is maintained at a normal level in only LVH. The three-dimensional data set acquired by cine MRI at many phases of the cardiac cycle can be used to construct and quantitate LV dimensions and function.

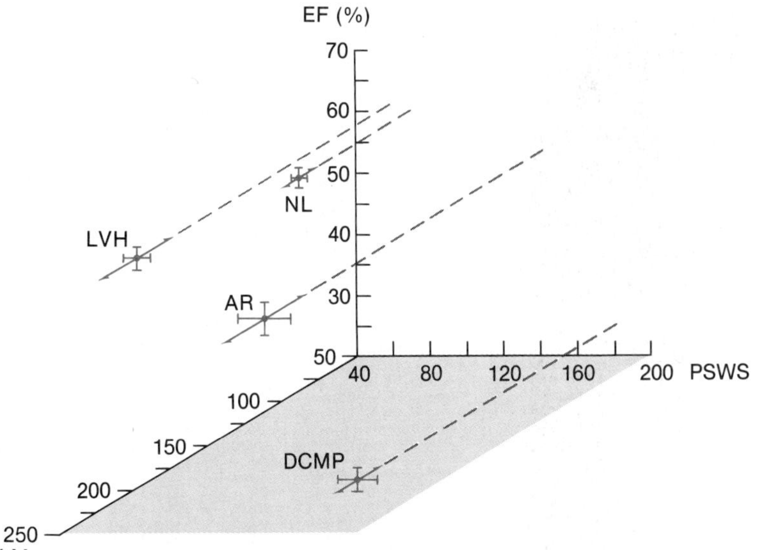

stress in patients with dilated cardiomyopathy[110,111] (Fig. 11-28). Cine MRI has demonstrated both a decrease in the extent of wall thickening and a change in the regional pattern of wall thickening in patients with dilated cardiomyopathy compared with normal subjects[108] (Fig. 11-29).

HYPERTROPHIC CARDIOMYOPATHY (see p. 1404). Because two-dimensional echocardiography provides excellent evaluation of hypertrophic cardiomyopathy, it is unlikely that it will be supplanted by MRI for the routine evaluation of these conditions. However, MRI has proved valuable in the evaluation of variant types of hypertrophic cardiomyopathy, such as the midventricular and apical forms.[102,103,112] It has also demonstrated abnormal signal intensity of the myocardium due to nonocclusive infarction of the left ventricular apical region as a complication of hypertrophic cardiomyopathy.[112]

RESTRICTIVE CARDIOMYOPATHY (see p. 1415). ECG-gated MRI has displayed features considered to be characteristic for restrictive cardiomyopathy.[113] There is substantial enlargement of the atria and the inferior vena cava, with usually less prominent ventricular enlargement. Because of resistance caused by the noncompliant ventricles to atrial emptying during diastole, prominent signal is observed in the atrial blood. Such intraatrial signal originates from slowly moving blood on spin-echo MR images. The major contribution of MRI for establishing the diagnosis of restrictive cardiomyopathy is the demonstration of normal pericardial thickness, which essentially excludes the alternate diagnosis of constrictive pericarditis. In *amyloid heart disease*, MRI has demonstrated thickened myocardial walls and diminished wall thickening during the cardiac cycle.[114,115] Cine MRI indicates apparent hypertrophy of the LV with normal or decreased LV contraction rather than hypercontractile LV contraction expected in LV hypertrophy (Fig. 11-30). MRI has also demonstrated infiltration of the myocardium by tumorous and inflammatory processes[116,117]; detection of such myocardial infiltrates can be useful for the diagnosis of specific forms of restrictive myocardial diseases.

The MRI findings in cardiomyopathies have thus far been limited to *anatomical and functional* abnormalities. No consistent changes in MRI relaxation times have been found for the myocardium in hypertrophic or congestive cardiomyopathies[118] or in amyloid heart disease.[115]

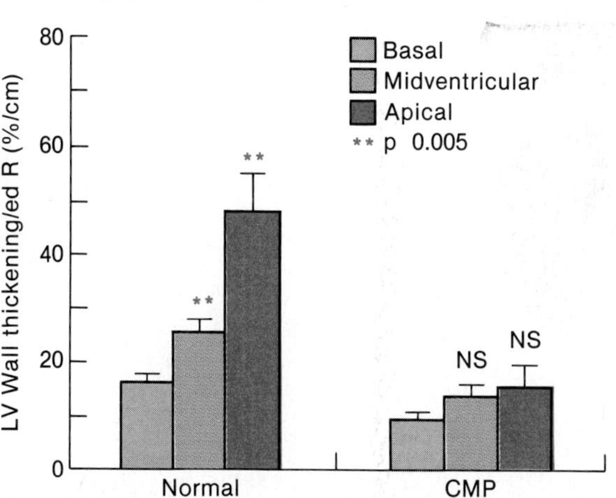

FIGURE 11-29. Block diagram showing the percentage wall thickening at the basal midventricular and apical layers of the left ventricle for normals and patients with dilated cardiomyopathy (CMP). The value for wall thickening at each layer represents the mean of measurements of wall thicknesses at four equidistant sites around the circumference of the left ventricle. Wall thickening is calculated as

$$WT = \frac{WT_{ES} - WT_{ED}}{WT_{ED}}$$

where WT_{ES} and WT_{ED} represent wall thickness at end-systole and end-diastole, respectively. There is a gradient in wall thickening from basal to apical layers in normals. Values are normalized to the end-diastolic radius, ed R. In CMP, the gradient is not evident and percentage wall thickening is decreased in all layers.

PERICARDIAL DISEASE

(See also Chap. 45)

Gated MRI provides direct visualization of the pericardium.[119-121] This technique is proving to be especially useful for the assessment of patients with known or suspected pericardial disease. Normal pericardium is composed primarily of fibrous tissue and has low MRI signal intensity (Fig. 11-31). The thickness of pericardial line measured in normal subjects was 1.5 ± 0.4 mm (S.D.) with a range from 0.8 to 2.6 mm.[120] A variation of thickness of the low-intensity line has been observed during the cardiac cycle in normal subjects. These latter observations, along with information from postmortem studies, indicate that the normal pericardium measures less than 1.0 mm; they suggest that the low-intensity pericardial line consists of pericardium and some adherent pericardial fluid. This is probably responsible for the pericardial line observed on CT as well, since normal CT measurements of pericardial thickness are similar to MRI measurements. Whereas pericardial fluid has a low signal intensity as well, it can usually be distinguished from the pericardium (Fig. 11-32). The distinction between the pericardium itself and normal fluid can also be achieved on cine MR images, in which the fluid has bright signal and the pericardium is a dark line (Fig. 11-33). MRI has been used to establish the diagnosis of congenital absence of the left pericardium.[122] Pericardial thickening and effusions are characteristic features of acute pericarditis (Fig. 11-32).

Gated MRI has been useful for demonstrating pericardial

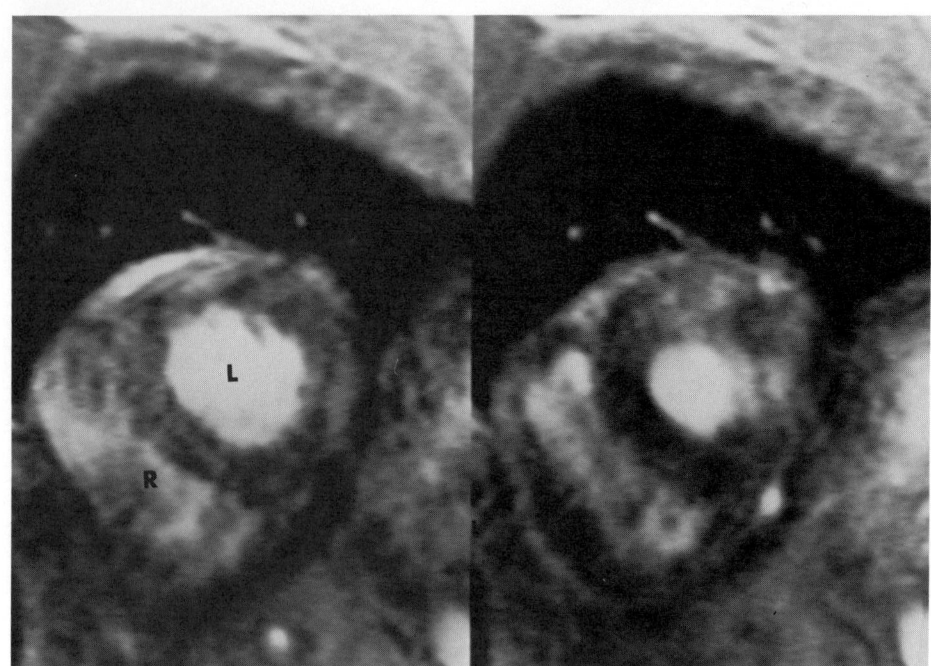

FIGURE 11-30. Two cine MR images at end diastole *(left)* and end systole *(right)* in a patient with cardiac amyloidosis. There is reduced systolic thickening of the septal and posterior regions of the left ventricle and an ejection fraction which is mildly reduced. L = left ventricle; R = right ventricle.

thickness in patients with suspected *constrictive pericarditis.*[119,121,123] The signal intensity of the thickened pericardium is variable. The purely fibrous or calcified pericardium in chronic constrictive pericardial disease has low signal intensity (Fig. 11-31). However, in subacute forms of constrictive pericarditis caused by irradiation, surgical trauma, or uremia, the thickened pericardium has moderate to high intensity on spin-echo images.[119,121] The effusive-constrictive form of pericardial disease involves thickened pericardium and pericardial effusion (Fig. 11-34).

MRI demonstrates even the small amount of pericardial fluid present in normal subjects. Fluid in the superior pericardial recesses is commonly seen even when fluid is not evident posterior to the left ventricle. The appearance of pericardial fluid is different on spin-echo and cine MRI (gradient-echo) images (Figs. 11-32 and 11-33). Nonhemorrhagic fluid shows low intensity on short TR, short TE sequences (T1-weighted) and has increased intensity on long TR, long TE sequences (T2-weighted). On the other hand, pericardial hematoma has high intensity on T1-weighted images (Fig. 11-35) and may have high intensity on T2-weighted images, depending upon the age of the hematoma and magnetic field strength of the imager.[124] On cine MRI, the nonhemorrhagic effusion is bright and the hemorrhagic one may be low intensity.

In pericardial disease the role of MRI must be considered in the light of the established effectiveness of echocardiography (pp. 1473 and 1477). An advantage of MRI over echocardiography is the capability to differentiate pericardial hematoma from other types of effusions. Also, because of the wide field of view, MRI seems to be useful in locating loculated effusions. Determination of pericardial thickening seems to be a clear indication for the use of MRI.

NEOPLASTIC DISEASE

(See also Chap. 44)

Several reports have documented the clinical utility of gated MRI for the evaluation of intracardiac[105,125-129] and paracardiac masses.[119,125,128-130] Because of the unequivocal delineation of the pericardium, myocardial walls, and chambers of

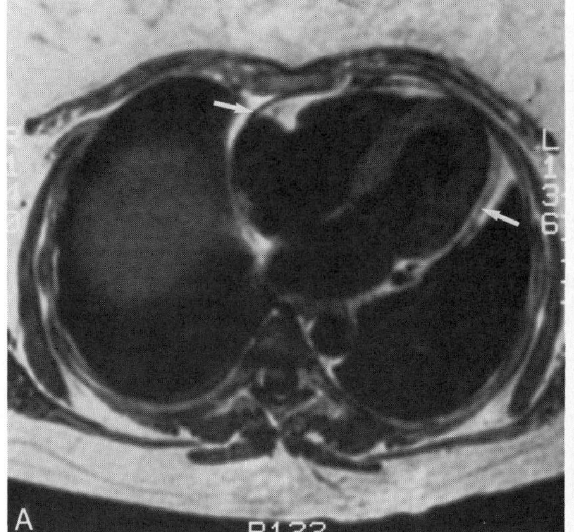

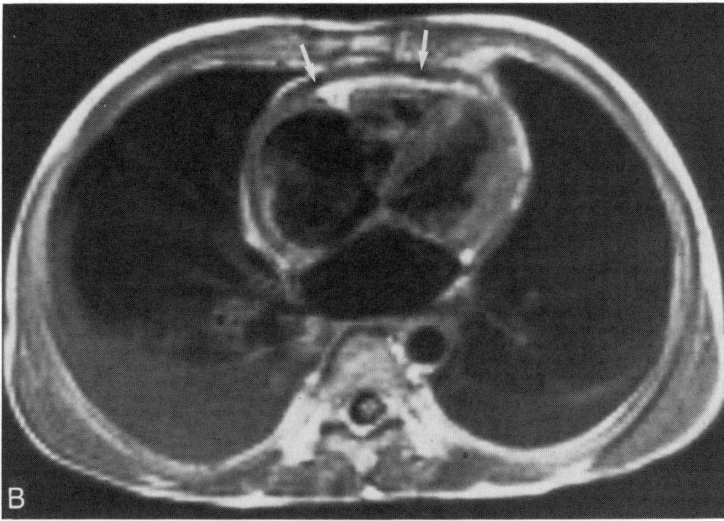

FIGURE 11-31. ***A,*** **Normal pericardium shown on transverse ECG-gated spin-echo images. Normal pericardial line in this subject can be seen over the right and left sides of the heart. Pericardial line (arrows) is visible due to the high-intensity pericardial fat and epicardial fat. Pericardial line is composed of parietal and visceral pericardia and a thin layer of adherent pericardial fluid between them.** ***B,*** **Constrictive pericarditis is indicated by marked thickening of the pericardium over the right and anterior aspects of the heart. Note the dark layer of tissue (arrows) separating the pericardial and epicardial fat layers over the anterior aspect of the right ventricle.**

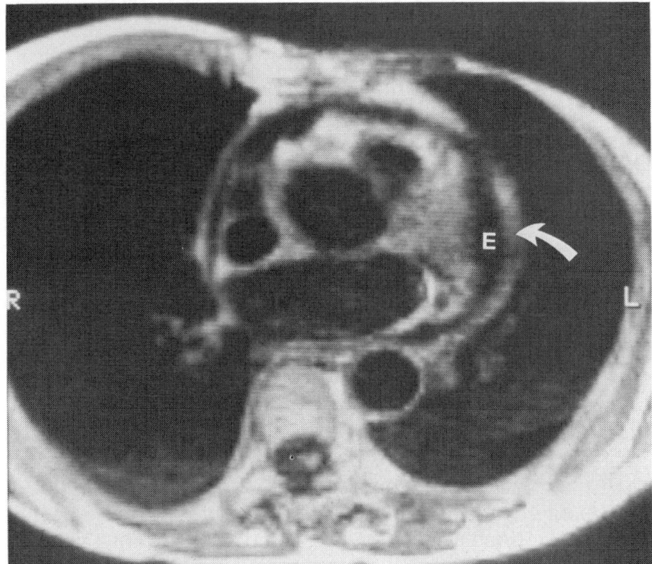

FIGURE 11–32. ECG-gated spin-echo image in pericarditis shows a pericardial effusion (E) and thickened parietal pericardium (curved arrow). The effusion shows low signal intensity on the spin-echo image with a short TE value (30 msec).

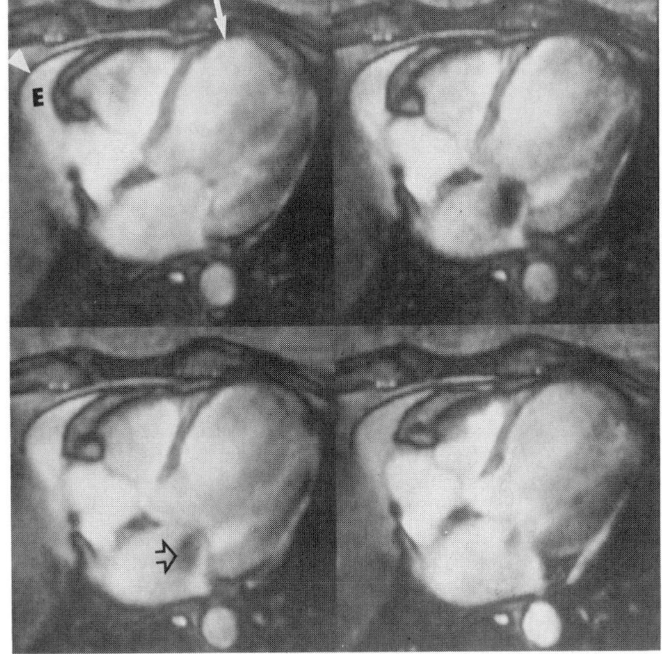

FIGURE 11–33. Cine MR images at four phases of the cardiac cycle in a patient show severe wall thinning at the site of an anteroseptal myocardial infarction (arrow) and pericardial effusion (E). The effusion is represented by a region of bright signal between the pericardium (arrowhead) and the right ventricular wall. The signal void (open black arrow) in the left atrium represents mitral regurgitation.

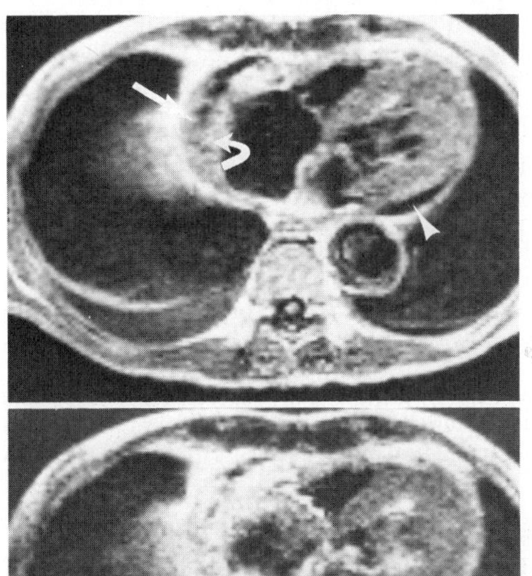

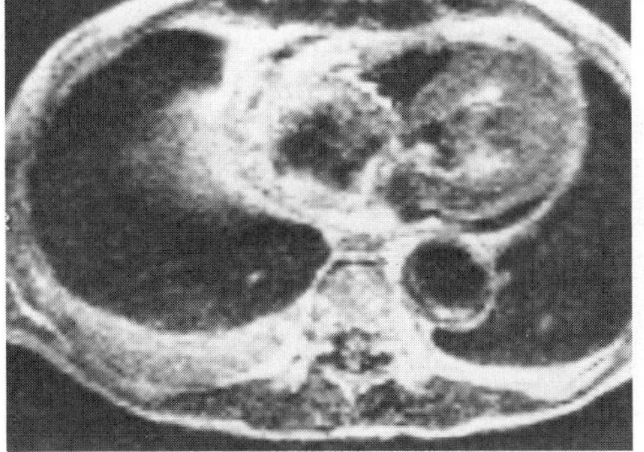

FIGURE 11–34. Effusive-constrictive pericarditis due to uremia. First *(top)* and second *(bottom)* echo images. Thickening of the visceral (curved arrow) and parietal pericardia (arrow) with inflammatory adhesions between them is evident. Pericardial fluid has low signal intensity. Both the thickened pericardium and fluid show a relative increase of intensity on the second echo image. Note the small posterior pericardial effusion on the right (arrowhead at top).

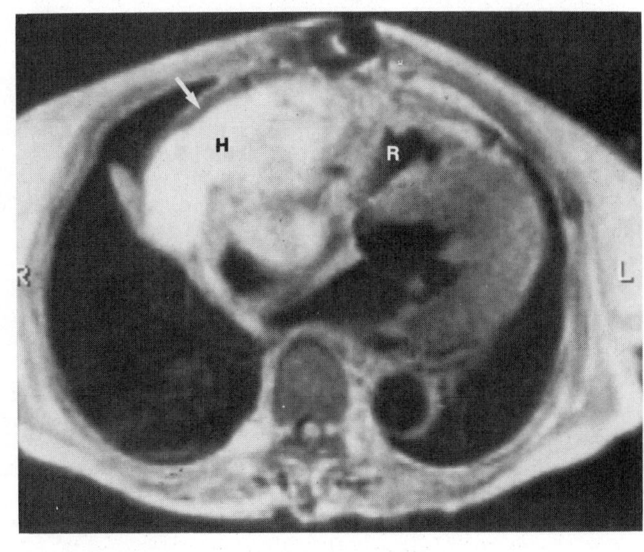

FIGURE 11–35. ECG-gated spin-echo images show a pericardial hematoma (H). The hemorrhagic pericardial effusion causes bright signal intensity on the T1-weighted (TE = 30 msec) image. The right atrium and right ventricle are compressed by the hematoma. Pericardium (arrow) is thickened. R = right ventricle.

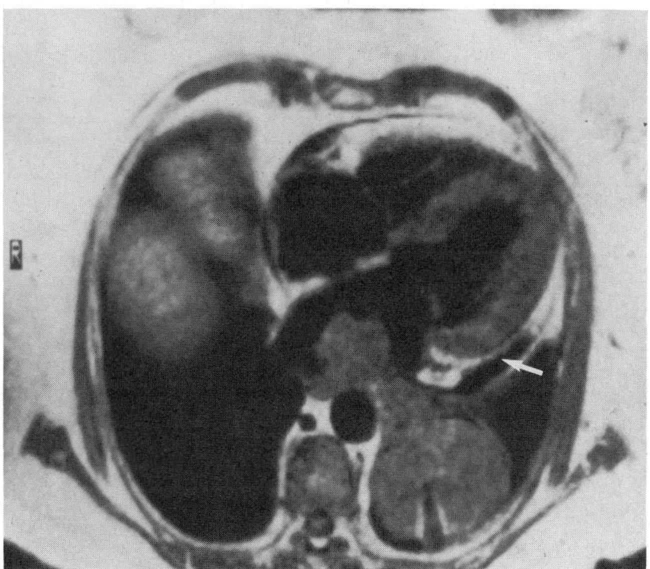

FIGURE 11–36. ECG-gated spin-echo image shows a lung tumor extending through the pericardium and into the left atrial chamber. The MR image clearly displays the extra- and intracardiac parts of the mass and a small pericardial effusion (arrow).

the heart on MR images, the precise relationship of tumors to cardiovascular structures can be defined. Tumors within the myocardial wall may be identified by virtue of a difference in signal intensity (usually higher) compared with the myocardium. In this regard, MRI contrast media can be used in an attempt to accentuate differences in signal intensity between tumor and myocardium.

Secondary cardiac involvement by tumors is about 40 times more frequent than are primary tumors. Secondary involvement occurs by three routes: direct extension from the mediastinum and lungs (Fig. 11–36), metastasis to the pericardium or cardiac chambers, or direct extension of upper abdominal tumors through the inferior vena cava or lung tumors through the pulmonary veins. MRI appears to be superior to CT for assessing the extent and effect of mediastinal masses adjacent to cardiovascular structures.[129,130] Gated MRI is the imaging procedure of choice for identifying paracardiac masses, defining their nature, and determining invasion of the pericardium. The intensity on spin-echo images can be used to differentiate such masses from innocuous lipomas, the pericardial fat pad, pericardial cysts, loculated pericardial effusions, and unusual enlargement or displacement of cardiac chambers. Gated MRI has been extremely useful for demonstrating invasion of cardiac chambers by pulmonary and mediastinal malignancies. Metastases to the pericardium and the possibility of pericardial effusion can be readily established by gated MRI.

Intracardiac tumors can be clearly identified within the signal void of the cardiac blood pool. Because of its wide field of view, MRI is ideal for defining both the intracardiac and extracardiac extent of masses (Figs. 11–36 and 44–6, p. 1459). For the evaluation of intracardiac masses, it is advisable to acquire spin-echo and gradient-echo MR images and to obtain images with at least two planes perpendicular to each other. A recent investigation has suggested that intracardiac or intravascular tumors can be distinguished from thrombus using cine MRI in most instances[131] (Fig. 11–37). Tumors are represented by medium signal (higher signal or similar signal compared with myocardium), while thrombus produces very low signal (less than myocardium). This low signal is due to elements in the thrombus (hemosiderin, deoxyhemoglobin, and the like), which induce a magnetic susceptibility effect and vitiate signal from the region. The cine MRI sequence is quite sensitive to this effect. Some myxomas contains a considerable amount of iron and can show the same effect, so it appears that confident distinction between myxoma and clot may not always be possible. Differentiation between tumor and thrombus has not been possible using the ECG-gated spin-echo sequence.

CONGENITAL HEART DISEASE

Reports from several centers indicate encouraging results with MRI for the evaluation of patients with congenital heart disease.[132–144] In several studies in which the results of MRI were corroborated by angiography or two-dimensional echocardiography or both, accurate anatomical diagnosis of anomalies was achieved by MRI in over 90 per cent of patients.[134,140]

Visceroatrial situs, the type of ventricular loop, and the relationship of the great vessels could be identified in all patients in whom studies encompassing the entire heart were done.[140] The diagnostic accuracy of MRI exceeded 90 per cent for abnormalities of arterioventricular connections, great vessel anomalies such as coarctation and vascular rings, ventricular and atrial septal defects, and abnormalities of venous connections.[140] Likewise, determination of visceroatrial situs and type of ventricular loop reached an accuracy of nearly 100 per cent with MRI.[140] The major limitation of spin-echo MRI was the determination of stenosis and regurgitation of the semilunar and atrioventricular valves; however, valvular atresia was accurately defined. The limitation of spin-echo MRI for valvular disease probably can be overcome with the use of cine MRI; however, this supposition has not yet been confirmed.

In another report,[138] blinded analysis of MR images has shown a sensitivity and specificity of over 90 per cent for the identification of atrial level abnormalities, including ostia se-

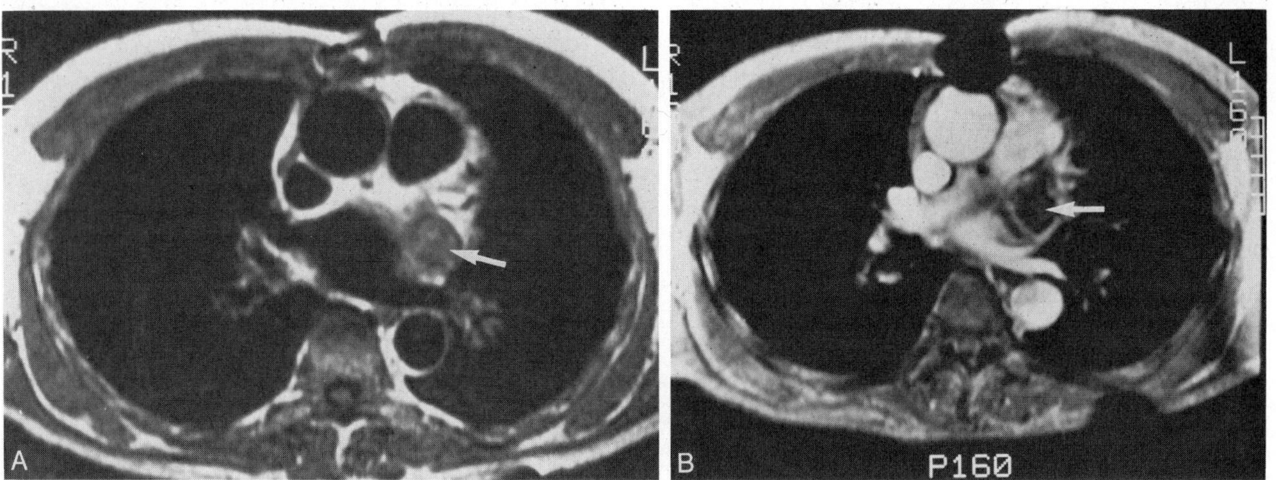

FIGURE 11–37. ECG-gated spin-echo (*A*) and cine (*B*) MR images of a patient with thrombus of the left atrial appendage. The thrombus (arrow) causes very low signal (nearly black) on the cine MR image.

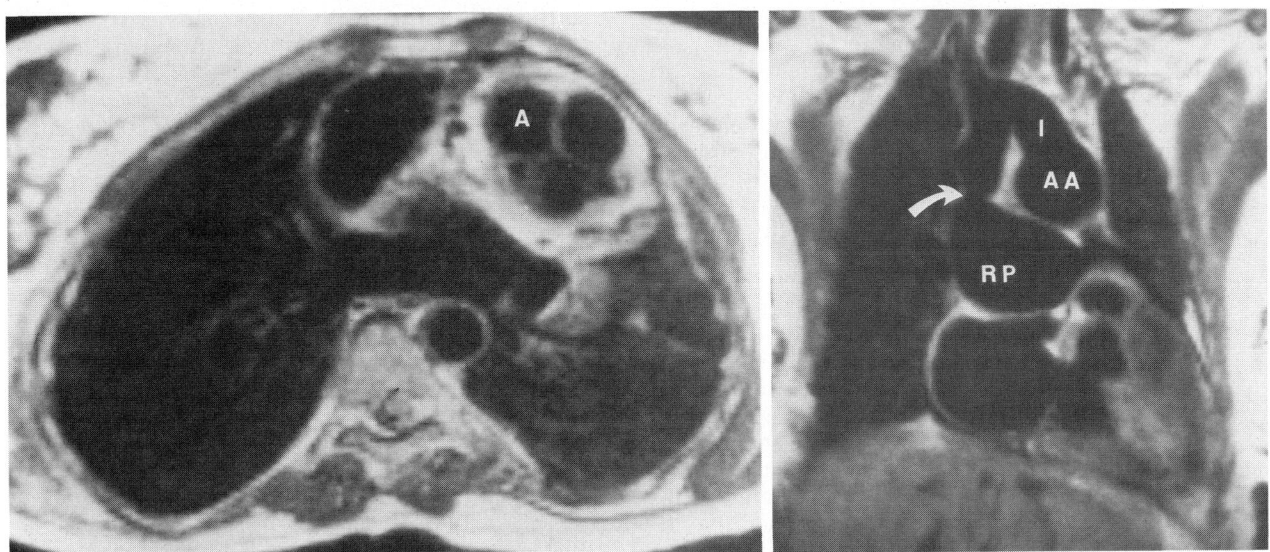

FIGURE 11–38. Transverse *(left)* and coronal *(right)* spin-echo images of a patient with transposition of the great arteries, pulmonary atresia, and ventricular septal defect. The transverse image acquired at the base of the heart shows only the aortic valve (A). Coronal image shows the right subclavian to pulmonary arterial anastomosis (curved arrow). The right pulmonary artery is aneurysmal while the left pulmonary artery is absent. The heart is shifted to the left due to decreased size of the left lung. AA = aortic arch; I = innominate artery; RP = right pulmonary artery.

cundum and primum atrial septal defects as well as anomalous pulmonary venous connection. However, another report had been less encouraging in this regard.[139] It is recognized that a thin fossa ovalis can be confused with an atrial septal defect on static MR images. It may be possible to avoid this misinterpretation using cine MRI techniques.

Much of the diagnostic information provided by MRI can also be shown by two-dimensional echocardiography (p. 76). Therefore, the role of MRI must be considered in respect to the established role of echocardiography. The unique capabilities of MRI in congenital heart disease are visualization of the central pulmonary arteries in cases of pulmonary atresia[144] (Fig. 11–38) and assessment of anomalies of the thoracic aorta[133,136] (Fig. 11–39), complete definition of complex anomalies involving both the great vessels and ventricles,[137,141] and postoperative evaluation of patients who have undergone complicated supracardiac operations for cyanotic congenital heart disease.[142,143] MRI has been shown to be reliable for both preoperative and postoperative evaluation of coarctation of the aorta;[133,136] angiography can usually be obviated in most patients. Two reports[142,143] have shown the effectiveness of MRI for the postoperative evaluation of the Fontan, Rastelli, Norwood, Damus, and Jatene procedures.

Therefore, the major indications for MRI in patients with congenital heart disease are: evaluation of thoracic aortic anomalies such as coarctation and aortic arch anomalies, determination of pulmonary arterial size in patients with pulmonary atresia or severe obstruction, definition of complex cyanotic lesions in which precise determination of septal size and chamber size are needed, and assessment of the status of surgically created shunts, anastomoses, and conduits. A recent study has shown that MRI depicts more completely the segmental anatomy of the heart and great vessels in patients with complex cyanotic anomalies than is possible with angiography.[141] In this regard, coronal images are particularly useful in providing a composite view of the ventricles and great vessels in complex anomalies such as a single ventricle. Likewise, a comparative study also showed that MRI was at least as

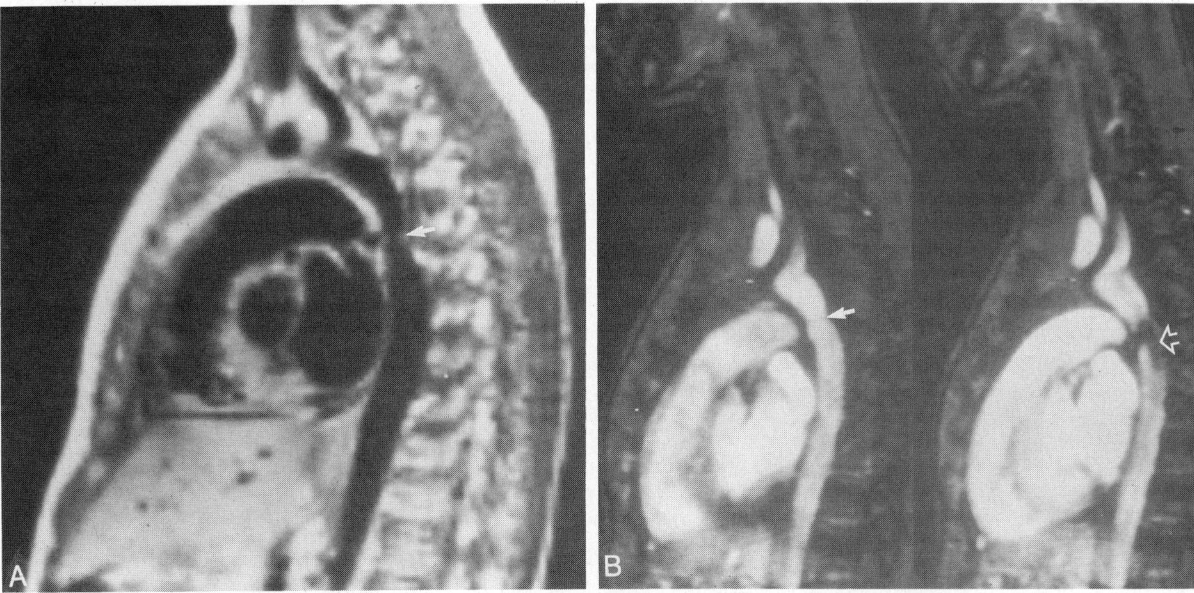

FIGURE 11–39. Spin-echo *(A)* and cine *(B)* MR sagittal images in two separate patients. Spin-echo image demonstrates a discrete coarctation (arrow) of the aorta. Cine MR images are acquired in diastole *(A)* and systole *(B)*. In diastole the thin membrane (arrow) is shown at the site of the coarctation and in systole a signal void (open arrow) is demonstrated emanating from the coarctation site due to high-velocity jet flow through the stenosis.

effective as angiography for demonstrating the anatomy and complications associated with surgical procedures involving supracardiac structures. Because echocardiography is limited to the demonstration of supracardiac anatomy, MRI may be the most effective technique for the monitoring of patients after various operations such as the Rastelli, Damus, Fontan, Jatene, and Norwood procedures.

The role of MRI in the evaluation of congenital heart disease is evolving rapidly and is not clearly defined as of this writing. Experience at many institutions in large numbers of patients has not been achieved, so widespread familiarity with the technique, its attributes, limitations, and indications does not exist. As reliance upon angiography as the definitive diagnostic procedure for congenital heart disease wanes, it seems likely that echocardiography and MRI will be used increasingly for this purpose and will eventually obviate angiography, both for preoperative analysis and postoperative monitoring of the morphology of congenital heart disease. Because the tomographic thickness can be reduced to 2 to 3 mm, MRI can be used to display morphology of the hearts of infants. However, limitations exist for its use in critically ill neonates because of lack of portability and difficulties in management of such patients.

The capability of MRI in congenital heart disease has been extended by cine MRI[145,146] and velocity-encoded cine MRI.[147-149] The former technique can provide multiple images per cardiac cycle so that ventricular function can be evaluated, while the latter technique permits measurement of blood flow in the aorta and pulmonary artery. High-velocity flow causes a signal void within the blood pool on cine MRI images; this enables the recognition of flow across atrial septal defects and through sites of stenosis, as well as depiction of valvular regurgitant flow. Velocity-encoded cine MRI can be used to measure stroke volume of each ventricle, volume of left-to-right shunt, and flow separately in the right and left pulmonary arteries. Velocity-encoded cine MRI has been shown to measure accurately flow velocities in excess of 5 m/sec in flow phantoms,[149] which indicates the ability of the technique to estimate the gradient across obstructed valves, conduits, and aortic coarctation.

DISEASES OF THE THORACIC AORTA

(See also Chap. 47)

MRI of the thoracic aorta is considerably improved by ECG gating. For imaging of the thoracic aorta, MRI appears to be superior to echocardiography and CT. A number of reports attest to its effectiveness for the evaluation of aortic dissection, true and false aneurysms, periaortic abscess and hematoma, aortic arch anomalies, and coarctation of the aorta.[150-154]

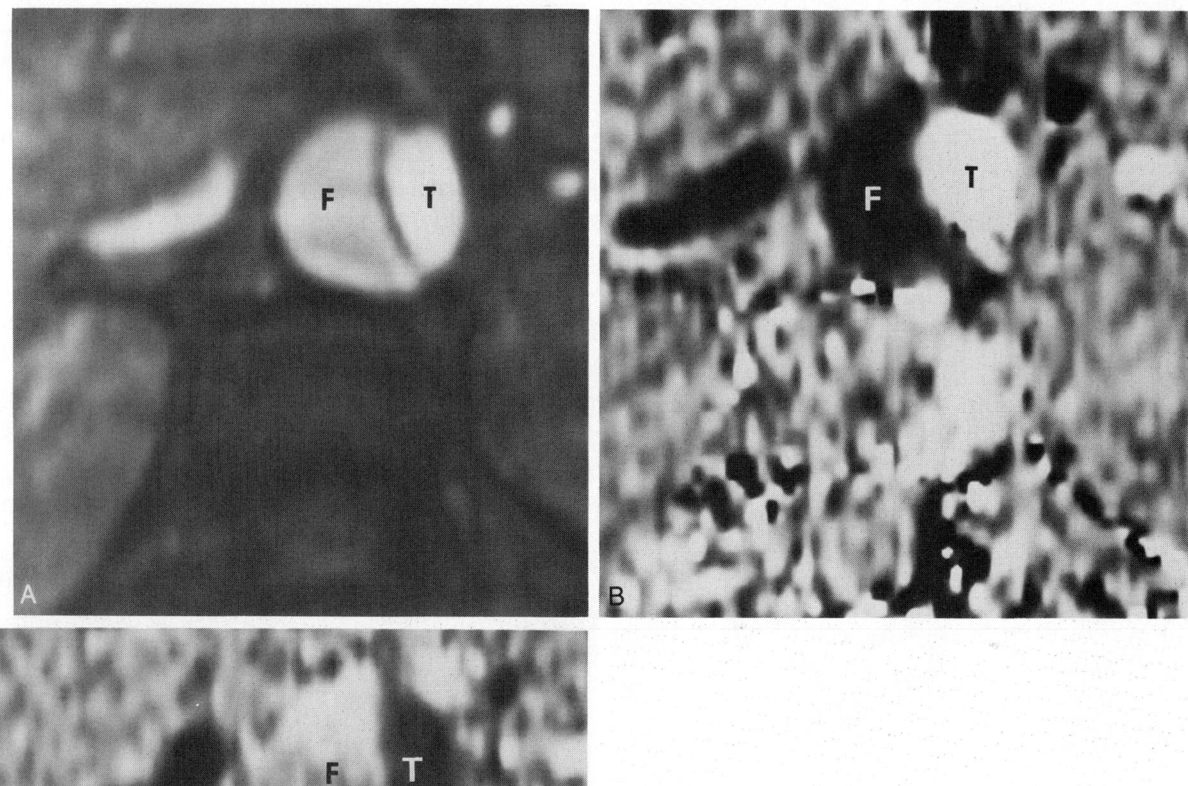

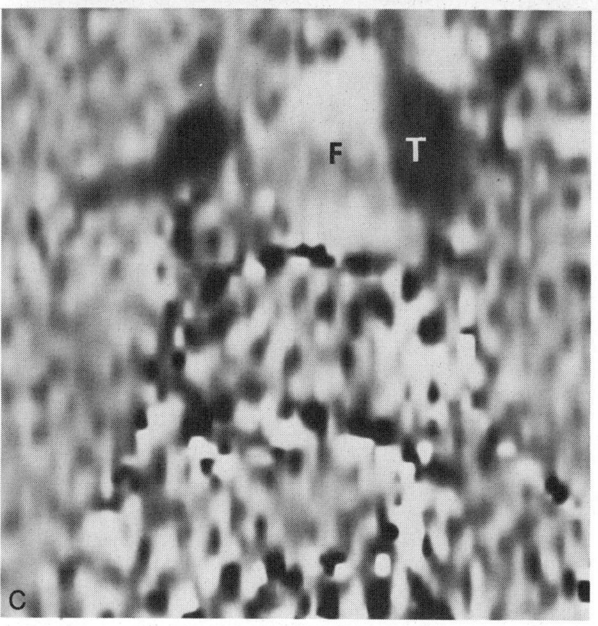

FIGURE 11-40. Patient with Type B chronic aortic dissection (see Chap. 47). *A,* Transaxial cine gradient-echo image showing the true (T) and false (F) channels. *B,* Phase-display image during systole shows forward velocity in the true channel (T) and retrograde velocity in the false channel (F). *C,* Phase-display image during diastole shows slow retrograde velocity in the true channel (T) and also slow forward velocity in the false channel (F).

In aortic dissection, MRI can depict the intimal flap and the proximal extent of the dissection, and it can distinguish true from false channel (Fig. 47–3, p. 1530). On spin-echo MR images, intraluminal signal is usually seen in the false channel due to thrombus or slow blood flow or both. Velocity-encoded cine MRI provides a measurement of the differential flow velocity in the true and false channels.[154] Using multiple images per cardiac cycle, a velocity-time curve can be generated that displays the disparate flow pattern in the two channels (Fig. 11–40).

MRI has been used to monitor the size of the thoracic aorta in patients with the Marfan syndrome and to exclude the presence of an occult dissection.[155] Dimensions at various segments of the thoracic aorta have been defined for normal subjects and patients with aneurysmal dilatation due to Marfan syndrome and other causes. Since MRI is a completely noninvasive technique, it is ideal for monitoring patients with aortic diseases and patients who have undergone surgical or medical treatment of aortic dissection.[156] MRI is also the most logical technique for the study of the patient whose chest roentgenogram suggests a substantial increase in the size of the thoracic aorta.

MRI has been used to detect periaortic abscess complicating bacterial endocarditis.[157] The three-dimensional tomographic nature of the technique permits precise localization of these abscesses. MRI can also demonstrate the presence of periaortic hematoma. With T1-weighted images, mediastinal or pericardial blood has high intensity.

It is necessary to reconsider the traditional reliance upon angiography for the evaluation of thoracic aortic disease. Recent studies indicate that MRI and CT are more effective for the diagnosis and monitoring of most thoracic aortic diseases.

EVALUATION OF CARDIOVASCULAR FUNCTION

(See also Chap. 15)

Because MRI is a three-dimensional imaging technique, it can provide most of the measurements upon which the evaluation of global left ventricular function is based. Using sets of images encompassing the left ventricle, it is possible to calculate end-diastolic, end-systolic, and stroke volumes, and ejection fraction. This can be done directly, without dependence on the geometric assumptions used for such measurements from angiograms. Even more important, MRI provides a three-dimensional direct visualization of the myocardium with excellent mural edge discrimination, thereby allowing quantitation of left ventricular mass.[158–160] MRI measurements have correlated closely with anatomical measurements of left ventricular mass[161,162] and the mass of acute myocardial infarctions.[159]

Since MRI also defines the right ventricular myocardium, it may serve as the preferred technique for the accurate determination of right ventricular mass; reasonable accuracy has been shown in the measurement of right ventricular end-diastolic, end-systolic, and stroke volumes as well as ejection fraction.[161,162] Moreover, comparison of right and left ventricular stroke volumes has been used to estimate the regurgitant fraction in patients with aortic and mitral regurgitation.[163] Stroke volumes of the two ventricles can also be quantified by time-integrated measurements of flow velocity in the aorta and pulmonary artery using velocity-encoded cine MRI.[147] Blood flow is the product of velocity and cross-sectional area, both of which can be measured at multiple phases of the cardiac cycle using this technique (described in detail below).

REGIONAL LEFT VENTRICULAR FUNCTION. Acquisition of MR images at various phases of the cardiac cycle provides a noninvasive method of assessing regional myocardial function.[114,164] Using a technique termed *rotating gated acquisition*, 10 transverse levels through the left ventricle are imaged at six sequential phases of the cardiac cycle. The 10 transverse levels (each approximately 10 mm in thickness) encompass the left ventricle; the six images at each transverse level start at end-diastole and then proceed in 100-msec intervals through the cardiac cycle. Thereby, the maximum extent of wall thickening may be calculated from the following formula:

$$\%\text{ wall thickening} = \frac{\text{WTes} = \text{WTed}}{\text{WTed}} \times 100 \text{ per cent}$$

where WTes = wall thickness at end-systole, and
WTed = wall thickness at end-diastole

Using this technique, the extent of regional thickening in normal subjects has been defined.[114,164] Diminished regional wall thickening has been demonstrated in patients with acute myocardial infarction, and generalized wall-thickening abnormalities have been demonstrated in patients with congestive cardiomyopathy and concentric left ventricular hypertrophy.[114] The unusual pattern, consisting of increased end-diastolic wall thickness and diminished wall thickening, was shown in amyloid heart disease.

Regional function usually is assessed with cine MRI because of the ability to segment the cycle into multiple frames (usually 16 to 30 per cycle) (Fig. 11–41). A study in normal persons and patients with prior myocardial infarction demonstrated that cine MRI in the transverse plane readily distinguished the site of previous injury by a diminution or absence of wall thickening during systole.[165] Systolic wall thickening of less than 2 mm was found in 31 of 40 abnormal segments (shown to be abnormal by angiography or echocardiography) and was found in only 3 of 78 segments of normal subjects. In addition, dyskinetic segments showed significantly thinned walls at end-diastole compared with normal values, whereas hypo- and akinetic segments did not show such severe wall thinning. Therefore, residual systolic wall thickening and nearly normal wall thickness at diastole may indicate the presence of residual viable myocardium in a previously infarcted region.

Theoretically, more accurate measurements of wall thickness should be accomplished using imaging planes perpendicular to the long axis of the left ventricular wall (cardiac short-axis plane) (Fig. 11–41). These cardiac imaging planes (short- or long-axis) can minimize the problem of overestimation of wall thickness caused by oblique sectioning of the heart using the standard transverse planes. However, because of the ellipsoid shape of the left ventricle, some obliquity is unavoidable even when planes oriented to the intrinsic axes

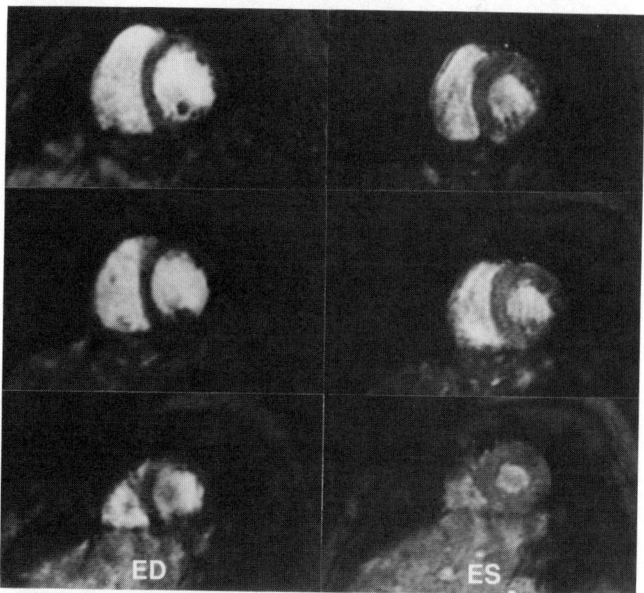

FIGURE 11–41. Cine MR images in the short-axis plane acquired at end diastole (ED) and end systole (ES) near the base (upper panels), middle (middle panels), and near the apex (lower panels) of the left ventricle (LV). These images demonstrate symmetrical wall thickening of the LV. From such images encompassing the length of both ventricles, measurement of ventricular volume and global function can be made.

of the left ventricle are used. This may be even more pronounced during systole because of shortening of the left ventricle along its long axis, resulting in possible overestimation of wall thickening at the apical level. A study with cine MRI acquired in short-axis planes showed a gradient of wall thickening increasing progressively from the base to the apex[108] (Fig. 11–29). The influence of the imaging plane on this finding is not clear, but a similar gradient in the extent of regional myocardial shortening has been observed using sonomicrometer measurements in dogs.[166]

Although cine MRI provides an accurate means to quantify wall thickening, the major limiting factor to its widespread clinical implementation will be the time required to create manually the ventricular epicardial and endocardial contours. In the future, with the development of a computerized automated contour detection algorithm, it may be possible to attain time-efficient, accurate, and clinically implemented analysis of wall thickening by cine MRI.

Myocardial Tagging. Recently, myocardial tagging, a new method for quantitation of myocardial motion with MRI, has been developed.[167,168] Specified regions of the myocardium can be labeled by restricted localized RF pulses; these are placed perpendicularly across the myocardial wall. These RF pulses are followed by a conventional imaging sequence after a short, specified delay. The labeled or "tagged" myocardial regions can be tracked precisely during systolic contraction. Myocardial motion occurring between RF excitation of the tag and image formation is expressed as the displacement and distortion of the tagged regions, which appear as dark stripes (Fig. 11–42). The extent of the displacement of the tagged myocardium can be measured as the distance between a given tag and its original position at end-diastole. Preliminary results showed heterogeneous myocardial motion of the left ventricle in normal subjects.[167] The longitudinal displacement of the tag during systole is significantly greater at the basal layer than at the mid or apical layers of the left ventricle. Short-axis images with tagging showed heterogeneous rotation of the wall with an increasing degree of counterclockwise rotation from the base to apex. This technique may provide the first noninvasive method for quantitating the complex multidirectional motion of myocardial segments.

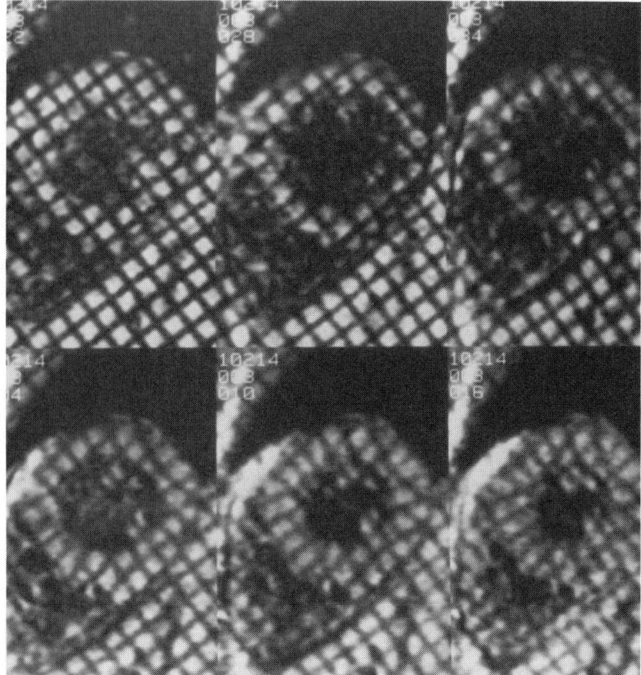

FIGURE 11–42. Composite of six short-axis views of the left ventricle (LV) from end diastole *(upper left)* to end systole *(lower right)* in a patient with LVH. The pattern of diagonal lines is a magnetic grid created in the tissue with spatial modulation of magnetization (SPAMM). Initially the grid moves with the underlying tissue, enabling analysis of regional wall motion within separate delineated elements of the wall. (Courtesy of Leon Axel, M.D., University of Pennsylvania Medical School.)

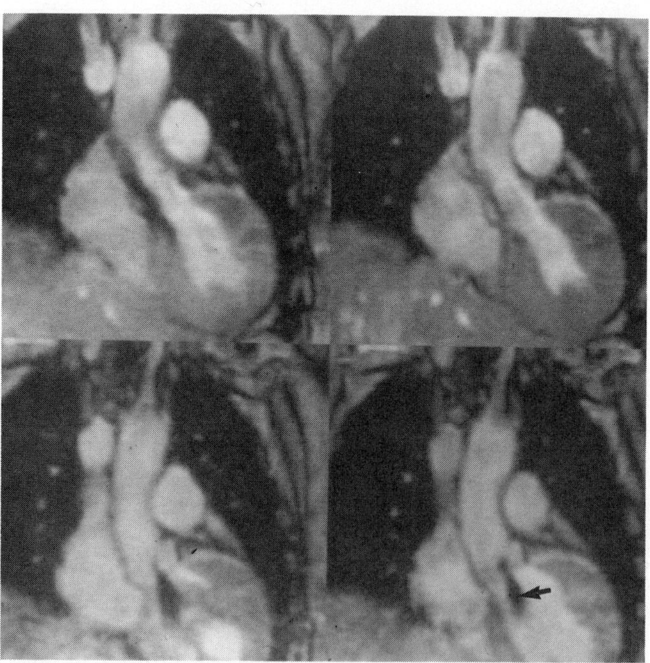

FIGURE 11–43. Series of cine MR images obtained in the coronal plane. Images in upper panels are from systole and those in the lower panels are from diastole. A signal void (arrow) originates from the closed aortic valve during diastole, indicating aortic regurgitation.

QUANTIFICATION OF VALVULAR REGURGITATION. Accurate determination of the severity of valvular regurgitation is important for the evaluation of medical therapy and timing of surgical interventions (Chap. 34). Among various methods, Doppler echocardiography has been utilized as the main diagnostic tool to detect valvular regurgitation because of its high sensitivity and specificity (p. 1025). However, quantification of severity has been less successful.[169] Mapping of the spatial extent of the disturbed flow in the regurgitant chamber with pulsed Doppler or color Doppler is useful for routine serial evaluation but provides only a semiquantitative estimate of the severity of valvular regurgitation. In this regard, cine MRI provides several methods for quantifying the extent of valvular regurgitation, including measurement of signal void on cine MRI, determination of the difference in stroke volumes of the two ventricles, and flow measurements at the ascending aorta or pulmonary artery using velocity-encoded cine MRI.

MEASUREMENTS OF SIGNAL VOID ON CINE MRI. The high-velocity jet caused by regurgitation can be readily identified on cine MR images because it produces a signal void in the recipient cardiac chamber[170] (Fig. 11–43). Mitral regurgitation causes a systolic signal void extending from the incompetent mitral valve into the left atrium, while aortic regurgitation causes a diastolic signal void extending from the aortic valve in the left ventricle. Measurements of the signal void have been used to provide a semiquantitative estimation of the severity of mitral or aortic regurgitation.[171,172] The area of signal loss corresponds approximately to the extent of turbulent retrograde flow and has been correlated with the severity of regurgitation established by angiography and echocardiography[171,172] or regurgitant volumes calculated as the difference between right and left ventricular stroke volumes using cine MRI[173] (Fig. 11–44).

Some possible pitfalls should be considered in measuring signal void on cine MRI. The size of the flow void can be affected by the relationship between the direction of regurgitant flow and orientation of the image voxel, because the degree of intravoxel dephasing can be influenced by the orientation and dimension of the voxel. In addition, the size of the

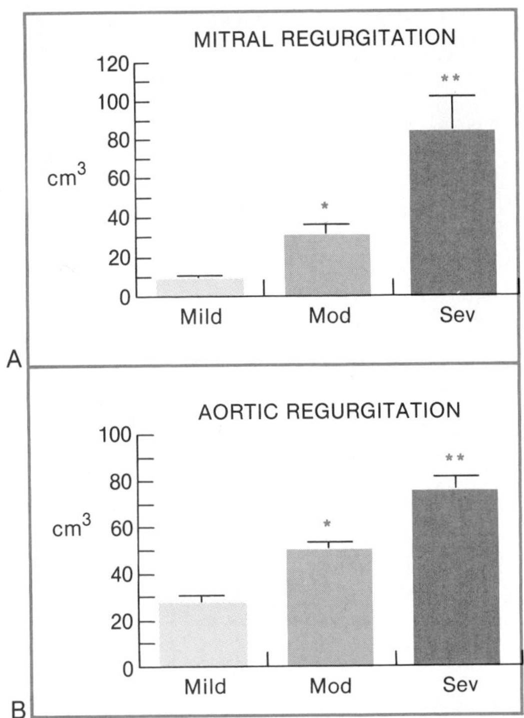

FIGURE 11-44. Block diagrams indicate the volume of the signal void measured on MR images in a group of patients with mitral *(upper)* and aortic *(lower)* regurgitation. The patients are separated into three groups of severity of regurgitation based upon Doppler echocardiographic and angiographic evaluation. * = $p < 0.05$, moderate vs. mild; ** $p < 0.01$, severe vs. mild and moderate. The volume of the signal void increased significantly with increasing severity of regurgitation.

void varies relative to the echo delay time (TE) used for imaging. With shortening of the TE, the size of the void is reduced. Therefore, serial quantification of valvular regurgitation or direct comparison of results among groups may be possible only if identical imaging parameters are utilized.

STROKE VOLUME RATIO AND REGURGITANT VOLUME. The differences between end-diastolic and end-systolic volume for a ventricle with a regurgitant valve include both the forward stroke volume and the regurgitant volume. Because the forward or net stroke volume is equal to the volume ejected from a normal ventricle, the difference in stroke volumes between a regurgitant ventricle (e.g., left ventricle with aortic and mitral regurgitation) and normal ventricle (e.g., right ventricle) is the regurgitant volume. The sum of the forward and regurgitant volumes is called total stroke volume of the regurgitant ventricle.

Several reports have verified that ventricular volume is accurately measured from cine MRI images.[174,175] In the absence of regurgitation, the stroke volumes of the right and left ventricle are nearly equal.[175] However, in patients with aortic and/or mitral regurgitation, the stroke volume of the left ventricle exceeds that of the right ventricle by a value equivalent to the regurgitant volume. The regurgitant fraction can be calculated as the regurgitant volume divided by the stroke volume of the regurgitant ventricle. The stroke volume ratio can also be calculated from the stroke volumes of the two ventricles. These measurements derived from cine or spin-echo MRI have differentiated patients with mild, moderate, and severe left-sided regurgitant lesions, as shown by independent imaging techniques.[163,176]

The major limitation of utilizing stroke volume difference for quantification of regurgitation is in the presence of multiple valve disease. If both aortic and mitral regurgitation are present, the calculation will determine only the total volume of regurgitation. If regurgitation coexists on both sides of the heart, this calculation will not be meaningful.

VELOCITY-ENCODED CINE MAGNETIC RESONANCE IMAGING. Forward stroke volume can be determined by measuring flow volume in the aorta or pulmonary artery throughout the cardiac cycle using velocity-encoded cine MRI (Figs. 11-45 and 11-46), because the volume ejected from the left or right ventricle is equal to the time-integrated flow volume measured at the ascending aorta or pulmonary artery, respectively.[147] Regurgitant volume can be measured as the difference between the net forward stroke volume measured by velocity-encoded cine MRI and the total stroke volume determined by volumetric measurements with cine MRI.

As discussed previously, the comparison of left and right stroke volumes determined by volumetric analysis with cine MRI is not meaningful in the presence of regurgitation on both sides of the heart. However, since velocity-encoded cine MRI can provide forward stroke volume ejected from one ventricle, regurgitant volume can be determined by subtracting this

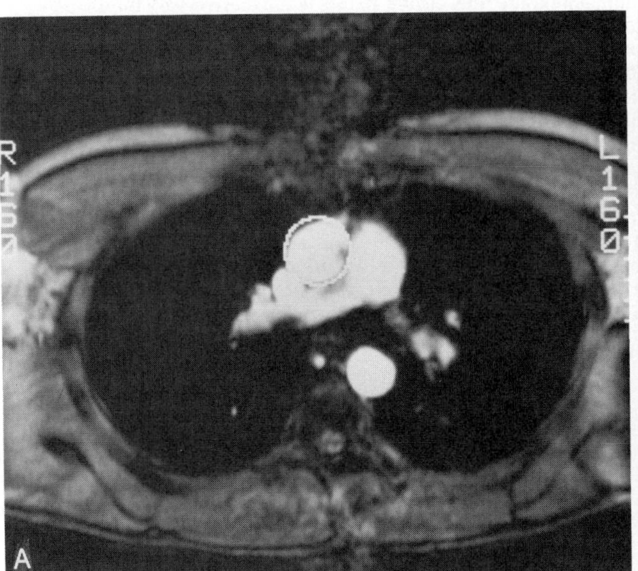

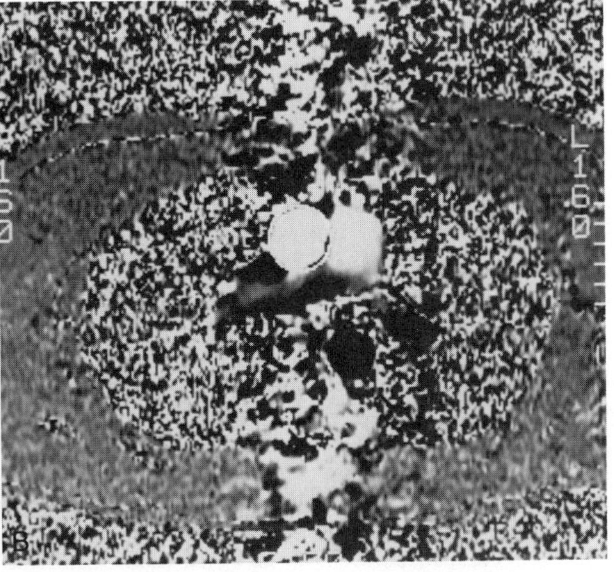

FIGURE 11-45. Magnitude *(left)* and phase *(right)* cine MR images acquired using the velocity-encoded cine MRI technique in a normal subject. From this pair of images, flow can be measured in the aorta and pulmonary artery. The voxels of the phase image have an intensity which is proportional to blood flow velocity. Note that the gray scale intensity is opposite in the ascending (white) and descending aortic (black), which occurs because flow is in opposite directions in the two. Magnitude image is used for dimension measurements. The mean velocity for the region of interest drawn around the ascending aorta is the spatial mean velocity.

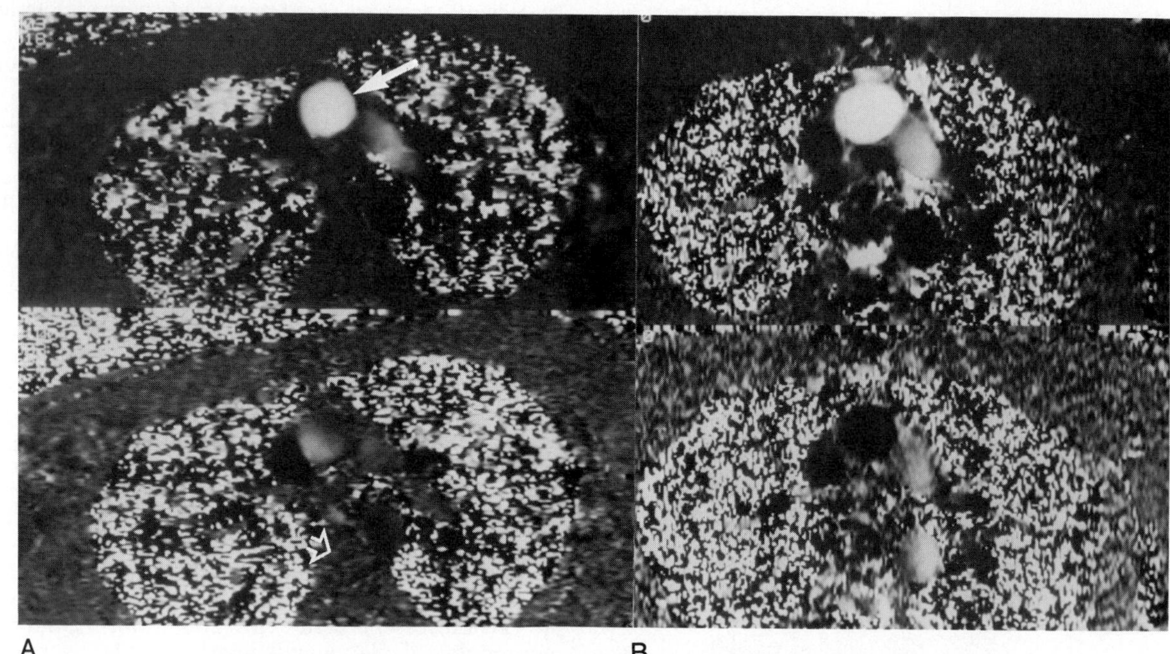

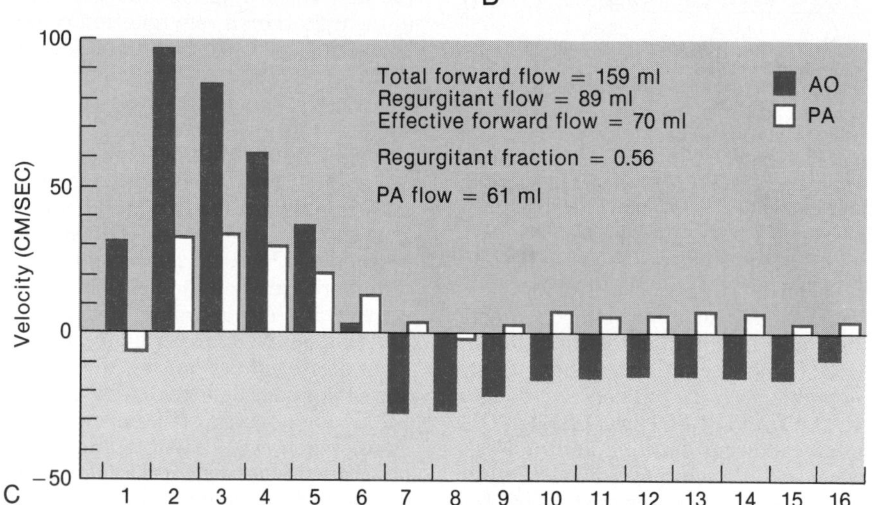

FIGURE 11–46. ***A,*** **Velocity images of ascending aorta in systole (*upper*) and diastole (*lower*) in a normal subject show white coloration in ascending aorta (arrow) indicating antegrade flow during systole while there is very little coloration in the ascending aorta in diastole indicating near-cessation of flow. *B,* Velocity images at same level in systole *(upper)* and diastole *(lower)* in a patient with aortic regurgitation show white coloration in the ascending aorta in systole and black coloration in diastole indicating retrograde flow (aortic regurgitation). The gray scale display is set so that increasing velocity in a caudal-to-cranial direction is indicated by increasing bright coloration while increasing velocity of cranial-to-caudal flow is shown by progressive darkening of the lumen. Cessation of flow causes a coloration similar to that of immobile structures such as the vertebral body (open arrow). *C,* Block diagram shows velocity from the aorta (AO) and pulmonary artery (PA) for each of 16 velocity images acquired at evenly spaced intervals during the cardiac cycle (plotted along the abscissa) in a patient with aortic regurgitation. Images progress from early systole *(left)* to late diastole *(right).* Note the presence of retrograde flow velocity during diastole in the ascending aorta while none exists in the pulmonary artery. Instantaneous flow is calculated for each frame as the product of cross-sectional areas of the vessel and flow velocity. Integration of all flow values during systole indicates forward flow, and integration of the values during diastole indicates retrograde flow (aortic regurgitation). These calculations can provide measures of total forward flow, effective forward flow, regurgitant flow, and regurgitant fraction.**

volume from the total stroke volume of the regurgitant ventricle. Moreover, because retrograde as well as antegrade flow can be determined from the instantaneous flow changes throughout the cardiac cycle using velocity-encoded cine MRI, the volume of aortic regurgitation or pulmonary regurgitation can be measured directly by the time integration of diastolic regurgitant flow (Fig. 11–46).

Blood Flow

The MR signal produced by flowing blood is variable and is determined by many factors, including the velocity and acceleration of blood flow, the flow profile (laminar or turbulent), the direction of flow in relation to the imaging, plane, even or odd spin-echo image, type of image, and the pulse sequence being applied. The appearance of flowing blood differs on spin-echo and gradient-echo (cine MR) images. Rapidly flowing blood is devoid of signal on spin-echo images but has bright signal on cine MR images. Cine MR images are now used to evaluate blood flow. Using cine MRI at very high velocities and with disturbed flow (nonlaminar), a signal void occurs in the blood pool. Such a signal void is caused by flow across stenotic and regurgitant valves and through septal defects and coarctation.

VELOCITY-ENCODED CINE MRI. Measurements of blood flow velocity with MRI have been achieved in several laboratories using a technique originally proposed by Moran[177] and introduced clinically by Longmore and associates.[178] The version used in the laboratory of the author is called "velocity-encoded cine MRI." This method principally is based on the phase shifts of moving spins in the magnetic field gradient.[179,180] The extent of phase shifts of moving spins is proportional to velocity along the direction of velocity encoding. Velocity encoding is performed by using bipolar gradient pulses. The direction of velocity encoding can be done in any orthogonal or oblique axis of the body.

Velocity encoding of blood flow in each pixel provides two-dimensional quantitative velocity mapping of the vascular system (Figs. 11–45 and 11–46). The instantaneous flow in the ascending aorta can be determined by the product of the cross-sectional area and mean velocity of the blood within the aorta. The integration of the instantaneous flow at the base of the aorta through the cardiac cycle provides a measure of left ventricular stroke volume, and the same done at the proximal pulmonary artery is a measure of right ventricular stroke volume (Fig. 11–46). The stroke volumes measured in this manner have correlated well with ventricular stroke volumes measured by planimetry of the multiple adjacent cine MR images.[147]

Measurement of flow by velocity-encoded cine MRI should be very accurate, provided that the flowing blood generates enough signal to calculate phase, the velocity phase-encoding gradients are calibrated accurately, and the correct range of velocity in the vessels being interrogated has been selected. The calculation of blood flow in the main pulmonary artery by the velocity-encoded cine MRI technique has shown nearly equivalent values to the sum of the flow in the right and left pulmonary arteries.[181] The technique can measure flow separately in the right and left pulmonary arteries.[181] Through the use of this technique a distinctly different flow pattern in the pulmonary artery has been observed in patients with pulmonary hypertension compared with normal subjects.[182]

CHARACTERIZATION OF MYOCARDIAL TISSUE

Characterization of myocardial tissue depends upon estimation of signal intensity on images with varying TR and TE values, hydrogen density, and T1 and T2 relaxation times. The measurements of relaxation times from gated images are approximations rendered inexact by cardiac and respiratory motion.[183,184] Despite these limitations, the T2 relaxation times have been found to discriminate between normal and pathological myocardium of the in situ beating heart.

Ex vivo measurements have revealed that several myocardial conditions, including ischemic myocardial injury,[185–187] cardiac transplant rejection,[187–189] and Adriamycin cardiomyopathy,[190] produce significant alteration of relaxation time. A number of experiments in the author's laboratory have been directed toward the identification and characterization of abnormal myocardium by MRI in vivo.

ACUTE MYOCARDIAL INFARCTION

This is characterized in vivo by increased signal intensity and prolonged T2 relaxation time.[191–193] Animals imaged before and during the first 5 hours after coronary occlusion showed regional increase in MRI signal intensity (prolongation of T2 relaxation time) in the jeopardized region by 3 hours after occlusion[191–192] (Fig. 11–47). In some animals, increased signal intensity was noted in the jeopardized region within the first hour after occlusion. Gated MRI of dogs with reperfused myocardial infarctions (1 hour of occlusion followed by reperfusion) showed significant alterations in regional signal intensity and T2 relaxation times by 30 minutes after reperfusion.[193] These studies show that MRI can potentially detect ischemically injured myocardium soon after coronary occlusion. MRI obtained in patients within 10 days after sustaining acute myocardial infarction has also shown that acutely infarcted myocardium is characterized by increased signal intensity and prolonged T2 relaxation time.[93,194] A regional decrease in signal intensity and decreased T2 relaxation time at the infarct site have been noted in some, but not all, patients with old myocardial infarctions.[89] These observations are consistent with fibrous replacement of myocardium.

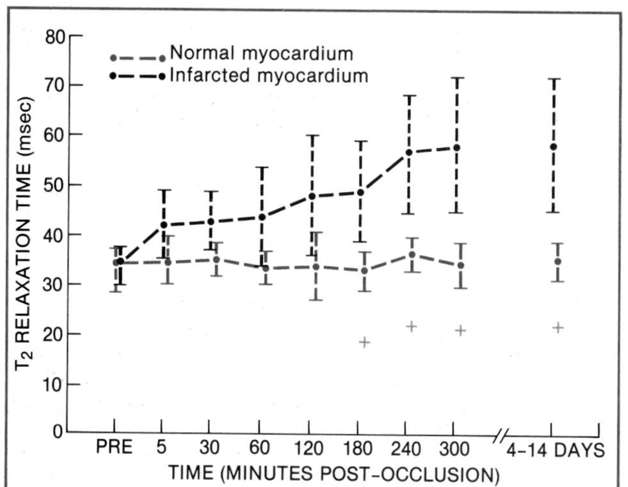

FIGURE 11–47. Graph displays the mean T2 relaxation times for normal and infarcted myocardium during the first 6 hours and at several days after acute occlusion of the left anterior descending coronary artery. Significant increases in T2 relaxation time of infarcted myocardium were present by 3 hours after occlusion. Crosses indicate the time intervals at which there were significant differences between normal and infarcted myocardium. (From Higgins, C. B.: MRI of the heart—1986. A.J.R. *146*:907, 1986.)

The wide range of MRI signal intensities among soft tissue present with MRI and the numerous parameters that potentially can be monitored from tissue protons during the MRI process suggest that this technique should be able to provide useful tissue characterization. Tissue characterization specific to disease processes is likely to depend on the recognition of new parameters for this purpose. Many features of the tissue appear to be evident in the proton MRI spectrum. In vivo proton spectroscopy is currently under study in several laboratories, and it will be of great interest to determine whether it can provide new parameters for the characterization of myocardial tissue.

MRI CONTRAST MEDIA FOR MYOCARDIAL ENHANCEMENT. ECG-gated spin-echo MRI can demonstrate the presence of acute myocardial infarction without the use of contrast agents. However, this ability to detect acute infarction depends on the prolongation of T1 and T2 relaxation times, which is caused by increased tissue water content and does not reach a detectable level until several hours after coronary artery occlusion. Therefore, acute ischemia is not visible until the onset of myocardial edema. Consequently, contrast agents seem to be necessary for identifying acute ischemia. Moreover, contrast agents may be useful to enhance the contrast between infarcted myocardial tissue and normal myocardium by a difference in the alteration of the relaxation times of the two regions.[195] The current status of myocardial contrast media has been reviewed recently.[196]

Contrast agents currently used can be classified by the mechanisms of action.[197] The first class of MRI contrast agents is relaxivity agents, which affect signal by enhancing relaxation of neighboring protons. In this class, paramagnetic compounds mainly decrease T1 relaxation time and thereby enhance the regional intensity of tissues. The effect is maximal on T1-weighted images. An example of a relaxivity agent is gadolinium-DTPA. The second class of MRI contrast media is magnetic susceptibility agents; these agents cause inhomogeneity in the local magnetic field within tissues and thereby decrease signal intensity. The effect of this agent is maximal on T2-weighted images. An example of a susceptibility agent is dysprosium-DTPA-BMA.[198]

Paramagnetic Agents. As of this writing, most MRI contrast agents used for myocardial imaging have been paramagnetic agents. They are soluble, aqueous substances much like x-ray contrast media. The magnitude of relaxation enhancement is influenced by magnetic field strength and the concentration of the paramagnetic agents. Although they can cause shortening of both T1 and T2 relaxation times, T1 shortening predominates at pharmacological doses and T2 effects are dominant at higher concentration.[199] Myocardial intensity after administration of a paramagnetic agent depends on myocardial perfusion as well as other factors, including diffusion of the agent through the capillaries, affinity of the agent to myocardial cells, volume of the interstitial space, and rate of elimination of the agent from myocardial tissue and bloodstream.[199]

GADOLINIUM-DTPA (Gd-DTPA). This agent has undergone laboratory and clinical testing extensively. This FDA-approved drug is a small molecular weight agent that diffuses rapidly from the vascular system into the extravascular interstitial space.[200] Several studies using Gd-DTPA as a myocardial contrast agent in humans have been reported.[201,202] Administration of Gd-DTPA was followed by an average 70 per cent increase in signal intensity within zones of acute infarction (5 to 10 days after infarc-

103. Higgins, C. B., Byrd, B. F., and Stark, D.: Magnetic resonance imaging of hypertrophic cardiomyopathy. Am. J. Cardiol. *55*:1121, 1985.
104. Wagner, S., Chew, W. M., Semelka, R., et al.: Integrative analysis of cardiac function and metabolism in patients with idiopathic hypertrophic cardiomyopathy with cine MR imaging and P-31 spectroscopy. Radiology *173*:238, 1989.
105. Suzuki, J-I., Chang, J-M., Caputo, G. R., and Higgins, C. B.: Evaluation of right ventricular early diastolic filling by cine nuclear magnetic resonance imaging in patients with hypertrophic cardiomyopathy. J. Am. Coll. Cardiol. *(in press).*
106. Suzuki, J. I., Sakamoto, T., Takenaka, K., et al.: Assessment of the thickness of the right ventricular free wall by MRI in patients with hypertrophic cardiomyopathy. Br. Heart J. *60*:440, 1988.
107. Byrd, B. F., Schiller, N. B., Botvinick, E. H., et al.: Magnetic resonance imaging and 2D echocardiography in dilated cardiomyopathy. Circulation *72*(Suppl. III):22, 1985.
108. Buser, P. T., Auffermann, W., Holt, W. W., et al.: Noninvasive evaluation of the global left ventricular function using cine MR imaging. J. Am. Coll. Cardiol. *13*:1294, 1989.
109. Semelka, R. C., Tomei, E., Wagner, S., et al.: Normal left ventricular dimensions and function: Interstudy reproducibility of measurements with cine MR imaging. Radiology *174*:763, 1990.
110. Semelka, R. C., Tomei, E., Wagner, S., et al.: Interstudy reproducibility of dimensional and functional measurements between cine magnetic resonance studies in the morphologically abnormal left ventricle. Am. Heart J. *119*:1367, 1990.
111. Wagner, S., Auffermann, W., Buser, P., et al.: Functional description of the left ventricle inpatients with volume overload, pressure overload and myocardial disease using cine nuclear magnetic resonance imaging (NMRI). Am. J. Cardiac Imaging *(in press).*
112. Farmer, D., Higgins, C. B., Yee, E., et al.: Tissue characterization by magnetic resonance imaging in an unusual case of hypertrophic cardiomyopathy. Am. J. Cardiol. *55*:230, 1985.
113. Sechtem, U., Higgins, C. B., Sommerhoff, B. A., et al.: Magnetic resonance imaging of restrictive cardiomyopathy: A report of 3 cases. Am. J. Cardiol. *59*:480, 1987.
114. Sechtem, U., Sommerhoff, B. A., Markiewicz, W., et al.: Assessment of regional left ventricular wall thickening by MRI. Am. J. Cardiol. *59*:149, 1987.
115. O'Donnell, J. K., Go, R. T., Bolt-Silverman, C., et al.: Cardiac amyloidosis: comparison of MR imaging and echocardiography. Radiology *153*:261, 1984 (Abs.).
116. Riedy, K., Fisher, M. Belic, N., and Koenignberg, D. I.: MR imaging of myocardial sarcoidosis. A.J.R. *151*:915, 1988.
117. Shiraiski, H., Yanazesawa, M., Kuramatsu, T., et al.: Cardiac tumor in a neonate with tuberous sclerosis: Echocardiographic demonstration and magnetic resonance imaging. Eur. J. Pediatr. *148*:50, 1988.
118. Caputo, G., Fisher, M. R., McNamara, M. T., et al.: Myocardial tissue characterization with the use of magnetic resonance imaging (Abs.). Circulation *72*(Suppl III:23), 1985.
119. Stark, D. D., Higgins, C. B., Lanzer, P., et al.: Magnetic resonance imaging of the pericardium: normal and pathologic findings. Radiology *150*:469, 1984.
120. Sechtem, U., Tscholakoff, D., and Higgins, C. B.: MRI of normal epicardium. Am. J. Roentgenol. *147*:245, 1986.
121. Sechtem, U., Tscholakoff, D., and Higgins, C. B.: Pericardial disease. Diagnosis by MRI. Am. J. Roentgenol. *147*:245, 1986.
122. Guttierrez, F. R., Shackleford, G. D., McKnight, R. L., et al.: Diagnosis of congenital absence of left pericardium by MR imaging. J. Comput. Assist. Tomogr. *9*:551, 1985.
123. Soulen, R. L., Stark, D. D., and Higgins, C. B.: Magnetic resonance imaging of constrictive pericardial disease. Am. J. Cardiol. *55*:480, 1985.
124. Rubin, J. I., Gomori, J. M., Grossman, R. I., et al.: High field MR imaging of extracranial hematomas. A.J.R. *148*:813, 1987.
125. Amparo, E. G., Higgins, C. B., Farmer, D., et al.: Gated MRI of cardiac and paracardiac masses: Initial experiment. Am. J. Roentgenol. *143*:1151, 1984.
126. Go, R. T., O'Donnell, J. K., Underwood, D. A., et al.: Comparison of gated cardiac MRI and 2D echocardiography of intracardiac neoplasms. Am. J. Roentgenol. *145*:21, 1985.
127. Conces, D. J., Vox, V. A., and Klatte, E. C.: Gated MR imaging of left atrial myxomas. Radiology *156*:445, 1985.
128. Fisher, M. R., Higgins, C. B., and Andereck, W.: Magnetic resonance imaging of an intrapericardial pheochromocytoma. J. Comput. Assist. Tomogr. *9*:1103, 1985.
129. Barakos, J. A., Brown, J. J., and Higgins, C. B.: Magnetic resonance imaging of secondary cardiac and paracardiac masses. A.J.R. *153*:48, 1989.
130. von Schulthess, G. K., Higashino, S. M., Higgins, S. S., et al.: Coarctation of the aorta: MR imaging. Radiology *158*:289, 1986.
131. Seelos K., Caputo, G. R., Higgins, C. B.: Differentiation of intravascular tumor and clot using gradient echo cine MR imaging. A.J.R. (submitted)
132. Higgins, C. B., Byrd, B. F., III, Farmer, D., et al.: Magnetic resonance imaging in patients with congenital heart disease. Circulation *70*:851, 1984.
133. Rees, S., Sommerville, J., Ward, C., et al.: Coarctation of the aorta: MR imaging in late postoperative assessment. Radiology *173*:499, 1989.
134. Didier, D., and Higgins, C. B., Fisher, M. R., et al.: Congenital heart disease in 72 patients. Radiology *158*:227, 1986.
135. Didier, D., and Higgins, C. B.: Identification and localization of ventricular septal defects by gated magnetic resonance imaging. Am. J. Coll. Cardiol. *57*:1363, 1986.
136. von Schulthess, G. K., Higashino, S. M., Higgins, S. S., et al.: Coarctation of the aorta: MR imaging. Radiology *158*:474, 1986.
137. Peshock, R. M., Parrish, M, Fixler, D., et al.: MR imaging in the evaluation of single ventricle. Radiology *158*:474, 1986.
138. Diethelm, L., Dery, R., Lipton, M. J., and Higgins, C. B.: Atrial level shunts: Sensitivity and specificity of MR diagnosis. Radiology *162*:181, 1987.
139. Lowell, D. G., Turner, D. A., Smith, S. M., et al.: The detection of atrial and ventricular septal defects with electrocardiographically synchronized MRI. Circulation *73*:89, 1986.
140. Kersting-Sommerhoff, B. A., Diethelm, L., Teitel, D. F., et al.: Magnetic resonance imaging of congenital heart disease: Sensitivity and specificity using receiver operating characteristic curve analysis. Am. Heart J. *118*:155, 1989.
141. Kersting-Sommerhoff, B. A., Diethelm, L., Stanger, P., et al.: Evaluation of complex congenital ventricular anomalies with magnetic resonance imaging. Am. Heart J. *120*:133, 1990.
142. Kersting-Sommerhoff, B. A., Seelos, K. C., Hardy, C., et al.: Evaluation of surgical procedures for cyanotic congenital heart disease using MR imaging. A.J.R. *155*:259, 1990.
143. Julsrud, P. P., Ehman, R. L., Hagler, D. J., and Ilstrup, D. M.: Extracardiac vasculature in candidates for Fontan surgery: MR imaging. Radiology *173*:503, 1989.
144. Sommerhoff, B. K., Sechtem, U. P., and Higgins, C. B.: Evaluation of pulmonary blood supply by nuclear magnetic resonance imaging in patients with pulmonary atresia. J. Am. Coll. Cardiol. *11*:166, 1988.
145. Sechtem, U., Pflugfelder, P., Cassidy, M. C., et al.: Ventricular septal defect: Visualization of shunt flow and determination of shunt size by cine magnetic resonance imaging. A.J.R. *149*:689, 1987.
146. Chung, K. J., Simpson, I. A., Glass, R. F., et al.: Cine MRI after surgical repair in patients with transposition of the great arteries. Circulation *77*:104, 1988.
147. Kondo, C., Caputo, G. R., Semelka, R., and Higgins, C. B.: Right and left ventricular stroke volume measurements with velocity encoded cine NMR imaging: In vitro and in vivo validation. AJR (In Press).
148. Firmin, D. N., Naigler, G. L., Klipstein, R. H., et al.: In vivo validation of MR velocity mapping. J. Comput. Assist. Tomogr. *11*:751, 1987.
149. Kilner, P. J., Firmin, D. N., Rees, R.S.O., et al.: Clinical assessment of stenosis using short echo cine MR velocity mapping. Mag. Reson. Imag. *8*(Suppl. I):90, 1990.
150. Amparo, E. G., Higgins, C. B., Hricak, H., and Sollitto, R.: Aortic dissection: Magnetic resonance imaging. Radiology *155*:399, 1985.
151. White, R. C., Dooms, G. C., and Higgins, C. B.: Advances in imaging thoracic aortic disease. Invest. Radiol. *21*:761, 1986.
152. Dinsmore, R. E., Liberthson, R. R., Wismer, G. L., et al.: Magnetic resonance imaging of thoracic aortic aneurysms. A.J.R. *146*:309, 1986.
153. Kersting-Sommerhoff, B. A., Higgins, C. B., White, R. D., et al.: Aortic dissection: Sensitivity and specificity of MR imaging. Radiology *3*(166):651, 1988.
154. Chang, J-M., Friese, K., Caputo, G. R., et al.: MR measurement of blood flow in the true and false channel in chronic aortic dissection. Submitted for publication.
155. Sommerhoff, B. A., Sechtem, U. P., and Schiller, N. B.: MRI of thoracic aorta in Marfan patients. J. Comput. Assist. Tomogr. *11*:633, 1987.
156. White, R. D., Ullyot, D. J., and Higgins, C. B.: MR imaging of the aorta after surgery for aortic dissection. A.J.R. *150*:87, 1988.
157. Winkr, M. L., and Higgins, C. B.: Magnetic resonance imaging of perivalvular infectious pseudoaneurysms. Am. J. Roentgenol. *147*:153, 1986.
158. Caputo, G. R., Tscholakoff, D., Sechtem, U., and Higgins, C. B.: Measurement of canine left ventricular mass using gated magnetic resonance imaging. Am. J. Roentgenol. *148*:33, 1987.
159. Caputo, G. R., Sechtem, U., Tscholakoff, D., and Higgins, C. B.: Measurement of canine myocardial infarct size at early and late time intervals using MRI. Am. J. Roentgenol. *148*:33, 1987.
160. Maddahi, J., Drues, J., Berman, D. S., et al.: Noninvasive quantitation of left ventricular mass by gated proton NMR imaging. J. Am. Coll. Cardiol. *10*:682, 1987.
161. Markiewicz, W., Sechtem, U., Kirby, R., et al.: Measurement of ventricular volumes in the dog by MRI. J. Am. Coll. Cardiol. *10*:170, 1987.
162. Underwood, S. R., Firmin, D. N., Klipstein, H., et al.: Rapid measurement of left ventricular volume from single oblique MR images. Radiology *157*:309, 1986.
163. Sechtem, U., Pflugfelder, P. W., Cassidy, M. W., et al.: Mitral or aortic regurgitation: Quantification of regurgitant volumes with cine MR imaging. Radiology *167*:425, 1988.
164. Fisher, M. R., von Schulthess, G. K., and Higgins, C. B.: Quantitation of regional left ventricular wall thickness using rotated gated magnetic resonance imaging. Am. J. Roentgenol. *142*:661, 1984.
165. Pflugfelder, P. W., Sechtem, U. P., White, R. D., and Higgins, C. B.: Quantification of regional myocardial function by rapid (cine) magnetic resonance imaging. A.J.R. *150*:523, 1988.
166. LeWinter, M. M., Kent, R. S., Kroener, J. M., et al.: Regional differences in myocardial performance in the left ventricle of the dog. Circ. Res. *37*:191, 1975.
167. Zerhouni, E. A., Parish, D. M., Roger, W. J., et al.: Human heart: Tagging with MR imaging—a method for noninvasive assessment of myocardial motion. Radiology *169*:59, 1988.
168. Axel, L., and Dougherty, L.: MR imaging of motion with spatial modulation of magnetization. Radiology *171*:841, 1989.
169. Monaghan, M. J., and Mills, P.: Doppler color flow mapping: technology in search of an application? Br. Heart J. *61*:133, 1989.

170. Sechtem, U., Pflugfelder, P. W., White, R. D., et al.: Cine MRI: potential for the evaluation of cardiovascular function. A.J.R. *148*:239, 1987.
171. Pflugfelder, P. W., Sechtem, U. P., White, R. D., et al.: Noninvasive evaluation of mitral regurgitation by analysis of left atrial signal loss in cine magnetic resonance. Am. Heart J. *117*:1113, 1989.
172. Pflugfelder, P. W., Landzberg, J. S., Cassidy, M. M., et al.: Comparison of cine MR imaging with Doppler echocardiography for the evaluation of aortic regurgitation. A.J.R. *152*:729, 1989.
173. Wagner, S., Auffermann, W., Buser, P., et al.: Diagnostic accuracy and estimation of the severity of valvular regurgitation from the signal void on cine magnetic resonance images. Am. Heart J. *118*:760, 1989.
174. Buser, P. T., Auffermann, W., Holt, W. W., et al.: Noninvasive evaluation of global left ventricular function with use of cine nuclear magnetic resonance. J. Am. Coll. Cardiol. *13*:1294, 1989.
175. Sechtem, U., Pflugfelder, P., Gould, R., et al.: Measurement of right and left ventricular volumes in healthy individuals with cine MR imaging. Radiology *163*:697, 1987.
176. Underwood, S. R., Klipstein, P. H., Firmin, D. N., et al.: Magnetic resonance assessment of aortic and mitral regurgitation. Br. Heart J. *56*:455, 1986.
177. Moran, P. R.: A flow zeugomatographic interface for NMR imaging in humans. Mag. Res. Imaging *1*:197, 1982.
178. Underwood, S. R., Firmin, D. N., Klipstein, R. H., et al.: Magnetic resonance velocity mapping: Clinical application of a new technique. Br. Heart J. *57*:404, 1987.
179. Meier, D., Meier, S., and Böseger, P.: Quantitative flow measurements on phantoms and on blood vessels with MR. Magn. Reson. Med. *8*:25, 1988.
180. Moran, P. R., Moran, R. A., and Karstaedt, N. K.: Verification and evaluation of internal flow and motion. Radiology *154*:433, 1985.
181. Kondo, C., Caputo, G. R., Masui, T., et al.: Determination of pulmonary blood flow by velocity encoded cine NMR. Society of Magnetic Resonance in Medicine. New York, NY, 1990 (Abs.).
182. Bogren, H. G., Klipstein, R. H., Mohiaddin, R. H., et al.: Pulmonary artery distensibility and blood flow patterns: a magnetic resonance study of normal subjects and of patients with pulmonary arterial hypertension. Am. Heart J. *118*:990, 1989.
183. Ehman, R. L., McNamara, M. T., Brasch, R. C., et al.: Influence of physiologic motion on the appearance of tissue in MR images. Radiology *159*:777, 1986.
184. Ehman, R. L., McNamara, M. T., Brasch, R. C., et al.: Influence of physiologic motion on the appearance of tissue in MR images. Radiology *159*:777, 1986.
185. Williams, E. S., Kaplan, J. L., Thatcher, F., et al.: Prolongation of proton spin lattice relaxation times in regionally ischemic tissue from dog hearts. J. Nucl. Med. *21*:449, 1980.
186. Higgins, C. B., Herfkens, R., Lipton, M. J., et al.: Nuclear magnetic resonance imaging of acute myocardial infarction in dogs: Alterations in magnetic relaxation times. Am. J. Cardiol. *52*:184, 1983.
187. Johnston, D. L., Brady, T. J., Ratner, A. V., et al.: Assessment of myocardial ischemia with proton magnetic resonance: Effects of a three-hour coronary occlusion with and without perfusion. Circulation *71*:595, 1985.
188. Ratner, A. V., Barrett, L. V., Okada, R. D., and Gang, D. L.: Alterations of the proton nuclear magnetic resonance spin-lattice relaxation time (T1) in rejecting cardiac allografts. J. Am. Coll. Cardiol. *3*:538, 1984 (Abs.).
189. Tscholakoff, D., Aherne, T., Yee, E. S., et al.: Cardiac transplantation in dogs: Evaluation with MRI. Radiology *157*:697, 1985.
190. Ratner, A. V., Okada, R. D., Thompson, R. D., et al.: Characterization of myocardium using proton NMR relaxation times (Abs.). Proc. Scientific Progr. New York, MR Med, August, 1983, p. 291.
191. Tscholakoff, D., Higgins, C. B., McNamara, M. T., and Derugin, N.: Early phase myocardial infarction: Evaluation by magnetic resonance imaging. Radiology *159*:667, 1986.
192. Pflugfelder, P. W., Wisenberg, G., Prato, F. S., et al.: Early detection of canine myocardial infarction by magnetic resonance imaging in vivo. Circulation *71*:587, 1985.
193. Tscholakoff, D., Higgins, C. B., Sechtem, U., et al.: MRI of reperfused myocardial infarctions. Am. J. Roentgenol. *146*:925, 1986.
194. Dinsmore, R. E., John, J. A., Yasuda, T., et al.: Characterization of myocardial signal intensity in normal and infarcted left ventricular segments of MR imaging. Radiology *157*(P):147, 1985.
195. Eichstaedt, H. W., Felix, R., Dougherty, F. C., et al.: Magnetic resonance imaging (MRI) in different stages of myocardial infarction using the contrast agent gadolinium-DTPA. Clin. Cardiol. *9*:527, 1986.
196. Brown, J. J., and Higgins, C. B.: Myocardial paramagnetic contrast agents for MR imaging. A.J.R. *15*:865, 1988.
197. Rosen, B. R.: Basics of contrast agents: Mechanisms and potential application to the measurement of microcirculation. *In* MR Imaging of Blood Flow. Berkeley, Society of Magnetic Resonance in Medicine, Inc., 1989, pp. 32–33.
198. Saeed, M., Wendland, M. F., and Tomei, E.: Demarcation of myocardial ischemia: Magnetic susceptibility effect of contrast medium in MR imaging. Radiology *173*:763, 1989.
199. Engelstad, B. L., and Wolf, G. L.: Contrast agent. *In* Stark, D. D., and Bradley, W. G., Jr., (eds.): Magnetic Resonance Imaging. St. Louis, C. V. Mosby, 1988, pp. 161–179.
200. Weinmann, H. J., Brasch, R. C., Press, W. R., and Wesbey, G. E.: Characteristics of gadolinium-DTPA complex: A potential NMR contrast agent. A.J.R. *142*:619, 1984.
201. Eichstaedt, H. W., Felix, R., Dougherty, F. C., et al.: Magnetic resonance imaging (MRI) in different stages of myocardial infarction using the contrast agent gadolinium-DTPA. Clin. Cardiol. *9*:527, 1986.
202. de Roos, A., van Rossum, A. C., van der Wall, E., et al.: Reperfused and nonreperfused myocardial infarction: Diagnostic potential of Gd-DTPA-enhanced MR imaging. Radiology *172*:717, 1989.
203. Wesbey, G. E., Higgins, C. B., McNamara, M. T., et al.: Effect of gadolinium-DTPA on the magnetic relaxation times of normal and infarcted myocardium. Radiology *153*:165, 1984.
204. Tscholakoff, D. T., Higgins, C. B., Sechtem, U., and McNamara, M. T.: Occlusive and reperfused myocardial infarcts: Effect of Gd-DTPA on ECG-gated MR imaging. Radiology *160*:515, 1986.
205. Schmiedl, U., Ogan, M., Paajanen, H., et al.: Albumin labelled with Gd-DTPA as an intravascular, blood pool-enhancing agent for MR imaging: Biodistribution and imaging studies. Radiology *162*:205, 1987.
206. Schmiedl, U., Sievers, R. E., Brasch, R. C., et al.: Acute myocardial ischemia and reperfusion: MR imaging with albumin-Gd-DTPA. Radiology *170*:351, 1989.
207. Wolfe, C. L., Moseley, M. E., Wikstrom, M. G., et al.: Assessment of myocardial salvage after ischemia and reperfusion using magnetic resonance imaging and spectroscopy. Circulation *80*:969, 1989.
208. Pflugfelder, P. W., Wendland, M. F., Holt, W. W., et al.: Acute myocardial ischemia: MR imaging with Mn-TP. Radiology *167*:129, 1988.
209. Saeed, M., Wagner, S., Wendland, M. F., et al.: Occlusive and reperfused myocardial infarcts: Differentiation with Mn-DPDP-enhanced MR imaging. Radiology *172*:59, 1989.

12

Relative Merits of Imaging Techniques

by DAVID J. SKORTON, M.D., HEINRICH R. SCHELBERT, M.D., GERALD L. WOLF, PH.D., M.D., and MELVIN L. MARCUS, M.D.*

The contemporary clinician may apply an astonishingly broad variety of methods (described in the first 11 chapters of this book) to the evaluation of the patient with known or suspected cardiovascular disease. The process of diagnosis in the 1990's still begins with a careful and thorough history (Chap. 1) and physical examination (Chaps. 2 and 3). Often, these are followed by a resting 12-lead electrocardiogram (Chap. 5). At this point in the diagnostic process, the clinician usually forms presumptive diagnostic hypotheses. To confirm or refute these hypotheses, the clinician can turn to a range of laboratory examinations, including measurements made on blood or urine, exercise electrocardiographic testing (Chap. 6), electrophysiological monitoring or testing, and a large number of imaging techniques. Currently, with the exception of evaluating dysrhythmias and conduction disturbances, methods of imaging the heart are the predominant laboratory diagnostic methods in cardiology.[1-3] Thus, clinicians need to be conversant with the several methods of imaging the heart and circulation and to be cognizant of the relative strengths and weaknesses of these techniques under particular clinical circumstances. In Chapters 4, 8 through 11, and 38, details regarding the use and interpretation of each of the imaging techniques are presented. It is the purpose of this chapter to offer some insights into the relative advantages and disadvantages of these several modalities, both in theory and as they may be used in clinical practice.

SCOPE OF CARDIAC IMAGING

The several available and developing methods of cardiac imaging may be categorized in various ways; we choose to divide them, somewhat arbitrarily, into "standard" and "evolving" methods (Table 12–1). The basis of this distinction is the general availability of and experience with the methods. Only a few investigative centers have all of these methods available for clinical use. In general, those we classify as *standard* are widely available and thus are methods with which most clinicians have at least some experience. Those modalities classified as *evolving* are available to a lesser degree or, if available, are quite new, so that most clinicians have little direct experience with them.

Projection Versus Tomographic Imaging

The distinction between *projection* and *tomographic* imaging is also of importance. The standard chest roentgenogram is a good example of a projection imaging method. The patient is placed between an x-ray source and an x-ray detector (a film-screen system). The x-rays are launched; they pass through the patient and are then received and detected on film. Thus, the imaging energy is *projected* through the patient, so that attenuation of x-rays occurs not only by the structure of interest (e.g., the heart) but also by other structures interposed along the path taken by the x-rays (such as chest wall and lung). Because of this projection phenomenon, x-ray shadows in the resulting roentgenogram represent a superimposition of wanted and unwanted information. Projection radionuclide images are usually referred to as *planar*. In the case of planar radionuclide images (p. 278), the basic data consist of photons emitted by the injected radionuclide; these photons are de-

TABLE 12–1 STANDARD AND EVOLVING METHODS OF CARDIAC IMAGING

STANDARD METHODS
Chest roentgenography
Echocardiography
Radionuclide methods: Planar and single-photon emission computed tomography
Thallium-201 scintigraphy
Technetium-99m blood pool scans
Technetium-99m pyrophosphate scans
Selective angiography
Ventriculography/aortography
Pulmonary angiography
Coronary angiography
EVOLVING METHODS
Computer-assisted echocardiography
Perfusion (contrast) studies
Ultrasound tissue characterization
Three-dimensional reconstructions
Radionuclide methods
Newer imaging tracers
Positron emission tomography
Digital angiography
Rapid-acquisition computed tomography
Magnetic resonance methods
Magnetic resonance imaging
Magnetic resonance spectroscopy

* Deceased.

tected externally by a gamma camera. The resulting images may be degraded by interactions of the photons with other tissues interposed along the paths taken by the photons as they travel from the tissue of interest to the gamma camera.

The other basic approach to imaging is the selective depiction of a slice or *tomogram* through the patient. For example, in the case of x-ray computed tomography (Chap. 11), this is accomplished by acquiring x-ray attenuation measurements from many different angles around the patient. At each angle, x-rays are sent from an x-ray source through the patient and are then received by a detector on the opposite side of the patient. This process is repeated for many angles around the patient, yielding a set of x-ray attenuation profiles. By computer reconstruction methods,[4] these many x-ray attenuation profiles are combined to produce an image depicting the two-dimensional distribution of x-ray attenuation data for a slice, or tomogram, through the patient. Since the resulting data selectively represent x-ray attenuation only in the "slice" under study, the superimposition problem found in projection methods does not occur. Thus, the tomographic imaging techniques permit clearer delineation of physical characteristics and anatomical features of selected body regions than is possible with nontomographic, projection methods. Many of the evolving imaging methods are tomographic in nature, and virtually all depend upon digital computer image processing methods for image generation and analysis.

Standard Imaging Methods

Standard, widely available imaging methods include chest roentgenography, echocardiography, thallium-201 (Tl-201) scans (including both planar scintigraphy and single-photon emission computed tomography), technetium-99m (99mTc) blood pool scans and infarct scans, and selective angiocardiography. The information content of these several imaging methods varies widely, since the method of image formation is different in each type of technique. Each imaging method represents the use of a particular energy source to produce an image containing anatomical and/or physiological information. As the energy sources vary, so do the types of information that may be extracted by application of the different methods. Table 12–2 lists the basic energy forms utilized to produce medical image data with an indication of some of the biophysical bases of image formation by each technique. Standard radiographic techniques (including chest roentgenography and selective angiocardiography) are based on differential attenuation of x-rays by tissues of varying density and atomic number. Attenuation of x-rays by blood is increased selectively by the administration of iodinated contrast media. Ultrasonographic imaging is based on differential reflection and absorption of ultrasound (mechanical) energy by strutures of varying density and elasticity. Finally, the determinants of radionuclide image data depend on both the radioisotope used as a label and the biologically relevant compound to which the label is attached. In a given radionuclide scan, regional image intensity reflects the regional distribution of that particular radiotracer at the time of the scan.

TABLE 12–2 SOME DETERMINANTS OF IMAGE INTENSITY

ENERGY FORM	IMAGE INTENSITY DETERMINANTS
• X-ray based methods • Plain-film radiography • Angiography • Computed tomography	• Density of tissue • Atomic number • Local contrast (iodine) concentration
• Ultrasound	• Acoustic velocity • Density of tissue • Tissue elasticity
• Radionuclides	• Tracer concentration (depends upon biological activity of ligand) • Photon energy
• Magnetic resonance methods	• Proton (spin) density (i.e., water content) • Blood flow • Nuclear magnetic resonance relaxation times

Evolving Imaging Methods

Evolving imaging methods include computer-assisted ultrasound applications (including contrast-based perfusion imaging, tissue characterization, and three-dimensional reconstruction), positron emission tomography (PET) (Chap. 38), digital angiography (Chap. 8), rapid-acquisition x-ray computed tomography (CT), and magnetic resonance methods (both imaging [MRI] and spectroscopy [Chap. 11]). As discussed already for standard imaging methods, the information content of the evolving methods also varies widely and is based on the energy form used to produce the image. The computer-assisted ultrasound applications depend on standard ultrasound interactions with tissue and therefore share the determinants of image intensity noted for standard echocardiography. Similarly, PET image data are related to the radionuclide and biologically relevant ligand. Rapid CT and digital angiography are x-ray–based techniques in which image intensity is related to tissue density and atomic number. MRI intensity (for proton images, the only widely available type) is a complex function of several variables, including regional water content, flow, motion, so-called nuclear magnetic resonance (NMR) relaxation times (both spin-lattice or T1 and spin-spin or T2 relaxation times), and possibly other factors not fully understood (Chap. 11). To summarize, the evolving and standard imaging methods are based on production of pictures using a wide variety of energy forms and biophysical determinants. Thus, these methods should be considered potentially complementary in the information they may offer.

A final general point to be emphasized is that the evolving imaging methods depend to a greater degree than do the standard methods on digital computer image processing technology for data acquisition, image production, storage, and analysis.[5,6] For example, chest roentgenography and selective angiocardiography may be performed without the aid of computer storage or manipulation of image data. However, computed tomographic techniques (including x-ray CT, single-photon emission computed tomography [SPECT], and PET) depend on computer technology for acquisition of basic image data and reconstruction of these data into tomographic images. Similarly, modern echocardiographic and MRI systems depend upon computer methods for image generation and display. Once images are produced, digital computer technology is widely used for image enhancement and quantitative analyses.

MEETING THE GOALS OF CARDIAC IMAGING

The complete assessment of a patient with heart disease should ideally include information on cardiac anatomy (including the detailed anatomy of the coronary ateries); the function of the heart chambers and valves; myocardial perfusion and metabolism and their responses to stress; and tissue characteristics, such as the replacement of normal myocardium by scar or infiltration by abnormal substances. Standard imaging methods give very useful information on cardiovascular anatomy and on chamber and valvular function (Table 12–3). In addition, information on relative regional deficits in myocardial perfusion is offered by thallium-201 scintigraphy. However, none of the standard imaging methods offers information on the *absolute* level of regional myocardial perfusion, the details of regional myocardial metabolism, or the definition of tissue characteristics. Thus, development of the evolv-

TABLE 12-3 RELATIVE USEFULNESS OF CONVENTIONAL IMAGING TECHNIQUES IN ACHIEVING DIAGNOSTIC GOALS*

DIAGNOSTIC GOAL	CXR	ANGIO	ECHO	PLANAR RNV	SPECT RNV	PLANAR PERFUSION IMAGING	SPECT PERFUSION IMAGING
Cardiac Anatomy							
Chamber size	+	+++	+++	++	++	+	+
Myocardial mass	0	+	+++	+	++	+	+
Intracardiac masses	0	++	++++	+	+	0	0
Valvular anatomy	0	++	++++	0	0	0	0
Pericardial disease	+	++	+++	0	0	0	0
Coronary anatomy	0	++++	+	0	0	0	0
Graft patency	0	++++	+	0	0	+	+
Cardiac Physiology							
Ventricular systolic function	+	+++	+++	+++	++++	0	0
Ventricular diastolic function	0	+++	++	+++	+++	0	0
Valvular stenosis/insufficiency	+	++++	+++	+	+	0	0
Intracardiac shunt	+	++++	+++	+++	+++	0	0
Myocardial blood flow	0	+	+	0	0	++	++
Tissue characterization	0	0	+	0	0	0	0
Myocardial metabolism	0	0	0	0	0	0	0

0, no information; ++++, maximum information; angio, angiography; CXR, chest roentgenogram; echo, echocardiography; RNV, radionuclide ventriculography; SPECT, single photon emission computer tomography.

* Modified from Grover-McKay, M., and Skorton, D.J.: Comparative aspects of modern imaging techniques. *In* Zipes, D.P., and Rowlands, D.J. (eds.): Progress in Cardiology. Philadelphia, Lea & Febiger, 1990; p. 3.

ing imaging methods has been based in part upon the perceived need to realize all the goals of cardiac imaging in clinical practice (Table 12–4). No single standard or evolving imaging modality is likely to be capable of optimal achievement of all the goals of cardiac imaging. Conversely, several techniques permit assessment of cardiac anatomy and function; therefore, redundant information will be obtained if these techniques are used additively without consideration of their relative strengths in the attainment of all imaging goals.

ASSESSMENT OF ANATOMY

Cardiac chamber and great vessel anatomy can be evaluated accurately with the use of several imaging techniques, including echocardiography, selective angiocardiography, rapid CT, and MRI. An estimate of chamber size and shape can also be obtained from radionuclide ventriculograms. However, because of relatively coarse spatial resolution (on the order of several millimeters to 1 centimeter), the radionuclide techniques are not the methods of choice for assessing the detailed aspects of cardiac morphology. Selective angiocardiography has long been the standard for chamber volume against which other techniques were judged. Tomographic methods, however, are superior in assessment of cardiac size and shape because of their ability to delineate wall thickness clearly and because of their relative freedom from problems caused by superimposition. Thus, echocardiography, rapid CT, and MRI are the best methods for determining chamber and great vessel morphology. Presently, rapid CT appears to be slightly more accurate than the other methods.[7] However, it has the disadvantages of being expensive, of not being portable, and of having the problems associated with iodinated

TABLE 12-4 RELATIVE USEFULNESS OF EVOLVING IMAGING TECHNIQUES IN ACHIEVING DIAGNOSTIC GOALS*

DIAGNOSTIC GOAL	DIGITAL ANGIO	COMPUTER-ASSISTED ECHO	MRI	MRS	RCT	PET
Cardiac Anatomy						
Chamber size	+++	+++	++++	0	++++	++
Myocardial mass	+	+++	++++	0	++++	++
Intracardiac masses	++	++++	+++	0	++++	0
Valvular anatomy	++	++++	+++	0	+++	0
Pericardial disease	++	+++	++++	0	++++	0
Coronary anatomy	++++	++	++	0	++	0
Graft patency	++++	+	++	0	+++	++
Cardiac Physiology						
Ventricular systolic function	+++	+++	+++	0	++++	++
Ventricular diastolic function	+++	++	+	0	+++	0
Valvular stenosis/insufficiency	++++	+++	++	0	++	0
Intracardiac shunt	++++	+++	++	0	+++	0
Myocardial blood flow	++	++	+	0	++	++++
Tissue characterization	0	++	++	+++	+	+++
Myocardial metabolism	0	0	0	++++	0	++++

0: no information; ++++: maximum information; angio, angiography; echo, echocardiography; MRI, magnetic resonance imaging; MRS, magnetic resonance spectroscopy; PET, positron emission tomography; RCT, rapid computed tomography.

*Modified from Grover-McKay, M., and Skorton, D.J.: Comparative aspects of modern imaging techniques. In: Zipes, D.P. and Rowlands, D.J. eds.: Progress in Cardiology. Philadelphia, Lea & Febiger, 1990, p. 3.

contrast medium and radiation exposure. In the patient who can lie relatively still for several minutes, MRI can produce exquisitely detailed images of cardiac anatomy. However, it too is not portable and requires a substantial expenditure. Because of these considerations, echocardiography is often considered the initial procedure of choice for the assessment of chamber and great vessel morphology in patients in whom studies of diagnostic quality can be achieved. Particularly with the advent of transesophageal echocardiography (p. 69), it is possible to assess accurately cardiac chamber and great vessel anatomy in the vast majority of patients by using ultrasound methods.

The detailed anatomy of the coronary arteries continues to be the domain of selective coronary arteriography (Chap. 9). Whether recorded on 35 mm cine film or in digital format, selective coronary angiograms exhibit the high spatial and temporal resolution necessary to image the coronary arteries, particularly the distal portions of the coronary vasculature in which vessel diameters may be 1 mm or smaller. Transesophageal echocardiography,[8] rapid CT,[9] and MRI[10] show promise in visualization of selected portions of the proximal coronary arteries. However, in the near future, it is unlikely that any technique other than selective coronary angiography will be capable of defining the details of coronary anatomy throughout the epicardial coronary tree.

Delineation of the anatomy of coronary bypass grafts (whether of internal mammary or saphenous vein origin) is also best done using angiography with selective graft injections. However, CT and MRI have substantial utility in identification of bypass graft patency (Fig. 11–6, p. 316).[11,12]

EVALUATION OF CHAMBER AND VALVULAR FUNCTION

LEFT VENTRICULAR FUNCTION. Global systolic and diastolic function of the left ventricle can be assessed with echocardiography, radionuclide ventriculography, selective angiocardiography, rapid CT, and MRI. Because of its portability, safety, and high patient acceptance, echocardiography is commonly used as the initial tool to assess left ventricular global and regional function. Echocardiography permits accurate assessment of left ventricular function[13] in patients in whom studies of adequate quality can be achieved. With the advent of transesophageal echocardiography, this should include the great majority of patients. Nonetheless, echocardiography has some inherent problems that limit its ability to define precisely left ventricular volume, mass, and ejection fraction. Among these is the fact that the echocardiographic images are not acquired in mutually parallel or perpendicular orientations but are obtained at somewhat arbitrary angles, dictated by the constraints of the intercostal spaces and other aspects of thoracic anatomy. As opposed to these problems of echocardiography, the newer methods of rapid CT and MRI permit the acquisition of multiple parallel high-resolution tomograms from the apex to the base of the left ventricle, yielding quite precise and accurate assessment of chamber volume,[14,15] mass,[7,16] and function. Whether the additional precision and accuracy afforded by CT and MRI justify the additional expense of these techniques and the biological hazards of CT (radiation exposure) remains to be proved. Nonetheless, in terms of theoretical and practical experience, the newer tomographic methods should be considered the most precise and accurate in this application.

Radionuclide methods, while not extremely precise for the calculation of left ventricular mass or volume, nonetheless offer acceptable accuracy for the determination of left ventricular systolic and diastolic performance (p. 298).[17] Radionuclide determinations of left ventricular function are achieved without the necessity of the geometric assumptions common to echocardiography and without the requirement for detailed definition of endocardial and epicardial contours (by hand or computer tracing) that are characteristic of echocardiographic, CT, and MRI methods.

In *summary*, echocardiographic or radionuclide techniques can be utilized at the bedside and thus are the techniques of choice in the assessment of left ventricular function in the intensive care unit or the emergency department. Overall, radionuclide techniques appear to offer a good balance of accuracy, ease of use, portability, and cost-effectiveness for the determination of left ventricular function. In situations in which extremely precise determinations of left ventricular mass or volume are desired, the use of rapid CT or MRI may be justified.

RIGHT VENTRICULAR FUNCTION. Assessment of right ventricular function is more difficult than that of the left ventricle because of the complex shape of the right ventricle, which defies easy representation by simple geometric models. Although echocardiographic methods of assessing right ventricular function have been proposed,[18] there has not been widespread validation or use of these techniques. CT methods are extremely precise and accurate in the derivation of right ventricular volumes[19] and stroke volumes,[14] and MRI methods probably will prove to have similar accuracy. Gated first-pass radionuclide ventriculography[20] (p. 298) is a relatively inexpensive and simple method that can determine right ventricular ejection fraction accurately at the bedside or in the clinical imaging area.

VALVULAR FUNCTION. A complete assessment of valvular function requires determining the characteristics of the valve itself (such as the degree of narrowing or regurgitation) as well as defining the effect of the valvular abnormality on ventricular or atrial anatomy and performance. For the determination of valvular anatomy, transvalvular gradient, and the severity of valvular regurgitation, echocardiographic methods are the current procedures of choice.[21] Particularly with the wide availability of high-quality pulsed, continuous-wave, and color flow Doppler systems, coupled with transesophageal echocardiography in selected patients, the assessment of valvular heart disease in general falls within the domain of echocardiography. With regard to determining the effect of the valvular abnormality on chamber size and function, the previous comments concerning the relative precision and accuracy of radionuclide, ultrasound, CT, and MRI methods apply.

ASSESSMENT OF MYOCARDIAL PERFUSION

At present, the only widely available clinical method used to identify regional deficits in perfusion is thallium-201 scintigraphy, or recently developed scintigraphy using ^{99m}Tc-labeled perfusion agents (p. 277) performed at rest and with exercise stress or pharmacological vasodilation. Unfortunately, these techniques have shortcomings, both in terms of the physics of thallium-201 as an imaging agent and the inability of the method to determine *absolute* levels of regional myocardial perfusion. Therefore, several additional methods of determining perfusion are being developed. As shown in Figure 12–1, the various methods of assessing perfusion can be considered systematically on the basis of the anatomical level at which data are acquired, beginning at the level of the epicardial coronary arteries. Clinicians commonly interpret the severity of a particular coronary artery narrowing on the cineangiogram as an indicator of the likelihood of hypoperfusion distal to that stenosis. Thus, arterial stenoses in excess of 50 to 75 per cent diameter narrowing are commonly assumed to represent hydraulically significant stenoses, capable of limiting flow at high rates.[22] Unfortunately, percentage diameter stenosis is proving to be an imperfect estimator of the functional significance of coronary lesions.[23] Further, this approach gives no information on *absolute* levels of regional perfusion. Videodensitometric techniques evaluate transit time or other measures of flow rate through an epicardial coronary artery based on angiograms and have shown some potential.[24,25] However, due in part to the relative complexity of the measurements, quantitative assessment of angiographic transit time has not gained widespread acceptance. Doppler ultra-

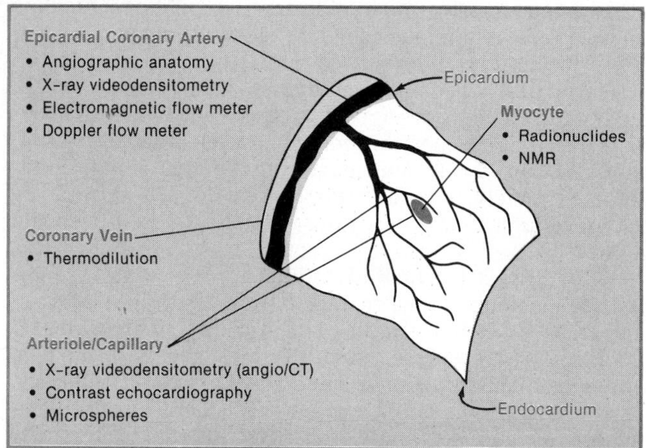

FIGURE 12-1. Approaches to the assessment of coronary artery flow and myocardial perfusion. A schematic cross-section of the left ventricular wall is shown, along with an indication of the anatomical levels at which various methods are used to assess perfusion. At the level of the epicardial coronary arteries, angiographic anatomy is commonly used to identify hydraulically significant stenoses, thereby inferring the potential for hypoperfusion with stress. X-ray videodensitometry and electromagnetic and Doppler flow meters may also be used to assess perfusion at the level of the coronary arteries. (Some of these methods can be used only with an open chest.) Coronary venous thermodilution methods offer some insight into global or regional perfusion. At the arteriolar/capillary level, x-ray videodensitometry, contrast echocardiography, and microspheres may be employed. Finally, radionuclide and nuclear magnetic resonance (NMR) methods can assess perfusion at the level of the myocyte. Angio: angiography; CT: computed tomography.

sound devices, either mounted on intracoronary catheters[26] or placed directly on the epicardial coronaries[27] in the operating room, have been utilized to measure velocity of coronary flow. These devices have been used to estimate relative coronary flow at rest and after a hyperemic stimulus, giving a measure of coronary flow reserve. Once again, these methods do not yield absolute measures of myocardial perfusion or regional perfusion data.

The next anatomical level to consider is that of the coronary microvasculature. Several densitometric methods utilize various indicators and the principles of indicator-dilution theory to assess myocardial perfusion. Thus, the kinetics of indicator entry into and washout from the myocardium may be assessed utilizing angiography[28] or rapid CT[29] (in which an iodinated contrast medium is the indicator), or echocardiography[30] (in which "microbubbles" or other echogenic material is used as the indicator). Most relevant to the clinician and physiologist would be the determination of nutrient flow at the level of the myocyte, utilizing indicators that are taken up by normally perfused cells. Thus, radionuclides such as Tl-201 have shown promise for the assessment of regional perfusion because of their relatively avid uptake by myocardial cells. Unfortunately, the low energy (80 keV mercury x-rays) and low photon flux of thallium-201 limit the accuracy of thallium data.

These problems of thallium scintigraphy have resulted in the development of myocardial perfusion tracers labeled with technetium-99m (p. 277). The higher energy photons released on decay of technetium (140 keV) and higher photon flux should permit the development of better quality images. Early experience with such agents as the technetium-99m isonitriles[31,32] tend to support an improvement in image quality with these agents.

The most promising radionuclide approach to myocardial perfusion imaging is PET.[32a] The combination of the high-energy photons released during positron annihilation (511 keV) and the method of coincidence detection for image formation permit high-resolution depiction of the distribution of a perfusion tracer. Extremely promising data on assessment of absolute levels of myocardial perfusion have been obtained with these methods.[33-35]

MRI methods, coupled with paramagnetic contrast agents, also show promise for the delineation of myocardial perfusion (p. 321). For example, regional myocardial concentration of manganese has been shown to correlate with microsphere-determined blood flow.[36]

As of this writing, radionuclide methods, particularly PET, appear to be the most likely to yield accurate, absolute measurements of regional myocardial perfusion at rest and with stress.

ASSESSMENT OF MYOCARDIAL METABOLISM

Two general approaches to the assessment of myocardial metabolism appear to be possible through imaging techniques: MR spectroscopy and PET. These two methods should be viewed as complementary, since they offer different insights into the biochemistry of the myocardium. MR spectroscopy can be performed utilizing a variety of nuclei including protons (hydrogen nuclei), phosphorus-31,[37] carbon-13, fluorine-19, and sodium-23 (p. 337). Currently, whole-body spectroscopy seems most feasible with phosphorus-31 or proton methods. Phosphorus-31 spectroscopy allows quantitation of the relative amounts of myocardial high-energy phosphates including phosphocreatine, inorganic phosphate, and the alpha, beta, and gamma phosphates of adenosine triphosphate.[38-43] In addition to a "snapshot" assessment of the relative amounts of differing high-energy phosphate compounds at a given point in time, magnetization transfer techniques[44] show promise for the assessment of enzyme kinetics in vivo. For example, quantitative aspects of the creatine kinase reaction have been studied in isolated hearts utilizing magnetic resonance spectroscopy (p. 321).[45] Finally, phosphorus-31 spectroscopy offers the potential of assessing intracellular pH based on the relative position of the inorganic phosphate resonance in the spectrum. MR spectroscopy using carbon-13 or protons offers insights into aspects of intermediary metabolism.

PET also offers a wide range of metabolic insights, chief among which are studies of the uptake of fuel substrates such as glucose[46,47] and fatty acids[48,49] (p. 302). Studies of oxidative metabolism,[50] of receptor density and function,[51] and of other aspects of intermediary metabolism may also be performed utilizing PET.

DELINEATION OF TISSUE CHARACTERISTICS

After assessment of anatomy, function, perfusion, and metabolism, the clinician will sometimes wish to have additional information on the physical characteristics or composition of the myocardium. For example, the identification of the amount of scar tissue versus viable myocardium present after myocardial infarction would be of great clinical interest. Similarly, knowledge of the degree of myocardial fibrosis attendant to longstanding volume overload in aortic regurgitation would be of use in the timing of valve replacement. The two techniques that appear to be most promising in the assessment of tissue characteristics are ultrasonography and MRI.

Myocardial reflection or absorption of ultrasound depends in part upon tissue composition. Since injury to tissue may alter underlying density or elasticity, acoustic characteristics of injured tissue will also vary in comparison with those of normal myocardium. Thus, edema related to acute ischemia and infarction, necrosis attendant on acute infarction, and collagen deposition in chronic infarction have all been identified and quantified utilizing acoustic ultrasonographic analyses.[52] Further, diffuse cardiomyopathies, such as amyloidosis and hypertrophic cardiomyopathy, have been identified and differentiated from each other and from left ventricular hypertrophy[53] utilizing ultrasonographic tissue characterization methods. Although many technical problems related to the acquisition of ultrasound data remain to be solved before these methods will be widely useful clinically, the general approach appears promising.

MR techniques may also identify alterations of tissue composition based on differing image brightness in appropriately weighted images or on measurement of tissue NMR relaxation times. For example, alterations in image intensity, in myocardial T1 and T2, or in proton spectra have been demonstrated in infarction,[54,55] scar,[56] and "stunned" myocardium.[57] Paramagnetic contrast agents such as gadolinium[58,59] appear to accentuate the image intensity and relaxation time differences and thus improve identification of myocardial abnormalities with MRI.

EVALUATING SPECIFIC CATEGORIES OF CARDIAC DISEASE WITH IMAGING METHODS

In Table 12–5 and the following paragraphs, we summarize our opinions on the relative current utility of the various imaging methods in specific patient groups.

Ischemic Heart Disease (see also Chaps. 39 and 40)

ACUTE TRANSIENT ISCHEMIA. Coronary atherosclerosis can be most definitively characterized utilizing selective coronary angiography. Particularly in the present era of aggressive interventional techniques to reduce the severity of coronary atherosclerotic narrowing, a large percentage of patients with ischemic heart disease will continue to be candidates for selective coronary angiography. As sophisticated methods of analyzing coronary arteriograms are further developed and validated, some advantages may accrue to the acquisition of coronary arteriographic data in digital format, so that the newer computer analysis algorithms may be easily applied.

In many patients with ischemic heart disease, however, coronary angiography is not indicated, particularly upon initial presentation. Thus, methods of identifying transient ischemia, particularly exercise or pharmacologically induced ischemia, are of great interest to clinicians. Stress ^{201}Tl scintigraphy (p. 1300) remains a useful procedure for the identification of regional myocardial ischemia including the approximate severity of ischemia and, in some patients, the identification of multivessel disease. The newer ^{99m}Tc-based myocardial perfusion tracers and PET[60] will ensure a continued important role for radionuclide methods in the assessment of transient ischemia.

Exercise or pharmacological stress radionuclide ventriculography and echocardiography offer an indirect but especially useful marker for acute ischemia: the production of new regional wall motion disturbances attendant on acute hypoperfusion of the myocardium. Although it does not give direct information on myocardial perfusion, the delineation of new regional wall motion disturbances (particularly ventricular wall thinning) will likely make stress echocardiography a more widely used technique in the future (p. 96). CT methods are of less use in the identification of transient ischemia. MRI may prove useful in the diagnosis of ischemia if paramagnetic contrast agents are found to be efficacious and safe enough for general application. However, MRI probably will *not* be a first-line method for assessing acute or transient ischemia in the near future.

INFARCTION/REPERFUSION (see Chap. 38). The only currently available imaging methods capable of directly identifying acutely necrotic myocardium are Tc-99m pyrophosphate scintigraphy and labeled monoclonal antimyosin-specific antibody[61] scintigraphy. Although these methods permit the identification of acute necrosis, their clinical applicability is somewhat limited by their poor spatial resolution, which precludes detailed assessment of the size of myocardial infarction. Nonetheless, infarct-avid scintigraphy is, in selected patients, a useful method of infarct identification. Metabolic imaging with PET and MRI (particularly phosphorus-31 spectroscopy), (p. 1221) shows great promise in the identification and quantitation of acute myocardial infarction. Less useful but showing some promise is echocardiographic wall motion analysis. If a patient is known to have had normal wall motion in a particular region before an infarction, echocardiographic estimates of regional wall motion disturbances in that region permit some assessment of the size of infarction, as do similar wall motion analyses utilizing radionuclide, rapid CT, or MRI techniques. However, the parameter of regional wall motion abnormalities is plagued by the inherent biological heterogeneity of contraction in normal subjects[62] and by the fact that regional wall motion patterns appear to be load dependent.[63] Thus, in the future, these indirect techniques may have a lesser place in the identification of infarction than more direct radionuclide methods.

Discrimination between reperfused, nonreperfused but viable, and irreversibly injured tissue is important, particularly with the availability of potent thrombolytic agents and other interventional procedures. The reversal of a regional wall motion disturbance identified by echocardiography, radionuclide ventriculography, CT, or MRI is a good marker for reperfusion of viable myocardium. Wall motion may not immediately return to normal, however, as the myocardium may be "stunned" (p. 1176) or "hibernating" (p. 1330). The most direct methods likely to help the clinician negotiate this quandary are metabolic imaging with PET and/or MR spectroscopy. For example, the combination of PET scans of fuel substrate uptake and perfusion offers a unique strategy to differentiate viable from irreversibly injured myocardium. Fatty acids are the preferred substrate for normal myocardium; nonetheless, normal myocardium does take up glucose. Ischemic but viable myocardium may take up increased amounts of glucose as it operates in an oxygen-limited environment. Thus, the combination of a PET scan showing preserved or *increased* glucose uptake in a region of *decreased* perfusion suggests that the region is, in fact, potentially viable. A concordant decrement in perfusion and fuel substrate uptake identifies irreversibly injured myocardium.[64]

The assessment of high-energy phosphate stores by MR spectroscopy also offers the potential for identification of the presence and extent of irreversibly injured myocardial tissue.

CHRONIC INFARCTION/SCAR FORMATION (see Chap.

TABLE 12–5 RELATIVE USEFULNESS OF CARDIAC IMAGING METHODS IN SPECIFIC PATIENT GROUPS

DISORDER	CXR	ECHO/DOPPLER	ANGIO	RADIONUCLIDES	RCT	MRI
Ischemic	+	++	++++	+++	++	++
Valvular	++	++++	++++	++	+++	+++
Congenital	++	++++	++++	++	+++	+++
Traumatic	++	++	+++	++	++	++
Cardiomyopathy	+	++++	+++	++	+++	+++
Pericardial	+	+++	++	0	++++	++++
Endocarditis	+	++++	++	0	++	+++
Masses	0	++++	+++	0	++++	+++

0: no information; ++++: maximum information; CXR, chest x-ray; echo, echocardiography; angio, angiography; RCT, rapid computed tomography; MRI, magnetic resonance imaging.

40). As already described, the combination of lack of perfusion and lack of fuel substrate uptake on PET identifies a region as infarcted, although scar tissue from earlier infarction may produce the same pattern. Fibrosis may be identified in the future by the use of MRI and/or echocardiographic tissue characterization techniques. As of this writing, however, no available imaging method is capable of identifying directly the presence and extent of myocardial fibrosis in the clinical setting. Thus, clinicians must depend upon persistent abnormalities of regional contraction (as delineated by echocardiography, radionuclide ventriculography, rapid CT, or MRI) to identify chronic infarction.

Valvular Heart Disease (see also Chap. 34)

Echocardiography remains the procedure of choice for the initial assessment of patients with valvular heart disease. In selected patients, angiography and cardiac catheterization are still quite useful, particularly in the identification of concomitant coronary artery disease and in cases of Doppler examinations with equivocal results. CT and MRI methods offer the ability to determine more precisely left ventricular mass (pp. 314 and 333), than does echocardiography. This may prove useful in selected patients with valvular heart disease.

Congenital Heart Disease (see also Chaps. 31 and 32)

Clinicians caring for patients with congenital heart disease need precise information on cardiac morphology, often in settings of extremely complex spatial relationships among atria, ventricles, and great vessels. Thus, methods capable of high-resolution anatomical assessment are of paramount importance in congenital heart disease. Currently, echocardiography is the initial method of choice in evaluating the anatomy of the heart and great vessels, whether in fetus, newborn, child, adolescent, or adult with established or suspected congenital heart disease. In addition to echocardiography, first-pass radionuclide angiography also offers information of use in congenital heart disease by permitting accurate noninvasive quantitation of cardiac shunts (p. 298). CT[65] and MRI[66] also permit shunt identification and quantitation.

Echocardiographic methods (especially using Doppler techniques), in combination with the other noninvasive methods, frequently yield diagnostic information of sufficient reliability to obviate the need for cardiac catheterization in patients with congenital heart disease. This is particularly true in relatively simple abnormalities, such as atrial septal defects in patients younger than 40 years of age. Invasive angiographic, oximetric, and hemodynamic studies will, however, be needed in most complex anomalies before surgical intervention. Further, a growing number of disorders have been found to be amenable to catheter-based interventions (Chap. 41), thus making the argument over the necessity of an invasive study somewhat superfluous. For abnormalities of the great vessels, particularly disorders of the aorta and pulmonary arteries, rapid CT (Fig. 11–16, p. 320) and MRI (Fig. 11–39, p. 321) offers extremely useful information in selected patients. Finally, assessment of patients who have undergone complex repairs, particularly those involving the placement of conduits or baffles, is greatly aided by CT and MRI studies.

Traumatic Heart Disease (see also Chap. 46)

Assessment of the patient after trauma generally involves a search for myocardial contusion, for deceleration injuries (chordal rupture, aortic dissection), and, in the case of penetrating wounds, an unpredictable variety of problems (including hemopericardium, tricuspid valve damage, and coronary artery laceration). While echocardiography is of use in the identification of acute valvular disruption, it may be difficult to perform after major thoracic trauma. Transesophageal echocardiography, rapid CT, and MRI are useful in identifying acute aortic dissection; of these three methods, only echocardiography can be performed at the bedside (Fig. 47–10, p. 1538).

Technetium-99m pyrophospate scintigraphy identifies myocardial contusion directly but has a temporal limitation: the need to wait at least 24 hours after injury for acceptable scan sensitivity. PET and NMR spectroscopy may in the future offer insight into the type and severity of cardiac injury.

Cardiac catheterization may be required to assess the conditions of selected patients after trauma. Most, however, will be evaluated adequately using echocardiography, rapid CT, and/or MRI.

Cardiomyopathies (see also Chap. 43)

Although echocardiography is capable in most patients of differentiating among dilated, hypertrophic, and restrictive cardiomyopathies, it offers limited insight into the specific causes of these disorders. Observations of unusual echocardiographic textural appearance of the myocardium in amyloidosis (p. 1753) and hypertrophic cardiomyopathy have led to successful quantitative approaches to discrimination among these disorders with ultrasound tissue characterization methods.[53] Although as of this writing these are not clinically applicable, these methods show promise for the future. Perhaps even more promising will be metabolic studies with PET and NMR spectroscopy. As of this writing, invasive studies, including hemodynamic evaluation and sometimes endomyocardial biopsy, also are required in selected cases for complete characterization of the type and severity of cardiomyopathy.

Pericardial Disease (see also Chap. 45)

Echocardiographic methods can ascertain the presence of pericardial effusion as well as give some indication of the existence of tamponade; therefore, echocardiography is the initial procedure of choice in investigating the patient with suspected pericardial effusion (Fig. 4–99, p. 102). In selected cases, echocardiography may be supplemented by rapid CT or MRI. Due to the wider field of view of these latter methods, in some patients, a better appreciation of the quantity and anatomical distribution of the effusion may be gained. However, echocardiography, rapid CT, and MRI give limited information on the cause of the effusion. PET and NMR spectroscopy may *eventually* offer assistance in this regard.

Echocardiographic images are of only limited value in identifying pericardial thickening and delineating the physiology of constrictive pericarditis. CT and MRI offer excellent visualization of the pericardium (Fig. 11–9, p. 317) and are more useful than echocardiography in precise measurement of the thickness of the pericardium. MRI and rapid CT, however, also are limited in the ability to diagnose constrictive physiology, which remains in general a hemodynamic diagnosis best made in the catheterization laboratory. Recent investigations with Doppler echocardiography[67,68] and CT[69] suggest that noninvasive assessment of ventricular filling dynamics may be performed with these methods. Precise and accurate assessment of diastolic filling may offer some help in the diagnosis of constrictive pericarditis, but these methods are not as well established as hemodynamic data obtained at cardiac catheterization (p. 187).

Infective Endocarditis (see also Chap. 35)

The presence of vegetations may be established in the majority of patients by using echocardiography (Fig. 4–60, p. 88). The advent of transesophageal echocardiography has substantially improved the sensitivity of ultrasonic identification of vegetations.[70] Thus, ultrasound is the initial imaging technique of choice in the patient suspected of having infective endocarditis. It should be emphasized, however, that failure to identify a vegetation by echocardiography should not be

TABLE 12-6 SOME COSTS ASSOCIATED WITH CARDIAC IMAGING METHODS

Purchase price of system
Site preparation
Power, water, and environmental costs
Personnel
Physicians
Nurses
Technicians
Support personnel (physicists, engineers, pharmacists, others)

used to exclude definitively a diagnosis of endocarditis, as false-negative examination results do occur, even with transesophageal echocardiography.

The complications of endocarditis, including valve disruption and abscess formation, can often be identified with echocardiography, rapid CT, or MRI. Catheterization and angiocardiography are necessary in some cases to identify either the presence of endocarditis or its attendant complications.

Intracardiac Masses (see also Chap. 44)

In addition to vegetations, clinicians will encounter many other varieties of intracardiac mass lesions, including thrombi, myxomata, and metastatic tumors. Once again, echocardiography is quite useful in assessment of these patients. Transesophageal echocardiography has proved particularly useful in identifying thrombi in the left atrial appendage in patients with a suspected cardiogenic source of cerebral emboli.[71] CT and MRI are also excellent methods of identifying intracardiac masses (Fig. 44-5, p. 1458, Fig. 11-36, p. 330) and should be considered when echocardiography is equivocal. The determination of the nature of an intracardiac mass is best made currently by indirect evidence, such as the anatomical position and attachment of the mass, but such methods as characterization of the tissue by ultrasonography and MRI may prove helpful in this regard in the future.

COST CONSIDERATIONS IN CARDIAC IMAGING

The several methods of imaging the heart and circulation vary widely in their costs. In considering these variations, several types of expense should be considered (Table 12-6). These expenses include the initial purchase price of the system and any necessary expenditures for site preparation.

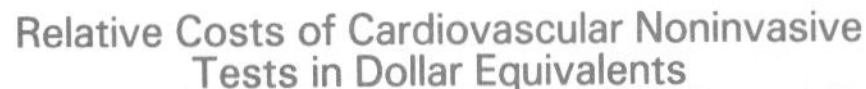

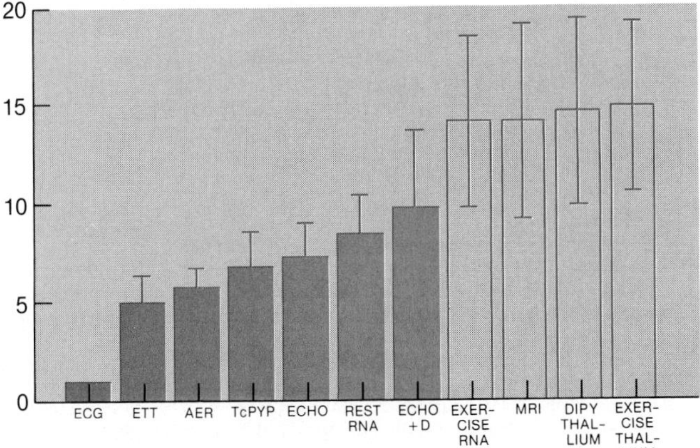

FIGURE 12-2. Relative costs of cardiovascular diagnostic tests. The cost of each test has been calculated relative to that of a resting electrocardiogram, to correct for geographical differences in specific fees. ECG, electrocardiography; ETT, exercise treadmill test; AER, ambulatory electrocardiography recording; TcPYP, technetium pyrophosphate scan; ECHO, echocardiography; RNA, radionuclide angiography; D, Doppler ultrasound; MRI, magnetic resonance imaging; DIPY, dipyridamole. (Reproduced with permission from O'Rourke, R. A.: Cost considerations. In: Pohost, G. M., O'Rourke, R. A. Principles and Practice of Cardiovascular Imaging. Boston, Little, Brown, Inc., 1991.)

Once the system is installed, consideration must be given to power and environmental costs. Personnel costs to be considered include the physicians, technicians, and nurses who deal with the day-to-day operation of the system, as well as support personnel for maintenance and quality control testing.

Two very different types of cost should be distinguished in considering the relative expense of the imaging methods. First is the set of costs already discussed. In terms of establishing and operating a particular imaging system, excluding chest roentgenography, echocardiography falls at the least expensive end of the spectrum, although a complete modern echocardiographic system costs about $200,000. At the other end of the spectrum are rapid CT, MRI, and PET, all of which cost in excess of $1,000,000; in the case of PET, including the purchase of a cyclotron to produce specific radionuclides, the expense may be closer to $4,000,000.

Although these costs vary tremendously, it is of interest that the cost of a single examination to the patient does not vary over as wide a range. Whereas the imaging methods vary over more than an order of magnitude in their purchase prices, the expense of an examination to the patient or third-party payor varies over a substantial but narrower range. An interesting analysis of these examination costs was completed recently by O'Rourke[72] and is presented in Figure 12-2.

REFERENCES

SCOPE OF CARDIAC IMAGING

1. Skorton, D. J., and Collins, S. M.: New directions in cardiac imaging. Ann. Intern. Med. *102*:795, 1985.
2. Miller, D. D., (ed.): Clinical Cardiac Imaging. New York, McGraw-Hill Book Co., 1988.
3. Marcus, M. L., Schelbert, H. R., Skorton, D. J., and Wolf, G. L., (eds.): Cardiac Imaging. Philadelphia, W. B. Saunders Company, 1991.
4. Hounsfield, G. N.: Computed medical imaging. Nobel Lecture, December 8, 1979. J. Comput. Assist. Tomogr. *4*:665, 1980.
5. Collins, S. M., and Skorton, D. J., (eds.): Cardiac Imaging and Image Processing. New York, McGraw-Hill Book Co., 1986.
6. Buda, A. J., and Delp, E. J.: Digital Cardiac Imaging. Boston, Martinus Nijhoff, 1985.

MEETING THE GOALS OF CARDIAC IMAGING

7. Feiring, A. J., Rumberger, J. A., Reiter, S. J., et al.: Determination of left ventricular mass in dogs with rapid-acquisition cardiac computed tomographic scanning. Circulation *72*:1355, 1985.
8. Zwicky, P., Daniel, W. G., Mugge, A., and Lichtlen, P. R.: Imaging of coronary arteries by color-coded transesophageal Doppler echocardiography. Am. J. Cardiol. *62*:639, 1988.
9. Spyra, W. J. T., Bell, M. R., Bove, A. A., et al.: Detection and localization of moderate coronary stenoses by fast CT with a single nonselective angiogram. Circulation *78*(Suppl. II):398, 1988.
10. Zerhouni, E. A.: New directions in cardiac magnetic resonance imaging. Top. Magn. Resonance Imag. *2*:67, 1990.
11. Stanford, W., Brundage, B. H., MacMillan, R., et al.: Sensitivity and specificity of assessing coronary bypass graft patency with ultrafast computed tomography: Results of a multicenter study. J. Am. Coll. Cardiol. *12*:1, 1988.
12. White, R. D, Caputo, G. R., Mark, A. S., et al.: Coronary artery bypass graft patency: Noninvasive evaluation with MR imaging. Radiology *164*:681, 1987.
13. Parisi, A. F., Moynihan, P. F., Feldman, C. L., et al.: Approaches to determination of left ventricular volumes and ejection fraction by real-time two-dimensional echocardiography. Clin. Cardiol. *2*:257, 1979.
14. Reiter, S. J., Rumberger, J. A., Feiring, A. J., et al.: Precision of measurements of right and left ventricular volume by cine computed tomography. Circulation *74*:890, 1986.
15. Rehr, R. B. Malloy, C. R., Filipchuck, N. G., and Peshock, R. M.: Left ventricular volumes measured by MR imaging. Radiology *156*:717, 1985.
16. Florentine, M. S., Grosskreutz, C. L., Chang, W., et al.: Measurement of left ventricular mass in vivo using gated nuclear magnetic resonance imaging. J. Am. Coll. Cardiol. *8*:107, 1986.
17. Gibbons, R. J.: Equilibrium radionuclide angiography. *In* Marcus, M. L., Schelbert, H. R., Skorton, D. J., Wolf, G. L. (eds.): Cardiac Imaging. Philadelphia, W. B. Saunders Company, 1991, p. 1027.
18. Aebischer, N. M., and Czegledy, F.: Determination of right ventricular volume by two-dimensional echocardiography with a crescentic model. J. Am. Soc. Echo. *2*:110, 1989.
19. Mahoney, L. T., Smith, W., Noel, M. P., et al.: Measurement of right ventricular volume using cine computed tomography. Invest. Radiol. *22*:451, 1987.

20. Rezai, K., Weiss, R., Stanford, W., et al.: Relative accuracy of three scintigraphic methods for determination of right ventricular ejection fraction: A correlative study with ultrafast CT. J. Nucl. Med. (in press).
21. Otto, C. M., and Pearlman, A. S.: Doppler echocardiography in adults with symptomatic aortic stenosis: diagnostic utility and cost-effectiveness. Arch. Intern. Med. *148*:2553, 1988.
22. Gould, K. L., and Lipscomb, K.: Effects of coronary stenoses on coronary flow reserve and resistance. Am. J. Cardiol. *34*:48, 1974.
23. White, C. W., Wright, C. B. Doty, D. B., et al.: Does the visual interpretation of the coronary arteriogram predict the physiological importance of a coronary stenosis? N. Engl. J. Med. *310*:819, 1984.
24. Rutishauser, W., Noseda, G., Bussman, W. D., and Preter, B.: Blood flow measurements through single coronary arteries by roentgen densitometry. Part II. Right coronary artery flow in conscious man. A. J. R. *109*:21, 1970.
25. Smith, H. C., Sturm, R. E., and Wood, E. H.: Videodensitometric system for measurement of vessel blood flow, particularly in the coronary arteries, in man. Am. J. Cardiol. *32*:144, 1973.
26. Wilson, R. F., Laughlin, D. E., Ackell, P. H., et al.: Transluminal subselective measurement of coronary artery blood flow velocity and vasodilator reserve in man. Circulation *72*:82, 1985.
27. Marcus, M. Wright, C., Doty, D., et al.: Measurements of coronary velocity and reactive hyperemia in the coronary circulation of humans. Circ. Res. *49*:877, 1981.
28. Hodgson, J. McB., LeGrand, V., Bates, E. R., et al.: Validation in dogs of a rapid digital angiographic technique to measure relative coronary blood flow during routine cardiac catheterization. Am. J. Cardiol. *55*:188, 1985.
29. Wolfkiel, C., Ferguson, J. L., Chomka, E. V., et al.: Measurement of myocardial blood flow by ultrafast computed tomography. Circulation *76*:1262, 1987.
30. Feinstein, S. B., Lang, R. M., Dick, C., et al.: Contrast echocardiography during coronary arteriography in humans: Perfusion and anatomic studies. J. Am. Coll. Cardiol. *11*:59, 1988.
31. Sporn, V., Perez-Balino, N., Holman, B. L., et al.: Simultaneous measurement of ventricular function and myocardial perfusion using the technetium 99m isonitriles. Clin. Nucl. Med. *13*:77, 1988.
32. Taillefer, R., Lambert, R., Dupras, G., et al.: Clinical comparison between thallium-201 and Tc-99m-methoxy isobutyl isonitrile (hexaMIBI) myocardial perfusion imaging for detection of coronary artery disease. Eur. J. Nucl. Med. *15*:280, 1989.
32a. Chan, S. Y., Brunken, R. C., and Buxton, D. B.: Cardiac positron emission tomography: The foundations and clinical applications. J. Thorac. Imaging *5*:9, 1990.
33. Shah, A., Schelbert, H. R., Schwaiger, M., et al.: Measurement of regional myocardial blood flow with N-13 ammonia and positron-emission tomography in intact dogs. J. Am. Coll. Cardiol. *5*:92, 1985.
34. Bergmann, S. R., Herrero, P., Markham, J., et al.: Noninvasive quantitation of myocardial blood flow in human subjects with oxygen-15-labeled water and positron emission tomography. J. Am. Coll. Cardiol. *14*:639, 1989.
35. Krivokapich, J., Smith, G. T., Huang, S. C., et al.: N-13 ammonia myocardial imaging at rest and with exercise in normal volunteers: Quantification of absolute myocardial perfusion with dynamic positron emission tomography. Circulation *80*:1328, 1989.
36. Schaefer, S., Lange, R. A., Kulkarni, P. V., et al.: In vivo nuclear magnetic resonance imaging of myocardial perfusion using the paramagnetic contrast agent manganese gluconate. J. Am. Coll. Cardiol. *14*:472, 1989.
37. Bottomley, P. A.: Noninvasive study of high-energy phosphate metabolism in human heart by depth-resolved P-31 NMR spectroscopy. Science *229*:769, 1985.
38. Osbakken, M. D., Mitchell, M. D.: Magnetic resonance spectroscopy to study myocardial metabolism and cellular function. *In* Marcus, M. L., Schelbert, H. R., Skorton, D. J., Wolf, G. L. (eds.): Cardiac Imaging. Philadelphia, W. B. Saunders Company, 1991, p. 841.
39. Kantor, H. L., Briggs, R. W., Metz, K. R., and Balaban, R. S.: Gated in vivo examination of cardiac metabolites with ^{31}P nuclear magnetic resonance. Am. J. Physiol. *251*:H171, 1986.
40. Schaefer, S., Camacho, A., Gober, J., et al.: Response of myocardial metabolites to graded regional ischemia: ^{31}P NMR spectroscopy of porcine myocardium in vivo. Circ. Res. *64*:968, 1989.
41. Osbakken, M. D., Pigott, J., Ligett, L., et al.: Myocardial bioenergetics of chronic volume overload studied with ^{31}P MRS. J. Appl. Cardiol. *5*:39, 1990.
42. Schaefer, S., Gober, J., Valenza, M., et al.: Nuclear magnetic resonance imaging-guided phosphorus-31 spectroscopy of the human heart. J. Am. Coll. Cardiol. *12*:1449, 1988.
43. Camacho, S. A., Lanzer, P., Toy, B. J., et al.: In vivo alterations of high-energy phosphates and intracellular pH during reversible ischemia in pigs: A ^{31}P magnetic resonance spectroscopy study. Am. Heart J. *116*:701, 1988.
44. Ugurbil, K.: Magnetization transfer measurements of individual rate constants in the presence of multiple reactions. J. Magn. Resonance *64*:207, 1985.
45. Neubauer, S., Hamman, B. L., Perry, S. B., et al.: Velocity of the creatine kinase reaction decreases in postischemic myocardium: A ^{31}P-NMR magnetization transfer study of the isolated ferret heart. Circ. Res. *63*:1, 1988.
46. Ratib, O., Phelps, M. E., Huang, S. C., et al.: Positron tomography with deoxyglucose for estimating local myocardial glucose metabolism. J. Nucl. Med. *23*:577, 1982.
47. Gambhir, S. S., Schwaiger, M., Huang, S. C., et al.: Simple noninvasive quantification method for measuring myocardial glucose utilization in humans employing positron emission tomography and Fluorine-18 deoxyglucose. J. Nucl. Med. *30*:359, 1989.
48. Schon, H. R., Schelbert, H. R., Robinson, G., et al.: C-11 labeled palmitic acid for the noninvasive evaluation of regional myocardial fatty acid metabolism with positron-computed tomography. I. Kinetics of C-11 palmitic acid in normal myocardium. Am. Heart J. *103*:532, 1982.
49. Schelbert, H. R., Henze, E., Sochor, H., et al.: Effects of substrate availability on myocardial C-11 palmitate kinetics by positron emission tomography in normal subjects and patients with ventricular dysfunction. Am. Heart J. *111*:1055, 1986.
50. Armbrecht, J. J., Buxton, D. B., Brunken, R. C., et al.: Regional myocardial oxygen consumption determined noninvasively in humans with [1-^{11}C] acetate and dynamic positron tomography. Circulation *80*:863, 1989.
51. Delforge, J., Nakajima, K., Syrota, A., et al.: PET investigation of β-adrenergic receptors using CGP 12177. J. Nucl. Med. *30*:825, 1989.
52. Miller, J. G., Perez, J. E., and Sobel, B. E.: Ultrasonic characterization of myocardium. Prog. Cardiovasc. Dis. *28*:85, 1985.
53. Chandrasekaran, K., Aylward, P. E., Fleagle, S. R., et al.: Feasibility of identifying amyloid and hypertrophic cardiomyopathy with the use of computerized quantitative texture analysis of clinical echocardiographic data. J. Am. Coll. Cardiol. *13*:832, 1989.
54. Rokey, R., Verani, M. S., Bolli, R., et al.: Myocardial infarct size quantification by MR imaging early after coronary occlusion in dogs. Radiology *158*:771, 1986.
55. Bouchard, A., Reeves, R. C., Cranney, G., et al.: Assessment of myocardial infarct size by means of T2-weighted ^{1}H nuclear magnetic resonance imaging. Am. Heart J. *117*:281, 1989.
56. Wisenberg, G., Prato, F. S., Carroll, S. E., et al.: Serial nuclear magnetic resonance imaging of acute myocardial infarction with and without reperfusion. Am. Heart J. *115*:510, 1988.
57. Reeves, R. C., Evanochko, W. T., Canby, R. C., et al.: Demonstration of increased myocardial lipid with postischemic dysfunction ("myocardial stunning") by proton nuclear magnetic resonance spectroscopy. J. Am. Coll. Cardiol. *13*:739, 1989.
58. Eichstaedt, H. W., Felix, R., Dougherty, F. C., et al.: Magnetic resonance imaging (MRI) in different stages of myocardial infarction using the contrast agent gadolinium-DTPA. Clin. Cardiol. *9*:527, 1986.
59. Miller, D. D., HolmVang, G., Gill, J. B., et al.: MRI detection of myocardial perfusion changes by gadolinium-DTPA infusion during dipyridamole hyperemia. Magn. Resonance Med. *10*:246, 1989.

EVALUATING SPECIFIC CATEGORIES OF CARDIAC DISEASE WITH IMAGING METHODS

60. Demer, L. L., Gould, K. L., Goldstein, R. A., et al.: Assessment of coronary artery disease severity by positron emission tomography: Comparison with quantitative arteriography in 193 patients. Circulation *79*:825, 1989.
61. Khaw, B. A., Gold, H. K., Yasuda, T., et al.: Scintigraphic quantification of myocardial necrosis in patients after intravenous injection of myosin-specific antibody. Circulation *74*:501, 1986.
62. Pandian, N. G., Skorton, D. J., Collins, S. M., et al.: Heterogeneity of left ventricular segmental wall thickening and excursion in two-dimensional echocardiograms of normal human subjects. Am. J. Cardiol. *51*:1667, 1983.
63. Weiss, R. M., Shonka, M. D., Kinzey, J. E., et al.: Effects of loading alterations on the pattern of heterogeneity of regional left ventricular function (abstract). FASEB J *2*:1494A, 1988.
64. Tillisch, J., Brunken, R., Marshall, R., et al.: Reversibility of cardiac wall-motion abnormalities predicted by positron tomography. N. Engl. J. Med. *314*:884, 1986.
65. Garrett, J. S., Jaschke, W., Aherne, T., et al.: Quantitation of intracardiac shunts by cine-CT. J. Comput. Assist. Tomogr. *12*:82, 1988.
66. Sechtem, U., Pflugfelder, P., Cassidy, M. C., et al.: Ventricular septal defect: Visualization of shunt flow and determination of shunt size by cine MR imaging. A. J. R. *149*:689, 1987.
67. Appleton, C. P., Hatle, L. K., and Popp, R. L.: Central venous flow velocity patterns can differentiate constrictive pericarditis from restrictive cardiomyopathy (Abstract). J. Am. Coll. Cardiol. *9*(Suppl. A):119A, 1987.
68. King, S. W., Pandian, N. G., and Gardin, J. M.: Doppler echocardiographic findings in pericardial tamponade and constriction . Echocardiography *5*:361, 1988.
69. Stanford, W. Rooholamini, S. A., and Galvin, J. R.: Assessment of intracardiac masses and extracardiac abnormalities by ultrafast computed tomography. *In* Marcus, M. L., Schelbert, H. R., Skorton, D. J., Wolf, G. L., (eds.): Cardiac Imaging. Philadephia, W. B. Saunders Company, 1991, p. 703.
70. Erbel, R., Rohmann, S., Drexler, M., et al.: Improved diagnostic value of echocardiography in patients with infective endocarditis by transesophageal approach. A prospective study. Eur. Heart J. *9*:43, 1988.
71. Zenker, G., Erbel, R., Kramer, G., et al.: Transesophageal two-dimensional echocardiography in young patients with cerebral ischemic events. Stroke *19*:345, 1988.

COST CONSIDERATIONS IN CARDIAC IMAGING

72. O'Rourke, R. A.: Cost considerations. *In* Pohost, G. M., O'Rourke, R. A: Principles and Practice of Cardiovascular Imaging. Boston, Little, Brown, Inc., 1991.

PART II

NORMAL AND ABNORMAL CIRCULATORY FUNCTION

13

Mechanisms of Cardiac Contraction and Relaxation

by EUGENE BRAUNWALD, M.D., EDMUND H. SONNENBLICK, M.D., and JOHN ROSS, Jr., M.D.

The function of the heart is to propel unoxygenated blood to the lungs and oxygenated blood to the peripheral tissues in accordance with their metabolic requirements. Heart failure may therefore be defined as the pathophysiological state in which an abnormality of *cardiac* function is responsible for the heart's failure to pump blood at a rate commensurate with these requirements and/or when it can do so only from an elevated filling pressure. Congestive heart failure describes the clinical syndrome that results from central heart failure and the compensatory responses of the peripheral organs and circulation. To comprehend the disturbances in cardiac contraction that characterize heart failure, described in Chapter 14, it is necessary to understand the structure and function of the normal cardiac cell and of the normal contractile process, described in this chapter.

Cellular Mechanisms

STRUCTURE OF THE MYOCYTE

MYOCYTES, MYOFIBRILS, AND SARCOMERES (Table 13–1). Ventricular myocytes (myocardial cells or fibers) are normally 100 to 120 μ in length and 15 to 25 μ in diameter (Fig. 13–1). Atrial myocytes are smaller while myocytes from the conduction system (Purkinje cells) are larger in both dimensions (p. 354). Numerous cross-banded strands or bundles, termed myofibrils, traverse the length of the fiber and, unlike skeletal muscle, are incompletely separated by clefts of cytoplasm that contain mitochondria and membranous tubules (Fig. 13–1*B*).[1–4]

Myofibrils are composed of longitudinally repeating sarcomeres separated by two adjacent dark lines—the Z lines (Fig. 13–1*B* and *C*).[4] *Sarcomeres* occupy about 50 per cent of the mass of the cardiac cells[5] and are aligned so that the ends of adjacent myofibrils are in register, giving the fiber its striated appearance.[1] The length of the sarcomere ranges from 1.6 to 2.2 μ, depending in part on the tension exerted on the muscle. The center of the sarcomere is occupied by a dark band, the A band (the anisotropic or birefringent band that rotates polarized light), and is 1.5 μ in length. The A band is flanked by two lighter bands, termed I (isotropic) bands, which vary in length depending on the length of the sarcomere. The bands of the

TABLE 13–1 CHARACTERISTICS OF CARDIAC CELLS, ORGANELLES, AND CONTRACTILE PROTEINS

A. MICROANATOMY OF HEART CELLS

	Ventricular myocyte[1,2]	Atrial myocyte[1,3]	Purkinje cells[1,4]
Shape	Long and narrow	Elliptical	Long and broad
Length, μm	50–100	About 20	150–200
Diameter, μm	10–25	5–6	35–40
T tubules	Plentiful	Rare or none	Absent
Intercalated disc	Prominent end-to-end transmission	Side-to-side as well as end-to-end transmission	Very prominent; abundant gap functions; fast end-to-end transmission
General appearance	Mitochondria and sarcomeres very abundant; rectangular, branching bundles with little interstitial collagen	Bundles of atrial tissue separated by wide areas of collagen	Fewer sarcomeres, more glycogen

B. COMPOSITION AND FUNCTION OF RAT VENTRICULAR CELL

Organelle	Percentage of cell volume	Function
Myofibril	About 50%[5]	Interaction of thick and thin filaments during contraction cycle
Mitochondria	16% in neonate[5] 33% in adult[5]	Provide ATP chiefly for contraction
T system	1%[6]	Transmits electrical signal from sarcolemma to cell interior
Sarcoplasmic reticulum	33% in neonate[5] 2% in adult[5]	Takes up and releases Ca^{++} during contraction cycle
Terminal cisternae	0.33% in adult[6]	? site of calcium storage and release[7] ? site of calcium uptake en route to cisternae
Rest of network	Rest of volume	
Sarcolemma	Very low	Control of ionic gradients; channels for ions (action potential); maintenance of cell integrity; receptors for drugs and hormones
Nucleus	5%	Protein synthesis
Lysosomes	Very low	Intracellular digestion and proteolysis
Sarcoplasmic (= cytoplasm) (+ nuclei + other structures)	12%	Provides cytosol in which rise and fall of ionized calcium occurs; contains other ions and small molecules

C. THE PROTEINS OF MYOFIBRILS

Function	Location	% of myofibrillar protein	Molecular weight
Contractile			
Myosin	Thick filaments	55–60	500,000
Actin	Thin filaments	20	43,000
Regulatory			
Tropomyosin	Thin filaments	5	70,000
Troponin I	Thin filaments		
Troponin C	Thin filaments	7	86,000
Troponin T	Thin filaments		
Structural			
C protein	Thick filaments		
alpha-actinin	Thick filaments and Z lines		
beta-actinin	Thin filaments	8–13	40,000–750,000
M line proteins	M lines		
Other proteins	Various		

There are about 7 actins, 2 myosins, 1 tropomyosin, and 1 troponin in the myofibrils, but their different molecular weights account for the different picture given by the percentage contributions each makes to the total myofibrillar mass (third column). Part C partly from Perry, S. V.: Biochem. Soc. Trans. *7*:593, 1979.

[1] Legato: The Myocardial Cell for the Clinical Cardiologist, 1973.
[2] Laks et al.: Circ. Res. *21*:671,1967.
[3] McNutt and Fawcett: J. Cell. Biol. *42*:46, 1969.
[4] Sommer: J. Mol. Cell. Cardiol. 14 Suppl *3*:77, 1982.
[5] David et al.: J. Mol. Cell. Cardiol. *11*:631, 1979.
[6] Page and McCallister: Am. J. Cardiol. *31*:172, 1973.
[7] Page and Surdyk-Droske: Circ. Res. *45*:260, 1979.
Part B modified from Page and McCallister, 1973.
From Opie, L.: The Heart. New York, Grune and Stratton, 1984, pp. 16 and 98.

sarcomere reflect the disposition of interdigitating myofilaments made up of contractile proteins (Figs. 13–1C and 13–2). *Thin filaments* composed of actin are attached to each Z line and project longitudinally into the middle of the sarcomere, where they interdigitate with an array of *thicker filaments* composed of myosin molecules.[1,4] Interactions between the thick and thin myofilaments in the A band generate force and shortening of the myocardium, with the myofilaments sliding past one another while maintaining a fixed length. Ultra-thin filaments composed of titin and possibly nebulin connect Z line discs and may serve to limit sarcomere distention and may affect the filaments themselves.[6,7]

The nucleus is centrally placed within the myocardial cell. Among adult myocytes, binucleate cells are the rule.[2] Mitochondria, which comprise about 20 per cent of cell volume,[5] are elliptically shaped, approximately 2 to 5 μ by 0.5 μ, and are situated between and in close apposition to the myofibrils as well as just beneath the sarcolemma.[4] Their platelike foldings,

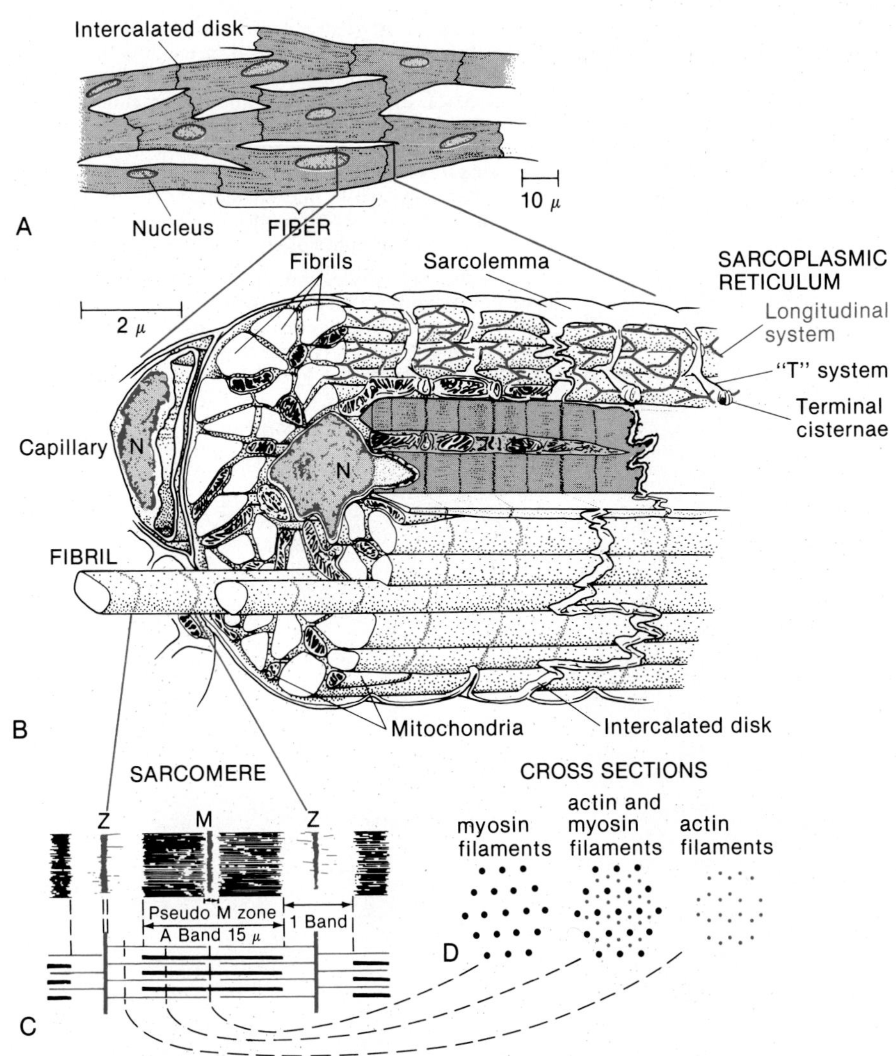

FIGURE 13-1. Schematic diagram of the microscopic structure of heart muscle.

***A,* Myocardium as seen under the light microscope. Branching of fibers is evident, with each containing a centrally located nucleus. Fibers or cells are connected across intercalated disks.**

***B,* A myocardial cell or fiber reconstructed from electron micrographs, showing the arrangement of multiple parallel fibrils that compose the cell and of serially connected sarcomeres that compose the individual fibril. N = nucleus. The sarcotubular system, which mediates activation, includes the sarcolemma and sarcoplasmic reticulum. An intercalated disk in the center of the reconstruction serves to separate two cells.**

***C,* An individual sarcomere from a myofibril. Diagrammatic representation of the arrangement of myofilaments that make up the sarcomere. Thick filaments, approximately 1.5 microns in length, composed of myosin, are localized to the A band, while thin filaments, 1.0 μ in length, composed primarily of actin, extend from the Z line through the I band into the A band, ending at the edges of the central H zone. The H zone is the central area of the A band where thin filaments are absent. Thick and thin filaments overlap only in the A band.**

***D,* Diagrammatic cross section of the sarcomere showing the specific lattice arrangements of the myofilaments. In the center of the sarcomere (*left*), only the thick (myosin) filaments arranged in a hexagonal array are seen. In the distal portions of the A band (*center*), both thick and thin (actin) filaments are found, each thick filament surrounded by six thin filaments. In the I band, only thin filaments are present. (From Braunwald, E., et al.: Mechanisms of Contraction of the Normal and Failing Heart. 2nd ed. Boston, Little, Brown, 1976.)**

or cristae, which contain the enzymes of the tricarboxylic acid cycle, project inward from the surface membrane. The close proximity of the mitochondria, the organelles in which ATP is produced, to the contractile filaments may facilitate the transfer of ATP from its site of production to its site of utilization during contraction. Lysosomes, membrane-limited vesicles about 0.1 μ in diameter and located near the pole of the nucleus, contain latent hydrolytic enzymes capable of lysing cellular membranes as well as other cellular components.[2]

Myocardial cells that initiate intrinsic activity in the heart, i.e., pacemaker or automatic cells (Chap. 22), are somewhat smaller than ventricular fibers[4] (Table 13-1A). Those that are specialized for conduction and the spread of excitation, i.e., Purkinje fibers, are very large when compared with contractile fibers; they contain fewer myofibrils and greater quantities of clear cytoplasm, fine intracellular noncontractile filaments, and glycogen in addition to having a rich external investment of capillaries and small nerves.[8]

Myocardial fibers are surrounded by a rich capillary network, and small, nonmyelinated nerves are found lying free in the extracellular space.[3] These nerves have no specific junctions with cardiac cells but do exhibit bulbous ends bearing granules that contain neurotransmitter substances. The most important of these are acetylcholine, located primarily in the

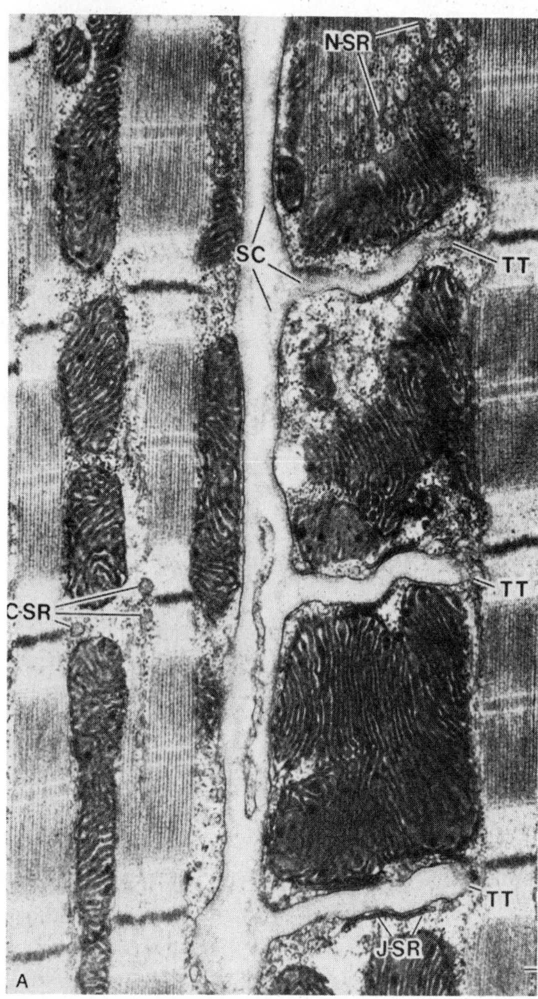

FIGURE 13-2. *A,* Ventricular myocardial cells from dog right ventricular wall. The sarcolemma of the right-hand cell forms three transverse tubules (TT) oriented in register with Z bands of the nearest myofibrils. The substance of the myocardial surface coat (SC) can be seen both in association with the surface sarcolemma and within the T tubules' lamina. Three categories of sarcoplasmic reticulum can be discerned: network SR (N-SR) on the face of one myofibril; junctional SR (J-SR), flattened saccules apposed to the T tubules; and corbular SR (C-SR). Note mitochondria, either arranged in intermyofibrillar row or located just beneath the surface sarcolemma. Scale bar represents 0.5 μm. (From Forbes, M. S., and Sperelakis, N.: *In* Physiology and Pathophysiology of the Heart. Boston, Martinus Nijhoff, 1984, p. 21.)

B, Schematic of T tubules and sarcoplasmic reticulum of mammalian cardiac muscle. Note how the diffuse tubular network of the sarcoplasmic reticulum forms saccular expansions, the subsarcolemmal cisternae, which are in close apposition to the sarcolemma and T tubules. (From Fawcett, D. W., and McNutt, N. S.: The ultrastructure of the cat myocardium. I. Ventricular papillary muscle. J. Cell Biol. *42:*1, 1969.)

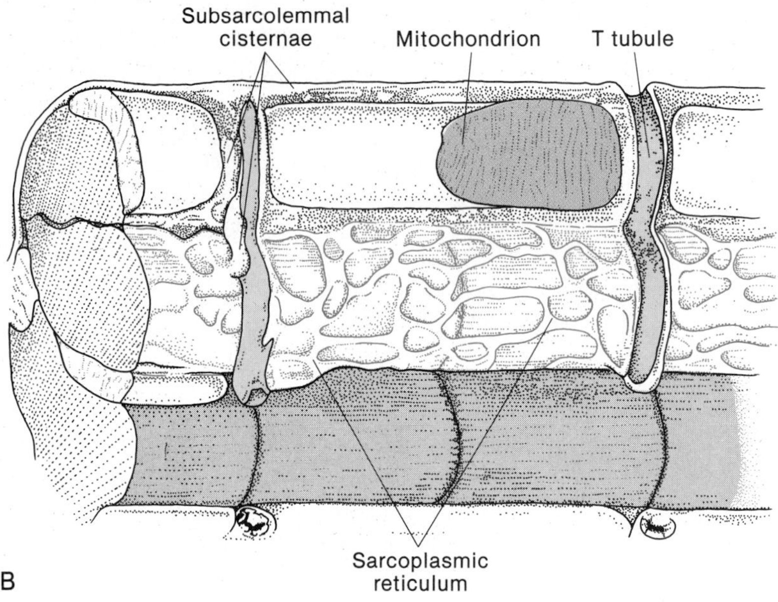

atria and in automatic and conduction tissues, and norepinephrine, found in these tissues but also in the ventricles; both can be released to act on membrane surface receptors of adjacent cells.

Unlike ventricular myocytes, atrial myocytes contain specific dense granules[1,9] (Fig. 62–4, p. 1859), the source of atrial natriuretic hormone,[10] which may play an important role in salt and water metabolism and thus in the control of blood pressure.[10,11]

SARCOLEMMA, INTERCALATED DISCS, AND SARCOPLASMIC RETICULUM. A surface membrane, the *sarcolemma,* surrounds the myocardial cells and invaginates at the Z lines of the sarcomere.[2,12,13] It is composed of a thin (7 to 9 nm), bimolecular phospholipid layer, the *plasmalemma,* which is the site of electrical polarization (Fig. 22–9, p. 593), and just exterior to the plasmalemma, the *basement membrane,* a glycocalyx approximately 50 nm in thickness, which in turn is composed of an inner and an outer coat. The plasmalemma is the major semipermeable membrane between the intracellular cytoplasm and the negatively charged glycocalyx to which Ca^{++} may be bound and which separates the cell from the extracellular matrix. Adjacent myocardial cells are connected end-to-end by a thickened portion of the sarcolemma, termed the *intercalated disc,*[1-4] a segment of which—the gap junction—represents a low-resistance pathway to the propagation of electrical activity between cells.[14]

Myocardial fibers are also invested with an extensive network of collagen fibers, fine microfibrils, and microthreads[15,16] (Fig. 13–3), which play an important role in cell orientation, tissue compliance in diastole, and intercellular force transmission in systole. The elastic fibers are composed of microfilaments of glycoprotein and amorphous elastin.[17] This "skeleton" contributes importantly to the diastolic properties of the ventricle, including distensibility and diastolic recoil, and limits the extent to which the heart can be dilated and hence the sarcomeres overstretched by a volume overload.

The hydrophobic phospholipid bilayer of the plasmalemma (Fig. 22–9, p. 593) acts as an ionic barrier and maintains higher intracellular than extracellular potassium [K^+] concentrations and lower intracellular than extracellular sodium

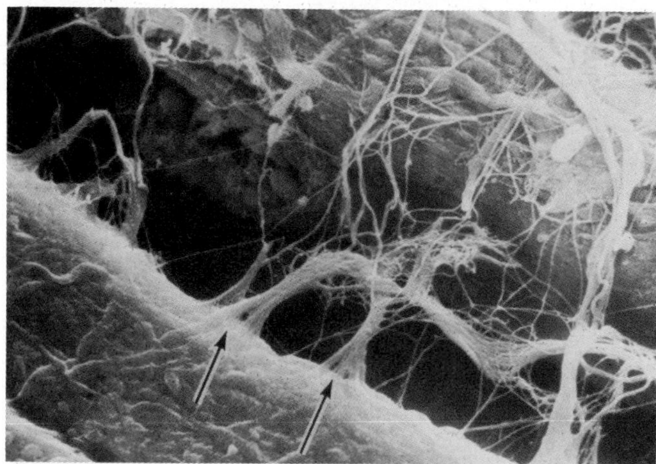

FIGURE 13-3. A scanning electron micrograph from a normal canine heart reveals complex connective tissue struts extending between and tethering two myocytes. The struts can be observed to attach to the sarcolemmal surface by root-like projections (arrows) (original magnification, × 1980). (From van Hoeven, K. H., and Factor, S. M.: Pathology of the cardiac collagen matrix: Mechanical and functional effects. *In* Hori, M., et al. [eds.]: Cardiac Mechanics and Function in the Normal and Diseased Heart. New York, Springer-Verlag, 1989, p. 51.)

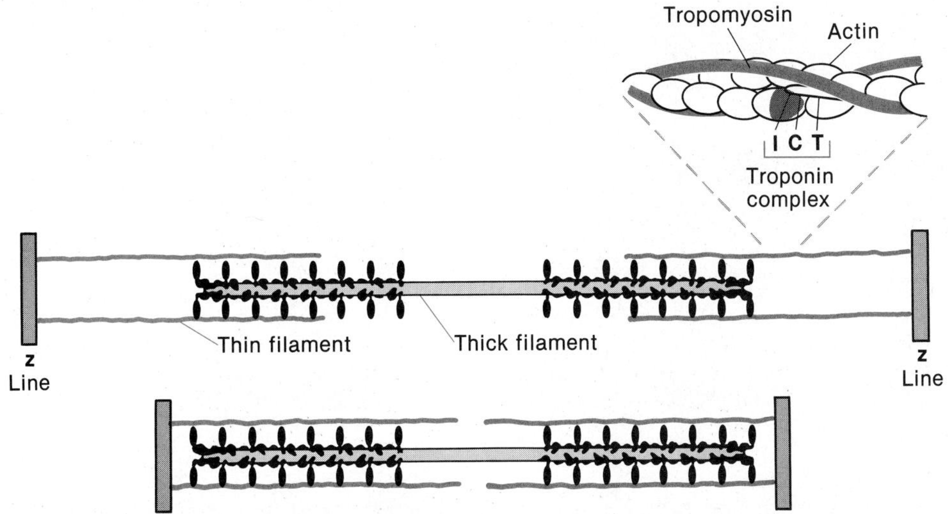

FIGURE 13–4. Schematic diagram of a single sarcomere of rabbit muscle showing the interdigitating thin (actin-containing) and thick (myosin-containing) filaments and how these filaments slide relative to one another during contraction. The expanded area (*upper right*) shows the arrangements of the regulatory proteins tropomyosin and troponin on the actin filaments. These proteins are present in a molar ratio of 1:1:7, respectively. Note that troponin is composed of 3 polypeptide subunits termed troponin I, troponin C and troponin T. Smooth muscles bear a distinct resemblance to skeletal muscles in that they also have interdigitating thick and thin filaments; however, the arrangement is not nearly so precise. The actin filaments in smooth muscle appear to be attached to dense bodies in the cytoplasm and in the membrane. Smooth muscle does not contain troponin. (From Adelstein, R. S., and Sellers, S. R.: Effects of calcium on vascular smooth muscle contraction. Am. J. Cardiol. *59:*4B, 1987.)

$[Na^+]$ and calcium $[Ca^{++}]$ concentrations. Cytoplasmic $[Ca^{++}]$ is of the order of 10^{-7} M; extracellular $[Ca^{++}]$ is 10^{-3} M.[18] Transmembrane ionic gradients are maintained by at least three systems in the sarcolemma, two of which require energy from ATP: (1) the Na^+-K^+ pump, which is an ATPase that exchanges intracellular Na^+ (Na^+_i) for extracellular K^+ (K^+_o); (2) the Na^+-Ca^{++} exchange, which normally extrudes intracellular calcium (Ca^{++}_i) for extracellular Na^+ (Na^+_o); and (3) an ATP-dependent pump that extrudes Ca^{++}_i. Voltage-sensitive ion channels mediate action potentials that are central to control excitation-contraction coupling.[19,20]

Near the Z lines the sarcolemma contains wide invaginations, the *T system,* which branch, both longitudinally and transversely, through the cell (Fig. 13–2). Closely coupled to but not continuous with the T system is the *sarcoplasmic reticulum* (SR),[21,22] a complex network of anastomosing, membrane-limited intracellular tubules, approximately 30 nm in diameter, which surrounds each myofibril and plays a critical role in excitation of the muscle.[23] Unlike the T system, the SR is not continuous with the extracellular space. Where the SR approaches the T tubules or the sarcolemma, it widens into flattened saclike enlargements (cisternae). At their junction, the SR and T tubules are separated by gaps of 10 to 12 nm.[4] In skeletal muscle, but probably not in the heart, depolarization of the sarcolemma may be channeled through the T system to release Ca^{++} from the SR, which mediates myofibrillar activa-

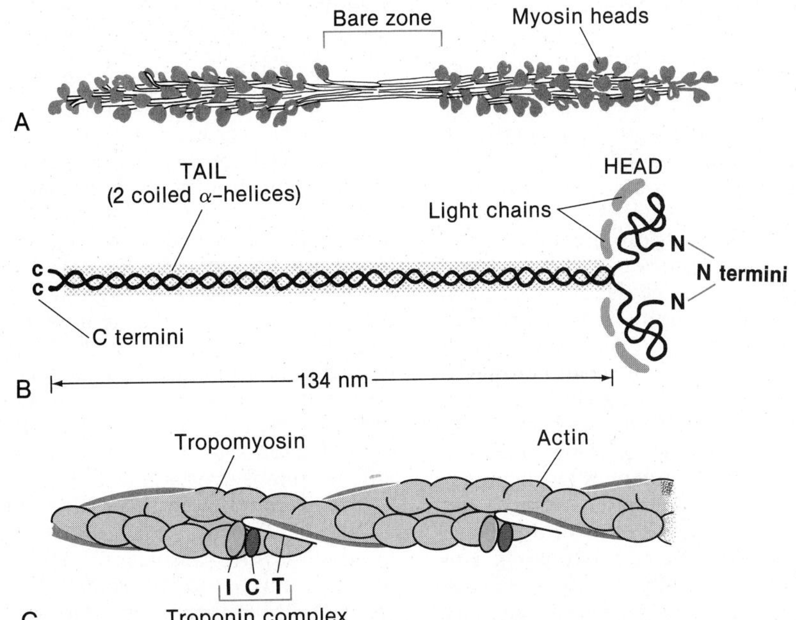

FIGURE 13–5. *A,* Schematic diagram of a myosin thick filament from skeletal muscle; *B,* schematic diagram of a myosin molecule showing the two heavy chains and four light chains of which it is composed. *C,* Schematic diagram of a muscle thin filament showing the position of tropomyosin and troponin along the actin filament. (From Pattison, C. W., Cumming, D.V.E., Clayton Jones, D. G., et al.: Variable adaptation of molecular mechanisms in relation to the use of autologous striated muscle to augment myocardial function. Cardiovasc. Res. *23:*593, 1989.)

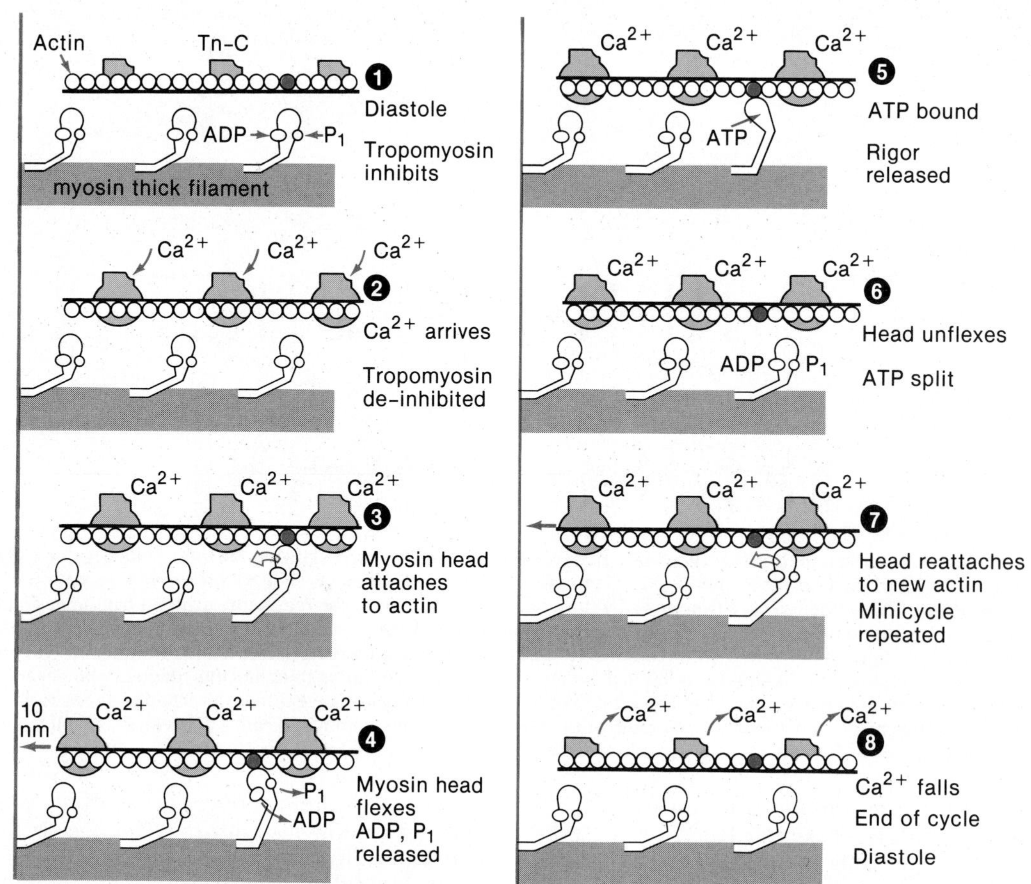

FIGURE 13-6. Contractile events in heart muscle. The cross-bridge cycle starts with relaxation in diastole (Step 1) when tropomyosin (Tm), the solid black horizontal line, "blocks" the myosin heads from binding to actin. At the start of systole (Step 2), Ca^{++} combines with troponin C (Tn-C) so that Tm no longer blocks the actin and so that myosin heads can bind and then "flex," whereupon ADP and inorganic phosphate (P_1) are released (Step 3). The "rigor state" develops transiently (Step 4). ATP moves in to the same binding site on the myosin head vacated by ADP, to "release" the myosin head (Step 5). After ATP has been split to ADP and P_1 by the myosin ATPase, the head extends (Step 6) to rebind to another actin 2 to 4 units "downstream" (Step 7). Steps 1 to 7 are repeated until [Ca^{++}] at the myofiber decreases at the start of diastole (Step 8). (From Opie, L.: The Heart, 2nd ed. New York, Raven Press, 1991, p. 184.)

tion (see below). Like the sarcolemma, the SR has a bilayer matrix consisting principally of phospholipids.

Contractile Proteins

The contractile apparatus consists of partially overlapping, rodlike myofilaments that are fixed in length, both at rest and during contraction (Figs. 13-1C and 13-4).[24,25]

MYOSIN. The thicker filaments, composed of myosin molecules, are limited to the A band, are about 100 to 150 nm in diameter with tapered ends, and measure 1.5 to 1.6 μ in length.[26] Each thick filament is composed of an orderly aggregation of 300 longitudinally stacked molecules of myosin proteins with a molecular weight of approximately 500,000 daltons, held parallel and in register by centrally located connections at the M line. A rodlike tail, approximately 130 nm in length, lies along the filament, and a globular bilobed head forms bridgelike outcroppings from the filament in groups of 3, each group 14.3 nm from the next. Thus, there are 50 such sets on each half of the thick filament, rotating so that a head appears in line every 43 nm. With activation of the muscle, these heads form attachments or cross bridges with actin filaments[27-32] to generate force and shortening (Fig. 13-5). Myosin by itself splits ATP; i.e., it acts as a weak ATPase that is activated by small amounts of Ca^{++}[33] and inhibited by Mg^{++}. When myosin combines with actin, an actomyosin complex is formed that is enzymatically even more active in its ability to split ATP and is stimulated primarily by Mg^{++}. The actomyosin ATPase constitutes the physiological enzyme in force development. The myosin molecule can be broken down by the proteolytic enzyme trypsin into two fragments, *light* and *heavy meromyosin*. The latter contains the bilobed globular heads and is the site of ATPase activity.[33]

Myosin itself can be separated into three isoenzyme components—V_1, V_2 and V_3—which have a different heavy-chain composition[34-36] (p. 1658). Only two chemically distinct heavy-chain subunits exist, α and β.[36] V_1 and V_3 comprise $\alpha\alpha$ and $\beta\beta$, respectively, while V_2 is a heterodimer, $\alpha\beta$. Myosin ATPase and intrinsic muscle speed (V_{max}) depend on the proportions of these isoenzymes that are present, V_1 being fast and V_3 being slow.[37-39] Hypertrophied heart muscle in small animal models has a lowered V_{max} and a greater proportion of V_3.[38] Similar shifts in the V_1/V_3 ratio also occur in experimental diabetes,[39] in altered thyroid states,[40] and with aging.[33] In humans, V_3 is normally the predominant isoenzyme.[41]

ACTIN. The thin filament, 1.0 μ in length and 55 nm in diameter, is a double alpha-helix consisting of two strands of actin with a molecular weight of 47,000 daltons.[26] Actin filaments course from the Z line through the I band and into the A band (Fig. 13-1C). The A band is the region of the sarcomere where there is overlapping of thick and thin filaments, while the I band contains only thin filaments. Polarity of actin determines the direction of the cross-bridge stroke when actin functions in the sarcomere.[27] Thin actin filaments from the opposite ends of the sarcomere inhibit cross-bridge formation when the thin filaments are double overlapped at short sarcomere lengths.[28]

TROPONIN AND TROPOMYOSIN. These are regulatory proteins that constitute about 10 per cent of total myofibrillar protein and are associated with the thin filament.[42,43] Tropomyosin is a rodlike protein, 400 nm in length and 20 to 30 nm in width, with a molecular weight of 70,000 daltons.[25] It comprises two helices, each of which lies slightly off the groove between the actin chains (Fig. 13–4*B*). Tropomyosin forms a continuing strand through the center of the thin filament, while the troponin complex is located at intervals of 365 nm. Troponin can be separated into three components[44]: (1) troponin C, a "calcium-sensitizing factor" that binds Ca^{++}[32]; (2) troponin I, an "inhibitory factor" that inhibits the Mg^{++}-stimulated ATPase of actomyosin; and (3) troponin T, which is necessary for the entire complex to function and serves to allow attachment of the troponin complex to actin and tropomyosin.

In the absence of troponin and tropomyosin, the contractile proteins actin and myosin interact and are fully activated, requiring the presence of only Mg^{++} and ATP to initiate the reaction leading to muscular contraction. When these two regulatory proteins are present, however, cross-bridge formation between myosin and actin is inhibited[43] (Fig. 13–6). In relaxed muscle, tropomyosin blocks the active sites of actin that react to form cross bridges with myosin. When Ca^{++} is bound to troponin C, the binding of troponin I to actin is inhibited, which in turn causes a conformational change in tropomyosin, so that the latter, instead of inhibiting, now enhances cross-bridge formation. Ca^{++} may thus be considered to be a "derepressor," since it inactivates an inhibitor of the reaction between actin and myosin. Inhibition of the interaction between actin and myosin is mediated by the ability of the Ca^{++}-troponin complex to alter the configuration of tropomyosin, which in turn changes the exposure of active sites all along the thin filaments.

With cellular depolarization, the myoplasmic [Ca^{++}] rises from 10^{-7} to about 10^{-5} M. Ca^{++} is bound to troponin, and the actin rods are drawn toward the center of the sarcomere.[31,32] Once each such cross-bridge "stroke" is completed, an attached myosin head ejects its ATP hydrolysis products, binds another ATP molecule, and detaches from the actin site. The myosin head then returns to its original orientation and the cycle is repeated, the head attaching to a different actin monomer farther along the thin filament (Fig. 13–6). Thus, shortening of cardiac muscle involves a relative change in position of these two sets of filaments; i.e., actin filaments are displaced by the force-generating process at many cross-bridge sites.[4] If the activated muscle is not permitted to shorten, i.e., during isometric contraction, the heavy meromyosin does not undergo a conformational change, the cross bridges between actin and myosin are maintained, and ADP rather than ATP remains bound to myosin.[31] The force that is developed is related to the quantity of Ca^{++} which is bound to troponin C, which in turn is related to the intracellular [Ca^{++}][18] and, as will be discussed further, the initial sarcomere length. Removal of Ca^{++} from troponin results in relaxation.

Smaller proteins, termed "light chains," are located on the heads of myosin and can be phosphorylated to produce changes in the enzymatic activity of myosin.[42] It has also been suggested that the actomyosin ATPase activity can be increased by increments in intracellular cyclic adenosine monophosphate (cyclic AMP),[46] a possible mechanism by which beta-adrenergic stimulation exerts a positive inotropic effect. Such a change would be consonant with the mechanical response of heart muscle to catecholamines to produce increments in the unloaded velocity of shortening ($\dot{V}_{max}$) (p. 364).

EXCITATION-CONTRACTION COUPLING: THE ROLE OF CALCIUM

In 1882, Ringer concluded that cardiac contraction depends on the presence of Ca^{++}[47] (Fig. 13–7). Heart muscle contains 2.5 mmol of Ca^{++} per liter of water, which is several hundred times higher than the concentration required for activation. However, the sarcoplasmic [Ca^{++}] within the relaxed cell is not directly available to initiate contraction but is bound to many structures, most notably the SR. Calcium triggers contraction by repressing troponin, the inhibitor of the actin-myosin interaction. The key event in the initiation of contraction then is the rise in sarcoplasmic [Ca^{++}].[19,22,48–50] Direct evidence for this in cardiac muscle was provided by Allen, Blinks, and Morgan, who used the photoprotein aequorin as an intracellular indicator of [Ca^{++}][51,52] (Fig. 13–8).

The source of activating Ca^{++} is not certain and may differ in the myocardium of different species.[55,55a] Extracellular Ca^{++}

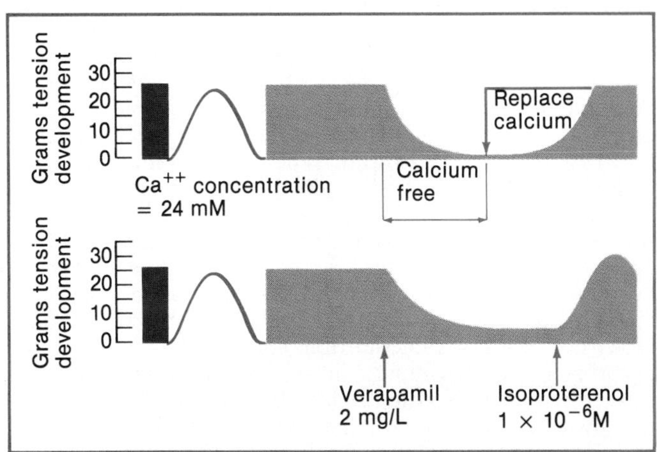

FIGURE 13–7. Diagram of effects on cardiac muscle contractility of altering extracellular Ca^{++} ion concentration (upper panel) or administration of calcium channel entry blocker (lower panel). Removal of Ca^{++} from extracellular fluid leads to rapid decrease in cardiac muscle force development by uncoupling the electrical event of membrane depolarizaton to the mechanical event of muscle shortening. Full contractility is restored on readmission of Ca^{++} ion to the extracellular environment. Lower panel illustrates action of a calcium channel entry blocker on cardiac muscle contractile activity in which there is dose-dependent decrease in inotropic activity. Reversal of negative-inotropic action of calcium entry blocker can be achieved by stimulation of cardiac beta-adrenoceptors, and the latter can alter contractile state by indirectly modulating the function of gating activity of the slow inward calcium channel. (From Lucchesi, B. R.: Role of calcium on excitation-contraction coupling in cardiac and vascular smooth muscle. Circulation *80*:IV1, 1989, by permission of the American Heart Association, Inc.)

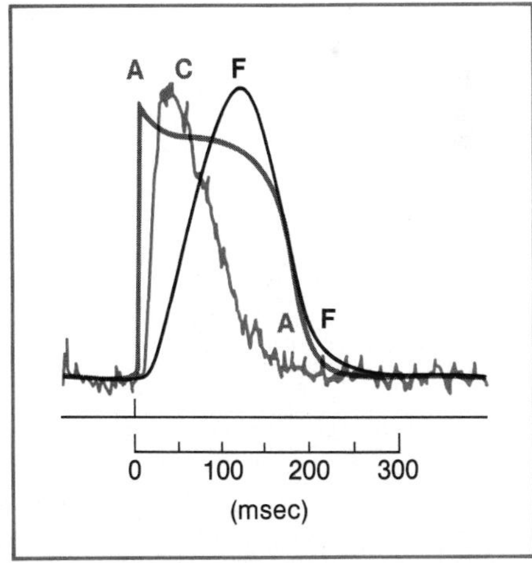

FIGURE 13–8. Schematic illustration of the approximate time course of excitation-activation-contraction coupling. The transients are the cell membrane action potential (A), the myoplasmic [Ca^{++}] as measured by the photoprotein aequorin (C), and myocardial force developed during an isometric contraction (F). Note the sequence of events: the action potential precedes the rise in myoplasmic free [Ca^{++}], which in turn precedes the onset of force development. The decline in myoplasmic [Ca^{++}] precedes the fall-off in force. Relationship between the time courses of the action potential, Ca^{++} transient, and developed tension in mammalian ventricular muscle. Schematic drawings: A, action potential; C, calcium transient (aequorin light signal); F, tension. (From Akera, T.: Pharmacological agents and myocardial calcium. *In* Langer, G. A. [ed.]: Calcium and the Heart, New York, Raven Press, 1990, p. 312.)

can enter via voltage-dependent gated "slow channels" (p. 361) or via a Na^+-Ca^{++} exchange mechanism.[19,20] Depolarization of the membrane caused by the upstroke of the action potential opens the ion channels that carry the inward Ca^{++} current.[53,54] During the plateau of the action potential, Ca^{++} that flows into the cell through the Ca^{++} channels does not activate the contractile system directly but appears to trigger a subsequent release of the large stores of Ca^{++} in the SR, a process termed "calcium-induced calcium release."[55–58] The Ca^{++} that actually activates the contractile system appears to be stored in the cisternae of the SR, which have the capacity to bind Ca^{++} actively and to store it in a bound form within their lumina.[49,50] Ca^{++} is released from a store, SR_1 (the terminal cisternae of the SR), into the cytoplasm. The amount of Ca^{++} release is graded according to the rate of rise and magnitude of the inward Ca^{++} current, larger and faster current transients causing more Ca^{++} release. Ca^{++} binding by troponin molecules results in contractile activity; relaxation is brought about by the active uptake of Ca^{++} into the temporary store, SR_2 (area of the SR adjacent to the contractile proteins), and from there the Ca^{++} eventually returns to SR_1. Thus SR_1 is considered to be a labile store, the Ca^{++} content of which determines the inotropic state of the muscle.[58,60]

The Ca^{++} current in cardiac fibers reaches its peak rapidly and then slowly decays. Fabiato[48] used repeated microinjection-aspiration sequences to simulate the time course of the Ca^{++} current in cardiac fibers from which the sarcolemma had been removed (skinned fibers). This technique mimicked the changes in cytoplasmic $[Ca^{++}]$ that would be produced by the native Ca^{++} current in fibers with intact sarcolemmas. The initial fast component of the simulated Ca^{++} current triggered a tension transient caused by Ca^{++}-induced release of Ca^{++} from the SR. In contrast, the subsequent slow component of decay of the simulated Ca^{++} current did not affect the first tension transient provoked by the fast component but did potentiate the subsequent tension transients.

Thus, the fast initial component of the Ca^{++} current triggers release of Ca^{++}, whereas the slow component loads the SR with Ca^{++} that becomes available for release during subsequent beats.[60,61] The extent of contraction can be directly related to the amplitude of the inward calcium current. The precise mechanism by which Ca^{++} is released by the SR is uncertain, although Na^+ influx may play an important role.[62] One suggestion is that the rise in cytoplasmic Ca^{++} activates a channel in the membrane of the SR that permits Ca^{++} efflux.[58,59] The Ca^{++} release channels in the SR bind ryanodine, which inhibits this action.

Studies with the calcium-sensitive photoprotein aequorin and more recently with the calcium-sensitive dyes Fura-2 and Indo have shown that changes in the rate or pattern of stimulation of heart muscle, in extracellular $[Ca^{++}]$, and in catecholamines all produce increases in cytoplasmic $[Ca^{++}]$[51,52,63,64] (Fig. 13–9). Catecholamines differ from the other inotropic interventions in that they produce a smaller increase in tension than would be expected from the increase in the cytoplasmic $[Ca^{++}]$, presumably by reducing the sensitivity of the contractile system to Ca^{++}. This decrease in sensitivity may result from an increase in the degree of phosphorylation of a serine residue on troponin I that is brought about by the cyclic AMP–induced activation of a protein kinase, but this is controversial.[65]

THE CARDIAC ACTION POTENTIAL. As presented in detail on pages 592 to 603 and in Figure 22–11, p. 595, the action potential for cardiac cells is generated by a sequence of voltage- and time-dependent changes in the permeability of the sarcolemma to ions.[66] The action potential of ventricular myocardium has three phases: (1) a rapidly rising upstroke (phase 0), generated by a large inward Na^+ current; (2) a plateau (phase 2) caused by a balance between inward Ca^{++} and outward K^+ currents; and (3) a repolarization (phase 3) due to an outward K^+ current.[67,68] The Ca^{++} channels that open during the plateau are blocked by the organic Ca^{++} antagonists such as verapamil, nifedipine, diltiazem, and their analogs[67–73] (p. 362) and by manganese ion, lanthanum ion, and acidosis; additional Ca^{++} channels are recruited by beta-adrenergic stimulation.[67]

The major portion of the Ca^{++} that activates the contractile proteins is stored within the cell, largely in the SR, in its subsarcolemmal cisternae, and on the inner surface of the sarcolemma itself.[74] This Ca^{++} diffuses toward the myofibrils and binds to troponin, which, together with tropomyosin (but in the absence of Ca^{++}), prevents the interaction between heavy

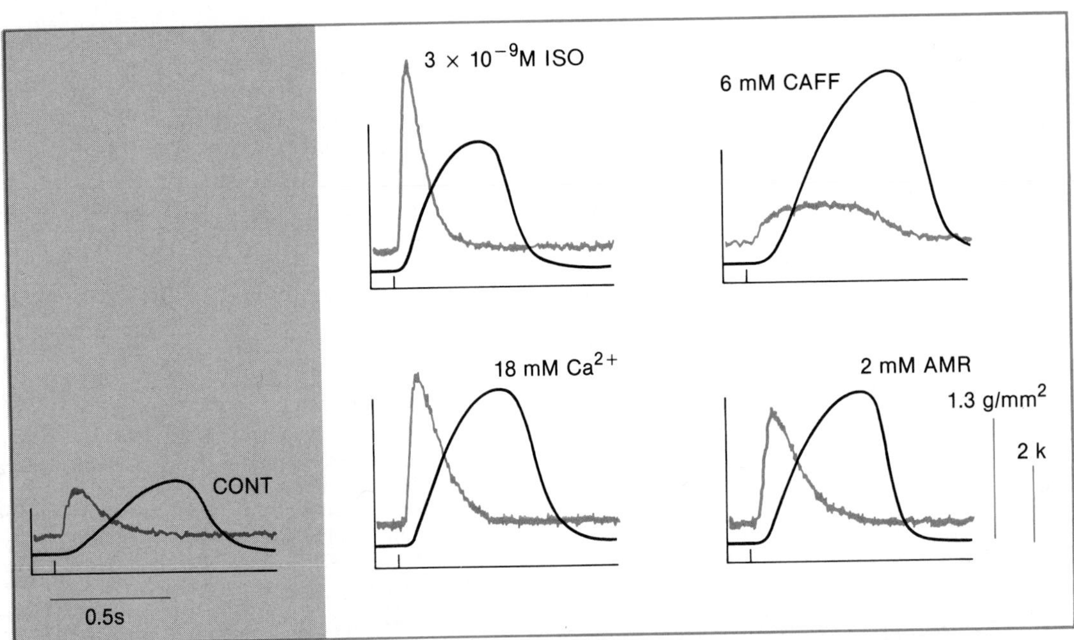

FIGURE 13–9. Comparative effects of agents producing response patterns I through IV in an isometric cat papillary muscle preparation. The red, noisy trace in each panel is the aequorin signal, and the black, smooth trace is the tension trace. Each trace represents 64 averaged responses at 4-second intervals of stimulation; temperature was 38° C. CONT = control; ISO = isoproterenol; CAFF = caffeine; AMR = amrinone. (From Morgan, J. P., and Morgan, K. G.: Calcium and cardiovascular function: Intracellular calcium levels during contraction and relaxation of mammalian cardiac and vascular smooth muscle as detected with aequorin. Am. J. Med. *77*:5A:33, 1984.)

meromyosin and actin. The number of contractile sites activated and therefore the force generated are directly related to the quantity of Ca^{++} present in the vicinity of the myofibrils, which in turn ultimately depends on the influx of Ca^{++} that accompanied the action potential, and the binding affinity of troponin for Ca^{++}.[75] This influx of Ca^{++}, in turn, is a function of the extracellular [Ca^{++}], the duration of the action potential, and the number of action potentials per unit time.

The total Ca^{++} within the myocyte available for activation is related to the amount of Ca^{++} that enters the cell across the sarcolemma.[74-79] During the plateau of the action potential (phase 2), there are two known mechanisms for calcium entry: (1) Ca^{++} influx via the inward voltage-dependent Ca^{++} channel, and (2) Ca^{++} influx via electrogenic Na^+-Ca^{++} exchange, wherein 3 Na^+ leave the cell for each Ca^{++} entry.

SODIUM-CALCIUM EXCHANGE. The activity of the Na^+-Ca^{++} exchange is closely linked to the Na^+-K^+ pump because the transmembrane electrochemical gradient of Na^+ provides the energy needed for Na^+-Ca^{++} exchange.[63a,63b] The electrochemical gradient for Na^+, in turn, is maintained by the Na^+-K^+ pump. Therefore, interventions that inhibit the Na^+-K^+ pump, such as digitalis glycosides or low K^+, alter the function of the Na^+-Ca^{++} exchange (Fig. 17–11, p. 481). Under such conditions intracellular Na^+ uses a charge that causes the Na^+-Ca^{++} exchange to extrude less Ca^{++} leading to an increased intracellular Ca^{++} and a positive inotropic effect.

CARDIAC RELAXATION. This results predominantly from a cessation of the inward slow Ca^{++} current coupled with the uptake and storage of Ca^{++} by the SR. Embedded in the latter is a 100,000-dalton membrane-bound protein, phospholamban, which spans the lipid bilayer. This protein, a Ca^{++}-stimulated Mg-ATPase, has a very high affinity for Ca^{++} and is responsible for the active transport of Ca^{++} from the cytoplasm into the lumen of the SR. Thus, during repolarization, the SR in the presence of ATP avidly accumulates myoplasmic Ca^{++} against a concentration gradient, so that intracellular [Ca^{++}] falls to 5 to 100×10^{-7} M and Ca^{++} detaches from the troponin, resulting in inhibition of the interactions between actin and myosin and hence in relaxation.[68] Further, the process of shortening itself reduces Ca^{++} binding to the contractile protein (troponin C).[80,81]

INOTROPIC EFFECTS AND CALCIUM KINETICS. There is evidence that (1) the total tension developed, (2) the rate of tension development, and (3) the rate of tension decline during relaxation are related, respectively, to (1) the quantity of Ca^{++} available for binding to troponin, (2) the rate of Ca^{++} delivery to troponin, and (3) the rate at which Ca^{++} is removed from troponin.[67,80] The extent of Ca^{++} binding to troponin also depends on muscle length as discussed on p. 368. Many interventions that augment or depress the contractile state of heart muscle are associated with—and indeed are caused by—alterations in Ca^{++} movement and concentrations in heart muscle[68] (Fig. 13–10). These include: (1) the force-frequency relation,[82] i.e., the increase in contractility resulting from an increase in the frequency of contraction,[83,84]; (2) postextrasystolic potentiation (a special instance of the force-frequency relation);[85-87] and (3) pharmacological agents such as the cardiac glycosides (p. 479), sympathomimetic amines[88,89] (p. 500), and phosphodiesterase inhibitors[88]—all of which improve contractility—and agents such as beta-adrenoceptor blockers, Ca^{++} antagonists, quinidine and other Type I antiarrhythmic agents, and barbiturates—all of which depress it.

In skinned cardiac cells, even moderate acidosis causes reductions in the quantity of Ca^{++} released from the SR of cardiac muscle,[90] and of Ca^{++} binding by troponin,[90-92] accounting in part for its negative inotropic effect. Hypo- and hyperthyroidism are associated with either slowed or accelerated contraction. Hypothyroidism is associated with slowed release and uptake of Ca^{++},[93] whereas hyperthyroidism has the opposite action. In experimental animals, hypothyroidism is also associated with synthesis of slower myosin isoenzymes, whereas hyperthyroidism is associated with synthesis of faster myosin isoenzymes.[93,94] Studies on Ca^{++} transients in

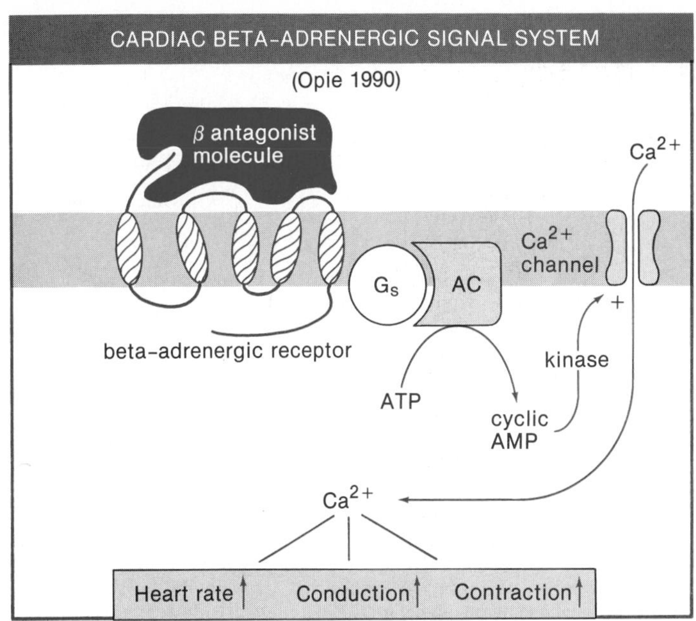

FIGURE 13–10. The cardiac beta-adrenoceptor and signaling system. The beta-antagonist molecule interacts with the beta-receptor, whose molecular structure recently has been revealed and its amino acid sequence characterized. In the presence of the stimulatory form the G protein (Gs), adenylate cyclase (AC) converts ATP to cyclic AMP, which, acting via a protein kinase, enhances phosphorylation of the calcium channel and permits more calcium to enter through the calcium channel during voltage-induced depolarization. Such calcium releases much more calcium from the sarcoplasmic reticulum (calcium-induced calcium release) to increase cytosolic calcium, heart rate, conduction and contraction, as well as the rate of relaxation (the latter of phosphorylation of the protein phospholamban in the sarcoplasmic reticulum). (From Opie, L. H., Sonnenblick, E. H., Kaplan, N. M., and Thadani, U: β-Blocking Agents. *In* Opie, L. H. [ed.]: Drugs for the Heart. 3rd ed. Philadelphia, W.B. Saunders Co., 1991, p. 3.)

the intact heart with rate, catecholamines, and caffeine confirm these general conclusions.[95]

ACTION OF BETA-ADRENOCEPTOR AGONISTS ON CALCIUM. Sympathomimetic amines, as shown in Figure 13–10, are thought to act on beta receptors on the cardiac sarcolemma.[96-99] This leads to the activation of a membrane-bound enzyme, adenylate cyclase, that catalyzes the production of cyclic AMP from ATP in the presence of Ca^{++}. The action of adenylate cyclase is modulated by both inhibitory and stimulatory subunits of guanine nucleotide-binding regulatory proteins (G proteins) (Figs. 13–11 and 13–12), which are heterodimer proteins in the cell membrane modulated by guanine nucleotides (e.g., guanosine triphosphate).[98-102] The stimulating subunit is inactive as a heterodimer, but in the presence of a guanine nucleotide, the stimulating subunit dissociates from its "repressor" subunit to activate adenyl cyclase. Multiple receptors on the sarcolemma can interact with these G proteins. The beta-adrenoceptor with a molecular weight of 60,000 to 69,000 dissociates when a $beta_1$-agonist occupies the receptor in the presence of a guanine nucleotide (Fig. 13–9).[103] When activated in this manner, this stimulatory subunit interacts with adenylate cyclase to increase its activity.

CYCLIC AMP, THE SECOND MESSENGER. Cyclic AMP, in turn, activates a class of enzymes, the cyclic AMP–dependent protein kinases, which phosphorylate a number of intracellular proteins.[104-106] This results in an increase in the transsarcolemmal influx of Ca^{++} through the voltage-dependent Ca^{++} current[73,100,107] channels (Fig. 13–10). At the same time, activity of the SR is enhanced, as characterized by accelerated release and more rapid uptake of Ca^{++}.[108] Activation of a protein kinase by an increase in cyclic AMP resulting from beta-adrenergic stimulation may induce phosphorylation of a protein located near the Ca^{++} channel and thus enhance its open state. Such Ca^{++} channels, which are recruited by beta-

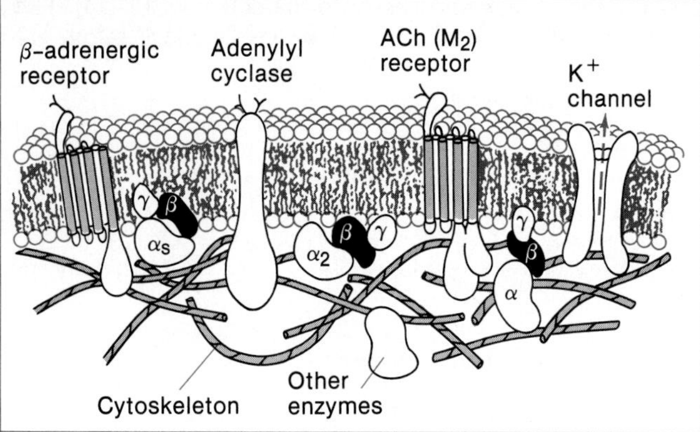

FIGURE 13-11. Schematic view of the organization of receptors, G proteins, and effectors in the plasma membrane. All receptors so far isolated are transmembrane glycoproteins. Receptors that work through the G proteins such as rhodopsin, beta-adrenergic receptors, and muscarinic receptors have a similar structure that appears to include seven transmembrane helices and regions of homology in the cytoplasmic loop. Adenylyl cyclase is a transmembrane glycosylated enzyme whose active site is on the cytoplasmic side of the membrane. The structure of the muscarinic K^+ channel is not yet known, although other ion channels are complex multimeric proteins. Three possible arrangements of α and $\beta\gamma$ subunits are illustrated. The α and/or $\beta\gamma$ subunits may interact with the cytoskeleton (From Neer, E. J., and Clapham, D. E.: Roles of G protein subunits in transmembrane signalling. Nature *333*:129, 1988.)

adrenergic agonists, are termed "receptor-operated channels." Another protein in the membrane of the SR, phospholamban, when phosphorylated by cyclic AMP-dependent protein kinase, stimulates the rate of Ca^{++} uptake by increasing the ATP-dependent calcium pump in the SR.[104] There is also some evidence that beta-adrenergic agonists decrease the sensitivity of the contractile system to Ca^{++} as a consequence of phosphorylation of troponin-I by a cyclic AMP-activated protein kinase.[89] The reactions resulting from myocardial beta-receptor stimulation increase the rate of Ca^{++} transport by the SR, which in turn is responsible for both enhancement of tension development and an increased rate of relaxation.

In *summary*, beta-adrenergic agonists augment Ca^{++} influx across the sarcolemma by recruiting additional voltage-dependent Ca^{++} channels. These agonists do not appear to affect the *rate* at which the Ca^{++} channels open but rather they increase the *number* of open channels.[67] The increase in the

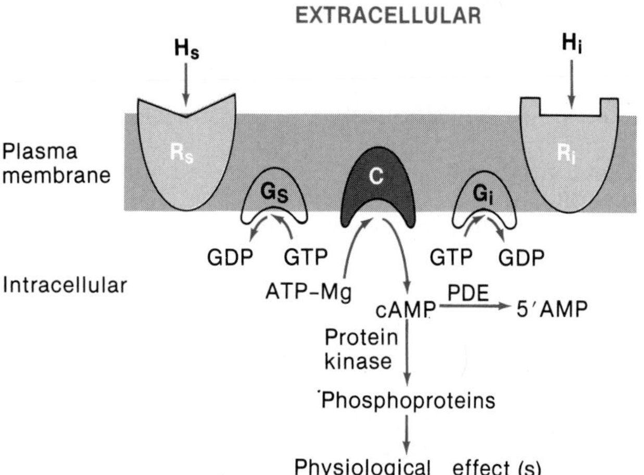

FIGURE 13-12. Schematic outline of the adenylate cyclase-G protein-cyclic AMP system. H_2 and H_1 denote stimulatory and inhibitory agents, respectively; R_s and R_i stimulatory and inhibitory receptors; and G_s and G_i the stimulatory and inhibitory guanine nucleotide-binding proteins. C = the catalytic unit of adenyate cyclase; PDE = phosphodiesterase; cAMP = cyclic AMP. (Reprinted by permission from Spiegel, A. M., Gierschik, P., Levine, M. A., and Downs, R. W., Jr.: Clinical implications of guanine nucleotide-binding proteins as receptor-effector couplers. N. Engl. J. Med. *312*:26, 1985.)

rate of relaxation of tension produced by cyclic AMP appears to be caused by enhancement of Ca^{++} accumulation by the SR[109] and a secondary effect of decreased sensitivity of the myofilament to Ca^{++}, as discussed below. Theophylline and related xanthines inhibit phosphodiesterase, an enzyme responsible for the breakdown of cyclic AMP, which has an effect similar to that of catecholamines. In addition, xanthines may increase the sensitivity of the contractile system to a given amount of Ca^{++}.[51]

Another cyclic nucleotide, *cyclic 3′,5′-guanosine monophosphate* (GMP), has been identified in the myocardium. The reduction of the contractile state induced by acetylcholine is accompanied by significant increases in cyclic GMP, which appears to mediate effects opposing those of cyclic AMP by stimulating an inhibitory G protein.[103,110,111]

CONTROL OF CYTOPLASMIC [Ca^{++}]: A SUMMARY. As already indicated, cytoplasmic [Ca^{++}] is critical to the contractile state of the heart. Therefore, it is useful to recapitulate the determinants of myoplasmic [Ca^{++}].[70] At least seven mechanisms have been identified, and these are shown diagrammatically in Figure 13-13.

1. The inward movement of Ca^{++} along its concentration gradient, across the sarcolema, i.e., the slow inward current through the Ca^{++} channels (Fig. 13-13, Mechanism 1A and 1B).[61,95] Ca^{++} antagonists (and agonists) act at these sites.[73]
2. Since small quantities of Ca^{++} enter the cardiac cell with each contraction, there must be some mechanism to restore Ca^{++} to its normal diastolic level. A bidirectional Na^+-Ca^{++} exchange system mediates Ca^{++} movement across the sarcolemma.[68] Energy required by this system for moving Ca^{++} out of the cell against a concentration gradient may be provided by the downhill movement of Na^+ into the cell along its electrochemical gradient. The direction of this exchange depends upon the relative concentrations of extracellular and intracellular Na^+ and Ca^{++}. Thus, when cardiac glycosides inhibit Na^+, K^+-ATPase and thereby inhibit the pump responsible for Na^+-K^+ exchange (Fig. 13-13, Mechanism 2A), intracellular [Na^+] is elevated. Ca^{++} enters the cell as a consequence of Na^+-Ca^{++} exchange, and this brings about a positive inotropic effect.[113,114] Prolongation of depolarization will decrease Ca^{++} extrusion.
3. The sarcolemma possesses a Ca^{++}-ATPase that extrudes Ca^{++} from the cell in an energy-requiring process (Fig. 13-13, Mechanism 3).[19,115]
4. A Ca^{++}-stimulated Mg-ATPase in the membrane of the SR (Fig. 13-13, Mechanism 4) transports Ca^{++} into the lumen of the SR and sequesters it there through an energy-requiring process.[104]
5. Ca^{++} can also be taken up and released by other intracellular structures, particularly the mitochondria (Fig. 13-13, Mechanism 5), and by the internal aspect of the sarcolemma. When intracellular [Ca^{++}] rises, ATP, generated by the mitochondria, is involved in the uptake of Ca^{++} by these organelles; excess uptake of mitochondrial Ca^{++} in turn interferes with mitochondrial function.[116] This mechanism is relatively slow and its relation to activating Ca^{++} is unclear.
6. A variety of ionophores can effect the selective movement of Ca^{++} along its concentration gradient directly across the sarcolemma, i.e., not through the slow channels (Fig. 13-13, Mechanism 6).
7. The buffering of Ca^{++} by intracellular proteins such as calmodulin, troponin C, and myosin-P light chains also regulates myoplasmic [Ca^{++}].

Since cardiac contraction and relaxation are critically dependent on precisely timed modulations of cytoplasmic [Ca^{++}], it is evident that abnormalities of any of the systems just described can affect myocardial performance.[68]

While an increase in the cytoplasmic [Ca^{++}] is necessary to activate contraction in myocardial cells and the force of contraction is modulated by the cytoplasmic [Ca^{++}], when [Ca^{++}] increases above a certain level, muscle function deteriorates. This excessive increase in myoplasmic Ca^{++} has been called

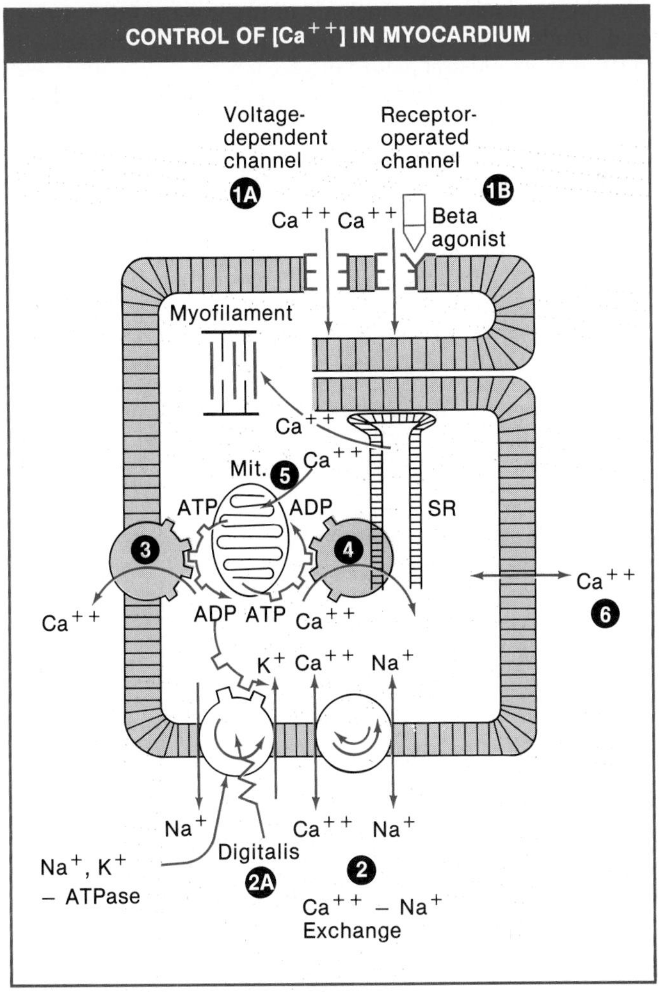

CONTROL OF [Ca^{++}] IN MYOCARDIUM

FIGURE 13–13. Determinants of [Ca^{++}] in myocardium. Numbers in circles denote the mechanisms affecting intracellular [Ca^{++}] described in the text. SR = sarcoplasmic reticulum; Mit = mitochondrion. (Reprinted by permission, Braunwald, E.: Mechanisms of action of calcium channel blocking agents. N. Engl. J. Med. *307*:1618, 1982.)

"calcium overload." For example, in skinned cardiac cells under certain conditions the level of tension development decreases when the myoplasmic [Ca^{++}] is raised above pCa 5.5 and increasing free [Ca^{++}] above the optimal level can inactivate Ca^{++}-induced release of Ca^{++}.[58] Digitalis intoxication can be associated with a decrease in force to values below the control level.[117] Another important pathophysiological consequence of raising cytoplasmic [Ca^{++}] beyond a certain level is the development of spontaneous mechanical and electrical oscillations, which could lead to arrhythmias through the development of delayed afterdepolarizations and triggered activity (p. 605). Suboptimal amounts of activating Ca^{++} may be associated with depressed myocardial contractility in some pathological states (p. 397).

CALCIUM CHANNELS

Increasing information is being acquired about the structure of ion channels in the sarcolemma.[20] This should provide insight into the structural basis for the ionic selectivity of transmembrane channels (Fig. 13–14). The channels have intracellular voltage sensors, i.e., charged regions of the channel proteins that determine the state of channel "gates" as open or shut.[118]

VOLTAGE-DEPENDENT CHANNELS. When a propagated wave of depolarization approaches the membrane region containing the Ca^{++} channel, a reduction of membrane potential (i.e., a decrease in the electronegativity of the cell interior) causes the activation gate to open, permitting Ca^{++} to cross the membrane and pass into the cell (Fig. 13–14). The gate closes when the interior of the cell has again become electronegative, i.e., when the resting level of transmembrane potential has been restored. Since the movement of Ca^{++} through these channels is controlled by electrical potentials, they have been termed *voltage-dependent channels* (Fig. 13–13, Mechanism 1A).

RECEPTOR-OPERATED CHANNELS. Many Ca^{++} channels are also sensitive to control by sarcolemmal receptors. $Beta_1$-agonists in cardiac muscle (and alpha-adrenoceptor agonists in vascular smooth muscle and to a lesser extent in heart muscle) increase Ca^{++} influx via the inward Ca^{++} current, thereby enhancing contractility in the case of $beta_1$ receptors in heart muscle, and the degree of contraction of arterioles in the case of alpha receptors on vascular smooth muscle. Activation of adrenoceptors appears to recruit an additional number of active channels and does not appear to increase Ca^{++} influx by increasing the size of the Ca^{++} channels nor the rates at which their gates open or close.[119,120] The transfer of charge of phosphate groups from ATP to the calcium channel produces a change in the channel's molecular configuration that increases the likelihood that it will open during depolarization. It has been proposed that when endogenous adrenergic nervous activity is low or is blocked by an adrenoceptor blocker, a certain proportion of the Ca^{++} channels is unable to open in response to a depolarizing stimulus. According to this theory, physiological stimuli or drugs that activate adrenoceptors elevate cyclic AMP levels in the myocardium. The latter in turn facilitates transfer of a phosphate in ATP to form a phosphoester bond with one of the proteins in

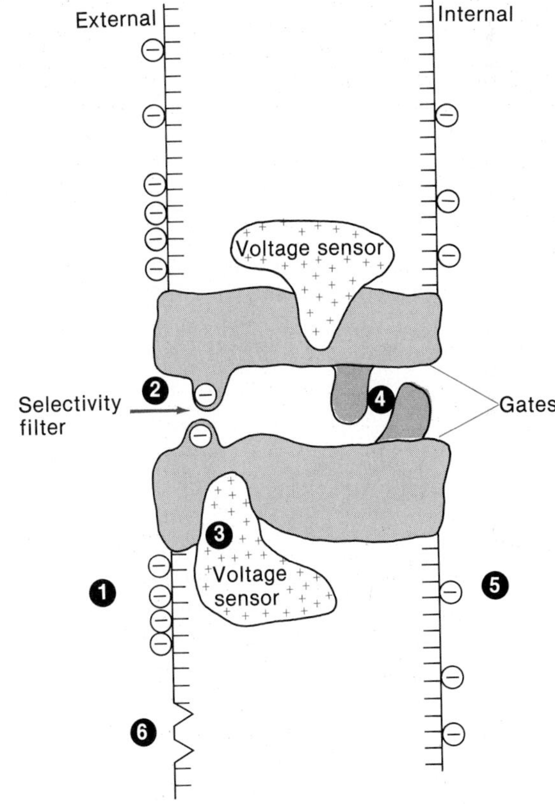

FIGURE 13–14. A calcium channel depicted as a membrane pore containing within it a negatively charged site (2) of dimensions and charge density appropriate to act as a "selectivity filter" to distinguish between different cations. Voltage sensor components (3) confer voltage dependence on channel opening and closing, and channel gates (4) determine the open or shut character of the channel. Negatively charged sites on the external (1) and internal (5) membrane surfaces serve as cation binding sites, particularly for divalent cations, by which transmembrane potential detected by voltage sensor components may be modulated. A receptor site (6) is shown adjacent to the channel. (From Triggle, D. J.: *In* Flaim, S. F., and Zelis, R. [eds.]: Calcium Channel Blockers: Mechanism of Action and Clinical Applications. Baltimore, Urban and Schwarzenberg, 1982.)

an inactive Ca^{++} channel, permitting the channel to participate in Ca^{++} entry into the cell. As a consequence, adrenergic influences increase Ca^{++} influx across the sarcolemma; the channels acted upon by receptor-mediated events are termed receptor-operated channels (Fig. 13–13, Mechanism 1B).

CALCIUM ANTAGONISTS

(See also pp. 1172 to 1173)

A number of inorganic cations such as manganese, cobalt, and lanthanum can function as general Ca^{++} antagonists and are effective in blocking a wide variety of Ca^{++}-dependent processes.[118] This nonselectivity of action probably arises from the ability of these cations to block directly the channels for Ca^{++} entry into the cell.[67,115] Of far more significance to clinical medicine are the organic Ca^{++} agonists. The pioneering work of Fleckenstein[121] revealed that these compounds can produce selective blockade of the inward Ca^{++} current and produce electromechanical uncoupling primarily in heart and vascular smooth muscle.

Since organic Ca^{++} antagonists exert their actions at nanomolar concentrations and exhibit stereospecificity, it appears likely that they are recognized by specific structures of the Ca^{++} channel[69,70,121–124] (Figs. 13–15 and 13–16). However, the diversity of molecular structures of Ca^{++} antagonists is consistent with differing modes and sites of action[118] rather than with the tight binding of these drugs to a specific receptor, analogous to the receptor that binds beta-adrenoceptor blockers.[122]

The action of dihydropiridine Ca^{++} antagonists such as nifedipine is consistent with the drug actually "plugging" Ca^{++} channels and decreasing the number of functional Ca^{++} channels that open[70] (Fig. 13–17). In contrast, verapamil, and to a lesser extent diltiazem, are "use-dependent"; i.e., their Ca^{++}-blocking activities are a function of the frequency of contrac-

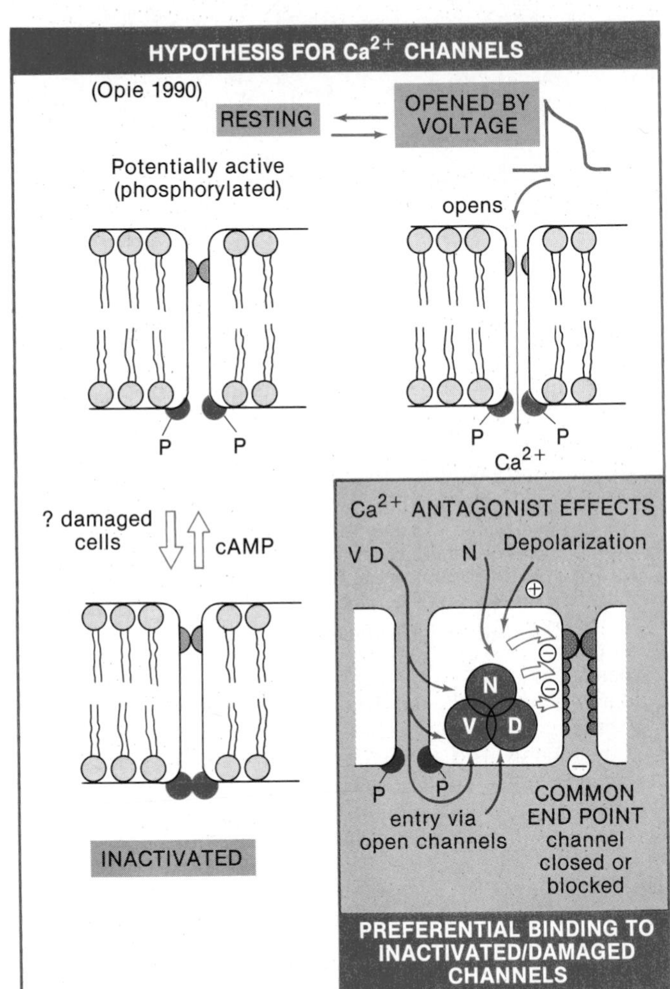

FIGURE 13–15. Postulated arrangement of calcium channel, modified from Sperelakis[1] and Bean et al.[2] Note the proposed role for phosphorylation (P) of Ca channel in changing inoperative channels to operative channels. Operative channels can change from the resting (*top left*) to the activated state (*top right*) in which the depolarization of the cell membrane has opened the outer (activation) gate and Ca^{++} enters the cell and then reverts spontaneously to the inactivated state (*bottom left*) when the inner (inactivation) gate is closed. During recovery, i.e., repolarization, the activation gate closes and the inactivation gate opens, returning the channel to the resting state and once again available for activation (*top left*). It is postulated that beta-adrenergic stimulation acts by its second messenger cyclic AMP (cAMP) to transfer charged phosphate groups (P) from ATP to the Ca channel so that there is a molecular change which allows a greater probability of the channels being open during depolarization. Ca^{++} antagonists interfere with the passage of Ca^{++} through the channel by causing a change in molecular configuration of the channel and/or gates (*bottom right*). N = nifedipine binding site; V = verapamil binding site; D = diltiazem binding site. (From Opie, L: Drugs for the Heart. 3rd ed. Grune & Stratton, 1990, p. 43.)

[1]Sperelakis, N.: *In* Opie, L. H. (ed.): Antagonists and Cardiovascular Disease. New York, Raven Press, 1984, pp. 277–291.

[2]Bean, B. P., et al.: Beta-adrenergic modulation of calcium channels in frog ventricular heart cells. Nature *307*:371, 1984.

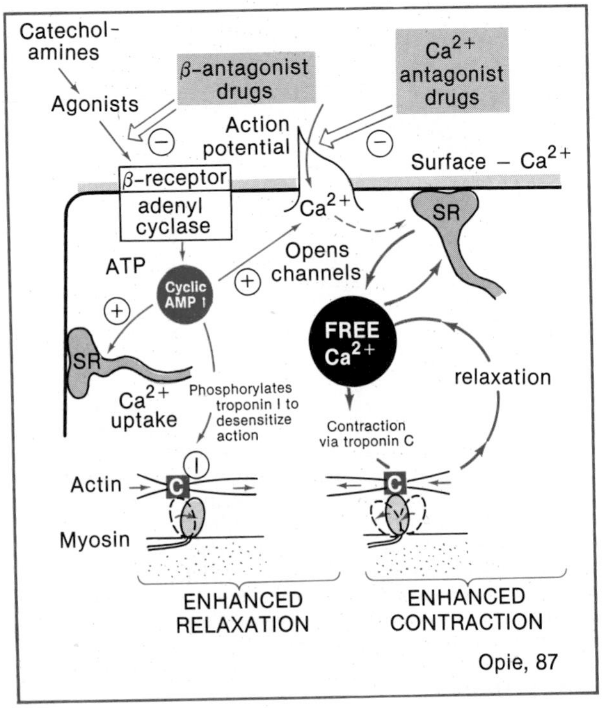

FIGURE 13–16. Schematic representation of different intracellular effects of calcium antagonists vs. beta-antagonist drugs inhibiting formation of cyclic AMP with consequent effects on all aspects of intracellular calcium ion movements (calcium ion entry, calcium ion uptake into the SR, and contraction-relaxation cycle). Calcium antagonist drugs act on only one of these aspects, namely, calcium ion entry. (From Opie, L. H.: Clinical Use of Calcium Channel Antagonist Drugs. 2nd ed. Boston, Kluwer, 1990, p. 38.)

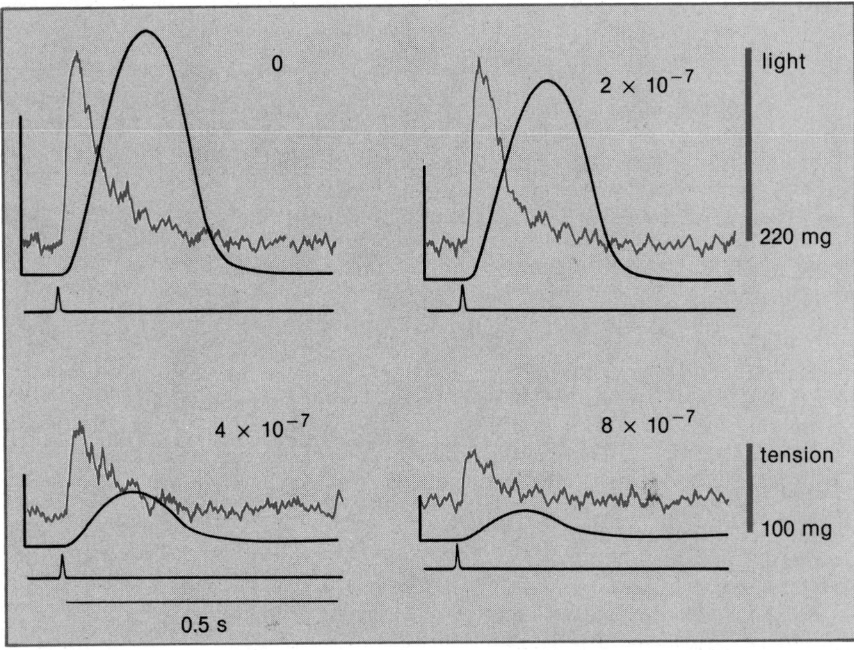

FIGURE 13–17. Effects of nifedipine on the Ca^{++} transient (red) and developed tension (black) in a cat papillary muscle. Ca^{++} concentration was estimated from aequorin light signal. Tension, in milligrams. Lower trace, Stimulus artifact. Numbers indicate molar concentrations of nifedipine. Note that nifedipine reduces the light signal and tension development is unchanged. (From Akera, T.: Pharmacological agents and myocardial calcium. *In* Langer, G. A. [ed.]: Calcium and the Heart. New York, Raven Press, 1990, p. 324.)

tion so that they cause an inversion of the myocardium's normal force-frequency relationship, an increase in contraction frequency reducing rather than increasing contraction.[122] This situation is analogous to the better-investigated, frequency-dependent inhibition of Na^+ channels by local anesthetics and Type I antiarrhythmic drugs and suggests that verapamil interacts preferentially with the depolarized, inactivated state of the Ca^{++} channel.

The clinical use of calcium antagonists is discussed on pp. 1310–1314 and 1238.

CARDIAC ADRENOCEPTORS

In 1948, Ahlquist introduced the concept of dual receptors, alpha and beta adrenoreceptors, and in 1967 Lands et al. demonstrated that beta-adrenoceptors could be further divided into two subtypes: $beta_1$ receptors, which mediate cardiac stimulation and lipolysis, and $beta_2$ receptors, which mediate relaxation of vascular and bronchial smooth muscle.[125,126] The effects of catecholamines on the contractile and electrical properties of the heart are mediated predominantly by the beta-adrenoceptors, embedded in the sarcolemma (Fig. 17–9, p. 480). As determined by physiological and radioligand-binding studies, the large majority of myocardial beta receptors are of the $beta_1$ subtype; likewise, the inotropic effects of beta-adrenoceptor agonists are mediated predominantly, if not exclusively, by $beta_1$ receptors.[101,127,128] However, chronotropy, i.e., sinoatrial rate, may be mediated by $beta_2$ receptors located in the sinoatrial node.[130] $Beta_1$-adrenoceptors are located on effector cells in proximity to adrenergic synapses, while $beta_2$ receptors are located at some distance from the synapses.[131] $Beta_1$ receptors appear to respond primarily to neuronally released norepinephrine, whereas $beta_2$ receptors respond preferentially to circulating epinephrine from the adrenal medulla (and to exogenously injected beta antagonists). Also, as in the case of alpha-adrenoceptors, beta-adrenoceptors located presynaptically on the nerve fiber regulate norepinephrine release. However, as opposed to presynaptic alpha receptors,[23] which have an inhibitory role, stimulation of presynaptic beta receptors produces release of norepinephrine.[132] Whereas ventricular receptors are exclusively $beta_1$,[133] approximately 25 per cent of atrial receptors are $beta_2$, presumably located within the sinoatrial node, and contribute to mediating the chronotropic effects of catecholamines.

Catecholamines appear to exert at least some of their effects through myocardial alpha-adrenoceptors[134,135] (Fig. 13–18). As with myocardial beta-adrenoceptors, stimulation of myocardial alpha receptors augments myocardial contractility.[134,136] The subtype of myocardial alpha-adrenoceptors is somewhat controversial, although most evidence favors the presence of $alpha_1$ receptors only. A number of observations suggest that the molecular mechanism by which alpha-adrenoceptors exert a positive inotropic effect is different from that of beta receptors. Whereas stimulation of beta-adrenoceptors increases intracellular cyclic AMP, which is thought to mediate subsequent events, stimulation of alpha-adrenoceptors appears to have no effect on cyclic AMP production in myocardium. Alpha-adrenoceptors appear to mediate an increase in inotropy almost exclusively by means of an increase in Ca^{++} influx[137] (Fig. 13–18).

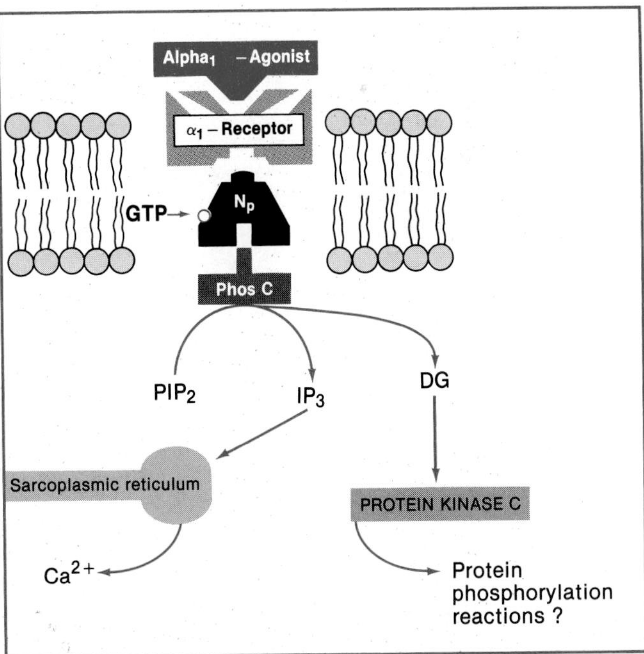

FIGURE 13–18. Diagram of response to α_1 adrenoceptor stimulation of intracellular Ca^{++} ion mobilization through activation of phospholipase C (Phos C) and subsequent mobilization of membrane phosphoinositides. N_p represents GTP-dependent protein (G protein) that couples membrane receptor to Phos C. (From Lucchesi, B. R.: Role of calcium on excitation-contraction coupling in cardiac and vascular smooth muscle. Circulation *80:*IV1. 1989, by permission of the American Heart Association, Inc.)

ISOMETRIC CONTRACTION

Cardiac contraction can be readily studied in vitro by mounting a mammalian papillary muscle, trabeculae carneae, or strip of atrial myocardium in an oxygenated, physiological salt solution.[138-142] When the ends of the muscle are fixed and the muscle is activated by electrical stimulation, the strength of individual isometric cardiac contractions is modified by two major influences: (1) a change in initial muscle length, or preload, induced by a change in the passive stretch of the muscle; and (2) a change in contractility or inotropic state at any given length.[139]

The relationship between the actively developed tension (the total tension minus resting tension) during the isometric contraction and the initial muscle length at which contraction occurred constitutes the length-active tension curve (Fig. 13–19). When contractility is altered at any given muscle length by an inotropic intervention such as the addition of Ca^{++}, digitalis, or norepinephrine to the medium, the rate of force development rises, the peak force developed increases, and the time to reach peak force shortens. Inotropic interventions do not generally alter the relationship between the preload (the tension placed on the resting muscle) and the length of the muscle, i.e., the length-resting tension relation, an expression of the resting stiffness (diastolic compliance or distensibility).[141] When the frequency of stimulation is altered, contractility is also changed; the pattern of the change depends on conditions and species. In the cat, dog, and human, increased stimulation frequency, within limits, increases the rate of force development and developed force and shortens the time to peak tension with accelerated relaxation. This response is termed the *force-frequency relation* (see also pp. 380 and 381); this positive inotropic action of frequency presumably results from the increased intramyocardial $[Ca^{++}]$ resulting from the increased frequency of depolarizations.[143]

As the nonstimulated muscle is stretched, the resting tension rises progressively and a point is reached at which actively developed tension is maximal; this length has been termed L_{max}. At this point resting tension rises very rapidly. Lengths beyond L_{max} are poorly tolerated and associated with very high resting tensions.

By definition, the length-active tension curve at lengths below L_{max} is termed the ascending limb of the curve and the portion above L_{max}, the descending limb. When initial muscle length is altered slightly on either side of L_{max}, active tension is altered substantially; a 10 per cent reduction in muscle length below L_{max} may be responsible for a 30 per cent decrease in actively developed tension.[144]

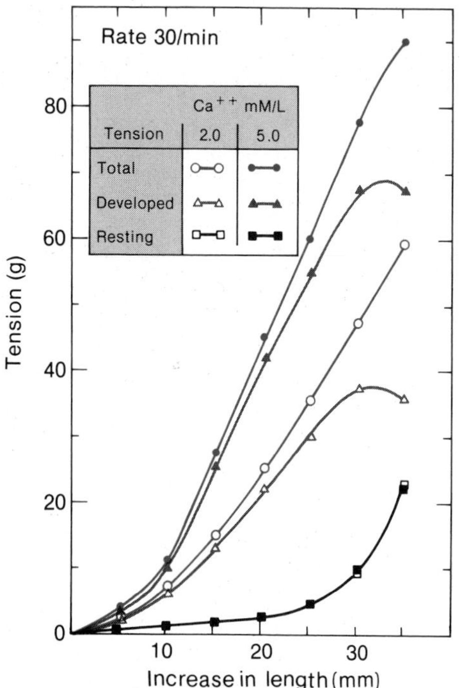

FIGURE 13–19. Effects of increased $[Ca^{++}]$ on the relation between muscle length and tension in an isolated cat papillary muscle. The $[Ca^{++}]$ in the perfusing medium was increased from 2.0 mM to 5.0 mM. The relation between resting muscle length and tension is not altered. However, the development of tension at any given muscle length is increased at the higher $[Ca^{++}]$ concentration, although L_{max} is not altered. Total tension is the sum of developed and resting tension.

ISOTONIC CONTRACTION: THE FORCE-LENGTH AND THE FORCE-VELOCITY RELATION

In order to analyze not only isometric contractions but also the physiologically pertinent shortening characteristics of the muscle, one end of the muscle is attached to a lever system and its degree of shortening is measured (Fig. 13–20*A*). The *preload,* a small weight placed on the opposite end of the lever, stretches the passive muscle to a length determined by the length-resting relation; a stop is then adjusted above the tip of the lever and any weight added to the lever over and above the preload, termed the afterload, may be sensed by the muscle after the onset of contraction (Fig. 13–20*B*). The extent and maximum velocity of shortening for each contraction depend on the load (Fig. 13–20*C*), and the inverse relation between the tension (force) developed and the velocity of contraction constitutes the force-velocity relation (Fig. 13–20*D*). When the load is greatest, there is no shortening, i.e., the muscle develops maximal force during isometric contraction (P_o). Conversely, when the load is smallest, the velocity of shortening is greatest. The velocity of shortening with zero load cannot be measured directly. However, extrapolation of the curve back to zero load allows approximation of this maximum velocity of unloaded shortening, termed V_{max}.[138-141,145-147]

When the initial muscle length is altered by increasing the preload, the force-velocity curve is shifted characteristically (Fig. 13–21); the velocity of shortening at any given load is increased, as is P_o. However, V_{max} is little altered by a change in initial muscle length. In contrast, when the contractility is augmented (Fig. 13–22), the rate of tension development is increased, as are the velocity and extent of shortening with a given load.[142,144] The entire force-velocity curve is shifted upward and to the right with increases in both P_o and V_{max}.

The length–active tension curve can also be constructed from isotonic contraction with increasing afterloads. The preload represents one point on the resting length-tension curve. When activated, the muscle will first develop an isometric force equal to the afterload that is imposed and then shorten isotonically to a length that corresponds to the length–active tension curve for that given state of contractility. As the afterload is increased, shortening decreases until only isometric force is generated (Fig. 13–20C). The same length–active tension curve is generated whether developed isotonically or isometrically, except under some conditions in which the muscle is very depressed and the isotonic points may fall to the right of the isometric ones.[146,147] Thus, the contraction reaches the same length–active tension curve, independent of the starting length of the muscle (preload) and the load carried (afterload).[147]

MUSCLE MODELS

Models of muscle contraction provide a method for analyzing contraction of heart muscle[148] as well as some insight into the complexities of ventricular function.[145] Current working models include a contractile element (CE), which represents the actively contracting portion of the muscle, arranged in series with a passive elastic component, the series elastic element (SE). At rest, CE is considered to be freely extensible, so that

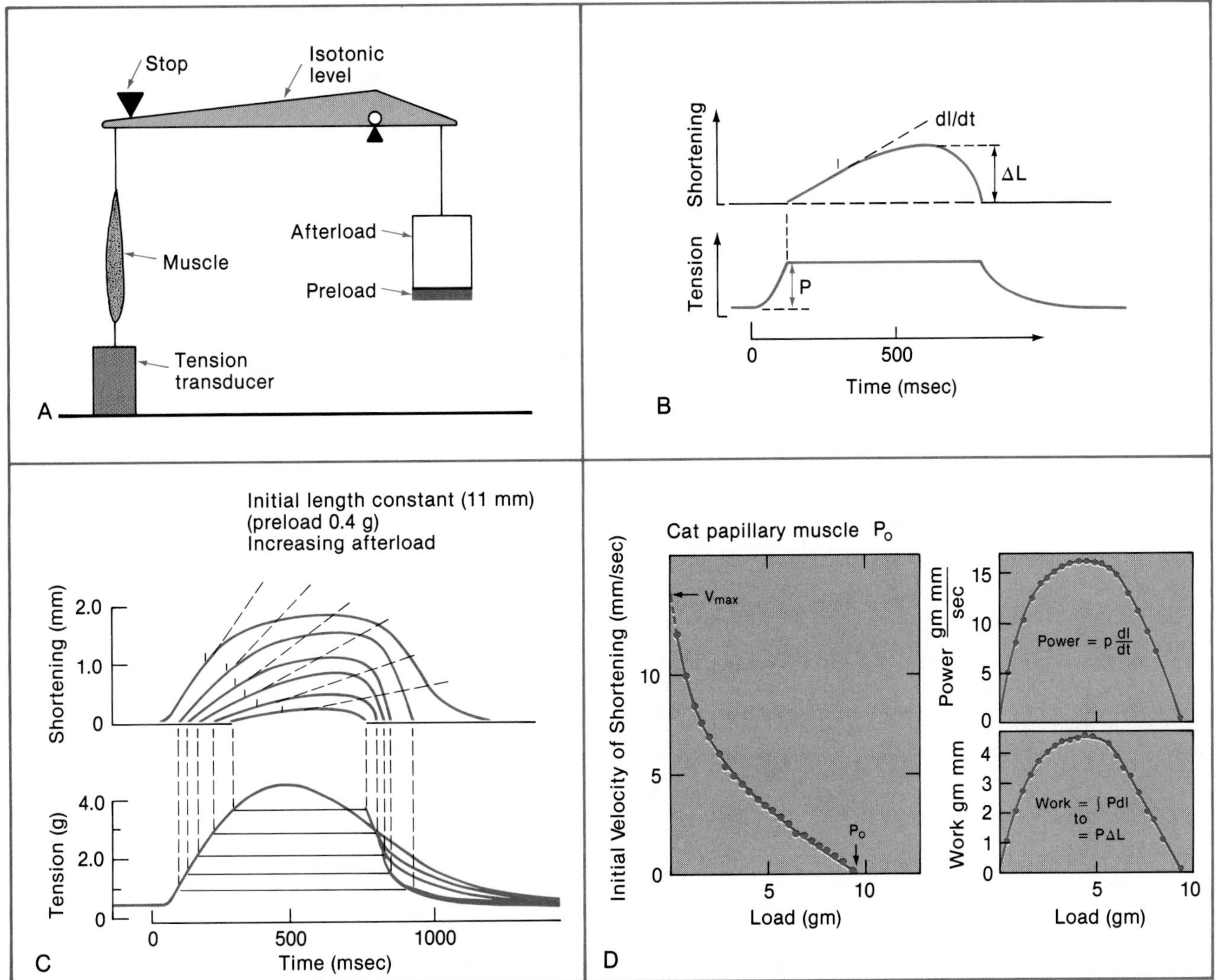

FIGURE 13-20. Use of afterloaded isotonic contractions to obtain force-velocity relations.

A, Diagrammatic representation of an isotonic lever system. A papillary muscle is placed in a bath (not shown) of Krebs-Ringer solution and stimulated by electrodes along its lateral aspect. The lower end of the muscle is attached to an extension from a tension transducer while the upper, free end is attached to the end of a lever system that is free to move. The fulcrum of the lever system is shown toward the right. Initially the stop is not above the tip of the lever, which is above the muscle. A small weight, termed a "preload," is placed on the opposite end of the lever; this preload will stretch the muscle to a length consistent with its resting length-tension relation. The stop is then fixed above the tip of the lever, so that any added weight above the preload will not be sensed by the muscle until it attempts to contract. Additional loads can be added to the preload (i.e., afterloads). Total load equals the sum of the preload and the afterload.

B, Tracings of an afterloaded isotonic contraction. The contraction is shown as a function of time, plotted along the abscissa. After stimulation at time zero, there is a short latent period followed by the generation of isometric force. When the force (P) equals the load, shortening begins, as shown in the upper half of the panel. Maximum velocity is reached shortly after shortening commences, and the tangent to this slope (dl/dt) approximates the maximum velocity of shortening with this particular load. ΔL denotes the extent of shortening. Subsequently the muscle elongates and then relaxes isometrically.

C, Effects of increasing afterloads on the course of tension development and subsequent shortening. Several superimposed contractions are displayed. The muscle develops a force equal to the afterload and thereafter shortens. As the afterload is increased, the velocity of shortening (dashed lines) and the extent of shortening decline.

D, Velocity of shortening plotted as a function of load: the force-velocity relation. As the load is increased, the velocity of shortening decreases. When the load is so high that no external shortening is recorded, velocity is zero, and the force is equivalent to the isometric contraction (P_0). When the curve is extrapolated back to zero load, V_{max} is obtained. Also shown at right are power (*top*) and work (*bottom*) curves as a function of increasing afterloads. Both power and work are zero when the load is zero or with isometric contractions, and both curves peak at an intermediate load. (From Braunwald, E., et al.: Mechanisms of Contraction of the Normal and Failing Heart. 2nd ed. Boston, Little, Brown, 1976.)

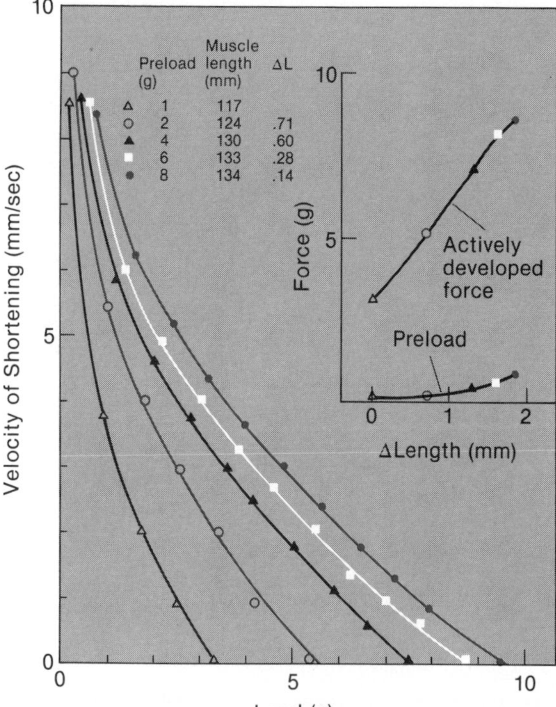

FIGURE 13-21. Relation between peak velocity of afterloaded, isotonic shortening and total load at several initial muscle lengths in a cat papillary muscle. The inset at the right shows the resting and developed active force at these various lengths. When initial muscle length is increased, the actively developed force is augmented, as is the velocity of shortening at any individual load. The maximum velocity of shortening with the preload alone is little altered. Moreover, if these curves were to be extrapolated back to zero load (V_{max}), this value would also show little or no change.

resting tension is sustained by another elastic component arranged in parallel, the *parallel elastic component* (PE). Depending on the model chosen, PE spans both CE and SE (Maxwell model) or CE alone (Voight model).

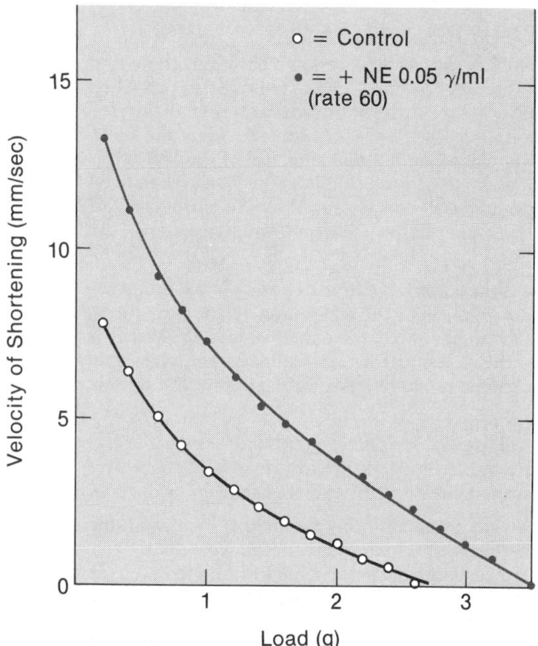

FIGURE 13-22. Effects of the addition of norepinephrine (NE) on the force-velocity relation of the cat papillary muscle. NE induces an increase in the velocity of shortening at any load, in the maximum force and isometric contraction (P_0), and in the maximum velocity of zero load shortening (V_{max}).

RESTING MUSCLE STIFFNESS

The resting stiffness of cardiac muscle is greater than that of skeletal muscle, but the reasons for this difference are not clear.[144] Myocardial cells are smaller than skeletal muscle cells and therefore possess a relatively greater proportion of stiff sarcolemma per unit weight of tissue; intercellular collagen is also more abundant in heart muscle.[15,149] The sarcomeres of cardiac muscle resist stretching beyond 2.2 μ, which may also be a factor in the stiffness of PE of heart muscle.[150] Minute intermediate filaments in the sarcomere of heart muscle may also contribute to its resting stiffness.[151]

The characteristics of muscular contraction are determined by the time course of activation of CE, its force-generating and shortening properties, and the stiffness of SE. The SE is a "lumped" elasticity, most of it being in elastic connections of the muscle to its points of fixation. In an isolated muscle, this would comprise the damaged ends of the muscle, while in the intact heart it would be any extraneous extensile tissue including the atrioventricular valves. Following contraction, elastic energy stored during contraction may lead to CE reextension, especially at short muscle lengths.

In the simplest model of an isometric contraction, with activation of the muscle, the CE shortens, stretching the springlike SE, and the force builds up at the ends of the system in a manner dependent upon the interaction of the shortening properties of the CE and compliance of the SE. On the other hand, in an afterloaded isotonic contraction, force is developed as shortening of the CE stretches the SE, until the force equals the load, and the load is then lifted. Muscle shortening occurs with the SE at a fixed length, and the subsequent course of shortening reflects shortening of the CE alone. Viscous elements are identified in the PE of resting heart muscle by the presence of stress relaxation, i.e., a fall in resting tension following a sustained stretch to a long length.

The mechanical activity of the CE reflects the summated contribution of cross bridges between myosin and actin and some form of conformational changes in the heads of the cross bridges, which then generate displacement of the actin filaments[42] (Fig. 13-6). Active state, a term adapted from skeletal muscle physiology, has been used to describe the capacity of the CE to shorten in accordance with the force-velocity relation.[146,150] It is a mechanical measure of the chemical processes in the CE that generate both force and shortening.

RESTING LENGTH-TENSION RELATIONS

When relaxed heart muscle is stretched progressively, its resting tension increases slightly at first and then rises more markedly (Fig. 13-19). The stiffness of the resting muscle is represented by the slope of the curve relating the change in resting tension (ΔP) to the change in length (ΔL), which is approximately exponential. The resting length-tension relation is not generally altered by interventions that acutely alter the length-active tension curve or the force-velocity length relation except that ischemia increases the apparent stiffness of the resting muscle, presumably by interfering with relaxation. Marked tachycardia also tends to increase the resting length-tension relation, because relaxation is not complete at the termination of diastole.[152] Aging also causes a significant increase in stiffness; less stress relaxation is exhibited by muscles from old adult rats compared with young adult ones, which may account, at least in part, for the age-associated changes in the resting length-tension curve[153] (p. 1657).

FORCE-VELOCITY CURVES

While force-velocity curves (Figs. 13-21 and 13-22) appear to provide valid descriptors of the contractile state in a wide variety of circumstances, an important theoretical limitation of such curves must be appreciated; the measurements to obtain each point in the curve are not made at the same time during contraction, so that the intensity of the active state might differ for each point. Thus, when the afterload is increased, velocity is measured later in time after the stimulus for contraction, and these measurements may occur at differing lengths of CE, thus distorting the enscribed curve from the "true" force-velocity curve.[146] The extrapolated V_{max} therefore could have been misleading. However, when the effects of these variables have been considered carefully, with unloading of the muscle to near zero external load once contraction has begun, the conclusions previously reached from simple afterloaded contractions have been supported.[154] Since initial length and end-systolic length can often be measured, indices of the end-systolic length allow one to approach the three-dimensional force-velocity-length relation. The assumption is made that the force-velocity-length relation moves symmetrically when contractility is altered.

When initial muscle length is reduced by 10 per cent, actively developed tension falls about 30 per cent, but unloaded velocity does not change. In intact muscle this dependency of force development on the length of heart muscle is related to the compliance of SE.[147] When cardiac muscle is activated and made to contract isometrically, the development of force is accompanied by an internal shortening, so that when maximal isometric force is reached, the CE (sarcomeres) is actually substantially shorter and the SE is longer than before activation. Indeed, sarcomeres actually do shorten substantially during "apparent" isometric contraction.[158-161] In contrast, isotonic contractions against very small loads do not involve the development of force, stretching of SE, and shortening of CE at the expense of SE; hence, shortening of CE is translated directly into shortening of the muscle, and velocities are measured at longer sarcomere lengths.[158] In studies in which sarcomere dynamics have been measured directly,[159] it appears that only a small fraction of the SE is associated with the contractile machinery and cross bridges in heart muscle and that the effective SE largely reflects external elastic connections.

THE ULTRASTRUCTURAL BASIS OF STARLING'S LAW OF THE HEART

The capacity of the intact ventricle to vary its force of contraction on a beat-to-beat basis as a function of its preload, reflected in the initial (end-diastolic) size, constitutes one of the major principles of cardiac function and is generally referred to as the *Frank-Starling phenomenon*, or *Starling's Law of the Heart*.[162,163] This fundamental property of the heart is based on the myocardial length–active tension relation, in which force of contraction and/or extent of shortening at any given tension depends on initial muscle length, which in turn is dependent on the ultrastructural disposition of thick and thin myofilaments within the sarcomeres.[164,165] As has already been pointed out (p. 351), the sarcomere is composed of an array of partially overlapping thick and thin filaments. A change in the length of the sarcomeres in striated muscle, whether skeletal or cardiac, creates a predictable change in the extent of overlapping between the two sets of filaments. The critical relation between sarcomere length and isometric tension development was defined for skeletal muscle by A. F. Huxley and associates[164] (Fig. 13–23), who found that developed tension was constant with a sarcomere length between 2.0 and 2.2 μ but that when sarcomeres were shortened to less than 2.0 μ, the developed force fell. These changes in force development were explained by the relative position of the two sets of myofilaments within the sarcomere. The thick filaments are about 1.5 μ in length while the thin filaments measure 1.0 μ.[26]

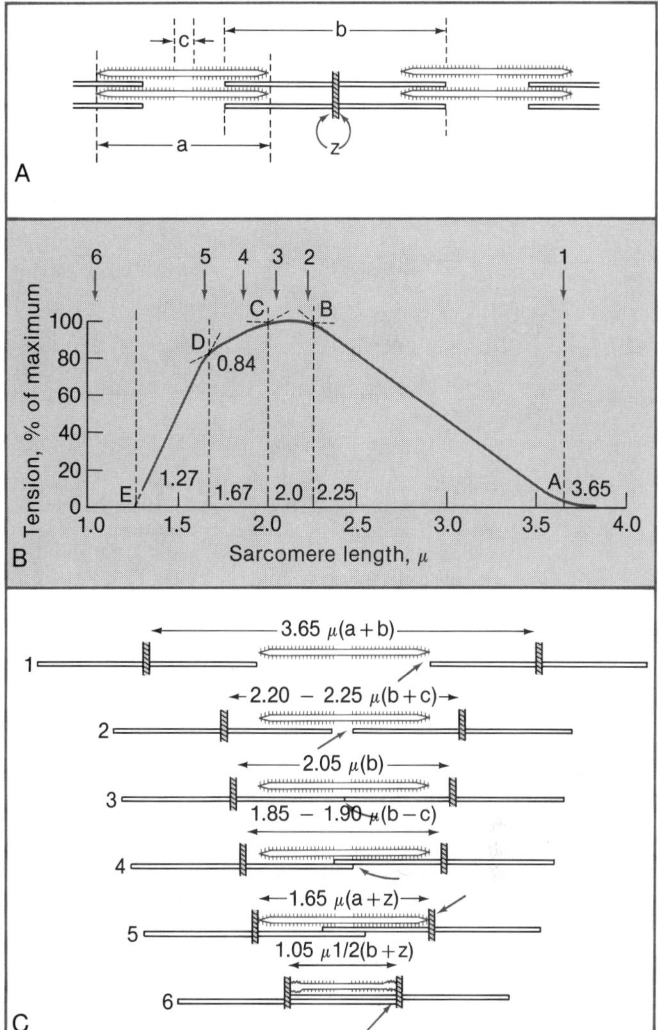

FIGURE 13–23. Relation between myofilament disposition and tension development in striated muscle. *A,* Diagram of myofilaments of the sarcomere drawn to scale. Thin filaments are 1.0 μ and thick filaments 1.6 μ in length. *B,* Relation between the tension development as percentage of maximum and the sarcomere length in single fibers of skeletal muscle. Numbers shown with arrows at top denote break points on the curve and correspond to the sarcomere lengths depicted diagrammatically in C. *C,* Myofilament overlap shown as a function of sarcomere length. At 3.65 μ (1) there is no overlap of myofilaments. The optimal overlap of myofilaments occurs at a sarcomere length of 2.05 to 2.25 μ (between 2 and 3). At a sarcomere length shorter than 2.0 μ (4), thin filaments pass into the opposite half of the sarcomere, and a double overlap occurs (5 and 6). Note that the central 0.2 μ of the thick filament is devoid of cross-bridges that could interact with sites on the thin filaments. (Adapted from Gordon, A. M., et al.: The variation in isometric tension with sarcomere length in vertebrate muscle fibers. J. Physiol. [Lond.] *184:*170, 1966.)

THE SLIDING FILAMENT THEORY OF STRIATED MUSCLE

According to this theory, the length of both sets of filaments remains constant, both at rest and during contraction. The central region of the thick filaments contains an area approximately 0.2 μ in width that is devoid of cross bridges for the formation of force-generating cross links between myosin heads and actin (Fig. 13–23). The optimal overlap of the 1.0 μ thin filaments with thick filaments occurs in sarcomeres between 2.0 and 2.2 μ In this range of sarcomere lengths, the number of force-generating cross links that can be formed and the resultant developed force are maximal and constant in skeletal fibers. With sarcomeres longer than 2.2 μ, the fall in developed force may be directly related to the widening H zone and the resultant decrease in overlap between thick and thin filaments, thereby reducing the potential for cross bridge formation. At 3.65 μ, no overlap of filaments remains, and force generation ceases.[164]

When sarcomere lengths are progressively reduced below 2.0 μ, a reduction in tension development also occurs, presumably because, as pointed out earlier, thin filaments of 1.0 μ meet in the center of the sarcomere and bypass one another as sarcomere length is decreased further, resulting in a double overlap of filaments. This may interfere with the formation of cross bridges, alter the ability of the filaments to bind Ca^{++} for activation, reduce the sensitivity of the overlapping filaments to Ca^{++},[166] and also generate significant internal loads that might impair shortening of the sarcomere.[166,167] As discussed below, troponin C serves as the "Ca^{++} switch" for activation as shown by direct exchange of troponin C in skinned fibers.[169] Thus, the Ca^{++} sensitivity of cardiac myofilaments is length dependent (Fig. 13–24) and that length dependence is greater with cardiac troponin C than with skeletal troponin C (Fig. 13–25). In general, the concept of cross bridges between thick and thin filaments also provides a useful working model that satisfactorily explains most of the observations of a variety of interventions involving cardiac contraction.

LENGTH-DEPENDENT ACTIVATION AND THE LENGTH-TENSION RELATION

In the prior discussion of the mechanics of muscular contraction, it generally was assumed that inotropic interventions and changes in muscle length are totally independent regulators of myocardial performance. However, it is now clear that both inotropic interventions and changes of muscle length may act primarily through mechanisms that involve Ca^{++} activation,[160,161,167-172] although the mechanism and resultant mechanical correlate may differ. The traditional view that length and inotropic state are independent regulators of myocardial performance was based on the observation that a decline of tension production occurs at short muscle lengths; this would be expected because tension is lost as a consequence of the double overlap of the thin filaments in the central region of each sarcomere, resulting in interference with normal cross-bridge formation.

The inotropic effect of changes in extracellular [Ca^{++}] depends on muscle length; the mechanical performance of cardiac muscle is more sensitive to changes in extracellular [Ca^{++}] at longer than at shorter muscle lengths.[166,167] In cardiac muscle (and to a lesser extent in skeletal muscle), the affinity of troponin for Ca^{++} is length dependent.[169,171] Although the quantity of Ca^{++} released remains the same when muscle length is altered,[167] more is actively bound at longer sarcomere lengths than at

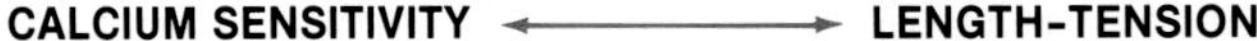

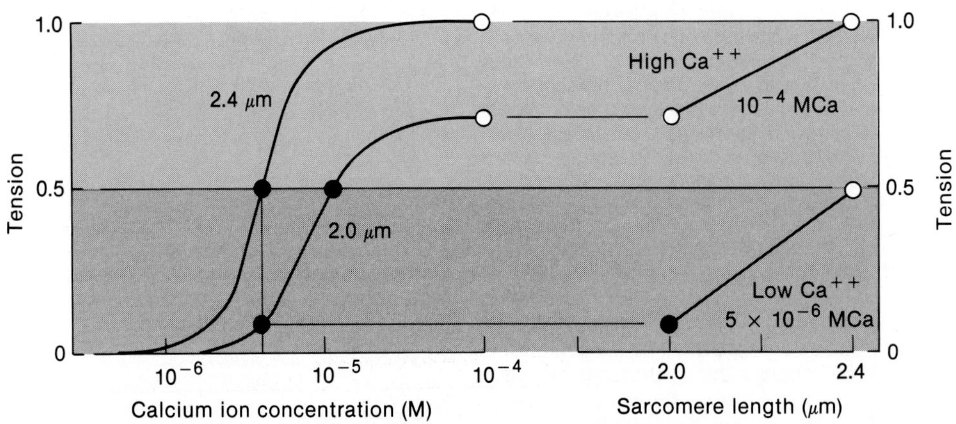

FIGURE 13-24. The length-dependency of Ca^{++} sensitivity of cardiac muscle and the resultant activation dependency of the length-tension relation. The left panel shows the contractile force produced by a segment of the heart muscle that has been "skinned," i.e., made permeable to Ca^{++} as a function of increasing amounts of Ca^{++}. The curve is shown at two fixed sarcomere lengths, 2.0 and 2.4 μ. Force increases with increasing Ca^{++}. Moreover, the Ca^{++} responsiveness is greater in the longer than the shorter sarcomere. When converted to the length-tension relation (*right panel*), the length tension curve is steeper when activation is less than maximal.

shorter ones. An increase in muscle length (1) does not change or actually decreases the transsarcolemmal influx of Ca^{++}, (2) may increase the release of Ca^{++} triggered by the transsarcolemmal Ca^{++} influx,[169] and (3) increases the sensitivity of the myofilaments to Ca^{++}.[169,171]

Thus, all changes in contractile behavior may result primarily from alterations in the degree of activation of the contractile system, and therefore contractility and muscle length (preload) should not be regarded as totally independent regulators of myocardial performance. While a change in contractility relates to changes in the quantity and rate of Ca^{++} made available to troponin C, a change in muscle length alters the sensitivity of the sarcomere to Ca^{++}. However, the distinct differences in the effects of changes in preload and of contractility on V_{max}, on the duration of the active state, and on the rate of tension development and decline all indicate that, regardless of the similarity in the fundamental molecular mechanism, consideration of preload and contractility as separate determinants of cardiac performance remains an extremely useful working model.

Although a change in initial length may alter the binding of Ca^{++} to the regulatory protein troponin C and thus alter the number of contractile bridges, one would expect the maximum velocity of cross bridge interactions, V_{max}, to remain constant, and force to be altered; indeed, this is the case.[160] However, when contractility is altered by inotropic interventions such as catecholamines, V_{max} rises.[139,160] Indeed, beta-adrenoceptor acti-

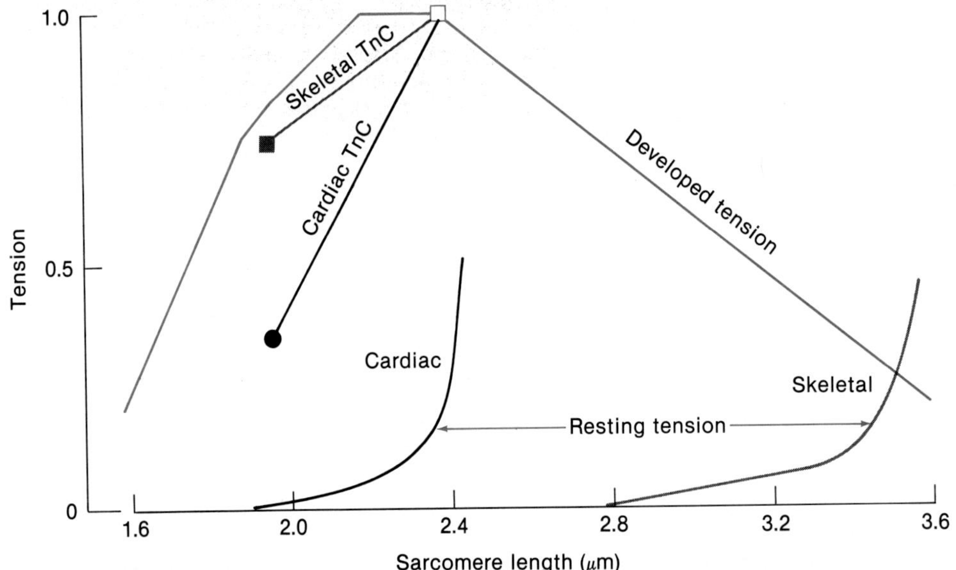

FIGURE 13-25. Relation between tension development and sarcomere length for cardiac and skeletal muscle. Data were obtained by fixing cat papillary muscles with glutaraldehyde at various diastolic lengths relative to the length-tension curve and determining the average sarcomere length with the tissue using electron microscopic methods. The relation between tension development and sarcomere length obtained with skeletal fibers has been superimposed for comparison. In cardiac muscle, peak tension occurs with a diastolic sarcomere length of 2.2 μ. In skeletal muscle, there is a plateau of developed tension between sarcomere lengths of 2.2 and 2.0 μ, whereas in cardiac muscle this is not the case, and developed tension falls as sarcomere length is decreased below 2.2 μ. Furthermore, the shortest diastolic sarcomere length obtained in cardiac muscle in the absence of activation is 1.8 μ. As the papillary muscle is stretched beyond 2.2 μ, resting tension rises substantially, while actively developed tension falls precipitously. In contrast, in skeletal muscle, actively developed tension falls in a linear fashion between a sarcomere length of 2.2 and 3.6 μ. When cardiac troponin C (C Tn C) is replaced by skeletal troponin C (S Tn C), the extreme length dependency of force present in the cardiac fibers (●) is markedly reduced (■). Note that the resting stiffness of cardiac muscle far exceeds that of skeletal muscle. (Modified from Sonnenblick, E. H., and Skelton, C. L.: Reconsideration of the ultrastructural basis of cardiac length-tension relations. Circ. Res. *35:*517, 1974, by permission of the American Heart Association, Inc.)

vation, acting through cyclic AMP, can apparently stimulate the enzymatic activity of actin-activated ATPase acutely in heart muscle.[46] This does not exclude an effect of increased activation to produce force to overcome any internal loads as well.

RELATION BETWEEN SARCOMERE LENGTH AND THE LENGTH-ACTIVE TENSION CURVE OF HEART MUSCLE

At L_{max}, the length of sarcomeres in mammalian ventricular myocardium fixed for electronmicroscopy averages 2.2 μ[150] (Fig. 13–24). Fixation results in about 5 per cent shrinkage so that measurements made during life need to be scaled upward somewhat.[158,159] As the resting muscle is shortened to about 85 per cent of L_{max}, sarcomere lengths decrease as a linear function of muscle length.[150,160,166] With further passive shortening of myocardium, however, the tissue becomes slack and little additional passive shortening of sarcomeres occurs, with diastolic sarcomere length remaining at 1.9 μ. Indeed, when sarcomeres shorten below this length, they extend in diastole, providing evidence for elastic recoils at short muscle lengths.[166]

DIFFERENCES BETWEEN CARDIAC AND SKELETAL MUSCLE. Although the structure of sarcomeres is similar in cardiac and skeletal muscle, important specialized differences permit cardiac muscle to function on the ascending portion of the length-active tension curve and maintain a length-dependent relation between sarcomere length and force development. First, the greater stiffness of the passive elastic component of cardiac muscle compared with skeletal muscle is such that diastolic sarcomere length is prevented from exceeding 2.3 μ,[176,177] thus preventing disengagement of the myofilaments[177] (Fig. 13–25). Second, the series elastic component is so compliant that during isometric contraction of cardiac muscle, substantial shortening of the sarcomeres occurs on the steep portion of their length-active tension curve.[175] Third, as already noted, the very high length dependency for development of tension results from the specified properties of cardiac troponin C.[169]

When cardiac muscle is stretched beyond L_{max}, resting tension rises to extremely high levels, while, by definition, actively developed tension rises no further. However, in contrast to skeletal muscle, sarcomeres in cardiac muscle resist overstretching. With extension of the muscle to 20 per cent beyond L_{max}, sarcomeres elongate only slightly beyond 2.2 μ, but developed tension falls substantially. A decrease in overlap between thick and thin filaments, i.e., disengagement of myofilaments, cannot explain the substantial decrements in developed force observed under these conditions; cellular damage occurs in cardiac muscle with this degree of overstretching and presumably is responsible, at least in part, for the reduction of tension development.[175]

SARCOMERE LENGTH–VENTRICULAR PERFORMANCE RELATION. Figure 13–26 shows the relation between average midwall sarcomere length and filling pressure for the left ventricles of the dog and cat.[177] When the left ventricle is empty, sarcomere length averages 1.9 μ, but as the left ventricle is filled, sarcomere lengths increase, so that at a filling pressure of 12 mm Hg the sarcomere length reaches 2.2 μ. With further ventricular distention, filling pressure rises markedly for small increments in ventricular volume, and only small increases in sarcomere length accompany large increases in intraventricular pressure. The same relation holds for the right ventricle but is scaled to lower filling pressures. The relation between tensions developed by the cat papillary muscle over a range of sarcomere lengths has been superimposed on the sarcomere resting length-tension relation in Figure 13–25. The optimal sarcomere length for maximum tension development (i.e., 2.2. μ) corresponds to the upper limits of normal ventricular filling pressure. When diastolic sarcomere length is related simultaneously to ventricular filling pressure and to active tension development, it becomes apparent that the apex of the sarcomere length–active tension curve and the normal upper limit of ventricular filling pressure coincide. Thus, the ventricle normally starts to contract when end-diastolic sarcomere lengths are along the upper half of the ascending portion of the sarcomere length–active tension curve.

In studies of the relation between sarcomere length and ventricular performance in the intact ejecting heart, the canine left ventricle was fixed in situ during end diastole and end systole.[178,179] Diastolic sarcomere lengths in the midwall of the left ventricle averaged 2.07 μ when filling pressure ranged from 6 to 8 mm Hg.[179] At end systole, when the ventricle had ejected about two-thirds of its end-diastolic volume, the average sarcomere length shortened to 1.8 μ, and when contractility of the ventricle was augmented by postextrasystolic potentiation, maximum systolic emptying was increased substantially and end-systolic sarcomere lengths were 1.6 μ. During relaxation, these sarcomeres will elongate to 1.9 to 2.0 μ, generating a restoring force that provides "suction" in early diastole to enhance early ventricular filling.

Sarcomeres tend to be longest in the midwall of the ventricle and reach a maximal length (2.25 μ) at filling pressures of about 10 mm Hg, when subendocardial and subepicardial sarcomeres are shorter. As filling pressure is raised further, sarcomere length increases across the entire wall; this recruitment of shorter sarcomeres from across the wall may constitute a further functional reserve of the Frank-Starling mechanism.[180]

The relative degree of sarcomere shortening cannot be the same across the ventricular wall during ejection; geometrical considerations dictate that epicardial fibers must shorten relatively less than endocardial fibers.[182,183] Nevertheless, when sarcomere lengths obtained from the intact heart are superimposed on the initial sarcomere length–tension curve (Fig. 13–

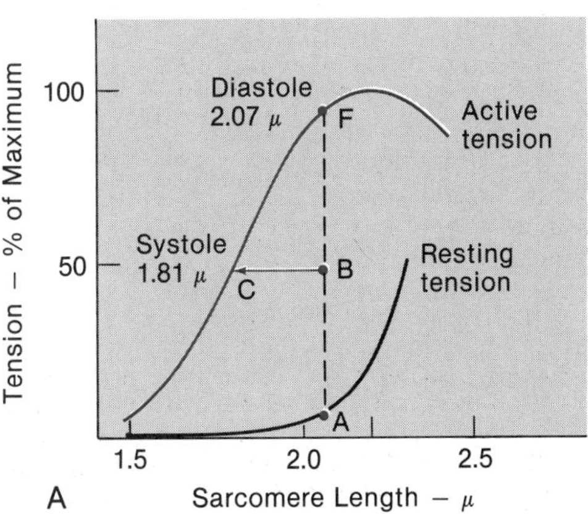

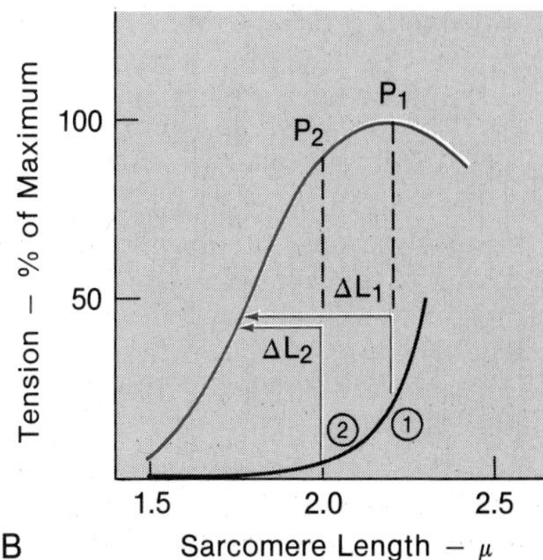

FIGURE 13–26. ***A,*** **Relation between average diastolic sarcomere lengths as noted in the midwall of the normal diastolic and systolic left ventricle of the dog and the sarcomere length-tension curve of the isolated cat papillary muscle. In the intact dog, normal diastole is associated with a diastolic sarcomere length of 2.07 μ. During systole, sarcomeres in the intact heart shorten to an average of 1.81 μ. This provides for a 13 per cent change in sarcomere length, which would produce an ejection fraction of 55 per cent when considered in terms of a thick-walled model of the left ventricle.**

B, **Effects of altering initial muscle lengths on shortening of afterloaded sarcomeres. During an afterloaded isotonic contraction (1), the sarcomere begins to shorten from a diastolic length of 2.20 μ (point 1) and to become 1.81 μ (ΔL_1). The isometric force associated with this sarcomere length is noted at P_1. When diastolic sarcomere length is reduced to 2.0 μ (point 2), the sarcomere with the same afterload will shorten to the same point on the length–active tension curve (ΔL_2). This will result in a shortening from 2.00 to 1.81 μ. In this instance the associated isometric force occurs at P_2. Note that despite a minor change in peak developed isometric force, a substantial change in afterloaded isotonic shortening occurs at the same afterload. This would produce a substantial change in the stroke volume when extrapolated to the intact heart; e.g., in a 100-gram canine left ventricle, a change in diastolic sarcomere length from 2.0 to 2.2 μ in the midwall would increase stroke volume from 17 to 42 ml, with end-diastolic volume increasing from 40 to 65 ml. (From Ross, J., Jr., et al.: Architecture of the heart in systole and diastole: Technique of rapid fixation and analysis of left ventricular geometry. Circ. Res. *21:*409, 1967, by permission of the American Heart Association, Inc.)**

26A), the normal sarcomere might be considered to start to contract at point A. Were the ends of the muscle fixed, the isometric force at point F would be developed. With an afterload, force is developed to point B, after which shortening occurs between points B and C from a sarcomere length of 2.07 μ to 1.81 μ. As diastolic sarcomere length is altered along the ascending limb of the sarcomere length-active tension curve, both peak isometric force development and the extent of shortening at any given load are changed (Fig. 13–26B). The extent of this shortening is of great physiological importance because it ultimately determines the quantity of blood ejected by the intact ventricle at any given diastolic fiber length. The basis for the Frank-Starling mechanism in the intact heart (discussed in the next section) is apparent in Fig. 13–26B, in which it is clear that small changes in diastolic sarcomere length can mediate relatively large changes in the extent of sarcomere shortening at any afterload.

Determinants of Contraction of the Intact Heart

Although the geometry of the intact ventricle is far more complex than that of papillary muscle with its parallel, longitudinally disposed fibers, if certain analogies are drawn and assumptions made, the basic mechanisms that influence the contraction of isolated cardiac muscle described above appear to affect the performance of the whole heart in a similar manner.[184–187] However, in the whole heart, the shapes of the ventricles, the angles of the adjacent muscle fibers, the wall thickness, and the developed and passive intracavitary pressure levels all affect the active and passive wall forces, and each importantly influences the characteristics of ventricular ejection and filling.

CHANGES IN VENTRICULAR SIZE AND SHAPE DURING THE CARDIAC CYCLE

In addition to the changes in ventricular size and shape that occur normally during the cardiac cycle and the additional alterations produced by acute physiological stresses, the shape of the ventricles often undergoes major alterations consequent to chronic cardiac disorders, such as valvular abnormalities, heart failure, or local scarring due to myocardial infarction (p. 1210). The model often applied in considering the left ventricle is a thick-walled ellipsoid of revolution, which has practical utility in the calculation of left ventricular volume (p. 423). The geometry of the right ventricle is more complex, and often nongeometric methods (such as measurement of ejection fraction by radionuclide ventriculography coupled with a separate method for determining the stroke volume) are used to determine right ventricular volumes and the ejection fraction.

The myocardial fibers are arranged in a spiral fashion around the central cavity of the left ventricle. The subendocardial and subepicardial fibers run largely parallel to the long axis of the cavity, and the midwall fibers are mostly circumferential, i.e., perpendicular to the long axis. All the fibers tend to be perpendicular to the radius of the cavity. During ventricular ejection contraction, the myocardial fibers shorten and thicken, and as the left ventricular cavity decreases circumferentially and longitudinally, the inner surface decreases more than the external surface, as dictated by the geometry of the heart. Because muscle mass remains constant, an increase in wall thickness must occur. Direct measurements of left ventricular wall thickness in intact animals,[188] as well as cineangiography in human subjects,[189] have confirmed that left ventricular wall thickness increases by 25 to 35 per cent during normal systole (Fig. 13–27). The generation of intraventricular pressure and the displacement of blood from the left ventricular cavity are produced by a combination of fiber shortening and wall thickening.

During isovolumetric left ventricular contraction, the chordae tendineae become tense, the mitral valve closes, and the ellipsoidal left ventricle becomes more spherical, with slight apex-to-base shortening and a small increase in the minor ventricular diameter whereas ellipticalization occurs during isovolumetric relaxation. During ejection, the internal major (longitudinal) axis shortens by only 9 per cent.[189] Shortening of the internal minor axis diameter by about 25 per cent accounts for approximately 80 to 90 per cent of the normal stroke volume.

DIASTOLIC PROPERTIES OF THE VENTRICLES

(See also pp. 402, 438, and 446)

A number of factors determine the filling of the ventricles during diastole.[192–194] These include the relaxation period of the ventricle, which primarily affects early ventricular filling and involves active relaxation (related to Ca^{++} reuptake by the sarcoplasmic reticulum). The relaxation rate is influenced by the level of inotropic state, by nonuniformity of relaxation, and by the load-dependent properties of relaxation that, in turn, affect ventricular "suction or restoring forces." In addition, the gradient from the atrium to ventricle importantly influences the early filling rate. During later phases of diastole (diastasis), as well as during atrial systole, the dimensions of the ventricular cavities, the thickness of the ventricular walls, and the intrinsic mechanical properties of cardiac tissue are the main determinants of the passive ventricular filling properties. Before these mechanisms are considered in more de-

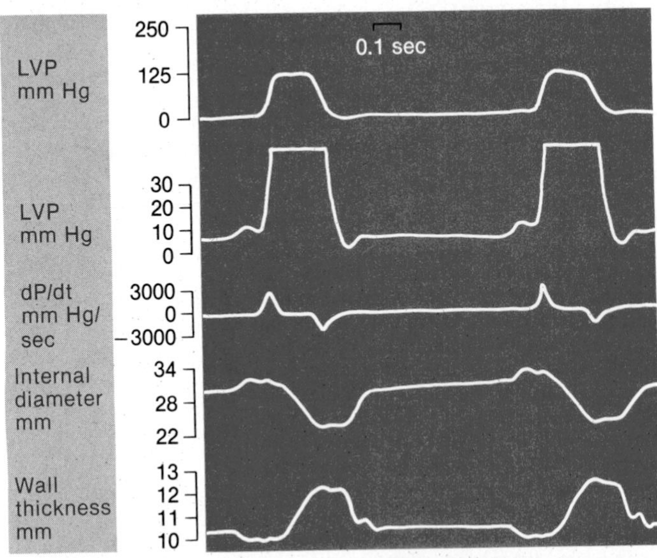

FIGURE 13–27. High-speed tracings obtained in a normal conscious, chronically instrumented dog with sinus arrhythmia. LVP = left ventricular pressure (in the top two tracings at high and low amplification). dP/dt = the first derivative of left ventricular pressure. The internal diameter of the left ventricle was measured by means of a pair of ultrasonic crystals placed on the endocardium near the minor equator. The wall thickness of the left ventricle was measured by means of a pair of miniature ultrasonic crystals juxtaposed across the free wall near the minor equator. Note presystolic wall thinning with atrial systole, followed by wall thickening during ejection, with mirror image changes of the internal diameter. (From Theroux, P., Ross, J., Jr., et al.: Unpublished observations.)

tail, some of the definitions commonly used for describing such properties are discussed below.

DEFINITIONS

Certain terms are commonly used to describe the mechanical properties of cardiac muscle.[195-198] Because there has been confusion about their meaning, they will be defined explicitly here. *Stress* is the force per unit of cross-sectional area, frequently expressed as gm/cm^2; *strain* is the fractional (or percentage of) change in dimension or size from the unstressed dimension that results from the application of stress; *elasticity* is the property of recovery of a deformed material after removal of the stress; *creep* is the time-dependent strain of tissue maintained at a constant level of stress after a rapid change in stress; *stress relaxation* is the time-dependent reduction of stress when tissue is maintained at a constant level of strain after a rapid change in strain. Like most biological materials, cardiac muscle exhibits a curvilinear relation between passive (diastolic) stress and strain (Fig. 13–19); this property is responsible for the nonlinear pressure-volume curve (Fig. 13–28) and stress-strain relation of the intact ventricle. *Elastic stiffness* defines the ratio of stress to strain at any defined point of the curve relating these two variables. The *elastic stiffness constant* is the slope of the straight line relating elastic stiffness to the corresponding stress. The term elastic stiffness, sometimes called *volume stiffness* or *chamber stiffness,* has also been used to refer to the stiffness of the ventricular chamber and, by simplification, has been defined as the ratio of the change in pressure (dP) to the change in volume (dV). When the stress-strain relation is analyzed, the term *myocardial stiffness* has been employed to differentiate those effects due to changes in the stiffness properties of each unit of muscle as opposed to those due to increased muscle mass alone, which can affect *chamber stiffness;* thus, in some patients with concentric left ventricular hypertrophy, chamber stiffness is increased and myocardial stiffness is normal, whereas in others, both are elevated.[195] The terms *compliance* and *distensibility* represent the inverse of elastic stiffness; i.e., in referring to isolated muscle it is the ratio of a change in strain relative to a change in stress (d_e/d_s). In the ventricle these terms have been used to refer to the ratio dV/dP. The term *specific compliance* introduces a correction for the initial volume. Efforts to correct this value for ventricles of different sizes have also led to such expressions as $\frac{dV/dP}{V}$ where V in the denominator represents end-diastolic volume.

The diastolic pressure-volume relation of the normal mammalian left ventricle is curvilinear (Fig. 13–28).[196] At a low ventricular end-diastolic pressure there is a relatively shallow slope, with large changes in volume being accompanied by small changes in pressure. At the upper limits of normal end-diastolic pressure, the curve becomes steeper[196] and approximates an exponential relation, so that as the chamber becomes progressively filled during each diastole, instantaneous ventricular compliance (dV/dP) decreases; the inverse of compliance, i.e., elastic stiffness (dP/dV), bears a linear relation to the pressure in left ventricle at diastolic pressures exceeding 3 mm Hg in the normal dog.[195] The slope of the line relating dP/dV to P represents the elastic stiffness constant of the chamber; it is relatively independent of ventricular shape and therefore may be useful for detecting changes in wall stiffness.[195,199] However, caution must be used in drawing conclusions from measuring these variables in one ventricle when the effects of changes in the volume of the other ventricle and the elastic limits of the pericardium cannot be excluded. Also, in comparing a normal chamber with a dilated one, identical chamber elastic stiffness constants might be obtained, and a definition of volume elasticity at a common pressure in which the different volumes are taken into account is needed to describe the properties of the two chambers.[200]

Although by definition, and as is apparent from Figure 13–29, the compliance of the ventricle changes as it fills, an alteration of the compliance of the chamber as a whole can be identified by a change in the shape and position of the curve relating ventricular diastolic volume or dimensions to pressure[196] (Fig. 13–29). Excluding the incomplete relaxation that occurs in tachycardia and myocardial ischemia, interventions that alter myocardial contractility acutely do not cause significant shifts in the ventricle's diastolic pressure-volume relation. The small changes in the relation reported in some studies may be secondary to effects on time-dependent, inertial,

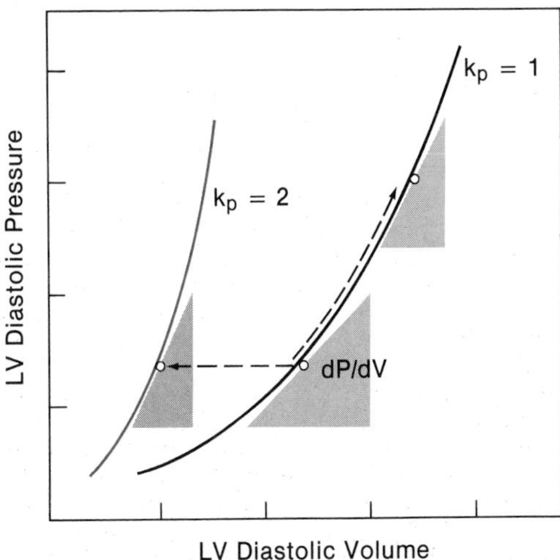

FIGURE 13–28. Diagrammatic representation of left ventricular (LV) diastolic pressure–volume relationships. *Right,* An increase in operative chamber stiffness (dp/dV) occurs in the absence of any change in the modulus of chamber stiffness (K_p). *Left,* an increase in operative chamber stiffness (relative to the curve on the right). Because operative chamber stiffness depends on the modulus of stiffness and the level of operative filling pressure, this comparison is made at equivalent levels of pressure. (From Gaasch, W. H., et al.: Left ventricular compliance: Mechanisms and clinical implications. Am. J. Cardiol. *38:*645, 1976.)

and viscous properties and to the influence of filling of the opposite ventricle. Since the diastolic pressure-volume relation is curvilinear, left ventricular diastolic compliance is determined by both the diastolic pressure-volume relation and the level of diastolic pressure at any instant, the so-called operating diastolic pressure (Fig. 13–28).[201] Therefore, ventricular compliance declines; i.e., the chamber elastic stiffness increases as it fills. Increased diastolic filling, for example, as occurs with acute aortic regurgitation, and, conversely, reduced ventricular preload, for example, as occurs after administration of nitroglycerin, result in increased and reduced stiffness, respectively, as the ventricle moves up or down its pressure-volume curve.

In the intact heart, *stress relaxation* is of significance only when large increases in ventricular diastolic pressure and volume occur abruptly. For example, there is a small drop in ventricular end-diastolic pressure (about 1 mm Hg) when systolic pressure is suddenly elevated by 70 to 80 per cent in the isovolumetrically contracting left ventricle, which is held at a constant volume. This suggests the presence of viscous elements, but these changes are of relatively minor significance in the intact heart.[202] *Creep,* a time-dependent shift of the left ventricular diastolic pressure–volume relation, has also been documented in the conscious dog after large increases in systolic and diastolic pressures (ventricular diastolic volume being larger at the same levels of diastolic pressure).[203]

The normal *right ventricle is more compliant than the left,* not because of any intrinsic difference in muscle stiffness but because of its thinner wall. In the isolated, nonbeating normal dog heart, when the left and right ventricles are filled simultaneously to a pressure of 10 mm Hg, the volume of the right ventricle is about 35 per cent greater than that of the left,[204] and the upper limit of normal for right ventricular end-diastolic pressure in humans is about one-half (6 mm Hg) that of the left ventricle (12 mm Hg). In humans, the end-diastolic volumes of the two ventricles are approximately equal,[205] and therefore the ejection fractions of the two ventricles are normally similar as well.

DETERMINANTS OF VENTRICULAR DIASTOLIC PROPERTIES AND VENTRICULAR FILLING (Table 13–2). The ventricular relaxation rate, an important determinant of early filling, is influenced by several factors. Inotropic stimulation of the heart affects the relaxation rate (the latter is sometimes termed as "lusitropic" effect),[206] a positive inotropic influence both shortening systole and increasing the rate of relaxation,

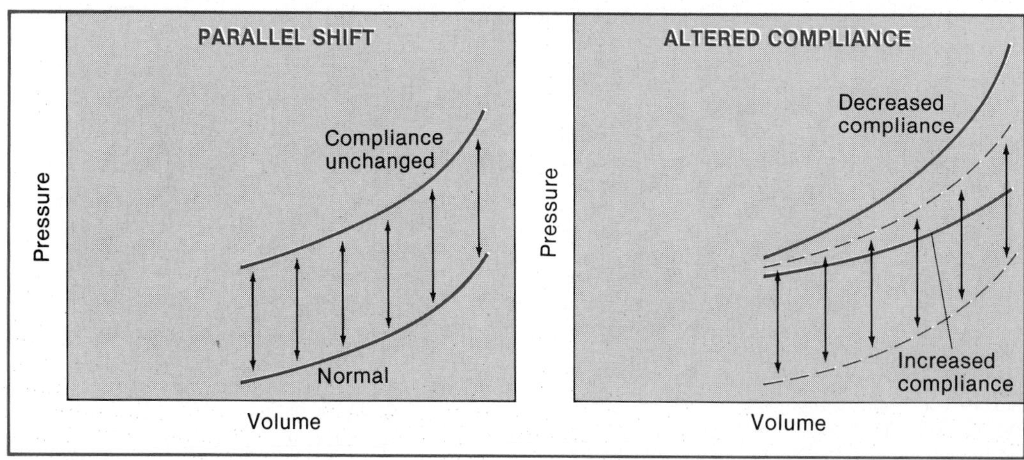

FIGURE 13–29. Schematic illustration of the difference between diastolic distensibility and altered compliance. On the left, the left ventricular diastolic pressure–volume relation has undergone a parallel upward shift. Distensibility is decreased (higher diastolic pressure required to fill the ventricle to the same chamber volume), although compliance (the slope of the pressure-volume relation) is unchanged. On the right, superimposed on the parallel upward shift are curves whose slopes are steeper (decreased compliance) or less steep (increased compliance) than either of the two parallel pressure-volume curves. This illustrates the importance of distinguishing distensibility from compliance, because the curve labeled "increased compliance" nevertheless exhibits decreased distensibility compared with the normal pressure volume relation. (From Grossman, W.: Relaxation and diastolic distensibility of the regionally ischemic left ventricle. *In* Grossman, W. H., and Lorell, B. H. [eds.]: Diastolic Relaxation of the Heart. Boston, Martinus-Nijhoff, 1988, p. 197.)

whereas negative inotropic stimulation produces opposite effects.[194,206] Increases in heart rate also can effect relaxation rate through the positive inotropic effect of the force-frequency relation (p. 380).[208] The rate of relaxation is sometimes measured as peak negative left ventricular dP/dT, or as a time constant, *tau;* such variations in the rate of ventricular relaxation can influence diastolic properties well into the early filling period of the ventricles.[194,206] Another factor affecting relaxation is nonuniformity, which can result from abnormal electrical excitation (as by electrically pacing the ventricle) or from regional variations in contractility.[192,209] Load-dependent relaxation is a well known phenomenon in isolated cardiac muscle,[192] and it has recently been demonstrated in the whole heart.[210–212] If load is increased early in systole, up to the time of mid ejection, an increase in active tension is accompanied by an increase in the duration of systole and delayed relaxation, whereas if load is increased later in contraction (by rapidly increasing ventricular volume), active tension

TABLE 13–2 FACTORS THAT INFLUENCE DIASTOLIC VENTRICULAR PROPERTIES

I. FACTORS EXTRINSIC TO THE VENTRICULAR CHAMBER
- A. Pericardial properties
- B. Loading of the contralateral ventricle
- C. Coronary vascular turgor (erectile effect)
- D. Extrinsic compression by tumor, pleural pressures etc.

II. FACTORS INTRINSIC TO THE VENTRICULAR CHAMBER
- A. Passive elasticity of the ventricular wall (stiffness or compliance when myocytes are completely relaxed)
  1. Thickness of ventricular wall, and composition of ventricular wall (muscle, fibrosis, amyloid, hemosiderin), including both endocardium and myocardium
  2. Temperature, osmolality
- B. Active elasticity of ventricular wall due to residual cross-bridge activation (cycling and/or latch state) through part or all of diastole
  1. Slow relaxation affecting early diastole only
  2. Incomplete relaxation affecting early, mid- and end-diastolic distensibility
  3. Diastolic tone, contracture, or rigor
- C. Elastic recoil (diastolic suction)
- D. Viscoelasticity (stress relaxation, creep)

From Grossman, W.: Relaxation and diastolic distensibility of the regionally ischemic left ventricle. *In* Grossman, W. H., and Lorell, B. H. (eds.): Diastolic Relaxation of the Heart. Boston, Martinus-Nijhoff, 1988, p. 196.

is lowered and relaxation is more rapid.[210] Such effects may relate to availability of free Ca^{++} to bind at muscle cross bridges adequate Ca^{++} being available for binding when muscle is stretched early in the contraction cycle, whereas late in the cycle Ca^{++} is being rapidly removed and cross bridges are broken by increased muscle stretch.[192]

Evidence for ventricular suction has been provided by demonstration of negative diastolic pressures during filling, such as with strenuous exercise[208] or volume clamping of the ventricle,[193] and by recording pressure gradients within the left ventricle early in diastole.[213] The level of left atrial pressure at the time of mitral valve opening also importantly influences early filling, a higher left atrial pressure augmenting the rate of filling.[214]

Changes in *ventricular chamber* geometry and wall thickness affect the passive filling properties of the ventricles (affecting *chamber* compliance) and should be distinguished from the intrinsic mechanical properties of cardiac *muscle,*[215] as well as from a continued influence on left ventricular pressure of incomplete ventricular relaxation into early diastole; models have been developed for assessing the influence of early incomplete ventricular relaxation, as well as the filling rate–dependent viscous properties of the walls on the dynamics of early ventricular filling.[215] Doppler echocardiographic studies in human subjects with and without chronic changes in myocardial properties have shown relatively characteristic patterns of early and late filling velocities, the latter related to atrial systole, as shown in Figure 13–30.[198,216] Abnormalities of *relaxation* primarily influence early diastolic filling velocity, slowed or delayed relaxation reducing the peak early filling velocity, often accompanied by a compensatory increase in the peak late filling velocity during atrial contraction (Fig. 13–30*A*). Such an effect may *not* be associated with shift in the left ventricular diastolic pressure-volume relation (Fig. 13–30*A*), although with pronounced positive inotropic stimulation (such as during exercise) a downward shift of the early portion of the diastolic pressure volume relation may be observed.[208] In contrast, changes in ventricular chamber stiffness can produce different responses, increased stiffness causing a reduction in the peak early filling velocity, and the associated increased impedance to atrial emptying causing a decrease in peak filling velocity during atrial contraction (Fig. 13–30*B*). The latter effects are usually associated with an upward displacement of the left ventricular diastolic pressure–volume curve (Fig. 13–30*B*).[216]

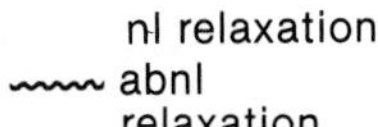

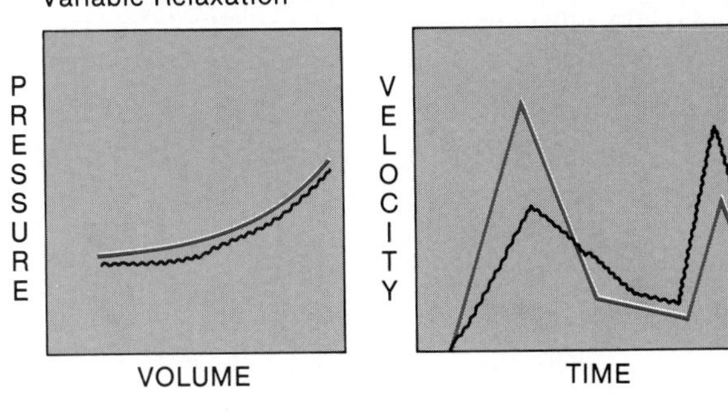

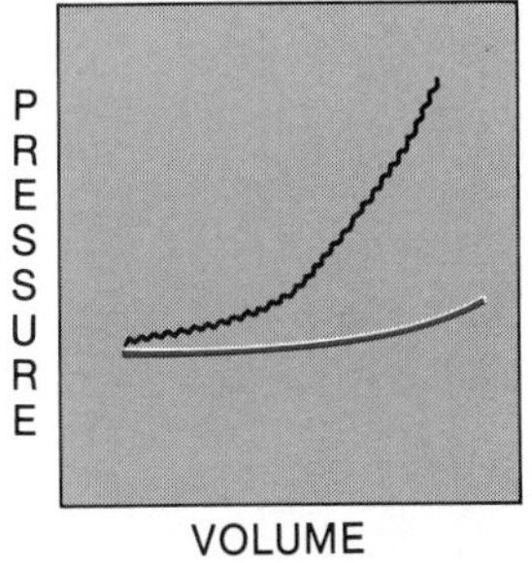

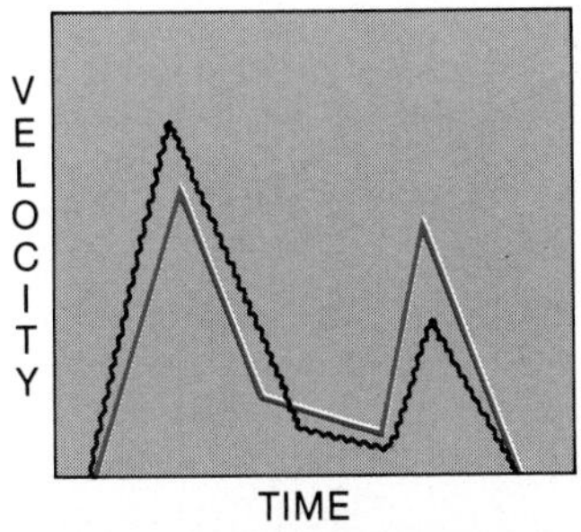

FIGURE 13-30. *A,* Effect of increased chamber stiffness on diastolic filling. Schematic of left ventricular pressure-volume relation (*left*) and Doppler transmitral velocity tracing (*right*) for ventricle with normal (nl) and abnormal (abnl) stiffness. As chamber stiffness increases and other factors that influence the filling pattern remain constant (for example, relaxation), early filling increases and atrial contribution is diminished. *B,* Effect of slowed relaxation on diastolic filling. Schematic of left ventricular pressure-volume relation (*left*) and Doppler transmitral velocity tracing (*right*). Impairment in relaxation with constant chamber stiffness decreases early filling with a compensatory increase in the atrial contribution to filling. In some circumstances, delayed relaxation can shift the initial portion of the diastolic pressure-volume relation upward (not shown). (Modified from Stoddard, M. F., et al.: Left ventricular diastolic function: Comparison of pulsed Doppler echocardiographic and hemodynamic indexes in subjects with and without coronary artery disease. J. Am. Coll. Cardiol. *13:*327, 1989.)

As mentioned, ventricular chamber stiffness can be a function of intrinsic muscle stiffness, as well as the wall thickness and geometry of the ventricle. If the intrinsic stiffness of cardiac tissue (muscle stiffness) is increased (as may occur in a fibrous scar or with infiltration by amyloid), even if the thickness of the ventricular wall remains normal the ventricular chamber stiffness will be increased. However, an increase in chamber stiffness also can occur if the thickness of each unit of muscle is augmented while intrinsic muscle stiffness remains normal, as in ventricular hypertrophy. Diastolic viscous properties[217] and the coronary venous pressure [218] both can affect left ventricular diastolic properties.

Effects of Exercise on Ventricular Filling. Studies in strenuously exercising normal dogs indicate that a considerable increase in the volume of left ventricular filling occurs during each beat, despite marked shortening of the diastolic filling period. Such effects are accomplished by marked enhancement of the ventricular relaxation rate, reduction of the early diastolic filling pressure to below zero, with a shift downward of the early portion of diastolic-pressure-volume curve (Fig. 13-31*B*), and augmentation of the atrial contribution to ventricular filling without significant elevation of the left ventricular end-diastolic pressure.[208] This response is similar to that observed in human subjects without significant cardiac disease, in whom a downward shift of the diastolic pressure-volume relation with an increased slope was observed during exercise; the increased slope was suggested to reflect increased chamber stiffness caused by higher passive filling rates and increased visoelastic resistance.[219]

During exercise in the presence of ischemia, ventricular relaxation becomes markedly impaired, with a shift upward of the minimum diastolic pressure and of the *early* portion of the ventricular diastolic pressure-volume curve[208] (Fig. 13-31*B*).

Left ventricular diastolic filling has been shown to be impaired at rest in patients with hypertension and left ventricular hypertrophy, and the abnormal ejection fraction response to exercise in such patients had been attributed to the greater left ventricular mass, leading to impaired diastolic filling during exercise and inability to maintain an adequate stroke volume.[220]

ROLE OF THE PERICARDIUM

(See also pp. 1465 to 1468)

Experimental data indicate that the normal pericardium has an important effect on the diastolic properties of the ventricles during acute volume overload and therefore could be important during acute heart failure. During acute volume

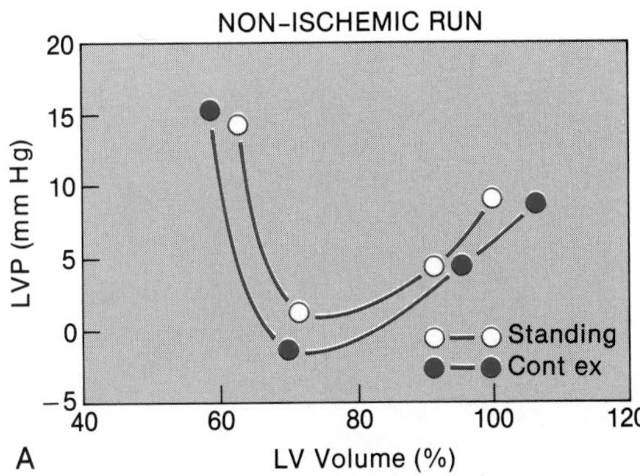

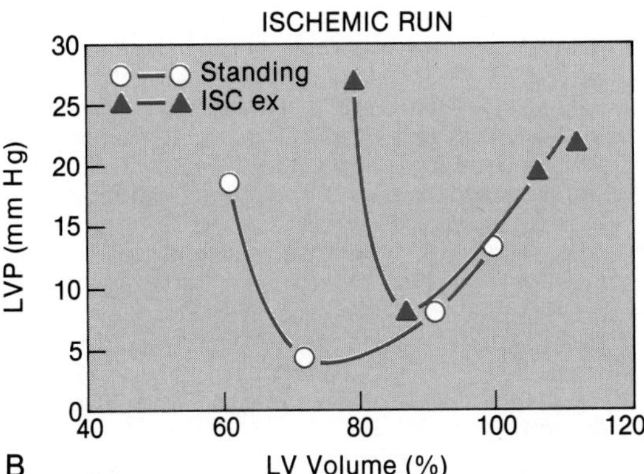

FIGURE 13-31. Averaged left ventricular (LV) diastolic pressure-volume curves. Volumes are expressed as percentage of resting and end-diastolic volume. *A,* Before (standing) and during normal strenuous running (Cont ex) in dogs without ischemia. *B,* Before (standing) and during running in which regional ischemia was induced during the exercise. Note that the diastolic pressure percentage volume curve is shifted downward and leftward during normal exercise (*A*). During exercise with ischemia, (ISC ex) the early portion of the curve is shifted rightward and upward (*B*). (From Miyazaki, S., et al.: Changes of left ventricular diastolic function in exercising dogs without and with ischemia. Circulation *81:*1058, 1989, by permission of the American Heart Association, Inc.)

loading in the dog, intrapericardial pressure rises when overall cardiac volume (both right and left heart chambers) is increased beyond the limit of pericardial distensibility, i.e., when the pericardium becomes restrictive.[221] This factor may also play a role in the large decreases in left ventricular filling pressures that are observed during nitroprusside vasodilator therapy in human heart failure (Fig. 17–19, p. 495) when the heart size decreases within the pericardial sac, which is no longer restrictive.

EFFECT OF PERICARDIUM ON VENTRICULAR LENGTH-PRESSURE RELATIONS. In a chronic volume overload model in the dog (arteriovenous fistula), little effect of the pericardium on the left ventricular diastolic pressure–volume relation was noted, since the pericardial sac gradually enlarged to accommodate the dilated heart.[222] However, in a similar model studied at an earlier time (average 2½ weeks after operation), a mild upward shift of the left ventricular diastolic pressure–volume relation was demonstrated using nitroprusside infusion, indicating a restrictive effect of the pericardium. This effect was absent after pericardiectomy.[223]

THE PERICARDIUM IN CHANGES IN CARDIAC COMPLIANCE. A reduction of left ventricular compliance occurs during angina pectoris (p. 1293), presumably as a consequence of impaired ventricular relaxation,[224] but whether or not the pericardium can contribute to the elevated left ventricular diastolic pressures and upward shift of the left ventricular diastolic pressure–volume curve under these conditions is not yet clear. Evidence suggests that during ischemia developing after pacing, changes in right heart diastolic pressures are not sufficient to account for such a shift.[225] Also, in animals a shift is seen during postpacing ischemia when the pericardium is absent.[226] Experimental work in hearts with the pericardium intact in which both the right atrium and the right ventricle were distended, while the left heart volume was constant at a relatively normal level, indicates that a 50 per cent increase in right heart volume accounts for an approximately 5 mm upward shift of the left ventricular diastolic pressure–volume relation.[227] When intrapericardial pressures were subtracted to yield transmural pressures, no such shifts were evident. Thus, substantial increases in right heart volume, as in the overtransfusion studies cited above,[221] appear to be required to affect the left ventricular diastolic pressure. The degree of filling of the atria at end diastole, which depends on whether or not atrial contraction occurs (e.g., atrial fibrillation) or the timing of atrial systole, can affect the left ventricular end-diastolic pressure–volume relation (and hence shift the standard ventricular function curve) by affecting intrapericardial pressure.[228] Further research is needed to establish the importance of the pericardium in human subjects. There is evidence, however, that acute right ventricular infarction can lead to elevated intrapericardial pressure, with increased right ventricular and left ventricular diastolic pressure.[229–232]

VENTRICULAR INTERACTION. Studies in isolated hearts (without the pericardium) in which the two ventricles were filled separately have shown that the filling of one chamber affects the properties of the other.[204] Other experiments in intact animals with the pericardium in place have shown that increased right ventricular filling not only can increase the left ventricular diastolic pressure but also can change the shape of the left ventricle, with displacement of the interventricular septum to the left.[233] Conversely, with alterations in left ventricular loading, changes in the right ventricular diastolic pressure–volume relation may not reflect an alteration of the right ventricular myocardial or chamber stiffness but rather may be secondary to left ventricular volume changes with elevation of the intrapericardial pressure in a pericardial sac that restrains changes in volume of the entire heart.[234,235] Evidence for a chronic effect of right heart overload on left ventricular function has also been obtained in studies after surgical thromboendarterectomy for chronic thromboembolic pulmonary hypertension. Following operation, Doppler measures of left ventricular diastolic function improved and correlated with a change in the position of the interventricular septum.[236]

In conscious dogs, changes in left ventricular shape and septal position appear to have only minor effects on the function of the left ventricle.[237] Thus, average fiber length rather than left ventricular shape or diastolic pressure was found to be the main determinant of performance. As might be expected, however, changes in the volume of the right ventricle importantly affect stroke output of the left ventricle in the same direction, as the two ventricles function in series.[237]

PERFORMANCE OF THE INTACT VENTRICLE

The traditional determinants of the performance of isolated cardiac muscle, i.e., the preload, the afterload, the inotropic state, and the frequency of contraction, also influence in major ways the performance of the intact ventricle, and when three of these factors are held constant, the fourth can be shown to affect ventricular performance significantly.[182,185] A fifth factor that can influence systolic contractile function (as well as ventricular relaxation) is the degree of electrical and mechanical uniformity of contraction. This factor can have particular importance in the presence of myocardial or coro-

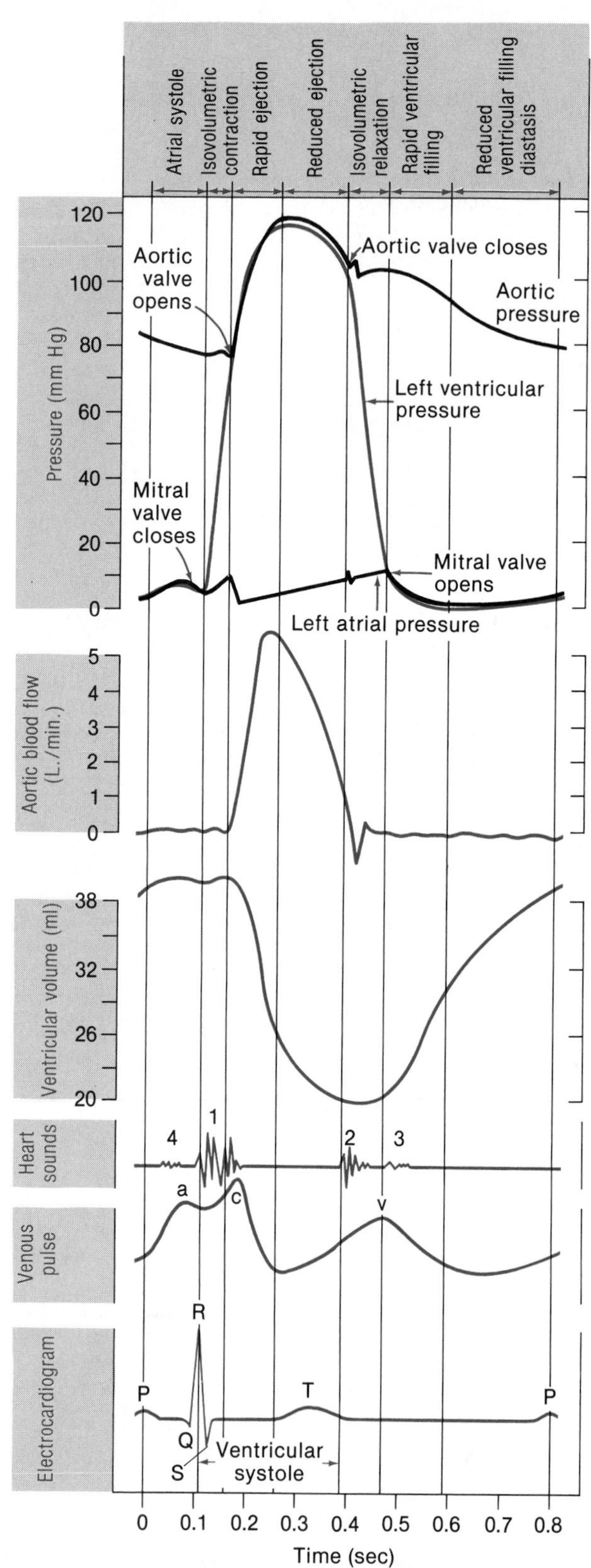

FIGURE 13–32. Events of the cardiac cycle. Left atrial, aortic, and left ventricular pressure pulses are correlated in time with aortic flow, ventricular volume, heart sounds, venous pulse, and electrocardiogram to provide a complete cardiac cycle in the dog. (From Berne, R. M., and Levy, M. N.: Cardiovascular Physiology. 3rd ed. St. Louis, The C. V. Mosby Co., 1977.)

nary heart disease.[238] Also, increased synchrony of systolic performance is important during positive inotropic stimulation, and nonuniformity of contraction in one region can impair function in other (normal) regions.[238] Nonuniformity of performance across the wall of the normal left ventricle has been demonstrated, with increased function of the inner wall compared with the outer wall,[239] and dispersion of sarcomere lengths varies across the left ventricular wall depending upon the ventricular volume.[240] When the ventricle is electrically paced from an abnormal site during exercise, the marked increase of peak left ventricular peak(+) dP/dT that normally occurs is greatly reduced, reflecting impairment of the increased synchrony of contraction that normally accompanies exercise.[241]

INTERRELATIONS OF FACTORS DETERMINING VENTRICULAR PERFORMANCE. While it will be convenient to consider separately the factors that influence cardiac performance, it should be understood that this approach represents an oversimplification since alterations in the length of cardiac muscle (as occur during alterations in preload and afterload in the intact heart) produce length-dependent activation, with a change in the Ca^{++} sensitivity of the myofilaments and hence a change in inotropic state or myocardial contractility. Thus, following an increase in muscle length, a gradual further augmentation of active force occurs in isolated cardiac muscle by this mechanism.[242,243] Such *time-dependent* changes in left ventricular contractility have been described during volume loading in the intact canine ventricle as well[244] and probably are the basis for the observation in the isolated heart that end-systolic pressure is higher in ejecting than in isovolumic beats originating at the same volume.[245,246] The persistence of such length-dependent activation over several beats in the whole heart is probably responsible for observations that the function of prior beats influences that of subsequent beats.[186,245] Length-dependent activation is probably also implicated in "homeometric autoregulation," a time-dependent increase in myocardial contractility after a sudden pressure load,[247] although it has been suggested that the response might represent recovery from transient insufficiency of blood flow to the inner wall of the heart caused by the sudden severe pressure change.[248]

THE CARDIAC CYCLE. The relations between left ventricular pressure, the diameter of the minor equator at the endocardial surface of the left ventricular wall, and the wall thickness in a conscious dog are shown in Figure 13–27, and the events of the cardiac cycle are shown diagrammatically in Figure 13–32. Ventricular end diastole is followed by a brief period of isovolumetric left ventricular contraction, the maximum rate of pressure change (peak dP/dt) occurring just before the onset of ejection.[184] The onset of inward motion of the ventricular wall then commences as blood is ejected into the aorta, and the rate of wall shortening becomes maximal near the middle of ejection. Wall thickness increases during shortening, becoming maximal at the end of ejection. Following isovolumetric relaxation, during which peak negative dP/dt is reached, a rapid increase in the diameter of the ventricle occurs during early diastole, followed by a slow phase of filling in mid-diastole (diastasis); a second, rapid increase in diame-

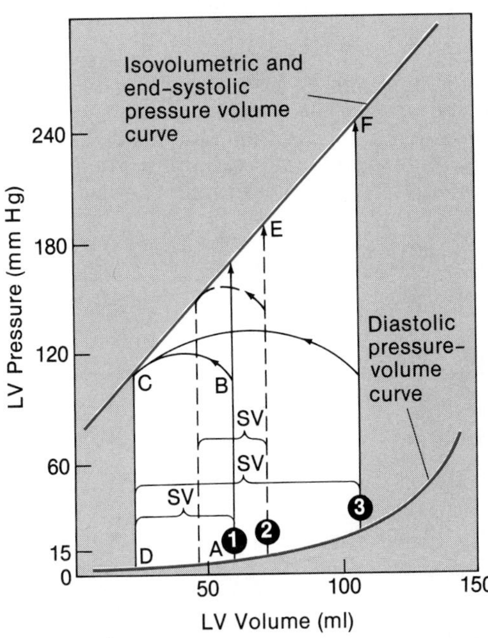

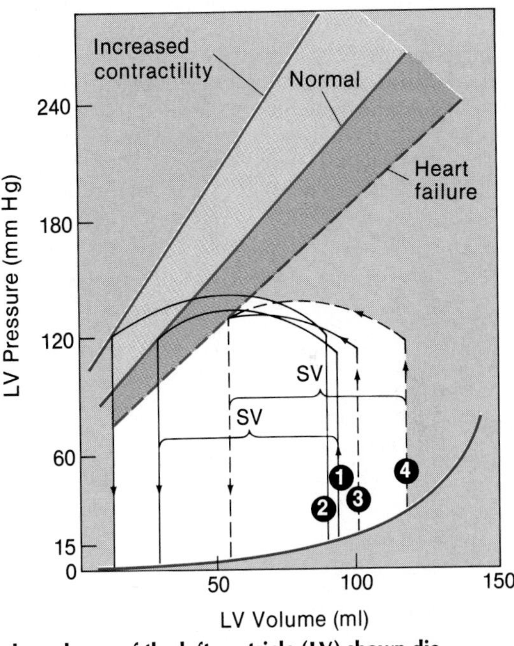

FIGURE 13–33. **Effects of several interventions on pressure-volume loops of the left ventricle (LV) shown diagrammatically. *Left,* Effects of varying preload and afterload (with level of contractility remaining constant). Contraction 1 commences at end diastole (A) and is isovolumetric (arrow A to B) until the onset of ejection (B); the end of ejection or end-systolic volume (C) is followed by isovolumetric relaxation (C to D), and then filling of the ventricle occurs along the diastolic pressure-volume curve (from D to A). When a contraction originating from the same diastolic volume as contraction 1 is forced to contract isovolumetrically (top arrows), a point on the volume-isovolumetric systolic pressure curve is generated; if beats originating at larger end-diastolic volumes (contractions 2 and 3) are forced to contract isovolumetrically, points E and F are generated on that curve. This active pressure-volume curve provides the limit for the end-systolic volume of ejecting contractions. Ejecting contraction 3 shows that increasing end-diastolic volume causes an increase in stroke volume (SV) when aortic pressure is relatively constant. Ejecting contraction 2 (dashed lines) shows the effect of increasing systolic aortic pressure; when compared with contraction 1, SV is actually less, despite an increased end-diastolic volume, because of the higher level of aortic pressure or afterload.**

***Right,* Effects of increasing contractility (positive inotropic agent) and decreasing contractility (heart failure) on left ventricular pressure–volume loops. Contraction 1 is a normal pressure–volume loop, at a normal level of contractility. Contraction 2 shows that when contractility is increased, a larger stroke volume is generated from a similar or even slightly reduced end-diastolic volume, aortic pressure being relatively constant. In the presence of heart failure, SV may be diminished despite a slightly larger end-diastolic volume at a comparable level of aortic pressure (dashed line, contraction 3); however, SV may be restored if end-diastolic volume is further increased (contraction 4).**

ter takes place in late diastole, as a consequence of atrial contraction. The time course of changes in ventricular volume closely parallels those shown for ventricular internal diameter during each cardiac cycle.

THE PRESSURE-VOLUME LOOP. The relation between ventricular pressure and volume can also be plotted as a pressure-volume loop (Fig. 13–33) in a manner analogous to that used in plotting the sarcomere length-tension (Fig. 13–26) relations. This provides a convenient framework for understanding the responses of individual left ventricular contractions to alterations in preload, afterload, and contractility.

The pressure-volume loop of the left ventricle can be related to the performance of isolated cardiac muscle, in which the active isometric length-tension curve provides the limit of shortening for isotonic contractions (Fig. 13–26). The relation between the end-systolic volume and the end-systolic pressure of the left ventricle is nearly linear, is analogous to this length-tension relation, and has been well defined in the isolated heart preparation[249] (Fig. 13–34, left). It can be shifted by inotropic influences without a change in the volume intercept in the isolated heart, thereby providing a load-independent measure of contractility.[250]

THE END-SYSTOLIC PRESSURE-VOLUME RELATION (see also p. 428). In the intact animal, linear end-systolic pressure–volume relations can be produced by altering loading conditions with infusion of a vasopressor which has no appreciable inotropic effects, such as angiotensin (Fig. 28–13, p. 830),[251] or by vena caval obstruction.[252] In humans, the end-systolic ventricular volume is determined by obtaining two or more angiocardiograms during infusion of phenylephrine, and the end-systolic values are then related to the corresponding ventricular or aortic pressure at the end of ventricular ejection.[253] Noninvasive techniques for measuring ventricular dimensions or volume (echocardiography and radionuclide methods)[254] can also be employed. The linear end-systolic pressure–volume relation of the human left ventricle has been found to shift downward and to the right in the presence of myocardial disease (Fig. 13–34, right) and to shift upward and to the left (with steepening of its slope) during acute positive inotropic interventions (Fig. 13–34, right).

This relation is of particular importance because it defines the level of inotropic state under acutely changing conditions *independent* of the end-diastolic volume (preload) and the systolic pressure (as a measure of afterload). It is analogous to the length–active tension curve of isolated muscle. Thus, for practical purposes, a given cardiac cycle arrives at end ejection and falls into this linear relation, regardless of the starting point for end-diastolic volume and the level of aortic pressure encountered during ejection, and the entire end-systolic pressure–volume relation is shifted acutely by a change in inotropic state (Fig. 13–32). Use of the end-systolic pressure–volume relation for comparing ventricles in different patients still has not been completely standardized,[255] although experimental work indicates that both the slope of the relation (E_{max}, or systolic elastance, which can be determined from the maximum instantaneous ratio of pressure to volume occurring near end-ejection) and its volume intercept are functions of body and left ventricular weight.[256] Although this relation is relatively linear, in more recent studies curvilinearity has been described during changes in loading conditions[228] and inotropic state.[229] Despite such curvilinearity, the slope of the relation was found useful for assessing changes in contractility in intact animals over a limited range of loading conditions, produced by vena caval obstruction.

Under conditions in which there are *chronic* changes in the shape and size of the ventricle or in the thickness of its wall, systolic pressure is not indicative of the level of afterload; under these conditions the end-systolic pressure–volume relation or E_{max} does not define the level of inotropic state. For example, in animals with compensated pressure-overload hypertrophy of the concentric type, the end-systolic pressure–volume relation was shifted upward (indicating hemodynamic hyperfunction), but when wall stress was used instead of pressure (to account for the increased wall thickness), the wall force–volume relation fell into the same relation as the normal ventricle, indicating normal contractility.[230] On the

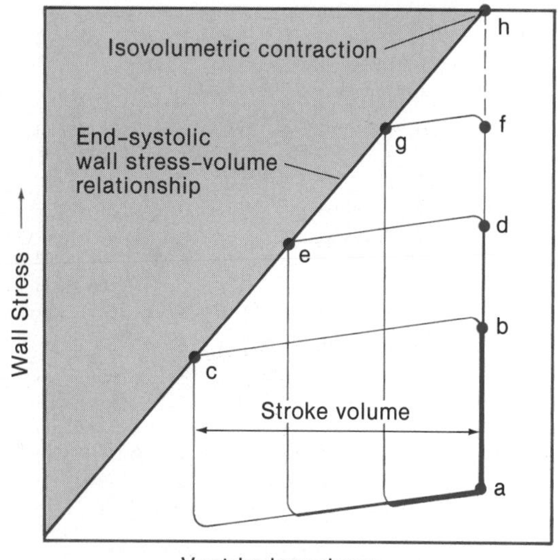

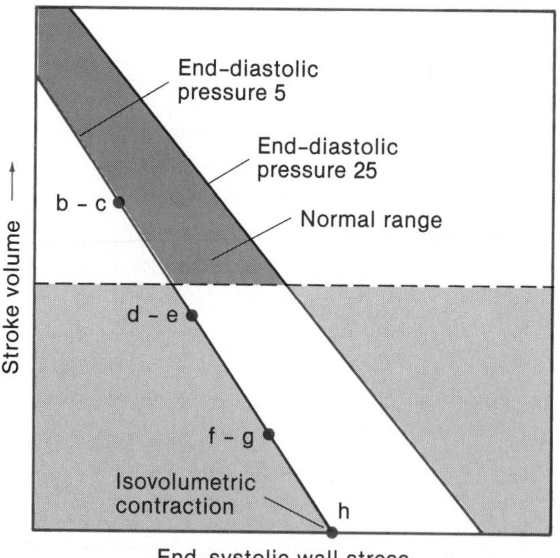

FIGURE 13–34. ***Left,* Loops showing the relation between left ventricular volume and wall stress during contractions in which the end-diastolic volume is held constant, and progressive increases in afterload are induced. In the initial contraction, beginning from end diastole (point A), the ventricle initially develops pressure volumetrically (points A and B) and the ejection volume (point B to C) is indicated as the stroke volume. The effects of progressively higher afterloads to reduce the stroke volume are shown (point D to E, and point F to G). Finally, at point H an isovolumetric contraction results at the same end-diastolic volume. *Right,* Inverse relation between end-systolic wall stress and stroke volume showing that progressively increased systolic wall stress causes a drop in stroke volume and vice versa, with zero stroke volume at point H. The left-hand inverse relation originates from a normal left ventricular end-diastolic pressure of 5 mm Hg, whereas the right-hand relation originates from an elevated end-diastolic pressure of 25 mm Hg, showing the effect of increased preload to shift the inverse end-systolic wall stress-stroke volume relation. Within the shaded range, the preload reserve can maintain the stroke volume at a normal level, despite increasing end-systolic wall stress. (Modified from Weber, K. T., et al.: The mechanics of ventricular function. Hosp. Pract. *18:*113, 1983.)**

other hand, studies in patients with chronically dilated hearts suggest that correction of E_{max} for ventricular volume may not be necessary to separate patients with depressed contractility from those with normal function.[231]

LAPLACE'S LAW. In comparing the whole heart to isolated muscle, heart volume and pressure are analogous to muscle length and tension. More complex formulations have also been developed; thus, the average circumferential wall stress (force per unit of cross-sectional area of wall) is related directly to the product of intraventricular pressure and internal radius and inversely to wall thickness. In the simplest version of Laplace's law for a spherical ventricle, $\sigma = Pa/2h$ and for an ellipsoidal ventricle, $\sigma = \frac{Pb}{h} \cdot \frac{1 - b^2}{2c^2}$ where σ = average circumferential wall stress, a = radius at the endocardial surface, P = intraventricular pressure, h = wall thickness; and b and c = the semiminor and semimajor axes at the endocardial surface.[170] In the ejecting ventricle, their extent and rate of wall shortening—and thus indirectly the stroke volume—are analogous to the extent and velocity of shortening of isolated muscle. The ventricular pressure during ventricular ejection is closely related to the afterload, although geometrical factors must be considered in order to calculate wall forces in the heart.

PRELOAD

In the intact heart, ventricular end-diastolic wall stress or tension is analogous to the preload of isolated muscle and ultimately determines the resting length of the sarcomeres (Fig. 13-26).

PRELOAD RESERVE. As a consequence of the exponential shape of the left ventricular diastolic pressure-volume curve (Fig. 15-27, p. 440), there is considerably less preload reserve beyond the upper limit of normal for ventricular filling pressure than below it. However, studies in conscious resting dogs (without the pericardium) under basal conditions indicate that with volume loading alone there is a stroke volume reserve of approximately 13 per cent.[262] With further volume loading, the left ventricular end-diastolic volume increases by an additional 3 or 4 per cent, and a theoretical stroke volume reserve of 31 per cent was calculated assuming an unchanged left ventricular systolic pressure.[262] Experiments in conscious dogs suggest that the preload reserve may be lower.[263]

Preload reserve is especially great in human subjects, in whom the basal resting end-diastolic volume is reduced by the pooling of blood in the lower extremities. Of course, a considerable further stroke volume reserve can be made available by enhanced inotropic state, which increases the ejection fraction and ventricular emptying.

During upright exercise in normal human subjects, in which radionuclide ventriculography was used to determine left ventricular volumes, it was found that preload reserve is utilized during low levels of exercise, increased left ventricular end-diastolic volume accompanying the augmentations of heart rate and stroke volume.[264,265] However, at high levels of exercise, as heart rate increased further, ventricular end-diastolic volume was shown to decrease, and stroke volume was maintained by a reduction of ventricular end-systolic volume.[264,265]

In addition to some preload reserve available during stress, variations on the performance of both ventricles due to alterations in preload occur on a beat-to-beat basis in maintaining balanced outputs from the right and left heart during normal respiration, with abrupt changes in body position, as well as during other changing physiological conditions.

INFLUENCE OF PRELOAD ON VENTRICULAR CONTRACTION. The effect of alterations in preload independent of alterations in frequency, afterload, and inotropic state for the left ventricle is shown diagrammatically in Figure 13-33, left. Increases in preload augment the stroke volume as well as the extent and velocity of wall shortening. This preload effect is operative at all levels of systolic pressure or afterload. From Figure 13-34, it can be seen that an inverse relation between systolic wall stress and stroke volume applies if the preload is constant, and that this entire relation is shifted upward by an increase in preload (Fig. 13-34, right panel)[266] and downward by diminished preload. If ejection is prevented and the ventricle contracts isovolumetrically, a direct correlation between preload, as reflected in the end-diastolic volume, and peak left ventricular systolic pressure or calculated wall stress can also be shown (analogous to the length-active tension curve of isolated muscle).

These relationships constitute expressions of the Frank-Starling mechanism and provide the basis for ventricular function curves in the normally ejecting heart, which relate ventricular end-diastolic volume or pressure to stroke volume and stroke work.[267] Any of the curves already discussed can, of course, be shifted up or down by positive and negative inotropic influences, respectively.

ATRIAL CONTRIBUTION TO PRELOAD. Like ventricular muscle, atrial muscle responds to increasing stretch with a more forceful contraction. When properly timed, atrial contraction augments ventricular filling and preload. Rapid ventricular filling induced by atrial contraction at the end of diastole abruptly elevates ventricular end-diastolic pressure and volume. This allows a lower mean atrial pressure to exist throughout most of diastole than would be the case if atrial contraction were ineffective (as in atrial fibrillation) or ill-timed (as in nodal rhythm or atrioventricular dissociation).[268] The atrial contribution to ventricular filling is of particular importance in the presence of ventricular hypertrophy and other states of reduced ventricular compliance. In these conditions, the loss of atrial systole reduces ventricular end-diastolic pressure and volume, ultimately impairing ventricular performance.[269]

DESCENDING LIMB OF STARLING'S CURVE. The question of whether a descending limb of cardiac function due to excessive increase in ventricular diastolic volume exists in the whole left ventricle has been of interest. In the isovolumetrically contracting isolated canine left ventricle, no reduction of developed wall stress or systolic pressure occurred until the ventricular end-diastolic pressure exceeded 60 mm Hg; when diastolic ventricular pressure was further elevated to 100 mm Hg, developed pressure declined by only 7.5 per cent. At these extremely high end-diastolic pressures, sarcomere lengths averaged 2.27 to 2.30 μ.[270] Based on this and other work showing that midwall sarcomere lengths did not exceed 2.27 μ at left ventricular end-diastolic pressure up to 40 mm Hg,[271] it may be postulated that the descending limb of ventricular performance, when observed in the ejecting ventricle, is *not* caused by operation of the heart on a descending limb of the sarcomere length-tension relation; i.e., it is not a consequence of overstretch with the disengagement of actin and myosin myofilaments.

APPARENT DESCENDING LIMB. However, a descending limb of curves that relate left ventricular end-diastolic pressure to stroke work, was demonstrated in dogs when volume loading was carried out to achieve end-diastolic pressures exceeding 30 mm Hg, after mean aortic pressure had initially been elevated.[272] Under these circumstances, slight further increases in aortic pressure occurred during the volume loading, which elevated left ventricular filling pressures above 30 mm Hg. It was concluded that the descending limb of function in the ejecting ventricle is only apparent and actually results from reduced myocardial wall shortening due to an increased afterload, when the ventricle is unable to compensate by further increases in sarcomere length.[272] It has also been proposed that the descending limb of function induced in the failing human heart by infusion of a vasopressor agent[273] is due to such an effect of augmented afterload, when preload reserve is absent.[274] The development of mitral regurgitation consequent to ventricular dilatation can also depress forward stroke volume and result in an *apparent* depression of ventricular performance as preload is elevated to very high levels.

Another cause for an *apparent* descending limb of the relationship between left ventricular end-diastolic pressure (or volume) and the stroke volume has also been described. Excessive afterload produced by angiotensin infusion in the normal, conscious dog resulted in an inability of the ventricle to maintain the stroke volume despite an increase in the ventricular end-diastolic pressure and volume.[262] If volume loading was then produced by fluid infusion and the angiotensin infusion repeated, such a descending limb occurred at higher levels of stroke volume. Thus, originating from the basic Frank-Starling curve relating left ventricular end-diastolic volume to stroke volume, a series of descending limbs can be demonstrated when pressure loading is carried out at various levels of left ventricular end-diastolic volume. Such responses explain how the entire function curve can be shifted downward by increased afterload and upward by reduced afterload, as with a vasodilator. Such *apparent* descending limbs of left ventricular function due to pressure loading are due to insufficient venous return. This inadequate venous return prevents the left ventricle from compensating and increasing left ventricular end-diastolic volume to the level required to meet the increased afterload.[262]

In *summary*, alterations in preload, operating through changes in end-diastolic fiber length, serve as an important determinant of the performance of the intact ventricle and provide the basis for the function curves of the intact ventricle. The ability to augment preload provides a functional reserve to the heart in situations of acute stress and exercise, and variations in preload operate on a beat-to-beat basis in maintaining balanced outputs of the two ventricles during such normal maneuvers as respiration.

Control of Preload in the Intact Organism

In the intact organism, preload is determined largely by venous return and total blood volume and its distribution[275] as well as by the activity of the atrium.

VENOUS RETURN. In the absence of heart failure in the intact organism, most changes in cardiac output can be accounted for largely by changes in the *return* of blood to the heart, which in turn alters the preload. In the absence of heart failure, simple augmentation of myocardial contractility, as occurs with administration of a cardiac glycoside or institution of sustained postextrasystolic potentiation (paired electrical stimulation), or cardiac pacing has little effect on cardiac output.[276] In contrast, relatively major changes in output occur during maneuvers that alter venous return, such as lower body positive or negative pressure, positive-pressure respiration, a sudden change in posture, and rapid changes in blood volume.

Conditions that lower peripheral vascular resistance are among the most important of those augmenting venous return and include the opening of arteriovenous fistulas and conditions that mimic the latter, such as patent ductus arteriosus, fever, beriberi, pregnancy, and Paget's disease. (These and other chronic high-output states are discussed in Chapter 16.) A reduction in vascular resistance also occurs during *exercise*, when the arterioles supplying the exercising muscle dilate; in severe *anoxia*, when generalized vascular dilation occurs; and in the presence of *anemia*, when blood viscosity and hence resistance to flow in the vascular bed are reduced.

EFFECTS OF VENODILATION. If nitroprusside is administered intravenously in the relatively normal circulation of the anesthetized dog, the cardiac output falls, despite lowered vascular resistance and hence more favorable afterloading conditions on the normal left ventricle. This response takes place because nitroprusside induces dilation of the venous bed as well as arteriolar dilation, and the venodilation is only partially compensated for by a modest shift of blood volume from the central to the peripheral circulation.[277] The ensuing reduction of venous return to the right heart produces a reduction in right ventricular output and hence in left ventricular output via the Frank-Starling mechanism. Thus, a fall in cardiac output occurs because of the limited venous return, despite a reduction of the afterload on the left ventricle.[277]

If nitroprusside is administered in the presence of acute experimental left ventricular failure (produced by multiple coronary artery ligations), in which the left ventricular end-diastolic pressure is elevated to more than 20 mm Hg, an *opposite* effect occurs and the cardiac output increases. Again, nitroprusside produces venodilation in the peripheral circulation, but in the setting of heart failure there is more than a threefold greater shift of blood volume from the distended central circulation to the peripheral bed.[277] This presumably occurs because the failing left ventricle is able to unload more effectively against the lowered systemic arteriolar resistance, thereby allowing a release of blood stored within the heart and lungs. Under these conditions, the shift of blood volume from the central circulation exactly counterbalances the effect of nitroprusside to reduce the effective systemic blood volume. The correction of excessive afterload (afterload mismatch)[274] on the failing left ventricle can then be expressed as an increase in the cardiac output. Under these conditions the failing left ventricle (not the venous return) becomes the limiting factor for cardiac output.[277] These observations explain the clinical effects of vasodilators in the treatment of heart failure (p. 491).

TOTAL BLOOD VOLUME. When blood volume is rapidly reduced, cardiac output and particularly stroke volume decline. However, in the intact organism, small (less than 15 per cent of control) or gradual reductions in blood volume can be tolerated with barely perceptible changes in cardiac output, as a consequence of a number of compensatory mechanisms resulting from activation of the adrenergic nervous system.

DISTRIBUTION OF BLOOD VOLUME. At any given total blood volume, the ventricular end-diastolic volume is a function of the distribution of blood between the intra- and extrathoracic compartments. The principal determinants of this distribution are described below.

Body Position. Gravitational forces pool blood in the dependent portions of the body; therefore, assumption of the upright posture increases extrathoracic blood volume at the expense of intrathoracic and ventricular end-diastolic volumes, thereby reducing preload and cardiac output. The effects of negative pressure (suction) applied to the lower extremities and trunk with the subject supine mimic those of assumption of the upright posture, while inflation of a lower-body positive-pressure suit, immersion of the lower extremities and trunk into water, or the absence of gravitational force during space flight increases intrathoracic blood volume and preload.

Intrathoracic Pressure. The negative intrathoracic pressure normally increases thoracic blood volume, improving cardiac filling and augmenting preload and thereby cardiac performance. The intrathoracic pressure becomes more negative during inspiration and approximates atmospheric pressure during expiration. Accordingly, the gradient for venous return (and therefore right ventricular stroke volume) rises during inspiration when the intrathoracic pressure declines. Elevation of mean intrathoracic pressure, as occurs with the application of positive-pressure respiration or the development of pneumothorax, tends to impede total venous return to

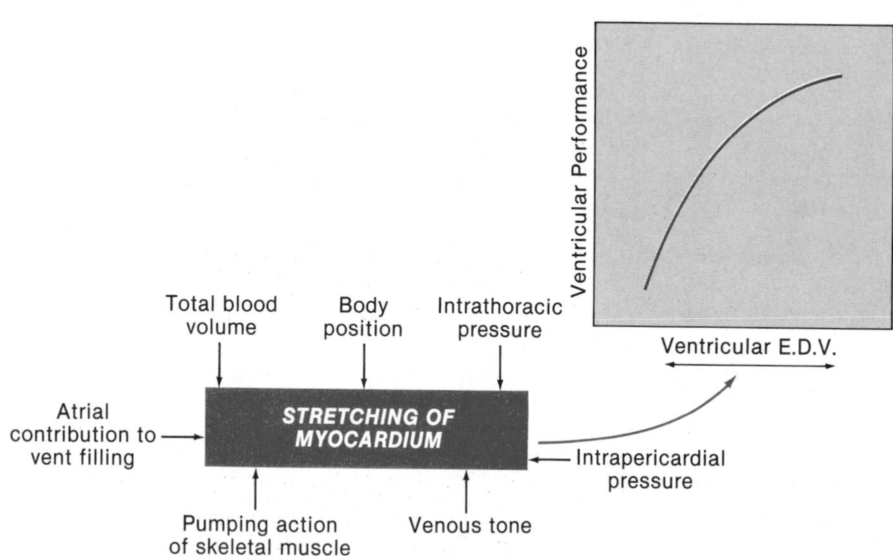

FIGURE 13–35. ***Bottom left,*** **Major influences that determine the degree of stretching of the myocardium, i.e., the magnitude of end-diastolic volume (E.D.V.).** ***Top right,*** **Diagram of a Frank-Starling curve, relating ventricular E.D.V. to ventricular performance. (From Braunwald, E., et al.: Mechanisms of Contraction of the Normal and Failing Heart, 2nd ed. Boston, Little, Brown, 1976.)**

the heart, diminishes intrathoracic blood volume, and ultimately reduces ventricular performance.[278]

Intrapericardial Pressure (see Chapter 45). When pericardial pressure is elevated, as occurs in pericardial effusion, there is interference with cardiac filling, and the resultant reduction in ventricular diastolic volume (preload) reduces ventricular performance. With marked elevations of intrapericardial pressure, cardiac tamponade may occur, which is characterized by marked lowering of stroke volume and arterial pressure with circulatory collapse. Chronic constrictive pericarditis also impedes ventricular filling and thereby lowers stroke volume.[279]

Venous Tone. Smooth muscle in the walls of the veins responds to a variety of neural and humoral stimuli; venoconstriction occurs during exercise, anxiety, deep respiration, or marked hypotension, tending to augment intrathoracic blood volume. A variety of drugs act on venous smooth muscle. Thus, sympathomimetic agents produce venoconstriction, while ganglionic blocking agents and sympatholytic and norepinephrine-depleting drugs or agents such as nitroglycerin that are direct venodilators produce extrathoracic pooling and thereby ultimately reduce preload and cardiac output.[280] Extravascular compression of the veins by skeletal muscle plays an important role in augmenting venous return by exercising skeletal muscle.[278]

ATRIAL CONTRIBUTION TO VENTRICULAR FILLING. A vigorous, appropriately timed atrial contraction augments ventricular filling and end-diastolic volume.[268]

AFTERLOAD

When applied to the intact ventricle, afterload may be defined as the tension, force, or stress (force per unit of cross-sectional area) acting on the fibers in the ventricular wall *after* the onset of shortening. It is influenced importantly by the arterial pressure and is a key determinant of the quantity of blood ejected by the ventricle. In the intact heart, abrupt alterations in the impedance to left ventricular ejection when the preload is constant cause reciprocal changes in wall shortening and the stroke volume of the left ventricle[281] (Fig. 13–33, left). As the left ventricle becomes smaller in size during normal ejection of blood into the aorta, its wall thickens, and despite a small rise in the aortic pressure during ejection, the afterload or wall stress falls during ejection (that is, the normal heart "unloads itself" as it ejects) (Fig. 15–11, p. 428).

VENTRICULOARTERIAL COUPLING. The coupling between the left ventricle and the arterial system depends on the independent properties of each (Fig. 13–36). At any equilibrium point, the inverse linear relation between the left ventricular systolic pressure and stroke volume or cardiac output resulting from the effect of afterload on shortening will intersect with the positive linear relation between stroke volume and the systolic arterial pressure.[185,266] This reflects the increased arterial pressure as flow through the arteries is increased. If vascular resistance is increased, for example, the slope of the relation between cardiac output and arterial pressure will decrease (i.e., pressure will be higher at any cardiac output). At equilibrium, the ability of the heart to generate systolic pressure just balances the pressure needed to push blood through the arterial system.[185,266]

The influence of variations in afterload on the systolic performance of the intact ventricle also can be studied using the isotonically contracting heart preparation in which preload, contractility, and heart rate are held constant. Increasing the afterload reduces both stroke volume and the extent and velocity of wall shortening. Curves showing inverse relationships between afterload (systolic pressure or wall stress) and stroke volume, extent of wall shortening (Fig. 13–34, right panel), and velocity of shortening can be constructed.[266,272,281]

BASIS FOR USE OF AFTERLOAD REDUCTION (see Chap. 17). The low impedance to left ventricular ejection (reduction in afterload) produced by mitral regurgitation,[282] patent ductus arteriosus, ventricular septal defect, or arteriovenous fistula can increase the extent of shortening and the ejection fraction. In the acutely pressure- and/or volume-overloaded ventricle, when sarcomere length is optimal and there is no preload reserve, any alteration in afterload causes a reciprocal change in stroke volume.[281] It is clear that the more severely depressed the inotropic state of the heart, the greater the influence of a change in afterload on the extent of myocardial fiber shortening, as evidenced by the decreased slope of the end-systolic pressure-volume relation in heart failure (Fig. 13–33, right). These considerations are relevant to the use of vasodilating agents to augment cardiac output in patients with left ventricular failure (Fig. 17–14, p. 492) and the use of pressor agents in the assessment of left ventricular function.

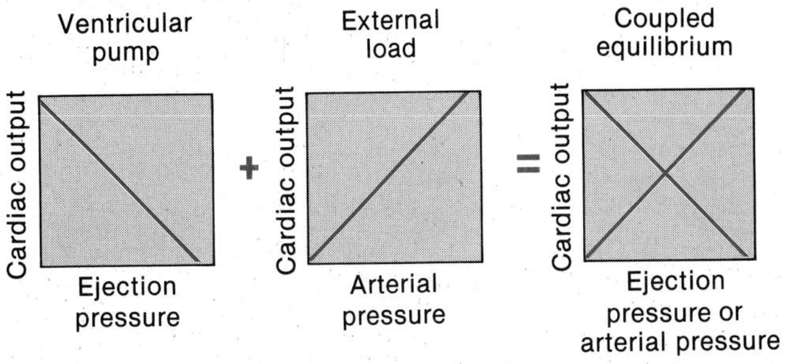

ARTERIAL COUPLING

FIGURE 13–36. The functional coupling of the left ventricular pump to the arterial system. *Left,* The ventricular pump responds to an increase in ejection pressure (afterload) with a reciprocal reduction of cardiac output. *Center,* The arterial pressure rises directly with an increase in cardiac output. *Right,* The intersection of these two relations leads to unique values for arterial pressure and cardiac output (at any level of preload and myocardial contractility). (From Weber, K. T.: The contractile behavior of the heart and its functional coupling to the circulation. Prog. Cardiovasc. Dis. *24*:389, 1982, by permission of Grune and Stratton.)

When the ventricle is not operating along the steep portion of its diastolic pressure–volume curve, i.e., when there is still some preload reserve, an elevation of afterload often results in a compensatory elevation of ventricular end-diastolic volume, i.e., a rise in ventricular preload, which enhances myocardial contraction. However, as a consequence of the operation of Laplace's law (p. 377), this compensatory elevation of preload elevates myocardial tension development (afterload) further, and this in turn reduces myocardial fiber shortening. However, geometrical considerations dictate that the relative extent of myocardial fiber shortening required to maintain stroke volume constant is less in the larger ventricle. Hence, stroke volume may remain constant even though myocardial fiber shortening declines. If afterload rises, and if inflow into the ventricle is not restricted and preload can also rise, stroke volume can be maintained. In accord with these considerations, the normal subject responds to a modest rise in arterial pressure by maintaining stroke volume and increasing stroke work while augmenting left ventricular end-diastolic pressure and volume; i.e., the increase in afterload is met by an increase in preload (Fig. 13–33, left), whereas in the diseased heart stroke volume and stroke work tend to fall because there is little, if any, preload reserve.[273,274] Thus, the response to increased aortic pressure is dependent in significant measure both on the level of myocardial contractility and on the preload, in that a moderate pressor stress will ordinarily produce little change in stroke volume in the normal heart but will diminish stroke volume in heart failure. When there is relative hypovolemia or the pressor stress is substantial, and preload cannot rise, an increase in afterload will reduce the stroke volume in the normal heart (Fig. 13–33, left, beat 2).[262]

In patients with congestive heart failure, the systemic vascular resistance and ventricular filling pressures are generally increased. In this setting, a mixed arteriolar and venodilator (such as nitroprusside, an angiotensin-converting enzyme inhibitor, or combined hydralazine and nitrates) usually is administered to reduce the afterload on the left ventricle (p. 482), yielding opposite effects to those already described for administration of a vasopressor agent. Vasodilator therapy causes a fall in systemic vascular resistance and the accompanying venodilation produces a shift of blood volume from the central to the peripheral circulation (as already discussed);[277]

these changes, in turn, cause ventricular volume to fall, with a reduction of left ventricular end-diastolic pressure and systolic wall stress. The latter can occur even when the change in systolic arterial pressure is minimal, and this reduction in afterload on the failing left ventricle allows an increase in the stroke volume and cardiac output.[187]

Control of Afterload in the Intact Organism

In the intact organism, afterload is determined largely by peripheral vascular resistance, the physical charateristics of the arterial tree, and the volume of blood that it contains at the onset of ejection. The critical role played by ventricular afterload in cardiovascular regulation is summarized in Figure 13–37. While increases in both preload and contractility increase myocardial fiber shortening, increases in afterload reduce it; myocardial fiber shortening and left ventricular size determine stroke volume. Arterial pressure, in turn, is related to the product of cardiac output and systemic vascular resistance, while afterload is a function of left ventricular size and arterial pressure. For example, when vasoconstriction raises arterial pressure, afterload is also augmented, which, through a negative feedback, reduces myocardial fiber shortening, stroke volume, and cardiac output; the fall of the latter, in turn, acts to restore arterial pressure to its previous level.

When ventricular function is impaired, afterload becomes an increasingly important determinant of cardiac performance. In the case of the left ventricle, afterload may rise as a consequence of vasoconstriction resulting from the influence on the arterial bed of neural, humoral, and structural changes that occur in response to a fall in cadiac output. This increased afterload may reduce cardiac output further; on the other hand, pharmacological reductions of afterload may be beneficial in elevating cardiac output.

In *summary*, when acute changes in arterial pressure occur, the resultant alteration in afterload has an important effect on cardiac performance. An understanding of the effects of changes in afterload is central to an appreciation of the effects of conditions such as systemic or pulmonary arterial hypertension and obstruction to ventricular ejection by valvular disease (aortic and pulmonic stenosis), which increase afterload, and of mitral regurgitation and ventricular septal defect, which reduce it. Adaptation to a chronic increase in afterload by hypertrophy, in which a gradual increase in wall thickness occurs and tends to return wall stress and wall shortening characteristics toward normal, is discussed in Chapter 14.

CONTRACTILITY (INOTROPIC STATE)

The terms "contractile state" and "inotropic state" may be used interchangeably but have different connotations. A change in performance is generally considered to indicate a change in cardiac function regardless of the mechanism (such as moving up or down on a single ventricular function curve, or a shift of the entire function curve). On the other hand, a change in myocardial contractility or in the inotropic state is generally considered to describe the changes in cardiac performance that are observed after sympathetic stimulation, administration of positive or negative inotropic agents, or the depressed function of myocardial disease, as reflected by a shift of the entire ventricular function curve. When loading conditions remain constant, an improvement in contractility augments cardiac performance (a positive inotropic effect), while a depression in contractility lowers cardiac performance (a negative inotropic effect). In the intact heart, inotropic influences generally act through altered Ca^{++} availability to the myofilaments or through an alteration in myofilament Ca^{++} sensitivity.

The effects of an increase in contractility induced by a positive inotropic agent such as a beta-adrenoceptor agonist have been studied in isotonically contracting hearts in which the other determinants of performance (preload, afterload, and contraction frequency) can be held constant. As in isolated muscle, increases in the velocity and extent of wall shortening and increased stroke volume occur while the duration of contraction is shortened and the rate of relaxation increases.[283,284] The force-velocity relation is shifted upward, P_o and V_{max} both increase (Fig. 13–22), and curves relating diastolic volume to active peak isovolumetric pressure and ventricular function curves are shifted upward (Fig. 13–33, right). Acute administration of negative inotropic agents produces the opposite effects.[284a]

THE INTERVAL-STRENGTH (FORCE-FREQUENCY) RELATION (see also p. 364). In the intact ventricle, as in isolated cardiac muscle, premature depolarization results in a reduced mechanical contraction, the extent of the reduction being directly proportional to the degree of prematurity. However, the ensuing contraction is then more forceful than normal, a phenomenon termed "postextrasystolic potentiation." When studied in the isovolumetrically beating heart with preload held constant to exclude loading effects, the degree of augmentation of the postextrasystolic beat (increased contractility, manifested by increased dP/dt) is related in a positive exponential manner to the prematurity (coupling interval) of the extra electrical stimulus (within limits, the earlier the stimulus, the greater the potentiation), and in an inverse exponential manner to the delay in the occurrence of the next (postextrasystolic) beat. The effect is related to the quantity of Ca^{++} released from an internal store during the postextrasystolic beat.[285] In the intact organism, when the premature beat is followed by a compensatory pause, the ventricular end-diastolic volume may be augmented, and this increased preload may contribute along with the greater contractility to the enhanced performance that characterizes the postextrasystolic contraction. Postextrasystolic potentiation can be sustained and results in a striking augmentation of myocardial contractility when pairs of stimuli are delivered repetitively to the intact ventricle. In this technique, termed "paired electrical stimulation,"[286] the second stimulus is placed immediately after the electrical refractory period and results in only a small secondary contraction.

Pulsus alternans (alternating weak and strong beats) sometimes is observed experimentally when cardiac contractility has deteriorated and the heart rate is rapid, and can be noted

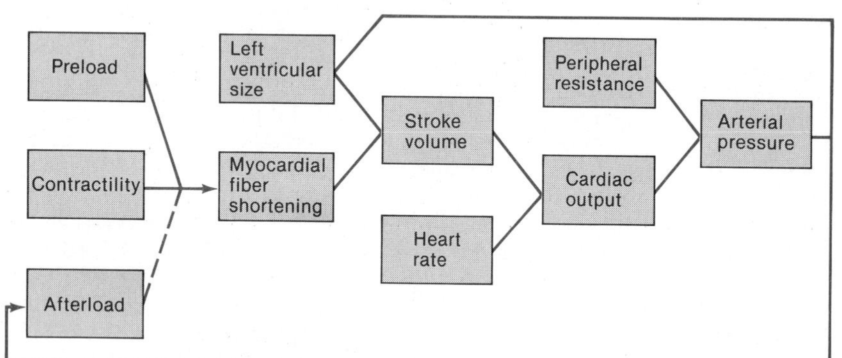

FIGURE 13–37. Schema showing interactions between various components regulating cardiac activity. Solid lines indicate an increasing effect; broken line represents a depressing effect. Note that left ventricular size is a determinant of both stroke volume and afterload. (Reprinted by permission from Braunwald, E.: Regulation of the circulation. N. Engl. J. Med. *290:*1124, 1974.)

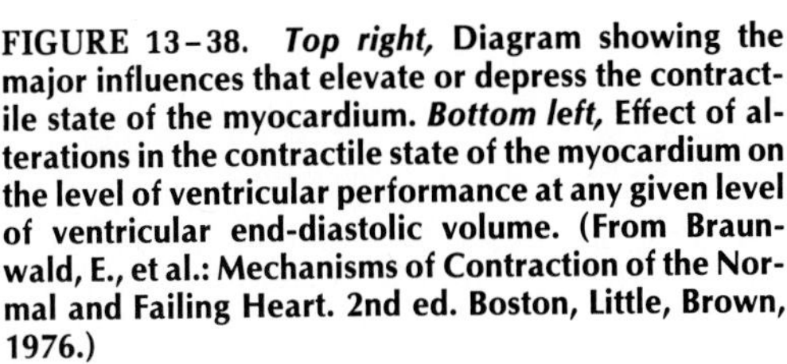

FIGURE 13–38. *Top right,* **Diagram showing the major influences that elevate or depress the contractile state of the myocardium.** ***Bottom left,*** **Effect of alterations in the contractile state of the myocardium on the level of ventricular performance at any given level of ventricular end-diastolic volume. (From Braunwald, E., et al.: Mechanisms of Contraction of the Normal and Failing Heart. 2nd ed. Boston, Little, Brown, 1976.)**

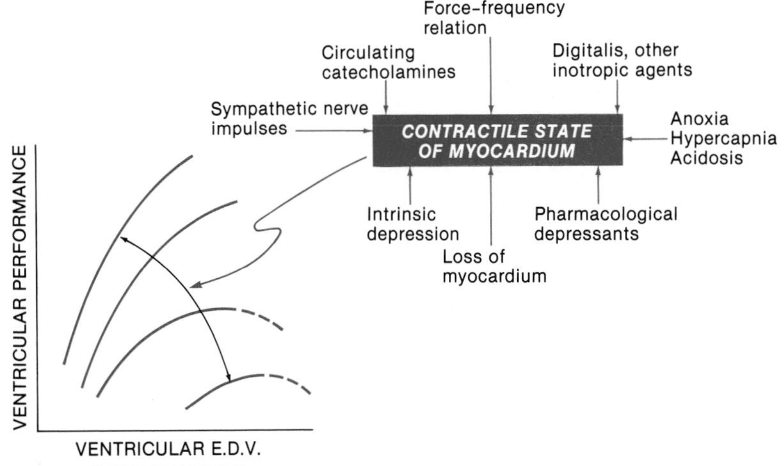

in patients with severe myocardial disease (p. 454). Its basic cause is uncertain, but experimental studies indicate that alternating changes in contractility occur in addition to accompanying alterations of preload and afterload.[287]

Control of Contractility in the Intact Organism

The factors that modify the contractility of the myocardium may be considered to operate by modifying the level of ventricular performance at any given ventricular end-diastolic volume, i.e., the relative position of the entire Frank-Starling curve (Fig. 13–38).

SYMPATHETIC NERVE ACTIVITY. The quantity of norepinephrine (NE) released by sympathetic nerve endings in the heart is probably the most important factor regulating myocardial contractility under physiological conditions. Rapid changes in contractility in the intact organism are effected by variations in the impulse traffic in the cardiac adrenergic nerves. Beta-adrenoceptor blocking agents and NE-depleting drugs interfere with the myocardial response to sympathetic nerve stimuli.

Prejunctional alpha-adrenergic receptors are important in regulating norepinephrine release to the myocardium during enhanced sympathetic nerve activity, such as with exercise, and they exert a negative feedback control by increasing norepinephrine reuptake under such conditions. This effect can be demonstrated by administration of an α_2-adrenergic blocking agent (such as yohimbine) during exercise, which causes pronounced increases in myocardial contractility, heart rate, and norepinephrine release from the heart.[288] Recent evidence indicates that alpha-adrenergic blockade produces similar effects during exercise, most likely also by a prejunctional mechanism.[289]

CIRCULATING CATECHOLAMINES. When stimulated by nerve impulses, the adrenal medulla releases epinephrine, which is carried by the bloodstream to the myocardium, where it stimulates beta receptors and augments contractility. This mechanism is slower than the response to NE release by cardiac nerves but may be of physiological importance in conditions such as hypovolemia and a variety of chronic stresses, including congestive heart failure.

FORCE-FREQUENCY RELATION. The inotropic effect of changing the frequency of contraction, which also alters the amount of Ca^{++} available to the myofilaments, is often termed the "force-frequency relation". Increases in heart rate augment contraction velocity and shorten the duration of contraction and vice versa.[183] A ventricular extrasystole augments contractility, although to a decreasing extent, for several cardiac cycles. A simple increase in frequency in the physiological range also augments cardiac contractility, but this effect is more prominent in isolated heart muscle or in the intact heart with depressed function than it is in the normal heart of the intact organism.

EXOGENOUS INOTROPIC AGENTS. The cardiac glycosides, sympathomimetic agents, caffeine, theophylline, amrinone, and their derivatives (Chap. 17) all augment cardiac contractility. Changes in blood ionized [Ca^{++}] also produce significant effects on myocardial contractility, as demonstrated by shifts in the relatively load-independent relation between left ventricular wall stress and shortening velocity in patients during variations in blood Ca^{++} levels caused by hemodialysis.[290]

PHYSIOLOGICAL AND PHARMACOLOGICAL DEPRESSANTS. These include anoxia,[291] ischemia (Chap. 38),[292] acidosis,[292] and local anesthetics (Chap. 28), barbiturates, and most general anesthetics.

LOSS OF CONTRACTILE MASS. When a portion of the ventricle becomes necrotic, as occurs in ischemic heart disease, the overall performance of the ventricle at any given end-diastolic volume is reduced, even though the contractility of the remaining myocardium may be normal (Chap. 39).

INTRINSIC MYOCARDIAL DEPRESSION. Although, as indicated in Chapter 14, the fundamental mechanism responsible for depression of myocardial contractility in heart failure still remains to be elucidated, it is now apparent that the contractile state of each unit of myocardium is depressed in this condition.

HEART RATE

(See also pp. 385 and 386)

Accelerating the frequency of contraction generally does not induce a shift of the ventricular function curve, i.e., the relation between ventricular end-diastolic pressure and stroke work, in the open-chest anesthetized dog; however, it does increase stroke power (rate of performance of stroke work) at any given level of filling pressure,[293] a finding consistent with improvement of myocardial contractility and with observations on the effects of increases in the frequency of contraction in isolated cardiac muscle. Pacing-induced increases in contraction frequency, unaccompanied by sympathetic stimulation of the ventricle, also increase the calculated V_{max} and elevate the force-velocity relation of the ventricle in the anesthetized open-chest dog, and augment the relaxation rate.

The positive inotropic effect resulting from an increase in the frequency of contraction is more prominent in the anesthetized animal, in the depressed heart, and in isolated cardiac muscle than in the normal heart of the intact, conscious dog. In the conscious state at rest, venous return to the heart is reflexly and metabolically stabilized, so that artificially varying heart rate between about 60 and 160 beats/min has little effect on cardiac output, despite the aforementioned modest changes in contractility that accompany changes in heart rate.[294] However, if the diastolic volume of the left ventricle is maintained by increasing venous return as heart rate is increased, an elevation of frequency will augment cardiac output, and during exercise, tachycardia normally plays the major role in increasing cardiac output.[264,265] Under these circumstances, the speed of ventricular contraction and relaxation are markedly augmented, atrial contraction is enhanced, and the increased venous return can be accommodated, despite the rapid heart rate and reduced diastolic filling time.[208]

When the heart is paced at a very rapid rate by electrical stimulation of the atrium, with the subject or experimental animal at rest, there is much less inotropic effect on contraction velocity and the duration of contraction, so that diastolic filling time per minute is much less. Therefore, with rapid pacing (and with tachyarrhythmias) the short duration of diastole can lead to interference with the ventricular filling, with a fall in cardiac output when rates approach 180 to 200 min.[293]

Since, at a constant stroke volume, cardiac output is a linear function of heart rate, the ability to alter the latter is a critically important mechanism in the adjustment of cardiac output. The importance of heart rate in the maintenance of cardiac output is reflected in the inability of patients or experimental animals with fixed heart rates to elevate cardiac output appropriately, even when myocardial function is entirely normal.[295,296] Under normal circumstances, heart rate is determined largely by the slope of phase 4 (spontaneous depolarization) of the sinoatrial node; the intrinsic rhythmicity may be altered by a variety of influences, such as temperature and metabolism, rising with fever and thyrotoxicosis and falling with hypothermia and hypothyroidism. The two neurotransmitters released by autonomic nerves innervating the sinoatrial node play a critical role in the control of heart rate; acetylcholine slows while NE accelerates the slope of diastolic depolarization.

RIGHT VENTRICULAR FUNCTION

The right ventricle responds to the same determinants of contraction as the left ventricle (preload, afterload, contractility), and it can exhibit a normal ventricular function curve when the left ventricular function curve is depressed, or vice versa. Under normal conditions, the right ventricle is not required for maintenance of pulmonary blood flow, arterial pressure, and cardiac output, as demonstrated by right ventricular bypass models.[297] Although there is a mild increase in the venous pressure at rest when the right ventricle is excluded, the left ventricle is capable of mantaining the circulation. Normally, however, the right ventricle serves to maintain a low pressure in the systemic veins so that peripheral edema does not occur,[298] and its function becomes highly important during exercise, hypovolemia, or when the pulmonary vascular resistance is elevated.[301] Also, the right ventricle undergoes hypertrophy in chronic pulmonary hypertension (p. 159), an adaptation that allows maintenance of a normal stroke volume.[301]

Neural Control of Cardiac Contraction

The autonomic nervous system is of critical importance in the moment-to-moment regulation of heart rate and contractility and of the capacitance and resistance of the vascular bed, thereby controlling cardiac output, blood flow distribution, and arterial pressure.[299] Neural regulation is capable of producing considerable changes in cardiocirculatory function within seconds, before more slowly acting mechanisms, such as those mediated by metabolic stimuli, circulating catecholamines, and the renin-angiotensin system, exert any effect. The basic function of cardiovascular reflexes is to integrate the function of the heart with the physiological demands of the peripheral circulation in the rest of the body.

Studies of control mechanisms have been greatly aided by observations of instrumented, conscious animals. Many of their responses are substantially different, even opposite, from those observed during study of anesthetized open-chest animals.[294] One major difference is that conscious animals (and humans) in the basal state have reduced sympathetic and augmented parasympathetic tone compared with that seen in the study of anesthetized and particularly anesthetized, open-chest animals.

ANATOMICAL CONSIDERATIONS

(Fig. 13–39)

Sympathetic and parasympathetic preganglionic cells represent the final common pathways of neural impulses to the cadiovascular system. These cells receive both excitatory and inhibitory impulses from all levels of the central nervous system but most importantly from the cardiovascular center in the medulla and from spinal neurons. The medullary cardiovascular centers, operating independently of higher structures, are capable of regulating cardiac contractility and rate, arterial pressure, and even blood flow distribution, but under normal conditions their activity is regulated by influences from higher centers, notably the cerebral cortex, especially its cingulate gyrus, the hypothalamus, and the reticular substance in the pons and the mesencephalon. The impulse traffic from the vasomotor center is heightened by wakefulness, pain, mental and muscular effort, or emotional stress. Tonic activity in the medullary cardiovascular-excitatory center is constantly inhibited by impulses from the cardiovascular mechanoreceptors (both the high-pressure receptors in the carotid sinuses, aorta, and left ventricle and the low-pressure receptors in the atria, pulmonary vascular bed, and ventricles). However, the medullary centers also receive input from chemoreceptors in skeletal muscle, skin, the viscera, and the special senses. An increased activity of nerve impulse traffic in the carotid sinus and aortic nerves as well as in vagal afferent fibers from the heart reflexly reduces neural activity in efferent sympathetic fibers and augments efferent vagal discharges. As a result, vasomotor tone in resistance and capacitance vessels and heart rate are reduced, AV conduction is prolonged, and contractility of the atria and ventricles is reduced.

The cell bodies of the sympathetic preganglionic neurons lie in the intermediolateral horns of the spinal cord; most of their axons leave the spinal cord through the anterior roots of the thoracic and first two lumbar spinal nerves, synapse with postganglionic neurons in the chains of ganglia on each side of the spinal cord or in the peripheral sympathetic ganglia, and then traverse peripheral sympathetic nerves or spinal nerves to the heart and blood vessels. Some preganglionic sympathetic nerve fibers pass directly through the sympathetic chains, through the splanchnic nerves, and into the adrenal medulla where they synapse with secretory cells, which are analogous to postganglionic neurons. Catecholamines (predominantly epinephrine) may be released thereby from the adrenal medulla into the bloodstream at times when sympathetic efferent activity involving other organs is heightened. These two means of sympathetic stimulation (neural and humoral) supplement each other, the former acting rapidly but often briefly and the latter acting slowly but in a more sustained manner.

While considerable overlap of autonomic innervation exists within most portions of the heart, certain regions receive their major supply from restricted sources. The sympathetic nerves originating from the right stellate ganglion are distributed primarily to the sinoatrial node and the right atrium, while the left ventrolateral cardiac nerve provides the primary supply to the posterolateral surfaces of the left atrium and ventricle; the central representation of these nerves may allow selective and rapid regulation of cardiac function. Contractility of both the epicardial and endocardial surfaces of the left ventricle can be independently altered, and it is now clear that certain nerves preferentially supply nodal tissues while others innervate contractile tissues.[299] The sympathetic nerve endings in the atria and ventricles are interposed between muscle bundles. The terminal sympathetic innervation of the heart is a plexiform structure, the so-called *perimuscular* or *perimysial plexus,* which extends around the muscle cells in close apposition to, but without penetrating, the myocardial cells. The cardiac muscle cells and innervating fibers might be considered to be analogous to a neuromuscular unit in skeletal muscle. When the rate of liberation of the neurotransmitter exceeds the capacity of the enclosed units to utilize or metabolize it, it may overflow into vascular channels.[300]

NOREPINEPHRINE, THE ADRENERGIC NEUROTRANSMITTER (Fig. 13–39)

The norepinephrine (NE) present in the heart is synthesized and then stored in the sympathetic nerve fibers rather than in the myocardial cells per se. Chemical sympathectomy with 6-hydroxydopamine, surgical denervation, and treatment with catecholamine-depleting drugs such as reserpine all result in a striking reduction in NE content of the heart as well as in the disappearance of histochemical fluorescence. Sympathetic nerve endings contain neurosecretory granules ranging in size from 400 to 700 nm, and the depolarization of the neurons causes release of intraneuronal Ca^{++}, which in turn causes the NE-containing granules to migrate to the cell membrane of the neuron, there to liberate NE.

The effects of released NE are terminated by three mechanisms[301]: (1) approximately 75 per cent is taken back into the adrenergic neuron (reuptake) by means of an energy-dependent pump; once inside the neuron, much of the transmitter is again taken up into the neurosecretory granules and is available for subsequent release;[302] (2) escape of NE into the circulation is metabolized by catechol-*O*-methyltransferase (COMT) to normetanephrine, some of which is further converted into vanillylmandelic acid (VMA) via the action of monoamine oxidase (MAO); and finally (3) conversion of NE intraneuronally to 3,4-dihydroxymandelic acid by MAO and then to VMA by COMT. The heart and other organs exhibit supersensitivity to NE after surgical denervation or the administration of cocaine and tricyclic antidepressants. These interventions prevent the neuronal uptake of NE, thus making a larger quantity of neurotransmitter available for binding to the receptor sites, and augment the response to NE. The denervated heart also exhibits hyperresponsiveness to circulating catecholamines, principally epinephrine, because of an increase in beta-adrenoceptor density.[302]

The peripheral effects mediated by NE and epinephrine have been classified as alpha or beta. An important effect of NE is to cause vasoconstriction, an action on postsynaptic $alpha_1$ receptors on vascular smooth muscle. The mechanisms by which NE acts upon cardiac beta and alpha receptors are discussed on page 363. Adrenergic neurons contain a variety of presynaptic receptors (Fig. 13–40). Circulating epinephrine acts on presynaptic beta receptors, enhancing the release of NE. On the other hand, the released NE acts on presynaptic $alpha_2$ receptors, thereby inhibiting its own release (feedback inhibition). Acetylcholine (released from vagal nerve endings) acts on muscarinic receptors on adrenergic neurons, inhibiting the release of NE.

As we have seen, NE, the natural transmitter for sympathetic neurons, has both alpha and beta receptor–stimulating properties. When NE is given systemically, the alpha vasoconstrictor action predominates, and the elevation of arterial pressure results in reflex bradycardia and an increase in stroke volume and coronary blood flow but no change in cardiac output. *Epinephrine*, synthesized only in the adrenal medulla, also has combined alpha and beta actions, but its beta effects are more striking than those of NE, especially in low doses; therefore, it produces tachycardia and an elevation of

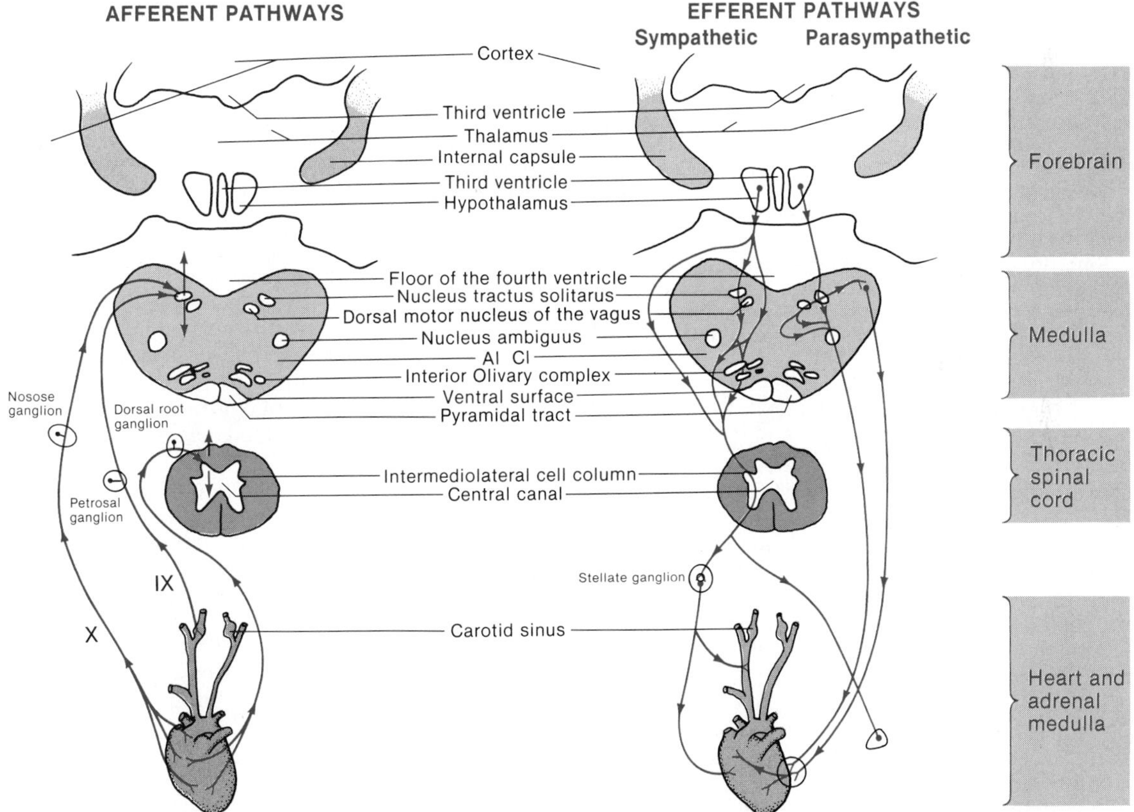

FIGURE 13–39. Schematic diagram of cardiovascular reflex pathways through the central nervous system. *Left,* Afferent limb of the supraspinal and spinal reflex arcs originating from the sensory receptors of the heart and vasculature. The site of the first synapse in the supraspinal arc is at the nucleus tractus solitarius (NTS). *Right,* Efferent sympathetic (left side of diagram) and parasympathetic (right side) pathways. The sympathetic pathway between NTS and the intermediolateral cell column of the spinal cord, which contains the cell bodies of the proganglionic sympathetic efferent fibers, may include synapses at a variety of medullary sites. The medulla depicted here is a composite diagram, because all of the structures, as drawn here, do not exist together in any one given section of the brain stem. The parasympathetic pathway between NTS and nucleus ambiguus, which contains the cell bodies of the preganglionic parasympathetic efferent fibers, may include synapses at a variety of sites, including the dorsal motor nucleus of the vagus, the midline raphe nuclei, or the external cuneate nucleus. Forebrain areas, such as the hypothalamus, may influence autonomic outflow. (From Corr, P. B., Yamada, K. A., and Witkowski, F. X.: Mechanisms controlling cardiac autonomic function and their relation to arrhythmogenesis. *In* Fozzard, H. A., et al. [eds.]: The Heart and Cardiovascular System. New York, Raven Press, 1986, p. 1357.)

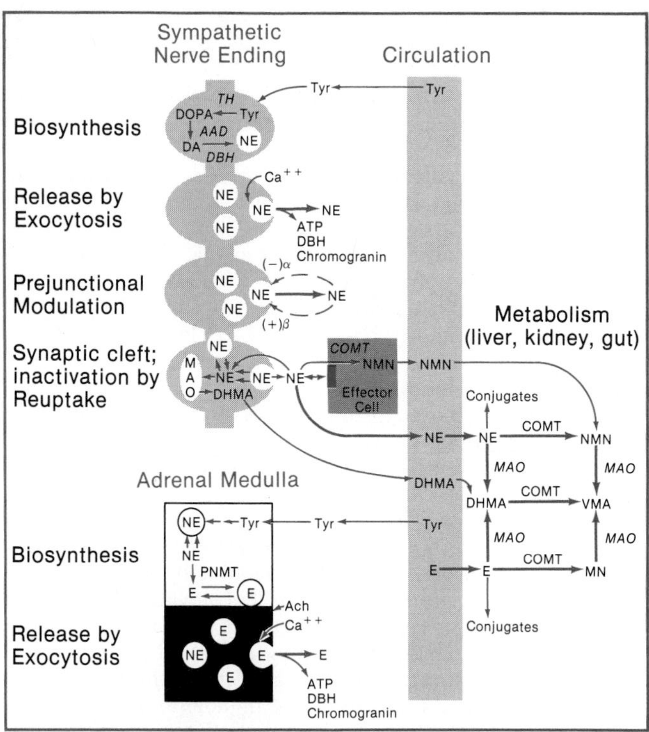

FIGURE 13–40. Catecholamine biosynthesis, release, and metabolism. Schematic representation of a peripheral sympathetic nerve ending is shown at the top; the bulbous areas on the terminal fiber represent varicosities identified by histochemical fluorescence techniques as areas of high neurotransmitter concentration. The processes of biosynthesis, release, modulation, and reuptake are shown sequentially for demonstration purposes only; in vivo they proceed concurrently. Adrenal medullary chromaffin cells are shown at the bottom of the diagram. TH = tyrosine hydroxylase, AAD = aromatic-L-amino acid decarboxylase, DA = dopamine, DBH = dopamine-beta-hydroxylase, NE = norepinephrine, PNMT = phenylethanolamine-N-methyltransferase, E = epinephrine, COMT = catechol-O-methyltransferase, NMN = normetanephrine, MAO = monoamine oxidase, DHMA = 3,4-dihydroxymandelic acid, VMA = 3-methoxy-4-hydroxymandelic acid. (From Landsberg, L., and Young, J. B.: Physiology and pharmacology of the autonomic nervous system. *In* Wilson, J., Braunwald, E., Isselbacher, K., et al.: Harrison's Principles of Internal Medicine. 12th ed. New York, McGraw-Hill, 1991, p. 381.)

cardiac output. *Dopamine* is the third naturally occurring catecholamine that subserves a transmitter function in the central nervous system. When infused, it has both alpha and beta effects and in addition acts on what appear to be specific dopamine receptors. At low doses (1 to 5 $\mu g/kg/min$, administered intravenously), it dilates mesenteric and renal vessels, producing increased renal blood flow and sodium excretion by its action on dopamine receptors. At slightly higher doses (5 to 10 $\mu g/kg/min$), beta stimulation increases cardiac output with relatively little tachycardia. At even higher doses (> 10 $\mu g/kg/min$), tachycardia and alpha stimulation occur. *Isoproterenol* is a synthetic compound with pure beta-agonist activity, causing a reduction in peripheral vascular resistance with an increase in heart rate and contractility and thus an increase in cardiac output.

When sympathetic nerves to the heart are stimulated, arterial NE concentrations rise, proportional to the workload and heart rate achieved during exercise. Also, coronary sinus catecholamine concentrations exceed those in arterial blood, indicating that the heart liberates large quantities of NE consequent to activation of sympathetic fibers, and that this NE exceeds the capacity for reuptake and local metabolism, resulting in a "spillover" into the circulation.[304,305]

THE PARASYMPATHETIC SYSTEM

The vagi provide rich parasympathetic innervation of the sinoatrial and A-V nodes, and, to a slightly lesser extent, of the myocardium. The parasympathetic neurotransmitter acetylcholine has a very brief duration of action, since it is rapidly hydrolyzed by the large quantities of acetylcholinesterase in the heart. The ventricular myocardium is only sparsely innervated by parasympathetic efferent nerves. There is some functional parasympathetic innervation of the ventricles, because when heart rate, preload, afterload, atrial function, and coronary perfusion pressure are all held constant, vagal stimulation depresses ventricular contractility. In the basal state, sympathetic activity is low and parasympathetic restraint is dominant. For this reason, beta-adrenoceptor blockade has relatively little effect on sinoatrial automaticity or A-V conduction of a human or animal in the basal state, while cholinergic blockade with atropine causes an increase in heart rate and acceleration of A-V conduction. In addition, cholinergic blockade does not alter heart rate during maximal exercise, consistent with the hypothesis that there is little if any parasympathetic tone during exercise.

CARDIAC CONTROL IN THE INTACT ORGANISM

(Figs. 13–41 and 13–42)

In the normal state, there are several redundant mechanisms that contribute to cardiac performance, and interference with one or even more of them may not influence the resting cardiac output. For example, a moderate reduction of blood volume or loss of the atrial contribution to ventricular contraction can ordinarily be sustained without a reduction of cardiac output in the resting state. Presumably, other factors such as an increase in adrenergic nerve impulse traffic, which augments contractility, and venoconstriction, which increases ventricular filling, can compensate for this depression.[306] Mechanisms are also available to prevent unnecessary elevation of cardiac output. For example, in normal subjects, expansion of blood volume, a simple increase in heart rate induced by atropine or electrical pacing, or augmentation of myocardial contractility by means of cardiac glycosides does not increase cardiac output.[307,308] Some of these stimuli may reduce the frequency of adrenergic nerve impulses to the heart, thereby tending to oppose the direct inotropic effect.[309] More importantly, since the normal heart is capable of expelling all of the blood returned to it under most physiological conditions, cardiac output is ordinarily a function of venous return, not of the level of contractility. Since the latter does not limit the volume of blood ejected by the heart in the normal subject except perhaps under severe stress, stimulation of myocardial contractility would not be expected to elevate cardiac output in a normal subject at rest or during mild activity unless there is a simultaneous reduction in peripheral arterial resistance (as occurs with isoproterenol administration),[310] or when this increased contractility is accompanied by an augmentation of venous return. In the presence of congestive heart failure, on the other hand, cardiac output is usually limited by the contractile state of the myocardium, and a positive inotropic influence or reduction of afterload raises cardiac output.[286]

CIRCULATORY ADJUSTMENT DURING EXERCISE

During maximal exercise, total body oxygen consumption may increase ten- to twelvefold, cardiac output four- to fivefold, and the arteriovenous–mixed venous oxygen difference may more than double. There is a redistribution of blood flow from nonexercising areas such as the splanchnic bed, with an enormous increase in flow to the exercising muscles. Despite this, the oxygen extraction by skeletal muscle rises to very high levels.

PERIPHERAL CIRCULATORY RESPONSES. As important as the heart may be in mediating the body's response to isotonic exercise, alterations in the peripheral circulation are of at least equal significance. Indeed, the elevation of cardiac output achieved in the resting state through infusion of a

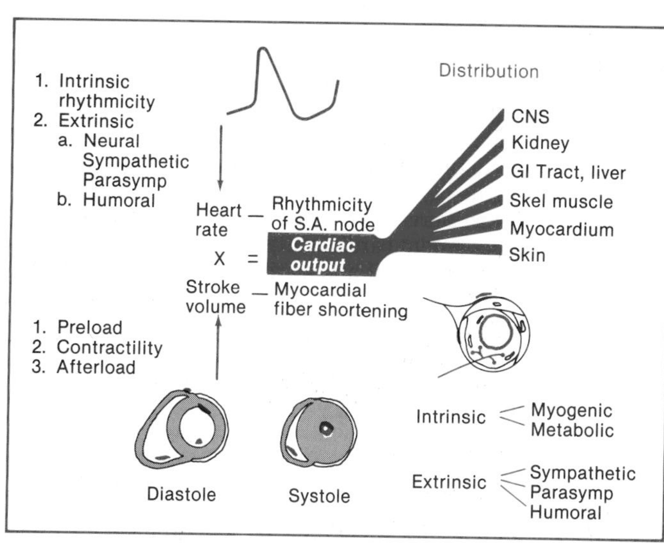

FIGURE 13-41. Schema of factors affecting systemic circulation. In the center, cardiac output is shown with its two determinants, heart rate and stroke volume; the former is a function of the automaticity of the sinoatrial (S. A.) node, while the latter is dependent on the extent of myocardial fiber shortening. The principal determinants of heart rate and stroke volume are listed at the extreme left. Distribution of cardiac output through various vascular beds is shown at the upper right (CNS = central nervous system). The two principal influences (intrinsic and extrinsic) on the lumen of the peripheral resistance vessels and their major determinants are shown at the lower right. (Reprinted by permission from Braunwald, E.: Regulation of the circulation. N. Engl. J. Med. *290*:1124, 1974.)

maximal dose of isoproterenol, which greatly augments cardiac rate and contractility, does not approach the level commonly observed during exercise. Changes in the peripheral circulation act in concert to augment the capacity of the vascular bed to return blood to the heart.[311] Perhaps the most important of these is the vasodilation that takes place in the blood vessels supplying the exercising muscles, resulting primarily from metabolic stimuli such as adenosine (p. 1168) and the release of endothelin-derived relaxing factor (EDRF) as a consequence of the increased shear stress acting on the endothelium by increased blood flow (p. 1170), but perhaps also through the activation of cholinergic nerves innervating arterioles that supply skeletal muscle. The marked reduction in systemic vascular resistance acts in a manner analogous to the opening of a large arteriovenous fistula and greatly reduces the resistance to the return of blood ejected from the left ventricle back to the right atrium. Despite profound vasodilation in the metabolizing muscles during exercise, arterial pressure tends to rise in normal subjects, primarily as a consequence of the marked elevation of cardiac output but also as a result of vasoconstriction, which occurs in many vascular beds other than in the heart and the exercising limbs.[312] This elevation of arterial pressure enhances perfusion of the exercising muscle. Failure of arterial pressure to rise during exercise usually signifies severe impairment of left ventricular function and reflects an inadequate rise of cardiac output. Among patients with ischemic heart disease, it identifies a subgroup of patients at higher risk of poor outcome. Other factors that facilitate venous return during exercise include the rhythmic tensing of the skeletal muscles, not only of the exercising limbs but of the abdomen and thorax as well, which compresses the veins and displaces blood centrally.[311] In addition, during exercise, sympathetic impulses to capacitance vessels further augment venous return.[313]

VENTRICULAR VOLUMES AND DIMENSIONS. The cardiac response to exercise is complex and involves the interaction of all four determinants of ventricular performance, i.e., heart rate, contractility, preload, and afterload. In humans, the elevation of cardiac output that occurs during mild exercise in the *supine* position results almost exclusively from an increase in heart rate, with stroke volume and end-systolic volume showing little change.[314] During maximal exercise in the supine position, stroke volume and end-diastolic volume increase slightly.[315,316] In contrast, in individuals at rest in the *erect* position blood pooling below the heart reduces ventricular end-diastolic and stroke volumes at rest. These variables increase markedly during strenuous exertion; the increases in stroke volume contribute substantially to the elevation of cardiac output. Indeed, during maximal treadmill exercise, stroke volume increases to approximately twice the levels present at rest in the upright position.[317,318] Radionuclide ventriculography obtained at rest and during exercise in normal subjects has shown increases in ejection fraction, stroke volume, left ventricular end-diastolic volume, and cardiac output, with a reduction of end-systolic volume.

The effects of *light* muscular exercise in the supine position on ventricular dimensions have been studied in patients by determining the distances between radiopaque markers sewn onto the epicardium.[319] End-diastolic dimensions in both ventricles decreased slightly[320,321] while myocardial contractility rose, as attested to by a shift of the force-velocity relation.[321] Maximal exercise in the dog[303] also results in an increase in end-diastolic dimensions.

HEART RATE (see also p. 381). The ability to alter heart rate is an extremely important mechanism for the adjustment of cardiac output during exercise. Indeed, changes in heart rate account in large measure for changes in cardiac output occurring under most circumstances in everyday life. The increase in cardiac output that occurs in humans during light to moderate exercise in the supine position is accompanied by a

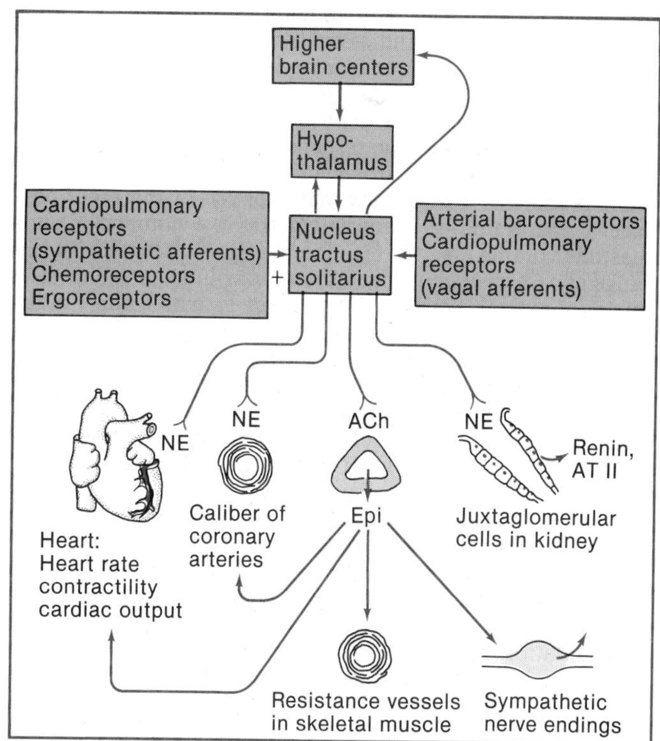

FIGURE 13-42. Neurohumeral control of the circulation. NE = Norepinephrine, Epi = epinephrine, ACh = acetylcholine, APII = angiotensin II. (From Shepherd, J. T.: Circulatory response to exercise in health. Circulation *76*(Suppl. VI):3, 1987, by permission of the American Heart Association, Inc.)

In Levy, M. N., and Vassale, M. (eds.): Excitation and Neural Control of the Heart. Baltimore, Williams and Wilkins, 1982, pp. 79–92.
13. Katz, A. M.: Membrane structure. *In* Fozzard, H. A., et al. (eds.): The Heart and Cardiovascular System. New York, Raven Press, 1986, p. 101.
14. Spray, D. C., and Bennett, M.V.L.: Physiology and pharmacology of gap junctions. Ann. Rev. Physiol. *47*:281, 1985.
15. Robinson, T. F., Geraci, M. A., Sonnenblick, E. H., and Factor, S. M.: Coiled perimysial fibers of papillary muscle in rat heart. Circ. Res. *63*:577, 1988.
16. Bong, T. K., and Caulfield, J. B.: The collagen matrix on the heart. Fed. Proc. *40*:2037–2041, 1981.
17. Sato, S., Ashrof, M., Millard, R. W., et al.: Connective tissue changes in early ischemia of porcine myocardium: An ultrastructural study. J. Mol. Cell. Cardiol. *15*:261, 1983.
18. Langer, G. A.: Calcium at the sarcolemma. J. Mol. Cell. Cardiol. *16*:147, 1984.
19. Carafoli, E.: Intracellular calcium homeostasis. Ann. Rev. Biochem. *56*:375, 1987.
20. Catterall, W. A.: Structure and function of voltage-sensitive ion channels. Science *242*:50, 1988.
21. Jones, L. R.: Subcellular fractionation of cardiac sarcolemma and sarcoplasmic reticulum. *In* Fozzard, H. A., et al. (eds.): The Heart and Cardiovascular System. New York, Raven Press, 1986, p. 253.
22. Rappaport, L., and Samuel, J. L.: Microtubules in cardiac myocytes. Int. Rev. Cytol. *113*:101, 1988.
23. Fabiato, A.: Calcium-induced release of calcium from the cardiac sarcoplasmic reticulum. Am. J. Physiol. *245*:Cl, 1983.
24. Huxley, H. E.: The double array of filament in cross-striated muscle, J. Biophys. Biochem. Cytol. *3*:631, 1957.
25. Warber, K. D., and Potter, J. D.: Contractile proteins and phosphorylation. In Fozzard, H. A., et al. (eds.): The Heart and Cardiovascular System. New York, Raven Press, 1986, pp. 779.
26. Page, S.: Management of structural parameters in cardiac muscle. CIBA Foundation Symposium 24 (New Series), Amsterdam, Elsevier, 1974, p. 13.
27. Toyoshima, Y. Y., Toyoshima, C., and Spudich, J. A.: Bidirectional movement of actin filaments of tracks of myosin heads. Nature *341*:154, 1989.
28. Trombitas, K., and Tigyi-Sebes, A.: Cross-bridge interaction with oppositely polarized actin filaments in double-overlap zones of insect flight muscle. Nature *309*:168, 1984.
29. Gevers, W.: The mechanism of myocardial-contraction. *In* Opie, L. (ed.): The Heart. New York, Grune and Stratton, 1986, pp. 98–107.
30. Murphy, R. A.: Contraction of muscle cells. *In* Berne, R. M., and Levy, M. N. (eds.): Physiology. St. Louis, C. V. Mosby, 1983, pp. 359–386.
31. Eisenberg, E., and Hill, J. L.: Muscle contraction and free energy transduction in biological systems. Science *277*:999, 1985.
32. Tao, T., Gong, B-J., and Leavis, P. C.: Calcium-induced movement of Troponin I relative to actin in skeletal muscle thin filaments. Science *247*:1339, 1990.
33. Scheuer, J., and Bhan, A. K.: Cardiac contractile proteins. Adenosine triphosphatase activity and physiological function. Circ. Res. *45*:1, 1979.
34. Morano, I., Bletz, C., Wojciechowski, R., and Ruegg, J. C.: Modulation of crossbridge kinetics by myosin isoenzymes in skinned human heart fibers. Circ. Res. *68*:614,1991.
35. Mahdavi, V., Izumo, S., and Nadal-Ginard, B.: Developmental and hormonal regulation of sarcomeric myosin heavy chain gene family. Circ. Res. *60*:804, 1987.
36. Sirovy, I.: Isoforms of contractile proteins. Prog. Biophys. Mol. Biol. *49*:1, 1987.
37. Swynghedauw, B.: Developmental and functional adaptation of contractile proteins in cardiac skeletal muscles. Physiol. Rev. *66*:710, 1966.
38. Schwartz, K., Lecarpentier, Y., Martin, J. L., et al.: Myosin isoenzymic distribution correlates with speed of myocardial contraction. J. Mol. Cell. Cardiol. *13*:1071, 1981.
39. Malhotra, A., Penpargkus, S., Fein, F. S., et al.: The effect of streptozotocin-induced diabetes in rats on cardiac contractile proteins. Circ. Res. *49*:1243, 1981.
40. Capelli, V., Bottinelli, R., Pogessi, C., et al.: Shortening velocity and myosin and myofibrillar ATPase activity related to myosin isoenzyme composition during postnatal development in rat myocardium. Circ. Res. *65*:446, 1989.
41. Morano, I., Arndt, H., Gartner, C., and Ruegg, J. C.: Skinned fibers of human atrium and ventricle: Myosin isoenzymes and contractility. Circ. Res. *62*:632, 1988.
42. Eisenberg, E., and Greene, L. E.: The relation of muscle biochemistry to muscle physiology. Ann. Rev. Physiol. *42*:293, 1980.
43. Ebashi, S.: Regulatory mechanism of muscle contraction with special reference to Ca-troponin-tropomyosin system. Essays Biochem. *10*:1, 1974.
44. Herzig, J. W., Ruegg, J. C., and Solaro, R. J.: Myocardial excitation-contraction coupling as influenced through modulation of the calcium sensitivity of the contractile proteins. Heart Failure *6*:244, 1991.
45. Goldman, Y. E.: Kinetics of the actomyosin ATPase in muscle fibers. Ann. Rev. Physiol. *49*:637, 1987.
46. Winegrad, S., Weisberg, A., Lin, E. L., and McClellan, G.: Adrenergic regulation of myosin adenosine triphosphatase activity. Circ. Res. *58*:83, 1986.
47. Ringer, S.: A further contribution regarding the influence of the different constituents of the blood on the contraction of the heart. J. Physiol. (Lond.) *4*:30, 1982.
48. Fabiato, A., and Fabiato, F.: Calcium and cardiac excitation muscle. Mayo Clin. Proc. 57 (Suppl.): 6, 1982.
49. McDonald, T. F.: Excitation-contraction coupling: Relationship of the slow inward current to contraction. *In* Sperelakis, N. (ed.): The Physiology and Pathophysiology of the Heart. Boston, Martinus Nijhoff, 1984, p. 187.
50. Jorgensen, A. D., Broderick, R., Somlyo, A. P., and Somlyo, A. V.: Two structurally distinct calcium storage sites in rat cardiac sarcoplasmic reticulum: An electron microprobe analysis study. Circ. Res. *63*:1060, 1988.
51. Blinks, J. R.: Intracellular [Ca^{2+}] measurements. *In* Fozzard, H. A., et al. (eds.): The Heart and Cardiovascular System. New York, Raven Press, 1986, p. 671.
52. Morgan, J. P., Perreault, C. L., and Morgan, K. G.: The cellular basis of contraction and relaxation in cardiac and vascular smooth muscle. Am. Heart J. *121*:961, 1991.
53. Barcenas-Ruiz, L., Beuckelmann, D. J., and Weir, W. G.: Sodium-calcium exchange in heart: Membrane currents and changes in $[Ca^{2+}]_i$. Science *238*:1719, 1987.
54. Bean, B. P.: Classes of calcium channels in vertebrate cells. Ann. Physiol. *51*:367, 1989.
55. London, B., and Krueger, J. W.: Contraction in voltage-clamped, internally perfused single heart cells. J. Gen. Physiol. *84*:475. 1986.
55a. Klitzner, T. S.: Maturational changes in excitation-contraction coupling in mammalian myocardium. J. Am. Coll. Cardiol. *17*:218, 1991.
56. Beuckelmann, D. J., and Weir, W. G.: Mechanism of release of calcium from sarcoplasmic reticulum of guinea-pig cardiac cells. J. Physiol. *404*:233, 1988.
57. Tada, M., Shigekawa, M., and Nimura, Y.: Uptake of calcium by the sarcoplasmic reticulum and its regulation and functional consequences. *In* Sperelakis, N. (ed.): Physiology and Pathophysiology of the Heart. Boston, Martinus Nijhoff, 1984, p. 255.
58. Fabiato, A.: Simulated calcium current can both cause calcium loading in and trigger calcium release from the sarcoplasmic reticulum of a skinned canine cardiac Purkinje cell. J. Gen. Physiol. *85*:291, 1985.
59. Lederer, W. J., Niggli, E., and Hadley, R. W.: Sodium-calcium exchange in excitable cells; fuzzy space. Science *248*:283, 1990.
60. Fabiato, A.: Time and calcium dependence of activation and inactivation of calcium-induced release of calcium from the sarcoplasmic reticulum of a skinned canine cardiac Purkinje cell. J. Gen. Physiol. *85*:247, 1985.
61. Nabauer, M., Callewaert, G., Cleemann, L., and Morad, M.: Regulation of calcium release is gated by calcium current, not gating charge, in cardiac myocytes. Science *244*:800, 1989.
62. Leblanc, N., and Hume, J. R.: Sodium current-induced release of calcium from cardiac sarcoplasmic reticulum. Science *248*:372, 1990.
63. Barcenas-Ruiz, L., and Wier, W. G.: Voltage dependence of intracellular $[Ca^{2+}]_i$ transients in guinea pig ventricular myocytes. Circ. Res. *61*:148, 1987.
64. Williamson, J. R., and Monck, J. R.: Hormonal effects on cellular Ca^{++} fluxes. Annu. Rev. Physiol. *51*:107, 1989.
65. Watanabe, A. M., and Lindemann, J. P.: Mechanisms of adrenergic and cholinergic regulation of myocardial contractility. J. Gen. Physiol. *85*:377, 1985.
66. DiFrancesco, D., and Noble, D.: A model of cardiac electrical activity incorporating ionic pumps and concentration changes. Philosoph. Trans. Roy. Soc. (Lond.) Series B *307*:353, 1985.
67. Reuter, H.: Calcium channel modulation by neurotransmitters, enzymes and drugs. Nature *301*:569, 1983.
68. Sperelakis, N.: Role of the sarcolemma in excitation-contraction coupling in cardiac muscle. Heart Failure *6*:212, 1991.
69. Flaim, S. F., and Zelis, R. (eds.): Calcium Blockers. Baltimore, Urban and Schwartzenberg, 1982, pp. 303.
70. Braunwald, E.: Mechanisms of action of calcium channel blocking agents. N. Engl. J. Med. *307*:1618, 1982.
71. Keung, E.C.H., and Aronson, R. S.: Physiology of calcium current in cardiac muscle. Prog. Cardiovas. Dis. *25*:279, 1983.
72. Triggle, D. J., and Jans, R. A.: Calcium channel ligands. Ann. Rev. Pharmacol. Toxicol. *27*:347, 1987.
73. Speralakis, N.: The slow action potential and properties of the myocardial slow channels. J. Gen. Physiol. *85*:159, 1985.
74. McDonald, T.: Excitation-contraction coupling: Relation of the slow inward current to contraction. J. Gen. Physiol. *85*:187, 1985.
75. McDonald, T. F., Pelzer, D., and Trautwein, W.: Does the calcium current modulate the contraction of the accompanying beat? A study of E-C coupling in mammalian ventricular muscle using cobalt ions. Circ. Res. *49*:576, 1981.
76. Crespo, L. M., Grantham, C. J., and Cannell, M. B.: Kinetics, stoichiometry and role of the Na-Ca exchange in isolated cardiac myocytes. Nature *345*:618, 1990.
77. Bers, D. M., Lederer, W. J., and Berlin, J. R.: Intracellular Ca transients in rat cardiac myocytes: Role of Na-Ca exchange in excitation-contraction coupling. Am. J. Physiol. *258* (Cell Physiol 27):C944, 1990.
78. Sheu, S-S., Sharma, V. K., and Uglesity, A.: Na^+-Ca^{2+} exchange contributes to increase of cytosolic Ca^{2+} concentration during depolarization in heart muscle. Am. J. Physiol. *250*:C651, 1986.
79. Sutko, J. L., Bers, D. M., and Reeves, J. P.: Postrest inotropy in rabbit ventricle: Na^+-Ca^{2+} exchange determines sarcoplasmic reticulum Ca^{2+} content. Am. J. Physiol. *250*:H654, 1986.
80. Housmans, P. K., Lee, N. K., and Blinks, J. P.: Active shortening retards the decline of intracellular calcium transient in mammalian heart muscle. Science *221*:159, 1983.
81. Lab, M. J., Allen, D. G., and Orchard, C. H.: The effects of shortening on myoplasmic calcium concentration and on the action potential in mammalian ventricular muscle. Circ. Res. *55*:825, 1984.
82. Johnson, E. A.: Force-interval relationship of cardiac muscle. *In* Berne, R. M. (ed.): Handbook of Physiology. Section 2, The Cardiovascular Sys-

tem, Vol. I, The Heart. Bethesda, American Physiological Society, 1979, pp. 475–496.
83. Covell, J. W., Ross, J., Jr., Taylor, R., et al.: Effects of increasing frequency of contraction of force-velocity relation of left ventricle. Cardiovasc. Res. *1*:2, 1967.
84. Higgins, C. B., Vatner, S. F., Franklin, D., and Braunwald, E.: Extent of regulation of the heart's contractile state in the conscious dog by alteration in the frequency of contraction. J. Clin. Invest. *52*:1187, 1973.
85. Hoffman, B. F., Bindler, E., and Suckling, E. E.: Postextrasystolic potentiation of contraction in cardiac muscle. Am. J. Physiol. *185*:95, 1956.
86. Ross, J., Jr., Sonnenblick, E. H., Kaiser, G. A., et al.: Electroaugmentation of ventricular performance and oxygen consumption by repetitive application of paired electrical stimuli. Circ. Res. *16*:332, 1965.
87. Cranefield, P. F.: The force of contraction of extrasystoles and the potentiation of force of the post-extrasystolic contraction: A historical review. Bull. N. Y. Acad. Med. *41*:419, 1965.
88. Colucci, W. S., Wright, B. F., and Braunwald, E.: New positive inotropic agents in the treatment of congestive heart failure. N. Engl. J. Med. *314*:290, 349, 1986.
89. Hicks, M. J., Shigekawa, M., and Katz, A. M.: Mechanism by which cyclic adenosine 3′:5′-monophosphate-dependent protein kinase stimulates calcium transport in cardiac sarcoplasmic reticulum. Circ. Res. *44*:384, 1979.
90. Solaro, R. J., Lee, J. A., Kentish, J. C., and Allen, D. G.: Effects of acidosis on ventricular muscle from adult and neonatal rats. Circ. Res. *63*:779, 1988.
91. Fabiato, A., and Fabiato, F.: Effects of pH on the myofilaments and sarcoplasmic reticulum of skinned cells from cardiac and skeletal muscles. J. Physiol. *276*:233, 1976.
92. Kohmoto, O., Spitzer, K. W., Movsesian, M. A., and Barry, W. H.: Effects of intracellular acidosis on $[Ca^{2+}]i$ transients, transsarcolemmal Ca^{2+} fluxes, and contraction in ventricular myocytes. Circ. Res. *60*:622, 1990.
93. MacKinnon, R., Gwathmey, J. K., Allen, P. D., et al.: Modulation by the thyroid state of intracellular calcium and contractility in ferret ventricular muscle. Circ. Res. *63*:1080, 1988.
94. Morkin, E., and Flink, I. L.: Biochemical and physiological effect of thyroid hormone on cardiac performance. Prog. Cardiovasc. Dis. *25*:434, 1983.
95. Lee, H. C., Smith, N., Mohabir, R., and Clusier, W.T.: Cytosolic calcium transients from the beating mammalian heart. Proc. Nat. Acad. Sci. *84*:7793, 1987.
96. Katz, A. M.: Cyclic adenosine monophosphate effects on the myocardium: A man who blows hot and cold with one breath. J. Am. Coll. Cardiol. *2*:143, 1983.
97. Spiegel, A. M., Gierschik, P., Levine, M., and Downs, R. W., Jr.: Clinical implications of guanine nucleotide-binding proteins as receptor-effector couplers. N. Engl. J. Med. *312*:26, 1988.
98. Gilman, A. G.: Guanine nucleotide-binding regulatory proteins and dual control of adenylate cyclase. J. Clin. Invest. *73*:1, 1984.
99. Gilman, A. G.: G Proteins: Transducers of receptor-generated signals. Annu. Rev. Biochem. *56*:615, 1987.
100. Yatani, A., and Brown, A. M.: Rapid B-adrenergic modulation of cardiac calcium channel currents by a fast G protein pathway. Science *245*:71, 1989.
101. Lefkowitz, R. J., and Caron, M. G.: Adrenergic receptors. Models for the study of receptors coupled to guanine nucleotide regulatory proteins. J. Biol. Chem. *263*:4993, 1988.
102. Robishaw, J. D., and Foster, K. A.: Role of G proteins in regulation of the cardiovascular system. Am. Rev. Physiol. *51*:229, 1989.
103. Neer, E. J., and Clapham, D. E.: Roles of G protein subunits in transmembrane signalling. Nature *333*:129, 1988.
104. Tada, M., and Katz, A.: Phosphorylation of the sarcoplasmic reticulum and sarcolemma. Ann. Rev. *44*:401, 1982.
105. Barany, K., Barany, M., Hager, S., and Sayers, S. T.: Myosin, light chain and membrane protein phosphorylation in various muscles. Fed. Proc. *42*:27, 1983.
106. Winegrad, S., McClellan, G., Horowitz, R., et al.: Regulation of cardiac contractile proteins by phosphorylation. Fed. Proc. *42*:39, 1983.
107. Sperelakis, N.: Cyclic AMP and phosphorylation in regulation of Ca^{++} influx into myocardial cells and blockade by calcium antagonistic drugs. Am. Heart J. *107*:347, 1984.
108. Kranias, E. G., and Solaro, J.: Coordination of cardiac sarcoplasmic reticulum and myofibrillar function by protein phosphorylation. Fed. Proc. *42*:33, 1983.
109. Fabiato, A., and Fabiato, F.: Cyclic AMP-induced enhancement of calcium accumulation by the sarcoplasmic reticulum with no modification of the sensitivity of the myofilaments to calcium in skinned fibres from a fast skeletal muscle. Biochim. Biophys. Acta *539*:253, 1978.
110. Nawrath, H.: Does cyclic GMP mediate the negative inotropic effect of acetylcholine in the heart? Nature *267*:72, 1977.
111. Freissmuth, M., Casey, P. J., and Gilmau, A. G.: G proteins control diverse pathways of transmembrane signaling. FASEB J. *3*:2125, 1989.
112. Carmeliet, E.: The slow inward current: Nonvoltage-clamp studies. *In* Zipes, D. P., Bailey, J. C., and Elharrar, V. (eds.): The Slow Inward Current and Cardiac Arrhythmias. The Hague, Martinus Nijhoff, 1980.
113. Barry, W. H., Biedert, S., Miura, D. S., and Smith, T. W.: Changes in cellular Na, K, and Ca contents, monovalent cation transport rate, and contractile state during washout of cardiac glycosides from cultured chick heart cells. Circ. Res. *49*:141, 1981.
114. Mullins, L. J.: The role of Na-Ca exchange in heart. *In* Sperelakis, N. (ed.): Physiology and Pathophysiology of the Heart. Boston, Martinus Nijhoff, 1984, p. 199.
115. Dhalla, N. S., Smith, C. I., Pierce, G. N., et al.: Heart sarcolemmal cation pumps and binding sites. *In* Rupp, H. (ed.): The Regulation of Heart Function. New York, Thieme Inc., 1986, p. 121.
116. Solaro, R. J.: The role of calcium in the contraction of the heart. *In* Flaim, S. F., and Zelis, R. (eds.): Calcium Blockers. Baltimore, Urban and Schwarzenberg, 1982, pp. 21–36.
117. Wier, W. G., and Hess, P.: Excitation-contraction coupling in cardiac Purkinje fibers. Effects of cardiotonic steroids of intracellular $[Ca^{++}]$ transient membrane potential and contraction. J. Gen. Physiol. *83*:395, 1984.
118. Reuter, H.: Ion channels in cardiac cell membrane. Ann. Rev. Physiol. *46*:473, 1984.
119. Hurwitz, L., Partridge, L. D., and Leach, J. K. (eds.): Calcium channels: Their Properties, Functions, Regulation, and Clinical Relevance. Boca Raton, CRC Press, 1991.
120. Trautwein, W., and Cavalie, A.: Cardiac calcium channels and their control by neurotransmitters and drugs. J. Am. Coll. Cardiol. *6*:1409, 1985.
121. Fleckenstein, A.: Calcium Antagonism in Heart and Smooth Muscle. New York, John Wiley and Sons, 1983.
122. Hondeghem, L. M., and Katzung, B. G.: Control of vascular smooth muscle contractility and the action of calcium channel blockers. *In* Rupp, H. (ed.): The Regulation of Heart Function. New York, Thieme Inc., 1986, pp. 38–52.
123. Stone, P. H., Antman, E. M., Muller, J. E., and Braunwald, E.: Calcium channel blocking agents in the treatment of cardiovascular disorders. Part II. Hemodynamic effects and clinical applications. Ann. Intern. Med. *93*:886, 1989.
124. Mikami, A., Imoto, K., Tanabe, T., et al.: Primary structure and functional expression of the cardiac dihydropyridine-sensitive calcium channel. Nature *340*:230, 1989.
125. Lands, A. M., Arnold, A., McAuliff, J. P., et al.: Differentiation of receptor systems activated by sympathomimetic amines. Nature *214*:597, 1967.
126. Kobinger, W., and Alquirst, R. P. (eds.): Alpha and Beta Adrenoceptors and the Cardiovascular System. Princeton, NJ., Excerpta Medica, 1984.
127. Watanabe, A. M.: Recent advances in knowledge about beta-adrenergic receptors: Application to clinical cardiology. J. Am. Coll. Cardiol. *1*:82, 1983.
128. Homcy, J. C., and Graham, R. M.: Molecular characterization of adrenergic receptors. Circ. Res. *56*:635, 1985.
129. Strader, C. D., Sigal, I. S., and Dixon, R.A.F.: Structural basis of β-adrenergic receptor function. FASEB J. *3*:1825, 1989.
130. Carlsson, E., Dahlot, C. G., Hedberg, A., et al.: Differentiation of cardiac chronotropic and inotropic effects of beta adrenoceptor agonists. Naunyn-Schmiedeberg's Arch. Pharmacol. *300*:101, 1977.
131. Wilffart, B., Tummermans, P.B.M.W.M., and van Zwieten, P.A.: Extrasynaptic location of alpha-2 and non-innervated beta-2 adrenoceptors in the vascular system in the pithed normotensive rat. J. Pharmacol. Exp. Ther. *221*:762, 1982.
132. Langer, S. Z.: Presynaptic regulation of catecholamines. Pharmacol. Rev. *32*:337, 1981.
133. Hedberg, A., Minneman, K. P., and Molinoff, P. B.: Differential distribution of beta-1 and beta-2 adrenergic receptors in cat and guinea-pig heart. J. Pharmacol. Exp. Ther. *213*:503, 1980.
134. Schumann, H. J.: What role do alpha and beta adrenoceptors play in the regulation of the heart? Eur. Heart J. *4* (Suppl. A):55, 1983.
135. Benfey, B. G.: Function of myocardial α-adrenoceptors. Life Sciences *46*:743, 1990.
136. Colucci, W. S., and Braunwald, E.: Adrenergic receptors: New concepts and implications for cardiovascular therapeutics. *In* Conti, C. R. (ed.): Cardiac Clinics. Philadelphia, F. A. Davis, 1983.
137. Wagner, J., and Schumann, H. J.: Different mechanisms underlying the stimulation of myocardial alpha- and beta-adrenoceptors. Life Sci. *24*:2045, 1979.

MECHANICS OF CARDIAC CONTRACTION

138. Abbott, B. C., and Mommaerts, W.F.H.M.A.: A study of inotropic mechanisms in the papillary muscle preparation. J. Gen. Physiol. *42*:533, 1959.
139. Sonnenblick, E. H.: Force-velocity relations in mammalian heart muscle. Am. J. Physiol. *202*:931, 1962.
140. Gwathmey, J. K., and Hajjar, R. J.: Relation between steady-state force and intracellular $[Ca^{++}]$ in intact human myocardium: Index of myofibrillar responsiveness to Ca^{2+}. Circulation *82*:1266, 1990.
141. Brutsaert, D. L., and Sonnenblick, E. H.: Force-velocity length-time rations of the contractile elements in heart muscle of the cat. Circ. Res. *24*:137, 1969.
142. Ford, L. E.: Mechanical manifestations of activation in cardiac muscle. Circ. Res. *68*:621, 1991.
143. Weir, W., and Yue, D. T.: Intracellular $[Ca^{++}]$ transients underlying the short-term force-interval relationship in ferret ventricular myocardium. J. Physiol. (Lond.) *376*:507, 1986.
144. Sonnenblick, E. H., and Skelton, C. L.: Reconsideration of the ultrastructural basis of the cardiac length-tension relation. Circ. Res. *35*:517, 1974.
145. Ross, J.: Mechanical performance of isolated cardiac muscle. In West, J. B. (ed.): Best and Taylor's Physiological Basics of Medical Practice. 11th ed. Baltimore, Williams and Wilkins, 1985, pp. 197–206.
146. Brutsaert, D. L., and Sonnenblick, E. H.: Cardiac muscle mechanics in the evaluation of myocardial contractility and pump function: Problems, concepts and directions. Prog. Cardiovasc. Dis. *16*:337, 1973.
147. Strobeck, J. E., Krueger, J. W., and Sonnenblick, E. H.: Load and time considerations in the force-length relation of cardiac muscle. Fed. Proc. *39*:175, 1980.

148. Parmley, W. W., and Sonnenblick, E. H.: Series elasticity: In relation to contractile element velocity and proposed muscle models. Circ. Res. *20*:112, 1967.
149. Robinson, T. F., Cohen-Gould, F., and Factor, S. M.: Skeletal framework of mammalian heart muscle. Lab. Invest. *49*:482, 1983.
150. ter Keurs, H.E.D.J.: Rijnsburger, W. H., van Heuningen, R., and Negelsmit, M. J.: Tension development and sarcomere length in rat cardiac trabeculae. Circ. Res. *46*:703, 1980.
151. Price, M. G.: Molecular analysis of intermediate filament cytoskeleton: A putative load-bearing structure. Am. J. Physiol. *246*:4566, 1984.
152. Braunwald, E., Frye, R. L., and Ross, J., Jr.: Studies on Starling's Law of the Heart: Determinants of the relationship between end-diastolic pressure and circumference. Circ. Res. *8*:1254, 1960.
153. Lakatta, E. G.: Cardiac muscle changes in senescence. Ann. Rev. Physiol. *49*:519, 1987.
154. Henderson, A. H., Van Ocken, E., and Brutsaert, D. L.: A reappraisal of force-velocity measurements in isolated heart muscle preparation. Eur. J. Cardiol. *1*:105, 1973.
155. Grossman, W., Braunwald, E., Mann, T., et al.: Contractile state of the left ventricle in man as evaluated from endsystolic pressure-volume relations. Circulation *56*:845, 1977.
156. Suga, H., and Yamakoshi, K.: Effects of stroke volume and velocity of ejection on end-systolic pressure on canine left ventricle. Circ. Res. *40*:445, 1977.
157. Sagawa, K., Sanagawa, K., and Maughan, W. L.: Ventricular end-systolic pressure-volume relations. *In* Levine, H. J., and Gaaschi, W. H. (eds.): The Ventricle: Basic and Clinical Aspects. Boston, Martinus Nijhoff, 1985, pp. 79–103.
158. Krueger, J. W., and Pollack, G. H.: Myocardial sarcomere dynamics during isometric contraction. J. Physiol. *251*:627, 1973.
159. Pollack, G. H., and Huntsman, L. L.: Sarcomere length-active force relations in living mammalian cardiac muscle. Am. J. Physiol. *227*:383, 1974.
160. ter Keurs, H.E.D.J.; Bucx, J.J.J.; de Tombe, P. P., et al.: The effects of sarcomere length and Ca^{++} on force and velocity of shortening in cardiac muscle. *In* Sugi, H, and Pollack, G. H. (eds.): Molecular Mechanism of Muscle Contraction. New York, Plenum, 1988, pp. 581–593.
161. Van Henningen, R., Rijnsburger, W. H., and ter Keurs, H.E.D.J.: Sarcomere length control in striated muscle. Am. J. Physiol. *242*:H411, 1982.
162. Frank, O.: On the dynamics of cardiac muscle. (Transl. by C. B. Chapman and E. Wasserman). Am. Heart J. *58*:282 and 467, 1959.
163. Starling, E. H.: Linacre Lecture on the Law of the Heart (1915). London, Longmans, Green and Co., Ltd., 1918.
164. Gordon, A. M., Huxley, A. F., and Julian, F. J.: The variation in isometric tension with sarcomere length in vertebrate muscle fibers. J. Physiol. (Lond.) *184*:170, 1966.
165. Lakatta, E. G.: Starling's law of the heart is explained by an intimate interaction of muscle length and myofilament calcium activation. J. Am. Coll. Cardiol. *10*:1157, 1987.
166. Krueger, J. W., and Tsujioka, K.: Sarcomere mechanics: Towards a physical basis for cardiac contraction. *In* Mura, R. (ed.): Some Mathematical Questions in Biology. Lectures on Mathematics in the Life Sciences. Vol. 16, 1986, p. 1.
167. Fabiato, A., and Fabiato, F.: Dependence of calcium release, tension generation, and restoring forces on sarcomere length in skinned cardiac cells. Eur. J. Cardiol. *4* (Suppl.):13, 1976.
168. Babu, A., Scoidilis, S. P., Sonnenblick, E. H., and Gulati, J.: The control of myocardial contraction with fast muscle troponin C. J. Biol. Chem. *262*:5815, 1987.
169. Allen, D. G., and Kentish, J. C.: The cellular basis of the length-tension relation in cardiac muscle. J. Mol. Cell. Cardiol. *17*:821, 1985.
170. Babu, A., Sonnenblick, E. H., and Gulati, J.: Molecular basis for the influence of muscle length on myocardial performance. Science *240*:74, 1988.
171. Gordon, A. M., and Pollack, G. H.: Effects of calcium on the sarcomere length-tension relation in rat cardiac muscle. Circ. Res. *47*:610, 1980.
172. Gillebert, T. C., Sys, S. U., and Brutsaert, D. L.: Influence of loading patterns on peak length–tension relation and on relaxation in cardiac muscle. J. Am. Coll. Cardiol. *13*:483, 1989.
173. Chiu, Y. C., Walley, K. R., and Ford, L. E.: Comparison of the effects of different inotropic interventions on force, velocity, and power in rabbit myocardium. Circ. Res. *65*:1161, 1989.
174. Gulati, J.: The length-sensor in Starling's law of the heart and characterization of the cardiac Ca^{+++}-switch. In Roberts, R., and Sambrook, J. (eds.): Molecular Biology of the Cardiovascular System. Vol. 132. N.Y., Alan R. Liss, 1989.
175. Sonnenblick, E. H., Spiro, D., and Cottrell, J. S.: Fine structural changes in heart muscle in relation to the length-tension curve. Proc. Natl. Acad. Sci. (USA) *49*:193, 1963.
176. Pollack, G. H., and Krueger, J. W.: Sarcomere dynamics in intact cardiac muscle. Eur. J. Cardiol. *4*:53, 1976.
177. Sonnenblick, E. H., Skelton, C. L., Spotnitz, W. D., and Feldman, D.: redefinition of the ultrastructural basis of cardiac length-tension relations. Circulation *48* (Suppl. 4):65, 1973.
178. Ross, J., Jr., Sonnenblick, E. H., Covell, J. W., et al.: Architecture of the heart in systole and diastole: Technique of rapid fixation and analysis of left ventricular geometry. Circ. Res. *21*:409, 1967.
179. Sonnenblick, E. H., Ross, J. Jr., Covell, J. W., et al.: Ultrastructure of the heart in systole and diastole. Circ. Res. *21*:423, 1967.
180. Yoran, C., Covell, J. W., and Ross, J. Jr.: Structural basis for ascending limb of left ventricular function. Circ. Res. *32*:297, 1973.
181. Ross, J., Jr., Sonnenblick, E. H., Covell, J. W., et al.: Architecture of the heart in systole and diastole: Technique of rapid fixation and analysis of left ventricular geometry. Circ. Res. *21*:409, 1967.
182. Sonnenblick, E. H., Ross, J., Jr., Covell, J. W., et al.: Ultrastructure of the heart in systole and diastole. Circ. Res. *21*:423, 1967.
183. Ross, J., Jr.: The Cardiac Pump. *In* West, J. B. (ed.): Best and Taylor's Physiological Basis of Medical Practice. 12th ed. Baltimore, Williams and Wilkins. (In press.)

DETERMINANTS OF CONTRACTION OF THE INTACT HEART

184. Strobeck, J. E., and Sonnenblick, E. H.: Myocardial and ventricular function. Cardiovasc. Rev. Rep. *4*:568, 1983.
185. Weber, K. T., Janicki, J. S., Hunter, W. C., et al.: The contractile behavior of the heart and its functional coupling to the circulation. Prog. Cardiovasc. Dis. *4*:375, 1982.
186. Slinker, B. K., and Glantz, S. A.: Beat-to-beat regulation of left ventricular function in the intact cardiovascular system. Am. J. Physiol. *256*:R962, 1989.
187. Ross, J., Jr.: Cardiac function and myocardial contractility: A perspective. J. Am. Coll. Cardiol. *1*:52, 1983.
188. Sasayama, S., Franklin, D., Ross., J., Jr., et al.: Dynamic changes in left ventricular wall thickness and their use in analyzing cardiac function in the conscious dog. Am. J. Cardiol. *38*:870, 1976.
189. Sandler, H., and Alderman, E.: Determination of left ventricular size and shape. Circ. Res. *34*:1, 1974.
190. Karliner, J. S., Bouchard, R. J., and Gault, J. H.: Dimensional changes of the human left ventricle prior to aortic valve opening: A cineangiographic study in patients with and without left heart disease. Circulation *44*:312, 1971.
191. Rankin, J. S., McHale, P. A., Arentzen, C. E., et al.: The three dimensional dynamic geometry of the left ventricle in the conscious dog. Circ. Res. *39*:304, 1976.
192. Brutsaert, D. L., and Sys, S. U.: Relaxation and diastole in the heart. Physiol. Rev. *69*:1228, 1989.
193. Nikolie, S. Yellin, E. L., Tamura, K., et al.: Passive properties canine left ventricle: Diastolic stiffness and restoring forces. Circ. Res. *62*:1210, 1988.
194. Gilbert, J. C., and Glantz, S. A.: Determinants of left ventricular filling and of the diastolic pressure-volume relation. Circ. Res. *64*:827, 1989.
195. Mirsky, I.: Elastic properties of the myocardium: A quantitative approach with physiological and clinical applications. *In* Berne, R. M. (ed.): Handbook of Physiology. Section 2, The Cardiovascular System. Vol. I, The Heart. Bethesda, Md., American Physiological Society, 1979, pp. 497–532.
196. Grossman, W., and McLaurin, L. P.: Diastolic properties of the left ventricle. Ann. Intern. Med. *84*:316, 1976.
197. Zile, M. R.: Diastolic dysfunction: Detection, consequences, and treatment. Part 1: Definition and determinants of diastolic function. Mod. Conc. Cardiovas. Dis. *58*:67, 1989.
198. Nishimura, R. A., Housmans, P. R., Hatle, L. K., and Tajik, A. J.: Assessment of diastolic function of the heart: Background and current applications of Doppler echocardiography. Mayo Clin. Proc. *64*:71, 1989.
199. Kurnik, M. S., Courtois, M. A., and Ludbrook, P.A.: Effects of nifedipine on intrinsic myocardial stiffness in man. Circulation *74*:126, 1986.
200. Mirsky, I.: Assessment of diastolic function: Suggested methods and future considerations. Circulation *69*:836, 1984.
201. Gaasch, W. H., Levine, H. J., Quinones, M. A., and Alexander, J. K.: Left ventricular compliance: Mechanisms and clinical implications. Am. J. Cardiol *38*:645, 1976.
202. Pouleur, H., Karliner, J. S., LeWinter, M. M., and Covell, J. W.: Diastolic viscous properties of the intact canine left ventricle. Circ. Res. *45*:410, 1979.
203. LeWinter, M. M., Engler, R., and Pavelec, R. S.: Time-dependent shifts of the left ventricular diastolic filling relationship in conscious dogs. Circ. Res. *45*:641, 1979.
204. Taylor, R. R., Covell, J. W., Sonnenblick, E. H., and Ross, J., Jr.: The independence of ventricular distensibility in the filling of the opposite ventricle. Am. J. Physiol. *213*:711, 1967.
205. Gentzler, R. D., II, Briselli, M. F., and Gault, J. H.: Angiographic estimate of right ventricular volume in man. Circulation *50*:324, 1974.
206. Katz, A. M.: Influence of altered inotropy and lusitropy on ventricular pressure-volume loops. J. Am. Coll. Cardiol. *11*:438, 1988.
207. Lew, W.Y.W.: Evaluation of left ventricular diastolic function. Circulation *79*:1393, 1989.
208. Miyazaki, S., Guth, B. D., Miura, T., et al.: Changes of left ventricular diastolic function in exercising dogs without and with ischemia. Circulation *81*:1058, 1990.
209. Lew, W.Y.W., and Rasmussen, C. M.: Influence of nonuniformity on rate of left ventricular pressure fall in the dog. Heart Circ. Physiol. *25*:H222, 1989.
210. Ariel, Y., Gaasch, W.H.L., Bogden, D. K., et al.: Load-dependent relaxation with late systolic volume steps: Servo-pump studies in the intact canine heart. Circulation *75*:1287, 1987.
211. Cheng, C-P., Freeman, G. L., Santamore, W. P., et al.: Effect of loading conditions, contractile state, and heart rate on early diastolic left ventricular filling in conscious dogs. Circ. Res. *66*:814, 1990.
212. Nikolic, S. Yellin, E. L., Tamura, K., et al.: Effect of early diastolic loading on myocardial relaxation in the intact canine left ventricle. Circ. Res. *66*:1217, 1990.
213. Courtois, M., Kovács, S. J., Jr., and Ludbrook, P. A.: Transmitral pressure-

flow velocity relation: Importance of regional pressure gradients in the left ventricle during diastole. Circulation 78:661, 1988.
214. Ishida, Y., Meisner, J. S., Tsujioka, K., et al.: Left ventricular filling dynamics: Influence of left ventricular relaxation and left atrial pressure. Circulation 74:187, 1986.
215. Pasipoularides, A., Mirsky, I. Hess, O. M., et al.: Myocardial relaxation and passive diastolic properties in man. Circulation 74:991, 1986.
216. Stoddard, M. F., Pearson, A. C., Kern, M. J., et al.: Left ventricular diastolic function: Comparison of pulsed Doppler echocardiographic and hemodynamic indexes in subjects with and without coronary artery disease. J. Am. Coll. Cardiol. 13:327, 1989.
217. Nikolic, S. D., Tamura, K., Tamura, T., et al.: Diastolic versus properties of the intact canine left ventricle. Circ. Res. 67:352, 1990.
218. Watanabe, J., Levine, M. J., Bellotto, F., et al.: Effects of coronary venous pressure on left ventricular diastolic distensibility. Circ. Res. 67:923, 1990.
219. Nonogi, H., Hess, O. M., Ritter, M., and Krayenhuehl, H. P.: Diastolic properties of the normal left ventricle during supine exercise. Br. Heart J. 60:30, 1988.
220. Cuocolo, A., Sax, F. L., Brush, J. E., et al.: Left ventricular hypertrophy and impaired diastolic filling in essential hypertension: diastolic mechanisms for systolic dysfunction during exercise. Circulation 81:978, 1990.
221. Shirato, K., Shabetai, R., Bhargava, V., et al.: Alteration of the left ventricular diastole pressure-segment length relation produced by the pericardium: Effects of cardiac distention and afterload reduction in conscious dogs. Circulation 57:1191, 1978.
222. LeWinter, M. M., and Porsche, R.: Influence of the pericardium on left ventricular end-diastolic pressure-segment relations during early and late stages of experimental chronic volume overloads in dogs. Circ. Res. 50:501, 1981.
223. Bhargava, V., Shabetai, R., Ross, J., Jr., et al.: Influence of the pericardium on left ventricular diastolic pressure-volume curves in dogs with sustained volume overload. Am. Heart. J. 105:95, 1983.
224. Bourdillon, P. D., Lorell, B. H., Mirsky, I., et al.: Increased regional myocardial stiffness of the left ventricle during pacing-induced angina in man. Circulation 67:316, 1983.
225. Mann, T., Goldberg, S., Mudge, G. A., Jr., and Grossman, W.: Factors contributing to altered left ventricular diastolic properties during angina pectoris. Circulation 59:14, 1979.
226. Serizawa, T., Carabello, B. A., and Grossman, W.: Effect of pacing-induced ischemia on left ventricular diastolic pressure-volume relations in dogs with coronary stenosis. Circ. Res. 46:430, 1980.
227. Hess, O. M., Bhargava, V., Ross, J., Jr., and Shabetai, R.: The role of pericardium in interactions between the cardiac chambers. Am. Heart. J. 106:1377, 1983.
228. Linderer, T., Chatterjee, K., Parmley, W. W., et al.: Influence of atrial systole on the Frank-Starling relation and the end-diastolic pressure-diameter relation of the left ventricle. Circulation 67:1045, 1983.
229. Jensen, D. P., Goolsby, J. P., Jr., and Oliva, P. B.: Hemodynamic pattern resembling pericardial constriction after acute myocardial infarction with right ventricular infarction. Am. J. Cardiol. 42:858, 1978.
230. Smiseth, O. A., Frais, M. A., Kingma, I., et al.: Assessment of pericardial constraint in dogs. Circulation 71:158, 1985.
231. Smiseth, O. A., Frais, M. A., Kingma, L., et al.: Assessment of pericardial constraint: The relation between right ventricular filling pressure and pericardial pressure measured after pericardiocentesis. J. Am. Coll. Cardiol. 7:307, 1986.
232. Regan, D. M.: Calculation of left ventricular wall stress. Circ. Res. 67:245, 1990.
233. Bemis, C. E., Serur, J. R., Korkenhagen, D., et al. Influence of right ventricular filling pressure on left ventricular pressure and dimension. Circ. Res. 34:498, 1974.
234. Glantz, S. A., and Parmley, W. W.: Factors which affect the diastolic pressure volume curve. Circ. Res. 42:171, 1978.
235. Ross, J., Jr.: Acute displacement of the diastolic pressure-volume curve of the left ventricle. Role of the pericardium on the right ventricle. Circulation 59:32, 1979.
236. Dittrich, H. C., Chow, L. C., and Nicod, P. H.: Early improvement in left ventricular diastolic function after relief of chronic right pressure overload. Circulation 80:823, 1989.
237. Olsen, G. O., Tyson, G. S., Maier, G. W., et al.: Dynamic ventricular interaction in the conscious dog. Circ. Res. 51:85, 1983.
238. Brutsaert, D. L.: Nonuniformity: A physiologic modulator of contraction and relaxation of the normal heart. J. Am. Coll. Cardiol. 9:341, 1987.
239. Gallagher, K. P., Osakada, G., Kemper, W. S., et al.: Cyclical coronary flow reductions in conscious dogs equipped with ameroid constrictors to produce severe coronary narrowing. Basic Res. Cardiol. 80:100, 1985.
240. Yoran, C., Covell, J. W., and Ross J., Jr.: Rapid fixation of the left ventricle: Continuous angiographic and dynamic recordings. J. Appl. Physiol. 35:155, 1973.
241. Heyndrickx, G. R., Villiane, J.-P., Knight, D. R., et al.: Effects of altered site of electrical activation on myocardial performance during inotropic stimulation. Circulation 71:1010, 1985.
242. Allen, D. G., and Kentish, J. C.: The cellular basis of the length-tension relation in cardiac muscle. J. Mol. Cell Cardiol. 17:821, 1985.
243. Lakatta, E. G.: Starling's Law of the Heart is explained by an intimate interaction of muscle length and myofilament calcium activation. J. Am. Coll. Cardiol. 10:1157, 1987.
244. Lew, W.Y.W.: Time-dependent increase in left ventricular contractility following acute volume loading in the dog. Circ. Res. 63:635, 1988.
245. Sugiura, S., Hunter, W. C., and Sagawa, K.: Long-term versus intrabeat history of ejection as determinants of canine ventricular end-systolic pressure. Circ. Res. 64:255, 1989.
246. Hunter, W. C.: End-systolic pressure as a balance between opposing effects of ejection. Circ. Res. 64:265, 1989.
247. Sarnoff, S. J., Mitchell, J. H., Gilmore, J. P., et al.: Homeometric autoregulation of the heart. Circ. Res. 8:1077, 1960.
248. Monroe, R. G., Gamble, W. J., LaFarge, C. G., et al.: Homeometric autoregilation. In The Physiological Basis of Starling's Law of the Heart. CHBA Foundation Symposium No. 27. Amsterdam, Elsevier/North Holland Biomedical Press, 1974, p. 257.
249. Sagawa, K.: The end systolic pressure-volume relation of the ventricle: Definition, modifications and clinical use. Circulation 63:1223, 1981.
250. Suga, H., Sagawa, K., and Shoukas, A. A.: Load independence of the instantaneous pressure-volume ratio of the canine left ventricle and effects of epinephrine and heart rate on the ratio. Circ. Res. 32:214, 1973.
251. Lee, J., Tajimi, T., Widmann, T. F., and Ross, J., Jr.: Application of end-systolic pressure-volume and pressure-wall thickness relations in conscious dogs. J. Am. Coll. Cardiol. 9:136, 1987.
252. Kaseda, S., Tomoike, H., Ogaa, I., and Nakamura, M.: End-systolic pressure-volume, pressure-length, and stress-strain relations in canine hearts. Am. J. Physiol. 18:H648, 1985.
253. Mehmel, H. C., Stocking, B., Ruffmann, K., et al.: The linearity of the end-systolic pressure-volume relationship in man and its sensitivity for assessment of left ventricular function. Circulation 63:1216, 1981.
254. McKay, R. G., Aroesty, J. M., Heller, G. V., et al.: Left ventricular pressure-volume diagrams and end-systolic pressure-volume relations in human beings. J. Am. Coll. Cardiol. 3:301, 1984.
255. Sagawa, K.: End-systolic pressure-volume relationship in retrospect and prospect. Fed. Proc. 43:2399, 1984.
256. Belcher, P., Boerboom, L. E., and Olinger, G. N.: Standardization of end-systolic pressure-volume relation in the dog. Am. J. Physiol 18:H547, 1985.
257. Bo Su, J., Crozatier, B.: Preload-induced curvilinearity of left ventricular end-systolic pressure-volume relations: Effects on derived indexes in closed-chest dogs. Circulation 79:431, 1989.
258. Kass, D. A., Beyar, R., Lankford, E., et al.: Influence of contractile state on curvilinearity of in situ end-systolic pressure-volume relations. Circulation 79:167, 1989.
259. Little, W. C., Cheng, C., Peterson, T., et al.: Response of the left ventricular end-systolic pressure-volume relation in conscious dogs to a wide range of contractile states. Circulation78:736, 1988.
260. Ross J., Jr.: Applications and limitations of end-systolic measures of ventricular performance. Fed. Proc. 43:2418, 1984.
261. Hsia, H. H., and Starling, M. R.: Is standardization of left ventricular chamber elastance necessary? Circulation 81:1826, 1990.
262. Lee, J. D., Tajimi, T., Patritta, J., and Ross, J., Jr.: Preload reserve and mechanisms of afterload mismatch in the normal conscious dog. Am. J. Physiol. 19:H464, 1986.
263. Boettcher, D. H., Vatner, S. F., Heyndrikx, G. R., and Braunwald, E.: Extent of utilization of the Frank-Starling mechanisms in conscious dogs. Am. J. Physiol. 3:338, 1978.
264. Higginbotham, M. B., Morris, K. G., Williams, R. S., et al.: Regulation of stroke volume during submaximal and maximul upright exercise in normal man. Circ. Res. 58:281, 1986.
265. Plotnick, G. D., Becker, L. C., Fisher, M. L., et al.: Use of the Frank-Starling mechanism during submaximal versus maximal upright exercise. Am. J. Physiol. 251:H1101, 1986.
266. Weber, K. T., Janicki, J. S., Shroff, S. G., and Laskey, W.: The mechanics of ventricular function. Hosp. Pract. 18:113, 1983.
267. Ross, J., Jr., Covell, J. W.: Chapter 17. Frameworks for analysis of ventricular and circulatory function: Integrated responses. In J. B. West (ed.): Best and Taylor's Physiological Basis of Medical Practice. 12th ed. Baltimore, Williams and Wilkins (In press).
268. Braunwald, E., and Frahm, C. J.: Studies on Starling's law of the heart. IV. Observations on hemodynamic functions of left atrium in man. Circulation 24:633, 1961.
269. Linderer, T., Chatterjee, K., Parmley, W. W., et al.: Influence of atrial systole on the Frank-Starling relation and the end-diastolic pressure-diameter relation of the left ventricle. Circulation 67:1045, 1983.
270. Monroe, R. G., Gamble, W. J., LaFarge, C. G., et al.: Left ventricular performance at high-end diastolic pressures in isolated, perfused dog heart. Circ. Res. 26:85, 1970.
271. Ross, J., Jr., Sonnenblick, E. H., Taylor, R. R., et al.: Diastolic geometry and sarcomere lengths in the chronically dilated canine left ventricle. Circ. Res. 28:49, 1971.
272. MacGregor, D. C., Covell, J. W., Mahler, F., et al.: Relations between afterload, stroke volume, and the descending limb of Starling's curve. Am. J. Physiol. 227:884, 1974.
273. Ross, J., Jr., and Braunwald, E.: The study of left ventricular function in man by increasing resistance to ventricular ejection with angiotensin. Circulation 29:739, 1964.
274. Ross, J., Jr.: Afterload mismatch and preload reserve: a conceptual framework for the analysis of ventricular function. Progr. Cardiovasc. Dis. 18:255, 1976.
275. Guyton, A. C., ed. Textbook of Medical Physiology. 8th ed. Philadelphia, W. B. Saunders Company, 1991, p. 227.
276. Braunwald, E.: Editorial—On the difference between the heart's output and its contractile state. Circulation 43:171, 1971.
277. Pouleur, H., Covell, J. W., and Ross, J., Jr.: Effects of nitroprusside on venous return and central blood volume in the absence and presence of acute heart failure. Circulation 61:328, 1980.

278. Braunwald, E., Binion, J. T., Morgan, W. L., Jr., and Sarnoff, S. J.: Alterations in central blood volume and cardiac output induced by positive pressure breathing and counteracted by metaraminol (Aramine). Circ. Res. *5*:670, 1957.
279. Shabetai, R.: The Pericardium. New York, Grune & Stratton, 1981, p. 154.
280. Shepherd, J. T., and Vanhoutte, P. M.: Veins and Their Control. Philadelphia, W. B. Saunders Company, 1975, 269 pp.
281. Ross, J., Jr., Covell, J. W., Sonnenblick, E. H., and Braunwald, E.: Contractile state of heart characterized by force-velocity relations in variably afterloaded and isovolumic beats. Circ. Res. *18*:149, 1966.
282. Urschel, C. W., Covell, J. W., Sonnenblick, E. H., et al.: Myocardial mechanics in aortic and mitral valvular regurgitation: The concept of instantaneous impedance as a determinant of the performance of the intact heart. J. Clin. Invest. *47*:867, 1968.
283. Weber, K. T., Janicki, J.S., and Shroff, S. G.: Measurement of ventricular function in the experimental laboratory. *In* Fozzard, H. M., et al. (eds.): The Heart and Cardiovascular System. New York, Raven Press, 1986, p. 865.
284. Katz, A. M.: Regulation of myocardial contractility 1958–1983. J. Am. Coll. Cardiol. *1*:126, 1983.
284a. Ross, J., Jr., Covell, J. W., and Sonnenblick, E. H.: The mechanics of left ventricular contraction in acute experimental cardiac failure. J. Clin. Invest. *46*:299, 1967.
285. Yue, D. T., Burkhoff, D., Franz, M. R., et al.: Postextrasystolic potential of the isolated canine left ventricle: Relationship to mechanical restitution. Circ. Res. *56*:340, 1985.
286. Frommer, P. L., Robinson, B. F., and Braunwald, E.: Paired electrical stimulation. A comparison of the effects on performance of the failing and nonfailing heart. Am. J. Cardiol. *18*:738, 1966.
287. McGaughey, M. D., Maughan, W. L., Sunagawa, K., and Sagawa, K.: Alternating contractility in pulsus alternans studied in the isolated canine heart. Circulation *71*:357, 1985.
288. Heyndrickx, G. R., Vilaine, J. P., Moerman, E. J., et al.: Role of prejunctional $\alpha 2$-adrenergic receptors in the regulation of myocardial performance during exercise in conscious dogs. Circ. Res. *54*:683, 1984.
289. Guth, B. D., Thaulow, E., Heusch, G., et al.: Myocardial effects of selective α-adrenoceptor blockade during exercise in dogs. Circ. Res. *66*:1703, 1990.
290. Lang, R. M., Fellner, S. K., and Neumann, A.: Left ventricular contractility varies directly with blood ionized calcium. Ann Intern. Med. *108*:524, 1988.
291. Beierholm, E. A., Grantham, R. N., O'Keefe, D. D., et al.: Effects of acid-base changes, hypoxia, and catecholamines on ventricular performance. Am. J. Physiol. *228*:1555, 1975.
292. Williamson, J. R., Schaffer, S. W., Ford, C., and Safen, B.: Contribution of tissue acidosis to ischemic injury in the perfused rat heart. Circulation *53* (Suppl. 1):3, 1976.
293. Mitchell, J. H., Wallace, A. G., and Skinner, N. S., Jr.: Intrinsic effects of heart rate on left ventricular performance. Am. J. Physiol. *205*:41, 1963.
294. Vatner, S. F., and Braunwald, E.: Cardiovascular control mechanisms in the conscious state. N. Engl. J. Med. *293*:970, 1975.
295. Narahara, K. A., and Blettel, M. L.: Effect of rate on left ventricular volumes and ejection fraction during chronic ventricular pacing. Circulation *67*:323, 1983.
296. Ross, J., Jr., Linhart, J. W., and Braunwald, E.: Effects of changing heart rate in man by electrical stimulation of the right atrium: Studies at rest, during exercise and with isoproterenol. Circulation *32*:549, 1965.
297. Weber, K. T., Janicki, J. S., Shroff, S. G., et al.: The right ventricle: Physiologic and pathophysiologic considerations. Crit. Care Med. *11*:323, 1983.
298. Furey, S. A., III., Zieske, H. A., and Levy, M. N.: The essential function of the right ventricle. Am. Heart J. *107*:404, 1984.

NEURAL CONTROL OF CARDIAC CONTRACTION

299. Randall, W. C. (ed.): Neural Regulation of the Heart. New York, Oxford University Press, 1977, 440 pp.
300. Yamaguchie, N., de Champlain, J., and Nadeau, R.: Correlation between the response of the heart to sympathetic stimulation and the release of endogenous catecholamines into the coronary sinus of the dog. Circ. Res. *36*:662, 1975.
301. Landsberg, L., and Young, J. B.: Catecholamines and the adrenal medulla. *In* Wilson, J. D., Foster, D. W. (eds.): Williams' Textbook of Endocrinology. Philadelphia, W. B. Saunders, 1985, p. 891.
302. Goldstein, D. S., Brush, J. E. Jr., Eisenhofer, G., et al.: In vivo measurement of neuronal uptake of norepinephrine in the human heart. Circulation *78*:41, 1988.
303. Fujii, I., and Vatner, S. F.: Sympathetic mechanisms regulating myocardial contractility in conscious animals. *In* Fozzard, H. A., et al. (eds.): The Heart and Cardiovascular System. New York, Raven Press, 1986, pp. 1119–1132.
304. Cousineau, D., Ferguson, R. J., DeChamplain, J., et al.: Catecholamines in coronary sinus during exercise in man before and after training. J. Appl. Physiol. *43*:801, 1977.
305. Hasking, G. J., Esler, M. D., Jennings, G. L., et al.: Norepinephrine spillover to plasma during steady-state supine bicycle exercise: Comparison of patients with congestive heart failure and normal subjects. Circulation *78*:516, 1988.
306. Martin, R. H., Lim, S. T., and VanCitters, R. L.: Atrial fibrillation in the intact anesthetized dog: Hemodynamic effects during rest, exercise, and beta-adrenergic blockade. J. Clin. Invest. *46*:205, 1967.
307. Frye, R. L., and Braunwald, E.: Studies on Starling's law of the heart. I. The circulatory response to acute hypervolemia and its modification by ganglionic blockade. J. Clin. Invest. *39*:1043, 1960.
308. Sonnenblick, E. H., Williams, J. F., Jr., Glick, G., et al.: Studies on digitalis. XV. Effects of cardiac glycosides on myocardial force-velocity relations in nonfailing human heart. Circulation *34*:532, 1966.
309. Daggett, W. M., and Weisfeldt, M. L.: Influence of sympathetic nervous system on response of normal heart to digitalis. Am. J. Cardiol. *16*:394, 1965.
310. Liedtke, A. M., Buoncristiani, J. F., Kirk, E. S., et al.: Regulation of cardiac output after administration of isoproterenol and ouabain. Cardiovasc. Res. *6*:325, 1972.
311. Guyton, A. C.: The relationship of cardiac output and arterial pressure control. Circulation *64*:1079, 1981.
312. Vatner, S. F., Higgins, C. B., White, S, et al.: The peripheral vascular response to severe exercise in untethered dogs before and after complete heart block. J. Clin. Invest. *50*:1950, 1971.
313. Rothe, C. F.: Physiology of venous return: An unappreciated boost to the heart. Arch. Intern. Med. *146*:977, 1986.
314. Ross, J., Jr., Gault, J. H., Mason, D. T., et al.: Left ventricular performance during muscular exercise in patients with and without cardiac dysfunction. Circulation *34*:597, 1966.
315. Poliner, L. R., Dehmer, G. J., Lewis, S. E., et al.: Left ventricular performance in normal subjects: A comparison of the responses to exercise in the upright and supine positions. Circulation *62*:528, 1980.
316. Iskandrian, A. S., Hakki, A. H., DePase, N. L., et al.: Evaluation of left ventricular function by radionuclide angiography during exercise in normal subjects and in patients with chronic coronary heart disease. J. Am. Coll. Cardiol. *1*:1518, 1983.
317. Epstein, S. E., Robinson, B. F., Kahler, R. L., and Braunwald, E.: Effects of beta-adrenergic blockade on the cardiac response to maximal and submaximal exercise in man. J. Clin. Invest. *44*:1745, 1965.
318. Robinson, B. F., Epstein, S. E., Kahler, R. L., and Braunwald, E.: Circulatory effects of acute expansion of blood volume: Studies during maximal exercise and at rest. Circ. Res.*19*:26, 1966.
319. Braunwald, E., Goldblatt, A., Harrison, D. C., and Mason, D.T.: Studies on cardiac dimensions in intact, unanesthetized man. III. Effects of muscular exercise. Circ. Res. *13*:460, 1963.
320. Caldwell, J. H., Stewart, D. K., Dodge, H. T., et al.: Left ventricular volume during maximal supine exercise. A study using metallic epicardial markers. Circulation *58*:732, 1978.
321. Sonnenblick, E. H., Braunwald, E., Williams, J. F., Jr., and Glick, G.: Effects of exercise on myocardial force-velocity relations in intact unanesthetized man: Relative roles of changes in heart rate, sympathetic activity, and ventricular dimensions. J. Clin. Invest. *44*:2051, 1965.
322. Hammond, H. K., White, F. C., Brunton, L. L., and Longhurst, J. C.: Association of decreased myocardial β-receptors and chronotropic response to isoproterenol and exercise in pigs following chronic dynamic exercise. Circ. Res. *60*:720, 1987.
323. Bevilacqua, M., Savonitto, S., Bosiso, E., et al.: Role of the Frank-Starling mechanism in maintaining cardiac output during increasing levels of treadmill exercise in beta-blocked normal men. Am. J. Cardiol. *63*:853, 1989.
324. Bruce, T. A., Chapman, C. P., Baker, O., and Fisher, J. N.: Role of autonomic and myocardial factors in cardiac control. J. Clin. Invest. *42*:721, 1963.
325. Saltin, B., and Astrand, P. O.: Maximal oxygen uptake in the athlete. J. Appl. Physiol. *23*:353, 1967.
326. Morganroth, J., Maron, B. J., Henry, W. L., and Epstein, S. E.: Comparative left ventricular dimensions in trained athletes. Ann. Intern. Med. *82*:521, 1975.
327. Roeske, W. R., O'Rourke, R. A., Klein, A., Leopold, G., and Karliner, J. S.: Noninvasive evaluation of ventricular hypertrophy in professional athletes. Circulation *53*:286, 1976.
328. Resink, T. J., Gevers, W., Noakes, T. D., and Opie, L. H.: Increased cardiac myosin ATPase activity as biochemical adaptation to running training: Enhanced response to catecholamines and a role for myosin phosphorylation. J. Mol. Cell. Cardiol. *13*:679, 1981.
329. Mitchell, J. H., Payne, F. C., Saltin, B., and Schibye, B.: The role of muscle mass in the cardiovascular response to static conditions. J. Physiol. *309*:45, 1980.
330. Hintze, T. H., and Vatner, S. F.: Cardiac dynamics during hemorrhage: Relative unimportance of adrenergic inotropic response. Circ. Res. *50*:705, 1982.
331. Bainbridge, F. A.: The influence of venous filling upon the rate of the heart. J. Physiol. (Lond.) *50*:65, 1915.
332. Vatner, S. F., Boettcher, D. H., Heyndrickx, G. R., and McRitchie, R. J.: Reduced baroreflex sensitivity with volume loading in conscious dogs. Circulation Res. *37*:236, 1975.
333. Vatner, S. F., and Boettcher, D. H.: Regulation of cardiac output by stroke volume and heart rate in conscious dogs. Circ. Res. *42*:557, 1978.
334. Vatner, S. F., and Rutherford, J. D.: Control of the myocardial contractile state of carotid chemo- and baroreceptor and pulmonary inflation reflexes in conscious dogs. J. Clin. Invest. *61*:1593, 1978.
335. Levy, M. N., and Martin, P. J.: Neural control of the heart. *In* Sperelakis, N. (ed.): Physiology and Pathophysiology of the Heart. Boston, Martinus Nijhoff, 1984, pp. 337–354.
336. Watanabe, A. M., and Lindemann, J. P.: Mechanism of adrenergic and cholinergic regulation of myocardial contractility. *In* Sperelakis, N. (ed.): Physiology and Pathophysiology of the Heart. Boston, Martinus Nijhoff, 1984, pp. 337–404.

14

Pathophysiology of Heart Failure

by EUGENE BRAUNWALD, M.D.

Heart (or cardiac) failure (the pathophysiological state in which an abnormality of *cardiac* function is responsible for failure of the heart to pump blood at a rate commensurate with the requirements of the metabolizing tissues, or to do so only from an elevated filling pressure) is frequently, but not always, caused by a defect in myocardial contraction, i.e., by *myocardial failure.* However, in some patients with heart failure, a similar clinical syndrome is present, but there is no detectable abnormality of *myocardial* function; in many such cases heart failure may be brought about by conditions in which the normal heart is suddenly presented with a load that exceeds its capacity or in which ventricular filling is impaired.[1] Heart failure must be distinguished from conditions in which there is circulatory congestion consequent to abnormal salt and water retention (the so-called congested state) but in which there is no disturbance of cardiac function per se.[2] A distinction must also be made between heart failure and *circulatory failure,* in which an abnormality of some component of the circulation—the heart, the blood volume, the concentration of oxygenated hemoglobin in the arterial blood, or the vascular bed—is responsible for inadequate cardiac output.

Thus, myocardial failure, heart failure, and circulatory failure are not synonymous but refer to progressively more inclusive entities. Myocardial failure, when sufficiently severe, always produces heart failure, but the converse is not necessarily the case, since a number of conditions in which the heart is suddenly overloaded (e.g., acute aortic regurgitation secondary to acute infective endocarditis) can produce heart failure in the presence of normal myocardial function, at least early in the course of the illness. Also, conditions such as tricuspid stenosis and constrictive pericarditis, which interfere with cardiac filling, can produce heart failure without myocardial failure. Heart failure, in turn, always produces circulatory failure, but again the converse is not necessarily the case, since a variety of noncardiac conditions, e.g., hypovolemic shock (Chap. 21) or extremely severe anemia, beriberi, and other high-output states (Chap. 16), can produce circulatory failure at a time when cardiac function is normal or only modestly impaired.

The hemodynamic, contractile, and wall motion disorders in heart failure are discussed in the chapters on echocardiography (Chap. 4), exercise (Chap. 6), cardiac catheterization (Chap. 7), radionuclide imaging (Chap. 10), and assessment of cardiac function (Chap. 15). In this chapter, the focus is on the anatomical, biochemical, cellular, and neurohormonal changes characteristic of heart failure.

ADAPTIVE MECHANISMS

In the presence of a primary disturbance in myocardial contractility or an excessive hemodynamic burden placed on the ventricle, or both, the heart depends on a number of adaptive mechanisms for maintenance of its pumping function[3] (Table 14–1). Most important among these are: (1) the Frank-Starling mechanism, in which an increased preload (i.e., lengthening of sarcomeres to provide optimal overlap between thick and thin myofilaments and thereby enhance contraction) brought about in part by salt and water retention helps to sustain cardiac performance (p. 420); (2) myocardial hypertrophy with or without cardiac chamber dilatation, in which the mass of contractile tissue is augmented (p. 395); and (3) increased release of catecholamines by adrenergic cardiac nerves and the adrenal medulla, which augment myocardial contractility, activation of the renin-angiotensin-aldosterone system, and other neurohumoral adjustments that act to maintain arterial pressure and perfusion of vital organs (p. 383). Initially, especially in acute heart failure, these adaptive mechanisms may be adequate to maintain the overall pumping performance of the heart at relatively normal levels. However, the capacity of each of these mechanisms to sustain cardiac performance in the face of hemodynamic overload relative to myocardial contractility is finite and often has adverse consequences. The clinical syndrome of heart failure, described in Chapter 16, is determined by an interaction between cardiac damage, hemodynamic overload, and these secondary compensating effects.[4,5]

Cardiac output is often depressed in the basal state in patients with the common forms of heart failure secondary to ischemic heart disease, hypertension, primary myocardial disease, valvular disease, and pericardial disease (so-called low-output heart failure). It tends to be elevated in patients with heart failure associated with conditions of reduced afterload and/or hypermetabolism (such as hyperthyroidism, anemia, arteriovenous fistula, beriberi, and Paget's disease), so-called high-output heart failure (Chap. 16). The mechanisms responsible for the development of heart failure in patients whose cardiac output is initially high are complex and depend on the specific underlying disease process and its effect on the myocardium. In most of these conditions, the heart is called upon to pump an abnormally large volume of blood in order to deliver an adequate quantity of oxygen to the metabolizing tissues. This increased volume load exerts an effect on the myocardium resembling that produced by regurgitant valvular lesions or congenital left-to-right shunts.

TABLE 14-1 SHORT-TERM AND LONG-TERM RESPONSES TO IMPAIRED CARDIAC PERFORMANCE

RESPONSE	SHORT-TERM EFFECTS*	LONG-TERM EFFECTS†
Salt and water retention	Augments preload	Causes pulmonary congestion, anasarca
Vasoconstriction	Maintains blood pressure for perfusion of vital organs (brain, heart)	Exacerbates pump dysfunction (afterload mismatch); increases cardiac energy expenditure
Sympathetic stimulation	Increases heart rate and ejection	Increases energy expenditure
Sympathetic desensitization	—	Spares energy
Hypertrophy	Unloads individual muscle fibers	Leads to deterioration and death of cardiac cells; cardiomyopathy of overload
Capillary deficit	—	Leads to energy starvation
Mitochondrial density	Increase in density helps meet energy demands	Decrease in density leads to energy starvation
Appearance of slow myosin	—	Increases force, decreases shortening velocity and contractility; is energy-sparing
Prolonged action potential	—	Increases contractility and energy expenditure
Decreased density of sarcoplasmic reticulum calcium-pump sites	—	Slows relaxation; may be energy-sparing
Increased collagen	May reduce dilatation	Impairs relaxation

* Short-term effects are mainly adaptive and occur after hemorrhage and in acute heart failure.
† Long-term effects are mainly deleterious and occur in chronic heart failure.
Reprinted by permission from Katz, A. M.: Cardiomyopathy of overload: A major determinant of prognosis in congestive heart failure. N. Engl. J. Med. *322*:100, 1990.

In the absence of the shunting of blood in the periphery, the inadequate delivery of oxygen to the metabolizing tissues characteristic of heart failure is reflected in an abnormally widened arterial-mixed venous oxygen difference (Fig. 15-1, p. 420). In cases of mild heart failure this abnormality may not be present in the basal state and may become evident only during increased activity. In the presence of the peripheral arteriovenous shunting of blood and heart failure (e.g., congenital arteriovenous fistula or beriberi heart disease, p. 461), although the arterial-mixed venous oxygen difference may be normal or even narrowed, the venous oxygen content *proximal* to the entry of the shunt—if it could be measured—would be reduced, reflecting an augmented extraction of oxygen by inadequately perfused tissues and a reduced partial pressure of oxygen in the peripheral tissues.

When the volume of blood delivered into the systemic vascular bed is chronically reduced, and/or when one or both ventricles has an elevated filling pressure, a complex sequence of adjustments occurs that ultimately results in an abnormal accumulation of fluid. These adjustments are described on page 453. Although many of the clinical manifestations of heart failure are secondary to this excessive retention of fluid (see Chap. 16), the expansion of blood volume also constitutes an important compensatory mechanism that tends to maintain arterial pressure[6] and cardiac output by elevating ventricular preload, since the myocardium operates on the ascending limb of a depressed function curve[7-9] (Fig. 14-24, p. 412). Except in the terminal stages of heart failure, the augmented ventricular end-diastolic volume must be regarded as helping to maintain cardiac output. Elevation of ventricular end-diastolic volume and pressure, in accordance with the Frank-Starling mechanism, raises ventricular performance but at the same time causes venous congestion and promotes the formation of pulmonary or peripheral edema.

REDISTRIBUTION OF LEFT VENTRICULAR OUTPUT. Maintenance of arterial pressure despite reduction of cardiac output is a primitive but effective compensatory mechanism.[10] In hypovolemia and heart failure this important mechanism is brought into play in order to conserve the limited cardiac output. Vasoconstriction, mediated largely by the adrenergic nervous system, is primarily responsible for this redistribution of peripheral blood flow, which occurs when an additional burden (such as exercise, fever, or anemia) is imposed on the circulation in the presence of impaired myocardial function, preventing cardiac output from rising normally. As cardiac performance declines, redistribution of left ventricular output ultimately occurs, even in the basal state[11-14] (Fig. 14-1). This redistribution maintains the delivery of oxygen to vital organs such as the brain and heart, whereas blood flow to less critical areas such as the skin, skeletal muscle, and kidney is reduced.[15,16] This underperfusion has been reported to cause metabolic changes in skeletal muscle leading to anaerobic metabolism.[17] Occasionally, serious complications can result from the redistribution and the resulting severe reduction of blood flow. These include marked sodium and nitrogen retention as a consequence of diminished renal perfusion and, very rarely, gangrene of the tips of the phalanges and mesenteric infarction.

AUTONOMIC CONTROL OF THE HEART AND PERIPHERAL CIRCULATION. In the early stages of heart failure, activation of the adrenergic nervous system maintains cardiac output by increasing contractility and raising heart rate; in severe heart failure, vasoconstriction mediated by the sympathetic nervous system and circulating angiotensin II tends to sustain arterial pressure and redistributes cardiac output.[18] In advanced stages of heart failure the excessive afterload secondary to vasoconstriction may reduce cardiac output and have other deleterious consequences, as discussed on page 379[19,20] (Fig. 14-2).

OTHER ADJUSTMENTS. Increased vascular sodium content and raised interstitial pressure resulting from sodium and water retention lead to stiffening, thickening, and compression of the blood vessel walls, which prevents normal vasodilation during exercise.[13] Inadequate perfusion of skeletal muscle, in turn, leads to earlier dependence on anaerobic metabolism, lactic acidemia, an excessive oxygen debt, weakness, and fatigue. The veins in the extremities of patients with heart failure are constricted by circulating venoconstrictors (norepinephrine and angiotensin II) and by the activity of the adrenergic nervous system as well as a consequence of compression by increased interstitial volume. Constriction of the veins in the extremities and abdominal viscera results in displacement of blood to the heart and lungs.

A progressive *decline in the affinity of hemoglobin for oxygen* due to an increase in 2,3-diphosphoglycerate (DPG) also occurs in heart failure.[21] This rightward shift in the oxygen-hemoglobin dissociation curve represents a compensatory mechanism that facilitates oxygen transport; increased DPG, tissue acidosis, and the slow circulation time characteristic of heart failure act synergistically to maintain the delivery of oxygen to the metabolizing tissues in the face of a reduced cardiac output.

Heart failure is accompanied by a rise in the transcapillary oncotic pressure gradient consequent to low tissue oncotic

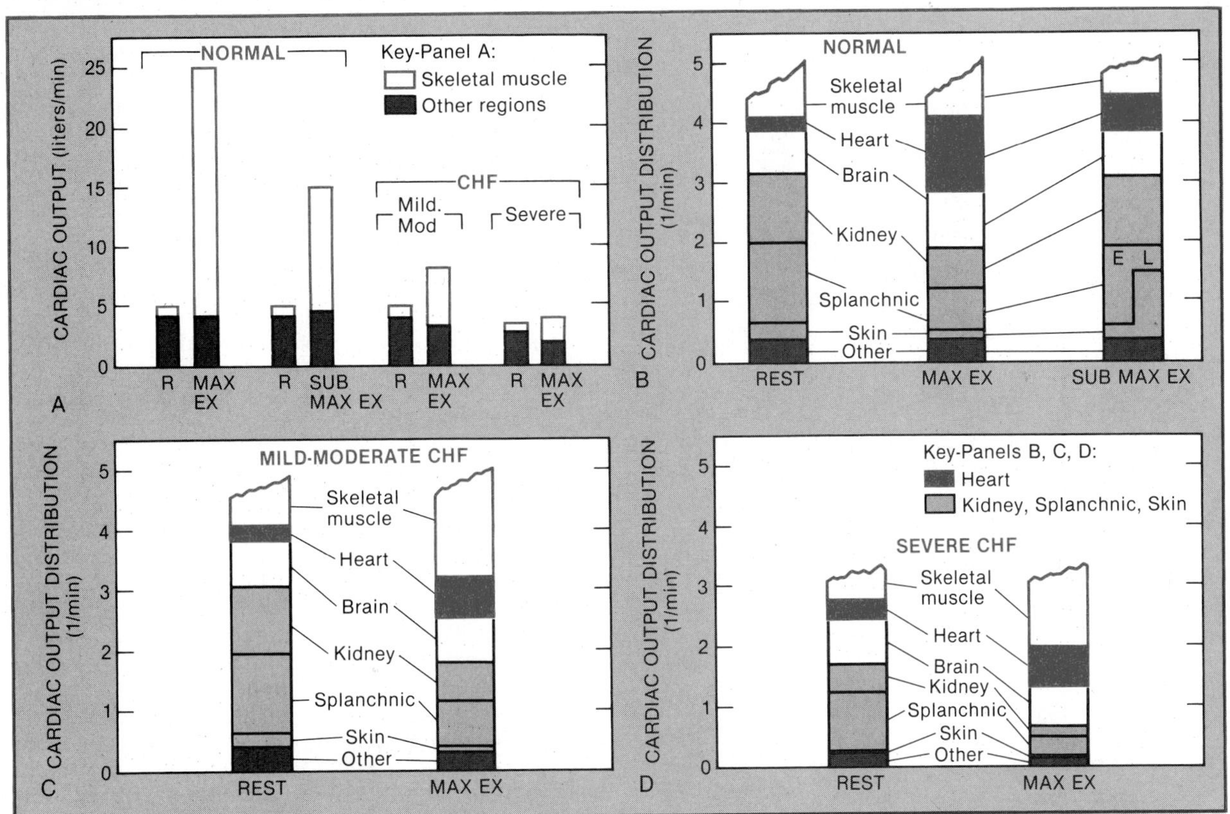

FIGURE 14–1. Regional distribution of the cardiac output at rest (R) and during exercise (EX) in normal subjects and in patients with congestive heart failure (CHF). These data are estimates from limited quantitative data in humans and are supplemented by directional changes in regional blood flow from animal studies. A, Total cardiac output and its distribution to skeletal muscle (open red bars) and all other regions (black bars). B, C, and D, Distribution of blood flow to the circulations exclusive of skeletal muscle. Attention is called to blood flow to the heart and to the circulations with high vasoconstrictor potential (kidney, skin, splanchnic) (key in D). E = distribution of cardiac output to the splanchnic and cutaneous circulations early during submaximal exercise in normals; L = late response. MAX-EX = maximal exercise; SUB MAX-EX = submaximal exercise at 50 to 60 per cent of maximum. (From Zelis, R., and Flaim, S. F.: Alterations in vasomotor tone in congestive heart failure. Prog. Cardiovasc. Dis. *24*:437, 1982.)

pressure, thereby limiting the formation of edema at any level of hydrostatic capillary pressure.[22]

CONTRACTILITY OF HYPERTROPHIED AND FAILING MYOCARDIUM

When an excessive pressure or volume load is imposed on a ventricle, myocardial hypertrophy develops, providing one of the aforementioned fundamental compensatory mechanisms that permits the ventricle to sustain this burden.[23] A ventricle subjected to an abnormally elevated load for a prolonged period, however, may fail to maintain compensation despite the presence of ventricular hypertrophy, and pump failure may ultimately occur, as discussed on page 397.

STUDIES ON ISOLATED MUSCLE. Cardiac muscle isolated from animals in which the heart was subjected to a controlled major stress has been carefully studied. One convenient experimental model of ventricular pressure overload is the cat or ferret with sudden pulmonary artery constriction. Papillary muscles are removed from the right ventricles in which either hypertrophy or overt failure has developed, and the excised muscle is then studied in vitro.[24,25] Right ventricu-

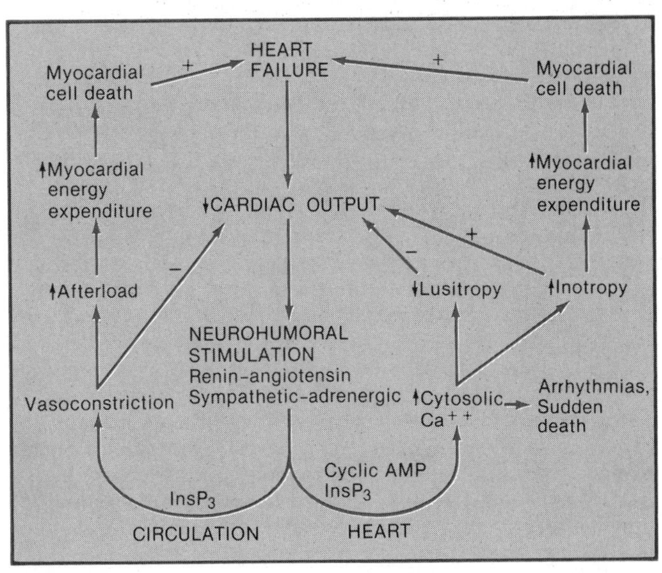

FIGURE 14–2. The low-output state can accelerate the rate of cell death in the failing heart by stimulating the renin-angiotensin and sympathetic-adrenergic systems, which act on both the circulation and the heart. Vasoconstriction increases afterload, which further decreases cardiac output; the increased afterload may also accelerate the rate of myocardial cell death by increasing the work of the heart. In the heart, increased concentrations of cyclic AMP and inositol-1,4,5-tris phosphate ($InsP_3$) promote calcium entry, augmenting contractility; along with a chronotropic response (not shown), this inotropic response increases cardiac output and is thus compensatory. However, the increased amount of calcium that enters the cytosol can overload the systems that pump this ion out of the cell during diastole, thus impairing relaxation. Calcium overload may also induce arrhythmias and lead to sudden death. Because the inotropic and chronotropic responses to sympathetic-adrenergic stimulation increase myocardial energy expenditure, they may also accelerate the rate of cell death in the failing heart. Thus, when the initial adaptive responses of both the circulation and the heart to a chronic low-output state become sustained, they can have deleterious long-term effects in patients with congestive heart failure. (Reprinted with permission from Katz, A. M.: Cardiomyopathy of overload: A major determinant of prognosis in congestive heart failure. N. Engl. J. Med. *322*:100, 1990.)

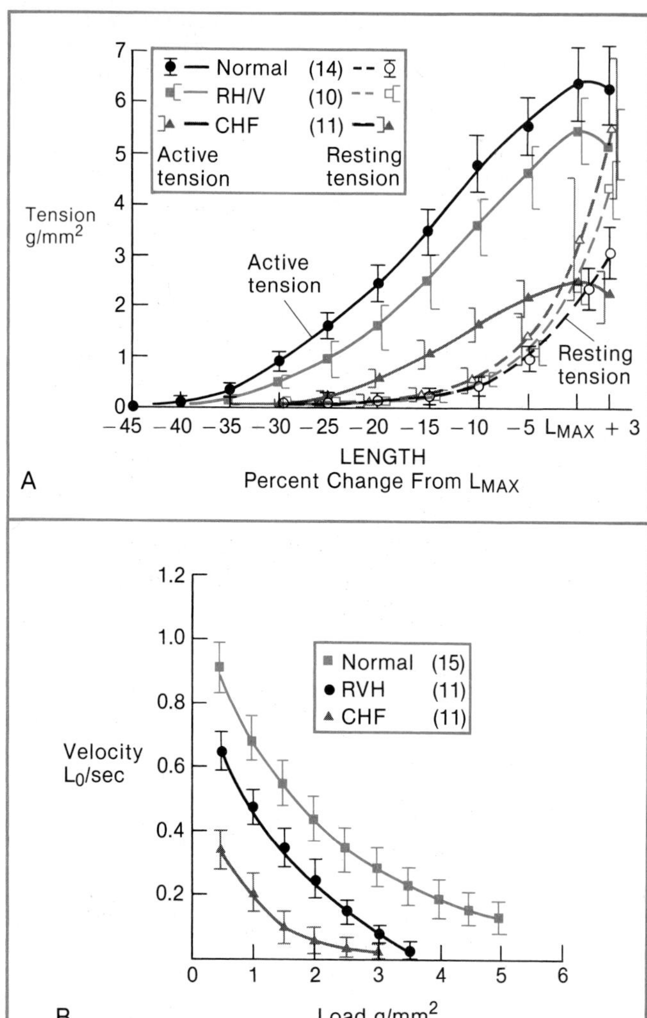

FIGURE 14–3. *A*, **Relation between muscle length and tension of papillary muscles from normal (circles), hypertrophied (squares), and failing (triangles) right ventricles. Open symbols = resting tension; filled symbols = actively developed tension. Tension is corrected for cross-sectional area (g/mm²). Numbers in parentheses = number of animals.** *B*, **Force-velocity relations of the three groups of cat papillary muscles. Average values ± SEM are given for each point. Velocity has been corrected to muscle lengths per second (L_0/sec). (From Spann, J. F., Jr., Buccino, R. A., Sonnenblick, E. H., and Braunwald, E.: Contractile state of cardiac muscle obtained from cats with experimentally produced ventricular hypertrophy and heart failure. Circ. Res. *21*:341, 1967, by permission of the American Heart Association, Inc.)**

lar hypertrophy and failure both reduce the maximum velocity of unloaded shortening (V_{max}, Fig. 13–21, p. 366) below the values observed in muscles obtained from normal cats; the changes are more marked in muscles obtained from animals in which heart failure was present than in those with hypertrophy alone (Fig. 14–3). The depression of contractility in hypertrophic myocardium is less marked or even absent entirely when the stress is imposed slowly, and when the measurements are made during the second, or stable, phase of the ventricular hypertrophic response to overload.[26] Heart failure depresses the maximal isometric tension, but hypertrophy without failure produces only borderline depression of this variable.

The findings just summarized are, in general, consonant with those of a number of other investigations on cardiac muscle isolated from animals with experimentally produced pressure overload. For example, the trabecular or papillary muscles removed from the left ventricles of the rat in which left ventricular hypertrophy has been created by aortic constriction or by renovascular hypertension also exhibit a depression in the velocity of isotonic shortening and a prolongation of the action potential, of the duration of isometric contraction, and of the time-to-peak tension even in the absence of a reduction in the development of isometric tension.[27] The force and rate of force development are also depressed in muscles obtained from hearts with totally different forms of heart failure, i.e., from Syrian hamsters with hereditary cardiomyopathy, as well as in papillary muscles removed from the left ventricles of patients with heart failure due to chronic valvular disease.[28]

In contrast to the depressed performance of cardiac muscle removed from cardiomyopathic or pressure-overloaded hearts, contractility has been found to be normal in papillary muscles removed from cats with a volume overload resulting from an experimentally produced atrial septal defect.[29] On the other hand, papillary muscles obtained from the left ventricles of dogs with heart failure produced by large infrarenal aortocaval fistulas show reduced maximum force development.[30] It should be noted that although the length–active tension curve, the maximal rate of isometric force development, and force-velocity relations are all significantly depressed in cat papillary muscles removed 6 weeks after pulmonary artery banding, in some,[31] but not all,[25] studies these variables returned to normal when the elevated pressure was maintained for prolonged periods. With even longer periods of pressure overload, isometric force declined a second time.[32] These observations emphasize the important temporal relationships between the imposition of a load, its nature (volume or pressure), severity, time, and the resultant depression of the contractile state. However, the available data are consonant with Meerson's concept of three stages of hypertrophy in response to an acutely induced pressure overload[33] (Table 14–2). The first stage reflects the initial myocardial damage as a consequence of the imposition of the load; during the second stage there is a recovery period of stable hyperfunction, followed by late deterioration during the stage of "exhaustion," the third stage.

Electron microscopic studies of myocardium removed from overloaded, dilated hearts fixed at the elevated filling pressures that existed during life have revealed sarcomere lengths averaging 2.2 μm—no longer than those at the apex of the length–active tension curve of normal cardiac muscle.[34] This indicates that the depressed contractility of failing heart muscle is *not* due to an enlarging H zone, i.e., the disengagement of actin and myosin filaments. Thus, the depression of contractility in failing heart muscle appears to be related to an *intrinsic defect of the muscle* rather than to its operation on the descending limb of the Frank-Starling curve.

In rats with pulmonary artery constriction, the diameter of individual right ventricular myocytes is increased, with proportional expansion of mitochondria and myofibrils. In this

TABLE 14–2 THREE STAGES IN THE RESPONSE TO A SUDDEN HEMODYNAMIC OVERLOAD

Stage 1: (Days) Transient breakdown	
Circulatory:	**Acute heart failure; pulmonary congestion, low output**
Cardiac:	**Acute left ventricular dilatation, early hypertrophy**
Myocardial:	**Increased content of mitochondria relative to myofibrils**
Stage 2: (Weeks) Stable hyperfunction	
Circulatory:	**Improved pulmonary congestion and cardiac output**
Cardiac:	**Established hypertrophy**
Myocardial:	**Increased content of myofibrils relative to mitochondria**
Stage 3: (Months) Exhaustion and progressive cardiosclerosis	
Circulatory:	**Progressive left ventricular failure**
Cardiac:	**Further hypertrophy with progressive fibrosis**
Myocardial:	**Cell death**

From Katz, A. M.: Energy requirements of contraction and relaxation: Implications of inotropic stimulation of the failing heart. *In* Just, H., Holubarsch, C., and Scholz, H. (eds.): Inotropic Stimulation and Myocardial Energetics. New York, Springer-Verlag, 1989, p. 49.

model, as well as in rats with renal hypertension,[35] there may be some increase in cell number (hyperplasia).[36] While it is not clear whether hyperplasia can occur with postnatal hemodynamic stress in other species, it does not play a significant role in humans. Dalen et al. have described a number of ultrastructural features of myocardial cells in hypertrophied human myocardium.[37] These include abnormal Z-band patterns, multiple intercalated discs, and prominent collagen fibrils connecting adjacent myocardial cells. Nuclei are enlarged and lobulated and contain well-developed nucleoli, together with an abundance of ribosomes, presumably reflecting enhanced protein synthesis.

STUDIES ON INTACT HEARTS. Immediately after imposition of a volume overload (such as an aortocaval fistula), contractility—as reflected in the end-systolic stress-circumference relationship—may increase. However, it then declines, while overall hemodynamic performance is sustained.[38] Later in the course of a large-volume overload, overt clinical heart failure develops,[30] accompanied by increases in left ventricular end-diastolic volume and left ventricle body weight ratio and depressed indices of left ventricular contractility[39] (Chap. 15). Changes in performance of the intact heart are, in general, similar to those observed in isolated cardiac tissue obtained from hearts subjected to abnormal hemodynamic loads. Thus, the contractile performance of the intact right ventricles of cats with pulmonary artery constriction reveals a marked depression paralleling that observed in the isolated papillary muscles removed from these ventricles.[40] When compared with normal values, the active tension developed by the right ventricle at equivalent end-diastolic fiber lengths is markedly reduced in cats with heart failure (Fig. 14-4). Studies involving manipulations of end-diastolic volume revealed that these failing hearts ordinarily function on the *ascending* limb of a *depressed* length–active tension curve rather than on the descending limb of a normal curve.

As the ventricle fails, it moves to the right along a depressed length–active tension curve, so that it requires an abnormally elevated end-diastolic volume (and often an elevation of end-diastolic pressure as well) to generate a level of tension equal to that achieved by the normal heart at a normal end-diastolic volume. The similar level of active tension at spontaneously

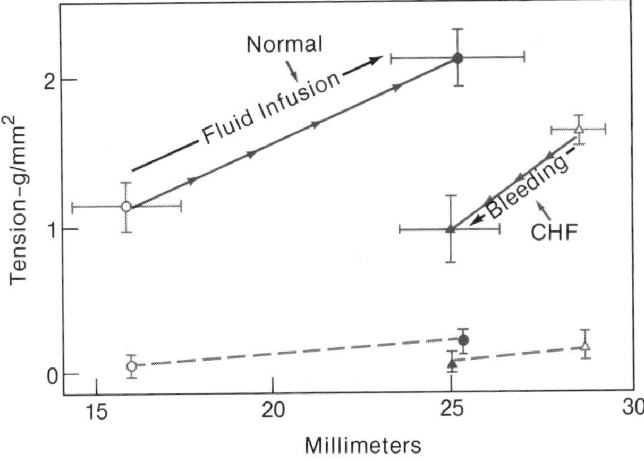

FIGURE 14–4. Length-tension relationships in the intact ventricle. Acute manipulation of end-diastolic volume to obtain ventricular Frank-Starling curves. Lines represent segments of active and resting length-tension curves (Frank-Starling relationship) of five normal (circles) and five failing (triangles) ventricles. Solid lines represent active tension, whereas dashed lines refer to resting or diastolic tension. Open symbols refer to values obtained at spontaneously occurring end-diastolic volume, whereas solid symbols refer to values obtained after volume infusion in normal cats and bleeding of cats with heart failure. Average values ± SEM are shown. Active and resting tensions are expressed on the ordinate, and normalized end-diastolic circumference, or muscle length, on the abscissa. (From Spann, J. F., Jr., Covell, J. W., Eckberg, D. L., Sonnenblick, E. H., Ross, J., Jr., and Braunwald, E.: Contractile performance of the hypertrophied and chronically failing cat ventricle. Am. J. Physiol. *223*:1150, 1972.)

occurring end-diastolic volumes in normal and failing cat hearts is evidence of the compensation afforded the depressed myocardium by cardiac dilatation. Contractile tension is thus preserved, but at the expense of an increased end-diastolic pressure and volume. However, the velocity of myocardial fiber shortening and the velocity of contraction at any given load are depressed despite the normal levels of tension development.

Although cardiac output and left ventricular end-diastolic pressure are normal at rest in spontaneously hypertensive rats with chronic pressure overload, the left ventricular ejection fraction is depressed.[41–43] When such rats are stressed with infusions of fluid, the stroke volume and cardiac output rise subnormally. A depression of contractility, as reflected in the relationship between ejection fraction and afterload, occurs before the deterioration of ventricular performance as reflected in baseline and maximal cardiac indices.[43] Renal hypertension in rats causes an elevation of left ventricular end-diastolic pressure and a depression of both +dp/dt and −dp/dt.[44] As already noted,[30,39] chronic left ventricular volume overload, produced by creating a large anteriovenous fistula, causes depression of a variety of indices of contractility.[45] Thus, there is substantial evidence that both chronic pressure and volume overload depress contractility and performance of the intact heart. In addition, left ventricular function has also been found to be depressed in isolated but intact hearts removed from rats with experimentally induced diabetes mellitus.[46]

MANIFESTATIONS OF DEPRESSED CONTRACTILITY. When the various studies on isolated muscle and intact hearts are taken together, it may be concluded that the depression of the cardiac contractile state observed in the hypertrophied and failing ventricle, however caused, represents an *intrinsic* property of the muscle. Since this depression is evident in vitro, when the muscle's physical and chemical milieu is controlled, it is not dependent on any altered humoral or other environmental factors or abnormal loading conditions existing in vivo. Although contractility may be markedly depressed in the intact ventricle and in isolated muscles of many preparations subjected to pressure overload, the cardiac index and stroke volume in the basal state are often maintained.

It appears, then, that when the ventricle is stressed, by either a pressure or a volume overload, the initial response is an increase in the length of sarcomeres, so that the overlap between myofilaments is optimal, i.e., approximately 2.2 μm (p. 369). This is followed by an increase in the total muscle mass, although the pattern of hypertrophy differs depending on whether the stress is a pressure load or a volume load (p. 400). If the overload is not extreme, this adaptation at first can allow maintenance of an elevated ventricular systolic pressure (in the case of a pressure overload) or augmented cardiac output (in the case of a volume overload) without a depression of contractility. If the intrinsic contractile state of the myocardium then becomes depressed, the increased muscle mass, operating in conjunction with increased sympathetic stimulation may, for a period, maintain overall circulatory compensation. If severe overload persists, Meerson has proposed (p. 399) that some of the hypertrophied cells become necrotic,[33] which places an additional load on the surviving cells and may thereby result in a vicious circle, ultimately causing heart failure.

In its mildest form, the depression of contractility is manifested by a reduction in the maximal velocity of shortening of unloaded myocardium (V_{max}) or by a reduction in the rate of force development during isometric contraction,[27] but by little, if any, decrease in the development of maximal isometric force (P_0) or in the extent of shortening of afterloaded ischemic contractions. As the intrinsic contractility of the myocardium becomes further depressed, a more extensive reduction in V_{max} occurs, and this is now accompanied by a decline in P_0 and shortening. At this point, circulatory compensation may still be provided by an increase in muscle mass and cardiac dilation, which tend to maintain wall stress at normal levels.

Cardiac output and stroke volume are maintained in the basal state, but ejection fraction is depressed, as are the maximal levels of cardiac output and/or left ventricular systolic pressure that can be attained during stress. As contractility declines further, overt congestive heart failure, as indicated by a depression of cardiac output and work and/or an elevation of ventricular end-diastolic volume and pressure, occurs.

Reversibility of Cardiac Depression. The depression of myocardial contractility in papillary muscles removed from cats with pressure overload–induced hypertrophy is reversible when the hypertrophy is reversed by unbanding the pulmonary artery.[32,47] Sustained treatment of hypertension also reverses the impairment of contractility caused by that condition.[41]

CAUSES OF HYPERTROPHY

The character of the stress (increased preload, increased afterload, primary loss of myocytes as in myocardial infarction, or primary depression of contractility as in cardiomyopathy) responsible for inciting the hypertrophy appears to play a critical role in determining the nature of the response.[42] After the neonatal period, an increase in myocardial mass is associated with a proportional increase in the size of individual cells, i.e., hypertrophy, with at most a slight increase in the number of cells, i.e., without hyperplasia.

One of the early cellular changes that occurs after the stimulus for hypertrophy is applied is a preferential synthesis of mitochondria; presumably the expanded mitochondrial mass provides sufficient adenosine triphosphate (ATP) to meet the increased energy demands of the hypertrophying cell. As the myofibrillar mass increases, there is an increase in the number of myofibrils laid down in parallel while sarcomeres are also added in series. There is evidence that with continued pressure overload the mitochrondrial/myofibrillar mass relationship becomes inadequate, ultimately interfering with myocardial function.[48] This is accompanied by the development of cytoskeletal connections between "Z" lines and the laying down of interstitial collagen.[37] Cardiac hypertrophy can take place only when the DNA in the myocyte nucleus is derepressed, allowing DNA replication to occur.[49] There has been much debate about the nature of the stimulus that activates the DNA.[50,50a] The following possible stimuli have been suggested[48]: (1) depletion of ATP; (2) stretch of myocytes caused by a sustained increase in preload or afterload; (3) accumulation of products of cell degeneration caused by "wear and tear"; and (4) humoral stimuli, such as thyroid hormone. While the specific stimulus (or stimuli) for derepression of DNA has not yet been identified, it could operate at various levels, including mRNA transcription, translation, or protein formation.

VOLUME OVERLOAD. When volume overload is produced by the creation of an aortocaval fistula, sarcomere length initially rises to the optimal level of 2.2 μm. Then progressive left ventricular dilatation and moderate left ventricular hypertrophy occur without clinical evidence of heart failure, and the length–active tension relations of the dilated, hypertrophied ventricle remain essentially normal.[51] Within one week of the creation of such a fistula, left ventricular end-diastolic pressure rises and then remains constant, whereas the left ventricular end-diastolic diameter continues to increase progressively, indicating a change in the ventricle's diastolic properties. Following chronic adjustment to the shunt, the end-diastolic volume increases at any given end-diastolic pressure (Fig. 14–5); left ventricular function, as reflected in the velocity of circumferential fiber shortening, may be normal or depressed. The performance of the chronically volume-overloaded ventricle is characterized by normal or nearly normal performance of each unit of myocardium, allowing delivery of a greater-than-normal stroke volume. The chronic ventricular dilatation is associated with diastolic sarcomere lengths that are optimal (2.2 μm). Thus, despite the augmented volumes and filling pressures, there is *no* disengagement of thick and thin myofilaments.

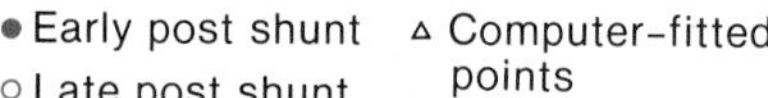

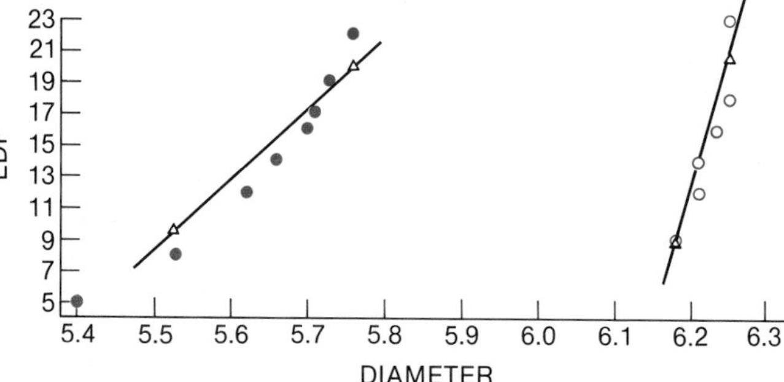

FIGURE 14–5. Relations between left ventricular end-diastolic pressure (EDP, mm Hg) and left ventricular diameter at end diastole (cm) in one dog studied early and late during the course of chronic volume overloading by means of an arteriovenous fistula. Each curve relating end-diastolic pressure to end-diastolic diameter was obtained by acute transfusion and bleeding. The shift to the right and increase in the slope of the pressure-diameter relation between the early postshunt study (closed circles) and the study many weeks after the occurrence of chronic cardiac dilatation (closed triangles) are apparent; the slope change reflects a reduction in diastolic compliance. (From McCullagh, W. H., et al.: Left ventricular dilatation and diastolic compliance changes during chronic volume overloading. Circulation *45*:943, 1972, by permission of the American Heart Association, Inc.)

Following the initial increase in stroke volume, mediated by increased sarcomere length during the acute phase of volume overloading, progressive cardiac dilatation subsequently occurs, whereas end-diastolic sarcomere lengths remain relatively constant. Cardiac dilatation presumably results from an increase in the size of myocardial cells or from a greater number of sarcomeres developing in series during the process of hypertrophy, causing a lengthening of myocytes and perhaps slippage between adjacent fibers and fibrils.[52] In addition, the myocardial capillary network may not increase in proportion to myocardial mass. These changes may be irreversible[45] and may impair further contractile performance.[52] Thus, in summary, the ventricle ordinarily compensates for a volume overload with both a change in ventricular geometry and an increase in the number of sarcomeres, resulting in an augmented stroke volume. In the compensated state of chronic volume overloading, the combination of ventricular dilata-

TABLE 14–3 ECHOCARDIOGRAPHIC CHANGES IN ISOTONIC AND ISOMETRIC ATHLETES*

	ISOTONIC	ISOMETRIC
Left ventricular end-diastolic diameter	↑	↑, no Δ
Left ventricular end-diastolic diameter per square meter or per kilogram	↑	no Δ
Left ventricular end-systolic diameter	↑, ↓, no Δ	↑, ↓, no Δ
Left ventricular end-diastolic volume	↑	no Δ
Left ventricular posterior wall thickness	↑	↑
Left ventricular mass	↑	↑
Left ventricular mass, per square meter or per kilogram	↑	no Δ
Interventricular septal thickness	↑	↑
Interventricular-septum/posterior wall ratio	↑, no Δ	↑, no Δ
Right ventricular diameter	↑	—
Left atrial diameter	↑	—
Ejection fraction	no Δ	no Δ
Cardiac output (resting)	no Δ	no Δ
Stroke volume	↑	↑, no Δ
Velocity of circumferential fiber shortening	↑, ↓, no Δ	no Δ

* ↑ = increase, ↓ = decrease, and no Δ = no change. (Reprinted by permission from Huston, T. P., Puffer, J. C., and Rodney, W. M.. The athletic heart syndrome. N. Engl. J. Med. *313*:29, 1985.)

tion and hypertrophy allows enhancement of overall cardiac performance, with normal function of each unit of an enlarged ventricle operating at an optimal sarcomere length. However, in the presence of a very large volume overload and clinical evidence of congestive heart failure, myocardial contractility does become seriously depressed.[45]

PRESSURE OVERLOAD. More is known about this form of overload, especially in animal models in which the aorta or pulmonary artery is abruptly constricted, than of other forms. As described by Meerson[33] (Table 14–2), immediately upon imposition of a large pressure load, the increase in work performed by the ventricle exceeds the augmentation of cardiac mass and the heart hyperfunctions and then dilates. As a consequence, hypertrophy develops,[53] a compensatory phase sets in, and the contractile function returns to approximately normal levels. Myofibrils are laid down in parallel so that the cross-sectional diameter of myocytes is increased.[52] Later, alterations in cellular organization take place, and during the "exhaustion" phase there is lysis of myofibrils, lysosomes increase in number, presumably to digest worn-out cell constituents,[37] the sarcoplasmic reticulum becomes distorted, the surface densities of the key tubular system are reduced,[54] and fibrous tissue takes the place of the cardiac cells.[55] In addition, capillary density[56,57] and coronary reserve, as reflected in the increase in coronary blood flow during adenosine reperfusion, become reduced.[54] The resulting ischemia, most severe in the subendocardium, might contribute further to the impairment of cardiac function. Myocardial failure occurs in the stage of "exhaustion" when cellular function deteriorates. Some cells drop out and the remainder function abnormally and are forced to sustain an even greater burden, leading to a vicious circle (Fig. 14–6).

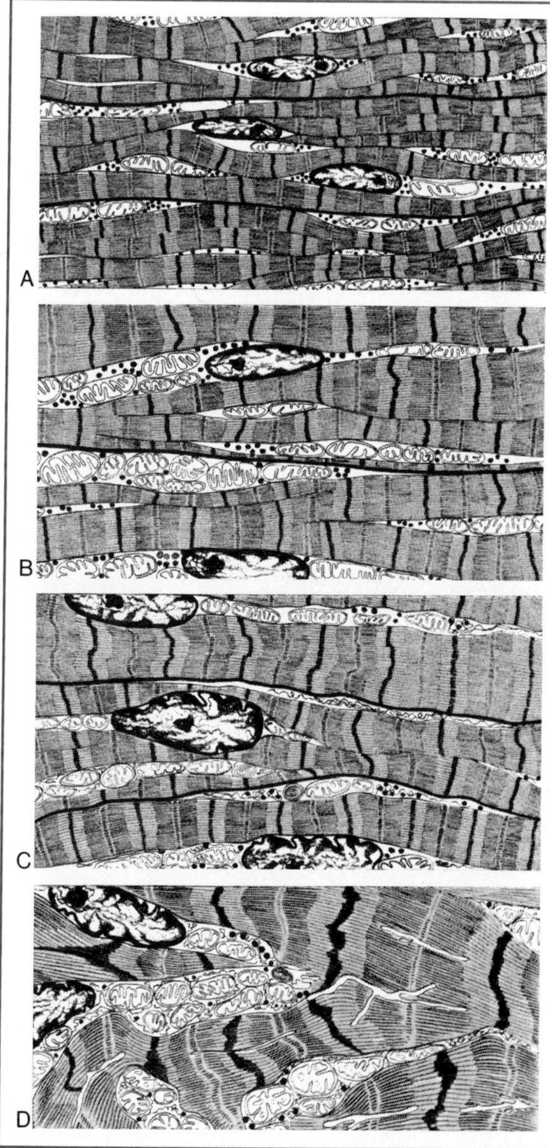

FIGURE 14–6. The early stage of cardiac hypertrophy (A) is characterized morphologically by increases in the number of myofibrils and mitochondria as well as enlargement of mitochondria and nuclei. Muscle cells are larger than normal, but cellular organization is largely preserved. At a more advanced stage of hypertrophy (B), preferential increases in the size or number of specific organelles, such as mitochondria, as well as irregular addition of new contractile elements in localized areas of the cell, result in subtle abnormalities of cellular organization and contour. Adjacent cells may vary in their degree of enlargement. Cells subjected to longstanding hypertrophy (C) show more obvious disruptions in cellular organization, such as markedly enlarged nuclei with highly lobulated membranes, which displace adjacent myofibrils and cause breakdown of normal Z-band registration. The early preferential increase in mitochondria is supplanted by a predominance by volume of myofibrils. The late stage of hypertrophy (D) is characterized by loss of contractile elements with marked disruption of Z bands, severe disruption of the normal parallel arrangement of the sarcomeres, deposition of fibrous tissue, and dilation and increased tortuosity of T tubules. (From Ferrans, V. J.: Morphology of the heart in hypertrophy. Hosp. Pract. *18*:69, 1983.)

OTHER FORMS OF HYPERTROPHY. A mild form of cardiac hypertrophy is seen in athletes[57–59,59a] (Table 14–3). Prolonged athletic training causes a moderate increase in myocardial mass. Isotonic exercise, such as long-distance running or swimming, resembles volume overload and causes an increase in left ventricular diastolic volume; isometric exercise, such as weightlifting or wrestling, resembles pressure overload and causes an increase in wall thickness. Neither form of hypertrophy appears to be deleterious in the absence of disease and rapidly disappears when training is discontinued.

Following myocardial infarction, there is hypertrophy of the spared myocytes with an increase of both myocyte diameter, as in pressure overload, and in myocyte length, as in volume overload.[52,59b]

Endomyocardial biopsies in patients with heart failure of diverse etiologies are consistent with the formulation presented above. Myocyte hypertrophy and fibrosis tend to be worse in patients with more severe forms of heart failure.[60] Patients in whom myocytes are composed of a reduced fraction of myofibrils appear to exhibit a particularly poor prognosis.[61]

The experimentally produced dilated cardiomyopathy induced by rapid right ventricular pacing[62] (which has its clinical counterparts[63]) is one form of stress placed on the myocardium that is *not* accompanied by ventricular hypertrophy.

EFFECTS OF DEPRESSED CONTRACTILITY. The effects of depression of myocardial contractility on the myocardial force-velocity relations are shown schematically in Figure 14–7.[64] Mild depression of contractility permits a normal extent and velocity of shortening of cardiac muscle through operation of the Frank-Starling mechanism, i.e., from an augmented end-diastolic fiber length, and the stress of any augmentation of afterload can be met only with even further augmentation of preload. When contractility is markedly depressed, no preload reserve is available, and any augmentation of afterload results in a marked reduction in the extent and velocity of shortening, a condition that Ross has referred to as "afterload mismatch."[64] Under these circumstances, a reduction of afterload will improve ventricular performance while a reduction of preload will depress it (although such a reduction may be helpful clinically by reducing ventricular filling pressure and thereby reducing the symptoms of pulmonary congestion [Fig. 17–14, p. 492].)

CARDIAC RESPONSE IN VARIOUS FORMS OF VOLUME AND PRESSURE OVERLOADING

Since alterations in preload and afterload are important determinants of the dynamics of cardiac contraction, it is not surprising that cardiac performance differs in various cardiac abnormalities depending on alterations in pressure and vol-

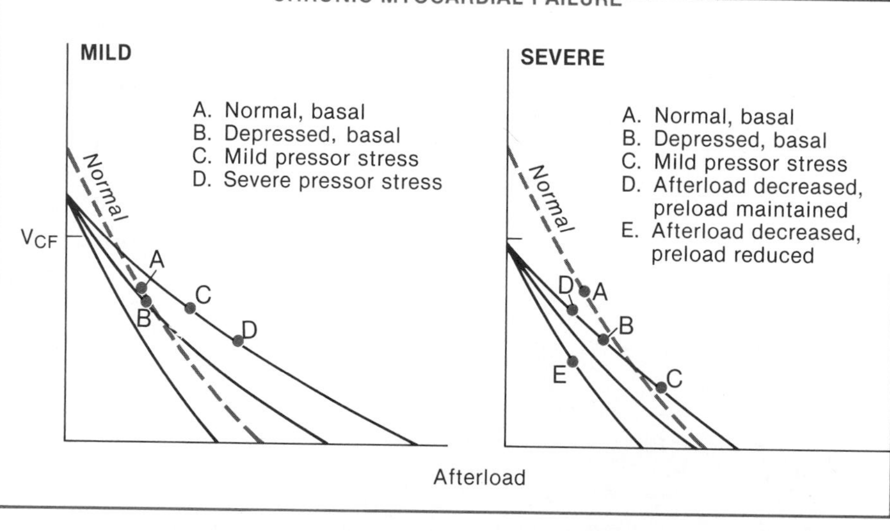

FIGURE 14–7. Alterations of force-velocity relations during afterload changes in the presence of left ventricular failure. *Left panel,* A normal force-velocity curve is indicated by the dashed line, and the normal basal state by point A. With mild depression of the inotropic activity in the basal state, through some encroachment on the Frank-Starling reserve, V_{CF} can be maintained near normal (point B). Some preload reserve may remain, and a mild pressor stress produced by infusion of a peripheral vasoconstrictor may cause little reduction in V_{CF} (point C). However, a more marked increase in afterload will result in a substantial drop in V_{CF} and stroke volume (point D). *Right panel,* With severe depression of the myocardial inotropic activity under basal conditions, V_{CF} is depressed to below the normal range (point B). Since the preload reserve has been fully utilized in the basal state, any afterload increase of even moderate degree will result in a marked drop in V_{CF} and stroke volume (point C). A reduction in afterload with preload maintained constant results in restoration of V_{CF} or stroke volume to near normal (point D), but if preload is allowed to fall substantially, such an afterload reduction may result in no change or even a fall in V_{CF} and stroke volume (point E). (From Ross, J., Jr.: Afterload mismatch and preload reserve: A conceptual framework for the analysis of ventricular function. Prog. Cardiovasc. Dis. *18*:255, 1976, by permission of Grune and Stratton.)

ume overloading. For example, with equivalent total and effective stroke volumes, left ventricular function is more severely stressed, with greater end-diastolic pressure and volume, in aortic than in mitral regurgitation.[65-67] In the former, the regurgitant volume is delivered into the high-pressure aorta whereas in the latter it must be ejected into the low-pressure left atrium. For similar reasons, left ventricular function appears to be less impaired in ventricular septal defect than in patent ductus arteriosus with similar degrees of left-to-right shunt.[68] Ventricular septal defect resembles mitral regurgitation in that the shunted blood is ejected directly into the low-pressure right ventricle, and there is a rapid fall in tension during systole as the result of a greater reduction in instantaneous impedance to left ventricular emptying. Patent ductus arteriosus is similar to aortic regurgitation in that the entire left ventricular stroke volume, including the shunted blood, is ejected into the high-pressure aorta. Furthermore, conditions in which the impedance to ejection is considerably reduced, such as mitral regurgitation and ventricular septal defect, impose a smaller demand on myocardial oxygen requirements than those such as patent ductus arteriosus and aortic regurgitation, in which it is not.[69]

PATTERNS OF VENTRICULAR HYPERTROPHY

The development of ventricular hypertrophy constitutes one of the principal mechanisms by which the heart compensates for an increased load. Grossman et al. examined systolic and diastolic wall stresses in normal subjects and in well-compensated patients with chronically pressure- and volume-overloaded left ventricles.[70] Left ventricular systolic stress, end-diastolic pressure, and mass were increased approximately equally in both the pressure- and volume-overloaded groups. There was a substantial increase in wall thickness in the pressure-overloaded ventricles, but only a mild increase in wall thickness in the volume-overloaded ventricles (Fig. 14–8). The latter was just sufficient to counterbalance the increased radius, so that the ratio of wall thickness (h) to radius (R) remained normal for the patients with volume-overloaded hypertrophy, while it was substantially increased in patients with pressure-overloaded hypertrophy, in whom there was disproportionate thickening of the ventricular wall.

The aforementioned observations are in concert with those of other investigators who have indicated that myocardial hypertrophy develops in a manner that maintains systolic stress within normal limits.[71-73] When the primary stimulus to hypertrophy is pressure overload, the resultant acute increase in systolic wall stress leads to parallel replication of myofibrils, wall thickening of individual myocytes[52] and of the ventricular wall, and concentric hypertrophy (Fig. 14–9). The wall thickening is just sufficient to maintain a normal level of systolic stress. The importance of preventing the development of excessive levels of ventricular wall stress is illustrated in Figure 14–10, obtained from a series of patients with hyperten-

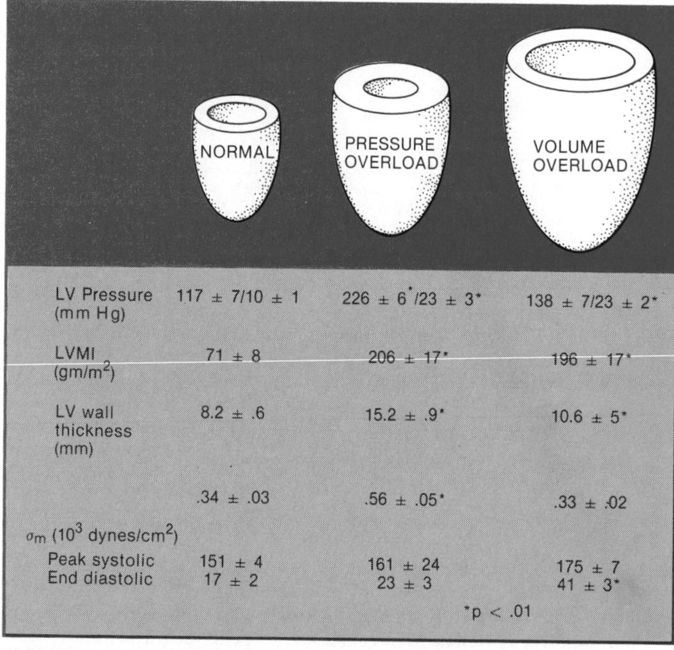

	NORMAL	PRESSURE OVERLOAD	VOLUME OVERLOAD
LV Pressure (mm Hg)	117 ± 7/10 ± 1	226 ± 6*/23 ± 3*	138 ± 7/23 ± 2*
LVMI (gm/m²)	71 ± 8	206 ± 17*	196 ± 17*
LV wall thickness (mm)	8.2 ± .6	15.2 ± .9*	10.6 ± 5*
	.34 ± .03	.56 ± .05*	.33 ± .02
σ_m (10³ dynes/cm²)			
Peak systolic	151 ± 4	161 ± 24	175 ± 7
End diastolic	17 ± 2	23 ± 3	41 ± 3*

*p < .01

FIGURE 14–8. Mean values for left ventricular (LV) pressure, mass index (LVMI), left ventricular wall thickness, the ratio of wall thickness to radius (h/R), and peak systolic and end-diastolic meridional wall stress in patients with normal (6 subjects), pressure-overloaded (6 subjects), and volume-overloaded (18 subjects) ventricles. Although mass is increased similarly in both pressure- and volume-overloaded groups, the increase is accomplished primarily by wall thickening in the pressure-overloaded group. The h/R ratio is normal in volume-overload hypertrophy, indicating a "magnification" type of growth. In pressure overload, concentric hypertrophy is quantified by the increase in h/R. Patients were compensated with respect to heart failure, and peak systolic tension (σ_m) was not statistically different from normal. However, end-diastolic stress was consistently elevated in the volume-overloaded group. See text for details. (Reproduced from Grossman, W., et al.: Wall stress and patterns of hypertrophy in the human left ventricle. J. Clin. Invest. *56*:56, 1975, by copyright permission of the American Society for Clinical Investigation.)

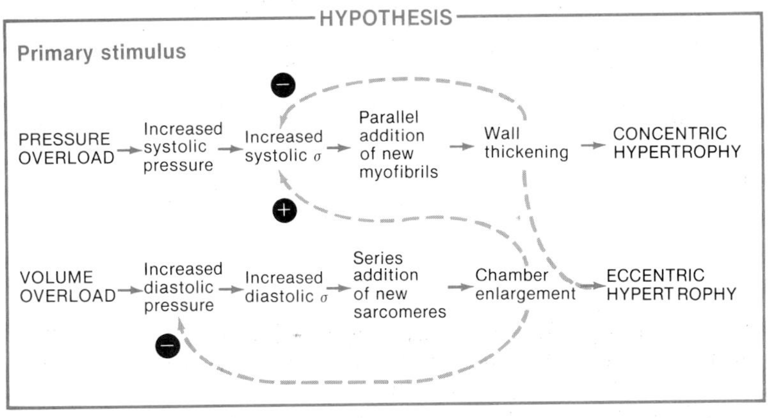

FIGURE 14–9. Hypothesis relating wall stress and patterns of hypertrophy. (Reproduced from Grossman, W., et al.: Wall stress (σ) and patterns of hypertrophy in the human left ventricle. J. Clin. Invest. *56*:56, 1975, by copyright permission of the American Society for Clinical Investigation.)

sion. As might be anticipated from the inverse relationship between afterload and shortening, as ventricular wall stress increased to excessive levels, both the extent and shortening of velocity declined. When the primary stimulus is ventricular volume overload, increased diastolic wall stress leads to replication of sarcomeres in series, elongation of myocytes, and ventricular dilatation. This, in turn, results in a modest increase in systolic stress[73a] (by the Laplace relationship); this causes wall thickening that again tends to maintain a normal level of systolic stress. Thus, in compensated subjects, both volume and pressure overload alter ventricular geometry and wall thickness, so that systolic stress is not changed greatly.

An inverse correlation between circumferential wall stress and both ejection fraction and velocity of fiber shortening has

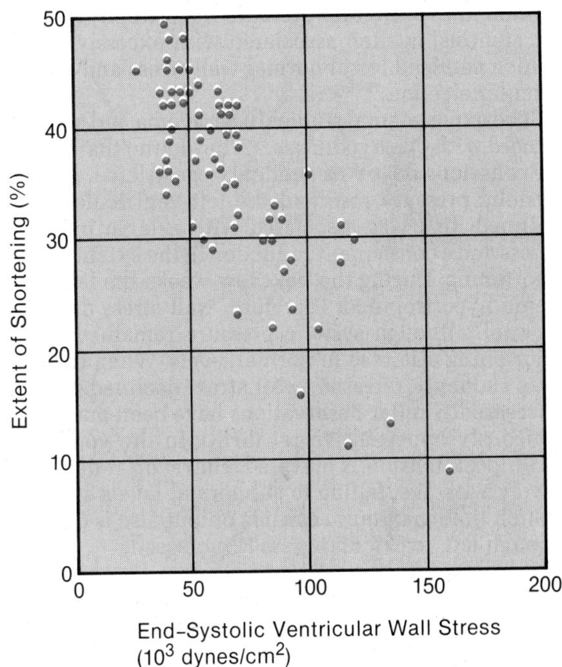

FIGURE 14–10. In a study of hypertensive patients, calculated end-systolic ventricular wall stress (indicative of afterload during ventricular ejection) correlated closely with ventricular performance. A consistent relationship occurred with extent of circumference shortening in the left ventricular wall. A similar relationship was observed between end-systolic ventricular wall stress and the velocity of shortening. (From Tarazi, R. C.: The progression from hypertrophy to heart failure. Hosp. Pract. *18*:104, 1983.)

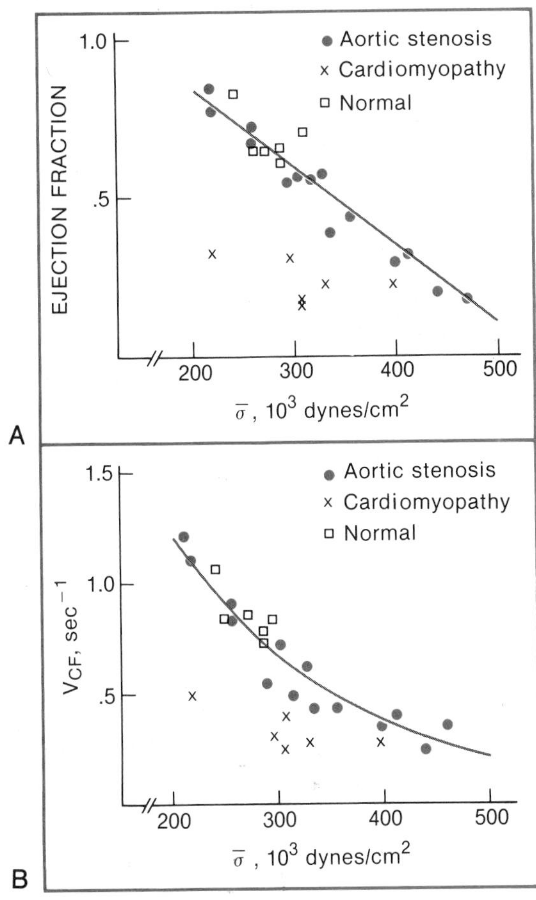

FIGURE 14–11. Relationship between mean wall stress ($\bar{\sigma}$) and muscle fiber shortening characteristics. *A*, Ejection fraction. The line represents the best curve derived from linear regression analysis of the data for patients with aortic stenosis. In these patients, normal values for ejection fraction are associated with normal levels of wall stress, whereas decreasing values for ejection fraction are associated with increasing levels of wall stress. Values for normal controls fall on or near the regression line for the aortic stenosis group. Patients with cardiomyopathy, however, have depressed ejection fractions, regardless of the level of stress. *B*, Mean midwall velocity of circumferential fiber shortening (V_{CF}). Values for patients with aortic stenosis are well approximated as an exponential function of wall stress. Normal patients, again, exhibit a relationship similar to those with aortic stenosis. Patients with cardiomyopathy show depressed values for V_{CF} for any corresponding wall stress. σ = Mean midwall circumferential stress. (From Gunther, S., and Grossman, W.: Determinants of ventricular function in pressure overload hypertrophy in man. Circulation *59*:679, 1979, by permission of the American Heart Association, Inc.)

phy,[93] even at a time when systolic function is normal. However, a reduced rate of relaxation is not an inevitable accompaniment of all forms of ventricular hypertrophy; for example, it is not observed in athletes who have eccentric hypertrophy (volume overload hypertrophy).[94]

Marked dilation of the left ventricles of patients with *chronic* volume overload, with congestive cardiomyopathy, or following large transmural infarction may be associated with little elevation of the left ventricular end-diastolic pressure, indicating a shift of the pressure-volume curve to the right, along its volume axis (Fig. 14–5). In contrast, concentric left ventricular hypertrophy, as occurs in aortic stenosis, hypertension, and hypertrophic cardiomyopathy, frequently changes the shape and position of the normal pressure-volume relation, so that at any diastolic volume ventricular diastolic pressure is abnormally elevated, representing a shift of the pressure-volume relation to the left along the volume axis.[87,95,96] *Myocardial* stiffness (in contrast to *ventricular* distensibility) may or may not be altered in the presence of myocardial hypertrophy secondary to pressure overload.[97]

ISCHEMIC HEART DISEASE. Marked changes can occur in the diastolic properties of the left ventricle in ischemic heart disease. First, as already pointed out, ventricular relaxation may be slowed and myocardial wall stiffness increased in the presence of acute, reversible myocardial ischemia.[98,98a,98b] Myocardial infarction causes complex changes in ventricular pressure-volume relations,[98c] depending on: (1) whether just the infarcted tissue or the entire ventricle is studied, (2) the size of the infarct, and (3) the time following infarction at which the study is carried out. Initially, infarcted muscle exhibits reduced stiffness.[98d–98f] Then the development of edema, fibrocellular infiltration, and scar contribute to stiffening of the necrotic tissue.[99] Later still, left ventricular remodeling causes a rightward displacement of the pressure-volume curve. In a rat model of well-healed infarction, the left ventricular diastolic volume is increased at any diastolic pressure, the extent of displacement of the pressure-volume curve being a function of infarct size.[100] In addition, the diastolic pressure-volume relationship of the entire ventricle is shifted so that volume is increased at low distending pressures—i.e., the chamber displays decreased stiffness—whereas at higher pressures the slope of the pressure-volume curve is normal. In addition to the fibrous tissue replacement of the ventricle in ischemic heart disease, the restrictive cardiomyopathies (p. 1415), the dilated cardiomyopathies with extensive interstitial fibrosis,[101] and the transplanted heart during rejection episodes[102] all exhibit upward and leftward displacement of the diastolic pressure-volume relation.

ROLE OF COLLAGEN IN VENTRICULAR DYSFUNCTION. The ventricle is composed not only of myocytes but also of the coronary vessels, nerves, fibroblasts, and types I and III fibrillar collagen.[103–105] The latter provide struts along which the myocytes are aligned. Branches of collagen fibers course at right angles to connect and align muscle bundles. Weber has pointed out that the passive properties of the ventricle depend on the quantity of the collagen relative to the myocytes, its elastic properties, and its physical disposition.[105] The left ventricular concentration of collagen has been shown to be increased in chronic pressure overload hypertrophy[106] induced experimentally or occurring in diseased patients. The messenger RNA for types I and III collagen that is present in fibroblasts increases markedly after aortic banding.[107,108] Less information is available on the role of collagen in volume overload hypertrophy, but the increase in diastolic stiffness sometimes seen in this condition has been associated with increased cross-linking of types I and III collagens.[107,108]

Clinical Implications

Changes in the diastolic properties of the ventricular chambers are of clinical as well as theoretical importance. Thus, impairment of cardiac relaxation and leftward displacement of the ventricular diastolic pressure-volume curve can interfere with ventricular filling. This situation constitutes a major hemodynamic abnormality in hypertrophic cardiomyopathy[96] as well as in other conditions characterized by concentric ventricular hypertrophy, such as aortic stenosis and hypertension. Impaired cardiac relaxation occurs also in reversible myocardial ischemia. The subendocardial ischemia that is characteristic of severe concentric hypertrophy (even in the presence of a normal coronary circulation) intensifies the failure of relaxation,[88,92] and when coronary artery obstruction accompanies severe hypertrophy, this abnormality may be particularly severe.[84] At any given diastolic volume, ventricular end-diastolic pressure and pulmonary venous pressures rise. Tachycardia, by reducing the duration of diastole and under some circumstances causing or intensifying ischemia, exaggerates this diastolic abnormality and may raise ventricular diastolic pressure, even while reducing diastolic ventricular volume; bradycardia has the opposite effect. When the left ventricular pressure-volume curve is shifted leftward by ischemia, successful treatment of the ischemia improves diastolic relaxation and lowers ventricular diastolic (and pulmonary venous) pressure.

Although a defect in ventricular emptying (systolic dysfunction) is the most common form of heart failure, there is increasing evidence that in the presence of ventricular hypertrophy diastolic dysfunction may play a dominant role. Topol et al. have described a group of elderly patients with hypertension and clinical evidence of severe heart failure with excessive left ventricular emptying and marked prolongation of early diastolic filling.[109] Sometimes isolated diastolic dysfunction can be severe enough to be responsible for advanced, even terminal, heart failure. Diastolic abnormalities also contribute to subclinical impairment of left ventricular function in patients with diabetes mellitus.[110,111] There is evidence that many patients with the usual forms of clinical heart failure have normal or near-normal systolic function, with symptoms related primarily to diastolic dysfunction.[112] The contribution of atrial contraction to ventricular filling is particularly important in conditions in which ventricular stiffness is increased. Thus, loss of a properly synchronized atrial contraction, as occurs in atrial fibrillation or atrioventricular dissociation in patients with leftward displacement of the ventricular pressure-volume curve (higher pressure at any volume), raises atrial pressure or lowers cardiac output or both. Pericardial tamponade and constrictive pericarditis also change the apparent diastolic properties of the heart. Early filling is unimpaired in constrictive pericarditis because the myocardium is normal. However, filling is abruptly halted in mid-diastole by the constricted pericardium, which imposes its mechanical properties on those of the ventricle in the latter half of diastole (Fig. 14–13*B*).

Since the normal left ventricle operates below the bend of the pressure-volume curve, an acute volume overload or an acute impairment of contractility may result in a marked rise in left ventricular diastolic pressure. The latter in turn can lead to pulmonary edema as the ventricle moves up along the steep portion of its pressure-volume curve. The rightward displacement of the curve—i.e., an increase in volume at any level of pressure—as occurs with chronic volume overload or dilated cardiomyopathy (Fig. 14–5), is helpful, because it lowers the pressure necessary to provide the preload (myocardial distension) required by the diseased left ventricle.

MECHANISMS RESPONSIBLE FOR DEPRESSED CONTRACTILITY

Considerable effort has been and continues to be directed toward elucidating the fundamental mechanism responsible for the contractile abnormality; this abnormality is ultimately expressed in a reduction in the work of the myocardium in the common forms of low-output heart failure.[112a,112b] The available evidence for the mechanism of myocardial failure, analyzed in terms of energy supply, production, storage, and utilization (as well as the structure and function of the contractile proteins), is conflicting. Although a number of metabolic alterations have been identified in the failing, hemodynamically overloaded heart, it is not clear which, if any, is the *primary* defect responsible for heart failure and which are *secondary* mechanisms that either aid the heart in coping with the overload or are contributory and deleterious but occur consequent to another primary abnormality. A *single unifying* biochemical defect responsible for the common forms of heart failure occurring secondary to myocardial hemodynamic overload, or the overloading of remaining viable myocytes following myocardial infarction, has not been identified. However, there is increasing evidence for several possible defects that might be responsible. Some of the confusion in this field results undoubtedly from the various models of experimental heart failure employed, from species differences, from the rate and severity of application of the myocardial overload, and from the time interval following the inciting stimulus at which the observations are made.

MYOCARDIAL ENERGY PRODUCTION

Heart failure, especially acute heart failure, can certainly occur as a consequence of impaired perfusion, as in ischemic heart failure, but chronic heart failure also frequently occurs in the *presence* of adequate myocardial perfusion, oxygen, and substrate. In early studies, measurement of coronary blood flow utilizing coronary sinus catheterization, both in humans and in dogs with chronic heart failure, showed that the coronary blood flow per gram of myocardium does not differ significantly from normal.[113] Several preparations of failing heart muscle have actually been shown to require less oxygen than does normal muscle. When contractility becomes acutely depressed, myocardial oxygen consumption also declines.[114] Similarly, patients with chronic impairment of left ventricular performance and reduction of the velocity of myocardial fiber shortening also exhibit reduction of coronary blood flow and myocardial oxygen consumption per unit of muscle.[115] Marked reductions in myocardial oxygen consumption have been described in the Syrian hamster with hereditary cardiomyopathy.[116] Papillary muscles removed from cats with pressure overload–induced right ventricular hypertrophy exhibit a depression of both contractility and oxygen consumption per unit of tension development.[25] These lowered energy needs of the failing heart may actually serve a protective function.

MITOCHONDRIAL FUNCTION

Considerable dispute has centered on the question of whether or not mitochondrial oxidative phosphorylation, i.e., energy production, is abnormal in heart failure. Some investigators have shown that experimentally produced heart failure is characterized by a defect in mitochondrial energy production.[116] The mitochondrial respiratory control index, i.e., the ratio of active phosphorylating respiration by mitochondria (the rate of oxygen uptake), in the presence of ADP added to the rate of oxygen uptake after phosphorylation of all ADP (normally greater than 4:1) and the number of atoms of inorganic phosphate esterified with ADP to form ATP per atom of oxygen consumed (normally 3:1), have been reported to be markedly abnormal in mitochondria obtained from hearts with experimentally produced failure. Similarly, mitochondria isolated from the hearts of hamsters with hereditary cardiomyopathy[117] and the cardiomyopathy produced by potassium depletion[118] exhibit depression of respiratory activity. Homogenates prepared from hamster hearts with hereditary cardiomyopathy have severe depression of the ability to oxidize fatty acids and acetate.[119] Mitochondria obtained from failing *human* cardiac muscle have also shown reduced oxygen consumption during active phosphorylation and reduced rates of NADH-linked respiratory activity.[116] In contrast to these observations, other data indicate that electron transport and the tightness of respiratory control are *normal* in mitochondria obtained from failing human hearts[120] and cat hearts with experimental heart failure produced by pressure overload.[121]

MITOCHONDRIAL FUNCTION IN HYPERTROPHY. Mitochondria obtained from hypertrophied, nonfailing rabbit hearts have shown significantly *increased* respiratory activity compared with those of normal hearts, without a change in the ADP/O ratio, i.e., in the rate of energy production to oxygen consumption, or in the respiratory control index, permitting an *increase* in the capacity to synthesize ATP. In contrast, mitochondria obtained from rabbit hearts with congestive heart failure have shown respiratory rates near or below normal, a decreased respiratory control index, and some lowering of the ADP/O ratio.[120] In the phase of compensatory hypertrophy the ability of mitochondria to generate ATP is increased, due at least in part to the increased mitochondrial mass. However, in the late phase of hypertrophy there is a reduction in the quantity of mitochondria to generate ATP. According to this concept, a cause of contractile failure of the hypertrophic heart might be an inability of the energy-producing system, that is, the mitochondria, to keep pace with the needs of the contractile apparatus.

MITOCHONDRIAL FUNCTION IN HEART FAILURE. Failing muscles removed from cats subjected to an acute pressure overload exhibit decreased efficiency–increased oxygen uptake for any level of tension development. The mitochondria from these papillary muscles exhibit an increase in the rate of oxygen consumption in state 4—basal respiration (so-called nonphosphorylating respiration).[122,123] Ruthenium red, a compound that blocks the mitochondrial uptake of Ca^{++}, reduces the rate of state 4 respiration to normal in these mitochondria. This suggests that nonphosphorylating mitochondrial respiration, linked to Ca^{++} transport and perhaps due to increased cycling of Ca^{++} across the mitochondrial membranes, is responsible for the abnormal myocardial oxygen consumption and the reduced external efficiency that characterizes hypertrophy induced by the acute imposition of a pressure load. Following unbanding of the pulmonary artery, myocardial hypertrophy, the accompanying depression of contractility, and the abnormality of state 4 mitochondrial function have been observed in hypertrophy produced by moderately severe volume overload.[29]

In one study in which mitochondria were studied in the hearts of patients with end-stage dilated cardiomyopathy, a decrease in cytochrome *a* content and in cytochrome-dependent enzyme activity was reported.[124] The cytochromes are located in the inner mitochondrial membrane and are constituents of the respiratory chain that couples oxidation to the synthesis of chemical energy. The nucleotide-transporting protein located on the inner mitochondrial membrane, the so-called ADP-ATP carrier, has been identified as an autoantigen in viral myocarditis and dilated cardiomyopathy. In guinea pigs immunized to this carrier protein, both myocardial oxygen consumption and cardiac work fell.[125] These findings are compatible with the hypothesis that the impaired cardiac performance in some cases of myocarditis (and dilated cardiomyopathy) may be secondary to an imbalance between energy delivery and demand.

The creatine kinase reaction catalyzes the transfer of high-energy phosphate groups between creatine phosphate and ATP. ^{31}P nuclear-magnetic resonance techniques in intact hearts have shown that this reaction is coupled to mitochondrial energy production and that it regulates the rate of oxidative phosphorylation. Hearts from old spontaneously hypertensive rats may exhibit a marked reduction of mitochondrial creatine kinase activity, which could be responsible for the abnormalities of contraction and relaxation observed in this muscle.[126]

CONCLUSIONS. The explanation for the conflicting data on mitochondrial respiration in experimental heart failure, summarized above, is not clear. It may be related to differences in species or in the nature, severity, and rate of application of the inciting stimulus. However, since, in some studies, oxidative phosphorylation appears to be sustained until very late in the course of heart failure, it is unlikely that the observed changes in mitochondrial function are causally related to the development of heart failure. However, they may well be important to contributing to and *perpetuating* chronic heart failure.

MYOCARDIAL ENERGY SUPPLIES

As is the case for mitochondrial function, the data concerning myocardial energy supplies in heart failure are conflicting. As myocardial hypertrophy occurs, the number of capillaries does not increase and the inter-capillary distances increase with resultant impairment of diffusion of oxygen and substrates to the center of the enlarged myocytes. This may be a special problem in the subendocardium, which is particularly vulnerable to ischemia.[92,127] In the cardiomyopathic Syrian hamster, there is a reduction in high-energy phosphate stores and a depression in the free energy of ATP hydrolysis and augmented levels of lactate and inorganic phosphate.[116] Whether these changes are *causally* related to the impairment of contractility is not clear.

In order to determine whether energy supplies are adequate in cardiac hypertrophy and failure, the contents of high-energy phosphates were compared in the papillary muscles of normal cats, cats with hypertrophy without failure, and cats with overt right ventricular failure induced by pulmonary artery constriction. Both the ATP and the creatine phosphate (CP) concentrations were normal in the papillary muscles removed from failing hearts and from nonfailing hypertrophied hearts studied in vitro. Because, as already pointed out (Fig. 14–3), the mechanical performance of these isolated muscles was impaired, *their depression of contractility could not be attributed to a reduction of total myocardial high-energy stores.*[128] In addition, there appear to be no reductions of ATP and CP concentrations in papillary muscles removed from failing human hearts.[120] On the other hand, a reduction of CP concentrations was found in the hypertrophied and failing right ventricle studied in vivo.[128] Thus, it would appear that just as is the case for mitochondrial function, defects both in energy production and in the total reserve of high-energy phosphate compounds are not *primarily* responsible for the reduced contractility of the hypertrophied or failing heart. However, it is possible that reduction of ATP in a specific compartment of the cell that is required for control of some vital function such as ionic movement does play a key role in the depression of contractility characteristic of heart failure.

One unusual form of heart failure which is *primarily* related to a reduction of myocardial energy stores is that due to phosphate deficiency. Chronic hypophosphatemia induced by dietary means is associated with reversible depression of myocardial performance in isolated muscle as well as in the intact heart of animals and humans, presumably as a consequence of reduced ATP stores.[129,130]

MYOCARDIAL ENERGY UTILIZATION

External efficiency, i.e., the ratio of work performed to oxygen utilized, is usually depressed in chronic myocardial failure, probably as a consequence of an abnormality in the conversion of metabolic energy to contractile work. However, other possibilities must also be considered, such as abnormalities of cellular alignment (including slippage between adjacent myocytes) as well as disruptions in the intercellular tethering by collagen with ineffective coordination of contraction.

ALTERATIONS OF CONTRACTILE PROTEINS

As already noted, in a model of stable pressure-induced hypertrophy, the fraction of cell volume composed of myofibrils is initially increased.[48,131] Patients with aortic stenosis *without* heart failure exhibit a normal fraction of myofibrils per cell, whereas those with left ventricular failure show a significant reduction in cell volume occupied by myofibrils, suggesting that this decrease in the quantity of the contractile machinery may play a role in the development of cardiac decompensation.[132] In end-stage heart failure in the human there is a reduction of myofibrillar protein (per gram wet weight ventricle). This is consistent with electron microscopic observations showing a reduction of ventricular myofibrillar protein in heart failure.[133,134]

Cardiac hypertrophy occurs largely in response to hemodynamic overload and primarily causes enlargement of individual myocytes (Fig. 14–6). The increase in protein synthesis (and the reduction of protein breakdown) in cardiac hypertrophy is associated with an increase in total RNA and messenger RNA. Animal studies have indicated that, when the adult heart hypertrophies, fetal and neonatal forms of contractile proteins (termed isoforms) and other proteins (such as atrial natriuretic peptide) reappear, signifying reexpression of the genes for these fetal and neonatal isoforms. Thus, hemodynamic overload leads to enhanced overall protein synthesis (Fig. 14–16) but alters the proteins qualitatively, i.e., it leads to the synthesis of protein isoforms that were present during fetal and neonatal life when protein synthesis in the heart was also rapid. Altered isoforms of cardiac proteins may arise from the expression of different members of a multigene family or from the assembly of the same gene in a different pattern.

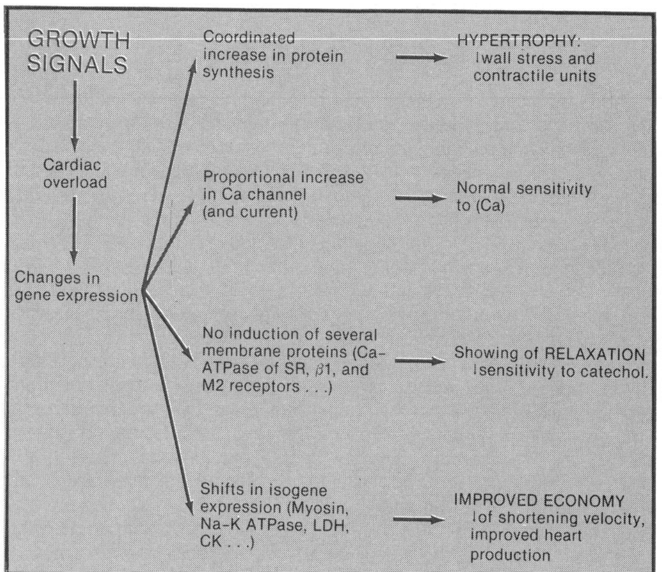

FIGURE 14–16. Main permanent changes in gene expression occurring during compensatory cardiac hypertrophy. Catechol = Catecholamines; SR = sarcoplasmic reticulum; LDH and CK = lactate dehydrogenase and creatine kinase. (From Swynghedauw, B.: Heart failure: A disease of adaptation. Heart Failure 6:57, 1990.)

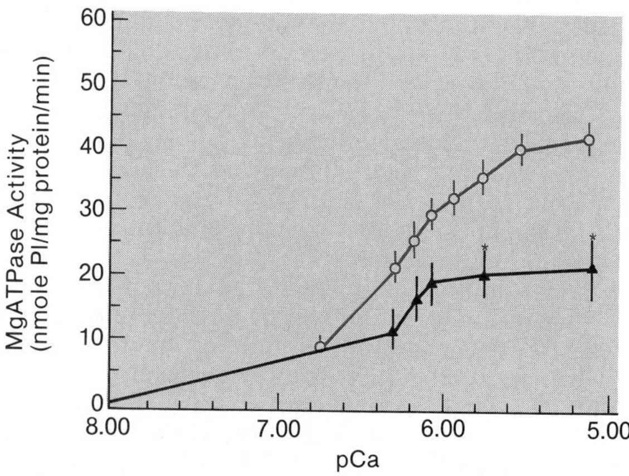

FIGURE 14–17. Myofibrillar Ca^{++}-dependent Mg-ATPase activity in normal hearts and hearts of patients with mitral regurgitation. Normal (red); mitral regurgitation (black) (n = 3); *$p < 0.05$. Each point and bar represents mean ± SEM. (From Pagani, E. D., Alousi, A. A., Grant, A. M., et al.: Changes in myofibrillar content and Mg-ATPase activity in ventricular tissues from patients with heart failure caused by coronary artery disease, cardiomyopathy, or mitral valve insufficiency. Circ. Res. *63*:380–385, 1988. Reprinted by permission of the American Heart Association, Inc.)

REDUCTION OF MYOSIN ATPase. Considerable data suggest that alterations of contractile proteins occur in heart failure. First, the finding that the reduced velocity of contraction of failing myocardium occurs in chemically skinned ventricular fiber suggests that this change reflects *intrinsic* alterations in the contractile apparatus. Early studies showed that the activity of myofibrillar ATPase is reduced in the hearts of patients who died of heart failure[135,136] (Fig. 14–17) and in dogs with naturally occurring heart failure.[137] Furthermore, reductions in the activities of myofibrillar ATPase, actomyosin ATPase, or myosin ATPase have been demonstrated in heart failure induced in cats by pulmonary artery constriction,[138] in guinea pigs with constriction of the ascending aorta,[139] in dogs with constriction of the pulmonary artery or aorta,[140] and in rats with renovascular hypertension.[141] These depressions of enzymatic activity could occur if an altered subunit of the myosin molecule, i.e., the portion of the molecule responsible for the ATPase activity, were produced in the overloaded heart and if it reduced contractility by lowering the rate of interaction between actin and myosin filaments. Reduction in the Mg-ATPase activity of myofibrils (which expresses the response of myofibrils to Ca^{++}) of patients with end-stage heart failure and in less sick patients who undergo valve replacement has been demonstrated. This may cause an abnormal interaction between thick and thin filaments. However, most investigators have not found an MHC switch in the ventricle in human heart failure. Consequently, while there has been a reduction in myofibrillar ATPase activity, no change has been detected in myosin ATPase activity.

MYOSIN ISOFORM SWITCH (see also p. 352). The heavy chains of cardiac myosin (myosin heavy chains, MHC) are composed of several polymorphic forms, termed *isoforms* or *isoenzymes*.[142,143,143a] Adaptation of cardiac performance may be mediated by changes in the characteristics of this myosin. Normally, alpha MHC (fast MHC, the V_1 isoform with high ATPase activity) is the myosin isoform that predominates in the rat. Aortic banding causes a rapid induction of beta-MHC RNA and beta-MHC protein (slow MHC, the V_3 isoform with low ATPase activity). A similar switch from V_1 to V_3 myosin occurs in the rat with myocardial infarction and heart failure.[144] These myosin isoform changes are not uniform through the ventricular wall of the rat, with greater concentrations of V_3 occurring in the subendocardium, possibly related to the increased wall tension of the subendocardial layers.[145,145a] Thyroxine, administered to rats with pressure overload, caused a deinduction of beta-MHC and reinduction of alpha-MHC (Fig. 50–13, p. 1615).[146]

The molecular mechanism(s) by which hemodynamic overload induces isoform switching is not known.[147] It is likely that the switch of cardiac MHC during pressure overload is induced in some manner by the stress imposed directly on the individual myocytes. The changes in MHC gene expression and myosin isoform synthesis produced by one-sided ventricular overload are limited to the involved ventricle and therefore are not related to the action of circulating hormones.[148] Perhaps the hemodynamic load causes some mechanical deformation of the myocyte, which in turn ultimately affects the cells' genetic machinery. $Alpha_1$ adrenoceptors appear to be molecular mediators of isogene expression in myocyte hypertrophy.[149] Waspe et al. have found that activation of the alpha-adrenergic receptors is a signal for increased beta-MHC isogene expression in cell culture.[150] Another fetal gene that is reexpressed in hypertrophy is the gene for alpha (skeletal sarcomeric) actin, which can also be induced by $alpha_1$-adrenergic receptor stimulation.

Another possible mechanism responsible for the switches of MHC gene expression in cardiac hypertrophy is overexpression of proto-oncogenes (Chap. 50). A proto-oncogene is a segment of DNA that is homologous to the genes of acute transforming viruses during periods of rapid growth. Both the c-*myc* and c-*fos* proto-oncogenes are induced in ventricular myocardium within 1 hour after induction of a pressure load.[151] The inherited idiopathic cardiomyopathy in the Syrian hamster is associated with the over-expression of the c-*myc* proto-oncogene, a finding not observed in normal hamsters; this overexpression may alter protein biosynthesis and may be related to the pathogenesis of this cardiomyopathy.[152] Proto-oncogenes act by encoding growth factors that control cellular proliferation. Cardiac myocytes might be the targets of heparin-binding and other peptide growth factors that provoke the expression of contractile protein genes.[153] Thus, transforming growth factor beta-1 and basic fibroblast growth factor cause upregulation of beta MHC myosin, similar to pressure overload hypertrophy.[153]

The composition of the myosin heavy chains determines the rate of energy liberation by myosin, i.e., the myosin ATPase activity. Replacement of fast (alpha, V_1) MHC by slow (beta, V_3) myosin isoforms reduces the rate of cross-bridge cycling (contractility) but prolongs ejection and reduces energy costs of contraction and thereby enhances myocardial efficiency. The synthesis of a myosin with abnormally low intrinsic ATPase activity could explain many of the functional changes in failing heart muscle, such as depression of the force-velocity curve (Fig. 14–2). However, it has also been proposed that such a biochemical abnormality might actually be beneficial in heart failure (Table 14–1). It would be expected to *increase* the quantity of mechanical energy derived from each mole of ATP utilized, i.e., it would increase the efficiency of cardiac muscle, albeit at the expense of a slowing of the maximum rate at which blood is ejected.[154] This suggestion is compatible with the finding of reduced oxygen consumption per unit of tension development of papillary muscles obtained from cats with pressure overload[25] and the other evidence of reduced oxygen requirements of failing heart muscle discussed on p. 405. In the human heart, a shift to the V_3 isozyme has been observed in hypertrophied left atria,[155,156] but the situation in the ventricles is less clear because normally the V_3 (beta MHC) isoform already predominates. However, there is one report that in the human with heart failure there is a reduction in the number of cells containing alpha MHC.[157] Also, increases in myosin *light-chain* isoforms have been observed in the ventricles of patients subjected to increased mechanical stress.[158]

A variety of other abnormalities in contractile protein have been reported in the ventricle in human and experimentally induced heart failure; these include upregulation of alpha skeletal actin (X-1, X-12) and changes in the myosin light chain and in the troponin-tropomyosin[159,160] system; any of these may be responsible for the aforementioned reductions in myofibrillar ATPase activity observed in human heart failure.

EXCITATION-CONTRACTION COUPLING AND THE ROLE OF Ca^{++}

Given the critical role played by Ca^{++} in the contractile process (p. 357), it is not surprising that considerable attention has been devoted to the role of this ion and of excitation-coupling in the etiology of heart failure.[160a] It has been noted that hypocalcemia (secondary to hypoparathyroidism and a variety of other conditions) can cause heart failure that is responsive to the infusion of Ca^{++}.[161,162] In contrast, elevation of serum ionized [Ca^{++}] augments contractility in patients with renal failure undergoing dialysis[163] as well as in patients with severe heart failure secondary to cardiomyopathy who have downregulation of beta receptors (p. 411) and whose condition is not responsive to sympathomimetic amines.[164]

Studies of a number of in vitro systems indicate that the delivery of Ca^{++} for activation of the contractile process is impaired in heart failure.[165,165a] A variety of cellular structures and membranes, including the sarcolemma, sarcoplasmic reticulum, and mitochondria, affect the myoplasmic [Ca^{++}] (Fig. 13–13, p. 361). It has been proposed that damage or impairment of function of these structures, or changes in the intracellular concentrations of other cations, adenonucleotides, or free fatty acids, may interfere with mechanisms regulating myoplasmic [Ca^{++}] and thereby participate in the production of heart failure.

Abnormalities of Uptake of Ca^{++} by Sarcoplasmic Reticulum

The uptake of Ca^{++} by the sarcoplasmic reticulum (SR) depends on a Ca^{++}-activated ATPase. Depressed activity of this enzyme, leading to defects in Ca^{++} accumulation by the SR, could certainly play a role in the development of slowed and inadequate relaxation, i.e., diastolic heart failure (p. 403). Relaxation is caused by ATP-dependent uptake of calcium by the SR.[166] This is reduced in the human with heart failure as well as in the rat and rabbit with pressure overload ventricular hypertrophy.[167–169] Figure 14–14 shows intracellular Ca^{++} transients recorded with aqueorin (see also Fig. 13–9, p. 358). Prolongations of the action potential, of the Ca^{++} transients (with delayed return to baseline), and prolonged contraction were observed in heart failure.[170] With less Ca^{++} bound to the SR, less Ca^{++} might be available for "regenerative release" (p. 358) for the contractile process (Fig. 14–18), thereby also causing systolic failure.[171] Reduced uptake of Ca^{++} by homogenates of SR prepared from patients with cardiomyopathy has been demonstrated. Similar changes were found in the hearts of hamsters with hereditary dilated cardiomyopathy; interestingly, no such defect was observed in the hearts of hypertrophic hamsters.[172] A cDNA encoding cardiac Ca^{++} ATPase of the rat SR has been isolated. Reductions of the mRNA for this ATPase have been found after aortic constriction, and the density of ATPase on the sarcoplasmic reticulum is reduced. Also, the transsarcolemmal Na^+/Ca^{++} exchange is slowed in hypertrophied myocardium.

That an abnormality in the handling of Ca^{++} by the SR occurs in heart failure is also supported by the finding that the ATPase isolated from the SR obtained from the ventricles of dogs with heart failure is depressed.[173] Also, in failing calf hearts the rate of Ca^{++} uptake by the SR and the activity of microsomal Ca^{++}-activated ATPase obtained are reduced to about 50 per cent of normal. These findings are compatible with the earlier observation that the rate of Ca^{++} uptake by the SR obtained from failing heart muscle in humans,[174] rabbits,[175] and hamsters[176] is slowed.

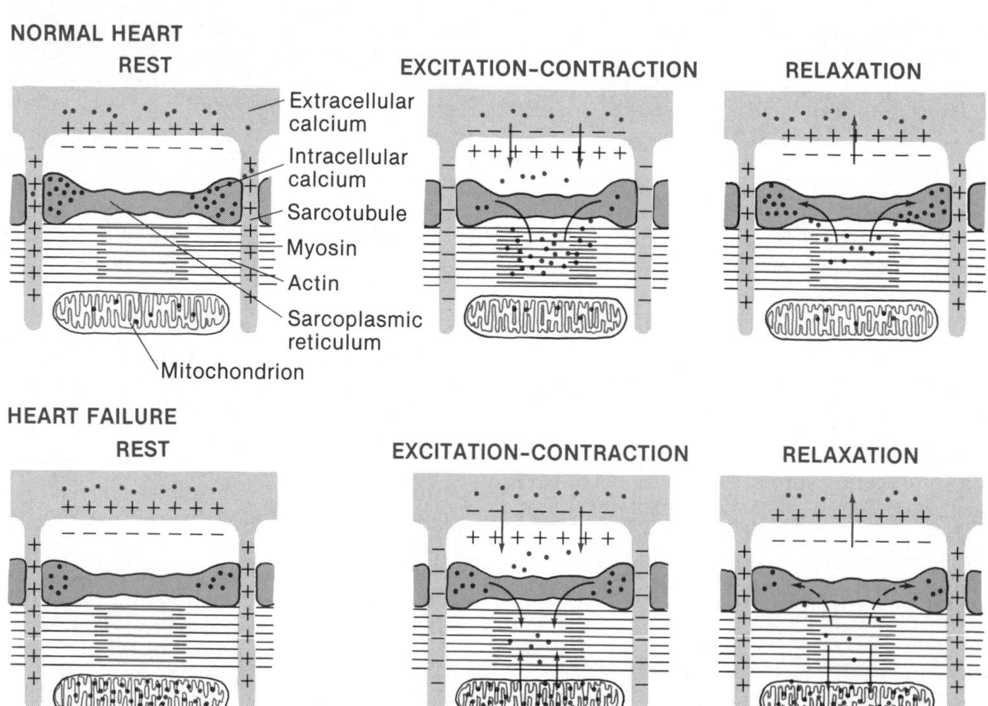

FIGURE 14–18. Hypothetical abnormality in excitation-contraction in heart failure. In the *normal heart* at rest, extracellular calcium is concentrated in the region of the sarcolemmal membrane and its invaginations (sarcotubular system); intracellular calcium sequestered chiefly in the sarcoplasmic reticulum is awaiting delivery to the contractile apparatus. With excitation of the cell membrane and depolarization, there is rapid entry of extracellular calcium; spread of electrical activity via the sarcotubules causes release of intracellular calcium and activation of contraction. For muscle to relax, intracellular calcium must be recaptured by the sarcoplasmic reticulum; efflux of calcium across the cell membrane probably also occurs. In contrast, according to the sequence of events postulated to occur in *heart failure,* ineffective calcium pumping by the sarcoplasmic reticulum may alter the normal relaxation process, rendering the mitochondria the dominant calcium uptake mechanism and a source of activator calcium for contraction. If so, in resting muscle, relatively little calcium would be available for release from the sarcoplasmic reticulum to activate contraction. Although the mitochondria may contain an ample amount, it is likely to be released slowly; thus, with depolarization, a diminished amount of calcium might be supplied to the contractile proteins. Whether the depressed myocardial contractility characteristic of heart failure develops on this basis remains to be determined. (From Chidsey, C. A.: Calcium metabolism in the normal and failing heart. *In* Braunwald, E. [ed.]: The Myocardium: Failure and Infarction. New York, HP Publishing Co., 1974, p. 37.)

The aforementioned reduction in contractility of papillary muscle obtained from cats with constriction of the pulmonary artery (Fig. 14–2) may be accompanied by reductions in the muscle's resting membrane potential, maximum rate of rise, and overshoot, as well as prolongation in the duration of the action potential.[177] Prolongation of the action potential has also been observed in myocytes obtained from rats with renovascular hypertension.[178] Although the precise mechanism responsible for these changes in electrical properties is unknown, the prolongation of the action potential may be related to delayed inactivation of L type calcium channels. It represents a compensatory mechanism for failing or hypertrophied myocardium; by augmenting the sarcolemmal flux of Ca^{++} it could result in an increase in the release of Ca^{++} from the SR to activate the increased volume of myofibrils of hypertrophied myocardium.[178]

When all of the available information on the subject is taken together, an abnormality in the SR's handling of Ca^{++} appears to be central to the development of heart failure in a wide variety of circumstances.

NEUROHORMONAL ADJUSTMENTS IN HEART FAILURE

A complex series of neurohormonal changes takes place consequent to the two principal hemodynamic alterations in heart failure—i.e., reduction of cardiac output and atrial hypertension. Many of these neurohumoral changes occur in response to the inadequate arterial volume characteristic of systolic heart failure (Fig. 14–1). In the early stages of acute systolic heart failure, these changes—heightened adrenergic drive, activation of the renin-angiotensin-aldosterone axis, and the augmented release of vasopressin—are truly compensatory and act to maintain perfusion to vital organs and to expand the inadequate arterial blood volume. However, each of these mechanisms may be thought of as a "double-edged sword." As heart failure becomes chronic, these three compensatory mechanisms can cause undesirable effects such as excessive vasoconstriction, increased afterload, excessive retention of salt and water, electrolyte abnormalities, and arrhythmias (Fig. 14–19). In contrast, the release of atrial natriuretic peptide (ANP) in response to atrial distention acts as a counter-regulatory hormone, which causes vasodilation and increased excretion of salt and water.

THE ADRENERGIC NERVOUS SYSTEM

ALTERATIONS IN NOREPINEPHRINE. Measurements of the concentration of the adrenergic neurotransmitter norepinephrine (NE) in arterial blood provide an index of the activity of this system, which is critical to the normal regulation of cardiac performance (p. 381). At rest, in patients with advanced heart failure, the circulating NE concentration is much higher, generally two to three times the level found in normal subjects[179–184] and is accompanied by elevation of circulating dopamine[184] and sometimes by epinephrine as well; the latter reflects increased adrenomedullary activity.[180] The elevation of NE results from a combination of increased release of NE from adrenergic nerve endings and its "spillover" into plasma[185] as well as reduced uptake of NE by adrenergic

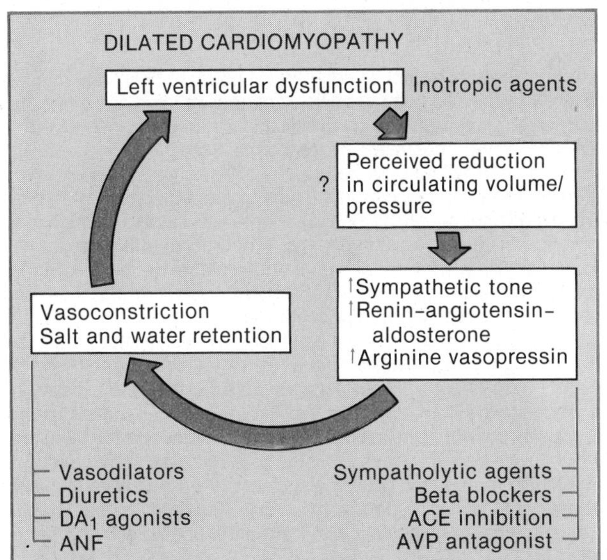

FIGURE 14–19. Circle of congestive heart failure. Heart failure is a complex clinical syndrome characterized by a sequence of neuroendocrine responses in an attempt to maintain circulatory homeostasis. Blocking the heightened sympathetic response with β-blockers, sympatholytic agents (bromocriptine, methyldopa, and clonidine), angiotensin-converting enzyme (ACE) inhibitors, and arginine vasopressin (AVP) antagonists is often useful. Dopaminergic receptor (DA_1) agonists (fenoldopam and ibopamine) and atrial natriuretic factor (ANF) are under investigation as therapeutic agents. (From Francis, G. S.: Neuroendocrine manifestations of congestive heart failure. Am. J. Cardiol. *62*:9A, 1988.)

nerve endings. In failing hearts, coronary sinus NE levels exceed arterial levels, while nonfailing hearts usually extract NE. Measurement of 24-hour urinary NE excretion has also revealed marked elevations in patients with heart failure,[186] confirming that the activity of the adrenergic nervous system (and the closely related secretion of catecholamines by the adrenal medulla) is augmented at rest. During comparable levels of exercise, much greater elevations in circulating NE occur in patients with heart failure than in normal subjects. Presumably this reflects greater activation of the adrenergic nervous system during exercise in these patients.[179,187,188] However, during *maximal* exercise, normal subjects exhibit higher levels of NE than do patients with heart failure.[182]

The extent of elevation of plasma NE concentration that occurs in patients with heart failure correlates directly with the severity of their left ventricular dysfunction[189]; the latter may be reflected in the height of the pulmonary capillary wedge pressure and depression of the cardiac index[190–192] and with cardiac mortality[183] (Fig. 14–20). It is not clear whether the elevated levels of NE in patients who subsequently die of heart failure are causally related to death as a consequence of their vasoconstrictor, arrhythmogenic, or other actions or whether they represent an "epiphenomenon" which merely reflects the severity of the underlying heart failure. The augmented adrenergic outflow from the central nervous system may trigger ventricular tachycardia or even sudden cardiac death, particularly in the presence of myocardial ischemia (perhaps accounting for the antiarrhythmic actions of beta blockers, which are potent antiischemic agents). As already suggested, the heightened activity of the adrenergic nervous system that leads to stimulation of alpha$_1$ adrenoceptors in the periphery may be harmful in advanced heart failure, since it intensifies vasoconstriction and thereby augments left ventricular afterload. Postsynaptic alpha-$_2$ adrenoceptors do *not* appear to be downregulated despite increased sympathetic activity and high circulating NE levels.[193] Stimulation of myocardial alpha$_1$ receptors in the myocardium may elicit a modest positive inotropic effect and may be responsible for myocyte hypertrophy.[194] These receptors are of low density in the human heart and appear to be unchanged in number in human heart failure.[195] The elevated levels of circulating epinephrine in advanced heart failure may also contribute to the development of hypokalemia and arrhythmias.[196]

Another abnormality of the adrenergic nervous system in heart failure is the extremely low concentration of NE in atrial[186] and ventricular myocardium[28] removed at operation from patients with heart failure.[186] NE concentrations are also markedly depressed in dogs with right ventricular failure produced by the creation of pulmonary stenosis and tricuspid regurgitation.[187] In patients it has been reported that cardiac NE content determined from endomyocardial biopsies correlates directly with the ejection fraction and inversely with plasma epinephrine concentration.[188,189]

In NE-depleted failing hearts, fluorescence is absent in the terminal varicosities of adrenergic fibers that are in close association to cardiac muscle cells. ^{131}I-labeled metaiodobenzylguanidine (MTBG) is a radiopharmaceutical that is taken up by adrenergic nerve endings and has been used to image the adrenergic nervous system (p. 301). Patients with cardiomyopathy do not retain the agent normally in their adrenergic nervous systems. This provides a noninvasive approach to assessing disturbances in adrenergic function in heart failure.

Following relief from pulmonary artery constriction, many indices of contractile function of the hypertrophied or failing cat right ventricle return to normal, but NE depletion persists.[190] It should be noted that local NE stores do *not* play any role in the *intrinsic* contractile state of cardiac muscle. Thus, no differences were found in papillary muscles removed from normal cats and from cats with NE depletion produced by chronic cardiac denervation or reserpine pretreatment.[191] Length-tension curves, force-velocity relations, and the augmentation of isometric tension achieved by postextrasystolic potentiation and by increasing the frequency of contraction were not altered from the normal state in NE-depleted muscles.

The mechanism responsible for cardiac NE depletion in severe heart failure is not clear; it may be an "exhaustion" phenomenon from the prolonged adrenergic activation of the cardiac adrenergic nerves in mild to moderate heart failure. Reductions in the activity of tyrosine hydroxylase,[192] which catalyzes the rate-limiting step in the biosynthesis of NE, and in the rate at which noradrenergic vesicles can take up dopamine[193] have been incriminated.

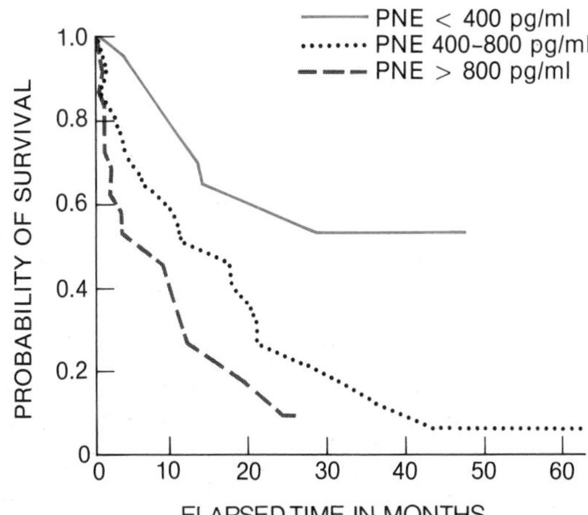

FIGURE 14–20. Life-table analysis of survival, according to tercile based on level of plasma norepinephrine (PNE). Group 1 (<400 pg/ml) contained 27 patients, group 2 (400 to 800 pg/ml) 49 patients, and group 3 (>800 pg/ml) 30 patients. The probability of survival in each group was significantly different from the probabilities in the other two groups. (Reprinted with permission from Cohn, J. N., Levine, T. B., Olivari, M. T., et al.: Plasma norepinephrine as a guide to prognosis in patients with chronic congestive heart failure. N. Engl. J. Med. *311*:822, 1984.)

CONSEQUENCES OF CARDIAC NE DEPLETION. In view of the strongly positive inotropic effect exerted by the NE released from its nerves, the adrenergic nervous system may be considered to provide important potential support to the failing myocardium. However, with supramaximal stimulation of the cardiac sympathetic nerves, the increments in heart rate and contractile force that occur in animals with heart failure and cardiac NE depletion are abolished or are much smaller than those in normal dogs.[194] The reduction in beta-adrenoceptor density in failing heart muscle and the increase in the inhibitory G protein (see below) further limit the response. While cardiac stores of NE are not fundamental to maintenance of the *intrinsic* contractile state of the myocardium, diminished release of the neurotransmitter and of beta-adrenoceptor density (see below) in heart failure may be responsible for loss of the much-needed adrenergic support of the failing heart and therefore could intensify the severity of the congestive heart failure state.

ADRENERGIC SUPPORT OF THE FAILING HEART. The importance of the adrenergic nervous system in maintaining ventricular contractility when myocardial function is depressed in congestive heart failure is demonstrated by the effects of adrenergic blockade. Pharmacological blockade of the sympathetic nervous system may cause sodium and water retention as well as intensification of heart failure.[195,196] Therefore, caution must be exercised in using beta-adrenoceptor blocking agents in the treatment of patients with limited cardiac reserve. Indeed, severe heart failure and occasionally even life-threatening pulmonary edema may be precipitated by the administration of a beta-adrenoceptor blocker in heart failure, attesting to the importance of the adrenergic drive in these patients. Additional evidence indicating that the NE-depleted failing heart is supported by circulating catecholamines comes from experiments on calves with experimentally produced heart failure and cardiac NE depletion in which beta-adrenoceptor blockade intensifies heart failure, presumably by blocking the inotropic action of circulating epinephrine.[197] Thus, the increased adrenergic drive presumably serves as a valuable compensatory mechanism in heart failure, stimulating cardiac contractility, redistributing blood flow from nonvital beds, and maintaining arterial pressure in the face of a limited cardiac output.

ADVERSE EFFECTS OF ADRENERGIC STIMULATION. However, the aforementioned compensatory mechanism in early heart failure may become deleterious in the late stages of severe failure by increasing afterload, precipitating cardiac arrhythmias, and perhaps exerting a toxic effect on the failing myocardium. Thus it has been postulated that in heart failure there actually may be a positive feedback loop causing a vicious circle. According to this concept, heart failure activates the sympathetic nervous system (as well as the renin-angiotensin system and stimulates the release of vasopressin); this causes increases in preload and afterload that intensify heart failure.[199] Administration of drugs such as the $alpha_2$ agonist guanabenz (which reduces sympathetic nerve impulse traffic[200]) and bromocriptine (a presynaptic dopamine-2 agonist[201]) reduces plasma NE, indicating that there is a potent presynaptic control mechanism in the heightened sympathetic nervous activity of heart failure.[199] It has been suggested that treatment with such agents might be useful in interrupting the vicious circle referred to above.[199]

ABNORMALITIES OF ADRENERGIC CONTROL IN HEART FAILURE

The possibility of defective adrenergic control of heart rate in patients with heart failure has been studied by observing the reflex chronotropic responses to stimuli such as upright tilt and to nitroglycerin-induced hypotension.[202,202a] An attenuation of the normal increase in heart rate in patients with heart failure both before and after administration of atropine confirmed that a defect exists in the adrenergic component of baroreceptor-mediated control of heart rate in patients with cardiac dysfunction; the severity of this defect was, in general, proportional to the impairment of cardiac reserve. In addition, during upright tilt there is a blunted response of the normal rise of plasma NE, of forearm vascular resistance, and of hepatic vascular resistance in patients with heart failure.[203,204] Some patients with heart failure exhibit a major reduction in arterial pressure during tilting, analogous to what is observed in idiopathic orthostatic hypotension[205] (p. 877). In such patients, not surprisingly, exercise capacity in the upright position is markedly reduced.[206] Further evidence for impairment of baroreflex control of the systemic circulation comes from investigations in which lower body negative pressure fails to cause normal reflex augmentation of forearm vascular resistance and from studies showing an impaired chronotropic response to exercise. The latter appears to be due to postsynaptic downregulation of beta adrenoceptors in the sinoatrial node.[207,208]

In dogs with experimental heart failure, carotid occlusion elicits a blunted reflex response of heart rate, arterial pressure, and vascular resistance.[209,210] An inappropriately depressed increase in heart rate in humans[211] and in dogs with heart failure was also observed when arterial pressure was reduced through administration of vasodilators. While the changes in mean arterial pressure observed in response to the vasodilators were similar in patients with heart failure and in control subjects, the changes in heart rate after vasodilators correlated significantly with the changes in concentration of circulating NE and with the sum of circulating NE and epinephrine. In normal individuals, both heart rate and catecholamine concentrations rose, whereas in patients with heart failure, in whom resting catecholamine levels were increased, cardiac acceleration was blunted, and catecholamine concentration failed to rise normally.[211,212]

ADRENERGIC NERVOUS FUNCTION IN THE PERIPHERAL CIRCULATION. Substantial changes also occur in heart failure in the function of the adrenergic nerves that innervate peripheral blood vessels.[212a–d] Thus, while adrenergically mediated vasoconstriction normally occurs in the vessels supplying the splanchnic viscera and kidneys during exercise, neurogenic vasoconstriction is even more important and much more marked when augmentation of cardiac output is seriously limited, as occurs in heart failure. Thus, it has been shown that exercise induces a much more marked reduction in mesenteric blood flow and elevation of mesenteric vascular resistance in dogs with heart failure produced experimentally by inducing tricuspid regurgitation and constric-

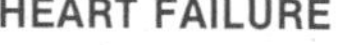

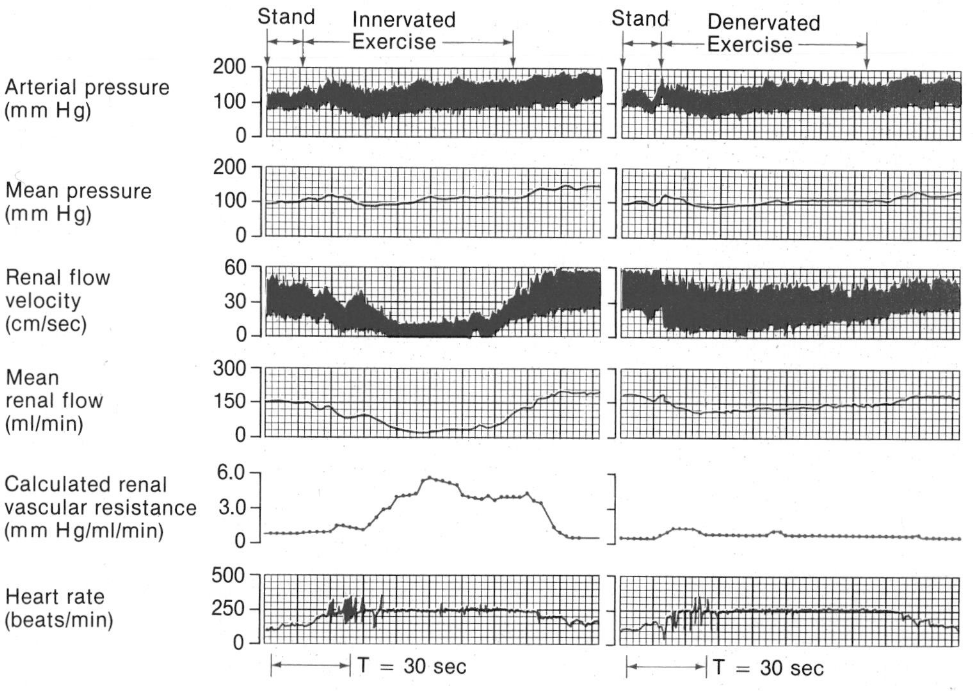

FIGURE 14–21. Tracings comparing the alterations in renal hemodynamics during exercise in the innervated kidney and contralateral denervated kidney in a dog with experimental heart failure. (From Higgins, C. B., et al.: Alterations in regional hemodynamics in experimental heart failure in conscious dogs. Trans. Assoc. Am. Physicians *85*:267, 1972.)

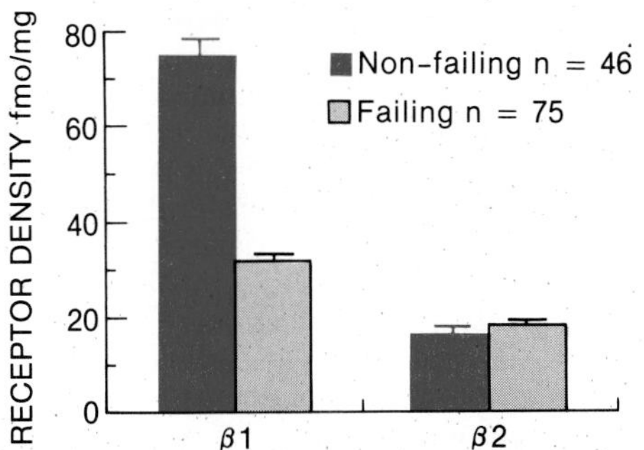

FIGURE 14–22. Bar graphs of β_1- and β_2-adrenergic receptor measurements in membranes extracted from failing and nonfailing human left and right ventricular myocardium, with approximately equal numbers of left ventricle and right ventricle in each group. Values are $p < 0.0001 \pm$ SEM for β_1, p = NS for B_2. (From Bristow, M. R., Hershberger, R. E., Port, J. D., et al.: β-Adrenergic pathways in nonfailing and failing human ventricular myocardium. Circulation *82*:(Suppl 1):12, 1990, reprinted by permission of the American Heart Association, Inc.)

tion of the pulmonary artery than in normal dogs.[12] Similar changes during exercise were observed in other major visceral vascular beds, such as the renal bed. Evidence that this intense vasoconstriction during exercise is mediated by the adrenergic nervous system is provided by observations on dogs with experimentally produced heart failure in which one kidney was denervated. Blood flow through the normal kidney declined precipitously during exercise, and calculated renal vascular resistance increased markedly. In contrast, little change in renal blood flow and calculated renal vascular resistance occurred in the denervated kidney[12] (Fig. 14–21). This intensive visceral vasoconstriction during exercise diverts cardiac output to exercising muscle.

DOWNREGULATION OF CARDIAC BETA-ADRENOCEPTORS. In patients with heart failure, beta-adrenoceptors on circulating lymphocytes[213] and alpha$_2$ receptors on platelets[214] are "downregulated," presumably as a consequence of prolonged elevation of circulating NE. More important is the finding that ventricles obtained from patients with heart failure demonstrated a *marked* reduction in beta-adrenoceptor density, in isoproterenol-mediated adenylate cyclase stimulation, and in myocardial contractility[215,216] (Fig. 14–22). This finding is consistent with an elevation of the concentration of NE in the synaptic clefts in the immediate vicinity of the cardiac beta-adrenoceptors.[216] Downregulation of beta receptors deprives the failing heart of an important compensatory mechanism. In patients with dilated cardiomyopathy, this reduction in receptor density is proportional to the severity of heart failure[217] and involves primarily beta$_1$ but *not* beta$_2$ adrenoceptors, thus shifting the ratio of beta$_1$ and beta$_2$ receptors from a normal of 77/23 to 60/40 (Fig. 14–23).[218] The beta$_2$ receptor, while not downregulated, becomes partially "uncoupled" from its effector enzyme (adenylate cyclase),[219] producing a similar effect.

Downregulation of myocardial beta adrenoceptors has been observed not only in heart failure but also in the hypertrophied left ventricle of renal hypertensive rats; when nephrectomy caused regression of ventricular hypertrophy, both receptor density and responsiveness to isoproterenol were restored.[220] Downregulation of beta$_1$ receptors in heart failure may be reversed by the administration of metoprolol, a relatively specific beta$_1$ antagonist, an action that may account for its value in low doses in the treatment of heart failure (p. 505). This reversal of downregulation of beta$_1$ receptors can restore responsiveness to adrenergic inotropic stimulation. The long-term clinical benefit of beta blockade in heart failure has been reported to be associated with a restoration of myocardial beta receptor density and restoration of the contractile response to administered catecholamines.[221] The downregulation of beta$_1$ receptors could cause inadequate production of cyclic AMP. Alteration in sarcolemmal G proteins (p. 359) may have a similar effect and intensify the failure of production of cyclic AMP.[222]

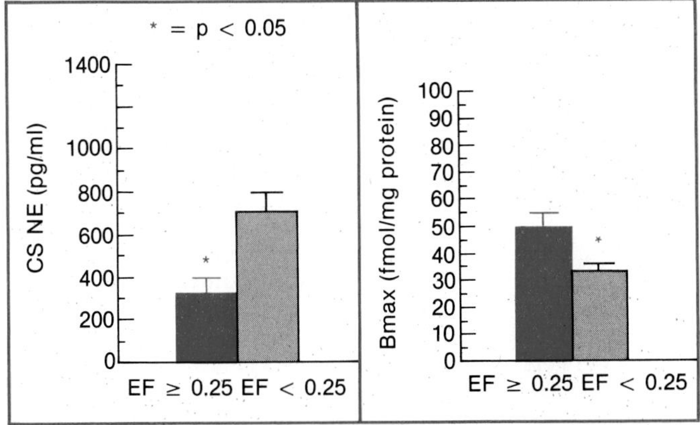

FIGURE 14–23. Bar graphs of coronary sinus norepinephrine (CS NE left) and right ventricular endomyocardial biopsy β-receptor density (βmax, right) in 47 patients with idiopathic dilated cardiomyopathy divided into patients with mild-to-moderate left ventricular ejection fraction (EF) (≥0.25, Av. = 0.31, red) and severe left ventricular EF (<0.25, Av. = 0.15, gray) ventricular dysfunction (values ± SEM). CS NE, coronary sinus norepinephrine. (From Bristow, M. R., Hershberger, R. E., Port, J. D., et al.: β-Adrenergic pathways in nonfailing and failing human ventricular myocardium. Circulation *82*(Suppl 1):12, 1990, reprinted by permission of the American Heart Association, Inc.)

GUANINE NUCLEOTIDE REGULATORY (G) PROTEINS. The critical role played by G proteins in coupling receptors, including beta adrenoceptors, to effector enzymes such as adenylate cyclase is discussed elsewhere (Fig. 13–10, p. 359). Cardiac cells contain at least two types of G proteins: (1) G_s, which mediates the *stimulation* of adenylate cyclase (and thereby causes a rise in intracellular cyclic AMP, which in turn stimulates Ca^{++} influx into the myocyte through Ca^{++} channels in the sarcolemma, and the more rapid uptake of Ca^{++} by the sarcoplasmic reticulum); and (2) G_i, which mediates the *inhibition* of adenylate cyclase and has the opposite effect on the movements of Ca^{++}.

Heart failure caused by dilated cardiomyopathy is associated with an increase in G_i in heart muscle,[223,224] which may be accompanied by a reduction in the activity of adenylate cyclase.[225] A reduction in the function of G_s has also been reported in dogs with chronic pressure overload as well as in the Syrian hamster with dilated cardiomyopathy.[226] Overall, heart failure is characterized by an increase in the ratio of G_i/G_s.[224]

The end results of three processes described in this section —i.e., (1) the reduction of NE stores in cardiac adrenergic stores; (2) the reduction in beta adrenoceptor density; and (3) the changes in G proteins—reduce, sometimes profoundly, the capacity of the failing heart to produce cyclic AMP. As a consequence, the inotropic response to beta-adrenoceptor agonists and to phosphodiesterase inhibitors (p. 503) is markedly reduced in myocardium obtained from patients with end-stage heart failure. However, the same muscle responds normally to raising extracellular [Ca^{++}], to a cardiac glycoside and to forskolin—a compound that activates adenylate cyclase directly (without requiring the activation of beta receptor or the transduction of G proteins). This reduction in the ability of the failing heart to produce cyclic AMP may diminish the inotropic effectiveness of drugs such as beta-adrenoceptor agonists and of phosphodiesterase inhibitors in heart failure, which require the production of cyclic AMP for their action.

THE RENIN-ANGIOTENSIN SYSTEM

(See also pp. 829 to 831)

In low cardiac output states there is activation of the renin-angiotensin-aldosterone axis, which operates in concert with the activated adrenergic nervous-adrenal medullary system to maintain arterial pressure. These two compensatory sys-

TABLE 14-4 FACTORS THAT STIMULATE OR SUPPRESS RENIN-ANGIOTENSIN-ALDOSTERONE SYSTEM ACTIVITY IN CHRONIC HEART FAILURE

FACTORS THAT STIMULATE RENIN RELEASE
Decreased renal perfusion
Decreased delivery of sodium to the macula densa
Enhanced sympathetic activity
Aberrant reflex regulation
Reduction of intracellular calcium
Pharmacological therapy
Diuretics
Some vasodilators
FACTORS THAT SUPPRESS RENIN RELEASE
Sodium repletion
Digoxin therapy
Atrial natriuretic factor

From Cody, R. J., and Laragh, J. H.: The renin-angiotensin-aldosterone system in chronic heart failure: Pathophysiology and implications for treatment. In Cohn, J. N. (ed.): Drug Treatment of Heart Failure, 2nd ed. Secaucus, NJ, ATC, 1988, p. 81.)

tems are clearly coupled; stimulation of beta$_1$-adrenoceptors in the juxtaglomerular apparatus as a consequence of heightened adrenergic drive is a principal mechanism responsible for the release of renin in acute heart failure. Activation of the baroreceptors in the renal vascular bed by a reduction of renal blood flow is also responsible for the release of renin, and in patients with severe chronic heart failure following salt restriction and diuretic treatment, reduction of the sodium presented to the macula densa also contributes to the release of renin (Table 14-4). Thus, elevated plasma renin activity is a common, although not universal, finding in heart failure.[191,192,226a-228] Renin may also be released from blood vessels, and the released angiotensin II can exert local vasoconstrictor effects.[229]

Angiotensin II is a potent peripheral vasoconstrictor (Fig. 14-24) and contributes, along with increased adrenergic activity, to the excessive elevation of systemic vascular resistance and the vicious circle already referred to[199] in patients with heart failure. Angiotensin II also enhances the adrenergic nervous system's release of NE; it constricts efferent renal arterioles and thereby increases glomerular filtration pressure. Aldosterone, on the other hand, has potent sodium-retaining properties (p. 474). Therefore, it is not surprising that interruption of the renin-angiotensin-aldosterone axis by means of an angiotensin-converting enzyme inhibitor reduces systemic vascular resistance, diminishes afterload, and thereby elevates cardiac output in heart failure (p. 1857). In some patients these compounds also elicit a mild diuretic action, presumably by lowering angiotensin II-stimulated production of aldosterone.

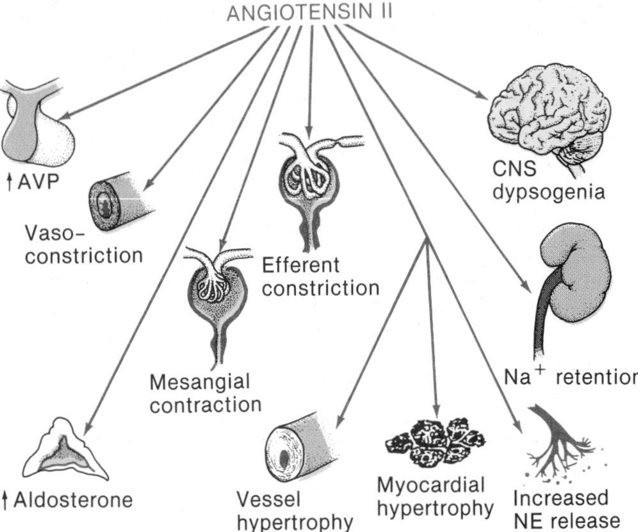

FIGURE 14-24. The activities of angiotensin II. This peptide can act on (1) the adrenal cortex to release aldosterone, (2) the posterior pituitary to release arginine vasopressin (AVP), (3) resistance arterioles to produce vasoconstriction, (4) the renal mesangial tissue to reduce filtration coefficient (K_f), and (5) the efferent glomerular arteriole to increase intraglomerular pressure and filtration. It probably contributes to vascular and myocardial hypertrophy (in some species), increases norepinephrine (NE) biosynthesis, facilitates release of NE from sympathetic nerve endings, promotes sodium (Na^+) retention directly by acting on renal tubules, and is a potent dipsogenic amine when experimentally placed in the central nervous system (CNS). (From Francis, G. S.: The relationship of the sympathetic nervous system and the renin-angiotensin system in congestive heart failure. Am. Heart J. *118*:642, 1989.)

ARGININE VASOPRESSIN (AVP)

Circulating AVP is elevated to approximately twice normal levels in many patients with heart failure,[230-232] even after correction for plasma osmolality. Patients with acute heart failure secondary to massive myocardial infarction may have particularly elevated levels,[233] which are usually associated with elevated concentrations of catecholamines and renin. Perhaps the *decreased* sensitivity of atrial stretch receptors, which normally inhibits AVP release with atrial distension (discussed below), contributes to the elevation of circulating AVP.[234-236] AVP is a potent endogenous vasoconstrictor, and the elevated levels may cause systemic vasoconstriction and perhaps contribute to the hyponatremia sometimes observed in advanced chronic congestive heart failure.

Control of circulating AVP concentration is abnormal in patients with heart failure who fail to show the normal reduction of AVP with a reduction of osmolality.[237] This may contribute to their inadequate ability to excrete free water and hence the hypoosmolarity in some patients with heart failure.[230] In addition, patients with heart failure exhibit failure of normal suppression of AVP following administration of ethanol,[238] as well as failure of the normal augmentation of circulating AVP in response to orthostatic stress.[231]

Administration of AVP antagonists reduces systemic vascular resistance and increases cardiac output in patients with heart failure and elevated AVP. These responses are analogous to the salutary effects evoked by converting enzyme inhibitors in patients with elevated plasma renin activity.

ATRIAL NATRIURETIC PEPTIDE (ANP)

The structure, biosynthesis, release, and physiological effects of ANP are discussed on pp. 1858 to 1860 and are illustrated in Figures 62-5, 62-7, and 62-8. An increase in atrial distending pressure, however produced, leads to the release of ANP. The latter is a counterregulatory hormone that opposes many of the vasoconstrictor and salt- and water-retaining effects of the adrenergic, renin-angiotensin-aldosterone, and arginine vasopressor systems. Therefore, ANP may protect the central circulation from volume overload. In addition, ANP reduces tachycardia by modulating baroreceptor function. The level of circulating ANP reflects the severity of heart failure and shows a positive correlation with plasma renin activity and plasma norepinephrine concentration, as well as with mortality.[239] Successful treatment of heart failure with reduction of atrial distention tends to normalize ANP levels.

In *acute* heart failure, ANP reduces the formation of renin, opposes angiotensin II's vasoconstrictor effects and its stimulation of the secretion of aldosterone and vasopressin, and enhances the renal excretion of salt and water. In *chronic* heart failure, while the circulating levels of ANP usually remain elevated, they often decline from the values reached in the acute stage. In chronic heart failure the response of atrial myocytes to atrial distention appears to be attenuated, as does the effect of ANP on the secretion of renin from the juxtaglomerular cells and on sodium and water excretion.[229]

ANP is normally expressed in fetal but not adult ventricles. However, in chronic heart failure (both in patients and in a variety of forms of experimental failure[240–243]), ANP is synthesized in the ventricles as well as the atria, and in this state the ventricles become an important source of circulating ANP.

Considerable effort is under way to attempt to take advantage of the favorable physiological effects of ANP in heart failure, i.e., vasodilation and enhanced salt and water excretion, by the development of cogeners of ANP and by drugs designed to reduce the metabolism of ANP or to interfere with its clearance.[244]

PARASYMPATHETIC FUNCTION IN HEART FAILURE

Cardiac enlargement, with or without heart failure, is associated with marked disturbances of parasympathetic as well as sympathetic function.[245,246] The parasympathetic restraint on sinoatrial node automaticity is markedly reduced in patients with heart disease, who also exhibit less heart rate slowing for any given elevation of systemic arterial pressure than do normal subjects. The sensitivity of the baroreceptor reflex to increase in pressure has also been shown to be significantly reduced in dogs with heart failure.[209] Cardiomyopathic hamster hearts display a reduction in the activity of choline acetyltransferase, an enzyme that provides an estimate of the density of parasympathetic innervation.[246,247]

There is evidence that the impairment of parasympathetic activity is related to a reduction in density of high-affinity muscarinic receptors in the heart.[248] This disturbance may be of considerable functional importance, since the ability to alter heart rate constitutes an extremely important mechanism for the adjustment of cardiac output; indeed, in normal subjects alterations in heart rate account to a large extent for changes in cardiac output. In patients with heart failure, exercise does not elevate stroke volume normally. When this limitation of stroke volume is combined with defective control of heart rate as a consequence of abnormalities of both the sympathetic and the parasympathetic limbs of the autonomic nervous system, cardiac output fails to rise appropriately.

ABNORMALITIES IN AFFERENT IMPULSES

Heart failure also interferes with the afferent limbs of cardiovascular reflexes. According to the schema proposed by Gauer and Henry,[249] under normal circumstances, elevated left atrial pressure increases left atrial stretch and stimulates left atrial stretch receptors.[250] The increased activity of both myelinated and nonmyelinated (C-fiber) afferents[251] normally inhibits the release of ADH, thereby increasing water excretion, which in turn reduces plasma volume and would act to restore left atrial pressure to normal. In addition, enhanced left atrial stretch receptor activity depresses renal efferent sympathetic nerve activity and increases renal blood flow and glomerular filtration rate, thereby enhancing the ability of the kidney to reduce plasma volume. Indeed, in patients with myocardial infarction and acute heart failure, urine flow and glomerular filtration rate (and sometimes even sodium excretion) are increased despite the decline in arterial pressure. Presumably, activation of atrial or ventricular receptors from a rise in left atrial pressure or bulging left ventricle is responsible.[252]

With continued stimulation of these afferents there is desensitization of atrial (and arterial) baroreceptors.[229] Zucker et al.[253] observed that the decreased sensitivity of left atrial stretch receptors in dogs with heart failure is the result of cardiac dilatation and alterations in atrial compliance and is reversible following reversal of heart failure.[254] This resetting of atrial receptors may be responsible for the inappropriately high plasma ADH levels in heart failure[255] and may contribute to the renal vasoconstriction, peripheral edema, ascites, and hyponatremia often seen in patients with chronic heart failure. With chronic heart failure and its attendant cardiac distention and decreased sensitivity of cardiac receptors, the reflex inhibition of adrenergic activity disappears, and the adrenergic drive to the heart, the peripheral vascular bed, and the adrenal medulla is enhanced, resulting in the sodium retention, tachycardia, and the vasoconstricted state characteristic of heart failure (p. 409).

CONCLUSIONS

It may be useful to consider normal and impaired myocardial function, whatever the etiology and pathogenesis, within the framework of the familiar Frank-Starling mechanism. The normal relationship between ventricular end-diastolic volume and performance is shown in Figure 14–25, curve 1. Normally, assumption of the upright posture reduces venous return; as a consequence, at any specific level of exercise, cardiac output tends to be lower in the upright than in the

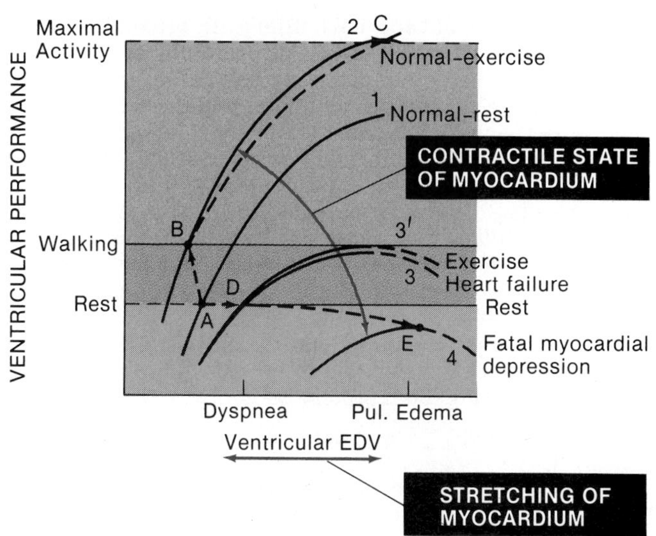

FIGURE 14–25. Diagram showing the interrelationship of influences on ventricular end-diastolic volume (EDV) through stretching of the myocardium and the contractile state of the myocardium. Levels of ventricular EDV associated with filling pressures that result in dyspnea and pulmonary edema are shown on the abscissa. Levels of ventricular performance required during rest, walking, and maximal activity are designated on the ordinate. The dotted lines are the descending limbs of the ventricular performance curves, which are rarely seen during life but which show what the level of ventricular performance would be if end-diastolic volume could be elevated to very high levels. (Modified from Braunwald, E., Ross, J., Jr., and Sonnenblick, E. H.: Mechanisms of Contraction of the Normal and Failing Heart. Boston, Little, Brown and Co., 1968.)

recumbent position. On the other hand, the hyperventilation of exercise, the pumping action of the exercising muscle, and the venoconstriction that occur all tend to augment ventricular filling. Simultaneously, the increase in adrenergic nerve impulses to the myocardium and in the contraction of circulating catecholamines and the tachycardia that occur during exercise all augment myocardial contractility and the stroke volume, with little change in end-diastolic pressure and volume. This state is represented by a shift from point A to point B in Figure 14–25. Vasodilation occurs in the exercising muscles, reducing peripheral vascular resistance and aortic impedance. This ultimately allows achievement of a greatly elevated cardiac output during exercise at an arterial pressure only slightly greater than that in the resting state. During intense exercise, cardiac output can rise to a maximal level if use is made of the Frank-Starling mechanism, as reflected in increases in the left ventricular end-diastolic volume and pressure (Fig. 14–25, point C).

In heart failure, the underlying abnormality resides in depressions of the length–active tension curve and of the myocardial force-velocity relation, reflecting reductions in the myocardial contractile state. In many cases, such as those represented by Figure 14–25, curve 3, cardiac output and external ventricular performance at rest are within normal limits but are maintained at these levels only because the end-diastolic fiber length and the ventricular end-diastolic volume are elevated, i.e., through the operation of the Frank-Starling mechanism. The elevations of left ventricular end-diastolic volume and pressure are associated with greater than normal levels of the pulmonary capillary pressure, contributing to the dyspnea experienced by patients with heart failure (Fig. 14–25, point D).

Since heart failure is frequently accompanied by reductions in (1) cardiac NE stores, (2) myocardial beta-adrenoceptor density, (3) catecholamine sensitivity, and (4) inotropic response to impulses in the cardiac adrenergic nerves, ventricular performance curves cannot be elevated to normal levels by the adrenergic nervous system, and the normal improvement of contractility that takes place during exercise is attenuated or even prevented (Fig. 14–25, curves 3 and 3′). The factors that tend to augment ventricular filling during exercise in the normal subject push the failing myocardium even farther along its flattened length–active tension curve, and there is an inordinate elevation of ventricular end-diastolic volume and pressure and therefore of pulmonary capillary pressure. The elevation of the latter intensifies dyspnea and therefore plays an important role in limiting the intensity of exercise that the patient can perform. According to this concept, left ventricular failure becomes fatal when the myocardial length–active tension curve becomes depressed (Fig. 14–25, curve 4) to the point at which either cardiac performance fails to satisfy the requirements of the peripheral tissues even at rest or the left ventricular end-diastolic and pulmonary capillary pressures are elevated to levels that result in pulmonary edema, or both (Fig. 14–25, point E).

REFERENCES

ADAPTIVE MECHANISMS

1. Braunwald, E., Mock, M. B., and Watson, J. (eds.): Congestive Heart Failure: Current Research and Clinical Applications. New York, Grune and Stratton, 1982, 384 pp.
2. Eichna, L. S.: Circulatory congestion and heart failure. Circulation *22*:864, 1960.
3. Katz, A. M.: Cardiomyopathy of overload: A major determinant of prognosis in congestive heart failure. N. Engl. J. Med. *322*:100, 1990.
4. Jennings, G. L., and Esler, M. D.: Circulatory regulation at rest and exercise and the functional assessment of patients with congestive heart failure. Circulation *81*(Suppl. II):5, 1990.
5. Braunwald, E.: The Myocardium: Failure and Infarction. New York, H. P. Publishing Co., 1974, 409 pp.
6. Anand, I. S., Ferrari, R., Kalra, G. S., et al.: Studies of body water and sodium, renal function, hemodynamic indexes, and plasma hormones in untreated congestive heart failure. Circulation *80*:299, 1989.
7. Guyton, A. C.: The relationship of cardiac output and arterial pressure control. Circulation *64*:1079, 1981.
8. Ross, J., Jr., and Braunwald, E.: Studies on Starling's law of the heart. IX. The effects of impeding venous return on performance of the normal and failing human left ventricle. Circulation *30*:719, 1964.
9. Braunwald, E., Ross, J., Jr., and Sonnenblick, E. H.: Mechanisms of Contraction of the Normal and Failing Heart. 2nd ed. Boston, Little, Brown and Co., 1976, 417 pp.
10. Harris, P.: Congestive cardiac failure: Central role of the arterial blood pressure. Br. Heart J. *58*:190, 1987.
11. Vanhoutte, P. M.: Adjustments in the peripheral circulation in chronic heart failure. Eur. Heart J. *4*(Suppl. A):67, 1983.
12. Higgins, C. B., Vatner, S. F., Millard, R. W., et al.: Alterations in regional hemodynamics in experimental heart failure in conscious dogs. Trans. Assoc. Am. Physicians *85*:267, 1972.
13. Zelis, R., Mason, D. T., and Braunwald, E.: A comparison of the effects of vasodilator stimuli on peripheral resistance vessels in normal subjects and in patients with congestive heart failure. J. Clin. Invest. *47*:960, 1968.
14. Zelis, R., Mason, D. T., and Braunwald, E.: Partition of blood flow to the cutaneous and muscular beds of the forearm at rest and during leg exercise in normal subjects and in patients with heart failure. Circ. Res. *24*:799, 1969.
15. Zelis, R., Sinoway, L. I., Musch, T. I., et al.: Regional blood flow in congestive heart failure: Concept of compensatory mechanisms with short and long time constants. Am. J. Cardiol. *62*:2E, 1988.
16. Wilson, J. R., Mancini, D. M., McCully, K., et al.: Noninvasive detection of skeletal muscle underperfusion with near-infrared spectroscopy in patients with heart failure. Circulation *80*:1668, 1989.
17. Mancini, D. M., Coyle, E., Coggan, A., et al.: Contribution of intrinsic skeletal muscle changes to ^{31}P NMR skeletal muscle metabolic abnormalities in patients with chronic heart failure. Circulation *80*:1338, 1989.
18. Zelis, R., and Flaim, S. F.: Peripheral vascular mechanisms mediating vasoconstriction. *In* Braunwald, E., Mock, M. B., and Watson, J. (eds.): Congestive Heart Failure: Current Research and Clinical Applications. New York, Grune and Stratton, 1982, p. 115.
19. Creager, M. A., Hirsch, A. T., Dzau, V. J., et al.: Baroreflex regulation of regional blood flow in congestive heart failure. Am. J. Physiol. *258*:H1409, 1990.
20. Kassis, E.: Cardiovascular response to orthostatic tilt in patients with congestive heart failure. Cardiovasc. Res. *21*:362, 1987.
21. Woodson, R. D., Torrance, J. D., Shappell, S. D., and Lenfant, C.: The effect of cardiac disease on hemoglobin-oxygen binding. J. Clin. Invest. *49*:1349, 1970.
22. Kwan, T., Pintea, M., Morino, F. G., et al.: Transcapillary oncotic pressure in the edema of congestive heart failure. Nephron *54*:21, 1990.

CONTRACTILITY OF HYPERTROPHIED AND FAILING MYOCARDIUM

23. Krayenbuehl, H. P., Hess, O. M., Schneider, J., and Turina, M.: Physiologic or pathologic hypertrophy. Eur. Heart J. *4*(Suppl. A):29, 1983.
24. Spann, J. F., Jr., Buccino, R. A., Sonnenblick, E. H., and Braunwald, E.: Contractile state of cardiac muscle obtained from cats with experimentally produced ventricular hypertrophy and heart failure. Circ. Res. *21*:341, 1967.
25. Cooper, G., IV, Tomanek, R. J., Ehrhardt, J. D., and Marcus, M. L.: Chronic progressive pressure overload of the cat right ventricle. Circ. Res. *48*:488, 1981.
26. Crozatier, B., and Hittinger, L.: Mechanical adaptation to chronic pressure overload. Eur. Heart J. *9*:E-7, 1988.
27. Capasso, J. M., Aronson, R. S., and Sonnenblick, E. H.: Reversible alterations in excitation-contraction coupling during myocardial hypertrophy in rat papillary muscle. Circ. Res. *51*:189, 1982.
28. Chidsey, C. A., Sonnenblick, E. H., Morrow, A. G., and Braunwald, E.: Norepinephrine stores and contractile force of papillary muscle from the failing human heart. Circulation *33*:43, 1966.
29. Cooper, G., IV, Puga, F., Zujko, K. J., et al.: Normal myocardial function and energetics in volume-overload hypertrophy in the cat. Circ. Res. *32*:140, 1973.
30. Legault, F., Rouleau, J. L., Juneau, C., et al.: Functional and morphological characteristics of compensated and decompensated cardiac hypertrophy in dogs with chronic infrarenal aorto-caval fistulas. Circ. Res. *66*:846, 1990.
31. Williams, J. F., Jr., and Potter, R. D.: Normal contractile state of hypertrophied myocardium following pulmonary artery constriction in the cat. J. Clin. Invest. *54*:1266, 1974.
32. Williams, J. F., Matthew, B., Hern, D. L., et al.: Myocardial hydroxyproline and mechanical response to prolonged pressure loading followed by unloading in the cat. J. Clin. Invest. *72*:1910, 1983.
33. Meerson, F. Z.: The myocardium in hyperfunction, hypertrophy, and heart failure. Circ. Res. *25*(Suppl. 2):1, 1969.
34. Ross, J., Jr., Sonnenblick, E. H., Taylor, R. R., and Covell, J. W.: Diastolic geometry and sarcomere length in the chronically dilated canine left ventricle. Circ. Res. *28*:49, 1971.
35. Anversa, P., Palackal, T., Sonnenblick, E. H., et al.: Hypertensive cardiomyopathy: Myocyte nuclei hyperplasia in the mammalian rat heart. J. Clin. Invest. *85*:994, 1990.
36. Olivetti, G., Ricci, R., Lagrasta, C., et al.: Cellular basis of wall remodeling in long-term pressure overload-induced right ventricular hypertrophy in rats. Circ. Res. *63*:648, 1988.
37. Dalen, H., Saetersdal, T., Odegarden, S.: Some ultrastructural features of the myocardial cells in the hypertrophied human papillary muscle. Virchows Arch. A. *410*:281, 1987.
38. Alyono, D., Ring, W. S., Anderson, M. R., and Anderson, R. W.: Left ventricular adaptation to volume overload from large aortocaval fistula. Surgery *96*:360, 1984.
39. Carabello, B. A., Nakano, K., Corin, W., et al.: Left ventricular function in experimental volume overload hypertrophy. Am. J. Physiol. *256*:H974, 1989.
40. Spann, J. F., Jr., Covell, J. W., Eckberg, D. L., et al.: Contractile performance of the hypertrophied and chronically failing cat ventricle. Am. J. Physiol. *223*:1150, 1972.
41. Pfeffer, J. M., Pfeffer, M. A., Mirsky, E., and Braunwald, E.: Regression of left ventricular hypertrophy and prevention of left ventricular dysfunction by captopril in the spontaneously hypertensive rat. Proc. Natl. Acad. Sci. *79*:3310, 1982.
42. Morgan, H. E., and Baker, K. M.: Cardiac hypertrophy: Mechanical, neural and endocrine dependence. Circulation *83*:13, 1991.
43. Mirsky, I., Pfeffer, J. M., Pfeffer, M. A., and Braunwald, E.: The contractile state as the major determinant in the evolution of left ventricular dysfunction in the spontaneously hypertensive rat. Circ. Res. *53*:767, 1983.
44. Capasso, J. M., Palackal, T., Olivetti, G., and Anversa, P.: Left ventricular failure induced by long-term hypertension in rats. Circ. Res. *66*:1400, 1990.
45. Pinsky, W. W., Lewis, R. M., Hartley, C. J., and Entman, M. L.: Permanent changes of ventricular contractility and compliance in chronic volume overload. Am. J. Physiol. *237*:H575, 1979.
46. Penpargkul, S., Schaible, T., Yipintsoi, T., and Scheuer, J.: The effect of diabetes on performance and metabolism of rat hearts. Circ. Res. *47*:911, 1980.
47. Cooper, G., IV, Satava, R. M., Harrison, C. E., and Coleman, H. N.: Normal myocardial function and energetics after reversing pressure-overload hypertrophy. Am. J. Physiol. *226*:1158, 1974.
48. Zak, R.: Cardiac hypertrophy: Biochemical and cellular relationships. Hosp. Prac. *18*:85, 1983.
49. Pritzl, N., and Zak, R.: Molecular biology of myocardial proteins. Circulation *75*(Suppl. I):85, 1987.
50. Tan, E., and Taegtmeyer, H.: Mechanisms of cardiac hypertrophy in systemic hypertension: A critical review. J. Appl. Cardiol. *1*:329, 1986.
50a. Buttrick, P., Malhotra, A., Factor, S., et al.: Effect of aging and hypertension on myosin biochemistry and gene expression in the rat heart. Circ Res. *68*:645, 1991.
51. McCullagh, W. H., Covell, J. W., and Ross, J., Jr.: Left ventricular dilatation and diastolic compliance changes during chronic volume overloading. Circulation *45*:943, 1972.
52. Anversa, P., Ricci, R., and Olivetti, G.: Quantitative structural analysis of the myocardium during physiologic growth and induced cardiac hypertrophy: A review. J. Am. Coll. Cardiol. *7*:1140, 1986.
53. Pearson, A. C., Pasierski, T., and Labovitz, A. J.: Left ventricular hypertrophy: Diagnosis, prognosis and management. Am. Heart J. *121*:148, 1991.
54. Breisch, E. A., White, F. C., and Bloor, C. M.: Myocardial characteristics of

pressure overload hypertrophy: A structural and functional study. Lab. Invest. *51*:333, 1984.

55. Ferrans, V. J.: Morphology of the heart in hypertrophy. Hosp. Pract. *18*:67, 1983.
56. Huston, T. P., Puffer, J. C., and Rodney, W. M.: The athletic heart syndrome. N. Engl. J. Med. *313*:24, 1985.
57. Strauer, B. E.: Significance of coronary circulation in hypertensive heart disease for development and prevention of heart failure. Am. J. Cardiol. *65*:34G, 1990.
58. Colan, S. D., Sanders, S. P., and Borow, K. M.: Physiologic hypertrophy: Effects on left ventricular systolic mechanics in athletes. J. Am. Coll. Cardiol. 9:776, 1987.
59. Maron, B. J.: Structural features of the athlete heart as defined by echocardiography. J. Am. Coll. Cardiol. *7*:190, 1986.
59a. Pelliccia, A., Maron, B. J., Spataro, A., et al.: The upper limit of physiologic cardiac hypertrophy in highly trained elite athletes. N. Engl. J. Med. *324*:295, 1991
59b. Olivetti, G., Capasso, J. M., Meggs, L. G., et al.: Cellular basis of chronic ventricular remodeling after myocardial infarction in rats. Circ. Res. *68*:856, 1991.
60. Unverferth, D. V., Fetters, J. K., Unverferth, B. J., et al.: Human myocardial histologic characteristics in congestive heart failure. Circulation *2*:1194, 1983.
61. Figulla, H. R., Rahlf, G., Nieger, M., Luig, H., and Kreuzer, H.: Spontaneous hemodynamic improvement or stabilization and associated biopsy findings in patients with congestive cardiomyopathy. Circulation *71*:1095, 1985.
62. Armstrong, P. W., Howard, R. J., and Moe, G. W.: Clinical lessons learned from experimental heart failure. Int. J. Cardiol. *24*:133, 1989.
63. Incalzi, R. A., Gemma, A., Frustaci, A., et al.: Low atrial tachycardia as primary cause of the heart failure complicating congestive cardiomyopathy. Acta Cardiologica *44*:335, 1989.
64. Ross, J., Jr.: Afterload mismatch and preload reserve: A conceptual framework for the analysis of ventricular function. Prog. Cardiovasc. Dis. *18*:255, 1976.
65. Braunwald, E., Welch, G. H., Jr., and Sarnoff, S. J.: Hemodynamic effects of quantitatively varied experimental mitral regurgitation. Circ. Res. *5*:539, 1957.
66. Welch, G. H., Jr., Braunwald, E., and Sarnoff, S. J.: Hemodynamic effects of quantitatively varied experimental aortic regurgitation. Circ. Res. *5*:546, 1957.
67. Urschel, C. W., Covell, J. W., Sonnenblick, E. H., et al.: Myocardial mechanics in aortic and mitral valvular regurgitation: The concept of instantaneous impedance as a determinant of the performance of the intact heart. J. Clin. Invest. *47*:867, 1968.
68. Mason, D. T.: Regulation of cardiac performance in clinical heart disease: Interactions between contractile state, mechanical abnormalities and ventricular compensatory mechanisms. Am. J. Cardiol. *32*:437, 1973.
69. Urschel, C. W., Covell, J. W., Graham, T. P., et al.: Effects of acute valvular regurgitation on the oxygen consumption of the canine heart. Circ. Res. *23*:33, 1968.
70. Grossman, W., Jones, D., and McLaurin, L. P.: Wall stress and patterns of hypertrophy in the human left ventricle. J. Clin. Invest. *56*:56, 1975.
71. Gunther, S., and Grossman, W.: Determinants of ventricular function in pressure overload hypertrophy in man. Circulation *59*:679, 1979.
72. Donner, R., Carabello, B. A., Black, I., and Spann, J. F.: Left ventricular wall stress in compensated aortic stenosis in children. Am. J. Cardiol. *51*:946, 1983.
73. Spann, J. F., Bove, A. A., Natarajan, G., and Kreulen, T.: Ventricular performance, pump function and compensatory mechanisms in patients with aortic stenosis. Circulation *62*:576, 1980.
73a. Hayashida, W., Kumada, T., Nohara, R., et al.: Left ventricular regional wall stress in dilated cardiomyopathy. Circulation, *82*:2075, 1990.
74. Al-Nouri, M. B., Ford, L. E., and Wix, H.: Dimensional correlates of left ventricular dilation in the presence of hypertrophy. Chest *83*:43, 1983.
75. Leman, R. B., Spinale, F. G., Dorn, G. W., et al.: Supranormal ejection performance is isolated to the ipsilateral congenitally pressure-overloaded ventricle. J. Am. Coll. Cardiol. *13*:1314, 1989.
76. Sasayama, S., Ross, J., Jr., Franklin, D., et al.: Adaptations of the left ventricle to chronic pressure overload. Circ. Res. *38*:172, 1976.
77. Zile, M. R.: Diastolic dysfunction: Detection, consequences, and treatment. Part 1: Definition and determinants of diastolic function. Mod. Concepts Cardiovasc. Dis. *58*:67, 1989.
78. Heyndrickx, G. R., and Paulus, W. J.: Effect of asynchrony on left ventricular relaxation. Circulation *81*(Suppl. III):41, 1990.
79. Bonow, R. O.: Regional left ventricular nonuniformity: Effects of left ventricular diastolic function in ischemic heart disease, hypertrophic cardiomyopathy, and the normal heart. Circulation *81*(Suppl. III):54, 1990.
80. Gaasch, W. H., Levine, H. J., Quinones, M. A., and Alexander, J. K.: Left ventricular compliance: Mechanisms and clinical implications. Am. J. Cardiol. *38*:645, 1976.
81. Brutsaert, D. L., Rademakers, F. E., and Sys, S. U.: Triple control of relaxation: Implications in cardiac disease. Circulation *69*:190, 1984.
82. Morgan, J. P., and Morgan, K. G.: Calcium and cardiovascular function: Intracellular calcium levels during contraction and relaxation of mammalian cardiac and vascular smooth muscle as detected with aequorin. Am. J. Med. *77*(Suppl. 5A):33, 1984.
83. Gwathmey, J. K., and Morgan, J. P.: Altered calcium handling in experimental pressure-overload hypertrophy in the ferret. Circ. Res. *57*:836, 1985.
84. Lorell, B. H., Wexler, L. F., Momomura, S., et al.: The influence of pressure overload left ventricular hypertrophy on diastolic properties during hypoxia in isovolumetrically contracting rat hearts. Circ. Res. *58*:683, 1986.
85. Braunwald, E., and Ross, J., Jr.: The ventricular end-diastolic pressure: Appraisal of its value in the recognition of ventricular failure in man (Editorial). Am. J. Med. *34*:147, 1963.
85a. Corin, W. J., Murakami, T., Monrad, E. S., et al.: Left ventricular passive diastolic properties in chronic mitral regurgitation. Circulation *83*:797, 1991.
86. Mirsky, I., and Laks, M. M.: Time course of changes in the mechanical properties of the canine right and left ventricles during hypertrophy caused by pressure overload. Circulation *46*:530, 1980.
87. Lecarpentier, Y., Waldenstrom, A., Clergue, M., et al.: Major alterations in relaxation during cardiac hypertrophy induced by aortic stenosis in guinea pig. Circ. Res. *61*:107, 1987.
88. Shepherd, R.F.J., Zachariah, P. K., and Shub, C.: Hypertension and left ventricular diastolic function. Mayo Clin. Proc. *64*:1521, 1989.
89. Cuocolo, A., Sax, F. L., Brush, J. E., et al.: Left ventricular hypertrophy and impaired diastolic filling in essential hypertension: Diastolic mechanisms for systolic dysfunction during exercise. Circulation *81*:978, 1990.
90. Diver, D. J., Royal, H. D., Aroesty, J. M., et al.: Diastolic function in patients with aortic stenosis: Influence of left ventricular load reduction. J. Am. Coll. Cardiol. *12*:642, 1988.
91. Fifer, M. A., Borow, K. M., Colan, S. D., and Lorell, B. H.: Early diastolic left ventricular function in children and adults with aortic stenosis. J. Am. Coll. Cardiol. *5*:1147, 1985.
92. Smith, V. E., Schulman, P., Karimeddini, M. K., et al.: Rapid ventricular filling in left ventricular hypertrophy: II. Pathologic hypertrophy. J. Am. Coll. Cardiol. *5*:869, 1985.
93. Papademetriou, V., Gottdiener, J. S., Fletcher, R. D., and Freis, E. D.: Echocardiographic assessment by computer-assisted analysis of diastolic left ventricular function and hypertrophy in borderline or mild systemic hypertension. Am. J. Cardiol. *56*:546, 1985.
94. Granger, C. B., Karimeddini, M. K., Smith, V. E., Shapiro, H. R., Katz, A. M., and Riba, A. L.: Rapid ventricular filling in left ventricular hypertrophy. I. Physiologic hypertrophy. Am. J. Cardiol. *5*:862, 1985.
95. Warren, S. E., Cohn, L. H., Shoen, F. J., et al.: Advanced diastolic heart failure in familial hypertrophic cardiomyopathy managed with cardiac transplantation. J. Applied Cardiol. *3*:415, 1988.
96. Douglas, P. S., Berko, B., Lesh, M., and Reichek, N.: Alterations in diastolic function in response to progressive left ventricular hypertrophy. J. Am. Coll. Cardiol. *13*:461, 1989.
97. Williams, J. F., Jr., Potter, R. D., Hern, D. L., et al.: Hydroxyproline and passive stiffness of pressure-induced hypertrophied kitten myocardium. J. Clin. Invest. *69*:309, 1982.
98. Vatner, S. F., Shannon, R., and Hittinger, L.: Reduced subendocardial coronary reserve: A potential mechanism for impaired diastolic function in the hypertrophied and failing heart. Circulation *81*(Suppl. III):8, 1990.
98a. Serizawa, T., Carabello, B. A., and Grossman, W.: Effect of pacing-induced ischemia on left ventricular diastolic pressure-volume relations in dogs with coronary stenosis. Circ. Res. *46*:430, 1980.
98b. Hess, O. M., Osakada, G., Lavelle, J. F., et al.: Diastolic myocardial wall stiffness and ventricular relaxation during partial and complete coronary occlusions in the conscious dog. Circ. Res. *52*:387, 1983.
98c. Forrester, J., Diamond, C., Parmley, W. W., and Swan, H.J.C.: Early increase in left ventricular compliance following myocardial infarction. J. Clin. Invest. *51*:598, 1972.
98d. Pirzada, F. A., Ekong, E. A., Vokonas, P. S., et al.: Experimental myocardial infarction. XIII. Sequential changes in left ventricular pressure-length relations in the acute phase. Circulation *53*:970, 1976.
98e. Swan, H.J.C., Forrester, J. S., Diamond, G., et al.: Hemodynamic spectrum of myocardial infarction and cardiogenic shock. Circulation *40*:1097, 1972.
98f. Farhi, E. R., Canty, J. J., and Klocke, F. J.: Effects of graded reductions in coronary perfusion pressure on the diastolic pressure-segment length relation and the rate of isovolumic relaxation in the resulting conscious dog. Circulation *80*:1458, 1989.
99. Diamond, C., and Forrester, J. S.: Effect of coronary artery disease and acute myocardial infarction on left ventricular compliance in man. Circulation *45*:11, 1972.
100. Fletcher, P. J., Pfeffer, J. M., Pfeffer, M. A., and Braunwald, E.: Left ventricular diastolic pressure-volume relations in rats with healed myocardial infarction. Effects on systolic function. Circ. Res. *49*:618, 1981.
101. Bortone, A. S., Hess, O. M., Chiddo, A., et al.: Functional and structural abnormalities in patients with dilated cardiomyopathy. J. Am. Coll. Cardiol. *14*:613, 1989.
102. Amende, I., Simon, R., Seegers, A., et al.: Diastolic dysfunction during acute cardiac allograft rejection. Circulation *81*(Suppl. III):66, 1990.
103. Lorell, B. M., Turi, Z., and Grossman, W.: Modification of left ventricular response to pacing tachycardia by nifedipine in patients with coronary artery disease. Am. J. Med. *71*:667, 1981.
104. Weber, K. T., Pick, R., Silver, M. A., et al.: Fibrillar collagen and remodeling of dilated canine left ventricle. Circulation *82*:1387, 1990.
105. Weber, K. T., Jalil, J. E., Janicki, J. S., and Pick, R.: Myocardial collagen remodeling in pressure overload hypertrophy. Am. J. Hypertension *2*:931, 1989.
106. Weber, K. T., Nanicki, J. S., Schroff, S. G., Pick, R., et al.: Collagen remodeling of the pressure-overloaded, hypertrophied nonhuman primate myocardium. Circ. Res. *62*:757, 1988.

107. Iimoto, D. S., Covell, J. W., and Harper, E.: Increase in cross-linking of Type I and Type III collagens associated with volume-overload hypertrophy. Circ. Res. *63*:399, 1988.
108. Chapman, D., Weber, K. T., and Eghbali, M.: Regulation of fibrillar collagen Types I and III and basement membrane Type IV collagen gene expression in pressure-overloaded rat myocardium. Circ. Res. *67*:787, 1990.
109. Topol, E. J., Traill, T. A., and Fortuin, N. J.: Hypertensive hypertrophic cardiomyopathy of the elderly. N. Engl. J. Med. *312*:277, 1985.
110. Park, J. W., Ziegler, A. G., Janka, H. U., et al.: Left ventricular relaxation and filling pattern in diabetic heart muscle disease: An echocardiographic study. Klin. Wochenschr. *66*:773, 1988.
111. Danielsen, R., Nordrehaug, J. E., and Vik-Mo, H.: Left ventricular diastolic function in young long-term type 1 insulin (insulin-dependent) diabetic men during exercise assessed by digitalized echocardiography. Eur. Heart J. *9*:395, 1988.
112. Aguirre, F. V., Pearson, A. C., Lewen, M. K., et al.: Usefulness of Doppler echocardiography in the diagnosis of congestive heart failure. Am. J. Cardiol. *63*:1098, 1989.
112a. Mann, D. L., Urabe, Y., Kent, R. L., et al.: Cellular versus myocardial basis for the contractile dysfunction of hypertrophied myocardium. Circ. Res. *68*:402, 1991.
112b. Holt, W., Auffermann, W., Wu, S. T., et al.: Mechanism for depressed cardiac function in left ventricular volume overload. Am. Heart J. *121*:531, 1991.

MECHANISMS RESPONSIBLE FOR DEPRESSED CONTRACTILITY

113. Bing, R. L.: The biochemical basis of myocardial failure. Hosp. Pract. *18*:93, 1983.
114. Graham, T. P., Jr., Ross, J., Jr., and Covell, J. W.: Myocardial oxygen consumption in acute experimental cardiac depression. Circ. Res. *21*:123, 1967.
115. Henry, P. D., Eckberg, D., Gault, J. H., and Ross, J., Jr.: Depressed inotropic state and reduced myocardial oxygen consumption in the human heart. Am. J. Cardiol. *31*:300, 1973.
116. Sievers, R., Parmley, W. W., James, T., and Coffelt-Wilman, J.: Energy levels at systole vs. diastole in normal hamster hearts vs. myopathic hamster hearts. Circ. Res. *53*:759, 1983.
117. Schwartz, A., Lindenmayer, G. E., and Harigaya, S.: Respiratory control and calcium transport in heart mitochondria from the cardiomyopathic Syrian hamster. Trans. N.Y. Acad. Sci. *30*(Suppl. II):951, 1968.
118. Harrison, C. E., Jr., Cooper, G., IV, Zujko, K. J., and Coleman, H. N., III: Myocardial and mitochondrial function in potassium depletion cardiomyopathy. J. Mol. Cell. Cardiol. *4*:633, 1972.
119. Kako, K. J., Thornton, M. J., and Hegtveit, H. A.: Depressed fatty acid and acetate oxidation and other metabolic defects in homogenates from hearts of hamsters with hereditary cardiomyopathy. Circ. Res. *34*:570, 1974.
120. Chidsey, C. A., Weinbach, E. C., Pool, P. E., and Morrow, A. G.: Biochemical studies of energy production in the failing human heart. J. Clin. Invest. *45*:40, 1966.
121. Sobel, B. E., Spann, J. F., Jr., Pool, P. E., et al.: Normal oxidative phosphorylation in mitochondria from the failing heart. Circ. Res. *21*:355, 1967.
122. Sordahl, L. A.: Some biochemical lesions in myocardial disease. Tex. Rep. Biol. Med. *38*:121, 1979.
123. Cooper, G., IV, Satava, R. M., Harrison, C. E., and Coleman, H. N.: Mechanisms for the abnormal energetics of pressure-induced hypertrophy of cat myocardium. Circ. Res. *33*:213, 1973.
124. Buchwald, A., Till, H., Unterberg, C., et al.: Alterations of the mitochondrial respiratory chain in human dilated cardiomyopathy. Eur. Heart J. *11*:509, 1990.
125. Schulze, K., Becker, B. F., Schauer, R., and Schultheiss, H. P.: Antibodies to ADP-ATP carrier—an autoantigen in myocarditis and dilated cardiomyopathy—impair cardiac function. Circulation *81*:959, 1990.
126. Bittl, J. A., and Ingwall, J. S.: Intracellular high-energy phosphate transfer in normal and hypertrophied myocardium. Circulation *75*(Suppl. I):96, 1987.
127. Katz, A. M.: Cellular mechanisms in congestive heart failure. Am. J. Cardiol. *62*:3A, 1988.
128. Pool, P. E., Spann, J. F., Jr., Buccino, R. A., et al.: Myocardial high energy phosphate stores in cardiac hypertrophy and heart failure. Circ. Res. *21*:365, 1967.
129. Capasso, J. M., Aronson, R. S., Strobeck, J. E., and Sonnenblick, E. H.: Effects of experimental phosphate deficiency on action potential characteristics and contractile performance of rat myocardium. Cardiovasc. Res. *16*:71, 1982.
130. Davis, S. V., Olichwier, K. K., and Chakko, S. C.: Reversible depression of myocardial performance in hypophosphatemia. Am. J. Med. Sci. *295*:183, 1988.
131. Page, E., and McCallister, L. P.: Quantitative electron microscopic description of heart muscle cells. Application to normal, hypertrophied and thyroxin-stimulated hearts. Am. J. Cardiol. *31*:172, 1973.
132. Schwarz, F., Schaper, J., Kittstein, D., et al.: Reduced volume fraction of myofibrils in myocardium of patients with decompensated pressure overload. Circulation *63*:1299, 1981.
133. Pagani, E. D., Alousi, A. A., Grant, A. M., et al.: Changes in myofibrillar content and Mg-ATPase activity in ventricular tissues from patients with heart failure caused by coronary artery disease, cardiomyopathy, or mitral valve insufficiency. Circ. Res. *63*:380, 1988.
134. Hammond, E. H., Anderson, J. L., and Menlove, R. L.: Prognostic significance of myofilament loss in patients with idiopathic cardiomyopathy determined by electron microscopy. J. Am. Coll. Cardiol. *7*:204A, 1986.
135. Alpert, N. R., and Gordon, M. S.: Myofibrillar adenosine triphosphate activity in congestive failure. Am. J. Physiol. *202*:940, 1962.
136. Gordon, M. S., and Brown, A. L.: Myofibrillar adenosine triphosphate activity of human heart tissue and congestive failure: Effects of ouabain and calcium. Circ. Res. *19*:534, 1966.
137. Luchi, R. J., Dritcher, E. M., and Thyrum, P. T.: Reduced cardiac myosin adenosine triphosphate activity in dogs with spontaneously occurring heart failure. Circ. Res. *24*:513, 1969.
138. Chandler, B. M., Sonnenblick, E. H., Spann, J. R., Jr., and Pool, P. E.: Association of depressed myofibrillar adenosine triphosphatase and reduced contractility in experimental heart failure. Circ. Res. *21*:717, 1967.
139. Draper, M., Taylor, N., and Alpert, N. R.: Alteration in contractile protein in hypertrophied guinea pig hearts. *In* Alpert, N. (ed.): Cardiac Hypertrophy. New York, Academic Press, 1971, pp. 315–331.
140. Wikman-Coffelt, J., Kamiyama, T., Salel, A. F., and Mason, D. T.: Differential responses of canine myosin ATPase activity and tissue gases in the pressure-overloaded ventricle dependent upon degree of obstruction —mild versus severe pulmonic and aortic stenosis. *In* Kobayashi, T., Yoshio, I., and Rona, G. (eds.): Recent Advances in Studies on Cardiac Structure and Metabolism. Vol. 12. Cardiac Adaption. Baltimore, University Park Press, 1978, pp. 367–372.
141. Scheuer, J., Malhotra, A., Hirsch, C., et al.: Physiologic cardiac hypertrophy corrects contractile protein abnormalities associated with pathologic hypertrophy in rats. J. Clin. Invest. *70*:1300, 1983.
142. Wikman-Coffelt, J., Parmley, W. W., and Mason, D. T.: Relation of myosin isozymes to the heart as a pump. Am. Heart J. *103*:934, 1982.
143. Gorza, L., Pauletto, P., Pessina, A. C., et al.: Isomyosin distribution in normal and pressure-overloaded rat ventricular myocardium. An immunohistochemical study. Circ. Res. *49*:1003, 1981.
143a. Walsh, R. A., Henkel, R., and Robbins, J.: Cardiac myosin heavy- and light-chain gene expression in hypertrophy and heart failure. Heart Failure *6*:238, 1991.
144. Geenen, D. L., Malhotra, A., Scheuer, J.: Ventricular function and contractile proteins in the infarcted rat heart exposed to chronic pressure overload. Am. J. Physiol. *256*:H745–50, 1989.
145. Bugaisky, L. B., Anderson, P. G., Hall, R. S., and Bishop, S. P.: Differences in myosin isoform expression in the subepicardial and subendocardial myocardium during cardiac hypertrophy in the rat. Circ. Res. *66*:1127, 1990.
145a. Scheuer, J.: Cardiac contractile proteins and congestive heart failure. J. Appl. Cardiol. *4*:407, 1989.
146. Izumo, S., Lompre, A-M, Matsuoka, R., et al.: Myosin heavy chain messenger RNA and protein isoform transitions during cardiac hypertrophy. J. Clin. Invest. *79*:970, 1987.
147. Komuro, I., Shibazaki, Y., Kurabayashi, M., et al.: Molecular cloning of gene sequences from rat heart rapidly responsive to pressure overload. Circ. Res. *66*:979, 1990.
148. Imamura, S-i, Matsuoka, R., Hiratsuka, E., et al.: Local response to cardiac overload on myosin heavy chain gene expression and isozyme transition. Circ. Res. *66*:1067, 1990.
149. Bishopric, N. H., Simpson, P. C., and Ordahl, C. P.: Induction of the skeletal α-Actin gene in α_1-adrenoreceptor-mediated hypertrophy of rat cardiac myocytes. J. Clin. Invest. *80*:1194, 1987.
150. Waspe, L. E., Ordahl, C. P., and Simpson, P. C.: The cardiac β-myosin heavy chain isogene is induced selectively in α-adrenergic receptor-stimulated hypertrophy of cultured rat heart myocytes. J. Clin. Invest. *85*:1206, 1990.
151. Izumo, S., Nadal-Ginard, B., Mahdavi, V.: Proto-oncogene induction and reprogramming of cardiac gene expression produced by pressure overload. Proc. Natl. Acad. Sci. USA. *85*:339, 1988.
152. Deguchi, Y., Azuma, J., Hamaguchi, T., et al.: Cellular oncogene expression in the idiopathic cardiomyopathic hamster heart during the growing process. J. Mol. Cell. Cardiol. *20*:801, 1988.
153. Parker, T. G., Packer, S. E., and Schneider, M. D.: Peptide growth factors can provoke "fetal" contractile protein gene expression in rat cardiac myocytes. J. Clin. Invest. *85*:507, 1990.
154. Katz, A. M.: Biochemical "defect" in the hypertrophied and failing heart. Circulation *47*:1076, 1973.
155. Gorza, L., Mercadier, J. J., Schwartz, K., et al.: Myosin types in the human heart: An immunofluorescence study of normal and hypertrophied atrial and ventricular myocardium. Circ. Res. *54*:694, 1984.
156. Bouvagnet, P., Leger, J., Dechesne, C. A., et al.: Local changes in myosin types in diseased human atrial myocardium: A quantitative immunofluorescence study. Circulation *72*:272, 1985.
157. Bouvagnet, P., Mairhofer, H., Leger, J.O.C., et al.: Distribution of pattern of and myosin in normal and diseased human ventricular myocardium. Basic Res. Cardiol. *84*:91, 1989.
158. Hirzel, H. O., Tuchschmid, C. R., Schneider, J., et al.: Relationship between myosin isoenzyme composition, hemodynamics and myocardial structure in various forms of human cardiac hypertrophy. Circ. Res. *57*:729, 1985.
159. Malhotra, A., and Scheuer, J.: Troponin-tropomyosin dysfunction in cardiomyopathy. Circulation *78*(Suppl. II):179, 1988.
160. Malhotra, A.: Regulatory proteins in hamster cardiomyopathy. Circ. Res. *66*:1302, 1990.
160a. Mann, D. L.: Pathophysiology of valvular heart disease: basic mechanisms. Curr. Opin. Cardiol. *6*:191–196, 1991.
161. Connor, T. B., Rosen, B. L., Blaustein, M. P., et al.: Hypocalcemia precipitating congestive heart failure. N. Engl. J. Med. *307*:869, 1982.

162. Levine, S. N., and Rheams, C. N.: Hypocalcemic heart failure. Am. J. Med. *78*:1033, 1985.
163. Henrich, W. L., Hunt, J. M., and Nixon, J. V.: Increased ionized calcium and left ventricular contractility during hemodialysis. N. Engl. J. Med. *310*:19, 1984.
164. Ginsburg, R., Esserman, L. J., and Bristow, M. R.: Myocardial performance and extracellular ionized calcium in a severely failing human heart. Ann. Intern. Med. *98*:603, 1983.
165. Fleckenstein, A.: Calcium Antagonism in Heart and Smooth Muscle. New York, John Wiley and Sons, 1983.
165a. Herzig, J. W., Ruegg, J. C., and Solaro, R. J.: Myocardial excitation-contraction coupling as influenced through modulation of the calcium sensitivity of the contractile proteins. Heart Failure *6*:244, 1991.
166. Mercadier, J-J, Lompre, A-M, Duc, P., et al.: Altered sarcoplasmic reticulum Ca^{2+}-ATPase gene expression in the human ventricle during end-stage heart failure. J. Clin. Invest. *85*:305, 1990.
167. de la Bastie, D., Levitsky, D., Rappaport, L., et al.: Function of the sarcoplasmic reticulum and expression of its Ca^{2+}-ATPase gene in pressure overload-induced cardiac hypertrophy in the rat. Circ. Res. *66*:554, 1990.
168. Dhalla Das, P. K., and Sharma, G. P.: Subcellular basis of cardiac contractile failure. J. Mol. Cell Cardiol. *10*:363, 1978.
169. Ito, Y., Suko, J., and Chidsey, C. A.: Intracellular calcium and myocardial contractility: Calcium uptake of sarcoplasmic reticulum fractions in hypertrophied and failing rabbit hearts. J. Mol. Cell Cardiol. *6*:237, 1974.
170. Gwathmey, J. K., Copelas, L., MacKinnon, R., et al.: Abnormal intracellular calcium handling in myocardium from patients with end-stage heart failure. Circ. Res. *61*:70, 1987.
171. Edes, I., Talosi, L., and Kranias, E. G.: Sarcoplasmic reticulum function in normal heart and in cardiac disease. Heart Failure *6*:221, 1991.
172. Whitmer, J. T., Kumar, Pl, and Solaro, R. J.: Calcium transport properties of cardiac sarcoplasmic reticulum from cardiomyopathic syrian hamsters (BIO 53.58 and 14.6): Evidence for a quantitative defect in dilated myopathic hearts not evident in hypertrophic hearts. Circ. Res. *62*:81, 1988.
173. Mead, R. J., Peterson, M. B., and Welty, J. D.: Sarcolemmal and sarcoplasmic reticular ATPase activities in the failing canine heart. Circ. Res. *29*:14, 1971.
174. Harigaya, S., and Schwartz, A.: Rate of calcium binding and uptake in normal animal and failing human cardiac muscle. Circ. Res. *25*:781, 1969.
175. Sordahl, L. A., Wood, W. G., and Schwartz, A.: Production of cardiac hypertrophy and failure in rabbits with ameroid clips. J. Mol. Cell. Cardiol. *1*:341, 1970.
176. McCollum, W. B., Crow, C., Harigaya, S., et al.: Calcium binding by cardiac relaxing system isolated from myopathic Syrian hamsters. J. Mol. Cell. Cardiol. *1*:445, 1970.
177. Gelband, H., and Bassett, A. L.: Depressed transmembrane potentials during experimentally induced ventricular failure in cats. Circ. Res. *32*:625, 1973.
178. Keung, E. C.: Calcium current is increased in isolated adult myocytes from hypertrophied rat myocardium. Circ. Res. *64*:753, 1989.

NEUROHORMONAL ADJUSTMENTS IN HEART FAILURE

179. Chidsey, C. A., Harrison, D. C., and Braunwald, E.: Augmentation of plasma norepinephrine response to exercise in patients with congestive heart failure. N. Engl. J. Med. *267*:650, 1962.
180. Hasking, G. J., Esler, M. D., Jennings, G. L., et al.: Norepinephrine spillover to plasma in patients with congestive heart failure: Evidence of increased overall and cardiorenal sympathetic nervous activity. Circulation *73*:615, 1986.
181. Minami, M., Yasuda, H., Yamazaki, N., et al.: Plasma norepinephrine concentration and plasma dopamine-beta-hydroxylase activity in patients with congestive heart failure. Circulation *67*:1324, 1983.
182. Francis, G. S., Goldsmith, S. R., Ziesche, S., et al.: Relative attenuation of sympathetic drive during exercise in patients with congestive heart failure. J. Am. Coll. Cardiol. *5*:832, 1985.
183. Cohn, J. N., Levine, T. B., Olivari, M. T., et al.: Plasma norepinephrine as a guide to prognosis in patients with chronic congestive heart failure. N. Engl. J. Med. *311*:819, 1984.
184. Viquerat, C. E., Daly, P., Swedberg, K., et al.: Endogenous catecholamine levels in chronic heart failure: Relation to the severity of hemodynamic abnormalities. Am. J. Med. *78*:455, 1985.
185. Rose, C. P., Burgess, J. H., and Cousineau, D.: Tracer norepinephrine kinetics in coronary circulation of patients with heart failure secondary to chronic pressure and volume overload. J. Clin. Invest. *76*:1740, 1985.
186. Chidsey, C. A., Braunwald, E., and Morrow, A. G.: Catecholamine excretion and cardiac stores of norepinephrine in congestive heart failure. Am. J. Med. *39*:442, 1965.
187. Henderson, E. B., Kahn, J. K., Corbett, J. R., et al.: Abnormal I-123 Metaoidobenzylguanidine myocardial washout and distribution may reflect myocardial adrenergic derangement in patients with congestive cardiomyopathy. Circulation *78*:1192, 1988.
187. Maurer, W., Ablasser, A., Tschada, R., et al: Myocardial catecholamine metabolism in patients with chronic aortic regurgitation. Circulation *66*(Suppl. 1):139, 1982.
188. Schoffer, J., Tews, A., Langes, K., et al.: Relationship between myocardial norepinephrine content and left ventricular function—an endomyocardial biopsy study. Eur. Heart J. *8*:748, 1987.
188. Malliani, A., and Pagani, M.: The role of the sympathetic nervous system in congestive heart failure. Eur. Heart J. *4*(Suppl. A):49, 1983.
189. Thomas, J. A., and Marks, B. H.: Plasma norepinephrine in congestive heart failure. Am. J. Cardiol. *41*:233, 1978.
190. Coulson, R. L., Yazdanfar, S., Rubio, E., et al.: Recuperative potential of cardiac muscle following relief of pressure overload hypertrophy and right ventricular failure in the cat. Circ. Res. *40*:41, 1977.
191. Spann, J. F., Jr., Sonnenblick, E. H., Cooper, T., et al.: Cardiac norepinephrine stores and the contractile state of heart muscle. Circ. Res. *19*:317, 1966.
192. Pool, P. E., Covell, J. W., Levitt, M., et al.: Reduction of cardiac tyrosine hydroxylase activity in experimental congestive heart failure. Its role in depletion of cardiac norepinephrine stores. Circ. Res. *20*:349, 1967.
193. Sole, M. J.: Alterations in sympathetic and parasympathetic neurotransmitter activity. *In* Braunwald, E., Mock, M. B., and Watson, J. (eds.): Congestive Heart Failure: Current Research and Clinical Applications. New York, Grune and Stratton, 1982, p. 101.
194. Covell, J. W., Chidsey, C. A., and Braunwald, E.: Reduction of the cardiac response to postganglionic sympathetic nerve stimulation in experimental heart failure. Circ. Res. *19*:51, 1966.
195. Gaffney, T. E., and Braunwald, E.: Importance of the adrenergic nervous system in the support of circulatory function in patients with congestive heart failure. Am. J. Med. *34*:320, 1963.
196. Epstein, S. E., and Braunwald, E.: The effect of beta-adrenergic blockade on patterns of urinary sodium excretion: Studies in normal subjects and in patients with heart disease. Ann. Intern. Med. *75*:20, 1966.
197. Vogel, J.H.K., and Chidsey, C. A.: Cardiac adrenergic activity in experimental heart failure assessed with beta-receptor blockade. Am. J. Cardiol. *24*:198, 1969.
198. Colucci, W. S., Leatherman, G. F., Ludmer, P. L., and Gauthier, D. F.: β-adrenergic inotropic responsiveness of patients with heart failure: Studies with intracoronary dobutamine infusion. Circ. Res. *61*(Suppl. I):8, 1987.
199. Francis, G. S., Goldsmith, S. R., Levine, T. B., et al.: The neurohumoral axis in congestive heart failure. Ann. Intern. Med. *101*:370, 1984.
200. Van Zweeten, P. A., and Timmermans, P. B.: Cardiovascular alpha-2 receptors. J. Mol. Cell. Cardiol. *15*:717, 1983.
201. Francis, G. S., Parks, R., and Cohn, J. N.: The effects of bromocriptine in patients with congestive heart failure. Am. Heart J. *106*:100, 1983.
202. Goldstein, R. E., Beiser, G. D., Stampfer, M., and Epstein, S. E.: Impairment of autonomically mediated heart rate control in patients with cardiac dysfunction. Circ. Res. *36*:571, 1975.
202a. Marin-Neto, J. A., Pintya, A. O., Gallo, L. Jr., and Maciel, B. C.: Abnormal baroreflex control of heart rate in decompensated congestive heart failure and reversal after compensation. Am. J. Cardiol. *67*:604, 1991.
203. Levine, T. B., Francis, G. S., Goldsmith, S. R., and Cohn, J. N.: The neurohumoral and hemodynamic response to orthostatic tilt in patients with congestive heart failure. Circulation *67*:1070, 1983.
204. Goldsmith, S. R., Francis, G. S., Levine, T. B., and Cohn, J. N.: Regional blood flow response to orthostasis in patients with congestive heart failure. J. Am. Coll. Cardiol. *1*:1391, 1983.
205. Kubo, S. H., and Cody, R. J.: Circulatory autoregulation in chronic congestive heart failure: Responses to head-up tilt in 41 patients. Am. J. Cardiol. *52*:512, 1983.
206. Stone, G. W., Kubo, S. H., and Cody, R. J.: Adverse influence of baroreceptor dysfunction on upright exercise in congestive heart failure. Am. J. Med. *80*:799, 1986.
207. Colucci, W. S., Rebeiro, J. P., Rocco, M. B., et al.: Impaired chronotropic response to exercise in patients with congestive heart failure. Role of postsynaptic beta-adrenergic desensitization. Circulation *80*:314, 1989.
208. Ferguson, D. W., Abboud, F. M., and Mark, A. L.: Selective impairment of baroreflex-mediated vasoconstrictor responses in patients with ventricular dysfunction. Circulation *69*:451, 1984.
209. Higgins, C. B., Vatner, S. F., Eckberg, D. L., and Braunwald, E.: Alterations in the baroreceptor reflex in conscious dogs with heart failure. J. Clin. Invest. *51*:715, 1972.
210. White, C. W.: Reversibility of abnormal arterial baroreflex control of heart rate in heart failure. Am. J. Physiol. *241*(Heart Circ. Physiol. 10):H778, 1981.
211. Cohn, J. N., Taylor, N., Vrobel, T., and Moskowitz, R..: Contrasting effect of vasodilators on heart rate and plasma catecholamines in patients with hypertension and heart failure. Clin. Res. *26*(Abstr.):547A, 1978.
212. Levine, T. B., Olivari, T., and Cohn, J. N.: Dissociation of the responses of the renin-angiotensin system and sympathetic nervous system to a vasodilator stimulus in congestive heart failure. Int. J. Cardiol. *12*:165, 1986.
212a. Kubo, S. H., Rector, T. S., Heifets, S. M., and Cohn, J. N.: α_2-receptor-mediated vasoconstriction in patients with congestive heart failure. Circulation *80*:1660, 1989.
212b. Leier, C. V., Binkley, P. F., and Cody, R. J.: α-adrenergic component of the sympathetic nervous system in congestive heart failure. Circulation *82*(Suppl):168, 1990.
212c. Bristow, M. R., Minobe, W., Rasmussen, R., et al.: Alpha-1 adrenergic receptors in the nonfailing and failing human heart. J. Pharmacol. Exp. Ther. *247*:1039, 1988.
212d. Francis, G-S: Interaction of the sympathetic nervous system and electrolytes in congestive heart failure. Am. J. Cardiol. *65*:24E, 1990.
213. Colucci, W. S., Alexander, R. W., Williams, G. H., et al.: Decreased lymphocyte beta-adrenergic-receptor density in patients with heart failure and tolerance to the beta-adrenergic agonist pirbuterol. N. Engl. J. Med. *305*:185, 1981.
214. Weiss, R. J., Tobes, M., Wertz, C. E., and Smith, C. B.: Platelet $alpha_2$ adrenoreceptors in chronic congestive heart failure. Am. J. Cardiol. *52*:101, 1983.

215. Bristow, M. R., Ginsburg, R., Minobe, W., et al.: Decreased catecholamine sensitivity and beta-adrenergic-receptor density in failing human hearts. N. Engl. J. Med. *307*:205, 1982.
216. Bristow, M. R.: The adrenergic nervous system in heart failure. N. Engl. J. Med. *311*:850, 1984.
217. Fowler, M. B., Laser, J. A., Hopkins, G. L., et al.: Assessment of the β-adrenergic receptor pathway in the intact failing human heart. Circulation *74*:1290, 1986.
218. Port, J. D., Larabee, P., Wiederin, J., et al.: Differences in ventricular myocardial beta receptor expression in ischemic versus idiopathic dilated cardiomyopathy. Circulation *80*(Suppl. IV):8, 1989.
219. Bristow, M. R., Hershberger, R. E., Port, J. D., and Rasmussen, R.: $Beta_1$ and $Beta_2$ adrenergic receptor-mediated adenylate cyclase stimulation in nonfailing and failing human ventricular myocardium. Mol. Pharmacol. *35*:295, 1989.
220. Ayobe, M. H., and Tarazi, R. C.: Reversal of changes in myocardial beta-receptors and inotropic responsiveness with regression of cardiac hypertrophy in renal hypertensive rats (RHR). Circ. Res. *54*:125, 1984.
221. Heilbrunn, S. M., Shah, P., Bristow, M. R., et al.: Increased β-receptor density and improved hemodynamic response to catecholamine stimulation during long-term metoprolol therapy in heart failure from dilated cardiomyopathy. Circulation *79*:483, 1989.
222. Feldman, M. D., Copelas, L., Gwathmey, J. K., et al.: Deficient production of cyclic AMP: Pharmacologic evidence of an important cause of contractile dysfunction in patients with end-stage heart failure. Circulation *75*:331, 1987.
223. Feldman, A. M., Gates, A. E., Veazey, W. B., et al.: Increase of the 40,000-mol wt pertussis toxin substrate (G protein) in the failing human heart. J. Clin. Invest. *82*:189, 1988.
224. Neumann, J., Schmitz, W., Scholz, H., et al.: Increase in myocardial G_1 proteins in heart failure. Lancet *22*:936, 1988.
225. Denniss, A. R., Marsh, J. D., Quigg, R. J., et al.: β-adrenergic receptor number and adenylate cyclase function in denervated transplanted and cardiomyopathic human hearts. Circulation *79*:1028, 1989.
226. Feldman, A. M., Tena, R. G., Kessler, P. D., et al.: Diminished β-adrenergic responsiveness and cardiac dilatation in hearts of myopathic syrian hamsters (BIO 53,58) are associated with a function abnormality of the G stimulatory protein. Circulation *81*:1341, 1990.
226a. Levine, T. B., Francis, G. S., Goldsmith, S. R., et al.: Activity of the sympathetic nervous system and renin-angiotensin system assessed by plasma hormone levels and their relation to hemodynamic abnormalities in congestive heart failure. Am. J. Cardiol. *49*:1659, 1982.
226b. Kluger, J., Cody, R. J., and Laragh, J. H.: The contributions of sympathetic tone and the renin-angiotensin system to severe chronic congestive heart failure: Response to specific inhibitors (prazosin and captopril). Am. J. Cardiol. *49*:1667, 1982.
227. Pedersen, E. B., Danielson, H., Jensen, T., et al.: Angiotensin II, aldosterone and arginine vasopressin in plasma in congestive heart failure. Eur. J. Clin. Invest. *16*:56, 1986.
228. Mettauer, B., Rouleau, J.-L., Bichet, D., et al.: Sodium and water excretion abnormalities in congestive heart failure: Determinant factors and clinical implications. Ann. Intern. Med. *105*:161, 1986.
229. Packer, M.: Neurohormonal interactions and adaptations in congestive heart failure. Circulation *77*:721, 1988.
230. Goldsmith, S. R., Francis, G. S., and Cowley, A. W.: Arginine vasopressin and the renal response to water loading in congestive heart failure. Am. J. Cardiol. *58*:295, 1986.
231. Goldsmith, S. R., Francis, G. S., Levine, T. B., et al.: Impaired response of plasma vasopressin to orthostatic stress in patients with congestive heart failure. J. Am. Coll. Cardiol. *2*:1080, 1983.
232. Broqvist, M., Dahlstrom, U., Karlberg, B. E., et al.: Neuroendocrine response in acute heart failure and the influence of treatment. Eur. Heart J. *10*:1075, 1989.
233. Schaller, M-D, Nussberger, J., Feihl, F., et al.: Clinical and hemodynamic correlates of elevated plasma arginine vasopressin after acute myocardial infarction. Am. J. Cardiol. *60*:1178, 1987.
234. Belleau, L., Mion, H., Simard, S., et al.: Studies on the mechanism of experimental congestive heart failure in dogs. Can. J. Physiol. Pharmacol. *48*:450, 1970.
235. Zehr, J. E., Hawe, A., Tsakiris, A. G., et al.: ADH levels following nonhypotensive hemorrhage in dogs with chronic mitral stenosis. Am. J. Physiol. *221*:312, 1971.
236. Greenberg, T. T., Richmond, W. H., Stocking, R. A., et al.: Impaired atrial receptor responses in dogs with heart failure due to tricuspid insufficiency and pulmonary artery stenosis. Circ. Res. *32*:424, 1973.
237. Pruszczynski, W., Vahanian, A., Ardaillou, R., and Acar, J.: Role of antidiuretic hormone in impaired water excretion of patients with congestive heart failure. J. Clin. Endocrinol. Metab. *58*:599, 1984.
238. Goldsmith, S. R., and Dodge, D.: Response of plasma vasopressin to ethanol in congestive heart failure. Am. J. Cardiol. *55*:1354, 1985.
239. Gottlieb, S. S., Kukin, M. L., Ahern, D., and Packer, M.: Prognostic importance of atrial natriuretic peptide in patients with chronic heart failure. J. Am. Coll. Cardiol. *13*:1535, 1989.
240. Cantin, M., Thibault, G., Ding, J., et al.: ANF in experimental congestive heart failure. Am. J. Pathol. *130*:552, 1988.
241. Saito, Y., Nakao, K., Arai, H., et al.: Augmented expression of atrial natriuretic polypeptide gene in ventricle of human failing heart. J. Clin. Invest. *83*:298, 1989.
242. Takemura, G., Fujiwara, H., Korike, K., et al.: Ventricular expression of atrial natriuretic polypeptide and its relation with hemodynamics and histology in dilated human hearts. Circulation *80*:1137, 1989.
243. Franch, H. A., Dixon, R.A.F., Blaine, E. H., and Siegel, P. K. S.: Ventricular atrial natriuretic factor in the cardiomyopathic hamster model of congestive heart failure. Circ. Res. *62*:31, 1988.
244. Burnett, J. C.: Atrial natriuretic factor: Is physiologically important? Circulation *82*:1523, 1990.
245. Eckberg, D. L., Drabinsky, M., and Braunwald, E.: Defective cardiac parasympathetic control in patients with heart disease. N. Engl. J. Med. *285*:877, 1971.
246. Roskoski, R., Jr., Schmid, P. G., Mayer, H. E., and Abboud, F. M.: In vitro acetylcholine biosynthesis in normal and failing guinea pig hearts. Circ. Res. *36*:547, 1975.
247. Schmid, P. G., Lund, D. D., and Roskoski, R., Jr.: Efferent autonomic dysfunction in heart failure. *In* Abboud, F. M., Fozzard, H. A., Gilmore, J. P., and Reis, D. J. (eds.): Disturbances in Neurogenic Control of the Circulation. Bethesda, Md., American Physiological Society, 1981, p. 138.
248. Vatner, D. E., Lee, D. L., Schwarz, K. R., et al.: Impaired cardiac muscarinic receptor function in dogs with heart failure. J. Clin. Invest. *81*:1836, 1988.
249. Gauer, O. H., and Henry, J. P.: Neurohumoral control of plasma volume. *In* Guyton, A. C., and Cowley, A. W. (eds.): International Review of Physiology. Cardiovascular Physiology II. Baltimore, University Park Press, 1976, pp. 145–190.
250. Nonidez, J. F.: Identification of the receptor areas in the venae cavae and pulmonary veins which initiate reflex cardiac acceleration (Bainbridge's reflex). Am. J. Anat. *61*:203, 1937.
251. Thoren, P., and Ricksten, S.-E.: Cardiac C-fiber endings in cardiovascular control under normal and pathophysiological conditions. *In* Abboud, F. M., Fozzard, H. A., Gilmore, J. P., and Reis, D. J. (eds.): Disturbances in Neurogenic Control of the Circulation. Bethesda, Md., American Physiological Society, 1981, p. 17.
252. Abboud, F. M., Thames, M. C., and Mark, A. L.: Role of cardiac afferent nerves in regulation of circulation during coronary occlusion and heart failure. *In* Abboud, F. M., Fozzard, H. A., Gilmore, J. P., and Reis, D. J. (eds.): Disturbances in Neurogenic Control of the Circulation. Bethesda, Md., American Physiological Society, 1981, p. 65.
253. Zucker, I. H., Earle, A. M., and Gilmore, J. P.: The mechanism of adaptation of left atrial stretch receptors in dogs with chronic congestive heart failure. J. Clin. Invest. *60*:323, 1977.
254. Zucker, I. H., Earle, A. M., and Gilmore, J. P.: Changes in the sensitivity of left atrial receptors following reversal of heart failure. Am. J. Physiol. *237*:H555, 1979.
255. Riegger, G.A.J., Leibau, G., and Kocksiek, K.: Antidiuretic hormone in congestive heart failure. Am. J. Med. *72*:49, 1982.

15

Assessment of Cardiac Function

by EUGENE BRAUNWALD, M.D.

THEORETICAL CONSIDERATIONS

Assessment of ventricular performance, function, and contractility is a critically important task in the evaluation of many patients with known or suspected heart disease. *Ventricular performance* is related to the simple pumping function of the ventricle, as reflected in the cardiac output or cardiac work, expressed per stroke or per minute. *Ventricular function* relates these parameters of ventricular performance to some measure of preload, such as end-diastolic volume, dimension, pressure, or wall stress. *Myocardial contractility*, also called the contractile or inotropic state, refers to a fundamental property of cardiac muscle which reflects, in the final analysis, the level of activation of cross-bridge formation and the rapidity of cross-bridge cycling (p. 357).

LIMITATIONS OF CARDIAC OUTPUT IN ASSESSING CARDIAC FUNCTION. Because the heart's prime function is to deliver sufficient oxygenated blood to meet the metabolic requirements of the tissues, it is understandable that measurement of cardiac output has been a time-honored method of assessing cardiac performance and function and that therapeutic interventions in patients with heart disease frequently are evaluated in terms of their effects on this variable. Determination of cardiac output does indeed provide a useful measure of the pumping ability of the heart. However, cardiac output is critically dependent on preload and afterload* in addition to myocardial contractility. As a consequence, measurement of cardiac output alone provides a quite limited and insensitive assessment of ventricular function or of myocardial contractility.[1]

At any level of contractility, the extent of myocardial fiber shortening varies directly with the preload and inversely with the afterload.[2] In the intact organism, afterload is closely related to *aortic impedance*, which is defined as the sum of the external factors that oppose ventricular ejection. Aortic impedance is the ratio of pressure to flow in the aorta and is determined by the physical properties of blood and the vascular wall; it includes the viscosity and density of blood, the diameter of the aorta, the viscoelasticity of the aortic wall, and the reflected pressure and flow waves generated in the distal part of the arterial tree. Aortic impedance usually is expressed as the sum of a series of sinusoidal functions of pressure and flow waves ("harmonics") superimposed on the mean pressure and flow.[3] When aortic impedance is progressively raised, an increasing proportion of the muscle's contractile activity is expressed in the generation of tension and a correspondingly smaller fraction in myocardial fiber shortening (Fig. 13–20C, p. 365). For example, if ventricular end-diastolic volume (preload) is held constant, while left ventricular afterload (aortic impedance) is raised progressively, stroke volume declines until a level of impedance is reached at which the maximum force-generating capacity of the myocardium is exceeded and ventricular ejection ceases; i.e., the contraction becomes isovolumetric. Conversely, when at a constant preload, the aortic impedance falls; i.e., when afterload is reduced, stroke volume rises.

From these considerations it is clear that when afterload is altered, reciprocal changes occur in cardiac output (and in related measures, such as stroke volume, ventricular fiber shortening, and its velocity) and that such reciprocal changes do *not* reflect changes in myocardial contractility (Fig. 13–37, p. 380). For example, an increase in cardiac output in a patient with heart failure after relief of severe aortic stenosis or the successful treatment of hypertension may be due to a reduction in afterload, an improvement in contractility, or both. Similarly, the elevated cardiac output associated with severe anemia (low blood viscosity), fever (arteriolar dilatation), or patent ductus arteriosus (arteriovenous fistula) may be explained in part or entirely by a reduction in aortic impedance, which reduces afterload (p. 379); an augmentation of contractility need not be invoked.

The effects of simple alterations of preload on cardiac output are well known. Thus, the depression of cardiac output that occurs with hypovolemia (e.g., hemorrhagic shock), displacement of blood from the thorax (e.g., positive-pressure ventilation), or cardiac compression (e.g., pericardial tamponade) may be explained by a reduction of preload. The elevation of cardiac output that occurs in patients with hypervolemia, including patients with polycythemia vera and acute glomerulonephritis, does *not* reflect an augmentation of contractility, but rather indicates a higher preload resulting from the hypervolemia.

THE RELATION BETWEEN CARDIAC OUTPUT AND CONTRACTILITY. When myocardial contractility is not depressed, cardiac output depends less on myocardial contractility than on peripheral factors and their influence on ventricular preload and afterload. For example, both digitalis glycosides and paired electrical stimulation exert powerful inotropic influences yet do *not* raise cardiac output in normal human subjects or laboratory animals. By contrast, in the

* Heart rate, the fourth fundamental determinant of cardiac performance (p. 381), is so easily measurable that it will not be considered further, although it is recognized that changes in heart rate exert an important effect on myocardial contractility.

presence of myocardial failure, these stimuli do elevate cardiac output significantly.[4]

The relationship between a chain and its several links may be a useful, although obviously oversimplified, analogy for explaining the relation between cardiac output and myocardial contractility. The total weight that the chain can support (analogous to the cardiac output) will increase only if its weakest link is strengthened. Thus, in a patient with myocardial failure, stimulation of contractility, which may be thought of as strengthening the weakest link in the chain of factors controlling this patient's cardiac output, will elevate cardiac output. On the other hand, when contractility is normal and is not the limiting factor, it is not surprising that stimulation of myocardial contractility often will not elevate cardiac output. When reduced preload is the limiting factor, as in hypovolemia, restoration of blood volume will restore cardiac output; when increased afterload is limiting, as in critical aortic stenosis, relief of the obstruction will elevate cardiac output.

From the foregoing discussion and Figure 13–37 (p. 380), it is evident that cardiac output can be lowered by a reduction of contractility and preload and by an elevation of afterload—operating singly or in combination. Therefore, it is not possible to deduce from the finding of a reduced cardiac output that contractility is depressed. Conversely, cardiac output may be within normal limits when depression of contractility is accompanied by an optimal preload and/or a reduced afterload. (Indeed, such manipulation of loading is an important goal in the management of heart failure with vasodilators [p. 491].) Therefore, although assessment of cardiac function should certainly include measurement of cardiac output, it must not be limited to this. Rather, it also should provide an analysis both of the heart's loading conditions and of contractility.

THE NEED FOR ASSESSING MYOCARDIAL CONTRACTILITY. It often is helpful to assess the level of myocardial contractility in the basal state and to determine how it may be influenced by therapeutic interventions, such as a drug or an operation. In isolated cardiac muscle or in the isolated heart, loading can be readily controlled and the effects of the intervention on the extent and velocity of muscle shortening can be determined. It is more difficult to make analogous measurements in patients in whom preload, afterload, or both may be abnormal and cannot be readily controlled or held constant. For example, it often is desirable to ascertain in a patient with valvular heart disease, ventricular hypertrophy, and symptoms of heart failure whether it is the abnormality in loading produced by the valvular lesion or a depression of myocardial contractility (or a combination) that is responsible for the clinical manifestations of heart failure. Similarly, many drugs that affect myocardial contractility also act on the arterial and/or venous beds, and therefore may change cardiac loading. These considerations have led to the search for methods of evaluating cardiac function that go beyond simple analysis of the pumping function of the ventricle and that are directed toward an assessment of contractility. Although a number of indices of contractility have been proposed and investigated empirically, conclusions drawn about them have involved an element of circular reasoning. Unfortunately there is no *absolute* hemodynamic or mechanical measure of this property of the myocardium; i.e., there is no gold standard with which these indices can be compared.

THE FRANK-STARLING MECHANISM AND THE VENTRICULAR FUNCTION CURVE

The earliest efforts to separate loading conditions from contractility in assessing ventricular performance used the Frank-Starling relation, i.e., the relation between ventricular end-diastolic pressure (or volume) and ventricular mechanical activity, as expressed in the pressure generated, the volume output, or the product of these two variables—that is, stroke work. It was shown early in this century in the heart–lung preparation that stroke volume is a function of both diastolic fiber length (i.e., of preload) and contractility. The failing heart was found to deliver a smaller than normal stroke volume from a normal or elevated end-diastolic volume.[5] Later, Sarnoff and his collaborators examined ventricular stroke work over a range of mean atrial or ventricular end-diastolic pressures, and termed the resulting relation the "ventricular function curve."[6] A family of such curves reflects a spectrum of contractile states, and the position of a given curve provides a description of ventricular contractility. Movement along a single curve (Fig. 13–35, p. 378), represents the operation of the Frank-Starling principle, which indicates that stroke work or volume varies with changes in preload. By contrast, upward or downward displacement of the curve represents a positive or negative inotropic effect, i.e., an augmentation or depression of contractility, respectively (Fig. 15–1).

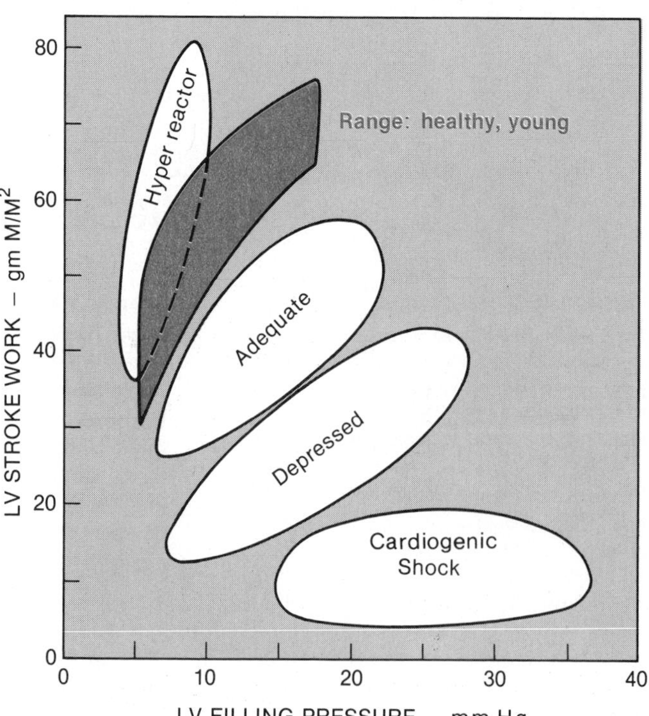

FIGURE 15–1. Hemodynamic consequences of myocardial infarction expressed as varying levels of left ventricular function. The red area represents the range of left ventricular (LV) function in healthy, young people. After acute myocardial infarction, there is wide variability in the hemodynamic response. Some patients with small infarcts and increased sympathetic tone may be in the normal or supernormal range. As the size of the infarct increases, function is progressively shifted down and to the right, so that all patients with cardiogenic shock fall in the lower right-hand group. (From Parmley, W. W.: Hemodynamic monitoring in acute ischemic disease. *In* Fishman, A. P. [ed.]: Heart Failure. New York, McGraw-Hill Book Co., 1978, p. 114.)

At any contractility and preload, stroke work also is influenced by the afterload, being low when outflow pressure is depressed, increasing to a maximal level as pressure is raised, and declining to zero when the afterload is high enough to prevent ventricular ejection (i.e., when ventricular contraction becomes isovolumetric).[7] Even when arterial pressure is held constant, the standard ventricular function curve (Fig. 13–35, p. 378) represents a complex interaction of preload and afterload. This is because as preload is augmented and heart size increases, according to Laplace's law (p. 377), afterload rises at a constant aortic pressure.

ASSESSMENT OF CARDIAC PERFORMANCE BASED ON PRESSURES, FLOWS, VOLUMES, AND DIMENSIONS

Despite the several theoretical limitations already discussed, the simplest, most straightforward approaches for assessing cardiac function are still based on analyzing the pumping function of the ventricles by measuring intravascular and intracardiac pressures, stroke volume (or cardiac output), and ventricular volume and/or dimensions.

CARDIAC OUTPUT. Basal State. The normal range for the cardiac index, i.e., the cardiac output corrected for body size, in the basal (resting) state and the supine position is wide —between 2.5 and 4.2 liters/min/m^2—making this variable relatively insensitive in the assessment of cardiac function. Therefore, it is possible for cardiac output to decline by almost 40 per cent as a consequence of myocardial failure and still remain within normal limits. Consequently, when the cardiac output falls below normal, it usually represents a marked disturbance in *circulatory* (although not necessarily *cardiac*) performance. Such a degree of impairment often is readily detectable clinically. (Hypovolemia secondary to hemorrhage or dehydration is the most common noncardiac circulatory cause of a depressed cardiac output.) The aforementioned limitations notwithstanding, measurement of cardiac output in the basal state is valuable because it provides an assessment of the most critical circulatory function, i.e., the delivery of blood to the metabolizing tissues.

Exercise (see also p. 161). A measurement that detects milder degrees of cardiac impairment with greater sensitivity than does the cardiac output in the basal state is the cardiac output in response to the stress of exercise. Most commonly, the effect of exercise on cardiac output is determined in the cardiac catheterization laboratory as the patient pedals a stationary bicycle in the supine position, and both oxygen consumption and cardiac output are measured at rest and during exercise (p. 195). It also can be determined during treadmill exercise testing (see Fig. 15–22). The increase in cardiac output is a function not only of the heart's pumping capacity but also of the intensity of exercise, which can be expressed by the patient's total oxygen consumption. The increase in cardiac output normally exceeds 6 ml/min for each milliliter increase in oxygen consumption per minute.

ARTERIOVENOUS OXYGEN DIFFERENCE. The pumping action of the heart is reflected not only in the cardiac output but also in the latter's reciprocal, i.e., the arterio–mixed venous O_2 difference. Transposing the Fick equation shown on p. 190:

$$CO = \frac{\dot{V}O_2}{AVO_2} \qquad AVO_2 = \frac{\dot{V}O_2}{CO}$$

where CO = cardiac output; $\dot{V}O_2$ = total O_2 consumption; AVO_2 = arteriovenous O_2 difference. The latter (reflecting the O_2 extraction by the peripheral tissues) indicates the extent to which the circulating blood actually satisfies the metabolic needs of the body. The normal AVO_2 in adults in the basal state ranges from 30 to 50 ml O_2 (average, 40 ml O_2/liter). As cardiac output declines in the resting state, AVO_2 rises in heart failure to levels as high as 120 ml/liter (Fig. 15–2). During exercise, as $\dot{V}O_2$ rises, so does O_2 extraction, and AVO_2 reaches similar maximal levels of about 120 ml/liter in patients with various degrees of impaired left ventricular function as well as in normal subjects and well-trained athletes. In the latter, cardiac output can rise about sixfold (from 3 to 18 liters/min/m^2), which, together with a tripling of the arteriovenous O_2 difference (from 40 to 120 ml/liter), can account for about an 18-fold increase in maximal O_2 consumption. On the other hand, in patients with varying degrees of cardiac dysfunction, cardiac output fails to rise as much as it does in normal subjects, but as just pointed out, the O_2 extraction reaches the same ceiling of about 120 ml/liter. Such a high O_2 extraction accompanied by lower levels of cardiac output and total $\dot{V}O_2$ reflects the inadequate delivery of O_2 to the metabolizing tissues characteristic of heart failure.

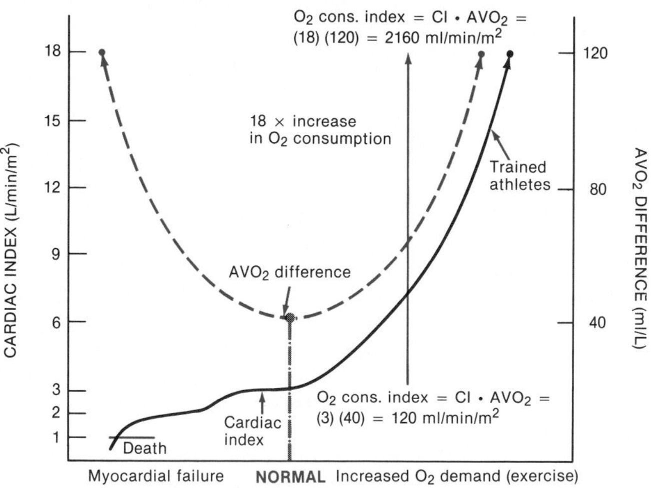

FIGURE 15–2. Relation between arteriovenous oxygen (AVO_2) difference (broken line) and cardiac index (solid curve) in normal subjects at rest (center) and during exercise (right), and in the patient with progressively worsening myocardial failure (left). (From Grossman, W.: Blood flow measurement: The cardiac output. *In* Grossman, W., and Baim, D. S.: Cardiac Catheterization, Angiography and Intervention. 4th ed. Philadelphia, Lea and Febiger, 1990, p. 106.)

INTRACARDIAC PRESSURES. The assessment of cardiac performance can be greatly increased by adding measurement of the ventricular filling pressure* to that of cardiac (or stroke) output. In the basal state, when the ventricular end-diastolic volume is abnormally elevated *and* cardiac performance (expressed as cardiac [or stroke] index or work) is depressed, myocardial contractility is impaired. An elevation of ventricular filling *pressure* does not necessarily indicate an elevation of end-diastolic volume, since ventricular distensibility may be reduced (Fig. 13–28, p. 371; see also p. 402). Such a reduction of compliance may be caused by pericardial disease, restrictive endocardial or myocardial disease, cardiac hypertrophy, or myocardial ischemia; it can be responsible for an elevation of the ventricular filling pressure while end-diastolic volume remains normal. Therefore, an abnormally elevated left ventricular filling pressure in the presence of a normal cardiac index or stroke work does not necessarily signify an impairment of contractility. Conversely, chronic volume overload may displace the ventricular diastolic pressure-volume curve so that volume is elevated at a normal end-diastolic pressure (Fig. 14–5, p. 398). Thus changes in the ventricle's diastolic pressure-volume relations can complicate interpretation of ventricular filling pressure and thereby the assessment of cardiac function on the basis of the relation between filling pressure and cardiac output or work.

Despite these problems, the combination of ventricular end-diastolic pressure and cardiac output or work often is helpful in assessing ventricular function (Fig. 15–1). For example, the combination of a normal cardiac index (>2.5 liters/min/m^2) and ventricular filling pressure (<12 mm Hg) is a far more accurate indicator of normal contractility than is either measurement alone. An obvious limitation of this combination of measurements emerges when cardiac output (or work) is depressed while left ventricular filling pressure is within the normal range. Such findings could reflect either a depression of contractility or a reduction of preload, perhaps caused by hypovolemia, in the presence of normal contractility.

---

* Ventricular filling pressure refers to ventricular end-diastolic pressure, or an index thereof. In the absence of disease of the atrioventricular valve, this is reflected in the mean atrial or, preferably, the atrial pressure at the onset of ventricular contraction, often termed the z point. In the case of the left ventricle, the mean pulmonary capillary wedge pressure or, in the case of the right ventricle, the central venous pressure provides a reasonably accurate approximation of ventricular end-diastolic pressure. When there is a tall *a* wave, the ventricular end-diastolic pressure exceeds the mean atrial pressure, and when there is a tall *v* wave, the mean atrial pressure exceeds the ventricular end-diastolic pressure. When pulmonary vascular resistance is normal, the pulmonary artery diastolic pressure is similar to the pulmonary capillary wedge pressure.

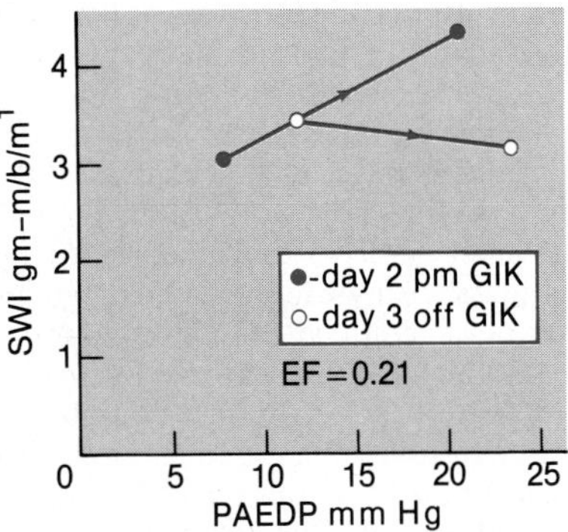

FIGURE 15-3. The hemodynamic effect of glucose-insulin-potassium (GIK) solution on left ventricular (LV) function is shown by the slope of the ventricular function curve in a patient with acute myocardial infarction. After the patient had been on the GIK solution for 2 days, the slope of the function curve was steeper than on day 3, 24 hours after the GIK solution had been discontinued. These changes indicate the positive inotropic effect of the metabolic solution on the viable and/or marginally ischemic myocardium surrounding the infarction site. Ventricular function is expressed as the relation between pulmonary artery end-diastolic pressure (PAEDP), reflecting left ventricular filling pressure and left ventricular stroke work index (SWI). (From Rackley, C. E., Russell, R. O., Jr., Rogers, W. J., et al.: Clinical experience with glucose-insulin-potassium therapy in acute myocardial infarction. Am. Heart J. *102*:1038, 1981.)

One approach to overcoming these problems is to measure cardiac performance (cardiac or stroke index or work) both in the basal state and after preload has been raised by an increase in intravascular volume. An elevation of preload normally is accompanied by an increase in cardiac output or cardiac work, i.e., the product of cardiac output and the difference between arterial and atrial pressures. In addition, the effects of an intervention on the slope of the relation between filling pressure and cardiac work can be evaluated. For example, as shown in Figure 15-3, in a patient recovering from myocardial infarction, cessation of the infusion of glucose-insulin-potassium depressed the slope of the line relating an index of ventricular filling pressure to the stroke work index,[8] a change that may be interpreted as a depression of contractility. This approach to the assessment of ventricular function commonly is used in the intensive care unit. In patients who have low cardiac output and/or hypotension, determining the response of the cardiac output, arterial pressure, and pulmonary capillary wedge pressure to a rapid expansion of blood volume will indicate whether the depression of ventricular performance is due to hypovolemia or left ventricular failure.

MEASUREMENTS OF VENTRICULAR VOLUME

Given the importance of changes in the diastolic properties of the ventricle to analyses of the pumping function of the ventricle in many circumstances, it is of importance that measurement of ventricular end-diastolic *volume* may be required in addition to that of *filling pressure* in the assessment of left ventricular function. Angiographic techniques, described below, provide the most widely accepted means for measuring ventricular cavity volumes as well as wall thickness. They allow calculation of the extent and velocity of wall shortening and the assessment of regional wall motion. When they are combined with measurements of intraventricular pressure and wall thickness, wall tension can be calculated and both ventricular stiffness and afterload (i.e., the force acting within the wall that opposes shortening) can be determined. Such calculations permit left ventricular performance to be analyzed in terms used for describing isolated heart muscle (Chap. 13). When the results are expressed in units corrected for muscle length or circumferences of the ventricle, comparisons can be made between patients with widely differing heart sizes. Although noninvasive techniques are now widely used in the assessment of ventricular volume or dimensions, their application to the assessment of cardiac function is based on the earlier work using ventricular angiography, which remains the benchmark and standard for these measurements.

Quantitative Angiocardiography

Angiography can be carried out using either large cut films or, much more commonly, cineangiograms (single-plane or biplane).[9] Cineangiography provides a larger number of sequential observations per unit of time (30 to 60 frames per second), whereas the large cut films produce sharper margins of the opacified chambers with improved edge detection but are exposed less frequently (6 to 12 per second). Although contrast material can be injected into the pulmonary artery and left atrium, the left ventricle is outlined more clearly by means of direct injection into its cavity. Therefore, this latter mode is used in most patients, except in those with severe aortic regurgitation in whom the contrast material may be injected into the aorta, with the resultant reflux outlining the left ventricular cavity. Digital subtraction angiography utilizing injections into a peripheral vein, pulmonary artery, or left ventricle also may be used.[10,11]

Unless the effects of premature contractions and of the resultant postextrasystolic potentiation are to be examined specifically,[12] ventricular irritability should be avoided during injection of the contrast material. Contact should be avoided between the tip of the catheter and the myocardium, and a multiholed catheter used to diminish the impact of the jet of contrast agent striking the endocardium. If premature contractions are induced, the results are subject to serious misinterpretation, since the premature contraction itself and the first and second postpremature beats may exhibit marked changes in cardiac function. The premature ventricular contraction also may induce mitral and/or tricuspid regurgitation. However, because the contrast material usually is injected within 2 or 3 seconds and filming is carried out for 5 to 8 seconds, one or two cardiac cycles usually are available for analysis, even if a single premature contraction occurs at the beginning of the injection. Multiple premature contractions during filming make the angiogram virtually useless in assessing ventricular performance. Injections usually are made at 10 to 15 ml/sec using a total volume of contrast of 30 to 55 ml, depending on the estimated ventricular size.

Injection of the contrast agent does not begin to produce hemodynamic changes (except for premature beats) until about the sixth beat after injection.[13] The hyperosmolarity produced by the contrast agent increases the blood volume, which begins to raise preload and heart rate within 30 seconds of the injection, an effect that may persist for as long as 2 hours. Regular contrast agents (so-called ionic agents, such as meglumine diatrizoate) also depress contractility directly; newer nonionic agents such as iohexol are useful in minimizing these adverse effects and should be used in patients with marked elevations of left ventricular end-diastolic pressures (>25 mm Hg). Digital subtraction techniques also are useful, since they allow the injection of much smaller quantities of contrast agent and still provide excellent resolution.[10]

When multiple observations made under comparable conditions are desired, it is essential to monitor hemodynamics to ensure that they have returned to control levels before the angiogram is repeated. Ordinarily, the exposure of each cineangiographic frame is recorded and related to a simultaneously recorded electrocardiogram and intracardiac pressure pulse.

In calculating ventricular volumes or dimensions from angiograms, it is essential to take into account and apply appropriate correction factors for magnification as well as for distortion resulting from nonparallel x-ray beams (pincushion distortion).[14,15] To apply these correction factors, care must be exercised to determine with accuracy the tube-to-patient and tube-to-film distances. With cine technique, correction is best accomplished by filming a calibrated grid at the position of the ventricle.[16]

Noninvasive Methods

Cardiac catheterization and quantitative selective angiography are the standard tools for evaluating the function and contractility of the heart, but these invasive procedures are not free of discomfort or slight risk and, most important, they usually are not suitable for repeated application at intervals in the same patient. Therefore, a continuing search has been made for reliable noninvasive methods of assessing cardiac performance.[17] Such methods are needed particularly for detecting *serial* changes in cardiac function and in evaluating both acute and chronic effects of interventions such as drug therapy and cardiac operations. Discussed elsewhere in this book are the four principal noninvasive methods for assessing cardiac performance: echocardiography (p. 64),[18,21a] radionuclide angiography (p. 204),[22-23a] ultrafast computed tomography (CT scanning) (p. 11),[24,24a] and gated magnetic resonance imaging (MRI).[25,25a] All of these are alternatives to contrast angiography for measurement of ventricular volumes and/or dimensions, and therefore permit the noninvasive estimation of ejection phase indices (see below). Other than in patients with obstruction to left ventricular outflow, wall stress (afterload) can be estimated from a combination of systemic arterial pressure, ventricular radius, and wall thickness. All four noninvasive imaging methods allow estimation of ventricular systolic and diastolic volumes and both global and regional ejection fraction (EF).

Mean velocity of circumferential fiber shortening (V_{CF}), a useful index of contractility, especially when combined with a simultaneous estimation of wall stress (p. 379), can be determined simply from measurements of end-diastolic and end-systolic dimensions by echocardiography, CT scanning, or MRI. Because the ventricle is approximately circular at its minor axis, the circumference is equal to diameter (D) $\cdot\ \pi$. Mean V_{CF} (in circumferences per second) is therefore the difference between end-diastolic and end-systolic circumferences (in centimeters) divided by the product of the duration of ejection (in seconds) and the end-diastolic circumference. Values of V_{CF} obtained by echocardiography compare closely with those determined from cineangiograms.

Thus, although the discussion in this chapter refers primarily to measurements made with angiography, they can be readily modified and applied to noninvasive techniques for imaging the ventricles.

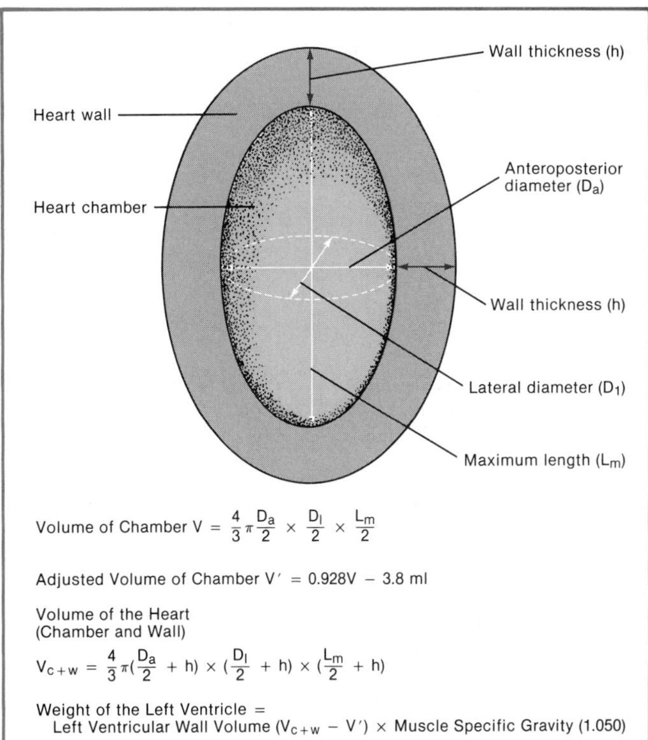

FIGURE 15–4. Diagram showing the approach used to calculate left ventricular volume by means of quantitative angiocardiography. Margins of the projected image of the left ventricular chamber are traced, and maximum length is measured in the anteroposterior and lateral views. Minor axes are derived from the planimetered areas of the chamber in both views; all dimensions are corrected to allow for distortion caused by nonparallel x-rays. Left ventricular volumes are calculated using the formula for the volume of an ellipsoid, since (with regression-equation adjustment) this has given results that tally closely with directly measured ventricular volume. To determine left ventricular mass, volume of the ventricular chamber is subtracted from volume of chamber plus wall; multiplying wall volume by the specific gravity of cardiac muscle converts volume to heart weight or mass. (From Dodge, H. T.: Hemodynamic aspects of cardiac failure. *In* Braunwald, E. [ed.]: The Myocardium: Failure and Infarction. New York, HP Publishing Co., 1974, p. 70.)

Left Ventricular Volume, Mass, and Force

The area-length method developed by Dodge remains the most useful for calculating left ventricular volume (Fig. 15–4).[14] The longest length (L) of the ventricular chamber, i.e., from the apex to the root of the aortic valve, is measured, and the diameter (D) of the ventricle is calculated from the formula $D = 4A/L$, where A = area of left ventricular cavity determined by planimetry. Ordinarily this calculation is made for images exposed in both anteroposterior (AP) and lateral projections. The shape of the left ventricle usually resembles a prolate ellipsoid with one major and two minor diameters.[14,26] With this assumption, left ventricular volume is calculated from the formula

$$V = 4/3\pi\ (L/2) \cdot (D_{AP}/2) \cdot (D_{lat}/2)$$

where V = volume in ml; L = longest length in centimeters in the AP or lateral projections; and D_{AP} and D_{lat} = the diameters (minor axes) calculated from the AP and lateral projections, respectively. These diameters in turn are calculated from the formula for the area of an ellipse (A) as follows:

$$D = \frac{4A}{\pi L}$$

A, the area of the opacified ventricle, can be conveniently determined by a hand or electronic planimeter and an X-Y plotter. The actual ventricular volume is determined from the calculated volume using a regression formula that takes into account the volume occupied by the papillary muscles and chordae tendineae within the ventricular chamber as well as corrections for distortion of x-ray beams (Fig. 15–4). Studies based on human autopsy specimens as well as on models and casts thereof have proved the accuracy of this approach.[9]

It is customary to obtain biplane angiograms in the 30-degree right anterior oblique (RAO) and 60-degree left anterior oblique (LAO) projections. Ventricular volume is calculated using a formula derived elsewhere:[16,27]

$$V = \frac{8}{3\pi} \cdot \frac{A_{RAO} - A_{LAO}}{L_{min}}$$

where L_{min} is the shorter L in the RAO or LAO projections.

Biplane angiographic methods are superior to single-plane methods for the calculation of left ventricular volumes. However, in patients without serious regional wall motion disorders, ventricular aneurysm, or distortion of the ventricular cavity, a reasonable estimate of ventricular volume can be obtained by utilizing either the AP or the RAO projection. Assuming that the two diameters of the left ventricle are equal, ventricular volume is calculated from the formula

$$V = L \cdot D^2 \cdot CF^3 \cdot \pi/6$$

where CF represents a one-dimensional correction factor.[9] Standardization of the degree of obliquity—usually 30-degree RAO and 60-degree LAO—is required for application of any particular correction factor in the calculation of ventricular volume. A close correlation has been found between left ventricular volume determined in the RAO projection and

TABLE 15–1 LEFT VENTRICULAR VOLUME DATA IN PATIENTS

GROUP	NUMBER OF PATIENTS	END-DIASTOLIC VOLUME (ml/m²)	STROKE VOLUME (ml/m²)	MASS (gm/m²)	EJECTION FRACTION
Normal*	—	70 ± 20.0	45 ± 13.0	92 ± 16.0	0.67 ± 0.08
AS	14	84 ± 22.9	44 ± 10.1	172 ± 32.7	0.56 ± 0.17
AR	22	193 ± 55.4	92 ± 30.9	223 ± 73.0	0.56 ± 0.13
AS and AR	13	138 ± 36.5	75 ± 19.1	231 ± 56.9	0.53 ± 0.10
MS	37	83 ± 21.2	43 ± 11.9	98 ± 24.1	0.57 ± 0.14
MR	29	160 ± 53.1	87 ± 21.3	166 ± 49.9	0.47 ± 0.10
MS and MR	29	106 ± 34.4	58 ± 14.7	119 ± 27.8	0.57 ± 0.12
A and M combined	45	130 ± 55.8	69 ± 25.5	156 ± 55.9	0.55 ± 0.12
Myocardial disease	15	199 ± 75.7	44 ± 14.5	145 ± 27.6	0.25 ± 0.09

* Normal values from Kennedy, J. W., et al.: Quantitative angiocardiography. The normal left ventricle in man. Circulation *34*:272, 1966.
AS = aortic valve stenosis with peak systolic pressure gradient > 30 mm Hg.
AR = aortic valve insufficiency with regurgitant flow > 30 ml per beat.
MS = mitral valve area < 1.5 sq cm.
MR = mitral valve regurgitant flow > 20 ml per beat.
A and M combined = combined aortic and mitral valve disease.
Myocardial disease = primary cardiomyopathy or myocardial disease secondary to coronary atherosclerosis.
From Dodge, H. T., and Baxley, W. A.: Left ventricular volume and mass and their significance in heart disease. Am. J. Cardiol. *23*:528, 1969.

true cardiac volume; however, the overestimation of true volume is greater than with the biplane oblique volume method, and appropriate corrections must be made.[16,28]

The normal left ventricular end-diastolic volume averages 70 ± 20 (SD) ml/m² (Table 15–1).[16,29] Left ventricular function ordinarily is considered to be depressed when ventricular end-diastolic volume is clearly elevated (i.e., >110 ml/m², or >2 SD's above the normal average) and *total* stroke volume and/or cardiac index and work are either reduced or within normal limits, while heart rate and arterial pressure are normal.

Left ventricular stroke volume (SV) is calculated as the difference between end-diastolic volume (EDV) and end-systolic volume (ESV). An important validation of the angiographic method for measuring ventricular volume in any laboratory is provided by ensuring that SV, calculated by angiocardiography, correlates closely with that determined by an independent measurement using the Fick or indicator dilution method. When the total SV, determined by angiocardiography, and the effective forward SV, determined by the Fick or indicator dilution method, are not equal, as occurs with aortic or mitral valvular regurgitation or with certain cardiac shunts, the difference between the two represents the regurgitant (or shunt) flow per cardiac cycle.

The ejection fraction (EF) represents the ratio between SV and EDV:

$$EF = \frac{(EDV - ESV)}{EDV} = SV/EDV$$

In the presence of valvular regurgitation, the total SV ejected by the ventricle, i.e., the sum of forward and regurgitant volumes, is used in this calculation. The regurgitant fraction (RF) represents the ratio of regurgitant flow per stroke to the total left ventricular SV:

$$RF = \frac{SV\ total - SV\ forward}{SV\ total}$$

where SV total is determined by angiography and SV forward by the Fick or indicator dilution method.

Because there are errors in both techniques for measuring SV, these errors may summate in the calculation of the regurgitant volume and the regurgitant fraction. Also, when mitral and aortic regurgitation coexist, the regurgitant fraction reflects the sum of the two regurgitant volumes and does not distinguish between them.

Just as the prolate ellipsoid provides a frame of reference for the shape of the left ventricle, the *right ventricle* is shaped like a pyramid with a triangular base, and the formula for deriving the volume of this geometrical figure should be used in the calculation of right ventricular volume.[30] The atria resemble ellipsoids, and their volumes can be determined using the area-length method.[31]

Two-dimensional echocardiography can readily be used to calculate left ventricular end-diastolic volume (EDV). In one approach,[19] $EDV = (D_{max} \times L_{max}/4 \times 4.35) - 6.44$, where D_{max} is the longest minor diameter determined from the parasternal long axis and the apical four-chamber and two-chamber views, and L_{max} is the major long axis derived from the apical views. The EDV, ESV, and EF calculated using this method correlate well with those obtained by biplane angiography.

LEFT VENTRICULAR MASS. This value also can be determined by angiocardiography. Wall thickness, h, as visualized and measured along the free lateral wall of the left ventricle just below the equator at end-diastole (best measured on the AP or RAO projections), is added to the major and minor semiaxes to obtain the sum of volumes of the chamber and wall. This volume minus the chamber volume equals the volume of the wall. The product of wall volume and the specific gravity of heart muscle (1.050) equals left ventricular mass.[29] Thus, left ventricular mass (M) in grams can be calculated from the formula

$$M = \left(\left[4/3 \cdot \pi \frac{(L + 2h)}{2} \cdot \frac{(D_{AP} + 2h)}{2} \cdot \frac{(D_{lat} + 2h)}{2}\right] - V\right) \cdot (1.050)$$

where h = ventricular wall thickness in centimeters; 1.050 = specific gravity of heart muscle; D_{AP} and D_{lat} = the ventricular diameters in centimeters in the AP and lateral views, respectively; and V = left ventricular volume in milliliters. In addition, the ventricular volume must be corrected for the volume of the papillary muscles and trabeculae. A major assumption made with this method and one that undoubtedly introduces some inaccuracy is that left ventricular wall thickness is uniform around the entire left ventricular cavity. However, this method has been appropriately validated by postmortem studies comparing actual and projected left ventricular weights.[16] When single-plane methods are applied, it may be assumed that $D_{AP} = D_{lat}$ and the formula for ventricular mass is

$$M = \frac{\pi}{6} (L + 2h) \frac{4A}{\pi L} + 2h)^2 - V \cdot (1.050)$$

where A = single-plane silhouette area.

Left ventricular mass also can be determined by two-dimensional echocardiography as the difference between total ventricular volume (estimated from the product of the epicardial left ventricular length and the area of the left ventricle in the short axis) and the volume of the left ventricular cavity. This method, too, has been validated against actual ventricular mass.[20] CT scanning and MRI also are useful in determining left ventricular mass.

Left ventricular wall thickness normally averages 10.9 ± 2.0 (SD) mm and left ventricular mass, 92 ± 16 gm/m² (Table

15–1).[9,29] Chronic cardiac dilatation secondary to volume overload or primary myocardial disease increases left ventricular mass, as does chronic pressure overload. Hypertrophy caused by pressure overload is characterized by an increased muscle mass resulting from an augmentation of wall thickness with, at first, little change in ventricular chamber volume (concentric hypertrophy). In contrast, hypertrophy caused by volume overload or by primary myocardial disease is characterized by an increased muscle mass resulting from ventricular dilatation, with only a slight increase in wall thickness (eccentric hypertrophy) (Fig. 14–8, p. 400). There often is a correlation between left ventricular stroke work and left ventricular mass in chronic valvular heart disease, but no such relation exists in primary myocardial disease (Table 15–1).

LEFT VENTRICULAR FORCES. To assess myocardial function, it is necessary to calculate the forces acting on the myocardial fibers within the ventricular wall. This requires knowledge of the dimensions of the left ventricular cavity, wall thickness, and intraventricular pressure.[32] *Tension* (force/cm), which, according to Laplace's law, is a product of the intraventricular pressure and radius (p. 377), may be defined as the force acting on a hypothetical slit in the ventricular wall that would tend to pull its edges apart. *Wall stress*, designated σ, is the force or tension (in dynes) per unit of cross-sectional area of the ventricular wall in square centimeters. Wall stress may be considered to act in three directions—circumferential, meridional, and radial (Fig. 15–5). The most useful calculation is that of *circumferential wall stress*, which is the strongest force generated and supported within the ventricular wall at the equator:

$$\mathrm{CWS} = \frac{(\mathrm{P} \cdot \mathrm{b})}{\mathrm{h}}\left(1 - \frac{\mathrm{h}}{2\mathrm{b}}\right)\left(1 - \frac{\mathrm{hb}}{2\mathrm{a}^2}\right)$$

where CWS = circumferential wall stress in dynes per square centimeter $\times 10^3$; P = left ventricular pressure in dynes per square centimeter; a and b are major and minor semiaxes (i.e., half the longest lengths), respectively, in centimeters, and h = left ventricular wall thickness in square centimeters.[33] Also of value clinically is *meridional wall stress* (MWS), which is calculated as[34]

$$\mathrm{MWS} = \frac{\mathrm{P} \cdot \mathrm{r}}{2\mathrm{h}\,(1 + \mathrm{h}/2\mathrm{r})}$$

where r is the internal radius of the ventricle in centimeters.

Simultaneous recording of an angiogram (preferably biplane) and intraventricular pressure pulse recorded with a high-fidelity micromanometer to avoid the artifacts inherent in the usual catheter–external manometer systems allows

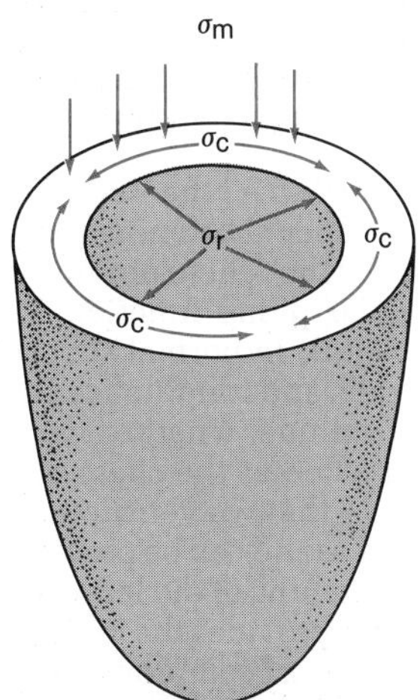

FIGURE 15–5. Circumferential (σ_c), meridional (σ_m), and radial (σ_r) components of left ventricular wall stress from an ellipsoid model. The three components of wall stress are mutually perpendicular. (From Grossman, W.: Pressure measurement. *In* Grossman, W. and Baim, D. S. [ed.]: Cardiac Catheterization and Angiography. 4th ed. Philadelphia, Lea and Febiger, 1990, p. 293.)

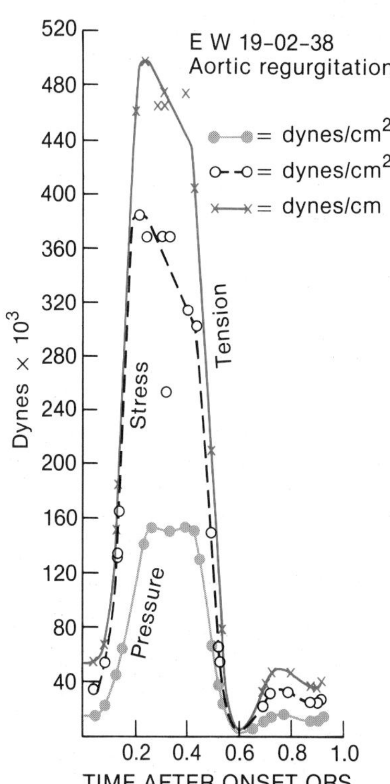

FIGURE 15–6. Sequential changes in left ventricular tension, stress, and pressure are shown throughout the cardiac cycle in a patient with aortic regurgitation. Note that tension, but particularly stress, declines during ejection (i.e., while the left ventricular volume decreases), although left ventricular pressure is maintained. (From Rackley, C. E.: Quantitative evaluation of left ventricular function by radiographic techniques. Circulation *54*:862, 1976, by permission of the American Heart Association, Inc.)

calculation of *left ventricular tension* and *stress* throughout the cardiac cycle.

A simpler method of analyzing the instantaneous left ventricular tension throughout the cardiac cycle consists of recording left ventricular pressure simultaneously with left ventricular diameter across the minor axis of the left ventricle determined by echocardiography. This combination of measurements provides the data necessary to calculate ventricular circumferential fiber shortening (at either the endocardium or the midwall) and midwall circumferential stress, using minor modifications of the equations presented above.[35] However, the use of echocardiography, especially M-mode, for these calculations is based on the assumption of uniform wall motion. This assumption can be made with reasonable assurance only in conditions that affect left ventricular function relatively uniformly, such as dilated cardiomyopathy or aortic or mitral regurgitation. It cannot be made in conditions that produce localized or regional dysfunction, such as ischemic heart disease.

Ventricular *preload* may be expressed as end-diastolic wall stress, and *afterload* as peak or mean systolic wall stress. During ejection, as the left ventricular cavity decreases in size and wall thickness increases, systolic wall stress and tension decline rapidly even though pressure is maintained (Fig. 15–6). *Left ventricular power* can be calculated as the product of intracavitary pressure and the rate of change of ventricular volume. Simultaneously recorded ventricular volumes and pressures during diastole allow the calculation of *left ventricular chamber and muscle compliance* (Fig. 13–28, p. 371).[36]

The use of automated methods has greatly simplified the calculations of all of these variables. For example, videodensitometric analysis of digital subtraction angiograms obtained after intravenous injection can provide in a simple manner an accurate measurement of EF.[10]

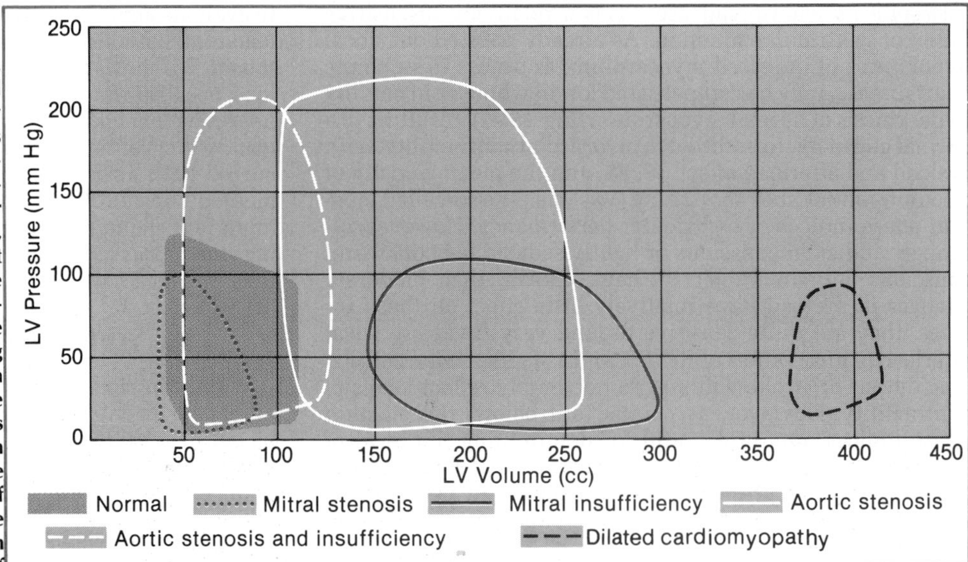

FIGURE 15–10. Left ventricular pressure-volume curves from patients with different varieties of heart disease. The height of each curve is determined by systolic pressure and the width by stroke volume. The two smallest curves —one from a patient with mitral stenosis, the other from a patient with primary cardiomyopathy—indicate similar stroke volumes; however, in the latter, the dilated left ventricle is functioning at an inappropriately large volume, and the ejection fraction is low. The curve in mitral insufficiency demonstrates volume overload by the large excursion along the volume axis and the absence of an isovolumetric contraction period. The shape of the curve in aortic stenosis shows the effect of pressure overload. In aortic stenosis and insufficiency, the curve demonstrates the influence of pressure and volume overload, with the large area subtended by the curve. (From Dodge, H. T.: Hemodynamic aspects of cardiac failure. *In* Braunwald, E. [ed.]: The Myocardium: Failure and Infarction. New York, HP Publishing Co., 1974, p. 70.)

stolic properties.[16] Characteristic changes in the left ventricular pressure-volume loops occur in various disease states (Fig. 15–10).

The left ventricular pressure-volume curve usually is based on ventricular volume measurements using cineventriculography. The use of radionuclide ventriculography,[22,23] or an impedance catheter,[50,51] for the continuous (or almost continuous) measurement of ventricular volume has greatly facilitated the construction of pressure-volume loops, and therefore their application in the assessment of left ventricular function.

VENTRICULAR END-SYSTOLIC PRESSURE-VOLUME RELATIONS

The extent of myocardial fiber shortening reflects the interactions among preload, afterload, and contractility. As already noted, at a constant preload, fiber shortening varies inversely with afterload (Fig. 13–20, p. 365), whereas end-systolic fiber length varies directly with afterload.[52] There is little difference between the end-systolic pressure-volume relation in isovolumetric and ejecting contractions. Indeed, the virtual identity of isometric and isotonic length-tension curves has been demonstrated in isolated cat papillary muscle (Fig. 15–11)[53,54] and in the intact heart (Fig. 13–33, p. 375),[55–57] and forms the basis for evaluating contractility.[58] Thus, at any level of contractility, end-systolic fiber length is a direct function of and varies inversely with afterload and myocardial contractility can be assessed by making use of this fundamental property of heart muscle. This is accomplished in the intact heart by focusing attention on the relationship between the end-systolic volume (ESV), and the simultaneous ventricular pressure, i.e., the end-systolic pressure (ESP). These two measurements are inscribed in the left upper corner of the pressure-volume loop. Because ESV varies inversely and ESP directly with contractility, the latter may be defined by the line relating these two variables.

The end-systolic pressure-volume relations can be obtained from the pressure-volume loop at different loading conditions (Fig. 13–34, p. 376).[59] In laboratory animals, this usually is

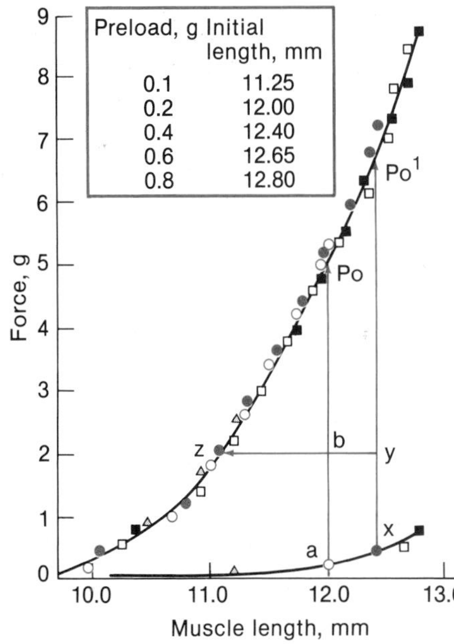

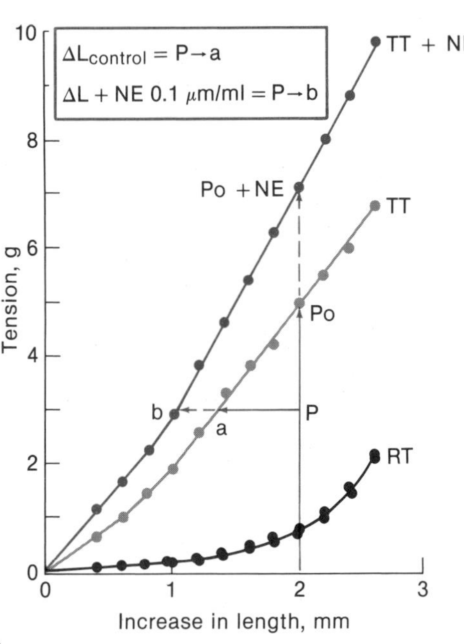

FIGURE 15–11. *A*, Length-tension curve of cat papillary muscle constructed by establishing the initial muscle length with a preload, and recording the extent of shortening against increasing afterloads. Po = total tension developed from initial length, a *(left)*, when the afterload was of such magnitude that shortening did not occur; Po[1] similar to Po but from initial length, x. Note that the muscle shortens to the same point on the active tension curve (z) independent of its initial length so long as the load is constant. Thus the isometric and isotonic length-tension curves are virtually identical. *B, (right)*, Length-tension curves of cat papillary muscle before and after the addition of norepinephrine (NE). The resting length-tension curve is unchanged by the intervention. The extent of isotonic shortening at load P is increased from a to b with addition of NE, while total isometric tension is increased from Po to Po + NE. (From Downing, S. E., and Sonnenblick, E. H.: Cardiac muscle mechanics and ventricular performance: Force and time parameters. Am. J. Physiol. *207*:705, 1964.)

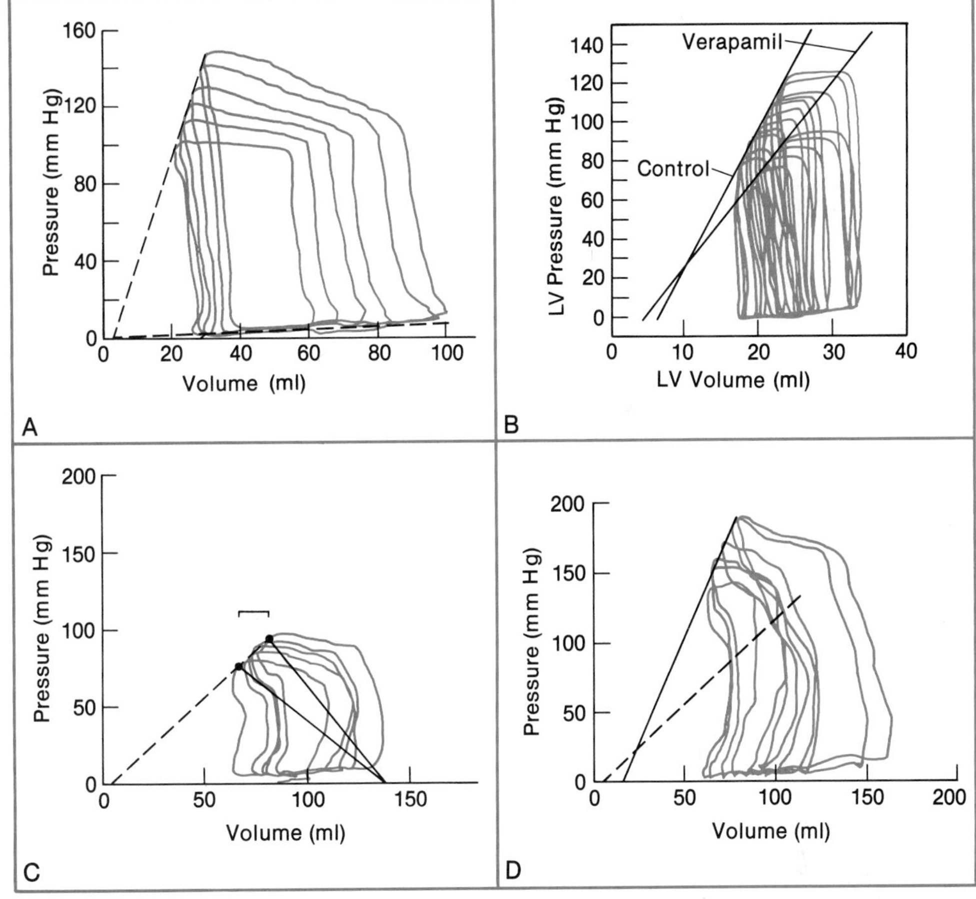

FIGURE 15-12. *A*, Multiple pressure-volume loops obtained during inferior vena cava occlusion in a patient. Pressure volume loops and end-systolic pressure-volume relation (ESPVR). (From Kass, D. A., and Maughan, W. L.: From "Emax" to pressure-volume relations: A broader view. Circulation *77*:1203, 1988.) *B*, Left ventricular pressure-volume loops obtained during caval occlusion during control and with verapamil. After verapamil, the ESPVR is shifted toward the right with a decreased slope. (From Little, W. C., Cheng, C-P., Peterson, T., and Vinten-Johansen, J.: Response of the left ventricular end-systolic pressure-volume relation in conscious dogs to a wide range of contractile states. Circulation *78*:736, 1988.) *C*, Example of use of pressure-volume relations and ESPVR to predict response to vasodilator therapy in a patient with dilated cardiomyopathy. There is a shallow ESPVR slope (1.3 mm Hg/ml), and a 35 per cent reduction in afterload resistance (solid lines) predicted a near 30 per cent increase in stroke volume (indicated by solid brackets above the loops), with little change in systolic pressure. *D*, Response of patient to intravenous dobutamine (10 μg/kg/min). There was a marked shift of the ESPVR (solid line) to the left and a steepening of the slope, consistent with substantial acute contractile reserve. The dashed line represents the control ESPVR. (From Kass, D. A., and Maugham, W. L.: From "Emax" to pressure-volume relations: A broader view. Circulation *77*:1203, 1988, by permission of the American Heart Association, Inc.).

accomplished by volume expansion and vena caval occlusion. In intact human subjects, loading may be altered by infusion of a noninotropic vasoconstrictor such as phenylephrine and/or a vasodilator such as nitroglycerin, or by transient occlusion of the inferior vena cava.

The end-systolic pressure-volume relation (ESPVR) for both isovolumetric and ejecting contractions can be expressed as $P_{es} = E_{es} (V_{es} - V_d)$, where P_{es} and V_{es} are the end-systolic pressure and end-systolic volume, respectively. E (not in the equation) is the ratio of ventricular pressure/volume (systolic ventricular elastance) at any time during the cardiac cycle; the maximum value for E, i.e., E_{max}, occurs near end-systole. E_{es} is the slope of the line joining E_{max} at various loading conditions (the oblique lines in Fig. 15-12); V_d is the intercept of this line on the volume (x) axis. Thus E_{es} is a numerical expression of myocardial contractility; a higher value, i.e., a steeper slope, indicates a smaller end-systolic volume, i.e., more complete systolic emptying, at any given end-systolic pressure. (There is controversy concerning the interpretation of the intercept on the volume axis of the line relating end-systolic pressure to volume.[60]) E_{es} can be measured by rearranging the equation as follows:

$$E_{es} = P_{es}/(V_{es} - V_d)$$

P_{es} and V_{es} can be measured relatively easily in patients; the determination of V_d requires measurement of P_{es} and V_{es} from contractions at a constant contractility but at different afterloads.

Although measurements of P_{es} appear to be useful clinically,[52] pressure is not an accurate estimate of end-systolic afterload. Rather, it is more accurate to use end-systolic wall

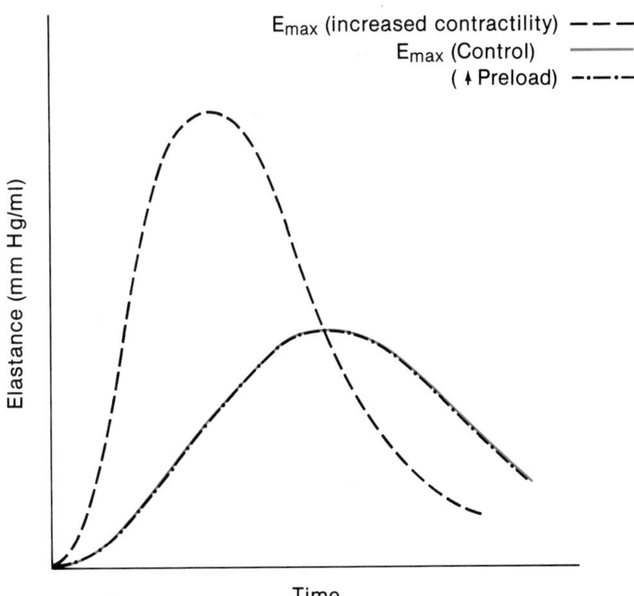

FIGURE 15-13. Plot of the ratio of pressure to volume (elastance) in a series of contractions that demonstrate the sensitivity of this index to increases in contractility (dashed lines) and insensitivity of the index to increases of preload (dot-dash line). Note that the amplitude of peak elastance in a given contraction increases with increases in contractility, and the time to peak elastance is shortened. (From Strobeck, J. E., and Sonnenblick, E. H.: Pathophysiology of heart failure. *In* Cohn, J. N.: Drug Treatment of Heart Failure. 2nd ed. Secaucus, NJ, Advanced Therapeutics Communications International, 1988, p. 31.)

intraventricular pressure, cavity diameter, and thickness.[69] The instantaneous ratio of ventricular pressure to volume (also termed the systolic ventricular elastance, E) varies throughout systole and is expressed in mm Hg/ml.[71–73] The maximum level of E (E_{max}),[75–77] i.e., the peak of the time-elastance curve, occurs near the end of systole and provides the basis for determining the end-systolic pressure–volume relation (ESPVR) (Figs. 15–12 and 15–13). E_{max} is insensitive to ventricular preload,[78,79] incorporates afterload, and is exquisitely sensitive to changes in contractility.[80–82] This provides a useful approach to assessing myocardial contractility. There are some limitations to the use of E_{max}, including slight dependency on ventricular size, cavity shape, and slight nonlinearity of the ESPVR,[80–82] as well as measurement variability.[75–77] Nonetheless, the ESPVR provides a useful clinical method for the assessment of myocardial contractility because it permits loading factors to be *relatively* well separated from the ventricle's intrinsic contractility.

Figure 15–12*A* demonstrates multiple pressure-volume loops obtained with a conductance catheter in a patient in whom a primary reduction in preload was achieved by progressive occlusion of the inferior vena cava; the linear nature of the ESPVR is evident. Figure 15–14 *A* shows the effects of occlusion of the distal left anterior descending coronary artery on pressure-volume relations in the intact canine heart. Rightward displacement of the ESPVR is evident. Figure 15–14 *B* demonstrates how the ESPVR can be used to grade the depression of contractility; with increasing ischemia, produced by occlusion of coronary arteries perfusing progressively larger segments of myocardium, the ESPVR becomes progressively more depressed and curvilinear.[82a]

Figure 15–15 shows left ventricular pressure-volume loops in a normal subject and in a patient with a dilated cardiomyopathy. The slope of the ESPVR in the latter was reduced.

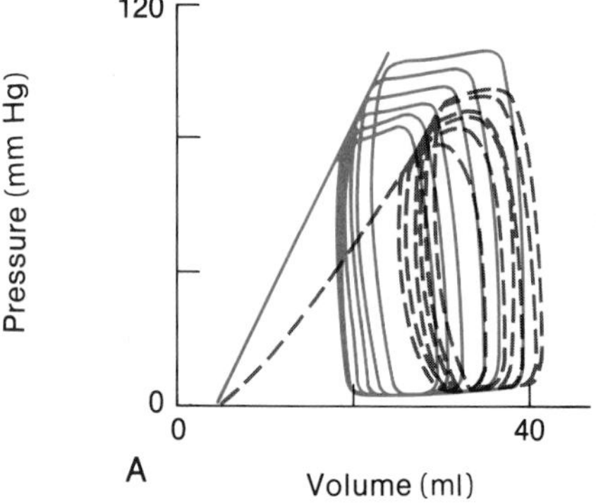

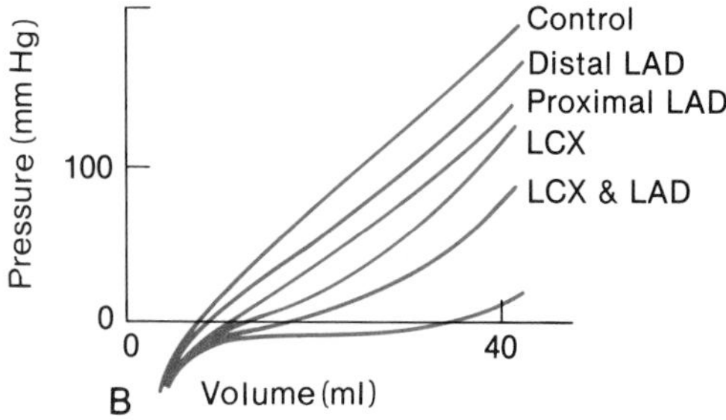

FIGURE 15–14. ***A,*** **Intact canine heart data displaying shift in ESPVR with distal LAD occlusion. Over the range of data obtained, the ESPVR appears shifted rightward with little change in Ees. The dashed line represents the theoretical ESPVR based on isolated heart data. LCX = left circumflex artery.** ***B,*** **Isolated canine heart data showing the effects of regional ischemia on ESPVR. With increasing extents of ischemia, the ESPVR becomes more curvilinear. (*****A*** **from Kass, D. A., and Maugham, W. L.: From "Emax" to pressure-volume relations: A broader view. Circulation** ***77*****:1203, 1988;** ***B*** **from Sunagawa, K., Maugham, W. L., and Sagawa, K.: Effect of regional ischemia on the left ventricular end-systolic pressure-volume relationship of isolated canine hearts. Circ. Res.** ***52*****:170, 1983, by permission of the American Heart Association, Inc.)**

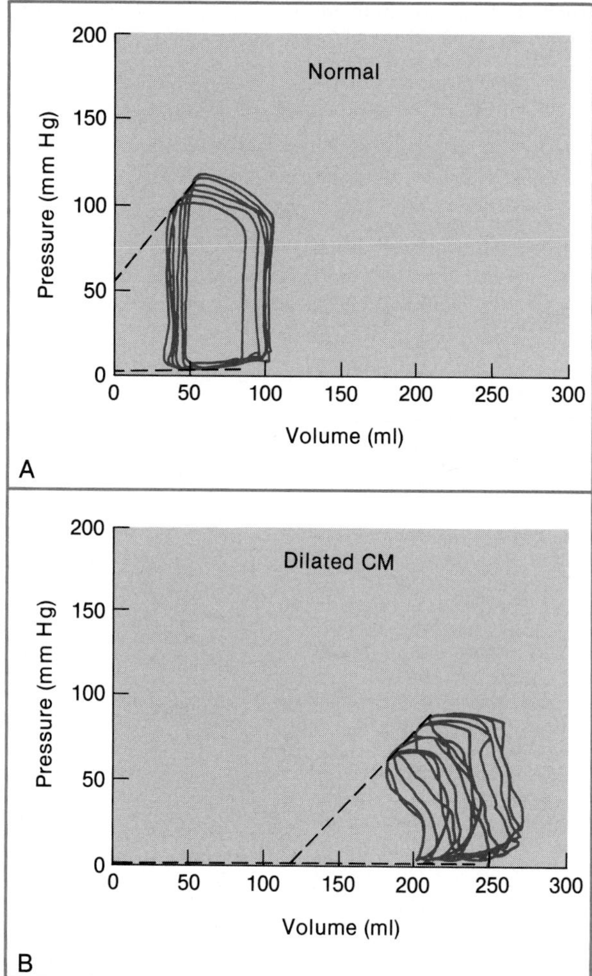

FIGURE 15–15. Examples of pressure-volume relations (PVR) in three patients. ***Panel A,*** **A typical relation in a healthy person with a flat diastolic PVR, and moderately steep end-systolic pressure-volume relation (ESPVR).** ***Panel B,*** **A patient with dilated cardiomyopathy. The loops are shifted to high volumes, with a flat ESPVR and steeper EDPVR. (From Kass, D. A.: Evaluation of left ventricular systolic function. Heart Failure** ***4*****:198, 1988.)**

Figure 15–12*D* demonstrates the improvement in myocardial contractility that occurs with an infusion of dobutamine. In contrast, Figure 15–12*B* shows the effects of the infusion of large doses of verapamil in intact conscious dogs by caval occlusion. A depression of the ESPVR is evident.

There appear to be a number of theoretical advantages to the use of the slope of the end-systolic pressure-(stress)-volume (dimension) relation (E_{es}) in assessment of myocardial contractility.[60,82b] First, because afterload is already incorporated into the calculation of E_{es}, any observed changes in this variable assess contractility directly; in contrast, the ejection phase indices provide a complex mixture of contractility and afterload. Second, because E_{es} is independent of preload, difficulties with the ejection phase indices that are affected by end-diastolic volume are obviated. This is especially the case in the presence of mitral regurgitation, with its marked changes in afterload and preload.[61,68]

SIMPLIFICATIONS. The use of the slope of the end-systolic pressure volume relation for the assessment of myocardial contractility can be further simplified by determining V_{es} noninvasively. Radionuclide angiography,[22,23] an impedance (volume) catheter technique,[50,51] and M-mode or two-dimensional echocardiography[18,21,69,83,84] have been used. In the absence of obstruction to left ventricular outflow, cuff pressure can be used to estimate ventricular systolic pressure. An indirect carotid pulse can indicate end-systole, and, together with cuff pressure, provides a noninvasive assessment of the end-systolic pressure.

This approach can be simplified further by determining the ratio of peak systolic pressure to end-systolic volume, the numerator determined by sphygmomanometry and the denominator by radionuclide ventriculography.[85] In normal subjects, this ratio rises markedly during exercise but fails to do so in patients with left ventricular dysfunction.[86] An even simpler, albeit less accurate, assessment of contractility may be provided by the end-systolic volume (or end-systolic dimension) at the operating end-systolic pressure, if the latter is normal or almost so. Under these circumstances, the end-systolic volume (corrected for body surface area) correlates inversely with contractility.[52,57] Indeed, end-systolic volume has been reported to be the major determinant of survival after recovery from myocardial infarction.[62]

Recording of serial pressure-volume loops, using first-pass radionuclide left ventriculography, has been found to be useful in the postoperative state.[63] Noninvasively determined end-systolic pressure (or stress)-volume (or dimension) relations have been found to be useful in defining patients with congestive heart failure[64,87] and in providing information of prognostic value.[65] Left ventricular pressure-volume loops also can be recorded by means of an impedance catheter and preload varied by transient inferior vena caval occlusion.[66,67]

ISOVOLUMETRIC PHASE INDICES OF CONTRACTILITY

VENTRICULAR dP/dt

Changes in the maximum rate of rise of ventricular pressure (peak dP/dt) are highly sensitive to acute *changes* in contractility (Fig. 15–16).[88–90] Therefore, measurement of this variable may be used along with ventricular end-diastolic volume and filling pressure in the assessment of *directional changes* in contractility. Peak dP/dt cannot be reliably measured with the catheter-manometer systems ordinarily used during cardiac catheterization, unless special precautions are taken to prevent artifacts and the frequency response of the system is carefully determined.[91] High-fidelity catheter-tip micromanometers should be used, but even with these, great care must be taken to avoid artifacts caused by flicking catheter motion during the cardiac cycle.

Peak dP/dt is largely independent of changes in afterload, provided that it occurs *before* aortic valve opening.[48,92] Studies in dogs[93] and humans[94] have shown that peak dP/dt is little changed by steady-state alterations in aortic pressure, and although it appears to be much more markedly affected by changes in contractility than by alterations in preload, the influence of the latter cannot be disregarded. Therefore, even when contractility is constant, major changes in preload can cause modest alterations in dP/dt in the same direction. Another difficulty with the use of peak dP/dt as an index of contractility is that it cannot be corrected for changes in muscle mass produced by ventricular hypertrophy. This difficulty can be surmounted, however, by calculating the peak rate of stress development ($d\sigma/dt$).[95] Although the absolute level of peak dP/dt correlates with the basal level of contractility, it is not as useful for assessing this property of cardiac function as are the ejection phase indices (see below). Instead, peak dP/dt is more useful in assessing *directional* changes in contractility with acute interventions. Significant increases in peak left ventricular dP/dt have been demonstrated with isometric and dynamic exercise,[95] with tachycardia produced by atrial pacing and atropine,[97] by beta adrenoceptor agonists, and by digitalis glycosides.[98]

OTHER ISOVOLUMETRIC PHASE INDICES (Table 15–2). V_{max}, the maximum velocity of shortening of the unloaded contractile elements (CE) (p. 364), theoretically provides a measure of myocardial contractility which is independent of preload or afterload. Controversy continues to surround calculation of CE V_{max}, in isolated muscle and even more so in the intact heart, in which the calculation must be based on many assumptions.[99] Despite these difficulties, observations in the intact left ventricle (p. 380) indicate that its V_{max}, determined by extrapolation of the force-velocity relation derived from multiple variably afterloaded beats, is, like the V_{max} of isolated cardiac muscle, not altered significantly by changes of preload within the physiological range, but is markedly sensitive to inotropic stimuli (Figs. 13–21 and 13–22, p. 366).[94]

V_{max}. It is obviously impractical in patients to determine V_{max} in either variably afterloaded or completely isovolumetric beats. However, a mathematical derivation of CE V_{max}, V_{CE}, can be obtained in the normally ejecting heart using only the isovolumetric phase of contraction and using one of the isovolumetric phase indices described below. In one approach that has been applied clinically,[100] V_{CE} is calculated as dP/dt/KP, (where K is an assumed stiffness constant for the series elastic element (p. 366) and is plotted against instantaneous wall stress. Instantaneous wall stress is calculated from intraventricular pressure, volume, and wall thickness) during the isovolumetric phase of left ventricular systole, and the curve is then extrapolated to zero stress to obtain V_{max}. If it is further assumed that contraction of the myocardium during isovolumetric contraction is truly isometric, then pressure and wall stress are linearly related to each other, and no calculation of wall stress is required to determine V_{max}[101]; calculated V_{CE} is simply plotted against the instantaneous intraventricular pressure and extrapolated to zero pressure. This index of V_{max} is relatively independent of acute changes in preload at low left ventricular end-diastolic pressure,[102] but declines at end-diastolic pressures exceeding 10 mm Hg.[103]

Relation Between dP/dt and Developed Pressure. Some of the difficulties cited above involving the calculation of V_{max} can be partially avoided by the selection of certain points on the curve relating dP/dt to DP, where DP is the *developed* left ventricular pressure (i.e., left ventricular pressure minus end-diastolic pressure). The dP/dt at a DP of 40 mm Hg, a level of pressure which, in most clinical circumstances, occurs before the opening

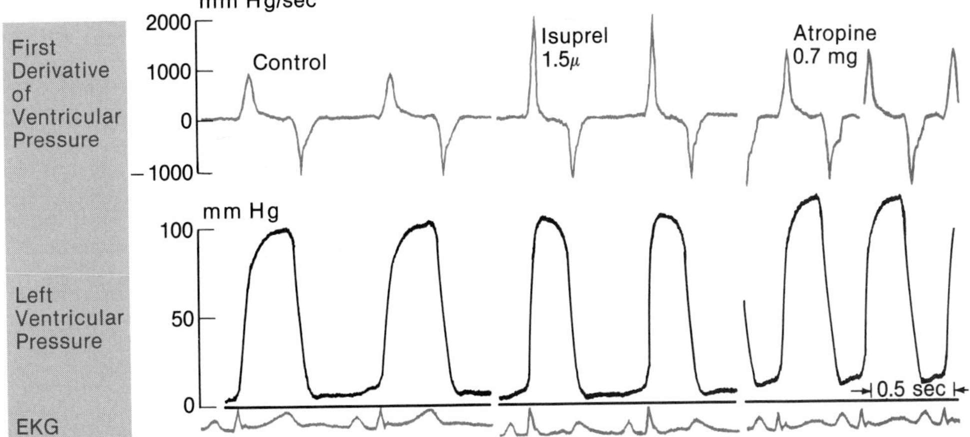

FIGURE 15–16. Serial recordings of left ventricular pressure and of the first derivative of left ventricular pressure (dP/dt) in a 12-year-old girl with mild pulmonic valvular stenosis. The first record (control) is in the basal state, the middle record after the administration of 1.5 µg isoproterenol, and the final record after 0.7 mg atropine. (Reproduced from Gleason, W. L., and Braunwald, E.: Studies on the first derivative of the ventricular pressure pulse in man. J. Clin. Invest. *41*:80, 1962, by copyright permission of the American Society for Clinical Investigation.)

TABLE 15-2 EVALUATION OF LEFT VENTRICULAR PERFORMANCE: NORMAL VALUES FOR SOME ISOVOLUMIC AND EJECTION PHASE INDICES

INDICES	NORMAL VALUES (MEAN ± SD)
SYSTOLE	
Isovolumic Indices:	
Maximum dP/dt	1650 ± 300
Maximum (dP/dt)/P)	$44 \pm 8.4\ sec^{-1}$
V_{PM} or peak $\left[\frac{dP/dt}{28P}\right]$	1.47 ± 0.19 ml/sec
(dP/dt)/DP at DP = 40 mm Hg	$37.6 \pm 12.2\ sec^{-1}$
Ejection Phase Indices:	
LVSW	81 ± 23 gm·m
LVSWI	$47 \pm 17\ gm \cdot m/m^2$
EF angio:	0.72 ± 0.08
MNSR angio:	3.32 ± 0.84 EDV/sec
echo:	2.29 ± 0.30 EDV/sec
Mean V_{CF} angio:	1.50 ± 0.27 ED circ/sec
echo:	1.09 ± 0.12 ED circ/sec
DIASTOLE	
Peak −dP/dt	1825-2900 ± 500 mm Hg/sec
T (tau) −logarithmic method:	34 ± 6 msec
−derivative method:	51 ± 11 msec
PFR	3.3 ± 0.6 EDV/sec
Time to PFR	136 ± 23 msec
Peak −dh/dt (posterior wall)	8.3 ± 3.4 cm/sec

dP/dt = rate of rise of left ventricular (LV) pressure; DP = developed LV pressure; ML = muscle lengths; MNSER = mean normalized systolic ejection rate; ED = end-diastolic; V = volume; circ = circumference; EF = ejection fraction.

Adapted from Grossman, W., and Baim, D.: Evaluation of systolic and diastolic function of the myocardium. *In* Grossman W., and Baim, D. (eds.): Cardiac Catheterization and Angiography. 4th ed. Philadelphia, Lea and Febiger, 1990, pp. 326-327. Original references for each item are given in Grossman and Baim, p. 307.

of the aortic valve is commonly used. Although somewhat less sensitive to acute changes in contractility than is simple peak dP/dt, dP/dt at a DP of 40 mm Hg, is, nonetheless, useful for assessing *directional* changes in contractility,[48,104,105] since it is unaffected by changes in afterload and is relatively insensitive to changes in preload. The maximum dP/dt/DP, termed V_{pm}, also is relatively independent of both preload and afterload but is quite insensitive to changes in the inotropic state.[106] It has been advocated as an index of the contractility in the basal state, as discussed further below.

Curves relating DP to dP/dt, and preferably developed stress (dσ) to the rate of stress development (dσ/dt) during isovolumetric contraction, are particularly useful isovolumetric indices of contractility.

ASSESSMENT OF CONTRACTILITY

DIRECTIONAL CHANGES IN CONTRACTILITY

When loading of the ventricle is constant, myocardial fiber shortening varies directly with and reflects myocardial contractility. Stated in another way, at constant levels of preload and afterload, various measures of left ventricular performance, such as the ejection phase indices (EF, peak and mean fiber shortening rate [FS] and the velocity of circumferential fiber shortening [V_{CF}]) as well as stroke volume, stroke work, and stroke power, all are functions of myocardial contractility. Thus, it is safe to conclude that an improvement in contractility has occurred if one of these indices increases while ventricular filling pressure or end-diastolic volume (reflecting preload) remains unchanged or declines and aortic pressure (reflecting afterload) remains unchanged or rises.

The absolute levels of ventricular filling pressure do not correlate with end-diastolic volume in *chronic* heart disease because of the effect of the latter on ventricular diastolic pressure-volume relations (Fig. 15-10).[29,107] *Acute* changes in ventricular filling pressure reflect directional changes in end-diastolic volume (except in the presence of acute myocardial ischemia or marked tachycardia). Therefore, when the effect

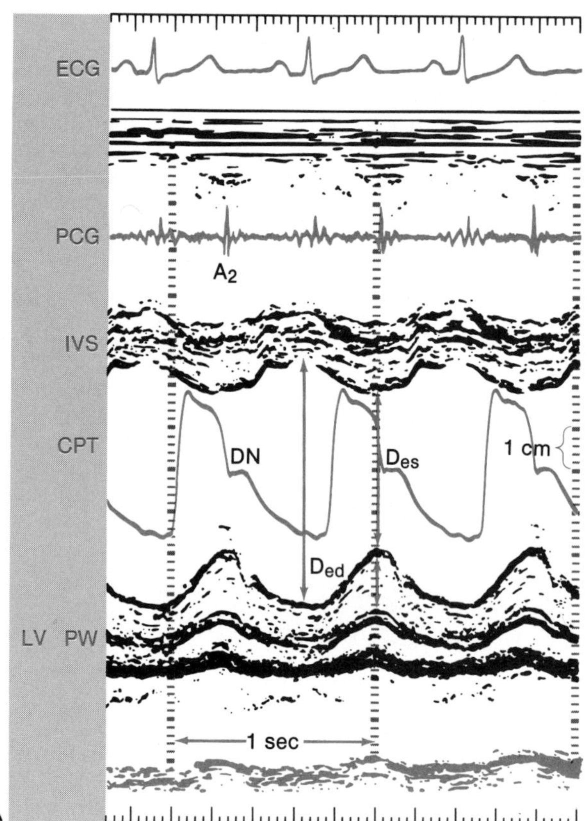

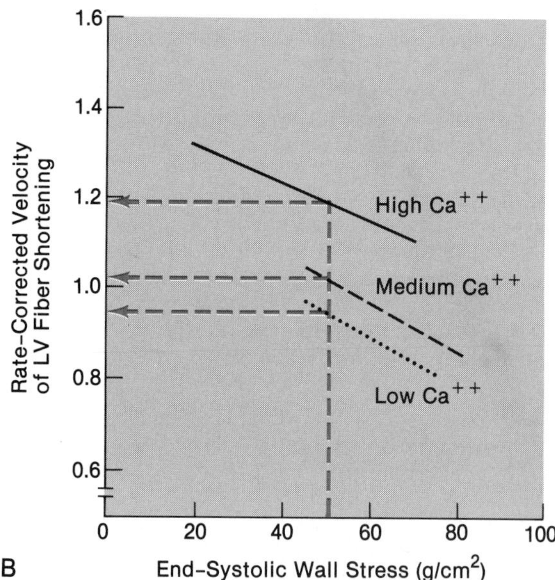

FIGURE 15-17. ***A,*** **Two-dimensionally-targeted M-mode echocardiogram from a representative patient. ECG = electrocardiogram; PCG = phonocardiogram; IVS = intraventricular septum; CPT = carotid pulse tracing; LV PW = left ventricular posterior wall; DN = dicrotic notch; D_{es} = end-systolic dimension; D_{ed} = end-diastolic dimension. *B,* Representative left ventricular end-systolic wall stress and rate-corrected velocity of fiber shortening in circ. (sec.) data showing method of data analysis. Low serum Ca^{++} concentration is represented by dotted line, medium Ca^{++} by dashed line, and high Ca^{++} by solid line. Correlation coefficient for each linear regression line was 0.90 or greater. (From Lang, R. M., Fellner, S. K., Neumann, A., et al.: Left ventricular contractility varies directly with blood ionized calcium. Ann. Intern. Med. *108*:524, 1988.)**

of an intervention is studied, a change in ventricular filling pressure may be related to a change in one of the hemodynamic measures of left ventricular performance enumerated above, to assess directional changes of contractility.[55,107] For instance, an intervention that is associated with a reduction of a constant filling pressure and an elevation of stroke work, while afterload remains constant, usually signifies an improvement in myocardial contractility; the converse also is true.

The end-systolic pressure (or stress) to end-systolic volume (or dimension) relation described above (Fig. 15–12) and the relation between ejection fraction (or the fractional shortening of the left ventricle) and left ventricular end-systolic wall stress (Fig. 15–17) are special cases of ejection phase indices. They are superior to the "classic" ejection phase indices, such as EF, FS, and V_{CF}, in that they correct, at least in part, for variations in loading conditions.

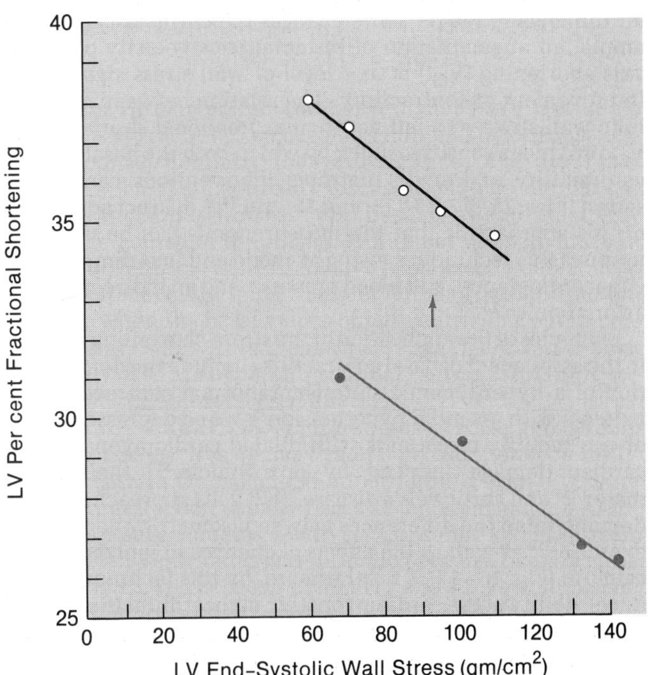

FIGURE 15–19. Comparison of the LV end-systolic wall stress-shortening lines joining points at different afterloads for control (closed circles) and increased (open circles) contractile states produced by dobutamine in a representative subject. With the dobutamine infusion, the percentage of ΔD is higher for any level of end-systolic wall stress. (From Borow, K. M., Green, L. H., Grossman, W., and Braunwald, E.: Left ventricular end-systolic stress-shortening and stress-length relations in humans. Am. J. Cardiol. *50*:1301, 1982.)

CONTRACTILITY IN THE BASAL STATE

ISOVOLUMETRIC PHASE INDICES. As already stated, these indices—peak dP/dt, $dP/dt/DP_{40}$, V_{pm}, and V_{max}—usually are of little value in assessing *basal levels* of contractility and in *comparing* contractility among different patients or in any given patient at different times.[108] However, they are exquisitely sensitive to *changes* in the inotropic state. V_{pm}, i.e., the maximum velocity of myocardial shortening, calculated at the maximum (dP/dt)DP, is superior to the others in separating *groups* of patients with normal or depressed contractility. However, even this index is not always reliable in establishing basal levels of contractility in individual patients.[109]

CONTRACTILITY INDICES BASED ON THE FORCE-VELOCITY RELATION. The myocardial force-velocity relation (Fig. 13–21, p. 366) provides a framework for the assessment of contractility of isolated cardiac muscle. Efforts have been made to apply this framework to clinical circumstances. The relation between percentage of fractional myocardial fiber shortening, determined noninvasively, and left ventricular end-systolic stress,[75] obtained in the basal state (Fig. 15–17), sometimes supplemented by the measurements made during a pharmacologically altered afterload (Fig. 15–18), provides a useful, practical framework for assessing the basal level of left ventricular contractility.[110–114] This relation is particularly useful in patients who have reduced ejection fraction indices and distinguishes between reduced myocardial shortening due to excessive afterload and that due to depressed myocardial contractility.

The end-systolic stress-mean V_{CF} relation at various levels of wall stress is preload-independent (and obviously incorporates afterload). Thus changes in the relation between the extent (or velocity) of myocardial wall shortening and the simultaneous ventricular wall stress σ (at any given ventricu-

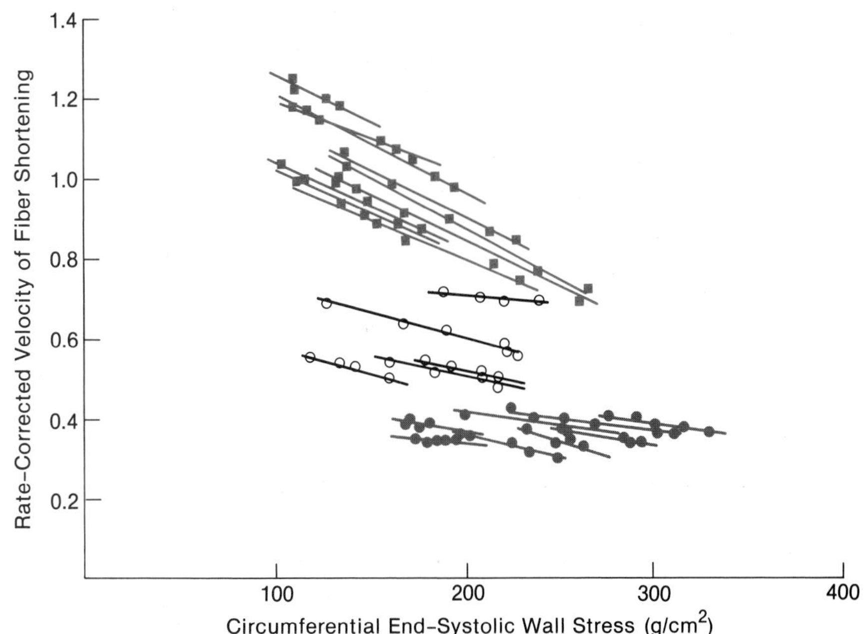

FIGURE 15–18. Plot of Vcf_c (velocity of fiber shortening) versus circumferential stress obtained over a wide range of left ventricular afterloads for normal subjects (■--■) and group 1 (○--○) and group 2 patients (●--●). At any level of σ_{es}, marked intergroup differences in Vcf_c are present. This is characteristic of a decrease in left ventricular contractility for the group 1 and group 2 patients independent of left ventricular loading conditions. (From Borow, K. M., Lang, R. M., Neumann, A., et al.: Physiologic mechanisms governing hemodynamic responses to positive inotropic therapy in patients with dilated cardiomyopathy. Circulation *77*:625, 1988, by permission of the American Heart Association, Inc.)

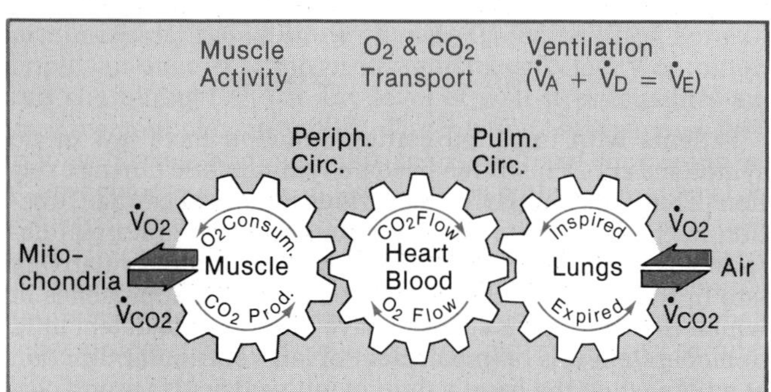

FIGURE 15–21. Diagram showing interaction of physiological mechanisms coupling external to cellular respiration. Central role of circulation explains why cardiovascular diseases cause abnormalities in O_2 transport and O_2 uptake kinetics. O_2 consum., O_2 consumption; CO_2 prod., CO_2 production; $\dot{V}_A$, alveolar ventilation; $\dot{V}_D$, physiological dead space ventilation; $\dot{V}_E$, expired ventilation; $\dot{V}O_2$, O_2 uptake; $\dot{V}CO_2$, CO_2 output. (From Wasserman, K.: Measures of functional capacity in patients with heart failure. Circulation *81*(Suppl. II):1, 1990, by permission of the American Heart Association, Inc.)

to remain constant or, at best, to rise less than in normal young subjects (Chap. 52). It is possible that stiffening of the arterial system with age results in a greater afterload during exercise, thereby reducing the ejection fraction.[132] Although both untrained and trained healthy young subjects develop an increased EF during supine exercise, this tends to be associated with an *increase* in end-diastolic volume in untrained subjects and a *reduction* in athletes.[133] These variations must be kept in mind in interpreting the results of exercise in patients with suspected heart disease.

ISOMETRIC EXERCISE. This form of exercise—most often sustained handgrip at a level between 20 per cent and 40 per cent of maximal—has the advantage over dynamic exercise in that it requires minimum movement of the patient, and therefore facilitates simultaneous recording of other variables such as those of the echocardiogram. It is a simple, convenient test of left ventricular function. The centrally mediated increases in heart rate, arterial pressure, and cardiac output appear to be designed to maintain flow in the compressed vascular bed of skeletal muscle. The normal left ventricle responds to the stress of isometric exercise with little or no change or a decline in filling pressure and end-diastolic volume, but with an increase in stroke work. In contrast, the ventricle with impaired function displays an increase in filling pressure and end-diastolic volume but little change or an actual fall in stroke work during isometric exercise.[134]

INCREASE IN AFTERLOAD. The response of stroke volume, stroke work, and ventricular end-diastolic pressure to an increase in left ventricular afterload induced by the infusion of a pressor agent such as angiotensin is another method for evaluating the response of the left ventricle to stress.[135] The normal left ventricle responds to this stress with little change in stroke volume, an increase in stroke work, and a small rise in ventricular end-diastolic pressure and volume. When left ventricular contractility is impaired, filling pressure rises markedly but stroke volume falls, so that stroke work either remains constant or declines. In noninvasive assessment of the end-systolic meridional wall stress (σ)-shortening relation, the stress of methoxamine infusion usually is used.

TACHYCARDIA. In normal subjects, cardiac output and arterial pressure remain constant during atrial pacing, and stroke volume varies inversely with heart rate,[136] while both end-diastolic and end-systolic volumes decline. In patients with coronary artery disease not severe enough to cause ischemia in the basal state, tachycardia may induce ischemia with impairment of wall motion in the distribution of the involved artery. If a sufficiently large area of the ventricle is involved, the left ventricular end-diastolic pressure will rise, primarily as a consequence of the ischemia-induced reduction of ventricular compliance.

CONCLUSIONS. The left ventricular response to various forms of stress is more sensitive than resting measurements in detecting mild impairment of myocardial functional reserve. It also is useful in expressing the severity of this impairment quantitatively and in determining the effects of therapeutic interventions such as drugs and operation on cardiac function. Substantial progress has been made in applying such stresses in a standardized manner, using noninvasive techniques to evaluate their effects on ventricular performance.

CARDIOPULMONARY EXERCISE TESTING

(See also p. 162, Fig. 6–1)

The heart and lungs play an integral role in the coupling of external respiration to cellular metabolism (Fig. 15–2).[137–141] For this reason, diseases of the cardiovascular system or pulmonary system cause reductions in O_2 uptake. In cardiopulmonary exercise testing, the two systems are ordinarily considered as a single unit.

A systematic approach to cardiopulmonary exercise testing allows the noninvasive assessment of total oxygen uptake ($\dot{V}O_2$) and carbon dioxide production ($\dot{V}CO_2$).[137–141] Progressively increasing isotonic exercise is carried out on a treadmill or bicycle ergometer. End tidal O_2 and CO_2 concentrations and ventilation are measured continuously, allowing the monitoring of $\dot{V}O_2$ and $\dot{V}CO_2$ on a breath-by-breath basis. This permits determination of (1) the maximal oxygen uptake ($\dot{V}O_{2max}$, or aerobic capacity), defined as the value achieved when $\dot{V}O_2$ remains stable *despite* an increase in the intensity of exercise (Figs. 15–22*A* and 15–23), and (2) the *anaerobic threshold*. The latter is reached during the course of progressive exercise when the O_2 available to the tissues becomes inadequate. At this point, energy is generated inefficiently by anaerobic metabolism, a process producing lactate, which is buffered by bicarbonate, leading to the production of CO_2. This can be recognized by a rise in $\dot{V}CO_2$ which exceeds the rise in $\dot{V}O_2$ and a rise in the respiratory quotient (R), i.e., the ratio $\dot{V}CO_2/\dot{V}O_2$ (Fig. 15–22*B*). The anaerobic threshold indicates the maximum level of physical activity and O_2 uptake at which the cardiopulmonary system is able to provide sufficient O_2 to maintain aerobic metabolism in skeletal muscle. These two endpoints—the $\dot{V}O_{2max}$ and the anaerobic threshold—can be determined objectively and are not affected by the bias of patient or examiner, which may limit the value of exercise tests. Although exercise capacity correlates with maximal $\dot{V}O_2$, these correlations are not good enough to allow the former to serve as a substitute for the latter. The reproducibility of $\dot{V}O_{2max}$ and the anaerobic threshold, when measured days or weeks apart in subjects whose condition has not changed in the interim, is excellent.[139] Normal values of $\dot{V}O_{2max}$ and of the anaerobic threshold decline with age after 20 years, are higher in men than in women, and exceed 20 and 14 ml/min/kg, respectively. Functional capacity has been conveniently categorized into five classes by Weber and his associates (A to E)[139]; impairment in group E is so severe that the patients cannot (or should not) exercise (Table 15–3).

The $\dot{V}O_{2max}$ is a function of both the maximal cardiac output and the maximal extraction of O_2 by the tissues (maximal A-$\dot{V}$[O_2]). The latter does not vary systematically in patients of various classes and usually exceeds 70 per cent at $\dot{V}O_{2max}$ (Fig. 15–2). Therefore, $\dot{V}O_{2max}$ reflects the maximum cardiac output, which is a far more sensitive measurement than is the resting cardiac output in discriminating among patients in different degrees of cardiac disability.

When $\dot{V}O_{2max}$ is reduced, it is probably due to pulmonary dysfunction if O_2 saturation declines markedly during exercise. Conversely, cardiac dysfunction can be recognized as the cause of reduced $\dot{V}O_{2max}$ by measuring pulmonary capillary wedge pressure together with arterial pressure, cardiac output, and gas exchange at each stage of exercise. A triple-lumen balloon flotation thermodilution catheter can be used conveniently to make these measurements. As function deterio-

FIGURE 15-22. O_2 uptake ($\dot{V}O_2$) plotted as a function of work rate *(A)* and CO_2 output ($\dot{V}CO_2$) as function of $\dot{V}O_2$ (V-slope plot) *(B)* of 64-year-old patient with shortness of breath at high altitude and ST segment changes consistent with myocardial ischemia at 120 W cycle ergometer exercise but without pain. Because of flattened $\dot{V}O_2$ response *(panel A)* but continued steep rise in $\dot{V}CO_2$ above anaerobic threshold, upper-component slope of $\dot{V}CO_2$-$\dot{V}O_2$ plot *(panel B)* is pathologically steep. Steep upper-component slope with a value of 3.3 suggests an exceptionally high rate of lactate release during exercise. Slope of 1 is drawn in panel B to provide visualization of steepening in the $\dot{V}CO_2$-$\dot{V}O_2$ plot reflecting the start of HCO_3^- buffering of lactic acid. (From Wasserman, K., Beaver, W. L., and Whipp, B. J.: Gas exchange theory and the lactic acidosis (anaerobic) threshold. Circulation *81* (Suppl. II):14, 1990, by permission of the American Heart Association, Inc.)

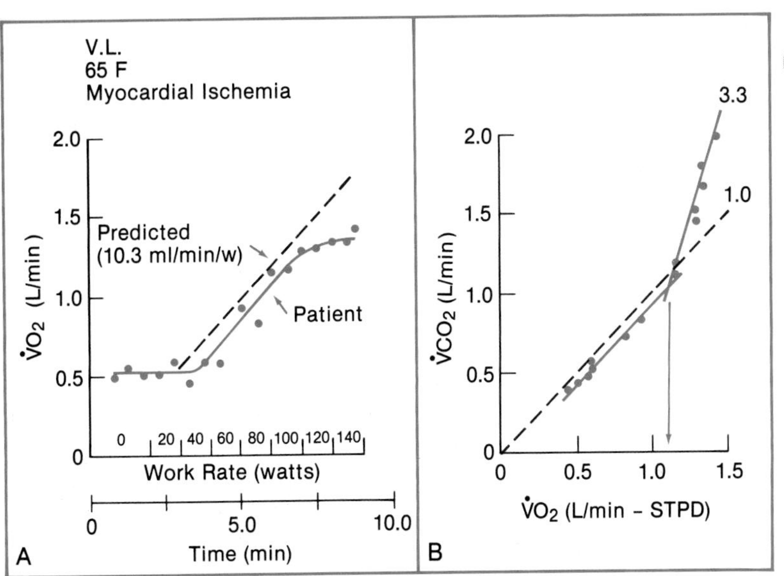

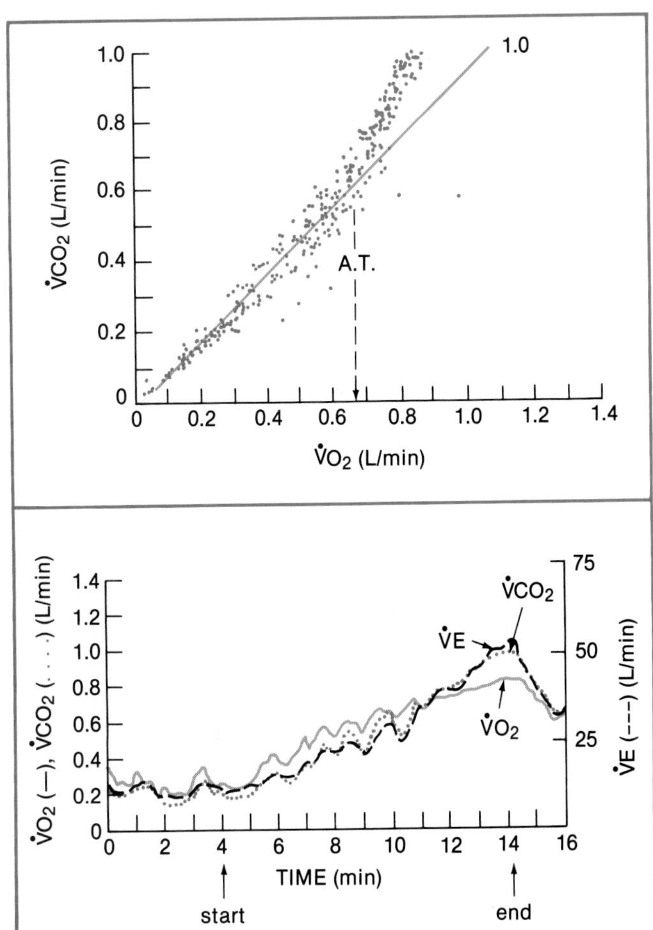

FIGURE 15-23. Graph (lower panel) of $\dot{V}O_2$, $\dot{V}CO_2$, and $\dot{V}E$ in adult male patient with heart failure in response to incremental work rate (ramp pattern) cycle ergometer exercise test, showing irregularity of breathing in patient. Plot of $\dot{V}CO_2$ as function of $\dot{V}O_2$ (V-slope analysis is shown in upper panel). Line with slope 1.0 is the approximate mean of data points up to the point where $\dot{V}CO_2$ breaks away and rises rapidly. $\dot{V}O_2$ where data points rise more steeply than a slope of 1.0 is theoretically the $\dot{V}O_2$ at which HCO_3^- starts buffering lactic acid, or anaerobic threshold. (From Wasserman, K., Beaver, W. L., and Whipp, B. J.: Gas exchange theory and the lactic acidosis (anaerobic) threshold. Circulation *81*(Suppl. II):14, 1990, by permission of the American Heart Association, Inc.)

rates, wedge pressure rises and cardiac output declines at peak exercise. The response of systolic arterial pressure to peak exercise is a function of the increment in cardiac output, rising substantially in class A, progressively less in classes B and C, and remaining virtually unchanged in class D.

Cardiopulmonary exercise testing is of clinical value in objectively assessing exercise tolerance and functional capacity, in evaluating the possible causes of exertional dyspnea and fatigue, in determining the severity of disability, in following its progress, and in assessing the response to therapy.[143,144] Impairment of pulmonary and/or musculoskeletal function can interfere with oxygen uptake during exertion. Therefore, in a patient with a reduced $\dot{V}O_{2max}$ and clinical manifestations of lung disease, pulmonary function should be evaluated.[145]

A *disadvantage* of cardiopulmonary exercise testing is that many patients with heart disease, particularly ischemic heart disease, cannot attain a level of exercise in which $\dot{V}O_2$ remains stable despite further increase in the intensity of exercise. The *peak* $\dot{V}O_2$ which they achieve is not the same and should not be confused with the $\dot{V}O_{2max}$, which by definition fails to rise despite a further increase in the intensity of exercise. Peak $\dot{V}O_2$ depends on the motivations of the patient as well as of the examiner.[142] On the other hand, the anaerobic threshold, which requires a lower level of activity than the $\dot{V}O_{2max}$, can be more readily determined in patients with cardiac dysfunction and is quite reproducible.[146,147] Alterations in the anaerobic threshold reflect changes in the underlying condition.

ASSESSMENT OF RIGHT VENTRICULAR FUNCTION

The systolic and diastolic volumes and ejection fraction of the right ventricle are exquisitely sensitive to right ventricular afterload. However, the right ventricular dilatation in response to increased afterload is limited by the tethering of the right ventricle to the much thicker left ventricle and the limitations imposed by the pericardium. With increased afterload, the thin-walled right ventricle dilates, causing functional tricuspid regurgitation.[148] In using the ejection fraction to estimate right ventricular function, the results will be influenced importantly by the presence and severity of such regurgitation, and it has been suggested that the regurgitant volume should be added to the stroke volume in the estimation of ejection fraction.

The most widely used technique for assessing right ventricular function is the thermodilution method, in which iced

TABLE 15-3 FUNCTIONAL IMPAIRMENT IN AEROBIC CAPACITY AND ANAEROBIC THRESHOLD AS MEASURED DURING INCREMENTAL TREADMILL CPX

CLASS	DEGREE OF IMPAIRMENT	$\dot{V}O_2$ MAX (ml/min/kg)	ANAEROBIC THRESHOLD (ml/min/kg)
A	Mild to none	> 20	> 14
B	Mild to moderate	16 to 20	11 to 14
C	Moderate to severe	10 to 16	8 to 11
D	Severe	6 to 10	5 to 8
E	Very severe	< 6	< 4

From Weber, K. T., Janicki, J. S., and McElroy, P. A.: Cardiopulmonary exercise (CPX) testing. *In* Weber, K. T., and Janicki, J. S. (eds.): Cardiopulmonary Exercise Testing. Philadelphia, W. B. Saunders Company, 1986, p. 153.

saline solution is injected into the right atrium and the temperature in the pulmonary artery is recorded using a rapidly responding thermistor mounted on a catheter.[149] This technique, commonly used in intensive care units, allows serial measurements of cardiac output and right ventricular ejection fraction, and the calculation of stroke volume as well as right ventricular end-diastolic and end-systolic volumes. It is convenient and reproducible and reasonably accurate when compared with measurement of the same variables by biplane angiocardiography[149] or first-pass radionuclide angiography.[150] Alternatively, right ventricular ejection fraction also can be estimated from two-dimensional echocardiography.

The right ventricular end-systolic pressure-volume relation (RVESPVR, like the LVESPVR, p. 376) can be determined with a manometer-tipped catheter in the right ventricle and either an impedance catheter or a radionuclide ventriculogram to provide simultaneous measurements of right ventricular volume. By varying right ventricular afterload, the RVESPVR has been found to be quite linear; it can be shifted upward and leftward by the positive inotropic agent dobutamine.[151,152]

ASSESSMENT OF DIASTOLIC FUNCTION

(Table 15-4)

The properties of the heart change during diastole as they do during systole. As Katz has pointed out,[58] the pressure-volume loop during diastole reflects the *lusitropic state* of the heart, as the systolic portion of the loop represents the *inotropic state* (Fig. 15-9). The diastolic properties of the heart are based on a complex series of interrelated events which include the speed and synchrony of myocardial relaxation, loading conditions, the viscoelastic properties of the ventricle, heart rate, the force of atrial contraction, ventricular interaction, pericardial restraint, and their effect on the position of the interventricular septum.[153,154] Grossman has classified the factors that influence the diastolic properties of the heart into those extrinsic and intrinsic to the left ventricle (Table 15-4).

The terms used to describe the diastolic properties of cardiac muscle and of the left ventricle are many, and are presented and defined on p. 371; the mechanism of cardiac relaxation is discussed on p. 359, changes in ventricular diastolic properties in cardiac hypertrophy and heart failure are described on p. 402, and the effects of these changes on the clinical manifestations of heart failure are described on p. 446. Here we deal with *methods* for assessing left ventricular diastolic function.

RATE OF VENTRICULAR RELAXATION (Table 15-4). This may be estimated from the maximum rate of pressure fall, i.e., the peak $-dP/dt$. However, just as the peak $+dP/dt$ is influenced by ventricular loading as well as contractility, so is the peak $-dP/dt$ affected by ventricular loading, as well as the rate of ventricular relaxation, thereby limiting its value as

TABLE 15-4 FACTORS THAT INFLUENCE LEFT VENTRICULAR DIASTOLIC CHAMBER DISTENSIBILITY

I. FACTORS EXTRINSIC TO THE LV CHAMBER
- **A. Pericardial restraint**
- **B. Right ventricular loading**
- **C. Coronary vascular turgor (erectile effect)**
- **D. Extrinsic compression by tumor, pleural pressure, etc.**

II. FACTORS INTRINSIC TO LV CHAMBER
- **A. Passive elasticity of LV wall (stiffness or compliance when myocytes are completely relaxed)**
  - **1. Thickness of LV wall**
  - **2. Composition of LV wall (muscle, fibrosis, edema, amyloid, hemosiderin) including both endocardium and myocardium**
  - **3. Temperature, osmolality**
- **B. Active elasticity of LV wall due to residual cross-bridge activation (cycling and/or latch state) through part or all of diastole:**
  - **1. Slow relaxation affecting early diastole only**
  - **2. Incomplete relaxation affecting early, mid-, and end-diastolic distensibility**
  - **3. Diastolic tone, contracture, or rigor**
- **C. Elastic recoil (diastolic suction)**
- **D. Viscoelasticity (stress relaxation, creep)**

From Grossman, W.: Evaluation of systolic and diastolic function of the myocardium. *In* Grossman, W., and Baim, D. S. (eds.): Cardiac Catheterization, Angiography and Intervention. 4th ed. Philadelphia, Lea and Febiger, 1990, p. 333.

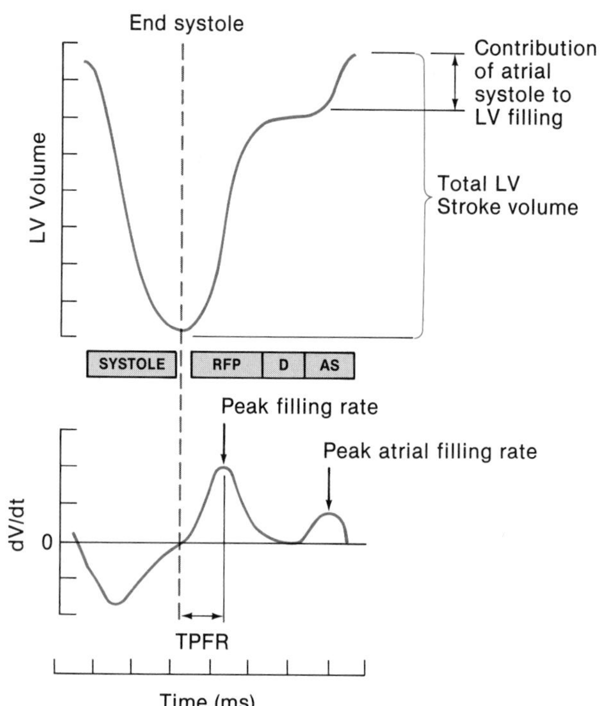

FIGURE 15-24. **Idealized plot of left ventricular volume versus time *(top)* and the rate of change of volume (dV/dt) versus time *(bottom)* as might be obtained from contrast or radionuclide ventriculography. The representative cardiac cycle begins at end diastole. Subsequent events as depicted by the bars in the center of the figure are: (1) systole, during which left ventricular volume decreases to a minimum and dV/dt reaches its maximum, and (2) diastole, the beginning of which is signaled by the opening of the mitral valve and the onset of left ventricular filling. Diastole has three distinct phases in normal individuals: (1) the rapid filling phase (RFP) during which the left ventricle fills rapidly, but passively, and the peak filling rate occurs; (2) diastasis (D) during which relatively little left ventricular volume change occurs; and (3) atrial systole (AS) in which active atrial contraction fills the left ventricle to its end-diastolic volume. The diastolic parameters that have been derived from such analysis are the peak filling rate, the time to peak filling rate (TPFR), the per cent contribution of atrial systole, and the first third filling fraction. (From Labovitz, A. J., and Pearson, A. C.: Evaluation of left ventricular diastolic function: Clinical relevance and recent Doppler echocardiographic insights. Am. Heart J. *114*:836, 1987.)**

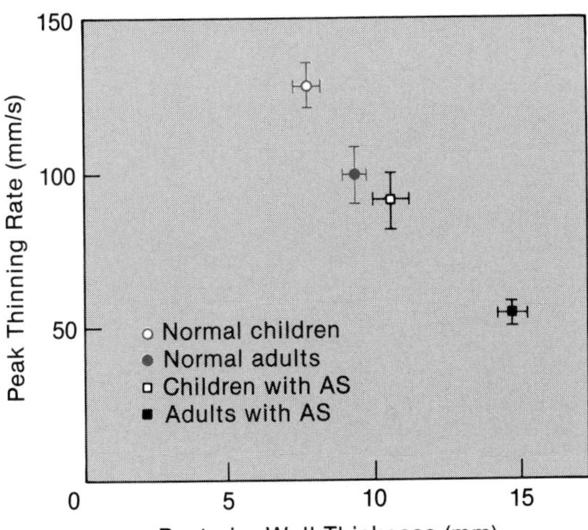

FIGURE 15–25. Relation between left ventricular end-diastolic posterior wall thickness and peak left ventricular early diastolic wall thinning rate for the four groups of subjects. Means and standard errors of the mean are shown. AS = aortic stenosis. (From Fifer, M. A., Borow, D. M., Colan, S. D., and Lorell, B. H.: Early diastolic left ventricular function in children and adults with aortic stenosis. Reprinted by permission of The American College of Cardiology. J. Am. Coll. Cardiol. 5:1151, 1985.)

a measure of the rate of relaxation. On the other hand, τ (tau), the time constant of pressure decline during isovolumetric relaxation, provides an accurate measure of the rate of relaxation.[155–158] Prolongation of the monoexponential decay in ventricular pressure (τ) occurs in conditions that slow and/or cause *asynchronous* ventricular relaxation. Three methods of calculating τ have been described[156]; τ is independent of ventricular volume, loading, systolic or diastolic pressure, and stroke volume. However, τ shortens with beta adrenoceptor stimulation of the myocardium, and is prolonged with beta blockade, during postischemic reperfusion, and with advanced age.[156]

PEAK FILLING RATE AND TIME TO PEAK FILLING (Fig. 15–24). After completion of isovolumetric relaxation, the mitral valve opens and left ventricular filling commences; it is most rapid early in diastole. In the absence of mitral stenosis, the peak filling rate (PFR) of the left ventricle reflects a composite of preload, left atrial pressure, ventricular wall thickness, external forces acting on the ventricle, the viscoelasticity of the myocardium, and the extent of filling of the coronary vascular bed.[158a] The absolute value of PFR usually is corrected for ventricular volume and is expressed in end-diastolic volumes per second. PFR is reduced when left ventricular inflow is reduced; in hypovolemia, when relaxation is slowed, as occurs in myocardial ischemia; with concentric hypertrophy secondary to hypertension or aortic stenosis; and especially in hypertrophic cardiomyopathy.[153] In the last condition, it may be shortened by calcium antagonists.

The PFR and the time from mitral valve opening to the PFR usually vary inversely with one another. These variables can be measured by determining the rate of change of left ventricular volume; the latter may be determined cineangiographically,[159] by radionuclide ventriculography or by two-dimensional or M-mode echocardiography.

Although the PFR reflects global ventricular diastolic properties, a closely related variable, the peak rate of wall thinning (peak negative dh/dt), can be determined regionally. This measurement is most commonly made clinically by determining the thickness of the interventricular septum and posterior ventricular wall continuously by two-dimensional or M-mode echocardiography and obtaining the first derivative of its rate of change during diastole. Myocardial ischemia reduces the rate of diastolic thinning, and this may be either global or regional, depending on the nature of the ischemic process. Ventricular hypertrophy also reduces peak negative dh/dt (Fig. 15–25).

LEFT VENTRICULAR FILLING MEASURED BY DOPPLER ECHOCARDIOGRAPHY. Left ventricular filling rate is reflected in the velocity of transmitral blood flow, which can be measured by pulsed Doppler echocardiography.[160] The early peak flow (E) (Fig. 15–26) coincides with the PFR, normally ranges from 50 to 80 cm/sec, and exceeds the peak late or atrial systolic flow (A), which normally ranges from 35 to 50 cm/sec. The peak E/A ratio ranges from 1.0 to 2.0. The pattern of diastolic inflow into the left ventricle has been demonstrated to be abnormal, with reduced early and accelerated late ventricular filling (E/A <1.0) in hypertension, aortic stenosis, hypertrophic cardiomyopathy, and, in some patients, ischemic heart disease. This abnormal inflow

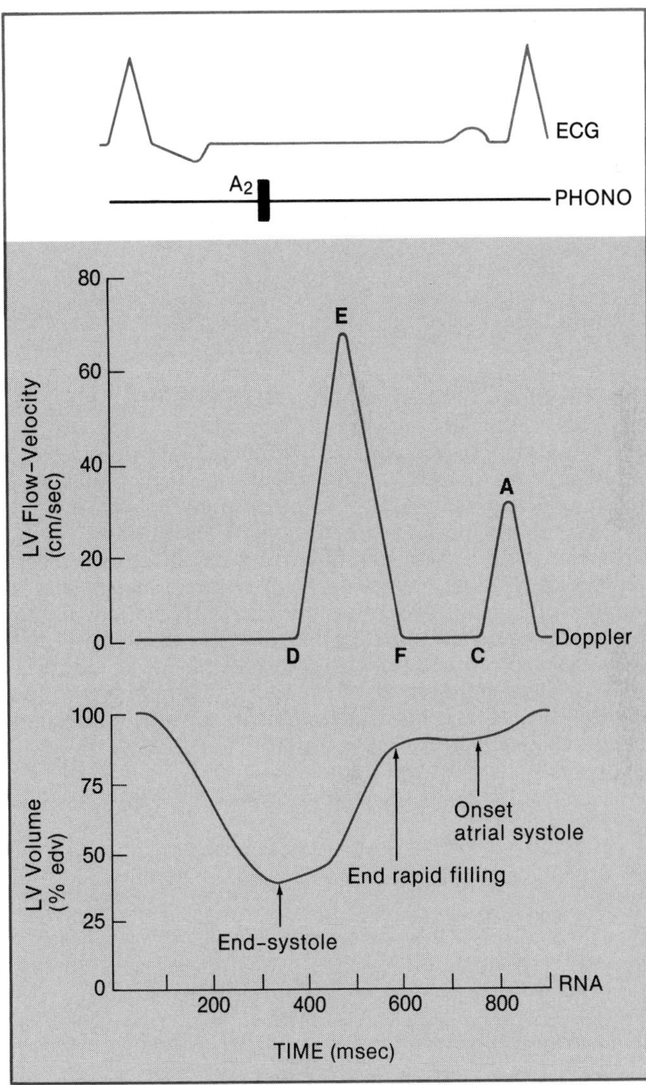

FIGURE 15–26. Superimposed Doppler left ventricular (LV) diastolic flow velocity waveform *(middle)* and radionuclide angiographic (RNA) time-activity curve *(bottom)*, obtained in a normal subject. Cycle length (878 milliseconds) was identical in the two studies. Changes in flow velocity appear to occur at the same time as changes in relative volume. The early diastolic flow velocity peak occurs during the period of LV rapid filling. At the end of rapid filling, flow velocity begins to decrease and reaches zero baseline at the beginning of diastasis. At the end of diastasis and after atrial systole (A), both flow velocity and filling rate increase again. A_2, aortic component of the second heart sound in the phonocardiograms (PHONO); ECG, electrocardiogram; edv, end-diastolic volume. (From Spirito, P., Maron, B. J., and Bonow, R. O.: Noninvasive assessment of left ventricular diastolic function: Comparison of Doppler echocardiographic and radionuclide angiographic techniques. Reprinted by permission of the American College of Cardiology. J. Am. Coll. Cardiol. 7:518, 1986.)

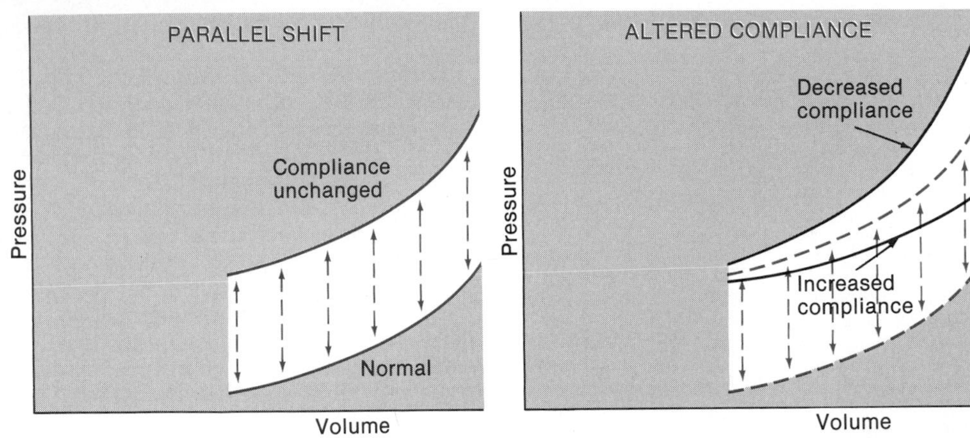

FIGURE 15–27. Schematic illustration of the difference between diastolic distensibility and compliance. On the left, the ventricular diastolic pressure-volume relation has undergone a parallel upward shift. Distensibility is decreased (higher diastolic pressure required to fill the ventricle to the same chamber volume), although compliance, defined as the slope of the pressure-volume relation, is unchanged. On the right, superimposed on the parallel upward shift, are curves whose slopes are steeper (decreased compliance) or less steep (increased compliance) than either of the two parallel pressure-volume curves. This illustrates the importance of distinguishing distensibility from compliance because the curve labeled "increased compliance" nevertheless exhibits decreased diastolic distensibility in comparison to the normal pressure-volume relation. (Reproduced, with permission, from Grossman, W.: Relaxation and diastolic distensibility of the regionally ischemic left ventricle. *In* Grossman, W. and Lorell, B. H. [eds.]: Diastolic Relaxation of the Heart. Boston, Martinus Nijhoff Publishing, 1988, pp. 193–203.)

reflects the increased resistance to early passive ventricular filling and the secondary augmentation of the atrial contribution to ventricular filling in these conditions.

DIASTOLIC VENTRICULAR PRESSURE-VOLUME RELATION. This relation represents the portion of the ventricular pressure-volume loop during diastole.[161–163] Pressure ordinarily is measured by a catheter-tip micromanometer, and volume by cineangiography, two-dimensional echocardiography, or radionuclide angiography, or with an impedance catheter. An upward displacement of the diastolic pressure-volume curve (higher pressure at any volume) represents a reduction of ventricular distensibility.[164] Ventricular compliance, defined as the *slope* (rather than the position) of the diastolic pressure-volume curve, is reduced when diastolic pressure rises more for any given increment in volume (Fig. 15–27). Displacement of the diastolic pressure-volume curve can occur by any of the mechanisms listed in Table 15–4.

REFERENCES

THEORETICAL CONSIDERATIONS

1. Braunwald, E.: On the difference between the heart's output and its contractile state (Editorial). Circulation *43*:171, 1971.
2. Ross, J., Jr.: Cardiac function and myocardial contractility: A perspective. J. Am. Coll. Cardiol. *1*:52, 1983.
3. Nichols, W. W., Conti, C. R., Walker, W. E., and Milnor, W. R.: Input impedance of the systemic circulation in man. Circ. Res. *40*:451, 1977.
4. Frommer, P. L., Robinson, B. F., and Braunwald, E.: Paired electrical stimulation. A comparison of the effects on performance of the failing and nonfailing heart. Am. J. Cardiol. *18*:738, 1966.
5. Starling, E. H.: Linacre Lecture on the Law of the Heart (1915). London, Longmans, 1918.
6. Sarnoff, S. J., and Mitchell, J. H.: Control of function of heart. *In* Hamilton, W. F., and Dow, P. (eds.): Handbook of Physiology. Section 2. Circulation, Vol. 1. Washington, D.C., American Physiological Society, 1962, pp. 489–532.
7. Suga, H., Sagawa, K., and Demer, L.: Determinants of instantaneous pressure in canine left ventricle: Time and volume specification. Circ. Res. *46*:256, 1980.

ASSESSMENT OF CARDIAC PERFORMANCE BASED ON PRESSURES, FLOWS, VOLUMES, AND DIMENSIONS

8. Rackley, C. E., Russell, R. O., Jr., Rogers, W. J., et al.: Clinical experience with glucose-insulin-potassium therapy in acute myocardial infarction. Am. Heart J. *102*:1038, 1981.
9. Rackley, C. E.: Quantitative evaluation of left ventricular function by radiographic techniques. Circulation *54*:862, 1976.
10. Tobis, J. Nalcioglu, O., Seibert, A., et al.: Measurement of left ventricular ejection fraction by videodensitometric analysis of digital subtraction angiograms. Am. J. Cardiol. *52*:871, 1983.
11. Kronenberg, M. W., Price, R. R., Smith, C. W., et al.: Evaluation of left ventricular performance using digital subtraction angiography. Am. J. Cardiol. *51*:837, 1983.
12. Popio, K. A., Gorlin, R., Bechtel, D., and Levine, J. A.: Postextrasystolic potentiation as a predictor of myocardial viability: Preoperative analyses compared with studies after coronary bypass surgery. Am. J. Cardiol. *39*:944, 1977.
13. Vine, D. L., Hegg, T. D., Dodge, H. T., et al.: Immediate effect of contrast medium injection of left ventricular volumes and ejection fraction. Circulation *56*:379, 1977.
14. Dodge, H. T., and Sheehan, F. H.: Quantitative contrast angiography for assessment of ventricular performance in heart disease. J. Am. Coll. Cardiol. *1*:73, 1983.
15. Rackley, C. E., and Hood, W. P., Jr.: Quantitative angiographic evaluation and pathophysiological mechanisms in valvular heart disease. Prog. Cardiovasc. Dis. *15*:427, 1973.
16. Fifer, M. A., and Grossman, W.: Measurement of ventricular volumes, ejection fraction, mass and wall stress. *In* Grossman, W. (ed.): Cardiac Catheterization and Angiography. 4th ed. Philadelphia, Lea and Febiger, 1991, pp. 300–318.
17. Luisada, A. A., Singhal, A., and Portaluppi, F.: Assessment of left ventricular function by noninvasive methods. Adv. Cardiol. *32*:111, 1985.
18. Borow, K. M., Green, L. H., Grossman, W., and Braunwald, E.: Left ventricular end-systolic stress-shortening and stress-length relations in humans: Normal values and sensitivity to inotropic state. Am. J. Cardiol. *50*:1301, 1982.
19. Tortoledo, F. A., Quinones, M. A., Fernandez, G. C., et al.: Quantification of left ventricular volumes by two-dimensional echocardiography: A simplified and accurate approach. Circulation *67*:579, 1983.
20. Reichek, N., Helak, J., Plappert, T., et al.: Anatomic validation of left ventricular mass estimates from clinical two-dimensional echocardiography: Initial results. Circulation *67*:348, 1983.
21. Borow, K. M., Come, P. C., Neumann, A., et al.: Physiological assessment of the inotropic, vasodilator and afterload reducing effects of milrinone in subjects without cardiac disease. Am. J. Cardiol. *55*:1204, 1985.
21a. Force, T. L., Folland, E. D., Aebischer, N., et al.: Echocardiographic assessment of ventricular function. *In* Marcus, M. L., Skorton, D. J., Schelbert, H. R., and Wolf, G. L. (eds.): Cardiac Imaging: A Companion to Braunwald's Heart Disease. Philadelphia, W. B. Saunders Company, 1991, pp. 374–401.
22. McKay, R. G., Aroesty, J. M., Heller, G. V., et al.: Left ventricular pressure-volume diagrams and end-systolic pressure-volume relations in human beings. J. Am. Coll. Cardiol. *3*:301, 1984.
23. Kronenberg, M. W., Parrish, M. D., Jenkins, D. W., Jr., et al.: Accuracy of radionuclide ventriculography for estimation of left ventricular volume changes and end-systolic pressure volume relations. J. Am. Coll. Cardiol. *6*:1064, 1985.
23a. Gibbons, R. J.: Equilibrium radionuclide angiography. *In* Marcus, M. L., Skorton, D. J., Schelbert, H. R., and Wolf, G. L. (eds.): Cardiac Imaging: A Companion to Braunwald's Heart Disease. Philadelphia, W. B. Saunders Company, 1991, pp. 1027–1046.
24. Rich, S., Chomka, E. V., Stagl, R., et al.: Determination of left ventricular

ejection fraction using ultrafast computed tomography. Am. Heart J. *112*:392, 1986.

24a. Marcus, M. L., and Weiss, R. M.: Evaluation of cardiac structure and function with ultrafast computed tomography. *In* Marcus, M. L., Skorton, D. J., Schelbert, H. R., and Wolf, G. L. (eds.): Cardiac Imaging: A Companion to Braunwald's Heart Disease. Philadelphia, W. B. Saunders Company, 1991, pp. 669–681.

25. Osbakken, M., and Yuschok, T.: Evaluation of ventricular function with gated cardiac magnetic resonance imaging. Catheter. Cardiovasc. Diag. *12*:156, 1986.

25a. Peshock, R. M.: Magnetic resonance imaging of the heart: Quantitation. *In* Marcus, M. L., Skorton, D. J., Schelbert, H. R., and Wolf, G. L. (eds.): Cardiac Imaging: A Companion to Braunwald's Heart Disease. Philadelphia, W. B. Saunders Company, 1991, pp. 811–827.

26. Herman, H. J., and Bartle, S. H.: Left ventricular volumes by angiocardiography: Comparison of methods and simplification of techniques. Cardiovasc. Res. *4*:404, 1968.

27. Dodge, H. T., Hay, R. E., and Sandler, H.: An angiocardiographic method for directly determining left ventricular stroke volume in man. Circ. Res. *11*:739, 1962.

28. Wynne, J., Green, L. H., Mann, T., et al.: Estimation of left ventricular volumes in man from biplane cineangiograms filmed in oblique projections. Am. J. Cardiol. *41*:726, 1978.

29. Dodge, H. T.: Hemodynamic aspects of cardiac failure. *In* Braunwald, E. (ed.): The Myocardium: Failure and Infarction. New York, H P Publishing Co., 1974, pp. 70–79.

30. Sandler, H., and Dodge, H. T.: Angiographic methods for determination of left ventricular geometry and volume. *In* Mirsky, I., Ghista, D. N., and Sandler, H. (eds.): Cardiac Mechanics: Physiological, Clinical and Mathematical Considerations. New York, John Wiley and Sons, 1974.

31. Graham, T. P., Jr., Atwood, G. F., Faulkner, S. L., and Nelson, J. H.: Right atrial volume measurements from biplane cineangiocardiography. Circulation *49*:709, 1974.

32. Yin, F.C.P.: Ventricular wall stress. Circ. Res. *49*:829, 1981.

33. Mirsky, I.: Elastic properties of the myocardium: A quantitative approach with physiological and clinical applications. *In* Berne, R. M. (ed.): Handbook of Physiology. Section 2, The Cardiovascular System. Vol. 1, Heart. Bethesda, Md., American Physiological Society, 1979, p. 501.

34. Grossman, W., Jones, D., and McLaurin, L. P.: Wall stress and patterns of hypertrophy in the human left ventricle. J. Clin. Invest. *56*:56, 1974.

35. Peterson, K. L.: Instantaneous force-velocity-length relations of the left ventricle: Methods, limitations and applications in humans. *In* Fishman, A. P. (ed.): Heart Failure. Washington, D.C., Hemisphere Publishing Co., 1978, pp. 121–132.

36. Smith, M., Russell, R. O., Jr., Feild, B. J., and Rackley, C. E.: Left ventricular compliance and abnormally contracting segments in post-myocardial infarction patients. Chest *65*:368, 1974.

37. Herman, M. V., Heinle, R. A., Klein, M. D., and Gorlin, R.: Localized disorders in myocardial contraction: Asynergy and its role in congestive heart failure. N. Engl. J. Med. *277*:222, 1967.

38. Dodge, H. T., Stewart, D. K., and Frimer, M.: Implications of shape, stress and wall dynamics in clinical heart disease. *In* Fishman, A. P. (ed.): Heart Failure. Washington, D.C., Hemisphere Publishing Co., 1978, p. 43.

39. Sheehan, F. H., Dodge, H. T., Mathey, D. G., et al.: Application of the centerline method: Analysis of change in regional left ventricular wall motion in serial studies. IEEE Comput. Cardiol., 1982, p. 9.

40. Sheehan, F. H., Stewart, D. K., Dodge, H. T., et al.: Variability in the measurement of regional left ventricular wall motion from contrast angiograms. Circulation *68*:550, 1983.

41. Tsakiris, A. G., Donald, D. E., Sturm, R. E., and Wood, E. H.: Volume, ejection fraction, and internal dimensions of left ventricle determined by biplane videometry. Fed. Proc. *28*:1358, 1969.

42. Marving, J., Hoilunk-Carlsen, P. F., Chraemmer-Jorgensen, B., and Gadsboll, N.: Are right and left ventricular ejection fractions equal? Ejection fractions in normal subjects and in patients with first acute myocardial infarction. Circulation *72*:502, 1985.

43. Stamm, R. B., Carabello, B. A., Mayers, D. L., and Martin, R. P.: Two-dimensional echocardiographic measurement of left ventricular ejection fraction: Prospective analysis of what constitutes an adequate determination. Am. Heart J. *104*:136, 1982.

44. Quinones, M. A., Waggoner, A. D., Reduto, L. A., et al.: A new simplified and accurate method for determining ejection fraction with two-dimensional echocardiography. Circulation *64*:744, 1981.

45. Zimpfer, M., and Vatner, S. F.: Effects of acute increases in left ventricular preload on indices of myocardial function in conscious, unrestrained and intact, tranquilized baboons. J. Clin. Invest. *67*:430, 1981.

46. Nixon, J. V., Murray, R. G., Leonard, P. D., et al.: Effect of large variations in preload on left ventricular performance characteristic in normal subjects. Circulation *65*:698, 1982.

47. Braunwald, E., Goldblatt, A., Harrison, D. C., and Mason, D. T.: Studies on cardiac dimensions in intact unanesthetized man. III. Effects of muscular exercise. Circ. Res. *13*:460, 1963.

48. Quinones, M. A., Gaasch, W. H., and Alexander, J. K.: Influence of acute changes in preload, afterload, contractile state and heart rate on ejection and isovolumic indices of myocardial contractility in man. Circulation *53*:293, 1976.

49. Grossman, W.: Evaluation of systolic and diastolic function of the myocardium. *In* Grossman, W., and Baim, D. (eds.): Cardiac Catheterization and Angiography. 4th ed. Philadelphia, Lea and Febiger, 1990, pp. 319–342.

50. McKay, R. G., Spears, J. R., Aroesty, J. M., et al.: Instantaneous measurement of left and right ventricular stroke volume and pressure-volume relationships with an impedance catheter. Circulation *69*:703, 1984.

51. Kass, D. A., Yamazaki, T., Burkhoff, D., et al.: Determination of left ventricular end-systolic pressure-volume relationships by the conductance (volume) catheter technique. Circulation *73*:586, 1986.

VENTRICULAR END-SYSTOLIC PRESSURE-VOLUME RELATIONS

52. Grossman, W., Braunwald, E., Mann, T., et al.: Contractile state of the left ventricle in man as evaluated from end-systolic pressure-volume relations. Circulation *56*:845, 1977.

53. Noble, M. I. M.: Problems concerning the application of concepts of muscle mechanics to the determination of contractile state of the heart. Circulation *45*:252, 1972.

54. Downing, S. E., and Sonnenblick, E. H.: Cardiac muscle mechanics and ventricular performance. Force and time parameters. Am. J. Physiol. *207*:705, 1964.

55. Suga, H., Katabatake, A., and Sagawa, K.: End-systolic pressure determines stroke volume from fixed end-diastolic volume in the isolated canine left ventricle under a constant contractile state. Circ. Res. *44*:238, 1979.

56. Weber, K. T., and Janicki, J. S.: Muscle-pump function of the intact heart. *In* Fishman, A. P. (ed.): Heart Failure. Washington, D.C., Hemisphere Publishing Co., 1978, pp. 29–42.

57. Mahler, F., Covell, J. W., and Ross, J., Jr.: Systolic pressure-diameter relations in the normal conscious dog. Cardiovasc. Res. *9*:447, 1975.

58. Katz, A. M.: Influence of altered inotropy and lusitropy on ventricular pressure-volume loops. J. Am. Coll. Cardiol. *11*:438, 1988.

59. Spratt, J. A., Tyson, G. S., Glower, D. D., et al.: The end-systolic pressure-volume relationship in conscious dogs. Circulation *75*:1295, 1987.

60. Carabello, B. A., and Spann, J. F.: The uses and limitations of end-systolic indexes of left ventricular function. Circulation *69*:1058, 1984.

61. Berko, B., Gaasch, W. H., Tanigawa, N., et al.: Disparity between ejection and end-systolic indexes of left ventricular contractility in mitral regurgitation. Circulation *75*:1310, 1987.

62. White, H. D., Norris, R. M., Brown, M. A., et al.: Left ventricular end-systolic volume as the major determinant of survival after recovery from myocardial infarction. Circulation *76*:44, 1987.

63. Purut, C. M., Sell, T. L., and Jones, R. H.: A new method to determine left ventricular pressure-volume loops in the clinical setting. J. Nucl. Med. *29*:1492, 1988.

64. Binkley, P. F., Lewe, R. F., Unverferth, D. F., and Leier, C. V.: Late systolic indices of ventricular function: Noninvasive derivation in congestive heart failure. Am. Heart J. *116*:1276, 1988.

65. Roman, M. J., Devereux, R. B., and Cody, R. J.: Ability of left ventricular stress-shortening relations, end-systolic stress/volume ratio and indirect indexes to detect severe contractile failure in ischemic or idiopathic dilated cardiomyopathy. Am. J. Cardiol. *64*:1338, 1989.

66. McKay, R. G., Miller, M. J., Ferguson, J. J., et al.: Assessment of left ventricular end-systolic pressure-volume relations with an impedance catheter and transient inferior vena cava occlusion: Use of this system in the evaluation of the cardiotonic effects of dobutamine, milrinone, posicor and epinephrine. J. Am. Coll. Cardiol. *8*:1152, 1986.

67. Kass, D. A., Midei, M., Graves, W., et al.: Use of a conductance (volume) catheter and transient inferior vena caval occlusion for rapid determination of pressure-volume relationships in man. Cathet. Cardiovasc. Diagn. *15*:192, 1988.

68. Carabello, B. A., Nolan, S. P., and McGuire, L. B.: Assessment of preoperative left ventricular function in patients with mitral regurgitation: Value of the end-systolic wall stress-end-systolic volume ratio. Circulation *64*:1212, 1981.

69. Reichek, N., Wilson, J., Sutton, M. St.J., et al.:Noninvasive determination of left ventricular end-systolic stress: Validation of the method and initial application. Circulation *65*:99, 1982.

70. Sagawa, K.: The end-systolic pressure-volume relation of the ventricle: Definition, modifications and clinical use (Editorial). Circulation *63*:1223, 1981.

71. Nakano, K., Sugawara, M., Ishihara, K., et al.: Myocardial stiffness derived from end-systolic wall stress and logarithm of reciprocal of wall thickness: Contractility index independent of ventricular size. Circulation *82*:1352, 1990.

72. McKay, R. G., Aroesty, J. M., Heller, G. V., et al.: Assessment of the end-systolic pressure-volume relationship in human beings with the use of a time-varying elastance model. Circulation *74*:97, 1986.

73. Starling, M. R., Walsh, R. A., Dell'Italia, L. J., et al.: The relationship of various measures of end-systole to left ventricular maximum time-varying elastance in man. Circulation *76*:32, 1987.

74. Borow, K. M., Green, L. H., Grossman, W., and Braunwald, E.: Left ventricular end-systolic stress-shortening and stress-length relations in humans. Am. J. Cardiol. *50*:1301, 1982.

75. Colan, S. D., Borow, K. M., and Neumann, A.: Left ventricular end-systolic wall stress-velocity of fiber shortening relation: A load independent index of myocardial contractility. J. Am. Coll. Cardiol. *4*:715, 1984.

76. Kass, D. A., and Maugham, W. L.: From Emax to pressure volume relations: A broader view. Circulation *77*:1203, 1988.

77. Lang, R. M., Fellner, S. K., Neumann, A., et al.: Left ventricular contractility varies directly with blood ionized calcium. Ann. Intern. Med. *108*:524, 1988.

78. Baan, J., and van der Velde, E. T.: Sensitivity of left ventricular end-sys-

16

Clinical Aspects of Heart Failure

by EUGENE BRAUNWALD, M.D., and WILLIAM GROSSMAN, M.D.

A principal complication of virtually all forms of heart disease is heart failure, defined as the *pathophysiological state in which an abnormality of cardiac function is responsible for the failure of the heart to pump blood at a rate commensurate with the requirements of the metabolizing tissues and/or to be able to do so only from an elevated filling pressure* (p. 393). An alternative definition, which focuses more on the clinical consequences of heart failure, has been offered by Packer as follows: "Congestive heart failure represents a complex clinical syndrome characterized by abnormalities of left ventricular function and neurohormonal regulation, which are accompanied by effort intolerance, fluid retention, and reduced longevity."[1] Included in these two definitions is a wide spectrum of clinicophysiological states, ranging from the rapid impairment of pumping function (occurring when, for example, a massive myocardial infarction, tachyarrhythmia, or bradyarrhythmia develops suddenly) to the gradual but progressive impairment of myocardial function, observed only during stress occurring in a patient whose heart sustains a pressure or volume overload for a prolonged period. Congestive heart failure is a relatively common disorder; it has been estimated that 2 million persons in the United States are being treated for heart failure and that there are 400,000 new cases each year.[2]

TABLE 16–1 FRAMINGHAM CRITERIA FOR CONGESTIVE HEART FAILURE

MAJOR CRITERIA
- Paroxysmal nocturnal dyspnea or orthopnea
- Neck-vein distention
- Rales
- Cardiomegaly
- Acute pulmonary edema
- S_3 gallop
- Increased venous pressure >16 cm of water
- Circulation time >25 sec
- Hepatojugular reflux

MINOR CRITERIA
- Ankle edema
- Night cough
- Dyspnea on exertion
- Hepatomegaly
- Pleural effusion
- Vital capacity decreased 1/3 from maximum
- Tachycardia (rate of >120/min)

MAJOR OR MINOR CRITERION
- Weight loss >4.5 kg in 5 days in response to treatment

For establishing a definite diagnosis of congestive heart failure in this study, two major or one major and two minor criteria had to be present concurrently.

From McKee, P. A., Castelli, W. P., McNamara, P. M., and Kannel, W. B.: The natural history of congestive heart failure, the Framingham Study. N. Engl. J. Med. *285*:1441, 1971.

The clinical manifestations of heart failure vary enormously and depend on a variety of factors, including the age of the patient, the extent and rate at which cardiac performance becomes impaired, the etiology of the heart disease, the precipitating causes of heart failure, and the specific ventricle initially involved in the disease process.[3,4] It must also be emphasized that there is a broad spectrum of severity of impairment of cardiac function, ranging from the mildest, which is manifest clinically only during marked stress, to the most advanced form, in which cardiac pump function is unable to sustain life without external support.

Useful criteria for the diagnosis of heart failure emerged from the Framingham study[5,6] (Table 16–1).

FORMS OF HEART FAILURE

FORWARD VS. BACKWARD HEART FAILURE

The clinical manifestations of heart failure arise as a consequence of inadequate cardiac output and/or damming up of blood behind one or both ventricles. These two principal mechanisms are the basis of the so-called forward and backward pressure theories of heart failure. The *backward failure hypothesis*, first proposed in 1832 by James Hope, contends that when the ventricle fails to discharge its contents, blood accumulates and pressure rises in the atrium and the venous system emptying into it.[7] There is substantial physiological evidence in favor of this theory. As discussed on page 396, the inability of cardiac muscle to shorten against a load alters the relationship between ventricular end-systolic pressure and volume, so that end-systolic (residual) volume rises. The following sequence then occurs that at first maintains cardiac output at a normal level: (1) ventricular end-diastolic volume and pressure increase; (2) the volume and pressure rise in the atrium behind the failing ventricle; (3) the atrium contracts more vigorously (a manifestation of Starling's Law, operating on the atrium)[8]; (4) the pressure in the venous and capillary beds behind (upstream to) the failing ventricle rises; and (5) transudation of fluid from the capillary bed into the interstitial space (pulmonary or systemic) increases. Many of the symptoms characteristic of heart failure can be traced to this sequence of events and the resultant increase in fluid in the interstitial spaces of the lungs, liver, subcutaneous tissues, and serous cavities.

Cardiac output in the resting (basal) state is a relatively *insensitive* index of cardiac function (p. 419). In many patients the entire sequence of events outlined above may transpire while cardiac output *at rest* is still within normal limits. Indeed, the backward pressure theory of heart failure reflects one of the principal compensatory mechanisms in heart failure, i.e., the operation of Starling's Law of the Heart (p. 367) in which distention of the ventricle helps to maintain cardiac output. The failing ventricle operates on an ascending, albeit depressed and flattened, function curve[9] (Fig. 15–1, p. 420), and the augmented ventricular end-diastolic volume and pressure characteristic of heart failure must be regarded as aiding in the maintenance of cardiac output. When this compensatory mechanism is interfered with (e.g., by means of dietary sodium restriction and treatment with diuretics), the patient may be less symptomatic owing to loss of extracellular fluid volume, with its accompanying reduction in congestion of the lungs, liver, and lower extremities. However, at the same time cardiac output may decline,[10] and symptoms secondary to a reduction of cardiac output, such as fatigue, may actually intensify. Thus, although many of the clinical manifestations of heart failure are secondary to excessive retention of extracellular fluid, the elevation of ventricular preload associated with this excess fluid constitutes an important adaptive mechanism.

"BACKWARD" FAILURE. Hope's backward pressure theory of cardiac failure incorporates the concept that the cardiac chambers may fail independently and that an imbalance in performance of the ventricles may result. If one considers, for simplicity, the development of left ventricular failure consequent to aortic stenosis or of right ventricular failure secondary to pulmonic stenosis, the initial clinical manifestations of each relate primarily to the damming up of blood behind the affected ventricle. An important extension of the backward failure theory is the development of right ventricular failure as a consequence of left ventricular failure. According to this concept, the elevation of left ventricular diastolic, left atrial, and pulmonary venous pressures results in backward transmission of pressure and leads to pulmonary hypertension, which ultimately causes right ventricular failure. Often, pulmonary vasoconstriction plays a part in this form of pulmonary hypertension as well (p. 790).

"FORWARD" FAILURE. Eighty years after publication of Hope's work, Mackenzie proposed the *forward failure hypothesis*, which relates clinical manifestations of heart failure to inadequate delivery of blood into the arterial system.[11] According to this hypothesis, the principal clinical manifestations of heart failure are due to reduced cardiac output, which results in diminished perfusion of vital organs, including the brain, leading to mental confusion; skeletal muscles, leading to weakness; and kidneys, leading to sodium and water retention through a series of complex mechanisms[12] (Chap. 62). This retention of sodium and water, in turn, augments extracellular fluid volume and ultimately leads to symptoms of heart failure which are caused by congestion of organs and tissues.

Although these two seemingly opposing views concerning the pathogenesis of heart failure led to lively controversy during the first half of this century, it no longer seems fruitful to make a rigid distinction between backward and forward heart failure, since *both* mechanisms appear to operate in the majority of patients with *chronic* heart failure.[12a] Exceptions may occur, however, and some patients, particularly those with *acute* decompensation, develop relatively pure forms of forward or backward failure. An example of relatively pure forward failure occurs in the patient with acute right ventricular failure secondary to massive pulmonary embolism in whom shock—perhaps even death—owing to inadequate cardiac output may ensue within minutes. Although right ventricular diastolic pressure and volume and right atrial and systemic venous pressure all rise markedly, the patient may succumb before sufficient extracellular fluid has accumulated to produce symptoms of systemic venous congestion. This presentation may be contrasted with that of the patient who develops chronic cor pulmonale as a result of multiple pulmonary emboli with organization and gradually rising pressures in the pulmonary artery, right side of the heart, and systemic venous bed. Cardiac output and perfusion of the renal bed may be normal, at least in the resting state, but abnormal retention of extracellular fluid volume, with congestive hepatomegaly, ankle edema, and ascites, may occur. Such a patient manifests relatively pure backward failure.

Similar considerations apply to disorders affecting the left ventricle. For instance, a massive myocardial infarction may result in either (1) forward failure with a marked reduction of left ventricular output and cardiogenic shock (p. 579) and clinical manifestations secondary to impaired perfusion (hypotension, mental confusion, oliguria, and so on) or (2) backward failure with a transient inequality of output between the two ventricles, resulting in acute pulmonary edema. More commonly, patients with large myocardial infarctions develop a combination of forward and backward failure, with symptoms resulting from both inadequate cardiac output and pulmonary congestion. Early in the course of acute myocardial infarction, patients might succumb long before renal retention of salt and water can occur. However, if the patients survive the acute insult, expansion of the extracellular fluid volume and manifestations resulting therefrom usually occur.

The relative importance of forward and backward failure in the genesis of the clinical manifestations of heart failure also depends on the specific anatomical abnormality. For instance, in conditions in which the filling of the right side of the heart is interfered with, such as tricuspid stenosis or constrictive pericarditis, systemic venous pressure is markedly elevated; one can readily appreciate how this leads to capillary transudation, hepatomegaly, edema, and ascites (i.e., to backward heart failure). Some patients with chronic left ventricular failure secondary to coronary artery disease or hypertension may exhibit marked accumulation of sodium and water in the systemic venous bed with little elevation of systemic venous pressure. In such patients, accumulation of fluid is largely due to impairment of renal perfusion (i.e., forward heart failure accompanied by excessive renal tubular sodium reabsorption).

There is general agreement that fluid retention in heart failure, regardless of the transudation of fluid from the capillary bed, is caused ultimately in part by reduction in glomerular filtration rate and in part by activation of the renin-angiotensin-aldosterone system. Reduced cardiac output is associated with a lowered glomerular filtration rate and an increased elaboration of renin, which, through the activation of angiotensin, results in the release of aldosterone. The combination of impaired hepatic function, owing to hepatic venous congestion, and reduced hepatic blood flow interferes with the metabolism of aldosterone,[12] further raising its plasma concentration and augmenting the retention of sodium and water.

As already noted, cardiac output (and glomerular filtration rate) may be normal in many patients with heart failure, particularly when they are at rest. However, during stress, such as physical exercise and fever, the cardiac output fails to rise normally, the glomerular filtration rate declines, and the renal mechanisms for salt and water retention described above come into play. In addition, ventricular filling pressure, and therefore pressures in the atrium and systemic veins behind (upstream to) the ventricle, may be normal at rest, only to rise abnormally during the stress. This, in turn, may cause transudation and symptoms of tissue congestion (pulmonary in the case of the left ventricle and systemic in the case of the right) during exercise. For this reason simple rest may induce diuresis and relieve symptoms in many patients with mild heart failure.

RIGHT-SIDED VS. LEFT-SIDED HEART FAILURE

Implicit in the backward failure theory is the idea that fluid localizes behind the specific cardiac chamber that is *initially* affected. Thus, symptoms secondary to pulmonary congestion initially predominate in patients with left ventricular infarction, hypertension, and aortic and mitral valve disease, i.e., they manifest *left heart failure*. With time, however, fluid accumulation becomes generalized, and ankle edema, congestive hepatomegaly, ascites, and pleural effusion occur (i.e., the patients later exhibit *right heart failure* as well). Less commonly, prolonged right ventricular failure with massive accumulation of extracellular fluid may be associated with dyspnea, particularly when the patient is in the supine position and when large pleural effusions are present.

Although a disturbance of contractile function initially takes place in the ventricle subjected to the abnormal burden, with the passage of time the other ventricle undergoes changes as well. For example, the depletion of norepinephrine that occurs in experimental animals subjected to ventricular pressure overload is not confined to the stressed ventricle, but also involves the opposite ventricle.[13] Similarly, alterations in the activity of actomyosin ATPase have been described in both ventricles of animals in which the hemodynamic burden was placed on only one.[14] These findings are not surprising when one considers that both ventricles share a common wall — the interventricular septum — and that the muscle bundles constituting the ventricles are continuous. In addition, all four cardiac chambers are enclosed within and share space within the pericardial sac. As a consequence, when cardiac expansion is limited by the pericardium, as occurs in pericardial constriction, with large pericardial effusions, or even with a normal pericardium when the size of one side of the heart suddenly increases (e.g., the left ventricle and atrium in acute severe aortic regurgitation), the opposite chambers are compressed, and the filling pressure of the normal ventricle rises. This condition is called *ventricular interdependence*.

ACUTE VS. CHRONIC HEART FAILURE

The clinical manifestations of heart failure depend importantly on the *rate* at which the syndrome develops and specifically on whether sufficient time has elapsed for compensatory mechanisms to become operative and for fluid to accumulate in the interstitial space. For example, when a previously normal person suddenly develops a serious anatomical or functional abnormality of the heart (such as massive myocardial infarction, heart block with a very slow ventricular rate [$<$35/min], a tachyarrhythmia with a very rapid rate [$>$180/min], rupture of a valve secondary to infective endocarditis, or occlusion of a large segment of the pulmonary vascular bed by a pulmonary embolus), a marked, sudden reduction in cardiac output with symptoms due to inadequate organ perfusion and/or acute congestion of the venous bed behind the affected ventricle will occur. If the same anatomical abnormality develops gradually, or if the patient survives the acute insult, a number of adaptive mechanisms become operational, especially cardiac hypertrophy, and these allow the patient to adjust to and tolerate not only the anatomical abnormality, but also a reduction in cardiac output, with less difficulty. Frequently, the important clinical manifestations of chronic heart failure secondary to tissue congestion may be suppressed by dietary sodium restriction and diuretics. Cardiac function may not have been improved, and such patients still are in "heart failure," albeit with fewer clinical manifestations thereof. Under these circumstances, an acute event such as an infection, an arrhythmia, or discontinuation of therapy may precipitate manifestations of acute heart failure.

LOW-OUTPUT VS. HIGH-OUTPUT HEART FAILURE

Low cardiac output at rest, or in milder cases only during exertion and other stresses, characterizes heart failure occurring in most forms of heart disease (i.e., congenital, valvular, rheumatic, hypertensive, coronary, and cardiomyopathic). A variety of high-output states, including thyrotoxicosis, arteriovenous fistulas, beriberi, Paget's disease of bone, anemia, and pregnancy (discussed later in this chapter), may lead to heart failure as well. Low-output heart failure is characterized by clinical evidence of impairment of the peripheral circulation, with systemic vasoconstriction and cold, pale, and sometimes cyanotic extremities; in advanced forms of low-output failure, as the stroke volume declines, the pulse pressure narrows.[15] In contrast, in high-output heart failure (pp. 458 to 462) the extremities are usually warm and flushed, and the pulse pressure is widened or at least normal. The ability of the heart to deliver the quantity of oxygen required by the metabolizing tissues is reflected in the arterial-mixed venous oxygen difference, which is abnormally widened (i.e., $>$5.0 ml/liter in the resting state) in patients with low-output heart failure. This difference may be normal or even reduced in high-output states, owing to elevation of the mixed venous oxygen saturation by the admixture of blood that has been shunted away from metabolizing tissues. However, regardless of the absolute level of the arterial-mixed venous oxygen (high in low-output heart failure and normal or low in high-output heart failure) in the presence of heart failure, this difference still exceeds the level that existed *before* the development of heart failure, and cardiac output, regardless of its absolute level, is lower than it had been before the development of heart failure.

SYSTOLIC VS. DIASTOLIC HEART FAILURE

(Fig. 16–1)

Implicit in the physiological definition of heart failure (inability to pump an adequate volume of blood and/or to do so only from an abnormally elevated filling pressure) is that heart failure can be caused by an abnormality in systolic function leading to a defect in the expulsion of blood (i.e., *systolic heart failure*), or by an abnormality in diastolic function leading to a defect in ventricular filling (i.e., *diastolic heart failure*). The former is the more familiar, classic heart failure in which an impaired inotropic state is responsible. Less familiar, but perhaps just as important, is diastolic heart failure, in which the ability of the ventricle(s) to accept blood is impaired. This may be due to slowed or incomplete ventricular relaxation which may be transient, as occurs in acute ischemia, or sustained, as in concentric myocardial hypertrophy or restrictive cardiomyopathy secondary to infiltrative conditions such as amyloidosis. The principal clinical manifestations of systolic failure result from an inadequate forward cardiac output, while the major consequences of diastolic failure relate to elevation of the ventricular filling pressure and the high venous pressure upstream to the ventricle, causing pulmonic and/or systemic congestion.

There are many examples of pure systolic or diastolic heart failure. Examples of the former are patients with acute massive pulmonary embolism or dilated cardiomyopathy, while examples of the latter are patients with hypertrophic cardiomyopathy or subendocardial fibrosis. However, in many patients systolic and diastolic heart failure coexist. The most common form of heart failure, that caused by coronary atherosclerosis, is an example of combined systolic and diastolic failure. Systolic failure is caused by both the chronic loss of contracting myocardium secondary to myocardial necrosis resulting from previous infarction and the acute loss of myocardial contractility induced by a transient episode of ischemia. Diastolic failure is due to the ventricle's reduced compliance caused by replacement of normal, distensible myocardium with nondistensible fibrous scar tissue and by the acute reduction of diastolic distensibility of reversibly injured myocardium during a transient episode of ischemia.

HEART FAILURE IN THE NEONATE AND INFANT

Heart failure in the neonate and infant has a different clinical expression from that in the older child and adult.[16] Feeding difficulties, failure to gain weight and grow, tachypnea, and excessive diaphoresis are manifestations of heart failure occurring in the first year of life. Obstruction of the airways because of enlargement of the left atrium and main pulmonary artery may result in either emphysematous expansion of the left lung or, in severer cases, atelectasis. Excessive sweat-

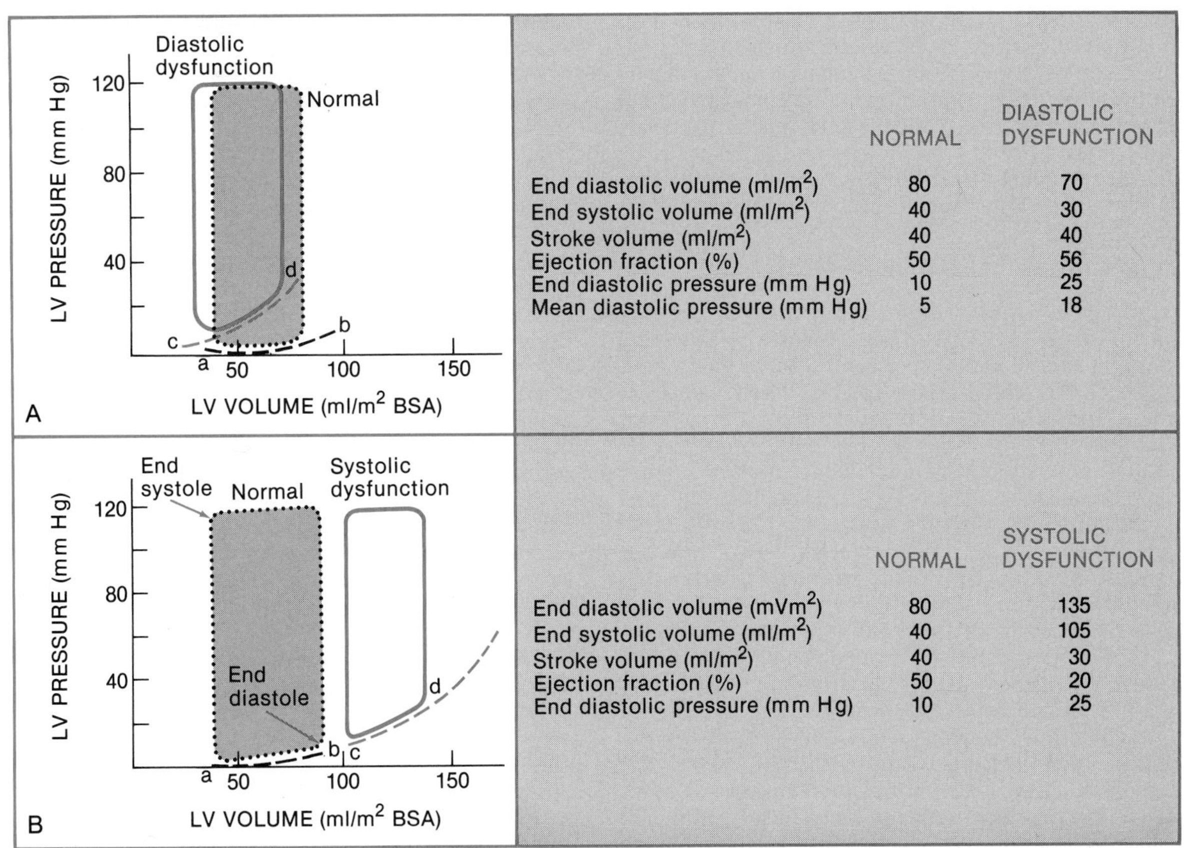

	NORMAL	DIASTOLIC DYSFUNCTION
End diastolic volume (ml/m²)	80	70
End systolic volume (ml/m²)	40	30
Stroke volume (ml/m²)	40	40
Ejection fraction (%)	50	56
End diastolic pressure (mm Hg)	10	25
Mean diastolic pressure (mm Hg)	5	18

	NORMAL	SYSTOLIC DYSFUNCTION
End diastolic volume (mVm²)	80	135
End systolic volume (ml/m²)	40	105
Stroke volume (ml/m²)	40	30
Ejection fraction (%)	50	20
End diastolic pressure (mm Hg)	10	25

FIGURE 16–1. ***A,*** **Schematic of a pressure-volume loop from a normal subject (dotted line) and a patient with diastolic dysfunction (solid line). Dashed lines represent the diastolic pressure-volume relation. Isolated diastolic dysfunction is characterized by a shift in pressure-volume loop to the left. Contractile performance is normal (normal or increased ejection fraction, normal or slightly decreased stroke volume). However, LV pressures throughout diastole are increased; at a common diastolic volume = 70 ml/m². LV diastolic pressure is 25 mm Hg in the patient with diastolic failure compared with a diastolic pressure of 5 mm Hg in normal subject. Thus, diastolic dysfunction increases modulus of chamber stiffness. LV, left ventricular.** ***B,*** **Schematic of pressure-volume loop from a normal subject (dotted line) and a patient with systolic dysfunction (solid line). Dashed line represents diastolic pressure-volume relation. Systolic dysfunction is characterized by displacement of pressure-volume loop to the right. Despite compensatory dilation, stroke volume or ejection fraction remains low. LV diastolic pressures are increased as a result of large LV volume. LV, left ventricular. (From Zile, M.R.: Diastolic dysfunction: Detection, consequences, and treatment. Part 2: Diagnosis and treatment of diastolic dysfunction. Mod. Concepts Cardiovasc. Dis. 59:1, 1990.)**

ing and repeated pulmonary infections are common features of heart failure in infants. Interstitial pulmonary edema causes a reduction in tidal volume; this in turn causes tachypnea, increased work of breathing, increased total metabolism, and tachycardia. Respiratory distress is manifested by flaring of the alae nasi, grunting, and retraction of the ribs, features seldom seen in adults. Peripheral perfusion is poor, with cool limbs and delayed capillary filling. Hepatomegaly is a common manifestation of both left and right heart failure in infants, as is a paradoxical pulse secondary to wide variations in ventricular filling as a consequence of marked swings in intrapulmonary pressure. Peripheral edema, ascites, and pulsus alternans occur *far less frequently* in infants than in older children or adults with heart failure. On the other hand, facial edema, an uncommon finding in adults with heart failure, is more common than peripheral edema in infants.

Because of infants' short necks, distention of the jugular veins is difficult to detect. However, prominence of the veins on the back of the hand may be a valuable sign of systemic venous congestion. Although most neonates and infants (as well as adults) with cardiac failure have heart disease that is obvious on clinical examination, sometimes it is difficult to distinguish respiratory distress arising from cardiac disease from that associated with primary pulmonary disorders. Specifically, heart failure may be confused with bronchiolitis, asthma, or pneumonia. The presence of cyanosis and heart murmurs on physical examination and of cardiomegaly and pulmonary congestion on radiological examination are helpful although not decisive signs in the differential diagnosis.

CAUSES OF HEART FAILURE

From a clinical viewpoint, it is useful to classify the causes of heart failure into three broad categories: (1) *underlying causes*, comprising the structural abnormalities—congenital or acquired—that affect the peripheral and coronary vessels, pericardium, myocardium, or cardiac valves and lead to the increased hemodynamic burden or myocardial or coronary insufficiency responsible for heart failure; (2) *fundamental causes*, comprising the biochemical and physiological mechanisms through which either an increased hemodynamic burden or a reduction in oxygen delivery to the myocardium results in impairment of myocardial contraction (Chap. 14); and (3) *precipitating causes*, including the specific causes or incidents that precipitate heart failure in 50 to 90 per cent of episodes of clinical heart failure.

It is helpful to recognize both the underlying and the precipitating causes of heart failure. Appropriate management of the underlying heart disease (e.g., surgical correction of a congenital defect or an acquired valvular abnormality, or pharmacological management of hypertension) may prevent the development or recurrence of heart failure. Similarly, treatment of the precipitating cause will usually rapidly terminate an episode of heart failure and may be life-saving. More important, *prevention* of a precipitating cause can prevent heart failure.

Overt heart failure may, of course, also be precipitated if there is progression of the underlying heart disease. A previously stable, compensated patient may develop heart failure that is apparent clinically for the first time when the intrinsic process has advanced to a critical point, such as with progressive obliteration of the pulmonary vascular bed in a patient with cor pulmonale or further narrowing of a stenotic aortic valve. Alternatively, decompensation may occur as a result of failure or exhaustion of the compensatory mechanisms but without any change in the volume load on the heart, or by progressive depression of intrinsic myocardial contractility which occurs with persistent severe pressure or volume overload.

PRECIPITATING CAUSES OF HEART FAILURE

In one study of 101 patients admitted to an inner city municipal hospital with the diagnosis of heart failure, precipitating factors could be identified in 93 per cent[17] (Table 16–2).

INAPPROPRIATE REDUCTION OF THERAPY. Perhaps the most common cause of decompensation in a previously compensated patient with heart failure is inappropriate reduction in the intensity of treatment—be it dietary sodium restriction, reduced physical activity, a drug regimen, or, most commonly, a combination of these measures. Many patients with serious underlying heart disease, regardless of whether they previously experienced heart failure, may be relatively asymptomatic for as long as they carefully adhere to their treatment regimen. However, without appropriate and reinforced instruction, the patient who has become asymptomatic may incorrectly assume that the underlying condition has been "cured" and may voluntarily diminish the intensity of therapy, precipitating recurrent heart failure. Perhaps the most serious example of this situation is the patient who adjusts his digitalis dosage on the basis of symptoms of heart failure, discontinuing the drug when these have diminished but taking three, four, or even more times the maintenance dose when symptoms of heart failure are present. Obviously this practice can lead to wide swings in digitalis levels, exacerbation of heart failure, and digitalis intoxication. Dietary excesses of sodium, incurred frequently on vacations or holidays or during an illness of the spouse responsible for preparing the patient's meals, are frequent causes of sudden cardiac decompensation. Careful and repeated instruction of the patient is a simple yet effective measure to prevent this common clinical problem.

ARRHYTHMIAS (see also Chap. 24). Cardiac arrhythmias are far more common in patients with underlying structural heart disease than in normal subjects and commonly precipitate or intensify heart failure. The development of arrhythmias may precipitate heart failure through several mechanisms: (1) *Tachyarrhythmias*, most commonly atrial fibrillation (Table 16–2), reduce the time available for ventricular filling. When there is already an impairment of ventricular filling, as in mitral stenosis, or reduced ventricular compliance (diastolic failure, see below), tachycardia will raise atrial pressure and reduce cardiac output further. In addition, tachyarrhythmias increase myocardial oxygen demands and, in a patient with obstructive coronary artery disease, may induce or intensify myocardial ischemia, which, in turn, impairs both cardiac relaxation and systolic function, thereby raising left atrial and pulmonary capillary pressure further and causing symptoms secondary to pulmonary congestion. (2) *Marked bradycardia* in a patient with underlying heart disease usually depresses cardiac output, since stroke volume may already be maximal and cannot rise further to maintain cardiac output. (3) *Dissociation between atrial and ventricular contraction*, which occurs in many arrhythmias, results in loss of the atrial booster pump mechanism, which impairs ventricular filling, lowers cardiac output, and raises atrial pressure.[18] This loss is particularly deleterious in patients with impaired ventricular filling due to concentric cardiac hypertrophy (e.g., in systemic hypertension, aortic stenosis, and hypertrophic cardiomyopathy). (4) *Abnormal intraventricular conduction*, which occurs in many arrhythmias such as ventricular tachycardia, impairs myocardial performance because of loss of the normal synchronicity of ventricular contraction. In addition to precipitating heart failure, arrhythmias—sometimes fatal—may be *caused* by heart failure.

SYSTEMIC INFECTION. Although patients with congestive heart failure are particularly susceptible to pulmonary infections, presumably because of the diminished ability of congested lungs to expel respiratory secretions, *any* infection may precipitate cardiac failure. The mechanisms include increased total metabolism as a consequence of fever, discomfort, and cough, which increase the hemodynamic burden on the heart; the accompanying sinus tachycardia, secondary to fever and discomfort, plays an additional adverse role.

PULMONARY EMBOLISM. Patients with congestive heart failure, particularly when confined to bed, are at high risk of developing pulmonary emboli. Such emboli may increase the hemodynamic burden on the right ventricle by elevating right ventricular systolic pressure further and may cause fever, tachypnea, and tachycardia (Chap. 48), the deleterious effects of which have already been discussed.

PHYSICAL, ENVIRONMENTAL, AND EMOTIONAL EXCESSES. Intense, prolonged exertion or severe fatigue, such as may result from prolonged travel or emotional crises, and a severe climatic change, such as to a hot, humid environment, are relatively common precipitants of cardiac decompensation.

CARDIAC INFECTION AND INFLAMMATION. Myocarditis owing to a recurrence of acute rheumatic fever (Chap. 56) or to infective endocarditis (Chap. 35) or as a consequence of a variety of allergic inflammatory or infectious processes (including viral myocarditis) may impair myocardial function directly and exacerbate existing heart disease. The anemia, fever, and tachycardia that frequently accompany these processes are also deleterious. In patients with infective endocarditis, additional valvular damage may also precipitate cardiac decompensation.

DEVELOPMENT OF AN UNRELATED ILLNESS. Heart failure may be precipitated in patients with compensated heart disease when an unrelated illness develops. For example, the development of intrinsic renal disease may impair further the ability of patients with heart failure to excrete sodium and thus may intensify the accumulation of fluid. Similarly, blood transfusion or the administration of sodium-containing fluid after a noncardiac operation may result in sudden heart failure in patients with underlying heart disease. Prostatic obstruction in the elderly male, parenchymal liver disease, and the administration of corticosteroids or estrogens with sodium-retaining properties may also precipitate heart failure in patients with underlying heart disease.

TABLE 16–2 PRECIPITATING FACTORS IN CHRONIC HEART FAILURE

	NO. OF PATIENTS
Lack of compliance	64
With diet	22
With drugs	6
With both (diet and drugs)	37
Uncontrolled hypertension	44
Cardiac arrhythmias	29
Atrial fibrillation	20
Atrial flutter	7
Multifocal atrial tachycardia	1
Ventricular tachycardia	1
Environmental factors	19
Inadequate therapy	17
Pulmonary infection	12
Emotional stress	7
Administration of inappropriate medications or fluid overload	4
Myocardial infarction	6
Endocrine disorders (thyrotoxicosis)	1

Adapted from Ghali, J. K., Kadakia, S., Cooper, R., and Ferlinz, J.: Precipitating factors leading to decompensation of heart failure: Traits among urban blacks. Arch. Intern. Med. *148*:2013, 1988.

ADMINISTRATION OF CARDIAC DEPRESSANTS OR SALT-RETAINING DRUGS. A variety of drugs depress myocardial function; among these are alcohol, beta-adrenoceptor blocking agents, many antiarrhythmic agents,[19] verapamil, and antineoplastic drugs such as doxorubicin (Adriamycin) and cyclophosphamide. Others, such as estrogens, androgens, glucocorticoids, and nonsteroidal antiinflammatory agents, may cause salt and water retention. Any of these drugs when administered to a patient with heart disease can precipitate or aggravate heart failure.

HIGH-OUTPUT STATES. Acute heart failure may be precipitated in patients with underlying heart disease who develop one of the hyperkinetic circulatory states (pp. 458–462).

DEVELOPMENT OF A SECOND FORM OF HEART DISEASE. Patients with one form of heart disease often remain compensated until they develop a second form. For example, a patient with chronic hypertension and left ventricular hypertrophy but without left ventricular failure may be asymptomatic until a myocardial infarction (which may be silent) develops and precipitates heart failure.

It is essential to search for these precipitating causes carefully and systematically in all patients with congestive heart failure, since lack of recognition or treatment or both may be responsible for otherwise refractory heart failure. In most instances they can be treated effectively, after which appropriate measures should be instituted to avoid recurrence. When a precipitating cause of heart failure can be identified, it generally signifies a better prognosis than when a similar degree of heart failure is due simply to progression of the underlying cardiac disease.

SYMPTOMS OF HEART FAILURE

RESPIRATORY DISTRESS

Breathlessness, a cardinal manifestation of left ventricular failure,[20,21] may present with progressively increasing severity as (1) exertional dyspnea, (2) orthopnea, (3) paroxysmal nocturnal dyspnea, (4) dyspnea at rest, and (5) acute pulmonary edema.

EXERTIONAL DYSPNEA (see also p. 2). The principal difference between exertional dyspnea in normal subjects and in patients with heart failure is the degree of activity necessary to induce the symptom. Indeed, as heart failure first develops, exertional dyspnea may simply appear to be an aggravation of the breathlessness that occurs in normal subjects during activity. Because dyspnea occurs on exertion in all individuals, normal and abnormal, an effort should be made to elicit in the history whether or not a *change* in the extent of exertion which causes dyspnea has actually occurred. It is also important to attempt to distinguish dyspnea secondary to poor conditioning from that caused by cardiac (or pulmonary) disease. Patients usually report that a specific task which they were able to carry out without difficulty for many years (e.g., climbing two flights of stairs) evokes more breathlessness than previously or requires them to stop midway or both. As left ventricular failure advances, the intensity of exercise resulting in breathlessness declines progressively. However, there is no close correlation between subjective exercise capacity and objective measures of left ventricular performance at rest in patients with heart failure.[21] It is obvious that exertional dyspnea can occur only in patients who exert themselves. This cardinal symptom of left ventricular failure may be absent in patients who are sedentary for a variety of reasons—habit, the presence of a cardiovascular disease (e.g., severe angina or intermittent claudication) or a noncardiovascular disease (e.g., crippling arthritis).

ORTHOPNEA. This symptom may be defined as dyspnea that develops in the recumbent position and is relieved by elevation of the head with pillows. Again, as in the case of exertional dyspnea, it is a *change* in the number of pillows required that is important, since many normal individuals prefer to sleep with their heads elevated by two or three pillows. In the recumbent position there is reduced pooling of fluid in the lower extremities and abdomen; blood is displaced from the extrathoracic to the thoracic compartment. The failing left ventricle, operating on the flat portion of its depressed Starling curve (Fig. 15–1, p. 420), cannot accept and pump out the extra volume of blood delivered to it by the competent right ventricle without dilating, and pulmonary venous and capillary pressures rise further, causing interstitial edema, reduced pulmonary compliance, increased airway resistance, and dyspnea. In contrast to paroxysmal nocturnal dyspnea (see below), orthopnea occurs rapidly, often within a minute or two of assuming recumbency, and develops when the patient is awake. It is an important symptom of heart failure but is far from specific and may occur in any condition in which vital capacity is low; dyspnea is exacerbated when recumbency elevates the diaphragm, reducing vital capacity even further. Marked ascites, whatever its etiology, is an important cause of orthopnea.

The patient with orthopnea generally elevates his head and chest on several pillows to prevent nocturnal breathlessness and the development of paroxysmal nocturnal dyspnea (see below); in fact, the severity of orthopnea is conveniently estimated from the number of pillows required. Patients frequently awaken short of breath if the head has slipped off the pillows, and they then often seek and find relief by sitting in front of an open window. In advanced left ventricular failure, orthopnea may be so severe that the patient cannot lie down and must spend the night in the sitting position. Often such patients are observed sitting at the side of the bed, slumped over a bedside table.

Cough may be caused by pulmonary congestion, occurs under the same circumstances as dyspnea (i.e., during exertion or recumbency), and is relieved by treatment of heart failure. Thus a nonproductive *cough* in patients with heart failure is often a "dyspnea equivalent," whereas a nocturnal cough may be considered an "orthopnea equivalent." Patients with severe chronic obstructive lung disease sometimes complain of orthopnea. These patients, whose lungs are hyperinflated, rely on their accessory muscles of respiration. Orthopnea is related to loss of the support provided by these muscles in the recumbent position. *Trepopnea* is a rare form of orthopnea limited to one lateral decubitus position. It has been attributed to distortions of the great vessels in one position but not in the other.

PAROXYSMAL NOCTURNAL DYSPNEA. Attacks of paroxysmal dyspnea usually occur at night. The patient awakens, often quite suddenly, and with a feeling of severe anxiety and suffocation, sits bolt upright, and gasps for breath. Bronchospasm, which may be caused by congestion of the bronchial mucosa and by interstitial pulmonary edema compressing the small bronchi, increases ventilatory difficulty and the work of breathing and is a common complicating factor of paroxysmal nocturnal dyspnea. The commonly associated wheezing is responsible for the alternate name of this condition, *cardiac asthma*. In contrast to orthopnea, which may be relieved immediately by sitting upright at the side of the bed with the legs dependent, attacks of paroxysmal nocturnal dyspnea may require 30 minutes or longer in this position for relief. Episodes of paroxysmal nocturnal dyspnea may be so frightening that the patient may be afraid to go back to sleep, even after the symptoms have abated.

The reason for the common occurrence of these episodes at night is not clear, but it seems likely that the combination of (1) the slow resorption of interstitial fluid from the dependent portion of the body and the resultant expansion of thoracic blood volume, (2) sudden elevation of thoracic blood volume and of the diaphragm which occurs immediately on assuming recumbency (as described above for orthopnea), (3) reduced adrenergic support of left ventricular function during sleep, and (4) normal nocturnal depression of the respiratory center plays a major role. Attacks of paroxysmal dyspnea seldom occur during the daytime and are provoked by effort or excitement. When accompanied by chest heaviness, these episodes

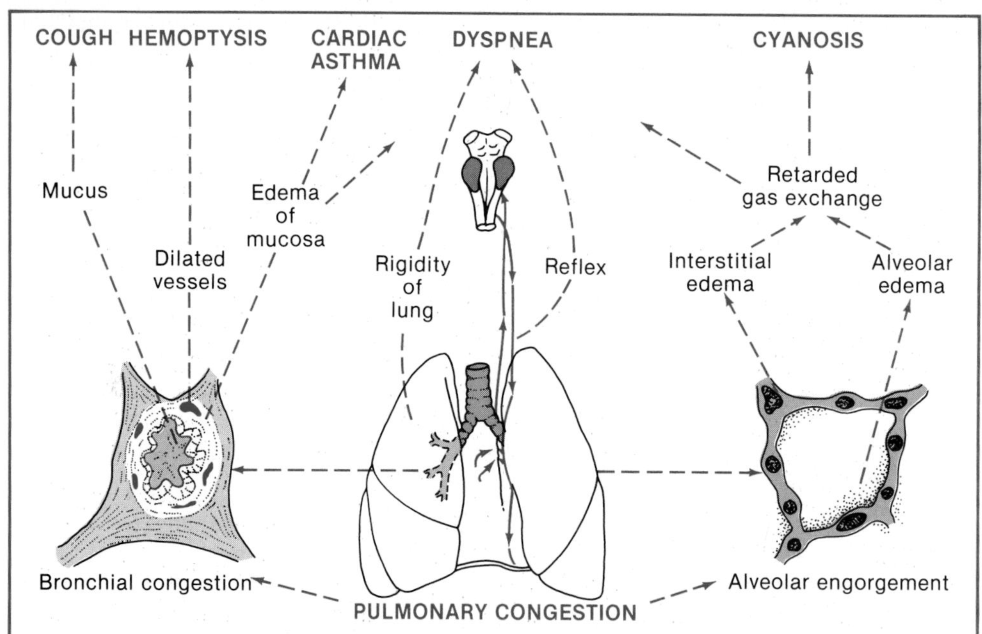

FIGURE 16–2. Etiology of respiratory symptoms from pulmonary congestion. Since most bronchial capillaries drain by way of the pulmonary veins, congestion develops simultaneously in alveolar and bronchial vascular networks. Bronchial congestion tends to stimulate production of mucus, leading to a productive cough. The distended bronchial capillaries may rupture, causing the patient to cough up blood-tinged sputum (hemoptysis). Edema of the bronchial mucosa increases resistance to air flow, producing respiratory distress similar to asthma. Dyspnea results primarily from reflexes initiated by vascular distention but may be supplemented by increased rigidity of the lungs and by impaired gas exchange resulting from interstitial edema and the accumulation of fluid in alveolar sacs. (From Rushmer, R. F.: Cardiac compensation, hypertrophy and myopathy and congestive heart failure. *In* Rushmer, R. F. [ed.]: Cardiovascular Dynamics. Philadelphia, W. B. Saunders Company, 1976, p. 532.)

may be "anginal equivalents" and caused by myocardial ischemia.

PULMONARY EDEMA. The most severe form of breathlessness, pulmonary edema, is associated with a number of unique pathophysiological and clinical features and is described in Chap. 20.

Mechanisms of Dyspnea

Increased awareness of respiration or difficulty in breathing is commonly associated with pulmonary capillary hypertension caused by an elevation of left atrial or left ventricular filling pressure. Patients with left ventricular failure typically exhibit a restrictive ventilatory defect, characterized by a reduction of vital capacity as a consequence of the replacement of the air in the lungs with blood or interstitial fluid or both. Consequently, the lungs become stiffer, air trapping occurs because of earlier than normal closure of dependent airways,[22] and the work of breathing is increased because higher intrapleural pressures are needed to distend the stiff lungs. Tidal volume is reduced, and respiratory frequency rises in a compensatory fashion. Engorgement of blood vessels may reduce the caliber of the peripheral airways, increasing airway resistance. In addition, there are alterations in the distribution of ventilation and perfusion, resulting in widened alveolar–arterial differences for oxygen, hypoxemia, and an increased ratio of dead space to tidal volume. Thus, dyspnea (during exertion or at rest) and orthopnea are clinical expressions of pulmonary venous and capillary congestion. Paroxysmal nocturnal dyspnea reflects the presence of primarily *interstitial* edema, whereas pulmonary edema, in which there is transudation and expectoration of blood-tinged fluid (Chap. 20), is often a manifestation of *alveolar* edema.

Whatever abnormalities in mechanics and gas exchange function of the lung that exist at rest are aggravated during exercise (and sometimes during recumbency) when pulmonary venous and capillary pressures rise further. Transudation of fluid from the intravascular to the extravascular space results in greater stiffening of the lungs, an augmentation in the work of breathing, and increased resistance to air flow.[23] There is an increased ventilatory drive, as a consequence of the stimulation of stretch receptors in the pulmonary vessels and interstitium, as well as a result of hypoxemia and metabolic acidosis. The increased work of breathing, combined with a low cardiac output and resulting impaired perfusion of the respiratory muscles, causes fatigue[24] and ultimately the sensation of dyspnea.[25]

The *precise* mechanism (or mechanisms) responsible for the respiratory distress of heart failure has not been definitively elucidated,[26] but a number of factors may be in operation (Fig. 16–2). Dyspnea occurs whenever the work of respiration is excessive. Increased force generation is required for the respiratory muscles to move a given volume of air if the compliance of the lungs is reduced or the resistance to air flow is increased; both of these changes occur in left heart failure. Although patients are more likely to become dyspneic when the work of respiration is augmented, this increased work does not account for the perceptual difference between a deep breath with a normal mechanical load and a normal-sized breath with an increased mechanical load. The amount of work may be the same with both breaths, but the normal breath with the increased load will be associated with discomfort.

A more appealing theory of the mechanism of dyspnea involves an inappropriate relation between length and tension in the respiratory muscles. It has been proposed that discomfort arises when there is misalignment of the nerve spindles, which sense tension, in relation to muscle length. This misalignment could lead to the sensation of getting an insufficient breath for the tension generated by the respiratory muscles.[27] Dyspnea at rest may also occur in the late stages of heart failure when the combination of very low cardiac output, hypoxemia, and acidosis conspires to reduce the delivery of oxygen to the respiratory muscle.[28] Dyspnea may occur without pulmonary congestion in patients with right ventricular failure, a fixed low cardiac output, and/or a right-to-left shunt.

Differentiation Between Cardiac and Pulmonary Dyspnea

In most patients with dyspnea there is obvious clinical evidence of disease of either the heart *or* the lungs, but in some the differentiation between cardiac and pulmonary dyspnea may be difficult.[21] The dyspnea of chronic obstructive lung disease tends to develop more gradually than that of heart disease; exceptions, of course, occur in patients with *obstructive lung disease* who experience episodes of infectious bronchitis, pneumonia, or pneumothorax or an exacerbation of asthma. Like patients with heart failure, patients with chronic obstructive lung disease may also waken at night with dyspnea, but this is usually associated with sputum production; the dyspnea is relieved after the patient rids himself of secretions by coughing rather than specifically by sitting up. When the dyspnea arises after a history of intensified cough and expectoration, it is usually primarily pulmonary in origin.

Acute cardiac asthma (paroxysmal nocturnal dyspnea with prominent wheezing) usually occurs in patients who have obvious clinical evidence of heart disease and may be further differentiated from acute bronchial asthma by diaphoresis, bubblier airway sounds, and the more common occurrence of cyanosis. The difficulty in distinguishing between cardiac and pulmonary dyspnea may be compounded by the coexistence of diseases involving both organ systems. Thus, patients with a history of chronic bronchitis or asthma who develop left ventricular failure tend to develop particularly severe bronchoconstriction and wheezing in association with bouts of paroxysmal nocturnal dyspnea and pulmonary edema. Airway obstruction and dyspnea that respond to bronchodilators or smoking cessation favor a pulmonary origin of the dyspnea, while the response of these manifestations to diuretics supports heart failure as the cause of dyspnea.

PULMONARY FUNCTION TESTING. This testing should be carried out in patients in whom the etiology of dyspnea is unclear despite detailed clinical evaluation. The results may be helpful in determining whether dyspnea is produced by heart disease, lung disease, a combination of the two, or neither. In the last case, it may be a manifestation of anxiety.

The major alterations in pulmonary function tests in congestive heart failure are reductions of vital capacity, total lung capacity, pulmonary diffusion capacity at rest and particularly during exercise, and pulmonary compliance; resistance to air flow is moderately increased; residual volume and functional residual volume are normal. Often there is hyperventilation at rest and during exercise, an increase in dead space, and some abnormalities of ventilation-perfusion relations with slight reductions in arterial P_{CO_2} and P_{O_2}. With pulmonary capillary hypertension, pulmonary compliance decreases and there is air trapping because of earlier than normal closure of dependent airways. The airway resistance rises,[29] as does the work of breathing.

Rarely, it may be difficult to differentiate among cardiac dyspnea, dyspnea based on *malingering*, and dyspnea caused by an *anxiety neurosis*. Careful observation for the appearance of effortless or irregular respiration during exercise testing often helps to identify the patient in whom dyspnea is related to the latter two noncardiac causes. Patients whose anxiety neurosis focuses on the heart may fear the presence of heart disease and may exhibit sighing respiration and difficulty in taking a deep breath as well as dyspnea at rest. Their breathing patterns are not rapid and shallow, as in cardiac dyspnea. Rarely a "therapeutic test" is helpful, and amelioration of dyspnea, accompanied by a weight loss exceeding 2 kg induced by administration of a diuretic, supports a cardiac origin for the dyspnea. Conversely, failure of these measures to achieve weight reduction in excess of 2 kg and to diminish dyspnea weighs heavily against a cardiac origin.

Exercise Testing

(See also Chap. 6 and p. 436)

Exercise stress testing may be an exceedingly useful adjunct in the *clinical* assessment of patients with suspected or known heart failure.[30,31] With use of a bicycle ergometer or treadmill with a progressively increasing load, the maximum level of exercise which can be achieved can be determined; the latter correlates closely with the total oxygen uptake ($\dot{V}O_2$). Close observation of the patient during an exercise test may disclose obvious difficulty in breathing at a low level of exercise (or the opposite). Thus, this simple test may be considered to be an extension of the clinical examination.

A more formal assessment in which $\dot{V}O_2$ is measured at each stage of exercise, or preferably in which $\dot{V}O_2$ and $\dot{V}CO_2$ are measured continuously, allows determination of maximum $\dot{V}O_2$ and the anaerobic threshold (i.e., the point during the exercise test at which the respiratory quotient rises as a consequence of the production of excess lactate)[29] (Figs. 6–1 and 6–2). When a progressive exercise test is carried out until (1) $\dot{V}O_2$ fails to rise with further increases in activity or (2) the patient is limited by severe dyspnea and/or fatigue, a $\dot{V}O_2$ less than 25 mg/kg/min represents a reduction of maximum $\dot{V}O_2$. When this reduction is caused by a cardiac abnormality (rather than by pulmonary disease, anemia, peripheral vascular disease, skeletal muscle deformity, marked obesity, severe deconditioning, or malingering), it may be used to classify the severity of heart failure, to follow the progress of the patient, and to assess the efficacy of therapeutic maneuvers.[31,32]

OTHER SYMPTOMS

FATIGUE AND WEAKNESS. These symptoms, often accompanied by a feeling of heaviness in the limbs, are generally related to poor perfusion of the skeletal muscles in patients with a lowered cardiac output. They may be associated with impaired vasodilation and altered metabolism in skeletal muscle.[28] Fatigue and weakness, of course, are notoriously nonspecific and may be caused by a variety of noncardiopulmonary diseases as well as by neurasthenia; they may be caused by sodium depletion, hypovolemia, or both, as a consequence of excessive treatment with diuretics and restriction of dietary sodium. Beta-adrenoreceptor blockers, administered for hypertension, angina, or following myocardial infarction, may cause fatigue.

URINARY SYMPTOMS. *Nocturia* may occur relatively early in the course of heart failure. Urine formation is suppressed during the day when the patient is upright and active; this is due, at least in part, to a redistribution of blood flow away from the kidneys during activity[33] (Fig. 14–21, p. 410). When the patient rests in the recumbent position at night, the deficit in cardiac output in relation to oxygen demands is reduced, renal vasoconstriction diminishes, and urine formation increases. Nocturia may be troublesome in that it prevents the patient with heart failure from obtaining much-needed rest. The diurnal pattern of urine flow characteristic of heart failure contrasts sharply with that existing in renal failure, in which urine formation occurs at a reasonably constant rate, both day and night. *Oliguria* is a sign of late cardiac failure and is related to the suppression of urine formation as a consequence of severely reduced cardiac output.

CEREBRAL SYMPTOMS. Confusion, impairment of memory, anxiety, headache, insomnia, bad dreams or nightmares, and, rarely, psychosis with disorientation, delirium, and even hallucinations may occur in elderly patients with advanced heart failure, particularly in those with accompanying cerebral arteriosclerosis.

SYMPTOMS OF PREDOMINANT RIGHT HEART FAILURE. Breathlessness, the cardinal manifestation of left ventricular failure, is not as prominent in isolated right ventricular failure as it is in left heart failure because pulmonary congestion is usually absent. Indeed, when a patient with mitral stenosis or left ventricular failure develops right ventricular failure, the severer forms of dyspnea (i.e., paroxysmal nocturnal dyspnea and episodic pulmonary edema) tend to diminish in frequency and intensity. This reduction results from inability of the right ventricle to augment its output which prevents the temporary imbalance between blood flow into and out of the pulmonary vascular bed. On the other hand, when cardiac output becomes markedly reduced in patients with terminal right heart failure, as may occur in isolated right ventricular infarction and in the late stages of primary pulmonary hypertension and of pulmonary thromboembolic disease, severe dyspnea (air hunger) may occur, presumably as a consequence of the reduced cardiac output, poor perfusion of respiratory muscle, hypoxemia, and metabolic acidosis. In addition, dyspnea may be a prominent symptom in some patients with right ventricular failure and anasarca, hydrothorax, and ascites as a consequence of lung compression; such patients may even have orthopnea.

As in patients with predominant left ventricular failure, fatigue, a sense of heaviness of the limbs, and anorexia may be troubling symptoms in patients with predominant right heart failure. In patients with severe obstruction of right ventricular outflow of any cause and right ventricular failure, right ventricular stroke volume cannot be augmented, and dizziness and syncope may occur on exertion, just as in patients with aortic stenosis.

Congestive hepatomegaly may produce discomfort, generally described as a dull ache or heaviness, in the right upper quadrant or epigastrium. This discomfort, which is caused by stretching of the hepatic capsule, may be severe when the liver enlarges rapidly, as in acute right heart failure. In contrast, chronic, slowly developing hepatic enlargement is generally painless. Other gastrointestinal symptoms, including anorexia, nausea, bloating, a sense of fullness after meals, and constipation, occur owing to congestion of the liver and gastrointestinal tract. In severe, preterminal heart failure, inadequate bowel perfusion can cause abdominal pain, distention, and bloody stools. Nausea, anorexia, and emesis may also be due to cardiac drugs, particularly digitalis (p. 481) and quinidine (p. 633).

Functional Classification

A classification of patients with heart disease based on the relation between symptoms and the amount of effort required to provoke them has been developed by the New York Heart Association.[34] Although there are obvious limitations to assigning numerical values to subjective findings, this classification is nonetheless useful in comparing groups of patients as well as the same patient at different times.

Class I—*No limitation:* Ordinary physical activity does not cause undue fatigue, dyspnea, or palpitation.

Class II—*Slight limitation of physical activity:* Such patients are comfortable at rest. Ordinary physical activity results in fatigue, palpitation, dyspnea, or angina.

Class III—*Marked limitation of physical activity:* Although patients are comfortable at rest, less than ordinary activity will lead to symptoms.

Class IV—*Inability to carry on any physical activity without discomfort:* Symptoms of congestive failure are present even at rest. With any physical activity, increased discomfort is experienced.

As discussed on page 12, the accuracy and reproducibility of this classification are limited. To overcome these limitations, Goldman et al. have developed a useful classification based on the estimated metabolic cost of various activities[35] (Table 1–6, p. 11).

PHYSICAL FINDINGS

GENERAL APPEARANCE. Patients with mild or moderate heart failure appear to be in no distress after a few minutes of rest. However, they may be obviously dyspneic during and immediately after activity, such as walking to the physician's office or even after undressing. Patients with left ventricular failure may become uncomfortable if they lie flat without elevation of the head for more than a few minutes. Those with severe heart failure appear anxious and may exhibit signs of air hunger in this position. Patients with heart failure of recent onset appear acutely ill but are usually well nourished, whereas those with chronic cardiac failure often appear malnourished and sometimes even cachectic. Chronic, marked elevation of systemic venous pressure may produce exophthalmos and severe tricuspid regurgitation and may lead to visible systolic pulsation of the eyes[36] and of the neck veins. Cyanosis, icterus, and a malar flush may be evident in patients with severe heart failure.

In mild or moderately severe heart failure, stroke volume is normal at rest; in severe heart failure, it is reduced, and this is reflected in a diminished pulse pressure and dusky discoloration of the skin. With very severe failure, particularly if cardiac output has declined acutely, systolic arterial pressure may be reduced. The pulse may be rapid, weak, and thready. The proportional pulse pressure (pulse pressure/systolic pressure) correlates reasonably well with cardiac output. In one study,[15] when it was less than 25 per cent, it usually reflected a cardiac index of less than 2.2 liters/min/sq meter.

EVIDENCE OF INCREASED ADRENERGIC ACTIVITY. Increased activity of the adrenergic nervous system is an important accompaniment of heart failure. It is responsible for a number of physical signs, including peripheral vasoconstriction, which is manifested as pallor and coldness of the extremities and cyanosis of the digits. There may be diaphoresis with sinus tachycardia, loss of normal sinus arrhythmia, and obvious distention of the peripheral veins secondary to venoconstriction. Diastolic arterial pressure may even be slightly elevated.

PULMONARY RALES. Moist rales result from the transudation into the alveoli of fluid, which then moves into the airways. Rales are heard over the lung bases and are often accompanied by some dullness to percussion. They are characteristic of congestive heart failure of at least moderate severity. In acute pulmonary edema, coarse, bubbling rales and wheezes are heard over both lung fields and are accompanied by the expectoration of frothy, blood-tinged sputum (p. 551). However, the absence of rales by no means excludes considerable elevation of pulmonary capillary pressure.[15] With congestion of the bronchial mucosa, excessive bronchial secretions or bronchospasm or both may give rise to rhonchi and wheezes. Rales are usually heard at both lung bases, but if unilateral, they occur more commonly on the right side. When rales are audible *only* over the left lung in a patient with heart failure, they may signify the presence of pulmonary embolism to that lung.

SYSTEMIC VENOUS HYPERTENSION (see also p. 18). This can be detected more readily by inspection of the jugular veins, which provides a useful index of right atrial pressure. The upper limit of normal of the jugular venous pressure is approximately 4 cm above the sternal angle when the patient is examined at a 45-degree angle. When tricuspid regurgitation is present, the *v* wave and *y* descent are most prominent; however, with impedance to right ventricular filling (tricuspid stenosis) or right ventricular emptying (pulmonary hypertension, pulmonic stenosis), the *a* wave is most prominent. The jugular venous pressure normally declines on exertion, but in patients with heart failure (and in those with constrictive pericarditis, p. 1483) it rises, a finding known as *Kussmaul's sign.* Rarely, venous pressure may be so high that the peripheral veins on the dorsum of the hands or in the temporal region are dilated.

HEPATOJUGULAR REFLUX (see also p. 19). In patients with mild right heart failure, the jugular venous pressure may be normal at rest but rises to abnormal levels with compression of the right upper quadrant, a sign known as the *hepatojugular reflux.* To elicit this sign, the right upper quadrant should be compressed firmly, gradually, and continuously for 1 minute while the veins of the neck are observed. The patient should be advised to avoid straining, holding the breath, or carrying out a Valsalva maneuver. A positive test (i.e., expansion of the jugular veins during and immediately after compression) usually reflects the combination of a congested abdomen (particularly liver) and inability of the right side of the heart to accept or reject the transiently increased venous return. Thus, a positive abdominojugular reflux is helpful in differentiating hepatic enlargement caused by heart failure from that caused by other conditions.

CONGESTIVE HEPATOMEGALY. The liver often enlarges *before* overt edema develops, and it may remain so even after other symptoms of right-sided heart failure have disappeared. Inspection of the abdomen may reveal epigastric fullness and, on percussion, dullness in the right upper quadrant. If hepatomegaly has occurred rapidly and relatively recently, the liver is usually tender, owing to stretching of its capsule. In longstanding heart failure this tenderness disappears, even though the liver remains enlarged.

In patients with tricuspid regurgitation, the prominent right atrial *v* wave may be transmitted to the liver, which pulsates during systole (Fig. 16–3). A prominent presystolic pulsation

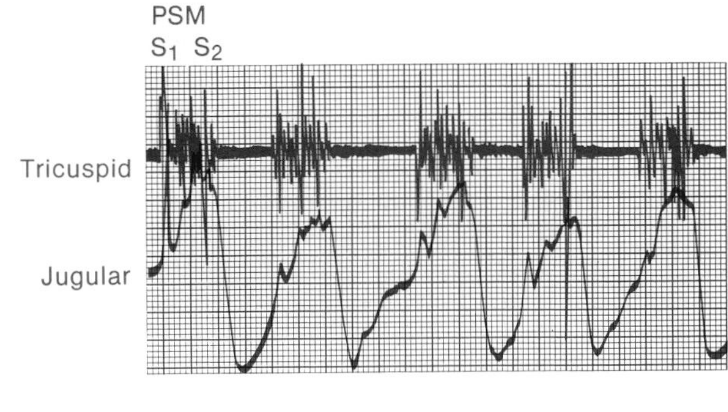

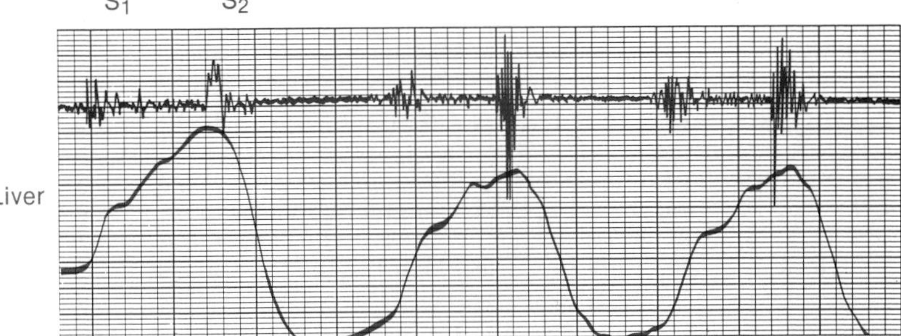

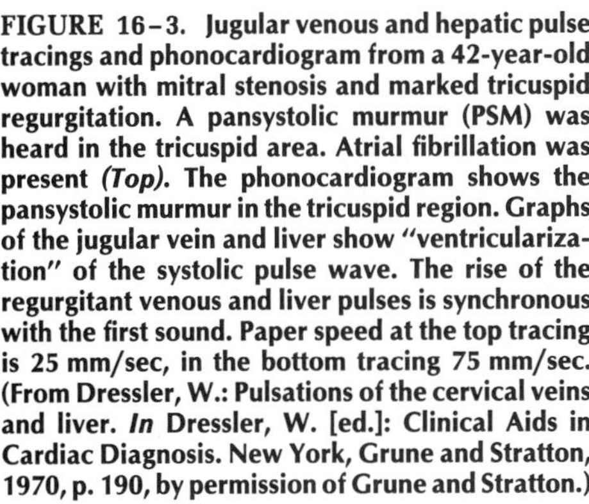
FIGURE 16-3. Jugular venous and hepatic pulse tracings and phonocardiogram from a 42-year-old woman with mitral stenosis and marked tricuspid regurgitation. A pansystolic murmur (PSM) was heard in the tricuspid area. Atrial fibrillation was present *(Top)*. The phonocardiogram shows the pansystolic murmur in the tricuspid region. Graphs of the jugular vein and liver show "ventricularization" of the systolic pulse wave. The rise of the regurgitant venous and liver pulses is synchronous with the first sound. Paper speed at the top tracing is 25 mm/sec, in the bottom tracing 75 mm/sec. (From Dressler, W.: Pulsations of the cervical veins and liver. *In* Dressler, W. [ed.]: Clinical Aids in Cardiac Diagnosis. New York, Grune and Stratton, 1970, p. 190, by permission of Grune and Stratton.)

in the liver owing to an enlarged right atrial *a* wave can occur in tricuspid stenosis, constrictive pericarditis, restrictive cardiomyopathy involving the right ventricle, pulmonary hypertension, and pulmonic stenosis.

EDEMA. Although a cardinal manifestation of congestive heart failure, edema does not correlate well with the level of systemic venous pressure. In patients with chronic left ventricular failure and a low cardiac output, extracellular fluid volume may be sufficiently expanded to cause edema in the presence of only slight elevations of systemic venous pressure. A substantial gain of extracellular fluid volume, a minimum of 5 liters in adults, must usually take place before peripheral edema is manifested. Therefore, edema may develop over a number of days and may not be present initially in patients with acute heart failure and marked systemic venous hypertension.

Edema is usually symmetrical, pitting, and generally occurs first in the dependent portions of the body, where the systemic venous pressure rises to its highest levels. Accordingly, cardiac edema in ambulatory patients is usually first noted in the feet or ankles at the end of the day and generally resolves after a night's rest. In bedridden patients it is most commonly found over the sacrum. Facial edema seldom appears in adults with heart failure but, as mentioned earlier, may occur in infants and young children. Late in the course of heart failure, edema may become massive and generalized (anasarca); it can involve the upper extremities, the thoracic and abdominal walls, and particularly the genital area. Rarely, when edema is severe and develops suddenly, it may cause rupture of the skin and extravasation of fluid. Longstanding edema results in pigmentation, reddening, and induration of the skin of the lower extremities, usually the dorsum of the feet and the pretibial areas. In patients with hemiplegia, edema is usually more marked on the paralyzed side. Unilateral edema of the lower extremity may be secondary to unilateral venous obstruction or a cerebrovascular accident.

HYDROTHORAX (PLEURAL EFFUSION). Because the pleural veins drain into both the systemic and the pulmonary venous beds, hydrothorax is observed most commonly in patients with hypertension involving both venous systems, but it may also occur when there is marked elevation of pressure in either venous bed. An increase in capillary permeability probably also plays a role in the pathogenesis of cardiac hydrothorax, since the protein content of the pleural fluid may be significantly greater (2 to 3 gm/dl) than that found in edema fluid (0.5 gm/dl). A "pseudoexudate," i.e., a concentration of solutes in the pleural fluid, may occur when pleural effusion begins to be resorbed in the early stages of treatment of heart failure.[37] Hydrothorax is usually bilateral, but when unilateral it is usually confined to the right side of the chest and is caused most commonly by severe systemic venous hypertension, as occurs in tricuspid stenosis or constrictive pericarditis. If pleural effusion is limited to the left side, it should suggest pulmonary embolism, a common complication of heart failure. When hydrothorax develops, dyspnea usually intensifies, owing to a further reduction in vital capacity. Although the excess fluid in hydrothorax is usually resorbed as heart failure improves, sometimes interlobar effusions persist.

ASCITES. This finding occurs in patients with increased pressure in the hepatic veins and in the veins draining the peritoneum. Ascites usually reflects longstanding systemic venous hypertension. In patients with organic tricuspid valve disease and chronic constrictive pericarditis, ascites may be more prominent than subcutaneous edema. As in the case of hydrothorax, there is increased capillary permeability because the protein content is similar to that of hepatic lymph (i.e., four to six times that of edema fluid). Protein-losing enteropathy may occur in patients with visceral congestion,[38] and the resultant reduced plasma oncotic pressure may lower the threshold for the development of ascites.

Cardiac Findings

The presence of cardiac disease is usually readily evident on clinical examination of patients with congestive heart failure.

CARDIOMEGALY. This finding is nonspecific and occurs in the majority of patients with chronic heart failure. Notable exceptions are heart failure associated with chronic constrictive pericarditis, restrictive cardiomyopathy, and a variety of acute insults such as acute myocardial infarction, the sudden development of tachyarrhythmias or bradyarrhythmias, or rupture of a valve or chordae tendineae; in such circumstances heart failure may develop before the heart has had a chance to enlarge.

GALLOP SOUNDS. Protodiastolic sounds, generally emanating from the left ventricle (but occasionally from the right) and occurring 0.13 to 0.16 second after the second heart sound, are common findings in healthy children and young adults. Such physiological sounds are seldom audible in healthy persons after the age of 40 years but occur in patients of all ages with heart failure and are referred to as protodiastolic, or S_3, gallops. In older adults they generally signify the presence of heart failure (p. 32). Protodiastolic gallops are caused by the sharp deceleration of ventricular inflow that occurs immediately after the early filling phase; a reduction in ventricular distensibility, i.e., the ventricle operating on the steep portion of its diastolic pressure-volume curve (Fig. 13–28, p. 371), may contribute to their genesis. In patients with mitral or tricuspid regurgitation or left-to-right shunts, rapid (torrential) flow into the ventricle in early diastole contributes to the generation of an S_3 (p. 32), but under these conditions this sound is *not* to be interpreted as signifying the presence of heart failure. In heart failure the atrioventricular pressure gradient during early filling may be high as a consequence of elevated atrial pressure, and the distensibility of the ventricle may be altered, resulting in a protodiastolic gallop. Thus, a protodiastolic gallop sound is an excellent sign of heart failure when other causes, such as a physiological S_3 occurring in a healthy child or young adult, constrictive pericarditis, mitral and tricuspid regurgitation, or a left-to-right shunt, can be excluded.

Left ventricular protodiastolic gallop sounds are best heard at the apex with the patient in the left lateral recumbent position and are frequently palpable, whereas right ventricular protodiastolic gallop sounds are best heard at the left sternal edge in the fourth or fifth interspace with the patient supine. Protodiastolic gallop sounds originating from the left ventricle tend to be louder *after* inspiration, whereas those originating from the right ventricle are best heard *during* inspiration. Gallop sounds are more readily audible in the presence of a rapid heart rate and sometimes may be elicited by a brief bout of exercise (repetitive sit-ups, or handgrip).

PULSUS ALTERNANS (see also p. 24). This sign is characterized by a regular rhythm with alternating strong and weak ventricular contractions. It should be distinguished from the alternation of strong and weak beats that occurs in pulsus bigeminus, in which the weak beat follows the strong beat by a shorter time interval than the strong beat follows the weak, whereas in pulsus alternans they are equally spaced or the weak beat is slightly closer to the succeeding than to the preceding beat. Severe pulsus alternans may be detected either by palpation of the peripheral pulses (the femoral more readily than the brachial, radial, or carotid) or by sphygmomanometry. As the cuff is slowly deflated, only alternate beats are audible for a variable number of millimeters of mercury below the systolic level, depending on the severity of the alternans, and then all beats are heard. Rarely the weak beat is so small that the aortic valve is not opened, and this results in an apparent halving of the pulse rate, a condition referred to as *total alternans*. Pulsus alternans may be accompanied by alternation in the intensity of the heart sounds and of existing heart murmurs. With total alternans there is a first heart sound for each contraction, but the second heart sound may be absent with the weak contractions owing to failure of the semilunar valves to open.

Pulsus alternans occurs most commonly in heart failure secondary to increased resistance to left ventricular ejection, as occurs in systemic hypertension and aortic stenosis, as well as in coronary atherosclerosis and dilated cardiomyopathy. It is usually associated with a ventricular protodiastolic gallop sound (S_3), signifies advanced myocardial disease, and often disappears with treatment of heart failure. In patients with heart failure, pulsus alternans can often be elicited by reduction in systemic venous return, as occurs with assumption of the erect posture or application of venous tourniquets, and it is reduced by an increase in venous return, as in recumbency or with exercise. Pulsus alternans tends to be present during tachycardia and is often initiated by a premature beat.

Pulsus alternans is attributed to an alternation in the stroke volume ejected by the left ventricle[39] and, ultimately, to a deletion in the number of contracting cells in every other cycle, presumably owing to incomplete recovery. Alternans is almost always concordant in the two sides of the circulation, i.e., the strong and weak beats occur simultaneously in the two ventricles. Rarely, pulsus alternans is accompanied by *electrical alternans*; however, the latter condition is usually not due to mechanical alternans, but to alternating positions of the heart within the fluid-filled pericardial sac (Fig. 4–100, p. 102).

ACCENTUATION OF P_2 AND SYSTOLIC MURMURS. With the development of left ventricular failure pulmonary artery pressure rises and P_2 becomes accentuated—often louder than A_2—and more widely transmitted. As left ventricular failure improves, P_2 becomes softer. *Systolic murmurs* are common in heart failure owing to the relative mitral or tricuspid regurgitation that may occur secondary to ventricular dilatation. Often these murmurs diminish or disappear when compensation is restored.

FEVER. A low-grade temperature (<38°C), which results from cutaneous vasoconstriction and therefore impairment of heat loss, may occur in severe heart failure; fever usually subsides when compensation is restored. Greater elevations of temperature usually signify the presence of an infection, pulmonary infarction, or infective endocarditis.

CARDIAC CACHEXIA. Longstanding, severe congestive heart failure, particularly of the right ventricle, may lead to anorexia, owing to hepatic and intestinal congestion and sometimes to digitalis intoxication. Occasionally there is impaired intestinal absorption of fat[40] and rarely protein-losing enteropathy.[38] Patients with heart failure may also exhibit increased total metabolism, secondary to (1) an augmentation of myocardial oxygen consumption, as occurs in patients with aortic stenosis and hypertension; (2) excessive work of breathing; (3) low-grade fever; and (4) elevated levels of circulating tumor necrosis factor.[41] This cytokine is produced by monocytes and causes cachexia and anorexia. The combination of reduced caloric intake and increased caloric expenditure, however produced, may lead to a reduction of tissue mass and, in severe cases, to cardiac cachexia.[42,43] In some patients the cachexia may be severe enough to suggest the presence of disseminated malignant disease. In others, the loss of lean body mass may be masked by the accumulation of edema.

CHEYNE-STOKES RESPIRATION. Also known as periodic or cyclic respiration, Cheyne-Stokes respiration is characterized by the combination of depression in the sensitivity of the respiratory center to carbon dioxide and left ventricular failure.[44] During the apneic phase, arterial P_{O_2} falls and P_{CO_2} rises; this combination excites the depressed respiratory center, resulting in hyperventilation and, subsequently, hypocapnia, followed by another period of apnea. The principal causes of depression of the respiratory center in patients with Cheyne-Stokes respiration are cerebral lesions such as cerebral arteriosclerosis, stroke, or head injury. These causes are often exaggerated by sleep, barbiturates, and narcotics, all of which further depress the sensitivity of the respiratory center. Left ventricular failure, which prolongs the circulation time from the lung to the brain, results in a sluggish response of the system and is responsible for the oscillations between apnea and hyperpnea and prevents return to a steady state of ventilation and blood gases. Usually patients are not aware of Cheyne-Stokes respiration. However, it can be readily observed in a sleeping patient, or a history can be elicited from the patient's bed partner. Occasionally the patient with heart failure awakens at night with dyspnea precipitated by Cheyne-Stokes respiration.[45]

PATHOLOGICAL FINDINGS

LUNGS. In patients who have died of left ventricular failure the lungs are enlarged, firm, and dark and may be filled with bloody fluid. With longstanding pulmonary congestion they are brown with deposition of hemosiderin and usually do not seep edema fluid. On microscopic examination, the capillaries are engorged, and there is thickening of the alveolar septa as well as extravasation of large mononuclear cells containing red blood cells or hemosiderin granules or both.[46] Often the pulmonary vessels show medial hypertrophy and intimal hyperplasia.

LIVER. In acute right heart failure, the liver is enlarged, firm, and filled with fluid. On microscopic examination, the central hepatic veins and sinusoids are dilated.[47,48] With longstanding right heart failure, the liver returns to normal size, subsequently atrophies, and becomes "nutmeg" in appearance as a consequence of the dark red areas of central venous congestion and the lighter, fatty area in the periphery of the lobule. Cardiac cirrhosis is characterized by central lobular necrosis and atrophy as well as extensive fibrous retraction; sometimes there is sclerosis of the hepatic veins. Because cardiac cirrhosis is a function of the level of hepatic venous pressure and the duration of its elevation, it is not surprising that it occurs most commonly in patients with chronic constrictive pericarditis and organic tricuspid valve disease and in children after a Fontan procedure for tricuspid atresia (p. 938),[49,49a] who often have prolonged elevation of systemic venous pressure. In patients with left ventricular failure, central hepatic necrosis without evidence of passive congestion may be present.[50,51]

Liver biopsies in patients with acute heart failure exhibiting fulminant hepatic failure showed replacement of hepatocytes by red blood cells. Presumably, the hypoxia caused by hypoperfusion produces hepatocyte necrosis[52,53]; erythrocytes may then enter the space of Disse between damaged endothelial cells. These changes resulting from acute heart failure may be transient if there is hemodynamic recovery.

OTHER VISCERA. Patients with chronic hepatic venous hypertension develop portal hypertension that results in congestive splenomegaly. On microscopic examination, the spleen shows dilatation of the sinusoids and fibrosis, and there is chronic passive congestion of the pancreas and of the veins and capillaries of the gastrointestinal tract. Rarely, intense mesenteric vasoconstriction without thrombotic or embolic occlusion of a mesenteric artery may lead to a hemorrhagic, nonbacterial enterocolitis, with hemorrhagic necrosis.

Chronic venous congestion also occurs in the kidney and brain, with dilatation and engorgement of the capillaries. Small infarcts are frequently observed in the spleen and kidneys of patients with longstanding atrial fibrillation.

LABORATORY FINDINGS

Proteinuria and a high urine specific gravity are common findings in heart failure. Blood urea nitrogen and creatinine levels are often moderately elevated secondary to reductions in renal blood flow and glomerular filtration rate[12] (prerenal azotemia). The erythrocyte sedimentation rate is usually quite low, presumably secondary to impaired fibrinogen synthesis and resultant decreased fibrinogen concentrations.

SERUM ELECTROLYTES. Serum electrolyte values are generally normal in patients with mild or moderate heart failure before treatment. However, in severe heart failure, prolonged, rigid sodium restriction, coupled with intensive diuretic therapy as well as the inability to excrete water, commonly leads to dilutional hyponatremia, which occurs because of substantial expansion of extracellular fluid volume and a normal or increased level of total body sodium. It may be accompanied by, and presumably is caused in part by elevated concentrations of circulating vasopressin.[54] Serum potassium levels are usually normal, although the prolonged administration of kaliuretic diuretics, such as the thiazides or loop diuretics, may result in hypokalemia (p. 860). Hyperkalemia may occur in patients with severe heart failure[55] who show marked reductions in glomerular filtration rate and inadequate delivery of sodium to the distal tubular sodium-potassium exchange sites, particularly if such patients are also receiving potassium-retaining diuretics and/or converting enzyme.

Congestive hepatomegaly and cardiac cirrhosis are often associated with impaired hepatic function, characterized by abnormal values of aspartate aminotransferase (AST), alanine aminotransferase (ALT), lactic dehydrogenase (LDH), and other liver enzymes.[56,57] Hyperbilirubinemia, secondary to an increase in both the directly and the indirectly reacting bilirubins, is common, and in severe cases of acute (right or left) ventricular failure, frank jaundice may occur. *Acute* hepatic venous congestion can result in severe jaundice with a bilirubin level as high as 15 to 20 mg/dl, elevation of AST to more than 10 times the upper limit of normal, and elevation of the serum alkaline phosphatase level, as well as prolongation of the prothrombin time. Both the clinical and the laboratory pictures may resemble viral hepatitis, but the impairment of hepatic function is rapidly ameliorated by successful treatment of heart failure. In patients with longstanding cardiac cirrhosis, albumin synthesis may be impaired, with resultant hypoalbuminemia, intensifying the accumulation of fluid. Hepatic hypoglycemia, fulminant hepatic failure, and hepatic coma are uncommon, late, and sometimes terminal complications of cardiac cirrhosis.[58,59] In general, disturbances of hepatic function are frequent when right atrial pressure rises above 10 mm Hg and cardiac index declines below 1.5/min/sq meter.[57]

Venous pressure can be conveniently measured with a spinal fluid manometer with the patient in the recumbent position and the arm abducted. The baseline for the measurement should be 5 cm below the sternal angle (i.e., the estimated position of the right atrium). The venous pressure is often elevated (i.e., >12 cm H_2O) at rest, but in mild or borderline cases it may be normal at rest but rises with hepatic compression or during exercise.

Circulation time can be measured by rapid intravenous injection of 3 to 5 ml of 20 per cent dehydrocholic acid (Decholin), with a bitter taste designating the endpoint. The normal range in adults is 9 to 16 seconds. Regrettably, this simple and useful test has fallen out of favor. Circulation time varies directly with the volume of blood in which the indicator is diluted and inversely with the velocity of blood flow. Therefore, pulmonary and/or systemic venous congestion, as well as reduced cardiac output, cause prolongation. Because of the high velocity of blood flow, circulation time tends to be normal or even shortened in patients with high-output heart failure. Although circulation time is not a particularly sensitive test for heart failure, it may be useful in differentiating between pulmonary and cardiac dyspnea and between low- and high-output cardiac failure.

THE VALSALVA MANEUVER. Performance of this maneuver—forced expiration against a closed glottis—is helpful in the diagnosis of heart failure.[60] The test has been standardized. The patient is asked to blow against an aneroid manometer and maintain a pressure of 40 mm Hg for 30 seconds. During the Valsalva maneuver, intrathoracic pressure rises, venous return to the heart diminishes, stroke volume falls, and venous pressure rises. Arterial pressure tracings normally show four distinct phases (Fig. 16–4*A*): (1) an initial rise in arterial pressure, which represents transmission to the periphery of the increased intrathoracic pressure; (2) with continuation of the strain and the accompanying reduction of venous return, reductions in systolic, diastolic, and pulse pressures accompanied by a reflex increase in heart rate; (3) on release of the strain, a sudden drop of arterial pressure equivalent to the fall in intrathoracic pressure; and (4) an overshoot of arterial pressure to above control levels, with a wide pulse pressure and bradycardia due to the combination of the inrush into the heart of blood that had been dammed up in the venous bed and reflex vasoconstriction and tachycardia secondary to the low perfusion pressure of the carotid and baroreceptors during phase 3.

In heart failure (Fig. 16–4*B*), phases 1 and 3 are normal; that is, there is normal transmission of the elevated intrathoracic pressure into the arterial tree during phase 1 and sudden loss of this with the release of the strain during phase 3. However, because the heart operates on the flat portion of its Starling curve (Fig. 14–4, p. 397), the impedance of venous return during phase 2 does not affect stroke volume. Therefore, the baroreceptor reflex is not activated, and there is no overshoot on release of the strain. This results in a "square-wave" appearance of the tracing. Although the Valsalva maneuver can be recorded most accurately through an indwelling needle, careful palpation of the pulse in normal individuals allows detection of phases 2 and 4 and their absence, and slowing of the pulse in phase 4.[61]

THE CHEST ROENTGENOGRAM

(See also Chap. 8)

Two principal features of the chest roentgenogram are useful in the patient with congestive heart failure.

The *size and shape of the cardiac silhouette* provide important information concerning the precise nature of the under-

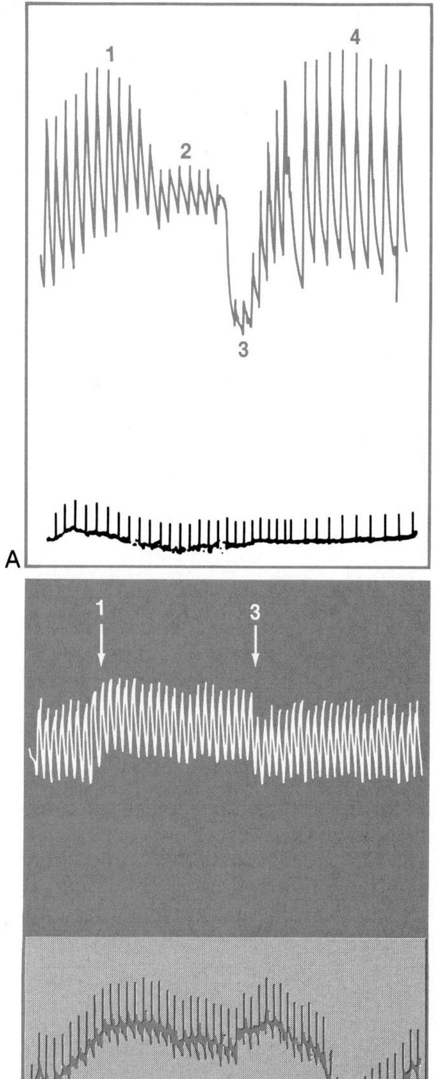

FIGURE 16–4. *A*, Intraarterial pressure tracing demonstrating normal response to Valsalva maneuver. Baseline heart rate is 60 beats/min (R-R interval, 1000 ms). Phase 1 demonstrates transient increase in blood pressure associated with onset of straining. During phase 2, blood pressure and pulse pressure decrease, and a reflex increase in heart rate occurs (R-R interval, 800 ms). Phase 3 consists of the initial release of straining, which causes a further transient decrease in blood pressure. Phase IV is characterized by an arterial pressure overshoot and reflex bradycardia (R-R interval, 1300 ms). Valsalva ratio (longest to shortest R-R interval) is 1.6. Numbers denote the four different phases. *B*, Intraarterial pressure tracing during Valsalva maneuver in patient with severe left ventricular dysfunction and left ventricular end-diastolic pressure of 35 mm Hg demonstrates square-wave response (absence of decreased pulse pressure and stroke volume normally seen in phase 2) and loss of arterial pressure overshoot in phase 4. R-R intervals do not change during the four phases, and the Valsalva ratio is 1.0. (From Nishimura, R. A., and Tajik, A. J.: The Valsalva maneuver and response revisited. Mayo Clin. Proc. *61*:211, 1986.)

lying heart disease. Both the cardiothoracic ratio (Fig. 8–19, p. 215) and the heart volume determined on the plain film[62] are relatively specific but insensitive indicators of increased left ventricular end-diastolic volume.

In the presence of normal pulmonary capillary and venous pressure in the erect position, the lung bases are better perfused than the apices, and the vessels supplying the lower lobes are significantly larger than are those supplying the upper lobes.[62a] With elevation of left atrial, pulmonary venous, and capillary pressures, interstitial and perivascular edema develops and is most prominent at the lung bases because hydrostatic pressure is greater there. When pulmonary capillary pressure is slightly elevated, i.e., approximately 13 to 17 mm Hg,[63] the resultant compression of pulmonary vessels in the lower lobes causes equalization in size of the vessels to the apices and bases. With greater pressure elevation (approximately 18 to 23 mm Hg), actual pulmonary vascular redistribution occurs (i.e., further constriction of vessels leading to the lower lobes and dilatation of vessels leading to the upper lobes). When pulmonary capillary pressures exceed approximately 20 to 25 mm Hg, interstitial pulmonary edema occurs. This may be of several varieties: (1) *septal*, producing Kerley's lines (i.e., sharp, linear densities of interlobular interstitial edema); (2) *perivascular*, producing loss of sharpness of the central and peripheral vessels; and (3) *subpleural*, producing spindle-shaped accumulations of fluid between the lung and adjacent pleural surface. When pulmonary capillary pressure exceeds 25 mm Hg, alveolar edema, with a cloudlike appearance and concentration of the fluid around the hili in a "butterfly pattern," and large pleural effusions may occur. With elevation of systemic venous pressure, the azygos vein and superior vena cava may enlarge.[64]

PROGNOSIS

A large number of factors have been found to correlate with mortality in patients with congestive heart failure (Table 16–3).[65] These fall into four major categories:

1. *Clinical.* In general, the presence of coronary artery disease as the etiology of heart failure, the presence of an audible S_3, low pulse and systolic arterial pressures, a high New York Heart Association Class, and reduced exercise capacity (Fig. 16–5*A*) have each been shown to be associated with a high mortality. When the NYHA Class is integrated with the maximal O_2 consumption determined during exercise, the mortality is 20 per cent per year in patients in Class III with a $\dot{V}O_{2\,max}$

TABLE 16–3 FACTORS AFFECTING SURVIVAL IN PATIENTS WITH CONGESTIVE HEART FAILURE

1. **CLINICAL**
   - Coronary artery disease etiology
   - New York Heart Association Class
   - Exercise capacity
   - Heart rate at rest
   - Systolic arterial pressure
   - Pulse pressure
   - S_3
2. **HEMODYNAMIC**
   - L.V. ejection fraction
   - R.V. ejection fraction
   - L.V. stroke work index
   - L.V. filling pressure
   - Right atrial pressure
   - Maximal O_2 uptake
   - L.V. systolic pressure
   - Mean arterial pressure
   - Cardiac index
   - Systemic vascular resistance
3. **BIOCHEMICAL**
   - Plasma norepinephrine
   - Plasma renin
   - Plasma vasopressin
   - Plasma atrial natriuretic peptide
   - Serum sodium
   - Serum potassium
   - Total potassium stores
   - Serum magnesium
4. **ELECTROPHYSIOLOGICAL**
   - Frequent ventricular asystole
   - Complex ventricular arrhythmias
   - Ventricular tachycardia
   - Atrial fibrillation/flutter

Modified from Cohn, J. N., and Rector, T. S.: Prognosis of congestive heart failure and predictors of mortality. Am. J. Cardiol. *62*:25A, 1988.

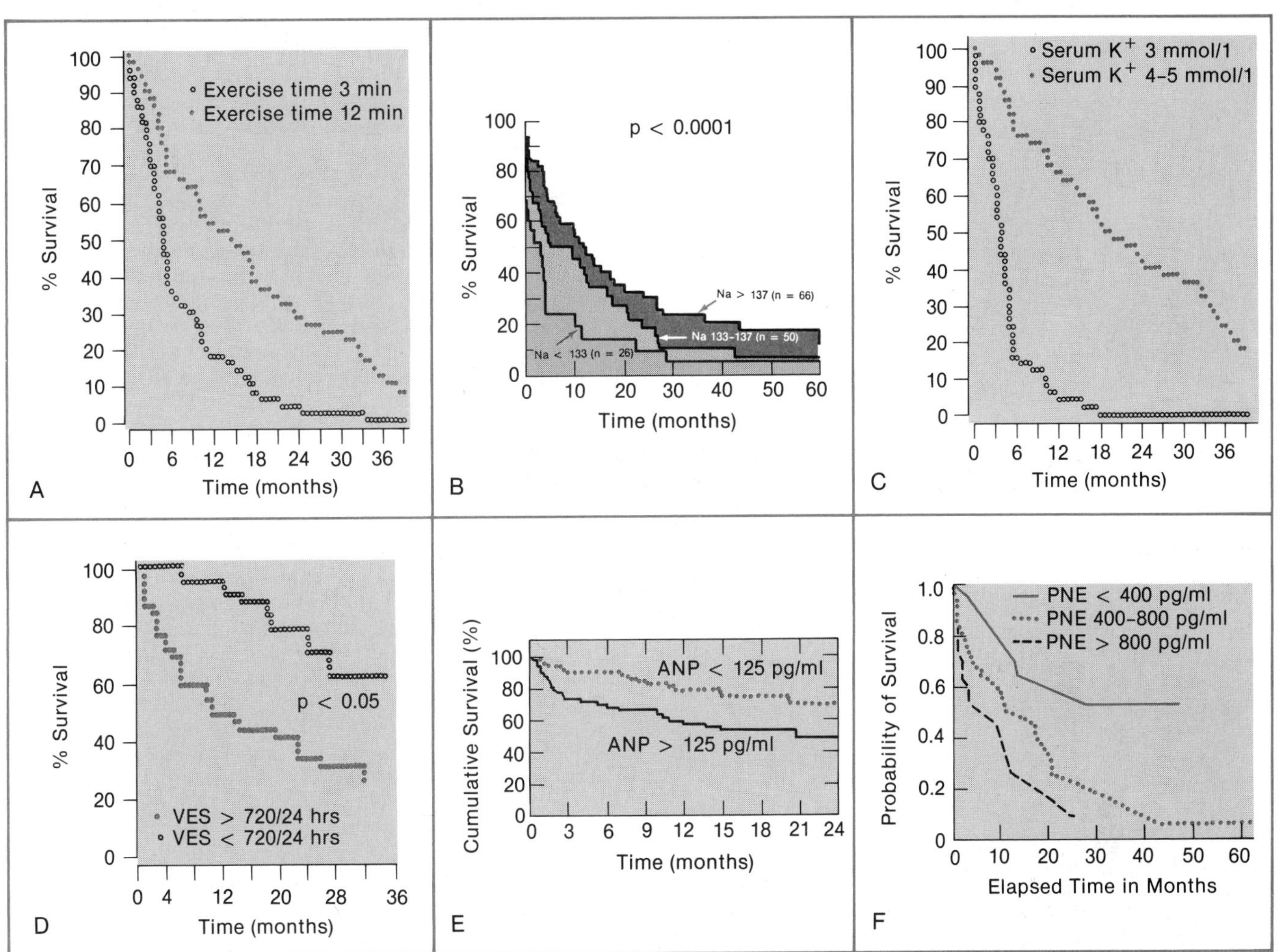

FIGURE 16–5. ***A,*** **Estimated survival curve for patients with a short or a long exercise time in the modified Bruce protocol. Values were chosen arbitrarily. Patients had other important prognostic factors fixed at median values and were assumed to have coronary artery disease but not to be taking amiodarone. (From Cleland, J.G.F., Dargie, H. J., and Ford, I.: Mortality in heart failure: Clinical variables of prognostic value. Br. Heart J.** ***58*****:572, 1987.)** ***B,*** **Kaplan-Meier analysis showing cumulative rates of survival in patients with severe chronic heart failure stratified into three groups based on pretreatment serum sodium concentration. Hyponatremic patients fared significantly worse than patients with a normal serum sodium concentration ($p < .0001$, Mantel-Cox). (From Packer, M., et al.: Role of neurohormonal mechanisms in determining survival in patients with severe chronic heart failure. Circulation** ***75*****:(Suppl. 4)80, 92, 1987, by permission of the American Heart Association, Inc.)** ***C,*** **Estimated survival curve for patients with a high or a low initial mean serum concentration of potassium. Values were chosen arbitrarily. Patients had other important prognostic factors fixed at median values and were assumed to have coronary artery disease but not to be taking amiodarone (From Cleland, J.G.F., Dargie, H. J., and Ford, I.: Mortality in heart failure: Clinical variables of prognostic value. Br. Heart J.** ***58*****:572, 1987.)**

D, **Relation between ventricular arrhythmia and survival in heart failure. VES = ventricular ectopic activity. (From Dargie, H. J., et al.: Relation of arrhythmias and electrolyte abnormalities to survival in patients with severe chronic heart failure. Circulation** ***75*****:98, 1987, by permission of the American Heart Association, Inc.)** ***E,*** **Kaplan-Meier analysis of cumulative rates of survival in patients with heart failure stratified into two groups on the basis of median plasma concentration of atrial natriuretic peptide (ANP) (125 pg/ml). (From Gottlieb, S. S., et al.: Prognostic importance of atrial natriuretic peptide in patients with chronic heart failure. Reprinted with permission from the American College of Cardiology. J. Am. Coll. Cardiol.** ***13*****:1534, 1989.)** ***F,*** **Life-table analysis of survival, according to Tercile, based on level of plasma norepinephrine (PNE). Group 1 (<400 pg/ml) contained 27 patients, group 2 (400 to 800 pg/ml) 49 patients, and group 3 (>800 pg/ml) 30 patients. The probability of survival in each group was significantly different from the probabilities in the other two groups. (From Cohn, J. N., et al.: Plasma norepinephrine as a guide to prognosis in patients with chronic congestive heart failure. N. Engl. J. Med.** ***311*****:822, 1984.)**

of 10 to 15 ml/kg/min and rises to 60 per cent in patients in Class IV with a $\dot{V}O_{2\,max}$ less than 10 ml/kg/min.[66–68]

2. *Hemodynamic.* Variables such as cardiac index, stroke work index, and especially ejection fraction[69] (Fig. 16–6*A*) have been shown to correlate directly with survival in patients with heart failure, while systemic vascular resistance and heart rate correlate inversely. Combinations of hemodynamic abnormalities, such as depression of stroke work associated with elevation of filling pressure and systemic vascular resistance, are associated with a poor prognosis.[69]

3. *Biochemical.* The observation that there is activation of the neurohormonal axis in heart failure has prompted examination of the relations between a variety of biochemical measurements and clinical outcome. Strong inverse correlations have been reported between survival and plasma norepinephrine (Fig. 16–5*F*)[1,65,70,71] plasma renin,[65,72,73] vasopressin,[73] and atrial natriuretic peptide concentrations[74] (Fig. 16–5*E*). The concentrations of these substances reflect the severity of the underlying impairment of circulatory function. In addition, these substances per se may exert adverse hemodynamic effects; norepinephrine, angiotensin II (the consequence of increasing renin concentration), and arginine vasopressin are potent vasoconstrictors, augmenting ventricular afterload and thereby reducing the shortening of myocardial fibers. Furthermore, they may be directly responsible for adverse biochemical effects on the myocardium. For example, the

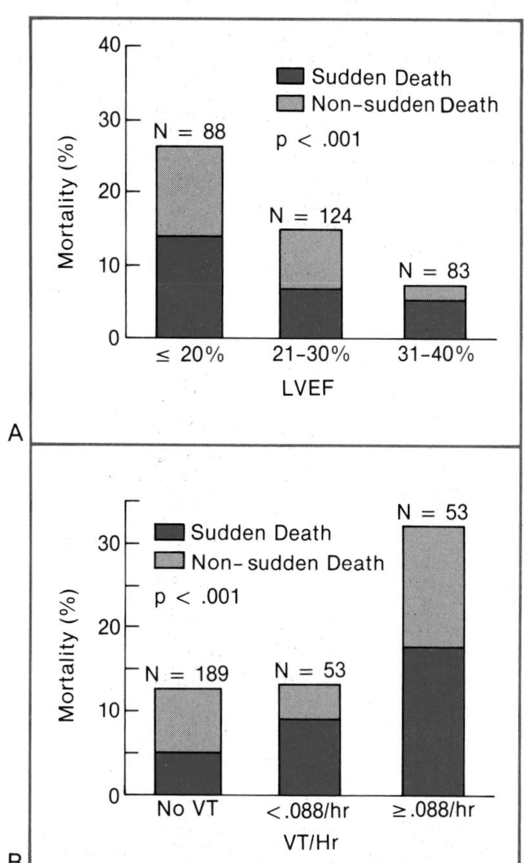

FIGURE 16-6. ***A*, Relation between baseline left ventricular ejection fraction (LVEF) and subsequent mortality rate. The average follow-up period was 16 months. *B*, Relation between baseline ventricular tachycardia (VT) event rate and subsequent mortality rate. (From Gradman, A., et al.: Predictors of total mortality and sudden death in mild to moderate heart failure. Reprinted with permission from the American College of Cardiology. J. Am. Coll. Cardiol. *14*:564, 1989.)**

elevated norepinephrine concentration may be directly responsible for ventricular tachyarrhythmias,[70] as may the hypokalemia (Fig. 16-5C) and reduction of total body potassium stores resulting from the activation of the renin-angiotensin-aldosterone axis (and the administration of potassium-losing diuretics).[75] Hyponatremia also correlates well with high mortality[73] (Fig. 16-5*B*), but it is likely that this variable reflects activation of the renin-angiotensin-aldosterone axis; hyponatremic patients appear to be especially helped by angiotensin-converting enzyme inhibitors (p. 496).

In most studies the above-mentioned variables have been assessed in a univariate manner, i.e., independently of one another, and there is still disagreement regarding whether each provides *independent* prognostic information. However, Cohn and Rector have shown that while ventricular function, as expressed in ejection fraction, appears to have the most profound effect on survival in patients with advanced heart failure, exercise tolerance (as reflected in peak O_2 consumption during a progressive exercise test) and activation of the sympathetic nervous system (as reflected in the plasma norepinephrine concentration) *each* provided important independent information.[65]

4. *Electrophysiological.* Death in patients with severe congestive heart failure occurs either by progressive pump failure or, in as many as one-half of all patients, suddenly and unexpectedly, presumably from an arrhythmia. When present, a variety of arrhythmias—especially frequent ventricular extrasystoles (Fig. 16-5*D*), ventricular tachyarrhythmias (Fig. 16-6*B*), left intraventricular conduction defects, as well as atrial flutter and fibrillation[65]—have been shown to be predictors of mortality. What is not yet clear is whether these arrhythmias are simply indicators of the severity of left ventricular dysfunction or whether they are responsible for and trigger fatal arrhythmias.[1] While there is some evidence that ventricular arrhythmias confer independent adverse prognostic effects,[70] routine treatment of patients with heart failure-associated arrhythmias with antiarrhythmic drugs has not yet been shown to exert a protective effect and reduce mortality. It has been speculated that repletion of potassium and magnesium stores will modify favorably the outcome in these patients.[1]

The administration of angiotensin-converting enzyme inhibitors to block aldosterone-induced potassium loss, may reduce mortality in advanced congestive heart failure by restoring intracellular and extracellular potassium stores. Similarly, the beneficial actions of beta-adrenoceptor blockers in patients with dilated cardiomyopathy and in postmyocardial infarction patients with heart failure are compatible with this hypothesis.

High-Output Heart Failure

Although high-cardiac output states by themselves are seldom responsible for heart failure, their development in the presence of underlying heart disease often precipitates heart failure.[76] In these conditions, which are often characterized by arteriovenous shunting, the requirements of the peripheral tissues for oxygen can be satisfied only by an increase in cardiac output. While the normal heart is capable of augmenting its output on a long-term basis, this may not be true of the diseased heart. The development of a high-output state as a precipitant of heart failure has already been described (Ch. 14). Here we discuss the clinical manifestation of the conditions responsible for high-output cardiac heart failure.

ANEMIA

(See also p. 1742)

HISTORY. Chronic anemia in the absence of underlying heart disease produces surprisingly few symptoms, which may consist of easy fatigability, mild exertional dyspnea, and occasionally palpitations and cardiac awareness. If heart failure or angina pectoris is present, it is likely that the high cardiac output is superimposed on some specific cardiac abnormality, such as valvular stenosis or regurgitation, or ischemic heart disease.

PHYSICAL EXAMINATION. The anemic patient generally has a pale, "pasty" appearance; in black, brown, or tanned persons in whom examination of the skin color is of little help, the finding of paleness of the conjunctivae, mucous membranes, and palmar creases is helpful. Arterial pulses are bounding, "pistol shot" sounds can be heard over the femoral arteries (Duroziez's sign), and subungual capillary pulsations (Quincke's pulse) are present, as in patients with aortic regurgitation. A medium-pitched, midsystolic murmur along the left sternal border, generally Grade 1/6 to 3/6 in intensity (seldom accompanied by a thrill), is common. Heart sounds are accentuated, and the pulmonic component of the second heart sound may be particularly prominent in patients with sickle cell anemia and pulmonary hypertension; in such patients a right ventricular lift can usually be palpated. Elevation of the cardiac output and the physical findings characteristic of anemia are present in patients with sickle cell anemia and hemoglobin SC disease (p. 1744) at *higher* hemoglobin levels than in patients with other forms of anemia. A mid-diastolic flow murmur secondary to augmented blood flow across the mitral orifice, holosystolic murmurs resulting from tricuspid and mitral regurgitation secondary to ventricular dilatation, and rarely diastolic murmurs resulting from aortic and pulmonic valve incompetence secondary to dilatation of these vessels may be heard. A protodiastolic gallop sound (S_3) frequently is audible at the cardiac apex. Jugular venous distention is uncommon, and although peripheral edema and hepatomegaly are occasionally present, they may be due not only to heart failure, but also to accompanying abnormalities such as hypoproteinemia and nutritional deficiency.

Laboratory findings in patients with severe chronic anemia without underlying heart disease usually include mild to moderate cardiomegaly on the chest roentgenogram. The electrocardiogram usually does not show any specific changes, but may show T-wave inversions in lateral precordial leads. The echocardiogram generally shows a modest and symmetrical increase in the size of all chambers, with large systolic excursions of the septal and posterior left ventricular walls. These findings are superimposed on those resulting from the underlying heart disease. Hematological and blood chemical findings reflect the specific type of anemia present.

MANAGEMENT OF HIGH-OUTPUT FAILURE DUE TO ANEMIA. Treatment of heart failure associated with severe anemia should be specific for the anemia (e.g., iron, folate, vitamin B_{12}, and so forth). When congestive heart failure is present, diuretics and cardiac glycosides are advisable, although some clinicians believe that the latter drugs are not helpful in this condition.

When both heart failure and anemia are severe, treatment must be carried out on an urgent basis and presents a difficult challenge. On the one hand, correction of the anemia is desirable to increase oxygen delivery to metabolizing tissues and thereby decrease the need for a sustained high cardiac output. On the other hand, a too-rapid expansion of the blood volume could intensify the manifestations of heart failure, and an increase in hematocrit will potentially depress cardiac output because of increased blood viscosity. The diagnostic steps for determining the etiology of the anemia should be taken immediately (e.g., blood drawn for serum iron, folate, and vitamin B_{12} measurements). The patient should be placed at bed rest and given supplementary oxygen. *Packed red blood cells* should then be transfused slowly (250 to 500 ml/24 hr), preceded or accompanied by vigorous diuretic therapy (e.g., furosemide, 40 mg intravenously immediately followed by 40 mg orally every 8 hours), and the patient should be observed closely for the development or exacerbation of dyspnea and pulmonary rales, so that the transfusion can be discontinued immediately to avoid precipitating pulmonary edema. Vasodilator therapy is seldom helpful, since impedance to left ventricular emptying is already markedly reduced in most cases.

HYPERTHYROIDISM

(See also p. 1832)

The principal findings on the physical examination of the cardiovascular system are tachycardia, a widened pulse pressure, brisk carotid and peripheral arterial pulsations, a hyperkinetic cardiac apex, and loud first heart sound. A midsystolic murmur along the left sternal border, secondary to increased flow, is common; occasionally this murmur has an unusual scratchy component (the so-called Means-Lerman scratch) thought to be due to the rubbing together of normal pleural and pericardial surfaces as a consequence of hyperkinetic heart action. Rarely, systolic murmurs of mitral and tricuspid regurgitation, presumably secondary to papillary muscle dysfunction, may occur.

In patients with hyperthyroidism without heart disease, the *chest roentgenogram* is usually normal, although the *echocardiogram* may show increased left ventricular wall thickness and chamber dimensions and a normal or increased ejection fraction and velocity of shortening.[77] The *electrocardiogram* often shows widespread but nonspecific ST-segment elevation and upward coving, with terminal T-wave inversion in about one-fourth of patients and shortening of the Q-T interval.[78] Atrial fibrillation may occur and is often associated with an unusually rapid ventricular response (i.e., 170 to 220 beats/min). There is relative resistance to slowing of the ventricular rate with digitalis.[79] Spontaneous reversion to sinus rhythm is common when euthyroidism is restored.

Thyrotoxic Heart Disease

As in many other high-output states, the hyperkinetic state of hyperthyroidism does not usually lead to heart failure in the absence of underlying cardiac or coronary artery disease; the normal heart appears capable of tolerating the burden imposed by hyperthyroidism simply by means of dilatation and hypertrophy. A rare exception is the development of heart failure in patients with neonatal thyrotoxicosis without underlying heart disease.[80] However, when the elevated flow load of hyperthyroidism is superimposed on a reduced cardiovascular reserve (i.e., asymptomatic or only mildly symptomatic heart disease), congestive heart failure is likely to ensue. Similarly, in patients with obstructive coronary artery disease who are asymptomatic or who have only mild evidence of ischemia in the euthyroid state, the demand for increased coronary blood flow with hyperthyroidism frequently leads to an exacerbation of angina.

Beta-adrenoceptor blockade may be both helpful and harmful in patients with thyrotoxic heart disease and heart failure. Although it may be beneficial by lowering the ventricular rate, particularly by prolonging the refractory period of the atrioventricular conduction system in patients with atrial fibrillation, it may also diminish myocardial contractility by blocking the adrenergic support of the heart. Therefore it must be administered cautiously to the patient with thyrotoxic heart disease and heart failure and only after treatment with a digitalis glycoside, with the patient at rest and under careful observation. The initial dose should be small (e.g., propranolol, 0.5 mg intravenously or 10 mg orally), and the patient should be observed after the administration to be sure that heart failure is not intensified.

It is particularly important to recognize so-called *apathetic hyperthyroidism*, a condition in the elderly in which the usual clinical manifestations of thyrotoxicosis, such as palpitations, tachycardia, and moist skin, are not present. In such patients the first clinical signs of hyperthyroidism may be unexplained heart failure, an exacerbation of angina pectoris, or unexplained atrial fibrillation, usually but not always with a rapid ventricular rate.

SYSTEMIC ARTERIOVENOUS FISTULAS

Systemic arteriovenous fistulas may be congenital or acquired; the latter are either post-traumatic or iatrogenic. Increased cardiac output associated with such fistulas depends on the size of the communication and the magnitude of the resultant reduction in systemic vascular resistance. An increased right atrial pressure does not seem to be necessary to maintain the high-output state, although plasma volume is generally increased.

The *physical findings* depend on the underlying disease, and the location and size of the shunt. In general, a widened pulse pressure, brisk carotid and peripheral arterial pulsations, and mild tachycardia are present. *Branham's sign* (also called *Nicaladoni-Branham's sign*), which consists of slowing of the heart after manual compression of the fistula,[81,82] is present in the majority of cases; this maneuver also raises arterial and lowers venous pressure. It appears to result from the operation of a cardioaccelerator reflex with both afferent and efferent pathways in the vagus nerves.[83]

The skin overlying the fistula is warmer than normal, and a

continuous "machinery" murmur and thrill are usually present over the lesion. Third and fourth heart sounds are commonly heard, as well as a precordial midsystolic murmur secondary to increased cardiac output. The electrocardiographic changes of left ventricular hypertrophy are often seen. Rarely, the fistula may become infected, leading to bacterial endarteritis.

CONGENITAL ARTERIOVENOUS FISTULAS. Congenital arteriovenous fistulas result from arrest of the normal embryonic development of the vascular system and are structurally similar to embryonic capillary networks. They range from barely noticeable strawberry birthmarks to enormous clusters of engorged vascular channels that may deform an entire extremity. Most frequently, the vessels of the lower extremities are involved (i.e., femoral, iliac, and popliteal), and the resultant clinical manifestations vary enormously.[84] When fistulas are large, patients generally complain of disfigurement as well as swelling and pain in the limb. On examination, erythema and cyanosis are usually apparent, as are venous varices, a continuous murmur, and thrill. *Left heart failure* occurs, particularly in patients with larger lesions that involve the pelvis as well as the extremities.[85,86] Physical examination shows hemangiomatous changes associated with venous distention, deformity, and increased limb length. The fistulous connection may involve any vascular bed, including an internal mammary artery–pulmonary artery connection. Angiography is useful in confirming the diagnosis and in determining the physical extent of the anomaly.

Surgical excision is the ideal treatment,[87] but in many instances the lesions are not sufficiently localized to permit this.[88] The results of ligation and excision have been unsatisfactory in the majority of cases, since the congenital arteriovenous communications are usually not confined to a single anatomical segment or to a circumscribed anatomical region. Complete cure of these lesions is possible in only a few instances. Embolization of Gelfoam pellets delivered through a catheter has been reported to obliterate multiple systemic arteriovenous fistulas and thereby diminish high-output heart failure.[87]

Hereditary Hemorrhagic Telangiectasia. Also known as Osler-Weber-Rendu disease, this condition may be associated with arteriovenous fistulas, particularly in the lungs and liver; the latter condition can produce a hyperkinetic circulation,[88,88a,89] with heart failure as well as hepatomegaly with abdominal bruits. Because of the presence of oxygenated blood in the inferior vena cava and right atrium, this condition may be misdiagnosed as atrial septal defect.

The congenital arteriovenous communications resulting from *hemangioendothelioma of the liver* are commonly associated with marked increases in cardiac output, sometimes as high as 10.5 liters/min/sq meter, and congestive heart failure.[90] These lesions, which are extremely difficult to treat surgically, may be quite large, increase in size with time, and lead to heart failure even in infancy. They are often associated with sizable cutaneous hemangiomas, which should alert the clinician to the possibility of their presence.

ACQUIRED ARTERIOVENOUS FISTULAS. Acquired arteriovenous fistulas occur most frequently after such injuries as gunshot wounds and stab wounds and may involve any part of the body, most frequently the thigh.[91] Blood flow in the affected limb distal to the fistula diminishes after the creation of the fistula but then returns to normal and often increases with the passage of time. As a consequence, the affected limb is usually larger than its opposite member, and the overlying skin is warmer; cellulitis, venostasis, edema, and dermatitis with pigmentation frequently occur, in part as a consequence of chronically elevated venous pressure. Surgical repair or excision is generally advisable in fistulas that develop after gunshot wounds or trauma.

A rare form of acquired arteriovenous fistula results from spontaneous rupture of an aortic aneurysm into the inferior vena cava. This usually produces an enormous arteriovenous shunt and rapidly progressive left ventricular failure. On physical examination a pulsating mass can be readily palpated superficially in the abdomen, and a continuous bruit is audible.

Massive fistulas may be associated with Wilms' tumors of the kidney, and these have been reported to cause high-output cardiac failure in children.[92]

High-output congestive heart failure resulting from the arteriovenous shunts surgically constructed for vascular access in patients undergoing long-term hemodialysis is not uncommon.[93,94] Cardiac outputs as high as 10 liters/min/sq meter, which decrease substantially during temporary occlusion of the shunt, have been found in such patients. These values undoubtedly also reflect the chronic anemia present in many of these patients, but it is clear that it is the added hemodynamic burden imposed by the shunt that precipitates heart

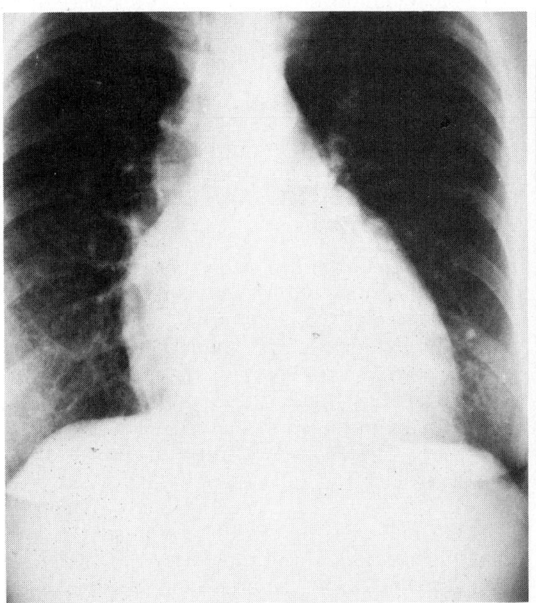

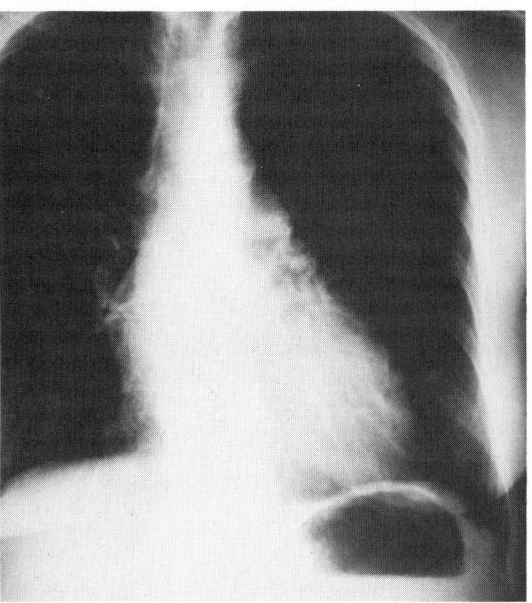

FIGURE 16–7. *Left,* Chest roentgenogram demonstrating cardiomegaly and pulmonary vascular congestion in patient with high-output cardiac failure attributable to end-to-side cephalic vein-radial artery fistula in wrist. *Right,* One month after banding of vein, cardiomegaly has decreased and pulmonary vascular congestion has improved. (From Anderson, C. B., et al.: Cardiac failure and upper extremity arteriovenous dialysis fistulas. Arch. Intern. Med. *136*:292, 1976, Copyright 1976, American Medical Association.)

failure in patients who had previously tolerated chronic anemia without apparent impairment of cardiac function. It is usually possible to revise or band the fistula to reduce it to the appropriate size for dialysis without compromising cardiac function[95] (Fig. 16–7).

BERIBERI HEART DISEASE

PATHOGENESIS AND CLINICAL CONSIDERATIONS. This condition is due to severe thiamine deficiency persisting for at least 3 months. Clinical beriberi is found most frequently in the Far East, although even in that part of the world it is far less prevalent now than in the past. It occurs predominantly in those individuals whose staple diet consists of polished rice, which is deficient in thiamine but high in carbohydrates. The presence of thiamine in the enriched flour used in white bread has virtually eradicated this disease in the United States and Western Europe, where beriberi is found most commonly in diet faddists and alcoholics; like polished rice, alcohol is low in vitamin B_1 but has a high carbohydrate content. In the West, alcoholics become thiamine deficient not only because of a low intake of the vitamin but also because they eat "junk" foods or drink large quantities of beer, with their high carbohydrate content and therefore their great demand for thiamine.

Patients in the Orient present with edema ("wet beriberi"), general malaise and fatigue. The elevation of cardiac output[96–100] is presumably secondary to the reduced systemic vascular resistance and augmented venous return. Hemodynamic findings in those studied before and after treatment with thiamine are presented in Figure 16–8.

Physical findings in most cases in Western countries are those of the high-output state and usually of severe generalized malnutrition and vitamin deficiency. Evidence of peripheral neuropathy with sensory and motor deficits is common (so-called dry beriberi), as is the presence of nutritional cirrhosis characterized by paresthesias of the extremities, absence of decreased knee and ankle jerks, painful glossitis, the anemia of combined iron and folate deficiency, and hyperkeratinized skin lesions.

Beriberi heart disease[99–104] is characterized by evidence of biventricular failure, sinus rhythm, and marked edema (so-called wet beriberi). There is arteriolar vasodilatation, and the cutaneous vessels may be dilated, or in later cases with congestive heart failure, they may be constricted. Therefore, the absence of warm hands does not exclude the diagnosis of beriberi. A third heart sound and an apical systolic murmur are heard almost invariably, and there is a wide pulse pressure characteristic of the hyperkinetic state.

The *electrocardiogram* characteristically exhibits low voltage of the QRS complex, prolongation of the Q-T interval, and low voltage or inversion of T waves. The chest roentgenogram usually shows biventricular enlargement, pulmonary congestion, and pleural effusions. In alcoholics with beriberi heart disease, the left ventricular ejection fraction and peak left ventricular dP/dt are usually reduced.[99] The role played by alcoholic cardiomyopathy (p. 1819) in this hemodynamic picture is not clear. The cardiac output falls, and the peripheral resistance rises acutely when thiamine is administered in the catheterization laboratory.[100]

Laboratory diagnosis can be made by demonstration of increased serum pyruvate and lactate levels in the presence of a low red blood cell transketolase level.[105] The thiamine concentration may be determined in biological fluids to confirm the diagnosis.[106–108]

At *postmortem examination* the heart usually shows simple dilation without other changes. On microscopic examination, there is sometimes edema and hydropic degeneration of the muscle fibers. Nonspecific but abnormal histological and electron microscopic changes have been found in cardiac biopsy specimens.

Heart failure may develop explosively in beriberi, and some patients succumb to the illness within 48 hours of the onset of symptoms. So-called Shoshin beriberi, seen most frequently

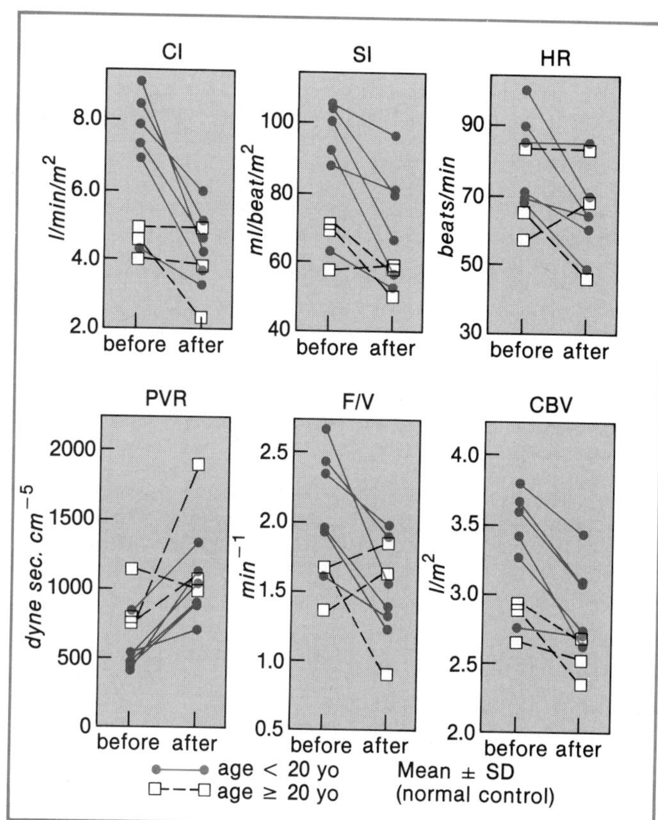

FIGURE 16–8. **Changes in cardiac index (CI), stroke index (SI), heart rate (HR), peripheral vascular resistance (PVR), blood turnover rate (F/V), and circulatory blood volume (CBV) in patients treated for beriberi in Kyoto, Japan. (From Kawai, C., et al.: Reappearance of beriberi heart disease in Japan. Am. J. Med. *69*:383, 1980.)**

in the Orient and Africa,[101,102] is a fulminating form of the disease[109] characterized by hypotension, tachycardia, and lactic acidosis; if left untreated, the patients die of pulmonary edema. Thus, since the course of the disease may advance rapidly, treatment must be begun immediately once the diagnosis has been established. In the Western world this fulminant form of the disease is uncommon.

TREATMENT. Akbarian and coworkers have reported careful hemodynamic studies which suggest that vasomotor depression or paralysis may be responsible for the depressed vascular resistance.[98] They studied four patients in whom ethanol excess was responsible for the thiamine deficiency. All had increased heart rate and cardiac output (averaging 6 liters/min/sq meter) and reduced arterial–mixed venous oxygen difference and systemic vascular resistance. Right and left ventricular filling pressures and blood volume were also elevated.

Patients with beriberi heart disease fail to respond adequately to digitalis and diuretics alone. However, improvement after the administration of thiamine (up to 100 mg intravenously followed by 25 mg per day orally for 1 to 2 weeks) may be dramatic. Marked diuresis, decrease in heart rate and size, and clearing of pulmonary congestion may occur within 12 to 48 hours.[98,109,110] However, the acute reversal of the vasodilation induced by correction of the deficiency may cause the unprepared left ventricle to go into low-output failure. Therefore, patients should receive a glycoside and diuretic therapy along with thiamine.

Latent beriberi deficiency may occur in conditions such as alcoholic cardiomyopathy and in other forms of refractory congestive heart failure. The possibility of thiamine deficiency should be considered in many patients with heart failure of obscure origin, and patients with heart failure from other causes could develop superimposed beriberi heart disease unless adequate thiamine intake is maintained.

PAGET'S DISEASE

PATHOGENESIS. Paget's disease of bone is an asymmetrical process characterized by extremely rapid bone formation and resorption of the involved areas. Because of the increased vascularity of bone affected by Paget's disease, it has been assumed that this high flow occurred through the involved bone. However, it appears that the additional blood flow through an affected, resting limb passes through the *cutaneous tissue* overlying the involved bone, possibly secondary to local heat production resulting from the increased metabolic activity of affected bone.[111]

Clinical findings are a function of the extent of the disease and the specific bones involved. Involvement of at least 15 per cent of the skeleton by Paget's disease in an active stage, accompanied by a high alkaline phosphatase level, is necessary before a clinically significant augmentation of cardiac output is observed.

Such a high-output state may be well tolerated for years with the patient remaining asymptomatic. However, if a specific cardiac disorder (e.g., valvular disease, coronary stenosis) is present, the combination may cause rapid clinical deterioration.

The cardiovascular findings are not distinguishable from those in other conditions with high-output states. However, metastatic calcifications are characteristic. If they involve the heart, they may lead to sclerosis and calcification of the valve rings, with extension into the interventricular septum, and may produce abnormalities of atrioventricular or interventricular conduction.

OTHER CAUSES OF HIGH-CARDIAC OUTPUT FAILURE

FIBROUS DYSPLASIA (ALBRIGHT SYNDROME). This condition, in which there is proliferation of fibrous tissue in bone, may also be associated with an elevated cardiac output, especially when multiple bones are involved.[112,113]

MULTIPLE MYELOMA. High-output heart failure has also been described in this condition.[114] The mechanism is not clear; it may be due to the associated anemia and/or hyperperfusion of the neoplastic tissue.

High-cardiac output failure also occurs in pregnancy (Chap. 59), renal disease, especially glomerulonephritis (Chap. 62), cor pulmonale (Chap. 45), polycythemia vera (Chap. 57), the carcinoid syndrome (Chap. 44), and obesity (Chap. 37).

REFERENCES

1. Packer, M.: Survival in patients with chronic heart failure and its potential modification by drug therapy. *In* Cohn, J. N. (ed.): Drug Treatment of Heart Failure, 2nd ed. Secaucus, N.J., ATC International, 1988, p. 273.
2. Kannel, W. B.: Epidemiologic aspects of heart failure. *In* Weber, K. T. (ed.): Heart Failure: Current Concepts and Management. Cardiology Clinics Series 7/1, Philadelphia, W. B. Saunders Co, 1989.
3. Braunwald, E., Mock, M. B., and Watson, J. (eds.): Congestive Heart Failure. Current Research and Clinical Applications. Orlando, Fla., Grune and Stratton, 1982.
4. Cohn, J. N. (ed.): Drug Treatment of Heart Failure, 2nd ed. Secaucus, N.J., ATC International, 1988, 310 pp.
5. McKee, P. A., Castell, W. P., McNamara, P. M., and Kannel, W. B.: The natural history of congestive heart failure, the Framingham Study. N. Engl. J. Med. *285*:1441, 1971.
6. Marantz, P. R., Tobin, J. N., Wassertheil-Smoller, S., et al.: The relationship between left ventricular systolic function and congestive heart failure diagnosed by clinical criteria. Circulation *77*:607, 1988.

FORMS AND CAUSES OF HEART FAILURE

7. Hope, J. A.: Treatise on the Diseases of the Heart and Great Vessels, London, Williams-Kidd, 1832.
8. Williams, J. F., Jr., Sonnenblick, E. H., and Braunwald, E.: Determinants of atrial contactile force in intact heart. Am. J. Physiol. *209*:1061, 1965.
9. Ross, J., Jr., and Braunwald, E.: Studies on Starling's law of the heart. IX. The effects of impeding venous return on performance of the normal and failing human left ventricle. Circulation *30*:719, 1964.
10. Stampfer, M., Epstein, S. E., Beiser, G. D., and Braunwald, E.: Hemodynamic effects of diuresis at rest and during intense upright exercise in patients with impaired cardiac function. Circulation *37*:900, 1968.
11. Mackenzie, J.: Disease of the Heart, 3rd ed. London, Oxford University Press, 1913.
12. Moe, G. W., Legault, L., and Skorecki, K. L.: Control of extracellular fluid volume and pathophysiology of edema formation. *In* Brenner, B. M., and Rector, F. C. Jr. (eds.): The Kidney, 4th ed. Philadelphia, W. B. Saunders Company, 1991, pp. 623–676.
12a. Braunwald, E.: The Pathogenesis of Heart Failure: Then and Now. Medicine *70*:68, 1991.
13. Chidsey C. A., Kaiser, G. A., Sonnenblick, E. H., et al.: Cardiac norepinephrine stores in experimental heart failure in the dog. J. Clin. Invest. *43*:2386, 1964.
14. Chandler, B. M., Sonnenblick, E. H., Spann, J. F., and Pool, P. E.: Association of depressed myofibrillar adenosinetriphosphate and reduced contractility in experimental heart failure. Circ. Res. *21*:717, 1967.
15. Stevenson, L. W., and Perloff, J. K.: The limited reliability of physical signs for estimating hemodynamics in chronic heart failure. J.A.M.A. *261*:884, 1989.
16. Artman, M., and Graham, T. P., Jr.: Congestive heart failure in infancy: Recognition and management. Am. Heart J. *103*:1040, 1982.
17. Ghali, J. K., Kadakia, S., Cooper, R., and Ferlinz, J.: Precipitating factors leading to decompensation of heart failure: Traits among urban blacks. Arch. Intern. Med. *148*:2013, 1988.
18. Braunwald, E., and Frahm, C. J.: Studies on Starling's law of the heart: IV. Observations on the hemodynamic functions of the left atrium in man. Circulation *24*:633, 1961.
19. Gottlieb, S. S., Kukin, M. L., Yushak, M., et al.: Adverse hemodynamic and clinical effects of encainide in severe chronic heart failure. Ann. Intern. Med. *110*:505, 1989.

SYMPTOMS AND PROGNOSIS IN HEART FAILURE

20. Srebro, J., and Karliner, J. S.: Congestive heart failure. Curr. Probl. Cardiol. *23*:1, 1986.
21. Geltman, E. M.: Mild heart failure: Diagnosis and treatment. Am. Heart J *118*:1277, 1989.
22. Collins, J. V., Clark, T.J.H., and Brown, D. J.: Airway function in healthy subjects and in patients with left heart disease. Clin. Sci. Molec. Med. *49*:217, 1975.
23. Fishman, A. P. (ed.): Pulmonary Diseases and Disorders, 2nd ed. New York, McGraw-Hill Book Co., 1988.
24. Macklem, P. T.: Respiratory muscles: The vital pump. Chest *78*:753, 1980.
25. Turino, G. M.: Origins of cardiac dyspnea. Primary Cardiol. *7*:76, 1981.
26. Fishman, A. P., and Ledlie, J. F.: Dyspnea. Bull. Eur. Physiopathol. Resp. *15*:789, 1979.
27. Campbell, E.J.M., Agostoni, E., and Newsom Davis, J.: The Respiratory Muscles: Mechanisms and Neural Control, 2nd ed. Philadelphia, W. B. Saunders Company, 1970.
28. Poole-Wilson, P. A., and Buller, N. P.: Causes of symptoms in chronic congestive heart failure and implications for treatment. Am. J. Cardiol. *62*:31A, 1988.
29. Petermann, W., Barth, J., and Entzian, P.: Heart failure and airway obstruction. Int. J. Cardiol. *17*:207, 1987.
30. Franciosa, J. A.: Exercise testing in chronic congestive heart failure. Am. J. Cardiol. *53*:1447, 1984.
31. Weber, K. T., and Janicki, J. S.: Cardiopulmonary Exercise Testing. Philadelphia, W. B. Saunders Company, 1986.
32. Wasserman, D.: Dyspnea on exertion: Is it the heart or the lungs? J.A.M.A. *248*:2042, 1982.
33. Higgins, C. B., Vatner, S. F., Franklin, D., and Braunwald, E.: Effects of experimentally produced heart failure on the peripheral vascular response to severe exercise in conscious dogs. Circ. Res. *31*:186, 1972.
34. Criteria Committee, New York Heart Association, Inc.: Diseases of the Heart and Blood Vessels. Nomenclature and Criteria for Diagnosis, 6th ed. Boston, Little, Brown and Co., 1964, p. 114.
35. Goldman, L., Hasimoto, B., Cook, E. F., and Loscalzo, A.: Comparative reproducibility and validity of symptoms for assessing cardiovascular functional class. Advantages of a new specific activity scale. Circulation *64*:1227, 1981.
36. Earnest, D. L., and Hurst, J. W.: Exophthalmos, stare and increase in intraocular pressure and systolic propulsion of the eyeballs due to congestive heart failure. Am. J. Cardiol. *26*:351, 1970.
37. Chakko, S. C., Caldwell, S. H., and Sforza, P. P.: Treatment of congestive heart failure: Its effect on pleural fluid chemistry. Chest *95*:798, 1989.
38. Strober, W., Cohen, L. S., Waldmann, T. A., and Braunwald, E.: Tricuspid regurgitation: A newly recognized cause of protein-losing enteropathy, lymphocytopenia and immunologic deficiency. Am. J. Med. *44*:842, 1968.
39. Gleason, W. L., and Braunwald, E.: Studies on Starling's law of the heart: VI. Relationships between left ventricular end-diastolic volume and stroke volume in man with observations on the mechanism of pulsus alternans. Circulation *25*:841, 1962.
40. Berkowitz, D., Croll, M. N., and Likoff, W.: Malabsorption as a complication of congestive heart failure. Am. J. Cardiol. *11*:43, 1963.
41. Levine, B., Kalman, J., Mayer, L., et al.: Elevated circulating levels of tumor necrosis factor in severe chronic heart failure. N. Engl. J. Med. *323*:236, 1990.
42. Carr, J. G., Stevenson, L. W., Walden, J. A., and Heber, D.: Prevalence and hemodynamic correlates of malnutrition in severe congestive heart failure secondary to ischemic or idiopathic dilated cardiomyopathy. Am. J. Cardiol. *63*:709, 1989.
43. Pittman, J. G., and Cohen, P.: The pathogenesis of cardiac cachexia. N. Engl. J. Med. *27*:403, 1964.
44. Lange, R. L., and Hecht, H. H.: The mechanism of Cheyne-Stokes respiration. J. Clin. Invest. *41*:42, 1962.
45. Rees, P. J., and Clark, T.J.H.: Paroxysmal nocturnal dyspnoea and periodic respiration. Lancet *2*:1315, 1979.
46. Friedman-Mor, Z., Chalon, J., Turndorf, H., and Orkin, L. R.: Cardiac index and incidence of heart failure cells. Arch. Pathol. Lab. Med. *102*:418, 1978.
47. Wolke, A. M., Brooks, K. M., and Schaffner, F.: The liver in congestive heart failure. Primary Cardiol. *8*:130, 1982.

48. Blasco, V. V.: Features of hepatic involvement in congestive heart failure. Cardiovasc. Rev. Rep. 4:963, 1983.
49. Lemmer, J. H., Coran, A. G., Behrendt, D. M., et al.: Liver fibrosis (cardiac cirrhosis) five years after modified Fontan operation for tricuspid atresia. J. Thorac. Cardiovasc. Surg. *86*:757, 1983.
49a. Matsuda, H., Covino, E., Hirose, H., et al.: Acute liver dysfunction after modified Fontan operation for complex cardiac lesions. J. Thorac. Cardiovasc. Surg. *96*:219, 1988.
50. Mace, S., Borkat, G., and Liebman, J.: Hepatic dysfunction and cardiovascular abnormalities: Occurrence in infants, children and young adults. Am. J. Dis. Child. *139*:60, 1985.
51. Kanel, G. C., Ucci, A. A., Kaplan, M. M., and Wolfe, H. J.: A distinctive perivenular hepatic lesion associated with heart failure. Am. J. Clin. Pathol. *73*:235, 1980.
52. Nouel, O., Henrion, J., Bernuau, J., et al.: Fulminant hepatic failure due to transient circulatory failure in patients with chronic heart disease. Dig. Dis. Sci. *25*:49, 1980.
53. Jenkins, J. G., Lynn, A. M., Wood, A. E., et al.: Acute hepatic failure following cardiac operation in children. J. Thorac. Cardiovasc. Surg. *84*:865, 1982.
54. Szatalowicz, V. L., Arnold, P. E., Chaimovitz, C., et al.: Radioimmunoassay of plasma arginine vasopressin in hyponatremic patients with congestive heart failure. N. Engl. J. Med. *305*:263, 1981.
55. Chakko, S. C., Frutchey, J., and Gheorghiade, M.: Life-threatening hyperkalemia in severe heart failure. Am. Heart J. *117*:1083, 1989.
56. Kaplan, M. M.: Liver dysfunction secondary to congestive heart failure. Practical Cardiol. *6*:39, 1980.
57. Kubo, S. H., Walter, B. A., John, D.H.A., et al.: Liver function abnormalities in chronic heart failure: Influence of systemic hemodynamics. Arch. Intern. Med. *147*:1227, 1987.
58. Kisloff, B., and Schaffer, G.: Fulminant hepatic failure secondary to congestive heart failure. Am. J. Dig. Dis. *21*:895, 1976.
59. Kaymakcalan, H., Dourdourekas, D., Szanto, P. B., and Steigmann, F.: Congestive heart failure as cause of fulminant hepatic failure. Am. J. Med. *65*:384, 1978.
60. Gorlin, R., Knowles, J. H., and Storey, C. F.: The Valsalva maneuver as a test of cardiac function. Pathologic physiology and clinical significance. Am. J. Med. *22*:197, 1957.
60a. Schmidt, D., and Shah, P. K.: Simple bedside application of Valsalva maneuver, accurately detects elevated left ventricular filling pressures in patients with normal or depressed ejection fraction. J. Am. Coll. Cardiol. (abstr.) *17*:28A, 1991.
61. Elisberg, E. I.: Heart rate response to the Valsalva maneuver as a test of circulatory integrity. J.A.M.A. *186*:200, 1963.
62. Baron, M. G.: Radiological and angiographic examination of the heart. *In* Braunwald, E. (ed.): Heart Disease, 3rd ed., Philadelphia, W. B. Saunders Company, 1988, p. 148.
62a. Chakko, S., Woska, D., Martinez, H., et al.: Clinical, radiographic, and hemodynamic correlations in chronic congestive heart failure: Conflicting results may lead to inappropriate care. Am. J. Med. *90*:353, 1991.
63. Evaluating the radiographic assessment of pulmonary venous hypertension in chronic heart disease. AJR *142*:877, 1984.
64. Daves, M. L.: Cardiac Roentgenology. Chicago, Year Book Medical Publishers, 1981, pp. 78–86.
65. Cohn, J. N., and Rector, T. S.: Prognosis of congestive heart failure and predictors of mortality. Am. J. Cardiol. *62*:25A, 1988.
66. Sziachic, J., et al.: Correlates and prognostic implications of exercise capacity in chronic congestive heart failure. Am. J. Cardiol. *55*:1037, 1986.
67. Rahimtoola, S. H.: The pharmacologic treatment of chronic congestive heart failure. Circulation *80*:693, 1989.
68. Murali, S., and Thompson, M. E.: Pathophysiology and drug therapy in congestive heart failure. Cardiology *7*:41, 1990.
69. Gradman, A., Deedwania, P., Cody, R., et al.: Predictors of total mortality and sudden death in mild to moderate heart failure. J. Am. Coll. Cardiol. *14*:564, 1989.
70. Cleland, J.G.F., and Dargie, H. J.: Arrhythmias, catecholamines and electrolyte. Am. J. Cardiol. *62*:55A, 1988.
71. Cleland, J.G.F., Dargie, H. J., and Ford, I.: Mortality in heart failure: Clinical variables of prognostic value. Br. Heart J. *58*:572, 1987.
72. Packer, M., Gottlieb, S. S., and Blum, M. A.: Immediate and long-term pathophysiologic mechanisms underlying the genesis of sudden cardiac death in patients with congestive heart failure. Am. J. Med. *82*(Suppl. 3a):4, 1987.
73. Packer, M., Lee, W. H., Kessler, P. D., et al.: Role of neurohormonal mechanisms in determining survival in patients with severe chronic heart failure. Circulation *75*:(Suppl. 4)80, 1987.
74. Gottlieb, S. S., Kukin, M. L., Ahern, D., and Packer, M.: Prognostic importance of atrial natriuretic peptide in patients with chronic heart failure. J. Am. Coll. Cardiol. *13*:1534, 1989.
75. Packer, M.: Potential role of potassium as a determinant of morbidity and mortality in patients with systemic hypertension and congestive heart failure. Am. J. Cardiol. *65*:45E, 1990.
76. Hyperdynamic States. *In* Fowler, N.O.: Diagnosis of Heart Disease. New York, Springer-Verlag, 1991, pp. 389–399.

HIGH OUTPUT HEART FAILURE

77. Lewis, B. S., Ehrenfelk, E. N., Lewis, N., and Gotsman, M. S.: Echocardiographic left ventricular function in thyrotoxicosis. Am. Heart J. *97*:460, 1979.
78. Hoffman, I., and Lowrey, R. D.: The electrocardiogram in thyrotoxicosis. Am. J. Cardiol. *8*:893, 1960.
79. Braunwald, E., Mason, D. T., and Ross, J., Jr.: Studies of the cardiocirculatory actions of digitalis. Medicine *44*:233, 1965
80. Shapiro, S., Steiner, M., and Dimich, I.: Congestive heart failure in neonatal thyrotoxicosis. A curable cause of heart failure in the newborn. Clin. Pediatr. *14*:1155, 1975.
81. Nicoladoni, C.: Phlebarteriectasie der rechten oberen Extermitat. Arch. Klin. Chir. *18*:252, 1875.
82. Branham, H. H.: Aneurysmal varix of the femoral artery and vein following a gunshot wound. Int. J. Surg. *3*:250, 1890.
83. Gupta, P. D., and Singh, M.: Neural mechanism underlying tachycardia induced by non-hypotensive A-V shunt. Am. J. Physiol. *236*:H35, 1979.
84. Szilagyi, D. E., Smith, R. F., Elliott, J. P., and Hageman, J. H.: Congenital arteriovenous anomalies of the limbs. Arch. Surg. *111*:423, 1976.
85. Becker, D. G., Fish, C. R., and Juergen, S.J.L.: Arteriovenous fistulas of the female pelvis. Obstet. Gynecol. *31*:799, 1968.
86. Price, A. C., Coran, A. G., and Mattern, A. L.: Hemangioendothelioma of the pelvis: A cause of cardiac failure in the newborn. N. Engl. J. Med. *286*:647, 1972.
87. Coel, M. N., and Alksne, J. F.: Embolization to diminish high output failure secondary to systemic angiomatosis (Ullman's syndrome). Vasc. Surg. *12*:336, 1978.
88. Vaksmann, G., Rey, C., Marache, P., et al.: Severe congestive heart failure in newborns due to giant cutaneous hemangiomas. Am. J. Cardiol. *60*:392, 1987.
88a. Gong, B., Baken, L. A., Julian, T. M., and Kubo, S. H.: High-output heart failure due to hepatic arteriovenous fistula during pregnancy: A case report. Obstet. Gynecol. *72*:440, 1988.
89. Baranda, M. M., Perez, M., DeAndres, J., et al.: High-output congestive heart failure as first manifestation of Osler-Weber-Rendu disease. J. Vasc. Dis. *35*:568, 1984.
90. Zavota, L., Bini, F., Carano, N., et al.: Hepatic hemangiomatosis with congestive cardiac failure and development into a cholostatic hepatopathy. Pediatr. Med. Chir. *6*:621, 1984.
91. Dorney, E. R.: Peripheral AV fistula of fifty-seven years' duration with refractory heart failure. Am. Heart J. *54*:778, 1957.
92. Sanyal, S. K., Saldivar, V., Coburn, T. P., et al.: Hyperdynamic heart failure due to A-V fistula associated with Wilms' tumor. Pediatrics *57*:564, 1976.
93. Ingram, C. W., Satler, L. F., and Rackley, C. E.: Progressive heart failure secondary to a high output state. Chest *92*:1117, 1987.
94. Fee, H. J., Levisman, J., Doud, R. B., and Golding, A. L.: High output congestive failure from femoral arteriovenous shunts for vascular access. Ann. Surg. *183*:321, 1976.
95. Anderson, C. B., Codd, J. R., Graff, R. A., et al.: Cardiac failure and upper extremity arteriovenous dialysis fistulas. Arch. Intern. Med. *136*:292, 1976.
96. Weiss, S., and Wilkinson, R. W.: The nature of the cardiovascular disturbances in nutritional deficiency states (beriberi). Ann. Intern. Med. *11*:104, 1937.
97. Burwell, C. S., and Dexter, L.: Beriberi heart disease. Trans. Assoc. Am. Physicians *60*:59, 1947.
98. Akbarian, M., Yankopoulos, N. A., and Abelmann, W. H.: Hemodynamic studies in beriberi heart disease. Am. J. Med. *41*:197, 1966.
99. Ayzenberg, O., Silber, M. H., and Bortz, D.: Beriberi heart disease. A case report describing the hemodynamic features. S. Afr. Med. J. *68*:263, 1985.
100. Akram, H., Maslowski, A. H., Smith, B. L., and Nichols, M. G.: The haemodynamic, histopathological and hormonal features of alcoholic beriberi. Q. J. Med. *50*:359, 1981.
101. Naidoo, D. P.: Beriberi heart disease in Durban. S. Afr. Med. J. *72*:241, 1987.
102. Naidoo, D. P., Rawat, R., Dyer, R. B., et al.: Cardiac beriberi: A report of four cases. S. Afr. Med. J. *72*:283, 1987.
103. Carson, P.: Alcoholic cardiac beriberi. Br. Med. J. *284*:1817, 1982.
104. Cardiovascular beriberi (editorial). Lancet *1*:1287, 1982.
105. Akbarian, M., and Dreyfus, P. M.: Blood trans-ketolase activity in beriberi heart disease. JAMA *203*:23, 1968.
106. Baker, H., quoted in Sauberlich, H. E.: Biochemical alterations in thiamine deficiency—their interpretation. Am. J. Clin. Nutr. *20*:543, 1967.
107. Brin, M.: Erythrocyte transketolase in early thiamine deficiency. Ann. N.Y. Acad. Sci. *98*:528, 1962.
108. Baker, H., and Frank, O.: Clinical Vitaminology: Methods and Interpretation. New York, Wiley Interscience, 1968.
109. Jeffrey, F. E., and Abelmann, W. H.: Recovery of proved Shoshin beriberi. Am. J. Med. *50*:123, 1971.
110. Whittemore, R., and Caddell, J. L.: Metabolic and nutritional diseases. *In* Moss, A. J., et al. (eds.): Heart Disease in Infants, Children and Adolescents, 2nd ed. Baltimore, Williams and Wilkins Co., 1977, pp. 590 and 591.
111. Heistad, D. D., Abboud, F. M., Schmid, P. G., et al.: Regulation of blood flow in Paget's disease of the bone. J. Clin. Invest. *55*:69, 1975.
112. Rutishauser, E., Veyrat, R., and Rouiller, C.: La vascularization de l'os pagé tique, étude anatomo-pathologique. Presse Méd. *62*:654, 1954.
113. Lequime, J., and Denolin, H.: Circulatory dynamics in osteitis deformans. Circulation *12*:215, 1955.
114. McBride, W., Jackman, J. D., Jr., Gammon, R. S., and Willerson, J. T.: High-output cardiac failure in patients with multiple myeloma. N. Engl. J. Med. *319*:1651, 1988.

17

The Management of Heart Failure

by THOMAS W. SMITH, M.D., EUGENE BRAUNWALD, M.D., and RALPH A. KELLY, M.D.

Therapeutic Strategy

The goals of treatment of patients with heart failure are to improve the quality and quantity of life, i.e., survival. Three general approaches are employed.

1. **REMOVAL OF THE UNDERLYING CAUSE. (see p. 447).** This—the most desirable approach—involves the surgical correction of structural abnormalities responsible for heart failure, such as congenital malformations, acquired valvular lesions, or, on occasion, left ventricular aneurysm, and effective medical treatment of conditions such as infective endocarditis or hypertension. When symptoms such as dyspnea on exertion or orthopnea are due to impairment of ventricular diastolic relaxation rather than to diminished systolic contraction, specific measures to reduce left ventricular hypertrophy or myocardial ischemia, if present, are in order.

2. **REMOVAL OF THE PRECIPITATING CAUSE(S).** The recognition, prompt treatment, and, whenever possible, prevention of the specific cause(s) or incidents that produce or exacerbate heart failure, such as infections, arrhythmias, and pulmonary emboli, are critical to the successful management of heart failure.

3. **CONTROL OF CONGESTIVE HEART FAILURE STATE.** This approach, which constitutes the subject of this chapter, may in turn be divided into three categories (Table 17–1):

A. *Reduction of the heart's workload*, which involves reduction of the demand placed on the heart to generate pressure and/or to pump blood.

B. *Improvement of the heart's pumping performance*, which consists of efforts to restore the contractility of the failing heart toward normal.

C. *Control of excessive salt and water retention*, i.e., control of the expansion of extracellular fluid volume, which is the principal cause of many manifestations of heart failure, such as dyspnea and edema.

In each of these three categories, a number of therapeutic measures are available. As outlined in Table 17-2, numbers *1* (restriction of physical activity) *4* (vasodilators), and *7C* (assisted circulation) involve reducing the heart's workload; numbers *5* (digitalis glycosides) and *6* (other inotropic agents) contribute to the direct improvement of the heart's pumping performance; while numbers *2* (restriction of sodium intake) and *3* (diuretics) involve elimination of excess salt and water.

TABLE 17–1 CONTROL OF CONGESTIVE HEART FAILURE

1. *REDUCTION OF WORKLOAD*
   - (A) Physical and emotional rest
   - (B) Treatment of obesity
   - (C) Vasodilator therapy
   - (D) Assisted circulation
2. *IMPROVEMENT OF PUMPING PERFORMANCE*
   - (A) Digitalis glycoside
   - (B) Sympathomimetic agents
   - (C) Other positive inotropic agents
   - (D) Pacemaker
3. *CONTROL OF EXCESSIVE SALT AND WATER RETENTION*
   - (A) Low-sodium diet
   - (B) Diuretics
   - (C) Mechanical removal of fluid
     - (1) Thoracentesis
     - (2) Paracentesis
     - (3) Dialysis
     - (4) Ultrafiltration

TABLE 17-2 OUTLINE OF TREATMENT OF OVERT CHRONIC CONGESTIVE HEART FAILURE

1. *RESTRICTION OF PHYSICAL ACTIVITY*
   (A) Discontinue exhausting sports and heavy labor
   (B) Discontinue full-time work or equivalent activity, introduce rest periods during the day
   (C) Confine to house
   (D) Confine to bed, chair
2. *RESTRICTION OF SODIUM INTAKE*
   (A) Eliminate saltshaker at table (Na = 1.6 to 2.8 gm)
   (B) Eliminate salt in cooking and at table (Na = 1.2 to 1.8 gm)
   (C) Institute A and B above plus low-sodium diet (Na = 0.2 to 1.0 gm)
3. *DIURETICS*
   (A) Moderately effective diuretics (thiazide*)
   (B) Loop diuretic (ethacrynic acid, furosemide, or bumetanide)
   (C) Loop diuretic plus distal tubular (potassium-sparing) diuretic
   (D) Loop diuretic plus thiazide and distal tubular diuretic
4. *VASODILATORS*
   (A) ACE inhibitor, or combination of hydralazine plus isosorbide dinitrate
   (B) Intensification of oral vasodilator regimen
   (C) Intravenous nitroprusside
5. *DIGITALIS GLYCOSIDES*
   (A) Usual maintenance dose
   (B) Maximum tolerable dose
6. *OTHER INOTROPIC AGENTS* (dopamine, dobutamine, amrinone)
7. *SPECIAL MEASURES*
   (A) Cardiac transplantation
   (B) Dialysis
   (C) Assisted circulation (intraaortic balloon, left ventricular assist device, artificial heart)

* Thiazide or a diuretic of approximately equal potency, such as metalazone.

APPROACH TO THE PATIENT WITH HEART FAILURE

EVALUATION. The first step in the care of a patient with known or suspected heart failure is a thorough evaluation, the elements of which have been covered in Chap. 16.

Formulation of the prognosis in a given patient will also challenge the clinician at the time of initial evaluation and as the response to treatment becomes apparent. Table 16–3 (p. 456) lists prognostic determinants.

While much emphasis is placed on the limited prognosis of patients with overt congestive heart failure (see p. 456), the current therapeutic armamentarium, carefully tailored to the individual patient, can yield noteworthy results. Stevenson and colleagues, for example, report that of 50 inpatients transferred to their care from other hospitals for urgent cardiac transplantation, intensive treatment with intravenous and subsequently oral vasodilators, as well as appropriate use of diuretics and digoxin, permitted hospital discharge without surgery in 40 of 50 patients.[1] Sixty per cent of patients referred could be kept stably compensated by means of tailored medical therapy, without transplantation, for at least 1 month, and at 6-month follow-up the improvement in exercise capacity was not significantly different between survivors of cardiac transplantation and survivors of sustained medical therapy, despite a marked improvement in left ventricular ejection fraction in the transplanted group (62 ± 7 per cent vs. 22 ± 9 per cent).[2] While this does not, of course, address the issue of long-term survival in the two groups, it does indicate the potential for symptomatic improvement with judiciously aggressive medical management in many patients considered to have end-stage heart failure.

CHRONIC HEART FAILURE. A condition as variable as congestive heart failure cannot be treated according to a simple formula. Intelligent management depends not only on an appreciation of the nature of the underlying condition but also on its rapidity of progression; the presence of associated illnesses; the patient's age, occupation, personality, life style, family setting, and ability and motivation to cooperate with treatment; and, importantly, the response to the therapeutic measures. With the recognition that wide differences exist among individual patients, Figure 17–1 is presented as a general guide to the therapy of adult patients with chronic congestive heart failure due primarily to systolic dysfunction, in whom the underlying disease is not amenable to further treatment and in whom the precipitating cause has been eliminated to the maximum extent possible. A guide to the assessment of the efficacy of treatment is shown in Table 17–3. The course of heart failure is rarely smoothly progressive; rather, it is usually punctuated by a series of abrupt downward steps due to acute decompensation (Fig. 17–2), generally as a consequence of one of the precipitating causes of heart failure described on page 477. When the precipitating cause has been removed and treatment has been intensified, the patient's previous condition is often restored. In other patients there are long periods—many months or even years—when the course is stable without any discernible deterioration.

In asymptomatic patients with left ventricular dysfunction secondary to coronary artery disease, emphasis is placed on reduction of risk factors (Chap. 37). Angiotensin-converting enzyme inhibitors have been shown to diminish ventricular dilatation in patients who have suffered myocardial infarction,[3,4] and they are useful in such patients because they may delay the development of heart failure. Ongoing trials are examining the effects on survival when administration of these drugs is begun in asymptomatic patients with impaired left

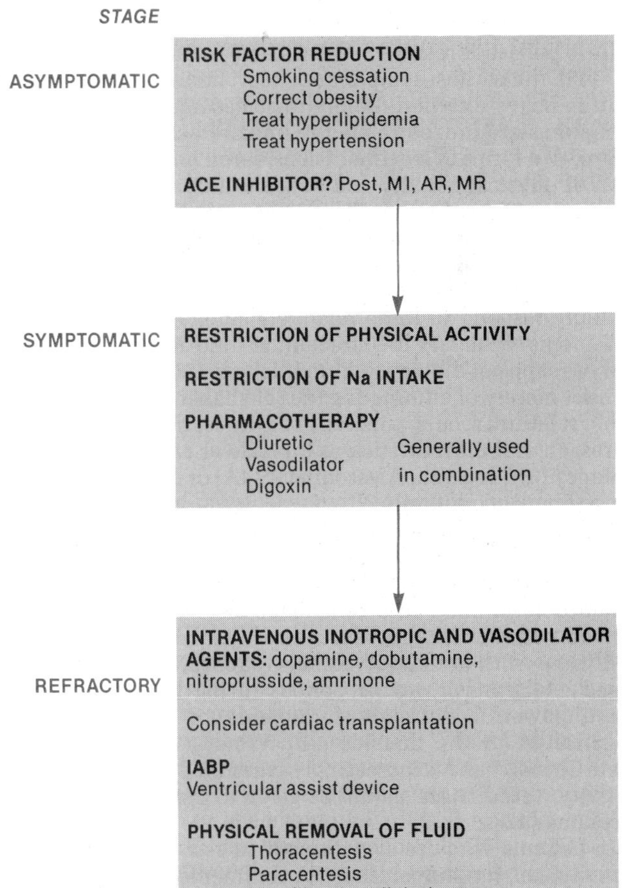

FIGURE 17–1. **Approach to treatment of ventricular dysfunction according to the severity of heart failure. ACE, angiotensin converting enzyme; MI, myocardial infarction; AR, aortic regurgitation; MR, mitral regurgitation; IABP, intraortic balloon counterpulsation.**

continue routine tasks. Insofar as recreation is concerned, again, minor adjustment, such as the use of a golf cart, may allow the patient many hours of pleasurable activity. As is the case in patients with angina pectoris, regular physical activity to a level that does not regularly produce symptoms is desirable in patients with congestive heart failure. Properly supervised graded exercise programs have been used with gratifying results in appropriately selected groups of patients.[13]

In patients with more severe heart failure, i.e., those in functional Class III, the problem of continued employment becomes more difficult. Such patients are usually unable, and should not be encouraged, to work full time, even in a relatively sedentary job. This should not mean, however, that cessation of employment is necessary or desirable. Often adjustment of the work schedule is feasible, e.g., reduction of the working day from 8 to 5 hours, with two mandatory 1-hour rest periods, or a 4-day work week, with a day in the middle of the week during which the patient remains home at rest. Evening activities should be curtailed. Even some patients who are in functional Class IV and confined to the home are able to lead more satisfying and productive lives by working for 2 or 3 hours a day at a desk.

In contrast to the situation in chronic congestive heart failure in which the patient is urged to remain active short of becoming symptomatic, physical activity should be rigidly restricted in the presence of acute myocardial decompensation. Under these circumstances, it is almost always desirable to hospitalize the patient, since this will facilitate the search for a precipitating cause and will allow adjustment of medications and institution of additional therapeutic measures while the patient is under observation. Hospitalization also usually allows more rigid restriction of physical activity. Although physical rest plays an important role in the treatment of heart failure, complete physical rest does not mean complete bed rest. Indeed, patients are usually more comfortable and the venous return (and therefore the cardiac preload) is lower when the patient is sitting rather than supine. Also, patients should not be forced to use the bedpan, and trips to the bathroom can usually be allowed. On the other hand, too much relaxation of the rules of restricting physical activity can obviate the value of physical rest.

The hazards of phlebothrombosis and pulmonary embolization should be recognized, and deep-breathing exercises, leg exercises, and wearing of elastic stockings are advisable. The use of anticoagulants (minidose heparin, coumadin) should be considered in patients with heart failure with or without a previous history of thromboembolic disease. Patients with marked impairment of ventricular function (e.g., ejection fraction $<$20 per cent) are at particularly high risk for both systemic and pulmonary emboli, and long-term anticoagulation with coumarin-type drugs should be considered for outpatient use if contraindications do not exist.

Emotional and mental rest are as important as physical rest. Hospitalization is often beneficial because it removes the patient from a situation that is anxiety-provoking. Since emotional stress can retard convalescence from an episode of acute congestive heart failure, visitors and incoming telephone calls should be limited. The physician should serve as a thoughtful, sympathetic listener with whom the patient can discuss a variety of problems. In particular, the patient must be given a realistic appraisal of the prognosis, and it must be emphasized that if a precipitating cause of heart failure can be identified, acute cardiac decompensation does not signify a hopeless outlook. It is important that the patient sleep well each night, and the use of flurazepam (15 to 30 mg) or triazolam (0.125 to 0.25 mg) as a hypnotic may be advisable. Diazepam (2 to 5 mg twice a day) may be helpful as well in patients with marked anxiety.

There is no formula for deciding on the duration of rigid restriction of physical activity for patients who are being treated for *acute* cardiac decompensation. It should depend principally on the patient's response to the overall treatment program. As a general rule, it is advisable to maintain the patient at rest as long as edema or moist pulmonary rales persist. Although the restriction of physical activity can be relaxed as these other clinical manifestations of heart failure abate, it should continue in a modified form for 2 to 4 weeks, depending on the course of the patient's convalescence.

DIET. Before effective oral diuretics were available, diet played a more important role in the control of salt and water retention than it does today. It is now possible to recommend only modest restriction of sodium intake in most patients with heart failure, with intensification of the diuretic regimen to prevent accumulation of extracellular fluid. Nonetheless, restriction of sodium intake remains one of the cornerstones of the treatment of congestive heart failure. The normal daily sodium content of the unrestricted American diet ranges from 3.0 to 6.0 gm; simple elimination of the saltshaker at the table and of some common foods such as pretzels, popcorn, salted nuts, potato chips, candy bars, smoked and salt-cured meats (including ham, bacon, and sausage), delicatessen meats, salt-cured fish, and condiments such as olives and pickles will reduce this to approximately half (1.5 to 3.0 gm). Potassium chloride (salt substitute) may be used in place of ordinary table salt. There is no need to eliminate salt in cooking and to make the diet unpalatable unless fluid retention occurs despite intensive use of diuretics. Indeed, the monotony and unpalatability of a low-sodium diet has caused unnecessary hardship to patients and their families and can interfere with adequate nutrition.

Reduction of sodium intake to 1.2 to 1.5 gm/day can be achieved by simply eliminating all salt from cooking and from the table. If it is necessary to reduce sodium intake to 0.2 gm daily in patients with Class IV congestive heart failure, many common foods must be eliminated. Spices and herbs can be used to flavor the food in place of sodium chloride, and as a wide variety of foods as possible should be employed to diminish monotony. A variety of books and pamphlets are available to aid in the preparation of salt-poor diets. It must be recognized that while the elimination of dietary salt may be necessary in patients with severe heart failure, this can result in anorexia and a marked reduction of caloric intake, contributing to malnutrition and cardiac cachexia (p. 1848).

While it is usually advisable simply to leave water intake to the patient's own desire, in far-advanced congestive heart failure the concentration of circulating antidiuretic hormone may be increased and the ability to excrete a free-water load may be impaired, with resulting dilutional hyponatremia (p. 479). Only under these circumstances is it desirable to restrict water intake so that the serum sodium concentration does not fall below approximately 130 mEq/liter.

OXYGEN. The use of oxygen in patients with pulmonary edema and with acute myocardial infarction is discussed elsewhere (pp. 562 and 1225). Oxygen inhalation, most conveniently by means of nasal prongs at 4 to 6 liters/min, should be employed in patients with other forms of congestive heart failure if the arterial oxygen saturation falls below 90 per cent. Oxygen therapy is useful in patients with heart failure precipitated by pulmonary infection or pulmonary infarction. The pulmonary vasorelaxant effect observed when hypoxemia is corrected is particularly valuable in reducing right ventricular afterload in the presence of right-sided failure.

PHYSICAL REMOVAL OF FLUID. Ordinarily, mechanical removal of fluid from the pleural and abdominal cavities is unnecessary in patients with congestive heart failure, because these collections are generally easily mobilized and eliminated with effective diuresis. Occasionally, patients with advanced congestive heart failure who have become resistant to diuretic therapy may regain their sensitivity following mechanical removal of fluid. In some patients with acute respiratory distress in whom the lungs are compressed by large pleural effusion(s) and/or by diaphragms elevated by ascites, mechanical removal of the effusions can bring rapid relief of dyspnea. Mechanical removal of fluid may be associated with a risk, albeit a small one in experienced hands, of pneumothorax or infection. Drainage of ascitic fluid should be carried out slowly, i.e., not more than 200 ml/hr, and the total quantity of pleural fluid removed on a single occasion should usually not exceed 1500 ml; otherwise, fluid may move rapidly from the circulation into the abdominal or pleural cavity and cause cardiovascular collapse.

Removal of excess fluid by *peritoneal dialysis* or, preferably, *hemodialysis with ultrafiltration* has been employed successfully in patients with congestive heart failure resistant to diuretic therapy.

Severe constipation and consequent straining at stool should be avoided in patients with heart failure. Dioctyl sodium sulfosuccinate, 50 to 200 mg daily, is useful as a softener. In addition, a mild laxative may be necessary in patients whose physical activity has been restricted.

Diuretics

The high efficacy and relatively low and predictable toxicity of "loop" diuretics have made them among the most commonly prescribed medicines. Indeed, bed rest, combined with modest salt restriction and a diuretic alone, may result in a clinically important degree of fluid loss and a decline in ventricular filling pressures in most patients with advanced congestive failure. In addition, vasodilators may be ineffective if not administered appropriately with a diuretic.

The importance of diuretics in the treatment of the syndrome of congestive heart failure relates to the central role of the kidney as the target organ of many of the neurohumoral and hemodynamic changes that occur in response to a failing myocardium[13a–14a] (p. 455). Reduced perfusion leads to activation of the renin-angiotensin system within the kidney, which decreases renal blood flow and increases the glomerular filtration fraction, leading to enhanced resorption of solute and water by the proximal tubules (p. 394) (Fig. 17–4). An elevated plasma angiotensin II level contributes to a rise in systemic vascular resistance and also causes release from the adrenal gland of the potent mineralocorticoid aldosterone. Enhanced renal sympathetic nerve activity also reduces renal blood flow, releases renin from macula densa cells, and directly augments sodium resorption along the nephron. Renal blood flow is directed away from superficial cortical nephrons to the more efficient solute-resorbing juxtamedullary nephrons that rely upon the high capacity of the ion transport carriers in their long loops of Henle and the countercurrent mechanism of the medulla to allow the formation of concentrated urine. Plasma antidiuretic hormone (ADH) levels are also elevated in many patients with congestive heart failure (p. 1858), which causes further reductions in free water clearance by the kidney. This, coupled with the increased thirst of many patients with advanced heart failure (perhaps caused by their high angiotensin II levels), often leads to a hypotonic edematous state. As with other complex biological systems, countervailing humoral responses also occur, including increased prostaglandin E_2 and prostacyclin levels within the kidney (tubuloglomerular feedback), and the release of humoral natriuretic

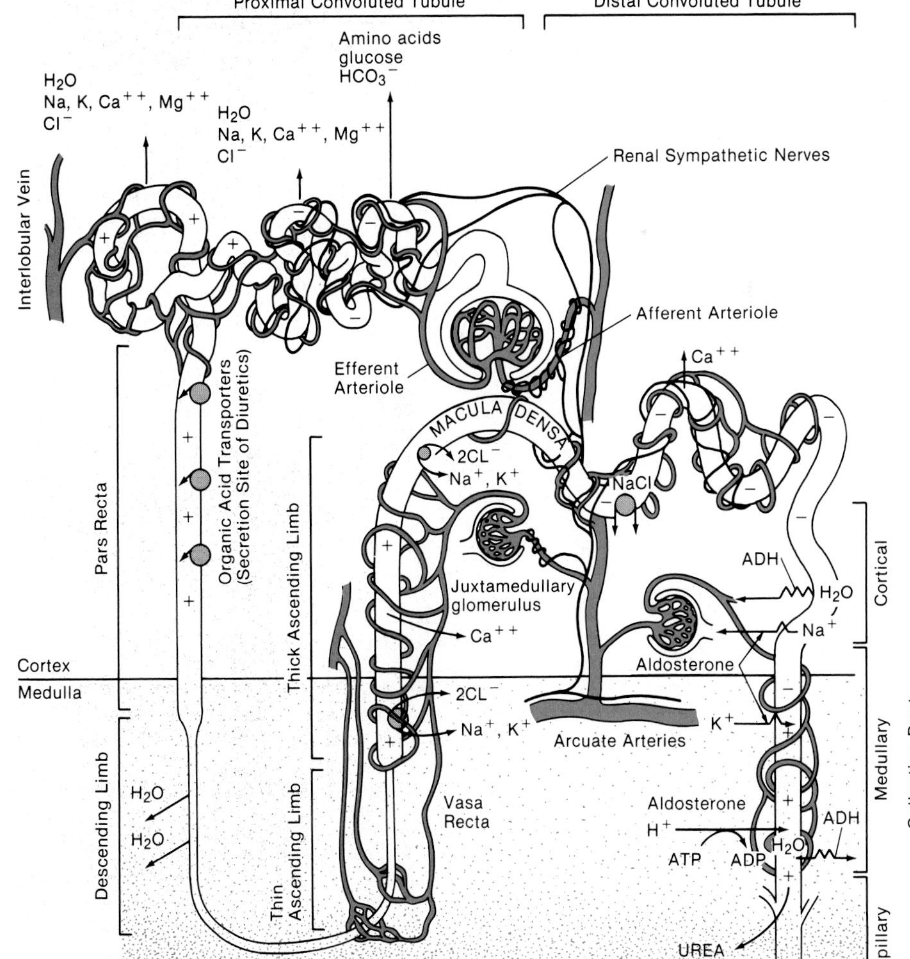

FIGURE 17–4. Transport functions of the anatomical segments of the mammalian nephron. Renal circulation in red.

factors, including atrial natriuretic peptide (ANP; p. 412).

The net effect of all the hemodynamic, hormonal, and neuronal influences on the kidney induced by the failing myocardium is retention of solute and water and expansion of extracellular volume. This may serve in the short run to sustain cardiac output and, therefore, tissue perfusion by allowing the ventricle to operate higher on its function curve. However, increasing cardiac filling pressures may lead to progressive cardiac dilation and worsening congestive symptoms. Therefore, although diuretics may not influence the natural history of the primary disease process responsible for myocardial dysfunction, they can improve symptoms of congestive failure by acting directly on solute and water resorption by the nephron and may slow the progression of cardiac chamber dilation by reducing ventricular filling pressure (preload).

A diuretic is any drug that increases urine flow. However, the term "diuretic" commonly is used to refer to agents that enhance the delivery into the urine of sodium chloride and the other principal small ions that form the extracellular milieu, along with water. Certain agents indirectly increase urine production by enhancing renal blood flow and the rate of glomerular filtration, thereby promoting a fall in the filtration fraction and diminished water and solute resorption by the proximal tubule. In patients with decompensated congestive heart failure, digitalis, by improving cardiac output, may enhance renal blood flow. In addition, the improved cardiac output will lead to withdrawal of elevated renal sympathetic tone and reduced angiotensin II production by the kidney. Dopamine, in doses ranging from 1 to 3 μg/kg/min, induces renal vasodilatation by stimulation of renal vascular dopaminergic receptors.

Most diuretics, however, act directly on the kidney to inhibit solute and water reabsorption. There are a number of classification schemes for diuretics, based upon their mechanism of action, their anatomical locus of action in the nephron, and the form of diuresis they elicit. Most diuretics can be classified according to whether they induce a "solute" or "water" diuresis. Of the latter ("aquaretics"), only three agents are of clinical relevance: demeclocycline, lithium, and vasopressin antagonists, each of which, by differing mechanisms, inhibits the action of ADH on the collecting duct, thereby increasing free water clearance. Drugs that cause solute diuresis are subdivided into two types: those that inhibit active transport of ions across tubular epithelia (the majority of potent, clinically useful diuretics) and those that are nonresorbable solutes that osmotically retain water and other solutes within the tubular lumen.

SITES AND MECHANISMS OF ACTION

(Fig. 17–4 and Table 17–4)

THE PROXIMAL TUBULE

Fluid resorption across the proximal tubule is isosmotic and accounts for approximately two-thirds of the resorption of filtered Na^+ and H_2O. The active resorption of sodium bicarbonate by carbonic anhydrase activity raises the intraluminal chloride concentration, allowing further isosmotic resorption of NaCl along the proximal tubule. Although active transport processes are important in solute resorption by this segment of the nephron, the most significant influences on the absolute quantity of solute and water resorbed in the proximal tubule are the volume of glomerular filtrate (a function of glomerular capillary permeability and filtration pressure) and the net effect of the physical forces that govern solute and water movement across and between tubular epithelial cells into peritubular capillaries. A variety of neuronal, hormonal, and hemodynamic factors, both extrinsic and intrinsic to the kidney, affect the volume and content of urine by altering the rate of formation of glomerular filtrate for a given renal blood flow (filtration fraction), which in turn directly alter the balance of physical forces between the proximal tubule and postglomerular peritubular capillaries.

Agents that alter the intrarenal regulation of formation of glomerular filtrate, such as angiotensin-converting enzyme inhibitors, may enhance the delivery of solute and water to more distal segments of the nephron that are sensitive to diuretics that inhibit ion transport. Predictably, other drugs, such as nonsteroidal antiinflammatory drugs, may diminish glomerular filtrate formation, thus reducing the flow of urine to distal diuretic-sensitive portions of the nephron. Clearly, a reduction in systemic blood pressure (or in renal artery pressure distal to a stenotic lesion) below that necessary for formation of glomerular filtrate will render the kidney refractory to any diuretic.

The *pars recta* section of the proximal tubule does resorb some of the glomerular filtrate and is important to the understanding of diuretic pharmacology because the organic anion secretory transport system exists here. Many diuretics that are not freely filtered at the glomerulus are actively secreted by the tubular cells of the pars recta. In patients with chronic renal failure, in whom the absolute number of transporters is diminished because of nephron loss, high concentrations of endogenous organic acids may compete with diuretics for secretion into the tubular lumen of the pars recta of the remaining functioning nephrons. This is clearly one cause of "diuretic resistance" in these patients.

THE LOOP OF HENLE

About one-third of the glomerular filtrate arrives at the descending limb of Henle's loop; no active transport of solute occurs here, although the tubular epithelium is highly permeable to water, which leaves the nephron for the hyperosmotic medullary interstitium. The generation of a hyperosmolar milieu is accomplished as the glomerular filtrate rounds the bend into the thin ascending limb. Most of the solute transport responsible for maintaining the hypertonicity of the medullary interstitium occurs in the water-impermeable thick ascending limb of Henle's loop. Here, a sodium-potassium cotransport system in the luminal membrane is coupled to the uptake of two chloride ions, an electroneutral process.[15] This process is dependent upon the electrochemical gradient for Na^+, and the energy is derived from ATP by Na^+,K^+-ATPase on the basolateral cell membrane. This Na/K/2Cl cotransport system serves mainly to resorb NaCl from the tubular lumen, as most of the resorbed K^+ is recycled back to the lumen as a result of the high K^+ conductivity of the luminal membrane. This recycled K^+ is responsible for the lumen-positive potential in this nephron segment. Substantial amounts of Ca^{++} and Mg^{++} are also resorbed in this segment, largely due to passive transport along with Na^+ through the "leaky" epithelial tight junctions driven by the lumen-positive potential difference. This cation flux mechanism depends upon the negative transepithelial electrical potential. The Na/K/2Cl cotransport system is the receptor for the loop diuretics (furosemide, bumetanide, piretanide, ethacrynic acid, torasemide, muzolimine) and is illustrated in Figure 17–5.

ACTION OF LOOP DIURETICS. Inhibition of cation transport by loop diuretics has two effects. First, it prevents the normal generation of the hypertonic medullary interstitium, thus reducing the osmotic gradient for free water reabsorption by ADH-sensitive epithelium in the collecting duct. Second, it causes delivery of large amounts of solute and water to the distal nephron, thus overwhelming distal Na^+ and Cl^- resorption sites and dramatically affecting K^+ secretion and urinary acidification. However, the efficacy of loop diuretics depends upon the delivery of a threshold amount of NaCl, at an adequate flow rate, to this nephron segment. This precondition may not be present in severe prerenal azotemia because of factors

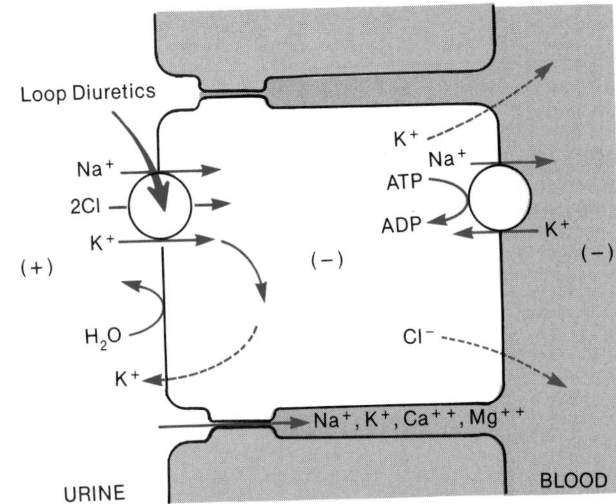

FIGURE 17–5. A medullary thick ascending limb (TAL) cell. The loop diuretics, furosemide, bumetanide, and piretanide, are all known to inhibit the Na/K/2Cl cotransporter in this epithelium. The loop diuretics also decrease the absorption of Ca^{++} and Mg^{++} by TAL cells, absorption that is indirectly linked to NaCl uptake. Inhibition of NaCl transport in this segment secondarily impairs urinary concentrating ability by preventing the formation of a hypertonic medullary interstitium.

TABLE 17–4 DIURETICS: ACTION, DOSAGE, AND DRUG INTERACTIONS

DIURETIC	BRAND NAME	PRINCIPAL SITE AND MECHANISM OF ACTION	EFFECTS ON URINARY ELECTROLYTES	EFFECTS ON BLOOD ELECTROLYTES AND ACID-BASE BALANCE	EXTRARENAL EFFECTS	USUAL DOSAGE*	DRUG INTERACTIONS
Thiazides and Related Compounds							
Chlorothiazide	Diuril	*Distal Tubule:* Inhibit NaCl reabsorption and Ca++ excretion	↑ Na+ ↑ Cl− ↑ K+ ↑ H+	↓ Na+, particularly in elderly patients	↑ Glucose ↑ LDL/triglycerides (may be dose related)	50–100 mg IV or p.o.	Efficacy reduced by prostaglandin inhibitors
Hydrochlorothiazide	Hydrodiuril					25–100 mg/d	Reduces renal clearance of lithium
Trichlormethiazide	Metahydrin					2–8 mg/d	
Chlorthalidone	Hygroton		↑ Mg^{++} ↓ Ca^{++}	↓ Cl, ↑ HCO_3^-, mild metabolic alkalosis ↑ Uric acid ↑ Ca^{++} ↓ K^+, ↓ Mg^{++}		25–100 mg/d	Additive effect on NaCl and K+ excretion with loop diuretics
Metolazone	Zaroxolyn					5–10 mg/d	
Cyclothiazide	Anhydron					2–6 mg/d	
Hydroflumethiazide	Diucardin					25–200 mg/d	
Polythiazide	Renese					1–4 mg/d	
Quinethazone	Hydromox					50–100 mg/d	
Methyclothiazide	Enduron					2.5–10 mg/d	
	Aquatensen						
Benzthiazide	Aquatag					50–200 mg/d	
	Exna				Extrarenal effects less marked with indapamide		
Bendroflumethiazide	Naturetin					2.5–30 mg/d	
Indapamide	Lozol	Vasodilator				2.5–5 mgd	
Carbonic Anhydrase Inhibitors							
Acetazolamide	Diamox	*Proximal Tubule:* Carbonic anhydrase inhibition	↑ NA+ ↑ K^+ ↑ HCO_3^-	Metabolic acidosis	↑ Ventilatory drive ↓ Intraocular pressure	250–500 mg/d	May be useful in alkalemia due to other diuretics
Osmotic Diuretics							
Mannitol	Osmitrol	*Proximal Tubule* (Primarily)	↑ Na+ ↑ Cl^- ↑ H_2O	↑ Extracellular volume transiently	↓ Intracranial pressure ↓ Intraocular pressure	50–200 gm/d IV	May enhance loop diuretic effectiveness by maintaining GFR
Glycerol	Glyrol					1–1.5 gm/kg	
Loop Diuretics							
Furosemide	Lasix	*Thick Ascending Limb of Loop of Henle:* Inhibition of Na/K/Cl cotransport	↑ Na^+ ↑ Cl^-	Hypochloremic alkalosis ↑ HCO3 ↓ K^+, ↓ Na^+ ↓ Cl^-, ↓ Mg^{++} ↑ Uric acid less than thiazides	*Acute:* ↑ Venous capacitance ↑ Systemic vascular resistance *Chronic:* ↓ Cardiac preload	20–1000 mg/d p.o./IV	Tubular secretion delayed by competing organic acids (renal failure) and some drugs
Bumetanide	Bumex					0.5–20.0 mg/d	
Piretanide†	Arelix					6–20 mg/d	Effectiveness reduced by prostaglandin inhibitors
	Diumax						
	Tauliz						
Ethacrynic Acid	Edecrin				Ototoxicity	50–200 mg/d IV	Additive ototoxicity with aminoglycosides
Mefruside†	Baycaron					25–50 mg/d	Longer duration of action than furosemide
Muzolimine†						2.5–5 mg/d	
Torasemide†							
Potassium-Sparing Diuretics							
Spironolactone	Aldactone	*Collecting Duct:* Aldosterone antagonists	↓ K+ ↑ Na+ ↑ Cl^- ↑ HCO_3^-	↑ K^+, particularly in patients with ↓ GFR; metabolic acidosis ↑ Mg^{++}	Gynecomastia	25–100 mg/d	Useful adjunct to therapy with K+ wasting diuretics; triamterene with indomethacin may cause abrupt ↓GFR
Canrenoate†							
Triamterene	Dyrenium	Inhibit apical membrane Na^+ conductance				100–300 mg/d	
Amiloride	Midamor					5–10 mg/d	

* Dosages are p.o. unless otherwise stated.
† Not yet licensed for use in the United States.

controlling the formation of glomerular filtrate and proximal tubular resorption, as already noted.

THE DISTAL TUBULE

The thick ascending limb approaches its own glomerulus as it reenters the cortex and passes between the afferent and efferent arterioles to form the juxtaglomerular apparatus (JGA), the tubular contribution to which is termed the macula densa. Loop diuretics may directly stimulate the release of renin by the JGA, an action that may contribute to the extrarenal vascular effects of these drugs.[16] The distal convoluted tubule begins beyond the macula densa. Na^+ and Cl^- as well as other ions (e.g., Ca^{++}) are resorbed in this segment, which is largely ADH insensitive and impermeable to water. The benzothiadiazides (i.e., commonly used thiazide diuretics) and related drugs inhibit NaCl uptake in this segment by blocking the coupled reabsorption of Na^+/Cl^-. They also enhance Ca^{++} resorption by epithelial cells in this segment. NaCl resorption by this distal water-impermeable portion of the nephron allows the formation of dilute urine, hence the term "cortical diluting segment." Thiazide-induced inhibition of resorption in this segment therefore may lead to hyponatremia, particularly when accompanied by elevated ADH levels and increased thirst.

THE COLLECTING DUCT

This structure is divided into three segments: the cortical, medullary, and papillary collecting ducts. The cortical collecting duct actively resorbs sodium via an aldosterone-sensitive mechanism. The primary effect is to increase the permeability of the apical membrane to sodium; the increased sodium entering into the cell is then pumped out by the Na^+,K^+-ATPase on the basolateral membrane. Aldosterone binds to a specific soluble cytoplasmic receptor protein leading to the sequence of events, including synthesis of specific proteins, that leads to the modulation of cation transport in the luminal membrane. The synthesis of new Na^+, K^+-ATPase units is probably secondary to the increase in intracellular Na^+ concentration, although aldosterone may also directly induce or facilitate expression of this gene in collecting duct epithelial cells. The increasing resorption of Na^+ from the tubule leads to a lumen-negative potential difference that favors the secretion of K^+ and H^+ ions. Thus, reduction of Na^+ delivery to the cortical collecting duct reduces the Na^+ linked secretion of K^+ down its electrochemical gradient into the tubular lumen. Conversely, increased Na^+ concentrations and high flow rates in the cortical collecting duct, as after loop or thiazide diuretic administration, leads to enhanced passive K^+ secretion, but only if Na^+ is being absorbed by epithelial cells in this segment. Blockade of apical membrane Na^+ conductance by amiloride reduces the lumen-negative potential to zero and greatly reduces the electrochemical driving force for K^+ (and H^+) secretion. Although amiloride also can block luminal Na^+/H^+ antiporters in the collecting duct and in proximal tubular epithelium, this occurs only at high, nonphysiological concentrations.

Antialdosterone drugs, such as spironolactone, competitively inhibit aldosterone's binding to its receptor and thereby limit Na^+ permeability by the apical membrane and reduce the negative lumen potential. It follows that reduced Na^+ entry into cortical collecting duct epithelial cells will reduce the active flux of Na^+ out of the cell into the blood via the Na^+, K^+-ATPase, which, in turn, will necessarily reduce the amount of K^+ available for secretion into the tubular lumen.

THE MEDULLARY COLLECTING DUCT

This portion of the duct is not a major site of action of any diuretic. It is important for the active secretion of H^+ via a H^+-ATPase, a Na^+-independent process. This proton pump is aldosterone sensitive and can be inhibited by aldosterone antagonists. The entire collecting duct is permeable to water in the presence of ADH; the final osmolality of the urine will depend upon the concentration of solute remaining in the collecting duct, the osmolality of the medullary interstitium, and the responsiveness of the tubular epithelium to ADH. Drugs such as demeclocycline and lithium may directly antagonize the effects of ADH, leading to diabetes insipidus. Atrial natriuretic peptide (ANP) may also act directly on inner medullary collecting duct cells to decrease solute and water formation in this portion of the nephron.

BLOOD SUPPLY TO THE NEPHRON

As illustrated in Figure 17–4, the blood supply to each nephron is derived from several sources. The *afferent arteriole* that enters the vascular pole of the glomerulus is a branch of an interlobular artery and is richly innervated with sympathetic nerve endings, particularly as it enters the glomerulus at its vascular pole within the juxtaglomerular apparatus. In the case of a superficial cortical nephron, as illustrated here, the efferent arteriole from the glomerulus perfuses segments of proximal and distal convoluted tubules. Tubular segments lying deeper in the cortex and medulla are perfused by efferent arterioles from juxtamedullary nephrons and include the long, unbranched peritubular vasa recta.

INNERVATION OF RENAL VESSELS. Postganglionic sympathetic nerves extend from the celiac and aortorenal ganglia along the renal nerves into the hilus of the kidney and then traverse, and innervate, successive branches of the renal arteries, with a concentration of sympathetic fibers surrounding the afferent arteriole and the juxtaglomerular apparatus. Direct sympathetic innervation of proximal and distal tubular epithelia has been described; increased sympathetic discharge to the kidney results in increased net NaCl resorption even in the absence of changes in glomerular hemodynamics. Increased efferent sympathetic activity, as in decompensated congestive heart failure, thus would be expected to result in avid retention of solute due to reduced renal perfusion, increased renin release, and enhanced tubular resorption of solute.

Dopamine is a potent renal vasodilator and may directly affect tubular epithelia to reduce NaCl resorption, thus acting as a natriuretic agent. Although dopaminergic innervation to the kidney has been described, most renal dopamine is produced locally by the action of dopa decarboxylase in tubular epithelial cells. Exogenously administered dopamine, particularly when infused at rates of 3 μg/kg/min (based on lean body mass) or less, may be a useful adjunct to diuretic therapy in selected patients with advanced congestive heart failure.

PHARMACOLOGY

The pharmacology of diuretic agents that is relevant to cardiovascular medicine is discussed below. For a more extensive review of the pharmacology of these drugs, several reviews are available.[17–22]

LOOP DIURETICS

The loop diuretics are among the most potent diuretic agents known, capable of inducing natriuresis of up to 20 per cent of the filtered load of sodium for a short period. Ethacrynic acid, a phenoxyacetic acid derivative, was the first loop diuretic to become available. Following shortly thereafter was the sulfonamide derivative of anthranilic acid, furosemide.[23] More potent congeners of furosemide include bumetanide and piretanide.[24] Piretanide, although not yet licensed in the United States, appears to have a similar pharmacokinetic and pharmacodynamic profile to furosemide aside from its greater potency and perhaps some potassium-sparing effects.[25–28a] Other loop diuretics that have reached the clinical testing stage and have not been licensed in the United States include the long-acting loop diuretic muzolimine, which has a terminal half-life of 10 to 20 hours in normal volunteers (compared with 1 to 2 hours for furosemide and bumetanide).[29] Torasemide is a loop diuretic that appears to have a sustained antihypertensive effect compared with the standard loop diuretics, despite a similar pharmacokinetic profile, and is effective in the treatment of edema due to congestive heart failure.[30–31a]

Although the precise site of action of ethacrynic acid in the ascending limb of Henle's loop is not yet known, it is presumed to be similar to that of furosemide and its congeners: the Na/K/2Cl transport system, an apical transmembrane protein responsible for the majority of solute resorption in the thick ascending limb (Fig. 17–5).[15,32–34b] In addition, torasemide is thought to inhibit Cl^- channels in the basolateral membranes of thick ascending limb epithelial cells, thus inhibiting salt reabsorption from both the luminal and peritubular surfaces. These drugs maintain solute loss even in the presence of a declining glomerular filtration rate (GFR) and reduced renal perfusion. Unlike thiazides and other diuretics, the loop-active agents do not induce a compensatory decline in GFR via tubuloglomerular feedback mechanisms, perhaps because the drugs themselves inhibit the flow of NaCl into macula densa cells. Loop diuretics do reduce medullary blood flow, however, an effect that is inhibited by angiotensin II antagonists.[35] Each of these drugs is secreted into the tubular lumen by the organic acid secretory pathway. Their pharmacological effect may therefore be delayed or diminished by exogenous (e.g., probenecid, indomethacin) or endogenous (e.g., metabolic byproducts in uremia) competitive inhibitors of the transporter.

ABSORPTION. The absorption of orally administered furosemide is highly variable even among normal subjects; the drug has an average bioavailability of 60 per cent that is markedly reduced when it is given with meals,[36] unlike bumetanide. Both bumetanide and furosemide, when administered orally, have reduced natriuretic effects in patients with congestive heart failure, in part because of delayed intestinal reabsorption and delivery of the drug to its tubular site of action, although absolute bioavailability (absorption) is little affected.[37–40] This lag time from administration of the drug to its natriuretic effect, which is exacerbated by decompensated congestive heart failure, not only delays the onset of the natriuresis but may prevent a sufficient amount of drug from arriving at its receptor in the loop of Henle to produce a clinically adequate natriuretic effect.

DOSE-RESPONSE RELATIONS. Even when furosemide is administered intravenously, the dose-response relationship between its urinary levels and sodium excretion rates is shifted to the right in patients undergoing long-term diuretic therapy or who have refractory edema formation, a reflection of enhanced proximal and distal solute resorption in the kidney.[37,39] To a certain extent, these problems can be overcome simply by giving more drug or by adding a diuretic active at another nephron site (see below). Extremely high dose furosemide regimens (0.25 to 4 gm/day) have also been advocated for patients with severe refractory cardiac failure but conserved renal function, to avoid some of the potential toxicity of a second drug.[41–42a] Ideally, however, optimal dosing of any loop diuretic would result in sustained tubular (urinary) levels of drug close to the drug concentration that is most effective in increasing urinary sodium excretion.[18,43] Typically, intravenous bolus doses of diuretic increase drug levels rapidly above the tubular drug concentration that results in maximal natriuresis, followed by a rapid decline. Only the relative absence of clinically significant toxicity allows this strategy to be employed, although toxicity has become an issue at intravenous doses above 0.5 gm. Slow-release formulations of furosemide have been shown to be efficacious in hypertension and may prove useful in the treatment of congestive heart failure.[44] Although loop diuretics given over a long time may induce hypochloremic metabolic alkalosis, resistance to these agents is not normally affected by arterial pH,[45] although advanced respiratory acidosis combined with hypoxemia may substantially reduce urinary clearance of these drugs,[46] thereby limiting their natriuretic effect.

INTERACTION WITH ANTIINFLAMMATORY DRUGS. The nonsteroidal antiinflammatory drugs (NSAIDs), including aspirin, blunt the natriuretic response to all the loop diuretics. Given alone, the NSAIDs may reduce glomerular filtration and cause sodium retention, particularly in patients with diminished renal perfusion (e.g., in congestive heart failure). The predominant effect of these agents in limiting the response to loop diuretics is to prevent the prostaglandin-induced rise in renal blood flow that accompanies and sustains the natriuretic response to loop diuretics.[47–49] Clinically, not all the NSAIDs are of equivalent potency in inducing this interaction; indomethacin competitively inhibits both furosemide and hydrochlorothiazide excretion into the proximal tubule in addition to inhibiting renal cyclooxygenase, but sulindac, a pro-drug that is not excreted into the renal tubule in its active form, has much less effect on acute diuretic-induced natriuresis or chronic diuretic antihypertensive effects.[50,51] Low-dose aspirin, in the dosage range that inhibits platelet production of thromboxane A_2 (<1.0 mg/kg/day), has no effect on enhanced urinary prostaglandin production or the natriuresis induced by furosemide.[52]

EFFECTS ON SYSTEMIC HEMODYNAMICS. All loop diuretics cause changes in systemic hemodynamics that are initially unrelated to the degree and extent of the natriuresis they induce. Short-term administration of furosemide, the best studied of these agents, results in a rapid increase in venous capacitance and a decline in cardiac filling pressures.[53] This effect is coincident with a rise in plasma renin activity, is blunted by prostaglandin synthesis inhibitors or a high dietary salt intake, and is abolished in anephric subjects.[54] Short-term furosemide administration also can result in a rise in systemic vascular resistance, both in normal volunteers and in patients with compensated congestive heart failure, an effect that is blocked by drugs that inhibit renin release (e.g., propranolol) or angiotensin II formation (e.g., captopril).[55] Indeed, this increase in left ventricular afterload can induce worsening congestive symptoms in patients with compensated but borderline systolic function and can also be detrimental to patients with acute myocardial ischemia but without signs or symptoms of congestive heart failure. In patients given 40 mg of intravenous furosemide prophylactically after acute myocardial infarction, both heart rate and systemic vascular resistance increased while stroke volume and pulmonary artery diastolic pressure fell.[56] All of these hemodynamic effects are presumed to be due to the rapid release of renin by the juxtaglomerular apparatus following an intravenous dose of furosemide. This results in arteriolar vasoconstriction due to increases in angiotensin II levels and an increase in venous capacitance due to angiotensin II-mediated vasodilatory prostaglandin release.[54] However, in patients with decompensated congestive heart failure or frank pulmonary edema, in whom systemic vascular resistance is already high, the venodilator effects of furosemide tend to predominate and may be prolonged (hours).[57] Unlike the natriuretic effect of furosemide, which increases almost linearly with dose above a threshold within the usual dose range given clinically, there is little further effect on systemic vascular resistance or venous capacitance above a 20-mg intravenous dose.[58] Nevertheless, diuretics may improve venous capacitance and systemic vascular resistance over days because of loss of salt and water and the induction of a negative sodium balance.[59] Dosages of bumetanide that result in a natriuretic effect equivalent to that of furosemide appear to have diminished vascular effects, both arteriolar and venous, at least in salt-depleted normal subjects.[60]

Furosemide may also have direct effects on arterial oxygen saturation in models of acute pulmonary edema characterized by increased capillary permeability. This effect is apparently due to a redistribution of pulmonary blood flow away from "flooded" alveoli and provides a rationale for use of furosemide in noncardiogenic pulmonary edema, although its clinical use remains controversial for this indication.[61,62] Interestingly, furosemide delivered by inhalation prevents exercise- and allergen-induced asthma, an effect that presumably is due to blockade of ion channels in bronchial epithelial or inflammatory cells.[63]

ADVERSE EFFECTS. Although the loop diuretics are potent inhibitors of Na/K/2Cl cotransport, inhibition of this transporter, which exists in most cells, is probably clinically unimportant in most nonrenal cells except in the inner ear. All the loop diuretics possess some toxicity for the eighth nerve, with ethacrynic acid being the most ototoxic.[64,65] Sensorineuronal hearing loss usually occurs at doses greater than 1 gm/day; transient hearing loss may occur in patients receiving bolus injections of furosemide because of a reversible decrease in endocochlear potential and the eighth nerve action potential.[66] Loop diuretic ototoxicity is synergistic with that of aminoglycoside antibiotics.[67] The mechanism of the rare syndrome of furosemide-induced exocrine pancreatitis is unknown but may have to do with increased pancreatic secretion due to amplified secretin release. Despite the structural similarity between furosemide and many thiazide diuretics, the etiology of thiazide-induced pancreatitis is presumed to be related to hypercalcemia.[68]

EFFICACY. All the loop diuretics are roughly equivalent in terms of their efficacy. There is little justification for the use of ethacrynic acid because of its increased ototoxicity, except in patients with a drug allergy or interstitial nephritis due to sulfonamides. Bumetanide and piretanide both have higher bioavailability and greater potency (40:1 and 6:1, respectively) than furosemide and may be slightly less ototoxic. Other differences among these drugs are small and probably clinically insignificant. Muzolimine and torasemide do offer significantly different pharmacokinetic or pharmacodynamic profiles, but it is unclear what if any advantages these drugs may have over the currently marketed loop diuretics, particularly in the treatment of congestive heart failure.

THIAZIDE DIURETICS

The thiazide diuretics include a number of agents that are chemically and pharmacologically similar, the prototype of which is chlorothiazide.[69] Chlorthalidone, indapamide, mefruside, quinethazone, and metolazone are heterocyclic variants of the basic benzothiadiazine nucleus. All of these drugs inhibit NaCl resorption in the distal tubule, an effect that is independent of the weak carbonic anhydrase inhibitory activity most of these drugs possess. Although these sulfonamide derivatives are the oldest orally effective diuretics in common use, their fundamental cellular mechanism of action remains unclear. By inhibiting NaCl transport in the distal tubule, they prevent dilution of the tubular fluid and augment the delivery of solute and water to the H^+- and K^+-secreting sites in the collecting duct. Recent evidence suggests that high-affinity metolazone-binding sites can be demonstrated in distal tubular epithelial cells in the rat, possibly a luminal Na^+/Cl^- cotransport channel.[70,71] The thiazides also promote Ca^{++} resorption, probably by directly enhancing Ca^{++} entry into distal tubular epithelial cells and by inducing mild volume depletion, thus increasing Ca^{++} resorption at several sites in the nephron. These effects appear to be largely independent of PTH or 1,25-dihydroxyvitamin D_3.[72] Although hypercalcemia complicating chronic thiazide administration is uncommon and should alert the clinician to other subclinical disorders of calcium homeostasis, long-term thiazide use has recently been implicated in reduced osteoporosis in the elderly by retrospective analyses.[73] Additional randomized prospective trials will be required to document the efficacy of thiazide diuretics and their safety for the prevention of osteoporosis and hip fracture in the elderly.

The thiazides are useful in the management of mild to moderate hypertension (p. 860) and as single agents in the initial management of mild congestive heart failure. However, their utility is limited by avidity of solute resorption by more proximal nephron segments. They are largely ineffective when the GFR is less than 30 ml/min. They may be useful for refractory edema in combination with loop diuretics, as discussed below. Metolazone may cause a smaller reduction in GFR than other drugs of this class, but it is unclear whether this is a clinically important distinction. Metolazone does inhibit proximal tubular sodium-dependent phosphate transport and perhaps other sodium-dependent transport pathways in this portion of the nephron, although, again, it is unclear whether the magnitude of these effects is sufficient to result in a more clinically effective natriuretic response.[70]

Indapamide is structurally related to the thiazides and has both a vasodilatory and diuretic effect, making it particularly useful in the treatment of hypertension.[74,74a] At doses of indapamide of less than 0.04 mg/kg, a long-term reduction in blood pressure that is equipotent with that of other thiazide diuretics can be documented with no natriuretic effect, implying that potassium and magnesium losses will also be minimized, as potentially may other metabolic side effects of chlorothiazide use.[75-77] Indeed, indapamide has been reported to cause little or no rise in total cholesterol or triglyceride levels.[76] Whether this would continue to be the case at the higher doses required in the long-term treatment of heart failure is unclear. Mefruside is a benzene sulfonamide heterocyclic thiazide derivative currently undergoing clinical testing. Structurally it is a cross between the thiazides and furosemide, but pharmacologically in humans it resembles a longer-acting thiazide. Whether it will offer any pharmacokinetic advantages or have a novel profile in terms of its metabolic side effects remains to be seen.

POTASSIUM-SPARING DIURETICS

Two classes of agents fall into this group of diuretic drugs: (1) the aldosterone antagonists and (2) the direct inhibitors of collecting duct sodium conductance, amiloride and triamterene (Fig. 17–6). The aldosterone antagonist in common use is spironolactone, although the spironolactone congener potassium canrenoate, which has been tested in clinical trials in the United States, and their common pharmacologically active metabolic byproduct, canrenone, are both available commercially in Europe. The aldosterone antagonists competitively bind to a cytoplasmic receptor protein in aldosterone-responsive cells, leading to enhanced transcription of mRNA and production of new cation-transporting proteins.[78,79] As single-diuretic therapy, their efficacy is enhanced in conditions characterized by high aldosterone levels, such as ascites due to cirrhosis. They are relatively ineffective in the therapy of heart failure unless combined with a second diuretic. Amiloride and triamterene are structurally related to one another; they inhibit Na^+ uptake into collecting duct epithelia by reducing Na^+ conductance of the apical membrane.[80-82] Amiloride has been the better studied of the two agents, although it is presumed that triamterene works via a similar mechanism.

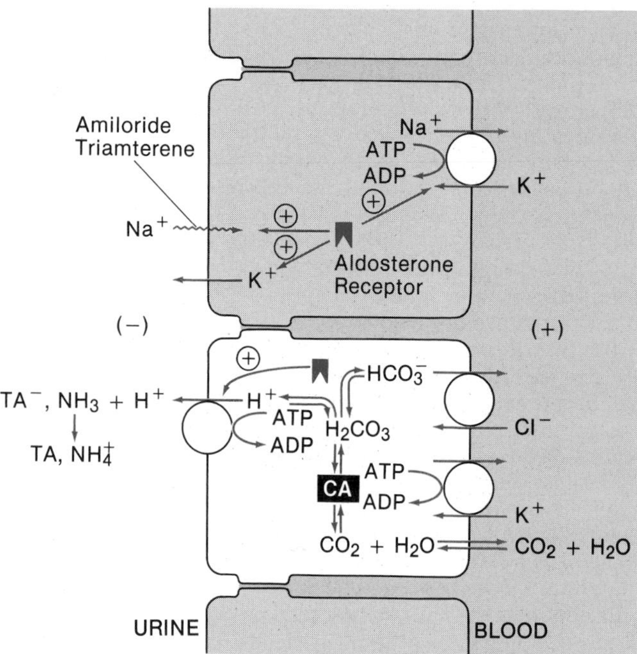

FIGURE 17–6. Diuretics acting in the cortical collecting duct. Aldosterone enhances apical membrane permeability by increasing conductance of sodium through the tubular membrane; aldosterone also increases H^+ secretion in intercalated cells by enhancing proton pump activity (TA = titratable acid; CA = carbonic anhydrase).

A major effect of these drugs is to diminish renal K^+ secretion, which may lead to clinically important hyperkalemia, particularly in patients with renal insufficiency.[83] These drugs also cause a mild metabolic acidosis due to reduced H^+ secretion into the urine by collecting duct epithelial cells. In patients with chronic obstructive pulmonary disease, potassium-sparing diuretics, alone or in combination with other diuretics, may be preferred to diuretics that enhance renal H^+ wasting and secondarily diminish ventilatory drive.

Despite the additional cost and modest risks of adding a second drug, the utility and relative safety of potassium-sparing diuretics in combination with loop diuretics, or in combination with a thiazide, have led to acceptance of their routine use in hypertension and congestive heart failure.[84] This is due in large part to the growing consensus that potassium and magnesium depletion should be avoided in patients with underlying coronary artery disease (discussed later) and, to a lesser degree, to new information about possible peripheral actions of spironolactone[84-86] and the potential contribution of additional potassium intake (or reduced excretion) on blood pressure control.

COMBINED DIURETIC REGIMENS

LOOP DIURETICS COMBINED WITH THIAZIDES. In patients with edema refractory to high doses of loop diuretics or with side effects from these agents, combinations of diuretics may result in clinically desirable diuresis at lower doses of both drugs. Indeed, the combination of a loop diuretic with a thiazide often results in a synergistic effect on solute and water excretion.[87,88] This may be due in part to an "unmasking" of the proximal tubular effects of thiazides due to inhibition of NaCl resorption in the loop of Henle, although additive effects in the distal tubule are also important.[89] Treatment of refractory edema due to cardiac failure is also enhanced in children with a combination of a thiazide and loop diuretic.[90] Severe hypoalbuminemia or chronic renal insufficiency (creatinine clearance <25 ml/min/1.73 m^2) will diminish the natriuretic response to this combination.

Although this combination of diuretics may be very efficacious in selected patients with refractory edema, profound intravascular volume depletion and electrolyte disturbances may complicate its use. K^+ wasting is severe and potentially life-threatening unless serum K^+ is carefully monitored. Advanced prerenal azotemia may occur, leading to irreversible renal insufficiency in some patients. A rapid reduction in GFR will directly affect the clearance of many drugs, and hypokalemia enhances the toxicity of cardiac glycosides. Consequently, this combination of diuretics should be initiated only with careful observation, preferably in a hospital setting. Subsequent outpatient therapy should be regulated carefully by monitoring of daily weights and appropriate checks of serum electrolytes and, when indicated, digoxin levels.

LOOP AND THIAZIDE DIURETICS IN COMBINATION WITH POTASSIUM-SPARING AGENTS. A potassium-sparing diuretic with a more proximally acting diuretic is the most commonly prescribed diuretic combination. The rationale for limiting potassium losses with routine diuretic administration is discussed subsequently. All the potassium-sparing diuretics limit K^+, Mg^{++}, and H^+ loss induced by diuretics acting more proximally. However, some combinations of these drugs may lead to a less than additive effect on NaCl excretion. Triamterene, but not amiloride or spironolactone, inhibits the tubular secretion of furosemide, thus delaying and possibly limiting its pharmacological effect. In addition, loop diuretics tend to attenuate the inhibitor effect of amiloride or triamterene on collecting duct Na^+ conductance because of the high luminal sodium concentration present in the collecting duct during furosemide natriuresis. Nevertheless, these combinations of agents are useful in selected patients with congestive heart failure,[91-91b] provided that a careful watch is kept for the development of hyperkalemia and metabolic acidosis, particularly in patients with renal insufficiency[91c] and those receiving other drugs (principally angiotensin-converting enzyme inhibitors) that might raise the serum potassium level.

CARBONIC ANHYDRASE INHIBITORS

Although all of the sulfonamide diuretics, including furosemide and the thiazides, are weak carbonic anhydrase inhibitors, only acetazolamide is used clinically for this purpose. Short-term administration of acetazolamide results in bicarbonaturia until the plasma bicarbonate falls to the point at which renal tubular bicarbonate resorption (both proximal and distal) exceeds the filtered lead of bicarbonate at the glomerulus (Fig. 17-7). This renal loss of bicarbonate can be used to alkalinize the urine transiently to enhance dissolution of uric acid crystals or the clearance of certain drugs. Maintenance of urinary alkalinization with these drugs requires long-term bicarbonate infusion; otherwise, a mild hyperchloremic (non-anion gap) metabolic acidosis develops, accompanied by a small contraction of extracellular volume and hypokalemia.[92,93]

Inducing metabolic acidosis with acetazolamide may be of use in edematous patients with hyperchloremic metabolic alkalosis due to long-term use of loop diuretics, particularly if the acid-base status of these patients is complicated by hypercarbia (either "primary" as in severe chronic obstructive pulmonary disease with cor pulmonale or "compensatory" respiratory acidosis due to the diuretic-induced alkalosis, or both).[94] In these patients, a fall in the renal threshold for bicarbonate resorption will often stimulate ventilatory drive. However, acetazolamide should be considered only if a patient is not intravascularly volume depleted and cannot tolerate infusions of NaCl or KCl. Careful monitoring of arterial pH and pCO_2 is necessary to insure that increased minute ventilation does occur; otherwise, metabolic acidosis will be added to an already complex acid-base disturbance. Renal potassium losses can be rapid and substantial and may be partially masked by intracellular to extracellular K^+ shifts induced by mild acidemia.

Another indication for use of acetazolamide is in the prevention of acute mountain sickness, including noncardiogenic pulmonary edema (p. 560) and cerebral edema.[95,96] The acute metabolic acidosis induced by the bicarbonaturia presumably stimulates the respiratory drive and prevents hypoxemia.

OSMOTIC DIURETICS

Any agent may act as an "osmotic diuretic" if it is freely filtered by the glomerulus, is neither resorbed nor metabolized in the renal tubule, and is relatively inactive pharmacologically to allow the intravenous administration of sufficiently large quantities of the drug to affect both plasma and urine osmolality. By these criteria, endogenous products of metabolism such as glucose and urea may act as osmotic diuretics, but only if the tubular capacity for resorption of these solutes is exceeded. Of the agents currently licensed for use as osmotic diuretics in the United States—mannitol, urea, glycerine, and isosorbide—only mannitol is likely to be used in the setting of cardiovascular therapeutics, while the others are reserved for the rapid reduction of intracranial or intraocular pressure.

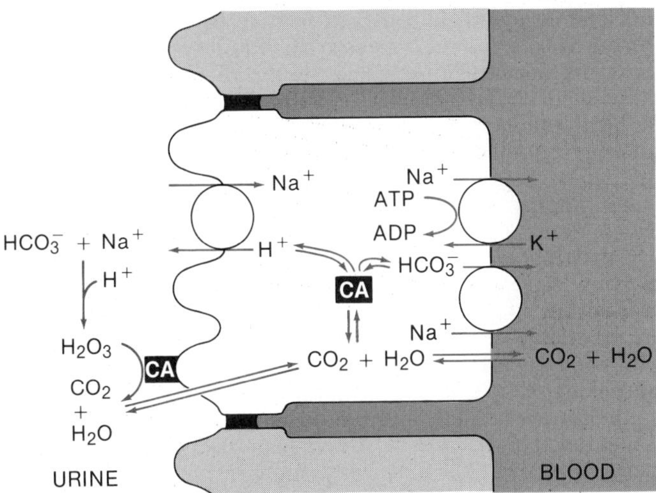

FIGURE 17-7. A proximal tubular cell, the primary site of action of carbonic anhydrase inhibitors. Inhibition of carbonic anhydrase (CA) will lead to a decrease in bicarbonate and Na^+ resorption, eventually producing hyperchloremic metabolic acidosis. Osmotic diuretics also reduce proximal tubular sodium resorption; the reduction in water flow through the epithelium dilutes luminal solute and favors back-leak of Na^+ into the tubular lumen.

Radiographic contrast dyes are also filtered by the glomerulus and are not resorbed by renal tubules; therefore, they act as osmotic diuretics, increasing urinary losses of salt and water. The diuresis induced by these agents is short-lived but may be intense, particularly in the setting of underlying renal disease, when the contrast agent must be cleared by a reduced number of functioning nephrons.

An important characteristic of osmotic diuretics is their ability to maintain urine flow even at very low glomerular filtration rates, as occurs in hypotension or dehydration. As long as perfusion pressure in the glomerular capillaries is sufficient to sustain filtration, and the tubular epithelium remains relatively impermeable, mannitol infusions will maintain a flow of salt and water to the distal nephron. This effect of mannitol, glycerol, and related agents is superior to that of resorbable solutes such as NaCl that are avidly absorbed by the proximal tubule in these clinical settings. Mannitol, as an inert extracellular osmotic agent, will increase the extracellular fluid volume; consequently, the drug is contraindicated in patients with decompensated congestive heart failure.

ATRIAL NATRIURETIC PEPTIDE (see also p. 412)

Considerable advances have been made in understanding the physiological actions of atrial natriuretic peptide (ANP) within the kidney, although pharmaceutical agents that act at ANP receptors to induce a natriuretic effect—aside from the synthetic hormone itself—remain in the developmental stages. ANP belongs to a family of related polypeptides, of which ANP, normally made in the adult atria, and brain natriuretic peptide (BNP) are the most abundant forms.[97] There is also evidence that BNP is produced within the heart, perhaps predominantly in the left ventricle, and plasma levels of BNPare increased in patients with heart failure.[97a] Two classes of receptors have been identified, a signal-transducing "B" receptor linked to the generation of cGMP, and a "C" receptor whose purpose appears to be to clear these peptides from the circulation.[98,98a] ANP acts on two distinct areas of the nephron: the glomerulus and tubular epithelial cells in the collecting duct. ANP also reduces renin and aldosterone secretion.[98] It augments glomerular filtration by increasing glomerular perfusion pressure and perhaps by reducing glomerular mesangial cell tone. This leads to an increase in filtration fraction with increased distal delivery of solute and water to the more distal nephron segments.

Although still somewhat controversial, ANP appears to have a direct effect on sodium resorption in epithelial cells in the inner medullary collecting duct and inhibits the rise in cAMP observed with vasopressin, thus increasing water, as well as solute, excretion. Although these actions of ANP clearly contribute to the balance of neurohormonal and physical forces that control salt and water homeostasis, the high ANP levels that are often observed in heart failure patients[99-101b] indicate that the kidney remains largely refractory to the action of this peptide in advanced congestive heart failure. The increased resistance to the action of ANP may be due to downregulation (homologous desensitization) of ANP receptors, as well as the enhanced countervailing activity of neurohumoral and glomerulotubular factors, particularly angiotensin II, that respond to the reduced cardiac output and decline in renal blood flow.[99,102] In addition to its direct renal actions, recent data suggest that the high systemic ANP levels may modulate baroreceptor function, principally by attenuating baroreflex-mediated cardioacceleration, while both the sustained natriuretic and vasodilatory actions of the peptide induce a moderate fall in blood pressure.[102a,102b] ANP may also directly reduce sympathetic nervous system activity centrally in humans.[102c] Although infusions of ANP to heart failure patients will reduce cardiac filling pressures and blood pressure, usually without an associated increase in sympathetic tone (or other endogenous vasoconstrictors), much of this hemodynamic effect may be due to a shift in plasma solutes and water into the extravascular space, thus limiting the peptide's effectiveness in the long term.[102d] Regardless, ANP, either as the synthetic peptide in a form suitable for intravenous administration or as a high-affinity analog that binds selectively to the "B" class of receptors, will likely find a role in the future as adjunctive pharmacotherapy in the treatment of selected patients with congestive heart failure.

ACID-BASE AND ELECTROLYTE DISORDERS IN HEART FAILURE: COMPLICATIONS OF DIURETIC THERAPY

POTASSIUM HOMEOSTASIS. All of the diuretics discussed in this chapter affect renal potassium handling.[103] In patients with congestive heart failure, both hypokalemia due to potassium-wasting diuretics and hyperkalemia due to potassium supplements, potassium-sparing diuretics, or angiotensin-converting enzyme inhibitors may contribute to morbidity and mortality. Renal potassium losses due to diuretic use can be exacerbated by hyperaldosteronism and persistent chloride depletion with the development of metabolic alkalosis. Dietary salt intake may also contribute to the extent of renal potassium wasting with diuretics. Very high salt diets increase delivery of NaCl to distal tubular K^+ secretory sites, while very low salt diets may stimulate aldosterone-induced K^+ secretion (Fig. 17–6). Extrarenal regulators of the serum potassium concentration may also produce effects additive with renal losses of K^+, such as the shift of K^+ into cells accompanying release of epinephrine in response to stress, myocardial ischemia, pulmonary edema, or the administration of insulin, whether or not glucose is given concurrently.[104]

Need for Treatment. The controversy whether diuretic-induced hypokalemia justifies therapy with oral potassium or potassium-sparing diuretics has been summarized.[105–107] Patients with congestive heart failure, a majority of whom have underlying ischemic heart disease, are a population at risk for malignant ventricular arrhythmias.[106,108,108a] Many of these patients are receiving maintenance cardiac glycosides.[109] The enhanced automaticity of cardiac tissue in response to toxic levels of digoxin is increased by hypokalemia. Caution should be exercised in giving additional potassium to any patient with digoxin-induced AV block, particularly if the serum potassium is in the normal range. However, KCl supplementation may aid in reversing digoxin-induced AV block at serum K^+ concentrations below 3.0 mmol/liter. Thus, there is a bimodal effect of potassium on A-V conduction; hypokalemia may exacerbate digitalis-induced AV block, whereas hyperkalemia may worsen A-V junctional conduction delays of any etiology. Potassium is often effective in treating digoxin-induced ventricular arrhythmias and may be effective even when the serum K^+ concentration is 4.0 mmol/liter or greater. Therefore, it is prudent to administer potassium supplements or a potassium-sparing diuretic to patients with hypokalemia with abnormal resting or exercise electrocardiograms or a history of ventricular arrhythmias or to any patient with hypokalemia receiving a cardiac glycoside. In patients with hepatic dysfunction due to advanced right heart failure or to other causes, K^+ supplements should be considered to reduce hepatic (and renal) ammonia production. Hypokalemia may also exacerbate glucose intolerance in certain patients.

There is less justification for treating other subsets of patients receiving diuretic therapy, including those with mild congestive heart failure and hypertension treated with a diuretic alone, with costly potassium supplements. Furthermore, there is a small but definite risk of inducing hyperkalemia with its attendant cardiovascular morbidity, particularly in patients with reduced renal function (which includes a majority of geriatric patients).[110] One should remember that concomitant administration with diuretics of prostaglandin synthetase inhibitors, beta blockers, and angiotensin-converting enzyme inhibitors may result in a rise in serum potassium levels. Oral potassium supplements in the form of potassium chloride extended-release tablets (10 mEq three times daily) or liquid concentrate should be used whenever possible. Intravenous potassium is potentially hazardous and should be avoided except in emergencies.

In summary, recent evidence supports the use of KCl supplements or potassium-sparing diuretics in most patients with congestive heart failure or ischemic heart disease receiving long-term diuretic therapy, although the link between drug-induced hypokalemia and cardiovascular mortality has yet to be definitively proven. There is also clinical and experimental evidence to support the use of KCl supplements in selected patients with essential hypertension (e.g., in blacks or elderly patients with a poor dietary potassium intake) with or without concomitant diuretic therapy. Nevertheless, these associations remain to be established with certainty, and the risk of hyperkalemia, with its attendant cardiovascular morbidity, is real.

HYPOMAGNESEMIA. The problem of magnesium depletion has received growing attention as a potential major contributor to cardiovascular morbidity (Table 17–5) in patients

TABLE 17–5 HYPOMAGNESEMIA-INDUCED CARDIAC EFFECTS

Ventricular premature contractions and ventricular tachyarrhythmia
Prolonged P-R and Q-T intervals
T-wave flattening
Atrial fibrillation and supraventricular tachycardia
Torsades de pointes
Coronary artery spasm
Increased sensitivity to digitalis
More extensive myocardial infarction
Possibly increased sensitivity to ventricular fibrillation and sudden death in ischemic heart disease

From Iseri, L. T.: Role of magnesium in cardiac tachyarrhythmias. Am. J. Cardiol. *65*:47K, 1990.

with congestive heart failure,[111,111a] both as a result of numerous clinical studies documenting the efficacy of magnesium replacement in selected patients with cardiac arrhythmias and as a result of much-improved understanding of the molecular and cellular actions of Mg^{++} in normal and abnormal physiology. Unlike urinary excretion of calcium, which is enhanced only by loop diuretics in volume-replete subjects, urinary magnesium wasting occurs with both thiazide and loop diuretics (although predominantly the latter), although not with potassium-sparing diuretics.[111b,112] Magnesium deficiency is more commonly detected in patients with poor dietary magnesium intake (e.g., the elderly) or increased renal magnesium wasting due to diuretic use as well as to lengthy exposure to other drugs that exacerbate renal Mg^{++} loss, including most commonly ethyl alcohol, but also *cis*-platinum, amphotericin B, and certain aminoglycoside antibiotics, including gentamicin and tobramycin.[113,114] Ironically, digitalis preparations, the toxicity of which can be exacerbated by hypomagnesemia,[109] also potentiate renal magnesium wasting.[115]

The Serum Magnesium Level. Unfortunately, the serum magnesium often does not correlate well with other measures for determining magnesium homeostasis, as would be expected for this divalent cation that is largely bound to intracellular buffers or to bone (31 per cent and 67 per cent, respectively, of total body magnesium) with only approximately 1 per cent in the extracellular space.[116,117] Although skeletal and cardiac muscle biopsies and/or measurements of free or total magnesium in circulating mononuclear cells are more reliable than serum magnesium levels,[117–119a] these measures are not readily available. Nevertheless, serial measurements of serum magnesium in a given patient reflect changes in total body magnesium homeostasis. For the clinician, a high index of suspicion (for example, a cachetic, elderly congestive heart failure patient receiving digoxin and chronic loop diuretic therapy) coupled with a low normal serum magnesium level may be sufficient to warrant beginning magnesium replacement therapy. If the total daily urinary magnesium excretion is less than 1 mEq/day (in the absence of diuretics), this also strongly increases the likelihood of clinically important magnesium depletion. Interestingly, hypermagnesemia (defined as a serum magnesium level greater than 2.1 mEq/liter) was as predictive of a poor prognosis in a prospective study of congestive heart failure patients as hypomagnesemia (i.e., a serum magnesium level less than 1.6 mEq/liter).[111a] While the latter correlated best with the presence of documented ventricular ectopic activity and dysrhythmias, hypermagnesemic patients tended to be older, have more severe symptoms, and demonstrated greater "neurohormonal" activation based on measurement of plasma renin, vasopressin, and catecholamine levels. Although serum creatinine levels were not higher than in hypomagnesemic patients, hypermagnesemic patients had higher BUN levels, suggestive of reduced renal perfusion due to declining cardiac output, relative intravascular volume depletion, or both.[111a] Tissue magnesium levels and urinary magnesium excretion were not measured, and therefore it is not known whether the hypermagnesemic patients had depleted or normal total body magnesium stores.

Magnesium Replacement. Awareness of the importance of magnesium supplementation or rapid replacement therapy in patients with chronic congestive heart failure and/or ongoing myocardial ischemia has come from a number of recent prospective studies in patients as well as animal experiments that have documented the efficacy of magnesium in the suppression of ventricular and atrial arrhythmias.[120–123] In the clinical trials that examined the effect of magnesium on acute myocardial infarction, no attempt was made to define the presence of hypomagnesia or total body magnesium deficiency before treating with magnesium or placebo, and yet arrhythmias and, most important, cardiovascular mortality at 1 year were lower in the magnesium-treated group. Regardless of a given patient's magnesium status, intravenous magnesium may also be of value in the treatment of selected arrhythmias, including long Q-T–related arrhythmias and nonhypomagnesemic torsades de pointes, multifocal atrial tachycardia,[123–126a] and digoxin-related ventricular arrhythmias.[109]

Although patients who have clinically important hypomagnesemia also often have abnormalities of potassium and calcium homeostasis, experimental hypomagnesemia is characterized by an increased sinus nodal discharge rate and abnormal atrial and ventricular impulse generation with prolongation of the P-R and Q-T intervals.[126] Conversely, intravenous magnesium administration has electrophysiological and hemodynamic effects that resemble those of several classes of commonly available calcium antagonists (e.g., verapamil, diltiazem): a slowed sinus node rate, prolonged atrioventricular conduction time, and increased AV node refractoriness, without important effects on normal ventricular electrophysiology and with a reduction in coronary and peripheral vascular resistance.[117,127–129]

Isolated magnesium deficiency is rare, particularly in congestive heart failure patients receiving diuretics. Hypokalemia and often hypochloremic metabolic alkalosis are common additional metabolic abnormalities.[113,117] It is now recognized that magnesium replacement must precede or accompany potassium repletion to normalize serum potassium levels, as magnesium facilitates potassium entry into cells. The concomitant hypochloremic metabolic alkalosis due to chronic diuretic-induced chloride and potassium loss, as well as the effect of secondary hyperaldosteronism due to congestive heart failure, also must be treated to allow restoration of magnesium and potassium levels.[113,117,130] Therefore, the chloride (or hydrochloride) salts of magnesium and potassium are preferred for long-term oral replacement of hypomagnesemia and hypokalemia, since this will also treat the metabolic alkalosis.[113] For short-term treatment of atrial or ventricular arrhythmias that may be magnesium responsive, 1 gm of magnesium can be given intravenously over 20 minutes in the treatment of torsades de pointes, while up to 12 gm of magnesium can be given safely over 5 to 6 hours (assuming adequate blood pressure monitoring) for treatment of multifocal atrial tachycardia.[120,125] For the treatment of documented magnesium deficiency, which usually will be found with concomitant potassium deficiency, enteric-coated tablets, up to 0.5 gm $MgCl_2$ six times a day for several months, in addition to KCl supplementation, may be necessary and safely given.

Hypermagnesemia is less common than hyperkalemia but can occur in the setting of renal insufficiency following vigorous magnesium replacement and/or magnesium-containing antacid therapy. If a patient has symptoms suggestive of hypermagnesia—sedation, nausea, muscle weakness, hypotension, and serum levels greater than 5 mEq/liter—intravenous calcium will temporarily reduce serum magnesium levels and often dramatically improve symptoms until definitive therapy with either peritoneal dialysis or hemodialysis can be initiated.[116]

HYPONATREMIA. This is a common complication of diuretic therapy in patients with congestive heart failure. The origin of hyponatremia in these patients is multifactorial and includes diuretic-induced defects in renal diluting ability, inappropriately high vasopressin levels due to reduced cardiac output and high angiotensin II levels, and excessive thirst.[131] Hyponatremic patients tend to have high plasma renin activity, elevated norepinephrine and epinephrine levels, and reduced renal plasma flows when compared with nonhyponatremic (≥135 mEq/liter) patients.[132–135] Indeed, hyponatremia per se is a powerful predictor of cardiovascular mortality, as one would expect if it were the result of increasing and relatively ineffective diuretic therapy along with heightened stimulation of neurohumoral compensatory systems due to worsening myocardial failure.[136] Mild hyponatremia (between 120 and 135 mEq/liter) generally responds to fluid restriction below urinary and insensible losses, usually less than 1000 ml/day, coupled with moderate (not severe) salt restriction.[137] More severe hyponatremia (<120 mEq/liter) should be treated more rapidly but cautiously, with a combination of loop diuretics and administration of 0.9 per cent NaCl (or, rarely, 3 per cent NaCl) administered intravenously. This may require concomitant monitoring of cardiac filling pressures. Combined therapy with angiotensin-converting enzyme inhibitors (but not other vasodilators) and a loop diuretic often results in improved control of hyponatremia in these patients.[136] This subset of patients with more advanced congestive heart failure may be the group that is at greatest risk for developing "functional" renal insufficiency with an angiotensin-converting enzyme inhibitor, presumably due to the loss of efferent arteriolar tone in the glomerulus and/or a concomitant fall in renal blood flow that prevents normal autoregulation of the glomerular filtration rate.[136–138]

ACID-BASE DISTURBANCES. These may be seen with any diuretic[139,140] and have been discussed previously, with the description of individual diuretics. Metabolic acidosis is an unusual complication of therapy with potassium-sparing diuretics but is a consistent outcome of acetazolamide administration. Thiazide diuretics may cause mild "contraction" alkalosis, while loop diuretics typically induce more severe hypochloremic alkalosis, particularly in salt-restricted, potassium-depleted patients. Loop diuretics also increase ammonium secretion, probably by stimulating ammonium production from glutamine in proximal tubular cells owing to chronic diuretic-induced hypokalemia, by reducing the urinary pH and by increasing the luminal flow rate in the distal tubule and collecting duct, both of which would favor NH_3 diffusion from the interstitium into the urine.[141,142] Because diuretics are commonly utilized in patients with multiple metabolic and respiratory acid-base problems, a mixed acid-base disorder tends to be the rule, and the contribution of diuretics to the clinical problem requires careful analysis. Of importance is the assessment of volume status, which may require invasive hemodynamic monitoring, particularly in the edematous heart failure patient continuously treated with diuretics who nevertheless displays several signs of intravascular volume depletion, including hypochloremic metabolic alkalosis and mild orthostatic hypotension. Severe volume depletion with marked hypochloremic alkalosis may require the administration of intravenous saline, with potassium chloride and magnesium chloride supplements as needed. Acetazolamide in relatively small doses (e.g., 250 mg twice daily) may gradually reverse the metabolic alkalosis if saline infusion is contraindicated, although potassium and magnesium repletion will still be required.

ADVERSE EFFECTS OF DIURETIC THERAPY (OTHER THAN ELECTROLYTE ABNORMALITIES)

CARBOHYDRATE INTOLERANCE

For many years thiazide diuretics have been known to induce a mild form of carbohydrate intolerance, with the development of the typical clinical pattern of adult-onset diabetes in those individuals genetically predisposed to this disease. Ketoacidosis is rare in these patients, although nonketotic hyperosmolar coma may develop in volume-depleted type II diabetics receiving thiazide diuretics. Although the development of clinically important diabetes may be unusual, it is now clear that some degree of insulin resistance can be documented in many patients receiving thiazide diuretics.[143]

In a comparison of hydrochlorothiazide and captopril in middle-aged Caucasian patients with essential hypertension tested in a double-blind, prospective crossover trial, Pollare and colleagues documented that hydrochlorothiazide (25 mg daily) increased basal insulin levels and the late insulin response to glucose, but decreased the glucose disposal rate, indicating some degree of peripheral insulin resistance.[143a,143b] In contrast, captopril improved peripheral glucose utilization with only minimal effects on insulin secretion. Although impaired insulin release from the pancreas, possibly as a result of hypokalemia, has been identified as one cause of carbohydrate intolerance in patients taking thiazides, none of the patients in this study was severely hypokalemic ($K^+ < 3.2$ mmol/liter).[143b] Nevertheless, repletion of potassium losses has been shown to improve carbohydrate tolerance in more severely potassium-depleted patients. The peripheral resistance to insulin in diuretic-treated patients may be limited to those receiving thiazides,[144] since hemoglobin A_{1C} levels were reported to be normal in patients receiving furosemide as opposed to those treated with hydrochlorothiazide.[144a]

HYPERLIPIDEMIA WITH DIURETICS

Since the early 1980's, studies on the drug therapy of hypertension have documented an unfavorable effect of thiazide diuretics on plasma lipid levels.[145,145a] Nevertheless, the early studies remained inconclusive, in part because of the small numbers of patients in some trials and the relatively small increases in plasma lipids (e.g., 5 to 7 per cent increase in total cholesterol), and in part because the doses of diuretics used (up to 100 mg of hydrochlorothiazide per day) were higher than are typically recommended today.[144a,145b,146] A subgroup of patients randomized to receive special intervention (SI), including thiazide diuretics, for aggressive management of hypertension in the Multiple Risk Factor Intervention Trial (MRFIT) had higher cardiovascular mortality than the usual care (UC) group. This experience focused intense scrutiny on the possible detrimental effects of long-term thiazide use on cardiac arrhythmias (see above) and abnormal lipid metabolism.[147,148] While the data from the MRFIT study that implicate thiazide diuretics in increased cardiovascular morbidity are inconclusive,[149] data from other studies supporting an effect of thiazide diuretics on increased plasma triglycerides, total cholesterol, and (when measured) LDL cholesterol are stronger. In the Veterans Administration–NHLBI Cooperative Trial, mean increases in triglyceride levels of 8 per cent and total cholesterol of 5 per cent were seen in 302 men treated with chlorthalidone for 1 year.[150]

It has been argued that the moderate elevations in serum cholesterol and triglyceride levels that are apparent at 6 months disappear during longer therapy.[147,151] At a 6-year follow-up of the MRFIT patients receiving a diet low in saturated fat and cholesterol, although all patients had a fall in total cholesterol and LDL cholesterol levels regardless whether or not they were receiving diuretics, the decrease in total cholesterol was significantly less in the diuretic-treated group, and triglyceride levels (VLDL-C) actually increased.[152] Finally, advocates for the thiazide diuretics, noting their proven efficacy, relative safety, and low cost, question whether the modest changes in total cholesterol, triglyceride levels, and/or LDL-cholesterol of, at most, 5 to 6 per cent are of clinical importance.[149] Here the evidence is less controversial: From the Lipid Research Clinics Primary Prevention Trial[153] and the Helsinki Heart Study,[154] lowering the total cholesterol by each 1 per cent increment reduced cardiovascular events by 2 to 4 per cent.

The mechanism of the increase in total cholesterol and triglycerides with thiazide diuretics is unknown. The thiazide-related vasodilator diuretic indapamide causes less perturbation of the serum lipid profile. A diet low in cholesterol and saturated fat will minimize or prevent the hyperlipidemia associated with thiazide diuretics.[155–156] Also, $alpha_1$-antagonists such as prazosin[157] or terazosin[158] (which have additive antihypertensive effects when given with a thiazide diuretic) appear to block or reverse the hyperlipidemic effects of the thiazides. Conversely, propranolol, in combination with a thiazide, does not reverse the hyperlipidemic effects of thiazides[157] and has also been shown to exacerbate the change in glucose tolerance with diuretic treatment.

Although most of the data reported above on the effects of diuretic agents on serum lipid levels have come from trials explicitly studying hypertension, the implications of these data are of immediate relevance to congestive heart failure patients, many of whom have known coronary artery disease. As these patients live longer, the cumulative additional risk of adding a potentially atherogenic drug becomes greater. Therefore, if issues of efficacy or cost mandate the use of a thiazide diuretic in the hypertensive patient with mild congestive heart failure, available data indicate that attention to a low cholesterol and low saturated fat diet and/or the addition of other cardiovascular drugs that block the hyperlipidemic effects of the thiazides (such as alpha 1-antagonists[157,158] or angiotensin-converting enzyme inhibitors[143]) or specific lipid-lowering agents should be considered.

HYPERURICEMIA WITH DIURETICS

This is a common complication of long-term diuretic therapy with all loop, potassium-sparing, and thiazide diuretics, except the ethacrynic acid derivative *indacrinone,* which has uricosuric properties but has not been licensed for clinical use. Competition by diuretics for the proximal tubular organic acid secretory pathway and diuretic-enhanced proximal and distal tubular resorption of uric acid causes the hyperuricemia.[159] Although sustained plasma urate levels of up to 13 mg/dl may sometimes occur, attacks of gout or uric acid nephropathy are rarely a problem clinically. However, if higher levels of hyperuricemia occur, or if moderate hyperuricemia occurs in a patient with a history of gouty arthritis, allopurinol should be prescribed.[159a]

SPECIAL USES OF DIURETICS

DIURETIC USE IN INFANTS AND CHILDREN (see also Table 33-3, p. 1002)

The treatment of pulmonary and peripheral edema due to heart failure as a consequence of pressure or volume loads or cardiomyopathy has traditionally been administration of digoxin and diuretics, with the more recent addition of angiotensin-converting enzyme inhibitors.[160] The loop diuretics are the most common class of diuretic agents used in the treatment of congestive heart failure in infants and children, and furosemide and bumetanide are the best studied of these. The oral bioavailability of furosemide and bumetanide is not importantly different from that in the adult. However, in premature infants and neonates, the normalized volume of distribution is larger, and both renal and hepatic drug elimination pathways are immature, leading to markedly prolonged elimination half-lives (often exceeding 24 hours in premature infants, compared with less than 1 hour in the older child or adult).[161] The administration of large doses of furosemide in premature infants with hyperbilirubinemia may displace bilirubin from albumin-binding sites and worsen kernicterus.[161,161a] Furosemide or bumetanide is not contraindicated at the usual doses in hyperbilirubinemic neonates, however, but should be used with caution at bilirubin levels above 10 mg/dl.

Most of the other metabolic consequences of loop diuretic administration are similar to those seen in adults, with the caveat that renal concentrating and diluting functions are impaired in the neonate and infant compared with the older child or adult.[161,162] This, combined with a longer elimination half-life, can lead to substantial losses of Na^+, K^+, Cl^-, Mg^{++}, and free water, resulting in significant volume contraction and hypochloremic and hypokalemic alkalosis. Furosemide is also more likely to induce significant calciuria in infants, contributing to nephrocalcinosis and calcium nephrolithiasis. This may lead to secondary hyperparathyroidism and pathological fractures.[161a,163]

The thiazide diuretics and potassium-sparing diuretics are also widely used in pediatric cardiology. As with furosemide, their elimination half-lives are significantly increased in premature and neonatal infants. Metolazone is the thiazide that has been most often used in this age group, usually in combination with a loop diuretic to enhance urine output in refractory congestive heart failure or the nephrotic syndrome.[161a] The thiazides reduce renal calcium excretion and can prevent or reverse furosemide-induced hypercalciuria and secondary hyperparathyroidism. Spironolactone is relatively well tolerated with a loop diuretic in the treatment of congestive heart failure in children. Hyperkalemia, especially in the setting of mild renal insufficiency, remains the most important adverse effect of spironolactone, triamterene, and amiloride in either young children or adults.

DIURETIC USE IN GERIATRIC PATIENTS

In general, absorption of oral agents is delayed and renal clearance rates are lower in the elderly, thus slowing delivery of active drug to its renal tubular site of action.[164] The decline in renal function that naturally occurs with aging diminishes the effectiveness of the thiazide diuretics earlier than the loop diuretics, since the thiazides are virtually ineffective at creatinine clearance rates below 30 to 40 ml/min.[165] Amiloride also loses effectiveness as a natriuretic agent in this range of creatinine clearance, although its potassium-sparing effects may be maintained.[165] The elderly also have decreased baroreceptor responsiveness, reduced cerebral, renal, coronary, and splanchnic blood flow, and a tendency to electrolyte depletion.[164,166,167]

Elderly patients with congestive heart failure, with or without concomitant hypertension, require long-acting thiazides or multiple daily doses of loop diuretics, thus necessitating potassium and magnesium replacement.[168,169] Another important problem, for which the elderly are probably at greater risk, is hyponatremia. Although hyponatremia can occur with any diuretic, whether or not congestive heart failure is present, the longer-acting thiazide diuretics or a thiazide in combination with a potassium-sparing diuretic appears to pose an unusually high risk. The decline in serum sodium is often exacerbated by poor dietary sodium and excessive free water intake and an inability to increase free water clearance (i.e., to dilute the urine appropriately), in part because of diuretic-induced hypovolemia. Hyponatremia may occur insidiously over weeks, unassociated with any change in serum potassium levels and, if accompanied by diuretic-induced volume contraction, results in improvement in congestive heart failure symptoms. Mild confusion may go unnoticed in the elderly, but can rapidly degenerate into dementia, convulsions, and coma, even at serum sodium values near 130 mEq/liter, particularly if the fall in serum sodium has been rapid. Long-term administration of loop diuretics also leads to significant degrees of calcium depletion. Consequently, calcium supplements are recommended in elderly patients receiving these drugs. Magnesium losses, which occur with both thiazide and loop diuretics, may need to be replaced to increase serum ionized calcium levels.

DIURETICS AND RENAL INSUFFICIENCY (see also Chap. 62)

Many patients with congestive heart failure manifest some degree of renal insufficiency as a consequence of hypertensive glomerulosclerosis and/or atherosclerotic disease. Renal dysfunction will necessarily result in a decline in efficacy and often an increase in toxicity of diuretics. Nevertheless, they remain valuable agents in the management of heart failure in patients with all but end-stage renal insufficiency.[21,170,171]

As already pointed out, the thiazide diuretics are of little use below a GFR of 30 to 40 ml/min and may actually reduce the GFR further. The loop diuretics remain the most effective class of diuretics in chronic renal failure, although their effectiveness is diminished by both pharmacokinetic and pharmacodynamic mechanisms. One potential exception is the new loop diuretic, muzolimine, now in clinical trials in the United States, which may not depend entirely upon secretion into the tubular lumen to reach its site of action. One useful approach to establishing an effective dose of a loop diuretic in congestive heart failure patients with chronic renal failure is to double the intravenous dose successively (i.e., from 40 mg furosemide or 1 mg bumetanide intravenously) until a plateau or "ceiling" is reached in NaCl excretion and urine volume.[171] Further increases in dose will not yield any greater immediate diuresis, although the duration of the natriuretic effect may be extended, albeit at increased risk of neurotoxicity. If one assumes a bioavailability of about 50 per cent for furosemide and 80 per cent for bumetanide, the oral dose can readily be calculated from the maximally effective intravenous dose.[171] The frequency of oral dosing can usually be diminished because of the prolonged elimination half-life of these drugs in chronic renal failure. As ethacrynic acid is more ototoxic than other loop diuretics, there is little justification for its use in the treatment of congestive failure in chronic renal failure patients. Bumetanide and piretanide may be less ototoxic than furosemide. Potassium-sparing diuretics should not be used in these patients. Although the combination of a loop diuretic and a thiazide diuretic may be efficacious in selected patients with refractory edema and chronic renal failure, it must be used cautiously since potassium wasting can be severe even in advanced renal insufficiency, and excessive intravascular volume depletion can contribute to irreversible loss of remaining functioning nephrons.

EXTRACORPOREAL ULTRAFILTRATION

In refractory heart failure, extracorporeal ultrafiltration has a place as a useful and relatively safe mechanism for removing fluid and electrolytes in a controlled fashion,[172-174] whether or not there is underlying renal insufficiency. Ultrafiltration also usually avoids the adverse hemodynamic effects of hemodialysis that can be difficult to manage in patients with heart failure and underlying ischemic heart disease. Ultrafiltration is far less effective in relieving symptoms attributable to uremia per se than is hemodialysis but is very effective in removing solutes and water. Concurrent invasive hemodynamic monitoring is desirable, especially in unstable patients. The maximal rate of loss of fluid should be around 500 ml/hr, with careful monitoring of plasma electrolytes and the hematocrit (which should not exceed 50 per cent). Replacement electrolyte solutions are usually not necessary unless removal of intravascular volume has been excessive, or a specific electrolyte defect is being corrected (e.g., hyponatremia or hypokalemia). An improved response to diuretics has been reported following ultrafiltration, an effect that might be due to improved cardiac output with a subsequent decline in the neurohumoral sodium-retaining signals to the kidney. Continuous hemofiltration has also been used successfully in pediatric patients with postoperative congestive heart failure.[175,176]

Digitalis Glycosides

For more than 200 years, digitalis glycosides have occupied a prominent place in the management of congestive heart failure and certain arrhythmias. Withering recognized in 1785 that optimal use of digitalis requires considerable knowledge and skill on the part of the physician because of the unusually narrow therapeutic/toxic dose ratio of this group of drugs.[177] A sound understanding of the actions and pharmacokinetics of these drugs is essential to provide maximum benefit to the patient and minimize the ever present risk of toxicity.

In the discussion that follows, the term digitalis is used to refer to any of the steroid or steroid glycoside compounds that exert typical positive inotropic and electrophysiological effects on the heart. Although there are important differences in pharmacokinetics among the more than 300 known compounds with these properties, their pharmacological actions are fundamentally similar, and detailed consideration will therefore be limited to those agents that are in current clinical use.

SOURCES. The majority of digitalis drugs that have been used clinically are steroid glycosides derived from the leaves of the common flowering plant known as foxglove, or *Digitalis purpurea* (digitoxin, gitalin, digitalis leaf), or from the leaves of *D. lanata* (digoxin, lanatoside C, deslanoside). Ouabain, an exception, is obtained from seeds of *Strophanthus gratus.*

STRUCTURE. The steroid nucleus common to all cardiac glycosides contains an α, β-unsaturated lactone ring attached at the C-17 position. Without attached sugars, the steroid and unsaturated lactone part of the molecule is called *genin* or *aglycone.* Genins are usually less potent and have more transient actions than do the parent glycosides. Figure 17-8 shows the structure of digoxin; digitoxin differs from digoxin only in the absence of the hydroxyl group at C-12. Research continues in the quest for improved cardiac glycoside molecules with reduced adverse side effects and enhanced selectivity of action.[178]

MECHANISMS OF ACTION

INOTROPY. The entire spectrum of myocardial cellular activity has been studied in search of the cellular or molecular mechanism underlying the positive inotropic action of digitalis.[179,180] Any comprehensive model of cardiac glycoside-induced inotropy must take into account several fundamental observations, including the following[180,181]: (1) glycosides increase the force and velocity of contraction of the normal as well as the failing heart; (2) digitalis glycosides exert a positive inotropic effect on cardiac muscle but not on skeletal muscle; (3) the extent of the positive inotropic response is dependent on contraction frequency, declining on either side of an optimum value; and (4) the magnitude and rate of onset of positive inotropy are dependent on the concentration of a number of ions, including potassium, sodium, calcium, and magnesium.

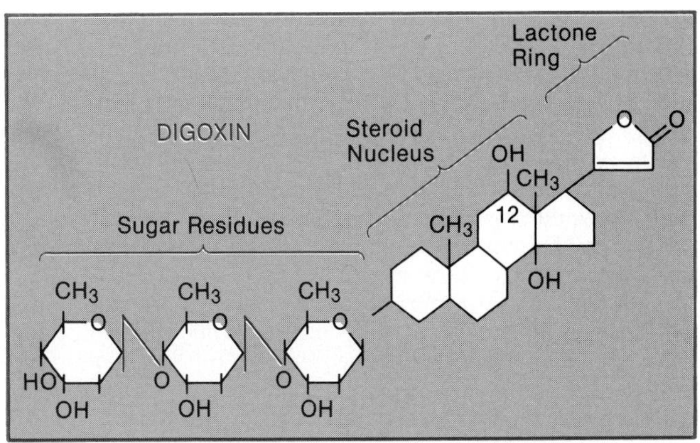

FIGURE 17-8. Chemical structure of digoxin.

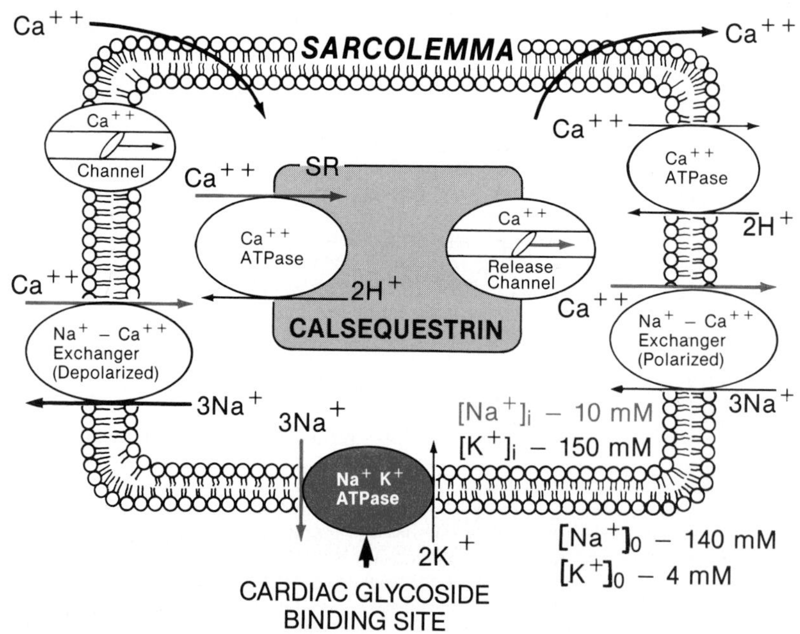

FIGURE 17–9. **Selected components regulating cellular calcium homeostasis in cardiac myocytes. Structures on the left side of the diagram depict pathways of transmembrane calcium entry. From the upper left, the slow calcium channel, a voltage-sensitive protein complex, carries the slow inward calcium current during phase 2 of the cardiac action potential and provides the pulse of intracellular calcium that triggers calcium-induced release of a larger amount of activator calcium from stores in the sarcoplasmic reticulum (SR). The arrow indicates the principal direction of ion movement when the channel is activated. Depolarization of the cell, activating the slow calcium channel, occurs by opening of the fast sodium channel (not shown).**

The Na^+-Ca^{++} exchanger is a membrane component that mediates the facilitated bidirectional exchange of Na^+ for Ca^{++} across the sarcolemmal membrane. This process is sensitive to membrane potential because of the asymmetry of charge movement inherent in the stoichiometry of the process (3 Na^+ ions for every Ca^{++} ion). Depolarization of the membrane favors the inward movement of Ca^{++} in exchange for outward movement of Na^+. At the bottom of the diagram is shown the Na^+,K^+-ATPase, or sodium pump, that maintains the normal distribution of Na^+ and K^+ across the sarcolemmal membrane as shown at the lower right. The cardiac glycoside-binding site is located on the outward-facing aspect of the alpha subunit of this enzyme complex.

In the center of the diagram is shown the SR with its ATP-driven Ca^{++} pump on the left and the ryanodine-sensitive calcium release channel on the right. On the right side of the diagram are shown the pathways for calcium extrusion across the sarcolemmal membrane, including the low-capacity, high-affinity, ATP-dependent ion-transport Ca^{++} ATPase that extrudes Ca^{++} from cardiac cells against a large electrochemical gradient and helps to maintain the low levels of free intracellular Ca^{++} that prevail during diastole. The Na^+-Ca^{++} exchanger extrudes Ca^{++} from the cell in exchange for Na^+ entry under conditions of normal diastolic polarization of the cell. Arrows or concentrations shown in red denote pathways that increase or decrease in magnitude in the presence of cardiac glycosides. When a cardiac glycoside binds to the Na^+,K^+-ATPase, that pump site is inactivated, and intracellular free Na^+ ($[Na^+]_i$) tends to increase. This results in an increase in intracellular Ca^{++}, mediated by reduced Ca^{++} extrusion via the Na^+-Ca^{++} exchanger and probably by an increase in Ca^{++} entry via this exchanger as well. The increased intracellular Ca^{++} content is largely stored in the SR via the SR Ca^{++} ATPase, and is thus available to be released through the Ca^{++} release channel at the time of excitation-contraction coupling.

Positive inotropic effects persist in the presence of full beta-adrenoceptor blockade. Therefore, the major inotropic effects of cardiac glycosides are not mediated by catecholamine release or increased sensitivity to catecholamines. Adenylyl cyclase activity, known to participate in the mediation of positive inotropic effects of beta-adrenoceptor agonists and glucagon, is not influenced by digitalis glycosides.

There is no evidence that digitalis has a direct effect on the contractile proteins, intermediary metabolism, or myocardial energetics, although cardiac glycosides share with other positive inotropic agents the tendency to increase myocardial oxygen consumption in isolated muscle. In the failing heart, digitalis may actually reduce myocardial oxygen consumption by decreasing heart size and hence wall tension through the Laplace relation.[182]

CARDIAC GLYCOSIDES, CALCIUM, AND EXCITATION-CONTRACTION COUPLING. Central to understanding the mechanism by which digitalis exerts its positive inotropic effect is the process of myocardial excitation-contraction coupling. As discussed on page 357, the slow inward current that occurs during the plateau phase of the myocardial action potential has been well documented to be carried, in large part, by Ca^{++}; this influx of Ca^{++} is ultimately related to excitation-contraction coupling. An increase in the magnitude of slow inward current in cardiac Purkinje and myocardial fibers exposed to cardiotonic steroids has been reported and may be related, at least in part, to inhibition of the Na pump, as discussed below.[183] Most investigators agree that cardiac glycosides, by some mechanism, increase the availability of Ca^{++} to the contractile element at the time of excitation-contraction coupling. As shown in Figure 17–9, this could be brought about by an increase in the steady-state contractile Ca^{++} pool as a result of increased influx or decreased efflux of Ca^{++}. The inotropic response requires an intact sarcolemma, and cardiac glycoside–induced increases in a rapidly exchangeable Ca^{++} pool linked to the contractile state of the cell have been reported.[184] Direct evidence for an increase in the intracellular Ca^{++} transient following exposure to digitalis is now available from studies using the photoactive calcium-sensitive protein aequorin (Fig. 13–8, p. 357).[185] Figure 17–10 shows aequorin signals together with action potential and tension recordings illustrating control and therapeutic responses.[186] In these studies using a canine Purkinje fiber, a 26-minute exposure to 10^{-7} M ouabain (*B*) results in little if any change in the action potential, but systolic aequorin luminescence (reflecting the Ca^{++} transient) and tension are markedly increased.

INHIBITION OF Na^+,K^+-ATPase BY CARDIAC GLYCOSIDES. All cardioactive steroids share the property of being potent and highly specific inhibitors of the intrinsic membrane monovalent cation active transport protein Na^+,K^+-ATPase, the enzymatic equivalent of the sodium pump. This Mg^{++} and ATP-dependent, Na^+- and K^+-activated transport enzyme complex consists of two polypeptide subunits, termed α (about 100 kd) and β (a sialoglycoprotein with a mass of approximately 50 kd), that occur in a 1:1 stoichiometry. The complete primary structure of both α and β subunits has now been deduced from the base sequence of cDNA clones, and chemical modification[188] and site-directed mutagenesis studies[189] are elucidating details of the monovalent cation transport process and its inhibition by cardiac glycosides. At least four genes coding for the α subunit have been identified, with distinct differences in their cardiac glycoside–binding properties.[190] One cardiac glycoside–binding site facing the extracellular surface is present per α chain. Optimal binding requires Na^+, Mg^{++}, and ATP and is inhibited by extracellular K^+. Cardiac glycoside binding results in complete inhibition of enzymatic and transport functions of each Na^+,K^+-ATPase site occupied. Na^+,K^+-ATPase is now generally agreed to be the receptor for the biological actions of digitalis glycosides. A wealth of circumstantial evidence supporting this conclusion has been reviewed,[178,180,191] and inhibition of the Na pump in atrial tissue of patients treated with conventional doses of digoxin has been demonstrated by Rasmussen et al.[192]

The normal biological role of the cardiac glycoside inhibitory site on the α subunit of Na^+,K^+-ATPase, implied by its

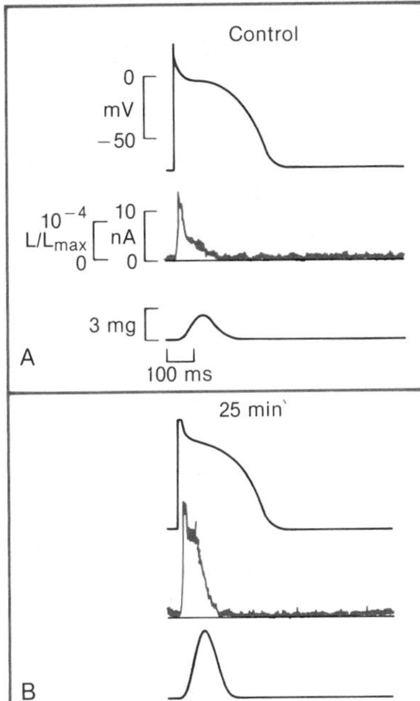

FIGURE 17–10. Calcium transients measured with aequorin during exposure to digitalis. Simultaneous signal-averaged recordings of membrane potential, aequorin luminescence (in red), and tension in a canine cardiac Purkinje fiber before (*A*) and during (*B*, 25 min); cardiac glycoside exposure. (From Wier, W. G., and Hess, P.: Excitation-contraction coupling in cardiac Purkinje fibers. Effects of cardiotonic steroids on the intracellular [Ca^{++}] transient, membrane potential, and contraction. J. Gen. Physiol. *83*:395, 1984.)

conservation over many phyla and millenia, remains speculative (and thus far inconclusive) despite extensive searches for an endogenous ligand[193,194] in mammalian species.

MONOVALENT CATION TRANSPORT INHIBITION AND INOTROPY

Studies with isotopic uptake and washout techniques have documented that positive inotropic responses are accompanied by a net loss of K^+ and a net uptake of Na^+, accompanied by a net uptake of cellular Ca^{++}.[184] The appearance of toxic manifestations, such as ectopic beats and contracture, is accompanied by further changes of still greater magnitude. Compelling direct evidence supporting cardiac glycoside–induced increases in intracellular [Na^+] is now available from impalement of cardiac cells with Na^+-sensitive microelectrodes.[195] The relation of $[Na]_i$ to tension development is direct and remarkably steep.

Data from these and other experiments support the view that inhibition of active cellular Na^+ transport results in augmentation of myocyte Ca^{++} content, which in turn produces a positive inotropic response analogous to that which follows an increase in contraction frequency in the *treppe* or *Bowditch staircase phenomenon.*[196] The mechanism of this effect appears to involve enhanced exchange of intracellular Na^+ for extracellular Ca^{++} (Fig. 17–9). This sequence is shown in schematic form in Figure 17–11. The transmembrane Na^+ influx occurring with each action potential, in the presence of diminished outward Na^+ pumping, would lead to the increased intracellular Na^+ concentration proposed to promote transmembrane exchange of Na^+ and Ca^{++}.[196a–196c] Another way in which digitalis could produce an increase in intracellular [Ca^{++}] is by increasing Ca influx through sarcolemmal Ca channels (Fig. 17–9). Marban and Tsien have proposed a mechanism for the increase in I_{Ca}: a small increase in intracellular free [Ca^{++}] (by sodium pump inhibition or any other mechanism) acts as a positive feedback signal to increase I_{Ca}.[183]

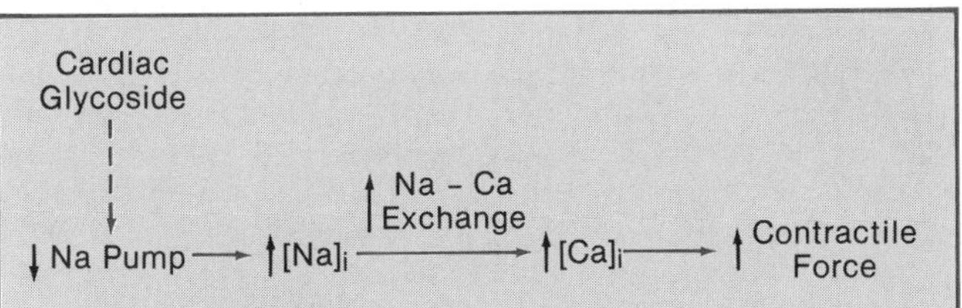

FIGURE 17–11. Schematic representation of the mechanism of inotropic action of cardiac glycosides. Binding of digitalis to the sodium pump, i.e., Na^+,K^+-ATPase, inhibits this enzyme and hence the active outward transport of Na^+ across the myocardial cell membrane. Na^+ pump inhibition thus leads to increased intracellular Na^+ $[Na^+]_i$ content and activity, which in turn enhances Na-Ca exchange with consequent increase in Ca influx, decrease of Ca efflux, or both. The resulting increase in intracellular $[Ca]_i$ is presumed to mediate the observed increase in myocardial contractile force.

ELECTROPHYSIOLOGICAL EFFECTS

(See also p. 606)

Major electrophysiological effects of digitalis on the heart are summarized in Table 17–6. The 80- to 90-mV transmembrane resting potential of cardiac cells (Fig. 22–10, p. 594) is maintained by Na^+ and K^+ gradients (particularly the latter), which in turn are dependent upon the integrity of the active Na^+-K^+ pump mechanism. It is therefore not surprising that agents such as cardiac glycosides that inhibit the pump mechanism have profound effects on the electrophysiology of the intact heart as well as on isolated muscle preparations. There is general agreement that inhibition of Na^+,K^+-ATPase underlies direct toxic effects on cardiac rhythm and thus represents an extension of the therapeutic (inotropic) effect. Cells in various parts of the heart show differing sensitivities to digitalis (Table 17–6), and both direct and neurally mediated effects must be dissected before conclusions can be drawn about the mechanisms involved.[197,198] Although usually absent or clinically inapparent at conventional doses, glycoside-induced depression of intraatrial conduction, manifested by increases in P-A interval and atrial effective and functional refractory periods, has been documented.[199]

ANTIARRHYTHMIC ACTIONS. Most of the antiarrhythmic effects of digitalis are the result of its action on the atria and atrioventricular junction. Within specialized conduction tissues of the heart, the refractory period is increased by digitalis, and conduction velocity is diminished, tending to slow the ventricular response to atrial fibrillation and atrial flutter or to prolong the P-R interval in the presence of normal sinus rhythm. In atrial and ventricular myocardium, the refractory period tends to be shortened, and the more rapid recovery time is reflected in a shortening of the Q-T

TABLE 17–6 SOME MAJOR EFFECTS OF DIGITALIS ON THE ELECTROPHYSIOLOGICAL PROPERTIES OF THE HEART

PROPERTY	EFFECT
Pacemaker Automaticity	
SA node	→ ↓ (↑ after atropine or toxic doses)
Purkinje fibers	↑
Excitability	
Atrium	→ *
Ventricle	Variable*
Purkinje fibers	↑ *
Membrane Responsiveness	
Atrium	Variable* (↓ after atropine)
Ventricle	↓ (toxic doses)
Purkinje fibers	↓ (toxic doses)
Conduction Velocity	
Atrium, ventricle	↑ (slight)*
AV node	↓
Purkinje fibers	↓
Effective Refractory Period	
Atrium	↓ (↑ after atropine)
Ventricle	↓
AV node	↑
Purkinje fibers	↑ *

From Moe, G. K., and Farah, A. E.: Digitalis and allied cardiac glycosides. In Goodman, L. S., and Gilman, A. (eds.): The Pharmacological Basis of Therapeutics, 5th ed. New York, Macmillan, 1975, p. 661.

↑ = increased; ↓ = decreased; → = no significant change.

* Decreased with high toxic doses of digitalis.

interval. Effects of digitalis on A-V conduction occur predominantly at the level of the AV node rather than more distally in the His-Purkinje system.[200]

At low concentrations, the resting potential, action potential amplitude, and time course of depolarization and repolarization of the mammalian ventricular Purkinje fiber remain unchanged at a time when inotropic effects are first apparent. At higher concentrations of cardiac glycosides and particularly at more rapid rates of stimulation, there is progressive loss of resting potential. Changes occur in the time course of depolarization and repolarization, including decreased slope of the upstroke of the action potential, shortening of the plateau phase, and increased rate of spontaneous diastolic depolarization.

Further details concerning the electrophysiological effects of cardiac glycosides may be found elsewhere.[198-201]

NEURALLY MEDIATED EFFECTS

Substantial progress has been made in recent years in the delineation of neurally mediated effects of cardiac glycosides.[197,202] Direct nerve recordings have shown that cardiac glycosides can influence preganglionic cardiac sympathetic nerve activity in anesthetized cats.[202] In the cat an important locus of neural augmentation of digitalis-induced arrhythmias lies within an area of the medulla 2 mm above to 2 mm below the obex,[203] a finding that implicates the area postrema as a likely site of digitalis-induced neural activation. Neurally mediated effects of cardiac glycosides are discussed in greater detail elsewhere,[197] and interactions with the autonomic nervous system are usefully reviewed by Rosen[204] and Watanabe.[205]

EFFECTS ON AUTONOMIC BALANCE. Substantial interest has been focused recently on the role of abnormal autonomic balance in general and abnormal baroreflex activity in particular in the clinical syndrome of congestive heart failure. Baroreceptors in the heart, lungs, and great vessels normally modulate neurohormonal activation to maintain blood pressure and volume status in response to physiological stimuli such as postural changes. An important end result of the disturbances evident in patients with heart failure is an increase in sympathetic outflow.

Stimulation of the baroreceptors normally inhibits sympathetic outflow as well as renin and vasopressin release while increasing parasympathetic activity. Marked desensitization of normal baroreflex activity occurs in heart failure[206,207] and contributes to augmented sympathetic outflow, vasopressin release, and renin secretion. The short-term effect leads to enhanced stroke volume and cardiac output by the failing heart,[208] but the longer-term consequences of these compensatory mechanisms are believed to be deleterious.[209] These changes are reversible, as shown dramatically following successful cardiac transplantation.[210,210a]

Ferguson et al. have obtained direct evidence from sympathetic neural recordings that digitalis in clinically relevant doses produces marked sympathoinhibitory action in patients with heart failure. They suggest that this effect probably cannot be ascribed solely to an inotropic action of the drug but rather results from afferent activation of low- or high-pressure baroreceptor mechanisms by digitalis.[211] Wang et al. have obtained experimental evidence that attenuation of baroreceptor discharge sensitivity from the carotid sinus is related to augmented Na^+,K^+-ATPase activity in these baroreceptor cells in a canine heart failure model, thus providing a plausible mechanism by which cardiac glycosides could resensitize this mechanism, restoring more normal autonomic tone.[212]

The entire field of sympathetic autonomic nervous system and adrenergic receptor function in heart failure is reviewed extensively in a recent series of monographs.[213]

HEMODYNAMIC EFFECTS

MYOCARDIAL CONTRACTILITY. The experiments of Cattell and Gold in 1938 showed directly that ouabain increased the force of contraction in isolated, electrically driven cat papillary muscles.[214] The inotropic action of digitalis is manifest in normal as well as in failing heart muscle.[215]

The effect of digitalis on the intact heart is reflected in the ventricular function curve (Fig. 17–3), in which glycoside administration causes the curve to shift upward and to the left, so that at any given ventricular filling pressure more stroke work is generated in the presence of digitalis than in control circumstances. Experimental studies of the velocity of contraction at varying loads demonstrate a shift in the force-velocity relation (p. 433) such that the velocity of muscle shortening is greater at any given load imposed.

Administration of cardiac glycosides results in no change or a slight decline in cardiac output in normal subjects. This is not surprising, since cardiac output is determined not only by contractile state but also by preload, afterload, and heart rate. Although digitalis augments the contractile state of the nonfailing myocardium in the intact human heart, adjustments in other determinants of cardiac output prevent any appreciable increase.[182]

DIGITALIS IN HEART FAILURE. The foregoing observations provide a basis for understanding the mechanisms whereby digitalis ameliorates the signs and symptoms of congestive heart failure. As various pathological processes (such as ischemia, volume or pressure loading, or intrinsic cardiac muscle defects) decrease contractility, compensatory mechanisms are brought into play. Elevations in end-diastolic pressure and volume result in increased contractile force through the Frank-Starling mechanism; increased sympathetic tone tends to increase the contractile state; and ventricular hypertrophy may provide more contractile elements. The renin-angiotensin system increases in activity in response to reduced cardiac output. However, each of these compensatory mechanisms has a price: Pulmonary or peripheral edema occurs when ventricular end-diastolic pressures rise excessively; tachycardia may be an undesirable effect of excessive sympathetic tone; increased activity of both sympathetic and renin-angiotensin systems increases peripheral vascular resistance; and increased myocardial oxygen consumption tends to occur with all of these compensatory mechanisms. If cardiac disease progresses and contractility continues to diminish, the consequences of one of these compensatory mechanisms will become dominant (e.g., pulmonary edema) or the compensatory mechanisms will become insufficient to maintain cardiac output.

Under these circumstances, administration of cardiac glycosides will improve the depressed contractile state, decreasing encroachment on compensatory mechanisms and improving cardiac reserve. The ventricular function curve is shifted upward (Fig. 17–3), so that for any given ventricular end-diastolic pressure, cardiac output is greater. The clinical consequence is a reduction in end-diastolic volume and pressure (and hence diminished pulmonary and systemic venous pressure) and increased cardiac output.[216] As would be expected, the favorable hemodynamic effects of digoxin are additive to those of the vasodilator captopril[228] (Fig. 17–20, p. 500) and also to those of the beta-adrenoceptor agonist prenalterol.[218]

Therapeutic Goals. The selection of appropriate endpoints or therapeutic goals is important in the clinical use of digitalis. Although experimental studies have indicated that the positive inotropic action of cardiac glycosides increases progressively until toxic arrhythmias appear, the limited clinical evidence available suggests that little if any further benefit is to

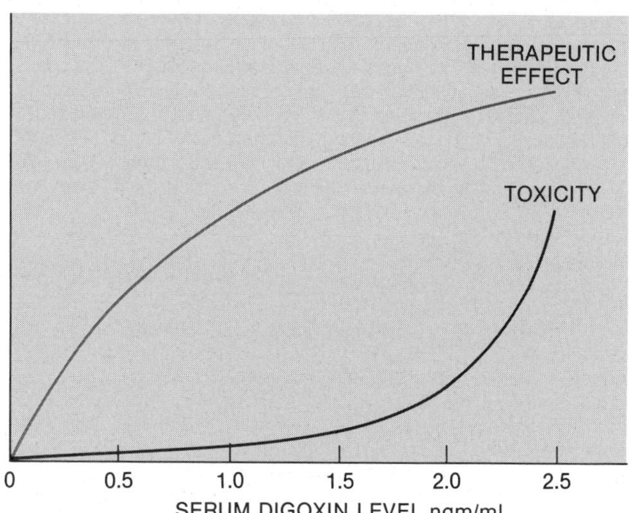

FIGURE 17–12. Schematic illustration of relationship between the therapeutic and toxic effects of digoxin and the serum digoxin level. Above a level of 2.0 ng/ml, there are minimal additional therapeutic effects and a dramatic increase in the toxic effect. (From Lewis, R. P.: Digitalis. *In* Leier, C. V. [ed.]: Cardiotonic Drugs: A Clinical Survey. New York, Marcel Dekker, 1987, pp. 85–150.)

be expected by increasing digoxin doses to levels resulting in serum concentrations in excess of about 1.5 to 2.0 ng/ml in patients with congestive heart failure and normal sinus rhythm[212,219] (Fig. 17–12). Nevertheless, digitalization is not an all-or-none state, and the degree of positive inotropic action of the drug increases in a graded manner with increasing dose, at least to the point where steady-state serum digoxin levels are in the range usually considered to be therapeutic. The clinician's task is to determine the appropriate dose consistent with an adequate margin of safety.

In mitral stenosis, cardiac glycosides are clearly beneficial in slowing the ventricular response to atrial fibrillation, thereby allowing more complete diastolic filling of the left ventricle. In the presence of right ventricular failure, benefit results from increased contractility and reduced end-diastolic pressure. However, in patients with mitral stenosis and normal sinus rhythm who were studied during maximal exercise, ouabain produced no significant change in heart rate and had no beneficial effect on cardiac output, oxygen consumption, or severity of pulmonary hypertension.[220]

THE NONFAILING HEART. The therapeutic value of digitalis in the hypertrophied or dilated nonfailing heart remains unclear. With the development of hypertrophy, and before the onset of overt failure, the work capacity of the myocardium at any given left ventricular end-diastolic pressure tends to be decreased, and digitalis exerts a positive inotropic action, augments the capacity for performance or cardiac work, and reduces end-diastolic volume and end-diastolic pressure.[182] If cardiac output has not been reduced, it does not increase as a result of digitalis administration, but the same stroke work and cardiac output can be delivered from a lower ventricular filling pressure. Thus, digitalis should provide a greater inotropic reserve.

EXTRACARDIAC HEMODYNAMIC EFFECTS

Although the direct cardiac effects of digitalis are of primary importance to an understanding of the hemodynamic effects of the drug, it is clear that extracardiac effects are also involved. Digitalis glycosides constrict isolated arterial and venous segments, and arteriolar and venous constriction has been demonstrated in intact laboratory animals. These effects appear to be mediated both by the local action of digitalis on vascular smooth muscle and indirectly through the sympathetic nervous system.[221]

Peripheral vasoconstrictor effects of ouabain have also been documented clinically, including observations in patients with cardiogenic shock in whom the vasoconstrictor effect preceded the positive inotropic effect.[22a] In some cases this effect was associated with increased left ventricular end-diastolic pressures. These observations indicate the need for caution when digitalis glycosides are administered rapidly, particularly in situations in which transient increases in peripheral resistance would be deleterious. There is also evidence that increased mesenteric vascular resistance can compromise splanchnic blood flow, possibly subjecting the patient with marginal perfusion to increased risk of ischemic bowel necrosis.[221]

In clinical circumstances in which the intravenous use of digitalis is required, gradual administration of glycosides over several minutes is preferred to a rapid bolus injection.[222]

Digitalis produces generalized vasoconstriction in the normal dog. This action is particularly marked in the hepatic veins and leads to pooling of blood in the portal venous system and consequently diminished venous return. Effects are probably less striking in man. Extracardiac and coronary vascular effects of digitalis are considered in further detail in the reviews by Longhurst and Ross[223] and by Blatt et al.[221]

In congestive heart failure, sympathetic augmentation of contractility is important in maintaining cardiac output, as discussed in Chap. 14. This increase in sympathetic nervous activity, producing systemic arteriolar and venous constriction, may serve to maintain blood pressure in the face of diminished cardiac output and redistribute this reduced output among various regional circulations. When digitalis is given to patients with heart failure, generalized vasodilation typically occurs instead of the vasoconstriction observed in normal persons[224]—an effect presumably related to increased cardiac output mediated by positive inotropic action of the drug and direct baroreflex-mediated withdrawal of sympathetic vasoconstriction. This withdrawal may account for the observation that venous pressure is often lowered *before* diuresis occurs after the administration of digitalis.[224] Digoxin has been shown to suppress plasma renin activity and also to reduce plasma aldosterone activity in patients with chronic congestive heart failure.[224]

DIURESIS. This is a characteristic and important manifestation of digitalis action in edematous patients with congestive heart failure. Digitalis has been shown to inhibit tubular reabsorption of sodium, and direct infusion of ouabain into the renal artery produces substantial inhibition of renal Na^+,K^+-ATPase and impairment of both concentrating and diluting ability. However, relatively large doses are needed to demonstrate these effects, and it is unlikely that any direct renal action of digitalis plays an important part in the diuresis that occurs in the treatment of congestive heart failure. Rather, it is through an improvement of cardiac output and therefore in renal hemodynamics that glycosides induce diuresis.

SLOWING OF VENTRICULAR RATE. Finally, a major hemodynamic effect of digitalis in enhancing cardiac performance lies in its ability to slow the ventricular response to supraventricular tachyarrhythmias, particularly in conditions such as mitral valve stenosis. Slowing of sinus tachycardia in patients with congestive heart failure is often pronounced, through withdrawal of enhanced sympathetic tone, when the failure state is ameliorated by virtue of increased cardiac contractility and baroreflex sensitivity. In usual doses, digitalis has no pronounced direct effect on sinoarterial pacemaker automaticity.

CLINICAL TRIALS WITH CARDIAC GLYCOSIDES

The effects of digoxin on cardiac function in patients in normal sinus rhythm have undergone considerable study. Studies using both noninvasive and invasive methods have documented sustained improvement in cardiac performance of patients with chronic congestive heart failure.[216,219,225–231a] In general, patients with more severe contractile dysfunction demonstrated the most pronounced beneficial response to digoxin. This is especially apparent in the study of Gheorghiade et al.,[227] in which marked improvements in mean cardiac output (+48 per cent), left ventricular filling pressure (−36 per cent), and ejection fraction (20 to 28 per cent) were observed in the subset of patients who remained in overt failure after diuretic and vasodilator treatment, while no significant further improvement was observed in the subset who were compensated at the completion of the diuretic-vasodilator treatment period.

Data from randomized, controlled trials of digoxin in patients with heart failure and normal sinus rhythm are still somewhat limited, but eight studies meeting customary criteria for such investigations have been published since 1980. Five smaller trials using a crossover design involved 22 to 44 patients with observations, including clinical endpoints and follow-up, for 7 to 12 weeks.[217,232–235] The studies of Lee et al.,[217] Guyatt et al.,[233] and Pugh et al.[234] showed significant clinical and/or hemodynamic benefit in digoxin-treated patients, while the studies of Fleg et al.[232] and Taggart et al.[235] found no clear evidence of benefit. Entry criteria, dosing regimen, and other aspects of trial design vary widely among these studies, probably accounting for the variation in conclusions reached. Again, the impression is that not all patients with a history of heart failure show obvious benefit from digoxin in these studies, and that patients with more advanced systolic ventricular dysfunction are more likely to benefit than those with less severe systolic dysfunction; in some instances, patients with normal left ventricular ejection fractions were included and almost invariably failed to show clinical improvement.[217]

Three larger multicenter trials have appeared since 1988. Of these, the digoxin-xamoterol study by a German and Austrian study group[236] is the most difficult to assess because the 433 patients entering the trial were not completely characterized at entry; indeed, 106 were stated to be NYHA Class I. Digoxin did not improve exercise duration and work done on a bicycle ergometer. However, significant improvement in symptoms was demonstrated with digoxin compared with placebo using the Likert functional scale. (Xamoterol was subsequently shown to increase mortality in patients with heart failure.)

The captopril-digoxin trial[231] compared captopril, digoxin, and placebo during maintenance diuretic therapy in 196 patients, 85 per cent of whom were judged to be in NYHA Class I or II. Three major conclusions emerged from this trial, as summarized in Figure 17–13. First, digoxin, but not captopril,

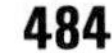

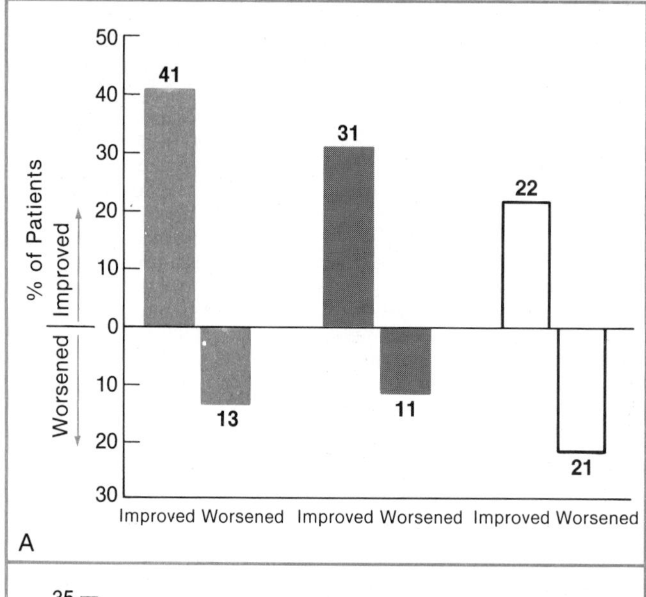

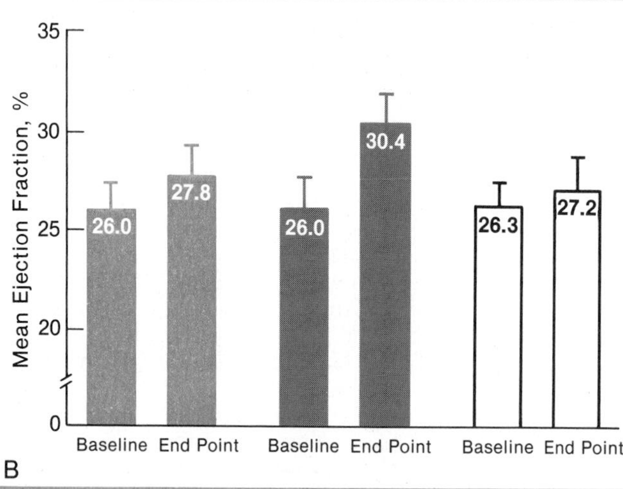

FIGURE 17-13. ***A,*** **Percentage of patients improving and worsening in functional class from baseline at endpoint. Captopril group (red solid bars) had significantly greater proportion of improvement compared with placebo group (open bars) ($P < .01$). Black solid bars indicate digoxin group.** ***B,*** **Mean (SEM) ejection fraction at baseline and endpoint. Digoxin group had significantly greater change compared with placebo ($P < .01$) and captopril ($P < .05$) groups. (From The Captopril-Digoxin Multicenter Research Group: Comparative effects of therapy with captopril and digoxin in patients with mild to moderate heart failure. JAMA** ***259:*****539, 1988.)**

significantly improved the left ventricular ejection fraction. Second, captopril significantly prolonged exercise time by 14 per cent compared with 6 per cent for placebo; digoxin was intermediate with 10 per cent improvement, not significantly different from either captopril or placebo. Third, and probably most important, compared with placebo, digoxin and captopril were both similarly effective in reducing morbidity in terms of increased diuretic requirements and hospitalization and emergency room visits (Fig. 17-13).

The milrinone-digoxin trial[230] randomly assigned 230 patients in sinus rhythm with moderately severe heart failure to treatment with digoxin, milrinone, both drugs, or placebo added to baseline diuretic therapy. After 3 months, digoxin improved ejection fraction by +1.7 per cent compared with −2 per cent in the placebo group ($p < 0.01$), while exercise tolerance improved by 14 per cent ($p < 0.05$) compared with placebo. There was marked benefit of digoxin over placebo or milrinone as judged by decompensation within 2 weeks and 3 months, and a significantly lower incidence of increased ventricular ectopy in the digoxin-treated group than in those receiving milrinone.

None of these trials had sufficient power to approach any assessment of the effects of digoxin on mortality, a goal that is likely to require the randomization of 5,000 to 10,000 patients with left ventricular dysfunction and symptoms of heart failure if a 10 to 15 per cent alteration in mortality is to be discerned.

PHARMACOKINETICS AND BIOAVAILABILITY

Table 17-7 summarizes data related to absorption, onset of action, and excretion times and patterns for cardiac glycosides available in the United States. It is important to recognize that the values cited are averages and that substantial individual variation is to be expected.

DIGOXIN. This glycoside has become the predominant preparation used, principally because of the flexibility in its route of administration and its intermediate duration of action. Digoxin is excreted exponentially, with a half-life of about 36 to 48 hours in subjects with normal renal function, resulting in the loss of about one-third of body stores daily.[237] Although the drug is excreted for the most part in unchanged form, some patients excrete appreciable quantities of the relatively inactive metabolite dihydrodigoxin, which arises through bacterial biotransformation in the gut lumen.[238] Renal excretion of digoxin is proportional to glomerular filtration rate (and hence to creatinine clearance) and is largely independent of rate of urine flow in patients with reasonably intact renal function.[237] In patients with prerenal azotemia, digoxin clearance correlates more closely with urea clearance than with creatinine clearance, suggesting that digoxin may undergo some degree of tubular reabsorption under these circumstances.[239] For patients not previously given digitalis, institution of daily maintenance therapy without a loading dose results in development of steady-state plateau concentrations after four to five half-lives, or about 7 days, in subjects with normal renal function. If the half-life of the drug is prolonged, the length of time before a steady state is reached with a daily maintenance dose is prolonged accordingly. Because of the high degree of tissue binding of digoxin, the drug is not effectively removed from the body by dialysis.[240] Similarly, it has been shown that cardiopulmonary bypass and exchange transfusion remove only minor amounts of digoxin from the body. Acute vasodilator therapy with nitroprusside or hydralazine tends to increase renal digoxin clearance without changing glomerular filtration rate and may necessitate adjustment of maintenance digoxin dosage.[241]

Infants and children absorb and excrete digoxin in much the same way as adults do,[242] although secretion at the renal tubular level may be quantitatively more important in prepubertal subjects.[243] Digoxin doses in neonates and infants are substantially larger than those in adults when calculated on the basis of body weight or body surface area.[244] These higher doses result in relatively higher serum digoxin concentrations, which are generally well tolerated. Digoxin concentrations at term in fetal umbilical-cord venous blood have been found to be similar to those in the venous blood of the mother maintained with digoxin, documenting transplacental passage of the drug.[242]

An important interaction between digoxin and quinidine has been described that leads to an approximately twofold increase in serum digoxin concentration when conventional quinidine doses are added to a standard maintenance digoxin regimen.[245] This increase is associated in some instances with the development of digoxin-toxic rhythm disturbances. A decrease in digoxin dosage, in addition to frequent assessment of serum digoxin concentration and clinical status, is advisable when quinidine is given concurrently. Interactions of digoxin with quinidine, verapamil, and amiodarone (among other drugs) are considered on page 634 and in Table 17-8.

DIGITOXIN. This cardiac glycoside is the least polar and most slowly excreted of the cardiac glycosides available for clinical use. It constitutes the principal active agent in digitalis leaf. Gastrointestinal absorption of digitoxin is a passive process and is thought to be essentially complete.

TABLE 17-7 CARDIAC GLYCOSIDE PREPARATIONS

AGENT	GASTRO-INTESTINAL ABSORPTION	ONSET OF ACTION* (MIN)	PEAK EFFECT (HR)	AVERAGE HALF-LIFE†	PRINCIPAL METABOLIC ROUTE (EXCRETORY PATHWAY)	AVERAGE DIGITALIZING DOSES§ Oral‡	Intravenous‡	USUAL DAILY ORAL MAINTENANCE DOSES‖
Ouabain	Unreliable	5 to 10	½ to 2	21 hours	Renal; some gastrointestinal excretion	—	0.3 to 0.50 mg	—
Deslanoside	Unreliable	10 to 30	1 to 2	33 hours	Renal	—	0.80 mg	—
Digoxin	55 to 75%¶ 90 to 100%**	15 to 30	1½ to 5	36 to 48 hours	Renal; some gastrointestnal excretion	1.25 to 1.50 mg**	0.75 to 1.00 mg**	0.25 to 0.50 mg
Digitoxin	90 to 100%	25 to 120	4 to 12	4 to 6 days	Hepatic#; renal excretion of metabolites	0.70 to 1.20 mg	1.00 mg	0.10 mg

Modified from Smith, T. W.: Drug therapy: Digitalis glycosides. N. Engl. J. Med. *288*:719, 1973.
* For intravenous dose.
† For normal subjects (prolonged by renal impairment with digoxin, ouabain, and deslanoside and probably by severe hepatic disease with digitoxin).
‡ Divided doses over 12 to 24 hours at intervals of 6 to 8 hours.
§ Given in increments for initial subcomplete digitalization, to be supplemented by further small increments as necessary.
‖ Average for adult patients without renal or hepatic impairment; varies widely among individual patients and requires close medical supervision.
¶ For tablet form of administration (may be less in malabsorption syndromes and in formulations with poor bioavailability).
# Enterohepatic cycle exists.
** Ninety to 100 per cent gastrointestinal absorption has been reported for the encapsulated gel formulation. Lanoxicaps® available in capsules containing 0.05, 0.10, and 0.20 mg. When this product is used, the average digitalizing dose should be lowered about 20 per cent.

TABLE 17-8 PHARMACOKINETIC DRUG INTERACTIONS WITH DIGOXIN

DRUG	MECHANISM OF INTERACTION EFFECT ON DIGOXIN	MEAN MAGNITUDE OF INTERACTION*	TYPE OF STUDY Single-Dose Digoxin	Steady State	SUGGESTED INTERVENTION
Cholestyramine	Absorption of digoxin	↓ 25%		×	1. Give digoxin 8 hours before cholestyramine 2. Use solution or capsule form of digoxin
Antacids	Unclear	↓ 25%	×		Temporal separation of time of administration
Kaolin-pectin	Adsorption of digoxin	?	×		1. Give digoxin 2 hours before kaolin-pectin 2. ? Use solution or capsule form of digoxin
Bran	Adsorption of digoxin	↓ 20%	×		Temporal separation of time of administration
Neomycin	Unknown	↓ 28%	×		Increase dose of digoxin
Sulfasalazine	Unknown	↓ 18%	×		
PAS	Unknown	↓ 22%	×		
Bepridil	Unknown	↑ 34%		×	None
Phenytoin	Unknown	↓ 30%		×	↑ Dose
Propafenone	Unknown	↑ 100%		×	Same as for quinidine
Erythromycin Tetracycline (in <10% of subjects)	↑ Bioavailability by ↓ intestinal metabolism of digoxin by certain gut flora	↑ 43 to 116%		×	1. Measure serum digoxin concentration 2. Decrease digoxin dose 3. Use solution or capsule form of digoxin
Quinidine	? ↓ Bioavailability, ↓ volume of distribution, ↓ renal and nonrenal clearance	↑ 100%	×	×	1. Decrease dose by 50% 2. Measure serum digoxin concentration
Amiodarone	↓ Renal and nonrenal clearance	↑ 70 to 100%		×	Same as for quinidine
Verapamil	↓ Renal and nonrenal clearance	↑ 70 to 100%		×	Same as for quinidine
Diltiazem	? ↓ Renal clearance	Zero to small ↑		×	None
Nicardipine	Unknown	↑ 15%		×	None
Tiapamil	Unknown	↑ 60%		×	Same as for quinidine
Spironolactone	↓ Renal and nonrenal clearance	↑ 30%	×		Measure serum digoxin concentration
Triamterene	↓ Nonrenal clearance	↑ 20%	×		Measure serum digoxin concentration
Indomethacin (preterm infants)	? ↓ Renal clearance	↑ 50%		×	Decrease dose by 25%

Adapted, with minor modification, from Marcus, F. I.: Pharmacokinetic interactions between digoxin and other drugs. J. Am. Coll. Cardiol., 5:82A, 1985, where relevant references not otherwise specified are found.
↑ = increased; ↓ = decreased; ? = questionable.
* Alteration in bioavailability or serum concentration. For single-dose studies, the magnitude of the anticipated change in serum digoxin concentration was estimated from pharmacokinetic data, particularly the change in total body clearance. Drugs reported to show no significant interaction at clinically relevant doses include ethmozine,[597] milrinone,[598] and isradipine.[599]
† Also see study of Elkayam, et al.[600].

Digitoxin binds avidly to human serum albumin, and about 97 per cent of the serum or plasma content of the drug is bound to albumin at clinically relevant concentrations.[237] It therefore differs considerably in this respect from digoxin, which is only about 23 per cent bound to plasma proteins.[237] Renal clearance of the native compound is relatively minor compared with digoxin, and extensive metabolism of digitoxin occurs, presumably in the liver. An enterohepatic cycle exists for digitoxin and can be interrupted by resins such as cholestyramine, which bind digitoxin in the gut lumen.

Half-times of digitoxin in plasma appear to vary relatively little from patient to patient, with most studies reporting mean values in the range of 4 to 6 days. Administration of daily maintenance doses of digitoxin without a loading dose will result in gradual digitalization, with the 4- to 6-day half-life of the drug resulting in establishment of the final steady-state plateau after 3 to 4 weeks.

OUABAIN. This is the most polar and rapidly acting of the cardiac glycosides currently available for clinical use. Like the other cardiac glycosides, its excretion from the body follows first-order pharmacokinetics, with a fixed portion of the residual drug in the body being excreted each day. For ouabain, the plasma half-life in normal subjects is about 21 hours —similar to the half-life of positive inotropic effect and of ventricular rate slowing in patients with atrial fibrillation.[246] Impairment of renal function prolongs the half-life of ouabain and also the period during which accumulation will continue. Although ouabain is predominantly excreted unchanged via the renal route, its gastrointestinal excretion is substantial after intravenous administration in both dog and man.[247] It is poorly absorbed from the gastrointestinal tract and is not available for oral use. Detailed reviews of pharmacokinetics and metabolism of these and other cardiac glycosides are available.[237,248]

BIOAVAILABILITY

Numerous studies over several decades have documented incomplete absorption of digoxin from the gastrointestinal tract.[249] The bioavailability of tablet preparations of digoxin averages about 67 to 75 per cent. Individual patient variation, circumstances of drug administration, and characteristics of the pharmaceutical preparation ingested are all known to affect digoxin bioavailability. Patients with malabsorption syndromes may absorb digoxin poorly and erratically. However, patients with maldigestion due to pancreatic insufficiency, despite comparable degrees of steatorrhea, appear to absorb the drug more normally. Administration of digoxin after meals is likely to decrease peak serum levels achieved, but total absorption is not affected to any noteworthy degree. Absorption of digoxin tends to be enhanced by drugs that decrease gastrointestinal motility and to be reduced by drugs that increase motility, particularly if the preparations have limited bioavailability. In addition, nonabsorbed substances such as cholestyramine, colestipol, kaolin and pectin (Kaopectate), and nonabsorbable antacids, when taken concurrently, can interfere with gastrointestinal absorption of digoxin; neomycin has also been shown to interfere with digoxin absorption. Because of previously documented variations in the bioavailability of commercially available digoxin preparations,[250] bioavailability specifications provided by the FDA and USP are in effect.[250,251]

DIGOXIN. Biological availability uniformly approaching 100 per cent probably cannot be achieved with any oral digoxin preparation, but an encapsulated gel preparation is reported to have 90 to 100 per cent bioavailability and reduced variability of absorption.[252] Digoxin elixir is somewhat more bioavailable than the tablet form. Intramuscular digoxin causes severe pain at the injection site, and bioavailability is only 83 per cent that of intravenous digoxin.

DIGITOXIN. Oral absorption of digitoxin is generally considered to be virtually 100 per cent. As with digoxin, binding to nonabsorbable substances such as cholestyramine can interfere with initial absorption. Patients receiving such anion-exchange resins in addition to cardiac glycoside should be instructed to ingest the cardiac glycoside 2 hours before the resin to minimize this effect.

CLINICAL USE OF DIGITALIS

A sound working knowledge of the pharmacokinetics of the commonly used cardiac glycosides is essential to the optimal use of these drugs. Computer programs and nomograms[253,254] can provide initial approximations of optimal dose, but further dosage adjustments based on close clinical observation of the patient are often required. In many cases, the variability in serum digoxin concentrations among different patients remains unexplained even after adjustments for dose, body size, and renal function have been made. Measurement of serum digoxin concentrations and their use for feedback dosage adjustments have been suggested.[254]

The clinical use of cardiac glycosides is complicated by the absence of a readily measurable therapeutic objective (except in certain atrial arrhythmias), the lack of a reliable means to predict individual cardiac responses, and the difficulty in defining proximity to toxicity.

CONGESTIVE HEART FAILURE. Cardiac glycosides are of potential value in most patients with symptoms and signs of congestive heart failure due to ischemic, valvular, hypertensive, or congenital heart disease, dilated cardiomyopathies, and cor pulmonale. Improvement of depressed myocardial contractility increases cardiac output, promotes diuresis, and reduces the filling pressure of the failing ventricle(s), with the consequent reduction of pulmonary vascular congestion and central venous pressure.

Although few clinicians would challenge the efficacy of cardiac glycosides in patients with congestive heart failure complicated by supraventricular tachyarrhythmias such as atrial fibrillation, the efficacy of digitalis in the management of heart failure in the presence of normal sinus rhythm has been called into question. Studies based on invasive as well as noninvasive measurements have documented sustained improvement in cardiac performance in patients with chronic congestive heart failure and sinus rhythm.[216–219,225–235] However, the clinical response is critically dependent on patient selection, with particular regard to the nature and extent of ventricular dysfunction. A consensus now exists that patients with dilated, failing hearts and impaired systolic function, often manifesting an S_3 gallop, have subjective and objective improvement after receiving digitalis, whereas patients with elevated filling pressures due to reduced ventricular compliance, but with preserved systolic function at rest, are not usually appropriate candidates for digitalis therapy unless supraventricular tachycardia is a concomitant problem. Griffiths et al.,[225] Murray and colleagues,[226] and the captopril-digoxin multicenter trial group[231] all reported sustained improvement in contractile function response to maintenance digoxin. Among 21 infants with congestive heart failure due to ventricular septal defects, 12 (57 per cent) were judged to have benefited from digoxin administration.[244] The beneficial hemodynamic effects of digoxin are additive to those of the vasodilator captopril and also to those of the beta-adrenergic agonist prenalterol.[218] Among patients with Class IV heart failure and sinus rhythm treated to the point of optimum benefit with diuretics and vasodilator, digoxin administration resulted in incremental mean increases of 27 per cent in the cardiac index and 50 per cent in the left ventricular stroke-work index, together with 29 per cent decrease in mean pulmonary capillary wedge pressure and an increase from a mean of 21 per cent to 29 per cent in the left ventricular ejection fraction.[227] Patients in this series with marked persisting abnormalities of cardiac function after diuretic and vasodilator treatment had greater hemodynamic improvement with digoxin than the subset with relatively normal values for pulmonary capillary wedge pressure and cardiac index. It is of interest that severely failing myocardium from hearts of cardiac transplant recipients showed markedly reduced responsiveness to beta-adrenergic agonists and phosphodiesterase inhibitors, but the effectiveness of inotropic stimulation with the cardioactive steroid acetylstrophanthidin was preserved.[255]

Advances in diuretic and vasodilator therapy, as well as in hemodynamic monitoring of critically ill patients, have made it increasingly inappropriate to use the largest dose of digitalis that can be tolerated without the emergence of overt toxicity, particularly in view of the narrow margin between therapeutic and toxic doses and the marked variation in individual sensitivity. Although the ventricular rate serves as an appropriate guide to determining doses of cardiac glycosides for patients with atrial fibrillation or flutter, overly aggressive use of digitalis can render electrical cardioversion hazardous.

As previously noted, digitalis is of no demonstrable benefit in isolated *mitral stenosis* with normal sinus rhythm unless right ventricular failure has supervened. Similarly, little benefit may result in patients with *pericardial tamponade* or *con-*

strictive pericarditis except when there is invasion of the myocardium in the latter. Hypertrophic obstructive cardiomyopathy represents another process in which digitalis is often of little value and may actually be deleterious because it can increase left ventricular outflow obstruction by augmenting the contractility of the hypertrophic outflow tract segment. There is no objective evidence that patients with left ventricular hypertrophy and well-preserved left ventricular ejection fraction, in the presence of symptoms related to filling pressures, benefit from digitalis. In the later stages of hypertrophic cardiomyopathy, in which ventricular dilation and congestive problems may predominate over obstructive hemodynamics, cardiac glycosides may be beneficial.

Patients who develop congestive heart failure with systolic dysfunction in response to a specific precipitating stress may benefit from temporary use of digitalis but will not necessarily require long-term maintenance digitalization. The risk/benefit ratio must be assessed with any change in clinical status and will often be found to favor discontinuation of digitalis when an acute stress such as infection, anemia, or thyrotoxicosis is no longer present.

Digitalis glycosides may improve symptoms of angina pectoris when it coexists with cardiomegaly and congestive heart failure. As discussed subsequently, however, an increase in angina may occur unless the tendency toward increased oxygen consumption is offset by decreased ventricular size and wall tension.

Prophylactic digitalization of the patients with diminished cardiac reserve about to undergo major stress such as surgery remains controversial (p. 1714). In the absence of obvious cardiomegaly or other evidence of overt congestive heart failure, most clinicians prefer to withhold digitalis until a specific indication arises. Prophylactic digitalization has been recommended for patients undergoing aortocoronary bypass surgery on the basis of a significant reduction in supraventricular arrhythmias.[256] Evidence of a difference in ultimate outcome between digitalized and nondigitalized patients was not documented, however, and another study of 140 consecutive patients undergoing myocardial revascularization showed a *higher* incidence of supraventricular tachyarrhythmias in patients receiving prophylactic digitalis.[257]

The availability of reliable pervenous catheter endocardial pacing techniques has helped to resolve the problem of digitalis use in patients with marginal atrioventricular conduction or established atrioventricular block. One can now carry out pacemaker implantation at minimal risk even in severely ill patients and then give digitalis without fear of aggravating conduction problems.

Clinical use of cardiac glycosides in congestive heart failure has been considered in further detail by Marsh and Smith[258] and by Kelly and Smith.[258a]

ARRHYTHMIAS (See also Chap. 24 and ref. 259)

Digitalis is of potential use in the management of four types of supraventricular tachyarrhythmias.

PAROXYSMAL SUPRAVENTRICULAR TACHYCARDIA (p. 1684). Whether of atrial or atrioventricular junctional origin, this arrhythmia usually responds to digitalization when simpler measures such as carotid sinus pressure alone have failed. Many clinicians now prefer to use verapamil or adenosine in this clinical setting. When digitalis is used, carotid sinus pressure should be repeated during the course of digitalization, since the combination of partial digitalization and carotid sinus pressure will often succeed when neither measure alone suffices. Maintenance digitalization usually abolishes or reduces the frequency of recurrent attacks. Use of digitalis in the setting of paroxysmal supraventricular tachycardia demands that digitalis intoxication be excluded as a cause of the arrhythmia.

ATRIAL FIBRILLATION. This arrhythmia with rapid ventricular response is one of the most common indications for the use of digitalis. Both vagal and direct mechanisms result in increased blockade of impulses arriving at the atrioventricular junction, with slowing of the ventricular rate. Conversion to normal sinus rhythm may occur in the course of digitalization, but a placebo-controlled trial did not demonstrate an increased likelihood of this outcome with acute administration of digoxin to patients with recent-onset atrial fibrillation.[260] There is a growing consensus that digitalis does not decrease the incidence of episodes of paroxysmal atrial fibrillation[261] and often is insufficiently effective in controlling the ventricular rate in atrial fibrillation when used alone.[262,263] Addition of beta-adrenoceptor blocking agents[264,265] or verapamil[265] may be useful in circumstances in which the ventricular rate is difficult to control without the emergence of toxic symptoms (e.g., untreated thyrotoxicosis) and congestive heart failure is absent or minimal. Cowan et al. have reported that patients with acute myocardial infarction complicated by atrial fibrillation showed a tendency toward earlier reversion to sinus rhythm when randomized to amiodarone treatment compared with digoxin.[266]

ATRIAL FLUTTER. This arrhythmia, usually accompanied by 2 : 1 atrioventricular block in untreated cases, can often be managed with digitalis in doses sufficient to produce a degree of atrioventricular blockade that results in a ventricular rate in the range of 70 to 100/min. This effect may require doses considerably in excess of the usual range.

WOLFF-PARKINSON-WHITE SYNDROME. Tachyarrhythmias associated with this form of conduction (p. 693) may be terminated or prevented by digitalis in cases in which preferential effects on conduction or refractoriness in the normal or anomalous conduction pathways result in interruption of the reentrant circus movement. Other antiarrhythmic drugs may be more effective in other cases. Digitalis exerts a variety of electrophysiological effects in patients with Wolff-Parkinson-White syndrome, the sum of which renders these drugs potentially hazardous in patients with a history of atrial fibrillation or flutter.

DOSAGE SCHEDULES

(Table 17–7)

Specific recommendations for digoxin dosage have been developed on the basis of the pharmacokinetic principles previously discussed. Usually there is no reason to use a loading dose in excess of what the steady-state body content will be with the usual maintenance dose. Patients with entirely normal renal function who excrete 37 per cent of the digoxin in their bodies each day will, with a maintenance dose of 0.25 or 0.50 mg/day, have a steady-state total body content of about 0.67 or 1.35 mg, respectively. If a reasonable estimation of 75 per cent absorption of the tablet form of digoxin is made, estimates for the oral loading dose are about 0.9 and 1.8 mg, respectively, corresponding to maintenance doses of 0.25 and 0.50 mg/day. This amount can be given over a period of a day or so in several increments, or the same level of digitalization can be achieved over a period of about a week in a patient with normal renal function by administration of the daily maintenance dose without any loading dose. Severe renal impairment will prolong the half-life of digoxin to a maximum of about 4.4 days and hence extend the period required to reach a steady-state plateau to a maximum of about 3 weeks. In adults, intravenous loading doses of about 0.50 to 0.75 mg/45 kg (100 lb) of body weight, given in increments, are unlikely to cause toxicity and can be supplemented by further increments if indicated by the clinical course.

The maintenance digoxin dose required to replace daily losses will vary from about 37 per cent of the total body content in patients with normal renal function to nonrenal losses averaging about 14 per cent in patients who are essentially anephric. Between the extremes of normal renal function and no renal function, digoxin excretion is linearly related to glomerular filtration rate or creatinine clearance (C_{cr}). A reasonable approximation of daily percentage of loss of digoxin is as follows[267]:

$$\%\ \text{daily loss (men)} = 11.6 + \frac{20}{C}$$

and

$$\%\ \text{daily loss (women)} = 12.6 + \frac{16}{C}$$

where C is a stable serum creatinine in milligrams per 100 ml.

The recommended oral loading dose of digoxin, based on lean body weight and administered in the form of digoxin elixir, is 25 to 35 μg/kg for full-term infants; 35 to 60 μg/kg for infants from 1 to 24 months; 30 to 40 μg/kg for ages 2 to 5 years; 20 to 35 μg/kg for 5 to 10 years; and 10 to 15 μg/kg for children over 10 years. For premature infants a loading dose of 20 to 30 μg/kg is recommended. Daily maintenance doses for patients with normal renal function are estimated as 20 to 30 per cent of the oral loading dose for premature infants and 25 to 35 per cent of the loading dose for full-term infants through children of 10 years of age and older. Parenteral (intravenous) loading and maintenance dose recommendations are approximately 75 per cent of the oral dosages.[267] Hougen has reviewed digoxin use in the young.[244] Digitoxin dosing is discussed in the third edition of this text.[191]

THERAPEUTIC ENDPOINTS

The optimal dose of digitalis is not necessarily the largest dose that can be tolerated without the emergence of overt toxicity. The ratio of toxic to therapeutic effect for cardiac glycosides is small, and the availability of other measures of treating heart failure, particularly potent oral diuretics and vasodilators, usually obviates balancing therapy at the edge of toxicity. Electrocardiographic ST-segment and T-wave changes and slowing of sinus tachycardia are of little value in gauging the adequacy of digitalis dosage.

In patients with atrial flutter or fibrillation, control of the ventricular response provides a relatively straightforward endpoint.

When congestive heart failure is the indication for use of digitalis, it is helpful to remember that positive inotropy is a graded response that is appreciable at doses well short of "maximally tolerated doses." As already stated, available data suggest that further inotropic benefit may not occur clinically beyond serum digoxin levels in the range of 1.5 to 2.0 ng/ml. Carotid sinus massage can provide useful bedside clues to impending digitalis excess. Rhythm disorders such as second-degree atrioventricular block, accelerated atrioventricular junctional rhythm, and ventricular premature beats or bigeminy may emerge in response to carotid sinus stimulation before they occur spontaneously.[268]

INDIVIDUAL SENSITIVITY TO DIGITALIS. A number of factors influencing individual sensitivity to cardiac glycosides are listed in Table 17–9.

ELECTROLYTE AND ACID-BASE DISTURBANCES. Disturbances of potassium homeostasis clearly influence the action of digitalis.[109] Myocardial concentrations of digoxin tend to decrease with increasing serum potassium concentration. Furthermore, hypokalemia has primary arrhythmogenic effects, both decreasing the effective refractory period of Purkinje cells and shortening the coupling interval for ventricular premature beats. Depression of atrioventricular nodal conduction can occur with both digitalis excess and either a very low or extremely high level of serum K^+.[200] Diuretic therapy, catecholamine administration, insulin administration or carbohydrate loading, renal disease, and acid-base disturbances must all be borne in mind as potential causes of clinically significant alterations in potassium homeostasis, which can, in turn, affect importantly the response to cardiac glycosides.

Administration of Mg^{++} salts suppresses digitalis-induced arrhythmias while hypomagnesemia appears to predispose to digitalis toxicity.[109,191] There is some evidence that the digitalis-induced K^+ efflux from the myocardium is reduced by Mg^{++} salts.[191] Magnesium depletion may become clinically important with the long-term administration of diuretic agents[112,116,118] and with gastrointestinal disease, diabetes mellitus, or poor nutritional states. Moreover, in patients with congestive heart failure, significant depletion of total body Mg^{++} stores may occur owing to prolonged secondary aldosteronism.[111,111a,113] Although the clinical importance of Mg^{++} depletion in digitalis therapy remains unresolved, it appears to be a frequent occurrence, with a reported incidence of 19 per cent in one recent series.[111] Poor or no correlation was found between serum and tissue Mg in patients with heart failure, leaving unsolved the problem of clinical assessment of Mg^{++} stores.[111,111a,115,270]

Elevated serum Ca^{++} levels increase ventricular automaticity, and this effect is at least additive to and perhaps synergistic with the effects of digitalis. The clinician should be alert for the possibility of enhanced digitalis sensitivity when treating hypercalcemic patients or when administering calcium parenterally to digitalized patients.

TABLE 17–9 FACTORS INFLUENCING INDIVIDUAL SENSITIVITY TO DIGITALIS

Type and severity of underlying cardiac disease
Serum electrolyte derangements
Hypokalemia or hyperkalemia
Hypomagnesemia
Hypercalcemia
Hyponatremia
Acid-base imbalance
Concomitant drug administration
Anesthetics
Catecholamines and sympathomimetics
Antiarrhythmic agents
Thyroid status
Renal function
Autonomic nervous system tone
Respiratory disease

TYPE AND SEVERITY OF UNDERLYING HEART DISEASE. The effects of digitalis on the heart are modified by the type and severity of the underlying heart disease. This is dramatically demonstrated in otherwise healthy subjects who ingest massive doses of digitalis. Toxicity in such situations is frequently manifested by progressively impaired atrioventricular conduction or by sinoatrial exit block, rather than by enhanced automaticity and ventricular ectopic activity as seen in patients with underlying heart disease.[272,273] In many patients with ischemic, myocardial, or valvular heart disease, the effects of digitalis are superimposed on an electrophysiologically unstable condition with preexisting abnormalities of impulse formation and conduction. The more severe and advanced the heart disease, the more likely the occurrence of focal ischemia, myocardial fibrosis, and ventricular dilation with stretching of the Purkinje fibers and resultant tendency toward increased automaticity. The observation that digitalis toxicity is particularly common in patients with amyloidosis involving the heart may be accounted for, at least in part, by digoxin binding by amyloid fibrils.[274]

DIGITALIS IN ISCHEMIC HEART DISEASE. Changes in myocardial oxygen consumption are always the net result of two opposing effects of digitalis: a potential reduction in wall tension and an increase in contractility. The increase in oxygen consumption in response to digitalis in the normal heart results from increased velocity of contraction with little change in wall tension. In the failing heart, decreased oxygen consumption typically occurs and can be explained by a decrease in left ventricular end-diastolic pressure and volume and, consequently, on the basis of the Laplace relation, a decline in intramyocardial tension.

These considerations are of clinical importance when a decision must be made whether to use digitalis in patients with coronary disease. Angina pectoris has been observed to improve after digitalization in patients with heart failure but occasionally to worsen in those who are well compensated. An objective study of the effects of ouabain on the response of the left ventricle in patients with angina pectoris showed that the depressed myocardial performance noted on exercise was improved by digitalization in the majority of patients studied.[275] Despite these beneficial effects on left ventricular performance, however, there was no consistent alteration in exercise tolerance or the pressure-rate product at which angina occurred. Improved myocardial perfusion judged by means of thallium-201 scans was found in response to maintenance doses of digoxin in patients with coronary artery disease and left ventricular dysfunction.[276] The combination of propranolol and digoxin in patients with angina pectoris appears to be advantageous in the subgroup with angina pectoris and abnormal ventricular function or large hearts.[277]

ACUTE MYOCARDIAL INFARCTION. There are still unanswered questions concerning the role of digitalis therapy after acute myocardial infarction (Chap. 39). There is little to be gained from administration of the drug to patients who have uncomplicated infarction without signs or symptoms of heart failure. There is limited clinical documentation of its value in cardiogenic shock, except in the management of supraventricular arrhythmias. Small increases in cardiac index and stroke work, as well as a reduction in left ventricular end-diastolic pressure, have been observed after digitalization in patients with left ventricular failure following myocardial infarction.[278] Although ouabain did not alter cardiac output in another series of patients with acute myocardial infarction,[279] it caused significant improvement in other indices of left ventricular performance, such as end-diastolic pressure and stroke work.

While the issue has been long debated, there appears to be no convincing evidence for an increased incidence of arrhythmias complicating digitalization in patients with acute infarction when serum levels do not exceed the conventional therapeutic range.[280] The clearest indication for digitalis after acute myocardial infarction is in the treatment of atrial fibrillation with a rapid ventricular rate. Electrical cardioversion may be preferred in the treatment of other supraventricular tachyarrhythmias.[281]

Evidence based on retrospective analysis by Moss et al.[282] and Bigger and colleagues[283] suggests that mortality within the first several months after myocardial infarction may be increased in a high-risk subset of patients with congestive heart failure and ventricular arrhythmias. However, four other large retrospective data base studies demonstrated the expected increased mortality after myocardial infarction among patients with chronic heart failure or cardiac arrhythmias, with no statistically significant increment in mortality attributable to digoxin.[284–287] We believe that the available data do not support the assertion that digoxin therapy is excessively hazardous after infarction, but the existence of an undetected harmful effect can be excluded only with a randomized study.

In summary, current evidence indicates that digitalis has no well-defined role in the management of acute myocardial infarction without congestive heart failure or supraventricular tachyarrhythmias. Judicious patient selection, management of drug doses, and careful monitoring will minimize the potentially deleterious effects of digitalis in acute myocardial infarction.

At present, we recommend a three-part approach: (1) careful consideration whether any treatment of ventricular dysfunction is needed, (2) consideration of alternatives to digoxin therapy, and (3) restriction of digoxin use to the subgroup of patients with chronic congestive heart failure and a dilated left ventricle previously shown to benefit clinically.

ADVANCED AGE. The diminished glomerular filtration rate with age will lead to a prolonged half-life of digoxin and increased serum levels and an increased probability of toxicity on a given dosage regimen. Advanced age is frequently associated with other factors that increase the likelihood of digitalis intoxication, including more severe heart disease; impairment of pulmonary, renal, and neurological function; and an increased number of concurrent medications.

RENAL FAILURE (see also p. 1861). The marked diminution of glomerular filtration rate with renal failure prolongs the half-life of digoxin and thus increases serum digoxin levels. Toxicity from this predictable response can be avoided by careful and frequent adjustments of dosage to correlate with the level of renal function present. Less predictably, dialysis can cause at least a transient decrease in serum potassium that will increase the tendency toward digitalis-induced arrhythmias. Depending on the magnesium content of the dialysate and the use of magnesium-containing antacids by the patients, there may be significant aberrations of serum magnesium levels in patients undergoing dialysis.[269] The clinician is advised to use the minimum drug dosage that produces the desired clinical effects in this condition noted for its extreme fluctuations in fluid and electrolyte balance.

THYROID DISEASE. In hypothyroid patients the serum digoxin half-life is consistently prolonged, while in those with hyperthyroidism, serum digoxin levels tend to be decreased.[288] An increased distribution space for digoxin may exist in hyperthyroid patients. This is of interest in light of experimental findings indicating higher levels of Na^+,K^+-ATPase activity in the myocardium[289] of hyperthyroid animals and increased tolerance to cardiac glycosides in heart cells grown in culture in the presence of high thyroid hormone concentrations, associated with an increased number of Na^+,K^+-ATPase sites and enhanced monovalent cation transport capacity.[290] Thus, the apparent resistance or sensitivity to digitalis in thyroid disease probably depends on changes in target organ responsiveness as well as in the pharmacokinetics of digoxin.

PULMONARY DISEASE. Ventricular ectopic activity consistent with digitalis toxicity frequently occurs in patients with respiratory disease who are receiving digitalis.[291] However, respiratory failure and hypoxemia frequently provoke arrhythmias indistinguishable from those associated with digitalis excess. A population of 931 patients admitted consecutively to a medical service and studied prospectively demonstrated an increased incidence of rhythm disturbance consistent with digitalis toxicity among patients with acute or chronic lung disease.[292] Excessive sensitivity to digitalis in patients with pulmonary disease generally correlates with overt cor pulmonale, hypercapnia, and hypoxemia. From the data available, it is reasonable to anticipate that patients with a variety of pulmonary diseases may be sensitive to the arrhythmogenic effects of digitalis at relatively low serum concentrations.[293]

DRUG INTERACTIONS

Concomitant drug administration may interact with the effects of digitalis through several mechanisms. Clinically important interactions are summarized in Table 17–8, updated from the review of Marcus.[294] As already noted, certain drugs such as cholestyramine, neomycin, nonabsorbable antacids, and Kaopectate may decrease oral absorption of digoxin.

Quinidine reduces both the renal and nonrenal elimination of digoxin and also appears to decrease the apparent volume of distribution of this glycoside.[295] The net result is an increase in serum digoxin concentration that averages twofold in patients in whom conventional doses of quinidine are added to a maintenance digoxin regimen; unfortunately, individual responses to quinidine may vary substantially, and close surveillance of clinical status (and, if possible, serum digoxin concentration) is needed to reduce the risk of precipitating overt digoxin toxicity. Procainamide and disopyramide do not appear to alter serum digoxin levels, but verapamil does increase serum digoxin concentration by an average of 35 per cent[296,599] by decreasing volume of distribution and clearance of digoxin. Both short- and long-term amiodarone administration has been found to increase steady-state serum digoxin concentration.[297,298] Nifedipine appears to produce no clinically significant change in digoxin disposition.

Diuretic agents potentially enhance the occurrence of digitalis toxicity both by decreasing glomerular filtration rate and through a variety of electrolyte disturbances, including hypokalemia, hypomagnesemia, and (for thiazide diuretics) hypercalcemia.

Several anesthetic agents are arrhythmogenic, and experimental studies suggest that this effect may be synergistic with digitalis enhancement of ventricular automaticity in the case of cyclopropane and succinylcholine. Experimental studies demonstrate that catecholamine-induced increases in ventricular automaticity can add to the arrhythmogenic effects of digitalis. It is reasonable for the clinician to assume that sympathomimetic agents increase the likelihood of enhanced automaticity of ectopic pacemakers in patients receiving digitalis.

Drug interactions with digitalis glycosides are considered in further detail elsewhere.[294–295a]

SERUM OR PLASMA CONCENTRATIONS OF DIGITALIS GLYCOSIDES

CLINICAL CORRELATIONS. Mean serum digoxin concentrations in groups of patients without evidence of toxicity average about 1.4 ng/ml. As would be expected, increasing digoxin doses or decreasing renal function is correlated with higher mean levels. Mean serum digoxin concentrations tend to be two to three times higher in patients with clinical evidence of digoxin toxicity, and the difference in mean levels is statistically significant in the vast majority of studies. However, overlap of levels exists between groups with and without evidence of toxicity and tends to be more pronounced in prospective blind studies than in retrospective studies.[292] Despite this overlap, use of serum digoxin concentration measurements to guide therapy is associated with a reduction in the incidence of digitalis toxicity.[299] It is more difficult to correlate therapeutic effects with serum levels in patients.[299a]

Analogous data correlating serum digitoxin concentrations with clinical state[197] indicate that although levels average about 10 times higher than those of digoxin because of digitoxin binding to serum proteins, patients with clinical evidence of toxicity again have mean levels about two times higher than those without evidence of a toxic response.

Measurement of serum cardiac glycoside concentrations is indicated whenever an unanticipated response to these drugs (either suspected toxicity or absence of an expected therapeutic effect) is encountered.

DIGITALIS TOXICITY

Toxic manifestations of digitalis persist as common adverse drug reactions in clinical practice.[197,292]

MECHANISMS. The major manifestations of digitalis intoxication include gastrointestinal and central nervous system symptoms and disturbances of cardiac rhythm. Anorexia, nausea, and vomiting are mediated by chemoreceptors located in the area postrema of the medulla rather than by a direct irritant effect of the drug on the gastrointestinal tract.[300] Digitalis-induced disturbances of impulse formation and conduction are conventionally explained in terms of alterations in refractory period, impulse transmission, and automaticity of cardiac tissues. Alterations in sympathetic activity and changes in vagal tone may also be of considerable importance in some situations, as discussed elsewhere.

Regarding the cellular mechanism of digitalis toxicity, until relatively recently most investigators favored a sequence in which digitalis-induced inhibition of Na^+ and K^+ transport caused increased intracellular [Na^+], decreased intracellular [K^+], and gradual depolarization. This in turn led to increased automaticity, conduction disturbances, and finally inexcitability. Subsequent experimental evidence suggests that cardiac glycosides promote a hitherto unrecognized mechanism of spontaneous activity in specialized cardiac conducting tissue. The underlying cellular event involves depolarizing afterpotentials most often referred to as "transient depolarizations,"[301] or "oscillatory afterpotentials" (p. 604). Potential or overt effects of digitalis on electrophysiology of the intact heart have been reviewed[197] and can be summarized as follows.

SINUS NODE AND ATRIUM. Digitalis-induced slowing of the sinus rate in patients without congestive heart failure is usually minor in degree and is largely mediated by vagal effects on the sinoatrial node. Patients with transplanted, denervated hearts do not respond to conventional doses of digoxin with any change in sinus rate.[302] A combination of vagal and direct effects on the sinus node contributes to sinus bradycardia as well as to occasional cases of sinoatrial arrest or exit block seen in digitalis intoxication. This bradycardia predisposes to the emergence of junctional ventricular escape rhythms. Digitalis, even in therapeutic doses, can impair sinoatrial conduction. Although usually tolerated in patients with sick sinus syndrome, occasionally sinus node dysfunction is precipitated by digoxin, even in doses not usually associated with toxicity.

ATRIOVENTRICULAR NODE. The effective refractory period of the atrioventricular node is prolonged by digitalis. As with the sinus node, this longer period is in part related to increased vagal activity and in part to direct action on nodal fibers, although the vagal effect predominates in subjects without intrinsic disease of the cardiac conduction system.

The therapeutic effect of digitalis in slowing ventricular response in atrial flutter or fibrillation depends in part on the entry of concealed atrial impulses into the atrioventricular node, with failure to reach the His-Purkinje system by virtue of decremental conduction within the node (p. 606). When atrioventricular block of second or third degree occurs as a result of digitalis intoxication, however, the principal mechanism is failure of propagation within the atrioventricular node.

HIS-PURKINJE SYSTEM. Digitalis-induced increases in the automaticity of the His-Purkinje system may come about because of enhanced spontaneous diastolic (phase 4) depolarization or the more recently described transient depolarization mechanism discussed above and elsewhere.[196a,301] The appearance of new pacemakers is manifest clinically by premature junctional or ventricular beats or by accelerated junctional or ventricular rhythms. The nonuniform effect of digitalis on ventricular and Purkinje fibers and simultaneous enhancement of automaticity, depression of conduction velocity, and local block may also predispose to arrhythmias based on reentry mechanisms that may progress to ventricular tachycardia and fibrillation.

CLINICAL MANIFESTATIONS OF DIGITALIS TOXICITY

GASTROINTESTINAL SYMPTOMS. Anorexia is often an early manifestation of digitalis intoxication; nausea and vomiting follow as clear consequence of digitalis overdose and result from central nervous system mechanisms.[300]

NEUROLOGICAL SYMPTOMS. These include headache, fatigue, malaise, neuralgic pain, disorientation, confusion, delirium,[303] and seizures. Visual symptoms are not infrequent[304] and include scotomas, flickering, halos, and changes in color perception.

CARDIAC TOXICITY (see also p. 604). Cardiac toxicity manifested by arrhythmias can take the form of most known rhythm disturbances.[197] Common arrhythmias include atrioventricular junctional escape rhythms, ventricular bigeminy or trigeminy, nonparoxysmal atrioventricular junctional tachycardias, unifocal or multifocal ectopic ventricular beats, and ventricular tachycardia. Atrioventricular junctional exit block, paroxysmal atrial tachycardia with atrioventricular block, sinus arrest, and Mobitz type I (Wenckebach) second-degree atrioventricular block also occur. This list should not be considered exhaustive. There are no unequivocal electrocardiographic features that distinguish digitalis-toxic rhythm disturbances from arrhythmias due to intrinsic cardiac disease, although rhythms combining features of increased automaticity of ectopic pacemakers with impaired conduction, such as paroxysmal atrial tachycardia with atrioventricular dissociation and an accelerated atrioventricular junctional pacemaker, strongly suggest digitalis toxicity. However, even rhythms such as atrial tachycardia with atrioventricular block, considered typical of digitalis toxicity, are frequently due to underlying heart disease rather than digitalis excess.[305] The cause of an arrhythmia may at times be clarified (but not defined with complete certainty) by demonstration of reversion to normal rhythm when the drug is withheld. Clinical and electrocardiographic findings associated with digitalis toxicity have been reviewed extensively.[198a,306–309]

OTHER MANIFESTATIONS. Allergic skin lesions are rare but have been reported.[310] Gynecomastia is occasionally induced in men, and sexual dysfunction has been reported.[311,312]

MASSIVE CARDIAC GLYCOSIDE OVERDOSE

Digitalis overdose, either suicidal or accidental, is occasionally encountered as a life-threatening problem. Patients without underlying heart disease tend to tolerate large doses, with serum digoxin concentrations ranging as high as 10 to 15 ng/ml. The principal manifestations in patients without intrinsic heart disease are most often sinus bradycardia; atrioventricular block of first, second, or third degree; or sinoatrial exit block.[197–198a] Atropine alone is often successful in reversing these manifestations but is not invariably effective.[197] Ventricular pacing with a pervenous endocardial catheter electrode is usually successful, although ventricular standstill unresponsive to pacing has been reported.[272,314]

The condition in patients with preexisting disease tends to be more difficult to manage, in that ectopic ventricular arrhythmias are frequently the initial manifestation of digitalis intoxication.

Refractory hyperkalemia can occur at extremely high digoxin doses and serum concentrations.[315] Greater elevations of serum K^+ concentration were associated with worsening prognosis in a large series of patients after massive doses, usually of digitoxin.[316] Elevation of serum potassium is a consequence of inhibition of Na^+,K^+-ATPase throughout the body, with consequent impairment of monovalent cation transport across cell membranes.

The half-time for digoxin clearance from plasma is shortened when levels are very high.[272,317] This effect may be related to an altered ratio between plasma and tissue concentrations, allowing a relatively large quantity of the drug to be presented to the kidney for excretion.

TREATMENT OF DIGITALIS INTOXICATION

The key to successful treatment is early recognition that an arrhythmia is related to digitalis intoxication.[315] The more common manifestations—including occasional ectopic beats, marked first-degree atrioventricular block, or atrial fibrillation with a slow ventricular response—require only temporary withdrawal of the drug, electrocardiographic monitoring (if indicated) until the arrhythmia has disappeared, and subsequent adjustment of the dosage schedule to prevent recurrence. Rhythm disturbances that impair cardiac output because of too rapid or too slow ventricular rates, or those that portend ventricular fibrillation, require more active intervention. Ventricular tachycardia due to digitalis intoxication demands immediate vigorous treatment. Sinus bradycardia, sinoatrial arrest, and atrioventricular block of second or third degree are sometimes treated effectively with atropine, as previously indicated. Occasionally, electrical pacing will be required. It has been recommended that nonparoxysmal atrioventricular junctional rhythms with rates greater than 90 or with exit block be treated actively.[318] Atrioventricular junctional escape rhythms may simply be monitored if the rate is satisfactory.

In an extensive experience with acute pediatric digoxin ingestion in 41 patients aged 15 months to 16 years, Lewander et al. found that symptoms and signs typically responded well to conventional therapeutic measures. None of the patients in this report required digoxin-specific Fab treatment.[319]

PHENYTOIN AND LIDOCAINE (see also pp. 641 and 639). Phenytoin and lidocaine are useful drugs in the treatment of ectopic arrhythmias due to digitalis toxicity.[315] They have little adverse effect on the sinoatrial rate, atrial conduction, atrioventricular conduction, or conduction in the His-Purkinje system. Indeed, phenytoin may improve sinoatrial block and atrioventricular conduction under some circumstances. A recommended regimen for phenytoin is 100 mg administered by slow intravenous infusion every 5 minutes until onset of toxicity or control of the arrhythmia, followed by an oral maintenance dose of 400 to 600 mg/day if control of the arrhythmia is achieved. Lidocaine is given intravenously in 100-mg bolus doses every 3 to 5 minutes, followed by continuous infusion of 15 to 50 μg/kg of body weight/min as required to maintain control of the rhythm disturbances.

POTASSIUM. Therapy with potassium is recommended for ectopic tachyarrhythmias when hypokalemia is present, but it must be used with caution in other circumstances because of the risks associated with hyperkalemia. Particular care is necessary when conduction disturbances are present, since elevations of plasma potassium concentrations may impair atrioventricular conduction.

BETA-ADRENERGIC BLOCKADE. Beta blockers are useful in the treatment of some digitalis-toxic arrhythmias. They cause decreases in automaticity, shorten the refractory period of atrial muscle, ventricular muscle, and Purkinje fibers, and slow the conduction velocity. Potential undesirable effects include depression of atrioventricular conduction and of sinoatrial and atrioventricular junctional pacemakers with asystole or marked bradycardia, and depression of myocardial contractility with hemodynamic deterioration. Use of a beta blocker with a short duration of action, such as esmolol, may be preferable as an initial step when this therapeutic approach is attempted.

DIRECT-CURRENT COUNTERSHOCK (see also p. 1248). Whereas countershock is generally inadvisable in the presence of digitalis intoxication because of the severe arrhythmias that may ensue, it must occasionally be used when all other methods have failed in the face of a life-threatening rhythm disturbance. The risk is decreased when lower energy levels are employed.[315]

CARDIAC GLYCOSIDE–BINDING RESINS AND HEMOPERFUSION. As previously noted (p. 486), digitoxin undergoes some enterohepatic circulation, and agents that bind the drug within the gastrointestinal lumen should shorten its half-life. Cholestyramine induced a modest reduction in serum half-life from 6.0 to 4.5 days after tritiated digitoxin administration in humans, and colestipol appears to have a similar effect.[320] These effects may provide a means of reducing the duration of digitoxin toxicity but are probably not of sufficient magnitude or rapidity to be of great importance in the management of severe, life-threatening toxicity. Limited clinical experience with extracorporeal hemoperfusion through columns containing immobilized antidigoxin antibodies has been reported.[321]

REVERSAL OF TOXICITY BY SPECIFIC ANTIBODY. The mechanism for the reversal of both inotropic and arrhythmogenic effects of cardiac glycosides with the use of cardiac glycoside–specific antibodies and their Fab fragments was suggested in experiments demonstrating that high-affinity cardiac glycoside–specific antibodies are able to reverse established glycoside-induced inhibition of myocardial Na^+,K^+-ATPase[322] and monovalent cation active transport.[323]

Fab fragments provide advantages over purified intact antibodies as therapeutic agents. Each intact IgG antibody molecule of molecular weight 150,000 yields two Fab fragments, each of which contains a specific binding site and has a molecular weight of 50,000. This smaller molecular species has a greater rate and volume of distribution after intravenous infusion and reverses experimentally induced digoxin-toxic arrhythmias more rapidly than does intact antibody.[324] Fab fragments are excreted to an appreciable extent in the urine, but intact IgG is not.[325] Rapid reversal of otherwise lethal experimentally induced digitoxin toxicity with specific antibodies and Fab fragments has been demonstrated,[326] together with substantial acceleration by Fab of the renal excretion of digitoxin. This rapid renal excretion of Fab fragments may be of importance in reducing the immunogenicity of the foreign protein.[325]

Several thousand patients with potentially life-threatening digoxin or digitoxin toxicity have been treated with purified digoxin-specified Fab fragments, the first 150 of whom have been reported in detail.[313] Nearly all of these patients had advanced cardiac rhythm disturbances, and in 56 cases hyperkalemia was present as well, due in many to ingestion of very large digitalis doses accidentally or with suicidal intent. All but 15 patients treated had an initial favorable response to intravenously administered Fab, and the diagnosis of digitalis toxicity was doubtful in at least 9 of these 15. In the remaining cases, cardiac arrhythmias and hyperkalemia were fully (119 patients) or partially (14 patients) reversed. This therapeutic approach has been approved by the FDA and is commercially available.[327] Postmarketing surveillance data on 717 patients treated, most in community hospital settings, confirms the findings in the 150 patients treated in the initial multicenter trial.[328]

The safety and efficacy of this approach, in our view, are such that it is recommended in cases of actual or potentially life-threatening digitalis toxicity.

Vasodilators

PATHOPHYSIOLOGICAL CONSIDERATIONS. Cardiac performance can be affected profoundly by alterations in the resistance and capacitance of the peripheral vascular bed. The response of the left ventricle to an augmentation of afterload is a direct function of myocardial contractility. When contractility is normal, elevating afterload leads to an increase in stroke work, with little elevation of ventricular end-diastolic volume or pressure and with little decline in stroke volume. In patients with left ventricular dysfunction, as afterload is increased further, stroke work fails to rise and stroke volume declines, while left ventricular end-diastolic pressure and volume rise even further.

In patients with congestive heart failure the arterial and venous beds are often inappropriately constricted.[329] The vasoconstriction is related to the same phenomenon observed in other conditions, such as hypovolemic shock, in which there is a reduction of cardiac output; the survival value of this fundamental response is to maintain perfusion of vital organs, such as the brain and the heart, at the expense of less immediately essential vascular beds, such as skin, gut, and kidney. While this maintenance of perfusion pressure may be a desirable evolutionary development insofar as the stress of hypovolemia is concerned, it is of little value and actually may be deleterious in patients with heart failure. (Presumably there is little evolutionary advantage to the survival of individuals with heart failure.) At least five mechanisms appear to be involved in the inappropriate vasoconstriction in heart failure: (1) increased adrenergically mediated vasoconstrictor tone; (2) elevated concentrations of circulating catecholamines; (3) increased elaboration of renin, with resultant increases in the potent vasoconstrictor angiotensin II; (4) elevated levels of circulating arginine vasopressin; and (5) increased thickness of arteriolar walls, presumably related to extracellular fluid accumulation in the blood vessels themselves.[330]

Venoconstriction tends to displace blood into the thorax, causing pulmonary congestion, while *arteriolar constriction* increases the impedance to left ventricular emptying. The combination of ventricular dilation induced by the cardiac lesion (augmented by the blood volume redistribution resulting from venoconstriction) and elevated vascular resistance, operating through Laplace's law (p. 377), increases the afterload on the failing myocardium, which is operating on the flat portion of its function curve (Fig. 17–14). Under these circumstances further elevation of preload increases pulmonary congestion but fails to raise cardiac output. Instead, the augmented afterload reduces myocardial fiber shortening and reduces stroke volume further, leading to a vicious circle (Fig. 17–15).

Eichna et al. were the first to demonstrate the effects of vasodilatation (by means of the intravenous infusion of the ganglionic blocking agent trimethaphan (Arfonad) in patients with heart failure.[331] Cardiac output rose and pulmonary capillary pressure fell. These investigators appreciated the significance of this observation when they noted, "Presumably, lowering the pressure against which the heart must eject blood permits an impaired myocardium to expel more blood without an intrinsic improvement in myocardial activity. Such a result may be of advantage to the circulation where a failing myocardium is not capable of improvement and greater work."

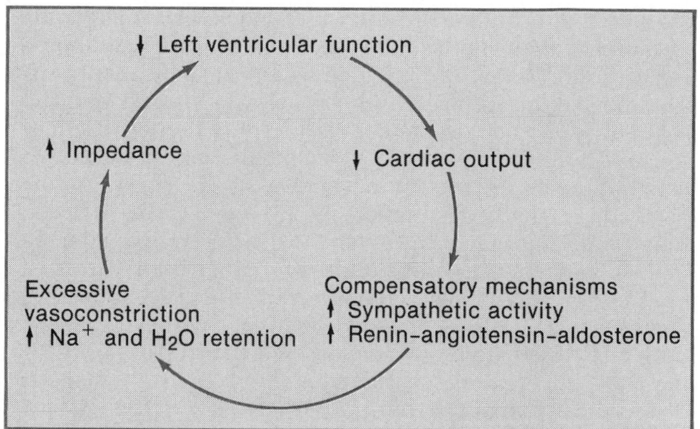

FIGURE 17–15. Compensatory mechanisms in congestive heart failure. H_2O, water; Na^+, increased sodium. (From Helfant, R. H.: Short- and long-term mechanisms of sudden cardiac death in congestive heart failure. Am. J. Cardiol. *65:*41K, 1990, p. 42.)

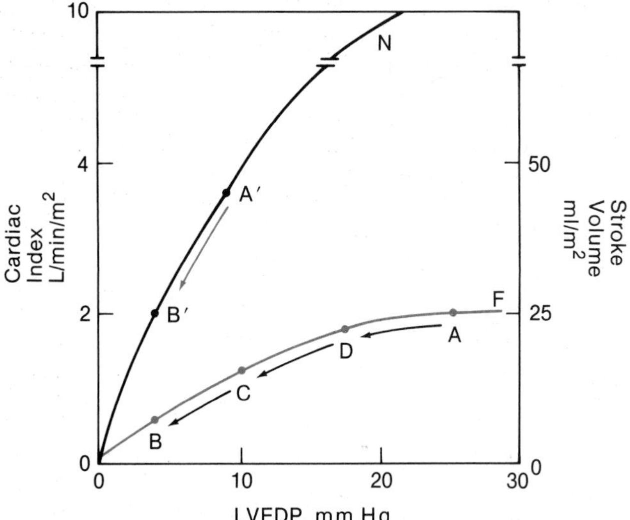

FIGURE 17–14. Effect of venodilator or diuretic therapy in a normal (N) subject (A′ → B′) and in a patient with heart failure (F) and markedly elevated left ventricular filling pressure (A → D), moderately elevated filling pressure (D → C), and normal filling pressure (C → B). In all instances venodilators or diuretic therapy results in a decline in filling pressure; except in the patient with marked elevation of filling pressure, cardiac output declines.

Intraarterial counterpulsation, a mechanical technique that reduces left ventricular afterload (p. 379), appears to have been the first deliberate clinical use of afterload reduction in the treatment of left ventricular failure,[332] although effective treatment of hypertension with antihypertensive drugs undoubtedly had also achieved this goal. Majid et al. then infused the alpha-adrenoceptor blocking agent phentolamine into normotensive patients with persistent left ventricular dysfunction after myocardial infarction and demonstrated that the induced fall in systemic vascular resistance was accompanied by considerable elevation of cardiac output and reduction in pulmonary artery pressure.[333] Since that report, vasodilators have achieved wide use in the treatment of heart failure.[335–344]

With few exceptions, vasodilators do not exert a direct effect on myocardium (phosphodiesterase inhibitors such as amrinone are both potent vasodilators and positive inotropic agents [p. 503]), but their ability to relax vascular smooth muscle, directly or indirectly, can result in marked improvement in both the clinical and hemodynamic state of the patient. By dilating arterioles and/or veins, these agents have the capacity to alter profoundly the loading conditions on the heart and thereby to modify cardiac performance. Arteriolar dilation results in a reduction in afterload and may augment cardiac output, while venodilation tends to produce a reduction in preload, to lower ventricular filling pressure, and to reduce symptoms of pulmonary congestion. Patients with mitral or tricuspid regurgitation derive particular benefit[345,346] that is sustained during upright exercise.[347]

VENODILATORS. Vasodilators with a venodilator action reduce toward normal the elevated intrathoracic blood volume characteristic of heart failure. Since the capacity of the venous bed (also referred to as the capacitance bed) is large, a relatively small reduction in venous tone can result in the pooling of substantial quantities of blood in this bed and its redistribution from the pulmonary to the systemic circuit.[344]

The acute hemodynamic effects of a pure systemic venodilator resemble those of a diuretic (Fig. 17–14) and cause a shift to the left along a given ventricular function curve. In a normal subject this reduction in preload can result in an undesirable decline in cardiac output (A′ → B′) and can cause postural hypotension, which is in fact often observed in patients without heart failure who take large doses of nitrates. In contrast, patients with heart failure and elevated filling pressures generally tolerate venodilators, such as nitrates, quite well. In patients with heart failure but normal filling pressure, perhaps from previous diuresis, venodilation may also result in a decline in cardiac output (C → B). In patients with heart failure and an elevated filling pressure, venodilation can reduce filling pressure and thereby relieve symptoms of pulmonary congestion without depressing cardiac output (A → D). Intermediate responses are observed in patients with moderate elevation of filling pressures (D → C).

Despite the impressive hemodynamic benefits that accompany vasodilator administration, especially in acute studies of supine patients, accumulating evidence supports the view that amelioration of the hemodynamic derangements that accompany left ventricular dysfunction is not the only important element in the treatment of heart failure.[348] Neurohormonal activation (p. 408) clearly plays an important part in the syndrome of congestive heart failure. Hence, the choice of vasodilator should take into account long-term effects on the neurohormonal milieu. Most important, of course, will be data from well-designed clinical trials testing safety, symptomatic efficacy, and survival effects of candidate drugs.

EFFECTS ON SURVIVAL. In addition to the well-recognized beneficial effects on signs and symptoms of heart failure, at the time of this writing improved survival has been demonstrated in three controlled clinical trials of vasodilator therapy. The VHeFT-I trial compared the survival of 642 patients with mild to moderate heart failure maintained on a regimen of diuretics and digoxin and then randomized to the combination of hydralazine (up to 300 mg daily) plus isosorbide dinitrate (up to 40 mg four times a day), the alpha$_1$-adrenergic blocking agent prazosin, or placebo.[11,349] The hydralazine–isosorbide dinitrate combination produced a modest but clinically significant improvement in survival at 6 months and 1 year that was sustained at 42 months. The benefit of treatment with hydralazine and isosorbide dinitrate was particularly prominent in younger patients with a lower ejection fraction, those with a history of hypertension, and those without a history of alcohol abuse.[349]

The CONSENSUS trial[12] tested the effect of the angiotensin-converting enzyme (ACE) inhibitor enalapril against a placebo control in a randomized, double-blind trial in 253 patients with advanced (NYHA Class IV) heart failure, who were also maintained on a regimen of diuretics and digoxin. The positive effect of enalapril on survival is summarized in Figure 17–16*A*; the beneficial effect of captopril on survival in patients with less severe heart failure is shown in Figure 17–16*B*.

The second Veterans Affairs Cooperative Vasodilator-Heart Failure Trial (VHeFT-II) was completed in February 1991 after a 6-month to 5-year follow-up of 804 patients with stable congestive heart failure.[5a] The patients were treated with digoxin and diuretic and were randomized double-blind to treatment with the converting enzyme inhibitor enalapril 20 mg daily (403 patients) or the vasodilator combination of hydralazine 300 mg daily and isosorbide dinitrate 160 mg daily (401 patients). Annual mortality rate in the enalapril group was 11.4 per cent compared with 14.0 per cent in the vasodilator com-

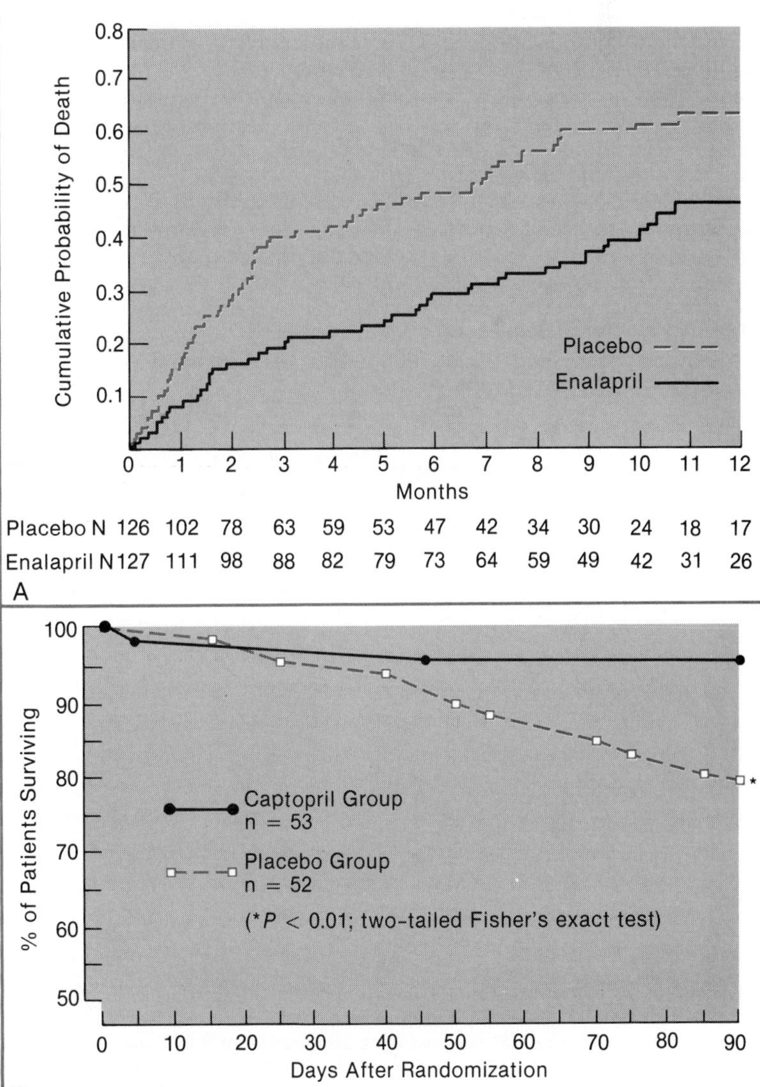

FIGURE 17–16. ***A,*** **Cumulative probability of death in the placebo and enalapril groups in the CONSENSUS trial** ***B,*** **Influence of converting-enzyme inhibition (with captopril) on mortality in moderately severe chronic congestive heart failure: The Captopril Multicenter Heart Failure Trial. (Reprinted by permission from CONSENSUS Trial Study Group: Effects of enalapril on mortality in severe congestive heart failure: Results of the Cooperative North Scandinavian Enalapril Survival Study [CONSENSUS].** ***316:*** **1429, 1987.)**

bination group. Survival on enalapril treatment was significantly ($p < 0.05$) better than on hydralazine-isosorbide dinitrate during the first 2 years after randomization. Since annual mortality rate in a placebo-treated group of similar patients in VHeFT-I was 20 per cent,[4] it can be inferred that both treatment regimens in VHeFT-II had a favorable effect on survival. An important finding in this trial is that the ACE inhibitor was superior to the combination of nonspecific vasodilators insofar as survival was concerned. It should be noted that the design of this trial tended to exclude patients with active ischemic heart disease, both in terms of the exercise capacity entry criterion and the exclusion of patients receiving beta blockers.

The SOLVD trial[5] randomized 2569 patients with moderate to moderately severe heart failure (87 per cent were in NYHA Classes II and III) and an ejection fraction <35 per cent to standard treatment plus placebo or enalapril. During a follow-up averaging 41 months there was a significant (16 per cent) reduction in mortality (from 39.7 per cent to 35.2 per cent) in the enalapril-treated group.

Treatment with vasodilators of asymptomatic patients or those with mild symptoms has been controversial.[350,351] The argument in favor of such treatment, which by definition can have no effect on symptoms, rests on the hypothesis that vasodilator therapy can alter the natural history of the syndrome in patients with left ventricular dysfunction. Several trials are currently under way to test this hypothesis.

CHOICE OF VASODILATOR. From a theoretical point of view, the administration of a pure vasodilator whose principal action is on the *venous system* is (1) desirable in patients whose principal clinical manifestation of heart failure is pulmonary congestion secondary to elevated left ventricular filling pressure; (2) undesirable in patients in whom the preload or filling pressure has already been restored to normal by means of diuretic therapy and/or dietary sodium restriction; and (3) useful in combination with arteriolar dilators in patients whose clinical manifestations of failure are related to both reduction of perfusion and pulmonary congestion.[352]

Arteriolar Dilators. These agents, exemplified by hydralazine or prazosin, act as afterload-reducing agents. As shown in Figure 17–17, at any level of preload and myocardial contractility, the extent of myocardial fiber shortening (and therefore stroke volume) is inversely related to the afterload. Afterload is related to the instantaneous stress in the muscle fibers of the ventricle (p. 379), which is also closely related to

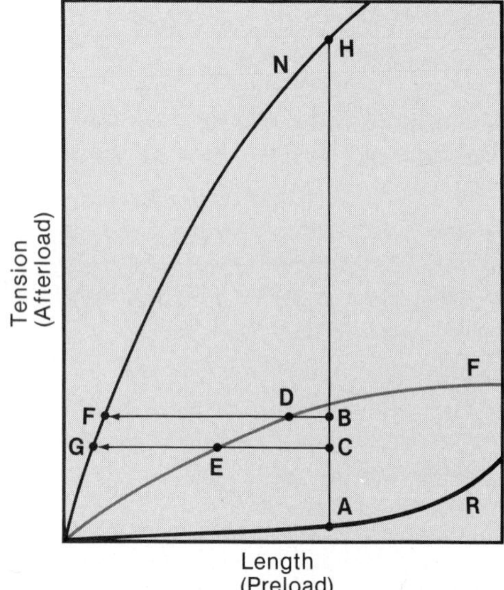

FIGURE 17–17. Length-tension relations in normal (N) and failing (F) heart muscle. R = length-resting tension curve for both normal and failing heart muscle. The effects of reducing afterload from B to C on shortening are contrasted. In the normal muscle, shortening increases only slightly (from B → F to C → G). In failing muscle, there is substantial enhancement of shortening (B → D to C → E). H represents isometric tension development by normal muscle.

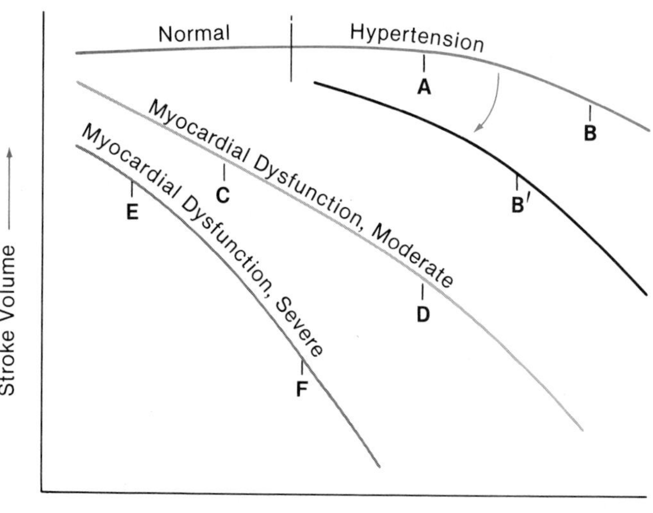

FIGURE 17–18. Relation of left ventricular stroke volume to systemic outflow resistance in normal and diseased hearts. A family of curves may be described, depending on the severity of the myocardial disease. If cardiac function is normal, a rise in resistance results in hypertension, since cardiac output remains fairly constant. Heart failure in a hypertensive patient could be shown by a move to either point B, a high resistance with normal function, or point B′, which represents a shift to a slightly depressed ventricular function curve. When myocardial dysfunction is more severe, as shown by the lower two curves, blood pressure is no longer directly determined by resistance, since stroke volume and resistance are inversely related. Consequently, arterial pressure may be similar at points E and F despite marked differences in cardiac output and resistance. It is also apparent that a reduction in outflow resistance will not affect significantly the stroke volume of the normal ventricle. However, it can produce a marked increase in the stroke volume on the failing ventricle (F → E). (Reproduced with permission from Cohn, J. N., and Franciosa, J. A.: Vasodilator therapy of cardiac failure. N. Engl. J. Med. *297:*27, 1977.)

the aortic impedance, i.e., the instantaneous relationship between pressure and flow in the aorta during ejection, and, in turn, to systemic vascular resistance. Just as hemodynamic and clinical effects of venodilation and the resultant reduction of ventricular preload depend on the filling pressure, so do the effects of afterload depend on myocardial contractility. Figure 17–17 displays, in schematic form, the acute effects of afterload reduction on ventricular fiber shortening in normal and failing hearts. In the normal heart a reduction in afterload (B → C) results in only minor augmentation of myocardial fiber shortening (B → F to C → G). In contrast, an identical reduction in afterload in the failing heart causes substantial augmentation of myocardial fiber shortening (B → D to C → E). The reduction of stroke volume caused by an increased afterload is substantially greater in the presence of myocardial dysfunction than in the normal heart (Fig. 17–18). A corollary is that any given reduction of afterload will cause a greater increase in stroke volume in the failing than in the normal heart.

In patients with heart failure the reduction in systemic vascular resistance induced by vasodilators is usually offset by an increase in cardiac output, and arterial pressure may decline only slightly or not at all. Since the reduction of systemic vascular resistance induced by arteriolar vasodilators in normal subjects is associated with no or only small increases in cardiac output (Fig. 17–19) (A′ → H′), their administration to normotensive subjects without heart failure may cause postural hypotension accompanied by reflex tachycardia. In patients with depressed contractility without elevation of filling pressure, arteriolar dilation may produce a small augmentation of cardiac output (C → H″). However, in contrast to the situation existing in patients with markedly elevated preload, arterial pressure may decline.

Balanced Vasodilators. Many vasodilators, such as angiotensin-converting enzyme inhibitors, and the combination of hydralazine and isosorbide dinitrate, act on both the arterial and the venous beds (so-called balanced vasodilators), and their actions are intermediate between those of pure venous and pure arterial dilators and resemble those of a combination (Fig. 17–19). In normal subjects (A′ → P′) and in patients with heart disease but without elevated ventricular filling pressure (C → P″), balanced dilators usually cause reductions in filling pressure, arterial pressure, and cardiac output. Patients with heart failure and pulmonary congestion who are given balanced vasodilators display favorable effects (A → P), with augmentation of cardiac output and reduction of capillary pressure but little decline in arterial pressure or elevation of heart rate.

From these considerations, it is apparent that patients with depressed myocardial contractility and elevation of filling pressure are likely to show hemodynamic benefit from vasodilator therapy. Arterial dilators cause an increase in cardiac output, while venodilators reduce pulmonary congestion and balanced dilators cause a combination of these effects. Patients with heart disease and left ventricular dysfunction without elevated vascular resistance, depressed cardiac output, and elevated filling pressures are unlikely to benefit immediately from the use of vasodilators, although, as stated earlier, the effects long term — reducing the incidence of heart failure and cardiac dilation — as well as on survival, may prove to be beneficial. It must be also recognized that improvement in cardiac output in short-term studies is not always predictive of improved blood flow to relevant regional vascular beds, especially in long-term use.[353] ACE inhibitors have shown the most consistently beneficial effects on skeletal muscle blood flow during exercise in heart failure patients.[354]

Although classification of vasodilators as arterial, venous, or balanced has proved to be useful in understanding their actions and sometimes in the selection of a particular agent for a specific patient, the intimate interactions between cardiac preload and afterload that exist in the intact circulation must be considered. Since afterload is a function of intraventricular pressure and ventricular volume, a pure venodilator would be expected, by reducing ventricular volume, to also lower afterload. Conversely, an arterial dilator, by enhancing stroke volume and ventricular emptying, will reduce ventricular volume (preload). This reduction in ventricular size combines with lowering arterial pressures to cause a proportionately greater reduction of systolic wall tension (afterload) than of arterial pressure.

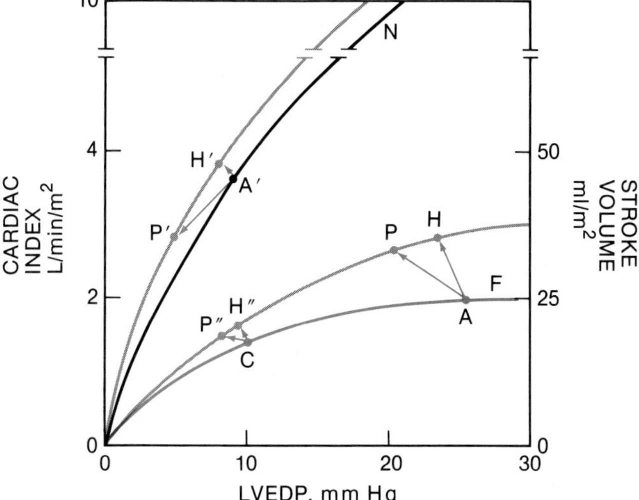

FIGURE 17–19. Effects of various vasodilators on the relationship between left ventricular end-diastolic pressure (LVEDP) and cardiac index or stroke volume in normal (N) and failing (F) hearts. H represents hydralazine or any other pure arterial dilator. It produces only a minimal increase in cardiac index in the normal subject (A′ → H′) or in the patient with heart failure with normal LVEDP (C → H″). In contrast, it elevates output in the patient with heart failure and elevated LVEDP (A → H). P represents a balanced vasodilator, such as sodium nitroprusside or prazosin. It reduces filling pressure in all patients, elevates cardiac output in patients with heart failure and elevated LVEDP (A → P), lowers cardiac output in normal subjects (A′ → P′), and has little effect on cardiac output in heart failure patients with normal filling pressures (C → P″).

Because wall tension is a principal determinant of myocardial oxygen consumption ($M\dot{V}O_2$) (p. 1162) and because vasodilators reduce wall tension in patients with heart failure, they also reduce $M\dot{V}O_2$ while increasing cardiac output. These actions of vasodilators compare favorably with those of positive inotropic agents or beta-adrenoceptor blocking agents. The former (like vasodilators) augment cardiac output but either increase $M\dot{V}O_2$ or at least maintain it at a constant level; the latter (like vasodilators) reduce $M\dot{V}O_2$ but depress cardiac performance.

MONITORING. The monitoring of vasodilators when they are used in the treatment of acute myocardial infarction is discussed on page 499. When drugs are given to patients with critical coronary artery obstructions, particularly with acute ischemia, reductions in coronary perfusion pressure in the face of critical coronary obstruction can further impair blood flow through narrowed coronary arteries and through collateral vessels, and thereby this therapy can intensify ischemia. Therefore, vasodilator therapy must be employed cautiously in patients with severe obstructive coronary artery disease, particularly in those with acute myocardial infarction or other acute ischemic syndromes. Arterial pressure should be monitored carefully during intravenously administered vasodilator therapy, particularly in patients with severe coronary artery disease. In view of the importance of ventricular filling pressure as a determinant of the response to a vasodilator (Figs. 17–14 and 17–19), the monitoring of pulmonary capillary wedge or pulmonary artery pressure by means of a Swan-Ganz catheter is helpful in regulating dosage of vasodilator during intravenous therapy. Because in addition to the reduction in pulmonary wedge pressure, the increase of cardiac output is an important endpoint, it is often desirable to make serial measurements of cardiac output in acutely ill patients receiving intravenous vasodilators.

In patients without ischemic heart disease, monitoring of intraarterial pressure during intravenous vasodilator therapy is desirable but is not essential as long as indirect pressure is measured at frequent intervals. Invasive monitoring is not necessary in patients treated for prolonged periods with agents administered orally, sublingually, or transdermally. However, it is desirable to make frequent measurements of arterial pressure in the supine and upright positions when therapy is initiated or the dosage is being adjusted.

VASODILATOR AGENTS

(Table 17–10)

SODIUM NITROPRUSSIDE. Probably the most widely used vasodilator in the treatment of acute congestive heart failure, sodium nitroprusside is extremely short acting and must be given as a continuous intravenous infusion. It acts directly to relax vascular smooth muscle in both arterioles and veins. Sodium nitroprusside had been employed successfully for many years to treat hypertensive crisis (p. 871) and subsequently was introduced for the treatment of congestive heart failure.[355] Since sodium nitroprusside is a balanced dilator, its hemodynamic action in the presence of severe impairment of left ventricular failure is both to increase cardiac output and reduce pulmonary congestion (Fig. 17–19). It is particularly useful in patients with severe hypertension associated with left ventricular failure, severe heart failure associated with mitral and/or aortic regurgitation, acute myocardial infarction, acute heart failure following cardiac surgery, and in patients with acute intensification of chronic heart failure. It should *not* be administered to patients with hypotension. The initial infusion rate in adults is usually 10 μg/min, and this may be increased by increments of 5 to 10 μg/min every 5 minutes until the desired effect is achieved, until hypotension or other side effects limit further dose increments, or a maximum dose of 300 μg/min is achieved.

TABLE 17-10 MAJOR VASODILATOR DRUGS*

DRUG	MECHANISM OF ACTION	VENOUS DILATING EFFECT (PRELOAD REDUCTION)	ARTERIOLAR DILATING EFFECT (AFTERLOAD REDUCTION)	USUAL DOSAGE	COMMENTS
Nitroglycerin	Direct	+++	+	25–500 μg/min IV 5–60 mg transdermal	Tolerance may be a problem with sustained continuous use.
Isosorbide dinitrate	Direct	+++	+	5–20 mg q 2 hr SL 10–60 mg q 4 hr p.o.	Improved survival shown in chronic CHF when used with hydralazine.
Nitroprusside	Direct	+++	+++	5–150 μg/min IV	Used IV only. Drug is light sensitive
Hydralazine	Direct	–	+++	10–100 mg q 6 hr p.o.	Sustained benefit in heart failure not shown when used as sole vasodilator.
Prostacyclin	Direct	+++	+++	5–15 ng/kg/min IV	Investigational use only.
Phenoxybenzamine	Alpha-adrenoceptor blockade (nonselective)	++	++	10–20 mg q 8 hr p.o.	Limited current use.
Phentolamine	Alpha-adrenoceptor blockade (nonselective)	++	++	50 mg q 4–6 hr p.o.	Limited current use.
Prazosin	Alpha-adrenoceptor blockade (α selective)	+++	++	1–5 mg q 6 hr p.o.	Extra caution required with initial doses.
Trimazosin	Alpha-adrenoceptor blockade plus undetermined mechanism	+++	++	50–450 mg b.i.d. p.o.	Investigational use only.
Captopril	Angiotensin-converting enzyme inhibitor	++	++	6.25–25.0 mg q 6–8 hr p.o.	Approved by FDA for use in chronic CHF. Acute renal failure can occur with initial doses; initiate use with extra caution.
Enalapril	Angiotensin-converting enzyme inhibitor	++	++	2.5 mg q.i.d. to 15 mg p.o. b.i.d.	Approved by FDA for treatment of hypertension and CHF.
Lisinopril	Angiotensin-converting enzyme inhibitor	++	++	5–40 mg q.i.d.	Approved by FDA for treatment of hypertension.
Nifedipine	Calcium channel blockade	+	++	10–40 mg q 6 hr p.o. 10–40 mg q 6 hr SL	Negative inotropic effect may be unmasked in severe CHF.

* All of these agents may cause severe hypotension, and special caution is required with initial use, particularly in patients with severe CHF.
SL = sublingual.

The most important adverse side effect of sodium nitroprusside is hypotension, an extension of its therapeutic action, which is typically reversed within 10 minutes after discontinuation of the drug. If this waiting period poses a danger, hypotension can be treated more rapidly by infusion of a vasoconstrictor such as phenylephrine or norepinephrine. Nitroprusside releases hydrocyanic acid, which could lead to cyanide poisoning.[355] However, this is an extremely uncommon complication, since hydrocyanic acid is converted to thiocyanate in the presence of thiosulfate. Thiocyanate is excreted by the kidney, and in the presence of renal insufficiency the infusion of large doses of nitroprusside for a prolonged period may lead to thiocyanate toxicity, which is characterized by convulsions, psychosis, abdominal pain, hypothyroidism, muscle twitching, and dizziness. Therefore, when patients receive nitroprusside for more than a few days, serum levels of thiocyanate should be measured and not allowed to exceed 6 mg/100 ml. Methemoglobinemia and vitamin B_{12} deficiency are two other rare complications of nitroprusside therapy. In patients with chronic pulmonary disease, nitroprusside can cause hypoxia due to pulmonary vascular dilation and perfusion of poorly ventilated alveoli.

As described later, for enhanced effect, nitroprusside may be infused in combination with positive inotropic agents such as dobutamine.

ANGIOTENSIN-CONVERTING ENZYME (ACE) INHIBITORS. The renin-angiotensin-aldosterone axis is activated in patients with overt congestive heart failure, and circulating levels of all three substances are often elevated. This has led to the use of captopril,[336,338,356,357] enalapril,[337,358-360] and lisinopril,[361-364] orally active drugs that block the enzymatic conversion of angiotensin I to angiotensin II, in the management of heart failure. ACE inhibitors are balanced vasodilators with actions on both the arteriolar and venous beds, and in sufficient doses they cause reductions in systemic vascular resistance and arterial pressure. ACE inhibition is particularly marked in arterioles that are highly sensitive to angiotensin II, such as those in the renal arterial bed.

ACE inhibitors depress circulating levels of angiotensin II and markedly elevate plasma renin activity. Also, by interfering with the breakdown of bradykinin, ACE inhibitors increase the circulating level of this vasodilator; this action, as well as possible increases in circulating prostaglandins, may play a role in the vasodilator action of these drugs.[365,366] Effects on tissue as well as plasma ACE may be important in the overall effects of ACE inhibitors.[367] Interestingly, it appears that the major pathway in human myocardium for angiotensin II formation from angiotensin I is not blocked by ACE inhibitors, suggesting a sustained or even enhanced positive inotropic effect of angiotensin in patients receiving ACE inhibitors.[368] In addition, ACE inhibitors tend to decrease circulating catecholamine concentrations at rest and particularly with exercise[369-371] and to restore toward normal downregulated beta-adrenergic receptors on lymphocytes of patients with chronic heart failure.[372] The latter effect was accompanied by an increase in levels of the stimulatory guanine nucleotide regulatory protein (G protein) that couples agonist occupancy of the beta receptor to an increase in adenylyl cyclase activity.[372]

In patients with heart failure, ACE inhibition causes left and right ventricular filling pressures to decline and cardiac output may rise modestly, but there is usually little or no change in the heart rate and arterial pressure. With captopril, the action begins $\frac{1}{2}$ hour after ingestion, is maximal at 1 to $1\frac{1}{2}$

hours, and persists for 6 to 8 hours. Treatment is usually begun with 12.5 mg three times a day; maximal effects are observed with 50 mg three times a day. The action of enalapril resembles that of captopril except that it has a slower onset and a longer duration (12 to 24 hours), permitting twice- and, in some patients, even once-a-day dosing.[373] The pro-drug enalapril is deesterified in the liver to the active form, enalaprilat. Enalaprilat has been reported to have a negative inotropic effect when infused directly into the coronary artery,[374] but this has not proven to be a problem in clinical use. The initial dose, which rarely causes hypotension or renal failure, is 2.5 mg, and the maintenance dose ranges between 10 mg every day and 15 mg twice a day. With careful attention to patient selection and appropriately small starting doses, patient tolerance of enalapril in clinical trials has been good.[375,376] Lisinopril's action commences 1 hour after ingestion, is maximal at 6 hours, and persists for 24 hours. The starting dose is 5 mg/day; the average and maximum maintenance doses are 20 mg/day and 40 mg/day, respectively.

ACE inhibitors have been reported to improve hemodynamics in patients with congestive heart failure that is poorly controlled by digitalis and diuretics,[377–379] to restore responsiveness to diuretics, and to restore serum sodium levels in azotemic hyponatremic patients with heart failure.[380]

As is the case with hypertension, ACE inhibitors appear to be effective in heart failure, regardless of the level of plasma renin[381]; they have been shown to be effective clinically even in patients with low plasma renin activity. ACE inhibition augments skeletal muscle flow in normal subjects and, in response to exercise, in patients with severe chronic heart failure who respond positively to captopril.[382] It reduces renal and vascular resistance and increases renal blood flow in patients with heart failure.[383] By reducing arterial pressure without causing reflex tachycardia, captopril lowers myocardial oxygen demands and thereby may exert an antianginal effect.[384]

The clinical benefits of ACE inhibitors in heart failure are impressive. These drugs enhance the sense of well-being in the majority of patients. In double-blind, placebo-controlled trials, ACE inhibitors exert a number of salutary effects, including symptomatic improvement,[335,385] less frequent clinical deterioration during follow-up,[359] sustained improvement of exercise tolerance[10,335–337,360,386] (Fig. 17–13), and hemodynamic improvement and reduction in cardiac dimensions.[337,385] ACE inhibition is effective for relief of symptoms in patients with mild[358] as well as with severe heart failure.

In a randomized trial carried out on 253 patients with severe heart failure, the previously mentioned CONSENSUS trial,[11] the 6-month survival of patients who received enalapril, digitalis, and diuretics was 74 per cent, significantly greater than that of patients receiving diuretics and digitalis alone (56 per cent). Clinical symptoms were improved among survivors in the enalapril-treated group. The entire reduction in mortality was found in patients dying from progressive heart failure; no difference was observed in the incidence of sudden cardiac death.[11] In further follow-up for 8.5 months from the end of blinded therapy, all patients originally randomized were encouraged to begin or continue enalapril. Mortality was markedly lower in patients treated with enalapril than in those not started on the drug (16 per cent vs. 61 per cent).[387] Thus, further follow-up data from the CONSENSUS trial strongly support the original findings with respect to reduced mortality in enalapril-treated patients with severe heart failure maintained on a regimen of digoxin and diuretics. Retrospective review of data from the Captopril Multicenter Trial also found improved survival among NYHA Class II and III patients randomized to captopril (versus placebo) in addition to digitalis and diuretics.[388] These studies, together with SOLVD,[5] VHeFT-I[11] and VHeFT-II,[5a] indicate that survival of patients with heart failure can be improved with vasodilator therapy. VHeFT-II demonstrated the superiority of an ACE inhibitor over the combination of hydralazine and isosorbide dinitrate[5a] which had been shown in VHeFT-I to be superior to placebo insofar as survival is concerned.[11]

ACE inhibitors tend to increase serum potassium levels and must be used with caution, if at all, with potassium supplements and/or potassium-sparing diuretics (except in the presence of hypokalemia).[389] Excessive hypotension is the major hazard, especially in patients who are already being treated with diuretics. The best way to avoid this problem is to begin with one-half of the recommended starting dose, observing the patient, and if no postural hypotension occurs, increasing the next dose. ACE inhibitors are contraindicated in patients with intrinsic renal disease with renal failure, bilateral renal artery stenosis, and in patients with systemic hypotension. Adverse effects on renal function are well documented[390–392] and appear to be more likely to occur in patients with hyponatremia, diabetes mellitus, or markedly increased plasma renin activity, in patients who have received large doses of loop diuretics, and in those who have been treated with nonsteroidal antiinflammatory agents.[393] Other adverse effects that are quite uncommon include angioedema and neutropenia.[361–364,373,375,376,387–389,393–396] The lack of arterial unsaturation, regularly observed with the use of other vasodilators, suggests that ACE inhibitors do not produce significant pulmonary arteriovenous shunting.

NITRATES (see also p. 1304). Nitroglycerin and the closely related long-acting nitrates such as isosorbide dinitrate and pentaerythritol tetranitrate are vasodilators that act on vascular smooth muscle, principally on the venous bed, the pulmonary arterial bed, and, to a lesser extent, on the systemic arteriolar bed. These drugs are available in a variety of formulations[10,397,398] and can be administered by various routes (Table 40–2, p. 1306), making them useful in a number of situations. In normal individuals and in patients with heart failure but without elevated filling pressure, the prominent venodilator action results in reduction of cardiac output (Fig. 17–16) and often postural hypotension. However, in patients with heart failure and elevated pulmonary capillary pressure, even when secondary to myocardial infarction, nitroglycerin reduces ventricular filling pressure and relieves congestive symptoms. The pulmonary vasodilating and slight systemic arteriolar dilating effects of the drug are sufficient to cause a modest increase in cardiac output as well,[399] if ventricular filling pressures are maintained in an adequate range.

Nitroglycerin. When administered sublingually, nitroglycerin is useful in the treatment of acute congestive heart failure in the absence of hypotension. It is usually administered in a dose of 0.3 to 1.2 mg; the effect usually begins within 2 minutes, becomes maximal in 8 minutes, and persists for 15 to 30 minutes. In patients in whom left ventricular filling pressure is elevated to 20 mm Hg, it usually declines to approximately 10 mm Hg in 5 to 10 minutes following nitroglycerin use.[400] Although slight reduction of arterial pressure may be accompanied by a mild acceleration of heart rate, $M\dot{V}O_2$ declines, and this is a major mechanism for the antianginal effect of the drug (p. 1304). Since the absorption of sublingual nitroglycerin may be erratic, continuous intravenous infusion has been utilized to produce a sustained, controllable effect in patients with acute heart failure and pulmonary congestion in whom predominant venodilation is desired. The initial dose is 10 μg/min and may be increased by increments of 10 μg/min every 5 minutes to a maximal dose of 100 μg/min.

Topical Nitroglycerin. This may be used for a prolonged duration of action; effects of the ointment last at least 3 hours. Depending on the dose desired, a 0.5- to 4.0-inch strip is applied to the skin, usually on the chest. Although topical administration does not make nitroglycerin ointment convenient for ambulatory patients, an advantage of this formulation is that it can be removed readily in case of adverse effects. It can be applied conveniently before retiring and is useful to combat attacks of paroxysmal nocturnal dyspnea. Any of several available transdermal administration systems (nitroglycerin patches or discs) provide a steady rate of absorption and stable venous plasma level for 24 hours. They are more convenient than the ointment for ambulatory patients and allow showering.

Isosorbide Dinitrate. This long-acting nitrate is available in sublingual and oral formulations. The sublingual dose is 2.5 to 10 mg every 2 hours, and the oral dose is 20 to 60 mg every 4 hours. In addition, other long-acting nitrates such as oral pentaerythritol tetranitrate (10 to 40 mg four times a day) or oral controlled-release nitroglycerin preparations (one 6.5-mg capsule every 4 hours) have been employed to achieve a prolonged nitrate effect and have been found useful in the treatment of chronic heart failure.[401,402] The side effects of all nitrates include headache and postural hypotension, but these symptoms are more prominent in patients with mild than severe heart failure and can be controlled by decreasing the dose. Methemoglobinemia, an extremely rare complication, may occur with long-term use of large doses.

There is some evidence from controlled trials that long-term administration of long-acting nitrates reduces symptoms of heart failure and increases exercise tolerance,[398,403] although the available data are limited.[404,405] When used in combination with hydralazine, long-term administration of isosorbide dinitrate was found in the VHeFT-I trial to prolong survival in patients with heart failure.[10]

Nitrate Tolerance (see also p. 1238). An important problem with all sustained-use nitrate preparations in the treatment of heart failure is the development of tolerance.[406,407] The time-course of development of tolerance to a constant intravenous dose of nitroglycerin appears to be more rapid in the pulmonary than in the systemic circulation.[408] The loss of hemodynamic efficacy over time at sustained constant doses may be due to a combination of depletion of sulfhydryl groups in vascular smooth muscle and countervailing neurohormonal activation.[409] Cross-tolerance to different nitrate compounds is regularly observed. Intermittent therapy, allowing several hours each day without nitrate administration, can effectively obviate the problem of nitrate tolerance, permitting longer-term efficacy to be maintained.[403,409]

HYDRALAZINE (see also p. 866). This orally effective vasodilator acts directly on arteriolar smooth muscle.[410] Hydralazine's predominant action on the arterial bed results in an increase in cardiac output with relatively minor reductions in ventricular filling and arterial pressures and increases in heart rate in patients with heart failure.[411] The usual dosage ranges from 25 to 100 mg three to four times daily, and its effects commence within 30 minutes and persist for about 6 hours.

The degree of left ventricular enlargement[412] and the level of peripheral vascular resistance appear to be important determinants of the response of hydralazine in patients with chronic heart failure. Patients with marked cardiomegaly and markedly elevated systemic vascular resistance exhibit the most salutary responses. Long-term hydralazine treatment of minimally symptomatic patients with stable, moderate to severe aortic regurgitation was shown to reduce left ventricular size and to increase ejection fraction at 24 months in a double-blind placebo-controlled trial, suggesting a possible beneficial effect of such therapy on the natural history of the disease.[413]

Side effects include vascular headaches, flushing, nausea, and vomiting, which often disappear with continued therapy. Drug fever and skin rash are seen occasionally; fluid retention and increased edema occur commonly when this drug (as well as other vasodilators) is administered over the long term. The latter complication usually responds readily to an increase in the dose of diuretics. In addition to fluid retention, tolerance to the favorable hemodynamic effects of hydralazine develops in a minority of patients, apparently because of altered responsiveness of vascular smooth muscle to the drug.[414]

A more serious adverse effect, a lupus-like syndrome, is seen in approximately 15 per cent of patients receiving 400 mg of hydralazine daily, and an even higher percentage of patients develops circulating antinuclear antibodies. Although this syndrome is not usually observed in patients who receive less than 200 mg of the drug daily, the average dose required for effective afterload reduction is about 75 mg four times a day, making this complication significant among patients receiving hydralazine. Hydralazine is metabolized principally by acetylation, and patients in whom this process is slow are more likely to develop both the lupus-like syndrome and peripheral neuropathy due to pyridoxine deficiency. Fortunately, the lupus-like syndrome subsides when hydralazine is discontinued. The peripheral neuropathy can be treated or prevented by pyridoxine administration.

The ultimate role of hydralazine in the management of chronic congestive heart failure has been controversial, but recent data from the VHeFT-II trial point to a greater survival benefit of enalapril than of a hydralazine–isosorbide dinitrate combination in patients also treated with diuretics and digoxin.[5a] However, both groups had substantially improved survival compared with a very comparable group of patients followed in the placebo arm of the VHeFT-I trial.[10] Some studies have yielded favorable long-term results with improved exercise capacity and reduced cardiac size on X-ray examination,[415] especially when hydralazine is used in combination with nitrates.[416] Other trials have not demonstrated a difference between hydralazine alone and placebo in long-term treatment of chronic heart failure.[417]

PRAZOSIN (see p. 864). This antihypertensive drug, a quinazoline derivative, is a potent alpha-adrenoceptor blocking agent, the action of which is limited to the vascular adrenergic ($alpha_1$) receptors with little effect on the presynaptic ($alpha_2$) receptors[418] (Fig. 13–18, p. 363). As a consequence, neuronally released norepinephrine is available to act on the $alpha_2$ receptors, inhibiting its own release and preventing development of reflex tachycardia.

Prazosin is an orally effective, balanced vasodilator, equally effective on arterioles and veins, and its circulatory effects resemble those of intravenous nitroprusside. Oral doses show maximum effectiveness in 45 minutes that persists for 6 hours. Tolerance to the drug occurs,[419] and in a long-term comparison of prazosin and captopril the latter was found to be superior in terms of clinical benefit and long-term hemodynamic improvement.[419] As noted above, in the VHeFT-I trial prazosin did not improve long-term patient survival in comparison with placebo.[10] Despite the favorable acute hemodynamic effects exerted by prazosin in heart failure and its value as an antihypertensive the side effects, frequent development of tolerance, and the unimpressive long-term effects do not argue for its use in the long-term treatment of heart failure.

The $alpha_1$-adrenergic antagonist terazosin has also been shown to have favorable acute hemodynamic effects in patients with heart failure,[420] but evidence of long-term efficacy is not yet available.

CALCIUM ANTAGONISTS (see also pp. 683 and 1310). These drugs have potent vasodilator properties that have been found to be of value in patients with chronic coronary artery disease or hypertension. While nifedipine, diltiazem, and several of the newer dihydropyridine derivatives, including nicardipine, nitrendipine, felodipine, and isradipine, have been shown to produce short-term improvement in left ventricular function,[421,422] most studies to date have not shown impressive improvement in short-term or long-term exercise capacity or other evidence of sustained clinical benefit in patients with overt heart failure.[421–425] Even the agents most selective for vascular smooth muscle–relaxant effects have been shown to exert negative inotropic effects[422,424,426] that can lead to hemodynamic or clinical deterioration. In contrast to the generally disappointing results of administration of calcium antagonists to patients with overt congestive heart failure, over the long term beneficial effects have been reported for patients with asymptomatic aortic regurgitation treated for 12 months in a randomized, double-blind placebo-controlled trial of nifedipine.[427,428]

In longer-term use, this class of drugs may also exert adverse effects by activation of endogenous neurohormonal systems, including the sympathetic and particularly the renin-angiotensin systems.[422,425]

Thus, available clinical experience does *not* support the use of calcium channel blockers for long-term management of chronic congestive heart failure.

CLINICAL APPLICATIONS OF VASODILATOR THERAPY

The use of vasodilators in two specific situations, acute pulmonary edema (p. 810) and acute myocardial infarction (p. 1253), is discussed elsewhere.

LEFT VENTRICULAR FAILURE. Vasodilator therapy has proved to be very effective in patients with acute left ventricular decompensation. The intravenous infusion of so-

TABLE 17–11 GUIDELINES FOR INTRAVENOUS VASODILATOR THERAPY IN ACUTE PUMP FAILURE

1. **Determine initial hemodynamics.**
2. **Start therapy with low initial dose (nitroprusside 15 μg/min, phentolamine 0.1 mg/min, or nitroglycerin 10 μg/min).**
3. **Monitor changes in blood pressure, heart rate, left ventricular filling pressure, cardiac output, and systemic vascular resistance.**
4. **If cardiac output increases with decrease in systemic vascular resistance and left ventricular filling pressure, and little change in blood pressure, maintain same infusion rate.**
5. **If above hemodynamic changes do not occur and arterial pressure is maintained, gradually increase infusion rate (every 5 to 15 min).**
6. **If blood pressure decreases without change in cardiac output or left ventricular filling pressure, discontinue vasodilator and substitute or add inotropic agent (dopamine, dobutamine, or amrinone).**
7. **Monitor thiocyanate level during prolonged nitroprusside infusion.**
8. **Substitute oral vasodilator when long-term therapy is indicated.**

Modified from Chatterjee, K.: Digitalis and non-ACE inhibitor vasodilators in heart failure. Cardiol. Clin. 7:110, 1989.

dium nitroprusside is generally associated with clinical improvement, clearing of pulmonary rales, elevation of cardiac output, improvement of peripheral perfusion, and augmented responsiveness to diuretics (Table 17–11). When left ventricular filling pressure has declined to approximately 15 mm Hg and cardiac output has risen to above 2.0 liters/min/m^2, an attempt should be made to wean the patient from the intravenous vasodilator and to convert to one of the oral medications, usually an ACE inhibitor. Although infusion of sodium nitroprusside usually can be discontinued after 48 to 72 hours, it may be necessary to continue it for as long as 7 to 10 days in patients with severe heart failure. The major problem with sodium nitroprusside infusion is hypotension. If, in a previously normotensive patient, systolic arterial pressure falls to below 90 mm Hg or decreases by more than 30 mm Hg from the control level, the drug should be discontinued or the dosage reduced. In patients who become hypotensive but require vasodilator therapy to improve perfusion, a combination of nitroprusside and an inotropic agent (dopamine or dobutamine) should be considered (p. 502). Particular care must be taken to avoid hypotension (and therefore hypoperfusion of myocardium in the distribution of stenotic coronary vessels) in patients with known or suspected coronary artery disease.

Transient myocardial depression during the perioperative period in patients who have undergone cardiac surgery may be associated with increased systemic vascular resistance, and in such cases sodium nitroprusside may be useful. In patients with perioperative depression of cardiac function and hypotension, a sympathomimetic agent and/or intraaortic balloon counterpulsation usually is used in combination with the vasodilator.

Infusion of sodium nitroprusside may also be effective in chronic heart failure that has become refractory to therapy with digitalis and diuretics,[429] although such patients can usually be managed with one of the orally active vasodilators. Patients with borderline elevations of left ventricular filling pressure (12 to 15 mm Hg) derive little benefit from nitroprusside, because the venodilator action results in further reduction of filling pressure with little change, or even a decline, in cardiac output. When filling pressure has been reduced to normal by nitroprusside and the principal hemodynamic abnormality is low cardiac output, cautious intravenous expansion of blood volume and the simultaneous administration of nitroprusside can result in a striking increase in cardiac output.[406] Rebound increases in systemic vascular resistance above baseline, with consequent reduction in cardiac output, have been reported immediately after withdrawal of nitroprusside and are most pronounced in patients who developed tachycardia during infusion of the drug.[384] This phenomenon is presumably due to unopposed vasoconstrictor influences and can be managed by the gradual tapering of nitroprusside and the substitution of an orally effective vasodilator.

MECHANICAL LESIONS. In patients with mitral regurgitation or ventricular septal defect,[430] the abnormal regurgitant or shunt flow is a direct function of the systemic vascular resistance; reduction of the latter augments systemic output and diminishes the load on the left ventricle by reducing the abnormal flow. Ordinarily when these lesions are severe enough to cause heart failure, they should be treated surgically; however, when they occur in the course of acute myocardial infarction, it may be best to defer operation for several weeks if the patient's condition is stable. Treatment with a vasodilator, at first with sodium nitroprusside and then sustained with orally active drugs, may aid in stabilizing the patient's condition during this interval.[431] Patients with either primary or secondary mitral regurgitation appear to achieve benefit.[345,347]

Increased systemic vascular resistance also augments the regurgitant volume in patients with aortic regurgitation, and vasodilator therapy reduces the regurgitation and increases the forward stroke volume and cardiac output.[432] Sustained benefit and improved ventricular function in response to long-term vasodilator treatment are now well documented in patients with aortic regurgitation.[413,427,428] However, caution must be exercised in the treatment of aortic regurgitation with vasodilators, since these drugs may lower further the already depressed aortic diastolic pressure and interfere with coronary filling. Vasodilator therapy is of little benefit and generally should not be used in patients with obstructive valvular lesions.

Although systemic vasodilators often have relatively little effect on the pulmonary vascular bed, oral hydralazine has been reported to exert favorable hemodynamic effects in some patients with cor pulmonale.[433] As noted above, nitrates produce a vasodilator effect in the pulmonary circuit, but tolerance with sustained dosing and blood levels develops even more rapidly for the pulmonary than for the systemic circulation.[408] Prazosin can improve right ventricular function by lowering left ventricular diastolic pressure and, secondarily, pulmonary artery and right ventricular systolic pressure in patients with severe congestive heart failure.[434] Oxygen may also be considered to be a right ventricular afterload reducing agent, since high concentrations may be used to counteract the pulmonary vasoconstrictor effect of hypoxia.

LONG-TERM THERAPY WITH VASODILATORS

There is general agreement that patients with chronic left ventricular failure secondary to left ventricular dysfunction who have no contraindications (hypotension; renal failure) should receive prolonged therapy with an orally active vasodilator. Evidence of improvement in survival as a result of such therapy has been demonstrated with the combination of hydralazine and isosorbide dinitrate,[349] and with both enalapril (Fig. 17–16*A*; see also data from VHeFT-II trial, p. 466) and captopril (Fig. 17–16*B*). In addition, the available clinical and hemodynamic data with the use of ACE inhibitors are quite impressive. These drugs usually are well tolerated and increasingly are the agents of choice when long-term vasodilator therapy is indicated. There is sound rationale, based on both animal[437] and clinical[3] investigations, for reducing ventricular wall tension in patients who have cardiac dilation and/or reduced ejection fraction without overt heart failure, in an effort to delay deterioration of cardiac function and the development of heart failure. As already noted, the use of vasodilators prophylactically in this manner is currently under active investigation.

After individual consideration of the use of diuretics, vasodilators, and digitalis, some further discussion of combined therapy is in order. Briefly stated, the therapeutic goal of "triple" therapy with diuretics, vasodilators, and digitalis in patients with chronic congestive heart failure is to maintain compensation so that the patient's level of activity is maximal with the minimum cardiac workload and the greatest possible margin between the dose of each drug administered and its toxicity threshold. Such combination therapy, while frequently effective, does, however, make it difficult to distinguish the individual contribution of each form of therapy in the overall clinical response.

The systematic study of hemodynamic responses to the combined administration of inotropic and vasodilator drugs began in the late 1970's with observations of the acute effects of intravenous nitroprusside alone and in combination with dopamine[438,439] or dobutamine.[440,441] These studies clearly demonstrated additive effects of combined administration of the vasodilator and $beta_1$-adrenergic or dopaminergic agonists. Similar observations were made with the combination of dobutamine with captopril.[442]

Ribner et al. documented increases in cardiac output and stroke volume in response to the combination of hydralazine and digoxin that equaled the sum of the two drugs' individual effects, while reductions in ventricular filling pressure were similar to the single-drug responses.[443]

The combined hemodynamic effects of a cardiac glycoside and ACE inhibitor[444] are shown in Figure 17–20 and demonstrate the additive effects of the short-term administration of digoxin and captopril in patients with congestive heart failure.

Gheorghiade and colleagues have extended earlier observations to confirm additive favorable effects of digoxin and captopril at rest and during exercise in patients with severe chronic heart failure and sinus rhythm.[445] Although increases in maximum exercise time were observed in response to digoxin or captopril alone, the increase reached statistical significance (+40 per cent) only with the combined administration of digoxin and captopril.[445] This favorable additive effect can be achieved with easily administered regimens that have a low incidence of digitalis toxicity.[446]

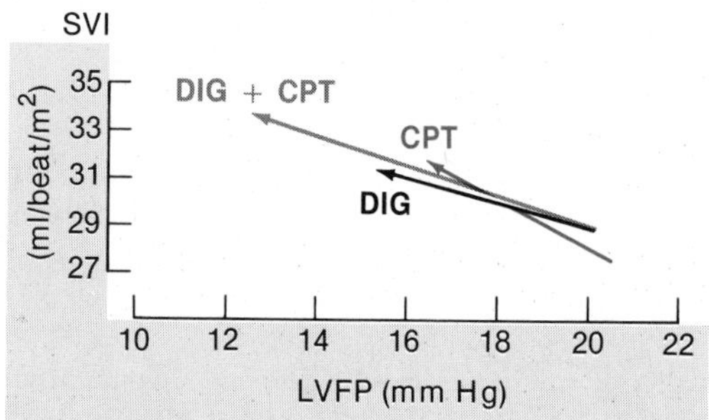

FIGURE 17–20. Combined hemodynamic effects of digoxin (DIG) and captopril (CPT) in patients with left ventricular failure. SVI, stroke volume index; LVFP, left ventricular filling pressure. (From Cantelli, I., Vitolo, A., Lombardi, G., et al.: Combined hemodynamic effects of digoxin and captopril in patients with congestive heart failure. Curr. Ther. Res. *36*:323, 1984.)

Data from several studies have found exercise capacity, left ventricular ejection fraction, and plasma norepinephrine concentration to be independent predictors of survival.[447,448] Although somewhat limited, available data indicate that each of these variables is improved by combined digitalis plus vasodilator therapy as much as or more than by either drug alone in patients with chronic heart failure. Taken together, and pending the availability of further information from controlled clinical trials, we view the available evidence as supporting the position that patients with symptomatic left ventricular dysfunction and depressed ejection fractions should be treated with combined diuretic, digitalis, and vasodilator therapy. It should be remembered that improved survival in the VHeFT-I and -II studies occurred in patients receiving combination therapy with diuretics and digoxin, when indicated, as well as vasodilators.

Nonglycoside Inotropic Agents

SYMPATHOMIMETIC AMINES

Catecholamines and other sympathomimetic amines exert potent inotropic effects by interacting with myocardial beta-adrenoceptors. For many years, attempts have been made to utilize these properties in the treatment of heart failure. However, these effects have been largely unsuccessful in long-term use because of the potent positive chronotropic, vasoconstrictor, or vasodilator actions of these agents (Tables 17–12 and 17–13), the development of tolerance to these agents, and downregulation of beta receptors with prolonged administration, causing reduced sensitivity of failing myocardium to beta-agonists (Fig. 14–22, p. 411). In addition, the norepinephrine depletion in cardiac sympathetic nerves reduces the response to indirectly acting sympathomimetic amines that act, in part, by releasing norepinephrine. Isoproterenol and, to a lesser extent, epinephrine cause tachycardia and hypotension by stimulating $beta_1$-adrenoceptors in the sinoatrial node and $beta_2$ receptors in the systemic vascular bed. Norepinephrine, on the other hand, a powerful stimulant not only of $beta_1$- but also of $alpha_1$-adrenoceptors, causes vasoconstriction and hypertension. Two sympathomimetic

TABLE 17–12 SOME RECEPTOR ACTIONS OF CATECHOLAMINES

ADRENOCEPTOR	SITE	ACTION
$Beta_1$	Myocardium	Increase atrial and ventricular contractility
	Sinoatrial node	Increase heart rate
	Atrioventricular conduction system	Enhance atrioventricular conduction
$Beta_2$	Arterioles	Vasodilation
	Lungs	Bronchodilation
Alpha	Peripheral arterioles	Vasoconstriction

From Sonnenblick, E. H., et al.: Dobutamine: A new synthetic cardioactive sympathetic amine. N. Engl. J. Med. *300*:18, 1979.

TABLE 17–13 ADRENERGIC RECEPTOR ACTIVITY OF SYMPATHOMIMETIC AMINES

	ALPHA PERIPHERAL	$BETA_1$ CARDIAC	$BETA_2$ PERIPHERAL
Norepinephrine	++++	++++	0
Epinephrine	++++	++++	++
Dopamine*	++++	++++	++
Isoproterenol	0	++++	++++
Dobutamine	+	++++	+
Methoxamine	++++	0	0

From Sonnenblick, E. H., et al.: Dobutamine: A new synthetic cardioactive sympathetic amine. N. Engl. J. Med. *300*:18, 1979.

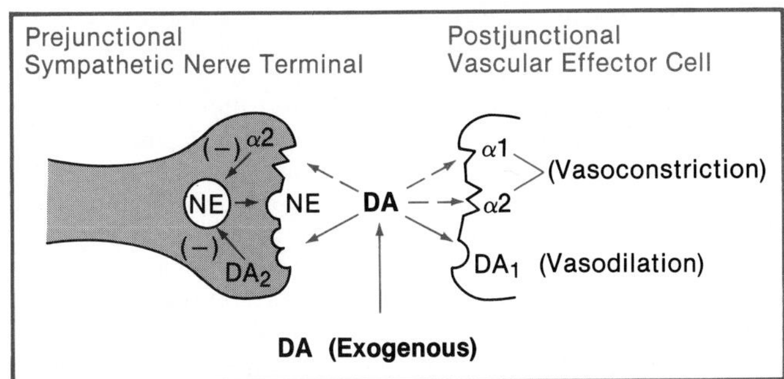

FIGURE 17–21. Location of dopamine-1 (DA_1) receptors, $alpha_1$- and $alpha_2$-adrenoceptors on postganglionic vascular effector cells, and DA_2 receptors and $alpha_2$-adrenoceptors on the prejunctional sympathetic nerve terminal. When dopamine is administered, activation of DA_1 receptors causes vasodilation and activation of DA_2 receptors causes inhibition (−) of norepinephrine (NE) release from storage granules. A larger dose of dopamine activates $alpha_1$- and $alpha_2$-adrenoceptors on the postjunctional effector cells to cause vasoconstriction and on $alpha_2$-adrenoceptors on the prejunctional sympathetic terminal to inhibit release of norepinephrine. Norepinephrine released from the prejunctional sympathetic terminal also acts on the two types of adrenoceptors. (From Goldberg, L. I., and Rajfer, S. I.: Dopamine receptors: Applications in clinical cardiology. Circulation *72*:245, 1985, by permission of the American Heart Association, Inc.)

agents, dopamine and dobutamine, cause less tachycardia and fewer systemic vascular effects. They are employed frequently by intravenous infusion and may be quite useful for short periods in the treatment of severe heart failure.

DOPAMINE

This endogenous catecholamine, the immediate biosynthetic precursor of norepinephrine, stimulates myocardial contractility by acting directly on $beta_1$-adrenoceptors in the myocardium and indirectly by releasing norepinephrine from sympathetic nerve terminals, which in turn also stimulates $beta_1$ receptors[449–451] (Tables 17–12 and 17–13 and Fig. 17–21). The cardiac effects of dopamine are antagonized by beta-adrenoceptor blockers. Dopamine-induced vasodilation is not blocked by propranolol and therefore is not related to activation of $beta_2$ receptors; also, it is not due to release of acetylcholine, histamine, or prostaglandin. However, dopaminergic vasodilation is antagonized by phenothiazines, such as chlorpromazine, and butyrophenones, such as haloperidol.[452,453] It is now clear that the vasodilation mediated by dopamine is secondary to activation of specific dopaminergic receptors, which exist in a variety of tissues, including blood vessels as well as the central and peripheral nervous systems.[453,454] Activation of $dopamine_1$ receptors cause vasodilation in the coronary, renal, mesenteric, and cerebral vascular beds (Fig. 17–22); these actions result from stimulation of adenylyl cyclase and increase of intracellular cyclic adenosine monophosphatase (AMP). The activation of $dopamine_2$ receptors is also responsible for vasodilation, but the mechanism is inhibition of the transmission of sympathetic nerve endings.[454] Dopamine-induced diuresis is a prominent and clinically important action in patients with heart failure[455] and is secondary to a combination of inotropic and, at lower doses, selective renal vasodilator effects.[450,454] Dopamine also preferentially dilates vessels in the renal cortex.[456]

When larger doses of dopamine are administered, the dilatation is reversed, and constriction occurs in both arterioles and veins in all vascular beds.[453] Although this vasoconstriction has been attributed to action of the drug on $alpha_1$-adrenoreceptors, the doses of the alpha-receptor blockers phentolamine and phenoxybenzamine required to prevent the dopamine-induced vasoconstriction are higher than those required to antagonize the vasoconstriction caused by other $alpha_1$-adrenoceptor agonists. Dopamine-induced contractions of isolated canine vessels can be attenuated by concentrations of the serotonin-blocking agent cyproheptadine that do not antagonize the actions of norepinephrine. These findings suggest that the vasoconstrictor action of larger doses of dopamine results from contraction of vascular smooth muscle, caused by its action on both serotonin and $alpha_1$ receptors.[455]

Effects of dopamine on vascular resistance and arterial pressure are dose dependent. With infusion rates below 2 μg/kg/min the major action of the drug is to reduce resistance in the renal, mesenteric, and coronary vascular beds. Doses of 2 to 5 μg/kg/min exert a positive inotropic effect; cardiac contractility and cardiac output increase, with little change in heart rate and either a reduction or no change in total peripheral resistance.[457] With higher infusion rates (5 to 10 μg/kg/min), arterial pressure, peripheral resistance, and heart rate increase and renal blood flow may decline.

Like other sympathomimetic amines that increase cardiac contractility, dopamine increases coronary blood flow[458] secondary to the increase in myocardial oxygen consumption that results from increased cardiac work.[459] Direct vasodilation mediated through action of dopaminergic receptors in the coronary arteries is an additional mechanism involved in the increase in coronary blood flow.[460] However, as is the case in other vascular beds, large doses of dopamine may increase coronary artery resistance by direct action on $alpha_1$-adrenergic and serotonergic receptors.[453] Ultimately, the effects of dopamine in patients with myocardial ischemia, like those of other catecholamines, depend on changes in the balance between myocardial oxygen utilization and coronary blood flow, which in turn are affected by the sum of its several actions. Augmented heart rate, contractility, and arterial pressure—all resulting from high doses of dopamine—increase oxygen utilization, whereas reduced peripheral resistance and heart size—caused by lower doses—reduce oxygen utilization. In addition, low doses of dopamine reduce coronary vascular resistance, while high doses increase it.

In early investigations, Goldberg et al. found that in patients with heart failure dopamine increased sodium excretion and cardiac output[461]; infusion rates of 2 to 6 μg/kg/min increased cardiac index (+26 per cent) without causing significant changes in heart rate or total body oxygen consumption. Peripheral resistance was reduced, and pulmonary vascular resistance, when elevated, also fell. Left ventricular dP/dt increased by 58 per cent, glomerular filtration rate by 38 per cent, renal plasma flow by 79 per cent, and sodium excretion by an average of 48 per cent. Thus, in patients with congestive heart failure, dopamine can exert important beneficial hemodynamic and renal effects. However, care must be taken to adjust the infusion rate carefully to prevent an excessive positive inotropic effect, tachycardia, and increased peripheral resistance.

In normotensive patients with refractory heart failure, infu-

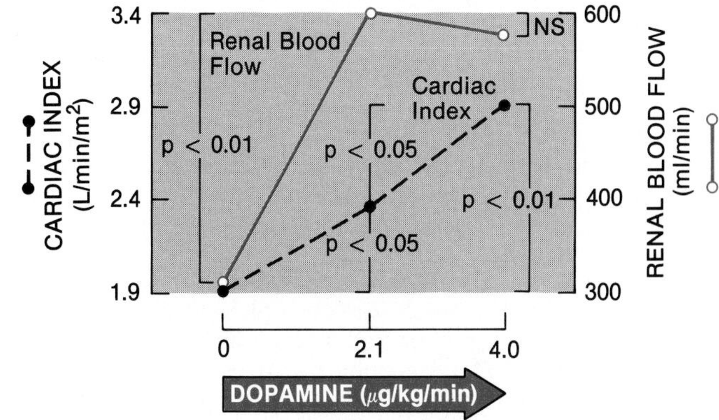

FIGURE 17–22. Changes in cardiac index and renal blood flow in response to ascending doses of dopamine. (From Maskin, C. S., Ocken, S., Chadwick, B., and LeJemtel, T. H.: Comparative systemic and renal effects of dopamine and angiotensin-converting enzyme inhibition with enalaprilat in patients with heart failure. Circulation *72*:846, 1985, by permission of the American Heart Association, Inc.)

sions should be begun at low rates (0.5 to 1.0 $\mu g/kg/min$) and should be gradually increased until cardiac output is augmented or until increments in diastolic pressure and heart rate are observed. After several hours, the infusion rate should be decreased and if possible discontinued. In patients with cardiogenic shock, both the vasoconstrictor and the more intense inotropic effects of higher doses may be desirable. When large doses of dopamine are required for its positive inotropic action, it may be infused together with nitroprusside[462] or nitroglycerin to counteract the vasoconstrictor action.

USE DURING AND FOLLOWING CARDIAC SURGERY. Dopamine is widely used for the treatment of acute heart failure following cardiopulmonary bypass.[463,464] In a comparison of the effects of three catecholamines in 22 patients with low cardiac output states following surgery, dopamine increased cardiac index by 1.1 liters/min/m^2, mean arterial pressure by 7 mm Hg, heart rate by 19 beats/min, and urine flow by 75 ml/hr. In contrast, norepinephrine increased cardiac index by much less (only 0.2 liter/min/m^2) and mean arterial pressure by much more (23 mm Hg), while heart rate rose by 9 beats/min and urine flow *decreased* by 8 ml/hr. The action of isoproterenol was similar to that of dopamine in that it increased cardiac index by 0.95 liter/min/m^2, but the former caused more severe tachycardia, increasing heart rate by 28 beats/min. Urine flow increased by 28 ml/hr, while mean arterial pressure decreased by 7 mm Hg. These observations demonstrate the superiority of dopamine over isoproterenol and norepinephrine in this common clinical setting. The use of dopamine (or dobutamine) sometimes combined with intraaortic balloon counterpulsation, permits the discontinuation of cardiopulmonary bypass in some patients with severe depression of cardiac function who cannot otherwise be weaned from the heart-lung machine.[465] Here also, dopamine appears to be superior to isoproterenol.

The low cardiac output state in the early postoperative period may be due to severe postischemic depression of myocardial contractility (myocardial stunning, p. 1329) resulting in a hemodynamic picture of cardiogenic shock. If the operation has successfully corrected the underlying mechanical defect(s), and no perioperative infarction has occurred, this depression of contractility is often reversible. Support with a sympathomimetic agent (dopamine or dobutamine) or with amrinone together with intraaortic balloon counterpulsation is often successful in tiding the patient over until myocardial function recovers.

DOBUTAMINE

Dobutamine is a synthetic cardioactive sympathomimetic amine that stimulates $beta_1$-, $beta_2$- and alpha-adrenoceptors.[465-468] Radioligand binding studies suggest that $beta_1$ activity predominates over $beta_2$, and that $alpha_1$- predominates over $alpha_2$-agonist activity of this drug.[469] Dobutamine is a racemic mixture; the (−) enantiomer is predominantly a potent $alpha_1$-agonist, while the (+) enantiomer is a potent stimulant of both $beta_1$ and $beta_2$ receptors.[468] Myocardial contractility is augmented by the stimulation of beta and $alpha_1$ receptors, while stimulation of each of these receptors in the systemic vascular bed counteracts the other so that there is little net effect. Dobutamine does *not* activate dopaminergic receptors and does not release norepinephrine from adrenergic nerve endings. At equivalent inotropic responses, dobutamine exerts a much weaker $beta_2$-adrenergic action than does isoproterenol and a much weaker $alpha_1$-adrenergic action than do either norepinephrine or dopamine. When given to patients with heart failure, dobutamine results in a reduction in systemic vascular resistance as cardiac output rises, and arterial pressure remains relatively constant.[470,471]

In contrast to dopamine, dobutamine is *not* a renal vasodilator. Also, it causes a redistribution of cardiac output in favor of the coronary and limb beds over the mesenteric and renal vascular beds.[472,473] However, it has been reported not to increase oxygen delivery to working skeletal muscle of patients with heart failure.[474] A low-dose infusion of dopamine may be added to dobutamine to obtain a renal vasodilator effect from the former and a positive inotropic effect from the latter.

Gillespie and colleagues administered dobutamine to patients with acute myocardial infarction and found that the drug improved hemodynamics without provoking undesirable side effects and without increasing the extent of myocardial injury.[475] Improvement in cardiac index (mean increase 54 per cent) and stroke-work index (mean increase 65 per cent) has been reported in response to dobutamine infusion in patients with chronic heart failure secondary to ischemic heart disease, with infrequent precipitation of overt myocardial ischemia.[476] Patients with dilated cardiomyopathy treated continuously for 2 or 3 days or on a weekly basis with intravenous dobutamine have been reported to exhibit favorable hemodynamic effects that were sustained for weeks to a few months.[477-480] Portable infusion devices have been used to administer intravenous dobutamine to ambulatory patients with severe heart failure awaiting cardiac transplantation.[481] Dobutamine, like dopamine, is also useful in the treatment of low cardiac output states following cardiac surgery.[463,464]

The usual dosage ranges from 2.5 to 10 $\mu g/kg/min$, although occasionally doses as low as 0.5 or as high as 40 $\mu g/kg/min$ have been used. It is important to be sure by clinical examination or invasive monitoring that hypovolemia is not present.

ADVERSE EFFECTS OF DOPAMINE AND DOBUTAMINE. Sinus tachycardia and other cardiac arrhythmias are important adverse effects developing from use of dopamine and dobutamine. The electrophysiological properties of these drugs resemble those of other sympathomimetic amines[473,482,483] and consist of acceleration of the spontaneous depolarization of sinoatrial cells (thereby increasing heart rate), acceleration of diastolic depolarization and facilitation of activation of latent pacemaker cells (thereby causing ectopic tachyarrhythmias), shortening of the refractory period of atrial and ventricular muscle, and speeding of atrioventricular conduction. They also cause a significant reduction of plasma potassium concentration[484]; ventricular arrhythmias have been observed with the use of both drugs.[450,485] In patients with coronary artery disease, both dobutamine and dopamine may precipitate overt myocardial ischemia by increasing myocardial oxygen needs.[453,485,486]

In patients with preexisting vascular disease, the vasoconstriction induced by high doses of dopamine may cause gangrene of the digits.[487] Tissue necrosis similar to that produced by norepinephrine can also occur if an infusion of dopamine extravasates into tissue; this can be prevented by infiltrating the area promptly with 5 to 10 mg of phentolamine diluted in saline. Dopamine differs from the other catecholamines in that it causes nausea and vomiting in some patients, a central nervous system effect more commonly observed with high dosage.[450,453]

COMPARISONS AMONG DOPAMINE, DOBUTAMINE, AND NITROPRUSSIDE

There has been considerable interest in comparing the effects of these drugs in patients with severe congestive heart failure.[457,488-490] In one study, dobutamine raised cardiac index while lowering left ventricular end-diastolic pressure and leaving mean aortic pressure unchanged. Dopamine also improved cardiac index but at the expense of a greater increase in heart rate than occurred with dobutamine. Dopamine increased mean aortic pressure but was ineffective in lowering left ventricular end-diastolic pressure. Both dopamine and dobutamine increase myocardial contractility and thereby augment myocardial oxygen consumption. Because dobutamine has little effect on two other major determinants of myocardial oxygen consumption, i.e., heart rate and aortic pressure, and reduces a third, ventricular filling pressure (a determinant of ventricular size), it may be superior to dopamine in patients with low cardiac output states associated with ischemic heart disease.[487] Dobutamine also effected a more favorable balance between myocardial oxygen supply and demand in patients with severe myocardial depression following cardiac surgery.[463,464]

In a study comparing the acute hemodynamic effects of dobutamine and dopamine in patients with chronic low-output cardiac failure, it was observed that at dosages adjusted to achieve similar increments in cardiac output, dobutamine reduced left ventricular filling pressure from an average of 25 to 17 mm Hg, while dopamine increased it to 30 mm Hg.[489] This response to dopamine was probably the result of its vasoconstrictor actions and illustrates the potential advantages of using a more cardioselective agent such as dobutamine when the desired goal of therapy is to improve ventricular function by direct inotropic stimulation.

In a comparison between these two sympathomimetic amines in patients with severe heart failure, dobutamine in doses up to 10 μg/kg/min progressively increased cardiac output while decreasing systemic and pulmonary vascular resistance and filling pressure, without a significant effect on heart rate and ventricular irritability. In contrast, dopamine at doses above 4 μg/kg/min increased not only cardiac output but also left ventricular filling pressure and ventricular ectopic activity; at doses greater than 6 μg/kg/min, dopamine also increased heart rate and systemic and pulmonary vascular resistance.[490] The heart rate–systolic pressure product, an index related to myocardial oxygen requirements, increases with both agents, but more so with dopamine than with dobutamine. Furthermore, at any increase in the heart rate–systolic pressure product, the increase in cardiac output with dobutamine is greater than with dopamine.

Thus, in normotensive patients with advanced heart failure, large doses of dopamine cause vasoconstriction and *raise* left ventricular filling pressure. However, filling pressures *decline* with dobutamine, or with a combination of dopamine or dobutamine and a vasodilator. The inotropic effects of dopamine are in part mediated by release of endogenous norepinephrine, which may be reduced in the hearts of patients with chronic heart failure[1]; low doses of this drug may be insufficient to achieve the desired inotropic effect of an increase in cardiac output, while larger doses may produce unwanted vasoconstriction.

Although dopamine can improve renal and mesenteric perfusion by selective dopaminergic vasodilation (a unique property of dopamine not shared by dobutamine), this beneficial effect on regional perfusion is often reversed when dopamine is given in the large doses sometimes required to achieve a sufficient inotropic effect. However, as already stated, it is possible to use dopamine in low doses (1.0 to 2.0 μg/kg/min) to provide selective vasodilation of mesenteric and renal vascular beds and combine it with dobutamine, or with a vasodilator, to achieve optimal hemodynamic improvement. In conclusion, both drugs are useful in the treatment of refractory heart failure; overall, dobutamine is preferred to dopamine, especially in normotensive patients with sinus tachycardia. However, in patients with heart failure and hypotension, dopamine, with its greater vasoconstrictor properties, may be the sympathomimetic of choice.

In a comparison between sodium nitroprusside and dobutamine, it was found that both drugs reduced systemic vascular resistance.[491] The reduction produced by dobutamine results primarily from withdrawal of compensatory vasoconstriction as a consequence of elevation of cardiac output. On the other hand, sodium nitroprusside infusion reduces systemic vascular resistance more than does dobutamine, suggesting that dobutamine might be preferable to nitroprusside for augmenting cardiac output in patients with borderline hypotension. When the major objective is to lower elevated filling pressure, especially in hypertensive patients, nitroprusside is superior to dobutamine.

DOPEXAMINE

This synthetic N-alkylated dopamine analog is a potent, intravenously active vasodilator, with both beta$_2$-adrenoceptor and dopaminergic-agonist activity. In contrast to dopamine, it has no alpha- or beta$_1$-adrenoceptor activity. In patients with heart failure its vasodilator action results in a reduction in filling pressures.[492–494] Like dopamine, dopexamine preferentially increased renal and hepatic-splanchnic blood flow. (It has not been approved by the FDA of the United States at the time of this writing.)

ORALLY ACTIVE SYMPATHOMIMETIC AMINES

Several orally active beta-adrenoceptor and dopaminergic agonists have undergone clinical study recently, although none has, at the time of this writing, been approved for clinical use in the United States.

LEVODOPA. This is the biosynthetic precursor of dopamine; when administered orally (with pyridoxine) it is decarboxylated to dopamine and exerts a similar salutary hemodynamic effect in heart failure[495]; this salutary effect may be sustained.[496–498] A central action may be responsible for the nausea, vomiting, and dyskinesia that are prominent side effects. Efforts are under way to find oral dopamine analogs that do not penetrate the blood-brain barrier and avoid these adverse effects.

IBOPAMINE. This synthetic, orally active pro-drug is hydrolyzed to epinine, a dopamine-like agent that stimulates beta$_1$-, beta$_2$-, and alpha$_1$-adrenoceptors as well as dopamine receptors. In short-term studies it raises cardiac output and reduces systemic vascular resistance, leaving arterial pressure unchanged.[499–501]

Other beta-adrenoceptor agonists originally introduced as bronchodilators, including *terbutaline* and *salbutamol* (albuterol),[502,503] have also been found to exert favorable hemodynamic effects consequent to vasodilator and/or positive inotropic activities.

XAMOTEROL. This is a synthetic, orally active sympathomimetic that is a beta$_1$-adrenoceptor partial agonist that also has beta-blocking properties. It has provided symptomatic benefit in patients with chronic congestive heart failure.[504] It was hoped that it would provide the correct degree of mild inotropic support to patients with congestive heart failure, without beta-adrenoceptor desensitization. However, it causes downregulation of beta$_1$ receptors on lymphocytes,[505,506] and recently a randomized controlled trial was discontinued early because of excess mortality[507]; 9.1 per cent of patients in the xamoterol group versus 3.1 per cent in the placebo group died within 100 days of randomization ($p = 0.02$).

At the time of this writing, while relatively brief (up to 72 hours) inotropic stimulation with dopamine and dobutamine has been found to be useful clinically in patients with chronic, but especially with acute, heart failure, there is no evidence that prolonged inotropic stimulation with any drug prolongs survival in patients with heart failure. Indeed, the aforementioned trial in which xamoterol increased mortality,[507] as well as a similar experience with oral milrinone,[508] lends credence to the idea that long-term stimulation of the myocardium with potent inotropic agents may actually be deleterious[509–511] despite initially favorable hemodynamic actions and symptomatic benefit.

PHOSPHODIESTERASE INHIBITORS

The action of this group of agents, which exert both positive inotropic and vasodilator effects, is through the inhibition of phosphodiesterase III.[510,511] This membrane-bound enzyme is responsible for the breakdown of cyclic AMP, and its inhibition raises intracellular cyclic AMP concentrations. The latter action appears to be responsible for both the positive inotropic and the vasodilator effects of these agents (Fig. 17–23). This mechanism is supported by the observation that the muscarinic agonist carbachol, which inhibits adenylate cyclase, interferes with the positive inotropic action of these agents.[512,513] As is the case for most other positive inotropic agents, an increased calcium flux into myocardial cells appears to be involved in the mechanism of action. It has been demonstrated that these drugs do not inhibit Na^+, K^+-ATPase, nor do they act on adrenergic or histaminergic receptors.

AMRINONE. This bipyridine is the only agent in this class that has been approved for clinical use in the United States (by intravenous administration).[514–516] Its administration to patients with heart failure causes dose-dependent increases in cardiac output and reductions in right- and left-sided filling pressures and systemic vascular resistance. Studies in isolated hearts and vascular beds have shown that amrinone exerts both direct positive inotropic and direct systemic vasodilator actions; it causes reductions in pulmonary vascular and coronary vascular resistances. Hemodynamic effects of amrinone (and its cogener milrinone) can be likened to those of a combination of dobutamine, a positive inotropic agent with little direct vascular action, and nitroprusside, a balanced arterial and venous dilator (Fig. 17–24). The drug's effects are additive

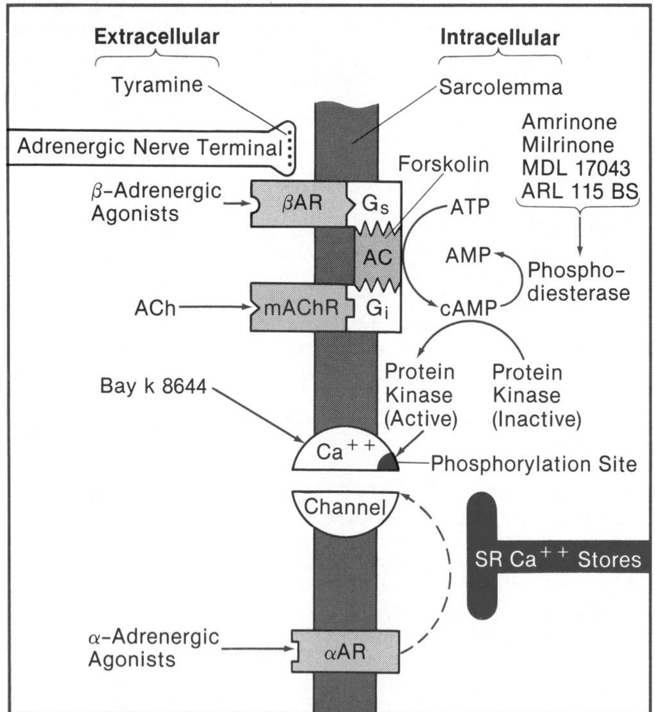

FIGURE 17–23. Diagram illustrating the sites of action of several positive inotropic agents. Circulating catecholamines, catecholamines released from adrenergic nerve terminals, and exogenous sympathomimetic drugs act on beta- and alpha-adrenoceptors (β-AR and α-AR, respectively). Stimulation of beta-adrenoceptors causes activation of adenylate cyclase (AC), resulting in increased cyclic AMP (cAMP) production, which in turn causes an increase in calcium influx through slow calcium channels, presumably due to the activation of protein kinases that phosphorylate the slow calcium channel. The mechanism by which stimulation of alpha-adrenoceptors causes an increase in myocardial contractility is not fully understood, but it may also involve an action on the slow calcium channel. Tyramine acts on adrenergic nerve terminals to release catecholamines, which then act on adrenoceptors. Calcium-channel agonists (e.g., the drug Bay K 8644) act directly on the calcium channel to increase calcium influx. Intracellular cAMP is degraded by phosphodiesterases; therefore, inhibition of cardiac phosphodiesterase results in an increase in intracellular cAMP levels. Several of the newer positive inotropic agents appear to act largely by this mechanism. cAMP can also be increased independently of beta-adrenoceptors by direct stimulation of adenylate cyclase with forskolin. G_S = guanine nucleotide stimulatory subunit, ACh = acetylcholine, mAChR = muscarinic ACh receptor, G_i = guanine nucleotide inhibitory subunit, and SR = sarcoplasmic reticulum. Schema prepared by Dr. T. Smith. (Reproduced with permission from Colucci, W. S., Wright, R. F., and Braunwald, E.: New positive inotropic agents in the treatment of congestive heart failure. N. Engl. J. Med. *314*:292, 1986.)

to those of the digitalis glycosides and are synergistic with direct-acting sympathomimetics. The development of tolerance has not been a problem as it has with the latter agents. The vasodilator action tends to offset the effects of the positive inotropic action, resulting in little change in myocardial oxygen consumption.[517] Therefore, amrinone tends not to intensify ischemia in patients with coronary artery disease. However, it facilitates atrioventricular conduction, causing an acceleration of ventricular rate in patients with atrial fibrillation; it is usually not otherwise arrhythmogenic.[518]

Amrinone, administered intravenously, is useful in the treatment of heart failure that is refractory to the combination of digitalis glycosides, diuretics, and vasodilators.[513,519] After an initial bolus of 0.75 mg/kg, it is infused intravenously at a dose of 5 to 10 μg/kg/min. Amrinone's vasodilator effects may cause hypotension in patients who are hypovolemic or who are already taking larger dosages of other vasodilators. It is useful when infused for several hours to several days in patients with severe heart failure in whom a reversible component is present. It is particularly helpful in patients with post-cardiac surgical myocardial depression,[520] in patients with acute exacerbation of chronic heart failure, and in some patients with myocardial infarction and left ventricular failure.[521]

While the mechanism of action of amrinone is quite different, its hemodynamic effects resemble those of dobutamine. However, several differences may confer some advantages on amrinone. First, it possesses a more potent direct vasodilator action, which is useful in patients with heart failure who are not hypotensive; indeed, the effects of amrinone resemble those produced by a combination of dobutamine and nitroprusside. Second, in contrast to dobutamine, amrinone does *not* appear to cause tolerance with prolonged infusion and perhaps has a lesser tendency to cause ischemia and ventricular tachyarrhythmias. Since amrinone is available only for intravenous use, it is *not* recommended for long-term management of heart failure, although it has been administered continuously for as long as 10 days. Amrinone has a favorable hemodynamic effect in patients with severe heart failure when it is combined with dopamine[522] or dobutamine[523] (Fig. 17–25). Amrinone has also been used to support the circulation in patients with severe heart failure awaiting cardiac transplantation.[524]

Amrinone is well absorbed from the gastrointestinal tract, and the hemodynamic effects produced after oral administration resemble those following intravenous infusion. However, it is *not* suitable for long-term oral administration because of the high incidence of adverse effects (gastrointestinal intolerance, fever, abnormalities in hepatic function, and reversible thrombocytopenia). While oral (and intravenous) amrinone initially improves exercise tolerance, there is controversy whether it delays or hastens deterioration of cardiac perform-

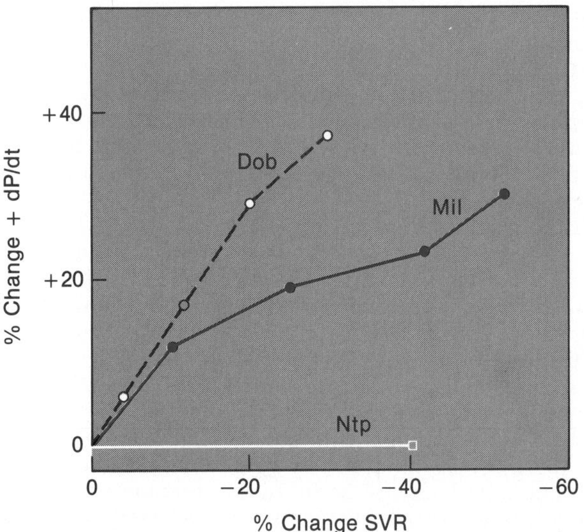

FIGURE 17–24. The relative effects of dobutamine (Dob), nitroprusside (Ntp), and milrinone (Mil) on systemic vascular resistance (SVR) and the peak positive rate of left ventricular pressure development (+dP/dt) in patients with severe congestive heart failure. Nitroprusside, a pure vasodilator agent, causes only a decrease in systemic vascular resistance, without evidence of a positive inotropic action. Dobutamine, a pure positive inotropic agent, causes a marked increase in +dP/dt, a measure of the myocardial inotropic state. In addition, there is a decrease in the systemic vascular resistance with dobutamine, which is most likely caused by reflex withdrawal of sympathetic tone. The new positive inotropic agent milrinone has an effect that is intermediate between those of nitroprusside and dobutamine, causing both a substantial increase in +dP/dt and a substantial reduction in systemic vascular resistance. Milrinone and several of the other new positive inotropic agents appear to exert both positive inotropic and direct vasodilator actions in patients with congestive heart failure, and both actions probably contribute markedly to the net hemodynamic response to the drug. (From Colucci, W. S., Wright, R. F., Jaski, B. E., Fifer, M. A., Braunwald, E.: Milrinone and dobutamine in severe heart failure: Differing hemodynamic effects and individual patient responsiveness. Circulation *73*[Suppl. 3]:178, 1986, by permission of the American Heart Association, Inc.)

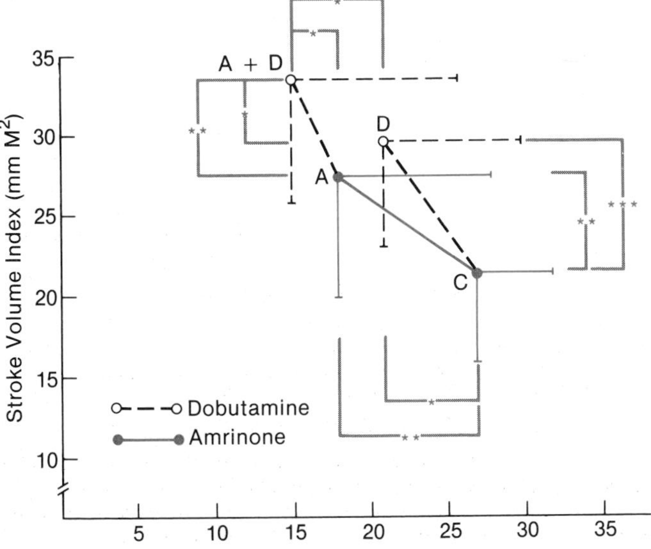

FIGURE 17–25. Stroke volume index and left ventricular end-diastolic pressure in 11 patients during the control periods (C), during administration of intravenous amrinone alone at a dose of 1.9 mg/kg (range 1.5 to 2.25) (A, solid line), during administration of dobutamine alone at a dose of 10.9 ug/kg/min (range 3 to 15) (D, broken line), and during combined administration of dobutamine (identical dose) and amrinone (A + D). ***$p < .001$, **$p < .01$, *$p < .05$. (From Gage, J., Rutman, H., Lucido, D., and LeJemtel, T. H.: Additive effects of dobutamine and amrinone on myocardial contractility and ventricular performance in patients with severe heart failure. Circulation *74*:367, 1986, by permission of the American Heart Association, Inc.)

ance, even among patients who tolerate long-term oral administration.

The following phosphodiesterase inhibitors are either currently in investigational use or have been approved for general clinical use in other countries.

MILRINONE. This congener of amrinone is 15 to 20 times as potent on a per milligram basis and except for a somewhat shorter duration of action has essentially identical pharmacological and hemodynamic effects when administered intravenously.[525–534] In contrast to amrinone, it is well tolerated when administered orally and exerts salutary effects in patients with refractory heart failure who *initially* exhibit striking clinical improvement with augmentation of maximum oxygen uptake, anaerobic threshold, and exercise capacity, which are sometimes sustained.[535] However, since it exerts a detrimental effect on patient survival[508] its use as a long-term oral inotropic agent has been abandoned.

The PROMISE trial was designed to evaluate the effect of milrinone on the survival of patients with chronic heart failure.[508] Patients were eligible for the study if they had Class III–IV symptoms despite treatment with digoxin, diuretics, and converting-enzyme inhibitors. A total of 1088 patients were randomly assigned to either milrinone (10 mg QID) or matching placebo. The trial was discontinued prematurely for the following reasons: (1) treatment with milrinone was associated with a 28 per cent increase in mortality compared with placebo ($p < 0.05$); (2) treatment with milrinone was associated with a 58 per cent increase in mortality in a prospectively defined subgroup, Class IV patients ($p = 0.007$); (3) treatment with milrinone was associated with a significantly higher incidence of serious (but nonfatal) adverse cardiovascular reactions (e.g., syncope, symptomatic hypotension, malignant ventricular arrhythmias) than placebo (all $p < 0.05$); and (4) milrinone appeared to have no beneficial effect on the clinical status of patients (as assessed by such criteria as quality-of-life tests and number of hospitalizations for worsening heart failure).

ENOXIMONE. This imidazole[532,536–541] is dissimilar chemically from the bipyridines (amrinone and milrinone) but has quite similar biochemical (they are all inhibitors of phosphodiesterase III) and pharmacological (positive inotropic and vasodilator) actions. When given intravenously it initially causes improvement in the clinical and hemodynamic manifestations of heart failure. Like intravenous amrinone and milrinone it may be useful in acute heart failure, particularly early postoperative cardiac depression. When administered orally it appears to reduce the symptoms of heart failure,[536,542] but the aforementioned deleterious effects of long-term milrinone therapy on survival[508] have dampened enthusiasm for the long-term administration of this (as well as other inotropic) agents.

NEW INOTROPIC AGENTS

PIMOBENDAN. This pyridazinone derivative is a phosphodiesterase inhibitor, which (like amrinone, milrinone, and enoximone) exerts both positive inotropic and vasodilating effects. It is active orally, appears to be well tolerated, and reverses the hemodynamic abnormalities of heart failure.[542–545] In contrast to the earlier phosphodiesterase inhibitors discussed above, pimobendan also sensitizes myofilaments to calcium.[546,546c] It is hoped that this important property may obviate the aforementioned harmful effects of inotropic agents.[547]

OPC-8212. This quinolinone derivative[547,548] also has positive inotropic and vasodilatory properties and is well tolerated. It, too, is thought to sensitize myofilaments (specifically troponin C) to calcium.[547,549]

DPI 201-106. This novel agent also exerts its positive inotropic action by enhancing myofilament sensitivity to calcium and augmenting the inward sodium current. Thus it appears to exert an additive effect with cardiac glycosides on cardiac muscle.[550] This agent, too, has produced favorable hemodynamic results in heart failure.[551]

Other Aspects of the Treatment of Heart Failure

BETA-ADRENOCEPTOR BLOCKERS IN HEART FAILURE

The premise that sympathetic nervous system hyperactivity may have deleterious long-term consequences in chronic heart failure,[213] particularly in dilated cardiomyopathy, has led to interest in the use of beta-adrenergic blocking drugs in these patients. Early reports from investigators in Gothenburg, Sweden,[552–555] indicating benefit of long-term beta-adrenergic blockade have been supported by some clinical studies,[556–559] while others of shorter duration have reported no evidence of benefit.[560–562] A recent study of long-term metoprolol therapy in patients with heart failure due to dilated cardiomyopathy[563] demonstrated an increase in myocardial beta-receptor density, improvement in resting cardiac output, and improved contractile response to catecholamine stimulation. While clinical benefit may be related to the observed upregulation of beta-adrenergic receptors[563] (Fig. 17–26), it is not clear that this mechanism accounts for the long-term benefit reported in some series.[564]

While the available data have generated the important and testable hypothesis that beta blockade is of benefit in chronic heart failure, this approach is clearly investigational at present, and beta-blocking agents must be used with extreme caution in patients with heart failure. We agree with Shanes[565] that beta-blocker therapy should not be considered part of the management of patients with heart failure until the results of larger randomized trials are available. Fortunately, such a large-scale, multicenter, placebo-controlled trial of metoprolol in dilated cardiomyopathy is in progress.

An additional layer of complexity exists with respect to drugs such as prenalterol, xamoterol, and pindolol that are partial beta-adrenergic agonists, also to be thought of as beta-adrenoceptor blockers with intrinsic sympathomimetic activity. Initially positive results of a clinical trial in patients with incompletely characterized but mainly mild heart failure treated with xamoterol[236] must be reconsidered in the light of the recently reported excess mortality among 516 patients with severe (NYHA Class III or IV) heart failure randomized to xamoterol or placebo for 13 weeks.[566]

MANAGEMENT OF ARRHYTHMIAS IN THE PATIENT WITH CONGESTIVE HEART FAILURE

The management of arrhythmias in patients with heart failure is difficult and remains far from satisfactory. Sudden death, presumably due to cardiac arrhythmia, occurs in ap-

heart failure. Dense areas on the chest roentgenogram may make it difficult or impossible to interpret lung scans, and a pulmonary angiogram may be required to establish the diagnosis. Although this procedure is not without risk, a positive result may lead to treatment with anticoagulants and/or vena cava interruption that could prevent further emboli and prove to be life saving.

5. Could pulmonary infection be present? Pneumonitis, a frequent complication of left ventricular failure, may be difficult to recognize in patients with chronic congestive heart failure who often have a chronic low-grade fever as well as increased interstitial markings on the chest roentgenogram and pulmonary rales on clinical examination. Is the suspicion of pulmonary infection high enough to warrant sputum culture and consideration of a course of antibiotics?

6. Could hyperthyroidism or infective endocarditis be present? Thyrotoxicosis (often apathetic in the elderly) and infective endocarditis may not have typical clinical manifestations in the presence of heart failure, but they can lead to refractory heart failure. Should tests, including an assessment of thyroid function and multiple blood cultures, be obtained?

7. Could alcohol, a potent myocardial depressant, be playing a role? In addition to producing cardiomyopathy (p. 1819), alcohol can contribute to heart failure even when it is not the primary cause but its use is superimposed on some other form of heart disease.

8. Does the patient have inappropriate bradycardia due to sinus node dysfunction or atrioventricular block that could be corrected by means of a pacemaker? Could AV sequential pacing restore atrial augmentation of ventricular stroke volume?

9. Is the patient receiving any medications with salt-retaining effects, such as corticosteroids, estrogens, or nonsteroidal antiinflammatory drugs, or drugs with negative inotropic actions, such as disopyramide, beta-adrenoceptor blocking agents, or verapamil (Table 17–15)?

10. Could vasodilator therapy be responsible for an increased tendency to salt and water retention?

11. Can any aspect of therapy be intensified without producing untoward effects?

12. Have the initial favorable hemodynamic effects of any drug in the regimen waned during long-term therapy (e.g., desensitization to an alpha-adrenergic blocking vasodilator or development of nitrate tolerance)?

TABLE 17–15 THERAPIES THAT MAY IMPAIR CARDIAC FUNCTION

1. **Agents causing water retention: estrogens, androgens, and chlorpropramide**
2. **Nonsteroidal anti-inflammatory agents, including ibuprofen, phenylbutazone, and indomethacin, may tend to cause water retention through impairment of renal prostaglandin synthesis**
3. **Calcium channel blocking agents, especially verapamil and occasionally diltiazem, may cause negative inotropic effects**
4. **Cardiac antiarrhythmic agents, such as disopyramide phosphate (Norpace), amiodarone, or flecainide, may cause or aggravate congestive failure**
5. **Adriamycin, especially in doses above 400 mg per square meter body surface area, may cause cardiomyopathy**
6. **Radiation therapy exceeding 4000 rads administered to the mediastinum may cause both myocardial and pericardial disease**
7. **In patients with obstructive cardiomyopathy, digitalis may worsen the outflow tract obstruction and actually cause congestive failure**
8. **Propranolol and other beta-adrenergic blocking agents may impair cardiac function**
9. **Sodium-retaining steroids, such as aldosterone or fludrocortisone, may cause sodium and water retention**
10. **Minoxidil, an antihyperensive drug, may cause water retention**
11. **Certain tricyclic psychotropic agents, e.g., Elavil, may cause or worsen congestive failure**
12. **The ingestion of ethyl alcohol may have a deleterious effect upon cardiac function**

From Fowler, N. O.: Diagnosis of Heart Disease. New York, Springer Verlag, 1991, p. 103.

TABLE 17–16 TAILORED THERAPY FOR ADVANCED HEART FAILURE

1. **Measurement of baseline hemodynamics**
2. **Intravenous nitroprusside and diuretics tailored to hemodynamic goals:**
   PCW ≤ 15 mm Hg
   SVR ≤ 1200 dynes · sec · cm^{-5}
   RA ≤ 8 mm Hg
   SBP ≥ 80 mm Hg
3. **Definition of optimal hemodynamics by 24–48 hours**
4. **Titration of high-dose oral vasodilators as nitroprusside weaned**
   Maximum doses: **captopril 400 mg/day**
   hydralazine 400 mg/day
   isosorbide 320 mg/day
5. **Monitored ambulation and diuretic adjustment for 24–48 hours**
6. **Maintain digoxin levels 1.0–2.0 ng/dL if no contraindication**
7. **Detailed patient education**
8. **Flexible outpatient diuretic regimen including prn metolazone**
9. **Progressive walking program**
10. **Vigilant follow-up**

PCW = pulmonary capillary wedge pressure; SVR = systemic vascular resistance; RA = right atrial pressure; SBP = systolic blood pressure.

From Stevenson, L. W., and Miller, L. W.: Cardiac transplantation as therapy for heart failure. Cur. Probl. Cardiol. *16*:233, 1991.

MANAGEMENT OF REFRACTORY HEART FAILURE

(Fig. 17–28, Table 17–16)

After any issues raised by the questions posed have been dealt with and refractory heart failure persists, both the nature and hemodynamic consequences of the underlying illness should be reassessed and surgical treatment should be considered or reconsidered; often cardiac catheterization and angiography should be carried out or repeated at this time. For example, resection of a large ventricular aneurysm might have been deferred as long as the patient responded to medical treatment for heart failure because of the surgical risk, but reconsideration might be in order when the response to medical therapy wanes. Similar considerations may apply to patients with known multivessel coronary artery disease or advanced valvular heart disease and poor left ventricular function. Elderly patients who might not have been considered to be suitable for surgical treatment when symptoms of heart failure were controlled might become surgical candidates, albeit at a significantly heightened risk. Other forms of heart disease that may lead to refractory heart failure and that may be amenable to surgical treatment, but which are not readily recognized on clinical examination, include cardiac tumors (Chap. 44), endomyocardial fibrosis (p. 1422), and constrictive pericarditis without calcification (Chap. 45). Such conditions should be considered and, if possible, excluded.

If every aspect of the diagnosis, including the underlying and precipitating causes of heart failure, has been carefully assessed, if every aspect of therapy has been meticulously reconsidered, if the patient has been placed at bed rest and has received optimal doses of cardiac glycosides, diuretics, and oral vasodilators, if any electrolyte imbalance has been corrected and large volumes of fluid in the serous cavities not mobilized by diuretics have been removed mechanically, then the patient should receive a course of intravenous therapy with a vasodilator, an inotropic agent (amrinone and/or dobutamine) (Fig. 17–25), or a combination of an inotropic agent and vasodilator for 2 to 3 days. Combinations of nitroprusside or nitroglycerin[591] with dobutamine or dopamine may be effective (Fig. 17–28). Such combined administration of a sympathomimetic amine and vasodilator may be of benefit in patients with severe heart failure in whom the use of one of these agents alone is insufficient. Thus, in one series of

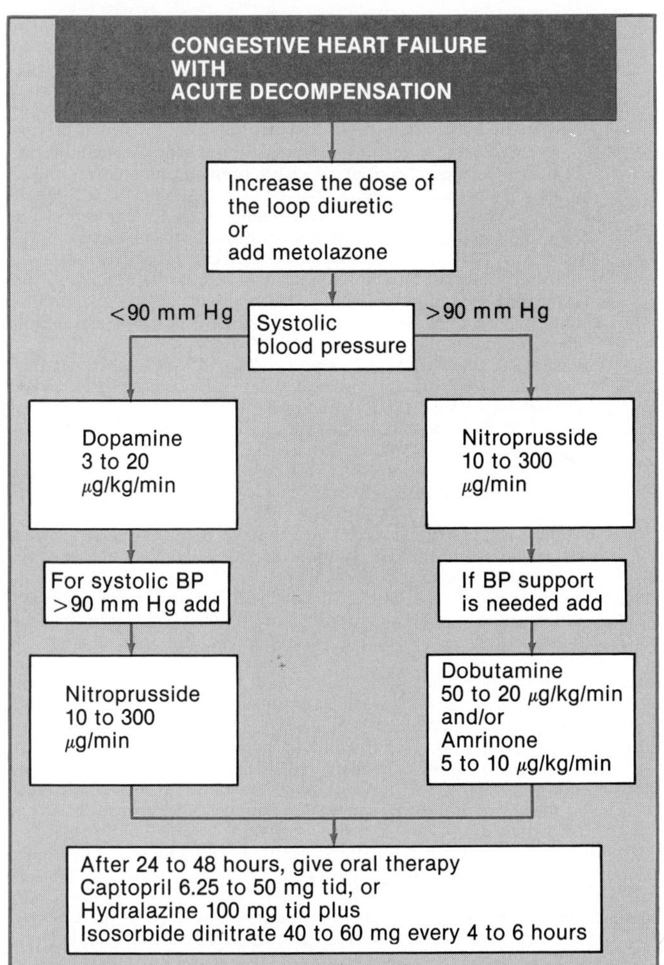

FIGURE 17-28. Flow diagram summarizing treatment of decompensated heart failure. (From Francis, G. S.: Inotropic agents in the management of heart failure. *In* Cohn, J. N.: Drug Treatment of Heart Failure. 2nd ed. Secaucus, NJ, ATC International, 1988.)

patients with severe chronic congestive heart failure, nitroprusside alone reduced left ventricular end-diastolic pressure from 25 to 14 mm Hg and increased cardiac index from 2.4 to 3.0 liters/min/m^2 but did not reduce end-diastolic pressure. Simultaneous infusion of the two agents resulted in favorable alterations in both hemodynamic variables: left ventricular end-diastolic pressure declined to 16 mm Hg and cardiac index rose to 3.5 liters/min/m^2.[592]

High-dose furosemide (250 to 4000 mg/day) may be utilized in patients with refractory heart failure.[42a] Ultrafiltration may be considered in patients with late-stage heart failure resistant to conventional treatment.[594,595] Experience with this technique suggests that sustained symptomatic improvement can be expected in properly selected patients, and the technique is relatively simple and cost-effective. Another supportive measure reported to be of benefit in the refractory heart failure patient with or at risk of cardiac cachexia is continuous nasogastric feeding.[596] The problem of Cheyne-Stokes respiration with severe sleep hypoxemia occurs relatively commonly in advanced heart failure. Supplemental oxygen therapy at night has been shown to confer benefit by reducing Cheyne-Stokes respiration, correcting hypoxemia, and consolidating sleep by reducing arousals caused by the hyperpneic phase of the Cheyne-Stokes cycle.[271]

Such treatment ordinarily can be carried out only in the hospital, with careful monitoring of filling pressure, cardiac output, and arterial pressure. If it is successful and the patient can be weaned from the intravenous therapy, larger doses of oral vasodilators and experimental drugs such as oral sympathomimetics or one of the new orally active phosphodiesterase inhibitors may provide benefit.

Heart failure can properly be termed intractable if it persists despite the judicious application of all of the aforementioned measures. Then the possibility of cardiac transplantation (Chap. 18) or assisted circulation (Chap. 19) may be considered in selected instances.

REFERENCES

THERAPEUTIC STRATEGY

1. Stevenson, L. W., Dracup, K. A., and Tillisch, J. H.: Congestive heart failure: Efficacy of medical therapy tailored for severe congestive heart failure in patients transferred for urgent cardiac transplantation. Am. J. Cardiol. *63*:461, 1989.
2. Stevenson, L. W., Sietsema, K., Tillisch, J. H., et al.: Exercise capacity for survivors of cardiac transplantation or sustained medical therapy for stable heart failure. Circulation *81*:78, 1990.
3. Pfeffer, M., Lamas, G. A., Vaughan, D. E., et al.: Effect of captopril on progressive ventricular dilatation after anterior myocardial infarction. N. Engl. J. Med. *319*:80, 1988.
4. Sharpe, N., Smith, H., Murphy, J., et al.: Treatments of patients with symptomless left ventricular dysfunction after myocardial infarction. Lancet *1*:255, 1988.
5. The SOLVD investigators: Effect of the angiotensin converting enzyme inhibitor enalapril on survival in patients with reduced left ventricular ejection fraction and congestive heart failure. N. Engl. J. Med. *325*:293, 1991.
5a. Cohn, J.N., Johnson, G., Ziesche, S., et al.: A comparison of enalapril with hydralazine-isosorbide dinitrate in the treatment of chronic congestive heart failure. N. Engl. J. Med. *325*:303, 1991.
6. Kubler, W., Manthey, J., and Osterziel, K. J.: Personal view. Congestive heart failure: How to evaluate efficacy of treatment. Eur. Heart J. *9*:602, 1988.
7. Francis, G. S.: Which drug for what patient with heart failure, and when? Cardiology *76*:374, 1989.
8. Cohn, J. N.: Current therapy of the failing heart. Circulation *78*:1099, 1988.
9. Jaeschke, R., and Guyatt, G. H.: Medical therapy for chronic congestive heart failure. Ann. Intern. Med. *110*:758, 1989.
10. Packer, M.: Therapeutic options in the management of chronic heart failure. Is there a drug of first choice? Circulation *79*:198, 1989.
11. Cohn, J. N., Archibald, D. G., Ziesche, S., et al.: Effect of vasodilator therapy on mortality in chronic congestive heart failure: Results of a Veterans Administration Cooperative Study. N. Engl. J. Med. *314*:1547, 1986.
12. The CONSENSUS Trial Group: Effects of enalapril on mortality in severe congestive heart failure: Results of the Cooperative North Scandinavian Enalapril Survival Study. N. Engl. J. Med. *316*:1429, 1987.
12a. The CONSENSUS Trial Study Group: Effects of enalapril and neuroendocrine activation on prognosis in severe congestive heart failure. Am. J. Cardiol. *66*:400, 1990.
12b. Braunwald, E.: ACE inhibitors—A cornerstone of the treatment of heart failure. N. Engl. J. Med. *325*:351, 1991.
13. Sullivan, M. J., Higginbotham, M. B., and Cobb, F. R.: Exercise training in patients with chronic heart failure delays ventilatory anaerobic threshold and improves submaximal exercise performance. Circulation *79*:324, 1989.

DIURETICS

13a. Anand, I., Ferrari, R., Kalra, G., et al.: Congestive heart failure: Edema of cardiac origin: Studies of body water and sodium, renal function, hemodynamic indexes, and plasma hormones in untreated congestive cardiac failure. Circulation *80*:299, 1989.
14. Anand, I., Veall, N., Kalra, G. S., et al.: Treatment of heart failure with diuretics: Body compartments, renal function and plasma hormones. Eur. Heart J. *10*:445, 1989.
14a. Cody, R. J., Ljungman, S., Covit, A. B., et al.: Regulation of glomerular filtration rate in chronic congestive heart failure patients. Kidney Int. *34*:361, 1988.
15. Haas, M.: Properties and diversity of (Na-K-Cl) cotransporters. Annu. Rev. Physiol. *51*:443, 1989.
16. Martinez-Maldonado, M., Gely, R., Tapia, E., and Benabe, J. E.: Role of macula densa in diuretics-induced renin release. Hypertension *16*:261, 1990.
17. Wilcox, C. S.: Diuretics. *In* Brenner, B. M. and Rector, F. C. (eds.): The Kidney, 4th ed. Philadelphia, W. B. Saunders Company, 1991, pp. 2123-2147.
18. Brater, D. C.: Drug-induced electrolyte disorders and use of diuretics. *In* Kokko, J. P., and Tannen, R. L. (eds.): Fluids and Electrolytes, 2nd ed. Philadelphia, W. B. Saunders Company, 1990.
19. Andreoli, T. E., and Weinman, E. J.: Diuretics: Physiology, biochemistry, and pharmacology. Semin. Nephrol. *8*:197, 1988.
20. Hollenberg, N.: Diuretics in congestive heart failure. *In* Messerli, F. H. (ed.): Cardiovascular Drug Therapy. Philadelphia, W. B. Saunders Company, 1990.
21. Wilcox, C. S.: Diuretics. *In* Brenner, B. M., and Rector, F. C. (eds.): The Kidney, 4th ed. Philadelphia, W. B. Saunders Company, 1991, pp. 2123-2147.

22. Rose, B. D.: Clinical Physiology of Acid Base Electrolyte Disorders, 3rd ed. New York, McGraw-Hill, 1989.

LOOP DIURETICS

23. Epstein, M., and Masterson, B. J.: Loop Diuretics: Furosemide. *In* Messerli, F. H. (ed.): Cardiovascular Drug Therapy. Philadelphia, W. B. Saunders Company, 1990, pp. 318–327.
24. Whelton, A., and Whelton, P. K.: Loop Diuretics: Bumetanide. *In* Messerli, F. H. (ed.): Cardiovascular Drug Therapy. Philadelphia, W. B. Saunders Company, 1990, pp. 328–336.
25. Sherman, L. G., Liang, C.-S., Baumgardner, S., et al.: Piretanide, a potent diuretic with potassium-sparing properties, for the treatment of congestive heart failure. Clin. Pharmacol. Ther. *40*:587, 1986.
26. Marone, C., Rivera, B., Zwahlen, H., et al.: Efficacy and pharmacokinetics of piretanide in patients with congestive heart failure. Eur. J. Clin. Invest. *19*:378, 1989.
27. Car, N., Skrabalo, Z., and Verho, M.: The effects of piretanide in patients with congestive heart failure and diabetes mellitus: A double-blind comparison with furosemide. Curr. Med. Res. Opin. *11*:133, 1988.
28. Hasenfuss, G., Holubarsch, C., Herzog, C., et al.: Influence of cardiac function on the diuretic and hemodynamic effects of the loop diuretic piretanide. Clin. Cardiol. *10*:83, 1987.
28a. Noormohamed, F. H., McNabb, W. R., Dixey, J. J., and Lant, A. F.: Renal responses and pharmacokinetics of piretanide in humans: Effect of route of administration, state of hydration and probenecid pretreatment. J. Pharmacol. Exp. Ther. *254*:992, 1990.
29. Beermann, B., and Grind, M.: Clinical pharmacokinetics of some newer diuretics. Clin. Pharmacokin. *13*:254, 1987.
30. Herchuelz, A., Deger, F., Douchamps, J., et al.: Comparative pharmacodynamics of torasemide and furosemide in patients with oedema. Arzneim. Forsch. Drug Res. *38*:180, 1988.
31. Reyes, A. J.: Formal comparison of the antihypertensive effects of torasemide and other diuretics by the Montevideo mathematical model. Arzneim. Forsch. Drug Res. *38*:194, 1988.
31a. Russo, D., Gazzotti, R. M., and Testa, A.: Torasemide, a new loop diuretic, in patients with chronic renal failure. Nephron *55*:141, 1990.
32. Reeves, W. B., and Molony, D. A.: The physiology of loop diuretic action. Semin. Nephrol. *8*:225, 1988.
33. Boles Ponto, L. L., and Schoenwald, R. D.: Furosemide (frusemide): I. A pharmacokinetic/pharmacodynamic review. Clin. Pharmacokinet. *18*:381, 1990.
34. Boles Ponto, L. L., and Schoenwald, R. D.: Furosemide (frusemide): II. A pharmacokinetic/pharmacodynamic review. Clin. Pharmacokinet. *18*:460, 1990.
34a. Staalsen, N. H., and Steiness, E.: Bumetanide-induced natriuresis and antinatriuresis in the proximal and distal parts of the human nephron. Investigations in acute and chronic bumetanide treatment. J. Pharmacol. Exp. Ther. *253*:1222, 1990.
34b. Park, C. S., Doh, P. S., Carraway, R. E., et al.: Stimulation of renin secretion by ethacrynic acid is independent of $Na^{(+)}$-$K^{(+)}$-$2Cl^{-}$ cotransport. Am. J. Physiol. *259*:F539, 1990.
35. Bock, H. A., and Stein, J. H.: Diuretics and the control of extracellular fluid volume: Role of counterregulation. Semin. Nephrol. *8*:264, 1988.
36. Beermann, B., and Midskov, C.: Reduced bioavailability and effect of furosemide given with food. Eur. J. Clin. Pharmacol. *29*:725, 1986.
37. Shammas, F. V., and Dickstein, K.: Clinical pharmacokinetics in heart failure. An updated review. Clin. Pharmacokinet. *15*:94, 1988.
38. Chaturvedi, P. R., O'Donnell, J. P., Nicholas, J. M., et al.: Steady state absorption kinetics and pharmacodynamics of furosemide in congestive heart failure. Int. J. Clin. Pharmacol. Therap. Toxicol. *25*:123, 1987.
39. Loon, N. R., Wilcox, C. S., and Unwin, R. J.: Mechanism of impaired natriuretic response to furosemide during prolonged therapy. Kidney Int. *36*:682, 1989.
40. Cook, J. A., Smith, D. E., Cornish, L. A., et al.: Kinetics, dynamics, and bioavailability of bumetanide in healthy subjects and patients with congestive heart failure. Clin. Pharmacol. Ther. *44*:487, 1988.
41. Kuchar, D. L., and O'Rourke, M. F.: High-dose furosemide in refractory cardiac failure. Eur. Heart J. *6*:954, 1985.
42. Gerlag, P. G., and van Meijel, J. J. M.: High-dose furosemide in the treatment of refractory congestive heart failure. Arch. Intern. Med. *148*:286, 1988.
42a. Marangoni, E., Oddone, A., Sarion, M., et al.: Effect of high-dose furosemide in refractory heart failure. Angiology *41*:862, 1990.
43. Alvan, G., Helleday, L., Lindholm, A., et al.: Diuretic effect and diuretic efficiency after intravenous dosage of frusemide. Br. J. Clin. Pharmacol. *29*:215, 1990.
44. Jorgensen, H., Anderssen, N., Silsand, T., and Peterson, L.-E.: Long-term treatment with slow-release frusemide compared with thiazide treatment in arterial hypertension. J. Int. Med. Res. *17*:552, 1989.
45. Colice, G. L., and Ramirez, G.: The effect of furosemide during normoxemia and hypoxemia. Am. Rev. Respir. Dis. *133*:279, 1986.
46. Babini, R., and du Souich, P.: Furosemide pharmacodynamics: Effects of respiratory and acid base disturbances. J. Pharmacol. Exp. Ther. *237*:623, 1987.
47. Nies, A. S., Gal, S., Fadul, S., and Gerker, J. G.: Indomethacin-furosemide interaction: The importance of renal blood flow. J. Pharmacol. Exp. Ther. *226*:27, 1983.
48. Webster, J.: Interactions of NSAIDs with diuretics and β-blockers. Mechanisms and clinical implications. Drugs *30*:32, 1985.
49. Furst, D. E.: Clinically important interactions of nonsteroidal antiinflammatory drugs with other medications. J. Rheumatol. *15*:58, 1988.
50. Koopmans, P. P., Thien, T. H., Thomas, C. M. G., et al.: The effects of sulindac and indomethacin on antihypertensive and diuretic action of hydrochlorothiazide in patients with mild to moderate essential hypertension. Br. J. Clin. Pharmacol. *21*:417, 1986.
51. Wong, D. G., Lamki, L., Spencer, J. P., et al.: Effect of non-steroidal antiinflammatory drugs on control of hypertension by beta-blockers and diuretics. Lancet *1*:997, 1986.
52. Wilson, T. W., McCauley, F. A., and Wells, H. D.: Effects of low-dose aspirin on responses to furosemide. J. Clin. Pharmacol. *26*:100, 1986.
53. Dikshit, K., Vyden, J. K., Forrester, J. S., et al.: Renal and extrarenal hemodynamic effects of furosemide in congestive heart failure after acute myocardial infarction. N. Engl. J. Med. *288*:1087, 1973.
54. Gerber, J. G.: Role of prostaglandins in the hemodynamic and tubular effects of furosemide. Fed. Proc. *42*:1707, 1983.
55. Francis, G. S., Siegel, R. M., Goldsmith, S. R., et al.: Acute vasoconstrictor response to intravenous furosemide in patients with chronic congestive failure. Ann. Intern. Med. *103*:1, 1985.
56. Larsen, F. F.: Haemodynamic effects of high or low doses of furosemide in acute myocardial infarction. Eur. Heart J. *9*:125, 1988.
57. Brater, D. C., Chennavasin, P., and Dehmer, G. J.: Prolonged hemodynamic effect of furosemide in congestive heart failure. Am. Heart J. *108*:1031, 1984.
58. Johnston, G. D., Nicholls, D. P., and Leahey, W. J.: The dose response characteristics of the acute non-diuretic peripheral vascular effects of furosemide in normal subjects. Br. J. Clin. Pharmacol. *18*:75, 1984.
59. Sinoway, L., Minotti, J., Musch, T., et al.: Enhanced metabolic vasodilation secondary to diuretic therapy in decompensated congestive heart failure secondary to coronary artery disease. Am. J. Cardiol. *60*:107, 1987.
60. Johnston, G. D., Nicholls, D. P., Kondowe, G. B., and Finch, M. B.: Comparison of the acute vascular effects of furosemide and bumetanide. Br. J. Clin. Pharmacol. *21*:359, 1986.
61. Ali, J., and Wood, L. D. H.: Pulmonary vascular effects of furosemide on gas exchange in pulmonary edema. Am. J. Physiol. *57*:160, 1984.
62. Lydon, J. C., Ebert, J. P., Grimes, B., and Niemann, K. M.: Furosemide may be detrimental in the treatment of pulmonary edema. Anesthesiology *64*:298, 1986.
63. Bianco, S., Pieroni, M. G., Refini, R. M., et al.: Protective effect of inhaled furosemide on allergen-induced early and late asthmatic reactions. N. Engl. J. Med. *321*:1069, 1989.
64. Norris, C. H.: Drugs affecting the inner ear. A review of their clinical efficacy, mechanisms of action, toxicity, and place in therapy. Drugs *36*:754, 1988.
65. Huang, M. Y., and Schacht, J.: Drug-induced ototoxicity. Pathogenesis and prevention. Med. Toxicol. Adverse Drug. Exp. *4*:452, 1989.
66. Rybak, L.: Furosemide ototoxicity: Clinical and experimental aspects. Laryngoscope *95*:1, 1985.
67. Mathog, R. H., and Klein, W. J.: Ototoxicity of ethacrynic acid and aminoglycoside antibiotics in uremia. N. Engl. J. Med. *280*:1223, 1989.
68. Scarpelli, D. G.: Toxicology of the pancreas. Toxicol. Appl. Pharmacol. *101*:543, 1989.

Thiazide Diuretics

69. Masterson, B. J., and Epstein, M.: Thiazide diuretics, chlorthalidone and metolazone. *In* Messerli, F. H. (ed.): Cardiovascular Drug Therapy. Philadelphia, W. B. Saunders Company, 1990, pp. 337–347.
70. Friedman, P. A.: Biochemistry and pharmacology of diuretics. Semin. Nephrol. *8*:198, 1988.
71. Ellison, D. H., Velazquez, H., and Wright, F. S.: Thiazide-sensitive sodium chloride cotransport in the early distal tubule. Am. J. Physiol. *253*(Renal Fluid Electrolyte Physiol.):F546, 1987.
72. Stier, C. T., and Itskovitz, H. D.: Renal calcium metabolism and diuretics. Ann. Rev. Pharmacol. Toxicol. *26*:101, 1986.
73. Ray, W. A., Downey, W., Griffin, M. R., and Melton, L. J., III: Long-term use of thiazide diuretics and risk of hip fracture. Lancet *1*:687, 1989.
74. Wilson, P. R., and Kem, D. C.: Thiazide diuretics and derivatives: Indapamide. *In* Messerli, F. H. (ed.): Cardiovascular Drug Therapy. Philadelphia, W. B. Saunders Company, 1990, pp. 348–356.
74a. Schaeffer, P., Vigne, P., Frelin, C., and Lazdunski, M.: Identification and pharmacological properties of binding sites for the atypical thiazide diuretic, indapamide. Eur. J. Pharmacol. *182*:503, 1990.
75. Leonetti, G., Rappelli, A., Salvetti, A., and Scapellato, L.: Long-term effects of indapamide: Final results of a two-year Italian multicenter study in systemic hypertension. Am. J. Cardiol. *65*:67H, 1990.
76. Aubert, I., Djian, F., and Rouffy, J.: Beneficial effects of indapamide on lipoproteins and apoproteins in ambulatory hypertensive patients. Am. J. Cardiol. *65*:77H, 1990.
77. Campbell, D. B., and Brackman, F.: Cardiovascular protective properties of indapamide. Am. J. Cardiol. *65*:11H, 1990.

Potassium-Sparing Diuretics

78. Fanestil, D. D.: Mechanism of action of aldosterone blockers. Semin. Nephrol. *8*:249, 1988.
79. Kim, K. E.: Potassium-sparing diuretics: Spironolactone. *In* Messerli, F. H.

(ed.): Cardiovascular Drug Therapy. Philadelphia, W. B. Saunders Company, 1990, pp. 382–391.
80. Kleyman, T. R., and Cragoe, E. J., Jr.: The mechanism of action of amiloride. Semin. Nephrol. *8*:242, 1988.
81. Eknoyan, G.: Potassium-sparing diuretics: Amiloride. *In* Messerli, F. H. (ed.): Cardiovascular Drug Therapy. Philadelphia, W. B. Saunders Company, 1990, pp. 368–381.
82. Rockstroh, J. K., Kasser, U. R., Losem, C. J., and Messerli, F. H.: Potassium-sparing diuretics. *In* Messerli, F. H. (ed.): Cardiovascular Drug Therapy. Philadelphia, W. B. Saunders Company, 1990, pp. 357–367.
83. Krishna, G. G., Shulman, M. D., and Narins, R. G.: Clinical use of the potassium-sparing diuretics. Semin. Nephrol. *8*:354, 1988.
84. Muller, J. E.: Spironolactone in the management of congestive heart failure. Am. J. Cardiol. *65*:51K, 1990.
85. Mironneau, J.: Calcium channel antagonist effects of spironolactone, an aldosterone antagonist. Am. J. Cardiol. *65*:7K, 1990.
86. Lagrue, G., Anaquer, J. C., and Meyer-Heine, A.: Peripheral action of spironolactone: Improvement in arterial elasticity. Am. J. Cardiol. *65*:9K, 1990.

Diuretic Combinations

87. Channer, K. S., Richardson, M., Crook, R., and Jones, J. V.: Thiazides with loop diuretics for severe congestive heart failure. Lancet *1*:922, 1990.
88. Kiyingi, A., Field, M. J., Pawsey, C. C., et al.: Metolazone in treatment of severe refractory congestive cardiac failure. Lancet *1*:29, 1990.
89. Loon, N. R., Wilcox, C. S., and Unwin, R. J.: Mechanism of impaired natriuretic response to furosemide during prolonged therapy. Kidney Int. *36*:682, 1989.
90. Arnold, W. C.: Efficacy of metolazone and furosemide in children with furosemide-resistant edema. Pediatrics *74*:872, 1984.
91. Allman, S., and Norris, R. J.: An open, parallel group study comparing a frusemide/amiloride diuretic and a diuretic containing cyclopenthiazide with sustained release potassium in the treatment of congestive cardiac failure—a multicenter general practice study. J. Int. Med. Res. *18*:17B, 1990.
91a. Schohn, D. C., and Jahn, H. A.: Effects of a potassium-sparing/thiazide diuretic combination on cardiovascular reactivity to vasopressor agents. Am. J. Cardiol. *65*:14K, 1990.
91b. Lipworth, B. J., McDevitt, D. G., and Struthers, A. D.: Hypokalemic and ECG sequelae of combined beta-agonist/diuretic therapy. Protection by conventional doses of spironolactone but not triamterene. Chest *98*:811, 1990.
91c. Ridgeway, N. A., Ginn, D. R., and Alley, K.: Outpatient conversation of treatment to potassium sparing diuretics. Am. J. Med. *80*:785, 1986.
92. Preisig, P. A., Toto, R. D., and Alpern, R. J.: Carbonic anhydrase inhibitors. Renal Physiol. *10*:136, 1987.
93. Eveloff, J., and Warnock, D. G.: Renal carbonic anhydrase. *In* Dirks, J. H., and Sutton, R. A. L. (eds.): Diuretics: Physiology, Pharmacology and Clinical Use. Philadelphia, W. B. Saunders Company, 1986, p. 49.
94. DuBose, T. D., Jr., and Good, D. W.: Effects of diuretics on renal acid-base transport. Semin. Nephrol. *8*:282, 1988.
95. Daniels, B. S., and Ferris, T. F.: The use of diuretics in nonedematous disorders. Semin. Nephrol. *8*:342, 1988.
96. Singh, M. V., Jain, S. C., Rawal, S. B., et al.: Comparative study of acetazolamide and spironolactone on body fluid components on induction to high altitude. Int. J. Biometeorol. *30*:33, 1986.

Atrial Natriuretic Peptide

97. Levin, E. R., Frank, H. J. L., Gelfand, R., et al.: Natriuretic peptide receptors in cultured rat diencephalon. J. Biol. Chem. *265*:10019, 1990.
97a. Mukoyama, M., Nakao K., Hosoda, K., et al.: Brain natriuretic peptide as a novel cardiac hormone in humans. J. Clin. Invest. *87*:1402–1412, 1991.
98. Zeidel, M. L.: Renal actions of atrial natriuretic peptide: Regulation of collecting duct sodium and water transport. Annu. Rev. Physiol. *52*:747, 1990.
98a. Nussenzveig, D. R., Lewicki, J. A., and Maack, T.: Cellular mechanisms of the clearance function of type C receptors of atrial natriuretic factor. J. Biol. Chem. *265*:20952, 1990.
99. Cody, R. J., Atlas, S. A., Laragh, J. H., et al.: Atrial natriuretic factor in normal subjects and heart failure patients. Plasma level and renal, hormonal and hemodynamic responses to peptide infusion. J. Clin. Invest. *78*:1362, 1986.
100. Burnett, J. C., Kao, P. C., Hu, D. C., et al.: Atrial natriuretic peptide elevation in congestive heart failure in the human. Science *231*:1145, 1986.
101. Raine, A. E. G., Phil, D., Erne, P., et al.: Atrial natriuretic peptide and atrial pressure in patients with congestive heart failure. N. Engl. J. Med. *315*:533, 1986.
101a. Northridge, D. B., Jardine, A. G., Findlay, I. N., et al.: Inhibition of the metabolism of atrial natriuretic factor causes diuresis and natriuresis in chronic heart failure. Am. J. Hypertens. *3*:682, 1990.
101b. Nakamura, M., Arakawa, N., and Kato, M.: Renal, hormonal, and hemodynamic effects of low-dose infusion of atrial natriuretic factor in acute myocardial infarction. Am. Heart J. *120*:1078, 1990.
102. Riegger, G. A. J., Elsner, D., Kromer, E. P., et al.: Atrial natriuretic peptide in congestive heart failure in the dog: Plasma levels, cyclic guanosine monophosphate, ultrastructure of atrial myoendocrine cells, and hemodynamic, hormonal, and renal effects. Circulation *77*:398, 1988.
102a. Curnett, J. C., Jr.: Atrial natriuretic factor. Is it physiologically important? Circulation *82*:1523, 1990.
102b. Volpe, M., Lembo, G., Condorelli, G., et al.: Converting enzyme inhibition prevents the effects of atrial natriuretic factor on baroreflex responses in humans. Circulation *82*:1214, 1990.
102c. Floras, J. S.: Sympathoinhibitory effects of atrial natriuretic factor in normal humans. Circulation *81*:1860, 1990.
102d. Münzel, T., Drexler, H., Holtz, J., et al.: Mechanism involved in the response to prolonged infusion of atrial natriuretic factor in patients with chronic heart failure. Circulation *83*:191, 1991.

Complications of Diuretic Therapy

103. Velazquez, H., and Giebisch, G.: Effect of diuretics on specific transport systems: Potassium. Semin. Nephrol. *8*:295, 1988.
104. Thier, S. O.: Potassium physiology. Am. J. Med. *80*:3, 1986.
105. Dyckner, T.: Relation of cardiovascular disease to potassium and magnesium deficiencies. Am. J. Cardiol. *65*:44K, 1990.
106. Freis, E. D.: Critique of the clinical importance of diuretic-induced hypokalemia and elevated cholesterol level. Arch. Intern. Med. *149*:2640, 1989.
107. Packer, M.: Potential role of potassium as a determinant of morbidity and mortality in patients with systemic hypertension and congestive heart failure. Am. J. Cardiol. *65*:45E, 1990.
108. Podrid, P. J.: Potassium and ventricular arrhythmias. Am. J. Cardiol. *65*:33E, 1990.
108a. Freis, E. D.: The cardiotoxicity of thiazide diuretics: Review of the evidence. J. Hypertens. *8*:S23, 1990.
109. Kelly, R. A.: Cardiac glycosides and congestive heart failure. Am. J. Cardiol. *65*:10E, 1990.
110. Chakko, S. C., Frutchey, J., and Gheorghiade, M.: Life-threatening hyperkalemia in severe heart failure. Am. Heart J. *117*:1083, 1989.
111. Gottlieb, S. S., Baruch, L., Kukin, M. L., et al.: Prognostic importance of the serum magnesium concentration in patients with congestive heart failure. J. Am. Coll. Cardiol. *16*:827, 1990.
111a. Ralston, M. A., Murnane, M. R., Unverferth, D. V., and Leier, C. V.: Serum and tissue magnesium concentrations in patients with heart failure and serious ventricular arrhythmias. Ann. Intern. Med. *113*:841, 1990.
111b. Dyckner, T., Wester, P.-O., and Widman, L.: Amiloride prevents thiazide-induced intracellular potassium and magnesium losses. Acta Med. Scand. *224*:25, 1988.
112. Kelepouris, E., and Agus, Z. S.: Effects of diuretics on calcium and phosphate transport. Semin. Nephrol. *8*:273, 1988.
113. Seelig, M.: Cardiovascular consequences of magnesium deficiency and loss: Pathogenesis, prevalence and manifestations—magnesium and chloride loss in refractory potassium repletion. Am. J. Cardiol. *63*:4G, 1989.
114. Mountakalakis, T. D.: Effects of aging, chronic disease, and multiple supplements on magnesium requirements. Magnesium *6*:5, 1987.
115. Gottlieb, S. S.: Importance of magnesium in congestive heart failure. Am. J. Cardiol. *63*:39G, 1989.
116. Cronin, R. E.: Magnesium disorders. *In* Kokko, J. P., and Tannen, R. L. (eds.): Fluids and Electrolytes, 2nd ed. Philadelphia, W. B. Saunders Company, 1990, p. 631.
117. Reinhart, R. A.: Magnesium metabolism. A review with special reference to the relationship between intracellular content and serum levels. Arch. Intern. Med. *148*:2415, 1988.
118. Dorup, I., Skajaa, K., Clausen, T., and Kjeldsen, K.: Reduced concentrations of potassium, magnesium, and sodium-potassium pumps in human skeletal muscle during treatment with diuretics. Br. Med. J. *296*:455, 1988.
119. Abraham, A. S., Rosenman, D., Meshulam, Z., et al.: Serum, lymphocyte, and erythrocyte potassium, magnesium, and calcium concentrations and their relation to tachyarrhythmias in patients with acute myocardial infarction. Am. J. Med. *81*:983, 1986.
119a. Reinhart, R. A., Marx, J. J., Broste, S. K., and Hass, R. G.: Myocardial magnesium: Relation to laboratory and clinical variables in patients undergoing cardiac surgery. J. Am. Coll. Cardiol. *17*:651, 1991.
120. Roden, D. M.: Magnesium treatment of ventricular arrhythmias. Am. J. Cardiol. *63*:43G, 1989.
121. Iseri, L. T.: Role of magnesium in cardiac tachyarrhythmias. Am. J. Cardiol. *65*:47K, 1990.
122. Rasmussen, A. S., McNair, P., Norregard, P., et al.: Intravenous magnesium in acute myocardial infarction. Lancet *1*:234, 1986.
123. Abraham, A. S., Rosenmann, D., Kramer, M., et al.: Magnesium in the prevention of lethal arrhythmias in acute myocardial infarction. Arch. Intern. Med. *147*:753, 1987.
123a. Tzivoni, D., Shmuel Banai, S., Schuger, C., et al.: Treatment of torsade de pointes with magnesium sulfate. Circulation *77*:392, 1988.
124. Kastor, J. A.: Multifocal atrial tachycardia. N. Engl. J. Med. *322*:1713, 1990.
125. Iseri, L. T., Fairshter, R. D., Hardemann, J. L., and Brodsky, M. A.: Magnesium and potassium therapy in multifocal atrial tachycardia. Am. Heart J. *110*:789, 1985.
126. Iseri, L. T.: Magnesium and cardiac arrhythmias. Magnesium 5:111, 1986.
126a. Perticone, F., Borelli, D., Ceravolo, R., et al.: Antiarrhythmic short-term protective magnesium treatment in ischemic dilated cardiomyopathy. J. Am. Coll. Nutr. *9*:492, 1990.

127. DiCarlo, L. A., Jr., Morady, F., DeButtleir, M., et al.: Effects of magnesium sulfate on cardiac conduction and refractoriness in humans. J. Am. Coll. Cardiol. 7:1356, 1986.
128. Kulick, D. L., Hong, R., Ryzen, E., et al.: Electrophysiologic effects of intravenous magnesium in patients with normal conduction systems and no clinical evidence of significant cardiac disease. Am. Heart J. 115:367, 1988.
129. White, R. E., and Hartzell, H. C.: Effects of intracellular free magnesium on calcium current in isolated cardiac myocytes. Science 239:778, 1988.
130. Hollifield, J. W.: Thiazide treatment of systemic hypertension: Effects on serum magnesium and ventricular ectopic activity. Am. J. Cardiol. 63:22G, 1989.
131. Nader, P. C., Thompson, J. R., and Alpern, R. J.: Complications of diuretic use. Semin. Nephrol. 8:365, 1988.
132. Packer, M., Lee, W. H., Kessler, P. D., et al.: Identification of hyponatremia as a risk factor for the development of functional renal insufficiency during converting-enzyme inhibition in severe chronic heart failure. J. Am. Coll. Cardiol. 10:837, 1987.
133. Nicholls, M. G.: Interaction of diuretics and electrolytes in congestive heart failure. Am. J. Cardiol. 65:17E, 1990.
134. Francis, G. S.: Interaction of the sympathetic nervous system and electrolytes in congestive heart failure. Am. J. Cardiol. 65:24E, 1990.
135. Dargie, H. J.: Interrelation of electrolytes and renin-angiotensin system in congestive heart failure. Am. J. Cardiol. 65:28E, 1990.
136. Packer, M.: Identification of risk factors predisposing to the development of functional renal insufficiency during treatment with converting-enzyme inhibitors in chronic heart failure. Cardiology 76:50, 1989.
137. Narins, R. G.: Therapy of hyponatremia. Does haste make waste? N. Engl. J. Med. 314:1573, 1986.
138. Packer, M., Lee, W. H., Medina, N., et al.: Functional renal insufficiency during long-term therapy with captopril and enalapril in severe chronic heart failure. Ann. Intern. Med. 106:346, 1987.
139. DuBose, T. D., Jr., and Good, D. W.: Effects of diuretics on renal acid-base transport. Semin. Nephrol. 8:282, 1988.
140. Wall, S. M., and Knepper, M. A.: Acid-base transport in the inner medullary collecting duct. Semin. Nephrol. 10:148, 1990.
141. Knepper, M. A., Packer, R., and Good, D. W.: Ammonium transport in the kidney. Physiol. Rev. 69:179, 1989.
142. Good, D. W., and Knepper, M. A.: Mechanisms of ammonium excretion: Role of the renal medulla. Semin. Nephrol. 10:166, 1990.
143. O'Byrne, S., and Feely, J.: Effects of drugs on glucose tolerance in non-insulin-dependent diabetics (Part I). Drugs 40:6, 1990.
143a. Pollare, T.: Insulin sensitivity and blood lipids during antihypertensive treatment with special reference to ACE inhibition. J. Diabet. Compl. 4:75, 1990.
143b. Pollare, T., Lithell, H., and Berne, C.: A comparison of the effects of hydrochlorothiazide and captopril on glucose and lipid metabolism in patients with hypertension. N. Engl. J. Med. 321:868, 1989.
144. Black, H. R.: The coronary artery disease paradox: The role of hyperinsulinemia and insulin resistance and implications for therapy. J. Cardiovasc. Pharmacol. 15:S26, 1990.
144a. Bloomgarden, Z. T., Ginsberg-Fellner, F., Rayfield, E. J., et al.: Elevated hemoglobin A_{1C} and low-density cholesterol levels in thiazide-treated diabetes. Am. J. Med. 77:823, 1984.
145. Raftery, E. B.: The metabolic effects of diuretics and other antihypertensive drugs: A perspective as of 1989. Int. J. Cardiol. 28:143, 1990.
145a. Thompson, W. G.: An assault on old friends: Thiazide diuretics under siege. Am. J. Med. Sci. 300:152, 1990.
145b. Ames, R.: Effects of diuretic drugs on the lipid profile. Drugs 36:33, 1988.
146. Johnson, B. F., and Danylchuk, M. A.: The relevance of plasma lipid changes with cardiovascular drug therapy. Med. Clin. North Am. 73:449, 1989.
147. Weinberger, M. H.: Diuretics and their side effects. Dilemma in the treatment of hypertension. Hypertension 11:II–16, 1988.
148. Multiple Risk Factor Intervention Trial Research Group: Multiple Risk Factor Intervention Trial: Risk factor changes and mortality results. J.A.M.A. 248:1465, 1982.
149. Freis, E. D.: Critique of the clinical importance of diuretic-induced hypokalemia and elevated cholesterol level. Arch. Intern. Med. 149:2640, 1989.
150. Goldman, A. I., Steele, B. W., Schnaper, H. W., et al.: Serum lipoprotein levels during chlorthalidone therapy—a Veterans Administration–National Heart, Lung, and Blood Institute cooperative study on antihypertensive therapy: Mild hypertension. J.A.M.A. 244:1691, 1980.
151. Williams, W. R., Scheider, K. A., Borhani, N. O., et al.: The relationship between diuretics and serum cholesterol in hypertension detection and follow-up program participants. Am. J. Prevent. Med. 2:248, 1986.
152. Linn, S., Fulwood, R., Rifkind, B., et al.: High density lipoprotein cholesterol levels among US adults by selected demographic and socioeconomic variables. Am. J. Epidemiol. 129:281, 1989.
153. Lipid Research Clinics Program. The Lipid Research Clinics Coronary Primary Prevention Trial results: I. Reduction in incidence of coronary heart disease. J.A.M.A. 251:351, 1984.
154. Frick, M. H., Elo, O., Haapa, K., et al.: Helsinki Heart Study: Primary prevention trial with gemfibrozil in middle-aged men with dyslipidemia. N. Engl. J. Med. 317:1237, 1987.
155. Samuelsson, O., Wilhelmsen, L., Andersson, O. K., et al.: Cardiovascular morbidity in relation to change in blood pressure and serum cholesterol levels in treated hypertension. J.A.M.A. 258:1768, 1987.
155a. Goldsmith, S. R., Francis, G., and Cohn, J. N.: Attenuation of the pressor response to intravenous furosemide by angiotensin converting enzyme inhibition in congestive heart failure. Am. J. Cardiol. 64:1382, 1989.
156. Ames, R. P.: The effects of antihypertensive drugs on serum lipids and lipoproteins: I. Diuretics. II. Non-diuretic drugs. Drugs 32:260, 1986.
157. Goto, Y., Tanabe, T., Ogasawara, Y., et al.: The effects of prazosin and propranolol in combination with thiazide diuretics on blood pressure and serum lipids: A multicenter study. Eur. J. Clin. Pharmacol. 33:339, 1987.
158. Luther, R. R., Glassman, H. N., Estep, C. B., et al.: The effects of terazosin and methyclothiazide on blood pressure and serum lipids. Am. Heart J. 117:842, 1989.
159. Kahn, A. M.: Effect of diuretics on the renal handling of urate. Semin. Nephrol. 8:305, 1988.
159a. Roubenoff, R.: Gout and hypertension. Rheum. Dis. Clin. North Am. 16:539, 1990.

SPECIAL USES OF DIURETICS

160. Kaplan, S.: New drug approaches to the treatment of heart failure in infants and children. Drugs 39:388, 1990.
161. Chemtob, S., Kaplan, B. S., Sherbotie, J. R., and Aranda, J. V.: Pharmacology of diuretics in the newborn. Pediatr. Clin. North Am. 36:1231, 1989.
161a. Wells, T. G.: The pharmacology and therapeutics of diuretics in the pediatric patient. Pediatr. Clin. North Am. 37:463, 1990.
162. Green, T. P.: The pharmacologic basis of diuretic therapy in the newborn. Clin. Perinatol. 14:951, 1987.
163. Vileisis, R. A.: Furosemide effect on mineral status of parenterally nourished premature neonates with chronic lung disease. Pediatrics 85:316, 1990.
164. Nicholls, M. G.: Age-related effects of diuretics in hypertensive subjects. J. Cardiovasc. Pharmacol. 12:S51, 1988.
165. Hulley, S. B., Furberg, C. D., Gurland, B., et al.: Systolic hypertension in the elderly program (SHEP): Antihypertensive efficacy of chlorthalidone. Am. J. Cardiol. 56:913, 1985.
166. Weinberger, M. H.: Diuretic responsiveness of blood pressure in the elderly. J. Cardiovasc. Pharmacol. 12:S60, 1988.
167. Moser, M.: Diuretics and alternative drugs in geriatric hypertension. Geriatrics 42:39, 1987.
168. McMurray, J., and McDevitt, D. G.: Treatment of heart failure in the elderly. Br. Med. Bull. 46:202, 1990.
169. Ikram, H.: Arrhythmias, electrolytes, and ACE inhibitor therapy in the elderly. Gerontology 33:42, 1987.
170. Kelly, R. A., and Mitch, W. E.: Diuretics in renal failure. In Messerli, F. H. (ed.): Cardiovascular Drug Therapy. Philadelphia, W. B. Saunders Company, 1990.
171. Brater, D. C.: Use of diuretics in chronic renal insufficiency and nephrotic syndrome. Semin. Nephrol. 8:333, 1988.
172. L'Abbate, A., Emdin, M., Piacenti, M., et al.: Ultrafiltration: A rational treatment for heart failure. Cardiology 76:384, 1989.
173. Rimondini, A., Cipolla, C. M., Della Bella, P., et al.: Hemofiltration as short-term treatment for refractory congestive heart failure. Am. J. Med. 83:43, 1987.
173a. Cipolla, C. M., Grazis, Rimondini, A., et al.: Changes in circulating norepinephrine with hemofiltration in advanced congestive heart failure. Am. J. Cardiol. 15:987, 1990.
174. Simpson, I. A., Simpson, K., Rae, A. P., et al.: Ultrafiltration in the management of refractory congestive heart failure. Renal Fail. 10:115, 1987.
175. Zobel, G., Beitzke, A., Stein, J. K., and Trop, M.: Continuous arteriovenous haemofiltration in children with postoperative cardiac failure. Br. Heart J. 58:473, 1987.
176. Simpson, I. A., Rae, A. P., Simpson, K., et al.: Ultrafiltration in the management of refractory congestive heart failure. Br. Heart J. 55:344, 1986.

DIGITALIS GLYCOSIDES

177. Withering, W.: An account of the foxglove and some of its medical uses, with practical remarks on dropsy, and other diseases. In Willis, F. A., and Keys, T. E. (eds.): Classics of Cardiology. New York, Henry Schuman, Inc., 1941, p. 231.
178. Thomas, R., Gray, P., and Andrews, J.: Digitalis: Its mode of action, receptor, and structure-activity relationships. In Testa, B. (ed.): Advances in Drug Research. Vol. 19. New York, Academic Press, 1989.
179. Kim, D., Barry, W. H., and Smith, T. W.: Kinetics of ouabain binding and changes in cellular sodium content, $^{42}K^+$ transport, and contractile state during ouabain exposure in cultured chick heart cells. J. Pharmacol. Exp. Ther. 231:326, 1984.
180. Marban, E., and Smith, T. W.: Digitalis. In Fozzard, H. M., et al. (eds.): The Heart and Cardiovascular System. New York, Raven Press, 1986.
181. Lee, C. O.: 200 years of digitalis: The emerging central role of the sodium ion in the control of cardiac force. Am. J. Physiol. 249:C367, 1985.
182. Braunwald, E.: Effects of digitalis on the normal and the failing heart. J. Am. Coll. Cardiol. 5:51A, 1985.
183. Marban, E., and Tsien, R. W.: Enhancement of cardiac calcium current during digitalis inotropy: Positive feedback regulation by intracellular calcium? J. Physiol. 329:589, 1982.
184. Langer, G. A., and Serena, S. D.: Effects of strophanthidin upon contraction and ionic exchange in rabbit ventricular myocardium: Relation to control of active state. J. Mol. Cell. Cardiol. 1:65, 1970.
185. Morgan, J. P., and Blinks, J. R.: Intracellular Ca^{++} transients in the cat papillary muscle. Can. J. Physiol. Pharmacol. 60:524, 1982.

186. Weir, W. G., and Hess, P.: Excitation-contraction coupling in cardiac Purkinje fibers. Effects of cardiotonic steroids on the intracellular [Ca^{2+}] transient, membrane potential, and contraction. J. Gen. Physiol. *83*:395, 1984.
187. Barry, W. H., Hasin, Y., and Smith, T. W.: Sodium pump inhibition, enhanced Ca-influx via Na-Ca exchange, and positive inotropic response in cultured heart cells. Circ. Res. *56*:231, 1985.
188. Pedemonte, C. H., and Kaplan, J. H.: Chemical modification as an approach to elucidation of sodium pump structure-function relations. Am. J. Physiol. *258*:C1, 1990.
189. Price, E. M., Rice, D. A., and Lingrel, J. B.: Site-directed mutagenesis of a conserved, extracellular aspartic acid residue affects the ouabain sensitivity of sheep Na,K-ATPase. J. Biol. Chem. *264*:21902, 1989.
190. Shull, M. M., and Lingrel, J. B.: Multiple genes encode the human Na^+,K^+-ATPase catalytic subunit. Proc. Natl. Acad. Sci. USA *84*:4039, 1987.
191. Smith, T. W., Braunwald, E., and Kelly, R.: Management of heart failure. *In* Braunwald, E. (ed.): Heart Disease, 3rd ed. Philadelphia, W. B. Saunders Company, 1988, pp. 485–543.
192. Rasmussen, H. H., Okita, G. T., Hartz, R. S., and Ten Eick, R. E.: Inhibition of electrogenic Na^+-pumping in isolated atrial tissue from patients treated with digoxin. J. Pharmacol. Exp. Ther. *252*:60, 1990.
193. Haddy, F. J.: Endogenous digitalis-like factor or factors. N. Engl. J. Med. *316*:621, 1987.
194. Kelly, R. A., and Smith, T. W.: The search for the endogenous digitalis: An alternative hypothesis. Am. J. Physiol. *256*:C937, 1989.
195. Grupp, I., Im, W. B., Lee, C. O., et al.: Relation of sodium pump inhibition to positive inotropy at low concentrations of ouabain in rat heart muscle. J. Physiol. *360*:149, 1985.
196. Langer, G. A.: Relationship between myocardial contractility and the effects of digitalis on ionic exchange. Fed. Proc. *36*:2231, 1977.
196a. Eisner, D. A., and Smith, T. W.: The Na-K pump and its effectors in cardiac muscle. *In* Fozzard HA, et al., (eds.): The Heart and Cardiovascular System. 2nd ed. New York, Raven Press. In press.
196b. Reuter, H.: Ins and outs of Ca^{2+} transport. Nature *349*:567, 1991.
196c. Niggli, E., and Lederer, W. J.: Molecular operations of the sodium-calcium exchanger revealed by conformation currents. Nature *349*:621, 1991.
197. Smith, T. W., Antman, E. M., Friedman, P. L., et al.: Digitalis glycosides: Mechanisms and manifestations of toxicity. Prog. Cardiovasc. Dis. *26*:413, 495, 1984; *27*:21, 1985.
198. Rosen, M. R.: Cellular electrophysiology of digitalis toxicity. J. Am. Coll. Cardiol. *5*:22A, 1985.
198a. Hoffman, B. F., and Bigger, J. T.: Digitalis and allied cardiac glycosides. *In* Gilman, A. F., et al. (eds.): The Pharmacologic Basis of Therapeutics. 8th ed. New York, Pergamon Press, 1990, p. 814.
199. Dhingra, R. C., Amat-Y-Leon, F., Wyndham, C., et al.: The electrophysiological effects of ouabain on sinus node and atrium in man. J. Clin. Invest. *56*:555, 1975.
200. Friedman, P. L.: Therapeutic and toxic electrophysiologic effects of cardiac glycosides. *In* Smith, T. W. (ed.): Digitalis Glycosides. Orlando, Grune & Stratton, 1985, p. 29.
201. Weingart, R.: Influence of cardiac glycosides on electrophysiologic processes. *In* Greeff, K. (ed.): Cardiac Glycosides. Vol. 56, Part I, Handbook of Experimental Pharmacology. Berlin, Springer-Verlag, 1981.
202. Gillis, R. A., and Quest, J. A.: The role of the nervous system in the cardiovascular effects of digitalis. Pharmacol. Rev. *31*:19, 1979.
203. Somberg, J. C., and Smith, T. W.: Localization of the neurally mediated arrhythmogenic properties of digitalis. Science *204*:321, 1979.
204. Rosen, M. R.: Interactions of digitalis with the autonomic nervous system and their relationship to cardiac arrhythmias. *In* Disturbances in Neurogenic Control of the Circulation. Bethesda, American Physiological Society, 1981, p. 251.
205. Watanabe, A. M.: Digitalis and the autonomic nervous system. J. Am. Coll. Cardiol. *5*:35A, 1985.
206. Porter, T. R., Eckberg, D. L., Fritsch, J. M., et al.: Autonomic pathophysiology in heart failure patients: Sympathetic-cholinergic interrelations. J. Clin. Invest. *85*:1362, 1990.
207. Creager, M. A., Hirsch, A. T., Dzau, V. J., et al.: Baroreflex regulation of regional blood flow in congestive heart failure. Am. J. Physiol. *258*:H1409, 1990.
208. Osterziel, K. J., Dietz, R., Manthey, J., et al.: Haemodynamic changes caused by alteration of autonomic activity in patients with heart failure. Br. Heart J. *63*:221, 1990.
209. Rea, R. F., and Berg, W. J.: Abnormal baroreflex mechanisms in congestive heart failure. Recent insights. Circulation *81*:2026, 1990.
210. Ellenbogen, K. A., Mohanty, P. K., Szentpetery, S., and Thames, M. D.: Studies after cardiac transplantation: Arterial baroreflex abnormalities in heart failure: Reversal after orthotopic cardiac transplantation. Circulation *79*:51, 1989.
210a. Marinnet, J. A., Pintya, A. O., Gallo, L., and Maciel, B. C.: Abnormal baroreflex control of heart rate in decompensated congestive heart failure and reversal after compensation. Am. J. Cardiol. *67*:604, 1991.
211. Ferguson, D. W., Berg, W. J., Sanders, J. S., et al.: Sympathoinhibitory responses to digitalis glycosides in heart failure patients: Direct evidence from sympathetic neural recordings. Circulation *80*:65, 1989.
212. Wang, W., Chen, J. S., and Zucker, I. H.: Carotid sinus baroreceptor sensitivity in experimental heart failure. Circulation *81*:1959, 1990.
213. Packer, M. (ed.): Role of the sympathetic nervous system in heart failure: Basic mechanisms and clinical directions. Circulation *82*(Suppl. 1):1, 1990.
214. Cattell, M., and Gold, H.: The influence of digitalis glycosides on the force of contraction of mammalian cardiac muscle. J. Pharmacol. Exp. Ther. *62*:116, 1938.
215. Braunwald, E., Bloodwell, R. D., Goldberg, L. I., and Morrow, A. G.: Studies on digitalis: IV. Observations in man on the effects of digitalis preparations on the contractility of the non-failing heart and on total vascular resistance. J. Clin. Invest. *40*:52, 1961.
216. Arnold, S. B., Byrd, R. C., Meister, W., et al.: Long-term digitalis therapy improves left ventricular function in heart failure. N. Engl. J. Med. *303*:1443, 1980.
217. Lee, D. C.-S., Johnson, R. A., Bingham, J. B., et al.: Heart failure in outpatients. A randomized trial of digoxin versus placebo. N. Engl. J. Med. *306*:699, 1982.
218. Bostrom, P. A., Andersson, J., Johansson, B. W., et al.: Haemodynamic effects of prenalterol and cardiac glycosides in patients with recent myocardial infarction. Eur. J. Clin. Invest. *14*:175, 1984.
219. Smith, T. W.: Medical treatment of advanced congestive heart failure: Digitalis and diuretics. *In* Braunwald, E., Moch, M. B., and Watson, J. T. (eds.): Congestive Heart Failure. New York, Grune & Stratton, 1982, p. 261.
220. Beiser, G. D., Epstein, S. E., Stampfer, M., et al.: Studies on digitalis: XVII. Effects of ouabain on the hemodynamic response to exercise in patients with mitral stenosis in normal sinus rhythm. N. Engl. J. Med. *278*:131, 1968.
221. Blatt, C. M., Marsh, J. D., and Smith, T. W.: Extracardiac effects of digitalis. *In* Smith, T. W. (ed.): Digitalis Glycosides. Orlando, Grune & Stratton, 1985, p. 209.
221a. Cohn, J. N., Tristani, F. E., and Khatril, M.: Cardiac and peripheral vascular effects of digitalis in clinical shock. Am. Heart J. *78*:318, 1969.
222. DeMots, H., Rahimtoola, S. H., McAnulty, J. H., and Porter, G. A.: Effects of ouabain on coronary and systemic vascular resistance and myocardial oxygen consumption in patients without heart failure. Am. J. Cardiol. *41*:88, 1978.
223. Longhurst, J. C., and Ross, J.: Extracardiac and coronary vascular effects of digitalis. J. Am. Coll. Cardiol. *5*:99A, 1985.
224. Covpit, A. B., Schaer, G. L., Scaley, J. E., et al.: Suppression of the renin-angiotensin system by IV digoxin in chronic congestive heart failure. Am. J. Med. *75*:445, 1983.
225. Griffiths, B. E., Penny, W. J., Lewis, M. J., and Henderson, A. H.: Maintenance of the inotropic effect of digoxin on long-term treatment. Br. Med. J. *284*:1819, 1982.
226. Murray, R. G., Tweddel, A. C., Martin, W., et al.: Evaluation of digitalis in cardiac failure. Br. Med. J. *284*:1526, 1982.
227. Gheorghiade, M., St. Clair, J., St. Clair, C., and Beller, G. A.: Hemodynamic effects of intravenous digoxin in patients with severe heart failure initially treated with diuretics and vasodilators. J. Am. Coll. Cardiol. *9*:849, 1987.
228. Gheorghiade, M., Hall, V., Lakier, J. B., and Goldstein, S.: Comparative hemodynamic and neurohormonal effects of intravenous captopril and digoxin and their combinations in patients with severe heart failure. J. Am. Coll. Cardiol. *13*:134, 1989.
229. Sullivan, M., Atwood, J. E., Myers, J., et al.: Increased exercise capacity after digoxin administration in patients with heart failure. J. Am. Coll. Cardiol. *13*:1138, 1989.
230. DiBianco, R., Shabetai, R., Kostuk, W., et al.: A comparison of oral milrinone, digoxin, and their combination in the treatment of patients with chronic heart failure. N. Engl. J. Med. *320*:677, 1989.
231. Captopril Digoxin Multicenter Research Group: Comparative effects of therapy with captopril and digoxin in patients with mild to moderate heart failure. J.A.M.A. *259*:539, 1988.
231a. Fleg, J. L., Fothfeld, B., Gottlieb, S. H., and Wright, J.: Effect of maintenance digoxin therapy on aerobic performance and exercise left ventricular function in mild-to-moderate heart failure due to coronary artery disease—a randomized, placebo controlled, crossover trial. J. Am. Coll. Cardiol. *17*:743, 1991.
232. Fleg, J. L., Gottlieb, S. H., and Lakatta, E. G.: Is digoxin really important in treatment of compensated heart failure? Am. J. Med. *73*:244, 1982.
233. Guyatt, G. H., Sullivan, M. J. J., Fallen, E. L., et al.: A controlled trial of digoxin in congestive heart failure. Am. J. Cardiol. *61*:371, 1988.
234. Pugh, S. E., White, N. J., Aronson, J. K., et al.: Clinical, haemodynamic, and pharmacological effects of withdrawal and reintroduction of digoxin in patients with heart failure in sinus rhythm after long-term treatment. Br. Heart J. *61*:529, 1989.
235. Taggart, A. J., Johnston, G. D., and McDevitt, D. G.: Digoxin withdrawal after cardiac failure in patients with sinus rhythm. J. Cardiovasc. Pharmacol. *5*:229, 1983.
236. German and Austrian Xamoterol Study Group: Double-blind placebo-controlled comparison of digoxin and xamoterol in chronic heart failure. Lancet *1*:489, 1988.
237. Antman, E. M., and Smith, T. W.: Pharmacokinetics of digitalis glycosides. *In* Smith, T. W. (ed.): Digitalis Glycosides. Orlando, Grune & Stratton, 1985, p. 45.
238. Lindebaum, J., Rund, D. G., and Butler, V. P., Jr.: Inactivation of digoxin by the gut flora: Reversal by antibiotic therapy. N. Engl. J. Med. *305*:789, 1981.
239. Halkin, H., Sheiner, L. B., Peck, C. C., and Melmon, K. L.: Determinants of the renal clearance of digoxin. Clin. Pharmacol. Ther. *385*:394, 1975.
240. Ackerman, G. L., Doherty, J. E., and Flanigan, W. J.: Peritoneal dialysis and hemodialysis of tritiated digoxin. Ann. Intern. Med. *67*:718, 1967.
241. Cogan, J. J., Humphreys, M. H., Carlson, C. J., et al.: Acute vasodilator therapy increases renal clearance of digoxin in patients with congestive heart failure. Circulation *64*:973, 1981.

364. Lewis, G. R.: Comparison of lisinopril versus placebo for congestive heart failure. Am. J. Cardiol. *63*:12D, 1989.
365. Lijnen, P., Fagard R., Staessen, J., et al.: Role of various vasodepressor systems in the acute hypotensive effect of captopril in man. Eur. J. Clin. Pharmacol. *20*:1, 1981.
366. Nishimura, H., Kubo, S., Ueyama, M., et al.: Peripheral hemodynamic effects of captopril in patients with congestive heart failure. Am. Heart J. *117*:100, 1989.
367. Dzau, V. J.: Mechanism of action of angiotensin-converting enzyme (ACE) inhibitors in hypertension and heart failure: Role of plasma versus tissue ACE. Drugs *39*(Suppl. 2):11, 1980.
368. Urata, H., Healey, B., Steward, R. W., et al.: Angiotensin II-forming pathways in normal and failing human hearts. Circ. Res. *66*:883, 1990.
369. Riegger, G. A. J., and Kochsiek, K.: Vasopressin, renin, and norepinephrine levels before and after captopril administration in patients with congestive heart failure due to idiopathic dilated cardiomyopathy. Am. J. Cardiol. *58*:300, 1986.
370. Mulligan, I. P., Fraser, A. G., Lewis, M. J., and Henderson, A. H.: Effects of enalapril on myocardial noradrenaline overflow during exercise in patients with chronic heart failure. Br. Heart J. *61*:23, 1989.
371. Corbalán, R., Jalil, J., Chamorro, G., et al.: Effects of captopril versus milrinone therapy in modulating the adrenergic nervous system response to exercise in congestive heart failure. Am. J. Cardiol. *65*:644, 1990.
372. Horn, E. M., Corwin, S. J., Steinberg, S. F., et al.: Reduced lymphocyte stimulatory guanine nucleotide regulatory protein and beta-adrenergic receptors in congestive heart failure and reversal with angiotensin converting enzyme inhibitor therapy. Circulation *78*:1373, 1988.
373. Francis, G. S., and Rucinska, E. J.: Long-term effects of a once-a-day versus twice-a-day regimen of enalapril for congestive heart failure. Am. J. Cardiol. *63*:17D, 1989.
374. Foult, J. M., Tavolaro, O., Antony, I., and Nitenberg, A.: Direct myocardial and coronary effects of enalaprilat in patients with dilated cardiomyopathy: Assessment by a bilateral intracoronary infusion technique. Circulation *77*:337, 1988.
375. Warner, N. J., Rush, J. E., and Keegan, M. E.: Tolerability of enalapril in congestive heart failure. Am. J. Cardiol. *63*:33D, 1989.
376. Kjekshus, J., Swedberg, K., and CONSENSUS Trial Study Group: Advances in Congestive Heart Failure: Tolerability of enalapril in congestive heart failure. Am. J. Cardiol. *62*:67A, 1988.
377. Kramer, B. L., Massie, B. M., and Topic, N.: Controlled trial of captopril in chronic heart failure: A rest and exercise hemodynamic study. Circulation *67*:807, 1983.
378. Awan, N. A., Amsterdam, E. A., Mermanovich, J., et al.: Long-term hemodynamic and clinical efficacy of captopril therapy in ambulatory management of severe chronic congestive heart failure. Am. Heart J. *103*:474, 1982.
379. DiCarlo, L., Chatterjee, K., Parmley, W. W., et al.: Enalapril: A new angiotensin-converting enzyme inhibitor in chronic heart failure. Acute and chronic hemodynamic evaluations. J. Am. Coll. Cardiol. *2*:865, 1983.
380. Packer, M., Medina, N., and Yushak, M.: Correction of dilutional hyponatremia in severe heart failure by converting-enzyme inhibition. Ann. Intern. Med. *100*:782, 1984.
381. Packer, M., Medina, N., Yushak, M., and Lee, W. H.: Usefulness of plasma renin activity in predicting hemodynamic and clinical responses and survival during long-term converting enzyme inhibition in severe chronic heart failure. Experience in 100 consecutive patients. Br. Heart J. *54*:298, 1985.
382. Mancini, D. M., Davis, L., Wexler, J. P., et al.: Dependence of enhanced maximal exercise performance on increased peak skeletal muscle perfusion during long-term captopril therapy in heart failure. J. Am. Coll. Cardiol. *10*:845, 1987.
383. Faxon, D. P., Creager, M. A., Halperin, J. L., et al.: Redistribution of regional blood flow following angiotensin-converting enzyme inhibition: Comparison of normal subjects and patients with heart failure. Am. J. Med. *76*:104, 1984.
384. Packer, M., and LeJemtel, T. H.: Physiologic and pharmacologic determinants of vasodilator response: A conceptual framework for rational drug therapy for chronic heart failure. Prog. Cardiovasc. Dis. *24*:275, 1982.
385. Brilla, C. G., Kramer, B., Hoffmeister, H. M., et al.: Low-dose enalapril in severe chronic heart failure. Cardiovasc. Drugs Ther. *3*:211, 1989.
386. Joy, M., Hubner, P. J., Thomas, R. D., et al.: Long-term use of enalapril in the treatment of patients with congestive heart failure. Int. J. Cardiol. *16*:137, 1987.
387. Swedberg, K., and Kjekshus, J.: Effect of enalapril on mortality in congestive heart failure. Follow-up survival data from the CONSENSUS trial. Drugs *39*:49, 1990.
388. Newman, T. J., Maskin, C. S., Dennick, L. G., et al.: Effects of captopril on survival in patients with heart failure. Am. J. Med. *84*:140, 1988.
389. Packer, M., and Lee, W. H.: Provocation of hyper- and hypokalemic sudden death during treatment with and withdrawal of converting-enzyme inhibition in severe chronic congestive heart failure. Am. J. Cardiol. *57*:347, 1986.
390. Cleland, J. G. F., Dargie, H. J., Gillen, G., et al.: Captopril in heart failure: A double-blind study of the effects on renal function. J. Cardiovasc. Pharmacol. *8*:700, 1986.
391. Packer, M., Lee, W. H., Medina, N., et al.: Functional renal insufficiency during long-term therapy with captopril and enalapril in severe chronic heart failure. Ann. Intern. Med. *106*:346, 1987.
392. Packer, M.: Identification of risk factors predisposing to the development of functional renal insufficiency during treatment with converting-enzyme inhibitors in chronic heart failure. Cardiology *76*(Suppl. 2):50, 1989.
393. Packer, M.: Why do the kidneys release renin in patients with congestive heart failure? A nephrocentric view of converting-enzyme inhibition. Am. J. Cardiol. *60*:179, 1987.
394. Packer, M., Lee, W. H., Kessler, P. D., et al.: Identification of hyponatremia as a risk factor for the development of functional renal insufficiency during converting enzyme inhibition in severe chronic heart failure. J. Am. Coll. Cardiol. *10*:837, 1987.
395. Swedberg, K., Kjekshus, J., and CONSENSUS Trial Study Group: Advances in congestive heart failure: Effects of enalapril on mortality in severe congestive heart failure: Results of the Cooperative North Scandinavian Enalapril Survival Study (CONSENSUS). Am. J. Cardiol. *62*:60A, 1988.
396. Packer, M., Lee, W. H., Medina, N., et al.: Influence of diabetes mellitus on changes in left ventricular performance and renal function produced by converting enzyme inhibition in patients with severe chronic heart failure. Am. J. Med. *82*:1119, 1987.
397. Jordan, R. A., Seth, L., Casebolt, P., et al.: Rapidly developing tolerance to transdermal nitroglycerin in congestive heart failure. Ann. Intern. Med. *104*:295, 1986.
398. Cohn, J. N.: Nitrates for congestive heart failure. Am. J. Cardiol. *56*:19A, 1985.
399. Packer, M.: Mechanisms of nitrate action in patients wtih severe left ventricular failure: Conceptual problems with the theory of venosequestration. Am. Heart J. *110*:259, 1985.
400. Williams, D. O., Amsterdam, E. A., and Mason, D. T.: Hemodynamic effects of nitroglycerin in acute myocardial infarction. Decrease in ventricular preload at the expense of cardiac output. Circulation *51*:421, 1975.
401. Franciosa, J. A., and Cohn, J. N.: Sustained hemodynamic effects without tolerance during long-term isosorbide dinitrate treatment of chronic left ventricular failure. Am. J. Cardiol. *45*:648, 1980.
402. Leier, C. V., Huss, P., Magorien, R. D., and Unverferth, D. V.: Improved exercise capacity and differing arterial and venous tolerance during chronic isosorbide dinitrate therapy for congestive heart failure. Circulation *67*:817, 1983.
403. Cohn, J. N.: Nitrates are effective in the treatment of chronic congestive heart failure: The protagonist's view. Am. J. Cardiol. *66*:444, 1990.
404. Leier, C. V., Huss, P., Margorien, R. D., and Unverfelt, D. V.: Improved exercise capacity and differing arterial and venous tolerance during chronic isosorbide dinitrate therapy for congestive heart failure. Circulation *67*:817, 1983.
405. Packer, M.: Are nitrates effective in the treatment of chronic heart failure? Antagonist's viewpoint. Am. J. Cardiol. *66*:458, 1990.
406. Jordon, R. A., Seith, L., Henry, D. A., et al.: Dose requirements and hemodynamic effects of transdermal nitroglycerin compared with placebo with congestive heart failure. Circulation *71*:980, 1985.
407. Armstrong, P. W.: Pharmacokinetic-hemodynamic studies of transdermal nitroglycerin in congestive heart failure. J. Am. Coll. Cardiol. *9*:420, 1987.
408. Makhoul, N., Dakak, N., Flugelman, M. Y., et al.: Nitrate tolerance in heart failure: Differential venous, pulmonary and systemic arterial effects? Am. J. Cardiol. *65*:28J, 1990.
409. Packer, M., Lee-Wai, H., Kessler, P. D., et al.: Prevention and reversal of nitrate tolerance in patients with congestive heart failure. N. Engl. J. Med. *317*:799, 1987.
410. Pierpont, G. L., Brown, D. C., Franciosa, J. A., and Cohn, J. N.: Effect of hydralazine on renal failure in patients with congestive heart failure. Circulation *61*:323, 1980.
411. Packer, M., Meller, J., Medina, N., et al.: Dose requirements of hydralazine in patients with severe chronic congestive heart failure. Am. J. Cardiol. *45*:655, 1980.
412. Packer, M., Meller, J., Medina, N., et al.: Importance of left ventricular chamber size in determining the response to hydralazine in severe chronic heart failure. N. Engl. J. Med. *303*:250, 1980.
413. Greenberg, B., Massie, B., Bristow, J. D., et al.: Long-term vasodilator therapy of chronic aortic insufficiency. A randomized double-blind, placebo-controlled clinical trial. Circulation *78*:92, 1988.
414. Packer, M., Meller, J., Medina, N., et al.: Hemodynamic characterization of tolerance to long-term hydralazine therapy in severe chronic heart failure. N. Engl. J. Med. *306*:57, 1982.
415. Conradson, T. B., Ryden, L., Ahlmark, G., et al.: Clinical efficacy of hydralazine in chronic heart failure: One-year double-blind placebo-controlled study. Am. Heart J. *108*:1001, 1984.
416. Massie, B., Ports, T., Chatterjee, K., et al.: Long-term vasodilator therapy for heart failure: Clinical response and its relationship to hemodynamic measurements. Circulation *63*:269, 1981.
417. Franciosa, J. A., Weber, K. T., Levin, T. B., et al.: Hydralazine in the long-term treatment of chronic heart failure: Lack of difference from placebo. Am. Heart J. *104*:587, 1982.
418. Colucci, W. S.: Alpha-adrenergic receptor blockage with prazosin: Consideration of hypertension, heart failure, and potential new applications. Ann. Intern. Med. *97*:67, 1982.
419. Packer, M., Meller, J., Gorlin, R., and Herman, H. V.: Hemodynamic and clinical tachyphylaxis to prazosin-mediated afterload reduction in severe congestive heart failure. Circulation *59*:531, 1979.
420. Magorien, R. D., Sinnathamby, S., Leier, C. V., et al.: Rest and exercise cardiovascular effects of terazosin in congestive heart failure. Am. J. Cardiol. *65*:638, 1990.

421. Colucci, W. S.: Usefulness of calcium antagonists for congestive heart failure. Am. J. Cardiol. *59*:52B, 1987.
422. Packer, M.: Second generation calcium channel blockers in the treatment of chronic heart failure: Are they any better than their predecessors? J. Am. Coll. Cardiol. *14*:1339, 1989.
423. Packer, M., Kessler, P. D., and Lee, W. H.: Calcium-channel blockade in the management of severe chronic congestive heart failure: A bridge too far. Circulation *75*:V56, 1987.
424. Schwinger, R. H. G., Bohm, M., and Erdmann, E.: Negative inotropic properties of isradipine, nifedipine, diltiazem, and verapamil in diseased human myocardial tissue. J. Cardiovasc. Pharmacol. *15*:892, 1990.
425. Packer, M.: Pathophysiological mechanisms underlying the adverse effects of calcium channel-blocking drugs in patients with chronic heart failure. Circulation *80*:IV-59, 1989.
426. Goldstein, R. E., Broccuzzi, S. J., Cruess, D., et al.: Diltiazem increases late-onset congestive heart failure in postinfarction patients with early reduction in ejection fraction. Circulation *83*:52, 1991.
426a. Francis, G. S.: Calcium channel blockers and congestive heart failure. *83*:336, 1991.
427. Scognamiglio, R., Fasoli, G., Ponchia, A., and Dalla-Volta, S.: Long-term nifedipine unloading therapy in asymptomatic patients with chronic severe aortic regurgitation. J. Am. Coll. Cardiol. *16*:424, 1990.
428. Rahimtola, S. H.: Vasodilator therapy in chronic severe aortic regurgitation. J. Am. Coll. Cardiol. *16*:430, 1990.
429. Franciosa, J. A.: Effectiveness of long-term vasodilator administration in the treatment of chronic left ventricular failure. Prog. Cardiovasc. Dis. *24*:319, 1982.
430. DiSegni, E., Kaplinsky, E., Klein, H. O., and Levy, M.: Treatment of ruptured interventricular septum with afterload reduction. Arch. Intern. Med. *138*:1427, 1978.
431. Greenberg, B. H., Massie, B. M., Brundage, B. H., et al.: Beneficial effects of hydralazine in severe mitral regurgitation. Circulation *58*:273, 1978.
432. Fioretti, P., Benussi, B., Scardi, S., et al.: Afterload reduction with nifedipine in aortic insufficiency. Am. J. Cardiol. *49*:1728, 1982.
433. Rubin, L. J., and Peter, R. H.: Hemodynamics at rest and during exercise after oral hydralazine in patients with cor pulmonale. Am. J. Cardiol. *47*:116, 1981.
434. Colucci, W. S., Holman, L., Wynne, J., et al.: Improved right ventricular function and reduced pulmonary vascular resistance during prazosin therapy of congestive heart failure. Am. J. Med. *71*:75, 1981.
435. Hamilton, M. A., Stevenson, L. W., Child, J. S., et al.: Sustained reduction in valvular regurgitation and atrial volumes with tailored vasodilator therapy in advanced congestive heart failure secondary to dilated (ischemic or idiopathic) cardiomyopathy. Am. J. Cardiol. *67*:259, 1991.
436. Pfeffer, M. A., Lamas, G. A., Vaughan, D. E., et al.: Effect of captopril on progressive ventricular dilatation after anterior myocardial infarction. N. Engl. J. Med. *319*:80, 1988.
437. Pfeffer, J. M., Pfeffer, M. A., and Braunwald, E.: Hemodynamic benefits and prolonged survival with long-term captopril therapy in rats with myocardial infarction and heart failure. Circulation *75*:I-1149, 1987.
438. Miller, R. R., Awan, N. A., Joye, J. A., et al.: Combined dopamine and nitroprusside therapy in congestive heart failure. Circulation *55*:881, 1977.
439. Stemple, D. R., Kleiman, J. H., and Harrison, D. C.: Combined nitroprusside-dopamine therapy in severe chronic congestive heart failure: Dose-related hemodynamic advantages over single drug infusions. Am. J. Cardiol. *42*:267, 1978.
440. Mikulic, E., Cohn, J. N., Franciosa, J. A.: Comparative hemodynamic effects of inotropic and vasodilator drugs in severe heart failure. Circulation *56*:526, 1977.
441. Cohn, J. N., and Franciosa, J. A.: Selection of vasodilator, inotropic or combined therapy for the management of heart failure. Am. J. Med. *65*:181, 1978.
442. Ibram, H., Maslowski, A. H., and Nicholls, M. G.: Hemodynamic effects of dobutamine in patients with congestive heart failure receiving captopril. Br. Heart J. *46*:528, 1981.
443. Ribner, H. S., Zucker, M. J., Stasior, C., et al.: Vasodilators as first-line therapy for congestive heart failure: A comparative hemodynamic study of hydralazine, digoxin, and their combination. Am. Heart J. *114*:91, 1987.
444. Cantelli, I., Vitolo, A., Lombardi, G., et al.: Combined hemodynamic effects of digoxin and captopril in patients with congestive heart failure. Curr. Ther. Res. *36*:323, 1984.
445. Gheorghiade, M., Hall, V., Lakier, J. B., and Colstein, S.: Comparative hemodynamic and neurohormonal effects of intravenous captopril and digoxin, and their combination in patients with severe heart failure. J. Am. Coll. Cardiol. *134*, 1989.
446. The Captopril-Digoxin Multicenter Research Group: Comparative effects of therapy with captopril and digoxin in patients with mild to moderate heart failure. J.A.M.A. *259*:539, 1988.
447. Cohn, J. N., and Rector, T. S.: Prognosis of congestive heart failure and predictors of mortality. Am. J. Cardiol. *62*:25A, 1988.
448. Packer, M. (ed.): Physiologic determinants of survival in congestive heart failure. Circulation *75*(Suppl. 4):1–111, 1987.

NONGLYCOSIDE INOTROPIC AGENTS

449. Port, J. D., Gilbert, E. M., Larrabee, P., et al.: Neurotransmitter depletion compromises the ability of indirect-acting amines to provide inotropic support in the failing human heart. Circulation *81*:929, 1990.
450. Goldberg, L. I.: Cardiovascular and renal actions of dopamine: Potential clinical applications. Pharmacol. Rev. *24*:1, 1972.
451. Rajfer, S. I., Borow, K. M., Lang, R. M., et al.: Effects of dopamine on left ventricular afterload and contractile state in heart failure: Relation to the activation of $beta_1$-adrenoceptors and dopamine receptors. J. Am. Coll. Cardiol. *12*:498, 1988.
452. Yeh, B. K., McNay, J. L., and Goldberg, L. I.: Attenuation of dopamine renal and mesenteric vasodilation by haloperidol: Evidence for a specific receptor. J. Pharmacol. Exp. Ther. *168*:203, 1969.
453. Hoffman, B. B., and Lefkowitz, R. J.: Catecholamines and sympathomimetic drugs. *In* Goodman, L. S., and Gilman, A. G. (eds.): The Pharmacological Basis of Therapeutics. New York, Pergamon Press, 1990, pp. 187–220.
454. Goldberg, L. I., and Rajfer, S. I.: Dopamine receptors: Applications in clinical cardiology. Circulation *72*:245, 1985.
455. Gilbert, J. C., and Goldberg, L. I.: Characterization by cyproheptadine of the dopamine-induced contraction in canine isolated arteries. J. Pharmacol. Exp. Ther. *193*:435, 1975.
456. Hollenberg, N. K., Adams, D. F., Mendell, P., et al.: Renal vascular responses to dopamine. Hemodynamics and angiographic observations in normal man. Clin. Sci. Mol. Med. *45*:733, 1973.
457. Goldberg, L. I.: Dopamine: Clinical uses of an endogenous catecholamine. N. Engl. J. Med. *291*:707, 1974.
458. Allwood, M. J., and Ginsburg, J.: Peripheral vascular and other effects of dopamine infusion in man. Clin. Sci. *27*:271, 1964.
459. Brooks, H. L., Stein, P. D., Matson, J. L., and Hyland, J. W.: Dopamine-induced alterations in coronary hemodynamics in dogs. Circ. Res. *24*:699, 1969.
460. Toda, N., and Goldberg, L. I.: Effects of dopamine on isolated canine coronary arteries. Cardiovasc. Res. *9*:384, 1975.
461. Goldberg, L. I., McDonald, R. H., Jr., and Zimmerman, A. M.: Sodium diuresis produced by dopamine in patients with congestive heart failure. N. Engl. J. Med. *269*:1060, 1963.
462. Miller, R. R., Awan, N. A., Joye, J. A., et al.: Combined dopamine and nitroprusside therapy in congestive heart failure. Circulation *55*:881, 1977.
463. van Trigt, P., Spray, T. L., Pasque, M. K., et al.: The comparative effects of dopamine and dobutamine on ventricular mechanics after coronary artery bypass grafting: A pressure-dimension analysis. Circulation *70*:(Suppl. 1):112, 1984.
464. Fowler, M. B., Alderman, E. L., Oesterle, S. N., et al.: Dobutamine and dopamine after cardiac surgery: Greater augmentation of myocardial blood flow with dobutamine. Circulation *70*(Suppl. 1):103, 1984.
465. Sturm, J. T., Guhrman, T. M., Sterling, R., et al.: Combined use of dopamine and nitroprusside therapy in conjunction with intra-aortic balloon pumping for the treatment of postcardiotomy low-output syndrome. J. Thorac. Cardiovasc. Surg. *82*:13, 1981.
466. Tuttle, R. R., and Mills, J.: Dopamine: Development of a new catecholamine to selectively increase cardiac contractility. Circ. Res. *36*:185, 1975.
467. Vatner, S. F., McRitchie, R. J., and Braunwald, E.: Effects of dobutamine on left ventricular performance, coronary dynamics, and distribution of cardiac output in conscious dogs. J. Clin. Invest. *53*:1265, 1974.
468. Majerus, T. C., Dasta, J. F., Bauman, J. L., et al.: Dobutamine: Ten years later. Pharmacotherapy *9*:245, 1989.
469. Williams, R. S., and Bishop, T.: Selectivity of dobutamine for adrenergic receptor subtypes. In vitro analysis by radioligand binding. J. Clin. Invest. *67*:1703, 1981.
470. Kenakin, T. P.: An in vitro quantitative analysis of the alpha adrenoceptor partial agonist activity of dobutamine and its relevance to inotropic selectively. J. Pharmacol. Exp. Ther. *9*:216, 1981.
471. Ruffolo, R. R., Jr., Sporadlin, T. A., Pollock, G. D., et al.: Alpha- and beta-adrenergic effects of the stereoisomers of dobutamine. J. Pharmacol. Exp. Ther. *219*:447, 1981.
472. Robie, N. W., and Goldberg, L. I.: Comparative systemic and regional hemodynamic effects of dopamine and dobutamine. Am. Heart J. *90*:340, 1975.
473. Magorien, R. D., Unverferth, D. V., Brown, G. P., and Leier, C. V.: Dobutamine and hydralazine: Comparative influences of positive inotropy and vasodilation on coronary blood flow and myocardial energetics in nonischemic congestive heart failure. J. Am. Coll. Cardiol. *1*:499, 1983.
474. Mancini, D. M., Schwartz, M., Ferraro, N., et al.: Effect of dobutamine on skeletal muscle metabolism in patients with congestive heart failure. Am. J. Cardiol. *65*:1121, 1990.
475. Gillespie, J. A., Ambros, H. D., Sobel, B. E., and Roberts, R.: Effects of dobutamine in patients with acute myocardial infarction. Am. J. Cardiol. *39*:588, 1977.
476. Bendersky, R., Chatterjee, K., Parmley, W. W., et al.: Dobutamine in chronic ischemic heart failure. Alterations in left ventricular function and coronary hemodynamics. Am. J. Cardiol. *48*:554, 1981.
477. Leier, C. V., Magorien, R. D., Altschuld, R., et al.: The hemodynamic and metabolic advantages gained by a three-day infusion of dobutamine in patients with congestive cardiomyopathy. Am. Heart J. *106*:29, 1983.
478. Applefeld, M. M., Newman, K. A., Grove, W. R., et al.: Intermittent, continuous outpatient dobutamine infusion in the management of congestive heart failure. Am. J. Cardiol. *51*:455, 1983.
479. Krell, M. J., Kline, E. M., Bates, E. R., et al.: Intermittent, ambulatory dobutamine infusions in patients with severe congestive heart failure. *112*:787, 1986.
480. Stecy, P., and Gunnar, R. M.: Is intermittent dobutamine infusion useful in the treatment of patients with refractory congestive heart failure? *In*

Cheitlin, M. (ed.): Dilemmas in Clinical Cardiology. Cardiology Clinics. Philadelphia, F. A. Davis Co., 1990, pp. 277–289.

481. Hodgson, J. M., Aja, M., and Sorkin, R. P.: Intermittent ambulatory dobutamine infusions for patients awaiting cardiac transplantation. Am. J. Cardiol. *53*:375, 1984.
482. Aronson, R. S., and Gelles, J. M.: Electrophysiologic effects of dopamine on sheep cardiac Purkinje fibers. J. Pharmacol. Exp. Ther. *188*:596, 1974.
483. Loeb, H. S., Sinno, M. Z., Saudye, A., et al.: Electrophysiologic properties of dobutamine. Circ. Shock *1*:217, 1974.
484. Goldenberg, I. F., Olivari, M. T., Levine, T. B., and Cohn, J. N.: Effect of dobutamine on plasma potassium in congestive heart failure secondary to idiopathic or ischemic cardiomyopathy. Am. J. Cardiol. *63*:843, 1989.
485. Loeb, H. S., Khan, M., Klodnycky, M. L., et al.: Haemodynamic effects of dobutamine in man. Circ. Shock *2*:29, 1975.
486. Pozen, R. G., DiBianco, R., Katz, R. J., et al.: Myocardial metabolic and hemodynamic effects of dobutamine in heart failure complicating coronary artery disease. Circulation *63*:1279, 1981.
487. Greene, S. I., and Smith, J. W.: Dopamine gangrene. N. Engl. J. Med. *294*:114, 1976.
488. Stoner, J. D., Bolen, J. L., and Harrison, D. C.: Comparison of dobutamine and dopamine in treatment of severe heart failure. Br. Heart J. *39*:536, 1977.
489. Loeb, H. S., Bredakis, J., and Gunnar, R. M.: Superiority of dobutamine over dopamine for augmentation of cardiac output in patients with chronic low output cardiac failure. Circulation *55*:375, 1977.
490. Leier, C. V., Heban, P. T., Huss, P., et al.: Comparative systemic and regional hemodynamic effects of dopamine and dobutamine in patients with cardiomyopathic heart failure. Circulation *58*:466, 1978.
491. Berkowitz, C., McKeever, L., Croke, R. P., et al.: Comparative responses to dobutamine and nitroprusside in patients wtih chronic low output cardiac failure. Circulation *56*:918, 1977.
492. Baumann, G., Felix, S. B., and Filcek, S. A. L.: Usefulness of dopexamine hydrochloride versus dobutamine in chronic congestive heart failure and effects of hemodynamics and urine output. Am. J. Cardiol. *65*:748, 1990.
493. Goldberg, L. I., and Rajfer, S. I.: Dopamine receptors: Applications in clinical cardiology. Circulation *72*:245, 1985.
494. Lang, R. M., Borow, K. M., Neumann, A., et al.: Role of the $beta_2$ adrenoceptor in mediating positive inotropic activity in the failing heart and its relation to the hemodynamic actions of dopexamine hydrochloride. Am. J. Cardiol. *62*:46C, 1988.
495. Rajfer, S. I., Anton, A. H., Rossen, J. D., and Goldberg, L. I.: Beneficial hemodynamic effects of oral levodopa in heart failure: Relation to the generation of dopamine. N. Engl. J. Med. *310*:1357, 1984.
496. Broderick, G., and Rajfer, S. I.: The use of levodopa, an oral dopamine precursor, in congestive heart failure. Basic Res. Cardiol. *84*(Suppl. 1):187, 1989.
497. Hasenfuss, G., and Just, H.: Clinical relevance of long-term therapy with levodopa and orally active dopamine analogues in patients with chronic congestive heart failure. Basic Res. Cardiol. *84*(Suppl. 1):191, 1989.
498. DeMarco, T., Daly, P. A., Chatterjee, K.: Congestive heart failure: Systemic and coronary hemodynamic and neurohormonal effects of levodopa in chronic congestive heart failure. Am. J. Cardiol. *62*:1228, 1988.
499. Opie, L. H.: Pharmacologic profile of ibopamine and related dopamine-like inodilators. Cardiovasc. Drugs Ther. *3*:1041, 1989.
500. Distante, A., Morales, M. A., Piacenti, M., et al.: An acute noninvasive study aimed at assessing the inotropic effect of oral ibopamine in patients with mild congestive heart failure. Cardiovasc. Drugs Ther. *3*:1025, 1989.
501. Lopez-Sendon, J.: Hemodynamic effects of ibopamine in congestive heart failure. Cardiovasc. Drugs Ther. *3*:1029, 1989.
502. Stoddard, M. F., Chaitman, B. R., Byers, S. L., et al.: Noninvasive assessment of diastolic and systolic properties of ibopamine in patients with congestive heart failure. Am. Heart J. *117*:395, 1989.
503. Fennell, W. H., Taylor, A. A., Young, J. B., et al.: Propylbutyldopamine: Hemodynamic effects in conscious dogs, normal human volunteers and patients with heart failure. Circulation *67*:829, 1983.
504. Sharma, B., and Goodwin, J. F.: Beneficial effects of salbutamol on cardiac function in severe congestive cardiomyopathy: Effect on systolic and diastolic function of the left ventricle. Circulation *58*:449, 1978.
505. Xamoterol, a β_1-adrenoceptor partial agonist: A new approach to heart failure. *In* Barnett, D. B., and Breckenridge, A. (eds.): Br. J. Clin. Pharmacol. *28*(Suppl. 1):1–92, 1989.
506. Brodde, O-E, Daul, A., Michel-Reher, M., et al.: Agonist-induced desensitization of β-adrenoceptor function in humans: Subtype-selective reduction in β_1- or β_2-adrenoceptor-mediated physiological effects by Xamoterol or Procaterol. Circulation *81*:914, 1990.
507. The Xamoterol in Severe Heart Failure Study Group: Xamoterol in severe heart failure. Lancet *2*:1, 1990.
508. Packer, M.: Personal communication.
509. Katz, A. M.: The myocardium in congestive heart failure. Am. J. Cardiol. *63*:12A, 1989.
510. Katz, A. M.: Changing strategies in the management of heart failure. J. Am. Coll. Cardiol. *13*:513, 1989.
511. Colucci, W. S., Wright, R. F., and Braunwald, E.: New positive inotropic agents in the treatment of congestive heart failure. Mechanisms of action and recent clinical developments. N. Engl. J. Med. *314*:349, 1986.
512. Evans, D. B.: Modulation of cAMP: Mechanism for positive inotropic action. J. Cardiovasc. Pharmacol. *8*(Suppl. 9):22, 1986.
513. van der Leyen, H.: Phosphodiesterase inhibition by new cardiotonic agents: Mechanism of action and possible clinical relevance in the therapy of congestive heart failure. Klin. Wochenschr. *67*:605, 1989.
514. Braunwald, E.: A Symposium on Amrinone. Am. J. Cardiol. *56*:1B, 1985.
515. Honerjäger, P., Schäfer-Koeting, M., and Reiter, M.: Involvement of cyclic AMP in the direct inotropic action of amrinone: Biochemical and functional evidence. Naunyn Schmiedebergs Arch. Pharmacol. *318*:112, 1981.
516. Benotti, J. R., Grossman, W., Braunwald, E., et al.: Hemodynamic assessment of amrinone: A new inotropic agent. N. Engl. J. Med. *299*:1373, 1978.
517. Benotti, J. R., Grossman, W., Braunwald, E., and Carabello, B. A.: Effects of amrinone on myocardial energy metabolism and hemodynamics in patients with severe congestive heart failure due to coronary artery disease. Circulation *62*:28, 1980.
518. Naccarelli, G. V., Gray, E. L., Dougherty, A. H., et al.: Amrinone: Acute electrophysiologic and hemodynamic effects in patients with congestive heart failure. Am. J. Cardiol. *54*:600, 1984.
519. Hartman, A., and Saeed, M.: Phosphodiesterase inhibition in positive inotropic therapy of congestive heart failure. J. Appl. Cardiol. *1*:361, 1986.
520. Goenen, M., Pedemonte, O., Baele, P., and Col, J.: Amrinone in the management of low cardiac output after open heart surgery. Am. J. Cardiol. *56*:33B, 1985.
521. Taylor, S. H., Verma, S. P., Hussain, M., et al.: Intravenous amrinone in left ventricular failure complicated by acute myocardial infarction. Am. J. Cardiol. *56*:29B, 1985.
522. Olsen, K. H., Kluger, J., and Fieldman, A.: Combination high dose amrinone and dopamine in the management of moribund cardiogenic shock after open heart surgery. Chest *94*:503, 1988.
523. Uretsky, B. F., Lawless, C. E., Verbalis, J. G., et al.: Combined therapy with dobutamine and amrinone in severe heart failure: Improved hemodynamics and increased activation of the renin-angiotensin system with combined intravenous therapy. Chest *92*:657, 1987.
524. Deeb, G. M., Bolling, S. F., Guynn, T. P., and Nicklas, J. M.: Amrinone versus conventional therapy in pulmonary hypertensive patients awaiting cardiac transplantation. Ann. Thorac. Surg. *48*:665, 1989.
525. Massie, B., Bourassa, M., DiBianco, R., et al.: Long-term oral administration of amrinone for congestive heart failure: Lack of efficacy in a multicenter controlled trial. Circulation *71*:963, 1985.
525a. Pflugfelder, P. W., O'Neill, B. J., Ogilvie, R. I., et al.: A Canadian multicentre study of a 48h infusion of milrinone in patients with severe heart failure. Can. J. Cardiol. *7*:5, 1991.
526. Monrad, E. S., Baim, D. S., Smith, H. S., et al.: Effects of milrinone on coronary hemodynamics and myocardial energetics in patients with congestive heart failure. Circulation *71*:972, 1985.
527. Jaski, B. E., Fifer, M. A., Wright, R. F., et al.: Positive inotropic and vasodilator actions of milrinone in patients with severe congestive heart failure: Dose-response relationships and comparison to nitroprusside. J. Clin. Invest. *75*:643, 1985.
528. Grose, R., Strain, J., Greenberg, M., and LeJemtel, T. H.: Systemic and coronary effects of intravenous milrinone and dobutamine in congestive heart failure. J. Am. Coll. Cardiol. *7*:1107, 1986.
529. Cody, R. J., Kubo, S. H., Covit, A. B., et al.: Regional blood flow and neurohumoral responses to milrinone in congestive heart failure. Clin. Pharmacol. Ther. *39*:128, 1986.
530. Sonnenblick, E. H., Grose, R., Strain, J., et al.: Effects of milrinone on left ventricular performance and myocardial contractility in patients with severe heart failure. Circulation *73*(Suppl. 3):162, 1986.
531. Braunwald, E. (ed.): Newer positive inotropic agents. Circulation *73*(Suppl. 3):237, 1986.
532. Schlepper, M., Thormann, J., Kremer, P., et al.: Present use of positive inotropic drugs in heart failure. J. Cardiovasc. Pharmacol. *14*(Suppl. 1):9, 1989.
533. Bohm, M., Diet, F., Kemkes, B., and Erdmann, E.: Enhancement of the effectiveness of milrinone to increase force of contraction by stimulation of cardiac beta-adrenoceptors in the failing human heart. Klin. Wochenschr. *66*:957, 1988.
534. Anderson, J. L., Baim, D. S., Fein, S. A., et al.: Efficacy and safety of sustained (48 hour) intravenous infusions of milrinone in patients with severe congestive heart failure: A multicenter study. J. Am. Coll. Cardiol. *9*:711, 1987.
535. DiBianco, R., Shabetai, R., Kostuk, W., et al.: A comparison of oral milrinone, digoxin, and their combination in the treatment of patients with chronic heart failure. N. Engl. J. Med. *320*:677, 1989.
536. Cowley, A. J., Stainer, K., Wynne, R. D., et al.: Comparison of the effects of captopril and enoximone in patients with severe heart failure: A placebo controlled double-blind study. Int. J. Cardiol. *24*:311, 1989.
537. Petein, M., Levine, T. B., and Cohn, J. N.: Persistent hemodynamic effects without long-term clinical benefits in response to oral piroximone (MDL 19,205) in patients with congestive heart failure. Circulation *73*(Suppl. 3):230, 1986.
538. Foex, P., and Davidson, I. A. (eds.): Acute heart failure in intensive care: A new approach. Proceedings of a symposium. Cardiology *77*:S3, 1990.
539. Cowley, A. J., Stainer, K., Fullwood, L., et al.: Effects of enoximone in patients with heart failure uncontrolled by catopril and diuretics. Int. J. Cardiol. *28*:Suppl 1:S45, 1990.
540. Vincent, J.-L., Madhoun, P., Primo, G., and Kahn, R. J.: Potentiation of the effects of enoximone by a dobutamine infusion. Intens. Care Med. *15*:530, 1989.
541. Narahara, K. A., and the Western Enoximone Study Group. Oral enoximone therapy in chronic heart failure; a placebo-controlled randomized trial. Am. Heart J. *121*:1471, 1991.
542. Hauf, G. F., Grom, E., Jahnchen, E., and Roskamm, H.: Acute and long-

term hemodynamic effects of pimobendan (UD-CG 115 BS) in comparison with captopril. J. Cardiovasc. Pharmacol. 14(Suppl. 2):49, 1989.
543. Endoh, M., Shibasaki, Satoh, H., et al.: Different mechanisms involved in the positive inotropic effects of benzimidazole derivative UD-CG 115 BS (Pimobendan) and its demethylated metabolite UD-CG 212 Cl in canine ventricular myocardium. J. Cardiovasc. Pharmacol. 17:365, 1991.
544. Baumann, G., Ningel, K., and Permanetter, B.: Clinical efficacy of pimobendan (UD-CG 115 BS) in patients with chronic congestive heart failure. J. Cardiovasc. Pharmacol. 14(Suppl. 2):23, 1989.
545. Hagemeijer, F., Brand, H. J., and van Mechelen, R.: Congestive heart failure: Hemodynamic effects of pimobendan given orally in congestive heart failure secondary to ischemic or idiopathic dilated cardiomyopathy. Am. J. Cardiol. 63:571, 1989.
546. Bohm, M., Morano, I., Pieske, B., et al.: Contribution of cAMP-phosphodiesterase inhibition and sensitization of the contractile proteins for calcium to the inotropic effect of pimobendan in the failing human myocardium. Circ. Res. 68:689, 1991.
547. Asanoi, H., Sasayama, S., Iuchi, K., and Kameyama, T.: Acute hemodynamic effects of a new inotropic agent (OPC-8212) in patients with congestive heart failure. J. Am. Coll. Cardiol. 9:865, 1987.
548. Futaki, S., Nozawa, T., Yasamura, Y., et al.: A new cardiotonic agent, OPC-8212, elevates the myocardial oxygen consumption versus pressure-volume area (PVA) relation in a similar manner to catecholamines and calcium in canine hearts. Heart Vessels 4:153–161, 1988.
549. Feldman, A. M., Becker, L. C., Llewellyn, M. P., and Baughman, K. L.: Clinical investigations: Evaluation of a new inotropic agent, OPC-8212, in patients with dilated cardiomyopathy and heart failure. Am. Heart J. 116:771, 1988.
550. Scholtysik, G., Salzmann, R., and Gerber, W.: Interaction of DPI 201-106 with cardiac glycosides. J. Cardiovasc. Pharmacol. 13:342, 1989.
551. Kostis, J. B., Lacy, C. R., Raia, J. J., et al.: Congestive heart failure: DPI 201-106 for severe congestive heart failure. Am. J. Cardiol. 60:1334, 1987.

OTHER ASPECTS OF TREATMENT OF HEART FAILURE

Beta-Adrenoceptors in Heart Failure

552. Waagstein, F., Hjalmarson, A., Varnauskas, E., and Wallentin, I.: Effect of chronic beta-adrenergic receptor blockade in congestive cardiomyopathy. Br. Heart J. 37:1022, 1975.
553. Swedberg, K., Waagstein, F., Hjarlmarson, A., and Wallentin, I.: Prolongation of survival in congestive cardiomyopathy by beta-receptor blockade. Lancet 1:1374, 1979.
554. Swedberg, K., Hjalmarson, A., Waagstein, F., and Wallentin, I.: Beneficial effects of long-term beta-blockade in congestive cardiomyopathy. Br. Heart J. 44:117, 1980.
555. Swedberg, K., Hjalmarson, A., Waagstein, F., and Wallentin, I.: Adverse effects of beta-blockade withdrawal in patients with congestive cardiomyopathy. Br. Heart J. 44:134, 1980.
556. Engelmeier, R. S., O'Connell, J. B., Walsh, R., et ol.: Improvement in symptoms and exercise tolerance by metoprolol in patients with dilated cardiomyopathy: A double-blind, randomized, placebo-controlled trial. Circulation 72:536, 1985.
557. Gilbert, E. M., Anderson, J. L., Deitchman, D., et al.: Long-term β-blocker vasodilator therapy improves cardiac function in idiopathic dilated cardiomyopathy: A double-blind, randomized study of bucindolol versus placebo. Am. J. Med. 88:223, 1990.
558. Eichhorn, E. J., Bedotto, J. B., Malloy, C. R., et al.: Effect of β-adrenergic blockade on myocardial function and energetics in congestive heart failure. Circulation 82:473, 1990.
559. Waagstein, F., Caidahl, K., Wallentin, I., et al.: Long-term beta-blockade in dilated cardiomyopathy. Effects of short- and long-term metoprolol treatment followed by withdrawal and readministration of metoprolol. Circulation 80:551, 1989.
560. Sethi, K. K., Nair, M., Arora, R., and Khalilullah, M.: Oral metoprolol therapy in dilated cardiomyopathy: Hemodynamic evidence for improved diastolic function accompanying amelioration of symptoms. Int. J. Cardiol. 29:317, 1990.
561. Binkley, P. F., Lewe, R. F., Lima, J. J., et al.: Hemodynamic-inotropic response to β-blocker with intrinsic sympathomimetic activity in patients with congestive cardiomyopathy. Circulation 74:1390, 1986.
562. Ikram, H., and Fitzpatrick, D.: Double-blind trial of chronic oral beta-blockade in congestive cardiomyopathy. Lancet 2:490, 1981.
563. Heilbrunn, S. M., Shah, P., Bristow, M. R., et al.: Increased beta-receptor density and improved hemodynamic response to catecholamine stimulation during long-term metoprolol therapy in heart failure from dilated cardiomyopathy. Circulation 79:483, 1989.
564. Packer, M.: Pathophysiological mechanisms underlying the effects of β-adrenergic agonists and antagonists on functional capacity and survival in chronic heart failure. Circulation 82:I-77, 1990.
565. Shanes, J. G.: β-Blockade—rational or irrational therapy for congestive heart failure? Circulation 76:971, 1987.

Arrhythmia Management in Heart Failure

567. Francis, G. S.: Development of arrhythmias in the patient with congestive heart failure: Pathophysiology, prevalence, and prognosis. Am. J. Cardiol. 57:3B, 1986.
568. Packer, M.: Sudden unexpected death in patients with congestive heart failure: A second frontier. Circulation 72:681, 1985.
569. Parmley, W. W., and Chatterjee, K.: Congestive heart failure and arrhythmias: An overview. Am. J. Cardiol. 57:34B, 1986.
570. Unverferth, D. V., Magorien, R. D., Moeschberger, M. L., et al.: Factors influencing the one-year mortality of dilated cardiomyopathy. Am. J. Cardiol. 54:147, 1984.
571. Bigger, J. T., Jr.: How to study cardiac death as an endpoint in congestive heart failure trials. In Morganroth, J., and Moore, E. N. (eds.): Congestive Heart Failure; Proceedings of the Symposium on New Drugs and Devices, 1986, Martinus Nijhoff, 1987.
572. Holmes, J., Kubo, S. H., Cody, R. J., et al.: Arrhythmias in ischemic and nonischemic dilated cardiomyopathy: Prediction of mortality by ambulatory electrocardiography. Am. J. Cardiol. 55:146, 1985.
573. Fenoglio, J. J., Jr., Pham, T. D., Harken, A. H., et al.: Recurrent sustained ventricular tachycardia: Structure and ultrastructure of subendocardial regions in which tachycardia originates. Circulation 68:518, 1983.
574. Cohen, M., Wiener, I., Pichard, A., et al.: Determinants of ventricular tachycardia in patient with coronary artery disease and ventricular aneurysm. Clinical, hemodynamic and angiographic factors. Am. J. Cardiol. 51:61, 1983.
575. Levy, D., Anderson, K. M., Savage, D. D., et al.: Risk of ventricular arrhythmias in left ventricular hypertrophy: The Framingham Heart Study. Am. J. Cardiol. 60:560, 1987.
576. Packer, M., Gottlieb, S. S., and Blum, M. A.: Immediate and long-term pathophysiologic mechanisms underlying the genesis of sudden cardiac death in patients with congestive heart failure. Am. J. Med. 82:4,]F1987.
577. Dargie, H. J., Cleland, J. G., Leckie, B. J., et al.: Relation of arrhythmias and electrolyte abnormalities to survival in patients with severe chronic heart failure. Circulation 75(Suppl. 4):98, 1987.
578. Packer, M., Gottlieb, S. S., and Kessler, P. D.: Hormone-electrolyte interactions in the pathogenesis of lethal cardiac arrhythmias in patients with congestive heart failure. Basis of a new physiologic approach to control of arrhythmia. Am. J. Med. 80:23, 1986.
579. Dyckner, T., and Wester, P. O.: Relation between potassium, magnesium and cardiac arrhythmias. Acta Med. Scand. 647(Suppl.):163, 1981.
580. Parmley, W. W.: Factors causing arrhythmias in chronic congestive heart failure. Am. Heart J. 114:1267, 1987.
581. Bigger, J. T., Jr.: Left ventricular arrhythmias after myocardial infarction. Am. J. Cardiol. 57:8B, 1986.
582. Woosley, R. L.: Pharmacokinetics and pharmacodynamics of antiarrhythmic agents in patients with congestive heart failure. Am. Heart J. 114:1280, 1987.
583. Williams, R. L., and Benet, L. Z.: Drug pharmacokinetics in cardiac and hepatic diseases. Ann. Rev. Pharmacol. Toxicol. 20:389, 1980.
584. Gottlieb, S. S., Kukin, M. L., Medina, N., et al.: Comparative hemodynamic effects of procainamide, tocainide, and encainide in severe chronic heart failure. Circulation 81:860, 1990.
584a. Hammermeister, K. E.: Adverse hemodynamic effects of antiarrhythmic drugs in congestive heart failure. Circulation 81:1151, 1990.
585. Marcus, F. I.: Pharmacokinetic interactions between digoxin and other drugs. J. Am. Coll. Cardiol. 5L82A, 1985.
586. Parmley, W. W., and Chatterjee, K.: Congestive heart failure and arrhythmias: An overview. Am. J. Cardiol. 57:34B, 1986.
587. Wilson, J. R.: Use of antiarrhythmic drugs in patients with heart failure: Clinical efficacy, hemodynamic results, and relation to survival. Circulation 75(Suppl. 4):64, 1987.
588. De Paola, A., Horowitz, L., Spellman, S. R., et al.: Development of congestive heart failure and alterations in left ventricular function in patients with sustained ventricular tachyarrhythmias treated with amiodarone. Am. J. Cardiol. 60:276, 1987.
589. Cleland, J. G. F., Dargie, H. J., Findlay, I. N., et al.: Clinical, hemodynamic and antiarrhythmic effects of long-term treatment with amiodarone of patients in heart failure. Br. Heart J. 57:436, 1987.
590. Neri, R., Mestroni, L., Salvi, A., et al.: Ventricular arrhythmias in dilated cardiomyopathy. Efficacy of amiodarone. Am. Heart J. 113:707, 1987.
591. Setaro, J. F., Zaret, B. L., Schulman, D. A., et al.: Usefulness of verapamil for congestive heart failure associated with abnormal left ventricular diastolic filling and normal left ventricular systolic performance. Am. J. Cardiol. 66:981, 1990.

Refractory Heart Failure

592. Gagnon, R. M., Fortin, L., Boucher, R., et al.: Combined hemodynamic effects of dobutamine and IV nitroglycerin in congestive heart failure. Chest 78:694, 1980.
593. Miller, R. R., Awan, N. A., Joye, J. A., et al.: Combined dopamine and nitroprusside therapy in congestive heart failure. Circulation 55:881, 1977.
594. Simpson, I. A., Prae, A., Simpson, K., et al.: Ultrafiltration in the management of refractory congestive heart failure. Br. Heart J. 55:344, 1986.
595. Abbate, A., Emdin, M., Piacenti, M., et al.: Ultrafiltration: A rational treatment for heart failure. Cardiology 76:384, 1989.
596. Heymsfield, S. B., and Casper, K.: Congestive heart failure: Clinical management by use of continuous nasoenteric feeding. Am. J. Clin. Nutr. 50:539, 1989.
597. Kennedy, H. L., Sprague, M. K., Redd, R. M., et al.: Serum digoxin concentrations during ethmozine antiarrhythmic therapy. Am. Heart J. 111:667, 1986.
598. Ferrick, K. J., Ferrick, A. M., Fein, S. A., and Doyle, J. T.: Effect of milrinone on steady-state digoxin levels in congestive heart failure. Am. J. Cardiol. 64:1057, 1989.
599. Rodin, S. M., Johnson, B. F., Wilson, J., et al.: Comparative effects of verapamil and isradipine on steady-state digoxin kinetics. Clin. Pharmacol. Ther. 43:668, 1988.
600. Elkayam, U., Parikh, K., Torkan, B., et al.: Effect of diltiazem on renal clearance and serum concentrations of digoxin in patients with cardiac disease. Am. J. Cardiol. 55:1393, 1985.

18

Heart and Heart-Lung Transplantation

by BRUCE A. REITZ, M.D.

Although cardiac transplantation in humans was first carried out in 1967, it is only since the early 1980's that it has established itself as an accepted treatment for end-stage heart disease. The advances in immunosuppression and transplant management that have made this possible also have led to successful heart-lung and lung transplantation, which are continuing to evolve. The increasingly widespread application of thoracic organ transplantation has brought this therapy to many centers around the world and to an ever-increasing patient population.

The Registry of the International Society for Heart Transplantation lists more than 13,000 cardiac transplant procedures performed in more than 230 transplant centers.[1] The number of transplant centers by the year of onset of the program is shown in Figure 18–1. The recent expansion of heart transplantation is emphasized by the fact that before 1980, fewer than 360 transplantations had been performed. More than 85 per cent of all heart transplantations have occurred since 1985. The management philosophies and strategies discussed in this chapter are based in part on the experience of the Johns Hopkins Hospital team, and have been reviewed in a recent book on heart and heart-lung transplantation.[2]

There are several mentions of heart transplantation in ancient Chinese mythology and biblical reference, but not until the pioneering work of Alexis Carrel at the beginning of the 20th century did surgeons have the ability to transplant organs such as the heart.[3] In a number of imaginative experiments, Carrel demonstrated that a heart could be transplanted and resume functioning in the new host. Not only did Carrel transplant hearts, but he also suggested and performed the en bloc transplantation of heart and lungs,[4] both of these procedures being heterotopic transplants into the necks of recipient dogs.

The next reported heart transplantations were those of Mann at the Mayo Clinic in 1933.[5] These heterotopic dog heart transplants were able to function until the onset of allograft rejection at 8 days. After these experiments, there was a 20-year period without progress until the late 1940's and early 1950's. V. P. Demikhov, a Russian surgeon, initiated a series of ingenious experiments on the technical feasibility of both intrathoracic heterotopic heart transplants[6] as well as heart-lung transplantation, although his work was not reported in the West until 1962. With the advent of techniques for successful cardiac surgery in the 1950's, major attention finally was directed to the problem of transplantation of the heart. Various experiments using either hypothermia and circulatory arrest or the early cardiopulmonary bypass machines permitted a number of ingenious laboratory studies to be performed.[7–9]

The currently used surgical technique for heart transplantation originated with the work of Lower and Shumway in 1959.[10] A number of important questions about transplants, including protocols for immunosuppression,[11] correlation of the surface electrocardiogram with allograft rejection,[12] and reversal of these changes with augmented immunosuppression, were subjects of early laboratory study. Despite this prior laboratory work, many were surprised when the first human heart transplant was performed by Christian Barnard in Capetown, South Africa, in December 1967.[13] This transplant initiated a great amount of interest at other centers around the world, with 170 transplants by 65 surgical teams between December 1967 and March 1971. The 1-year survival was only 15 per cent, and because of this, enthusiasm for heart transplantation rapidly waned by the end of 1971.

Only at Stanford University in Stanford, California, and the Medical College of Virginia in Richmond, Virginia, did surgical teams continue with programs in heart transplantation. Working virtually alone through the decade of the 1970's, these investigators refined recipient selection criteria,[14] saw the development of the transvenous endomyocardial biopsy for diagnosing allograft rejection,[15] developed rabbit antithymocyte globulin as an effective treatment of acute rejection,[16] and defined many of the late, post-transplant complications and management principles.[17]

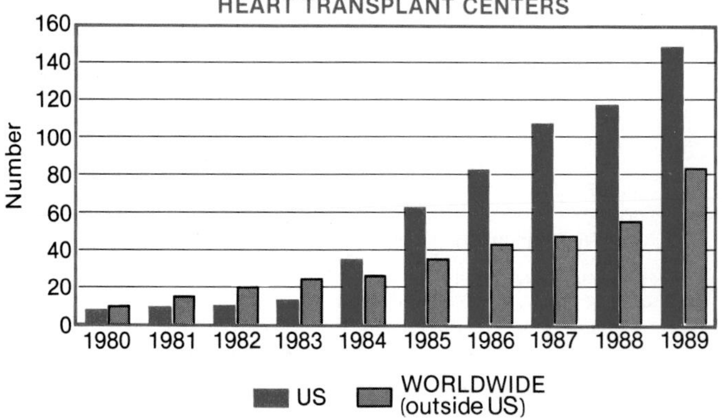

Year	U.S.	Worldwide (outside US)
1980	8	10
1981	9	15
1982	10	20
1983	13	24
1984	35	26
1985	63	35
1986	83	43
1987	108	47
1988	118	55
1989	149	83

FIGURE 18–1. Number of Centers Performing Heart Transplants by Year. (Adapted from Kriett, J. M., and Kaye, M. P.: The Registry of the International Society for Heart Transplantation: Seventh Official Report—1990. J. Heart Transplant. 9:323, 1990.)

IMMUNOSUPPRESSIVE THERAPY

Widespread application of heart transplantation depended on development of better immunosuppressive therapy. This goal was reached with the discovery that cyclosporin A, a novel polypeptide of fungal origin, could selectively block the effect of interleukin-2 (IL-2) in stimulating T cells.[18-20] The rapid development and introduction of this compound to clinical transplantation resulted in superior results. It was first used for heart transplantation in December 1980[21] and for successful heart-lung transplantation in March 1981.[22] Then followed the rapid development of heart transplant centers and the marked increase in the number of procedures indicated earlier.

A good deal of additional progress has been made based on the rapidly accumulating experience. Other immunosuppressive protocols have been developed. A number of promising new immunosuppressive drugs are being studied experimentally, and heart transplantation has been extended to a large number of additional recipients, including neonates with hypoplastic left heart syndrome and patients with primary lung disease, such as emphysema and cystic fibrosis.

ORGANIZATIONAL ASPECTS OF A TRANSPLANT PROGRAM. In the last 5 years more than 140 new cardiac transplant programs have been instituted in the United States. A similar large number of programs have begun at centers in other countries. Experience has shown that a successful program depends on both institutional commitment and commitment on the part of multiple professional groups within the institution that must work together in caring for the patient. Careful attention to detail in organizing a transplant program is crucial in obtaining and sustaining good outcomes in transplant patients.

The development of an effective cardiac transplant program requires compulsive organization and cooperation from both clinical and nonclinical personnel. Some states require a certificate of need to initiate a new program of heart transplantation, whereas other states have no such requirements. The National Organ Transplantation Act of 1984 established certain minimum criteria for transplant programs to enroll in the nationwide computerized matching system.[23] To encourage excellent patient care and to eliminate centers with suboptimal results, the act established the United Network for Organ Sharing (UNOS), with membership limited to those centers that perform a minimum of 12 transplant procedures per year and that obtain a 1-year survival rate of at least 70 per cent. In addition to these performance criteria, the center must have adequate operating room facilities and trained physicians and nursing personnel and be a participating member in a local organ procurement organization. The program must have established protocols and procedures for the selection of patients, the evaluation and distribution of donor organs, and postoperative management and long-term follow-up. Both surgeons and physicians involved in the care of the patient must meet certain criteria in terms of training and prior experience. The ability of an individual center to obtain funding from Medicare depends on similar criteria.[24]

TABLE 18–1 DEATHS OF POTENTIAL HEART TRANSPLANT RECIPIENTS (1979)

AGE	NO. OF POTENTIAL RECIPIENTS (U.S.)
10–54	14,085
55–59	18,925
60–64	30,115
65–69	132,055
70–74	135,485

From Evans, R. W., Manninan, D. L., Overcast, T. D., et al.: The National Heart Transplant Study: Final Report. Vol. 2, Table 13–A-30. Seattle, Battelle Human Affairs Research Centers, 1984.

TABLE 18–2 DIAGNOSES OF PATIENTS UNDERGOING TRANSPLANTATION

	ISHT (%)*	JHH (%)†
Cardiomyopathy	49	61
Coronary artery disease	41	31
Valvular disease	4	1
Retransplantation	3	1
Congenital	2	5
Other	1	1

ISHT, International Society for Heart Transplantation; JHH, Johns Hopkins Hospital.

* Data from Kriett, J. M., and Kaye, M. P.: The Registry of the International Society for Heart Transplantation: Seventh Official Report—1990. J. Heart Transplant. 9:323, 1990.

† July 1983 to June 1990 (n = 120 patients).

TABLE 18–3 CONTRAINDICATIONS TO HEART TRANSPLANTATION

Advanced age (greater than 60 years)
Irreversible hepatic or renal dysfunction
Severe vascular disease
Insulin-requiring diabetes mellitus
Active infection
Recent cancer with uncertain status
Psychiatric illness, poor medical compliance
Systemic disease which will significantly limit survival or rehabilitation

RECIPIENT SELECTION

With improved outcomes in both quality of life and percentage of patients surviving, cardiac transplantation has become accepted therapy for a number of patients with end-stage heart disease. A fairly rigid selection process is required in order to obtain excellent results in individual patients. Although in recent years there has been a tendency to relax these criteria in an effort to extend the benefits of transplantation to a larger number of patients, this needs to be balanced by the knowledge that donor organs are scarce. The number of potential recipients rises exponentially with an extension of the upper age accepted, as shown in Table 18–1. The diagnoses of patients undergoing heart transplantation are listed in Table 18–2. The most frequent indication is cardiomyopathy. Contraindications vary somewhat by program but are listed in Table 18–3.

An important aspect of evaluation is a comprehensive psychosocial evaluation by a clinical social worker or psychologist. The ability of the patient to follow a complex medical regimen is extremely important, as is the family support necessary to help the patient through multiple medical procedures and evaluations and to maintain the essential medical regimen after transplant.

All conventional medical or surgical therapies should be used before consideration of transplantation. Evaluation might reasonably include endomyocardial biopsy to rule out other treatable causes of cardiomyopathy, especially for patients without ischemic heart disease. Occasionally, unsuspected sarcoidosis or myocarditis is detected that might respond favorably to corticosteroids or immunosuppressive therapy, and some patients with recurrent life-threatening arrhythmias may be best treated initially by placement of an automatic implantable cardiac defibrillator (p. 749).

Although it may be easy to identify the most severely ill patients with a poor prognosis for 6-month survival, there is a large group of patients with symptomatic cardiomyopathy and poor objective findings (ejection fraction <20 per cent, stroke volume ≤40 ml, severe ventricular arrhythmias) for whom timing may be somewhat difficult. A further consideration may be the quality of life, which is a judgment of the patient and the physicians caring for the patient. This comes into play in patients who have been transplanted who have severe angina and unbypassable vessels.

One of the most controversial aspects of patient selection is the upper age limit for cardiac transplantation. The initial Stanford University criteria considered an upper age limit of 50 years. This was modified to include patients older than 55, and up to 60 years of age during the era of improving results in the early 1980's because of cyclosporine therapy. Sufficient additional experience has now been reported in patients over age 55 to indicate that a strict chronologic age criteria is not appropriate.[25-27] Older people can undergo transplantation with good expectation of survival and improvement in quality of life, although these patients should be optimum in every other respect. Some evidence has been reported suggesting that older patients may experience less rejection than younger patients.[28] The additional relative contraindication of diabetes or other systemic disease such as chronic pulmonary disease probably would eliminate most patients over 60 as potential candidates.

Pulmonary vascular disease is an important consideration. Orthotopic cardiac transplantation requires that the pulmonary vascular resistance be low, so that the normal right ventricle of the donor heart can adequately support the recipient's circulation after transplant. A great deal of controversy has developed over the optimal measure of pulmonary vascular resistance. Most programs use the measurement of the traditional Wood unit, and limit the value to less than or equal to 6 units at rest. Other centers use the pulmonary vascular resistance index (Wood units × body surface area) or transpulmonary pressure gradient (mean pulmonary artery pressure minus mean pulmonary capillary wedge pressure).[29] Whatever measure of resistance is used, in those patients with values toward the upper limits, it is imperative to demonstrate in the catheterization laboratory that the resistance can be manipulated with either oxygen or vasodilators with or without inotropic agents.[30] If the pulmonary vascular resistance measurements remain elevated, strong consideration should be given to either heterotopic cardiac transplantation, which leaves the recipient's heart intact, or heart-lung transplantation. Because patients may remain on a waiting list for more than 6 months, repeat cardiac catheterization may be necessary to determine if the pulmonary vascular resistance has increased. Significantly elevated pulmonary vascular resistance and right heart failure remain problems after orthotopic cardiac transplantation and are major causes of early postoperative mortality.

Although the evaluation of potential candidates for cardiac transplantation is difficult, these established criteria have led to certain predictable outcomes in terms of quality of life and actuarial survival. The result of deviations from these protocols is not as well defined but clearly is less favorable. As with any medical or surgical procedure, the final decision ultimately rests with the patient, in accordance with the concept of informed consent.

MANAGEMENT OF PATIENTS AWAITING TRANSPLANTATION

Because there are a number of patients awaiting transplantation at any point in time, their management is important. The UNOS patient waiting list for needed organs at the time of this writing lists 1700 patients awaiting heart transplantation and 260 United States patients awaiting heart-lung transplantation (June 1990). Because the current yearly number of procedures performed is about 1700, with about 60 heart-lung transplants, a number of awaiting recipients will not survive to receive a needed organ. Most centers experience between 20 per cent and 30 per cent mortality of patients on the waiting list.

The mainstay of management of end-stage congestive heart failure is diuretic therapy. The use of many currently available agents is described in Chapter 17. In addition, a number of potential vasodilator therapies for end-stage heart disease have been developed in the 1980's.

Some patients require inpatient therapy with use of inotropic agents. Although digitalis remains the only generally available oral inotropic agent, the use of intravenous low-dose dopamine or dobutamine has been a helpful tool for managing some of these patients.[31] In addition, amrinone has been reported to be specifically helpful in maintaining patients awaiting transplantation, especially in reducing pulmonary vascular resistance.[32]

Patients in whom conventional medical therapy fails may require intraaortic balloon counterpulsation, or possibly a mechanical assist device for bridging to transplantation (Chap. 19).[33-35] Growing experience has demonstrated that for short-term bridging, up to 1 week, the use of a centrifugal pump similar to types used during routine cardiac surgery can be effective. For longer-term mechanical support, ventricular assist devices have been successful. The use of the totally implantable heart has resulted in poor bridging to transplantation, with multiple complications owing to infections and/or thromboemboli.[36] Long-term mechanical support currently is limited to ventricular assist devices such as the Novacor electrically powered and implantable device[34] or the Pierce-Donachy prosthetic ventricle, which is a pneumatic-powered pump.[35] A recent report[35] indicated that 20 of 21 patients were successfully bridged to be able to receive a transplant and were discharged alive from the hospital, a remarkable accomplishment, given the complex technology required.

EVALUATION AND MANAGEMENT OF THE HEART DONOR

The limiting factor to the number of heart transplants performed is the availability of donor organs. Thus, it is imperative to obtain as high a percentage of potential donor organs as possible by increasing the donation rate, and also to consider all donor organs which might possibly be suitable for transplantation. The cardiologist frequently is asked to take part in the donor evaluation process, so that the adequate function of the graft can be predicted before transplantation.

The specific neurological catastrophe which has resulted in brain death may include blunt traumatic injury to the head, intracranial hemorrhage, and penetrating traumatic injury. The characteristics of cardiac donors are listed in Table 18–4. Until fairly recently, heart and heart-lung transplant donor criteria were very selective. The upper age limit usually was 35 years of age, and there were a number of other criteria.[37] With the need to increase the number of transplants, these criteria have been extended.[38,39] Most centers evaluate any potential donor up to as high as 55 years of age. Especially with the older or less optimum donor, careful cardiac history must be obtained from the next of kin and adequate cardiac function ensured, including potential evaluation with coronary arteriography. The use of "on the operating table" coronary arteriography has been suggested because of the logistic requirements for performing coronary arteriography in a brain-dead patient.[40] Alternatively, simple inspection of the graft with palpation of the coronary arteries at the time of harvesting has been used by some groups to rule in or out the presence of significant atherosclerosis. Sweeney and colleagues have reported on the use of hearts from donors who did not meet the standard criteria.[38] Recipients received grafts from older donors (more than 40 years of age) or from patients with a history of prolonged cardiac arrest or septicemia. Their results indicate that selective use of such donors is possible with reasonable outcomes.

The evaluation of potential donors includes obtaining an adequate history from next of kin, physical examination, a

TABLE 18–4 CAUSES OF DEATH IN DONORS* FOR HEART TRANSPLANT PROCEDURES IN THE JOHNS HOPKINS SERIES (JULY 1983–JUNE 1990)

CAUSE OF DEATH	NO. OF DONORS
Head trauma	68
Gunshot wound	21
Cerebrovascular accident	23
Asphyxiation	5
Brain tumor	1
Liver failure	1
Heart-lung recipient	1

* Age, 24 years mean (0.7–47); sex, 92 males/28 females.

12-lead electrocardiogram, and an echocardiogram. Brain death and increased intracranial pressure often result in nonspecific ST and T wave changes. These also may be seen with hypothermia. The echocardiogram has assumed an even greater role in recent years in evaluating cardiac function. This evaluation should be done at a time when intravenous inotropic agents have been lowered to as low a dose as is compatible with adequate blood pressure and cardiac output, and after adequate fluid resuscitation.

Current matching criteria of donors and recipients include only ABO compatibility and appropriate size match. A prospective specific crossmatch between donor and recipient is performed only when recipients have been identified who have more than 5 per cent of reactivity when evaluated against a panel of random donors. When heart transplantation has been performed across the ABO blood barrier, there is a significant risk of hyperacute rejection.[41]

With respect to size, fairly wide limits are acceptable, although donors who weigh less than 80 per cent of the recipient's weight should not be accepted for those patients who have higher levels of pulmonary vascular resistance. Similarly, hearts with ischemic times over 2 hours should be avoided in this situation.

Patients with brain death usually are unstable and require close attention to fluid balance, owing to diabetes insipidus. This necessitates monitoring of central venous pressure and adequate fluid resuscitation, administration of vasopressin, and replacement of fluid lost through urine output. If hypotension occurs despite adequate volume replacement, a vasopressor is infused. Dopamine is the standard inotropic agent used, but some donors will be better maintained on an alpha-adrenergic agent such as aramine.

Donor evaluation currently also includes various serology results. These are for human immunodeficiency virus (HIV), hepatitis B antigen, cytomegalovirus (CMV), and toxoplasmosis. The finding of HIV+ antibody rules out a potential donor, and the presence of CMV antibody may disqualify a potential heart-lung donor for a CMV (−) recipient by some centers.

Distant procurement of the heart and heart-lung for transplantation is now routine in almost all transplant centers.[42] The technique for heart preservation remains quite simple, with a cold crystalloid or blood cardioplegia infusion combined with topical cold for extended preservation. Average ischemic times are between 3 and 4 hours, with excellent function in most cases. Data from the Registry of the International Society for Heart Transplantation show some relation between ischemic time and survival, although most experienced centers see no particular relation for up to 6 hours of ischemia.[43] Although laboratory work has shown satisfactory preservation using various techniques for up to 24 hours of ischemia, these have not been clinically applied.[44] The longest ex vivo preservation of the human heart has been 16 hours, but the heart was implanted heterotopically, so it did not supply all of the recipient's cardiac output immediately.[45]

Techniques for distant heart-lung procurement and preservation of isolated lung grafts include flush solutions in the pulmonary artery with potent pulmonary vasodilators,[46] the use of cold blood for flush,[47] placing the donor on cardiopulmonary bypass,[48] and the use of an autoperfusing heart-lung preparation for maintaining the organs at normothermia in a working state.[49] Again, distant procurement is limited to 6 hours or less, with most procurements having an ischemic period between 3 and 4 hours.

This length of allowable ischemic time usually has kept procurement between centers of not more than 1000 miles distance. The tendency to use donor organs within the local region also has limited ischemic times.

OPERATIVE TECHNIQUE

The current technique for orthotopic heart transplantation was described in 1960 by Lower and Shumway.[10] The method involves retaining a large portion of the posterior wall of the right and left atrium in the recipient and implanting the donor heart with relatively long suture lines in the atria, together with direct end-to-end anastomoses of the aorta and the pulmonary artery. The operation is performed by way of a median sternotomy incision, with routine cannulation of the aorta and both venae cavae. Cardiopulmonary bypass usually is performed with moderate hypothermia of between 28° and 30°C. The implantation procedure usually requires from 45 to 60 minutes, and after careful attention to de-airing maneuvers and resuscitation of the heart, cardiopulmonary bypass is weaned. After placement of temporary pacing wires and chest drainage catheters, the incision is routinely closed.

RIGHT VENTRICULAR FAILURE. Because the pulmonary vascular resistance of the recipient may be elevated, acute right ventricular failure is a frequent cause of early morbidity and mortality. The normal donor right ventricle may be unable to meet the elevated resistance, and there is a high degree of both pulmonary and tricuspid valve insufficiency in the early post-transplant period.[50] This problem may be exacerbated by a relatively long ischemic time or if the donor heart is somewhat smaller than that of the recipient. Isoproterenol often is routinely given, for its chronotropic and inotropic effects as well as for its beneficial lowering of pulmonary vascular resistance. Armitage and associates reported that elevated pulmonary vascular resistance could be successfully treated with an infusion of prostaglandin E_1.[51] Support of the transplanted heart with a right ventricular assist device also has been helpful in overcoming this early postoperative problem.[52]

Multiple types of congenital anomalies have been dealt with during cardiac transplantation. For example, absence of the right superior vena cava or persistent left superior vena cava can easily be accommodated.[53] Corrected transposition of the great vessels requires extra length of the donor aorta and pulmonary artery.[54]

HETEROTOPIC HEART TRANSPLANTATION. For certain rather limited indications, cardiac transplantation can be performed as a heterotopic graft. This procedure was first described by Demikhov[6] and in early experimental work performed by McGough and colleagues.[55] It was introduced into clinical practice by Barnard in 1974, with the placement of a heterotopic heart in the right lower thorax, and the donor heart anastomosed in parallel with the retained recipient heart.[56] In cases in which the pulmonary vascular resistance remains severely elevated, the recipient's right heart can continue to function while the left heart is bypassed with the transplant. Other indications include a patient with a relatively small donor heart, a donor heart with a long ischemic time and anticipated poor early function, and a patient who has a reversible type of heart disease in which the graft may be removed when the native heart recovers. Heterotopic transplants account for about 2.5 per cent of the cardiac transplants currently performed. The operative technique includes left atrial-to-left atrial anastomosis, aorta-to-aorta anastomosis, superior vena cava-to-right atrium, and pulmonary artery-to-pulmonary artery connection, as shown in Figure 18-2.

EARLY POSTOPERATIVE RECOVERY

Much of the early postoperative management is similar to that of other patients recovering from cardiac surgical procedures. Strict isolation precautions are no longer considered mandatory. The patient is weaned from the ventilator and

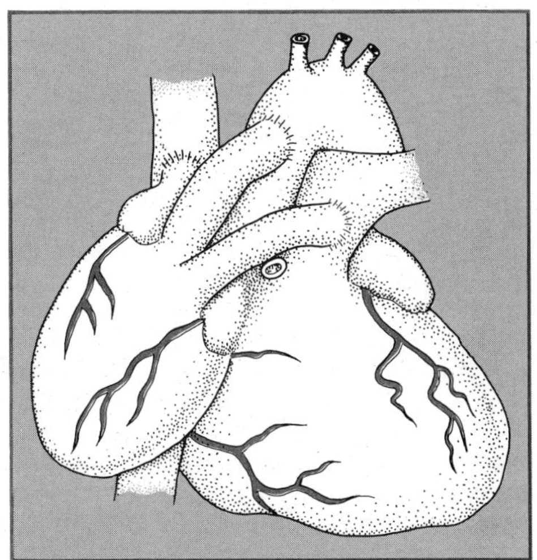

FIGURE 18-2. Diagram showing the position and anastomoses in heterotopic heart transplantation. The donor heart is placed parallel to the recipient's heart.

TABLE 18–5 IMMUNOSUPPRESSION FOR HEART TRANSPLANTATION—TRIPLE-DRUG PROTOCOL

DRUG	PREOPERATIVE OR PERIOPERATIVE	POSTOPERATIVE	
		Early	Late
Cyclosporine	6 mg/kg PO	6–10 mg/kg/day PO* or 0.5–2 mg/kg/day IV	4–6 mg/kg/day PO
Methylprednisolone		500 mg IV after cardiopulmonary bypass 125 mg q 8 h × 3	
Prednisone		1 mg/kg/day PO tapered to 0.4 mg/kg	0.2 mg/kg/day PO
Azathioprine		2 mg/kg/day PO	1–2 mg/kg/day PO

* Omit if preoperative serum creatinine level is greater than 1.5 mg/dl and use IV.

from inotropic drugs as tolerated. Early mobilization and use of physical therapy are begun as soon as tolerated.

The most important feature of early management is the institution of the immunosuppressive regimen which will be continued throughout the patient's lifetime. Numerous protocols exist for maintenance immunosuppression, and these protocols are continually changing. Most patients receive cyclosporine in combination with several other medications. Currently, the most common protocol involves triple-drug therapy of cyclosporine, azathioprine, and prednisone. Most of these medications are given in higher doses in the early post-transplant period, with weaning to lower and less toxic levels for chronic administration. A typical protocol for immunosuppression is shown in Table 18–5. At the Johns Hopkins Hospital, patients are given cyclosporine, 6 to 10 mg/kg of body weight preoperatively, and 500 mg of methylprednisolone intraoperatively. Postoperatively, patients receive cyclosporine at 10 mg/kg/day in divided doses, depending on serum levels and renal function, and an early tapering course of methylprednisolone. After the third dose of methylprednisolone, oral prednisone is begun in doses of 1 mg/kg of body weight and is tapered to 0.4 mg/kg over 2 weeks. Azathioprine is given at about 2 mg/kg and is lowered if the white blood cell count falls below 4000/mm.[3]

The demonstration of certain advantages has popularized prophylactic induction therapy.[57] The Utah transplant group showed that the monoclonal antibody directed against the T3 (helper) lymphocyte (orthoclone, OKT3) results in excellent early renal function and almost a complete absence of early acute rejection, allowing the patient to recover from the surgical procedure and begin rehabilitation. There is a low incidence of sensitization against the mouse monoclonal antibody, so early prophylactic administration does not preclude later use of OKT3 for treatment of acute rejection, if necessary.[58]

Chronic maintenance immunosuppression usually consists of either cyclosporine, azathioprine, and prednisone or cyclosporine and azathioprine alone.

DETECTION OF REJECTION

Detection and treatment of allograft rejection remain perhaps the most crucial aspects of transplant management. The most reliable and frequent technique to assess allograft rejection is the endomyocardial biopsy. Other less invasive techniques have relied on the detection of activated circulating lymphoblasts,[59] changes in the appearance of the heart by echocardiography[60] or in the voltage of the electrocardiogram,[61] and experimental techniques looking at the energy state of the myocardium by nuclear magnetic resonance (NMR) spectroscopy.[62]

Almost all of these techniques rely on measurement of myocardial depression as a result of injury from the rejection process. Myocyte necrosis is a relatively late manifestation of rejection, emphasizing the need for more sensitive and specific early signs.

In 1965, Lower and associates noted a consistent drop in the *summed values of electrocardiographic voltage,* coincident with rejection in 20 untreated dogs with heart transplants.[12] Later, electrocardiographic monitoring was used for patients treated with prednisone and azathioprine, and found to be helpful. A decrease in the summed QRS voltage by 20 per cent was thought to be indicative of rejection.[63] However, a number of other conditions influence the QRS voltage, including myocardial and pulmonary edema, pulmonary infiltrates owing to a variety of causes, and pericardial effusion. Furthermore, cyclosporine-treated patients have less cardiac tissue edema, and thus the standard electrocardiogram is less sensitive. A directly implanted epicardial electrode with a telemetry monitoring system for following heart transplant patients' electrocardiograms has been successfully used by the Berlin transplant group, but it has not been widely adopted because of the need to implant electrodes and to maintain equipment for telemetry.

Echocardiographic studies of transplant recipients are suggestive of rejection episodes. Dubroff and others have shown that there is an increase in left ventricular wall thickness during episodes of cardiac rejection.[60] Further studies have shown this is a relatively insensitive technique. Dawkins and coworkers demonstrated that the appearance of rejection can be diagnosed by an increase in the isovolumetric relaxation time.[64] Thus, changes associated with rejection are an increase in posterior wall thickness, an increase in left ventricular mass, and decreased diastolic compliance. Unfortunately, most of these changes are indicative of rather advanced stages of rejection, and thus the finding has limited usefulness. Echocardiograms currently are obtained as baseline studies early after transplantation, and are correlated with those during moderate or severe rejection to assess left ventricular performance during treatment and to ensure that left ventricular function is stable or improving. Patients' echocardiograms are recorded on their own individual tapes, which allows easy review of serial evaluation of left ventricular performance.

Among radionuclide tests, *technetium-99m pyrophosphate scintigraphy* (p. 315) is a sensitive and specific indicator of myocardial injury caused by ischemia. With increasingly severe cardiac rejection, there is a progressive increase in myocardial uptake in laboratory animals.[65] Other studies with thallium-201 or indium-111 have suggested some usefulness in experimental laboratory studies, but none of the nuclear scans are used clinically on a routine basis.[66]

Antimyosin antibodies (p. 292), which are monoclonal Fab fragments directed against myosin, can be used to evaluate myosin exposure during the cell death associated with cardiac rejection. This has been demonstrated both in rejecting dog hearts and in patients.[67]

Nuclear magnetic resonance spectroscopy is a recent noninvasive technique for evaluating tissue biochemical characteristics. In rejecting dog and human hearts there is a decline in phosphocreatine detected by NMR spectroscopy during the course of allograft rejection. The ratio of phosphocreatine to inorganic phosphorus declines, and these changes occur 24 to 48 hours before appearance of myocyte necrosis on endomyocardial biopsies.[62] Although these techniques hold promise for a less invasive measure, and would be particularly helpful in pediatric recipients, a low-cost, sensitive, and reliable technique has yet to be developed.

Other investigators have examined urinary byproducts of cellular degradation. Foegh and colleagues examined urinary *thromboxane* B_2 as a noninvasive indicator for cardiac rejection.[68] Another compound is *putrescine*, a naturally occurring polyamine, stimulated by T cell proliferation. Putrescine is excreted by cells undergoing mitosis. Levels will rise before histological rejection in untreated dogs after heterotopic heart transplantation and fall despite presumed continued rejection.[69] This finding has been confirmed in patients by the Tucson, Arizona, transplant group.[70] However, these studies show minimal changes in cyclosporine-treated patients, and the technique is not widely used.

Measurement of lymphocyte subsets has been a potentially attractive method for detecting rejection. In general, these techniques have not been sensitive or specific, as demonstrated by the studies of O'Toole and associates.[71] Recipients receiving heart and heart-lung transplants and immunosuppression with cyclosporine, prednisone, and antithymocyte globulin (ATG) were followed for 1 year, but demonstrated no reproducible correlation of T4-T8 ratios with rejection episodes. These lymphocyte subsets were found to be affected more by viral infections than by rejection episodes.

ENDOMYOCARDIAL BIOPSY

With the inadequacy of these noninvasive tests, the endomyocardial biopsy remains the standard method for the detection of rejection and its effective treatment with augmented immunosuppression. The endomyocardial biopsy technique was introduced for cardiac transplantation by Caves and associates in 1973.[72] They proved the efficacy of monitoring the heart by a biopsy technique in canine laboratory studies. The relatively diffuse interstitial infiltrate associated with rejection makes it possible for the focal biopsy to be a good reflection of events throughout the myocardium.[73] Although the endomyocardial biopsy is an invasive procedure, it seems relatively well tolerated and can be performed in a sequential manner. Complications usually are mild, and include pneumothoraces, transient rhythm disturbances, and a rare instance of myocardial perforation. Because it is a percutaneous and transvenous technique, there is no operative incision and only local anesthetic is required with minimal discomfort. The procedure is rapidly performed, usually through the right internal jugular vein, and can be repeated on many occasions through the same access site. The most common site for placement of the bioptome is the right internal jugular vein, but it can be placed from the left jugular vein, from the subclavian vein, and from the femoral veins, as shown in Figure 18-3. Fluoroscopy usually is used, although some operators prefer the echocardiogram to guide the bioptome within the heart.

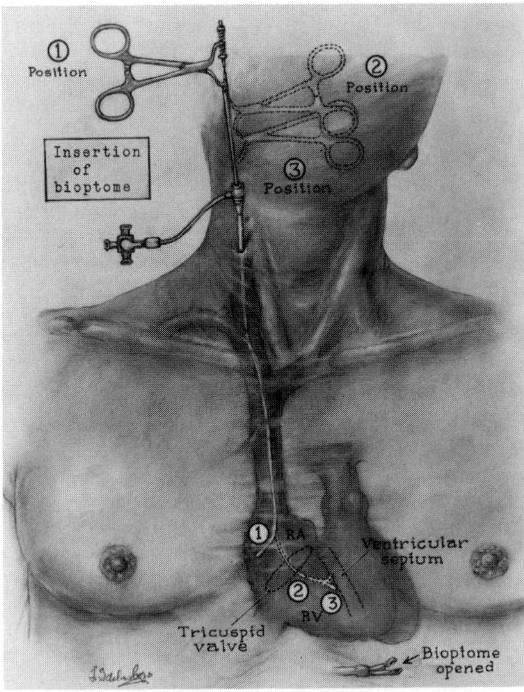

FIGURE 18-3. Positioning of the bioptome for endomyocardial biopsy. 1. Bioptome is inserted with the tip pointed toward the lateral wall of the right atrium. 2. At the level of the mid-right atrium, the bioptome is rotated anteriorly about 180 degrees and is advanced through the tricuspid valve apparatus toward the right ventricle. 3. The bioptome is advanced to the interventricular septum with the jaws opened. (From Baughman, K. L.: History and current techniques of endomyocardial biopsy. *In* Baumgartner, W. A., Reitz, B. A., and Achuff, S. A. [eds.]: Heart and Heart-Lung Transplantation. Philadelphia, W. B. Saunders Company, 1990.)

TABLE 18-6 RECOMMENDED FREQUENCY OF ENDOMYOCARDIAL BIOPSY FOR ROUTINE MONITORING OF HEART TRANSPLANT REJECTION*

TIME AFTER TRANSPLANT	INTERVAL	NO. OF BIOPSIES
0-6 wk	Every 10 days	4
6 wk to 3 mo	Every 2 wk	2
3-6 mo	Every mo	3
6 mo to indefinite	Every 3 mo	3
	Total yr 1	12

* Rebiopsy if indeterminate and 10 days after conclusion of rejection treatment.

Adapted from Baughman, K. L.: Monitoring of allograft rejection. *In* Baumgartner, W. A., Reitz, B. A., and Achuff, S. A. (eds.): Heart and Heart-Lung Transplantation. Philadelphia, W. B. Saunders Company, 1990, p. 162.

To get an adequate sample for examination, four to six biopsy specimens are taken at each examination.[73] These specimens are stained with hematoxylin and eosin. A typical post-transplant biopsy schedule is shown in Table 18-6. Patients who demonstrate allograft rejection are treated with an appropriate immunosuppressive regimen and repeat endomyocardial biopsy is performed 7 to 10 days later. Biopsies performed during the course of treatment for acute rejection are difficult to interpret. Therefore, the effect of rejection treatment usually is followed by echocardiographic examination of left ventricular function, and biopsy is performed 7 to 10 days after the completion of a planned immunosuppressive course.

The variety and significance of the observed histological changes in cardiac allografts have now been reasonably well defined. Multiple grading systems have been advocated by different transplant groups, but recently the International Society for Heart Transplantation has attempted to adopt more uniform criteria.[73] The preparation of biopsy specimens includes taking an adequate number of fragments, usually a minimum of four. The tissue fragments are imbedded together in a single block, processed, and sectioned. Most biopsies are assessed using standard hematoxylin and eosin stains, but other, special stains may be useful for additional information, such as the amount of collagen present or identification of specific subtypes of infiltrating lymphocytes.

The most important feature of most post-transplant biopsies is the detection of lymphocyte infiltration and the presence of myocyte necrosis. The continuum of histological findings from a normal biopsy to one showing severe acute rejection will include a variety of subtle findings, which are listed in Table 18-7. The histological characteristics together with their approximate frequency in a large number of post-transplant biopsies are shown in the table. Figure 18-4*A* is an example of early interstitial infiltrate in a patient with no evidence of myocyte necrosis, and Figure 18-4*B* is an example of further infiltrate and definite evidence of myocyte cell injury. The former is cause for a follow-up biopsy, and the latter for antirejection treatment.

A certain number of confusing histopathological changes

TABLE 18-7 HISTOPATHOLOGICAL GRADING SYSTEM FOR ACUTE REJECTION

GRADE	MORPHOLOGY	TREATMENT RESPONSE
Mild acute rejection	Perivascular and/or sparse interstitial infiltrate of mononuclear cells; very focal necrosis occasionally	Follow-up biopsy
Moderate acute rejection	Perivascular and interstitial infiltrates of mononuclear (eosinophils with CyA) and myocyte necrosis	Treatment indicated; intravenous or oral prednisone
Severe acute rejection	Diffuse mixed infiltrate (neutrophils, eosinophils, and lymphocytes) myocyte necrosis, hemorrhage, and vasculitis	Treatment indicated; intravenous prednisone or "rescue" therapy
Resolving rejection	Diminished infiltrate of small lymphocytes, hemosiderin-laden macrophages, fibroblasts, and new collagen formation	Complete course of treatment or follow-up biopsy
Resolved rejection	Mature focal scars, which may include "trapped" lymphocytes	Usual surveillance protocol

Adapted from Billingham, M. E.: The pathology of transplanted hearts. Semin. Thorac. Cardiovasc. Surg. *2*:223, 1990.

can be seen in some biopsy specimens and be unrelated to rejection. For example, in specimens taken early after transplantation, there may be necrotic myocytes undergoing macrophagic removal because of ischemia at the time of the transplant procedure itself. Necrosis also may be secondary to infectious agents such as CMV and toxoplasmosis. Occasional infections with these agents have been first diagnosed by the endomyocardial biopsy. Perhaps the most frequent abnormality is a biopsy taken from a previous biopsy site which may contain contraction bands and evidence of inflammation and collagen formation as a result of healing of the previous biopsy site. The subtle findings associated with previous biopsy site histology are described in more detail in a recent review.[74]

TREATMENT OF ACUTE REJECTION

Immunosuppression to prevent allograft rejection begins at the time of the transplant procedure and continues throughout the life of the recipient. Although a number of strategies are being developed to enhance the induction of immunosuppression and to maximize the potential for developing tolerance in the recipient, virtually every patient probably experiences some acute allograft rejection during the first posttransplant year. The balance between effective immunosuppression and excess immunosuppression and the possibility of multiple opportunistic infections requires careful tailoring of the immunosuppressive therapy to the specific needs of the individual recipient. Although a number of new immunosuppressive agents will probably become available in the next few years, as of this writing acute rejection episodes are treated by a relatively small number of standard therapies.

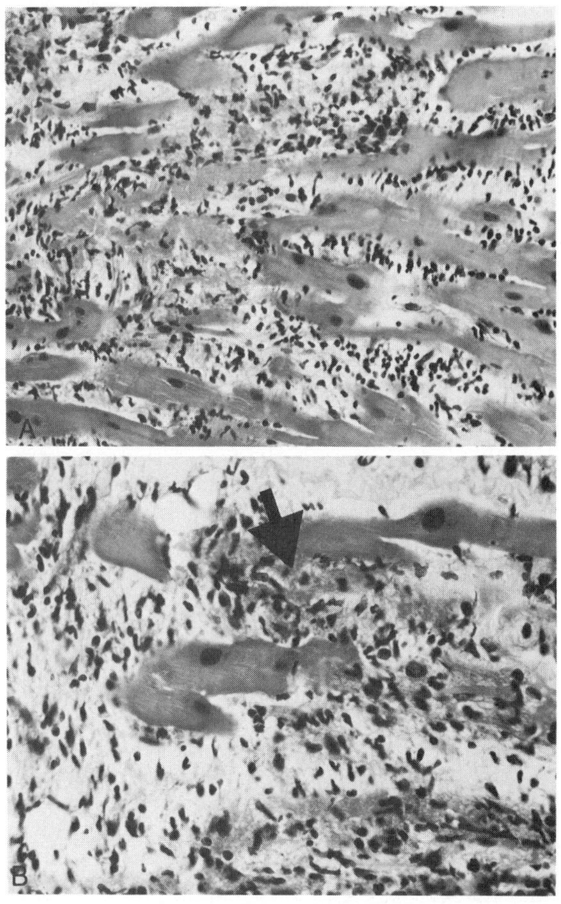

FIGURE 18-4. Photomicrographs of endomyocardial biopsy taken from a patient with early acute rejection. *A*, Diffuse interstitial infiltrate of mononuclear cells. *B*, Higher-power view showing associated myocardial necrosis (arrow).

The highest incidence of acute rejection occurs within the first 3 months after transplantation. Of patients receiving standard triple-drug therapy that includes cyclosporine, azathioprine, and prednisone, we have found that 84 per cent have at least one episode of rejection during the first 3 months. After 3 months, the incidence of rejection diminishes significantly to about one episode per patient-year. Those patients with a relatively good match between donor and recipient, and who do not experience rejection within the first 3 months, usually have a lower incidence of late rejection.

The timing and severity of rejection episodes dictate the appropriate therapy. A representative algorithm for treatment is shown in Figure 18-5. Episodes that occur within the first 3 months or that are moderate to severe are best treated by pulse therapy with methylprednisolone. Methylprednisolone sodium succinate is administered at a dose of 1000 mg/day, given intravenously for 3 consecutive days. Rejection that occurs later than 1 month may be treated by augmenting oral steroid intake to 100 mg of prednisone per day for 3 consecutive days, tapered gradually back to a baseline over 2 weeks. Several studies have demonstrated that an equivalent oral dose of prednisone may be as effective as intravenous methylprednisolone in early acute rejection.[75] In children or small adults the dose of methylprednisolone and prednisone should be decreased proportionate to body size.

Because of the side effects of increased corticosteroid therapy, the patient should be carefully monitored for infections, increased fluid retention, glucose intolerance, and psychological or mood changes. When prednisone treatment has been ineffective for reversing the rejection, or in particularly severe cases of rejection associated with hemodynamic changes, more aggressive therapy is given. The use of ATGAM (horse antithymocyte globulin), rabbit ATG, or OKT3 monoclonal antibody constitutes rescue therapy after unsuccessful use of prednisone or methylprednisolone. Unfortunately, the availability of commercial preparations of ATGAM is limited. Similarly, the availability of rabbit ATG preparations is limited because such preparations are not commercially obtained and require special local arrangements for preparation. Consequently OKT3 therapy is probably the most frequent type of rescue therapy being used, and is an effective treatment for most resistant rejection episodes.[76,77]

Additional strategies for treatment of early or mild rejection have been advocated. Kobashigawa and associates treated patients with mild acute rejection with increases in oral cyclosporine, treating 40 episodes in 28 patients.[78] In their study, in

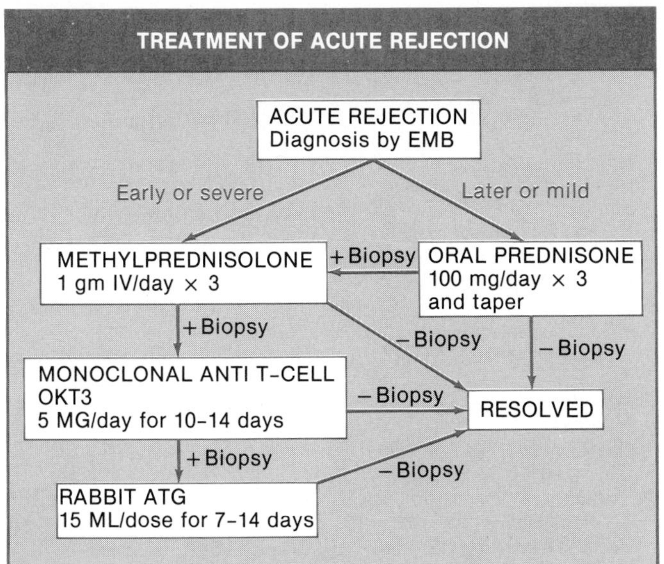

FIGURE 18–5. Algorithm for determining treatment of acute allograft rejection. EMB = endomyocardial biopsy; ATG = antithymocyte globulin.

those patients with an actual increase in serum cyclosporine levels, 90 per cent had no progression of rejection or clearing of rejection, whereas 37 per cent of those who had no increase in levels progressed with more evidence of acute rejection requiring treatment. Olsen and coworkers from the University of Utah, reported using methotrexate in the treatment of persistent low-grade rejection.[79] Methotrexate was given three times a week for an average of 8 weeks to 16 patients. All rejections were reversed, and the dose of prednisone could be reduced. There were no infections, but azathioprine dosage had to be reduced in 10 patients because of leukopenia.

For patients with persistent recurrent rejection episodes, the use of total lymphoid irradiation has recently been advocated. Hunt and colleagues, from Stanford University, reported the use of this modality in patients who were unresponsive to multiple courses of conventional therapy.[80] Total lymphoid irradiation was given according to standard protocols, with doses ranging from 240 to 640 rads. The amount of radiation was determined by the absolute T lymphocyte count. This treatment was remarkably effective in preventing further rejection and in being able to lower the maintenance doses of immunosuppression. The only side effect was mild, transient neutropenia. This is a promising modality for patients who experience repeated rejection, and may be considered in the future for other patients who could benefit from reduction in maintenance therapy because of side effects of corticosteroids or cyclosporine.

NEW IMMUNOSUPPRESSIVE AGENTS

The introduction of cyclosporine in the early 1980's was the stimulus for the tremendous growth in heart transplantation. The mode of action of cyclosporine was more specific, interfering with several steps in the allograft response, rather than a generalized depression of all immune-competent cells. Attention subsequently had focused on a variety of other agents, which also have selective effects and which may have fewer side effects than cyclosporine. The first of these new agents to be introduced into clinical practice is the macrolide antibiotic compound FK-506, identified in 1984 by the Fujisawa Company of Japan.[81] This compound is produced by *Streptomyces tsukubaensis.* It appears to be about 100 times more effective at the same dosage range than cyclosporine. It acts by suppressing IL-2 production by T cells by inhibiting expression of both IL-2 receptors on T cells and the generation of cytotoxic killer T cells, and achieves these results at dosages which do not interfere with bone marrow function.

FK-506 for cardiac transplantation currently has been restricted to a series of patients at the University of Pittsburgh. After encouraging results in liver transplantations at that center, FK-506 has been given as the sole immunosuppressive agent in about 30 patients undergoing heart or lung transplantation.[82] Ten heart transplants and four patients with lung grafts had minimal rejection within the first 30 days. Sixty-three per cent were rejection free during the initial hospitalization. The role of this and other new agents remains to be established by prospective randomized trials, the determination of long-term side effects, and the incidence of graft atherosclerosis when compared with conventional treatments. The availability of multiple agents for selective immunosuppression will almost certainly enhance the early and late acceptance of cardiac allografts, minimize toxicities, and increase the safety of cardiac transplantation.

Infectious Complications After Cardiac Transplantation

In most centers, infectious complications are the most common cause of death after transplantation. Despite the fact that more effective immunosuppressive therapy has reduced the incidence and severity of infectious complications, they still remain a major problem.[83] The overall incidence of infectious complications ranges from 41 per cent to 71 per cent in various series, and multiple infections are frequent.

With the extensive experience now available from both kidney, liver, and heart transplant recipients, certain typical infection patterns can be described. Infections in the first postoperative month tend to involve bacterial pathogens encountered in surgical patients in general. Infections in the time from 1 to 4 months after surgery usually involve opportunistic pathogens, especially CMV. After this period a mixture of both conventional and opportunistic infections are found.

In contradistinction to renal transplant recipients, cardiac recipients must receive somewhat higher levels of pharmacological immunosuppression, which cannot be significantly reduced at the time of infectious complications. This emphasizes the need for early diagnosis and aggressive therapy for any type of infection.

EARLY INFECTION. Infections in the first month after transplantation are commonly bacterial and most frequently in the lung. This is especially true for patients with lung transplants in addition to heart. Typically, nosocomial organisms such as *Pseudomonas aeruginosa, Proteus, Klebsiella,* and *Escherichia coli* are encountered. The incidence of significant mediastinitis is between 0.4 per cent and 4.5 per cent in heart transplant recipients. Treatment includes prolonged courses of antibiotics, debridement of devitalized bone, and the use of vascularized muscle flaps for subsequent wound closure. Other typical causes of early postoperative infection, such as urinary tract infections, bacteremias, and pneumonia, should be suspected. The clinical diagnosis of pneumonia is made on the basis of typical clinical features, including cough, fever, sputum production, and chest x-rays showing a new pulmonary infiltrate. An aggressive approach to early diagnosis is recommended. This may include transtracheal aspiration for culture or bronchoscopy with washings and culture. The results of these cultures will determine specific antibiotic therapy, but early, aggressive broad-spectrum coverage started immediately after obtaining appropriate cultures is recommended.

LATE INFECTION. Late post-transplant infections are more diverse. These are frequently of the opportunistic variety, including virus *Pneumocystis carinii, Aspergillus,* and *Nocardia* species. The variety of late post-transplant pneumonias may vary from center to center, depending on local prevalences and the use of prophylactic treatments. For example, in some series *Pneumocystis carinii* is the most common late pulmonary infection, whereas in other series it is absent. The regular prophylactic administration of trimethoprim and sulfamethoxazole on a long-term basis is recommended by a number of heart transplant teams.

CYTOMEGALOVIRUS INFECTION. CMV infection is the most frequent and important viral infection in transplant recipients, with an incidence in cardiac recipients of between 73 per cent and 100 per cent.[84,85] This can be minimized in CMV-negative patients by the use of CMV-negative blood products, but a CMV-positive donor will invariably transmit infection. This organism results in a number of potentially important clinical problems, including pneumonitis, hepatitis, chorioretinitis, and fever with leukopenia, which additionally predisposes to other infectious complications. Fortunately current prophylactic and antiviral therapy will help to minimize the effects of CMV infection. 9-(1,3-dihydroxy-2-propoxymethyl) Guanine (DHPG), or ganciclovir, is the current treatment for acute symptomatic CMV infections. Early prophylaxis in the setting of a positive CMV graft into a negative recipient includes the use of ganciclovir and hyperimmune globulin for 6 to 8 weeks post transplant.

The importance of CMV infection cannot be overemphasized because of its relation to the development of late graft atherosclerosis, discussed on p. 528. The availability of newer antiviral treatments may help to minimize the complications of this particular infection in the future.

OTHER COMPLICATIONS OF IMMUNOSUPPRESSION

The cardiologist following cardiac transplant patients should be aware of the multiple complications of the immunosuppressive drugs. All of the commonly used drugs increase

TABLE 18–8 COMPLICATONS OF CYCLOSPORINE ADMINISTRATION

COMPLICATION	PATHOGENESIS	DIAGNOSIS	TREATMENT
Nephrotoxicity	↓ Renal blood flow and glomerular filtration rate	↑ BUN ↑ Creatinine Hyperkalemia Hyperchloremic acidosis	↓ Dosage of cyclosporine
Hepatotoxicity	Unclear Centrilobular fatty change	↑ SGPT ↑ SGOT ↑ Bilirubin	↓ Dosage of cyclosporine
Neoplasms	Overimmunosuppression when combined with other agents	Usually B cell lymphoma	↓ Dosage of cyclosporine
Hypertension	Nephrotoxicity ? Renin release	Mild to moderately elevated blood pressure	↓ Dosage of cyclosporine Conventional antihypertensive medications
Neurological	Unknown, potentiated by hypomagnesemia	Hand tremors Seizures	↓ Dosage of cyclosporine
Hypertrichosis	Unknown, exacerbated by concomitant use of minoxidil	Excessive hair growth in preexisting hair growth areas	↓ Dosage of cyclosporine
Gingival hyperplasia	Unclear	Develops slowly over several months	Good oral hygiene ↓ Dosage of cyclosporine

the risk of infectious complications and are associated with neoplasia, because immunocompromised patients are more susceptible to various cancers.[86]

CYCLOSPORINE TOXICITY. Cyclosporine is associated with a number of complications, which are summarized in Table 18–8. The most clinically significant effects of cyclosporine involve the kidneys. Almost all patient groups receiving cyclosporine have a fall in creatinine clearance, an increase in serum creatinine level, associated fluid retention and edema, and significant hypertension.[87,88] Histopathological changes after chronic administration are found in the proximal convoluted tubule and in the distal tubules, and consist of vacuolization of cells, epithelial swelling, hydropic degeneration, and necrosis. There is increasing clinical and experimental evidence that cyclosporine produces a derangement in the prostaglandin system in the renal tubules. Indomethacin exacerbates renal dysfunction after cyclosporine administration. Cyclosporine may act by increasing urinary thromboxane B_2 levels in a dose-dependent manner, with local vasoconstriction, platelet aggregation, and release of platelet-produced thromboxane. This may explain the development of hypertension, renal ischemia, and the dysfunction that is seen clinically. Early after transplant, many patients have oliguria. Thus, many transplant groups restrict the use of cyclosporine to continuous intravenous administration with careful control of serum levels during the early post-transplant period, or omit cyclosporine altogether and use induction therapy with monoclonal antibody (OKT3), until serum creatinine is normal and the patient has recovered from the effects of cardiopulmonary bypass.[88–90]

Hepatotoxicity is evidenced by an increase in bilirubin and by increases in liver enzymes. There are no characteristic cellular pathological alterations for centrilobular fatty changes. The hepatotoxicity is dose-related and reverts to normal after the dose of cyclosporine is lowered or eliminated. In general, hepatotoxicity is uncommon after cardiac transplantation, and so far no long-term sequelae of cyclosporine on liver function have been reported.

Neurotoxic reactions are manifested by a fine tremor, paresthesias, and, occasionally, seizures. Most of these events are dose-related and reversible but are certainly bothersome to some patients. Other unusual side effects include the development of hirsutism, or hypertrichosis, observed in almost all patients who receive cyclosporine. These effects tend to regress as the dosage of cyclosporine is lowered. Similarly, gingival hyperplasia has been observed with no particular morbidity. A combination of cyclosporine and nifedipine has resulted in an increased rate of gingival hyperplasia (51 per cent) when compared with cyclosporine alone (8 per cent).[91]

CORTICOSTEROID TOXICITY. Perhaps the most troublesome side effects of immunosuppressive therapy are associated with long-term administration of corticosteroids. In patients who require relatively high doses of steroids, these can be especially severe, and include peptic ulcers, aseptic necrosis of bone, weight gain, psychiatric effects, diabetes, elevated serum lipid levels, and heightened susceptibility to infection of all types. Perhaps the major advance in transplantation will come when corticosteroid therapy can be completely eliminated.

AZATHIOPRINE TOXICITY. The major morbidity of long-term azathioprine administration is bone marrow suppression. It also is associated with hepatotoxicity in some patients, which may be so severe that the drug must be discontinued with substitution of an antimetabolite such as cyclophosphamide.

NEOPLASIA IN IMMUNOSUPPRESSED CARDIAC TRANSPLANT RECIPIENTS

Cancer is an unfortunate consequence of chronic immunosuppression.[86] In general, transplant recipients have a threefold increase in the incidence in various cancers when compared with age-matched controls. Some specific cancers are more than 100 times more frequent in immunosuppressed patients than in the general population. For all tumors, the average time of appearance of the cancer after transplantation is 58 months, although some tumors may characteristically appear at other intervals. Cardiac transplant recipients have a somewhat higher incidence of cancer than do renal transplant patients, perhaps because of the higher levels of immunosuppression. The most common tumors among transplant patients are those of the skin and lips, non-Hodgkin lymphomas, Kaposi sarcomas, and uterine, cervical, vulval, and perineal neoplasms.[86]

Perhaps the most important neoplasms are the lymphoproliferative tumors that occur early after transplantation, more frequently in younger recipients. Most of these tumors are thought to be the result of Epstein-Barr viral infection and consist of B cell proliferation because of T cell suppression or depletion.[92] These B cell proliferations result in tumors that cannot be treated well by conventional surgical or radiotherapy treatments. The most effective approach is to discontinue or at least reduce immunosuppressive treatment. Antiviral chemotherapy is ineffective because the virus usually is in a latent phase and no longer replicating. There are multiple reports of regression of these tumors in patients whose immunosuppression has been reduced.[93]

GRAFT ATHEROSCLEROSIS

The major long-term problem after cardiac transplantation, assuming greater importance as the number of survivors increases, is the development of significant coronary artery disease in the transplanted heart. Graft atherosclerosis was first observed by Thomson in 1969, in the first long-term survivor reported from South Africa.[94] Nineteen months after transplantation for ischemic cardiomyopathy, the patient died with extensive coronary artery disease. Of the first 18 orthotopic transplant patients at Stanford, 7 died within a 2-year period of graft atherosclerosis.[95] By 1979 the role of lipids, donor age, and the possible use of antiplatelet therapy was recognized, and the incidence of significant graft atherosclerosis in long-term survivors was 38 per cent at 5 years.[96] A variety of reports show an incidence of between 20 per cent and 50 per cent at 5 years.[97–100,100a]

With the advent of protocols using cyclosporine for immunosuppression, there has been no significant decline in the incidence of this disease. A recent report of the long-term survivors from the Stanford series shows that at 1 year, 6.2 per cent of cyclosporine-treated patients have angiographic or autopsy evidence of disease, and at 5 years the incidence is 24 per cent.[101]

The cause of graft atherosclerosis remains controversial and is probably multifactorial.[102] Vascular endothelium is known to be immunologically active, and similar vascular changes are seen late after kidney and liver transplantation. The early stages of cardiac allograft rejection are characterized by lymphocytic perivascular infiltration, and vasculitis frequently is a prominent part of moderate to severe allograft rejection. Vascular changes with deposition of immunoglobulin, complement, and fibrin have been demonstrated both in patients and in animals. Platelet-derived growth factor producing activation and aggregation of platelets as well as proliferation of mononuclear cells has been demonstrated to occur during acute rejection. These data strongly support a complex immune mechanism for the development of graft atherosclerosis.

Several clinical studies have attempted to identify risk factors. In the most comprehensive report of patients treated with prednisone and azathioprine, the only significant clinical factors were donor age over 35, incompatibility at the HLA-A1 and A2 loci, and serum triglyceride concentration greater than 280 mg/dl.[96] In reports from other centers, which include experience with cyclosporine, the development of graft atherosclerosis was correlated with two or more rejection episodes, but not with lipid levels or donor age.[97]

Several recent reports emphasize the possible role of CMV infection in atherogenesis in general[103] and graft atherosclerosis in particular. In a recent review of 301 cardiac transplant recipients during the cyclosporine era, the Stanford group divided patients into two groups based on freedom from CMV infection.[104] Two hundred ten patients were included in this group and 91 patients in the CMV infection group. The incidence of graft rejection was significantly higher in the CMV infection group, and using angiographic criteria or autopsy examination, graft atherosclerosis was found to be significantly more severe. Surprisingly, actuarial 5-year survival in the CMV infection–free group was 68.3 per cent, compared with only 32.2 per cent for the CMV infection group. Data from Johns Hopkins Hospital indicate that the presence of CMV infection and donor age were the two factors in a multifactorial analysis which correlated with the development of graft atherosclerosis.[105]

In addition to measures to limit CMV, strategies have been directed toward limiting the amount of steroid administered. Hypercholesterolemia is a known risk factor for the development of coronary artery disease in general, and the use of prednisone is correlated with significantly elevated serum cholesterol levels in cardiac transplant recipients.[106] A number of centers have tried to maintain as many patients as possible on long-term cyclosporine and azathioprine alone to reduce lipid levels. It is hoped that newer immunosuppressive drugs, such as FK-506, may allow steroid-free treatment, and thus have a positive impact on the development of this significant complication.

Most centers use some preventive measures in the hopes of reducing the incidence of graft atherosclerosis. These measures include modification of known risk factors, maintenance of ideal body weight through dietary restriction, reduced intake of cholesterol and saturated fats, cessation of smoking, regular exercise, and the use of an antiplatelet agent such as low-dose aspirin.

Graft atherosclerosis has been observed as an incidental finding at autopsy as early as 3 months after transplantation. Significant coronary disease may produce arrhythmias, myocardial infarction, sudden death, or impaired left ventricular function with congestive heart failure.[107] It is extremely rare to develop angina pectoris because the cardiac allograft remains essentially denervated, although a patient has been reported who had angina pectoris in the presence of coronary artery disease.[108] The disease tends to be rather diffuse and concentric, and coronary angiograms must be closely inspected and compared with previous studies to appreciate the reduction in coronary diameter. The existence of more discrete proximal lesions has been treated by percutaneous transluminal coronary angioplasty in some cases, and even coronary artery bypass grafting has been reported.[109,110] However, retransplantation is the major alternative once diffuse graft atherosclerosis develops. The results of retransplantation are less good than for the primary procedure, with a reported patient survival rate of 44 per cent at 1 year among 23 patients treated in the cyclosporine era.[111]

LATE FOLLOW-UP

The late follow-up of cardiac transplant recipients requires a coordinated and systematic approach. Because the two leading causes of morbidity and mortality are rejection and infection, surveillance should focus on these two possibilities in addition to the other problems of graft atherosclerosis and cancer. The frequency and timing of transplant follow-up visits are determined by the general condition of the patient and the time after transplant. The commonly performed tests for following heart transplant recipients and their frequency are shown in Table 18–9. Endomyocardial biopsy remains a necessity and is performed on an every 3- to 4-month interval indefinitely. The author currently recommends performing coronary arteriography on a yearly basis, although some programs alternate this with less invasive studies of myocardial ischemia, such as exercise stress thallium study.

In addition to the objective laboratory data, a detailed interval history and physical examination are important to detect other complicating illnesses at an early stage. Patients may minimize new symptoms, and the physician must be constantly alert to the possibility of an occult but potentially life-threatening infectious complication. A detailed inquiry into all medications that the patient is taking should be performed

TABLE 18–9 COMMONLY PERFORMED TESTS FOR HEART TRANSPLANT FOLLOW-UP

PROCEDURE OR BLOOD TEST	FREQUENCY
Endomyocardial biopsy	See Table 18–6
Electrolytes, BUN, creatinine, glucose, magnesium	q visit
Complete blood count, platelets	q visit
Cyclosporine levels (trough)	q visit
Lipid profile	q 3–6 mo
Complete chemistry profile	q 3–6 mo
Chest x-ray, posteroanterior and lateral	q 6 mo + PRN
Echocardiogram	q 1 yr + PRN
Electrocardiogram	q 1 yr + PRN
24-hour urine for creatinine, protein	q 1 yr
Coronary angiography	q 1 yr

Adapted from Achuff, A. C., and Augustine, S. M.: Outpatient management of the heart transplant patient. *In* Baumgartner, W. A., Reitz, B. A., and Achuff, S. A. (eds.): Heart and Heart-Lung Transplantation. Philadelphia, W. B. Saunders Company, 1990, p. 263.

TABLE 18-10 TYPICAL DRUG REGIMEN FOR HEART TRANSPLANT PATIENT

MEDICATION	DOSAGE
Prednisone	0.2 mg/kg/day
Cyclosporine	4-6 mg/kg/day
Azathioprine	1-2 mg/kg/day
Enalapril	5-20 mg q P.M.
Furosemide	40 mg q.d., or b.i.d. with K^+
Aspirin (buffered or coated)	325 mg q.d.
Antacid	1 h p.c. and h.s.

Adapted from Achuff, A. C., and Augustine, S. M.: Outpatient management of the heart transplant patient. *In* Baumgartner, W. A., Reitz, B. A., and Achuff, S. A. (eds.): Heart and Heart-Lung Transplantation. Philadelphia, W. B. Saunders Company, 1990, p. 264.

to avoid errors of omission, dosage misunderstanding, or unexplained additions that might interfere with other drugs. A typical drug regimen for the long-term recipient is listed in Table 18-10.

SURVIVAL EXPECTATIONS

Long-term survival and complete rehabilitation can be attained by most patients currently undergoing heart transplantation. Several studies have attempted to define the rehabilitation potential of surviving patients. In a reported series of 56 patients at Stanford, 51 (91 per cent) were classified as successfully rehabilitated. However, only 26 out of 51 patients (46 per cent of the total) returned to full-time work.[112] This may reflect the attitude of employers or the planned early retirement of the surviving patient, rather than any physical limitation. In another study, 90 per cent of surviving patients were judged to be in a functional New York Heart Association Class 1.[113] In a study by Lough and associates, a measure of life satisfaction demonstrated that 89 per cent of recipients rated their quality of life as good to excellent.[114]

Simple survival statistics as reported by the International Society for Heart Transplantation indicate a 1-year actuarial survival of 83 per cent.[1] Individual programs may report survivals up to 90 per cent to 95 per cent at 1 year. The current data from the International Society are shown in Figure 18-6. Another actuarial curve recently reported[111] as contemporary results in cyclosporine-treated patients is shown in Figure 18-7. This latter figure compares patients treated with cyclosporine with the immediate preceding group of 100 patients in the precyclosporine era. Although survival is about 20 per cent better at each interval, the slopes of the curve are essentially identical out to 8 years, indicating that long-term morbidity and mortality are relatively constant and the advantages of cyclosporine-based protocols are primarily in the first 6 to 12 months after the transplantation. In this particular group of patients, those older than age 50 had a significantly lower survival than patients between 20 and 49 years of age.[111] This negative effect of age on survival has not been seen in other groups, as, for example, the Berlin Heart Transplant Group, although follow-up is shorter in this report.[27]

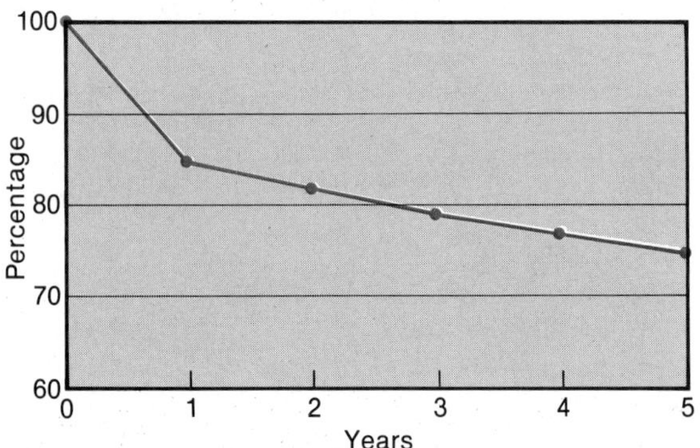

FIGURE 18-6. Heart transplant survival as reported to the Registry of the International Society for Heart Transplantation. (Adapted from Kriett, J. M., and Kaye, M. P.: The Registry of the International Society for Heart Transplantation: Seventh Official Report—1990. J. Heart Transplant. 9:323, 1990.) Triple Therapy refers to a combination of prednisone, cyclosporine, and azathioprine.

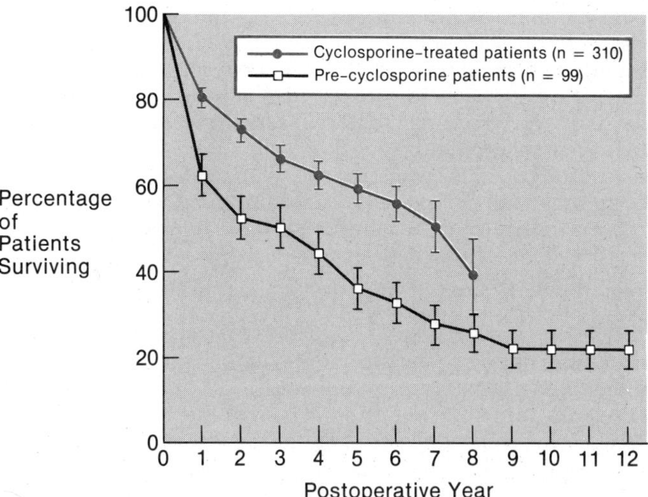

FIGURE 18-7. Patients treated with cyclosporine had a significantly higher survival rate than had patients not treated with cyclosporine ($p < .005$). Survival of patients treated with cyclosporine compared with patients receiving conventional immunosuppression before cyclosporine. (From Grattan, M. T., Moreno-Cabral, C. E., Starnes, V. A., et al.: Eight-year results of cyclosporine-treated patients with cardiac transplants. J. Thorac. Cardiovasc. Surg. 99:500, 1990.)

PHYSIOLOGY OF THE TRANSPLANTED HEART

The heart transplant remains largely[115] but not entirely[115a] denervated throughout the life of the recipient. A variety of studies document the response of the transplanted heart to exercise or stress, which is less than normal but adequate for almost all activities.[116-118] The heart rate accelerates slowly during the first stages of exercise, accompanied by an immediate increase in filling pressures as a result of augmented venous return from exercising muscles. The more gradual increase of heart rate with exercise parallels the rise in circulating catecholamines, which also leads to an increase in the inotropic state of the myocardium. With augmented venous return and higher filling pressures, the stroke volume increases, contributing to the necessary increase in cardiac output during exercise. Because of the dependence on circulating catecholamines, the exercise capacity and heart rate response of recipients are reduced by beta blockade.

Cardiac denervation results in an increase in beta-adrenergic receptor density.[119] In laboratory animals, denervation results in an increased sensitivity to noradrenaline and isoproterenol. This supersensitivity appears to be due both to up-regulation of beta receptors and to a loss of norepinephrine uptake in postganglionic sympathetic neurones. In a study by Borow and associates, the heart rate response to dobutamine was compared with that of normal subjects pretreated with atropine and found to be greater in the transplanted group.[120] In other studies, infusions of isoproterenol produced a greater increase in heart rate than in normal controls.[121] This slight supersensitivity of the chronically denervated heart may be important in maintaining the cardiac response to exercise and other stresses. All of the mechanisms underlying this supersensitivity have not been fully defined.

With respect to the coronary circulation, it has been shown that coronary vasodilator reserve of the transplanted heart is normal in the absence of rejection, hypertrophy, or regional wall motion abnormalities. During periods of acute rejection, coronary flow reserve is impaired. A recent study of coronary reactivity to ergonovine showed that 5 to 10 subjects responded with vasoconstriction.[122] Interestingly, four of these five patients subsequently developed angiographic evidence of coronary artery disease, whereas none of the five nonresponders developed coronary disease. The vasoconstrictor response may thus be a marker for development of endothelial damage and subsequent coronary atherosclerosis in the cardiac allograft.

HEART TRANSPLANTATION IN CHILDREN

Although the total number of heart transplant procedures has remained relatively constant since 1988, the number of children undergoing heart transplantation is increasing yearly. About 220 patients under the age of 18 years received a heart transplant in 1989, with 120 being less than 4 years of age. The most common indication for heart transplantation in children has been cardiomyopathy, although congenital heart disease is rapidly increasing as an indication. The largest segment of children with congenital defects are those with hypoplastic left heart syndrome. The use of heart transplantation for this group was pioneered by the work of Leonard Bailey, who initially began with a xenograft procedure using a donor baboon.[123] Human heart donors subsequently have been found to be available with reasonable frequency, and the number of procedures performed has gone up accordingly.[124] Although the longest surviving patient is just over 4 years, early results have been encouraging. A 1-year survival of about 85 per cent has been reported, with excellent early growth and development. There is some evidence that rejection complications are less frequent in children in whom transplant occurs before 1 month of age. After that time rejection is clearly common and appears to be no less than in adult patients. A major drawback to transplantation in children is the need for invasive endomyocardial biopsy to monitor the function of the transplanted heart. Because of these difficulties, Bailey and coworkers have advocated clinical signs together with echocardiography as a means of diagnosing and treating rejection episodes.

Rejection in neonatal patients may be associated with fever, fussiness, and difficulty feeding, together with thickening of the left ventricular free wall on echocardiogram and slight depression of function. There has not been a good study of concomitant endomyocardial biopsy and clinical events such as these to in fact prove the utility of this approach. The lack of careful monitoring and treatment of rejection may result in an increased incidence of graft coronary artery disease in these patients, but the frequency of this complication has yet to be determined in the neonatal transplants.

Various other indications have been treated, including severe Ebstein's anomaly, single ventricle, and tricuspid and pulmonary atresia with coronary artery sinusoids. Another use of cardiac transplantation in infants has been following palliative procedures for hypoplastic left heart syndrome, so-called bridging-to-transplantation procedures, such as the Norwood type I. Patients with hypoplastic left heart may develop cardiomyopathy or tricuspid valve insufficiency that makes them inappropriate candidates for the second-stage Fontan procedure. Cardiac transplantation has been successful in several patients with this indication.[125]

With continual improvements in immunosuppression, the consequence of long-term administration of these drugs may be lessened, and the need for retransplantation later in life also may be improved. These issues, together with limited donor resources, remain the major stumbling blocks to more widespread use of transplantation in infants and children.

RETRANSPLANTATION PROCEDURES

An important consideration in cardiac transplantation is the question of retransplantation. The major indications are (1) the development of graft coronary atherosclerosis, (2) treatment of severe acute early rejection, and (3) treatment of early acute right heart failure owing to an inadequate donor heart. All of these patient groups are less than optimum potential recipients than are primary transplant candidates, either because of chronic immunosuppression or the circumstances surrounding early graft failure. Fairly strict patient selection criteria should be followed to assure that the donor hearts are best utilized.

Patients should meet standard criteria as candidates. These include lack of evidence of systemic infection, no other major organ system failure which is thought to be irreversible, and the potential for adequate rehabilitation. Recipients should be screened for the presence of preexisting cytotoxic antibodies; if a sufficient percentage is determined against a panel of random donor cells, a specific crossmatch will be required for the retransplantation procedure.

A variety of reports have demonstrated that the survival of retransplant procedures is less than for primary procedures. Survival has been reported from between 0 per cent and 75 per cent, depending on the center, the number of patients treated, and the indication for retransplantation.[126,127] In the largest report, 41 patients underwent 44 retransplantations out of 487 total procedures at Stanford Medical Center. Thirteen patients were treated for early rejection and 31 patients for development of coronary artery disease. Causes of death were similar to those for other transplant recipients, and late survival was 11 patients, or 26 per cent.[128] A comparison of the actuarial survival of retransplant procedures reported to the Registry of the International Society for Heart Transplantation is shown in Figure 18–8. One-year survival in this group of 220 patients is 48 per cent, contrasted with 83 per cent at 1 year in primary procedures.

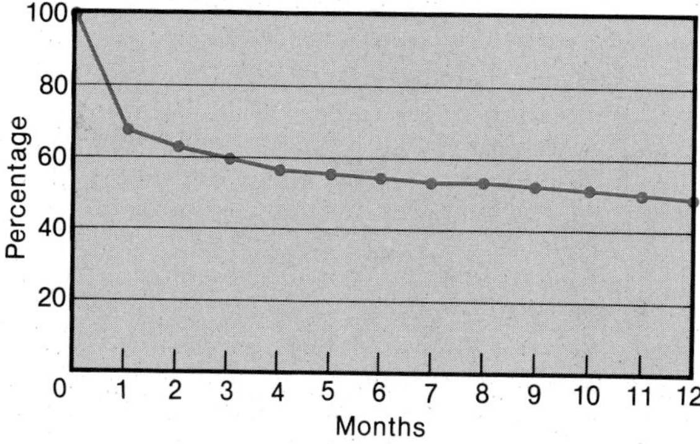

FIGURE 18–8. Actuarial survival of patients undergoing retransplantation as reported to the Registry for the International Society of Heart Transplantation (ISHT). (Reprinted by permission.)

HEART AND LUNG TRANSPLANTATION

The technical ease of transplanting the entire cardiopulmonary axis was accomplished experimentally even before orthotopic heart transplantation.[6,129] Despite early experimental attempts, it was a difficult clinical endeavor because of problems inherent with lung transplantation. The rather diffuse and nonspecific immunosuppression available before cyclosporine therapy led to major problems with pulmonary infections and delayed healing of the trachea or bronchus such that no truly therapeutic and extended lung transplant had been reported.[130] The availability of cyclosporine-based protocols led to success in primate allografts in the laboratory,[131] and then a clinical series initiated at Stanford Medical Center. The first patient in 1981 was the first reported therapeutic success in a lung transplantation.[22]

The indications for heart-lung transplantation initially were severe pulmonary vascular disease, either primary or secondary to congenital heart disease. Later, heart-lung transplantation was extended to patients with a variety of diffuse pulmonary diseases, such as emphysema, lymphangioleiomyomatosis, diffuse pulmonary arteriovenous fistulas, and cystic fibrosis.[132,133]

SINGLE LUNG TRANSPLANTATION

Based on work with cyclosporine-based immunosuppressive protocols, single lung transplantation has been reported for interstitial pulmonary fibrosis[134] and double lung transplantation for emphysema and cystic fibrosis, among other indications.[135] Lung transplantation currently is undergoing a widespread renaissance with ever-increasing survival expectations. A number of centers are offering lung transplant procedures, and the availability of organ donors also is improving with an increasing awareness of the value and success in lung transplantation.

Current data show that the most frequent indication for single lung transplantation is interstitial pulmonary fibrosis, with the second indication being emphysema. More diffuse pulmonary diseases are being treated by either bilateral single lung transplantation, en bloc double lung transplantation, or heart-lung transplantation in which the recipient's relatively normal heart is used as a donor for a second recipient (the "domino donor" procedure).[136,137]

INDICATIONS. Patient selection for lung transplantation follows the guidelines for heart transplants. Most patients over age 60 are excluded, as are patients who are ventilator-dependent or who have irreversible hepatic or renal disease, insulin-dependent diabetes, or a history of cancer or other systemic diseases that might limit rehabilitation. Chronic pulmonary disease is somewhat difficult to gauge for potential timing of transplantation, but patients who are severely oxygen-dependent and demonstrate a course of clinical deterioration should be considered. A good indication of disability suggesting need for transplant is a marked decrease in oxygen saturation with exercise.

THE DONOR LUNGS. Potential donors for lung transplant procedures must be infection-free, have good pulmonary gas exchange, lack a significant smoking history, and have a lung volume similar to or less than that of the intended recipient. Lung volumes can be judged by measurements on the chest x-ray or by the lung volume determined by standard tables of lung volumes based on weight and height, comparing them with ideal similar measurements of lung volume for the intended recipient. In bilateral lung transplants, the volume of donor lungs should be the same or less than that of the intended recipient, although larger lungs in single lung transplantation can be placed on the left side, where the diaphragm has the potential to descend because of the absence of the liver under the left hemidiaphragm. Infection remains a major consideration, since this is the greatest source of morbidity and mortality. The presence of CMV in the donor, when transplanted into a CMV recipient, has resulted in significant morbidity.[138–140] Other donor-transmitted pathogens are frequent as well.

PREVENTION OF REJECTION. Immunosuppression protocols are similar to those for cardiac transplantation, with the exception that prednisone often is omitted for the first several weeks. Induction therapy with polyclonal ATG preparations or monoclonal OKT3 prophylaxis is advocated by some groups to allow for a rejection-free interval without the use of steroids, which might delay bronchial healing. Ultimately, most patients are maintained on triple-drug therapy, which has been shown to correlate with better long-term survival and a reduced incidence of bronchiolitis obliterans.[141]

The diagnosis of rejection remains somewhat imprecise and based in large degree on clinical grounds. The use of fiberoptic bronchoscopy with transbronchial parenchymal lung biopsy has been most successful in following recipients.[142] Transbronchial biopsy usually can differentiate infection from rejection. It is performed in a prospective surveillance manner as well as for specific indications. When used for specific indications, it usually gives a higher percentage of positive results, which are about equally divided between the diagnosis of infection or rejection.[143,144] When cardiac biopsies and transbronchial biopsies are compared, pulmonary and cardiac rejection were present synchronously on 6 occasions and asynchronously on 16 occasions (9 pulmonary and 7 cardiac). Thus, cardiac biopsy alone is insufficient to follow the heart-lung transplant patient.

Early acute pulmonary rejection usually is manifested by an interstitial infiltrate, a decrease in lung volume and in pulmonary compliance, a low-grade fever, cough, and a feeling of breathlessness. These changes can all be rapidly reversed by using intravenous methylprednisolone, usually 1 gm IV daily for 3 days. It is not uncommon for recipients to undergo two or three rejection episodes in the first month after transplantation. Later, more chronic episodes of rejection may present without a pulmonary infiltrate on x-ray film, and long-term follow-up requires careful attention to pulmonary function testing. Patients will need a home spirometer to check for expiratory indices such as the forced expiratory volume at 1 second, which will show a decline as a consequence of chronic rejection. When suspected, these changes need to be followed up by transbronchial parenchymal biopsy or a therapeutic trial of immunosuppression, to preserve pulmonary function as much as possible.

OTHER COMPLICATIONS. Infection is an important complication of lung transplantation. Pulmonary infection is at least three times more frequent than in heart transplant recipients, and is the major cause of death in long-term surviving patients.[145] The transplanted lung may have deficiencies in lymphatic drainage, especially early after transplant, and ciliary function may be depressed. Patients frequently develop chronic bronchitis and may lack bronchus-associated lymphatic tissue as a result of chronic rejection.[146]

The late development of bronchiolitis obliterans limits the results in long-term surviving patients.[143,147] The incidence was reported as high as 50 per cent from the initial Stanford series, and is 20 per cent to 30 per cent in most recent reports. The causes are almost certainly immunologic; there is a demonstrated higher incidence in patients with a poor human leukocyte antigen match and in patients treated with a two-drug protocol as compared with a three-drug protocol. Bronchiolitis obliterans is partially reversed or arrested by an aggressive increase in immunosuppression. This complication has been reported to occur both after isolated single-lung and double-lung transplantation as well as after heart-lung transplantation.[148]

The therapeutic potential of lung transplant procedures is readily apparent. Patients are able to exercise without oxygen, to have a much greater feeling of well-being, and to resume active life styles. Late pulmonary function usually is quite satisfactory. Most reports show a progressive improvement in pulmonary function over time, and gas exchange and ventilation are essentially normal at 1 and 2 years.[149] Continuing improvement in immunosuppressive protocols will certainly lead to an even more reliable and safer long-term result in such patients.

REFERENCES

1. Kriett, J. M., and Kaye, M. P.: The Registry of the International Society for Heart Transplantation: Seventh Official Report—1990. J. Heart Transplant. *9*:323, 1990.
2. Baumgartner, W. A., Reitz, B. A., and Achuff, S. A.: Heart and Heart-Lung Transplantation. Philadelphia, W. B. Saunders Company, 1990.
3. Carrel, A., and Guthrie, C. C.: The transplantation of veins and organs. Am. J. Med. *10*:1101, 1905.
4. Carrel, A.: The surgery of blood vessels. Johns Hopkins Hosp. Bull. *18*:18, 1907.
5. Mann, F. C., Priestley, J. T., Markowitz, J., et al.: Transplantation of the intact mammalian heart. Arch. Surg. *26*:219, 1933.
6. Demikhov, V. P.: Experimental Transplantation of Vital Organs. New York, Consultants Bureau, 1962.
7. Neptune, W. B., Cookson, B. A., Bailey, C. P., et al.: Complete homologous heart transplantation. Arch. Surg. *66*:174, 1953.
8. Goldberg, M., Berman, E. F., and Akman, O. C.: Homologous transplantation of the canine heart. J. Int. Coll. Surg. *30*:575, 1958.
9. Cass, M. H., and Brock, R.: Heart excision and replacement. Guy's Hosp. Rep. *108*:285, 1958.
10. Lower, R. R., and Shumway, N. E.: Studies on the orthotopic homotransplantation of the canine heart. Surg. Forum *11*:18, 1960.
11. Lower, R. R., Dong, E., and Shumway N. E.: Long-term survival of cardiac homografts. Surgery *58*:110, 1965.
12. Lower, R. R., Dong, E., and Shumway N. E.: Suppression of rejection crises in the cardiac homograft. Ann. Thorac. Surg. *1*:645, 1965.
13. Barnard, C. N.: A human cardiac transplant: An interim report of a successful operation performed at Groote Shuur Hospital, Capetown. S. Afr. Med. J. *41*:1271, 1967.
14. Griepp, R. B., Stinson, E. B., Dong, E., et al.: Determinants of operative risk in human heart transplantation. Am. J. Surg. *122*:192, 1971.
15. Caves, P. K., Stinson, E. B., Billingham, M. E., et al.: Percutaneous endomyocardial biopsy in human heart recipients. Ann. Thorac. Surg. *16*:325, 1973.
16. Bieber C. P., Griepp, R. B., Oyer, P. E., et al.: Use of rabbit antithymocyte globulin in cardiac transplantation: Relationship of serum clearance rates in clinical outcomes. Transplantation *22*:478, 1976.
17. Baumgartner, W. A., Reitz, B. A., Oyer, P. E., et al.: Cardiac homotransplantation. Curr. Prob. Surg. *16*:24, 1979.
18. Kostakis, A. J., White, D.J.G., and Calne, R. Y.: Prolongation of the rat heart allograft survival by cyclosporine-A. IRCS Med. Sci. *5*:280, 1977.
19. Borel, J. F.: The history of cyclosporine-A and its significance. *In* White, D.J.G. (ed.): Cyclosporine-A: Proceedings of an International Conference on Cyclosporin-A. New York, Elsevier North-Holland, Inc., 1982.
20. Calne, R. Y., Rolles, K., White, D.J.G., et al.: Cyclosporin-A initially as the only immunosuppressant in 34 recipients of cadaveric organs: Thirty-two kidneys, two pancreases, two livers. Lancet *2*:1033, 1979.

21. Oyer, P. E., Stinson, E. B., Jamieson, S. W., et al.: Cyclosporine in cardiac transplantation: A two and a half year follow-up. Transplant. Proc. *15*:2546, 1983.
22. Reitz, B. A., Wallwork, J. L., Hunt, S. A., et al.: Heart-lung transplantation: Successful therapy for patients with pulmonary vascular disease. N. Engl. J. Med. *306*:557, 1982.
23. Annas, G. J.: Regulating the introduction of heart and liver transplantation. Am. J. Public Health *75*:93, 1985.
24. Medicare Program: Criteria for Medicare coverage of heart transplants. Fed. Reg. *52*:10935, 1987.
25. Miller, L. W., Vitale-Noedel, N., Pennington, D. G., et al.: Heart transplantation in patients over age 55 years. J. Heart Transplant. *7*:254, 1988.
26. Olivari, M. T., Antolick, A., Kaye, M. P., et al.: Heart transplantation in elderly patients. J. Heart Transplant. *7*:258, 1988.
27. Loebe, M., Schueler, S., Warnecke, H., et al.: The effect of older age on the outcome of heart transplantation. J. Heart Transplant. *8*:107, 1989.
28. Renlund, D. G., Gilbert, E. M., O'Connell, J. B., et al.: Age-associated decline in cardiac allograft rejection. Am. J. Med. *83*:391, 1987.
29. Murali, S., Uretsky, B. F., Reddy, P. S., et al.: The use of transpulmonary pressure gradient in the selection of cardiac transplantation candidates. J. Am. Coll. Cardiol. *11*:45, 1988.
30. Deeb, G. M., Bolling, S. F., Guynn, T. P., et al.: Amrinone versus conventional therapy in pulmonary hypertensive patients awaiting cardiac transplantation. Ann. Thorac. Surg. *48*:665, 1989.
31. Applefeld, M. M., Newman, K. A., Grove, W. R., et al.: Intermittent, continuous outpatient dobutamine infusion in the management of congestive heart failure. Am. J. Cardiol. *51*:455, 1983.
32. Bolling, S. F., Deeb, G. M., Crowley, D. C., et al.: Prolonged amrinone therapy prior to orthotopic cardiac transplantation in patients with pulmonary hypertension. Transplant. Proc. *20*:753, 1988.
33. Miller, C. A., Pae, W. E., and Pierce, W. S.: Combined registry for the clinical use of mechanical ventricular assist pumps and the total artificial heart in conjunction with heart transplantation; 4th official report —1989. J. Heart Transplant. *9*:453, 1990.
34. Shumway, S. J., and Bolman, R. M. III: Cardiac transplantation and ventricular assist devices. Curr. Opin. Cardiol. *6*:269, 1991.
35. Farrar, D. J., Hill, J. D., Gray, L. A., et al.: Heterotopic prosthetic ventricles as a bridge to cardiac transplantation: A multi-center study in 29 patients. N. Engl. J. Med. *318*:33, 1988.
36. Griffith, B. P., Kormos, R. L., Hardesty, R. L., et al.: The artificial heart: Infection-related morbidity and its effect on transplantation. Ann. Thorac. Surg. *45*:409, 1988.
37. Griepp, R. B., Stinson, E. B., Clark, D. A., et al.: The cardiac donor. Surg. Gynecol. Obstet. *133*:792, 1971.
38. Sweeney, M. S., Lammermeier, D. E., Frazier, O. H., et al.: Extension of donor criteria in cardiac transplantation: Surgical risk vs. supply-side economics. Ann. Thorac. Surg. *50*:7, 1990.
39. Schueler, S., Warnecke, H., and Loeb, E. M., et al.: Extended donor age in cardiac transplantation. Circulation *3*:133, 1989.
40. Robicsek, F. R.: On the table coronary arteriography in the evaluation of the cardiac transplant donor. J. Thorac. Cardiovasc. Surg. *(in press)*.
41. Cooper, D.K.C., Human, P. A., Rose, A. G., et al.: Can cardiac allografts and xenografts be transplanted against the ABO blood group barrier? Transplant. Proc. *21*:549, 1989.
42. Baumgartner, W. A.: Evaluation and management of the heart donor. *In* Baumgartner, W. A., Reitz, B. A., and Achuff, S. A. (eds.): Heart and Heart-Lung Transplantation. Philadelphia, W. B. Saunders Company, 1990, p. 86.
43. Kaye, M. P.: The Registry of the International Society for Heart Transplantation: Fourth Official Report—1987. J. Heart Transplant. *6*:63, 1987.
44. Yacoub, M., Mancad, P., and Ledingham, S.: Donor procurement and surgical techniques for cardiac transplantation. Semin. Thorac. Cardiovasc. Surg. *2*:153, 1990.
45. Wicomb, W. N., Cooper, D.K.C., Novitsky, D., et al.: Cardiac transplantation following storage of the donor heart by a portable hypothermic perfusion system. Ann. Thorac. Surg. *37*:243, 1984.
46. Baldwin, J. C., Frist, W. H., Starkey, T. D., et al.: Distant graft procurement for combined heart and lung transplantation using pulmonary artery flush and simple topical hypothermia for graft preservation. Ann. Thorac. Surg. *43*:670, 1987.
47. Wallwork, J., Jones, K., Cavarocchi, N., et al.: Distant procurement of organs for clinical heart-lung transplantation using a single flush technique. Transplantation *44*:654, 1987.
48. Hardesty, R. L., and Griffith, B. P.: Autoperfusion of the heart and lungs for preservation during distant procurement. J. Thorac. Cardiovasc. Surg. *93*:11, 1987.
49. Baumgartner, W. A., Williams, G. M., Fraser, C. D., et al.: Cardiopulmonary bypass with profound hypothermia: An optimal preservation method for multi-organ procurement. Transplantation *47*:123, 1989.
50. Bhatia, S. J. S., Kirshenbaum, J. M., Shemin, R. J., et al.: Time course of resolution of pulmonary hypertension and right ventricular remodelling after orthotopic cardiac transplantation. Circulation *76*:819, 1987.
51. Armitage, J. M., Hardesty, R. L., and Griffith, B. P.: Prostaglandin E_1: An effective treatment of right heart failure after orthotopic heart transplantation. J. Heart Transplant. *6*:348, 1987.
52. Fonger, J. D., Borkon, A. M., Baumgartner, W. A., et al.: Acute right ventricular failure following heart transplantation: Improvement with prostaglandin E_1 and right ventricular assist. J. Heart Transplant. 5:317, 1986.
53. McGriffin, D. C., and Carp, R. B.: Cardiac transplantation in a patient with a persistent left superior vena cava and an absent right superior vena cava. J. Heart Transplant. *3*:115, 1984.
54. Reitz, B. A., Jamieson, S. W., Gaudiani, V. A., et al.: Method for cardiac transplantation in corrected transposition of the great arteries. J. Cardiovasc. Surg. (Torino) *23*:293, 1982.
55. McGough, E. C., Brener, P. L., and Reemstma, K.: The parallel heart studies of intrathoracic auxiliary cardiac transplants. Surgery *60*:153, 1966.
56. Barnard, C. N., and Losman, J. G.: Left ventricular bypass. S. Afr. Med. J. *49*:303, 1985.
57. Renlund, D. G., O'Connell, J. B., and Bristow, M. R.: Early rejection prophylaxis in heart transplantation: Is cytolytic therapy necessary? J. Heart Transplant. *8*:191, 1989.
58. First, M. R., Schroeder, T. J., Hurtubise, P. E., et al.: Successful retreatment of allograft rejection with OKT3. J. Transplant. *47*:88, 1989.
59. Reichenspurner, H., Ertel, W., Hammer, C., et al.: Immunologic monitoring of heart transplant patients under cyclosporine immunosuppression. Transplant. Proc. *16*:1251, 1984.
60. Dubroff, J. M., Clark M. B., Wong, C. Y. H., et al.: Changes in left ventricular mass associated with the onset of acute rejection after cardiac transplantation. J. Heart Transplant. *3*:105, 1984.
61. Haberl, R., Weber, M., Reichenspurner, H., et al.: Frequency analysis of the surface electrocardiogram for recognition of acute rejection after orthotopic cardiac transplantation in man. Circulation *76*:101, 1987.
62. Fraser, C. D., Jr., Chacko, V. P., Jacobus, W. E., et al.: Evidence of 31p nuclear magnetic resonance studies of cardiac allografts that early rejection is characterized by reversible biochemical changes. Transplantation *48*:1068, 1989.
63. Griepp, R. B., Stinson, E. B., Dong, E., Jr., et al.: Acute rejection of the allografted human heart: Diagnosis and treatment. Ann. Thorac. Surg. *12*:1113, 1971.
64. Dawkins, K. D., Oldershaw, P. J., Billingham, M. E., et al.: Changes in diastolic function as a noninvasive marker of cardiac allograft rejection. J. Heart Transplant. *3*:286, 1984.
65. Golitsin, A., Pinedo, J. I., Cienfuegos, J. A., et al.: Thallium-201 uptake: A useful method for assessing heart transplantation. Transplant. Proc. *16*:1262, 1984.
66. McKillop, J. H., McDougall, I. R., Goris, M. L., et al.: Failure to diagnose cardiac transplant rejection with Tc-99m-pyp images. Clin. Nucl. Med. *6*:375, 1981.
67. Schutz, A., Fritsch, S., Weiler, A., et al.: Antimyosin monoclonal antibodies for early detection of mild cardiac rejection. J. Heart Transplant. *8*:88, 1989.
68. Foegh, M. L., Khirabadi, B. S., Shapiro, R., et al.: Monitoring of rat heart allograft rejection by urinary thromboxane. Transplant. Proc. *16*:1606, 1984.
69. Carrier, M., Russell, D. H., Davis, T. P., et al.: Value of urinary polyamines as non-invasive markers of cardiac allograft rejection in the dog. Ann. Thorac. Surg. *45*:158, 1988.
70. Womble, J. R., Larson, D. F., Copeland J. G., et al.: Urinary polyamine levels are markers of altered T lymphocyte proliferation/loss and rejection in heart transplant patients. Transplant. Proc. *16*:1573, 1984.
71. O'Toole, C. M., Maher, P., Spiegelhalter, D., et al.: "Rejection or Infection" predictive value of T-cell subject ratio before and after heart transplantation. Heart Transplant. 4:518, 1985.
72. Caves, P. K., Billingham, M. E., Schulz, W. P., et al.: Transvenous biopsy from canine orthotopic heart allografts. Am. Heart J. *85*:525, 1973.
73. Billingham, M. E.: The pathology of transplanted hearts. Sem. Thorac. Cardiovasc. Surg. *2*:233, 1990.
74. Hutchins, G. M.: The pathology of heart transplantation. *In* Baumgartner, W. A., Reitz, B. A., and Achuff, S. A. (eds.): Heart and Heart-Lung Transplantation. Philadelphia, W. B. Saunders Company, 1990, p. 183.
75. Michler, R. E., Smith, C. R., Drusin, R. E., et al.: Reversal of cardiac transplant rejection without massive immunosuppression. Circulation *74*:III-68, 1986.
76. Gilbert, E. M., DeWitt, C. W., Eiswirth, C. C., et al.: Treatment of refractory cardiac allograft rejection with OKT3 monoclonal antibody. Am. J. Med. *82*:202, 1987.
77. O'Connell, J. B., Renlund, D. G., Gay, W. A., Jr., et al.: Efficacy of OKT3 retreatment for refractory cardiac allograft rejection. Transplantation *47*:788, 1989.
78. Kobashigawa, J., Stevenson, L. W., Moriguchi, J., et al.: Randomized study of high dose oral cyclosporine therapy for mild acute cardiac rejection. J. Heart Transplant. *8*:53, 1989.
79. Olsen, S. L., O'Connell, J. B., Bristow, M. R., et al.: Methotrexate in the treatment of persistent cardiac allograft rejection. J. Heart Transplant. *8*(abstr.):96, 1989.
80. Hunt, S., Strober, S., Hoppe, R., et al.: Use of total lymphoid irradiation for therapy of intractable cardiac allograft rejection. J. Heart Transplant. *8*(abstr.):104, 1989.
81. Todo, S., Fung, J. J., Demetris, A. J., et al.: Early trials with FK 506 as primary treatment in liver transplantation. Transplant. Proc. *22*:13, 1990.
82. Armitage, J., Fung, J., Kormos, R., et al.: Preliminary experience with FK506 in thoracic transplantation. Transplant. Proc. *(in press)*.
83. Horn, J. E., and Bartlett, J. G.: Infectious complications following heart transplantation. *In* Baumgartner, W. A., Reitz, B. A., and Achuff, S. A. (eds.): Heart and Heart-Lung Transplantation. Philadelphia, W. B. Saunders Company, 1990, p. 220.
84. Dummer, J. S., Gardy, A., Poorsattar, A., et al.: Early infections in kidney, heart and liver transplant recipients on cyclosporine. Transplantation *36*:259, 1983.

85. Onorato, I. M., Morens, D. M., Martone, W. J., et al.: Epidemiology of cytomegaloviral infections: Recommendations for prevention and control. Rev. Infect. Dis. *7*:479, 1985.
86. Penn, I., and Brunson, M. E.: Cancers after cyclosporine therapy. Transplant. Proc. *20*:85, 1988.
87. Myers, B. D., Ross, J., Newton, L., et al.: Cyclosporine-associated chronic nephropathy. N. Engl. J. Med. *311*:699, 1984.
88. McGiffin, D. C., Kirklin, J. K., and Naftel, D. C.: Acute renal failure after heart transplantation and cyclosporine therapy. J. Heart Transplant. *4*:396, 1985.
89. Renlund, D. G., O'Connell, J. B., Gilbert, E. M., et al.: A prospective comparison of murine monoclonal CD-3 antibody-based and equine antithymocyte globulin-based rejection prophylaxis in cardiac transplantation: Decreased rejection and less corticosteroid use with OKT3. Transplantation *47*:599, 1989.
90. Copeland, J. G., Emery, R. W., Levinson, M. M., et al.: Cyclosporine: An immunosuppressive panacea? J. Thorac. Cardiovasc. Surg. *91*:26, 1986.
91. Slavin, J., and Taylor, J.: Cyclosporine, nifedipine, and gingival hyperplasia. Lancet *2*:739, 1987.
92. Hanto, D. W., Frizzera, G., Gajl-Peczalska, K. J., et al.: Epstein-Barr virus, immunodeficiency, and B-cell lymphoproliferation. Transplantation *39*:461, 1985.
93. Hanto, D. W., Frizzera, G., Gajl-Peczalska, K. J., et al.: Epstein-Barr virus–induced B-cell lymphoma after renal transplantation: A cyclovir therapy and transition from polyclonal to monoclonal B-cell proliferation. N. Engl. J. Med. *306*:913, 1982.
94. Thomson, J. G.: Production of severe atheroma in a transplanted human heart. Lancet *2*:1088, 1969.
95. Beiber, C. P., Stinson, E. B., Payne, R., et al.: Cardiac transplantation in man. VII. Cardiac allograft pathology. Circulation *41*:753, 1970.
96. Beiber, C. P., Hunt, S. A., Schwinn, D. A., et al.: Complications in long-term survivors of cardiac transplantation. Transplant. Proc. *13*:207, 1981.
97. Billingham, M. E.: Cardiac transplant atherosclerosis. Transplant. Proc. *19* (Suppl. 5):19, 1987.
98. Hess, M. L., Hastillo, A., Thompson, J. A., et al.: Lipid mediators in organ transplantation: Does cyclosporine accelerate coronary atherosclerosis? Transplant. Proc. *19* (Suppl. 5):71, 1987.
99. Uretsky, B. F., Murali, S., Reedy, S., et al.: Development of coronary artery disease in cardiac transplant patients receiving immunosuppressive therapy with cyclosporine and prednisone. Circulation *76*:827, 1987.
100. Nitkin, R. S., and Schroeder, J. S.: Accelerated coronary artery disease risk in heart transplant patients. J. Am. Coll. Cardiol. *5* (Suppl. II):535, 1985.
100a. Johnson, D. E., Alderman, E. L., Schroeder, J. S., et al.: Transplant coronary artery disease: Histopathologic correlations with angiographic morphology. J. Am. Coll. Cardiol. *17*:449, 1991.
101. Grattan, M. T., Moreno-Cabral, C. E., Starnes, V. A., et al.: Eight-year results of cyclosporine-treated patients with cardiac transplants. J. Thorac. Cardiovasc. Surg. *99*:500, 1990.
102. Gao, S., Hunt, S. A., and Schroeder, J. S.: Accelerated transplant coronary artery disease. Semin. Thorac. Cardiovasc. Surg. *2*:241, 1990.
103. Melnick, J. L., Adam, E., and DeBakey, M. E.: Possible role of cytomegalovirus in atherogenesis. J.A.M.A. *263*:2204, 1990.
104. Grattan, M. T., Moreno-Cabral, C. E., Starnes, V. A., et al.: Cytomegalovirus infection is associated with cardiac allograft rejection and atherosclerosis. J.A.M.A. *261*:3561, 1989.
105. Cameron, D. E., Greene, P. S., Alejo, D., et al.: Postoperative cytomegalovirus (CMV) infection and older donor age predispose to coronary atherosclerosis after heart transplantation. Circulation *(in press)*.
106. Butman, S. M.: Hyperlipidemia after cardiac transplantation: Be aware and possibly wary of drug therapy for lowering of serum lipids. Am. Heart J. *121*:1585, 1991.
107. Gao, S. Z., Schroeder, J. S., Hunt, S. A., et al.: Myocardial infarction in cardiac transplant recipients: A clinicopathologic correlation. Am. J. Cardiol. *64*:1093, 1989.
108. Banner, N. R., and Yacoub, M. H.: Physiology of the orthotopic cardiac transplant recipient. Semin. Thorac. Cardiovasc. Surg. *2*:259, 1990.
109. Vetrovec, G. W., Cowley, M. J., Newton, C. M., et al.: Applications of percutaneous transluminal coronary angioplasty in cardiac transplantation: Preliminary results in 5 patients. Circulation *78*:III83, 1988.
110. Copeland, J. G., Butman, S. M., and Cethi, G.: Successful coronary artery bypass grafting for high-risk left main coronary artery atherosclerosis after cardiac transplantation. Ann. Thorac. Surg. *49*:106, 1990.
111. Dein, J. R., Oyer, P. E., Stinson, E. B., et al.: Cardiac retransplantation in the cyclosporine era. Ann. Thorac. Surg. *48*:350, 1989.
112. Christopherson, L. K., Griepp, R. B., and Stinson, E. B.: Rehabilitation after heart transplantation. J.A.M.A. *236*:2082, 1976.
113. Hunt, S. A., Rider, A. K., Stinson, E. B., et al.: Does cardiac transplantation prolong life and improve its quality? Cardiovasc. Surg. *54*:56, 1975.
114. Lough, M. E., Lindsey, A. M., Shinn, J. A., et al.: Life satisfaction following heart transplantation. J. Heart Transplant. *4*:446, 1985.
115. Mason, J. W., and Harrison, D. C.: Electrophysiology and electropharmacology of the transplanted human heart. *In* Narula, O. S. (ed.): Cardiac Arrhythmias: Electrophysiology, Diagnosis, Management. Baltimore, Williams and Wilkins, 1979, p. 66.
115a. Wilson, R. F., Christensen, B. V., Olivari, M. T., et al.: Evidence for structural sympathetic reinnervation after orthotopic cardiac transplantation in humans. Circulation *83*:1210, 1991.
116. Banner, N. R., Lloyd, M. H., Hamilton, R. D., et al.: Cardiopulmonary response to dynamic exercise after heart and combined heart-lung transplantation. Br. Heart J. *61*:215, 1989.
117. Kavanagh, T., Yacoub, M. H., Mertens, D. J., et al.: Cardiorespiratory responses to exercise training after orthotopic cardiac transplantation. Circulation *77*:162, 1988.
118. von Scheidt, W., Neudert, J., Erdmann, E., et al.: Contractility of the transplanted, denervated human heart. Am. Heart J. *121*:1480, 1991.
119. Naurie, K. G., Bristow, M. R., and Reitz, B. A.: Increased beta adrenergic receptor density in an experimental model of cardiac transplantation. J. Thorac. Cardiovasc. Surg. *86*:195, 1983.
120. Borow, K. M., Neumann, A. A., Arensman, F. W., et al.: Cardiac and peripheral vascular responses to adrenoceptor stimulation and blockage after cardiac transplantation. J. Am. Coll. Cardiol. *14*:1229, 1989.
121. Yusuf, S., Theodoropoulos, S., Mathias, C. J., et al.: Increased sensitivity of the denervated transplanted human heart to isoprenaline both before and after beta-adrenergic blockade. Circulation *75*:696, 1987.
122. Cushwaha, S., Lythall, D. L., Maseri, A., et al.: Coronary reactivity to ergonovine—possible relationship to accelerated coronary sclerosis in cardiac transplant recipients. *(Submitted)*
123. Bailey, L. L., Nehlsen-Cannarella, S. L., Concepcion, W., et al.: Baboon to human cardiac xenotransplantation in a neonate. J.A.M.A. *254*:3321, 1985.
124. Boucek, M. M., Kanakriyeh, M. S., Mathis, C. M., et al.: Cardiac transplantation in infancy: Donors and recipients. J. Pediatr. *116*:171, 1990.
125. Cameron, D. E., and Gardner, T. J.: Heart transplantation in children. *In* Baumgartner, W. A., Reitz, B. A. and Achuff, S. A. (eds.): Heart and Heart-Lung Transplantation. Philadelphia, W. B. Saunders Company, 1990, p. 293.
126. Watson, D. C., Reitz, B. A., Oyer, P. E., et al.: Sequential orthotopic heart transplantation in man. Transplantation *30*:401, 1980.
127. Novitsky, D., Cooper, D. K. C., Brink, J. G., et al.: Sequential second and third transplants in patients with heterotopic heart allografts. Clin. Transplant. *1*:57, 1987.
128. Baumgartner, W. A.: Retransplantation of the heart. *In* Baumgartner, W. A., Reitz B. A., and Achuff, S. A. (eds.): Heart and Heart-Lung Transplantation. Philadelphia, W. B. Saunders Company, 1990, p. 282.
129. Neptune, W. B., Cookson, B. A., Bailey, C. P., et al.: Complete homologous heart transplantation. Arch. Surg. *66*:174, 1953.
130. Veith, F. J.: Lung transplantation. Surg. Clin. North Am. *58*:357, 1978.
131. Reitz, B. A., Burton, N. A., Jamieson, S. W., et al.: Heart and lung transplantation, autotransplantation, and allotransplantation in primates with extended survival. J. Thorac. Cardiovasc. Surg. *80*:360, 1980.
132. Wellens, F., Estenne, M., deFrancquen, P., et al.: Combined heart-lung transplantation for terminal pulmonary lymphangioleiomyomatosis. J. Thorac. Cardiovasc. Surg. *89*:872, 1985.
133. Jones, D. K., Higgenbottam, T. W., and Wallwork, J.: Long-term survival after heart-lung transplantation in cystic fibrosis. Chest *93*:644, 1988.
134. Toronto Lung Transplant Group: Experience with single lung transplantation for pulmonary fibrosis. J.A.M.A. *259*:2258, 1988.
135. Cooper, J. D., Patterson, G. A., Grosman, R., et al.: Double lung transplant for advanced chronic obstructive lung disease. Am. Rev. Respir. Dis. *139*:303, 1989.
136. Baumgartner, W. A., Traill, T. A., Cameron, D. E., et al.: Unique aspects of heart and lung transplantation exhibited in the "domino-donor" operation. J.A.M.A. *261*:3121, 1989.
137. Yacoub, M. H., Banner, N. R., Khaghani, A., et al.: Heart-lung transplantation for cystic fibrosis and subsequent domino heart transplantation. J. Heart Transplant. *9*:459, 1990.
138. Burke, C. M., Glanville, A. R., Macoviak, J. A., et al.: The spectrum of cytomegalovirus infection following human heart-lung transplantation. J. Heart Transplant. *5*:267, 1986.
139. Dummer, J. S., White, L. T., Monto, H. O., et al.: Morbidity of cytomegalovirus infection in recipients of heart or heart-lung transplants who received cyclosporine. J. Infect. Dis. *152*:1182, 1985.
140. Hutter, J. A., Scott, J. P., Wreghitt, T., et al.: The importance of cytomegalovirus in heart-lung transplantation. Chest. *95*:627, 1989.
141. McCarthy, P. M., Starnes, V. A., Theodore, J., et al.: Improved survival after heart-lung transplantation. J. Thorac. Cardiovasc. Surg. *99*:54, 1990.
142. Higgenbottam, T., Stewart, S., Penketh, A., et al.: Transbronchial lung biopsy for the diagnosis of rejection in heart-lung transplant patients. Transplantation *46*:532, 1988.
143. Starnes, V. A., Theodore, J., Oyer, P. E., et al.: Pulmonary infiltrates after heart-lung transplantation: Evaluation by serial transbronchial biopsies. J. Thorac. Cardiovasc. Surg. *98*:945, 1989.
144. Starnes, V. A., Theodore, J., Oyer, P. E., et al.: Evaluation of heart-lung transplant recipients with prospective, serial, transbronchial biopsies in pulmonary function studies. J. Thorac. Cardiosvasc. Surg. *98*:683, 1989.
145. Dummer, J. S., Montero, C. G., Grifith, B. P., et al.: Infections in heart-lung recipients. Transplantation *41*:725, 1986.
146. Ren, H., Hruban, R. H., Baumgartner, W. A., et al.: Hemorrhagic infarction of hilar lymph nodes associated with combined heart-lung transplantation. J. Thorac. Cardiovasc. Surg. *99*:861, 1990.
147. Allen, M. D., Burke, C. M., McGregor, C.G.A., et al.: Steroid-responsive bronchiolitis after human heart-lung transplantation. J. Thorac. Cardiovasc. Surg. *92*:449, 1986.
148. LoCicero, J., Robinson, P. G., and Fisher, M.: Chronic rejection in single lung transplantation manifested by obliterative bronchiolitis. J. Thorac. Cardiovasc. Surg. *99*:1059, 1990.
149. Theodore, J., Morris, A. J., Burke, C. M., et al.: Cardiopulmonary function at maximum tolerable constant work rate exercise following human heart-lung transplantation. Chest *92*:433, 1987.

19

Assisted Circulation and Mechanical Hearts

by D. GLENN PENNINGTON, M.D., and MARC T. SWARTZ

HISTORY

Researchers and clinicians have long sought a reliable method to mechanically support the circulation. Initial efforts were centered on the development of devices that would temporarily support the circulation during intracardiac repair. This early work resulted in the first successful clinical use of cardiopulmonary bypass by Gibbon in 1952.[1] The system could temporarily support part of or the entire circulation during cardiac operations. Within a few years, cardiopulmonary bypass was used as a temporary device in a variety of clinical situations which were associated with severe cardiopulmonary decompensation. For example, cardiopulmonary bypass was used by Cooley and coworkers to treat patients with massive pulmonary embolus,[2] and by Stuckey and associates to treat several patients in acute myocardial infarction shock.[3]

It was soon apparent that a temporary mechanical circulatory assist device was needed to support patients long enough to allow myocardial recovery. The temporary use of cardiopulmonary bypass required total heparinization and, in the early days, an operating room environment. This method was thought to be ineffective, since cardiac decompression could not be accomplished by closed-chest cannulation techniques. Additionally, most patients in cardiogenic shock did not require pulmonary support with an in-line oxygenator. For this reason, cardiopulmonary bypass was essentially abandoned as a mechanism to treat cardiogenic shock. Investigators began to develop methods of isolated ventricular support. Dennis and colleagues introduced a method of left heart bypass in 1962,[4] a concept that was later modified and used successfully by DeBakey, who implanted a left atrial-aortic bypass pump in patients who could not be weaned from cardiopulmonary bypass.[5]

In the early 1960's, the theory of counterpulsation was introduced. An early method of counterpulsation called for withdrawal of arterial blood from the patient during systole and rapid reinfusion during diastole,[6] resulting in systolic unloading and diastolic augmentation. The system was composed of an external pumping chamber and a reservoir. This concept eventually led to the work by Moloupolous, who introduced counterpulsation by means of an intraaortic balloon (IAB).[7] Kantrowitz and coworkers reported the first successful clinical application of IAB counterpulsation in 1968.[8] Other methods of mechanical circulatory support, such as external counterpulsation, also were investigated with limited clinical success, and were soon abandoned.[9]

During the 1950's, work was begun in several laboratories to develop an artificial heart. During the 1960's, the National Heart, Lung and Blood Institute (NHLBI) began a formal program for the development of mechanical circulatory support. In July 1964, the first congressionally approved allocation for support of artificial heart research was made. The initial NHLBI plan for the artificial heart program was to develop a family of devices for emergency use—devices for temporary support until the heart recovered, for short- and long-term ventricular assistance (VADs), and for cardiac replacement devices.[10]

During the 1970's, more sophisticated and innovative devices were developed that were capable of providing assistance to a failing ventricle for a longer period of time with less damage to blood components.[11-14] These systems included external and internal pneumatic VADs. During this period, the IAB pump remained the primary method of mechanical circulatory support, and VADs were used only if balloon pumping failed.[15,16] During the 1980's, technological developments as well as improvements in clinical management were made. Pneumatic total artificial hearts, electrical left VADs, percutaneous cardiopulmonary bypass, and other innovative devices such as the Hemopump found their way to the clinical arena.[17-20]

Improved technology and clinical results have led to a widespread growth of mechanical circulatory support. Survival rates have increased and morbidity rates are on the decline. Several patients have been supported for longer than 1 year with different devices, and successful perfusions of longer than 1 month are now commonplace. The indications for mechanical circulatory support are varied, and various devices are now available either commercially or with special exemption from the Food and Drug Administration (FDA) for investigational use. Some devices have been designed for particular circumstances, whereas others are capable of multiple applications.

RATIONALE FOR CIRCULATORY SUPPORT

The consequences of cardiac failure occur because, despite adequate loading, the heart cannot pump enough blood to supply the metabolic needs of the body. In severe cardiac failure, the heart shows little or no response to the Frank-Starling mechanism, so that cardiac output cannot be increased by volume loading (Chap. 14). The two primary goals of mechanical circulatory support are to decrease cardiac work and to restore adequate perfusion of vital organs. If successful, mechanical support may decrease myocardial oxygen consumption, increase systemic and coronary perfusion, and allow the ventricles to function under more physiologic conditions. Of the two primary benefits, the authors believe that the more crucial is the restoration of adequate perfusion. Total systemic blood flow (pump output plus natural heart output) must be sufficient to provide rapid reversal of systemic acidosis, hypoxia, vasoconstriction, hypotension, and poor peripheral perfusion, as well as to reduce the possibility of major organ dysfunction.

Reversal of major organ dysfunction will be partially determined by whether the low cardiac output state is acute or chronic. The restoration of normal perfusion can almost immediately correct such conditions in patients with acute cardiogenic shock, whereas patients who have suffered from a chronic low cardiac output state may require several weeks of normal perfusion before the function of vital organs returns to normal. Cardiogenic shock (pp. 576 and 1251) affects virtually every organ system negatively and progressively. Prolonged mechanical circulatory support is a substantial undertaking, because most defense mechanisms have been activated, and insertion of a mechanical assist device may activate additional mechanisms. Often a large physiological deficit must be corrected in addition to providing adequate circulation. Once adequate perfusion is restored, the progressive deterioration of vital organ function usually ceases, and organs that have not suffered irreversible damage recover. Most of the currently used devices provide flows in excess of 2 liters/m²/min, and thereby completely support a resting patient's circulation. If mechanical circulatory support is initiated early, ischemic damage to major organs should be reversible.

REVERSAL OF CARDIAC DAMAGE. The question of whether cardiac damage can be reversed by circulatory support is problematic. Circulatory support may be carried out in patients in whom cardiac recovery is not expected. For example, patients with severe cardiac damage and longstanding cardiac failure may be supported before heart transplantation. It is hoped that the future will provide the opportunity to replace such damaged hearts with mechanical artificial hearts as well. In some patients, reversal of cardiac dysfunction and cardiac injury may be a realistic goal. Unfortunately, in the clinical setting, at the time when the decision must be made to place an assist device, the determination of whether cardiac injury is reversible often is difficult or impossible.

Indeed, the specific factors responsible for the recovery from cardiac injury are not well understood. It is thought that the duration and severity of myocardial ischemia determine the extent of myocardial recovery and the rate at which recovery will occur. Apparently, recovery takes place in two stages. Initially, there is rapid functional recovery of cells in marginally ischemic areas. Next, there is a slower process of hypertrophy of normal and recovering myofibrils.[21] The healing process of necrotic myocardium is slow, and little healing occurs during brief periods of circulatory support, since irreversibly damaged necrotic myocardium benefits little, if any, from improved perfusion. Recovery, therefore, involves resolving interstitial or intercellular myocardial edema in areas of viable myocardium or halting the extension of necrosis into reversibly ischemic areas.

Cardiac failure often is a result of depressed myocardial contractility and/or decreased myocardial compliance. The presence of ischemia or edema may aggravate either type of impairment. The period for recovery of myocardial contractility after temporary ischemia is short, usually 3 to 7 days.[22] Previous studies indicate that after uncomplicated coronary artery bypass grafting, left ventricular function is depressed and shows spontaneous improvement within 3 days.[23] Clinical data from the use of circulatory support devices in postcardiotomy patients suggest that myocardial recovery occurs within 1 week and that if it has not occurred within 2 weeks, myocardial recovery is unlikely.[24] Patterns of recovery and the question of whether longer circulatory support perfusion will enhance recovery have not been fully determined.[25]

Recent studies of a series of postcardiotomy patients treated with circulatory support devices at St. Louis University suggest that myocardial recovery is much more likely in patients with a "stunned" (p. 1329) rather than an acutely infarcted myocardium. When 12 survivors were compared with 34 nonsurvivors, it was apparent that only one of the survivors had suffered a perioperative infarction, whereas among nonsurvivors the instance of perioperative infarction was 70 per cent. Examination of the infarcts at autopsy in the nonsurvivors demonstrated that most of them had biventricular infarctions, that is, infarctions of the left and right ventricles or infarctions of the left ventricle and the interventricular septum. From these data, it became apparent that a clinically significant perioperative infarction with biventricular failure had a strong negative impact on survival.[26] Unfortunately, the diagnosis of perioperative infarction could not be made in the operating room unless it had been detected before operation. Therefore, the criteria used to decide whether patients have suffered reversible or irreversible injury often are subjective, and the estimation of the extent of likely ventricular recovery often cannot be determined at the time of placement of the device.

EFFECTS ON MYOCARDIAL METABOLISM AND HEMODYNAMICS. Mechanical circulatory support is known to benefit myocardial metabolism. Diastolic augmentation with an infraaortic balloon (IAB) reduces myocardial oxygen demand by decreasing afterload and increases myocardial oxygen supply by improving coronary diastolic flow. These changes usually result in an increase in cardiac output.[27] The ability of IAB counterpulsation to aid in the recovery of ischemic myocardium after myocardial infarction or cardiac surgery is well known. VADs provide an even greater degree of support, since they provide more ventricular decompression.[28-30] Myocardial recovery frequently has occurred in postcardiotomy patients supported with VADs after failure to improve with IAB and inotropic drugs.[31,32] Animal investigations have shown that left ventricular bypass reduces myocardial oxygen consumption in the nonischemic heart[33,34] and has a beneficial effect on myocardial ischemia and evolving infarction.[35] The degree of left ventricular decompression correlates well with the decrease in myocardial oxygen consumption.[34]

Circulatory support devices also have the capability of dramatically affecting cardiac hemodynamics, particularly in terms of preload and afterload. The effects of devices operating in a nonsynchronized mode on left and right ventricular loading conditions are outlined in Table 19–1. Venoarterial bypass systems and VADs compete with the natural heart for volume, resulting in a substantial decrease in preload of the assisted ventricle. The type of device used, method of cannulation, and mode of operation all affect natural heart preload and afterload. In addition, the decrease in preload is partially dependent on the degree of unloading desired, and this can be regulated, depending on the patient's clinical condition. Heterotopic assist devices decrease preload of the assisted ventricle but may increase preload to the opposite ventricle. Biventricular assist devices can simultaneously increase and decrease ventricular preload. Most assist devices can maintain device flows at 2.5 liters/m²/min or greater with atrial pressures in the range of 10 to 15 mm Hg. Myocardial recovery is enhanced while pulmonary and hepatic congestion are diminished by these devices' ability to decrease and maintain preload while providing adequate perfusion.

However, many circulatory support devices increase the afterload of the supported ventricle. This has been shown clinically[36] and experimentally[37] with extracorporeal membrane oxygenators (ECMOs) and clinically with the Pierce-Donachy VAD, using atrial cannulation.[38] In the latter studies, aortic and/or pulmonary artery pressures were consistently higher when the device was activated. Nuclear multigated

TABLE 19–1 EFFECTS OF NONSYNCHRONIZED MECHANICAL CIRCULATORY ASSIST DEVICES ON CARDIAC PHYSIOLOGY*

	LEFT VENTRICLE		RIGHT VENTRICLE	
	Preload	**Afterload**	**Preload**	**Afterload**
LVAD	↓	↑	↑	↓
RVAD	↑	—	↓	↑
BVAD	⇃↾	↑	⇅	⇅
ECMO	↓	↑	↓	↓

LVAD, left ventricular assist device; RVAD, right ventricular assist device; BVAD, biventricular assist device; ECMO, extracorporeal membrane oxygenation.

* Normal pulmonary vascular resistance.

acquisition studies documented a lower left ventricular ejection fraction when the device was active as compared with when the device was inactive. This effect coincided with a decrease in diastolic volume and left atrial pressure, resulting in a reduction in preload and a simultaneous increase in afterload. These data demonstrate that atrial cannulation techniques used in conjunction with asynchronous pumping do not effectively decompress the ventricle and that the ventricle may actually be subjected to increased afterload. Despite these apparently adverse effects, the survival rate in patients supported with such techniques is significant. Historically, it was believed that ventricular recovery would occur more rapidly if the ventricle was decompressed, but clinically, the degree of decompression has not correlated with survival.

CRITERIA FOR PATIENT SELECTION

During the 1980's, three major categories of patients evolved as the most likely to require circulatory support. These are patients with cardiogenic shock owing to postcardiotomy heart failure, patients who develop cardiogenic shock while awaiting cardiac transplantation (bridge-to-transplant group; Chap. 18), or patients with cardiogenic shock after acute myocardial deterioration, with or without infarction. There is considerable overlap between these three groups, particularly between the bridge-to-transplant group and the acute deterioration group. However, the hemodynamic criteria for patient selection can be applied generically and are useful in all three categories. The hemodynamic protocols for patient selection are based on the work of Norman and associates, who described hemodynamic criteria for postcardiotomy patients with cardiogenic shock unresponsive to drug therapy and IABs.[16] These criteria are outlined in Table 19–2 and were reasonably well tested during the 1980's. In addition to the hemodynamic criteria, it is assumed in these guidelines that optimal pharmacological support is being supplied, and that blood gas abnormalities, hypovolemia, cardiac arrhythmias, and hypothermia all have been corrected. Although the hemodynamic criteria are extremely useful, it is now apparent that some patients may be better served by the insertion of assist devices before they reach all of the limits described by these criteria. It also is important to note how long patients must be maintained in a borderline state and the regimen necessary to maintain them in marginal condition. For example, many patients who require high doses of inotropic drugs or an IAB pump for more than 48 hours are considered for insertion of an assist device, even though they are able to maintain adequate or marginal hemodynamic parameters. Certainly, if patients are to be maintained on balloon pumps and high-dose inotropic drugs for longer than 1 week, the authors would favor insertion of assist devices.[39]

The criteria for excluding patients from circulatory support are outlined in Table 19–3. In general, the authors have found that the most common reasons to exclude patients from cardiac support are severe bleeding, renal failure requiring dialysis, irreversible major organ injury such as cerebrovascular accident, and unacceptable psychosocial history, particularly when considering patients for cardiac transplantation. Further discussion of the patient selection criteria appears later in this chapter in the section on determinants of success. The results presented in this chapter are based, to some extent, on patient data obtained using the hemodynamic criteria outlined in Table 19–2. These criteria were by no means uniform, and therefore the results include instances in which patients were supported who would not have met the criteria as indicated here.

TABLE 19–2 HEMODYNAMIC CRITERIA FOR MECHANICAL CIRCULATORY SUPPORT

A. Cardiac index <1.8 liters /m²/min
B. Systolic arterial pressure <90 mm Hg
C. Left and/or right atrial pressure >20 mm Hg
D. Urine output <20 ml/hr (adult)
E. Systemic vascular resistance >2100 dynes-sec-cm^{-5}
F. Metabolic acidosis

Despite
Adequate preload, maximal pharmacological support, corrected metabolism, and intraaortic balloon pumping

TABLE 19–3 EXCLUSION CRITERIA FOR MECHANICAL CIRCULATORY SUPPORT

A. Renal failure (BUN >100 mg/dl, creatinine >5 mg/dl)
B. Severe peripheral vascular disease
C. Symptomatic cerebrovascular disease
D. Cancer with metastasis
E. Severe hepatic disease
F. Coagulopathy
G. Severe infections resistant to therapy

DESCRIPTION OF DEVICES

A number of devices are now available[39a] which can be classified in several ways (Table 19–4). There currently is no universal method of classification for mechanical circulatory support devices. They may be classified according to their availability, in that some are investigational and require special approval by the FDA, whereas others can be obtained commercially. The position of the device can be described as extracorporeal, paracorporeal, heterotopic (internal or external), or orthotopic. Devices also can be classified according to their intended use (i.e., resuscitation or long-term support), or they may be classified according to their source of energy. In this chapter, we describe seven separate classes which include the devices currently being used clinically.

INTRAAORTIC BALLOON COUNTERPULSATION

Counterpulsation or diastolic augmentation is the most commonly used method of mechanical circulatory support. Except for improvements in the devices and methods of insertion, the techniques of IAB counterpulsation have not changed substantially since their first successful application in 1968.[8] For this technique, a balloon is positioned within the thoracic aorta distal to the left subclavian artery and proximal to the renal arteries (Fig. 19–1). The IAB is synchronized with left ventricular contraction by means of the electrocardiogram. A predetermined volume of gas is pumped into the balloon during cardiac diastole and withdrawn during systole. As a result, there is a dual hemodynamic response: a reduction in systolic blood pressure, which reduces the resistance against which the left ventricle contracts, and an increase of diastolic blood pressure, which results in an increase in coronary artery perfusion pressure and, possibly, coronary blood flow. The hemodynamic effects of IAB pumping are outlined in Table 19–5. Although the cardiac output may increase 10 to 40 per cent,[40] the magnitude of increase usually is only 10 to 20 per cent depending on the contractility of the ventricle and the extent of myocardial infarction and ischemia. Perhaps the more significant effect of IAB assist is to improve the myocardial oxygen supply/demand ratio. On the one hand, there frequently is evidence of increased myocardial blood flow, depending on the extent of collateral circulation, and on the other, there is a reduction in left ventricular wall tension, sometimes accompanied by a decrease in heart rate. If the IAB assist improves the patient's condition enough to allow inotropic agents to be reduced, there also may be a decrease in the oxygen needs of the myocardium. Recent experimental studies have demonstrated that an IAB alone significantly reduced

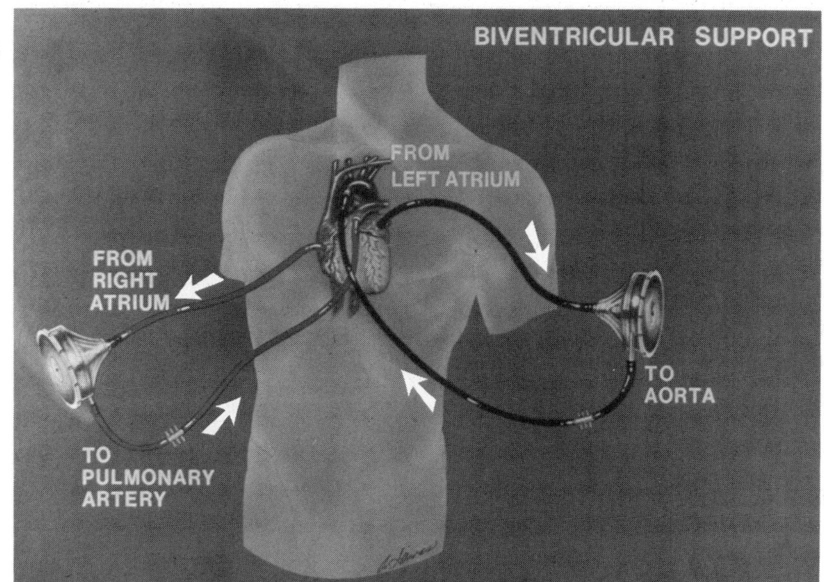

FIGURE 19–3. **Biventricular support with Biomedicus pumps with atrial pump inflow. (Courtesy of Biomedicus Inc., Eden Prairie, MN.)**

scending aorta. The current survival rate in patients with the Hemopump pending myocardial recovery is 20 to 25 per cent. With design modifications, this device could be used for longer durations as a bridge to cardiac transplantation or even as a permanent device. This device also can be implanted into the iliac artery or into the ascending aorta. It currently is used for left ventricular support only, but it could be adapted for right ventricular support as well.

EXTERNAL CENTRIFUGAL AND ROLLER PUMPS

External centrifugal pumps and roller pumps are commercially available and do not require special FDA approval. These devices have been used extensively for postcardiotomy myocardial recovery and as bridges to transplantation.[31,55–58] These pumps are positioned extracorporeally and can be connected to cannulae that are placed in any of the cardiac chambers to provide the desired type of support. For right ventricular support, blood is withdrawn from the right atrium and returned to the pulmonary artery. For left ventricular support, blood is removed from the left atrium or left ventricle and returned to the ascending aorta (Fig. 19–3). Of all the devices discussed, these are the least expensive. In addition, insertion of a centrifugal or roller pump does not necessitate cardiopulmonary bypass in all patients, although a sternotomy or thoracotomy is necessary. Patient mobility usually is impaired because of the extracorporeal position and size of these devices, although greater mobility may be possible with improved designs. These pumps are best suited to short durations of support (less than 1 week); however, there has been at least one case of support for longer than 30 days before cardiac transplantation was performed.[59] Results of the clinical use of centrifugal pumps for postcardiotomy shock and as a bridge to transplantation are included in Tables 19–6 and 19–7.

EXTERNAL PULSATILE VENTRICULAR ASSIST DEVICES

External pulsatile assist devices have had fairly extensive worldwide use. The Pierce-Donachy Thoratec VAD (Fig. 19–4) has been used successfully in both bridge-to-transplant and postcardiotomy cardiogenic shock patients.[32,60] The Pierce-Donachy Sarns pulsatile VAD, which is similar in design to the Thoratec VAD, has had limited clinical applications. The Symbion device, known as the AVAD (acute ventricular assist device), is similar to one ventricle of the Symbion J-7 artificial heart, which is discussed on p. 541. The Thoratec VAD, Sarns VAD, and Symbion AVAD are similar in that they all are powered by compressed air, they all contain mechanical valves, and they all can provide biventricular support. Cannulation for the Thoratec VAD, Symbion AVAD, and Sarns VAD is the same as for centrifugal pumps, except left ventricular cannulation is not available when using the Symbion AVAD, since it is designed for left atrial cannulation only. The Pierce-Donachy Thoratec VAD and Symbion AVAD have proved effective in providing intermediate-term support for patients for as long as 163 days. Because these devices require transcutaneous cannulae and large pneumatic power supplies, it is doubtful whether they will ever be used as permanent systems.

The Abiomed device (the BVS 5000, or biventricular support system) is different in configuration from the other devices discussed in this section.[61] It is located extracorporeally, and significantly impairs patient mobility. It also can provide right, left, or biventricular support. Cannulation options include right atrial–to–pulmonary artery and left atrial–to–ascending aortic support. This device contains polyurethane valves. Patients have been supported successfully with this device both as a bridge to cardiac transplantation and for post-cardiotomy recovery. The clinical results of these pneumatic devices are shown in Tables 19–6, 19–7, and 19–8.

TABLE 19–8 RESULTS OF MECHANICAL CIRCULATORY SUPPORT FOR POSTCARDIOTOMY CARDIOGENIC SHOCK* (N = 451)

TYPE OF SUPPORT	NO. OF PATIENTS	MEAN DURATION OF SUPPORT (DAYS)	NO. WEANED	NO. DISCHARGED	LEVEL OF SIGNIFICANCE†
LVAD	239	3.0 ± 0.1	111 (46%)	61 (26%)	NS
RVAD	60	2.8 ± 0.1	28 (47%)	17 (28%)	NS
BVAD	152	3.4 ± 0.1	64 (42%)	29 (19%)	NS
Total	451	3.3 ± 0.1	203 (45%)	107 (24%)	

LVAD, left ventricular assist device; RVAD, right ventricular assist device; BVAD, biventricular assist device; NS, not significant.
*ASAIO/ISHT Registry.
†Chi square.

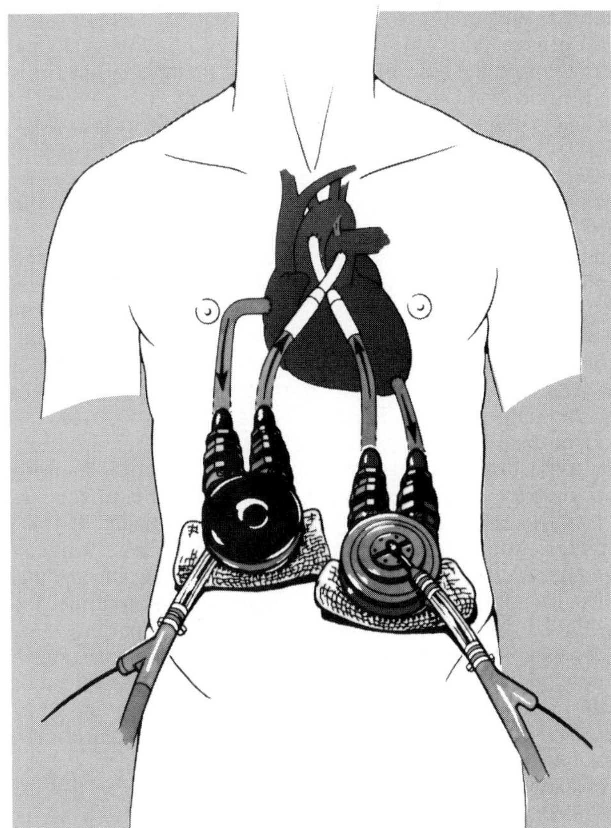

FIGURE 19–4. Biventricular support with Pierce-Donachy ventricular assist device. Right atrial–to–pulmonary artery and left ventricular–to-aortic cannulation.

IMPLANTABLE LEFT VENTRICULAR ASSIST SYSTEMS

Implantable left ventricular assist systems are particularly important since these devices are prototypes of permanent nontethered systems which will provide an alternative to cardiac transplantation for patients with end-stage heart disease. Several manufacturers are developing permanent implantable systems. Two devices (Novacor LVAS [Fig. 19–5] and Thermocardiosystems LVAS [Fig. 19–6]) currently are in clinical studies in tethered configurations.[18,62] Both devices have been used in postcardiotomy and bridge-to-transplant patients. These devices, however, may not be well suited for postcardiotomy use, as they are designed for left ventricular cannulation only and require removal of a portion of ventricular tissue at insertion. In these devices, blood is withdrawn from the apex of the left ventricle into the pump and pumped to the ascending aorta. Only left-sided support can be provided with these devices, and biventricular failure has been shown to be prevalent in postcardiotomy patients.[63] The Novacor LVAS currently is the only electrical system available. An external power cable is the only element traversing the skin, allowing for excellent patient mobility. One patient at St. Louis University successfully underwent transplant after 370 days of support with this device.

The Thermocardiosystems LVAS is similar to the Novacor, except that as of this writing it uses compressed air as its power source. It has a unique feature in that it uses a textured rather than a smooth blood-contacting surface, which promotes the development of a viable biological lining. Patients have been successfully supported with this device for up to 271 days before successful transplantation. The results of these tethered configurations as bridges to cardiac transplantation are included in Table 19–7. A small number of postcardiotomy patients have been supported with these devices with poor results.

ORTHOTOPIC BIVENTRICULAR REPLACEMENT PROSTHESES (ARTIFICIAL HEARTS)

Orthotopic biventricular replacement prostheses are perhaps the most publicized devices available. The Symbion Jarvik-7 TAH (Fig. 19–7) has been used worldwide. It is pneumatically powered and requires removal of the patient's ventricles. Polyurethane cuffs are sewn to the native atria. These atrial cuffs as well as the grafts that are sewn to the pulmonary artery and aorta contain connections which quickly snap onto the prosthetic ventricles. Blood flow through this device is the same as that through the normal heart. It has had limited use as a permanent implant and has been used since the mid-1980's only as a bridge to transplantation.[64,65] Two drive lines exit the chest, so patient mobility is not severely restricted. Clinical results with this device are shown in Table 19–7.

PERMANENT DEVICES

Two types of mechanical circulatory support devices for permanent use are under development. The first type of device is the implantable left ventricular assist system. Two such devices, the Novacor and the Thermocardiosystems, currently are being used in a temporary tethered configuration as a bridge to cardiac transplantation. The initial clinical results with these two devices have been excellent, with a low incidence of thromboembolism and mechanical failure documented. It is anticipated that permanent implantations with the Novacor LVAS will begin shortly. Permanent implantation with the Thermocardiosystems device will, it is hoped, follow within a few years. The second type of system being

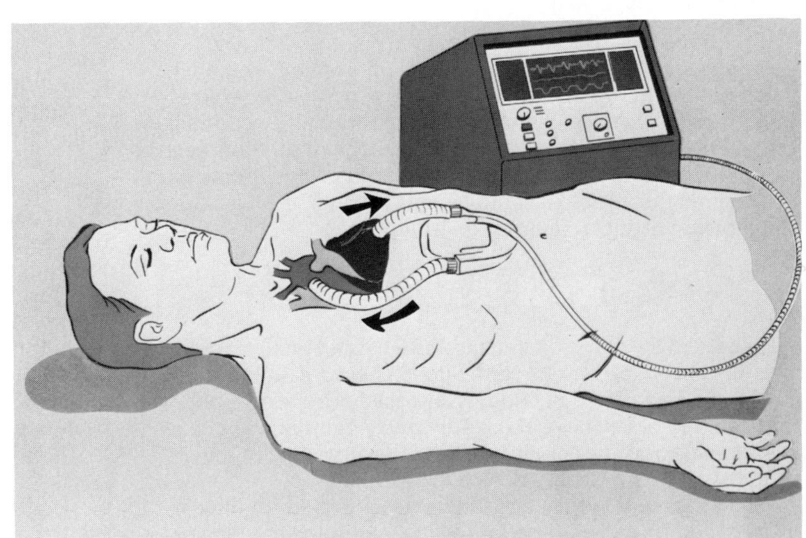

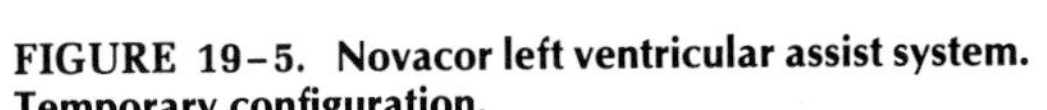

FIGURE 19–5. Novacor left ventricular assist system. Temporary configuration.

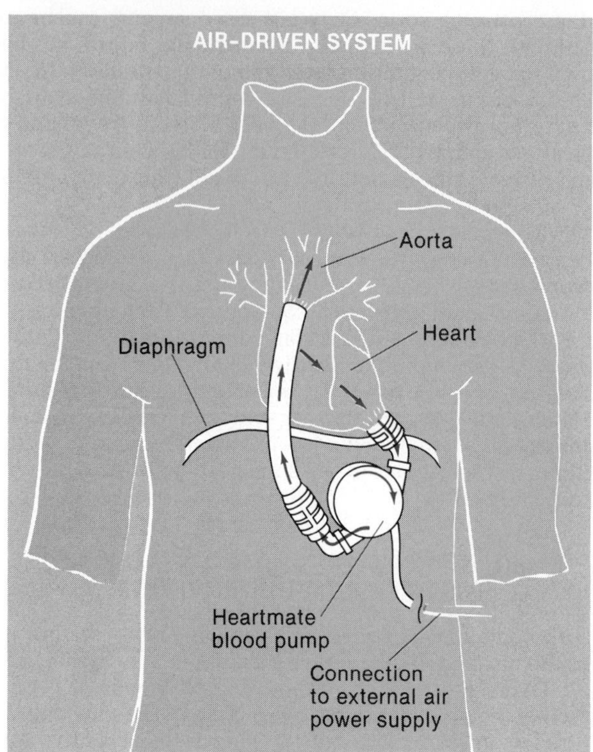

FIGURE 19-6. Thermocardiosystems left ventricular assist system. Temporary pneumatic configuration. (Courtesy of Thermocardiosystems Inc., Woburn, MA.)

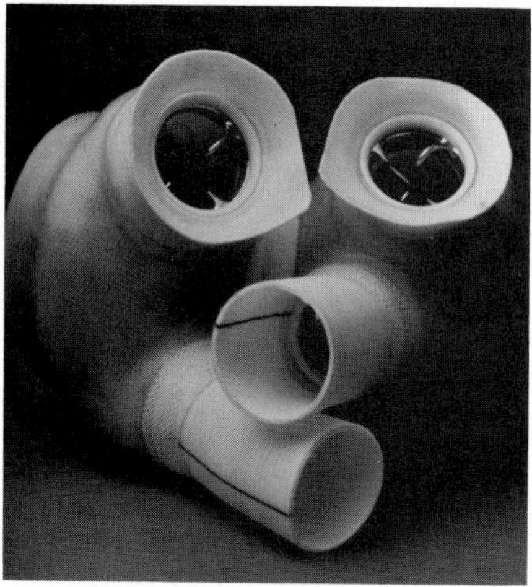

FIGURE 19-7. Symbion Jarvik-7 (70 ml) artificial heart. (Courtesy of Symbion Inc., Tempe, AZ.)

developed is a biventricular replacement system, which will be composed of either implantable orthotopic or heterotopic biventricular devices. Bench testing and animal experimentation are ongoing with both these types of devices. It has been estimated that anywhere from 17,000 to 35,000 patients per year below the age of 70 could benefit from an effective fully implantable artificial heart or assist device.

DEVICE SELECTION

Proper device selection depends on a careful analysis of the circumstances leading to cardiogenic shock. Although it is advantageous to have the optimal device for a given application, few centers have all of the previously mentioned devices at their disposal. In actual practice, the investigator's decisions often are limited by device availability.

When a patient suffers a cardiac arrest, perhaps in the cardiac catheterization laboratory or in the emergency department, the immediate concern is to restore perfusion to the vital organs. Therefore, it is necessary to have a system that allows rapid access to the circulatory system. All of the systems mentioned in this section on resuscitative devices have this advantage and would, therefore, be appropriate choices. The transseptal left atrial–femoral artery and Hemopump systems require insertion under fluoroscopic guidance. If cardiac arrest occurs outside the cardiac catheterization laboratory, these systems may be more difficult to insert than the femorofemoral ECMO systems. It is now thought that femorofemoral ECMO systems are not effective for support longer than 48 hours. Prolonged support with ECMO is associated with bleeding and infectious complications. In addition, femorofemoral systems have been shown to inhibit ventricular function; support for longer than 24 hours may worsen the cardiac condition.[36,37] ECMO systems, however, allow a period of stabilization, which allows for further evaluation. Some of the resuscitated patients may be candidates for cardiac surgery, especially those having undergone unsuccessful percutaneous transluminal coronary angioplasty. If the patient is a candidate for surgery, cardiac transplantation may be considered if the patient meets the transplant criteria. Because it is doubtful that a donor organ would be immediately available, it would be necessary to switch the patient to some other system that could provide intermediate- or long-term support. Conversely, the Hemopump has been used successfully in patients for 4 to 5 days and has been shown to have favorable effects on myocardial function during coronary occlusion.[66]

Postcardiotomy ventricular failure has been the most widely used application of mechanical circulatory support. Several factors affect the decision as to which device would best fit the patient's needs, but the most important is the probability of cardiac recovery. If the patient has not suffered a large perioperative myocardial infarction or had previous extensive myocardial damage, the possibility for recovery should be assumed. For this reason, an artificial heart would not be an appropriate choice. The ECMO systems have little positive effect on myocardial recovery, and are not as effective for postcardiotomy cardiogenic shock, since continuous anticoagulation is required and support frequently is required for more than 48 hours. External centrifugal or roller pumps or external pulsatile assist devices are appropriate devices for this application, since they can provide right, left, or biventricular support, often allow the discontinuance of anticoagulants, allow for atrial rather than ventricular cannulation, and may be used for at least a week. External pulsatile pumps are more likely to allow for ambulation and have more favorable margins of safety when anticoagulation is discontinued. When myocardial damage is severe and is believed to preclude recovery, transplantation may be considered. Fortunately, the external pulsatile assist devices are effective for use as bridges to transplantation as well as for postcardiotomy recovery. Centrifugal pumps may not be desirable if the wait for a donor heart is extended beyond 1 week.

Another circumstance that may lead to the institution of mechanical support is the patient whose condition deteriorates after having been evaluated and accepted for cardiac transplantation. In these patients, myocardial recovery need not be considered. Therefore, the primary concern in the selection of the device is the ability to support the patient for intermediate to long terms (greater than 30 days). Because the waiting time for donor organs lengthens annually, it is important to support transplant candidates on devices that will be effective for the necessary period of time. Minimal monitoring and adjustments and reduced impairment of patient mobility are other desirable attributes for devices intended for intermediate- and long-term support. A number of patients have been supported for 80 to 440 days with the Pierce-Donachy VAD, Novacor LVAS, Thermocardiosystems VAS, Symbion Jarvik-7 TAH, and Symbion AVAD. All these devices would be possible options for bridge-to-transplantation support. In smaller patients and in those with biventricular failure, the

Novacor and Thermocardiosystems devices may not be useful. If there is extensive intracardiac thrombus, an orthotopic replacement device such as a total artificial heart is preferred.

CLINICAL RESULTS

The clinical data presented in this chapter are a compilation of information derived from a variety of sources, including communications from investigators and manufacturers as well as from the Registry for Mechanical Assist Devices and Artificial Hearts sponsored by the American Society for Artificial Internal Organs (ASAIO) and the International Society for Heart Transplantation (ISHT). Although it is by no means complete, the ASAIO/ISHT Registry currently is the most readily available and reliable source of data concerning patients who have undergone mechanical circulatory support. Participation in this registry is voluntary; therefore, not all cases are reported. Because uniform criteria for complications have not yet been developed, comparisons between devices or patients in this chapter must be kept in perspective. The clinical results in this chapter are divided into three patient groups: postcardiotomy cardiogenic shock, bridge to transplantation, and acute deterioration requiring mechanical support.

POSTCARDIOTOMY CARDIOGENIC SHOCK

Table 19–8 shows the results for 451 patients who received mechanical circulatory support for postcardiotomy cardiogenic shock.[24] There is no significant difference in the mean duration of support or in the percentage of patients weaned between the left ventricular assist device, right ventricular assist device, or biventricular assist device patients. The best survival (28 per cent) is in those patients who received isolated right ventricular support. The right ventricular assist device patient group is the smallest, comprising only 13 per cent of the total patient population. The largest patient group (52 per cent) are those who received isolated left ventricular support, of whom 26 per cent survived. Of the 152 patients who received biventricular assist devices, 19 per cent were discharged. These data support the contention that isolated ventricular dysfunction in postcardiotomy patients is more likely to be reversible than biventricular dysfunction. Thirty-four per cent of these 451 patients received biventricular assist devices. It also can be assumed that a certain percentage of patients receiving isolated left or right ventricular support suffered biventricular failure. From these data, it may be deduced that at least one in three postcardiotomy patients who require ventricular support will suffer biventricular failure severe enough to require biventricular support. The mean duration of support for all patients was 3.3 days, and most patients who were able to be weaned from the devices were supported less than 5 days. Some patients required longer periods of support to allow for cardiac recovery. The amount of time necessary for cardiac recovery is related to the nature and extent of the injury. Ischemic injury usually allows myocardial recovery in less than 5 days, whereas injuries involving necrosis require longer durations of support. The overall survival rate of 24 per cent is consistent with published reports from smaller series. There was no significant difference in the percentage of patients weaned or discharged when comparing patients who received pneumatic devices with patients who received centrifugal devices (Table 19–6).

Morbidity rates were high. Data concerning the five most commonly reported complications associated with postcardiotomy support are included in Table 19–9. Bleeding was the most common complication, occurring in 45 per cent of all patients. Renal failure, which developed in 38 per cent of patients, was a common and often devastating complication. The incidence of biventricular failure (32 per cent) is consistent with the number of patients receiving biventricular support. The incidences of infection and thrombosis/embolus also are high (15 and 17 per cent). The most striking result from this table is the relation between survivors and nonsurvivors who suffered either renal failure or biventricular failure. Both of these complications were much more prevalent in the nonsurvivors than in the survivors. This information has been substantiated in reports identifying these two complications as predictors of nonsurvival.[63,67]

Important factors in evaluating the clinical results of postcardiotomy circulatory support are the length of survival and functional status. In a multiinstitutional study of clinical VADs, 15 survivors of postcardiotomy shock supported by VADS were followed for periods up to 4 years.[68] Although 13 were in New York Heart Association Class III or IV preoperatively, only two were Class III or IV postoperatively. Six of the 13 patients with improved cardiac function were working full-time, and all but 2 of the others chose retirement but had no physical limitations. Moreover, of the 15 survivors, almost half had normal cardiac function. Several other long-term follow-up studies have verified these results.[69,70] Therefore, it is clear that these severely dysfunctional hearts have a remarkable capability to recover functional capacity, and cardiac function of many survivors returns to normal after a brief period of circulatory support.

BRIDGE TO TRANSPLANTATION

The results of bridging to transplantation with some of the most commonly used devices are shown in Table 19–7. The percentage of survival after transplantation ranges from 40 to 89 per cent, depending on the type of device used. The overall survival rate of 379 patients known to be bridge-to-transplant candidates (excluding Symbion AVAD and Abiomed patients) was 77 per cent, a rate comparable to survival for routine cardiac transplantation. Specific data for the Symbion AVAD and Abiomed patients are not available to determine how many were recovery or transplant candidates. The overall survival rate of these 379 patients was 54 per cent. The percentage of patients transplanted (excluding the Symbion AVAD and Abiomed groups) ranged from 62 to 78 per cent for individual devices. From these data the following generalizations may be made. If a patient undergoes mechanical circulatory support as a bridge to cardiac transplantation, the overall chance of hospital discharge is 54 per cent. The patient would have a 70 per cent chance if undergoing cardiac transplantation, and if transplantation is performed, a 75 to 80 per cent 2-year survival rate can be anticipated.

TABLE 19–9 COMPLICATIONS OF POSTCARDIOTOMY SHOCK* (N = 448)

	NO. OF PATIENTS AFFECTED		
COMPLICATION	Survivors (N = 107)	Nonsurvivors (N = 341)	LEVEL OF SIGNIFICANCE†
Bleeding	45 (42%)	160 (47%)	NS
Renal failure	16 (15%)	153 (45%)	$p < .0001$
Infection	15 (14%)	51 (15%)	NS
Thrombus embolus	15 (14%)	58 (17%)	NS
Biventricular failure	22 (21%)	122 (36%)	$p < .005$

NS, not significant.
*ASAIO/ISHT Registry.
†Chi square.

TABLE 19–10 COMPLICATIONS OF BRIDGE TO TRANSPLANTATION* (N = 216)

COMPLICATION	NO. OF PATIENTS AFFECTED Survivors (N = 106)	Nonsurvivors (N = 110)	LEVEL OF SIGNIFICANCE†
Bleeding	29 (27%)	61 (55%)	$p < .0001$
Renal failure	3 (3%)	42 (38%)	$p < .0001$
Infection	15 (14%)	32 (29%)	$p < .05$
Thrombosis/embolus	8 (8%)	11 (10%)	NS

NS, not significant.
*ASAIO/ISHT Registry.
† Chi square.

As with the postcardiotomy patients, complications were common in this group of patients awaiting donor hearts. Table 19–10 shows the complications associated with bridging to transplantation with VADs and artificial hearts. Bleeding was the most common complication, occurring in 42 per cent of patients. Fifty-five per cent of nonsurvivors had bleeding complications, as compared with 27 per cent of survivors. Although renal failure occurred in 21 per cent of all patients, it occurred in only 3 per cent of the survivors, as opposed to 38 per cent of nonsurvivors. The incidence of infection was twice as high in nonsurvivors as in survivors. Thromboembolic events occurred in 9 per cent of the patients and were about equal between survivors and nonsurvivors. Many of these thromboembolic events were in the early bridge-to-transplantation experience before the development of more effective anticoagulation regimens as well as better device regulation. The incidence of thromboembolism has dropped, despite the fact that the duration of perfusion has increased.

ACUTE DETERIORATION

Early clinical experience with closed-chest methods of cardiopulmonary bypass proved unsuccessful.[3] In recent years, there has been a resurgence of the use of ECMO as a resuscitative system to temporarily support patients until further intervention can be accomplished. Data from patients undergoing ECMO for cardiac failure are not included in information collected by the ASAIO/ISHT Registry. There have been several reports on the use of femorofemoral ECMO in groups of 20 or more patients. Survival rates in these reports ranged from 17 to 22 per cent.[19,51,52] These studies contained a heterogeneous patient population, with the cause of cardiac failure and/or arrest ranging from hypothermia to postcardiac transplant graft failure. It is believed that as patient selection criteria are refined, the survival rates for these techniques should improve. No specific data are available on the exact number or types of complications encountered in these patients, but bleeding, infection, renal failure, and neurological injury all must be considered complications which will be encountered in a significant percentage.

SPECIAL PROBLEMS

RIGHT VENTRICULAR FAILURE

Right ventricular failure is a problem commonly encountered in patients supported with LVADs after cardiac surgery and in bridge to transplantation. Mechanisms of right ventricular failure are not clear. Right ventricular dysfunction usually is a component of biventricular failure, but it occasionally occurs as an isolated phenomenon despite good left ventricular function. It is not understood why certain patients who are supported with LVADs develop right ventricular failure whereas others do not. Some experimental studies have demonstrated deterioration of right ventricular function in dogs during left ventricular bypass,[71] but in other studies this negative effect was offset by decreasing right ventricular afterload.[72,73] Clinically, no decrease in right ventricular function has been shown in patients with isolated LVAD support.[74,75] The severity of biventricular dysfunction is a factor which strongly influences survival of patients receiving isolated ventricular support.

During LVAD support, three factors may significantly influence right ventricular function: (1) as a result of LVAD flow, venous return increases to the right ventricle; (2) a decrease in left ventricular filling pressure in patients with normal pulmonary vascular resistance reduces right ventricular afterload; and (3) decreased left ventricular pressure may shift the interventricular septum to the left, reducing the septal contribution to right ventricular contraction. Pulmonary vascular resistance is an important variable in determining the right ventricular response to these events. The ability of the right heart to tolerate LVAD-induced increase in preload frequently is determined by the degree of the decrease in right ventricular afterload. Elevated pulmonary vascular resistance negatively affects the right heart's capacity to tolerate increased volume. When pulmonary hypertension is present, lowering left ventricular pressure will not reduce right ventricular afterload.

Hershon and colleagues found that in patients undergoing left ventricular support, left ventricular decompression did not lead to right ventricular failure.[74] In fact, in patients with left ventricular dysfunction, decompression of the left ventricle with a LVAD resulted in progressive improvement of right ventricular function.[75] Therefore, it seems that in postcardiotomy patients supported with LVADs, the development of right heart failure usually can be attributed to increased pulmonary vascular resistance and/or right ventricular ischemia.

BLEEDING AND THROMBOEMBOLISM

Mechanical circulatory support devices are associated with significant and often detrimental effects on other body systems. Bleeding and thromboembolism are recognized as major complications associated with these devices. The incidence and severity of life-threatening bleeding complications have decreased considerably with increasing clinical experience. Thromboembolism, transient ischemic attacks, and cerebrovascular accidents remain major concerns, but the incidence of thromboembolism has decreased significantly since the late 1980's.

The causative factors involved in blood coagulation and thrombus formation in mechanical circulatory devices are just beginning to be understood. A complex series of reactions occurs when blood comes in contact with an artificial surface. This reaction activates platelets and white blood cells, the blood coagulation/fibrinolytic system, and the complement system.[76–78] These initial reactions are followed by progressive "passivation" of the device surfaces, probably as a result of protein absorption and protein-protein interaction.[79] The exact mechanism of passivation is not known. However, it is believed that passivation is a process in which layers of protein accumulate on the artificial surface of the device. After passivation, the circulation "sees" protein rather than an artificial surface, resulting in less platelet surface interaction and a reduced risk of thrombus formation. Before passivation can occur, these interactions may lead to thrombus formation, thromboembolic complications, consumption coagulopathy, and excessive bleeding. Platelets become refractory and dysfunctional as a result of interaction with artificial surfaces.[80] This transient platelet dysfunction is related to selective alpha granule release. The amount of time that platelets are in contact with an artificial surface is important with respect to their hemostatic function. Platelet activation also results in platelet-platelet interaction or platelet aggregation.[81] When platelets come in contact with a foreign surface, especially at high shear rates, they undergo conformational changes associated with pseudopod formation, a reaction called platelet spreading. Platelet adherence, which includes contact and spreading, leads to the release of adenosine diphosphate, which attracts other platelets streaming close to the adherent platelet. Patients with mechanical circulatory support devices have continued activation of platelets until passivation of the artificial surface takes place. Platelet activation often is associated with thrombocytopenia, which persists for several days after device implantation, and platelet transfusions may be necessary.

Increased clinical experience, improved anticoagulation protocols, and more physiological biomaterials have significantly decreased the incidence of thromboembolic complications. Despite these improvements, a small percentage of patients continue to suffer thromboembolic events, the mechanisms of which have not been clearly elucidated. Preliminary studies suggested an important role of infection in promoting thromboembolic complications or initiating hemostatic system alterations, such as the activation of platelets, coagulation, or the complement system.[82]

HEMOLYSIS

Hemolysis is a potential complication for patients undergoing mechanical support with a device that involves blood and artificial surface interaction. The erythrocytes are damaged primarily by shear stresses; however, blood contact with an unphysiological surface often contributes to hemolysis. Cell damage results in either immediate lysis with release of free hemoglobin or a shortened life span and delayed hemolysis. It has been shown that the level of hemolysis is directly related to shear rates.[83] If hemolysis occurs, it usually is shortly after placement of a mechanical support device. If the plasma hemoglobin level exceeds 100 mg/dl, the likelihood of renal insufficiency and increased serum potassium levels increases. Increased serum potassium levels resulting from hemolysis may lead to an increased incidence of arrhythmias. Even serum hemoglobin levels less than 100 mg/dl are associated with a loss of red cell mass and anemia, which requires transfusions. Some of the simpler circulatory support systems, such as centrifugal pumps, roller pumps, and routine cardiopulmonary bypass, produce a low to moderate degree of hemolysis (less than 100 mg/dl). Because support with these devices usually lasts less than 7 days, many patients tolerate this level of hemolysis with no renal or metabolic complications. The more sophisticated systems designed for longer-term use (more than 1 week) have a much lower propensity for hemolysis. If hemolysis does occur, it is possible to decrease the shear rate by decreasing device dP/dt, device flow, and/or negative pressure on the control console, thereby avoiding hepatic and renal dysfunction as well as coagulopathies and severe anemia related to hemolysis.[84] The patient should be closely monitored with determination of serum hemoglobins and serum haptoglobins, since hemoglobinuria is not always apparent at the lower levels of hemolysis.

COMPLEMENT ACTIVATION

The complement system is known to be activated during cardiopulmonary bypass, hemodialysis, and circulatory support with mechanical devices.[85,86] Numerous factors, including the interaction of blood with artificial surfaces and increased shear rates in mechanical devices, are responsible for this activation. As a result of complement activation, serum complement components are consumed. Because the complement system contributes to the immunological defense mechanisms, a decrease in circulating complement levels may increase the risk of infection. There also is evidence that complement activation results in the formation of several anaphylatoxins (C3a and C5a)[87]; C5a is suspected of being a potent pulmonary vasoconstrictor. Complement activation has been associated with a variety of clinical problems, including pulmonary dysfunction, acute respiratory distress syndrome, increased infection, myocardial ischemia, and heparin–protamine complex–induced hypotension.[86,88–91] Despite studies that have shown complement activation during cardiopulmonary bypass, few, if any, related clinical complications have been documented. Complement activation may be similar to other blood surface interactions, in that after passivation of the surface or clinical stabilization, complement activation ceases. More work is required to document the role of complement activation in mechanical circulatory support physiology.

INFECTION

Infection also is one of the common complications seen in patients with mechanical circulatory support devices. Infection and renal failure often occur simultaneously, and this combination often is lethal. Most of the infections are nosocomial bacterial infections similar to those that occur after routine cardiac surgery.[92] Pneumonia is especially prevalent. Bacteremia usually is the result of contaminated intravascular lines. However, many patients develop infections which are directly related to the mechanical support devices. Infections may originate at the exit sites of cannula or transcutaneous power cables and migrate along the prosthetic materials to invade the mediastinum or pump pocket. If such infections are detected early and treated aggressively with wound drainage and antibiotics, mediastinitis may be avoided. The shorter the duration of support, the less likely infection will occur.

Discussion continues over how best to handle the threat of infections in patients who require prolonged support. Continuous antibiotics do not prevent infection, and may create the problem of superinfection. Therefore, only specific antibiotic therapy for proven clinically significant infections should be used. Infections are also less likely if the patients are hemodynamically stable and have good nutritional status. It should be noted that few patients develop opportunistic infections while being supported with mechanical devices. If an opportunistic infection occurs, it usually is in patients who have had prolonged multiple antibiotic therapy. It is known that cardiopulmonary bypass significantly depresses T cell function. However, in patients undergoing routine cardiopulmonary bypass, T cell function returns to normal within 48 to 72 hours. A recent study of T cell lymphocytes in patients with mechanical circulatory support devices at St. Louis University revealed marked depression of the total lymphocyte count and the T cell lymphocytes during the early days of support.[93] In patients whose conditions were stabilized and who went on to survive, this rather marked immunosuppression disappeared within 5 days. In nonsurvivors, especially patients who developed renal failure or infectious complications, the immunosuppression continued until their death.

Since it is clear that externally driven assist devices will always carry the risk of bacterial infection, permanent systems are designed to be totally implantable, eliminating any need for lines or cables to traverse the body wall. It is hoped that elimination of these external routes of infection will greatly diminish the risk of infection, but whether or not this hope is realized will await the beginning of the clinical use of totally implantable LVAS devices.

OTHER HOST–DEVICE INTERACTIONS

Surface interactions occur between the artificial surfaces of the device and the body. These host–device interactions result in a series of events which have been labeled "the race to the surface."[94] In the early postoperative period, healthy tissue and bacterial cells compete for the surfaces of the implanted device. If bacteria win the race for the biomaterial surface over the host tissue cells, antibiotic-resistant infections may occur. If tissue cells are the first to attach to the artificial surface, pathogens arriving later encounter living cells, which provide various defense mechanisms, including the opportunity to deliver antibiotics to the site of threatened bacterial invasion.

The selection of appropriate biomaterials is difficult, since the materials must all be compatible with blood or tissue. Many devices contain several polymers as well as stainless steel or titanium. There currently are two types of blood sacs used in clinical devices—smooth and textured surfaces. The Novacor, Thoratec, and Sarns pulsatile VADs all contain blood sacs and cannulae coated with a smooth polyurethane (Biomer). At this time, the only clinically used device with a textured blood sac is the Thermocardiosystems LVAS. This system's blood sac and cannula are textured to induce the formation and adherence of a biological lining. Initial clinical reports have identified what may be the presence of a few endothelial cells within the cellular coating of the blood sac. To date, there have been no reported incidences of thromboembolism in more than 3.5 patient years of support with the Thermocardiosystems LVAS.

A broad spectrum of bacteria are attracted to these materials, particularly in the early period after implantation. Recent studies suggest that some bacteria are "material specific,"[95,96] creating a high propensity for specific infections. If specific bacteria arrive at a susceptible surface before healthy tissue integration, infection will develop which will be extremely difficult to eradicate.

HORMONAL RESPONSES

In patients with cardiogenic shock, impaired cardiac function results in high cardiac filling pressures with atrial distention, which may cause the release of atrial natriuretic factor (ANF) (see p. 829).[97] ANF is produced by the atrial myocytes and is stored in the Pallade bodies of the left and right atria. Elevation of atrial wall tension is known to stimulate the release of ANF, part of the endocrine blood pressure–regulating mechanism and functionally an antagonist of aldosterone. It induces sodium and water excretion and mild vasodilatation.[98] In patients with mechanical circulatory support devices in whom the atrial tissue is left intact, the secretion of ANF is normal. It is apparent that implantation of a total artificial heart as well as cardiac transplantation reduces ANF levels, and renin and aldosterone levels return to normal within 5 days of total artificial heart implantation.[99,100] However, studies investigating the human hormonal responses to mechanical circulatory support have been limited to patients receiving artificial hearts. Since ventricular assist devices require the removal of little myocardial tissue and the neurohumoral system is intact, it is likely that hormonal responses will return to normal once the manifestations of cardiogenic shock or other forms of pump failure are corrected with ventricular assist devices. However, further studies are necessary to confirm these suspicions and to relate hormonal levels to atrial pressures.

DETERMINANTS OF SURVIVAL

Mechanical circulatory support, while gratifying when successful, is expensive and demanding of personnel and resources. Therefore, it is critical that every effort be made to determine the likelihood of survival before initiating support. Although prediction of success in any individual patient may be impossible, some guidelines can be offered which aid in the selection process.

Most postcardiotomy patients are considered for support with the expectation of myocardial recovery. Although it is possible to provide support for postcardiotomy patients until successful transplantation is accomplished, many of these patients develop complications which preclude successful transplantation. Because myocardial recovery is the most likely chance for success, one of the most important determinants is whether or not the surgery was successful. Patients undergoing coronary artery bypass grafting should have adequate flow through all bypass grafts. Valve replacements should be functional, and if an aneurysm resection has been performed, enough myocardial tissue must remain to allow for recovery and survival. A particularly difficult group are patients who suffer an acute perioperative myocardial infarction within 24 to 48 hours of operation, a complication that has been shown to be an important determinant of death.[26] The diagnosis may be quite difficult to make if the infarction occurs perioperatively, but it often is diagnosed preoperatively.

Another important factor to consider in the survival of postcardiotomy patients who require mechanical support is the patient's age. The overall hospital discharge rate for patients less than 59 years of age is 34 per cent, whereas patients older than 70 years of age have a hospital discharge rate of only 10 per cent.[24] This disadvantage of the elderly is probably related to a higher incidence of concomitant disease.

Intraoperative bleeding associated with the inability to maintain adequate systemic pressure on cardiopulmonary bypass is a relative contraindication. Many assist devices (Thoratec, Sarns, Novacor, Thermocardiosystems, Biomedicus) allow for the reversal of heparinization and a better opportunity to obtain hemostasis once the device is implanted and cardiopulmonary bypass is no longer required. Of course, major surgical bleeding unrelated to coagulopathy must be controlled. In Table 19–9 data are presented which compare survival with nonsurvival in postcardiotomy patients based on the development of individual complications. Unfortunately, most patients develop a combination of complications, and to date a multivariate analysis of these factors has not been performed in a large group of patients. Although bleeding, thromboembolism, and infection are not factors which by themselves primarily affect survival, they frequently occur in combinations that do affect survival. For postcardiotomy patients, there is a statistically significant difference in the occurrence of renal failure in survivors versus nonsurvivors ($p < .0001$), and biventricular failure was more prevalent in the nonsurvivors than in the survivors ($p < .005$). Undoubtedly some of the patients suffering biventricular failure were supported inadequately with only univentricular devices. However, many patients who were supported adequately failed to survive. Unfortunately, many postcardiotomy patients who develop severe biventricular failure have suffered large, irreversible myocardial injuries which make them unsalvageable. It often is impossible to make this determination at the time of VAD placement.

BRIDGE TO TRANSPLANTATION

Selection criteria for bridge-to-transplantation patients often differ from those for patients in the other two groups. Most bridge-to-transplant candidates are relatively stable and do not require cardiopulmonary bypass at the time the decision to provide prolonged circulatory support must be made. The adverse effects of prolonged cardiopulmonary bypass[87,101] are not present to force a rapid decision, as often is the case in postcardiotomy patients. The condition of many bridge-to-transplant candidates can be stabilized with IAB pump and pharmacological support. Although they may have deteriorating hemodynamic function, their clinical condition usually allows time for a thorough evaluation.

Hemodynamic criteria for patient selection for mechanical circulatory support have been used successfully beginning in the 1980's. However, these criteria were developed for patients with cardiogenic shock immediately after or within 24 hours of cardiac surgery, and therefore they often are not directly applicable to bridge-to-transplant candidates. Because myocardial recovery is not the issue, the question becomes how long the patient can be effectively maintained while waiting for a donor heart. With the increasing popularity of cardiac transplantation, the time to locate donor hearts is increasing (Chap. 18). Waiting periods of weeks or months are now the rule, even for patients in the most urgent category. Therefore, the decision of when to intervene in the severely compromised patient is crucial. In the authors' experience, some patients who were initially rejected as candidates because they were hemodynamically stable later developed complications that excluded them from transplantation. It was concluded that hemodynamic stability per se should not exclude patients from mechanical assistance. The amount of pharmacological, respiratory, and IAB pump support necessary to keep them stable must be taken into account. If these supportive measures cannot be reduced within 24 to 48 hours, mechanical support with a more sophisticated device should be considered. Although the authors and others have successfully supported patients with IAB pumps for several weeks, this may not be an adequate length of time to locate a heart. Therefore, in most cases, the authors prefer to insert a more sophisticated device, which would provide sufficient levels of cardiac output to allow discontinuation of all inotropic support. Such patients may safely have all intravenous lines removed, take oral medications, and begin regular ambulation and muscle-strengthening exercises. Therefore, the devices (Novacor, Thoratec, Sarns, Thermocardiosystems, Symbion AVAD and TAH) offer the potential for rehabilitation of the patients, changing them from questionable transplant candidates to vigorous recipients with the potential for an excellent outcome.

Patients whose conditions are so unstable that they require immediate implantation of an assist system are at a higher risk of developing complications than the stabilized patient in whom device implantation is performed under more controlled conditions. Several strict criteria *preclude* patients for circulatory support before cardiac transplantation: (a) unresolved pulmonary emboli, (b) renal failure requiring dialysis, (c) irreversible cerebrovascular accident, (d) unacceptable psychosocial history, and (e) severe bleeding. Ideally, patients selected for mechanical circulatory support before transplantation should meet the normal criteria for transplantation to ensure that donor hearts are not wasted. It is not essential that patients meet *all* transplantation criteria at the time of device insertion. Complications such as acute oliguric renal failure, infection, and hypoxia often can be more effectively treated if the patients receive circulatory support, allowing the conversion of a nontransplant candidate to a transplant candidate. Unfortunately, in some patients, complications worsen after support is initiated. Because of the considerable expenditure of money and resources for a bridge-to-transplantation procedure, candidates for assistance must be carefully chosen, and many of those who develop multiple complications during mechanical support must be rejected for transplantation.

In the authors' experience, most of the patients who were refused mechanical circulatory support before cardiac transplantation were rejected on the basis of infection or renal failure. Infections are problematic, since immunosuppression after transplantation may worsen the problem. On the other hand, when adequate perfusion is established with mechanical circulatory support, patients with infectious complications may respond better to antibiotics and have a better chance for eradication of the infection. Patients with superficial wound or skin infections, urinary tract infections, or mild pneumonia with low-grade fever and minimal elevation in white blood cell count should be considered reasonable candidates for mechanical circulatory support. Increased cardiac output, nutrition, and mobility aid in clearing up the infections. At St. Louis University, six patients supported with mechanical circulatory support devices had positive sputum cultures and mildly elevated white blood cell counts, and were treated with intravenous antibiotics before insertion of the device. Five underwent heart transplantation and survived. These data are in contrast to those of Griffith and coworkers, who believe that preexisting subclinical pneumonia often leads to mediastinitis after total artificial heart implantation.[102] Other factors, such as large amounts of prosthetic material and the need for invasive monitoring lines, also may play a role. Patients who have a combination of infectious and renal complications that originated before device insertion are at much higher risk, and patients with sepsis and positive blood cultures should be excluded.

In the authors' experience, a pre-device serum creatinine level higher than 2.5 mg/dl is highly predictive of nonsurvival. For that reason, most patients who have a drastic increase in blood urea nitrogen and/or creatinine with a decrease in urine output and increased resistance to diuretic therapy are excluded for insertion of an assist device at St. Louis University. Unfortunately, it has been found that establishing normal perfusion does not always improve renal function. In many cases, renal function actually deteriorated after the devices were implanted.[67] Cardiopulmonary bypass and bleeding complications at the time of device insertion may have further aggravated the renal insufficiency.

Other factors that influence survival to a lesser degree are the number of hospitalization days, the number of days the patient requires inotropic support, and whether or not IAB pump support is necessary. Hemodynamic parameters such as cardiac index, right atrial pressure, and pulmonary capillary wedge pressure were not predictors of survival in the authors' bridge-to-transplant patient population.[39]

The four most commonly reported complications of patients with mechanical circulatory support devices awaiting cardiac transplantation are shown in Table 19–10. Biventricular failure is not considered a critical factor in the bridge-to-transplant population, since myocardial recovery is not expected and is not necessary for survival. If the biventricular failure is correctly supported, the results in the bridge-to-transplant patient population should be the same whether the patient suffers univentricular or biventricular failure.[103,104] As with the postcardiotomy group, renal failure is highly predictive of nonsurvival ($p < .0001$). In the bridge-to-transplant population, infection plays an important role in determining success of the procedure. For this reason, infections which develop before device insertion and/or before transplantation need to be carefully evaluated. Thromboembolism was not a predictor of survival. Many of the patients in this category had thrombi confined to the device (all types) which did not embolize. Many of the patients who suffered thromboemboli did not have permanent damage and recovered before transplantation.

Because donor hearts are at such a premium, the development of any complication during the interval of circulatory support may reduce the patient's eligibility for transplantation. Complications such as serious bleeding, renal failure, or infection usually eliminate a patient as a candidate for transplantation until the problem has been resolved.

ACUTE DETERIORATION

Many of the patients who develop cardiogenic shock secondary to acute myocardial infarction may qualify for circulatory support. These patients may be hospitalized, or arrive in the emergency department, intensive care unit, or cardiac catheterization laboratory with acute massive infarcts and cardiogenic shock without previous evaluation of cardiac function. Many of these patients are rapidly deteriorating or being actively resuscitated when the mechanical circulatory support team is notified. It often is necessary to institute circulatory support before evaluating ventricular function. However, it is possible to establish a diagnosis after circulatory assistance has begun. Endomyocardial biopsy, cardiac catheterization, echocardiograms, and nuclear multigated acquisition scans can all be obtained while the patient is being supported with the device. It may be possible to wean some of these patients from mechanical support after a period of recovery. Others may benefit from corrective surgery once their hemodynamics have been stabilized. Most of these patients have not been evaluated for transplantation before the need for circulatory assistance. Many have a better chance for survival *after* transplantation, since they have not had a progressive chronic illness which has left them debilitated. If the detrimental effects of cardiogenic shock can be rapidly reversed by medical therapy or circulatory assistance, many of these patients are excellent cardiac transplant recipients.

It is imperative in this group of patients that mechanical circulatory support be initiated as soon as possible. Mechanical assist devices that require insertion in the operating room are not practical under these circumstances. An ECMO system, whether percutaneous or by cutdown cannulation, allows placement of cardiopulmonary bypass within 30 minutes and can be readily applied in the emergency department, cardiac catheterization laboratory, or medical or surgical intensive care unit. Candidates for this therapy have included patients suffering from postcardiotomy cardiogenic shock while in the intensive care unit, failed coronary angioplasty myocardial infarction with cardiogenic shock, massive pulmonary embolus, deterioration after cardiac transplantation, cardiomyopathy with acute shock, aortic stenosis, hypothermia, traumatic injury, and refractory ventricular fibrillation.[19,51,52]

ASAIO/ISHT Registry information is not available on patients who suffer acute deterioration that requires mechanical circulatory support with resuscitative devices such as the ECMO circuits described in this chapter. Patients with acute myocardial infarction shock who ultimately were supported with VADs or artificial hearts would be included in the Registry. Unfortunately, there are insufficient clinical data available to assess the impact that various factors have on survival in this group. There are, however, some general beliefs that will probably be supported: (1) patients who have suffered large, irreversible myocardial insults and are not cardiac transplant candidates have a small chance of survival; and (2) patients who undergo conventional cardiopulmonary resuscitation for extended periods (greater than 1.5 hours) are at considerable risk for neurological injury, and thus have a greatly reduced opportunity for survival. As with the other groups, patients with coagulopathy or infection before the initiation of mechanical support would be expected to have a higher risk of complications.

OTHER FACTORS THAT AFFECT SURVIVAL

There are insufficient data to determine whether the type of device significantly affects survival. It has been shown in postcardiotomy patients that there is no difference in survival whether the patient is supported with a pneumatic or a centrifugal device (Table 19–6). This also holds true, for the most part, for the bridge-to-transplantation experience (Table 19–7). The amount of time required for myocardial recovery or location of a donor organ plays an important role, and indirectly influences results according to the type of device. For example, centrifugal pumps and resuscitative devices such as ECMO will permit the best survival rate if perfusion is limited to less than 3 to 4 days. The Pierce-Donachy has been effective for at least 3 months, and the Novacor, Thermocardiosystems, and Symbion TAH have been effective for periods of 9 months to 1 year. The durations of support (<10 days) for postcardiotomy patients have remained relatively constant, based on the concept that myocardial recovery should occur within 7 to 10 days. There are, however, few clinical data to verify this theory. It is unknown whether myocardial recovery might occur if support is continued beyond 2 weeks.

Recent clinical experience has resulted in dramatic improvements in patient and device management. At St. Louis University, the average duration of support for the last 20

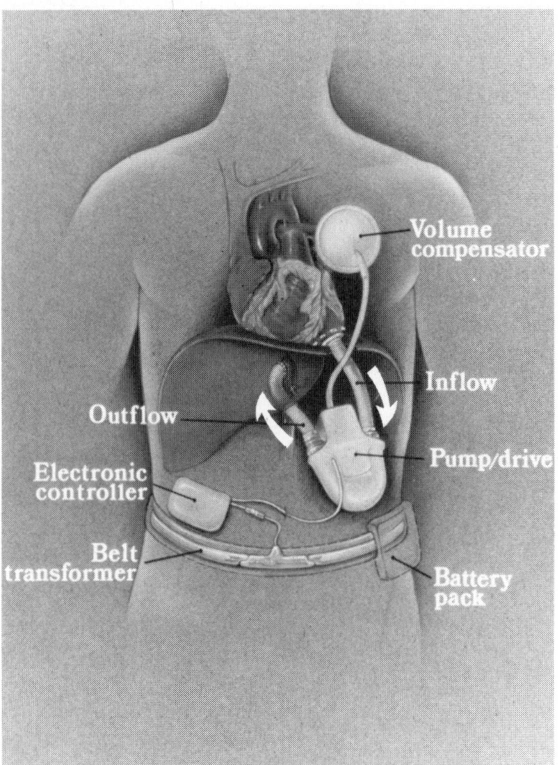

FIGURE 19–8. Novacor left ventricular assist system. Permanent configuration. (Courtesy of Novacor Division, Baxter Healthcare Corp., Oakland, CA.)

patients (at the time of this writing) was 33 days, as opposed to 15 days for the previous 20 patients. Of seven patients supported longer than 50 days, six survived, five of whom received transplants. As the durations of support continue to lengthen in the bridge-to-transplant population, some of this experience will undoubtedly be transferred to the postcardiotomy and acute deterioration patient groups, allowing longer durations of support in these patients as well.

Age is a factor that is likely to affect survival in all patient groups, owing to the presence of concomitant disease. The effects of age on survival in postcardiotomy patients have been documented. There are inadequate data to determine the results in bridge-to-transplantation patients older than 60 years of age.

The most important frontiers of circulatory support are in the use of totally implantable systems that do not require external power lines to transverse the skin and body wall. Most investigators agree that the externally powered systems will ultimately fail because of infection from the driveline site or endogenous seeding of foreign materials. In the experience at St. Louis University with seven patients supported more than 50 days, six patients had at least one episode of device-related infection. Until a totally implantable system is available, no implantations can be considered permanent. The development of permanent totally implantable biventricular support or replacement devices is being explored in the laboratory. The development of a permanent totally implantable LVAS has been completed (Fig. 19–8), and early human implantations are planned. If these clinical trials prove successful during the 5 years' study, it may be possible to begin implantations on a broader scale by the late 1990's. It is hoped that these devices will make it possible to offer a therapeutic alternative to the majority of patients with heart failure in the United States. Estimates of numbers of candidates for such devices range from 10,000 to 30,000 patients per year.[105] Although it is unlikely that circulatory support device applications will substantially affect these numbers in the first half of the 1990's, it is a realistic hope that the feasibility and efficacy of the devices will be well demonstrated during this time.

REFERENCES

1. Gibbon, J. H., Jr.: Application of a mechanical heart and lung apparatus to cardiac surgery. Minn. Med. *37*:171, 1954.
2. Cooley, D. A., Beall, A. C., Jr., and Alexander, J. L.: Acute massive pulmonary embolism: Successful surgical treatment using temporary cardiopulmonary bypass. JAMA *177*:283, 1961.
3. Stuckey, J. H., Newman, M. M., Dennis, C., et al.: The use of the heart-lung machine in selected cases of acute myocardial infarction. Surg. Forum *8*:342, 1957.
4. Dennis, C., Carlens, E., Senning, A., et al.: Clinical use of a cannula for left heart bypass without thoracotomy. Ann. Surg. *156*:623, 1962.
5. DeBakey, M. E.: Left ventricular bypass pump for cardiac assistance. Clinical experience. Am. J. Cardiol. *27*:3, 1971.
6. Clauss, R. H., Birtwell, W. C., Albertal, G., et al.: Assisted circulation. I. The arterial counterpulsator. J. Thorac. Cardiovasc. Surg. *41*:447, 1961.
7. Moulopoulos, S. D., Topaz, S., and Kolff, W. J.: Diastolic balloon pumping (with carbon dioxide) in the aorta. Mechanical assistance of the failing circulation. Am. Heart J. *63*:669, 1962.
8. Kantrowitz, A., Tjonneland, S., Freed, P. S., et al.: Initial clinical experience with intra-aortic balloon pumping in cardiogenic shock. JAMA *203*:135, 1968.
9. Mueller, H., Ayres, S., Grace, W., and Giannelli, S.: External counterpulsation—noninvasive method to protect ischemic myocardium in man. Circulation *45*, *46* (Suppl. 2):195, 1972.
10. The Working Group on Mechanical Circulatory Support of the National Heart, Lung and Blood Institute. Artificial Heart and Assist Devices: Directions, needs, costs, societal, and ethical issues. U.S. Department of Health and Human Services. Public Health Service, National Institutes of Health. NIH publication No. 85–2723, p. 9.
11. Bernhard, W. F., Poirier, V., LaFarge, C. G., and Carr, J. G.: A new method for temporary left ventricular bypass: Preclinical appraisal. J. Thorac. Cardiovasc. Surg. *70*:880, 1975.
12. Pierce, W. S., Brighton, J. A., O'Bannon, W., et al.: Complete left ventricular bypass with paracorporeal pump: Design and evaluation. Ann. Surg. *180*:418, 1974.
13. Norman, J. C.: Intracorporeal partial artificial hearts: Initial results in ten patients. Artif. Organs *1*:41, 1977.
14. Boretos, J. W., and Pierce, W. S.: Segmented polyurethane: A new elastomer for biomedical applications. Science *158*:1481, 1967.
15. McEnany, M. T., Kay, H. R., Buckley, M. J., et al.: Clinical experience with intra-aortic balloon pump support in 728 patients. Circulation *58* (Suppl. I):124, 1978.
16. Norman, J. C., Cooley, D. A., Igo, S. R., et al.: Prognostic indices for survival during postcardiotomy intra-aortic balloon pumping. J. Thorac. Cardiovasc. Surg. *74*:709, 1977.
17. DeVries, W. C., Anderson, J. L., Joyce, L. D., et al.: Clinical use of the total artificial heart. N. Engl. J. Med. *310*:273, 1984.
18. Portner, P. M., Oyer, P. E., Pennington, D. G., et al.: Implantable electrical ventricular assist system: Bridge-to-transplantation and the future. Ann. Thorac. Surg. *47*:142, 1989.
19. Phillips, S. J., Zeff, R. H., Kongtahworn, C., et al.: Percutaneous cardiopulmonary bypass: Application and indication for use. Ann. Thorac. Surg. *47*:121, 1989.
20. Frazier, O. H., Nakatani, T., Duncan, J. M., et al.: Clinical experience with the Hemopump. Trans. Am. Soc. Artif. Intern. Organs *35*:604, 1989.
21. Anversa, P., Beghi, C., Kikkawa, Y., and Olivetti, G.: Myocardial response to infarction in the rat. Morphometric measurement of infarct size and myocyte cellular hypertrophy. Am. J. Pathol. *118*:484, 1985.
22. Rich, G. F., Smith, K. W., Murashita, J., et al.: Ischemic dysfunction: Relationship to mechanical rest. Trans. Am. Soc. Artif. Intern. Organs *29*:88, 1983.
23. Gray, R., Maddahi, J., Berman, D., et al.: Scintigraphic and hemodynamic demonstration of transient left ventricular dysfunction immediately after uncomplicated coronary artery bypass grafting. J. Thorac. Cardiovasc. Surg. *77*:504, 1979.
24. Miller, C. A., Pae, W. E., and Pierce, W. S.: Combined registry for the clinical use of mechanical ventricular assist devices: Postcardiotomy cardiogenic shock. Trans. Am. Soc. Artif. Intern. Organs *36*:43, 1990.
25. Termuhlen, D. F., Swartz, M. T., Pennington, D. G., et al.: Predictors for weaning patients from ventricular assist devices. Trans. Am. Soc. Artif. Intern. Organs *34*:131, 1988.
26. Pennington, D. G., McBride, L. R., Kanter, K. R., et al.: The effect of perioperative myocardial infarction on survival of postcardiotomy patients supported with ventricular assist devices. Circulation *78* (Suppl. III):110, 1988.
27. Scheidt, S., Collins, M., Goldstein, J., and Fisher, J.: Mechanical circulatory assistance with intra-aortic balloon pump and other counterpulsation devices. Prog. Cardiovasc. Dis. *25*:55, 1982.
28. Pierce, W. S., Aaronson, A. E., Prophet, G. A., et al.: Hemodynamic and metabolic studies during two types of left ventricular bypass. Surg. Forum *23*:176, 1972.
29. Laks, H., Hahn, J. W., Blair, O., et al.: Cardiac assistance and infarct size: Left atrial-to-aortic vs left ventricular-to-aortic bypass. Surg. Forum *27*:226, 1976.
30. Takanashi, Y., Campbell, C. D., Laas, J., et al.: Reduction of myocardial infarction size in swine: A comparative study of intra-aortic balloon pumping and transapical left ventricular bypass. Ann. Thorac. Surg. *32*:475, 1981.
31. Magovern, G. J., Park, S. B., and Maher, T. D.: Use of a centrifugal pump

without anticoagulants for postoperative left ventricular assist. World J. Surg. 9:25, 1985.
32. Pennington, D. G., McBride, L. R., Swartz, M. T., et al.: Use of the Pierce-Donachy ventricular assist device in patients with cardiogenic shock after cardiac operations. Ann. Thorac. Surg. 47:130, 1989.
33. Dennis, C., Hall, D. P., Moreno, J. R., and Senning, A.: Reduction of the oxygen utilization of the heart by left heart bypass. Circ. Res. 10:298, 1962.
34. Watanabe, K., Kabei, N., McRea, J., and Peters, J.: Continuous measurement of oxygen consumption (MVO_2) and hemodynamic response during transapical left ventricular bypass (TALVB). Trans. Am. Soc. Artif. Intern. Organs 21:566, 1975.
35. Pennock, J., Pierce, W. S., and Waldhausen, J. A.: Quantitative evaluation of left ventricular bypass in reducing myocardial ischemia. Surgery 79:523, 1976.
36. Martin, G. R., and Short, B. L.: Doppler echocardiographic evaluation of cardiac performance in infants on prolonged extracorporeal membrane oxygenation. Am. J. Cardiol. 62:929, 1988.
37. Bavaria, J. E., Ratcliffe, M. B., Gupta, K. B., et al.: Changes in left ventricular systolic wall stress during biventricular circulatory assistance. Ann. Thorac. Surg. 45:526, 1988.
38. Pennington, D. G., Samuels, L. D., Williams, G., et al.: Experience with Pierce-Donachy ventricular assist device in postcardiotomy patients with cardiogenic shock. World J. Surg. 9:37, 1985.
39. Reedy, J. E., Swartz, M. T., Pennington, D. G., et al.: Bridge-to-cardiac transplantation—importance of patient selection. J. Heart Transplant. 9:473, 1990.
39a. Shumway, S. J., and Bolman, R. M. III: Cardiac transplantation and ventricular assist devices. Curr. Opin. Cardiol. 6:269, 1991.
40. Bolooki, H.: Physiology of balloon-pumping. In Bolooki, H. (ed.): Clinical Application of Intra-aortic Balloon Pump. Mount Kisco, NY, Futura, 1984, pp. 57–126.
41. Bavaria, J. E., Furukawa, S., Kreiner, G., et al.: Effect of circulatory assist devices on stunned myocardium. Ann. Thorac. Surg. 49:123, 1990.
42. Pennington, D. G., Swartz, M. T., Codd, J. E., et al.: Intra-aortic balloon pumping in cardiac surgical patients: A nine-year experience. Ann. Thorac. Surg. 36:125, 1983.
43. DiLello, F., Mullen, D. C., Flemmon, R. J., et al.: Results of intra-aortic balloon pumping after cardiac surgery: Experience with the Percor balloon catheter. Ann. Thorac. Surg. 46:442, 1988.
44. Downing, T. P., Miller, D. C., Stofer, R., and Shumway, N. E.: Use of the intra-aortic balloon pump after valve replacement. J. Thorac. Cardiovasc. Surg. 92:210, 1986.
45. Bregman, D., Nicholas, A. B., Weiss, M. B., et al.: Percutaneous intra-aortic balloon insertion. Am. J. Cardiol. 46:261, 1980.
46. McBride, L. R., Miller, L. W., Naunheim, K. S., and Pennington, D. G.: Axillary artery insertion of an intra-aortic balloon pump. Ann. Thorac. Surg. 48:874, 1989.
47. Hardesty, R. L., Griffith, B. P., Trento, A., et al.: Mortally ill patients and excellent survival following cardiac transplantation. Ann. Thorac. Surg. 41:126, 1986.
48. Reedy, J. E., Pennington, D. G., Miller, L. W., et al.: Status I heart transplant patients—conventional vs ventricular assist device support (Abst). J. Heart Transplant. 10:159, 1991.
49. Laschinger, J. C., Cunningham, J. N., Catinella, E. P., et al.: "Pulsatile" left atrial femoral artery bypass: A new method of preventing extension of myocardial infarction. Arch. Surg. 118:965, 1983.
50. Pennington, D. G., Merjavy, J. P., Codd, J. E., et al.: Extracorporeal membrane oxygenation for patients with cardiogenic shock. Circulation 70 (Suppl. I):130, 1984.
51. Reichman, R. T., Joyo, C. I., Dembitsky, W. P., et al.: Improved patient survival after cardiac arrest using a cardiopulmonary support system. Ann. Thorac. Surg. 49:101, 1990.
52. Raithel, S. C., Swartz, M. T., Braun, P. R., et al.: Experience with an emergency resuscitation system. Trans. Am. Soc. Artif. Intern. Organs 35:475, 1989.
53. Pennington, D. G., Codd, J. E., Merjavy, J. P., et al.: The expanded use of ventricular bypass systems for severe cardiac failure and as a bridge to cardiac transplantation. J. Heart Transplant. 3:170, 1984.
54. Wampler, R. K., Moise, J. C., Frazier, O. H., and Olsen, D. B.: In "vivo" evaluation of a peripheral vascular access axial flow blood pump. Trans. Am. Soc. Artif. Intern. Organs 34:450, 1988.
55. Golding, L. R., Groves, L. K., Peter, M., et al.: Initial clinical experience with a new temporary left ventricular assist device. Ann. Thorac. Surg. 29:66, 1980.
56. Pennington, D. G., Merjavy, J. P., Swartz, M. T., and Willman, V. L.: Clinical experience with a centrifugal pump ventricular assist device. Trans. Am. Soc. Artif. Intern. Organs 28:93, 1982.
57. Bolman, R. M., Spray, T. L., Cox, J. L., et al.: Heart transplantation in patients requiring preoperative mechanical support. J. Heart Transplant. 6:273, 1987.
58. Joyce, L. D., Emery, R. W., Eales, F., et al.: Mechanical circulatory support as a bridge-to-cardiac transplantation. J. Thorac. Cardiovasc. Surg. 98:935, 1989.
59. Golding, L.A.R., Stewart, R. W., Sinkewich, M., et al.: Nonpulsatile ventricular assist bridging to transplantation. Trans. Am. Soc. Artif. Intern. Organs 34:476, 1988.
60. Farrar, D. J., Hill, D. J., Gray, L. A., et al.: Heterotopic prosthetic ventricles as a bridge-to-cardiac transplantation. N. Engl. J. Med. 318:333, 1988.
61. Champsaur, G., Ninet, J., Vigneron, M., et al.: Use of the Abiomed BVS 5000 System as a bridge to cardiac transplantation. J. Thorac. Cardiovasc. Surg. 100:122, 1990.
62. McGee, M. C., Parnis, S. M., Nakatani, T., et al.: Extended clinical support with an implantable left ventricular assist device. Trans. Am. Soc. Artif. Intern. Organs 35:614, 1989.
63. Pennington, D. G., Merjavy, J. P., Swartz, M. T., et al.: The importance of biventricular failure in patients with postoperative cardiogenic shock. Ann. Thorac. Surg. 39:16, 1985.
64. DeVries, W. C.: The permanent artificial heart—four case reports. JAMA 259:849, 1988.
65. Joyce, L. D., Johnson, K. E., Toninato, C. J., et al.: Results of the first 100 patients who received Symbion total artificial hearts as a bridge-to-cardiac transplantation. Circulation 80 (Suppl. III):192, 1989.
66. Merhige, M. E., Smalling, R. W., Cassidy, D., et al.: Effect of the Hemopump left ventricular assist device on regional myocardial perfusion and function. Reduction of ischemia during coronary occlusion. Circulation 80 (Suppl. II):III–158, 1989.
67. Kanter, K. R., Swartz, M. T., Pennington, D. G., et al.: Renal failure in patients with ventricular assist devices. Trans. Am. Soc. Artif. Intern. Organs 33:426, 1987.
68. Pennington, D. G., Bernhard, W. F., Golding, L. R., et al.: Long-term follow-up of postcardiotomy patients with profound cardiogenic shock treated with ventricular assist devices. Circulation 72 (Suppl. II):216, 1985.
69. Rose, D. M., Colvin, S. B., Culliford, A. T., et al.: Long-term survival with partial left heart bypass following perioperative myocardial infarction and shock. J. Thorac. Cardiovasc. Surg. 83:483, 1982.
70. Pae, W. E., Pierce, W. S., Pennock, J. L., et al.: Long-term results of ventricular assist pumping in postcardiotomy cardiogenic shock. J. Thorac. Cardiovasc. Surg. 93:434, 1978.
71. Miyamoto, A. T., Tanaka, S., and Matloff, J. M.: Effects of left heart bypass on right ventricular function. Trans. Am. Soc. Artif. Intern. Organs 28:543, 1982.
72. Farrar, D. J., Compton, P. G., Dajee, H., et al.: Right heart function during left heart assist and the effects of volume loading in a canine preparation. Circulation 70:708, 1984.
73. Farrar, D. J., Compton, P. G., Hershon, J. J., et al.: Right ventricular pressure dimension relationship during left ventricular assistance in dogs. Trans. Am. Soc. Artif. Intern. Organs 30:121, 1984.
74. Hershon, J. J., Farrar, D. J., Compton, P. G., and Hill, J. D.: Right ventricular dimensions with transesophageal echocardiography during an operating room model of left heart assist. Trans. Am. Soc. Artif. Intern. Organs 30:129, 1984.
75. Kormos, R. L., Borovetz, H. S., Gasior, T., et al.: Experience with univentricular support in mortally ill cardiac transplant candidates. Ann. Thorac. Surg. 49:261, 1990.
76. Anderson, J. M., and Kottke-Marchant, K.: Platelet interactions with biomaterials and artificial devices. CRC Crit. Rev. Biocompatibility 1:111, 1985.
77. Salzman, E. W., and Merrill, E. W.: Interaction of blood with artificial surfaces. In Colman, R. W., Hirsh, J., Marder, V. J., and Salzman, E. W. (eds.): Hemostasis and Thrombosis. Philadelphia, J. B. Lippincott Company, 1987, p. 1335.
78. Chenoweth, D. E.: Complement activation produced by biomaterials. Trans. Am. Soc. Artif. Intern. Organs 32:226, 1986.
79. Matsuda, T., and Iwata, H.: Mechanistic aspects of in vivo antithrombogenicity of segmented polyurethane. In Akutsu, T. (ed.): Artificial Heart 1. Berlin, Springer-Verlag, 1986, pp. 11–22.
80. Turitto, T., and Baumgartner, H. R.: Platelet-surface interactions. In Colman, R. W., Hirsh, J., Marder, V. J., and Salzman, E. W. (eds.): Hemostasis and Thrombosis. Philadelphia, J. B. Lippincott Company, 1987, p. 555.
81. Joist, J. H., and Pennington, D. G.: Platelet reactions with artificial surfaces. Trans. Am. Soc. Artif. Intern. Organs 33:341, 1987.
82. Didisheim, P., Olsen, D. B., Farrar, D. J., et al.: Infections and thromboembolism with implantable cardiovascular devices. Trans. Am. Soc. Artif. Intern. Organs 35:54, 1989.
83. Monit, R.: Extracorporeal oxygenators. In Hwang, N.H.L., Gross, D. R., and Patel, D. J. (eds.): Quantitative Cardiovascular Studies: Clinical and Research Applications of Engineering Principles. Baltimore, University Park, 1979, p. 593.
84. Levinson, M. M., Copeland, J. G., Smith, R. G., et al.: Indexes of hemolysis in human recipients of the Jarvik-7 total artificial heart: A cooperative report of 15 patients. J. Heart Transplant. 5:236, 1986.
85. Boralessa, H., Shifferli, J. A., Zaime, F., et al.: Perioperative changes in complement associated with cardiopulmonary bypass. Br. J. Anaesth. 54:1047, 1982.
86. Craddock, P. R., Fehr, J., Brigham, K. L., et al.: Complement and leukocyte-mediated pulmonary dysfunction in hemodialysis. N. Engl. J. Med. 196:769, 1977.
87. Chenoweth, D. E., Cooper, S. W., Hugli, T. E., et al.: Complement activation during cardiopulmonary bypass: Evidence for generation of C3a and C5a anaphylatoxins. N. Engl. J. Med. 304:497, 1981.
88. Weaver, L. J., Hudson, L. D., Craddock, P. R., and Jacob, H. S.: Association of complement activation and elevated plasma-C5a with adult respiratory distress syndrome. Lancet 1:947, 1980.
89. Lyakhov, N. T., Zhivoderov, V. M., and Belobrzhek, L. M.: Immunological changes in postoperative myocardial infarction. Khirurgiaa (Mosk) 1:21, 1979.
90. Crawford, M. H., Grover, F. L., O'Rourke, R. A., et al.: Preservation of jeopardized myocardium by C3 depletion in the baboon. Am. Fed. Clin. Res. 27:160A, 1979.

91. Chiu, R. C., and Samson, R.: Complement (C3, C4) consumption in cardiopulmonary bypass, cardioplegia and protamine administration. Ann. Thorac. Surg. *37*:229, 1984.
92. McBride, L. R., Ruzevich, S. A., Pennington, D. G., et al.: Infectious complications associated with ventricular assist device support. Trans. Am. Soc. Artif. Intern. Organs *33*:201, 1987.
93. Termuhlen, D. F., Pennington, D. G., Roodman, S. T., et al.: T-cells in ventricular assist device patients. Circulation *80*(Suppl. III):174, 1989.
94. Gristina, A. G.: Biomaterial-centered infection; microbial adhesion versus tissue integration. Science *237*:1588, 1987.
95. Gristina, A. G., Dobbins, J. J., Giammara, B., et al.: Biomaterial-centered sepsis and the total artificial heart. JAMA *259*:870, 1988.
96. Kunin, C. M., Dobbins, J. J., Melo, J. C., et al.: Infectious complications in four long-term recipients of the Jarvik-7 artificial heart. JAMA *259*:860, 1988.
97. Tikkanen, I., Fyhrquist, F., Metsarenni, K., and Leidenius, R.: Plasma atrial natriuretic peptide in cardiac disease and during infusion in healthy volunteers. Lancet *2*:66, 1985.
98. Cantin, M., and Genest, J.: The heart and the atrial natriuretic factor. Endocrinol. Rev. *6*:107, 1985.
99. Murray, K. D., Myerowitz, P. D., Watson, K. M., et al.: Effect of a total artificial heart on adaptive hormonal responses in humans with end-stage heart failure. Trans. Am. Soc. Artif. Intern. Organs *35*:229, 1989.
100. Trubel, W., Wieselthaler, G., Buxbaum, P., et al.: Atrial natriuretic factor production and secretion during clinical artificial heart bridge-to-transplantation. Trans. Am. Soc. Artif. Intern. Organs *35*:718, 1989.
101. Harker, L. A., Malpass, T. W., Branson, H. E., et al.: Mechanism of abnormal bleeding in patients undergoing cardiopulmonary bypass: Acquired transient platelet dysfunction associated with selective α-granule release. Blood *56*:284, 1980.
102. Griffith, B. P., Kormos, R. L., Hardesty, R. L., et al.: The artificial heart: Infection-related morbidity and its effect on transplantation. Ann. Thorac. Surg. *45*:409, 1988.
103. Farrar, D. J., Lawson, J. H., Litwak, P., and Cederwall, G.: Thoratec VAD system as a bridge to heart transplantation. J. Heart Transplant. *9*:415, 1990.
104. Swartz, M. T., Pennington, D. G., Ruzevich, S. A., et al.: The incidence of isolated left ventricular failure in bridge-to-transplant patients. Trans. Am. Soc. Artif. Intern. Organs *35*:730, 1989.
105. Evans, R. W., Mannion, D. L., Garrison, L. P., Jr., and Maier, A. M.: Donor availability as the primary determinant of the future of heart transplantation. JAMA *255*:1892, 1986.

Pulmonary Edema: Cardiogenic and Noncardiogenic

by ROLAND H. INGRAM, Jr., M.D., and EUGENE BRAUNWALD, M.D.

THE ALVEOLAR-CAPILLARY MEMBRANE AND PULMONARY EDEMA

Pulmonary edema develops when the movement of liquid from the blood to the interstitial space and in some instances to the alveoli exceeds the return of liquid to the blood and its drainage through the lymphatics.[1] Integral to an understanding of the pathogenesis of pulmonary edema is a comprehension of the structure of the alveolar-capillary membrane.[1a]

STRUCTURE OF THE ALVEOLAR-CAPILLARY MEMBRANE

The barrier between pulmonary capillaries and alveolar gas consists of a series of three anatomical layers with distinct structural characteristics (Figs. 20–1 and 20–2).

(1) The cytoplasmic projections of the *capillary endothelial cells* join by abutment or interdigitation or overlap to form a continuous cytoplasmic tube. At the overlapping junctions of these cytoplasmic projections are clefts of varying sizes, averaging approximately 4 nm in width, which provide communication between pulmonary capillaries and the interstitial space. Because these clefts can be widened with relatively small increases in vascular pressure, they are referred to as "loose" junctions. Although thin cytoplasmic projections result in maximal area for gas exchange with minimal tissue mass, these tenuous projections and junctions may be unusually vulnerable to disruption.[2] One side of the pulmonary capillary generally abuts the interalveolar septum (Fig. 20–2); with elevation of pressure, the pulmonary capillary endothelial cells may swell.[1]

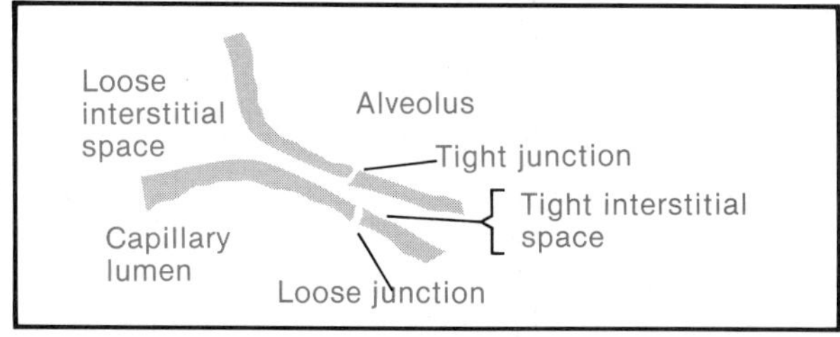

FIGURE 20–1. Schematic representation of the ultrastructure of the alveolar-capillary membrane. (Labeling corresponds to the discussion in the text.)

(2) The *interstitial space* varies in thickness and may contain connective tissue fibrils, fibroblasts, and macrophages between the capillary endothelium and the alveolar epithelium. There are no lymphatics in the alveolar-capillary interstitium. This interstitial space of the alveolar-capillary septum is continuous with the wider and more compliant space sur-

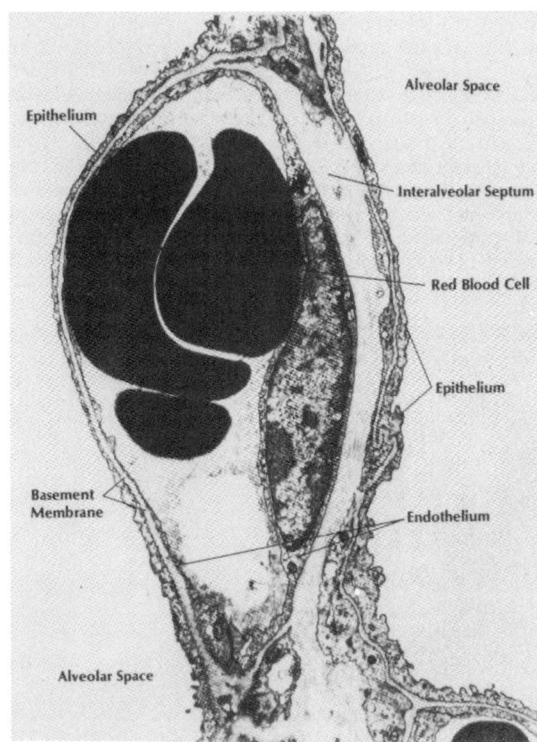

FIGURE 20–2. Electrophotomicrograph showing alveolar-capillary function. Capillaries in alveolar wall are arranged to create a "thin" portion of the alveolar-capillary barrier on one side *(left);* alveolar epithelium, basement membrane, and endothelium are attenuated in this region and air-to-blood gas diffusion distance is less than 1 μm. The "thick" side of the capillary in the alveolar wall *(right)* faces the interalveolar septum and contains abundant interstitial connective tissue fibrils, ground substance, and cells. (From Murray, J. F.: The lungs and heart failure. Hosp. Pract. *20*:63, 1985.)

rounding terminal bronchioles, small arteries, and veins, and it is in this latter portion of the interstitial space that lymphatic channels first appear. The lymphatics serve to remove solutes, colloids, and liquid derived from the blood vessels. Because of a more negative pressure in the peribronchial and perivascular interstitial space and the increased compliance of this nonalveolar interstitium, liquid is more likely to increase here once the pumping capacity of the lymphatic channels is exceeded. As a consequence of the development of interstitial edema, small airways and blood vessels may become compressed.

(3) The *lining of the alveolar wall*, which is continuous with the bronchial epithelium, is composed predominantly of large squamous cells (Type I) with thin cytoplasmic projections. Many fewer granular pneumocytes (Type II) join with the Type I cells to form the alveolar epithelium. Similar to the junctions of capillary endothelium, the projections of the alveolar cells abut and overlap. In contrast to the endothelial junctions, which allow for variable continuity between blood vessels and interstitial space, the alveolar epithelial clefts are obliterated by complete fusion of the membranes of the adjacent cells. Because the alveolar intercellular unions require much greater distending forces for their disruption than do the capillary endothelial connections, the former are referred to as "tight" junctions. The *tightness* of these junctions helps to forestall alveolar flooding, which represents the third and final stage of pulmonary edema. Although its principal function is to maintain alveolar stability, surfactant, the hydrophobic lipoprotein that lines the alveoli, may represent an additional mechanism for maintaining a dry alveolus.

CAPILLARY-INTERSTITIAL LIQUID EXCHANGE IN THE LUNG (THE STARLING RELATIONSHIP). As in other tissues, there is normally a continuous exchange of liquid, colloid, and solutes between the vascular bed and interstitium[3,4] (Fig. 20–3). A pathological state exists only when there is an increase in the net flux of liquids, colloids, and solutes from the vasculature into the interstitial space (Fig. 20–4). Experimental studies have confirmed that the basic principles outlined in the classic Starling equation apply to the lung as well as to the systemic circulation. The equation describes the net flux of liquid between capillaries and interstitium in terms of hydraulic conductance (K_f), which is a function of area and conductivity per unit area, and the balance of the total forces tending to move liquid out of the capillary into the interstitial space and those that act to move liquid into the capillary from the interstitial space. Liquid accumulation in the lung is determined by the net flux between the vascular and interstitial spaces (which is in turn determined by the algebraic sum of vascular and interstitial hydrostatic and colloid osmotic pressures) and the rate of lymphatic drainage. That is to say, there will be an undetectable net accumulation of liquid in the lung with time if the rate of transudation of

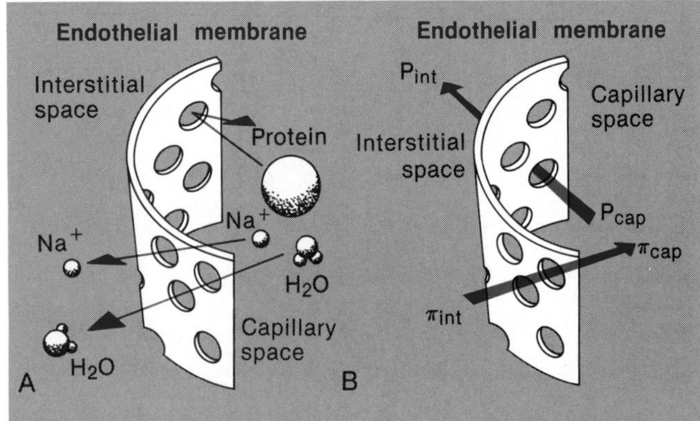

FIGURE 20–3. ***A,*** **The lung endothelial membrane is permeable to water and electrolytes, but less permeable to macromolecules.** ***B,*** **The Starling equation: $\dot{Q}_f = K(P_{cap} - P_{int}) - K\sigma(\pi_{cap} - \pi_{int})$ where $\dot{Q}_f$ is the net fluid filtration rate, K is the filtration coefficient, σ is the reflection coefficient. $(P_{cap} - P_{int})$ is the hydrostatic pressure gradient from the capillary lumen to interstitial space, and $(\pi_{cap} - \pi_{int})$ is the oncotic pressure difference across the capillary membrane. (From Prichard, J. S., Lee, G. de J.: Pulmonary Oedema, in Weatherall, D. J., Ledingham, J. G. G., Warrell, D. A., (eds.): Oxford Textbook of Medicine, 2nd ed., Oxford, Oxford University Press, 1987.)**

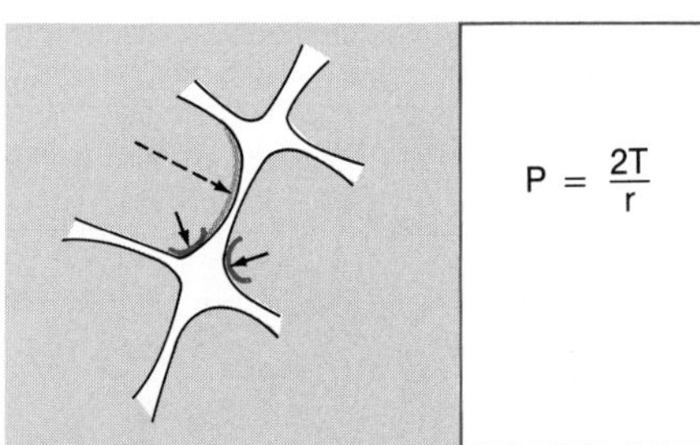

FIGURE 20–4. Schematic representation of the junction of several alveoli. The radii of curvature of a single alveolus vary considerably. The portion of the alveolar wall at which the radius of curvature is small (solid arrows) will tend toward greater local recoil pressures according to the Laplace relationship (P = 2T/r, where P = transmural pressure, T = surface tension, and r = the local radius of curvature). Since pressure in communicating alveoli is the same relative to atmospheric pressure, differences in transmural pressure result in different local interstitial pressures. It is in that portion of the interstitial space beneath smaller radii that liquid would first accumulate under conditions of increased transduction. These portions of the wall with greater radii of curvature (dashed arrow) would have smaller transmural pressures and hence would accumulate less liquid.

liquid from the blood vessels to the interstitial space is equal to the rate of removal of liquid from the interstitial space by way of the lymphatics ($\dot{Q}_{lymph}$). The rate of transudation from blood vessels can be expressed either as the balance of those forces acting to move liquid out of and those acting to move liquid into the vessels (Eq. 1) or as the balance of hydrostatic and colloid osmotic forces (Eq. 2) (Fig. 20–5):

$$\dot{Q}_{(iv\text{-}int)} \propto K_f[\underbrace{(P_{iv} + \Pi_{int})}_{\text{Outward force}} - \underbrace{(P_{int} + \Pi_{iv})}_{\text{Inward force}}] \quad (1)$$

$$\dot{Q}_{(iv\text{-}int)} = K_f[\underbrace{P_{iv} - P_{int})}_{\text{Hydrostatic force}} - \underbrace{\sigma_f(\Pi_{iv} - \Pi_{int})}_{\text{Colloid osmotic force}}] \quad (2)$$

where

$\dot{Q}$ = net rate of transudation (flow of liquid from blood vessels to interstitial space)
P_{int} = interstitial hydrostatic pressures
P_{iv} = intravascular hydrostatic pressures
Π_{int} = interstitial colloid osmotic pressure
Π_{iv} = intravascular colloid osmotic pressure
σ_f = reflection coefficient for proteins
K_f = hydraulic conductance. Thus, the Starling relationship is analogous to Ohm's law, because transvascular flow equals conductance times driving pressure.

Although the traditional Starling relationship has in the past been considered to apply to the transfer of liquid between pulmonary vasculature

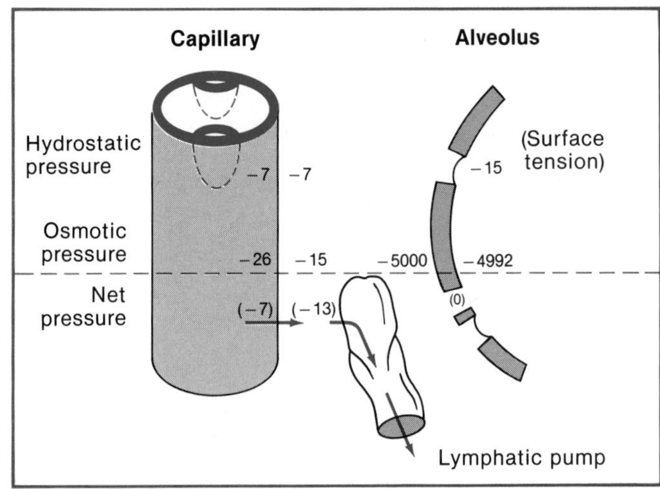

FIGURE 20–5. Pressures causing fluid movement between lung water compartments. Pressures are expressed as mm Hg. (From Prichard, J. S.: Edema of the Lung. Springfield, Ill., Charles C Thomas, 1982.)

and alveolar space, it is clear from both the structural and the functional standpoints outlined above that this relationship applies mainly to the transfer between blood vessels and interstitial space. Although the equations are straightforward and set the stage for designating cardiogenic versus noncardiogenic pulmonary edema, there are many specific points to be made with regard to quantitative assessments.

VARIABLES AMENABLE TO MEASUREMENT. An estimate of pulmonary capillary pressure (P_{iv}) can be obtained from capillary wedge or left atrial pressure measurements.

Pulmonary artery wedge or left atrial pressures. These are equal to pulmonary capillary pressures only if venous resistance is assumed to be negligible. It has been estimated that 40 per cent of the pulmonary vascular resistance resides in the veins in normal lungs. To the extent that the venous system contributes to the pressure drop across the pulmonary circulation from the main pulmonary artery to the left atrium, both wedge and left atrial pressures will be lower than the true capillary filtration pressure. Holloway and colleagues devised a method to calculate capillary pressure by analyzing the pressure-time plot of the fall in pulmonary arterial pressure following balloon occlusion.[5] The initial, rapid pressure fall is thought to represent the discharge of elastic energy stored in the large pulmonary arteries through the arteriolar bed and the second, slow component is the discharge of elastic energy stored in the capillaries through the venous resistance. This indirect technique produced capillary pressures quite close to those determined by isogravimetric techniques. In a clinical setting this technique has been used to show that the wedge pressure underestimates the capillary pressure by a mean of 7 mm Hg.[6]

Plasma colloid osmotic pressure. (Π_{iv}) This can be determined by means of an osmometer. However, accurate measurements of interstitial colloid osmotic pressures (Π_{int}) and interstitial hydrostatic pressures (P_{int}) continue to be elusive. With regard to Π_{int}, it has been frequently assumed in experimental studies that values obtained for lymph or for the free space of implanted capsules are representative of interstitial liquid. However, Staub has pointed out that such assumptions are ill-founded, since interstitial liquid is not homogeneous, and lymph from the lung collected experimentally may be contaminated with lymph from other tissues. Interstitial hydrostatic pressure is equally elusive, but the assumption is often made that pleural pressures or hydrostatic pressures in implanted capsules are closely related to interstitial pressure. Direct measurements using micropipettes inserted into the perivascular interstitium of hilar vessels of dog lungs indicate, indeed, that P_{int} is more negative than pleural pressure and that the difference increases at higher lung volumes.[7] However, the difference is small, and pleural pressure is probably sufficiently close to interstitial hydrostatic pressure to be useful as a clinical index.

The reflection coefficient (σ_f in Equation 2 above) is often considered to be 1.0 in experimental studies, i.e., the capillary membrane does not allow colloids to pass. In fact, as can be anticipated from the existence of the clefts between cells (loose junctions) described above and possibly through pinocytotic vesicles in the capillary endothelial projections, macromolecules can and do pass into the interstitial space. This is reflected by the fact that the mean lymph to plasma protein ratio is 0.75 in experimental animals. The larger the molecule, the higher the reflection coefficient and the smaller the lymph to plasma ratio.[8] Hence the lymphatic proteins are predominantly of the smaller variety. Any disruption of the endothelial barrier produced either by increasing P_{iv} or by direct toxins will result in greater passage of macromolecules into the interstitium, which in turn increases Π_{int} and results in the passage of greater quantities of liquid.

ROLE OF LYMPHATICS IN THE LUNGS. As stated above, the lymphatics play a key role in removing liquid from the interstitial space, and unless the pumping capacity of the lymphatic channels is exceeded, edema will occur.

$$\dot{Q}_{(iv\text{-}int)} - \dot{Q}_{lymph} = \text{Rate of accumulation} \qquad (3)$$

where $\dot{Q}$ = flow, iv = intravascular, and int = interstitial.

Although there is no direct way to measure lymph flow in humans, on the basis of extrapolation from animal data, Staub has estimated that an average 70-kg person at rest has a $\dot{Q}_{lymph}$ of approximately 20 ml per hour.[9] Experimentally, lymph flow rates of up to 10 times control values have been reported. Thus, it is possible that lymphatic pumping capacity can be as much as 200 ml per hour in an average-sized adult. It is probable that there would be some measurable accumulation of liquid in the lung before this capacity were reached, but it should be clear that there is an enormous lymphatic reserve. Given the capacity of lymphatic pumping, it can readily be comprehended that complete interruption of lymph flow, as with experiments on isolated lungs or in animals that have had surgical excision and reimplantation of the lung,[10] would result in much more rapid accumulation of interstitial liquid at any given rate of transudation from vessels.

Studies in the dog have shown that with chronic elevations of left atrial pressure, the pulmonary lymphatic system hypertrophies and is able to transport greater quantities of capillary filtrate during acute edematogenic incidents, thus prolonging survival.[11] On the basis of these experimental findings it is tempting to speculate that chronic increases in left atrial pressure in human disease might result in the same adaptive changes in the lymphatics that protect the lungs from edema during acute insults. A sudden marked increase in pulmonary capillary pressure can be rapidly fatal in a patient or animal not preconditioned by growth of the lymphatic drainage system. The same hemodynamic abnormality may be well tolerated in the presence of well-developed lymphatics. Also, since pulmonary lymph drains into the thoracic duct and from these into the systemic venous bed, when systemic venous pressure is elevated, lymph flow is impeded and the formation of pulmonary edema at any given level of pulmonary microvascular pressure is enhanced.[12]

Since the lymphatic channels are so important in determining the net accumulation of interstitial liquid in the lung, it is worthwhile to consider how liquids and colloids get into these channels and the manner by which they are then transferred to the systemic circulation. Normally, filtered liquid does not accumulate in the less compliant interstitial space of the alveolar-capillary septum but moves into the more compliant interstitial space that surrounds the bronchioles, venules, and arterioles. As noted earlier, it is in this latter interstitial space that the lymphatic channels are found.

MOVEMENT OF LIQUIDS AND COLLOIDS FROM THE TIGHT INTERSTITIUM OF THE ALVEOLAR-CAPILLARY SEPTUM TO THE MORE COMPLIANT INTERSTITIAL SPACE. It has been suggested that the forces resulting from the geometrical configuration of adjacent alveoli serve as a means of collecting liquid.[13] Figure 20–4 shows this configuration schematically. Through the Laplace relationship, the smaller radius of curvature at the corners results in greater local recoil pressures (hence more negative interstitial pressures) than occur at portions with greater radii of curvature. The resulting hydrostatic gradient would result in transfer of liquid to those junctions with smaller radii of curvature. Indeed, after subpleural injections of dye-containing saline into cat lung, rapid accumulation of dye at such corners has been demonstrated. Within several minutes, the dye appears in the loose connective tissue spaces where the lymph capillaries are located. The more negative pressure and the greater compliance of this loose interstitial space favor collection of liquid here. Thus, there is a relatively direct pathway from the alveolar-capillary septum to the site of lymphatic channels. How liquids and colloids get into the lymphatic channels is not known. Increased permeability of the lymphatic walls with passive movement according to hydrostatic pressure gradients has been suggested,[14] yet with no experimental support. It has also been suggested that the pinocytotic vesicles within the lymphatic capillary endothelium serve to transfer liquid and protein into these channels; however, two studies have failed to demonstrate active transport.[15] Some structural data have supported the proposition that the fine fibrillar attachments of connective tissue to the edges of the cytoplasmic projections at points of juncture serve as one-way valve mechanisms.[16] These fibrils are thought to expand the lymph-capillary lumen and open junctions during tissue swelling, thus opening the drainage pathway when tissue pressure rises. Conversely, as lymph pressure rises, the junctions close.

MOVEMENT THROUGH THE LYMPHATICS. Once inside the lymphatic channels, liquids and colloids are driven to major channels and ultimately to the systemic venous circulation. It had long been thought that only extrinsic forces were responsible for the propulsion of lymph through these valved channels, i.e., respiratory movements and vascular pulsations were thought to massage the lymphatics and result in unidirectional movement due to the valves in the lymphatic capillaries. Although there is no doubt that extrinsic forces influence the rate of lymph movement, it is now well established in experimental animals that lymphatic capillaries are actively contractile. Factors that control or regulate contraction of lymphatic capillaries and any change in their contractile properties under conditions of increased liquid and colloid filtration remain to be elucidated.

SEQUENCE OF LIQUID ACCUMULATION DURING PULMONARY EDEMA

Whether initiated by an imbalance of Starling forces or by primary damage to the various components of the alveolar-capillary membranes, the sequence of liquid exchange and accumulation in the lungs is the same (Fig. 20–6). It can be represented as three separate stages, the last of which has two substages that occur closely in time,[17,18] and two possible routes; one direct and the other indirect. These 3 stages of liquid accumulation in the lungs are shown schematically in Figure 20–7. As just discussed, the top portion demonstrates that normally there is continuous movement of liquid and colloid from the vessels to the interstitial space and that lymphatic channels constantly pump this liquid and colloid into the systemic venous system to maintain a constant interstitial volume.

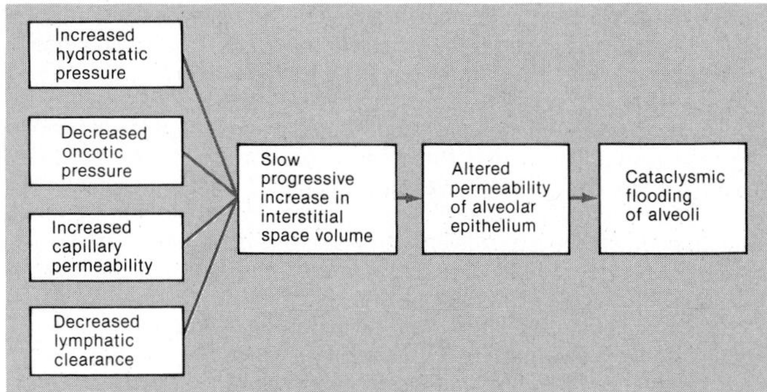

FIGURE 20-6. The initiation of pulmonary edema and the sequence of development. (From Prichard, J. S., and Lee, G. de J.: Pulmonary oedema. *In* Weatherall, D. J., et al.: Oxford Textbook of Medicine. 2nd ed. Oxford, Oxford University Press, 1987.)

In *Stage 1*, there is an increase in mass transfer of liquid and colloid from blood capillaries through the interstitium. The pulmonary capillary endothelial junctions may have been widened by an increase in filtrative forces or by toxic damage. Despite the increased filtration, there is no measurable increase in interstitial volume because there is an equal increase in lymphatic outflow. The stimulus or mechanism for increased lymph flow is not clear, yet it is possible that small increases in interstitial volume that defy detection by present techniques stimulate stretch receptors, resulting in tachypnea and, in turn, extrinsically augmenting lymphatic pumping.[2] Furthermore, it is possible that the same stimulus somehow augments the intrinsic lymphatic pumping capacity.

When the filtered load from the pulmonary capillaries is sufficiently large, the pumping capacity of the lymphatics is approached or exceeded, and liquid and colloid then begin to accumulate in the more compliant interstitial compartment surrounding bronchioles, arterioles, and venules. This is designated *Stage 2*.

With further increments in filtered load, the volume limits of the loose interstitial spaces are exceeded, causing distention of the less compliant interstitial space of the alveolar-capillary septum. As already mentioned, there are two possible roles for alveolar flooding. The first is *indirect* due to overflow from bronchioles, whose epithelium provides less of a barrier to liquid and solutes, into alveoli. This is the overflow, or "bathtub hypothesis" of Staub. The second is *direct* with pressures sufficient to disrupt the tight junctions of the alveolar membranes so that alveolar edema results. In early alveolar edema (*Stage 3A*), liquid accumulates at the corners of alveolar-capillary membranes where the radii of curvature are the smallest. Alveolar flooding (*Stage 3B*) occurs when alveoli reach a critical configuration at which inflation pressures can no longer maintain the existing configuration, and the alveolar gas volume rapidly decreases, being replaced by liquid and macromolecules. At this final stage of alveolar flooding, disruption of all components of the alveolar-capillary membrane occurs, irrespective of the initiating events. If the major route of flooding is via the overflow, or indirect, route, alveolar-capillary membranes would be intact and active resorption of liquid and solutes by alveolar epithelium would occur more readily and quickly. The rapidity of clearing of cardiogenic or hemodynamic pulmonary edema could be explained by there being minimal, if any, damage to the alveolar epithelium.

Indeed the intact alveolar epithelium appears to play an extremely important and *active* role in clearing liquid from the alveolar surface. It is well known that the fetal alveolar membrane actively secretes liquid into the alveoli and that this process is both active and rapid in the reverse direction at birth.[19] This solute coupled liquid transport is mainly through a Na^+, K^+-ATPase mechanism that pumps liquid from the alveoli to the interstitial space in the immediate postnatal period and continues to function into adulthood. Experimental data indicate that this mechanism can be modulated by beta-adrenergic stimulation and is important for maintenance of a dry alveolar surface.[20]

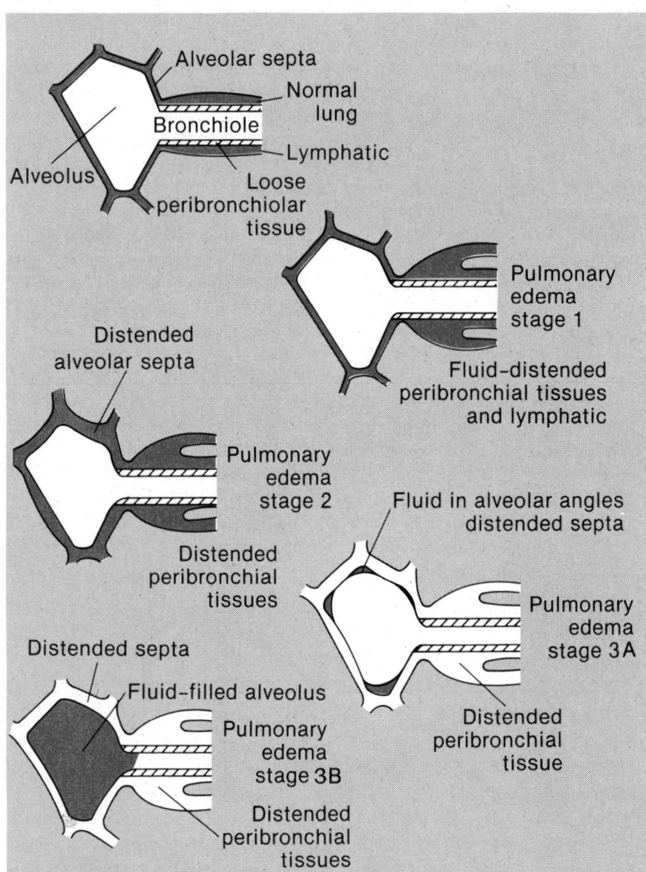

FIGURE 20-7. Stages in the development of pulmonary edema. Stage 1-peribronchial swelling: stage 2-distended alveolar septa; stage 3A-limited accumulation of fluid in alveolar angles; stage 3B-alveolar flooding. (From Prichard, J. S.: Edema of the lung. Springfield, Charles C Thomas, 1982.)

GRAVITY-DEPENDENT DISTRIBUTION OF PULMONARY EDEMA AND PULMONARY BLOOD FLOW

The foregoing discussion dealt with the forces across the alveolar-capillary membranes as if they were homogeneously distributed throughout the lung. However, it is well known that neither lung tissue forces nor intravascular pressures are homogeneous and that major interregional nonhomogeneities exist owing to the differential effects of gravity on blood, gas-containing lung tissue, and air. Since blood is more dense (i.e., heavier) than gas-containing lung, the effects of gravity are much greater on the distribution of blood flow than on the distribution of tissue forces in the lung. From apex to base, the effective perfusion pressure of the pulmonary circulation (P_{pa}) increases by approximately 1.00 cm H_2O/cm vertical distance, whereas pleural pressures (P_{pl}) increase by only 0.25 cm H_2O/cm vertical distance.[21] Pulmonary capillaries (or alveolar vessels) are exposed to alveolar pressure (P_{alv}), which does not vary from apex to base. In contrast, pulmonary arteries, arterioles, veins, and venules (extraalveolar vessels) are exposed to pleural pressure, which does vary from apex to base. The consequences of these differences in forces on ventilation-perfusion relationships have been well described.

ZONE 1. As shown in Figure 20-8, in Zone 1, pulmonary arterial pressure is less than alveolar pressure; thus there is no flow. Indeed, rapid-freezing techniques in animals have confirmed that apical capillaries are bloodless.[22] On the other hand, gamma-emitting isotope studies in normal humans in-

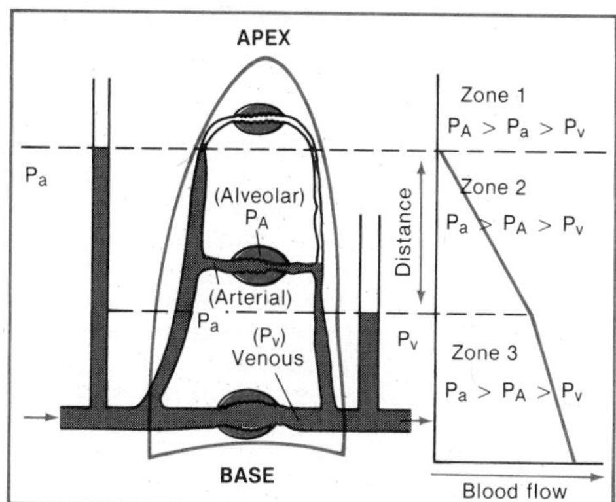

FIGURE 20-8. Schematic representation of the gravity-dependent, apex-to-base distribution of pulmonary blood flow in an upright lung. Pulmonary artery pressure (P_a) and pulmonary venous pressure (P_v) increase on a hydrostatic basis as the base is approached. Alveolar pressure (P_A) is constant with vertical distance. (The three zones are described at length in the text.)

dicate that, although blood flow is strikingly diminished at the apex, no *true* Zone 1 (with total absence of flow) exists.[23]

ZONE 2. In this zone, arterial pressure exceeds alveolar pressure, which in turn exceeds venous pressure. Here, each vessel is similar to a collapsible tube in a pressure chamber. An analogy has been drawn between these vessels and a Starling resistor, which has the following interesting property: When chamber pressure (analogous to alveolar pressure) exceeds the downstream pressure (analogous to venous pressure), the pressure drop for flow is not equal to the difference between upstream (arterial) and downstream (venous) pressures but rather to the difference between upstream (arterial) and chamber (alveolar) pressures. It is in this zone that large increases in flow occur per unit of distance of descent down the lung. These are due to significant increases in perfusing pressures with no change in alveolar pressures.

ZONE 3. In this zone, venous pressure exceeds alveolar pressure, resulting in distention of collapsible capillaries. Mean intravascular pressures are greatest in this zone; hence, with elevations of venous pressure or with disruption of alveolar-capillary membranes, edema formation is both more rapid and greatest here. It is only in this zone that the usual calculation of pulmonary vascular resistance is valid, and it is the only zone in which a valid pulmonary capillary wedge pressure measurement can be obtained. Increases in blood flow with increasing distance from the apex are more gradual in this zone because increases in pulmonary arterial pressures are offset by identical increases in venous pressures. The basis for the increase in flow with distance is the greater mean distending intravascular pressure with greater distention of the vessels as the base is approached.

VASCULAR REDISTRIBUTION. Thus, in normal, erect humans, perfusion is greater in the basilar lung regions than in the more apical ones. Deviation from this gravity-dependent pattern has been called vascular redistribution. There are several ways to view the phenomenon of redistribution. Any encroachment of Zone 1 upon Zone 2 secondary to increased pulmonary venous pressure is, in a sense, redistribution, since regional blood flow is distributed differently after such a change. In like manner, greater relative perfusion of Zone 2 with increases in pulmonary artery pressure distributes more blood to the apex. However, true redistribution is generally considered to be a relative reduction in perfusion of the bases with a relative increase in apical perfusion. This phenomenon is most likely due to compression of the lumina of basilar vessels secondary to the greater and more rapid formation of edema at the lung bases and the tendency for extravascular liquid formed elsewhere to gravitate toward the bases. In addition, pulmonary arteriolar constriction secondary to alveolar hypoxia, which may also contribute to this redistribution, is more prominent at the lung bases. Several experimental studies either imply[24] or demonstrate[25] that vascular redistribution occurs only *after* the acute onset of alveolar edema. If this were the case in human disease, as it seems likely to be, redistribution should be no more subtle a finding than auscultatory abnormalities.

The situation with *chronic* elevations of left atrial pressure, as in mitral stenosis or chronic congestive heart failure, should be contrasted with that of *acute* pulmonary edema. Clinical experience with such chronic conditions suggests that redistribution of flow does occur with minimal or no evidence of interstitial edema and in the absence of alveolar edema. Because of the pathological changes found in such lungs at postmortem examination,[26] i.e., interstitial fibrosis of basilar lung regions and narrowing of basilar arteries and arterioles by lesions that often occur with pulmonary hypertension (p. 790), it is more likely that redistribution is secondary to such changes.

CLASSIFICATION OF PULMONARY EDEMA

The two most common forms of pulmonary edema are those initiated by an imbalance of Starling forces and those initiated by disruption of one or more components of the alveolar-capillary membrane (Table 20-1).[27-29] Less often, lymphatic insufficiency can be involved as a predisposing, if not initiating, factor in the genesis of edema. Although the initiating or primary mechanism may be clearly identifiable, multiple factors come into play during the development of edema, and irrespective of the initiating event, the stage of alveolar flooding is characterized to some degree by disruption of the alveolar-capillary membrane.

IMBALANCE OF STARLING FORCES

Increased pulmonary capillary pressure is a straightforward initiating event, whether due to mitral stenosis, left ventricular failure, or pulmonary venoocclusive disease. It has been found in experimental animals that pulmonary edema will occur only when the pulmonary capillary pressure rises to values exceeding the plasma colloid osmotic pressure, which is approximately 28 mm Hg in the human. Since the normal pulmonary capillary pressure is about 8 mm Hg, there is a margin of safety of approximately 20 mm Hg in the development of pulmonary edema.[4] Although pulmonary capillary wedge pressures must be abnormally high to increase the flow of interstitial liquid, at a time when edema is clearly present, these pressures may not correlate with the severity of pulmonary edema.[30] In fact, pulmonary capillary wedge pressures may have returned to normal at a time when there is still considerable pulmonary edema, since time is required for removal of both interstitial and alveolar edema. Other factors obscure the relationship between the severity of edema and measured pulmonary capillary pressures in addition to slower rates of removal after edema has collected. The rate of increase in lung liquid at any given elevation of capillary pressure is related to the functional capacity of lymphatics,[31] which may vary from patient to patient, and to variations in interstitial oncotic and hydrostatic pressures.

The question of increased capillary pressures secondary to increased pulmonary artery pressure due to overperfusion is difficult to place in a clinical context.[32] Indeed, experimental resection of well over half the pulmonary capillary bed has been required to produce pulmonary edema.[33] The most relevant clinical observation has been the description of pulmonary edema in one lung or lobe following the creation of an end-to-end shunt from a systemic artery to a single pulmonary artery for the treatment of cyanotic congenital heart disease.[34] The question might be raised of why pulmonary edema does not occur with severe pulmonary hypertension (e.g., primary pulmonary hypertension). The obvious answer is that the arteriolar bed is severely narrowed in the latter instance, and thus capillaries are not exposed to the increased pressure, whereas in the former instance, the arteriolar bed is not narrowed, and increased pressures are found in the pulmonary capillaries.

HYPOALBUMINEMIA. This is well known to produce dependent systemic edema without elevations of systemic venous pressures. In contrast, pulmonary edema does *not* develop with hypoalbuminemia alone. Hypoalbuminemia may alter the fluid conductivity of the interstitial gel so that liquid moves more easily between capillaries and lymphatics to add to the lymphatic safety factor.[35] Thus, there must be, in addition to hypoalbuminemia, some elevations of pulmonary capillary pressure, albeit only small increases are necessary before pulmonary edema ensues. Indeed, in such patients, only moderate fluid overload can precipitate overt pulmonary edema in the absence of left ventricular failure.

INCREASED NEGATIVITY OF INTERSTITIAL PRESSURE. When this is due to rapid removal of pleural air for relief of a relatively complete pneumothorax, it may be associated with pulmonary edema. Usually, the pneumothorax has been present for several hours to days, allowing time for alterations in surfactant, so that large negative pressures are necessary to open collapsed alveoli.[36] In this instance the edema is unilateral and is most often only a radiographic finding with few clinical findings.

Large negative pleural pressures thought to approximate interstitial pressures have been shown experimentally to increase the rate of edema formation in sheep.[37] It has been shown that the degree of negativity of the mean intrapleural pressure in asthma correlates with the severity of an attack and speculated that there might be associated pulmonary edema, although it is radiographically inapparent owing to the hyperinflation of the lung in this condition. This interesting hypothesis should be tested, since asthma is a common condition that is often treated with large volumes of intravenous fluids. Animal experiments involving inspiratory loading and increased lung volume as a means of increasing pleural pressure swings have demonstrated increases in left atrial transmural pressures along with diminution in left ventricular end-diastolic dimensions and decreases in cardiac output.[38-40] Thus, it is possible that diminution of left ventricular diastolic filling and an elevation of left atrial pressures accompany such large negative intrapleural pressures.

INCREASED INTERSTITIAL ONCOTIC PRESSURE. There is no known clinical or experimental example of pulmonary edema initiated by this mechanism. However, after the appearance of increased concentrations of macromolecules in the liquid of the interstitium or in alveoli, extravascular oncotic forces undoubtedly serve to intensify and perpetuate the process of edema formation.

TABLE 20-1 CLASSIFICATION OF PULMONARY EDEMA BASED UPON INITIATING MECHANISM

I. Imbalance of Starling Forces
- A. Increased pulmonary capillary pressure
  1. Increased pulmonary venous pressure without left ventricular failure (e.g., mitral stenosis)
  2. Increased pulmonary venous pressure secondary to left ventricular failure
  3. Increased pulmonary capillary pressure secondary to increased pulmonary arterial pressure (so-called overperfusion pulmonary edema)*
- B. Decreased plasma oncotic pressure
  1. Hypoalbuminemia secondary to renal, hepatic, protein-losing enteropathic, or dermatological disease or nutritional causes†
- C. Increased negativity of interstitial pressure
  1. Rapid removal of pneumothorax with large applied negative pressures (unilateral)
  2. Large negative pleural pressures due to acute airway obstruction along with increased end-expiratory volumes (asthma)*
- D. Increased interstitial oncotic pressure
  1. No known clinical or experimental example

II. Altered Alveolar-Capillary Membrane Permeability (Adult Respiratory Distress Syndrome)
- A. Infectious pneumonia—bacterial, viral, parasitic
- B. Inhaled toxins (e.g., phosgene, ozone, chlorine, Teflon fumes, nitrogen dioxide, smoke)
- C. Circulating foreign substances (e.g., snake venom, bacterial endotoxins, alloxan‡, alpha-naphthyl thiourea‡)
- D. Aspiration of acidic gastric contents
- E. Acute radiation pneumonitis
- F. Endogenous vasoactive substances (e.g., histamine, kinins*)
- G. Disseminated intravascular coagulation
- H. Immunological-hypersensitivity pneumonitis, drugs (nitrofurantoin), leukoagglutinins
- I. Shock lung in association with nonthoracic trauma
- J. Acute hemorrhagic pancreatitis

III. Lymphatic Insufficiency
- A. Post lung transplant
- B. Lymphangitic carcinomatosis
- C. Fibrosing lymphangitis (e.g., silicosis)

IV. Unknown or Incompletely Understood
- A. High-altitude pulmonary edema
- B. Neurogenic pulmonary edema
- C. Narcotic overdose
- D. Pulmonary embolism
- E. Eclampsia
- F. Post cardioversion
- G. Post anesthesia
- H. Post cardiopulmonary bypass

* Not certain to exist as a clinical entity.
† Not certain that this, as a single factor, leads to clinical pulmonary edema.
‡ Predominantly an experimental technique.

PRIMARY ALVEOLAR-CAPILLARY MEMBRANE DAMAGE

Many diverse medical and surgical conditions are associated with pulmonary edema that appears to be due not to primary alteration in Starling forces but rather to damage of the alveolar-capillary membrane (Table 20-1). These conditions include acute pulmonary infections and pulmonary effects of gram-negative septicemia and nonthoracic trauma as well as any condition associated with disseminated intravascular coagulation.[27,28,41-43] Despite the diversity of underlying causes, once diffuse alveolar-capillary injury has occurred, the pathophysiological and clinical sequence of events is quite similar in most patients. Because of the resemblance of the clinical picture to that seen with respiratory distress of the neonate, these conditions have been referred to as the *adult respiratory distress syndrome* (ARDS). This similarity includes the superimposition of secondary factors, either occurring spontaneously or induced by therapeutic interventions, that serve to perpetuate or worsen the clinical course. An example of a spontaneously occurring secondary factor is the appearance of left ventricular failure with elevation of pulmonary capillary pressure during the course of the illness; a frequent consequence of therapeutic intervention is liquid overload of the patient due to the administration of excessive volumes of intravenous liquids.

Direct evidence for increased capillary permeability has come mainly from experimental studies in which pulmonary edema has been produced by endotoxin infusion[44]; hemorrhagic shock[45]; infusion of oleic acid[46,47]; ethchlorvynol, alloxan, thiourea, phorbol myristate acetate, complement fragments, cobra venom factor[47-51]; freebase cocaine smoking[52]; and inhalation of high concentrations of oxygen[53] or toxic gases, such as phosgene,[54] ozone,[55] and nitrogen dioxide.[56] Reliable clinical data are far more difficult to obtain, since (1) macromolecules in alveolar liquid may be diluted by tracheobronchial secretion, resulting in an underestimation of the extent of the alveolar-capillary leak, and (2) such macromolecules, secondary to previously elevated capillary pressures, can be present at a time when intravascular pressures have returned to normal levels, hence leading to the erroneous conclusion that alveolar-capillary membrane damage was the primary event. Nonetheless, clinical studies of ARDS with normal pulmonary capillary wedge pressures have been reported and have shown either an elevation of protein in the liquid aspirated from the tracheobronchial tree[57,58] or appearance in this liquid of foreign macromolecules injected intravenously.[59] Thus, it is probable, though not yet proved, that

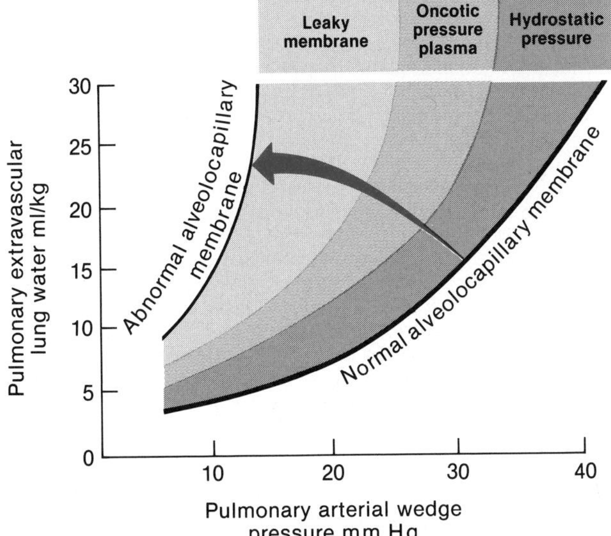

FIGURE 20-9. Relationship between pulmonary capillary wedge pressure and extravascular lung water when the alveolocapillary membrane is normal (gray, right) when there is increased permeability (light pink, left) and the range (pink) of pressures at which a diminished intravascular colloid osmotic pressure might make a measurable difference. Note that this is a continuum, which is indicated by the arrow going from right to left, and not a series of firmly established dividing lines. These data are plotted from several sources and have been adapted to the format shown here for illustrative purposes.

TABLE 20-2 THEORIES OF PATHOGENESIS OF SHOCK LUNG

- **I. Hemodynamic**
  - A. Backward theory—pulmonary venular constriction (? centrally mediated; ? cerebral hypoxia)
  - B. Forward theory—pulmonary hypertension. See IV, Microemboli (below)
- **II. Circulating humoral agent(s)**
  - A. Soluble factor(s) released from extrapulmonary cells injures vascular endothelium
- **III. Cellular agent(s)**
  - A. Locally released in lung injuries vascular endothelium
- **IV. Microemboli—altered permeability arises from diffuse microembolization of lung**
  - A. Subtheories: why emboli form
    1. Exogenous from transfusions
    2. Increased rate of formation (platelet, leukocyte, or erythrocyte aggregates)
    3. Decreased breakdown (altered fibrinolysis)
    4. Decreased removal by reticuloendothelial system (liver)
       a. Humoral—deficient opsonin
       b. Decreased hepatic phagocytosis
  - B. Mechanism of injury
    1. Hemodynamic (forward theory—severe, unevenly distributed pulmonary arterial hypertension transmitted to pulmonary capillaries, leading to shear stress and mechanical injury)
    2. Chemical (endothelium is injured by clot products: platelet, leukocyte, or erythrocyte aggregates)

From Robin, E. D.: Permeability pulmonary edema. *In* Fishman, A. P., and Renkin, E. M. (eds.): Pulmonary Edema. Bethesda, American Physiological Society, 1979, p. 217.

increased permeability of the alveolar-capillary membrane is an initiating event in most of the cases designated as ARDS. There is some experimental evidence that electrical charge of the involved membranes (the pulmonary capillary endothelium and alveolar basement membrane are negatively charged while capillary basement membrane is positively charged) and of macromolecules can affect the movement of the latter into the alveolar space.[60] The relationship between pulmonary capillary pressures and lymph flow and extracellular lung water (Fig. 20-9) differs in cardiogenic pulmonary edema from that edema caused primarily by alveolar capillary damage. In the former, both lymph flow and lung water increase modestly, as a consequence of a large increase in microvascular hydrostatic pressure; in the latter, lymph flow and lung water increase markedly in the absence of or with only a slight rise in hydrostatic pressure.

There are many similarities between ARDS from diverse etiologies and the respiratory distress syndrome seen in infants, which is due only to immaturity of the surfactant system. Although surfactant deficiency cannot be assigned a *primary* role in the pathogenesis of ARDS, there are many data to support the idea that changes in the properties of surfactant are added to the initial impairment and serve to perpetuate pulmonary dysfunction. Impairment of surfactant has been shown to occur with cardiogenic pulmonary edema, exposure to various plasma constituents,[61] and high concentrations of oxygen[62] and in association with systemic hypotension.[63] Closely related to the pulmonary edema in the ARDS is that which is commonly associated with all forms of shock—the so-called "shock lung." The theories of pathogenesis of shock lung are shown in Table 20-2. (For further discussion of ARDS and shock lung, see p. 556.)

ROLE OF POLYMORPHONUCLEAR LEUKOCYTES (PMN's). Experimental and clinical data strongly imply a major role for interaction of polymorphonuclear leukocytes in the blood and circulating or cellular chemotactic macromolecules for the initiation, perpetuation, or amplification of lung injury leading to most forms of ARDS. There is a preponderance of PMN's in the bronchoalveolar lavage liquid of patients with ARDS and their secretory products (electases, collagenases) are found in abundance. The precise sequence of events is not truly settled but comprises some combination of items II, III, IVA, and B in Table 20-2. Figure 20-10 gives the elements of the potential role of leukocytes and chemotactic agents. Chemotaxins in the circulating blood (e.g., the fifth component of complement, C5a) or from alveolar macrophages can recruit polymorphonuclear leukocytes, cause them to adhere to the pulmonary capillary endothelium, and activate them to produce several toxic substances that alter alveolar-capillary membrane permeability or cause circulatory changes or both. Because of the location of the polymorphonuclear leukocytes, their peripheral depletion and pulmonary vascular sequestration in many forms of acute lung injury, and their ability, when activated, to produce arachidonic acid metabolites (by both cyclo- and lipo-oxygenase pathways), oxygen radicals, proteases, and other mediators that alter permeability and influence vasomotoricity, the hypothesis is an appealing, though not unchallenged,[64] one. Experimental challenge, mainly in sheep, has been based upon PMN depletion studies which have shown for some agents (e.g.,

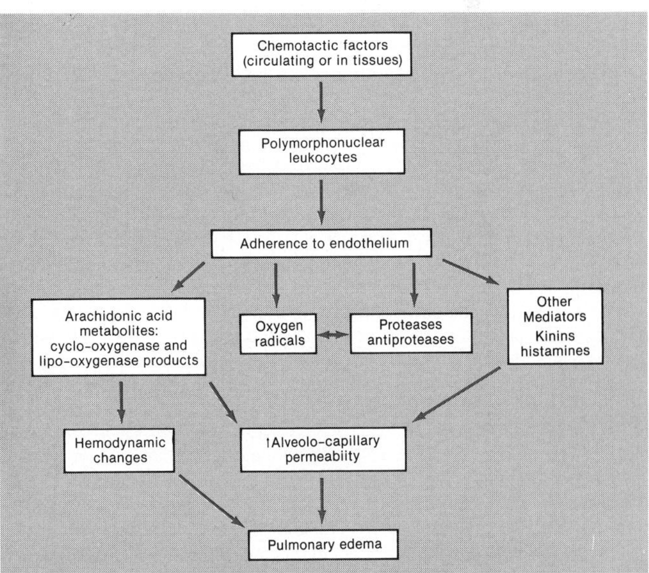

FIGURE 20-10. Flow chart showing the proposed mechanisms for chemotaxin and leukocyte interactions to produce alveolar-capillary membrane damage and pulmonary edema. (Adapted from Repine, J. E., Bowman, C. M., and Tate, R. M.: Neutrophils and lung edema. Chest *81*(Suppl.):5, 1982.)

phorbol myristate acetate)[65] that PMN's play a minimal role. However, granulocyte depletion is never complete, and extremely toxic drugs, which may alter a series of responses, are used to produce the leukopenic state. In addition, the sheep may be a poor species for assessment of the role of granulocytes in lung injury because their pulmonary endothelium has many phagocytic cells that can initiate and perpetuate injury (see below). Hence at this stage of knowledge it is believed that the balance is strongly in favor of a role for the polymorphonuclear leukocyte in clinically important forms of ARDS.

Since chemotaxins can arrive from distal sources in the body to inflict injury or can be derived from the alveolar macrophages of the alveolar side, systemic events such as gram-negative septicemia, distal events such as pancreatitis, and local pulmonary events such as inhalational injury can all be accommodated by this hypothesis.[66,67] Moreover, since the leukocyte aggregates often include platelets, the thrombocytopenic and consumptive coagulopathic states often accompanying ARDS can be explained. Clinical studies appear to support this hypothesis.[66] Bronchoalveolar lavage liquid from patients with ARDS has shown a predominance of neutrophils, leukocytic elastase, and partially inactivated alpha$_1$ antitrypsin.[68–70] Further, there is a strong correlation between neutrophil-aggregating activity in the plasma and the subsequent development of ARDS in clinical conditions that are often associated with this syndrome. In addition, the numbers of neutrophils obtained by bronchoalveolar lavage correlate strongly with abnormalities in gas exchange and indices of permeability.[70] To date, no observations are available to negate this hypothesis, yet the many potential and complex interactions await elucidation before preventive or therapeutic measures can be devised and translated into clinical practice for the avoidance or arrest of lung injury.

ROLE OF MONOCYTIC CELLS. Another group of cells that appears to play an important pathogenic and/or amplification role in ARDS, especially when sepsis or endotoxemia is a causal or complicating factor, is the monocytic group of cells including circulating monocytes and lymphocytes, macrophages within the tissues, and phagocytic cells along the vascular endothelium (reticuloendothelial cells). In bovine and ovine species the vascular reticuloendothelial cells predominate in the lung, whereas in humans the liver and spleen are the major locations for these cells. These are prime locations for cell stimulation by endotoxin from the intestine. Upon being stimulated with several agents, e.g., endotoxin, these cells release several cytokines including interleukin-1 (IL-1), interleukin-6 (IL-6), and tumor necrosis factor (TNF).[71] There are several observations that support the theory that these cytokines may play a role in ARDS. First, greater plasma levels of endotoxin have been found in intensive care unit patients who either had or subsequently developed ARDS than in those patients considered at risk for this syndrome but who did not develop it.[72] Of the cytokines monitored, TNF has been best studied in the context of ARDS associated with sepsis. Endotoxin causes TNF expression and TNF alone given to animals causes the same ARDS picture seen following endotoxin.[73] Plasma TNF levels are elevated in approximately one-third of patients with septic shock, in over 50 per cent of that subgroup who had or developed ARDS and in over 80 per cent of the subsubgroup who died.[74] While these laboratory and clinical observations only raise possibilities, the development of monospecific antibodies against endotoxin and against each of the cytokines will allow assessment of the pathogenesis of this syndrome and might provide useful therapies for the future.

ROLE OF PLATELETS. While considerable data, both clinical and experimental, suggest a role for platelets in altering vascular permeability,[75] their role in lung injury is not well demonstrated. It is clear, however, that thrombin-stimulated platelets can release many vasoactive substances that are injurious to cultured endothelial cells. In an experimental rat model of endotoxin induced lung injury, a specific platelet activating factor antagonist has been shown to have some protective effect.[76] Furthermore, the frequency of thrombocytopenia in association with worsening of lung injury is also suggestive. Nonetheless, heterologous platelet transfusions given to patients with ARDS and thrombocytopenia have no adverse effects on the extent or degree of lung injury.[77] To date it has not been possible to ascribe a major pathogenetic role to platelets, yet a secondary role seems probable.

QUANTITATION OF ALVEOLAR-CAPILLARY MEMBRANE DAMAGE. The problems with measurement of extravascular lung water just described multiply when the task is to measure both increased liquid accumulation *and* increased permeability of the alveolar-capillary membrane. All of the principles and techniques described for quantitation of pulmonary edema can be applied *in addition to* a macromolecular marker for vascular and even alveolar membrane leak. Combined techniques involve obtaining multiple indicator dilution curves using large intravascular markers (e.g., ^{51}Cr-labeled erythrocytes) for blood volume, smaller intravascular markers (e.g., ^{125}I labeled albumen) for measuring increased permeability, a diffusion barrier limited compound (e.g., ^{14}C-labeled urea) for measuring permeability surface area and a freely diffusible marker (^{3}H-labeled water) for measuring extravascular lung water.[78] Using these combined markers for simultaneous indicator dilation studies, Harris et al. have shown that more severe damage is associated with increased edema and poorer clinical outcome.[79] While the development of such techniques is of importance and interest for the future assessment of treatments in this most often fatal syndrome, they require such great technical expertise and elaborate equipment that their general clinical use is not practical at this point.

Some techniques assess only alveolar capillary membrane leak with no quantitation of the resulting edema. One such radioactive emission technique is the clearance ^{99M}Tc-labeled diethylenetriamine pentaacetate (DTPA) from the lung after its administration by inhalation as an aerosol. By external counting, the time course of clearance from the thorax can be measured. In the presence of lung injury its rate of clearance is increased. Unfortunately, the rate of DTPA is also increased by smoking, histamine, increases in lung volume, and in the asthmatic lung.[80] Thus it appears too sensitive and nonspecific to be of clinical use. The most direct technique for assessing Stage 3 edema is to sample liquid either by deep suction or from lavage using a wedged bronchoscope. Both liquid composition and cellular elements can be assessed from lavage and the degree of permeability can be inferred.

LYMPHATIC DYSFUNCTION. Abnormalities in pulmonary lymphatics can produce abnormalities of liquid transport in the lung. However, the question remains whether such alterations alone ever account for pulmonary edema. Experimental studies have been in direct conflict on this point.[81] However, in the presence of experimental lung injury, impeding lymphatic flow clearly increases the degree of edema that develops.[82] From the clinical standpoint there are clear examples to suggest the importance of pulmonary lymphatics. In silicosis, with the invariably associated obliterative lymphangitis, only moderate elevations of left atrial pressures result in impressive pulmonary edema.[31] Similar observations have been made following lung transplantation with complete disruption of lymphatics[10] and in association with obstruction of lymphatics due to lymphangitic carcinomatosis.[83]

There are experimental studies showing that lymphatic dysfunction can be present *without structural abnormalities.* For example, the normal rhythmic contractions of pulmonary lymphatic vessels in sheep disappear when the animals are anesthetized. Furthermore, lymphatic flow is significantly impaired following endotoxin infusion in sheep.[84] Cessation of lymphatic pumping would be expected to result in a net gain of interstitial liquid, and this may leave a clinical counterpart of pulmonary edema following anesthesia or sedative drug overdose. More importantly, the paralytic effect following endotoxin infusion suggests that lymphatic dysfunction may play a significant role in a common cause or propagator of lung injury. Impairment of lymphatic flow with a net gain of lung liquid content has also been shown to occur in sheep given continuous positive airway pressure.[85] The clinical occurrence or importance of this finding has yet to be established, but the question is a significant one, since both continuous positive airway pressure and positive end-expiratory pressure with mechanical ventilation are often used to improve gas exchange in patients with pulmonary edema.

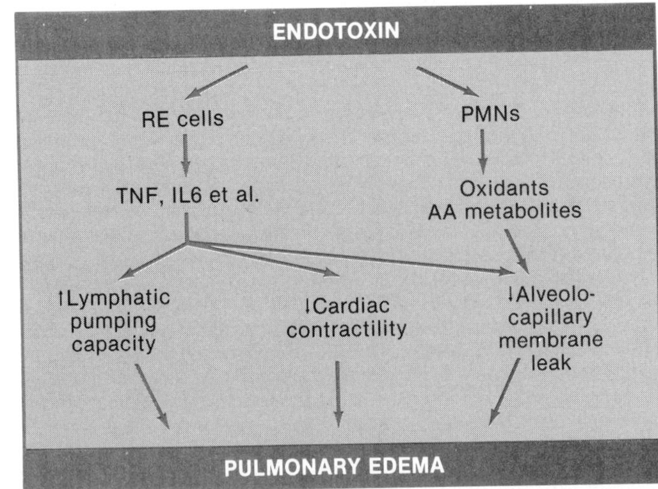

FIGURE 20–11. Schematic showing that multiple mechanisms for increasing pulmonary edema can come into play during septicemia. Each pathway has been demonstrated in an experimental setting and inferred in the clinical area as indicated in the text. Therefore, decreased clearance of edema liquid by lymphatic dysfunction along with increased liquid accumulation, both pressure- and leak-induced, occur.

COMBINATIONS OF MECHANISMS. In certain clinical settings, typified by gram-negative sepsis, several mechanisms combine to increase pulmonary edema. A potential sequence supported by clinical and experimental data is shown in Figure 20–11. The effects of endotoxin on reticuloendothelial cells with release of cytokines and on polymorphonuclear leukocytes with oxidant and arachidonic acid metabolites have been discussed already, as has the effect on lymphatic pumping capacity. What is not often recognized is the onset of cardiac dysfunction that occurs with septicemia. This responds to inotropic agents, which have been used with some success in lowering wedge pressures already in the normal range.[86]

PULMONARY EDEMA OF UNKNOWN PATHOGENESIS

HIGH-ALTITUDE PULMONARY EDEMA (HAPE). Victims of this disorder are usually persons mostly in their teens or early twenties who have quickly ascended to altitudes in excess of 2700 meters and who then engage in strenuous physical exercise at that altitude before they have become acclimatized.[57,87–89] At one time this syndrome was considered to be rare; however, recent estimates place the incidence at 6.4 clinically apparent cases per 100 exposures to high altitude in persons less than 21 years of age and 0.4 case per 100 exposures in those older than 21 years. Gradual ascent, allowing time for acclimatization, and limiting physical exertion upon more rapid ascent are thought to be preventive. Usually within one day of ascent, affected patients complain of cough, dyspnea, and, in some cases, chest pain in association with tachycardia, bilateral rales, and cyanosis accompanied by radiographic evidence of discrete patches of pulmonary infiltrate (Fig. 20–12).

Reversal of this syndrome is both rapid (less than 48 hours) and certain either by returning the patient to a lower altitude and/or by administering a high inspiratory concentration of oxygen. Sleeping below 8000 ft, gradual acclimatization, and avoidance of heavy exertion for the first 2 or 3 days at high altitude appear to be preventive. Although formerly thought to occur only in persons from low altitudes who ascend quickly for mountaineering or skiing, it has now been documented to occur among natives of high-altitude regions upon their return from altitudes below 2200 meters.[90]

Although no single mechanism satisfactorily explains the pathogenesis of HAPE, several possible mechanisms have been proposed. Although most patients have shown pulmonary arterial hypertension, the pulmonary capillary wedge pressures have been near normal,[91] a finding which has led to the suggestion that direct disruption of the walls of small arteries proximal to the hypoxically constructed arterioles in patients with hyperresponsive pulmonary vessels with resultant leakage of liquid may be responsible. Subjects with a previous history of HAPE have been compared with those having a similar high altitude experience but who did not experience HAPE. Those susceptible to HAPE have a depressed hypoxic ventilatory drive and an exaggerated pulmonary vasoconstrictor response to hypoxia but no elevation of wedge pressure at rest or exercise with exposure to either normobaric or hypobaric hypoxia.[92,93] No hemodynamic data have been obtained during the development of, nor at the peak of, pulmonary edema, so that transitory elevations of pulmonary capillary pressures could have been present and could have returned to normal at the time of measurement. However, in view of the existing data showing normal pulmonary capillary wedge pressures, other mechanisms have been proposed. The direct effect of alveolar hypoxia on increasing alveolar-capillary membrane permeability was initially considered, yet data do not support that idea. Transient intravascular coagulation with hypoxic sequestration of platelets in the pulmonary circulation has also been implicated in the past; however, more recent prospective study with sea level control periods and non-HAPE control subjects has shown that increased fibrin levels and decreased fibrinolytic activity do not precede or accompany HAPE.[94] At this point, it is fair to state that the pathogenesis is unknown,[95] but the response to simple treatment is dramatic.

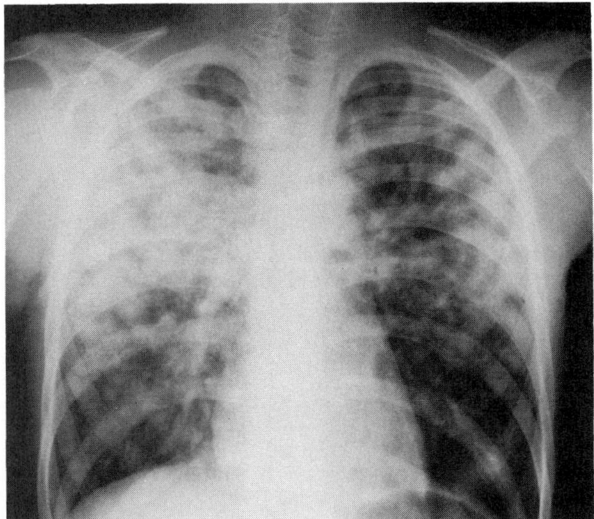

FIGURE 20–12. Chest x-ray of a 10-year-old boy in whom pulmonary edema developed on his return to his home at an elevation of 3100 meters after a visit to low altitude. Note patchy infiltrates scattered throughout both lung fields. Normal heart size indicates absence of left heart failure. (From Grover, R. F., et al.: High-altitude pulmonary edema. *In* Fishman, A. P., and Renkin, E. M. [eds.]: Pulmonary Edema. Bethesda, American Physiological Society, 1979, p. 229.)

NEUROGENIC PULMONARY EDEMA. Central nervous system disorders ranging from head trauma to grand mal seizures can be associated with acute pulmonary edema (without detectable left ventricular disease).[96] An early experimental model for this syndrome, consisting of fibrin injections into the fourth ventricle of dogs, has been used to show that sympathectomy completely prevented the accumulation of lung liquid. Indeed, observation that a variety of sympatholytic drugs serve to prevent neurogenic pulmonary edema makes it likely that the sympathetic nervous system plays a key role. Although not completely supported by direct measurements, the current idea is that sympathetic overactivity produces shifts of blood volume from the systemic to the pulmonary circulation, with secondary elevations of left atrial and pulmonary capillary pressures. Thus, it would appear that an imbalance of Starling forces is the basis for this form of pulmonary edema, although capillary pressure quickly returns to normal after the acute and transitory sympathetic discharge. There is a sound experimental basis for this proposal.[97] In addition, an unusually timely set of observations made on a patient with a pulmonary arterial catheter who experienced a grand mal seizure lent support to this idea. Wray and Nicotra observed transitory and severe elevations of pulmonary capillary wedge pressure in this patient during and immediately following the seizure.[98] Pulmonary edema diagnosed by both radiographic and clinical criteria was clearly present after wedge pressures had returned to normal levels. It should be emphasized that although sympatholytics prevent neurogenic pulmonary edema, they appear to have no place in the *treatment* of this syndrome, since it appears that pulmonary capillary pressures have returned to near normal by the time the syndrome is diagnosed.

The idea of a transitory sympathetic neural discharge of sufficient magnitude to account for high-pressure pulmonary edema as the basis for the neurogenic variety has not gone without challenge. It has been shown that modest increases in pulmonary endothelial permeability can be produced by stellate ganglion stimulation in dogs without elevation of pressures.[99] Also, neurally mediated elevations in permeability during status epilepticus in anesthetized and paralyzed sheep, also without elevations of pulmonary capillary pressures,[100] have been demonstrated. Both of these observations, although demonstrating only a modest effect, suggest that neural mechanisms can alter membrane permeability.[100a] However,

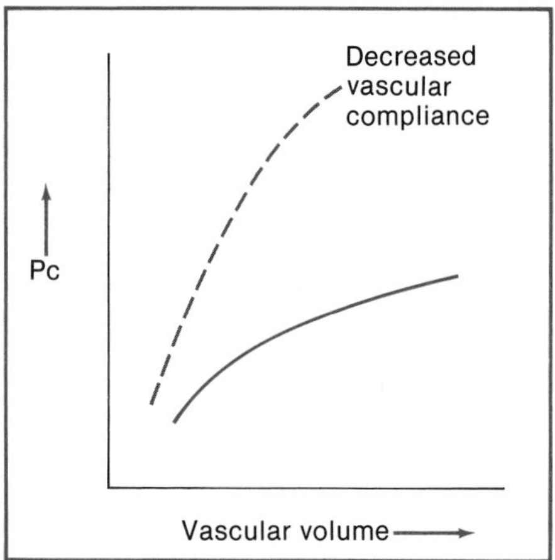

FIGURE 20-13. The relationship between vascular volume and the pulmonary capillary hydrostatic pressure (Pc) in the normal lung (—) and the lung with decreased vascular compliance (-----). For a given increase in blood volume, the increase in Pc is greater in the lung with reduced vascular compliance. (From Malik, A. B.: Mechanisms of neurogenic pulmonary edema. Circ. Res. *57*:10, 1985, by permission of the American Heart Association, Inc.)

whether these changes are of sufficient magnitude to produce pulmonary edema is open to question. Recently Malik[101] reviewed the combined experimental and clinical data and concluded that a combination of hemodynamic and permeability changes probably contributes to the genesis of pulmonary edema of neurogenic origin. While both factors undoubtedly contribute, it is believed that the major alteration is due to hemodynamics. One way that sympathetic stimulation can magnify the hydrostatic gradient is by decreasing the capacitance of the vasculature which, at any given blood volume, would increase pressures dramatically, as illustrated in Figure 20-13. This implies intact nerves to the pulmonary vessels, yet it has been shown in denervated lobes that similar changes occur due to circulating catecholamines with venoconstriction accounting for 75 per cent[102] of the pressure increase. Given the discussion on p. 553 dealing with the effect of venoconstriction on wedge pressure measurements, it seems likely that capillary pressures are much higher than was thought in previous studies.

NARCOTIC OVERDOSE PULMONARY EDEMA. Acute pulmonary edema is a well-recognized sequela of heroin overdose.[103] Because of the illicit traffic in this drug, which is given by the intravenous route, the syndrome was initially thought to be due to injected impurities rather than to the heroin itself. However, since oral methadone and dextropropoxyphene can also be associated with pulmonary edema,[104,105] the syndrome cannot be attributed entirely to injected impurities.

The well-known respiratory depressant effects of opiates lead to severe hypoxemia and hypercapnia with respiratory acidosis, which may account for the cerebral edema seen in many of these patients.[106] Cerebral edema, along with opiate-induced hypothalamic dysfunction, raises the possibility of a neurogenic mechanism. Transient impairment of lymphatic pumping capacity may be a contributory factor. The fact that edema fluid contains protein concentrations nearly identical to those found in plasma[107] and that pulmonary capillary wedge pressures, when measured, are normal[108] argues for an alveolar-capillary membrane leak as the initiating cause. In animal experiments, histamine has been shown to be released in the lung after both heroin and morphine administration.[109] Thus, it is possible that the well-known effects of histamine on increasing vascular permeability might play a role in this syndrome. However, there is not sufficient experimental or clinical evidence in support of such a role. As with several other pulmonary edema syndromes of uncertain etiology that develop quickly, the possibility must be considered that transitory pulmonary capillary pressure elevations account in part for the edema and that the reported normal measurements were made during the phase of resolution.

PULMONARY EMBOLISM. Acute pulmonary edema in association with either a massive embolus or multiple smaller emboli has been well described and most often attributed to concomitant left ventricular dysfunction due to a combination of hypoxemia and encroachment of the interventricular septum on the left ventricular cavity. Although this sequence is quite likely to be applicable in the case of massive embolism, whether it applies equally well to instances of multiple small emboli or microemboli is open to question. There are data to suggest, in the latter instance, that an increase in permeability of the alveolar-capillary membrane occurs.[42] It has been suggested that both clotting factors and formed elements act in the pathogenesis of a pulmonary capillary leak.[110] Thrombin generated by the clotting process and in association with the embolus causes aggregation of platelets, complement activation, and leukostasis. It is proposed that the sequence then follows that outlined in Figure 20-14. Experimental support for this notion comes from the blunting of the capillary leak process following defibrinogenation[111] or leukocyte depletion.[112]

ECLAMPSIA. Acute pulmonary edema frequently complicates eclampsia.[113] Multiple factors such as cerebral dysfunction with massive sympathetic discharge, left ventricular dysfunction secondary to acute systemic hypertension, hypervolemia, hypoalbuminemia (secondary to renal losses), and disseminated intravascular coagulation probably play a role in the pathogenesis.

POST CARDIOVERSION. Although pulmonary edema has been documented to occur after cardioversion,[114] the mechanism is poorly understood. Ineffective left atrial function immediately following cardioversion has been suggested as a contributing factor, yet left ventricular dysfunction and neurogenic mechanisms are also possible.

POST ANESTHESIA. In previously healthy subjects, pulmonary edema has been found in the early postanesthesia period without a clear relationship to fluid overload or any subsequent evidence of left ventricular disease. The basis for this disorder is unknown, but it is tempting to invoke some role for temporary lymphatic dysfunction under anesthesia, as previously shown in sheep.

POST CARDIOPULMONARY BYPASS. Although all patients who undergo cardiopulmonary bypass obviously have significant heart disease, the development of edema has been associated with normal left atrial pressures.[115,116] Alterations of surfactant due to prolonged collapse of the lung during the procedure, with subsequent need to apply high negative intrapleural pressures for reexpansion, and release of toxic substances have been suggested as mechanisms. Some data suggest that anaphylactic reactions to fresh frozen plasma may account for some episodes.[115] The matter is far from settled, but the syndrome is fortunately rare.

DIFFERENTIAL DIAGNOSIS

The differentiation between the two principal forms of pulmonary edema, i.e., cardiogenic (hemodynamic) and noncar-

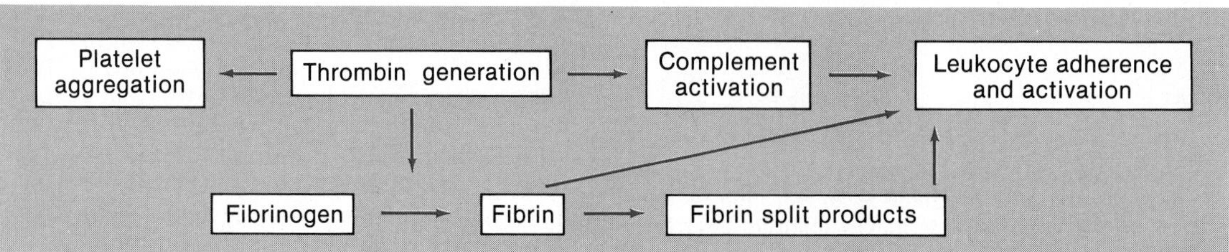

FIGURE 20-14. Flow chart showing the proposed mechanism for microembolic generation of increased permeability through the route shown in Figure 20-10. (Adapted from Malik, A. B.: Pulmonary microembolism. Physiol. Rev. *63*:1114, 1983.)

TABLE 20–3 INITIAL DIFFERENTIATION OF CARDIOGENIC FROM NONCARDIOGENIC PULMONARY EDEMA

CARDIAC PULMONARY EDEMA	NONCARDIAC PULMONARY EDEMA
History	
Acute cardiac event	Acute cardiac event is uncommon in immediate history (but possible!)
	Underlying disease? (Table 20–1)
Clinical Examination	
Low flow state = cool periphery	Usually high flow state = warm periphery
S_3 gallop/cardiomegaly	Bounding pulses
Jugular venous distention	No gallop
Crackles (wet)	No jugular venous distention
	Crackles (dry)
	Evidence of underlying disease (e.g., peritonitis)
Laboratory Tests	
ECG, ischemia/infarct?	ECG, usually normal
CXR, perihilar distribution	CXR, peripheral distribution
Cardiac enzymes may be ↑	Cardiac enzymes usually normal
PCWP > 18 mm Hg	PCWP < 18 mm Hg
Intrapulmonary shunting: small ↑	Intrapulmonary shunting: large↑
Edema fluid/serum protein < 0.5	Edema fluid/serum protein > 0.7

From Sibbald, W. J., Cunningham, D. R., and Chin, D. N.: Noncardiac or cardiac pulmonary edema? A practical approach to clinical differentiation in critically ill patients. Chest 84:460, 1983.

diogenic (caused by alterations in the pulmonary capillary membrane) can usually be made through assessment of the clinical context in which it occurs and through examination and consideration of the clinical data as shown in Table 20–3. Although the approach taken in that table suggests an either/or situation, this is not quite the case in reality. For example, sudden and large increases in intravascular pressure may disrupt the capillary and alveolar membranes leading to interstitial edema and alveolar flooding with macromolecules that produce an edema liquid more compatible with noncardiogenic causes. Thus a primary hemodynamic event can cause an alveolar-capillary membrane leak. Furthermore, high, normal, or only mild elevations in capillary hydrostatic pressures in the presence of alveolar capillary damage can cause an increase in the rate and extent of edema formation. Hence hemodynamic factors can and do play a role in increasing and perpetuating increased permeability edema. A reasonable example of a combination of hemodynamic and increased permeability has been provided by the study of experimental pulmonary edema produced by smoke inhalation.[117] Leakage of macromolecules following smoke inhalation was intermediate between that which occurred following increases in left atrial pressure and that found after alloxan. In all three cases the amount of edema, measured as extravascular lung water, was the same.

CARDIOGENIC PULMONARY EDEMA

CLINICAL MANIFESTATIONS. It would be satisfying to relate signs, symptoms, radiographic changes, and measurable dysfunction to all three stages of pulmonary edema. Unfortunately, there is currently no reliable way to detect pulmonary edema clinically or to quantitate it in its earliest stage—i.e., increased lymph flow without net gain of interstitial liquid. If the process is initiated by an increase in left atrial or pulmonary venous pressures, prominent pulmonary veins with secondary prominence of pulmonary arteries would be an expected radiographic finding. Although earlier studies were able to relate vascular dimensions to intravascular pressures, those measurements were made only under conditions of *chronic* pressure elevation.[118] However, it is likely, given the pressure-diameter characteristics of both pulmonary veins and pulmonary arteries, that acute changes could be easily detectable radiographically, especially if serial films were available. Hogg and coworkers have demonstrated in animal studies an increase in resistance of peripheral airways during pulmonary venous hypertension and have shown that this finding could be attributed to competition for space between vessels and airways within the bronchovascular sheaths, with consequent compression of small airways.[119] The same phenomenon may occur in human disease in which there is increased pulmonary blood volume.[120] Compromise of the lumina of small airways, predominantly in the more dependent portions of the lung, would be expected to increase both the alveolar-to-arterial difference for oxygen and the wasted ventilation ratio.

Stage 1. The distention and recruitment of small pulmonary vessels in Stage 1 edema may actually improve gas exchange in the lung and augment slightly the diffusing capacity for carbon monoxide.[121] Since such mild changes in other settings rarely lead to symptoms, it is doubtful that any symptoms, except for exertional dyspnea, would accompany these abnormalities in Stage 1 edema. In like manner, physical findings in the lungs would be scarce except for mild inspiratory rales due to opening of closed airways.

Stage 2. In this stage interstitial edema presents similar problems, in that correlative studies are scarce or nonexistent. Radiographic changes have been attributed to the increase in liquid in the loose interstitial space contiguous with the perivascular tissue of larger vessels and containing venules and arterioles. These changes (Figs. 8–23 and 24, pp. 217 and 218) are a loss of the normally sharp radiographic definition of pulmonary vascular markings, haziness and loss of demarcation of hilar shadows, and thickening of interlobular septa (Kerley B lines). Competition for space between vessels, airways, and increased liquid within the loose interstitial space produces greater compromise of small airway lumina, particularly in the dependent portions of the lungs, than does Stage 1 edema. There may also be reflex bronchoconstriction.[121] A mismatch exists between ventilation and perfusion that results in hypoxemia and more wasted ventilation. Indeed, in the setting of acute myocardial infarction, the degree of hypoxemia correlates with the degree of elevation of the pulmonary capillary wedge pressure.[122] *Tachypnea* is a frequent finding with interstitial edema and has been attributed to stimulation by the edema of interstitial J-type receptors or to stretch receptors in the interstitium rather than to hypoxemia, which is rarely of sufficient magnitude to stimulate breathing.[2] Although the tachypnea itself is a sign of dysfunction, it augments the pumping action of lymphatic vessels and may serve to minimize or delay the increase in interstitial liquid. There are few changes in the standard spirometric indices.

Stage 3. With the onset of alveolar flooding, or Stage 3 edema, gas exchange is extremely abnormal, with severe hypoxemia and hypocapnia. Alveolar flooding can proceed to such a degree that many large airways are filled with blood-tinged foam that can be expectorated. Vital capacity and other lung volumes are, of course, markedly reduced. A right-to-left intrapulmonary shunt develops as a consequence of perfusion of the flooded alveoli. Although hypocapnia is the rule, it has been well documented that hypercapnia with acute respiratory acidemia can occur in more severe cases. It is in such instances that morphine, with its well-known respiratory depressant effects, should be used with caution.

As already indicated, pulmonary edema developing during acute myocardial infarction most often is thought to be due to pulmonary capillary hypertension, yet experimental data in dogs with acute ligation of coronary arteries indicate another possible contributory mechanism. Edema developing after coronary artery ligation occurred when pulmonary capillary pressures were normal and the increases in lung water were blocked when animals were pretreated with indomethacin.[123] This finding suggests that inhibition of cyclooxygenase or cyclic nucleotide phosphodiesterase reduced pulmonary edema secondary to increased permeability of the alveolar-capillary membrane. Whether and to what extent these findings will apply to the human illness must await further study. Occasionally, patients with acute myocardial infarction and pulmonary edema present with normal pulmonary capillary wedge pressures.[124] It is possible that delay in radiographing clearance after a fall in pulmonary venous pressure is responsible, but it is also possible that in some patients an increase in permeability of the alveolar-capillary membrane secondary to low cardiac output, i.e., a form of "cardiogenic shock" lung, causes the pulmonary edema.

DIAGNOSIS. Acute cardiogenic pulmonary edema is the most dramatic symptom of left heart failure. Impaired left ventricular systolic and/or diastolic function, mitral stenosis, or whatever cause of elevated left atrial and pulmonary capillary pressures leading to cardiogenic pulmonary edema, interferes with oxygen transfer in the lungs and, in turn, depresses arterial oxygen tension. At the same time the sensation of suffocation and oppression in the chest intensifies the patient's fright, elevates heart rate and blood pressure, and further restricts ventricular filling. The increased discomfort and work of breathing place an additional load on the heart, and cardiac function becomes depressed further by the hypoxia. If this vicious circle is not interrupted, it may lead rapidly to death.

Acute cardiogenic pulmonary edema differs from orthopnea and paroxysmal nocturnal dyspnea in the more *rapid* development of severe pulmonary capillary hypertension. Acute pulmonary edema is a terrifying experience for the patient and often the bystander as well. Usually extreme breathlessness develops suddenly, and the patient becomes extremely anxious, coughs, and expectorates pink, frothy liquid, causing him to feel as if he is literally drowning. The patient sits bolt upright, or may stand, exhibits air hunger, and may thrash about. The respiratory rate is elevated, the alae nasi are dilated, and there is inspiratory retraction of the intercostal spaces and supraclavicular fossae that reflects the large negative intrapleural pressures required for inspiration. The patient often grasps the sides of the bed in order to allow use of the accessory muscles of respiration. Respiration is noisy, with loud inspiratory and expiratory gurgling sounds that are often easily audible across the room. Sweating is profuse, and the skin is usually cold, ashen, and cyanotic, reflecting low cardiac output and increased sympathetic drive.

On auscultation the lungs are noisy, with rhonchi, wheezes, and moist and fine crepitant rales that appear at first over the lung bases but then extend upward to the apices as the condition worsens. Cardiac auscultation may be difficult because of the respiratory sounds, but a third heart sound and an accentuated pulmonic component of the second heart sound are frequently present.

The patient may suffer from intense precordial pain if the pulmonary edema is secondary to acute myocardial infarction. Unless cardiogenic shock is present, arterial pressure is usually elevated above the patient's normal level as a result of excitement and sympathetic vasoconstriction. Because of the presence of this systemic hypertension, it may be inappropriately suspected that the pulmonary edema is due to hypertensive heart disease. However, it should be noted that the latter condition is now quite rare, and if arterial pressure is elevated, examination of the fundi will usually indicate whether or not hypertensive heart disease is actually present. Obviously, if the attack is not terminated, arterial pressure declines preterminally.

Differentiation from Bronchial Asthma. It may be difficult to differentiate severe bronchial asthma from acute pulmonary edema, since both conditions may be associated with extreme dyspnea, pulsus paradoxicus, demands for an upright posture, and diffuse wheezes that interfere with cardiac auscultation. In bronchial asthma, there is most often a history of previous similar episodes, and the patient is frequently aware of the diagnosis. During the acute attack, the asthmatic patient does not usually sweat profusely, and arterial hypoxemia, although present, is not usually of sufficient magnitude to produce cyanosis. In addition, the chest is hyperexpanded and hyperresonant, and use of accessory muscles is most prominent during respiration. The wheezes are more high-pitched and musical than in pulmonary edema, and other adventitious sounds such as rhonchi and rales are less prominent in asthma.

The patient with acute cardiogenic pulmonary edema most often perspires profusely and is frequently cyanotic owing to desaturation of arterial blood *and* decreased cutaneous blood flow. The chest is often dull to percussion, there is no hyperexpansion, accessory muscle use is less prominent than in asthma, and moist, bubbly rales and rhonchi are heard in addition to wheezes. The radiological changes in pulmonary edema are illustrated in Figures 8–24 (p. 218) and 20–12. As the patient recovers, the radiological appearance of pulmonary edema usually resolves *more slowly* than the elevated pulmonary capillary wedge pressure.

Pulmonary Artery Wedge Pressure Measurements. Measurement of pulmonary artery wedge pressure by means of a Swan-Ganz catheter may be critical to the differentiation between pulmonary edema secondary to an imbalance of Starling forces, i.e., cardiogenic pulmonary edema, and that secondary to alterations of the alveolar-capillary membrane. Specifically, a pulmonary capillary wedge or pulmonary artery diastolic pressure exceeding 25 mm Hg in a patient without previous pulmonary capillary pressure elevation (or exceeding 30 mm Hg in a patient with chronic pulmonary capillary pressure elevation) and with the clinical features of pulmonary edema strongly suggests that the edema is cardiogenic in origin.

Following effective treatment of the pulmonary edema, patients are often restored rapidly to the condition that existed before the attack, although they usually feel exhausted; between attacks of pulmonary edema there may be few symptoms or signs of heart failure.

TREATMENT

In the treatment of acute pulmonary edema, the physician normally cannot work alone, since multiple simultaneous maneuvers are required. Therefore, if logistics and time permit, the patient should be transferred to an intensive care unit, and cardiac rhythm should be monitored.[125] However, it is important to emphasize that transfer of the patient and institution of monitoring *must not delay initial therapy,* which must often be begun in the home or ambulance. While initial treatment is under way, and if it is logistically feasible, it is frequently helpful to place an arterial catheter to record intra-arterial pressure and obtain frequent samples for arterial blood gas measurements. If possible, a Swan-Ganz catheter should be inserted, so that pulmonary arterial and capillary wedge pressures can be measured and monitored.

The strategy of treatment of cardiogenic pulmonary edema is threefold: (1) a series of nonspecific measures is applied; (2) the precipitating factor is identified, if possible, and treated; and (3) attention is directed to the underlying condition, which is then corrected, if possible.

Nonspecific Measures

1. *Inhalation of oxygen-enriched inspired gas,* often with the aid of mechanical ventilation, is useful, as discussed below (p. 565).

2. The patient should be placed in the *sitting position.* Usually this is not necessary, because patients recognize that distress is increased when they lie down and that they are more

comfortable sitting up. However, it is often helpful to seat the patient at the side of the bed or in a chair in order to lower the feet and thereby diminish further the venous return.

3. *Morphine sulfate* remains an extremely valuable drug in the treatment of cardiogenic pulmonary edema. By its narcotic action it diminishes the patient's distress, reduces the work of breathing, and, perhaps most importantly, diminishes the central sympathetic outflow which causes venous and arteriolar constriction. Thus, even though morphine does not relax vascular smooth muscle directly, in the setting of acute pulmonary edema it results ultimately in arteriolar and especially in venous dilation.[126]

Three to 5 mg of morphine sulfate may be injected intravenously over a 3-minute period, while the patient is observed for both its beneficial action (i.e., relief of pulmonary edema) and its principal adverse effect (i.e., respiratory depression). This dose may usually be repeated two or three times at 15-minute intervals, if necessary. When the situation is somewhat less urgent, 8 to 15 mg of morphine sulfate may be injected subcutaneously or intramuscularly, and this dose can be repeated every 3 to 4 hours. Morphine antagonists should be readily available whenever morphine is administered. Morphine should be avoided if acute pulmonary edema is associated with intracranial bleeding, disturbed consciousness, bronchial asthma, chronic pulmonary disease, or reduced ventilation, as reflected in an elevated arterial Pco_2.

4. *Furosemide,* 40 to 60 mg injected intravenously over a 2-minute period, is another mainstay of therapy. With furosemide, diuresis commences within 5 minutes, reaches a peak effect at approximately 30 minutes, and lasts for approximately 2 hours.[127] However, pulmonary edema is relieved even before diuresis has occurred, suggesting that the initial effect of furosemide is not on the kidney but on the venous bed, causing dilatation.[128] In addition, there is evidence that furosemide reduces afterload and may act in part to relieve pulmonary edema by improving left ventricular emptying (p. 472).[129]

5. *Reduction of preload* can be accomplished by applying rotating tourniquets of wide, soft rubber tubing or blood pressure cuffs to the extremities. These should be placed several inches below the groin and shoulders, and the cuffs should be inflated to approximately 10 mm Hg below diastolic pressure, thus permitting arterial inflow to the limbs but restricting venous outflow. Only three of the four extremities should be compressed at one time, and every 15 to 20 minutes one of the tourniquets should be released and rotated to the free extremity. Rotating tourniquets are used less frequently than previously because of the effectiveness of the intravenously administered diuretics, described above.

6. Acute cardiogenic pulmonary edema, even in patients without hypertensive heart disease, is frequently associated with elevation of systemic vascular resistance and of arterial and left ventricular end-diastolic pressures, and with depression of cardiac output. Diuretic therapy, although of considerable value in reducing pulmonary capillary pressure, often does little to elevate cardiac output. *Vasodilators* promptly reduce systemic and pulmonary vascular pressures and relieve symptoms of acute pulmonary edema. A most appropriate vasodilator is *nitroprusside* (p. 495), which has a dual action: (1) it lowers systemic vascular resistance (afterload), thereby elevating cardiac output; and (2) it produces venodilatation (preload), thereby reducing pulmonary capillary pressure. A useful regimen is as follows: an initial dose of 40 to 80 μg/min can be employed, with the dose increased by increments of 5 μg/min every 5 minutes until pulmonary edema is relieved or until systemic arterial systolic pressure falls below approximately 100 mm Hg. If possible, arterial pressure should be recorded directly by means of an indwelling cannula during administration of this agent.

Nitroglycerin, 0.3 to 0.6 mg sublingually, also reduces ventricular preload by inducing venous dilation. The difficulty with this drug is that buccal absorption may be erratic; some patients develop marked reductions in arterial pressure. The hypotensive effect may be beneficial in patients with acute cardiogenic pulmonary edema and hypertension. However, it may be hazardous in patients with pulmonary edema secondary to acute myocardial infarction in whom arterial pressure is normal or reduced. Arterial pressure usually declines little in patients with hypervolemia and systemic edema. Nitroglycerin, like nitroprusside, may be given intravenously at a dose of 5 μg/min titrated upward in 5 μg/min increments at 3-minute intervals until pulmonary edema is relieved or until systolic arterial pressure falls below approximately 100 mm Hg.

7. The combination of morphine, rotating tourniquets, a diuretic, and sublingual nitroglycerin and/or intravenous nitroprusside or nitroglycerin generally diminishes preload sufficiently to obviate *phlebotomy.* Although the removal of approximately 500 ml of blood certainly diminishes preload, it is a time-consuming and often cumbersome procedure for an acutely ill patient, and it is therefore rarely, if ever, necessary to employ this technique.

8. In a patient known *not to* be receiving *digitalis,* a rapidly acting cardiac glycoside given intravenously may be helpful, depending on the etiology of the pulmonary edema. It is most useful in patients in whom pulmonary edema is secondary to severe mitral stenosis, in whom atrial fibrillation or other supraventricular tachycardias and an excessive ventricular rate have developed, and in whom the abbreviated diastolic filling period has caused increased left atrial pressure (Chap. 34). The slowing of ventricular rate accomplished by the glycoside, either by conversion of the arrhythmia to sinus rhythm or by increasing the effective refractory period of the atrioventricular conduction system, can exert a rapid and salutary effect. Specific glycosides and dosages are discussed in Chapter 17. Digitalis is also useful in patients with sinus rhythm, who are known not to be taking glycosides and who have impaired systolic function of the left ventricle, such as those with acute pulmonary edema secondary to severe aortic valve disease and hypertension.

The problem is much more difficult in patients with acute pulmonary edema with sinus rhythm who have been taking an unknown dose of digitalis. Time usually does not allow one to wait for a serum glycoside level, and one must decide on the basis of clinical examination and the electrocardiogram (p. 218) whether the pulmonary edema has been precipitated by digitalis intoxication or whether the patient requires more drug. A history of previous digitalis intoxication and/or nausea, vomiting, paroxysmal atrial tachycardia with atrioventricular block, nonparoxysmal atrioventricular junctional tachycardia, frequent ventricular premature contractions, ventricular tachycardia, and hypokalemia all imply digitalis intoxication. If these signs are absent, it is well to remember that when patients on a maintenance dose of a cardiac glycoside suddenly develop atrial fibrillation or other supraventricular tachycardia, the ventricular rate may be almost as rapid as if they had not been receiving the glycoside previously, and almost full doses may be required to slow the ventricular rate.

9. *Aminophylline* (theophylline ethylenediamine) is particularly useful when bronchospasm complicates pulmonary edema or in the occasional patient in whom it is not clear whether the attack of breathlessness is due to bronchial or cardiac asthma. Aminophylline is useful because it exerts a direct myocardial stimulating effect, analogous to that of caffeine. The reduction of ventricular filling pressure induced by aminophylline is caused not only by its positive inotropic effect but by mild venodilatation as well. In addition, it is a central nervous system stimulant, although less so than caffeine, and it exerts mild diuretic and bronchodilator effects.

The usual dose is 5 mg/kg intravenously in 10 minutes, followed by a constant infusion of 0.5 mg/kg/hr. This dose should be decreased in older persons and in those with hepatic or renal dysfunction.[130] After 12 hours the dose should be reduced to 0.1 mg/kg/hr. Optimal blood levels range from 10 to 20 mg/liter. Measurements of blood levels are important in the clinical use of this drug, since there are surprisingly wide individual variations in the kinetics of aminophylline degradation and since symptoms of nausea and vomiting are frequently due to other drugs used in the treatment of pulmonary edema rather than to aminophylline. Other side effects include headache, flushing, palpitations, precordial pain, hypotension, and, rarely, convulsions. The more serious side effects are sudden death from ventricular arrhythmias and hypotension due to vasodilation. Arterial unsaturation may occur owing to pulmonary vasodilatation and perfusion of poorly ventilated alveoli in patients with pulmonary edema.[131]

10. In patients who do not respond quickly to the aforementioned measures and in whom myocardial failure is deemed responsible for the pulmonary edema, three positive inotropic agents can be administered intravenously. The use and dosages of amrinone (a phosphodiesterase inhibitor that acts simultaneously as a vasodilator and positive inotropic agent, p. 503, and dobutamine, p. 502, and dopamine, p. 501), two sympathomimetics, are discussed elsewhere.

IDENTIFICATION AND TREATMENT OF PRECIPITATING FACTORS. In most patients with pulmonary edema, it is possible to identify one or more precipitating factors, similar to those that exacerbate congestive heart failure. Most frequently, pulmonary edema is brought on by acute myocardial ischemia or infarction,[132] the development of a tachyarrhythmia, fluid overloading, an infection in a patient with established underlying heart disease, pulmonary embolism (Chap. 48), thyrotoxicosis (Chap. 62), or severe anemia (Chap. 58).

In addition to applying the nonspecific measures for the treatment of pulmonary edema outlined above, additional attention must be directed to identifying and treating the precipitating factors (e.g., lowering body temperature in a patient with a high fever or treating thyroid storm or severe anemia). If acute pulmonary edema has been precipitated by a *tachyarrhythmia* that does not respond to appropriate pharmacological therapy (Chap. 23) and does not appear to be secondary to digitalis intoxication, it may be necessary to institute cardioversion with direct-current countershock (p. 491). On the other hand, if acute pulmonary edema occurs in a patient with a *bradyarrhythmia* that does not respond to appropriate pharmacotherapy, a temporary pacemaker should be inserted and the heart rate restored to normal (Chap. 25).

If acute pulmonary edema is precipitated or aggravated by a *hypertensive crisis*, treatment of the pulmonary edema clearly requires a rapidly acting hypotensive drug such as sodium nitroprusside (as discussed above). Alternatively, diazoxide, 300 mg as an intravenous bolus, or other vasodilators (Table 29–12, p. 870) may be employed.

RECOGNITION AND TREATMENT OF THE UNDERLYING CONDITION. After emergency therapeutic measures have been instituted, the underlying cardiac disorder responsible for the pulmonary edema must be diagnosed rapidly, when this is not already clear. Obviously, the history, physical examination, chest x-ray, and electrocardiogram are of great value. The echocardiogram may be helpful in the diagnosis of mitral valve disease, particularly silent mitral stenosis, as well as in the recognition of left atrial myxoma, which may be responsible for acute pulmonary edema. The diagnosis of congestive cardiomyopathy and of hypertrophic obstructive cardiomyopathy, both of which may be responsible for pulmonary edema, can also be strongly suggested by the echocardiogram. Although the echocardiogram may be enormously helpful in establishing an anatomical diagnosis, it must be recognized that the *quality* of echocardiographic tracings may be poor in patients who are acutely ill, thrashing about, and unable to cooperate fully.

Catheterization of the right side of the heart and pulmonary artery with a Swan-Ganz catheter is useful not only in the diagnosis of pulmonary edema, as already indicated, but also in aiding in the recognition of underlying cardiac disorders such as ventricular septal defect and mitral regurgitation, which may be responsible for pulmonary edema in patients with acute myocardial infarction. In addition, blood cultures for infective bacterial endocarditis and emergency creatine kinase isoenzyme (CK-MB) determinations for the diagnosis of acute myocardial infarction are critical tests in a patient in whom the cause of the pulmonary edema is obscure. Radioisotope angiography (Chap. 10) may be helpful in revealing the status of left ventricular function.

Rarely, *surgical treatment* is necessary to relieve pulmonary edema in patients with acute infective endocarditis (Chap. 35), prosthetic valve dysfunction (Chap. 34), prolapsing atrial myxoma (Chap. 44), end-stage critically severe aortic or mitral stenosis, ventricular septal defect, or mitral regurgitation complicating acute myocardial infarction (Chap. 39). Whenever possible, the patient's condition should first be stabilized, so that operation is not carried out on an emergency basis. Occasionally, however, when pulmonary edema persists despite optimal application of the nonspecific measures and removal of the precipitating factors, preoperative stabilization is not possible, and emergency surgery must be employed as a life-saving maneuver. Balloon valvuloplasty (p. 931) may be employed in patients with aortic and/or mitral stenosis who are poor surgical candidates.

LONG-TERM MANAGEMENT. The initial management of pulmonary edema blends in with the long-term management of heart failure described in Chapter 17. If the nature of the patient's underlying heart disease is known, it is necessary to assess its severity, attempt to ascertain the precipitating cause of the pulmonary edema, and develop a therapeutic strategy to prevent its recurrence. In many instances this consists of instructing the patient to commence or remain on a salt-poor diet and to commence or continue administration of a cardiac glycoside, a diuretic, and a vasodilator. Often, higher doses must be given. In other instances, the development of pulmonary edema in a patient with chronic heart disease signals a process of such severity that, following recovery from the acute decompensation, it may be advisable to assess carefully the patient's hemodynamic status and consider or reconsider surgical treatment. If the patient is seen for the first time during an acute episode of pulmonary edema, and the nature of the underlying heart disease is not clear, a detailed cardiac work-up should be undertaken soon after recovery in order to evaluate the underlying disorder with a view to identifying a surgically correctable lesion.

PULMONARY EDEMA SECONDARY TO ALTERATIONS OF THE ALVEOLAR-CAPILLARY MEMBRANE

CLINICAL MANIFESTATIONS. Since the sequence of liquid accumulation is similar whether primary membrane damage or alteration of Starling forces is responsible, both radiographic and clinical signs described above for patients with cardiogenic pulmonary edema also apply in patients with pulmonary edema due to primary alterations of the alveolar-capillary membrane.[133] At the time of initial injury and for several hours thereafter, the patient may be free of respiratory symptoms or signs. The earliest sign is an increase in respiratory frequency followed shortly by dyspnea. Arterial blood gas measurement in the earlier period will disclose a depressed P_{O_2} despite a decreased P_{CO_2}, so that the alveolar-to-arterial difference for oxygen is increased. At this point, oxygen given by mask or nasal prongs results in a significant increase in the arterial P_{O_2}. Physical examination may be unremarkable, although a few fine inspiratory rales may be audible. With progression, the patient becomes cyanotic and increasingly dyspneic and tachypneic. Rales are more prominent and easily heard throughout both lung fields along with regions of tubular breath sounds. At this stage, hypoxemia cannot be corrected by the simple administration of oxygen, and mechanical ventilatory assistance or control must be initiated in order to provide adequate oxygenation of arterial blood. Should this more aggressive therapy be delayed, the combination of increasing tachypnea and smaller tidal volumes results in a rising P_{CO_2} and further fall in P_{O_2} to near fatal levels.

TREATMENT

Whatever the underlying cause of pulmonary edema, analysis of arterial blood to assess the type and degree of gas exchange abnormality is necessary, followed by institution of appropriate inhalation therapeutic measures. When there is hypoxemia ($Pa_{O_2} < 60$ mm Hg) without hypercapnia, oxygen enrichment of the inspired gas may suffice and can be given by nasal prongs, Venturi masks, or reservoir bag masks, depending upon the degree of oxygen enrichment required to elevate the Pa_{O_2} sufficiently. If arterial oxygen tensions cannot be maintained at or near 60 mm Hg despite inhalation of 100 per cent O_2 at 20 liters per minute, or if there is progressive hypercapnia, intubation and institution of mechanical ventilation are usually necessary.

MECHANICAL VENTILATION. In the instance of progressive hypoxemia without hypercapnia, the role of mechanical ventilation is not to increase alveolar ventilation but to increase mean lung volume during the respiratory cycle, which in turn opens more alveoli for gas exchange. When hypercapnia with respiratory acidosis is present, mechanical ventilatory support may be necessary for improving alveolar ventilation in addition to improving oxygenation. If hypoxemia is not corrected by mechanical ventilation or if toxic concentrations of oxygen are necessary for prolonged periods, further improvements in arterial oxygenation at the same inspired oxygen concentration or equivalent levels of arterial oxygenation at lower concentrations of oxygen can be achieved by increasing end-expiratory lung volumes by the addition of positive end-expiratory pressure (PEEP).[134] Early use of PEEP to avoid or delay the onset of more severe respiratory failure has not been found to be effective.[135] Since maintenance of oxygenation is absolutely necessary for survival, reports that mechanical ventilation with PEEP actually increases the liquid content of the lung[85] may unsettle physicians who must utilize these techniques but will make them aware that this form of treatment should be discontinued as soon as possible.

Two complications of mechanical ventilation with PEEP deserve special mention. The first is that high intrathoracic pressures and increasing lung volumes impede venous return and increase the afterload to the right ventricle, with attendant decreases in cardiac output.[38] In the case of cardiogenic pulmonary edema, the impedance of venous return may provide some benefit with decreases in pulmonary vascular pressures but no decline in cardiac output. However, in other forms of pulmonary edema, a fall in cardiac output may be detrimental to the oxygen transport system. A fall in blood pressure or urine output or both may indicate that a severe diminution in cardiac output has occurred unless cardiac output is monitored during this form of therapy. The predominant basis for the decrease in cardiac output is increased intrathoracic pressure, which directly impedes venous return.[38,39] An additional contribution may come from greater pulmonary vascular resistance due to increased lung volume.[38] The result of increased right ventricular afterload is a displacement of the interventricular septum, which impedes left ventricular diastolic filling.[40,136–138] It is also likely that direct compression of the left ventricle by the inflated lung also restricts diastolic filling.[139,140] The second complication of mechanical ventilation is barotrauma (pneumomediastinum, pneumothorax, and subcutaneous emphysema). Pneumothorax may require appropriate decompressive therapy by means of a chest tube.

OTHER MEASURES. When it is not possible to maintain oxygenation utilizing the above techniques, *extracorporeal membrane oxygenators* have been tried with the hope that life could be maintained during critical periods while reparative processes in the heart or lung or both are taking place. However, a National Heart, Lung, and Blood Institute trial designed to evaluate this heroic and costly form of life support has shown that it did not improve the clinical outcome.

There are recent data suggesting that extracorporeal membrane therapy should be reevaluated in light of new data, a different rationale, and new technology. On the basis of the experimental observation that high inflation pressures actually produce lung damage in the ventilated (less damaged) portion of the diseased lung,[141] the approach of using small tidal volumes at low frequencies to minimize peak inflation pressures was devised. Since small tidal volumes are insufficient to eliminate carbon dioxide, a venovenous bypass apparatus has been used to eliminate 25 to 30 per cent of the CO_2 output. Arterial oxygenation is maintained through the patient's own lungs using the small tidal volumes and direct insufflation of oxygen into the trachea (a variant of apneic oxygenation).[142] With use of this approach in Italy, a 77 per cent survival rate in ARDS has been achieved.[143] This contrasts with the current U.S. success rate of only 30 to 40 per cent; in the NIH trial already mentioned, the survival was only 10 per cent in each group. A cooperative multiinstitutional study on this mode of therapy is now under way in the U.S., with similar assessments either planned or in process elsewhere. Hence, data should be forthcoming soon.

Both human patient and animal data have shown abnormalities in surfactant activity, which is necessary in maintaining alveolar and terminal airway patency. Indeed, pulmonary edema can actually result from surfactant deficiency. These facts have raised the possibility that exogenously administered surfactant as an aerosol might be of some therapeutic benefit in ARDS as it is in neonatal RDS.[144] In the latter instance, there is clearly a deficiency in surfactant production, whereas in ARDS inactivation and altered composition of surfactant by the inflammatory process might play a greater role. Hence, the expected therapeutic benefit would be less than in the neonate. Although no prospective clinical trial has been undertaken in ARDS, the results with exogenous surfactant aerosols in experimental lung injury have not been encouraging.

An obvious and not often emphasized principle is to *maintain pulmonary capillary pressures at the lowest possible levels* (i.e., compatible with maintaining cardiac and urinary outputs and blood pressure) when there is increased permeability. Prewitt et al. have shown, using a dog model of oleic acid–induced pulmonary edema, that the rate of formation of pulmonary edema is cut to less than half when pulmonary capillary wedge pressures are decreased from 12 to 6 mm Hg.[145] More recently, using retrospective analysis, Humphrey et al.[146] have shown that further lowering of wedge pressures that began within the normal range improves survival in ARDS.

THE CASE AGAINST INTRAVENOUS COLLOIDS. Since both increases in pulmonary capillary pressure and primary alveolar-capillary damage result in interstitial edema and alveolar flooding with liquid containing erythrocytes and macromolecules, indicating severe membrane disruption, it is difficult to evolve a rationale for the use of intravenous colloids such as albumin or high molecular weight dextrans. In fact, high molecular weight compounds administered intravenously have been shown to appear rapidly in alveolar liquid.[59] Furthermore, there is experimental evidence that the administration of colloid to dogs with experimental lung injury actually *slows* the resolution of ultrastructural changes in the interstitium.[147] Since there is no firm clinical evidence that treatment with protein-containing solutions results in more rapid recovery from acute pulmonary edema, and since there are strong intuitive reasons and some experimental data to suggest detrimental results, the use of albumin and other colloids should generally be avoided. There are, however, two situations in which albumin can be reasonably considered. First, if hypoalbuminemia is present, administration of albumin in addition to interventions designed to lower pulmonary capillary pressures is rational. Second, it has been suggested that albumin might hasten the rate of resolution of pulmonary edema once alveolar-capillary membrane integrity has been reestablished.[148]

Measures aimed at combating increased capillary permeability in ARDS are nonspecific and have not been shown to alter the time course or outcome of the illness. A possible exception is the use of specific antibiotic therapy directed against a causative or complicating bacterial infection. Adrenal glucocorticosteroid therapy leads the list of nonspecific measures that have yet to be proved beneficial in properly designed prospective studies.[149] In cases of pulmonary edema related to or complicated by disseminated intravascular coagulation, low-molecular weight dextran and heparin have been used without any clear evidence of an effect on the severity of the lung lesion.

Based upon alterations of multiple models of lung injury, agents will undoubtedly be tried that reduce chemotaxis, adherence, and activation of polymorphonuclear leukocytes (e.g., prostaglandins of the E series), that inhibit the formation of cell membrane–derived arachidonic acid metabolites (e.g., cyclo-oxygenase, lipoxygenase, and thromboxane synthase inhibitors), that competitively inhibit the various products (e.g., leukotriene D_4, E_4 antagonists), that scavenge toxic metabolites of oxygen (e.g., glutathione, catalase) and antibodies that neutralize endotoxin or several of the cytokines thought to produce or perpetuate injury. The rationale for and effectiveness of each are well documented in various experimental systems. However, the ultimate safety of such agents and their efficacy against the onset or continuation of membrane leaks in the clinical setting must await prospective trials.

REFERENCES

THE ALVEOLAR-CAPILLARY MEMBRANE AND PULMONARY EDEMA

1. Harris, P., and Heath, D.: Pulmonary edema. *In* The Human Pulmonary Circulation, 3rd ed. New York, Churchill Livingstone, 1986, pp. 373–383.

1a. Taylor, A. E., Barnard, J. W., Barman, S. A., and Adkins, W. K.: Fluid balance. *In* Crystal, R. G., et al. [eds.]: The Lung: Scientific Foundations. New York, Raven Press, 1991, pp. 1156–1158.

2. Szidon, J. P., Pietra, G. G., and Fishman, A. P.: The alveolar-capillary membrane and pulmonary edema. N. Engl. J. Med. *286*:1200, 1972.
3. Guyton, A. C., Parker, J. C., Taylor, A. E., et al.: Forces governing water movement in the lung. *In* Fishman, A. P., and Renkin, E. M. (eds.): Pulmonary Edema. Bethesda, American Physiological Society, 1979, p. 70.
4. Guyton, A. C.: Textbook of Medical Physiology, 7th ed. Philadelphia, W. B. Saunders Company, 1986, p. 372.
5. Holloway, H., Perry, M., Downey, J., et al.: Estimation of effective pulmonary capillary pressure in intact lungs. J. Appl. Physiol. *54*:846, 1983.
6. Collee, C. G., Lynch, K. E., Hill, R. D., et al.: Bedside measurement of pulmonary capillary pressure in patients with acute respiratory failure. Anesthesiology *66*:614, 1987.
7. Lai-Fook, S. J.: Perivascular interstitial fluid pressure measured by micropipettes in isolated dog lung. J. Appl. Physiol. *52*:9, 1982.
8. Parker, J. C., Parker, R. E., Granger, D. N., and Taylor, A. E.: Vascular permeability and transvascular fluid and protein transport in the dog lung. Circ. Res. *48*:549, 1981.
9. Staub, N. C.: Pulmonary edema due to increased microvascular permeability to fluid and protein. Circ. Res. *43*:143, 1978.
10. Ersalan, S., Turner, M. D., and Hardy, J. D.: Lymphatic regeneration following lung reimplantation in dogs. Surgery *56*:970, 1964.
11. Sampson, J. J., Leeds, S. E., Uhley, H. N., and Friedman, M.: The lymphatic system and pulmonary disease. *In* Mayerson, H. S. (ed.): Lymph and the Lymphatic System. Springfield, Ill., Charles C Thomas, 1968, p. 200.
12. Laine, G. A., Allen, S. J., Katz, J., et al.: Effect of systemic venous pressure elevation on lymph flow and lung edema formation. J. Appl. Physiol. *61*:1634, 1986.
13. Bruderman, I., Somers, K., Hamilton, W. K., et al.: Effect of surface tension on circulation in the excised lungs of dogs. J. Appl. Physiol. *19*:707, 1964.
14. Yoffey, J. M., and Courtice, F. C.: Lymphatics, Lymph and the lymphomyeloid Complex. London, Academic Press, 1970.
15. Hammersen, F.: Ultrastructure and functions of capillaries and lymphatics. Arch. Physiol. *336* (Suppl.):S43, 1972.
16. Casley-Smith, J. R.: The role of the endothelial intercellular junctions in the functioning of the initial lymphatics. Angiologica *9*:106, 1972.
17. Fishman, A. P.: Pulmonary edema. *In* Fishman, A. P. (ed.): Pulmonary Diseases and Disorders. New York, McGraw-Hill Book Co., 2nd ed. 1988, p. 919.
18. Staub, N. C., Nagano, H., and Pearce, M. L.: Pulmonary edema in dogs, especially the sequence of fluid accumulation in lungs. J. Appl. Physiol. *22*:227, 1967.
19. O'Brodovich, H., Hannam, V., Seear, M., and Mullen, J. B. M.: Amiloride impairs lung water clearance in newborn pigs. J. Appl. Physiol. *68*:1758, 1990.
20. Saumon, G., Basset, G., Boncleonnet, F., and Crone, C.: Cellular effects of β-adrenergic and of cAMP stimulation on potassium transport in rat alveolar epithelium. Pfluegers Arch. *414*:340, 1989.
21. Agostoni, E.: Mechanics of the pleural space. Physiol. Rev. *52*:57, 1972.
22. Glazier, J. B., Hughes, J. M. B., Maloney, J. E., and West, J. B.: Measurements of capillary dimensions and blood volume in rapidly frozen lung. J. Appl. Physiol. *26*:65, 1969.
23. Dollery, C. T., Heimberg, P., and Hugh-Jones, P.: Relationships between blood flow and clearance rate of radioactive carbon dioxide and oxygen in normal and oedematous lungs. J. Physiol. (London) *162*:93, 1962.
24. Ritchie, B. C., Schauberger, G., and Staub, N. C.: Inadequacy of perivascular edema hypothesis to account for distribution of pulmonary blood flow in lung edema. Circ. Res. *24*:807, 1969.
25. Muir, A. L., Hogg, J. C., Naimark, A., et al.: Effect of alveolar liquid on distribution of blood flow in dog lungs. J. Appl. Physiol. *39*:885, 1975.
26. Parker, F., Jr., and Weiss, S.: The nature and significance of the structural changes in the lungs in mitral stenosis. Am. J. Pathol. *12*:573, 1936.

CLASSIFICATION OF PULMONARY EDEMA

27. Bernard, G. R., and Brigham, K. L.: Pulmonary edema. Pathophysiologic mechanisms and new approaches to therapy. Chest *89*:594, 1986.
28. Snapper, J. R., and Brigham, K. L.: Pulmonary edema. Hosp. Pract. *21*:87, 1986.
29. Sprung, C. L., Rackow, E. C., Fein, I. A., et al.: The spectrum of pulmonary edema: Differentiation of cardiogenic, intermediate, and noncardiogenic forms of pulmonary edema. Ann. Rev. Respir. Dis. *124*:718, 1981.
30. Minnear, F. L., Barie, P. S., and Malik, A. B.: Effects of large, transient increases in pulmonary vascular pressures on lung fluid balance. J. Appl. Physiol. *55*:983, 1983.
31. Cross, C. E., Shaver, J. A., Wilson, R. J., and Robin, E. D.: Mitral stenosis and pulmonary fibrosis: Special reference to pulmonary edema and lung lymphatic function. Arch. Intern. Med. *125*:248, 1970.
32. Landolt, C. C., Matthay, M. A., Albertine, K. H., et al.: Overperfusion, hypoxia, and increased pressure cause only hydrostatic pulmonary edema in anesthetized sheep. Circ. Res. *52*:335, 1983.
33. Hultgren, H. N., and Grover, R. F.: Circulatory adaptation to high altitude. Annu. Rev. Med. *19*:119, 1968.
34. Albers, W. H., and Nadas, A. S.: Unilateral chronic pulmonary edema and pleural effusion after systemic-pulmonary arterial shunts for cyanotic congenital heart disease. Am. J. Cardiol. *19*:861, 1967.
35. Kramer, G. C., Harms, B. A., Gunther, R. A., et al.: The effects of hypoproteinemia on blood-to-lymph fluid transport in sheep lung. Circ. Res. *49*:1173, 1981.
36. Mahfood, S., Hix, W. R., Aaron, B. L., et al.: Reexpansion pulmonary edema. Ann. Thorac. Surg. *45*:340, 1988.
37. Loyd, J. E., Nolop, K. B., Parker, R. E., et al.: Effects of inspiratory resistance loading on lung fluid balance in awake sheep. J. Appl. Physiol. *60*:198, 1986.
38. Scharf, S. M., Caldini, P., and Ingram, R. H., Jr.: Cardiovascular effects of increasing airway pressure. Am. J. Physiol. *1*:35, 1977.
39. Scharf, S. M., Brown, R., Saunders, N. A., et al.: Changes in left ventricular size and configuration with positive end-expiratory pressure. Circ. Res. *44*:672, 1979.
40. Scharf, S. M., and Brown, R.: Influence of the right ventricle on canine left ventricular function with PEEP. J. Appl. Physiol. *52*:254, 1982.
41. Malik, A. B., and Staub, N. C. (eds.): Mechanisms of Lung Microvascular Injury. New York, New York Academy of Sciences, 1982.
42. Staub, N. C.: Pulmonary edema due to increased microvascular permeability. Ann. Rev. Med. *32*:291, 1981.
43. Carlson, R. W., Schaeffer, R. C., Jr., Puri, V. K., et al.: Hypovolemia and permeability pulmonary edema associated with anaphylaxis. Crit. Care Med. *9*:883, 1981.
44. Snell, J. D., Jr., and Ramsey, L. H.: Pulmonary edema as a result of endotoxemia. Am. J. Physiol. *217*:170, 1969.
45. Ratliff, N. B., Wilson, J. W., Horckel, D. B., and Martin, A. M., Jr.: The lung in hemorrhagic shock. II. Observations on alveolar and vascular ultrastructure. Am. J. Pathol. *58*:353, 1970.
46. Henning, R. J., Heyman, V., Alcover, I., and Romeo, S.: Cardiopulmonary effects of oleic acid-induced pulmonary edema and mechanical ventilation. Anesth. Analg. *65*:925, 1986.
47. Glauser, F. L., Fairman, R. P., Miller, J. E., and Falls, R. K.: Indomethacin blunts ethchloryne induced pulmonary hypertension but not pulmonary edema. J. Appl. Physiol. *53*:563, 1982.
48. Havill, A. M., Gee, M. H., Washburne, J. D., et al.: Alpha naphthyl thiourea produces dose dependent lung vascular injury in sheep. Am. J. Physiol. *243*:505, 1982.
49. Weinberg, P. F., Mathey, M. A., Webster, R. O., et al.: Biologically active products of complement in acute lung injury in patients with sepsis syndrome. Am. Rev. Resp. Dis. *130*:791, 1984.
50. Rinaldo, J. E., Dauber, G. H., Christman, J., and Rogers, R. M.: Neutrophil alveolitis endotoxemia. Am. Rev. Respir. Dis. *130*:1065, 1984.
51. Biermann, G. J., Dockey, B. F., and Thrall, R. S.: Polymorphonuclear leukocyte participation in acute oleic acid induced lung injury. Am. Rev. Respir. Dis. *128*:845, 1983.
52. Kline, J. N., and Hirasuna, J. D.: Pulmonary edema after freebase cocaine smoking—not due to an adulterant. Chest *97*:1009, 1990.
53. Kapanci, Y., Weibel, E. R., Kaplan, H. P., and Robinson, P. V. M.: Pathogenesis and reversibility of the pulmonary lesions of oxygen toxicity in monkey. II. Ultrastructural and morphometric studies. Lab. Invest. *20*:101, 1969.
54. Cameron, G. R., and Courtice, F. C.: The production and removal of oedema fluid in the lungs after exposure to carbonyl chloride (phosgene). J. Physiol. (London) *105*:175, 1946.
55. Bils, R. F.: Ultrastructural alterations of alveolar tissue of mice. III. Ozone. Arch. Environ. Health *20*:468, 1970.
56. Sherwin, R. P., and Richters, V.: Lung capillary permeability: nitrogen dioxide exposure and leakage of tritiated serum. Arch. Intern. Med. *128*:61, 1971.
57. Schoene, R. B., Hackett, P. H., Henderson, W. R., et al.: High-altitude pulmonary edema. Characteristics of lung lavage fluid. J.A.M.A. *256*:63, 1986.
58. Sprung, C. L., Rackow, E. C., Fein, I. A., et al.: The spectrum of pulmonary edema: differentiation of cardiogenic, intermediate, and noncardiogenic forms of pulmonary edema. Am. Rev. Respir. Dis. *124*:718, 1981.
59. Robin, E. D., Carey, L. C., Grenvik, A., et al.: Capillary leak syndrome with pulmonary edema. Arch. Intern. Med. *130*:66, 1972.
60. Brady, J. S., Vaccara, C. A., Hill, N. S., and Rounds, S.: Binding of charged ferritin to alveolar wall components and charge selectivity of macromolecular transport in permeability pulmonary edema in rats. Circ. Res. *55*:155, 1984.
61. Said, S. I., Avery, M. E., Davis, R. K., et al.: Pulmonary surface activity in induced pulmonary edema. J. Clin. Invest. *44*:458, 1965.
62. Miller, W. W., Waldhausen, J. A., and Rashkind, W. J.: Comparison of oxygen poisoning of the lung in cyanotic and acyanotic dogs. N. Engl. J. Med. *282*:943, 1970.

63. Henry, J. H.: The effect of shock on pulmonary alveolar surfactant. Its role in refractory respiratory insufficiency of the critically ill or severely injured patient. J. Trauma *8*:756, 1968.
64. Glauser, F. L., and Fairman, R. P.: The uncertain role of the neutrophil in increased permeability pulmonary edema. Chest *88*:601, 1985.
65. Dyer, E. L., and Snapper, J. R.: Role of circulating granulocytes in sheep lung injury produced by phorbol myristate acetate. J. Appl. Physiol. *60*:576, 1986.
66. Rinaldo, J. E., and Rogers, R. M.: Adult respiratory-distress syndrome: Changing concepts of lung injury and repair. N. Engl. J. Med. *306*:900, 1982.
67. Brigham, K. L., Loyd, J. E., Newman, J. H., et al.: Granulocytes in acute lung vascular injury in unanesthetized sheep. Chest *81*(Suppl.):5, 1982.
68. Lee, C. T., Fein, A. M., Lippman, M., et al.: Elastolytic activity in pulmonary lavage fluid from patients with adult respiratory distress syndrome. N. Engl. J. Med. *304*:192, 1981.
69. Cohen, A. B., and Cochrane, C. G.: Studies on the pathogenesis of the adult respiratory distress syndrome. J. Clin. Invest. *69*:543, 1982.
70. Welland, J. E., David, W. B., Holter, J. F., et al.: Lung neutrophils in ARDS: Clinical and pathological significance. Am. Rev. Respir. Dis. *133*:218, 1986.
71. Kelly, J.: Cytokines and the lung: State of the art. Am. Rev. Resp. Dis. *141*:765, 1990.
72. Parsons, P. E., Worthen, G. S., Moore, E. E., et al.: The association of circulating endotoxin with the development of the adult respiratory distress syndrome. Am. Rev. Resp. Dis. *140*:294, 1989.
73. Wheeler, A. P., Jesmok, G., and Brigham, K. L.: Tumor necrosis factor's effects on lung mechanics, gas exchange and airway reactivity in sheep. J. Appl. Physiol. *68*:2542, 1990.
74. Marks, J. D., Marks, C. B., Luce, J. M., et al.: Plasma tumor necrosis factor in patients with septic shock: mortality rate, incidence of adult respiratory distress syndrome, and effects of methylprednisolone administration. Am. Rev. Resp. Dis. *141*:94, 1990.
75. Heffner, J. E., Cook, J. A., and Halushko, P. V.: Human platelets modulate edema formation in isolated rabbit lungs. J. Clin. Invest. *84*:757, 1989.
76. Chang, S. W., Fernyak, S., and Voelket, N. J.: Beneficial effect of a platelet-activating factor antagonist, WEB2086, on endotoxin-induced lung injury. Am. J. Physiol. *258*(Heart Circ. Physiol. 27):H153, 1990.
77. Eichacker, P. Q. Shelhamer, J. H., Brenner, M., Parillo, J. E.: The effects of heterologous platelet transfusion on pulmonary function during ARDS. Chest *97*:923, 1990.
78. Staub, N. C., Hyde, R. W., and Crandall, E.: Workshop on techniques to evaluate lung alveolar-microvascular injury. Am. Rev. Resp. Dis. *141*:1071, 1990.
79. Harris, T. R., Bernard, G. R., Brigham, K. L., et al.: Lung microvascular transport properties measured by multiple indicator dilution methods in patients with adult respiratory distress syndrome: A comparison between patients reversing respiratory failure and those failing to reverse. Am. Rev. Resp. Dis. *141*:272, 1990.
80. Ilowite, J. S., Bennett, W. D., Sheetz, M. S., et al.: Permeability of the bronchial mucosa to ^{99m}Tc-DTPA in asthma. Am. Rev. Resp. Dis. *139*:1139, 1989.
81. Magno, M., and Szidon, J. P.: Hemodynamic pulmonary edema in dogs with acute and chronic lymphatic ligation. Am. J. Physiol. *231*:1777, 1976.
82. Ando, F., Arakawa, M., Miyazaki, H., et al.: Effect of superior vena caval hypertension on alloxon-induced lung injury in dogs. J. Appl. Physiol. *68*:478, 1990.
83. Trapnell, D. H.: Radiological appearances of lymphangitis carcinomatosa of the lung. Thorax *19*:251, 1964.
84. Elias, R. M., and Johnston, M. G.: Modulation of lymphatic pumping by lymph borne factors after endotoxin administration in sheep. J. Appl. Physiol. *68*: 199, 1990.
85. Permutt, S.: Mechanical influences on water accumulation in the lungs. *In* Fishman, A. P., and Renkin, E. M. (eds.): Pulmonary Edema. Bethesda, American Physiological Society, 1979, p. 175.
86. Parillo, J. E., Parker, M. M., Nartanson, C., et al.: Septic shock in humans: advances in the understanding of pathogenesis, cardiovascular dysfunction and therapy. Ann. Intern. Med. *113*:227, 1990.
87. Naeije, R., Melot, C., and Lejeune, P.: Hypoxic pulmonary vasoconstriction and high altitude pulmonary edema. Am. Rev. Respir. Dis. *134*:332, 1986.
88. Sophocles, A. M., Jr.: High-altitude pulmonary edema in Vail, Colorado, 1975–1982. West. J. Med. *144*:569, 1986.
89. Lockhart, A., and Saiag, B.: Altitude and the human pulmonary circulation. Clin. Sci. *60*:599, 1981.
90. Harris, P., and Heath, D.: The pulmonary circulation at high altitude. *In* The Human Pulmonary Circulation. 3rd ed. New York, Churchill Livingstone, 1986, pp. 499–503.
91. Hultgren, H. N., Lopez, C. E., Lundberg, E., and Miller, H.: Physiologic studies of pulmonary edema at high altitude. Circulation *29*:393, 1964.
92. Matsuzawa, Y., Fujimoto, K., Kobayaoshi, T., et al.: Blunted hypoxic ventilatory drive in subjects susceptible to high altitude pulmonary edema. J. Appl. Physiol. *66*:1152, 1989.
93. Kawashima, A., Kubo, K., Kobayashi, T., and Sekiguchi, M.: Hemodynamic responses to acute hypoxia, hypobaria and exercise in subjects susceptible to high-altitude pulmonary edema. J. Appl. Physiol. *67*:1982, 1989.
94. Bortsch, P., Haeberli, A., Franciolli, M., et al.: Coagulation and fibrinolysis in acute mountain sickness and beginning pulmonary edema. J. Appl. Physiol. *66*:2136, 1989.
95. Grover, R. F., Hyers, R. M., McCurty, I. F., and Reeves, J. T.: High-altitude pulmonary edema. *In* Fishman, A. P., and Renkin, E. M. (eds.): Pulmonary Edema. Bethesda, American Physiological Society, 1979, p. 229.
96. Yabumoto, M., Kuriyama, T., Iwamoto, M., and Kinoshita, T.: Neurogenic pulmonary edema associated with ruptured intracranial aneurysm: Case report. Neurosurgery *19*:300, 1986.
97. Maron, M. B.: Effect of elevated vascular pressure transients on protein permeability in the lung. J. Appl. Physiol. *67*:305, 1989.
98. Wray, N. P., and Nicotra, M. B.: Pathogenesis of neurogenic pulmonary edema. Am. Rev. Respir. Dis. *118*:783, 1978.
99. Hakim, T. S., van der Zee, H., and Malik, A. B.: Effects of sympathetic nerve stimulation on lung fluid and protein exchange. J. Appl. Physiol. *47*:1025, 1979.
100. Simon, R. P., Bayne, L. L., Tranbaugh, R. F., and Lewis, F. R.: Elevated pulmonary lymph flow and protein content during status epilepticus in sheep. J. Appl. Physiol. *52*:91, 1982.
100a. Humbert, V. H. Jr., Munn, N. J., and Hawkins, R. F.: Noncardiogenic pulmonary edema complicating massive diltiazem overdose. Chest *99*:258, 1991.
101. Malik, A. B.: Mechanisms of neurogenic pulmonary edema. Circ. Res. *57*:1, 1985.
102. Maron, M. B.: Pulmonary vasoconstriction in a canine model of neurogenic pulmonary edema. J. Appl., Physiol. *68*:912, 1990.
103. Steinberg, A. D., and Karliner, J. S.: The clinical spectrum of heroin pulmonary edema. Arch. Intern. Med. *122*:122, 1968.
104. Fraser, D. W.: Methadone overdose: Illicit use of pharmaceutically prepared narcotics. J.A.M.A. *217*:1387, 1971.
105. Bogartz, L. J., and Miller, W. C.: Pulmonary edema associated with propoxyphene intoxication. J.A.M.A. *215*:259, 1971.
106. Richter, R. W., Baden, M. N., and Pearson, J.: Cerebral edema seen in many "sudden death" heroin victims. J.A.M.A. *212*:967, 1970.
107. Katz, S., Aberman, A., Frand, U. I., et al.: Heroin pulmonary edema: Evidence for increased pulmonary capillary permeability. Am. Rev. Respir. Dis. *106*:472, 1972.
108. Gopinathan, K., Saroja, D., Spears, J. R., et al.: Hemodynamic studies in heroin induced acute pulmonary edema. Circulation *42* (Suppl. 3):44, 1970.
109. Brashear, R. E., Kelly, M. T., and White, A. C.: Elevated plasma histamine after heroin and morphine. J. Lab. Clin. Med. *83*:451, 1974.
110. Malik, A. B., Tahamont, M. V., Minnear, F. L., et al.: Lung fluid and protein exchange after pulmonary vascular thrombosis. Chest *81*:5, 1982.
111. Johnson, A., and Malik, A. B.: Effect of defibrinogenation on lung water accumulation after pulmonary microembolism in dogs. J. Appl. Physiol. *49*:841, 1980.
112. Flick, M. R., Perel, A., and Staub, N. C.: Leukocytes are required for increased lung microvascular permeability after microembolization in sheep. Circ. Res. *48*:344, 1981.
113. Rovinsky, J. J., and Guttmacher, A. F.: Medical, Surgical, and Gynecologic Complications of Pregnancy. 2nd ed. Baltimore, Williams and Wilkins Co., 1965.
114. Goldbaum, T. S., Bacos, J. M., and Lindsay, J., Jr.: Pulmonary edema following conversion of tachyarrhythmia. Chest *89*:465, 1986.
115. Hashim, S. E., Kay, H. R., Hammond, G. L., et al.: Noncardiac pulmonary edema after cardiopulmonary bypass. Am. J. Surg. *147*:560, 1984.
116. Culliford, A. T., Thomas, S., and Spencer, F. C.: Fulminating noncardiogenic pulmonary edema: A newly recognized hazard during cardiac operations. J. Thorac. Cardiovasc. Surg. *80*:868, 1980.
117. Clark, W. R., Nieman, G., and Hakim, T. S.: Distribution of extravascular lung water after acute smoke inhalation. J. Appl. Physiol. *68*:2394, 1990.
118. Teichmann, V., Jezek, V., and Herles, F.: Relevance of width of right descending branch of pulmonary artery as a radiological sign of pulmonary hypertension. Thorax *25*:91, 1970.
119. Hogg, J. C., Agarawal, J. B., Gardiner, A. J. S., et al.: Distribution of airway resistance with developing pulmonary edema in dogs. J. Appl. Physiol. *32*:20, 1972.
120. DeTroyer, A., Yernault, J., and Englert, M.: Mechanics of breathing in patients with atrial septal defect. Am. Rev. Respir. Dis. *115*:413, 1977.
121. Murray, J. F.: The lungs and heart failure. Hosp. Prac. *20*:55, 1985.
122. Fillmore, S. J., Giumaraes, A. C., Scheidt, S. S., and Killip, T.: Blood gas changes and pulmonary hemodynamics following acute myocardial infarction. Circulation *45*:583, 1972.
123. Richeson, J. F., Paulshock, C., and Yu, P. N.: Non-hydrostatic pulmonary edema after coronary artery ligation in dogs. Circ. Res. *50*:301, 1982.
124. Timmis, A. D., Fowler, M. B., Burwood, R. J., et al.: Pulmonary oedema without critical increase in left atrial pressure in acute myocardial infarction. Br. Med. J. *283*:636, 1981.
125. Donat, W. E., and Weiner, B. H.: Syndromes of left ventricular failure. *In* Rippe, J. M., Irwin, R. S., and Alpert, J. S. (eds.): Intensive Care of Medicine. Boston, Little, Brown and Co., 1985, pp. 322–336.
126. Vismara, L. A., Leaman, D. M., and Zelis, R.: The effects of morphine on venous tone in patients with acute pulmonary edema. Circulation *54*:335, 1976.
127. Iff, H. W., and Flenley, D. C.: Blood-gas exchange after furosemide in acute pulmonary edema. Lancet *1*:616, 1971.
128. Dikshit, K., Vyden, J. K., Forrester, J. S., et al.: Renal and extrarenal hemodynamic effects of furosemide in congestive heart failure after acute myocardial infarction. N. Engl. J. Med. *288*:1087, 1973.
129. Wilson, J. R., Reichek, N., Dunkman, W. B., and Goldberg, S.: Effect of diuresis on the performance of the failing left ventricle in man. Am. J. Med. *70*:234, 1981.

130. Mitenko, P. A., and Ogilvie, R. I.: Rational intravenous doses of theophylline. N. Engl. J. Med. *289*:600, 1973.
131. Tai, E., and Read, J.: Response of blood gas tensions to aminophylline and isoprenaline in patients with asthma. Thorax *22*:543, 1967.
132. Goldberger, J. J., Peled, H. B., Stroh, J. A., et al.: Prognostic factors in acute pulmonary edema. Arch. Intern. Med. *146*:489, 1986.
133. Hildner, F. J.: Pulmonary edema associated with low left ventricular filling pressures. Am. J. Cardiol. *44*:1410, 1979.
134. Rizk, N. W., and Murray, J. F.: PEEP and pulmonary edema. Am. J. Med. *72*:381, 1982.
135. Pepe, P. E., Hudson, L. D., and Carrico, C. J.: Early application of PEEP in patients at risk for the adult respiratory distress syndrome. N. Engl. J. Med. *311*:281, 1984.
136. Cassidy, S. S., and Mitchell, J. H.: Effects of positive pressure breathing on right and left ventricular preload and afterload. Fed. Proc. *40*:2178, 1981.
137. Jardin, F., Farcot, J.-C., Boisante, L., et al.: Influence of positive end-expiratory pressure on left ventricular performance. N. Engl. J. Med. *304*:387, 1981.
138. Lorell, B. H., Palacios, I., Daggett, W. M., et al.: Right ventricular distension and left ventricular compliance. Am. J. Physiol. *240*:H87, 1981.
139. Wead, W. B., and Norton, J. F.: Effects of intrapleural pressure changes on canine left ventricular function. J. Appl. Physiol. *50*:1027, 1981.
140. Fewell, J. E., Abendschein, D. R., Carlson, C. J., et al.: Continuous positive-pressure ventilation does not alter ventricular pressure-volume relationship. Am. J. Physiol. *240*:H821, 1981.
141. Kolobow, T., Moretti, M. P., Fumagalli, R., et al.: Severe impairment in lung function induced by high peak airway pressure during mechanical ventilation: An experimental study. Am. Rev. Resp. Dis. *135*:312, 1987.
142. Borelli, M., Kolobow, T., Spatola, R., et al.: Severe acute respiratory failure managed with continuous positive airway pressure and partial extracorporeal carbon dioxide removal by an artificial membrane lung: a controlled, randomized animal study. Am. Rev. Resp. Dis. *138*:1480, 1988.
143. Gattinoni, L., Pesenti, A., Caspani, M. L., et al.: The role of total static lung compliance in the management of severe ARDS unresponsive to conventional treatment. Int. Care Med. *10*:121–126, 1984.
144. Zelter, M., Escudier, B. J., Hoeffel, J. M., and Murray, J. F.: Effects of aerosolized artificial surfactant on repeated oleic acid injury in sheep. Am. Rev. Resp. Dis. *141*:1014, 1990.
145. Prewitt, R. M., McCarthy, J., and Wood, L. D. H.: Treatment of acute low pressure pulmonary edema in dogs: Relative effects of hydrostatic and oncotic pressure, nitroprusside, and positive end-expiratory pressure. J. Clin. Invest. *67*:409, 1981.
146. Humphrey, H., Hall, J., Sznajder, I., et al.: Improved survival in ARDS patients associated with a reduction in pulmonary capillary wedge pressure. Chest *97*:1176, 1990.
147. Lowe, R. J., and Moss, G. S.: Pulmonary failure after trauma. Surg. Annu. *8*:63, 1976.
148. Tullis, J. L.: Albumin, I. Background and use. J.A.M.A. *237*:355 and 460, 1977.
149. Andreadis, N., and Petty, T. L.: Adult respiratory distress syndrome: Problems and prognosis. Am. Rev. Respir. Dis. *132*:1344, 1985.

Acute Circulatory Failure (Shock)

by MAX HARRY WEIL, M.D., PhD., MARTIN von PLANTA, M.D., and ERIC C. RACKOW, M.D.

Pathophysiology

DEFINITIONS

Acute circulatory failure, for purposes of this chapter, encompasses the syndromes associated with an acute reduction in effective blood flow with failure to maintain the transport and delivery of essential substrates to sustain the function of vital organ systems.[1,2] The fully developed syndrome is clinically recognized as circulatory shock. There is usually little controversy regarding the serious clinical status of the patient who presents with prostration, hypotension, pallor, coldness and moistness of the skin, collapse of superficial veins, suppression of the formation of urine, and mental obtundation. The term "shock" of itself is descriptive of these signs and spotlights the dire threat of a critical reduction in systemic blood flow.

A WORKING MODEL OF THE CIRCULATION

For purposes of defining primary hemodynamic mechanisms of circulatory shock and implications for its management, conceptualization of a simple working model of the circulatory system is likely to be helpful (Fig. 21-1). Eight primary components of the circulatory system may be identified. The first component is the *intravascular volume,* which moderates the venous return or preload. The second, the *heart,* serves as the pump and provides contractile power for circulation. Contractility, rate (and rhythm), and loading conditions determine cardiac output (p. 375). Third is the *resistance circuit,* which includes the arteries and arterioles. It is the mainstream by which blood is carried from the heart to the capillary beds; changes in arteriolar resistance moderate the afterload on the heart. The fourth component is the *capillary exchange bed,* a largely passive circuit which provides for exchange of fluid and metabolites between the intravascular and extravascular compartments. The fifth is the *venous resistance bed,* which includes the postcapillary venules and probably the small veins. Blood flow through the capillary bed and both fluid and substrate filtration between the intravascular and interstitial fluid compartments are largely regulated by humoral and neurogenic controls on precapillary arterioles and postcapillary venules.[3-5] The sixth component is represented by *metarterioles* that bridge the arterial resistance and postcapillary venous vessels. Blood may be shunted through these vessels from the resistance to the capacitance circuits.[6] It thereby bypasses the capillary exchange vessels. The seventh extends from the medium-sized veins to the large veins, including the cavae. This venous capacitance bed acts as the primary storage reservoir for the intravascular compartment. Approximately 70 to 80 per cent of the total blood volume is contained within the venous capacitance bed.[7,8] Changes in venous compliance moderate venous capacitance. This, in turn, regulates the "effective circulating volume" and therefore the venous return of blood to the heart. Accordingly, it is the major determinant of preload. The eighth component represents obstruction in the mainstream of blood flow. Such obstruction may be due to vena caval or pericardial compression, mechanical obstruction in the heart or pulmonary circulation, or dissection or compression of the aorta.

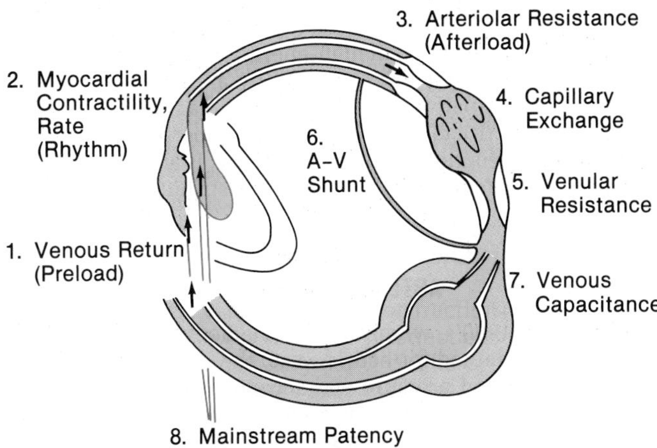

FIGURE 21-1. Functional components of the circulatory system of import in the regulation of systemic perfusion.

Goldfarb[50] implicated L-leucine as a cardiodepressant during shock. A high-molecular-weight cardiodepressive has also been described.[51] Its effects are reversed by intravenous infusion of a glucose-insulin-potassium mixture.[51] Perhaps most persuasive have been the investigations by Parrillo and his associates,[52,53] who identified a myocardial depressant substance in the serum of patients with septic shock. Decreases in ejection fraction of patients with systemic sepsis were correlated with reductions in the in vitro contractility of beating rat myocardial cells when exposed to the serum of the same patients. After endotoxin administration, left ventricular function is impaired and this is independent of changes in either preload or afterload.[54] Meningococcal bacteremia is associated with reversible myocardial depression, including reductions in cardiac output and increases in left ventricular filling pressure.[55] During experimental hemorrhagic shock in dogs, perfusion of the anterior and posterior papillary muscles is impaired.[56] Histologically, myocyte injury with "zonal lesions," including fragmentation of Z bands, distortion of microfilaments, and displacement of mitochondria away from the intercalated discs, is observed after hemorrhagic shock.[57]

Impaired ventricular function during shock is associated with substantial decreases in left ventricular compliance, together with decreases in end-diastolic volume.[58] Such diastolic dysfunction may be due to myocardial fluid retention with swelling of myocytes.[59] Glucose-insulin-potassium dilution may also minimize such cell swelling and improve compliance after endotoxin shock.[60]

Aerobic myocardial metabolism is required for efficient generation of energy to maintain contraction of myofibrillar proteins.[61] Anaerobic metabolism yields lactic acid with reduced adenosine triphospate (ATP) production. Without regeneration of high-energy phosphate, ion pump function and myocardial contractility are impaired. The inorganic phosphate concentration of myocardium increases. There is impaired cation transport, with an efflux of potassium and an influx of sodium. Consequently, myocytes swell and the compliance of the myocardium is decreased.[62] Although oxygen supply to the myocardium is decreased, the oxygen requirements of the myocardium are augmented because of increased beta$_1$ adrenergic activity and increases in afterload because of arterial constriction.[63] As myocardial ischemia and cell swelling progress, maldistribution of blood flow is intensified. As the heart becomes less compliant, myocardial contractility becomes less efficient and the imbalance between myocardial oxygen requirements and oxygen delivery increases.

Reflex increases in heart rate and the onset of cardiac arrhythmias may of themselves curtail cardiac output. The problem may be further complicated in patients with preexisting heart disease and especially in patients who are treated with digitalis glycosides. During shock there is decreased myocardial clearance of the glycoside, and hence substantially greater risk of digitalis toxicity and, therefore, ectopic dysrhythmia.[64]

OXYGEN CONSUMPTION AND ANAEROBIC METABOLISM

Fundamental to the understanding of metabolic defects during the low perfusion state is the critical reduction in cardiac output and the reduced delivery of oxygen stemming therefrom.[64a] A decline in oxygen consumption is an almost inevitable feature of fatal progression of shock states. This also applies to high or normal cardiac output states during septic shock in which disproportionate increases in oxygen consumption accompany the low-resistance, hyperdynamic state.[65] More precisely, however, the fundamental defect stems from failure to maintain oxygen delivery in amounts which fulfill the oxygen requirements of the organism.

The metabolic requirements for oxygen are contingent on the metabolic state of the patient, which reflects the underlying illness, the presence or absence of fever, effects of both endogenous and exogenous hormones (especially adrenergic agonists and thyroid hormones), and the physical activity status of the patient. Accordingly, the oxygen consumption during shock is highly variable and not of itself a clinically useful measurement for diagnosis or prognosis.[66] A substantial reduction in oxygen consumption during the more advanced stages of perfusion failure is almost always preceded by a major deterioration of hemodynamic status. This does not detract from the fact that a marked decline in oxygen consumption often ushers in the terminal course of perfusion failure. Experimentally, there is a close relationship between the cumulative oxygen deficit during hemorrhagic shock and survival. When oxygen deficit increases from 100 to 150 ml/kg during hemorrhage in dogs, survival declines from 100 to 0 per cent[13] (Fig. 21–3).

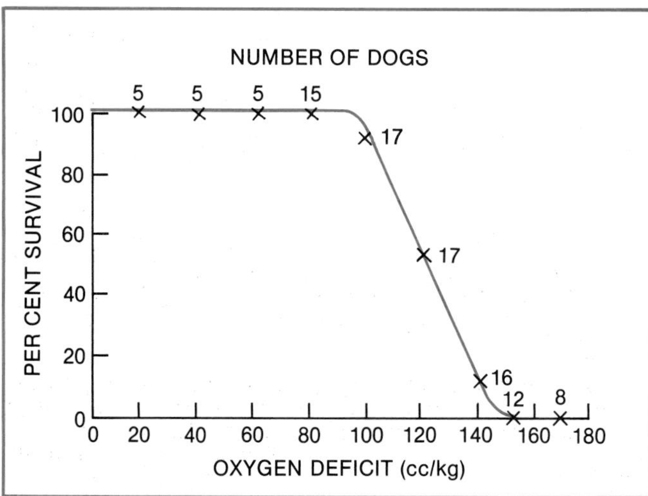

FIGURE 21–3. The relationship between oxygen deficit and survival during experimental shock produced by hemorrhage. (From Crowell, J. W., and Smith, E. E.: Oxygen deficit and irreversible hemorrhagic shock. Am. J. Physiol. *206*:313, 1964.)

When oxygen delivery is critically reduced, the regeneration of high-energy phosphate compounds is impaired. For oxidation of pyruvate derived from carbohydrates, amino acids, and fatty acids, the final common pathway of aerobic energy production by mitochondria is aerobic oxidation by way of the citric acid (Krebs) cycle (Fig. 21–4). Electron

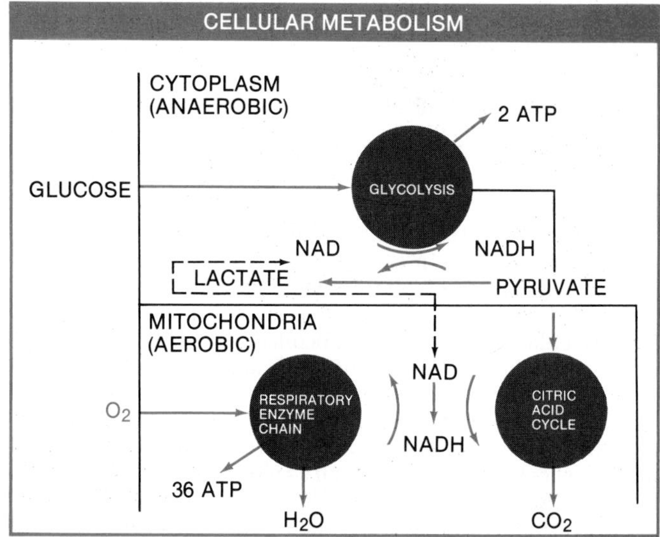

FIGURE 21–4. Inefficient extramitochondrial anaerobic metabolism has lactate as its end product. This contrasts with mitochondrial aerobic metabolism through the citric acid (Krebs) cycle with production of carbon dioxide and water.

transfer occurs through pyridine nucleotides and flavoproteins. Final electron transfer is to oxygen, which is then converted to water. This produces ATP, which is the energy source for the cell. During shock, however, oxidation through the citric acid cycle is inhibited because of the lack of an external electron acceptor (i.e., oxygen). Therefore, ATP is produced only by anaerobic glycolysis in cytoplasm, which cannot proceed beyond the metabolism of pyruvate to lactate. The pyruvate-to-lactate shunt is then activated as an emergency pathway of anaerobic metabolism. Anaerobic metabolism of 1 mole of glucose provides less than 10 per cent of the amount of ATP which would be generated by aerobic metabolism of the same quantity of glucose.

ELEVATIONS OF BLOOD LACTATE. The quantitative increases in blood lactate of the intact organism are in turn related to the oxygen deficit.[24] When lactic acid concentration increases from 2 to 8 mM/liter in human patients during circulatory shock, survival progressively decreases from approximately 90 to 10 per cent (Fig. 21–5). The lactate concentration, measured in either arterial or mixed venous blood, therefore reflects the cumulative oxygen deficit and serves as a close correlate of survival. This is of great practical moment in the clinical setting, since the measurement of blood lactate, which can now be performed with technical ease and rapidity as part of blood gases by an electrode technique,[67] serves as an objective measure of both the presence and the severity of the shock state.[24,68,69] The clinical diagnosis of perfusion failure (shock) is confirmed only if the blood lactate exceeds 1.5 mM/liter. Reversal of the perfusion deficit is accompanied by a reduction in arterial blood lactate, and the effectiveness of therapy may therefore be gauged by repetitive measurement of blood lactic acid concentration. Transient increases in blood lactate occur during hyperventilation, physical exertion, shivering, and convulsive seizures.[70] Accordingly, the activity status of the patient at the time of measurement should be taken into account in the interpretation of the lactate measurement.

When lactate is generated during exertion under physiologic conditions, it is cleared over an interval of minutes by liver, skeletal muscle, and myocardium when physical exertion ceases. However, lactate is cleared much more slowly (over periods of hours) during recovery from circulatory shock. After cardiac arrest and resuscitation, substantial but transient increases in blood lactate are observed more like those which occur during physical exertion.[71]

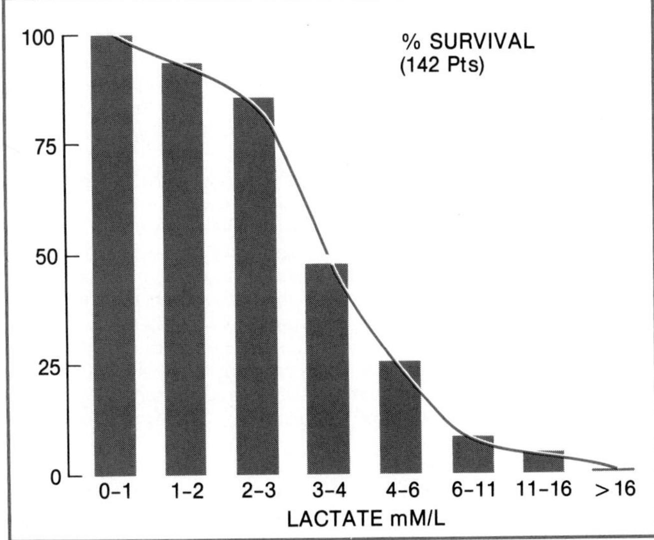

FIGURE 21–5. Relationship between concentrations of arterial blood lactate and survival in clinical shock states. (From Weil, M. H., and Shubin, H.: Metabolic consequences of cardiogenic shock. *In* Meltzer, L. E., and Dunning, A. J. (eds.): Textbook of Coronary Care. Amsterdam, Excerpta Medica, 1972, p. 634).

Exercise physiologists have traditionally measured both lactate and pyruvate and computed the lactate : pyruvate ratio (L/P) as a correlate of oxygen deficit. Huckabee[72] proposed the concept of excess lactate (XL) as a preferred quantitator of the severity of the perfusion defect. Both L/P and XL are based on the assumption that increases in "metabolic" lactate are accompanied by corresponding increases in pyruvate in the absence of anaerobic metabolism. Such may occur during infusions of glucose, bicarbonate, and pyruvate. However, both experimental and clinical investigations fail to confirm that, in the setting of circulatory shock, either the diagnostic or the prognostic value of the lactate measurement is enhanced by the concurrent measurement of pyruvate.[24,73]

Increases in blood lactate are also observed after major vascular obstruction and especially after aortic occlusion in which there is so-called *regional shock*.[74] It is assumed that restoration of blood flow is accompanied by a "washout" of lactate, with transient elevations in systemic lactate during restoration of more normal perfusion.[75] There is rapid diffusion of lactate throughout the central circulation. Even in the setting of regional shock due to aortic obstruction, the lactate concentrations measured in carotid artery blood are essentially the same as those of blood simultaneously sampled from a femoral vein.

METABOLIC AND ENDOCRINE ABNORMALITIES

Other abnormalities of carbohydrate and lipid metabolism accompany circulatory shock. Hyperglycemia during the initial stages of shock is attributed to increased secretion of catecholamines, glucagon, and glucocorticoids.[76] When glycogen stores are depleted, in the more advanced stages of perfusion failure, hypoglycemia is more likely.[76] Increased lipolysis is also attributed to excessive catecholamine secretion together with reduced lipoprotein lipase activity. This accounts for hypertriglyceridemia.[77] The concentration of fatty acids is inversely related to increases in blood lactate, presumably because of reduced perfusion of adipose tissue.[78]

A large number of humoral substances have been identified, both experimentally and clinically, during the low-flow states. Among hormones, increases in epinephrine, norepinephrine, atrial natriuretic factor,[79] renin-angiotensin-aldosterone, glucocorticoids, and vasopressin levels have already been cited. The actions of these hormones account for vasoconstriction, inotropic and chronotropic effects on the myocardium, expansion and contraction of intravascular volume, and altered glucose, fat, and protein metabolism.

Critical reductions in cardiac output are accompanied by increases in the arteriovenous gradients of pH and PCO_2 both in the experimental setting[80] and in human patients.[81] Measurements of venous blood gases during circulatory failure may therefore serve as an indication of acid-base changes in tissues. During canine hemorrhagic shock[82] and cardiac tamponade[83] and during porcine[84] and human cardiopulmonary resuscitation,[85] hypercarbic acidosis of mixed venous blood is consistently observed even though arterial blood PCO_2 may be normal or even decreased. These increases in venous PCO_2 are best explained by both decreases in pulmonary CO_2 excretion[80,84,86] and increases in the production of CO_2 in underperfused tissues.[87]

OTHER MEDIATORS IN SHOCK

Increased release of *histamine* in part related to a reduction in histaminase has been identified in shock states and particularly during the course of sepsis and anaphylaxis.[88] *Kinins* are released by the action of a group of enzymes termed kallikreins acting on kininogen, a plasma globulin.[89] The predominant vasoactive peptide is bradykinin, which mediates vasodilation and increases vascular permeability. It also accounts for margination of leukocytes at local sites of inflammation, where kinins are released from granulocytes.[90] Serotonin is a potentially potent vasoconstrictor found in large concentrations in circulating platelets. Rapid destruction of platelets, especially in the settings of septic (endotoxin) shock and anaphylactic shock, is accompanied by *serotonin* release.[91] Serotonin increases pulmonary vascular resistance and therefore has been implicated in the development of pulmonary hypertension after sepsis and trauma.[92] It has also been implicated in the development of adult respiratory distress syndrome (ARDS).[93]

The products of the *arachidonic acid* cascade have been implicated in cellular injury of a variety of causes. The concentrations of various prostanoids in blood are increased in shock, but the precise role of prostanoids in the pathophysiology of shock is as yet unclear. The vasoconstrictor actions of thromboxane are prevented after injection of endotoxin when rats are pretreated with a thromboxane synthetase inhibitor such as imidazole.[94] The vasodilator effects of prostaglandins, and more specifically prostaglandin E_2 (PGE_2) and prostacyclin (PGI_2), may, at least in part, account for the typical hyperdynamic abnormalities characteristic of septic shock.[95] The hyperdynamic state is reversed by the administration of indomethacin and ibuprofen, which inhibit prostaglandin synthesis.[96]

Increases in *endorphins,* endogenous opiates liberated from the pituitary gland, have been implicated in the progression of septic shock.[36,97] These peptides are regarded as mediators of hypotension during sepsis and hemorrhage. Naloxone, an antagonist to endogenous opiates, has reversed endotoxin-mediated hypotension and increased survival. However, it has not as yet proved to have long-term survival benefits in patients.[98]

The primary toxic component of gram-negative lipopolysaccharides is *lipid-A.*[99] When endotoxin is administered to laboratory animals, diffuse endothelial cell damage occurs. There is abrupt onset of thrombocytopenia and granulocytopenia.[100]: A variety of *lysosomal enzymes* and especially proteases, serotonin, epinephrine, and thromboxanes are released. Antiproteases are disabled and there is lipid peroxidation of cell membranes. Among cytotoxic products, *free oxygen radicals* are liberated. There is lipid peroxidation of cell membranes and fragmentation of the interstitial hyaluronic acid lattices. Consequently, both proteases and free oxygen radicals cause diffuse tissue injury.[101-103]

The *complement system* is activated directly by endotoxin, chiefly through the intrinsic coagulation cascade. This accounts for intravascular coagulation with consumption of clotting factors, fibrinolysis with generation of fibrin monomers and fibrin split products.[104] Together with progressive thrombocytopenia and fibrinogen depletion, this characterizes the clinical syndrome of disseminated intravascular coagulation.

These injuries are additive to those of tissue hypoxia and impaired mitochondrial capability for oxidative phosphorylation. The therapeutic administration of an exogenous high-energy phosphate source, ATP magnesium chloride, has been proposed as an adjunct for treatment of shock with the anticipation that it would restore more normal membrane permeability, decrease cellular edema, reduce enzyme leakage, and thereby improve cell function.[105] However, confirmation of its efficacy and safety for clinical management is still required.

IMMUNOLOGICAL MECHANISMS

Altered immunological function is in evidence during circulatory shock. It is the primary cause of anaphylaxis, which is mediated by antigen-antibody reactions with IgE antibody. This antibody, also known as reagin, acts directly on tissue-bound mast cells and circulatory basophils to release primary mediators, including histamine, slow-reacting substances of anaphylaxis, eosinophil chemotactic factor of anaphylaxis, and a platelet-activating factor.[106,107] The activation of complement by classic and alternative pathways generates the kinins from platelets, eosinophils, and neutrophils. The kinins increase capillary permeability and stimulate mast cells and basophils to increase their release of primary mediators. Complement fractions also act as opsonins, which facilitate phagocytosis.[108] These cascading reactions trigger the release of Hageman factor (factor XII), and therefore the intrinsic coagulation cascade. The end result is bronchoconstriction, increased capillary permeability with pulmonary and systemic edema, increased leukocyte aggregation, release of lysosomal enzymes, intravascular coagulation, thrombocytopenia, and progressive hypovolemia with perfusion failure. These pathophysiological processes are of major importance in anaphylactic shock (p. 581).

Although the side effects of complement activation are detrimental, the more fundamental biological role of complement may be beneficial for enhancing phagocytosis and curtailing infection. However, the reticuloendothelial system (RES), and therefore the capability for clearing circulating microorganisms from the bloodstream, is impaired during shock states.[109] The principal components of the RES, which is made up of tissue-based phagocytes, include macrophages in the lung, spleen, lymph nodes, and Kupffer cells of the liver.[110] RES function is impaired during both hypovolemic and endotoxin shock. Both histamine and serotonin reduce the capability of the RES to clear particulate matter, and a dialyzable RES-depressant substance has been described.[111] In the clinical setting in which the RES is impaired, as it is in debilitated patients after cytotoxic or radiation therapy, in patients with neoplastic diseases, or in patients with hepatic cirrhosis, the mortality from shock, and particularly septic shock, is increased. Cytokines such as tumor necrosis factor alpha (TNF-α) or interleukines are released from macrophages and T lymphocytes after stimulation with endotoxin.[112] Increases in TNF-α levels are correlated with greater mortality.[113,114] Experimentally, pretreatment with neutralizing monoclonal anti-TNF-α antibodies protects against lethal shock[115] as does pretreatment with cyclo-oxygenase inhibitors such as ibuprofen.[116]

Secondary Effects of Shock

HEART

Except in instances of cardiogenic shock in which primary abnormalities in cardiac function are responsible, the heart, like the brain, is remarkably accommodating to decreases in systemic blood flow during the early stages of shock.[117] In the late stages of shock, the decreases in left ventricular compliance which are associated with cellular injury and particularly cell swelling may be important. However, these are not likely to be the major causes for fatal progression of shock. The same applies to the as-yet-not-fully-elucidated role of several myocardial depressant substances.

KIDNEYS (see also Ch. 62)

Renal failure is a major complication of circulatory shock. It typically appears within an interval of 36 to 72 hours after the onset of acute circulatory failure and in close association with other manifestations of tissue catabolism.

PATHOPHYSIOLOGY. During low-perfusion states, and most especially during hypovolemic shock, renal blood flow may be reduced to as low as 10 per cent of normal. There is redistribution of renal blood flow with diminished cortical blood flow. Such redistribution of renal blood flow is in part attributed to endogenous alpha$_1$ adrenergic action and accentuated by renal sympathetic nerve activity. it is accentuated by the vasoconstrictor actions of exogenous administration of predominant alpha$_1$-adrenergic agonists and probably by angiotensin II, especially when cardiac output and arterial perfusion pressures are critically reduced. Renal tubular injury progresses to cell necrosis with tubular obstruction. Proteinaceous and cellular debris accumulates within the tubular lumina. There is back diffusion and ultimately leakage of the glomerular filtrate, which, together with peritubular interstitial edema, may cause tubular collapse.[118] Contrary to earlier reports, there is rather good correlation between histological changes in the kidney and renal function.[119]

Under conditions of extremely low flow, there may be critical limitations in renal tissue oxygen tension, especially in the medullary thick ascending limb of the nephron.[120,121] During the low-flow state there is initial increase in sodium and free water reabsorption, in part caused by increases in the secretion of aldosterone and ADH, which may enhance back diffusion. Nevertheless, the mineralocorticoids and ADH subsequently fail to maintain sodium reabsorption. Both sodium and urea concentration in the medulla are reduced so that the hypertonic gradient for reabsorption of water by the countercurrent mechanism is disabled. The capability of renal solute concentration is therefore rapidly lost.[122]

CLINICAL FEATURES. In acute renal failure, clinical features include proteinuria, hematuria, isosthenuria, and iso-osmolality with plasma. Progressive increases in serum urea nitrogen, creatinine, potassium, phosphate, and sulfate are frequently observed, together with decreases in serum sodium, calcium, and bicarbonate. Initial reduction in urine output to volumes of less than 400 ml per day ushers in the oliguric phase. The urine typically contains protein, red cells, epithelial cells, and characteristic brown granular casts of renal failure. *Hypertension* frequently develops during the recovery stage of acute renal failure. It is important to adjust potassium intake to avoid hyperkalemia and consequent cardiac arrhythmias and neuromuscular depression. In the absence of dialysis, the onset of the diuretic phase between 6 days and 2 weeks after the clinical shock state signals recovery, but renal concentration capability returns much more slowly.[123]

The typical laboratory findings of acute renal failure include urine osmolality of less than 350 mOsm, urine : plasma urea ration of less than 10, urine : plasma creatinine ratio of less than 20, and urinary sodium concentration of greater than 40 mEq/liter. Renal failure indices based on measurements of urine flow and either renal clearance of creatinine and sodium or both may increase precision for purposes of monitoring and prognosis.[124] When renal failure occurs as part of multisystemic failure, the prognosis diminishes contingent on the number of major organ systems that fail.[125] However, when renal failure occurs after reversal of shock, it does not of itself prognosticate an unfavorable outcome. With the availability of intermittent dialysis or hemofiltration, recovery of essentially normal renal function is the rule.[126]

MANAGEMENT. Management is directed to the treatment of the shock state, control of infection, appropriate nutrition, careful control of fluid intake, and appropriate electrolyte replacement. Hemodialysis, peritoneal dialysis, and hemofiltration are liberally used for the control of uremia and for fluid and electrolyte management. The routine use of diuretic agents for reversal of oliguria is not advised, not only because it is unlikely to be effective but also because it invalidates both diagnostic and prognostic measurement of renal function and particularly the tests of urea, creatinine, sodium, and osmolal clearance.

LUNGS (see also p. 564)

Early changes of pulmonary function include increases in ventilation so that the ventilation-perfusion ratio is markedly increased, with augmented physiological dead space and alveolocapillary gradients for oxygen. Pulmonary vascular resistance is usually only mildly elevated except for disproportionate increases in patients with arterial hypoxemia.

Progressive pulmonary injury, associated with circulatory shock, termed the adult respiratory distress syndrome (ARDS), represents impairment of alveolocapillary membrane integrity.[127,127a] This is attributed to injury of alveolocapillary endothelium. Injury to Type 2 pneumocytes contributes to permeability defects and accounts for reduced synthesis of surfactin. There is sequestration of platelets and neutrophils in the pulmonary capillaries with liberation of proteases. Macrophage-mediated neutrophil sequestration is associated with complement activation and generation of lipid peroxidases from oxygen free radicals. The RES response is blunted and immunological resistance to infection is decreased.[128] An increase in T lymphocyte killer cells has been identified with decreases in fibronectin and immunoglobulin (IgG).[129] Perivascular leakage, potentiated by histamine and bradykinin, augments the increases in extravascular lung water produced by increased capillary permeability. In advanced stages of pulmonary failure, there is more extensive loss of capillary endothelial integrity with perivascular interstitial and intraalveolar hemorrhage.

Pulmonary failure is much more often observed in the setting of hypovolemic and septic shock and after pulmonary embolization; it is relatively uncommon in patients with cardiogenic shock. There is some hope that prostaglandin E may curtail pulmonary injury.[130] However, objective clinical studies have given contradictory results after high-dose glucocorticoid therapy.[127,131]

THERAPY. Treatment is largely supportive. Positive end-expiratory pressure (PEEP) improves oxygenation such that FIO_2 of more than 0.6 may be avoided. Prolonged administration of higher concentrations of inspired oxygen may be an iatrogenic cause of pulmonary damage owing to oxygen toxicity.[132] When continuous positive airway pressure (CPAP) or PEEP is used at levels of 5 to 10 cm H_2O, it does not usually impede venous return (i.e., preload). When CPAP or PEEP of larger magnitudes is used, especially in patients with hypovolemia, venous return is impeded such that cardiac output is further reduced.[133,134] A careful balance between volume expansion and positive airway pressure is therefore required (see p. 565). Positive airway pressure usually reduces the magnitude of pulmonary arteriovenous shunts, most likely by preventing collapse of alveoli, but increases the risk of barotrauma and especially pneumothorax, pneumomediastinum, and subcutaneous emphysema.

SKELETAL MUSCLE

With decreases in cell muscle blood flow, the resting transmembrane potential declines and there is impaired membrane transport. Respiratory muscle function, and particularly that of the diaphragm, may be compromised, accounting for decreased efficiency and increased oxygen requirements of breathing.[135] This in part accounts for respiratory muscle fatigue. When metabolic demands are increased and oxygen delivery is severely curtailed, the increased work requirements of breathing may exceed the patient's capability, leading to alveolar hypoventilation with hypercarbia and hypoxemia.[136] The clinician may then have little option other than to intubate the trachea and mechanically assist or control ventilation.

LIVER

Isolated zones of centrilobular necrosis are observed in laboratory animals and in humans, but massive hepatic necrosis is uncommon except when circulatory shock occurs in patients with underlying hepatocellular disease. Nonspecific increases in aspartate aminotransferase (SGOT, AST), alanine aminotransferase (SGPT, ALT), and lactic dehydrogenase (LDH) appear early in patients with circulatory shock of diverse causes.[137] Cytoplasmic lysosomal enzymes increase and RES function decreases, accounting for decreases in circulating opsonins and $alpha_2$-glycoproteins.[109] The decreased efficiency of protein and carbohydrate metabolism disables the detoxification function of the liver.[138] This may account for impaired coagulation because of inadequate regeneration of essential clotting factors. Nevertheless, liver failure is a late complication of shock, even though subtle changes in liver architecture are seen early on electron microscopy.[139] Increases in serum bilirubin, in part caused by intravascular hemolysis, are more often observed in patients with septic shock.

STOMACH AND INTESTINE

Mucosal congestion and bleeding of the stomach and intestines may account for hypermotility and hypomotility. Submucosal hemorrhage, particularly in the colon, with progressive hemorrhagic necrosis and ulceration is commonly observed on autopsy after hemorrhagic and endotoxic shock, especially in dogs. Similar lesions have been observed in humans.[140] The barrier function of the gut may be decreased so that gram-negative bacilli or their endotoxins may enter the circulation.[141] There is sequestration of blood in the portal venous system. Splanchnic ischemia is attributed to alpha-adrenergically induced vasoconstriction with disproportionate reduction in mucosal blood flow. Elderly patients are likely to exhibit a higher incidence of intestinal ischemia because of preceding atherosclerotic disease of the splanchnic arteries. Nevertheless, transmural infarction complicated by perforation is an uncommon complication. However, mucosal necrosis may cause pseudomembraneous enterocolities during recovery.

The intestinal tract, like many other systems or organs, has been cited as responsible for irreversibility of shock.[142] However, such hypotheses of "irreversibility" have not proved to be clinically applicable and do not currently call for specific prophylactic or therapeutic interventions.

PANCREAS

Blood flow to the pancreas is markedly reduced during shock,[143] and this may account for pancreatic sources of proteases, especially the cathepsins.[144] Experimentally, the pancreas has also been viewed as the source of the myocardial depressant factor, which decreases contractility of an isolated papillary muscle preparation.[145] Subcellular alterations in the pancreas, including dilated endoplasmic reticulum and swollen mitochondria, are reversible.[146] Local areas of necrosis have been observed in the pancreas. Although this organ is also cited as a primary shock organ which determines reversibility,[147] an important limiting role of the pancreas, or of toxic substances produced by it during clinical shock states, has not been established.

BLOOD

With slowing of blood flow, there is intravascular aggregation and clumping of red cells, leukocytes, and platelets, called sludging. Although this process of itself may increase vascular resistance, it is usually reversible. However, a serious complication of shock is *disseminated intravascular coagulation* (DIC). It results from intravascular activation of the coagulation process by infection, by the abnormal production or liberation of coagulant tissue factors such as endotoxin, amniotic fluid, snake bites, or by generation of procoagulants in the blood as may be the case during hemolytic transfusion reactions.[148] *Purpura fulminans* is an uncommon and extreme complication of DIC and may cause extensive tissue necrosis with gangrene of extremities. Microthrombi are formed within small blood vessels by fibrin deposition, and this triggers fibrinolysis. High levels of fibrin split products have of themselves antihemostatic properties, and they act as circulating anticoagulants and impair platelet function with enhancement of bleeding. The microthrombi and the intravascular fibrin strands associated with them obstruct blood flow so as to produce microangiopathic hemolysis caused by sheer damage to red cells. Both injured endothelium and microthrombi activate fibrinolysis. The fibrinogen concentration of plasma is reduced. There is diffuse tissue injury because of small vessel obstruction by thrombosis, embolization, and bleeding into tissues.[104] The contact of blood with subendothelial components such as collagen may activate factor XII, the Hageman factor, and trigger coagulation through the intrinsic pathway. Plasma levels of the various plasma serum protease inhibitors, such as antithrombin III, $alpha_2$ macroglobulin, and $alpha_2$ antiplasma, are decreased. Sustained release of vonWillebrand factor was observed in vivo after administration of *Escherichia coli* endotoxin.[149]

Typical laboratory findings include thrombocytopenia, prolongation of prothrombin time and partial thromboplastin time, decreased factors V and VIII and fibrinogen concentrations, and increased concentration of fibrin monomers and fibrin split products.

Therapy is directed first at the control of the underlying cause of the shock state, particularly sepsis. If bleeding and thrombosis are mild, no specific therapy is advised. If bleeding is serious, replacement of clotting factors with fresh frozen plasma, cryoprecipitate, and platelet transfusions may be required in conjunction with heparin. If the primary defect is thrombosis in contrast to bleeding, the administration of a therapeutic anticoagulant loading dose of heparin followed by continuous infusion is advocated to interrupt the cycle of coagulation and fibrinolysis.[150] Replacement of fibrinogen and antithrombin III by the administration of fresh frozen plasma may also be indicated when the fibrinogen level is decreased to less than 150 mg/dl. Fresh frozen plasma replaces depleted clotting factors and serum protease inhibitors. Cryoprecipitate contains a high concentration of fibrinogen and may be used when fibrinogen levels decrease to less than 100 mg/dl.

The role of altered oxyhemoglobin dissociation is unclear. During shock states the affinity of hemoglobin for oxygen is decreased such that the P_{50} (the oxygen tension at which 50 per cent of hemoglobin is saturated with oxygen) is increased[151] (see Fig. 57–2, p. 1743). This facilitates the unloading of oxygen at tissue levels. However, when the blood pH is decreased with metabolic acidosis, the erythrocyte 2,3-diphosphoglycerate (2,3-DPG) declines, which decreased P_{50}. At the present time there are no indications for routine measurement or treatment of abnormalities of either P_{50} or 2,3-DPG.[152]

BRAIN

The cerebral circulation is remarkably well protected in shock.[153] Except when there is intrinsic cerebrovascular disease, there is preferential flow to the cerebral circuit in a manner analogous to that which occurs during cardiac arrest. Autoregulation maintains constancy of cerebral blood flow.[154] During hypotension there is a reduction in cerebrovascular resistance associated with cerebral vasodilation. Symptoms of ischemia emerge only when cerebral blood flow decreases to less than 50 per cent of normal values, and this is not likely until mean arterial pressure decreases to less than 50 mm Hg.[155]

The arterial carbon dioxide tension exerts a profound effect on cerebral blood flow.[156] Cerebral blood flow is reduced when Pa_{CO_2} declines because of cerebral vasoconstriction and increases when arterial P_{CO_2} increases because of cerebral arterial vasodilation. The response is highly sensitive; for each 1 mm Hg change, cerebral blood flow normally changes by approximately 4 per cent. Alterations in arterial oxygen tension also affect cerebral blood flow. When arterial P_{O_2} declines, there is progressive cerebral vasodilation. Cerebral blood flow may increase fivefold when arterial P_{O_2} falls below 50 mm Hg.

Clinical Shock States

CLASSIFICATION

Earlier classifications of circulatory shock related etiology and hemodynamic mechanisms.[1] A widely used classification included hypovolemic, cardiogenic, hypersensitivity (anaphylactic), bacteremic, neurogenic, obstructive, and endocrine types of shock.[1] Subsequent investigations, however, indicated that anaphylactic shock is predominantly hypovolemic shock and that shock associated with major neurological defects, such as transection of the spinal cord, in fact represented increases in venous capacitance. Endocrine types of shock such as those which occur in the course of pheochromocytoma were demonstrated to be caused by hypovolemia.[33] Consequently, a classification[157] based on four discrete hemodynamic defects was evolved. These defects are shown in Figure 21–6.

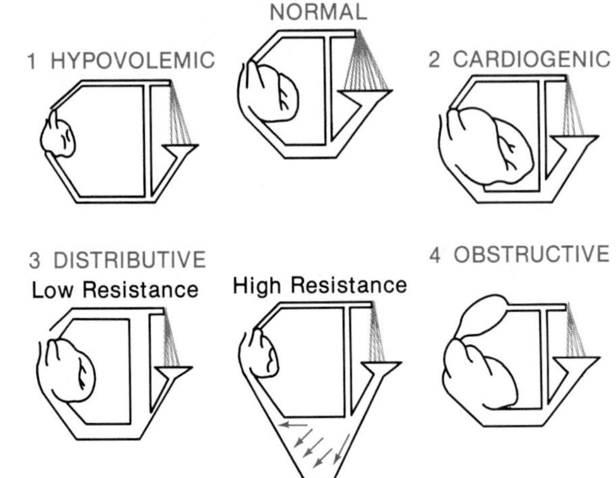

FIGURE 21–6. Hemodynamic classification of circulatory shock states. The common denominator is a critical reduction in blood flow.

The most common cause of reduced systemic blood flow is *hypovolemia,* which results from a reduction of volume within the intravascular compartment. *Cardiogenic shock* represents failure of the cardiac pump to maintain systemic blood flow in amounts that will fulfill metabolic requirements. *Obstruction* may occur in the great veins, including the vena cava, by compression caused by the gravid uterus (the supine hypotensive syndrome [p. 1790]); in the heart itself owing to pericardial tamponade (p. 1473), ball valve thrombi, or pulmonary embolism (Chap. 48); or in the aorta owing to dissection and may physically impede the main stream of blood flow (Chap. 47). This represents obstructive shock. The important new category is that of distributive shock, which represents major alterations in the distribution of blood flow without critical decreases in intravascular volume, cardiac function, or obstruction of blood flow. Abnormalities in distribution may be due to either low arterial resistance in association with inflammatory vasodilation or arteriovenous shunting as in hyperdynamic states of septic shock. In the more advanced stages of gram-negative sepsis with shock, there is an increase in arterial resistance and a concomitant increase in venous capacitance with decreased venous return. This also applies to shock states which are associated with altered neural control, including barbiturate intoxication, ganglionic blockade, or spinal shock resulting from transection of the spinal cord. In Table 21–2 the hemodynamic classification is related to commonly encountered clinical circulatory shock states.

In the instance of low-resistance distributive shock, the cardiac output may be normal or increased, yet the blood pressure is low. Accordingly, the shock state represents a failure to maintain capillary perfusion, which, in the instance of low-resistance distributive states, is largely independent of cardiac output. The common denominator is *failure of tissue perfusion*

TABLE 21–2 CLASSIFICATION OF SHOCK STATES

TYPE OF SHOCK	PRIMARY MECHANISM	CLINICAL CAUSES
1. Hypovolemic	Volume loss	Exogenous blood, plasma, fluid, or electrolyte loss Endogenous extravasation
2. Cardiogenic	Pump failure	Myocardial infarction, cardiac arrhythmias Intracardiac obstruction, heart failure
3. Distributive (vasomotor dysfunction) (1) High or normal resistance	Expanded venous capacitance	Hypodynamic late septic shock Autonomic blockade, spinal shock Drug overdose
(2) Low resistance	Arteriovenous shunting	Pneumonia, peritonitis, abscess
4. Obstructive	Extracardiac obstruction of main channel of blood flow	Vena caval obstruction (supine hypotensive syndrome) Pericarditis (tamponade) Pulmonary embolism Dissecting aneurysm or compression of aorta

so that oxygen delivery is not sufficient to sustain normal aerobic metabolism. Consequently, it is lactic acidosis, as the metabolic consequence of anaerobic metabolism, which is the sine qua non of the low-perfusion state, regardless of cause.

GENERAL PRINCIPLES OF DIAGNOSIS AND MANAGEMENT: THE VIPS

For the patient who presents with clinical signs of shock, a useful guide to initial evaluation and management is provided by the acronym VIP.[158] "V" refers to ventilation to ensure adequate pulmonary exchange of oxygen and carbon dioxide. "I" refers to infusion and, in turn, the adequacy of intravascular volume. "P" refers to pump function, and therefore cardiac competence. These priorities apply to the initial management of patients with circulatory shock, regardless of cause.

VENTILATION

In addition to overt physical signs which indicate inadequate chest movement or respiratory distress, analysis or arterial blood gases provides quantitative measurement of the adequacy of both ventilation and acid-base status. When hypoxemia appears in the absence of hypercarbia and respiratory acidosis, the initial intervention is that of increasing inspired concentrations of oxygen. Oxygen therapy by mask or nasal catheter may suffice. If alveolar ventilation is impaired, arterial blood gas measurements will demonstrate respiratory acidosis with substantial increases in arterial carbon dioxide tension.

Either failure to reverse hypoxemia ($Pa_{O_2} < 60$ mm Hg) by increasing the concentration of oxygen in inspired gas to 60 per cent or progressive respiratory acidosis ($Pa_{CO_2} > 60$ mm Hg would ordinarily require endotracheal intubation and mechanical ventilation with a volume-controlled respirator. Positive pressure ventilation is likely to overcome life-threatening hypoxemia, especially in patients with reduced pulmonary compliance caused by pulmonary edema or pneumonia. Intubation of the airway facilitates suctioning and therefore control of secretions. Mechanical ventilation is also likely to decrease the oxygen cost owing to the work of breathing.[159] When pulmonary compliance is decreased in the absence of hypoxemia and hypercarbia, the increased oxygen requirement for breathing nevertheless augments the oxygen deficit and therefore the severity of the shock state. Ventilation may be either assisted or intermittent so that it is coordinated with the voluntary ventilatory drive of the patient. Fully controlled ventilation in patients who "fight" the ventilator is facilitated by the administration of tranquilizer-sedatives (e.g., diazepam) in intravenous doses of 5 to 20 mg at intervals of 1 to 3 hours or by narcotic drugs. In extreme cases, when mechanical ventilation is opposed by spontaneous ventilation of the patient, neuromuscular blockade with an agent such as pancuronium in initial doses of 0.1 mg/kg and subsequently 0.01 to 0.02 mg/kg, which are repeated at intervals of 20 to 60 minutes as required in addition to the tranquilizer-sedative or narcotic. The frequency and minute volume of mechanical ventilation are adjusted to maintain physiological levels of arterial blood gases.

With decreases in pulmonary compliance, increasingly larger airway pressures are required to maintain adequate minute volumes. When patients develop ARDS (shock lung), PEEP or CPAP improves the patency of small airways, recruits alveoli, and decreases pulmonary arterial venous shunting.[160] Because increases in airway pressure produced by mechanical ventilation, PEEP, and CPAP are accompanied by corresponding increases in intrathoracic pressure, these mechanical interventions impede venous return and therefore preload and cardiac output (p. 379). Accordingly, the clinician is required to balance the effects of positive airway pressures on cardiac output and, more specifically, oxygen delivery.[134] The computation of oxygen transport, represented by the product of cardiac output and arterial oxygen content, is useful for this purpose. Decreases in venous return, and therefore cardiac output, which stem from increases in intrathoracic pressure are usually overcome by expansion of the intravascular volume by judicious fluid challenge.

INFUSION

It is not only true that hypovolemia is the most common cause of shock, but progression of shock states, regardless of cause, is likely to be accompanied by reductions in intravascular volume owing to increased hydrostatic pressure and increased permeability of capillary exchange vessels. Volume expansion is therefore routinely required to increase oxygen delivery, not only during hypovolemic shock but in all shock states, including cardiogenic and distributive (septic) shock states.[14]

In the absence of impaired left heart function, the central venous pressure may serve as an appropriate monitor for volume infusion.[161] The changes in central venous pressure parallel those of the pulmonary artery occlusive (wedge) pressure, the pulmonary artery diastolic pressure, and the left ventricular end-diastolic pressure in the normal heart (Fig. 21–7). However, this clearly does not apply in patients (especially after acute myocardial infarction) with impaired left ventricular function, in whom changes in left ventricular filling pressure are not reflected in the central venous pressure (Fig. 21–8).[162] Nevertheless, it is important to monitor routinely right-sided filling pressure in addition to left-sided pressures, which is easily accomplished through the right atrial port of the conventional flow-directed, balloon-tipped (Swan-Ganz) catheter. Increases in right-sided filling pressures are of import in the diagnosis and management of right ventricular failure from a diversity of causes in the setting of circulatory shock, including right ventricular infarction with cardiogenic shock, right and left ventricular failure in the late stages of distributive shock resulting from sepsis, or with pulmonary embolism, primary pulmonary hypertension, and ARDS.

The pulmonary diastolic pressure is typically between 1 and 5 mm Hg less than the pulmonary artery occlusive pressure, except in patients who have increased pulmonary vascular resistance and when pulmonary systolic pressures exceed 45 mm Hg.[163] Because changes in pulmonary artery diastolic pressure usually reflect those of the left-sided filling pressure, they provide a useful check on the validity of the pulmonary artery occlusive pressure. Monitoring of the pulmonary diastolic pressure makes it possible to avoid repetitive inflation of the distal balloon for measurement of pulmonary artery occlusive pressure during fluid challenge. Minute-to-minute monitoring of pulmonary diastolic pressure allows for only intermittent measurement of occlusive (wedge) pressure

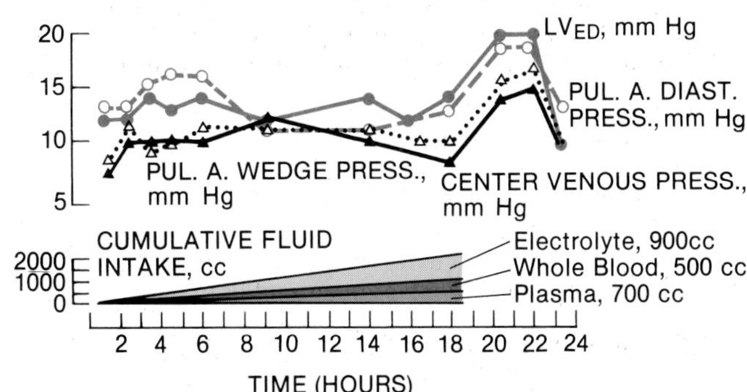

FIGURE 21–7. Parallel changes in right ventricular and left ventricular filling pressures during fluid challenge in the absence of myocardial impairment in a 67-year-old woman who had hypovolemia following total hip replacement.

shock occurs predominantly in the setting of anterior and anteroseptal myocardial infarction with recent or old infarction of the apex. This typically follows proximal obstruction of the left anterior descending coronary artery. However, a majority of patients in cardiogenic shock secondary to myocardial infarction present with three-vessel coronary artery disease and with acute infarction of more than 40 per cent of the left ventricular myocardium.[184] In a minority of instances, cardiogenic shock may occur in patients with inferior myocardial infarction after infarction of the right ventricle. Approximately 25 per cent of patients who sustain inferior myocardial infarction also have associated right ventricular infarction. However, isolated infarction of the right ventricle is uncommon.[185]

Specific hemodynamic complications, in addition to loss of viable myocardium, may trigger the onset of shock. These include major cardiac arrhythmias with excessively rapid or slow heart rates and loss of atrial transfer function with atrial arrhythmias, atrioventricular block, perforation of the interventricular septum, papillary muscle dysfunction or rupture, myocardial rupture with consequent pericardial tamponade, and pulmonary embolism. Congestive heart failure may progress to cardiogenic shock.

HEMODYNAMIC FEATURES. Routine bedside hemodynamic measurements in cardiogenic shock demonstrate increases in left ventricular filling pressure, as reflected in pulmonary artery occlusive pressure, to levels greater than 18 mm Hg in combination with a decline in the cardiac index to less than 2.2 liters/min/M^2. Except in the setting of right ventricular infarction, pulmonary embolism, cardiac tamponade, or pulmonary hypertension induced by hypoxemia or preexisting pulmonary heart disease, the right-sided filling pressures are normal or only slightly increased.

DIFFERENTIAL DIAGNOSIS. Hemodynamic diagnosis of complications of acute myocardial infarction which may usher in or increase the severity of cardiogenic shock is also facilitated by measurements obtained with the flow-directed, balloon-tipped thermodilution catheter (Table 21–6). Papillary muscle dysfunction is characterized by prominent *v* waves with characteristic morphology in pressure waveforms obtained from the pulmonary artery occlusive and pulmonary artery sites. Septal perforation is characterized by arterialization of blood sampled from the right ventricle and pulmonary artery. Pulmonary hypertension and pulmonary embolism are characterized by disproportionate increases in right-sided pressures, including the pulmonary artery pressure. With right ventricular infarction in the setting of inferior myocardial infarction, there is selective increase in right ventricular filling pressure and typically lower pulmonary artery occlusive pressure. For the diagnosis of pericardial tamponade, the right atrial pressure pulse demonstrates a characteristic steep *y* descent, with equilibration of mean right atrial, pulmonary artery diastolic, and pulmonary artery occlusive pressures (p. 1476). These hemodynamic abnormalities complement characteristic physical signs, together with electrocardiographic, radiographic, and echocardiographic findings.

TABLE 21–6 CARDIAC CAUSES OF SHOCK BY HEMODYNAMIC DIAGNOSIS

	FLOW	INTRACARDIAC PRESSURES				SATURATION
MECHANISM	CO	RA	$RV_{S/D}$	$PA_{S/D}$	PA_O	SaO_2
LV failure	↓	—↑	—↑	↑	↑↑	—
Mitral regurgitation	↓	—↑	—↑	↑("V wave")		—
VSD	±	—↑	↑	↑	—↑	↑(RV, PA)
Pulmonary hypertension pulmonary embolism	↓	↑	↑	↑	—	—
RV (Infarction)	↓	↑	↑	↓↑	↓↑	—
Tamponade	↓	↑	↑	↑	↑	—

CO, cardiac output, SaO_2, arterial oxygen saturation. See also Table 21–5.

PROGNOSIS. Of the correlates of survival, measurements of blood flow and perfusion have been substantially better than those of arterial pressure. Arterial blood lactate, cardiac output or stroke work, and arterial pressure are prognostic of outcome, in that order.[68] There is substantial variability in the reported acute mortality in cardiogenic shock because of differences in definition of this condition. When lactate is increased to levels exceeding 4 mM/liter, cardiac index is reduced to less than 2.2 liters/min/M^2, arterial resistance is increased to more than 2,000 dyne/sec/cm^{-5}, left ventricular filling pressure exceeds 18 mm Hg, mean arterial pressure is less than 60 mm Hg, and there is no prompt reversal after fluid challenge, mortality approaches 100 per cent. With less rigorous criteria, mortality is generally stated to be between 85 and 95 per cent with medical management, and there has been little improvement over the past 30 years.[186]

MANAGEMENT. Routine measures include the amelioration of pain by the intravenous administration of morphine in titrated doses of 2 to 5 mg at intervals of 30 minutes to 1 hour. Morphine may increase venous capacitance, and therefore decrease preload and ventricular filling pressures, but this is readily reversed with fluid challenge. Morphine may also provoke increased vagal activity, which may be controlled by the intravenous injection of 0.5 to 1.0 mg of atropine sulfate. Anxiety may be relieved by slow intravenous bolus injection of diazepam in doses of 3 to 5 mg repeated as frequently as necessary, usually at intervals of 30 to 60 minutes.

Optimization of preload by fluid challenge provides the single best option for improving left ventricular performance (Table 21–3). If pulmonary artery occlusion pressure is less than 18 mm Hg, 50-ml fluid challenges by standard protocol with either physiological salt solution or 6 per cent hydroxyethyl starch should be undertaken.[187] If the safe limits of fluid challenge have been exceeded, and provided that mean arterial pressure is not reduced to less than 50 mm Hg, vasodilator therapy with sodium nitroprusside in amounts of 15 to 400 μg/min by continuous intravenous infusion is titrated to maintain constancy of arterial perfusion pressure.

INOTROPIC AGENTS. These drugs, including digitalis glycosides, dopamine, dobutamine, and amrinone, may be tried in unresponsive patients in whom fluid challenge and afterload reduction are of no avail.[187a] However, *digitalis glycosides* are not generally effective and increase the risk of dysrhythmias. Nevertheless, digitalis may be used judiciously for the treatment of atrial fibrillation with rapid ventricular rates. *Dopamine*, when used in doses which exceed 6 μg/kg/min, has a predominant $alpha_1$-adrenoceptor effect, and therefore increases afterload, but may be used for transient vasopressor support when marked reduction in arterial pressure with ventricular ectopy threatens immediate survival. However, this agent should be used only for brief periods with the understanding that increases in cardiac output and coronary blood flow are likely to be transient and at the risk of increased ischemic injury and depletion of plasma volume. *Dobutamine* is an effective inotropic agent with predominant $beta_1$-adrenoceptor inotropic effect but potentially at the cost of increased myocardial oxygen requirements, and therefore the risk of extending the infarction. The benefits of nonadrenergic inotropic agents like amrinone or milrinone are not well defined. Except for the temporary management of bradycardia resulting from heart block, the $beta_{1,2}$-adrenoceptor agonist *isoproterenol* is contraindicated because its conjoint chronotropic and inotropic effects extract disproportionately large myocardial oxygen requirements which are likely to increase myocardial ischemic injury.[175]

MYOCARDIAL REPERFUSION. Improved outcome after reperfusion, whether induced by pharmacological thrombolysis and/or percutaneous transluminal coronary angioplasty or emergency coronary artery bypass, has been suggested but has not been well documented.[188–190]

INTRAAORTIC BALLOON COUNTERPULSATION (see also Chap. 19). There is increasing enthusiasm for mechanical support of the failing pump. The largest experience has been gained with intraaortic counterpulsation. Although the technique, first described in the early 1960s, was slow to gain acceptance, there is little doubt that it provides an effective option for *temporary* hemodynamic stabilization. With the development of percutaneous techniques for balloon insertion through the femoral artery, mechanical support need not be delayed when pharmacological interventions have failed. The outcome is generally more favorable if counterpulsation is initiated early.[191]

Technique. (Fig. 19–1, p. 538). The balloon is advanced into the thoracic aorta just distal to the left subclavian artery with the aid of an image intensifier. The controller is adjusted so that the balloon is immediately inflated after closure of the aortic valve so that diastolic aortic runoff is decreased and diastolic aortic pressure is augmented. This increases coronary perfusion. Deflation is initiated just before the onset of systole so that there is systolic unloading with decreased aortic impedance to left ventricular ejection. The mechanically induced increases in diastolic aortic pressure are counterbalanced by decreases in aortic systolic pressure so that there is relatively little change in mean aortic pressure. Left ventricular pressure is decreased by approximately 20 per cent and cardiac output is typically increased by 40 per cent (Table 21–7). Decreases in coronary venous and systemic lactate concentrations, together with improvements in systemic perfusion with increases in urine output, are typically observed.[192]

However, the benefits of balloon counterpulsation are primarily those of gaining time for more definitive interventions. This technique stabilizes the patients, who may then be taken to the invasive laboratory on an urgent basis for diagnosis with view to surgical or other mechanical intervention. Contingent on the angiographic findings, early revascularization, resection of ventricular aneurysm, repair of ruptured ventricular septum, and mitral valve replacement for control of valvular insufficiency stemming from rupture or dysfunction of papillary muscle may then be undertaken. If the patient is stabilized by balloon counterpulsation, both the timing and the preparations for surgical intervention may be optimized with a generally more favorable outcome.[191] However, if surgical intervention is indicated and hemodynamic stability cannot be maintained, surgical operation should not be deferred.

In patients in whom there has been an orderly sequence of intraaortic balloon pumping, invasive diagnosis, and appropriate surgical intervention, the outcome may be more favorable, and immediate survival of between 30 and 75 per cent of patients has been reported.[191,192] However, the benefits of balloon pumping are not without cost. One or more complications of balloon counterpulsation have been reported in 36 per cent of patients, especially during *insertion* of the aortic balloon.[193] Complications, occasionally fatal, are due to perforation of the aorta, aortic dissection, ischemic injury to the lower extremities caused by critical reduction in femoral blood flow, embolism, thrombocytopenia, and hemolysis.[194] A minority of complications are due to mechanical failure of the counterpulsation system or rupture of the intraaortic balloon. However, infection at the site of balloon insertion constitutes a significant problem.[194] Increased incidence of left ventricular rupture has been reported in patients maintained on aortic counterpulsation. However, this may be due to more protracted survival of patients with extensive infarction attributable to counterpulsation rather than an adverse effect of counterpulsation itself.[192]

Contraindications. These include aortic regurgitation, aortic aneurysm, and major rhythm defects which preclude synchronization of the patient's rhythm with inflation and deflation of the balloon. Inotropic therapy, and particularly dobutamine, may be used in conjunction with counterpulsation to augment cardiac output with lesser risk of extending myocardial infarction.[195]

For management of cardiogenic shock associated with *right ventricular infarction,* fluid challenge without other intervention has high likelihood of reversing the clinical signs of shock. When right ventricular infarction is unresponsive to fluids, intraaortic balloon counterpulsation is an appropriate option, followed by invasive diagnosis and surgical intervention, which may include tricuspid valve replacement. Alternative cardiac assist techniques include ventricular assist pumping (left atrial or left ventricular bypass;[196,197] or percutaneous cardiopulmonary bypass.[198] These have not yet come into routine use.

TABLE 21–7 EFFECTS OF INTRAAORTIC BALLOON PUMPING (IABP) IN 35 PATIENTS WITH CARDIOGENIC SHOCK

	BEFORE	IABP	CHANGE (%)
Pulmonary artery occlusive pressure mm Hg	24	19	− 21
Aortic systolic/diastolic mm Hg	78/55	68/95	− 13/+ 73
Cardiac index l/min/M²	1.7	2.4	+ 41

Adapted from Resnekov, L.: Cardiogenic shock. Chest 83:893, 1983.

Causes of cardiogenic shock, other than myocardial infarction, include extremes of tachycardia, in which there is inadequate diastolic filling time; extremes of bradycardia, with inadequate cardiac output; and ventricular ectopic rhythms, with disorganized or asynchronous myocardial contraction for which pharmacological, electrical, and surgical interventions are indicated.

Intracardiac obstruction may be due to valvular obstruction, with marked reductions in cardiac output of either congenital or acquired cause. Newly developed techniques of balloon valvuloplasty (p. 1376) may be useful for emergency intervention,[199–202] although the long-term benefits have not been secured.[203,204] Intracardiac obstruction caused by ball valve thrombus or atrial myxoma may now be diagnosed at the bedside with conventional echocardiographic techniques; urgent surgery may be lifesaving. Previously undetected hypertrophic obstructive cardiomyopathies may present with cardiogenic shock, especially when provoked by the administration of beta-adrenoceptor agents, inotropic drugs, or vasodilator agents. Beta-adrenoceptor blockade and calcium channel blocking agents may be lifesaving. Acute pump failure may also threaten immediate survival after open heart surgery as a complication of prolonged cardiopulmonary bypass or impairment of contractility owing to incision or resection of myocardium. Temporary inotropic support with beta-adrenoceptors such as dobutamine, epinephrine, dopamine, and isoproterenol is appropriate for improving contractility, especially when coronary blood flow is not compromised.

HYPOVOLEMIC SHOCK

ETIOLOGY. Intravascular volume is depleted by overt or occult extravasation of blood, by increases in capillary permeability after traumatic injuries, by infection, or by hypersensitivity reactions with extravasation of plasma and hemoconcentration. Low-perfusion states may also be due to marked increases in capillary hydrostatic pressure with extravasation of plasma water, and therefore hemoconcentration. Water and electrolyte losses from the gastrointestinal tract, the skin, the airways, and the kidneys account for hypovolemia with hemoconcentration. Hemoconcentration is characterized by increases in hemoglobin and hematocrit and in the concentration of plasma proteins, and therefore oncotic pressure. These parameters should be measured at intervals to follow the response to therapy.

COMPENSATORY VOLUME SHIFTS. When intravascular volume is depleted in the absence of protein depletion or marked increases in capillary permeability, lowering of capillary hydrostatic pressure increases the effective capillary oncotic pressures. Consequently, fluid diffuses into the vascular compartment from the interstitial and intracellular compartments. This compensatory restoration of intravascular volume is known as "transcapillary refill" and accounts for the usual reductions in hematocrit and hemoglobin, together with transient reductions in plasma oncotic pressure. However, when intravascular volume is depleted by the selective loss of plasma water with or without protein, the vascular volume deficit is initially accompanied by hemoconcentration. Such hemoconcentration is observed after protracted vomiting and diarrhea, renal losses of water in association with osmolar diuresis owing to hyperosmolar states and especially diabetes mellitus, endocrine abnormalities including diabetes insipidus, adrenocortical insufficiency, pheochromocytoma, and primary renal diseases with impaired salt and water conservation.

ANAPHYLAXIS. Significant quantities of plasma water may also be lost during acute hypersensitivity reactions, especially anaphylaxis. Giant urticaria and angioneurotic edema represent localized extravasations of plasma water and protein. The shock state which accompanies systemic anaphylaxis may occur with or without respiratory distress. Respiratory distress is due to mucosal edema of the airway with the clinical manifestation of stridor and/or by bronchiolar constriction with clinical manifestations of acute asthma. Perfusion failure is usually of later onset than the respiratory distress, which typically occurs within 3 minutes. The onset of shock is associated with a marked decrease in cardiac output and arterial pressure. This is now known to be due to loss of plasma volume with a concurrent increase in the hematocrit and hemoglobin. The features of perfusion failure are usually characteristic of hypovolemic shock with a reduction in right heart filling pressure, marked increases in arterial resistance, decreased peripheral blood flow, anuria, and lactic acidosis. Shock is promptly reversed by the administration of large volumes of fluid. There may be evidence of bleeding owing to disseminated intravascular coagulation. The immediate administration of epinephrine in amounts of 0.5 mg (5 ml of 1/10,000 concentration) intravenously or 1.0 mg (10 ml) into the trachea, if an intravenous route is not immediately available, remains the therapy of choice for reversal of the respiratory defect. It is possible that epinephrine also ameliorates the circulatory defect of anaphylaxis.

CLINICAL FEATURES. Except for the history and for external signs of bleeding or other fluid loss, the physical findings in patients with hypovolemic shock are not specific. Pallor and postural hypotension may be useful, but sinus tachycardia is not of itself a reliable sign of volume depletion. Reduction in arterial blood pressure is a relatively late manifestation of hypovolemia. With progressive reduction in blood volume by bleeding to approximately 50 per cent of normal, there is a progressive decline in cardiac output to less than 50 per cent of control (Fig. 21–11).[205] Mean arterial pressure is maintained by compensatory increases in peripheral vascular resistance. Consequently, decreases in cardiac output are compensated for by arterial vasoconstriction. Lactic acidosis usually occurs only after more than 20 per cent of the blood volume has been depleted and cardiac output is reduced by approximately 50 per cent. Transcapillary refill mitigates decreases in intravascular volume, but this compensatory process occurs over hours and is of little event during rapid blood loss.

Bedside hemodynamic measurements disclose decreases in both right and left ventricular filling pressures, the pulmonary artery pressures, and cardiac output (Table 21–5).

MANAGEMENT. Rapid repletion of intravascular volume by fluid challenge is likely to be curative. General guidelines for the selection of appropriate fluids has already been discussed (p. 578). For practical purposes, red cell mass is most efficiently repleted with type-specific, washed red blood cells. Five per cent human serum albumin is the colloid of choice, but its use is restricted by high cost and limited availability. A 6 per cent solution of hydroxyethyl starch is a satisfactory alternative and generally is preferred over Dextran 70, which has somewhat less favorable effects on blood coagulation and may interfere with cross matching of blood because of red cell agglutination. If blood loss is associated with a coagulation defect, a specific diagnosis of the defect guides component therapy with platelet concentrates, fresh frozen plasma, and cryoprecipitate. Under most conditions, initial volume repletion is carried out with crystalloid solutions and, more specifically, physiological salt or lactated Ringer's solution. However, for treatment of hypovolemic shock, especially in the setting of massive body burns or during advanced stages of hemorrhagic shock, early administration of hypertonic saline solutions containing up to 7.5 per cent sodium chloride have been well tolerated.[206–208]

Citrate is used as an anticoagulant for liquid storage of red blood cells. Infusion of citrate may induce hypocalcemia after the administration of multiple units of citrate-phosphate-dextrose, but this is an unusual complication. It may be recognized by prolongation of the electrocardiographic Q-T interval and confirmed by measurement of plasma-ionized calcium.

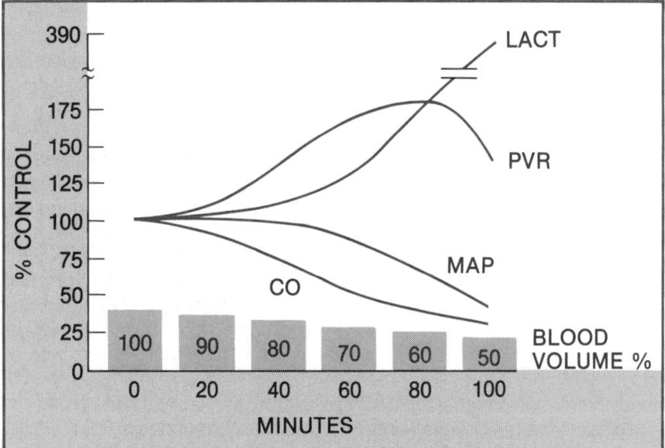

FIGURE 21–11. Relationship between percentage of changes in cardiac output, mean arterial pressure, computed peripheral (arterial) resistance, and lactate concentrations during graded hemorrhage in dogs. (From the data of Nelimarkka, O., et al.: Effect of graded hemorrhage on renal cortical perfusion in dogs. Am. J. Surg. *141*:235, 1981.)

There is controversy regarding the benefits of glucocorticoids administered in pharmacological doses for ancillary treatment of hypovolemic shock. Except in the setting of iatrogenic adrenal insufficiency and, rarely, when addisonian crises masquerade as hypovolemic shock after trauma or surgical operation, there is no specific indication for the administration of glucocorticoids.[209]

DISTRIBUTIVE SHOCK

ETIOLOGY. This form of shock is due to alterations in the distribution of blood flow such that tissue perfusion is compromised in the setting of infection or altered neurological function, or due to the effects of drugs and other substances which alter vascular reactivity. The predominant cause of distributive types of shock, however, is bacterial sepsis and particularly infections caused by gram-negative enteric bacilli.[210] The second most common cause is altered arterial resistance and venous capacitance produced by overdoses of barbiturate, narcotic, sedative-tranquilizer, and some anesthetic agents. Neurogenic causes include transection of the spinal cord and ganglionic blockade.

A diversity of microorganisms and toxic substances derived from them have been implicated as causative agents of septic shock, and the hemodynamic, metabolic, and immunological disturbances which accompany the septic shock state are complex. Accordingly, the pathophysiological mechanisms and clinical features are variable, depending on the causative organism, the host, and the magnitude and site of the primary infectious process. This contrasts with either neurological injury or drug-induced alterations of vasomotor function in which the predominant defect is decreased arterial resistance or, more frequently, expanded venous capacitance. Such defects of vasomotion are fully reversed with a high level of predictability by conventional fluid challenge to expand intravascular volume.

Gram-Negative Sepsis

The most frequent cause of septic shock is bacteremia caused by gram-negative enteric bacilli, and these constitute approximately two-thirds of clinical cases of septic shock.[211,211a] Between one-fourth and one-half of patients with such bacteremia develop shock.[212] These organisms are largely hospital acquired and often gain entrance into the bloodstream at sites of instrumentation or injury. Accordingly, a majority of instances are related to invasive procedures. In the case of arterial catheters, for instance, there is a progressive increase in the incidence of subcutaneous infection at the site of catheterization so that pathogenic bacteria are recovered from one-third of the patients by the fifth day; approximately one-third of these patients develop bacteremias.[213] The morbidity and mortality stemming from protracted vascular catheterizations are therefore substantial.

The incidence of bacteremia and shock is greatly increased when immunological competence is compromised by neoplastic disease, malnutrition, cytotoxic agents, or radiation therapy. Bacteremia caused by gram-negative bacilli has substantially increased in incidence over the past 30 years partly because of more extensive surgical procedures, the much greater use of invasive diagnostic and therapeutic interventions, and the proliferation of gram-negative enteric organisms which are resistant to commonly used antimicrobial drugs in the hospital setting. Most gram-negative infections that occur in the urinary tract are caused by *Escherichia coli,* and bacteremia follows invasion of the urinary tract by catheterization, cystoscopy, or urological surgery. Invasion of the airway by endotracheal tubes or tracheostomy, or seeding of the airway with organisms from contaminated mechanical ventilators and aerosols, accounts for respiratory infections by gram-negative enteric bacilli, especially the *Pseudomonas* and *Klebsiella* species. Surgical manipulation in the gastrointestinal and genitourinary tracts provokes bacteremia resulting from Bacteroides. Contaminations at the site of skin penetration of intravenous catheters or needles, infusion of contaminated solutions, including blood and drugs, and decubitus ulcers occur in the hospital setting.[214] In the community setting such contamination is found in intravenous drug abusers and in patients with long-term indwelling catheters. The primary site of infection may be a surgical skin wound of the vagina or uterus after vaginal delivery or abortion. Specific species of opportunistic bacteria are predominant causes in given hospital locales, but these change from time to time, in part related to the local preferences for antimicrobial agents.

DIAGNOSIS OF GRAM-NEGATIVE SEPSIS. A characteristic sequence of clinical events follows bloodstream invasion by gram-negative bacilli. The onset is usually heralded by a teeth-chattering chill, typically but not inevitably followed by an increase in body temperature to levels of as high as 41°C (106°F). This typically occurs between 2 and 24 hours after a surgical procedure or mechanical invasion of an infected site. Hyperventilation and therefore respiratory alkalosis occur in the early stages of shock followed by metabolic (lactic) acidosis. Because the skin is warm and dry during the early hyperdynamic stage of septic shock, the physician may not suspect that the blood pressure is falling. An early clue to shock is a relatively abrupt alteration in mental status often with inappropriate behavior, presumably caused by reduction in cerebral blood flow. The cause becomes apparent as soon as the blood pressure is measured. An average fall in arterial pressure from 138/70 to 70/36 mm Hg was observed in one series.[215] When the hemodynamic defect becomes more profound over the subsequent 12 to 24 hours, the skin may become pale, cool, and moist. Approximately one-half of the patients present with gastrointestinal signs, including hyperperistalsis, followed by vomiting and diarrhea, often with green and sometimes bloody stools which have a characteristic "laundry room" odor.

LABORATORY FINDINGS. At the time of onset of hypotension, laboratory findings include abrupt reduction in the white blood cell count to levels as low as 1,000/mm^3, primarily caused by reduction in the number of polymorphonuclear cells. This is followed within 4 hours by an overall increase in white cells, typically to levels exceeding 20,000 mm^3, with a marked increase in the number of polymorphonuclear cells and immature forms. Increases in serum enzymes, including AST (SGOT), ALT (SGPT), and LDH, reflect nonspecific cellular injury associated with perfusion failure.[137] An increase in blood sugar is most likely caused by increased secretion of catecholamines from the adrenal medulla. Urine flow is decreased, together with decreased renal clearance of amylase such that serum amylase may be increased in the absence of pancreatic injury. The electrocardiographic findings should be interpreted with caution, since T-wave and ST-segment abnormalities are not unusual in older patients after the onset of shock.[25] In the absence of antibiotic therapy, gram-negative enteric organisms are likely to be recovered from the bloodstream with three cultures of more than 10 ml of blood in approximately 99 per cent of patients with bacteremia.[215]

HEMODYNAMIC MEASUREMENTS. Bedside hemodynamic measurements usually demonstrate normal or increased cardiac output with decreased arterial resistance in the absence of increases in either right or left ventricular filling pressure. In the setting of fever, hypotension with normal or increased cardiac output, together with lactic acidosis, distinguishes this type of shock from low-output states associated with hypovolemia, cardiogenic causes, and vascular obstruction. Fatal progression of shock is associated with decreases in cardiac output and decreases in both right and left ventricular stroke work.[45] Decreases in cardiac output in the later stages of shock are highly correlated with mortality.[216] Such decreases in cardiac output are, in turn, associated with rather striking impairment of both left and right ventricular function.[216a] In Figure 21–12 fatal progression of sepsis is associated with decreases in the left ventricular stroke work and increases in pulmonary artery occlusive pressure. Comparable changes were observed in right ventricular function.[45]

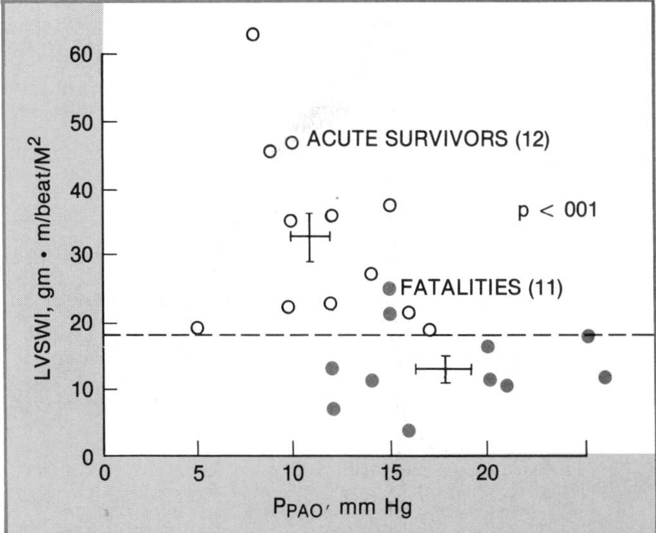

FIGURE 21–12. Stroke work index vs. left ventricular filling pressure at 24 hours in patients with purulent peritonitis. (From Vincent, J.-L., et al.: Circulatory shock associated with purulent peritonitis. Am. J. Surg. *142*:262, 1981.)

Reductions in intravascular volume occur during progression of the shock state. As the total blood volume decreases, mortality strikingly increases.[16] Accordingly, this type of septic shock is characterized by vasodilation with decreased peripheral arterial resistance during the hyperdynamic stage of shock and vasoconstriction, with more typical physical signs of circulatory shock during the late hypodynamic state. However, many patients succumb in the hyperdynamic stage of shock.[17]

The reason for the hyperdynamic state is not fully understood. Experimentally, the injection of live organisms produces vasodilation, and lipopolysaccharides (endotoxins) derived from these organisms produce vasoconstriction. As in shock states resulting from other causes, there is progressive lactic acidosis even though total oxygen consumption remains at near normal levels.[15] However, it is not known whether this represents an inadequate capability to augment oxygen delivery when oxygen requirements are increased, whether there is a reduced capability for oxygen utilization at the exchange site, or whether there is anatomical bypass of the capillary exchange vessels by arteriovenous shunts. Because the mixed venous oxygen content during the hyperdynamic septic state is maintained at relatively high levels, the concept of arteriovenous shunting with "wasted flow" predominates. Yet measurements of capillary blood flow through muscle during the hyperdynamic shock state have failed to demonstrate reductions in capillary flow in support of this hypothesis.[217] However, there is evidence of splanchnic and renal shunting during shock produced by endotoxin.[8]

MANAGEMENT. As in other shock states, therapy is primarily directed to management of the underlying cause: in this instance, the control of infection. There is a close relationship between the concentration of bacteria in the bloodstream and the outcome.[218] Both the fatality of bacteremia and the incidence of shock are reduced by one-half if appropriate antibiotic therapy is instituted promptly.[212] When the source of infection is due to continuous seeding of organisms from an open viscus, an abscess, or necrotic tissue, antibiotic therapy is not likely to suffice. Prompt surgical drainage or control with excision of nonviable tissue is lifesaving. Supportive therapy, as in other shock states, includes attention to ventilation and blood gas exchange and adequacy of intravascular volume. Although vasopressor agents continue to be widely used, their efficacy is unproven and they may accentuate the shock state by their vasoconstrictor action. Consequently, they may further compromise tissue perfusion, reduce intravascular volume, and increase the workload on the heart when left ventricular function is already compromised. On the contrary, there is more persuasive evidence favoring the use of vasodilator agents and particularly alpha-adrenoceptor drugs.[178,219]

Glucocorticoids in high doses increase cardiac output and decrease arterial resistance in both normal subjects and in patients.[220] In laboratory animals they uniformly protect against the fatal effects of endotoxins and, when used in conjunction with antibiotic therapy, improve outcome when bacteremia is experimentally produced by live gram-negative organisms.[221] Nevertheless, a prospective study suggests that glucocorticoid therapy may only prolong initial survival without benefit of improved hospital survival.[222] Two relatively recent multicenter randomized trials of glucocorticoids for management of septic shock failed to confirm benefit, although selective improvement in outcomes for patients with gram-negative bacteremia have not been excluded.[223,224]

Passive immunotherapy may be more promising. Human antiserum to the lipopolysaccharide core of endotoxin from heat-killed *E. coli* have decreased mortality caused by bacteremia and shock.[231] With better understanding that the predominant lethal substance of the bacterial cell wall is lipid-A, immunotherapy may have special promise.

Disseminated intravascular coagulation (DIC) is a major complication of gram-negative sepsis. While thrombocytopenia occurs in a majority of patients, gross bleeding is observed in only about 3 per cent of patients.[212] Except in patients with uncontrolled bleeding caused by DIC who fail to respond to replacement of clotting factors, or in rare instances of ischemic necrosis caused by thrombosis with purpura, anticoagulation with heparin is not likely to be redeeming.

PROGNOSIS. The mortality of shock complicating gram-negative sepsis ranges from 25 to 90 per cent.[25, 211,227] This large range reflects not only the age of the patients, but also, more important, the severity of the underlying diseases. This was documented by Kreger and his colleagues,[212] who observed increasing mortality of gram-negative bacteria in close relationship to the estimated severity of the underlying diseases.

Septic Shock Caused by Other Organisms

In approximately one-third of the patients in whom shock is of infectious cause, the causative organisms are gram-positive cocci, meningococci, clostridia, or fungi. Primary treatment in such cases is also directed to control of the infection. In contrast to gram-negative sepsis, shock more often occurs as a final event, except for toxic shock.

Toxic Shock

The syndrome now termed "toxic shock" may be indistinguishable from shock associated with gram-negative sepsis except for a characteristic rash. It was initially described as a febrile illness in children with an exanthematous rash complicated by hypotension. The rash was typically diffuse and macular with blanching on pressure. The syndrome was further characterized by marked neutrophilia, mucosal hyperemia, and nonpurulent conjunctivitis. Multisystem dysfunction with early renal and hepatic impairment was observed.[228] An adult form of toxic shock was identified in 1980 in menstruating women averaging 25 years in age and related to the use of vaginal tampons. Since then, between 10 and 20 per cent of instances of toxic shock have been identified in nonmenstruating women and in men.[229] The causative organism is *Staphylococcus aureus*, and toxic shock is believed to be due to a pyrogenic exotoxin produced by some strains of this bacterial species.[230] However, a recent report documented severe streptococcal A infection associated with the toxic shock syndrome.[231]

The staphylcoccal infection occurs typically in a closed space, such as in the vagina and uterus or in the nares, in a surgical wound, or in a joint after arthroscopy.[232–234] Progression is characterized by multiorgan failure with high concentrations of creatine phosphokinase. Because the organism may not be recovered in smear and culture, differential diagnosis includes serological tests for streptococci, Rocky Mountain spotted fever, leptospirosis, and measles. Toxic shock, like gram-negative sepsis, is often complicated by thrombocytopenia and sometimes by DIC.

The most immediate intervention is removal of packing in closed spaces, such as in the nose and in the vagina, and vigorous therapy with antistaphylococcal antimicrobials. Within 1 to 2 weeks after recovery, there is typically desquamation of skin.

Obstructive Shock

The primary causes of obstructive shock have already been reviewed (p. 576). The management of obstructive shock states is singularly directed to rapid reestablishment of patency of the mainstream of blood flow. Thrombolysis with streptokinase, urokinase, or tissue plasminogen activator, or transvenous removal of emboli after major pulmonary artery obstruction may be attempted.[235] Pericardial tamponade may be relieved by conventional pericardiocentesis. For practical purposes, however, the successful management of obstructive shock states requires early diagnosis and intervention, often surgical, for prompt restoration of blood flow.

REFERENCES

PATHOPHYSIOLOGY

1. Weil, M. H.: Bacterial shock. *In* Weil, M. H., and Shubin, H. (eds.): Diagnosis and Treatment of Shock. Baltimore, Williams and Wilkins Co., 1967, p. 10.
2. Weil, M. H.: Current understanding of mechanisms and treatment of circulatory shock caused by bacterial infections. Ann. Clin. Res. *9*:181, 1977.
3. Zweifach, B. W.: Quantitative studies of microcirculatory structure and function. I. Analysis of pressure distribution in the terminal vascular bed in cat mesentery. Circ. Res. *34*:843, 1974.
4. Abboud, F. M., Heistad, D. D., Mark, A. L., and Schmid, P. G.: Reflex control of the peripheral circulation. Prog. Cardiovasc. Dis. *18*:371, 1976.
5. Bond, R. F., and Johnson, G. S.: Vascular adrenergic interactions during hemorrhagic shock. Fed. Proc. *44*:281, 1985.
6. Hinshaw, L. B., and Owen, S. E.: Correlation of pooling and resistance changes in the canine forelimb in septic shock. J. Appl. Physiol. *30*:331, 1971.
7. Wiedeman, M. P.: Dimensions of blood vessels from distributing artery to collecting vein. Circ. Res. *12*:375, 1963.
8. Kerr, A. R., and Kirklin, J. W.: Changes in canine venous volume and pressure during hemorrhage. Surgery *68*:3, 1970.
9. Scheidt, S., Arscheim, R., and Killip, T., III: Shock after acute myocardial infarction. Am J. Cardiol. *26*:556, 1970.
10. Diamond, G., and Forrest, J. S.: Effect of coronary artery disease and acute myocardial infarction on left ventricular compliance in man. Circulation *45*:11, 1972.
11. Parker, M. M., and Parillo, J. E.: Septic shock. Hemodynamics and pathogenesis. J.A.M.A. *250*:3324, 1983.
12. Ellrodt, A. G., Riedinger, M. S., Kimchi, A., et al.: Left ventricular performance in septic shock: Reversible segmental and global abnormalities. Am. Heart J. *110*:402, 1985.
13. Crowell, J. W., and Smith, E. E.: Oxygen deficit and irreversible hemorrhagic shock. Am. J. Physiol. *206*:313, 1964.
14. Kaufman, B. S., Rackow, E. C., and Falk, J. L.: The relationship between oxygen delivery and consumption during fluid resuscitation of hypovolemic and septic shock. Chest *85*:336, 1984.
15. Houtchens, B. A., and Westenskow, D. R.: Review article. Oxygen consumption in septic shock: Collective review. Circ. Shock *13*:361, 1984.
16. Weil, M. H., and Nishijima, H.: Cardiac output in bacterial shock. Am. J. Med. *64*:920, 1978.
17. Groeneveld, A. B. J., Bronsveld, W., and Thijs, L. G.: Hemodynamic determinants of mortality in human septic shock. Surgery *99*:140, 1984.
18. Hinshaw, L. B., Gilbert, R. P., Kuida, H., and Visscher, M. B.: Peripheral resistance changes and blood pooling after endotoxin in eviscerated dogs. Am J. Physiol. *195*:631, 1958.
19. Cohn, J. N.: Blood pressure measurement in shock: Mechanism of inaccuracy in auscultatory and palpatory methods. J.A.M.A. *199*:118, 1967.
20. Kazamias, T. M., Gander, M. P., Franklin, D. L., and Ross, J., Jr.: Blood pressure measurement with doppler ultrasonic flow meter. J. Appl. Physiol. *30*:585, 1971.
21. Weil, M. H., Shubin, H., and Carlson, R. W.: Treatment of circulatory shock: Use of sympathomimetic and related vasoactive agents. J.A.M.A. *231*:1280, 1975.
22. Henning, R. J., Wiener, F., Valdes, S., and Weil, M. H.: Measurement of toe temperature for assessing the severity of acute circulatory failure. Surg. Gynecol. Obstet. *149*:1, 1979.
23. Shoemaker, W. C., Fink, S., Ray, C. W., and McCartney, S.: Effect of hemorrhagic shock on conjunctival and transcutaneous oxygen tensions in relation to hemodynamic and oxygen transport changes. Crit. Care Med. *12*:949, 1984.
24. Weil, M. H., and Afifi, A. A.: Experimental and clinical studies on lactate and pyruvate as indicators of the severity of acute circulatory failure (shock). Circulation *41*:989, 1970.
25. Weil, M. H., Shubin, H., and Biddle, M.: Shock caused by gram-negative microorganisms. Analysis of 169 cases. Ann. Intern. Med. *60*: 384, 1964.
26. Terradellas, J. B., Bellot, J. F., Saris, A. B., et al.: Acute and transient ST segment elevation during bacterial shock in seven patients without apparent heart disease. Chest *81*:444, 1982.
27. Thomas, F., Smith, J. L., Orme, J. F., Jr., et al.: Reversible segmental myocardial dysfunction in septic shock. Crit. Care Med. *14*:587, 1986.
28. Ollodart, R., and Mansberger, A. R.: The effect of hypovolemic shock on bacterial defense. Am. J. Surg. *110*:302, 1965.
29. Chien, S.: Role of the sympathetic nervous system in hemorrhage. Physiol. Rev. *47*:214, 1967.
30. Rutherford, R. B., Balis, J. V., Trow, R. S., and Graves, G. M.: Comparison of hemodynamic and regional blood flow changes at equivalent stages of endotoxin and hemorrhagic shock. J. Trauma *16*:886, 1976.
31. DelGuercio, L. R., Cohn, S. D., Feins, N. R., et al.: Pulmonary and systemic arteriovenous shunting in clinical septic shock. *In* Third International Conference on Hyperbaric Medicine. Washington, D.C., National Academy of Sciences, 1966, p. 337.
32. Jardin, F., Eveleigh, M. C., Gurdjian, F., et al.: Venous admixture in human septic shock. Comparative effects of blood volume expansion, dopamine infusion and isoproterenol infusion on mismatching of ventilation and pulmonary blood flow in peritonitis. Circulation *60*:155, 1979.
33. Brunjes, S., Johns, V. J., Jr., and Crane, M. G.: Pheochromocytoma: Postoperative shock and blood volume. N. Engl. J. Med. *262*:393, 1960.
34. Henning, R. J., Shubin, H., and Weil, M. H.: Afterload reduction with phentolamine in patients with acute pulmonary edema. Am. J. Med *63*:568, 1977.
35. Zucker, I. H., Earle, A. M., and Gilmore, J. P.: The mechanism of adaptation of left atrial stretch receptors in dogs with chronic congestive heart failure. J. Clin. Invest. *60*:323, 1977.
36. Feuerstein, G., Johnson, A. K., Zerbe, R. L., et al.: Anteroventral hypothalamus and hemorrhagic shock: Cardiovascular and neuroendocrine responses. Am. J. Physiol. *246*:551, 1984.
37. Henrich, W. L., Berl, T., McDonald, K. M., et al.: Angiotensin II, renal nerves, and prostaglandins in renal hemodynamics during hemorrhage. Am. J. Physiol. *235*:F46, 1978.
38. Scriven, T. A., and Burnett, J. C.: The natriuretic response to atrial natriuretic peptide is attenuated in acute low output failure. Clin. Res. *33*:498, 1985.
39. Carlson, E. L., Selinger, S. L., Utley, J., and Hoffman, J. I. E.: Intramyocardial distribution of blood flow in hemorrhagic shock in anesthetized dogs. Am. J. Physiol. *230*:41, 1976.
40. Hackel, D. B., Ratliff, N. B., and Mikat, E.: The heart in shock. Circ. Res. *35*:805, 1974.
41. Schenk, E. A., and Moss, A. J.: Cardiovascular effects of sustained norepinephrine infusions. II. Morphology. Circ. Res. *18*:605, 1966.
42. Greenhout, J. H., and Reichenbach, D. D.: Cardiac injury and subarachnoid hemorrhage. J. Neurosurg. *30*:521, 1969.
43. Nickerson, M., and Gourzis, J. T.: Blockade of sympathetic vasoconstriction in the treatment of shock. J. Trauma *2*:399, 1962.
44. Crowell, J. W., and Guyton, A. C.: Further evidence favoring a cardiac mechanism in irreversible hemorrhagic shock. Am. J. Physiol. *203*:248, 1962.
45. Vincent, J.-L., Weil, M. H., Puri, V., and Carlson, R. W.: Circulatory shock associated with purulent peritonitis. Am. J. Surg. *142*:262, 1981.
46. Guntheroth, W., Warren, G., Jacky, J. P., et al.: Left ventricular performance in endotoxin shock in dogs. Am. J. Physiol. *242*:H172, 1982.
47. Lee, J. C., and Downing, S. E.: Myocardial oxygen availability and cardiac failure in hemorrhagic shock. Am. Heart J. *92*:201, 1976.
48. Cunnion, R. E., Schaer, G. L., Parker, M. M., et al.: The coronary circulation in human septic shock. Circulation *73*:637, 1986.
49. Lefer, A. M.: Blood-borne humoral factors in the pathophysiology of circulatory shock. Circ. Res. *32*:129, 1973.

50. Goldfarb, R. D.: Characteristics of shock-induced circulating cardiodepressant substances: A brief review. Circ. Shock (Suppl.) *1*:23, 1979.
51. McConn, R., Greineder, J. K., Wasserman, F., and Clowes, G. H. A., Jr.: Is there a humoral factor that depresses ventricular function in sepsis? Circ. Shock (Suppl.) *1*:9, 1979.
52. Parrillo, J. E., Burch, C., Shelhamer, J. H., et al.: A circulating myocardial depressant substance in humans with septic shock. J. Clin. Invest. *76*:1539, 1985.
53. Reilly, J. M., Cunnion, R. E., Burch-Whitman, C., et al.: A circulating myocardial depressant substance is associated with cardiac dysfunction and peripheral hypoperfusion (lactic acidemia) in patients with septic shock. Chest *95*:1072, 1989.
54. Suffredini, A. F., Fromm, R. E., Parker, M. M., et al.: The cardiovascular response of normal humans to the administration of endotoxin. N. Engl. J. Med. *321*:280, 1989.
55. Monsalve, F., Rucabado, L., Salvador, A., et al.: Myocardial depression in septic shock caused by meningococcal infection. Crit. Care Med. *12*:1021, 1984.
56. Jones, C. E., Smith, E. E., DuPont, E., and Williams, R. D.: Demonstration of nonperfused myocardium in late hemorrhagic shock. Circ. Shock *5*:97, 1978.
57. Geft, I. L., Fishbein, M. C., Ninomiya, K., et al.: Intermittent brief periods of ischemia have a cumulative effect and may cause myocardial necrosis. Circulation *66*:1150, 1982.
58. Horton, J. W., Coln, D., and Mitchell, J. H.: Left ventricular volumes and contractility during hemorrhagic hypotension. Dimensional analysis and biplane cinefluorography. Circ. Shock *11*:73, 1983.
59. Willerson, J. T., Scales, F., Mukherjee, A., et al.: Abnormal myocardial fluid retention as an early manifestation of ischemic injury. Am. J. Pathol. *87*:159, 1977.
60. Bronsveld, W., van Lambalgen, A. A., van den Bos, G. C., et al.: Effects of glucose-insulin-potassium (GIK) on myocardial blood flow and metabolism in canine endotoxin shock. Circ. Shock *13*:325, 1984.
61. Braunwald, E., and Kloner, R. A.: The stunned myocardium: Prolonged, postischemic ventricular dysfunction. Circulation *66*:1146, 1982.
62. Jennings, R. B.: Early phase of myocardial ischemic injury and infarction. Am. J. Cardiol. *24*:753, 1969.
63. Udhoji, V. N., and Weil, M. H.: Circulatory effects of angiotensin, levarterenol and metaraminol in the treatment of shock. N. Engl. J. Med. *270*:501, 1964.
64. Lloyd, B. L., and Taylor, R. R.: Augmentation of myocardial digoxin concentration in hemorrhagic shock. Circulation *51*:718, 1975.
64a. Edwards, J. D.: Practical application of oxygen transport principles. Crit. Care Med. 18:545, 1990.
65. Cohn, J. D., Greenspan, M., Goldstein, C. R., et al.: Arteriovenous shunting in high cardiac output shock syndromes. Surg. Gynecol. Obstet. *127*:282, 1968.
66. Hillir, C., Bone, R., Wilson, F.: Comparison of tissue and mixed venous oxygen tension in endotoxic shock. Am. Rev. Resp. Dis. *119a*:127, 1979.
67. Weil, M. H., Leavy, J. A., Rackow, E. C., et al.: Validation of a semi-automated technique for measurement of whole blood lactate. Clin. Chem. *32*:2175, 1986.
68. Afifi, A. A., Chang, P. C., Liu, V. Y., et al.: Prognostic indexes in acute myocardial infarction complicated by shock. Am. J. Cardiol. *33*:826, 1974.
69. Weisel, R. D., Vito, L., Dennis, R. C., et al.: Myocardial depression during sepsis. Am. J. Surg. *133*:512, 1977.
70. Orringer, C. E., Eustace, J. C., Wunsch, C. D., and Gardner, L. B.: Natural history of lactic acidosis after grand-mal seizure. A model for the study of an anion-gap acidosis not associated with hyperkalemia. N. Engl. J. Med *297*:796, 1977.
71. Weil, M. H., Ruiz, C. E., Michaels, S., Rackow, E. C.: Acid-base determinants of survival after cardiopulmonary resuscitation. Crit. Care Med. *13*:888, 1985.
72. Huckabee, W. E.: Relationship of pyruvate and lactate during anaerobic metabolism. V. Coronary adequacy. Am. J. Physiol. *200*:1169, 1961.
73. Blair, E., Cowley, R. A., and Tait, M. K.: Refractory septic shock in men. Role of lactate and pyruvate metabolism and acid-base balance in prognosis. Am. Surg. *31*:537, 1965.
74. Puri, V. K., Schaeffer, R. C., Carlson, R. W., and Weil, M. H.: Experimental aortic occlusion: A model for the study of regional shock with specific reference to blood lactate. Circ. Shock *7*:447, 1980.
75. Levy, J. A., Weil, M. H., Rackow, E. C.: "Lactate washout" following circulatory arrest. J.A.M.A. *260*:662, 1988.
76. Naylor, J. M., and Kronfeld, D. S.: In vivo studies of hypoglycemia and lactic acidosis in endotoxic shock. Am. J. Physiol. *248*:E309, 1985.
77. Bagby, G. J., and Spitzer, J. A.: Decreased rat heart and skeletal muscle lipoprotein lipase activity following endotoxin administration. Circ. Shock *6*:170, 1979.
78. Daniel, A. M., Pierce, C. H., Shizgal, H. M., and MacLean, L. D.: Protein and fat utilization in shock. Surgery *84*:588, 1978.
79. Robalino, B. D., Petrella, R. W., Jubran, F. J., et al.: Atrial natriuretic factor in patients with right ventricular infarction. J. Am. Coll. Cardiol. *15*:546, 1990.
80. Adrogué, H. J., Rashad, M. N., Gorin, A. B., et al.: Arteriovenous acid-base disparity in circulatory failure: Studies on mechanism. Am. J. Physiol. *257*:F1087, 1989.
81. Adrogué, H. J., Rashad, M. N., Gorin, A. B., et al.: Assessing acid-base status in circulatory failure: Differences in arterial and central venous blood. N. Engl. J. Med. *320*:1312, 1989.
82. Benjamin, E., Paluch, T. A., Berger, S. R., et al.: Venous hypercarbia in canine hemorrhagic shock. Crit. Care Med. *15*:516, 1987.
83. Mathias, D. W., Clifford, P. S., and Klopfenstein, H. S.: Mixed venous blood gases are superior to arterial blood gases in assessing acid-base status and oxygenation during acute cardiac tamponade in dogs. J. Clin. Invest. *82*:833, 1988.
84. von Planta, M., Weil, M. H., Gazmuri, R. J., et al.: Myocardial acidosis associated with CO_2 production during cardiac arrest and resuscitation. Circulation *80*:684, 1989.
85. Weil, M. H., Rackow, E. C., Trevino, R., et al.: Difference in acid-base state between venous and arterial blood during cardiopulmonary resuscitation. N. Engl. J. Med. *315*:153, 1986.
86. Falk, J. L., Rackow, E. C., and Weil, M. H.: End-tidal carbon dioxide during cardiopulmonary resuscitation. N. Engl. J. Med. *318*:607, 1988.
87. Kette, F., Weil, M. H., Gazmuri, R. J., et al.: Increases in myocardial PCO_2 during CPR correlate inversely with coronary perfusion pressures (CPP) and resuscitability (abstract). Circulation *80*(Suppl. II):494, 1989.
88. David, R. B., Bailey, W. L., and Hanson, N. P.: Modification of serotonin and histamine release after *E. coli* endotoxin administration. Am. J. Physiol. *205*:560, 1963.
89. Miller, R. L., Reichgott, M. J., and Melmon, K. L.: Biochemical mechanisms of generation of bradykinin by endotoxin. J. Infect. Dis. *128*:S144, 1973.
90. Hallett, J. W., Jr., Sneiderman, C. A., and Wilson, J. W.: Pulmonary effects of arterial infusion of filtered blood in experimental hemorrhagic shock. Surg. Gynecol. Obstet. *138*:517, 1974.
91. Davis, R. B., Meeker, W. R., and Bailey, W. L.: Serotonin release by bacterial endotoxin. Proc. Soc. Exp. Biol. Med. *108*:774, 1961.
92. Glazier, J. C., and Murray, J. F.: Sites of pulmonary vasomotor reactivity in the dog during alveolar hypoxia and serotonin and histamine infusion. J. Clin. Invest. *50*:2550, 1971.
93. Brigham, K. L., and Owen, P. J.: Mechanism of the serotonin effect on lung transvascular fluid and protein movement in awake sheep. Circ. Res. *36*:761, 1975.
94. Cook, J. A., Wise, W. C., and Halushka, P. V.: Elevated thromboxane levels in the rat during endotoxic shock. Protective effects of imidazole 13-azaprostanoic acid, or essential fatty acid deficiency. J. Clin. Invest. *65*:227, 1980.
95. Carmona, R. H., Tsao, T. C., and Trunkey, D. D.: The role of prostacyclin and thromboxane in sepsis and septic shock. Arch. Surg. *119*:189, 1984.
96. Fink, M. P., MacVittie, T. J., and Casey, L. C.: Inhibition of prostaglandin synthesis restores normal hemodynamics in canine hyperdynamic sepsis. Ann. Surg. *200*:619, 1984.
97. Gurll, N. J., Reynolds, D. G., and Holaday, J. W.: Evidence for a role of endorphins in the cardiovascular pathophysiology of primate shock. Crit. Care Med. *16*:521, 1988.
98. Rock, P., Silverman, H., Plump, D., et al.: Efficacy and safety of naloxone in septic shock. Crit. Care Med. *13*:28, 1985.
99. Kalter, E. S., Jaspers, F. C., van Dijk, W. C., et al.: Induction of the early hypotensive phase by *Escherichia coli*: Role of bacterial surface structures and inflammatory mediators. J. Infect. Dis. *152*:493, 1985.
100. Krausz, M. M., Utsunomiya, T., Feuerstein, G., et al.: Prostacyclin reversal of lethal endotoxemia in dogs. J. Clin. Invest. *67*:1118, 1981.
101. Weissman, G., Smolen, J. E., and Korchak, H. M.: Release of inflammatory mediators from stimulated neutrophils. N. Engl. J. Med. *303*:27, 1980.
102. Casey, L. C., Fletcher, J. R., Zmudka, M. I., and Ramwell, P. W.: The role of thromboxane in primate endotoxin shock. J. Surg. Res. *39*:140, 1985.
103. Zimmerman, J. J., Shelhamer, J. H., and Parrillo, J. E.: Quantitative analysis of polymorphonuclear leukocyte superoxide anion generation in critically ill children. Crit. Care Med. *13*:143, 1985.
104. Siegal, T., Seligsohn, U., Aghai, E., and Modan, M.: Clinical and laboratory aspects of disseminated intravascular coagulation (DIC): A study of 118 cases. Thromb. Haemost. *39*:122, 1978.
105. Chaudry, I. H.: Cellular mechanisms in shock and ischemia and their correction. Am. J. Physiol. *245*:R117, 1983.
106. Cusack, N. J.: Platelet-activating factor. Nature *285*:193, 1980.
107. Creticos, P. S., Peters, S. P., Adkinson, F., Jr., et al.: Peptide leukotriene release after antigen challenge in patients sensitive to ragweed. N. Engl. J. Med. *310*:1626, 1984.
108. McCafferty, M. H., and Saba, T. M.: Influence of septic peritonitis on circulating fibronectin, immunoglobulin, and complement: Relationship to reticuloendothelial phagocytic function. Adv. Shock Res. *9*:241, 1983.
109. Loegerling, D. J.: Humoral factor depletion and reticuloendothelial depression during hemorrhagic shock. Am. J. Physiol. *232*:H283, 1977.
110. Carlson, R. P., and Lefer, A. M.: Hepatic cell integrity in hypodynamic states. Am. J. Physiol. *231*:1408, 1976.
111. Blattberg, B., and Levy, M. N.: Vasoactive substances and reticuloendothelial function. Am. J. Physiol. *210*:569, 1966.
112. Michie, H. R., Manogue, K. R., Spriggs, D. R., et al.: Detection of circulating tumor necrosis factor after endotoxin administration. N. Engl. J. Med. *318*:1481, 1988.
113. Girardin, E., Grau, G. E., Dayer, J. M., et al.: Tumor necrosis factor and interleukin-1 in the serum of children with severe infectious purpura. N. Engl. J. Med. *319*:397, 1988.
114. Grau, G. E., Taylor, T. E., Molyneux, M. E., et al.: Tumor necrosis factor and disease severity in children with falciparum malaria. N. Engl. J. Med. *320*:1586, 1989.
115. Tracey, K. J., Fong, Y., Hesse, D. G., et al.: Anti-cachectin/TNF monoclonal antibodies prevent septic shock during lethal bacteremia. Nature *330*:662, 1987.

116. Okusawa, S., Gelfand, J. A., Ikejima, T., et al.: Interleukin-1 induces a shock-like state in rabbits. Synergism with tumor necrosis factor and the effect of cyclooxygenase inhibition. J. Clin. Invest. *81*:1162, 1988.

SECONDARY EFFECTS OF SHOCK

117. Mosher, P., Ross, J., Jr., McFate, P. A., and Shaw, R. F.: Control of coronary blood flow by an autoregulatory mechanism. Circ. Res. *14*:250, 1964.
118. Donohoe, J. F., Venkatachalam, M. A., Bernard, D. B., and Levinsky, N. G.: Tubular leakage and obstruction after renal ischemia: Structural-functional correlations. Kidney Int. *13*:208, 1978.
119. Solez, K.: Pathogenesis of acute renal failure. Int. Rev. Exp. Pathol. *24*:277, 1983.
120. Brezis, M., Rosen, S., Silva, P., and Epstein, F. H.: Renal ischemia: A new perspective. Kidney Int. *26*:375, 1984.
121. Brezis, M., Rosen, S., Spokes, K., et al.: Transport-dependent anoxic cell injury in the isolated perfused rat kidney. Am. J. Pathol. *116*:327, 1984.
122. Brown, R., Babcock, R., Talbert, J., et al.: Renal function in critically ill postoperative patients: Sequential assessment of creatinine osmolar and free water clearance. Crit. Care Med. *8*:68, 1980.
123. Lucas, C. E., Harrigan, C., Denis, R., and Ledgerwood, A. M.: Impaired renal concentrating ability during resuscitation from shock. Arch. Surg. *118*:642, 1983.
124. Miller, T. R., Anderson, R. J., Stuart, L., et al.: Urinary diagnostic indices in acute renal failure. A prospective study. Ann. Intern. Med. *89*:47, 1978.
125. Knaus, W. A. Draper, E. Wagner, D. P., and Zimmerman, J. E.: Prognosis in acute organ-system failure. Ann. Surg. *202*:685, 1985.
126. Finn, W. F.: Recovery from renal failure. *In* Brenner, B. M., and Lazarus, J. M. (eds.): Acute Renal Failure. Philadephia, W. B. Saunders Company, 1983, p. 753.
127. Rinaldo, J. E., and Rogers, R. M.: Adult respiratory-distress syndrome. Changing concepts of lung injury and repair. N. Engl. J. Med. *306*:900, 1982.
127a. Pulmonary Edema. *In* Crystal, R. G., et al. (eds.): The Lung: Scientific Foundations. New York, Raven Press, 1991, p. 2190.
128. Dillon, B. C., and Saba, T. M.: Fibronectin deficiency and intestinal transvascular fluid balance during bacteremia. Am. J. Physiol. *242*:H557, 1982.
129. Saba, T. M., and Jaffe, E.: Plasma fibronectin (opsonic glycoprotein): Its synthesis by vascular endothelial cells and role in cardiopulmonary integrity after trauma as related to reticuloendothelial function. Am. J. Med. *68*:577, 1980.
130. Holcroft, J. W., Vassar, M. J., and Weber, C. J.: Prostaglandin E_1 and survival in patients with the adult respiratory distress syndrome. Ann. Surg. *203*:371, 1986.
131. Nicholson, D. P.: Corticosteroids in the treatment of septic shock and the adult respiratory distress syndrome. Med. Clin. North Am. *67*:717, 1983.
132. Hackney, J. D., Evans, M. J., Spier, C. E., et al.: Effect of high concentrations of oxygen on reparative regeneration of damaged alveolar epithelium in mice. Exp. Mol. Pathol. *34*:338, 1981.
133. Lutch, J. S., and Murray, J. F.: Continuous positive-pressure ventilation: Effects on systemic oxygen transport and tissue oxygenation. Ann. Intern. Med. *76*:193, 1972.
134. Suter, P. M., Fairley, H. B., and Isenberg, M. D.: Optimum end-expiratory airway pressure in patients with acute pulmonary failure. N. Engl. J. Med. *292*:284, 1975.
135. Johnson, G., III, Henderson, D., and Bond, R. F.: Morphological differences in cutaneous and skeletal muscle vasculature during compensatory and decompensatory hemorrhagic hypotension. Circ. Shock *15*:111, 1985.
136. Henning, R. J., Shubin, H., and Weil, M. H.: The measurement of the work of breathing for the clinical assessment of ventilator dependence. Crit. Care Med. *5*:264, 1977.
137. Shubin, H., and Weil, M. H.: Acute elevation of serum transaminase and lactic dehydrogenase during circulatory shock. Am. J. Cardiol. *11*:327, 1963.
138. Bor, N. M., Alvur, M., Ercan, M. T., and Bekdik, C. F.: Liver blood flow rate and glucose metabolism in hemorrhagic hypotension and shock. J. Trauma *22*:753, 1982.
139. Cowley, R. A., Mergner, W. J., Fisher, R. S., et al.: The subcellular pathology of shock in trauma patients: Studies using the immediate autopsy. Am. Surg. *45*:255, 1979.
140. Bhagwat, A. G., and Hawk, W. A.: Terminal hemorrhagic necrotizing enteropathy (THNE). Am. J. Gastroenterol. *45*:163, 1966.
141. Cuevas, P., and Fine, J.: Demonstration of a lethal endotoxemia in experimental occlusion of the superior mesenteric artery. Surg. Gynecol. Obstet. *133*:81, 1971.
142. Lillehei, R. C., and MacLean, L. D.: The intestinal factor in irreversible endotoxin shock. Ann. Surg. *148*:513, 1958.
143. Spath, J. A., Jr., Gorczynski, R. J., and Lefer, A. M.: Pancreatic perfusion in the pathophysiology of hemorrhagic shock. Am. J. Physiol. *226*:443, 1974.
144. Hock, C. E., Su, J., and Lefer, A,. M.: Role of AVP in maintenance of circulatory homeostasis during hemorrhagic shock. Am. J. Physiol. *246*:H174, 1984.
145. Lefer, A. M.: Pharmacologic and surgical modulation of myocardial depressant factor formation and action during shock. Prog. Clin. Biol. Res. *111*:111, 1983.
146. Jones, R. T., and Linhardt, G. E.: Pathology and pathophysiology of the exocrine pancreas in shock. *In* Cowley, R. A., and Trump, B. F. (eds.): Pathophysiology of Shock, Anoxia, and Ischemia. Baltimore, Williams and Wilkins Co., 1982, p. 309.
147. Herlihy, B. L., and Lefer, A. M.: Alterations in pancreatic acinar cell organelles during circulatory shock. Circ. Shock *2*:143, 1975.
148. McManus, W. F., Eurenius K., and Pruitt, B. A.: Disseminated intravascular coagulation in burned patients. J. Trauma *13*:416, 1973.
149. Gralnick, H. R., McKeown, L. P., Wilson, O. M., et al.: Von Willebrand factor release induced by endotoxin. J. Lab. Clin. Med. *113*:118, 1989.
150. Feinstein, D. I.: Diagnosis and management of disseminated intravascular coagulation: The role of heparin therapy. Blood *60*:284, 1982.
151. da Luz, P. L., Cavanilles, J. M., Michaels, S., et al.: Oxygen delivery, anoxic metabolism and hemoglobin-oxygen affinity (P_{50}) in patients with acute myocardial infarction and shock. Am. J. Cardiol. *36*:148, 1975.
152. Kalter, E. S., Henning, R. J., Thijs, L., et al.: Effects of methylprednisolone on P_{50}, 2,3-diphosphoglycerate and arteriovenous oxygen difference in acute myocardial infarction. Circulation *62*:970, 1980.
153. Tindall, G. T., Greenfield, J. C., Jr., Dillon, M. L., and Odom, G. L.: Effect of hemorrhage on blood flow in the carotid arteries. Studies in ten rhesus monkeys. J. Neurosurg. *21*:763, 1964.
154. Johansson, B., Strandgaard, S., and Lassen, N. A.: On the pathogenesis of hypertensive encephalopathy. The hypertensive "breakthrough" of autoregulation of cerebral blood flow with forced vasodilatation, flow increase, and blood-brain-barrier damage. Circ. Res. *35*:167, 1974.
155. Harper, A. M.: Autoregulation of cerebral blood flow: Influence of the arterial blood pressure on the blood flow through the cerebral cortex. J. Neurol. Neurosurg. Psychiatry *29*:398, 1966.
156. Lambertson, C. J., Semple, S. J. G., Smyth, M. G., and Gelfand, R.: H+ and pCO_2 as chemical factors in respiratory and cerebral circulatory control. J. Appl. Physiol. *16*:473, 1967.

CLINICAL SHOCK STATES

157. Hinshaw, L. B., and Cox, B. G.: The fundamental mechanisms of shock. New York, Plenum Press, 1972, p. 13.
158. Weil, M. H., and Shubin, H.: The "VIP" approach to the bedside management of shock. J.A.M.A. *207*:337, 1969.
159. Viires, N., Sillye, G., Auber, M., et al.: Regional blood flow distribution in dog during induced hypotension and low cardiac output: Spontaneous breathing versus artificial ventilation. J. Clin. Invest. *72*:935, 1983.
160. Kumar, A., Falke, K. J., Geffin, B., et al.: Continuous positive-pressure ventilation in acute respiratory failure. N. Engl. J. Med. *283*:1430, 1970.
161. Weil, M. H., and Henning, R. J.: New concepts in the diagnosis and fluid treatment of circulatory shock. Anesth. Analg. *58*:124, 1979.
162. Forrester, J. S., Diamond, G., McHugh, T. J., and Swan, H. J. C.: Filling pressures in the right and left sides of the heart in acute myocardial infarction. N. Engl. J. Med. *285*:190, 1971.
163. Hanashiro, P. K., and Weil, M. H.: Reliability of central venous pressure as a measure of changes in left sided intracardiac pressures. Chest *62*:479, 1972.
164. Forrester, J. S., Diamond, G., Chatterjee, K., and Swan, H. J. C.: Medical therapy of acute myocardial infarction by application of hemodynamic subsets (first of two parts). N. Engl. J. Med. *295*:1356, 1976.
165. Forrester, J. S., Diamond, G., Chatterjee, K., and Swan, H. J. C.: Medical therapy of acute myocardial infarction by application of hemodynamic subsets (second of two parts). N. Engl. J. Med. *295*:1404, 1976.
166. Lamke, L. O., and Liljedahl, S. O.: Plasma volume changes after infusion of various plasma expanders. Resuscitation *5*:93, 1976.
167. Weil, M. H.: Pulmonary edema. *In* Parmley, W., and Chatterjee, K. (eds.): Cardiology. Philadelphia, J. B. Lippincott, 1988, pp. 1–12.
168. Mazzoni, M. C., Borgstrom, P., Arfors, K. E., and Intaglietto, M.: Dynamic fluid redistribution in hyperosmotic resuscitation of hypovolemic hemorrhage. Am. J. Physiol. *255*:H629, 1988.
169. Moylan, J. A., Jr., Reckler, J. M., and Mason, A. D., Jr.: Resuscitation with hypertonic lactate saline in thermal injury. Am. J. Surg. *125*:580, 1973.
170. Nakayama, S., Sibley, L., Gunther, R. A., et al.: Small-volume resuscitation with hypertonic saline (2,400 mOsm/liter) during hemorrhagic shock. Circ. Shock *13*:149, 1984.
171. Shoemaker, W. C.: Evaluation of colloids, crystalloids, whole blood and red cell therapy in the critically ill patients. Clin. Lab. Med. *2*:35, 1982.
172. Holcroft, J. W., Link, D. P., Lantz, B. M. T., et al.: Venous return and the pneumatic antishock garment in hypovolemic baboons. J. Trauma *24*:928, 1984.
173. Mackersie, R. C., Christensen, J. M., and Lewis, F. R.: The prehospital use of external counterpressure: Does MAST make a difference? J. Trauma *24*:882, 1984.
174. Mattox, K. L., Bickell, W. H., Pepe, P. E., and Mangelsdorff, A. D.: Prospective randomized evaluation of antishock MAST in post-traumatic hypotension. J. Trauma *26*:779, 1986.
175. Mueller, H., Ayres, S. M., Gregory, J. J., et al.: Hemodynamics, coronary blood flow, and myocardial metabolism in coronary shock; response to L-norepinephrine and isoproterenol. J. Clin. Invest. *49*:1885, 1970.
176. Nasraway, S. A., Rackow, E. C., Astiz, M. A., et al.: Inotropic response to digoxin and dopamine in patients with severe sepsis, cardiac failure, and systemic hypoperfusion. Chest *95*:612, 1989.
177. DiBianco, R., Shabetai, R., Kostuk, W., et al. for the milrinone multicenter trial group: A comparison of oral milrinone, digoxin, and their combination in the treatment of patients with chronic heart failure. N. Engl. J. Med. *320*:677, 1989.

178. Nicolas, F., Villers, D., and Blanloeil, Y.: Hemodynamic pattern in anaphylactic shock with cardiac arrest. Crit. Care Med. *12*:144, 1984.
179. Ruiz, C. E., Weil, M. H., and Carlson, R. W.: Treatment of circulatory shock with dopamine. J.A.M.A. *242*:165, 1979.
180. Da Luz, P. L., Shubin, H., and Weil, M. H.: Effectiveness of phentolamine for reversal of circulatory failure (shock). Crit. Care Med. *1*:135, 1973.
181. Guiha, N. H., Cohen, J. N., Mikulic, E., et al.: Treatment of refractory heart failure with infusion of nitroprusside. N. Engl. J. Med. *291*:587, 1974.

CARDIOGENIC SHOCK

182. Sonnenblick, E. H., Frishman, W. H., and LeJemtel, T. H.: Dobutamine: A new synthetic cardioactive sympathetic amine. N. Engl. J. Med. *300*:17, 1979.
183. Page, D. L., Caulfield, J. B., Kastor, J. A., et al.: Myocardial changes associated with cardiogenic shock. N. Engl. J. Med. *285*:133, 1971.
184. Wackers, F. J., Lie, K. I., Becker, A. E., et al.: Coronary artery disease in patients dying from cardiogenic shock or congestive heart failure in the setting of acute myocardial infarction. Br. Heart J. *38*:906, 1976.
185. Roberts, N., Harrison, D. G., Reimer, K. A., et al.: Right ventricular infarction with shock but without significant left ventricular infarction: A new clinical syndrome. Am. Heart J. *110*:1047, 1985.
186. Gunnar, R. M., Cruz, A., Boswell, J., et al.: Myocardial infarction with shock. Hemodynamic studies and results of therapy. Circulation *33*:753, 1966.
187. Da Luz, P., Weil, M. H., Liu, V. Y., and Shubin, H.: Plasma volume prior to and following volume loading during shock complicating acute myocardial infarction. Circulation *49*:98, 1974.
187a. Lollgen, H., and Drexler, H.: Use of inotropes in the critical care setting. Crit. Care Med. 18:556, 1990.
188. Lew, A. S., Weiss, A. T., Shah, P, K., et al.: Extensive myocardial salvage and reversal of cardiogenic shock after reperfusion of the left main coronary artery by intravenous streptokinase. Am. J. Cardiol. *54*:450, 1984.
189. Lee, L., Bates, E. R., Pitt, B., et al.: Percutaneous transluminal coronary angioplasty improves survival in acute myocardial infarction complicated by cardiogenic shock. Circulation *78*:1345, 1988.
190. Guyton, R. A., Arcidi, J. M., Langford, D. A., et al.: Emergency coronary bypass for cardiogenic shock. Circulation *76*:V22, 1987.
191. DeWood, M. A., Notske, R. N., Hensley, G. R., et al.: Intra-aortic balloon counterpulsation with and without reperfusion for myocardial infarction shock. Circulation *61*:1105, 1980.
192. Scheidt, S., Wilner, G., Mueller, H., et al.: Intra-aortic balloon counterpulsation in cardiogenic shock. N. Engl. J. Med. *288*:979, 1973.
193. Isner, J. M., Cohen, S. R., Virmani, R., et al.: Complications of the intraaortic balloon counterpulsation device: Clinical and morphologic observations in 45 necropsy patients. Am. J. Cardiol. *45*:260, 1980.
194. McCabe, J. C., Abel, R. M., Subramanian, V. A., and Gay, W. A., Jr.: Complications of intra-aortic balloon insertion and counterpulsation. Circulation *57*:769, 1978.
195. Iqbal, M. Z., and Liebson, P. R.: Counterpulsation and dobutamine. Their use in treatment of cardiogenic shock due to right ventricular infarct. Arch. Intern. Med. *141*:247, 1981.
196. Bernhard, W. F., Poirer, B. S., La-Farge, G., and Carr, J.: A new method for temporary left ventricular bypass. J. Thorac. Cardiovasc. Surg. *70*:880, 1975.
197. Pierce, W. S., Parr, G. V. S., Myers, J. L., et al.: Ventricular-assist pumping in patients with cardiogenic shock after cardiac operations. N. Engl. J. Med. *305*:1606, 1981.
198. Shawl, F. A., Domanski, M. J., Hernandez, T. J., and Punja, S.: Emergency percutaneous cardiopulmonary bypass support in cardiogenic shock from acute myocardial infarction. Am. J. Cardiol. *64*:967, 1989.
199. Inoue, K., Owaki, T., Nakamura, T., et al.: Clinical application of transvenous mitral commissurotomy by a new balloon catheter. J. Thorac. Cardiovasc. Surg. *87*:394, 1984.
200. McKay, R. G., Safian, R. D., Lock, J. E., et al.: Balloon dilatation of calcific aortic stenosis in elderly patients: Postmortem, intraoperative, and percutaneous valvuloplasty studies. Circulation *74*:119, 1986.
201. McKay, R. G., Lock, J. E., Keane, J. F., et al.: Percutaneous mitral valvuloplasty in an adult patient with calcific rheumatic mitral stenosis. J. Am. Coll. Cardiol. *7*:1410, 1986.
202. Palacios, I. F., Lock, J. E., Keane, J. F., and Block, P. C.: Percutaneous transvenous balloon valvotomy in a patient with severe calcific mitral stenosis. J. Am. Coll. Cardiol. *7*:1416, 1986.
203. Palacios, I. F., Block, P. C., Wilkins, G. T., and Weyman, A. E.: Follow-up of patients undergoing percutaneous mitral balloon valvotomy. Analysis of factors determining restenosis. Circulation *79*:573, 1989.
204. Safian, R. D., Berman, A. D., Diver, D. J., et al.: Balloon aortic valvuloplasty in 170 consecutive patients. N. Engl. J. Med. *329*:125, 1988.
205. Nelimarkka, O., Halkola, L., and Ninikoski, J.: Effect of graded hemorrhage on renal cortical perfusion in dogs. Am. J. Surg. *141*:235, 1981.
206. Rackow, E. C., Mecher, C., Astiz, M. E., et al.: Effects of pentastarch and albumin infusion on cardiorespiratory function and coagulation in patients with severe sepsis and systemic hypoperfusion. Crit. Care Med. *17*:394, 1989.
207. Maningas, P. A., and Bellamy, R. F.: Hypertonic sodium chloride solutions for the prehospital management of traumatic hemorrhagic shock: A possible improvement in the standard of care? Ann. Emerg. Med. *15*:1411, 1986.
208. Gross, D., Landau, E. H., Klin, B., and Krausz, M. M.: Treatment of uncontrolled hemorrhagic shock with hypertonic saline solution. Surg. Gynecol. Obstet. *170*:106, 1990.
209. Shubin, H., and Weil, M. H.: Failure of corticosteroid to potentiate sympathomimetic pressor response during shock. J.A.M.A. *197*:808, 1966.
210. Shubin, H., and Weil. M. H.: Bacterial shock. J.A.M.A. *235*:421, 1976.
211. Hruska, J. F., and Hornick, R. B.: Treatment of infection in septic shock. *In* Cowley, R. A., and Trump, B. F. (eds.): Pathophysiology of Shock, Anoxia, and Ischemia. Baltimore, Williams and Wilkins Co., 1982, p. 482.
211a. Vincent, J. L., and Van der Linden, P.: Septic shock: Particular type of acute circulator failure. Crit. Care Med. *18*:S70, 1990.
212. Kreger, B. E., Craven, D. E., and McCabe, W. R.: Gram-negative bacteremia. IV. Re-evaluation of clinical features and treatment in 612 patients. Am. J. Med. *68*:344, 1980.
213. Band, J. D., and Maki, D. G.: Infections caused by arterial catheters used for hemodynamic monitoring. Am. J. Med. *67*:735, 1979.
214. Goldmann, D. A., Maki, M. G., Rhame, F. S., et al.: Guidelines for infection control in intravenous therapy. Ann. Intern. Med. *79*:848, 1973.
215. Washington, J. A., II, and Ilstrup, D. M.: Blood cultures: Issues and controversies. Rev. Infect. Dis. *8*:792, 1986.
216. Nishijima, H., Weil, M. H., Shubin, H., and Canavilles, J.: Hemodynamic and metabolic studies on shock associated with gram-negative bacteremia. Medicine *52*:287, 1973.
216a. Schremmer, B., and Dhainaut, J-F.: Heart failure in septic shock: Effects of inotropic support. Crit. Care Med. *18*:S49, 1990.
217. Finley, R. J., Duff, J. H., Holliday, R. L., et al.: Capillary muscle blood flow in human sepsis. Surgery *78*:87, 1975.
218. Kreger, B. E., Craven, D. E., Carling, P. C., and McCabe, W. R.: Gram-negative bacteremia. III. Reassessment of etiology, epidemiology and ecology in 612 patients. Am. J. Med. *68*:332, 1980.
219. Weil, M. H., and Allen, K. S.: Comparison of sympathetic blocking drugs in prevention of lethal effects of endotoxin. Proc. Soc. Exp. Biol. Med. *115*:627, 1964.
220. Sambhi, M. P., Weil, M. H., and Udhoji, V. N.: Acute pharmacodynamic effects of glucocorticoids: Cardiac output and related hemodynamic changes in normal subjects and patients in shock. Circulation *31*:523, 1965.
221. Hinshaw, L. B., Solomon, L. A., Holmes, D. D., and Greenfield, J. L.: Comparison of canine responses to *Escherichia coli* organisms and endotoxin. Surg. Gynecol. Obstet. *127*:981, 1968.
222. Sprung, C. L., Caralis, P. V., Marcial, E. H., et al.: The effects of high-dose corticosteroids in patients with septic shock. N. Engl. J. Med. *311*:1137, 1984.
223. Bone, R. C., Fisher, C. F., Clemmer, T. P., et al.: A controlled clinical trial of high-dose methylprednisolone in the treatment of severe sepsis and septic shock. N. Engl. J. Med. *317*:653, 1987.
224. Veterans Administration Systemic Sepsis Cooperative Study Group: Effect of high-dose glucocorticoid therapy on mortality in patients with clinical signs of systemic sepsis. N. Engl. J. Med. *317*:659, 1987.
225. Ziegler, E. J., McCutchan, J. A., Fierer, J., et al.: Treatment of gram-negative bacteremia and shock with human antiserum to a mutant *Escherichia coli*. N. Engl. J. Med., *307*:1225, 1982.
226. Teng, N. N. H., Kaplan, H. S., Hebert, J. M., et al.: Protection against gram-negative bacteremia and endotoxemia with human monoclonal IgM antibodies. Proc. Natl. Acad. Sci. USA *82*:1790, 1985.
227. Ledingham, I., McA., McArdle, C. S., and Macdonald, R. C.: Septic shock. *In* Ledingham, I., McA. (eds.): Recent Advances in Intensive Therapy. New York, Churchill Livingstone, 1977, p. 161.
228. Todd, J. K., Ressman, M., Caston, S. A., et al.: Corticosteroid therapy for patients with toxic shock syndrome. J.A.M.A. *252*:3399, 1984.
229. Todd, J.: Toxic shock syndrome. Disease-a-Month. *32*(2):82, 1986.
230. Hayes, P. S., Graves, L. M., Feeley, J. C., et al.: Production of toxic-shock-associated protein(s) in *Staphylococcus aureus* strains isolated from 1956 through 1982. J. Clin. Microbiol. *20*:43, 1984.
231. Stevens, D. L., Tanner, M. H., Winship, J., et al.: Severe group A streptococcal infections associated with a toxic shock-like syndrome and scarlet fever toxin A. N. Engl. J. Med. *321*:1, 1989.
232. Hull, H. F., Mann, J. M., Sands, C. J., et al.: Toxic shock syndrome related to nasal packing. Arch. Otolaryngol, *109*:624, 1983.
233. Toback, J., and Fayerman, J. W.: Toxic shock syndrome following septorhinoplasty. Arch. Otolaryngol. *109*:627, 1983.
234. Farber, B. F., Broome, C. V., and Hopkins, C. C.: Fulminant hospital-acquired toxic shock syndrome. Am. J. Med. *77*:331, 1984.
235. A Collaborative Study by the PIOPED Investigators: Tissue plasminogen activator for the treatment of acute pulmonary embolism. Chest *97*:528, 1990.

22

Genesis of Cardiac Arrhythmias: Electrophysiological Considerations

by DOUGLAS P. ZIPES, M.D.

ANATOMY OF THE CARDIAC CONDUCTION SYSTEM

SINUS NODE

In humans, the sinus node is a spindle-shaped structure composed of a fibrous tissue matrix with closely packed cells. It is 10 to 20 mm long, 2 to 3 mm wide, and thick, tending to narrow caudally toward the inferior vena cava. It lies less than 1 mm from the epicardial surface, laterally in the right atrial sulcus terminalis, at the junction of the superior vena cava and right atrium (Figs. 22–1 and 22–2). The artery supplying the sinus node branches from the right (55 to 60 per cent of the time) or the left circumflex (40 to 45 per cent) coronary artery, approaching the node from a clockwise or counterclockwise direction around the superior vena caval-right atrial junction.

CELLULAR STRUCTURE. Cell types in the sinus node include nodal cells, transitional cells, and atrial muscle cells. *Nodal cells,* also called P cells, thought to be the source of normal impulse formation in the sinus node, are small (5 to 10 μm), ovoid, primitive-appearing cells with cytoplasm that contains relatively few organelles and myofibrils. The few mitochondria are distributed randomly and are variable in size and shape. No transverse tubular system exists. Nodal cells stain poorly, have a pale appearance on light and electron microscopy, and are grouped in elongated clusters located centrally in the sinus node. Contact between nodal cells appears to occur via nexus connections.

Transitional Cells. Also known as T cells, these are elongated cells intermediate in size and complexity between nodal cells and atrial muscle cells. These plentiful cells have large numbers of myofibrils and are heterogeneous, with some T cells more organized and complex than others. T cells near nodal cells have simple intercellular connections, while more fully developed intercalated discs exist between T cells and atrial myocardium. Since nodal cells make contact only with each other or T cells, the latter may provide the only functional pathway for distribution of the sinus impulse formed in the nodal cells to the rest of the atrial myocardium. T cells constitute a spectrum of morphologies ranging from "typical" nodal cells on the one hand and "typical" working atrial myocardium on the other.

The third cell type present in the sinus node is the working *atrial myocardial cell.* These cells extend as peninsulas into the nodal boundaries, with overlapping zones of sinus and atrial cells most prominent on the nodal surface that abuts the crista terminalis. These three cell types have been identified in freshly excised human myocardium.[1]

Very probably there is no single cell in the sinus node that serves as *the* pacemaker. Rather, sinus nodal cells function as electrically coupled oscillators, discharging synchronously because of mutual entrainment. Thus, faster discharging cells are slowed by cells firing more slowly, while they themselves are sped so that a "democratically derived" discharge rate occurs.[2] Digitalis-induced arrhythmias in the sinus node may result from cell-to-cell uncoupling and loss of synchrony.[3] In humans, sinus rhythm results from impulse origin at widely separated sites, creating two or three individual wavefronts that merge to form a single widely disseminated wavefront,[4] and shifts in the sinus node pacemaker complex occur spontaneously.[5] Modulated parasystole has been described in the human sinus node.[6]

INNERVATION. The sinus node is richly innervated with postganglionic adrenergic and cholinergic nerve terminals. Discrete vagal efferent pathways innervate both the sinus and atrioventricular (AV) regions of the dog and nonhuman primate.[7] The concentration of norepinephrine is two

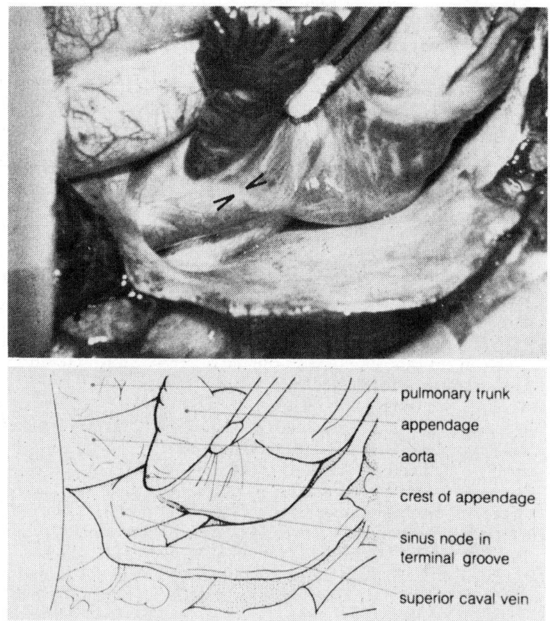

FIGURE 22–1. The human sinus node. This photograph taken in the operating room shows the location of the normal cigar-shaped sinus node along the lateral border of the terminal groove at the superior vena cava–atrial junction (arrowheads). (From Anderson, R. H., Wilcox, B. R., and Becker, A. E.: Anatomy of the normal heart. *In* Hurst, J. W., Anderson, R. H., Becker, A. E., and Wilcox, B. R. [eds.]: Atlas of the Heart. New York, Gower Medical Publishing, 1988, p. 1.2.)

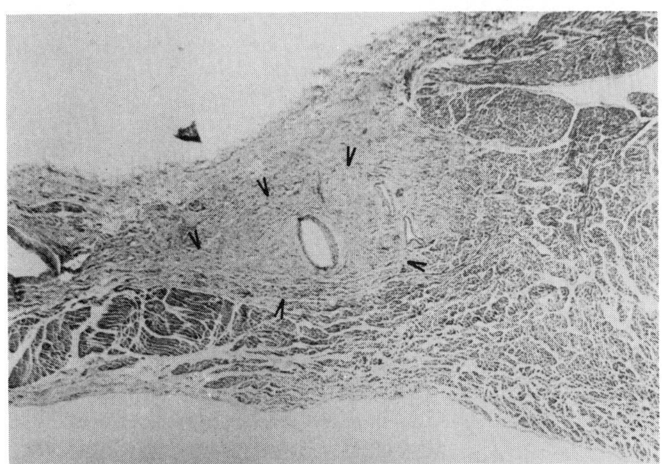

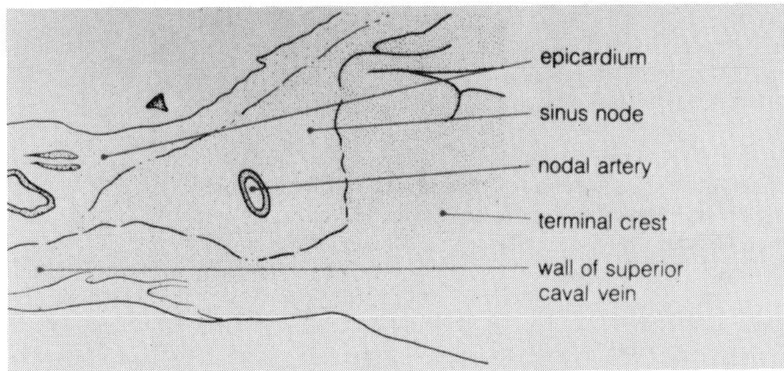

FIGURE 22-2. Histological section taken at right angles to the cigar-shaped sinus node shows how, in short axis, the node is a wedge-shaped structure located between the wall of the superior vena cava and the terminal crest. Discrete boundaries between the sinus node and atrial muscle are noted (arrowheads). The node is penetrated by the sinus nodal artery. (From Anderson, R. H., Wilcox, B. R., and Becker, A. E.: Anatomy of the normal heart. *In* Hurst, J. W., Anderson, R. H., Becker, A. E., and Wilcox, B. R. [eds.]: Atlas of the Heart. New York, Gower Medical Publishing, 1988, p. 1.2.)

to four times higher in atrial than in ventricular tissue in canine and guinea pig hearts. Although the sinus nodal region contains amounts of norepinephrine equivalent to those in other parts of the right atrium, acetylcholine, acetylcholinesterase, and choline acetyltransferase (the enzyme necessary for the synthesis of acetylcholine) have all been found in greatest concentration in the sinus node, with the next highest concentration in the right and then the left atrium. The concentration of acetylcholine in the ventricles is only 20 to 50 per cent of that in the atria.

Vagal stimulation, by releasing acetylcholine, slows sinus nodal discharge rate and prolongs intranodal conduction time, at times to the point of sinus nodal exit block. Adrenergic stimulation speeds sinus discharge rate. The phase (timing) in the cardiac cycle at which vagal discharge occurs and the background sympathetic tone importantly influence vagal effects on sinus rate and conduction (see below).[8] Acetylcholine increases and norepinephrine decreases refractoriness in the center of the sinus node. Negative chronotropic effects of acetylcholine are due to inhibition of the hyperpolarization-activated pacemaker current, i_f[9-11] probably mediated by a G protein[12,13] (p. 359). Acetylcholine also activates the muscarinic m_2 receptor in the pacemaker cell which in turn activates a specific G protein that activates the K channel which also modulates discharge rate.[13] After cessation of vagal stimulation, sinus nodal automatically may accelerate transiently (postvagal tachycardia).

INTERNODAL AND INTERATRIAL CONDUCTION

Whether impulses travel from the sinus to the AV node over preferentially conducting pathways has been contested.[14] Anatomical evidence has been interpreted to indicate the presence of three pathways. The *anterior internodal pathway* begins at the anterior margin of the sinus node and curves anteriorly around the superior vena cava to enter the anterior interatrial band, called *Bachmann's bundle.* This band continues to the left atrium, with the anterior internodal pathway entering the superior margin of the AV node. *Bachmann's bundle* is a large muscle bundle that appears to conduct the cardiac impulse preferentially from right to left atrium. The *middle internodal tract* begins at the superior and posterior margins of the sinus node and travels behind the superior vena cava to the crest of the interatrial septum, descending in the interatrial septum to the superior margin of the AV node. The *posterior internodal tract* starts at the posterior margin of the sinus node and travels posteriorly around the superior vena cava and along the crista terminalis to the eustachian ridge and then into the interatrial septum above the coronary sinus, joining the posterior portion of the AV node. Some fibers from all three tracts bypass the crest of the AV node and enter its more distal segment. These groups of internodal tissue are best referred to as internodal atrial myocardium, not tracts, because they do not appear to be histologically discrete specialized tracts, only plain atrial myocardium.

The basis for specialized tracts stems from finding cell types in the atrium that differ electrophysiologically and anatomically, but it is not clear that these different cells are responsible for more rapid conduction velocity. Also, differential sensitivity of atrial fibers to potassium, giving rise to an apparent sinoventricular rhythm (i.e., impulse propagation from the sinus node to the ventricle without activating atrial myocardium), and activation changes following localized surgical lesions designed to interrupt discrete pathways provide further functional data to support the presence of specialized tracts. However, the *weight of evidence does not support the presence of specialized internodal tracts resembling the bundle branches, i.e., discrete histologically identifiable tracts of tissue.* Preferential internodal conduction, i.e., more rapid conduction velocity between the nodes in some parts of the atrium compared to other parts, probably does exist and may be due to fiber orientation, size, geometry, or other factors rather than to specialized tracts located between the nodes.[15]

THE ATRIOVENTRICULAR JUNCTIONAL AREA AND INTRAVENTRICULAR CONDUCTION SYSTEM

The normal AV junctional area (Figs. 22-3 and 22-4) can be divided into distinct regions: transitional cell zone, also called nodal approaches; compact portion, or the AV node itself; and the penetrating part of the AV bundle (His bundle), which continues as a nonbranching portion. Some investigators consider the branching portion of the AV bundle (i.e., the bundle branches) to be part of the AV junctional area anatomically, while others, relying more on electrophysiological function, separate the branching from the nonbranching portion.[16]

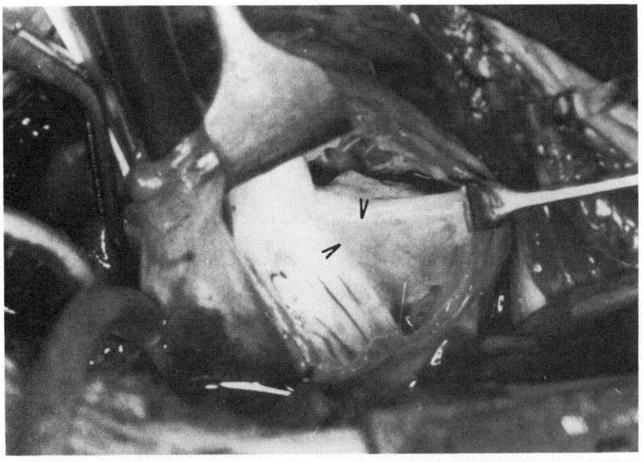

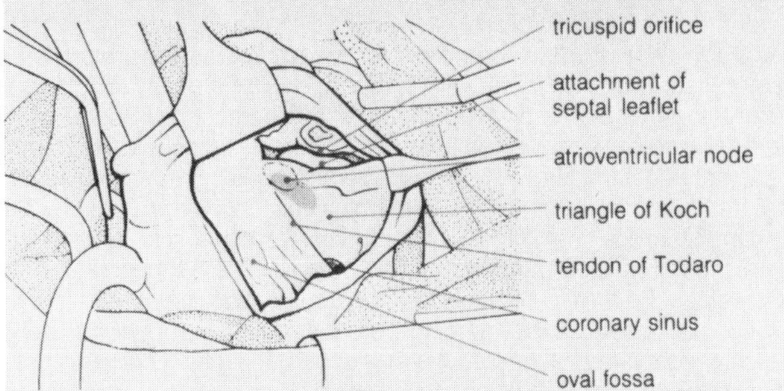

FIGURE 22-3. The human atrioventricular node lies at the apex of the triangle of Koch, which is delimited by the septal leaflet of the tricuspid valve (arrowhead) and tendon of Todaro (arrowhead). The atrioventricular node itself is not visible since it lies beneath the endocardium. (From Anderson, R. H., Wilcox, B. R., and Becker, A. E.: Anatomy of the normal heart. *In* Hurst, J. W., Anderson, R. H., Becker, A. E., and Wilcox, B. R. [eds.]: Atlas of the Heart. New York, Gower Medical Publishing, 1988, p. 1.2.)

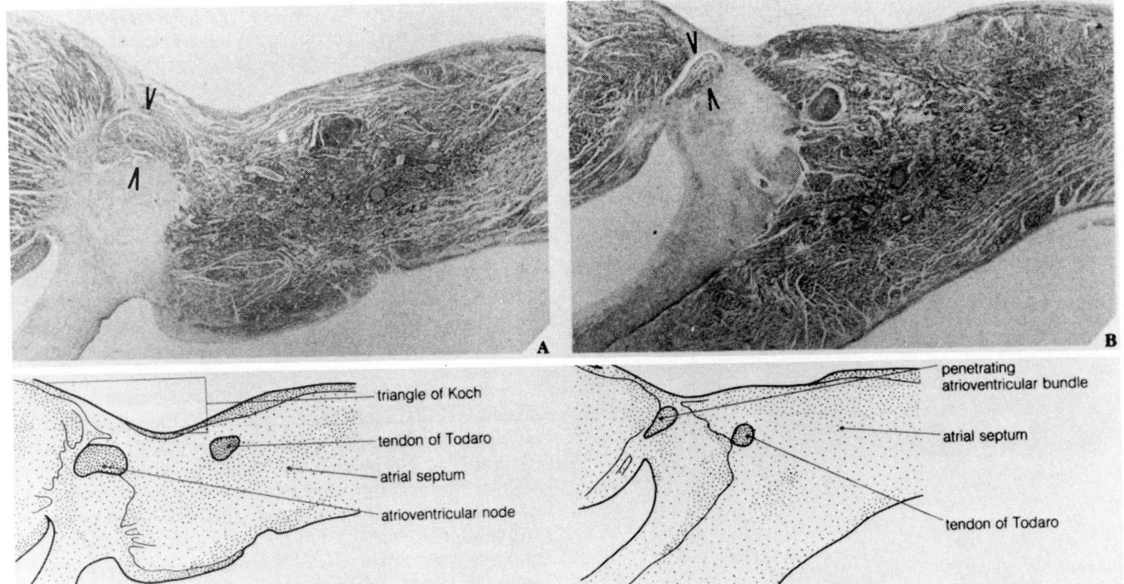

FIGURE 22–4. Sections through the atrioventricular junction show the position of the atrioventricular node (arrowhead) within the triangle of Koch *(A)* and the penetrating atrioventricular bundle of His (arrowheads) within the central fibrous body *(B)*. (From Anderson, R. H., Wilcox, B. R., and Becker, A. E.: Anatomy of the normal heart. *In* Hurst, J. W., Anderson, R. H., Becker, A. E., and Wilcox, B. R. [eds.]: Atlas of the Heart. New York, Gower Medical Publishing, 1988, p. 1.2.)

TRANSITIONAL CELL ZONE. In the rabbit AV node, the transitional cells or nodal approaches are located in posterior, superficial, and deep groups of cells. They differ histologically from atrial myocardium and connect the latter with the compact portion of the AV node. Some fibers may pass from the posterior internodal tract to the distal portion of the AV node or His bundle and provide the anatomical substrate for conduction to bypass AV nodal slowing. However, the importance of this structure is unclear (see p. 692).

THE AV NODE. The compact portion of the AV node is a superficial structure, lying just beneath the right atrial endocardium, anterior to the ostium of the coronary sinus, and directly above the insertion of the septal leaflet of the tricuspid valve. It is at the apex of a triangle formed by the tricuspid annulus and the tendon of Todaro, which originates in the central fibrous body, and passes posteriorly through the atrial septum to continue with the eustachian valve (Figs. 22–3 and 22–4). The compact portion of the AV node is divided from and becomes the penetrating portion of the His bundle at the point where it enters the central fibrous body. In 85 to 90 per cent of human hearts, the arterial supply to the AV node is a branch from the right coronary artery that originates at the posterior intersection of the AV and interventricular grooves (crux). A branch of the circumflex coronary artery provides the AV nodal artery in the remaining hearts. Fibers in the lower part of the AV node may exhibit automatic impulse formation electronically depressed by the connecting myocardium.[17] Similarly, atrial myocardium may depress automaticity in border zone of the sinus node.[18]

THE BUNDLE OF HIS, OR PENETRATING PORTION OF THE AV BUNDLE. This connects with the distal part of the compact AV node and perforates the central fibrous body, continuing through the annulus fibrosis, where it is called the nonbranching portion as it penetrates the membranous septum (Fig. 22–4). Proximal cells of the penetrating portion are heterogeneous, resembling those of the compact AV node, while distal cells are similar to cells in the proximal bundle branches. Connective tissue of the central fibrous body and membranous septum encloses the penetrating portion of the AV bundle, which may send out extensions into the central fibrous body. However, large well-formed fasciculoventricular connections between the penetrating portion of the AV bundle and the ventricular septal crest are rarely found in adult hearts. Branches from the anterior and posterior descending coronary arteries supply the upper muscular interventricular septum with blood, making the conduction system at this site more impervious to ischemic damage unless the ischemia is extensive.

THE BUNDLE BRANCHES, OR BRANCHING PORTION OF THE AV BUNDLE. These structures begin at the superior margin of the muscular interventricular septum, immediately beneath the membranous septum, with the cells of the left bundle branch cascading downward as a continuous sheet onto the septum beneath the noncoronary aortic cusp (Fig. 22–5). The AV bundle then may give off other left bundle branches, sometimes constituting a true bifascicular system with an anterosuperior branch, in other hearts giving rise to a group of central fibers, and in still others appearing more as a network without a clear division into a fascicular system. The right bundle branch continues intramyocardially as an unbranched extension of the AV bundle down the right side of the interventricular septum to the apex of the right ventricle and base of the anterior papillary muscle. In some human hearts, the His bundle traverses the right interventricular crest, giving rise to a right-sided narrow stem

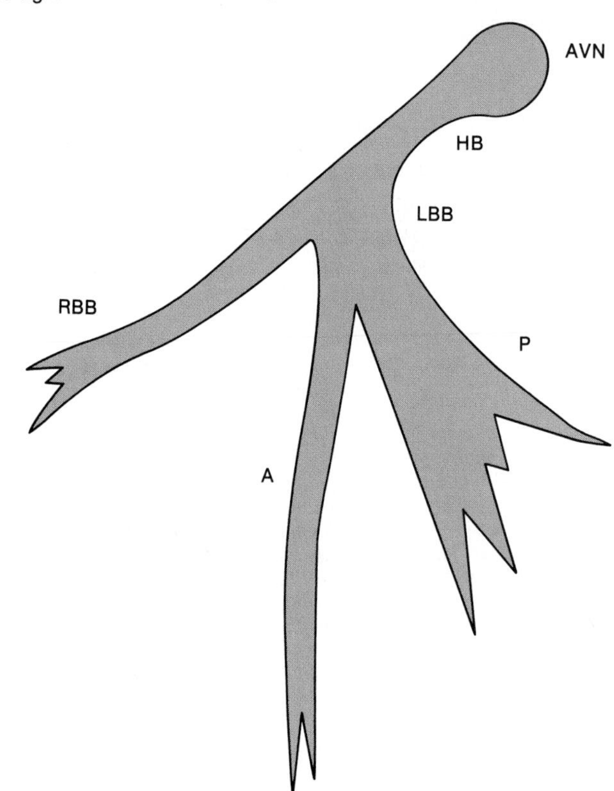

FIGURE 22–5. Schematic representation of the trifascicular bundle branch system. AVN, atrioventricular node; HB, His bundle; LBB, main left bundle branch; A, anterosuperior fascicle of the left bundle; P, posteroinferior fascicle of the left bundle branch; RBB, right bundle branch. (Modified from Rosenbaum, M. B., Elizari, M. V., and Lazzari, J. O.: The Hemiblocks. Oldsmar, FL, Tampa Tracings, 1970, cover illustration.)

origin of the left bundle branch. The anatomy of the left bundle branch system may be variable and may not conform to a constant bifascicular division. However, the concept of a trifascicular system remains useful to both the electrocardiographer and the clinician (Fig. 22–5).[19]

TERMINAL PURKINJE FIBERS. These fibers connect with the ends of the bundle branches to form interweaving networks on the endocardial surface of both ventricles that transmit the cardiac impulse almost simultaneously to the entire right and left ventricular endocardium. Purkinje fibers tend to be less concentrated at the base of the ventricle and at the papillary muscle tips. They penetrate the myocardium for varying distances depending on the animal species; in humans, they apparently penetrate only the inner third of the endocardium, while in the pig they almost reach the epicardium. Such variations could influence changes produced by myocardial ischemia, for example, since Purkinje fibers appear more resistant to ischemia than are ordinary myocardial fibers.

CELLULAR COMPOSITION OF THE AV JUNCTIONAL AREA. Transitional cells in the rabbit are elongated, smaller than atrial cells, stain more palely, and are separated by numerous strands of connective tissue. They merge at the entrance of the compact portion of the AV node, where the cells are small and spherical, not separated by muscle or connective tissue, and have very few nexuses. They interweave in interconnecting whorls of fasciculi. The AV node is divided, based on electrophysiological characteristics, into AN, N, and NH regions[20] (Fig. 22–6). In the rabbit, the AN region corresponds to the transitional cell groups of the posterior portion of the node, the NH region to the anterior portion of the bundle of lower nodal cells, and the N region to the small enclosed node where transitional cells merge with midnodal cells. *Dead-end pathways*—groups of cells that form an apparent electrophysiological cul-de-sac that does not contribute to overall conduction in the node—are also found at several sites. Cells in the penetrating bundle remain similar to compact AV nodal cells. In the dog, P cells, similar to those found in the sinus node, and several types of transitional cells have been noted and related to the automaticity and conduction properties of the AV node. Sinus and AV nodal cells have a distinct type of myosin heavy chain (MHC) immunologically related to atrial MHC. This alpha MHC is found in about half of the myofibers of the ventricular conduction tissue.[21–23]

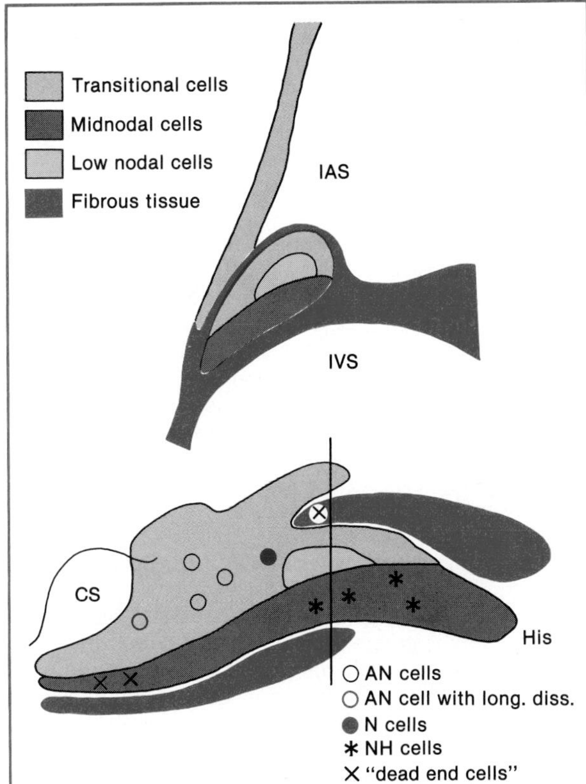

FIGURE 22–6. Diagram showing distribution of morphologically different cell types in AV node. Upper panel, Transverse section showing trilaminar appearance of the interior part of the node. The level of sectioning is indicated by the vertical dark line in the lower panel. Lower panel, Diagram of the AV node indicating the different sites identified histologically after recording typical action potentials. (From Janse, M. J., et al.: Electrophysiology and structure of the atrioventricular node of the isolated rabbit heart. *In* Wellens, J. H. H., et al. [eds.]: The Conduction System of the Heart. Philadelphia, Lea and Febiger, 1976, p. 296.)

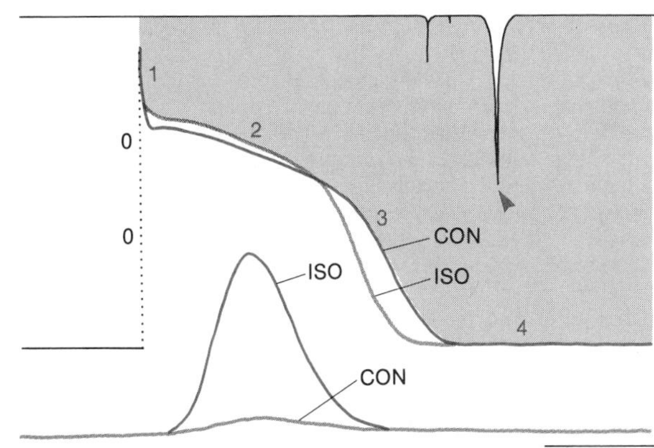

FIGURE 22–7. Recordings of canine Purkinje fiber action potential and developed tension before and during isoproterenol administration. Tracings from above downward show upstroke velocity of phase 0 (Vmax, arrowhead), action potential configuration of Purkinje fiber, and developed tension in the Purkinje fiber bundle during control (CON) and after exposure to isoproterenol (ISO, 0.1 ml/10^{-5} M, added directly to the tissue bath). The five phases of the action potential are indicated by the large numerals. The short horizontal line to the left with a zero near the peak of the action potential indicates the zero voltage potential. Vertical calibration: 400 V/sec for Vmax/sec, 50 mV for action potential amplitude, and 400 mg for the developed tension, respectively. Horizontal calibration: 4 msec for the upper record and 100 msec for the middle and lower records. (V = volts; mV = millivolts; msec = milliseconds.) Isoproterenol increased plateau height of the action potential and developed tension and decreased action potential duration during the terminal phase of repolarization, without significantly affecting resting membrane potential or phase 0. (From Gilmour, R. F., Jr., and Zipes, D. P.: Basic electrophysiology of the slow inward current. *In* Antman, E., and Stone, P. [eds.]: Calcium Blocking Agents in the Treatment of Cardiovascular Disorders. Mt. Kisco, N.Y., Futura Publishing Co. Inc., 1983, pp. 1–37.)

Purkinje cells are found in the His bundle and bundle branches, cover much of the endocardium of both ventricles, and align to form multicellular bundles in longitudinal strands separated by collagen. They are large, clear cells (10 to 30 μm in diameter, 20 to 50 μm long) with loosely arrayed mitochondria distributed between few linearly aligned myofibrils that have few myofilaments. Round nuclei occupy the center of the cell. Although conduction of the cardiac impulse appears to be their major function, free-running Purkinje fibers, sometimes called *false tendons,* which are composed of many Purkinje cells in a series, are capable of contraction (Fig. 22–7). While also exhibiting side-to-side connections, the major intercellular connection of Purkinje fibers is end-to-end through well-developed intercalated discs (see p. 593) that may facilitate rapid longitudinal conduction.

Innervation of AV Node and His Bundle

PATHWAYS OF INNERVATION. The AV node and His bundle region are innervated by a rich supply of cholinergic and adrenergic fibers with a density exceeding that found in the ventricular myocardium. Nerve fibers showing substance P–like immunoreactivity are found in abundance in the AV node.[24] Ganglia, nerve fibers, and nerve nets lie close to the AV node. Parasympathetic nerves to the AV node region enter the canine heart at the junction of the inferior vena cava and the inferior left atrium, adjacent to the coronary sinus entrance.[7] Nerves in direct contact with AV nodal fibers have been noted, along with agranular and granular vesicular processes, presumably representing cholinergic and adrenergic processes. Acetylcholine release may be concentrated around the N region of the AV node.[24a]

In general, autonomic neural input to the heart exhibits some degree of "sidedness," with the right sympathetic and vagal nerves affecting the sinus node more than the AV node and the left sympathetic and vagal nerves affecting the AV node more than the sinus node. The distribution of the neural input to the sinus and AV nodes is complex because of substantial overlapping innervation. Despite the overlap, specific branches of the vagal and sympathetic nerves can be shown to innervate certain regions preferentially, and sympathetic or vagal nerves to the sinus node can be interrupted discretely without affecting AV nodal innervation. Similarly, vagal or sympathetic neural input to the AV node can be interrupted without affecting sinus innervation.[7] Supersensitivity to acetylcholine follows vagal denervation.[25] Stimulation of the right stellate ganglion produces sinus tachycardia with less effect on AV nodal conduction, while stimulation of the left stellate ganglion generally produces a shift in the sinus pacemaker to an ectopic site and consistently shortens AV nodal conduction time and refractoriness, but inconsistently speeds the sinus nodal discharge rate. Stimulation of the right cervical vagus nerve primarily slows the sinus nodal discharge rate, while stimulation of the left vagus primarily prolongs AV nodal conduction time and refractoriness when "sidedness" is present. While neither sympathetic nor vagal stimulation affects normal conduction in the His bundle, either can affect abnormal AV conduction.[26]

Most efferent sympathetic impulses reach the canine ventricles over the ansae subclaviae, branches from the stellate ganglia. Sympathetic nerves then synapse primarily in the caudal cervical ganglia and form individual cardiac nerves that innervate relatively localized parts of the ventricles. On the right side, the major route to the heart is the recurrent cardiac nerve, and on the left, the ventrolateral cardiac nerve. In general, the right sympathetic chain shortens refractoriness primarily of the anterior portion of the ventricles while the left affects primarily the posterior surface of the ventricles, although overlapping areas of distribution occur.

The intraventricular route of sympathetic nerves generally follows coronary arteries. Functional data suggest that afferent and efferent sympathetic nerves travel in the superficial layers of the epicardium and dive to innervate the endocardium,[27] and anatomical observations support that conclusion.[28] Vagal fibers travel intramurally or subendocardially, rising to the epicardium at the AV groove[27] (Fig. 22–8).

EFFECTS OF VAGAL STIMULATION. The vagus modulates cardiac sympathetic activity at prejunctional and postjunctional sites by regulating the amount of norepinephrine released and by inhibiting cyclic AMP-induced phosphorylation of cardiac proteins such as phospholamban. The latter inhibition occurs at more than one level in the series of reactions comprising the adenylate cyclase, cyclic AMP-dependent, protein kinase system.[29,30] Neuropeptides released from nerve fibers of both autonomic limbs also modulate autonomic responses. For example, neuropeptide Y released from sympathetic nerve terminals inhibits cardiac vagal effects.[31]

Tonic vagal stimulation produces a greater absolute reduction in sinus rate in the presence of tonic background sympathetic stimulation, a sympathetic-parasympathetic interaction termed *accentuated antagonism.*[31] In contrast, changes in AV conduction during concomitant sympathetic and vagal stimulation are essentially the *algebraic sum* of the individual AV conduction responses to tonic vagal and sympathetic stimulation alone.[32] In puppies, sympathetic stimulation exerts greater effects on improving AV conduction than vagal stimulation does on retarding it.[33] Cardiac responses to brief vagal bursts begin after a short latency and dissipate quickly; in contrast, cardiac responses to sympathetic stimulation commence and dissipate slowly. The rapid onset and offset of responses to vagal stimulation allow for dynamic vagal modulation of heart rate and AV conduction (phase-dependent), whereas the slow temporal response to sympathetic stimulation precludes any beat-to-beat regulation by sympathetic activity (phase-independent). Periodic vagal bursting (as may occur each time a systolic pressure wave arrives at the baroreceptor regions in the aortic and carotid sinuses) induces phasic changes in sinus cycle length and can entrain the sinus node to discharge faster or slower at periods that are identical to those of the vagal burst. In a similar phasic manner, vagal bursts prolong AV nodal conduction time and are influenced by background levels of sympathetic tone. Because the peak vagal effects on sinus rate and AV nodal conduction occur at differrent times in the cardiac cycle, a brief vagal burst can slow the sinus rate without affecting AV nodal conduction or can prolong AV nodal conduction time and not slow the sinus rate.[8] Shifts in pacemaker location can occur.

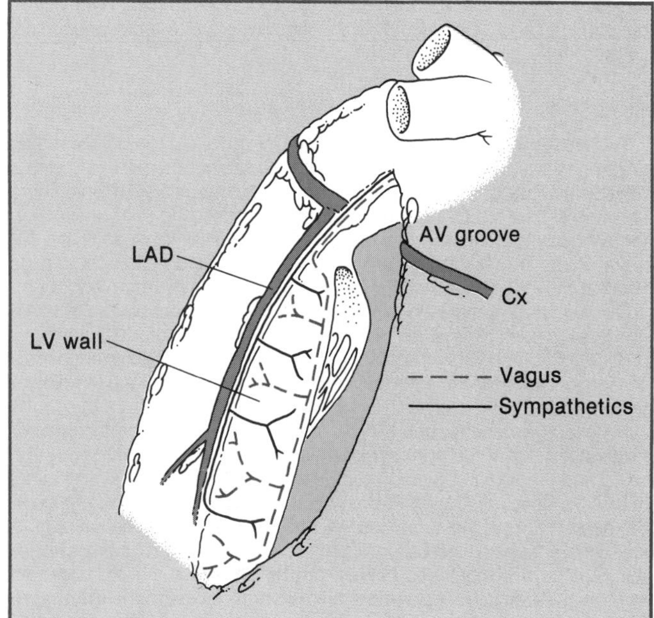

FIGURE 22–8. Intraventricular route of sympathetic and vagal nerves.

EFFECTS OF SYMPATHETIC STIMULATION. Stimulation of sympathetic ganglia shortens the refractory period equally in the epicardium and underlying endocardium of the left ventricular free wall, although dispersion of recovery properties occurs, i.e., different degrees of shortening of refractoriness occur when measured at different epicardial sites.[27] Nonuniform distribution of norepinephrine may, in part, contribute to some of the nonuniform electrophysiological effects following sympathetic neural stimulation, since the ventricular content of norepinephrine, for example, is greater at the base than at the apex of the heart, with greater distribution to muscle than to Purkinje fibers.[27] Afferent vagal activity appears to be greater in the posterior ventricular myocardium.[34] This may account for the vagomimetic effects of inferior myocardial infarction.[35]

The vagi exert minimal but measurable effects on ventricular tissue, decreasing the strength of myocardial contraction and prolonging refractoriness.[27] Under some circumstances, acetylcholine can cause a positive inotropic effect.[36] It is now clear that the vagus (acetylcholine) can exert direct effects on some types of ventricular fibers,[37] as well as exert indirect effects by modulating sympathetic influences.

ARRHYTHMIAS AND THE AUTONOMIC NERVOUS SYSTEM. Alterations in vagal and sympathetic innervation can influence the development of arrhythmias. Damage to nerves extrinsic to the heart, such as the stellate ganglia, as well as to intrinsic cardiac nerves from diseases that may affect nerves primarily, e.g., viral infections, or secondarily, from diseases that cause cardiac damage, may produce cardioneuropathy.[38] Such neural changes may create electrical instability via a variety of electrophysiological mechanisms. For example, myocardial infarction can interrupt afferent[39] and efferent[40a] neural transmission and create areas of sympathetic supersensitivity[41,42] that may be conducive to the development of arrhythmias.[43–45]

BASIC ELECTROPHYSIOLOGICAL PRINCIPLES

CELL MEMBRANE (SARCOLEMMA) (see also p. 354)

The cell membrane constitutes a bilayer boundary of phospholipid molecules (Fig. 22–9). The tail end of the phospholipid molecules is nonpolar and hydrophobic, pointing toward the center of the membrane, while the head end is polar and hydrophilic, pointing toward the outer and inner layers of the membrane, in contact with the aqueous extracellular and intracellular environment. The sarcolemma, particularly the hydrophobic core, provides a high-resistance, insulated wrapping around the cell that exhibits selective permeability to ions—a property responsible for creating an electrical potential across the cell membrane. Ions are positively (cations) or negatively (anions) charged atoms such as Na^+, K^+, Ca^{++}, or Cl^- and other molecules whose movement inside the cell or across the cell membrane constitutes a flow of current that generates signals in excitable membranes. At rest, the resistance to ion flow is greater across the cell membrane than in the cytoplasm of the cell interior. The cell membrane has openings called channels that span the cell membrane and serve as conduits through which ions move. The different protein or phospholipoprotein channels are selective, favoring passage of one ion over another. In contrast to the membrane lipids that act primarily as inert barriers, membrane proteins appear to be responsible for most of the known biological activities of membranes. Some kinds of channels open as a result of a neurotransmitter binding to their extracellular site and are called *receptor-operated channels.* Others open in response to a voltage change and are called *voltage-operated channels.* Gates, influenced by the electric field and by time, control ion movement through the channels and, when opened or closed, permit or prevent ion travel. Drugs can bind to sites within the channel and prevent ion passage.[46–49]

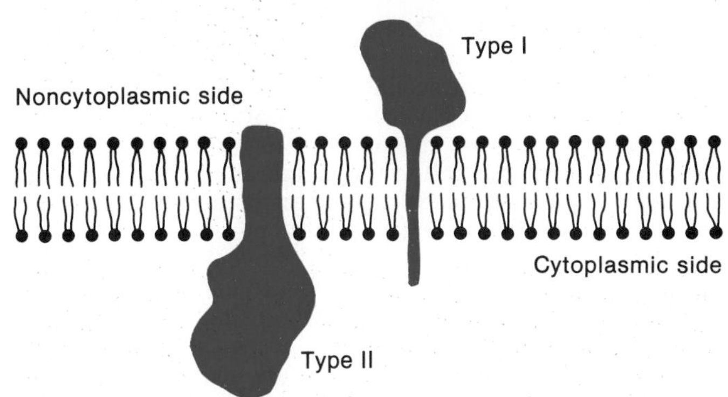

FIGURE 22-9. **Arrangement in the membrane of two classes of intrinsic membrane proteins, type I, which have most of their mass and all of their functional properties in the aqueous environment outside the cytoplasm with the internal membrane portion serving only to anchor the protein to the membrane, and type II, which has the major part of the polypeptide mass in the cytoplasm with a very small fraction of the amino acid residue exposed to the noncytoplasmic side of the bilayer. (From Guidotti, G.: Membrane proteins. Structure, arrangement and disposition in the membrane. *In* Andreoli, T. E., Hoffman, J. F., Fanestil, B. D., and Schultz, S. G., [eds.]: Physiology of Membrane Disorders. New York, Plenum Medical Book Company, 1986, p. 48.)**

In addition to the channels, other protein complexes serve as a major supplementary transport system through the cell membrane and provide for neutral exchange of some ions and small organic molecules along their concentration gradients (passive ion transport) and for transporting ions against their electrochemical energy gradients (active ion transport). Some protein complexes penetrate only the outer cell membrane and may serve as receptor sites for neurotransmitters and hormones, while others, such as the adenylate cyclase system, protrude through the inner cell membrane and may be involved in various enzymatic activities. Protein molecules protruding through the entire cell membrane, such as the Na-K pump, may help regulate the ionic fluxes that determine the electrical status of the resting and excited membrane.[50] The Na-K pump requires adenosine triphosphate (ATP) to extrude intracellular Na against its concentration and electrical gradients and to move K intracellularly, against its concentration gradient, resulting in high concentrations of K inside and of Na outside the cell (Table 22-1).

INTERCALATED DISCS. The cell membranes of some types of adjacent cells form close margins called *intercalated discs* (p. 354). Three types of specialized junctions make up each intercalated disc. The macula adherens or desmosome and fascia adherens form the areas of strong adhesions between cells and may provide a linkage for the transfer of mechanical energy from one cell to the next. The *nexus*, also called *tight* or *gap junction*, is a region in the intercalated disc where cells are in functional contact with each other. Membranes at these junctions are separated by only about 10 to 20 Å and are connected by a series of hexagonally packed subunit bridges. Gap junctions probably provide low-resistance electrical coupling between adjacent cells[51-55] at their longitudinal ends, reducing cell-to-cell resistance. The presence of true lateral gap junctions has been challenged.[51] The gap junctions allow movement of ions and perhaps of small molecules between cells. They link interiors of adjacent cells and are stable in their open state, closing when intracellular calcium rises. The gap junctions permit a multicellular structure such as the heart to function electrically like an orderly, synchronized, interconnected unit and are probably responsible in part for the fact that conduction in the myocardium is *anisotropic;* that is, its anatomical and biophysical properties vary according to the direction in which they are measured.[56] Usually, conduction velocity is two to three times faster horizontally, i.e., in the direction of the long axis of the fiber, than it is transversely, i.e., in the direction perpendicular to this long axis. Resistivity is lower longitudinally than transversely. Interestingly, the safety factor for propagation is greater transversely than horizontally. Conduction delay or block occurs more commonly,[57] but not always,[58] in the horizontal direction than it does transversely. Because of anisotropy, propagation is discontinuous[59] and can be a cause of reentry.[56] Gap junctions may also provide "biochemical coupling" that might permit cell-to-cell movement of ATP or other high-energy phosphates and can change their electrical resistance, controlled in part by calcium.[60] When intracellular calcium rises, as in myocardial infarction, the gap junction may close to help "seal off" the effects of injured from noninjured cells. Acidosis increases and alkalosis decreases gap junctional resistance. Increased gap junctional resistance tends to slow the rate of action potential propagation, a condition that could lead to conduction delay or block.

In ventricular muscle cells, but apparently not in atrial or His-Purkinje cells, the cell membrane invaginates to form a transverse tubular system that introduces the cell membrane and extracellular space deep into the cells. Because of reduced diffusion in that space, ions, metabolites, or other constituents may be present in greater or lower concentrations than are found intracellularly or extracellularly. Such surface scalloping can greatly increase the surface area of the ventricular cell.

TABLE 22-1 INTRACELLULAR AND EXTRACELLULAR ION CONCENTRATIONS IN CARDIAC MUSCLE

ION	EXTRACELLULAR CONCENTRATION	INTRACELLULAR CONCENTRATION	RATIO OF EXTRACELLULAR TO INTRACELLULAR CONCENTRATION	E_i
Na	145 mM	15 mM	9.7	+60 mV
K	4 mM	150 mM	0.027	−94 mV
Cl	120 mM	5 mM	24	−83 mV
Ca	2 mM	10^{-7} M	2×10^4	+129 mV

E_i = equilibrium potential for a particular ion.

Although intracellular Ca content is about 2 mM/kg, most of this is bound or sequestered in intracellular organelles (mitochondria and sarcoplasmic reticulum). For the same reason, the actual free Na concentration may be less. Intracellular Cl concentration depends on the average membrane potential, if Cl is passively distributed, and therefore on heart rate.

From Sperelakis, N.: Origin of the cardiac resting potential. *In* Berne, R. M., et al. (eds.): Handbook of Physiology, The Cardiovascular System, Bethesda, Md., American Physiological Society, 1979, p. 193.

PHASES OF THE CARDIAC ACTION POTENTIAL

The cardiac transmembrane potential consists of five phases: phase 0—the upstroke or rapid depolarization; phase 1—early rapid repolarization; phase 2—plateau; phase 3—final rapid repolarization; phase 4—resting membrane potential and diastolic depolarization (Fig. 22-7). These phases are the result of ion fluxes that are passive: Ions move down electrochemical gradients established by active ion pumps and exchange mechanisms. Each ion moves primarily through its own ion-specific channel. Impulses spread from one cell to the next without requiring neural input. The transplanted heart dramatically demonstrates this fact. The following discussion will explain the electrogenesis of each of these phases. For in-depth coverage, the reader is referred to other reference sources.[61-63]

Phase 4—The Resting Membrane Potential (see also p. 601)

Intracellular electrical activity can be recorded by inserting a glass microelectrode with a tip diameter less than 0.5 μm into a single cell. The electrode produces minimal damage, its entry point apparently being sealed by the cell. The transmembrane potential is recorded using this electrode in reference to an extracellular ground electrode placed in the tissue bath near the cell membrane and represents the potential difference between intracellular and extracellular voltages (Fig. 22–10 *Left*). A variety of other techniques, including voltage and patch clamp procedures, can be used to study the passage of individual ionic species across specific channels in the cell membrane (Fig. 22–10 and 22–11).

Intracellular potential during electrical quiescence in diastole is −50 to −95 mV, depending on the cell type (Table 22–2). This means that the inside of the cell is 50 to 95 mV negative relative to the outside of the cell owing to the distribution of ions such as K^+, Na^+, Cl^-, and Ca^{++} across the cell membrane.

K^+ is the major ion determining the resting potential. During diastole the cell membrane is quite permeable to K^+ and relatively impermeable to Na^+. Because of the Na-K pump, which pumps Na^+ out of the cell against its electrochemical gradient and simultaneously pumps K^+ into the cell against its chemical gradient, intracellular K^+ concentration remains high and intracellular Na^+ concentration remains low. This pump, fueled by an Na^+, K^+-ATPase enzyme that hydrolyzes ATP for energy, is bound to the membrane. It requires both Na^+ and K^+ to function and can transport three Na^+ outward for two K^+ ions inward. Therefore the pump can be electrogenic, generating a net outward movement of positive charges. The rate of Na^+-K^+ pumping to maintain the same ionic gradients must increase as heart rate increases, since the cell gains a slight amount of Na^+ and loses a slight amount of K^+ with each depolarization. Heart rate becomes important when we consider the electrophysiological basis of some types of digitalis-induced cardiac arrhythmias, because cardiac glycosides block this pump.

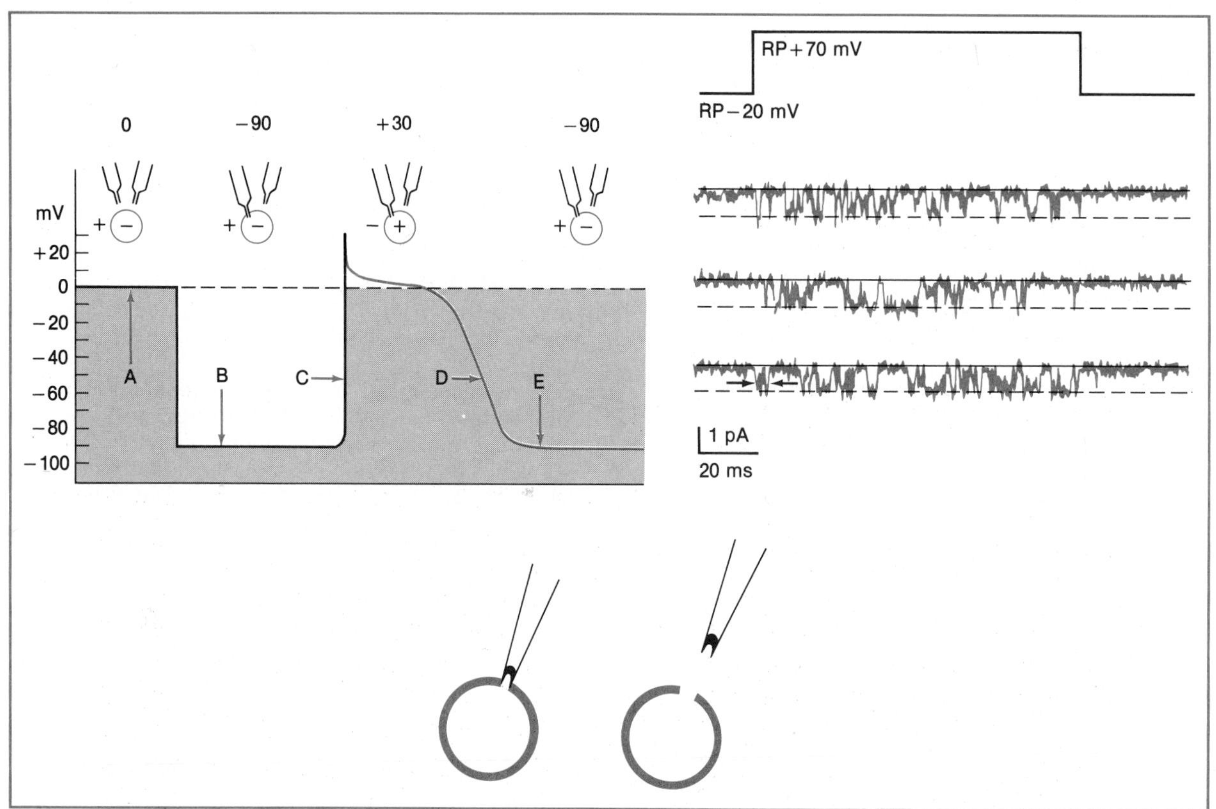

FIGURE 22–10. ***Left,*** **A demonstration of action potentials recorded during impalement of a cardiac cell. The upper row of diagrams shows a cell (circle), two microelectrodes, and stages during impalement of the cell and its activation and recovery. *A,* Both microelectrodes are extracellular, and no difference in potential exists between them (0 potential). The environment inside the cell is negative and the outside is positive, since the cell is polarized. *B,* One microelectrode has pierced the cell membrane to record the intracellular resting membrane potential, which is −90 mV with respect to the outside of the cell. *C,* The cell has depolarized and the upstroke of the action potential is recorded. At its peak voltage, the inside of the cell is about +30 mV with respect to the outside of the cell. *D,* Phase of repolarization, returning the membrane to its former resting potential *(E)* (From The Conduction of the Cardiac Impulse. Mt. Kisco, N.Y., Futura Publishing Co. Inc., 1975.)**

Right, **Calcium channel recording. A portion or patch of the sarcolemmal membrane from a single guinea pig ventricular muscle cell is sucked up into a micropipette to record the opening and closing of single calcium channels. The pipette is filled with 110 mM Ba^{++}. The Ba^{++} crosses the membrane through the calcium channel when it opens and generates a current, recorded as the large downward pulses that reach the interrupted line (first in the bottom tracing). The solid line indicates average baseline current while the interrupted line (about 1 pA) indicates average single channel current. The channel stays open for brief but varied durations and then closes (upward deflection back to solid line, second). Three sequentially obtained current records are shown. Resting membrane potential (RP) was near −60 mV by addition of 10 mM [K]o. The RP was then reduced by 20 mV (RP −20 mV) and virtually no Ca^{++} channel openings occurred. When RP was made 70 mV more positive (RP + 70 mV) Ca^{++} channel activity was generated. (Square wave-shaped tracing at very top indicates RP changes). Thus, this figure illustrates opening and closing of single calcium channels when the RP is reduced to the range at which the slow inward current functions. (From Tsien, R.: Excitable tissues: The heart. *In* Andreoli, T. E., et al. [eds.]: Physiology of Membrane Disorders. New York, Plenum, 1986, p. 478.)**

Bottom insert shows micropipette technique used to study single channels in a portion of the membrane still attached to the cell *(left).* Membrane studied after being detached from the rest of the cell *(right).*

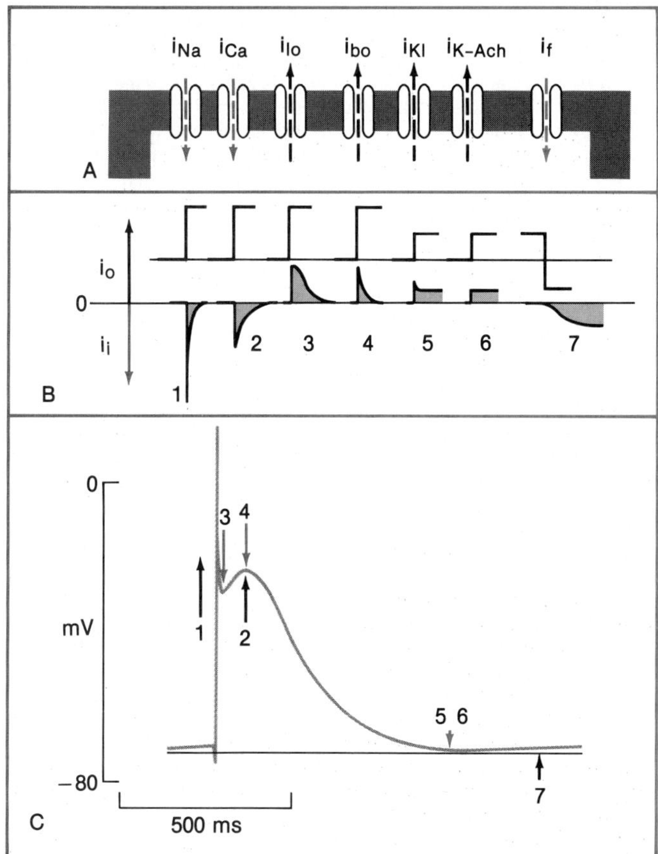

FIGURE 22-11. Schematic diagram of ionic channels *(A)* and corresponding transmembrane currents *(B)* presently known in human atrial myocardium and their influences on development of cellular action potential *(C)*. *A,* Currents crossing different channels under normal conditions are either inward (downward arrows) and therefore depolarize the membrane or outward (upward arrows) and therefore repolarize the membrane. i_{Na}, sodium current; i_{ca}, calcium current; i_{lo} and i_{bo}, long-lasting and brief transient potassium currents; i_{K1}, background potassium current; $i_{K\text{-}ACh}$, potassium current flowing through muscarinic cholinergic receptor channels; i_f, pacemaker current carried by both sodium and potassium ions. *B,* Time course of different transmembrane ionic currents (hatched areas) occurring when the membrane is submitted to rectangular (top traces) depolarizing pulses (1–6) or repolarizing pulses (7). Currents i_{Ki} and $i_{K\text{-}ACh}$ are shown here as outward currents, but because of the inward rectification, they are much smaller in the outward than in the inward direction. i_o, outward current; i_i, inward current. C, 1–7 correspond to the currents shown in *A* and *B,* and arrows indicate effect of each ionic current on the action potential; upward arrows, depolarizing effect; downward arrows, repolarizing or hyperpolarizing effects. (From Coraboeuf, E., and Escande, D.: Ionic currents in the human myocardium. NIPS *5*:28, 1990.)

THE NERNST EQUATION. Little Na^+, despite its concentration gradient, can diffuse into the cell, owing to the relative impermeability to Na^+ of the polarized cell membrane. However, K^+ can diffuse freely out of the cell down its concentration gradient, and does so, removing with it a positive charge and leaving the inside of the cell more negative. Negative intracellular charges, presumably due to large polyvalent ions such as proteins, do not cross the membrane and help maintain intracellular negativity. K^+ continues to leave the cell until the forces driving it down its concentration gradient are balanced by the negative intracellular electrical charges that attract K^+ back into the cell. The transmembrane voltage at which the electrical gradient is equal and opposite to the concentration gradient, so that the algebraic sum of these two passive forces equals zero, is the K^+ electrochemical equilibrium potential E_k, and is described by the Nernst equation

$$E_k = \frac{RT}{F} \ln \frac{[K^+]_o}{[K^+]_i} \tag{1}$$

where R is the gas constant, T is the absolute temperature, F is the Faraday number, ln is the logarithm to the base E, $[K^+]_o$ is the extracellular K^+ concentration and $[K^+]_i$ the intracellular K^+ concentration.

Solving this equation predicts a transmembrane voltage of about −96 mV in cardiac muscle, which is very near the observed voltages. However, certain factors make the equation an approximation. Because the $[K^+]_o/[K^+]_i$ ratio primarily determines transmembrane voltage, the cell membrane is said to behave as a K^+ electrode during diastole, and more closely follows the values predicted by the Nernst equation at $[K^+]_o$ greater than 10 mM. When $[K^+]_o$ is reduced, membrane permeability to K^+ also decreases, the small inward movement of Na^{-1}, negligible at high $[K^+]_o$, becomes more important, and the actual resting membrane voltage becomes less than that predicted by the Nernst equation for a K^+ electrode. The difference between predicted and observed voltages increases as $[K^+]_o$ is reduced further. The contribution of the minimal inward movement of Na^{-1} to the resting membrane potential can be incorporated into an equation called the Goldman constant-field equation and is a slight modification of the Nernst equation. If one assumes that the membrane is permeable to only Na^{-1} and K^+, the resting membrane potential (V_r) would be

$$V_r = \frac{RT}{F} \ln \frac{[K^+]_o + P_{Na}/P_K\,[Na]_o}{[K^+]_i + P_{Na}P_K\,[Na]_i} \tag{2}$$

where P_{Na}/P_K is the ratio of the sodium to the potassium permeability coefficient of the cell membrane, $[Na]_o$ is the extracellular sodium concentration, and $[Na]_i$ is the intracellular sodium concentration. The equation can be modified further to include the minimal contributions of other ions.

Calcium contributes little to the resting membrane potential, although changes in Ca concentration can affect the permeability of the cell membrane to other ions. An increase in $[Ca]_i$ increases potassium conductance. Ca^{++} is handled by several mechanisms, including uptake by the sarcoplasmic reticulum. Also, there appears to be a passive transsarcolemmal Ca^{++}-Na^{-1} exchange reaction. This exchange depends in part on maintenance of the Na^{-1} concentration gradient by the Na^{-1}-K^+ pump. Under normal conditions, one internal Ca^{++} ion is probably exchanged for three or more external Na^{-1} ions. $Na^{-1}Ca^{++}$ exchange generates a current across the cell membrane.[64] Under some pathological conditions or drug actions when $[Na^+]_i$ is abnormally high, external Ca^{++} may be exchanged for internal Na^{-1}. Cells that gain Na^+, in general, gain Ca^{++}—a reaction important to the genesis of some digitalis-induced arrhythmias. The role of Ca^{++} is further considered on page 357.

TABLE 22-2 PROPERTIES OF TRANSMEMBRANE POTENTIALS IN MAMMALIAN HEARTS

	SINUS NODAL CELL	ATRIAL MUSCLE CELL	AV NODAL CELL	PURKINJE FIBER	VENTRICULAR MUSCLE CELL
Resting potential (mV)	−50 to −60	−80 to −90	−60 to −70	−90 to −95	−80 to −90
Action potential					
Amplitude (mV)	60 to 70	110 to 120	70 to 80	120	110 to 120
Overshoot (mV)	0 to 10	30	5 to 15	30	30
Duration (msec)	100 to 300	100 to 300	100 to 300	300 to 500	200 to 300
Vmax (V/S)	1 to 10	100 to 200	5 to 15	500 to 700	100 to 200
Propagation velocity (M/sec)	<0.05	0.3 to 0.4	0.1	2 to 3	0.3 to 0.4
Fiber diameter (μm)	5 to 10	10 to 15	5 to 10	100	10 to 16

Modified from Sperelakis, N.: Origin of the cardiac resting potential. *In* Berne, R. M., Sperelakis, N., and Geiger, S. R. (eds.): Handbook of Physiology, The Cardiovascular System, Bethesda, Md., American Physiological Society, 1979, p. 190.

Phase 0 – Upstroke or Rapid Depolarization

A stimulus delivered to excitable tissue evokes an action potential characterized by a sudden voltage change due to transient depolarization followed by repolarization. The action potential is conducted throughout the heart and is responsible for initiating each "heart beat." Electrical changes of the action potential follow a relatively fixed time and voltage relationship that differs according to specific cell types (Fig. 22–11 and 22–12). In nerve, the entire process takes several milliseconds, while action potentials in cardiac fibers last several hundred milliseconds. Normally the action potential is independent of the size of the depolarizing stimulus, if the latter exceeds a certain threshold potential. Small subthreshold depolarizing stimuli depolarize the membrane in proportion to the strength of the stimulus. However, once the stimulus is sufficiently intense to reduce membrane potential to a threshold value in the range of −70 to −65 mV for normal Purkinje fibers, more intense stimuli do not produce larger action potential responses, and an "all-or-none" response results. In contrast, hyperpolarizing pulses, i.e., stimuli that render the membrane potential more negative, elicit a response proportional to the strength of the stimulus.

MECHANISM OF PHASE 0. The upstroke of the cardiac action potential in atrial and ventricular muscle and His-Purkinje fibers is due to a sudden increase in membrane conductance to Na^+. An externally applied stimulus, or a spontaneously generated local membrane circuit current in advance of a propagating action potential, depolarizes a sufficiently large area of membrane at a sufficiently rapid rate to open the Na^+ channels and depolarize the membrane further. When the membrane voltage reaches threshold, Na^+ rushes through ion-specific channels into the cell, down its electrochemical gradient—i.e., Na^+ is "drawn" into the cell by the low $[Na^+]_i$ and the negatively charged intracellular environment. The excited membrane no longer behaves like a K^+ electrode, i.e., exclusively permeable to K^+, but more closely approximates an Na^+ electrode, and the membrane moves toward the Na^+ equilibrium potential.

The rate at which depolarization occurs during phase 0, i.e., the maximum rate of change of voltage over time, is indicated by the expression dV/dt_{max} or V_{max} (Table 22–2), which is a reasonable approximation of the rate and magnitude of Na^+ entry into the cell and a determinant of conduction velocity for the propagated action potential. The transient increase in sodium conductance lasts 1 to 2 msec. The action potential, or more properly the Na^+ current, is said to be regenerative; that is, intracellular movement of a little Na^+ depolarizes the membrane more, which increases conductance to Na^+ more, which allows more Na^+ to enter, and so on. As this is occurring, however, $[Na^+]_i$ and positive intracellular charges increase and reduce the driving force for Na^+. When the equilibrium potential for Na^+ (E_{Na}) is reached, Na^+ no longer enters the cell, i.e., when the driving force acting on the ion is zero, no current will flow. In addition, Na^+ conductance is time dependent so that when the membrane spends some time at voltages less negative than the resting potential, Na^+ conductance decreases. Therefore an intervention that reduces membrane potential for a time—but not to threshold—partially inactivates Na^+ channels, so that if threshold is now achieved, the magnitude and rate of Na^+ influx are reduced.

In cardiac Purkinje fibers and to a lesser extent in ventricular muscle, two different populations of Na^+ channels, or two different modes of operation of the same Na^+ channel, exist. One is responsible for the brief Na^+ current of phase 0, while the other, which is longer lasting, participates in the action potential plateau. Tetrodotoxin (TTX) and local anesthetics block both types of channels, diminishing the rate of rise of phase 0 and shortening action potential duration.[65]

At this point, several concepts need to be expanded. Ohm's law states that voltage equals current times resistance. The term conductance (g) is the inverse or reciprocal of resistance and is related to the ease with which ions can cross the cell membrane when driven by a potential difference across the membrane. As resistance of the membrane to passage of an ion increases, conductance decreases. Membrane permeability or conductance of the Na^+ channel during phase 0 is regulated hypothetically by two types of gates, the "m" gate and the "h" gate, which modulate Na ion passage through the channel (Fig. 22–13).

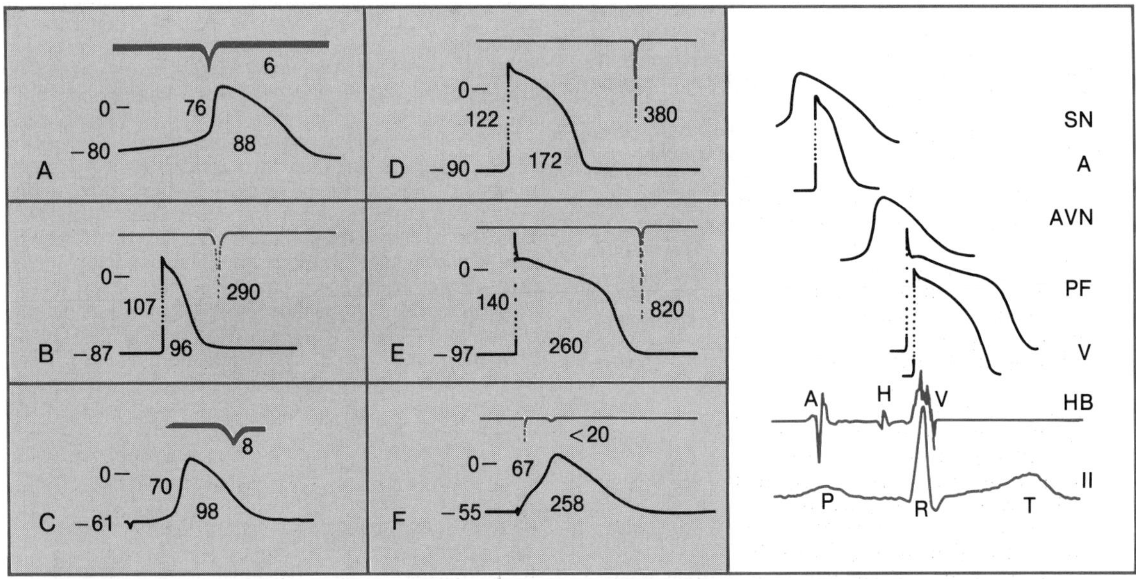

FIGURE 22–12. Action potentials recorded from different tissues in the heart *(left),* remounted along with a His bundle recording and scalar ECG from a patient *(right)* to illustrate the timing during a single cardiac cycle. In panels *A* to *F*, the top tracing is dV/dt of phase 0 and the second tracing is the action potential. For each panel, the numbers (from left to right) indicate maximum diastolic potential (mV), action potential amplitude (mV), action potential duration at 90 per cent of repolarization (msec), and Vmax of phase 0 (V/sec). Zero potential is indicated by the short horizontal line next to the zero on the upper left of each action potential. *A*, Rabbit sinoatrial node; *B*, canine atrial muscle; *C*, rabbit atrioventricular node; *D*, canine ventricular muscle; *E*, canine Purkinje fiber; *F*, diseased human ventricle. Note that the action potentials recorded in *A*, *C*, and *F* have reduced resting membrane potentials, amplitudes, and Vmax compared with the other action potentials. In the right panel, SN = sinus nodal potential; A = atrial muscle potential; AVN = atrioventricular nodal potential; PF = Purkinje fiber potential; V = ventricular muscle potential; HB = His bundle recording; II = lead II. Horizontal calibration on the left: 50 msec for *A* and *C*, 100 msec for *B*, *D*, *E*, and *F*; 200 msec on the right. Vertical calibration on the left: 50 mV. Horizontal calibration on the right: 200 msec. (Modified from Gilmour, R. F., Jr., and Zipes, D. P.: Basic electrophysiology of the slow inward current. *In* Antman, E., and Stone, P. H. [eds.]: Calcium Blocking Agents in the Treatment of Cardiovascular Disorders. Mt. Kisco, N.Y., Futura Publishing Co. Inc., 1983, pp. 1–37.)

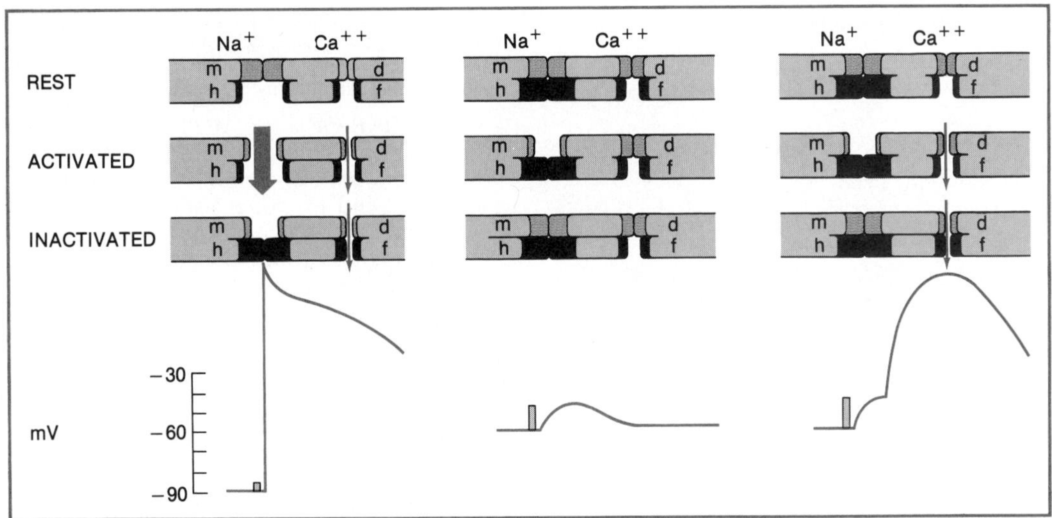

FIGURE 22–13. Schematic representation of membrane channels for rapid and slow inward currents at resting membrane potential *(top row),* during the activated state *(middle row),* and during the inactivated state *(bottom row).* Vertically separated panels depict fibers with a normal resting potential of −90 mV *(left),* with resting membrane potential reduced to less than −60 mV *(middle),* and after stimulation of the cell with catecholamines *(right).* The activation (m) and inactivation (h) gates of the fast channel and the activation (d) and inactivation (f) gates of the slow channel are depicted.

During the resting state *(left panel),* the activation gates of both channels are closed while the inactivation gates are open. When the cell is stimulated, the m gates of the fast channel open, and for a brief period of time, the open m gates and h gates allow inward sodium current to flow, depolarize the cell, and produce its upstroke. The action potential is depicted below. The h gates then close the channel and inactivate sodium conductance. When the upstroke of the action potential exceeds the threshold for activation of the slow inward current, the d gates open, allowing ingress of the slow inward current that contributes to the plateau phase of the action potential. The f gates of the slow channel close more slowly than the h gates. Although the slow inward channel remains open longer than does the fast channel, less total current flows.

When the resting membrane potential is reduced below −60 mV by increasing $[K]_o$ from 4.0 to 14.0 mm *(middle panel),* the cell depolarizes to −60 mV and the fast channel becomes inactivated because the h gates remain closed. Even though the m gate may open during activation, the amount of sodium current is too small to elicit an action potential. The inactivation gates of the slow channel (f gates) are only partially closed, and when the cell is excited after addition of catecholamine *(right panel),* the d gates open and permit flow of a slow inward current that causes a slow-response action potential. This action potential resembles those in panels *A, C,* and *F* of Figure 22–12. (From Wit, A. L., and Bigger, J. T., Jr.: Possible electrophysiological mechanisms for lethal arrhythmias accompanying myocardial ischemia and infarction. Circulation *52* (Suppl. 3):96, 1975, by permission of the American Heart Association, Inc.)

THE GATED SYSTEM - A HYPOTHETICAL MODEL. In this hypothetical model, three m (activation) gates and one h (inactivation) gate can be considered to be lined up in series in the membrane Na channel (Fig. 22–13), with the m gate on the extracellular side and the h gate on the intracellular side of the membrane. When the membrane is in a resting polarized state, the m gates are almost completely closed, the h gate is open, and no Na^+ can cross the membrane. Although depolarization of the membrane opens the m gates and closes the h gate, the m gates open faster than the h gate closes, i.e., activation of the channel proceeds faster than inactivation can occur, and Na^+ flows through the Na^+ channel for about 1 msec while both gates are open simultaneously. When the membrane repolarizes to fairly high negative values, i.e., membrane potential becomes more negative than about −60 mV, the gates shut rapidly, the h gate opens more slowly (reactivation or recovery from inactivation), and the membrane is once again capable of depolarization. Until that time, the cell is absolutely refractory, i.e., no stimulus, regardless of intensity, can activate the cell. If the membrane is activated a second time before reaching a large negative value, all the h gates have not yet reopened so that the maximum number of Na^+ channels that can open is reduced. The resulting action potential will have reduced V_{max}, amplitude, duration, and conduction velocity. The state of the gates at any time depends on the membrane potential and the length of time the potential has been maintained.

The three distinct states in this Hodgkin-Huxley model—closed resting, open activated, and closed inactivated—may not be applicable to mammalian cells. When single Na^+ channel currents are studied, Na channels are noted to open only once and rapidly move from the open to the inactivated state.[46] Thus, true inactivation may be faster than the model predicts. Calcium channels have three modes of gating behavior: brief openings, no openings because of channel unavailability, and long-lasting openings with rare, very brief closings.[47]

However, using this model, the amount of current (I) generated by a specific ion (I_i) equals the membrane conductance for the ion (g_i) multiplied by the driving force for that ion. The driving force is the difference between the actual membrane voltage (V_m) and the equilibrium potential for that ion (E_i). Thus

$$I_i = g_i (V_m - E_i)$$

Conductance can be determined by rearranging the equation:

$$g_i = (V_m - E_i)$$

The equations indicate that the current flow is voltage dependent, i.e., as the voltage of the membrane (V_m) changes relative to the equilibrium potential (E_i), the electrical driving force for an ion ($V_m - E_i$) changes and so does the current. The relationship between membrane voltage, V_m, at the time of depolarization, and I_{Na}, measured in terms of V_{max} (maximum rate of rise of phase 0), is indicated by the so-called membrane responsiveness curve. Depolarization results in decreased I_{Na} and V_{max} when it occurs at reduced membrane potentials.

Membrane voltage may also regulate current flow by altering the status of the channel gates, thereby altering conductance. For the Na^+ channel,

$$gi_{Na} = \bar{g}_{Na}\, m^3 h$$

where gi_{Na} is the conductance of the Na^+ channel at a given voltage, $\bar{g}_{Na}$ is the maximum possible conductance of the channel, m^3 represents the status of the activation gate (m = 1, the gate is open; m = 0, the gate is closed) and h represents the status of the inactivation gate (h = 1, gate open; h = 0, gate closed). Since the opening and closing of the gates are voltage and time dependent, the conductance of the channel (g) will be some fraction of the maximum possible conductance ($\bar{g}_{Na}$), depending on membrane voltage and the period during which the membrane has been at that voltage. V_{max} in Purkinje fibers approximates the Na^+ current. The state of the channel influences the effects of drugs (Fig. 22–14, see also Chap. 23).

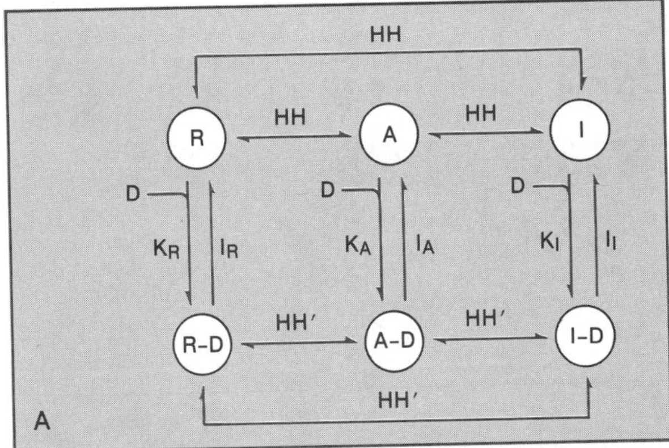

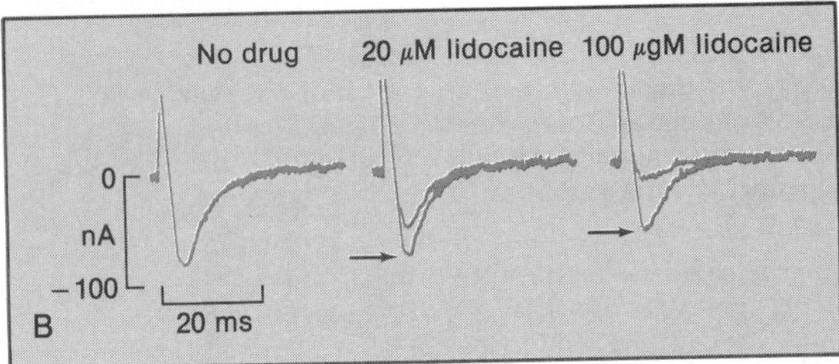

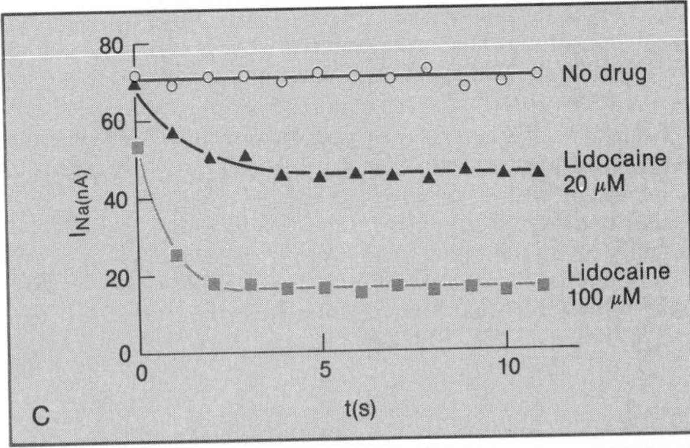

FIGURE 22–14. Interaction between sodium channels and lidocaine. *A*, **Schematic of the modulated receptor hypothesis is presented. Sodium channel gating is represented by transitions between a resting state (R), an open state (A), and an inactivated state (I). The rate constants for binding and unbinding of drug to the channel (k's, l's) depend on the gating state. The presence of bound drug alters the gating transitions from their normal kinetics (HH for Hodgkin-Huxley) to modified kinetics (HH′). Application of this hypothesis explains why some drugs affect cardiac electrophysiological properties according to different channel states, e.g., depolarized or repolarized conditions. (From Hondeghem, L. M., and Katzung, B. G.: Antiarrhythmic agents: The modulated receptor mechanism of action of sodium and calcium-blocking drugs. Ann. Rev. Pharmacol. Toxicol.** ***24***:**387, 1984).**

B, **An example of use dependent block of I_{Na} by lidocaine is demonstrated. I_{Na} was measured (nA) during trains of 500 msec pulses when the cell was depolarized from a holding potential of −105 mV to −35 mV at 1 Hz following a period of rest. The traces show membrane currents associated with the 1st and 12th pulses superimposed, and the graph** *(C)* **plots measured I_{Na} amplitudes for each of the 12 pulses. Lidocaine exerted relatively little effect on the first inward current signal following the rest period (arrows B), but it substantially reduced peak I_{Na} following repetitive depolarizations. Lidocaine exerted a greater effect at the higher concentration. This figure illustrates that lidocaine blocks the sodium channel and reduces I_{Na} to a greater degree after repeated depolarizations of the cell compared with the first depolarization when the cell has been resting (use-dependence). (From Bean, B. P., Cohen, C. J., and Tsien, R. W.: Lidocaine block of cardiac sodium channels. J. Gen. Physiol.** ***81***:**613, 1983.)**

More recent evidence suggests the "ball and chain" explanation for channel inactivation. Essentially, a protein ball dangles on a chain of protein. When it dangles free, ions can move in or out of the channel. When the protein ball plugs the mouth of the pore, ion flow stops.[65b]

UPSTROKE OF THE ACTION POTENTIAL. In normal atrial and ventricular muscle and in the fibers in the His-Purkinje system, action potentials have very rapid upstrokes with a large V_{max} and are called fast responses. Action potentials in the normal sinus and atrioventricular (AV) nodes have very slow upstrokes with a reduced V_{max} and are called slow responses[66] (Fig. 22–12). Upstrokes of "slow responses" are mediated by a slow inward, predominantly Ca^{++} current rather than the fast inward Na^+ current.[47,66] These potentials received the name *slow response* because the time required for activation and inactivation of the slow inward current (I_{si}) is approximately an order of magnitude slower than that for the fast inward Na^+ current (I_{Na}). Recovery from inactivation also takes longer. Calcium entry and $[Ca^{++}]_i$ help promote inactivation. Thus the slow channel opens (activation gates "d") and closes (inactivation gates "f") more slowly than the fast channel, remains open for a longer time, and requires more time following a stimulus to be reactivated (Fig. 22–13). In fact, recovery of excitability outlasts full restoration of maximum diastolic potential. This means that even though the membrane potential has returned to normal, the cell has not recovered excitability completely because the latter depends on elapse of a certain amount of time (i.e., is time dependent) and not just on recovery of a particular membrane potential (i.e., voltage dependence).

Calcium channels are much more selective for Ca^{++} than sodium channels are for Na^+. Selectivity results from the presence of binding sites for which the permeant ions must compete, and under physiological conditions, more than 90 per cent of the inward current through the calcium channel is carried by Ca^{++}. Other divalent cations such as barium and strontium may also carry I_{si}. The magnitude of I_{si} is determined by the probability of calcium channel opening (P), the current through an open channel (i) and the number of channels (N): $I_{si} = N \cdot P \cdot i$. There are estimated to be 1 to 10 functional Ca^{++} channels/μM^2 surface area. At 3mM$[Ca^{++}]_o$ and a membrane potential of 0mV, i approximates 0.05 pA.[67]

The threshold for activation of I_{si}, i.e., the voltage the cell must reach to "turn on" the slow inward current, is about −30 to −40 mV. In fast-response type fibers, I_{si} is normally activated during phase 0 by the regenerative depolarization caused by the fast sodium current. Current flows through both fast and slow channels during the latter part of the action potential upstroke. However, I_{si} is much smaller than the peak Na^+ current and therefore contributes little to the action potential until the fast Na^+ current is inactivated, after completion of phase 0. Thus, I_{si} affects mainly the plateau of action potentials recorded in atrial and ventricular muscle and His-Purkinje fibers. When the fast Na^+ current inactivates rapidly, such as in frog ventricle, I_{si} may contribute noticeably to the peak of phase 0. In addition, I_{si} can be activated and may play a prominent role in partially depolarized cells in which the fast Na^+ channels have been inactivated, if conditions are appropriate for slow-channel activation.

Two types of calcium currents exist: a slowly inactivating high-threshold dihydropyridine-sensitive current (slow or L current) and a fast inactivating low-threshold dihydropyridine-insensitive current (fast or T current).[68] The L-type calcium channel represents the major entry pathway of extracellular calcium[69] and is sensitive to β adrenoceptor stimulation as well as to glucagon.[70]

Other significant differences exist between the fast and slow channels (Table 22–3). The following features are of some clinical relevance (Table 22–4). Drugs that elevate cyclic AMP levels such as beta-adrenoceptor agonists, phosphodiesterase inhibitors such as theophylline and the lipid-soluble derivative of cyclic AMP, dibutyryl cyclic AMP, increase I_{si} via the L-type channel. The beta-adrenoceptor agonist,

TABLE 22-3 CHARACTERISTICS OF FAST AND SLOW INWARD CURRENTS IN CARDIAC TISSUE

	FAST	SLOW
Primary charge carrier	Na	Ca (Na)
Activation threshold	−70 to −55 mV	−55 to −30 mV
Magnitude	1 to 30 μA	0.1 to 3.0 μA
Time constant of Activation	<1 msec	10 to 20 msec
Inactivation	< 1 msec	50 to 500 msec
Inhibitors	Tetrodotoxin, local anesthetics, sustained depolarization at < −40 mV	Verapamil, D-600, nifedipine, diltiazem, Mn, Co, Ni, La
Resting membrane potential	−80 to −95 mV	−40 to −70 mV
Conduction velocity	0.3 to 3.0 M/sec	0.01 to 0.10 M/sec
Rate of rise ($\dot{V}_{max}$) of action potential upstroke	200 to 1000 V/sec	1 to 10 V/sec
Action potential amplitude	100 to 130 mV	35 to 75 mV
Response to stimulus	All-or-none	Affected by characteristics of stimulus
Recovery of excitability	Prompt, ends with repolarization	Delayed, outlasts full repolarization
Safety factor for conduction	High	Low
Major current of action potential upstroke in the following:		
SA node	−	+
Atrial myocardium	+	−
AV node (N region)	−	+
His-Purkinje system	+	−
Ventricular myocardium	+	−
Neurotransmitter influence		
Beta-adrenergic	−	↑↑
Alpha-adrenergic	−	↑
Muscarinic cholinergic	−	↓ in atrium ↓ in ventricle

binding to specific sarcolemmal receptors, facilitates the dissociation of two subunits of a regulatory protein (G protein, p. 359), one of which (G_s) activates adenylate cyclase and thus increases intracellular levels of cyclic AMP. The latter binds to a regulatory subunit of a cyclic AMP–dependent protein kinase that promotes phosphorylation of specific membrane proteins controlling the permeability of the slow channel. This putative conformational change in the channel increases the magnitude of the current or the conductance to the ion, presumably by increasing the amount of time the individual channels are open, without increasing the total number of calcium channels. The probability of channel opening increases.[71] The alpha subunit of the regulatory protein G_s can activate Ca channels directly.[13,72] Acetylcholine reduces I_{si} by decreasing adenylate cyclase activity. However, acetylcholine stimulates cGMP accumulation. cGMP has negligible effects on the basal I_{si} but decreases I_{si} that has been elevated by beta-adrenoceptor agonists. This effect is mediated by cAMP hydrolysis via a cGMP-stimulated cyclic nucleotide phosphodiesterase.[73]

Fast and slow channels can be differentiated on the basis of their pharmacological sensitivity. Drugs that block the slow channel with a *fair* degree of specificity include verapamil, nifedipine, diltiazem, D-600 (a methoxy derivative of verapamil), and compounds such as manganese, lanthanum, nickel, and cobalt. D-600 reduces I_{si} by reducing open-channel probability, as does nifedipine. Other drugs of the same dihydropyridine family as nifedipine can enhance I_{si} by stabilizing the channel in the open mode. Antiarrhythmic agents such as lidocaine, quinidine, procainamide, and disopyramide (see Chap. 23) affect the fast channel and not the slow channel. The puffer fish poison tetrodotoxin (TTX), which is too toxic to be used clinically, blocks the fast channel with considerable specificity.

While fast-response action potentials are characteristic of atrial and ventricular muscle and His-Purkinje tissue, slow-response type action potentials are found in the normal sinus and AV nodes and many kinds of diseased tissue (Table 22–4). Normal action potentials recorded from the sinus node and the N region of the AV node have a reduced resting membrane potential, action potential amplitude, overshoot, upstroke, and conduction velocity compared to action potentials in muscle or Purkinje fibers (Fig. 22–12).

Slow-channel blockers, but not TTX, suppress sinus and AV nodal action potentials. The prolonged time for reactivation of the I_{si} probably accounts for the fact that these cells remain refractory longer than the time it takes for full voltage repolarization to occur. Thus, premature stimulation immediately after the membrane potential reaches full repolarization leads to action potentials with reduced amplitudes and upstroke velocities. Therefore, slow conduction and prolonged refractoriness are characteristic features of nodal cells. These cells also have a reduced "safety factor for conduction," which means that the stimulating efficacy of the propagating impulse is low and conduction block occurs easily. Membranes of nodal cells probably do have Na channels that are inactivated by the relatively depolarized range of potentials over which activity takes place. Hyperpolarization exposes a fast TTX-sensitive sodium current in nodal cells.

These and many other observations support the conclusion that, in the *normal* heart, the I_{si} mediates not only the plateau but also the upstroke of the action potential in the sinus and AV nodes. A small current called i_f, an inward Na^+ and K^+ current that turns on at voltages more negative than −40mV, initiates sinus nodal discharge. Catecholamines increase the probability of channel opening, with no change in single channel amplitude, and increase the discharge rate.[74,75]

A variety of manipulations, including those that block or inactivate the fast inward current (such as administration of TTX or depolarization of the cell membrane with K^+), combined with those that increase the slow current (such as administration of Ca^{++} or catecholamines), or those that decrease the outward potassium currents (such as barium), can transform a fast-channel–dependent fiber (e.g., a Purkinje fiber) to a slow-channel–dependent fiber. Whether these artificial in vitro alterations have clinical relevance is not known, but it is possible that myocardial ischemia or infarction, for example, can produce this transformation (Fig. 22–12*F*). Current data suggest that the electrophysiological changes accompanying *acute* myocardial ischemia represent a depressed form of a fast response rather than a slow response. However, probable slow-response activity has been shown in myocardium resected from patients undergoing surgery for recurrent ventricular tachyarrhythmias (Fig. 22–15). Whether these responses play a role in the genesis of ventricular arrhythmias in these patients has not been established.

Phase 1 — Early Rapid Repolarization

Following phase 0, the membrane repolarizes rapidly and transiently to near 0 mV, partly owing to inactivation of I_{Na} or activation of a transient outward current carried mostly by K ions. Two different types of transient outward currents have

TABLE 22-4 IONIC CURRENTS

TISSUE TYPE	I_{Na}	I_{si}	I_{k_1}	$I_K(I_x)$	I_{to}	$I_f(I_h)$	I_{TI}
Atrial and ventricular myocardium	Responsible for action potential upstroke	Responsible for action potential plateau, excitation contraction coupling, activation in depolarized cells exhibiting the slow response; inactivates to terminate plateau; increased by beta stimulation inhibited by ACh	Responsible for resting potential; repolarizing current in last phase of action potential. Exhibits inward rectification. Time independent, voltage dependent	Responsible for duration of plateau; time-dependent rate-limiting effect; increased by beta stimulation	Responsible for early, transient repolarization preceding plateau; two separate components, I_{to1} and I_{to2}	Not prominent but may be present	Responsible for delayed afterdepolarization; carried by influx of Na due to increase in [Ca]; easily produced with digitalis
His-Purkinje tissue	As in myocardium	As in myocardium; can be responsible for automaticity in all cells that are sufficiently depolarized	As in myocardium	As in myocardium	Prominent; causes phase I; modulates action potential duration in Purkinje fibers	Responsible for automaticity; prominent; increased by beta stimulation	Prominent
SA node and AV node	If present, largely inactivated at reduced membrane potentials	Responsible for action potential upstroke in normal SA and AV nodes. Probably contributes to automaticity	Not prominent	Decay important for normal automaticity	Present	May contribute to automaticity	Present

Abbreviations
I_{Na}, sodium current, I_{si}, slow inward current two components: L type and T type (see text); I_{k_1}, time independent inwardly rectifying potassium current; I_K, delayed rectifier, time-dependent potassium current; I_{to}, transient outward current; I_f (also called I_h), pacemaker current; I_{TI}, Ca^{+2}, calcium activated transient inward current. (See also Fig. 22-11.)

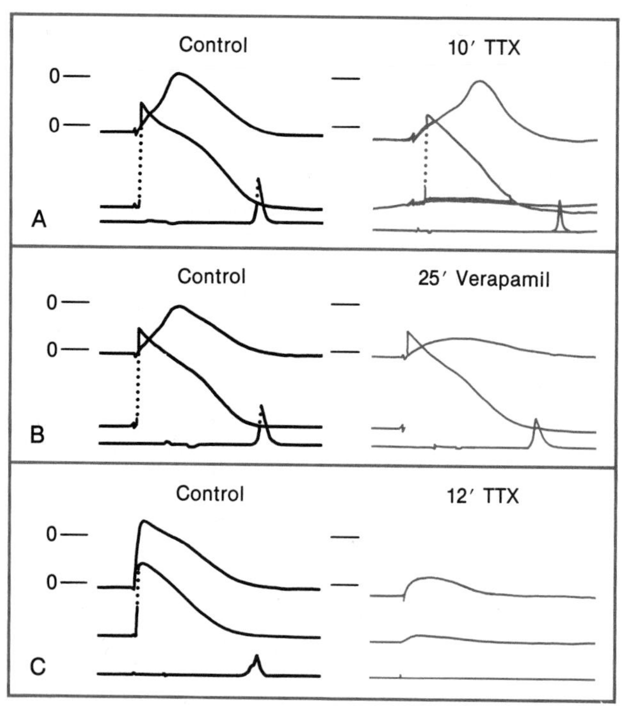

FIGURE 22-15. Effects of tetrodotoxin (TTX) and verapamil on action potentials in diseased human ventricle, removed from a patient at the time of endocardial resection for recurrent ventricular tachycardia. *A*, Action potentials and upstroke velocity recordings from an abnormal cell (upper action potential recording) and a relatively normal cell (lower action potential recording) before *(left)* and after *(right)* exposure to TTX for 10 minutes. Vmax for the lower cell is shown in the bottom tracing. TTX produced activation delay and intermittent conduction block in the normal cell but had little effect on the action potential of the abnormal cell *(right panel)*. Two consecutive cycles are superimposed in the right panel. *B*, after washout of TTX, the same two cells were exposed to verapamil for 25 minutes. Verapamil reduced both the action potential and the amplitude of the abnormal cell without affecting its resting membrane potential and slightly reduced both the action potential amplitude and Vmax in the normal cell *(right panel)*. *C*, Effects of TTX on a different specimen of myocardium from the same patient. Control recordings are shown on the left. In these cells, TTX markedly reduced action potential amplitude and Vmax *(right panel)* while verapamil only slightly reduced action potential amplitude (not shown). (From Gilmour, R. F., Jr., et al.: Cellular electrophysiological abnormalities of diseased human ventricular myocardium. Am. J. Cardiol. *51*:137, 1983.)

been described in human atrial cells. A long-lasting outward current (i_{lo})[76] and a brief outward current (i_{bo}) overlap the inward calcium current and modulate the amplitude of the plateau phase and therefore the amount of calcium entering the cell through calcium channels (Fig. 22–11).[65] Cl^- moving intracellularly through a Cl channel may also affect the plateau. Beta-adrenoceptor stimulation via cyclic AMP–dependent protein kinase,[77] activation of adenylate cyclase,[78] and histamine[79] activate the chloride current. The increase in intracellular negative ions reduces the positive membrane voltage, and the membrane potential returns to near 0 mV, from which the plateau, or phase 2, arises. Sometimes a slight transient depolarization follows phase 1 repolarization. Phase 1 is well defined and separated from phase 2 in Purkinje fibers and some muscle fibers.

Phase 2 – Plateau

During the plateau phase, which may last several hundred milliseconds, membrane conductance to all ions falls to rather low values. Potassium conductance (g_K) falls almost immediately upon depolarization, in spite of the large electrochemical gradient for K^+, owing to "inward-going rectification" (sometimes called "anomalous rectification," since it is opposite to that observed in the squid giant axon). This ponderous term simply means that when the membrane depolarizes it passes inward current more easily than it passes outward current, or, in this instance, K^+ can enter the cell more easily than it can exit, and therefore, despite at least three important outward K^+ currents and a large electrochemical gradient, g_K is low and few K^+ ions leave the cell. Sodium conductance (g_{Na}) is low because of inactivation of sodium channels. Minor contributions to repolarization include a small inward Cl^- flux and electrogenic Na^+-K^+ exchange, pumping out 3 Na^+ in exchange for 2 K^+. The Na^+-K^+ exchange does not turn on and off with each single action potential but restores the ionic gradient over a cumulative time period. The slow inward current, active during the plateau, supplies a small (compared to the Na^+ or fast current) inward current and balances these outward currents, and membrane voltage remains near zero for more than 100 msec. An inward Na^+ current, mentioned earlier, is blocked by tetrodotoxin, and also contributes to the plateau.[65] A transient outward current exists in ventricular epicardium but not endocardium[80] and may be more prominent in some fibers ("M cells") than in others.[81]

Phase 3 – Final Rapid Repolarization

In this portion of the action potential, repolarization proceeds rapidly, owing at least in part to two currents: time-dependent inactivation of the slow inward current, so that intracellular movement of positive charges decreases, and activation of an outward K^+ current (reversal of "inward-going rectification"), so that extracellular movement of positive charges increases. The outward K^+ current is called I_x (or I_K). The net membrane current becomes more outward, and the membrane potential shifts in a negative direction. As repolarization continues, g_K increases, and these repolarization changes self-perpetuate in a regenerative manner.

Phase 4 – Diastolic Depolarization (see also p. 596)

Under normal conditions, the membrane potential of atrial and ventricular muscle cells remains steady throughout diastole. Factors responsible for this resting membrane potential were described earlier. In other fibers found in certain parts of the atria, in the muscle of the mitral and tricuspid valves,[82] in His-Purkinje fibers, and in the sinus node and distal portion of the AV node,[17] the resting membrane potential does not remain constant in diastole but gradually depolarizes (Fig. 22–12*A*). If a propagating impulse does not depolarize the cell or group of cells, it may reach threshold by itself and produce a spontaneous action potential. The property possessed by spontaneously discharging cells is called phase 4 diastolic depolarization; when it leads to initiation of action potentials, automaticity results. The discharge rate of the sinus node normally exceeds the discharge rate of other potentially automatic pacemaker sites and thus maintains dominance of the cardiac rhythm. Discharge rate of the sinus node is more sensitive to the effects of norepinephrine and acetylcholine than is the discharge rate of ventricular muscle cells.[83] Normal or abnormal automaticity at other sites may discharge at rates faster than the sinus nodal discharge rate and may usurp control of the cardiac rhythm for one cycle or many. This will be discussed subsequently.

NORMAL AUTOMATICITY

The ionic basis of automaticity must be explained by a net gain in intracellular positive charges during diastole. Until recently it was believed that cardiac Purkinje fibers experienced a decrease in an outward K^+ current (I_{K2}) during a relatively constant background inward current that caused pacemaker activity. It is now thought that all cardiac pacemaker cells exhibit a voltage-dependent channel that is activated by potentials negative to −50 to −60 mV, i.e., a hyperpolarization-activated inward pacemaker current.[74] At this potential an inward current becomes activated and is carried by a channel relatively nonselective for monovalent cations. Hyperpolarization increases its rate of activation and, at −70 mV, the time constant ranges from 2 to 4 sec. This pacemaker current (I_h or I_f) probably underlies the slow diastolic depolarization that occurs between −90 and −60 mV in Purkinje fibers. Although either K^+or Na^+ can serve as ion transporters, I_f carries largely Na^+ at the more negative intracellular voltages. Extracellular K^+ ions activate I_f, but $[Na^+]_o$ does not influence its conductance. Reduction in K^+ conductance by barium or amantidine seemingly can unmask I_f in ventricular muscle to produce automaticity at relatively normal membrane potentials.[84]

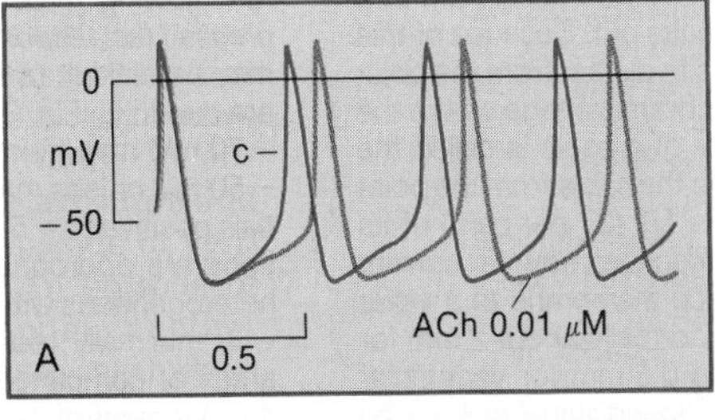

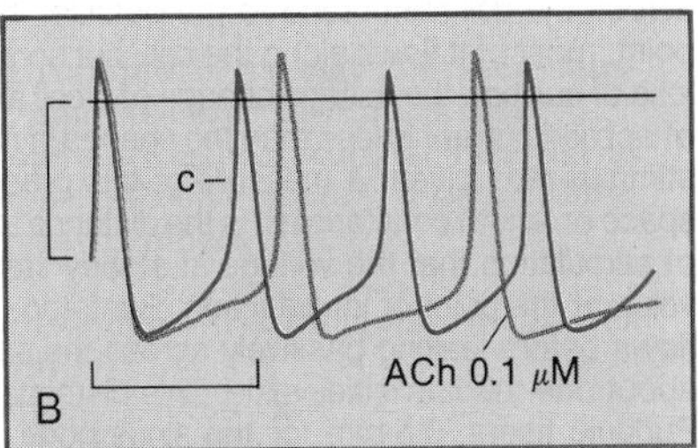

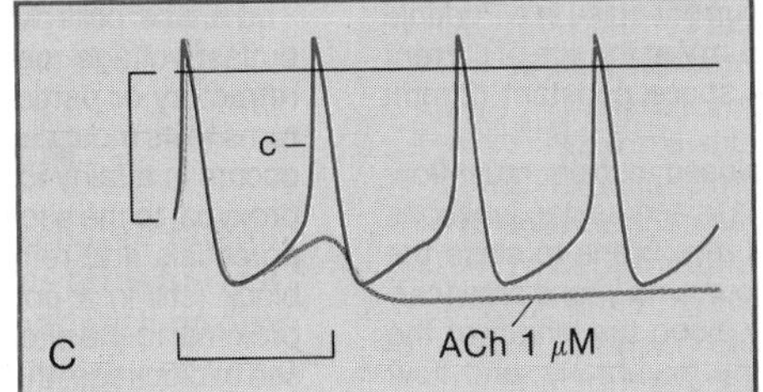

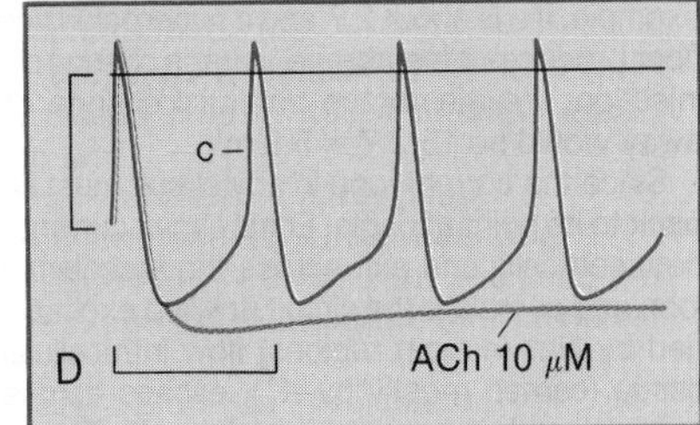

FIGURE 22–16. **Effects of different doses of ACh on spontaneous activity in single S-A node cell. *A–D*, Activity in the control Tyrode solution (*C*) is compared with that in the presence of 0.01, 0.1, 1.0, and 10 μM ACh, respectively. Each concentration of ACh was perfused for about 20 sec. Note that slowing occurred with 0.01 and 0.1 μM ACh and that the cell ceased to beat at higher concentrations, at which point hyperpolarization of the maximum diastolic depolarization also clearly appeared. (From DiFrancisco, O.: Current i_f and the neuronal modulation of heart rate. *In* Zipes, D. P., and Jalife, J. (eds.): Cardiac Electrophysiology. From Cell to Bedside. Philadelphia, W. B. Saunders Co., 1990.)**

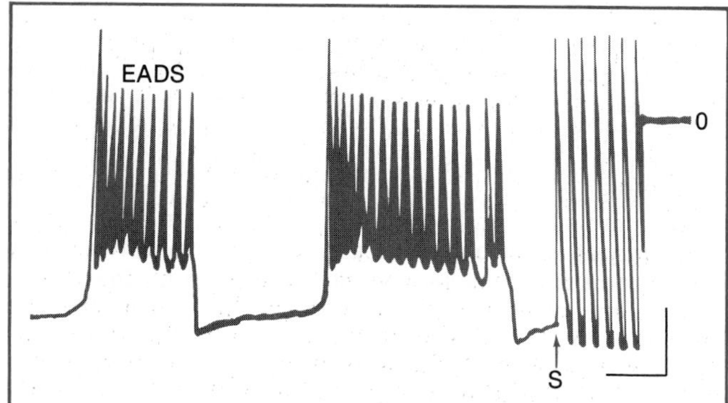

FIGURE 22-18. Early afterdepolarizations (EADs). Early afterdepolarizations occur spontaneously in an isolated canine cardiac Purkinje fiber when exposed to reduced extracellular potassium concentration. Note spontaneous phase four diastolic depolarization is present. In the initial two action potentials, a series of spontaneous depolarizations (EADs) result before the membrane returns to its maximum diastolic potential. Following the second series of EADs, pacing is begun (S) and normal action potentials follow. Horizontal calibration bar = 5 seconds, vertical bar = 25 mV. (From Kovacs, R. J., Bailey, J. C., and Zipes, D. P.: Mechanisms of cardiac arrhythmias. *In* Parmley, W. W., et al. [eds.]: Cardiology. Philadelphia, J.B. Lippincott Co., 1989.)

mal sinus rhythm by a premature ventricular complex or a burst of ventricular tachycardia. It is important to remember that such disorders of impulse formation can be due to a speeding or slowing of a *normal* pacemaker mechanism (e.g., phase 4 diastolic depolarization that is ionically normal for the sinus node or for an ectopic site such as a Purkinje fiber but occurs inappropriately fast or slow) or due to an ionically *abnormal* pacemaker mechanism. The patient with persistent sinus tachycardia at rest or sinus bradycardia during exertion exhibits inappropriate sinus nodal discharge rates, but the ionic mechanisms responsible for sinus nodal discharge may still be normal, although the kinetics or magnitude of the currents may be altered. Conversely, when a patient experiences ventricular tachycardia during an acute myocardial infarction, ionic mechanisms ordinarily not involved in formation of spontaneous impulses for this fiber type may be operative to generate this tachycardia. For example, although pacemaker activity generally is not found in ordinary working myocardium, the effects of myocardial infarction perhaps can depolarize these cells to membrane potentials at which inactivation of I_K and activation of I_{si} cause automatic discharge. Experimental evidence suggests, however, that *acute* myocardial ischemia does not enhance, but may actually suppress, automaticity and after depolarizations.[112,113] Enhanced automaticity[98,99] and after depolarizations have been found in depolarized Purkinje fibers surviving myocardial infarction. Areas of conduction block that may produce entrance block to the automatic focus may protect it from the effects of overdrive suppression and favor the development of automatic discharge. Because the maximum rate that can be achieved by adrenergic stimulation of normal automaticity is generally less than 200 beats/min, it is likely that episodes of faster tachycardia are not due to enhanced normal automaticity.

ABNORMAL AUTOMATICITY. Mechanisms responsible for *normal* automaticity were described earlier. *Abnormal* automaticity may arise from cells that have reduced maximum diastolic potentials, often at membrane potentials positive to −50 mV, when I_K and I_{si} may be operative.

Automaticity at membrane potentials more negative than −70 mV may be due to I_f. When the membrane potential is between −50 and −70 mV the cell may be quiescent. Electrotonic effects from surrounding normally polarized or more depolarized myocardium will influence the development of automaticity. Abnormal automaticity has been found in Purkinje fibers removed from dogs subjected to myocardial infarction, in rat myocardium damaged by epinephrine, in human atrial samples, and in ventricular myocardial specimens from patients undergoing aneurysmectomy and endocardial resection for recurrent ventricular tachyarrhythmias. Abnormal automaticity can be produced in normal muscle or Purkinje fibers by appropriate interventions such as current passage that reduces diastolic potential. Automatic discharge rate speeds up with progressive depolarization, while hyperpolarizing pulses slow the spontaneous firing. Other interventions, such as barium administration, produce automaticity during which action potentials are similar to those produced by current passage. Both may be due to I_K and I_{si}. It is possible that partial depolarization and failure to reach normal maximal diastolic potential can induce automatic discharge in most if not all cardiac fibers. Although this type of spontaneous automatic activity has been found in human atrial and ventricular fibers, its relation to the genesis of clinical arrhythmias has not been established.

Rhythms due to automaticity may be slow atrial, junctional and ventricular escape rhythms, certain types of atrial tachycardias (such as those produced by digitalis), accelerated junctional (nonparoxysmal junctional tachycardia), and idioventricular rhythms and parasystole[114] (see Chap. 24).

TRIGGERED ACTIVITY

The demonstration of triggered activity requires a more precise consideration of the term "automaticity." Triggered activity is pacemaker activity that results *consequent to* a preceding impulse or series of impulses, without which electrical quiescence occurs (Figs. 22-18 and 22-19). Technically, that is not an automatic self-generating mechanism.[63] *Automaticity* is the property of a fiber to initiate an impulse *spontaneously,* without need for prior stimulation, so that electrical

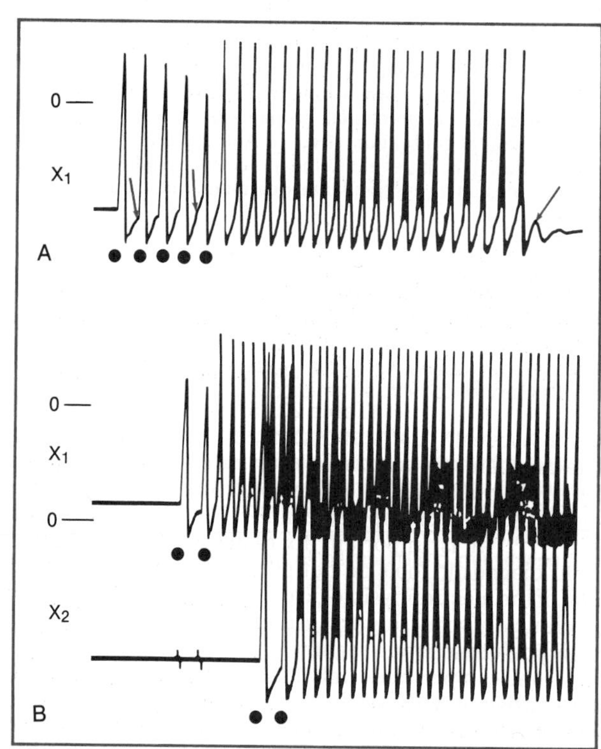

FIGURE 22-19. Triggered sustained rhythmic activity and delayed afterdepolarizations in diseased human ventricle. *A,* Spontaneous activity triggered by a series of driven action potentials (indicated by the dots) at a recording site X1. Note the gradual increase in the size of the delayed afterdepolarizations (arrows) until the afterdepolarization reaches threshold and maintains sustained rhythmic activity after cessation of pacing. The sustained rhythmic activity finally terminates when the last afterdepolarization fails to reach threshold (arrow). *B,* Initiation of triggered activity by intracellular current injection (indicated by dots beneath the respective action potential recordings) at sites X1 and X2, which lie along the same trabeculum. Although sites X1 and X2 were only about 4 mm apart, triggered sustained rhythmic activity from one site did not propagate to the other site, indicating complete dissociation between these two sites. For current pulses, cycle length = 2000 msec; pulse duration = 10 msec; pulse intensity = 200 na. Vertical calibration: 50 mV. Horizontal calibration: 10 sec. (From Gilmour, R. F., Jr., et al.: Cellular electrophysiological abnormalities of diseased human ventricular myocardium. Am. J. Cardiol. *51:*137, 1983.)

TABLE 22-6 DETERMINANTS OF THE AMPLITUDE OF AFTERDEPOLARIZATIONS

INTERVENTION	EFFECT ON AMPLITUDE OF EADs	DADs
Long cycles (Basic and Premature)	↑	↓
Long action potential duration	↑	↑
Reduced membrane potential	↑	↓
Na channel blockers	No effect	↓
Ca channel blockers	↓	↓
Catecholamines	↑	↑

↑ Increase amplitude
↓ Decrease amplitude
EADs = Early afterdepolarizations
DADs = Delayed afterdepolarizations

quiescence does not occur. *Triggered activity* is initiated by afterdepolarizations. These depolarizations may occur before (Fig. 22-18) or after (Fig. 22-19) full repolarization of the fiber and are best termed *early afterdepolarizations* (EADs) when they arise from a reduced level of membrane potential during phases 2 and 3 of the cardiac action potential, and *late* or *delayed afterdepolarizations* (DADs) when they occur after completion of repolarization (phase 4) generally at a more negative membrane potential than from which EADs arise (Table 22-6). All afterdepolarizations may not reach threshold potential, but if they do, they can trigger another afterdepolarization and thus self-perpetuate.

EARLY AFTERDEPOLARIZATIONS (EADS). A variety of interventions can produce EADs. Each results in some reperfusion arrhythmias[116a] and an increase in intracellular positivity.[115,116] EADs may be responsible for the lengthened repolarization time and ventricular tachyarrhythmias in some patients with the long Q-T syndrome.[117-123] Left ansae subclaviae stimulation (Fig. 22-20) increases the amplitude of cesium-induced EADs and the prevalence of ventricular tachyarrhythmias more than does right ansae subclaviae stimulation.[124] These differences may be due to a greater quantitative effect that the left stellate ganglion exerts on the left ventricle compared with the right stellate ganglion. It is possible that patients with the idiopathic congenital long Q-T syndrome have a myocardial defect in repolarization, for example involving an outward potassium current or an inward slow calcium current, rather than "sympathetic imbalance."[124] Sympathetic stimulation, primarily left, could periodically increase the EAD amplitude to provoke ventricular tachyarrhythmias (Fig. 22-20). Alpha-adrenoceptor stimulation also increases the amplitude of cesium-induced EADs and the prevalence of ventricular tachyarrhythmias,[125,126] both of which are suppressed by magnesium.[127] Alpha-adrenoceptor blockade may be helpful in suppressing arrhythmias in some of these patients.

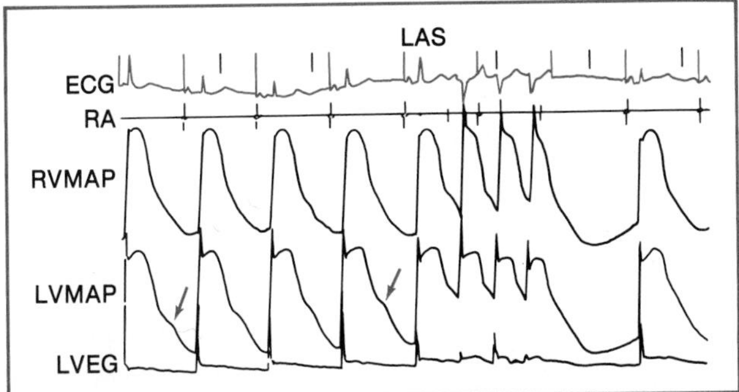

FIGURE 22-20. Following cesium administration during left ansae subclaviae stimulation (LAS), early afterdepolarizations increase in amplitude (arrows), culminating in a short run of nonsustained ventricular tachycardia. RVMAP, right ventricular monophasic action potential recording; LVMAP, left ventricular monophasic action potential recording; LVEG, left ventricular electrograms; time lines, one second. (From Ben-David, J., and Zipes, D. P.: Differential response to right and left stellate stimulation of early afterdepolarizations and ventricular tachycardia in the dog. Circulation *78:*1241, 1988, with permission of the American Heart Association.)

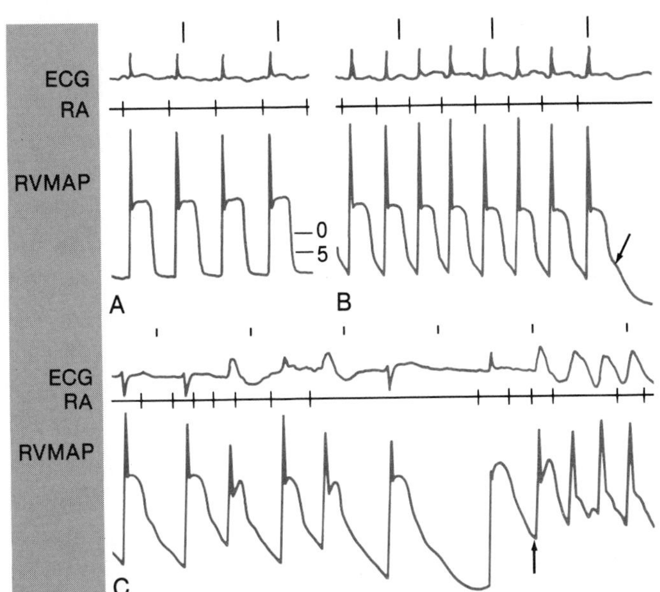

FIGURE 22-21. Induction of early afterdepolarizations in the dog by cesium chloride. Monophasic action potentials recorded from the right ventricle (RVMAP) initially show uniform contour with rapid upstroke, plateau, smooth continuous repolarization, and isoelectric interval for the resting potential (*panel A,* control). A prominent early afterdepolarization is apparent several seconds after cesium administration (*panel B,* arrow). *Panel C* shows development of premature ventricular complexes and long-short RR cycle grouping, culminating in the onset of ventricular tachycardia. A particularly prominent early afterdepolarization (arrow) follows a QRS complex that terminates the long cycle. Paper speed, 50 mm per second; time lines, one second intervals; ECG, electrocardiogram lead II; RA, right atrial electrogram; RVMAP, monophasic action potentials recorded from the apex of the right ventricle. Numbers in millivolts. (From Baillie, D. S., Inoue, H., Kaseda, S., et al.: Magnesium suppresses early depolarizations and ventricular tachyarrhythmias induced in dogs by cesium. Circulation *77:*1395, 1989, with permission of the American Heart Association.)

In patients with the acquired long Q-T syndrome and torsades de pointes due to drugs such as quinidine, N-acetyl procainamide, and some class III antiarrhythmic agents, EADs also may be responsible.[128] Such drugs easily elecit EADs experimentally,[129-131] while magnesium suppresses them[127,130] (Figs. 22-21 and 22-22). The potassium channel activators pinacidil and chromakalim can eliminate EADs.[130a]

DELAYED AFTERDEPOLARIZATIONS (DADs). DADs and triggered activity have been demonstrated in Purkinje fibers, specialized atrial fibers and ventricular muscle fibers exposed to digitalis preparations and in normal Purkinje fibers exposed to Na-free surperfusates from the endocardium of the intact heart,[131a] and from endocardial preparations 1 day after a myocardial infarction.[131b] When fibers in the rabbit, canine, simian, and human mitral valves and in the canine tricuspid valve and coronary sinus are superfused with norepinephrine, they exhibit the capacity for sustained triggered rhythmic activity. In general, the fibers exhibit delayed afterhyperpolarizations (i.e., membrane potential following depolarization transiently becomes more negative than the resting potential), followed by DADs capable of reaching threshold and triggering sustained rhythmic activity. Quinidine enhances these DADs.[132] Triggered activity not requiring norepinephrine for initiation has been recorded in the rabbit atrial pectinate muscle. Triggered activity due to DADs has also been noted in diseased human atrial and ventricular fibers (Fig. 22-19) studied in vitro.[133,134] Left stellate ganglion stimulation can elicit DADs in canine ventricles.[135] In vivo, atrial and ventricular arrhythmias apparently due to triggered activity have been reported in the dog[136,137] and possibly in humans. However, as indicated earlier, it is very difficult to be certain that a particular mechanism is operative in vivo, given our present state of knowledge. It is tempting to ascribe certain clinical arrhythmias to DADs, such as some arrhythmias precipitated by digitalis. The accelerated idioventricular rhythm one day after experimental canine myocardial infarction may be due to DADs.[138]

IONIC BASIS OF DELAYED AFTERDEPOLARIZATIONS. DADs appear to be caused by a transient inward current (I_{TI}) that is small or absent under normal physiological conditions.[139,140] When intracellular calcium overload occurs, as during extensive sympathetic stimulation, high $[Ca^{++}]_o$, or after large doses of digitalis, oscillatory release of Ca^{++} from the sarcoplasmic reticulum activates a nonselective cation channel (or an

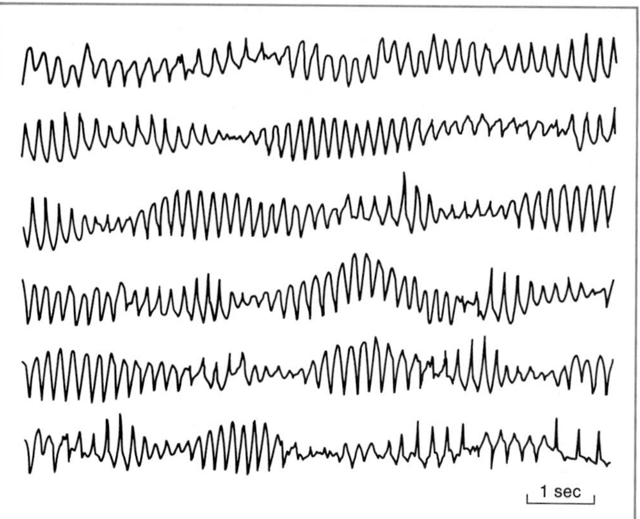

FIGURE 22-22. Torsades de pointes. Ventricular tachycardia initiated in Figure 22-21 continued, with varying morphology characteristic of torsades de points. Continuous recording of lead II. (From Zipes, D. P., and Ben-David, J.: Autonomic neural modulation of cardiac rhythm. Part 2. Mechanisms and examples. Mod. Concepts Cardiovasc. Dis. *57:*47, 1988. Reprinted by permission of the American Heart Association, Inc.)

electrogenic Na^+-Ca^{++} exchange). This results in a transient inward current, carried primarily by Na^+, that generates the DAD. Drugs that block the diastolic Ca^{++} transient, by reducing Ca^{++} overload (e.g., Ca^{++} channel blockers, beta receptor blockers) or by inhibiting Ca^{++} release from the sarcoplasmic reticulum (caffeine, ryanodine), inhibit the DAD. Drugs that reduce the Na^+ current also reduce $[Na^+]_i$ (tetrodotoxin, lidocaine, phenytoin), relieve the Ca^{++} overload, and also can abolish DADs.[67]

DADs due to *digitalis toxicity* (p. 490) behave differently from DADs due to catecholamines. Catecholamine-induced triggering often slows slightly after initiation, then regularizes but slows still further prior to termination, without a progressive increase in maximum diastolic potential. A subthreshold DAD often follows termination of triggered activity. Spontaneous termination may be due, in part, to an increase in the rate of electrogenic sodium extrusion. Termination of digitalis-induced triggering is often characterized by speeding of the rate, decrease in action potential amplitude, and decrease in membrane potential, possibly due to $[Na^+]_i$ or $[Ca^{++}]_i$ accumulation.

Short coupling intervals or pacing at rates more rapid than the triggered activity rate (overdrive pacing) increases the amplitude and shortens the cycle length of the DAD following cessation of pacing (overdrive acceleration) rather than suppressing and delaying the escape rate of the afterdepolarization, as in normal automatic mechanisms (Table 22-7). Premature stimulation exerts a similar effect; the shorter the premature interval, the larger the amplitude and shorter the escape interval of the triggered event. Digitalis and catecholamine-induced DADs behave slightly differently. The amplitude of catecholamine-induced DADs progressively increases as the coupling interval for the DAD shortens, while the amplitude of digitalis-induced DADs increases to a maximum and then decreases at very short coupling intervals. The mechanisms responsible for overdrive acceleration are not clear but may relate to steepening of the slope of diastolic depolarization and the influence of Na/K electrogenic pumping. The clinical implication might be that tachyarrhythmias due to DAD-triggered activity may not be suppressed easily or, indeed, may be precipitated by rapid rates, either spontaneous (such as a sinus tachycardia) or pacing induced. Finally, because a single premature stimulus can both initiate and terminate triggered activity, differentiation from reentry (see below) becomes quite difficult. The response to overdrive pacing may help separate triggered arrhythmias from reentrant ones.[141]

TABLE 22-7 EFFECTS OF ELECTRICAL STIMULATION ON AUTOMATICITY AND TRIGGERED ACTIVITY

	NORMAL AUTOMATICITY	EADs	DADs
Suppressed by overdrive pacing	Yes	Not usually	Not usually
Terminated by premature stimulation	Not usually	Not usually	Usually

EADs = early afterdepolarizations; DADs = delayed afterdepolarizations

PARASYSTOLE

Classically, parasystole has been likened to the function of a fixed-rate asynchronously discharging pacemaker: Its timing is not altered by the dominant rhythm, it produces depolarization when the myocardium is excitable, and the intervals between discharges are multiples of a basic interval. Complete *entrance block*, constant or intermittent, insulates and protects the parasystolic focus from surrounding electrical events and accounts for such behavior. Occasionally the focus may exhibit *exit block*, during which it may fail to depolarize excitable myocardium.[142,143] Data from recent experiments indicate that, in fact, the dominant cardiac rhythm may modulate parasystolic discharge to speed up or slow down its rate.[144,145] Experimental simulations of parasystole demonstrate that the discharge rate of an isolated, "protected" focus can be modulated by electrotonic interactions with the dominant rhythm across an area of depressed excitability. Brief subthreshold depolarizations induced during the first half of the cardiac cycle of a spontaneously discharging pacemaker will delay the subsequent discharge, while similar depolarizations induced in the second half of the cardiac cycle will accelerate it (Fig. 22-23). The ionic basis for these rate changes is not totally established, but it is probable that early depolarizing stimuli reactivate outward potassium currents and retard depolarization while late stimuli contribute depolarizing current that enables the cell to reach threshold more quickly. Early hyperpolarizing subthreshold stimuli accelerate, while late hyperpolarizing stimuli retard discharge. Complex interactions of complete silence, concealed or manifest bigeminy, trigeminy, quadrigeminy, and periods of more complex group beating may occur owing to the entraining effects of the dominant rhythm on the ectopic focus. Similar examples have been noted in human ventricular tissue and interactions may be predicted according to the general rules of biological oscillators. Numerous clinical examples have been published to support these experimental observations[144-148] (see p. 717). Ventricular parasystole may not always be the benign rhythm disorder previously thought.[149]

DISORDERS OF IMPULSE CONDUCTION

Conduction delay and block can result in bradyarrhythmias or tachyarrhythmias, the former when the propagating impulse blocks and is followed by asystole or a slow escape rhythm, and the latter when the delay and block produce reentrant excitation (see below). Various factors, involving both active and passive membrane properties, determine the conduction velocity of an impulse and whether or not conduction is successful. Among these factors are the stimulating efficacy of the propagating impulse, which is related to the amplitude and rate of rise of phase 0, the excitability of the tissue into which the impulse conducts and the geometry of the tissue.[150]

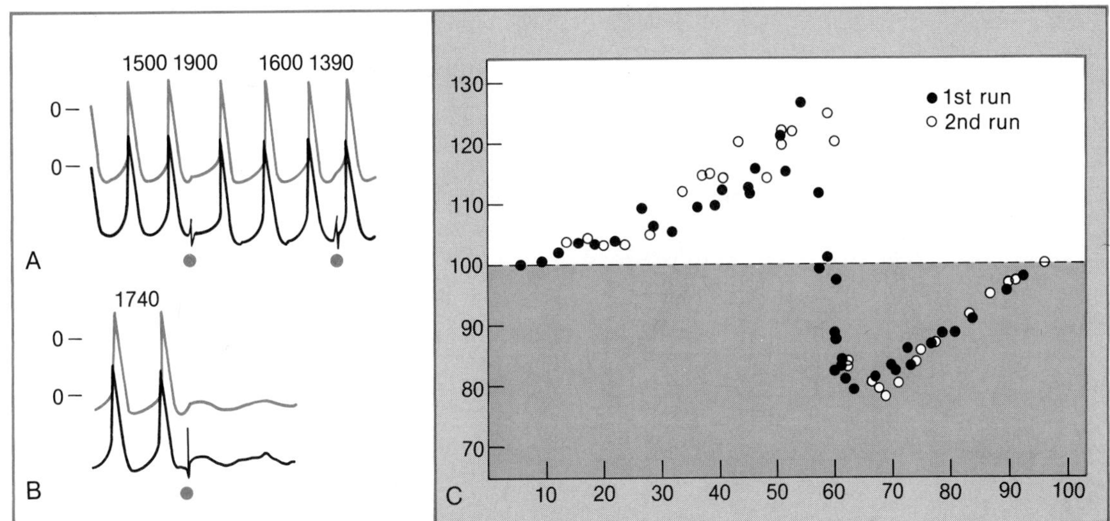

FIGURE 22–23. *Left,* Modulation of pacemaker activity by subthreshold current pulses in diseased human ventricle. *Panel A,* two recording sites along the same trabeculum in a spontaneously active preparation. Current pulses (indicated by the dots) of 30 msec duration were injected through the lower microelectrode at various times. The interval between the spontaneous action potentials is given in milliseconds above each cycle. Injection of a subthreshold current pulse through the lower microelectrode relatively early in the spontaneous cycle (about 680 msec after initiation of the rapid portion of the preceding action potential upstroke) produced a subthreshold depolarization in the upper recording and delayed the next spontaneous discharge by 400 msec to 1900 msec. This response curve would fall in the first half of the curve indicated in panel C. The current pulse of the same intensity and duration delivered later in the spontaneous cycle (950 msec after the preceding upstroke) accelerated the next discharge by 210 msec to 1390 msec, relative to the previous two action potentials. The response to this current injection falls in the second half of the graph depicted in panel C.

Panel B, A stimulus at a precise interval in the cardiac cycle (called the singular point, in this example, 930 msec after the preceding action potential upstroke) abolishes pacemaker activity. (From Gilmour, R. F., Jr., et al.: Cellular electrophysiological abnormalities of diseased human ventricular myocardium. Am. J. Cardiol. *51:*137, 1983.) *Panel C,* Phase response curves from experimental data obtained in canine Purkinje fibers in a manner similar to the human experiment shown in panels A and B. Two different runs are shown. Ordinate: Percentage increase or decrease in the spontaneous cycle length of the "parasystolic focus" (control cycle length equals 100 per cent), Abscissa: Percentage of the "parasystolic focus" spontaneous cycle length during which stimulation was performed. The spontaneous cycle length was maximally prolonged (by 26 per cent) or shortened (by 20 per cent) by subthreshold depolarizations that entered the "parasystolic focus" after approximately 50 and 60 per cent of cycle had elapsed, respectively. Very similar curves can be plotted for patients with parasystole (for example, see figures 9 and 10 from reference 45).(From Jalife, J., and Moe, G. K.: Effect of electronic potentials on pacemaker activity of canine Purkinje fibers and relation to parasystole. Circ. Res. *39:*801, 1976, by permission of the American Heart Association.)

DECELERATION-DEPENDENT BLOCK. Diastolic depolarization has been suggested as a cause of conduction block at slow rates, so-called bradycardia or deceleration-dependent block.[151] Yet excitability increases as the membrane depolarizes until about −70 mV, despite a reduction in action potential amplitude and V_{max}. Evidently depolarization-induced inactivation of fast Na channels is offset by other factors such as reduction in the difference between membrane potential and threshold potential. A more probable explanation of deceleration-dependent block is the reduction in action potential amplitude and excitability at long diastolic intervals in continuously depolarized Purkinje fibers and atrial muscle. Rapid pacing also can produce overdrive suppression of conduction, with a mechanism related to the depression of action potential amplitude and excitability noted above.[152]

DECREMENTAL CONDUCTION. This term is used commonly in the clinical literature but often is misapplied to describe any Wenckebach-like conduction block, i.e., responses similar to block in the AV node during which progressive conduction delay precedes the nonconducted impulse (p. 711). Correctly used, decremental conduction refers to the situation in which the properties of the fiber change along its length so that the action potential loses its efficacy as a stimulus to excite the fiber ahead of it. Thus the stimulating efficacy of the propagating action potential diminishes progressively, possibly as a result of its decreasing amplitude and V_{max}. Wenckebach block results from slow recovery of excitability that produces postrepolarization refractoriness.[153]

REENTRY

Electrical activity during each normal cardiac cycle begins in the sinus node and continues until the entire heart has been activated. Each cell becomes activated in turn and the cardiac impulse dies out when all fibers have been discharged and are completely refractory. During this absolute refractory period, the cardiac impulse has "no place to go." It must be extinguished and restarted by the next sinus impulse. If, however, a group of fibers not activated during the initial wave of depolarization recovers excitability in time to be discharged before the impulse dies out, they may serve as a link to reexcite areas that were just discharged and have now recovered from the initial depolarization. Such a process is given various names, all meaning approximately the same thing: reentry, reentrant excitation, circus movement, reciprocal or echo beat, or reciprocating tachycardia.

ANATOMICAL REENTRY. The earliest studies on reentry were with models that had anatomically defined separate pathways in which it could be shown that there was (1) an area of unidirectional block, (2) recirculation of the impulse to its point of origin, and (3) elimination of the arrhythmia by cutting the pathway. In models with anatomically defined pathways,[154–157] because the two (or more) pathways have different electrophysiological properties, e.g., a refractory period longer in one pathway than the other, the impulse (1) blocks in one pathway (site A in Fig. 22–24*A*) and (2) propagates slowly in the adjacent pathway (serpentine arrow, D to C, Fig. 22–

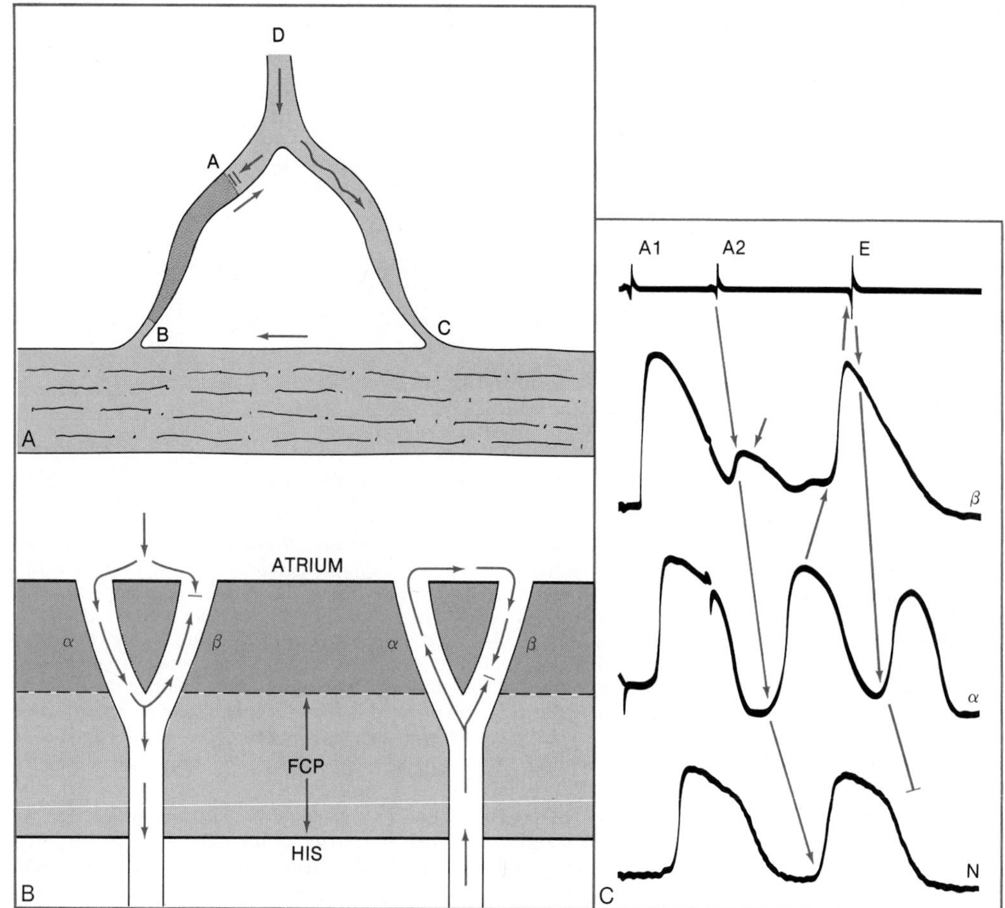

FIGURE 22–24. ***Top,*** **A diagram of reentry published by Schmitt and Erlanger in 1928. A Purkinje fiber (D) divides into two pathways (B and C), both of which join ventricular muscle. It is assumed that the original impulse travels down D, blocks in its anterograde direction at site A (arrow followed by double bar), but continues slowly down C (serpentine arrow) to excite ventricular muscle. The impulse then reenters the Purkinje twig at B and retrogradely excites A and D. If the impulse continues to propagate through D to the ventricular myocardium and elicits ventricular depolarization, a reentrant ventricular extrasystole results. Continued reentry of this type would produce ventricular tachycardia.**

Center, **Atrial echoes.** ***Left,*** **Schematic representation of intranodal dissociation responsible for an atrial echo. A premature atrial response fails to penetrate the beta pathway, which exhibits unidirectional block, but propagates anterogradely through the alpha pathway. Once the final common pathway (FCP) is engaged, the impulse may return to the atrium via the now recovered beta pathway to produce an atrial echo. The neighboring diagram illustrates the pattern of propagation during generation of a ventricular echo. A premature response in the His bundle traverses the final common pathway, encounters a refractory beta pathway (unidirectional block), reaches the atrium over the alpha pathway, and returns through a now recovered beta pathway to produce a ventricular echo.**

Bottom, C, Right, **Actual recordings from the atrium (top tracing), cells impaled in the beta region (second tracing), alpha region (third tracing), and N portion of the AV node (bottom tracing) in an isolated rabbit preparation. The basic response to A_1 activated both alpha and beta pathways and the N cell (first tier of action potentials). The premature atrial response, A_2, caused only a local response in the beta cell (heavy arrow), was delayed in transmission to the alpha cell, and was further delayed in propagation to the N cell. Following the alpha response, a retrograde spontaneous response occurred in the beta cell and propagated to the atrium (E). This atrial response represents an atrial echo. The echo returned to stimulate the alpha cell but was not propagated to the N cell. (From Mendez, C., and Moe, G. K.: Demonstrations of a dual AV nodal conduction system in the isolated rabbit heart. Circ. Res.** ***19:*****378, 1966, by permission of the American Heart Association, Inc.)**

24*A*). If conduction in this alternative route is sufficiently depressed, the slowly propagating impulse excites tissue beyond the blocked pathway (horizontal lined area in Fig. 22–24*A*) and returns in a reversed direction along the pathway initially blocked (B to A in Fig. 22–24*A*) to (3) reexcite tissue proximal to the site of block (A to D in Fig. 22–24*A*). For reentry of this type to occur, the time for conduction within the depressed but unblocked area and for excitation of the distal segments must exceed the refractory period of the initially blocked pathway (A in Fig. 22–24*A*) and the tissue proximal to the site of block (D in Fig. 22–24*A*). Stated another way, continuous reentry requires the anatomical length of the circuit traveled to equal or exceed the reentrant wavelength. The latter is equal to mean conduction velocity of the impulse multiplied by the longest refractory period of the elements in the circuit.

The length of the pathway is fixed and determined by the anatomy. Conditions that depress conduction velocity or abbreviate the refractory period will promote the development of reentry in this model, while prolonging refractoriness and speeding conduction velocity will hinder its onset. For example, if conduction velocity (0.30 M/sec) and refractoriness (350 M/sec) for ventricular muscle were normal, a pathway of 105 mm (0.30 M/sec × 0.35 sec) would be necessary for reentry to occur. However, under certain conditions, conduction velocity in ventricular muscle and Purkinje fibers can be very slow (0.03 M/sec), and if refractoriness is not greatly prolonged (600 msec), a pathway of only 18 mm (0.03 M/sec × 0.60 sec) may be necessary. It frequently exhibits an excitable gap, i.e., a time interval between the end of refractoriness from one cycle and beginning of depolarization in the next, when tissue in the circuit is excitable.[158,159] This results because the wavelength of the reentrant circuit is less than the pathway length. Electrical stimulation during this time period can invade the reentrant circuit and reset its timing[160,161] or terminate the tachycardia. Rapid pacing can entrain the tachycardia,[162] i.e., continuously reset it by entering the circuit and propagating around it in the same way as the reentrant impulse, increasing the tachycardia rate to the pacing rate without terminating the tachycardia. In reentrant circuits with an excitable gap, conduction velocity determines the revolution time of the impulse around the circuit and hence the rate of the tachycardia. Prolongation of refractoriness, unless it is great enough to eliminate the excitable gap and make the impulse propagate in relatively refractory tissue, will not influence the revolution time around the circuit or the rate of the tachycardia. Conceivably, anatomical reentry may have a very small or even absent excitable gap in some instances. Anatomical reentry occurs in patients with the Wolff-Parkinson-White syndrome and probably in AV nodal reentry and in some ventricular tachycardias (Fig. 22–24*B*).

FUNCTIONAL REENTRY. Reentry without anatomical boundaries can occur in contiguous fibers that exhibit functionally different electrophysiological properties and is exemplified by the leading circle hypothesis, which may be important in atrial flutter and atrial fibrillation.[163] According to the leading circle hypothesis, the reentrant circuit propagates around a functionally refractory core and follows a course along fibers that have a shorter refractory period, blocking in one direction in fibers with a longer refractory period (Fig. 22–25). The pathway length of a functional circuit is determined by the smallest circuit in which the leading wavefront is just able to excite tissue ahead that is still relatively refractory. If these parameters change, the size of the circuit may change also, altering the rate of the tachycardia.[164] Shorter wavelengths may predispose to fibrillation. No excitable gap exists, and the duration of the refractory period of the tissue in the circuit primarily determines the cycle length of the tachycardia. Propagating impulses originating outside the circuit cannot easily enter the circuit to reset, entrain, or terminate the reentry.

Theoretically, drugs that prolong refractoriness and do not delay conduction would slow tachycardia due to the leading circle mechanism and not affect tachycardia with an excitable gap until the prolongation of refractoriness exceeded the duration of the excitable gap. Drugs that primarily slow conduction would have major effects on tachycardia with an excitable gap and not on tachycardias due to the leading circle concept. Mixed circuits with both anatomical and functional pathways obfuscate these differences, and circuits due to the leading circle phenomenon also may have an excitable gap.

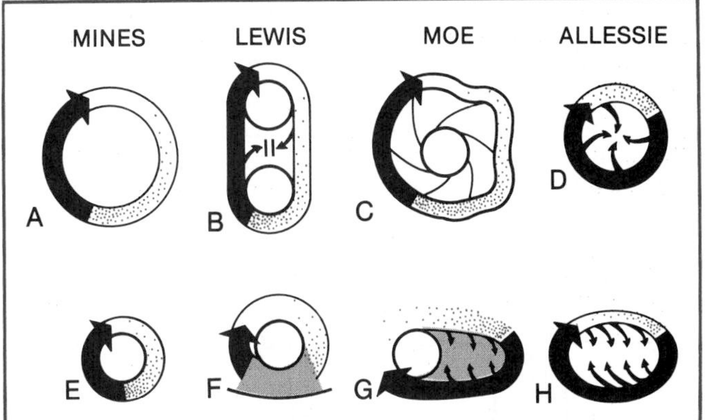

FIGURE 22–25. Schematic representation of various types of reentry. The large arrows represent the crest of a circulating depolarization wave and the absolute refractory phase. The dotted area indicates the tail of relatively refractory tissue. Panel A shows the earliest model of circus movement as introduced by Mines in 1913. A large excitable gap (white part of the circuit) exists between the crest of the excitation wave and its tail of relative refractoriness (dotted area). In panel B circus movement around two obstacles (such as the venae cavae), as popularized by Sir Thomas Lewis, is shown. Panel C is drawn to indicate rapidly conducting muscle bundles such as the internodal bands and Bachmann's bundle that form closed loops to serve as preferential circuits through which excitation waves may circulate. Panel D indicates the leading circle type reentry as described by Allessie et al.[163] In panel E, reentry is facilitated by shortening the wave length of the impulse. Panel F exhibits an area of depressed conduction between two anatomical boundaries and produces an excitable gap in this circuit. Panel G portrays an area of prolonged refractoriness near an anatomical obstacle. Panel H is the diagram of anisotropic reentry. Panel A (excitable gap of anatomic reentry), panel D (functional leading circle reentry), and panel H (anisotropic reentry) depict forms of reentry considered relevant. Reflection is not shown. (From Allessie, M. A., Lammers, W. J. E. P., Rensma, P. L., et al.: Determinant reentry in cardiac muscle. Progr. Cardiol. *1*-2:3, 1988.)

ANISOTROPIC REENTRY. Anisotropic reentry is due to the structural features responsible for variations in conduction velocity and time course of repolarization that can result in block and slowed conduction causing reentry (Fig. 22–25).[56,69,165] Even in normal cardiac tissue showing normal transmembrane potentials and uniform refractory periods, conduction can block in the direction parallel to the long axis of fiber orientation, propagate slowly in the direction transverse to the long axis of fiber orientation, and reenter the area of block. Such anisotropic reentry has been shown in atrial[59] and ventricular[56] muscle, and may be responsible for ventricular tachycardia in epicardial muscle surviving myocardial infarction.[166,167] An excitable gap may be present.

REFLECTION. This can be considered a special subclass of reentry.[168] As in reentry, an area of conduction delay is required, and the total time for the impulse to leave and return to its site of origin must exceed the refractory period of the proximal segment.

Reflection differs from reentry in that the impulse does not require a circuit but appears to travel along the *same* pathway in both directions. The impulse travels in one direction and meets an area of impaired conduction where active transmission pauses. Electrotonically, the impulse spans the zone of impairment, activates the distal segment, and returns electrotonically across the zone of impaired conduction to reexcite the proximal segment. A single reflection could cause a coupled premature complex, while continued reflection back and forth across an inexcitable zone could cause a tachycardia.

Tachycardias Due to Reentry

Reentry is probably the cause of many tachyarrhythmias, including various kinds of supraventricular and ventricular tachycardias, flutter, and fibrillation. However, in complex preparations, such as large pieces of tissue in vitro or the intact heart, it becomes much more difficult to prove unequivocally that reentry exists. In addition, many other factors, such as stretch,[169–175,175a] autonomic stimulation,[27] tissue hyperplasia due to genetic abnormalities,[176] and a host of other modulating influences can act on these electrophysiological mechanisms, obscuring the cause of many arrhythmias. Initiation or termination of tachycardia by pacing stimuli, the demonstration of electrical activity bridging diastole, fixed coupling, and a variety of other clinically used techniques such as entrainment and resetting curves,[176a] while consistent with reentry, do not constitute proof of its existence.

ATRIAL FLUTTER. Reentry is the most likely cause of atrial flutter, with the wavefront traveling a pathway established by atrial anatomy, distribution of refractoriness, and conduction delay.[177–180] Entrainment of atrial flutter, i.e., an increase to the pacing rate of all tissue responsible for sustaining the tachycardia, with resumption of the intrinsic rate of the tachycardia upon either abrupt cessation of pacing or slowing of the pacing rate below the intrinsic rate of the tachycardia, strongly supports a reentrant mechanism with an excitable gap. Constant fusion beats (except for the last captured beat after cessation of pacing, which is entrained but is not a fusion beat), different degrees of fusion at different paced rates, and interruption of tachycardia during rapid pacing with localized conduction block are other features of entrainment and are influenced by the pacing site.

ATRIAL AND VENTRICULAR FIBRILLATION. A critical mass of myocardium, either atrial or ventricular, is required to maintain fibrillation. For example, ventricular myocardium cut into small pieces ceases fibrillating when the pieces reach a critically small size, a concept that has led to a corrective surgical procedure (see p. 656).

Ventricles of small animals stop fibrillating spontaneously, while that seldom occurs in the canine or human heart. In the canine ventricle, the left ventricular free wall and septum appear to be required as a critical mass to maintain fibrillation, since, if they are depolarized, the right ventricle stops fibrillating spontaneously. Fibrillation in the atrial appendage stops when it is clamped off from the rest of the atria in which fibrillation is induced by rapid atrial pacing and vagal stimulation. These observations support Moe's hypothesis that multiple wavelets of reentry, influenced by the mass of the tissue, refractory periods, and conduction velocity, maintain fibrillation. These factors influence the number of wavelets present, which determines the likelihood of the fibrillation to continue. Elegant atrial map-

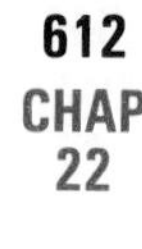

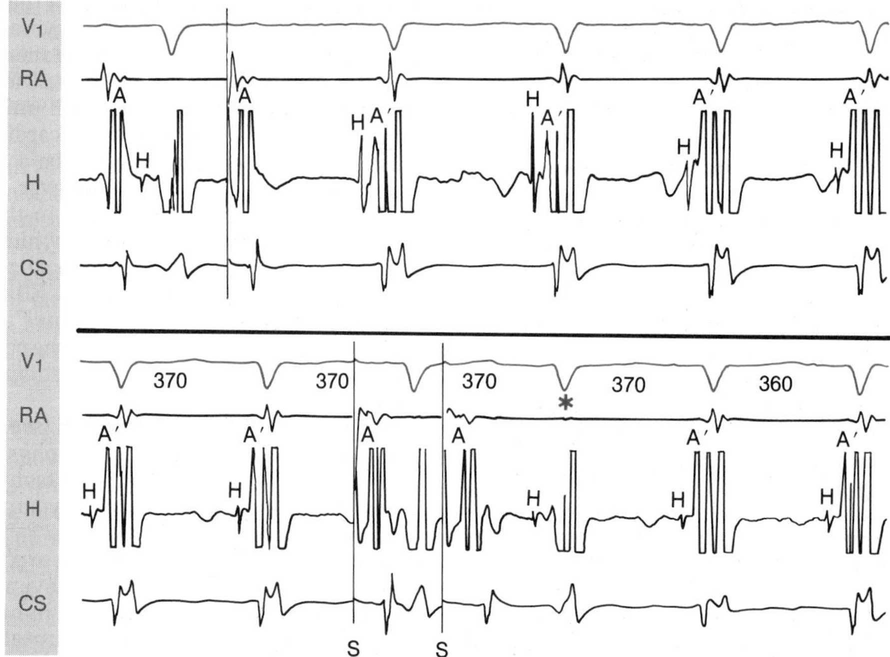

FIGURE 22–28. Dissociation of atria from ventricles without interrupting AV nodal reentrant supraventricular tachycardia. During sinus rhythm, a single premature atrial complex (S, *top panel*) was conducted with AV nodal delay (prolonged A-H interval) and initiated an AV nodal reentrant supraventricular tachycardia. Note that retrograde atrial activation (A′) occurred prior to onset of the QRS complex. Two premature atrial stimuli (S-S, *bottom panel*) captured the atria on both occasions without altering the regular cycle length of the AV nodal reentrant supraventricular tachycardia. Note that the QRS complex marked by an asterisk has no accompanying atrial complex, suggesting that atrial participation in the reentrant circuit was not required. V_1 = scalar lead; RA = right atrial electrogram; H = His bundle electrogram; CS = coronary sinus electrogram.

ally, the activation wave travels in a reverse (antidromic) direction to the ventricles over the accessory pathway and to the atria retrogradely up the AV node. Two accessory pathways may form the circuit in some patients with antidromic AVRT.[196] In some patients, the accessory pathway may be capable only of retrograde conduction, but the circuit and mechanism of tachycardia remain the same. Less commonly, the accessory pathway may conduct only anterogradely. The reentrant loop can be interrupted by oblation of the normal AV node–His bundle pathway or the accessory pathway.[197,198]

Other pathways, such as those having an unusual accessory pathway with AV nodal–like electrophysiological properties, nodofascicular or nodoventricular fibers, may constitute the circuit for reciprocating tachycardias in patients who have some form of the Wolff-Parkinson-White syndrome. Tachycardia in patients with nodoventricular fibers may be due to reentry using these fibers as the anterograde pathway and the His-Purkinje fibers and a portion of the AV node retrogradely.[199–202] In the Lown-Ganong-Levine syndrome (short P-R interval and normal QRS complex), conduction over a James fiber that connects atrium to the distal portion of the AV node and His bundle has been proposed, although little functional evidence to support the presence of this entity has been published, except in a rare patient with an unusual atrio His connection[203] (p. 697).

VENTRICULAR REENTRY (see also p. 703). Reentry in the ventricle as a cause of sustained ventricular tachycardia has been supported by many animal[56,165–167,204] and clinical[205–207,207a] studies. Bundle branch reentry has been demonstrated to occur in dogs and humans, and appears to be a more common cause of sustained ventricular tachycardia than previously thought, particularly in patients with dilated cardiomyopathy.[155] Reentry in ventricular muscle, with or without contribution from specialized tissue, is responsible for many or most ventricular tachycardias in patients with ischemic heart disease. The area of reentry appears to be less than 1.4 cm^2 and only uncommonly is a macroreentry around the infarct scar.[206] In a recent electrophysiological-histological study of Langendorff-perfused human hearts removed from patients undergoing heart transplant in which ventricular tachycardia was induced, surviving myocardial tissue (Fig. 22–30) separated by connective tissue provided serpentine routes of activation that could establish reentry pathways. In two hearts, such tissue constituted a continuous trail that traversed the infarct.[206a]

Complete coronary occlusion in the dog results in a surviving epicardial layer of tissue—almost two-dimensional—in which electrical activity can be mapped accurately during normal sinus rhythm and during ventricular tachycardia induced by premature ventricular stimulation. Both figure-of-eight (Fig. 22–31)[208] and single circle[56] reentrant loops have been described, circulating around an area of functional block in a manner consistent with the leading circle hypothesis or conducting slowly across an apparent area of block created by anisotropy.[56,167] The location of the infarction and structure of surviving myocardium importantly influence the development of reentry as well as the location of the circuit. When intramural myocardium survives, it may form part of the reentrant loop. Structural discontinuities that separate muscle bundles, owing to naturally occurring myocardial fiber orientation and anisotropic conduction as well as to collagen matrices formed from the fibrosis after a myocardial infarction, establish the basis for slowed conduction, fragmented electrograms, and continuous electrical activity that can lead to reentry.[209] After the infarction, action potential recordings from surviving cells return to normal, suggesting that depressed activity in these cells does not account for the slowed conduction.[56] During acute ischemia, however, a variety of factors, including elevated $[K]_o$ and reduced pH, combine to create depressed action potentials in ischemic cells that retards conduction and can lead to reentry.[210,211]

Ventricular myocardium resected from humans with recurrent ventricular tachycardia demonstrates abnormal action potentials, suggesting that causes of depressed conduction in humans may be multifactorial (Figs. 22–17 and 22–19). In addition, since endocardial resection often eliminates ventricular tachycardia in patients with coronary artery disease, it is likely that the origin of the tachycardia, part of its reen-

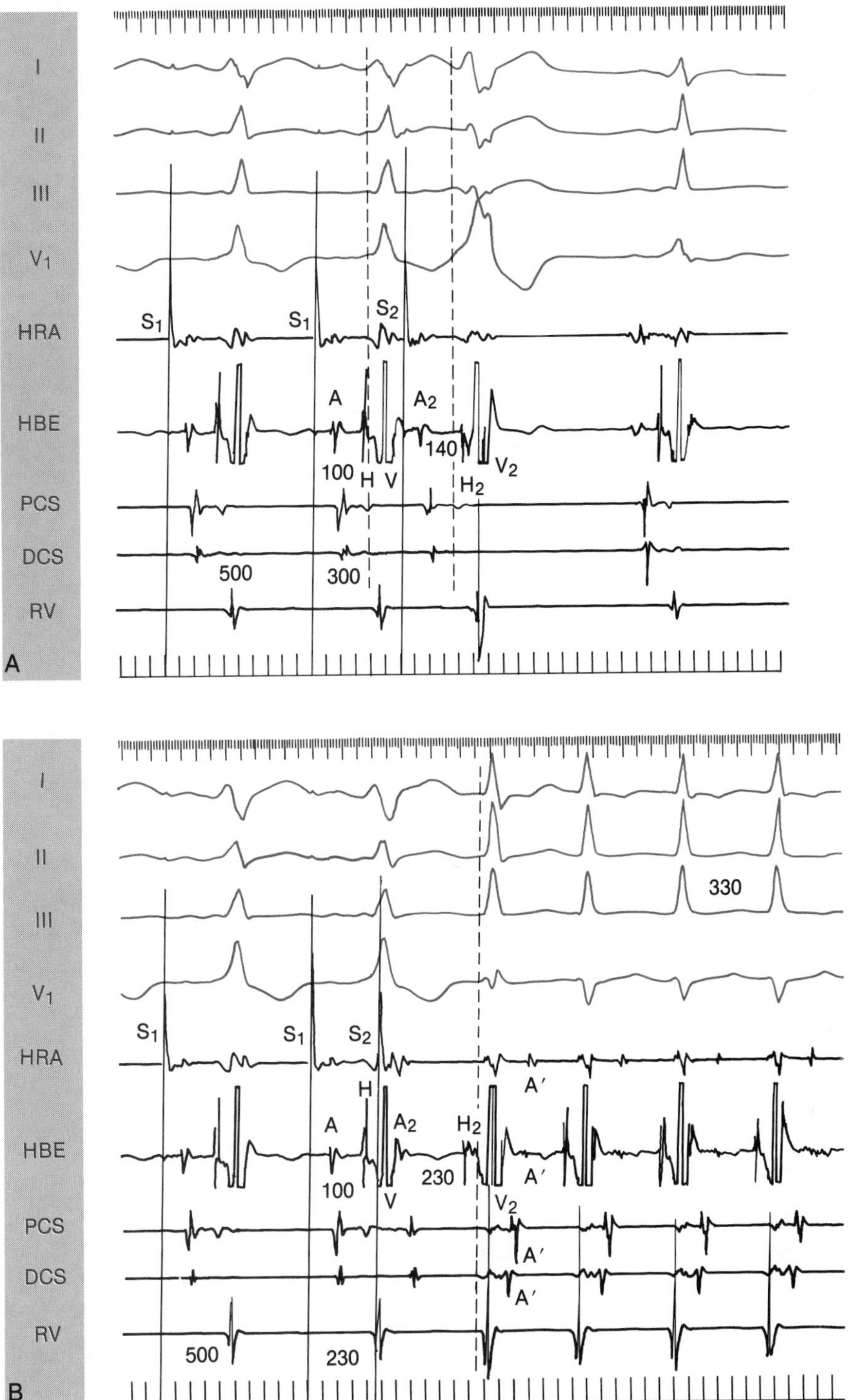

FIGURE 22–29. *A*, Wolff-Parkinson-White syndrome. Following high right atrial pacing at a cycle length of 500 msec (S_1-S_1), premature stimulation at a coupling interval of 300 msec (S_1-S_2) produces physiological delay in AV nodal conduction resulting in an increase in the AH interval from 100 to 140 msec but no delay in the AV interval. Consequently, activation of the His bundle occurs following activation of the QRS complex (second interrupted line) and the QRS complex becomes more anomalous in appearance due to increased ventricular activation over the accessory pathway. I, II, III, and V_1 are scalar leads. HRA, high right atrium; HBE, His bundle electrogram; PCS, proximal coronary sinus electrogram; DCS, distal coronary sinus electrogram; RV, right ventricular electrogram. Time lines 50 and 10 msec intervals. S_1, stimulus of the drive train; S_2, premature stimulus. A, H. V, atrial His bundle, and ventricular activation during the drive train. A_2, H_2, V_2, atrial His bundle, and ventricular activation during the premature stimulus.

B, Induction of reciprocating atrioventricular tachycardia. Premature stimulation at a coupling interval of 230 msec prolongs the AH interval to 230 msec and results in anterograde block in the accessory pathway and normalization of the QRS complex (slight functional aberrancy in the nature of incomplete right bundle branch block occurs). Note that H2 precedes the onset of the QRS complex (interrupted line). Following V_2, the atria are excited retrogradely (A′) beginning in the distal coronary sinus, then followed by atrial activation in leads recording from the proximal coronary sinus, His bundle, and high right atrium. A supraventricular tachycardia is initiated at a cycle length of 330 msec. Conventions as in panel A. (From Zipes, D. P., Mahomed, Y., King, R. D., et al.: Wolff-Parkinson-White syndrome: Cryosurgical treatment. Indiana Med. *89:*432, 1986.)

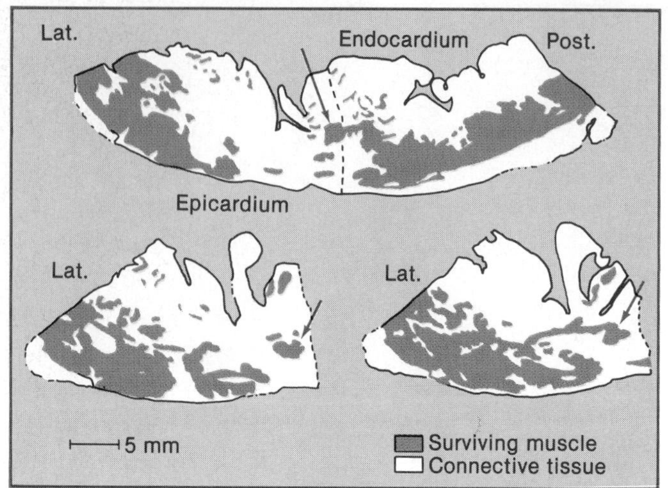

FIGURE 22–30. Top panel is a schematic drawing illustrating left ventricular myocardial sections of a human heart studied electrophysiologically and histologically after removal for cardiac transplant. Dark areas mark surviving cardiac tissue, while light areas point to fibrotic and fatty tissue. Note the irregularity of the surviving cardiac tissue interspersed with fibrotic tissue. Lower two panels are schematic drawings of sections from the lateral left ventricular wall 500 *(left)* and 1000 *(right)* μm, respectively, beneath the level of those shown in the top panel. Note that bulge of viable tissue at the left of the surviving posterior wall (arrow in the top panel) becomes isolated in the lower left panel (arrow). In the lower right panel, this isolated area merges with the bulk of surviving tissue in the lateral wall (arrow). (From deBakken, J. M. T., Coronel, R., Tisserons, S., et al.: Ventricular tachycardia in the infarcted Langendorff-perfused human heart: Role of the arrangement of surviving cardiac fibers. J. Am. Coll. Cardiol. *15:*1594, 1990.)

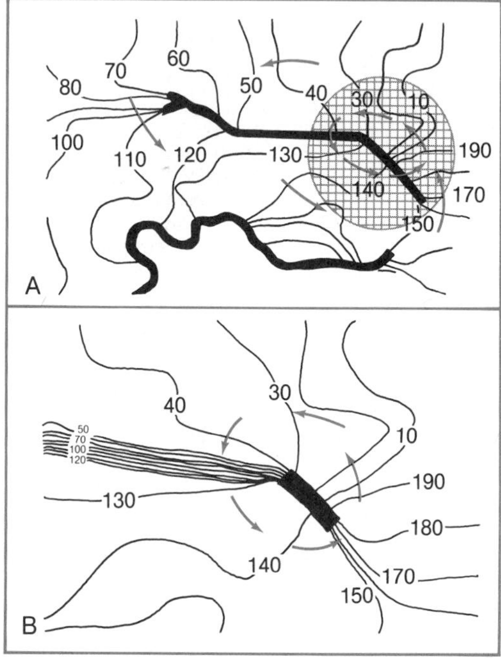

FIGURE 22–31. Model of anisotropic reentry in the epicardial border zone. *A,* The activation map of the single reentrant circuit is shown. The large arrows point out the general activation pattern; activation appears to occur around a long line of block. However, parallel isochrones adjacent to the line (isochrones 130 and 140) suggest that activation is also occurring across the line, resulting in the smaller circuit shown by the small arrows. *B,* This circuit is shown enlarged. Rapid activation occurs parallel to the long axis of the fiber orientation (isochrones 10–40 and at 130–150), whereas very slow activation (closely bunched isochrones 50–120) occurs transverse to fiber orientation in the circuit. The dark black rectangle is an area of either functional or anatomical block that forms the fulcrum of the circuit. (From Wit, A. L., and Dillon, S. M.: Anisotropic reentry. *In* Zipes, D. P., and Jalife, J. (eds.): Cardiac Electrophysiology. From Cell to Bedside. Philadelphia, W. B. Saunders Company, 1990.)

trant loop, or a necessary pathway for its exit to the rest of the ventricle resides in the endocardium after myocardial infarction.

APPROACH TO THE DIAGNOSIS OF CARDIAC ARRHYTHMIAS

It is important to remember that the physician evaluates a *patient* who has a rhythm disturbance and does not evaluate a rhythm disturbance in isolation. Some arrhythmias are hazardous to the patient regardless of the clinical setting, while others are hazardous *because* of the clinical setting. Evaluation of the patient should usually progress from the simplest to the most complex test, from the least invasive and safest to the most invasive and risky, and from the least expensive out-of-hospital evaluations to those that require hospitalization and sophisticated, costly procedures. Occasionally, depending on the clinical circumstances, the physician may wish to proceed directly to a high-risk, expensive procedure, such as an electrophysiological study, prior to obtaining a 24-hour electrocardiographic (ECG) recording.

Patients with cardiac rhythm disturbances may present with a variety of complaints, but commonly symptoms such as palpitations, syncope, presyncope, or congestive heart failure cause them to seek a physician's help. Their awareness of regular or irregular cardiac rhythm varies greatly. Some patients perceive slight variations in their heart rhythm with uncommon accuracy, while others are oblivious even to sustained episodes of ventricular tachycardia; still others complain of palpitations when they actually have regular sinus rhythm. The following tests can be used to evaluate patients who have cardiac arrhythmias.

EXERCISE TESTING

(See also Chap. 6)

About one-third of normal subjects develop ventricular ectopy in response to exercise testing. Ectopy is more likely to occur at faster heart rates, usually in the form of occasional premature ventricular complexes (PVCs) of constant morphology, or even pairs of PVCs, and is often not reproducible from one stress test to the next. Three to six beats of nonsustained ventricular tachycardia can occur in normal patients, especially the elderly, and its occurrence does not establish the existence of ischemic or other forms of heart disease or predict increased cardiovascular morbidity or mortality. Supraventricular premature complexes are often more common during exercise than at rest and increase in frequency with age; their occurrence does not suggest the presence of structural heart disease.

Approximately 50 per cent of patients who have coronary artery disease develop PVCs in response to exercise testing. Ventricular ectopy appears in these patients at lower heart rates (less than 130 beats/min) than in the normal population and often occurs in the early recovery period as well. The prognostic importance of exercise-provoked ventricular arrhythmias in patients with coronary artery disease is unsettled.

Patients who have symptoms consistent with an arrhythmia induced by exercise (e.g., syncope, sustained palpitation) should be considered for stress testing. Stress testing may be indicated to uncover more complex grades of ventricular arrhythmia,[212-214] to provoke supraventricular arrhythmias,[215] to determine the relationship of the arrhythmia to activity, to aid in choosing antiarrhythmic therapy and uncovering proarrhythmic responses,[216,217] and possibly to provide some insight into the mechanism of the tachycardia.[218] The test can be performed safely[219] and appears more sensitive than a standard 12-lead resting ECG to detect ventricular ectopy. However, prolonged ambulatory recording is more sensitive than exercise testing in detecting ventricular ectopy. Since either technique may uncover serious arrhythmias that the other technique misses, both examinations may be indicated for selected patients.

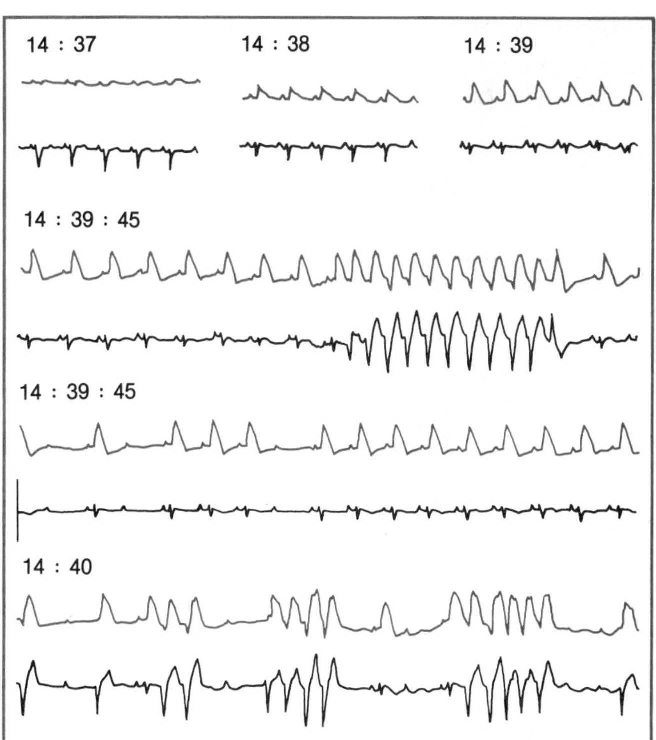

FIGURE 22–32. Long-term ECG recording in a patient with atypical angina. The top channel reflects an inferior lead while the bottom channel records an anterior lead. Note progressive ST segment elevation in the inferior lead, eventually resembling a monophasic action potential. Bursts of nonsustained ventricular tachycardia result. Then, sinus slowing and Wenckebach AV block occur from a vasodepressor reflex response elicited by ischemia of the inferior myocardial wall, or possibly caused by ischemia of the sinus and AV nodes. In the bottom tracing, both AV block and ventricular arrhythmias are apparent. Numbers indicate time, e.g., 2:37 PM. (Tracing of a patient of D. A. Chilson, M.D.)

LONG-TERM ELECTROCARDIOGRAPHIC RECORDING

Prolonged ECG recording in patients engaged in normal daily activities is the most useful noninvasive method to document and quantitate frequency and complexity of arrhythmia, correlate arrhythmia with the patient's symptoms, and evaluate the effect of antiarrhythmic therapy on spontaneous arrhythmia. For example, recording normal sinus rhythm during the patient's typical symptomatic episode effectively excludes cardiac arrhythmia as a cause. In addition, some recorders can document alterations in QRS, ST, and T contours (Fig. 22–32).

Several modes of recordings are available[220]: (1) A recording can be continuous. If a tape recorder is used, every beat is recorded and is available for analysis. A real-time analysis device can also be used. (2) A recording can be patient activated. This is useful if the patient is able to perceive symptoms of the arrhythmia and activate the recorder. (3) A recording can be arrhythmia (event) activated. This is an effective mode, but it depends on the accuracy and reliability of the device's arrhythmia-detection algorithm.

Transmitters that send an electrocardiographic signal transtelephonically[221] to a receiver unit can be used to transmit on-line or stored electrocardiographic information. Such an instrument converts the patient's electrocardiogram to an audiotone, which, when transmitted to a recorder-receiver, is converted back to an electrocardiographic signal for interpretation. This device may be indicated when the rhythm disturbance is sufficiently infrequent and short lasting that continuous ECG recording is impractical. The arrhythmia must be of sufficient duration to permit real-time actual transmission or for storage and later transmission. It must not be associated with syncope or other symptoms that prevent the patient from transmitting or recording, or the patient must have another individual available to record the event. A disadvantage is that this approach relies on the patient's perception of a cardiac rhythm disturbance, and many patients may be unaware of significant or serious bradyarrhythmias and tachyarrhythmias. In addition, the technique requires access to a receiver 24 hours a day. Such an approach can be adapted for continuous monitoring.

Home monitoring systems, presently not widely available, operate in a fashion similar to telemetry monitoring in hospital, but transmit ECG data over telephone lines. Effective use of this system may shorten hospital stay and provide safer home care for many patients with cardiac arrhythmias.

HOLTER MONITORING. Continuous ECG tape recorders represent the traditional Holter "monitor" and typically record on tape two ECG channels for 24 hours. Interpretative accuracy of long-term tape recordings varies with the system used but most computers that scan the tapes are sufficiently accurate to meet clinical needs. All systems can potentially record more information than the physician needs or can assimilate. So long as the system detects important episodes of ectopic activity, ventricular tachycardia, or asystolic intervals and semiquantitates those abnormalities, the physician probably receives all the clinical information that is needed. Approximately 25 to 50 per cent of patients experience a complaint during a 24-hour recording, caused by an arrhythmia in 2 to 15 per cent.[220]

Significant rhythm disturbances are fairly uncommon in healthy young persons. However, sinus bradycardia with heart rates of 35 to 40 beats/min, sinus arrhythmia with pauses exceeding 3 secs, sinoatrial exit block, Wenckebach second-degree AV block (often during sleep), a wandering atrial pacemaker, junctional escape complexes, and premature atrial complexes (PACs) and PVCs are not necessarily abnormal. Frequent and complex atrial and ventricular rhythm disturbances are less commonly observed, however, and type II second-degree AV conduction disturbances are not recorded in normal patients. Elderly patients may have a greater prevalence of arrhythmias,[222] some of which may be responsible for neurological symptoms. The long-term prognosis in asymptomatic healthy subjects with frequent and complex PVCs resembles that of the healthy U.S. population without an increased risk of death.[220]

A majority of patients who have ischemic heart disease, particularly those after myocardial infarction, exhibit PVCs when monitored for periods of 6 to 24 hours (p. 1245). The frequency of PVCs progressively increases over the first several weeks, decreasing at about 6 months after infarction. Frequent and complex PVCs are an independent risk factor and are associated with a two- to fivefold increased risk of cardiac or sudden death in patients after myocardial infarction. Recent evidence from the Cardiac Arrhythmia Suppression Trial (CAST) raises the possibility that the ventricular ectopy may be a *marker* identifying the patient at risk rather than being *causally related* to sudden death. In that trial,[223] which followed a feasibility study called the Cardiac Arrhythmia Pilot Study (CAPS),[224] antiarrhythmic therapy of patients with asymptomatic or minimally symptomatic ventricular arrhythmias after myocardial infraction was evaluated. During an average of 10 months of follow-up, patients treated with flecainide and encainide had an excess of deaths from arrhythmia and nonfatal cardiac arrests (4.5 per cent versus 1.2 per cent taking placebo) and had a higher total mortality (7.7 per cent versus 3.0 per cent taking placebo), despite having suppression of spontaneous ventricular ectopy. Thus, the PVC may be an *innocent bystander*, unrelated to the tachyarrhythmia producing sudden death. Encainide and flecainide suppressed the PVCs and nonsustained ventricular tachycardia in the CAST patients but apparently exacerbated the incidence of ventricular tachyarrhythmias, resulting in an increased mortality.[225–227] Although the mechanism responsible for this exacerbation is not clear, it may relate to a drug-induced increase in ischemia-produced conduction delay.[225,226]

Recently, Holter recordings have been used to assess heart rate variability measured as the standard deviation of sinus cycle lengths, as a measure of vagal input to the sinus node. Decreased heart rate variability correlates with an increased risk of sudden cardiac death.[228–231,231a] Alternation in wave form morphology may be another clue to cardiac electrical instability detectable by Holter recordings.[232]

Long-term ECG recording has also exposed potentially serious arrhythmias and complex ventricular ectopy in patients with hypertrophic cardiomyopathy (p. 1404), mitral valve prolapse (p. 1029), in patients who have otherwise unexplained syncope (Chap. 34) or transient vague cerebrovascular symptoms, in patients with conduction disturbances,[233] sinus node dysfunction, the bradycardia-tachycardia syndrome, the Wolff-Parkinson-White syndrome, or pacemaker malfunction (p. 745).

In patients with ventricular arrhythmias, programmed stimulation studies commonly provoke ventricular arrhythmias not found on the long-term ECG recording, but it has not yet been clearly established which technique is more useful for predicting therapeutic response to pharmacological therapy. It is important to remember that in normal subjects and in patients with serious rhythm disturbances, the cardiac rhythm may vary markedly from one recording period to the next.

INVASIVE ELECTROPHYSIOLOGICAL STUDIES

An invasive electrophysiological procedure involves introducing multipolar catheter electrodes into the venous and/or arterial system, positioning the electrodes at various intracardiac sites to record electrical activity from portions of the atria or ventricles, from the region of the His bundle, bundle branches, accessory pathways, and stimulating the atria or ventricles electrically. Such studies are performed *diagnostically* to provide information on the type of rhythm disturbance and insight into its electrophysiological mechanism; *therapeutically* to terminate a tachycardia by electrical stimulation or electroshock, to evaluate effects of therapy by determining whether a particular intervention prevents electrical induction of a tachycardia or whether an electrical device properly senses and terminates an induced tachyarrhythmia, and to ablate myocardium involved in the tachycardia. Finally, these tests have been used *prognostically* to identify patients at risk for sudden cardiac death. The study may be helpful in patients who have AV block, intraventricular conduction disturbance, sinus node dysfunction, tachycardia, and unexplained syncope or palpitations.[234]

False-negative responses—not finding a particular electrical abnormality known to be present—as well as false-positive ones—induction of a nonclinical arrhythmia—may complicate interpretation of the results, as may lack of reproducibility.[235] Altered autonomic tone in a supine patient undergoing study, hemodynamic or ischemic influences, changing anatomy (e.g., new infarction) after the study, day-to-day variability,[236] and the fact that the test employs an artificial "trigger" (electrical stimulation) to induce the arrhythmia[237] are several of many factors that may explain the disparity between test results and spontaneous clinical occurrences. Overall, these studies are quite safe when performed by skilled physicians.

AV BLOCK (see also pp. 684, and 710 to 715). In patients with AV block, the site of block usually dictates the clinical course of the patient and whether or not a pacemaker is needed. Generally the site of AV block can be determined from an analysis of the scalar ECG. When the site of block cannot be determined from such an analysis, and when knowing the site of block is imperative for patient management, an invasive electrophysiological study is indicated. Candidates include symptomatic patients in whom His-Purkinje block is suspected but not established and patients with AV block treated with a pacemaker who continue to be symptomatic, to search for a causal ventricular tachyarrhythmia. Possible candidates are those with second- or third-degree AV block in whom knowledge of the site of block or its mechanism may help direct therapy or assess prognosis, and patients suspected of having concealed His extrasystoles (Fig. 22–33).[234] Patients with block in the His-Purkinje system more commonly become symptomatic because of periods of bradycardia or asystole and require pacemaker implantation than do patients who have AV nodal block. Wenckebach (type I) AV block in older patients may have clinical implications similar to type II AV block.

INTRAVENTRICULAR CONDUCTION DISTURBANCE. For patients with an intraventricular conduction disturbance, an electrophysiological study provides information on the duration of the H-V interval, which can be prolonged with a normal P-R interval or normal with a prolonged P-R interval. A prolonged H-V interval (>55 msec) is associated with a greater likelihood of developing trifascicular block (but the rate of progression is slow, 2 to 3 per cent annually), having organic disease, and higher mortality. Some data suggest that finding very long H-V intervals (>80 to 90 msec) identifies patients at significant risk of developing AV block. The H-V interval has a high specificity (about 80 per cent) but low sensitivity (about 66 per cent) for predicting the development of complete AV block. During the study, atrial pacing is used to uncover abnormal His-Purkinje conduction. A positive response is provocation of distal His block during 1:1 AV nodal conduction. Once again, sensitivity is low but specificity is high. Functional His-Purkinje block due to normal His-Purkinje refractoriness is not a positive response. Drug infusion, such as with procainamide or ajmaline, sometimes exposes abnormal His-Purkinje conduction. Ajmaline can cause arrhythmias and should be used cautiously.

An electrophysiological study is indicated in the patient with symptoms (syncope or presyncope) that appear to be related to a bradyarrhythmia or tachyarrhythmia when no other cause of symptoms is found. For many of these patients, ventricular *tachyarrhythmias* rather than AV block might be the cause of their symptoms.[234]

SINUS NODAL DYSFUNCTION. The demonstration of slow sinus rates, sinus exit block, or sinus pauses temporally related to symptoms suggests a causal relationship and usually obviates further diagnostic studies. Carotid sinus pressure that results in complete cardiac asystole or AV block with the patient's usual symptoms exposes the presence of a hypersensitive carotid sinus reflex (p. 676). Carotid sinus massage must be done cautiously. Rarely, carotid sinus massage can precipi-

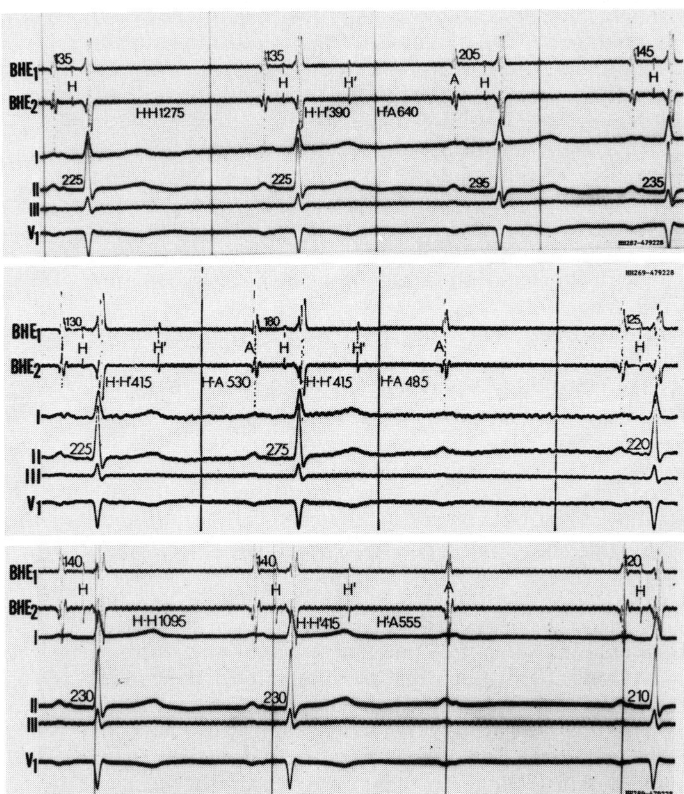

FIGURE 22–33. Concealed discharge from the bundle of His mimicking first-degree *(top)*, type I *(middle)*, and type II *(bottom)* second-degree AV block. Numbers are in milliseconds. Time lines are one second. (Magnification differs in the three panels.) Numbers in the bipolar His electrogram (BHE_1) indicate A-H intervals; the H-V interval is constant. Numbers in lead II indicate the P-R interval. H-H = interval between His responses in normal conducted cycles. H-H' = interval between the last normal His discharge and the premature His discharge. H'-A = interval between the premature His depolarization and the next normal sinus-initiated atrial discharge. H' invaded the AV node and lengthened the A-H interval or produced AV nodal block of the next atrial depolarization. (From Bonner, A. J., and Zipes, D. P.: Lidocaine and His bundle extrasystoles. His bundle discharge conducted normally, conducted with functional right or left bundle branch block, or blocked entirely (concealed). Arch. Intern Med. *136:*, 700, 1976.)

tate a stroke. Neurohumoral agents or stress testing may be employed to evaluate effects of autonomic tone on sinus node automaticity and sinoatrial conduction time. Electrophysiological studies should be considered in patients who have symptoms attributable to bradycardia or asystole, such as presyncope or syncope, and for whom noninvasive approaches have provided no explanation for the symptoms.[234]

Sinus Node Recovery Time (SNRT). This technique can be a useful and sensitive test to evaluate sinus node function. The interval between the last paced high right atrial response and the first spontaneous (sinus) high right atrial response after termination of pacing is measured to determine the *sinus node recovery time* (SNRT). Because the spontaneous sinus rate influences the SNRT, the value is corrected by subtracting the spontaneous sinus node cycle length (prior to pacing) from the sinus recovery time (CSNRT) (Fig. 22–34). Normal CSNRT values are generally less than 525 msec. Prolonged CSNRT has been found in patients suspected of having sinus node

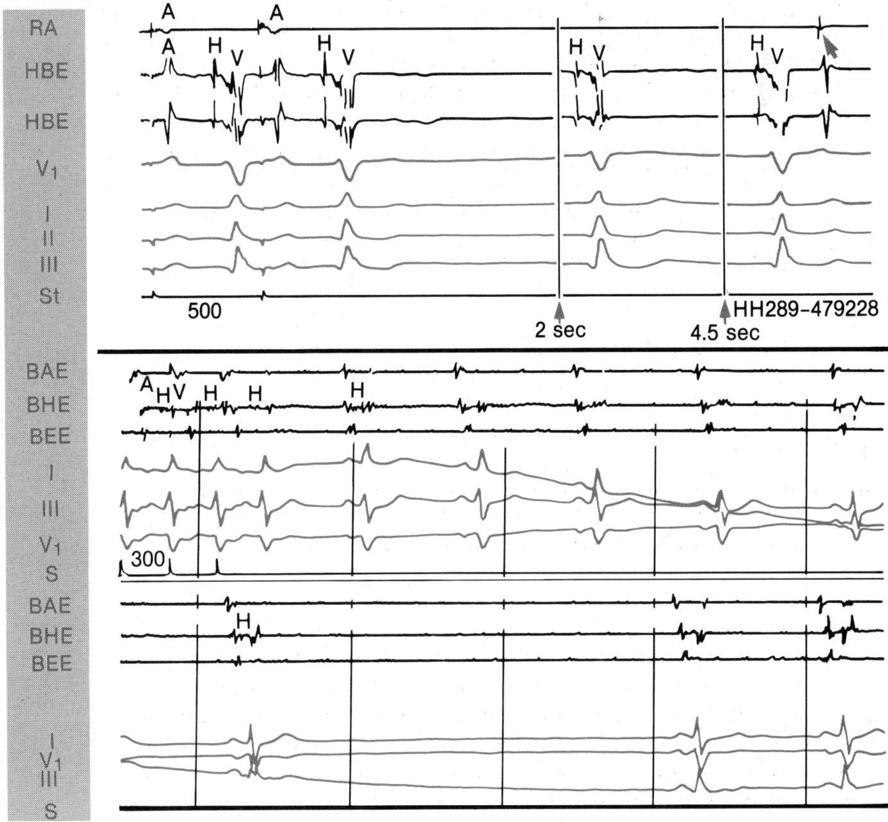

FIGURE 22–34. Abnormal response of sinus node to overdrive pacing. *Top,* After 30 sec of right atrial pacing at a cycle length of 500 msec, sinus nodal discharge where is suppressed for more than 8 sec. (Sections of 2 sec and 4.5 sec removed for mounting.) *Bottom,* Right atrial pacing at a cycle length of 300 msec was followed by initial P waves occurring at an appropriate rate. The rate then slowed progressively, with P-P prolongation reaching 3 seconds and reproducing the patient's symptoms. Continuous recording; time lines = 1 sec. RA and BAE = bi-polar right atrial electrogram; HBE and BHE = bi-polar His electrogram; BEE = bipolar esophageal electrogram; I, II, III, and V = scalar leads; St and S = stimulus. (Modified from Zipes, D. P., and Noble, R. J.: Assessment of electrical abnormalities. *In* Hurst, J. W. [ed.]: The Heart. 5th ed. New York, McGraw-Hill Book Co., 1982, pp. 333–357.)

dysfunction. Direct recordings of sinus node electrogram have documented that SNRT is influenced by prolongation of sinoatrial conduction time, as well as by changes in sinus nodal automaticity, especially in the first beat after cessation of pacing. After cessation of pacing, the first return sinus cycle can be normal and can be followed by secondary pauses (Fig. 22–34). Secondary pauses appear to be more common in patients whose sinus node dysfunction is caused by sinoatrial exit block. Sinoatrial exit block can cause some sinus pauses. It is important to evaluate AV nodal and His-Purkinje function in patients with sinus node dysfunction, since many also exhibit impaired AV conduction.

Sinoatrial Conduction Time (SACT). This time can be estimated, based on the assumptions that (1) conduction times into and out of the sinus node are equal, (2) no depression of sinus node automaticity occurs, and (3) the pacemaker site does not shift following premature stimulation. These assumptions may be erroneous, particularly in patients with sinus nodal dysfunction; SACT can be measured directly with extracellular electrodes placed in the region of the sinus node and correlates well with the CSACT measured indirectly in patients with normal sinus node function. The sensitivity of the SACT and SNRT tests is only about 50 per cent for each test alone and about 65 per cent when combined. The specificity, when combined, is about 88 per cent, with a low predictive value. Thus, if they are abnormal, the likelihood of the patient having sinus nodal dysfunction is great. However, the fact that they are normal does not exclude the possibility of sinus node disease. Candidates for invasive electrophysiological study are symptomatic patients in whom sinus node dysfunction has not been established as a cause of the symptoms. Potential candidates are those requiring pacemakers to determine the pacing modality, patients with sinus node dysfunction to determine the mechanism and response to therapy, and patients in whom other causes of symptoms, e.g., tachyarrhythmias, are to be excluded.[234]

TACHYCARDIA. In patients with tachycardias, an electrophysiological study may be used to diagnose the arrhythmia, determine and deliver therapy, determine anatomical site(s) involved in the tachycardia, identify patients at high risk for developing serious arrhythmias, and gain insights into mechanisms responsible for the arrhythmia. For example, results of the study can differentiate aberrant supraventricular conduction from ventricular tachyarrhythmias. Since all the electrocardiographic manifestations of ventricular tachycardia[238] can be mimicked, under certain circumstances, by aberrantly conducted supraventricular tachycardia, exceptions exist to the criteria that help to differentiate supraventricular tachyarrhythmias with abnormal QRS complexes from ventricular tachyarrhythmias. A *supraventricular tachycardia* is recognized electrophysiologically by the presence of an H-V interval equaling or exceeding that recorded during normal sinus rhythm (Fig. 22–35). In contrast, during *ventricular tachycardia*, the H-V interval is shorter than normal or, more commonly, the His deflection cannot be recorded clearly. Only two situations exist when a consistently short H-V interval occurs: during retrograde activation of the His bundle from activation originating in the ventricle or during conduction over an accessory pathway (preexcitation syndrome). Only in bundle branch reentry will the HV interval resemble the normal sinus HV interval during ventricular tachycardia, but His activation will be in the retrograde direction. Atrial pacing at rates exceeding the tachycardia rate can demonstrate ventricular origin of the wide QRS tachycardia by producing fusion and capture beats and normalization of the H-V interval (Fig. 22–36).

An electrophysiological study should be carried out in patients with frequent or poorly tolerated episodes of *supraventricular tachycardia* not responding adequately to drug therapy in whom information about the tachycardia is essential for choosing proper therapy and in patients in whom nonpharmacological therapy is preferred over drug management. Patients with the WPW syndrome may be studied to help guide future participation in high-risk activities or to guide therapy in those who have a family history of sudden cardiac death.[234] Studies are performed in patients with wide-QRS complex tachycardias that are sustained or symptomatic when the diagnosis is unclear and is necessary for appropriate care, and in patients surviving an episode of cardiac arrest occurring ≥48 hours after an acute myocardial infarction or without evidence of an acute Q wave myocardial infarction.[234,239] Electrophysiological studies are generally *not* indicated in patients with the long Q-T syndrome and torsades de pointes, although recent information about early afterdepolarizations (p. 605) may make such studies useful in the future.

The process of initiation and termination with programmed electrical stimulation of supraventricular or ventricular tachycardia to test the potential efficacy of pharmacological, electrical, or surgical therapy represents an important application of electrophysiological studies in patients with tachycardia. Determination of drug efficacy based on results from long-term ECG recordings may be insufficient to predict a

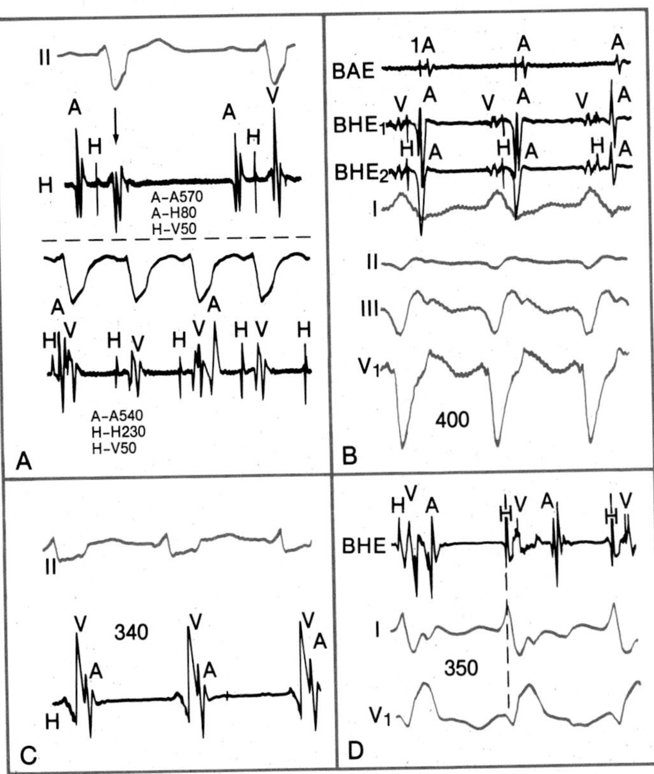

FIGURE 22–35. His bundle recording in four different patients with tachycardias. *A*, The top portion of the tracing shows His bundle recording during sinus rhythm. The H-V interval is 50 msec. The bottom portion shows His bundle recording during tachycardia. Since the QRS complex and H-V interval are the same as those recorded during sinus rhythm, this is a supraventricular tachycardia. Of note is the fact that the atria discharged at a rate that was different from (not a multiple of) the ventricular rate. Thus, AV dissociation is present during this supraventricular tachycardia. *B*, His bundle activity occurred after the onset of the QRS complex, during ventricular tachycardia. (WPW had been excluded.) The R-P interval remained constant, and the atria were captured retrogradely from the ventricles. Thus, AV dissociation is not present during this ventricular tachycardia. *C*, His bundle activity was not recorded despite careful exploration of the His bundle area with the catheter electrode tip. This most likely represents ventricular tachycardia with 1:1 retrograde atrial capture, but the diagnosis cannot be as clear as in panels *B* and *D*, In panel D His bundle activity (interrupted line) preceded the onset of ventricular septal depolarization but followed the onset of the QRS complex. Thus, this must be ventricular tachycardia. Retrograde (VA) Wenckebach conduction (not shown in its entirety) was also present. (From Zipes, D. P., et al.: Clinical electrophysiology and electrocardiography. *In* Willerson, J. T., and Sanders, C. A. [eds.]: The Science and Practice of Clinical Medicine. Clinical Cardiology. New York, Grune and Stratton, 1977, pp. 235–248.)

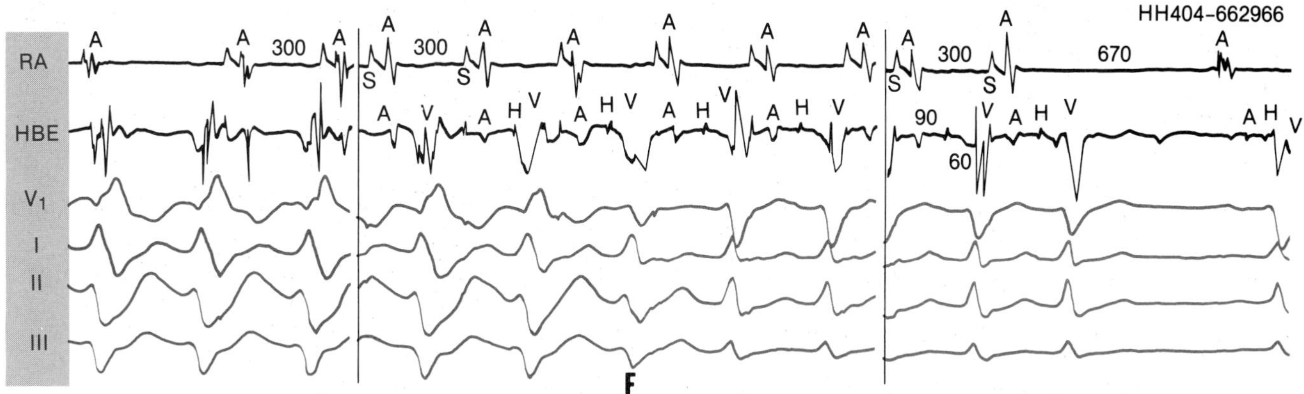

FIGURE 22–36. Termination of ventricular tachycardia by rapid atrial pacing. Ventricular tachycardia *(left panel)* with AV dissociation became captured by rapid atrial pacing (200 bpm) *(middle panel)* and was terminated after cessation of atrial pacing *(right panel)*. Note fusion beat (F) in the midportion of panel 2 and normalization of the H-V interval. (From Foster, P. R., and Zipes, D. P.: Pacing and cardiac arrhythmias. *In* Mandel, W. J. [ed.]: Cardiac Arrhythmias. Their Mechanisms, Diagnosis and Management. Philadelphia, J. B. Lippincott Co., 1980, pp. 605–624.)

patient's therapeutic response, particularly in the patient with a low frequency of spontaneous ventricular arrhythmias.[240] A drug that prevents electrical induction of a sustained monomorphic ventricular tachycardia that was induced during the predrug control state has a high probability of achieving long-term successful suppression of spontaneous episodes. A drug that fails to prevent electrical induction may still prevent spontaneous clinical episodes, but in a lesser percentage of patients.[241] The patient's hemodynamic response to the tachycardia can be assessed. Often, drugs slow the rate of a tachycardia, even though they fail to prevent its induction, and the patient may have a better hemodynamic response to the tachycardia. Electrical therapy also can be delivered via the catheter electrode (pacing, cardioversion, defibrillation, ablation; see p. 653).

INDICATIONS. An electrophysiological study should be considered (1) in patients who have symptomatic, recurrent, or drug-resistant supraventricular or ventricular tachyarrhythmias, particularly when the tachycardia produces hemodynamically significant consequences; (2) in patients with tachyarrhythmias occurring too infrequently to permit adequate diagnostic or therapeutic assessment; or (3) to differentiate supraventricular tachycardia and aberrant conduction from ventricular tachycardia; (4) whenever nonpharmacological therapy such as the use of electrical devices, catheter ablation, or surgery is contemplated.[234]

Patients with Unexplained Syncope (see p. 879). The three common arrhythmic causes of syncope include sinus node dysfunction, tachyarrhythmias, and AV block. Of the three, tachyarrhythmias are most reliably initiated in the electrophysiology laboratory, followed by sinus node abnormalities and then His-Purkinje block.[242–244]

The cause of syncope goes undetected in up to 50 per cent of patients, depending in part on the extent of the evaluation.[245] A careful, accurately performed history and physical examination begin the evaluation, followed by noninvasive tests, including a 12-lead and 24-hour ECG recording. An arrhythmic cause of syncope can produce motor activity similar to that accompanying epilepsy.[246] The 1-year mortality is about 6 per cent in patients with unknown cause, 1 to 12 per cent in patients with noncardiovascular causes, but 19 to 30 per cent in patients with cardiovascular causes. The incidence of sudden death is also higher in patients with a cardiovascular cause of syncope. A small percentage (<5 per cent) of patients develop an arrhythmia coincident with syncope or presyncope during a 24-hour ECG recording, while a large percentage (15 per cent) have symptoms without an arrhythmia, excluding an arrhythmic cause. Prolonged ECG monitoring with patient-activated transtelephonic event recorders that have memory loops may increase the yield.[245] Signal averaging (p. 620) has a high sensitivity (about 75 per cent) and specificity (about 90 per cent) for predicting patients with syncope in whom ventricular tachycardia can be induced at electrophysiological study.[247,248] Administration of isoproterenol during tilt testing has an overall sensitivity of 73 per cent, specificity of 85 per cent and positive predictive accuracy of 69 per cent in inducing vasodepressor responses in vasodepressor-prone patients.[249] Stress testing can be helpful in evaluating some patients.

The electrophysiological study helps explain the cause of syncope or palpitations when it induces an arrhythmia that replicates the patient's symptoms. Syncopal patients with a nondiagnostic electrophysiological study have a low incidence of sudden death and 80 per cent remission rate. In those with recurrent syncope, the test is falsely negative in ≥20 per cent, due to failure to find AV block or sinus node dysfunction.[250]

Syncopal patients considered for electrophysiological study are those whose spells remain undiagnosed despite general, neurological, and noninvasive cardiac evaluation, particularly if the patient has structural heart disease. The diagnostic yield is about 70 per cent in that group but only about 12 per cent in patients without structural heart disease. Mortality and incidence of sudden cardiac death are mainly determined by the presence of underlying heart disease.[251] Syncopal patients with a nondiagnostic electrophysiological study have a low incidence of sudden death and 80 per cent remission rate. In those with recurrent syncope, the test is falsely negative in ≥20 per cent due to failure to find AV block or sinus node dysfunction.[250] Therapy of a putative cause found during electrophysiological testing prevents recurrence of syncope in about 80 per cent of patients. At times, empiric pacing is justified.[252]

Palpitations. An electrophysiological study is indicated in patients with palpitations[253] who have had a pulse rate that medical personnel documented to be inappropriately rapid without electrocardiographic recording or in those suspected of having clinically significant palpitations without ECG documentation.[234]

In patients with syncope or palpitation, the sensitivity of the electrophysiological test may be very low, but may be increased at the expense of specificity. For example, more aggressive pacing techniques (e.g., using three or four premature stimuli), administration of drugs (e.g., isoproterenol), or left ventricular pacing can increase the success rate of ventricular tachycardia induction, but by precipitating nonclinical ventricular tachyarrhythmias such as nonsustained polymorphic or monomorphic ventricular tachycardia or ventricular fibrillation. Similarly, aggressive techniques during atrial pacing can induce nonspecific episodes of atrial flutter or atrial fibrillation. A diagnostic dilemma arises when the patient's clinical, symptom-producing arrhythmia is one of these nonspecific arrhythmias that can be produced in the normal patient who has no arrhythmia. Induction of *sustained* supraventricular (e.g., AV nodal reentry, AV reciprocating tachycardia) or monomorphic ventricular tachycardia in patients who are not subject to the spontaneous development of the tachycardia appears to be uncommon and provides important information that the induced tachyarrhythmia may be clinically significant and responsible for the patient's symptoms. Generally, other abnormalities such as prolonged sinus pauses following overdrive atrial pacing or His-Purkinje AV block are not induced in patients who do not or may not experience these abnormalities spontaneously. Induction of these arrhythmias has a high degree of specificity.

COMPLICATIONS OF ELECTROPHYSIOLOGICAL STUDIES. The risks of these studies are small. Five deaths have been noted in 4015 patients (0.12 per cent) undergoing 8545 studies (0.06 per cent) in six major institutions; 19 patients had cardiac perforation, 4 had major hemorrhage, 8 had arterial injury, and 20 had major venous thromboses.[254] Adding therapeutic maneuvers, e.g., ablation, to the procedure may increase the incidence of complications.

OTHER DIAGNOSTIC ELECTROCARDIOGRAPHIC TECHNIQUES

ESOPHAGEAL ELECTROCARDIOGRAPHY. Esophageal electrocardiography is a useful noninvasive technique to diagnose arrhythmias.[255,256] The esophagus is adjacent to the posterior atria, and an electrode inserted into the esophagus can record atrial potentials. Bipolar recording is superior to unipolar recording. In addition, atrial and occasionally ventricular pacing can be performed via a catheter electrode inserted into the esophagus, and initiation and termination of tachycardias can be accomplished. Optimal electrode position for pacing correlates with patient height and is within about 1 cm of the site at which the maximum amplitude of the atrial electrogram is recorded. No serious immediate complications of transesophageal pacing have been reported. A capsule electrode that is easily swallowed has been used to record continuous atrial electrograms from the esophagus.

The esophageal atrial electrogram is useful to differentiate supraventricular tachycardia with aberrancy from ventricular tachycardia. During a wide QRS tachycardia when the ventricular rate exceeds the atrial rate, AV dissociation is often present, and the most likely diagnosis is ventricular tachycardia (see p. 703). If each ventricular depolarization is coupled to an atrial depolarization, either supraventricular tachycardia or ventricular tachycardia with 1:1 ventriculoatrial conduction may be present. Uncommonly, junctional tachycardia with aberrancy can mimic ventricular tachycardia, and His bundle recordings are needed for a definitive diagnosis. When the same number of atrial and ventricular depolarizations occurs, vagal maneuvers can be used to evoke AV nodal block or slow the supraventricular rate to differentiate ventricular tachycardia from supraventricular tachycardia.

Esophageal atrial electrograms are also helpful to define the mechanism of supraventricular tachycardias. For example, a narrow QRS tachycardia with a ventricular rate of 150 beats/min can be due to atrial flutter with a 2:1 ventricular response, confirmed by finding an atrial rate of 300 beats/min. If atrial and ventricular depolarization occur simultaneously during paroxysmal supraventricular tachycardia, reentry utilizing an accessory AV pathway (Wolff-Parkinson-White) can be excluded, and AV nodal reentry is the most likely mechanism for the tachycardia (p. 688).

BODY SURFACE MAPPING. Isopotential body surface maps are used to provide a complete picture of the effects of the currents from the heart on the body surface. The potential distributions are represented by contour lines of equal potential, and each distribution is displayed instant by instant throughout activation or recovery, or both.

Body surface maps have been used clinically to localize and size areas of myocardial ischemia,[257,258] localize ectopic foci or accessory pathways,[259,260] differentiate aberrant supraventricular conduction from ventricular origin, recognize the patient prone to developing arrhythmias,[261,262] and possibly understand the mechanisms involved.[263] Although these procedures are of interest, their clinical utility has not yet been established.

DIRECT CARDIAC MAPPING: RECORDING POTENTIALS DIRECTLY FROM THE HEART. Cardiac mapping is a method whereby potentials recorded directly from the heart are spatially depicted as a function of time in an integrated manner. The location of recording electrodes (epicardial, intramural, or endocardial) and the recording mode used (unipolar versus bipolar) as well as the method of display (isopotential versus isochrone maps) depend upon the problem under consideration.

Direct cardiac mapping via catheter electrodes or at the time of cardiac surgery can be used to localize accessory pathways associated with the Wolff-Parkinson-White syndrome, to delineate the anatomical course of the His bundle during open-heart surgery to avoid injury during procedures to correct congenital heart defects, and to identify the site of rhythm disturbances in patients with supraventricular and ventricular tachyarrhythmias for electrical or surgical ablation, isolation, or resection. These approaches are discussed in greater detail in Chap. 23 under "surgical approaches" and in Chap. 24 under the "individual arrhythmias".

SIGNAL-AVERAGING TECHNIQUES. Signal averaging is a method that improves signal-to-noise ratio when signals are recurrent and the noise is random.[264,265] In conjunction with appropriate filtering and other methods of noise reduction, signal averaging can detect cardiac signals of a few microvolts in amplitude, reducing noise amplitude, such as muscle potentials that are typically 5 to 25 μV, to less than 1 μV. With this method, electrical potentials generated by the sinus and AV nodes, His bundle, and bundle branches are detectable at the body surface.

Signal averaging has been applied clinically most often to detect late ventricular potentials of 1 to 25 μV, which are microvolt waveforms continuous with the QRS complex, probably corresponding to delayed and fragmented conduction in the ventricle[266] (Fig. 22–37). Criteria for late potentials are: (1) filtered QRS complex duration $>$114 to 120 msec, (2) $<$20 μV of signal in the last 40 msec of the filtered QRS complex, and (3) the terminal filtered QRS complex remains below 40 μV for longer than 39 msec.[264,265] These late potentials have been recorded in 73 to 92 per cent of patients with sustained and inducible ventricular tachycardia after myocardial infarction, in only 0 to 6 per cent of normal volunteers, and in 7 to 15 per cent of patients after myocardial infarction who do not have ventricular tachycardia.[265–267] Late potentials can be detected as early as three hours after the onset of chest pain and increase in prevalence in the first week after infarction and may disappear in some patients after one year. If not present initially, late potentials usually do not appear later.[268–271] Early use of thrombolytic agents may reduce the prevalence of late potentials after coronary occlusion.[272] They have also been recorded in patients with ventricular tachycardia not related to ischemia, such as dilated cardiomyopathies.[273] Successful surgical control of the ventricular tachycardia can eliminate late potentials but is not necessary to effect tachycardia suppression.[274] Antiarrhythmic drug therapy, on the other hand, decreases the amplitude of the late potentials without abolishing them.[275–277] Late potentials after myocardial infarction are an independent risk factor that identifies patients prone to develop ventricular tachycardia and can be combined with other data such as ejection fraction, spontaneous ventricular ectopy on a 24-hour ECG recording, or response to stress testing to recognize with high sensitivity and specificity patients at risk for ventricular tachycardia or sud-

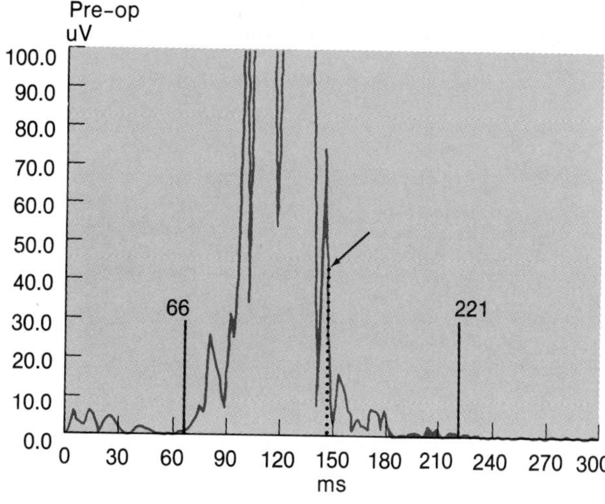

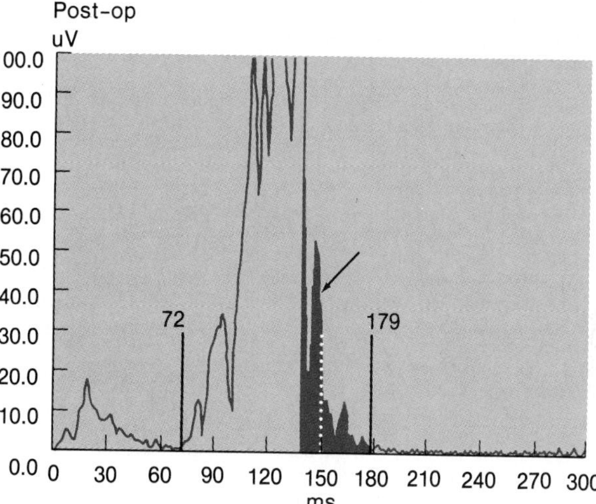

FIGURE 22–37. Signal-averaged ECG showing the presence of prolonged QRS duration due to late potentials (dark filled components in the terminal portion of the complex) present preoperatively but not postoperatively. RMS, root mean square (in mV); IN, integral of wave form delineated by the onset and offset markers; LAS, low amplitude signal. MN, mean value in the terminal QRS. Arrow indicates the 40mV mark, after which the presence of low amplitude signals is determined. Scale = number of mV per notch.

den cardiac death.[278–280a] It can also be used to identify patients with nonsustained ventricular tachycardia or syncope who may develop sustained ventricular tachycardia at electrophysiological study.[281–285]

The high pass filtering used to record late potentials meeting the criteria just noted is called *time domain analysis* because the filter output corresponds in time with the input signal. Since late potentials are high-frequency signals, Fourier transform can be applied to extract high-frequency content from the signal-averaged ECG, so-called *frequency-domain analysis*.[265] Some[286–288] but not all[289–291] data suggest that frequency domain analysis provides useful information not available in the time domain analysis. The preferable alternative has not been determined.

UPRIGHT TILT TESTING (see also p. 882). The tilt test is used to identify patients who have a vasodepressor and/or a cardioinhibitory response as a cause of syncope. Patients are positioned on a tilt table in the supine position and are tilted upright to a maximum of 60° to 80° for 20 to 45 minutes, or longer if necessary. A bolus of isoproterenol may be injected to provoke syncope in patients asymptomatic after initial upright tilt testing or after just several minutes of tilt to shorten the time of the test necessary to produce a positive response. An initial intravenous isoproterenol dose of 2 μg can be increased in 2 μg steps until symptoms occur or a maximum of 8 μg is given. Isoproterenol produces a vasodepressor response in upright susceptible patients generally consisting of a decrease in heart rate and blood pressure along with near syncope or syncope. Atropine can block the early bradycardia but not the hypotension. Propranolol inhibits the latter. Tilt test results correlate reasonably well with the presence or absence of a history of vasodepressor response or syncope.[292,293]

Vasodepressor reactions, which are thought to be caused by activation of unmyelinated left ventricular vagal C fibers, can be excited by a variety of substances, including increased left ventricular pressure. Stimulation of C fibers from vigorous left ventricular contraction on an empty cavity reduces efferent sympathetic tone while increasing efferent vagal tone, possibly producing vasodepression and paradoxic bradycardia. Isoproterenol increases left ventricular contractility while reducing left ventricular volume. A passive upright tilt exaggerates these responses because the tilt also reduces venous return and prevents isoproterenol from increasing cardiac output. Isoproterenol often results in symptom-producing hypotension before the onset of bradycardia. Some patients may experience profound bradycardia while others may have a prominent vasodepressor component.[294,295]

Acknowledgment

The author thanks Robert F. Gilmour, Jr., Ph.D., Lawrence S. Klein, M.D., and William M. Miles, M.D., for critical review of this chapter.

REFERENCES

ANATOMY OF THE CONDUCTION SYSTEM

1. Lowe, J. E., Hartwich, T., Takla, M., and Schaper, J.: Ultrastructure of electrophysiologically identified human sinoatrial nodes. Basic Res. Cardiol. *83*:401, 1988.
2. Michaels, D. C., Matyas, E. P., and Jalife, J.: Mechanisms of sinoatrial pacemaker synchronization: A new hypothesis. Circ. Res. *61*:704, 1987.
3. Takayanagi, K., and Jalife, J.: Effects of digitalis intoxication on pacemaker rhythm and synchronization in rabbit sinus node. Am. J. Physiol. *250*:H567, 1986.
4. Boineau, J. P., Canavan, T. E., Schuessler, R. B., et al.: Demonstration of a widely distributed atrial pacemaker complex in the human heart. Circulation *77*:1221, 1988.

5. Gomes, J. A., and Winters, S. L.: The origins of the sinus node pacemaker complex in man: Demonstration of dominant and subsidiary foci. J. Am. Coll. Cardiol. *9*:45, 1987.
6. Jalife, J., Michaels, D. C., and Langendorf, R.: Modulated parasystole originating in the sinoatrial node. Circulation *74*:945, 1986.
7. Billman, G. E., Hoskins, R. S., Randall, D. C., et al.: Selective vagal postganglionic innervation of the sinoatrial and atrioventricular nodes in the non-human primate. J. Auton. Nerv. Syst. *26*:27, 1989.
8. Salata, J. J., Gill, R. M., Gilmour, R. F., Jr., and Zipes, D. P.: Effects of sympathetic tone on vagally-induced phasic changes in heart rate and A-V nodal conduction in the anesthetized dog. Circ. Res. *58*:584, 1986.
9. DiFrancesco, D., and Tromba, C.: Inhibition of the hyperpolarization-activated current (i_f) induced by acetylcholine in rabbit sino-atrial node myocytes. J. Physiol. (Lond.) *405*:477, 1988.
10. DiFrancesco, D., and Tromba, C.: Muscarinic control of the hyperpolarization-activated current (i_f) in rabbit sino-atrial node myocytes. J. Physiol. (Lond.) *405*:493, 1988.
11. DiFrancesco, D., Ducouret, P., and Robinson, R. B.: Muscarinic modulation of cardiac rate at low acetylcholine concentrations. Science *243*:669, 1989.
12. Molyvdas, P. A., and Sperelakis, N.: Acetylcholine inhibition in rabbit sinoatrial node is prevented by pertussis toxin. Can. J. Physiol. Pharmacol. *67*:522, 1989.
13. Brown, A. M., and Birnbaumer, L.: Direct G protein gating of ion channels. Am. J. Physiol. *23*:H401, 1988.
14. Racker, D. K.: Atrioventricular node and input pathways: A correlated gross anatomical and histological study of the canine atrioventricular junctional region. Anat. Rec. *224*:336, 1989.
15. Spach, M. S., Dolber, P. C., and Heidlage, J. F.: Resolution of discontinuous versus continuous propagation: Microscopic mapping of the derivatives of extracellular potential waveforms. *In* Zipes, D. P., and Jalife, J., (eds.): Cardiac Electrophysiology. From Cell to Bedside. Philadelphia, W.B. Saunders Company, 1990.
16. Meijler, F. L., and Janse, M. J.: Morphology and electrophysiology of the mammalian atrioventricular node. Physiol. Rev. *68*:608, 1988.
17. Kirchhof, C. J., Bonke, F. I., and Allessie, M. A.: Evidence for the presence of electrotonic depression of pacemakers in the rabbit atrioventricular node. The effects of uncoupling from the surrounding myocardium. Basic Res. Cardiol. *83*:190, 1988.
18. Kirchhof, C. J., Bonke, F. I., Allessie, M. A., and Lammers, W. J.: The influence of the atrial myocardium on impulse formation in the rabbit sinus node. Pflugers Arch. *410*:198, 1987.
19. Rosenbaum, M. B., Elizari, M. V., and Lazzari, J. O.: The Hemiblocks. Oldsmar, FL. Tampa Tracings, 1970.
20. Paes de Carvalho, A., and de Almeida, D. F.: Spread of activity through the atrioventricular node. Circ. Res. *8*:801, 1960.
21. Gorza, L., Sartore, S., Thornell, L. E., and Schiaffino, S.: Myosin types and fiber types in cardiac muscle. III. Nodal conduction tissue. J. Cell Biol. *102*:1758, 1986.
22. Kuro-o, M., Tsuchimochi, H., Ueda, S., et al.: Distribution of cardiac myosin isozymes in human conduction system. Immunohistochemical study using monoclonal antibodies. J. Clin. Invest. *77*:340, 1986.
23. Gorza, L., Thornell, L. E., and Schiaffino, S.: Nodal myosin distribution in the bovine heart during prenatal development: An immunohistochemical study. Circ. Res. *62*:1182, 1988.
24. Forsgren, S.: The distribution of nerve fibers showing substance P-like immunoreactivity in the conduction system of the bovine heart: Dense innervation in the atrioventricular bundle. Anat. Embryol. (Berl.) *179*:485, 1989.
24a. Imaizumi, S., Mazgalev, T., Dreifus, L., et al.: Morphological and electrophysiological correlates of atrioventricular nodal response to increased vagal activity. Circulation *82*:951, 1990.
25. Kaseda, S., and Zipes, D. P.: Supersensitivity to acetylcholine of canine sinus and atrioventricular nodes after parasympathetic denervation. Am. J. Physiol. *24*:H534, 1988.
26. Markel, M. L., Miles, W. M., Zipes, D. P., and Prystowsky, E. N.: Parasympathetic and sympathetic alterations of Mobitz II heart block. J. Am. Coll. Cardiol. *11*:271, 1988.
27. Zipes, D. P.: Influence of myocardial ischemia and infarction on autonomic innervation of the heart. Circulation *82*:1095, 1990.
28. Ursell, P. C., Ren, C. L., and Danilo, P.: Anatomic distribution of autonomic neural tissue in the developing dog heart: I. Sympathetic innervation. Anat. Rec. *222*:71, 1990.
29. Pappano, A.: Parasympathetic control of cardiac electrical activity. *In* Zipes, D. P., and Jalife, J. (eds.): Cardiac Electrophysiology. From Cell to Bedside. Philadelphia, W.B. Saunders Company, 1990, p. 271.
30. Lindemann, J. P., and Watanabe, A. M.: Sympathetic control of cardiac electrical activity. *In* Zipes, D. P., and Jalife, J. (ed.): Cardiac Electrophysiology. From Cell to Bedside. Philadelphia, W.B. Saunders Company, 1990, p. 277.
31. Warner, M. R., and Levy, M. N.: Role of neuropeptide Y in neural control of the heart. J. Cardiovasc. Electrophys. *1*:80, 1990.
32. Inoue, H., and Zipes, D. P.: Changes in atrial and ventricular refractoriness and in atrioventricular nodal conduction produced by combinations of vagal and sympathetic stimulation that result in a constant spontaneous sinus cycle length. Circ. Res. *60*:942, 1987.
33. Urthaler, F., Neely, B. H., Hageman, G. R., and Smith, L. R.: Differential sympathetic-parasympathetic interactions in sinus node and AV junction. Am. J. Physiol. *250*:H43, 1986.
34. Inoue, H., and Zipes, D. P.: Increased afferent vagal responses produced by epicardial application of nicotine on the canine posterior left ventricle. Am. Heart J. *114*:757, 1987.
35. Thames, M. D., and Minisi, A. J.: Reflex responses to myocardial ischemia and reperfusion. Role of prostaglandins. Circulation *80*:1878, 1989.
36. Zipes, D. P., and Miyazaki, T.: The autonomic nervous system and the heart: Basis for understanding interactions and effects on arrhythmia development. *In* Zipes, D. P., and Jalife, J. (eds.): Cardiac Electrophysiology. From Cell to Bedside. Philadelphia, W.B. Saunders Company, 1990, p. 312.
37. Litovshy, S. H., and Antzelevitch, C.: Differences in the electrophysiologic response of canine ventricular subendocardium and subepicardium to acetylcholine and isoproterenol. A direct effect of acetylcholine in ventricular myocardium (abstract). PACE *13*:499, 1990.
38. Kulbertus, H. E., and Frank, G. (eds.): Neurocardiology. Mt. Kisco, NY, Futura Publishing Company, 1988.
39. Inoue, H., Skale, B., and Zipes, D. P.: Effects of ischemia on cardiac afferent sympathetic and vagal reflexes in dogs. Am. J. Physiol. *255*:H26, 1988.
40. Inoue, H., and Zipes, D. P.: Time course of denervation of efferent sympathetic and vagal nerves after occlusion of the coronary artery in the canine heart. Circ. Res. *62*:1111, 1988.
40a. Herre, J. M., Wetstein, L., Lin, Y. L., et al.: Effect of transmural versus nontransmural myocardial infarction on inducibility of ventricular arrhythmias during sympathetic stimulation in dogs. J. Am. Coll. Cardiol. *11*:414, 1988.
41. Kammerling, J. M., Green, F. J., Watanabe, A. M., et al.: Denervation supersensitivity of refractoriness in noninfarcted areas apical to transmural myocardial infarction. Circulation *76*:383, 1987.
42. Minardo, J. D., Tuli, M. M., Mock, B. H., et al.: Scintigraphic and electrophysiologic evidence of canine myocardial sympathetic denervation and reinnervation produced by myocardial infarction or phenol application. Circulation *78*:1008, 1988.
43. Inoue, H., and Zipes, D. P.: Results of sympathetic denervation in the canine heart: Supersensitivity that may be arrhythmogenic. Circulation *75*:877, 1987.
44. Stanton, M. S., Tuli, M. M., Radtke, N. L., et al.: Regional sympathetic denervation following myocardial infarction in humans detected noninvasively using I-123 metaiodobenzylguanidine. J. Am. Coll. Cardiol. *14*:1519, 1989.
45. Zipes, D. P.: Plenary lecture. Cardiac electrophysiology: Promises and contributions. J. Am. Coll. Cardiol. *13*:1329, 1989.

BASIC ELECTROPHYSIOLOGICAL PRINCIPLES

46. Kirsch, G. E., and Brown, A. M.: Cardiac sodium channels. *In* Zipes, D. P., and Jalife, J. (eds.): Cardiac Electrophysiology. From Cell to Bedside. Philadelphia, W.B. Saunders Company, 1990, p. 1.
47. Hess, P.: Cardiac calcium channels. *In* Zipes, D. P., and Jalife, J. (eds.): Cardiac Electrophysiology. From Cell to Bedside. Philadelphia, W.B. Saunders Company, 1990, p. 10.
48. Pennefather, P., and Cohen, I. S.: Molecular mechanisms of cardiac K^+ channel regulation. *In* Zipes, D. P., and Jalife, J. (eds.): Cardiac Electrophysiology. From Cell to Bedside. Philadelphia, W.B. Saunders Company, 1990, p. 17.
49. Clapham, D.: Intracellular regulation of ion channels. *In* Zipes, D. P., and Jalife, J. (eds.): Cardiac Electrophysiology. From Cell to Bedside. Philadelphia, W.B. Saunders Company, 1990, p. 85.
50. Gadsby, D. C.: The Na/K pump of cardiac myocytes. *In* Zipes, D. P., and Jalife, J. (eds.): Cardiac Electrophysiology. From Cell to Bedside. Philadelphia, W.B. Saunders Company, 1990, p. 35.
51. Hoyt, R. H., Cohen, M. L., and Saffitz, J. E.: Distribution and three-dimensional structure of intercellular junctions in canine myocardium. Circ. Res. *64*:563, 1989.
52. Veenstra, R. D.: Physiology of cardiac gap junction channels. *In* Zipes, D. P., and Jalife, J. (eds.): Cardiac Electrophysiology. From Cell to Bedside. Philadelphia, W.B. Saunders Company, 1990, p.62.
53. Pressler, M. L.: Passive electrical properties of cardiac tissue. *In* Zipes, D. P., and Jalife, J. (eds.): Cardiac Electrophysiology. From Cell to Bedside. Philadelphia, W.B. Saunders Company, 1990, p. 108.
54. Weingart, R., Rudisuli, A., and Maurer, P.: Cell to cell communication. *In* Zipes, D. P., and Jalife, J. (eds.): Cardiac Electrophysiology. From Cell to Bedside. Philadelphia, W.B. Saunders Company, 1990, p. 122.
55. Beyer, E. C., and Vallano, M. L.: Molecular structure of cardiac gap junctions. *In* Zipes, D. P., and Jalife, J. (eds.): Cardiac Electrophysiology. From Cell to Bedside. Philadelphia, W.B. Saunders Company, 1990, p. 235.
56. Wit, A. L., and Dillon, S. M.: Anisotropic reentry. *In* Zipes, D. P., and Jalife, J. (eds.): Cardiac Electrophysiology. From Cell to Bedside. Philadelphia, W.B. Saunders Company, 1990, p. 353.
57. Kadish, A. H., Spear, J. F., Levine, J. H., and Moore, E. N.: The effects of procainamide in anisotropic canine ventricular myocardium. Circulation *74*:616, 1986.
58. Delmar, M., Michaels, D. C., Johnson, T., and Jalife, J.: Effects of increasing intercellular resistance on transverse and longitudinal propagation in sheep epicardial muscle. Circ. Res. *60*:780, 1987.
59. Spach, M. S., Dolber, P. C., and Heidlage, J. F.: Resolution of discontinuous versus continuous propagation: Microscopic mapping of the derivatives of extracellular potential waveforms. *In* Zipes, D. P., and Jalife, J. (eds.): Cardiac Electrophysiology. From Cell to Bedside. Philadelphia, W.B. Saunders Company, 1990, p. 139.

60. Noma, A., and Tsuboi, N.: Dependence of junctional conductance on proton, calcium and magnesium ions in cardiac paired cells of guinea-pig. J. Physiol. (Lond.) *382*:193, 1987.
61. Fozzard, H. M., Haber, E., Jennings, R. B., et al. (eds.): The Heart and Cardiovascular System. New York, Raven Press, 1986.
62. Zipes, D. P., and Jalife, J. (eds.): Cardiac Electrophysiology. From Cell to Bedside. Philadelphia, W.B. Saunders Company, 1990.
63. Cranefield, P. F., and Aronson, R. S.: Cardiac Arrhythmias: The Role of Triggered Activity and Other Mechanisms. Mt. Kisco, NY, Futura Publishing Company, 1988.
64. Mechmann, S., and Pott, L.: Identification of Na-Ca exchange current in single cardiac myocytes. Nature *319*:597, 1986.
65. Coraboeuf, E., and Escande, D.: Ionic currents in the human myocardium. New in Physiol Sciences *5*:28, 1990.
65a. Hoshi, T., Zagotta, W. N., and Aldrich, R. W.: Biophysical and molecular mechanisms of *Shaker* potassium channel inactivation. Science *250*:533, 1990.
65b. Zagotta, W. N., Hoshi, T., and Aldrich, R. W.: Restoration of inactivation in mutants of *Shaker* potassium channels by a peptide derived from SLB. Science *250*:568, 1990.
66. Irisawa, H., and Giles, W. R.: Sinus and atrioventricular node cells: cellular electrophysiology. *In* Zipes, D. P., and Jalife, J. (eds.): Cardiac Electrophysiology. From Cell to Bedside. Philadelphia, W.B. Saunders Company, 1990, p. 95.
67. Tsien, R. W., and Hess, P.: Excitable tissues. The Heart. *In* Andreoli, T. E., et al. (eds.): Physiology of Membrane Disorders. New York, Plenum Publishing Co., 1986, p. 469.
68. Hagiwara, N., Irisawa, H., and Kameyama, M.: Contribution of two types of calcium currents to the pacemaker potentials of rabbit sino-atrial node cells. J. Physiol. (Lond.) *395*:233, 1988.
69. Mikami, A., Imoto, K., Tanabe, T., et al.: Primary structure and functional expression of the cardiac dihydropyridine-sensitive calcium channel. Nature *340*:230, 1989.
70. Mery, P. F., Brechler, V., Pavoine, C., et al.: Glucagon stimulates the cardiac Ca^{2+} current by activation of adenyl cyclase and inhibition of phosphodiesterase. Nature *345*:158, 1980.
71. Hofmann, F., Oeken, H. J., Schneider, T., and Sieber, M.: The biochemical properties of L-type calcium channels. J. Cardiovasc. Pharmacol. *12*:S25, 1988.
72. Yatani, A., and Brown, A. M.: Rapid alpha-adrenergic modulation of cardiac calcium channel currents by a fast G protein pathway. Science *245*:71, 1989.
73. Hartzell, H. C., and Fischmeister, R.: Opposite effects of cyclic GMP and cyclic AMP on Ca^{2+} current in single heart cells. Nature *323*:273, 1986.
74. DiFrancesco, D.: The cardiac hyperpolarizing-activated current, i_f. Origins and development. Prog. Biophys. Mol. Biol. *46*:163, 1985.
75. DiFrancesco, D.: Current i_f and the neuronal modulation of heart rate. *In* Zipes, D. P., and Jalife, J. (eds.): Cardiac Electrophysiology. From Cell to Bedside. Philadelphia, W.B. Saunders Company, 1990.
76. Escande, D., Coulombe, A., Fairre, J. F., et al.: Two types of transient outward currents in adult human atrial cells. Am. J. Physiol. (Heart Circ. Physiol.) *21*:H142, 1987.
77. Bahinski, A., Nairn, A. C., Greengard, P., and Gadsby, D. C.: Chloride conductance regulated by cyclic AMP-dependent protein kinase in cardiac myocytes. Nature *340*:718, 1989.
78. Harvey, R. D., and Hume, J. R.: Autonomic regulation of a chloride current in the heart. Science *244*:983, 1989.
79. Harvey, R. D., and Hume, J. R.: Histamine activates the chloride current in cardiac ventricular myocytes. J. Cardiovasc. Electrophysiol *1*:309, 1990.
80. Litovsky, S. H., and Antzelevitch, C.: Transient outward current prominent in canine ventricular epicardium but not endocardium. Circ. Res. *62*:116, 1988.
81. Sicouri, S., and Antzelevitch, C.: Drug-induced early after-depolarizations and triggered activity in deep subepicardium of the canine ventricle (abstract). PACE *13*:520, 1990.
82. Rozanski, G. J.: Electrophysiological properties of automatic fibers in rabbit atrioventricular valves. Am. J. Physiol. *253*:H720, 1987.
83. Atkins, D. L., and Marvin, W. J., Jr.: Chronotropic responsiveness of developing sinoatrial and ventricular rat myocytes to autonomic agonists following adrenergic and cholinergic innervation in vitro. Circ. Res. *64*:1051, 1989.
84. Gilmour, R. F., Jr., and Zipes, D. P.: Abnormal automaticity and related phenomena. *In* Fozzard, H. M., et al. (eds.): The Heart and Cardiovascular System. New York, Raven Press, 1986, p. 1239.
85. Kreitner, D.: Electrophysiological study of the two main pacemaker mechanisms in the rabbit sinus node. Cardiovasc. Res. *19*:304, 1985.
86. Watanabe, I., Johnson, T. A., Buchanan, J., et al.: Effect of graded coronary flow reduction on ionic, electrical, and mechanical indexes of ischemia in the pig. Circulation *76*:1127, 1987.
87. Wolleben, C. D., Sanguinetti, M. C., and Siegl, P. K.: Influence of ATP-sensitive potassium channel modulators on ischemia-induced fibrillation in isolated rat hearts. J. Mol. Cell. Cardiol. *21*:783, 1989.
88. Orchard, C. H., Houser, S. R., Kort, A. A., et al.: Acidosis facilitates spontaneous sarcoplasmic reticulum Ca^{2+} release in rat myocardium. J. Gen. Physiol. *90*:145, 1987.
89. Lee, H. C., Mohabir, R., Smith, N., et al.: Effect of ischemia on calcium-dependent fluorescence transients in rabbit hearts containing indo 1. Correlation with monophasic action potentials and contraction. Circulation *78*:1047, 1988.
90. Corr, P. B., Creer, M. H., Yamada, K. A., et al.: Prophylaxis of early ventricular fibrillation by inhibition of acylcarnitine accumulation. J. Clin. Invest. *83*:927, 1989.
91. Creer, M. H., Dobmeyer, D. J., and Corr, P. B.: Amphipathic lipid metabolites and arrhythmias during myocardial ischemia. *In* Zipes, D. P., and Jalife, J. (eds.): Cardiac Electrophysiology. From Cell to Bedside. Philadelphia, W.B. Saunders Company, 1990, p. 417.
92. Kaneko, M., Elimban, V., and Dhalla, N. S.: Mechanism for depression of heart sarcolemmal Ca^{2+}-pump activity by oxygen free radicals. Am. J. Physiol. *257*:H804; 1989.
93. Kaneko, M., Beamish, R. E., and Dhalla, N. S.: Depression of heart sarcolemmal Ca^{2+}-pump activity by oxygen free radicals. Am. J. Physiol. *256*:H368, 1989.
94. Janse, M. J.: Electrophysiology and electrocardiology of acute myocardial ischemia. Can. J. Cardiol. *Suppl A*:46A, 1986.
95. Wilensky, R. L., Tranum-Jensen, J., Coronel, R., et al.: The subendocardial border zone during acute ischemia of the rabbit heart: An electrophysiologic, metabolic, and morphologic correlative study. Circulation *74*:1137, 1986.
96. Kimura, S., Bassett, A. L., Kohya, T., et al.: Simultaneous recording of action potentials from endocardium and epicardium during ischemia in the isolated cat ventricle: Relation of temporal electrophysiologic heterogeneities to arrhythmias. Circulation *74*:401, 1986.
97. Kleber, A. G., Riegger, C. B., and Janse, M. J.: Electrical uncoupling and increase of extracellular resistance after induction of ischemia in isolated, arterially perfused rabbit papillary muscle. Circ. Res. *61*:271, 1987.
98. Kimura, S., Bassett, A. L., Kohya, T., et al.: Automaticity, triggered activity, and responses to adrenergic stimulation in cat subendocardial Purkinje fibers after healing of myocardial infarction. Circulation *75*:651, 1987.
99. Dangman, K. H., Dresdner, K. P., Jr., and Zaim, S.: Automatic and triggered impulse initiation in canine subepicardial ventricular muscle cells from border zones of 24-hour transmural infarcts. New mechanisms for malignant cardiac arrhythmias? Circulation *78*:1020, 1988.
100. Rosenthal, J. E.: Reflected reentry in depolarized foci with variable conduction impairment in 1 day old infarcted canine cardiac tissue. J. Am. Coll. Cardiol. *12*:404, 1988.
101. Lazzara, R., and Scherlag, B. J.: Generation of arrhythmias in myocardial ischemia and infarction. Am. J. Cardiol. *61*:20A, 1988.
102. Levine, J. H., Moore, E. N., Weisman, H. F., et al.: Depression of action potential characteristics and a decreased space constant are present in postischemic, reperfused myocardium. J. Clin. Invest. *79*:107, 1987.
103. Nayler, W. G., Panagiotopoulos, S., Elz, J. S., and Daly, M. J.: Calcium-mediated damage during post-ischaemic reperfusion. J. Mol. Cell. Cardiol. *20* (Suppl 2):41, 1988.
104. Opie, L. H.: Reperfusion injury and its pharmacologic modification. Circulation *80*:1049, 1989.
105. Lukas, A., and Ferrier, G. R.: Interaction of ischemia and reperfusion with subtoxic concentrations of acetylstrophanthidin in isolated cardiac ventricular tissues: Effects on mechanisms of arrhythmia. J. Mol. Cell. Cardiol. *18*:1143, 1986.
106. Zipes, D. P.: Targeted drug therapy. (Editorial) Circulation *81*:1139, 1990.

MECHANISMS OF ARRHYTHMOGENESIS

107. Brugada, P., and Wellens, H. J. J. (eds.): Cardiac Arrhythmias. Where Do We Go From Here? Mt. Kisco, NY, Futura Publishing Company, 1987.
108. Ward, D. E., and Camm, A. J.: Clinical Electrophysiology of the Heart. New York, Edward Arnold Publishers, 1987.
109. Rosen, M. R.: Mechanisms for arrhythmias. Am. J. Cardiol. *61*:2a, 1988.
110. Akhtar, M., Tchou, P. J., and Jazayeri, M.: Mechanisms of clinical tachycardias. Am. J. Cardiol. *61*:9a, 1988.
111. Pogwizd, S. M., and Corr, P. B.: Reentrant and nonreentrant mechanisms contribute to arrhythmogenesis during early myocardial ischemia: Results using three-dimensional mapping. Circ. Res. *61*:352, 1987.
112. Gilmour, R. F., Jr., and Zipes, D. P.: Effects of myocardial ischemia on triggered activity in hamster atrial transplants. J. Cardiovasc. Electrophysiol. *1*:139, 1990.
113. Coetzee, W. A., and Opie, L. H.: Effects of components of ischemia and metabolic inhibition on delayed afterdepolarizations in guinea pig papillary muscle. Circ. Res. *61*:157, 1987.
114. Gilmour, R. F., Jr., and Zipes, D. P.: Pathophysiology of cardiac arrhythmias. *In* Andreoli, T. E., et al. (eds.): Physiology of Membrane Disorders. New York, Plenum Publishing Company, 1986, p. 841.
115. January, C. T., and Shorofsky, S.: Early afterdepolarizations: Newer insights into cellular mechanisms. J. Cardiovasc. Electrophysiol. *1*:161, 1990.
116. El-Sherif, N., Craelius, W., Boutjdir, M., and Gough, W. B.: Early afterdepolarizations and arrhythmogenesis. J. Cardiovasc. Electrophysiol. *1*:145, 1990.
116a. Priori, S. G., Mantica, M., and Napolitano, C.: Early afterdepolarizations induced in vivo by reperfusion of ischemic myocardium. A possible mechanism for reperfusion arrhythmias. Circulation *81*:1911, 1990.
117. Jackman, W. M., Friday, K. J., Anderson, J. L., et al.: The long QT syndromes: A critical review, new clinical observations and a unifying hypothesis. Prog. Cardiovasc. Dis. *31*:115, 1988.
118. Jackman, W. M., Szabo, B., Friday, K. J., et al.: Ventricular tachyarrhythmias related to early afterdepolarizations and triggered firing: Relationship to QT interval prolongation and potential therapeutic role for cal-

cium channel blocking agents. J. Cardiovasc. Electrophysiol. *1*:170, 1990.

119. El-Sherif, N., Bekheit, S., and Henkin, R.: Quinidine-induced long QTU interval and torsades de pointes: Role of bradycardiac-dependent early afterdepolarizations. J. Am. Coll. Cardiol. *14*:252, 1989.
120. Zipes, D. P.: Monophasic action potentials in the diagnosis of triggered arrhythmias. Prog. Cardiovasc. Dis (*in press*).
121. Zipes, D. P.: Autonomic innervation of the heart: Role in arrhythmia development during ischemia and in the long QT syndrome. In Fozzard, H.A., et al. (eds.): Heart and Cardiovascular System. New York, Raven Press, 1991.
122. Bonatti, V., Rolli, A., and Botti, G.: Monophasic action potential studies in human subjects with prolonged ventricular repolarization and long QT syndromes. Am. Heart J. *6*(Suppl D):131, 1985.
123. Schwartz, P. J., Locati, E., Priori, S. G., and Zaza, A.: The long Q-T syndrome. *In* Zipes, D. P., and Jalife, J. (eds.): Cardiac Electrophysiology. From Cell to Bedside. Philadelphia, W.B. Saunders Company, 1990.
124. Ben-David, J., and Zipes, D. P.: Differential response to right and left stellate stimulation of early afterdepolarizations and ventricular tachycardia in the dog. Circulation *78*:1241, 1988.
125. Kaseda, S., and Zipes, D. P.: Effects of alpha adrenoceptor stimulation and blockade on early afterdepolarizations and triggered activity induced by cesium in canine cardiac Purkinje fibers. J. Cardiovasc. Electrophysiol. *1*:31, 1990.
126. Ben-David, J., and Zipes, D. P.: Alpha adrenoceptor stimulation and blockade modulated cesium-induced early afterdepolarizations and ventricular tachyarrhythmias in dogs. Circulation *82*:225, 1990.
127. Bailie, D. S., Inoue, H., Kaseda, S., et al.: Magnesium suppresses early afterdepolarizations and ventricular tachyarrhythmias induced in dogs by cesium. Circulation *77*:1395, 1988.
128. El-Sherif, N., Bekheit, S. S., and Henkin, R.: Quinidine-induced long QTU interval and torsade de pointes: Role of bradycardia-dependent early afterdepolarizations. J. Am. Coll. Cardiol. *14*:252, 1989.
129. Roden, D. M., and Hoffman, B. F.: Action potential prolongation and induction of abnormal automaticity by low quinidine concentrations in canine Purkinje fibers. Relationship to potassium and cycle length. Circ. Res. *56*:857, 1985.
130. Kaseda, S., Gilmour, R. F., Jr., and Zipes, D. P.: Depressant effect of magnesium on early afterdepolarizations and triggered activity induced by cesium quinidine and 4-aminopyridine in canine cardiac Purkinje fibers. Am. Heart J. *118*:458, 1989.
130a. Fish, F. A., Prakash, C., and Rodin, D. M.: Suppression of repolarization related arrhythmias in vitro and in vivo by low-dose potassium channel activators. Circulation *82*:1362, 1990.
131. Davidenko, J. M., Cohen, L., Goodrow, R., and Antzelevitch, C.: Quinidine-induced action potential prolongation, early afterdepolarizations, and triggered activity in canine Purkinje fibers. Effects of stimulation rate, potassium and magnesium. Circulation *79*:674, 1989.
131a. Furukawa, T., Kimura, S., and Castellanas, A.: In vivo induction of "focal" triggered ventricular arrhythmias and responses to overdrive pacing in the canine heart. Circulation *82*:549, 1990.
131b. Boutjdir, M., El-Sherif, N., and Gough, W. B.: Effects of caffeine and ryanodine on delayed afterdepolarizations and sustained rhythmic activity in 1-day-old myocardial infarction in the dog. Circulation *81*:1393, 1990.
132. Wit, A. L., Tseng, G., Henning, B., and Hanna, M. S.: Arrhythmogenic effects of quinidine on catecholamine-induced delayed afterdepolarizations in canine atrial fibers. J. Cardiovasc. Electrophysiol. *1*:15, 1990.
133. Dangman, K. H., Dresdner, K. P., Jr., and Zaim, S.: Automatic and triggered impulse initiation in canine subepicardial ventricular muscle cells from border zones of 24-hour transmural infarcts. New mechanisms for malignant cardiac arrhythmias. Circulation *78*:1020, 1988.
134. Gough, W. B., and El-Sherif, N.: Dependence of delayed afterdepolarizations on diastolic potentials in ischemic Purkinje fibers. Am. J. Physiol. *257*:H770, 1989.
135. Priori, S. G., Mantica, M., and Schwartz, P. J.: Delayed afterdepolarizations elicited in vivo by left stellate ganglion stimulation. Circulation *78*:178, 1988.
136. Iinuma, H., Sekiguchi, A., and Kato, K.: The response of digitalized canine ventricle to programmed stimulation: A study on triggered activity arrhythmias in the whole heart. PACE *12*:1331, 1989.
137. Vos, M. A., Gorgels, A. P., Leunissen-Beekman, J. D., et al.: The effect of an entrainment protocol on ouabain-induced ventricular tachycardia. PACE *12*:1485, 1989.
138. Boutjdir, M., El-Sherif, N., Gough, W. R.: Effects of caffeine and ryanodine on delayed afterdepolarizations and sustained rhythmic activity in 1-day-old myocardial infarction in the dog. Circulation *81*:1393, 1990.
139. Stern, M. D., Capogrossi, M. C., and Lakatta, E. G.: Spontaneous calcium release from the sarcoplasmic reticulum in myocardial cells: Mechanisms and consequences. Cell Calcium *9*:247, 1988.
140. Berlin, J. R., Cannell, M. B., and Lederer, W. J.: Cellular origins of the transient inward current in cardiac myocytes. Role of fluctuations and waves of elevated intracellular calcium. Circ. Res. *65*:115, 1989.
141. Malfatto, G., Rosen, T. S., and Rosen, M. R.: The response to overdrive pacing of triggered atrial and ventricular arrhythmias in the canine heart. Circulation *77*:1139, 1988.
142. Rosenthal, J. E.: Exit block: Cellular mechanisms. *In* Zipes, D. P., and Jalife, J. (eds.): Cardiac Electrophysiology. From Cell to Bedside. Philadelphia, W.B. Saunders Company, 1990, p. 409.
143. Fisch, C.: Electrocardiographic manifestations of exit block. *In* Zipes, D. P., and Jalife, J. (eds.): Cardiac Electrophysiology. From Cell to Bedside. Philadelphia, W.B. Saunders Company, 1990, p. 628.
144. Castellanos, A., Moleiro, F., Saoudi, N. C., and Myerburg, R. J.: Parasystole. *In* Zipes, D. P., and Jalife, J. (eds.): Cardiac Electrophysiology. From Cell to Bedside. Philadelphia, W.B. Saunders Company, 1990, p. 619.
145. Courtemanche, M., Glass, L., Rosengarten, M. D., and Goldberger, A. L.: Beyond pure parasystole: Promises and problems in modeling complex arrhythmias. Am. J. Physiol. *257*:H693, 1989.
146. Gordon, D., Scagliotti, D., Courtemanche, M., and Glass, L.: A clinical study of the dynamics of parasystole. PACE *12*:1412, 1989.
147. Ahlfeldt, H., Nilsson, G., Bandh, S., et al.: Deduction of triphasic phase response curves from ventricular parasystole. PACE *12*:1104, 1989.
148. Robles de Medina, E. O., Delmar, M., Sicouri, S., and Jalife, J.: Modulated parasystole as a mechanism of ventricular ectopic activity leading to ventricular fibrillation. Am. J. Cardiol. *63*:1326, 1989.
149. Davidenko, J. M., and Nau, G. J.: Parasystole. Prog. Cardiol. *1/2*:171, 1988.
150. Inoue, H., and Zipes, D. P.: Conduction over an isthmus of atrial myocardium in vivo. A model of Wolff-Parkinson-White syndrome. Circulation *76*:637, 1987.
151. Fisch, C.: Electrocardiography of Arrhythmias. Philadelphia, Lea and Febiger, 1990, p. 46.
152. Gilmour, R. L., and Zipes, D. P.: Rate-related suppression and facilitation of conduction. *In* Zipes, D. P., and Jalife, J. (eds.): Cardiac Electrophysiology. From Cell to Bedside. Philadelphia, W.B. Saunders Company, 1990, p. 610.
153. Delmar, M., Michaels, D. C., and Jalife, J.: Slow recovery of excitability and the Wenckebach phenomenon in the single guinea pig ventricular myocyte. Circ. Res. *65*:761, 1989.
154. Tchou, P., Jazayeri, M., Denker, S., et al.: Transcatheter electrical ablation of right bundle branch. A method of treating macroreentrant ventricular tachycardia attributed to bundle branch reentry. Circulation *78*:246, 1988.
155. Caceres, J., Jazayeri, M., McKinnie, J., et al.: Sustained bundle branch reentry as a mechanism of clinical tachycardia. Circulation *79*:256, 1989.
156. Frame, L. H., Page, R. L., Boyden, P. A., et al.: Circus movement in the canine atrium around the tricuspid ring during experimental atrial flutter and during reentry in vitro. Circulation *76*:1155, 1987.
157. Boyden, P. A., Frame, L. H., and Hoffman, B. F.: Activation mapping of reentry around an anatomic barrier in the canine atrium. Observations during entrainment and termination. Circulation *79*:406, 1989.
158. Kay, G. N., Epstein, A. E., and Plumb, V. J.: Incidence of reentry with an excitable gap in ventricular tachycardia: A prospective evaluation utilizing transient entrainment. J. Am. Coll. Cardiol. *11*:530, 1988.
159. Schuger, C. D., Steinman, R. T., and Lehmann, M. H.: The excitable gap in atrioventricular nodal reentrant tachycardia. Characterization with ventricular extrastimuli and pharmacologic intervention. Circulation *80*:324, 1989.
160. Stevenson, W. G., Weiss, J. N., Weiner, I., et al.: Resetting of ventricular tachycardia: Implications for localizing the area of slow conduction. J. Am. Coll. Cardiol. *11*:522, 1988.
161a. Gottlieb, C. D., Rosenthal, M. E., Stamato, N. J., et al.: A quantitative evaluation of refractoriness within a reentrant circuit during ventricular tachycardia. Relation to termination. Circulation *82*:1289, 1990.
161. Stamato, N. J., Frame, L. H., Rosenthal, M. E., et al.: Procainamide-induced slowing of ventricular tachycardia with insights from analysis of resetting response patterns. Am. J. Cardiol. *63*:1455, 1989.
162. Almendral, J. M., Gottlieb, C. D., Rosenthal, M. E., et al.: Entrainment of ventricular tachycardia: Explanation for surface electrocardiographic phenomena by analysis of electrograms recorded within the tachycardia circuit. Circulation *77*:569, 1988.
163. Allessie, M. A., Rensma, P. L., Brugada, J., et al.: Pathophysiology of atrial fibrillation. *In* Zipes, D. P., and Jalife, J. (eds.): Cardiac Electrophysiology. From Cell to Bedside. Philadelphia, W.B. Saunders Company, 1990, p. 548.
164. Rensma, P. L., Allessie, M. A., Lammers, W. J., et al.: Length of excitation wave and susceptibility to reentrant atrial arrhythmias in normal conscious dogs. Circ. Res. *62*:395, 1988.
165. Lesh, M. D., Spear, J. F., and Moore, E. N.: Myocardial anisotropy: Basic electrophysiology and role in cardiac arrhythmias. *In* Zipes, D. P., and Jalife, J. (eds.): Cardiac Electrophysiology. From Cell to Bedside. Philadelphia, W.B. Saunders Company, 1990, p. 364.
166. Dillon, S. M., Allessie, M. A., Ursell, P. C., and Wit, A. L.: Influences of anisotropic tissue structure on reentrant circuits in the epicardial border zone of subacute canine infarcts. Circ. Res. *63*:182, 1988.
167. Cardinal, R., Vermeulen, M., Shenasa, M., et al.: Anisotropic conduction and functional dissociation of ischemic tissue during reentrant ventricular tachycardia in canine myocardial infarction. Circulation *77*:1162, 1988.
167a. Brugada, J., Boersma, L., Kirchhof, C. et al.: Double-wave reentry as a mechanism of acceleration of ventricular tachycardia. Circulation *81*:1633, 1990.
168. Lukas, A., and Antzelevitch, C.: Reflected reentry, delayed conduction, and electrotonic inhibition in segmentally depressed atrial tissues. Can. J. Physiol. Pharmacol. *67*:757, 1989.
169. Kaseda, S., and Zipes, D. P.: Contraction-excitation feedback in the atria. A cause of changes in refractoriness. J. Am. Coll. Cardiol. *11*:1327, 1988.
170. Levine, J. H., Guarnieri, T., Kadish, A. H., et al.: Changes in myocardial repolarization in patients undergoing balloon valvuloplasty for congenital pulmonary stenosis: Evidence for contraction-excitation feedback in humans. Circulation *77*:70, 1988.

171. Calkins, H., Maughan, W. L., Kass, D. A., et al.: Electrophysiological effect of volume load in isolated canine hearts. Am. J. Physiol. *256*:H1697, 1989.
172. Gornick, C. C., Tobler, H. G., Tuna, I. C., and Benditt, D. G.: Electrophysiological effects of left ventricular free wall traction in intact hearts. Am. J. Physiol. *257*:H1211, 1989.
173. Calkins, H., Maughan, W. L., Weisman, H. F., et al.: Effect of acute volume load on refractoriness and arrhythmia development in isolated, chronically infarcted canine hearts. Circulation *79*:687, 1989.
174. Klein, L. S., Miles, W. M., and Zipes, D. P.: Effect of the atrioventricular interval during pacing or reciprocating tachycardia on atrial size, pressure and refractory period: Contraction-excitation feedback in human atrium. Circulation *82*:60, 1990.
175. Reiter, M. J., Synhorst, D. P., and Mann, D. E.: Electrophysiological effects of acute ventricular dilatation in the isolated rabbit heart. Circ. Res. *62*:554, 1988.
175a. Hansen, D. E., Craig, C. S., and Hondeghem, L. M.: Stretch-induced arrhythmias in the isolated canine ventricle. Circulation *81*:1094, 1990.
176. Field, L. J.: Atrial natriuretic factor-SV40 T antigen transgenes produce tumors and cardiac arrhythmias in mice. Science *239*:1029, 1988.
176a. Bernstein, R. C., and Frame, L. H.: Ventricular reentry around a fixed barrier: Resetting with advancement in an in vitro model. Circulation *81*:267, 1990.
177. Smith, J. M., Kaplan, D. T., and Cohen, R. J.: The physics of reentry and fibrillation. *In* Zipes, D. P., and Jalife, J. (eds.): Cardiac Electrophysiology. From Cell to Bedside. Philadelphia, W.B. Saunders Company, 1990, p. 215.
178. Waldo, A. L., Carlson, M. D., and Henthorn, R. W.: Atrial flutter: Transient entrainment and related phenomena. *In* Zipes, D. P., and Jalife, J. (eds.): Cardiac Electrophysiology. From Cell to Bedside. Philadelphia, W.B. Saunders Company, 1990, p. 530.
179. Boineau, J. P., Schuessler, R. B., Cain, M. E., et al.: Activation mapping during normal atrial rhythms and atrial flutter. *In* Zipes, D. P., and Jalife, J. (eds.): Cardiac Electrophysiology. From Cell to Bedside. Philadelphia, W.B. Saunders Company, 1990, p. 537.
180. Boyden, P. A.: Activation sequence during atrial flutter in dogs with surgically induced right atrial enlargement: I. Observations during sustained rhythms. Circ. Res. *62*:596, 1988.
181. Bonke, F. I. M., Kirchhof, C. J. H. J., and Allessie, M. A.: Sinus node reentry. *In* Zipes, D. P., and Jalife, J. (eds.): Cardiac Electrophysiology. From Cell to Bedside. Philadelphia, W.B. Saunders Company, 1990, p. 526.
182. Gillette, P. C., Crawford, F. C., and Zeigler, V. L.: Mechanisms of atrial tachycardias. *In* Zipes, D. P., and Jalife, J. (eds.): Cardiac Electrophysiology. From Cell to Bedside. Philadelphia, W.B. Saunders Company, 1990, p. 559.
183. Sung, R. J., Huycke, E. C., Keung, E. C., et al.: Atrioventricular node reentry: Evidence of reentry and functional properties of fast and slow pathways. *In* Zipes, D. P., and Jalife, J. (eds.): Cardiac Electrophysiology. From Cell to Bedside. Philadelphia, W.B. Saunders Company, 1990, p. 513.
184. Schmitt, C., Miller, J. M., and Josephson, M. E.: Atrioventricular nodal supraventricular tachycardia with 2:1 block above the bundle of His. PACE *11*:1018, 1988.
185. Johnson, D. C., Nunn, G. R., Richards, D. A., et al.: Surgical therapy for supraventricular tachycardia, a potentially curable disorder. J. Thorac. Cardiovasc. Surg. *93*:913, 1987.
186. Epstein, L. M., Scheinman, M. M., Langberg, J. J., et al.: Percutaneous catheter modification of the atrioventricular node. A potential cure for atrioventricular nodal reentrant tachycardia. Circulation *80*:757, 1989.
186a. Wilensky, R. L., Miles, W. M., Klein, L. S., et al.: Effects of surgery for AV nodal reentry on AV nodal physiology. Clin. Res. *37*:886A, 1989 (abstract).
187. Guiraudon, G. M., Klein, G. J., Sharma, A., et al.: Skeletonization of atrioventricular node: Surgical alternatives for AV nodal reentry tachycardia experienced with 32 patients. Ann. Thorac. Surg. *49*:565, 1990.
188. Cox, J. L., and Ferguson, T. B., Jr.: Surgery for atrioventricular node reentry tachycardia: The discrete cryosurgical technique. Semin. Thorac. Cardiovasc. Surg. *1*:47, 1989.
189. Yee, R., Klein, G. J., Sharma, A. D., et al.: Tachycardia associated with accessory atrioventricular pathways. *In* Zipes, D. P., and Jalife, J. (eds.): Cardiac Electrophysiology. From Cell to Bedside. Philadelphia, W.B. Saunders Company, 1990, p. 463.
190. Prystowsky, E. N., and Packer, D. L.: Pre-excited tachycardias. *In* Zipes, D. P., and Jalife, J. (eds.): Cardiac Electrophysiology. From Cell to Bedside. Philadelphia, W.B. Saunders Company, 1990, p. 472.
191. Gallagher, J. J., Selle, J. G., Sealy, W. C., et al.: Variants of pre-excitation: Update 1989. *In* Zipes, D. P., and Jalife, J. (eds.): Cardiac Electrophysiology. From Cell to Bedside. Philadelphia, W.B. Saunders Company, 1990, p. 480.
192. Jackman, W. W., Kuck, K. H., Friday, K. J., and Lazzara, R.: Catheter recordings of accessory atrioventricular pathway activation. *In* Zipes, D. P., and Jalife, J. (eds.): Cardiac Electrophysiology. From Cell to Bedside. Philadelphia, W.B. Saunders Company, 1990, p. 491.
193. Kuck, K. H., Jackman, W. M., Friday, K. J., et al.: Sites of conduction block in accessory atrioventricular pathways: Basis for concealed accessory pathways. *In* Zipes, D. P., and Jalife, J. (eds.): Cardiac Electrophysiology. From Cell to Bedside. Philadelphia, W.B. Saunders Company, 1990, p. 503.
194. Kent, A. F. S.: Researches on the structure and function of mammalian heart. J. Physiol. *14*:233, 1893.
195. Kent, A. F. S.: Observation on the auriculo-ventricular junction of the mammalian heart. Q. J. Exp. Physiol. *7*:193, 1913.
196. Lehmann, M. H., Tchou, P., Mahmud, R., et al.: Electrophysiological determinants of antidromic reentry induced during atrial extrastimulation. Insights from a pacing model of Wolff-Parkinson-White syndrome. Circ. Res. *65*:295, 1989.
197. Ferguson, T. B., Jr., and Cox, J. L.: Surgical treatment for the Wolff-Parkinson-White syndrome: The endocardial approach. *In* Zipes, D. P., and Jalife, J. (eds.): Cardiac Electrophysiology. From Cell to Bedside. Philadelphia, W.B. Saunders Company, 1990, p. 897.
198. Guiraudon, G. M., Klein, G. J., Sharma, A. D., et al.: Surgery for the Wolff-Parkinson-White syndrome: The epicardial approach. *In* Zipes, D. P., and Jalife, J. (eds.): Cardiac Electrophysiology. From Cell to Bedside. Philadelphia, W.B. Saunders Company, 1990, p. 907.
199. Tchou, P., Lehmann, M. H., Jazayeri, M., and Akhtar, M.: Atriofascicular connection or a nodoventricular Mahaim fiber? Electrophysiologic elucidation of the pathway and associated reentrant circuit. Circulation *77*:837, 1988.
200. Klein, G. J., Guiraudon, G. M., Kerr, C. R., et al.: "Nodoventricular" accessory pathway: Evidence for a distinct accessory atrioventricular pathway with atrioventricular node-like properties. Angiology *39*:307, 1988.
201. Leitch, J., and Klein, G. J.: New concepts on nodoventricular accessory pathways. J. Cardiovasc. Electrophysiol *1*:220, 1990.
202. Benditt, D. G., and Milstein, S.: Nodoventricular accessory connections: A misnomer or a structural/functional spectrum. J. Cardiovasc. Electrophysiol *1*:231, 1990.
203. Finzi, A., Rossi, L., Pagnoni, F., et al.: Permanent form of junctional reciprocating tachycardia involving an atrio-hisian accessory pathway: Electrophysiologic and histologic correlations. PACE *10*:1331, 1987.
204. Hanich, R. F., de Langen, C. D., Kadish, A. H., et al.: Inducible sustained ventricular tachycardia 4 years after experimental canine myocardial infarction: Electrophysiologic and anatomic comparisons with early healed infarcts. Circulation *77*:445, 1988.
205. Morady, F., Frank, R., Kou, W. H., et al.: Identification and catheter ablation of a zone of slow conduction in the reentrant circuit of ventricular tachycardia in humans. J. Am. Coll. Cardiol. *11*:775, 1988.
206. deBakker, J. M., van Capelle, F. J., Janse, M. J., et al.: Reentry as a cause of ventricular tachycardia in patients with chronic ischemic heart disease: Electrophysiologic and anatomic correlation. Circulation *77*:589, 1988.
206a. deBakker, J. M., Coronel, R., Tasserson, S., et al.: Ventricular tachycardia in the infarcted Langendorff-perfused human heart: Role of the arrangement of surviving cardiac fibers. J. Am. Coll. Cardiol. *15*:1594, 1990.
207. Downar, E., Harris, L., Mickleborough, L. L., et al.: Endocardial mapping of ventricular tachycardia in the intact human ventricle: Evidence for reentrant mechanisms. J. Am. Coll. Cardiol. *11*:783, 1988.
207a. Kay, G. N., Epstein, A. E., and Plumb, J. J.: Resetting of ventricular tachycardia by single extrastimuli. Circulation *81*:1507, 1990.
208. El Sherif, N.: The figure 8 model of reentrant excitation in the canine postinfarction heart. *In* Zipes, D. P., and Jalife, J. (eds.) *Electrophysiology and arrhythmias*. New York, Grune and Stratton, 1985, p. 363.
209. Zipes, D. P.: Antiarrhythmia uncoupling (Editorial). PACE *11*:127, 1988.
210. Buchanan, J. W., and Gettes, L. S.: Ionic environment and propagation. *In* Zipes, D. P., and Jalife, J. (eds.): Cardiac Electrophysiology. From Cell to Bedside. Philadelphia, W.B. Saunders Company, 1990, p. 149.
211. Kleber, A. G., and Janse, M. J.: Impulse propagation in myocardial ischemia. *In* Zipes, D.P., and Jalife, J. (eds.): Cardiac Electrophysiology. From Cell to Bedside. Philadelphia, W.B. Saunders Company, 1990, p. 156.

APPROACH TO DIAGNOSIS OF ARRHYTHMIAS

212. Allen, B. J., Casey, T. P., Brodsky, M. A., et al.: Exercise testing in patients with life-threatening ventricular tachyarrhythmias: Results and correlation with clinical and arrhythmia factors. Am. Heart J. *116*:997, 1988.
213. Podrid, P. J., Venditti, F. J., Levine, P. A., and Klein, M. D.: The role of exercise testing in evaluation of arrhythmias. Am. J. Cardiol. *62*:24H, 1988.
214. Saini, V., Graboys, T. B., Towne, V., and Lown, B.: Reproducibility of exercise-induced ventricular arrhythmia in patients undergoing evaluation for malignant ventricular arrhythmia. Am. J. Cardiol. *15*:697, 1989.
215. Yeh, S. J., Lin, F. C., and Wu, D. L.: The mechanisms of exercise provocation of supraventricular tachycardia. Am. Heart J. *117*:1041, 1989.
216. Ranger, S., Talajic, M., Lemery, R., et al.: Amplification of flecainide-induced ventricular conduction slowing by exercise. A potentially significant clinical consequence of use-dependent sodium channel blockade. Circulation *79*:1000, 1989.
217. Falk, R. H.: Flecainide-induced ventricular tachycardia and fibrillation in patients treated for atrial fibrillation. Ann. Intern. Med. *111*:107, 1989.
218. Sokoloff, N. M., Spielman, S. R., Greenspan, A. M., et al.: Plasma norepinephrine in exercise-induced ventricular tachycardia. J. Am. Coll. Cardiol. *8*:11, 1986.
219. McHenry, P. L.: Clinical role of exercise testing for detection, evaluation, and treatment of ventricular arrhythmias. *In* Zipes, D. P., and Jalife, J. (eds.): Cardiac Electrophysiology. From Cell to Bedside. Philadelphia, W.B. Saunders Company, 1990, p. 832.
220. Kennedy, H. L.: Long-term (Holter) electrocardiogram recordings. *In* Zipes, D. P., and Jalife, J. (eds.): Cardiac Electrophysiology. From Cell to Bedside. Philadelphia, W.B. Saunders Company, 1990, p. 791.

221. Pritchett, E. L., McCarthy, E. A., and Lee, K. L.: Clinical behavior of paroxysmal atrial tachycardia. Am. J. Cardiol. *62*:3D, 1988.
222. Fleg, J. L.: Ventricular arrhythmias in the elderly: Prevalence, mechanisms, and therapeutic implications. Geriatrics *43*:23, 1988.
223. The Cardiac Arrhythmia Suppression Trial (CAST) Investigators: Effect of encainide and flecainide on mortality in a randomized trial of arrhythmia suppression after myocardial infarction. N. Engl. J. Med. *321*:406, 1989.
224. The Cardiac Arrhythmia Pilot Study (CAPS) Investigators: Effects of encainide, flecainide, imipramine and moricizine on ventricular arrhythmias during the year after acute myocardial infarction: The CAPS. Am. J. Cardiol. *61*:501, 1988.
225. Akhtar, M., Breithardt, G., Camm, A. J., et al.: CAST and beyond. Implications of the Cardiac Arrhythmia Suppression Trial. Circulation *81*:1123, 1990.
226. Pratt, C. M., Brater, D. C., Harrele, F. E., et al.: Clinical and regulatory implications of the Cardiac Arrhythmia Suppression Trial. Am. J. Cardiol *65*:103, 1990.
227. Kowey, P. R., Marinchak, R. A., and Rials, S. J.: The Cardiac Arrhythmia Suppression Trial: How has it impacted on contemporary arrhythmia management? J. Cardiovasc. Electrophysiol *1*:457, 1990.
228. Kleiger, R. E., Miller, J. P., Bigger, J. T., Jr., and Moss, A. J.: Decreased heart rate variability and its association with increased mortality after acute myocardial infarction. Am. J. Cardiol. *59*:256, 1987.
229. Martin, G. J., Magid, N. M., Myers, G., et al.: Heart rate variability and sudden death secondary to coronary artery disease during ambulatory electrocardiographic monitoring. Am. J. Cardiol. *60*:86, 1987.
230. Saul, J. P., Berger, R. D., Chen, M. H., and Cohen, R. J.: Transfer function analysis of autonomic regulation. II. Respiratory sinus arrhythmia. Am. J. Physiol. *256*:H153, 1989.
231. Appel, M. L., Berger, R. D., Saul, J. P., et al.: Beat or beat variability in cardiovascular variables: Noise or music? J. Am. Coll. Cardiol. *14*:1139, 1989.
231a. Billman, G. E., and Hoskins, R. S.: Time-series analysis of heart rate variability during submaximal exercise. Evidence for reduced cardiac vagal tone in animals susceptible to ventricular fibrillation. Circulation *80*:146, 1990.
232. Smith, J. M., Clancy, E. A., Valeri, C. R., et al.: Electrical alternans and cardiac electrical instability. Circulation *77*:110, 1988.
233. Dewey, R. C., Capeless, M. A., and Levy, A. M.: Use of ambulatory electrocardiographic monitoring to identify high-risk patients with congenital complete heart block. N. Engl. J. Med. *316*:835, 1987.
234. Zipes, D. P., Akhtar, M., Denes, P., et al.: ACC/AHA guidelines for clinical intracardiac electrophysiologic studies. J. Am. Coll. Cardiol. *14*:1827, 1989 and Circulation *80*:1925, 1989.
235. Cooper, M. J., Hunt, L. J., Richards, D. A., et al.: Effect of repetition of extrastimuli on sensitivity and reproducibility of mode of induction of ventricular tachycardia by programmed stimulation. J. Am. Coll. Cardiol. *11*:1260, 1988.
236. Cooper, M. J., Hunt, L. J., Palmer, K. J., et al.: Quantitation of day to day variability in mode of induction of ventricular tachyarrhythmias by programmed stimulation. J. Am. Coll. Cardiol. *11*:101, 1988.
237. Berger, M. D., Waxman, H. L., Buxton, A. E., et al.: Spontaneous compared with induced onset of sustained ventricular tachycardia. Circulation *78*:885, 1988.
238. Akhtar, M., Shenasa, M., Jazayeri, M., et al.: QRS complex tachycardia: Reappraisal of a common clinical problem. Ann. Intern. Med. *109*:905, 1988.
239. Wilber, D. J., Garan, H., Finkelstein, D., et al.: Out-of-hospital cardiac arrest. Use of electrophysiologic testing in the prediction of long-term outcome. N. Engl. J. Med. *318*:19, 1988.
240. The ESVEM Investigators: The ESVEM trial. Electrophysiologic study versus electrocardiographic monitoring for selection of antiarrhythmic therapy of ventricular tachyarrhythmias. Circulation *79*:1354, 1989.
241. Kuchar, D. L., Garan, H., and Ruskin, J. N.: Electrophysiologic evaluation of antiarrhythmic therapy for ventricular tachyarrhythmias. Am. J. Cardiol. *62*:39H, 1988.
242. Fujimura, O., Yee, R., Klein, G. J., et al.: The diagnostic sensitivity of electrophysiologic testing in patients with syncope caused by transient bradycardia. N. Engl. J. Med. *321*:1703, 1989.
243. Brooks, R., Garan, H., and Ruskin, J. N.: Evaluation of the patient with unexplained syncope. *In* Zipes, D. P., and Jalife, J. (eds.): Cardiac Electrophysiology. From Cell to Bedside. Philadelphia, W.B. Saunders Company, 1990, p. 646.
244. Camm, A. J., and Lau, C. P.: Syncope of undetermined origin: Diagnosis and management. Prog. Cardiol. *1/2*:139, 1988.
245. Manolis, A. S., Linzer, M., Salem, D., and Estes, N. A. M. III: Syncope: Current diagnostic evaluation and management. Ann. Intern. Med. *112*:850, 1990.
246. Aminoff, M. J., Scheinman, M. M., Griffin, J. C., and Herre, J. M.: Electrocerebral accompaniments of syncope associated with malignant ventricular arrhythmias. Ann. Intern. Med. *108*:791, 1988.
247. Winters, S. L., Stewart, D., and Gomes, J. A.: Signal averaging of the surface QRS complex predicts inducibility of ventricular tachycardia in patients with syncope of unknown origin: A prospective study. J. Am. Coll. Cardiol. *10*:775, 1987.
248. Kuchar, D. L., Thorburn, C. W., and Sammel, N. L.: Late potentials detected after myocardial infarction: Natural history and prognostic significance. Circulation *74*:1280, 1986.
249. Waxman, M. B., Yao, L., Cameron, D. A., et al.: Isoproterenol induction of vasodepressor-type reaction in vasodepressor-prone persons. Am. J. Cardiol. *63*:58, 1989.
250. Kushner, J. A., Kou, W. H., Kadish, A. H., and Morady, F.: Natural history of patients with unexplained syncope and a nondiagnostic electrophysiologic study. J. Am. Coll. Cardiol. *14*:391, 1989.
251. Kapoor, W. N., Hammill, S. C., and Gersh, B. J.: Diagnosis and natural history of syncope and the role of invasive electrophysiological testing. Am. J. Cardiol. *63*:730, 1989.
252. Rattes, M. F., Klein, G. J., Sharma, A. D., et al.: Efficacy of empirical cardiac pacing in syncope of unknown cause. Can. Med. Assoc. J. *140*:381, 1989.
253. Ruffy, R., Roman-Smith, P., and Barbey, J. T.: Palpitations: Evaluation and Management. *In* Zipes, D. P., and Rowlands, D. J. (eds.): Progress in Cardiology, Vol 1/2. Philadelphia, Lea and Febiger, 1988, p. 131.
254. Horowitz, L. N.: Safety of electrophysiologic studies. Circulation *73*:II28, 1986.

OTHER DIAGNOSTIC ELECTROCARDIOGRAPHIC TECHNIQUES

255. Guarnieri, T.: Esophageal recording and pacing. *In* Zipes, D. P., and Rowlands, D. J. (eds.): Progress in Cardiology, Vol 1/2. Philadelphia, Lea and Febiger, 1988, p. 305.
256. Levine, J. H., Kadish, A. H., and Reiter, M. J.: Transesophageal pacing and recording. *In* Zipes, D. P., and Jalife, J. (eds.): Cardiac Electrophysiology. From Cell to Bedside. Philadelphia, W.B. Saunders Company, 1990, p. 858.
257. Mirvis, D. M.: Detection of experimental right ventricular infarction by isopotential body surface mapping during sinus rhythm and during ectopic ventricular pacing. J. Am. Coll. Cardiol. *10*:157, 1987.
258. Hirai, M., Burgess, M. J., and Haws, C. W.: Effects of coronary occlusion on cardiac and body surface PQRST isoarea maps of dogs with abnormal activation simulating left bundle branch block. Circulation *77*:1414, 1988.
259. Kamakura, S., Shimomura, K., Ohe, T., et al.: The role of initial minimum potentials on body surface maps in predicting the site of accessory pathways in patients with Wolff-Parkinson-White syndrome. Am. J. Physiol. *250*:H736, 1986.
260. Nadeau, R., Ackaoui, A., Giorgi, C., et al.: PQRST isoarea maps from patients with Wolff-Parkinson-White syndrome: An index for global alterations of ventricular repolarization. Circulation *77*:499, 1988.
261. Gardner, M. J., Montague, T. J., Armstrong, C. S., et al.: Vulnerability to ventricular arrhythmia: Assessment by mapping of body surface potential. Circulation *73*:684, 1986.
262. Hanashima, K., Ikeda, K., Yamaki, M., et al.: Clinical significance of body surface isochrone maps for predicting ventricular arrhythmias in patients with previous myocardial infarction. Jpn. Circ. J. *52*:203, 1988.
263. DeAmbroggi, L., Bertoni, T., Locati, E., et al.: Mapping of body surface potentials in patients with the idiopathic long QT syndrome. Circulation *74*:1334, 1986.
264. Breithardt, G., Borggrefe, M., Martinez-Rubio, A., and Podczeck, A.: Signal averaging. Prog. Cardiol. *1/2*:257, 1988.
265. Simson, M. B.: Signal-averaged electrocardiography: Methods and clinical applications. *In* Braunwald, E. (ed.): Heart Disease, A Textbook of Cardiovascular Medicine, 3rd ed. Philadelphia, W.B. Saunders Company. Update No. 7, 1990.
266. Mehta, D., McKenna, W. J., Ward, D. E., et al.: Significance of signal-averaged electrocardiography in relation to endomyocardial biopsy and ventricular stimulation studies in patients with ventricular tachycardia without clinically apparent heart disease. J. Am. Coll. Cardiol. *14*:372, 1989.
267. Denniss, A. R., Richards, D. A., Cody, D. V., et al.: Prognostic significance of ventricular tachycardia and fibrillation induced at programmed stimulation and delayed potentials detected on the signal-averaged electrocardiograms of survivors of acute myocardial infarction. Circulation *74*:731, 1986.
268. Denniss, A. R., Ross, D. L., Richards, D. A., and Uther, J. B.: Changes in ventricular activation time on the signal-averaged electrocardiogram in the first year after acute myocardial infarction. Am. J. Cardiol. *60*:580, 1987.
269. McGuire, M., Kuchar, D., Ganis, J., et al.: Natural history of late potentials in the first 10 days after acute myocardial infarction and relation to early ventricular arrhythmias. Am. J. Cardiol. *61*:1187, 1988.
270. Turitto, G., Caref, E. B., Macina, G., et al.: Time course of ventricular arrhythmias and the signal averaged electrocardiogram in the post-infarction period: A prospective study of correlation. Br. Heart J. *60*:17, 1988.
271. El-Sherif, N., Ursell, S. N., Bekheit, S., et al.: Prognostic significance of the signal-averaged ECG depends on the time of recording in the postinfarction period. Am. Heart J. *118*:256, 1989.
272. Gang, E. S., Lew, A. S., Hong, M., et al.: Decreased incidence of ventricular late potentials after successful thrombolytic therapy for acute myocardial infarction. N. Engl. J. Med. *321*:712, 1989.
273. Fauchier, J. P., Cosnay, P., Moquet, B., et al.: Late ventricular arrhythmias in dilated or hypertrophic cardiomyopathies. A prospective study about 83 patients. PACE *11*:1974, 1988.
274. Denniss, A. R., Johnson, D. C., Richards, D. A., et al.: Effect of excision of ventricular myocardium on delayed potentials detected by the signal-averaged electrocardiogram in patients with ventricular tachycardia. Am. J. Cardiol. *59*:591, 1987.
275. Denniss, A. R., Ross, D. L., Richards, D. A., et al.: Effect of antiarrhythmic

therapy on delayed potentials detected by the signal-averaged electrocardiogram in patients with ventricular tachycardia after acute myocardial infarction. Am. J. Cardiol. *58*:261, 1986.
276. Breithardt, G., Borggrefe, M., Karbenn, U., and Schwarzmaier, J.: Effects of pharmacological and non-pharmacological interventions on ventricular late potentials. Eur. Heart J. *8* Suppl *A*:97, 1987.
277. Borbola, J., and Denes, P.: Oral amiodarone loading therapy. I. The effect on serial signal-averaged electrocardiographic recordings and the QTc in patients with ventricular tachyarrhythmias. Am. Heart J. *115*:1202, 1988.
278. Kuchar, D. L., Thorburn, C. W., and Sammel, N. L.: Prediction of serious arrhythmic events after myocardial infarction: Signal-averaged electrocardiogram, Holter monitoring and radionuclide ventriculography. J. Am. Coll. Cardiol. *9*:531, 1987.
279. Cripps, T., Bennett, D., Camm, J., and Ward, D.: Prospective evaluation of clinical assessment, exercise testing and signal-averaged electrocardiogram in predicting outcome after acute myocardial infarction. Am. J. Cardiol. *62*:995, 1988.
280. Gomes, J. A., Winters, S. L., Martinson, M., et al.: The prognostic significance of quantitative signal-averaged variables relative to clinical variables, site of myocardial infarction, ejection fraction and ventricular premature beats: A prospective study. J. Am. Coll. Cardiol. *13*:377, 1989.
280a. Vatterott, P. J., Bailey, K. R., and Hammill, S. C.: Improving the predictive ability of the signal-averaged electrocardiogram with a linear logistic model incorporating clinical variables. Circulation *81*:797, 1990.
281. Nalos, P. C., Gang, E. S., Mandel, W. J., et al.: The signal-averaged electrocardiogram as a screening test for inducibility of sustained ventricular tachycardia in high risk patients: A prospective study. J. Am. Coll. Cardiol. *9*:539, 1987.
282. Buxton, A. E., Simson, M. B., Falcone, R. A., et al.: Results of signal-averaged electrocardiography and electrophysiologic study in patients with nonsustained ventricular tachycardia after healing of acute myocardial infarction. Am. J. Cardiol. *60*:80, 1987.
283. Winters, S. L., Stewart, D., Targonski, A., and Gomes, J. A.: Role of signal averaging of the surface QRS complex in selecting patients with nonsustained ventricular tachycardia and high grade ventricular arrhythmias for programmed ventricular stimulation. J. Am. Coll. Cardiol. *12*:1481, 1988.
284. Turitto, G., Fontaine, J. M., Ursell, S. N., et al.: Value of the signal-averaged electrocardiogram as a predictor of the results of programmed stimulation in nonsustained ventricular tachycardia. Am. J. Cardiol. *61*:1272, 1988.
285. Cripps, T., Bennett, E. D., Camm, A. J., and Ward, D. E.: Inducibility of sustained monomorphic ventricular tachycardia as a prognostic indicator in survivors of recent myocardial infarction: A prospective evaluation in relation to other prognostic variables. J. Am. Coll. Cardiol. *14*:289, 1989.
286. Lindsay, B. D., Ambos, H. D., Schechtman, K. B., and Cain, M. E.: Improved selection of patients for programmed ventricular stimulation by frequency analysis of signal-averaged electrocardiograms. Circulation *73*:675, 1986.
287. Lindsay, B. D., Markham, J., Schechtman, K. B., et al.: Identification of patients with sustained ventricular tachycardia by frequency analysis of signal-averaged electrocardiograms despite the presence of bundle branch block. Circulation *77*:122, 1988.
288. Haberl, R., Jilge, G., Pulter, R., and Steinbeck, G.: Comparison of frequency and time domain analysis of the signal-averaged electrocardiogram in patients with ventricular tachycardia and coronary artery disease: Methodologic validation and clinical relevance. J. Am. Coll. Cardiol. *12*:150, 1988.
289. Peirce, D. L., Easley, A. R., Jr., Windle, J. R., and Engel, T. R.: Fast Fourier transformation of the entire low amplitude late QRS potential to predict ventricular tachycardia. J. Am. Coll. Cardiol. *14*:1731, 1989.
290. Worley, S. J., Mark, D. B., Smith, W. M., et al.: Comparison of time domain and frequency domain variables from the signal-averaged electrocardiogram: A multivariable analysis. J. Am. Coll. Cardiol. *11*:1041, 1988.
291. Machac, J., Weiss, A., Winders, S. L., et al.: A comparative study of frequency domain and time domain analysis of signal-averaged electrocardiograms in patients with ventricular tachycardia. J. Am. Coll. Cardiol. *11*:284, 1988.
292. Almquist, A., Goldenberg, I. F., Milstein, S., et al.: Provocation of bradycardia and hypotension by isoproterenol and upright posture in patients with unexplained syncope. N. Engl. J. Med. *320*:346, 1989.
293. Waxman, M. B., Yao, L., Cameron, D. A., et al.: Isoproterenol induction of vasodepressor-type reaction in vasodepressor-prone persons. Am. J. Cardiol. *63*:58, 1989.
294. Chen, M. Y., Goldenberg, I. F., Milstein, S., et al.: Cardiac electrophysiologic and hemodynamic correlates of neurally mediated syncope. Am. J. Cardiol. *63*:66, 1989.
295. Kenney, R. A., Ingram, A., Bayliss, J., and Sutton, R.: Head-up tilt: A useful test for investigating unexplained syncope. Lancet *1*:1352, 1986.

23

Management of Cardiac Arrhythmias: Pharmacological, Electrical, and Surgical Techniques

by DOUGLAS P. ZIPES, M.D.

Pharmacological Therapy

PRINCIPLES OF CLINICAL PHARMACOKINETICS

Pharmacological treatment of a patient with a cardiac arrhythmia has as its primary objective to reach an effective and well-tolerated plasma drug concentration as rapidly as possible and to maintain this concentration for as long as required without producing adverse effects. In many but not all situations and not with all drugs, plasma concentration after equilibration correlates with the antiarrhythmic as well as adverse effects of the drug. Therapeutic serum concentrations for the most important available antiarrhythmic agents are listed in Table 23–1 and are based on concentrations of drugs that exert therapeutic effects on often benign arrhythmias such as premature ventricular complexes (PVCs), without adverse effects in a majority of patients. However, the therapeutic concentration for any individual patient is the amount of drug required *for that patient* to suppress or terminate the specific cardiac arrhythmia requiring treatment without producing adverse effects. For a specific patient, one must consider the response both of the patient and of the arrhythmia to the drug; the actual plasma concentration of the drug is often of secondary importance. Low drug concentrations can exert a therapeutic or toxic effect in some patients, while drug concentrations higher than the normal range may be needed and tolerated in another patient. In some patients measured plasma concentrations can be useful to establish concentrations needed for prophylaxis, to judge the sensitivity or resistance of the arrhythmia to the drug, and to evaluate symptoms that suggest drug toxicity. Plasma concentrations can also be used to determine the effects of changing physiological states on drug concentrations, establish drug compliance or abuse, search for drug interactions, and establish the importance of physiologically active metabolites of the parent compound. Active metabolites may be suspected when the clinical effect of the drug outlasts the therapeutic serum concentration of the drug or when results immediately following intravenous drug administration differ from those after oral administration of the drug.[1]

Normally, because antiarrhythmic agents have a narrow toxic-therapeutic relationship, important complications of therapy can result from amounts of drug that only slightly exceed the amount necessary to produce beneficial effects; lesser concentrations are often subtherapeutic. It is obvious that careful dosing with these agents is essential to maintain adequate but nontoxic amounts of drug in the body, a task facilitated by understanding drug pharmacokinetics. The latter consists of a quantitative assessment of drug dose-concentration factors, including drug absorption, distribution, metabolism, and excretion. Alterations in the rate of any of these processes can account for significant intra- and interpatient variations in plasma concentrations.[2] In addition, changes in the functional status of any of the organs involved, e.g., the heart, liver or kidneys, can significantly alter dose requirements in a given patient. The latter concerns a study of pharmacodynamics, or drug concentration-response issues.

ABSORPTION. Drug absorption from the intestinal tract occurs for most drugs with a half-time of absorption in the range of 20 to 30 minutes. Completeness of absorption can vary between 50 and over 90 per cent, depending on the drug, with most absorption occurring in the small intestine. Different preparations of the same drug, e.g., digoxin or phenytoin, can undergo different rates of absorption in the same patient because the tablet preparations have different dissolution rates. Thus, two brands of drug may not result in the same serum concentration. By altering the properties of the tablet, a slow release form of a drug ordinarily rapidly absorbed and metabolized, such as procainamide, can be developed. Large amounts of some orally administered drugs, such as propranolol or verapamil, are transformed to inactive metabolites in the liver before they reach the systemic circulation—the so-called first-pass hepatic effect. For such an agent, much more drug must be administered orally than intravenously to achieve the same physiological effect.

Disease states and other factors can alter the rate and completeness of drug absorption. For example, heart failure can cause mucosal edema of the gut and impair the absorption of orally administered drugs, as can decreased intestinal blood flow. Renal or hepatic hypoperfusion can reduce drug elimination and metabolism. Reduced volume of distribution and impaired clearance can increase elimination half-life, requiring a reduction in loading and maintenance doses[3] (Table 23–2). Malabsorption syndromes, concomitant use of other drugs, or changes in gut motility or flora caused by diarrheal states, antibiotics, or the use of cathartics can alter absorption. Since most antiarrhythmic agents are basic compounds, they are ionized and poorly absorbed at normal gastric pH, and some drugs can decompose at gastric pH. Conditions that delay gastric emptying increase the absorption lag phase between ingestion of these drugs and their arrival in the small intestine, where most absorption takes place, and therefore can decrease absorption. In patients with severe hypotension, shock , or cardiac arrest, impaired tissue perfusion prevents reliable absorption of intramuscularly administered agents; these patients should receive all medications by the intravenous (IV) route.

BIOAVAILABILITY. The rate of drug absorption, determined by the time required to achieve maximum plasma concentration, and the fraction of drug absorbed influence the drug's *bioavailability*, which is a measure of the amount of drug that reaches the systemic circulation intact. Bioavailability of a drug is influenced by factors such as pill dissolution, metabolism by gut mucosa, hepatic metabolism and binding, and absorption. It is a most important property of the drug. Absorption is thus only one component affecting bioavailability. The fraction of an orally administered drug reaching the systemic circulation intact, or *systemic availability*, can be calculated (assuming equal clearances for IV and oral forms of drug) by comparing the area under the plasma concentration curve achieved with oral and intravenous administrations from the following relationship. Systemic availability equals the area under the plasma concentration curve following oral administration/the area under the plasma concentration curve following IV administration times 100 (assuming equal IV and oral doses).

DRUG DISTRIBUTION. Most antiarrhythmic drugs in the therapeutic range are eliminated according to *first-order kinetics*, which means that the amount of drug eliminated per unit time is directly proportional to the amount (or concentration) of drug in the body. More drug in the body results in more drug excreted by the kidneys or metabolized by the liver, so that the *fraction* of drug eliminated per unit of time remains constant regardless of the amount of drug in the body. For example, one-half the drug may be eliminated in 6 hours whether the total amount of drug in the body is 4 gm or 10 gm, resulting in elimination of 2 gm in the first example and 5 gm in the second. As a consequence, the elimination half-life, or time required to eliminate half the body load (or to halve the plasma concentration) of such a drug is constant and independent of the total body load. The following discussion will assume first-order kinetics unless otherwise stated. (*Zero-order kinetics* indicates that the reaction occurs at a constant, usually maximal, rate and cannot increase further despite increased drug concentrations. Such nonlinear or saturable kinetics can occur at high concentrations of a drug that at usual concentrations exhibits first-order kinetics.)

THE ONE-COMPARTMENT MODEL

Generally two models, a *one-compartment open model* and a *two-compartment open model*, are used with relative accuracy to describe and predict serum concentrations at a given time for a variety of dose regimens. Even though these models are oversimplified representations of drug disposition, they provide guidelines for choosing loading doses and maintenance dose schedules for a given patient. In the one-compartment open model, drugs are considered to enter and to be eliminated from a single homogeneous unit that represents the entire body. Drugs entering the compartment are considered to be distributed immediately throughout the compartment, making the concentration of the drug equal to the amount of drug in the compartment divided by the volume of the compartment. The latter equals the amount of the drug in the compartment divided by the drug concentration.

In reality, a one-compartment open model is not entirely appropriate because a certain amount of time is needed to distribute the drug throughout the volume of the compartment. However, the one-compartment model predicts plasma concentration as a function of time and dose, if distribution is significantly faster than the rate of administration or of excretion, which is the case for many antiarrhythmic drugs.

THE TWO-COMPARTMENT MODEL

If the rate of drug administration is rapid in relation to drug distribution (e.g., intravenous administration), a two-compartment open model more accurately predicts drug concentrations (Fig. 23–1). In this model the drug enters the system by the central compartment and can leave the system only by distribution into a peripheral compartment or elimination from the central compartment. The central compartment, in dynamic equilibrium with the more slowly equilibrating peripheral compartment, is assumed to consist of the blood volume and extracellular fluid of highly perfused tissues such as heart, lungs, kidneys, and liver, while the peripheral compartment, acting as a reservoir, consists of less well perfused tissue such as muscle, skin, and adipose tissue. The first-order rate constants $K_{1 \rightarrow 2}$ and $K_{2 \rightarrow 1}$ determine the rate of transfer of drug between the central and peripheral compartments or vice versa, with K_β representing the overall elimination rate constant. K_β relates the sum of all methods of irreversible drug elimination from the central compartment to the concentration of drug in that compartment (Fig. 23–1). For antiarrhythmic drugs, the peripheral compartment is generally larger than the central compartment. The concepts of distribution volumes and drug movement are more complex in the two-compartment open model than in the one-compartment open model. The two-compartment model may behave similarly to the one-compartment model when drugs are infused slowly or given orally and K_1 approximates K_2, but pronounced differences exist when injections are given rapidly.

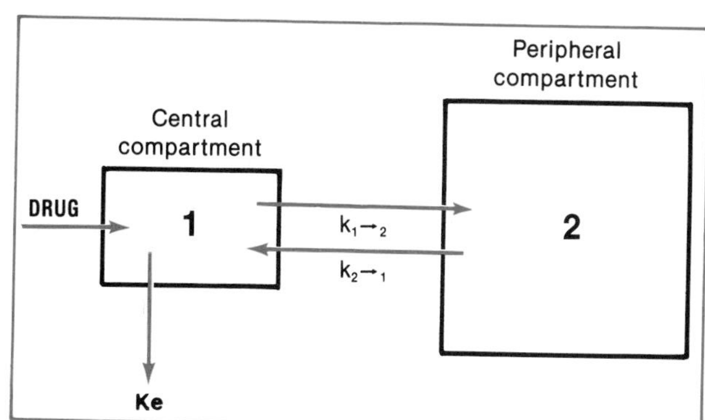

FIGURE 23–1. Two-compartment open model. A smaller central compartment into which drug is administered and from which it is eliminated (K_e) connects in dynamic equilibrium with a larger peripheral compartment.

Following administration of drugs for which the kinetics are described by a two-compartment model, the curve of plasma drug concentration demonstrates two distinct phases: an early phase (alpha, or distribution phase), characterized by rapidly falling plasma drug concentrations due to distribution between the central compartment and the peripheral compartment, and a second phase (beta, or elimination phase) of slower decline in plasma drug concentration, representing primarily elimination of drugs from the central compartment (Fig. 23–2). *Alpha* is often referred to as the *rate constant for distribution* and *beta* as the *rate constant for elimination.* During the latter beta phase, when the drug is in distribution equilibrium, serum concentrations correlate with the pharmacological effects of the drug. The distribution of quinidine is shown in Figure 23–3.

The extent of extravascular distribution of a drug is obtained by measuring the apparent *volume of distribution*, which is the hypothetical volume into which a dose of drug would have to be diluted to give the observed plasma concentration. It is determined by the dose administered divided by the plasma concentration at time 0. The latter equals the sum of A and B on the logarithmic plasma concentration axis obtained by extrapolating the alpha and beta phases back to 0 time (Fig. 23–2). It is also calculated by dividing the systemic clearance of the drug by beta, the rate constant of elimination. A large volume of distribution indicates a wide distribution and extensive tissue uptake of the drug and often exceeds by several times the actual amount of total body water. The large volume of distribution for most antiarrhythmic agents indicates that they are present in higher concentrations in some tissues than in the plasma. The volume of

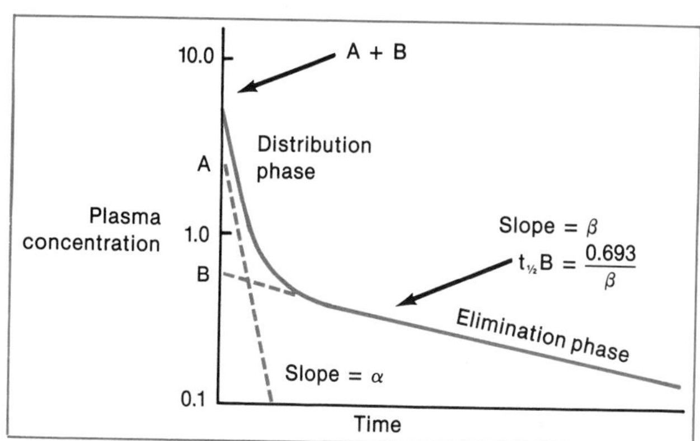

FIGURE 23–2. Schematic diagram of the semilogarithmic plot of drug plasma concentration as a function of time following rapid intravenous injection, according to the principles outlined for a two-compartment open model. (From Gibaldi, M., and Perrier, D.: Drugs and the pharmaceutical sciences. *In* Pharmacokinetics, Vol. 1. New York, Marcel Dekker, 1975.)

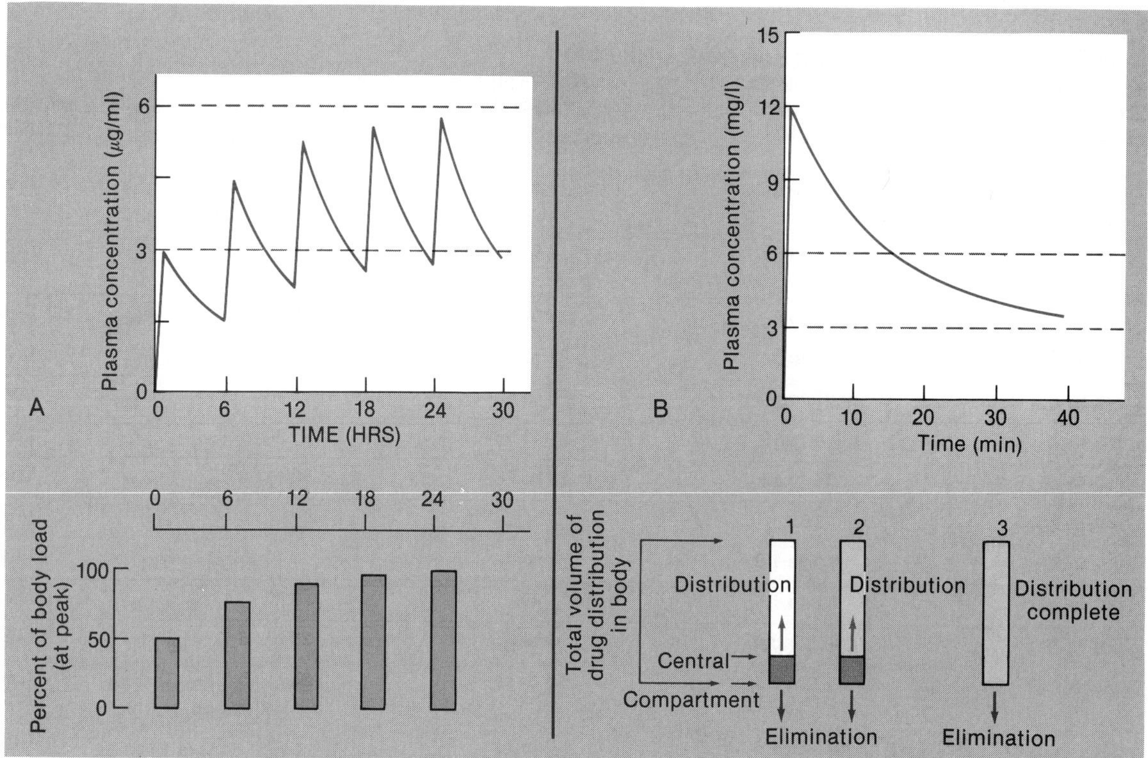

FIGURE 23–3. ***A,*** **Changes in plasma concentration over time after beginning treatment with quinidine.** ***Top,*** **Quinidine plasma concentration over time, with the dashed line indicating the therapeutic range.** ***Bottom,*** **The hatched bars represent the body load immediately after each dose of quinidine, expressed as a percentage of the load after a dose when a steady state has been achieved. Quinidine is administered every 6 hours (the half-life in this case). Four half-lives, or 24 hours, are required to achieve a body load of quinidine that exceeds 90 per cent of the load at steady state.** ***B, Top,*** **Plasma concentrations produced by administering a full intravenous loading dose of quinidine as a bolus, with the therapeutic range shown by a dashed line.** ***Bottom,*** **The numbered vertical boxes indicate the volume of distribution of quinidine. Just after the drug is given, it is dissolved only in the small central compartment, as in box 1, and very high peak concentrations are achieved (in the toxic range). The drug then distributes throughout the rest of the body. Distribution has a half-life of about 8 minutes and is complete by 30 minutes (box 3). Quinidine concentration is now in the therapeutic range, and further decreases in plasma concentration are due solely to drug elimination. (From Nattel, S., and Zipes, D. P.: Clinical pharmacology of old and new antiarrhythmic drugs. Cardiovasc. Clin.** ***11*****:221, 1980.)**

Class IC. Drugs that reduce $\dot{V}_{max}$, primarily slow conduction and can prolong refractoriness minimally: flecainide, encainide, propafenone; slow onset and offset kinetics (10 to 20 sec).

Class II drugs that block beta-adrenergic receptors are: Propranolol, timolol, metoprolol, and others.

Class III drugs that block potassium channels and prolong repolarization are: sotalol, amiodarone, bretylium, N-acetylprocainamide.

Class IV drugs that block the slow calcium channel are: verapamil, diltiazem, nifedipine, and others.

A recently proposed model suggests that antiarrhythmic drugs cross the cell membrane and interact with receptors in the membrane channels when the latter are in the rested, activated, or inactivated states and that each of these interactions is characterized by a different association and dissociation rate constant (Fig. 22–14, p. 598). Such interactions are voltage- and time-dependent. Transitions among rested, activated, and inactivated states are governed by standard Hodgkin-Huxley–type equations. When the drug is bound (associated) to a receptor site at or very close to the ionic channel (the drug probably does not actually plug the channel), the latter cannot conduct, even in the activated state.[6]

USE DEPENDENCE. Some drugs exert greater inhibitory effects on the upstroke of the action potential at more rapid rates of stimulation and after longer periods of stimulation, a characteristic called *use dependence*. Use-dependence means that depression of $\dot{V}_{max}$ is greater after the channel has been "used," i.e., after action potential depolarization rather than after a rest period. It is possible that this use-dependence results from preferential interaction of the antiarrhythmic drug with either the open or the inactive channel and little interaction with the resting channels of the unstimulated cell. Agents in class IB exhibit fast kinetics of onset and offset or use-dependent block of the fast channel; that is, they bind and dissociate quickly from the receptors. Class IC drugs have slow kinetics, and class IA drugs are intermediate. With increased time spent in diastole (slower rate), a greater proportion of receptors become drug-free and the drug exerts less effect. Cells with reduced membrane potentials recover more slowly from drug actions than cells with more negative membrane potentials (Fig. 22–14, p. 598).

Given the fact that enhanced automaticity or reentry can cause cardiac arrhythmias, mechanisms by which antiarrhythmic agents suppress arrhythmias can be postulated. Antiarrhythmic agents can slow the spontaneous discharge frequency of an automatic pacemaker by depressing the slope of diastolic depolarization, shifting the threshold voltage toward zero, or hyperpolarizing the resting membrane potential. Mechanisms by which different drugs suppress normal or abnormal automaticity may not be the same. In general, however, most antiarrhythmic agents in therapeutic doses depress the automatic firing rate of spontaneously discharging ectopic sites while minimally affecting the discharge rate of the normal sinus node. Slow-channel blockers like verapamil, beta blockers like propranolol, and some antiarrhythmic agents like amiodarone also depress spontaneous discharge of the normal sinus node, while drugs that exert vagolytic effects, such as disopyramide or quinidine, can increase the sinus discharge rate. Drugs can also suppress early or delayed afterdepolarizations (p. 605) and eliminate arrhythmias due to these mechanisms.

As mentioned earlier, reentry depends critically on the tim-

TABLE 23-2 KNOWN INFLUENCE OF DISEASE STATES AND OTHER CONDITIONS ON ANTIARRHYTHMIC DRUG PHARMACOKINETICS

DISEASE OR CONDITION	EFFECTS
Congestive heart failure	**Reduced clearance of:** lidocaine, procainamide, flecainide **Reduced volume of distribution of:** lidocaine
Liver disease	**Reduced clearance of:** lidocaine, disopyramide, phenytoin, propranolol
Renal disease	**Reduced clearance of:** disopyramide, procainamide, bretylium, tocainide, flecainide **Altered protein binding (with usually unchanged drug requirements) of:** phenytoin
Postmyocardial infarction	**Reduced clearance of:** procainamide **Altered protein binding of:** lidocaine, quinidine
Prolonged administration	**Reduced clearance of:** lidocaine
Obesity	**Increased volume of distribution of:** lidocaine

From Roden, D.: New concepts in antiarrhythmic drug pharmacokinetics Progr. Cardiol. *15*:19, 1987.

ing interrelationships between refractoriness and conduction velocity, the presence of unidirectional block in one of the pathways, and other factors that influence refractoriness and conduction, such as excitability. An antiarrhythmic agent can stop reentry that is already present or prevent it from starting if the drug improves or depresses conduction. For example, *improved conduction* can (1) eliminate the unidirectional block so that reentry cannot begin or (2) facilitate conduction in the reentrant loop so that the returning wavefront reenters too quickly, encroaches on fibers still refractory, and becomes extinguished. A drug that *depresses conduction* can transform the unidirectional block to bidirectional block and thus terminate reentry or prevent it from occurring by creating an area of complete block in the reentrant pathway. Conversely, a drug that slows conduction without producing block or lengthening refractoriness significantly can promote reentry. Finally, most antiarrhythmic agents share the ability to prolong refractoriness relative to their effects on action potential duration, i.e., the ratio of effective refractory period to action potential duration exceeds 1.0. If a drug *prolongs refractoriness* of fibers in the reentrant pathway, the pathway may not recover excitability in time to be depolarized by the reentering impulse, and the reentrant propagation ceases. The different types of reentry influence the effects of a drug.

When one is discussing any of the properties of a drug, it is important that the situation and/or model from which conclusions are drawn be defined with care. Electrophysiological, hemodynamic, autonomic, pharmacokinetic, and adverse effects all may differ in normal subjects compared to patients, in normal tissue compared to abnormal tissue, in muscle compared to specialized fibers, and in different species.

STEREOSELECTIVITY. Drug interactions with a channel, receptor, or enzyme may depend on the three-dimensional geometry of the drug.[1] Many drugs have stereoisomers, molecules with the same atomic composition but different spatial arrangement, that can influence drug effects, metabolism binding, clearance, and excretion. Most drugs are prescribed as 50/50 mixtures of their two forms (racemates), which may make 50 per cent of the dose ineffective for some drugs. Except for timolol, virtually all beta blockers are racemates. d-Propranolol exerts antiarrhythmic actions unrelated to beta-adrenoceptor blockade,[7] while l-propranolol blocks the beta receptor. Both enantiomers (mirror images) of sotalol block the potassium channel to prolong action potential duration and suppress arrhythmias equally, but d-sotalol does not block the beta adrenoceptor. Racemic propafenone exhibits beta blocking actions due to the s-enantiomer.[8] Other drugs with notable stereoselective differences include disopyramide with one form (S (+)) prolonging repolarization and having greater antiarrhythmic effects than R (−), which shortens repolarization. The latter form has less anticholinergic effects.[9] The (−) enantiomer of verapamil exerts much more negative inotropic and dromotropic effects than does the (+) form and may have more potent antiarrhythmic actions.[10] Stereoselectivity affects sodium channel blocking drugs less than it affects beta adrenoceptor, potassium, and calcium blockers.

DRUG METABOLITES. Drug metabolites may add to or alter the effects of the parent compound by exerting similar actions, competing with the parent compound, or mediating drug toxicity.[1] Quinidine has at least four active metabolites, but none with a potency exceeding the parent drug, and none preliminarily implicated in causing torsades de pointes.[11] Encainide has at least two active metabolites, one of which is threefold as potent as the parent drug. About 50 per cent of procainamide is metabolized to NAPA. Only the parent drug blocks cardiac sodium channels and slows impulse propagation in the His-Purkinje system. NAPA is a less effective antiarrhythmic drug but competes with procainamide for renal tubular secretory sites and can increase the parent's elimination half-life.[12] Lidocaine's metabolite can compete with lidocaine for sodium channels and partially reverse block produced by lidocaine.[13]

Genetically determined metabolic pathways account for many of the differences in patients' responses to some drugs. The genetically determined activity of hepatic *N*-acetyltransferase regulates the development of antinuclear antibodies and development of the lupus syndrome in response to procainamide. Slow acetylator phenotypes appear more prone to develop lupus than do rapid acetylators.[1] About 7 per cent of white and black subjects lack debrisoquin 4-hydroxylase. This enzyme is needed to metabolize debrisoquin (an antihypertensive drug), encainide, propafenone, to hydroxylate several beta blockers, and to biotransform flecainide.[14] The gene coding for this enzyme (termed $P450_{dbl}$) is on human chromosome 22.[15] Lack of this enzyme reduces metabolism of the parent compound, leading to increased plasma concentrations of the parent drug and reduced concentrations of metabolites. Quinidine in low doses can inhibit this enzyme and thereby alter concentrations of the drugs and metabolites given in combination that are affected by the $P450_{db1}$ enzyme, such as encainide, propafenone, or flecainide.[16] Understanding stereoselectivity and pharmacogenetics can provide major clues to understanding differences in drug efficacy and toxicity from one patient to the next. Cimetidine and ranitidine also affect drug metabolism, probably by inhibiting hepatic P-450–metabolizing enzymes[17] (Table 23–3).

SIDE EFFECTS. Antiarrhythmic drugs produce one group of side effects that relate to excessive dosage and plasma concentrations, resulting in both noncardiac (e.g., neurological) and cardiac (e.g., heart failure, some arrhythmias) toxicity, and another group of side effects unrelated to plasma concentrations, termed idiopathic. Examples of the latter include procainamide-induced lupus syndrome, amiodarone-induced pulmonary toxicity (although a recent publication[18] relates maintenance dose to this side effect) and some arrhythmias such as quinidine-induced torsades de pointes.[19]

TABLE 23-5 IN VITRO ELECTROPHYSIOLOGICAL CHARACTERISTICS OF ANTIARRHYTHMIC DRUGS

DRUG	APA	APD	dV/dt	MDP	ERP	CONDUCTION VELOCITY	PF NODAL PHASE 4	SINUS NODAL AUTOMATICITY
Quinidine	↓	↑	↓	0	↑	↓	↓	0
Procainamide	↓	↑	↓	0	↑	↓	↓	0
Disopyramide	↓	↑	↓	0	↑	↓	↓	↑ 0 ↓
Lidocaine	0 ↓	↓	0 ↓	0	↓	0 ↓	↓	0
Mexiletine	0	↓	0 ↓	0	↓	↓	↓	0
Tocainide	0	↓	0 ↓	0	↓	↓	0	↓
Phenytoin	0	↓	↑ 0 ↓	0	↓	0	↓	0
Moricizine	↓	↓	↓	0	↓	↓	0	0
Encainide	↓	0 ↑	↓	0	↑	↓↓	↓	0
Flecainide	↓	0 ↑	↓	0	↑	↓↓	↓	0
Propafenone	↓	0 ↑	↓	0	↑	↓↓	↓	↓
Propranolol	0 ↓	0 ↓	0 ↓	0	↓	0	↓*	↓
Amiodarone	0	↑	0 ↓	0	↑	↓	↓	↓
Bretylium	0	↑	0	0	↑	0	0 ↓*	0 ↓
Verapamil	0	↓	0	0	0	0	↓*	↓
Adenosine	0	0	0	0	0	0	0	↓

* With a background of sympathetic activity.
Key: APA = action potential amplitude; APD = action potential duration; dV/dt = rate of rise of action potential; MDP = maximum diastolic potential; ERP = effective refractory period; PF = Pukinje fibers; ET = excitability threshold; VFT = ventricular fibrillation threshold.

Q-T interval, such as lidocaine or phenytoin, can be tried. When pacing is not available, isoproterenol can be given *with caution*. Magnesium given intravenously (2 gm over 1 to 2 min, followed by an infusion of 3 to 20 mg/min) has been successful in suppressing quinidine-induced torsades de pointes.[38,52]

Drugs that induce hepatic enzyme production, such as phenobarbital and phenytoin, can shorten the duration of quinidine's action by increasing its rate of elimination. Quinidine may elevate serum digoxin and digitoxin concentrations by decreasing total body clearance of digitoxin and by decreasing the clearance, volume of distribution, and affinity of tissue receptors for digoxin (see p. 484).

PROCAINAMIDE

ELECTROPHYSIOLOGICAL ACTIONS (Tables 23–4 and 23–5). The cardiac actions of procainamide on automaticity, conduction, excitability, and membrane responsiveness resemble those of quinidine.[5,6] Like quinidine, procainamide usually prolongs the effective refractory period (ERP) more than it prolongs the action potential duration (APD). When the ERP duration/APD exceeds 1.0, the earliest premature impulse that can be initiated during repolarization arises when the cell has returned to its most negative potential. Premature responses induced at this potential are more likely to have greater $\dot{V}_{max}$ and amplitude, presumably establishing better conduction. Thus the antiarrhythmic agent prevents early responses, arising from less negative resting potentials, that might conduct slowly or block, thereby potentiating the development of arrhythmias. Compared with disopyramide and quinidine, procainamide exerts the least anticholinergic effects but does produce more local anesthetic effects than quinidine. It does not affect normal sinus nodal automaticity. In vitro, procainamide decreases abnormal automaticity, with less effect on triggered activity or catecholamine-enhanced normal automaticity.[53] It prolongs the QRS duration and electrograms recorded from normal and chronically infarcted human myocardium to the same degree; lidocaine has no effect on electrograms in either situation.[54]

The electrophysiological effects of NAPA, procainamide's major metabolite, differ from those of the parent compound. NAPA (10 to 40 mg/liter) does not suppress the rate of phase 4 diastolic depolarization of Purkinje fibers and does not alter resting membrane potential, action potential amplitude, or $\dot{V}_{max}$ of phase 0 of the action potential of Purkinje fibers or ventricular muscle. However, NAPA exerts a class III action and prolongs the action potential duration of ventricular muscle and Purkinje fibers in a dose-dependent manner. Toxic doses produce early afterdepolarizations, triggered activity, and ventricular tachyarrhythmias. Torsades de pointes due to NAPA has been recorded in patients. Procainamide appears to exert greater electrophysiological effects than NAPA.

HEMODYNAMIC EFFECTS. Procainamide can depress myocardial contractility in high doses. It does not produce alpha blockade but can result in peripheral vasodilation via a mild ganglionic blocking action that impairs cardiovascular reflexes. It produces less hemodynamic depression than do eucainide and tocainide.[54a]

PHARMACOKINETICS (Table 23–1). Oral administration produces peak plasma concentration in about one hour. Absorption may be reduced in the first week after myocardial infarction. Approximately 80 per cent of oral procainamide is bioavailable, with 20 per cent bound to serum proteins. The overall elimination half-life for procainamide is 3 to 5 hours, with 50 to 60 per cent of the drug eliminated by the kidney and 10 to 30 per cent eliminated by hepatic metabolism. A prolonged-release form of procainamide given every 6 hours provides steady-state plasma levels of the drug equivalent to an equal total daily dose of short-acting procainamide given every 3 hours.

The drug is acetylated to NAPA, which is excreted almost exclusively by the kidneys. As renal function decreases and in patients with heart failure, procainamide levels—and particularly NAPA levels—increase and, because of the risk of serious cardiotoxicity, need to be carefully monitored in such situations. NAPA has an elimination half-life of 7 to 8 hours but exceeds 10 hours if high doses are used. Small amounts of procainamide are present in patients receiving NAPA because of deacetylation. Increased age, congestive heart failure, and reduced creatinine clearance lower the procainamide clearance.[55]

DOSAGE AND ADMINISTRATION (Table 23–1). Procainamide can be given by the oral, intravenous, or intramuscular routes to achieve plasma concentrations that produce an antiarrhythmic effect in the range of 4 to 10 μg/ml. Occasionally plasma concentrations exceeding 10 μg/ml have been required, but the probability of adverse effects generally preclude long-term administration at these higher plasma concentrations. Several intravenous regimens have been used to administer procainamide. Twenty-five to 50 mg can be given

MEMBRANE RESPONSIVENESS	ET	VFT	CONTRACTILITY	SLOW INWARD CURRENT	AUTONOMIC NERVOUS SYSTEM	LOCAL ANESTHETIC EFFECT
↓	↑	↑	0	0	Antivagal; alpha blocker	Yes
↓	↑	↑	0	0	Slight antivagal	Yes
↓	↑	↑	↓	0	Central: antivagal, antisympathetic	Yes
0 ↓	0 ↑	↑	0	0	0	Yes
↓	↑	↑	↓	0	0	Yes
↓	↑	↑	0	0	0	Yes
0 ↑	0			0	0	No
↓	↑	0		0	0	No
↓	↑		↓	0	0	Yes
↓			↓	0	0	Yes
↓	↑	↑	↓	May inhibit	Antisympathetic	Yes
↓			↓	0 ↓	Antisympathetic	No
0	0	↑	0 ↑	0	Antisympathetic	Yes
0 ↑	0	0 ↑	↓	0	Antisympathetic	Yes
0	0	0	↓	Inhibit	? Block alpha receptors; enhance vagal	Yes
0	0	0	0	May inhibit	Vagomimetic	No

over a one-minute period and then repeated every 5 minutes until the arrhythmia is controlled, hypotension results, or the QRS complex is prolonged more than 50 per cent. Doses of 10 to 15 mg/kg at 50 mg/min are commonly used during electrophysiological testing. Using this method, plasma concentration falls rapidly during the first 15 minutes after the loading dose, with parallel effects on refractoriness and conduction.[56] A constant-rate intravenous infusion of procainamide can be given at a dose of 2 to 6 mg/min. The upper limits regarding total IV dose are flexible and range between 1000 and 2000 mg, depending upon the patient's response.

Oral administration of procainamide requires a 3- or 4-hour dosing interval at a total daily dose of 2 to 6 gm, with a steady state reached within one day. When a loading dose is used, it should be twice the maintenance dose. Frequent dosing is required because of the short elimination half-life in normal subjects. For the prolonged-release form of procainamide, dosing is at 6-hour intervals. While a longer half-life may be seen in some cardiac patients, allowing longer intervals between drug administration, this needs to be documented for the individual patient. Procainamide is well absorbed after intramuscular injection, with virtually 100 per cent of the dose bioavailable. The plasma concentration of procainamide required to suppress complex ventricular ectopy is usually less than that required to suppress simple premature ventricular complexes (PVCs). PVCs of one morphology can be suppressed while those of another remain.[57]

CLINICAL INDICATIONS. Procainamide is used to treat both supraventricular and ventricular arrhythmias in a manner comparable to that of quinidine. Although both drugs have similar electrophysiological actions, either drug can effectively suppress a supraventricular or ventricular arrhythmia that is resistant to the other drug.

Procainamide can be used to convert atrial fibrillation of recent onset to sinus rhythm and may render persistent atrial fibrillation difficult to detect by arrhythmia recognition algorithms because of changes in the electrograms.[58] As with quinidine, prior treatment with digitalis, propranolol, or verapamil is recommended to prevent acceleration of the ventricular response following procainamide therapy. In patients with paroxysmal supraventricular tachycardia, procainamide can inhibit the induction of sustained AV nodal reentrant tachycardia as a result of selective depression of retrograde AV nodal conduction in the fast pathway. Procainamide can block conduction in the accessory pathway of patients with the Wolff-Parkinson-White syndrome. Whether it can be used intravenously to identify those patients who have a short anterograde effective refractory period is not resolved.[59,60] It can produce His-Purkinje block.[61] (p. 711).

Procainamide has been only partially effective in preventing the induction of ventricular tachycardia by programmed stimulation during electrophysiological studies in patients with a history of ventricular tachycardia or ventricular fibrillation, but is more effective than lidocaine.[62] It is also more effective than lidocaine in acutely terminating sustained ventricular tachycardia.[63] The electrophysiological response to procainamide given intravenously appears to predict the response to the drug given orally. Patients with ejection fractions ≥ 40 per cent whose ventricular tachycardia procainamide renders noninducible have a high likelihood of responding to the drug given orally.[64] High doses, 500 to 1000 mg orally every 4 hours, resulting in a plasma concentration exceeding 10.0 μg/ml, may be necessary to suppress ventricular tachycardia in some patients. Most consistently, procainamide slows the rate of the induced ventricular tachycardia,[65] a change correlated with the increase in QRS duration.[66] Adding amiodarone to procainamide slows the ventricular tachycardia cycle length further but increases the noninducibility success rate only slightly.[67] Procainamide appears to affect preferentially the reentrant circuit of the ventricular tachycardia compared with other areas of myocardium.[68] The antiarrhythmic response to procainamide does not predict the response to NAPA.

ADVERSE EFFECTS. Multiple adverse noncardiac effects have been reported with procainamide administration and include skin rashes, myalgias, digital vasculitis, and Raynaud's phenomenon. Gastrointestinal side effects are less frequent than with quinidine, and adverse central nervous system side effects are less frequent than with lidocaine. Procainamide can cause giddiness, psychosis, hallucinations, and depression. Toxic concentrations of procainamide can diminish myocardial performance and promote hypotension. A variety of conduction disturbances[61] or ventricular tachyarrhythmias can occur similar to those produced by quinidine, including prolonged Q-T syndrome and polymorphous ventricular tachycardia.[26,27,41] NAPA can also induce Q-T prolongation and a polymorphous ventricular tachycardia.[69] In the absence of sinus node disease, procainamide does not adversely affect sinus node function. In patients with sinus dysfunction, procainamide tends to prolong corrected sinus node recovery time and can worsen symptoms in some patients who have the bradycardia-tachycardia syndrome. Fever and agranulocytosis may be due to hypersensitivity reactions, and white blood cell and differential blood counts should be performed at regular intervals. Procainamide does not increase the serum digoxin concentration.

Arthralgia, fever, pleuropericarditis, hepatomegaly, and hemorrhagic pericardial effusion with tamponade have been described in a systemic lupus erythematosus (SLE)-like syndrome. The syndrome can occur more frequently and earlier in patients who are "slow acetylators" of procainamide. The aromatic amino group on procainamide appears important for induction of SLE syndrome, since acetylating this amino group to form NAPA appears to block the SLE-inducing effect. Sixty to 70 per cent of patients who receive procainamide on a chronic basis develop antinuclear antibodies, with clinical symptoms in 20 to 30 per cent, but this is reversible when procainamide is stopped. When symptoms occur, SLE cell preparations are often positive. Positive serological tests are not necessarily a reason to discontinue drug therapy; however, the development of symptoms or a positive anti-DNA antibody is, except for patients whose life-threatening arrhythmia is controlled only by procainamide. Steroid administration in those patients may eliminate the symptoms. In contrast to naturally occurring SLE, the brain and kidney are spared and there is no predilection for females.

DISOPYRAMIDE

Disopyramide has been approved in the United States for oral but not intravenous administration to treat patients with ventricular arrhythmias.

ELECTROPHYSIOLOGICAL ACTIONS (Tables 23–4 and 23–5). Although structurally different from quinidine and procainamide, disopyramide produces similar electrophysiological effects in vitro.[5,6] It decreases the slope of phase 4 diastolic depolarization in Purkinje fibers, produces a rate-dependent depression of V_{max} of phase 0, prolongs the effective refractory period more than it prolongs the action potential duration, lengthens conduction time in normal and depolarized Purkinje fibers, and does not affect calcium-dependent action potentials, except possibly at very high concentrations. Disopyramide, like procainamide, reduces the differences in action potential duration between normal and infarcted tissue by lengthening the action potential of normal cells more than it lengthens the action potential of cells from infarcted regions of the heart.

Stereochemical properties influence the effects of disopyramide.[1] Racemic (clinically used) and (+) disopyramide prolong canine Purkinje fiber action potential, while (−) disopyramide shortens it. The (+) isomer exerts approximately three times more vagolytic effects than does the (−) isomer. Disopyramide can speed the sinus nodal discharge rate and shorten AV nodal conduction time and refractoriness when the nodes are restrained by cholinergic influences. Atropine tends to nullify or even reverse this effect. Disopyramide also can slow the sinus nodal discharge rate by a direct action when given in high concentration and can significantly depress sinus nodal activity in patients with sinus node dysfunction. Disopyramide exerts greater anticholinergic effects than quinidine and does not appear to affect alpha- or beta-adrenoceptors.

Atrial and ventricular refractory periods increase, as do conduction time and refractoriness of the accessory pathway in patients with the Wolff-Parkinson-White syndrome.[70] Disopyramide's effect on AV nodal conduction and refractoriness in vivo is not consistent. Disopyramide prolongs His-Purkinje conduction time, but infra-His block results infrequently. Disopyramide can be administered safely to patients who have first degree AV block and narrow QRS complexes.

HEMODYNAMIC EFFECTS. Disopyramide administered intravenously reduces systemic blood pressure, cardiac and stroke index, and increases right atrial pressures and total peripheral resistance. Profound hemodynamic deterioration can occur, and patients who have abnormal ventricular function tolerate the negative inotropic effects of IV and oral disopyramide quite poorly. In these patients the drug should be used with extreme caution or not at all.

PHARMACOKINETICS (Table 23–1). Disopyramide is 80 to 90 per cent absorbed, with a mean elimination half-life of 8 to 9 hours in healthy volunteers but almost 10 hours in patients with heart failure and sometimes longer in some patients with ventricular arrhythmias. Total body clearance and volume of distribution decrease in patients, and mean serum concentration is higher than reported in normal subjects. Renal insufficiency prolongs the elimination time. Thus, in patients who have renal, hepatic, or cardiac insufficiency, loading and maintenance doses need to be reduced. Peak blood levels after oral administration result in 1 to 2 hours, and bioavailability exceeds 80 per cent. The fraction of disopyramide bound to serum protein varies inversely with the total plasma concentration of the drug but may be more stable (30 to 40 per cent) at clinically relevant concentrations of 3 μg/ml. About half an oral dose is recovered unchanged in the urine, with about 30 per cent as the mono N-dealkylated metabolite. The metabolites appear to exert less effect than the parent compound.

DOSAGE AND ADMINISTRATION (Table 23–1). Doses are generally 100 to 200 mg orally every 6 hours with a range of 400 to 1200 mg/day. The intravenous (investigational) dose is 1 to 2 mg/kg as an initial bolus given over 5 to 10 minutes, which may be followed by an infusion of 1 mg/kg/hour.

CLINICAL INDICATIONS. Disopyramide appears comparable to quinidine and procainamide in reducing the frequency of premature ventricular complexes and effectively prevents recurrence of ventricular tachycardia in selected patients. Disopyramide has been combined with other drugs such as mexiletine to treat patients who do not respond or only partially respond to one drug.

Disopyramide terminates and prevents recurrent episodes of paroxysmal supraventricular tachycardia due to AV and AV nodal reentry. It prolongs the anterograde and retrograde refractory period of the accessory pathway in patients with the Wolff-Parkinson-White syndrome,[70] helps prevent recurrence of atrial fibrillation after successful cardioversion as effectively as quinidine, and may terminate atrial flutter. In treating patients with atrial fibrillation, and particularly atrial flutter, the ventricular rate must be controlled prior to administering disopyramide, or the atrial rate may decrease sufficiently, aided by the vagolytic effects of disopyramide, to create 1:1 conduction during atrial flutter. Disopyramide has been shown effective for preventing inducible and spontaneous neurally mediated syncope.[71]

ADVERSE EFFECTS. Three categories of adverse effects are seen following disopyramide administration. The most common adverse effect relates to the drug's potent parasympatholytic properties and includes urinary hesitancy or retention, constipation, blurred vision, closed-angle glaucoma, and dry mouth. Symptoms may be minimized by concomitant administration of pyridostigmine.[72] Second, disopyramide can produce ventricular tachyarrhythmias that are commonly associated with Q-T prolongation and torsades de pointes.[69] Some patients can have "cross sensitivity" to both quinidine and disopyramide and develop torsades de pointes while receiving either drug. When drug-induced torsades de pointes occur, agents that prolong the Q-T interval should be used very cautiously or not at all.[26,27] Finally, disopyramide can reduce contractility of the normal ventricle but the depression of ventricular function is much more pronounced in patients with preexisting ventricular failure. Occasionally, cardiovascular collapse can result.

CLASS IB ANTIARRHYTHMIC AGENTS

LIDOCAINE

ELECTROPHYSIOLOGICAL ACTIONS (Tables 23–4 and 23–5). Lidocaine does not affect normal sinus nodal automaticity but does depress both normal and abnormal forms of automaticity,[73] as well as early and late afterdepolarizations in Purkinje fibers in vitro. External environment significantly influences the effects of lidocaine. It exhibits only a modest depressant effect on V_{max} and has no effect on maximal diastolic potential of normal muscle and specialized tissue in concentrations of about 1.5 μg/ml. However, faster rates of stimulation, reduced pH,[74] increased extracellular K^+ concentration, and reduced membrane potential—all changes that can result from ischemia—increase the ability of lidocaine to block the fast sodium channels, perhaps in part accounting for its efficacy in patients with acute myocardial infarction (Ch. 39).

Lidocaine can increase refractoriness in partially depolarized fibers. Lidocaine appears to have greatest affinity for open channels but dissociates rapidly from them when membrane potential returns to its maximum diastolic value. Both non-use-dependent (tonic) and use-dependent block are greater and develop more rapidly in Purkinje fibers from old dogs as compared with young dogs. Fibers from young dogs recover more quickly. Lidocaine reduces intracellular sodium activity and the magnitude of the transient inward current responsible for some forms of afterdepolarizations. Intracellular calcium activity may be reduced because of the sodium-calcium exchange mechanism. Lidocaine can convert areas of unidirectional block into bidirectional block during ischemia and prevent development of ventricular fibrillation by preventing fragmentation of organized large wavefronts into heterogeneous wavelets. Lidocaine may be arrhythmogenic if it depresses conduction but not to the point of bidirectional block. For example, it can create an area of unidirectional block and another area of conduction delay and promote reentry.

Lidocaine, except in very high concentrations, does *not* affect slow-channel-dependent action potentials despite its moderate suppression of the slow inward current. In fact, its depressant effect on electrical potentials from ischemic myocardium supports the notion that these ischemic potentials are depressed fast responses rather than slow responses.[75,76] Lidocaine significantly reduces the action potential duration and the effective refractory period of Purkinje fibers and ventricular muscle due to blocking of tetrodotoxin-sensitive sodium channels, and decreasing entry of sodium into the cell.[77] It has little effect on atrial fibers and does not affect conduction in accessory pathways. In some in vitro preparations, lidocaine can improve conduction by hyperpolarizing tissues depolarized as a result of stretch or low external potassium concentration.

In vivo, lidocaine has a minimal effect on automaticity or conduction except in unusual circumstances. Patients with preexisting sinus nodal dysfunction, abnormal His-Purkinje conduction, or junctional or ventricular escape rhythms may develop depressed automaticity or conduction. Part of its effects may be to inhibit cardiac sympathetic nerve activity.

HEMODYNAMIC EFFECTS. Clinically significant adverse hemodynamic effects are rarely noted at usual drug concentrations unless left ventricular function is severely impaired.

PHARMACOKINETICS (Table 23–1). Lidocaine is used only parenterally because oral administration results in extensive first-pass hepatic metabolism and unpredictable, low plasma levels with excessive metabolites that can produce toxicity. Hepatic metabolism of lidocaine depends greatly on hepatic blood flow, so that clearance of this drug almost equals (and can be approximated by) measurements of this flow. Severe hepatic disease or reduced hepatic blood flow, as in heart failure or shock, can markedly decrease the rate of lidocaine metabolism. Prolonged infusion can reduce lidocaine clearance. Its elimination half-life averages about 1 to 2 hours in normal subjects, more than 4 hours in patients after relatively uncomplicated myocardial infarction, more than 10 hours in patients after myocardial infarction complicated by cardiac failure, and even longer in the presence of cardiogenic shock. Maintenance doses should be reduced by one-third to one-half for patients with low cardiac output. Intravenous infusions should be discontinued as far in advance of electrophysiological studies as possible to avoid residual lidocaine effects.[78]

DOSAGE AND ADMINISTRATION (Table 23–1). Although lidocaine may be given intramuscularly, the intravenous route is most commonly used (Fig. 23–4). Intramuscular lidocaine is given in doses of 4 to 5 mg/kg (250 to 350 mg), resulting in effective serum levels at about 15 minutes and lasting for about 90 minutes. Intravenously, lidocaine is given as an initial bolus of 1 to 2 mg/kg body weight at a rate of approximately 20 to 50 mg/min, with a second injection of one-half the initial dose 20 to 40 minutes later. Patients treated with an initial bolus followed by a maintenance infusion may experience transient subtherapeutic plasma concentrations at 30 to 120 minutes after initiation of therapy. A second bolus of about 0.5 mg/kg without increasing the maintenance infusion rate reestablishes therapeutic serum concentrations. If recurrence of arrhythmia appears after a steady state has been achieved (e.g., 6 to 10 hours after starting therapy), a similar bolus should be given and the maintenance infusion rate increased. Increasing the maintenance infusion rate alone without an additional bolus results in a very slow increase in plasma lidocaine concentrations, reaching a new plateau in over 6 hours (four elimination half-lives), and is therefore not recommended. Another recommended intravenous dosing is 1.5 mg/kg initially and 0.8 mg/kg at 8-minute intervals for three doses. Doses are reduced by about 50 per cent for patients with heart failure.

If the initial bolus of lidocaine is ineffective, up to two more boluses of 1 mg/kg may be administered at 5-minute intervals. Patients who require more than one bolus to achieve a therapeutic effect have arrhythmias that respond only to higher lidocaine plasma concentrations, and a greater maintenance dose may be necessary to sustain these higher concentrations. Patients requiring only a single initial bolus of lidocaine should probably receive a maintenance infusion of 30 μg/kg/min, while those requiring two or three boluses may need infusions at 40 to 50 μg/kg/min. Loading doses may also be administered by rapid infusion and a constant-rate intravenous infusion may be used to maintain an effective concentration. Maintenance infusion rates in the range of 1 to 4 mg/min produce steady-state plasma levels of 1 to 5 μg/ml in patients with uncomplicated myocardial infarction, but these rates must be reduced during heart failure or shock because of concomitant reduced hepatic blood flow. A loading dose in the range of 75 mg followed by an initial infusion rate of 5.33 mg/min that declines exponentially to 2 mg/min with a half-life of 25 min also has been recommended.

CLINICAL INDICATIONS. Lidocaine demonstrates great efficacy against ventricular arrhythmias of diverse etiology, the ability to achieve effective plasma concentrations rapidly, and a fairly wide toxic-to-therapeutic ratio with a low incidence of hemodynamic complications and other side effects. However, its first-pass hepatic effect precludes oral use, and it is generally ineffective against supraventricular arrhythmias. In patients with the Wolff-Parkinson-White syndrome, when the effective refractory period of the accessory pathway is relatively short, lidocaine generally has no significant effect and may even accelerate the ventricular response during atrial fibrillation.

Lidocaine is used primarily for patients with acute myocardial infarction or recurrent ventricular tachyarrhythmias. In patients resuscitated from out-of-hospital ventricular fibrillation, lidocaine is comparable to bretylium in preventing recurrent episodes of ventricular tachyarrhythmia. Lidocaine prophylaxis in patients with acute myocardial infarction is

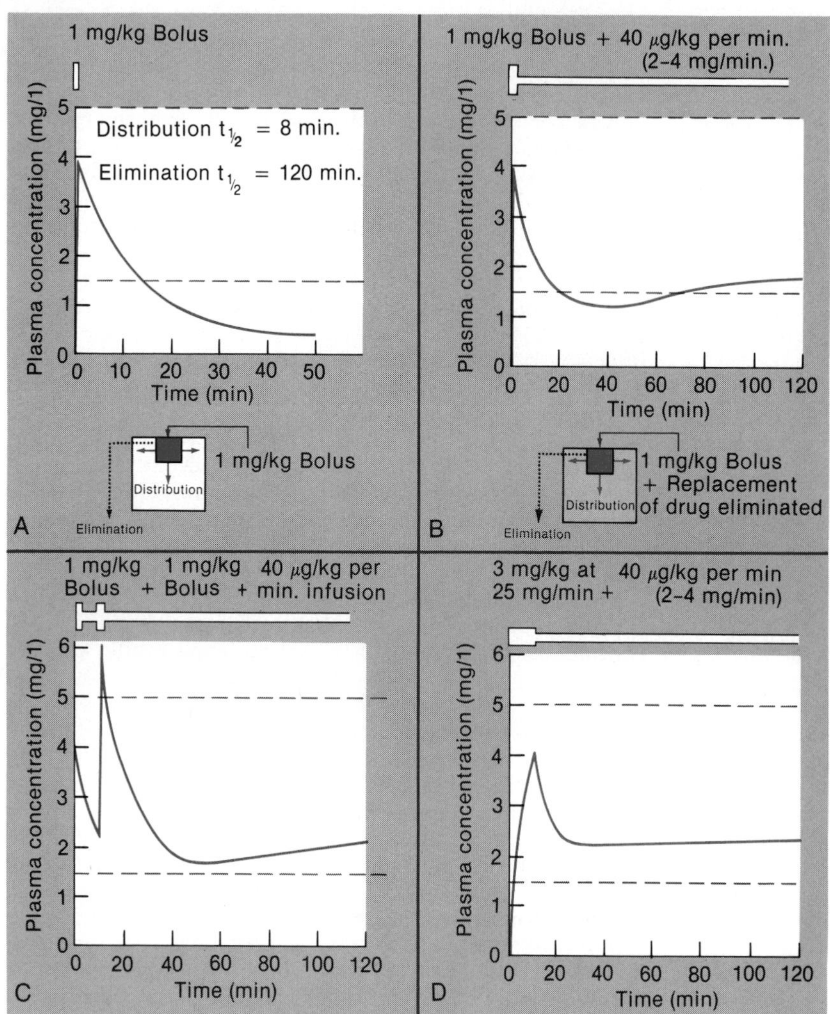

FIGURE 23-4. ***A, Top,*** **Plasma concentrations after a bolus of lidocaine, with the therapeutic range indicated by a dashed line.** ***Bottom,*** **The disposition of the drug in the body, with the larger box indicating the total volume of distribution and the smaller box the central compartment. The bolus initially produces therapeutic lidocaine concentrations in the small central compartment. Rapid distribution of the drug to the rest of the body produces subtherapeutic concentrations within 15 minutes.** ***B,*** **Lidocaine is administered by an initial bolus as in** ***A,*** **with a maintenance infusion begun just after the bolus. The maintenance infusion replaces drug eliminated from the body, but drug is also lost from the central compartment by distribution, which is more rapid than elimination. As a result, plasma concentrations decrease transiently. In this instance, lidocaine concentration is subtherapeutic between 30 and 70 minutes after initiation of therapy.** ***C,*** **Subtherapeutic lidocaine concentrations after an initial bolus (as in** ***B*****) can be prevented by giving a second lidocaine bolus 10 minutes after the first. A maintenance infusion should be started after the second bolus rather than after the first, as shown here. This will prevent excessive lidocaine concentrations after the second bolus.** ***D,*** **An alternative method to produce therapeutic lidocaine concentrations rapidly. This illustration indicates plasma concentrations after the administration of a loading dose of lidocaine given over 10 minutes. A maintenance infusion is begun after the loading dose has been given. (From Nattel, S., and Zipes, D. P.: Clinical pharmacology of old and new antiarrhythmic drugs. Cardiovasc. Clin.** ***11*****:221, 1980.)**

controversial. However, most data suggest that the benefits of prophylactic lidocaine therapy in reducing the incidence of ventricular fibrillation in hospitalized patients who have had acute myocardial infarction have not been clearly established. Drug-induced side effects and a possible increase in the risk of developing asystole lead to the conclusion that prophylaxis is probably not indicated for all patients.[79,80]

ADVERSE EFFECTS. The most commonly reported adverse effects of lidocaine are dose-related manifestations of central nervous system toxicity: dizziness, paresthesias, confusion, delirium, stupor, coma, and seizures. Occasional sinus node depression and His-Purkinje block have been reported. In patients with atrial tachyarrhythmias, ventricular rate acceleration has been noted.

MEXILETINE

Mexiletine, a local anesthetic congener of lidocaine with anticonvulsant properties, is approved by the FDA for oral treatment of patients with symptomatic ventricular arrhythmias.

ELECTROPHYSIOLOGICAL ACTIONS (Tables 23-4 and 23-5). Mexiletine is similar to lidocaine in many of its electrophysiological actions. In vitro, mexiletine shortens the duration of the action potential and refractory period of Purkinje fibers and to a lesser extent of ventricular muscle. It depresses V_{max} of phase 0 by blocking the fast sodium channel, especially at faster rates, and depresses automaticity of Purkinje fibers but not of the normal sinus node. Its onset and offset kinetics are rapid. Hypoxia or ischemia can increase its effects on V_{max}. Mexiletine suppresses digitalis-induced triggered activity.[81]

Mexiletine can result in severe bradycardia and abnormal sinus nodal recovery time in patients with sinus node disease but not in patients with a normal sinus node. It does not affect AV nodal conduction and can depress His-Purkinje conduction, but not greatly, unless conduction was abnormal initially. Mexiletine does not appear to affect the refractory period of human atrial and ventricular muscle. The duration of the Q-T interval does not increase. Because of its rate-dependent effects, theoretically mexiletine might be expected to suppress closely coupled rather than late coupled ventricular extrasystoles or faster tachycardias.

HEMODYNAMIC EFFECTS. Mexiletine exerts no major hemodynamic effects. It does not depress myocardial performance when given orally, although intravenous administration can produce hypotension.

PHARMACOKINETICS. Mexiletine has been reported to be rapidly and almost completely absorbed after oral ingestion by volunteers, with peak plasma concentrations attained in 2 to 4 hours. Elimination half-life in healthy subjects is approximately 10 hours and in patients after myocardial infarction, 17 hours. Therapeutic plasma levels of 1 to 2 μg/ml are maintained by oral doses of 200 to 300 mg every 6 to 8 hours. Absorption with less than 10 per cent first-pass hepatic effect occurs in the upper small intestine and is delayed and incomplete in patients who have myocardial infarction and in patients receiving narcotic analgesics, antacids, or atropine-like drugs that retard gastric emptying. Bioavailability of orally administered mexiletine is approximately 90 per cent, and about 70 per cent of the drug is protein-bound. The apparent volume of distribution is large, reflecting extensive tissue uptake. Normally, mexiletine is eliminated metabolically by the liver, with less than 10 per cent excreted unchanged in the urine. Doses probably should be reduced in patients with cirrhosis and those with left ventricular failure. Renal clearance of mexiletine decreases as urinary pH increases. Known metabolites exert no electrophysiological effects.

DOSAGE AND ADMINISTRATION. Recommended starting dose is 200 mg orally every 8 hours when rapid arrhythmia control is not essential. Doses may be increased or decreased by 50 to 100 mg every 2 to 3 days, and are better tolerated when given with food. Total daily dose should not exceed 1200 mg. In some patients, administration every 12 hours can be effective. For rapid loading, 400 mg followed in 8 hours by a 200 mg dose is suggested.

CLINICAL INDICATIONS. Mexiletine is an effective antiarrhythmic agent for treating patients with both acute and chronic ventricular tachyarrhythmias but not with supraventricular tachycardias.[82] Success rates vary from 6 to 60 per cent. Mexiletine combined with other drugs such as procainamide, beta blockers, quinidine,[83] disopyramide,[84] or amiodarone may become a major use of the drug. Most studies show no clear superiority of mexiletine over other class I agents. It may be very useful in children with congenital heart disease and serious ventricular arrhythmias.[85] In treating patients with a long Q-T interval, mexiletine probably would be safer than drugs such as quinidine that increase the Q-T interval further. It does not appear to alter the prognosis of patients with inducible ventricular tachyarrhythmias after myocardial infarction.[86]

ADVERSE EFFECTS. Thirty to 40 per cent of patients may require a change in dose or discontinuation of mexiletine therapy as a result of adverse effects, including tremor, dysarthria, dizziness, paresthesia, diplopia, nystagmus, mental confusion, anxiety, nausea, vomiting, and dyspepsia. Cardiovascular side effects are most often seen after intravenous dosing and include hypotension, bradycardia, and exacerbation of arrhythmia. Adverse effects of mexiletine appear to be dose-related, and toxic effects occur at plasma concentrations only slightly higher than therapeutic levels. Therefore, effective use of this antiarrhythmic drug requires careful titration of dose and monitoring of plasma concentration.

TOCAINIDE

Tocainide is a primary amine analog of lidocaine that lacks two ethyl groups; this characteristic protects it from first-pass hepatic elimination and makes it effective orally.[87]

ELECTROPHYSIOLOGICAL AND HEMODYNAMIC ACTIONS (Tables 23-4 and 23-5). Electrophysiological effects are virtually the same as those exerted by lidocaine and mexiletine. In patients with compensated left ventricular dysfunction, intravenous infusion of tocainide moderately decreases mean arterial pressure and slightly increases pulmonary and systemic vascular resistance and left ventricular end-diastolic pressure without altering heart rate, cardiac index, or left ventricular dP/dt. It has a small negative inotropic effect and increases peripheral vascular resistance slightly. Oral administration in patients after myocardial infarction does not appear to affect hemodynamic compensation adversely.

PHARMACOKINETICS. Bioavailability of tocainide is almost 100 per cent. The drug is rapidly and completely absorbed, yielding peak plasma concentrations 0.5 to 2 hours after oral ingestion. Approximately 40 per cent is excreted unchanged in the urine. It is not extensively bound by plasma proteins and there are no known active metabolites. Enantiomers may be more effective than the racemic mixture.[88,89] Mean elimination half-life is 11 hours in normal volunteers, possibly longer in patients. There appears to be no pharmacokinetic interaction with other drugs,[87] but caution must be used when combining drugs because of additive antiarrhythmic effects.

DOSAGE AND ADMINISTRATION. Oral regimens of 400 to 600 mg every 8 hours produce therapeutic plasma concentrations of 4 to 10 μg/ml. Dosing increases should not be made more often than every 3 or 4 days. Twice daily doses can be tried in patients who respond to dosing three times a day. Doses should be reduced in patients with heart failure, liver, or renal disease.

CLINICAL INDICATIONS. Although tocainide effectively reduces the frequency of premature ventricular complexes, it has been less effective in preventing chronic recurrent ventricular tachycardia-ventricular fibrillation in some but not all studies. Tocainide may be effective when mexiletine is not. Response to intravenous lidocaine may help predict an individual's response to oral tocainide. A recent study of 82 patients with drug-resistant ventricular tachyarrhythmias showed that tocainide was not very useful because of limited effectiveness and side effects.[90] Tocainide and mexiletine may be acceptable choices for patients with ventricular arrhythmias in whom the Q-T interval is prolonged.

ADVERSE EFFECTS. Adverse effects are dose-related, similar to those produced by lidocaine, and include nausea, vomiting, anorexia, tremulousness, memory impairment, skin rash, sweating, paresthesia, diplopia, dizziness, anxiety, and tinnitus. Dosing with meals may reduce side effects, possibly by reducing peak serum concentrations of the drug. Occasionally, tocainide may produce pulmonary fibrosis or induce or aggravate ventricular arrhythmias. Hematological disorders including agranulocytosis, bone marrow depression, leukopenia, hypoplastic anemia, and thrombocytopenia have been reported with an estimated incidence of 0.18 per cent and may seriously limit the use of tocainide.

PHENYTOIN (DIPHENYLHYDANTOIN)

Phenytoin was employed originally to treat seizure disorders. Its value as an antiarrhythmic agent remains limited.

ELECTROPHYSIOLOGICAL ACTIONS (Tables 23-4 and 23-5). Therapeutic concentrations of phenytoin do not alter the discharge rate of rabbit sinus nodal tissue but may depress normal automaticity in cardiac Purkinje fibers in vitro or spontaneous ventricular rate in vivo. Phenytoin effectively abolishes abnormal automaticity caused by digitalis-induced delayed afterdepolarizations in cardiac Purkinje fibers and suppresses certain digitalis-induced arrhythmias in man. Similar to lidocaine, phenytoin abbreviates Purkinje fiber action potential duration more than it shortens the effective refractory period, thus increasing the ratio of effective refractory period to action potential duration. Phenytoin can cause depolarized cells to repolarize by increasing potassium conductance and, in so doing, may increase the $\dot{V}_{max}$ of phase 0 in Purkinje fibers, particularly when these are depressed by digitalis. The rate of rise of action potentials initiated early in the relative refractory period is increased, as is membrane responsiveness, possibly reducing the chance for impaired conduction and block. Phenytoin may slow conduction at high potassium concentrations but minimally affects sinus discharge rate and AV conduction in man. As with other Class IB agents, it has little effect on $\dot{V}_{max}$ in normally polarized fibers at slow rates, and shows use-dependence and rapid kinetics for onset and termination of effects.

Some of phenytoin's antiarrhythmic effects may be neurally mediated, since phenytoin may reduce the increase in impulse traffic in cardiac sympathetic nerves caused by ouabain toxicity and protect against some arrhythmias when it is injected into the central nervous system. The drug may also modulate vagal efferent activity centrally. It has no peripheral cholinergic or beta-adrenergic blocking actions.

Phenytoin exerts minimal *hemodynamic effects*.

PHARMACOKINETICS (Table 23-5). The pharmacokinetics of phenytoin are less than ideal. Absorption following oral administration is incomplete and delayed and varies with the brand of drug. Plasma concentrations peak 8 to 12 hours after an oral dose. Ninety per cent of the drug is protein-bound. Phenytoin has limited solubility at physiologic pH, and intramuscular administration is associated with pain, muscle necrosis, sterile abscesses, and variable absorption. Therapeutic serum concentrations of phenytoin (10 to 20 μg/ml) are similar for treating both cardiac arrhythmias and epilepsy. Lower concentrations can suppress certain digitalis-induced arrhythmias or other arrhythmias when decreased plasma protein binding occurs (as in uremia), since a larger fraction of drug is free and pharmacologically active.

Over 90 per cent of a dose is hydroxylated in the liver to presumably inactive compounds. Some families have a genetically determined inability to hydroxylate phenytoin, while others have a higher than usual capability for hydroxylation. Elimination half-time is about 24 hours and can be slowed in the presence of liver disease or when phenytoin is administered concomitantly with drugs such as phenylbutazone, dicumarol, isoniazid, chloramphenicol, and phenothiazines that compete with phenytoin for hepatic enzymes (Table 23-2). Because of the large number of medications that can increase or decrease phenytoin levels during chronic therapy, phenytoin plasma concentration should be determined frequently when changes are made in other medications. In some patients, maintenance dose regimens of phenytoin are difficult to predict because the enzyme system that metabolizes phenytoin becomes saturated at plasma concentrations within the therapeutic range. The half-life then increases with increasing phenytoin load. Above the saturation point, phenytoin elimination follows zero-order kinetics, so that only a fixed amount of drug is eliminated per unit time. These concentration-dependent kinetics for elimination can cause unexpected toxicity, since disproportionately large changes in plasma concentration can follow dose increases.

DOSAGE AND ADMINISTRATION (Table 23–5). To achieve therapeutic plasma concentration rapidly, 100 mg of phenytoin should be administered intravenously every 5 minutes until the arrhythmia is controlled, about 1 gm has been given, or adverse side effects result. Generally, 700 to 1000 mg will control the arrhythmia. A large central vein should be used to avoid pain and development of phlebitis produced by the severely alkalotic (pH 11.0) vehicle in which phenytoin is dissolved. Orally, phenytoin is given as a loading dose of approximately 1000 mg the first day, 500 mg on the second and third days, and 400 mg daily thereafter. All maintenance doses can be given once or twice daily, depending on the brand, because of the long half-life of elimination.

CLINICAL INDICATIONS. Phenytoin has been used successfully to treat atrial and ventricular arrhythmias caused by digitalis toxicity but is much less effective in treating ventricular arrhythmias in patients with ischemic heart disease or with atrial arrhythmias not due to digitalis toxicity. The drug has been somewhat more successful in treating ventricular arrhythmias associated with general anesthesia and cardiac surgery. It can be tried in patients with the long Q-T syndrome.

ADVERSE EFFECTS. The most common manifestations of phenytoin toxicity are central nervous system effects of nystagmus, ataxia, drowsiness, stupor, and coma. Progression of such symptoms can be correlated with increases in plasma drug concentration. Neurological signs, such as nystagmus on lateral gaze, develop at plasma drug levels of about 20 μg/ml. Nausea, epigastric pain, and anorexia are also relatively common effects of phenytoin. Long-term administration can result in hyperglycemia, hypocalcemia, skin rashes, megaloblastic anemia, gingival hypertrophy, lymph node hyperplasia (a syndrome resembling malignant lymphoma), peripheral neuropathy, and drug-induced systemic lupus erythematosus.

MORICIZINE HCl (ETHMOZINE)

Moricizine HCl is a phenothiazine developed in the Soviet Union that has been approved by the FDA for treatment of patients with ventricular tachyarrhythmias. It is being discussed as a IB antiarrhythmic drug because it shortens Purkinje fiber action potential. However, the intensity of its effect on the Na^+ channel is more like that of a IA antiarrhythmic drug.[90a]

ELECTROPHYSIOLOGICAL ACTIONS. Moricizine decreases I_{Na} and, therefore, $\dot{V}_{max}$ of phase 0, action potential amplitude and action potential duration in canine cardiac Purkinje fibers (Tables 23–4 and 23–5). Maximum diastolic potential is not changed.[91] In patients with ventricular tachycardia, moricizine prolongs AV nodal (about 10 per cent) and His-Purkinje (about 25 per cent) conduction time, and QRS duration (about 15 per cent). The J-T interval shortens slightly, while the $Q\text{-}T_c$ prolongs <5 per cent due to QRS prolongation. Ventricular refractoriness prolongs slightly with no consistent atrial change.[92] No alterations in sinus node automaticity result. In vitro, moricizine suppresses abnormal automaticity arising from depolarized fibers and delayed afterdepolarizations.

HEMODYNAMIC EFFECTS. Moricizine exerts minimal effects on cardiac performance in patients with impaired left ventricular function. Exercise tolerance and ejection fraction do not change. A small but consistent increase in blood pressure and heart rate result. An occasional patient with significant left ventricular dysfunction may have worsening of heart failure.[92,93]

PHARMACOKINETICS. Following oral ingestion, moricizine undergoes extensive first pass metabolism resulting in absolute bioavailability of 35 to 40 per cent. Peak plasma concentrations are reached in 0.5 to 2 hours and later if the drug is taken after meals. Extent of absorption is not changed. Proportionality exists between dose and plasma concentrations in the therapeutic range. Protein binding is 95 per cent. Antiarrhythmic and electrophysiological actions do not relate to plasma concentrations, or to any identified metabolite, of which there are more than 20. At least two metabolites are pharmacologically active but are in small concentrations. Moricizine induces its own metabolism, and plasma concentrations decrease with multiple dosing. Plasma half-life is 1.5 to 3.5 hours, with slightly more than half of the drug excreted in the feces and slightly less than half excreted in the urine.

DOSAGE AND ADMINISTRATION. The usual adult dose is 600 to 900 mg/day, given every 8 hours in three equally divided doses. Increments of 150 mg/day at 3-day intervals can be tried. Some patients may be treated every 12 hours. Dose reductions in patients with hepatic or neural disease, AV conduction disturbances, or sick sinus syndrome without a pacemaker and significant congestive heart failure should be observed.

CLINICAL INDICATIONS. Moricizine suppresses 50 to 70 per cent of spontaneous premature ventricular complexes (PVCs) in about 70 per cent of the patients treated. It exerts an efficacy comparable to quinidine and disopyramide. It prevents spontaneous ventricular tachycardia recurrence in about 50 per cent of patients[94] but is less effective in preventing ventricular tachycardia initiation at electrophysiologic study. In contrast to the effects of flecainide and encainide, moricizine did not lead to an increase in mortality in the Cardiac Arrhythmia Suppression Trial[29] and the study has been continued with this drug.

ADVERSE EFFECTS. Usually the drug is well tolerated. Noncardiac adverse effects primarily involve the nervous system and include tremor, mood changes, headache, vertigo, nystagmus, and dizziness. Gastrointestinal side effects include nausea, vomiting, and diarrhea. Worsening of congestive heart failure is uncommon. Proarrhythmic effects occurred in 3.2 per cent of 908 patients and appeared to be more common in patients with severe ventricular arrhythmias.[95]

CLASS IC ANTIARRHYTHMIC AGENTS

ENCAINIDE

Encainide has been approved by the FDA for treatment of patients with life-threatening ventricular arrhythmias.

ELECTROPHYSIOLOGICAL ACTIONS (Tables 23–4 and 23–5). Encainide resembles flecainide electrophysiologically. It produces more slowing of conduction and less prolongation of the refractory period than do Class IA drugs. The rate-dependent block of the fast sodium channel has slow onset and offset kinetics and is greater in depolarized fibers.[6,96–99] It shortens the action potential duration of Purkinje fibers but exerts little effect on atrial or ventricular muscle. It markedly slows conduction in all cardiac tissue, ischemic more than normal, at fast rates more than slow rates (use-dependent block). Encainide does not affect the slow response in vitro. Encainide is metabolized by debrisoquine-4 hydroxylase, the presence of which is genetically determined (see earlier discussion). It has several active metabolites that contribute to its antiarrhythmic efficacy[99] and proarrhythmic response.[97] Variation in the conversion of encainide to its active metabolites may be a source of interpatient differences in drug response. In patients, oral encainide prolongs atrial, ventricular, and accessory pathway refractory periods, A-H and H-V intervals, P-R, QRS, and Q-T intervals. Sodium loading can partially reverse the conduction slowing produced by o-desmethyl encainide acutely.[100]

HEMODYNAMIC EFFECTS. While most published studies[101] indicate that encainide exerts no important effects on cardiac dynamics, in a report on 30 patients with severe left ventricular failure (EF <40 per cent, NYHA Classes III and IV), investigators found that a single oral dose of 50 mg reduced stroke work and cardiac index and increased left ventricular filling pressure. Eight patients had worsening of symptoms. Therefore, encainide can cause adverse hemodynamic and clinical effects in patients with severe chronic heart failure.[102a]

PHARMACOKINETICS. Encainide exhibits a wide range of bioavailability and a relatively short half-life of 3 to 4 hours. However, the existence of at least two active metabolites (o-desmethyl and 3-methoxy-o-desmethyl encainide) permits a long interval between dosing during which the concentration of encainide metabolites exceeds that of the parent compound and is probably responsible for the prolonged antiarrhythmic action. Metabolism of encainide is genetically determined. Encainide and metabolites are more than 75 per cent protein bound. In patients with renal disease, the oral dosage should be reduced.

DOSAGE AND ADMINISTRATION. Encainide is generally administered beginning with 25 mg orally every eight hours, in increments until 35 mg tid and then 50 mg tid are reached. Daily dosage generally should not exceed 200 mg and dose changes should not be made more often than every 3 to 5 days, which is the time required to achieve steady state. Treatment should be done in hospital in a monitored area. Rapid dose escalation should be avoided.

CLINICAL INDICATIONS. Encainide is indicated for the treatment of patients with threatening ventricular tachyarrhythmias,[102b] but only a small percentage of patients have noninducible ventricular tachycardia after treatment.[102c] However, it is important to emphasize that in controlled trials, there are no data to indicate that this drug, nor any other class I antiarrhythmic agent, favorably affects survival or sudden cardiac death. Although not FDA-approved for treating patients with supraventricular tachyarrhythmias, encainide is effective in suppressing AV reciprocating tachycardias by prolonging conduction time and refractoriness in the AV node and accessory pathway,[102] for treating patients with atrial fibrillation and the WPW syndrome,[103] and for treating patients with AV nodal reentrant tachycardia.[104,105] Isoproterenol can reverse some of encainide's effects.[106] Encainide may also be useful in treating chronic ectopic atrial and junctional tachycardia[107] and supraventricular tachycardias in children.[108]

ADVERSE EFFECTS. Adverse effects include dizziness, diplopia, vertigo, paresthesia, leg cramps, and a metallic taste in the mouth. Sinus arrest[109] or AV block may occur. Most significant is encainide's potential to cause or exacerbate serious ventricular tachyarrhythmias in approximately 10 per cent of patients treated. Commonly, a polymorphous ventricular tachycardia not usually associated with marked Q-T prolongation ensues and may result in hemodynamic collapse. It may be difficult to terminate electrically. Ventricular proarrhythmia occurs more often in patients with a history of sustained ventricular tachycardia, structural heart disease, or congestive heart failure. In the Cardiac Arrhythmia Suppression Trial, patients treated with encainide experienced 9.6 per cent mortality or nonfatal cardiac arrest compared with 3.6 per cent in the placebo group over a period of 10 months.[24,29,110,111]

FLECAINIDE

Flecainide is approved by the FDA for the treatment of patients with life-threatening ventricular arrhythmias.

ELECTROPHYSIOLOGICAL ACTIONS. Flecainide exhibits marked use-dependent depressant effects on the rapid sodium channel, decreasing V_{max} with slow onset and offset kinetics. Drug dissociation from the sodium channel is very slow, with time constants of 10 to 30 sec (compared with 4 to 8 sec for quinidine and <1 second for lidocaine). Marked drug effects occur at physiological heart rates. Flecainide shortens the duration of Purkinje fiber action potential but prolongs it in ventricular muscle, actions that, depending on the circumstances, could enhance or reduce electrical heterogeneity and create or suppress arrhythmias. Flecainide profoundly slows conduction in all cardiac fibers, and, in high concentrations, inhibits the slow channel. Conduction time in the atria, ventricles, AV node, and His-Purkinje system is prolonged. Minimal increases in atrial or ventricular refractoriness, or in the Q-T interval, result. Anterograde and retrograde refractoriness in accessory pathways can increase by 100 msec or more. Normal sinus node function remains unchanged, but abnormal sinus node discharge may be depressed. Its actions are very similar to those of encainide.

HEMODYNAMIC EFFECTS. Flecainide depresses cardiac performance, particularly in patients with compromised myocardial function. Left ventricular ejection fraction decreases after oral (single dose of 200 to 250 mg) or intravenous (1 mg) administration. Caution is warranted, particularly in patients with a history of heart failure. Flecainide should be used cautiously, if at all, in patients with severely compromised cardiac function.

PHARMACOKINETICS. Flecainide is at least 90 per cent absorbed with peak plasma concentrations in 3 to 4 hours. Elimination half-life in patients with ventricular arrhythmias is 20 hours, 85 per cent of the drug being excreted unchanged or as an inactive metabolite in urine. Two major metabolites exert less effects than the parent drug. Rate of elimination is slower in patients with renal disease and heart failure and doses should be reduced in these situations. Therapeutic plasma concentrations range from 0.2 to 1.0 μg/ml. About 40 per cent of the drug is protein bound. Small increases in serum concentrations of digoxin (13 per cent) and propranolol (30 per cent) result during co-administration with flecainide. Propranolol may increase flecainide serum concentration and both drugs may produce combined detrimental hemodynamic effects. Five to 7 days of dosing may be required to reach steady-state in some patients.

DOSAGE AND ADMINISTRATION. Starting dose is 100 mg every 12 hours, increased in increments of 50 mg twice daily, no sooner than every 4 days, until efficacy is achieved, an adverse effect is noted, or to a maximum of 400 mg/day.

CLINICAL INDICATIONS. Flecainide is indicated for the treatment of life-threatening ventricular tachyarrhythmias. Therapy should begin in the hospital while the ECG is being monitored because of the high incidence of proarrhythmia events (see below). Serum concentration should not exceed 1.0 μg/ml. Flecainide is particularly effective, more so than quinidine, in almost totally suppressing premature ventricular complexes and short runs of nonsustained ventricular tachycardia,[112] although the importance of such a response on the subsequent outcome of the patient has not been established. As with encainide and all other class I antiarrhythmic drugs, there are no data from controlled studies to indicate that the drug favorably affects survival or sudden cardiac death. Flecainide prevents electrical induction of ventricular tachyarrhythmias in a small percentage of patients (10 to 30 per cent)[102c,113] and eliminates recurrence of life-threatening ventricular tachyarrhythmias in about 40 per cent. Flecainide may be very useful in patients with AV nodal reentry tachycardias and other supraventricular tachycardias.[114,115] Isoproterenol can reverse some of these effects.[116]

ADVERSE EFFECTS. Proarrhythmic effects are one of the most important adverse effects of flecainide.[102c] Its marked slowing of conduction precludes its use in patients with second degree AV block without a pacemaker and warrants cautious administration in patients with intraventricular conduction disorders. Aggravation of existing ventricular arrhythmias or onset of new ventricular arrhythmias can occur in 5 to 30 per cent of patients, the increased percentage in patients with preexisting sustained ventricular tachycardia, cardiac decompensation, and higher doses of the drug. Failure of the flecainide-related arrhythmia to respond to therapy, including electrical cardioversion-defibrillation, may result in a mortality as high as 10 per cent in patients who develop proarrhythmic events. Negative inotropic effects can cause or worsen heart failure. Patients with sinus node dysfunction may experience sinus arrest and those with pacemakers may develop an increase in pacing threshold. In the Cardiac Arrhythmia Suppression Trial, patients treated with flecainide had 5.1 per cent mortality or nonfatal cardiac arrest compared with 2.3 per cent in the placebo group over 10 months.[29] Exercise can amplify the conduction slowing in the ventricle produced by flecainide[117] and in some cases can precipitate a proarrhythmic response.[118] Central nervous system complaints, including confusion and irritability, represent the most frequent noncardiac adverse effect.

PROPAFENONE

Propafenone has recently been approved by the FDA for treatment of patients with life-threatening ventricular tachyrhythmias.[119]

ELECTROPHYSIOLOGICAL ACTIONS (Tables 23–4 and 23–5). Propafenone blocks the fast sodium current in a use-dependent manner, as well as at rest, in Purkinje fibers and to a lesser degree in ventricular muscle. The dissociation constant is slow, like that of encainide and flecainide. Effects are greater in ischemic than normal tissue and at reduced membrane potentials. Propafenone decreases excitability and suppresses spontaneous automaticity and triggered activity. Effects on action potential duration are variable in that guinea pig action potential duration is shortened while rabbit action potential duration is prolonged. Although ventricular refractoriness increases, conduction slowing is the major effect. The active metabolites of propafenone exert important actions,[120] reducing $\dot{V}_{max}$, action potential amplitude, and duration in canine Purkinje fibers.[121] In contrast to propafenone and the N-depropylpropafenone metabolite, the 5-hydroxypropafenone metabolite suppressed ventricular tachycardia in the postinfarct canine model.[121] Propafenone depresses sinus nodal automaticity. In patients, the A-H, H-V, P-R, and QRS intervals increase, as do refractory periods of the atria, ventricles, AV node and accessory pathways.[119] The corrected Q-T interval increases only as a function of increased QRS duration.

HEMODYNAMIC EFFECTS. Propafenone and 5-hydroxypropafenone exhibit negative inotropic properties at high concentrations in vitro, and large doses depress left ventricular function in vivo.[119] In patients with ejection fractions exceeding 40 per cent, the negative inotropic effects are well tolerated, but patients with preexisting left ventricular dysfunction and congestive heart failure may have symptomatic worsening of their hemodynamic status.

PHARMACOKINETICS. With more than 95 per cent of the drug absorbed, propafenone's maximum plasma concentration occurs in 2 to 3 hours. Systemic bioavailability is dose dependent and ranges from 3 to 40 per cent due to extensive presystemic clearance. Bioavailability increases as the dose increases and plasma concentration is therefore nonlinear. A threefold increase in dosage (300 to 900 mg/day) results in a tenfold increase in plasma concentration, presumably due to saturation of hepatic metabolic mechanisms. Propafenone is 97 per cent bound to alpha$_1$-acid glycoprotein with an elimination half-life of 5 to 8 hours. Maximum therapeutic effects occur at serum concentrations of 0.2 to 1.5 μg/ml. Marked interpatient variability of pharmacokinetics and pharmacodynamics may be due to genetically determined differences in metabolism. About 93 per cent of the population are extensive metabolizers and exhibit shorter elimination half-lives (5 to 6 hours), lower plasma concentration of the parent compound, and higher concentrations of metabolites. Poor metabolizers, due to diminished capacity of the microsomal cytochrome P-450 enzyme system in the liver (see earlier), exhibit an elimination half-life of 15 to 20 hours for the parent compound and virtually no 5-hydroxypropafenone. Low-dose quinidine may inhibit the metabolism of propafenone, and stereoselectivity may be important with the (+) -s enantiomer, providing nonspecific beta adrenergic receptor blockade[122] approximately 2.5 to 5 per cent the potency of propranolol. Poor metabolizers have a greater beta-adrenergic receptor blocking effect than extensive metabolizers.[123] Since plasma propafenone concentrations may be 50 times or more propranolol levels, these beta blocking properties may be relevant. Propafenone also blocks the slow calcium channel to a degree about 100 times less than verapamil.

DOSAGE AND ADMINISTRATION. Most patients respond to oral doses of 150 to 300 mg every 8 hours, not exceeding 1200 mg/day. Doses are similar for both phenotype patients. Concomitant food administration increases bioavailability, as does hepatic dysfunction. No good correlation between plasma propafenone concentration and arrhythmia suppression has been shown. Doses should not be increased more often than every 3 to 4 days. Propafenone increases plasma concentrations of warfarin, digoxin, and metoprolol.

CLINICAL INDICATIONS. Propafenone is indicated for the treatment of life-threatening ventricular tachyarrhythmias and effectively suppresses spontaneous premature ventricular complexes and nonsustained and sustained ventricular tachycardia.[119,124] Spontaneous sinus rate during exercise is reduced. Although propafenone has not been approved by the FDA for treatment of patients with supraventricular tachycardias, the drug is effective in patients with AV nodal reentry, AV reentry,[119,125] and atrial flutter/fibrillation.[126,127]

ADVERSE EFFECTS. Minor, noncardiac effects occur in about 15 per cent of patients, with dizziness, disturbances in taste, and blurred vision the most common, and gastrointestinal side effects next. Exacerbation of bronchospastic lung disease can occur. Cardiovascular side effects occur in 13 per cent of patients, including conduction abnormalities such as AV block, sinus node depression, and worsening of heart failure. Proarrhythmic responses, more often in patients with a history of sustained ventricular tachycardia and decreased ejection fractions, appear less common than with flecainide and encainide, and may be in the range of 5 per cent. The applicability of data from the Cardiac Arrhythmic Suppression Trial about flecainide and encainide to propafenone is not clear but limiting propafenone's application in a manner similar to other IC drugs seems prudent at present until more information is available.[24]

CLASS II ANTIARRHYTHMIC AGENTS

BETA-ADRENORECEPTOR BLOCKING AGENTS

Although 11 beta-adrenoreceptor blocking drugs have been approved for use in the United States (Table 40–3, p. 1308), only acebutolol (PVCs), esmolol (SVT), metoprolol (post myocardial infarction), propranolol (post myocardial infarction, SVT, VT) and timolol (post myocardial infarction) have been approved to treat arrhythmias or to prevent sudden death after myocardial infarction. While it is generally considered that no beta blocker offers distinct advantages over the others and that, when titrated to the proper dose, all can be used effectively to treat cardiac arrhythmias, hypertension, or other disorders, differences in pharmacokinetic or pharmacodynamic properties that confer safety, reduce adverse effects, or affect dosing intervals or drug interactions influence the choice of agent. Also, some beta blockers such as sotalol exert unique actions.

Beta receptors can be separated into those that affect predominantly the heart (beta$_1$) or the bronchi and blood vessels (beta$_2$). In low doses, selective beta blockers can block beta$_1$ receptors more than they block beta$_2$ receptors and might be preferable for treating patients with pulmonary or peripheral vascular diseases. In high doses, the selective beta$_1$ blockers also block beta$_2$ receptors.

Some beta blockers exert intrinsic sympathomimetic activity, i.e., they slightly activate the beta receptor. These drugs appear to be as efficacious as beta blockers without intrinsic sympathomimetic actions and may cause less slowing of heart rate at rest and less prolongation of AV nodal conduction time.[128] They have been shown to induce less depression of left ventricular function than beta blockers without intrinsic sympathomimetic activity. Beta blockers with intrinsic sympathomimetic activity have not been shown to reduce mortality in patients after myocardial infarction.

The following discussion will concentrate on the use of propranolol as a prototypical antiarrhythmic agent. Acebutolol and esmolol will be considered briefly under clinical indications.

ELECTROPHYSIOLOGICAL ACTIONS. Beta blockers may exert an electrophysiological action by competitively inhibiting catecholamine binding at beta-adrenoreceptor sites, an effect almost entirely due to the (−) levorotatory stereoisomer, or by their quinidine-like or direct membrane-stabilizing action. (Tables 23–4 and 23–5). The latter is a local anesthetic effect that depresses I_{Na} and membrane responsiveness in cardiac Purkinje fibers, occurs at concentrations generally 10 times that necessary to produce beta blockade, and most likely plays an insignificant antiarrhythmic role. At beta-blocking concentrations, propranolol slows spontaneous automaticity in the sinus node or in Purkinje fibers that are being stimulated by adrenergic tone. In the absence of adrenergic tone, only high concentrations of propranolol slow normal automaticity in Purkinje fibers, probably by a direct membrane action. Concentrations that cause beta-receptor blockade but no local anesthetic effects do not alter the normal resting membrane potential, maximum diastolic potential, amplitude, $\dot{V}_{max}$, repolarization, or refractoriness of atrial, Purkinje, or ventricular muscle cells when these tissues are not being superfused with catecholamines. However, in the presence of isoproterenol, a pure beta-receptor stimulator, beta blockers reverse isoproterenol's accelerating effects on repolarization; in the presence of norepinephrine, beta blockade permits unopposed alpha-adrenoreceptor stimulation to prolong action potential duration in Purkinje fibers. Propranolol (2×10^{-6}M) reduces the amplitude of digitalis-induced delayed afterdepolarizations and suppresses triggered activity in Purkinje fibers.

Propranolol up-regulates beta adrenoreceptors in part by externalizing receptors from a light vesicle fraction to the sarcolemma. Ischemia does not further alter receptor distribution and therefore propranolol-treated animals show blunting in externalization of beta receptors, which may contribute to propranolol's beneficial effects during ischemia.[129]

Concentrations exceeding 3 μg/ml are required to depress $\dot{V}_{max}$ action potential amplitude, membrane responsiveness, and conduction in normal atrial, ventricular, and Purkinje fibers without altering resting membrane potential. These effects probably result from depression of sodium conductance. The direct effect of propranolol shortens the action potential duration of Purkinje fibers and, to a lesser extent, of atrial and ventricular muscle fibers. Long-term administration of propranolol may lengthen action potential duration. Similar to the effects of lidocaine, acceleration of repolarization of Purkinje fibers is most marked in areas of the ventricular conduction system in which the action potential duration is greatest. The reduction in refractory period is not as great as the reduction in action potential duration (effective refractory period duration/action potential duration >1.0). At least one beta blocker, sotalol, markedly increases the time course of repolarization in Purkinje fibers and ventricular muscle (p. 1308). Smaller doses of propranolol are required to prevent sympathetically induced shortening of ventricular refractoriness than are required to prevent sympathetically induced sinus acceleration.[130]

Propranolol slows the sinus discharge rate in humans by 10 to 20 per cent, while severe bradycardia occasionally results if the heart is particularly dependent on sympathetic tone or if sinus node dysfunction is present. The slowing is probably due to beta blockade because D-propranolol does not significantly slow the sinus discharge rate in doses comparable to the racemic mixture. The P-R interval lengthens, as does AV nodal conduction time and refractoriness (if the heart rate is maintained constant), but refractoriness and conduction in the normal His-Purkinje system remain unchanged even after high doses of propranolol. Therefore, therapeutic doses of propranolol in humans do not exert a direct depressant or "quinidine-like" action but influence cardiac electrophysiology via a beta-blocking action. Beta blockers do not affect conduction in ventricular muscle, as evidenced by their lack of effect on the QRS complex, and they insignificantly prolong the right ventricular effective refractory period and uncorrected Q-T interval.

Because administration of beta blockers that do not have direct membrane action prevents many arrhythmias resulting from activation of the autonomic nervous system, it is thought that the beta-blocking action is responsible for their antiarrhythmic effects. However, the possible importance of direct membrane effect of some of these drugs cannot be discounted totally because beta blockers with direct membrane actions can affect transmembrane potentials of diseased cardiac fibers at much lower concentrations than are needed to affect normal fibers directly. In addition, the role of important metabolites of propranolol and other beta blockers that may exert electrophysiological actions is not clearly established. Finally, indirect actions on arrhythmogenic effects of ischemia[129,131] or the autonomic nervous system[132,132a] may be important.

HEMODYNAMIC EFFECTS. Beta blockers exert negative inotropic effects and can precipitate or worsen heart failure. By blocking beta receptors, these drugs may cause peripheral vasoconstriction and exacerbate coronary artery spasm in some patients.

PHARMACOKINETICS (Table 23–1). Although various types of beta blockers exert similar pharmacological effects, their pharmacokinetics differ substantially. Propranolol is almost 100 per cent absorbed, but the effects of first-pass hepatic metabolism reduce bioavailability to about 30 per cent and produce significant interpatient variability of plasma concentration for a given dose. Reduction in hepatic blood flow, as in patients with heart failure, decreases the hepatic extraction of propranolol, and in these patients propranolol may further decrease its own elimination rate by reducing cardiac output and hepatic blood flow. Beta blockers eliminated by the kidney tend to have longer half-lives and exhibit less interpatient variability of drug concentration than do those beta blockers metabolized by the liver.

DOSAGE AND ADMINISTRATION (Table 23–5). The appropriate dose of propranolol is best determined by a measure of the patient's physiological response, such as changes in resting heart rate or in the prevention of exercise-induced tachycardia, since wide individual differences exist between the observed physiological effect and plasma concentration. For example, intravenous dosing is best achieved by titrating the dose to a clinical effect, beginning with doses of 0.25 to 0.50 mg, increasing to 1.0 mg if necessary, and administering doses every 5 minutes until either a desired effect or toxicity is produced or a total of 0.15 to 0.20 mg/kg has been given. Orally, propranolol is given in four divided doses, usually ranging from 40 to 160 mg a day to more than 1 gram a day. Generally, if one agent in adequate doses proves to be ineffective, other beta blockers will be ineffective also.

CLINICAL INDICATIONS. Arrhythmias associated with thyrotoxicosis, pheochromocytoma, and anesthesia with cyclopropane or halothane or arrhythmias largely due to excessive cardiac adrenergic stimulation, such as those initiated by exercise or emotion, often respond to propranolol therapy. Beta-blocking drugs usually do not convert chronic atrial flutter or atrial fibrillation to normal sinus rhythm but may do so if the arrhythmia is of recent onset. The rate of the atrial flutter/fibrillation is not changed, but the ventricular response decreases because beta blockade prolongs AV nodal conduction time and refractoriness. For reentrant supraventricular tachycardias using the AV node as one of the reentrant pathways, such as AV nodal reentrant tachycardia and reciprocating tachycardias in Wolff-Parkinson-White syndrome, or for sinus reentrant tachycardia, propranolol may terminate the tachycardia and be used prophylactically to prevent a recurrence. Combining propranolol with digitalis, quinidine, or a variety of other agents may be effective when propranolol as a single agent fails. *Metoprolol* may be useful in patients with multifocal atrial tachycardia.[133]

Propranolol may be effective for digitalis-induced arrhythmias such as atrial tachycardia, nonparoxysmal AV junctional tachycardia, premature ventricular complexes, or ventricular tachycardia. If a significant degree of AV block is present during a digitalis-induced arrhythmia, lidocaine or phenytoin may be preferable to propranolol. Propranolol may also be useful to treat ventricular arrhythmias associated with the prolonged Q-T interval syndrome[134] and with mitral valve prolapse.[135] For patients with ischemic heart disease, propranolol generally does not prevent episodes of chronic recurrent ventricular tachycardia that occur in the absence of acute ischemia, but may be effective in some patients,[136] usually at a beta blocking concentration.[137] It is well accepted that propranolol, timolol and metoprolol reduce the incidence of overall death and sudden cardiac death after myocardial infarction. The mechanism of this reduction in mortality is not entirely clear and may relate to reduction in the extent of ischemic damage, autonomic effects, a direct antiarrhythmic effect, or combinations of these factors.[132a,138–140]

Acebutolol is a cardioselective (β_1) beta-adrenoreceptor blocker with mild intrinsic sympathomimetic activity demonstrated to reduce the incidence of premature ventricular complexes in controlled studies. *Esmolol* is an ultra-short-acting (elimination half-life 9 minutes) cardioselective beta-adrenoreceptor blocker useful for the rapid control of the ventricular rate in patients with atrial flutter/fibrillation.

ADVERSE EFFECTS. Adverse cardiovascular effects from propranolol include unacceptable hypotension, bradycardia, and congestive heart failure. The bradycardia may be due to sinus bradycardia or AV block. Sudden withdrawal of propranolol in patients with angina pectoris can precipitate worsening of angina, cardiac arrhythmias, and acute myocardial infarction, possibly owing to heightened sensitivity to beta agonists caused by previous beta blockade (up-regulation). Heightened sensitivity may begin several days after cessation of propranolol therapy and may last 5 or 6 days. Other adverse effects of propranolol include worsening of asthma or chronic obstructive pulmonary disease, intermittent claudication, Raynaud's phenomenon, mental depression, increased risk of hypoglycemia among insulin-dependent diabetic patients, easy fatigability, disturbingly vivid dreams or insomnia, and impaired sexual function.

CLASS III ANTIARRHYTHMIC AGENTS

AMIODARONE

Amiodarone is a benzofuran derivative approved by the FDA for the treatment of patients with life-threatening ventricular tachyarrhythmias when other drugs are ineffective or are not tolerated.

ELECTROPHYSIOLOGICAL ACTIONS (Tables 23–4 and 23–5). When chronically given orally, amiodarone prolongs action potential duration and refractoriness of all cardiac fibers[141] without affecting resting membrane potential. When acute effects are evaluated, amiodarone and its metabolite, desethylamiodarone, prolong the action potential duration of ventricular muscle but shorten the action potential duration of Purkinje fibers. Injected into the sinus and AV nodal arteries, amiodarone reduces sinus and junctional discharge rates and prolongs AV nodal conduction time. It decreases the slope of diastolic depolarization of the sinus node and markedly depresses $\dot{V}_{max}$ in guinea pig papillary muscle in a rate- or use-dependent manner. Such depression of $\dot{V}_{max}$ is caused by blocking of inactivated sodium channels, an effect that is accentuated by depolarized, and reduced by hyperpolarized, membrane potentials. Amiodarone also inhibits depolarization-induced automaticity. Amiodarone depresses conduction at fast rates more than at slow rates (use dependence),[142–144] not only by depressing $\dot{V}_{max}$ but also by increasing resistance to passive current flow.[145] Desethylamiodarone has relatively greater effects on fast channel tissue and probably contributes importantly to antiarrhythmic efficacy.[146,147] The delay to build up adequate concentrations of this metabolite may explain in part the delay in amiodarone's antiarrhythmic action.

In vivo, amiodarone noncompetitively antagonizes alpha and beta receptors and blocks conversion of thyroxine (T_4) to triiodothyronine (T_3), which may account for some of its electrophysiologic effects.[148] Amiodarone exhibits slow-channel blocking effects and chronic oral therapy slows the spontaneous sinus nodal discharge rate in anesthetized dogs even after pretreatment with propranolol and atropine. With oral administration it prolongs the Q-T interval, at times changing the contour of the T wave and producing U waves, and slows the sinus rate by 20 to 30 per cent. Effective refractory periods of all cardiac tissues are prolonged. His-Purkinje conduction time increases and QRS duration lengthens, especially at fast rates. Amiodarone given intravenously modestly prolongs the refractory period of atrial and ventricular muscle. P-R interval and AV nodal conduction time lengthen. The duration of the QRS complex lengthens at increased rates but less than after oral amiodarone. Thus, far less increase in prolongation of conduction time (except for the AV node), duration of repolarization, and refractoriness occur after intravenous administration, compared with the oral route. Considering these actions, it is clear that amiodarone has Class I (blocks Na channel), Class II (antiadrenergic), and Class IV (blocks Ca^{++} channel) actions,[148a] in addition to Class III effects. Amiodarone's actions approximate those of a theoretically ideal drug that exhibits use dependence of Na^+ channels with fast diastolic recovery from block and use-dependent prolongation of action potential duration.[46]

HEMODYNAMIC EFFECTS. Amiodarone is a peripheral and coronary vasodilator. When administered intravenously in doses of 2.5 to 10 mg/kg, amiodarone decreases heart rate, systemic vascular resistance, left ventricular contractile force, and left ventricular dP/dt. Left ventricular output may increase. Oral doses of amiodarone sufficient to control cardiac arrhythmias do not depress left ventricular ejection fraction, even in patients with reduced ejection fractions measured by radionuclide ventriculography. However, because amiodarone antiadrenergic actions may block I_{si} to some degree, and does exert some negative inotropic action, it should be given cautiously, particularly intravenously,[149] to patients with marginal cardiac compensation.

PHARMACOKINETICS. Amiodarone is slowly, variably, and incompletely absorbed, with systemic bioavailability of 35 to 65 per cent. Plasma concentrations peak 3 to 7 hours after a single oral dose. There is minimal first-pass effect, indicating little hepatic extraction. Elimination is by hepatic excretion into bile with some enterohepatic recirculation. Extensive hepatic metabolism occurs with desethylamiodarone as a major metabolite. The plasma concentration ratio of parent to metabolite is 3 : 2. Both extensively accumulate in liver, lung, fat, "blue" skin, and other tissues. Myocardium develops a concentration 10 to 50 times that found in the plasma. Plasma clearance of amiodarone is low and renal excretion negligible. Doses need not be reduced in patients with renal disease. Amiodarone and desethylamiodarone are not dialyzable. Volume of distribution is large but variable, averaging 60 liters/kg. Amiodarone is highly protein-bound (96 per cent), crosses the placenta (10 to 50 per cent), and is found in breast milk.

The onset of action after intravenous administration generally is within several hours.[149,150] Following oral administration the onset of action may require 2 to 3 days, often 1 to 3 weeks and, on occasion, even longer. Loading doses reduce this time interval. Plasma concentrations relate well to oral doses during chronic treatment, averaging about 0.5 μg/ml for each 100 mg/day at doses between 100 and 600 mg/day. Elimination half-life is multiphasic with an initial 50 per cent reduction in plasma concentration 3 to 10 days after cessation of drug ingestion (probably representing elimination from well-perfused tissues) followed by a terminal half-life of 26 to 107 days (mean 53 days), with most patients in the 40- to 55-day range. To achieve steady-state without a loading dose takes about 265 days. Interpatient variability of these pharmacokinetic parameters mandates close monitoring of the patient. Therapeutic serum concentrations range from 1 to 2.5 μg/ml. Greater suppression of arrhythmias may occur up to 3.5 μg/ml, but the risk of side effects increases.

DOSAGE AND ADMINISTRATION. An optimal dosing schedule for all patients has not been achieved. One recommended approach is to treat with 800 to 1600 mg daily for 1 to 3 weeks, reduced to 800 mg daily for the next 2 to 4 weeks, then 600 mg daily for 4 to 8 weeks, and finally, after 2 to 3 months of treatment, a maintenance dose of 400 mg or less per day. Maintenance drug can be given once or twice daily, and should be titrated to the *lowest effective dose* to minimize the occurrence of side effects. Regimens must be individualized for a given patient and clinical situation. Amiodarone may be administered intravenously (not approved for this route of administration by the FDA at the time of this writing) to achieve more rapid loading and effect in emergencies[149,150] at initial doses of 5 to 10 mg/kg over 20 to 30 minutes, followed by 1 gm/24 hours for several days. Additional boluses of 1 to 3 mg/kg may be given several hours after the first bolus if necessary. An alternative approach is to infuse 2.0 to 2.5 mg/min for 12 hours followed by a maintenance dose of 0.7 mg/min for the next 36 hours. Patients with depressed ejection fractions should receive intravenous amiodarone with great caution. High-dose oral loading (800 to 2000 mg two or three times a day to maintain trough serum concentrations of 2 to 3 μg/ml) may suppress ventricular arrhythmias in 1 to 2 days.

CLINICAL INDICATIONS. Amiodarone has been used to suppress a wide spectrum of supraventricular[150–153] and ventricular[154–157] tachyarrhythmias in adults and children,[158] including AV nodal and AV entry, atrial flutter and fibrillation, ventricular tachycardia and ventricular fibrillation associated with coronary artery disease, and hypertrophic cardiomyopathy. Success rates vary widely depending on patient population, arrhythmia, underlying heart disease, length of follow-up, definition and determination of success, and other factors. In general, however, amiodarone's efficacy equals[159] or exceeds that of all other antiarrhythmic agents, and may be in the range of 60 to 80 per cent for most supraventricular tachyarrhythmias (including those associated with the WPW syndrome) and 40 to 60 per cent for ventricular tachyarrhythmias. Amiodarone may be useful in improving survival in patients with hypertrophic cardiomyopathy,[160] asymptomatic ventricular arrhythmias after myocardial infarction[161] and after resuscitation for ventricular tachyarrhythmia.[162] Because of its long half-life and the difficulty involved in starting another antiarrhythmic drug (while not knowing if amiodarone's effects are still present), and its side effects profile, amiodarone is generally among the last antiarrhythmic agents tried.

Some controversy exists regarding the ability to predict effectiveness of amiodarone in patients with ventricular tachyarrhythmias. Clinical assessment, suppression of spontaneous ventricular arrhythmias as documented by 24-hour ECG recordings,[163] and response to electrophysiological testing have served as endpoints to judge therapy. In the patient with a history of sustained ventricular tachycardia or fibrillation and minimal spontaneous ventricular arrhythmias in between symptomatic episodes, an invasive electrophysiologic study is indicated to judge drug efficacy. The answer to when after amiodarone therapy is started such a study should be done is still not entirely resolved but probably should be 1 week or longer.[164–166] In the 10 to 40 per cent of patients whose electrically induced clinical ventricular tachyarrhythmias become no longer inducible while they are receiving amiodarone, the chances for a spontaneous recurrence of the arrhythmias are low while the patients are taking amiodarone, probably less than 5 to 10 per cent at 1 year. For those patients whose ventricular tachyarrhythmias are still inducible, the recurrence rate is 40 to 50 per cent at 1 year. However, in this latter group, greater difficulty in inducing the arrhythmias may predict a less likely possibility of a recurrence.[167] Patients' hemodynamic responses to the induced arrhythmia also may predict how they tolerate a spontaneous recurrence. It is important to remember, however, that the supine patient in the electrophysiology laboratory may tolerate the same tachycardia better than when in an erect position.

Because of the serious nature of the arrhythmias being treated, the unusual pharmacokinetics of the drug, and its adverse effects (see below), amiodarone therapy should be started with the patient hospitalized and monitored for generally a week or longer. Combining other antiarrhythmic agents with amiodarone may improve efficacy in some patients.[168–170]

ADVERSE EFFECTS. Adverse effects are reported by about 75 per cent of patients treated with amiodarone for 5 years[157] but compel stopping the drug in 18 per cent[156] to 37 per cent.[157] The most frequent side effects requiring drug discontinuation involve pulmonary and gastrointestinal complaints. Most adverse effects are reversible with dose reduction or cessation of treatment. Adverse effects become more frequent when therapy is continued long term. Of the noncardiac adverse reactions, pulmonary toxicity is the most serious; in one study it occurred between 6 days and 60 months of treatment in 33 of 573 patients, with 3 deaths.[171] The mechanism is unclear but may relate to a hypersensitivity reaction and/or widespread phospholipidosis. Dyspnea, nonproductive cough, and fever are common symptoms with rales, hypoxia, a positive gallium scan, reduced diffusion capacity, and radiographic evidence of pulmonary infiltrates noted. Amiodarone must be discontinued if such pulmonary inflammatory changes occur. Steroids can be tried but no controlled studies have been done to support their use. A 10 per cent mortality in patients with pulmonary inflammatory changes results, often in patients with unrecognized pulmonary involvement that is allowed to progress. Chest roentgenograms at 3-month intervals for a year and then twice a year have been recommended. At maintenance doses less than 300 mg daily, pulmonary toxicity is uncommon.[171] Advanced age, high drug maintenance dose and reduced predrug diffusion capacity (DL_{co}) are risk factors for developing pulmonary toxicity.[171] An unchanged DL_{co} volume may be a negative predictor of pulmonary toxicity.[172]

Although asymptomatic elevations of liver enzymes are found in most patients, the drug is not stopped unless values exceed two or three times normal in a patient with initially abnormal values. Cirrhosis occurs uncommonly but may be fatal. Neurological dysfunction, photosensitivity (perhaps minimized by sunscreens), bluish skin discoloration, corneal microdeposits (in almost 100 per cent of adults receiving the drug more than 6 months), gastroenterological disturbances, and hyperthyroidism (1 to 2 per cent) or hypothyroidism (2 to 4 per cent) can occur. Amiodarone appears to inhibit the peripheral conversion of T_4 to T_3 so that chemical changes result, characterized by a slight increase in T_4, reverse T_3 and TSH, and a slight decrease in T_3. Reverse T_3 concentration has been used as an index of drug efficacy. During hypothyroidism, TSH increases greatly while T_3 increases in hyperthyroidism.

Cardiac side effects include symptomatic bradycardias in about 2 per cent, aggravation of ventricular tachyarrhythmias (with occasional development of torsades de pointes) in 2 to 3 per cent, and worsening of congestive heart failure in 2 per cent. Possibly due to interactions with anesthetics, complications after open heart surgery have been noted, including pulmonary dysfunction, hypotension, hepatic dysfunction and low cardiac output.[173,174]

Important interactions with other drugs occur and, when given concomitantly with amiodarone, the dose of warfarin, digoxin, and other antiarrhythmic drugs should be reduced by one-third to one-half, and the patient watched closely.

Drugs with synergistic actions, such as beta blockers or calcium channel blockers, must be given cautiously.

BRETYLIUM TOSYLATE

Bretylium is a quaternary ammonium compound that is approved by the FDA for parenteral use only in patients with life threatening ventricular tachyarrhythmias.

ELECTROPHYSIOLOGICAL ACTIONS (Tables 23–4 and 23–5). Bretylium is selectively concentrated in sympathetic ganglia and their postganglionic adrenergic nerve terminals. After initially *causing* norepinephrine release, bretylium *prevents* norepinephrine release by depressing sympathetic nerve terminal excitability, without depressing pre- or postganglionic sympathetic nerve conduction, impairing conduction across sympathetic ganglia, depleting the adrenergic neuron of norepinephrine, or decreasing the responsiveness of adrenergic receptors. It produces a state resembling chemical sympathectomy. During chronic bretylium treatment, the beta-adrenergic responses to circulating catecholamines are increased. The initial release of catecholamines results in several transient electrophysiological responses such as an increase in the discharge rates of the isolated perfused sinus node and of in vitro Purkinje fibers, often making quiescent fibers automatic. Bretylium initially increases conduction velocity and excitability and decreases refractoriness in the rabbit atrium, and partially depolarized fibers may hyperpolarize. Pretreatment with reserpine or propranolol prevents these early changes. Initial catecholamine release can aggravate some arrhythmias, such as those caused by digitalis excess or myocardial infarction. Prolonged drug administration lengthens the duration of the action potential and refractoriness of atrial and ventricular muscle and Purkinje fibers, possibly by blocking one or more repolarizing potassium currents.[175] The ratio of effective refractory period to action potential duration does not change, nor do membrane responsiveness and conduction velocity. Bretylium exerts little effect on diastolic excitability but increases ventricular fibrillation thresholds significantly. Despite that action, it may not protect against some experimentally induced ischemic arrhythmias.[176] It is not clear whether the chemical sympathectomy-like state alone, or together with other actions, exerts the antifibrillatory effect. Reduced disparity between action potential duration and refractory period in regions of normal and infarcted myocardium may account for some of its antifibrillatory effects. Bretylium has no effect on vagal reflexes and does not alter the responsiveness of cholinergic receptors in the heart.

HEMODYNAMIC EFFECTS. Bretylium does not depress myocardial contractility. After an initial increase in blood pressure, the drug can cause significant hypotension by blocking the efferent limb of the baroreceptor reflex. Hypotension results most commonly when patients are sitting or standing but can also occur in the supine position in seriously ill patients. Bretylium reduces the extent of the vasoconstriction and tachycardia reflexes during standing. Orthostatic hypotension can persist for several days after the drug has been discontinued.

PHARMACOKINETICS (Table 23–1). Bretylium is effective orally as well as parenterally, but it is absorbed poorly and erratically from the gastrointestinal tract. Bioavailability may be less than 50 per cent and elimination is almost exclusively by renal excretion without significant metabolism or active metabolites being recognized. Elimination half-life is 5 to 10 hours but with fairly wide variability. Doses should be reduced in patients with renal insufficiency. In survivors of ventricular tachycardia or ventricular fibrillation, bretylium had an elimination half-life of 13.5 hours following single intravenous dosing, which was similar to previous results in normal subjects. Renal clearance accounted for virtually all elimination. Onset of action after intravenous administration occurs within several minutes, but full antiarrhythmic effects may not be seen for 30 minutes to 2 hours.

DOSAGE AND ADMINISTRATION (Table 23–1). Bretylium can be given intravenously in doses of 5 to 10 mg/kg body weight diluted in 50 to 100 ml of 5 per cent dextrose in water and administered over 10 to 20 minutes, or more quickly in a life threatening state. This dose can be repeated in 1 to 2 hours if the arrhythmia persists. The total daily dose should probably not exceed 30 mg/kg. A similar initial dose, but undiluted, can be given intramuscularly. The maintenance intravenous dose is 0.5 to 2.0 mg/min. Intramuscular injection during cardiopulmonary resuscitation from cardiac arrest and in shock states should be avoided because of unreliable absorption during reduced tissue perfusion. In this situation, bretylium should be given intravenously.

CLINICAL INDICATIONS. Bretylium is used in patients who are in an intensive care setting and who have life-threatening recurrent ventricular tachyarrhythmias that have not responded to lidocaine, quinidine, procainamide, or disopyramide. Bretylium has been effective in treating some patients with drug-resistant tachyarrhythmias and in treating victims of out-of-hospital ventricular fibrillation. It exerts no influence on the energy required for defibrillating dogs.

ADVERSE EFFECTS. Hypotension, most prominently orthostatic but also supine, appears to be the most significant side effect and can be prevented with tricyclic drugs such as protriptyline. Transient hypertension, increased sinus rate, and worsening of arrhythmias, often those due to digitalis excess or ischemia, may follow initial drug administration and may be due to initial release of catecholamines. Bretylium should be used cautiously or not at all in patients who have a relatively fixed cardiac output, such as those with severe aortic stenosis. Vasodilators or diuretics can enhance these hypotensive effects. Nausea and vomiting can occur following parenteral administration. Parotid pain primarily during meals commonly occurs after 2 to 4 months of oral therapy and is associated with increased salivation without parotid swelling or inflammation.

CLASS IV ANTIARRHYTHMIC AGENTS

THE CALCIUM CHANNEL ANTAGONISTS: VERAPAMIL AND DILTIAZEM

Verapamil, a synthetic papaverine derivative, is one of several drugs that, though heterogeneous in structure, block the slow calcium channel in cardiac muscle.[177] *Nifedipine* exhibits minimal electrophysiological effects at clinically used doses, and will not be discussed here (see p. 1311). Diltiazem has electrophysiological actions similar to those of verapamil.

ELECTROPHYSIOLOGICAL ACTIONS (Tables 23–4 and 23–5). By blocking the slow inward current in all cardiac fibers, verapamil reduces the plateau height of the action potential, slightly shortens muscle action potential, and slightly prolongs total Purkinje fiber action potential. It does not affect the action potential amplitude, $\dot{V}_{max}$ of phase 0, or resting membrane voltage in cells that have fast-response characteristics (atrial and ventricular muscle, the His-Purkinje system). Verapamil suppresses slow responses elicited by a variety of experimental methods and also triggered sustained rhythmic activity and early and late afterdepolarizations (see p. 605). Verapamil and other slow-channel blockers in concentrations that do not suppress action potentials of fast-channel dependent cells do so in the normal sinus and AV nodes. Verapamil depresses the slope of diastolic depolarization in sinus nodal cells, $\dot{V}_{max}$ of phase 0, maximum diastolic potential, and action potential amplitude in the sinus and AV nodal cells and prolongs conduction time and the effective and functional refractory periods of the AV node. The blocking effects of verapamil are more apparent at faster rates of stimulation (use-dependency) and in depolarized fibers (voltage-dependency). Verapamil probably slows the activation and delays recovery from inactivation of the slow channel. Unbinding of the drug from its receptor occurs more rapidly if this tissue is hyperpolarized. *Diltiazem* exerts similar effects on the AV node that are also rate dependent.[178a] Cocaine, which exerts Class I antiarrhythmic drug effects in vitro,[179] can produce ventricular fibrillation during ischemia which can be blocked by verapamil.

Verapamil does exert some local anesthetic activity because the dextrorotatory stereoisomer of the clinically used racemic mixture exerts slight blocking effects on the fast sodium current. The levorotatory stereoisomer blocks the slow inward current carried by calcium, as well as other ions, traveling through the slow channel. Verapamil does not modify calcium uptake, binding, or exchange by cardiac microsomes nor does it affect calcium-activated ATPase. Verapamil does not block beta receptors, but recent data suggest that it may block alpha receptors and potentiate vagal effects on the AV node.[181] Verapamil may also cause other effects that indirectly alter cardiac electrophysiology, such as decreasing platelet adhesiveness or reducing the extent of myocardial ischemia.[182,183]

In vivo, both in experimental animals and humans, verapamil prolongs conduction time through the AV node (the A-H interval) without affecting the P-A, H-V, or QRS intervals and lengthens the functional and effective refractory periods of the AV node. Spontaneous sinus rate may decrease slightly, an event only partially reversed by atropine. More commonly, the sinus rate does not change significantly in vivo because verapamil causes peripheral vasodilation, transient hypotension, and reflex sympathetic stimulation that mitigates any direct slowing effect verapamil may exert on the sinus node. If verapamil is given to a patient who is also receiving a beta blocker, the sinus nodal discharge rate may slow because reflex sympathetic stimulation is blocked.[184] Verapamil does not exert a direct effect on atrial or ventricular refractoriness or on antegrade or retrograde properties of accessory pathways. However, reflex sympathetic stimulation may increase the ventricular response over the accessory pathway during atrial fibrillation in patients with the Wolff-Parkinson-White syndrome.

HEMODYNAMIC EFFECTS. Since verapamil interferes with excitation-contraction coupling, it inhibits vascular smooth muscle contraction and causes marked vasodilation in coronary and other peripheral vascular beds. Propranolol does not block the vasodilation produced by verapamil. Reflex sympathetic effects may reduce in vivo the marked negative inotropic action of verapamil on isolated cardiac muscle, but direct myocardial depressant effects of verapamil may predominate when the drug is given in high doses. In patients with well-preserved left ventricular function, combined therapy with propranolol and verapamil appears to be well tolerated, but beta blockade can accentuate the hemodynamic depressant effects produced by oral verapamil. Patients who have reduced left ventricular function may not tolerate the combined blockade of beta receptors and of slow channels and the combined use of verapamil and propranolol in these patients must be undertaken cautiously or not at all. Verapamil decreases myocardial oxygen demand while decreasing coronary vascular resistance and reduces the extent of ischemic damage in experimental preparations. Such changes may be antiarrhythmic. Diltiazem also reduces ventricular arrhythmias during coronary occlusion in the dog, possibly by preventing calcium overload. In a hamster model of hereditary cardiomyopathy, verapamil prevents progression of the disease and the secondary heart failure.[185]

Peak alterations in hemodynamic variables occur 3 to 5 minutes after completion of the verapamil injection, the major effects being dissipated within 10 minutes. Mean arterial pressure decreases and left ventricular end-diastolic pressure increases; systemic resistance decreases and left ventricular dP/dt max decreases. Heart rate, cardiac index, left ventricular minute work, and mean pulmonary artery pressure do not change significantly. Thus, afterload reduction produced by verapamil significantly minimizes its negative inotropic action so that cardiac index may not be reduced. In addition, when verapamil slows the ventricular rate in a patient with a tachycardia, cardiac slowing may also improve hemodynamics. Nevertheless, caution should be exercised when giving verapamil to patients with severe myocardial depression or those receiving beta blockers or disopyramide, because hemodynamic deterioration may progress in some patients.

PHARMACOKINETICS (Table 23–1). Following single oral doses of verapamil, measurable prolongation of AV nodal conduction time occurs in 30 minutes and lasts 4 to 6 hours. After intravenous administration, AV nodal conduction delay occurs within 1 to 2 minutes and A-H interval prolongation is still detectable after 6 hours. Effective plasma concentrations necessary to terminate supraventricular tachycardia are in the range of 125 ng/ml following doses of 0.075 mg/kg to 0.150 mg/kg. After oral administration absorption is almost complete, but an overall bioavailability of 20 to 35 per cent suggests substantial first-pass metabolism in the liver, particularly of the l-isomer. The elimination half-life of verapamil is 3 to 7 hours, with up to 70 per cent of the drug excreted by the kidneys. Norverapamil is a major metabolite that may contribute to verapamil's electrophysiological actions. Serum protein binding is approximately 90 per cent.

DOSAGE AND ADMINISTRATION (Table 23–1). The most commonly used intravenous dose is 10 mg infused over 1 to 2 minutes while cardiac rhythm and blood pressure are monitored. A second injection of equal dose may be given 30 minutes later. The initial effect achieved with the first bolus injection, such as slowing of the ventricular response during atrial fibrillation, may be maintained by a continuous infusion of the drug at a rate of 0.005 mg/kg/min. The oral dose is 80 to 120 mg, given three or four times a day, usually not exceeding 480 mg/day. Various long-acting preparations exist that can be substituted on a milligram for milligram basis.

CLINICAL INDICATIONS. After simple vagal maneuvers have been tried, and probably adenosine given,[186] intravenous verapamil or diltiazem[187] is the next treatment of choice for terminating sustained sinus nodal reentry, AV nodal reentry, or reciprocating tachycardias associated with the Wolff-Parkinson-White syndrome, when one of the reentrant pathways is the AV node. Verapamil should definitely be tried prior to attempting termination by digitalis administration, pacing, electrical direct-current cardioversion, or acute blood pressure elevation with vasopressors. Verapamil and diltiazem terminate 60 to more than 90 per cent of episodes of paroxysmal supraventricular tachycardias within several minutes. Verapamil may be of use in some fetal supraventricular tachycardias as well.[188–190] Although intravenous verapamil has been given along with intravenous propranolol, this combination should be used only with great caution.

Verapamil and diltiazem decrease the ventricular response over the AV node during atrial fibrillation or atrial flutter, possibly converting a small number of episodes to sinus rhythm, particularly if the atrial flutter or fibrillation is of recent onset.[191–193] Some patients who exhibit atrial flutter may develop atrial fibrillation following verapamil administration. Quinidine, flecainide,[191] and esmolol[192] appear to be more effective than verapamil in establishing and maintaining sinus rhythm in patients with atrial fibrillation. As noted earlier, in patients with atrial fibrillation associated with the Wolff-Parkinson-White syndrome, intravenous verapamil may *accelerate* the ventricular response, and therefore the intravenous route is contraindicated in that situation.[194] Verapamil occasionally can terminate ectopic atrial tachycardias. Even though verapamil terminates a special kind of ventricular tachycardia,[195–197] hemodynamic collapse may occur if intravenous verapamil is given to patients with the more common forms of ventricular tachycardia.[198] A general rule of thumb to avoid complications is to not give intravenous verapamil to any patient with wide-QRS tachycardia, unless one is absolutely certain of the nature of the tachycardia and its response to verapamil.

Orally, verapamil or diltiazem may prevent the recurrence of AV nodal reentrant and reciprocating tachycardias associated with the Wolff-Parkinson-White syndrome as well as help maintain a decreased ventricular response during atrial flutter or atrial fibrillation in patients without an accessory pathway. In this regard, the effectiveness of verapamil appears to be enhanced when given concomitantly with digitalis or propranolol. Verapamil generally has not been effective in treating patients who have recurrent ventricular tachyarrhythmias, although it may suppress some forms of ventricular tachycardia as noted above. While data from animal models suggest that verapamil may be useful in reducing or preventing ventricular arrhythmias due to acute myocardial ischemia,[182,183] calcium antagonists have not been shown to reduce mortality or prevent sudden cardiac death in patients after acute myocardial infarction, except for diltiazem in patients with non-Qwave infarctions.

ADVERSE EFFECTS. Verapamil must be used cautiously in patients with significant hemodynamic impairment or in those receiving beta blockers, as previously noted. Hypotension, bradycardia, AV block, and asystole are more likely to occur when the drug is given to patients who are already receiving beta blocking agents. Hemodynamic collapse has been noted in infants, and verapamil should be used cautiously in patients less than 1 year old. Verapamil should also be used with caution in patients with sinus node abnormalities, since marked depression of sinus nodal function or asystole can result in some of these patients. Isoproterenol, calcium, glucagon infusion, or atropine (which may be only partially effective) or temporary pacing may be necessary to counteract some of the adverse effects of verapamil. Isoproterenol may be more effective for treating bradyarrhythmias and calcium for treating hemodynamic dysfunction secondary to verapamil. Verapamil can cause accelerated junctional discharge. Contraindications to the use of verapamil and diltiazem include the presence of advanced heart failure, second- or third-degree AV block without a pacemaker in place, atrial fibrillation and anterograde conduction over an accessory pathway, significant sinus node dysfunction, most ventricular tachycardias, cardiogenic shock, or other hypotensive states. While the drugs probably should not be used in patients with manifest heart failure, if the latter is due to one of the supraventricular tachyarrhythmias noted earlier, verapamil or diltiazem may restore sinus rhythm or significantly decrease the ventricular rate, leading to hemodynamic improvement. Finally, it is important to note that verapamil can decrease the excretion of digoxin by about 30 per cent. Hepatotoxicity may occur on occasion.

OTHER ANTIARRHYTHMIC AGENTS

ADENOSINE

Adenosine is an endogenous nucleoside present throughout the body and has been recently approved by the FDA to treat patients with supraventricular tachycardias.[199-202]

ELECTROPHYSIOLOGICAL ACTIONS (Tables 23–4 and 23–5). Adenosine interacts with A_1 receptors present on the extracellular surface of cardiac cells, activating K^+ channels in a fashion similar to that produced by acetylcholine. The increase in K^+ conductance shortens atrial action potential duration, hyperpolarizes the membrane potential, and decreases atrial contractility. Similar changes occur in the sinus and AV nodes. In contrast to these direct effects mediated through guanine nucleotide regulatory proteins G_i and G_o, adenosine antagonizes catecholamine-stimulated adenylate cyclase to decrease cyclic AMP accumulation and to decrease inward calcium conductance and the pacemaker current, i_f, in sinus nodal cells. V_{max} is reduced. Shifts in pacemaker site within the sinus node and sinus exit block may occur. Reflex-mediated sinus tachycardia can follow adenosine administration. In the N region of the AV node, conduction is depressed, along with decreases in action potential amplitude, duration, and V_{max}.[200] Adenosine slows the sinus rate in humans,[199] and is followed by a reflex increase in sinus discharge.[201] Transient prolongation of the AH interval results, often with transient first, second, or third degree AV nodal block.[199,201] His-Purkinje conduction is generally not directly affected.[203] Adenosine does not affect conduction in normal accessory pathways. Conduction may block in accessory pathways that have long conduction times or decremental conduction properties.[201] Patients with heart transplants exhibit a supersensitive response to adenosine.[201a] Adenosine plus lidocaine may limit myocardial reperfusion injury.[201b]

PHARMACOKINETICS. Adenosine is removed from the extracellular space by washout, enzymatically by degradation to inosine, phosphorylation to AMP, or by reuptake into cells via a nucleoside transport system. The vascular endothelium and the formed blood elements contain these elimination systems which result in very rapid clearance of adenosine from the circulation. Elimination half-life is 1 to 6 seconds. Most of adenosine's effects are produced during its first passage through the circulation. Important drug interactions occur. Methyl xanthines are competitive antagonists and therapeutic concentrations of theophylline totally block the exogeneous adenosine effect. Dipyridamole is a nucleoside transport blocker that blocks reuptake of adenosine, delaying its clearance from the circulation or interstitial space and potentiating its effect. Smaller adenosine doses should be used in patients receiving dispyridamole.[200,201]

DOSAGE AND ADMINISTRATION. To terminate tachycardia, a bolus of adenosine is injected intravenously rapidly into a central vein (if possible) at doses of 6 to 12 mg. Transient sinus slowing or AV nodal block results.[186,204-206]

CLINICAL INDICATIONS. Adenosine probably has become the drug of first choice to terminate acutely a supraventricular tachycardia such as AV nodal or AV reentry.[186,204-206] Doses as low as 2.5 mg terminate some tachycardias; 12 mg or less terminate 92 per cent of supraventricular tachycardias, usually within 30 seconds.[206] Central venous injections appear to require smaller doses than peripheral venous injections. Successful termination rates with adenosine are comparable or greater to those achieved with verapamil.[186,205,206] Adenosine may be preferable to verapamil in patients who previously have received intravenous beta adrenoceptor blockers, in those having poorly compensated heart failure or severe hypotension, and in neonates. Adenosine produces transient AV nodal block in patients with atrial flutter, atrial fibrillation, and some types of atrial tachycardia, facilitating the diagnosis.

Adenosine may be useful to help differentiate wide QRS tachycardias,[207-209] since it terminates many supraventricular tachycardias with aberrancy or reveals the underlying atrial mechanism, and it does not block conduction over the accessory pathway[210] or terminate most ventricular tachycardias. Adenosine does terminate some ventricular tachycardias.[211] This agent may predispose to the development of atrial fibrillation and possibly can increase the ventricular response in patients with atrial fibrillation conducting over an accessory pathway. Adenosine may also be useful in differentiating conduction over the AV node versus an accessory pathway during ablative procedures designed to interrupt the accessory pathway.[210] Endogenously released adenosine may be important in ischemia and hypoxia-induced AV nodal block[212] and in postdefibrillation bradyarrhythmias.[213]

ADVERSE EFFECTS. Transient side effects occur in almost 40 per cent of patients with supraventricular tachycardia given adenosine and are most commonly flushing, dyspnea and chest pressure. These symptoms are fleeting, generally less than 1 minute, and are well tolerated.

NEW ANTIARRHYTHMIC AGENTS

The following drugs are being evaluated at the time of this writing and have not yet been approved by the FDA.

SOTALOL

Electrophysiological Actions

Sotalol is a nonspecific beta-adrenoceptor blocking agent without intrinsic sympathomimetic activity. The D-isomer exhibits much less beta adrenoceptor blocking activity than does either the L-isomer or racemic mixture.[214,215] Sotalol does not block alpha-adrenoceptors and does not block the sodium channel (no membrane-stabilizing effects) but does prolong atrial and ventricular repolarization times by reducing the time-dependent outward potassium current activated during the plateau of the action potential. Action potential prolongation is greater at slower rates. Both D- and L- isomers exert Class III effects comparable to those observed with the racemic mixture. Resting membrane potential, action potential amplitude, and $\dot{V}_{max}$ are not significantly altered. Sotalol prolongs atrial and ventricular refractoriness, A-H, H-V, and Q-T intervals and sinus cycle length in humans.[214]

PHARMACOKINETICS AND PHARMACODYNAMICS. Sotalol is completely absorbed and not metabolized, making it 100 per cent bioavailable. It is not bound to plasma proteins, is excreted unchanged primarily by the kidneys, and has an elimination half-life of 10 to 15 hours. Peak plasma concentrations occur 2 to 3 hours after oral ingestion. Sotalol depresses myocardial contractility less than does propranolol. At an intravenous dose of 0.2 mg/kg, sotalol in humans significantly reduces heart rate, systolic pressure, cardiac output, and external cardiac work. Changes are those expected with beta-adrenoceptor blockade with little intrinsic negative inotropic effects.

DOSAGE AND CLINICAL INDICATIONS. Whereas the typical oral dose is 80 to 160 mg every 12 hours, doses of 640 mg or more daily have been administered. Sotalol effectively reduces the number of PVCs[216] and spontaneous and electrically induced episodes of ventricular tachyarrhythmias.[217-221] Sotalol is also effective in suppressing spontaneous and electrically induced AV nodal and AV reentrant tachycardias.[222,223] One of the most disturbing side effects is Q-T prolongation and torsades de pointes; the latter occurs in about 2 per cent of patients, usually those with severe underlying heart disease and prolonged Q-T interval initially.[102b,214]

PIRMENOL

Pirmenol is a class IA antiarrhythmic agent with electrophysiological actions similar to quinidine. In vitro it reduces action potential amplitude, duration, and $\dot{V}_{max}$ in canine Purkinje fibers and depresses ventricular and His-Purkinje conduction and membrane responsiveness. Pirmenol in vivo prolongs the P-R interval, QRS duration, QTc interval, H-V interval, sinus cycle length, and atrial and ventricular refractory periods. AV nodal function is unchanged.[224] Pirmenol suppresses ventricular tachyarrhythmias with a moderate adverse effect profile.[224-226]

CIBENZOLINE

Cibenzoline (cifenline in the United States) is a sodium-channel blocker and exerts primarily Class IA electrophysiological actions but also prolongs action potential duration (Class III) and may exhibit calcium-blocking effects as well (Class IV). Oral cibenzoline in humans prolongs His-Purkinje conduction time, QRS duration, and ventricular refractoriness. The Q-T remains unchanged. Cibenzoline is effective for some ventricular tachyarrhythmias.[227]

Recainam is a sodium-channel blocker with actions consistent with Class IC antiarrhythmic drugs and is presently undergoing testing.[228-230] *Ameloride,* a Class I antiarrhythmic agent,[232] and several new calcium antagonists, *nicardipine, nitrendipine,* and *bepridil,* are undergoing evaluation.[233]

Electrical Therapy of Cardiac Arrhythmias

DIRECT CURRENT CARDIOVERSION

Electrical cardioversion offers obvious advantages over drug therapy in terminating tachycardia. Under conditions optimal for close supervision and monitoring, a precisely regulated "dose" of electricity can restore sinus rhythm immediately and safely. The distinction between supraventricular and ventricular tachyarrhythmias—crucial to the proper medical management of arrhythmias—becomes less significant, and the time-consuming titration of drugs with potential side effects is abolished.[234]

MECHANISMS. Electrical cardioversion appears to terminate most effectively those tachycardias presumed to be due to reentry, such as atrial flutter and atrial fibrillation, AV nodal reentry, reciprocating tachycardias associated with Wolff-Parkinson-White syndrome, most forms of ventricular tachycardia, ventricular flutter, and ventricular fibrillation. The electric shock, by depolarizing all excitable myocardium, and possibly by prolonging refractoriness.[234a] interrupts reentrant circuits, discharges foci, and establishes electrical homogeneity that terminates reentry. A shock that does not end the tachycardia may fail to depolarize critical areas involved in the maintenance of the tachycardia, although the mechanism by which a shock successfully terminates ventricular fibrillation has not been completely explained.[235,236] A tachycardia that terminates and then restarts may be reinitiated by factors provoking the tachycardia in the first place. If the precipitating factors are no longer present, interrupting the tachyarrhythmia for only the brief time produced by the shock may prevent its return for long duration even though the anatomical and electrophysiological substrates required for the tachycardia are still present.

Tachycardias thought to be due to disorders of impulse formation (automaticity) include parasystole, some forms of atrial tachycardias, nonparoxysmal AV junctional tachycardia, and accelerated idioventricular rhythms. An attempt to cardiovert these tachycardias electrically is not indicated in most instances. It is possible that the shock can terminate tachycardias due to enhanced automaticity or triggered activity, but this notion is conjectural at present.

TECHNIQUE. Prior to elective cardioversion, a careful physical examination, including palpation of all pulses, should be performed. A 12-lead electrocardiogram is obtained before and after cardioversion as well as a rhythm strip during the electroshock. The patient, who should be informed completely about what to expect, is in a fasting state and "metabolically balanced," i.e., blood gases, pH, and electrolytes should be normal with no evidence of drug toxicity. Withholding digitalis for several days before elective cardioversion in patients without clinical evidence of digitalis toxicity is not necessary. Maintenance quinidine administration 1 to 2 days before electrical cardioversion of patients with atrial fibrillation may revert 10 to 15 per cent to sinus rhythm, may help prevent recurrence of atrial fibrillation once sinus rhythm is restored, and may help determine patient tolerance to the drug.

Self-adhesive pads applied in the standard apex-anterior or apex-posterior paddle positions have similar transthoracic impedances to paddles and are very useful in elective cardioversions or other situations in which there is time for their application, such as at the start of an electrophysiological study. Paddles 12 to 13 cm in diameter can be used to deliver maximum current to the heart, but the benefits of these paddles as compared with those of 8 to 9 cm diameter have not been clearly established. Larger paddles may distribute the intracardiac current over a wider area and may reduce shock-induced myocardial necrosis.

A synchronized shock, i.e., one delivered during the QRS complex, is used for all cardioversions except for very rapid ventricular tachyarrhythmias, such as ventricular flutter or fibrillation. Because myocardial damage increases directly with increases in applied energy, the minimum effective energy should be used. Therefore, shocks are "titrated" when the clinical situation permits. Except for atrial fibrillation, shocks in the range of 25 to 50 joules successfully terminate most supraventricular tachycardias and should be tried initially. If unsuccessful, a second shock of higher energy can be delivered. The starting level to terminate atrial fibrillation should probably be 50 to 100 joules. For patients with stable ventricular tachycardia, starting levels in the range of 25 to 50 joules can be employed. If there is some urgency to terminate the tachyarrhythmia, one can begin with higher energies. To terminate ventricular fibrillation, 200 to 400 joules generally are used, although much lower energies (<100 joules) terminate ventricular fibrillation when the shock is delivered at the *very onset* of the arrhythmia, using adhesive pads in the electrophysiology laboratory, for example.

During elective cardioversion, a short-acting barbiturate such as methohexital or an amnesic such as diazepam or midazolam can be used. A physician skilled in airway management should be in attendance, an intravenous route should be established, and all equipment necessary for emergency resuscitation should be immediately accessible. Before cardioversion, 100 per cent oxygen may be administered for 5 to 15 minutes and is continued throughout the procedure. Manual ventilation of the patient may be necessary to avoid hypoxia during periods of deepest sleep.

INDICATIONS. As a rule, any tachycardia that produces hypotension, congestive heart failure, or angina and does not respond promptly to medical management should be terminated electrically. Very rapid ventricular rates in patients with atrial fibrillation and the Wolff-Parkinson-White syndrome are often best treated by electrical cardioversion. In almost all instances, the patient's hemodynamic status improves after cardioversion. An occasional patient may develop hypotension, reduced cardiac output, or congestive heart failure following the shock. This may be related to complications of the cardioversion, such as embolic events, myocardial depression resulting from the anesthetic agent, hypoxia, lack of restoration of left atrial contraction despite return of electrical atrial systole, or postshock arrhythmias. Direct-current countershock of digitalis-induced tachyarrhythmias is contraindicated.

Favorable candidates for electrical cardioversion of atrial fibrillation include those patients who (1) have symptomatic atrial fibrillation of less than 12 months' duration and derive significant hemodynamic benefits from sinus rhythm; (2) have embolic episodes; (3) continue to have atrial fibrillation after the precipitating cause has been removed, e.g., following treatment of thyrotoxicosis, and (4) have a rapid ventricular rate that is difficult to slow.

Unfavorable candidates include patients with (1) digitalis toxicity, (2) no symptoms and a well-controlled ventricular rate without therapy, (3) sinus node dysfunction and various unstable supraventricular tachyarrhythmias or bradyarrhythmias (often the bradycardia-tachycardia syndrome) who finally develop and maintain atrial fibrillation (which in essence represents a "cure" of the sick sinus syndrome), (4) little or no benefit from normal sinus rhythm who promptly revert to atrial fibrillation after cardioversion despite drug therapy, (5) a large left atrium and long-standing atrial fibrillation, (6) infrequent episodes of atrial fibrillation that revert spontaneously to sinus rhythm, (7) no mechanical atrial systole after the return of electrical atrial systole, (8) atrial fibrillation and advanced heart block, (9) cardiac surgery planned in the near future, and (10) antiarrhythmic drug intolerance. Atrial fibrillation is likely to recur after cardioversion in patients who have significant chronic obstructive lung disease, congestive heart failure, or mitral valve disease, particularly mitral insufficiency.

In patients with atrial flutter, slowing the ventricular rate by administering digitalis or terminating the flutter with quinidine may be difficult, so that electrical cardioversion is often the initial treatment of choice. For the patient with other types of supraventricular tachycardia, electrical cardioversion may be employed when: (1) maneuvers to enhance vagal tone or simple medical management (e.g., intravenous verapamil) have failed to terminate the tachycardia and (2) the clinical setting indicates that fairly prompt restoration of sinus rhythm is desirable because of hemodynamic decompensation or electrophysiological consequences of the tachycardia. Similarly, in patients with ventricular tachycardia, the hemodynamic and electrophysiological consequences of the arrhythmias determine the need and urgency for direct current-cardioversion (p. 653). Electrical countershock is the *initial* treatment of choice for ventricular flutter or ventricular fibrillation.

If, after the first shock, reversion to sinus rhythm does not occur, a higher energy level should be tried. When transient ventricular arrhythmias result after an unsuccessful shock, a bolus of lidocaine can be given prior to delivering a shock at the next energy level. If sinus rhythm returns only transiently and is promptly supplanted by the tachycardia, a repeat shock can be tried, depending on the tachyarrhythmia being treated and its consequences. Administration of an antiarrhythmic agent intravenously may be useful prior to delivering the next cardioversion shock. After cardioversion, the patient should be monitored at least until full consciousness has been restored and preferably for several hours thereafter.

RESULTS. Cardioversion restores sinus rhythm in 70 to 95 per cent of patients, depending upon the type of tachyarrhythmia. However, sinus rhythm remains after 12 months in less than one-third to one-half the patients with chronic atrial fibrillation. Thus, maintenance of sinus rhythm once established is the difficult problem, not the immediate termination of the tachycardia, and depends on the particular arrhythmia, the presence of underlying heart disease, and the adequacy of antiarrhythmic drug therapy.

COMPLICATIONS. Arrhythmias induced by the cardioversion generally are caused by inadequate synchronization, with the shock occurring during the ST segment or T wave. Occasionally, a properly synchronized shock can produce ventricular fibrillation (Fig. 23–5). Post-shock arrhythmias usually are transient and do not require therapy. Embolic episodes are reported to occur in 1 to 3 per cent of the patients converted from atrial fibrillation to sinus rhythm. Prior anticoagulation for 1 to 2 weeks should be considered for patients who have no contraindication to such therapy and who are at high risk for emboli, such as those with mitral stenosis and atrial fibrillation of recent onset, a history of recent or recurrent emboli, a prosthetic mitral valve, enlarged hearts (including left atrial enlargement), or congestive heart failure. Anticoagulation with warfarin for several weeks afterward is recommended. However, it must be emphasized that few controlled studies to support this approach have been published.

Although direct-current shock has been demonstrated in

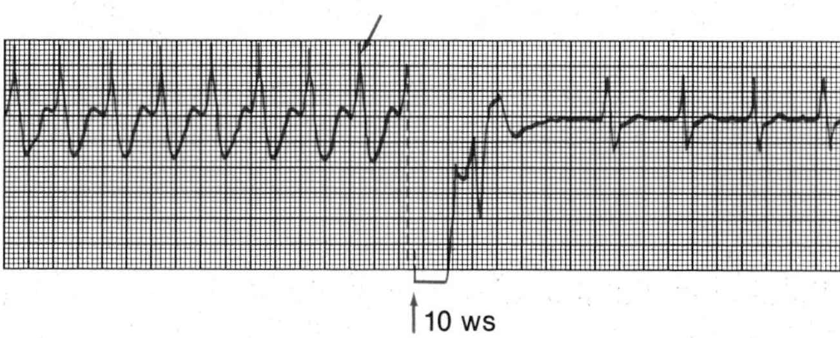

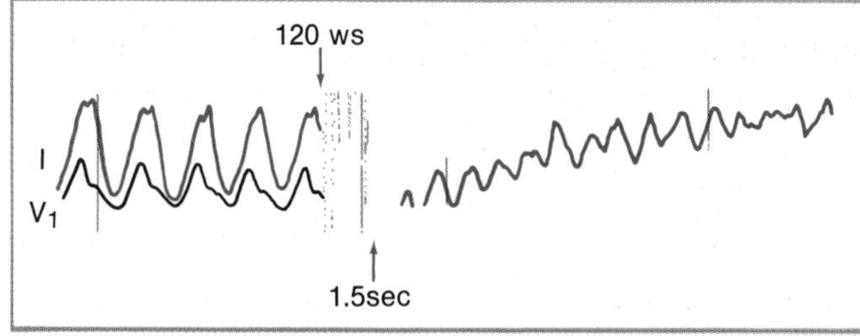

FIGURE 23–5. *Top,* A synchronized shock (note synchronization marks in the apex of the QRS complex [↓]) during ventricular tachycardia is followed by a single repetitive ventricular response and then normal sinus rhythm. *Bottom,* A shock synchronized to the terminal portion of the QRS complex in a patient with atrial fibrillation and conduction to the ventricle over an accessory pathway (WPW syndrome) results in ventricular fibrillation that was promptly terminated by a 400 watt-sec (or joule) shock. Recording was lost for 1.5 sec (↑) owing to baseline drift after the shock.

animals to cause cardiac injury, studies in man indicate that elevations of myocardial enzymes after cardioversion are not common. ST-segment elevation may occur with elective direct-current cardioversion, although cardiac enzymes and myocardial scintigraphy may be unremarkable.

Cardioversion of ventricular tachycardia can also be achieved by a chest thump. Its mechanism of termination probably relates to a mechanically induced premature atrial or ventricular complex that interrupts a tachycardia. The thump cannot be timed very well and is probably only effective when delivered during a nonrefractory part of the cardiac cycle. Care must therefore be taken, because the thump can alter a ventricular tachycardia and possibly induce ventricular flutter or fibrillation.

IMPLANTABLE ELECTRICAL DEVICES FOR TREATMENT OF CARDIAC ARRHYTHMIAS

Implantable devices that monitor the cardiac rhythm and can deliver competing pacing stimuli and low- and high-energy shocks have been used effectively in selected patients and are discussed fully in Chapter 25.

ABLATION THERAPY

The purpose of catheter ablation therapy is to destroy myocardial tissue[237] by delivering electrical energy in the form of a high energy direct current shock[238–241] or radiofrequency energy[242,243] over electrodes on a catheter placed next to an area of the endocardium integrally related to the arrhythmia. Lasers have also been used.[244,245] For direct current (DC) shock the intracardiac electrode can be the anode, to maximize the effects of the shock, with a large metal plate or conducting adhesive pad on the skin of the thorax serving as the cathode. The shock can also be given over the cathode in the heart or between two electrodes on the same or two separate intracardiac catheters. Energy is delivered from an external cardioverter-defibrillator and produces barotrauma, electrolysis, heat, and flow of current to destroy tissue. Radiofrequency ablation destroys tissue by controlled heat production and avoids the need for general anesthesia since pain is minimal and skeletal muscle contraction does not occur. Presently, catheter ablation is used to treat patients with four major tachyarrhythmias: atrial flutter/fibrillation, AV nodal reentry, AV reentry and ventricular tachycardia.

CREATION OF AV HEART BLOCK BY HIS BUNDLE ABLATION IN PATIENTS WITH ATRIAL FLUTTER/FIBRILLATION. The creation of complete AV block can be considered in patients with atrial flutter/fibrillation, and at times an atrial tachycardia, in whom the arrhythmia cannot be suppressed and the ventricular rate cannot be adequately controlled pharmacologically. The therapy makes the patient pacemaker-dependent and does not eliminate other consequences of the flutter/fibrillation such as the loss of sequential AV contraction (assuming DDD pacing is instituted postshock) or the possibility of emboli. It does, however, establish a more physiological ventricular rate.

For His bundle ablation to achieve complete AV block, the shock is delivered at a site where the largest His bundle potential amplitude is recorded (Fig. 23–6). Single shocks of 150 to 300 joules frequently are effective. An unreliable escape rhythm follows and pacemaker implantation is necessary.[246] Radiofrequency ablation may have a slightly lower success rate but probably should be tried first, and if unsuccessful, should be followed by DC ablation. Short-duration DC pulses may be safer than long-duration shocks.[247]

Approximately 65 per cent of patients receiving His bundle ablation develop chronic complete AV block, 8 per cent have intact AV conduction but do not require drugs for arrhythmia

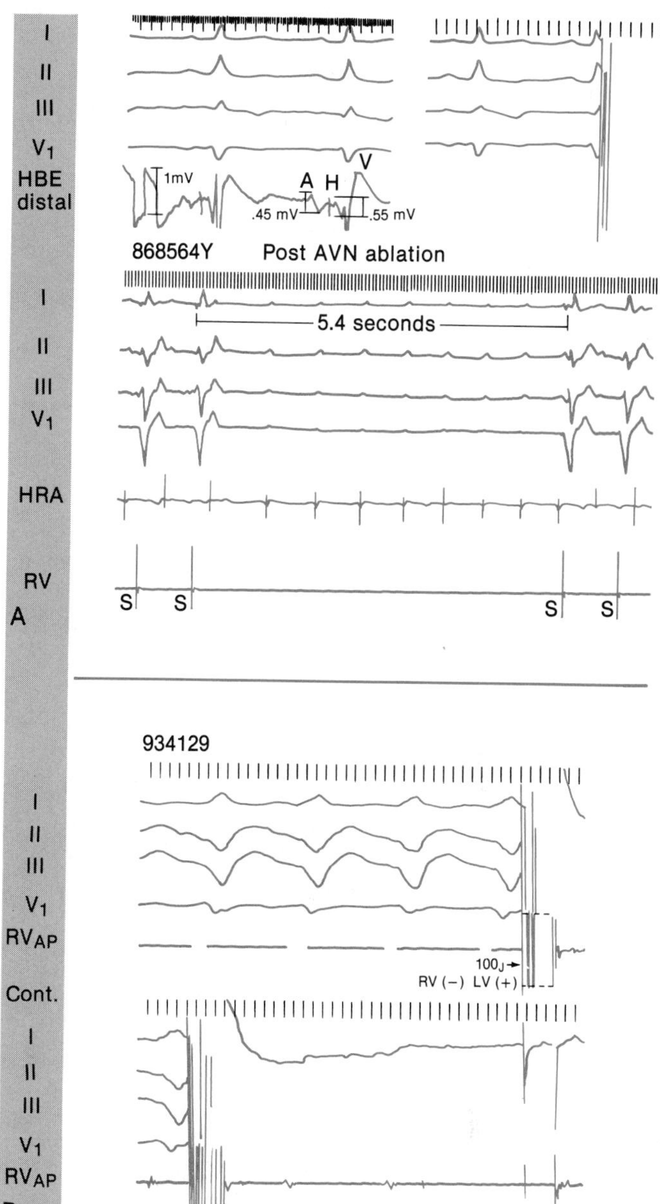

FIGURE 23–6. Electrical catheter ablation of AV conduction and of ventricular tachycardia. Panel A, *top*, illustrates leads I, II, III, and V_1 and a His bundle electrogram during sinus rhythm prior to the delivery of the shock. Amplitude of the atrial and His bundle electrogram is given. At the dark vertical line in the top panel, 200 joules are delivered between the cathodal electrode situated at the His bundle and an anodal patch on the patient's back. In the bottom of panel A, the rhythm immediately following the shock is displayed. The patient is now pacemaker-dependent; turning off the pacemaker for 5.4 seconds illustrates underlying complete AV heart block. HRA, high right atrial electrogram recording; RV, right ventricular electrogram recording; S, stimulus. Panel B illustrates an attempt at ablation of a ventricular tachycardia with the site of origin located near the apical portion of the interventricular septum. The first of several 100-joule shocks was delivered between the anodal electrode placed in the left ventricular apex and the cathodal electrode placed in the right ventricular apex. The delivery of the shock in the top right is reproduced in the bottom left of the panel. The ventricular tachycardia is terminated and the patient's dual chamber pacemaker paces the atrium and then the ventricle after a slight pause. RV_{AP} is the right ventricular electrocardiogram recorded at the apex. The electrocardiogram recording at the left ventricular apex occurred 40 msec in advance of the onset of the QRS complex (not shown).

control, and 12 per cent achieve arrhythmia control with drugs. About 15 per cent of patients show no improvement. Recovery of AV conduction has been observed up to a year after a successful attempt at His ablation while AV block can occur several weeks or months after an initially unsuccessful or partially effective attempt. A 1.8 per cent incidence of late sudden death occurs on long-term follow-up.[248] Immediate complications related to the shock include ventricular tachycardia and fibrillation, pericardial tamponade, and transient hypotension. In-hospital mortality related to DC shock ablation is 5.6 per cent and is more common in patients with ejection fractions $<$20 per cent.[249] Late complications include ventricular tachycardia and ventricular fibrillation, sepsis involving the pacemaker pocket, thrombophlebitis, and hemothorax. Catheter ablation can eliminate atrial flutter in some patients (Ch. 679).

AV NODAL MODIFICATION FOR PATIENTS WITH AV NODAL REENTRY. Careful titration of the dose of radiofrequency energy[250] and positioning of the ablation catheter can result in selective ablation of conduction over the slow or fast pathway involved in AV nodal reentry (AVNRT), with preservation of intact AV nodal conduction (Fig. 23–7).[243,251,251a] Successful elimination of AVNRT occurs in 80 to 90 per cent of patients with radiofrequency ablation, but the chance of creating complete heart block is about 10 per cent.[252,253] Catheter-induced AV nodal modification with radiofrequency ablation should be tried before surgery is considered. Complications from radiofrequency ablation appear relatively mild and include arrhythmias, occlusion of the coronary sinus, and the potential for embolic events from the site of ablation.

ABLATION OF THE ACCESSORY PATHWAY IN PATIENTS WITH THE WOLFF-PARKINSON-WHITE SYNDROME. In patients with WPW syndrome, an accessory pathway located in a posterior paraseptal position can be ablated by a quadripolar electrode catheter positioned within the os of the coronary sinus so that the proximal pair of electrodes is just outside the os. The shock is delivered to the proximal pair of electrodes.[254] Success rates are about 70 per cent but pericardial tamponade due to coronary sinus rupture (5 per cent) and complete heart block (2 per cent) are important risks.[240,255] More recent experience indicates that DC ablation can be applied to accessory pathways located in any position[256–259] with a success rate exceeding 90 per cent and an acceptable risk profile.[258] Radiofrequency ablation similarly achieves a high success rate and a low risk[259] (Fig. 23–8). For radiofrequency ablation the ablation electrode is positioned up under the tricuspid or mitral valve or on top of the AV ring, or along the top of the septum, at a site where activation from the accessory pathway or the shortest ventricular atrial interval during AVNRT is recorded. Twenty-five to 50 watts are delivered for 20 to 50 seconds using radiofrequency ablation.

ABLATION OF VENTRICULAR TACHYCARDIA. For patients with ventricular tachycardia, DC shocks are synchronized to the QRS complex during the ventricular tachycardia and are delivered through the tip electrode of the same cath-

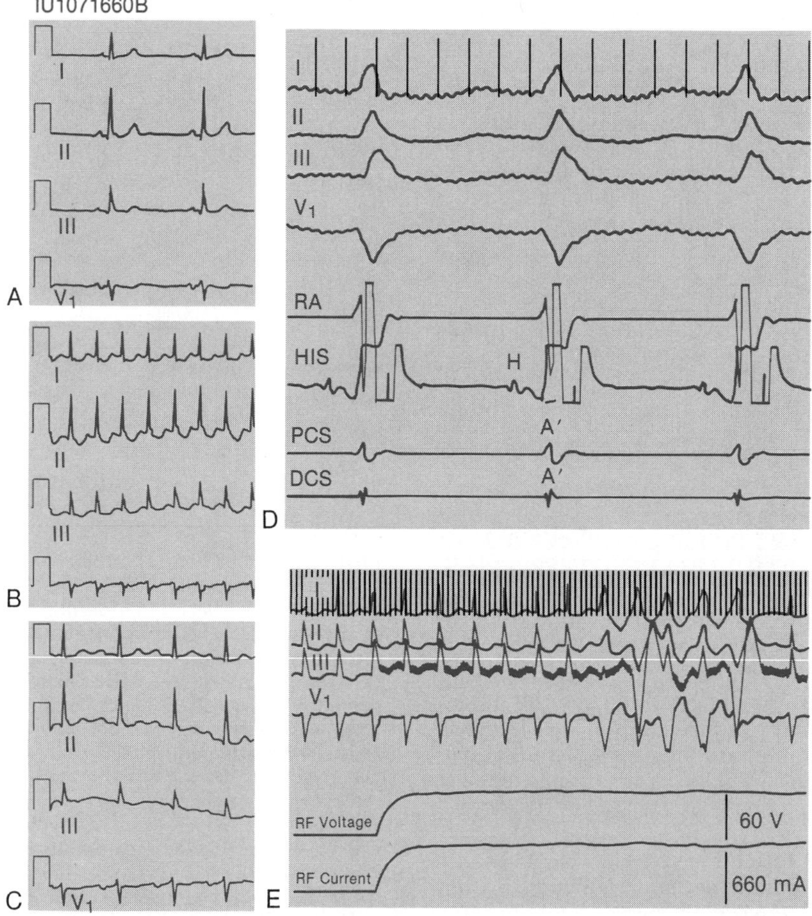

FIGURE 23–7. Radiofrequency (RF) A-V nodal modification for A-V nodal reentrant tachycardia. Panel A, Normal sinus rhythm. Panel B, A-V nodal reentrant tachycardia. Panel C, Normal sinus rhythm following A-V nodal ablation. Note prolonged P-R interval. Panel D, A-V nodal reentrant tachycardia with intracavitary recordings. Note virtual simultaneous activation of atria and ventricles, consistent with A-V nodal reentrant tachycardia. Panel E, Radiofrequency ablation with catheter placed in the anterior region of the A-V node producing selective ablation of the anterogradely conducting fast pathway. Leads 1, 2, 3, and V_1, scalar recordings. RA, right atrial electrogram; His, His bundle electrogram; PCS, electrogram recorded from the proximal electrodes of the coronary sinus catheter; DCS, electrogram recorded from the distal electrode of the coronary sinus catheter. Large time lines 50 msec; small time lines 10 msec. Vertical bars, calibration for RF voltage and current. Square wave for ECG = 1 mV, 200 msec.

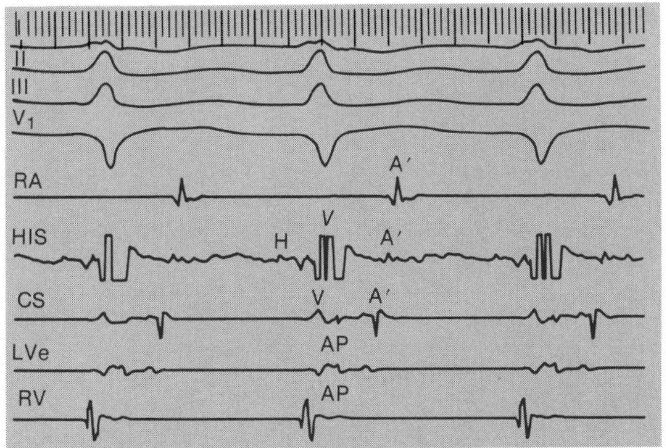

A

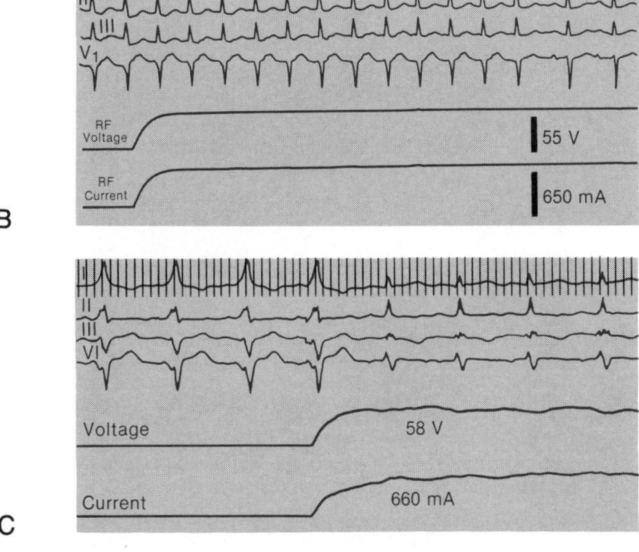

B

C

FIGURE 23-8. ***A* and *B*, Radiofrequency ablation of a left free-wall accessory pathway. *A,* depicts atrioventricular reentrant tachycardia with anterograde conduction over the normal pathway and retrograde conduction over the left free-wall accessory pathway. The electrodes in the coronary sinus (CS) record activation over the accessory pathway (AP), which is apposed by the catheter positioned in the left ventricular endocardium (LV_e). *B*, RF energy is delivered during the tachycardia and produces termination after 3.8 seconds. The delta wave has disappeared and tachycardia can no longer be initiated (not shown). Conventions as in 23-7. *C*, Radiofrequency catheter ablation of a right free-wall accessory pathway. Elimination of accessory pathway conduction almost immediately after delivery of radiofrequency energy indicates that the catheter is positioned virtually on the accessory pathway and best ensures a successful ablation. Leads I, II, III, V scalar recordings. (From Zipes, D. P., et al.: Nonpharmacologic therapy: Can it replace antiarrhymic drug therapy? J. Cardiovasc. Electrophysiol. *2:*S255, 1991.)**

eter that has been used to locate the "origin of the tachycardia."[260,261] Pace mapping can be used to locate the exit of the tachycardia to the myocardium (see below).[262] Shocks can be delivered over a balloon in the left ventricle studded with silver bead electrodes[263] and also between two catheters placed on either side of the interventricular septum.[264] More recently shocks have been delivered to sites where isolated mid-diastolic potentials[265] and areas of slow conduction in the reentrant circuit of the tachycardia have been recorded.[266,267] Since sustained bundle branch reentry can be responsible for some ventricular tachycardias,[268] ablation of the right bundle branch may be effective in these patients.[269] For patients with right ventricular dysplasia, shocks are delivered to the endocardium of the right ventricle.[270,271] Radiofrequency ablation can also be used (Fig. 23-9). In patients with scarred and thickened endocardium, it is questionable whether such electrical therapy can penetrate to the arrhythmogenic area (see below).

Several ablation attempts are required in some patients and, when ventricular tachycardias with different morphologies are present, multiple sites of ablation are necessary. Following ablation, attempts are made to reinitiate the tachycardia. Clinical success, i.e., no recurrence of ventricular tachycardia after ablation, averages rates of about 25 per cent for elimination of ventricular tachycardia without need for antiarrhythmic drugs and about 25 per cent for suppression with drugs previously ineffective. Procedure-related mortality is 7 per cent. The relatively low success rates and complications[248,260,261,272,273] have restrained enthusiastic acceptance of this approach, which should still be considered investigational. Complications are similar to those following His bundle ablation and have included pump failure, electromechanical dissociation, intractable ventricular tachyarrhythmias, myocardial perforation, and cerebrovascular accidents. The short- and long-term results of endocardial shocks, in terms of tissue damage and late sequelae, are still being investigated. Reported complications are very likely to be underestimated and events such as coronary artery spasm and subsequent damage to coronary arteries may go unnoticed.

CHEMICAL ABLATION. Chemical ablation with alcohol

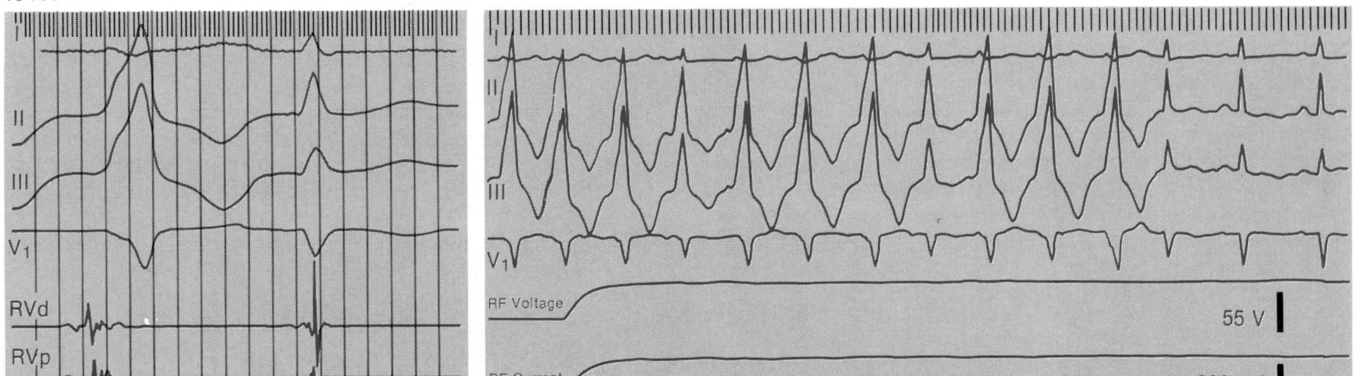

FIGURE 23-9. Radiofrequency ablation of ventricular tachycardia. Left panel demonstrates recordings during ventricular bigeminy. The distal right ventricular electrogram recorded from the right ventricular outflow tract (RV_d) occurred 30 msec prior to the onset of the QRS complex. The right panel demonstrates termination of the ventricular tachycardia by radiofrequency energy. Following this ablation, ventricular bigeminy resumed. A second ablation in the same area eliminated the premature ventricular complexes entirely. RV_d, distal right ventricular electrogram; RV_p, proximal right ventricular electrogram.

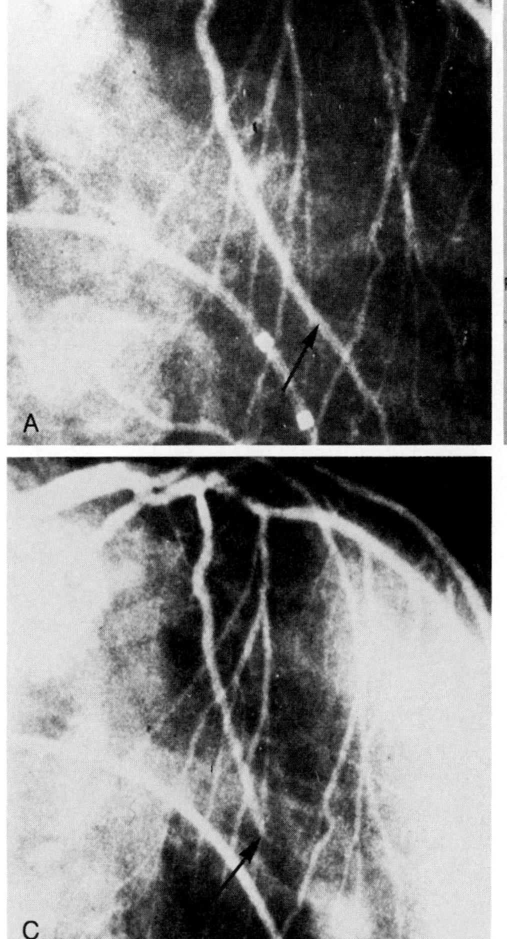

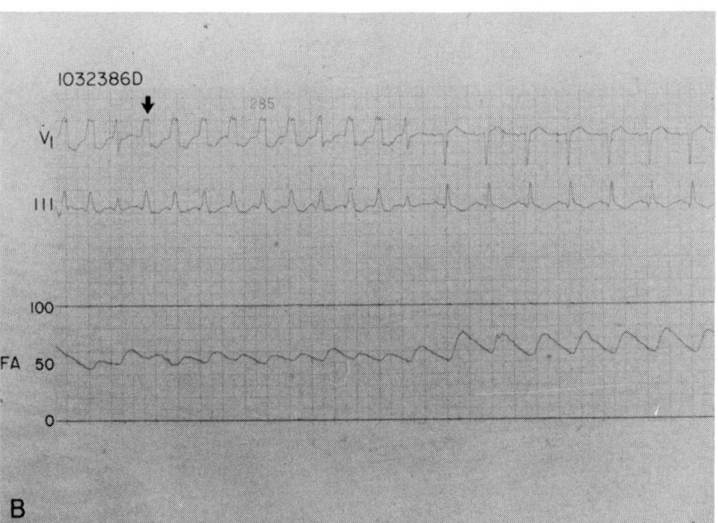

FIGURE 23–10. Alcohol ablation of ventricular tachycardia. Injection of dye into the posterolateral branch of the circumflex coronary artery (panel A) results in sudden termination of sustained ventricular tachycardia (panel B). Following alcohol injection, the distal portion of the posterolateral branch becomes occluded (panel C) and the ventricular tachycardia can no longer be induced. Arrow indicates site of occlusion in vessel after alcohol injection (C) and similar position prior to alcohol injection (A). (From Nora, M., Miles, W., Dillon, J., Klein, L., and Zipes, D. P.: Alcohol ablation of ventricular tachycardia. J. Cardiovasc. Electrophys. In press.)

or phenol of an area of myocardium involved in a tachycardia was first demonstrated in animals[274,275] and subsequently in patients with ventricular[276,277] and atrial[278] tachycardia. Angioplasty catheters are mandatory for cannulating the smallest vessel perfusing the site to be ablated in order to minimize the amount of myocardium exposed to the alcohol. Test injections with iced saline or lidocaine are carried out to determine whether the appropriate coronary artery is cannulated by noting whether the injectate terminates the sustained tachycardia is done before alcohol injection. Alcohol injected into the AV nodal artery has been used to create AV block in patients not responding to catheter ablation[279] (Fig. 23–10). Excessive myocardial necrosis is the major complication, and alcohol ablation should be considered only when other ablative approaches fail or cannot be done.[280] Infusion of drugs into the AV nodal artery can reversibly alter AV nodal function.[280a]

Surgical Therapy of Tachyarrhythmias

The objectives of a surgical approach to treating a tachycardia are to excise, isolate, or interrupt tissue in the heart critical for the initiation, maintenance, or propagation of the tachycardia, while preserving or even improving myocardial function. In addition to a direct surgical approach on the arrhythmia, indirect approaches such as aneurysmectomy, coronary artery bypass grafting, and relief of valvular insufficiency or stenosis can be useful in selected patients by improving cardiac hemodynamics and myocardial blood flow. Cardiac sympathectomy alters adrenergic influences on the heart and has been effective in some patients, particularly those who have recurrent ventricular tachycardia with the long Q-T syndrome.

SUPRAVENTRICULAR TACHYCARDIAS

Surgical candidates are patients with symptomatic, drug-resistant, recurrent supraventricular tachycardias for whom a surgical procedure exists that offers a high probability of success, minimal morbidity and virtually no mortality, and for whom alternative therapies are less desirable or have been unsuccessful.[281–283] Such patients include: (1) those with atrial tachycardias confined to a relatively localized area in the atrium, (2) those with the preexcitation syndrome or one of its variants, and (3) those with AV nodal entry. Electrical or alcohol ablation of AV conduction has virtually replaced open heart surgery to produce AV block in patients who have uncontrollably rapid ventricular rates during a supraventricular tachycardia such as atrial flutter or fibrillation. Probably, over the next several years, these mildly invasive catheter ablation techniques will obviate the need for arrhythmia surgery in all but a minority of patients. Selected patients with symptomatic, drug-resistant AV atrial flutter, and atrial fibrillation can be surgical candidates on occasion.

PREOPERATIVE MAPPING. Preoperatively a thorough cardiac evaluation using noninvasive and invasive means establishes whether concomitant nonarrhythmic cardiac surgery such as coronary artery bypass grafting or valve replacement may be necessary. At the electrophysiological study, the tachycardia is initiated, confirmed to be the "clinical tachycardia," and mapped to ascertain areas of the myocardium involved in the arrhythmia. Although more accurate intraoperative mapping refines the preoperative map, the latter is essential because general anesthesia, cooling of the heart when the chest is open, inadvertent trauma to pathways, and other factors can prevent induction of the tachycardia at surgery and preclude the opportunity for intraoperative mapping. (This is particularly true for ventricular tachycardias which, perversely, may not be initiated at surgery.) Also, for types of tachycardia that cannot be induced electrically, the preoperative electrophysiological study can be performed at a time when the tachycardia has begun spontaneously. *Mapping* in the present context is the term applied to the procedure during which the activation sequence—that is, the origin of and the pathways followed by the electrical impulse as it depolarizes the heart—is determined.

WOLFF-PARKINSON-WHITE SYNDROME (p. 693). In patients with the WPW syndrome, the electrophysiological study establishes the presence of preexcitation, the number, type, and location of accessory pathways, mechanism of the arrhythmia(s), participation of the accessory pathway in the arrhythmia, functional properties of the normal and accessory pathways, effect of drugs or other interventions, and presence of associated electrophysiological or anatomical anomalies. Catheter electrodes are positioned at various endocardial right atrial sites around the margin of the tricuspid ring, at the His bundle area, and along the length of the coronary sinus to obtain recording of left atrial activity at the region of the AV ring. The atrial insertion of the accessory pathway is determined by (1) locating the earliest site of atrial activation when the atrium is depolarized over the accessory pathway during ventricular pacing or (2) during reciprocating tachycardia characterized by anterograde conduction over the normal pathway and retrograde conduction over the accessory pathway. At times, the shortest absolute VA time may be an inaccurate measure of accessory pathway insertion.[283a] Specialized catheter recording techniques permit recording activation from the accessory pathway directly[284-287] positioning the electrode on top of the AV ring, beneath the valve leaflets, or in the coronary sinus (Fig. 23-8).

Atrial mapping during tachycardia rather than during ventricular pacing is preferable to be certain that the retrograde atrial activation is due solely to conduction over the accessory pathway and is not a retrograde fusion P wave from simultaneous activation over the accessory pathway and AV node. Adenosine, verapamil, propranolol, or reflex vagal activation from phenylephrine infusion can be used to prolong conduction time selectively over the AV node. Ten to 15 per cent of patients have multiple accessory pathways and the retrograde P wave may be a fusion of activation from two or more accessory pathways. The ventricular insertion can be determined by locating the earliest site of ventricular activation when the ventricle is depolarized over the accessory pathway during stable sinus rhythm, during atrial pacing from a site near the accessory pathway, or during stable (antidromic) reciprocating tachycardia characterized by anterograde conduction over the accessory pathway and retrograde conduction over the normal pathway.

Other information may be helpful. This includes the vectorial analysis of the delta wave, effect of functional bundle branch block or axis shift[288] on the V-A interval during orthodromic tachycardia, the V-A interval of right ventricular apical extrasystoles and bundle branch reentrant beats[289] ventricular coupling intervals required to produce atrial preexcitation during orthodromic tachycardia ("preexcitation index"),[289a] phase[290] and echo analysis, and finding the shortest interval between the stimulus applied to various atrial sites and the delta wave of the QRS complex all. Mapping is repeated at the time of operation with single or multiple bipolar and/or unipolar electrode probes (Fig. 23-11) to localize more precisely the site of the accessory pathway insertion in the atrium and ventricle. Atrial and ventricular insertions generally are less than 2 cm apart from each other. Usually, complete epicardial maps are not necessary unless a Mahaim connection is present.

FIGURE 23-11. See color plate 5.

SURGICAL TECHNIQUES. Two surgical techniques have evolved, an open heart endocardial[291,292] and a closed heart epicardial approach.[293-296] The open heart procedure is done after the map is completed, using hypothermic, cardioplegic arrest. An atrial endocardial incision above the annulus is extended to the AV groove fat pad, which is cleaned away; the incision interrupts the pathway. No electrophysiological data can be obtained until after rewarming the heart. If the pathway is not interrupted or a second pathway becomes manifest, the procedure is repeated.

For the closed heart approach normothermic cardiopulmonary bypass is used only in some patients to avoid hypotension when the heart is manipulated or tachycardia occurs or for anteroseptal pathways. The dissection begins at the atrial epicardium and is extended to the AV groove, which is frozen with the cryoprobe (Fig. 23-12). An atriotomy is required for right anteroseptal pathways but not for those in the posteroseptal or lateral positions. Electrophysiological assessment is continuous and on-line. The successful interruption of the accessory pathway can be pinpointed, damage to the AV node-His bundle (during paraseptal dissections) avoided, multiple pathways discovered, and interruption of tachycardia verified as the dissection is carried out.

In both approaches, after the accessory pathway has been interrupted, an attempt is made to reinitiate the tachycardia and another map is obtained to be certain that the operation was successful and that no other accessory pathways exist.

Both procedures have evolved to the point at which, in expert hands, mortality approaches zero (depending on associated cardiac abnormalities) and the success rate for interrupting the AV connection and eliminating the tachycardia approaches 100 per cent.

AV NODAL REENTRY. Three surgical approaches for patients with AV nodal reentry have evolved. Johnson et al.[297] open the right atrium, and during cold cardioplegia bypass incise the right atrial endocardium at a point behind the tricuspid valve annulus, inferolateral to the coronary sinus os and over the central fibrous body. For "type A" AV nodal reentry (p. 610) in which earliest retrograde atrial activation (during tachycardia) occurs superomedially to the AV node, the *tendon of Todaro* along with all muscle over the central fibrous body and interatrial septum superomedial to the AV node is resected down to the submucosa or fat in the atrial septum. For "type B," in which earliest retrograde atrial activation during AV nodal reentry occurs posterolaterally near the coronary sinus os, connections between the AV node and right atrium posterolateral to the AV node are divided.

Cox et al.[298] developed the second approach, which consists of delivering nine separate 3 mm cryolesions (−60°C, 2 min) around the triangle of Koch in the lower right atrial septum under normothermic cardiopulmonary bypass. AV conduction is monitored and freezing can be discontinued in most instances before the development of permanent AV block.

Finally, Giraudon et al.[299] developed a surgical dissection of the AV node that isolates it from right atrial and septal input, leaving connections to the left atrium.[300] This procedure involves more surgical dissection than does the one advanced by Johnson et al. Each of these approaches has a success rate of about 95 per cent. Heart block is a potential problem.

Less experience has been acquired with surgical treatment of other supraventricular tachycardias that include basically three types: focal atrial or junctional tachycardia, atrial flutter, and atrial fibrillation. When the atrial tachycardia can be well-mapped and is found to be localized to a portion of the atrium such as in the atrial appendage, focal excision[301] or ablation[302] has effectively removed the tachycardia. When precise mapping is impossible, when the tachycardia is lo-

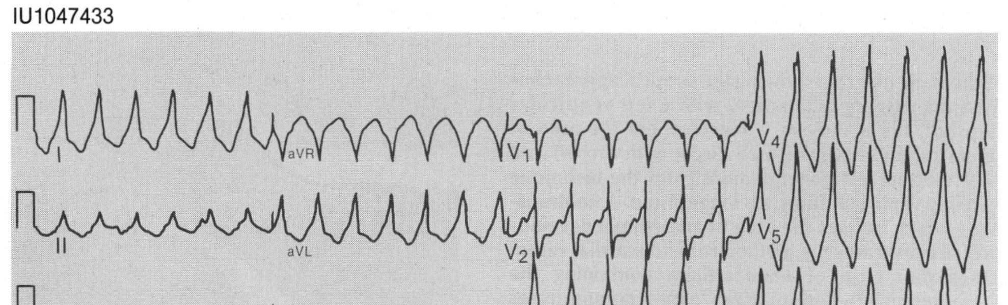

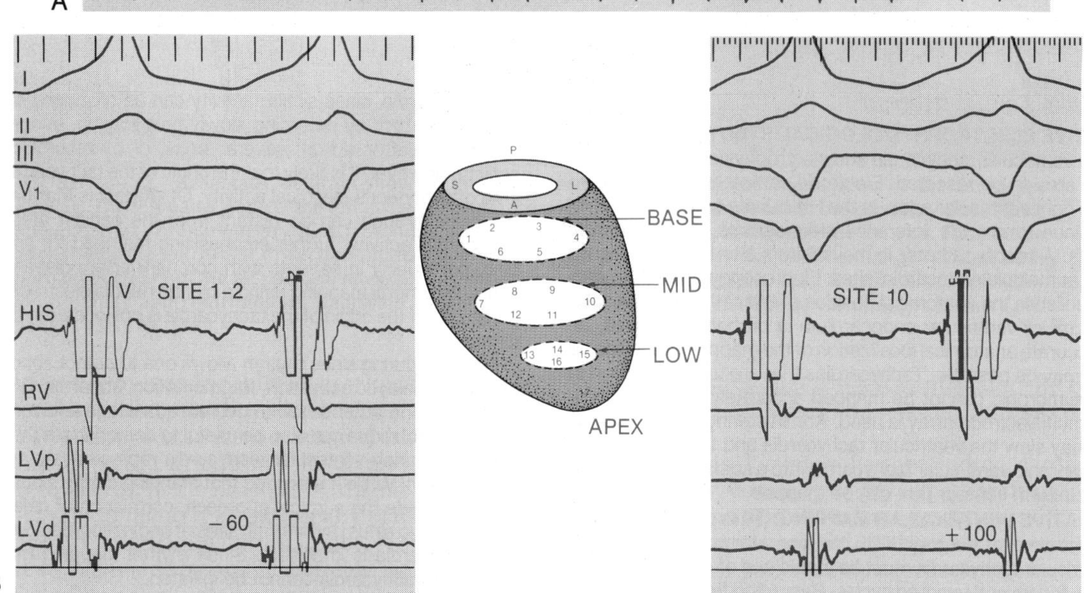

FIGURE 23-14. Mapping of a ventricular tachycardia. Figure 23-14*A*, The 12-lead ECG demonstrates a ventricular tachycardia with a normal axis and left bundle branch block contour. *B*, A left ventricular catheter placed in the posteroseptal region of the left ventricle (positions 1, 2 in the schematic insert) records electrical activity from the distal electrodes of the left ventricular catheter (LVd) 60 msec in advance of the onset of the QRS complex. This illustrates that the tip of the catheter is close to the "origin" of the ventricular tachycardia. Electrical activity in the proximal left ventricular electrodes (LVp) and in the right ventricular recording (RV) is quite late (left panel). In the right panel, electrical activity recorded at site 10 in the midlateral left ventricle occurs well after the onset of the QRS complex, indicating that it is far from the origin of the tachycardia.

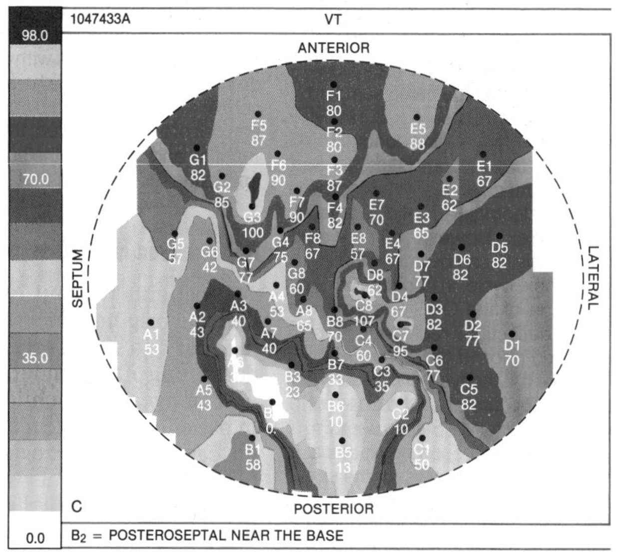

***C*, At the time of surgery, a balloon studded with electrodes was inflated in the left ventricle and recorded an isopotential map that confirmed the origin of the ventricular tachycardia at a posteroseptal position in the left ventricle (color print). (Schematic in B reproduced with permission from Dusman, R. E. et al.: Electrophysiological directed endocardial resection and cryoablation in the treatment of ventricular tachyarrhythmias. Indiana Med. *81*:242, 1988.)**

promising but still need improvement. Patients with prolonged Q-T or Q-U syndrome are thought to have arrhythmias due to preponderant left stellate sympathetic tone, and accordingly, left stellate ganglionectomy has been effective in some patients.[134] Valve replacement may eliminate the tachycardia in some patients with mitral valve prolapse and associated ventricular tachycardia.

Acknowledgments

The author thanks William M. Miles and Lawrence S. Klein for critical comments on this chapter. Some of the illustrations were taken from studies they performed.

REFERENCES

PHARMACOLOGICAL THERAPY

1. Turgeon, J., Murray, K., and Roden, D. M.: Effects of drug metabolism, metabolites and stereoselectivity on antiarrhythmic drug action. J. Cardiovasc. Electrophys. *1*:238, 1990.
2. Woosley, R.: Antiarrhythmic agents. *In* Zipes, D. P., and Jalife, J. (eds.): Cardiac Electrophysiology. From Cell to Bedside. Philadelphia, W. B. Saunders Company, 1990, p.872.
3. Shammas, F. V., and Dickstein, K.: Clinical pharmacokinetics in heart failure. An updated review. Clin. Pharmacokinet. *15*:94, 1988.
4. Woosley, R. L., and Funck-Brentano, C.: Overview of the clinical pharmacology of antiarrhythmic drugs. Am. J. Cardiol. *61*:61A, 1988.
5. Singh, B. N., and Courtney, K. P.: The classification of antiarrhythmic mechanisms of drug action: Experimental and clinical considerations. *In* Zipes, D. P., and Jalife, J., (eds.): Cardiac Electrophysiology. From Cell to Bedside. Philadelphia, W. B. Saunders Company, 1990, p. 882.
6. Hondeghem, L. M.: Molecular interactions of antiarrhythmic agents with their receptor sites. *In* Zipes, D. P., and Jalife, J., (eds.): Cardiac Electrophysiology. From Cell to Bedside. W. B. Saunders Company, 1990, p. 865.
7. Murray, K. T., Reilly, C., Koshakji, R. P., et al.: Suppression of ventricular arrhythmias in man by D-propranolol independent of beta-adrenergic receptor blockade. J. Clin. Invest. *85*:836, 1990.
8. Kroemer, H. K., Funck-Brentano, C., Silberstein, D. J., et al.: Stereoselective disposition and pharmacologic activity of propafenone enantiomers. Circulation *79*:1068, 1989.
9. Le Corre, P., Gibassier, B., desCaves, C., et al.: Clinical pharmacokinetics of levorotatory and racemic disopyramide, at steady state, following oral administration in patients with ventricular arrhythmias. J. Clin. Pharmacol. *29*:1089, 1989.
10. Curtis, M. J., and Walker, M. J. A.: The mechanism of action of the optical enantiomers of verapamil against ischemia-induced arrhythmias in the conscious rat. Br. J. Pharmacol. *89*:137, 1986.
11. Thompson, K. A., Murray, J. J., Blair, I. A., et al.: Plasma concentrations of quinidine, its major metabolites, and dihydroquinidine in patients with torsades de pointes. Clin. Pharmacol. Ther. *43*:636, 1988.
12. Funck-Brentano, C., Light, R. T., Lineberry, M. D., et al.: Pharmacokinetic and pharmacodynamic interaction of N-acetyl procainamide and procainamide in humans. J. Cardiovasc. Pharmacol. *14*:364, 1989.
13. Bennett, P. B., Woosley, R. L., and Hondeghem, L. M.: Competition between lidocaine and one of its metabolites, glycylxylidide, for cardiac sodium channels. Circulation *78*:692, 1988.
14. Eichelbaum, M., and Gross, A. S.: Genetic polymorphism of debrisoquine/sparteine metabolism-clinical aspects. Pharmacol. Ther. (In press.)
15. Skoda, R. C., Gonzalez, F. J., Demierre, A., and Meyer, U. S.: Two mutant alleles of the human cytochrome p-450db 1 gene (p450c2di) associated with genetically deficient metabolism of debrisoquine and other drugs. Proc. Natl. Acad. Sci. USA *85*:5240, 1988.
16. Turgeon, J., Pavlou, H. N., Wong, W, et al.: Genetically determined steady state interaction between encainide and quinidine in patients with arrhythmias. J. Pharmacol. Exp. Ther. (In press.)
17. Baciewicz, A. M., and Baciewicz, F. A., Jr.: Effect of cimetidine and ranitidine on cardiovascular drugs. Am. Heart J. *118*:144, 1989.
18. Dusman, R. E., Stanton, M. S., Miles, W. M., et al.: Clinical features of amiodarone-induced pulmonary toxicity. Circulation *82*:51, 1990.
19. Roden, D.: New concepts in antiarrhythmic drug pharmacokinetics. Prog. Cardiol. *15*:1987.
20. Horowitz, L. N., Zipes, D. P., Bigger, J. J., Jr., et al.: Proarrhythmia, arrhythmogenesis, or aggravation of arrhythmia—a status report 1987. Am. J. Cardiol. *59*:54E, 1987.
21. Zipes, D. P.: Proarrhythmia effects of antiarrhythmic drugs. Am. J. Cardiol. *59*:26E, 1987.
22. Rosen, M. R., and Wit, A. L.: Arrhythmogenic actions of antiarrhythmic drugs. Am. J. Cardiol. *59*:10E, 1987.
23. Josephson, M. E.: Antiarrhythmic agents and the danger of proarrhythmic events. Ann. Intern. Med. *111*:101, 1989.
24. Akhtar, M., Breithardt, G., Camm, A. J., et al.: CAST and beyond. Implications of the Cardiac Arrhythmia Suppression Trial. Circulation *81*:1123, 1990.
25. Rae, A. P., Kay, H. R., Horowitz, L. N., et al.: Proarrhythmic effects of antiarrhythmic drugs in patients with malignant ventricular arrhythmias evaluated by electrophysiologic testing. J. Am. Coll. Cardiol. *12*:131, 1988.
26. Stanton, M. S., Prystowsky, E. N., Fineberg, N. S., et al.: Arrhythmogenic effects of antiarrhythmic drugs: A study of 506 patients treated for ventricular tachycardia or fibrillation. J. Am. Coll. Cardiol. *14*:209, 1989.
27. Minardo, J. D., Heger, J. J., Miles, W. M., et al.: Clinical characteristics of patients with ventricular fibrillation during antiarrhythmic drug therapy. N. Engl. J. Med. *319*:257, 1988.
28. Bigger, J. T., Jr., Sahar, D. I.: Clinical types of proarrhythmic response to antiarrhythmic drugs. Am. J. Cardiol. *59*:2E, 1987.
29. The Cardiac Arrhythmia Suppression Trial (CAST) Investigators: Preliminary report: Effect of encainide and flecainide on mortality in a randomized trial of arrhythmia suppression after myocardial infarction. N. Engl. J. Med. *321*:406, 1989.
30. Wit, A. L., Tseng, G., Henning, B., and Hanna, M. S.: Arrhythmogenic effects of quinidine on catecholamine-induced delayed afterdepolarizations in canine atrial fibers. J. Cardiovasc. Electrophys. *1*:15, 1990.
31. Roden, D. M., and Hoffman, B. F.: Action potential prolongation and induction of abnormal automaticity by low quinidine concentrations in canine Purkinje fibers. Circ. Res. *56*:857, 1985.
32. Nattel, S., and Quantz, M. A.: Pharmacological response of quinidine-induced early afterdepolarizations in canine cardiac Purkinje fibres: Insights into underlying ionic mechanisms. Cardiovasc. Res. *22*:808, 1988.
33. Davidenko, J. M., Cohn, L., Goodrow, R., and Antzelevitch, C.: Quinidine-induced action potential prolongation, early afterdepolarizations, and triggered activity in canine Purkinje fibers. Effects of stimulation rate, potassium, and magnesium. Circulation *79*:674, 1989.
34. Kaseda, S., Gilmour, R. F., Jr., and Zipes, D. P.: Depressant effect of magnesium on early afterdepolarizations and triggered activity induced by cesium quinidine and 4-aminopyridine in canine cardiac Purkinje fibers. Am. Heart J. *118*:458, 1989.
35. El-Sherif, N., Bekheit, S. S., and Henkin, R.: Quinidine-induced long QTU interval and torsades de pointes: Role of bradycardia-dependent early afterdepolarizations. J. Am. Coll. Cardiol. *14*:252, 1989.
36. Hoffman, B. F., and Dangman, K. H.: The role of antiarrhythmic drugs in sudden cardiac death. J. Am. Coll. Cardiol. *8*:104A, 1986.
37. Leichter, D., Danilo, P., Jr., Boyden, P., et al.: A canine model of torsades de pointes. PACE *11*:2235, 1988.
38. Bailie, D. S., Inoue, H., Kaseda, S., et al.: Magnesium suppresses early afterdepolarizations and ventricular tachyarrhythmias induced in dogs by cesium. Circulation *77*:1395, 1988.
39. Ben-David, J., and Zipes, D. P.: Differential response to right and left stellate stimulation of early afterdepolarizations and ventricular tachycardia in the dog. Circulation *78*:1241, 1988.
40. Ben-David, J., and Zipes, D. P.: Alpha adrenoceptor stimulation and blockade modulates cesium-induced early afterdepolarizations and ventricular tachyarrhythmia in dogs. Circulation *82*:225, 1990.
41. Zipes, D. P.: Monophasic action potentials in the diagnosis of triggered arrhythmias. Prog. Cardiovasc. Dis. In press.
42. Scamps, F., Undrovinas, A., and Vassort, G.: Inhibition of ICa in single frog cardiac cells by quinidine, flecainide, ethmozin, and ethacizin. Am. J. Physiol. *256*:C549, 1989.
43. Nishimura, M., Huan, R. M., Habuchi, Y., et al.: Membrane actions of quinidine sulfate in the rabbit atrioventricular node studied by voltage clamp method. J. Pharmacol. Exp. Ther. *244*:780, 1988.
44. Morikawa, Y., and Rosen, M. R.: Effects of quinidine on the transmembrane potentials of young and adult canine cardiac Purkinje fibers. J. Pharmacol. Exp. Ther. *236*:832, 1986.
45. Imaizumi, Y., and Giles, W. R.: Quinidine-induced inhibition of transient outward current in cardiac muscle. Am. J. Physiol. *253* (Heart Circ. Physiol. 22): H704, 1987.
46. Hondeghem, L. M., and Snyders, D. J.: Class III antiarrhythmic agents have a lot of potential but a long way to go. Reduced effectiveness and dangers of reverse use dependence. Circulation *81*:686, 1990.
47. Swerdlow, C. D., and Liem, L. B.: Atrial and junctional tachycardias: Clinical presentation, course, and therapy. *In* Zipes, D. P., and Jalife, J., (eds.): Cardiac Electrophysiology. From Cell to Bedside. Philadelphia, W. B. Saunders Company, 1990, p. 742.
48. Wellens, H. J. J., Brugada, P., Penn, O. C., et al.: Pre-excitation syndromes. *In* Zipes, D. P., and Jalife, J., (eds.): Cardiac Electrophysiology. From Cell to Bedside. Philadelphia, W. B. Saunders Company, 1990, p. 691.
49. Stanton, M. S., Miles, W. M., and Zipes, D. P.: Atrial fibrillation and flutter. *In* Zipes, D. P., and Jalife, J. (eds.): Cardiac Electrophysiology. From Cell to Bedside, Philadelphia, W. B. Saunders Company, 1990, p. 735.
50. Coplen, S. E., Antman, E. M., Berlin, J. A., et al.: Efficacy and safety of quinidine therapy for maintenance of sinus rhythm after cardioversion: A metaanalysis of randomized trials. Circulation *82*:1106, 1990.
50a. Giardina, E. G., and Wechsler, M. E.: Low-dose quinidine-mexiletine combination therapy versus quinidine monotherapy for treatment of ventricular arrhythmias. J. Am. Coll. Cardiol. *15*:1138, 1990.
51. Selzer, A., and Wray, H. W.: Quinidine syncope: Paroxysmal ventricular fibrillation occurring during treatment of chronic atrial arrhythmias. Circulation *30*:17, 1964.
52. Tzivoni, D., Banai, S., Schuger, C., et al.: Treatment of torsades de pointes with magnesium sulfate. Circulation *77*:392, 1988.
53. Dangman, K. H.: Effects of procainamide on automatic and triggered impulse initiation in isolated preparations of canine cardiac Purkinje fibers. J. Cardiovasc. Pharmacol. *12*:78, 1988.

54. Schmitt C. G., Kadish A. H., Marchlinski F. E., et al.: Effects of lidocaine and procainamide on normal and abnormal intraventricular electrograms during sinus rhythm. Circulation *77*:1030, 1988.
54a. Gottlieb, S. S., Kukin, M. L., Medina, N. et al.: Comparative hemodynamic effects of procainamide, tocainide and encainide in severe chronic heart failure. Circulation *81*:860, 1990.
55. Bauer, L. A., Black, D., Gensler, A., and Sprinkle, J.: Influence of age, renal function and heart failure on procainamide clearance and N-acetylprocainamide serum concentrations. Int. J. Clin. Pharmacol. Ther. Toxicol. *27*:213, 1989.
56. Morady, F., Kou, W. H., Schmaltz, S., et al.: Pharmacodynamics of intravenous procainamide as used during acute electropharmacologic testing. Am. J. Cardiol. *61*:93, 1988.
57. Kessler, K. M., McAuliffe, D., Kozlovskis, P., et al.: QRS morphology-dependent pharmacodynamics in multiform ventricular ectopic activity. Am. J. Cardiol. *61*:563, 1988.
58. Ropella, K. M., Sahakian, A. V., Baierman, J. M., and Swiryn, S.: Effects of procainamide on intra-atrial electrograms during atrial fibrillation: Implications for detection algorithms. Circulation *77*:1047, 1988.
59. Fananapazir, L., Packer, D. L., German, L. D., et al.: Procainamide infusion test: Inability to identify patients with Wolff-Parkinson-White syndrome who are potentially at risk of sudden death. Circulation *77*:1291, 1988.
60. Boahene, K. A., Klein, G. J., Sharma, A. D., and Yee, R.: Value of a revised procainamide test in the Wolff-Parkinson-White syndrome. Am. J. Cardiol. *65*:195, 1990.
61. Twidale, N., Heddle, W. F., and Tonkin, A. M.: Procainamide administration during electrophysiology study—utility as a provocative test for intermittent atrioventricular block. PACE *11*:1388, 1988.
62. Iesaka, Y., Aonuma, K., Nitta, J., et al.: Effects of procainamide and lidocaine on electrically inducible ventricular tachycardia studied with programmed ventricular stimulation in postmyocardial infarction. Jpn. Circ. J. *52*:262, 1988.
63. Gorgels, A. P. M., van den Dool, A., Hofs, A., et al.: Procainamide is superior to lidocaine in terminating sustained ventricular tachycardia. Circulation *80*:652, 1989.
64. Kuchar, D. L., Rottman, J., Berger, E., et al.: Prediction of successful suppression of sustained ventricular tachyarrhythmias by serial drug testing from data derived at the initial electrophysiologic study. J. Am. Coll. Cardiol. *12*:982, 1988.
65. Stamato, N. J., Frame, L. H., Rosenthal, M. E., et al.: Procainamide-induced slowing of ventricular tachycardia with insights for analysis of resetting response patterns. Am. J. Cardiol. *63*:1455, 1989.
66. Marchlinski, F. E., Buxton, A. E., Josephson, M. E., and Schmitt, C.: Predicting ventricular tachycardia cycle length after procainamide by assessing cycle length-dependent changes in paced QRS duration. Circulation *79*:39, 1989.
67. Marchlinski, F. E., Buxton, A. E., Kindwall, K. E., et al.: Comparison of individual and combined effects of procainamide and amiodarone in patients with sustained ventricular tachyarrhythmias. Circulation *78*:583, 1988.
68. Kay, G. N., Epstein, A. E., and Plumb, V. J.: Preferential effect of procainamide on the reentrant circuit of ventricular tachycardia. J. Am. Coll. Cardiol. *14*:382, 1989.
69. Kadish, A. H., and Morady, F.: Torsades de Pointes. *In* Zipes, D. P., and Jalife, J., (eds.): Cardiac Electrophysiology. From Cell to Bedside. W. B. Saunders Company, 1990, p. 605.
70. Sharma, A. J., Yee, R., Guiraudon, G., and Klein, G. J.: Sensitivity and specificity of invasive and noninvasive testing for risk of sudden death in Wolff-Parkinson-White Syndrome. J. Am. Coll. Cardiol. *10*:373, 1987.
71. Milstein, S., Buetikofer, J., Dunnigan, A., et al.: Usefulness of disopyramide for prevention of upright tilt-induced hypotension-bradycardia. Am. J. Cardiol. *65*:1339, 1990.
72. Teichman, S. L., Ferrick, A., Kim, S. G., et al.: Disopyramide-pyridostigmine interaction: Selective reversal of anticholenergic symptoms with preservation of antiarrhythmic effect. J. Am. Coll. Cardiol. *10*:633, 1987.
73. Coraboeuf, E., Deroubaix, E., Escande, D., and Coulombe, A.: Comparative effects of three class I antiarrhythmic drugs on plateau and pacemaker currents of sheep cardiac Purkinje fibres. Cardiovasc. Res. *22*:375, 1988.
74. Nattel, S., Elharrar, V., Zipes, D. P., and Bailey, J. C.: The pH-dependent electrophysiological effects of quinidine and lidocaine on canine cardiac Purkinje fibers. Circ. Res. *48*:55, 1981.
75. Cardinal, R., Janse, M. J., vanEeden, I., et al.: The effects of lidocaine on intracellular and extracellular potentials, activation, and ventricular arrhythmias during acute regional ischemia in the isolated porcine heart. Circ. Res. *49*:792, 1981.
76. Gilmour, R. F., Jr., and Zipes, D. P.: Electrophysiological response of vascularized hamster cardiac transplants to ischemia. Circ. Res. *50*:599, 1982.
77. Colatsky, I.: Mechanisms of action of lidocaine and quinidine on action potential duration in rabbit cardiac Purkinje fibers. Circ. Res. *50*:17, 1982.
78. Estes, N. A., 3d, Manolis, A. S., Greenblatt, D. J., et al.: Therapeutic serum lidocaine and metabolite concentrations in patients undergoing electrophysiologic study after discontinuation of intravenous lidocaine infusion. Am. Heart J. *117*:1060, 1989.
79. Yusuf, S., Wittes, J., and Friedman, L.: Overview of results of randomized clinical trials in heart disease. 1. Treatments following myocardial infarction. J.A.M.A. *260*:2088, 1988.
80. MacMahon, S., Collins, R., Peto, R., et al.: Effects of prophylactic lidocaine in suspected acute myocardial infarction. J.A.M.A. *260*:1910, 1988.
81. Amerini, S., Bernabei, R., Carbonin, P., et al.: Electrophysiological mechanism for the antiarrhythmic action of propafenone: A comparison with mexiletine. Br. J. Pharmacol. *95*:1039, 1988.
82. Duke, M.: Chronic mexiletine therapy for suppression of ventricular arrhythmias. Clin. Cardiol. *11*:132, 1988.
83. Duff, H. J.: Mexiletine quinidine combination: Enhanced antiarrhythmic and electrophysiologic activity in the dog. J. Pharmacol. Exp. Ther. *249*:617, 1989.
84. Kim, S. G., Mercando, A. D., Tam, S., and Fisher, J. D.: Combination of disopyramide and mexiletine for better tolerance and additive effects for treatment of ventricular arrhythmias. J. Am. Coll. Cardiol. *13*:659, 1989.
85. Moak, J. P., Smith, R. T., and Garson, A., Jr.: Mexiletine: An effective antiarrhythmic drug for treatment of ventricular arrhythmias in congenital heart disease. J. Am. Coll. Cardiol. *10*:824, 1987.
86. Denniss, A. R., Ross, D. L., Cody, D. V., et al.: Randomized controlled trial of prophylactic antiarrhythmic therapy in patients with inducible ventricular tachyarrhythmias after recent myocardial infarction. Eur. Heart J. *9*:746, 1988.
87. Roden, D. M., and Woosley, R. L.: Tocainide. N. Engl. J. Med. *315*:41, 1986.
88. Block, A. J., Merrill, D., and Smith, E. R.: Stereoselectivity of tocainide pharmacodynamics in vivo and in vitro. J. Cardiovasc. Pharmacol. *11*:216, 1988.
89. Uprichard, A.C., Allen, J. D., and Harron, D. W.: Effects of tocainide enantiomers on experimental arrhythmias produced by programmed electrical stimulation. J. Cardiovasc. Pharmacol. *11*:235, 1988.
90. Adhar, G. C., Swerdlow, C. D., Lance, B. L., et al.: Tocainide for drug-resistant sustained ventricular tachyarrhythmias. J. Am. Coll. Cardiol. *11*:124, 1988.
90a. Biggêr, J. T., Jr.: Cardiac electrophysiologic effects of moricizine hydrochloride. Am. J. Cardiol. *65*:15D, 1990.
91. Arnsdorf, M. F., and Sawicki, G. J.: Effects of ethmozin on excitability in sheep Purkinje fibers: The balance among active and passive cellular properties which comprise the electrophysiologic matrix. J. Pharmacol. Exp. Ther. *248*:1158, 1989.
92. Dorian, P., Echt, D. S., Mead, R. H., et al.: Ethmozine: Electrophysiology, hemodynamics, and antiarrhythmic efficacy in patients with life-threatening ventricular arrhythmias. Am. Heart J. *112*:327, 1986.
93. Pratt, C. M., Podrid, P. J., Seals, A. A., et al.: Effects of ethmozine (moricizine HCl) on ventricular function using echocardiographic, hemodynamic and radionuclide assessments. Am. J. Cardiol. *60*:73F, 1987.
94. The Cardiac Arrhythmia Pilot Study (CAPS) Investigators: Effects of encainide, flecainide, imipramine and moricizine on ventricular arrhythmias during the year after acute myocardial infarction: The CAPS. Am. J. Cardiol. *61*:501, 1988.
95. Morganroth, J., and Pratt, C. M.: Prevalence and characteristics of proarrhythmia from moricizine (ethmozine). Am. J. Cardiol. *63*:172, 1989.
96. Mason, J. W.: Basic and clinical cardiac electrophysiology of encainide. Am. J. Cardiol. *58*:18C, 1986.
97. Hemsworth, P. D., and Campbell, T. J.: Depression of maximum rate of depolarization of guinea pig ventricular action potentials by metabolites of encainide. Br. J. Pharmacol. *97*:619, 1989.
98. Kinnaird, A. A., and Man, R. Y.: Electrophysiological effects of encainide and its metabolites in normal canine Purkinje fibers and Purkinje fibers surviving infarction. Can. J. Physiol. Pharmacol. *67*:751, 1989.
99. Roden, D. M., Lee, J. T., Woosley, R. L., and Echt, D. S.: Antiarrhythmic efficacy, clinical electrophysiology, and pharmacokinetics of 3-methoxy-o-desmethyl encainide (MODE) in patients with inducible ventricular tachycardia or fibrillation. Circulation *80*:1247, 1989.
100. Bajaj, A. K., Woosley, R. L., and Roden, D. M.: Acute electrophysiologic effects of sodium administration in dogs treated with o-desmethyl encainide. Circulation *80*:994, 1989.
101. The Encainide-Ventricular Tachycardia Study Group: Treatment of life-threatening ventricular tachycardia with encainide hydrochloride in patients with left ventricular dysfunction. Am. J. Cardiol. *62*:571, 1988.
102. Miles, W. M., Zipes, D. P., Rinkenberger, R. L., et al.: Encainide for treatment of atrioventricular reciprocating tachycardia in the Wolff-Parkinson-White syndrome. Am. J. Cardiol. *62*:20L, 1988.
102a. Gottlieb, S. S., Kukin, M. L., Yushak, M., et al.: Adverse hemodynamic and clinical effects of encainide in severe chronic heart failure. Ann. Intern. Med. *110*:505, 1989.
102b. Symposium on management of cardiac arrhythmias: The role of encainide and sotalol. Cardiovasc. Drugs Ther. *4*(Suppl. 3):531, 1990.
102c. Herre, J. M., Titus, C., Oeff, M., et al.: Inefficacy and proarrhythmic effects of flecainide and encainide for sustained ventricular tachycardia and ventricular fibrillation. Ann. Intern. Med. *113*:671, 1990.
103. Rinkenberger, R. L., Naccarelli, G. V., Miles, W. M., et al.: Encainide for atrial fibrillation associated with Wolff-Parkinson-White syndrome. Am. J. Cardiol. *62*:26L, 1988.
104. Naccarelli, G. V., Jackman, W. M., Akhtar, M., et al.: Efficacy and electrophysiologic effects of encainide for atrioventricular nodal reentrant tachycardia. Am. J. Cardiol. *62*:31L, 1988.
105. Chimienti, M., Li Bergolis, M., Moizi, M., and Salerno, J. A.: Electrophysiologic and clinical effects of oral encainide in paroxysmal atrioventricular node reentrant tachycardia. J. Am. Coll. Cardiol. *14*:992, 1989.
106. Niazi, I., Naccarelli, G., Dougherty, A., et al.: Treatment of atrioventricular node reentrant tachycardia with encainide: reversal of drug effect with isoproterenol. J. Am. Coll. Cardiol. *13*:904, 1989.
107. Kuck, K. H., Kunze, K. P., Schluter, M., and Duckeck, W.: Encainide versus

flecainide for chronic atrial and junctional ectopic tachycardia. Am. J. Cardiol. *62*:37L, 1988.

108. Strasburger, J. F., Smith, R. T., Jr., and Moak, J. P., et al.: Encainide for resistant supraventricular tachycardia in children: Follow-up report. Am. J. Cardiol. *62*:50L, 1988.

109. Lemery, R., Talajic, M., Nattel, S., et al.: Sinus node dysfunction and sudden cardiac death following treatment with encainide. PACE *12*:1607, 1989.

110. Pratt, C. M., Brater, D. C., Harrell, F. E., Jr., et al.: Clinical and regulatory implications of the cardiac arrhythmia suppression trial. Am. J. Cardiol. *65*:103, 1990.

111. Bigger, J. T., Jr.: The events surrounding the removal of encainide and flecainide from the Cardiac Arrhythmia Suppression Trial (CAST) and why CAST is continuing with moricizine. J. Am. Coll. Cardiol. *15*:243, 1990.

112. Multicenter trial of the Italian Study Group on the Electrophysiology of Arrhythmias: Efficacy and safety of flecainide in patients with stable ventricular ectopic beats. G. Ital. Cardiol. *19*:360, 1989.

113. Capparelli, E. V., Kluger, J., Regnier, J. C., and Chow, M. S.: Clinical and electrophysiologic effects of flecainide in patients with refractory ventricular tachycardia. J. Clin. Pharmacol. *28*:268, 1988.

114. Anderson, J. L., and Pritchett, E. L. C.: International symposium on supraventricular arrhythmias: Focus on flecainide. Am. J. Cardiol. *62*:1D, 1988.

115. Wafa, S. S., Ward, D. E., Parker, D. J., and Camm, A. J.: Efficacy of flecainide acetate for atrial arrhythmias following coronary artery bypass grafting. Am. J. Cardiol. *63*:1058, 1989.

116. Manolis, A. S., Estes, N. A., 3d: Reversal of electrophysiologic effects of flecainide on the accessory pathway by isoproterenol in the Wolff-Parkinson-White syndrome. Am. J. Cardiol. *64*:194, 1989.

117. Ranger, S., Talajic, M., Lemery, R., et al.: Amplification of flecainide-induced ventricular conduction slowing by exercise. A potentially significant clinical consequence of use-dependent sodium channel blockade. Circulation *79*:1000, 1989.

118. Falk, R. H.: Flecainide-induced ventricular tachycardia and fibrillation in patients treated for atrial fibrillation. Ann. Intern. Med. *111*:107, 1989.

119. Funck-Brentano, C., Kroemer, H. K., Lee, J. T., and Roden, D. M.: Propafenone. N. Engl. J. Med. *322*:518, 1990.

120. Thompson, K. A., Iansmith, D. H., Siddoway, L. A., et al: Potent electrophysiologic effects of the major metabolites of propafenone in canine Purkinje fibers. J. Pharmacol. Exp. Ther. *244*:950, 1988.

121. Malfatto, G., Zaza, A., Forster, M., et al.: Electrophysiologic, inotropic and antiarrhythmic effects of propafenone, 5-hydroxypropafenone and N-depropylpropafenone. J. Pharmacol. Exp. Ther. *246*:419, 1988.

122. Kroemer, H. K., Funck-Brentano, C., Silberstein, D. J., et al.: Stereoselective disposition and pharmacologic activity of propafenone enantiomers. Circulation *79*:1068, 1989.

123. Lee, J. T., Kroemer, H. K., Silberstein, D. J., et al.: The role of genetically determined polymorphic drug metabolism in the beta-blockade produced by propafenone. N. Engl. J. Med. *322*:1764, 1990.

124. Singh, B. N., Kaplinsky, E., Kirsten, E., and Guerrero, J.: Effects of propafenone on ventricular arrhythmias: Double-blind, parallel, randomized, placebo-controlled dose-ranging study. Am. Heart J. *116*:1542, 1988.

125. Musto, B., D'Onofio, A., Cavallaro, C., and Musto, A.: Electrophysiological effects and clinical efficacy of propafenone in children with recurrent paroxysmal supraventricular tachycardia. Circulation *78*:863, 1988.

126. Antman, E. M., Beamer, A. D., Cantillon, C., et al.: Long-term oral propafenone therapy for suppression of refractory symptomatic atrial fibrillation and atrial flutter (published erratum appears in J. Am. Coll. Cardiol. *13*:264, 1989). J. Am. Coll. Cardiol. *12*:1005, 1988.

127. Bianconi, L., Boccadamo, R., Pappalardo, A., et al.: Effectiveness of intravenous propafenone for conversion of atrial fibrillation and flutter of recent onset. Am. J. Cardiol. *64*:335, 1989.

128. Northcote, R. J., and Ballantyne, D.: The influence of beta-adrenoceptor blockers with and without intrinsic sympathomimetic activity on heart rate, arrhythmias and ST-T segments, using ambulatory electrocardiography. Br. J. Clin. Pharmaol. *25*:179, 1988.

129. Maisel, A. S., Motulsky, H. J., and Insel, P. A.: Propranolol treatment externalizes beta-adrenergic receptors in guinea pig myocardium and prevents further externalization by ischemia. Circ. Res. *60*:108, 1987.

130. Chang, M. S., and Zipes, D. P.: Differential sensitivity of sinus node, atrioventricular node, atrium and ventricle to propranolol. Am. Heart J. *116*:371, 1988.

131. Kinoshita, K., Hearse, D. J., Braimbridge, M. V., and Manning, A. S.: Ischemia- and reperfusion-induced arrhythmias in conscious rats—studies with prazosin and atenolol. Jpn. Circ. J. *52*:1384, 1988.

132. Inoue, H., and Zipes, D. P.: Results of sympathetic denervation in the canine heart: supersensitivity that may be arrhythmogenic. Circulation *75*:877, 1987.

132a. Zipes, D. P.: Influence of myocardial ischemia and infarction on autonomic innervation of the heart. Circulation *82*:1095, 1990.

133. Arsura, E., Lefkin, A. S., Scher, D. L., et al.: A randomized, double-blind, placebo-controlled study of verapamil and metoprolol in treatment of multifocal atrial tachycardia. Am. J. Med. *85*:519, 1988.

134. Schwartz, P. J., Locati, E., Priori, S. G., and Zaza, A.: The long Q-T syndrome. *In* Zipes, D. P., and Jalife, J., (eds.): Cardiac Electrophysiology. From Cell to Bedside. Philadelphia, W. B. Saunders Company, 1990, p. 589.

135. Boudoulas, H., Kolibash, A. J., Jr., Baker, P., et al.: Mitral valve prolapse and the mitral valve prolapse syndrome: A diagnostic classification and pathogenesis of symptoms. Am. Heart J. *118*:796, 1989.

136. Brodsky, M. A., Allen, B. J., Luckett, C. R., et al.: Antiarrhythmic efficacy of solitary beta-adrenergic blockade for patients with sustained ventricular tachyarrhythmias. Am. Heart J. *118*:272, 1989.

137. Duff, H. J., Mitchell, L. B., and Wyse, D. G.: Antiarrhythmic efficacy of propranolol: Comparison of low and high serum concentrations. J. Am. Coll. Cardiol. *8*:959, 1986.

138. Yusuf, S.: Early intravenous beta blockade in acute myocardial infarction. Postgrad. Med. *29*:(Spec No):90, 1988.

139. Hjalmarson, A.: International beta-blocker review in acute and postmyocardial infarction. Am. J. Cardiol. *61*:26B, 1988.

140. Furberg, C. D., and Byington, R. P.: Beta-adrenergic blockers in patients with acute myocardial infarction. Cardiovasc. Clin. *20*:235, 1989.

141. Gallagher, J. D., Bianchi, J., and Gessman, L. J.: A comparison of the electrophysiologic effects of acute and chronic amiodarone administration on canine Purkinje fibers. J. Cardiovasc. Pharmacol. *13*:723, 1989.

142. Nattel, S., Talajic, J., Quantz, M., and DeRoode, M.: Frequency-dependent effects of amiodarone on atrioventricular nodal function and slow-channel action potentials: evidence for calcium channel-blocking activity. Circulation *76*:442, 1987.

143. Anderson, K. P., Walker, R., Dustman, T., et al.: Rate-related electrophysiologic effects of long-term administration of amiodarone on canine ventricular myocardium in vivo. Circulation *79*:948, 1989.

144. Cascio, W. E., Woelfel, A., Knisley, S. B., et al.: Use dependence of amiodarone during the sinus tachycardia of exercise in coronary artery disease. Am. J. Cardiol. *61*:1042, 1988.

145. Levine, J. H., Moore, E. N., Kadish, A. H., et al.: Mechanisms of depressed conduction from long-term amiodarone therapy in canine myocardium. Circulation *78*:684, 1988.

146. Nattel, S., Davies, M., and Quantz, M.: The antiarrhythmic efficacy of amiodarone and desethylamiodarone, alone and in combination, in dogs with acute myocardial infarction. Circulation *77*:200, 1988.

147. Kato, R., Venkatesh, N., Kamiya, K., et al.: Electrophysiologic effects of desethylamiodarone, an active metabolite of amiodarone: Comparison with amiodarone during chronic administration in rabbits. Am. Heart J. *115*:351, 1988.

148. Talajic, M., Nattel, S., Davies, M., and McCans, J.: Attenuation of class 3 and sinus node effects of amiodarone by experimental hypothyroidism. J. Cardiovasc. Pharmacol. *13*:447, 1989.

148a. Takanaka, C., and Singh, B.: Barium-induced nondriven action potentials as a model of triggered potentials from early afterdepolarizations: Significance of slow channel activity and differing effects of quinidine and amiodarone. J. Am. Coll. Cardiol. *15*:213, 1990.

149. Klein, R. C., Machell, C., Rushforth, N., and Standefur, J.: Efficacy of intravenous amiodarone as short-term treatment for refractory ventricular tachycardia. Am. Heart J. *115*:96, 1988.

150. Ochi, R. P., Goldenberg, I. F., Almquist, A., et al.: Intravenous amiodarone for the rapid treatment of life-threatening ventricular arrhythmias in critically ill patients with coronary artery disease. Am. J. Cardiol. *64*:599, 1989.

151. Feld, G. K., Nademanee, K., Stevenson, W., et al.: Clinical and electrophysiologic effects of amiodarone in patients with atrial fibrillation complicating the Wolff-Parkinson-White syndrome. Am. Heart J. *115*:102, 1988.

152. Kopelman, H. A., and Horowitz, L. N.: Efficacy and toxicity of amiodarone for the treatment of supraventricular tachyarrhythmias. Prog. Cardiovasc. Dis. *31*:355, 1989.

153. Kouvaras, G., Cokkinos, D. V., Halal, G., et al.: The effective treatment of multifocal atrial tachycardia with amiodarone. Jpn. Heart J. *30*:301, 1989.

154. Kowey, P. R., Friehling, T. D., Marinchak, R. A., et al.: Safety and efficacy of amiodarone. The low-dose perspective. Chest *93*:54, 1988.

155. Primeau, R., Agha, A., and Giorgi, C., et al.: Long-term efficacy and toxicity of amiodarone in the treatment of refractory cardiac arrhythmias. Can. J. Cardiol. *5*:98, 1989.

156. Weinberg, B., Dusman, R., Stanton, M., et al.: Five year follow-up of 590 patients treated with amiodarone. PACE *12*:642, 1989 (abstract).

157. Herre, J. M., Sauve, M. J., Malone, P., et al.: Long-term results of amiodarone therapy in patients with recurrent sustained ventricular tachycardia or ventricular fibrillation. J. Am. Coll. Cardiol. *13*:442, 1989.

158. Ardura, J., Hermoso, F., and Bermejo, J.: Effect on growth of children with cardiac dysrhythmias treated with amiodarone. Pediatr. Cardiol. *9*:33, 1988.

159. Amiodarone vs Sotalol Study Group: Multicentre randomized trial of sotalol vs amiodarone for chronic malignant ventricular tachyarrhythmias. Eur. Heart J. *10*:685, 1989.

160. McKenna, W. J., Adams, K. M., Poloniecki, J. D., et al.: Long-term survival with amiodarone in patients with hypertrophic cardiomyopathy and ventricular tachycardia. Circulation *80*(Suppl. II):II7, 1989.

161. Burkart, F., Pfisterer, M., Kiowski, W., et al.: Improved survival of patients with asymptomatic ventricular arrhythmias after myocardial infarction with amiodarone: A randomized controlled trial. Circulation *80*(Suppl. II):II119, 1989.

162. Marks, M. L., Graham, E. L., Powell, J. L., et al.: Mortality and arrhythmia recurrence following amiodarone discontinuation. Circulation *80*(Suppl. II):II651, 1989.

163. Manolis, A. S., Uricchio, F., Estes, N. A., 3d: Prognostic value of early electrophysiologic studies for ventricular tachycardia recurrence in patients with coronary artery disease treated with amiodarone. Am. J. Cardiol. *63*:1052, 1989.

164. Krafchek, J., Lin, H. T., Beckman, K. J., et al.: Cumulative effects of amiodarone on inducibility of ventricular tachycardia: implications for electrophysiological testing. PACE *11*:434, 1988.

165. Rotmensch, H. H.: Amiodarone therapy: Role of early and late electrophysiologic studies. J. Am. Coll. Cardiol. *11*:117, 1988.
166. Greenberg, M. L., Lerman, B. B., Haines, D. E., et al.: Stability of electrophysiological parameters after acute amiodarone loading: Implications for patient management. PACE *12*:1038, 1989.
167. Klein, L. S., Fineberg, N., Heger, J. J., et al.: Prospective evaluation of a discriminant function for prediction of recurrent symptomatic ventricular tachycardia or ventricular fibrillation in coronary artery disease patients receiving amiodarone and having inducible ventricular tachycardia at electrophysiologic study. Am. J. Cardiol. *61*:1024, 1988.
168. Tonet, J., Frank, R., Fontaine, G., Grosgogeat, Y.: Efficacy and safety of low doses of beta-blocker agents combined with amiodarone in refractory ventricular tachycardia. PACE *11*:1984, 1988.
169. Marchlinski, F. E., Buxton, A. E., Kindwall, K. E., et al.: Comparison of individual and combined effects of procainamide and amiodarone in patients with sustained ventricular tachyarrhythmias. Circulation *78*:583, 1988.
170. Paul, V., Griffith, M., Ward, D. E., and Camm, A. J.: Adjuvant xamoterol or metoprolol in patients with malignant ventricular arrhythmia resistant to amiodarone. Lancet *2*:302, 1989.
171. Dusman, R. E., Stanton, M. S., Miles, W. M., et al.: Clinical features of amiodarone-induced pulmonary toxicity. Circulation *82*:51, 1990.
172. Gleadhill, I. C., Wise, R. A., Schonfeld, S. A., et al.: Serial lung function testing in patients treated with amiodarone: A prospective study. Am. J. Med. *86*:4, 1989.
173. Perkins, M. W., Dasta, J. F., Reilley, T. E., and Halpern, P.: Intraoperative complications in patients receiving amiodarone: Characteristics and risk factors. DICP *23*:757, 1989.
174. Kupferschmid, J. P., Rosengart, T. K., McIntocsh, C. L., et al.: Amiodarone-induced complications after cardiac operation for obstructive hypertrophic cardiomyopahty. Ann. Thorac. Surg. *48*:359, 1989.
175. Bacaner, M. B., Clay, J. R., Shrier, A., Brochu, R. M.: Potassium channel blockade: A mechanism for suppressing ventricular fibrillation. Proc. Natl. Acad. Sci. USA *83*:2223, 1986.
176. Kabell, G.: Ischemia-induced conduction delay and ventricular arrhythmias: Comparative electropharmacology of bethanidine sulfate and bretylium tosylate. J. Cardiovasc. Pharmacol. *13*:471, 1989.
177. Nademanee, K., and Singh, B. N.: Control of cardiac arrhythmias by calcium antagonism. Ann. NY Acad. Sci. *522*:536, 1988.
178. Talajic, M., Nayebpour, M., Jing, W., Nattel, S.: Frequency-dependent effects of diltiazem on the atrioventricular node during experimental atrial fibrillation. Circulation *80*:380, 1989.
178a. Talajic, M., Papadatos, D, Villemarie, C., et al.: Antiarrhythmic actions of diltiazem during experimental atrioventricular reentrant tachycardias. Circulation *81*:334, 1990.
179. Przywara, D. A., and Dambach, G. E.: Direct actions of cocaine on cardiac cellular electrical activity. Circ. Res. *65*:185, 1989.
180. Billman, G. E., and Hoskins, R. S.: Cocaine-induced ventricular fibrillation: Protection afforded by the calcium antagonist verapamil. FASEB J *2*:2990, 1988.
181. Wallick, D. W., Stuesse, S. L., and Crafford, W.: Verapamil potentiates vagally mediated atrioventricular chronotropic responses in dogs. J. Cardiovasc. Pharmacol. *12*:122, 1988.
182. Kabell, G.: Modulation of conduction slowing in ischemic rabbit myocardium by calcium-channel activation and blockade. Circulation *77*:1385, 1988.
183. Jenkins, M. G., Johnson, T. A., Engle, C., and Gettes, L.: Metabolic protection by verapamil during graded coronary flow reduction independent of effect on baseline systolic function. Circulation *80*:1870, 1989.
184. Qi, A. Z., Tuna, I. C., Gornick, C. C., et al.: Potentiation of cardiac electrophysiologic effects of verapamil after autonomic blockade or cardiac transplantation. Circulation *75*:888, 1987.
185. Factor, S. M., Cho, S. H., Scheuer, J., et al.: Prevention of hereditary cardiomyopathy in the Syrian hamster with chronic verapamil therapy. J. Am. Coll. Cardiol. *12*:1599, 1988.
186. Belhassen, B., Glick, A., and Laniado, S.: Comparative clinical and electrophysiologic effects of adenosine triphosphate and verapamil on paroxysmal reciprocating junctional tachycardia. Circulation *77*:795, 1988.
187. Huycke, E. C., Sung, R. J., Dias, V. C., et al.: Intravenous diltiazem for termination of reentrant supraventricular tachycardia: A placebo-controlled, randomized, double-blind multicenter study. J. Am. Coll. Cardiol. *13*:538, 1989.
188. Maxwell, D. J., Crawford, D. C., Curry, P. V., et al.: Obstetric importance, diagnosis, and management of fetal tachycardias. Br. Med. J. *297*:107, 1988.
189. Gembruch, U., Hansmann, M., Redel, D. A., and Bald, R.: Intrauterine therapy of fetal tachyarrhythmias: Intraperitoneal administration of antiarrhythmic drugs to the fetus in fetal tachyarrhythmias with severe hydrops fetalis. J. Perinat. Med. *16*:39, 1988.
190. Silberbach, M., Dunnigan, A., and Benson, D. W., Jr.: Effect of intravenous propranolol or verapamil on infant orthodromic reciprocating tachycardia. Am. J. Cardiol *63*:438, 1989.
191. Suttorp, M. J., Kingma, J. H., Lie-A-Huen, L., and Mast, E. G.: Intravenous flecainide versus verapamil for acute conversion of paroxysmal atrial fibrillation or flutter to sinus rhythm. Am. J. Cardiol. *63*:693, 1989.
192. Platia, E. V., Michelson, E. L., Porterfield, J. K., and Das, G.: Esmolol versus verapamil in the acute treatment of atrial fibrillation or atrial flutter. Am. J. Cardiol. *63*:925, 1989.
193. Lewis, R. V., McMurray, J., and McDevitt, D. G.: Effects of atenolol, verapamil, and xamoterol on heart rate and exercise tolerance in digitalized patients with chronic atrial fibrillation. J. Cardiovasc. Pharmacol. *13*:1, 1989.
194. Garratt, C., Antoniou, A., Ward, D., and Camm, A. J.: Misuse of verapamil in pre-excited atrial fibrillation. Lancet *1*(8634):367, 1989.
195. Sung, R. J., Keung, E. C., Nguyen, N. X., and Huycke, E. C.: Effects of beta-adrenergic blockade on verapamil-responsive and verapamil-irresponsive sustained ventricular tachycardias. J. Clin. Invest. *81*:688, 1988.
196. Miyajima, S., Aizawa, Y., Suzuki, K., et al.: Sustained ventricular tachycardia responsive to verapamil in patients with hypertrophic cardiomyopathy. Clinical and electrophysiological assessment of drug efficacy. Jpn. Heart J. *30*:241, 1989.
197. Okumura, K., Matsuyama, K., Miyagi, H., et al.: Entrainment of idiopathic ventricular tachycardia of left ventricular origin with evidence for reentry with an area of slow conduction and effect of verapamil. Am. J. Cardiol. *62*:727, 1988.
198. Rankin, A. C., Rae, A. P., and Cobbe, S. M.: Misuse of intravenous verapamil in patients with ventricular tachycardia. Lancet *2*:472, 1987.
199. Sharma, A. D., and Klein, G. J.: Comparative quantitative electrophysiologic effects of adenosine triphosphate on the sinus node and atrioventricular node. Am. J. Cardiol. *61*:330, 1988.
200. Bellardinelli, L., and Pelleg, A.: Cardiac electrophysiology and pharmacology of adenosine. J. Cardiovasc. Electrophysiol. *1*:327, 1990.
201. DiMarco J. P.: Electrophysiology of adenosine. J. Cardiovasc. Electrophys. *1*:340, 1990.
201a. Ellenbogen, K. A., Thames, M. D., and DiMarco, J. P.: Electrophysiological effects of adenosine in the transplanted human heart: Evidence of supersensitivity. Circulation *81*:821, 1990.
201b. Homeister, J. W., Hoff, P. T., and Fletcher, D. D.: Combined adenosine and lidocaine administration limits myocardial reperfusion injury. Circulation *82*:595, 1990.
202. Belardinelli, L., and Berne, R. M.: The cardiac effects of adenosine. Prog. Cardiovasc. Dis. *32*:73, 1989.
203. Lerman, B. B., Wesley, R. C., Jr., DiMarco, J. P., et al.: Antiadrenergic effects of adenosine on His-Purkinje automaticity. Evidence for accentuated antagonism. J. Clin. Invest. *82*:2127, 1988.
204. DiMarco, J. P., Miles, W., Akhtar, M., et al.: Adenosine for paroxysmal supraventricular tachycardia: Dose ranging and comparison with verapamil in placebo-controlled, multicenter trials. Ann. Intern. Med. (*In press*).
205. Overholt, E. D., Rheuban, K. S., Gutgesell, H. P., et al.: Usefulness of adenosine for arrhythmias in infants and children. Am. J. Cardiol. *61*:336, 1988.
205a. Belhassen, B., Glick, A., and Laniado, S.: Comparative clinical and electrophysiologic effects of adenosine triphosphate and verapamil on paroxysmal reciprocating junctional tachycardia. Circulation *77*:795, 1988.
206. DiMarco, J. P., Miles, W., Akhtar, M., et al.: Adenosine for paroxysmal supraventricular tachycardia: Dose ranging and comparison with verapamil. Ann. Intern. Med. *113*:104, 1990.
207. Griffith, M. J., Linker, N. J., Ward, D. E., and Camm. A. J.: Adenosine in the diagnosis of broad complex tachycardia. Lancet *1*:672, 1988.
208. Rankin, A. C., Oldroyd, K. G., Chong, E., et al.: Value and limitations of adenosine in the diagnosis and treatment of narrow and broad complex tachycardias. Br. Heart J. *62*:195, 1989.
209. Sharma, A. D., Klein, G. J., and Yee, R.: Intravenous adenosine triphosphate during wide QRS complex tachycardia: Safety, therapeutic efficacy and diagnostic utility. Am. J. Med. *88*:337, 1990.
210. Rinne, C., Sharma, A. D., Klein G. J., et al.: Comparative effects of adenosine triphosphate on accessory pathway and atrioventricular nodal conduction. Am. Heart J. *115*:1042, 1988.
211. Lerman, B. B., Belardinelli, L., West, G. A., et al.: Adenosine-sensitive ventricular tachycardia: evidence suggesting cyclic AMP-mediated triggered activity. Circulation *74*:270, 1986.
212. Clemo, H. F., and Belardinelli, L.: Effect of adenosine on atrioventricular conduction. I. Site and characterization of adenosine action in the guinea pig atrioventricular node. Circ. Res. *59*:427, 1986.
213. Wesley, R. C., Jr., and Belardinelli, L.: Role of endogenous adenosine in postdefibrillation bradyarrhythmia and hemodynamic depression. Circulation *80*:128, 1989.
214. Antonaccio, M. J., and Gomoll, A. W.: Sotalol—pharmacological and antiarrhythmic effects. Cardiovasc. Drug Rev. *6*:239, 1988.
215. McComb, J. M., McGovern, B., McGowan, J. B., et al.: Electrophysiologic effects of D-sotalol in humans. J. Am. Coll. Cardiol. *10*:211, 1987.
216. Petzl, D. H., Probst, P., Glogar, D., and Schuster, E.: The effect of sotalol on exercise-induced ventricular arrhythmias. Eur. Heart J. *9*:265, 1988.
217. Kopelman, H. A., Woosley, R. L., Lee, J. T., et al.: Electrophysiologic effects of intravenous and oral sotalol for sustained ventricular tachycardia secondary to coronary artery disease. Am. J. Cardiol. *61*:1006, 1988.
218. Singh, S. N., Cohen, A., Chen, Y. W., et al.: Sotalol for refractory sustained ventricular tachycardia and nonfatal cardiac arrest. Am. J. Cardiol. *62*:399, 1988.
219. Ruder, M. A., Ellis, T., Lebsack, C., et al.: Clinical experience with sotalol in patients with drug-refractory ventricular arrhythmias. J. Am. Coll. Cardiol. *13*:145, 1989.
220. Kuchar, D. L., Garan, H., Venditti, F. J., et al.: Usefulness of sotalol in suppressing ventricular tachycardia or ventricular fibrillation in patients with healed myocardial infarcts. Am. J. Cardiol. *64*:33, 1989.
221. Amiodarone vs Sotalol Study Group: Multicentre randomized trial of sotalol vs amiodarone for chronic malignant ventricular tachyarrhythmias. Eur. Heart J. *10*:685, 1989.

222. Mitchell, L. B., Wyse, D. G., and Duff, H. J.: Electropharmacology of sotalol in patients with Wolff-Parkinson-White syndrome. Circulation *76*:810, 1987.

223. Sahar, D. I., Reiffel, J. A., Bigger, J. T., Jr., et al.: Efficacy, safety, and tolerance of D-sotalol in patients with refractory supraventricular tachyarrhythmias. Am. Heart J. *117*:562, 1989.

224. Gold, R. L., Frumin, H., Haffajee, C. I., et al.: The efficacy, electrophysiologic and electrocardiographic effects of intravenous pirmenol, a new class I antiarrhythmic agent, in patients with ventricular tachycardia: Comparison with procainamide. PACE *11*:308, 1988.

225. Garg, D. C., Jallad, N. S., Singh, S., et al.: Efficacy and pharmacokinetics of oral pirmenol, a new antiarrhythmic drug. J. Clin. Pharmacol. *28*:812, 1988.

226. Reiter, M. J.: Clinical pharmacology and pharmacokinetics of pirmenol. Angiology *39*:293, 1988.

227. Mohiuddin, S. M., Woodruff, M. P., Esterbrooks, D. J., et al.: Crossover comparison of cibenzoline and quinidine in ambulatory patients with chronic ventricular arrhythmias. J. Cardiovasc. Pharmacol. *13*:525, 1989.

228. Colatsky, T. J., Bird, L. B., Jurkiewicz, N. K., and Wendt, R. L.: Cellular electrophysiology of the new antiarrhythmic agent recainam (Wy-42,362) in canine cardiac Purkinje fibers. J. Cardiovasc. Pharmacol. *9*:435, 1987.

229. Takikawa, R., Kamiya, K., Kato, R., and Singh, B. N.: Electrophysiologic effects of a new antiarrhythmic agent, recainam, on isolated canine and rabbit myocardial fibers. J. Am. Coll. Cardiol. *11*:875, 1988.

230. Kamiya, K., Takikawa, R., and Singh, B. N.: Frequency- and voltage-dependent effects of recainam on the upstroke velocity of action potential in rabbit ventricular muscle. J. Cardiovasc. Pharmacol. *13*:630, 1989.

231. Holland, D. R., Lacefield, W. B., Gonzales, C. R., et al.: Indecainide: Effects on arrhythmias, electrophysiology, and cardiovascular dynamics. J. Cardiovasc. Pharmacol. *14*:454, 1989.

232. Duff, H. J., Mitchell, L. B., Kavanagh, K. M., et al.: Amiloride. Antiarrhythmic and electrophysiologic actions in patients with inducible sustained ventricular tachycardia. Circulation *79*:1257, 1989.

233. Hasegawa, G. R.: Nicardipine, nitrendipine, and bepridil: New calcium antagonists for cardiovascular disorders. Clin. Pharm. *7*:97, 1988.

ELECTRICAL THERAPY

234. Kerber, R. E.: External direct current defibrillation and cardioversion. *In* Zipes, D. P., and Jalife, J. (eds.): Cardiac Electrophysiology. From Cell to Bedside. Philadelphia, W. B. Saunders Company, 1990, p. 954.

234a. Sweeney, R. J., Gill, R. M., and Skinberg, M. I.: Ventricular refractory period extension caused by defibrillation shocks. Circulation *82*:965, 1990.

235. Witkowski, F. X., Penkoske, P. A., and Plonsey, R.: Mechanisms of cardiac defibrillation in open-chest dogs with unipolar DC-coupled simultaneous activation and shock potential recordings. Circulation *82*:244, 1990.

236. Shibata, N., Chen, P. S., Dixon, E. G., et al.: Epicardial activation after unsuccessful defibrillation shocks in dogs. Am. J. Physiol. *255*:H902, 1988.

237. Bharati, S., and Lev, M.: Histopathologic changes in the heart including the conduction system after catheter ablation. PACE *12*:159, 1989.

238. Moore, E. N., Schafer, W., Kadish, A., et al.: Electrophysiological studies on cardiac catheter ablation. PACE *12*:150, 1989.

239. Mickleborough, L. L., Wilson, G. J., Harris, L., et al.: Balloon electric shock ablation. Effects on ventricular structure, function, and electrophysiology. J. Thorac. Cardiovasc. Surg. *97*:135, 1989.

240. Scheinman, M. M., and Morady, F.: Catheter ablation for treatment of supraventricular arrhythmias. *In* Zipes, D. P., and Jalife, J., (eds.): Cardiac Electrophysiology. From Cell to Bedside. Philadelphia, W. B. Saunders Company, 1990, p. 970.

241. Fontaine, G., Frank, R., Tonet, J., et al.: Fulguration of chronic ventricular tachycardia: Results of 47 consecutive cases with a follow-up ranging from 11 to 65. *In* Zipes, D. P., and Jalife, J., (eds.): Cardiac Electrophysiology. From Cell to Bedside. Philadelphia, W. B. Saunders Company, 1990, p. 978.

242. Huang, S. K., Graham, A. R., and Wharton, K.: Radiofrequency catheter ablation of the left and right ventricles: anatomic and electrophysiologic observations. PACE *11*:449, 1988.

243. Borggrefe, M., Hindricks, G., Haverkamp, W., et al.: Radiofrequency ablation. *In* Zipes, D. P., and Jalife, J., (eds.): Cardiac Electrophysiology. From Cell to Bedside. Philadelphia, W. B. Saunders Company, 1990, p. 997.

244. Weber, H., Enders, S., and Keiditisch, E.: Percutaneous Nd: YAG laser coagulation of ventricular myocardium in dogs using a special electrode laser catheter. PACE *12*:899, 1989.

245. Svenson, R. H., Littmann, L., Splinter, R., et al.: Application of lasers for arrhythmia ablation. In Zipes, D. P., and Jalife, J., (eds.): Cardiac Electrophysiology. From Cell to Bedside, Philadelphia, W. B. Saunders Company, 1990, p. 986.

246. Vijgen, J., Ector, H., and DeGeest, H.: Underlying heart rhythm after catheter ablation of the atrioventricular conduction system. J. Cardiovasc. Electrophys. *1*:209, 1990.

247. Holt, P. M., and Boyd, E. C. G.: A complete heart block using 0.6J ablation impulses (abstract). PACE *11*:489, 1988.

248. Evans, G. T., Scheinman, M. M., Zipes, D. P., et al.: The percutaneous cardiac mapping and ablation registry: Final summary of results. PACE *11*:1621, 1988.

249. Evans, G. T., Scheinman, M. M., Akhtar, M., et al.: In-hospital mortality after direct current catheter ablation of the atrioventricular junction: A prospective international multicenter study. Submitted for publication.

250. Huang, S. K., Bharati, S., Graham, A. R., et al.: Chronic incomplete atrioventricular block induced by radiofrequency catheter ablation. Circulation *80*:951, 1989.

251. Roman, C. A., Wang, X., Friday, K. J., et al.: Catheter technique for selective ablation of slow pathway in AV nodal reentrant tachycardia. PACE *13*:498, 1990 (abstract).

251a. Goy, J. J., Fromer, M., Schlaepfer, J., et al.: Clinical efficacy of radiofrequency current in the treatment of patients atrioventricular node reentrant tachycardia. J. Am. Coll. Cardiol. *16*:418, 1990.

252. Haissaguerre, M., Warin, J. F., Lemetayer, P., et al.: Closed-chest ablation of retrograde conduction in patients with atrioventricular nodal reentrant tachycardia. N. Engl. J. Med. *320*:426, 1989.

253. Epstein, L. M., Scheinman, M. M., Langberg, J. J., et al.: Percutaneous catheter modification of the atrioventricular node. Circulation *80*:757, 1989.

254. Morady, F., Scheinman, M. M., Kou, W. H., et al.: Long-term results of catheter ablation of a posterior accessory atrioventricular connection in 48 patients. Circulation *79*:1160, 1989.

255. Bardy, G. H., Ivey, T. D., Coltorti, F., et al.: Developments, complications and limitations of catheter-mediated electrical ablation of posterior accessory atrioventricular pathways. Am. J. Cardiol. *61*:309, 1988.

256. Ruder, M. A., Mead, R. H., Gaudiani, V., et al.: Transvenous catheter ablation of extranodal accessory pathways. J. Am. Coll. Cardiol. *11*:1245, 1988.

257. Bromberg, B. I., Dick, M., 2d, Scott, W. A., and Morady, F.: Transcatheter electrical ablation of accessory pathways in children. PACE *12*:1787, 1989.

258. Warin, J. F., and Haissaguerre, M.: Fulguration of accessory pathways in any location: Report of 70 cases. PACE *12*:215, 1989.

259. Roman, C. A., Friday, K. J., Wang, X., et al.: Ablation of simple multiple accessory pathways with radio frequency current. Circulation *80*(Suppl II):323, 1989 (abstract).

260. Garan, H., Kuchar, D., Freeman, C., et al.: Early assessment of the effect of map-guided transcatheter intracardiac electric shock on sustained ventricular tachycardia secondary to coronary artery disease. Am. J. Cardiol. *61*:1018, 1988.

261. Borggrefe, M., Breithardt, G., Podozeck, A., et al.: Catheter ablation of ventricular tachycardia using defibrillator pulses: Electrophysiological findings and long-term results. Eur. Heart J. *10*:591, 1989.

262. Stevenson, W. G., Weiss, U. N., Wiener, I., et al.: Fractionated endocardial eclectrograms are associated with slow conduction in humans: Evidence from pace-mapping. J. Am. Coll. Cardiol. *13*:369, 1989.

263. Harris, L., Mickleborough, L. L., Shaikh, N., et al.: Electrical ablation with a balloon electrode array: Chronic electrophysiologic response. PACE *11*:1262, 1988.

264. Davis, J. C., Finkebeiner, W., Ruder, M. A., et al.: Histologic changes and arrhythmogenicity after discharge through transseptal catheter electrode. Circulation *74*:637, 1986.

265. Fitzgerald, D. M., Friday, K. J., Lai Wah, J. A. Y., et al.: Electrogram patterns predicting successful catheter ablation of ventricular tachycardia. Circulation *77*:806, 1988.

266. Morady, F., Frank, R., Kou, W. H., et al.: Identification and catheter ablation of a zone of slow conduction in the reentrant circuit of ventricular tachycardia in humans. J. Am. Coll. Cardiol. *11*:775, 1988.

267. Okumura, K., Olshansky, B., Henthorn, R. W. et al.: Demonstration of the presence of slow conduction during sustained ventricular tachycardia in man: Use of transient entrainment of the tachycardia. Circulation *75*:369, 1987.

268. Caceres, J., Jazayeri, M., McKinnie, J., et al.: Sustained bundle branch reentry as a mechanism of clinical tachycardia. Circulation *79*:256, 1989.

269. Tchou, P., Jazayeri, M., Denker, S., et al.: Transcatheter electrical ablation of right bundle branch. A method of treating macroreentrant ventricular tachycardia attributed to bundle branch reentry. Circulation *78*:246, 1988.

270. Leclercq, J. F., Chouty, F., Cauchemez, B., et al.: Results of electrical fulguration in arrhythmogenic right ventricular disease. Am. J. Cardiol. *62*:220, 1988.

271. Fontaine, G., Frank, R., Rougier, I., et al.: Electrode catheter ablation of resistant ventricular tachycardia in arrhythmogenic right ventricular dysplasia: Experience of 13 patients with a mean follow-up of 45 months. Eur. Heart J. *10*(Suppl. D):74, 1989.

272. Morady, F., Scheinman, M. M., Lorenzo, M. D., et al.: Catheter ablation of ventricular tachycardia with intracardiac shocks: Results in 33 patients. Circulation *75*:1037, 1987.

273. Sellers, T. D., Dilorenzo, D., Primerano, P., et al.: Catheter ablation of resistant ventricular tachycardia: Immediate results and long-term follow-up. PACE *11*:920, 1988 (abstract).

274. Chilson, D. A., Peigh, P. S., Mahomed, Y., et al.: Chemical ablation of ventricular tachycardia in the dog. Am. Heart J. *111*:1113, 1986.

275. Inoue, H., Waller, B. E., and Zipes, D. P.: Intracoronary ethyl alcohol or phenol injection ablates aconitine-induced ventricular tachycardia in the dog. J. Am. Coll. Cardiol. *10*:1342, 1987.

276. Brugada, P., de Swart, H., Smeets, J., and Wellens, H. J. J.: Transcoronary termination and ablation of ventricular tachycardia. Circulation *79*:475, 1989.

277. Brugada, P., de Swart, H., Bar, F. W. H. M., et al.: Transcoronary termina-

tion and chemical ablation of arrhythmias. *In* Zipes, D. P., and Jalife, J. (eds.): Cardiac Electrophysiology. From Cell to Bedside. Philadelphia, W. B. Saunders Company, 1990, p. 1005.
278. Sosa, E. M., Arie, S., Scanavacca, M. I., et al.: Transcoronary chemical ablation of incessant atrial tachycardia. J. Cardiovasc. Electrophysiology *1*:116, 1990.
279. Brugada, P., de Swart, H., Smeets, J., and Wellens, H. J. J.: Transcoronary chemical ablation of atrioventricular conduction. Circulation *81*:757, 1990.
280. Zipes, D. P.: Targeted drug therapy. Circulation *81*:1139, 1990.
280a. Wang, P. J., Sosa-Suarez, G., and Friedman, P. L.: Modification of human atrioventricular nodal function by selective atrioventricular nodal artery catheterization. Circulation *82*:817, 1990.

SURGICAL THERAPY

281. Gallagher, J. J., Selle, J. G., Svenson, R. H., et al.: Surgical treatment of arrhythmias. Am. J. Cardiol. *61*:27A, 1988.
282. Garson, A., Jr., Moak, J. P., Friedman, R. A., et al.: Surgical treatment of arrhythmias in children. Cardiol. Clin. *7*:319, 1989.
283. Case, C. L., Crawford, F. A., Gillette, P. C., et al.: Management strategies for surgical treatment of dysrhythmias in infants and children. Am. J. Cardiol. *63*:1069, 1989.
283a. Smeets, J. L., Kirchhof, C., and Penn, O. C.: Epicardial high resolution mapping of retrograde conduction over the accessory pathway in patients with the Wolff-Parkinson-White syndrome. Circulation *82* (suppl. III):472, 1990 (abstract).
284. Jackman, W. M., Friday, K. J., Yeung-Lai-Wah, J. A., et al.: New catheter technique for recording left free-wall accessory atrioventricular pathway activation. Identification of pathway fiber orientation. Circulation *78*:598, 1988.
285. Jackman, W. M., Friday, K. J., Fitzgerald, D. M., et al.: Localization of left free-wall and posteroseptal accessory atrioventricular pathways by direct recording of accessory pathway activation. PACE *12*:204, 1989.
286. Jackman, W. W., Kuck, K. H., Friday, K. J., and Lazzara, R.: Catheter recordings of accessory atrioventricular pathway activation. *In* Zipes, D. P., and Jalife, J. (eds.): Cardiac Electrophysiology. From Cell to Bedside. Philadelphia, W. B. Saunders Company, 1990, p. 491.
287. Kuck, K. H., Jackman, W. M., Friday, K. J., et al.: Sites of conduction block in accessory atrioventricular pathways: Basis for concealed accessory pathways. *In* Zipes, D. P., and Jalife, J., (eds.): Cardiac Electrophysiology. From Cell to Bedside. Philadelphia, W. B. Saunders Company, 1990, p. 503.
288. Jazayeri, M. R., Caceres, J., Tchou, P., et al.: Electrophysiologic characteristics of sudden QRS axis deviation during orthodromic tachycardia. Role of functional fascicular block in localization of accessory pathway. J. Clin. Invest. *83*:952, 1989.
289. Jazayeri, M., Tchou, P., Caceres, J., et al.: Ventricular conduction time during bundle branch reentrant beat initiating orthodromic tachycardia: A simple and reliable method for localization of accessory pathways. J. Cardiovasc. Electrophys. *1*:121, 1990.
289a. Miles, W. M., Yee, R., Klein, G., et al.: The preexcitation index: An aid in determining the mechanism of supraventricular tachycardia and localizing accessory pathways. Circulation *74*:493, 1986.
290. Schechtmann, N., Botvinik, E. H., Dae, M., et al.: The scintigraphic characteristics of ventricular pre-excitation through Mahaim fibers with the use of phase analysis. J. Am. Coll. Cardiol. *13*:882, 1989.
291. Ferguson, T. B., Jr., and Cox, J. L.: Surgical treatment for the Wolff-Parkinson-White syndrome: The endocardial approach. *In* Zipes, D. P., and Jalife, J. (eds.): Cardiac Electrophysiology. From Cell to Bedside. Philadelphia, W. B., Saunders Company, 1990, p. 897.
292. Kirklin, J. K., McGiffin, D. C., Plumb, V. J., et al.: Intermediate-term results of the endocardial surgical approach for anomalous atrioventricular bypass tracts. Am. Heart J. *115*:444, 1988.
293. Guiraudon G. M., Klein, G. J., Sharma A. D., et al.: Surgery for the Wolff-Parkinson-White syndrome: The epicardial approach. *In* Zipes, D. P., and Jalife, J. (eds.): Cardiac Electrophysiology. From Cell to Bedside. Philadelphia, W. B. Saunders Company, 1990, p. 907.
294. Guiraudon, G. M., Klein, G. J., Sharma, A. D., et al.: "Atypical" posteroseptal accessory pathway in Wolff-Parkinson-White syndrome. J. Am. Coll. Cardiol. *12*:1605, 1988.
295. O'Neill, B. J., Klein, G. J., Guiraudon, G. M., et al.: Results of operative therapy in the permanent form of junctional reciprocating tachycardia. Am. J. Cardiol. *63*:1074, 1989.
296. Mahomed, Y., King, R. D., Zipes, et al.: Surgical division of Wolff-Parkinson-White pathways utilizing the closed heart technique; a 2 year experience in 47 patients. Ann. Thorac. Surg. *45*:495, 1988.
297. Johnson, D. C., Ross, D. L., Uther, J. B.: The surgical cure of atrioventricular junctional reentrant tachycardia. *In* Zipes, D. P., and Jalife J., (eds.): Cardiac Electrophysiology. From Cell to Bedside. Philadelphia, W. B. Saunders, 1990, p. 921.
298. Cox, J. L., Holman, W. L., and Cain, M. E.: Cryosurgical treatment of atrioventricular node reentrant tachycardia. Circulation *76*:1329, 1987.
299. Guiraudon, G. M., Klein, G. J., Sharma, A. D., et al.: Skeletonization of the atrioventricular node. Surgical alternative for AV nodal reentrant tachycardia. Experience with 32 patients. Ann. Thorac. Surg. *49*:565, 1990.
300. Gartman, D. M., Brady, G. H., Williams, A. B., and Ivey, T. D.: Direct surgical treatment of atrioventricular node reentrant tachycardia. J. Thorac. Cardiovasc. Surg. *98*:63, 1989.
301. Seals, A. A., Lawrie, G. M., Magro S., et al.: Surgical treatment of right atrial focal tachycardia in adults. J. Am. Coll. Cardiol. *11*:1111, 1988.
302. Kerr, C. R., Klein, G. G., Guiraudon, G. M., and Webb, J. G.: Surgical therapy for sinoatrial reentrant tachycardia. PACE *11*:776, 1988.
303. Harada, A., D'Agostino, H. J., Jr., Schuessler, R. B., et al.: Right atrial isolation: A new surgical treatment for supraventricular tachycardia. I. Surgical technique and electrophysiologic effects. J. Thorac. Cardiovasc. Surg. *95*:643, 1988.
304. Harada, A., D'Agostino, H. J., Jr., Boineau, J. P., and Cox, J. L.: Right atrial isolation: a new surgical treatment for supraventricular tachycardia. II. Hemodynamic effects. J. Thorac. Cardiovasc. Surg. *95*:651, 1988.
305. Guiraudon, G. M., Klein, G. J., Sharma, A. D., and Yee, R.: Surgery for atrial flutter, atrial fibrillation, and atrial tachycardia. *In* Zipes, D. P., and Jalife, J. (eds.): Cardiac Electrophysiology. From Cell to Bedside. Philadelphia, W. B. Saunders Company, 1990, p. 915.
306. Cox, J. L., Schuessler, R. B., Cain, M. E., et al.: Surgery for atrial fibrillation. Semin. Thorac. Cardiovasc. Surg. *1*:67, 1989.
307. Dapper, F., Gorlach, G., Hoffmann, C., et al.: Primary cardiac tumors—clinical experiences and late results in 48 patients. Thorac. Cardiovasc. Surg. *36*:80, 1988.
308. Hargrove, W. C., III: Surgery for ventricular tachycardia associated with ischemic heart disease: *In* Zipes, D. P., and Jalife, J. (eds.): Cardiac Electrophysiology. From Cell to Bedside. W. B. Saunders Company, 1990, p. 924.
309. Lawrie, G. M., and Pacifico, A.: Surgery for ventricular tachycardia unassociated with coronary artery disease: *In* Zipes, D. P., Jalife, J. (eds.): Cardiac Electrophysiology. From Cell to Bedside. Philadelphia, W. B. Saunders Company, 1990, p. 926.
310. Lawrie, G. M., Pacifico, A., and Kaushik, R.: Results of direct surgical ablation of ventricular tachycardia not due to ischemic heart disease. Ann. Surg. *209*:716, 1989.
311. Cox, J. L.: Patient selection criteria and results of surgery for refractory ischemic ventricular tachycardia. Circulation *79*:I163, 1989.
312. Brandt, B., III, Martins, J. B., and Kienzle, M. G.: Predictors of failure after endocardial resection for sustained ventricular tachycardia. J. Thorac. Cardiovasc. Surg. *95*:495, 1988.
313. Miller, J. M., Marchlinski, F. E., Buxton, A. E., and Josephson, M. E.: Relationship between the 12-lead electrocardiogram during ventricular tachycardia and endocardial site of origin in patients with coronary artery disease. Circulation *77*:759, 1988.
314. Kelly, P., Ruskin, J. N., Vlahakes, G. J., et al.: Surgical coronary revascularization in survivors of prehospital cardiac arrest: Its effect on inducible ventricular arrhythmias and long-term survival. J. Am. Coll. Cardiol. *15*:267, 1990.
315. Manolis, A. S., Rasteger, H., Payne, D., et al.: Surgical therapy for drug-refractory ventricular tachycardia: Results with mapping-guided subendocardial resection. J. Am. Coll. Cardiol. *14*:199, 1989.
315a. Page, P., Kaltenbrunner, W., and Dubric, M.: Epicardial/endocardial mapping of ventricular tachycardia in humans: Is the reentry substrate always subendocardially located? Circulation *82* (suppl. III):473, 1990 (abstract).
316. Guiraudon, G. M., Guiraudon, C. M., McLellan, D. G., and MacDonald, J. L.: Mitral valve function after cryoablation of the posterior papillary muscle in the dog. Ann. Thorac. Surg. *47*:872, 1989.
317. Page, P. L., Cardinal, R., Shenasa, M., et al.: Surgical treatment of ventricular tachycardia. Regional cryoablation guided by computerized epicardial and endocardial mapping. Circulation *80*:I124, 1989.
318. Svenson, R. H., Littmann, L., Gallagher, J. J., et al.: Termination of ventricular tachycardia with epicardial laser photocoagulation. J. Am. Coll. Cardiol. *15*:163, 1990.
319. Ayisi, K., Darup, J., Krebber, H. J., et al.: Alcohol-induced coagulation necrosis in cardiac tissue: A new concept in the surgical management of recurrent ventricular arrhythmias. Thorac. Cardiovasc. Surg. *37*:86, 1989.
320. Hargrove, W. C., III, Josephson, M. E., Marchlinski, F. E., and Miller, J. M.: Surgical decisions in the management of sudden cardiac death and malignant ventricular arrhythmias. Subendocardial resection, the automatic internal defibrillator, or both. J. Thorac. Cardiovasc. Surg. *97*:923, 1989.
321. Borggrefe, M., Podczeck, A., Ostermeyer, J., et al.: Long-term results of electrophysiologically guided antitachycardia surgery in ventricular tachyarrhythmias. A collaborative report on 665 patients. *In* Breithardt, G., Borggrefe, M., and Zipes, D. P. (eds.): Nonpharmacological therapy of tachyarrhythmias. Mt. Kisco, N. Y., Futura Publishing Co., 1987, p. 109.
322. Mickleborough, L. L., Harris, L., Downar, E., et al.: A new intraoperative approach for endocardial mapping of ventricular tachycardia. J. Thorac. Cardiovasc. Surg. *95*:271, 1988.
323. Haines, D. E., Lerman, B. B., Kron, I. L., and DiMarco, J. P.: Surgical ablation of ventricular tachycardia with sequential map-guided subendocardial resection: electrophysiologic assessment and long-term follow-up. Circulation *77*:131, 1988.
324. Zee-Cheng, C. S., Kouchoukos, N. T., Connors, J. P., and Ruffy, R.: Treatment of life-threatening ventricular arrhythmias with nonguided surgery supported by electrophysiologic testing and drug therapy. J. Am. Coll. Cardiol. *13*:153, 1989.
325. Guiraudon, G. M., Klein, G. J., Sharma, A. D., et al.: Surgical therapy for arrhythmogenic right ventricular adiposis. Eur. Heart J. *10*:(Suppl. D):82, 1989.

Specific Arrhythmias: Diagnosis and Treatment

by DOUGLAS P. ZIPES, M.D.

Diagnostic and Therapeutic Considerations

HISTORY

The initial evaluation of the patient suspected of having a cardiac arrhythmia begins by obtaining a careful history, specifically questioning the patient regarding the presence of palpitations,[1] syncope, spells of lightheadedness, chest pain, or symptoms of congestive heart failure. Palpitations, an awareness of the heartbeat (p. 8), may result from irregularities in cardiac rate or rhythm or a change in contractility of the heart. Some patients are able to reproduce this sensation by tapping their hand on their chest, knee, or a table top in a fashion similar to the perceived palpitation or recognize a cadence tapped out by a physician. Such a maneuver can help establish the rate and rhythm of the arrhythmia, narrowing it to a particular rate range, a regular or irregular arrhythmia, or one in which a regular rhythm is interrupted by premature beats. The latter often are perceived only upon the contraction that ends a pause following the premature beat, while the patient feels as if the heart has stopped for a moment. A rapid irregular tapping can suggest the ventricular response to atrial fibrillation while a rapid regular tapping can suggest an atrioventricular (AV) nodal reentrant supraventricular tachycardia, particularly in a young person, or ventricular tachycardia in an older person. Information regarding the nature of onset and termination of the rhythm disturbance is particularly important. Knowing the rate of the arrhythmia is crucial, and a brief demonstration by the physician of how to determine heart rate can yield important dividends. The patient, and sometimes a close relative, should be instructed in how to count the pulse.

Answers by the patient to key questions can provide clues to the type of rhythm disturbance, particularly if the physician has some additional information, such as physical findings and a 12-lead electrocardiogram. For example, a young adult with presyncope, normal physical findings, and electrocardiographic changes indicating Wolff-Parkinson-White (WPW) syndrome (p. 693) should be asked whether the palpitations are regular or irregular, how fast they are, and how they start and stop. If the tachycardia is regular, with a rate of approximately 200 beats per minute and of sudden onset and termination, it is likely that the patient is experiencing an AV reciprocating tachycardia (p. 692); on the other hand, if the rhythm is irregular, the patient may have atrial fibrillation, a potentially more serious arrhythmia in the presence of WPW syndrome. In an older patient with presyncope, especially with a history of myocardial infarction, the physician should suspect ventricular tachycardia (p. 703) if the ventricular rate is rapid and AV heart block (p. 711) or sinus nodal disease (p. 673) if the rate is slow. The ventricular rhythm can be regular or irregular. Premature atrial or ventricular beats, perceived as dropped or skipped beats by the patient, are probably the most common cause of palpitations.

The physician should inquire about circumstances that can trigger the tachycardia, such as emotionally upsetting events, ingestion of caffeine-containing beverages, cigarette smoking, exercise, excessive alcohol intake, or fatigue. A careful diet and drug history can be useful, for example, in revealing that the patient develops palpitations only after using a nasal decongestant that contains a sympathomimetic vasoconstrictor or that the patient has been exposed to "street" drugs such as cocaine.[2] States conducive to the genesis of arrhythmias should be considered, such as thyrotoxicosis, pericarditis, mitral valve prolapse, hypokalemia secondary to diuretics, and so forth. Family history can be helpful. A variety of familial disorders can result in arrhythmias,[3,4] including myotonic dystrophy,[5-7] Duchenne muscular dystrophy[8-10] (p. 1810), and dilated cardiomyopathy (p. 1398).[11] Congenital disorders of the conduction system can result in sudden death.[12]

PHYSICAL EXAMINATION

In addition to recording cardiac rate and rhythm, a number of physical findings can be helpful. For example, findings ac-

companying AV dissociation (p. 715) include variable peak systolic blood pressure as the atria alter their contribution to ventricular filling, variable intensity of the first heart sound as the P-R interval changes despite a regular ventricular rhythm, intermittent cannon *a* waves in the jugular venous pulse as atrial contraction occurs against closed AV valves, and apparent "intermittent" gallop sounds when atrial systole occurs at various times of the cardiac cycle. The *venous pulse* provides a window through which to judge atrial and ventricular rates and relative timing relationships. It is of interest that Wenckebach first noted the two types of second degree AV block that bear his name (p. 710) by recording the jugular phlebogram before the electrocardiogram was available.

Examining the *second heart sound* can be helpful (pp. 30 and 46). A paradoxically split second heart sound can occur during a QRS complex with a left bundle branch block contour that results from ventricular tachycardia or supraventricular tachycardia with aberration. A widely split second heart sound that does not become single during expiration can accompany right bundle branch block. Unfortunately, similar physical findings occur with different cardiac arrhythmias. For example, progressive diminution of the intensity of the first heart sound results as the P-R interval lengthens, which can occur during AV dissociation when the atrial rate exceeds the ventricular rate or during Wenckebach second degree AV block. Similarly, constant cannon *a* waves can occur with 1:1 atrioventricular relationships during ventricular or supraventricular tachycardia. Since AV dissociation can occur (uncommonly) during a supraventricular tachycardia and VA association can occur during a ventricular tachycardia, the clues provided by physical findings can be only suggestive.

CAROTID SINUS MASSAGE. The response to carotid sinus massage or the Valsalva maneuver provides important diagnostic information by increasing vagal tone and primarily slowing the rate of sinus nodal discharge and prolonging AV nodal conduction time and refractoriness.[13] Sinus tachycardia slows gradually during carotid massage and then returns to the previous rate when massage is discontinued; AV nodal reentry and AV reciprocating tachycardias that involve the AV node in one of its pathways sometimes slow slightly, terminate abruptly, or do not change; and the ventricular response to atrial flutter, atrial fibrillation, and some atrial tachycardias usually decreases (Table 24–1). Rarely, carotid sinus massage terminates a ventricular tachycardia.

To perform carotid massage, the patient is placed in a supine position, with the neck hyperextended and the head turned away from the side being tested, the sternocleidomastoid muscles relaxed or gently pushed out of the way, and the carotid impulse felt at the angle of the jaw. The carotid bifurcation is touched gently initially with the palmar portion of the fingertips to detect hypersensitive responses. Then, if no change in cardiac rhythm occurs, pressure is applied more firmly for approximately 5 seconds, first on one side and then on the other (*never* on both sides simultaneously) with a gentle rotating massaging motion. External pressure stimulates baroreceptors in the carotid sinus to trigger a reflex increase in vagal activity and sympathetic withdrawal. Responses can occur with right-sided massage and not left, or vice versa, so each side should be tested separately. Generally, the maximal response occurs with the first massage if repeated attempts are performed at short intervals. Some risk is associated with carotid sinus massage, particularly in older patients, and cerebral emboli can occur. Before massage, the carotid artery should be auscultated so that massage is not performed in patients who have carotid bruits indicative of carotid arterial disease.

ELECTROCARDIOGRAPHY

The ECG remains the most important and definitive single noninvasive diagnostic test. Initially, a 12-lead electrocardiogram is recorded and a long recording employing the lead that shows distinct P waves is obtained for proper analysis. If P waves are not clearly visible, atrial activity can be recorded by placing the right and left arm leads in various chest positions to discern P waves (so-called Lewis leads), using esophageal electrodes or intracavitary right atrial leads. An echocardiogram showing atrial contraction can be helpful.

Each arrhythmia must be approached in a systematic manner to answer the following questions: Are P waves present? What are the atrial and ventricular rates? Are they identical? Are the P-P and R-R intervals regular or irregular? If irregular, is it a consistent, repeating irregularity? Is there a P wave related to each ventricular complex? Does the P wave precede or follow the QRS complex? Is the resultant P-R or R-P interval constant? Is the R-P interval long and the P-R interval short, or vice versa? Are all P waves and QRS complexes identical and normal in contour? To determine the significance of changes in P-wave or QRS contour, or amplitude, one must know the lead being recorded. Are P, P-R, QRS, and Q-T durations normal? Considering the clinical setting, what is the significance of the arrhythmia? Should it be treated and, if so, how? For supraventricular tachycardias with a normal QRS complex, a branching decision tree may be useful (Table 24–2).

THE LADDER DIAGRAM. This is employed to depict depolarization and conduction schematically. Straight or slightly slanting lines drawn on a tiered framework beneath an ECG trace represent electrical events occurring in the various cardiac structures (Fig. 24–1*A* and *B*). Since the ECG and therefore the ladder diagram represent electrical activity against a time base, conduction is indicated by the lines of the ladder diagram sloping in a left to right direction. A less steep line depicts slower conduction. A short bar drawn perpendicular to a sloping line represents blocked conduction (Fig. 24–1*C*). On occasion, activity originating in an ectopic ventricular site is indicated in another tier drawn beneath the ventricular tier or from the sinus node in a tier drawn above the atrial tier. In general, atrial, AV junctional, or ventricular activity is diagrammed to begin in the appropriate tier. It is important to remember that sinus nodal discharge and conduction and, under certain circumstances, AV junctional discharge and conduction can only be assumed, since their activity is not recorded on the scalar ECG.

ELECTROPHYSIOLOGICAL STUDY. When this study is indicated,[14] it is performed by introducing multipolar catheter electrodes into the vascular system and positioning them in various parts of the heart. The catheters are used to record local electrical activity and to stimulate the heart. Multiple leads are recorded simultaneously, usually at a paper speed of 50 to 100 mm/sec. (Standard ECGs generally are recorded at a paper speed of 25 mm/sec.) Because of the rapid recording speed, intervals or complexes of normal duration may appear prolonged. An electrode positioned across the septal leaflet of the tricuspid valve records His bundle activity as well as low right atrial activity and high ventricular septal depolarization. Occasionally, a right bundle branch deflection also can be recorded. Three basic measurements are made using the ECG and the His bundle catheter recording: the P-A, A-H, and H-V intervals (Fig. 24–1*D*). The *P-A interval* is the time between the onset of the P wave in the surface tracing (which generally slightly precedes the onset of the high right atrial recording) and the low right atrial deflection, recorded in the His lead. This interval reflects intraatrial conduction and has not proved to be of much clinical value.

The A-H Interval. This is timed from the onset of the first rapid deflection recorded in the atrial electrogram (A) in the His bundle lead to the beginning of the His (H) deflection. Since the low right atrium and His bundle anatomically delimit the boundaries of the AV node, the A-H interval closely approximates AV nodal conduction time. The A-H interval is affected importantly by various interventions: atropine and isoproterenol shorten the A-H interval, while vagal maneuvers, digitalis, propranolol, verapamil, adenosine, and rapid or premature atrial pacing lengthen it. The normal range for the A-H interval is 55 to 130 msec, depending on heart rate, autonomic tone, and other factors.

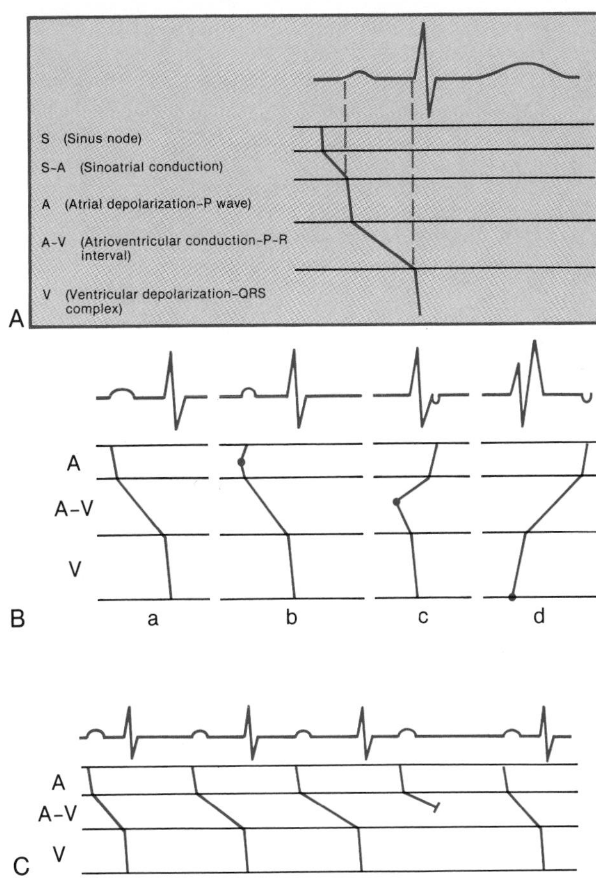

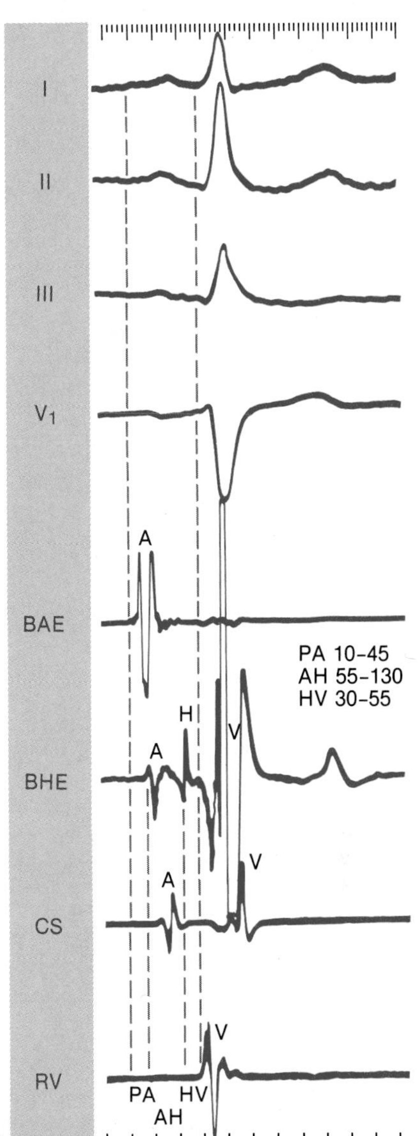

FIGURE 24-1. ***A,*** **Ladder diagram. Straight or slightly sloping lines beginning with the P wave and QRS complex indicate atrial and ventricular depolarization. The instants at which the sinus node discharges and the duration of sinoatrial conduction cannot be measured in the surface ECG and are therefore assumed. The sloping line connecting A and V, delimited by the interrupted lines, represents AV conduction.**

B, **Normal and ectopic beats. a = Normal sinus rhythm; b = ectopic atrial beat; c = AV junctional beat; d = ventricular ectopic beats. All are drawn with appropriate ladder diagrams beneath (T waves omitted). Retrograde atrial conduction is inscribed for the latter two beats. As with the sinus node, the exact discharge time of the AV junctional focus and conduction time from that point to the ventricles and atria are assumed.**

C, **Second degree Wenckebach type I AV block. The P-R interval lengthens progressively until finally the fourth P wave fails to reach the ventricles. As the P-R interval is prolonged, note decreasing slope of the line representing AV conduction and the small line perpendicular to the fourth sloping line indicating that the P wave is blocked. (*A* to *C* reproduced with permission from Zipes, D. P., and Fisch, C.: ECG Analysis. 1. Introduction. Premature ventricular complexes. Arch. Intern. Med. *128:*140, 1971.)**

D, **A single cardiac cycle showing the intervals measured during an electrophysiological study. In this and in similar subsequent figures, BAE indicates bipolar atrial electrogram recording high right atrial activity; BHE indicates the bipolar His electrogram recording low right atrial activity (A), His bundle activity (H), and ventricular septal activity (V); CS indicates bipolar electrogram recording of left atrial activity in coronary sinus lead; RV indicates right ventricular electrogram recording right ventricular activity; I = lead I; II = lead II; III = lead III; V_1 = lead V_1; PA = interval representing intraatrial conduction time; AH = interval representing AV nodal conduction time; HV = interval representing His-Purkinje conduction time. All values are in milliseconds. Normal values for P-A, A-H, and H-V intervals are given at the upper right. Paper speed = 100 mm/sec unless otherwise stated. Interrupted lines demarcate the various intervals. Note the normal sequence of atrial activation recorded with this technique: high right atrial activity (BAE) precedes low right atrial activity recorded in the BHE lead, which precedes left atrial activity recorded in the CS lead. Large time lines = 50 msec. Small time lines = 10 msec.**

The H-V Interval. This is the time from the beginning of the H deflection to the earliest onset of ventricular depolarization recorded in *any* lead. This interval represents conduction from the His bundle through the bundle branch–Purkinje system to the point of ventricular muscle activation and is usually constant—between 30 and 55 msec—regardless of heart rate or autonomic tone. Other intervals can be important and are discussed under the individual tachycardias.

CONSEQUENCES OF ARRHYTHMIAS. The ventricular rate and duration of an arrhythmia, its site of origin, and the

TABLE 24-2 ELECTROCARDIOGRAPHIC DIFFERENTIAL DIAGNOSIS OF SUPRAVENTRICULAR TACHYCARDIA WITH QRS DURATION <120 msec

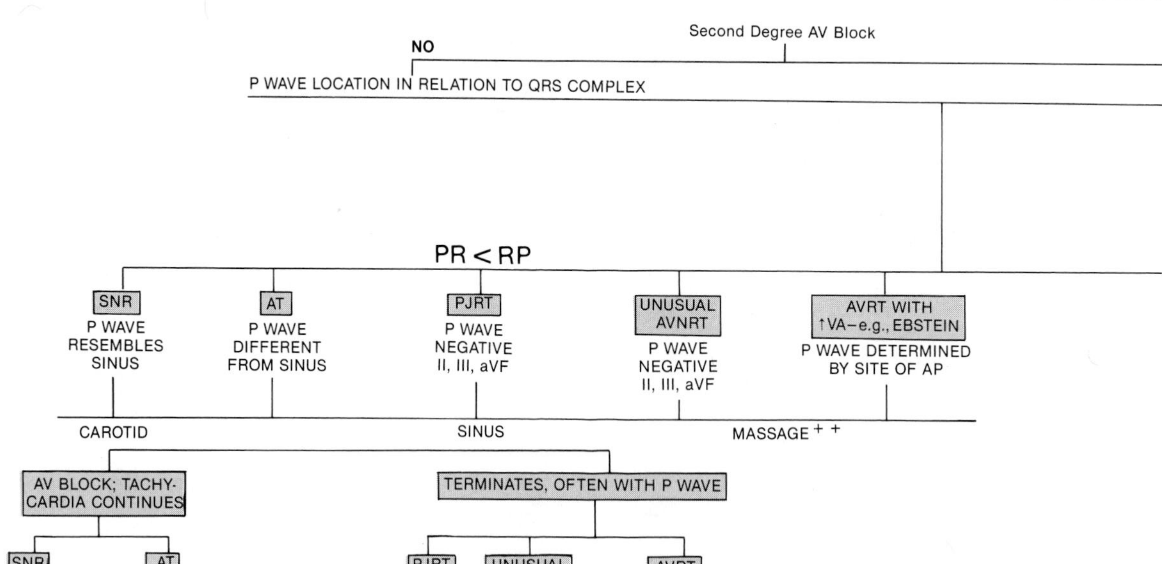

cardiovascular status of the patient primarily determine the electrophysiological and hemodynamic consequences of a particular rhythm disturbance. Electrophysiological consequences, often influenced by the presence of underlying heart disease such as acute myocardial infarction, include the development of serious arrhythmias as a result of rapid or slow rates, initiation of sustained arrhythmias by premature systoles, or the progression of rhythms such as ventricular tachycardia to ventricular fibrillation. Extremes of heart rate or loss of the atrial contribution to ventricular filling can alter circulatory dynamics. Rapid rates greatly shorten the diastolic filling time and, particularly in diseased hearts, the increased heart rate can fail to compensate for the reduced stroke output; as a consequence, arterial pressure, cardiac output, and coronary blood flow decline. Arrhythmias that prevent sequential AV contraction mitigate the hemodynamic benefits of the atrial booster pump, whereas atrial fibrillation causes complete loss of atrial contraction and can reduce cardiac output. Chronic tachycardias can cause cardiac dilation and heart failure from a tachycardia-induced cardiomyopathy.[15]

MANAGEMENT

The therapeutic approach to a patient with a cardiac arrhythmia begins with an accurate electrocardiographic *interpretation* of the arrhythmia and continues with determination of the *cause* of the arrhythmia (if possible), the nature of the underlying *heart disease* (if any), and the *consequences* of the arrhythmias in the individual patient. Thus, one does not treat arrhythmias as isolated events without having knowledge of the entire clinical situation. *Patients* who have arrhythmias, rather than the arrhythmias themselves, are treated.

When a patient develops a tachyarrhythmia, slowing the ventricular rate is the initial and often most important therapeutic maneuver. Therapy can differ radically for the same arrhythmia in two different patients because the consequences of tachycardia in individual patients differ. For example, a supraventricular tachycardia at a rate of 200 beats/min may produce few or no symptoms in a healthy young adult and therefore requires little or no therapy as it is usually self-limited. The same arrhythmia may precipitate pulmonary edema in a patient with mitral stenosis, syncope in a patient with aortic stenosis, shock in a patient with acute myocardial infarction, or hemiparesis in a patient with cerebrovascular disease. In these situations the tachycardia requires prompt electrical conversion.

The *cause* of the arrhythmia can influence therapy greatly. Electrolyte imbalance (potassium, magnesium, calcium), acidosis or alkalosis, hypoxemia, and many drugs may produce rhythm disturbances, and their identification and treatment can abolish or prevent these arrhythmias. Because heart failure can cause arrhythmias,[16–18] treatment of this condition with digitalis, diuretics, or vasodilators can suppress some of the arrhythmias that accompany cardiac decompensation.[19] Similarly, arrhythmias secondary to hypotension may respond to leg elevation or vasopressor therapy. Mild sedation or reassurance may be successful in treating some arrhythmias related to emotional stress. Precipitating or contributing disease states such as myocarditis,[20–22] infection, hypokalemia, anemia, and thyroid disorders should be sought and treated when possible.[23] Since therapy always involves some risk, one must be sure—particularly as the therapeutic regimen escalates—that the risks of *not* treating the arrhythmia continue to outweigh the risks of therapy with potentially hazardous antiarrhythmic measures.

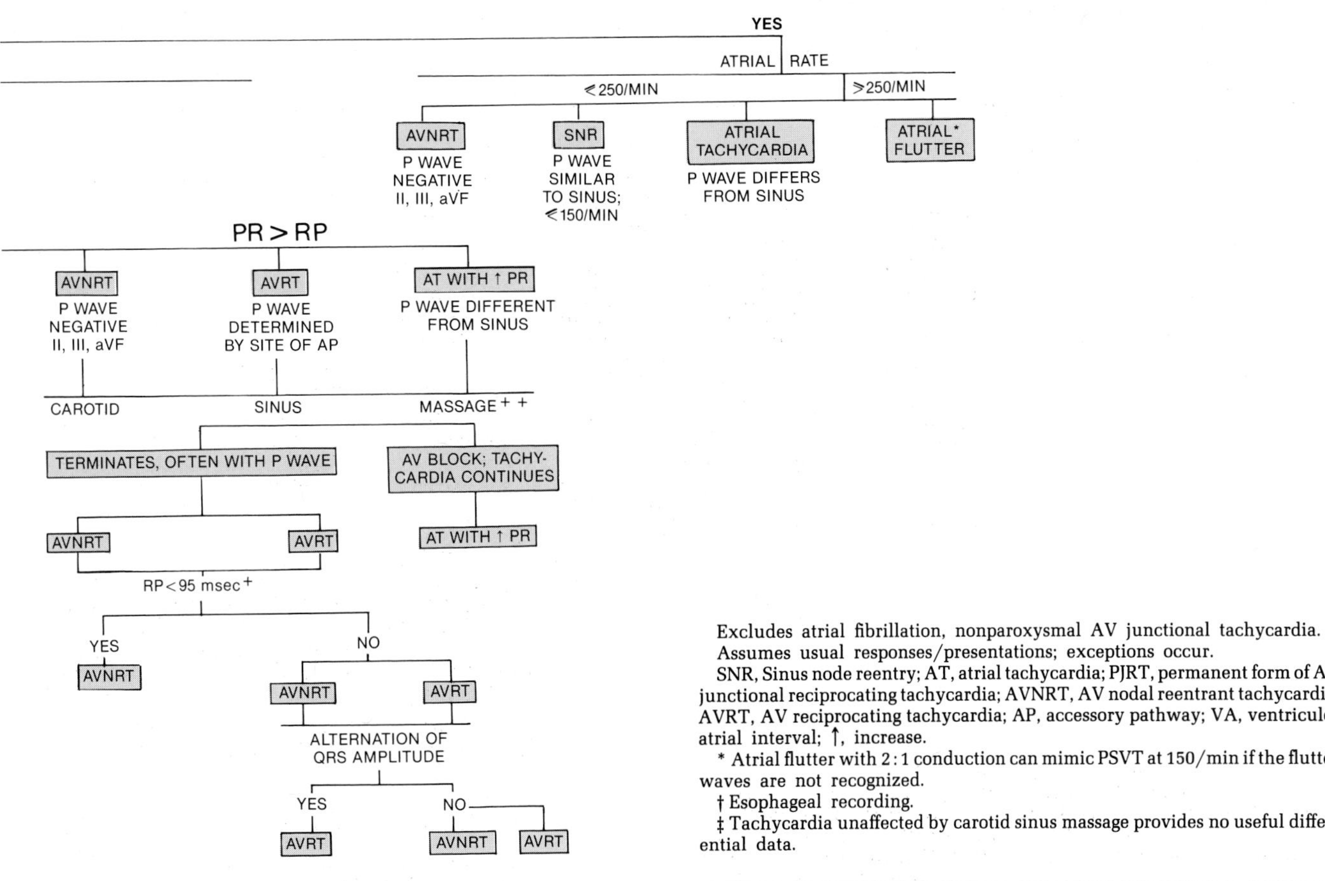

Excludes atrial fibrillation, nonparoxysmal AV junctional tachycardia. Assumes usual responses/presentations; exceptions occur.

SNR, Sinus node reentry; AT, atrial tachycardia; PJRT, permanent form of AV junctional reciprocating tachycardia; AVNRT, AV nodal reentrant tachycardia; AVRT, AV reciprocating tachycardia; AP, accessory pathway; VA, ventriculo-atrial interval; ↑, increase.

* Atrial flutter with 2:1 conduction can mimic PSVT at 150/min if the flutter waves are not recognized.

† Esophageal recording.

‡ Tachycardia unaffected by carotid sinus massage provides no useful differential data.

Individual Cardiac Arrhythmias

SINUS NODAL DISTURBANCES

NORMAL SINUS RHYTHM

Normal sinus rhythm is arbitrarily limited to impulse formation beginning in the sinus node at frequencies between 60 and 100 beats/min. Infants and children generally have faster heart rates than do adults, both at rest and during exercise. The P wave is upright in leads I, II, and aV_f and negative in lead aV_r, with a vector in the frontal plane between 0 and +90°. In the horizontal plane, the P vector is directed anteriorly and slightly leftward and therefore may be negative in leads V_1 and V_2 but positive in V_3 to V_6. The P-R interval exceeds 120 msec and may vary slightly with rate. If the pacemaker site shifts, a change in the morphology of the P wave may occur. The rate of sinus rhythm varies significantly and depends on many factors, including age,[24] sex, and physical activity.

The sinus nodal discharge rate responds readily to autonomic stimuli and depends on the effect of the two opposing autonomic influences.[25] Steady vagal stimulation decreases the spontaneous sinus nodal discharge rate and predominates over steady sympathetic stimulation, which increases the spontaneous sinus nodal discharge rate. Single or brief bursts of vagal stimulation can speed, slow, or entrain sinus nodal discharge. A given vagal stimulus produces a greater absolute reduction in heart rate when the basal heart rate has been increased by sympathetic stimulation, a phenomenon known as *accentuated antagonism*[26] (see p. 387).

SINUS TACHYCARDIA

ELECTROCARDIOGRAPHIC RECOGNITION (Fig. 24–2A). "Tachycardia" in the adult is defined as a rate exceeding 100 beats/min. During sinus tachycardia, the sinus node exhibits a discharge frequency between 100 and 180 beats/min but it may be higher with extreme exertion. The maximum heart rate achieved during strenuous physical activity decreases with age from near 200 beats/min to less than 140 beats/min (Chap. 52). Sinus tachycardia generally has a gradual onset and termination. The P-P interval can vary slightly from cycle to cycle. P waves have a normal contour but can develop a larger amplitude and become peaked. They appear before each QRS complex with a stable P-R interval unless concomitant AV block ensues.

Accelerated phase 4 diastolic depolarization of sinus nodal cells generally is responsible for sinus tachycardia. Rate changes can result from a shift in pacemaker cells to a different locus within the sinus node.[27,28] Carotid sinus massage and Valsalva or other vagal maneuvers gradually slow a sinus tachycardia, which then accelerates to its previous rate upon cessation of enhanced vagal tone. More rapid sinus rates can fail to slow in response to a vagal maneuver.

CLINICAL FEATURES. Sinus tachycardia is common in infancy and early childhood and is the normal reaction to a variety of physiological or pathophysiological stresses such as fever, hypotension, thyrotoxicosis, anemia, anxiety, exertion, hypovolemia, pulmonary emboli, myocardial ischemia, congestive heart failure, or shock. Drugs, such as atropine, catecholamines, thyroid, alcohol, nicotine, or caffeine, or inflammation can produce sinus tachycardia. Persistent sinus tachycardia can be a manifestation of heart failure. In patients with mitral stenosis or severe ischemic heart disease, sinus tachycardia can result in a reduced cardiac output or angina, or can precipitate another arrhythmia, in part related to the abbreviated ventricular filling time and compromised coronary blood flow. *Chronic nonparoxysmal sinus tachycardia* has been described in otherwise healthy persons, possibly owing to increased automaticity of the sinus node or an automatic atrial focus located near the sinus node. The abnormality may result from a defect in either sympathetic or vagal nerve

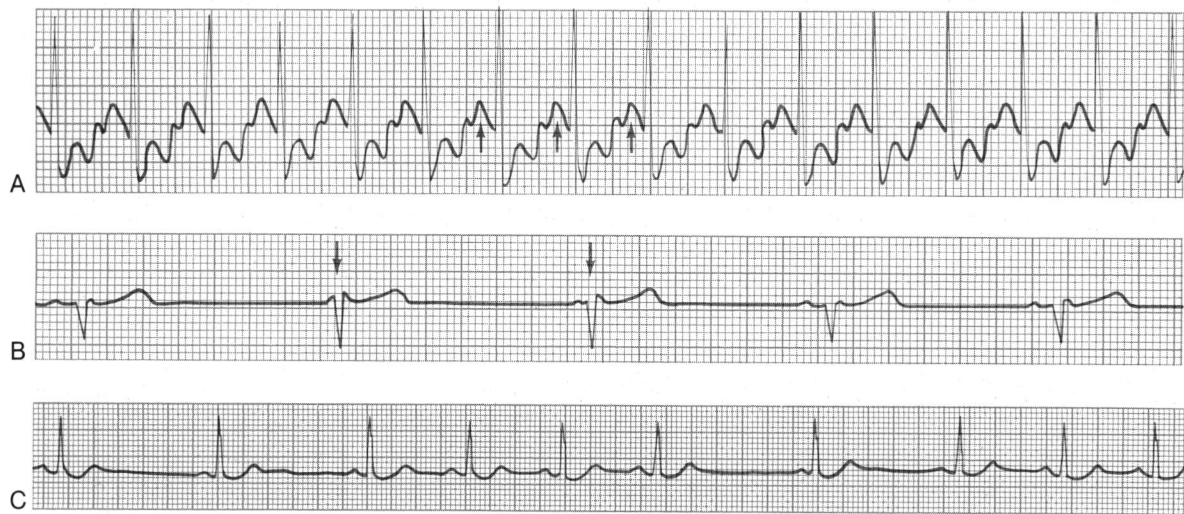

FIGURE 24-2. *A*, Sinus tachycardia (150 beats/min) in a patient during acute myocardial ischemia; note ST-segment depression. P waves are indicated by arrows. *B*, Sinus bradycardia at a rate of 40 to 48 beats/min. The second and third QRS complexes (arrows) represent junctional escape beats. Note P waves at onset of QRS complex. *C*, Nonrespiratory sinus arrhythmia occurring as a consequence of digitalis toxicity. Monitor leads.

control of sinoatrial automaticity, with or without an abnormality of intrinsic heart rate.

MANAGEMENT. This should focus on the *cause* of the sinus tachycardia. Elimination of tobacco, alcohol, coffee, tea, or other stimulants, such as the sympathomimetic agents in nose drops, may be helpful. Drugs such as propranolol or verapamil, or fluid replacement in a hypovolemic patient or fever reduction in a febrile patient, can be used to help slow the sinus nodal discharge rate.

SINUS BRADYCARDIA

ELECTROCARDIOGRAPHIC RECOGNITION (Fig. 24-2*B*). Sinus bradycardia exists in the adult when the sinus node discharges at a rate less than 60 beats/min. P waves have a normal contour and occur before each QRS complex with a constant P-R interval exceeding 120 msec unless concomitant AV block is present. Sinus arrhythmia often coexists.

CLINICAL FEATURES. Sinus bradycardia can result from excessive vagal or decreased sympathetic tone as well as from anatomical changes in the sinus node (see Sick Sinus Syndrome, p. 677). Sinus bradycardia frequently occurs in healthy young adults, particularly well-trained athletes,[29] (who can also have tachyarrhythmias[30]), and decreases in prevalence with advancing age. During sleep the normal heart rate can fall to 35 to 40 beats/min, especially in adolescents and young adults, with marked sinus arrhythmia sometimes producing pauses of 2 seconds or longer; REM sleep has been associated with sinus arrest. Eye surgery, coronary arteriography,[31] meningitis, intracranial tumors, increased intracranial pressure, cervical and mediastinal tumors, and certain disease states such as severe hypoxia,[32] myxedema, hypothermia, fibrodegenerative changes, convalescence from some infections, gram-negative sepsis, and mental depression can produce sinus bradycardia. Obstructive jaundice is considered to cause sinus bradycardia, but the evidence is not clear. Sinus bradycardia also occurs during vomiting or vasovagal syncope (p. 875) and can be produced by carotid sinus stimulation or by administration of parasympathomimetic drugs, lithium, amiodarone,[33] beta-adrenoceptor blocking drugs,[34] clonidine,[35] encainide,[36] propafenone[37] or calcium-antagonists (see Chap. 22). Conjunctival instillation of beta blockers for glaucoma can produce sinus or AV nodal abnormalities. In most instances sinus bradycardia is a benign arrhythmia and actually can be beneficial by producing a longer period of diastole and increasing ventricular filling time. Sinus bradycardia occurs in 10 to 15 per cent of patients with acute myocardial infarction and may be even more prevalent when patients are seen in the early hours of infarction. Unless accompanied by hemodynamic decompensation or arrhythmias, sinus bradycardia generally is associated with a more favorable outcome following myocardial infarction than is the presence of sinus tachycardia. It usually is transient[38] and occurs more commonly during inferior than anterior myocardial infarction; it has been noted during reperfusion with thrombolytic agents. Bradycardia following resuscitation from cardiac arrest is associated with a poor prognosis.

MANAGEMENT. Treatment of sinus bradycardia *per se* is usually not necessary. For example, if the patient with an acute myocardial infarction is asymptomatic, it is probably best not to speed up the sinus rate. If cardiac output is inadequate or if arrhythmias are associated with the slow rate, atropine (0.5 mg IV as an initial dose, repeated if necessary) is usually effective. Lower doses of atropine, particularly when given subcutaneously or intramuscularly, can exert an initial parasympathomimetic effect, possibly via a central action.[39] Ephedrine, hydralazine, or theophylline can be useful in managing some patients with symptomatic sinus bradycardia. These drugs should be given with caution, so as not to "overshoot" and produce too rapid a rate. In some patients who experience congestive heart failure or symptoms of low cardiac output as a result of chronic sinus bradycardia, electrical pacing may be needed.[40] Atrial pacing is usually preferable to ventricular pacing[41,42] in order to preserve sequential atrioventricular contraction and is preferable to drug therapy for long-term management of sinus bradycardia. As a general rule, no available drugs increase the heart rate reliably and safely over long periods without important side effects.

SINUS ARRHYTHMIA

Sinus arrhythmia (Fig. 24-2*C*) is characterized by a phasic variation in sinus cycle length[43] during which the maximum sinus cycle length minus minimum sinus cycle length exceeds 120 msec or the maximum sinus cycle length minus minimum sinus cycle length divided by the minimum sinus cycle length exceeds 10 per cent. It is the most frequent form of arrhythmia and is considered to be a normal event. P-wave morphology does not vary, and the P-R interval exceeds 120 msec and remains unchanged, since the focus of discharge remains relatively fixed within the sinus node. Occasionally the pacemaker focus can wander within the sinus node, or its exit to the atrium may change, producing P waves of slightly different contour (but not retrograde) and a slightly changing P-R interval that exceeds 120 msec.

Sinus arrhythmia commonly occurs in the young, especially with slower heart rates or following enhanced vagal tone, such as after the administration of digitalis or morphine, and decreases with age or with autonomic dysfunction such as diabetic neuropathy. Sinus arrhythmia appears in two basic forms. In the *respiratory* form, the P-P interval cyclically shortens during inspiration, primarily as a result of reflex inhibition of vagal tone, and slows during expiration; breath-holding eliminates the cycle-length variation.[43,44] Efferent vagal effects alone have been suggested as responsible for respiratory sinus arrhythmias. *Nonrespiratory* sinus arrhythmia is characterized by a phasic variation in P-P interval unrelated to the respiratory cycle and may be the result of digitalis intoxication. Loss of sinus rhythm variability is a risk factor for sudden cardiac death (see p. 705).

Symptoms produced by sinus arrhythmia are uncommon, but on occasion, if the pauses between beats are excessively long, palpitations or dizziness may result. Marked sinus arrhythmia can produce a sinus pause sufficiently long to produce syncope if not accompanied by an escape rhythm.

Treatment is usually unnecessary. Increasing the heart rate by exercise or drugs generally abolishes sinus arrhythmia. Symptomatic individuals may experience relief from palpitations with sedatives, tranquilizers, atropine, ephedrine, or isoproterenol administration, as in the treatment of sinus bradycardia.

VENTRICULOPHASIC SINUS ARRHYTHMIA. This arrhythmia occurs when the ventricular rate is slow. The most common example occurs during complete AV block, when P-P cycles that contain a QRS complex are shorter than P-P cycles without a QRS complex. Similar lengthening can be present in the P-P cycle that follows a premature ventricular complex with a compensatory pause. Alterations in the P-P interval are probably due to the influence of the autonomic nervous system responding to changes in ventricular stroke volume.

SINUS PAUSE OR SINUS ARREST

Sinus pause or sinus arrest[45,46] (Fig. 24–3) is recognized by a pause in the sinus rhythm. The P-P interval delimiting the pause does not equal a multiple of the basic P-P interval. Differentiation of sinus arrest, which is thought to be due to a slowing or cessation of spontaneous sinus nodal automaticity and therefore a disorder of impulse formation, from sinoatrial exit block (see below) in patients with sinus arrhythmia can be quite difficult without direct recordings of sinus node discharge.[47,48]

Failure of sinus nodal discharge results in absence of atrial depolarization, and in periods of ventricular asystole if escape beats initiated by latent pacemakers do not occur (Fig. 24–3). Involvement of the sinus node by acute myocardial infarction, degenerative fibrotic changes, effects of digitalis toxicity, stroke,[49] or excessive vagal tone all can produce sinus arrest. Transient sinus arrest may have no clinical significance by itself if latent pacemakers promptly escape to prevent ventricular asystole or the genesis of other arrhythmias precipitated by the slow rates.

Treatment is as outlined above for sinus bradycardia. In patients who have a chronic form of sinus node disease characterized by marked sinus bradycardia or sinus arrest, permanent pacing is often necessary.

SINOATRIAL (SA) EXIT BLOCK

This arrhythmia is recognized electrocardiographically by a pause due to the absence of the normally expected P wave (Fig. 24–4). The duration of the pause is a multiple of the basic P-P interval. SA exit block is due to a conduction disturbance during which an impulse formed within the sinus node fails to depolarize the atria or does so with delay.[47,48] An interval without P waves that equals approximately two, three, or four times the normal P-P cycle characterizes type II second degree SA exit block. During type I (Wenckebach) second degree SA exit block, the P-P interval progressively shortens prior to the pause, and the duration of the pause is less than two P-P cycles. (See p. 710 and Fig. 24–42, p. 711, for further discussion of Wenckebach intervals.) First degree SA exit block cannot be recognized electrocardiographically because SA nodal discharge is not recorded. Third degree SA exit block can present as complete absence of P waves and is difficult to diagnose with certainty without sinus node electrograms.[50]

Excessive vagal stimulation, acute myocarditis, infarction, or fibrosis involving the atrium as well as drugs such as quinidine, procainamide, or digitalis can produce SA exit block. SA exit block is usually transient. It may be of no clinical importance except to prompt a search for the underlying cause. Occasionally, syncope can result if the SA block is prolonged and unaccompanied by an escape rhythm.

Therapy for patients who have symptomatic SA exit block is as outlined for sinus bradycardia.

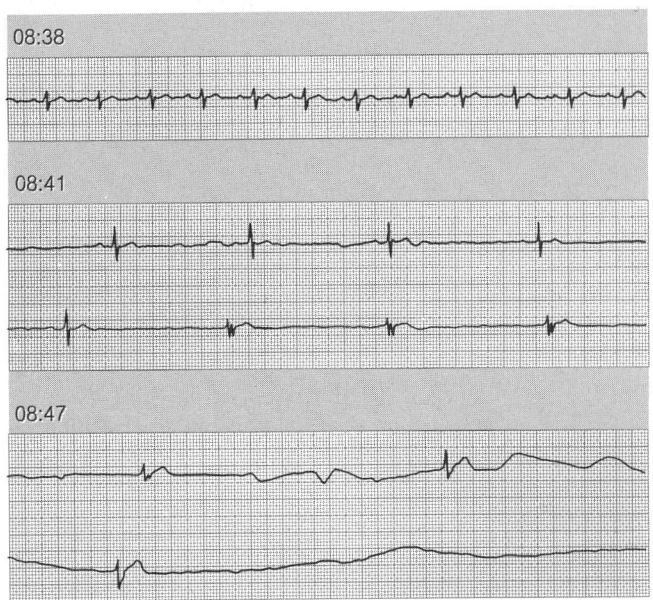

FIGURE 24–3. **Sinus arrest. The patient had a long-term ECG recorder connected when he died suddenly due to cardiac standstill. The rhythms demonstrate progressive sinus bradycardia and sinus arrest at 08:41. The rhythm then becomes a ventricular escape rhythm which progressively slows and finally ceases at 08:47. Monitor lead. Double ECG strips are continuous recordings.**

WANDERING PACEMAKER

This variant of sinus arrhythmia involves the passive transfer of the dominant pacemaker focus from the sinus node to latent pacemakers that have the next highest degree of automaticity located in other atrial sites or in AV junctional tissue. Thus, only one pacemaker at a time controls the rhythm, in sharp contrast to AV dissociation (p. 715). As with other forms of sinus arrhythmia, the change occurs in a gradual fashion over the duration of several beats. The ECG (Fig. 24–5) displays a cyclical increase in R-R interval; a P-R interval that gradually shortens and can become less than 120 msec; and a change in the P-wave contour, which becomes negative in lead I or II (depending on the site of discharge) or is lost within the QRS complex. Generally, these changes occur in reverse as the pacemaker shifts back to the sinus node. Rarely the rate may remain unchanged during these P-wave transitions.

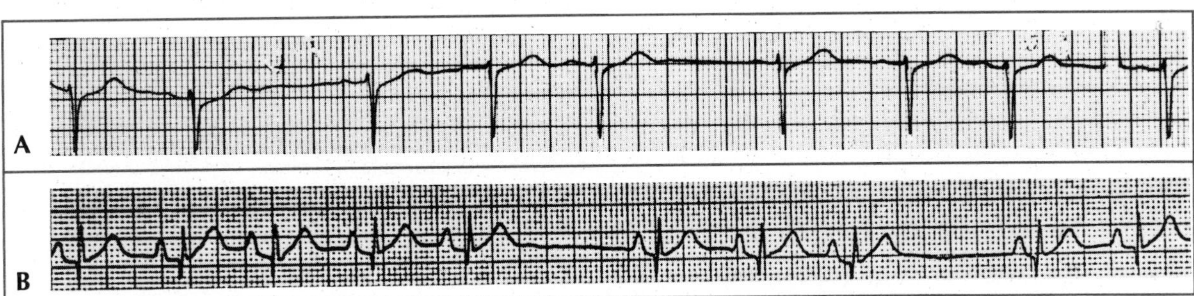

FIGURE 24–4. **Sinus nodal exit block. *A*, Type I SA nodal exit block has the following features: the P-P interval shortens from the first to the second cycle in each grouping, followed by a pause. The duration of the pause is less than twice the shortest cycle length, and the cycle after the pause exceeds the cycle before the pause. The P-R interval is normal and constant. Lead V_1. *B*, The P-P interval varies slightly because of sinus arrhythmia. Two pauses in sinus nodal activity occur, equalling twice the basic P-P interval and are consistent with type II 2 : 1 SA nodal exit block. The P-R interval is normal and constant. Lead III.**

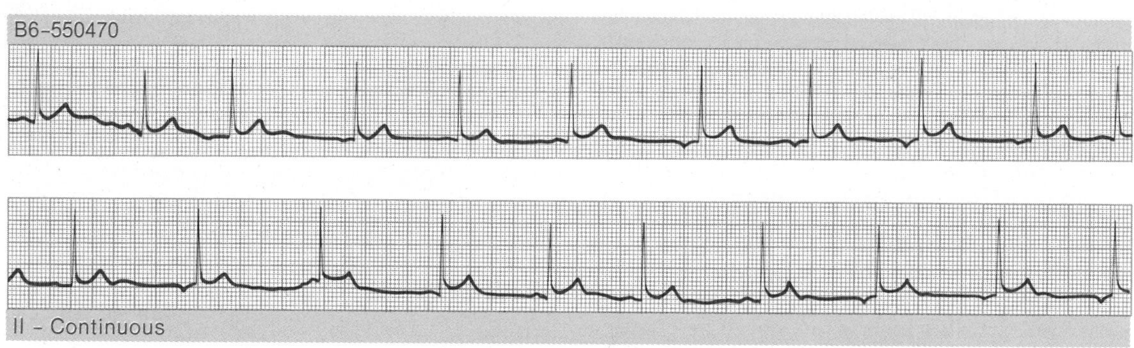

FIGURE 24-5. Wandering atrial pacemaker. As the heart rate slows, the P waves become inverted and then gradually revert toward normal when the heart rate speeds up again. The P-R interval shortens to 0.14 sec with the inverted P wave and is 0.16 sec with the upright P wave. This phasic variation in cycle length with varying P-wave contour suggests a shift in pacemaker site and is characteristic of wandering atrial pacemaker.

Wandering pacemaker is a normal phenomenon that often occurs in the very young and particularly in athletes, presumably because of augmented vagal tone. Persistence of an AV junctional rhythm for long periods of time, however, may indicate underlying heart disease. *Treatment* is usually not indicated but, if necessary, is the same as that for sinus bradycardia (see above).

HYPERSENSITIVE CAROTID SINUS SYNDROME

(See also p. 878)

ELECTROCARDIOGRAPHIC RECOGNITION (Fig. 24-6) This condition is most frequently characterized by ventricular asystole due to cessation of atrial activity from sinus arrest or SA exit block. AV block is observed less frequently, probably in part because the absence of atrial activity due to sinus arrest precludes the manifestations of AV block.[51] However, if an atrial pacemaker maintained an atrial rhythm during the episodes, a higher prevalence of AV block probably would be noted. In symptomatic patients, AV junctional or ventricular escapes generally do not occur or are present at very slow rates, suggesting that heightened vagal tone and sympathetic withdrawal can suppress subsidiary pacemakers located in the ventricles as well as supraventricular structures.

CLINICAL FEATURES. Two types of hypersensitive carotid sinus responses are noted. *Cardioinhibitory* carotid sinus hypersensitivity is generally defined as ventricular asystole exceeding 3 seconds during carotid sinus stimulation, although normal limits have not been carefully established. In fact, asystole exceeding 3 seconds during carotid sinus massage is not common but can occur in asymptomatic subjects. *Vasodepressor* carotid sinus hypersensitivity is generally defined as a decrease in systolic blood pressure of 50 mm Hg or more without associated cardiac slowing, or a decrease in systolic blood pressure exceeding 30 mm Hg when the patient's symptoms are reproduced.

Even if a hyperactive carotid sinus reflex is elicited in patients, particularly in older patients who complain of syncope or presyncope, the hyperactive reflex elicited with carotid sinus massage may not necessarily be responsible for these symptoms. Direct pressure or extension on the carotid sinus from head turning, neck tension, and tight collars can also be a source of syncope by reducing blood flow through the vertebral arteries.

Hypersensitive carotid sinus reflex is most commonly associated with coronary artery disease. The mechanism responsible for hypersensitive carotid sinus reflex is not known, but possibilities include a high level of resting vagal tone, hyperresponsiveness to acetylcholine, excessive release of acetylcholine, baroreflex hypersensitivity, inadequate cholinesterase activity to metabolize the acetylcholine released, and concomitant sympathetic abnormality. Carotid sinus receptors, autonomic centers of the brain stem, and the afferent limb of the reflex have all been incriminated.

TREATMENT. Atropine abolishes cardioinhibitory carotid sinus hypersensitivity. However, the majority of symptomatic patients require pacemaker implantation. It must be stressed that because AV block can occur during the periods of hypersensitive carotid reflex, some form of *ventricular* pacing, with or without atrial pacing, is generally required. Atropine does not prevent the decrease in systemic blood pressure in the vasodepressor form of carotid sinus hypersensitivity, which may result from inhibition of sympathetic vasoconstrictor nerves and possibly activation of

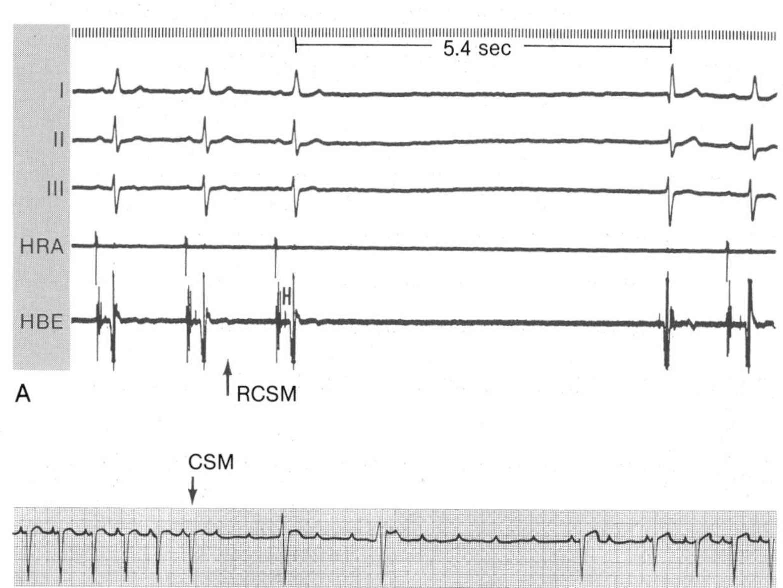

FIGURE 24-6. Panel A, Right carotid sinus massage (arrow, RCSM) results in sinus arrest and a ventricular escape beat (probably fascicular) 5.4 seconds later. Sinus discharge then resumes. In panel B (monitor lead) carotid sinus massage (see arrow, CSM) results in slight sinus slowing but, more importantly, advanced AV block. Obviously, an atrial pacemaker without ventricular pacing would be inappropriate for this patient.

cholinergic sympathetic vasodilator fibers. Combinations of vasodepressor and cardioinhibitory types can occur, and vasodepression may account for continued syncope after pacemaker implantation in some patients. Patients who have a hyperactive carotid sinus reflex that does not cause symptoms require no treatment. Drugs such as digitalis, alpha-methyldopa, clonidine, and propranolol can enhance the response to carotid sinus massage and be responsible for symptoms in some patients. Severe vasodepressor or mixed vasodepressor and cardioinhibitory responses may require treatment with either radiation therapy or surgical denervation of the carotid sinus. Elastic support hose and sodium-retaining drugs may be helpful in patients with vasodepressor responses.

SICK SINUS SYNDROME

This term is applied to a syndrome encompassing a number of sinus nodal abnormalities that include (1) persistent spontaneous sinus bradycardia not caused by drugs, and inappropriate for the physiological circumstance, (2) apparent sinus arrest or exit block, (3) combinations of SA and AV conduction disturbances, or (4) alternation of paroxysms of rapid regular or irregular atrial tachyarrhythmias and periods of slow atrial and ventricular rates (bradycardia-tachycardia syndrome, Fig. 24–7). More than one of these conditions can be recorded in the same patient on different occasions, and often their mechanisms can be shown to be causally interrelated and combined with an abnormal state of AV conduction or automaticity.[52–54]

More than one pathophysiological mechanism can produce the clinical manifestations of sick sinus syndrome. The spontaneous clinical arrhythmia and the response to electrophysiological testing (see Chap. 22) depend on the underlying mechanism of sinus nodal dysfunction. Patients who have sinus node disease can be categorized as having intrinsic sinus node disease unrelated to autonomic abnormalities or combinations of intrinsic and autonomic abnormalities.[53,54] Symptomatic patients with sinus pauses and/or SA exit block frequently show abnormal responses on electrophysiological testing and can have a relatively high incidence of life-threatening arrhythmias and/or embolic episodes. The total number of spontaneous complexes per 24 hours may be reduced.[55] In children, sinus node dysfunction most commonly occurs in those with congenital or acquired heart disease, particularly following corrective cardiac surgery.[56–58a] A familial disorder has been suggested.[59] However, sick sinus syndrome may occur in the absence of other cardiac abnormalities. The course of the disease is frequently intermittent and unpredictable, influenced by the severity of the underlying heart disease. Excessive physical training can heighten vagal tone and produce syncope related to sinus bradycardia or AV conduction abnormalities in otherwise normal individuals.

The anatomical basis of sick sinus syndrome can involve total or subtotal destruction of the sinus node, areas of nodal-atrial discontinuity, inflammatory or degenerative changes of the nerves and ganglia surrounding the node, and pathological changes in the atrial wall. Fibrosis and fatty infiltration occur, and the sclerodegenerative processes generally involve the sinus node and the AV node or the bundle of His and its branches or distal subdivisions.

TREATMENT. For patients with sick sinus syndrome, treatment depends on the basic rhythm problem but generally involves permanent pacemaker implantation when symptoms are manifested (p. 728). Pacing for the bradycardia combined with drug therapy to treat the tachycardia is required in those with the bradycardia-tachycardia syndrome. In these patients, drug therapy without pacing can aggravate the bradycardia. Digitalis and other drugs that can affect sinus discharge should be used cautiously in patients with sick sinus syndrome without a pacemaker. Prolonged sinoatrial conduction time or sinus nodal recovery time at electrophysiological study in the absence of symptoms is not an indication for prophylactic pacing, since therapy is directed toward control of symptoms.

SINUS NODAL REENTRY TACHYCARDIA

(See also p. 606)

The rate of sinus nodal reentrant tachycardia varies from 80 to 200 beats/min but is generally slower than the other forms of supraventricular tachycardia, with an average rate of 130 to 140 beats/min (Fig. 24–8). Electrocardiographically, P waves are identical or very similar to the sinus P wave morphologically; the P-R interval is related to the tachycardia rate, but generally the R-P interval is long, with a shorter P-R interval (Fig. 24–9*D*). AV block can occur without affecting the tachycardia, and vagal maneuvers can slow and then abruptly terminate the tachycardia. Electrophysiologically, the tachycardia can be initiated and terminated by premature atrial and, uncommonly, premature ventricular stimulation (Fig. 24–8). Initiation of sinus nodal reentry does not depend on a critical degree of intraatrial or AV nodal conduction delay, and the atrial activation sequence is the same as during sinus rhythm. AV nodal Wenckebach block during the tachycardia is common. The development of bundle branch block does not affect the cycle length or P-R interval during tachycardia. Prolongation of AV nodal conduction time or development of AV nodal block can occur prior to termination of the tachycardia but does not affect the sinus nodal reentry.[60]

Sinus nodal reentry may account for 5 to 10 per cent of cases of supraventricular tachycardia. It occurs in all age groups, without sex predilection. Patients may be slightly older and have a higher incidence of heart disease than patients with supraventricular tachycardia due to other mechanisms. Many may not seek medical attention because the relatively slow rate of the tachycardia does not result in serious symptoms. On the other hand, sinus nodal reentry may be responsible for apparent "anxiety-related sinus tachycardia" in some patients. Drugs such as propranolol, verapamil, and digitalis may be effective in terminating and preventing recurrences of sinus node reentrant tachycardia. Surgery to ablate the sinus node is rarely necessary.[61]

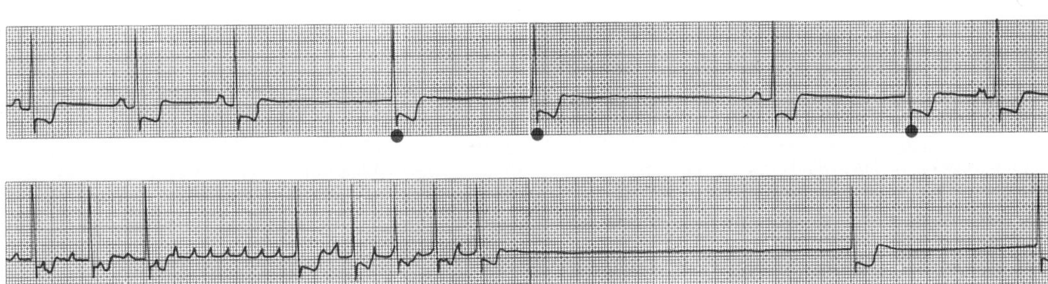

FIGURE 24–7. Sick sinus syndrome with bradycardia-tachycardia. Intermittent sinus arrest is apparent with junctional escape beats at irregular intervals (filled circles, top). In the bottom panel of this continuous monitor lead recording, a short episode of atrial flutter is followed by almost 5 sec of asystole before a junctional escape rhythm resumes. The patient became presyncopal at this point.

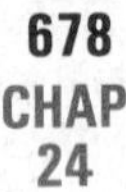

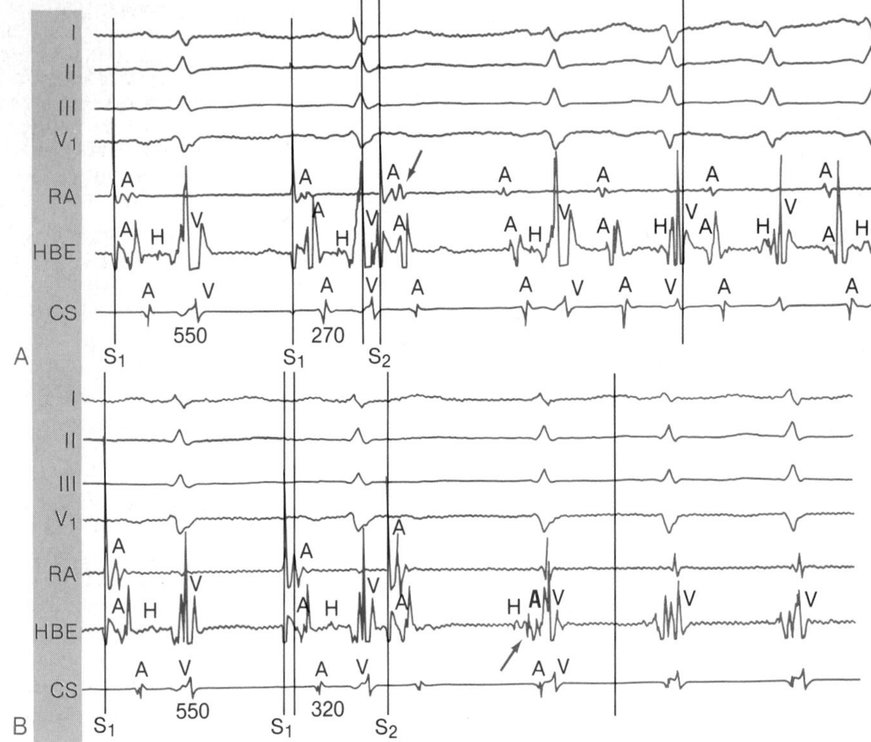

FIGURE 24–8. ***A, Sinoatrial nodal reentry.*** Premature stimulation of the high right atrium at an S_1-S_2 interval of 270 msec initiates an atrial tachycardia with an activation sequence similar to that occurring during high right atrial pacing. The premature P wave blocks proximal (arrow) to the His bundle but the tachycardia is still initiated. ***B, AV nodal reentry.*** Premature stimulation of the high right atrium at an S_1-S_2 interval of 320 msec results in a prolonged A-H interval and initiation of AV nodal reentry. Retrograde low right atrial activation recorded in the HBE lead occurs before ventricular activation and is followed by left atrial (CS) and high right atrial (arrow) activation. This is in sharp contrast to *A,* in which the atrial activation sequence begins in the high right atrium and then progresses to the low right atrium (HBE) and finally to the left atrium (CS).

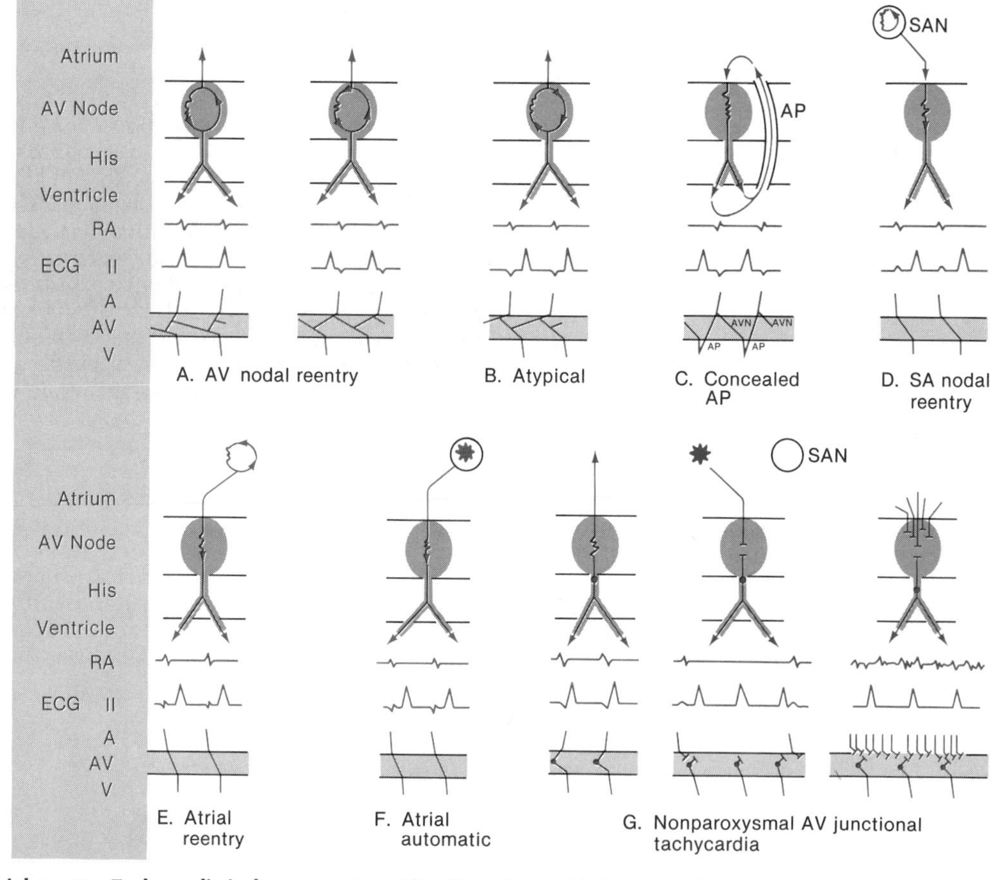

FIGURE 24–9. Diagrammatic representation of various tachycardias. In the top portion of each example, a schematic of the presumed anatomical pathways is drawn; in the bottom half, the ECG presentation and the explanatory ladder diagram are depicted. *A,* AV nodal reentry. In the left example, reentrant excitation is drawn confined to the AV node, with retrograde atrial activity occurring simultaneously with ventricular activity owing to anterograde conduction over the slow AV nodal pathway and retrograde conduction over the fast AV nodal pathway. In the right example, atrial activity occurs slightly later than ventricular activity, owing to retrograde conduction delay. *B,* Atypical AV nodal reentry due to anterograde conduction over a fast AV nodal pathway and retrograde conduction over a slow AV nodal pathway. *C,* Concealed accessory pathway. Reciprocating tachycardia is due to anterograde conduction over the AV node and retrograde conduction over the accessory pathway. Retrograde P waves occur after the QRS complex. *D,* Sinus nodal reentry. The tachycardia is due to reentry within the sinus node, which then conducts to the rest of the heart. *E,* Atrial reentry. Tachycardia is due to reentry within the atrium, which then conducts to the rest of the heart. *F,* Automatic atrial tachycardia. Tachycardia is due to automatic discharge in the atrium, which then conducts to the rest of the heart; it is difficult to distinguish from atrial reentry. *G,* Nonparoxysmal AV junctional tachycardia. Various presentations of this tachycardia are depicted with retrograde atrial capture, AV dissociation with the sinus node in control of the atria, and AV dissociation with atrial fibrillation.

DISTURBANCES OF ATRIAL RHYTHM

PREMATURE ATRIAL COMPLEXES

Premature complexes are one of the most common causes of an irregular pulse. They can originate from any area in the heart—most frequently from the ventricles, less often from the atria and from the AV junctional area, and rarely from the sinus node. Although premature complexes arise in normal hearts, they are more often associated with structural heart disease and increase in frequency with age.

ELECTROCARDIOGRAPHIC RECOGNITION (Fig. 24–10). The diagnosis of premature atrial complexes is indicated on the ECG by a premature P wave with a P-R interval exceeding 120 msec (except in WPW syndrome, in which the P-R interval is usually less than 120 msec). Although the contour of the premature P wave can resemble that of the normal sinus P wave, it generally differs. While variations in the basic sinus rate at times can make the diagnosis of prematurity difficult, differences in the contour of the P waves are usually apparent and indicate a different focus of origin. When a premature atrial complex occurs early in diastole, conduction may not be completely normal. The AV junction may still be refractory from the preceding beat and prevent propagation of the impulse (blocked or nonconducted premature atrial complex, Fig. 24–10*A*) or cause conduction to be slowed (premature atrial complex with a prolonged P-R interval). As a general rule, the R-P interval is inversely related to the P-R interval: thus, a short R-P interval produced by an early premature atrial complex occurring close to the preceding QRS complex is followed by a long P-R interval. When premature atrial complexes occur early in the cardiac cycle, the premature P waves may be difficult to discern because they are superimposed on T waves. Careful examination of tracings from several leads may be necessary before the premature atrial complex is recognized as a slight deformity of the T wave. Often such premature atrial complexes block before reaching the ventricle and can be misinterpreted as a sinus pause or sinus exit block (Fig. 24–10*A*).

The length of the pause following any premature complex or series of premature complexes is determined by the interaction of several factors. If the premature atrial complex occurs when the sinus node and perinodal tissue are not refractory, the impulse can conduct into the sinus node, discharge it prematurely, and cause the next sinus cycle to begin from that time. The interval between the two normal P waves flanking a premature atrial complex that has reset the timing of the basic sinus rhythm is less than twice the normal P-P interval and the pause after the premature atrial complex is said to be "noncompensatory." Referring to Figure 24–10*E*, reset (noncompensatory pause) occurs when A_1-A_2 interval + A_2-A_3 interval < two times the A_1-A_1 interval, and A_2-A_3 interval > A_1-A_1 interval. The interval between the premature atrial complex (A_2) and the following sinus-initiated P wave (A_3) exceeds one sinus cycle but is less than "fully compensatory" (see below), because the A_2-A_3 interval is lengthened by the time it takes the ectopic atrial impulse to conduct to the sinus node and depolarize it and then for the sinus impulse to return to the atrium. These factors lengthen the return cycle, i.e., the interval between the premature atrial complex (A_2) and the following sinus-initiated P wave (A_3) (Fig. 24–10*E*). Premature discharge of the sinus node by an early premature atrial complex can temporarily depress sinus nodal automatic activity, causing the sinus node to beat more slowly initially (Fig. 24–10*D*). Often when this happens, the interval between the A_3 and the next sinus-initiated P wave exceeds the A_1-A_1 interval.

Less commonly, the premature atrial complex encounters a refractory sinus node or perinodal tissue, in which case the timing of the basic sinus rhythm is not altered, since the sinus node is not reset by the premature atrial complex and the interval between the two normal, sinus-initated P waves flanking the premature atrial complex is twice the normal P-P interval. The interval following this premature atrial discharge is said to be a "full compensatory pause," i.e., of sufficient duration so that the P-P interval bounding the premature atrial complex is twice the normal P-P interval. However, sinus arrhythmia can lengthen or shorten this pause. Rarely, an *interpolated premature atrial* complex may occur. In this case, the pause after the premature atrial complex is very short and the interval bounded by the normal sinus-initiated P waves on each side of the premature atrial complex is only slightly longer than or equals one normal P-P cycle length. The interpolated premature atrial complex fails to affect the sinus nodal pacemaker, and the sinus impulse following the premature atrial complex is conducted to the ventricles, often with a slightly lengthened P-R interval. An interpolated premature complex of any type represents the only type of premature systole that does not actually replace the normally conducted beat. Premature atrial complexes can originate in the sinus node and are identified by premature P waves that have a contour identical to the normal sinus P wave.[62] The cycle after the premature sinus complex equals or is slightly shorter than the basic sinus cycle. Premature sinus complexes are not commonly recognized.

On occasion, when the AV node has had sufficient time to repolarize and conduct without delay, the supraventricular QRS complex initiated by the premature atrial complex can be aberrant in configuration because the His-Purkinje system or ventricular muscle has *not* completely repolarized and conducts with functional delay or block (Fig. 24–10*A*). It is important to remember that the refractory period of cardiac fibers is related directly to cycle length. (In the adult, AV nodal effective refractory period prolongs at shorter cycle lengths.) A slow heart rate (long cycle length) produces a longer His-Purkinje refractory period than does a faster heart rate. As a consequence, a premature atrial complex that follows a long R-R interval (long refractory period) can result in functional bundle branch block (aberrant ventricular conduction. Since the right bundle branch at long cycles has a longer refractory period than the left bundle branch, aberration with a right bundle branch block pattern at slow rates occurs more commonly than aberration with a left bundle branch block pattern. At shorter cycles, the refractory period of the left bundle branch exceeds that of the right bundle branch and a left bundle branch block pattern may be more likely to occur.

CLINICAL FEATURES. Premature atrial complexes can occur in a variety of situations, for example, during infection, inflammation, or myocardial ischemia, or they can be provoked by a variety of medications, by tension states, or by tobacco, alcohol, or caffeine.[63] Premature atrial complexes can precipitate or presage the occurrence of sustained supraventricular (Fig. 24–10*B* and C) and rarely ventricular tachyarrhythmias.

MANAGEMENT. Premature atrial complexes generally do not require therapy. In symptomatic patients or when the premature atrial complexes precipitate tachycardias, treatment with digitalis, a beta blocker, or a calcium antagonist can be tried.

ATRIAL FLUTTER

(See also p. 609)

ELECTROCARDIOGRAPHIC RECOGNITION (Fig. 24–11). The atrial rate during classical or type I atrial flutter is usually 250 to 350 beats/min, although antiarrhythmic drugs such as quinidine and amiodarone can reduce the rate to the range of 200 beats/min. If this occurs, the ventricles can respond in a 1:1 fashion to the slower atrial rate. Ordinarily the atrial rate is about 300 beats/min, and in untreated patients the ventricular rate is half the atrial rate, i.e., 150 beats/min (Fig. 24–11*A*). A significantly slower ventricular rate (in the absence of drugs) suggests abnormal AV conduction. In children, in patients with the preexcitation syndrome (p. 693), occasionally in patients with hyperthyroidism, and in those whose AV nodes conduct rapidly, atrial flutter can conduct to the ventricle in a 1:1 fashion, producing a ventricular rate of 300 beats/min. The rate in type II flutter is 350 to 450 beats/min.[64,65] Reentry is probably responsible for most atrial flutters.[65a]

The ECG reveals identically recurring regular sawtooth flutter waves (Figs. 24–10C and 24–11*B*) and evidence of continual electrical activity (lack of an isoelectric interval between flutter waves), often best visualized in leads II, III, aV_f, or V_1. The flutter waves are commonly inverted (negative) in these leads and less often are upright (positive). If the AV conduction ratio remains constant, the ventricular rhythm will be regular; if the ratio of conducted beats varies (usually the result of a Wenckebach AV block), the ventricular rhythm

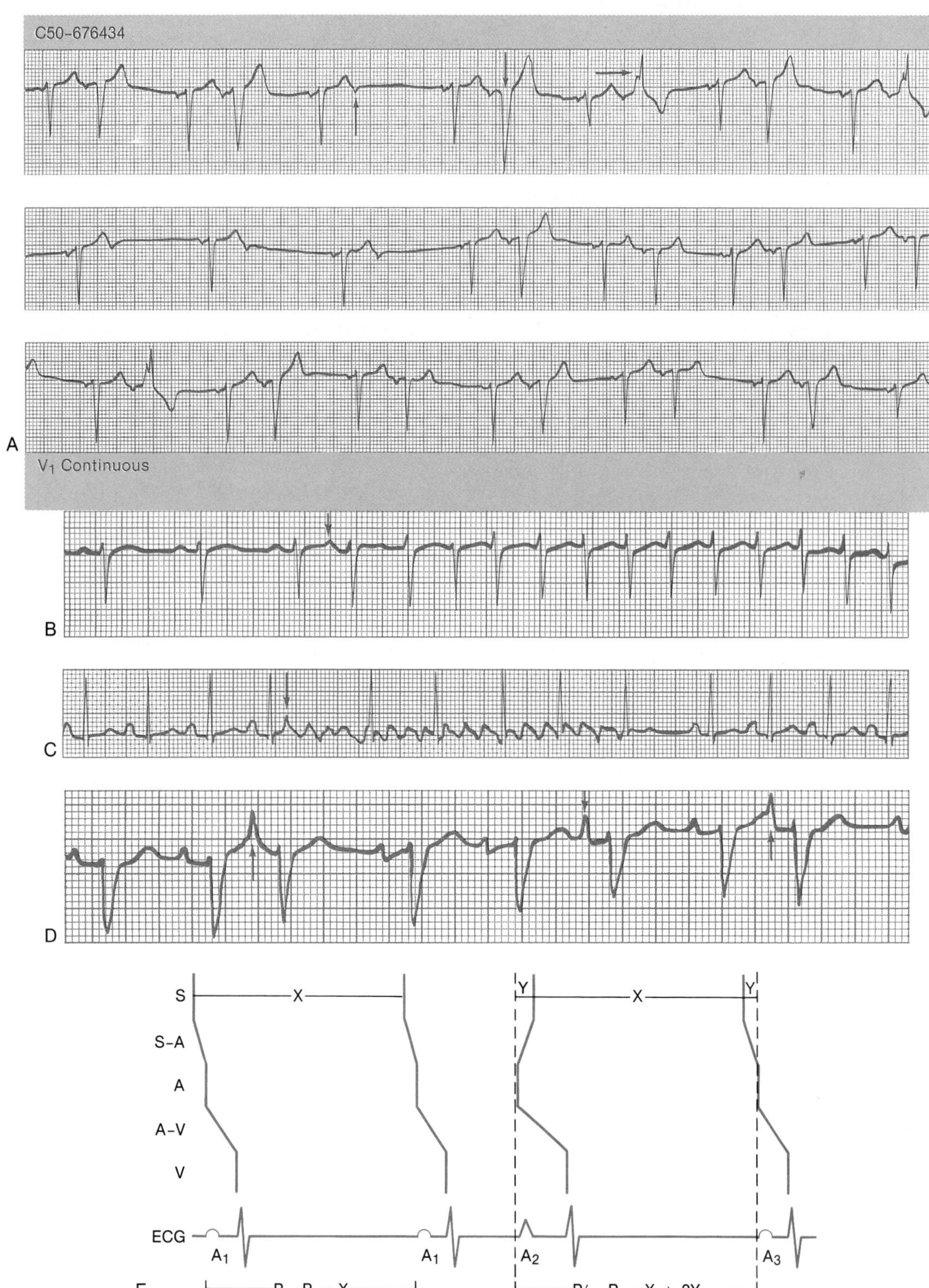

FIGURE 24-10. *A*, Premature atrial complexes that block entirely or conduct with functional right or functional left bundle branch block. Depending on preceding cycle length and coupling interval of the premature atrial complex, the latter blocks entirely in the AV node (↑) or conducts with functional left bundle branch block (↓) or functional right bundle branch block (→).

B, Premature atrial complex (↓) initiates a supraventricular tachycardia probably due to AV nodal reentry. Monitor lead.

C and *D*, A premature atrial complex (↓) initiating a short run of atrial flutter (*C*) and a premature atrial complex (↑) depressing the return of the next sinus nodal discharge (*D*). A slightly later premature atrial complex (↓) in *D* does not depress sinus nodal automaticity. Panels B-D Monitor leads.

E, Diagrammatic example of effects of a premature atrial complex. Sinus interval (A_1-A_1) equals X. Third P wave represents premature atrial complex (A_2) that reaches and discharges SA node, causing the next sinus cycle to begin at that time. Therefore, the P′-P (A_2-A_3) equals X + 2Y msec, assuming no depression of SA nodal automaticity. (Modified from Zipes, D. P., and Fisch, C.: Premature atrial contraction. Arch. Intern. Med. *128:*453, 1971.)

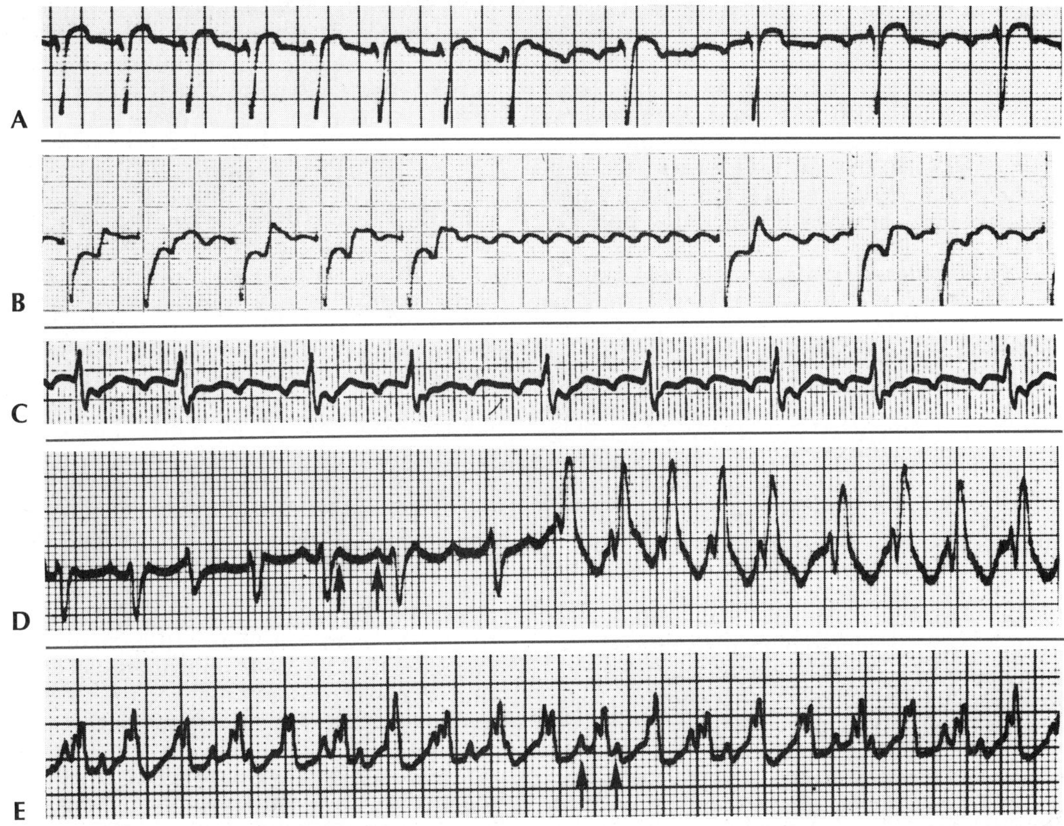

FIGURE 24–11. Various manifestations of atrial flutter. *A*, Atrial flutter at a rate of 300 beats/min conducts to ventricles with 2:1 block. In the midportion of the tracing, carotid sinus massage converts the block to 4:1 and the ventricular rate slows to 75 beats/min. *B*, Carotid sinus massage produces a transient period of AV block clearly revealing the flutter waves. *C*, Quinidine has slowed the atrial flutter rate to approximately 188 beats/min. The block is variable. *D*, Wide QRS complexes with an RSR′ configuration in V_1 begin after a short cycle that follows a long cycle in the midportion of the ECG strip. This represents functional right bundle branch block. Arrows indicate flutter waves. *E*, The QRS complexes are 0.12 sec in duration and have a regular interval at a rate of 200 beats/min. Atrial activity is also regular at a rate of 300 beats/min and independent from the ventricular activity (arrows). Thus, atrial flutter is present with a probable ventricular tachycardia, an example of complete AV dissociation. Monitor leads in *A*, *B*, *C*, and *E*.

will be irregular. Alternation between 2:1 and 4:1 VA conduction often occurs and may be due to two levels of block—2:1 high in the AV node and 3:2 lower down. The irregular ventricular response frequently has the structure that results from Wenckebach periodicity. Recurrent alternation of short and long ventricular intervals may be due to concealed conduction (p. 717). Various degrees of penetration into the AV junction by the flutter impulses can also influence AV conduction. The ratio of flutter waves to conducted ventricular complexes most often is an even number (e.g., 2:1, 4:1, and so on). Impure flutter (flutter-fibrillation or "flitter"), occurring at a rate faster than pure flutter, shows variability in the contour and spacing of the flutter waves and in some instances may represent dissimilar atrial rhythms, i.e., fibrillation in one atrium and a slower, more regular rhythm resembling atrial flutter in the opposite atrium. Prolonged atrial conduction time has been found to be a predisposing factor for the development of atrial flutter.

CLINICAL FEATURES. Atrial flutter is less common than atrial fibrillation. Paroxysmal atrial flutter can occur in patients without structural heart disease, while chronic (persistent) atrial flutter is usually associated with underlying heart disease such as rheumatic or ischemic heart disease or cardiomyopathy. It may occur as a result of atrial dilation from septal defects, pulmonary emboli, mitral or tricuspid valve stenosis or regurgitation, or chronic ventricular failure. Toxic and metabolic conditions that affect the heart, such as thyrotoxicosis, alcoholism, and pericarditis, can cause atrial flutter. Occasionally, it may be congenital or follow surgery for congenital heart disease,[66] or even occur in utero.[67,68] Atrial flutter tends to be unstable, reverting to sinus rhythm or degenerating into atrial fibrillation. Less commonly, the atria can continue to flutter for months or years. In atrial flutter the atria contract, which may, in part, account for fewer systemic emboli than in atrial fibrillation. In children, continued episodes of atrial flutter are associated with an increased possibility of sudden death.

Atrial flutter usually responds to carotid sinus massage with a decrease in ventricular rate in stepwise multiples, returning in a reverse manner to the former ventricular rate at the termination of carotid massage (Fig. 24–11*A*). Very rarely sinus rhythm follows carotid sinus massage. Exercise, by enhancing sympathetic or lessening parasympathetic tone, can reduce the AV conduction delay and produce a doubling of the ventricular rate.

Physical examination may reveal rapid flutter waves in the jugular venous pulse. If the relationship of flutter waves to conducted QRS complexes remains constant, the first heart sound will have a constant intensity. Occasionally, sounds caused by atrial contraction can be auscultated.

MANAGEMENT. Synchronous direct-current (DC) cardioversion (p. 651) is commonly the initial treatment of choice for atrial flutter, since cardioversion promptly and effectively restores sinus rhythm, often requiring relatively low energies (<50 joules). If the electrical shock results in atrial fibrillation, a second shock at a higher energy level is used to restore sinus rhythm or, depending on the clinical circumstances, the atrial fibrillation can be left untreated. The latter can revert to atrial flutter or sinus rhythm. If the patient cannot be electrically cardioverted or if electrical cardioversion is contraindicated—for example, after amounts of digitalis are administered—*rapid atrial pacing* with a catheter in the esophagus[69,70] or the right atrium[71] can terminate type I (but not type II) atrial flutter effectively in most patients producing sinus rhythm or atrial fibrillation with a slowing of the ventricular rate and concomitant clinical improvement. Termination of atrial flutter by atrial pacing can be associated with entrainment, whereby at critical rates of overdrive atrial pacing the flutter morphology changes but the flutter does not terminate.[64]

Verapamil (p. 648), given as an initial bolus of 5 to 10 mg IV, followed by a constant infusion at a rate of 5 μg/kg/min, or *diltiazem*, 0.25 mg/kg, to slow the ventricular response, can be tried. Calcium antagonists[72] can restore sinus rhythm in patients with atrial flutter of recent onset but less commonly terminate chronic atrial flutter. *Adenosine* produces transient AV block and can be used to reveal flutter waves if the diagnosis of the arrhythmias is in doubt. It generally will not terminate the atrial flutter.[73] Esmolol, a beta-adrenergic blocker with a 9-min elimination half-life, can be used in doses of 200 μg/kg/min[74] to slow the ventricular rate.

If the flutter cannot be electrically cardioverted, terminated by pacing, or slowed by drugs, or if it recurs at frequent intervals, a *short-acting digitalis preparation* (such as digoxin or deslanoside) can be tried. The dose of digitalis necessary to slow the ventricular response varies and at times can result in toxic levels because it is often difficult to slow the ventricular rate during atrial flutter. Frequently, atrial fibrillation develops after digitalis administration and can revert to normal sinus rhythm upon withdrawal of digitalis; occasionally, normal sinus rhythm may occur without intervening atrial fibrillation. *Propranolol* or other beta blockers[75] as well as calcium antagonists[72] (p. 648) effectively diminish the ventricular response to atrial flutter and can be used together with digitalis in patients whose ventricular rate is not decreased after digitalis alone. Beta blockers do not appear to affect the atrial rate during atrial flutter.

If the atrial flutter persists, class IA or IC (see Chap. 22) drugs can be tried to restore sinus rhythm and to prevent a recurrence of atrial flutter.[76-80] Amiodarone, also, especially in low doses of 200 mg/day, 5 days/week, can prevent recurrences. Side effects of these drugs,[81] especially proarrhythmic responses,[82-84] must be carefully considered and are dealt with at length in Chap. 22. Sometimes treatment of the underlying disorder, such as thyrotoxicosis, is necessary to effect conversion to sinus rhythm. In certain instances atrial flutter may continue, and if the ventricular rate can be controlled with digitalis, conversion to sinus rhythm may not be indicated. Classes I and III drugs should be discontinued if flutter remains.

It is important to reemphasize that class I drugs should *not* be used unless the ventricular rate during atrial flutter has been *slowed* with digitalis or a calcium antagonist or beta blocking drug. Because of the vagolytic action of quinidine, procainamide, and disopyramide (see Chap. 22) but primarily because of the ability of class I drugs to slow the flutter rate, AV conduction can be *facilitated* sufficiently to result in a 1:1 ventricular response to the atrial flutter.

Prevention of recurrent atrial flutter is often difficult to achieve but should be approached as outlined for the prevention of paroxysmal supraventricular tachycardia due to AV nodal reentry (p. 688). If recurrences cannot be prevented, therapy is directed toward controlling the ventricular rate when the flutter does recur, with digitalis alone or combined with beta blockers or calcium antagonists. Catheter ablation approaches are potential techniques to eliminate atrial flutter.[85,86] Surgery has a similar advantage.[87]

ATRIAL FIBRILLATION

(See also p. 653)

ELECTROCARDIOGRAPHIC RECOGNITION (Fig. 24–12). This arrhythmia is characterized by totally disorganized atrial depolarizations without effective atrial contraction. Electrical activity of the atrium can be detected electrocardiographically as small irregular baseline undulations of variable amplitude and morphology, called f waves, at a rate of 350 to 600 beats/min.[65,88] At times, small, fine, rapid f waves may occur and are detectable only by right atrial leads, or by intracavitary or esophageal electrodes. The ventricular response is grossly irregular ("irregularly irregular") and, in the untreated patient with normal AV conduction, is usually between 100 and 160 beats/min. In patients with the WPW syndrome (see p. 693), the ventricular rate during atrial fibrillation at times can exceed 300 beats/min and lead to ventricular fibrillation (see Fig. 24–23*B*). Atrial fibrillation should be suspected when the ECG shows supraventricular complexes at an irregular rhythm and no obvious P waves. The recognizable f waves probably do not represent total atrial activity but depict only the larger vectors generated by the multiple wavelets of depolarization that occur at any given moment.

Each recorded f wave is not conducted through the AV junction so that a rapid ventricular response comparable to the atrial rate does not occur. Many atrial impulses are canceled, owing to a collision of wavefronts, or are blocked in the AV junction without reaching the ventricles (i.e., concealed conduction [p. 717]), which accounts for the irregular ventricular rhythm. The refractory period and conductivity of the AV node are indicators of the ventricular rate.[88a] When the ventricular rate is very rapid or very slow, it may appear to be more regular. Even though the conversion of atrial fibrillation to atrial flutter is accompanied by slowing of the atrial rate, an increase in the ventricular response may result, since more atrial impulses are transmitted to the ventricle because of less concealed conduction. Also, it is easier to slow the ventricular rate during atrial fibrillation than during atrial flutter with drugs such as digitalis, calcium antagonists, and beta blockers, because the increased concealed conduction makes it easier to produce AV block.

Recent evidence raises the possiblity that transmission of impulses across the AV node during atrial fibrillation occurs electrotonically[89,89a] and that the distal portion of the AV node behaves as a pacemaker, producing the ventricular rhythm during atrial fibrillation.[90]

CLINICAL FEATURES. Atrial fibrillation is a common arrhythmia, found in 1 per cent of persons older than 60 years. The overall chance of atrial fibrillation developing over 2 decades in patients more than 30 years old, according to Framingham data, is 2 per cent. Its presence relates to left atrial size, underlying heart disease, and abnormal atrial electrophysiology.[91,92] The incidence increases with age and most affected people have underlying cardiac disease, including coronary artery disease, rheumatic heart disease, cardiomyopathy, hypertensive cardiovascular disease, and heart failure. Occult or manifest thyrotoxicosis should be considered in patients with

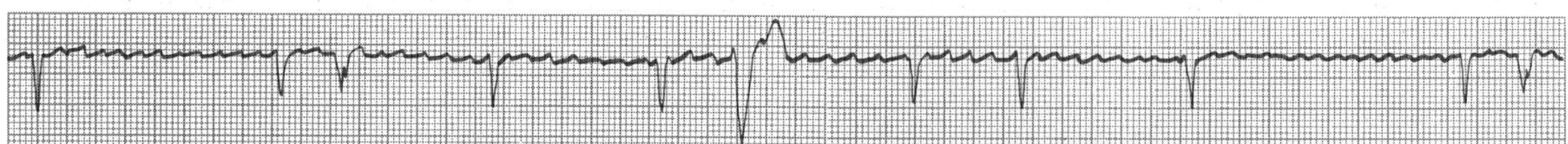

FIGURE 24–12. Atrial fibrillation with ventricular extrasystoles following the longer pauses (monitor lead). Fibrillatory waves are quite obvious. When the ventricular cycle lengths prolong, ventricular extrasystoles result. This phenomenon has been called the "rule of bigeminy."

recent-onset atrial fibrillation.[65] Atrial fibrillation can be intermittent[93] or chronic. Chronic atrial fibrillation carries greater risk than intermittent atrial fibrillation, doubling the risk of cardiovascular mortality.[93a]

Symptoms as a result of atrial fibrillation are determined by multiple factors, the most important of which is the cardiac status. The rapid ventricular rate and loss of atrial contraction adversely affect cardiac output.

Physical findings include a slight variation in the intensity of the first heart sound, absence of *a* waves in the jugular venous pulse, and an irregularly irregular ventricular rhythm. Often with fast ventricular rates a significant pulse deficit appears, during which the auscultated or palpated apical rate is faster than the rate palpated at the wrist (pulse deficit) because each contraction is not sufficiently strong to open the aortic valve or to transmit an arterial pressure wave through the peripheral artery. If the ventricular rhythm becomes regular in patients with atrial fibrillation, conversion to sinus rhythm, atrial tachycardia, atrial flutter with a constant ratio of conducted beats, or development of junctional or ventricular tachycardia, should be suspected.

RISK OF EMBOLIZATION. In addition to hemodynamic alterations, the risk of systemic emboli, probably arising in the left atrial cavity or appendage due to circulatory stasis, is an important consideration.[94,95] Nonvalvular atrial fibrillation is the most common cardiac disease associated with cerebral embolism.[96] In fact, 45 per cent of cardiogenic emboli in the United States occur in patients with nonvalvular atrial fibrillation; the rest occur in patients with acute myocardial infarction (15 per cent), chronic left ventricular dysfunction (10 per cent), rheumatic heart disease (10 per cent), prosthetic heart valves (10 per cent), and other conditions. The risk of stroke in patients with nonvalvular atrial fibrillation is 5 to 7 times greater than in controls without atrial fibrillation.[96a] Overall, about 15 per cent of ischemic strokes are due to cardiogenic emboli, totaling more than 75,000 cases per year.

Certain patients with atrial fibrillation appear at higher risk of emboli. For example, patients with mitral stenosis and atrial fibrillation have a 4 to 6 per cent incidence of embolism per year, an increase of 3- to 7-fold compared with those who have sinus rhythm.[97] The majority of these embolic events affect the brain. Cerebral emboli tend to recur in 30 to 75 per cent of patients at a rate of about 10 per cent per year, most frequently in the first year. Mitral valve prolapse also carries an increased risk of stroke, greater if atrial fibrillation is also present.

The risk of stroke in patients with *lone atrial fibrillation*, that is, idiopathic atrial fibrillation in the absence of any structural heart disease, is not clear. The Framingham Heart Study indicates an increased risk of stroke in these patients, while the Mayo Clinic Study does not.[98]

The risk of embolism following cardioversion to sinus rhythm in patients wtih atrial fibrillation varies from 0 to 7 per cent, depending on the underlying risk factors. Patients at high risk are those with prior embolism, mechanical valve prosthesis, or mitral stenosis. Low-risk patients are those younger than 60 without underlying heart disease. The high-risk group should receive chronic anticoagulation (see below), whether or not they will undergo cardioversion, while anticoagulation in the low-risk group may not be necessary.[97] However, the American College of Chest Physicians has suggested that patients with atrial fibrillation longer in duration than 3 days should receive warfarin (prothrombin time prolongation, 1.3–1.5 × control) for 3 weeks before elective cardioversion and for 2 to 4 weeks after reversion to sinus rhythm. Anticoagulation with heparin has been recommended for emergency cardioversion.[99]

ANTICOAGULANT THERAPY. The issue of chronic anticoagulation is not resolved. Very likely the high-risk group noted above should receive chronic warfarin therapy, while those with lone atrial fibrillation should not. In one study of patients with nonvalvular atrial fibrillation, comparing the effects of placebo, aspirin (75 mg once daily), and warfarin, thromboembolic complications were the same in patients receiving placebo and aspirin and were reduced only in the warfarin-treated group.[100] However, another study[101] comparing warfarin, placebo, and a higher dose of aspirin (325 mg once daily) found that event rates for ischemic stroke and systemic embolism in patients receiving aspirin were the same as for those taking warfarin and were both less than in the placebo group. There was no benefit shown with aspirin in patients older than 75 years, however.[101]

Therefore, on the basis of present data, it seems reasonable to recommend either long-term aspirin (325 mg daily) or warfarin for all patients with chronic atrial fibrillation and nonvalvular heart disease, favoring warfarin in the highest risk group and in those older than 75 years. The patient with lone atrial fibrillation could take aspirin or possibly nothing. Short-term anticoagulation before and after cardioversion, except possibly in the patient with lone atrial fibrillation, is reasonable. Conceivably, using transesophageal echocardiography to determine whether a left atrial thrombus is present could influence the decision of whether or not to give anticoagulants.

It is important to emphasize that these suggestions must be individualized for a given patient. For example, patients at risk of trauma by virtue of occupation, participation in sports, and episodes of dizziness or syncope are at increased risk of bleeding if given anticoagulants and probably should not receive warfarin. Patients should be warned about taking any new drugs, e.g., nonsteroidal antiinflammatory agents, if they are receiving warfarin.

For patients with intermittent atrial fibrillation, guidelines are unclear. A reasonable approach would be to treat them according to the recommendations noted above.

MANAGEMENT. The atria are often abnormal in patients with atrial fibrillation, showing increased conduction time[91,92] or enlargement.[102] Maintenance of sinus rhythm after cardioversion is influenced by the duration of atrial fibrillation[103,104] and, in some studies, atrial dilation. The latter can occur as a *consequence* of atrial fibrillation.[104a]

The patient with atrial fibrillation discovered for the first time should be evaluated for a precipitating cause, such as thyrotoxicosis, mitral stenosis, pulmonary emboli, or pericarditis. The patient's clinical status determines initial therapy, the objectives being to slow the ventricular rate and to restore atrial systole. If the sudden onset of atrial fibrillation with a rapid ventricular rate results in acute cardiovascular decompensation, electrical cardioversion is the treatment of choice.[104] High-energy shock over a right atrial catheter can be successful when transthoracic shocks fail.[105] Atrial contraction may not return immediately after restoration of electrical systole and clinical improvement may be delayed.[106,107] DC cardioversion establishes normal sinus rhythm in over 90 per cent of patients, but sinus rhythm remains for 12 months in only 30 to 50 per cent. Class IC drugs may be useful.[107a] Patients with atrial fibrillation of less than 12 months' duration have a greater chance of maintaining sinus rhythm after cardioversion. In the absence of decompensation, the patient can be treated with drugs such as digitalis, beta blockers,[108] or calcium antagonists[109,110] to maintain a resting apical rate of 60 to 80 beats/min that does not exceed 100 beats/min after slight exercise. The combined use of digitalis and a beta blocker or calcium antagonist can be helpful in slowing the ventricular rate.[111] Esmolol is more likely to terminate the atrial fibrillation than is verapamil,[108] which may actually prolong a paroxysm.[112]

Classes IA,[113] IC,[114–116] and III (amiodarone,[117] sotalol[117a]) agents can be used to prevent recurrences of atrial fibrillation. No one drug, with the possible exception of amiodarone, appears clearly superior, and selection is often based on side effect profile. In some patients with frequent recurrences and rapid ventricular rates not controlled by drugs, AV node–His bundle ablation and implantation of a rate-adaptive VVI (VVIR) pacemaker constitute acceptable therapy (see Ch. 23). Whenever possible, atrial or dual-chamber pacing is preferable, since the incidence of atrial fibrillation is reduced compared with VVI pacing.[118] Quinidine, given with digitalis, is often necessary to convert to sinus rhythm. The use of large doses of quinidine to produce reversion to normal sinus rhythm is no longer indicated. Before electrical cardioversion, maintenance doses of quinidine sulfate in the range of 800 to 1600 mg/day should be administered for a few days. Rapid atrial pacing will *not* terminate atrial fibrillation.

Many elderly patients tolerate atrial fibrillation well without therapy because the ventricular rate is slow as a result of concomitant AV nodal disease. These patients often have associated sick sinus syndrome, and the development of atrial fibrillation respresents a cure of sorts. Such patients may demonstrate serious supraventricular and ventricular arrhythmias or asystole after cardioversion, so that the likelihood of establishing and maintaining sinus rhythm should be weighed against the risks of cardioversion or other forms of therapy.

ATRIAL TACHYCARDIAS

ELECTROCARDIOGRAPHIC RECOGNITION (Fig. 24–13). In atrial tachycardia, sometimes called atrial tachycardia with block or paroxysmal atrial tachycardia with block (PAT with block), the atrial rate is generally 150 to 200 beats/min and the P-wave contour is different from that of the sinus P wave. When the tachycardia is due to digitalis excess, the atrial rate can increase gradually as the digitalis is continued (a similar response can occur in nonparoxysmal AV junctional tachycardia); this increase may be associated with gradual prolongation of the P-R interval. If the atrial rate is not excessive and AV conduction is not significantly depressed by the digitalis, each P wave may conduct to the ventricles. As the atrial rate increases and AV conduction becomes impaired, Wenckebach (Mobitz type I) second degree AV block (p. 710) can ensue—hence the term atrial tachycardia with block. Frequently, other manifestations of digitalis excess, such as premature ventricular complexes, are present. In nearly half the cases of atrial tachycardia with block, the atrial rate is irregular. Characteristic isoelectric intervals between P waves, in contrast to atrial flutter, are usually present in all leads. However, at rapid atrial rates the distinction between atrial tachycardia with block and atrial flutter can be difficult.[119]

The term "paroxysmal" is used to indicate a tachycardia of sudden onset that changes from sinus rhythm to a tachycardia in one beat—for example, a premature atrial complex precipitating a paroxysmal supraventricular tachycardia (Fig. 24–10*B*). In contrast, the term "nonparoxysmal" refers to a tachycardia that has a gradual onset and termination, similar to the warm-up phenomenon characteristic of automaticity (p. 601). Nonparoxysmal AV junctional tachycardia is such a tachycardia. Because the atrial tachycardia described above appears to be a "nonparoxysmal" variety, the term "paroxysmal atrial tachycardia with block" is inappropriate.

CLINICAL FEATURES. Atrial tachycardia with block occurs most commonly in patients with significant structural heart disease, such as coronary artery disease, with or without myocardial infarction, cor pulmonale, or digitalis intoxication. Potassium depletion can precipitate the arrhythmia in patients taking digitalis. The signs, symptoms, and prognosis are usually related to underlying cardiovascular status.

Physical findings include a variable rhythm and intensity of the first heart sound, owing to the varying AV block and P-R interval. An excessive number of *a* waves may be auscultated in the jugular venous pulse. Carotid sinus massage increases the degree of AV block by slowing the ventricular rate in a stepwise fashion without terminating the tachycardia as in atrial flutter. It should be performed cautiously in patients who have digitalis toxicity because serious ventricular arrhythmias can result.

MANAGEMENT. Atrial tachycardia with block in a patient not receiving digitalis is treated in a manner similar to other atrial tachyarrhythmias. Depending on the clinical situation, digitalis can be administered to slow the ventricular rate and then if atrial tachycardia with block remains, class IA, IC, or III (amiodarone) drugs can be added. Ablation procedures can be tried, including surgical isolation.[120] Tachycardias can recur at a different site following a successful ablation attempt. If atrial tachycardia with block appears in a patient receiving digitalis, the drug should initially be assumed to be responsible for the arrhythmia. Therapy includes cessation of digitalis and administration of potassium chloride orally or intravenously if serum [K^+] is not abnormally elevated, or a drug such as lidocaine, propranolol, and phenytoin while cardiac rhythm is monitored. Often, the ventricular response is not excessively fast and simply withholding digitalis is all that is necessary.

AUTOMATIC ATRIAL TACHYCARDIA

Two types of atrial tachycardias have been distinguished electrophysiologically: automatic and reentrant atrial tachycardia. While it is likely that one or both of these atrial tachycardias is responsible for atrial tachycardia with block (described above), the relationship, if any, is not clear at present, and these two tachycardias will be discussed separately.

ELECTROCARDIOGRAPHIC FEATURES (Fig. 24–9*F* and Table 24–2). Automatic atrial tachycardia is characterized electrocardiographically by a supraventricular tachycardia that generally accelerates after its initation, with heart rates less than 200 beats/min. The P-wave contour differs from the sinus P wave, the P-R interval is influenced directly by the tachycardia rate, and AV block can exist without affecting the tachycardia, i.e., it continues uninterrupted. Vagal maneuvers generally do not terminate the tachycardia, even though they can produce AV nodal block. Thus, pharmacological or physiological maneuvers that selectively result in AV block

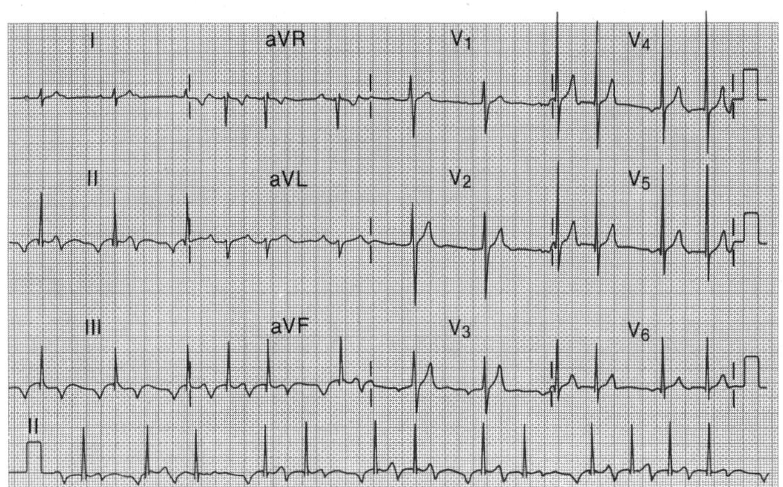

FIGURE 24–13. Atrial tachycardia. This 12-lead ECG and rhythm strip (bottom) demonstrate an atrial tachycardia at a cycle length of approximately 520 msec. Conduction varies between 3 : 2 and 2 : 1. Note the negative P waves in leads 2, 3, and aVF and, when consecutive P waves conduct, that the R-P interval exceeds the P-R interval. Note also that the tachycardia persists despite the development of AV block, an important finding that excludes the participation of an atrioventricular accessory pathway and sharply differentiates this tachycardia from the one shown in Figure 24–29*B*.

do not affect the automatic focus nor does the development of bundle branch block alter the P-R or R-P interval unless it is associated with prolongation of the H-V interval.

Electrophysiologically, initiation of tachycardia with premature atrial stimulation is generally not possible but is independent of intraatrial or AV nodal conduction delay when it occurs. The atrial activation sequence usually differs from a sinus-initiated P wave, and the A-H interval is related to the tachycardia rate. The first P wave of the tachycardia is the same as the subsequent P waves of the tachycardia in contrast to most forms of reentrant supraventricular tachycardias, in which the initial and subsequent P waves differ. Usually the tachycardia cannot be terminated by pacing, although it can exhibit overdrive suppression. The introduction of premature atrial complexes during tachycardia merely resets the timing of the tachycardia. It is very difficult to differentiate this mechanism from micro-reentry, using the leading circle concept (see p. 609).

CLINICAL FEATURES. Many supraventricular tachycardias associated with AV block are probably due to automatic atrial tachycardia, including atrial tachycardia with block due to digitalis intoxication (Fig. 24–13). Automatic atrial tachycardia occurs in all age groups; it is thought to be due to enhanced automaticity and is seen in settings of myocardial infarction, chronic lung disease (especially with acute infection), acute alcohol ingestion, and a variety of metabolic derangements. Rarely, swallowing can precipitate the tachycardia.[121] Digitalis appears to be a particularly important precipitating agent. Differentiation from other tachycardias such as sinus nodal reentry (if the P waves of the automatic atrial tachycardia resemble the sinus-initiated P waves), atrial reentry (particularly if caused by micro-reentry), and some other mechanisms can be difficult (Table 24–2). In view of the experimental findings of triggered activity from a variety of atrial fibers, including that of human mitral valve (see p. 604), it is possible that such activity also occurs in humans. However, many automatic atrial tachycardias are not suppressed by verapamil.

Management is as discussed under atrial tachycardia with block.

ATRIAL TACHYCARDIA DUE TO REENTRY

(See also p. 607)

ELECTROCARDIOGRAPHIC RECOGNITION (Fig. 24–9E). This arrhythmia presents electrocardiographically with a P wave that has a contour different from the sinus P wave, a P-R interval influenced directly by the tachycardia rate, and the ability to develop AV block without interrupting the tachycardia (Table 24–2). Electrophysiologically, initiation of the tachycardia occurs with premature stimulation during the atrial relative refractory period, resulting in a critical degree of intraatrial conduction delay, an atrial activation sequence different from that which occurs during sinus rhythm, and an AV nodal conduction time related to the tachycardia rate. Vagal maneuvers generally do not terminate the tachycardia and can produce AV block.

CLINICAL FEATURES. The relative infrequency of published reports suggests that atrial reentry is not a commonly recognized cause of supraventricular tachycardia. The tachycardia rate is about 130 to 150 beats/min, although a recent study reported rates of about 180 beats/min.[122] The tachycardia can be started and stopped by an atrial extrastimulus. Spontaneous termination can be either sudden, with progressive slowing, or with alternating long-short cycle lengths. Amiodarone can be effective.[122]

CHAOTIC ATRIAL TACHYCARDIA

Chaotic (sometimes called multifocal) atrial tachycardia is characterized by atrial rates between 100 and 130 beats/min, with marked variation in P-wave morphology and totally irregular P-P intervals (Fig. 24–14). Generally at least three P-wave contours are noted, with most P waves conducted to the ventricles. This tachycardia occurs commonly in older patients with chronic obstructive pulmonary disease and congestive heart failure[123] and may eventually develop into atrial fibrillation. Digitalis appears to be an unusual cause while theophylline administration has been implicated. Chaotic atrial tachycardia can occur in childhood.

MANAGEMENT. This is primarily directed toward the underlying disease. Antiarrhythmic agents are often ineffective in slowing either the rate of the atrial tachycardia or the ventricular response. Beta-adrenoreceptor blockers should be avoided in patients with bronchospastic pulmonary disease but can be effective if tolerated.[124] Verapamil and amiodarone[125] have been useful. Potassium and magnesium replacement may suppress the tachycardia.

AV JUNCTIONAL RHYTHM DISTURBANCES

AV JUNCTIONAL ESCAPE BEATS

MECHANISM. Automatic fibers that are prevented from initiating depolarization by a pacemaker such as the sinus node which possesses a more rapid rate of firing are called *latent pacemakers*. Such latent pacemakers are found in some parts of the atrium, in the AV node–His bundle area, in the right and left bundle branches, and in the Purkinje system. Under usual conditions automatic fibers are *not* found in atrial or ventricular myocardium. It is possible that the N region of the AV node is automatic, at least in some species, but is kept suppressed by neighboring atrial tissue.[126] A latent pacemaker can become the dominant pacemaker by default or usurpation, that is, by passive or active mechanisms. A decrease in the number of impulses arriving at a latent pacemaker site, the result of slowing of the sinus node or interrup-

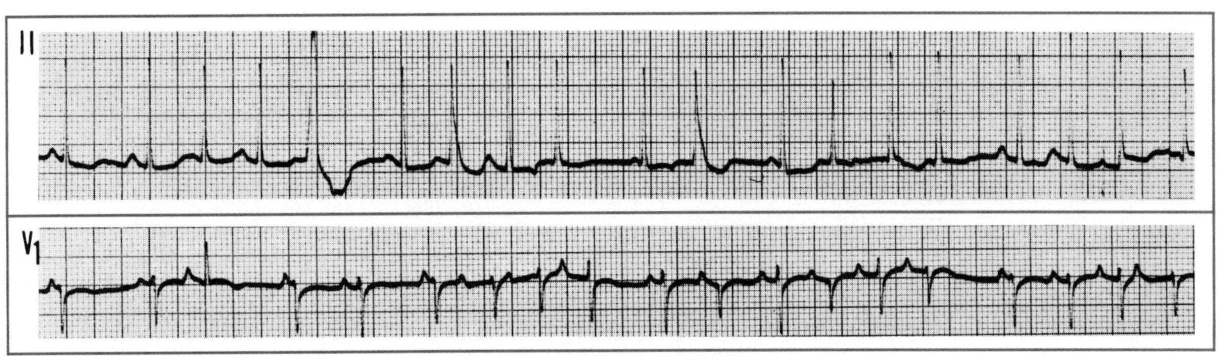

FIGURE 24–14. Chaotic (multifocal) atrial tachycardia. Premature atrial complexes occur at varying cycle lengths and with differing contours.

tion of the propagation of the normal impulse anywhere along its course, allows the latent pacemaker to escape and initiate depolarization passively, by default. An increase in the discharge rate of a latent pacemaker can capture pacemaker control actively, by usurpation. As will be seen, the implication of the two different mechanisms of ectopic impulse formation is important therapeutically. It is not clear whether premature escape beats are due to triggered activity[126a] or to normal automaticity.[126b]

ELECTROCARDIOGRAPHIC RECOGNITION. An AV junctional escape beat occurs when the rate of impulse formation of the primary pacemaker, generally the sinus node, becomes less than that of the AV junctional region, or when impulses from the primary pacemaker do not penetrate to the region of the escape focus and allow the AV junctional focus to reach threshold and discharge. The interval from the last normally conducted beat to the AV junctional escape beat is a measure of the initial discharge rate of the AV junctional focus and generally corresponds to a rate of 35 to 60 beats/min (Fig. 24–2*B*). Although an AV junctional escape rhythm is usually fairly regular, intervals between subsequent escape beats after the initial escape beat can gradually shorten as the rate of discharge of the escape focus increases, the so-called *rhythm of development* or *warm-up phenomenon.*

The electrocardiogram displays pauses longer than the normal P-P interval, interrupted by a QRS complex of supraventricular configuration with absent, retrograde, fusion, or sinus P waves that do not conduct to the ventricle. If P waves precede the QRS, they have a P-R interval generally less than 0.12 sec. The exact site of impulse formation (i.e., AN, N, or NH regions; low atrium; or His bundle) is not known and may differ from patient to patient and be influenced by the cause of the arrhythmia.

Treatment, if any, lies in increasing the discharge rate of the higher pacemakers and improving AV conduction and can require pacing. Frequently, no treatment is necessary.

PREMATURE AV JUNCTIONAL COMPLEXES

Premature AV junctional complexes are characterized by an impulse that arises prematurely in the AV junction (the exact site—i.e., AN, N, or NH regions; low atrium; or His bundle—is not known and may vary from patient to patient) and that attempts conduction in anterograde and retrograde directions. If unimpeded in its course, the impulse discharges at the atrium to produce a premature retrograde P wave and a premature QRS complex with a supraventricular contour. The retrograde P wave can occur before, during, or after the QRS complex. Alterations in conduction time may influence the P-R or R-P relationships without a change in the site of origin of the impulse. Premature AV junctional complexes that conduct aberrantly are difficult to distinguish from premature ventricular complexes using the scalar ECG (Fig. 24–15).

Treatment of premature AV junctional complexes is generally not necessary. However, since they may arise distal to the AV node, they can occur early in the cardiac cycle and can initiate a ventricular tachyarrhythmia in some instances. Under these circumstances therapy is approached as for premature ventricular complexes (see p. 701).

AV JUNCTIONAL RHYTHM

If the AV junctional escape beats continue for a period of time, the rhythm is called an AV junctional rhythm (Fig. 24–16). Since the inherent rate of the AV junctional tissue is 35 to 60 beats/min, the AV junctional tissue can assume the role of the dominant pacemaker at this rate only by passive default of the sinus pacemaker. The ECG displays a normally conducted QRS complex, which can conduct retrogradely to the atrium or can occur independently of atrial discharge, producing AV dissociation (see p. 715).

An AV junctional escape rhythm can be a normal phenomenon in response to the effects of vagal tone or it can occur during pathological sinus bradycardia or heart block. The

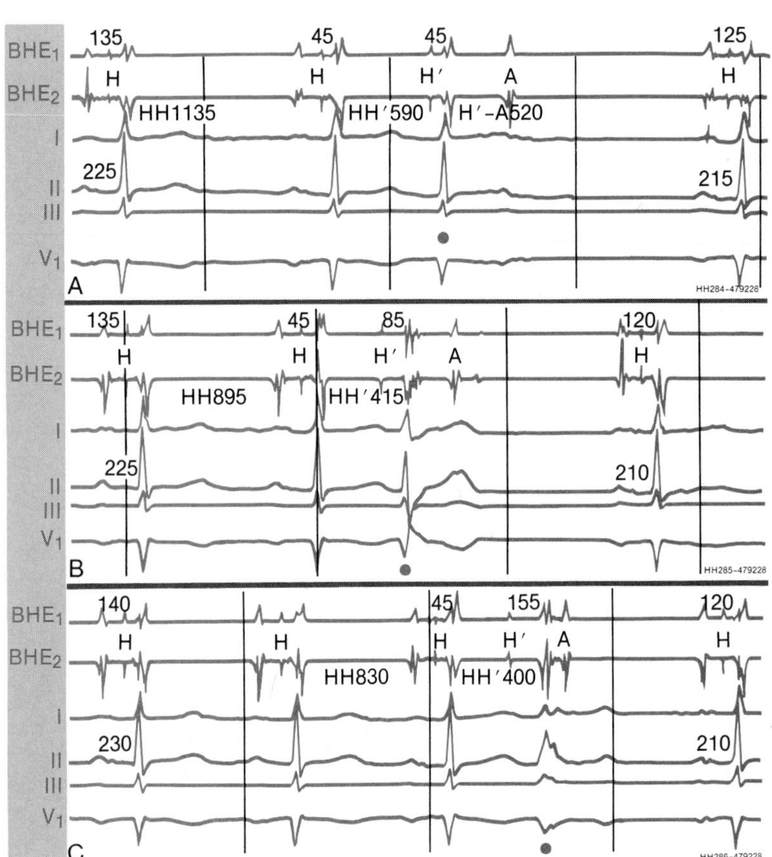

FIGURE 24–15. Premature AV junctional complexes arising in or near the bundle of His (H′) conduct normally (*A*) or with (*B*) functional right or (*C*) functional left bundle branch block. The filled circles indicate the premature junctional complex. Anterograde conduction of the premature junctional (H′) discharges depends on the coupling interval between the last normal His discharge (H) and H-H′ interval and the spontaneous cycle length (H-H) that preceded H′. When H′ follows a shorter preceding cycle length and occurs at longer coupling intervals, a normal QRS complex results. As the preceding H-H cycle lengthens or as the H-H′ interval shortens, a zone of functional right bundle branch block occurs, followed by a zone of functional left bundle branch block. Not shown are premature His discharges that fail to conduct entirely (Fig. 22–33, p. 618). Numbers in milliseconds. Time lines = 1 sec in each panel. (Magnification is not the same in all three panels.) (From Bonner, A. J., and Zipes, D. P.: Lidocaine and His bundle extrasystoles. His bundle discharge conducted normally, conducted with functional right or left bundle branch block, or blocked entirely [concealed]. Arch. Intern. Med. *136*:700, 1976.)

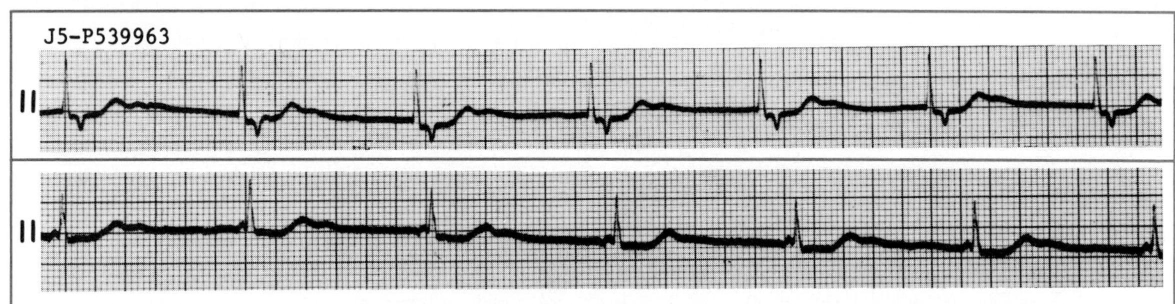

FIGURE 24-16. AV junctional rhythm. *Top,* AV junctional discharge occurs fairly regularly at a rate of approximately 50 beats/min. Retrograde atrial activity follows each junctional discharge. *Bottom,* Recording made on a different day in the same patient; the AV junctional rate is slightly more variable, and retrograde P waves precede the onset of the QRS complex. The positive terminal portion of the P wave gives the appearance of AV dissociation, which was not present.

escape beat or rhythm serves as a safety mechanism to prevent the occurrence of ventricular asystole. *Physical findings* vary depending on the P-QRS relationship. Large *a* waves in the jugular venous pulse and a loud, soft, or changing intensity of the first heart sound may be present if atrial contraction occurs when the tricuspid valve is shut.

Therapy is discussed under AV junctional escape beats (see above).

NONPAROXYSMAL AV JUNCTIONAL TACHYCARDIA

ELECTROCARDIOGRAPHIC RECOGNITION (Figs. 24-17 and 24-18). To usurp dominant pacemaker status, the AV junctional tissue must exhibit enhanced discharge rate such as during nonparoxysmal AV junctional tachycardia. The tachycardia is usually of gradual onset and termination hence the modifier "nonparoxysmal." On occasion, nonparoxysmal AV junctional tachycardia can become manifest abruptly because of slowing of the dominant pacemaker that may then allow sudden capture and control of the rhythm by the AV junctional focus.

Nonparoxysmal AV junctional tachycardia is recognized by a QRS of supraventricular configuration at a fairly regular rate of 70 to 130 beats/min but can be faster.[126,127] Accepted terminology assigns the label of tachycardia to rates exceeding 100 beats/min. The term nonparoxysmal AV junctional tachycardia, although not entirely correct when the rate is 70 to 100 beats/min, has generally been accepted, since rates exceeding 60 beats/min represent in effect a tachycardia for the AV junctional tissue. Enhanced vagal tone can slow while vagolytic agents can speed up the discharge rate. Although retrograde activation of the atria can occur, the atria commonly are controlled by an independent sinus, atrial, or on occasion a second AV junctional focus resulting in AV dissociation (Fig. 24-9G). The electrocardiographic diagnosis can be complicated by the presence of entrance and exit blocks at the AV junctional tissue level and incomplete forms of AV dissociation.

The cause of this arrhythmia probably is *accelerated automatic discharge* in or near the His bundle.[126-128] It is possible that nonparoxysmal AV junctional tachycardia originates in atrial fibers without recognition of the latter's role from analysis of the scalar ECG or on intracardiac electrograms, unless a careful search is made. Wenckebach periods can occur (Fig. 5-49, p. 148), but the presence of exit block has not yet been demonstrated by His bundle recording in humans, and the block can be in the AV node with the origin of the nonparoxysmal AV junctional tachycardia proximal to the site of the His bundle recording.

CLINICAL FEATURES. Nonparoxysmal AV junctional tachycardia occurs most commonly in patients with underlying heart disease, such as inferior infarction or myocarditis (often the result of acute rheumatic fever), or after open-heart surgery. Probably the most important cause is excessive digitalis, which may also produce the ECG manifestations of varying degrees of exit block (usually Wenckebach type) from the accelerated AV junctional focus. Nonparoxysmal AV junctional tachycardia can occur in otherwise healthy individuals without symptoms (Fig. 24-18) or can be a serious and difficult-to-control tachycardia, occasionally chronic, rapid, and long-lasting. It can occur congenitally in infants, with a relatively high mortality.[128a]

The clinical features vary depending on the rate of the arrhythmia and the underlying etiology and severity of heart disease. As in most arrhythmias, the physical signs are deter-

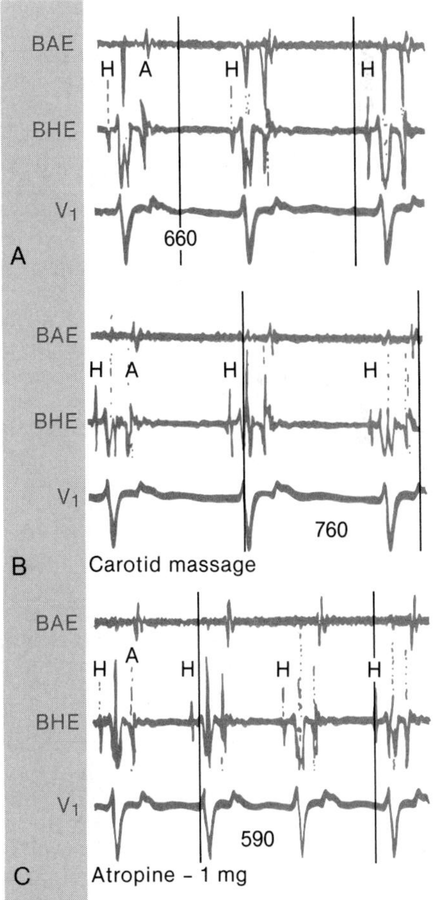

FIGURE 24-17. Nonparoxysmal AV junctional tachycardia. *A,* Control; *B,* response to carotid sinus massage; *C,* response to atropine, 1 mg intravenously. Note that His bundle depolarization is the earliest recordable electrical activity in each cycle. The atria are depolarized retrogradely (low right atrial activity recorded in BHE precedes high right atrial activity recorded in BAE). Note also that carotid sinus massage slows the junctional discharge rate while atropine speeds it up. From these tracings alone one could not distinguish the rhythm from some other types of supraventricular tachycardias. However, onset and termination of this tachycardia were typical of nonparoxysmal AV junctional tachycardia.

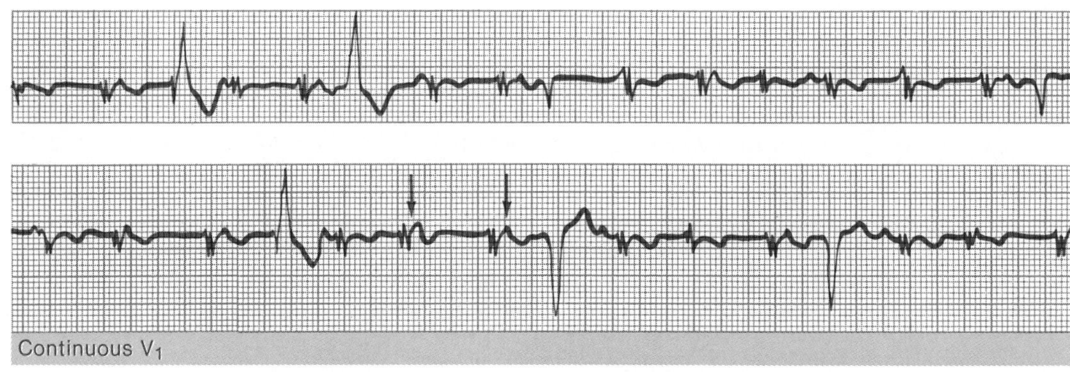

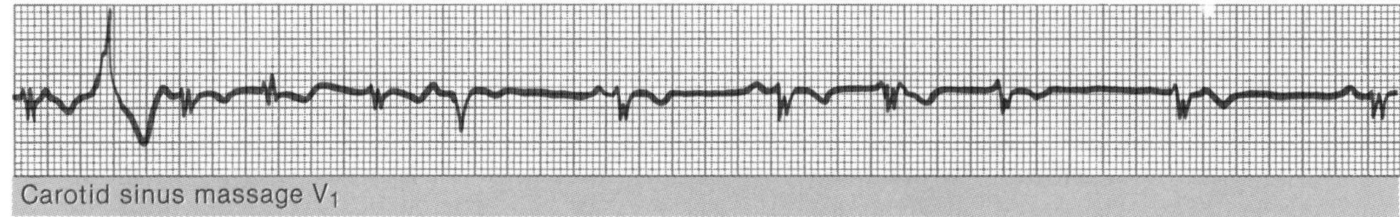

FIGURE 24–18. Nonparoxysmal AV junctional tachycardia in a healthy young adult. This tachycardia occurs at a fairly regular interval ("W-shaped" complexes) and is interrupted intermittently with sinus captures that produce functional right and left bundle branch block. Two P waves are indicated by arrows. The junctional discharge rate is approximately 120 beats/min (cycle length = 500 msec) and the rhythm irregular, sometimes shortened by sinus captures or delayed by concealed conduction that resets and displaces the junctional focus. In the bottom panel, carotid sinus massage slows the junctional as well as the sinus discharge rate.

mined by the relationship of the P wave to the QRS complex and the rate of atrial and ventricular discharge. The first heart sound can therefore be constant or varying, and cannon *a* waves may or may not occur in the jugular venous pulse.

The ventricular rhythm may be regular or irregular, often in a constant fashion. It is especially important to recognize slowing and regularization of the ventricular rhythm in a patient with atrial fibrillation as being caused by nonparoxysmal AV junctional tachycardia and as a possible early sign of *digitalis intoxication* (p. 490). Initially, during atrial fibrillation, the regular ventricular rhythm can result from an AV junctional escape rhythm because the depressed AV conduction caused by digitalis blocks the passage of impulses from the fibrillating atria (Fig. 24–9G). As digitalis administration is continued, the ventricular rate can then speed because of increased discharge of the AV junctional pacemaker but can still be regular. Further digitalis administration can produce a rate that is slow and irregular because of varying degrees of AV junctional exit block. The rhythm can be misdiagnosed as resumption of conduction from the fibrillating atria. The rate then can increase further because of development of a ventricular tachycardia.

MANAGEMENT. This is directed toward the underlying etiological factor and functional support of the cardiovascular system. If the rhythm is regular, the cardiovascular status is not compromised, and if the patient is not taking digitalis, digitalis administration should be considered. Cardioversion can be tried if necessary and if digitalis toxicity is excluded; theoretically, however, if the nonparoxysmal AV junctional tachycardia is due to enhanced automaticity, cardioversion may be ineffective. If the patient tolerates the arrhythmia well, careful monitoring and attention to the underlying heart disease is usually all that is required. The arrhythmia usually will abate spontaneously. If digitalis toxicity is the cause, the drug must be stopped and potassium, lidocaine, phenytoin, or propranolol administered. Drug therapy includes agents from classes IA, IC, and III (amiodarone). Catheter ablation of the junctional site can be effective.[126,127]

TACHYCARDIAS INVOLVING THE AV JUNCTION

Much confusion exists regarding the nomenclature of tachycardias characterized by a supraventricular QRS complex, a regular R-R interval, and no evidence of ventricular preexcitation. These tachycardias have often been called paroxysmal atrial tachycardia (PAT) if the P wave occurred in front of the QRS complex or paroxysmal nodal or junctional tachycardia (PJT) if the P wave occurred within or just following the QRS complex and exhibited a retrograde contour. Because it is now apparent that a variety of electrophysiological mechanisms can account for these tachycardias (Fig. 24–9 and Table 24–2), the nonspecific term paroxysmal supraventricular tachycardia (PSVT) has been proposed to encompass the entire group. This term may be inappropriate because tachycardias in patients with accessory pathways (see below) are no more supraventricular than they are ventricular in origin, since they may require participation of both the atria and the ventricles in the reentrant pathway, and they exhibit a QRS complex of normal contour and duration only because anterograde conduction occurs over the normal AV node–His bundle pathways (Fig. 24–9C). If conduction over the reentrant pathway reverses direction and travels in an "antidromic" direction—i.e., to the ventricles over the accessory pathway and to the atria over the AV node–His bundle—the QRS complex exhibits a prolonged duration, although the tachycardia is basically the same. The term *reciprocating tachycardia* has been offered as a substitute for paroxysmal supraventricular tachycardia, but use of such a term presumes the mechanism of the tachycardia to be reentrant (which is probably the case for many supraventricular tachycardias). Reciprocating tachycardia is probably the mechanism of many ventricular tachycardias as well. Thus, no universally acceptable nomenclature exists for these tachycardias. In this chapter, descriptive titles, although cumbersome, will be used for the sake of clarity. In addition, the mechanism of reentry will be assumed operative when the weight of evidence supports its presence even though unequivocal proof is lacking.

ATRIOVENTRICULAR (AV) NODAL REENTRANT TACHYCARDIA

ELECTROCARDIOGRAPHIC RECOGNITION. Reentrant tachycardia in the AV node is characterized by a tachycardia with a QRS complex of supraventricular origin, with sudden onset and termination generally at rates between 150 and 250 beats/min (commonly 180 to 200 beats/min in adults), and with a regular rhythm (Table 24–2). Uncommonly, the rate may be as low as 110 beats/min and occasionally, especially in children, may exceed 250. Unless functional aberrant ventricular conduction or a previous conduction defect exists, the QRS complex is normal in contour and duration. P waves are generally buried in the QRS complex (Table 24–2). AV nodal reentry recorded at the onset begins abruptly, usually following a premature atrial complex that conducts with a prolonged P-R interval (see Figs. 24–9*A* and 24–10*B* and Figs. 22–27 and 22–28, pp. 611 and 612). The abrupt termination is sometimes followed by a brief period of asystole or bradycardia. The R-R interval can shorten over the course of the first few beats at the onset or lengthen during the last few beats preceding termination of the tachycardia. Variation in cycle length is usually caused by variation in anterograde AV nodal conduction time. Carotid sinus massage can slow the tachycardia slightly prior to its termination or, if termination does not occur, can produce only slight slowing of the tachycardia.

ELECTROPHYSIOLOGICAL FEATURES. An atrial complex that conducts with a critical prolongation of AV nodal conduction time generally precipitates AV nodal reentry (see Figs. 24–19, 24–20, and 24–21*B*).[129] Premature ventricular stimulation also can induce AV nodal reentry in about one-third of patients. Several AV nodal pathways can be diagrammed to explain this tachycardia. In Figure 22–24*B* (p. 608), the atria are shown as a necessary link in the reentrant pathway, while in Figure 24–9*A* and *B* (p. 678), the atria are not incorporated in the circuit. In most examples, the retrograde P wave occurs at the onset of the QRS complex, clearly excluding the possibility of an accessory pathway. If an accessory pathway in the ventricle were part of the tachycardia circuit, the ventricles would have to be activated anterogradely before the accessory pathway could be activated retrogradely and depolarize the atria (see Preexcitation Syndrome, p. 693).

In approximately 30 per cent of instances, atrial activation begins at the end of, or just after, the QRS complex, giving rise to a discrete P wave on the surface ECG (often appearing as a nubbin of an R′ in V_1) (Fig. 24–9*B*), while in the majority of patients P waves are not seen, since they are buried within the inscription of the QRS complex (Fig. 24–9*A*). In the most common variety of AV nodal reentrant tachycardia, the V-A interval (i.e., interval between onset of QRS and onset of atrial activity) is less than 50 per cent of the R-R interval and the ratio of A-V to V-A interval exceeds 1.0. Most of these patients during tachycardia have a V-A minimum value of ≤61 msec measured to the earliest recorded atrial activity and of ≤95 msec measured to atrial activity recorded in the high right atrial electrogram. These V-A intervals are longer in patients with tachycardia related to accessory pathways as well as in atypical forms of AV nodal reentry (Fig. 24–9*B* and Table 24–2).

Slow and Fast Pathways. In the majority of patients, anterograde conduction occurs to the ventricle over the slow (alpha) pathway and retrograde conduction over the fast (beta) pathway (see Fig. 22–24*B*, and Fig. 24–9*A* and *B*). To initiate tachycardia, an atrial complex blocks in the fast pathway anterogradely, travels to the ventricle over the slow pathway, and returns to the atrium over the previously blocked fast pathway. The proximal and distal final pathways for this circus movement appear to be located within the AV node, so that, as currently conceived, the circus movement is located totally within the AV node (Fig. 24–9*A* and *B*). The reentrant loop is slow AV nodal pathway → final distal common pathway (probably distal AV node) → retrograde fast AV nodal pathway → final proximal common pathway (probably proximal AV node, possibly a portion of low atrium). In some patients, the His bundle may be incorporated in the reentrant circuit. The cycle length of the tachycardia generally depends on how well the slow pathway conducts, because the fast pathway usually exhibits excellent capability for retrograde conduction and has the shorter refractory period in the retrograde direction. Therefore, conduction time in the anterograde slow pathway is a major determinant of the cycle length of the tachycardia. The finding of an excitable gap supports the presence of reentry.[130]

The Dual Pathway Concept. The evidence supporting the dual pathway concept derives in part from the observation that in these patients, a plot of the A_1-A_2 versus the A_2-H_2 or A_1-A_2 versus the H_1-H_2 intervals shows a discontinuous curve (Fig. 24–20). The explanation is that, at a critical A_1-A_2 interval, the impulse suddenly blocks in the fast pathway and

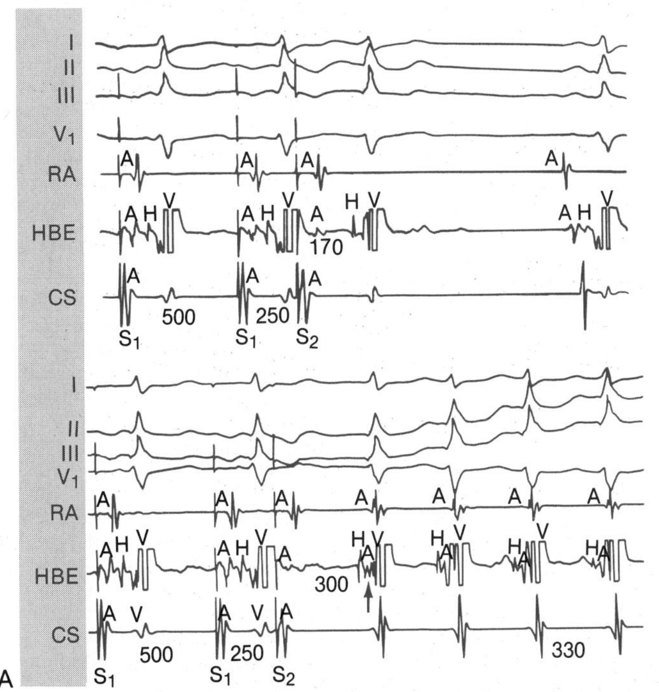

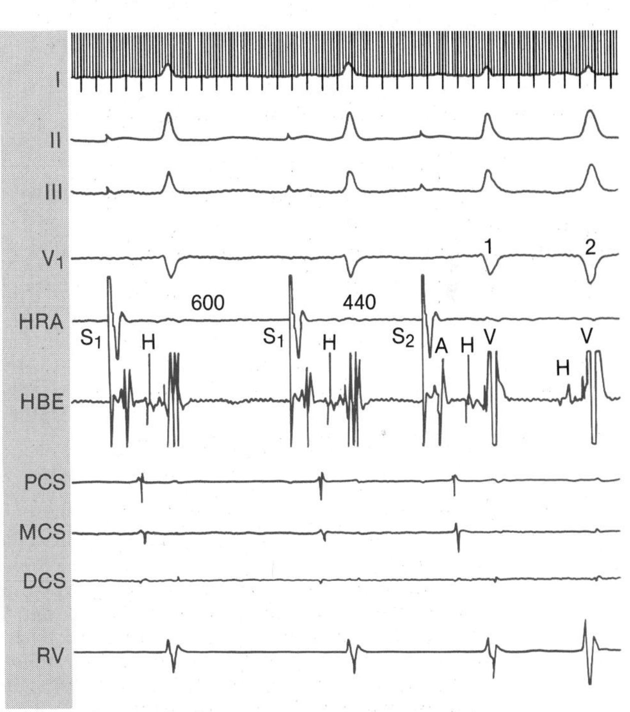

FIGURE 24–19. ***A,*** **Initiation of AV nodal reentrant tachycardia in a patient with dual atrioventricular nodal pathways. Upper and lower panels show the last two paced beats of a train of stimuli delivered to the coronary sinus at a pacing cycle length of 500 msec. The results of premature atrial stimulation at an S_1-S_2 interval of 250 msec on two occasions are shown. In the upper panel, S_2 was conducted to the ventricle with an A-H interval of 170 msec and then was followed by a sinus beat. In the lower panel, S_2 was conducted with an A-H interval of 300 msec and initiated AV nodal reentry. Note that the retrograde atrial activity occurs (arrow) prior to the onset of ventricular septal depolarization and is superimposed on the QRS complex. Retrograde atrial activity begins first in the low right atrium (HBE lead) and then progresses to the high right atrium (RA) and coronary sinus (CS) recordings.**

B, **Two QRS complexes in response to a single atrial premature complex. Following a basic train of S_1 stimuli at 600 msec, an S_2 at 440 msec is introduced. The first QRS complex in response to S_2 occurs following a short (95 msec) A-H interval due to anterograde conduction over the fast AV nodal pathway. The first QRS complex is labeled number 1 (in lead V_1). The second QRS complex in response to the S_2 stimulus (labeled number 2) follows a long A-H interval (430 msec) due to anterograde conduction over the slow AV nodal pathway.**

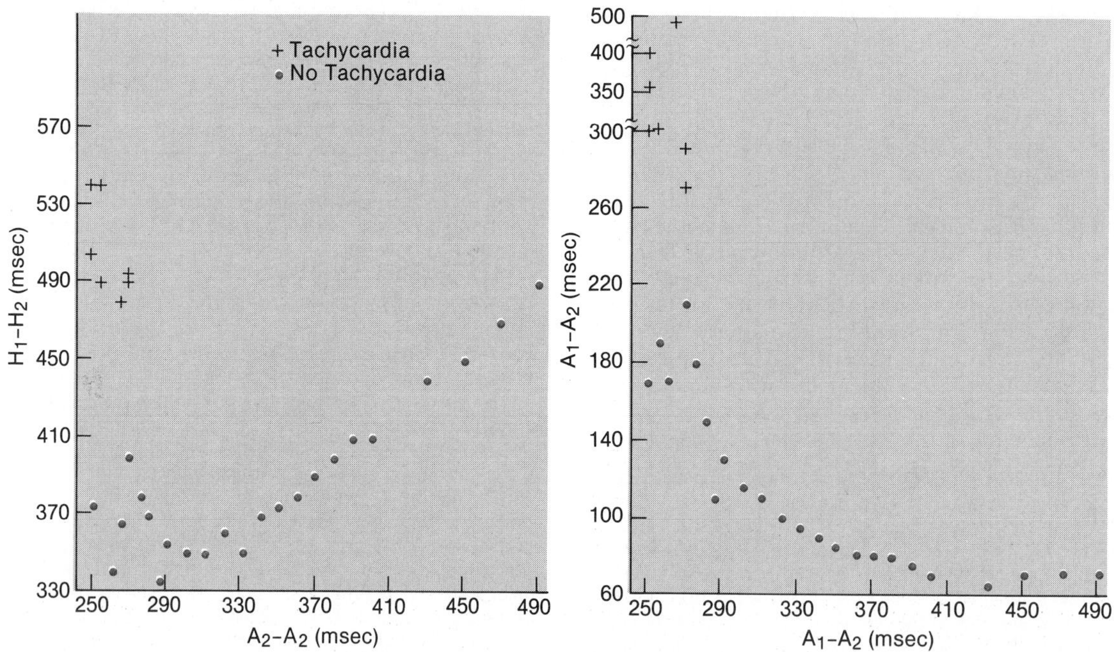

FIGURE 24-20. H_1-H_2 intervals *(left)* and A_2-H_2 intervals *(right)* at various A_1-A_2 intervals. Discontinuous AV nodal curve. At a critical A_1-A_2 interval the H_1-H_2 interval and the A_2-H_2 intervals increase markedly. At the break in the curves, AV nodal reentrant tachycardia is initiated.

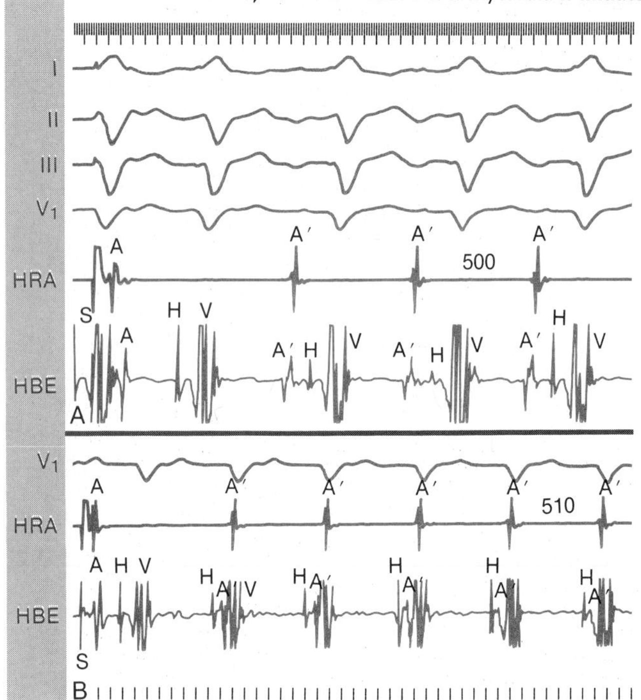

FIGURE 24-21. Unusual and usual forms of AV nodal reentry in the same patient. Panel A, Following the last atrial stimulus (S) of a train of rapid atrial pacing at an increasing rate, a supraventricular tachycardia occurs at a cycle length of 500 msec. The P-R interval is short and the R-P interval is long (see Table 24-2). The retrograde atrial activation sequence is recorded first in the low right atrium (A',HBE lead) and then in the high right atrium (A',HRA). Ventricular stimulation when the His bundle was refractory during the tachycardia did not preexcite the atrium (see Fig. 24-22). In panel B following the cessation of atrial pacing (S), a supraventricular tachycardia of identical QRS morphology (only V_1 is demonstrated) is initiated at a cycle length of 510 msec. Note, however, that the R-P interval is zero with a long P-R interval. The retrograde atrial activation occurs at the onset of the QRS complex and is recorded first in the low right atrium (A',HBE) and then in the high right atrium (A',HRA). Thus, panel A most likely represents anterograde conduction down the fast AV nodal pathway and retrograde conduction up the slow AV nodal pathway, while panel B represents anterograde conduction down the slow AV nodal pathway and retrograde conduction up the fast AV nodal pathway. Note also that the atrial activation sequence and PR-RP relationships in panel A are similar to that shown in Figure 24-29.

conducts with delay over the slow pathway, with sudden prolongation of the A_2-H_2 (or H_1-H_2) interval. Generally, the A-H interval increases at least 50 msec with only a 10 to 20 msec decrease in the coupling interval of the premature atrial complex. Less commonly, dual pathways may be manifested by different P-R or A-H intervals during sinus rhythm or at identical paced rates or by a sudden jump in the A-H interval during atrial pacing at a constant cycle length. Two QRS complexes in response to one P wave provide additional evidence (Fig. 24-19*B*). Some patients with AV nodal reentry may not have discontinuous refractory period curves, and some patients who do not have AV nodal reentry can exhibit discontinuous refractory curves. In the latter patients, dual AV nodal pathways can be a benign finding. Many of these patients also exhibit discontinuous curves retrogradely. Similar mechanisms of tachycardia can occur in children. Triple AV nodal pathways can be demonstrated in occasional patients. Virtually irrefutable proof of dual AV nodal pathways is the simultaneous propagation in opposite directions of two AV nodal wavefronts without collision (Fig. 22-26) or the production of two QRS complexes from one P wave (Fig. 24-19*B*) or two P waves from one QRS complex.

In fewer than 5 to 10 per cent of patients with AV nodal reentry, anterograde conduction proceeds over the fast pathway and retrograde conduction over the slow pathway (termed the unusual form of AV nodal reentry), causing atrial activation to begin *after* the QRS complex and producing a long V-A interval and a relatively short A-V interval (generally A-V/V-A $<$ 0.75, Figs. 24-9*B* and 24-21*A*). Finally, it is possible to have tachycardias that use either the anterograde slow or fast pathways and a retrograde concealed accessory pathway (see below).

Certainly the ventricles and possibly the atria (Fig. 22-28) are not needed to maintain AV nodal reentry in man, and spontaneous AV block has been noted on occasion, particularly at the onset of the arrhythmia. Such block can take place in the AV node distal to the reentry circuit, between the AV node and bundle of His, within the bundle of His, or distal to it (see Fig. 22-27). Rarely the block can be located between the reentry circuit in the AV node and the atrium. Most commonly when block appears, it is below the bundle of His. Termination of the tachycardia generally results from block in the anterogradely conducting slow pathway ("weak link"), so that a retrograde atrial response is not followed by a His or ventricular response.

Retrograde Atrial Activation. The sequence of retrograde atrial activation is normal during AV nodal reentrant supraventricular tachycardia. This means that the earliest site of atrial activation during retrograde conduction over the fast pathway is recorded in the His bundle electrogram followed by electrograms recorded from the os of the coronary sinus and then spreading to depolarize the rest of the right and left atria. During retrograde conduction over the slow pathway in the atypical type of AV nodal reentry, atrial activation recorded in the proximal coronary sinus can precede atrial activation recorded in the low right atrium, suggesting that the slow and fast pathways can enter the atria at slightly different positions. Mapping at the time of surgery confirms that conclusion.[131] Functional bundle branch block during AV nodal reentrant tachycardia does not modify the tachycardia significantly.

CLINICAL FEATURES. AV nodal reentry commonly occurs in patients who have no structural heart disease. Symptoms frequently accompany the tachycardia and range from feelings of palpitations, nervousness, and anxiety to angina, heart failure, syncope, or shock, depending on the duration and rate of the tachycardia and the presence of structural heart disease. Tachycardia can cause syncope because of the rapid ventricular rate, reduced cardiac output, and cerebral circulation, or because of asystole when the tachycardia terminates, owing to tachycardia-induced depression of sinus node automaticity. The prognosis for patients without heart disease is usually good. Recurrences occur according to common probability models like a Poisson process.[132]

Hemodynamic consequences of supraventricular tachyarrhythmias in patients with normal ventricular function are due primarily to a marked decrease in left ventricular end-diastolic and stroke volumes with an increase in ejection rate and cardiac output without a significant change in ejection fraction as heart rate is increased and the atrial contribution to ventricular filling is lost. Heart disease or tachycardia can reduce the ejection fraction. Initial hypotension during tachycardia can evoke a sympathetic response that increases blood pressure and in turn causes a rise in vagal tone that can terminate the tachycardia.

MANAGEMENT

The Acute Attack. This depends on the underlying heart disease, how well the tachycardia is tolerated, and the natural history of previous attacks in the individual patient. For some patients, rest, reassurance, and sedation may be all that are required to abort an attack. Vagal maneuvers, including carotid sinus massage, Valsalva and Mueller maneuvers, gagging, and occasionally exposure of the face to ice water serve as the first line of therapy. These maneuvers may slightly slow the tachycardia rate, which then may speed up to the original rate following cessation of the attempt, or may terminate it. Vagal maneuvers should be tried *again* after each pharmacological approach. Digitalis, calcium antagonists, beta-adrenoreceptor blockers, and adenosine normally depress conduction in the anterogradely conducting slow AV nodal pathway, while class IA and IC drugs depress conduction in the retrogradely conducting fast pathway.[129]

Adenosine, 6 to 12 mg given rapidly IV, is the initial drug of choice.[73,133-135] *Verapamil* (see p. 706), 5 to 10 mg IV, or diltiazem,[136] 0.25 to 0.35 mg/kg IV, terminates AV nodal reentry successfully in about 2 minutes in about 90 per cent of instances and is given when simple vagal maneuvers and adenosine fail.

Cholinergic drugs, such as *edrophonium chloride* (Tensilon), a short-acting cholinesterase inhibitor, can terminate AV nodal reentry when administered initially at a trial dose of 3 to 5 mg IV. If unsuccessful, a dose of 10 mg IV may be given. Edrophonium is infrequently needed. Similarly, *intravenous digitalis* administration is usually not necessary to terminate AV nodal reentry. If digitalis is used, one of the following short-acting preparations is recommended: ouabain, 0.25 to 0.5 mg IV, followed by 0.1 mg every 30 to 60 minutes, if needed, keeping the total dose less than 1.0 mg within a 24-hour period or 0.01 mg/kg as a single dose over 10 to 15 minutes; digoxin, 0.5 to 1.0 mg IV given over 10 to 15 min, followed by 0.25 mg every 2 to 4 hours, with a total dose less than 1.5 mg within any 24-hour period; or deslanoside, 0.8 mg IV, followed by 0.4 mg every 2 to 4 hours, restricting the total dose to less than 2.0 mg within a 24-hour period. *Oral digitalis* administration to terminate an acute attack is generally not indicated. Vagal maneuvers that were previously ineffective can terminate the tachycardia following digitalis administration and therefore should be repeated.

Propranolol given intravenously can be tried if digitalis administration is unsuccessful. Recommended IV dosing is best achieved by titrating the dose to the clinical effect, begun with doses of 0.25 to 0.5 mg, increasing to 1.0 mg if necessary, and administering doses every 5 minutes until either a desired effect or toxicity is produced or a total of 0.15 to 0.2 mg/kg is given. Propranolol must be used cautiously, if at all, in patients with heart failure, chronic lung disease, or a history of asthma because its beta-adrenoceptor blocking action depresses myocardial contractility and may produce bronchospasm. If a beta-adrenoreceptor antagonist is selected, esmolol (50 to 200 mcg/kg/min) would seem preferable because of its shorter duration of action.[74]

DC Cardioversion. Before digitalis or propranolol is administered, it is advisable to reassess the clinical status of the patient and consider whether DC cardioversion may be advisable. DC shock administered to patients who have received excessive amounts of digitalis can be dangerous and can result in serious post-shock ventricular arrhythmias (p. 652). Particularly if signs or symptoms of cardiac decompensation occur, DC electrical shock should be considered early. DC shock, synchronized to the QRS complex to avoid precipitating ventricular fibrillation, successfully terminates AV nodal reentry with energies in the range of 10 to 50 watt-seconds; higher energies may be required in some instances (p. 654).

In the event that digitalis has been given in large doses and DC shock is contraindicated, *atrial* or *ventricular pacing* may restore sinus rhythm.[137] In some instances, esophageal pacing may be useful (p. 727).

Class IA and IC drugs are usually not required to terminate AV nodal reentry. Unless contraindicated, DC cardioversion generally should be employed before using these agents, which are more often administered to prevent recurrences.

Pressor drugs can terminate AV nodal reentry by inducing reflex vagal stimulation mediated by baroreceptors in the carotid sinus and aorta when the systolic blood pressure is acutely elevated to levels of about 180 mm Hg. One of the following drugs, diluted in 5 to 10 ml of 5 per cent dextrose and water, may be given over 1 to 3 minutes: phenylephrine (Neo-Synephrine), 0.5 to 1.0 mg; methoxamine (Vasoxyl), 3 to 5 mg; or metaraminol (Aramine), 0.5 to 2.0 mg. Pressor drugs should be used cautiously or not at all in the elderly and in patients who have structural heart disease, significant hypertension, hyperthyroidism, or acute myocardial infarction. This potentially dangerous and almost always uncomfortable mode of therapy is rarely needed unless the patient is also hypotensive.

Prevention of Recurrences. This is often more difficult than terminating the acute episode. Initially, one must decide whether the frequency and severity of the attacks warrant long-term drug prophylaxis. If the attacks of paroxysmal tachycardia are infrequent, well tolerated, short lasting, and either terminate spontaneously or are easily terminated by the patient, no prophylactic therapy may be necessary. If the attacks are sufficiently frequent and/or long lasting to necessitate therapy, the patient can be treated with drugs empirically or on the basis of serial electrophysiological testing. Because drug responses are variable, serial electrophysiological testing of responses to multiple drugs appears reasonable in some patients with poorly tolerated tachycardias that recur only sporadically (p. 617).

If empirical testing is desirable, digitalis or a long-acting calcium antagonist or beta-adrenoreceptor blocker is a reasonable initial choice. The clinical situation and potential contraindications, e.g., beta blockers in an asthmatic, usually dictate the selection. If digitalis is used, rapid oral digitalization can be accomplished in 24 to 36 hours with digoxin at an initial dose of 1.0 to 1.5 mg, followed by 0.25 to 0.5 mg every 6 hours for a total dose of 2.0 to 3.0 mg. A less rapid oral regimen digitalizes in 2 to 3 days with an initial dose of 0.75 to 1.0 mg, followed by 0.25 to 0.50 mg every 12 hours for a total dose of 2.0 to 3.0 mg. Alternatively, digoxin administered as a maintenance dose of 0.125 to 0.500 mg achieves digitalization in about one week. Digitoxin, which has a longer duration of action, can be used instead of digoxin. Oral digitalization with digitoxin can be accomplished in 24 to 36 hours with an initial dose of 0.5 to 0.8 mg, followed by 0.2 mg every 6 to 8 hours until a total dose of 1.2 mg is reached. A slower approach involves administering 0.2 mg three times daily for 2 to 3 days. Complete digitalization can also be accomplished in about one month by simply giving a daily maintenance dose of 0.05 to 0.20 mg.

Sustained-release verapamil in the range of 240 mg per day, long-acting diltiazem 60 to 120 mg twice daily, or long-acting propranolol in doses of 80 to 120 mg per day can be tried. If these drugs are ineffective taken singly, combinations can be tested. Drugs such as flecainide,[138,139,139a] propafenone,[140] and encainide[141] also can be effective. Because of the successful nonpharmacological therapies available, extensive drug and combination trials usually are not necessary. Therefore, in some patients, pacemaker implantation provides acceptable treatment[137] (Chap. 23). Competitive atrial pacing promptly terminates AV nodal reentry, restoring sinus rhythm immediately or sometimes after a transient episode of atrial flutter or atrial fibrillation, and avoids the necessity of daily drug administration with potential side effects. However, the availability of effective and safe surgical[142] and catheter ablation techniques[143] makes antitachycardia pacing and complex drug regimens poor choices for patients with hard-to-control recurrent tachycardia. It is preferable to *cure* the patient of the tachycardia rather than to use potentially toxic drugs to suppress it or to implant a device that only terminates the tachycardia after its onset (Chap. 23).

REENTRY OVER A RETROGRADELY CONDUCTING (CONCEALED) ACCESSORY PATHWAY

ELECTROCARDIOGRAPHIC RECOGNITION (Fig. 24-22). The presence of an accessory pathway that conducts unidirectionally from the ventricle to the atrium but not in the reverse direction is not apparent by analysis of the scalar ECG during sinus rhythm because the ventricle is not preexcited. Therefore, the ECG manifestations of the Wolff-Parkinson-White (WPW) syndrome are absent and the accessory pathway is said to be "concealed." Since the mechanism responsible for most tachycardias in patients who have the WPW syndrome is macro-reentry caused by anterograde conduction over the AV node-His bundle pathway and retrograde conduction over an accessory pathway, the latter, even if it only conducts retrogradely, can still participate in the reentrant circuit to cause an *AV reciprocating tachycardia*. Electrocardiographically, a tachycardia due to this mechanism may be *suspected* when the QRS complex is normal and the retrograde P wave occurs *after* completion of the QRS complex, in the ST segment or early T wave (Fig. 24-9C and Table 24-2).[144]

MECHANISMS. The cause of unidirectional propagation is not clear and may relate to multiple factors.[145] During sinus rhythm, the atrial impulse probably enters the accessory pathway but blocks near the ventricular insertion site with both right- and left-sided concealed accessory pathways. During functional block in patients with anterograde conduction over accessory pathways, block occurs near the ventricular insertion site most commonly with left-sided pathways, but more often near the atrial insertion site with right-sided accessory pathways.[145]

The P wave follows the QRS complex during tachycardia because the ventricle must be activated before the propagating impulse can enter the accessory pathway and excite the atria retrogradely. Therefore, the retrograde P wave must occur after ventricular excitation, in contrast to AV nodal reentry, in which the atria can be excited during ventricular activation (Fig. 24-9*A*). Also, the contour of the retrograde P wave may differ from the usual retrograde P wave, since the atria may be activated eccentrically, i.e., in a manner other than the normal retrograde activation sequence, which starts at the low right atrial septum as in AV nodal reentry. This occurs because the concealed accessory pathway in most instances is left-sided, i.e., inserts into the left atrium, making the left atrium the first site of retrograde atrial activation and causing the retrograde P wave to be negative in lead I (Fig. 24-22). Finally, since the tachycardia circuit involves the ventricles, if functional bundle branch block occurs in the same ventricle in which the accessory pathway is located, the cycle length of the tachycardia can become longer. This important change ensues because the bundle branch block lengthens the reentrant circuit (see Preexcitation Syndrome). For example, the normal activation sequence for a reciprocating tachycardia circuit with a left-sided accessory pathway without functional bundle branch block progresses from atrium → AV node-His bundle → right and left ventricles → accessory pathway → atrium. However, during functional left bundle branch block as an example, the tachycardia circuit travels from atrium → AV node-His bundle → right ventricle → septum → left ventricle → accessory pathway → atrium. This response provides definitive proof that the ventricle and accessory pathway are part of the reentry circuit.

The additional time required for the impulse to travel across the septum from the right to the left ventricle before reaching the accessory pathway

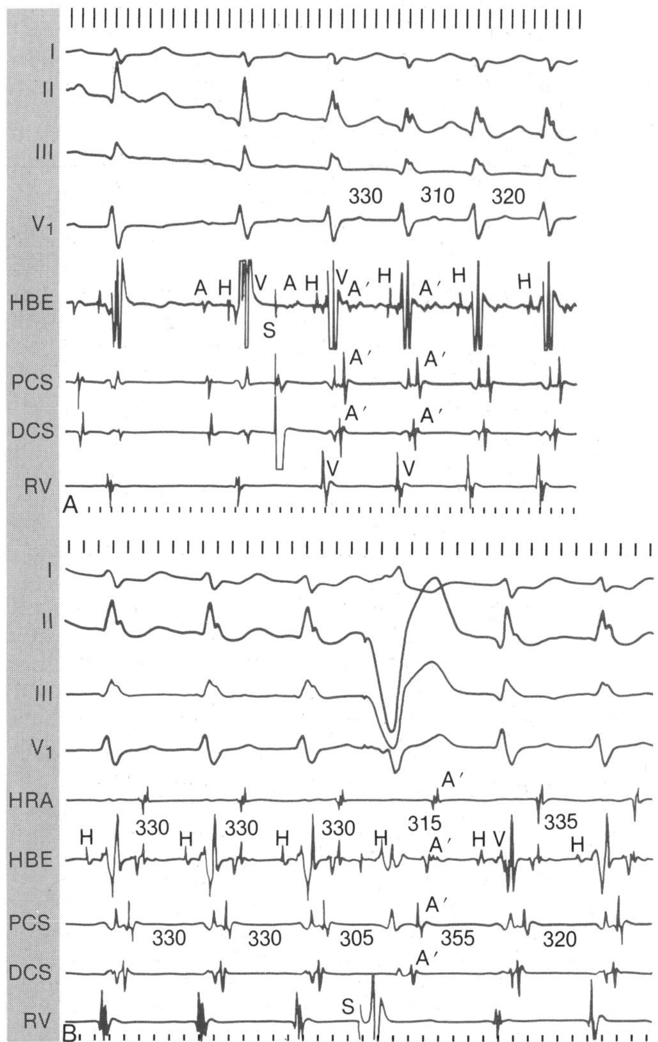

FIGURE 24-22. Atrial preexcitation during atrioventricular reciprocating tachycardia (AVRT) in a patient with a concealed accessory pathway. No evidence of an accessory pathway conduction is present in the two sinus-initiated beats shown in panel A. A premature stimulus in the coronary sinus (S) precipitates a supraventricular tachycardia at a cycle length of approximately 330 msec. The retrograde atrial activation sequence begins first in the distal coronary sinus (A',DCS), followed by activation recorded in the proximal coronary sinus (PCS), low right atrium (HBE), and then high right atrium (not shown). The QRS complex is normal and identical to the sinus-initiated QRS complex. (The terminal portion is slightly deformed by the superimposition of the retrograde atrial recording.) Note that the R-P interval is short and the P-R interval is long (see Table 24-2). The shortest V-A interval exceeds 65 msec, consistent with conduction over a retrogradely conducting atrioventricular pathway.

In panel B, premature ventricular stimulation at a time when the His bundle is still refractory from anterograde activation during tachycardia shortens the A-A interval from 330 to 305 msec without a change in the retrograde atrial activation sequence. (Note that no change occurs in the H-H interval when the right ventricular stimulus, S, is delivered. H-H intervals are in msec in HBE lead.) Thus the ventricular stimulus, despite His bundle refractoriness, still reaches the atrium and produces an identical retrograde atrial activation sequence. The only way this can be explained is via conduction over a retrogradely conducting accessory pathway. Therefore, the patient has a concealed accessory pathway with the Wolff-Parkinson-White syndrome.

and atrium lengthens the V-A interval, which lengthens the cycle length of the tachycardia by an equal amount, assuming no other changes in conduction times occur within the circuit. Thus, lengthening of the tachycardia cycle length by more than 35 msec during ipsilateral functional bundle branch block is diagnostic of a free wall accessory pathway if the lengthening can be shown to be due to V-A prolongation only and not to prolongation of the H-V interval (which can develop with the appearance of bundle branch block). In an occasional patient, the increase in cycle length due to prolongation of VA conduction may be nullified by a simultaneous decrease in the P-R (A-H) interval.

Septal Accessoory Pathway. An exception to these observations occurs in the patient with a concealed septal accessory pathway (see Preexcitation Syndrome, p. 693), in whom retrograde atrial activation is normal and the V-A interval and the cycle length of the tachycardia increase 25 msec or less with the development of ipsilateral functional bundle branch block. Functional bundle branch block in the ventricle contralateral to the accessory pathway does not lengthen the tachycardia cycle if the H-V interval does not lengthen. Functional bundle branch block, particularly functional left bundle branch block, during tachycardia occurs much more commonly in patients who have an accessory pathway than in those with AV nodal reentry, possibly because in the latter, slow pathway anterograde conduction allows for longer recovery time of the His-Purkinje system, while in tachycardias associated with accessory pathways, anterograde conduction over the AV node may be more rapid. Functional left bundle branch block may occur more commonly during rapid tachycardias, perhaps because the refractory period of the right bundle branch appears to be shorter than that of the left bundle branch at short cycle lengths. Premature right ventricular stimulation that starts an AV reciprocating tachycardia is more likely to induce functional left bundle branch block than is premature atrial stimulation.

Vagal maneuvers, by acting predominantly on the AV node, produce a response similar to AV nodal reentry, and the tachycardia can transiently slow and sometimes terminate. Generally, termination occurs in the anterograde direction, so that the last retrograde P wave fails to conduct to the ventricle.

ELECTROPHYSIOLOGICAL FEATURES. Electrophysiological criteria supporting the diagnosis of tachycardia involving reentry over a concealed accessory pathway include the fact that initiation of tachycardia depends on a critical degree of atrioventricular delay (necessary to allow time for the accessory pathway to recover excitability), but the delay can be in the AV node or His-Purkinje system, i.e., a critical degree of A-H delay is not necessary. Occasionally, a tachycardia can start with little or no measurable lengthening of AV nodal or His-Purkinje conduction time. The AV nodal refractory period curve is smooth, in contrast to the discontinuous curve found in many patients with AV nodal reentry. Dual AV nodal pathways occasionally can be noted as a concomitant but unrelated finding.

Diagnosis of Accessory Pathways. This can be accomplished by demonstrating that during ventricular pacing, premature ventricular stimulation activates the atria before retrograde depolarization of the His bundle, indicating that the impulse reached the atria before it depolarized the His bundle and must have traveled a different pathway to do so. Also, if the ventricles can be stimulated prematurely during tachycardia at a time when the His bundle is refractory, and the impulse still conducts to the atrium, this indicates that retrograde propagation traveled to the atrium over a pathway other than the bundle of His (Fig. 24–22*B*). If the premature ventricular complex depolarizes the atria without lengthening of the V-A interval and with the same retrograde atrial activation sequence, one assumes that the stimulation site (i.e., ventricle) is within the reentrant circuit without intervening His-Purkinje or AV nodal tissue that might increase the V-A interval and therefore the A-A interval. In addition, if a premature ventricular complex delivered at a time when the His bundle is refractory terminates the tachycardia without activating the atria retrogradely, an accessory pathway is most likely present.

The V-A interval (conduction over the accessory pathway) generally is constant over a wide range of ventricular paced rates and coupling intervals of premature ventricular complexes as well as during the tachycardia in the absence of aberration. Similar short V-A intervals can be observed in patients during AV nodal reentry, but if the VA conduction time or R-P interval is the same during tachycardia *and* ventricular pacing at comparable rates, an accessory pathway is almost certainly present. The V-A interval is usually less than 50 per cent of the R-R interval (Table 24–2). The tachycardia can be easily initiated following premature ventricular stimulation that conducts retrogradely in the accessory pathway but blocks in the AV node or His bundle. Atria and ventricles are required components of the macro-reentrant circuit, and therefore continuation of the tachycardia in the presence of AV or VA block excludes an accessory atrioventricular pathway as part of the reentrant circuit.

CLINICAL FEATURES. The presence of concealed accessory pathways is estimated to account for about 30 per cent of patients with apparent supraventricular tachycardia referred for electrophysiological evaluation. The great majority of these accessory pathways are located between left ventricle and left atrium and in the posteroseptal area, less commonly between right ventricle and right atrium. It is important to be aware of a concealed accessory pathway as a possible cause for apparently "routine" supraventricular tachycardia, since the therapeutic response at times may not follow the usual guidelines. Antiarrhythmic targeting may need to be directed toward drugs that affect the accessory pathway such as drugs in classes 1A and 1C, or amiodarone (Chap. 23). Also, surgical interruption or catheter ablation of the accessory pathway can be accomplished (p. 656). The tachycardia rates tend to be somewhat faster than those occurring in AV nodal reentry (≥200 beats/min), but a great deal of overlap exists between the two groups.

Paroxysmal supraventricular tachycardia can be followed by polyuria after termination due to atrial dilatation and release of antinatriuretic factor.[147] Syncope can occur because the rapid ventricular rate fails to provide adequate cerebral circulation or because the tachyarrhythmia depresses the sinus pacemaker, causing a period of asystole when the tachyarrhythmia terminates. Physical examination reveals an unvarying, regular ventricular rhythm with constant intensity of the first heart sound. The jugular venous pressure may be elevated, but the waveform generally remains constant.

MANAGEMENT. The therapeutic approach to terminate this form of tachycardia acutely is as outlined for AV nodal reentry (see p. 688). It is necessary to achieve block of a single impulse from atrium to ventricle or ventricle to atrium. Generally, the most successful method is to produce transient AV nodal block; therefore vagal maneuvers, IV adenosine, verapamil or diltiazem, digitalis, and beta blockers are acceptable choices. Conventional antiarrhythmic agents that prolong activation time or refractory period in the accessory pathway need to be considered for chronic prophylactic therapy, similar to that discussed for reciprocating tachycardias associated with the preexcitation syndrome. The presence of atrial fibrillation in patients with a *concealed accessory pathway* should not present a greater therapeutic challenge than it does in patients who do not have such a pathway, because anterograde AV conduction occurs over the AV node. Verapamil and digitalis are not contraindicated. However, it must be remembered that under some circumstances, such as catecholamine stimulation, anterograde conduction in the apparently concealed accessory pathway can occur.

PREEXCITATION SYNDROME

ELECTROCARDIOGRAPHIC RECOGNITION (Fig. 24–23). Preexcitation syndrome occurs when the atrial impulse activates the whole or some part of the ventricle, or the ventricular impulse activates the whole or some part of the atrium, earlier than would be expected if the impulse traveled by way of the normal specialized conduction system only. In the Wolff-Parkinson-White syndrome, muscular connections composed of working myocardial fibers exist outside the specialized conducting tissue, and connect atrium and ventricle. They are named *accessory atrioventricular pathways* or connections, commonly called *Kent bundles*, and are responsible for the most common variety of preexcitation (incidentally noted in other species such as monkeys, dogs, and cats). Three basic features typify the ECG abnormalities of patients with the usual form of WPW syndrome caused by an AV connection: (1) P-R interval less than 120 msec during sinus rhythm; (2) QRS complex duration exceeding 120 msec with a slurred, slowly rising onset of the QRS in some leads (delta wave) and usually a normal terminal QRS portion; and (3) secondary ST-T wave changes that are generally directed opposite to the major delta and QRS vectors.[148]

The term *Wolff-Parkinson-White* (WPW) *syndrome* is applied when the patient has symptoms, generally due to tachyarrhythmias. The most common tachycardia is characterized by a normal QRS, by ventricular rates of 150 to 250 beats/min

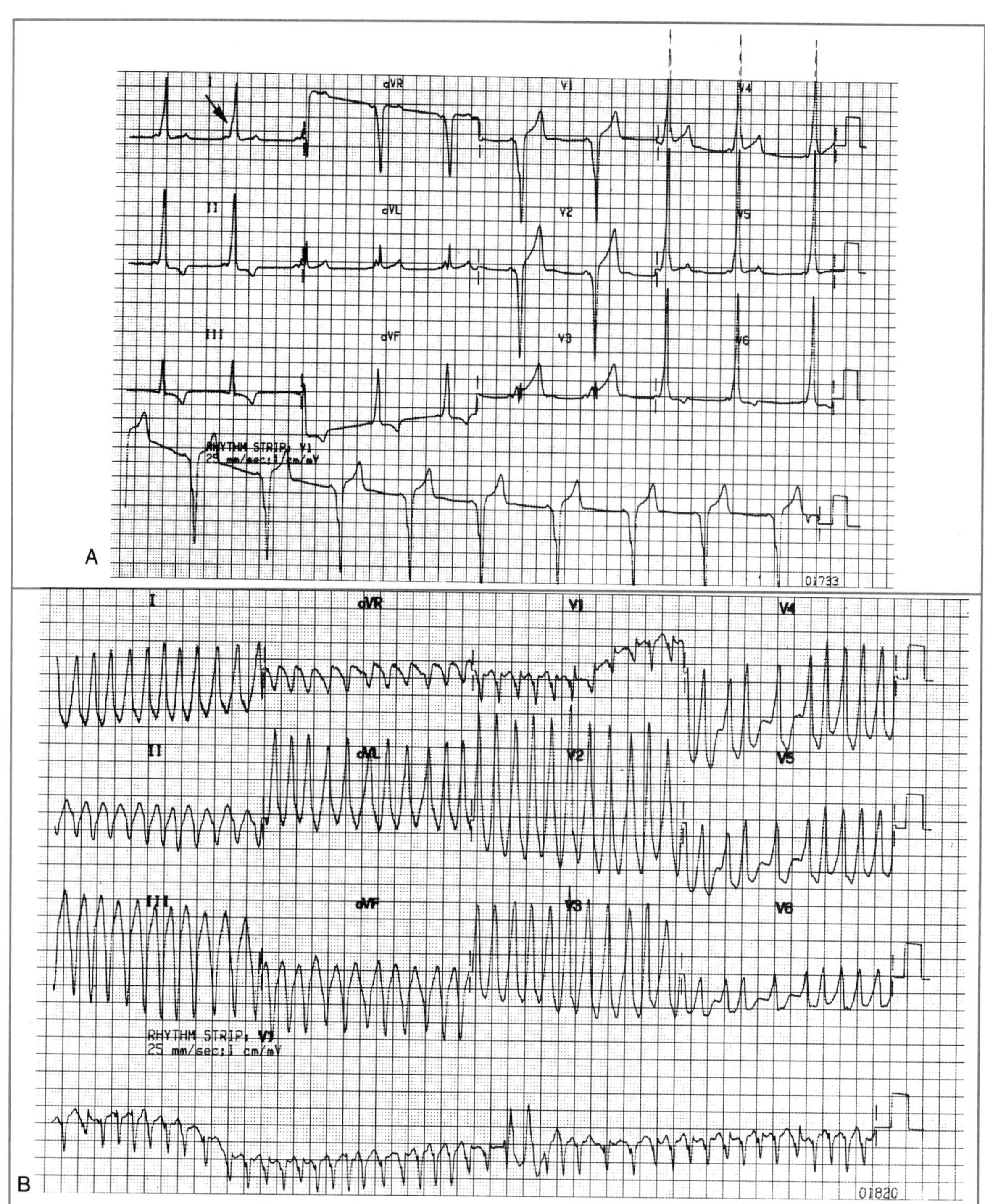

FIGURE 24–23. *A*, Right anteroseptal accessory pathway. The 12-lead ECG characteristically exhibits a normal to inferior axis. The delta wave is negative in V_1 and V_2, upright in leads I, II, AVL, and AVF, isoelectric in lead III, and negative in AVR. Location verified at surgery. Arrow indicates delta wave (lead I).

B, Right posteroseptal accessory pathway. Negative delta waves in leads II, III, and AVF, upright in I and AVL, localize this pathway to the posteroseptal region. The negative delta wave in V_1 with sharp transition to an upright delta wave in V_2 pinpoint it to the right posteroseptal area. Atrial fibrillation is present. Location verified at surgery. Arrow indicates delta wave (V_4).

C, Left lateral accessory pathway. Positive delta wave in the anterior precordial leads and in leads II, III, and AVF, positive or isoelectric in lead I and AVL, and isoelectric or negative in V_5 and V_6 are typical of a left lateral accessory pathway. Rapid coronary sinus pacing (450 msec cycle length) was used to enhance preexcitation (negative P wave I, II, III, aVf, V_{3-6}). Location verified at surgery. Arrow indicates delta wave (V_1).

D, Logic diagram to determine location of accessory pathways. Begin with analysis of V_1 to determine whether the delta wave and the QRS complex are negative or positive. That establishes the ventricle in which the accessory pathway is located. Next, determine whether the delta wave and QRS complex are negative in leads II, III and AVF. If so, then the accessory pathway is located in a posteroseptal position. If the accessory pathway is located in the right ventricle, an inferior axis indicates an anteroseptal location while left axis indicates a right free wall location. If the accessory pathway is located in the left ventricle, an isoelectric or negative delta wave and QRS complex in leads I, aVl, V_5, and V_6 indicate a left lateral (free wall) location.

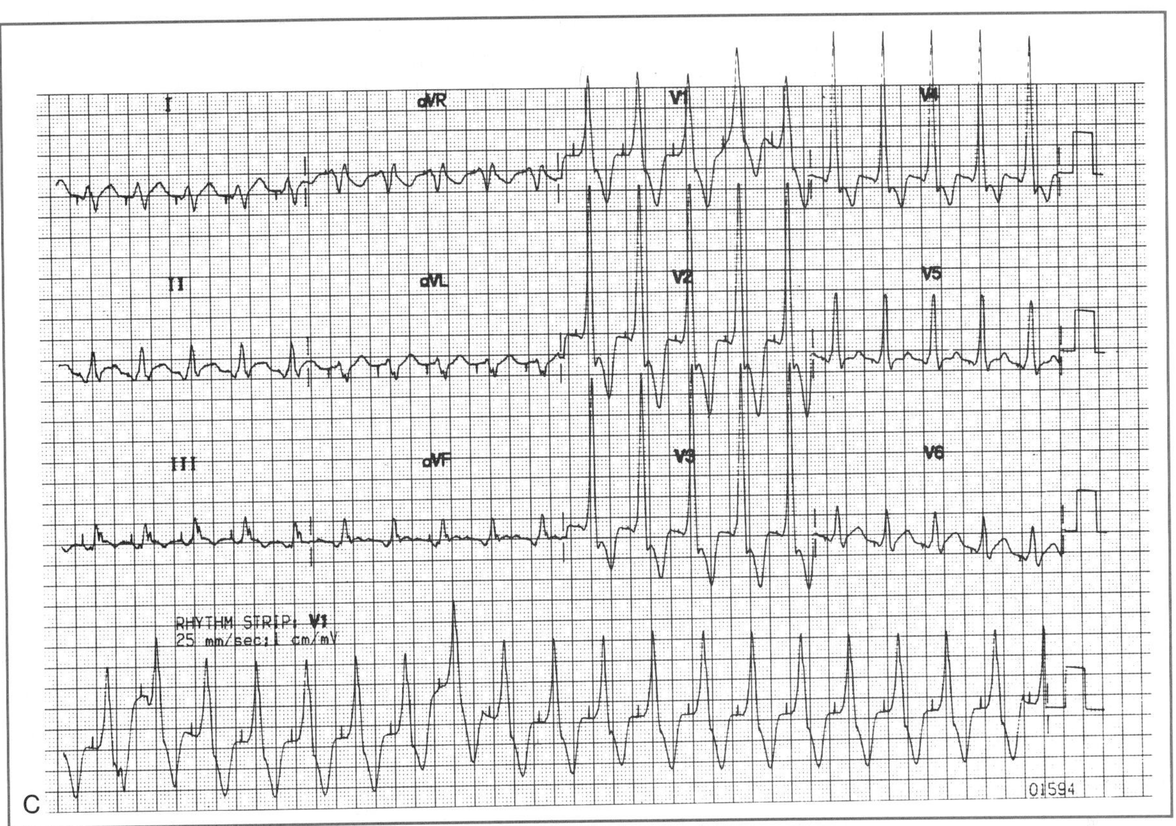

FIGURE 24-23*C*. *See legend on opposite page*

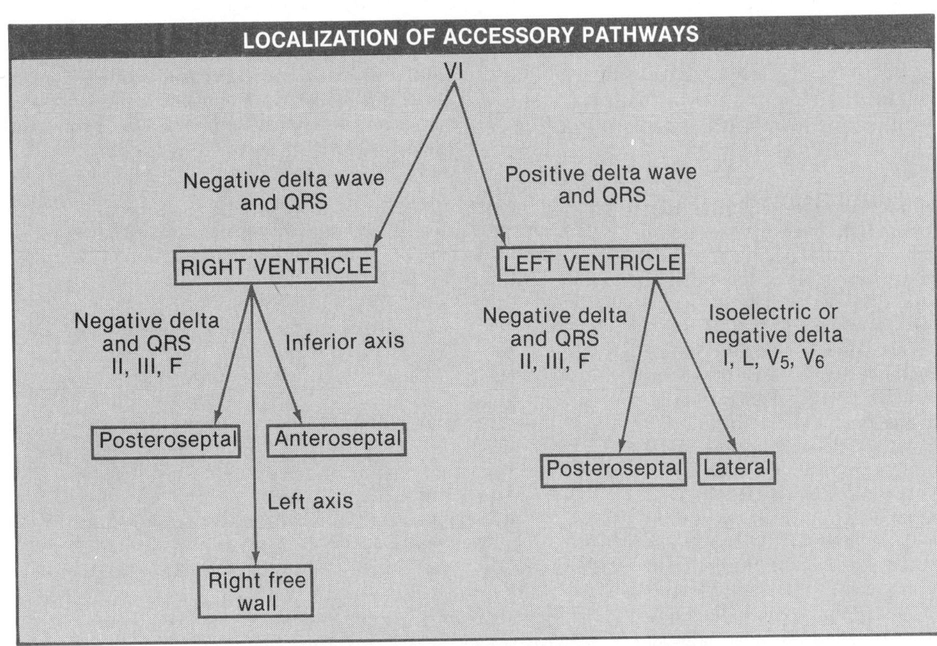

FIGURE 24-23*D*. *See legend on opposite page*

(generally faster than AV nodal reentry), and by sudden onset and termination, behaving in most respects like the tachycardia described for conduction utilizing a concealed pathway (p. 692). The major difference between the two is the capacity for anterograde conduction over the accessory pathway during atrial flutter or atrial fibrillation (see below).

A variety of other anatomical substrates exist that provide the basis for different ECG manifestations of several variations of the preexcitation syndrome (Fig. 24–24). Fibers from atrium to His bundle bypassing the physiological delay of the AV node are called *atriohisian tracts* (Fig. 24–24*B*) and are associated with a short P-R interval and a normal QRS complex. Although demonstrated anatomically (see below), the electrophysiological significance of these tracts in the genesis of tachycardias with a short P-R interval and a normal QRS complex (Lown-Ganong-Levine, or LGL, syndrome) remains to be established. Indeed, evidence does *not* support the presence of a specific LGL syndrome comprising a short P-R interval, normal QRS complex, and tachycardias related to an atriohisian bypass tract. Two varieties of Mahaim fibers include those passing from the AV node to the ventricle, called nodoventricular fibers (or nodofascicular if the insertion is into the right bundle branch rather than ventricular muscle) (Fig. 24–24*C* and *E*), and those arising in the His bundle or bundle branches and inserting in the ventricular myocardium, called fasciculoventricular fibers (Fig. 24–24*D*). For nodoventricular connections, the P-R interval may be normal or short, and the QRS complex is a fusion beat. Recent successful surgical interruption of accessory pathway conduction in patients with apparent nodoventricular or nodofascicular pathways has led to a reappraisal of the anatomy with the suggestion that there are right *atrioventricular* accessory pathways with AV nodal–like conducting properties. Tachycardia proceeds anterogradely over the accessory pathway and retrogradely over the normal pathway, making the atria a necessary part of the circuit. It is possible that other anatomical variants exist.[149–153] Fasciculoventricular connections create a normal P-R interval and a fixed, anomalous QRS complex and do not appear to be important in tachycardia development.

ELECTROPHYSIOLOGICAL FEATURES (Figs. 24–25 to 24–28; see also p. 692). If the Kent bundle accessory pathway is capable of anterograde conduction, two parallel routes of AV conduction are possible, one subject to physiological delay over the AV node and the other passing directly without delay from atrium to ventricle. This produces the typical QRS complex that is a fusion beat, due to depolarization of the ventricle in part by the wavefront traveling over the accessory pathway and in part by the wavefront traveling over the normal AV node–His bundle route. The delta wave represents ventricular activation from input over the accessory pathway. The extent of contribution to ventricular depolarization by the wavefront over each route depends upon their relative activa-

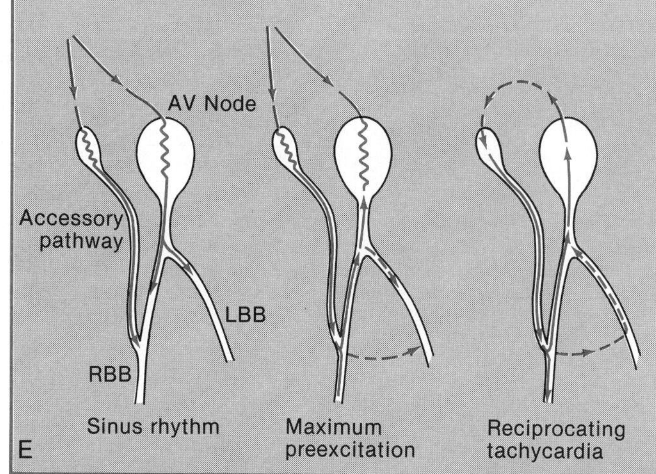

FIGURE 24–24. Schematic representation of accessory pathways. Panel A demonstrates the "usual" atrioventricular accessory pathway giving rise to most clinical presentations of tachycardia associated with Wolff-Parkinson-White syndrome. Panel B illustrates the very uncommon atriohisian accessory pathway. If the LGL syndrome exists, it would have this type of anatomy which has been demonstrated on occasion histopathologically. Panel C, nodoventricular pathways, original concept, in which anterograde conduction travels down the accessory pathway with retrograde conduction in the bundle branch–His bundle–AV node (see below). Panel D demonstrates the fasciculoventricular connections, not thought to play an important role in the genesis of tachycardias. Panel E illustrates the current concept of nodoventricular accessory pathway in which the accessory pathway is an atrioventricular communication with AV nodal–like properties. Sinus rhythm results in a fusion QRS complex, as in the usual form of WPW shown in panel A. Maximum preexcitation results in ventricular activation over the accessory pathway and the His bundle is activated retrogradely. During reciprocating tachycardia, anterograde conduction occurs over the accessory pathway with retrograde conduction over the normal pathway. (Panel E reproduced with permission from Benditt, D. G., and Milstein, S.: Nodoventricular accessory connection: A misnomer or a structural/functional spectrum. J. Cardiovasc. Electrophys. *1*:231, 1990.)

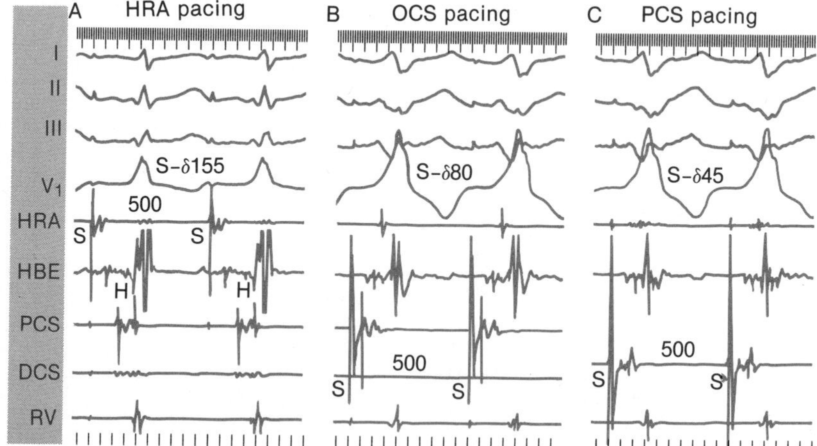

FIGURE 24–25. Atrial pacing at different atrial sites illustrating different conduction over the accessory pathway. In panel A, high right atrial pacing at a cycle length of 500 msec produces anomalous activation of the ventricle (note upright QRS complex in V_1) and a stimulus-delta interval of 155 msec. This indicates that the time from the onset of the stimulus to the beginning of the QRS complex is relatively long because the stimulus is delivered at a fairly large distance from the accessory pathway. Note that the His bundle activation (H) occurs at about the onset of the QRS complex. In panel B atrial pacing occurs through the distal coronary sinus electrode (DCS). At the same pacing cycle length, DCS pacing results in more anomalous ventricular activation and a shorter stimulus-delta interval (80 msec). His bundle activation is now buried within the inscription of the ventricular electrogram in the HBE lead. Panel C, Pacing from the proximal coronary sinus electrode (PCS) results in the shortest stimulus-delta interval (45 msec) indicating that the pacing stimulus is being delivered very close to the atrial insertion of the accessory pathway, which is located in the left posteroseptal region of the atrioventricular groove.

tion times. If AV nodal conduction delay occurs, for example, because of a rapid atrial pacing rate or premature atrial complex, more of the ventricle becomes activated over the accessory pathway, and the QRS complex becomes more anomalous in contour. Total activation of the ventricle over the accessory pathway can occur if the AV nodal delay is sufficiently long. In contrast, if the accessory pathway is relatively far from the sinus node, for example, a left lateral accessory pathway, or if AV nodal conduction time is relatively short, more of the ventricle may be activated by conduction over the normal pathway (Fig. 24–25). The normal fusion beat during sinus rhythm has a short H-V interval, or His bundle activation actually begins after the onset of ventricular depolarization, because part of the atrial impulse bypasses the AV node and activates the ventricle early, at a time when the atrial impulse traveling the normal route just reaches the His bundle. This finding of a short or negative H-V interval occurs *only* during conduction over an accessory pathway or from retrograde His activation during a complex originating in the ventricle, such as a ventricular tachycardia.

Pacing the atrium at rapid rates, at premature intervals, or from a site close to the atrial insertion of the Kent bundle accentuates the anomalous activation of the ventricles and shortens the H-V interval even more (His activation may become buried in the ventricular electrogram, as in Fig. 24–25). The position of the accessory pathway can be determined by a careful analysis of the spatial direction of the delta wave in the 12-lead ECG in maximally preexcited beats[154] (Fig. 24–26).

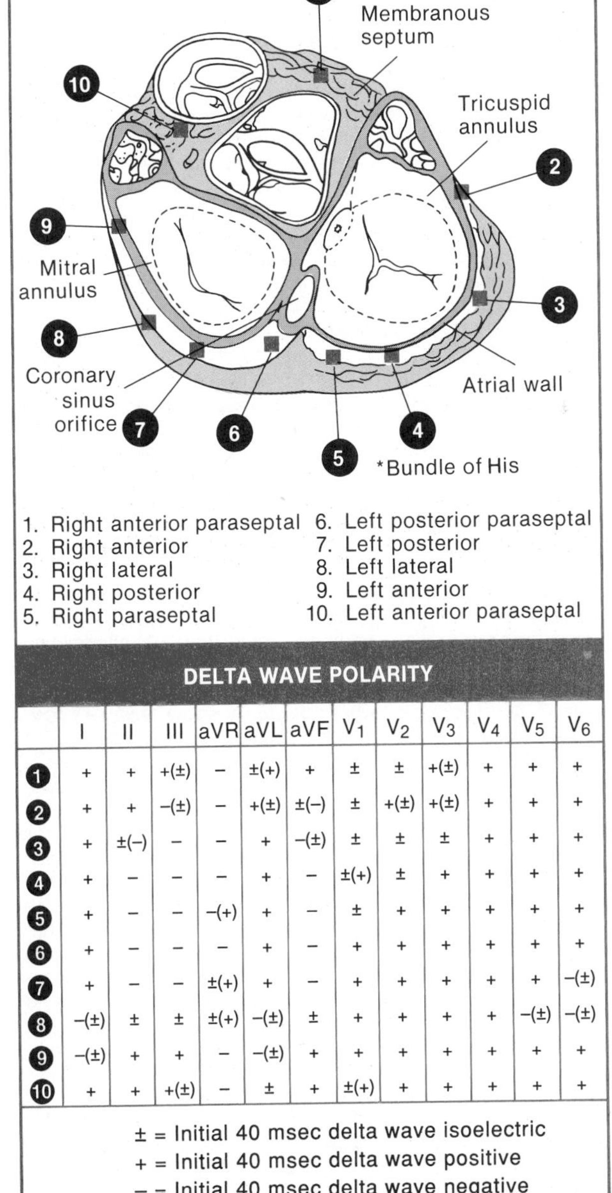

DELTA WAVE POLARITY

	I	II	III	aVR	aVL	aVF	V_1	V_2	V_3	V_4	V_5	V_6
1	+	+	+(±)	–	±(+)	+	±	±	+(±)	+	+	+
2	+	+	–(±)	–	+(±)	±(–)	±	+(±)	+(±)	+	+	+
3	+	±(–)	–	–	+	–(±)	±	±	±	+	+	+
4	+	–	–	–	+	–	±(+)	±	+	+	+	+
5	+	–	–	–(+)	+	–	±	+	+	+	+	+
6	+	–	–	–	+	–	+	+	+	+	+	+
7	+	–	–	±(+)	+	–	+	+	+	+	+	–(±)
8	–(±)	±	±	±(+)	–(±)	±	+	+	+	+	–(±)	–(±)
9	–(±)	+	+	–	–(±)	+	+	+	+	+	+	+
10	+	+	+(±)	–	±	+	±(+)	+	+	+	+	+

± = Initial 40 msec delta wave isoelectric
+ = Initial 40 msec delta wave positive
– = Initial 40 msec delta wave negative

FIGURE 24–26. **In this schematic representation *(top),* sites of the potential position of the accessory pathway are indicated by filled boxes numbered 1 through 10. The delta wave polarity in the 12-lead ECG for each of the 10 sites is depicted in the table at the bottom. (From Gallagher, J. J., et al.: The preexcitation syndromes. Progr. Cardiovasc. Dis. *20:*285, 1978.)**

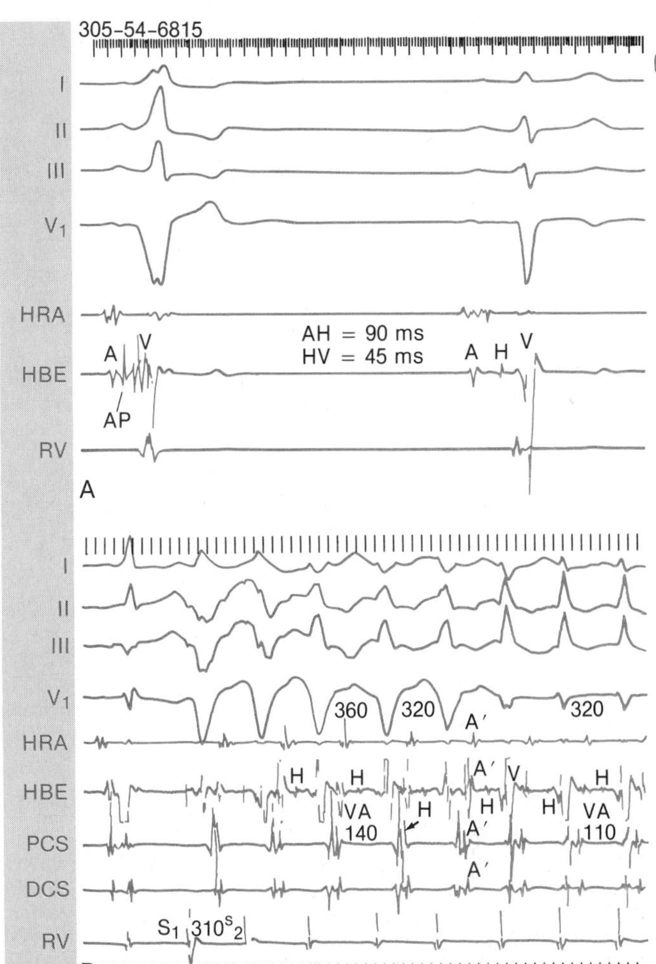

FIGURE 24–27. ***A,* Recording of depolarization of an accessory pathway (AP) with a catheter electrode. The first QRS complex illustrates conduction over the accessory pathway (AP). In the scalar ECG a short P-R interval and delta wave (best seen in leads I and V_1) are apparent. His bundle activation is buried within the ventricular complex. In the following complex, conduction has blocked over the accessory pathway and a normal QRS complex results. His bundle activation clearly precedes the onset of ventricular depolarization by 45 msec. The A-H interval for this complex is 90 msec. (From Prystowsky, E. N., Browne, K. F., and Zipes, D. P.: Intracardiac recording by catheter electrode of accessory pathway depolarization. J. Am. Coll. Cardiol. *1:*468, 1983.)**

***B,* Influence of functional ipsilateral bundle branch block on the V-A interval during an atrioventricular reciprocating tachycardia (AVRT). Partial preexcitation can be noted in the sinus-initiated complex (first complex). Two premature ventricular stimuli (S_1, S_2) initiate a sustained supraventricular tachycardia that persists with a left bundle branch block for several complexes, finally reverting to normal. The retrograde atrial activation sequence is recorded first in the proximal coronary sinus lead (arrow, PCS), then in the distal coronary sinus lead (DCS) and low right atrium (HBE) and then high right atrium (HRA). During the functional bundle branch block, the V-A interval in the PCS lead is 140 msec, shortening to 110 msec when the QRS complex reverts to normal. Such behavior is characteristic of a left-sided accessory pathway with prolongation of the reentrant pathway by the functional left bundle branch block.**

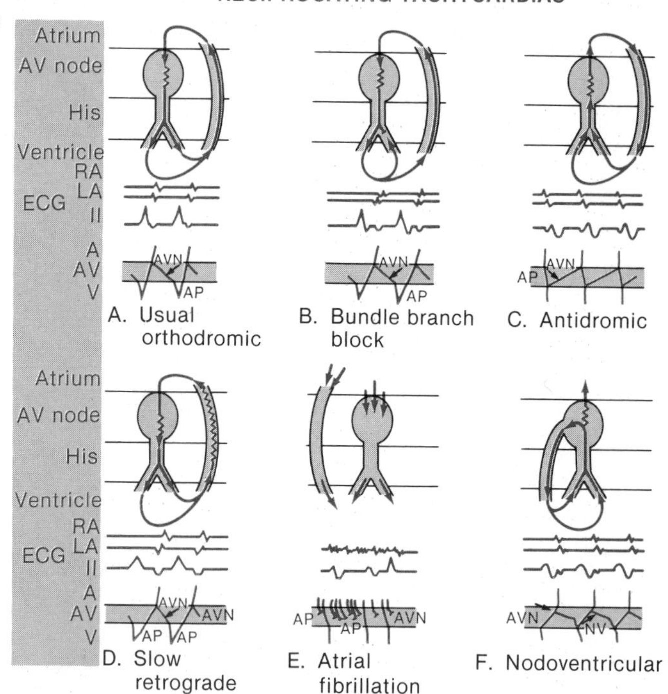

FIGURE 24–28. Schematic diagram of tachycardias associated with accessory pathways. Format as in Figure 24–9. *A*, Orthodromic tachycardia with anterograde conduction over the AV node–His bundle route and retrograde conduction over the accessory pathway (left-sided for this example as depicted by LA activation preceding RA activation). *B*, Orthodromic tachycardia and ipsilateral functional bundle branch block. *C*, Antidromic tachycardia with anterograde conduction over the accessory pathway and retrograde conduction over the AV node–His bundle. *D*, Orthodromic tachycardia with a slowly conducting accessory pathway. *E*, Atrial fibrillation with the accessory pathway as a bystander. *F*, Anterograde conduction over a portion of the AV node and a nodoventricular pathway and retrograde conduction over the AV node.

T-wave abnormalities can occur after disappearance of preexcitation with orientation of the T wave according to the site of preexcitation. A variety of electrical[155,156] (Fig. 24–27), radionuclide, and echocardiographic techniques can be used to localize the insertion site of the accessory pathway (Chap. 23).

ATRIOHISIAN TRACT. In patients who have an atriohisian tract, theoretically the QRS complex would remain normal and the short A-H interval fixed or show very little increase during atrial pacing at more rapid rates. The author has found this response to be uncommon. Rapid atrial pacing in patients who have nodoventricular or nodofascicular connections shortens the H-V interval and widens the QRS complex, producing a left bundle branch block contour, but, in contrast to the situation in patients who have an atrioventricular connection (Fig. 24–25), the A-V interval also lengthens.[157] In patients who have fasciculoventricular connections, the H-V interval remains short and QRS complex unchanged and anomalous during rapid atrial pacing.

KENT BUNDLE CONDUCTION. Even though the Kent bundle conducts more rapidly than does the AV node (conduction velocity is faster in the accessory pathway), the Kent bundle usually has a longer refractory period during long cycle lengths (e.g., sinus rhythm)—i.e., it takes longer for the accessory pathway to recover excitability than it does for the AV node. Consequently, a premature atrial complex[158,159] can occur sufficiently early to block anterogradely in the accessory pathway and conduct to the ventricle only over the normal AV node–His bundle (Fig. 24–28*A*,*B*). The resultant H-V interval and the QRS complex become normal. Such an event can initiate the most common type of reciprocating tachycardia, which is characterized by anterograde conduction over the normal pathway and retrograde conduction over the accessory pathway *(orthodromic AV reciprocating)* (Fig. 24–28). The accessory pathway, blocking in an anterograde direction, recovers excitability in time to be activated following the QRS complex, in a retrograde direction, completing the reentrant loop. Much less commonly, patients can have tachycardias called *antidromic* tachycardias during which anterograde conduction occurs over the accessory pathway and retrograde conduction over the AV node. The resultant QRS complex is abnormal owing to total ventricular activation over the accessory pathway (Fig. 24–28*C*). In both tachycardias the accessory pathway is an obligatory part of the reentrant circuit. In patients with bidirectional conduction over the accessory pathway, different fibers may be used anterogradely and retrogradely.[159a]

Ten to fifteen per cent of patients have multiple accessory pathways often suggested by various ECG clues,[160,160a] and on occasion tachycardia can be due to a reentrant loop conducting anterogradely over one accessory pathway and retrogradely over the other. Interestingly, 15 to 20 per cent of patients may exhibit AV nodal echoes or AV nodal reentry after interruption of the accessory pathway.[161]

PERMANENT FORM OF AV JUNCTIONAL RECIPROCATING TACHYCARDIA (PJRT). An incessant form of supraventricular tachycardia has been recognized that generally occurs with a long R-P interval that exceeds the P-R interval (Fig. 24–29 and Table 24–2).[148,153] A posteroseptal accessory pathway, usually right ventricular, rarely left ventricular, that conducts very slowly, possibly due to a long and tortuous route, appears responsible. Tachycardia is maintained by anterograde AV nodal conduction and retrograde conduction over the accessory pathway (Fig. 24–28*D*). While anterograde conduction over this pathway has been demonstrated, the long anterograde conduction time over the accessory pathway ordinarily may prevent ECG manifestations of accessory pathway conduction during sinus rhythm. Therefore, during sinus rhythm the QRS is prolonged from conduction over this accessory pathway only when conduction times through the AV node–His bundle exceed those in the accessory pathway.

RECOGNITION OF ACCESSORY PATHWAYS. When retrograde atrial activation during tachycardia occurs over an accessory pathway that connects the left atrium to the left ventricle, the earliest retrograde activity is recorded from a left atrial electrode usually positioned in the coronary sinus (Fig. 24–27*B*). When retrograde atrial activation during tachycardia occurs over an accessory pathway that connects the right ventricle to the right atrium, the earliest retrograde atrial activity generally is recorded from a lateral right atrial electrode. Participation of a septal accessory pathway creates earliest retrograde atrial activation in the low right atrium situated near the septum, anterior or posterior, depending on the insertion site. These mapping techniques with catheter electrodes and at the time of surgery (pp. 620 and 656) provide accurate assessments of the position of the accessory pathway, which can be anywhere in the AV groove except in the intervalvular trigone between the mitral valve and the aortic valve annuli (Fig. 24–26). Recording electrical activity directly from the accessory pathway obviously provides precise localization[145,162] (Fig. 24–27*A*).

It may be difficult to distinguish AV nodal reentry from participation of a septal accessory connection using the retrograde sequence of atrial activation because activation sequences during both tachycardias are similar. Other approaches to demonstrate retrograde atrial activation over the accessory pathway must be tried and can be accomplished by inducing premature ventricular complexes during tachycardia to determine whether retrograde atrial preexcitation can occur at a time when the His bundle is refractory (Fig. 24–27*B*). Since ventriculoatrial conduction cannot occur over the normal conduction system because the His bundle is refractory, an accessory pathway must be present for the atria to become preexcited and is most likely participating in the tachycardia circuit. No patient with a reciprocating tachycardia due to an accessory AV pathway has a V-A interval less than 70 msec measured from the onset of ventricular depolarization to the onset of the earliest atrial activity recorded on an esophageal lead or less than 95 msec when measured to the high right atrium. In contrast, in the majority of patients with reentry in the AV node, intervals from the onset of ventricular activity to the earliest onset of atrial activity recorded in the esophageal lead are less than 70 msec.

OTHER FORMS OF TACHYCARDIA IN PATIENTS WITH WPW SYNDROME. Patients can have other types of tachycardia during which the accessory pathway is a "bystander," i.e., uninvolved in the mechanism responsible for the tachycardia, such as AV nodal reentry or an atrial tachycardia that conducts to the ventricle over the accessory pathway. In patients with atrial flutter or atrial fibrillation, the accessory pathway is not a requisite part of the mechanism responsible for tachycardia, and the flutter or fibrillation occurs in the atrium unrelated to the accessory pathway (Fig. 24–28*E*). Propagation to the ventricle during atrial flutter or atrial fibrillation therefore can occur over the normal AV node–His bundle or accessory pathway. Patients with WPW syndrome who have atrial fibrillation almost always have inducible reciprocating tachycardias as well, which can develop into the atrial fibrillation[163] (Fig. 24–30). In fact, interruption of the accessory pathway and elimination of AV reciprocating tachycardia usually prevents recurrence of the atrial fibrillation. In some patients, atrial abnormalities independent of the accessory pathway can be important.[164] Atrial fibrillation presents a potentially serious risk because of the possibility for very rapid conduction over the accessory pathway. At more rapid rates, the refractory period of the accessory pathway can shorten significantly and permit an extremely rapid ventricular response during atrial flutter or atrial fibrillation (Figs. 24–23*B* and 24–30) that can lead to ventricular fibrillation. The rapid ventricular re-

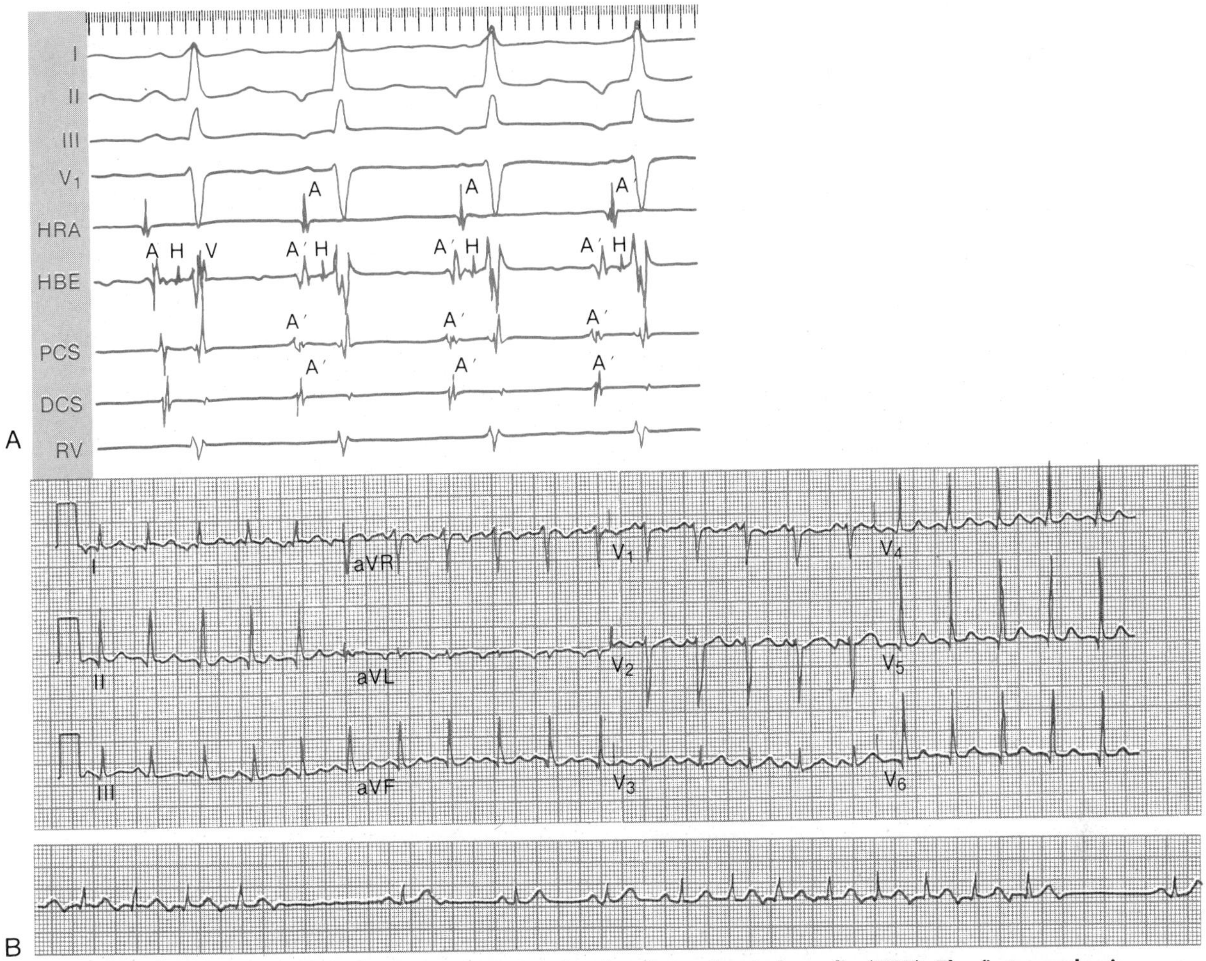

FIGURE 24–29. *A*, Permanent form of AV junctional reciprocating tachycardia (PJRT). The first complex is initiated by sinus discharge, while the morphology of the subsequent P waves changes. The high right atrium probably is still discharged by the sinus node for the second and third P, waves, which represent fusion P waves. The fourth P wave represents full activation of the atrium during the tachycardia. The atrial activation sequence during the tachycardia demonstrates initial activation in the proximal coronary sinus (PCS) followed by recording in the distal coronary sinus (DCS), then low right atrium (HBE), and finally high right atrium (HRA). Premature ventricular stimulation during tachycardia at a time when His bundle was refractory preexcited the atrium retrogradely (during isoproterenol infusion to shorten the refractory period of this slowly conducting accessory pathway), thus proving the existence of an accessory atrioventricular pathway. Note the PR-RP relationship and P-wave contour that resemble Figure 24–21*A*. Not shown, during retrograde conduction over the AV node His bundle axis, retrograde atrial activation was recorded first in the HBE lead.

B, Permanent form of junctional reciprocating tachycardia (PJRT) in a patient with a left-sided accessory pathway. The 12-lead ECG demonstrates a long R-P interval–short PR interval tachycardia, which, in contrast to the usual form of PJRT, exhibits negative P waves in leads I and aVL. The rhythm strips below (lead I) indicate that whenever a nonconducted P wave occurs, the tachycardia always terminates, only to begin again after several sinus beats. This is in marked contrast to Figure 24–13, in which the tachycardia continues despite nonconducted P waves.

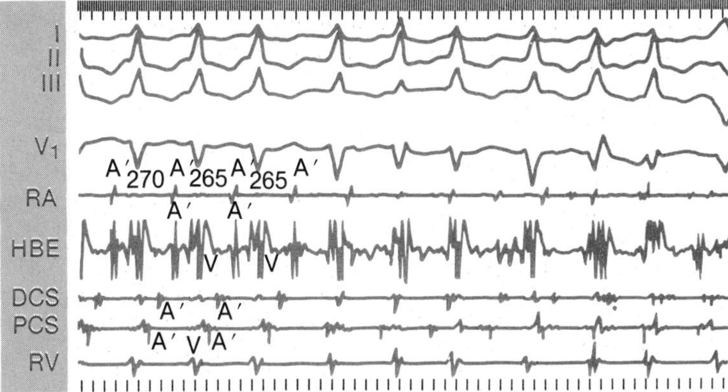

FIGURE 24–30. AV reciprocating tachycardia disorganizing into atrial fibrillation. Same patient as in Figure 24–23*B*. During sustained atrioventricular reciprocating tachycardia at a cycle length of approximately 265 msec, retrograde atrial activation sequence began first in the right paraseptal region (not shown in this example; location proven at surgery) and was then recorded in the proximal coronary sinus electrogram, followed by atrial activity in the distal coronary sinus, in the low right atrium recorded in the His bundle lead and then in the high right atrium. Spontaneously, the atrial activation sequence becomes irregular (after the last A′) and atrial fibrillation begins. Note that the last QRS complex reflects conduction over the accessory pathway. Such a transformation occurred repeatedly in this patient and was associated with a quickening of the ventricular rate. Atrial fibrillation did not recur following surgical interruption of the accessory pathway.

sponse probably exceeds the ability of the ventricle to follow in an organized manner, resulting in fragmented, disorganized ventricular activation and hypotension, and leads to ventricular fibrillation. Alternatively, supraventricular discharge bypassing AV nodal delay can activate the ventricle during the vulnerable period of the antecedent T wave and precipitate ventricular fibrillation. Patients who have had ventricular fibrillation have ventricular cycle lengths during atrial fibrillation in the range of 200 msec or less.

Patients with preexcitation syndrome can have other causes of tachycardia such as AV nodal reentry, sometimes with dual AV nodal curves, sinus nodal reentry, or even ventricular tachycardia unrelated to the accessory pathway. Accessory pathways can conduct anterogradely only as well as retrogradely only. If the pathway conducts only anterogradely, it cannot participate in the usual form of reciprocating tachycardia (Fig. 24–28*A*). It can, however, participate in antidromic tachycardia (Fig. 24–28*C*) as well as conduct to the ventricle during atrial flutter or atrial fibrillation (Fig. 24–28*E*). Some data suggest that the accessory pathway demonstrates automatic activity, which could conceivably be responsible for some instances of tachycardia.

"Wide QRS Tachycardias." In patients with the preexcitation syndrome, so-called wide QRS tachycardias can be due to multiple mechanisms including sinus or atrial tachycardias, AV nodal reentry, atrial flutter or fibrillation with anterograde conduction over the accessory pathway; orthodromic reciprocating tachycardia with functional or preexisting bundle branch block; antidromic reciprocating tachycardia; reciprocating tachycardia with anterograde conduction over one accessory pathway and retrograde conduction over a second one; tachycardias using Mahaim fibers; or ventricular tachycardia.[152,157]

CLINICAL FEATURES. The reported incidence of preexcitation syndrome depends in large measure on the population studied, varying from 0.1 to 3.0 per thousand in apparently healthy subjects, with an average of about 1.5 per thousand. Recent information suggests a higher incidence of 3.7 per thousand.[164a] The incidence of the electrocardiographic pattern of WPW conduction in 22,500 healthy aviation personnel was 0.25 per cent with a prevalence of documented tachyarrhythmias of 1.8 per cent. Left free wall accessory pathways are most common, followed in frequency by posteroseptal,[165] right free wall, and anteroseptal locations. WPW syndrome is found in all age groups, from fetal and neonatal periods[166] to the elderly, and in identical twins. The prevalence is higher in males and decreases with age, apparently due to loss of preexcitation. The majority of adults with preexcitation syndrome have normal hearts, although a variety of acquired and congenital cardiac defects have been reported, including Ebstein's anomaly, mitral valve prolapse, and cardiomyopathies. Patients with Ebstein's anomaly (p. 940) often have multiple accessory pathways, right-sided either in the posterior septum or posterolateral wall, with preexcitation localized to the atrialized ventricle. They often have reciprocating tachycardia with a long V-A interval and a right bundle branch block morphology.

The frequency of paroxysmal tachycardia apparently increases with age, from 10 per 100 patients with WPW syndrome in a 20- to 39-year age group to 36 per 100 in patients more than 60 years old. Approximately 80 per cent of patients with tachycardia have a reciprocating tachycardia, 15 to 30 per cent have atrial fibrillation, and 5 per cent atrial flutter. Ventricular tachycardia occurs uncommonly. The anomalous complexes can mask or mimic myocardial infarction (p. 144), bundle branch block, or ventricular hypertrophy, and the presence of the preexcitation syndrome can call attention to an associated cardiac defect. The prognosis is excellent in patients without tachycardia or an associated cardiac anomaly. For most patients with recurrent tachycardia the prognosis is good but sudden death occurs rarely. In one study, it occurred in 1 of 151 patients followed 1 to 11 years.

It is very likely that acquisition of an accessory pathway occurs congenitally, although its manifestations can be detected in later years and appear to be "acquired." Relatives of patients with preexcitation, particularly those with multiple pathways, have an increased prevalence of preexcitation, suggesting a hereditary mode of acquisition. Some children and adults can lose their tendency to develop tachyarrhythmias as they grow older, possibly owing to fibrotic or other changes at the site of the accessory pathway insertion.[167] Tachycardia beginning in infancy can disappear but frequently recurs. Tachycardia still present after age 5 years persists in 75 per cent of patients, regardless of accessory pathway location.[167a] Intermittent preexcitation during sinus rhythm and loss of conduction over the accessory pathway after intravenous ajmaline or procainamide and with exercise suggest that the refractory period of the accessory pathway is long and that the patient is not at risk of developing a rapid ventricular rate should atrial flutter or fibrillation develop. These approaches are relatively specific, but not very sensitive, with a low positive predictive accuracy.[168,169] Exceptions to these safeguards can occur.[170,171] Isoproterenol infusion is not helpful in identifying patients at risk of sudden death.[172]

TREATMENT. Patients with ventricular preexcitation may have no or only occasional tachyarrhythmias unassociated with significant symptoms. These patients do not require electrophysiological evaluation or therapy.[173] However, if a patient has frequent episodes of tachyarrhythmias and/or the arrhythmias cause significant symptoms, therapy should be initiated. Those who suffer significant hemodynamic consequences from the tachycardia should be considered for electrophysiological study (p. 616).

Three therapeutic options exist: electrical (p. 651), or surgical (p. 656) ablation, and pharmacological therapy. Drugs are chosen to prolong conduction time and/or refractoriness in the AV node, the accessory pathway, or both to prevent rapid rates from occurring[174] (Table 24–3). If successful, this would prevent maintenance of an AV reciprocating tachycardia or a rapid ventricular response to atrial flutter or atrial fibrillation. Some drugs might suppress premature complexes that precipitate the arrhythmias.

Adenosine, verapamil, propranolol, and digitalis all prolong conduction time and refractoriness in the AV node. Verapamil and propranolol do not directly affect conduction in the accessory pathway, while digitalis has had variable effects. Because digitalis has been reported to shorten refractoriness in the accessory pathway and speed the ventricular response in some patients with atrial fibrillation, it is advisable *not* to use digitalis as a single drug in patients with the WPW syndrome who have or may develop atrial flutter or atrial fibrillation. Since many patients can develop atrial fibrillation *during* the reciprocating tachycardia (Fig. 24–30), this caveat probably applies to *all* patients who have tachycardia and the WPW syndrome. Rather, drugs that prolong the refractory period in the accessory pathway such as class IA and IC drugs (Chap. 23) should be used. Class IC drugs and amiodarone can affect both the AV node and the accessory pathway. Lidocaine does not prolong refractoriness of the accessory pathway in patients whose effective refractory period is ≤300 msec. Verapamil and lidocaine IV can *increase* the ventricular rate during atrial fibrillation in patients with the WPW syndrome. Intravenous verapamil may precipitate *ventricular fibrillation* when given to a patient with the WPW syndrome who has a rapid ventricular rate during atrial fibrillation.[175] This does not appear to happen with *oral* verapamil. Catecholamines expose WPW syndromes, shorten the refractory period of the accessory pathway, and reverse the effects of some antiarrhythmic drugs.[176,176a] Resting vagal tone exerts a direct depressant effect on accessory AV connections.[176b]

TABLE 24-3 DRUGS THAT SLOW CONDUCTION IN, AND PROLONG REFRACTORINESS OF, ACCESSORY PATHWAY AND AV NODE

AFFECTED TISSUE	DRUGS
Accessory pathway	Class IA
AV node	Class II Class IV Adenosine Digitalis
Both	Class IC Class III (amiodarone)

Termination of the acute episode of reciprocating tachycardia, suspected electrocardiographically from a normal QRS complex, regular R-R intervals, a rate of about 200 beats/min, and a P wave in the ST segment, should be approached as for AV nodal reentry. After vagal maneuvers, adenosine followed by verapamil or a similar calcium antagonist is the initial treatment of choice. For atrial flutter or fibrillation, the latter suspected from an anomalous QRS complex and grossly irregular R-R intervals (Figs. 24–23*B* and 24–30), drugs that prolong refractoriness in the accessory pathway, often coupled with drugs that prolong AV nodal refractoriness (e.g., procainamide and propranolol), must be used. In many patients, particularly those with a very rapid ventricular response, electrical cardioversion is the *initial* treatment of choice.

Prevention. For long-term therapy to prevent a recurrence, it is not always possible to predict which drugs may be most effective for an individual patient. Some drugs actually can increase the frequency of episodes of reciprocating tachycardia by prolonging the duration of anterograde and not retrograde refractory periods of the accessory pathway, thereby making it easier for a premature atrial complex to block anterogradely in the accessory pathway and initiate tachycardia. Oral administration of two drugs, such as quinidine and propranolol or procainamide and verapamil, to decrease conduction capabilities in both limbs of the reentrant circuit, can be beneficial. Class IC drugs[177–179] and amiodarone, which prolong refractoriness in both the accessory pathway and the AV node, can be effective. Depending on the clinical situation, empirical drug trials or serial electrophysiological drug testing may be employed to determine optimal drug therapy for patients with reciprocating tachycardia. For patients who have atrial fibrillation with a rapid ventricular response, induction of atrial fibrillation while the patient is receiving therapy is essential to be certain that the ventricular rate is controlled.

Electrical or Surgical Ablation (Ch. 23). Ablation of the accessory pathway is advisable for patients with frequent symptomatic arrhythmias that are not fully controlled by drugs or with rapid AV conduction over the accessory pathway during atrial flutter or fibrillation and in whom significant slowing of the ventricular response during tachycardia cannot be obtained by drug therapy. Patients who have accessory pathways with very short refractory periods may be poor candidates for drug therapy, since the refractory periods may be prolonged insignificantly in response to the standard agents. Mahaim connections can also be ablated.[179a] *Pacing therapy*[137,180,181] may be useful on occasion, but precipitation of atrial flutter or atrial fibrillation can result in very rapid ventricular rates and clinical deterioration. Interruption of the accessory pathway should be considered before an antitachycardia device is implanted. The success of radiofrequency ablation is changing concepts about therapy because it offers patients a *curative* procedure with minimal morbidity. Hence it is being offered earlier in the course of therapy and eventually may supplant most drug therapy. Cure of a tachycardia is preferable to years of drug therapy.

SUMMARY. Electrocardiographic clues are often present that permit differentiation among the various supraventricular tachycardias (Table 24–2). P waves during tachycardia identical to sinus P waves and occurring with a long R-P interval and a short P-R interval are most likely due to sinus nodal reentry. Retrograde (inverted in II, III, and aV_f) P waves generally represent reentry involving the AV junction, either AV nodal reentry or reciprocating tachycardia using a paraseptal accessory pathway. Tachycardia without manifest P waves is probably due to AV nodal reentry (P waves buried in QRS), while a tachycardia with an R-P interval exceeding 60 to 70 msec may be due to an accessory pathway. The condition of multiple pathways can be recognized. AV dissociation or AV block during tachycardia excludes the presence of a functioning AV accessory pathway and makes AV nodal reentry less likely. Multiple tachycardias can occur at different times in the same patient. QRS alternans, thought to be a feature of AV reciprocating tachycardia (Table 24–2), is more likely a rapid rate-related phenomenon, independent of the tachycardia mechanism.[182]

VENTRICULAR RHYTHM DISTURBANCES

PREMATURE VENTRICULAR COMPLEXES

ELECTROCARDIOGRAPHIC RECOGNITION. A premature ventricular complex is characterized by the premature occurrence of a QRS complex that is bizarre in shape and has a duration usually exceeding the dominant QRS complex, generally greater than 120 msec. The T wave is commonly large and opposite in direction to the major deflection of the QRS. The QRS complex is not preceded by a premature P wave but can be preceded by a nonconducted sinus P wave occurring at its expected time. The diagnosis of premature ventricular complex can never be made with unequivocal certainty from the scalar electrocardiogram, since a supraventricular beat or rhythm can mimic the manifestations of ventricular arrhythmia (Figs. 24–15 and 24–31). Retrograde transmission to the atria from the premature ventricular complex occurs fairly frequently but is often obscured by the distorted QRS complex

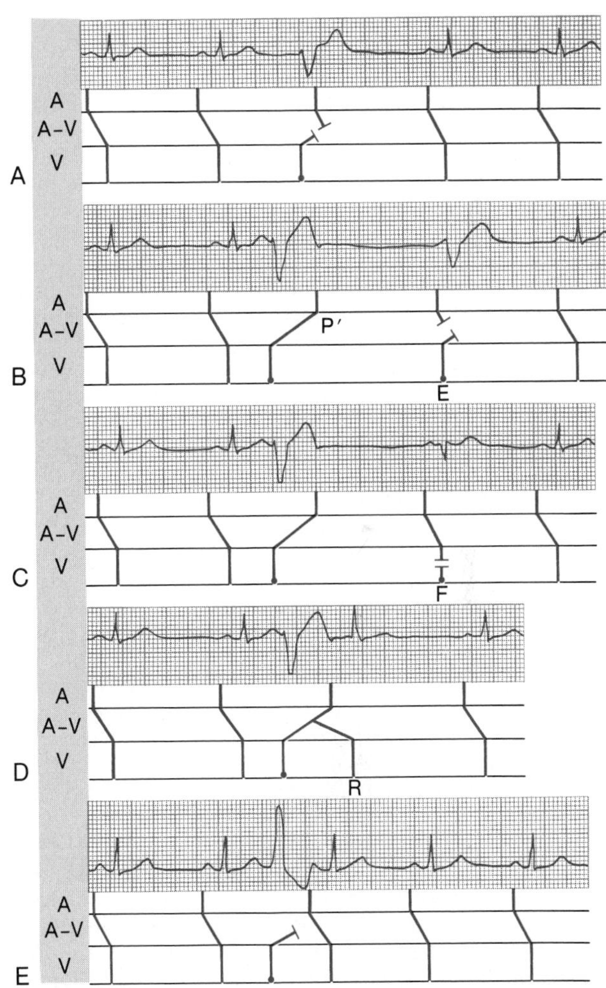

FIGURE 24–31. Premature ventricular complexes. *A* to *D* were recorded in the same patient. *A*, A late premature ventricular complex results in a compensatory pause. *B*, A slower sinus rate and a slightly earlier premature complex results in retrograde atrial excitation (P′). The sinus node is reset, producing a noncompensatory pause. Before the sinus-initiated P wave that follows the retrograde P wave can conduct to the ventricle, a ventricular escape (E) occurs. *C*, Events are similar to those in *B* except that a ventricular fusion beat (F) results following the premature ventricular complex owing to a slightly faster sinus rate. *D*, The impulse propagating retrogradely to the atrium reverses its direction after a delay and returns to reexcite the ventricles (R) to produce a ventricular echo. *E*, An interpolated premature ventricular complex is followed by a slightly prolonged P-R interval of the sinus-initiated beat. Lead II.

and T wave. If the retrograde impulse discharges and resets the sinus node prematurely, it produces a pause that is not fully compensatory. More commonly, the sinus node and atria are not discharged prematurely by the retrograde impulse, since interference of impulses frequently occurs at the AV junction (see p. 715), establishing a collision between the anterograde impulse conducted from the sinus node and the retrograde impulse conducted from the premature ventricular complex. Therefore, a fully compensatory pause usually follows a premature ventricular complex: the R-R interval produced by the two sinus-initiated QRS complexes on either side of the premature complex equals twice the normally conducted R-R interval. The premature ventricular complex may not produce any pause and may therefore be interpolated (Fig. 24–31), or it may produce a postponed compensatory pause when an interpolated premature complex causes P-R prolongation of the first post-extrasystolic beat to such a degree that the P wave of the second postextrasystolic beat occurs at a very short R-P interval and is therefore blocked.

Interference within the ventricle can result in *ventricular fusion beats* (p. 733), which may be narrower than the dominant beat, as when a right bundle branch block pattern of a premature ventricular complex arising in the left ventricle fuses with the sinus-initiated complex conducting through the AV junction with a left bundle branch block pattern, or when the ventricle with a bundle branch block pattern is paced artificially, producing a narrow ventricular fusion beat between the paced and the sinus-conducted beats. Narrow premature ventricular complexes also have been explained as originating at a point equidistant from each ventricle in the ventricular septum and by arising high in the fascicular system. Whether a compensatory or noncompensatory pause, retrograde atrial excitation, or an interpolated complex, fusion complex, or echo beat occurs (Fig. 24–31), it is merely a function of how the AV junction conducts and the timing of the events taking place.

The term *bigeminy* refers to pairs of complexes and indicates a normal and premature complex; *trigeminy* indicates a premature complex following two normal beats; a premature complex following three normal beats is called *quadrigeminy;* and so on. Two successive premature ventricular complexes are termed a pair or a couplet, while three successive premature ventricular complexes are called a triplet. Arbitrarily, three or more successive premature ventricular complexes are termed ventricular tachycardia. Premature ventricular complexes can have different contours and often are called multifocal (Fig. 24–32). More properly they should be called "multiform," "polymorphic," or "pleomorphic," since it is not known whether multiple foci are discharging or whether conduction of the impulse originating from one site is merely changing. A broadly notched PVC exceeding 160 msec in duration is often associated with a dilated, globally hypokinetic left ventricle while a smooth, narrow-notched PVC of short duration often reflects a normal-sized heart.[182a]

Premature ventricular complexes may exhibit fixed or variable coupling, i.e., the interval between the normal QRS complex and the premature ventricular complex can be relatively stable or variable. Fixed coupling can be due to reentry, triggered activity (p. 604), or other mechanisms. Variable coupling can be due to parasystole (p. 717), to changing conduction in a reentrant circuit, or to changing discharge rates of triggered activity. Usually, it is difficult to determine the precise mechanism responsible for the premature ventricular complex with either constant or variable coupling intervals.

CLINICAL FEATURES. The prevalence of premature complexes increases with age. Symptoms of palpitations or discomfort in the neck or chest can result because of the greater-than-normal contractile force of the postextrasystolic beat or the feeling that the heart has stopped during the long pause after the premature complex. Long runs of frequent premature ventricular complexes in patients with heart disease can produce angina or hypotension. Frequent interpolated premature ventricular complexes actually represent a doubling of the heart rate and can compromise the patient's hemodynamic status. Activity that increases the heart rate can decrease the patient's awareness of the premature systoles or reduce their number. Exercise can increase the number of premature complexes in other patients. Premature systoles can be quite uncomfortable in patients who have aortic regurgitation because of the large stroke volume. Sleep is usually associated with a decrease in the frequency of ventricular arrhythmias,[183] but some patients can experience an increase.

Premature ventricular complexes occur in association with a variety of stimuli and can be produced by direct mechanical, electrical, and chemical stimulation of the myocardium. Often they are noted in patients with left ventricular false tendons,[184,185] during infection, in ischemic or inflamed myocardium, and during hypoxia, anesthesia, or surgery. They can be provoked by a variety of medications, by electrolyte imbalance,[186,187] by tension states, and by excessive use of tobacco, caffeine, or alcohol. Both central and peripheral autonomic stimulation have profound effects on heart rate, which can produce or suppress premature complexes.[188]

Physical examination reveals the presence of a premature beat followed by a pause that is longer than normal. A fully compensatory pause can be distinguished from one that is not fully compensatory, since the former does not change the timing of the basic rhythm. The premature beat is often accompanied by a decrease in intensity of the heart sounds, often with auscultation of just the first heart sound, which can be sharp and snapping, and a decreased or absent peripheral (e.g., radial) pulse. The relationship of atrial to ventricular systole determines the presence of normal *a* waves or giant *a* waves in the jugular venous pulse, and the length of the P-R interval determines the intensity of the first heart sound. The second heart sound can be abnormally split, depending on the origin of the ventricular complex.

The importance of premature ventricular complexes varies depending on the clinical setting. In the absence of underlying heart disease, the presence of premature ventricular complexes usually has no impact on longevity or limitation of activity; antiarrhythmic drugs are not indicated. The patient should be reassured if he or she is symptomatic (see Chap. 22, Exercise Testing and Long-Term ECG Recording). In middle-aged men, premature ventricular systoles and complex ventricular arrhythmias are associated with the presence of coronary heart disease and with a greater risk of subsequent death from coronary heart disease. However, it has not been demonstrated that premature ventricular systoles or complex ventricular arrhythmias play a *precipitating* role in the genesis of sudden death in these patients, and the arrhythmias may simply be a marker of heart disease. Results from electrophysiological testing suggest that patients with premature ventricular complexes who do not have ventricular tachycardia induced at electrophysiological study have a low incidence of subsequent sudden death.[189,190] Antiarrhythmic therapy given to suppress the premature ventricular systoles or complex ventricular arrhythmias has not been shown to reduce the incidence of sudden death in such apparently healthy men.

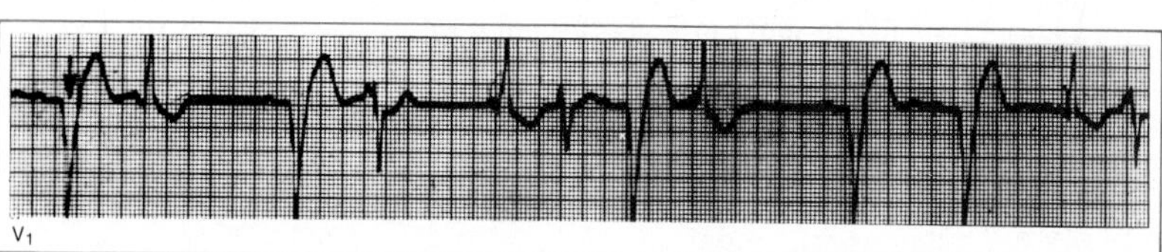

FIGURE 24–32. Multiform premature ventricular complexes. The normally conducted QRS complexes exhibit a left bundle branch block contour (arrow) and are followed by premature ventricular complexes with three different morphologies.

In patients suffering from acute myocardial infarction, premature ventricular complexes considered to presage the onset of ventricular fibrillation, such as those occurring close to the preceding T wave, more than five or six per minute, bigeminal or multiform complexes, or those occurring in salvoes of two, three, or more, do not occur in about half the patients who develop ventricular fibrillation, and about half of those patients who have these premature ventricular complexes do not develop ventricular fibrillation. Thus, these premature ventricular complexes are not particularly helpful prognostically. Electrophysiological testing may be useful to identify patients at increased risk of developing ventricular tachycardia or sudden cardiac death after myocardial infarction, although use of such studies is currently controversial.[14,191,192]

MANAGEMENT. Both fast and slow heart rates can provoke the development of premature ventricular complexes. Premature ventricular complexes accompanying slow ventricular rates can be abolished by increasing the basic rate with atropine or isoproterenol or by pacing, whereas slowing the heart rate in some patients with sinus tachycardia can eradicate premature ventricular complexes. In the hospitalized patient, intravenous lidocaine (p. 639) is generally the initial treatment of choice to suppress premature ventricular complexes. If maximum dosages of lidocaine are unsuccessful, then procainamide given intravenously can be tried. Quinidine can be given intravenously slowly and cautiously. The use of disopyramide and amiodarone given intravenously is still investigational. Propranolol can be tried if the other drugs have been unsuccessful. For long-term oral maintenance, a variety of classes I and II drugs may be useful, as for the prevention of ventricular tachycardia (p. 634). Class IC drugs seem particularly successful in suppressing premature ventricular complexes, but flecainide and encainide have been shown to increase mortality in patients treated after myocardial infarction.[82] Amiodarone may be quite effective.[192a] Because of spontaneous variability, it is often difficult to judge whether an antiarrhythmic regimen is beneficial or harmful.[192b]

VENTRICULAR TACHYCARDIA

ELECTROCARDIOGRAPHIC RECOGNITION. Ventricular tachycardia arises distal to the bifurcation of the His bundle, in the specialized conduction system, in ventricular muscle, or in combinations of both tissue types. The mechanisms include disorders of impulse formation and conduction considered earlier[193–200] (Chap. 20). Autonomic modulation may be important.[201–203] The electrocardiographic diagnosis of ventricular tachycardia is suggested by the occurrence of a series of three or more bizarrely shaped premature ventricular complexes whose duration exceeds 120 msec, with the ST-T vector pointing opposite to the major QRS deflection.[157,204] The R-R interval can be exceedingly regular or can vary. Many patients have ventricular tachycardia with multiple morphologies originating at the same or closely adjacent sites, probably with different exit paths. Others have multiple sites of origin. Atrial activity can be independent of ventricular activity (AV dissociation, p. 715), or the atria may be depolarized by the ventricles retrogradely (VA association). Depending on the particular type of ventricular tachycardia, the rates range from 70 to 250 beats/min, and the onset can be paroxysmal (sudden) or nonparoxysmal. QRS contours during the ventricular tachycardia can be unchanging (uniform, monomorphic), can vary randomly (multiform, polymorphic, or pleomorphic[205]), vary in a more or less repetitive manner (torsades de pointes), vary in alternate complexes (bidirectional ventricular tachycardia), or vary in a stable but changing contour (i.e., right bundle branch contour changing to left bundle branch contour). Ventricular tachycardia can be sustained, defined arbitrarily as lasting longer than 30 sec or requiring termination because of hemodynamic collapse, or nonsustained (unsustained), when it stops spontaneously in less than 30 sec. Most commonly, very premature stimulation is required to initiate ventricular tachycardia electrically, while late coupled ventricular complexes usually initiate its spontaneous onset.[200]

TABLE 24–4 MAJOR FEATURES IN THE DIFFERENTIAL DIAGNOSIS OF WIDE QRS BEATS VERSUS TACHYCARDIA

SUPPORTS SVT	SUPPORTS VT
Slowing or termination by ↑ vagal tone	Fusion beats
Onset with premature P wave	Capture beats
RP interval ≤ 100 msec	AV dissociation
P and QRS rate and rhythm linked to suggest ventricular activation depends on atrial discharge, e.g., 2:1 AV block	P and QRS rate and rhythm linked to suggest atrial activation depends on ventricular discharge, e.g., 2:1 VA block
RSR′ V_1	
Long-short cycle sequence	"Compensatory" pause
	Left axis deviation;
	QRS duration > 140 msec
	Specific QRS contours (see text)

SVT = supraventricular tachycardia; VT = ventricular tachycardia.

Making the electrocardiographic distinction between supraventricular tachycardia with aberration and ventricular tachycardia can be difficult at times, since features of both arrhythmias overlap and under certain circumstances a supraventricular tachycardia can mimic the criteria established for ventricular tachycardia.[206–210] Ventricular complexes with bizarre or prolonged configuration indicate only that conduction through the ventricle is abnormal, and such complexes can occur in supraventricular rhythms due to preexisting bundle branch block, aberrant conduction during incomplete recovery of repolarization, conduction over accessory pathways, and several other conditions. These complexes do not necessarily indicate the origin of impulse formation or the reason for the abnormal conduction. Conversely, ectopic beats originating in the ventricle uncommonly can have a fairly normal duration and shape. However, it is important to emphasize that ventricular tachycardia is the most common cause of a wide QRS complex tachycardia. A past history of myocardial infarction makes the diagnosis even more likely.[207,208]

During the course of a tachycardia characterized by widespread, bizarre QRS complexes, the presence of fusion beats

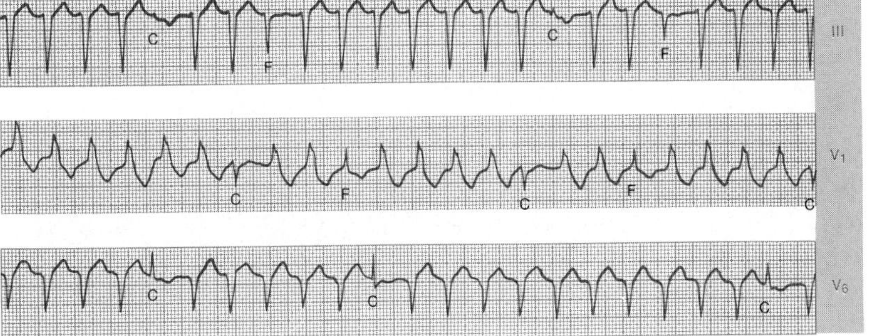

FIGURE 24–33. Fusion and capture beats during a probable ventricular tachycardia. The QRS complex is prolonged, and the R-R interval is regular except for occasional capture beats (C) that have a normal contour and are slightly premature. Complexes intermediate in contour represent fusion beats (F). Thus, even though atrial activity is not clearly apparent, it is likely that AV dissociation is present during a ventricular tachycardia and produces intermittent capture and fusion beats.

and capture beats provides maximum support for the diagnosis of ventricular tachycardia (Table 24–4). *Fusion beats* indicate activation of the ventricle from two different foci, implying that one of the foci had a ventricular origin. *Capture* of the ventricle by the supraventricular rhythm with a normal configuration of the captured QRS complex at an interval shorter than the tachycardia in question indicates that the impulse has a supraventricular origin (Fig. 24–33). Atrioventricular dissociation (p. 715) has long been considered a hallmark of ventricular tachycardia.[157,206] However, retrograde VA conduction to the atria from ventricular beats occurs in a large percentage of patients, and therefore ventricular tachycardia may not exhibit AV dissociation. Atrioventricular dissociation can occur uncommonly during supraventricular tachycardias. Even if a P wave appears to be related to each QRS complex it is at times difficult to determine whether the P wave is conducted anterogradely to the next QRS complex (i.e., supraventricular tachycardia with aberrancy and a long P-R interval) or retrogradely from the preceding QRS complex (i.e., a ventricular tachycardia). As a general rule, however, AV dissociation during a wide QRS tachycardia is strong presumptive evidence that the tachycardia is of ventricular origin.

Differentiation Between Ventricular and Supraventricular Tachycardia. Some electrocardiographic features characterizing supraventricular arrhythmia with aberrancy are (1) consistent onset of the tachycardia with a premature P wave, (2) a very short R-P interval (≤0.1 sec) often requiring an esophageal recording to visualize the P waves, (3) a QRS configuration the same as that which occurs from known supraventricular conduction at similar rates, (4) P-wave and QRS rate and rhythm linked to suggest that ventricular activation depends on atrial discharge (e.g., A-V Wenckebach block), and (5) slowing or termination of the tachycardia by vagal maneuvers.

Analysis of specific QRS contours also can be helpful in diagnosing ventricular tachycardia and localizing its site of origin.[209,210] For example, QRS contours suggesting a ventricular tachycardia include left-axis deviation in the frontal plane and a QRS duration exceeding 140 msec with a QRS of normal duration during sinus rhythm. During ventricular tachycardia with a right bundle branch block appearance, (1) the QRS complex is monophasic or biphasic in V_1 with an initial deflection different from sinus-initiated QRS complex, (2) the amplitude of the R wave in V_1 exceeds the R′, and (3) small R and large S wave or a QS pattern in V_6 may be present. With a ventricular tachycardia having a left bundle branch block contour, (1) the axis may be rightward with negative deflections deeper in V_1 than in V_6, (2) a broad prolonged (>40 msec) R wave in V_1, and (3) a small Q–large R wave or QS pattern in V_6 may exist. A QRS complex that is similar in V_1 through V_6, either all negative or all positive, favors a ventricular origin as does the presence of 2:1 ventriculoatrial block. (An upright QRS complex in V_1 through V_6 also may occur due to conduction over a left-sided accessory pathway.) Supraventricular beats with aberration often have a triphasic pattern in V_1, an initial vector of the abnormal complex similar to that of the normally conducted beats, and a wide QRS complex that terminates a short cycle length which follows a long cycle (long-short cycle sequence). During atrial fibrillation fixed coupling, short coupling intervals, a long pause after the abnormal beat, and runs of bigeminy rather than a consecutive series of abnormal complexes all favor ventricular origin of the premature complex rather than supraventricular origin with aberration. A grossly irregular, wide QRS tachycardia with ventricular rates faster than 200 beats/min should raise the question of atrial fibrillation with conduction over an accessory pathway (Figs. 24–23*B* and 24–30). In the presence of preexisting bundle branch block, a wide QRS tachycardia with a contour different from that which occurred during sinus rhythm is most likely a ventricular tachycardia. Exceptions exist to all the aforementioned criteria, especially in patients who have preexisting conduction disturbances or preexcitation syndrome; when in doubt, one must rely on sound clinical judgment, considering the ECG as only one of several helpful ancillary tests.

Termination of a tachycardia by triggering vagal reflexes is considered diagnostic of supraventricular tachycardias. However, ventricular tachycardia uncommonly can be stopped in a similar manner.

ELECTROPHYSIOLOGICAL FEATURES. Electrophysiologically, ventricular tachycardia can be distinguished by a short or negative H-V interval (i.e., H begins after the onset of ventricular depolarization) because of retrograde activation from the ventricles (see Fig. 22–35, p. 618). His bundle deflections usually are not apparent during ventricular tachycardia because they are obscured by simultaneous ventricular septal depolarization or because of inadequate catheter position. The latter must be determined during supraventricular rhythm before the onset or after the termination of ventricular tachycardia (Fig. 24–34). His bundle deflections dissociated from ventricular activation are diagnostic, with rare exception. Ventricular tachycardia can produce QRS complexes of narrow duration and of short H-V interval, most likely when the site of origin is close to the His bundle in the fascicles.

Successful electrical induction of ventricular tachycardia by premature stimulation of the ventricle (Fig. 24–34) depends on the characteristics of the ventricular tachycardia and the anatomical substrate. Patients with sustained ventricular tachycardia and ventricular tachycardia due to coronary artery disease[211] have ventricular tachycardia induced more frequently than patients who have nonsustained ventricular tachycardia and ventricular tachycardia due to noncoronary-related causes.[212] In general, it is more difficult to induce ventricular tachycardia with late premature ventricular stimuli compared with early premature stimuli, during sinus rhythm compared with ventricular pacing, and with one premature stimulus compared with two or three. The specificity of ventricular tachycardia induction using more than two premature ventricular stimuli begins to decrease (while the sensitivity increases), and nonsustained polymorphic ventricular tachycardia or ventricular fibrillation can be induced in patients who have no history of ventricular tachycardia. Occasionally, ventricular tachycardia can be initiated only from the left ventricle or from specific sites in the right ventricle. Multiple premature stimuli reduce the need for left ventricular stimulation. Drugs such as isoproterenol, various antiarrhythmic agents, and alcohol can facilitate the induction of

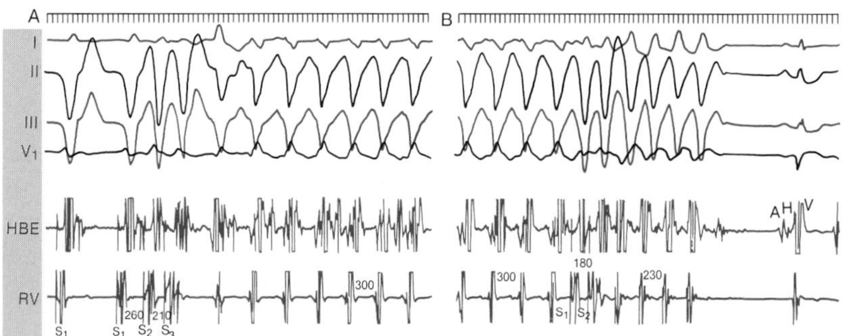

FIGURE 24–34. Initiation and termination of ventricular tachycardia using programmed ventricular stimulation. The last two ventricular-paced beats at a cycle length of 600 msec are shown in panel A. A premature stimulus (S_2) at an S_1-S_2 interval of 260 msec and another premature stimulus (S_3) at a cycle length of 210 msec initiate a sustained monomorphic ventricular tachycardia at a cycle length of 300 msec. Two premature ventricular stimuli (S_1-S_2) in panel B create an unstable ventricular tachycardia which persists for several beats at a shorter cycle length (230 msec) and then terminates, followed by sinus rhythm.

ventricular tachycardia. Coughing during ventricular tachycardia that causes hypotension can help to maintain blood pressure.[213]

Termination by pacing depends significantly on the rate of the ventricular tachycardia and the site of pacing. Slower ventricular tachycardias are terminated more easily and with fewer stimuli than are more rapid ones. An increasing number of stimuli are required to terminate more rapid ventricular tachycardias, which increases the risks of pacing-induced acceleration of the ventricular tachycardia. Subthreshold stimulation[214,215] and transthoracic stimulation[216,217] can terminate ventricular tachycardia. It can also be induced and terminated during atrial pacing.

CLINICAL FEATURES. Symptoms occurring during ventricular tachycardia depend on the ventricular rate, duration of tachycardia, the presence and extent of the underlying heart disease, and peripheral vascular disease.[218] The location of impulse formation and therefore the way in which the depolarization wave spreads across the myocardium may also be important. Physical findings depend in part on the P to QRS relationship. If atrial activity is dissociated from the ventricular contractions, the findings of AV dissociation (p. 715) are present. If the atria are captured retrogradely, regularly occurring cannon *a* waves appear when atrial and ventricular contractions occur simultaneously and the signs of AV dissociation are absent.

More than half of the patients treated for symptomatic recurrent ventricular tachycardia have ischemic heart disease. The next biggest group has cardiomyopathy (both congestive and hypertrophic), with lesser percentages divided among those with primary electrical disease, mitral valve prolapse, valvular heart disease, and miscellaneous causes.[218] Coronary artery spasm can cause transient myocardial ischemia with severe ventricular arrhythmias (during ischemia and during the apparent reperfusion period) in some patients. Complex ventricular arrhythmias can occur *after* coronary artery bypass grafting. In patients resuscitated from sudden cardiac death (Chap. 26) the majority (75 per cent) have severe coronary artery disease, and ventricular tachyarrhythmias can be induced by premature ventricular stimulation in approximately 75 per cent. When ventricular tachycardia occurs in the ambulatory patient, it is uncommonly induced by R-on-T premature ventricular complexes[200,219] (see Ventricular Fibrillation). Patients who have sustained ventricular tachycardia are more likely to have reduced ejection fraction, slowed ventricular conduction, left ventricular aneurysm, and previous myocardial infarction than are patients who have ventricular fibrillation, indicating different electrophysiological and anatomical substrates.[220,221] Similar results occur in dogs after myocardial infarction.[222] Young patients can also suffer cardiac arrest from ventricular tachycardia[223] or ventricular fibrillation, and persistent electrical inducibility of arrhythmia in these patients connotes a poor prognosis.

Many approaches have been used to assess prognosis in patients with ventricular tachyarrhythmias. Reduced baroreceptor sensitivity and heart period variability apparently due to reduced vagal activity may indicate an increased risk of ventricular tachycardia or sudden cardiac death.[224] Coronary artery disease is associated with reduction in cardiac vagal function,[224a] and baroreceptor control of heart rate is impaired early after myocardial infarction.[224b] Vagal stimulation protects against development of ventricular fibrillation in a number of animal models.[225] Findings of reduced left ventricular function,[226-228] spontaneous ventricular arrhythmias,[227] late potentials on signal-averaged ECG,[227,229-233] and inducible sustained ventricular tachyarrhythmias at electrophysiological study[234-239] all carry increased risk, further exaggerated when two or more of these features are present in the same patient.[227] Also, clinical presentation of cardiac arrest[240] during the first spontaneous episode of ventricular arrhythmia[241,242] identifies patients at increased risk. Electrophysiological testing can be useful to stratify patients according to risk and to help guide therapy in cardiac arrest survivors, patients with sustained or nonsustained ventricular tachycardia, unexplained syncope after myocardial infarction, and cardiomyopathy.[242a]

MANAGEMENT. The most important decision involves whether or not to treat. Because reduction in sudden death with antiarrhythmic drug therapy (excluding beta blockers) has not been demonstrated in controlled studies, therapy of asymptomatic patients should, in general, be discouraged. Treatment is reserved for prevention or reduction of symptoms produced by sustained and at times nonsustained ventricular tachyarrhythmias; it can be divided into approaches used to terminate sustained ventricular tachycardia and to prevent recurrences.

Termination of Sustained Ventricular Tachycardia. Ventricular tachycardia that does not cause hemodynamic decompensation can be treated medically to achieve acute termination by administering intravenous lidocaine or procainamide, followed by an infusion of the successful drug. Although quinidine can be used intravenously, great caution is needed because of hypotension. Amiodarone is effective intravenously, although this method of administration has not been approved by the FDA.

If the arrhythmia does not respond to medical therapy, electrical DC cardioversion can be employed. Ventricular tachycardia that precipitates hypotension, shock, angina, or congestive heart failure or symptoms of cerebral hypoperfusion should be treated *promptly* with DC cardioversion (p. 749). Very low energies can terminate ventricular tachycardia, beginning with a synchronized shock of 10 to 50 watt-seconds. Digitalis-induced ventricular tachycardia is best treated pharmacologically. After conversion of the arrhythmia to a normal rhythm, it is essential to institute measures to prevent a recurrence.

Striking the patient's chest, sometimes called "thumpversion," (p. 775) can terminate ventricular tachycardia by mechanically inducing a premature ventricular complex that presumably interrupts the reentrant pathway necessary to support it. Chest stimulation at the time of the vulnerable period during the arrhythmia may accelerate the ventricular tachycardia or possibly provoke ventricular fibrillation.

In patients with recurrent ventricular tachycardia, competitive ventricular pacing via a pacing catheter inserted into the right ventricle or transcutaneously can be used. This procedure incurs the risk of accelerating the ventricular tachycardia to ventricular flutter or ventricular fibrillation. Synchronized cardioversion via a catheter electrode in the ventricle can be performed. Intermittent ventricular tachycardia, interrupted by several supraventricular beats, is generally best treated pharmacologically (see Chap. 23).

A search for reversible conditions contributing to the initiation and maintenance of ventricular tachycardia should be made and the conditions corrected if possible. For example, ventricular tachycardia related to ischemia, hypotension, or hypokalemia at times may be terminated by antianginal treatment, vasopressors, or potassium, respectively. Correction of heart failure can reduce the frequency of ventricular arrhythmias.[243,244] Slow ventricular rates that are caused by sinus bradycardia or AV block may permit the occurrence of premature ventricular complexes and ventricular tachyarrhythmias that can be corrected by administering atropine, by temporary isoproterenol administration, or by transvenous pacing. Supraventricular tachycardia can initiate ventricular tachyarrhythmias[245,246] and should be prevented if possible.[247]

Prevention of Recurrences. This is generally more difficult than is terminating the acute episode, and there is no "right" drug to choose. Often, because of similar levels of efficacy, drugs are selected on the basis of poential side effects, e.g., avoiding procainamide for long-term therapy because of the development of drug-induced lupus; avoiding flecainide and disopyramide in patients with reduced left ventricular function; not giving disopyramide to patients with prostate enlargement; and withholding flecainide and encainide from patients after myocardial infarction. Positive attributes of

CLINICAL FEATURES. While many predisposing factors have been cited, the most common are congenital, severe bradycardia, potassium depletion, and use of class IA and some IC drugs.[318,330,331] Clinical features depend on whether the torsades de pointes is due to the acquired or congenital (idiopathic) long Q-T syndrome (see below).

MANAGEMENT. The approach to ventricular tachycardia with a polymorphic pattern depends on whether or not it occurs in the setting of a prolonged Q-T interval. For this practical reason and because the mechanism of the tachycardia can differ depending on whether or not a long Q-T interval is present, it is important to restrict the definition of torsades de pointes to the typical polymorphic ventricular tachycardia in the setting of a long Q-T and/or U wave in the basal complexes. In all patients with torsades de pointes, administration of class IA, possibly some class IC, and some class III antiarrhythmic agents can increase the abnormal Q-T interval and worsen the arrhythmia. Class IB drugs can be tried. Intravenous magnesium has been successful.[319,322,332] Temporary ventricular or atrial pacing suppresses the ventricular tachycardia, which often does not recur even after cessation of pacing.[318] Isoproterenol can be tried until pacing is instituted. The cause of the long Q-T should be determined and corrected if possible. When the Q-T interval is normal, polymorphic ventricular tachycardia *resembling* torsades de pointes is diagnosed, and standard antiarrhythmic drugs can be given. In borderline cases, the clinical context may help determine whether treatment should be initiated with antiarrhythmic drugs. In doubtful cases when the Q-T interval is at upper limits of normal, treatment with pacing is preferable.

Long Q-T Syndrome

ELECTROCARDIOGRAPHIC RECOGNITION (Fig. 24–36*B*). The upper limit for the duration of the normal Q-T interval *corrected* for heart rate (Q-Tc) is given as 0.44 sec.[333,334] However, the normal corrected Q-T interval actually may be longer,[333] 0.46 for men and 0.47 for women, with a normal range ±15 per cent of the mean value. The nature of the U-wave abnormality and its relationship to the long Q-T syndrome are not clear. It is possible that more subtle ST-T-U wave abnormalities might provide improved sensitivity and specificity in identifying patients with the long Q-T syndrome.[335] T wave alternans can occur.[334]

CLINICAL FEATURES. The long Q-T syndrome can be divided into idiopathic (congenital) and acquired forms. The idiopathic form is a familial disorder that can be associated with sensorineural deafness (Jervell and Lange-Nielsen syndrome, autosomal recessive) or normal hearing (Romano-Ward syndrome, autosomal dominant). A nonfamilial form with normal hearing has been called the sporadic form. Information supporting the hypothesis that the idiopathic long Q-T syndrome results from a preponderance of left sympathetic tone has been questioned,[336,337] and present data suggest that early afterdepolarizations may be important.[318–329] The acquired form has a long Q-T interval caused by various drugs such as quinidine, procainamide, N-acetylprocainamide, sotalol, amiodarone, disopyramide, phenothiazines, or tricyclic antidepressants; electrolyte abnormalities such as hypokalemia and hypomagnesemia; the results of the liquid protein diet and starvation; central nervous system lesions;[338,339] significant bradyarrhythmias; cardiac ganglionitis; or mitral valve prolapse; there is also a possible association with the sudden infant death syndrome.

Patients with long Q-T syndrome can present with syncope, at times misdiagnosed as epilepsy,[340] due to ventricular tachycardias that are often caused by torsades de pointes. Since sudden death can occur in this group of patients,[341,342] it is obvious that, in some, the ventricular arrhythmia becomes sustained and probably results in ventricular fibrillation. Patients with idiopathic long Q-T syndrome who are at increased risk for sudden death include those with family members who died suddenly at an early age and those who have experienced syncope. They commonly develop ventricular tachyarrhythmias during periods of adrenergic stimulation such as fright or exertion. Stress testing can prolong the Q-T interval and produce T wave alternans.[341] Electrocardiograms should be obtained for all family members when the propositus presents with symptoms. Patients should undergo prolonged ECG recording, with various stresses designed to evoke ventricular arrhythmias, such as auditory stimuli, psychological stress, cold pressor stimulation, and exercise. The Valsalva maneuver can lengthen the Q-T interval and cause T wave alternans and ventricular tachycardia in patients who have prolonged Q-T syndromes. Catecholamines may be infused in some patients, but this challenge must be performed cautiously, with resuscitative equipment along with alpha and beta antagonists close at hand. Stellate ganglion stimulation and blockade has been useful to provoke or abolish arrhythmias. Premature ventricular stimulation electrically generally does not induce arrhythmias in this syndrome. Patients with the acquired form commonly develop torsades de pointes during periods of bradycardia or after a long pause in the R-R interval.

MANAGEMENT. For patients who have the idiopathic long Q-T syndrome but do not have syncope, complex ventricular arrhythmias, or a family history of sudden cardiac death, no therapy is recommended. In asymptomatic patients with complex ventricular arrhythmias or a family history of early sudden cardiac death, beta-adrenoreceptor blockers at maximally tolerated doses are recommended. In patients with syncope, beta blockers at maximally tolerated doses, perhaps combined with a class IB antiarrhythmic drug, are suggested. For patients who continue to have syncope despite maximum drug therapy, left-sided cervicothoracic sympathetic ganglionectomy that interrupts the stellate ganglion and the first three or four thoracic ganglia may be helpful,[342] and permanent pacing has also been used. Implantation of a cardioverter-defibrillator seems advisable in patients who have syncope despite sympathetic interruption (Chap. 25). For patients with the acquired form and torsades de pointes, IV magnesium and atrial or ventricular pacing are initial choices. Class IB antiarrhythmic drugs or isoproterenol (cautiously) to increase heart rate can be tried. Avoidance of precipitating drugs is mandatory. Potassium channel–activating drugs such as pinacidil and cromakalim may become useful in the future.[343]

BIDIRECTIONAL VENTRICULAR TACHYCARDIA

This is an uncommon type of ventricular tachycardia characterized by QRS complexes with a right bundle branch block pattern, alternating polarity in the frontal plane from −60 to −90 degrees to +120 to +130 degrees, and a regular rhythm (Fig. 24–37). The ventricular rate is between 140 and 200 beats/min. Although the mechanism and site of origin of this tachycardia have remained somewhat controversial, most evidence supports a ventricular origin.

Bidirectional ventricular tachycardia is usually but not exclusively[195] a manifestation of digitalis excess, typically in older patients and in those with severe myocardial disease. When the tachycardia is due to digitalis, the extent of toxicity is often advanced, with a poor prognosis.

Drugs useful to treat digitalis toxicity such as lidocaine, potassium, phenytoin, and propranolol should be considered if excessive digitalis administration is suspected. Otherwise, the usual therapeutic approach to ventricular tachycardia (p. 705) is recommended.

REPETITIVE MONOMORPHIC VENTRICULAR TACHYCARDIA

Repetitive monomorphic ventricular tachycardia is defined as three or more consecutive premature ventricular complexes with only brief periods of intervening sinus complexes. Ventricular complexes generally occur in groups of 3 to 15, but occasionally the ventricular tachycardia can be almost continuous. Single premature ventricular complexes with the same contour can be present. All ventricular complexes have a uniform QRS morphology. Interectopic, sinus-conducted complexes have a normal QRS without intraventricular conduction delay or pathological Q waves in patients without structural heart disease (Fig. 24–38). Cycle lengths of the ventricular tachycardia are fairly regular, and the rate ranges between 100 and 150 beats/min, occasionally becoming as rapid as 250 beats/min. Episodes of ventricular tachycardia tend to cluster around certain time

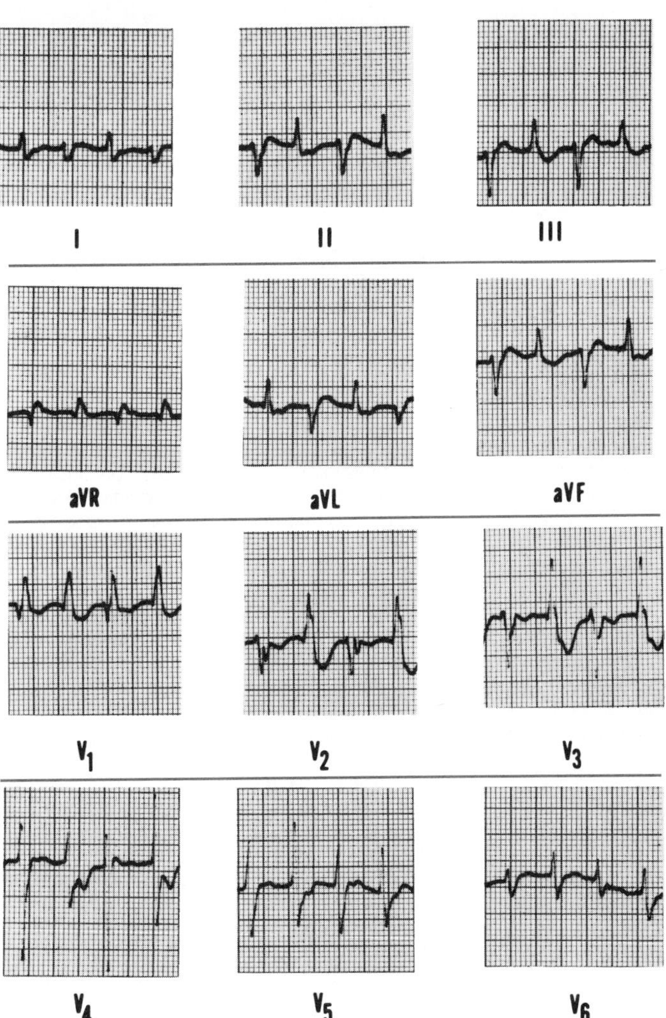

FIGURE 24–37. Bidirectional ventricular tachycardia. The mean frontal plane QRS axis alternates between −60° and +130° in successive beats and all complexes demonstrate a right bundle branch block pattern in V_1. R-R intervals are regular. The tachycardia was shown to be ventricular during an electrophysiological study. (From Morris, S. N., and Zipes, D. P.: His bundle electrocardiography during bidirectional tachycardia. Circulation *48*:32, 1973, by permission of the American Heart Association, Inc.)

periods in an individual patient. Late-cycle and variably coupled premature ventricular complexes are common. The tachycardia can be difficult to induce with premature electrical stimulation. Isoproterenol may be helpful in some patients. Electrophysiological parameters are normal in patients with structurally normal hearts. While some electrophysiological features suggest triggered activity, abnormal automaticity or reentry cannot be excluded.

This type of tachycardia is often associated with no or minimal structural heart disease and young age. When it occurs in patients who have normal, sinus-conducted QRS complexes and minimal or no structural heart disease, it may originate in the right ventricular outflow tract; it appears to be benign, and the prognosis is favorable. Occurring after myocardial infarction, it appears to originate near the border of the previous infarction. Arrhythmia-related deaths are reported infrequently. The arrhythmia may disappear with time, perhaps accounting for its reduced prevalence in older populations. The exact prevalence of the tachycardia is difficult to assess, since often it produces no symptoms and may be identified only during routine examination.

Therapy, as outlined on p. 705, is reserved for patients who are symptomatic from palpitations or have very rapid rates of the ventricular tachycardia. Recently, radiofrequency ablation has successfully eliminated this ventricular tachycardia (unpublished observations).

BUNDLE BRANCH REENTRANT TACHYCARDIA

Ventricular tachycardia due to bundle branch reentry is characterized by a QRS morphology determined by the circuit established over the bundle branches. Retrograde conduction over the left bundle branch system and anterograde conduction over the right bundle branch creates a QRS complex with a left bundle branch block contour. The frontal plane axis may be about +30 degrees. Conduction in the opposite direction produces a right bundle branch block contour. Electrophysiologically, bundle branch reentrant complexes are started after a critical S_2-H_2 or S_3-H_3 delay. The H-V interval of the bundle branch reentrant complex equals or exceeds the H-V interval of the spontaneous normally conducted QRS complex.

Bundle branch reentry has been clearly demonstrated to occur in animals and in humans, with sustained ventricular tachycardia appearing to be more prevalent in patients with dilated cardiomyopathy.[344]

The therapeutic approach is as for other types of ventricular tachycardia, except that creation of bundle branch block interrupts the reentry circuit and can eliminate the tachycardia.[279]

VENTRICULAR FLUTTER AND FIBRILLATION

(See also Chap. 26)

ELECTROCARDIOGRAPHIC RECOGNITION. These arrhythmias represent severe derangements of the heartbeat that usually terminate fatally within 3 to 5 minutes unless corrective measures are undertaken promptly. Ventricular flutter presents as a sine wave in appearance: regular large oscillations occurring at a rate of 150 to 300/min (usually about 200) (Fig. 24–39*A*). The distinction between rapid ventricular tachycardia and ventricular flutter can be difficult and is usually of academic interest only. Hemodynamic collapse is present with both. Ventricular fibrillation is recognized by the presence of irregular undulations of varying contour and amplitude (Fig. 24–39*B*). Distinct QRS complexes, ST segments, and T waves are absent. Fine-amplitude fibrillatory waves (<0.2 mV) are present when termination of ventricular fibrillation has been delayed, which identifies patients with worse survival rates, and are sometimes misdiagnosed as asystole.

MECHANISMS. Ventricular fibrillation occurs in a variety of clinical situations, most commonly associated with coronary artery disease and as a terminal event. Intracellular calcium accumulation,[345–348] effects of long-chain acylcarnitine and lysophosphatidylcholine,[349,350] action of free radicals,[351] metabolic alterations,[352] and autonomic modulation[353–358] are some important influences on development of ventricular fibrillation during ischemia. Thrombolytic agents reduce the incidence of ischemic ventricular fibrillation[359,360] and of inducible ventricular tachycardia after myocardial infarction.[360a] Cardiovascular events, including sudden cardiac death, occur most frequently in the morning[361,361a] and may be related to increased platelet aggregability.[362–365] Aspirin reduces this mortality.[366] Often, intramural reentry precipitates ventricular fibrillation during ische-

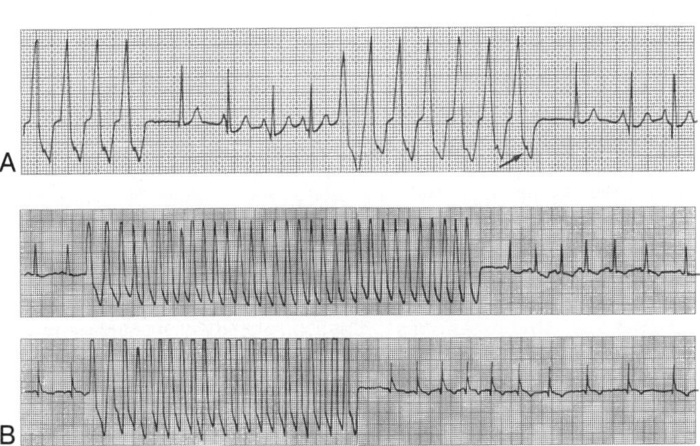

FIGURE 24–38. Panel *A*, Repetitive monomorphic ventricular tachycardia. Short episodes of a monomorphic ventricular tachycardia at a rate of 160 beats/min repeatedly interrupt the normal sinus rhythm. Retrograde atrial capture probably occurs (arrow points to the deflection in the ST segment) and the retrograde P wave of the last complex of the repetitive monomorphic ventricular tachycardia conducts over the normal pathway to produce a normal contour QRS complex. In panel B, short runs of a very rapid (260 beats/min) ventricular tachycardia of uniform contour occur. They probably provoke a compensatory sympathetic response because each is followed by a brief period of sinus tachycardia. The sinus pacemaker appears unstable as changes in P-wave morphology result.

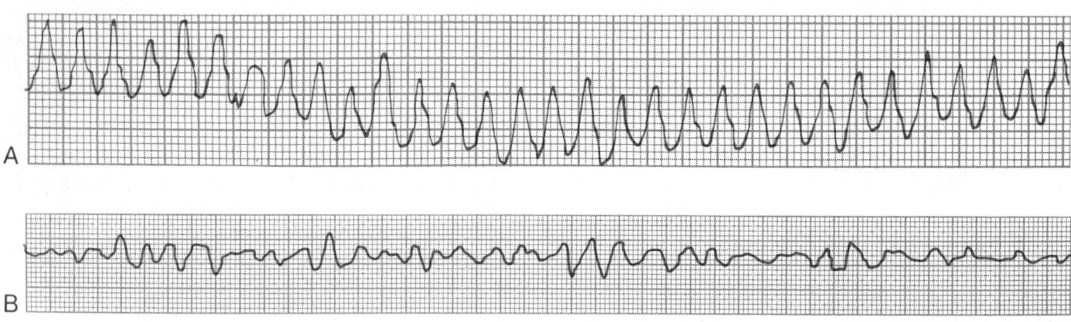

FIGURE 24-39. Ventricular flutter and ventricular fibrillation. *A*, The sine wave appearance of the complexes occurring at a rate of 300 beats/min is characteristic of ventricular flutter. *B*, The irregular undulating baseline typifies ventricular fibrillation.

mia.[366a] Ventricular fibrillation can occur during antiarrhythmic drug administration, hypoxia, ischemia, atrial fibrillation and very rapid ventricular rates in the preexcitation syndrome, after electrical shock administered during cardioversion or accidentally by improperly grounded equipment, and during competitive ventricular pacing to terminate ventricular tachycardia.

CLINICAL FEATURES. Ventricular flutter or ventricular fibrillation results in faintness, followed by loss of consciousness, seizures, apnea and eventually, if the rhythm continues untreated, death. The blood pressure is unobtainable and heart sounds are usually absent. The atria can continue to beat at an independent rhythm for a time or in response to impulses from the fibrillating ventricles. Eventually, electrical activity of the heart ceases.

In patients resuscitated from out-of-hospital cardiac arrest, 75 per cent have ventricular fibrillation. Bradycardia and asystole can occur in 15 to 25 per cent of these patients and is associated with a worse prognosis than is ventricular fibrillation. Ventricular tachycardia commonly precedes the onset of ventricular fibrillation,[367] although frequently no consistent premonitory patterns emerge.[219]

While 75 per cent of resuscitated patients exhibit significant coronary artery disease, only 20 to 30 percent develop acute transmural myocardial infarction. Those who do *not* develop a myocardial infarction have a recurrence rate for sudden cardiac death or nonfatal ventricular fibrillation of approximately 15 to 30 percent at 30 months.[368] The presence of congestive heart failure is an independent predictor of outcome.[368] There appears to be an overall decrease in the incidence of sudden cardiac death, parallel to the decrease in death from coronary heart disease.[369-372] Patients who have ventricular fibrillation and acute myocardial infarction have a recurrence rate at 1 year of 2 per cent. In some studies, patients at risk for sudden cardiac death have ischemia,[373-379] reduced left ventricular function,[368-378] 10 or more premature ventricular complexes/hr, spontaneous and induced ventricular tachycardia,[191,192] hypertension[380,381] and left ventricular hypertrophy,[382,383] obesity,[377,384] and elevated cholesterol levels; smoking, male sex, increased age, and excess alcohol consumption also predispose to sudden cardiac death. Predictors of death for resuscitated patients include reduced ejection fraction, abnormal wall motion, history of congestive heart failure, history of myocardial infarction but no acute event, and the presence of ventricular arrhythmias. Patients discharged after an anterior myocardial infarction complicated by ventricular fibrillation appear to represent a subgroup at high risk of sudden death. Ventricular fibrillation can occur in infants,[385-388] young people,[389-394] athletes,[395-398] persons without known structural heart disease,[304-308,399,400] and in unexplained syndromes.[401]

MANAGEMENT (see also pp. 651 and 749). *Immediate* nonsynchronized DC electrical shock using 200 to 400 joules is mandatory treatment for ventricular fibrillation and for ventricular flutter that has caused loss of consciousness. Cardiopulmonary resuscitation is employed only until defibrillation equipment is readied. *Time should not be wasted with cardiopulmonary resuscitation maneuvers if electrical defibrillation can be done promptly.* Defibrillation requires fewer joules if done early.[401a] If the circulation is markedly inadequate despite return to sinus rhythm, closed-chest massage with artificial ventilation as needed should be instituted. The use of anesthesia during electrical shock obviously is dictated by the patient's condition and is generally not required. After conversion of the arrhythmia to a normal rhythm, it is essential to monitor the rhythm continuously and to institute measures to prevent a recurrence.

Metabolic acidosis quickly follows cardiovascular collapse. If the arrhythmia is terminated within 30 to 60 seconds, significant acidosis does not occur. The use of sodium bicarbonate to reverse the acidosis may be necessary, but its efficacy is presently being reevaluated (p. 777). Intravenous calcium generally is recommended only for situations characterized by hypocalcemia, hyperkalemia, calcium-antagonist overdose, and possibly electromechanical dissociation.

In this short period of time, artificial ventilation by means of a tightly fitting rubber face mask and an Ambu bag is quite satisfactory and eliminates the delay attending intubation by inexperienced personnel. If such a mask and bag are not available, mouth-to-mouth or mouth-to-nose resuscitation is indicated. It is important to reemphasize that there should be *no delay in instituting electrical shock.* If the patient is not monitored and it cannot be established whether asystole or ventricular fibrillation caused the cardiovascular collapse, the electrical shock should be administered *without* wasting precious seconds attempting to obtain an electrocardiogram. The DC shock may cause the asystolic heart to begin discharging and also terminate ventricular fibrillation, if the latter is present. Lidocaine administration may be associated with asystole.[401b]

A search for conditions contributing to the initiation of ventricular flutter or fibrillation should be made and the conditions corrected, if possible. Initial medical approaches to prevent a recurrence of ventricular fibrillation include intravenous administration of lidocaine, bretylium, procainamide, quinidine, disopyramide, or amiodarone. (Disopyramide and amiodarone are not approved for IV use by the FDA at the time of this writing.) Beta blockers may reduce the incidence of ventricular fibrillation following acute myocardial infarction. Ventricular fibrillation rarely spontaneously terminates and death results unless countermeasures are instituted immediately. Subsequent therapy is necessary to prevent a recurrence.[402]

HEART BLOCK

Heart block is a disturbance of impulse conduction that can be permanent or transient, owing to anatomical or functional impairment. It must be distinguished from *interference*, a normal phenomenon that is a disturbance of impulse conduction caused by physiological refractoriness due to inexcitability from a preceding impulse. Either interference or block can occur at any site where impulses are conducted, but they are recognized most commonly between the sinus node and atrium (SA block), between the atria and ventricles (AV block), within the atria (intraatrial block), or within the ventricles (intraventricular block). During AV block, the block can occur in the AV node, His bundle, or bundle branches. In some instances of bundle branch block the impulse may only be delayed and not completely blocked in the bundle branch, yet the resulting QRS complex may be indistinguishable from a QRS complex generated by complete bundle branch block.

The conduction disturbance is classified by severity in three categories. During *first degree heart block*, conduction time is prolonged but all impulses are conducted. *Second degree heart block* occurs in two forms: Mobitz type I (Wenckebach) and type II. Type I heart block is characterized by a progressive lengthening of the conduction time until an impulse is not conducted. Type II heart block denotes occasional or repetitive sudden block of conduction of an impulse without prior measurable lengthening of conduction time. When no impulses are conducted, *complete* or *third degree block* is present. The degree of block may depend in part on the direction of impulse propagation. For unknown reasons, normal retrograde conduction can occur in the presence of advanced anterograde AV block. The reverse can also occur. Some electrocardiographers use the term *advanced heart block* to indicate blockage of two or more consecutive impulses.

Certain features of type I second degree block deserve special emphasis because when actual conduction times are not apparent in the electrocardiogram, for example, during SA, junctional, or ventricular exit block (see Fig. 24–42), type I conduction disturbance can be difficult to recognize. During typical type I block, the increment in conduction time is greatest in the second beat of the Wenckebach group, and the absolute *increase* in conduction time *decreases* progressively over subsequent beats. These two features serve to establish the characteristics of classic Wenckebach group beating: (1) the interval between successive beats progressively decreases, although the conduction time increases (but by a decreasing function); (2) the duration of the pause produced by the nonconducted impulse is less than twice the interval preceding the blocked impulse (which is usually the shortest interval); and (3) the cycle following the nonconducted beat (beginning the Wenckebach group) is longer than the cycle preceding the blocked impulse. Although much emphasis has been placed on this characteristic grouping of cycles, primarily to be able to diagnose Wenckebach exit block, this typical grouping occurs in fewer than 50 per cent of patients who have type I Wenckebach AV nodal block.

Differences in these cycle-length patterns can result from changes in pacemaker rate (e.g., sinus arrhythmia), in neurogenic control of conduction, and changes in the increment of conduction delay. For example, if the P-R increment in the last cycle *increases*, the R-R cycle of the last conducted beat may lengthen rather than shorten. In addition, since the last conducted beat is often at a critical state of conduction, it may become blocked, producing a 5:3 or 3:1 conduction ratio instead of a 5:4 or 3:2 ratio. During a 3:2 Wenckebach structure, the duration of the cycle following the nonconducted beat will be the same as the duration of the cycle preceding the nonconducted beat.

ATRIOVENTRICULAR (AV) BLOCK

AV block exists when the atrial impulse is conducted with delay or is not conducted at all to the venticle at a time when the AV junction is not physiologically refractory.

FIRST DEGREE AV BLOCK. During first degree AV block, every atrial impulse conducts to the ventricles, producing a regular ventricular rate, but the P-R interval exceeds 0.20 sec in the adult. P-R intervals as long as 1.0 sec have been noted and at times can exceed the P-P interval, a phenomenon known as "skipped" P waves. Clinically important P-R interval prolongation can result from conduction delay in the AV node (A-H interval), in the His-Purkinje system (H-V interval), or at both sites. Equally delayed conduction over both bundle branches uncommonly can produce P-R prolongation without significant QRS complex aberration. Occasionally, intraatrial conduction delay can result in P-R prolongation. If the QRS complex in the scalar ECG is normal in contour and duration, the AV delay almost always resides in the AV node, rarely within the His bundle itself. If the QRS complex shows a bundle branch block pattern, conduction delay may be within the AV node and/or His-Purkinje system (Fig. 24–40). In this latter instance, His bundle electrocardiography is necessary to localize the site of conduction delay. Acceleration of the atrial rate or enhancement of vagal tone by carotid massage may cause first degree AV nodal block to progress to type I second degree AV block. Conversely, type I second degree AV nodal block may revert to first degree block with deceleration of the sinus rate.

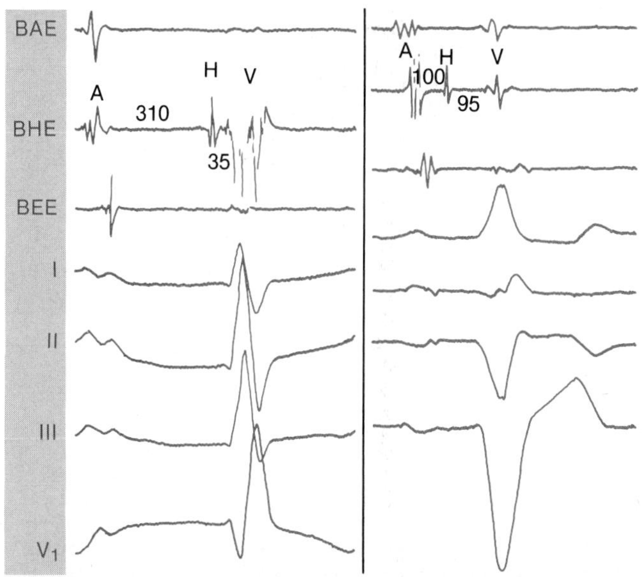

FIGURE 24–40. First degree AV block. One complex during sinus rhythm is shown. The P-R interval in the left panel measured 370 msec (P-A = 25 msec; A-H = 310 msec; H-V = 35 msec) during a right bundle branch block. Conduction delay in the AV node causes the first degree AV block. In the panel on the right, the P-R interval is 230 msec (P-A = 35 msec; A-H = 100 msec; H-V = 95 msec) during a left bundle branch block. The conduction delay in the His-Purkinje system causes the first degree AV block.

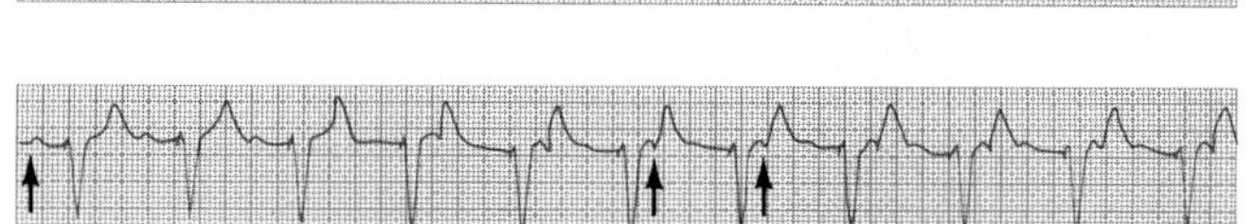

FIGURE 24–41. Unidirectional block. *Top,* During spontaneous sinus rhythm at a rate of 68 beats/min, 2:1 anterograde AV conduction occurs. In the bottom ECG, during ventricular pacing at a rate of 70 beats/min, 1:1 retrograde conduction is seen. P waves are indicated by arrows.

SECOND DEGREE AV BLOCK (Figs. 24–41, 24–42, and 24–43). The block of some atrial impulses conducted to the ventricle at a time when physiological interference is not involved constitutes second degree AV block. The non-

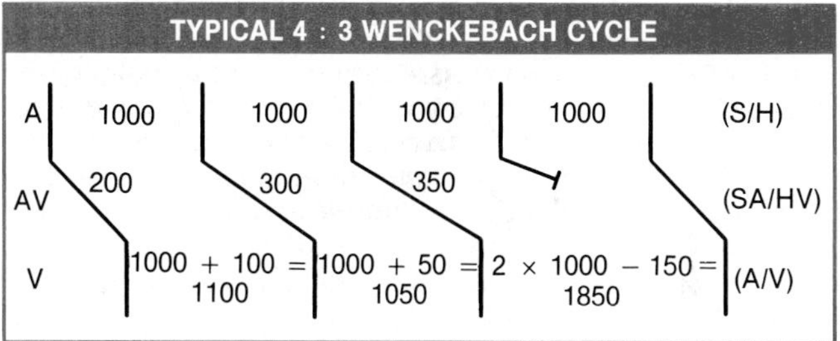

FIGURE 24–42. Typical 4:3 Wenckebach cycle. P waves ("A" tier) occur at a cycle length of 1000 msec. The P-R interval ("A-V" tier) is 200 msec for the first beat and generates a ventricular response ("V" tier). The P-R interval increases by 100 msec in the next complex, resulting in an R-R interval of 1100 msec (1000 + 100). The increment in the P-R interval is only 50 msec for the third cycle, and the P-R interval becomes 350 msec. The R-R interval shortens to 1050 msec (1000 + 50). The next P wave blocks, creating an R-R interval that is less than twice the P-P interval by an amount equal to the increments in the P-R interval. Thus, the Wenckebach features explained in the text can be found in this diagram. If the increment in the P-R interval of the last conducted complex *increased* rather than decreased (e.g., 150 msec rather than 50 msec) then the last R-R interval before the block would increase (1150 msec) rather than decrease and thus become an example of atypical Wenckebach (Fig. 24–43).

If this were a Wenckebach exit block from the sinus node to the atrium, the sinus node cycle length (S) would be 1000 msec, and the S-A interval would increase from 200 to 300 to 350 msec, culminating in block. These events would be inapparent in the scalar ECG. However, the P-P interval in the ECG would shorten from 1100 to 1050 msec and finally there would be a pause of 1850 msec (A) (Fig. 24–4). If this were a junctional rhythm arising from the His bundle and conducting to the ventricle, the junctional rhythm cycle length would be 1000 msec (H), and the H-V interval would progressively lengthen from 200 to 300 to 350 msec, while the R-R interval would decrease from 1100 to 1050 msec and then increase to 1850 msec (V). The only clue to the Wenckebach exit block would be the cycle length changes in the ventricular rhythm.

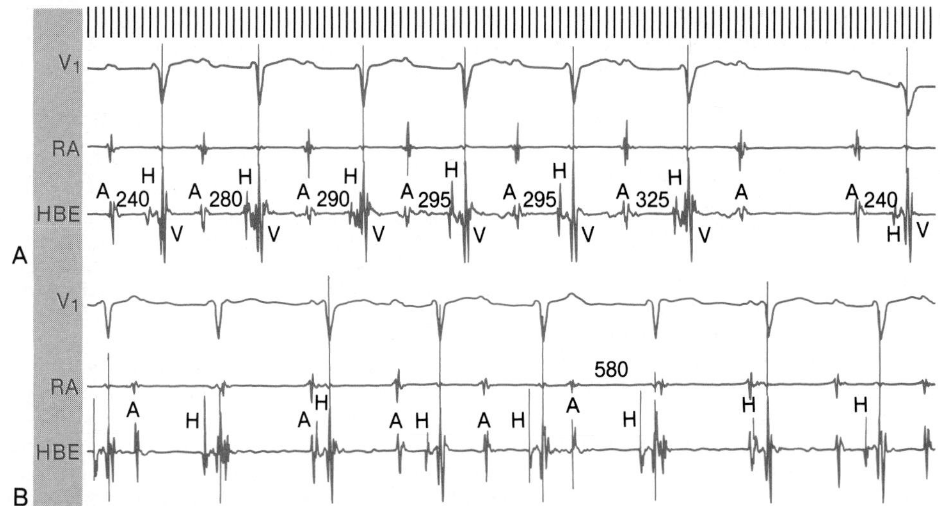

FIGURE 24–43. Type I (Wenckebach) atrioventricular nodal block (panel A). During spontaneous sinus rhythm, progressive P-R prolongation occurs, culminating in a nonconducted P wave. From the His bundle recording (HBE), it is apparent that the conduction delay and subsequent block occurs within the AV node. Since the increment in conduction delay does not consistently decrease, the R-R intervals do not reflect the classic Wenckebach structure diagrammed in Figure 24–42. Panel B was recorded 5 min following 0.6 mg IV atropine. Atropine has had its predominant effect on sinus and junctional automaticity at this time, with little improvement in AV conduction. Consequently, more P waves are blocked and AV dissociation, due to a combination of AV block and enhanced junctional discharge rate, is present. At 8 min (not shown) 1 : 1 atrioventricular conduction occurred, when atropine finally improved AV conduction.

conducted P wave can be intermittent or frequent, at regular or irregular intervals, and can be preceded by fixed or lengthening P-R intervals. A distinguishing feature is that conducted P waves relate to the QRS complex with recurring P-R intervals, i.e., the association of P with QRS is not random. Wenckebach and Hay, by analyzing the *a-c* and *v* waves in the jugular venous pulse, described two types of second degree AV block. After the introduction of the electrocardiograph, Mobitz classified them as type I and type II. Electrocardiographically, typical type I second degree AV block is characterized by progressive P-R prolongation culminating in a nonconducted P wave (Figs. 24–42 and 24–43), while in type II second degree AV block, the P-R interval remains constant prior to the blocked P wave (Fig. 24–44*A*). In both instances the AV block is intermittent and generally repetitive and can block several P waves in a row. Often, the eponyms Mobitz type I and Mobitz type II are applied to the two types of block, while the term "Wenckebach block" refers to type I block only. Wenckebach block in the His-Purkinje system in a patient with a bundle branch block can resemble AV nodal Wenckebach block very closely (Fig. 24–44*B*).

Although it has been suggested that type I and type II AV block may be different manifestations of the same electrophysiological mechanism, differing only quantitatively in the size of the increments, clinically separating second degree AV block into type I and type II serves a useful function and, in most instances, the differentiation can be made easily and reliably from the surface ECG. Type II AV block often antedates the development of Adams-Stokes syncope and complete AV block, while type I AV block with a normal QRS complex is generally more benign and does not progress to more advanced forms of AV conduction disturbance. In older people, type I AV block with or without bundle branch block has been associated with a clinical picture similar to that in type II AV block.

In the patient with an acute myocardial infarction, type I AV block usually accompanies inferior infarction (perhaps more often if a right ventricular infarction also occurs), is transient, and does not require temporary pacing, whereas type II AV block occurs in the setting of an acute anterior myocardial infarction, can require temporary or permanent pacing, and is associated with a high rate of mortality, generally due to pump failure. A high degree of AV block can occur in patients with acute inferior myocardial infarction and is associated with more myocardial damage and a higher mortality rate compared to those without AV block.

While type I conduction disturbance is ubiquitous and can occur in any cardiac tissue in vivo, as well as in vitro even in single cells,[402a] the site of block for the usual forms of second degree AV block can be judged from the surface ECG with sufficient reliability to permit clinical decisions without requiring invasive electrophysiological studies in most instances. Type I AV block with a normal QRS complex almost always takes place at the level of the AV node, proximal to the

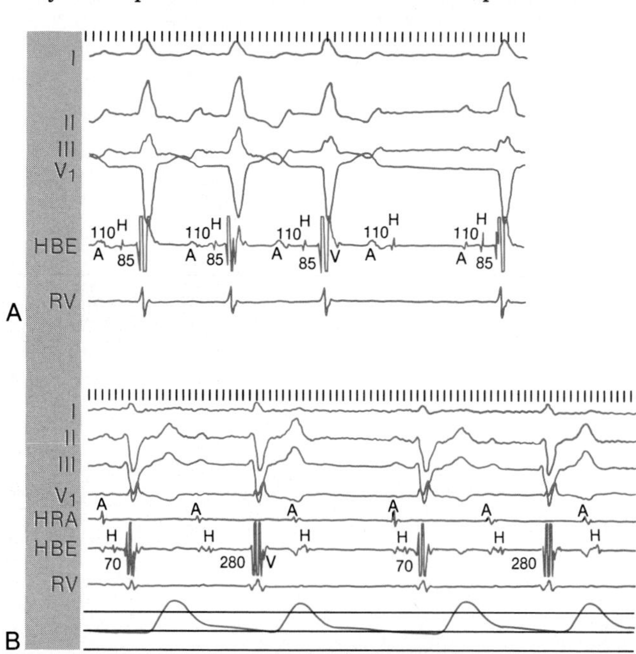

FIGURE 24–44. Type II AV block. *A,* Sudden development of His-Purkinje block is apparent. The A-H and H-V intervals remain constant, as does the P-R interval. Left bundle branch block is present. *B,* Wenckebach AV block in the His-Purkinje system. The QRS complex exhibits a right bundle branch block morphology. However, note that the second QRS complex in the 3 : 2 conduction exhibits a slightly different contour from the first QRS complex, particularly in V_1. This is the clue that the Wenckebach AV block might be in the His-Purkinje system. The HV interval increases from 70 msec to 280 msec, and then block distal to His results.

His bundle. An exception is the uncommon patient with type I intrahisian block. Type II AV block, particularly in association with a bundle branch block, is localized to the His-Purkinje system. Type I AV block in a patient with a bundle branch block can be due to block in the AV node or in the His-Purkinje system. Type II AV block in a patient with a normal QRS complex can be due to intrahisian AV block, but the block is likely to be type I AV nodal block, which exhibits small increments in AV conduction time.

DIFFERENTIATING TYPE I FROM TYPE II AV BLOCK

The above generalizations encompass the vast majority of patients who present with second degree AV block. However, certain caveats must be heeded to avoid misdiagnosis because of subtle ECG changes or exceptions:

1. The 2:1 AV block can be a form of type I or type II AV block (Fig. 24–45). If the QRS complex is normal, the block is more likely to be type I, located in the AV node, and one should search for a transition of the 2:1 block to 3:2 block, during which the P-R interval lengthens in the second cardiac cycle. If a bundle branch block is present, the block can be located either in the AV node or in the His-Purkinje system.
2. AV block can occur simultaneously at two or more levels and can cause difficulty in distinguishing between types I and II.
3. If the atrial rate varies, it can alter conduction times and cause type I AV block to simulate type II or change type II AV block into type I. For example, if the shortest atrial cycle length that just achieved 1:1 AV nodal conduction at a constant P-R interval is decreased by as little as 10 or 20 msec, the P wave of the shortened cycle can block at the level of the AV node without an apparent increase in the antecedent P-R interval. Apparent type II AV block in the His-Purkinje system can be converted to type I in the His-Purkinje system in some patients by increasing the atrial rate.
4. Concealed premature His depolarizations can create electrocardiographic patterns that simulate type I or type II AV block (see Fig. 22–33, p. 617).
5. Abrupt, transient alterations in autonomic tone can cause sudden block of one or more P waves without altering the P-R interval of the conducted P wave before or after block. Thus, apparent type II AV block would be produced at the AV node. Clinically, a burst of vagal tone usually lengthens the P-P interval as well as producing AV block.
6. The response of the AV block to autonomic changes, either spontaneous or induced to distinguish type I from type II AV block, can be misleading. Although vagal stimulation generally increases and vagolytic agents decrease the extent of type I AV block, such conclusions are based on the assumption that the intervention acts primarily on the AV node and fail to consider rate changes. For example, atropine can minimally improve conduction in the AV node and markedly increase the sinus rate, resulting in an *increase* in AV nodal conduction time and the degree of AV block as a result of the faster atrial rate (Fig. 24–43*B*). Conversely, if an increase in vagal tone minimally prolongs AV conduction time but greatly slows the heart rate, the net effect on type I AV block may be to improve conduction. In general, however, carotid sinus massage improves and atropine worsens AV conduction in patients with His-Purkinje block, while the opposite results are to be expected in patients who have AV nodal block. These two interventions can help differentiate the site of block without invasive study, although damaged His–Purkinje tissue may be influenced by changes in autonomic tone.
7. During type I AV block with high ratios of conducted beats, the increment in P-R interval can be quite small, suggesting type II AV block if only the last few P-R intervals before the blocked P wave are measured. By comparing the P-R interval of the first beat in the long Wenckebach cycle with that of the beats immediately preceding the blocked P wave, the increment in AV conduction becomes readily apparent.
8. The classic AV Wenckebach structure depends on a stable atrial rate and a maximal increment in AV conduction time for the second P-R interval of the Wenckebach cycle, with a progressive decrease in subsequent beats. Unstable or unusual alterations in the increment of AV conduction time or in the atrial rate, often seen with long Wenckebach cycles, result in atypical forms of type I AV block in which the last R-R interval can lengthen because the P-R increment *increases;* these are common.
9. Finally, it is important to remember that the P-R interval in the scalar ECG is made up of conduction through the atrium, the AV node, and the His-Purkinje system. An increment in HV conduction, for example, can be masked in the scalar ECG by a reduction in the A-H interval, and the resulting P-R interval will not reflect the entire increment in His-Purkinje conduction time. Very long P-R intervals (>200 msec) are more likely to

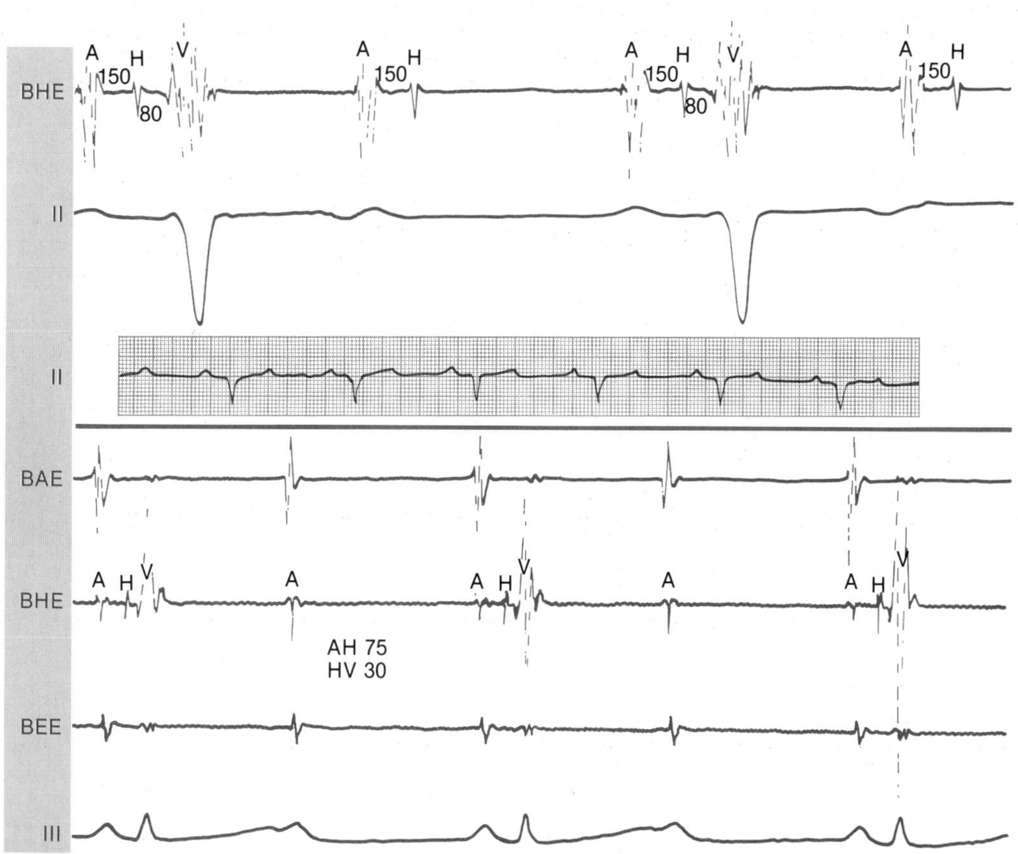

FIGURE 24–45. 2:1 AV block proximal and distal to the His bundle deflection in two different patients. ***Top,*** **2:1 AV block seen in the scalar ECG occurs distal to the His bundle recording site in a patient with right bundle branch block and anterior hemiblock. The A-H interval (150 msec) and H-V interval (80 msec) are both prolonged.** ***Bottom,*** **2:1 AV block occurs proximal to the bundle of His in a patient with a normal QRS complex. The A-H interval (75 msec) and the H-V interval (30 msec) remain constant and normal.**

result from AV nodal conduction delay (and block), with or without concomitant His-Purkinje conduction delay, although an HV interval of 350 msec is quite possible.

First degree and type I second degree AV block can occur in normal healthy children, and Wenckebach AV block can be a normal phenomenon in well-trained athletes, probably related to an increase in resting vagal tone. Occasionally, progressive worsening of the Wenckebach AV conduction disorder can result so that the athlete becomes symptomatic and has to decondition. In patients who have chronic second degree AV nodal block (proximal to the His bundle) without structural heart disease, the course is relatively benign (except in older age groups), while in those who have structural heart disease the prognosis is poor and related to underlying heart disease. *Advanced AV block* indicates block of two or more consecutive P waves.

COMPLETE AV BLOCK

ELECTROCARDIOGRAPHIC RECOGNITION. Complete AV block occurs when no atrial activity conducts to the ventricles and therefore the atria and ventricles are controlled by independent pacemakers. Thus, complete AV block is one type of complete AV dissociation (see p. 715). The atrial pacemaker can be sinus or ectopic (tachycardia, flutter, or fibrillation) or can result from an AV junctional focus occurring above the block with retrograde atrial conduction. The ventricular focus is usually located just below the region of block, which can be above or below the His bundle bifurcation. Sites of ventricular pacemaker activity that are in, or closer to, the His bundle appear to be more stable and may produce a faster escape rate than those located more distally in the ventricular conduction system. The ventricular rate in acquired complete heart block is less than 40 beats/min but may be faster in congenital complete AV block. The ventricular rhythm, usually regular, can vary owing to premature ventricular complexes, a shift in the pacemaker site, an irregularly discharging pacemaker focus, or autonomic influences.

CLINICAL FEATURES. Complete AV block can result from block at the level of the AV node (usually congenital) (Fig. 24–46), within the bundle of His, or distal to it in the Purkinje system (usually acquired) (Fig. 24–47). Block proximal to the His bundle generally exhibits normal QRS complexes and rates of 40 to 60 beats/min because the escape focus that controls the ventricle arises in or near the His bundle. In complete AV nodal block, the P wave is not followed by a His deflection, but each ventricular complex is preceded by a His deflection (Fig. 24–46). His bundle electrocardiography can be useful to differentiate AV nodal from intrahisian block, since the latter may carry a more serious prognosis than the former. Intrahisian block is recognized infrequently without invasive studies. In patients with AV nodal block, atropine usually speeds both the atrial and the ventricular rates. Exercise can reduce the extent of AV nodal block. Acquired complete AV block occurs most commonly distal to the bundle of His owing to trifascicular conduction disturbance. Each P wave is followed by a His deflection, and the ventricular escape complexes are not preceded by a His deflection (Fig. 24–47). The QRS complex is abnormal and the ventricular rate is usually less than 40 beats/min.

Unusual forms such as paroxysmal AV block or AV block following a period of rapid ventricular rate can occur. Paroxysmal AV block[403] in some instances can be due to hyperresponsiveness of the AV node to vagotonic reflexes. Surgery, electrolyte disturbances, endocarditis, tumors, Chagas' disease, rheumatoid nodules, calcific aortic stenosis, myxedema, polymyositis, infiltrative processes (such as amyloid, sarcoid, or scleroderma), and an almost endless assortment of common and unusual conditions can produce AV block. In the adult, drug toxicity, coronary disease, and degenerative processes appear to be the most common causes of AV heart block. The degenerative process produces partial or complete anatomical

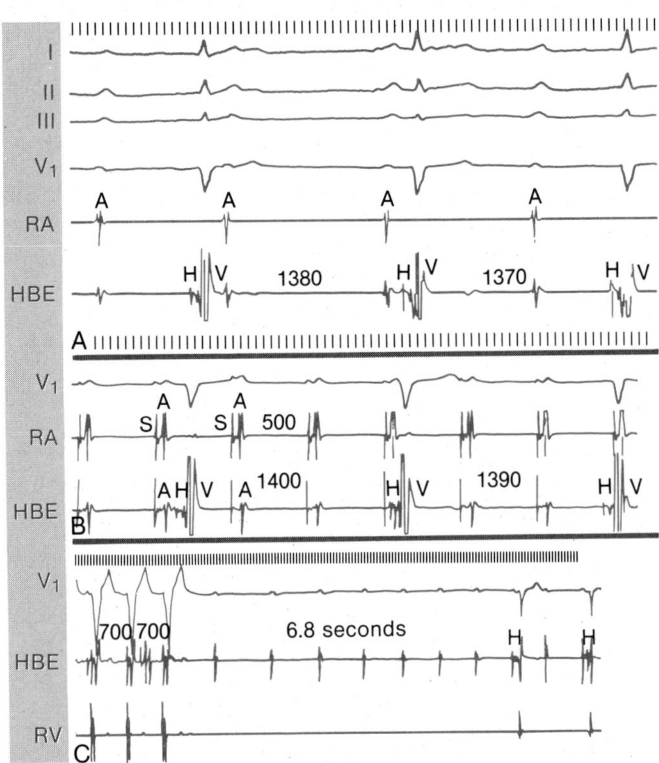

FIGURE 24–46. Congenital third degree AV block. In panel A, complete AV nodal block is apparent. No P wave is followed by a His bundle potential, while each ventricular depolarization is preceded by a His bundle potential. In panel B, atrial pacing (cycle length 500 msec) fails to alter cycle length of the functional rhythm. Still, no P wave is followed by a His bundle potential. In panel C, after 30 seconds of ventricular pacing (cycle length 700 msec), suppression of the junctional focus results for almost 7 sec (overdrive suppression of automaticity; see Chapter 20).

or electrical disruption within the AV nodal region, the AV bundle, or both bundle branches. Rapid rates can sometimes be followed by block, an event known as overdrive suppression of conduction. This form of block may be important as a cause of paroxysmal AV block after cessation of a tachycardia.[404]

AV Block in Children. In children, the most common etiological category of AV block is congenital (Chap. 31). Under such circumstances the AV block can be an isolated finding or associated with other lesions. Connective tissue disease (p. 1721) and the presence of anti–Rh_o negative antibodies in

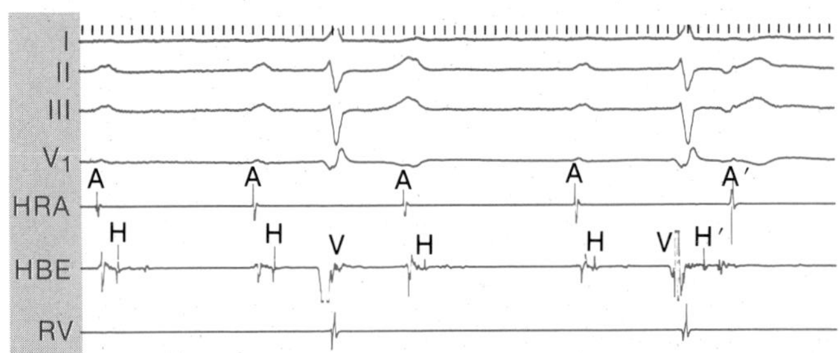

FIGURE 24–47. Complete anterograde AV block with retrograde VA conduction. All of the sinus P waves block distal to His, consistent with acquired complete AV block. The ventricles escape at a cycle length of approximately 1800 msec (33 beats/min) and are not preceded by His bundle activation. The ventricular escape rhythm produces a QRS contour with left axis deviation and right bundle branch block, possibly due to impulse origin in the posterior fascicle of the left bundle branch. Of interest is the fact that the second ventricular escape beat conducts retrogradely through His (H′) and to the atrium (note the low-high atrial activation sequence and the negative P wave in leads II and III). The first ventricular complex does not conduct retrogradely, probably because the His bundle is still refractory from the immediately atrial impulse.

maternal sera of patients with congenital complete AV block raise the possibility that placentally transmitted antibodies play a role in some instances. Anatomical disruption between the atrial musculature and peripheral parts of the conduction system, and nodoventricular discontinuity are two common histological findings. Children are most often asymptomatic; however, some may develop symptoms that require pacemaker implantation. Mortality from congenital AV block is highest in the neonatal period, is much lower during childhood and adolescence, and increases slowly later in life. Adams-Stokes attacks can occur in patients with congenital heart block at any age. It is difficult to predict the prognosis in the individual patient. A persistent heart rate at rest of 50 beats/min or less correlates with the incidence of syncope, and extreme bradycardia can contribute to the frequency of Adams-Stokes attacks in children with congenital complete AV block. The site of block may not separate symptomatic children who have congenital or surgically-induced complete heart block from those without symptoms. Prolonged recovery times of escape foci following rapid pacing (Fig. 24–46C) (see discussion of sinus node recovery time, p. 617) slow heart rates on 24-hour ECG recordings,[405] and the occurrence of paroxysmal tachycardias may be predisposing factors to the development of symptoms.

CLINICAL FEATURES. Many of the signs of AV block are demonstrated at the bedside. First degree AV block can be recognized by a long *a-c* wave interval in the jugular venous pulse and by diminished intensity of the first heart sound as the P-R interval lengthens. In type I second degree AV block, the heart rate may increase imperceptibly with gradually diminishing intensity of the first heart sound, widening the *a-c* interval terminated by a pause, and an *a* wave not followed by a *v* wave. Intermittent ventricular pauses and *a* waves in the neck not followed by *v* waves characterize type II AV block. The first heart sound maintains a constant intensity. In complete AV block, the findings are the same as those in AV dissociation (see below).

Significant clinical manifestations of first and second degree AV block usually consist of palpitations or subjective feelings of the heart "missing a beat." Persistent 2:1 AV block can produce symptoms of chronic bradycardia. Complete AV block can be accompanied by signs and symptoms of reduced cardiac output, syncope or presyncope, angina, or palpitations due to ventricular tachyarrhythmias.

MANAGEMENT. As discussed in detail in Chapter 25, drugs cannot be relied on to increase the heart rate for more than several hours to several days in patients with symptomatic heart block without producing significant side effects. Therefore, temporary or permanent pacemaker insertion is indicated in patients with symptomatic bradyarrhythmias. For short-term therapy when the block is likely to be evanescent but still requires treatment or until adequate pacing therapy can be established, vagolytic agents such as atropine are useful for patients who have AV nodal disturbances, while catecholamines such as isoproterenol can be used transiently to treat patients who have heart block at any site (see treatment for Sinus Bradycardia, above). Isoproterenol should be used with extreme caution or not at all in patients who have acute myocardial infarction. The use of transcutaneous pacing is preferable.[406]

ATRIOVENTRICULAR (AV) DISSOCIATION

CLASSIFICATION. As the term indicates, dissociated or independent beating of atria and ventricles defines AV dissociation. AV dissociation is never a *primary* disturbance of rhythm but is a "symptom" of an underlying rhythm disturbance produced by one of three causes or a combination of causes (Fig. 24–48), that prevent the normal transmission of impulses from atrium to ventricle, as follows:

1. Slowing of the dominant pacemaker of the heart (usually the sinus node), which allows escape of a subsidiary or latent pacemaker. AV dissociation by *default* of the primary pacemaker to a subsidiary one in this manner is often a normal phenomenon. It may occur during sinus arrhythmia or sinus bradycardia, permitting an independent AV junction rhythm to arise (see Fig. 24–2*B*).

2. Acceleration of a latent pacemaker that *usurps* control of the ventricles. Abnormally enhanced discharge rate of a usually slower subsidiary pacemaker is pathological and commonly occurs during nonparoxysmal AV junctional tachycardia or ventricular tachycardia without retrograde atrial capture (see Figs. 24–18 and 24–33).

3. Block, generally at the AV junction, that prevents impulses formed at a normal rate in a dominant pacemaker from reaching the ventricles and allows the ventricles to beat under the control of a subsidiary pacemaker. Junctional or ventricular escape rhythm during AV block, without retrograde atrial capture, is a common example in which block gives rise to AV

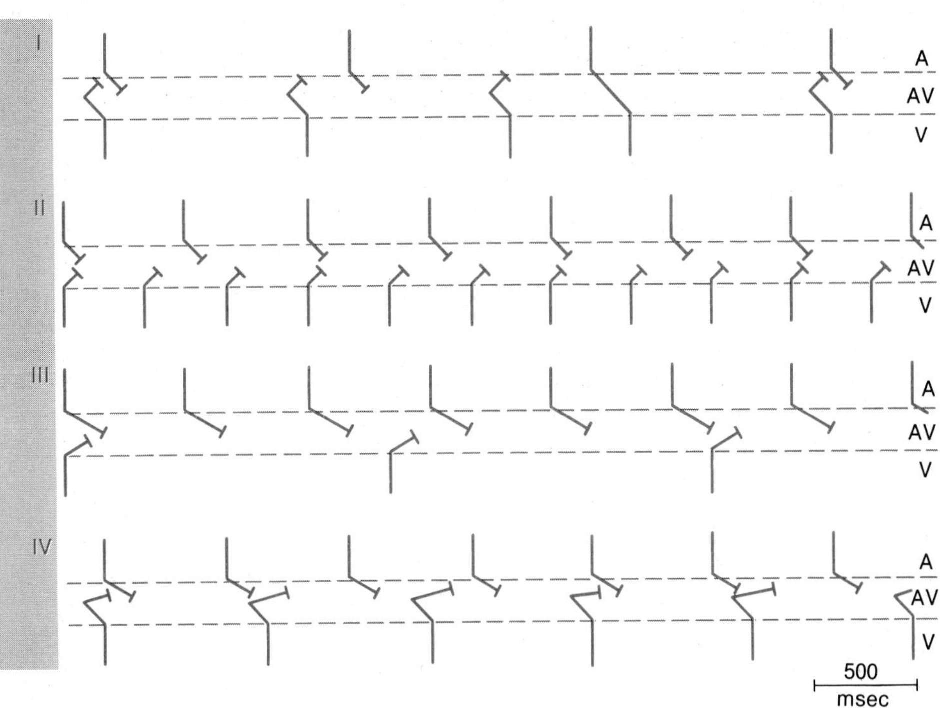

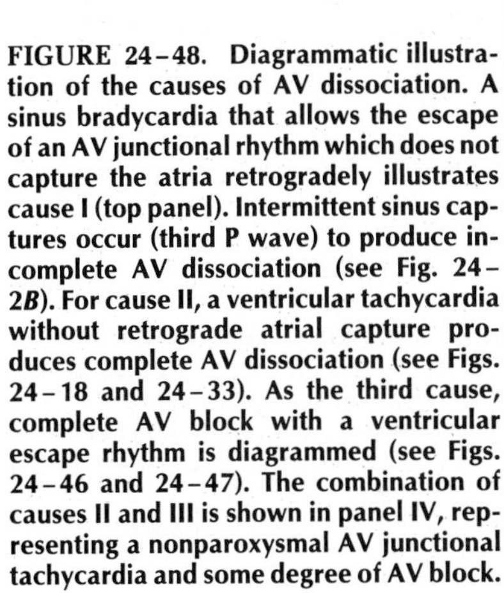
FIGURE 24–48. Diagrammatic illustration of the causes of AV dissociation. A sinus bradycardia that allows the escape of an AV junctional rhythm which does not capture the atria retrogradely illustrates cause I (top panel). Intermittent sinus captures occur (third P wave) to produce incomplete AV dissociation (see Fig. 24–2*B*). For cause II, a ventricular tachycardia without retrograde atrial capture produces complete AV dissociation (see Figs. 24–18 and 24–33). As the third cause, complete AV block with a ventricular escape rhythm is diagrammed (see Figs. 24–46 and 24–47). The combination of causes II and III is shown in panel IV, representing a nonparoxysmal AV junctional tachycardia and some degree of AV block.

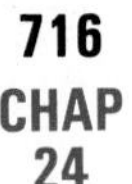

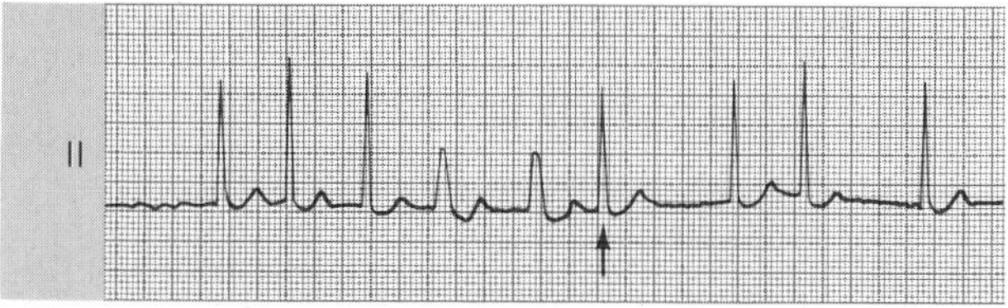

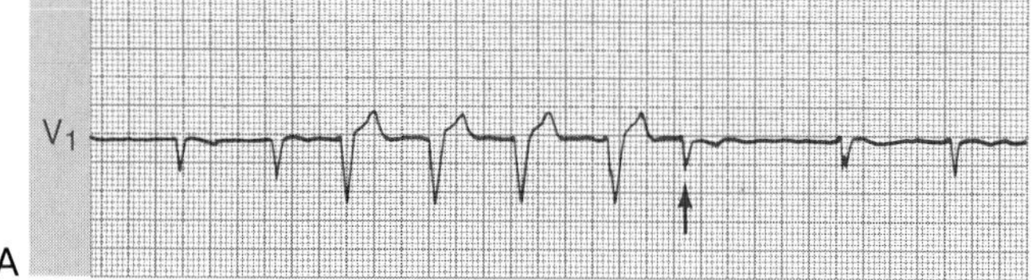

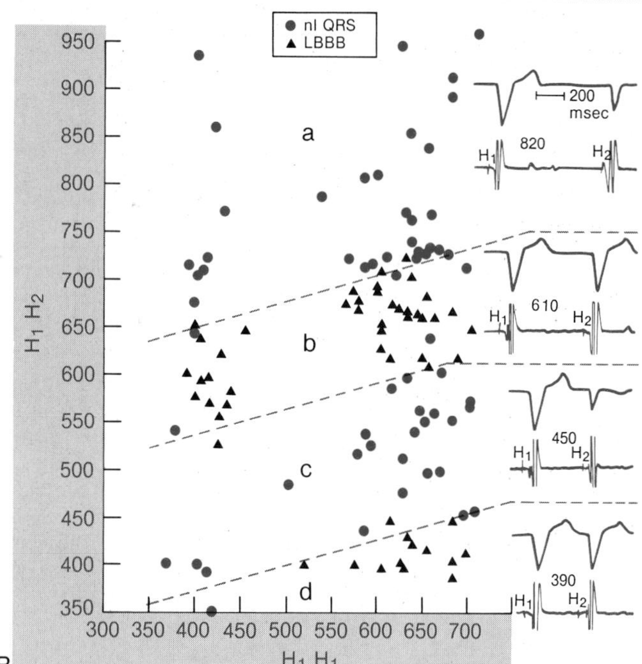

FIGURE 24–49. Supernormal conduction. Panel A illustrates atrial fibrillation with long-short R-R cycle sequences giving rise to QRS complexes conducted with a functional left bundle branch block. In each example, however, a shorter R-R cycle length is terminated by a normal QRS complex (arrow), an example of supernormal conduction.

Panel B shows a graph of the intervals and illustrative recordings during an electrophysiological study of the patient whose ECG is shown in panel A. The H-V interval of the complexes conducted with a left bundle branch block morphology is 45 msec, while the H-V interval of those conducted with a normal morphology is 35 msec. The graph indicates the premature interval (H_1-H_2, ordinate) plotted against the preceding cycle length (H_1-H_1, abscissa). All H_1-H_1 intervals were taken from complexes with a left bundle branch block morphology. Normal complexes are represented by filled circles and left bundle branch block contours by filled triangles. Four zones of conduction are identified, and illustrated by the four examples to the right. The longest H_1-H_2 intervals are followed by a normal intraventricular conduction (zone A), while at shorter intervals, left bundle branch block occurs (zone B). When the H_1-H_2 interval shortens further, normal intraventricular conduction returns and the H-V intervals shorten to 35 msec (zone C, supernormal conduction). At the shortest H_1-H_2 interval, left bundle branch block again appears (zone D). (From Miles, W. M., Prystowsky, E. N., Heger, J. J., and Zipes, D. P.: Evaluation of the patient with wide QRS tachycardia. Med. Clin. North Am. *68:*1015, 1984.)

dissociation. It is important to remember that complete AV block is *not* synonymous with complete AV dissociation: patients who have complete AV block have complete AV dissociation, but patients who have complete AV dissociation may or may not have complete AV block (see Figs. 24–46 and 24–47).

4. A combination of causes can exist, for example, when digitalis excess results in the production of nonparoxysmal AV junctional tachycardia associated with SA or AV block.

MECHANISMS. With this classification in mind, it is important to emphasize that the term "AV dissociation" is *not* a diagnosis and is analogous to the term "jaundice" or "fever." One must state that "AV dissociation is present *due to . . .*" and then give the cause. The accelerated rate of a slower, normally subsidiary pacemaker or the slower rate of a faster, normally dominant pacemaker that prevents conduction due to physiological collision and mutual extinction of opposing wavefronts (interference), or the manifestations of AV block, are the basic disturbances producing AV dissociation. The atria in all these cases beat independently from the ventricles, under control of the sinus node, ectopic atrial, or AV junctional pacemakers, and can exhibit any type of supraventricular rhythms. If a single pacemaker establishes control of both atria and ventricles for one beat (capture) or a series of beats (sinus rhythm, AV junctional rhythm with retrograde atrial capture, ventricular tachycardia with retrograde atrial capture, and so forth), AV dissociation is abolished for that period. Conversely, as stated above, whenever the atria and ventricles fail to respond to a single impulse for one beat (premature ventricular complex without retrograde capture of the atrium) or a series of beats (ventricular tachycardia without retrograde atrial capture), AV dissociation exists for that period. The interruption of AV dissociation by one or a series of beats under the control of one pacemaker, either anterogradely or retrogradely, indicates that the AV dissociation is incomplete. Complete or incomplete dissociation can also occur in association with all forms of AV block. Commonly, when AV dissociation occurs as a result of AV block the atrial rate exceeds the ventricular rate. For example, a subsidiary pacemaker with a rate of 40 beats/min can escape in the presence of a 2:1 AV block when the atrial rate is 78. If the AV block is bidirectional, AV dissociation results.

ELECTROCARDIOGRAPHIC AND CLINICAL FEATURES. The electrocardiogram demonstrates the independence of P waves and QRS complexes. The P-wave morphology depends on the rhythm controlling the atria (sinus, atrial tachycardia, junctional, flutter, or fibrillation). During complete AV dissociation both the QRS complex and the P waves appear regularly spaced without a fixed temporal relationship to each other. When the dissociation is incomplete, a QRS complex of supraventricular contour occurs early and is preceded by a P wave at a P-R interval exceeding 0.12 sec and within a conductable range. This indicates ventricular capture by the supraventricular focus. Similarly, a premature P wave with a retrograde morphology and a conductable R-P interval may indicate retrograde atrial capture by the subsidiary focus.

The physical findings include a variable intensity of the first heart sound as the P-R interval changes, atrial sounds, and *a* waves in the jugular venous pulse lacking a consistent relationship to ventricular contraction. Intermittent large (cannon) *a* waves may be seen in the jugular venous pulse when atrial and ventricular contraction occur simultaneously. The second heart sound can split normally or paradoxically, depending on the manner of ventricular activation. A premature beat representing a ventricular capture may interrupt a regular heart rhythm. When the ventricular rate exceeds the atrial rate, a cyclic increase in intensity of the first heart sound is produced as the P-R interval shortens, climaxed by a very loud sound (bruit de canon). This intense sound is followed by a sudden reduction in intensity of the first heart sound and the appearance of giant *a* waves as the P-R interval shortens and P waves "march through" the cardiac cycle.

MANAGEMENT. This is directed toward the underlying heart disease and precipitating cause. The individual components *producing the AV dissociation*—not the AV dissociation per se—determine the specific type of antiarrhythmic approaches. Therapy ranges from pacemaker insertion in a patient who has AV dissociation due to complete AV block to lidocaine administration in a patient who has AV dissociation due to a ventricular tachycardia.

OTHER ELECTROPHYSIOLOGICAL ABNORMALITIES LEADING TO CARDIAC ARRHYTHMIAS

SUPERNORMAL CONDUCTION AND EXCITATION

Supernormal Conduction. This is the term applied to situations characterized by conduction that is better than expected but generally not as good as normal. The phenomenon almost always occurs when conduction is depressed but can be present in normal cardiac tissues as well. It generally occurs when conduction takes place during the relative refractory period of the preceding complex (Fig. 24–49). The electrophysiological basis can relate, in some examples, to supernormal excitability (see below), but probably to other mechanisms as well. Supernormal conduction commonly has been invoked to explain AV (most probably His-Purkinje rather than AV nodal) conduction that is more rapid than expected or AV conduction that results when AV block is expected.

Supernormal Excitation. This phenomenon results when a stimulus, normally subthreshold, occurs during the supernormal period of recovery of the preceding complex and produces a propagated response. Stimuli occurring earlier or later fail to produce a propagated response. Demonstrated in vitro in Purkinje fibers[406a] but not ventricular muscle, supernormal excitation occurs during phase 3 of the cardiac action potential when the membrane potential, closer to threshold at the end of repolarization, requires less current to produce a propagated response. A similar phenomenon occurs during phase 4 diastolic depolarization or during afterdepolarizations that reduce the membrane potential closer to threshold. The phenomenon is most easily recognized when a non-sensing pacemaker, failing because of battery exhaustion and reduced output, produces a propagated response only when discharge falls during a specific time period in a cardiac cycle (Fig. 24–50). Similar phenomena probably occur spontaneously with "weak" automatic foci, but the recognition of these events clinically is difficult and often speculative.

CONCEALED CONDUCTION

Concealed conduction describes the phenomenon during which impulses penetrate an area of the conduction tissue, the AV node commonly but other areas as well, without emerging. Since the transmission of the impulse is concealed, that is, electrically silent in the standard electrocardiogram, concealed conduction becomes manifested only by its *effects* on the conduction and/or formation of subsequent impulses. The most common example follows a premature ventricular complex. Partial retrograde penetration of the AV node by the premature ventricular complex is *deduced* because the following sinus-initiated P wave blocks to produce a compensatory pause (Fig. 24–51) or conducts with a longer P-R interval if the premature ventricular complex is interpolated. The slower ventricular response when the atrial rate increases from atrial flutter to atrial fibrillation is due to a greater number of atrial impulses blocking (conducting into, without emerging) in the AV node and is a manifestation of concealed conduction. Concealed conduction occurs in WPW syndrome and can be manifested by unidirectional block anterogradely or retrogradely in an accessory pathway (p. 654). Concealed junctional extrasystoles (Fig. 22–33, p. 617) can create electrocardiographic manifestations of apparent AV block. Strict confirmation of concealed conduction should be the demonstration of conduction, such as in the form of conducted junctional extrasystoles (Fig. 24–15, p. 686).

PARASYSTOLE (Fig. 24–52)

This refers to a cardiac arrhythmia characterized electrocardiographically by: (1) varying coupling interval between the ectopic (parasystolic) complex and the dominant (generally, sinus-initiated) complex; (2) a common minimal time interval between interectopic intervals, with the longer interectopic intervals being multiples of this minimal interval; (3) fusion complexes; and (4) the presence of the parasystolic impulse whenever the cardiac chamber is excitable. Parasystole with exit block is suspected when the parasystolic discharge focus fails to appear even though cardiac tissue is excitable. The analogy commonly invoked to represent parasystole is the behavior of a fixed-rate non-sensing (VOO) pacemaker (Chap. 25). Parasystole can occur in the sinus and AV nodes, atrium and ventricle, and AV junction. The parasystolic mechanism presumably results from the regular discharge of an automatic focus that is independent of, and protected from, discharge by the dominant cardiac rhythm. A variety of mech-

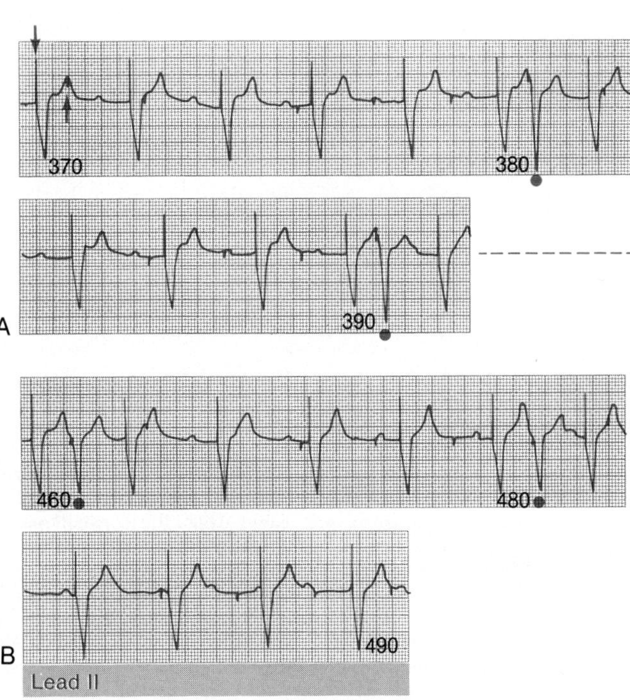

FIGURE 24–50. Supernormal excitation. Panels A and B represent noncontiguous portions of a continuous ECG recording with a middle segment removed (dotted line). The patient presented with a bipolar pacemaker that had exceeded end-of-life and was no longer consistently producing ventricular depolarization (small negative deflections indicated by the upright arrow). A temporary pacemaker was implanted and set at a fixed rate (asynchronous, V00). These large deflections are indicated by the inverted arrow. The numbers in msec indicate the interval between the onset of the QRS complex and the following subthreshold pacemaker stimulus. At intervals of 370 msec (beginning, panel A) and 490 msec (end, panel B), the subthreshold stimulus fails to produce a propagated ventricular response. However, at intervals between 380 and 480 msec, ventricular depolarizations result (filled circles). Thus, the period of supernormal excitation is 100 msec duration, from 380 to 480 msec after the onset of the QRS complex.

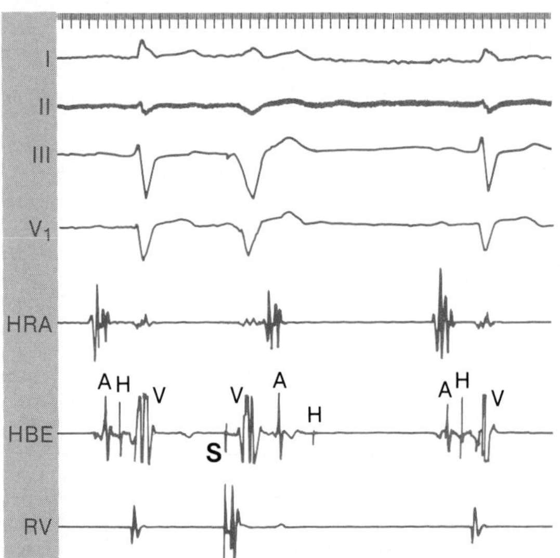

FIGURE 24–51. Concealed conduction. Following the first normally conducted sinus-initiated complex, a premature ventricular complex is stimulated (S). The next spontaneous sinus-initiated P wave blocks to produce a fully compensatory pause. The third sinus-initiated P wave conducts normally. From the His bundle recording it is obvious that the nonconducted sinus beat blocks distal to the His bundle recording site. Note that the A-H interval of the nonconducted sinus P wave beat is prolonged, suggesting that the premature ventricular complex retrogradely activated His and invaded the AV node, making it partially refractory to the next sinus beat. Since retrograde conduction into the AV node is not recorded, and can only be surmised on the basis of the increase in the following A-H interval, it is an example of concealed conduction. Further, since retrograde His and AV node activation by the premature ventricular complex would not be apparent in the scalar ECG but is responsible for the compensatory pause, the blocked P wave is an example of concealed conduction.

anisms have been postulated to explain the apparent protection enjoyed by the parasystolic rhythm.

These "classic" definitions of parasystole now need to be modified because it has been well established that the dominant sinus beats can modulate the discharge rate of the parasystolic rhythm despite entrance block.[62] Thus, wide variations in the modulated parasystolic cycle may occur. The "true" or unmodulated parasystolic cycle length can be determined by finding two consecutive parasystolic complexes without intervening beats. Phase response curves can be generated.[407,408] Fixed coupling between the dominant and parasystolic rhythms can occur due to a variety of mechanisms, including entrainment. It is possible that modulated parasystole in the presence of supernormal excitability can trigger ventricular fibrillation.[409]

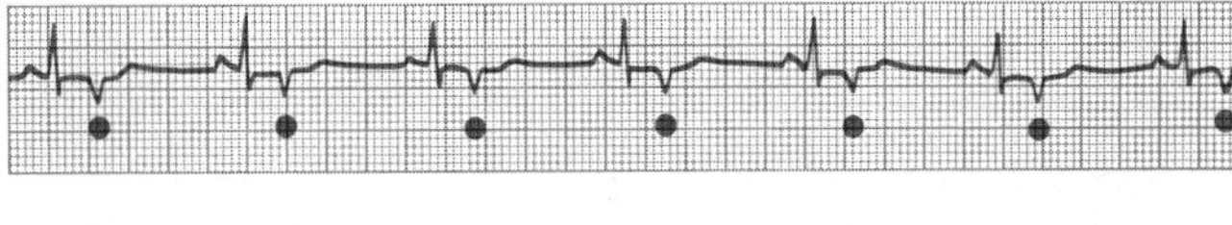

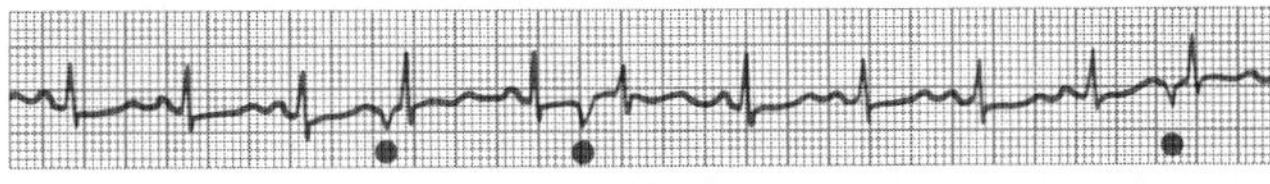

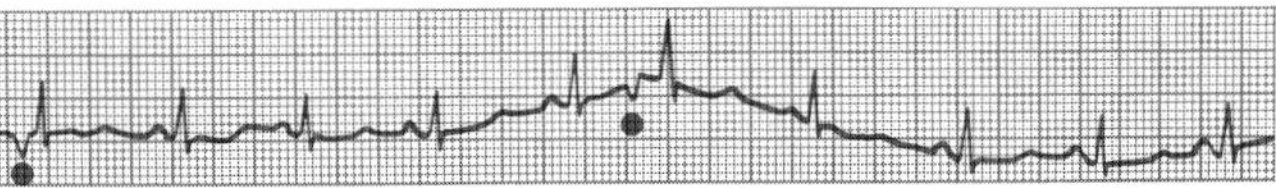

FIGURE 24–52. Atrial parasystole. Top panel, the atrial parasystolic impulses (filled circles under the negative P waves) are present at a fixed coupling interval to the dominant sinus rhythm. The reason for the fixed coupling is as follows: Each time the parasystolic impulse depolarizes the atrium, it also discharges the sinus node. Diastolic depolarization in the sinus node begins at that point (reset) and results in the following sinus P wave (positive P wave). Thus, the constant parasystolic discharge rate (interectopic interval approximately 960 msec), resetting of the sinus node, and constant phase 4 diastolic depolarization in the sinus node combine to result in fixed coupling. Bottom panel, the sinus discharge rate is slightly faster. It is no longer discharged by the parasystolic impulse which is still occurring at approximately 960 msec (slightly longer interval in the bottom tracing). Variable coupling, the usual presentation of parasystole, results. Lead II.

Acknowledgments

The author thanks William M. Miles, M.D. and Lawrence S. Klein, M.D. for critical comments and Joan Zipes and Shirley Myers for secretarial assistance.

REFERENCES

DIAGNOSTIC AND THERAPEUTIC CONSIDERATIONS

1. Ruffy, R., Roman-Smith, P., and Barbey, J. T.: Palpitations: Evaluation and treatment. Prog. Cardiol. *1/2*:131, 1988.
2. Vitullo, J. C., Karam, R., Mekhail, N. et al.: Cocaine-induced small vessel spasm in isolated rat hearts. Am. J. Pathol. *135*:85, 1989.
3. Barak, M., Herschkowitz, S., Shapiro, I., and Roguin, N.: Familial combined sinus node and atrioventricular conduction dysfunctions. Int. J. Cardiol. *15*:231, 1987.
4. Graber, H. L., Unverferth, D. V., Baker, P. B., et al.: Evolution of a hereditary cardiac conduction and muscle disorder: A study involving a family with six generations affected. Circulation *74*:21, 1986.
5. Hiromasa, S., Ikeda, T., Kubota, K., et al: Myotonic dystrophy: Ambulatory electrocardiogram, electrophysiologic study, and echocardiographic evaluation. Am. Heart J. *113*:1482, 1987.
6. Nguyen, H. H., Wolfe, J. T. 3rd, Holmes, D. R., Jr., and Edwards, W. D.: Pathology of the cardiac conduction system in myotonic dystrophy: A study of 12 cases. J. Am. Coll. Cardiol. *11*:662, 1988.
7. Olofsson, B. O., Forsberg, H., Andersson, S., et al.: Electrocardiographic findings in myotonic dystrophy. Br. Heart J. *59*:47, 1988.
8. D'Orsogna, L., O'Shea, J. P., and Miller, G.: Cardiomyopathy of Duchenne muscular dystrophy. Pediatr. Cardiol. *9*:205, 1988.
9. Miller, G., D'Orsogna, L., and O'Shea, J. P.: Autonomic function and the sinus tachycardia of Duchenne muscular dystrophy. Brain Dev. *11*:247, 1989.
10. Perloff, J. K., Roberts, W. C., DeLeon, A. C., Jr., and O'Doherty, D.: The distinctive electrocardiogram of Duchenne's progressive muscular dystrophy. Am. J. Med. *42*:179, 1967.
11. Schmidt, M. A., Michels, V. V., Edwards, W. D., and Miller, F. A.: Familial dilated cardiomyopathy. Am. J. Med. Genet. *31*:135, 1988.
12. Bharati, S., and Lev, M.: *Cardiac Conduction System in Unexplained Sudden Death.* Mt. Kisco, N.Y., Futura Publishing Company, 1990.
13. Mehta, D., Wafa, S., Ward, D. E., and Camm, A. J.: Relative efficacy of various physical manoeuvres in the termination of junctional tachycardia. Lancet *1*(8596):1181, 1988.
14. Zipes, D. P., Akhtar, M., Denes, P., et al.: ACC/AHA guidelines for clinical intracardiac electrophysiologic studies. J. Am. Coll. Cardiol. *14*:1827, 1989 and Circulation *80*:1925, 1989.
15. Packer, D. L., Bardy, G. H., Worley, S. J., et al.: Tachycardia-induced cardiomyopathy: A reversible form of left ventricular dysfunction. Am. J. Cardiol. *57*:563, 1986.
16. Stevenson, W. G., Stevenson, L. W., Weiss, J., and Tillisch, J. H.: Inducible ventricular arrhythmias and sudden death during vasodilator therapy of severe heart failure. Am. Heart J. *116*:1447, 1988.
17. Gradman, A., Deedwania, P., Cody, R., et al.: Predictors of total mortality and sudden death in mild to moderate heart failure. Captopril-Digoxin Study Group. J. Am. Coll. Cardiol. *14*:564, 1989.
18. Wesseling, H., de Graeff, P. A., van Gilst, W. H., and Kingma, J. H.: Cardiac arrhythmias—a new indication for angiotensin-converting enzyme inhibitors. J. Hum. Hypertens. 3(Suppl. I):79, 1989.
19. Swedberg, K., and Kjekshus, J.: Effects of enalapril on mortality in severe congestive heart failure: Results of the Cooperative North Scandinavian Enalapril Survival Study (CONSENSUS). Am. J. Cardiol. *62*:60A, 1988.
20. Acquatella, H., Catalioti, F., Gomez-Mancebo, J. R., et al.: Long-term control of Chagas disease in Venezuela: Effects on serologic findings, electrocardiographic abnormalities, and clinical outcome. Circulation *76*:556, 1987.
21. Inoue, S., Shinohara, F., Sakai, T., et al.: Myocarditis and arrhythmia: A clinico-pathological study of conduction system based on serial section in 65 cases. Jpn. Circ. J. *53*:49, 1989.
22. McAlister, H. F., Klementowicz, P. T., and Andrews, C.: Lyme carditis: An important cause of reversible heart block. Ann. Intern. Med. *110*:339, 1989.
23. Chan, K. Y., Yip, W. C., Tay, J. S., and Rajan, U.: Detection of cardiac problems among school children by health screening. J. Trop. Pediatr. *35*:221, 1989.

INDIVIDUAL CARDIAC ARRHYTHMIAS

24. de Marneffe, M., Jacobs, P., Haardt, R., et al.: Variations of normal sinus node function in relation to age: Role of autonomic influence. Eur. Heart J. *7*:662, 1986.
25. Randall, W. C., and Ardell, J. L.: Nervous control of the heart: Anatomy and pathophysiology. *In* Zipes, D. P., and Jalife, J. (eds.): Cardiac Electrophysiology: From Cell to Bedside. Philadelphia, W. B. Saunders Company, 1990, p. 291.
26. Morady, F., Kou, W. H., and Nelson, S. D.: Accentuated antagonism between beta-adrenergic and vagal effects on ventricular refractoriness in humans. Circulation *77*:289, 1988.

27. Gomes, J. A., and Winters, S. L.: The origins of the sinus node pacemaker complex in man: Demonstration of dominant and subsidiary foci. J. Am. Coll. Cardiol. *9*:45, 1987.
28. Boineau, J. P., Canavan, T. E., Schuessler, R. B., et al.: Demonstration of a widely distributed atrial pacemaker complex in the human heart. Circulation *77*:1221, 1988.
29. Northcote, R. J., Canning, G. P., and Ballantyne, D.: Electrocardiographic findings in male veteran endurance athletes. Br. Heart J. *61*:155, 1989.
30. Coelho, A., Palileo, E., Ashley, W., et al.: Tachyarrhythmias in young athletes. J. Am. Coll. Cardiol. *7*:237, 1986.
31. Arrowood, J. A., Mohanty, P. K., Hodgson, J. M., et al.: Ventricular sensory endings mediate reflex bradycardia during coronary arteriography in humans. Circulation *80*:1293, 1989.
32. Krause, P., Inoue, H., and Zipes, D. P.: Electrophysiologic alterations produced by hypoxia in the canine heart. Am. Heart J. *117*:550, 1989.
33. Kusniec, J., Strasberg, B., Sclarovsky, S., et al.: The effect of intravenous amiodarone on heart rate in patients with acute myocardial infarction or ischemia and sinus tachycardia. Chest *94*:584, 1988.
34. Tsuchioka, Y., Matsumoto, K., Fujii, H., et al.: Electrophysiological effects of propranolol in patients with sinus node dysfunction. Jpn. Heart J. *29*:319, 1988.
35. Schwartz, E., Friedman, E., Mouallem, M., and Farfel, Z.: Sinus arrest associated with clonidine therapy. Clin. Cardiol. *11*:53, 1988.
36. Lemery, R., Talajic, M., Nattel, S., and Theroux, P.: Sinus node dysfunction and sudden cardiac death following treatment with encainide. PACE *12*:1607, 1989.
37. Lee, P. K., Kerr, C. R., Vorderbrugge, S., et al.: Symptomatic sinus node dysfunction associated with the use of propafenone. Am. J. Cardiol. *62*:480, 1988.
38. Schuger, C. D., Tzivoni, D., Gottlieb, S., et al.: Sinus node and atrioventricular nodal function in 220 patients recovering from acute myocardial infarction. Cardiology *75*:274, 1988.
39. Epstein, A. E., Hirschowitz, B. I., and Kirklin, J. K.: Evidence for a central site of action to explain the negative chronotropic effect of atropine: Studies on the human transplanted heart. J. Am. Coll. Cardiol. *15*:1610, 1990.
40. Levander-Lindgren, M., and Lantz, B.: Bradyarrhythmia profile and associated diseases in 1,265 patients with cardiac pacing. PACE *11*:2207, 1988.
41. Rosenqvist, M., Brandt, J., and Schuller, H.: Long-term pacing in sinus node disease: effects of stimulation mode on cardiovascular morbidity and mortality. Am. Heart J. *116*:16, 1988.
42. Kallryd, A., Kruse, I., and Ryden, L.: Atrial inhibited pacing in the sick sinus node syndrome: Clinical value and the demand for rate responsiveness. PACE *12*:954, 1989.
43. Rawles, J. M., Pai, G. R., and Reid, S. R.: A method of quantifying sinus arrhythmia: parallel effect of respiration on P-P and P-R intervals. Clin. Sci. *76*:103, 1989.
44. Bernardi, L., Keller, F., Sanders, M., et al.: Respiratory sinus arrhythmia in the denervated human heart. J. Appl. Physiol. *67*:1447, 1989.
45. Choi, Y. S., Kim, J. J., Oh, B. H., et al.: Cough syncope caused by sinus arrest in a patient with sick sinus syndrome. PACE *12*:883, 1989.
46. Kofflard, M., De Boer, H., and van Mechelen, R.: Reflex cardiac asystole. PACE *9*:908, 1986.
47. Rosenthal, J. E.: Exit block: Cellular mechanisms. *In* Zipes, D. P., and Jalife, J. (eds.): Cardiac Electrophysiology: From Cell to Bedside. Philadelphia, W. B. Saunders Company, 1990, p. 409.
48. Fisch, C.: Electrocardiographic manifestations of exit block. *In* Zipes D. P., and Jalife, J. (eds.): Cardiac Electrophysiology: From Cell to Bedside. Philadelphia, W. B. Saunders Company, 1990, p. 628.
49. Bashour, T. T., Cohen, M. S., Ryan, C., and Antonini, C., Sr.: Sinus node suppression in acute strokes—case reports. Angiology *39*:1048, 1988.
50. Yeh, S. J., Lin, F. C., and Wu, D.: Complete sinoatrial block in two patients with bradycardia-tachycardia syndrome. J. Am. Coll. Cardiol. *9*:1184, 1987.
51. Huang, S. K., Ezri, M. D., Hauser, R. G., and Denes, P.: Carotid sinus hypersensitivity in patients with unexplained syncope: Clinical, electrophysiologic, and long-term follow-up observations. Am. Heart J. *116*:989, 1988.
52. Sasaki, Y., Shimotori, M., Akahane, K., et al.: Long-term follow-up of patients with sick sinus syndrome: A comparison of clinical aspects among unpaced, ventricular inhibited paced, and physiologically paced groups. PACE *11*:1575, 1988.
53. Kuga, K., Yamaguchi, I., Sugishita, Y., and Ito, I.: Assessment by autonomic blockade of age-related changes of the sinus node function and autonomic regulation in sick sinus syndrome. Am. J. Cardiol. *61*:361, 1988.
54. Piwowarska, W., Mroczek-Czernecka, D., and Bacior, B.: Diagnostic value of pharmacological autonomic blockade in patients with suspected sick sinus syndrome. Jpn. Heart J. *29*:639, 1988.
55. Shimizu, A., Fukatani, M., Kitano, K., et al.: The total heart beats per 24 hours by ambulatory electrocardiography and the changes of heart rate by treadmill exercise test in sick sinus syndrome. Jpn. Circ. J. *52*:139, 1988.
56. Ceithaml, E. L., Midgley, F. M., and Perry, L. W.: Long-term results after surgical repair of incomplete endocardial cushion defects. Ann. Thorac. Surg. *48*:413, 1989.
57. Bender, H. W., Jr., Stewart, J. R., Merrill, W. H., et al.: Ten years' experience with the Senning operation for transposition of the great arteries: Physiological results and late follow-up. Ann. Thorac. Surg. *47*:218, 1989.
58. Vetter, V. L., Tanner, C. S., and Horowitz, L. N.: Electrophysiologic consequences of the Mustard repair of d-transposition of the great arteries. J. Am. Coll. Cardiol. *10*:1265, 1987.
58a. Kürer, C. C., Tanner, C. S., and Vetter, V. L.: Electrophysiologic findings after Fontan repair of functional single ventricle. J. Am. Coll. Cardiol. *17*:174, 1991.
59. Onat, A.: Familial sinus node disease and degenerative myopia—a new hereditary syndrome? Hum. Genet. *72*:182, 1986.
60. Bonke, F. I. M., Kirchhof, C.J.H.S., and Allessie, M. A.: Sinus node reentry. *In* Zipes, D. P., and Jalife, J. (eds.): Cardiac Electrophysiology. From Cell to Bedside. Philadelphia, W. B. Saunders Company, 1990, p. 526.
61. Kerr, C. R., Klein, G. G., Guiraudon, G. M., and Webb, J. G.: Surgical therapy for sinoatrial reentrant tachycardia. PACE *11*:776, 1988.
62. Jalife, J., Michaels, D. C., and Langendorf, R.: Modulated parasystole originating in the sinoatrial node. Circulation *74*:945, 1986.
63. Wennmalm, A., and Wennmalm, M.: Coffee, catecholamines and cardiac arrhythmia. Clin. Physiol. *9*:201, 1989.
64. Waldo, A. L., Carlson, M. D., and Henthorn, R. W.: Atrial flutter: transient entrainment and related phenomena. *In* Zipes, D. P., and Jalife, J. (eds.): Cardiac Electrophysiology: From Cell to Bedside. Philadelphia, W. B. Saunders Company, 1990, p. 530.
65. Stanton, M. S., Miles, W. M., and Zipes, D. P.: Atrial fibrillation and flutter. *In* Zipes, D. P., and Jalife, J. (eds.): Cardiac Electrophysiology: From Cell to Bedside. Philadelphia, W. B. Saunders Company, 1990, p. 735.
65a. Olshansky, B., Okumura, K., Hess, P. G., et al.: Demonstration of an area of slow conduction in human atrial flutter. J. Am. Coll. Cardiol. *16*:1639, 1990.
66. Vetter, V. L., Tanner, C. S., and Horowitz, L. N.: Inducible atrial flutter after the Mustard repair of complete transposition of the great arteries. Am. J. Cardiol. *61*:428, 1988.
67. Gembruch, U., Hansmann, M., Redel, D. A., and Bald, R.: Intrauterine therapy of fetal tachyarrhythmias: Intraperitoneal administration of antiarrhythmic drugs to the fetus in fetal tachyarrhythmias with severe hydrops fetalis. J. Perinat. Med. *16*:39, 1988.
68. Maxwell, D. J., Crawford, D. C., Curry, P. V., et al.: Obstetric importance, diagnosis, and management of fetal tachycardias. Br. Med. J. *297*(6641):107, 1988.
69. Crawford, W., Plumb, V. J., Epstein, A. E., and Kay, G. N.: Prospective evaluation of transesophageal pacing for the interruption of atrial flutter. Am. J. Med. *86*:663, 1989.
70. Kaneda, S., Inoue, T., and Fukuzaki, H.: Treatment of atrial flutter and rapid atrial tachycardia with transesophageal atrial pacing. Jpn. Heart J. *30*:471, 1989.
71. Olshansky, B., Okumura, K., Hess, P. G., et al.: Use of procainamide with rapid atrial pacing for successful conversion of atrial flutter to sinus rhythm. J. Am. Coll. Cardiol. *11*:359, 1988.
72. Nademanee, K., and Singh, B. N.: Control of cardiac arrhythmias by calcium antagonism. Ann. N. Y. Acad. Sci. *522*:536, 1988.
73. Till, J., Shinebourne, E. A., Rigby, M. L., et al.: Efficacy and safety of adenosine in the treatment of supraventricular tachycardia in infants and children. Br. Heart J. *62*:204, 1989.
74. Das, G., Tschida, V., Gray, R., et al.: Efficacy of esmolol in the treatment and transfer of patients with supraventricular tachyarrhythmias to alternate oral antiarrhythmic agents. J. Clin. Pharmacol. *28*:746, 1988.
75. Sahar, D. I., Reiffel, J. A., Bigger, J. T., et al.: Efficacy, safety, and tolerance of d-sotalol in patients with refractory supraventricular tachyarrhythmias. Am. Heart J. *117*:562, 1989.
76. Fujimoto, T., Inoue, T., Ogawa, H., et al.: The effects of class IA antiarrhythmic drug on the common type of atrial flutter in combination with pacing therapy. Jpn. Circ. J. *53*:237, 1989.
77. Anderson, J. L., Jolivette, D. M., and Fredell, P. A.: Summary of efficacy and safety of flecainide for supraventricular arrhythmias. Am. J. Cardiol. *62*:62D, 1988.
78. Hellestrand, K. J.: Intravenous flecainide acetate for supraventricular tachycardias. Am. J. Cardiol. *62*:16D, 1988.
79. Strasburger, J. F., Smith, R. T., Jr., Moak, J. P., et al.: Encainide for resistant supraventricular tachycardia in children: Follow-up report. Am. J. Cardiol. *62*:50L, 1988.
80. Spinelli, W., and Hoffman, B. F.: Mechanisms of termination of reentrant atrial arrhythmias by class I and class III antiarrhythmic agents. Circ. Res. *65*:1565, 1989.
81. Lewis, J. H., Ranard, R. C., Caruso, A., et al.: Amiodarone hepatotoxicity: Prevalence and clinicopathologic correlations among 104 patients. Hepatology *9*:679, 1989.
82. Echt, D. S., Liebson, P. R., Mitchell, L. B., et al.: Mortality and morbidity in patients receiving encainide, flecainide, or placebo: The Cardiac Arrhythmia Suppression Trial. N. Engl. J. Med. *324*:781, 1991.
83. Falk, R. H.: Flecainide-induced ventricular tachycardia and fibrillation in patients treated for atrial fibrillation. Ann. Intern. Med. *111*:107, 1989.
84. Ranger, S., Talajic, M., Lemery, R., et al.: Amplification of flecainide-induced ventricular conduction slowing by exercise. A potentially significant clinical consequence of use-dependent sodium channel blockade. Circulation *79*:1000, 1989.
85. Saoudi, N., Atallah, G., Kirkorian, G., and Touboul, P.: Catheter ablation of the atrial myocardium in human type I atrial flutter. Circulation *81*:762, 1990.
86. Chauvin, M., and Brechenmacher, C.: A clinical study of the application of endocardial fulguration in the treatment of recurrent atrial flutter. PACE *12*:219, 1989.
87. Guiraudon, G. M., Klein, G. J., Sharma, A. D., and Yee, R.: Surgery for atrial flutter, atrial fibrillation, and atrial tachycardia. *In* Zipes, D. P., and

Jalife, J. (eds.): Cardiac Electrophysiology From Cell to Bedside. Philadelphia, W. B. Saunders Company, 1990, p. 915.

88. Slocum, J., Sahakian, A., and Swiryn, S.: Computer discrimination of atrial fibrillation and regular atrial rhythms from intra-atrial electrograms. PACE *11*:610, 1988.

88a. Toivonen, L., Kadish, A., Kou, W., and Morady, F.: Determinants of the ventricular rate during atrial fibrillation. J. Am. Coll. Cardiol. *16*:1194, 1990.

89. Meijler, F. L., and Fisch, C.: Does the atrioventricular node conduct? Br. Heart J. *61*:309, 1989.

89a. Wittkampf, F.H.M., de Jongste, M.J.L., and Meijler, F. L.: Atrioventricular nodal response to retrograde activation in atrial fibrillation. J. Cardiovasc. Electrophys. *1*:437, 1990.

90. Wittkampf, F.H.M., de Jongste, M.J.L., and Meijler, F. L.: Competitive anterograde and retrograde atrioventricular junctional activation in atrial fibrillation. J. Cardiovasc. Electrophys. *1*:448, 1990.

91. Simpson, R. J., Jr., Amara, I., Foster, J. R., et al.: Thresholds, refractory periods, and conduction times of the normal and diseased human atrium. Am. Heart J. *116*:1080, 1988.

92. Kawano, S., Hiraoka, M., and Sawanobori, T.: Electrocardiographic features of P waves from patients with transient atrial fibrillation. Jpn. Heart J. *29*:57, 1988.

93. Greer, G. S., Wilkinson, W. E., McCarthy, E. A., and Pritchett, E. L.: Random and nonrandom behavior of symptomatic paroxysmal atrial fibrillation. Am. J. Cardiol. *64*:339, 1989.

93a. Wolf, P. A., Abbott, R. D., and Kannel, W. B.: Atrial fibrillation: a major contributor to stroke in the elderly. The Framingham Study. Arch. Intern. Med. *147*:1561, 1987.

94. Yamanouchi, H., Tomonaga, M., Shimada, H., et al.: Nonvalvular atrial fibrillation as a cause of fatal massive cerebral infarction in the elderly. Stroke *20*:1653, 1989.

95. Lake, F. R., Cullen, K. J., de Klerk, N. H., et al.: Atrial fibrillation and mortality in an elderly population. Aust. N. Z. J. Med. *19*:321, 1989.

96. Sherman, D. G., Dyken, M. L., and Fisher, M.: Antithrombotic therapy for cerebrovascular disorders. Chest *95*(Supp. 1):140S, 1989.

96a. Petersen, P.: Thromboembolic complications in atrial fibrillation. Stroke *21*:4, 1990.

97. Stein, B., Halperin, J. L., and Fuster, V.: Should patients with atrial fibrillation be anticoagulated prior to and chronically following cardioversion? Cardiovasc. Clin. *21*:231, 1990.

98. Kopecky, S. L., Gersh, B. J., McGoon, M. D., et al.: The natural history of lone atrial fibrillation. A population-based study over 3 decades. N. Engl. J. Med. *317*:669, 1987.

99. Dunn, M., Alexander, J., de Silva, R., et al.: Antithrombotic therapy in atrial fibrillation. Chest *95*(Suppl.):118S, 1989.

100. Petersen, P., Boysen, G., Godtfredsen, J., et al.: Placebo-controlled, randomised trial of warfarin and aspirin for prevention of thromboembolic complications in chronic atrial fibrillation. The Copenhagen AFASAK study. Lancet *1*(8631):175, 1989.

101. Preliminary report of the stroke prevention in atrial fibrillation study. N. Engl. J. Med. *322*:863, 1990.

102. Brodsky, M. A., Allen, B. J., Capparelli, E. V., et al.: Factors determining maintenance of sinus rhythm after chronic atrial fibrillation with left atrial dilatation. Am. J. Cardiol. *63*:1065, 1989.

103. Dittrich, H. C., Erickson, J. S., Schneiderman, T., et al.: Echocardiographic and clinical predictors for outcome of elective cardioversion of atrial fibrillation. Am. J. Cardiol. *63*:193, 1989.

104. Kerber, R. E., Martins, J. B., and Kienzle, M. G.: Energy, current, and success in defibrillation and cardioversion: Clinical studies using an automated impedance-based method of energy adjustment. Circulation *77*:1038, 1988.

104a. Sanfilippo, A. J., Abascal, V. M., Sheehan, M., et al.: Atrial enlargement as a consequence of atrial fibrillation. A prospective echocardiographic study. Circulation *82*:792, 1990.

105. Levy, S., Lacombe, P., Cointe, R., and Bru, P.: High energy transcatheter cardioversion of chronic atrial fibrillation. J. Am. Coll. Cardiol. *12*:514, 1988.

106. Shapiro, E. P., Effron, M. B., Lima, S., et al.: Transient atrial dysfunction after conversion of chronic atrial fibrillation to sinus rhythm. Am. J. Cardiol. *62*:1202, 1988.

107. Lipkin, D. P., Frenneaux, M., Stewart, R., et al.: Delayed improvement in exercise capacity after cardioversion of atrial fibrillation to sinus rhythm. Br. Heart J. *59*:572, 1988.

107a. Suttorp, M. J., Kingma, J. H., Jessurun, E. R., et al.: The value of class IC antiarrhythmic drugs for acute conversion of paroxysmal atrial fibrillation or flutter to sinus rhythm. J. Am. Coll. Cardiol. *16*:1722, 1990.

108. Platia, E. V., Michelson, E. L., Porterfield, J. K., and Das, G.: Esmolol versus verapamil in the acute treatment of atrial fibrillation or atrial flutter. Am. J. Cardiol. *63*:925, 1989.

109. Talajic, M., Nayebpour, M., Jing, W., and Nattel, S.: Frequency-dependent effects of diltiazem on the atrioventricular node during experimental atrial fibrillation. Circulation *80*:380, 1989.

110. Salerno, D. M., Dias, V. C., Kleiger, R. E., et al.: Efficacy and safety of intravenous diltiazem for treatment of atrial fibrillation and atrial flutter. The Diltiazem-Atrial Fibrillation/Flutter Study Group. Am. J. Cardiol. *63*:1046, 1989.

111. Lewis, R. V., Laing, E., Moreland, T. A., et al.: A comparison of digoxin, diltiazem and their combination in the treatment of atrial fibrillation. Eur. Heart J. *9*:279, 1988.

112. Shenasa, M., Kus, T., Fromer, M., et al.: Effect of intravenous and oral calcium antagonists (diltiazem and verapamil) on sustenance of atrial fibrillation. Am. J. Cardiol. *62*:403, 1988.

113. van Wijk, L. M., den Heijer, P., Crijns, H. J., et al.: Flecainide versus quinidine in the prevention of paroxysms of atrial fibrillation. J. Cardiovasc. Pharmacol. *13*:32, 1989.

114. Antman, E. M., Beamer, A. D., Cantillon, C., et al.: Long-term oral propafenone therapy for suppression of refractory symptomatic atrial fibrillation and atrial flutter. J. Am. Coll. Cardiol. *12*:1005, 1988.

115. Suttorp, M. J., Kingma, J. H., Lie-A-Huen, L., and Mast, E. G.: Intravenous flecainide versus verapamil for acute conversion of paroxysmal atrial fibrillation or flutter to sinus rhythm. Am. J. Cardiol. *63*:693, 1989.

116. Chouty, F., and Coumel, P.: Oral flecainide for prophylaxis of paroxysmal atrial fibrillation. Am. J. Cardiol. *62*:35D, 1988.

117. Feld, G. K., Nademanee, K., Stevenson, W., et al.: Clinical and electrophysiologic effects of amiodarone in patients with atrial fibrillation complicating the Wolff-Parkinson-White syndrome. Am. Heart J. *115*:102, 1988.

117a. Juul-Moller, S., Edvardsson, N., and Rehnqvist-Ahlberg, N.: Sotalol versus quinidine for the maintenance of sinus rhythm after direct current conversion of atrial fibrillation. Circulation *82*:1932, 1990.

118. Langenfeld, H., Grimm, W., Maisch, B., and Kochsiek, K.: Atrial fibrillation and embolic complications in paced patients. PACE *11*:1667, 1988.

119. Swerdlow, C. D., and Liem, L. B.: Atrial and junctional tachycardias: clinical presentation, course, and therapy. *In* Zipes, D. P., and Jalife, J. (eds.): Cardiac Electrophysiology. From Cell to Bedside. Philadelphia, W. B. Saunders Company, 1990, p. 742.

120. Harada, A., D'Agostino, H. J., Jr., Schuessler, R. B., et al.: Right atrial isolation: A new surgical treatment for supraventricular tachycardia. I. Surgical technique and electrophysiologic effects. J. Thorac. Cardiovasc. Surg. *95*:643, 1988.

121. Morady, F., Krol, R. B., Nostrant, T. T., et al.: Supraventricular tachycardia induced by swallowing: A case report and review of the literature. PACE *10*:133, 1987.

122. Haines, D. E., and Di Marco, J. P.: Sustained intraatrial reentrant tachycardia: Clinical, electrocardiographic and electrophysiologic characteristics and long-term follow-up. J. Am. Coll. Cardiol. *15*:1345, 1990.

123. Scher, D. L., and Arsura, E. L.: Multifocal atrial tachycardia: mechanisms, clinical correlates and treatment. Am. Heart J. *118*:574, 1989.

124. Arsura, E., Lefkin, A. S., Scher, D. L., et al.: A randomized, double-blind, placebo-controlled study of verapamil and metoprolol in treatment of multifocal atrial tachycardia. Am. J. Med. *85*:519, 1988.

125. Kouvaras, G., Cokkinos, D. V., Halal, G., et al.: The effective treatment of multifocal atrial tachycardia with amiodarone. Jpn. Heart J. *30*:301, 1989.

126. Watanabe, Y., Nishimura, M., Noda, T., et al.: Atrioventricular junctional tachycardias. *In* Zipes, D. P., and Jalife, J. (eds.): Cardiac Electrophysiology. From Cell to Bedside. Philadelphia, W. B. Saunders Company, 1990, p. 564.

126a. Vos, M. A., Gorgels, A.P.M., de Wit, B., et al.: Premature escape beats: A model for triggered activity in the intact heart? Circulation *82*:213, 1990.

126b. Viamonte, V.A.M., and Rosen, M. R.: Premature escape beats induced by overdrive pacing in canine Purkinje fibers: Evidence for the role of normal automaticity as an underlying cellular mechanism. Circulation *82*:234, 1990.

127. Ruder, M. A., Davis, J. C., Eldar, M., et al.: Clinical and electrophysiologic characterization of automatic junctional tachycardia in adults. Circulation *73*:930, 1986.

128. Kirchhof, C. J., Bonke, F. I., and Allessie, M. A.: Evidence for the presence of electrotonic depression of pacemakers in the rabbit atrioventricular node. The effects of uncoupling from the surrounding myocardium. Basic Res. Cardiol. *83*:190, 1988.

128a. Villain, E., Vetter, V. L., Garcia, J. M., et al.: Evolving concepts in the management of congenital junctional ectopic tachycardia. Circulation *81*:1544, 1990.

129. Sung, R. J., Huycke, E. C., Keung, E. C., et al.: Atrioventricular node reentry: Evidence of reentry and functional properties of fast and slow pathways. *In* Zipes, D. P., and Jalife, J. (eds.): Cardiac Electrophysiology: From Cell to Bedside. Philadelphia, W. B. Saunders Company, 1990, p. 513.

130. Schuger, C. D., Steinman, R. T., Lehmann, M. H., et al.: The excitable gap in atrioventricular nodal reentrant tachycardia. Characterization with ventricular extrastimuli and pharmacologic intervention. Circulation *80*:324, 1989.

131. Johnson, D. C., Ross, D. L., and Uther, J. B.: The surgical cure of atrioventricular junctional reentrant tachycardia. *In* Zipes, D. P., and Jalife, J. (eds.): Cardiac Electrophysiology: From Cell to Bedside. Philadelphia, W. B. Saunders Company, 1990, p. 921.

132. Pritchett, E. L., McCarthy, E. A., and Lee, K. L.: Clinical behavior of paroxysmal atrial tachycardia. Am. J. Cardiol. *62*:30, 1988.

133. Rankin, A. C., Oldroyd, K. G., Chong, E., et al.: Value and limitations of adenosine in the diagnosis and treatment of narrow and broad complex tachycardias. Br. Heart J. *62*:195, 1989.

134. Garratt, C., Linker, N., Griffith, M., et al.: Comparison of adenosine and verapamil for termination of paroxysmal junctional tachycardia. Am. J. Cardiol. *64*:1310, 1989.

135. DiMarco, J. P.: Electrophysiology of adenosine. J. Cardiovasc. Electrophys. *1*:340, 1990.

136. Huycke, E. C., Sung, R. J., Dias, V. C., et al.: Intravenous diltiazem for termination of reentrant supraventricular tachycardia: A placebo-controlled, randomized double-blind, multicenter study. J. Am. Coll. Cardiol. *13*:538, 1989.

137. Schnittger, I., Lee, J. T., Hargis, J., et al.: Long-term results of antitachycardia pacing in patients with supraventricular tachycardia. PACE *12*:936, 1989.

138. Hoff, P. I., Tronstad, A., Oie, B., and Ohm, O. J.: Electrophysiologic and clinical effects of flecainide for recurrent paroxysmal supraventricular tachycardia. Am. J. Cardiol. *62*:585, 1988.
139. Neuss, H., and Schlepper, M.: Long-term efficacy and safety of flecainide for supraventricular tachycardia. Am. J. Cardiol. *62*:56D, 1988.
139a. Henthorn, R. W., Waldo, A. L., Anderson, J. L., et al.: Flecainide acetate prevents recurrence of symptomatic paroxysmal supraventricular tachycardia. Circulation *83*:119, 1991.
140. Musto, B., D'Onofrio, A., Cavallaro, C., and Musto, A.: Electrophysiological effects and clinical efficacy of propafenone in children with recurrent paroxysmal supraventricular tachycardia. Circulation *78*:863, 1988.
141. Miles, W. M., Chang, M., Heger, J. J., et al.: Electrophysiologic and antiarrhythmic effects of oral encainide in patients with atrioventricular nodal reentry or nodoventricular reentry. Am. Heart J. *114*:26, 1987.
142. Guiraudon, G. M., Klein, G. J., Sharma, A. D., et al.: Surgical alternatives for supraventricular tachycardias. Am. J. Cardiol. *64*:92J, 1989.
143. Epstein, L. M., Scheinman, M. M., Langberg, J. J., et al.: Percutaneous catheter modification of the atrioventricular node. Circulation *80*:757, 1989.
144. Yee, R., Klein, G. J., Sharma, A. D., et al.: Tachycardia associated with accessory atrioventricular pathways. *In* Zipes, D. P., and Jalife, J. (eds.): Cardiac Electrophysiology. From Cell to Bedside. Philadelphia, W. B. Saunders Company, 1990, p. 463.
145. Kuck, K. H., Friday, K. J., and Kunze, K. P.: Sites of conduction block in accessory atrioventricular pathways: Basis for concealed accessory pathways. Circulation *82*:407, 1990.
146. Kou, W. H., Morady, F., Dick, M., et al.: Concealed anterograde accessory pathway conduction during the induction of orthodromic reciprocating tachycardia. J. Am. Coll. Cardiol. *13*:391, 1989.
147. Burnett, J. C., Jr.: Importance of atrial natrimetic factor in cardiovascular volume regulation. Prog. Cardiol. *2/1*:183, 1989.
148. Wellens, H.J.J., Brugada, P. C., Penn, O. C., et al.: Pre-excitation syndromes. *In* Zipes, D. P., and Jalife, J. (eds.): Cardiac Electrophysiology: From Cell to Bedside. Philadelphia, W. B. Saunders Company, 1990, p. 691.
149. Tchou, P., Lehmann, M. H., Jazayeri, M., and Akhtar, M.: Atriofascicular connection or a nodoventricular Mahaim fiber? Electrophysiologic elucidation of the pathway and associated reentrant circuit. Circulation *77*:837, 1988.
150. Leitch, J., Klein, G. J., Yee, R., et al.: New concepts on nodoventricular accessory pathways. J. Cardiovasc. Electrophys. *1*:220, 1990.
151. Benditt, D. G., and Milstein, S.: Nodoventricular accessory connections: A misnomer or a structural functional spectrum? J. Cardiovasc. Electrophys. *1*:231, 1990.
152. Prystowsky, E. N., and Packer, D. L.: Pre-excited tachycardias. *In* Zipes, D. P., and Jalife, J. (eds.): Cardiac Electrophysiology: From Cell to Bedside. Philadelphia, W. B. Saunders Company, 1990, p. 472.
153. Gallagher, J. J., Selle, J. G., Sealy, W. C., et al.: Variants of pre-excitation: Update 1989. *In* Zipes, D. P., and Jalife, J. (eds.): Cardiac Electrophysiology: From Cell to Bedside. Philadelphia, W. B. Saunders Company, 1990, p. 480.
154. Szabo, T. S., Klein, G. J., Guiraudon, G. M., et al.: Localization of accessory pathways in the Wolff-Parkinson-White syndrome. PACE *12*:1691, 1989.
155. Miles, W. M., Yee, R., Klein, G. J., et al.: The preexcitation index: An aid in determining the mechanism of supraventricular tachycardia and localizing accessory pathways. Circulation *74*:493, 1986.
156. Jazayeri, M. R., Tchou, P., Caceres, J., et al.: Ventricular conduction time during bundle branch reentrant beat initiating orthodromic tachycardia: A simple and reliable method for localization of accessory pathways. J. Cardiovasc. Electrophys. *1*:121, 1990.
157. Miles, W. M., and Zipes, D. P.: Electrophysiology of wide QRS tachycardia. Prog. Cardiol. *1/2*:77, 1988.
158. Yeh, S. J., Lin, F. C., and Wu, D. L.: The mechanisms of exercise provocation of supraventricular tachycardia. Am. Heart J. *117*:1041, 1989.
159. Mahmud, R., Denker, S. T., Tchou, P. J., et al.: Modulation of conduction and refractoriness in atrioventricular junctional reentrant circuit. Effect on reentry initiated by atrial extrastimulus. J. Clin. Invest. *81*:39, 1988.
159a. Jackman, W., Margolis, D., Moulton, K., et al.: Antegrade and retrograde pathway conduction occurring over separate but close fibers: Evidence from RF catheter ablation. Circulation *82*(Suppl. III):317, 1990 (abstract).
160. Wellens, H.J.J., Atie, J., Smeets, J.L.R.M., et al.: The electrocardiogram in patients with multiple accessory atrioventricular pathways. J. Am. Coll. Cardiol. *16*:745, 1990.
160a. Fananapazir, L., German, L. D., Gallagher, J. J., et al.: Importance of preexcited QRS morphology during induced atrial fibrillation to the diagnosis and location of multiple accessory pathways. Circulation *81*:578, 1990.
161. Radtke, N. S., Miles, W. M., Klein, L. S., and Zipes, D. P.: Predictive value of inducible atrioventricular nodal reentry after surgery for Wolff-Parkinson-White syndrome. J. Am. Coll. Cardiol. *15*:174A, 1990.
162. Jackman, W. M., Kuck, K. H., Friday, K. J., and Lazzara, R.: Catheter recordings of accessory atrioventricular pathway activation. *In* Zipes, D. P., and Jalife, J. (eds.): Cardiac Electrophysiology: From Cell to Bedside. Philadelphia, W. B. Saunders Company, 1990, p. 491.
163. Klein, L. S., Miles, W. M., and Zipes, D. P.: Effect of atrioventricular interval during pacing or reciprocating tachycardia on atrial size, pressure and refractory period: Contraction-excitation feedback in human atrium. Circulation *82*:60, 1990.
164. Fujimura, O., Klein, G. J., Yee, R., and Sharma, A. D.: Mode of onset of atrial fibrillation in the Wolff-Parkinson-White syndrome: How important is the accessory pathway? J. Am. Coll. Cardiol. *15*:1082, 1990.
164a. Munger, T. M., Feldman, B. J., Hammill, S. C., et al.: The natural history of Wolff-Parkinson-White syndrome: A population study—Olmsted County, Minnesota: 1953–1989. Circulation *82*(Suppl. III):317, 1990 (abstract).
165. Guiraudon, G. M., Klein, G. J., Sharma, A. D., et al.: "Atypical" posteroseptal accessory pathway in Wolff-Parkinson-White syndrome. J. Am. Coll. Cardiol. *12*:1605, 1988.
166. Zales, V. R., Dunnigan, A., and Benson, D. W., Jr.: Clinical and electrophysiological features of fetal and neonatal paroxysmal atrial tachycardia resulting in congestive heart failure. Am. J. Cardiol. *62*:225, 1988.
167. Klein, G. J., Yee, R., and Sharma, A. D.: Longitudinal electrophysiologic assessment of asymptomatic patients with the Wolff-Parkinson-White electrocardiographic pattern. N. Engl. J. Med. *320*:1229, 1989.
167a. Perry, J. C., and Garson, A.: Supraventricular tachycardia due to Wolff-Parkinson-White syndrome in children: Early disappearance and late recurrence. J. Am. Coll. Cardiol. *16*:1215, 1990.
168. Sharma, A. D., Yee, R., Guiraudon, G., and Klein, G. J.: Sensitivity and specificity of invasive and noninvasive testing for risk of sudden death in Wolff-Parkinson-White syndrome. J. Am. Coll. Cardiol. *10*:373, 1987.
169. Gaita, F., Giustetto, C., Riccardi, R., et al.: Stress and pharmacologic tests as methods to identify patients with Wolff-Parkinson-White syndrome at risk of sudden death. Am. J. Cardiol. *64*:487, 1989.
170. Daubert, C., Ollitrault, J., Descaves, C., et al.: Failure of the exercise test to predict the anterograde refractory period of the accessory pathway in Wolff-Parkinson-White syndrome. PACE *11*:1130, 1988.
171. Fananapazir, L., Packer, D. L., German, L. D., et al.: Procainamide infusion test: Inability to identify patients with Wolff-Parkinson-White syndrome who are potentially at risk of sudden death. Circulation *77*:1291, 1988.
171a. Silka, M. J., Kron, J., Walance, C. G., et al.: Assessment and follow-up of pediatric survivors of sudden cardiac death. Circulation *82*:341, 1990.
172. Szabo, T. S., Klein, G. J., Sharma, A. D., et al.: Usefulness of isoproterenol during atrial fibrillation in evaluation of asymptomatic Wolff-Parkinson-White pattern. Am. J. Cardiol. *63*:187, 1989.
173. Klein, G. J., Prystowsky, E. N., Yee, R., Sharma, A. D., et al.: Asymptomatic Wolff-Parkinson-White. Should we intervene? Circulation *80*:1902, 1989.
173a. Leitch, J. W., Klein, G. J., Yee, R., and Murdock, C.: Prognostic value of electrophysiology testing in asymptomatic patients with Wolff-Parkinson-White pattern. Circulation *82*:1718, 1990.
174. Fujimura, O., Klein, G. J., Sharma, A. D., et al.: Acute effect of disopyramide on atrial fibrillation in the Wolff-Parkinson-White syndrome. J. Am. Coll. Cardiol. *13*:1133, 1989.
175. Garratt, C., Antoniou, A., Ward, D., Camm, A. J.: Misuse of verapamil in pre-excited atrial fibrillation. Lancet *1*(8634):367, 1989.
176. Morady, F., Kou, W. H., Kadish, A. H., et al.: Effects of epinephrine in patients with an accessory atrioventricular connection treated with quinidine. Am. J. Cardiol. *62*:580, 1988.
176a. Helmy, I., Scheinman, M. M., Herre, J. M., et al.: Electrophysiologic effects of isoproterenol in patients with atrioventricular reentrant tachycardia treated with isoproterenol. J. Am. Coll. Cardiol. *16*:1649, 1990.
176b. Morady, F., Kadish, A. H., Schmaltz, S., et al.: Effects of resting vagal tone on accessory atrioventricular connections. Circulation *81*:86, 1990.
177. Rinkenberger, R. L., Naccarelli, G. V., Miles, W. M., et al.: Encainide for atrial fibrillation associated with Wolff-Parkinson-White syndrome. Am. J. Cardiol. *62*:26L, 1988.
178. Kim, S. S., Smith, P., and Ruffy, R.: Treatment of atrial tachyarrhythmias and preexcitation syndrome with flecainide acetate. Am. J. Cardiol. *62*:29D, 1988.
179. Miles, W. M., Zipes, D, P., Rinkenberger, R. L., et al.: Encainide for treatment of atrioventricular reciprocating tachycardia in the Wolff-Parkinson-White syndrome: Electrophysiologic effects and long-term follow-up. Am. J. Cardiol. *62*:26L, 1988.
179a. Haissaguerre, M., Warin, J. F., and Le Metayer, P.: Catheter ablation of Mahaim fibers with preservation of atrioventricular nodal conduction. Circulation *82*:418, 1990.
180. Holmes, D. R., Jr.: Pacing for tachycardia. *In* Furman, S., Hayes, D. L., and Holmes, D. R., Jr. (eds.): A Practice of Cardiac Pacing. Mt. Kisco, N.Y., Futura Publishing Company, 1989, p. 457.
181. Kappenberger, L., Valin, H., and Sowton, E.: Multicenter long-term results of antitachycardia pacing for supraventricular tachycardias. Am. J. Cardiol. *64*:191, 1989.
182. Morady, F., DiCarlo, L. A., Jr., Baerman, J. M., et al.: Determinants of QRS alternans during narrow QRS tachycardia. J. Am. Coll. Cardiol. *9*:489, 1987.
182a. Moulton, K. P., Medcalf, T., and Lazzara, R.: Premature ventricular complex morphology. Circulation *81*:1245, 1990.
183. Lucente, M., Rebuzzi, A. G., Lanza, G. A., et al.: Circadian variation of ventricular tachycardia in acute myocardial infarction. Am. J. Cardiol. *62*:670, 1988.
184. Suwa, M., Hirota, Y., Kaku, K., et al.: Prevalence of the coexistence of left ventricular false tendons and premature ventricular complexes in apparently healthy subjects: A prospective study in the general population. J. Am. Coll. Cardiol. *12*:910, 1988.
185. Kudoh, Y., Hiraga, Y., and Iimura, O.: Benign ventricular tachycardia in systemic sarcoidosis—a case of false tendon. Jpn. Circ. J. *52*:385, 1988.
186. Holland, O. B., Kuhnert, L., Pollard, J., et al.: Ventricular ectopic activity with diuretic therapy. Am. J. Hypertens. *1*:380, 1988.
187. Garan, H., McGovern, B. A., Canzanello, V. J., et al.: The effect of potassium ion depletion on postinfarction canine cardiac arrhythmias. Circulation *77*:696, 1988.

188. Funck-Brentano, C., Coumel, P., Lorente, P., et al.: Rate dependence of ventricular extrasystoles: Computer identification and quantitative analysis. Cardiovasc. Res. *22*:101, 1988.

189. Kharsa, M. H., Gold, R. L., Moore, H., et al.: Long-term outcome following programmed electrical stimulation in patients with high-grade ventricular ectopy. PACE *11*:603, 1988.

190. El-Sherif, N., Turitto, G., and Fontaine, J. M.: Risk stratification of patients with complex ventricular arrhythmias. Value of ambulatory electrocardiographic recording, programmed electrical stimulation and the signal-averaged electrocardiogram. Herz *13*:204, 1988.

191. Wilber, D. J., Olshansky, B., Moran, J. F., and Scanlon, P. J.: Electrophysiological testing and nonsustained ventricular tachycardia. Circulation *82*:350, 1990.

192. Wellens, H.J.J.: The approach to nonsustained ventricular tachycardia after myocardial infarction. Circulation *82*:633, 1990.

192a. Burkart, F., Pfisterer, M., Kiowski, W., et al.: Effect of antiarrhythmic therapy on mortality in survivors of myocardial infarction with asymptomatic complex ventricular arrhythmias. Basel Antiarrhythmic Study of Infarct Survival (BASIS). J. Am. Coll. Cardiol. *16*:1711, 1990.

192b. Pratt, C. M., Hallstrom, A., Theroux, P., et al.: Avoiding interpretative pitfalls when assessing arrhythmia suppression after myocardial infarction: Insights from the long-term observations of the placebo-treated patients in the Cardiac Arrhythmia Pilot Study (CAPS). J. Am. Coll. Cardiol. *17*:1, 1991.

193. Lerman, B. B., Belardinelli, L., West, G. A., et al.: Adenosine-sensitive ventricular tachycardia: Evidence suggesting cyclic AMP-mediated triggered activity. Circulation *74*:270, 1986.

194. Stevenson, W. G., Weiss, J. N., Wiener, I., et al.: Resetting of ventricular tachycardia: Implications for localizing the area of slow conduction. J. Am. Coll. Cardiol. *11*:522, 1988.

195. Martini, B., Buja, G. F., Canciani, B., and Nava, A.: Bidirectional tachycardia. A sustained form, not related to digitalis intoxication, in an adult without apparent cardiac disease. Jpn. Heart J. *29*:381, 1988.

196. Kay, G. N., Epstein, A. E., and Plumb, V. J.: Region of slow conduction in sustained ventricular tachycardia: Direct endocardial recordings and functional characterization in humans. J. Am. Coll. Cardiol. *11*:109, 1988.

197. McComb, J. M., Gold, H. K., Leinbach, R. C., et al.: Electrically induced ventricular arrhythmias in acute myocardial infarction treated with thrombolytic agents. Am. J. Cardiol. *62*:186, 1988.

198. Stevenson, W. G., Weiss, J. N., Wiener, I., et al.: Fractionated endocardial electrograms are associated with slow conduction in humans: Evidence from pace-mapping. J. Am. Coll. Cardiol. *13*:369, 1989.

199. Kay, G. N., Epstein, A. E., and Plumb, V. J.: Entrainment of ventricular tachycardia by AV nodal reentrant tachycardia. PACE *12*:2, 1989.

200. Berger, M. D., Waxman, H. L., Buxton, A. E., et al.: Spontaneous compared with induced onset of sustained ventricular tachycardia. Circulation *78*:885, 1988.

201. Huikuri, H. V., Zaman, L., Castellanos, A., et al.: Changes in spontaneous sinus node rate as an estimate of cardiac autonomic tone during stable and unstable ventricular tachycardia. J. Am. Coll. Cardiol. *13*:646, 1989.

202. Schwartz, P. J., Vanoli, E., Stramba-Badiale, M., et al.: Autonomic mechanisms and sudden death. New insights from analysis of baroreceptor reflexes in conscious dogs with and without a myocardial infarction. Circulation *78*:969, 1988.

203. Zipes, D. P.: Influence of myocardial ischemia and infarction on autonomic innervation of the heart. Circulation *82*:1095, 1990.

204. Akhtar, M., Jazayeri, M., Avitall, B., et al.: Electrophysiologic spectrum of wide QRS complex tachycardia. *In* Zipes, D. P., and Jalife, J. (eds.): Cardiac Electrophysiology. From Cell to Bedside. Philadelphia, W. B. Saunders Company, 1990, p. 635.

205. Nguyen, P.T., Scheinman, M. M., and Seger, J.: Polymorphous ventricular tachycardia: clinical characterization, therapy, and the QT interval. Circulation *74*:340, 1986.

206. Curione, M., Fuoco, U., Borgia, C., et al.: An electrocardiographic criterion to detect AV dissociation in wide QRS tachyarrhythmias. Clin. Cardiol. *11*:250, 1988.

207. Akhtar, M., Shenasa, M., Jazayeri, M., et al.: Wide QRS complex tachycardia. Reappraisal of a common clinical problem. Ann. Intern. Med. *109*:905, 1988.

208. Steinman, R. T., Herrera, C., and Schuger, C. D.: Wide QRS tachycardia in the conscious adult. Ventricular tachycardia is the most frequent cause. JAMA *261*:1013, 1989.

209. Miller, J. M., Marchlinski, F. E., Buxton, A. E., and Josephson, M. E.: Relationship between the 12-lead electrocardiogram during ventricular tachycardia and endocardial site of origin in patients with coronary artery disease. Circulation *77*:759, 1988.

210. Kuchar, D. L., Ruskin, J. N., and Garan, H.: Electrocardiographic localization of the site of origin of ventricular tachycardia in patients with prior myocardial infarction. J. Am. Coll. Cardiol. *15*:893, 1989.

211. Josephson, M. E., and Gottlieb, C. D.: Ventricular tachycardias associated with coronary artery disease. *In* Zipes, D. P., and Jalife, J. (eds.): Cardiac Electrophysiology. From Cell to Bedside. Philadelphia, W. B. Saunders Company, 1990, p. 571.

212. Martins, J. B., Constantin, L., Kienzle, M. G., et al.: Mechanisms of ventricular tachycardia unassociated with coronary artery disease. *In* Zipes, D. P., and Jalife, J. (eds.): Cardiac Electrophysiology. From Cell to Bedside. Philadelphia, W. B. Saunders Company, 1990, p. 581.

213. Miller, B., Lesnefsky, E., Heyborne, T., et al.: Cough-cardiopulmonary resuscitation in the cardiac catheterization laboratory: Hemodynamics during an episode of prolonged hypotensive ventricular tachycardia. Cathet. Cardiovasc. Diagn. *18*:168, 1989.

214. Podczeck, A., Borggrefe, M., Martinez-Rubio, A., and Breithardt, G.: Termination of re-entrant ventricular tachycardia by subthreshold stimulus applied to the zone of slow conduction. Eur. Heart J. *9*:1146, 1988.

215. Shenasa, M., Cardinal, R., Kus, T., et al.: Termination of sustained ventricular tachycardia by ultrarapid subthreshold stimulation in humans. Circulation *78*:1135, 1988.

216. Klein, L. S., Miles, W. M., Heger, J. J., and Zipes, D. P.: Transcutaneous pacing: patient tolerance strength-interval relations and feasibility for programmed electrical stimulation. Am. J. Cardiol. *62*:1126, 1988.

217. Estes, N. A. 3d, Deering, T. F., Manolis, A. S., et al.: External cardiac programmed stimulation for noninvasive termination of sustained supraventricular and ventricular tachycardia. Am. J. Cardiol. *63*:177, 1989.

218. Marchlinski, F. E.: Ventricular tachycardia: Clinical presentation, course, and therapy. *In* Zipes, D. P., and Jalife, J. (eds.): Cardiac Electrophysiology. From Cell to Bedside. Philadelphia, W. B. Saunders Company, 1990, p. 756.

219. Bardy, G. H., and Olson, W. H.: Clinical characteristics of spontaneous-onset sustained ventricular tachycardia and ventricular fibrillation in survivors of cardiac arrest. *In* Zipes, D. P., and Jalife, J. (eds.): Cardiac Electrophysiology. From Cell to Bedside. Philadelphia, W. B. Saunders Company, 1990, p. 778.

220. Denniss, A. R., Ross, D. L., Richards, D. A., et al.: Differences between patients with ventricular tachycardia and ventricular fibrillation as assessed by signal-averaged electrocardiogram, radionuclide ventriculography and cardiac mapping. J. Am. Coll. Cardiol. *11*:276, 1988.

221. Adhar, G. C., Larson, L. W., Bardy, G. H., and Greene, H. L.: Sustained ventricular arrhythmias: Differences between survivors of cardiac arrest and patients with recurrent sustained ventricular tachycardia. J. Am. Coll. Cardiol. *12*:159, 1988.

222. Denniss, A. R., Richards, D. A., Waywood, J. A., et al.: Electrophysiological and anatomic differences between canine hearts with inducible ventricular tachycardia and fibrillation associated with chronic myocardial infarction. Circ. Res. *64*:155, 1989.

223. Akhtar, M.: Clinical spectrum of ventricular tachycardia. Circulation *82*:1561, 1990.

224. Bigger, J. T., Jr., La Rovere, M. T., Steinman, R. C., et al.: Comparison of baroreflex sensitivity and heart period variability after myocardial infarction. J. Am. Cardiol. *14*:1511, 1989.

224a. Hayano, J., Sakakibara, Y., Yamada, M., et al.: Decreased magnitude of heart rate spectral components in coronary artery disease. Circulation *81*:1217, 1990.

224b. Osculati, G., Giannattasio, C., Seravalle, G., et al.: Early alterations of the baroreceptor control of heart rate in patients with acute myocardial infarction. Circulation *81*:939, 1990.

225. Waxman, M. B., Sharma, A. D., Asta, J., et al.: The protective effect of vagus nerve stimulation on catecholamine-halothane-induced ventricular fibrillation in dogs. Can. J. Physiol. Pharmacol. *67*:801, 1989.

226. Hargrove, W. C., and Miller, J. M.: Risk stratification and management of patients with recurrent ventricular tachycardia and other malignant ventricular arrhythmias. Circulation *79*:I178, 1989.

227. Gomes, J. A., Winters, S. L., Stewart, D., et al.: A new noninvasive index to predict sustained ventricular tachycardia and sudden death in the first year after myocardial infarction: Based on signal averaged electrocardiograms, radionuclide ejection fraction and Holter monitoring. J. Am. Coll. Cardiol. *10*:349, 1987.

228. Trappe, H. J., Brugada, P., Talajic, M., et al.: Prognosis of patients with ventricular tachycardia and ventricular fibrillation: Role of the underlying etiology. J. Am. Coll. Cardiol. *12*:166, 1988.

229. Kuchar, D. L., Thorburn, C. W., Freund, J., et al.: Noninvasive predictors of cardiac events after myocardial infarction. Complementary value of exercise testing and signal-averaged electrocardiography. Cardiology *76*:18, 1989.

230. Breithardt, G., Borggrefe, M., Martinez-Rubio, A., and Podczeck, A.: Prognostic significance of ventricular late potentials in the postmyocardial infarction period. Herz *13*:180, 1988.

231. Lindsay, B. D., Markham, J., Schechtman, K. B., et al.: Identification of patients with sustained ventricular tachycardia by frequency analysis of signal-averaged electrocardiograms despite the presence of bundle branch block. Circulation *77*:122, 1988.

232. Simson, M. B.: Signal-averaged electrocardiography. *In* Zipes, D. P., and Jalife, J. (eds.): Cardiac Electrophysiology. From Cell to Bedside. Philadelphia, W. B. Saunders Company, 1990, p. 807.

233. Cain, M. E., Lindsay, B. D., Arthur, R. M., et al.: Noninvasive detection of patients prone to life-threatening ventricular arrhythmias by frequency analysis of electrocardiographic signals. *In* Zipes, D. P., and Jalife, J. (eds.): Cardiac Electrophysiology. From Cell to Bedside. Philadelphia, W. B. Saunders Company, 1990, p. 817.

234. Klein, R. C., and Machell, C.: Use of electrophysiologic testing in patients with nonsustained ventricular tachycardia: Prognostic and therapeutic implications. J. Am. Coll. Cardiol. *14*:155, 1989.

235. Vorperian, V. R., Gittelsohn, A. M., and Veltri, E. P.: Predictors of inducible sustained ventricular tachyarrhythmias in patients with coronary artery disease. J. Am. Coll. Cardiol. *13*:637, 1989.

236. McLaran, C. J., Gersh, B. J., Sugrue, D. D., et al.: Out-of-hospital cardiac arrest in patients without clinically significant coronary artery disease: Comparison of clinical, electrophysiological, and survival characteristics with those in similar patients who have clinically significant coronary artery disease. Br. Heart J. *58*:583, 1987.

237. Miller, J. M., Vassallo, J. A., Kussmaul, W. G., 3d, et al.: Anterior left ventricular aneurysm: Factors associated with the development of sustained ventricular tachycardia. J. Am. Coll. Cardiol. *12*:375, 1988.

238. Kadish, A. H., Rosenthal, M. E., Vasallo, J. A., et al.: Sinus mapping in patients with cardiac arrest and coronary disease—results and correlation with outcome. PACE *12*:301, 1989.
239. Buxton, A. E., Marchlinski, F. E., Flores, B. T., et al.: Nonsustained ventricular tachycardia in patients with coronary artery disease: role of electrophysiologic study. Circulation *75*:1178, 1987.
240. Saxon, L. A., Uretz, E. F., and Denes, P.: Significance of the clinical presentation in ventricular tachycardia/fibrillation. Am. Heart J. *118*:695, 1989.
241. Brugada, P., Talajic, M., Smeets, J., et al.: The value of the clinical history to assess prognosis of patients with ventricular tachycardia or ventricular fibrillation after myocardial infarction. Eur. Heart J. *10*:747, 1989.
242. Willems, A. R., Tijssen, J.G.P., vanCapelle, F.J.L., et al.: Determinants of prognosis in symptomatic ventricular tachycardia or ventricular fibrillation late after myocardial infarction. J. Am. Coll. Cardiol. *16*:521, 1990.
242a. Ruskin, J. N.: Identification of high risk patients: invasive methods. Circulation (*In press*).
243. Rehnqvist, N.: Arrhythmias and their treatment in patients with heart failure. Am. J. Cardiol. *64*:61J, 1989.
244. Chakko, S., de Marchena, E., Kessler, K. M., and Myerburg, R. J.: Ventricular arrhythmias in congestive heart failure. Clin. Cardiol. *12*:525, 1989.
245. Bekheit, S., Turitto, G., Fontaine, J., and El-Sherif, N.: Initiation of ventricular fibrillation by supraventricular beats in patients with acute myocardial infarction. Br. Heart J. *59*:190, 1988.
246. Hays, L. J., Lerman, B. B., and DiMarco, J. P.: Nonventricular arrhythmias as precursors of ventricular fibrillation in patients with out-of-hospital cardiac arrest. Am. Heart J. *118*:53, 1989.
247. Rinkenberger, R. L., Naccarelli, G. V., Berns, E., and Dougherty, A. H.: Efficacy and safety of class IC antiarrhythmic agents for the treatment of coexisting supraventricular and ventricular tachycardia. Am. J. Cardiol. *62*:44D, 1988.
248. Sung, R. J., Keung, E. C., Nguyen, N. X., and Huycke, E. C.: Effects of beta-adrenergic blockade on verapamil-responsive and verapamil-irresponsive sustained ventricular tachycardias. J. Clin. Invest. *81*:688, 1988.
249. Kasanuki, H., Ohnishi, S., and Hosoda, S.: Differentiation and mechanisms of prevention and termination of verapamil-sensitive sustained ventricular tachycardia. Am. J. Cardiol. *64*:46J, 1989.
250. Primeau, R., Agha, A., Giorgi, C., et al.: Long-term efficacy and toxicity of amiodarone in the treatment of refractory cardiac arrhythmias. Can. J. Cardiol. *5*:98, 1989.
251. Herre, J. M., Sauve, M. J., Malone, P., et al.: Long-term results of amiodarone therapy in patients with recurrent sustained ventricular tachycardia or ventricular fibrillation. J. Am. Coll. Cardiol. *13*:442, 1989.
252. Mitchell, L. B., Wyse, D. G., Gillis, A. M., and Duff, H. J.: Electropharmacology of amiodarone therapy initiation. Time course of onset of electrophysiologic and antiarrhythmic effects. Circulation *80*:34, 1989.
253. Weinberg, B., Dusman, R., Stanton, M., et al.: Five year follow-up of 590 patients treated with amiodarone (abstract). PACE *12*:642, 1989.
254. Dusman, R. E., Stanton, M. S., Miles, W. M., et al.: Clinical features of amiodarone-induced pulmonary toxicity. Circulation *82*:51, 1990.
255. Morady, F., Nelson, S. D., Kou, W. H., et al.: Electrophysiologic effects of epinephrine in humans. J. Am. Coll. Cardiol. *11*:1235, 1988.
256. Jazayeri, M. R., Van Wyhe, G., Avitall, B., et al.: Isoproterenol reversal of antiarrhythmic effects in patients with inducible sustained ventricular tachyarrhythmias. J. Am. Coll. Cardiol. *14*:705, 1989.
257. Morady, F., Kou, W. H., Kadish, A. H., et al.: Antagonism of quinidine's electrophysiologic effects by epinephrine in patients with ventricular tachycardia. J. Am. Coll. Cardiol. *12*:388, 1988.
258. Tonet, J., Frank, R., Fontaine, G., et al.: Efficacy and safety of low doses of beta-blocker agents combined with amiodarone in refractory ventricular tachycardia. PACE *11*:1984, 1988.
259. Marchlinski, F. E., Buxton, A. E., Kindwall, K. E., et al.: Comparison of individual and combined effects of procainamide and amiodarone in patients with sustained ventricular tachyarrhythmias. Circulation *78*:583, 1988.
260. Klein, L. S., Fineberg, N., Heger, J. J., et al.: Prospective evaluation of a discriminant function for prediction of recurrent symptomatic ventricular tachycardia or ventricular fibrillation in coronary artery disease patients receiving amiodarone and having inducible ventricular tachycardia at electrophysiologic study. Am. J. Cardiol. *61*:1024, 1988.
261. Borggrefe, M., Trampisch, H. J., and Breithardt, G.: Reappraisal of criteria for assessing drug efficacy in patients with ventricular tachyarrhythmias: Complete versus partial suppression of inducible arrhythmias. J. Am. Coll. Cardiol. *12*:140, 1988.
262. Manolis, A. S., Uricchio, F., Estes, N. A., 3d: Prognostic value of early electrophysiologic studies for ventricular tachycardia recurrence in patients with coronary artery disease treated with amiodarone. Am. J. Cardiol. *63*:1052, 1989.
263. Schoels, W., Brachmann, J., Schmitt, C., et al.: Conversion of sustained into nonsustained ventricular tachycardia during therapy assessment by programmed ventricular stimulation: Criterion for a positive drug effect? Am. J. Cardiol. *64*:329, 1989.
263a. Rosenbaum, M. S., Wilber, D. J., Finkelstein, D., et al.: Immediate reproducibility of electrically induced sustained monomorphic ventricular tachycardia before and during antiarrhythmic drug therapy. J. Am. Coll. Cardiol. *17*:133, 1991.
264. The ESVEM trial: Electrophysiologic study versus electrocardiographic monitoring for selection of antiarrhythmic therapy of ventricular tachyarrhythmias. The ESVEM investigators. Circulation *79*:1354, 1989.
265. Winkle, R. A., Mead, R. H., Ruder, M. A., et al.: Long-term outcome with the automatic implantable cardioverter-defibrillator. J. Am. Coll. Cardiol. *13*:1353, 1989.
266. Tchou, P. J., Kadri, N., Anderson, J., et al.: Automatic implantable cardioverter defibrillators and survival of patients with left ventricular dysfunction and malignant ventricular arrhythmias. Ann. Intern. Med. *109*:529, 1988.
267. Kalbfleisch, K. R., Lehmann, M. H., Steinman, R. T., et al.: Reemployment following implantation of the automatic cardioverter defibrillator. Am. J. Cardiol. *64*:199, 1989.
268. Saksena, S., and Parsonnet, V.: Implantation of a cardioverter/defibrillator without thoracotomy using a triple electrode system. JAMA *259*:69, 1988.
269. Mercando, A. D., Furman, S., Johnston, D., et al.: Survival of patients with the automatic implantable cardioverter defibrillator. PACE *11*:2059, 1988.
269a. Rosenthal, M. E., and Josephson, M. E.: Current status of antitachycardia devices. Circulation *82*:1889, 1990.
270. Haines, D. E., Lerman, B. B., Kron, I. L., and DiMarco, J. P.: Surgical ablation of ventricular tachycardia with sequential map-guided subendocardial resection: electrophysiologic assessment and long-term follow-up. Circulation *77*:131, 1988.
271. Garson, A., Jr., Smith, R. T., Jr., Moak, J. P., et al.: Incessant ventricular tachycardia in infants: Myocardial hamartomas and surgical cure. J. Am. Coll. Cardiol. *10*:619, 1987.
272. Manolis, A. S., Rastegar, H., Payne, D., et al.: Surgical therapy for drug-refractory ventricular tachycardia. Results with mapping-guided subendocardial resection. J. Am. Coll. Cardiol. *14*:199, 1989.
273. Hargrove, W. C., 3d, Josephson, M. E., Marchlinski, F. E., and Miller, J. M.: Surgical decisions in the management of sudden cardiac death and malignant ventricular arrhythmias. Subendocardial resection, the automatic internal defibrillator, or both. J. Thorac. Cardiovasc. Surg. *97*:923, 1989.
274. Borggrefe, M., Podczeck, A., Ostermeyer, J., and Breithardt, G.: Value of post-operative programmed ventricular stimulation after map-guided surgery for ventricular tachyarrhythmias—epicardial versus endocardial stimulation. Eur. Heart J. *9*:969, 1988.
275. Zee-Cheng, C. S., Kouchoukos, N. T., Connors, J. P., and Ruffy, R.: Treatment of life-threatening ventricular arrhythmias with nonguided surgery supported by electrophysiologic testing and drug therapy. J. Am. Coll. Cardiol. *13*:153, 1989.
276. Selle, J. G., Svenson, R. H., Gallagher, J. J., et al.: Laser ablation of ventricular tachycardia. Thorac. Cardiovasc. Surg. *36*(Suppl. 2):155, 1988.
277. Kleiman, R. B., Miller, J. M., Buxton, A. E., et al.: Prognosis following sustained ventricular tachycardia occurring early after myocardial infarction. Am. J. Cardiol. *62*(9):528, 1988.
278. Kelly, P., Ruskin, J. N., Vlahakes, G. J., et al.: Surgical coronary revascularization in survivors of prehospital cardiac arrest: Its effect on inducible ventricular arrhythmias and long-term survival. J. Am. Coll. Cardiol. *15*:267, 1990.
279. Tchou, P., Jazayeri, M., Denker, S., et al.: Transcatheter electrical ablation of right bundle branch. A method of treating macroreentrant ventricular tachycardia attributed to bundle branch reentry. Circulation *78*:246, 1988.
279a. Morady, F., Kadish, A., DiCarlo, et al.: Long-term results of catheter ablation of idiopathic right ventricular tachycardia. Circulation *82*:2093, 1990.
279b. Klein, L. S., Miles, W. M., Gering, L. E., et al.: Radiofrequency catheter ablation of ventricular tachycardia in patients without structural heart disease (abstract). J. Am. Coll. Cardiol. (*in press*).
280. Leclercq, J. F., and Coumel, P.: Characteristics, prognosis and treatment of the ventricular arrhythmias of right ventricular dysplasia. Eur. Heart J. *10*(Suppl. D):61, 1989.
281. Furlanello, F., Bettini, R., Bertoldi, A., et al.: Arrhythmia patterns in athletes with arrhythmogenic right ventricular dysplasia. Eur. Heart J. *10*(Suppl. D):16, 1989.
282. Strain, J.: Adipose dysplasia of the right ventricle: Is endomyocardial biopsy useful? Eur. Heart J. *10*(Suppl. D):84, 1989.
283. Buja, G. F., Nava, A., Martini, B., et al.: Right ventricular dysplasia: a familial cardiomyopathy? Eur. Heart J. *10*(Suppl. D):13, 1989.
284. Nava, A., Canciana, B., Daliento, L., et al.: Juvenile sudden death and effort ventricular tachycardias in a family with right ventricular cardiomyopathy. Int. J. Cardiol. *21*:111, 1988.
285. Nava, A., Thiene, G., Canciani, B., et al.: Familial occurrence of right ventricular dysplasia: A study involving nine families. J. Am. Coll. Cardiol. *12*:1222, 1988.
286. Martini, B., Nava, A., Thiene, G., et al.: Accelerated idioventricular rhythm of infundibular origin in patients with a concealed form of arrhythmogenic right ventricular dysplasia. Br. Heart J. *59*:564, 1988.
287. Lemery, R., Brugada, P., Janssen, J., et al.: Nonischemic sustained ventricular tachycardia: clinical outcome in 12 patients with arrhythmogenic right ventricular dysplasia. J. Am. Coll. Cardiol. *14*:96, 1989.
288. Satoh, M., Aizawa, Y., Murata, M., et al.: Electrophysiologic study of patients with ventricular dysrhythmias during long-term follow-up after repair of tetralogy of Fallot. Jpn. Heart J. *29*:69, 1988.
289. Perry, J. C., Moak, J. P., and Garson, A., Jr.: Pediatric arrhythmias. *In* Zipes, D. P., and Jalife, J. (eds.): Cardiac Electrophysiology. From Cell to Bedside. Philadelphia, W. B. Saunders Company, 1990, p. 678.
290. Kron, J., Hart, M., Schual-Berke, S., et al.: Idiopathic dilated cardiomyopathy. Role of programmed electrical stimulation and Holter monitoring in predicting those at risk of sudden death. Chest *93*:85, 1988.
291. Milner, P. G., DiMarco, J. P., and Lerman, B. B.: Electrophysiological eval-

uation of sustained ventricular tachyarrhythmias in idiopathic dilated cardiomyopathy. PACE *11*:562, 1988.
292. Constantin, L., Martins, J. B., Kienzle, M. G., et al.: Induced sustained ventricular tachycardia in nonischemic dilated cardiomyopathy: Dependence on clinical presentation and response to antiarrhythmic agents. PACE *12*:776, 1989.
293. Milechma, G., and Scheinman, M. M.: Ventricular dysrhythmias and sudden death in dilated cardiomyopathy. Prog. Cardiol. *2/1*:85, 1989.
294. Kuck, K. H., Kunze, K. P., Schluter, M., et al.: Programmed electrical stimulation in hypertrophic cardiomyopathy. Eur. Heart J. *9*:177, 1988.
295. von Dohlen, T. W. Prisant, L. M., Frank, M. J.: Significance of positive or negative thallium-201 scintigraphy in hypertrophic cardiomyopathy. Am. J. Cardiol. *64*:498, 1989.
296. Fananapazir, L., Tracy, C. M., Leon, M. B., et al.: Electrophysiologic abnormalities in patients with hypertrophic cardiomyopathy. A consecutive analysis in 155 patients. Circulation *80*:1259, 1989.
297. McKenna, W. J., Franklin, R. C., Nihoyannopoulos, P., et al: Arrhythmia and prognosis in infants, children and adolescents with hypertrophic cardiomyopathy. J. Am. Coll. Cardiol. *11*:147, 1988.
298. Cecchi, F., Maron, B. J., and Epstein, S. E.: Long-term outcome of patients with hypertrophic cardiomyopathy successfully resuscitated after cardiac arrest. J. Am. Coll. Cardiol. *13*:1283, 1989.
299. Miyajima, S., Aizawa, Y., Suzuki, Y., et al.: Sustained ventricular tachycardia responsive to verapamil in patients with hypertrophic cardiomyopathy. Clinical and electrophysiological assessment of drug efficacy. Jpn. Heart J. *30*:241, 1989.
300. Nienaber, C. A., Hiller, S., Spielmann, R. P., Geiger, M., Kuck, K. H.: Syncope in hypertrophic cardiomyopathy: Multivariant analysis of prognostic determinants. J. Am. Coll. Cardiol. *15*:948, 1990.
301. Cripts, T. R., Counihan, P. J., Frenneaux, M. P., et al.: Signal-averaged electrocardiography in hypertrophic cardiomyopathy. J. Am. Coll. Cardiol. *15*:956, 1990.
302. Kawano, T., Oki, T., Uchida, T., et al.: Innervation of the mitral valve in normal and prolapsed mitral valves. J. Cardiol. *19*(Suppl. 21):43, 1989.
303. Hauer, R.N.W., and Robles de Medina, E. O.: Cardiomyopathies and mitral valve prolapse. *In* Zipes, D. P., and Jalife, J. (eds.): Cardiac Electrophysiology. From Cell to Bedside. Philadelphia, W. B. Saunders Company, 1990, p. 685.
304. Ohe, T., Shimomura, K., Aihara, N., et al.: Idiopathic sustained left ventricular tachycardia: clinical and electrophysiologic characteristics. Circulation *77*:560, 1988.
305. Lemery, R., Brugada, P., Bella, P. D., et al.: Nonischemic ventricular tachycardia. Clinical course and long-term follow-up in patients without clinically overt heart disease. Circulation *79*:990, 1989.
306. Deal, B. J., Miller, S. M., Scagliotti, D., et al.: Ventricular tachycardia in a young population without overt heart disease. Circulation *73*:1111, 1986.
307. Belhassen, B., Shapira, I., Shoshani, D., et al.: Idiopathic ventricular fibrillation: inducibility and beneficial effects of class I antiarrhythmic agents. Circulation *75*:809, 1987.
308. Lemery, R., Brugada, P., Della Bella, P., et al.: Ventricular fibrillation in six adults without overt heart disease. J. Am. Coll. Cardiol. *13*:911, 1989.
309. Ritchie, A. H., Kerr, C. R., Qi, A., and Yeung-Lai-Wah, J. A.: Nonsustained ventricular tachycardia arising from the right ventricular outflow tract. Am. J. Cardiol. *64*:594, 1989.
310. Proclemer, A., Ciani, R., and Feruglio, G. A.: Right ventricular tachycardia with left bundle branch block and inferior axis morphology: Clinical and arrhythmological characteristics in 15 patients. PACE *12*:977, 1989.
311. Kasanuki, H., Ohnishi, S., Tanaka, E., and Hirosawa, K.: Idiopathic sustained ventricular tachycardia responsive to verapamil: clinical electrocardiographic and electrophysiologic considerations. Jpn. Circ. J. *50*:109, 1986.
312. Waxman, M. B., Cupps, C. L., and Cameron, D. A.: Modulation of an idioventricular rhythm by vagal tone. J. Am. Coll. Cardiol. *11*:1052, 1988.
313. Lerman, B. B., Wesley, R. C., Jr., DiMarco, J. P., et al.: Antiadrenergic effects of adenosine on His-Purkinje automaticity. Evidence for accentuated antagonism. J. Clin. Invest. *82*:2127, 1988.
314. Kadish, A. H., and Morady, F.: Torsade de pointes. *In* Zipes, D. P., and Jalife, J. (eds.): Cardiac Electrophysiology: From Cell to Bedside. Philadelphia, W. B. Saunders Company, 1990, p. 605.
315. Curtis, M. J., Bernier, M., and Szendey, G.: Torsades de pointes: a reevaluation. Cardiovasc. Drugs Ther. *4*:1169, 1990.
316. Opie, L. H.: Forum on torsades de pointes: introduction. Cardiovasc. Drugs Ther. *4*:1167, 1990.
317. Surawicz, B.: Electrophysiologic substrate of torsade de pointes: dispersion of repolarization or early afterdepolarizations? J. Am. Coll. Cardiol. *14*:172, 1989.
318. Jackman, W. M., Friday, K. J., Clark, M., Anderson, J., et al.: The long QT syndromes: a critical review, new clinical observations and unifying hypothesis. Prog. Cardiovasc. Dis. *31*:115, 1988.
319. Bailie, D. S., Inoue, H., Kaseda, S., et al.: Magnesium suppresses early afterdepolarizations and ventricular tachyarrhythmias induced in dogs by cesium. Circulation *77*:1395, 1988.
320. Ben-David, J., and Zipes, D. P.: Differential response to right and left stellate stimulation of early afterdepolarizations and ventricular tachycardia in the dog. Circulation *78*:1241, 1988.
321. El-Sherif, N., Bekheit, S. S., and Henkin, R.: Quinidine-induced long QTU interval and torsades de pointes: Role of bradycardia-dependent early afterdepolarizations. J. Am. Coll. Cardiol. *14*:252, 1989.
322. Kaseda, S., Gilmour, R. F., Jr., and Zipes, D. P.: Depressant effect of magnesium on early afterdepolarizations and triggered activity induced by cesium quinidine and 4-aminopyridine in canine cardiac Purkinje fibers. Am. Heart J. *118*:458, 1989.
323. El-Sherif, N., Craelius, W., Boutjdir, M., and Gough, W. B.: Early afterdepolarizations and arrhythmogenesis. J. Cardiovasc. Electrophys. *1*:145, 1990.
324. January, C. T., and Shorofsky, S.: Early afterdepolarizations: Newer insights into cellular mechanisms. J. Cardiovasc. Electrophys. *1*:161, 1990.
325. Jackman, W. M., Szabo, B., Friday, K. J., et al.: Ventricular tachyarrhythmias related to early afterdepolarizations and triggered firing: relationship to QT interval prolongation and potential therapeutic role for calcium channel blocking agents. J. Cardiovasc. Electrophys. *1*:170, 1990.
326. Ben-David, J., and Zipes, D. P.: Alpha adrenoceptor stimulation and blockade modulates cesium-induced early afterdepolarizations and ventricular tachyarrhythmias in dogs. Circulation *82*:225, 1990.
327. Kaseda, S., and Zipes, D. P.: Effects of alpha adrenoceptor stimulation and blockade on early afterdepolarizations and triggered activity induced by cesium in canine cardiac Purkinje fibers. J. Cardiovasc. Electrophys. *1*:31, 1990.
328. Miyazaki, T., Pride, H. P., and Zipes, D. P.: Prostaglandin modulation of early afterdepolarizations and ventricular tachyarrhythmias induced by cesium chloride combined with efferent cardiac sympathetic stimulation in dogs. J. Am. Coll. Cardiol. *16*:1287, 1990.
329. Zipes, D. P.: Monophasic action potentials in the diagnosis of triggered arrhythmias. Prog. Cardiovasc. Dis. *(In press).*
330. Stanton, M. S., Prystowsky, E. N., Fineberg, N. S., et al.: Arrhythmogenic effects of antiarrhythmic drugs: A study of 506 patients treated for ventricular tachycardia or fibrillation. J. Am. Coll. Cardiol. *14*:209, 1989.
331. Minardo, J. D., Heger, J. J., Miles, W. M., et al.: Clinical characteristics of patients with ventricular fibrillation during antiarrhythmic drug therapy. N. Engl. J. Med. *319*:257, 1988.
332. Tzivoni, D., Banai, S., Schugar, C., et al.: Treatment of torsade de pointes with magnesium sulfate. Circulation *77*:392, 1988.
333. Laks, M. M.: Long QT interval syndrome. A new look at an old electrophysiologic measurement—the power of the computer. Circulation *82*:1539, 1990.
334. Schwartz, P. J., Locati, E., Priori, S. G., and Zaza, A.: The long Q-T syndrome. *In* Zipes, D. P., and Jalife, J. (eds.): Cardiac Electrophysiology. From Cell to Bedside. Philadelphia, W. B. Saunders Company, 1990, p. 589.
335. Benhorin, J., Meru, M., Albert, M., et al.: Long QT syndrome. New electrocardiographic characteristics. Circulation *82*:521, 1990.
336. Puddu, P.E., Jouve, R., Langlet, F., et al.: Prevention of postischemic ventricular fibrillation late after right or left stellate ganglionectomy in dogs. Circulation *77*:935, 1988.
337. Zipes, D. P.: The long QT syndrome: A Rosetta stone for sympathetic related arrhythmias. (editorial). Circulation *(In press).*
338. Di Pasquale, G., Pinelli, G., Andreoli, A., et al.: Holter detection of cardiac arrhythmias in intracranial subarachnoid hemorrhage. Am. J. Cardiol. *59*:596, 1987
339. Andreoli, A., di Pasquale, G., Pinelli, G., et al.: Subarachnoid hemorrhage: Frequency and severity of cardiac arrhythmias. A survey of 70 cases studied in the acute phase. Stroke *18*:558, 1987.
340. Gospe, S. M., Jr., and Choy, M.: Hereditary long Q-T syndrome presenting as epilepsy. Electroencephalography laboratory diagnosis. Ann. Neurol. *25*:514, 1989.
341. Weintraub, R. G., Gow, R. M., and Wilkinson, J. L.: The congenital long QT syndromes in childhood. J. Am. Coll. Cardiol. *16*:674, 1990.
342. Schwartz, P. J., Locati, E., Moss, A. J., et al.: Left cardiac sympathetic denervation in the therapy of the congenital long QT syndrome: A world wide report. Circulation *(In press).*
343. Fish, F. A., Prakash, C., and Roden, D. M.: Suppression of repolarization-related arrhythmias in vitro and in vivo by low-dose potassium channel activators. Circulation *82*:1362, 1990.
344. Caceres, J., Jazayeri, M., McKinnie, J., et al.: Sustained bundle branch reentry as a mechanism of clinical tachycardia. Circulation *79*:256, 1989.
345. Lazzara, R., and Scherlag, B. J.: Generation of arrhythmias in myocardial ischemia and infarction. Am. J. Cardiol. *61*:20A, 1988.
346. Koretsune, Y., and Marban, E.: Cell calcium in the pathophysiology of ventricular fibrillation and in the pathogenesis of postarrhythmic contractile dysfunction. Circulation *80*:369, 1989.
347. Thandroyen, F. T., McCarthy, J., Burton, K. P., and Opie, L. H.: Ryanodine and caffeine prevent ventricular arrhythmias during acute myocardial ischemia and reperfusion in rat heart. Circ. Res. *62*:306, 1988.
348. Mohabir, R., Clusin, W. T., and Lee, H. C.: Intracellular calcium alternans and the genesis of ischemic ventricular fibrillation. *In* Zipes, D. P., and Jalife, J. (eds.): Cardiac Electrophysiology. From Cell to Bedside. Philadelphia, W. B. Saunders Company, 1990, p. 448.
349. Corr, P. B., Creer, M. H., Yamada, K. A., et al.: Prophylaxis of early ventricular fibrillation by inhibition of acylcarnitine accumulation. J. Clin. Invest. *83*:927, 1989.
350. Creer, M. H., Dobmeyer, D. J., and Corr, P. B.: Amphipathic lipid metabolites and arrhythmias during myocardial ischemia. *In* Zipes, D. P., and Jalife, J. (eds.): Cardiac Electrophysiology. From Cell to Bedside. Philadelphia, W. B. Saunders Company, 1990, p. 417.
351. Hearse, D. J.: Free radicals, membrane injury, and electrophysiological disorders. *In* Zipes, D. P., and Jalife, J. (eds.): Cardiac Electrophysiology. From Cell to Bedside. Philadelphia, W. B. Saunders Company, 1990, p. 442.
352. Opie, L. H., and Coetzee, W. A.: Metabolic components of ischemia and fibrillation. *In* Zipes, D. P., and Jalife, J. (eds.): Cardiac Electrophysiol-

ogy. From Cell to Bedside. Philadelphia, W. B. Saunders Company, 1990, p. 456.

353. Schwartz, P. J., Vanoli, E., Stramba-Badiale, M., et al.: Autonomic mechanisms and sudden death. New insights from analysis of baroreceptor reflexes in conscious dogs with and without a myocardial infarction. Circulation *78*:969, 1988.

354. Rosen, M. R., Danilo, P., Jr., Robinson, R. B., et al.: Sympathetic neural and alpha-adrenergic modulation of arrhythmias. Ann. N. Y. Acad. Sci. *533*:200, 1988.

355. Fedida, D., Shimoni, Y., and Giles, W. R.: A novel effect of norepinephrine on cardiac cells is mediated by alpha-1-adrenoceptors. Am. J. Physiol. *256*:H1500, 1989.

356. Corr, P. B., Heathers, G. P., and Yamada, K. A.: Mechanisms contributing to the arrhythmogenic influences of alpha-1-adrenergic stimulation in the ischemic heart. Am. J. Med. *87*:19S, 1989.

357. Heathers, G. P., Evers, A. S., and Corr, P. B.: Enhanced inositol triphosphate response to alpha-1-adrenergic stimulation in cardiac myocytes exposed to hypoxia. J. Clin. Invest. *83*:1409, 1989.

358. Singer, D. H., Martin, G. J., Magid, N., et al.: Low heart rate variability and sudden cardiac death. J. Electrocardiol. *21*(Suppl.):S46, 1988.

359. Gang, E. S., Lew, A. S., Hong, M., et al.: Decreased incidence of ventricular late potentials after successful thrombolytic therapy for acute myocardial infarction. N. Engl. J. Med. *321*:712, 1989.

360. Volpi, A., Cavalli, A., Santoro, E., et al.: Incidence and prognosis of secondary ventricular fibrillation in acute myocardial infarction. Evidence for a protective effect of thrombolytic therapy. Circulation *82*:1279, 1990.

360a. Bourke, J. P., Young, A. A., Richards, D. B., et al.: Reduction in incidence of inducible ventricular tachycardia after myocardial infarction by treatment with streptokinase during infarct evolution. J. Am. Coll. Cardiol. *16*:1703, 1990.

361. Muller, J. E., Tofler, G. H., and Stone, P. H.: Circadian variation and triggers of onset of acute cardiovascular disease. Circulation *79*:733, 1989.

361a. Muller, J. E., and Tofler, G. H.: Introduction. A symposium: triggering and circadian variation of onset of acute cardiovascular disease. Am. J. Cardiol. *66*:1G, 1990.

362. Brezinski, D. A., Tofler, G. H., Muller, J. E., et al.: Morning increase in platelet aggregability. Association with assumption of the upright posture. Circulation. *78*:35, 1988.

363. Falk, E.: Morphologic features of unstable atherothrombotic plaques underlying acute coronary syndromes. Am. J. Cardiol. *63*:114E, 1989.

364. Stein, B., Badimon, L., Israel, D. H., et al.: Thrombosis/platelets and other blood factors in acute coronary syndromes. Cardiovasc. Clin. *20*:105, 1989.

365. Willerson, J. T., Golino, P., Eidt, J., et al.: Specific platelet mediators and unstable coronary artery lesions. Experimental evidence and potential clinical implications. Circulation *80*:198, 1989.

366. Ridker, P. M., Manson, J. E., Buring, J. E., et al.: Circadian variation of acute myocardial infarction and the effect of low-dose aspirin in a randomized trial of physicians. Circulation *82*:897, 1990.

366a. Pogwizd, S. M., and Corr, P. B.: Mechanisms underlying the development of ventricular fibrillation during early myocardial ischemia. Circ. Res. *66*:672, 1990.

367. Bay es de Luna, A., Coumel, P., and Leclercq, J. F.: Ambulatory sudden cardiac death: mechanisms of production of fatal arrhythmia on the basis of data from 157 cases. Am. Heart J. *117*:151, 1989.

368. Poole, J. E., Mathisen, T. L., Kudenchuk, P. J., et al.: Long-term outcome in patients who survive out of hospital ventricular fibrillation and undergo electrophysiologic studies: Evaluation by electrophysiologic subgroups. J. Am. Coll. Cardiol. *16*:657, 1990.

369. Gillum, R. F.: Sudden coronary death in the United States: 1980–1985. Circulation *79*:756, 1989.

370. Kuller, L. H., Traven, N. D., Rutan, G. H., et al.: Marked decline of coronary heart disease mortality in 35–44-year-old white men in Allegheny County, Pennsylvania. Circulation *80*:261, 1989.

371. Kremers, M. S., Black, W. H., and Wells, P. J.: Sudden cardiac death: etiologies, pathogenesis, and management. DM *35*:381, 1989.

372. Hetzel, B. S., Charnock, J. S., Dwyer, T., and McLennan, P. L.: Fall in coronary heart disease mortality in U.S.A. and Australia due to sudden death: Evidence for the role of polyunsaturated fat. J. Clin. Epidemiol. *42*:885, 1989.

373. Holmes, D. R., Jr., Davis, K., Gersh, B. J., et al.: Risk factor profiles of patients with sudden cardiac death and death from other cardiac causes: A report from the Coronary Artery Surgery Study (CASS). J. Am. Coll. Cardiol. *13*:524, 1989.

374. Sheps, D. S., and Heiss, G.: Sudden death and silent myocardial ischemia. Am. Heart J. *117*:177, 1989.

375. Meldahl, R. V., Marshall, R. C., and Scheinmann, M. C.: Identification of persons at risk for sudden cardiac death. Med. Clin. North Am. *72*:1015, 1988.

376. Weiner, D. A., Ryan, T. J., McCabe, C. H., et al.: Risk of developing an acute myocardial infarction or sudden coronary death in patients with exercise-induced silent myocardial ischemia. A Report From the Coronary Artery Surgery Study (CASS) Registry. Am. J. Cardiol. *62*:1155, 1988.

377. Rapaport, E.: Sudden cardiac death. Am. J. Cardiol. *62*:3I, 1988.

378. Kannel, W. B., Plehn, J. F., and Cupples, L. A.: Cardiac failure and sudden death in the Framingham Study. Am. Heart J. *115*:869, 1988.

379. Marcus, F. I., Cobb, L. A., Edwards, J. E., et al.: Mechanism of death and prevalence of myocardial ischemic symptoms in the terminal event after acute myocardial infarction. Am. J. Cardiol. *61*:8, 1988.

380. Kannel, W. B., Cupples, L. A., D'Agostino, R. B., Stokes, J., 3d: Hypertension, antihypertensive treatment and sudden coronary death. The Framingham Study. Hypertension *11*:II45, 1988.

381. Le Heuzey, J. Y., and Guize, L.: Cardiac prognosis in hypertensive patients. Incidence of sudden death and ventricular arrhythmias. Am. J. Med. *84*:65, 1988.

382. Messerli, F. H., Oren, S., and Grossman, E.: Left ventricular hypertrophy and antihypertensive therapy. Drugs *35*(Suppl. 5):27, 1988.

383. Levy, D.: Left ventricular hypertrophy. Epidemiological insights from the Framingham Heart Study. Drugs *35*(Suppl. 5):1, 1988.

384. Messerli, F. H., Nunez, B. D., Ventura, H. O., and Snyder, D. W.: Overweight and sudden death. Increased ventricular ectopy in cardiopathy of obesity. Arch. Intern. Med. *147*:1725, 1987.

385. Kluge, K. A., Harper, R. M., Schechtman, V. L., et al.: Spectral analysis assessment of respiratory sinus arrhythmia in normal infants and infants who subsequently died of sudden infant death syndrome. Pediatr. Res. *24*:677, 1988.

386. Rajs, J., and Hammarquist, F.: Sudden infant death in Stockholm. A forensic pathology study covering ten years. Acta Paediatr. Scand. *77*:812, 1988.

387. Peirano, P., Lacombe, J., Kastler, B., et al.: Night sleep heart rate patterns recorded by cardiopneumography at home in normal and at-risk for SIDS infants. Early Hum. Dev. *17*:175, 1988.

388. Woolf, P. K., Gweitz, M. H., Preminger, T., et al.: Infants with apparent life threatening events. Cardiac rhythm and conduction. Clin. Pediatr. *28*:517, 1989.

389. Topaz, O., Perin, E., Cox, M., et al.: Young adult survivors of sudden cardiac arrest: Analysis of invasive evaluation of 22 subjects. Am. Heart J. *118*:281, 1989.

390. Kramer, M. R., Drori, Y., and Lev, B.: Sudden death in young soldiers. High incidence of syncope prior to death. Chest *93*:345, 1988.

391. Thiene, G., Nava, A., Corrado, D., et al.: Right ventricular cardiomyopathy and sudden death in young people. N. Engl. J. Med. *318*:129, 1988.

392. Corrado, D., Thiene, G., and Penneli, N.: Sudden death as the first manifestation of coronary artery disease in young people (less than or equal to 35 years). Eur. Heart J. *9*(Suppl. N):139, 1988.

393. Brookfield, L., Bharati, S., Denes, P., et al.: Familial sudden death. Report of a case and review of the literature. Chest *94*:989, 1988.

394. Raymond, J. R., van den Berg, E. K., Jr., and Knapp, M. J.: Nontraumatic prehospital sudden death in young adults. Arch. Intern. Med. *148*:303, 1988.

395. Lewis, J. F., Maron, B. J., Diggs, J. A., et al.: Preparticipation echocardiographic screening for cardiovascular disease in a large, predominantly black population of collegiate athletes. Am. J. Cardiol. *64*:1029, 1989.

396. Firor, W. B., and Faulkner, R. A.: Sudden death during exercise: how real a hazard? Can. J. Cardiol. *4*:251, 1988.

397. Marti, B., Goerre, S., Spuhler, T., et al.: Sudden death during mass running events in Switzerland 1978–1987: An epidemiologico-pathologic study. Schweiz. Med. Wochenschr. *119*:473, 1989.

398. Fontaine, G., Fontaliran, F., Frank, R., et al.: Causes of sudden death in athletes. Arch. Mal. Coeur *82* Spec No 2:107, 1989.

399. Kurita, A., Uehata, A., Nishioka, T., et al.: An investigation of sudden cardiac death in apparently healthy young men by annual health examination. Nippon Eiseigaku. Zasshi. *44*:739, 1989.

400. Rosman, H. S., Goldstein, S., Landis, J. R., et al.: Clinical characteristics and survival experience of out-of-hospital cardiac arrest victims without coronary heart disease. Eur. Heart J. *9*:17, 1988.

401. Melles, R. B., and Katz, B.: Night terrors and sudden unexplained nocturnal death. Med. Hypotheses. *26*:149, 1988.

401a. Winkle, R. A., Mead, H. R., and Ruder, M. A.: Effect of duration of ventricular fibrillation on defibrillation efficacy in humans. Circulation *81*:1477, 1990.

401b. Weaver, W. D., Fahrenbruch, C. E., and Johnson, D. D.: Effect of epinephrine and lidocaine therapy on outcome after cardiac arrest due to ventricular fibrillation. Circulation *82*:2027, 1990.

402. Horowitz, L. N.: Drug therapy for survivors of sudden cardiac death. PACE *11*:1960, 1988.

402a. Hoshino, K., Anumonwo, J., Delmar, M., and Jalife, J.: Wenckebach periodicity in single atrioventricular nodal cells from the rabbit heart. Circulation *82*:2201, 1990.

403. Medina-Ravell, V., Rodriguez-Salas, L., Castellanos, A., and Myerburg, R. J.: Death due to paroxysmal atrioventricular block during ambulatory electrocardiographic monitoring. PACE *12*:65, 1989.

404. Gilmour, R. F., Jr., and Zipes, D. P.: Rate-related suppression and facilitation of conduction. *In* Zipes, D. P., and Jalife, J. (eds.): Cardiac Electrophysiology. From Cell to Bedside. Philadelphia, W. B. Saunders, 1990, p. 610.

405. Nagashima, M., Nakashima, T., Asai, T., et al.: Study on congenital complete heart block in children by 24-hour ambulatory electrocardiographic monitoring. Jpn. Heart J. *28*:323, 1987.

406. Madsen, J. K., Meibom, J., Videbak, R., et al.: Transcutaneous pacing: experience with the Zoll noninvasive temporary pacemaker. Am. Heart J. *116*:7, 1988.

406a. Chialo, D. R., Michaels, D. C., and Jalife, J.: Supernormal excitability as a mechanism of chaotic dynamics of activation in cardiac Purkinje fibers. Circ. Res. *66*:525, 1990.

407. Castellanos, A., Moleiro, F., Saoudi, N. C., and Myerburg, R. J.: Parasysole. *In* Zipes, D. P., and Jalife, J. (eds.): Cardiac Electrophysiology. From Cell to Bedside. Philadelphia, 1990, p. 619.

408. Oreto, G., Satullo, G., Luzza, F., et al.: "Irregular" ventricular parasystole: the influence of sinus rhythm on a parasystolic focus. Am. Heart J. *115*:121, 1988.

409. Robles de Medina, E. O., Delmar, M., Sicouri, S., and Jalife, J.: Modulated parasystole as a mechanism of ventricular ectopic activity leading to ventricular fibrillation. Am. J. Cardiol. *63*:1326, 1989.

25

Cardiac Pacemakers and Antiarrhythmic Devices

by S. SERGE BAROLD, M.D., and DOUGLAS P. ZIPES, M.D.

Since the first pacemaker implantation in 1958, cardiac pacing has continued to grow so that presently more than 500,000 patients have pacemakers in the United States. In addition to pacemakers that treat bradyarrhythmias with the aim of restoring normal or near-normal hemodynamics at rest and exercise, electrical therapy of ventricular tachyarrhythmias with devices capable of pacing, cardioversion, and defibrillation has become very important.

A pacemaker is a device that delivers battery-supplied electrical stimuli over leads with electrodes in contact with the heart. Virtually all leads are inserted transvenously. Electronic circuitry regulates the timing and characteristics of the stimuli. The *power source* is usually a lithium-iodine battery that has a high-energy density (energy content/volume), low internal losses caused by self-discharge, and a long shelf life; it can be hermetically sealed to prevent ingress of body fluids. Importantly, the lithium-iodine battery retains a satisfactory voltage for 90 per cent of its life, and as the voltage decays at end-of-life, the pacing rate usually declines. For single-chamber pulse generators, the expected life is 7 to 12 years and for dual-chamber pulse generators 4 to 8 years, depending on pacemaker function.

Pacemaker Modalities and Function

Pacemakers are categorized with a three-letter identification code (recently expanded to five) according to the site of the pacing electrodes and the mode of pacing[1]: V = ventricle, A = atrium, D = dual (A and V), I = inhibited, T = triggered, and 0 = none (Table 25–1). The first position denotes the chamber paced and the second position indicates the chamber sensed. The third position indicates the response to sensing, if any, with "I" indicating an inhibited response (pacemaker discharge suppressed by a sensed signal), "T" indicating a triggered response (pacemaker discharge triggered by a sensed signal), and "D" indicating both inhibited and triggered functions. I and T responses reset the timing circuit controlling the pacemaker lower rate interval. Occasionally the letter "S" is used for the first or second position to indicate that a single-chamber device is suitable for either atrial or ventricular pacing depending on how its parameters are programmed. For most pacemakers, the first three positions contain all the information of practical importance. The fourth and fifth positions are available to describe additional functions; however, the letters are infrequently stated in practice except for "R", which indicates a rate-adaptive pulse generator driven by a sensor (Table 25–1).

USES FOR CARDIAC PACING

Cardiac pacing can be performed to treat patients who have bradyarrhythmias and tachyarrhythmias. Temporary pacing is used when an arrhythmia is transient and permanent pacing when an arrhythmia is likely to be recurrent or permanent.

TABLE 25-1 THE NASPE/BPEG GENERIC PACEMAKER CODE*

POSITION CATEGORY	I CHAMBER(S) PACED	II CHAMBER(S) SENSED	III RESPONSE TO SENSING	IV PROGRAMMABILITY, RATE MODULATION	V ANTITACHYARRHYTHMIA FUNCTION(S)
	O = None A = Atrium V = Ventricle D = Dual (A + V)	O = None A = Atrium V = Ventricle D = Dual (A + V)	O = None T = Triggered I = Inhibited D = Dual (T + I)	O = None P = Simple programmable M = Multiprogrammable C = Communicating R = Rate modulation	O = None P = Pacing (antitachyarrhythmia) S = Shock D = Dual (P + S)
MANUFACTURER'S DESIGNATION ONLY	S = single (A or V)	S = single (A or V)			

* NASPE: North American Society of Pacing and Electrophysiology; BPEG = British Pacing and Electrophysiology Group

TEMPORARY PACING

Temporary cardiac pacing can be accomplished transvenously, via the esophagus, transcutaneously, epicardially, and via a coronary artery. Transvenous pacing is done through percutaneous puncture of the internal jugular, subclavian, or femoral vein using balloon-tipped and semifloating catheters without fluoroscopy or stiffer catheters with fluoroscopy.[2] An electrode in the esophagus achieves atrial pacing. It is relatively noninvasive, safe, and simple and can be useful to initiate or terminate some supraventricular tachycardias, to treat sinus bradycardia or arrest, and to provide overdrive suppression of ventricular tachyarrhythmias such as torsades de pointes with Q-T prolongation.[3-6] Transcutaneous ventricular pacing is used during emergency treatment of asystole or severe bradycardia; it involves large surface area, high impedance electrodes on the anterior and posterior chest wall, stimuli of long duration (20 to 40 ms), and high current (50 to 100 mA).[7-8] Transcutaneous pacing produces a hemodynamic response similar to that of transvenous ventricular pacing and demand pacing can be accomplished by sensing the surface QRS complex. Many supraventricular and ventricular tachyarrhythmias can be initiated and terminated deliberately.[9-12] In some patients, severe pain from skeletal muscle stimulation requires analgesics. Transcutaneous pacing may be useful when endocardial pacing is contraindicated and avoids some of the possible complications associated with temporary endocardial pacing such as infection, phlebitis, venous thrombosis, and perforation of the right ventricle.[13] Epicardial pacing using ventricular and/or atrial pacing wires implanted at surgery is done in postoperative cardiac surgical patients (Chap. 53), while pacing via a coronary artery can be accomplished during percutaneous transluminal coronary angioplasty.

INDICATIONS. Temporary pacing is indicated prophylactically in patients with a high risk of developing high-degree AV block, severe sinus node dysfunction, or asystole in acute myocardial infarction (Chap. 39) after cardiac surgery (Chap. 53), during cardiac catheterization, and occasionally before implantation or replacement of a permanent pacemaker. Asymptomatic patients with bifascicular block only who undergo surgery with general anesthesia do *not* need prophylactic pacing. Pacing is also indicated when temporary bradycardia causes symptomatic, hemodynamic, or electrophysiological consequences as in acute myocardial infarction (discussed later), hyperkalemia, drug-induced bradycardia or toxicity (e.g., digitalis), bradycardia-dependent ventricular tachycardia, before implantation of a permanent pacemaker in a patient with unstable rhythm, and in myocarditis such as in Lyme disease.[14,15] Finally, rapid (burst) temporary pacing can be used to terminate tachycardias such as atrial flutter, AV nodal and AV reentry (Chap. 24), and sustained ventricular tachycardia. A transvenous lead designed for low-energy transvenous cardioversion can also terminate ventricular tachycardia.[16]

Atrial fibrillation, ventricular fibrillation, and very rapid ventricular tachycardia *cannot* be treated by pacing techniques. Pacing at rapid rates can prevent some ventricular tachycardias that are bradycardia-dependent or associated with Q-T prolongation and torsades de pointes. Less frequent uses include atrial pacing at a rate faster than the tachycardia to increase the degree of AV block, synchronized atrial pacing to restore AV synchrony during incessant ventricular tachycardia, and coupled ventricular pacing with an early stimulus timed to provide an electrical but not a mechanical response to slow the effective rate.[17]

TEMPORARY PACING IN ACUTE MYOCARDIAL INFARCTION (see also p. 1242). The role of temporary pacing in acute myocardial infarction is still controversial because the risk-to-benefit ratio is unclear. Death is generally not related directly to the conduction disturbance, and the prognosis depends more on the size of the myocardial infarction than the degree of AV block. AV block in *inferior infarction* is almost always localized in the AV node and is relatively benign. Most hemodynamically stable patients with second degree AV block can be treated without pacing but require monitoring. Pacing is rarely necessary in hemodynamically stable patients with complete AV block and a ventricular rate around 40 to 45 per minute in the absence of ventricular arrhythmia. Temporary pacing is indicated in second or third degree AV block only in the presence of an excessively slow ventricular rate, ventricular arrhythmia, hypotension, signs of hypoperfusion, or congestive heart failure. *Right ventricular infarction* causes an acute increase in diastolic compliance so that the right ventricle becomes far more dependent on preload and acts more or less as a passive conduit for the atrial pump. Right ventricular infarction can be associated with hypotension or shock, partly or entirely due to AV block and loss of AV synchrony. Ventricular pacing may not improve the hemodynamic state, but AV sequential pacing with restoration of AV synchrony can cause a dramatic increase in the blood pressure, cardiac output, and stroke volume.[18] AV synchrony also lowers intrapericardial pressure because of the appropriately timed decline in atrial volume during ventricular end-diastole, thereby providing space within the pericardium for additional filling of the atria and left ventricle.

The development of type II second degree or higher degree of AV block during *anterior myocardial infarction* necessitates temporary pacing, but the mortality is nonetheless quite high because these conduction disturbances generally occur in patients with very large infarcts. Prophylactic pacing is also generally recommended in the presence of new right bundle branch block with left axis deviation (left anterior hemiblock), right bundle branch block with right axis deviation (left posterior hemiblock), left bundle branch block with first degree AV block and alternating right and left bundle branch block because these patients are at higher risk of suddenly developing high degree AV block with catastrophic consequences.

The role of pacing for right bundle branch block with normal axis or left bundle branch block with normal P-R interval is more controversial. Preexisting right or left bundle branch

(*Text continued on page 730*)

higher rate of symptomatic remission and a better prognosis with a low risk of dying from an arrhythmia.[25] Obviously, a negative study does not exclude transient bradycardia as a cause of syncope[27] or possibly sudden death, although the risk is quite low[25] and recurrence of syncope does not correlate with a higher mortality or sudden death. An H-V interval ≥100 ms identifies patients with a higher risk of AV block who require pacing. Pacing can be considered in patients who have an H-V between 70 and 100 ms and no identifiable cause for syncope.

SICK SINUS SYNDROME. Sick sinus syndrome (p. 677) is the most common indication for cardiac pacing in the United States and Europe, accounting for 40 to 55 per cent of pacemaker implantations.[28,29] A pacemaker should be implanted only when a causal relationship has been demonstrated between bradycardia and symptoms, which may be difficult to accomplish in elderly patients with vague symptoms. If in doubt about the need for pacing, it is usually safe to wait, because arrhythmias associated with sick sinus syndrome rarely result in sudden cardiac death. In the bradycardia-tachycardia syndrome (Chap. 24), drugs alone may worsen the bradycardia; symptomatic patients are usually best managed by a combination of pacemaker and antiarrhythmic drugs. When bradycardia is secondary to necessary drug therapy, e.g., beta blocker or amiodarone, a pacemaker can be used to treat the consequences of the drug. Permanent pacing should *not* be considered when there is transient bradycardia due to an increase in vagal tone or from drug therapy that can be discontinued or reduced. In the sick sinus syndrome, pacing improves the quality of life and facilitates treatment of supraventricular tachycardias exhibited by half of the patients. Most patients have structural heart disease, and single-chamber ventricular pacing (as opposed to atrial pacing, discussed later) does not reduce the incidence of overall mortality or sudden death.

The role of prophylactic pacing in asymptomatic patients with ECG evidence of sick sinus syndrome has not been established. Asymptomatic patients should be followed closely; drugs that depress sinus node function should be avoided. Two-second pauses are usually harmless. During sleep, the sinus rate normally may fall to 30/min and exhibit pauses of 3 sec. While it is often stated that sinus pauses are abnormal if they exceed 3 sec without intervening escape beats, the validity of such a conclusion has not been established; neither has the validity of permanent pacing in these asymptomatic patients.

METHODS OF PACEMAKER IMPLANTATION

The Inter-society Commission for Heart Disease Resources (American Heart Association) published in 1983 the optimal resources for implantable cardiac pacemakers. Virtually all pacemakers are implanted transvenously under local anesthesia using either the cephalic vein exposed by cutdown or blind percutaneous puncture of the subclavian vein. The pacemaker pocket is fashioned over the pectoralis major muscle. The cephalic vein is often of sufficient size to accept one or two pacing leads.[30] If not, passage of a flexible guidewire followed by a standard subclavian vein introducer provides simple and direct access to the subclavian vein.[31] Although blind percutaneous subclavian vein puncture is potentially more dangerous than insertion through the cephalic vein, in skilled hands it is remarkably safe.[30,32,33] It reduces the time required for implantation, facilitates implanting two leads, reduces the need for surgical expertise (especially with peel-away sheaths), and has made the implantation of most sophisticated pacemakers a relatively simple surgical procedure. Many of the complications (some lethal) of blind subclavian puncture, which include pneumothorax, subclavian arterial puncture with hemothorax, air embolism, hemopneumomediastinum, subcutaneous emphysema, nerve injury, and thoracic duct injury, are preventable.

With contemporary transvenous leads, complications are related more to the skill and experience of the implanter and implantation technique than lead design because all leads now possess good performance characteristics.[34] Epicardial leads are used only if there is no venous access, in certain pediatric patients, or in patients undergoing open heart surgery. The operative techniques and intraoperative measurements necessary for safe and long-term pacing (Table 25–3) are straightforward compared with the technical knowledge required to understand the electrophysiology of pacing and follow-up of patients so as to make the best use of the important programmable functions.

CAPTURE THRESHOLDS, SENSING, AND LEADS

PACING THRESHOLD

DETERMINATION OF THE PACING THRESHOLD. This is crucial to optimize pacemaker longevity and is determined at the time of implanta-

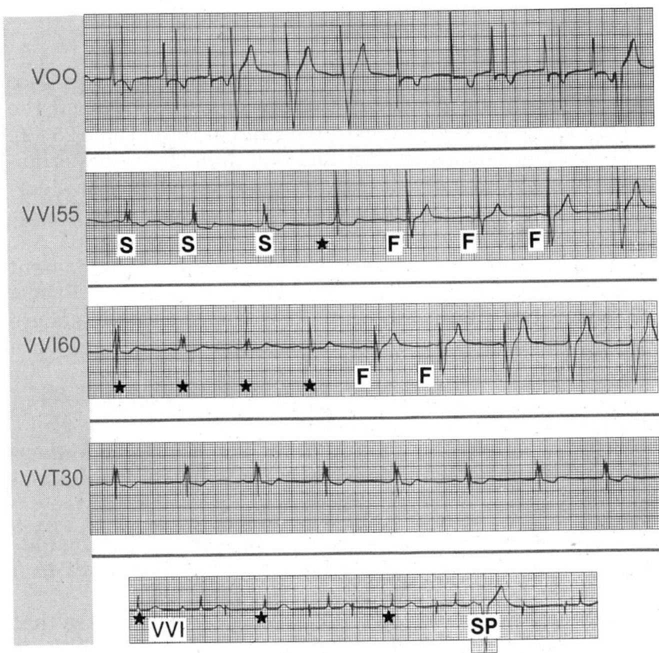

FIGURE 25–1. VOO, VVI, and VVT pacing. ***Top strip:*** **VOO pacing. The pacemaker competes with the spontaneous rhythm and stimuli capture the ventricle only beyond the myocardial refractory period.**

Second strip: **VVI pacemaker, rate = 55/min. The first three beats are sensed (S) and the 4th beat (star) is a ventricular pseudofusion beat. The 5th, 6th , and 7th complexes are ventricular fusion beats (F).**

Third strip: **VVI pacemaker, rate = 60/min. The first three beats (stars) are ventricular pseudofusion beats. The 4th beat (star) appears to be a ventricular pseudofusion beat because the initial QRS vector occurs just before the stimulus. The T wave of the 4th beat is identical to that of the previous beat, suggesting that depolarization was also identical, providing futher proof for pseudofusion. The 5th and 6th complexes are ventricular fusion beats (F) while the last three beats are pure ventricular-paced beats.**

Fourth strip: **Same patient as in third strip. The pacemaker was programmed to the VVT mode, rate = 30/min. The pacemaker emits or triggers a ventricular stimulus immediately upon sensing each QRS complex. Thus, the stimulus marks the precise time of sensing in the VVT mode. This may be correlated with the ventricular pseudofusion beats in the third strip where the first pseudofusion beat is deformed by a ventricular stimulus just before the R wave returns to the baseline, i.e., just before sensing would have occurred as determined from the VVT mode in the 4th strip.**

Bottom strip: **VVI pacemaker with ineffectual stimuli but normal sensing. The high pacing threshold was close to the output of the pulse generator. The 3rd to the last stimulus captures the ventricle in the supernormal phase (SP) when the excitability threshold attains its lowest value. Spontaneous QRS complexes falling within the pacemaker refractory period (for sensing—350 ms after the stimulus) are not sensed; those beyond the pacemaker refractory period are sensed and recycle the pacemaker.**

tion using an external testing device (pacing system analyzer, or PSA) with circuitry similar to that of the implantable pulse generator. Most implantable pulse generators are constant voltage sources: the leading edge of the voltage pulse remains constant regardless of the impedance (resistance). The threshold should be determined in volts at a given pulse width or duration. If only one measurement is made, it should be made at a pulse width of 0.5 to 0.6 msec. To measure the threshold, the PSA is set at 5 V (volts) and pulse width 0.5 msec (usually the nominal parameters of an implantable device). The pacing rate is increased until constant pacing capture is achieved. The voltage is then slowly reduced until loss of capture occurs outside the myocardial refractory period. The lowest voltage capable of causing consistent capture outside the myocardial refractory period defines the stimulation threshold (Fig. 25–1). Near threshold, ventricular capture may occur only when stimuli fall in the supernormal phase (Fig. 25–1).

The current delivered to the myocardium is determined by the impedance (resistance) according to Ohm's law. Normal lead impedance, ranging between 250 and 1000 ohms, typically is 500 to 700 ohms at the nominal output of 5 V. The relationship of threshold voltage and pulse width is not linear and establishes the strength-duration curve; the shorter the pulse width, the higher the voltage threshold (Fig. 25–2).

THE STRENGTH-DURATION CURVE. This is steep, with a short pulse width, and becomes essentially flat at a pulse width exceeding 2 msec (rheobase). The acute ventricular pacing threshold should be ≦ 0.8 V at 0.5 msec pulse width, and the acute atrial pacing threshold ≦ 1.5 V at 0.5 msec. Lower values are often obtained. A high initial threshold value requires lead repositioning. The lowest threshold possible at implantation should be sought because ultimately it may determine the threshold at maturity and hence the voltage required for long-term pacing.

After implantation, the output of the pulse generator is usually left at 5 V and 0.5 msec pulse width or longer for the first 8 weeks. At 8 weeks, when the chronic threshold has been attained in most cases, the output voltage and pulse width should be programmed to enhance pacemaker longevity and yet maintain an adequate margin of safety. The *safety margin* for capture is the amount by which the pulse generator output exceeds the chronic threshold value at a given pulse duration and should be about 3 times the chronic threshold value in terms of energy (microjoules) or 1.75 in terms of voltage, i.e., the output voltage should be at least 1.75 times chronic threshold voltage at the same pulse width. In practice, a voltage safety margin of 2 is often used, so that the output voltage is set at twice the chronic threshold voltage at the same pulse width. An output voltage exceeding 5 volts should not be used routinely because of reduced pulse generator efficiency and longevity.

If the pulse width is varied, without a programmable voltage output, it should be adjusted to 3 times the value at threshold provided that the pulse width at threshold is ≦ 0.2 msec. Because of the configuration of the strength-duration curve, with a pulse width at threshold ≧ 0.3 msec, tripling the pulse width (keeping the voltage constant) may or may not provide a voltage safety margin of 2 and probably should not be used in pacemaker-dependent patients.

The relatively flat characteristic of the voltage strength-duration curve from 0.5 to 1.5 msec means that an increase in the pulse width in this range will not provide a sufficient margin of safety in terms of volts. Therefore, when the voltage at threshold requires a pulse width ≧ 0.4 to 0.5 msec, an adequate safety margin cannot be obtained by programming pulse width alone. With a threshold of 2.5 V/0.1 msec, the pulse generator can be programmed to 2.5 V/0.3 msec or 5 V/0.1 msec to provide a voltage safety factor of at least 2. In terms of output energy (and battery current drain), multiplying the voltage output by 2 (keeping the pulse width constant) is equivalent to multiplying the pulse width by 4 (keeping the voltage constant). Consequently, if the pacemaker circuit is more efficient at 2.5 V than at 5 V, an output of 2.5 V/0.3 msec is preferable to 5.0 V/0.1 msec. With a voltage threshold of 2.5 V/0.3 msec, an output of 5.0 V/0.3 msec is recommended. With relatively high chronic thresholds exceeding 3 to 3.5 volts at pulse width of 0.5 msec at the time of pacemaker replacement or during follow-up, the output voltage should exceed 5 volts. In this situation, use of a new lead or (less preferably) a pulse generator programmable to a high voltage (10 volts) should be considered.

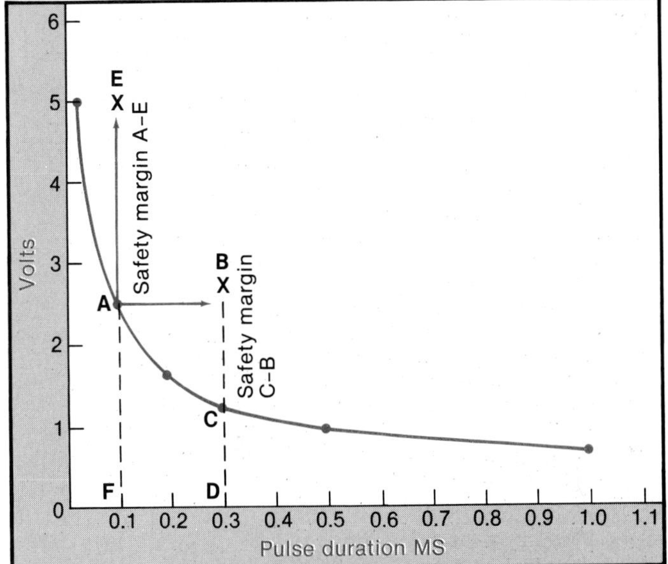

FIGURE 25–2. Strength-duration curve relating voltage and pulse width at the chronic pacing threshold. Values above the curve pace the heart while values below the curve fail to capture. The threshold for pacing at A is 2.5 V at a pulse width of 0.1 ms. Consequently, starting from the threshold at A, the output voltage of the pulse generator could be doubled to 5 V while the pulse is kept width constant at 0.1 ms, i.e., going to E. This would provide a voltage safety margin of EF/AF = 2. Alternatively, the output voltage could be left at 2.5 V and the pulse width increased to 0.3 ms to B. This would yield a voltage safety margin of BD/CD or slightly more than 2. The second option consumes less battery current and is to be preferred.

FUNCTION AND TESTING OF PACING LEADS

In addition to testing thresholds, the integrity of new and old leads can be evaluated by determining the voltage threshold and lead impedance either directly or by telemetry.[35] *Lead impedance* normally remains constant or falls slightly over time. *Lead fracture* (with apposed ends) elevates both the voltage threshold and lead impedance (>1000 ohms), while with an insulation defect the voltage threshold may be low or normal and the lead impedance will be low (<250 ohms). A high-voltage threshold due to lead displacement or an excessive tissue reaction around the electrode (exit block) is associated with a normal lead impedance.

THE PACING THRESHOLD. This variable rises shortly after implantation because edema and inflammation separate the tip from the myocardium. Most of the threshold increase appears to result from the formation of nonexcitable fibrous tissue around the electrode, increasing the effective size of the "virtual" electrode at the interface with the myocardium. The threshold reaches its maximum value 10 to 20 days after implantation and stabilizes to about 2 to 4 times the acute value at 1 to 2 months. Small electrodes have lower initial thresholds and a greater proportional rise during the initial reaction, but the chronic threshold is lower than that of larger electrodes. Threshold evolution sometimes takes longer than expected and on rare occasions the threshold continues to rise gradually with ultimate failure to capture. If there is no lead displacement, such failure to capture is often called *exit block;* this is a relatively rare complication. Exercise, sympathomimetic drugs, and glucocorticoids *decrease* the threshold while food, sleep, insulin, ischemia, hypothyroidism, hyperkalemia, mineralocorticoids, and certan antiarrhythmic agents *increase* the threshold. Type 1C antiarrhythmic drugs[36,37] (especially flecainide), toxic levels of type 1A antiarrhythmic agents, and hyperkalemia[38,39] may cause exit block. Isoproterenol infusion or systemic steroids[40] may be used to treat a high threshold temporarily until the underlying condition is corrected.

SENSING

A pacemaker *senses* the potential difference between the two electrodes (anode and cathode) used for pacing. In a bipolar system (two electrodes in the heart), the bipolar electrogram should be recorded to determine adequate electrode position for sensing. In a unipolar system (one electrode in the heart and the other being the pacemaker container itself), the unipolar electrogram is recorded from the tip electrode and closely reflects the cardiac signal because the anodal contribution from the pacemaker plate is generally negligible. The amplitude and slew rate (dV/dt) of the electrogram must exceed the sensitivity of the pulse generator to ensure reliable sensing.[41]

AMPLITUDE OF THE VENTRICULAR SIGNAL. This is often 6 to 15 mV, a range that exceeds the sensitivity threshold of a pulse generator. The atrial electrogram should measure at least 2 mV. A signal with a gradual slope (lower *slew rate*) is more difficult to sense than is a sharp upstroke signal. Determination of the slew rate may be useful when the signal is low or borderline (3 to 5 mV for ventricular signals) but is not necessary if the amplitude of the signal is large. A low electrographic signal may require repositioning of the lead. Rarely, unipolar and bipolar ventricular electrograms are too small for sensing at nominal sensitivity because of chronic ischemia or cardiomyopathy; in this situation a bipolar pulse generator programmable to a high sensitivity should be used.

Following initial lead placement, the ventricular electrogram shows an initial current of injury (ST-segment elevation) that reflects good endocardial contact and disappears after a few days.[41] Over the long term, the amplitude of the QRS signal diminishes slightly,[35] but the slew rate can diminish further (about 40 per cent). These changes normally are of no clinical importance for ventricular sensing but can be important in the case of smaller atrial signals, although recent studies with contemporary leads have documented the stability of the atrial signal chronically.[35,42]

LEAD DESIGN

New *lead* technology and design have improved bipolar leads sufficiently to eliminate the previous advantages of unipolar leads over bipolar leads. Generally, bipolar leads are preferred because of a greater signal-to-noise ratio, less sensitivity to extraneous interference (especially skeletal myopotentials), less frequent crosstalk (atrial stimulus sensed by ventricular lead in a dual-chamber system), and avoidance of muscle stimulation occasionally seen at the anodal site of unipolar pulse generators. Improvement in the design of lead fixation mechanisms has reduced the incidence of dislodgement to 1.5 per cent or less with ventricular leads and about 1 to 5 per cent with atrial leads.[43-46] Adhering leads utilize either passive fixation with tines or fins to enhance entanglement in trabeculae or active fixation with myocardial penetration by grasping screws or small jaws. Tined and screw-in leads are the most popular and exhibit equally good performance.[47] Active fixation leads are particularly useful in right ventricular dilatation, in tricuspid insufficiency, and when pacing of the right ventricular outflow tract is needed. Contemporary electrodes have a small surface area that reduces stimulation thresholds because of a higher current density.[48] Porous electrodes with a small surface area yield a low pacing threshold and yet provide a greater surface area for improved sensing.[48-50] Steroid-eluting leads have a reservoir within the electrode tip that elutes a trace of dexamethasone directly at the electrode-tissue interface and reduces the local tissue reaction and the thickness of the fibrous capsule surrounding the tip electrode.[51] Steroid-eluting leads are associated with very low pacing thresholds, and lack of initial peaking,[52] and have virtually eliminated so-called exit block with ineffectual pacemaker stimuli.[53-56]

TYPES OF PACEMAKERS

SINGLE-CHAMBER PACEMAKERS

AOO AND VOO MODES. In the AOO and VOO modes, the pacemaker stimuli are generated at a fixed rate (asynchronously) with no relationship to the spontaneous rhythm. Stimuli capture the atria or ventricles only when they fall outside the refractory period following spontaneous beats (Fig. 25–1). Ventricular fibrillation induced by a pacemaker stimulus falling in the ventricular vulnerable period is extremely rare unless myocardial ischemia or severe electrolyte abnormalities are present. AOO or VOO pacing is used only temporarily during pacemaker testing with application of the magnet or for competitive pacing to terminate some tachycardias (p. 747).

VVI MODE. A VVI (ventricular demand) pacemaker prevents the ventricular rate from decreasing below a predetermined programmed level (Fig. 25–1). If the spontaneous rate decreases below the set rate, the pacemaker paces at a cycle length appropriate to maintain the preset rate. A faster spontaneous rate inhibits pacemaker discharge. The timing cycle (or internal clock) of a VVI pulse generator begins with either a sensed or a paced ventricular event. The initial portion of the cycle consists of a refractory period (usually 200 to 350 msec) during which the pulse generator is insensitive to any signals so as to avoid sensing its own stimulus, the paced or spontaneous QRS complex, T waves, and the decaying residual voltage at the electrode-myocardial interface. Beyond the pacemaker refractory period, a sensed spontaneous QRS complex inhibits the pacemaker and its timing clock returns to the baseline: a new pacing cycle is initiated and the output circuit remains inhibited for a period equal to the programmed pacemaker interval. If no spontaneous QRS complex is sensed, the timing cycle ends with the delivery of a ventricular stimulus and a new cycle is started. The sensing function conserves energy and prevents competition between the pacemaker and the intrinsic rhythm. VVI (or VVIR, p. 742) pacing is by far the most common mode of pacing and still accounts for more than 70 per cent of new pacemaker implantations worldwide.[57] A VVI pacemaker is simple, inexpensive, reliable, and has a small size and long life. However, its inability to maintain AV synchrony and provide an increased rate on exercise constitutes an important disadvantage.

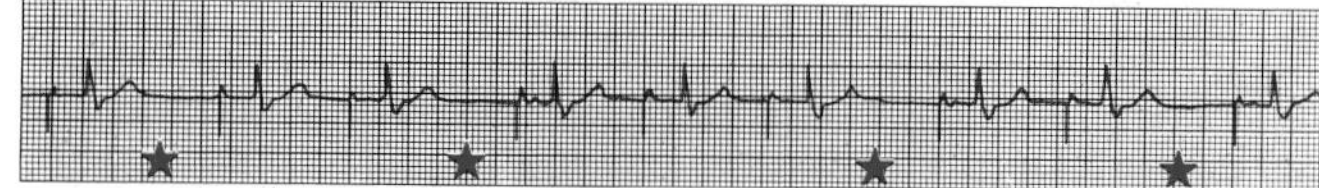

FIGURE 25–3. AAI pacemaker, rate = 70/min (automatic interval = 857 msec) and refractory period = 250 msec. There is intermittent prolongation of the interstimulus interval (stars) because the atrial lead senses the farfield QRS complex just beyond the 250 msec pacemaker refractory period. When the refractory period was programmed to 400 msec, the irregularity disappeared, with restoration of regular atrial pacing at a rate of 70/min.

AAI MODE. This (atrial demand) mode is similar to the VVI mode except that the pacemaker senses atrial electrical activity and paces the atrium (Fig. 25–3). AAI units must have a greater sensitivity than VVI units because the atrial electrogram is considerably smaller than the ventricular electrogram and the refractory period should be longer (400 msec) to avoid sensing the "farfield" ventricular electrogram via the atrial lead. AAI pacing is used for patients with sick sinus syndrome and intact AV conduction.

VVT MODE. In the VVT mode, upon sensing a spontaneous QRS complex, the pacemaker immediately discharges (rather than inhibits) its stimulus during the absolute refractory period of the ventricular myocardium (Fig. 25–1). If no QRS is sensed, the pacemaker delivers its impulse at the end of the interval corresponding to the programmed (lower) rate. The maximum pacing rate that can be generated by continual sensing is either factory set or programmable. The triggered mode can be used to activate discharge of an implanted pacemaker by the application of chest wall stimuli (generating signals for sensing) from an external pacemaker. In this way, appropriately timed stimuli to the chest wall can be used to initiate or terminate some tachycardias by triggering corresponding stimuli from the implanted pacemaker.[58]

Intervals and Rates

Three pacemaker intervals are important. The *automatic interval* is the time between two consecutive stimuli during continuous pacing. The *escape interval* is measured from the onset of the sensed surface QRS complex (in a ventricular pacemaker) to the following stimulus and exceeds the automatic interval by a few milliseconds to almost the duration of the entire QRS complex, depending on when during the surface QRS complex the intracardiac electrogram is sensed by the pacemaker. A special magnet held over a pulse generator closes a magnetic reed switch that eliminates the sensing function with conversion to the AOO/VOO mode. The *magnet interval* varies according to the manufacturer and is generally shorter than the automatic interval so as to override the spontaneous rhythm. The magnet interval is often used to assess battery status and lengthens with impending battery depletion.

Some pacemakers have a *hysteresis interval*, i.e., the escape interval is significantly longer than the automatic interval. Its purpose is to maintain sinus rhythm (and AV synchrony) by preventing the onset of pacing for as long as possible at a rate lower than the automatic rate of the pacemaker. However, hysteresis appears to have no advantage over a simple decrease in the pacing rate and its advantages are more theoretical than real.

Electrocardiogram During Pacing

Evaluation of the *pacemaker stimulus* recorded on digital ECG machines is meaningless because the recording circuitry distorts stimuli with striking changes in amplitude and polarity.[59] The vector of the pacemaker stimulus in the frontal plane when recorded with an analog ECG machine correlates with lead position, and amplitude changes are meaningful. A change from small bipolar stimuli to large amplitude spikes suggests an insulation defect, while spike attenuation of a unipolar stimulus in several ECG leads during held respiration suggests an increase in lead impedance due to a fracture or loose connection.

FUSION AND PSEUDOFUSION BEATS. During ventricular pacing, ventricular fusion beats occur when the ventricles are activated simultaneously by a spontaneous depolarization and a paced impulse. A ventricular fusion beat is often narrower than a pure paced beat and can exhibit various morphologies depending on the relative contribution of the two foci to ventricular depolarization (Fig. 25–1). *Pseudofusion beats* consist of the superimposition of an ineffectual pacemaker spike upon the spontaneous QRS complex originating from a single focus and represent a normal manifestation of VVI pacing. A large portion of the *surface* QRS complex may be inscribed before its *intracardiac* counterpart (electrogram) generates the necessary voltage (about 3 to 4 mV) capable of inhibiting a VVI pacemaker (Fig. 25–4). Therefore, a normally functioning VVI pacemaker can deliver its impulse within a spontaneous surface QRS complex (mimicking undersensing) before the pulse generator has the opportunity to sense the somewhat late intracardiac electrogram in the right ventricle.[41] In a pseudofusion beat, the pacemaker stimulus occurs too late to cause true fusion because it falls within the absolute refractory period of the myocardium initiated by the spontaneous depolarization. In the presence of normal sensing, striking examples of pseudofusion beats with pacemaker stimuli occurring late within the QRS complex can be seen in right bundle branch block, left ventricular extrasystoles, and any condition causing delayed intraventricular conduction. True sensing failure must be excluded whenever pseudofusion beats are observed. Pacemaker spikes falling clearly after termination of the surface QRS complex indicate sensing failure. Fusion and pseudofusion atrial beats can also occur with atrial pacing but are more difficult to recognize in view of the smaller size of the P wave in the ECG.

SITES OF PACING

LEFT VENTRICULAR PACING. Stimulation of the left ventricle produces late activation of the right ventricle and therefore a right bundle branch block pattern of depolarization. Conversely, right ventricular pacing produces a left bundle branch block pattern of depolarization. During right ventricular pacing, paced beats usually exhibit a typical left bundle branch block pattern in leads I and aV_l, but leads V_5 and V_6 sometimes show deep S waves because the main electrical forces may be moving away from the horizontal level where V_5 and V_6 are recorded. The mean electrical axis of the QRS complex in the frontal plane is oriented superiorly and leftward because the sequence of activation travels from apex to base, away from the inferior leads. As the pacing electrode moves toward the right ventricular outflow tract, activation travels simultaneously to the base superiorly and the apex inferiorly, and the mean frontal plane QRS electrical axis may point to the right lower quadrant. Right ventricular outflow tract stimulation immediately below the pulmonary valve causes right axis deviation of the QRS complex in the frontal plane because most of the activation travels from base to apex, but the pattern in the left precordial lead always remains that of left bundle branch block. Paced beats from the right ventricular ouflow tract not uncommonly exhibit qR, QR, or Qr configuration in leads I and aV_l, but the inferior leads show a dominant R wave. In this situation, the precordial leads do not exhibit Qr, qR, or QR complexes.

Because the QRS complex during right ventricular pacing resembles that of spontaneous left bundle branch block (except for the initial forces), the diagnosis of *myocardial infarction* often can be made during ventricular pacing by applying the criteria used in complete left bundle branch block.[60] An extensive anteroseptal myocardial infarction can cause an initial q in leads I, aV_l, V_5, and V_6, producing a qR pattern following the stimulus (not to be confused with a normal QS pattern). Although the sensitivity of the qR changes is low, its specificity approaches 100 per cent because it is *never* seen in V_5 and V_6 during uncomplicated right ventricular pacing. A QR or Qr complex in leads II, III, and aV_f is also diagnostic of an inferior myocardial infarction. Large unipolar stimuli can mask an initial Q wave. Also, an anterior myocardial infarction can be associated with late notching of the ascending limb of the QRS complex in the left precordial leads, indicating an extensive infarction.

RIGHT VENTRICULAR PACING. During right ventricular apical pacing, the inferior leads and the anterior leads (V_1 to V_3) often record secondary ST elevation. ST segment depression can occur as a normal finding in leads I, aV_l, V_5, and V_6. Relatively stable ST-T wave changes resembling primary abnormalities occasionally can be seen during uncomplicated right ventricular pacing. Discordant T waves are of no diagnostic value. Sequential electrocardiograms are often needed to determine the significance of the ST-T wave abnormalities.

ST-T wave abnormalities occur more commonly in acute myocardial infarction than the qR pattern or QRS notching noted earlier. Pronounced primary ST elevation with convex configuration clinches the diagnosis of myocardial infarction. When less obvious, the diagnosis becomes fairly certain only when the polarity of the T wave is opposite to that of the ST segment elevation.[60] ST depression concordant with the QRS complex can occasionally occur in V_3 to V_6 during uncomplicated RV pacing and rarely in leads V_1 and V_2. Consequently, obvious ST segment depression in leads V_1 and V_2 should be considered abnormal and indicative of anterior or inferior myocardial infarction (or ischemia). Inhibition of the VVI pacemaker by chest wall stimulation or by reduction of the rate of output may allow the emergence of the spontaneous rhythm and reveal diagnostic Q waves.

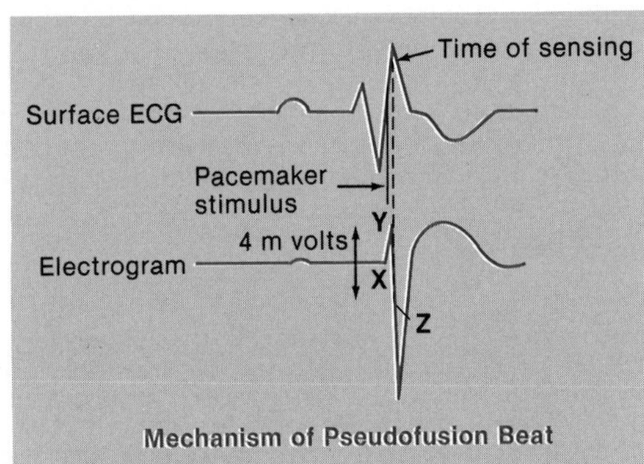

FIGURE 25–4. Mechanism of pseudofusion beat. The surface ECG and the ventricular electrogram are recorded simultaneously. The electrogram generates the necessary intracardiac voltage to inhibit the pacemaker (yz assumed at 4 mV) at a point corresponding with the descending limb of the surface QRS complex in its second half (dotted line). Consequently, it is possible for a pacemaker stimulus to occur at the apex of the R deflection just before the dotted line (which depicts the time of sensing) because the ventricular electrogram has not yet generated the required voltage to reach the sensitivity of the pulse generator and inhibit it. (From Barold, S. S., Falkoff, M. D., Ong, L. S., and Heinle, R. A.: Electrocardiographic analysis of normal and abnormal pacemaker function. Cardiovasc. Clin. *14*:97, 1983.)

DUAL-CHAMBER PACEMAKERS

Types, Rates, and Intervals

TIMING INTERVALS. In the various types of dual-chamber pacemakers the timing intervals are best understood by focusing first on the DDD mode. A DDD pulse generator paces and senses in both the atrium and the ventricle. Simpler dual-chamber pacing modes are then derived by the removal of "building blocks" from the DDD mode and equalization of the various timing intervals.[61,62] These simpler pacing modes are important because a DDD pacemaker may have to be downgraded for treatment of certain complications.

As in a standard VVI pacemaker, the ventricular channel of a DDD device requires two basic timing cycles: *the lower rate interval* and the ventricular refractory period. A simple DDD system consists of the VVI mode with an added atrial channel (Fig. 25–5). This arrangement necessitates two new intervals, an *atrioventricular (AV) interval* (the electronic analog of the P-R interval) and an *upper rate interval* (equal to the pacemaker total atrial refractory period, discussed later) to control the response of the ventricular channel to sensed atrial activity and maintain 1:1 AV synchrony between the lower and upper rates (Fig. 25–5). The atrial escape interval is obtained by subtracting the programmed AV delay from the lower rate

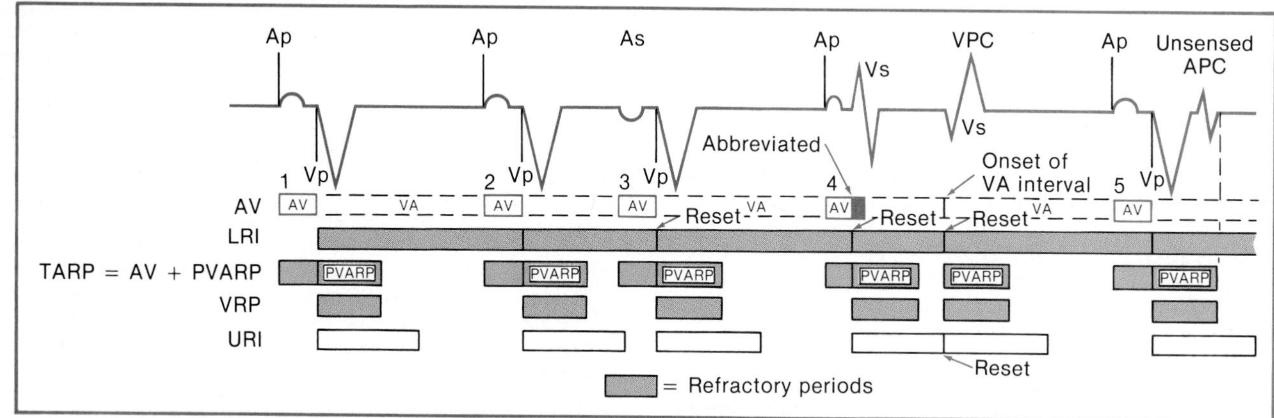

FIGURE 25–5. Diagram showing the function and timing intervals of a simple DDD pacemaker consisting of only four fundamental intervals: lower rate interval = LRI, ventricular refractory period = VRP, atrioventricular delay = AV, postventricular atrial refractory period = PVARP. These provide two derived intervals: atrial escape (pacemaker VA) interval = LRI - AV, and total atrial refractory period (TARP) = AV + PVARP. Ap = atrial paced beat, Vp = ventricular paced beat, As = atrial sensed event, Vs = ventricular sensed event. *Reset* refers to the termination and reinitiation of a timing interval before it has timed out to its completion according to its programmed duration. Premature termination of the programmed AV delay by a ventricular sensed event (Vs) is indicated by its abbreviation. The upper rate interval (URI) is equal to the total atrial refractory period. An atrial sensed event, As (third beat) initiates an AV interval terminating with a ventricular paced beat (Vp); As also aborts the atrial escape interval initiated by the second Vp. The third Vp resets the lower rate interval and starts the postventricular atrial refractory period, ventricular refractory period, and upper rate interval. The fourth beat consists of an atrial paced beat (Ap) that terminates the atrial escape interval initiated by the third ventricular paced beat (Vp). The atrial paced beat is followed by a sensed conducted QRS (Vs).

The AV interval is therefore abbreviated. The QRS of the fourth beat sensed (Vs) initiates the atrial escape interval, lower rate interval, postventricular atrial refractory period, ventricular refractory period, and upper rate interval. The fifth beat is a ventricular extrasystole (VPC) that initiates an atrial escape interval, postventricular atrial refractory period, and ventricular refractory period; it resets the lower rate interval and upper rate interval. The last beat is followed by an atrial extrasystole (APC), unsensed by the atrial channel because it falls within the postventricular atrial refractory period. Such a simple DDD pulse generator equipped with six timing cycles functions quite well provided that crosstalk (sensing of atrial stimulus by ventricular channel) does not occur.

interval. The atrial escape interval starts with a ventricular paced or sensed event and terminates with the release of an atrial stimulus.

Most dual-chamber pulse generators are designed with ventricular based (V-V) lower rate timing controlled by ventricular events[63] and a constant atrial escape interval. An atrial-sensed event *triggers* a ventricular stimulus after the completion of the AV interval (provided that no ventricular-sensed event occurs during the AV interval) and *inhibits* the release of the atrial stimulus expected at the completion of the atrial escape interval. A ventricular-sensed event beyond the AV interval inhibits both the atrial and ventricular channels and initiates new lower rate and atrial escape intervals. An atrial-paced or -sensed event initiates the atrial refractory period because the atrial channel must remain refractory during the AV interval to prevent initiation of a new AV interval when one is already in progress.[62,63] The AV interval must terminate with a paced or sensed ventricular event that continues the atrial refractory period. The second part, called the postventricular atrial refractory period (PVARP), must be programmed appropriately to prevent sensing of retrograde P waves due to ventriculoatrial (VA) conduction. The total atrial refractory period is equal to the sum of the AV delay and the PVARP. In a simple DDD pulse generator, the upper rate interval is equal to the total atrial refractory period. The AV interval, PVARP, and upper rate interval are interrelated according to the formula: upper rate (ppm) = 60/total atrial refractory period (sec). Consequently, a pacemaker with an upper rate of 120/min can sense atrial signals only 500 msec or longer apart.

CROSSTALK. Also known as self-inhibition, this refers to the inappropriate detection of the atrial stimulus by the ventricular channel.[62] Crosstalk depends on the amplitude of the atrial stimulus and the sensitivity of the ventricular channel and is less frequent with bipolar leads. Crosstalk can often be eliminated by reduction of the atrial output and/or ventricular sensitivity. The prevention of crosstalk also requires a ventricular blanking (refractory) period (10 to 60 msec) that starts coincidentally with the atrial stimulus[62] (Fig. 25–6). In some DDD pacemakers the first part of the A-V interval (beyond the blanking period) initiated by an atrial stimulus contains an additional backup system known as ventricular safety pacing (VSP) (Fig. 25–6). During the VSP interval (or its initial portion), any signal (atrial stimulus, QRS, and the like) sensed by the ventricular channel triggers a ventricular stimulus at the completion of the VSP period (usually 100 to 110 msec) producing characteristic abbreviation of the paced AV interval[64] (Fig. 25–7). Crosstalk without a VSP mechanism produces unexpected prolongation of the interval from atrial stimulus to succeeding spontaneous QRS complex (if any) to a value longer than the programmed AV interval (Fig. 25–8). In patients without underlying spontaneous rhythm, crosstalk can cause asystole (Fig. 25–8); however, with appropriate programming and the VSP mechanism, it is rarely a clinical problem.

UPPER RATE RESPONSE OF DDD PULSE GENERATORS

The programmed upper rate of a DDD pulse generator depends on the patient's activity level, age, left ventricular function, and the presence of coronary artery disease, atrial tachyarrhythmias and retrograde VA conduction. The maximal rate of a DDD pacemaker can be defined by either the duration of the total atrial refractory period (causing fixed-ratio pacemaker AV block such as 2:1, 3:1, and so on) or a separate upper rate timing circuit causing Wenckebach-like AV block (6:5, 5:4, and so on).[65]

FIXED RATIO AV BLOCK. This provides the simplest way of controlling the upper rate by programming the total atrial refractory period. The number of unsensed P waves depends on the atrial rate and where the P waves occur in the pacemaker cycle (Fig. 25-9). The AV interval always remains constant. This response is often called 2:1 AV block. Actually, the paced ventricular rate will be exactly half the atrial rate or equal to the lower rate of the pacemaker, whichever is higher. An upper rate using fixed-ratio AV block may be inappropriate in some patients, especially young and physically active individuals, because the sudden reduction of the ventricular rate with 2:1 AV block on exercise may be poorly tolerated.

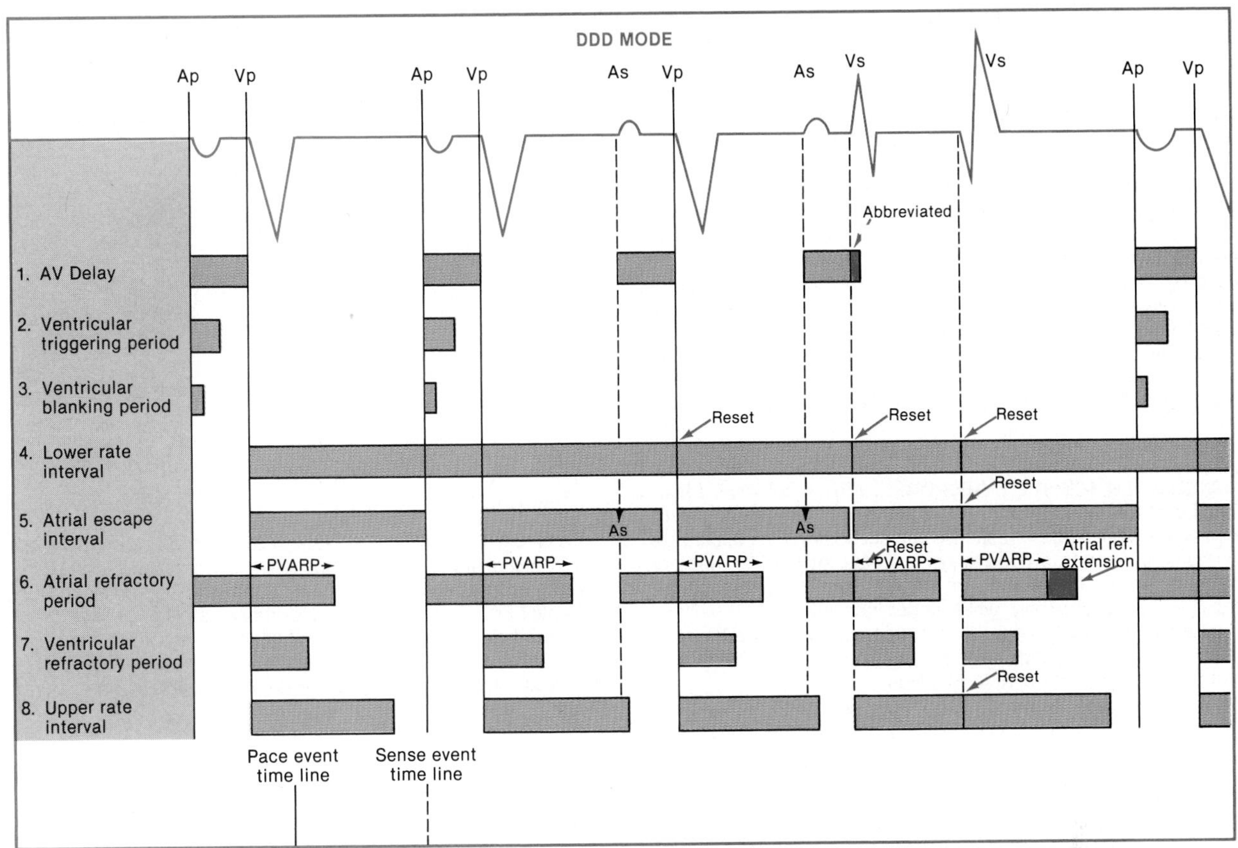

FIGURE 25-6. DDD mode. Diagrammatic representation of timing cycles. REF = refractory ventricular triggering period or ventricular safety pacing period. The second Vs (ventricular sensed event) is a ventricular extrasystole. The fourth AV interval initiated by As (atrial sensed event) is abbreviated because the conducted QRS (Vs) occurs before the AV interval has timed out. The postventricular atrial refractory period (PVARP) generated by the ventricular extrasystole is automatically extended by the atrial refractory period extension. (This design is based on the concept that most episodes of endless loop tachycardia are initiated by a ventricular extrasystole with retrograde ventriculoatrial conduction.) The arrow pointing down within the atrial escape (pacemaker VA) interval indicates that an atrial sensed event (As) has taken place; the atrial escape interval actually terminates at this point, but the atrial escape interval is depicted in its entirety (as if As had not occurred) for the sake of clarity. The signal As inhibits release of the atrial stimulus otherwise expected at the completion of the atrial escape interval. Ap = atrial paced beat, Vp = ventricular paced beat, As = atrial sensed event, Vs = ventricular sensed event. The abbreviations and format used in this illustration are the same for Figures 25-9 through 25-13 (From Barold, S. S. et al.: All dual-chamber pacemakers function in the DDD mode. Am. Heart J. *115:*1353, 1988.)

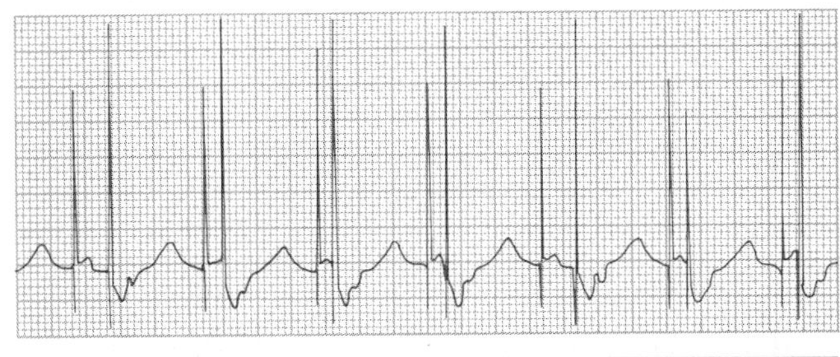

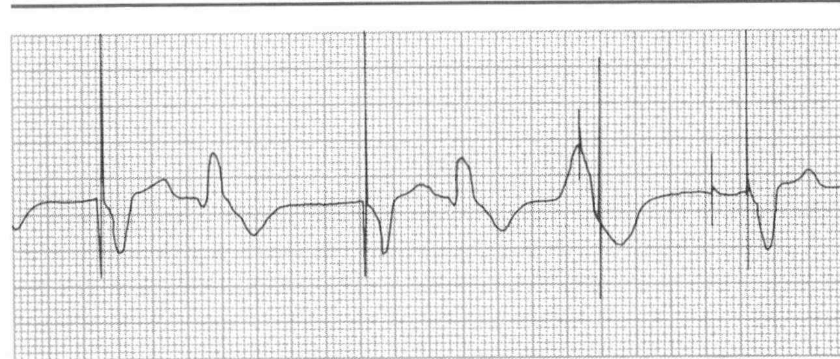

FIGURE 25-7. Ventricular safety pacing during DDD pacing. *Top,* In the absence of crosstalk, the first and fifth AV intervals are equal to the programmed value of 200 msec. Intermittent crosstalk leads to activation of the ventricular safety pacing mechanism so that the AV interval of the second, third, fourth, sixth, and seventh beats is abbreviated to 100 msec. In a DDD pulse generator with ventricular lower rate timing, activation of the ventricular safety pacing mechanism due to continual crosstalk leads to an increase in the pacing rate (although the atrial escape interval remains constant). *Bottom,* Activation of the ventricular safety pacing mechanism of DDD pulse generator by a sensed ventricular extrasystole. AV = 200 msec, lower rate interval = 857 msec. The first and second ventricular extrasystoles are sensed by the ventricular channel of the DDD pacemaker. The third ventricular extrasystole is deformed by an atrial stimulus falling at the apex of the R wave; the atrial stimulus occurs because the ventricular electrogram has not yet generated sufficient voltage for sensing by the ventricular channel to inhibit the atrial and ventricular channels. The mechanism is identical to that of ventricular pseudofusion beats (Fig. 25-4). This particular pseudofusion beat is created by events occurring in different chambers (atrial stimulus and ventricular depolarization). The ventricular channel senses the ventricular electrogram within the ventricular safety pacing period that follows the ventricular blanking period initiated by the atrial stimulus (at the apex of the R wave). The pacemaker therefore triggers a ventricular stimulus at the completion of the ventricular safety pacing period, producing an abbreviated AV interval of 100 msec. The ventricular stimulus falls at the end of the QRS complex. This ECG represents normal function of a DDD pacemaker with a ventricular safety pacing mechanism.

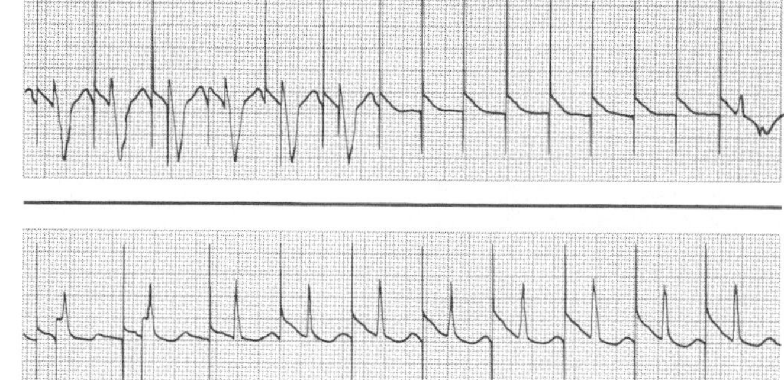

FIGURE 25-8. Crosstalk during DDD pacing without a ventricular safety pacing mechanism. *Top strip,* The lower rate was increased to test for crosstalk. Lower rate interval = 580 msec, AV = 170 msec. The interval between atrial stimuli on the right is shorter than the lower rate interval. Crosstalk therefore causes an increase in the atrial pacing rate faster than the freerunning (lower) AV sequential rate on the left. Continual crosstalk causes prolonged ventricular asystole. *Bottom strip,* Crosstalk with AV conduction. Lower rate interval = 857 msec, AV interval = 200 msec. Crosstalk occurs with the third atrial stimulus and produces characteristic prolongation of the interval between the atrial stimulus and the succeeding conducted QRS complex to a value longer than the programmed AV interval. The rate of atrial pacing increases because the sensed atrial stimulus by the ventricular channel initiates a new atrial escape interval just beyond the termination of the ventricular blanking period. Consequently, the interval between two consecutive atrial stimuli becomes equal to the atrial escape interval of 657 msec (857 − 200) plus the duration of the ventricular blanking period (50 msec), providing a total of about 700 msec.

WENCKEBACH UPPER RATE RESPONSE. This mode avoids sudden reduction of the paced ventricular rate and maintains some degree of AV synchrony. A Wenckebach response can occur only if the upper rate interval is programmed to a value longer than the total atrial refractory period (Fig. 25-10). Prolongation of the AV interval (atrial sensed–ventricular paced) occurs only when upper rate interval > P-P interval > total atrial refractory period. With a progressive increase in atrial rate, when P-P interval is < total atrial refractory period, the Wenckebach response switches to 2:1 fixed ratio AV block.

OTHER DUAL-CHAMBER PACING MODES

DVI MODE. The DVI mode can be considered as the DDD mode with the PVARP extending through the entire atrial escape interval.[61] No atrial sensing occurs because the total atrial refractory period extends through the entire lower rate interval. Asynchronous atrial pacing can precipitate atrial fibrillation. Three types of DVI function are possible: uncommitted, partially committed, and committed. In the *uncommitted DVI* mode, the ventricular channel can sense through the entire duration of the AV interval

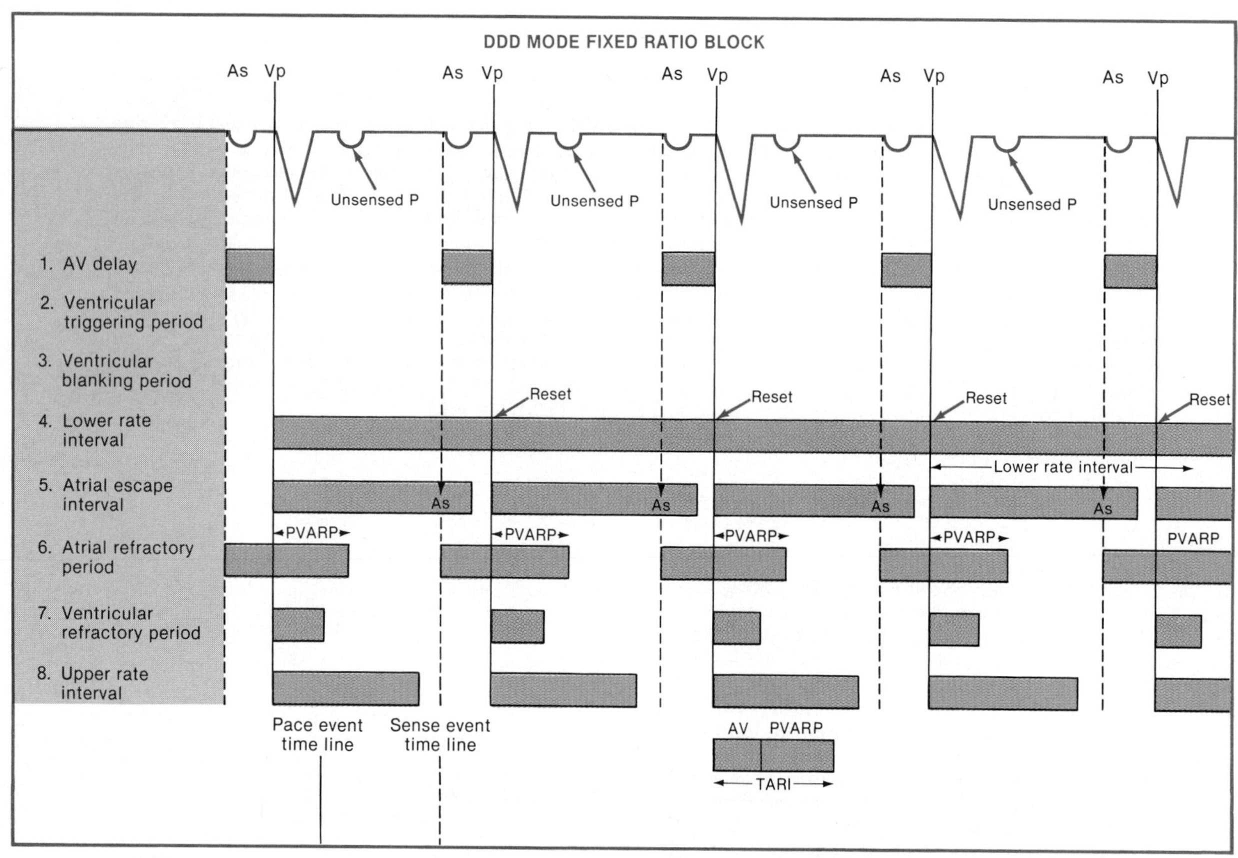

FIGURE 25-9. Upper rate response of DDD pacemaker with fixed ratio AV block. The upper rate interval is longer than the total atrial refractory period (AV + postventricular atrial refractory period or PVARP) and the P-P interval (As-As) is shorter than the total atrial refractory period. The arrow pointing down within the atrial escape (pacemaker VA) interval indicates that an atrial sensed event (As) has taken place; the atrial escape interval actually terminates at this point but the atrial escape interval is depicted in its entirety (as if As had not occurred) for the sake of clarity. Every second P wave falls within the postventricular atrial refractory period and is unsensed. The AV interval remains constant. An upper rate response with fixed ratio pacemaker AV block occurs in two types of DDD pacemakers. (1) A device without a separately programmable upper rate interval in which the total atrial refractory period is equal to the upper rate interval. (2) A device with a separately programmable upper rate interval (i.e., upper rate interval > total atrial refractory period) only when the P-P interval < total atrial refractory period as shown in this figure. In such a device, an upper rate response with pacemaker Wenckebach AV block can only occur when the P-P interval > total atrial refractory period as shown in Figure 25-10. (From Barold, S. S.: Management of patients with dual chamber pulse generators: Central role of pacemaker atrial refractory period. Learning Center Highlights, Heart House, American College of Cardiology 5:[4], 8, 1990, with permission.)

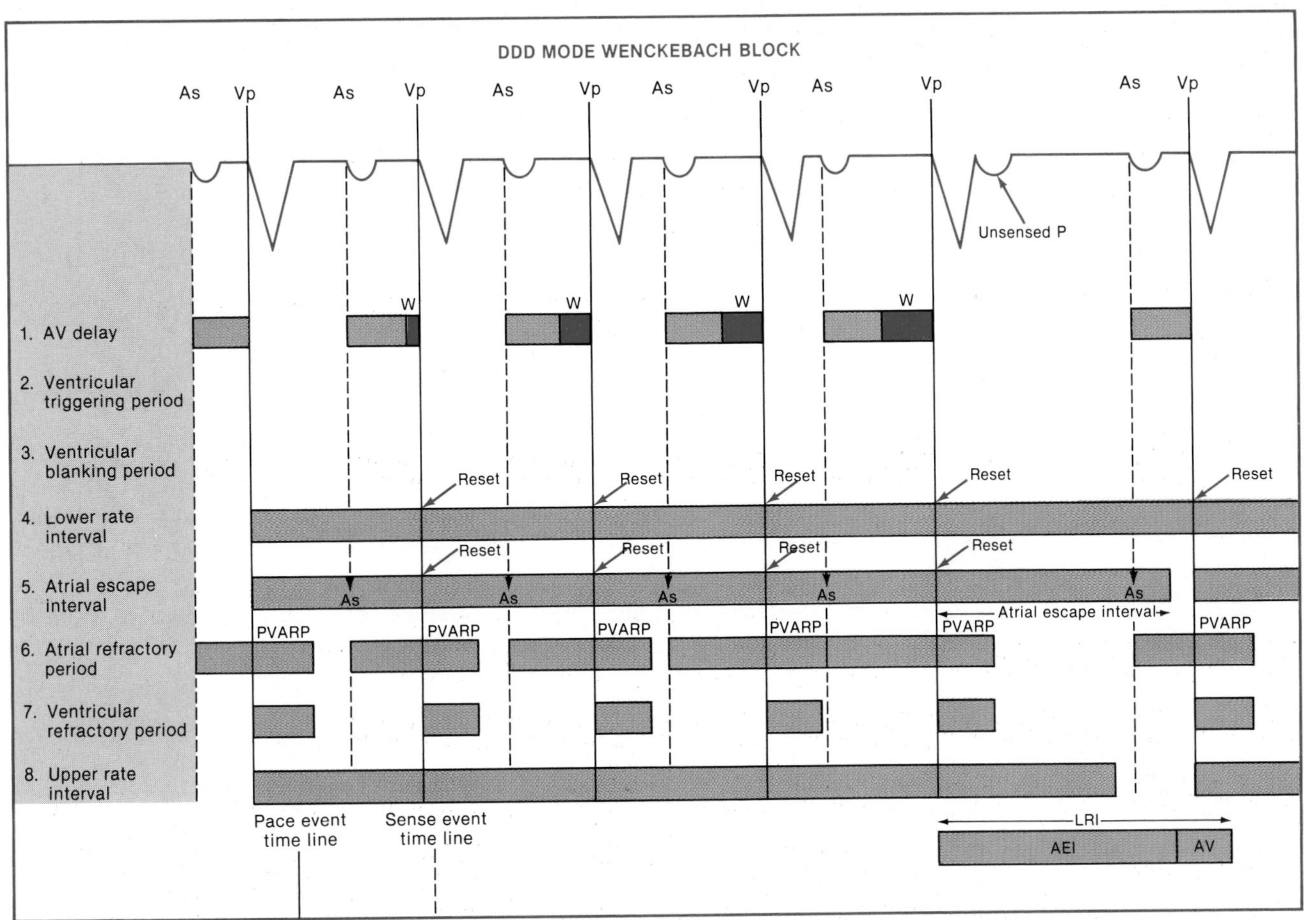

FIGURE 25–10. DDD mode. Upper rate response with pacemaker Wenckebach AV block. AEI = atrial escape interval. The upper rate interval is *longer* than the programmed total atrial refractory period, a mandatory prerequisite for a Wenckebach upper rate response. The P-P interval (As-As) is *longer* than the programmed total atrial refractory period. The As-Vp (atrial sensed–ventricular paced) interval lengthens by a varying period to conform to the upper rate interval. During the Wenckebach sequence, the pacemaker synchronizes a ventricular paced beat (Vp) to an atrial sensed event (As). Because the pacemaker cannot violate its programmed (ventricular) upper rate interval, the ventricular paced beat (Vp) can be released only at the completion of the upper rate interval. The AV delay (As-Vp) becomes progressively longer (than the programmed value) as the ventricular channel waits to deliver its ventricular stimulus (Vp) until the upper rate interval has timed out. The maximum prolongation of the AV interval represents the difference between the upper rate interval and the total atrial refractory period. The As-Vp (atrial sensed–ventricular paced) interval lengthens during the pacemaker Wenckebach sequence as long as the As-As interval (P-P) remains longer than the total atrial refractory period. The sixth P wave falls within the postventricular atrial refractory period (PVARP) and is unsensed and thus not followed by a ventricular stimulus (Vp). A pause occurs and the Wenckebach cycle restarts. In the first four pacing cycles, the intervals between pacemaker stimuli (Vp-Vp) are constant and equal to the upper rate interval. When the P-P interval becomes shorter than the programmed total atrial refractory period, Wenckebach pacemaker AV block cannot occur and fixed ratio pacemaker AV block, e.g., 2:1, will supervene as in Figure 25–9. The arrow pointing down within the atrial escape interval indicates that an atrial sensed event (As) has taken place; the atrial escape interval actually terminates at this point, but for the sake of clarity the atrial escape interval is depicted as if As had not occurred. (From Barold, S. S. et al.: All dual chamber pacemakers function in the DDD mode. Am. Heart J. *115:*1353, 1988.)

while in the *partially committed DVI* mode the ventricular channel can sense only beyond an initial ventricular blanking period.[61] In contrast, a *committed DVI* pacemaker possesses a ventricular blanking period encompassing the entire AV interval, making crosstalk impossible. In the committed DVI mode, AV sequential pacing occurs in an all-or-none manner; that is, sensing spontaneous ventricular activity inhibits both stimuli or two sequential stimuli occur together.

VDD MODE. The VDD mode functions like the DDD mode except that the generated atrial stimulus is diverted internally rather than emitted.[61] Therefore, *no atrial pacing occurs*. The absence of the atrial stimulus eliminates the need for crosstalk intervals (Fig. 25–11). The omitted atrial stimulus nevertheless begins an "implied" AV interval that must be refractory in its entirety so that in most contemporary designs a P wave occurring within the "implied" AV interval is not sensed. Without sensed atrial activity, the VDD mode paces effectively in the VVI mode at the lower rate of the pacemaker.

DDI MODE. The DDI mode has generally been described as an improved DVI mode or a hybrid of the DVI and DDD modes. Sensing and pacing occur in both atria and ventricles, and the DDI mode is best considered as a DDD mode with identical upper and lower rate intervals[61,66] (provided that the lower rate is controlled by ventricular events, i.e., V-V timing) (Fig. 25–12). Atrial sensing occurs beyond the PVARP. An atrial-sensed event initiates an AV interval that terminates (as in the DDD mode) only at the completion of the upper rate interval (identical to the lower rate interval). Although atrial sensing occurs, the pacemaker cannot increase the ventricular pacing rate in response to a faster atrial rate so that ventricular pacing always occurs at the programmed lower rate. For this reason, the DDI mode is useful in patients with the sick sinus syndrome and paroxysmal atrial tachyarrhythmias.[67] The DDI mode provides atrial pacing and AV synchrony (in the absence of atrial tachyarrhythmias) with the potential of preventing atrial tachyarrhythmias by overdrive suppression.[67] During atrial tachyarrhythmia, the DDI pacemaker simply paces the ventricle at its constant rate.

RETROGRADE CONDUCTION AND ENDLESS LOOP TACHYCARDIA. Pacemaker-mediated tachycardia or endless loop tachycardia is a well-known complication of dual-chamber pacing (DDD or VDD) and starts with sensing of a

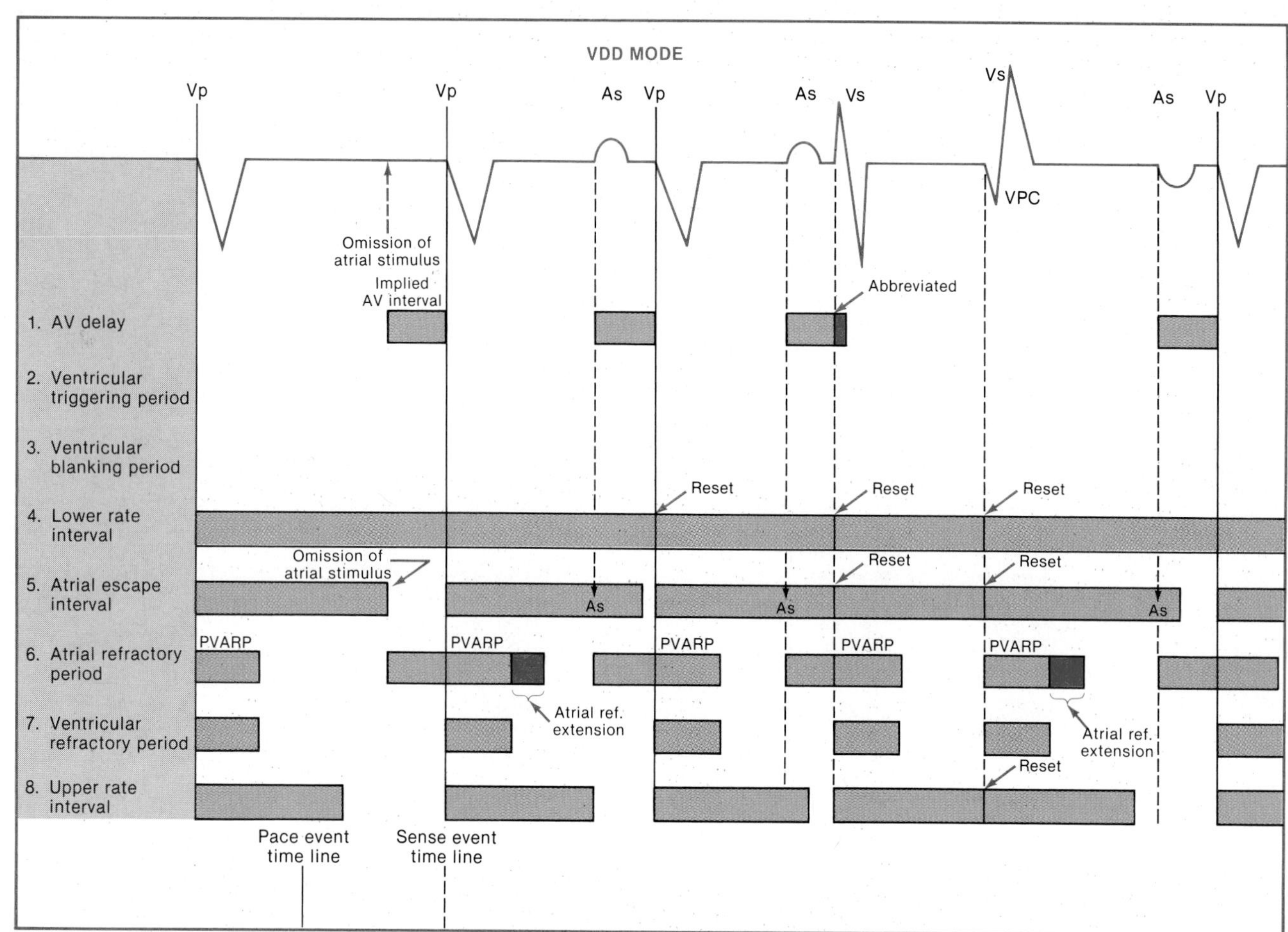

FIGURE 25–11. VDD mode. In the DDD mode, an atrial stimulus is released at the completion of the atrial escape interval whenever an atrial sensed event (As) does not occur within the atrial escape interval. This atrial stimulus is omitted in the VDD mode. Nevertheless the pulse generator initiates an implied AV interval with the same characteristics as in the DDD mode. In the first ventricular cycle (Vp-Vp) because the ventricular paced beat (Vp) terminating the implied AV interval is not preceded by an atrial paced beat or atrial sensed event (As), the post-ventricular atrial refractory period (PVARP) is automatically extended as occurs after a sensed ventricular extrasystole (depicted as VPC) (Fig. 25–6). Ventricular blanking and ventricular triggering (ventricular safety pacing) periods are not needed because there are no atrial stimuli in the VDD mode. In the absence of atrial sensed events (As), the pulse generator effectively paces in the VVI mode at the programmed lower rate interval (first cycle). The arrow pointing down within the atrial escape interval indicates that an atrial sensed event (As) has taken place; the atrial escape interval actually terminates at this point, but for the sake of clarity it is depicted as if As had not occurred. (From Barold, S. S. et al.: All dual chamber pacemakers function in the DDD mode. Am. Heart J. *115:*1353, 1988.)

retrograde P wave usually linked to a ventricular extrasystole[68,69] (Fig. 25–13). Endless loop tachycardia can be sustained or unsustained and often occurs at the programmed upper rate of the pacemaker. Intact retrograde VA conduction occurs in approximately two-thirds or more of patients with sinus node dysfunction and 15 to 35 per cent of patients with complete AV block.[41] Thus, 35 to 50 per cent of all patients receiving dual-chamber pacemakers may be susceptible to endless loop tachycardia. Absent retrograde VA conduction at the time of implantation or even later provides no guarantee of protection because a few patients may exhibit VA conduction subsequently, particularly during states of sympathetic stimulation.[68] Any condition capable of separating the sinus P wave from the QRS complex, coupled with retrograde VA conduction, can initiate endless loop tachycardia.[68,69] These include a ventricular extrasystole, loss of atrial capture, myopotential sensing by the atrial channel of unipolar devices, undersensing of sinus P waves (with preserved sensing of retrograde P waves), an excessively long AV interval, and application and removal of the magnet.

Endless loop tachycardia may be induced when the atrial output is programmed below the pacing threshold, PVARP at its minimum value, and lower rate above the spontaneous rate (Fig. 25–14). When atrial capture persists at the lowest output, endless loop tachycardia can be induced by chest wall stimulation (delivered by a temporary pacemaker) provided that the external signals are sensed selectively by the atrial channel.[58,70] Conversion to the asynchronous mode with the magnet over the pacemaker terminates endless loop tachycardia with rare exceptions.[71] *To prevent endless loop tachycardia,* the PVARP should be programmed to 50 msec beyond the duration of retrograde VA conduction determined noninvasively by pacemaker programming.[72] Other measures include a shorter AV interval, differential discrimination of the larger anterograde P wave from smaller retrograde atrial depolarization,[73] and activation of a special mechanism after a sensed ventricular event (outside AV delay) that is interpreted as a ventricular extrasystole: synchronous atrial stimulation (to preempt retrograde atrial depolarization) or automatic PVARP extension for one cycle[69,72] (Fig. 25–8). Some pacemakers possess an automatic tachycardia-terminating algorithm (e.g., omission of a ventricular stimulus or temporary PVARP prolongation) activated when ventricular pacing occurs at designated rates (usually the programmed upper rate) for a certain duration.

TACHYCARDIA DURING DDD PACING. Various types of tachycardia can occur during DDD pacing.[69] The diagnosis is usually simple and facilitated by telemetry of event markers

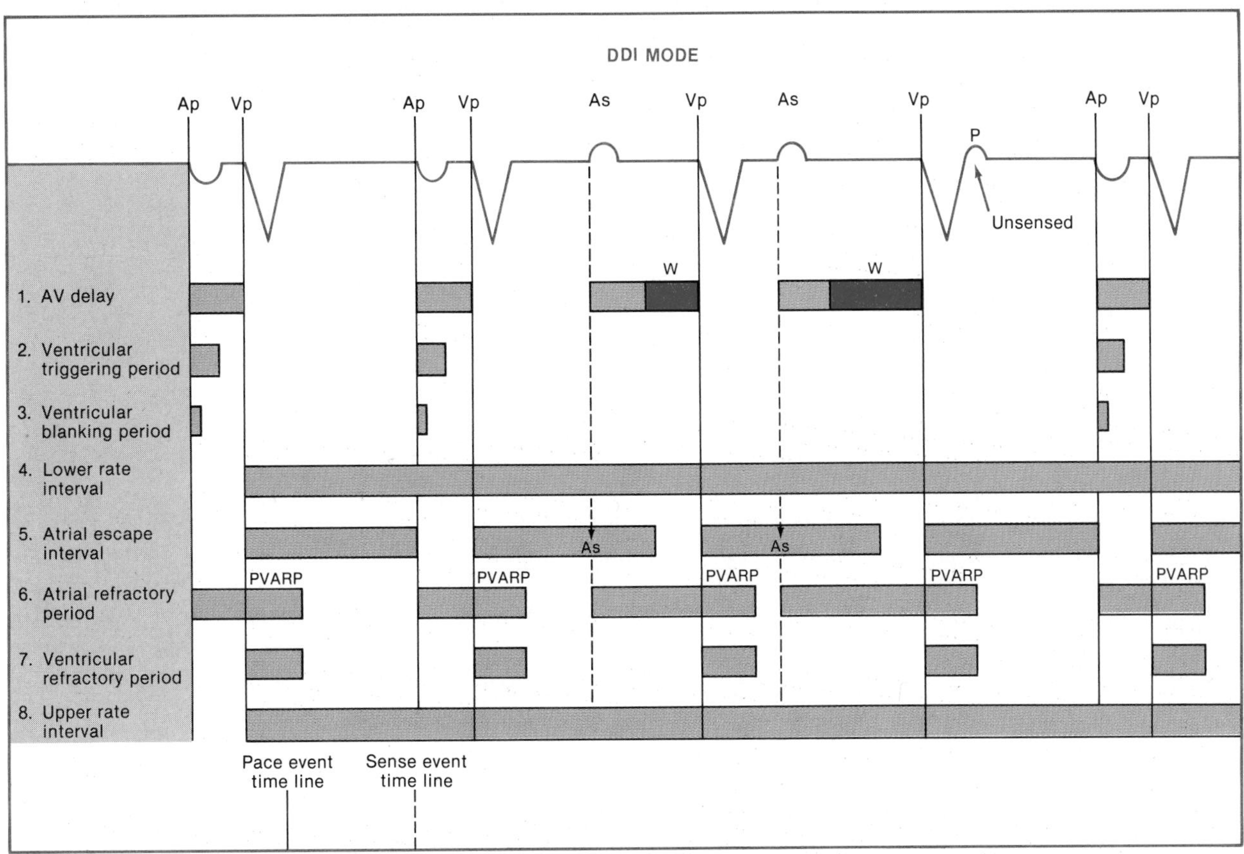

FIGURE 25–12. DDI mode. The DDI mode is equivalent to the DDD mode with identical lower rate interval and upper rate interval (provided the lower rate interval is controlled by ventricular events). In the diagram, the upper rate interval is *longer* than the programmed total atrial refractory period (postventricular atrial refractory period plus AV interval) so that the device will function as in Figure 25–10 with a Wenckebach AV block response. The P-P interval (As-As) is *shorter* than the upper rate interval but longer than the total atrial refractory period. As in Figure 25–10 in the DDD mode, P waves outside the postventricular atrial refractory period are sensed and initiate an AV interval. The As-Vp (atrial sensed–ventricular paced) interval lengthens by a varying period (W) to conform to the upper rate interval (which is equal to the lower rate interval in the DDI mode). As in the DDD mode (Fig. 25–10), the maximum prolongation of the As-Vp (atrial sensed–ventricular paced) interval during Wenckebach pacemaker AV block represents the difference between the upper rate interval and the programmed total atrial refractory period. When the P-P interval (As-As) becomes shorter than the programmed total atrial refractory period, the Wenckebach upper rate response will disappear and give rise to fixed-ratio pacemaker AV block. The arrow pointing down within the atrial escape interval indicates that an atrial sensed event (As) has taken place. Although the atrial escape interval actually terminates at this point, for the sake of clarity it is depicted as if As had not occurred. (From Barold, S. S. et al.: All dual chamber pacemakers function in the DDD mode. Am. Heart J. *115:*1353, 1988.)

or electrograms (discussed later). Tachycardias other than endless loop tachycardia return upon removal of the magnet. The magnet, by producing a slower rate in the DOO or VOO mode, permits identification of P or f waves. Programming to slow VVI pacing allows analysis of atrial activity. Atrial flutter or fibrillation can cause regular or irregular atrial and ventricular pacing due to intermittent lack of atrial sensing with consequent release of atrial stimuli. This response, coupled with periods of rapid ventricular pacing, produces a chaotic pattern virtually diagnostic of atrial fibrillation or flutter (Fig. 25–15). Tachycardia triggered by myopotentials sensed by the atrial channel of a unipolar device is easily reproducible with isometric exercise (Fig. 25–16).

MULTIPROGRAMMABILITY

A programmable pulse generator is capable of noninvasive adjustment of its function so that an appropriate pacemaker "prescription" can be "written" by the physician. The available technology, which is reliable and cost effective, is mandatory in modern pacemaker practice because it reduces the need for secondary interventions and increases the pulse generator longevity by optimizing pacemaker output.[74] The program change should always be confirmed by telemetry to reduce the likelihood of error and should be entered in the patient's chart. Programmability after pacemaker implantation is often underutilized. It offers the opportunity to create an optimal pacing system for a specific clinical situation. Like chronic pharmacological therapy requiring dosage adjustment according to changing circumstances, pacemaker parameters appropriate at the time of implantation may cease to be adequate in the future and may need modification. Programmability has simplified troubleshooting many pacemaker problems and often obviates operative revision to treat pacemaker complications.

SINGLE-CHAMBER PACEMAKERS. The three most important parameters for single-chamber pacing are rate, output (voltage and pulse width), and sensitivity. The ability to program other parameters such as refractory period, mode, polarity, and hysteresis is also desirable in certain clinical circumstances (Table 25–4).

Programming an increase in output may be necessary when the acute or chronic pacing thresholds rise disproportionately. When the pacing threshold has stabilized several weeks after implantation, decreasing output is important to conserve battery life and increase longevity of the pulse generator. For most patients, the nominal output delivered by the pacemaker is excessive and wasteful. Reducing voltage rather than pulse width often minimizes or eliminates undesirable diaphragmatic pacing or muscle stimulation at the anodal site of normally functioning unipolar pacemakers (in the absence of insulation leak).

Programming the output to subthreshold levels (or very low rate) permits study of the underlying rhythm. The pacemaker should be programmed to be twice as sensitive as the value of the sensing threshold. This corresponds to a numerical setting at least half the threshold value. For example, if the sensitivity threshold, i.e., the lowest setting associated

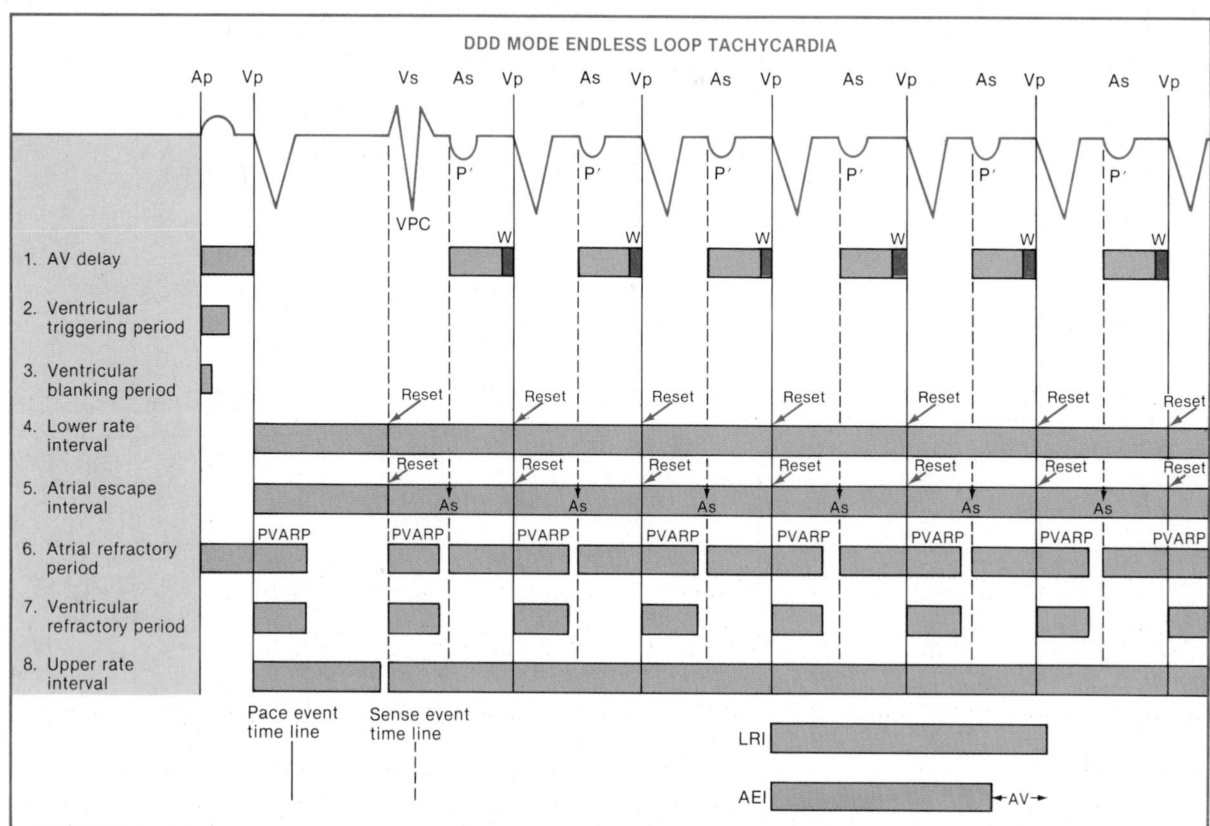

FIGURE 25-13. DDD mode. Endless loop (reentrant) tachycardia initiated by a ventricular extrasystole (VPC, second beat) with retrograde ventriculoatrial (VA) conduction (P′ or As). The atrial channel senses the retrograde P wave (P′) and a ventricular pacemaker stimulus (Vp) is issued after extension of the As-Vp (atrial sensed–ventricular paced) interval to conform to the supremacy of the upper rate interval (as in Fig. 25-10). The ventricular paced beat (Vp) generates another retrograde P wave, again sensed by the pulse generator outside its postventricular atrial refractory period (PVARP) and the process perpetuates itself. The pulse generator itself provides the anterograde limb of the macroreentrant process because it functions as an artificial AV junction. Retrograde VA conduction (P′) following a ventricular paced beat (Vp) provides the retrograde limb of the reentrant process. The cycle length of the endless loop tachycardia is equal to the upper rate interval. However, the cycle length of an endless loop tachycardia may occasionally be longer than the upper rate interval if retrograde VA conduction is prolonged. In this situation when the AV interval is *not* extended, the retrograde VA conduction time (as seen by the pacemaker) may be calculated by subtracting the AV interval from the cycle length of the tachycardia. Disruption of either the anterograde limb (by eliminating atrial sensing) or the retrograde limb (by eliminating retrograde VA conduction) terminates endless loop tachycardia. The arrow pointing down within the atrial escape interval indicates that an atrial sensed event (As) has taken place. Although the atrial escape interval actually terminates at this point, for the sake of clarity it is depicted as if As had not occurred. (From Barold, S. S. et al.: All dual chamber pacemakers function in the DDD mode. Am. Heart J. *115:*1353, 1988.)

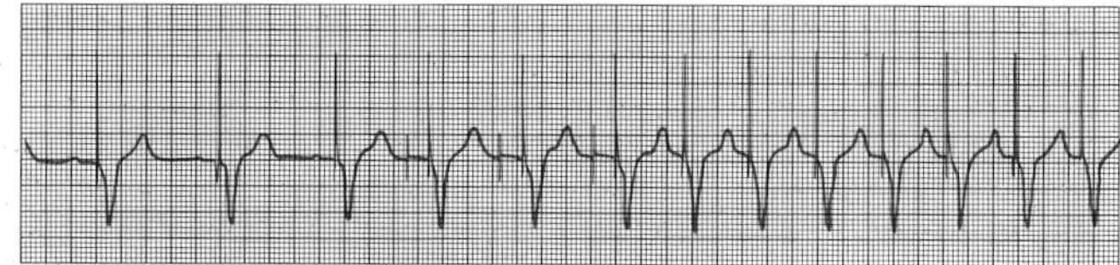

FIGURE 25-14. DDD pacing with subthreshold atrial stimulation precipitating endless loop tachycardia. Initial parameters: lower rate interval = 1000 msec, upper rate interval = 480 msec, postventricular atrial refractory period = 200 msec, AV interval = 180 msec. After the third beat, the lower rate interval was shortened to 750 ms (rate = 80/min) to test for retrograde VA conduction. Ineffectual subthreshold atrial stimulation is followed by a retrograde P wave seen as a notch on the ST segment of the fifth ventricular paced beat. However, this retrograde P wave is unsensed. The next ventricular paced beat gives rise to a retrograde P wave slightly later so that it is now sensed and initiates an endless loop tachycardia at the programmed upper rate of 125/min. When the postventricular atrial refractory period was programmed to 325 msec, subthreshold atrial stimulation no longer induced endless loop tachycardia.

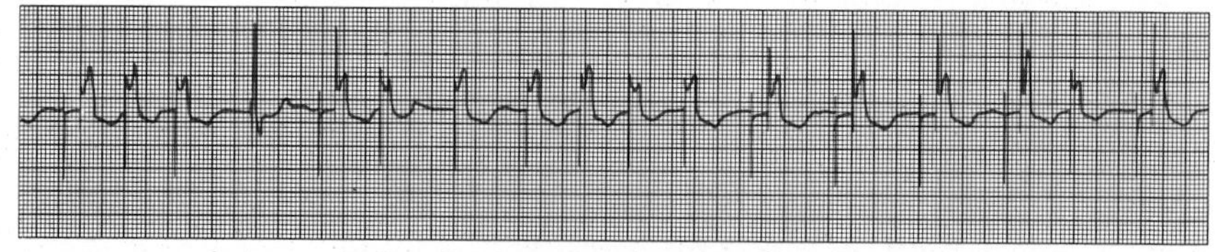

FIGURE 25-15. DDD pacing with atrial fibrillation. Programmed parameters: lower rate interval = 750 msec, upper rate interval = 375 msec, AV interval = 160 msec. The constantly changing pattern is due to intermittent sensing of f waves. When the f waves are not sensed, an atrial stimulus is delivered at the termination of the atrial escape interval. This chaotic pattern is virtually diagnostic of atrial fibrillation or flutter during DDD pacing. (From Barold, S. S., et al: Electrocardiography of contemporary DDD pacemakers. A. Basic concepts, upper rate response, retrograde ventriculoatrial conduction, and differential diagnosis of pacemaker tachycardias. *In* Saksena, S., and Goldschlager, N. [eds.]: Electrical Therapy for Cardiac Arrhythmias. Philadelphia, W. B. Saunders, 1990, p. 257.)

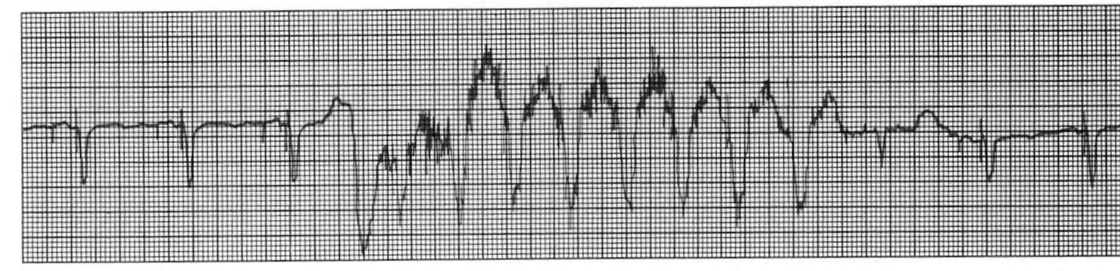

FIGURE 25–16. Unipolar DDD pacing with myopotential triggering. The atrial channel senses myopotentials whereupon ventricular stimulation is delivered at the programmed upper rate of 130/min. (From Barold, S. S. et al.: Function and electrocardiography of DDD pacemakers. *In* Barold, S. S. [ed.]: Modern Cardiac Pacing. Mt. Kisco, NY, Futura Publishing Co., 1985, p. 668.)

with regular sensing during deep respiration, is 8 mV, the sensitivity value should be programmed to 4 mV. Oversensing the T wave and/or residual voltage at the electrode-myocardial interface is easily remedied by decreasing the sensitivity (*increasing* the numerical value) and/or prolonging the refractory period. Oversensing myopotentials by a unipolar pacemaker requires reduction of sensitivity; however, if this is associated with undersensing the QRS, programming to the triggered (VVT, AAT) mode may be required.

DDD PACEMAKERS. The programming of DDD pacemakers requires special considerations. In addition to programming output voltage, pulse width, and sensitivity, the PVARP must be programmed to prevent sensing retrograde P waves and the possibility of endless loop tachycardia. The AV interval, upper and lower rates (intervals) must be programmed.[75] Programming the ventricular blanking period may be desirable to prevent crosstalk. The AV interval should be programmed to obtain maximum hemodynamic advantage. A relatively long AV interval may allow spontaneous AV conduction and provide better left ventricular function and conservation of battery life. Abnormal depolarization from ventricular pacing results in an altered contraction pattern that can decrease left ventricular function,[76] a response circumvented by an AV interval that allows spontaneous AV conduction. However, a long AV interval can facilitate the induction of endless loop tachycardia.

Many DDD pacemakers have identical AV intervals after atrial pacing and sensing. However, the AV interval during right atrial pacing may be too short to allow for propagation to the left atrium and left atrial contribution to left ventricular filling. It may be reasonable to prolong the AV interval after atrial pacing by 50 msec to produce basically the same effective AV interval as that initiated by atrial sensing.[77] Some pulse generators possess algorithms that shorten the AV interval during exercise as the normal heart does.[78] Two-dimensional and Doppler echocardiography can be useful to "fine-tune" and individualize the hemodynamic response at rest and on exercise.[79–81] The optimal AV interval can vary considerably from patient to patient and depends on many factors including left ventricular compliance, left ventricular filling pressure, atrial contractility, mitral valve function, and heart rate.

Most DDD pulse generators should remain in the DDD mode. However, programming the DDD unit to different modes may be necessary to respond to changing circumstances or complications. For example, VVI pacing may be necessary if permanent atrial fibrillation supervenes. If the patient develops frequent episodes of paroxysmal supraventricular tachyarrhythmias, the DDI mode is useful to provide atrial pacing and AV synchrony during sinus bradycardia and a constant ventricular pacing rate (lower rate) during atrial tachyarrhythmia. The VDD mode may be useful in patients with relatively normal atrial response to activity when atrial pacing is not functioning appropriately owing to a high pacing threshold or atrial lead displacement. If the VDD mode is not available, the DDD mode can be used with the atrial output programmed turned off or to the lowest value for subthreshold stimulation.

HEMODYNAMICS OF CARDIAC PACING

In the normal subject, increase in cardiac output with exercise is provided by rate increase (300 per cent) with only a modest contribution from increased stroke volume (50 per cent). Advancing age changes the relative contributions; however, increase in heart rate at age 70 still provides approxi-

TABLE 25–4 MULTIPROGRAMMABILITY

PARAMETER	VARIABILITY	PURPOSE
Rate	Increase	To optimize cardiac output, to overdrive or terminate tachyarrhythmias, to adapt pediatric needs, to test AV conduction with AAI pacemakers, to confirm atrial capture during AAI pacing by observing concomitant change in ventricular rate
	Decrease	To assess underlying rhythm and dependency status, to adjust rate below angina threshold, to allow emergence of normal sinus rhythm and preservation of atrial transport, to test sensing function
Output	Increase	To adapt to pacing threshold
	Decrease	To test threshold for pacing, to conserve battery longevity according to threshold for pacing, to reduce extracardiac stimulation (pectoral muscle, diaphragm), to assess underlying rhythm and dependency status
Sensitivity	Increase (Reduction of numerical value)	To sense low electrographic signals (P and QRS)
	Decrease (Increase of numerical value)	To test sensing threshold, to avoid T wave or afterpotential sensing (VVI pacing), to avoid sensing extracardiac signals, e.g. myopotentials
Refractory period	Increase	To minimize QRS sensing (AAI pacing), to minimize T wave or afterpotential sensing (VVI pacing)
	Decrease	To maximize QRS sensing (VVI pacing), to detect early premature ventricular complexes
Hysteresis		To delay onset of ventricular pacing to preserve atrial transport function
Polarity	Conversion to unipolar mode	To amplify the signal for sensing in the presence of a low bipolar electrogram, to compensate temporarily for lead fracture in the other electrode
	Conversion to bipolar mode	To decrease electromagnetic or myopotential interference, to evaluate oversensing, to eliminate extracardiac anodal stimulation
Mode	VVT/AAT	To perform noninvasive electrophysiological study and to terminate reentrant tachycardias (chest wall stimulation with external pacemaker), to prevent inhibition of unipolar pacemaker by extracardiac interference, to evaluate oversensing by "marking" sensed signals
	VOO/AOO	To prevent inhibition of pacemaker by interference when triggered mode is not available or is undesirable

mately two-thirds of the total increase in cardiac output with maximum exercise. Although patients with fixed-frequency pacing (VVI) may tolerate loss of AV synchrony, their effort tolerance is limited because in them cardiac output increase relies solely on an increase in stroke volume. This limitation is worse in patients with severe left ventricular dysfunction because their stroke volume is fixed, making an increase in cardiac output dependent solely on rate augmentation.

In the normal heart, AV synchrony at rest contributes about 20 to 30 per cent of the cardiac output. In some patients with congestive heart failure, atrial systole may contribute little to the resting cardiac output because of a substantial increase in left ventricular filling pressure. However, such patients should not be denied AV sequential pacing; medical therapy can improve their ventricular performance, reduce left ventricular filling pressure, and restore their responsiveness to the benefits of atrial systole. AV synchrony is quite important in patients with diastolic left ventricular dysfunction, contributing 30 to 40 per cent to end-diastolic volume and cardiac output at rest. Loss of AV synchrony in the presence of decreased left ventricular compliance leads to marked reduction in cardiac output and produces serious hemodynamic changes including pulmonary venous congestion. Consequently, AV sequential pacing should be used in all patients with diastolic left ventricular dysfunction (aortic stenosis, hypertrophic cardiomyopathy, and left ventricular hypertrophy secondary to hypertension).

The contribution of AV synchrony with exercise is difficult to quantitate. While some studies suggest that it is inconsequential and drops to 10 per cent or less,[82] others (particularly in patients with left ventricular dysfunction) suggest that AV synchrony with exercise further improves cardiac function and efficiency.[83]

Many studies have shown that during exercise an increase in the pacing rate provided by VVIR, VDD, DDD, or DDDR modes increases the cardiac output and duration of exercise more than does fixed-frequency VVI pacing.[84-89] In addition to superior hemodynamic effects, an increase in maximum O_2 consumption, reduced AV O_2 difference, and an increase in subjective well-being result. The hemodynamic advantage is retained on an ongoing basis, as studies have shown no difference between acute and long-term results. Furthermore, rate-responsive or adaptive pacemakers actually may lead to improved left ventricular function over time.[90]

PACEMAKER SYNDROME

Pacemaker syndrome is a clinical constellation of signs and symptoms produced by adverse hemodynamic and electrophysiological responses to a ventricular pacemaker. The pacemaker syndrome most commonly occurs in patients with normal or near-normal left ventricular function and retrograde ventriculoatrial (VA) conduction. Only about 15 to 20 per cent of patients with preserved VA conduction develop symptoms suggestive of the pacemaker syndrome, with about half exhibiting its full-blown form. Others may have subtle, unrecognized manifestations. Adverse responses include vague symptoms of low cardiac output generally more pronounced in the upright position, hypotension, orthostatic hypotension (especially in the first few seconds of ventricular pacing taking over from normal sinus rhythm), syncope or near-syncope (due to reduction in cerebral flow), fatigue, lightheadedness, malaise, weakness, lethargy, dyspnea, induction of congestive heart failure, patient awareness of beat-to-beat variations of cardiac response (from spontaneous to pacemaker beats), neck pulsations or pressure sensation of fullness in the chest, neck, or head, chest pain, and impaired exercise capacity.[91] Many nonspecific symptoms similar to those of the pacemaker syndrome are common in the elderly and complicate the diagnosis. Physical examination may show cannon waves in the jugular venous pulse and palpable liver pulsations.

LOSS OF AV SYNCHRONY. This can decrease cardiac output by 20 to 30 per cent at rest, but hemodynamic compromise in the pacemaker syndrome is more complex because retrograde VA conduction causes a "negative atrial kick" with more profound hemodynamic disadvantage than simple loss of AV synchrony. Atrial contraction against closed mitral and tricuspid AV valves causes systemic and pulmonary venous regurgitation and congestion (cannon *a* wave), sometimes leading to the development of congestive heart failure in previously compensated patients. In addition to the marked reduction in cardiac output,[92,93] retrograde VA conduction leads to atrial distension and activation of stretch receptors that produce a reflex vasodepressor effect probably mediated in part by atrial natriuretic factor.[94] Thus in the face of hypotension due to low cardiac output, compensatory mechanisms that ordinarily increase the peripheral resistance become attenuated. In some cases involving profound hypotension there can even be a net reduction in peripheral resistance, and for this reason concomitant treatment of congestive heart failure with vasodilators can precipitate the pacemaker syndrome.[95] The relatively small group of patients who have pacemaker syndrome without VA conduction often exhibit venous cannon *a* waves that probably are responsible for their symptoms.

Implantation of a VVIR pacemaker (see below) does not protect the patient from the development of the pacemaker syndrome.[96] Indeed, the pacemaker syndrome can occur during exercise if ventricular pacing with VA conduction persists. If VA block occurs, for example as a result of an increase in the ventricular pacing rate, pacemaker syndrome can disappear.

The pacemaker syndrome can be eliminated by restoring AV synchrony either with atrial pacing (if AV conduction is normal) or dual-chamber pacing with an appropriate AV delay. Occasionally, restoration of AV synchrony during VVI pacing can be achieved by reducing the ventricular pacing rate (or using hysteresis) to minimize competition with sinus rhythm. At the time of pacemaker implantation, if ventricular pacing produces a 20 mm Hg or more decrease in blood pressure, the likelihood of the pacemaker syndrome exists and use of a dual-chamber pacemaker should be considered.

RATE-ADAPTIVE PACEMAKERS

Atrial chronotropic incompetence is the inability to increase the heart rate to appropriate levels that satisfy body needs.[97] Guidelines such as the inability to achieve a heart rate exceeding 70 per cent of the maximum heart rate predicted for a given level of metabolic demand or the inability to reach a heart rate of 100/min on exercise provide practical definitions of atrial chronotropic incompetence. Testing can be by treadmill or long-term ambulatory ECG recordings during walking or ordinary activities. One-third or more of patients with sick sinus syndrome exhibit varying degrees of atrial chronotropic incompetence[98]; it is also found in some patients with AV block. A pacemaker that varies its rate in response to changes in the activity of a biological parameter that varies in parallel with the need for greater cardiac output can provide heart rate adaptability. Such a rate-responsive system is called rate-modulated, rate-adaptive, or sensor-driven and is designated by the letter "R" in the fourth position of the pacemaker code, e.g., VVIR is a rate-adaptive ventricular demand pacemaker and DDDR is a rate-adaptive DDD device. The magnitude and rate change of the sensor-driven response are programmable. The ideal sensor should be stable, reliable long-term, and easy to implant, program, and troubleshoot. It should also respond in direct proportion to metabolic demand, use a standard lead, be energy efficient, be autoprogrammable, respond quickly, and decelerate gradually at the end of exercise.

Of the many sensors in clinical use or investigation[99,100] (Table 25-5), currently approved devices in the United States respond to activity, temperature, or minute ventilation.[101]

Types of Rate-Adaptive Pacemakers

ACTIVITY-SENSING PACEMAKER. This is the most commonly used rate-adaptive system and employs a piezo-

TABLE 25–5 SENSORS INCORPORATED INTO RATE-ADAPTIVE PACEMAKERS

1. Activity
2. Respiration
   A. Respiratory rate
   B. Minute ventilation volume
3. Temperature
4. Ventricular repolarization: Q-T interval
5. Ventricular depolarization gradient
6. Myocardial contractility
   A. Stroke volume and rate of change of stroke volume (dV/dt)
   B. Rate of change of right ventricular pressure (dP/dt)
   C. Preejection interval
7. Oxygen saturation
8. Central venous pH

electric sensor bonded to the inner surface of the pacemaker to detect mechanical forces or vibrations (body movements but not myopotentials) that are transformed to electrical energy to control the pacing rate. The pacing rate is increased in proportion to the detected vibration. The sensor is nonmetabolic and therefore nonphysiological because it does not respond to an increase in metabolic demand such as with emotional stimuli that are unrelated to exercise. Nevertheless, it works well in practice.[86,101,102–104] The system is simple, reliable, stable, uses a standard lead, and exhibits a fast response to brief periods of exercise. Its main advantage is being able to recognize the precise onset and end of exercise, an important characteristic in older patients who do not exercise much and do so primarily in short bursts of physical work such as walking or climbing stairs. Other systems that exhibit a delayed response at the onset of exercise and reach a maximum rate after the end of the exercise are less desirable for the elderly. Several disadvantages exist. Pacing rate plateaus after the initial increase despite continued exercise. Rate change does not occur during mental exercise or emotional stress. Physical pressure on the pacemaker such as lying on it can cause an inappropriate rate increase during sleep. Pacing rate may be slower when stairs are climbed compared with when they are descended. External vibrations such as occurs when riding a vehicle in a rough terrain and in a train or a helicopter can increase the pacing rate. Generally these aberrations are innocuous.

OTHER TYPES OF SENSING

QT INTERVAL SENSING PACEMAKER. This operates on the principle that the Q-T interval shortens with physical exercise due to the release of catecholamines.[105,106] The QT system provides a stable, rugged sensor using a standard pacemaker lead. Its disadvantages include a relatively slow response, nonsustained rate changes, and some difficulty in ensuring reliable T wave sensing.

RESPIRATORY-DEPENDENT PACEMAKERS. Two basic systems are available. One measures the *respiratory rate* by detecting the electrical impedance between the pacemaker can and an additional subcutaneous auxiliary lead in the anterior chest wall and paces over a standard unipolar cardiac lead.[107] A small current creates the sensor impedance that varies with respiration. This system has been used successfully in Europe for several years but as of this writing is not available in the United States.[108] The second respiratory system calculates the *minute ventilation* volume (total volume times respiratory rate) by measuring the transthoracic impedance. The system injects a small current between the pacemaker casing and the proximal electrode of a standard bipolar lead and determines impedance between the tip electrode and the pacemaker casing. The transthoracic impedance increases with inspiration and decreases with expiration, and its amplitude varies according to the tidal volume. The calculated minute ventilation volume (and the generated pacing rate) correlates closely with metabolic demand or work load (Fig. 25–17). The system works well clinically.[109,110] Drawbacks include a delayed reaction to the onset of exercise, inappropriately fast rate after the end of exercise, additional energy required for sensor function that may reduce the life span of the pulse generator, and excessive pacing rates in patients with tachypnea from congestive heart failure or other causes, and also as a response to swinging of the arms, shoulder movements, or coughing.

TEMPERATURE-SENSING PACEMAKER. This pacemaker's operation is based on an increase in metabolic rate with activity that produces heat transported in the blood. A small thermistor totally incorporated into a special pacing lead can detect temperature change in the right ventricular blood.[111] A special algorithm compensates for the decrease in blood temperature at the onset of exercise as the cooler blood returns from the extremities. While clinical experience so far has been satisfactory,[112,113] disadvantages exist. Temperature acutely reflects O_2 consumption in the middle or late stage of exercise. Thus, while central venous temperature correlates well with metabolic demand at high work loads, the rate response is insufficient at low work loads such as brief everyday activities because of the relatively slow and minimal increase in central venous temperature. Also, heat dissipation mechanisms at the end of exercise are often impaired in patients with heart failure. Finally, the system requires a special lead with a thermistor that consumes additional energy, the long-term stability of which has not yet been established.

Despite drawbacks, each of the rate-adaptive units has made important contributions. Future pacemakers will combine two or more sensors that can overcome the drawbacks of each one alone.[114–116]

PROGRAMMING RATE-ADAPTIVE PACEMAKERS

The rate-adaptive pulse generator should be programmed so that a casual 2 to 3 minute walk increases the rate 10 to 25/min, to about 90/min, and a fast walk or stair climbing increments the rate 20 to 45/min, to about 100 to 120/min. Stress testing and Holter recordings can be useful to set appropriate functions, and pacer-derived histograms can help assess rate response. Very rapid rate increases and decreases generally should be avoided. Care should be taken that fast rates do not precipitate angina in patients with coronary artery disease, worsening of congestive heart failure, and hypotension in patients with cardiomyopathy[117] or atrial or ventricular tachyarrhythmias. Pacemaker syndrome may occur with both VVIR and AAIR modes. Rapid atrial pacing rates may prolong the P-R interval so much that the P wave follows close to the previous QRS complex, resulting in atrial contraction against a closed AV valve.[97,118,119] Care must be taken during therapeutic or diagnostic procedures: for example, electrocautery can increase the pacing rate of the minute ventilation sensor-driven pacemaker to its upper limit.[120]

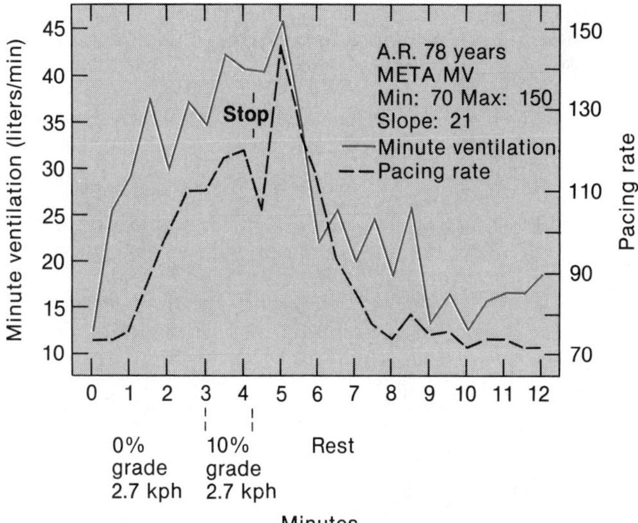

FIGURE 25–17. Exercise test (modified Bruce protocol) to demonstrate the close correlation between measured minute ventilation and pacing rate with a minute ventilation rate responsive pacemaker system. The patient at the end of exercise continues to hyperventilate, and the pacing rate rises to the upper rate limit. Then a physiological fall occurs in both minute ventilation and pacing rate. Tidal volume and respiratory rate were measured using a Fleisch Head Pneumotach with air flow converted to volume using a respiratory integrator. (From Mond, H. G., and Kertes, P. J.: Rate responsive cardiac pacing. Denver, Telectronics and Cordis Pacing Systems, 1988, p. 47.)

Atrial and AV Pacing

Atrial and AV pacing generally are preferable to single-chamber ventricular pacing because they reduce the incidence of chronic (and perhaps paroxysmal[121]) atrial fibrillation, particularly in patients with the bradycardia-tachycardia syndrome and probably in other forms of sinus node disease. They prevent retrograde VA conduction[122–129] and decrease the risk of embolization and stroke,[98,125–128] the incidence of congestive heart failure,[125] and overall mortality.[125,127,130] Single-chamber ventricular pacing should therefore be avoided in most patients with the bradycardia-tachycardia syndrome. Nevertheless, in the United States perhaps 1 per cent or less of patients requiring pacing receive a single-chamber atrial pacemaker.[33] AAI and AAIR pacemakers are underutilized despite the wealth of information showing their superiority over VVI pacing in the sick sinus syndrome.[98] Previous problems with atrial pacing such as lead instability have been resolved.[42] The concern that patients with AAI (AAIR) pacemakers may develop AV block is largely unfounded. Second or third degree AV block has an annual incidence of about 1.2 per cent in carefully selected patients with AAI (AAIR) pacemakers, and its occurrence is rarely catastrophic and often related to drug therapy.[42,98,131,132] Guidelines for selecting AAI or AAIR pacing include 1:1 AV conduction with atrial pacing to rates 120 to 140/min, P-R < 0.24 sec at rest, an H-V interval < 75 msec, and/or absence of bundle branch block. With careful patient selection, AAI or AAIR pacing could be used safely in probably half of those with sick sinus syndrome, and of these about 40 per cent may require rate-adaptive devices (AAIR) because of atrial chronotropic imcompetence.[98,133–136]

VVIR vs. DDD Pacing

In the United States only about one-third of the patients requiring pacemakers presently receive dual-chamber devices. A VVI pacemaker programmed to a low rate may be justified in the occasional patient with infrequent episodes of bradycardia and in selected inactive patients with a short life expectancy. The majority of patients with atria that can be paced should be considered for single-chamber atrial or dual-chamber pacing (AAI, AAIR, DDD, or DDDR).[89] VVI or VVIR pacing contributes to left ventricular dysfunction, pacemaker syndrome, atrial fibrillation, and systemic emboli and should be reserved primarily for patients with chronic atrial fibrillation and AV block.

In choosing between VVIR and DDD pacing, maintenance of AV synchrony at rest contributes more to quality of life than rate responsiveness with exercise. Most pacemaker patients spend their lives predominantly at rest, punctuated by relatively short periods of mild exercise during the course of the day when a moderate rate response would be clearly beneficial. Pacemaker function in elderly patients should be evaluated at low exercise loads to correspond with their activities of daily living and not with maximum exercise, which obviously represents an artificial situation. DDDR pacing will resolve the controversy of VVIR vs. DDD.[137] In a recent study, patients with atrial chronotropic incompetence performed better in the DDDR than in the VVIR mode.[138]

Individual Patient Considerations

When deciding the type of pacemaker to be used, the physician needs to determine whether the atrium can be paced, whether latent or overt AV block exists, and whether atrial chronotropic incompetence is present[139] (Fig. 25–18). It is also important to assess what is best for the patient's level of activity, whether there is underlying coronary artery disease or left ventricular function, what is affordable, what is the simplest system that will optimize hemodynamics, what is the natural history of the condition for which pacing is being used, and what is the impact of present and future drug therapy.

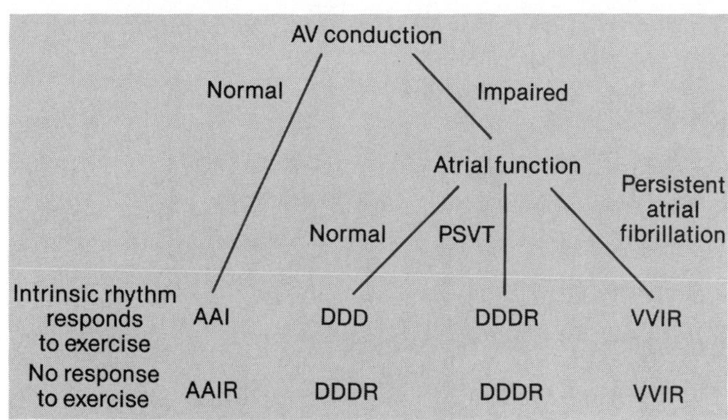

FIGURE 25–18. Algorithm for determining the optimal pacemaker mode for an individual patient. PSVT = paroxysmal supraventricular arrhythmias of all types including atrial fibrillation. A DDDR should be considered in patients with the bradycardia-tachycardia syndrome with intrinsic or drug-induced AV conduction delay to provide greater flexibility because (1) drug therapy of supraventricular tachyarrhythmias may further depress the atrial chronotropic response on exercise, and (2) troublesome paroxysmal atrial tachyarrhythmias may necessitate programming to the DDIR mode. (From Griffin, J. C.: The optimal pacing mode for the individual patient. The role of DDDR. *In* Barold, S. S., and Mugica, J. [eds.]: New Perspectives in Cardiac Pacing. 2. Mt. Kisco, NY, Futura Publishing Co., 1991, p. 325.)

A single-lead VDD pacing system may provide a relatively simple and less expensive VDD/VVIR pacemaker for patients with AV block and normal atrial chronotropic function.[140–142] Cost considerations aside, either a sensor-driven single-chamber or a sensor-driven dual-chamber pacemaker with extensive programmability of pacing modes would meet the needs of all patients. In the future, as costs decrease, virtually all patients will receive rate-adaptive pulse generators and the sensor (or combinations of sensors) will be just one of the many programmable functions. Indications for simple VVI pacemakers will dwindle as VVIR and other modes become more price competitive.

COMPLICATIONS OF PACEMAKERS

Complications of *venous entry* complications of *lead placement* and *pocket formation*, and *electrical complications* or *pacemaker malfunction* constitute three major groups of complications associated with permanent pacemaker implantation.

Complications of Lead Placement and Pocket Formation

Lead displacement can produce loss of pacing and sensing. Whereas myocardial perforation is rare with contemporary leads, it is more common with stiff temporary leads. Perforation may produce no symptoms or may cause intermittent or complete failure to pace and/or diaphragmatic pacing. A friction rub may be audible. If the lead has migrated to the left ventricle, paced beats can have a right bundle branch block contour in lead V_1. Echocardiography can be diagnostic. Although cardiac tamponade is rare, if it does occur it is usually at the time of lead insertion and rarely after the first 24 hours; at this time the lead may be withdrawn and safely repositioned under careful observation.

The incidence of symptomatic venous thrombosis is quite low despite the fact that contrast venography is abnormal in 30 to 45 per cent of patients, with total subclavian vein obstruction in 8 to 20 per cent.[143] Subclavian venous obstruction probably occurs gradually so that the development of collaterals makes symptomatic obstruction rare. Should symptoms occur, treatment with anticoagulants is required for several weeks. Superior vena caval obstruction is a rare complication and has been treated successfully with streptokinase, while superior vena caval stenosis has been treated successfully with balloon angioplasty.[144,145]

Contraction of the left diaphragm synchronously with a paced stimulus can occur with or without lead perforation and is generally eliminated or minimized by programming the pacemaker output to a lower value. Contraction of the right diaphragm is due to phrenic nerve stimulation from a malpositioned right atrial electrode. Invariably, left intercostal muscle stimulation is due to lead perforation of the right ventricle. An insulation break causing a current leak either from the extravascular portion of the lead or the pulse generator can be associated with pectoral muscle twitching at or near the site of implantation. Some normally functioning unipolar pulse generators can cause pectoral muscle stimulation by the indifferent (anodal) plate without an insulation leak, particularly if the pacemaker has flipped over in a large pocket.

Twiddler's syndrome usually occurs when there is a relatively large pacemaker pocket and the patient repeatedly rotates the implanted pulse generator under the skin. The lead may retract from the heart to produce pacemaker failure.[146] A pulse generator may erode through the skin or migrate, usually because of suboptimal implantation technique. Early infections are rare. *Staphylococcus aureus* is the most common offending organism in early infections and *Staphylococcus epidermidis* is most common in late infections. Eradication of infection often requires removal of the entire pacing system.[147]

Pacemaker Malfunction

LOSS OF CAPTURE. The causes of loss of capture by visible pacemaker stimuli and pacemaker failure with no stimuli are listed in Table 25–6. Many of the abnormalities with visible stimuli are due to changes in the electrode-tissue interface that can be overcome by reprogramming or correcting any reversible metabolic or drug-related abnormalities. In some cases of chronic progressive increases in pacing threshold, lead replacement can be required. Absence of stimuli usually is due to pulse generator failure (battery or component) or to interrruption of the electrical circuit with no current flow commonly due to a broken electrode with intact insulation. Wire breakage is not always evident radiologically. A tight ligature on polyurethane leads can compress the insulation and spread the coils of wire without interfering with function, giving the appearance of a fracture (pseudofracture) radiologically.

ABNORMAL PACING RATE. A change in the pacing rate or erratic pacing can occur due to normal function (Table 25–7). Abnormal causes due to pacemaker malfunction are often found by exclusion. A constantly changing spike-to-spike interval during pacing often is caused by oversensing and/or a problem with the electrode rather than component failure. "Runaway pacemakers" with very rapid, life-threatening rates of stimulation are now rare but can still occur.[148] At extremely rapid rates, stimulation is either ineffectual or can occur intermittently, producing bursts of tachycardia. This situation requires immediate disconnection and removal of the pacemaker.

UNDERSENSING. Low-amplitude electrograms represent the commonest cause of undersensing. Lead dislodgement, low-amplitude signal from premature ventricular complexes, and myocardial infarction are common causes, often correctable by programming sensitivity to a more sensitive value. Undersensing can also occur with component failure of a pulse generator, an abnormal (jammed) magnetic reed switch (that fails to restore sensing upon magnet removal), or inappropriate programming of sensitivity or refractory period. Asynchronous pacing can also occur at a preset rate as a protective response to continually sensed interference. Insulation or wire fracture defects can also attenuate the effective electrogram detected by a pulse generator. Hyperkalemia, toxic effects of antiarryhythmic drugs (especially antiar-

TABLE 25–6 CAUSES OF LOSS OF CAPTURE BY VISIBLE PACEMAKER STIMULI AND LOSS OF PACING STIMULI

LOSS OF CAPTURE

1. **ELECTRODE-TISSUE INTERFACE**
   Displacement or unstable position of pacing leads (commonest cause); perforation; malposition into coronary sinus or middle cardiac vein; elevated threshold (acute or chronic); inapparent displacement (exit block) and perforation; myocardial infarction, ischemia, or fibrosis; hypothyroidism; transient or chronic elevation of pacing threshold after defibrillation or cardioversion; electrolyte abnormalities, e.g., hyperkalemia; drug toxicity, e.g., type 1A antiarrhythmic agents or drug effect, e.g., 1C antiarrhythmic agents (flecainide, encainide, and propafenone)
2. **ELECTRODE**
   Fracture, short circuit, and insulation break
3. **PULSE GENERATOR**
   Normally functioning pulse generator: inappropriate programming of output parameters, spontaneous pacemaker failure due to battery exhaustion or component failure, component failure from iatrogenic causes such as defibrillation, therapeutic radiation, and electrocautery

LOSS OF PACING STIMULI

1. **NORMAL SITUATION: total inhibition of pulse generator when the intrinsic rate is faster than the preset pacemaker rate**
2. **PSEUDOMALFUNCTION: overlooking tiny bipolar pacemaker stimuli in the ECG**
3. **LEAD FRACTURE, loose connection, or set screw problem**
4. **PULSE GENERATOR: battery depletion, component failure, sticky magnetic reed switch (application of magnet produces no effect), poor anodal contact (air in pacemaker pocket or dry pocket)**
5. **EXTREME ELECTROMAGNETIC INTERFERENCE**
6. **OVERSENSING (signals originating from outside or inside the pulse generator)**

TABLE 25–7 CAUSES OF CHANGES IN PACING RATE

NORMAL FUNCTION

1. **Low programmed rate**
2. **Application of the magnet**
3. **Inaccurate speed of ECG machine drive**
4. **Apparent malfunction in special function pulse generators, e.g., hysteresis or triggered mode (AAT, VVT)**
5. **Reversion to interference rate (in response to electromagnetic or other signals) with either a faster or a slower rate than the spontaneous free-running or magnet rate (according to manufacturer)**

ABNORMAL FUNCTION

1. **Battery failure (slowing of rate)**
2. **Runaway pacemaker: spontaneous or due to therapeutic radiation**
3. **Component failure, e.g., erratic delivery of pacemaker stimuli: spontaneous or due to therapeutic radiation**
4. **Change in mode after defibrillation or electrocautery, e.g., DDD to VVI**
5. **Phantom reprogramming, misprogramming, and oversensing**

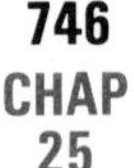

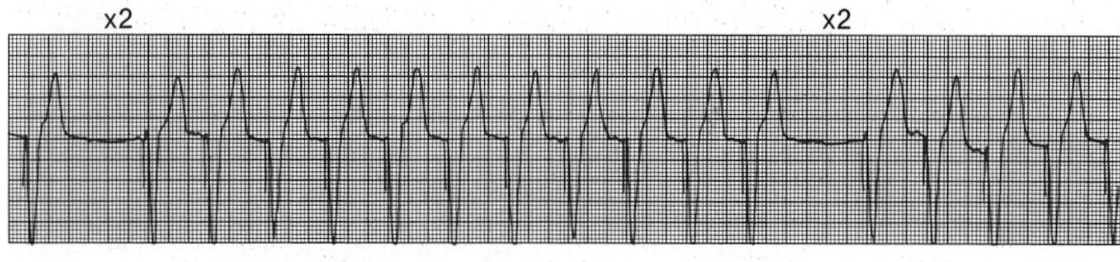

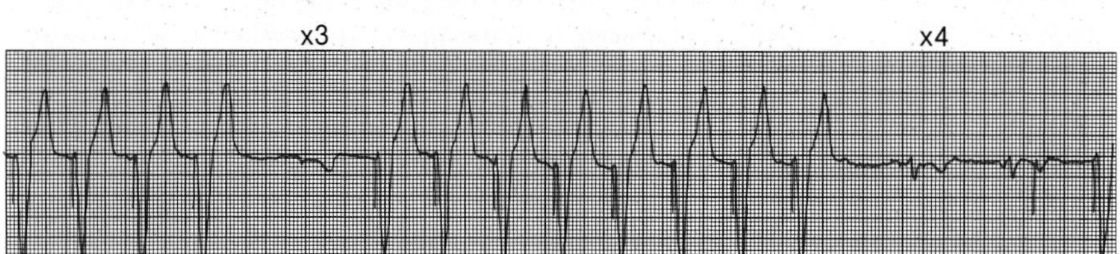

FIGURE 25–19. Electrocardiographic diagnosis of intermittent lead fracture or loose connection. During spontaneous pacing the electrocardiogram (not shown) revealed intermittent pacemaker pauses of varying duration. The ECG shows asynchronous pacing at 100/min upon application of the magnet over the pulse generator. Wriggling the pulse generator in its pocket produces pauses that are exact multiples of the magnet interval (×2, ×3, and ×4) a response diagnostic of an intermittent electrode problem because it reflects the correct timing of a normally functioning pulse generator delivering its impulse into a transiently disrupted circuit with high impedance. (From Barold, S. S. et al.: Differential diagnosis of pacemaker pauses. *In* Barold, S. S. [ed.]: Modern Cardiac Pacing. Mt. Kisco, NY, Futura Publishing Co., 1985, p. 592.)

rhythmic drugs in classes 1A and 1C) and cardioversion and defibrillation can also lead to transient undersensing. Oversensing of an extraneous signal that initiates a new refractory period can lead to undersensing if the electrogram falls within the refractory period initiated by the sensed extraneous event.

OVERSENSING. This is by far the most common cause of pacemaker pauses, that is, failure of delivery of a pacemaker stimulus at the anticipated time according to the programmed automatic (escape) interval; its occurrence is confirmed by magnet-induced conversion to the asynchronous mode.[149] Unwanted signals causing oversensing arise from several sources. For example, atrial depolarization can be sensed during VVI pacing when the ventricular lead becomes displaced toward the right ventricular inflow tract. The faster sinus rate can inhibit the VVI pacemaker and cause asystole if complete AV block is present. Emergency treatment consists of magnet application or programming to the VOO or VVT mode. T wave sensing often represents the detection of a combined voltage originating from both the residual voltage at the electrode-myocardial interface and the natural T wave and can be corrected by programming a lesser sensitivity and/or a longer pacemaker refractory period.

The pacemaker itself can generate signals that are sensed and inhibit delivery of the pacemaker stimulus. For example, the electrode-tissue interface can act as a capacitor that generates voltage (polarization voltage or afterpotential) that is subsequently dissipated over a relatively long period. The decay of the "afterpotential" constitutes a time changing voltage that can be sensed when the pacemaker refractory period terminates. Also, abrupt changes in resistance within a pacing system can produce corresponding voltage changes that generate signals often invisible on the surface ECG. Such "make-break" or false signals can occur from loose connections, wire fractures with intermittent contact, short circuits, insulation defects, or the interaction of two pacemaker catheters lying side by side and touching each other within the heart.

Intermittent electrode problems, especially oversensing due to an intermittent fracture, constitute the "great imitator" in cardiac pacing and often cause a chaotic pattern of pacing. Indeed, erratic behavior with pauses of varying length suggests a defective lead system rather than pacemaker component malfunction. False signals tend to occur at random, producing inhibition of stimuli for relatively long and constantly changing periods. Magnet application eliminates the pauses in pacing that are caused by oversensing. The demonstration of pacemaker pauses that are exact multiples of the magnet interval during asynchronous pacing is virtually diagnostic of an intermittent wire fracture (or electrode problem) (Fig. 25–19). Sometimes this irregularity can be demonstrated only by wriggling the pacemaker in its pocket.

Oversensing skeletal muscle potentials (myopotential interference) remains the most common cause of pacemaker pauses and occurs almost invariably with unipolar pulse generators[149,150] (Fig. 25–20). Although myopotential interference can be demonstrated in as many as 50 per cent of patients with unipolar pulse generators, only 10 per cent report symptoms and require pacemaker reprogramming. Oversensing of diaphragmatic potentials provoked by deep inspiration is uncommon.[149] Rarely, an atrial J lead in the right atrial appendage senses intercostal myopotentials on deep inspiration. Interestingly, the incidence of myopotential interference has remained unchanged over the last 19 years because absolute discrimination between the cardiac electrogram and myopotentials is difficult.[151] The problem will disappear as bipolar systems eventually replace unipolar ones. In the meantime, myopotential oversensing can be corrected by reducing the input sensitivity, converting to the triggered VVT (AAT) or VOO (AOO) mode, programming from unipolar to bipolar sensing, and, rarely, pacemaker replacement.[151]

INTERFERENCE

Electromagnetic or other signals from the environment can be sensed by a pacemaker.[152] For example, transthoracic *cardioversion* or *defibrillation* delivers a large amount of energy to the heart during a relatively brief period. Paddles or patches must be placed well away from the pacemaker along a line perpendicular to the axis of the ventricular lead inside the heart. Circuitry designed to protect the pulse generator shunts energy to the lead. Contemporary pacemaker design with large-scale integrated circuits and microprocessors has made pulse generators more susceptible than in the past to disturbance from this type of electrical discharge. Unipolar pacing systems are more susceptible than bipolar systems. The shock can damage circuitry, with partial or complete destruction of the pulse generator that can result in runaway state, induction of end-of-life behavior, and reversible or irreversible alteration of the microprocessor program. It can also cause an acute, temporary (usual) or chronic increase in the pacing threshold, probably due to myocardial burns; undersensing abnormalities, usually temporary but sometimes lasting as long as 10 days; reprogramming to another mode even with different parameters; and reset to the VOO or VVI mode as a normal response to high level interference.[153] Similar problems can occur during catheter ablation using energy from a standard defibrillator or possibly from discharge of an implanted cardioverter/defibrillator.

While thermal and electrical burns at the electrode-myocardial interface can theoretically precipitate ventricular fibrillation, this has not yet been clearly documented in man.

ELECTROCAUTERY. This is the most common form of interference in the hospital environment. Apart from the expected inhibition during its application, electrical and thermal burns at the electrode-myocardial interface can cause ventricular fibrillation or chronic elevation of pacing threshold.[152] Damage to the pulse generator can result with permanent loss of output, random failure, reprogramming, alteration of the random access

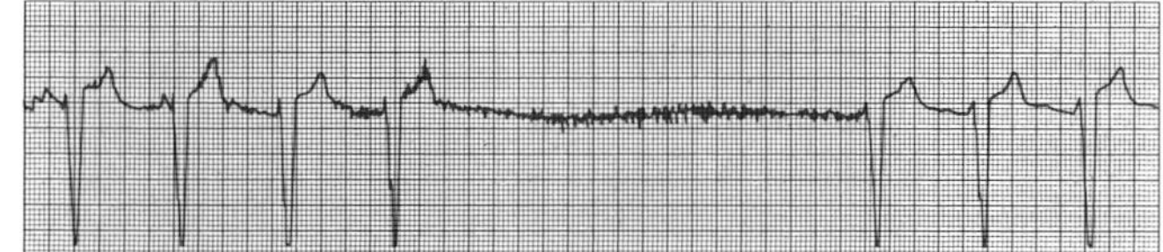

FIGURE 25–20. Prolonged inhibition of unipolar VVI pacemaker (rate = 70 ppm) from myopotential oversensing.

memory, and reset of the pulse generator to the VVI or VOO mode as a normal response to high-intensity interference.[153] Patients must be managed according to a careful protocol during electrocautery, with pacemaker testing before and after the procedure. Radiofrequency catheter ablation of arrhythmias (p. 653) can also cause similar severe disturbances of pacemaker behavior.[154]

Contemporary pulse generators are more sensitive to the effects of *radiation therapy* than were those used in the past. The damage to pacemaker electronics varies, occasionally is transient but often permanent, and the phenomenon is cumulative. The effect is similar whether the dose is given at one time or spread over several treatments. Given a sufficiently high cumulative absorbed dose, all pulse generators will fail catastrophically.[152,155] Appropriate shielding of the pulse generator during radiation therapy is mandatory.

MAGNETIC RESONANCE IMAGING (MRI). This can cause rapid pacing, inhibition, resetting of DDD pulse generators, and transient reed switch malfunction.[152,156] MRI is contraindicated in all patients with permanent pacemakers because serious malfunction with no output or rapid pacing may occur.

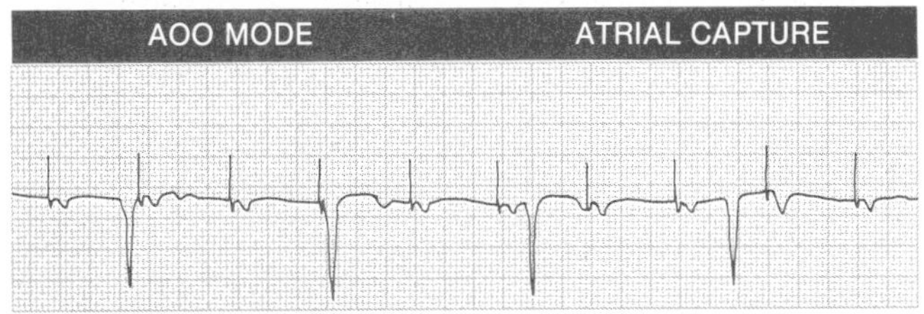

FIGURE 25-21. Determination of atrial capture in a patient with a DDD pulse generator and complete AV block. The pulse generator was first reprogrammed to the VVI mode and the rate was gradually decreased to 30/min, whereupon a ventricular escape rhythm at a rate of 45/min emerged. The pulse generator was then programmed to the AOO mode at a rapid rate. The atrial stimuli dissociated from the QRS complex demonstrate successful atrial capture. This maneuver is contraindicated in pacemaker-dependent patients.

PACEMAKER FOLLOW-UP

Despite the reliability of modern pacemakers, a follow-up program is mandatory because complications are not uncommon and pacemaker failure is ultimately inevitable. Good follow-up should provide improved pacemaker longevity by appropriate programming and should identify impending pacemaker failure in most instances. The frequency and type of follow-up depend on the projected battery life, type, mode, and programming of pulse generators, the stability of pacing and sensing, the need for programming changes, the underlying rhythm (pacemaker dependency), travel logistics, and the use of alternative methods of follow-up such as the telephone.[157]

Transtelephonic pacemaker monitoring is the simplest method of pacemaker follow-up, and its main function is to detect changes in pacemaker rate as an indirect reflection of battery depletion. Transtelephonic monitoring should complement and not replace comprehensive follow-up and is generally used to document satisfactory pacing function between visits. Transtelephonic monitoring usually is performed *every 2 to 3 months* until the first indication of battery depletion when it may be performed once a month. The ECG is recorded with and without magnet placement. Free-running and magnet intervals and pulse width are measured. In dual-chamber pacemakers, rate and pulse width are measured along with the AV interval. Complex ECGs from DDD pulse generators transmitted by phone are often uninterpretable. As a rule, transtelephonic follow-up does not allow programming or transmission of telemetry data.

When the patient is discharged after pacemaker implantation, the pulse generator is programmed to optimize function during the expected physiological changes in the early phase. The patient should be seen about 2 weeks after implantation, when the operative site is also inspected. The pacing system is evaluated 2 months after implantation when pacing and sensing thresholds have stabilized, and, in virtually all patients, definitive programming can be performed for long-term function. Follow-up in the clinic should be done every 6 to 12 months for single-chamber and every 3 to 6 months for dual-chamber pacemakers. Periodic transtelephonic pacemaker monitoring should supplement these visits. More frequent follow-up can become necessary when impending battery depletion is detected. Pacemaker follow-up requires equipment such as a three-channel ECG machine, magnet, digital counter for interval measurement, programmers, temporary pacemaker and chest electrodes for the chest wall stimulation,[58,70] echocardiography, long-term ECG recorders, and equipment for cardiopulmonary resuscitation. First, a 12-lead ECG is obtained with and without application of the magnet. Various intervals (lower rate, pulse width, and so on) are measured with an electronic counter. If telemetry is available, the pulse generator is interrogated to document initial pacemaker parameters. The following aspects of pacemaker function are then evaluated systematically.

Battery voltage can be evaluated indirectly. When it reaches a critical level, the elective replacement indicator (ERI) is activated and the pacing rate in the free-running and/or magnet mode slows.[158,159] This change can be gradual or stepwise (sudden). The ERI of some DDD pulse generators consists of reversion to the VVI or VOO mode.[153]

Ventricular pacing is documented from the control ECG and the ECG after application of the magnet. Ventricular pacing threshold is best determined in the VVI mode (or DDD with short AV interval to ensure ventricular capture) by programming voltage and/or pulse width until capture is lost. *Ventricular pacing* rate is also best confirmed in the VVI mode by reducing the pacing rate to allow the spontaneous rhythm to emerge. The ventricular sensing threshold can be determined by decreasing the ventricular sensitivity gradually until sensing failure occurs.

Using the AAI or AOO mode confirms *atrial capture* (Fig. 25-21). If the P wave is not visible with double standardization of the ECG, echocardiography or esophageal electrocardiography can be used to document atrial systole.[75,160] Evaluating *atrial sensing* is extremely important because atrial undersensing is one of the most common problems in DDD pacing.[161] To evaluate atrial sensing, the pacemaker lower rate should be reduced below that of spontaneous atrial activity and the AV delay shortened to 50 to 100 msec to guarantee that any sensed P wave will generate a ventricular stimulus. Atrial sensing can be assessed by decreasing the atrial sensitivity from the lowest numerical value (or most sensitive) to the highest numerical value (or least sensitive) until P wave tracking is lost (Fig. 25-22). The final programmed value should be double the atrial sensing threshold (half the numerical value). Telemetry when available provides proof of atrial sensing and its exact timing by transmitted event markers (Fig. 25-23). Random rather than sustained loss of atrial sens-

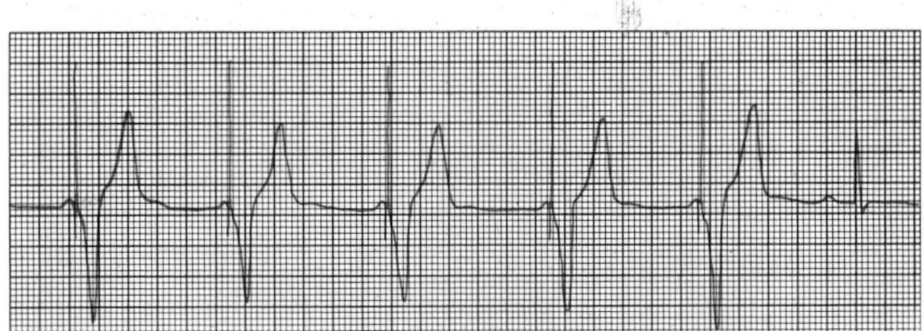

FIGURE 25-22. Semiquantitative assessment of atrial signal amplitude by programming the sensitivity of a DDD pulse generator. To demonstrate atrial sensing, the pulse generator was programmed to a lower rate of 50 ppm and AV = 50 msec. With an atrial sensitivity of 1.2 mV, all the P waves were sensed (not shown). At an atrial sensitivity of 1.6 mV, the tracing shows intermittent failure of atrial sensing (last P wave, i.e., if it had been sensed the ventricular stimulus would have occurred near the apex of the P wave). In this case, the lowest sensitivity (corresponding to the highest numerical value) causing consistent P wave sensing was 1.2 mV. Consequently, the atrial sensitivity should be programmed to 0.6 mV.

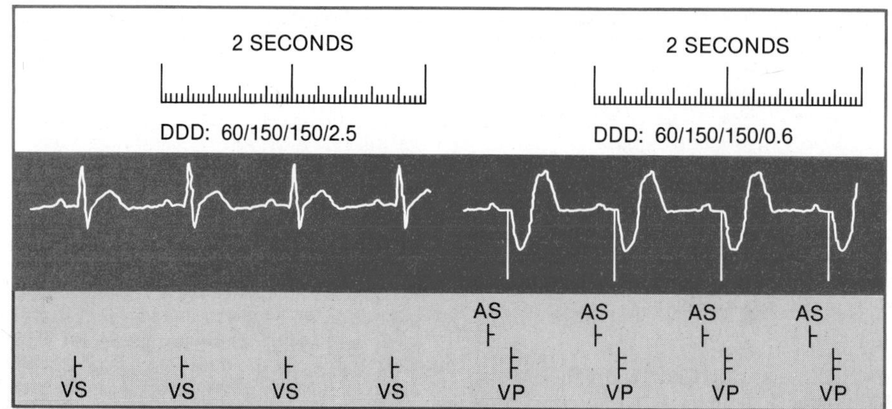

FIGURE 25–23. **Surface ECGs with annotated marker channel indicating sensing and pacing functions of an implanted DDD pacemaker. Left panel, The pacemaker has been programmed to the DDD mode with a lower rate of 60 bpm, and AV delay of 150 msec, an upper rate limit of 150 bpm, and an atrial channel sensitivity of 2.5 mV. The marker channel shows appropriate inhibition of ventricular stimulation by sensed ventricular depolarization (VS). Absence of a marker channel indicating atrial sensing confirms loss of atrial sensing function. (The atrial stimulus is inhibited because the VS-VS interval is shorter than the atrial escape interval, i.e., VS resets the atrial escape interval, and starts a new interval.)**

ing is not uncommon in Holter recordings but rarely is of any clinical significance. Changes in body position, respiration, congestive heart failure, and exercise may alter the amplitude of the P wave signal and affect sensing.[75]

Myopotential interference in unipolar pulse generators should be evaluated routinely with isometric exercise and 24-hour Holter recordings. In DDD pacing, myopotential interference can inhibit the ventricular channel (Fig. 25–20), can increase the ventricular pacing rate when the atrial channel senses myopotentials (Fig. 25–16), can cause the pacemaker to revert to the asynchronous interference mode at a predetermined rate, and can activate the ventricular safety pacing mechanism of dual-chamber devices with abbreviation of the paced AV delay.

Evaluating *retrograde VA conduction* is important in patients prone to development of endless loop tachycardia. Susceptibility to crosstalk should be determined as previously discussed.

Telemetry is an indispensable feature of sophisticated pulse generators and provides information on all programmed values as well as real-time or measured data on how the pacemaker is operating at the time of interrogation. These data include information on the output circuit, battery parameters, sensor activity for rate-adaptive pacemakers, diagnostic data about the interaction between the pulse generator and the patient over an extended period of time, and event markers and transmission of electrograms. Event markers depicting pacing and sensing are recorded simultaneously with the ECG and permit real-time evaluation of the pacing system and facilitate troubleshooting (Figs. 25–23 and 25–24). Although the actual sensed signal cannot be identified, event markers indicate how the pacemaker interprets a specific paced or sensed event and provide precise representation of timing intervals. While the telemetered endocardial electrogram is generally less useful than event markers, it may demonstrate the nature of a malfunction caused by lead displacement or fracture, undersensing due to a poor signal, or oversensing, especially when the nature of the signal cannot be determined from the ECG. The telemetered atrial electrogram or atrial event markers can easily document the existence of retrograde VA conduction and its precise duration.

Finally, long-term ECG recordings help to investigate pacemaker function and the significance of syncope, dizziness, and palpitations.[162]

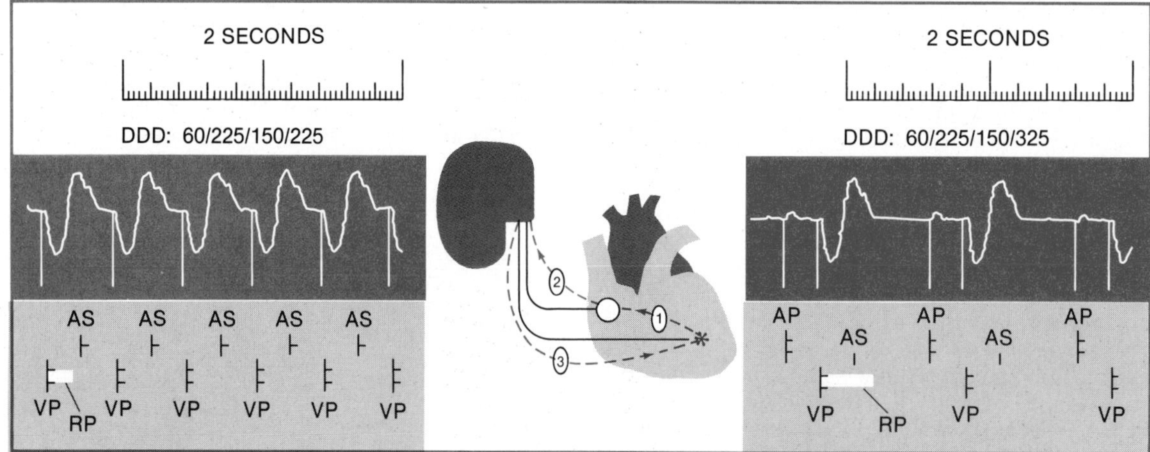

FIGURE 25–24. **Surface ECG and annotated marker channels from an implanted DDD pacemaker. Left panel, The pacemaker is programmed in the DDD mode with a lower rate of 60 bpm, an AV delay of 225 msec, an upper rate limit of 150 bpm, and a postventricular atrial refractory period of 225 msec (RP). Each ventricular stimulus (indicated in the marker channel as VP) results in retrograde atrial activation (dotted pathway 1 in center diagram), which is sensed by the pacemaker (dotted pathway 2 and indicated in the marker channel as AS), in turn triggering yet another ventricular stimulus (dotted pathway 3) and creating endless loop tachycardia. Right panel, The pacemaker postventricular atrial refractory period (RP) has been lengthened to 325 msec. Again, each ventricular stimulus produces a retrograde P wave, but these now occur during the pacemaker refractory period and do not trigger ventricular stimulation. Each retrograde P wave is indicated in the marker channel as having been sensed but not used as a trigger (AS). Thus, appropriate selection of the pacemaker atrial refractory period prevents endless loop tachycardia.**

Electrical Devices to Treat Tachycardias

Electrical devices can be used to treat tachycardias by preventing the tachycardia onset or terminating the tachycardia after it has developed (p. 651). Techniques to prevent tachycardia onset are applicable to a very small number of patients and include pacing at normal or increased rates to suppress bradycardia-dependent tachyarrhythmias such as torsades de pointes associated with the long Q-T syndrome.[163] In the absence of bradycardia, an increase in pacing rate rarely successfully suppresses refractory ventricular tachyarrhythmias chronically.[164] Dual-chamber pacing with a short AV interval can prevent some AV nodal or AV reciprocating tachycardias,[165,166] and rapid continuous atrial pacing can be used to produce a fast atrial tachycardia with a high degree of AV block to override a slower atrial tachycardia associated with a faster ventricular rate,[167] but ablative or surgical cures are preferable (see Chap. 23).

TERMINATION OF TACHYCARDIA

Rapid pacing and/or premature stimulation can be used to terminate AV nodal (Fig. 25–25) and AV reciprocating tachycardias, atrial flutter, some atrial tachycardias, and many ventricular tachycardias (Fig. 25–25).[168–184] Although trains or bursts of stimuli constitute the most effective way of terminating these tachycardias,[185] this method is also more likely to accelerate the tachycardia or cause fibrillation.[186–189] A preferable pacing approach that delivers initially four or five stimuli at progressively shorter intervals and then recycles to deliver the initial number of stimuli plus one or more at a still shorter interval seems to be quite effective and safe.[190–192] Originally employed in systems manually activated by the physician or patient, such approaches are now incorporated in implanted devices that function automatically[193] (Fig. 25–26).

The success of automatic antitachycardia pacing depends a great deal on the accuracy of the detection algorithm because paroxysmal tachycardia must be differentiated from sinus tachycardia, atrial fibrillation, and the like. Contemporary devices use a rate cutoff that exceeds a certain programmed value and can include suddenness of onset of the rate increase (to differentiate a pathological tachycardia with abrupt onset from sinus tachycardia with a gradual onset) and rate stability of the tachycardia (to exclude atrial fibrillation) before the device is triggered to deliver the electrical therapy.[194,195] Advantages of automatic pacemakers include (1) convenience, as there is no need for an external device, (2) automatic termination, which is important for patients who are confused, anxious, or seriously symptomatic at the onset of tachycardia, and (3) rapid activation of the system (within four to eight cycles) to avoid the development of compensatory cardiovascular reflexes that can make subsequent conversion more difficult. Most devices have bradycardia pacing (VVI or AAI) backup as well as memory capability to record device function and patient response. Generally such devices are no longer popular for most patients with supraventricular tachycardias because ablation and surgical procedures can be curative. Only when drug therapy is ineffective or not tolerated and the patient has undergone unsuccessful curative surgery, refuses surgery or when it is contraindicated should an antitachycardia pacemaker be considered.[196] Considering the fact that catheter ablative therapy and surgery successfully eliminates AV nodal and AV reentry in over 95 per cent of patients with a mortality close to zero, success rates of antitachycardia pacing are not impressive. In 291 patients receiving such a device for supra-

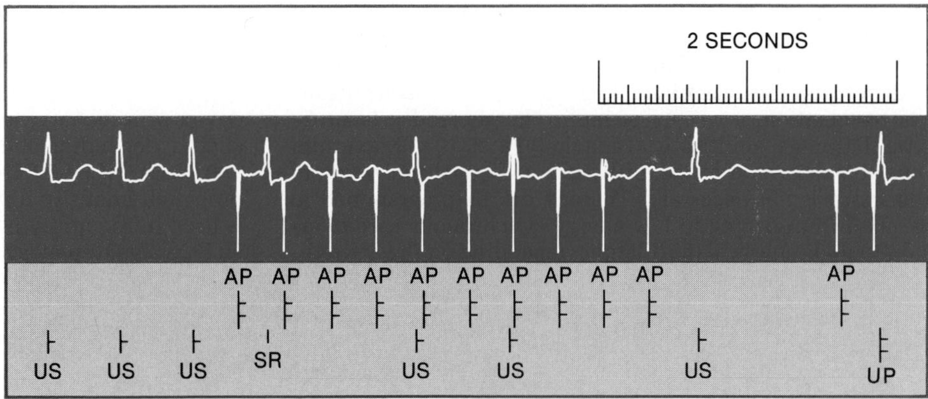

FIGURE 25–25. Pacing termination of atrial ventricular (AV) nodal reentry. The antitachycardia pacemaker performs in the DVI mode, responding spontaneously to the onset of AV nodal reentrant tachycardia (Medtronic Symbios). Termination of AV nodal reentry by 10 stimuli delivered to the atrium follows. The marker channel indicates ventricular sensing (VS), atrial pacing (AP), a sensed ventricular event in the refractory period of the ventricular amplifier (SR), and ventricular pacing (VP). After tachycardia termination, AV sequential pacing occurs for the last beat. (From Zipes, D. P. et al.: Initial experience with symbios Model 7008 Pacemaker. PACE *7*:1301, 1984.)

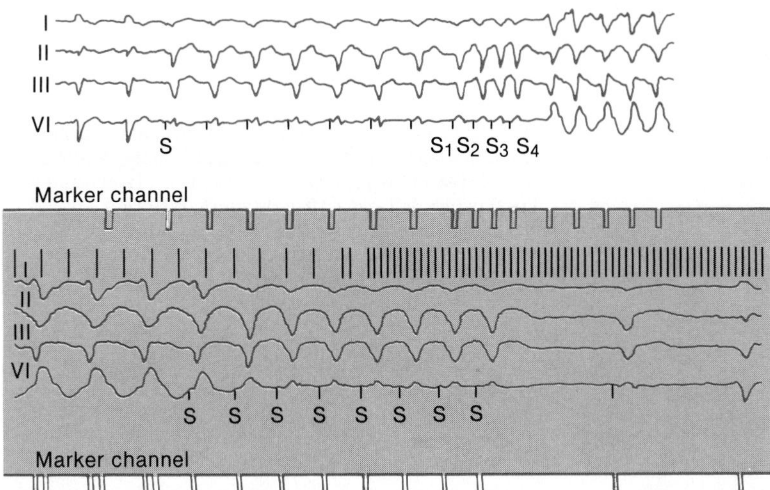

FIGURE 25–26. Pacing induction and termination of ventricular tachycardia by an implantable cardiovert defibrillator (ICD). The first two complexes in the top panel demonstrate spontaneous sinus rhythm. Eight paced complexes at a cycle length of 300 msec (S_1) follow, with three premature (S_2, S_3, S_4) stimuli initiating sustained monomorphic ventricular tachycardia. The marker channel exhibits a single large negative deflection illustrating ventricular pacing (V_p) and then a smaller negative potential illustrating ventricular sensing (V_s). The rapid rate has not yet been determined by the ICD to be ventricular tachycardia. In the bottom panel, the ICD has recognized the ventricular tachycardia (short negative pairs of stimuli, VT_s) and begins to deliver a decremental ramp of eight pacing stimuli, which terminate the ventricular tachycardia. A paced ventricular complex (S) and then a sinus beat (NSR) follow.

ventricular tachycardia, results were described as excellent in 51 per cent, good in 35 per cent, and poor in 5 per cent (unstated in 9 per cent).[182] At 5 years, only 60 to 80 per cent of the pacing systems remained effective and about 40 to 50 per cent of patients still required drugs.[182] Antitachycardia pacing for supraventricular tachycardia has had little growth in the past 10 years and is still not widely used (about 1 per cent of all pacemaker implantations).

A recent review of 195 patients with tachycardia terminating pacemakers for ventricular tachycardia revealed that 53 per cent of patients were thought to have an excellent response, 18 per cent a good response, and 3 per cent a poor response (unstated 14 per cent).[182] Slower ventricular tachycardias were more successfully terminated by pacing. Drug therapy by slowing the rate can facilitate tachycardia termination by pacing techniques. A faster ventricular tachycardia requires a more aggressive pacing protocol associated with a greater incidence of acceleration and degeneration into ventricular fibrillation. Automatic devices should not be used to treat ventricular tachycardia without "backup" defibrillation.[183,197-199]

TABLE 25-8 INDICATIONS FOR CARDIOVERTER-DEFIBRILLATOR IMPLANTATION

PRESENTLY APPROVED
Last-resort treatment for patients with documented life-threatening ventricular tachyarrhythmias or cardiac arrest not associated with acute myocardial infarction
Inducible ventricular tachyarrhythmias at electrophysiological study unresponsive to medical or surgical treatment, or the patient is not a candidate for such treatment
PROPOSED INDICATIONS
Patients with documented cardiac arrest or hypotensive ventricular tachycardia not associated with acute myocardial infarction (<48 hours), transient ischemic episode correctable by treatment, electrolyte imbalance or drug toxicity, even if ventricular tachyarrhythmia is not inducible by aggressive (three extra stimuli) electrophysiological testing. Life expectancy should exceed 6 months and patient should be psychologically capable of accepting such treatment.
Ventricular tachyarrhythmias still inducible after corrective surgery for ventricular tachycardia
Unexplained syncope in a patient with inducible hypotensive ventricular tachyarrhythmia
Symptomatic long Q-T syndrome despite medical treatment

IMPLANTABLE CARDIOVERTER/ DEFIBRILLATORS (ICD)

Table 25-8 outlines indications for cardioverter-defibrillator implantation. At the time of this writing, only one device is approved for implantation by the FDA. However, several devices are undergoing clinical testing and therefore this chapter will describe generically the capabilities of these devices rather than focus on any one unit. The ICDs weigh about 250 to 280 gm with a volume of 150 cc and are powered by lithium silver vanadium pentoxide cells. The sizes of the newer devices are progressively smaller. While longevity varies depending on the use of the ICD in an individual patient, it is in the range of 3 to 4 years, with an ability to deliver about 100 to 200 discharges. The more sophisticated ones are capable of pacing, cardioversion, and defibrillation.[200-203] Pacing therapy for bradycardia (VVI),[204] for electrophysiological studies (premature and rapid stimulation), and for ventricular tachycardia termination, a variety of ramps, bursts, and premature stimulation capabilities is available (Fig. 25-27). Maximum output is delivered for defibrillation, and synchronization of the shock is not necessary. Therapy can be programmed to escalate from pacing to low-energy synchronous cardioversion to high-energy defibrillation, depending on the arrhythmia and the patient's response. Shocks for cardioversion of ventricular tachycardia are synchronized to the onset of ventricular depolarization registered by special rate detector leads. Energy of the shocks is programmable, generally from 0.1 to 35 or 40 joules. The ICD can be interrogated for all its functions and is fully programmable. It has a memory that stores the number of arrhythmic episodes, successful responses, and cycle lengths of R-R intervals before and after therapy is delivered. The number of consecutive cycles before tachycardia recognition is programmable and therefore the time to respond with therapy is variable. Charging to about 30 joules takes 5 to 15 seconds (depending on circumstances). The number of times the device retries therapy is programmable. For ventricular fibrillation, if the first shock fails, the device will recharge and deliver up to three to six additional shocks, depending on the manufacturer.

ARRHYTHMIA SENSING. This is an evolving area. The probability density function (PDF), which was used initially, is used infrequently now. PDF evaluates the amount of time an ECG signal spends away from the baseline (zero potential).

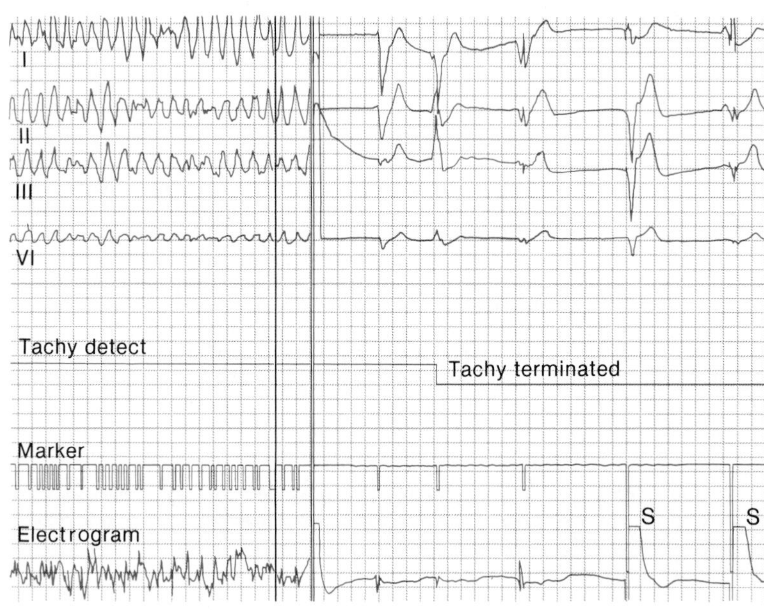

FIGURE 25-27. Termination of ventricular fibrillation followed by bradycardia requiring pacing. Ventricular fibrillation is recognized by the ICD (Telectronics 4203) which delivers a 10 joule shock, restoring a regular rhythm of ventricular complexes. A period of bradycardia initiates two ventricular paced complexes (S) before restoration of normal sinus rhythm.

During normal sinus rhythm, the ECG spends most of the time at the baseline while a sinusoidal rhythm such as ventricular fibrillation or a rapid ventricular tachycardia spends a high percentage of time away from the baseline. Most commonly, rate only is used for ventricular tachycardia and ventricular fibrillation detection. Rate sensing alone is quite sensitive but not specific because therapy can be delivered for a supraventricular tachycardia when the rate exceeds the programmed upper rate cutoff of the device. Future devices probably will include electrogram recognition, possibly the presence of AV dissociation, and a wide QRS tachycardia or even biosensors to discriminate a ventricular from a supraventricular tachycardia.[205]

IMPLANTATION. Several surgical approaches are used, including left lateral thoracotomy, median sternotomy (especially if other cardiac procedures are performed), and subxiphoid or subcostal incisions.[206] Two or three defibrillating patches are applied inside or outside the pericardium, the outside being more popular to facilitate coronary bypass surgery. The patches do not interfere with global or regional left ventricular function. Additional pacemaker electrodes for rate sensing are applied epicardially and less often transvenously. All leads are then tunneled subcutaneously to the device implanted in an abdominal pocket in the left upper quadrant. Preliminary experience with nonthoracotomy approaches involving right ventricular/superior vena caval/coronary sinus electrodes plus a subcutaneous extrathoracic electrode is encouraging.[207–209] Careful testing at the time of implantation must establish adequate electrograms for sensing during sinus rhythm, ventricular tachycardia, and fibrillation, as well as appropriate pacing thresholds. The minimum amount of energy required for successful and reliable defibrillation (defibrillation threshold, DFT) must be measured and should be 50 per cent or less of the maximum output of the device and is usually 15 to 18 joules.[210,211] Even if the device is being used to treat ventricular tachycardia alone, it must be shown to defibrillate as well. Antiarrhythmic drugs can alter the DFT. Amiodarone, class 1B agents (lidocaine, mexiletine) and class 1C agents (encainide, flecainide) can increase DFT, while class 1A agents have little effect. Bretylium and sotalol with class 3 properties decrease DFT.[212–216] Acceptable device function, including its ability to defibrillate, is tested after recovery from surgery before the patient is discharged. Continuing efficacy of the ICD should be reevaluated whenever antiarrhythmic therapy is altered.

COMPLICATIONS. The mortality of the implantation is about 1 to 3 per cent, partly due to the severity of the underlying cardiopulmonary disease and the risk of additional surgery such as coronary bypass surgery. The complications include those associated with thoracotomy, pericarditis (rarely constrictive[217]), postpericardiotomy syndrome, atrial fibrillation, cardiac tamponade, congestive heart failure, myocardial infarction, cardiogenic shock, postoperative stroke, erosion and extrusion, infection (in 2 to 3 per cent of implants and one of the most serious complications),[218] lead migration, and fracture.[219–221] Other complications consist of high DFT (sometimes due to drugs), premature battery depletion, component failure, undersensing, oversensing (P or T wave, fracture with or without myopotential oversensing), and other causes of inappropriate shocks. Psychological complications are important and include the fear of painful shocks, anxiety, and depression that may respond to psychological counseling and rarely may lead to explantation.[222,223]

FOLLOW-UP. After implantation, more than half the patients require antiarrhythmic drug therapy to control sustained or nonsustained ventricular tachycardia to avoid repeated device therapy. However, when an implanted ICD is in place, the number of drugs and dosage can be reduced to avoid side effects, with the knowledge that the ICD will adequately treat an occasional "breakthrough" tachycardia. Patients should be seen every 2 to 3 months, depending on individual responses. The capacitors of the device need periodic reformation (charged and discharged) for proper continuing function. At the time of each visit, the device is investigated to determine whether and what type of therapy has been delivered, the patient's response, adequate pacing and sensing, and the charge time of the capacitors. The elective replacement time of the device is indicated by an increase in the charge time. Multiple ICD discharges usually require hospitalization for further investigation. With current FDA-approved devices, appropriate discharges seem to occur in 33 to 62 per cent of the cases with a mean follow-up of 18 to 29 months and 80 per cent at 4 years.[201] The likelihood of appropriate discharges increases with decreasing left ventricular ejection, inducible sustained ventricular tachycardia before treatment, inducible sustained ventricular tachycardia while on drug therapy, and induction of ventricular tachycardia by only one or two stimuli.[224] Inappropriate shocks are not uncommon and can be due to sinus or supraventricular tachycardia that may be treated with beta blockers or digitalis for atrial fibrillation. Without a device memory, unless the patient develops syncope or near syncope, the appropriateness of a shock is difficult to determine.

IMPACT ON SURVIVAL. Although no randomized trials concerning the efficacy of the ICD have yet been published, it is generally considered that the device effectively reduces the incidence of sudden death[201,220,221,225–228] (p. 781). The 5-year rate of sudden death of 5 per cent compared with 20 per cent for similar drug refractory patients obtained from historical controls strongly suggests that the ICD is the most effective therapy for the prevention of sudden cardiac death in high-risk patients.[201,229] The patient population receiving ICDs is also at a higher risk of dying suddenly from asystole or arrhythmia, myocardial infarction, and congestive heart failure.[226–229] Some groups have shown total survival as high as 80 per cent (considering all causes of death) at 4 years while others have not observed such an optimistic prognosis. There is need for a stricter analysis of ICD benefit compared with other forms of therapy in terms of surgical mortality, patient selection, standardized methods of evaluating survival, and appropriateness of shock, bearing in mind that not all appropriate shocks prevent sudden death.[201,202,220,221,228,230–235]

REFERENCES

PACEMAKER MODALITIES AND FUNCTION

1. Bernstein, A. D., Camm, A. J., Fletcher, R. D. et al.: The NASPE/BPEG generic pacemaker code for antibradyarrhythmias and adaptive-rate pacing and antitachyarrhythmias devices. PACE *10*:794, 1987.
2. Bartecchi, C. E.: Temporary pacing catheter electrodes. *In* Bartecchi, C. E., and Mann, D. E. (eds.): Temporary Cardiac Pacing. Chicago, Precept Press, Inc., 1990, p. 268.
3. Jadvar, H., and Arzbaecher, R.: Temporary esophageal pacing. *In* Bartecchi, C. E., and Mann, D. E. (eds.): Temporary Cardiac Pacing. Chicago, Precept Press, Inc., 1990, p. 146.
4. Barold, S. S.: Transesophageal pacing. PACE *13*:1324, 1990.
5. Benson, D. W., Jr.: Transesophageal electrocardiography and cardiac pacing: State of the art. Circulation (Suppl. *75* III):86, 1987.
6. Santini, M., Ansalone, G., Cacciatore, G., and Turitto, G.: Transesophageal pacing, PACE *13*:298, 1990.
7. Bocka, J. J.: External transcutaneous pacemakers. Ann. Emerg. Med. *18*:1280, 1989.
8. Zoll, P. M.: Noninvasive temporary cardiac pacing. J. Electrophysiol. *1*:156, 1987.
9. Klein, L. S., Miles, W. M., Heger, J. J., and Zipes, D. P.: Transcutaneous pacing: Patient tolerance, strength interval relations and feasibility for programmed electrical stimulation. Am. J. Cardiol. *62*:1126, 1988.
10. Estes, N. A. M., III, Deering, T. F., Manolis, A. S. et al.: External cardiac programmed stimulation for noninvasive termination of sustained supraventricular and ventricular tachycardia. Am. J. Cardiol. *63*:177, 1989.
11. Luck, J. C., Grubb, B. P., Artman, S E. et al.: Termination of sustained ventricular tachycardia by external noninvasive pacing. Am. J. Cardiol. *61*:574, 1988.
12. Barold, S. S., Falkoff, M. D., Ong, L. S., and Heinle, R. A.: Termination of ventricular tachycardia by transcutaneous cardiac pacing. Am. Heart J. *114*:180, 1987.
13. Winner, S., and Boon, N.: Clinical problems with temporary pacemakers prior to permanent pacing. J. Roy. Coll. Phys. *23*:161, 1989.
14. McAllister, H. F., Klementowicz, P. T., Andrews, C. et al.: Lyme carditis:

An important cause of reversible heart block. Ann. Intern. Med. *110*:339, 1989.

15. Kimball, S. A., Janson, P. A., and LaRaia, P. J.: Complete heart block as the sole presentation of Lyme disease. Arch. Intern. Med. *149*:1897, 1989.
16. Zipes, D. P., Heger, J. J., and Prystowsky, E. N.: Synchronized low energy transvenous cardioversion. *In* Morganroth, J. (ed.): Sudden Cardiac Death. Orlando, Grune and Stratton, 1986, p. 285.
17. Lau, C. P., Leung, W. H., Wong, C. K. et al.: A new pacing method for rapid regularization and rate control in atrial fibrillation. Am. J. Cardiol. *65*:1198, 1990.
18. Matangi, M.: Temporary physiologic pacing in inferior wall acute myocardial infarction with right ventricular damage. Am. J. Cardiol. *59*:1207, 1987.
19. Dewey, R. C., Capeless, M. A., and Levy, A. M.: Use of ambulatory electrocardiographic monitoring to identify high risk patients with congenital heart block. N. Engl. J. Med. *316*:835, 1987.
20. Sholler, G. F., and Walsh, E. P.: Congenital complete heart block in patients without anatomic cardiac defects. Am. Heart J. *118*:1193, 1989.
21. Click, R. L., Gersh, B., Sugrue, D. D. et al.: Role of invasive electrophysiologic testing in patients with symptomatic bundle branch block. Am. J. Cardiol. *59*:817, 1987.
22. Petràc, D., Gjurović, J., Vukosavić, D., and Birtić, K.: Clinical significance and natural history of exercise-induced atrioventricular block. *In* Belhassen, B., Feldman, S., and Copperman, Y. (eds.): Cardiac Pacing and Electrophysiology. Jerusalem, Israel, R & L Creative Communications Ltd., 1987, p. 265.
23. Paillard, F., Mabo, P., BenSlimane, A. et al.: Les blocs auriculoventriculaire desmasqués à l'épreuve d'effort. Ann. Cardiol. Angeiol. *39*:55, 1990.
24. Kaul, U., Dev, V., Narula, J. et al.: Evaluation of patients with bundle branch block and "unexplained" syncope. A study based on comprehensive electrophysiologic testing and ajmaline stress. PACE *11*:289, 1988.
25. Denes, P., Uretz, E., Ezri, M. D., and Borbola, J.: Clinical predictors of electrophysiologic findings in patients with syncope of unknown etiology. Arch. Intern. Med. *148*:1922, 1988.
26. Bass, E. B., Elson, J. J., Fogoros, R. N. et al.: Long-term prognosis of patients undergoing electrophysiologic studies for syncope of unknown origin. Am. J. Cardiol. *62*:1186, 1988.
27. Fujimara, O., Yee, R., Klein, G. R. et al.: The diagnostic sensitivity of electrophysiologic testing in patients with syncope caused by transient bradycardia. N. Engl. J. Med. *321*:1703, 1989.
28. Feruglio, G. A., Rickards, A. F., Steinbach, K. et al.: Cardiac pacing in the world. A survey of the state of the art. PACE *10*:768, 1987.
29. Parsonnet, V., Bernstein, A. D., and Galasso, A. D.: Cardiac pacing practices in the United States, 1985. Am. J. Cardiol. *62*:71, 1988.
30. Furman, S: Venous cutdown for pacemaker implantation. Ann. Thorac. Surg. *41*:438, 1986.
31. Ong, L. S., Barold, S. S., Lederman, M. et al.: Cephalic vein guidewire technique for implantation of permanent pacemakers. Am. Heart J. *114*:753, 1987.
32. Furman, S: Subclavian puncture for pacemaker lead placement (editorial). PACE *9*:467, 1986.
33. Parsonnet, V., and Bernstein, A. D.: Pacing in perspective. Concepts and controversies. Circulation *73*:1087, 1986.
34. Parsonnet, V., Bernstein, A. D., and Lindsay, B.: Pacemaker implantation complication rates: An analysis of some contributing factors. J. Am. Coll. Cardiol. *13*:917, 1989.
35. Platia, E. V., and Brinker, J. A.: Time course of transvenous pacemaker stimulation impedance, capture threshold and electrogram amplitude. PACE *9*:620, 1986.
36. Montefoschi, N., and Boccadamo, R.: Propafenone-induced acute variation of chronic pacing threshold. A case report. PACE *13*:480, 1990.
37. Salel, A. F., Seagren, S. C., and Pool, P. E.: Effects of encainide on the function of implanted pacemakers. PACE *12*:1439, 1989.
38. Barold, S. S., Falkoff, M. D., Ong, L. S., and Heinle, R. A.: Hyperkalemia-induced failure of atrial capture during dual-chamber pacing. J. Am. Coll. Cardiol. *10*:467, 1987.
39. Bashour, T. T.: Spectrum of ventricular pacemaker exit block owing to hyperkalemia. Am. J. Cardiol. *57*:337, 1986.
40. Nagamoto, Y., Ogawa, T., Kumagae, H. et al.: Pacing failure due to markedly increased stimulation threshold 2 years after implantation: Successful management with oral prednisolone. A case report. PACE *12*:1034, 1989.
41. Furman, S.: Sensing and timing the cardiac electrogram. *In* Furman, S., Hayes, D. L., and Holmes, D. R., Jr. (eds.): 2nd ed. A Practice of Cardiac Pacing. Mt. Kisco, NY, Futura Publishing Co., 1989, p. 79.
42. Santini, M., Ansalone, G., Cacciatore, G., and Turitto, G.: Status of single chamber atrial pacing. *In* Barold, S. S., and Mugica, J. (eds.): New perspectives in Cardiac pacing. 2. Mt. Kisco, NY, Futura Publishing Co., 1991, p. 273.
43. Kruse, I. M., and Rydén, L.: Long-term follow-up of transvenous endocardial leads, PACE *10*:702, 1987.
44. Kerr, C. R., Tyers, F. O., and Vorderbrugge, S.: Atrial pacing: Safety and efficacy, PACE *12*:1049, 1989.
45. Lemke, B., Holtmann, B. F., Selbach, H., and Barmeyer, J.: The atrial pacemaker: Retrospective analysis of complications and life expectancy in patients with sinus node dysfunction. Int. J. Cardiol. *22*:185, 1989.
46. Brownlee, W. C., and Hirst, R. M.: Six years experience with atrial leads. PACE *9*:1239, 1986.
47. Emre, A., McAlister, H., Tuzcu, E. M., and Maloney, J. D.: Comparison of atrial leads: Importance of polarity and fixation mechanism. J. Interven. Cardiol. *2*:2, 1989.
48. Timmis, G. C.: The electrobiology and engineering of pacemaker leads. *In* Saksena, S., and Goldschlager, N. (eds.): Electrical Therapy for Cardiac Arrhythmias. Pacing. Antitachycardia Devices. Catheter Ablation. Philadelphia, W. B. Saunders Company, 1990, p. 35.
49. Mugica, J., Henry, L., Attuel, P. et al.: Clinical experience with 910 carbon tip leads. Comparison with polished platinum leads. PACE *9*:1230, 1986.
50. Djordjevic, M., Stojanov, P., and Velimirovic, D.: Target lead-low threshold electrode. PACE *9*:1206, 1986.
51. Radovsky, A. S., and VanVleet, J. F.: Effects of dexamethasone elution on tissue reaction around stimulating electrodes of endocardial pacing leads in dogs. Am. Heart J. *117*:1288, 1989.
52. Jones, B. R., Midei, M. G., and Brinker, J. A.: Does the long term performance of the target tip electrode justify reducing a pacemaker's nominal output? PACE *9*:299, 1986.
53. Klein, H. H., Steinberger, J., and Knake, W.: Stimulation characteristics of a steroid-eluting electrode compared with three conventional electrodes. PACE *13*:134, 1990.
54. Mond, H., Stokes, K., Helland, J. et al.: The porous titanium steroid eluting electrode: A double blind study assessing the stimulation threshold effects of steroid. PACE *11*:214, 1988.
55. Pirzada, F. A., Moschitto, L. J., Diorio, D.: Clinical experience with steroid-eluting unipolar electrodes. PACE *11*:1739, 1988.
56. Stokes, K., and Church, T.: The elimination of exit block as a pacing complication using transvenous steroid eluting lead. PACE *10*:748, 1987.

TYPES OF PACEMAKERS

57. Camm, A. J., and Katritsis, D.: Ventricular pacing for sick sinus syndrome. A risky business? PACE *13*:695, 1990.
58. Barold, S. S.: Clinical uses of chest wall stimulation in patients with DDD pulse generators. Intelligence Reports in Cardiac Pacing and Electrophysiology *7*:2, 1988.
59. Kleinfeld, M., Barold, S. S., and Rozanski, J. J.: Pacemaker alternans. A review. PACE *10*:924, 1987.
60. Barold, S. S., Falkoff, M. D., Ong, L. S., Heinle, R. A.: Electrocardiographic diagnosis of myocardial infarction during ventricular pacing. Cardiol. Clin. *5*:403, 1987.
61. Barold, S S., Falkoff, M. D., Ong, L. S., Heinle, R. A.: All dual-chamber pacemakers function in the DDD mode. Am. Heart J. *115*:1353, 1988.
62. Barold, S. S., Falkoff, M. D., Ong, L. S., and Heinle, R. A.: Timing cycles of DDD pacemakers. *In* Barold, S. S., and Mugica, J. (eds.): New Perspectives in Cardiac Pacing, Mt. Kisco, NY, Futura Publishing Co., 1988, p. 62.
63. Furman, S: Comprehension of pacemaker cycles. *In* Furman, S., Hayes, D. L., and Holmes, D. R., Jr. (eds.): A Practice of Cardiac Pacing. 2nd ed., Mt. Kisco, NY., Futura Publishing Co., 1989, p. 115.
64. Barold, S. S., and Belott, P.: Behavior of the ventricular triggering period of DDD pacemakers. PACE *10*:1237, 1987.
65. Barold, S. S., Falkoff, M. D., Ong, L. S., and Heinle, R. A.: Upper rate response of DDD pacemakers. *In* Barold, S. S., and Mugica, J. (eds.): New Perspectives in Cardiac Pacing. Mt. Kisco, NY, Futura Publishing Co., 1988, p. 121.
66. Barold, S. S.: The DDI mode of cardiac pacing. PACE *9*:480, 1987.
67. Sutton, R., Ingram, A., Kenny, R. A. et al.: Clinical experience of DDI pacing. *In* Belhassen, B., Feldman, S., and Copperman, Y. (eds.): Cardiac Pacing and Electrophysiology. Proceedings of the VIIIth World Symposium on Cardiac Pacing and Electrophysiology, Jerusalem, R & L Creative Communications, Ltd., 1987, p. 161.
68. Furman, S., and Gross, J.: Dual chamber pacing and pacemakers. Curr. Probl. Cardiol. *15*:119, 1990.
69. Barold, S. S., Falkoff, M. D., Ong, L. S., and Heinle, R. A.: Electrocardiography of contemporary DDD pacemakers. Basic concepts; upper rate response, retrograde ventriculoatrial conduction and differential diagnosis of pacemaker tachycardias. *In* Saksena, S., and Goldschlager, N. (eds.): Electrical Therapy for Cardiac Arrhythmias. Pacing, Antitachycardia Devices, Catheter Ablation. Philadelphia, W. B. Saunders Company, 1990, p. 225.
70. Barold, S. S., Falkoff, M. D., Ong, L. S., and Heinle, R. A.: Termination of ventricular tachycardia by chest wall stimulation during DDD pacing. Am. J. Med. *84*:549, 1988.
71. Barold, S. S., Falkoff, M. D., Ong, L. S., and Heinle, R. A.: Magnet unresponsive pacemaker endless loop tachycardia. Am. Heart J. *116*:726, 1988.
72. Barold, S. S.: Management of patients with dual chamber pacemakers. Central role of the atrial refractory period. American College of Cardiology Learning Center Highlights *5*:8, 1990.
73. Klementowicz, P. T., and Furman, S: Selective atrial sensing in dual chamber pacemakers eliminates endless loop tachycardia. J. Am. Coll. Cardiol. *7*:590, 1986.
74. Pless, P., Simonsen, E., Arnsbo, P., and Fabricius, J.: Superiority of multiprogrammable VVI pacing. A comparative study with special reference to management of pacing systems malfunctions. PACE *9*:739, 1986.
75. Barold, S. S., Falkoff, M. D., Ong, L. S., and Heinle, R. A.: Electrocardiography of contemporary DDD pacemakers. Multiprogrammability, follow-up, and troubleshooting. *In* Saksena, S., and Goldschlager, N. (eds.):

Electrical Therapy for Cardiac Arrhythmias, Pacing, Antitachycardia Devices, Catheter Ablation. Philadelphia, W. B. Saunders Company, 1990, p. 265.

76. Grines, C. L., Bashore, T. M., Boudoulas, H. et al.: Functional abnormalities in isolated left bundle branch block. The effect of interventricular asynchrony. Circulation *79*:845, 1989.
77. Alt, E. U., vonBibra, H., and Blömer, H.: Different benefit AV intervals with DDD pacing after sensed and paced atrial events. J. Electrophysiol. *1*:250, 1987.
78. Ritter, P., Daubert, C., and Mabo, P.: Haemodynamic benefit of a rate adapted A-V delay in dual chamber pacing, Eur. Heart J. *10*:637, 1989.
79. Iwase, M., Sotobatta, I., Yokota, M. et al.: Evaluation of pulsed Doppler echocardiography of the atrial contribution to left ventricular filling in patients with DDD pacemakers. Am. J. Cardiol. *58*:104, 1986.
80. Janosik, D. L., Pearson, A. C., Buckingham, T. A. et al.: The hemodynamic benefit of differential atrioventricular delay intervals for sensed and paced atrial events during physiological pacing. J. Am. Coll. Cardiol. *14*:499, 1989.
81. Wish, M., Gottdiener, J. S., Cohen, A. I., and Fletcher, R. D.: M-mode echocardiograms for determination of optimal left atrial timing in patients with dual chamber pacemakers. J. Am. Coll. Cardiol. *11*:317, 1988.

HEMODYNAMICS OF CARDIAC PACING

82. Rydén, L., Karlsson, O., and Kristensson, B. E.: The importance of different atrioventricular intervals for exercise capacity. PACE *11*:1051, 1988.
83. Mehta, D., Gilmour, S., Ward, D., and Camm, A. J.: Optimal atrioventricular delay at rest and during exercise in patients with dual chamber pacemakers: A noninvasive assessment by continuous wave Doppler. Br. Heart J. *61*:161, 1989.
84. Kristensson, B. E., Kruse, I., Nordlander, R., and Rydén, L.: Hemodynamics of cardiac pacing. *In* Barold, S. S., and Mugica, J. (eds.): Mt. Kisco, NY, Futura Publishing Co., 1991, p. 75.
85. Nordlander, R., Hedman, A., and Pehrsson, S. K.: Rate responsive pacing and exercise capacity. PACE *12*:749, 1989.
86. Benditt, D. G., Mianulli, M., Fetter, J. et al: Single chamber cardiac pacing with activity-initiated chronotropic response: Evaluation by cardiopulmonary exercise testing. Circulation *75*:184, 1987.
87. Rediker, D. E., Eagle, K. A., Homma, S. et al.: Clinical and hemodynamic comparison of VVI versus DDD pacing in patients with DDD pacemakers. Am. J. Cardiol. *61*:323, 1988.
88. Mitsuoka, T., Kenny, R. A., Yeung, T. A. et al.: Benefits of dual chamber pacing in sick sinus syndrome. Br. Heart J. *60*:338, 1988.
89. Tyers, G. F.: Current status of sensor-modulated rate-adaptive cardiac pacing. J. Am. Coll. Cardiol. *15*:412, 1990.
90. Sedney, M. I., Weijers, E. VanDerWall, E. E. et al.: Short-term and long-term changes of left ventricular volumes during rate-adaptive and single-rate pacing. PACE *12*:1863, 1989.
91. Parsonnet, V., Myers, M., and Perry, G. Y.: Paradoxical paroxysmal nocturnal congestive heart failure as a severe manifestation of the pacemaker syndrome. Am. J. Cardiol. *65*:683, 1990.
92. Stewart, W. J., Dicola, V. C., Harthorne, J. W. et al.: Doppler ultra-sound measurement of cardiac output in patients with physiological pacemakers. Effect of left ventricular function and retrograde ventriculoatrial conduction. Am. J. Cardiol. *54*:308, 1984.
93. Faerestrand, S., Ole, B., and Ohm, O. J.: Noninvasive assessment by Doppler and M-mode echocardiography of hemodynamic responses to temporary pacing and to ventriculoatrial conduction. PACE *10*:871, 1987.
94. Noll, B., Irappe, J., Goke, B., and Maisch, B.: Influence of pacing mode and rate on peripheral levels of atrial natriuretic peptide. PACE *12*:1763, 1989.
95. Toivonen, L. K., and Pohjola-Sintonen, S.: Vasodilator therapy-induced pacemaker syndrome. Chest *91*:919, 1987.
96. Liebert, H. P., O'Donoghue, S., Tullner, W. F., and Platia, E. V.: Pacemaker syndrome in activity-response VVI pacing. Am. J. Cardiol. *64*:124, 1989.
97. Daubert, C., Mabo, P. H., Pouillot, C. H., and Lelong, B.: Atrial chronotropic incompetence. Implications for DDDR pacing. *In* Barold, S. S., and Mugica, J. (eds.): New Perspectives in Cardiac Pacing 2. Mt. Kisco, NY, Futura Publishing Co., 1991, p. 251.
98. Rosenqvist, M.: Atrial pacing for sick sinus syndrome. Clin. Cardiol. *13*:43, 1990.
99. Fearnot, N. E., Smith, H. J., and Geddes, L. A.: A review of pacemakers that physiologically increase rate: The DDD and rate-responsive pacemakers. Prog. Cardiovasc. Dis. *29*:145, 1986.
100. Benditt, D. G., Milstein, S., Buetikofer, J. et al.: Sensor-triggered, rate-variable cardiac pacing. Current technologies and clinical implications. Ann. Intern. Med. *107*:714, 1987.
101. Maloney, J. D., Vaneiro, G., and Pashkow, F. J.: Single chamber rate modulated pacing AAIR-VVIR. Follow-up and complications. *In* Barold, S. S., and Mugica, J. (eds.): New Perspectives in Cardiac Pacing 2. Mt. Kisco, NY, Futura Publishing Co., 1991, p. 429.
102. Bloomfield, P., MacAreavey, D., Kerr, F., and Fananapazir, L.: Long-term follow-up of patients with the QT rate-adaptive pacemaker. PACE *12*:111, 1989.
103. Hedman, A., and Nordlander, R.: QT sensing rate responsive pacing compared to fixed rate ventricular inhibited pacing. A controlled clinical study. PACE *12*:374, 1989.
104. Faerestrand, S., Breivik, K., and Ohm, O. J.: Assessment of the work capacity and relationships between rate response and exercise tolerance associated with activity-sensing rate-responsive ventricular pacing. PACE *10*:1277, 1987.
105. Lipkin, D. P., Buller, N., Frenneaux, M. et al.: Randomised crossover trial of rate-responsive Activitrax and conventional fixed-rate ventricular pacing. Br. Heart J. *58*:613, 1987.
106. denDulk, K., Bouwels, L., Lindemans, F. et al.: The Activitrax rate responsive pacemaker system. Am. J. Cardiol. *61*:107, 1988.
107. Rossi, P., Prando, M. D., Magnani, A. et al.: Physiological sensitivity of respiratory dependent cardiac pacing: Four-year follow-up. PACE *11*:1267, 1988.
108. Lau, C. P., Ward, D. E., and Camm, A.: Rate-responsive pacing with a pacemaker that detects respiratory rate (Biorate). Clinical advantages and complications. Clin. Cardiol. *11*:318, 1988.
109. Lau, C. P., Antoniou, A., Ward, D. E., and Camm, A. J.: Initial clinical experience with a minute-ventilation sensing rate modulated pacemaker. Improvement in exercise capacity and symptomatology. PACE *11*:1815, 1988.
110. Mond, H., Strathmore, N., Kertes, P. et al.: Rate-responsive pacing using a minute ventilation sensor. PACE *11*:1866, 1988.
111. Alt, E., Hirgstetter, C., Heinz, M., and Blömer, H.: Rate control of physiologic pacemakers by central venous blood temperature. Circulation *73*:1206, 1986.
112. Platia, E. V., Waclawski, S., Fearnot, N., and the Kelvin 500 investigators: A temperature based, rate-responsive permanent pacing system: Temperature curves during exercise. *In* Belhassen, B., Feldman, S., and Copperman, Y. (eds.): Cardiac Pacing and Electrophysiology. Proceedings of the VIIIth World Symposium on Cardiac Pacing and Electrophysiology. Jerusalem, Israel, Keterpress Enterprises, 1987, p. 91.
113. Fearnot, N. E., Smith, H. J., Sellers, D., and Boal, B.: Evaluation of the temperature response to exercise testing in patients with single chamber, rate adaptive pacemakers. A multicenter study. PACE *12*:1806, 1989.
114. Mond, H. G.: Rate responsive cardiac pacing. A perspective. PACE *12*:1309, 1989.
115. Alt, E., Theres, H., Heinz, M. et al.: A new rate-modulated pacemaker optimized by combination of two sensors. PACE *11*:1119, 1988.
116. Paul, V., Garratt, C., and Camm, A. J.: Combination of sensors to provide optimal pacing rate response. Clin. Cardiol. *12*:400, 1989.
117. Moreira, L. F. P., Costa, R., Stolf, N. A. G., and Jatene, A. D.: Pacing rate increase as cause of syncope in a patient with severe cardiomyopathy. PACE *12*:1027, 1989.
118. Pouillot, C. H., Mabo, P. H., Lelong, B. et al.: Bénéfices et limites de la stimulation mono-chambre atriale à fréquence asservie. Arch. Mal. Coeur (*in press*).
119. DenDulk, K., Lindemans, F. W., Brugada, P. et al.: Pacemaker syndrome with AAI rate variable pacing: Importance of atrioventricular conduction properties, medication, and pacemaker programmability. PACE *11*:1226, 1988.
120. VanHemel, N. M., Hamerlijnck, R. P. H. M., Pronk, K. J., and VanDerVeen, E. P.: Upper limit ventricular stimulation in respiratory rate responsive pacing due to electrocautery. PACE *12*:1720, 1989.

SELECTION OF PACING MODE

121. Denjoy, I., Leclerq, J. F., Druelles, P. et al.: Comparative efficacy of permanent atrial pacing in vagal atrial arrhythmias and in bradycardia-tachycardia syndrome. PACE *12*:1236, 1989.
122. Langenfeld, H., Grimm, W., Maisch, B., and Kochsiek, K.: Atrial fibrillation and embolic complications in paced patients PACE *11*:1667, 1988.
123. Ebagosti, A., Gueunoun, M., Saadjian, A. et al.: Long term followup of patients with VVI pacing with special reference to VA retrograde conduction. PACE *11*:679, 1988.
124. Bianconi, L., Boccadamo, R., DiFlorio, A. et al.: Atrial versus ventricular stimulation in sick sinus syndrome. Effects on morbidity and mortality. PACE *12*:1236, 1989.
125. Rosenqvist, M., Brandt, J., and Schüller, H.: Long-term pacing in sinus node disease. Effects of stimulation mode on cardiovascular morbidity and mortality. Am. Heart J. *116*:16, 1988.
126. Sutton, R., and Kenny, R. A.: The natural history of sinus node disease. PACE *9*:1110, 1986.
127. Santini, M., Alexidou, G., Ansalone, G. et al.: Relation of prognosis in sick sinus syndrome to age, conduction defects and modes of permanent cardiac pacing. Am. J. Cardiol. *65*:729, 1990.
128. Sasaki, Y., Shimotori, M., Akahane, K. et al.: Long-term follow-up of patients with sick sinus syndrome: A comparison of clinical aspects among unpaced, ventricular inhibited paced and physiologically paced groups. PACE *11*:1575, 1988.
129. Feuer, J. M., Shandling, A. H., and Messenger, J. C.: Influence of cardiac pacing mode on long-term development of atrial fibrillation. Am. J. Cardiol. *64*:1376, 1989.
130. Alpert, M. A., Curtis, J. J., Sanfelippo, J. F. et al.: Comparative survival following permanent ventricular and dual chamber pacing for patients with chronic symptomatic sinus node dysfunction with and without congestive heart failure. Am. Heart J. *113*:958, 1987.
131. Rydén, L.: Atrial inhibited pacing—An underused mode of cardiac stimulation. PACE *11*:1375, 1988.
132. Rosenqvist, M., and Obel, I. P. W.: Atrial pacing and the risk for AV block. Time for a change in attitude? PACE *12*:97, 1989.
133. Kallryd, A., Kruse, I., and Rydén, L.: Atrial-inhibited pacing in the sick

sinus syndrome: Clinical value and the demand for rate responsiveness. PACE 12:954, 1989.
134. Johnston, F. A., Robinson, J. R., and Fyfe, T.: Exercise testing in the diagnosis of sick sinus syndrome in the elderly: Implication for treatment. PACE 10:831, 1987.
135. Brandt, J., Fåhraeus, T., and Schüller, H.: Rate adaptive atrial pacing (AAIR). Clinical aspects. In Barold, S. S., and Mugica, J. (eds.): New Perspectives in Cardiac Pacing. 2. Mt. Kisco, NY, Futura Publishing Co., 1991, p. 303.
136. Rogononi, G., Bolognese, L., Aina, F. et al.: Respiratory depend atrial pacing. Management of sinus node disease. PACE 11:1853, 1988.
137. Sutton, R.: DDDR pacing. PACE 13:385, 1990.
138. Landzberg, J. S., Franklin, J. O., Mahawar, S. K. et al.: Benefits of physiologic atrioventricular synchronization for pacing with an exercise rate response. Am. J. Cardiol. 66:193, 1990.
139. Griffin, J. C.: The optimal pacing mode for the individual patient: The role of DDDR. In Barold, S. S., and Mugica, J. (eds.): New Perspectives in Cardiac Pacing. 2. Mt. Kisco, NY., Futura Publishing Co., 1991, p. 325.
140. Cornacchia, D., Fabbri, M., Maresta, A. et al.: Clinical evaluation of VDD pacing with a unipolar single-pass lead. PACE 12:604, 1989.
141. Varriale, P., Pilla, A. G., and Tekriwal, M.: Single-lead VDD pacing system. PACE 13:757, 1990.
142. Longo, E., and Catrini, V.: Experience and implantation techniques with a new single-pass lead VDD pacing system. PACE 13:927, 1990.

COMPLICATIONS OF PACEMAKERS

143. Antonelli, D., Turgeman, Y., Kaveh, Z. et al.: Short-term thrombosis after transvenous permanent pacemaker insertion. PACE 12:280, 1989.
144. Spittell, P. C., Vliestra, R. E., Hayes, D. L., and Higano, S. T.: Venous obstruction due to permanent transvenous pacemaker electrodes. Treatment with percutaneous transluminal balloon venoplasty. PACE 13:271, 1990.
145. Blackburn, T., and Dunn, M.: Pacemaker-induced superior vena cava syndrome. Consideration of management. Am. Heart J. 116:893, 1988.
146. Lal, R. B., and Avery, R. D.: Aggressive pacemaker twiddler's syndrome. Dislodgement of an active fixation ventricular pacing electrode. Chest 97:756, 1990.
147. Wade, J. S., and Cobbs, C. G.: Infections in cardiac pacemakers. Curr. Clin. Top. Infect. Dis. 9:44, 1988.
148. Mickley, H., Andersen, C., and Nielsen, L. H.: Runaway pacemaker: A still existing complication and therapeutic guidelines. Clin. Cardiol. 12:412, 1989.
149. Barold, S. S., Falkoff, M. D., Ong., L. S., and Heinle, R. A.: Arrhythmias related to the sensing function of VVI pacemakers. Prac. Cardi. 12:115, 1986.
150. Barold, S. S., Falkoff, M. D., Ong, L. S., and Heinle, R. A.: Interference in cardiac pacemakers. Endogenous sources. Myopotentials. In El-Sherif, N., and Samet, P. (eds.): Cardiac Pacing and Electrophysiology. (3rd ed.) Philadelphia, W. B. Saunders Company, 1991, p. 634.
151. Lau, C. P., Linker, N. J., Butrous, G. S. et al.: Myopotential interference in unipolar rate responsive pacemakers. PACE 12:1324, 1989.
152. Barold, S S., Falkoff, M. D., Ong, L. S., and Heinle, R. A.: Interference in Cardiac Pacemakers. Exogenous sources. In El-Sherif, N., and Samet, P. (eds.): Cardiac Pacing and Electrophysiology. (3rd ed.). Philadelphia, W. B. Saunders Company, 1991, p. 608.
153. Sanders, R., and Barold, S. S.: Understanding elective replacement indicators and automatic parameter conversion mechanisms in DDD pacemakers. In Barold, S. S., Mugica, J. (eds.): New Perspectives in Cardiac Pacing. Mt. Kisco, NY, Futura Publishing Co., 1988, p. 203.
154. Chin, M. C., Rosenqvist, M., Lee, M. A. et al.: The effect of radiofrequency catheter ablation in permanent pacemakers. An experimental study. PACE 13:23. 1990.
155. Lee, R. W., Huang, S. K., Mechling, E., and Bazgan, L.: Runaway atrioventricular sequential pacemaker after radiation therapy. Am. J. Med. 81:833, 1986.
156. Hayes, D. L., Holmes, D. R., Jr., and Gray, J. E.: Effect of 1.5 Tesla nuclear magnetic resonance imaging scanner on implanted permanent pacemakers. J. Am. Coll. Cardiol. 10:782, 1987.
157. Griffin, J. C., Schunemeyer, T. D., Hess, K. R. et al.: Pacemaker follow-up: Its role in the detection and correction of pacemaker system malfunction. PACE 9:387, 1986.
158. Levine, P. A.: Magnet rates and recommended replacement time indicators of lithium pacemakers 1986. Clin. Prog. Electrophysiol. Pacing 4:608, 1986.
159. Barold, S. S., and Schoenfeld, M. H.: Pacemaker elective replacement indicators. PACE 12:990, 1989.
160. Schüller, H., Brandt, J., and Fåhraeus, T.: Determination of atrial depolarization during dual-chamber pacing. In Barold, S S., and Mugica, J. (eds.): New Perspectives in Cardiac Pacing, Mt. Kisco, NY, Futura Publishing Co., 1988, p. 319.
161. Byrd, C. L., Schwartz, S. J., Gonzales, M. et al.: DDD pacemakers maximize hemodynamic benefits and minimize complications for most patients. PACE 11:1911, 1988.
162. Janosik, D. L., Redd, R. M., Buckingham, T. A. et al.: Utility of ambulatory electrocardiography in detecting pacemaker dysfunction in the early post-implantation period. Am. J. Cardiol. 60:1030, 1987.

ELECTRICAL DEVICES TO TREAT TACHYCARDIAS

163. Eldar, M., Griffin, J. C., Abbott, J. A. et al: Permanent cardiac pacing in patients with the long QT syndrome. J. Am. Coll. Cardiol. 10:600, 1987.
164. Fisher, J. D., Teichman, S., Ferrick, A. et al.: Antiarrhythmic effects of VVI pacing at physiologic rates: A crossover controlled evaluation. PACE 10:822, 1987.
165. Attuel, P., Pellerin, D., Mugica, J., and Coumel, P. H.: DDD pacing: An effective treatment modality for recurrent atrial arrhythmias. PACE 11:1647, 1988.
166. Davies, C. W., Butrous, G. S., Spurrell, R. A. J., and Camm, A. J.: Pacing techniques in the prophylaxis of junctional reentry tachycardia. PACE 10:519, 1987.
167. Moreira, D. A., Shepard, R. B., and Waldo, A. L.: Chronic rapid atrial pacing to maintain atrial fibrillation: Use to permit control of ventricular rate in order to treat tachycardia induced cardiomyopathy. PACE 12:761, 1989.
168. Shandling, A. H., Li, C. K., and Thomas, L.: Sustained effectiveness of an atrial antitachycardia pacemaker during follow-up. PACE 13:833, 1990.
169. DenDulk, K., Brugada, P., Smeets, J. L. R. M., and Wellens, H. J. J.: Long-term antitachycardia pacing experience for supraventricular tachycardia. PACE 13:1020, 1990.
170. Fisher, J. D.: Clinical results with antitachycardia pacemakers. In Saksena, S., and Goldschlager, N. (eds.): Electrical Therapy for Cardiac Arrhythmias, Pacing, Antitachycardia Devices. Catheter Ablation, Philadelphia, W. B. Saunders, 1990, p. 525.
171. Falkoff, M. D., Barold, S. S., Goodfriend, M. A. et al.: Long-term management of ventricular tachycardia by implantable automatic burst tachycardia-terminating pacemakers. PACE 9:885, 1986.
172. Occhetta, E., Bolognese, L., Magnani, A. et al.: Clinical experience with Orthocor II antitachycardia pacing system for recurrent tachyarrhythmia termination. J. Electrophysiol. 3:289, 1989.
173. Moller, M., Simonsen, E., Arnsbo, P. I., Oxho, H.: Long-term follow-up of patients treated with automatic scanning antitachycardia pacemaker. PACE 12:425, 1989.
174. Schnittger, I., Lee, J. T., Hargis, J. et al.: Long-term results of antitachycardia pacing in patients with supraventricular tachycardia. PACE 12:936, 1989.
175. Fromer, M., Gloor, H., Kus, T., and Shenesa, M.: Clinical experience with a new software-based antitachycardia pacemaker for recurrent supraventricular and ventricular tachycardias. PACE 13:890, 1990.
176. Saksena, S., Pantopoulos, D., Parsonnet, V. et al.: Usefulness of an implantable antitachycardia pacemaker system for supraventricular or ventricular tachycardia. Am. J. Cardiol. 58:70, 1986.
177. Griffin, J. C., and Sweeney, M.: The management of paroxysmal tachycardias using the Cybertach-60. PACE 7:1291, 1987.
178. Palakurthy, P. R., and Slater, D.: Automatic implantable scanning burst pacemakers for recurrent tachyarrhythmias. PACE 11:185, 1988.
179. Kappenberger, L., Valin, H., and Sowton, E: Multicenter long-term results of antitachycardia pacing for supraventricular tachycardias. Am. J. Cardiol. 64:191, 1989.
180. Zipes, D. P.: Electrical treatment of tachycardia. Circulation 75 (Suppl. III):190, 1987.
181. Duffin, E., and Zipes, D. P.: Chronic electrical control of tachyarrhythmias, In Mandel, W. J. (ed.): Cardiac Arrhythmias: Their mechanism, diagnosis, and management. Philadelphia, J. B. Lippincott Co., 1987, p. 764.
182. Fisher, J. D., Kim, S. G., and Mercando, A. D.: Electrical devices for the treatment of arrhythmias. Am. J. Cardiol., 61:45A, 1988.
183. Newman, D. M., Lee, M. A., Herre, J. M. et al.: Permanent antitachycardia pacemaker therapy for ventricular tachycardia. PACE 12:1387, 1989.
184. Barold, S. S., Wyndham, C. R., Kappenberger, L. et al.: Implanted atrial pacemakers for paroxysmal atrial flutter. Long-term efficacy. Ann. Intern. Med. 107:44, 1987.
185. DeBelder, M. A., Malik, M., Ward, D. E., and Camm, A. J.: Pacing modalities for tachycardia termination. PACE 13:231, 1990.
186. Holley, L. K,. Cooper, M., Uther, J. B. , and Ross, D. A.: Safety and efficacy of pacing for ventricular tachycardia. PACE 9(II):1316, 1986.
187. Lau, C. P., Cornu, E., and Camm, A. J.: Fatal and nonfatal cardiac arrest in patients with an implanted antitachycardia device for the treatment of supraventricular tachycardia. Am. J. Cardiol. 61:919, 1988.
188. Waldecker, B., Brugada, P., Zehender, M. et al.: Importance of modes of electrical termination of ventricular tachycardia for the selection of implantable antitachycardia devices. Am. J. Cardiol 57:150, 1986.
189. Rosenthal, M. E., Marchlinski, F. E., and Josephson, M. E.: Complications of implantable antitachycardia devices. Diagnosis and management. In Saksena, S, and Goldschlager, N. (eds.): Electrical Therapy for Cardiac Arrhythmias. Pacing. Antitachycardia Devices. Catheter Ablation. Philadelphia, W. B. Saunders Company, 1990, p. 574.
190. Charos, G. S., Haffajee, C. I., Gold, R. L. et al.: A theoretically and practically more effective method for interruption of ventricular tachycardias: Self-adapting autodecremental overdrive pacing. Circulation 73:309, 1986.
191. denDulk, K., Bertholet, M., Brugada, P. et al.: A versatile pacemaker system for termination of tachycardias. Am. J. Cardiol. 57:950, 1986.
192. denDulk, K., Kersschot, I. E., Brugada, P., Wellens, H. J. J.: Is there a universal antitachycardia pacing mode? Am. J. Cardiol. 57:950, 1986.
193. deBelder, M. A., and Camm, A. J.: Devices for tachycardia termination. Am. J. Cardiol. 64:70J, 1989.

194. Pannizzo, F., Mercando, A. D., Fisher, J. D., and Furman, S.: Automatic methods for detection of tachyarrhythmias by antitachycardia devices. J. Am. Coll. Cardiol. *11*:308, 1988.
195. Camm, A. J., Davies, D. W., and Ward, D. E.: Tachycardia recognition by implantable electronic devices. PACE *10*:1175, 1987.
196. Li, C. K., Shandling, A. H., Norasco, M. et al.: Atrial automatic tachycardia-reversion pacemakers: Their economic viability and impact on quality-of-life. PACE *13*:639, 1990.
197. Manz, M., Gerckens, U., Funke, H. D. et al.: Combination of antitachycardia pacemaker and automatic implantable cardioverter/defibrillator for ventricular tachycardia. PACE *9*:676, 1986.
198. Luderitz, B., and Manz, M.: Role of antitachycardia devices in the treatment of ventricular tachyarrhythmias. Am. J. Cardiol. *64*:75J, 1989.
199. Greve, H., Koch, T., Gulker, H., and Heuer, H.: Termination of malignant ventricular tachycardias by use of an automatic defibrillator (AICD) in combination with an antitachycardia pacemaker. PACE *11*:2040, 1988.
200. DeBelder, M. A., and Camm, A. J.: Implantable cardioverter/defibrillators (ICDs) 1989. How close are we to ideal device? Clin. Cardiol. *12*:339, 1989.
201. Brooks, R., Garan, H., McGovern, B. A., and Ruskin, J. N.: The automatic implantable cardioverter/defibrillator. *In* Braunwald E. (ed.): Heart Disease: A Textbook of Cardiovascular Medicine, 3rd ed. Philadelphia, W. B. Saunders Company, Update No. 9, p. 193, 1990.
202. Winkle, R. A., and Cannom, D. S.: The automatic implantable cardioverter/defibrillator: Current applications and future directions. *In* Barold, S. S., and Mugica, J. (eds.): New Perspectives in Cardiac Pacing. 2. Mt. Kisco, NY, Futura Publishing Co., 1991, p. 405.
203. Troup, P. J.: Implantable cardioverters and defibrillators. Curr. Probl. Cardiol. *14*:679, 1989.
204. Waldecker, B., Brugada, P., Zehender, M. et al.: Dysrhythmias after direct-current cardioversion. Am. J. Cardiol. *57*:120, 1986.
205. Cohen, T. J., and Liem, L. D.: A hemodynamic responsive antitachycardia system: Development and basis for design in humans. Circulation *82*:394, 1990.
206. Thurer, R. J., Luceri, R. M., and Bolooki, H.: Automatic implantable cardioverter-defibrillator: Techniques of implantation and results. Ann. Thorac. Surg. *42*:143, 1986.
207. Saksena, S., and Parsonnet, V.: Implantation of a cardioverter-defibrillator without thoracotomy using a triple electrode system. JAMA, *259*:69, 1988.
208. Saksena, S., Tullo, N. G., Kroll, R. B., and Mauro, A. M.: Initial clinical experience with endocardial defibrillation using an implantable cardioverter-defibrillator with a triple-electrode system. Arch. Intern. Med. *149*:2333, 1989.
209. Mirowski, M., and Mower, M. M.: Transvenous catheter defibrillation for prevention of sudden cardiac death. J. Am. Coll. Cardiol. *11*:371, 1988.
210. Cannom, D. S., and Winkle, R. A.: Implantation of the automatic implantable cardioverter defibrillator (AICD): Practical aspects. PACE *9*:793, 1986.
211. Marchlinski, F. E., Flores, B., Miller, J. M. et al.: Relation of the intraoperative defibrillation threshold to successful postoperative defibrillation with an automatic implantable cardioverter-defibrillator. Am. J. Cardiol. *62*:393, 1988.
212. Fain, E. S., Lee, J. T., and Winkle, R. A.: Effect of acute intravenous and chronic oral amiodarone on defibrillation energy requirements. Am. Heart J. *114*:8, 1987.
213. Singer, I., Guanieri, T., and Kupersmith, J.: Implanted automatic defibrillators: Effects of drugs and pacemakers. PACE *11*:2250, 1988.
214. Guarnieri, T., Levine, J. H., Veltri, E. P. et al.: Success of chronic defibrillation and the role of antiarrhythmic drugs with the automatic implantable cardioverter-defibrillator. Am. J. Cardiol. *60*:1061, 1987.
215. Marinchak, R. A., Friehling, T. D., Kline, R. A. et al.: Effect of antiarrhythmic drugs on defibrillation threshold: Case report of an adverse effect of mexiletine and review of the literature. PACE *11*:7, 1988.
216. Haberman, R. J., Veltri, E. P., and Mowrer, M. M.: The effect of amiodarone on defibrillation threshold. J. Electrophysiol. *2*:415, 1988.
217. Goodman, L. R., Almassi, G. H., Troup, P. J. et al.: Complications of automatic implantable cardioverter-defibrillators: Radiographic, CT, and echocardiographic evaluation. Radiology *170*:447, 1989.
218. Kelly, P. A., Wallace, S., Tucker, B. et al.: Postoperative infection with the automatic implantable cardioverter-defibrillator: Clinical presentation and use of the gallium scan in diagnosis. PACE *11*:1220, 1988.
219. Marchlinski, F. E., Flores, B. T., Buxton, A. E. et al.: The automatic implantable cardioverter-defibrillator: Efficacy, complications, and device failures. Ann. Intern. Med. *104*:481, 1986.
220. Winkle, R. A., Mead, R. H., Rucer, M. A. et al.: Long-term outcome with the automatic implantable cardioverter-defibrillator. J. Am. Coll. Cardiol. *13*:1353, 1989.
221. Kelly, P. A., Cannom, D. S., Garan, H. et al.: The automatic implantable cardioverter-defibrillator: Efficacy, complications and survival in patients with malignant ventricular arrhythmias. J. Am. Coll. Cardiol. *11*:1278, 1988.
222. Fricchione, G. L., Olson, L. C., and Vlay, S. C.: Psychiatric syndromes in patients with the automatic internal cardioverter defibrillator: Anxiety, psychological dependence, abuse, and withdrawal. Am. Heart J. *117*:1411, 1989.
223. Tchou, P. J., Piasecki, E., Gutmann, M. et al.: Psychological support and psychiatric management of patients with automatic implantable cardioverter defibrillator. Int. J. Psychiatry *19*:393, 1989.
224. Kelly, P. A., Cannom, D. S., Garan, H. et al.: Predictors of automatic implantable cardioverter-defibrillator discharge for life-threatening ventricular arrhythmias. Am. J. Cardiol. *62*:83, 1988.
225. Kay, G. N., Vance, J. P., Dailey, S. M., and Epstein, A. E.: Current role of the automatic implantable cardioverter-defibrillator in the treatment of life-threatening ventricular arrhythmias. Am. J. Med. *88*:25N, 1990.
226. Fogoros, R. M., Fiedler, S. B., and Elson, J. J.: The automatic implantable cardioverter-defibrillator in drug-refractory ventricular tachyarrhythmias. Ann. Intern. Med. *107*:635, 1987.
227. Manolis, A. S., Rastegar, H., and Estes, N. A. M., III: Automatic implantable cardioverter defibrillator. Current status. J. A. M. A. *262*:1362, 1989.
228. Tchou, P. J., Kadri, N., Anderson, J. et al.: Automatic implantable cardioverter defibrillators and survival of patients with left ventricular dysfunction and malignant ventricular arrhythmias. Ann. Intern. Med. *109*:529, 1988.
229. Luceri, R. M., Habal, S. M., Castellanos, A. et al.: Mechanism of death in patients with the automatic implantable cardioverter defibrillator. PACE *11*:2015, 1988.
230. Gabry, M. D., Brodman, R., Johnston, D. et al.: Automatic implantable cardioverter defibrillators: Patient survival, battery longevity and shock delivery analysis. J. Am. Coll. Cardiol. *9*:1349, 1987.
231. Furman, S.: Implantable cardioverter defibrillator statistics. PACE *13*:1, 1990.
232. Furman, S.: AICD benefit. PACE *12*:399, 1989.
233. Fogoros, R. M., Elson, J. J., Bonnet, C. A. et al.: Efficacy of the automatic implantable cardioverter defibrillator in prolonging survival in patients with severe underlying cardiac disease. J. Am. Coll. Cardiol. *16*:381, 1990.
234. Fisher, J. D., Brodman, R. F., Kim, S. G. et al.: VT/VF: 6/60 Protection. PACE *13*:218, 1990.
235. Gross, J., Zilo, P., Ferrick, K. J. et al.: Sudden death mortality in AICD patients. Nice, France, RBM, Cardiostim 90, *12*:114, 1990.

26

Cardiac Arrest and Sudden Cardiac Death

by ROBERT J. MYERBURG, M.D., and AGUSTIN CASTELLANOS, M.D.

DEFINITION

Sudden cardiac death (SCD) is natural death due to cardiac causes, heralded by abrupt loss of consciousness within 1 hour of the onset of acute symptoms, in a person with or without known preexisting heart disease, but in whom the time and mode of death are unexpected. This definition reflects a view of the event which incorporates the key elements of "natural," "rapid," and "unexpected." It has been derived from definitions in the literature in the past,[1-20] which have conflicted, largely because the most useful operational definition of SCD differs for the clinician, the cardiovascular epidemiologist, the pathologist, and the scientist attempting to define pathophysiological mechanisms.

Four elements must be considered in the construction of a definition of SCD to satisfy medical, scientific, legal, and social disciplines: (1) prodromes, (2) onset, (3) cardiac arrest, and (4) biological death (Fig. 26–1). Because the proximate cause of SCD is a disturbance of cardiovascular function, which is incompatible with maintaining consciousness because of abrupt loss of cerebral blood flow, any definition must include the concept that a brief time interval exists between the onset of the mechanism directly responsible for cardiac arrest and the consequent loss of consciousness (Fig. 26–1*C*). The 1-hour definition, however, refers to the duration of the "terminal event" (Fig. 26–1*B*), which is the interval between the onset of symptoms signaling the presence of a pathophysiological disturbance which will lead to the cardiac arrest and the onset of the cardiac arrest itself (Fig. 26–1*B* and *C*).

Premonitory signs and symptoms, which may occur during a period of weeks before a cardiac arrest,[17] tend to be nonspecific for the impending event.[8] *Prodromes* (Fig. 26–1*A*) which may be specific for an imminent cardiac arrest are relatively abrupt changes that begin during an arbitrarily defined period of up to 24 hours before the cardiac arrest.[4,21] The fourth element, *biological death* (Fig. 26–1*D*), is not necessarily an immediate consequence of the clinical event, cardiac arrest. The latter point has been highlighted since the development of community-based intervention systems, in that patients may now remain biologically alive for a long period of time after the onset of a pathophysiological process which has caused irreversible damage and will ultimately lead to death.[18-20,22] In this circumstance, the causative pathophysiological and clinical event is the cardiac arrest itself, rather than the factors responsible for the delayed biological death. However, in legal, forensic, and certain social circumstances, biological death must continue to be used as the most relevant event. Finally, the pathologist and the epidemiologist studying *unwitnessed deaths* may use the definition of sudden death for a person known to be alive and functioning normally 24 hours before,[4] and this remains appropriate within its obvious limits because unwitnessed death cannot be ignored in their studies.[23] Thus the generally accepted clinical-pathophysiological definition of up to 1 hour between onset of the terminal event and biological death requires qualifications for specific circumstances and uses.

The development of community-based intervention systems also has led to inconsistencies in the use of terms considered absolute. *Death* is defined biologically, legally, and literally as an absolute and irreversible event. Thus SCD may be aborted, or a patient may survive cardiac arrest or cardiovascular collapse; however, survival after (sudden) death is a contradiction in terms. Table 26–1 provides definitions for events and terms related to the concept of SCD—death, cardiac arrest, and cardiovascular collapse.

EPIDEMIOLOGY AND CAUSES OF SUDDEN DEATH

EPIDEMIOLOGY

The worldwide incidence of SCD is difficult to estimate because it varies largely as a function of coronary heart disease prevalence in different countries.[24] Estimates for the United States range from 300,000 to nearly 400,000 SCDs annually,[25] the variation based in part on the definition of sudden death used in individual studies.[5,16] Most surveys and studies currently use the estimate of 300,000 SCDs annually,[26] a figure which represents 50 per cent or more of all cardiovascular deaths in the United States.[24-28]

The influence of the temporal definition of SCD on epidemiological data[4] is demonstrated by data derived from a retrospective death certificate study in a large metropolitan area in the United States reported by Kuller et al.[4] When the temporal definition was restricted to death less than 2 hours after the onset of symptoms, 12 per cent of all natural deaths were sudden, and 88 per cent of the sudden natural deaths were due to cardiac causes. This estimate is similar to observations in a large prospective cohort study—the Framingham study—in which 13 per cent of all deaths observed during a 26-year period were "sudden," defined as death within an hour of the onset of symptoms.[29,30] In contrast to deaths occurring less

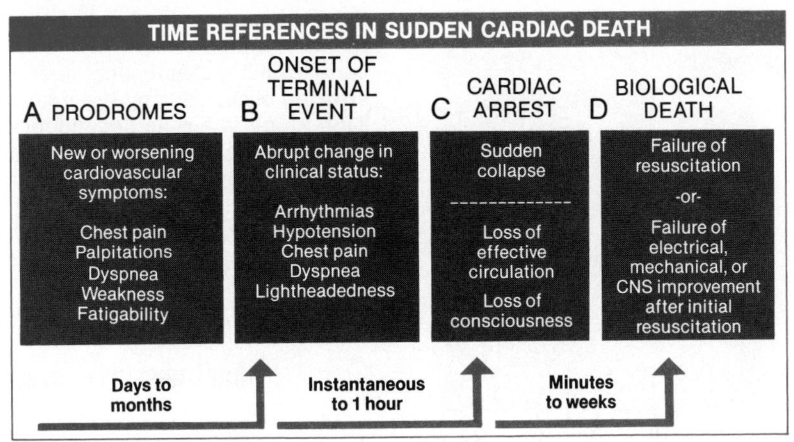

FIGURE 26–1. Sudden death, as defined by current investigators, has four temporal components: (*A*) prodromes, (*B*) onset of the terminal event, (*C*) the cardiac arrest itself, and (*D*) progression to biological death. Individual variability of the components influences the clinical expression: some cases have no prodromes, with onset leading almost instantaneously to cardiac arrest; others may have an onset which lasts up to 1 hour before clinical cardiac arrest; some patients may live weeks after the cardiac arrest before progression to biological death if there has been irreversible brain damage and life-support systems are used. These modifying factors influence application of the 1-hour definition. From the perspective of the clinician, the two most relevant factors are the onset of the terminal event (*B*) and the clinical cardiac arrest itself (*C*). In contrast, legal and social definitions focus on the time of biological death (*D*).

than 2 hours after the onset of symptoms, the application of the 24-hour definition of sudden death to the data from Kuller et al.[4] increased the fraction of all natural deaths falling into the "sudden" category to 32 per cent but reduced the proportion of all sudden natural deaths which were cardiac deaths to 75 per cent.

More recent prospective studies demonstrate that about 50 per cent of all coronary heart disease deaths are sudden and unexpected, occurring shortly (instantaneous to 1 hour) after the onset of symptoms. In the prospective combined Albany-Framingham study of 4120 males, sudden deaths within 1 hour of an observed collapse were analyzed for a population of men dying between 45 and 74 years of age.[9] During a 16-year follow-up, there were 234 total coronary deaths/1000 population observed, of which 109 (47 per cent) were sudden and unexpected. Because coronary heart disease dominates sudden and total cardiac deaths in the United States, the fraction of total cardiac deaths which are sudden is similar to the fraction of coronary heart disease deaths which are sudden, although there does appear to be a geographical variation in the fraction of coronary deaths which are sudden.[31] This 50 per cent fraction may not apply to other nations or to subcultures which have a lower prevalence of coronary heart disease. It also is of interest that the recent decline in coronary heart disease mortality in the United States[32] has not changed the fraction of coronary deaths that are sudden and unexpected,[33] even though there may be a decline in out-of-hospital deaths compared with emergency department deaths.[27]

POPULATION POOLS AND TIME-DEPENDENCE OF RISK

Two factors are of primary importance for identifying populations at risk and when considering strategies for primary prevention of SCD: (1) the size of denominators of population subgroups (Fig. 26–2*A*), and (2) time-dependence of risk (Fig. 26–2*B*).

POPULATION SUBGROUPS AND SCD. The more than 300,000 adult SCDs which occur annually in the United States can be viewed in toto as a derivation from an unselected population. Because of the large denominator which this population pool represents, the overall incidence is 1 to 2/1000 population (0.1–0.2 per cent) per year. This large population base contains both those victims whose SCDs occur as a first cardiac event and those whose SCDs may be predicted with greater accuracy because they come from higher-risk subgroups. Any intervention designed for the *general* population must, therefore, be applied to the 99/1000 who will *not* have an event to reach and possibly influence the 1/1000 who will. The cost and risk-to-benefit uncertainties limit the nature of such broad-based interventions, and demand a higher resolution of risk identification. Figure 26–2*A* highlights this problem by expressing the incidence (per cent/year) of SCD among various subgroups and contrasting the incidence to the total number of events/year which are represented by each subgroup. By moving from the total adult population to a subgroup with high risk because of the presence of selected coronary risk factors, there may be a ≥10-fold range of increases in the incidence of events annually, with the magnitude dependent on the number of risk factors operating in the subgroup. The size of the denominator pool, however, remains very large, and implementation of interventions remains problematic, even at this heightened level of risk. Higher resolution is desirable, and can be achieved by identification of more specific subgroups. The corresponding absolute number of deaths becomes progressively smaller as the subgroups become more focused (Fig. 26–2*A*), limiting the impact of interventions to the much smaller subgroups.

TIME-DEPENDENCE OF RISK. Risk of SCD is not linear as a function of time after a change in cardiovascular status.

TABLE 26–1 DEFINITION OF TERMS RELATED TO SUDDEN CARDIAC DEATH

TERM	DEFINITION	QUALIFIERS OR EXCEPTIONS
Death	Irreversible cessation of all biological functions	None
Cardiac arrest	Abrupt cessation of cardiac pump function which may be reversible by a prompt intervention but will lead to death in its absence	Rare spontaneous reversions; likelihood of successful intervention relates to mechanism of arrest and clinical setting
Cardiovascular collapse	A (sudden) loss of effective blood flow due to cardiac and/or peripheral vascular factors which may revert spontaneously (e.g., vasodepressor syncope) or only with interventions (e.g., cardiac arrest)	Nonspecific term which includes cardiac arrest and its consequences and also events which characteristically revert spontaneously

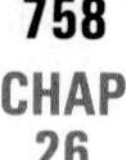

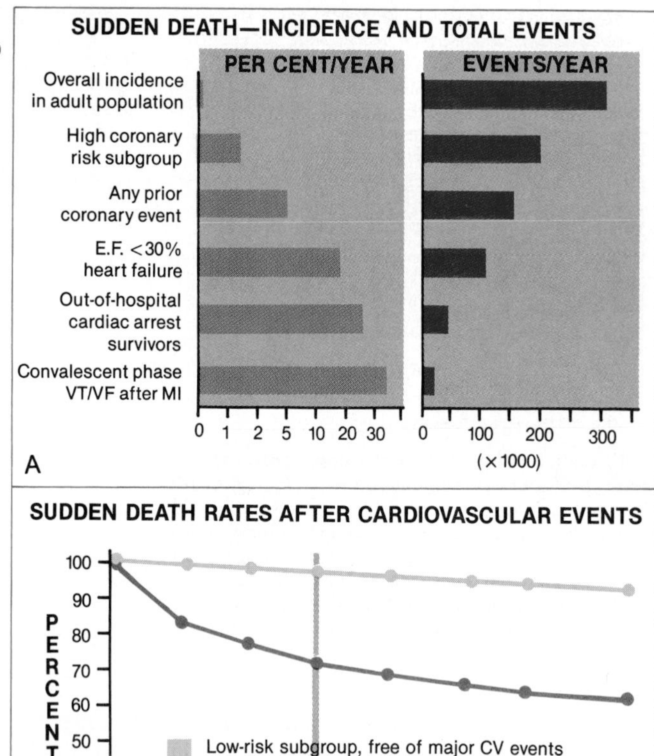

FIGURE 26-2. Impact of population pools and time-from-events on the clinical epidemiology of sudden cardiac death. The top panel (*A*) compares incidence and total numbers of sudden cardiac deaths in different subgroups; the lower panel (*B*) demonstrates time-dependence of risk after major cardiovascular events.

In the top panel, estimates of incidence figures (per cent/year) and the total number of events/year are shown for the overall adult population in the United States, and for increasingly higher-risk subgroups. The overall adult population has an estimated sudden death incidence of 0.1 to 0.2 per cent/year, accounting for a total number of events of more than 300,000/year. With the identification of increasingly powerful risk factors, the incidence *increases* progressively, but it is accompanied by a progressive *decrease* in the total number of patients identified. The inverse relation between incidence and total number of events occurs because of the progressively smaller denominator pool in the highest subgroup categories.

Successful interventions among larger population subgroups will require identification of specific markers to increase the ability to identify specific patients who will be at particularly high risk for a future event (Note: The horizontal axis for the incidence figures is not linear, and should be interpreted accordingly.)

In the lower panel (*B*), idealized survival curves are shown for a population of patients with known cardiovascular disease but at low risk because of freedom from major cardiovascular (C-V) events (top curve), and for populations of patients who have survived a major cardiovascular event (bottom curve). Attrition over time is accelerated in both absolute and relative terms for the initial 6 to 18 months after the major cardiovascular event. After the initial attrition, the slopes of the curves for the high-risk and low-risk populations parallel each other, highlighting both the early attrition and the attenuation of risk after 18 to 24 months.

These relations have been observed in diverse high-risk subgroups (cardiac arrest survivors, post-myocardial infarction patients with high-risk markers, recent onset of heart failure), and highlight the changing risk pattern as a function of time and the importance of the time dimension for recognition and intervention in strategies designed to alter outcome. (Modified from Myerburg, R. J., et al.: Sudden cardiac death: Structure, function and time-dependence of risk. Circulation [in press]. Reprinted with permission of the American Heart Association, Inc.)

Survival curves after major cardiovascular events, which identify populations at high risk for both sudden and total cardiac death, usually demonstrate that the most rapid rate of attrition occurs during the first 6 to 18 months (Fig. 26-2*B*). Thus there is a time-dependence of risk which focuses the opportunity for effective intervention to the early period after a conditioning event. Curves that have these characteristics have been generated from among survivors of out-of-hospital cardiac arrest, new onset of heart failure, unstable angina, and high-risk subgroups of patients having recent myocardial infarction. *The addition of time as a dimension for measuring risk may increase the resolution within subgroups.*

AGE, HEREDITY, GENDER, AND RACE

AGE. There are two ages of peak incidence of sudden death: between birth and 6 months of age (the sudden infant death syndrome) and between 45 and 75 years of age.[3] In the adult population the *incidence* of sudden death owing to coronary heart disease increases as a function of advancing age,[33-36] in parallel with the age-related increase in incidence of total coronary heart disease deaths.[32] However, the *proportion* of deaths caused by coronary heart disease that are sudden and unexpected decreases with advancing age.[9,33-36] Kuller et al.[37] reported that 76 per cent of coronary heart disease deaths in the 20-to-39-year age group were sudden and unexpected, and the Framingham data demonstrated that 62 per cent of all coronary heart disease deaths were sudden in the 45-to-54-year age group in men. The proportion fell progressively to 58 per cent in the 55-to-64-year age group and to 42 per cent in the 65-to-74-year age group.[34,35] Age also influences the proportion of cardiovascular causes among all causes of natural sudden death in that the proportion of coronary deaths and of all cardiac causes of death which are sudden is highest in the younger age groups, whereas the fraction of total sudden natural deaths which are due to any cardiovascular cause is higher in the older age groups.[38] In their study of sudden death in children and young adults, Neuspiel and Kuller[38] reported that only 19 per cent of sudden natural deaths in children between 1 and 13 years of age were cardiac deaths; the proportion increased to 30 per cent in the 14-to 21-year age group. All of these studies on age factors used a 24-hour definition of sudden death.

HEREDITY. To the extent that SCD is an expression of underlying coronary heart disease, hereditary factors that contribute to coronary heart disease risk operate nonspecifically for the SCD syndrome.[39]

Among the less common causes of SCD, hereditary patterns have been reported for some specific syndromes. Such patterns are described for some forms of congenital and hereditary Q-T interval prolongation (p. 708),[40] hypertrophic obstructive cardiomyopathy,[41] and familial SCD in children and young adults.[42] Although stable congenital conducting system abnormalities have a good prognosis,[43] progressive familial conducting system disease, which appears to have a hereditary pattern, carries an increased risk of SCD.[44] Familial sudden death associated with cardiac ganglionitis has been reported,[45] but an inheritance pattern has not been demonstrated in the reports to date.

GENDER. The SCD syndrome has a huge preponderance in males compared with females because of the protection females enjoy from coronary atherosclerosis before advanced years.[29,30,35] During the first 14 years of follow-up in the Framingham study, 59 of 66 (89 per cent) of sudden unexpected coronary deaths (< 1 hour) occurred in men.[8] The Framingham study at 20 years of follow-up demonstrated a 3.8-fold excess incidence of sudden coronary death in men compared with women.[35] This male:female ratio is similar to data recorded in three prospective studies of prehospital cardiac arrest in which the percentages of males observed were 75 per cent (mean age 63 years),[18] 85 per cent (mean age 60 years),[19] and 89 per cent (mean age 58 years),[45] respectively. In the study by Kuller et al.,[4] 75 per cent of all SCDs (using the 24-hour definition) in a 40-to-64-year-old population were in men. When the data in another study by Kuller et al. were analyzed for survival of less than 2 hours, the proportion of men increased to 80 per cent.[47] In the Framingham study[35] the excess risk in men peaked at 6.75:1 in the 55-to-64-year age group and then fell to 2.17:1 in the 65-to-74-year age group. Even though the overall risk is much lower in women, the classic coronary risk factors are expressed in them.[29,30,48,49] Cigarette smoking, diabetes, use of oral contraceptives,[50] and reduced vital capacity[30] are particularly strong factors.

RACE. A number of studies comparing racial differences and relative risk of SCD in whites and blacks with coronary heart disease in the United States have yielded inconclusive data.[4,26,51] However, data on the prevalence of coronary heart disease in Japanese men living in the United States have demonstrated that the low rates reported in those living in Japan tend to increase toward, but do not reach, levels observed in white men in the United States.[52] Thus, an interplay between race and environmental factors may be operative.

BIOLOGICAL CORONARY RISK FACTORS AND SUDDEN DEATH

The known coronary risk factors cannot be used to distinguish the patients at risk for SCD from those at risk for other manifestations of coronary heart disease.[9] Using a multivariate analysis of selected risk factors (i.e., age, systolic blood pressure, heart rate, ECG abnormalities, vital capacity, relative weight, cigarette consumption, and serum cholesterol) from the population in the Framingham data, Kannel and Schatzkin[33] determined that 53 per cent of the SCDs in men and 42 per cent of those in women occurred among the 10 per cent of the population in the highest risk decile (Fig. 26–3). The comparison of risk factors in the victims of SCD to those in people who developed any manifestations of coronary artery disease did not provide useful patterns, by either univariate or multivariate analyses, to distinguish victims of SCD from the overall pool.[9] In addition, data from 19,946 patients in the Coronary Artery Surgery Study identified no angiographic or hemodynamic patterns that discriminated sudden from nonsudden cardiac deaths.[36]

Hypertension is a clearly established risk factor for coronary heart disease and also emerges as a highly significant risk factor for incidence of SCD.[9] However, there is no influence of increasing systolic blood pressure levels on the ratio of sudden deaths to total coronary heart disease deaths.[34] No relationship has been observed between cholesterol concentration and the proportion of coronary deaths that were sudden.[35] Neither the ECG pattern of left ventricular hypertrophy nor nonspecific ST-T wave abnormalities influence the proportion of total coronary deaths that are sudden and unexpected[34]; *only intraventricular conduction abnormalities are suggestive of a disproportionate number of SCDs*.[35] A low vital capacity also suggests a disproportionate risk for sudden versus total coronary deaths.[35] This is of interest because such a relation was particularly striking in the analysis of data on women in the Framingham study who had died suddenly.[29,30] A high hematocrit also was predictive in women.[31]

LIFE STYLE AND PSYCHOSOCIAL FACTORS

LIFE STYLE. There is a strong association between *cigarette smoking* and all manifestations of coronary heart disease. The Framingham study demonstrates that cigarette smokers have a 2- to 3-fold increase in sudden death risk in each decade of life at entry between 30 and 59 years, and that this is one of the few risk factors in which the proportion of coronary heart disease deaths that are sudden increases in association with the risk factor.[35] In addition, in a study of 310 survivors of out-of-hospital cardiac arrest, Hallstrom et al.[53] observed a 27 per cent incidence of recurrent cardiac arrest at 3 years in those who continued to smoke after their index event, compared with 19 per cent in those who stopped ($p < .04$). Obesity is a second factor which appears to influence the proportion of coronary deaths that occur suddenly.[30,35] With increasing relative weight, the percentage of coronary heart disease deaths that were sudden in the Framingham study increased linearly from a low of 39 per cent to a high of 70 per cent. Total coronary heart disease deaths increased with increasing relative weight as well.

Epidemiological observations suggest a relationship between *low levels of physical activity* and increased coronary heart disease death risk.[54] The Framingham study, however, showed an *insignificant* relationship between low levels of physical activity and incidence of sudden death but a high proportion of sudden to total cardiac deaths at *higher* levels of physical activity.[35]

PSYCHOSOCIAL FACTORS. These appear to influence the risk for SCDs. Rahe and coworkers[55] recorded recent life changes in the realms of health, work, home and family, and personal and social factors, relating the magnitude of such changes to myocardial infarction and SCD. There was an association between significant elevations of life-change scores during the 6 months before a coronary event, and the association was particularly striking in victims of SCD. In a study of sudden death in women,[56] those who died suddenly were less often married, had fewer children, and had greater educational discrepancies with their spouses than did age-related controls living in the same neighborhood as the sudden death victims. A history of psychiatric treatment, cigarette smoking, and greater quantities of alcohol consumption than the controls also characterized the sudden death group.[56] Ruberman and coworkers reported on the influences of psychosocial factors on sudden and total death after myocardial infarction in 2320 male survivors of myocardial infarction.[57] Controlling for other major prognostic factors, including frequency of premature ventricular contractions, a greater than four-fold increase in risk of sudden and total deaths was predicted by *social isolation* and a *high level of life stress*. These psychosocial factors were inversely related to levels of education. In an earlier study, a more than 3-fold increase of sudden death risk during follow-up after myocardial infarction had been reported in men who had complex ventricular ectopy and low levels of education compared with better-educated men with the same arrhythmias.[58] Interestingly, there was no relation betwen educational level and recurrent myocardial infarction.

In a survey of life style, it was found that people with lower educational levels smoked more cigarettes, drank more alcohol, exercised less, and were more overweight.[59] The studies by Friedman and Rosenman[60] on the time-oriented, aggressive *type A personality* characteristics have suggested an increased incidence of all manifestations of coronary heart disease in such patients, including the incidence of sudden cardiac death. The validity of the discrimination of a high-risk subgroup based on type A personality characteristics has recently been challenged.[61]

FUNCTIONAL CLASSIFICATION AND SUDDEN DEATH. The Framingham study demonstrated a striking relation between functional classification and death during a 2-year follow-up period. However, the proportion of deaths that were sudden did not vary with functional classification, ranging from 50 to 57 per cent in all groups, ranging from those free of clinical heart disease to those in functional class IV.[35]

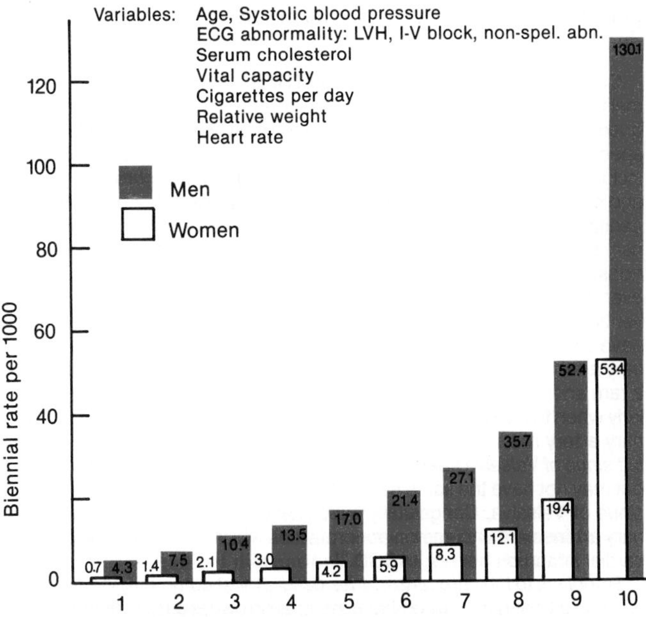

FIGURE 26–3. Risk of sudden death by decile of multivariant risk: 26-year follow-up, the Framingham Study. ECG = electrocardiographic; IV = intraventricular; LVH = left ventricular hypertrophy; Non-spec Abn = nonspecific abnormality. (From Kannel, W.B., and Shatzkin, A.: Sudden death: Lessons from subsets in population studies. Reprinted by permission of the American College of Cardiology. J. Am. Coll. Cardiol. *5*[Suppl 6]:141B, 1985.)

SUDDEN DEATH AND PREVIOUS CORONARY HEART DISEASE

Although SCD is the first clinical manifestation of coronary heart disease in 20 to 25 per cent or more of all coronary heart disease patients,[9,16,23,26] a previous myocardial infarction can be identified in as many as 75 per cent of patients who die suddenly. The high incidence of both clinical and unrecognized prior myocardial infarction in victims of SCD has led to a search for predictors of SCD in survivors of myocardial infarction, as well as in patients with other clinical manifestations of coronary heart disease.

LEFT VENTRICULAR EJECTION FRACTION IN CHRONIC ISCHEMIC HEART DISEASE. A marked depression of the left ventricular ejection fraction is the most powerful predictor of SCD in patients with chronic ischemic heart disease, as well as other causes (see below). Increased risk, independent of other risk factors, is measurable at ejection

TABLE 26-2 CAUSES AND CONTRIBUTING FACTORS IN SUDDEN CARDIAC DEATH *Continued*

IX. SUDDEN INFANT DEATH SYNDROME AND SUDDEN DEATH IN CHILDREN
  A. Sudden infant death syndrome
    1. Immature respiratory control functions
    2. Susceptibility to lethal arrhythmias
    3. Congenital heart disease
    4. Myocarditis
  B. Sudden death in children
    1. Eisenmenger syndrome, aortic stenosis, hypertrophic cardiomyopathy, pulmonary atresia
    2. After corrective surgery for congenital heart disease
    3. Myocarditis
    4. Unexplained

X. MISCELLANEOUS
  A. Sudden death during extreme physical activity
  B. Mechanical interference with venous return
    1. Acute cardiac tamponade
    2. Massive pulmonary embolism
    3. Acute intracardiac thrombosis
  C. Dissecting aneurysm of the aorta
  D. Toxic/metabolic disturbances
    1. Electrolyte disturbances
    2. Metabolic disturbances
    3. Proarrhythmic effects of antiarrhythmic drugs
    4. Proarrhythmic effects of noncardiac drugs
  E. Mimics of sudden cardiac death
    1. "Cafe coronary"
    2. Acute alcoholic states ("holiday heart")
    3. Acute asthmatic attacks
    4. Air or amniotic fluid embolism

in clinical settings, some observations have focused attention on the feasibility of such a mechanism.[88]

The *mucocutaneous lymph node syndrome* (Kawasaki's disease)[89] (p. 997) carries a risk of SCD in association with coronary arteritis. Polyarteritis nodosa and related vasculitis syndromes (p. 1735) can cause SCD presumably because of coronary arteritis,[90] as can coronary ostial stenosis in syphilitic aortitis[43] (p. 1548). The latter has become a very rare manifestation of syphilis.[91]

Several types of mechanical obstruction to coronary arteries must be listed among causes of SCD. Coronary dissection, with or without dissection of the aorta, occurs in the Marfan syndrome[92] (p. 1641) and has also been reported in the peripartum period of pregnancy.[93] Among the rare mechanical causes of SCD are prolapse of myxomatous polyps from the aortic valve into coronary ostia[94] as well as dissection or rupture of a sinus of Valsalva aneurysm, with involvement of the coronary ostia and proximal coronary arteries.[95]

Coronary artery spasm (p. 1342) may cause serious arrhythmias and SCD[96,97] with or without concomitant coronary atherosclerotic lesions.[96,98] Painless myocardial ischemia,[99] associated with either spasm or fixed lesions, may be a cause of heretofore unexplained sudden death.[100,101] Different patterns of silent ischemia (e.g., totally asymptomatic, post-myocardial infarction, and mixed silent/anginal pattern) may have different prognostic implications.[102] Finally, deep *myocardial bridges* over coronary arteries (p. 251) have been reported in association with SCD during strenuous exercise.[103]

VENTRICULAR HYPERTROPHY. Hypertrophic muscle is a common denominator among many causes of SCD,[104] has been identified as an independent risk factor for SCD,[6] and may be a factor in propensity to potentially lethal arrhythmias.[104-106] The underlying states resulting in hypertrophy include hypertensive heart disease with or without atherosclerosis, valvular heart disease, obstructive and nonobstructive hypertrophic cardiomyopathy, primary pulmonary hypertension with right ventricular hypertrophy, and advanced right ventricular overload secondary to congenital heart disease. Each of these conditions is associated with risk of SCD, and it has been suggested that patients with severely hypertrophic ventricles are particularly susceptible to arrhythmic death.[104]

HYPERTROPHIC OBSTRUCTIVE CARDIOMYOPATHY (p. 1404). Risk of SCD in hypertrophic obstructive cardiomyopathy was identified in the early clinical and hemodynamic studies of this entity.[107] Two subsequent large series have yielded similar data on the magnitude of this risk. Goodwin[108] observed 48 deaths, of which 36 (67 per cent) were sudden, among a cohort of 254 patients followed for a mean of 6 years, while Shah et al.[109] reported that 26 of 49 deaths (55 per cent) among 190 patients were sudden. Cardiac arrest survivors in this etiological group may have better long-term outcome than do survivors with other etiologies. In one report only 11/33 (33 per cent) had recurrent cardiac arrest or death during a mean follow-up of 7 years.[110] Specific clinical markers have not been especially predictive of SCD in individual patients, although young age,[108,111] strong family history,[41,108] and worsening symptoms[108] appear to indicate higher risk. In one study, however, 54 per cent of the sudden deaths occurred in patients without any functional limitations.[111] The mechanism of SCD in patients with hypertrophic obstructive cardiomyopathy was initially thought to involve outflow tract obstruction, possibly as a consequence of catecholamine stimulation, but more recent data have focused on cardiac arrhythmias as the more common mechanism of sudden death in this disease.[104,112-115a] These studies have demonstrated a high prevalence of high-risk or potentially lethal arrhythmias on ambulatory monitoring[112,114] or the inducibility of potentially lethal arrhythmias during programmed electrical stimulation.[115,116] The question of whether the pathogenesis of the arrhythmias represents an interaction between electrophysiological and hemodynamic abnormalities or is a consequence of electrophysiological derangement of hypertrophied muscle[104-106] is unanswered. The observation that patients with nonobstructive hypertrophic cardiomyopathy have high-risk arrhythmias and are at increased risk for SCD[112] suggests that an electrophysiological mechanism secondary to the hypertrophied muscle itself plays some role. Stafford and colleagues[117] reported exercise-related cardiac arrest in nonobstructive hypertrophic cardiomyopathy. Ventricular fibrillation (VF) was reproduced during electrophysiological testing after induction of atrial fibrillation with a rapid ventricular response. In athletes under 35 years of age, hypertrophic cardiomyopathy is the most common cause of SCD, in contrast to athletes over the age of 35, among whom ischemic heart disease is the most common cause.[85,86,118-120]

HEART FAILURE AND SUDDEN DEATH. The advent of therapeutic interventions which provide better long-term control of congestive heart failure has begun to improve long-term survival of such patients (p. 499). However, the proportion of heart failure patients with stable hemodynamics who die suddenly appears to be increasing.[121] In reports to date, as many as 47 per cent of deaths in heart failure patients are categorized as SCDs.

The interaction between post-myocardial infarction ventricular arrhythmia and depressed ejection fraction in determining risk for SCD has been described.[62,78] The majority of studies addressing the relation between chronic congestive heart failure and SCD focused on patients with ischemic, idiopathic, and alcoholic congestive cardiomyopathy.[71,121-124] A chronic myopathic syndrome after myocarditis has been cited as an infrequent but well-documented cause of SCD.[125] Peripartum cardiomyopathy (p. 1798) also may cause SCD.

Acute Heart Failure. All causes of acute cardiac failure, in the absence of prompt interventions, may result in SCD caused by either the circulatory failure itself or secondary arrhythmias. The electrophysiological mechanisms involved have been proposed to be related to acute stretching of myocardial fibers and/or the His-Purkinje system, with its experimentally demonstrated arrhythmogenic effect,[126] but the roles of neurohumoral mechanisms and acute electrolyte shifts have not been fully evaluated.[121] Among the causes of acute cardiac failure which are associated with SCD are massive acute myocardial infarction, acute myocarditis, acute alcoholic cardiac dysfunction, and a number of mechanical causes of heart failure such as massive pulmonary embolism, mechanical disruption of intracardiac structures secondary to infarction or infection, and ball-valve embolism in aortic or mitral stenosis (Table 26–2).

INFLAMMATORY, INFILTRATIVE, NEOPLASTIC, AND DEGENERATIVE DISEASES OF THE HEART. Almost all diseases in this category have been associated with SCD, with or without concomitant cardiac failure. Acute viral myocarditis with left ventricular dysfunction (p. 1426) is commonly associated with cardiac arrhythmias, including potentially lethal arrhythmias. It is now recognized that serious ventricular arrhythmias or SCD can occur in myocarditis in the absence of clinical evidence of left ventricular dysfunction.[43,125,127] In a report of 19 SCDs among 1,606,167 previously screened U.S. Air Force recruits, 8 of the 19 (42 per cent) had evidence of myocarditis (5 nonrheumatic, 3 rheumatic) at postmortem examination, and 15 (79 per cent) suffered their cardiac arrests during strenuous exertion.[128] Viral carditis also may cause damage isolated to the specialized conducting system and result in a propensity to arrhythmias; the rare association of this process with SCD has been reported.[129] The risk of potentially lethal arrhythmias is not limited to the acute phase of the disease.[125]

Myocardial involvement in collagen-vascular disorders, tumors, chronic granulomatous diseases, infiltrative disorders, and protozoan infestations varies widely, but in all instances SCD may be the initial or terminal manifestation of the disease process. Among the granulomatous diseases, *sarcoidosis* (p. 1420) stands out because of the frequency of SCD. Roberts et al.[130] reported that SCD was the terminal event in 67 per cent of sarcoid heart disease deaths; the occurrence of SCD has been related to the extent of cardiac involvement.[131] In a report on the pathological findings in nine patients who died of *progressive systemic sclerosis* (p. 1736), eight who died suddenly had evidence of transient ischemia and reperfusion histologically, suggesting that this might represent Raynaud-like involvement of coronary vessels.[132] In contrast, *arrhythmogenic right ventricular dysplasia* (p. 706) is associated with a high incidence of arrhythmias, particularly recurrent ventricular tachycardia, but the frequency of SCD appears to be relatively low.[133] Isolated *right ventricular cardiomyopathy* (p. 1404) has characteristics suggestive of an advanced form of right ventricular dysplasia, but carries a high risk of SCD.[134,135] *Amyloidosis* of the heart (p. 1753) may also cause sudden death. An incidence of 30 per cent has been reported[136]; diffuse involvement of ventricular muscle or of the specialized conducting system may be associated with SCD.

VALVULAR HEART DISEASE (Chap. 34). Before the advent of surgery for valvular heart disease, *aortic stenosis* was one of the more common noncoronary causes of SCD. Campbell reported in 1968 that 44 of 70 (73 per cent) deaths in patients with aortic stenosis were sudden.[138] The advent of safe and effective procedures for aortic valve replacement has reduced the incidence of this cause of sudden death,[139] but patients with prosthetic or heterograft aortic valve replacements remain at some risk for SCD caused by arrhythmias, prosthetic valve dysfunction, or coexistent coronary heart disease.[140] SCD has been reported to be the second most common mode of death after valve replacement surgery, accounting for 62 of 298 deaths (21 per cent).[141] The incidence peaked 3 weeks after operation and then plateaued after 8 months. Nonetheless, the risk is appreciably lower than in those patients who had not had the advantage of valvular surgery in prior years. In another report analyzing outcome in patients receiving prosthetic valves for pure severe aortic stenosis, SCD occurred at a rate of only 0.3 per cent/year, and was responsible for only 18 per cent of late deaths.[142] A high incidence of ventricular arrhythmia has been observed during follow-up of patients with valve replacement,[142,143] especially in those who had aortic stenosis, multiple valve surgery, or cardiomegaly.[143] Sudden death during follow-up was associated with ventricular arrhythmias and thromboembolism. Hemodynamic variables were less predictive. Although all valvular stenotic lesions are associated with some risk for SCD, valvular regurgitation, particularly chronic aortic regurgitation and acute mitral regurgitation, also may be associated with SCD.

Mitral valve prolapse (p. 1029) is prevalent and associated with a high incidence of cardiac arrhythmias; however, the incidence of SCD is quite low.[144] This uncommon complication appears to correlate with nonspecific ST-T wave changes in the inferior leads on the ECG.[145] In data reviewed from 17 reported instances of SCD in mitral valve prolapse patients, these nonspecific ST-T wave changes were present in 6 of 8 who had had prior electrocardiograms.[146] An association with redundancy of mitral leaflets on echocardiogram also has been suggested.[147] Reported associations between Q-T interval prolongation or preexcitation and SCD in mitral prolapse syndrome are less consistent.[144]

Endocarditis of the aortic and mitral valves (see Chap. 35) may be associated with rapid death resulting from acute disruption of the valvular apparatus, coronary embolism, or abscesses of valvular rings or the septum; however, such deaths are rarely true sudden deaths as conventionally defined.

CONGENITAL HEART DISEASE. The congenital lesions most commonly associated with SCD are aortic stenosis (p. 1035)[127,148,149] and communications between the left and right sides of the heart with Eisenmenger syndrome (p. 971).[150] In the latter the risk of SCD is a function of pulmonary vascular disease severity; also, there is an extraordinarily high risk of maternal mortality during labor and delivery in the pregnant patient with Eisenmenger syndrome (p. 1795).[151] Potentially lethal arrhythmias and SCD have been described as late complications after surgical repair of complex congenital lesions, particularly tetralogy of Fallot (p. 935),[152] transposition of the great arteries,[153] and atrioventricular canal.[154] These patients should be followed closely and treated aggressively when cardiac arrhythmias are identified.[154]

ELECTROPHYSIOLOGICAL ABNORMALITIES. Acquired disease of the AV node and His-Purkinje system and the presence of accessory pathways of conduction are two groups of structural abnormalities of specialized conduction which may be associated with SCD. Epidemiological studies have suggested that intraventricular conduction disturbances in coronary heart disease are one of the few factors that may increase the proportion of SCD in coronary heart disease.[35] A specific clinical example is the risk of VF during the first 30 days after myocardial infarction in patients with anterior infarctions and bundle branch block. Lie et al.[155] reported that 47 per cent of patients who had late hospital VF had had anteroseptal infarcts with bundle branch block, and that these 14 were from a total pool of only 40 patients with the combination of bundle branch block and anterior myocardial infarction. Thus there was a 35 per cent incidence of VF in this subgroup, which represented only 4.1 per cent of a total of 966 myocardial infarctions. This risk persists for 6 weeks after the infarction and then abates.[156] AV block or intraventricular conduction abnormalities were found in 9 of 10 patients who had recurrent VF during hospitalization after resuscitation from prehospital cardiac arrest.[20]

Primary fibrosis (Lenegre's disease)[157] or secondary mechanical injury (Lev's disease)[158] of the His-Purkinje system is commonly associated with intraventricular conduction abnormalities and symptomatic AV block, and less commonly with SCD. The identification of people at risk and the efficacy of pacemakers for preventing SCD, rather than only ameliorating systems, have been the subjects of debate.[159,160]

Survival may depend more on the nature and extent of the underlying disease than on the conduction disturbance itself.[161] Patients with congenital AV block (Chap. 31) or nonprogressive congenital intraventricular block usually have a low risk of SCD.[162] Progressive congenital intraventricular blocks predict a high risk,[162] and a hereditary form has been reported in association with a familial propensity to SCD.[44,162]

The anomalous pathways of conduction, bundles of Kent in the Wolff-Parkinson-White syndrome, and Mahaim fibers are commonly associated with nonlethal arrhythmias. However, when the anomalous pathways of conduction have short refractory periods, the occurrence of atrial fibrillation may allow the induction of VF during very rapid conduction across the bypass tract.[163] The incidence of SCD in patients with short refractory period bypass tracts is not yet known. Patients who have multiple pathways appear to be at higher risk of SCD,[163] as do patients with a familial pattern of anomalous pathways and premature SCD's.[164]

Q-T PROLONGATION (see also p. 708). The prolonged Q-T interval syndrome is a functional abnormality, perhaps associated with neurogenic influences, that may cause lethal arrhythmias.[165] In the hereditary *congenital form* two varieties have been reported: those with autosomal recessive inheritance and associated deafness, the Jervell and Lange-Nielsen syndrome,[166] and those without deafness, the Romano-Ward syndrome.[40] Some patients have prolonged Q-T intervals throughout life without any manifest arrhythmias, whereas others are highly susceptible to ventricular arrhythmias, particularly the torsades de pointes form of ventricular tachycardia;[167] SCD is a risk associated with the abnormality in these patients. Patients at higher risk are characterized by deafness, female gender, syncope, and documented torsades de pointes or prior ventricular fibrillation, and they require aggressive medical or surgical interventions.[168,169]

The *acquired form* of prolonged Q-T interval may be due to drug idiosyncrasies (particularly antiarrhythmics and psychotropic drugs), electrolyte abnormalities, hypothermia, toxic substances, and central nervous system injury.[169] It also has been reported both in intensive weight reduction programs that involve the use of liquid protein diets[170] and in anorexia nervosa.[171] Lithium carbonate may prolong the Q-T interval and has been reported to be associated with an increased incidence of SCD in cancer patients with preexisting heart disease.[172] Acquired prolonged Q-T intervals usually carry a risk of serious arrhythmias and SCD, but the risk is abolished when the inciting factor is removed. In acquired prolonged Q-T syndrome, as in the congenital form, the torsades de pointes form of VT is commonly the specific arrhythmia that triggers or degenerates into lethal VF.

ELECTRICAL INSTABILITY RESULTING FROM NEUROHUMORAL AND CENTRAL NERVOUS SYSTEM INFLUENCES. Catecholamine-dependent lethal arrhythmias in the absence of Q-T interval prolongation, with control by beta-adrenoreceptor blocking agents, have been described.[173] Several central nervous system–related interactions with cardiac electrical stability have been suggested. The hereditary forms of prolonged Q-T interval syndrome, discussed above, appear to have a relation to sympathetic nervous system imbalance.[165,174] Lown and coworkers identified psychic stress as a mediating factor for advanced cardiac arrhythmias and perhaps SCD.[175] Epidemiological data also suggest an association between behavioral abnormalities and the risk of SCD, particularly in women[56,57]; emotional extremes have been suggested as a triggering mechanism for SCD.[3,176] Associations between auditory stimulation[127] and auditory auras[177] and SCD have been reported.[127] The auditory abnormalities in some forms of congenital Q-T prolongation have already been cited.[166]

The syndrome of "voodoo death" in underdeveloped cultures was studied extensively.[178,178a] There appears to be an association between isolation from the tribe, a sense of hopelessness, severe bradyarrhythmias, and sudden death. With cultural changes in many of these areas, the syndrome has become less amenable to observation and study; however, there do remain pockets of cultural isolation in which the syndrome no doubt still exists.

SUDDEN INFANT DEATH SYNDROME AND SCD IN CHILDREN. The sudden infant death syndrome occurs between birth and 6 months of age, more commonly in males, and has an incidence of 0.1 to 0.3 per cent of live births.[179] Because of its abrupt nature, a cardiac mechanism had been suspected for many years,[180] but a variety of causes, with respiratory dysfunction playing a major role, are considered likely.[181] Many cases of the sudden infant death syndrome are believed to represent a form of "sleep apnea" which, if prolonged, may lead to hypoxia, cyanosis, and cardiac arrhythmias. Experience with "near-misses" and the results of respiratory monitoring, in conjunction with the propensity of the syndrome to occur in premature infants, all suggest impaired central nervous system respiratory control reflexes, possibly owing to immaturity.[179,181–184] There has recently been interest, however, in the possibility of obstructive apnea as another possible mechanism.[181] Identification of individual infants at risk is difficult, but the risk does not persist beyond the first 6 months of life.

Despite the current focus on the respiratory mechanisms involved in the syndrome, their role has not yet been explicitly established.[182] Furthermore, the question of whether or not an identifiable subset of infants who have apneic spells are particularly prone to genesis of cardiac arrhythmias remains conjectural.[183–185] A primary cardiac cause is still considered the basis of this syndrome in some victims.[181,185] Marino and Kane[186] observed either accessory pathways (two cases) or dispersed or immature AV nodal or bundle branch cells in the annulus fibrosis (four cases) among a group of seven sudden infant death syndrome victims studied by detailed histopathology.

Sudden death in children beyond the age group at risk for sudden infant death syndrome often is associated with identifiable heart disease,[126,187] although one study identified cardiac causes in only 25 per cent of sudden natural death victims between the ages of 1 and 21 years.[38] About 25 per cent of SCDs in children occur in those who have undergone previous surgery for congenital cardiac disease. Of the remaining 75 per cent, more than one-half occur in children who have one of four lesions: congenital aortic stenosis, Eisenmenger syndrome, pulmonary stenosis or atresia, and obstructive hypertrophic cardiomyopathy.[187] Neuspiel and Kuller[38] observed 14 cases of myocarditis among 51 SCDs in children (27 per cent).

OTHER CAUSES OF SUDDEN DEATH

SCD in athletes during or after extreme physical activity is infrequent but receives a great deal of attention when it does occur. The majority of such individuals have a previously unrecognized cardiac abnormality, with hypertrophic cardiomyopathy with or without obstruction, valvular aortic stenosis, and occult coronary artery disease as the most common causes identified after death.[86,118–120,188,189] A surprisingly large fraction of people who died suddenly during exertion had unsuspected myocarditis, according to a report of a large cohort of U.S. Air Force recruits.[128] A small group of such victims, however, have neither previously determined functional abnormality nor structural abnormalities at postmortem examination.[20,85,86,125,126]

There are rare instances of idiopathic VF causing SCD in the absence of any identifiable structural or functional abnormality of the heart.[190] Risk for recurrence may remain after surviving an initial event, although limited data suggest that risk persists only in patients with subtle cardiac abnormalities, in contrast to patients who are truly normal.[191] In addition, these events tend to occur in young, otherwise healthy people. A specific variation of this syndrome has been observed in southeast Asians. Many years ago syndromes referred to as *Bangungut* in young Filipino males,[192] *Pokkuri* in young Japanese males,[193] and *Nonlaitai* in young Laotian males[194] were reported. In each there was a tendency for sudden death to occur during sleep, and at one time a toxic cause was suspected.[192,193] Documented cases have now been reported in Laotians who came to the United States after the Vietnam war. The mechanism was identified to be VF in some of these cases; in at least one instance electrophysiological study demonstrated inducible ventricular arrhythmia by programmed electrical stimulation.[195] Pathological examinations have revealed a high incidence of mild to significant cardiomegaly (14 of 18) and a variety of structural abnormalities of specialized conducting tissue.[196] The fact that these cases continue to occur in a new cultural setting suggests that there may be a hereditary predisposition.

There also are a number of noncardiac conditions which *mimic* SCD. These include the so-called *cafe coronary,*[197,198] in which food, usually an unchewed piece of meat, lodges in the oropharynx and causes an abrupt obstruction at the glottis. The classic description of a cafe coronary is sudden cyanosis and collapse in a restaurant, during a meal accompanied by lively conversation. The *holiday heart syndrome* is characterized by cardiac arrhythmias, most commonly atrial, and other cardiac abnormalities associated with acute alcoholic states.[199] It has not been determined whether potentially lethal arrhythmias occurring in such settings account for reported sudden deaths associated with acute alcoholic states.[3] *Massive pulmonary embolism* (Chap. 48) may cause acute cardiovascular collapse and sudden death; sudden death in severe acute asthmatic attacks, without prolonged deterioration of the patient's condition, is well recognized.[200] Air or amnionic fluid embolism at the time of labor and delivery may cause sudden death on rare occasions, with the clinical picture mimicking sudden cardiac death.[201] Peripartum air embolism caused by an unusual sexual practice has been reported as a cause of such sudden deaths.[202]

Proarrhythmic effects of antiarrhythmic drugs have received particular attention,[203,204] but psychotropic drugs, arrhythmogenic effects of toxic substances, and electrolyte disturbances—particularly hypokalemia, hypocalcemia, and hypomagnesemia—also have been implicated.[169] The proarrhythmic effects resulting in worsening of arrhythmias are more commonly associated with normal than with prolonged Q-T intervals, and therefore are difficult to predict.[203,204] Classic proarrhythmia is an event which tends to appear within days after the initiation of antiarrhythmic therapy.[205] The pattern of SCD over time among patients treated with two of the drugs used in the Cardiac Arrhythmia Suppression Trial suggests the possibility that a different pattern of proarrhythmic risk, perhaps caused by a different mechanism,[77] may be a continuous function extending over 1 or more years of exposure.

Finally, a number of abnormalities that do not directly involve the heart may cause SCD or mimic it. These include aortic dissection (p. 1539), acute cardiac tamponade (p. 1473), and rapid exsanguination (p. 1521).

PATHOLOGY AND PATHOPHYSIOLOGY OF SUDDEN CARDIAC DEATH

Pathological observations in SCD victims reflect the epidemiological and clinical preponderance of coronary heart disease as the major structural predisposing factor.[206] Liberthson and coworkers[207] reported that 81 per cent of 220 autopsied victims of SCD had pathological findings of coronary heart disease as the major causative factor (i.e., more than one coronary vessel with more than 75 per cent stenosis). At least one vessel with more than 75 per cent stenosis was found in 94 per cent of victims, acute coronary occlusion in 58 per cent, healed myocardial infarction in 44 per cent, and acute myocardial infarction in 27 per cent. These observations are consistent with many other studies of the frequency of coronary disease in sudden death victims. The numerous other specific causes of SCD collectively account for no more than 10 to 20 per cent of cases, but they have provided a large base of enlightening pathological data.[43,125]

THE PATHOLOGY OF SUDDEN DEATH CAUSED BY CORONARY HEART DISEASE

THE CORONARY ARTERIES. Extensive atherosclerosis is the most common pathological finding in the coronary arteries of victims of SCD (Table 26–3). In postmortem examinations of 169 hearts, sites of 75 per cent or more stenosis were present in three or four of the major vessels in 61 per cent of the hearts studied; two vessels with at least 75 per cent stenosis were found in 15 per cent, and 24 per cent of the hearts had either single-vessel disease or no vessels having lesions producing 75 per cent stenosis.[208] A distinctly higher proportion of hearts having three or four vessels with 75 per cent stenotic lesions occurred in white males (70 per cent) compared with white females (34 per cent). In contrast, 58 per cent of the hearts of both black males and black females had three or four vessels with 75 per cent or more stenoses. Consistent with clinical findings in survivors of prehospital cardiac arrest,[20] there was no special predilection of disease distribution for any coronary artery, and there was no quantitative difference between proximal and distal distribution of disease. Kuller et al.[47] pointed out that 90 per cent or greater narrowing of at least one coronary artery was found in 77 per cent of autopsied victims of sudden *coronary* death, compared with 8 per cent of victims of other causes of sudden death. Davies[43] reported that 61 per cent of patients dying suddenly because of coronary heart disease had three vessels with 75 per cent or more stenosis at any one point; an additional 18 (23 per cent) had two vessels with 75 per cent or more stenosis. Among 100 age- and sex-matched controls who died of trauma or cerebral tumors, only 27 per cent had two- or three-vessel disease, and 52 per cent had no vessels with lesions of 75 per cent or more. In the same study the majority of sudden deaths caused by coronary heart disease were associated with at least one point of more than 85 per cent stenosis, and Davies suggested that this parameter provided the best discrimination between hearts of SCD victims and controls.

TABLE 26–3 PATHOLOGICAL FINDINGS IN SUDDEN DEATH DUE TO CORONARY HEART DISEASE

THE CORONARY ARTERIES	VENTRICULAR MYOCARDIUM
A. Chronic atherosclerosis	A. Healed myocardial infarction
B. Acute lesions	B. Left ventricular hypertrophy
1. Plaque fissuring	C. Ventricular aneurysm
2. Platelet aggregates	D. Acute myocardial infarction
3. Organizing thrombus	
4. Coronary artery spasm	

Roberts and colleagues[209] have quantitated coronary artery narrowing at postmortem examination of sudden coronary death victims and controls. Thirty-six per cent of 5-mm segments of the coronary arteries from the SCD group had 76 to 100 per cent cross-sectional area reductions compared with 3 per cent in the controls. An additional 34 per cent of the sections from the SCD group had 51 to 75 per cent reductions in cross-sectional areas. Only 7 per cent of the sections from the SCD patients had 0 to 25 per cent reductions in cross-sectional areas. The *distribution* of the lesions causing greater than 75 per cent narrowing was similar in the three major coronary arteries, but quantitative differences between proximal and distal halves of the vessels were inconsistent.[209] Similar conclusions resulted from pathological observations of prehospital cardiac arrest victims who were not successfully resuscitated.[207] These studies indicate that extensive coronary artery disease is the pathological hallmark of SCDs caused by coronary heart disease and that there is no specific anatomical pattern of distribution of the disease which preselects SCD victims.

The role of acute *coronary artery thrombosis* as a factor in precipitating SCD is less clear.[210–213] In one study of 100 consecutive sudden coronary death victims, 44 per cent had major (more than 50 per cent luminal occlusion) recent coronary thrombi, 30 per cent had minor occlusive thrombi, and 21 per cent had plaque fissuring.[210] Only 5 per cent had no acute coronary artery changes; 65 per cent of the thrombi occurred at sites of preexisting high-grade stenoses, and an additional 19 per cent were found at sites of more than 50 per cent stenosis. In a subsequent study by the same investigators, 50/168 victims (30 per cent) had occlusive intraluminal coronary thrombi, and 73 (44 per cent) had mural intraluminal thrombi.[211] Single-vessel disease, acute infarction at postmortem examination, and prodromal symptoms were associated with the presence of thrombi.

An overview of the major studies on the incidence of acute thrombotic occlusions, in which the definition of sudden death ranges from 15 minutes to 24 hours, reveals wide variation in the reported frequency of recent coronary thrombosis in sudden death. It ranges from 15 to 64 per cent, but the majority of studies which used 6 hours or less as the definition of "sudden" had frequencies of less than 40 per cent.[206,207,210-213] Factors which confound the analysis of such data include relations between platelet aggregates and thrombus formation and the spontaneous lysis of clots.

Baba et al.[213] reported the presence of *organizing* thrombus in about 31 per cent of 121 sudden coronary heart disease deaths. They were commonly associated with sites of more than 75 per cent chronic obstruction and with concomitant acute lesions at the same sites, leading to the speculation that clinical events 5 to 7 days before death might create a substrate for fatal acute coronal events. *Coronary artery spasm,* an established cause of acute ischemia, also may cause SCD, and is recognizable in rare instances at postmortem examination.[214]

THE MYOCARDIUM. Myocardial pathology in SCD caused by coronary heart disease reflects the extensive atherosclerosis which usually is present. Studies in nonsurvivors of prehospital cardiac arrest and from epidemiological sources indicate that healed myocardial infarction is a common finding in sudden coronary death victims, with most investigators reporting frequencies ranging from 40 to more than 70 per cent.[8,190,215,216] For example, Newman and coworkers[215,216] reported that 72 per cent of males in a 25-to-44-year age group who died suddenly (24 or fewer hours) with no previous clinical history of coronary heart disease had scars of large (63 per cent) or small (less than 1 cm cross-sectional area, 9 per cent) areas of healed myocardial necrosis. The incidence of acute myocardial infarction is considerably less, with cytopathological evidence of recent myocardial infarction averaging about 20 per cent. Even though the problem of cytopathological recognition of early acute myocardial infarction confounds some of these observations, the figures fit quite well with studies in out-of-hospital cardiac arrest survivors which suggest that the incidence of new myocardial infarction is in the range of only 20 to 30 per cent.

VENTRICULAR HYPERTROPHY AND SUDDEN DEATH

Myocardial hypertrophy may interact with acute or chronic ischemia, but the nature of the interaction in SCD is incompletely understood.[217] The correlation between increased heart weight and severity of coronary heart disease in SCD victims is not close[208]; heart weights are higher in SCD victims than in those with non–sudden death despite similar prevalence of history of hypertension before death.[8] Anderson[104] interprets these observations to suggest that left ventricular hypertrophy itself may be a predisposing factor to SCD. Although there are data to suggest increased susceptibility to potentially lethal ventricular arrhythmias in patients with left ventricular hypertrophy of many causes,[105,218] the study by Roberts and Podolak[219] on massively enlarged hearts (i.e., more than 1000 gm) did not indicate an excess incidence of SCD in such patients. However, the underlying pathology in that study was dominated by lesions that produce volume overload.

SPECIALIZED CONDUCTING SYSTEM IN SCD

Pathological data on the specialized conducting system of victims of SCD are relatively sparse. Lie[220] studied the specialized conducting system of 49 of 120 SCD patients with no previous history of coronary heart disease who died within 6 hours of onset of symptoms. Thirty-nine patients had acute myocardial infarction and 10 did not. Two patients with acute anteroseptal infarctions had hemorrhage and/or infarction involving the AV node and peripheral bundle branches. Luminal narrowing of the artery to the AV node was present in 50 per cent, but there were no thromboses of vessels to the specialized conducting system. Evidence of ischemic injury was present with an equal frequency in SCD[220] and myocardial infarction patients.[221]

TABLE 26–4 PATHOLOGICAL CHANGES IN THE CARDIAC CONDUCTION SYSTEM AND CARDIAC NERVES IN SUDDEN CARDIAC DEATH

SPECIALIZED CONDUCTION SYSTEM

A. Chronic fibrosis
   1. Primary
   2. Secondary
B. Acute ischemic injury
C. Inflammatory and infiltrative diseases
D. Focal diseases—granulomas, tumors
E. Arteritis
F. Abnormal postnatal morphogenesis

CARDIAC NERVES

A. Cardiac plexus disruption
B. Neural depletion in cardiomyopathy
C. Viral neuropathy
D. Neural ganglionitis
E. Neurotoxic injury
F. Hereditary neuropathy
G. Extrinsic nerve abnormalities

Fibrosis of the specialized conducting system is a common but nonspecific endpoint of multiple causes. Although this process is associated with AV block or intraventricular conduction abnormalities, its role in SCD is uncertain. Lev's and Lenegre's diseases, ischemic injury caused by small-vessel disease, and numerous infiltrative or inflammatory processes all may result in such changes (Table 26–4). In addition, active inflammatory processes such as myocarditis and infiltrative processes such as amyloidosis, scleroderma, hemochromatosis, and morbid obesity all may damage or destroy the AV node and/or bundle of His and result in AV block.[222] Focal diseases such as sarcoidosis, Whipple's disease, and rheumatoid arthritis also may involve the conducting system. These various categories of conducting system disease have been considered as possible pathological substrates for SCD which may be overlooked because of the difficulty in doing careful postmortem examinations of the conducting system routinely.[222] Focal involvement of conducting tissue by tumors (especially mesothelioma of the AV node but also lymphoma, carcinoma, rhabdomyoma, and fibroma) also has been reported,[222] and rare cases of SCD have been associated with these lesions. It has been suggested that abnormal postnatal morphogenesis of the specialized conducting system may be a significant factor in some SCD's in infants and children.[222]

CARDIONEUROPATHY AND SCD

Diseases of cardiac nerves have recently received attention for their possible role in SCD.[223,224] Cardiac neural involvement may be the result of random damage to neural elements within the myocardium (i.e., "secondary" cardioneuropathy), or may be "primary," such as in a selective cardiac viral neuropathy.[224] Secondary involvement may be a consequence of ischemic neural injury in coronary heart disease and has been postulated to result in autonomic destabilization, enhancing the propensity to arrhythmias. There are some experimental data in support of this hypothesis, and a new clinical technique for imaging cardiac neural fibers suggests a changing pattern over time after myocardial infarction.[225-228] Involvement of neural plexuses, with or without conducting system involvement, has been observed at necropsy in 54 per cent of patients who died within 24 hours of onset of myocardial infarction.[223] Specific causes for primary cardioneuropathies are less obvious. Viral, neurotoxic, and hereditary causes (e.g., progressive muscular dystrophy and Friedreich's ataxia) have been emphasized.

Disordered extrinsic neural involvement of the heart usually is considered to be functional, such as in prolonged Q-T interval syndrome; however, stellate ganglion inflammation has been observed in some tissues removed surgically for symptomatic Q-T prolongation in hereditary Q-T syndrome[229] or after myocardial infarction.[230] The possible significance of such extrinsic cardiac neural involvement is not yet clear.[230]

MECHANISMS AND PATHOPHYSIOLOGY OF CARDIAC ARREST

The occurrence of potentially lethal tachyarrhythmias, or of severe bradyarrhythmia or asystole, is the end of a cascade of pathophysiological abnormalities which result from com-

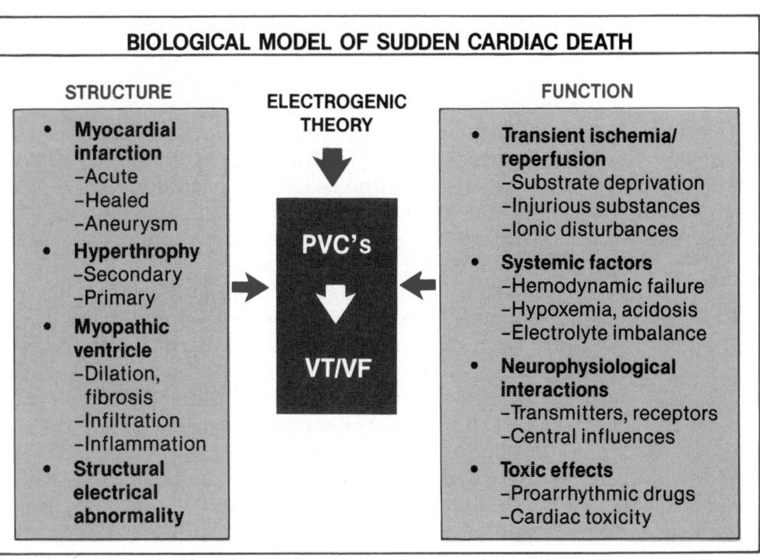

FIGURE 26-5. Biological model of sudden cardiac death. Structural cardiac abnormalities are commonly thought of as the causative basis for SCD. However, functional alterations of this substrate usually are required to alter stability of the myocardium, permitting a potentially fatal arrhythmia to be initiated. In this conceptual model, short- or long-term structural abnormalities interact with functional modulations to influence the propensity for premature ventricular contractions (PVCs) to initiate ventricular tachycardia or fibrillation (VT/VF). (From Myerburg, R.J., et al.: A biological approach to sudden cardiac death: Structure, function, and cause. Am. J. Cardiol. *63*:1512, 1989.)

plex interactions between coronary vascular events, myocardial injury, variations in autonomic tone, and/or the metabolic and electrolyte state of the myocardium. There is no uniform hypothesis regarding mechanisms by which these elements interact to lead to the final pathway of lethal arrhythmias. However, Figure 26-5 shows a model of the pathophysiology of SCD, in which the central event is the initiation of a potentially fatal arrhythmia. This event is predisposed to by a variety of *structural abnormalities* and modulated by *functional variations*.[231]

Pathophysiological Mechanisms of Lethal Tachyarrhythmias

CORONARY ARTERY STRUCTURE AND FUNCTION. In that large majority of SCDs associated with coronary atherosclerosis, the distribution of chronic arterial narrowing has been well defined by pathological studies.[43,206,207] However, the specific mechanisms by which these lesions lead to potentially lethal disturbances of electrical stability are poorly understood. Steady-state reductions in regional myocardial blood flow, in the absence of superimposed acute lesions, may create a setting in which alterations in the metabolic or electrolyte state of the myocardium, or neural fluctuations will result in loss of electrical stability.[121] Increased myocardial oxygen demand with a fixed supply may be the mechanism of exercise-induced arrhythmias and sudden death during intense physical activity in athletes or others whose heart disease had not previously become clinically manifested.[85,86,118-120,128,188,189,232] Vasoactive events leading to acute reduction in regional myocardial blood flow in the presence of a normal or previously compromised circulation constitute a common cause of transient ischemia, angina pectoris, arrhythmias, and perhaps SCD.[96,101] Coronary artery spasm or modulation of coronary collateral flow exposes the myocardium to the double hazard of transient ischemia and reperfusion.[233] The mechanism of production of spasm is unclear, although sites of endothelial disease appear to predispose.[234] A role of the autonomic nervous system, particularly mechanisms related to alpha-adrenoceptor activity, has been suggested[235-237]; vagal activity also may be involved in the production of spasm.[238] However, neurogenic influences do not appear to be a sine qua non for the production of spasm. Vessel susceptibility and humoral factors, particularly those related to platelet activation and aggregation,[239] also must be considered.

Recent studies have refocused attention on platelet aggregation or thrombosis or both as key events in the initiation of lethal arrhythmias.[206,210,211,240] Chronic stable atherosclerotic plaques appear to undergo endothelial damage, with plaque fissuring leading to platelet activation and aggregation, followed by thrombosis. In addition to initiating the thrombus, platelet activation produces a series of biochemical alterations which may enhance or retard susceptibility to VF by means of vasomotor modulation.[241] The frequency of VF induced by acute coronary occlusion in dogs has been markedly reduced by prostacyclin at doses sufficient to prevent platelet aggregation.[242] Hammon and Oates studied the effects of thromboxane synthetase inhibitors[241] and demonstrated protection against the induction of experimental VF, presumably by blocking conversion of PGH_2 to thromboxane A_2, which theoretically shunts accumulated PGH_2 to metabolic pathways that favor conversion to prostacyclin. Inhibition of cyclooxygenase by concurrent indomethacin administration gave further support to the hypothesis that PGH_2 shunting to other prostaglandin pathways might protect against VF by prostacyclin production. The possibility that inhibition of prostacyclin production might enhance the risk of VF[241] is supported by the finding from the Aspirin-Myocardial Infarction Study that the incidence of recurrent myocardial infarction was reduced by aspirin, but the relative and perhaps absolute numbers of SCD tended to increase.[243]

A number of pieces of indirect evidence support the possibility that more than the mechanical consequences to flow is involved in platelet-activated thrombosis of coronary arteries in SCD. Davies and Thomas[210] pointed out that 95 of 100 subjects who died suddenly (fewer than 6 hours after the onset of symptoms) had acute coronary thrombi, plaque fissuring, or both. This incidence was considerably higher than in many previous reports, but it is noteworthy that only 44 per cent of the patients had the largest thrombus occluding 51 per cent or more of the cross-sectional area of the involved vessel, and only 18 per cent of the patients had more than 75 per cent occlusion. This raises questions whether mechanical obstruction to flow was dominant, or whether the high incidence of nonoccluding thrombi simply reflected the state of activation of the platelets. The discrepancy between the relatively high incidence of acute thrombi in postmortem studies and the low incidence of evolution of new myocardial infarction among survivors of out-of-hospital VF[18-20,244] highlights this question. Spontaneous thrombolysis or a dominant role of spasm induced by platelet products, or a combination, may explain this discrepancy.

THE UNSTABLE MYOCARDIUM AND INITIATION OF LETHAL ARRHYTHMIAS. The onset of acute ischemia produces immediate electrical, mechanical, and biochemical dysfunction of cardiac muscle (Fig. 26-5). The specialized conducting tissue is more resistant to acute ischemia than is working myocardium, and therefore the electrophysiological consequences are less intense and delayed in onset in this tissue.[245] Experimental studies also have provided data on the long-term consequences of left ventricular hypertrophy and healed experimental myocardial infarction. Tissue exposed to chronic stress produced by long-term left ventricular pressure overload[246] and tissue which has healed after ischemic injury[247,248] both show lasting cellular electrophysiological abnormalities, including regional changes in transmembrane action potentials and refractory periods, which may establish a propensity to chronic lethal arrhythmias. In fact, these studies have demonstrated that acute ischemic injury or acute myocardial infarction in the presence of healed myocardial infarction is more arrhythmogenic than is the same extent of acute ischemia in previously normal tissue.[248,249] In addition to the direct effect of ischemia on normal or previously abnormal tissue, it is possible that reperfusion after transient ischemia may cause lethal arrhythmias.[250,251] Reperfusion of ischemic areas may occur by three mechanisms: (1) spontaneous thrombolysis, (2) collateral flow from other coronary vascular beds to the ischemic bed, and (3) reversal of vasospasm.

ELECTROPHYSIOLOGICAL EFFECTS OF ACUTE ISCHEMIA. Within the first minutes after experimental coronary ligation there is a propensity to ventricular arrhythmias which abates after 30 minutes and reappears after several hours.[252] The initial 30 minutes of arrhythmias is divided into two periods, the first of which lasts for about 10 minutes and is presumably directly related to the initial ischemic injury. The second period (20 to 30 minutes) may be related either to reperfusion of ischemic areas or to the evolution of differing injury patterns in the epicardial and endocardial muscle.[253,254] At a myocardial cellular level, the immediate consequences of ischemia, which include loss of integrity of cell membranes with efflux of K^+, influx of Ca^{++}, acidosis, reduction of transmembrane resting potentials, and enhanced automaticity in some tissues, are followed by a separate series of changes during reperfusion. Those of particular current interest are the possible continued influx of Ca^{++} which may produce electrical instability,[251,255] responses to alpha- and/or beta-adrenoceptor stimulation,[227,228,256–258] and neurophysiologically induced afterdepolarization as triggering responses for Ca^{++}-dependent arrhythmias.[255–262] Other possible mechanisms studied experimentally include formation of superoxide radicals in reperfusion arrhythmias,[259,260] a direct or indirect role of angiotensin-converting enzyme activity in potentially lethal arrhythmias,[261] and differential responses of endocardial and epicardial muscle activation times and refractory periods during ischemia or reperfusion.[253,263]

The importance of the myocardial response to the onset of ischemia has been emphasized, on the basis of the demonstration of dramatic cellular electrophysiological changes during the first 30 seconds after coronary occlusion.[264] However, the state of the myocardium at the time of onset of ischemia is a critical additional factor. Tissue healed after previous injury appears to be more susceptible to the electrical destabilizing effects of acute ischemia, as is chronically hypertrophied muscle. Of more direct clinical relevance is the suggestion that K^+ depletion by diuretics and clinical hypokalemia may make ventricular myocardium more susceptible to potentially lethal arrhythmias.[265–267] The association of metabolic and electrolyte abnormalities, as well as neurophysiological and neurohumoral changes,[121,262,268–271] with SCD emphasizes the importance of changes in the myocardial substrate in the propensity to lethal arrhythmias. Most direct among myocardial metabolic changes in response to ischemia are acute increase in interstitial K^+ levels to values exceeding 15 mM, a fall in tissue pH to below 6.0, changes in adrenoceptor activity, and alterations in autonomic nerve traffic,[126] all of which tend to create and maintain electrical instability, especially if regional in distribution. Other metabolic changes such as cyclic adenosine monophosphate elevation, accumulation of free fatty acids and their metabolites, formation of lysophosphoglycerides, and impaired myocardial glycolysis also have been suggested as myocardial destabilizing influences.[272]

THE TRANSITION FROM MYOCARDIAL INSTABILITY TO POTENTIALLY LETHAL ARRHYTHMIAS. *The combination of a triggering event and a susceptible myocardium is evolving as a fundamental electrophysiological concept for the mechanism of initiation of potentially lethal arrhythmias* (Fig. 26–5). The endpoint of their interaction is disorganization of patterns of myocardial activation, usually by premature impulses (i.e., the "trigger"), into multiple uncoordinated reentrant pathways (i.e., ventricular fibrillation). Clinical,[69,273] experimental,[274] and pharmacological[247] data all suggest that triggering events and the myocardial instability permitting the evolution of lethal arrhythmias may be dissociated from one another. In the absence of myocardial vulnerability, many triggering events, such as frequent and complex PVCs, may be innocuous.

The onset of ischemia is accompanied by abrupt reduction in transmembrane resting potential and amplitude and in duration of the action potential in the affected area,[264] with little change in remote areas. When ischemic cells depolarize to resting potentials less than −60 mV, they may become inexcitable and of little electrophysiological importance. As they are depolarizing to that range, however, or repolarizing as a consequence of reperfusion, the membranes pass through ranges of reduced excitability, upstroke velocity, and time courses of repolarization. These characteristics result in slow conduction and electrophysiological instability. These events that occur regionally in ischemic myocardium, adjacent to nonischemic tissue, create a setting for the key elements of reentry —slow conduction and unidirectional block—which makes them vulnerable to reentrant arrhythmias. When premature impulses are generated in this environment, they may further alter the dispersion of recovery between ischemic tissue, chronically abnormal tissue, and normal cells,[248,249] ultimately leading to complete disorganization and VF. VF is probably not a consequence only of reentry.[126] Rapid-enhanced automaticity caused by ischemic injury to the specialized conducting tissue, or slow-channel–triggered activity in partially depolarized tissue, may result in rapid bursts of automatic activity which also could lead to failure of coordinated conduction and VF.

The dispersion of refractory periods produced by acute ischemia, which provides the substrate for reentrant tachycardias and VF, may be further enhanced by a healed ischemic injury. The time course of repolarization is lengthened after healing of ischemic injury[247,248] and shortened by acute ischemia.[248,251,264] The coexistence of the two appears to make the ventricle more susceptible to sustained arrhythmias in some experimental models.[248]

Bradyarrhythmias and Asystolic Arrest

The basic electrophysiological mechanism in this form of arrest is failure of normal subordinate automatic activity to assume pacemaking function of the heart in the absence of normal function of the sinus node and/or AV junction. Bradyarrhythmic and asystolic arrests are more common in severely diseased hearts, and probably represent diffuse involvement of subendocardial Purkinje fibers. Systemic influences which increase extracellular K^+ concentration, such as anoxia, acidosis, shock, renal failure, trauma, and hypothermia, may result in partial depolarization of normal or already diseased pacemaker cells in the His-Purkinje system, with a decrease in the slope of spontaneous phase 4 depolarization, and ultimate loss of automaticity.[275] These processes usually produce global dysfunction of automatic cell activity, in contrast to the regional dysfunction more common in acute ischemia. Functionally depressed automatic cells (e.g., owing to increased extracellular K^+ concentration) are more susceptible to overdrive suppression. Under these conditions, brief bursts of tachycardia may be followed by prolonged asystolic periods, with further depression of automaticity by the consequent acidosis and increased local K^+ concentration or by changes in adrenergic tone. The ultimate consequence may be degeneration into VF or persistent asystole.

Electromechanical Dissociation

Electromechanical dissociation has been separated into *primary* and *secondary* forms. The common denominator in both is continued electrical rhythmicity of the heart in the absence of effective mechanical function. The secondary form includes those causes which result from an abrupt cessation of cardiac venous return, such as massive pulmonary embolism, acute malfunction of prosthetic valves, exsanguination, and cardiac tamponade from hemopericardium. The primary form is the more familiar; in it none of these obvious mechanical factors are present, but ventricular muscle fails to produce an effective contraction despite continued electrical activity (i.e., *failure of electromechanical coupling*). Although this usually occurs as an end-stage event in advanced heart disease, it may be seen in patients with acute ischemic events or, more commonly, after electrical resuscitation from a prolonged cardiac arrest. Although not thoroughly understood, it appears that global ischemia or diffuse disease, or both, provide the pathophysiological substrate and that the proximate mechanism for failure of electromechanical coupling may be abnormal intracellular Ca^{++} metabolism, intracellular acidosis, and perhaps adenosine triphosphate depletion.

CLINICAL CHARACTERISTICS OF THE PATIENT WITH CARDIAC ARREST

Before the development of coronary care units, the in-hospital mortality owing to acute myocardial infarction was in the range of 25 to 30 per cent.[277] The current in-hospital mortality rate (see Chap. 39) is lower in large part because of prevention of in-hospital sudden deaths, now that acute potentially lethal arrhythmias in this setting are preventable or reversible.[278] However, the prior relationship between acute myocardial infarction and SCD in the in-hospital setting ingrained the concept of the association between the two, which was then extrapolated to the setting of out-of-hospital cardiac arrests. With the advent of community-based emergency rescue systems, leading to cohorts of survivors of out-of-hospital cardiac arrest, it rapidly became apparent that the majority of these cardiac arrests were, in fact, not associated with the evolution of a new transmural myocardial infarction. Studies from Seattle[19] and from Miami[244] demonstrated that only a minority of survivors of out-of-hospital VF had clinical evidence indicating that a new transmural myocardial infarction was associated with the cardiac arrest. In the Seattle study only one of five survivors had new transmural infarctions.[19] These studies led to the conclusion that in the majority of such patients, transient pathophysiological events were responsible for cardiac arrest. That this conclusion is reasonable and has clinical relevance is supported by the fact that the recurrence rate in survivors of prehospital cardiac arrest is low in the subgroup of patients who had documentation of a new transmural myocardial infarction. It was found to be 30 per cent at 1 year and 45 per cent at 2 years in those survivors who did not have a new transmural myocardial infarction.[18,19] These recurrence rates have decreased more recently,[46] possibly owing in part to long-term interventions.

Clinical cardiac arrest and SCD are best described in the framework of the same four phases of the event used to establish definitions (see Fig. 26–1): prodromes, onset of the terminal event, the cardiac arrest, and progression to biological death or survival.

PRODROMAL SYMPTOMS

Patients at risk for SCD may have prodromes such as chest pain, dyspnea, weakness or fatigue, palpitations, and a number of nonspecific complaints. Several epidemiological and clinical studies demonstrated that such symptoms may presage coronary events, particularly myocardial infarction and SCD,[8,47,279] and result in contact with the medical system weeks to months before SCD.[279] In a prospective study in Edinburgh, Scotland, however, only 12 per cent of victims of SCD had consulted a physician because of new or worsening angina pectoris during periods of up to 6 months before death.[280] In contrast, 33 per cent of myocardial infarction patients had consulted their physicians for this complaint. Nonetheless, 46 per cent of victims of SCD had seen a physician within 4 weeks before death, but three-fourths of them had sought medical help for complaints which appeared to be unrelated to the heart. Liberthson et al.,[18] in a study of patients successfully resuscitated after prehospital cardiac arrest, noted that 28 per cent reported retrospectively that they had had new or changing angina pectoris or dyspnea in the 4 weeks before arrest, and that 31 per cent had seen a physician during this time but only 12 per cent because of these symptoms. Patients who have chest pain as a prodrome to SCD appear to have a higher probability of intraluminal coronary thrombosis at postmortem examination.[211] Attempts to identify early prodromal symptoms which are more specific for the patient at risk for SCD have not yet been successful. Fatigue has been a particularly common symptom in the days or weeks before SCD in a number of studies,[279] but this symptom is nonspecific. The prodromata that occur within the last hours or minutes before cardiac arrest are more specific for heart disease and may include symptoms of arrhythmias, ischemia, or heart failure.[21,281] Liberthson et al.[207] reported specific cardiac symptoms at a mean interval of about 3.8 hours before collapse in 24 per cent of victims of SCD. However, most studies have reported such symptoms even less commonly, particularly when victims whose deaths were instantaneous are included.[8]

ONSET OF THE TERMINAL EVENT

The period of 1 hour or less between acute changes in cardiovascular status and the cardiac arrest itself, which has been defined as the "onset of the terminal event," is a subject about which there is limited information. Reports from ambulatory monitor recordings fortuitously obtained at the time of unexpected cardiac arrest indicate dynamic change in cardiac electrical activity during the minutes or hours before the onset of cardiac arrest.[282–284] These reports suggest that increasing heart rate and advancing grades of ventricular ectopy—including R-on-T phenomenon and VT—are common antecedents of VF. Although these recordings suggest transient electrophysiological destabilization of the myocardium, the extent to which these objective observations are paralleled by clinical symptoms is less well documented. SCDs caused by either arrhythmias or acute circulatory failure mechanisms involve a high incidence of acute myocardial disorders at the onset of the terminal event; such disorders are more likely to be ischemic when the death is due to arrhythmias and to be associated with low-output states or myocardial anoxia when the deaths are due to circulatory failure.[21,285]

Abrupt, unexpected loss of effective circulation may be caused by cardiac arrhythmias or mechanical disturbances, but the majority of such events that terminate in SCD are arrhythmic in origin. Hinkle and Thaler[285] classified cardiac deaths among 142 subjects who died during a follow-up of 5 to 10 years. Class I was labeled arrhythmic death and Class II was death caused by circulatory failure. The distinction between the two classes was based on whether circulatory failure preceded (Class II) or followed (Class I) the disappearance of the pulse. Among deaths which occurred less than 1 hour after the onset of the terminal illness, 93 per cent were due to arrhythmias; in addition, 90 per cent of deaths caused by heart disease were initiated by arrhythmic events rather than circulatory failure. Table 26–5 demonstrates that deaths caused by circulatory failure occurred predominantly in patients who could be identified as having terminal illnesses (95 per cent were comatose), were associated more frequently with bradyarrhythmias than with VF as the terminal arrhythmias, and

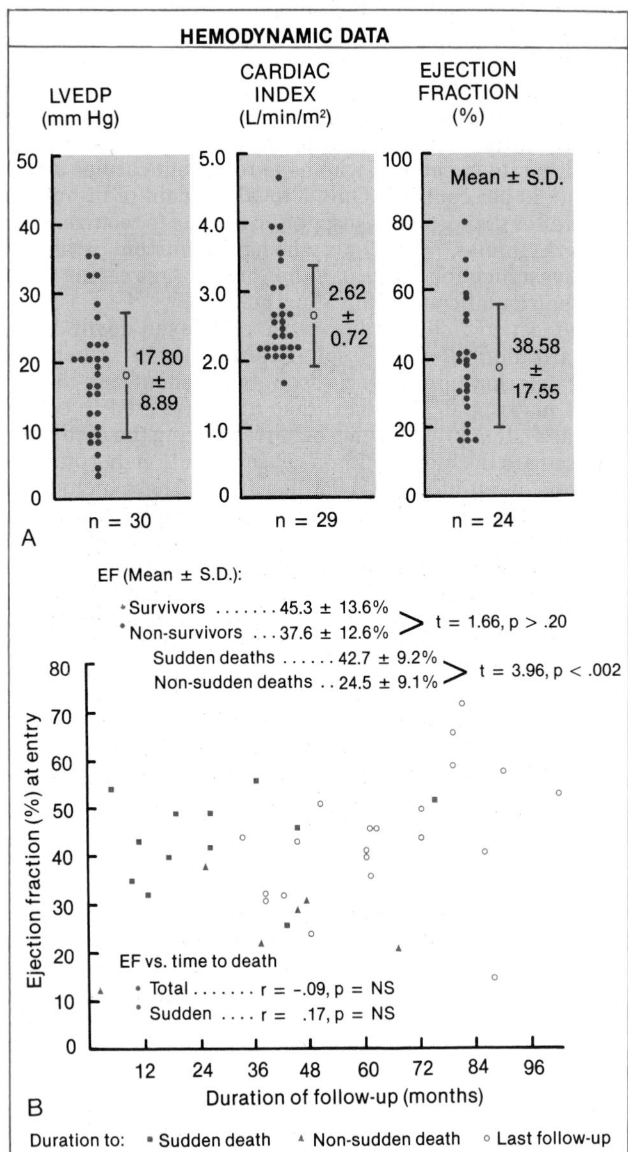

FIGURE 26–6. *A*, **Hemodynamic data from prehospital cardiac arrest victims studied during initial post-arrest hospitalization, and *B*, the relation between ejection fraction (EF) at initial study and long-term outcome. These data indicate a broad range of cardiac function (*A*), and a statistically insignificant difference between EF at entry in long-term survivors and in recurrent cardiac arrest victims (*B*). Severity of decreased EF was more predictive of non-sudden deaths. (*A*, From Myerburg, R.J., et al.: Clinical, electrophysiologic, and hemodynamic profile of patients resuscitated from prehospital cardiac arrest. Am. J. Med. *68*:568, 1980. *B*, From Myerburg, R. J., et al.: Long-term survival after prehospital cardiac arrest: Analysis of outcome during an 8-year study. Circulation *70*:538, 1984, by permission of the American Heart Association, Inc.)**

from severe dysfunction to normal or near-normal measurements in as many as 50 per cent of the survivors (Fig. 26–6*A*).[46] The author found that the ejection fraction of those who died during follow-up was lower than that of the long-term survivors (38 versus 45 per cent, respectively).[20,46] Patients who died of recurrent cardiac arrest had higher ejection fractions than those who died non–sudden cardiac deaths (43 versus 25 per cent) (Fig. 26–6*B*). Ritchie et al.[305] reported on studies of left ventricular function by radionuclide techniques in 154 survivors of out-of-hospital VF, 91 of whom had both rest and exercise studies. The mean ejection fraction at rest was 40 per cent, with 29 per cent having values greater than 50 per cent. Only 3 of 91 patients (3 per cent) studied had a normal increase (>5 per cent) in ejection fraction during exertion. Only 18 per cent had normal resting wall motion. The ejection fraction at rest was the best predictor of death during follow-up.[305] Fifty per cent of survivors studied by cardiac catheterization and angiography had ejection fractions below 50 per cent, and 30 per cent had left ventricular end-diastolic pressures greater than 15 mm Hg[306]; in this study, ejection fraction and severity of wall motion abnormality correlated with risk of recurrent cardiac arrest.

Coronary angiographic studies in survivors of out-of-hospital cardiac arrest have shown that as a group, this population tends to have extensive disease but no specific pattern of abnormalities. Moderate to severe stenosis of the left main coronary artery was present in only 8 per cent of the patients in one series,[306] and only 9 per cent in another,[20] frequencies not different from those in the overall population of coronary heart disease patients. Significant lesions in two or more vessels were present in 74 per cent of the patients who had any coronary lesions in one study,[20] and 94 per cent of the patients in another had 70 per cent or less stenosis in one or more arteries.[306] Among patients who had recurrent cardiac arrests, the incidence of triple-vessel disease was higher than among those who did not.

Exercise testing is commonly used to evaluate the need for and response to antiischemic therapy in survivors of prehospital cardiac arrest. The incidence of positive tests related to ischemia is relatively low, although termination of testing because of fatigue is common.[244,303,307] Mortality during follow-up is greater in patients who had angina or failure of a normal rise in systolic blood pressure occurring during exercise.[307]

Electrocardiographic observations in survivors of out-of-hospital cardiac arrest have proved of value only for discriminating risk of recurrence in those whose arrest was associated with new transmural myocardial infarction. Patients who develop documented new Q waves in association with cardiac arrest are at much lower risk for recurrence.[18,244,308] A higher incidence of repolarization abnormalities (ST-segment depression, flat T waves, prolonged QTc) occurs in out-of-hospital cardiac arrest survivors than in post-myocardial infarction patients, and these might be markers for increased risk.[309]

Lower serum K^+ levels were observed in survivors of cardiac arrest than in patients with acute myocardial infarction or stable coronary heart disease.[310] The investigators concluded that this was a consequence of resuscitation interventions, rather than a preexisting state owing to chronic diuretic use. Low ionized Ca^{++} levels, with normal total calcium levels, also were observed during resuscitation from out-of-hospital cardiac arrest.[311] Higher resting lactate levels have been reported in out-of-hospital cardiac arrest survivors than in normal subjects.[312] Lactate levels correlated inversely with ejection fractions and directly with PVC frequency and complexity.

Studies from the early 1970's in both Miami[18] and Seattle[19] indicated that the risk of recurrent cardiac arrest in the first year after surviving an initial event was about 30 per cent and at 2 years was 45 per cent. Total mortality at 2 years was about 60 per cent in both studies. In both of these studies, less than half of the patients followed were being treated with long-term antiarrhythmic therapy; beta-adrenoceptor blocker therapy was in its infancy, and Ca^{++}-entry blockers were not yet available. Thus these figures appear to be as close to valid natural history figures as possible. However, they can serve only as historical control figures for current observations, and thus are of limited value, since it is likely that risk of recurrent cardiac arrest is lower now than it was in the early 1970's.[313] Moreover, the risk of recurrent cardiac arrest/SCD appears to be lower for survivors with hypertrophic cardiomyopathy—about 33 per cent during a mean follow-up period of 7 years.[110] In a recent report of cardiac arrest survivors with and without successful medical and/or surgical antiarrhythmic end-points, the 1-year recurrent cardiac arrest rate was 14.5 per cent and the 2-year cumulative rate was 21.1 per cent, with a clustering of events within the first 6 to 12 months (i.e., time-dependent risk) (Fig. 26–7).[314]

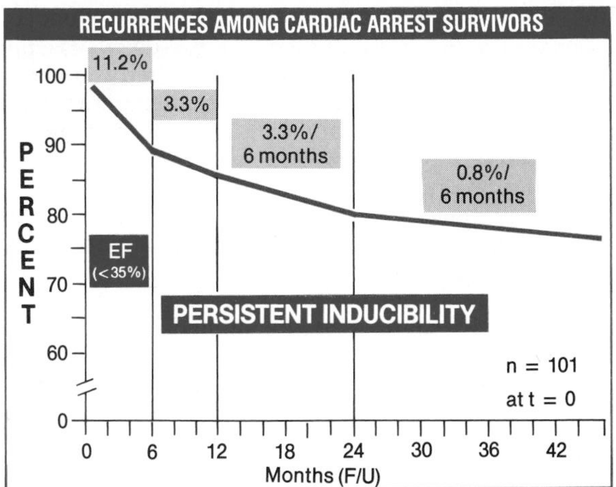

FIGURE 26-7. Time-dependence of recurrences among survivors of cardiac arrest. Actuarial analysis of occurrences among a population of 101 cardiac arrest survivors with coronary artery disease is demonstrated. The risk was highest in the first 6 months (11.2 per cent) and then fell to 3.3 per cent/6 months for the next three 6-month blocks. After 24 months the rate fell to 0.8 per cent/6 months. A low ejection fraction (EF) was the most powerful predictor of death during the first 6 months; subsequently, persistent inducibility during programmed stimulation, despite drug therapy or surgery, was the most powerful predictor. (Modified from Furukawa, T., et al.: Time-dependent risk of and predictors for cardiac arrest recurrence in survivors of out-of-hospital cardiac arrest with chronic coronary artery disease. Circulation *80*:599, 1989. The figure is reproduced from Myerburg, R. J., et al.: Sudden cardiac death: Structure, function and time-dependence of risk. Circulation [in press], permission of the American Heart Association, Inc.)

MANAGEMENT OF CARDIAC ARREST

COMMUNITY-BASED INTERVENTIONS IN OUT-OF-HOSPITAL CARDIAC ARREST

Systems for intervention in out-of-hospital cardiac arrest have their roots in the development of the coronary care unit (CCU) approach to the management of potentially lethal arrhythmias.[315] Previously, cardiac arrest in the setting of acute coronary events was almost uniformly fatal, wherever it occurred. With the development of the key elements of the CCU (i.e., continuous monitoring, CPR, effective acute drug therapy, and electrical management of tachycardias, bradycardias, and VF), there was a dramatic reduction in the immediate in-hospital mortality from potentially lethal arrhythmias occurring in the course of acute coronary events.[316] The next step toward the development of community-based intervention for cardiac arrest was the concept of the mobile coronary care unit,[317] which was based on the rationale of providing a CCU environment during the high-risk prehospital phase of acute myocardial infarction. Only a small extension in concept led to the development of community-based intervention systems designed to respond routinely to out-of-hospital cardiac arrests. The systems as developed in the United States are largely integrated into fire departments as emergency rescue systems. They employ paramedical personnel or emergency medical technicians trained in CPR and the use of telemetered monitoring equipment, defibrillators, and specific intravenous drug therapy. Although the initial prehospital intervention experience in Miami and Seattle[18,19] in the early 1970's yielded only 14 and 10 per cent survivals to discharge, respectively, later data indicate that such systems are becoming increasingly effective in saving lives.[292,308] By the mid-1970's, both had increased survival rates to about 25 per cent,[20,292] and by the early 1980's to 30 per cent or more.[292] Survival rates appear to have decreased since then, presumably because of the extension of rescue systems into less densely populated regions.[318]

IMPORTANCE OF ELECTRICAL MECHANISMS. The electrical mechanism of out-of-hospital cardiac arrest, as defined by the initial rhythm recorded by emergency rescue personnel, has a powerful impact on success of initial resuscitation and outcome, the latter measured in terms of patients discharged from the hospital alive. The subgroup of patients who are in sustained VT at the time of first contact, although the smallest group statistically, has the best outcome (Fig. 26–8). Eighty-eight per cent of patients in cardiac arrest due to VT were successfully resuscitated and admitted to the hospital alive, and 67 per cent were ultimately discharged alive.[20] However, this relatively low-risk group represents only 7 to 10 per cent of all cardiac arrests in studies reported to date. Because of the inherent time lag between collapse and initial recordings, it is possible that many more cardiac arrests begin as rapid sustained VT and degenerate into VF before arrival of emergency rescue personnel.

Patients who are in a bradyarrhythmia or asystole at initial contact have the worst prognosis; only 9 per cent of such patients in the Miami study were admitted to the hospital alive and none were discharged.[20] In a later experience there was some improvement in outcome, although it was strictly limited to those patients in whom the initial bradyarrhythmia recorded was an idioventricular rhythm which responded promptly to chronotropic agents in the field.[299] Bradyarrhythmias also have adverse prognostic implications after defibrillation from VF in the field. Patients who were defibrillated to an initial heart rate less than 60 beats/min, regardless of the specific bradyarrhythmic mechanism, had a poor prognosis, with 95 per cent of such patients dying either before hospitalization or in the hospital (Fig. 26–9).[18] In contrast, an initial heart rate in excess of 100 beats/min yielded a 43 per cent rate of discharge from hospital, with only 17 per cent of such patients dying before hospitalization, and 40 per cent during hospitalization. Heart rates between 60 and 100 beats/min after defibrillation yield intermediate results.

The outcome in the largest group of patients, those in whom VF is the initial rhythm recorded, is intermediate between sustained VT and bradyarrhythmia and asystole. Figure 26–8 demonstrates that 40 per cent of such patients were successfully resuscitated and admitted to the hospital alive, and 23 per cent were ultimately discharged alive.[20] More recent data indicate continued improvement in outcome. The proportion of each of the electrophysiological mechanisms responsible

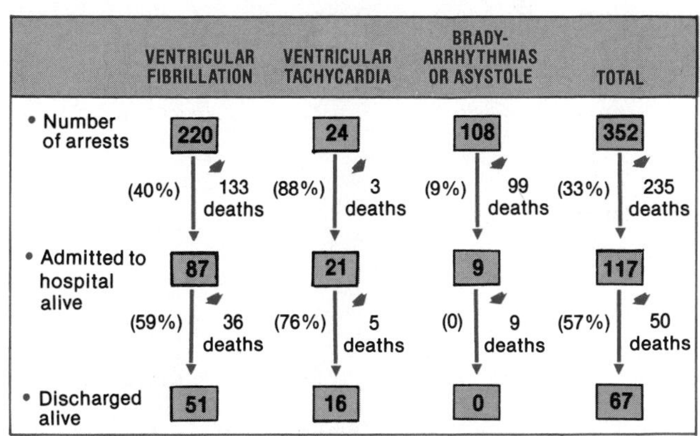

FIGURE 26-8. Survival related to initial electrophysiological mechanisms recorded during prehospital cardiac arrest. The figures highlighted by the boxes indicate the number of patients in each of three mechanism categories (ventricular fibrillation, ventricular tachycardia, and bradyarrhythmia/asystole), plus totals. In each category the data indicate the number of prehospital cardiac arrests (*top*), the number of patients successfully resuscitated in the field and transferred to the hospital alive (*middle*), and the number of patients who survived hospitalization and were discharged (*bottom*). The percentages in parentheses indicate survivals at each level of care for each category. (From Myerburg, R. J., et al.: Clinical, electrophysiologic, and hemodynamic profile of patients resuscitated from prehospital cardiac arrest. Am. J. Med. *68*:568, 1980.)

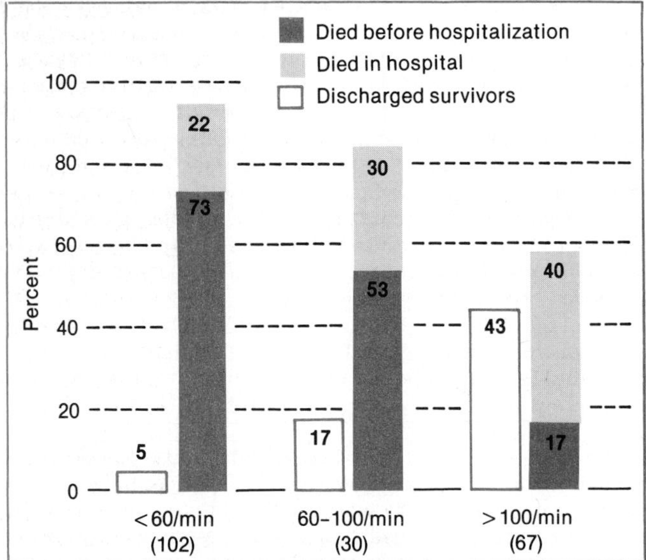

FIGURE 26–9. **Prognostic implication of initial heart rate after prehospital defibrillation. Prehospital and in-hospital deaths, and long-range survival (i.e., discharged survivors), are compared with the initial post-defibrillation heart rate: <60 beats/min, 60 to 100 beats/min, or >100 beats/min. (Modified from Liberthson, R. R., et al.: Prehospital ventricular fibrillation: Prognosis and follow-up course. Reprinted by permission of N. Engl. J. Med. *291*:317, 1974.)**

for cardiac arrest varies among the studies, with VF ranging from 65 to greater than 90 per cent of the study populations, and bradyarrhythmia and asystole ranging from 10 to 30 per cent.[20,281,292,308]

The factors which have contributed to improved outcome since the first observations in the early 1970's are incompletely understood. Both improved prehospital care and improvements in in-hospital technology and practices may contribute. Of these two general factors, the influence of prehospital care has been studied in more detail. Eisenberg and coworkers[319] compared initial resuscitation and ultimate discharge alive in two subgroups of patients, those who had standard CPR continuously from the arrival of emergency rescue personnel through transport to an emergency department where defibrillation took place, and another group in whom paramedics or emergency rescue personnel trained to defibrillate were allowed to do so at the scene of the cardiac arrest. The standard CPR technique resulted in only 23 per cent of patients arriving at the hospital alive and 7 per cent discharged alive, in contrast to the immediate defibrillation group in which 53 per cent arrived at the hospital alive and 26 per cent were discharged alive (Fig. 26–10). Subsequent data continue to support the concept that early defibrillation is a key element in improving survival rates.[292,298,320] Immediate defibrillation by ambulance technicians is especially important in rural communities, where it yields a 19 per cent survival, compared with only 3 per cent from standard CPR.[318]

A second element in prehospital care which appears to contribute to outcome is the role of bystander CPR by laypeople awaiting the arrival of emergency rescue personnel. It has been reported that although there was no significant difference in the percentage of patients successfully resuscitated and admitted to the hospital alive with (67 per cent) or without (61 per cent) bystander intervention, almost twice as many prehospital cardiac arrest victims were ultimately discharged alive when they had had bystander CPR (43 per cent) than when such support was not provided (22 per cent) (Fig. 26–11).[22] Central nervous system protection, expressed as early regaining of consciousness, appears to be the major protective element of bystander CPR.[22] The rationale for bystander intervention is further highlighted by the relation between time to defibrillation and survival, when analyzed as a function of time to initiation of basic CPR. It has been reported that more than 40 per cent of victims whose defibrillation and other advanced life support activities were instituted more than 8 minutes after collapse survived if basic CPR had been initi-

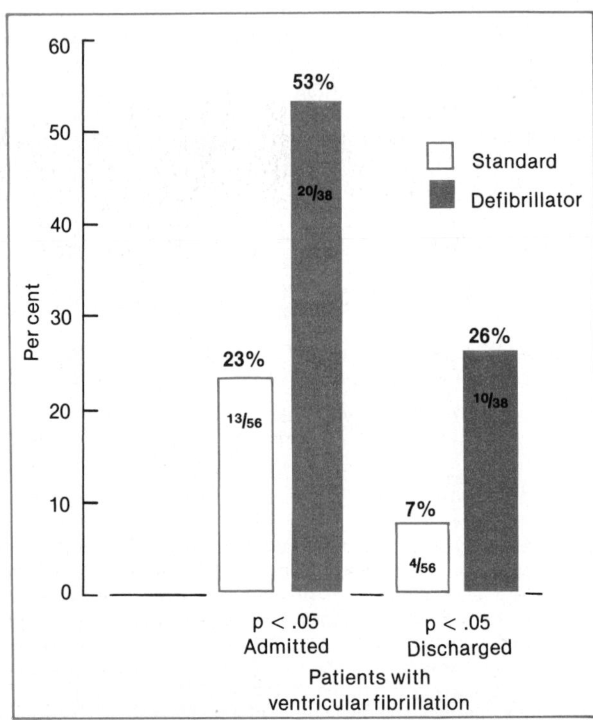

FIGURE 26–10. **Standard CPR by emergency medical technicians versus immediate defibrillation in the prehospital setting. Survival to admission and discharge with standard care versus early defibrillation. (Modified from Eisenberg, M. S., et al.: Treatment of out-of-hospital cardiac arrests with rapid defibrillation by emergency medical technicians. Reprinted by permission of N. Engl. J. Med. *302*:1379, 1980.)**

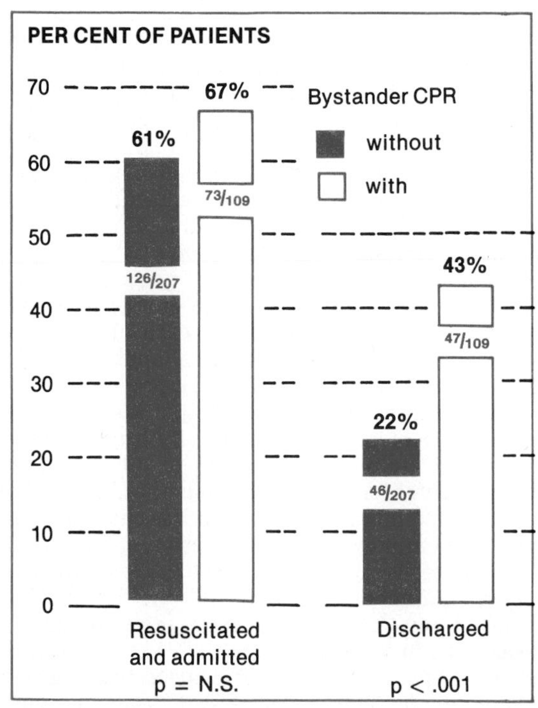

FIGURE 26–11. **Influence of lay bystander cardiopulmonary resuscitation (CPR) on outcome after prehospital cardiac arrest. There was no influence of bystander intervention on the proportion of victims resuscitated and admitted to the hospital alive, but those with bystander CPR had a significantly higher survival and rate of discharge than did those without bystander CPR. (From Myerburg, R. J., et al.: Survivors of prehospital cardiac arrest. J.A.M.A. *247*:1485, 1982. Copyright 1982, American Medical Association.)**

ated less than 2 minutes after onset of the arrest. A delay of more than 5 minutes to basic CPR was associated with no survivors.[292]

The time from onset of cardiac arrest to advanced life support influences outcome statistics. Mayer[321] reported improved short-term (to hospital admission) and long-term (to hospital discharge) survival rates for prehospital VF victims with short paramedic response times compared with those with long response times. Improvement in both early neurological status and survival occurs in the patients defibrillated by first responders, even if they are minimally trained emergency technicians allowed to carry out defibrillation as part of basic life support, compared with outcomes associated with awaiting more highly trained paramedics.[322] Thus the time to defibrillation plays a central role in determining outcome in cardiac arrest caused by VF. The development and deployment of automatic external defibrillators (p. 749) in the community hold promise for progress in the future.[323] This technology is a natural extension of lay bystander CPR.

The success of lidocaine in preventing primary VF in acute myocardial infarction in coronary care units[324] (p. 776) also led to the concept that routine prehospital administration of the drug might reduce prehospital cardiac arrests in these patients.[325] On the basis of encouraging results, its use by not only physicians and paramedics but also high-risk patients themselves has been suggested.[326]

MANAGEMENT OF THE INDIVIDUAL PATIENT

Management of the cardiac arrest victim is divided into five elements: (1) the initial response, (2) basic life support, (3) advanced life support and definitive resuscitative efforts, (4) post-cardiac arrest care, and (5) long-term management. The first of these can be applied by a broad population base, which includes physicians and nurses as well as paramedical personnel, emergency rescue technicians, and laypeople educated in bystander intervention. The requirements for specialized knowledge and skills become progressively more focused as the patient moves through post-cardiac arrest management and into long-term follow-up care.

INITIAL RESPONSE

This activity includes both diagnostic maneuvers and elementary interventions. The first action of the person(s) in attendance when an individual collapses unexpectedly must be *confirmation that collapse is due to a cardiac arrest.* A few seconds of observation for respiratory movements and skin color and simultaneous palpation of major arteries for the presence or absence of a pulse yields sufficient information to determine whether a life-threatening incident is in progress. The absence of carotid or femoral pulses, particularly if confirmed by the absence of an audible heartbeat, is the primary diagnostic criterion and can be performed accurately by trained laypeople. Skin color may be pale or intensely cyanotic. Absence of respiratory efforts, or the presence of only agonal respiratory efforts, in conjunction with an absent pulse, is diagnostic of cardiac arrest; however, respiratory efforts may persist for a minute or more after the onset of the arrest. In contrast, absence of respiratory efforts or severe stridor with persistence of a pulse suggests a primary respiratory arrest which will lead to a cardiac arrest in a short time. In the latter circumstance, initial efforts should include exploration of the oropharynx in search of a foreign body and the Heimlich maneuver, particularly if this occurs in a setting in which aspiration is likely (e.g., restaurant death or "cafe coronary").[197,198]

THUMPVERSION. Once the diagnosis of cardiac arrest is established, two immediate initial efforts are carried out: a blow to the chest (precordial thump, "thumpversion") and clearing the airway so that proper CPR can be carried out. Although the American Heart Association now recommends the use of precordial thumps only in monitored patients because of concern about converting VT to VF,[287,288] Caldwell and coworkers urged its continued use on the basis of a prospective study in 5000 patients.[327] In their study precordial thumps successfully reverted VF in 5 events, VT in 11, asystole in 2, and undefined cardiovascular collapse in 2 others in whom the electrical mechanism was unknown. In no instance was conversion of VT to VF observed. Because the latter is the major concern of the precordial thump technique, and electrical activity can be initiated by mechanical stimulation in the asystolic heart,[328] the technique may be used in the absence of monitoring when the diagnosis is clear and no other option is available. It should not be used unmonitored for the patient with a rapid tachycardia without complete loss of consciousness. For attempted thumpversion in cardiac arrest, one or two blows should be delivered firmly to the junction of the middle and lower thirds of the sternum from a height of 8 to 10 inches, but the effort should be abandoned if the patient does not immediately develop a spontaneous pulse and begin breathing. Another mechanical method, which requires that the patient is still conscious, is "cough-induced cardiac compression"[329] or "cough-version."[327,350] In the former a conscious act of forceful coughing by the patient in VF may support forward flow by cyclic increases in intrathoracic pressure[329]; the same act during sustained VT may cause conversion.[327,330]

AIRWAY. The next step is clearing the airway. This includes tilting the head backward and lifting the chin, in addition to seeking foreign bodies—including dentures—and removing them. The Heimlich maneuver should be performed if there is reason to suspect a foreign body lodged in the oropharynx. This entails wrapping the arms around the victim from the back and delivering a sharp thrust to the upper abdomen with a closed fist.[331] If it is not possible for the person in attendance to carry out the maneuver because of insufficient physical strength, mechanical dislodgment of the foreign body can sometimes be achieved by abdominal thrusts with the unconscious patient in a supine position. The Heimlich maneuver is not entirely benign: ruptured abdominal viscera in the victim have been reported,[332] as has an instance in which the rescuer disrupted his own aortic root and died.[333]

If there is strong suspicion that respiratory arrest precipitated cardiac arrest, particularly in the presence of a mechanical airway obstruction, a second precordial thump should be delivered after the airway is cleared.

BASIC LIFE SUPPORT

The goal of this activity is to maintain viability of the central nervous system, heart, and other vital organs until definitive intervention can be achieved. The activities included within basic life support encompass both the initial responses outlined above and their natural flow into establishing ventilation and perfusion.[334] This range of activities can be carried out not only by professional and paraprofessional personnel, but also by trained emergency technicians and laypeople. Time is the key issue, and there should be no delay between the diagnosis and preparatory efforts in the initial response and the institution of basic life support.

MOUTH-TO-MOUTH RESPIRATION. With the head properly placed and the oropharynx clear, mouth-to-mouth respiration can be initiated if no specific rescue equipment is available. To a large extent, the procedure used for establishing ventilation depends on the site at which the cardiac arrest occurs. A variety of devices are available, including plastic oropharyngeal airways, esophageal obturators, the masked AMBU bag, and endotracheal tubes. Intubation is the preferred procedure, but time should not be sacrificed even in the in-hospital setting while awaiting an endotracheal tube or a person trained to insert it quickly and properly. Thus, in the in-hospital setting, temporary support with AMBU bag venti-

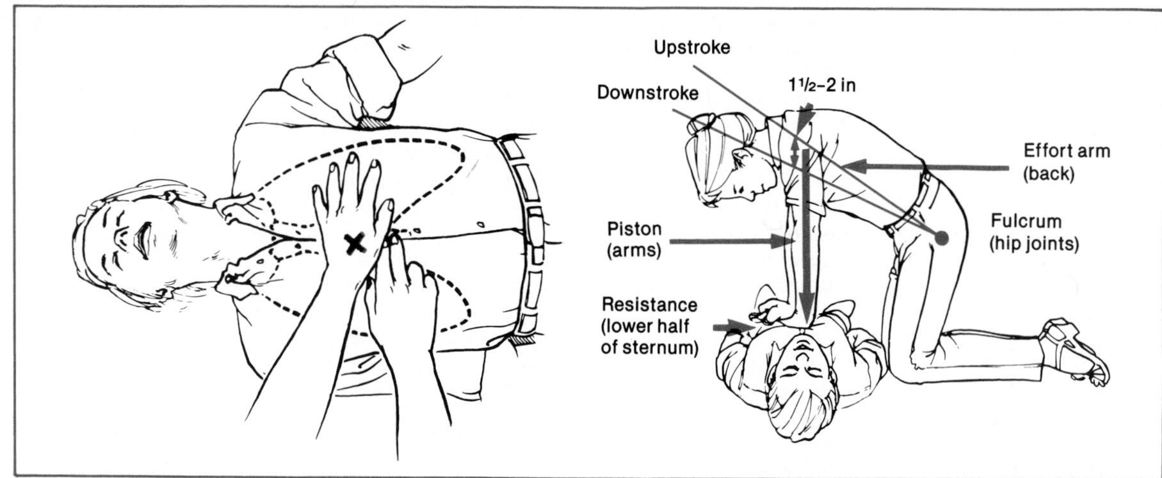

FIGURE 26-12. External chest compression. *Left,* Locating the correct hand position on the lower half of the sternum. *Right,* Proper position of the rescuer, with shoulders directly over the victim's sternum and elbows locked. (From Standards and guidelines for cardiopulmonary resuscitation [CPR] and emergency cardiac care [ECC].) JAMA *255:*2906, 1986. Copyright 1986, the American Medical Association.)

lation is the usual method until endotracheal intubation can be carried out, and in the out-of-hospital setting mouth-to-mouth resuscitation is used while awaiting emergency rescue personnel. The effect of the acquired immunodeficiency syndrome and hepatitis B transmission on attitudes toward mouth-to-mouth resuscitation by bystanders and even professional personnel in hospitals is an area of concern,[288] but no current data are available to assess the impact of this problem on the outcome of resuscitative efforts.

Conventional CPR techniques require that the lungs be inflated once every 5 seconds when two persons are available for the resuscitative effort and twice every 15 seconds when only one person is present to carry out both ventilation and chest wall compression.[334] A new technique of CPR, which is based on increased intrathoracic pressure as the prime mover of blood, rather than cardiac compression itself,[320,335] currently is being evaluated; the cyclic ventilatory techniques are altered in this procedure (see below).

CHEST COMPRESSION (Fig. 26-12). The second element of basic life support, chest compression, is intended to maintain blood flow until definitive steps can be taken. The rationale as originally developed was based on the hypothesis that cardiac compression allows the heart to maintain an externally driven pump function by sequential emptying and filling of its chambers, with competent valves favoring the forward direction of flow. In fact, the application of this technique has proved successful when used as recommended.[334] The palm of one hand is placed over the lower sternum and the heel of the other rests on the dorsum of the lower hand. The sternum is then depressed with the resuscitator's arms straight at the elbows to provide a less tiring and more forceful fulcrum at the junction of the shoulders and back (Fig. 26-12). Using this technique, sufficient force is applied to depress the sternum about 3 to 5 cm, with abrupt relaxation, and the cycle is carried out at a rate of about 80 to 100 compressions/min.[288] Despite the fact that this conventional technique produces measurable carotid artery flow and a record of successful resuscitations, the absence of a pressure gradient across the heart in the presence of an extrathoracic arterial-venous pressure gradient has lead to a concept that it is not cardiac compression per se, but rather a pumping action produced by pressure changes in the entire thoracic cavity that optimizes systemic blood flow during resuscitation.[220,335-337] Experimental work in which the chest is compressed during ventilations rather than between them (simultaneous compression-ventilation, SCV) demonstrates better extrathoracic arterial flow.[335,337-339] However, increased carotid artery flow does not necessarily equate with improved cerebral perfusion,[320,340,341] and the reduction in coronary blood flow caused by elevated intrathoracic pressures by certain techniques[320,342] may be too high a price for the improved peripheral flow. In addition, a high thoracoabdominal gradient has been demonstrated during experimental SCV,[343] which could divert flow from the brain in the absence of concomitant abdominal binding. Studies of comparative hemodynamics of models of conventional cardiac compression and techniques based on chest (thoracic) compression suggest that blood movement is based on fluctuations of intrathoracic pressure in both.[344]

ADVANCED LIFE SUPPORT AND DEFINITIVE RESUSCITATION

This next step in the sequence of resuscitative efforts is designed to achieve definitive support and stabilization of the patient.[334] The implementation of advanced life support does not indicate abrupt cessation of basic life support activities, but rather a transition from one level of activity to the next. In the past, advanced life support required judgments and technical skills which removed it from the realm of activity of lay bystanders and even emergency medical technicians, limiting these activities to specifically trained paramedical personnel, nurses, and physicians. With further education of emergency technicians, many community-based CPR programs now permit them to carry out advanced life support activities.[298,319] In addition, the development and testing of equipment which has the ability to sense and analyze air flow, sense cardiac electrical activity, and provide definitive electrical intervention[323,345] may eventually provide a limited role for lay bystanders in advanced life support.

The general goals of advanced life support are to optimize ventilation, revert the cardiac rhythm to one which is hemodynamically effective, and maintain and support the restored circulation. Thus, during advanced life support, the patient (1) will be intubated and well oxygenated, (2) will be defibrillated, cardioverted, or paced, and (3) will have an intravenous line established to deliver necessary medications. After intubation, the goal of ventilation is to reverse hypoxemia and not merely achieve a high alveolar pO_2. Thus oxygen rather than room air should be used to ventilate the patient; if possible, the arterial pO_2 should be monitored. Respirator support in hospital and AMBU bag by means of an endotracheal tube or face mask in the out-of-hospital setting usually are used.

DEFIBRILLATION-CARDIOVERSION (Fig. 26-13). Rapid conversion to an effective cardiac electrical mechanism is a key step for successful resuscitation.[292,308] Delay should be minimal, even when conditions for CPR are optimal. When VF or a rapid VT is recognized on a monitor or by telemetry, defibrillation should be carried out immediately with a shock of 200 joules. Up to 90 per cent of VF victims weighing up to 90 kg can be successfully resuscitated with a 200-joule shock,[346] and a 300- or 360-joule shock may be used if this is not successful. High-energy defibrillation has been suggested by some,[347] but not in excess of 360 joules; others have expressed caution about the use of high energies.[348] Failure of the initial one or two shocks to successfully cardiovert to an effective rhythm is a poor prognostic sign[288,334]; however, resuscitative efforts should not be abandoned. At this point the focus should be on ventilation and correcting the biochemistry of the blood, efforts which will render the heart more likely to reestablish a stable rhythm (i.e., improved oxygenation, reversal of acidosis, and improvement of the underlying electrophysiological condition). Although adequate oxygenation of the blood is crucial in managing the metabolic acidosis of cardiac arrest, additional correction may be achieved if necessary by intravenous administration of sodium bicarbonate. It is important to recognize, however, that much less sodium bicarbonate than was previously recommended is adequate for treatment of acidosis in this setting[349] and that excessive quantities can be deleterious.[349] Although some investigators question the use of sodium bicarbonate at all because risks of alkalosis, hypernatremia, and hyperosmolality may outweigh its benefits,[350] the acidotic patient (particularly if resistant to defibrillation) may benefit from administration of 1 mEq/kg of sodium bicarbonate while CPR is being carried out. Up to 50 per cent of this dose may be repeated every 10 to 15 minutes during the course of CPR.[351] When possible, arterial pH, pO_2, and pCO_2 should be monitored during the resuscitation.

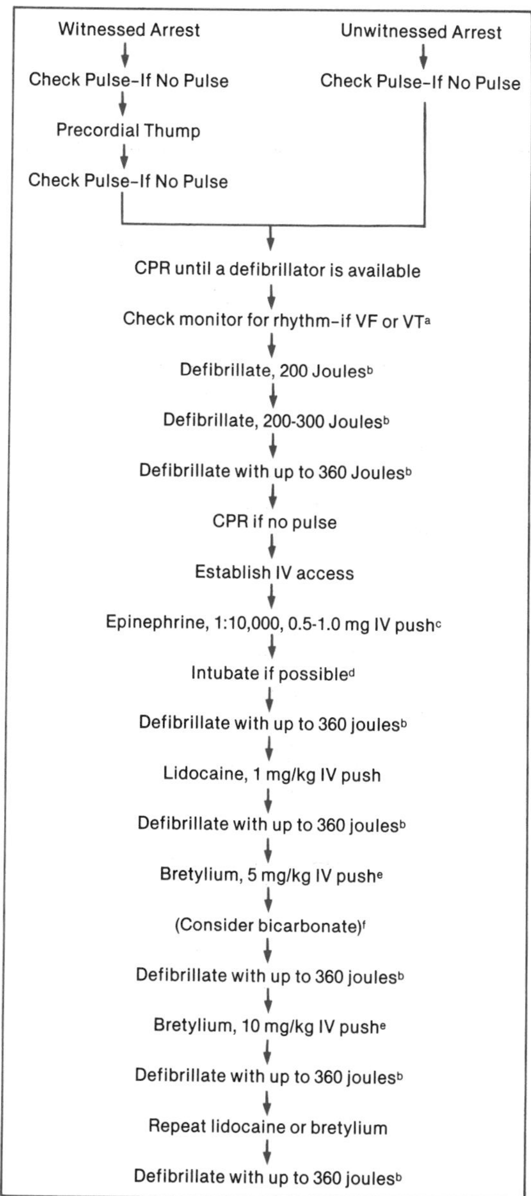

FIGURE 26–13. Algorithm for treatment of VF (and pulseless VT). This sequence was developed to assist in teaching how to treat a broad range of patients with VF and VT. Some patients may require care not specified herein; this algorithm should not be construed as prohibiting such flexibility. Flow of algorithm presumes that VF is continuing. CPR indicates cardiopulmonary resuscitation.

[a] Pulseless VT should be treated identically to VF.

[b] Check pulse and rhythm after each shock. If VF recurs after transiently coverting (rather than persists without ever converting), use whatever energy level has previously been successful for defibrillation.

[c] Epinephrine should be repeated every 5 minutes.

[d] Intubation is preferable. If it can be accomplished simultaneously with other techniques, the earlier the better. However, defibrillation and epinephrine are more important initially if the patient can be ventilated without intubation.

[e] Some may prefer repeated doses of lidocaine, which may be given in 0.5 mg/kg boluses every 8 minutes to a total dose of 3 mg/kg.

[f] Value of sodium bicarbonate is questionable during cardiac arrest, and it is not recommended for routine cardiac arrest sequence. Consideration of its use in a dose of 1 mEq/kg is appropriate at this point. Half of original dose may be repeated every 10 minutes if it is used. (From Standard and guidelines for cardiopulmonary resuscitation [CPR] and emergency cardiac care [ECC]. JAMA *255*:2905, 1986. Copyright 1986, the American Medical Association.)

PHARMACOTHERAPY. Electrical stability of the heart may be achieved by intravenous administration of *lidocaine* during resuscitation. As a matter of routine, all patients should receive a bolus of 1 mg/kg of lidocaine (p. 1246) intravenously, with the dose repeated in 2 minutes in those in whom resuscitation remains unsuccessful or unstable electrical activity persists. A continuous infusion of lidocaine follows, at a rate of 1 to 4 mg/min, depending on the patient's age and size and other factors.[352] The patient who remains in VF after these initial efforts should be given *epinephrine*, 0.5 to 1.0 mg (5 to 10 ml of a 1:10,000 solution) intravenously, and attempts at defibrillation should be repeated. This dose of epinephrine can be repeated every 5 minutes during the resuscitation. It may be given by the intracardiac route only in the absence of or inaccessibility of intravenous or endotracheal routes of administration.[288] Continued failure is an indication for other intravenous antiarrhythmic drugs, such as *procainamide hydrochloride* (p. 1246)[353] and *bretylium tosylate* (p. 1249).[354] Procainamide is administered as a series of 100-mg boluses every 5 minutes to a total dose of 500 to 1000 mg, followed by a constant infusion of 2 to 4 mg/min. Bretylium tosylate given in an initial dose of 5 mg/kg intravenously is followed by another attempt at defibrillation. Additional doses can be given every 15 minutes, to a maximum of 25 mg/kg. Intravenous amiodarone (p. 646), given as a 150- to 500-mg bolus and a 10 mg/kg/day infusion, also has been suggested for refractory VT and VF.[355] In patients in whom acute hyperkalemia is the triggering event for resistant VF, or who are hypocalcemic or toxic from Ca^{++}-entry blocking drugs, 10 per cent calcium gluconate, 5 to 20 ml infused at a rate of 2 to 4 ml/min, may be helpful.[288] Calcium should *not* be used routinely during resuscitation,[356] even though ionized Ca^{++} levels may be low during resuscitation from cardiac arrest.[311]

BRADYARRHYTHMIC AND ASYSTOLIC ARREST. The approach to the patient with bradyarrhythmic or asystolic arrest differs (Fig. 26–14). Once this form of cardiac arrest is recognized, efforts should focus on actions which are likely to favor the emergence of a stable spontaneous rhythm, or attempts should be made to pace the heart. Epinephrine (0.5 to 1.0 mg) and atropine, 0.6 to 2.0 mg intravenously, are commonly used in an attempt to elicit spontaneous electrical activity or increase the rate of a bradycardia. These have had only limited success, as has intravenous isoproterenol infusions in doses up to 15 to 20 μg/min. In the absence of an intravenous line, epinephrine (1 mg [i.e., 10 ml of a 1:10,000 solution]) may be given by the intracardiac route, but there is danger of coronary or myocardial laceration.

Pacing of the bradyarrhythmic or asystolic heart has been limited in the past by the unavailability of personnel capable

has passed through the early convalescent period (2 to 7 days), has awakened, and has stable cardiopulmonary dynamics, decisions must be made regarding the nature and extent of the work-up required to establish a long-term management strategy. The goals of the work-up are to identify the specific cause of the cardiac arrest (if not already evident), clarify the functional status of the patient's cardiovascular system, establish long-term therapy, and determine endpoints of antiarrhythmic, antiischemic, and hemodynamic therapy. The extent of the work-up is largely dictated by the degree of central nervous system recovery and the factors already known to have contributed to the cardiac arrest. For instance, patients who have limited return of central nervous system function usually do not undergo extensive work-ups, and patients whose cardiac arrests were triggered by an acute transmural myocardial infarction have work-ups similar to those for other patients with acute myocardial infarction.

Survivors of prehospital cardiac arrest not associated with acute myocardial infarction who have good return of neurological function undergo extensive diagnostic work-ups and carefully designed long-term therapy. The work-up normally includes cardiac catheterization with coronary angiography, an evaluation of functional significance of coronary lesions by stress-imaging techniques, and estimation of baseline susceptibility to life-threatening arrhythmias and of the expected response to long-term therapy.

GENERAL CARE. The general management of survivors of cardiac arrest is determined by the specific cause and the pathophysiology of the underlying process. For patients with ischemic heart disease (who form the vast majority of this population), control of episodes of myocardial ischemia, optimization of therapy for left ventricular dysfunction, and attention to general medical status are all addressed. Antiischemic therapy may be medical or surgical, depending on the anatomy and physiology of the disease process. Although there are limited data suggesting that coronary bypass surgery may improve the recurrence rate and total mortality rates after survival from prehospital cardiac arrest,[373] no properly controlled prospective studies have validated this impression. Therefore, indications for surgery are limited to two groups of patients: (1) those who have a generally accepted indication for surgery[228] (including a documented ischemic mechanism for the cardiac arrest), and (2) those who meet specific criteria for surgery directed to arrhythmia control.[374]

Medical antiischemic therapy includes nitrates, beta-adrenoceptor blocking agents, and Ca^{++}-entry blockers. Beta-adrenoceptors may have an antianginal effect and also influence the role of sympathetic nervous system activity on the genesis of potentially lethal arrhythmias. Although two studies could not establish a difference in long-term outcome between survivors receiving and those not receiving beta blockers,[46,293] Morady and colleagues[97] suggested that medical or surgical antiischemic therapy, rather than antiarrhythmic therapy, should be the primary approach to long-term management of the subgroup of prehospital cardiac arrest survivors in whom transient myocardial ischemia was the inciting factor. In a report from the Coronary Artery Surgery Study (CASS), Holmes et al.[375] compared sudden death rates in medically and surgically treated patients in the CASS registry. This study did not directly address the issue of surgery in survivors of out-of-hospital cardiac arrest, but there was a significant difference at 5 years, with a 98 per cent sudden death–free survival in the surgical group versus 94 per cent in the medical group ($p < .0001$). The differences were minimal in the groups with one- or two-vessel disease and no history of heart failure, but expanded to 91 and 69 per cent, respectively, in patients with three-vessel disease and a history of heart failure. The question of how to apply these data to indications for surgery for cardiac arrest survivors remains unanswered at this time. The problem is further confounded by the fact that assignment of the 13,476 analyzable patients to medical versus surgical groups was not randomized (i.e., it was based instead on clinical judgment). Further evaluation of the specific role of coronary surgery *after* out-of-hospital cardiac arrest is needed.

The long-term management of the consequences of left ventricular dysfunction by conventional means such as digitalis preparations and chronic diuretic use has been evaluated in several studies. Data from the Multiple Risk Factor Intervention Trial (MRFIT) suggested a higher mortality rate in the special intervention group,[376] presumably related to diuretic use and K^+ depletion, and other data regarding the relation between K^+ depletion and arrhythmias have focused attention on routine use of such drugs. Although the facts currently are far from conclusive,[265] use of such drugs should be accompanied by careful monitoring of electrolytes. Similar concerns have been raised in respect to digitalis use in high-risk patients after acute myocardial infarction.[377–381] As of this writing, use of digoxin in survivors of prehospital cardiac arrest should be tailored to specific indications for left ventricular dysfunction.

PREVENTION OF RECURRENT CARDIAC ARREST

Long-term therapeutic strategies intended to prevent recurrences of potentially lethal arrhythmias have been based on several medical approaches,[303,382–390a] on antiarrhythmic surgery, and on the use of implantable devices. Antiarrhythmic surgery[374,391,392] evolved in parallel with programmed stimulation approaches to management, and most recently antitachycardiac and antifibrillatory devices[391,393,394] have been developed for use in subgroups of these patients. A problem which impinges on all long-term strategies is the lack of a reliable current natural history denominator against which to compare the results of any intervention.

LONG-TERM ANTIARRHYTHMIC THERAPY. The antiarrhythmic approach to long-term management of survivors of prehospital cardiac arrest was devised on two assumptions: (1) that the high frequency of chronic PVCs identified in cardiac arrest survivors constitutes a triggering mechanism for potentially lethal arrhythmias, and (2) that electrophysiological instability of the myocardium predisposing to potentially lethal arrhythmias can be modified by antiarrhythmic drugs.[273,303] In an 8-year follow-up study of 61 survivors of prehospital cardiac arrest whose management was based on empirical dose titration to achieve stable high therapeutic plasma concentrations of antiarrhythmic agents, the recurrent cardiac arrest rate was 10 per cent at 1 year and 15 per cent at 2 years (Fig. 26–16), with 31 per cent of the recurrences occurring in patients whose drug had been stopped or changed without monitoring of the levels of the new drug.[46] With the development of more detailed methods of analysis of ambulatory monitoring recordings[382] and electrophysiological stimulation for testing inducibility of clinically significant arrhythmias, attention focused on these more specific and individualized means of evaluating drug therapy. Graboys et al.[382] reported the outcome in a group of 123 patients with malignant ventricular arrhythmias who had survived one or

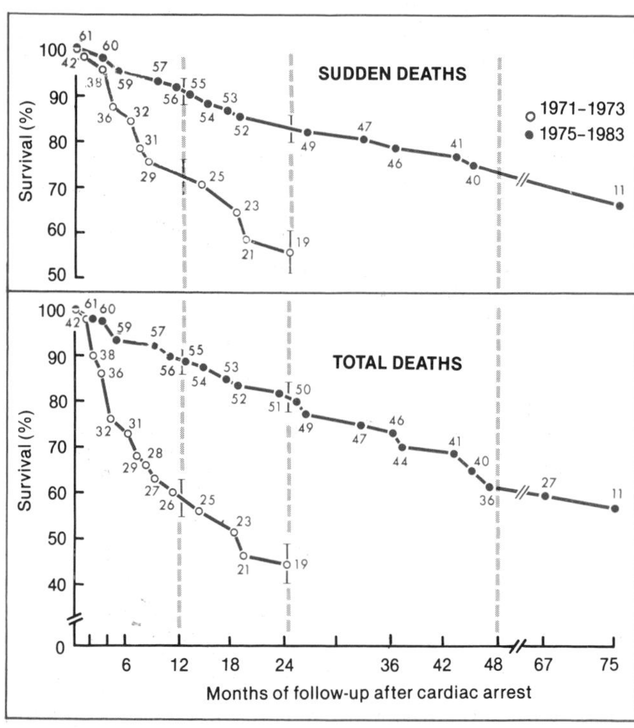

FIGURE 26–16. Sudden deaths and total deaths in survivors of prehospital cardiac arrest during an 8-year follow-up period (closed circles), compared with 1970–1973 historical experience during the initial Miami studies (open circles). The more recent experience indicates a 67 per cent reduction in recurrent cardiac arrest rate in the first year of followup. Whether this was due to aggressive antiarrhythmic therapy or other factors in the patient populations or their management cannot be determined from comparison to historical controls. However, the 10 per cent 1-year mortality rate is similar to outcome with other forms of antiarrhythmic intervention in recent years. (From Myerburg, R. J., and Kessler, K. M.: Management of patients who survive cardiac arrest. Mod. Concepts Cardiovasc. Dis. *55*:61, 1986.)

more cardiac arrests. Suppression of specific forms of ventricular ectopy (salvoes of three or more ectopic beats and early cycle PVCs) identified on ambulatory monitoring or exercise testing was accompanied by a significantly reduced mortality rate, compared with those in whom such suppression was not achieved. The mortality rate was more than 80 per cent at 3 years in patients whose complex forms could not be suppressed, compared with a nearly 90 per cent survival of those whose complex PVCs were suppressed.

The use of programmed electrophysiological stimulation for guiding therapy in survivors of out-of-hospital cardiac arrest has evolved as the preferred method of management, despite problems related to sensitivity and specificity of the various pacing protocols[395] and concerns about the extent to which the myocardial status at the time of electrophysiological stimulation reflects that at the time of the cardiac arrest. Imponderables such as the extent to which electrode catheter–stimulated extrasystoles mimic spontaneous PVCs, and the ischemic, autonomic, and biochemical status of the heart at the time of the study, may influence the data.[396] Nonetheless, among a series of 6 reports,[383–389] induction of sustained VT or VF at baseline study ranged from 31 to 79 per cent, and successful suppression of inducibility ranged from 18 to 78 per cent. The mortality rate during follow-up of those patients in whom inducibility was suppressed by antiarrhythmic therapy ranged from 0 to 22 per cent (mean 9 per cent), compared with a range of 22 to 78 per cent (mean 43 per cent) in those patients in whom VT or VF was still inducible on any antiarrhythmic therapy.

The evaluation of these data is significantly influenced by definitions of inducibility and noninducibility and also by the clinical details of the patient population in each of the studies, which varied considerably. In most reports VF or sustained VT could not be induced in 25 to 30 per cent of the patients. It is probable that differences are determined in part by the numbers of patients who have anatomically discrete versus ischemic substrates among various populations studied.[313] Careful attention to protocol details, anatomy of the disease processes, and definitions of inducibility may help to clarify these discrepancies in the future. For the present, however, 50 to 70 per cent of *unselected* survivors of cardiac arrest caused by VF or sustained VT can be anticipated to be inducible into sustained arrhythmias. For the subgroup with discrete ventricular aneurysms, more than 90 per cent may be inducible.[244,386]

Most investigators agree that inducibility into a *sustained* clinical arrhythmia provides an indication of risk and that its prevention is an endpoint for therapy, but the induction of *nonsustained* forms is more controversial. While it has been suggested that induction of nonsustained rhythms may indicate risk, it often is nonspecific if an aggressive protocol is used.[395] The use of the suppression of nonsustained arrhythmias as an endpoint of therapy is not considered valid. The significance of *noninducibility* at baseline electrophysiological stimulation testing in relation to risk and long-term management also is a controversial issue. Opinions range from the conclusion that patients showing noninducibility are not electrophysiologically unstable and require no long-term antiarrhythmic therapy[97,383,389,390] to the other extreme that such patients remain at risk but do not provide an objective endpoint of therapy by this method, and therefore must be treated by other techniques.[46,244,303,382] Some patients in this category have had cardiac arrest based on transient ischemia and require control with antiischemic therapy.[97] In the 6 reports, 24-month mortality in patients who had noninducibility ranged from 3 to 38 per cent, higher than in patients in whom inducibility could be suppressed by antiarrhythmic therapy (average 9 per cent) but lower than in those in whom inducibility could not be suppressed (average 43 per cent). In one study, left ventricular ejection fraction discriminated high risk from low risk in noninducible patients[384]; in another, reversible causes of the index event predicted noninducibility.[397]

SURGICAL MANAGEMENT (p. 1236)

Techniques initially conceived for control of recurrent sustained VT, map-guided endocardial resection,[398] and encircling endocardial ventriculotomy[399] also are used for selected survivors of out-of-hospital cardiac arrest. This approach is limited largely to those patients who have inducibility into sustained VT and VF during electrophysiological testing, are unresponsive to drug therapy, and have suitable ventricular and coronary artery anatomy. Unfortunately, most data available on this approach to management of cardiac arrest survivors are derived from broader studies of either mixed populations (i.e., recurrent VT and cardiac arrest survivors) or mixed therapeutic approaches (i.e., surgery after medical failure). Nonetheless, it appears that surgical intervention is successful in selected patients in whom medical therapy does not produce an acceptable endpoint,[388,389,392] even though statistics limited to out-of-hospital cardiac arrest survivors are difficult to derive from published data. Coronary revascularization alone may be useful in subsets of survivors of out-of-hospital cardiac arrest caused by an ischemic mechanism.[97,400]

IMPLANTABLE DEVICES (Chap. 25)

The development of a reliable implantable cardioverter-defibrillator has added a new dimension to the management of patients at high risk of cardiac arrest.[401] Mirowski and coworkers[393] evaluated the results in 52 patients who had survived an arrhythmic cardiac arrest plus at least one recurrence not associated with acute myocardial infarction. Other forms of preventive management had failed in all these patients, and the group had a mean of 3.9 cardiac arrests per patient. The analysis is complicated by the fact that concomitant cardiovascular surgical procedures were carried out in 15 patients, and about the same number had previous surgery, plus pacemaker implantation in 9. Although 12 of these 52 very high-risk patients died during a 14-month mean follow-up period, producing a 23 per cent 1-year total mortality rate, the 1-year sudden death rate was 8.5 per cent. Devices were triggered 62 times in 17 patients. Assuming death would have followed in these patients without the device, the total 1-year mortality rate would have been 48 per cent. Subsequently, Echt and colleagues[394] reported their experience in 70 patients. Because 35 of their patients (50 per cent) had had no previous cardiac arrests (14 patients with uncontrollable recurrent ventricular tachycardia) or only 1 previous arrest (21 patients), this population may have been less "unstable" than Mirowski's group.[393] There was a mean of 1.9 ± 1.7 cardiac arrests/patient, 3.1 ± 2.3 arrhythmic episodes/patient, and 4.0 ± 2.1 drug failures/patient. During an average follow-up period of 8.9 months (range, 1 to 33 months), 37 patients (53 per cent) received one or more shocks. The 12-month total death rate was 10 per cent, the sudden death rate was less than 2 per cent, and the complication rate was acceptably low. Subsequent reports have confirmed that implantable cardioverter-defibrillators can achieve sudden death rates consistently less than 5 per cent at 1 year, and total death rates in the 10 to 20 per cent range, among populations who have higher mortality risks, estimated by time to first appropriate shock.[402–405] Platia et al.[391] evaluated the concomitant use of the device with ventricular endocardial resection for refractory ventricular arrhythmias. During a mean 25-month follow-up, 4 of 25 patients (16 per cent) had recurrent tachycardia which was successfully reverted by the device, but 1 patient died because the device malfunctioned.

MANAGEMENT ALGORITHM

The options for diagnostic evaluation and long-term management of cardiac arrest survivors are complex, with specific problems unique both to patient subgroups and to the various therapeutic strategies. A two-tiered algorithm has been developed as a guide to management.[406] Management stage I (Fig. 26–17) addresses diagnostic evaluation and general management, and stage II (Fig. 26–18) is oriented to specific electrophysiological/pharmacological strategies for control of potentially lethal arrhythmias. Endpoints of management are reached in stage I for those patients in whom cardiac arrest was precipitated by acute myocardial infarction, those who have some form of non-coronary heart disease or cardiac arrest clearly related to transient ischemia, and those who have cardiac arrest caused by proarrhythmic factors, such as adverse drug effect or electrolyte imbalances. Patients with life-limiting concurrent morbid states and those who have major post-arrest residual damage of the central nervous system also reach their management endpoints in stage I.

Among the remainder, who constitute the majority of survivors and most commonly have chronic ischemic heart disease, electrophysiological stimulation studies should be performed (Fig. 26–18). In that subgroup of patients among whom

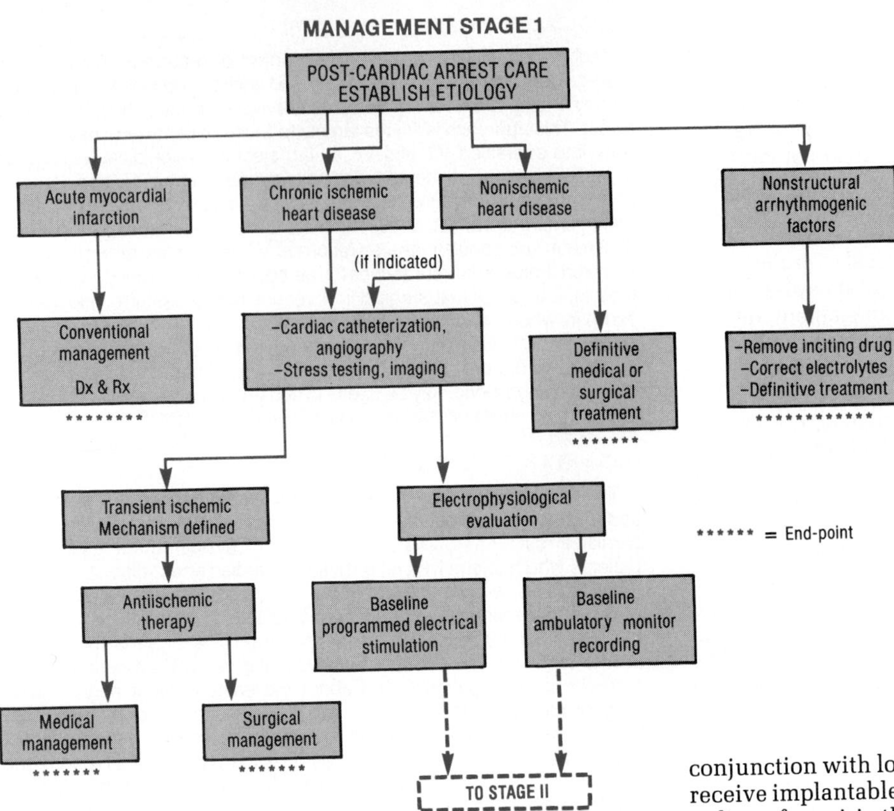

FIGURE 26–17. Management algorithm—stage I. Flow diagram for initial management and diagnostic activities in survivors of prehospital cardiac arrest. Patients whose arrests were associated with new acute transmural myocardial infarction or nonstructural arrhythmogenic factors are managed by conventional techniques. All patients with chronic ischemic heart disease, and many with nonischemic heart disease, enter a pathway which leads to advanced electrophysiological study and management. (From Myerburg, R. J., and Kessler, K. M.: Management of patients who survive cardiac arrest. Mod. Concepts Cardiovasc. Dis. *55*:61, 1986.)

sustained VT with or without degeneration to VF is inducible, the primary endpoint of therapy is prevention of inducibility by an appropriate antiarrhythmic agent or drug combination. Once identified, the plasma concentration required to achieve noninducibility should be noted and monitored periodically during follow-up. In those patients in whom this approach is not feasible because of noninducibility of sustained VT or VF, another objective approach should be used (Fig. 26–18). Some patients who have salvoes or nonsustained VT on ambulatory monitoring may be given antiarrhythmic drugs singly or in combination in an attempt to suppress repetitive forms[382] or treated with amiodarone empirically.[407,407a] If this is successful, it may be used as the endpoint of therapy.[408] Those patients who have neither inducibility by electrophysiological stimulation nor complex forms on ambulatory monitoring in conjunction with low (<35 per cent) ejection fractions should receive implantable cardioverter-defibrillator devices[391,393,394] in lieu of empiric therapy (Fig. 26–19).

Surgical intervention is preferred in patients who have discrete ventricular aneurysms, are inducible into sustained VT or VF, and cannot be managed by antiarrhythmic drugs. The results of surgery in such patients have been encouraging.[374] Implantable devices are the method of choice for patients who have survived a *recurrence on therapy predicted to be successful by one of the other endpoints*, and in most of those who fail the electrophysiological stimulation or ambulatory monitoring legs of the algorithm and are considered to be at high risk. Concomitant antiarrhythmic therapy after a device is implanted may reduce the number of shocks delivered.[394] Implantable devices also may have a role in conjunction with antiarrhythmic surgery, especially in those in whom inducibility into high-risk arrhythmias remains postoperatively (Fig. 26–19).[391,392]

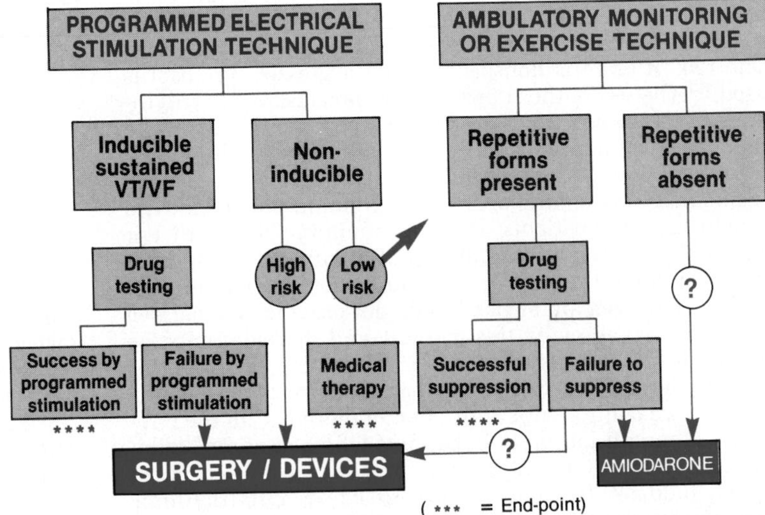

FIGURE 26–18. Management algorithm—stage II. Advanced electrophysiological evaluation of survivors of out-of-hospital cardiac arrest. Ideally, patients enter the programmed electrical stimulation pathway, and are initially evaluated by drug testing using this technique. If the heart is inducible into sustainted VT or VF (with some limitations of interpretation for the latter), and drug testing results in successful prevention of inducibility, an acceptable endpoint of therapy has been achieved (****). If the heart remains inducible (failure by programmed stimulation), antiarrhythmic surgery or an implantable device is considered (see Fig. 26–19). If the heart is noninducible at baseline and the patient is at low risk for recurrence because of either (1) an identifiable and controllable ischemic mechanism, (2) reversible metabolic mechanisms, or (3) no more than moderate depression of ejection fraction, the patient may be managed by appropriate medical therapy and by ambulatory monitoring techniques if repetitive forms are present.

When programmed stimulation is not available or not applicable to an individual patient, the ambulatory monitoring or exercise techniques may be used. For drug testing, repetitive forms must be identified as the target arrhythmia and successful suppression by conventional drug therapy is considered an acceptable endpoint. Failure to suppress repetitive forms in high-risk patients should lead to considerations for implantable devices and possibly some forms of surgical intervention. Among others in this category, amiodarone is an acceptable therapeutic approach. If repetitive forms are absent and the patient is at high risk (e.g., very low EF), amiodarone or implantable devices are the therapies of choice. (From Myerburg, R. J., and Kessler, K. M.: Management of patients who survive cardiac arrest. Med. Concepts Cardiovasc. Dis. *55*:61, 1986.)

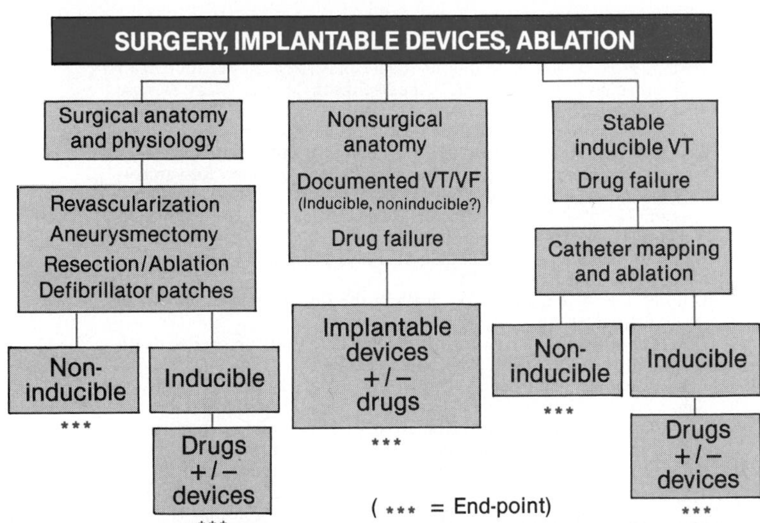

FIGURE 26–19. **Management algorithm—stage III. Therapy by surgery, implantable devices, or catheter ablation. Patients who do not achieve an acceptable endpoint by programmed electrical stimulation with drug testing and/or ambulatory monitoring techniques, and who have defined anatomical/physiological characteristics, require these higher-level interventions. In addition, patients who survive recurrences of out-of-hospital cardiac arrest on drug therapy deemed to be effective are candidates for these alternatives. Antiarrhythmic surgery requires appropriate anatomy and physiology, and a successful outcome requires the identification of noninducibility postoperatively. Patients whose hearts remain inducible may respond to drug therapy previously unsuccessful or require implantable devices. Primary use of implantable devices is indicated in patients with nonsurgical anatomy in whom drug therapy has failed, and who have documented survival from a potentially fatal arrhythmia. Antiarrhythmic drugs may be used in conjunction with implantable devices to limit the number of shocks if necessary, but many patients can be managed without drugs. Catheter ablation has had only limited success for primary management of recurrent ventricular arrhythmias in selected subsets. An evolving strategy is the use of catheter ablation as adjunctive therapy to an implantable device, to limit the number of recurrent defibrillator discharges without depending on successful long-term efficacy of the ablation procedure. (Modified from Myerburg, R. J., et al.: *In* Zipes, D. P., and Jalipe, J. [eds.]: Cardiac Electrophysiology: From Cell to Bedside. Philadelphia, W. B. Saunders Company, 1990, pp. 666–678.)**

When used according to defined indications, the recent statistics for each of the approaches outlined above are intriguing. Each method has now been recognized to yield a 1-year survival rate of 90 per cent or better, compared with the 70 per cent survival cited earlier. Whether this means that each of the methods is equally effective or whether some other uncontrolled factor is influencing outcome has not been defined and requires further evaluation. However, high risk is attendant on indiscriminate changes in pharmacological therapy which has been determined appropriate by any of the endpoints used. Swerdlow et al.[392] and Myerburg et al.,[46] using different therapeutic approaches, both have reported that arbitrary cessation, or changes in therapy without retesting for the endpoint used to establish the initial therapy, is accompanied by a high risk of recurrent cardiac arrest.

SUDDEN DEATH AND PUBLIC SAFETY

The unexpectedness of SCD has raised questions concerning secondary risk to the public created by people in the throes of a cardiac arrest. There are no controlled data available to guide public policy regarding people at high risk for potentially lethal arrhythmias and for abrupt incapacitation. Myerburg and Davis[409] reported observations on 1348 sudden deaths caused by coronary heart disease in people 65 years of age or less during a 7-year period in Dade County, Florida. One hundred one (7.5 per cent) of these deaths occurred in people who were engaged in activities at the time of death which were potentially hazardous to the public (e.g., 56 driving private automobiles or taxis, 15 driving trucks, 10 working at altitude, 2 piloting aircraft) and 122 (9.1 per cent) of the victims had occupations which could create potential hazards to others if an abrupt loss of consciousness had occurred while at work (e.g., 57 taxi and truck drivers, 8 aircraft pilots, 9 bus drivers, 9 policemen and firemen). There were no catastrophic events as a result of these cardiac arrests, only minor property damage in 19 and minor injuries in 5. Levy et al.[410] reported a case of a bus driver with a strong history of coronary heart disease who caused the deaths of himself and several others, but they did not conclusively demonstrate that unexpected cardiac arrest was the proximate cause of the accident. Furthermore, Waller et al.[411] studied an elderly population and demonstrated that cardiac disease alone was not responsible for a significant increase in accident risk: *senility, or senility plus cardiovascular disease, was much more important.* Several other studies also have led to the conclusion that risk to the public is small.[412] In specific reference to private automobile drivers, most of the data show that sudden death at the wheel usually involves enough of a prodrome to allow the driver to get to the roadside before losing consciousness.[409,412] Therefore, although there are likely to be isolated instances in which cardiac arrest causes public hazards in the future, the risk appears to be small, and because it is difficult to identify specific individuals at risk, sweeping restrictions to avoid such risks appear unwarranted. The exceptions are people with multisystem disease, particularly senility, and individual circumstances that require specific consideration, such as high-risk patients who have special responsibilities—school bus drivers, aircraft pilots, trainmen, and truck drivers.

REFERENCES

DEFINITION

1. Weiss, S.: Instantaneous "physiologic" death. N. Engl. J. Med. *223*:793, 1940.
2. Spain, D. M., Bradess, V. A., and Mohr, C.: Coronary atherosclerosis as a cause of unexpected and unexplained death: An autopsy study from 1949–1959. J.A.M.A. *174*:384, 1960.
3. Burch, G. E., and DePasquale, N. P.: Sudden, unexpected, natural death. Am. J. Med. Sci. *249*:86, 1965.
4. Kuller, L., Lilienfeld, A., and Fisher, R.: An epidemiological study of sudden and unexpected deaths in adults. Medicine *46*:341, 1967.
5. Paul, O., and Schatz, M.: On sudden death. Circulation *43*:7, 1971.
6. Gordon, T., and Kannel, W. B.: Premature mortality from coronary heart disease. The Framingham Study. J.A.M.A. *215*:1617, 1971.
7. Biorck, C., and Wikland, B.: Sudden death—what are we talking about? Circulation *45*:256, 1972.
8. Friedman, M., Manwaring, J. H., Rosenman, R. H., et al.: Instantaneous and sudden deaths: Clinical and pathological differentiation in coronary artery disease. J.A.M.A. *225*:1319, 1973.
9. Kannel, W. B., Doyle, J. T., McNamara, P. M., et al.: Precursors of sudden coronary death: Factors related to the incidence of sudden death. Circulation *51*:606, 1975.
10. Helmers, C., Lundman, T., Maasing, R., and Wester, P. O.: Mortality pattern among initial survivors of acute myocardial infarction using a life-table technique. Acta Med. Scand. *200*:469, 1976.
11. Mitchell, J.R.A., and Schwartz, C. J.: Arterial Disease. Oxford, Blackwell, 1965.
12. Ruberman, W., Weinblatt, E., Goldberg, J. D., et al.: Ventricular premature beats and mortality after myocardial infarction. N. Engl. J. Med. *297*:750, 1977.
13. Myerburg, R. J.: Sudden death. J. Cont. Ed. Cardiol. *14*:15, 1978.
14. Lovegrove, T., and Thompson, P.: The role of acute myocardial infarction in sudden cardiac death—a statistician's nightmare. Am. Heart J. *96*:711, 1978.
15. Thomas, A. C., Davies, M. J., and Popple, A. W.: A pathologist's view of sudden cardiac death. *In* Kulbertus, H. E., and Wellens, H.J.J. (eds.): Sudden Death. The Hague, Netherlands, Martinus Nijhoff, 1980, pp. 34–48.
16. Goldstein, S.: The necessity of a uniform definition of sudden coronary death: Witnessed death within 1 hour of the onset of acute symptoms. Am. Heart J. *103*:156, 1982.
17. Kuller, L. H.: Prodromata of sudden death and myocardial infarction. Adv. Cardiol. *25*:61, 1978.
18. Liberthson, R. R., Nagel, E. L., Hirschman, J. C., and Nussenfeld, S. R.: Prehospital ventricular fibrillation: Prognosis and follow-up course. N. Engl. J. Med. *291*:317, 1974.
19. Baum, R. S., Alvarez, H., and Cobb, L. A.: Survival after resuscitation from out-of-hospital ventricular fibrillation. Circulation *50*:1231, 1974.
20. Myerburg, R. J., Conde, C. A., Sung, R. J., et al.: Clinical, electrophysiologic, and hemodynamic profile of patients resuscitated from prehospital cardiac arrest. Am. J. Med. *68*:568, 1980.
21. Hinkle, L. E.: The immediate antecedents of sudden death. Acta Med. Scand. *210*:207, 1981.
22. Thompson, R. G., Hallstrom, A. P., and Cobb, L. A.: Bystander-initiated cardiopulmonary resuscitation in the management of ventricular fibrillation. Ann. Intern. Med. *90*:737, 1979.
23. Kuller, L. H.: Sudden death: Definition and epidemiologic considerations. Prog. Cardiovasc. Dis. *23*:1, 1980.

24. Epstein, F. H., and Pisa, Z.: International comparisons in ischemic heart disease mortality. Proc. Conf. on the Decline in Coronary Heart Disease Mortality. DHEW, NIH Publication No. 79–1610, Washington, D.C., U.S. Government Printing Office, 1979, pp. 58–88.
25. Report of the Working Group on Arteriosclerosis of the National Heart, Lung, and Blood Institute (Volume 2): Patient Oriented Research—Fundamental and Applied, Sudden cardiac death. DHEW, NIH Publication No. 82–2035, Washington, D.C., U.S. Government Printing Office, 1981, pp. 114–122.
26. Goldstein, S.: Sudden Death and Coronary Heart Disease. Mt. Kisco, N.Y., Futura Publishing Co., 1974.
27. Gillum, R. F.: Sudden coronary death in the United States; 1980–1985. Circulation *79*:756, 1989.
28. Epstein, S. E., Quyyumi, A. A., and Bonow, R. O.: Sudden cardiac death without warning: Possible mechanisms and implications for screening asymptomatic populations. N. Engl. J. Med. *321*:321, 1989.
29. Schatzkin, A., Cupples, L. A., Heeren, T., et al.: The epidemiology of sudden unexpected death: Risk factors for men and women in the Framingham Heart Study. Am. Heart J. *107*:1300, 1984.
30. Schatzkin, A., Cupples, L. A., Heeren, T., et al.: Sudden death in the Framingham Heart Study: Differences in incidence and risk factors by sex and coronary disease status. Am. J. Epidemiol. *120*:888, 1984.
31. Gillum, R. F.: Geographic variations in sudden coronary death. Am. Heart J. *119*:380, 1990.
32. Rosenberg, H. M., and Klebbs, A. J.: Trends in cardiovascular mortality with a focus on ischemic heart disease: United States, 1950–1976. Proc. Conf. Decline in Coronary Heart Disease Mortality. DHEW, NIH Publication No. 79–1610, Washington, D.C., U.S. Government Printing Office, 1979, pp. 11–41.
33. Kannel, W. B., and Schatzkin, A.: Sudden death: Lessons from subsets in population studies. J. Am. Coll. Cardiol. 5(Suppl. 6):141B, 1985.
34. Doyle, J. T., Kannel, W. B., McNamara, P. M., et al.: Factors related to suddenness of death from coronary disease: Combined Albany-Framingham studies. Am. J. Cardiol. *37*:1073, 1976.
35. Kannel, W. B., and Thomas, H. E.: Sudden coronary death: The Framingham study. Ann. N.Y. Acad. Sci., *382*:3, 1982.
36. Holmes, D. R., Davis, K., Gersh, B. J., et al.: Rich factor profiles of patients with sudden cardiac death and death from other cardiac causes: A report from the Coronary Artery Surgery Study (CASS). J. Am. Coll. Cardiol. *13*:524, 1989.
37. Kuller, L., Lilienfeld, A., and Fischer, R.: Sudden and unexpected deaths in young adults: An epidemiologic study. J.A.M.A. *198*:158, 1966.
38. Neuspiel, D. R., and Kuller, L. H.: Sudden and unexpected natural death in childhood and adolescence. J.A.M.A. *254*:1321, 1985.
39. Neufeld, H. N., and Goldbourt, V.: Coronary heart disease: Genetic aspects. Circulation *67*:943, 1983.
40. Garza, L. A., Vick, R. L., Nora, J. J., and McNamara, D. G.: Heritable Q-T prolongation without deafness. Circulation *41*:39, 1970.
41. Clark, C. E., Henry, W. L., and Epstein, S. E.: Familial prevalence and genetic transmission of idiopathic hypertrophic subaortic stenosis. N. Engl. J. Med. *289*:709, 1973.
42. Green, J. R., Krovetz, M. J., Shanklin, D. R., et al.: Sudden unexpected death in three generations. Arch. Intern. Med. *124*:359, 1969.
43. Davies, M. J.: Pathological view of sudden cardiac death. Br. Heart J. *45*:88, 1981.
44. Brookfield, L., Bharati, S., Denes, P., et al.: Familial sudden death: Report of a case and review of the literature. Chest *94*:989, 1988.
45. James, T. N., and MacLean, W.A.H.: Paroxysmal ventricular arrhythmias and familial sudden death associated with neural lesions in the heart. Chest *78*:24, 1980.
46. Myerburg, R. J., Kessler, K. M., Estes, D., et al.: Long-term survival after prehospital cardiac arrest: Analysis of outcome during an 8-year study. Circulation *70*:538, 1984.
47. Kuller, L., Cooper, M., and Perper, J.: Epidemiology of sudden death. Arch. Intern. Med. *129*:714, 1972.
48. Krueger, D. E., Ellenberg, S. S., Bloom, S., et al.: Risk factors for fatal heart attack in young women. Am. J. Epidemiol. *113*:357, 1981.
49. Wenger, N. K.: Coronary disease in women. Annu. Rev. Med. *36*:285, 1985.
50. Jick, H., Dinan, B., Herman, R., and Rothman, K. J.: Myocardial infarction and other vascular diseases in young women: Role of estrogens and other factors. J.A.M.A. *240*:2548, 1978.
51. Hagstrom, R. M., Federspiel, C. F., and Ho, Y. C.: Incidence of myocardial infarction and sudden death from coronary heart disease in Nashville, Tennessee. Circulation *44*:884, 1971.
52. Marmot, M. E., Syme, S. L., Kagan, A., et al.: Epidemiologic studies of coronary heart disease and stroke in Japanese men living in Japan, Hawaii, and California: Prevalence of coronary and hypertensive heart disease and associated risk factors. Am. J. Epidemiol. *102*:514, 1975.
53. Hallstrom, A. P., Cobb, L. A., and Ray, R.: Smoking as a risk factor for recurrence of sudden cardiac arrest. N. Engl. J. Med. *314*:271, 1986.
54. Paffenbarger, R. S., Hale, W. E., Brand, R. J., and Hyde, R. T.: Work energy level, personal characteristics, and fatal heart attack: A birth-cohort effect. Am. J. Epidemiol. *105*:200, 1977.
55. Rahe, R. H., Romo, M., Bennett, L., and Siltman, P.: Recent life changes, myocardial infarction, and abrupt coronary death. Arch. Intern. Med. *133*:221, 1974.
56. Talbott, E., Kuller, L. H., Petre, K., and Perper, J.: Biologic and psychosocial risk factors of sudden death from coronary disease in white women. Am. J. Cardiol. *39*:858, 1977.
57. Ruberman, W., Weinblatt, E., Goldberg, J. D., and Chaudhary, B. S.: Psychosocial influences on mortality after myocardial infarction. N. Engl. J. Med. *311*:552, 1984.
58. Weinblatt, E., Ruberman, W. Goldberg, J. D., et al.: Relation of education to sudden death after myocardial infarction. N. Engl. J. Med. *299*:60, 1978.
59. Lambert, C. A., Netherton, D. R., Finison, L. J., et al.: Risk factors and life style: A statewide health-interview survey. N. Engl. J. Med. *306*:1048, 1982.
60. Friedman, M., and Rosenman, R. H.: Association of specific overt behavior pattern with blood and cardiovascular findings. J.A.M.A. *169*:1286, 1959.
61. Shekelle, R. B., Gale, M., and Norosis, M.: Type A score (Jenkins Activity Survey) and risk of recurrent coronary heart disease in the aspirin–myocardial study. Am. J. Cardiol. *56*:221, 1985.
62. Bigger, J. T., Fleiss, J. L., Kleiger, R., et al.: The relationships among ventricular arrhythmias, left ventricular dysfunction, and mortality in the 2 years after myocardial infarction. Circulation *69*:250, 1984.
63. Kennedy, H. L., Whitlock, J. A., Sprague, M. K., et al.: Long-term follow-up of asymptomatic healthy subjects with frequent and complex ventricular ectopy. N. Engl. J. Med. *312*:193, 1985.
64. Chiang, B. N., Perlman, L., Ostrander, L. D., and Epstein, F.: Relation of premature systole to coronary heart disease and sudden death in the Tecumseh epidemiologic study. Ann. Intern. Med. *70*:1159, 1969.
65. Pratt, C. M., Theroux, P., Slymen, D., et al.: Spontaneous variability of ventricular arrhythmias in patients at increased risk for sudden death after acute myocardial infarction: Consecutive ambulatory electrocardiographic recordings of 88 patients. Am. J. Cardiol. *59*:278, 1987.
66. Moss, A. J., DeCamilla, J., and David, H.: Factors associated with cardiac death in the post-hospital phase of myocardial infarction. *In* Kulbertus, H. E., and Wellens, H. J. J. (eds.): Sudden Death. The Hague, Netherlands, Martinus Nijhoff, 1980, pp. 237–247.
67. Ruberman, W., Weinblatt, E., Goldberg, J. D., et al.: Ventricular premature complexes and sudden death after myocardial infarction. Circulation *64*:297, 1981.
68. Bigger, J. T., and Weld, F. M.: Analysis of prognostic significance of ventricular arrhythmias after myocardial infarction: Shortcomings of Lown grading system. Br. Heart J. *45*:717, 1981
69. Myerburg, R. J., Kessler, K. M., Luceri, R. M., et al.: Classification of ventricular arrhythmias based on parallel hierarchies of frequency and form. Am. J. Cardiol. *54*:1355, 1984.
70. Ruberman, W., Weinblatt, E., Frank, C. W., et al.: Repeated 1-hour electrocardiographic monitoring of survivors of myocardial infarction at 6-month intervals: Arrhythmia detection and relation to prognosis. Am. J. Cardiol. *47*:1197, 1981.
71. Follansbee, W. P., Michelson, E. L., and Morganroth, J.: Non-sustained ventricular tachycardia in ambulatory patients. Characteristics and association with sudden cardiac death. Ann. Intern. Med. *92*:741, 1980.
72. Lown, B., and Wolf, M.: Approaches to sudden death from coronary heart disease. Circulation *44*:130, 1971.
73. Bigger, J. T., Weld, F. M., and Rolnitzky, L. N.: Problems with the Lown grading system for observational and experimental studies in ischemic heart disease. *In* Harrison, D. C. (ed.): Cardiac Arrhythmias: A Decade of Progress. Boston, G. K. Hall, 1981, pp. 653–670.
74. Campbell, R. W. F.: Evaluation of antiarrhythmic drugs: Should the Lown classification be used as a measure of efficacy? *In* Morganroth, J., Moore, E. N., Dreifus, L. S., and Michelson, E. L. (eds.): The Evaluation of New Antiarrhythmic Drugs. The Hague, Netherlands, Martinus Nijhoff, 1981, pp. 113–121.
75. Myerburg, R. J., Zaman, L., Luceri, R., et al.: Antiarrhythmic drug therapy after myocardial infarction. *In* Kulbertus, H. E., and Wellens, H. J. J. (eds.): The First Year After Myocardial Infarction. Mt. Kisko, N.Y., Futura Publishing Co., 1983, pp. 321–339.
76. The Cardiac Arrhythmia Suppression Trial (CAST) Investigators: Preliminary report: Effect of encainide and flecainide on mortality in a randomized trial of arrhythmia suppression after myocardial infarction. N. Engl. J. Med. *321*:406, 1989.
77. Akhtar, M., Breithardt, G., Camm, A. J., et al.: CAST and beyond: Implications of the Cardiac Arrhythmia Suppression Trial. Circulation *81*:1123, 1990.
78. Schulze, R. A., Strauss, H. W., and Pitt, B.: Sudden death in the year following myocardial infarction: Relationship of ventricular premature contractions in the late hospital phase and left ventricular ejection fraction. Am. J. Med. *62*:192, 1977.
79. Maisel, A. S., Scott, N., Gilpin, E., et al.: Complex ventricular arrhythmias in patients with Q wave versus non-Q wave myocardial infarction. Circulation *72*:963, 1985.
80. Cobb, L. A., Baum, R. S., Alvarez, H., and Schaffer, W. A.: Resuscitation from out-of-hospital ventricular fibrillation: 4-year follow-up. Circulation *52*(Suppl 3):223, 1975.
81. Levin, D. C., Fellows, K. E., and Abrams, H. L.: Hemodynamically significant primary anomalies of the coronary arteries: Angiographic aspects. Circulation *58*:25, 1978.
82. Harthorne, J. W., Scannell, J. G., and Dinsmore, R. E.: Anomalous origin of the left coronary artery: Remedial cause of sudden death in adults. N. Engl. J. Med. *275*:660, 1966.
83. Benge, W., Martins, J. B., and Funk, D. C.: Morbidity associated with anomalous origin of the right coronary artery from the left sinus of Valsalva. Am. Heart J. *99*:96, 1980.
84. Roberts, W. C., Siegel, R. J., and Zipes, D. P.: Origin of the right coronary artery from the left sinus of Valsalva and its functional consequences: Analysis of 10 necropsy patients. Am. J. Cardiol. *49*:863, 1982.

85. Maron, B. J., Epstein, S. E., and Roberts, W. C.: Causes of sudden death in competitive athletes. J. Am. Coll. Cardiol. *7*:204, 1986.
86. Waller, B. F.: Exercise-related sudden death in young (age ≤ 30 years) and old (age > 30 years) conditioned subjects. *In* Wenger, N.K. (ed.): Exercise and the Heart. Philadelphia, F. A. Davis Co., 1985, pp. 9–73.
87. Roberts, W. C.: Coronary embolism: A review of causes, consequences, and diagnostic considerations. Cardiovasc. Med. *3*:699, 1978.
88. El Maraghi, N., and Genton, E.: The relevance of platelet and fibrin thromboembolism of the coronary microcirculation, with special reference to sudden cardiac death. Circulation *62*:936, 1980.
89. Kegel, S. M., Dorsey, T. J., Rowen, M., and Taylor, W. F.: Cardiac death in mucocutaneous lymph node syndrome. Am. J. Cardiol. *40*:282, 1977.
90. Thiene, G., Valente, M., and Rossi, L.: Involvement of the cardiac conduction system in panarteritis nodosa. Am. Heart J. *95*:716, 1978.
91. Heggveit, H. A.: Syphilitic aortitis–a clinicopathological autopsy of 100 cases. Circulation *29*:346, 1964.
92. Roberts, W. C., and Honig, H. S.: The spectrum of cardiovascular disease in the Marfan syndrome. Am. Heart J. *104*:115, 1982.
93. Shaver, P. J., Carrig, T. F., and Baker, W. P.: Postpartum coronary artery dissection. Br. Heart J. *40*:83, 1978.
94. Harris, L. S., and Adelson, L.: Fatal coronary embolism from a myxomatous polyp of the aortic valve. An unusual cause of sudden death. Am. J. Clin. Pathol. *43*:61, 1965.
95. Roberts, W. C.: Pathology of arterial aneurysms. *In* Bergan, J. J., and Yao, S. T. (eds.): Aneurysms, Diagnosis and Treatment. New York, Grune and Stratton, 1982, pp. 17–43.
96. Miller, D D., Waters, D. D., Szlachcic, J., and Theroux, P.: Clinical characteristics associated with sudden death in patients with variant angina. Circulation *66*:588, 1982.
97. Morady, F., DiCarlo, L., Winston, S., et al.: Clinical features and prognosis of patients with out-of-hospital cardiac arrest and a normal electrophysiologic study. J. Am. Coll. Cardiol. *4*:39, 1984.
98. Nakamura, M., Takeshita, A., and Nose, Y.: Clinical characteristics associated with myocardial infarction, arrhythmias, and sudden death in patients with vasospastic angina. Circulation *75*:1110, 1987.
99. Cohn, P. F.: Silent myocardial ischemia in patients with a defective anginal warning system. Am. J. Cardiol. *45*:697, 1980.
100. Sharma, B., Francis, G., Hodges, M., and Asinger, R.: Demonstration of exercise-induced ischemia without angina in patients who recover from out-of-hospital ventricular fibrillation. Am. J. Cardiol. *47*:445, 1981 (abstract).
101. Maseri, A., Severi, S., and Marzullo, P.: Role of coronary arterial spasm in sudden coronary ischemic death. Ann. N.Y. Acad. Sci. *382*:204, 1982.
102. Sheps, D. S., and Heiss, G.: Sudden death and silent myocardial ischemia. Am. Heart J. *117*:177, 1989.
103. Morales, A. R., Romanelli, R., and Boucek, R. J.: The mural left anterior descending coronary artery, strenuous exercise, and sudden death. Circulation *62*:230, 1980.
104. Anderson, K. P.: Sudden death, hypertension, and hypertrophy. J. Cardiovasc. Pharmacol. *6*(Suppl 3):S498, 1984.
105. Anderson, K. P.: Hypertension and sudden cardiac death. N.Z. Med. J. *95*:33, 1982.
106. Messerli, F. H., Ventura, H. O., Elizardi, D. J., et al.: Hypertension and sudden death: Increased ventricular ectopic activity in left ventricular hypertrophy. Am. J. Med. *77*:18, 1984.
107. Braunwald, E., Morrow, A. G., Cornell, W. P., et al.: Idiopathic hypertrophic subaortic stenosis: Clinical, hemodynamic, and angiographic manifestations. Am. J. Med. *29*:924, 1960.
108. Goodwin, J. F.: The frontiers of cardiomyopathy. Br. Heart J. *48*:1, 1982.
109. Shah, P. M., Adelman, A. G., Wigle, E. D., et al.: The natural (and unnatural) history of hypertrophic obstructive cardiomyopathy. Circ. Res. *35*(Suppl 2):179, 1974.
110. Cecchi, F., Maron, B. J., and Epstein, S. E.: Long-term outcome of patients with hypertrophic cardiomyopathy successfully resuscitated after cardiac arrest. J. Am. Coll. Cardiol. *13*:1283, 1989.
111. Maron, B. J., Roberts, W. C., and Epstein, S. E.: Sudden death in hypertrophic cardiomyopathy: A profile of 78 patients. Circulation *65*:1388, 1982.
112. Savage, D. D., Seides, S. F., Maron, B. J., et al.: Prevalence of arrhythmias during 24-hour electrocardiographic monitoring and exercise testing in patients with obstructive and non-obstructive hypertrophic cardiomyopathy. Circulation *59*:866, 1979.
113. Goodwin, J. F., and Krikler, D. M.: Arrhythmia as a cause of sudden death in hypertrophic cardiomyopathy. Lancet *2*:937, 1976.
114. Maron, B. J., Savage, D. D., Wolfson, J. K., and Epstein, S. E.: Prognostic significance of 24 hour ambulatory electrocardiographic monitoring in patients with hypertrophic cardiomyopathy: A prospective study. Am. J. Cardiol. *48*:252, 1981.
115. Fananapazir, L., and Epstein, S. E.: Hemodynamic and electrophysiologic evaluation of patients with hypertrophic cardiomyopathy surviving cardiac arrest. Am. J. Cardiol. *67*:280, 1991.
116. Kowey, P. R., Eisenberg, R., and Engel, T. R.: Sustained arrhythmias in hypertrophic obstructive cardiomyopathy. N. Engl. J. Med. *310*:1566, 1984.
117. Stafford, W. J., Trohman, R. G., Bilsker, M., et al.: Cardiac arrest in an adolescent with atrial fibrillation and hypertrophic cardiomyopathy. J. Am. Coll. Cardiol. *7*:701, 1986.
118. Maron, B. J., Epstein, S. E., and Roberts, W. C.: Hypertrophic cardiomyopathy: A common cause of sudden death in the young competitive athlete. Eur. Heart J. *4*(Suppl F):135, 1983.
119. Waller, B. F.: Sudden death in midlife. Cardiovasc. Med. *10*:55, 1985.
120. Northcote, R. J., Flannigan, C., and Ballantyne, D.: Sudden death and vigorous exercise: A study of 60 deaths associated with squash. Br. Heart J. *55*:198, 1986.
121. Packer, M.: Sudden unexpected death in patients with congestive heart failure: A second frontier. Circulation *72*:681, 1985.
122. Huang, S. K., Messer, J. V., and Denes, P.: Significance of ventricular tachycardia in idiopathic dilated cardiomyopathy: Observations in 35 patients. Am. J. Cardiol. *51*:507, 1983.
123. Meinertz, T., Hoffmann, T., Kasper, W., et al.: Significance of ventricular arrhythmias in idiopathic dilated cardiomyopathy. Am. J. Cardiol. *53*:902, 1984.
124. Poll, D. S., Marchinski, F. E., Buxton, A. E., et al.: Sustained ventricular tachycardia in patients with idiopathic dilated cardiomyopathy: Electrophysiologic testing and lack of response to antiarrhythmic drug therapy. Circulation *70*:451, 1984.
125. Warren, J. V.: Unusual sudden death. Cardiol. Ser. *8*(4):5, 1984.
126. Surawicz, B.: Ventricular fibrillation. J. Am. Coll. Cardiol. *51*(Suppl B):43, 1985.
127. Topaz, O., and Edwards, J. E.: Pathologic features of sudden death in children, adolescents, and young adults. Chest *87*:476, 1985.
128. Phillips, M., Rabinowitz, M., Higgins, J. R., et al.: Sudden cardiac death in air force recruits. J.A.M.A. *256*:2696, 1986.
129. Robboy, S. J.: Atrioventricular node inflammation: Mechanisms of sudden death in protracted meningococcemia. N. Engl. J. Med. *286*:1091, 1972.
130. Roberts, W. C., McAllister, H. A., and Farrans, V. J.: Sarcoidosis of the heart: A clinicopathologic study of 35 necropsy patients (group I) and review of 78 previously described necropsy patients (group II). Am. J. Med. *63*:86, 1977.
131. Silverman, K. J., Hutchins, G. M., and Bulkley, B. H.: Cardiac sarcoid: A clinicopathologic study of 84 unselected patients with systemic sarcoidosis. Circulation *58*:1204, 1978.
132. Bulkley, B. H., Klacsman, P. G., and Hutchins, G. M.: Angina pectoris, myocardial infarction and sudden cardiac death with normal coronary arteries: A clinicopathological study of nine patients with progressive systemic sclerosis. Am. Heart J. *95*:563, 1978.
133. Marcus, F. L., Fontaine, G. H., Guiraudon, G., et al.: Right ventricular dysplasia: A report of 24 adult cases. Circulation *65*:384, 1982.
134. Ibsen, H.H.W., Baandrup, U., and Simonsen, E. E.: Familial right ventricular dilated cardiomyopathy. Br. Heart J. *54*:156, 1985.
135. Thiene, G., Nava, A., Corrado, D., et al.: Right ventricular cardiomyopathy and sudden death in young people. N. Engl. J. Med. *318*:129, 1988.
136. Wright, J. R., and Calkins, E.: Clinical-pathologic differentiation of common amyloid syndromes. Medicine *60*:429, 1981.
137. Ridolfi, R. L., Bulkley, B. H., and Hutchins, G. M.: The conduction system in cardiac amyloidosis: Clinical and pathologic features of 23 patients. Am. J. Med. *62*:677, 1977.
138. Campbell, M.: Calcific aortic stenosis and congenital bicuspid aortic valves. Br. Heart J. *30*:606, 1968.
139. Smith, N., McAnulty, J. G., and Rahimtoola, S. H.: Severe aortic stenosis with impaired left ventricular function and clinical heart failure: Results of valve replacement. Circulation *58*:255, 1978.
140. Rahimtoola, S. H.: Valvular heart disease: A perspective. J. Am. Coll. Cardiol. *1*:199, 1983.
141. Blackstone, E. H., and Kirklin, J. W.: Death and other time-related events after valve replacement. Circulation *72*:753, 1985.
142. Gohlke-Barwolf, C., Peters, K., Petersen, J., et al.: Influence of aortic valve replacement on sudden death in patients with pure aortic stenosis. Eur. Heart J. *9*(Suppl E):139, 1988.
143. Konishi, Y., Matsuda, K., Nishiwaki, N., et al.: Ventricular arrhythmias late after aortic and/or mitral valve replacement. Jpn. Cir. J. *49*:576, 1985.
144. Chesler, E., King, R. A., and Edwards, J. E.: The myxomatous mitral valve and sudden death. Circulation *67*:632, 1983.
145. Campbell, R.W.F., Godman, M. G., Fiddler, G. I., et al.: Ventricular arrhythmias in the syndrome of balloon deformity of mitral valve: Definition of possible high-risk group. Br. Heart J. *38*:1053, 1976.
146. Pocock, W. A., Bosman, C. K., Chesler, E., et al.: Sudden death in primary mitral valve prolapse. Am. Heart J. *107*:378, 1984.
147. Nishimura, R. A., McGoon, M. D., Shub, C., et al.: Echocardiographically documented mitral valve prolapse: Long-term follow-up of 237 patients. N. Engl. J. Med. *313*:1305, 1985.
148. Glew, R. H., Varghese, P. J., Krovetz, L. J., et al.: Sudden death in congenital aortic stenosis: A review of 8 cases with an evaluation of premonitory clinical features. Am. Heart J. *78*:615, 1969.
149. Hoffman, J. I. E.: The natural history of congenital isolated pulmonic and aortic stenosis. Annu. Rev. Med. *20*:15, 1969.
150. Young, D., and Marks, H.: Fate of the patient with the Eisenmenger syndrome. Am. J. Cardiol. *28*:658, 1971.
151. Jones, A. M., and Howitt, G.: Eisenmenger syndrome in pregnancy. Br. Med. J. *1*:1627, 1965.
152. Garson, A., Nihill, M. R., McNamara, D. G., and Cooley, D. A.: Status of the adult and adolescent after repair of tetralogy of Fallot. Circulation *59*:1232, 1979.
153. Gillette, P. C., Kugler, J. D., Garson, A., et al.: The mechanism of cardiac dysrhythmia after Mustard operation for transposition of the great arteries. Am. J. Cardiol. *45*:1225, 1980.
154. Garson, A., and McNamara, D. G.: Sudden death in a pediatric cardiology population, 1958 to 1983: Relation to prior arrhythmias. J. Am. Coll. Cardiol. *5*(Suppl B):134B, 1985.
155. Lie, K. I., Leim, K. L., Schuilenberg, R. M., et al.: Early identification of patients developing late in-hospital ventricular fibrillation after discharge from the coronary care unit. Am. J. Cardiol. *41*:674, 1978.

(eds.): Textbook of Advanced Cardiac Life Support. Dallas, American Heart Association, Inc., 1983, pp. 89–96.

288. Standard and guidelines for cardiopulmonary resuscitation (CPR) and emergency cardiac care (ECC). J.A.M.A. *255*:290, 1986.
289. Lo, B., and Jonsen, A. R.: Clinical decisions to limit treatment. Ann. Intern. Med. *93*:764, 1980.
290. Lo, B., and Steinbrook, R. L.: Deciding whether to resuscitate. Arch. Intern. Med. *143*:1561, 1983.
291. Bedell, S. E., Delbanco, T. L., Cook, E. F., and Epstein, F. H.: Survival after cardiopulmonary resuscitation in the hospital. N. Engl. J. Med. *309*:569, 1983.
292. Cobb, L. A., and Hallstrom, A. P.: Community-based cardiopulmonary resuscitation: What have we learned? Ann. N.Y. Acad. Sci. *382*:330, 1982.
293. Cobb, L. A., Hallstrom, A. P., Weaver, W. D., et al.: Considerations in the long-term management of survivors of cardiac arrest. Ann. N.Y. Acad. Sci. *432*:247, 1984.
294. Goldstein, S., Landis, J. R., Leighton, R., et al.: Predictive survival models for resuscitated victims of out-of-hospital cardiac arrest with coronary heart disease. Circulation *71*:873, 1985.
295. Gulati, R. S., Bhan, G. L., and Horan, M. A.: Cardiopulmonary resuscitation of old people. Lancet *2*:267, 1983.
296. Taffet, G. E., Teasdale, T. A., and Luchi, R. J.: In-hospital cardiopulmonary resuscitation. J.A.M.A. *260*:2069, 1988.
297. Tresch, D. D., Thakur, R. K., Hoffmann, R. G., et al.: Should the elderly be resuscitated following out-of-hospital cardiac arrest? Am. J. Med. *86*:145, 1989.
298. Eisenberg, M. S., Bergner, L., and Hallstrom, A. P.: Cardiac resuscitation in the community: Importance of rapid provision and implications of program planning. J.A.M.A. *241*:1905, 1979.
299. Myerburg, R. J., Estes, D, Zaman, L., et al.: Outcome of resuscitation from bradyarrhythmic or asystolic prehospital cardiac arrest. J. Am. Coll. Cardiol. *4*:1118, 1984.
300. Jaggarao, N. S. V. Heber, M., Grainger, R., et al.: Use of an automated external defibrillator-pacemaker by ambulance staff. Lancet *2*:73, 1982.
301. Longstreth, W. T., Inui, T. S., Cobb, L. A., and Copass, M. K.: Neurologic recovery after out-of-hospital cardiac arrest. Ann. Intern. Med. *98*:588, 1983.
302. Longstreth, W. T., Diehr, P., and Inui, T. S.: Prediction of awakening after out-of-hospital cardiac arrest. N. Engl. J. Med. *308*:1378, 1983.
303. Myerburg, R. J., Conde, C. A., Sheps, D. S., et al.: Antiarrhythmic drug therapy in survivors of prehospital cardiac arrest: Comparison of effects on chronic ventricular arrhythmias and on recurrent cardiac arrest. Circulation *59*:855, 1979.
304. Weaver, W. D., Cobb, L. A., and Hallstrom, A. P.: Ambulatory arrhythmia in resuscitated victims of cardiac arrest. Circulation *66*:212, 1982.
305. Ritchie, J. L., Hallstrom, A. P., Troubaugh, G. B., et al.: Out-of-hospital sudden coronary death: Rest and exercise radionuclide left ventricular function in survivors. Am. J. Cardiol. *55*:645, 1985.
306. Weaver, W. D., Lorch, G. S., Alvarez, H. A., and Cobb, L. A.: Angiographic findings and prognostic indicators in patients resuscitated from sudden cardiac death. Circulation *54*:895, 1976.
307. Weaver, W. D., Cobb, L. A., and Hallstrom, A. P.: Characteristics of survivors of exertion- and nonexertion-related cardiac arrest: Value of subsequent exercise testing. Am. J. Cardiol. *50*:671, 1982.
308. Cobb, L. A., Werner, J. A., and Trobaugh, G. B.: Sudden cardiac death: I. A decade's experience with out-of-hospital resuscitation; and II. Outcome of resuscitation, management, and future directions. Mod. Concepts Cardiovasc. Dis. *49*:31, 1980.
309. Haynes, R. E., Hallstrom, A. P., and Cobb, L. A.: Repolarization abnormalities in survivors of out-of-hospital ventricular fibrillation. Circulation *57*:654, 1978.
310. Thompson, R. G., and Cobb, L. A.: Hypokalemia after resuscitation from out-of-hospital cardiac arrest. J.A.M.A. *248*:2860, 1982.
311. Urban, P., Scheidegger, D., Buchmann, B., and Barth, D.: Cardiac arrest and blood ionized calcium levels. Ann. Intern. Med. *109*:110, 1988.
312. Sheps, D. S., Conde, C., Cameron, B., et al.: Resting peripheral blood lactate elevation in survivors of prehospital cardiac arrest: Correlation with hemodynamic, electrophysiologic, and oxyhemoglobin dissociation indexes. Am. J. Cardiol. *44*:1276, 1979.
313. Myerburg, R. J., Kessler, K. M., Zaman, L., et al.: Factors leading to decreasing mortality among patients resuscitated from out-of-hospital cardiac arrest. *In* Brugada, P., and Wellens, H. J. J. (eds.): Cardiac Arrhythmias: Where to Go from Here? Mt. Kisko, N.Y., Futura, 1987, pp. 505–525.
314. Furukawa, T., Rozanski, J. J., Nogami, J., et al.: Time-dependent risk of and predictors for cardiac arrest recurrence in survivors of out-of-hospital cardiac arrest with chronic coronary artery disease. Circulation *80*:599, 1989.

MANAGEMENT OF CARDIAC ARREST

315. Goldman, L.: Coronary care units: A perspective on their epidemiologic impact. Int. J. Cardiol. *2*:284, 1982.
316. Killip, T., and Kimball, J. T.: Treatment of myocardial infarction in a coronary care unit: A two-year experience with 250 patients. Am. J. Cardiol. *20*:457, 1967.
317. Pantridge, J. F., and Adgey, A.A.J.: Pre-hospital coronary care. The mobile coronary care unit. Am. J. Cardiol. *24*:666, 1969.
318. Stults, K. R., Brown, D. D., Schug, V. L., and Bean, J. A.: Prehospital defibrillation performed by emergency medical technicians in rural communities. N. Engl. J. Med. *310*:219, 1984.
319. Eisenberg, M. S., Copass, M. K., Hallstrom, A. P., et al.: Treatment of out-of-hospital cardiac arrests with rapid defibrillation by emergency medical technicians. N. Engl. J. Med. *302*:1379, 1980.
320. Ewy, G. A.: Current status of cardiopulmonary resuscitation. Mod. Concepts Cardiovasc. Dis. *53*:43, 1984.
321. Mayer, J. D.: Paramedic response time and survival from cardiac arrest. Soc. Sci. Med. *13D*:267, 1979.
322. Weaver, W. D., Copass, M. K., Bufi, D., et al.: Improved neurologic recovery and survival after early defibrillation. Circulation *69*:943, 1984.
323. Weaver, W. D., Hill, D., Fahrenbruch, C. E., et al.: Use of the automatic external defibrillator in the management of out-of-hospital cardiac arrest. N. Engl. J. Med. *318*:661, 1988.
324. Lie, K. I., Wellens, H. J. J., van Capelle, F. J., and Durrer, D.: Lidocaine in the prevention of primary ventricular fibrillation. N. Engl. J. Med. *291*:1324, 1974.
325. Valentine, P. A, Frew, J. L., Mashford, M. L., and Sloman, J. G.: Lidocaine in the prevention of sudden death in the prehospital phase of acute infarction. N. Engl. J. Med. *291*:1327, 1974.
326. Koster, R. W., and Dunning, R. J.: Intramuscular lidocaine for prevention of lethal arrhythmias in the prehospitalization phase of acute myocardial infarction. N. Engl. J. Med. *313*:1105, 1985.
327. Caldwell, G., Miller, G., Quinn, E., et al.: Simple mechanical methods for cardioversion: Defense of the precordial thump and cough version. Br. Med. J. *291*:627, 1985.
328. Lown, B., and Taylor, J.: "Thumpversion" (editorial). N. Engl. J. Med. *283*:1223, 1970.
329. Criley, J. M., Blaufuss, A. N., and Kissel, J. L.: Cough-induced cardiac compression: Self-administered form of cardiopulmonary resuscitation. J.A.M.A. *263*:1246, 1976.
330. Wei, J. Y., Greene, H. L., and Weisfeldt, M. L.: Cough-facilitated conversion of ventricular tachycardia. Am. J. Cardiol. *45*:174, 1980.
331. Heimlich, H. J.: A life-saving maneuver to prevent food-choking. J.A.M.A. *234*:398, 1975.
332. Visintine, R. E., and Baick, C. H.: Ruptured stomach after Heimlich maneuver. J.A.M.A. *234*:415, 1975.
333. Feldman, T., Mallon, S. M., Bolooki, H., et al.: Fatal acute aortic regurgitation in a person performing the Heimlich maneuver (letter). N. Engl. J. Med. *315*:1613, 1986.
334. Standards and guidelines for cardiopulmonary resuscitation (CPR) and emergency cardiac care (ECC). J.A.M.A. *244*:453, 1980.
335. Weisfeldt, M. L., and Chandra, N.: Physiology of cardiopulmonary resuscitation. Annu. Rev. Med. *32*:435, 1981.
336. Weisfeldt, M. L., Chandra, N., and Tsitlik, J. E.: Increased intrathoracic pressure—not direct heart compression—causes the rise in intrathoracic vascular pressures during CPR in dogs and pigs. Crit. Care Med. *9*:377, 1981.
337. Rudikoff, M. T., Maughan, W. L., Effrom, M., et al.: Mechanisms of blood flow during cardiopulmonary resuscitation. Circulation *61*:345, 1980.
338. Niemann, J. T., Rosborough, J. P., Hausknecht, M., et al.: Pressure-synchronized cineangiography during experimental cardiopulmonary resuscitation. Circulation *4*:985, 1981.
339. Chandra, N., Rudikoff, M., and Weisfeldt, M. L.: Simultaneous chest compression and ventilation at high airway pressure during cardiopulmonary resuscitation. Lancet *1*:175, 1980.
340. Ditchey, R. V., and Lindenfeld, J.: Potential adverse effects of volume loading on perfusion of vital organs during closed-chest resuscitation. Circulation *69*:181, 1984.
341. Michael, J. R., Guerci, D., Koehler, R. C., et al.: Mechanisms by which epinephrine augments cerebral and myocardial perfusion during cardiopulmonary resuscitation in dogs. Circulation *69*:822, 1984.
342. Sanders, A. B., Ewy, G. A., Alferness, A., et al.: Failure of one method of simultaneous chest compression, ventilation, and abdominal binding during CPR. Crit. Care Med. *120*:509, 1982.
343. Ducas, J., Roussos, C. H., Karsaidis, C., and Magder, S.: Thoracoabdominal mechanisms during resuscitation maneuvers. Chest *84*:446, 1983.
344. Guerci, A. D., Halperin, H. R., Beyar, R., et al.: Aortic diameter and pressure-flow sequence identify mechanism of blood flow during external chest compression in dogs. J. Am. Coll. Cardiol. *14*:790, 1989.
345. Cummins, R. O., Eisenberg, M., Bergner, L., and Murray, J. A.: Sensitivity, accuracy, and safety of an automatic external defibrillator. Lancet *2*:318, 1984.
346. Gascho, J. A., Crampton, R. S., Cherwek, M. L., et al.: Determinants of ventricular defibrillation in adults. Circulation *60*:231, 1979.
347. Tacker, W. A., and Ewy, G. A.: Emergency defibrillation dose, recommendation and rationale. Circulation *60*:223, 1979.
348. Lown, B., Crampton, R. S., and DeSilva, R. A.: The energy for ventricular defibrillation: Too little or too much? N. Engl. J. Med. *298*:1252, 1978.
349. Sodium bicarbonate in cardiac arrest (editorial). Lancet *1*:946, 1976.
350. Weil, M. H., Trevino, R. P., and Rackow, E. C.: Sodium bicarbonate during CPR: Does it help or hinder? Chest *88*:487, 1985.
351. White, R. D.: Cardiovascular pharmacology: Part I. *In* McIntyre, K. M., and Lewis, A. J. (eds.): Textbook of Advanced Life Support. Dallas, American Heart Association, Inc., 1983, pp. 99–114.
352. Thompson, P. D., Melmon, K. L., Richardson, J. A., et al.: Lidocaine pharmocokinetics in advanced heart failure, liver disease, and renal failure in humans. Ann. Intern. Med. *78*:499, 1973.
353. Giardina, E G., Heissenbuttel, R. H., and Bigger, J. T.: Intermittent intravenous procainamide to treat ventricular arrhythmias. Correlation of plasma concentration with effect on arrhythmia, electrocardiogram, and blood pressure. Ann. Intern. Med. *78*:183, 1973.

354. Haynes, R. E., Chinn, T. L., Copass, M. K., and Cobb, L. A.: Comparison of bretylium tosylate and lidocaine in the resuscitation of patients from out-of-hospital ventricular fibrillation: A randomized clinical trial. Am. J. Cardiol. *487*:353, 1981.
355. Kutalek, S. P., Horowitz, L. N., Spielman, S. R., and Greenspan, A M.: Emergent use of intravenous amiodarone for refractory ventricular tachyarrhythmias. Circulation *72*(Suppl 3):274, 1985 (Abstract).
356. Hughes, W. G., and Ruedy, J. R.: Should calcium be used in cardiac arrest? Am. J. Med. *81*:285, 1986.
357. Zoll, P. M., Zoll, R. H., Clinton, J. E., et al.: External non-invasive temporary cardiac pacing: Clinical trials. Circulation *71*:937, 1985.
358. Knowlton, A. A., and Falk, R. H.: External cardiac pacing during in hospital cardiac arrest. Am. J. Cardiol. *51*:1295, 1986.
359. Lee, R. V., Rogers, B. D., White, L. M., and Harvey, R. C.: Cardiopulmonary resuscitation of pregnant women. Am. J. Med. *81*:311, 1986.
360. Holmes, H. R., Babbs, C. F., Voorhees, W. D., et al.: Influence of adrenergic drugs upon vital organ perfusion during CPR. Crit. Care Med. *8*:137, 1980.
361. Otto, C. W., Yakaitis, R. W., Redding, J. S., and Blitt, C. D.: Comparison of dopamine, dobutamine, and epinephrine in CPR. Crit. Care Med. *9*:366, 1981.
362. Ralston, S. H., Voorhees, W. D., and Babbs, C. F.: Intrapulmonary epinephrine during prolonged cardiopulmonary resuscitation: Improved regional blood flow and resuscitation in dogs. Ann. Emerg. Med. *13*:79, 1984.
363. Yakaitis, R. W., Otto, C. W., and Blitt, C. D.: Relative importance of alpha and beta-adrenergic receptors during resuscitation. Crit. Care Med. *7*:293, 1979.
364. Wyman, M. G., and Hammersmith, L.: Comprehensive treatment plan for the prevention of primary ventricular fibrillation in acute myocardial infarction. Am. J. Cardiol. *33*:661, 1974.
365. Conley, M. J., McNeer, J. F., Lee, K. L., et al.: Cardiac arrest complicating acute myocardial infarction: Predictability and prognosis. Am. J. Cardiol. *39*:7, 1977.
366. Vismara, L. A., Amsterdam, B. A., and Mason, D. T.: Relation of ventricular arrhythmias in the late-hospital phase of acute myocardial infarction to sudden death after hospital discharge. Am. J. Med. *59*:6, 1975.
367. Robinson, J. S., Sloman, G., Mathew, T. H., and Goble, A. J.: Survival after resuscitation from cardiac arrest in acute myocardial infarction. Am. Heart J. *69*:740, 1965.
368. Norris, R. M., and Mercer, C. J.: Significance of idioventricular rhythms in acute myocardial infarction. Prog. Cardiovasc. Dis. *16*:455, 1974.
369. Myerburg, R. J., Kessler, K. M., Cox, M. M., et al.: Reversal of proarrhythmic effects of flecainide acetate and encainide hydrochloride by propranolol. Circulation *80*:1571, 1989.
370. Bass, E.: Cardiopulmonary arrest: Pathophysiology and neurologic complications. Ann. Intern. Med. *103*:920, 1985.
371. Breivik, H., Safar, P., Sands, P., et al.: Clinical feasibility trials of barbiturate therapy after cardiac arrest. Crit. Care Med. *6*:228, 1978.
372. Brain Resuscitation Clinical Trial I Study Group: Randomized clinical study of thiopental loading in comatose survivors of cardiac arrest. N. Engl. J. Med. *314*:397, 1986.
373. Cobb, L. A., Hallstrom, A. P., Zia, M., et al.: Influence of coronary revascularization on recurrent sudden cardiac death syndrome. J. Am. Coll. Cardiol. *1*:688, 1983 (Abstract).
374. Harken, A. H., Wetstein, L., and Josephson, M. E.: Mechanisms and surgical management of ventricular tachyarrhythmias. *In* Josephson, M. E. (ed.): Sudden Cardiac Death. Philadelphia, F. A. Davis Co., 1985, pp. 287–300.
375. Holmes, D. R., Davis, K. B., Mock, M. B., et al.: The effect of medical and surgical treatment on subsequent sudden cardiac death in patients with coronary artery disease: A report from the Coronary Artery Surgery Study. Circulation *73*:1254, 1986.
376. Multiple Risk Factor Intervention Trial Research Group: Baseline rest electrocardiographic abnormalities, antihypertensive treatment, and mortality in the Multiple Risk Factor Intervention Trial. Am. J. Cardiol. *55*:1, 1985.
377. Moss, A. J., Davis, H. T., Conard, D. L., et al.: Digitalis-associated cardiac mortality after myocardial infarction. Circulation *64*:1150, 1981.
378. Bigger, J. T., Fleiss, J. L., Rolnitzky, L. M., et al.: Effect of digitalis treatment on survival after acute myocardial infarction. Am. J. Cardiol. *55*:623, 1985.
379. Ryan, T. J., Bailey, K. R., McCabe, C. H., et al.: The effects of digitalis on survival in high risk patients with coronary artery disease. The Coronary Artery Surgery Study (CASS). Circulation *67*:735, 1983.
380. Madsen, E. G., Gilpin, E., Henning, H., et al. Prognostic importance of digitalis after acute myocardial infarction. J. Am. Coll. Cardiol. *3*:681, 1984.
381. Muller, J. E., Turi, Z. G., Stone, P. H., et al.: Digoxin therapy and mortality after myocardial infarction: Experience in the MILIS study. N. Engl. J. Med. *314*:265, 1986.
382. Graboys, T. B., Lown, B., Podrid, P. J., and DeSilva, R.: Long-term survival of patients with malignant ventricular arrhythmias treated with antiarrhythmic drugs. Am. J. Cardiol. *50*:437, 1982.
383. Ruskin, J. N., DiMarco, J. P., and Garan, H.: Out-of-hospital cardiac arrest: Electrophysiologic observations and selection of long-term antiarrhythmic therapy. N. Engl. J. Med. *303*:607, 1980.
384. Wilber, D. J., Garan, H., Finkelstein, D., et al.: Out-of-hospital cardiac arrest: Use of electrophysiological testing in the prediction of long-term outcome. N. Engl. J. Med. *318*:19, 1988.
385. Josephson, M. E., Horowitz, L. N., Spielman, S. C., and Greenspan, A. M.: Electrophysiologic and hemodynamic studies in patients resuscitated from cardiac arrest. Am. J. Cardiol. *46*:948, 1980.
386. Roy, D., Waxman, H. L., Kienzle, M. G., et al.: Clinical characteristics and long-term follow-up in 119 survivors of cardiac arrest: Relation to inducibility at electrophysiologic testing. Am. J. Cardiol. *52*:969, 1983.
387. Benditt, D. G., Benson, D. W., Jr., Klein, G. J., et al.: Prevention of recurrent sudden cardiac arrest: Role of provocative electropharmacologic testing. J. Am. Coll. Cardiol. *2*:418, 1983.
388. Morady, F., Scheinman, M. M., Hess, D. S., et al.: Electrophysiologic testing in the management of survivors of out-of-hospital cardiac arrest. Am. J. Cardiol. *51*:85, 1983.
389. Skale, B. T., Miles, W. M., Heger, J. J., et al.: Survivors of cardiac arrest: Prevention of recurrence by drug therapy as predicted by electrophysiologic testing or electrocardiographic monitoring. Am. J. Cardiol. *57*:113, 1986.
390. Akhtar, M., Guran, H., Lehmann, M. H., and Troup, P. J.: Sudden cardiac death: Management of high-risk patients. Ann. Intern. Med. *114*:499, 1991.
391. Platia, E. V., Griffith, L. S. C., Watkins, L., et al.: Treatment of malignant ventricular arrhythmias with endocardial resection and implantation of the automatic cardioverter-defibrillator. N. Engl. J. Med. *314*:213, 1986.
392. Swerdlow, C. R., Winkle, R. A., and Mason, J. W.: Determinants of survival in patients with ventricular tachycardia. N. Engl. J. Med. *308*:1436, 1983.
393. Mirowski, M., Reid, P. R., Winkle, R. A., et al.: Mortality in patients with implanted automatic defibrillators. Ann. Intern. Med. *98*:585, 1983.
394. Echt, D S., Armstrong, K., Schmidt, P., et al.: Clinical experience, complications, and survival in 70 patients with the automatic implantable cardioverter/defibrillator. Circulation *71*:289, 1985.
395. Wellens, H. J. J., Brugada, P., and Stevenson, W. G.: Programmed electrical stimulation of the heart in patients with life-threatening ventricular arrhythmias: What is the significance of induced arrhythmias and what is the correct stimulation protocol? Circulation *72*:1, 1985.
396. Myerburg, R. J., and Zaman, L.: Indications for intracardiac electrophysiologic studies in survivors of prehospital cardiac arrest. Circulation *75*:151, 1987.
397. Zheutlin, T. A., Steinman, R. T., Mattioni, T. A., and Kehoe, R. F.: Long-term arrhythmic outcome in survivors of ventricular fibrillation with absence of inducible ventricular tachycardia. Am. J. Cardiol. *62*:1213, 1988.
398. Josephson, M. E., Harken, A. H., and Horowitz, L. N.: Endocardial excision: A new surgical technique for the treatment of recurrent ventricular tachycardia. Circulation *60*:1430, 1979.
399. Guiradon, G., Fontaine, G., Frank, R., et al.: Encircling endocardial ventriculotomy: A new surgical treatment for life-threatening ventricular tachycardias resistant to medical treatment following myocardial infarction. Ann. Thorac. Surg. *26*:438, 1978.
400. Kelly, P., Ruskin, J. N., Vlahakes, G. J., et al.: Surgical coronary revascularization in survivors of prehospital cardiac arrest. J. Am. Coll. Cardiol. *15*:267, 1990.
401. Mirowski, M., Reid, P. R., Mower, M. M., et al.: Termination of malignant ventricular arrhythmias with an implanted automatic defibrillator in human beings. N. Engl. J. Med. *303*:322, 1980.
402. Kelly, P. A., Cannom, D. S., Garan, H., et al.: The automatic implantable defibrillator (AICD): Efficacy, complications and survival in patients with malignant ventricular arrhythmias. J. Am. Coll. Cardiol. *11*:1278, 1988.
403. Tchou, P. J., Kadri, N., Anderson, J., et al.: Automatic implantable cardioverter-defibrillators and survival of patients with left ventricular dysfunction and malignant ventricular arrhythmias. Ann. Intern. Med. *109*:529, 1988.
404. Fogoros, R. N., Elson, J. J., and Bonnet, C. A.: Actuarial incidence and pattern of occurrence of shocks following implantation of the automatic implantable cardioverter-defibrillator. PACE *12*:1465, 1989.
405. Myerburg, R. J., Luceri, R. M., Thurer, R., et al.: Time to first shock and clinical outcome in patients receiving automatic implantable cardioverter-defibrillators. J. Am. Coll. Cardiol. *14*:508, 1989.
406. Myerburg, R. J., and Kessler, K. M.: Management of patients who survive cardiac arrest. Mod. Concepts Cardiovasc. Dis. *55*:61, 1986.
407. Herre, J., Sauve, M. J., Malone, P., et al.: Long-term results of amiodarone therapy in patients with recurrent sustained ventricular tachycardia or ventricular fibrillation. J. Am. Coll. Cardiol. *13*:442, 1989.
408. Kim, S. O., Seiden, S. W., Felder, S. D., et al.: Is programmed stimulation of value in predicting the long-term success of antiarrhythmic therapy for ventricular tachycardia? N. Engl. J. Med. *315*:356, 1986.
409. Myerburg, R. J., and Davis, J. H.: The medical ecology of public safety. I. Sudden death due to coronary heart disease. Am. Heart J. *68*:586, 1964.
410. Levy, R. L., De La Chapelle, C. E., and Richards, D. W.:Heart disease in drivers of public motor vehicles as a cause of highway accidents. J.A.M.A. *184*:143, 1963.
411. Waller, J. A.: Cardiovascular disease, aging, and traffic accidents. J. Chron. Dis. *20*:615, 1967.
412. Kerwin, A. J.: Sudden death while driving. Can. Med. Assoc. J. *131*:312, 1984.
413. Myerburg, R. J., Kessler, K. M., Interian, A., et al.: Clinical and experimental pathophysiology of sudden cardiac death. *In* Zipes, D. P., Jalife, J. (eds.): Cardiac Electrophysiology: From Cell to Bedside. Philadelphia, W. B. Saunders Company, 1990, pp. 666–678.

27

Pulmonary Hypertension

by WILLIAM GROSSMAN, M.D., and EUGENE BRAUNWALD, M.D.

Normal Pulmonary Circulation

During the passage of red blood cells through the lungs, hemoglobin is normally oxygenated to nearly full capacity and the blood is cleansed of much particulate matter and bacteria. The lungs, in addition to functioning as a blood oxygenator and filter, play a dominant role in achieving acid-base balance by excreting carbon dioxide, thereby helping to maintain an optimal blood pH.[1] Normally, the pulmonary vascular bed offers remarkably little resistance to flow. Pulmonary hypertension results when reductions in the caliber of the pulmonary vessels and/or increases in pulmonary blood flow occur.

PULMONARY BLOOD FLOW, PRESSURE, AND RESISTANCE

PULMONARY CIRCULATION IN THE NORMAL ADULT. *Pulmonary blood flow* refers to the volume of blood per unit of time that passes from the pulmonary artery through the capillary bed and into the pulmonary veins. However, it must be remembered that the lungs have a dual circulation and receive both systemic venous blood (the "pulmonary blood flow") through the pulmonary artery as well as arterial blood through the bronchial circulation. The bronchial arteries ramify normally into a capillary network drained by bronchial veins, some of which empty into the pulmonary veins, whereas the remainder empty into the systemic venous bed. Therefore, the bronchial circulation constitutes a physiological "right-to-left" shunt. The function of the bronchial circulation is to provide nutrition to the airways. Normally, blood flow through this system is quite low, amounting to approximately 1 per cent of cardiac output[2]; the resulting desaturation of left atrial blood is usually trivial. However, in some forms of pulmonary disease, e.g., severe bronchiectasis of cystic fibrosis, and in the presence of many congenital cardiovascular malformations that cause cyanosis, the blood flow through the bronchial circulation can increase significantly, account for nearly 30 per cent of the left ventricular output,[3] and produce a significant right-to-left shunt. In pulmonary disease, significant right-to-left shunting through the bronchial circulation may also result in arterial desaturation. In cyanotic congenital heart disease, bronchial blood is not fully oxygenated; it may participate in gas exchange and improve systemic oxygenation.

The normal pulmonary artery pressure in a person living at sea level has a peak systolic value of 18 to 25 mm Hg, an end-diastolic value of 6 to 10 mm Hg, and a mean value ranging from 12 to 16 mm Hg (Chap. 7).* Definite pulmonary hypertension is present when pulmonary artery systolic and mean pressures exceed 30 and 20 mm Hg, respectively. The normal mean pulmonary venous pressure is 6 to 10 mm Hg; therefore, the normal arteriovenous pressure difference, which moves the entire cardiac output across the pulmonary vascular bed, ranges from 2 to 10 mm Hg. This small pressure gradient is all the more remarkable when one considers that to move the same amount of blood per minute through the systemic vascular bed a pressure differential of approximately 90 mm Hg (systemic arterial mean pressure minus right atrial mean pressure) is required.

Thus, the normal pulmonary vascular bed offers less than one-tenth the *resistance* to flow offered by the systemic bed. *Vascular resistance* is generally quantified, by analogy to Ohm's law, as the ratio of pressure drop (ΔP in mm Hg) to mean flow (Q in liters/min). The ratio is commonly multiplied by 79.9 (or 80 for simplification) to express the results in dynes-seconds-centimeters^{-5}. This conversion to metric units may be avoided, i.e., resistance may be expressed in units of mm Hg/liter/min, which are sometimes referred to as hybrid units, PRU (peripheral resistance units), or Wood units (after the English cardiologist Paul Wood). The calculated pulmonary vascular resistance in normal adults[4] is 67 ± 23 (S.D.) dynes-sec-cm^{-5}.

Vascular resistance reflects a composite of variables that includes, but is not limited to, the cross-sectional area of small muscular arteries and arterioles. Other determinants are blood viscosity, the total mass of lung tissue (i.e., resistance is higher in infants and children than in adults), proximal vascular obstruction (e.g., pulmonary coarctation, pulmonary embolism, peripheral pulmonic stenosis), and extramural compression of vessels (perivascular edema).

Because the pulmonary vascular bed contains considerable elastic tissue, the cross-sectional area of the bed varies directly with transmural pressure and flow. Therefore, pulmonary vascular resistance decreases passively with increases in flow, as illustrated in Figure 49–3, p. 1583. The fall in resistance results in part from the increase in the radius of distensible vessels secondary to increased flow. From a consideration of the Poi-

*All pressures discussed here are in reference to atmospheric pressure at the level of the heart. True transmural pressures are more physiologically meaningful, especially when pulmonary parenchymal disease is present, but these are rarely measured.

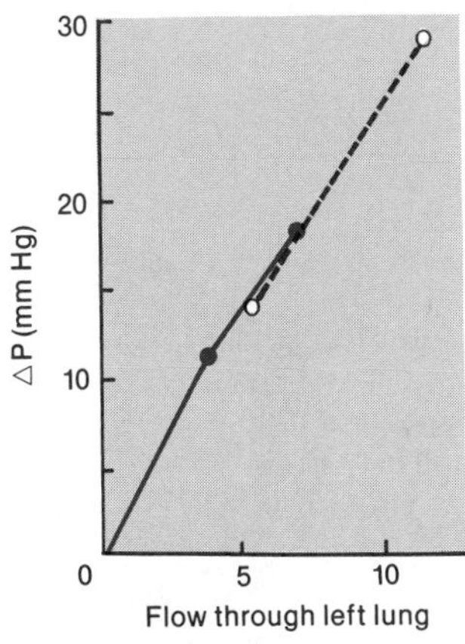

FIGURE 27-1. The relation between the drop in pressure (ΔP) and blood flow across the left lung in a supine normal human subject studied with and without occlusion of one pulmonary artery during rest (●-●) and exercise (○-○). In both states, rest and exercise, the lower circles indicate flow through the left lung without occlusion of the right pulmonary artery and the upper circles flow with the right pulmonary artery occluded. (From Harris, P., and Heath, D.: The Human Pulmonary Circulation. 2nd ed. New York, Churchill Livingstone, 1977.)

seuille relationship—in which $R = \Delta P/Q = 8\eta l/\pi r^4$, where R = resistance, ΔP = pressure drop, Q = flow, η = viscosity of fluid, and l and r = length and radius of the vessel, respectively—it is apparent that resistance can be effectively influenced by even small changes in the radius of the vessel. Recruitment of additional vascular channels will also contribute to the fall in resistance that characterizes increased flow through the pulmonary circuit. This phenomenon is particularly prominent in the upright position, when vessels in the upper parts of the lungs are in a partially collapsed state owing to low hydrostatic pressure (p. 554).

The reduction in resistance in a distensible vascular bed that occurs with increased flow has been offered as the explanation for the absence of pulmonary hypertension in many patients with large left-to-right intracardiac shunts, paticularly of the pretricuspid variety (e.g., atrial septal defect). However, it must be pointed out that the increased distensibility of pulmonary vessels in such situations has developed over years and that this principle is not necessarily applicable to acute increase in pulmonary blood flow.[5] In this regard, the results of studies with unilateral occlusion of a pulmonary artery using a balloon catheter are relevant.[6] Figure 27-1 illustrates the relationship between the flow and pressure drop, ΔP, across the left lung during balloon occlusion of the right pulmonary artery, at rest and during exercise, and under both conditions together. It is apparent that acute increases in flow in the supine position were associated with increases in ΔP, so that vascular resistance of the lung (the slope of the line relating ΔP to flow) remained unchanged. In the upright position, however, blood vessels in the upper part of the lung usually are in a partially or fully collapsed state (Fig. 20-8, p. 555) and with an increase in flow, these vessels may expand, thereby reducing vascular resistance.[5]

The influence of blood viscosity on pulmonary vascular resistance is also important, particularly in the cyanotic patient with hematocrit in excess of 60 per cent or in the severely anemic patient with hematocrit less than 20 per cent. In experiments in dogs in which pulmonary pressure-flow curves were constructed at varying hematocrits and rates of flow, ΔP doubled when the hematocrit was increased from 43 per cent to 64 per cent at a normal flow, indicating a doubling of effective pulmonary vascular resistance.[7]

FETAL AND NEONATAL CIRCULATIONS (see also p. 1582)

In the fetus, oxygenated blood enters the heart from the inferior vena cava and streams across the foramen ovale to the left atrium, left ventricle, ascending aorta, and cranial vessels. Desaturated blood returns from the superior vena cava and passes through the tricuspid valve into the right ventricle and pulmonary artery. Since the resistance of the pulmonary vascular bed in the collapsed fetal lung is extremely high, only 10 to 30 per cent of the total right ventricular output passes through the lungs, the remainder being shunted across the ductus arteriosus to the descending aorta and thence back to the placenta. At birth, there is an abrupt change in the pulmonary circulation. With the first breath of extrauterine life, expansion of the lungs and the abrupt rise in the Po_2 of blood lead to a release of pulmonary arteriolar vasoconstriction and a stretching and dilatation of muscular pulmonary arteries and arterioles, with a marked drop in vascular resistance.[8-10] This facilitates a large increase in pulmonary blood flow and results in an augmented left atrial volume and pressure. The latter closes the flap valve of the foramen ovale, so that interatrial right-to-left shunting ordinarily ceases within the first hour of life. Normally, the ductus arteriosus closes over the next 10 hours as a result of contraction of the thick smooth muscle bundles within its wall in response to a rising arterial oxygen tension and a change in the prostaglandin milieu.[11] Following the initial dramatic fall in pulmonary vascular resistance at birth, there is a continuous decline over the first few months of life associated with thinning of the media of muscular pulmonary arteries and arterioles until the normal adult pattern is achieved[2,12] (Fig. 27-2).

RESPONSE TO ANOXIA, DRUGS, AND NEURAL AND ENVIRONMENTAL FACTORS

HYPOXIA. It is well established that acute *hypoxia* elicits pulmonary vasoconstriction,[13-16] and there is general agreement that this response is part of a self-regulatory mechanism for adjusting capillary perfusion to alveolar ventilation. There appears to be an age dependency and a considerable species variability in the magnitude of this vasoconstrictor response, which is quite intense in cattle, intermediate in humans and the pig, and comparatively mild in dogs and sheep[17]; hypoxic vasoconstriction is more profound in the infant or young mammal than in the adult. Variability exists within a given species as well, and there is strong evidence for a genetic determination of individual reactivity to hypoxia in animals.[17,18] This finding, if it is applicable to humans, may be relevant to the occasional familial occurrence of primary pulmonary hypertension in humans (p. 804).

The mechanism of the acute pulmonary vasoconstriction that occurs in response to hypoxia is uncertain (Fig. 27-3). There is some evidence that hypoxia-induced local release of histamine may play an important role, with pulmonary vasoconstriction secondary to stimulation of pulmonary vascular H_1-receptors (cf. discussion of histamine below). There has

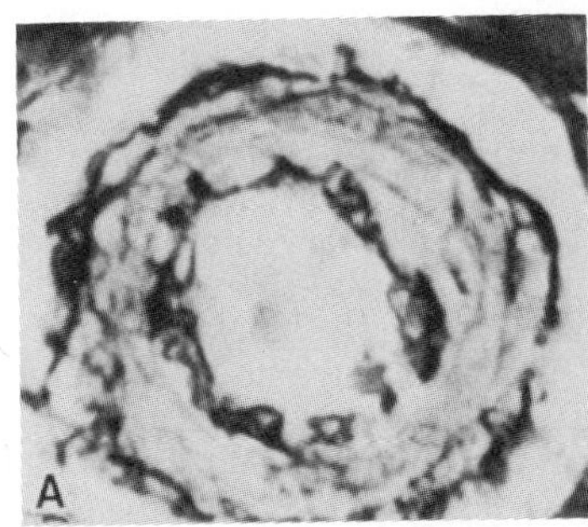

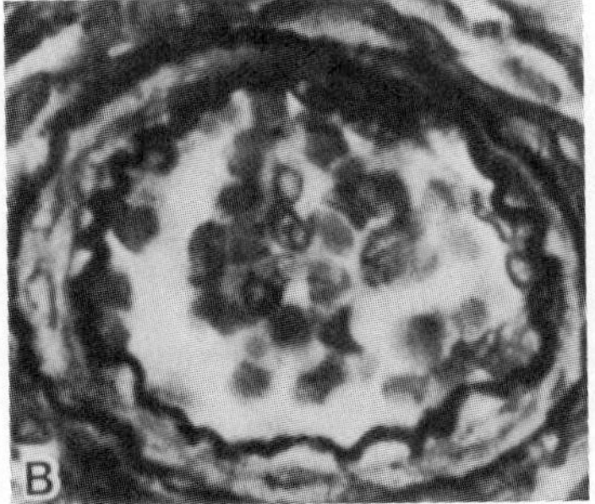

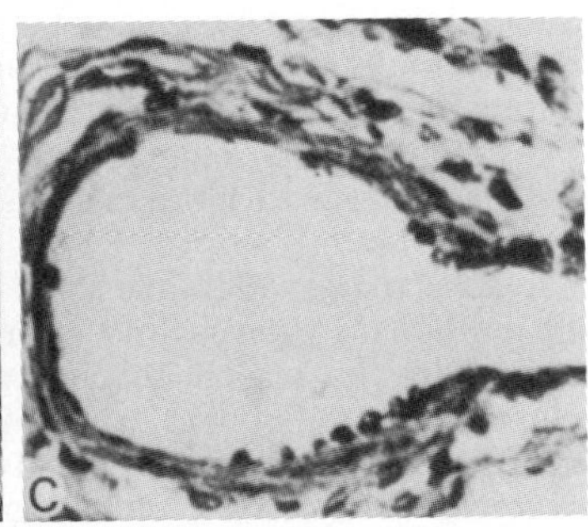

FIGURE 27-2. Changes in pulmonary arteries after birth. Comparison of relative medial thicknesses at birth *(A)*, at age 2 months *(B)*, and at age 7 months *(C)*. Elastic-van Gieson stain; magnification ×360; reduced 17 per cent.) (From Edwards, W. D.: Pathology of pulmonary hypertension. Cardiovasc. Clin. *18*:321, 1988.)

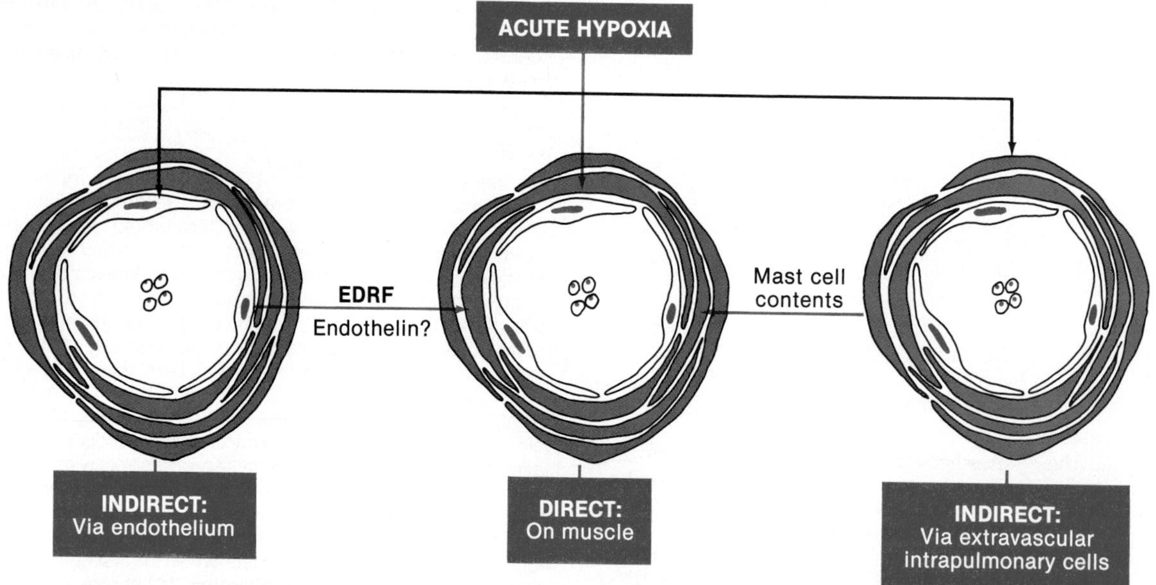

FIGURE 27-3. Possible mechanisms whereby acute hypoxia leads to pulmonary vasoconstriction. A small pulmonary artery can be affected in one of three ways: indirectly via the endothelium *(left)*, indirectly via extravascular cells in the lung *(right)*, or directly via an effect of hypoxia on vascular smooth muscle cells *(middle)*. (From Fishman, A. P.: The enigma of hypoxic pulmonary vasoconstriction. *In* Fishman, A. P. [ed.]: The Pulmonary Circulation: Normal and Abnormal. Philadelphia, University of Pennsylvania Press, 1990, pp. 109-129.)

been considerable speculation about the role of vascular endothelium as a mediator of hypoxia-induced pulmonary vasoconstriction.[19] This is based on recent findings concerning the role of vascular endothelium in the regulation of vascular smooth muscle contraction and relaxation.[20-24] Balanced release of endothelial-derived relaxing factor (EDRF)[21] and a potent vasoconstrictor peptide (endothelin)[23,23a] by endothelial cells plays a critical role in regulation of tone in systemic vascular resistance vessels and may be of considerable importance in the pulmonary circulation as well.

A role for increased Ca^{++} entry into vascular smooth muscle in mediating hypoxic pulmonary vasoconstriction is suggested by the observation that the Ca^{++} antagonist verapamil inhibits hypoxic pulmonary vasoconstriction.[25] The clinical relevance of this observation is supported by a study of the pulmonary vascular effects of nifedipine in patients with acute respiratory failure[26] in whom the Ca^{++} antagonist produced a reduction in pulmonary vascular resistance dependent on the severity of hypoxia.

The effects of chronic hypoxia on pulmonary hemodynamics and histology have been studied in the rat.[27] Mean pulmonary artery pressure rose substantially after 3 days of hypoxia and had doubled by day 14. These hemodynamic changes were associated with (1) extension of vascular smooth muscle into peripheral arteries where it is not normally present, (2) increased wall thickness of the muscular arteries, and (3) reduction in the number of arteries expressed as an increase in the ratio of alveoli to arteries. In a follow-up study,[28] it was found that these hypoxia-induced chronic vascular changes were more extensive in infants than in adult rats. Futhermore, after recovery under normoxic conditions for 3 months, residual vascular changes were present in all animals studied, but again were more marked in the younger rats.

Changes in alveolar oxygenation affect the oxygenation of blood in small pulmonary arteries and arterioles by direct gaseous diffusion from the alveoli, respiratory bronchioles, and alveolar ducts in the pulmonary arterioles, even though the latter are "upstream" in relation to the alveoli. This fact, taken together with evidence for a reduction in pulmonary arterial blood volume during hypoxia,[29] supports the view that the small pulmonary arteries and arterioles are the main sites of vasoconstriction and increased resistance during hypoxia.[29,30] While alveolar oxygen tension is a major physiological determinant of pulmonary arteriolar tone, a reduction in the oxygen tension in the mixed venous blood flowing through the small pulmonary arteries and arterioles may also lead to pulmonary arterial vasoconstriction.[15,31] *Acidemia* appears to potentiate the effects of hypoxemia (Fig. 49-4, p. 1585), whereas alkalosis may be protective.[32,33] Thus, two potent stimuli for vasodilatation in the systemic arteriolar bed cause constriction of pulmonary arteries and arterioles. Although *hypercapnia* can be shown to increase pulmonary vascular resistance in some experimental preparations, the effects are variable and probably not important in humans.[15]

NEURAL REGULATION. Morphological studies have demonstrated that the media and adventitia of the large elastic pulmonary arteries and of the large pulmonary veins are supplied by nerve fibers that may influence the distensibility of these capacitance vessels.[2,13] Although *neural regulation* of pulmonary vascular resistance can be demonstrated[34] and may be particularly important in fetal life, its importance in the normal human adult is uncertain. *Chemical and hormonal regulation* of pulmonary vascular resistance is a complex and as yet incompletely understood subject, with roles having been reported for catecholamines, acetylcholine, prostaglandins, histamine, bradykinin, serotonin, and angiotensin.[2,13,35-60] The exact site of action of these agents within the pulmonary vascular tree (i.e., arterioles, venules, capillaries, and so on) is uncertain at present.

DRUGS. There is controversy concerning the effects of *alpha-adrenergic agonists* on the pulmonary vascular bed. Some studies have shown that norepinephrine causes increases in pulmonary arterial and wedge pressures with no change in pulmonary blood flow or pulmonary vascular resistance.[49,50] In one study an increase in pulmonary vascular resistance with norepinephrine was reported,[51] and there is experimental evidence for alpha-adrenergic-mediated constriction of small pulmonary arteries and veins induced by the stimulation of sympathetic nerves.[52]

Both the alpha-adrenergic blocking agent phentolamine and tolazoline (Priscoline), which also exhibits alpha-adrenergic blocking action, can lower pulmonary vascular resistance. Tolazoline was first reported in the pharmacological literature as a vasodepressor agent having effects comparable to those of histamine. Subsequently, it was shown to antagonize the actions of alpha-adrenergic agonists. Like phentolamine, it is an imidazoline compound, and both these agents have vasodepressor effects independent of their alpha-adrenergic antagonistic properties. In fact, there is some evidence that the pulmonary vasodilator effect of tolazoline is mediated through histamine-2 receptors.[53] Tolazoline has been reported to produce a transient fall in pulmonary vascular resistance in patients with pulmonary hypertension having a major reversible component, including primary pulmonary hypertension.[54,55]

Beta-adrenergic stimulation with isoproterenol has been shown repeatedly to cause pulmonary *vasodilatation*. In contrast, beta-adrenergic blockade does not produce any change in pulmonary vascular resistance, suggesting that there is no tonic activation of beta receptors for maintenance of the normal low pulmonary vascular resistance. *Acetylcholine* is also a potent relaxant of pulmonary arteries and arterioles[35,36] and transiently lowers pulmonary vascular resistance in patients with elevated pulmonary vascular resistance with a major reversible component. Whether this effect of acetylcholine is mediated by release of EDRF from pulmonary vascular endothelium has not been determined.

Lung tissue is particularly active in the synthesis, metabolism, and release of a number of the *prostaglandins*, some of which may play a role in the regulation of pulmonary vascular resistance. Prostaglandins I_2 and E are active pulmonary vasodilators, whereas $F_2\alpha$ and A_2 are pulmonary vasoconstrictors.[37] The role of these prostaglandins and their precursors in the regulation of pulmonary vascular tone in humans is uncertain at present. However, the prostaglandin synthesis inhibitor indomethacin produced a substantial increase in pulmonary vascular resistance and a decline in cardiac output.[38] Furthermore, repeated indomethacin administration has been shown to lead to a progressive rise in pulmonary vascular resistance in chronically instrumented sheep.[38a] Thus, long-term indomethacin administration may be harmful in the setting of established pulmonary hypertension. If inhibition of prostaglandin synthesis leads to an *increase* in pulmonary vascular resistance, it might be expected that specific prostaglandin infusion might have a vasodilatory effect on the pulmonary vasculature. Such an effect has been noted in several studies of patients with pulmonary hypertension who have received either acute or chronic intravenous infusion of PGI_2 (prostacyclin).[39-43] These studies (see also p. 811) indicate that prostacyclin produces substantial vasodilatory effects in patients with primary pulmonary hypertension. These effects may be sustained in some patients for considerable periods of time during continuous intravenous administration by portable infusion pumps.[42]

Histamine, a vasodilator in the systemic circulation, is primarily a vasoconstrictor in the pulmonary vascular bed. Since large doses of histamine receptor blockers or histamine depletors attenuate the hypoxia-induced pulmonary vasoconstrictor response, it has been suggested that histamine may actually be the chemical mediator of hypoxia-induced vasoconstriction in animals.[44-48] This suggestion is supported by the observation that the periarterial mast cells in the rat and guinea pig lung lose their granules and apparently release histamine during hypoxia.[30] However, other experimental findings are contradictory,[13] and as a consequence, the role of histamine in the regulation of the pulmonary circulation in man remains unclear. Perhaps this confusion can be resolved by the finding that histamine may have both pulmonary vasoconstrictor (H_1-receptor) and vasodilator (H_2-receptor) actions.[56-58] In at least one study, histamine acted as a pulmonary vasoconstrictor in the presence of normal oxygenation and as a vasodilator under hypoxic conditions.[56] As mentioned above, tolazoline may act through stimulation of the H_2-receptors.[53]

Serotonin is a potent pulmonary vasoconstrictor in experimental animals[59] but apparently has little or no effect in humans.[60] In this regard, it should be noted that in patients with hepatic metastases of malignant carcinoid of the bowel, large quantities of serotonin are produced and changes in the endocardium and valves of the right side of the heart may occur, but these patients do not exhibit pulmonary hypertension. *Angiotensin II*, generated in the lung by means of enzymatic conversion of angiotensin I, is thought to be a potent pulmonary vasoconstrictor.[30] However, its role in the normal regulation of pulmonary vascular resistance in humans is unknown.

HIGH ALTITUDE. Life at high altitudes is associated with pulmonary hypertension of variable severity, reflecting the range of reactivities of different persons to the pulmonary vasoconstrictive effect of hypoxia.[15,61-64] As discussed earlier, pulmonary arterial pressure normally declines rapidly following birth at sea level. However, the fall in pulmonary artery pressure of infants born at high altitude may be slower in onset and of lesser magnitude.[64] Mean pulmonary arterial pressure in normal adults living 10,000 feet above sea level is approximately 25 mm Hg[65] and increases to over 50 mm Hg with exercise. The relationship between *cigarette smoking* and chronic obstructive lung diseases is clear.[66-68] Since many patients with chronic obstructive lung diseases exhibit pulmonary hypertension (Chap. 51),[69,70] cigarette smoking may be considered an *indirect* stimulus to the development of pulmonary hypertension.

Secondary Pulmonary Hypertension

Pulmonary hypertension results when there is increased resistance to blood flow at any of a number of sites within the circulation, the pulmonary vascular bed itself representing only one of these potential sites (Table 27–1).[70a] In addition to increased resistance to blood flow, markedly increased flow alone may cause pulmonary hypertension, even when resistance to flow is normal at every point in the circulation. Hypoventilation and its various causes are often considered to be a separate category of conditions associated with pulmonary hypertension, although this is somewhat arbitrary, and it might well be argued that these conditions all produce pulmonary hypertension by hypoxic pulmonary vasoconstriction and thus represent a subcategory of increased resistance to flow through the pulmonary vascular bed.

INCREASED RESISTANCE TO PULMONARY VENOUS DRAINAGE

PATHOPHYSIOLOGY. Increased resistance to pulmonary venous drainage is a mechanism common to several conditions of diverse causes in which pulmonary arterial hypertension occurs. Altered resistance to pulmonary venous drainage may be the result of diseases affecting the left ventricle or pericardium, mitral or aortic valvular disease, or rare entities such as cor triatriatum, left atrial myxoma, or pulmonary veno-occlusive disease (see below).

The magnitude of pulmonary hypertension depends, in part, on the performance of the right ventricle. In response to

(i.e., in the range of 200 to 300 dynes-sec-cm^{-5}) and moderately severe pulmonary hypertension (pulmonary artery systolic and mean pressures exceeding 60 and 40 mm Hg, respectively).

Decreased Left Ventricular Diastolic Distensibility. This may have a variety of causes and may be associated with elevation of left ventricular end-diastolic pressure, and passive increases in left atrial, pulmonary venous, and pulmonary arterial pressures.[84] Specific conditions associated with decreased left ventricular distensibility include concentric left ventricular hypertrophy from a variety of causes,[85,86] diffuse fibrosis as a consequence of ischemic disease,[87] and restrictive cardiomyopathy of various etiologies.[88-90] These causes of pulmonary arterial hypertension should be distinguished from those secondary to left ventricular systolic failure, since they do not respond to digitalis or other inotropic drugs. Usually, the levels of pulmonary hypertension in such patients are only moderate, and increases in pulmonary vascular resistance are less marked than with other causes of elevated pulmonary venous pressure.

Constrictive pericarditis (Chap. 45) is also associated with increased pulmonary artery pressures as a result of an increase in the resistance to pulmonary venous drainage into the left side of the heart. Pulmonary artery systolic pressure is usually only mildly increased in this condition, ranging from 35 to 45 mm Hg at rest,[90] but commonly exceeding 50 to 60 mm Hg in such patients during exertion.[91]

PULMONARY HYPERTENSION SECONDARY TO LEFT ATRIAL HYPERTENSION

Mitral Valve Disease (see also Chap. 34)

MITRAL STENOSIS. This valvular lesion represents an important cause of pulmonary hypertension. While the pulmonary hypertension associated with mitral stenosis is initially a result of an increase in resistance to pulmonary venous drainage and backward transmission of the elevated left atrial pressure, many patients subsequently exhibit marked pulmonary vasoconstriction and anatomical changes in vessels, so that the pulmonary hypertension is "reactive" as well as "passive." The elevation of pulmonary vascular resistance and the associated pulmonary hypertension may come to dominate the clinical picture in mitral stenosis (Fig. 27–5).[92-95] Thus, patients with mitral stenosis often develop what might be considered to be a more proximal obstruction at the level of the pulmonary arterioles and small muscular arteries (the "second stenosis"), with resultant pulmonary hypertension equal to or exceeding systemic arterial pressure during exertion and sometimes even at rest. The clinical picture in such patients is characterized by right ventricular failure with distended neck veins, hepatomegaly, and ascites (p. 1010). These patients exhibit marked fatigue, occasionally a more serious complaint than dyspnea. The murmur of mitral stenosis may be soft or even inaudible, and the opening snap of the stenotic mitral valve may be indistinguishable from a loud pulmonic component of S_2, owing to narrowing of the S_2-opening snap interval. Pulmonary congestion and edema may not be prominent clinically. Cardiac output is usually markedly reduced. This constellation of findings may obscure the underlying diagnosis of mitral stenosis and suggest instead either primary pulmonary hypertension or pulmonary hypertension secondary to some other disorder, such as chronic recurrent pulmonary embolism.

Diagnostic Studies. These usually permit identification of the cause of the severe pulmonary hypertension. The echocardiogram shows left atrial enlargement and thickened mitral valve leaflets whose mobility is markedly reduced (p. 1013). At cardiac catheterization, the pulmonary arterial hypertension is associated with substantial elevations of the pulmonary wedge pressure, and there is generally a sizable (>10 mm Hg) pressure gradient between pulmonary capillary wedge and left ventricular diastolic pressures. The latter findings are of key importance in distinguishing mitral stenosis from primary pulmonary hypertension, a condition in which left atrial size and the wedge pressure are normal and in which there is no diastolic pressure gradient between the wedge and left ventricular pressures.

Protection Against Pulmonary Edema. In general, acute elevations of pulmonary venous pressure equal to or greater than 25 mm Hg result in the formation of pulmonary edema. However, pulmonary venous pressure may rise gradually to levels of 35 mm Hg or more without the development of gross pulmonary edema.[93,95-98] At least three mechanisms that tend to protect against pulmonary edema formation are operative in patients with mitral stenosis and chronic elevations of pulmonary venous pressure in excess of 25 mm Hg (Chap. 20). First, lymphatic drainage of the pulmonary interstitium increases abruptly when pulmonary venous pressure is increased to 25 mm Hg.[99,100] Acute increases in pulmonary lymph flow of up to eight times the resting level will occur when pulmonary venous pressure is raised to 30 mm Hg for a 10-minute interval, and the increased lymphatic flow will persist at high levels for 30 to 60 minutes after pulmonary venous pressure has returned to normal.[99] In models of *chronic* pulmonary venous pressure elevation, increases in pulmonary lymph flow of up to 28 times normal have been observed.[100] Histological evidence of marked dilatation of the pulmonary lymphatics has been observed in some patients with chronic left atrial pressure overload.[2,5,101] Thus, despite the imbalance of Starling forces at the capillary level, the edema fluid may be drained away as rapidly as it is formed, and as a result chronic elevation of pulmonary venous pressure to levels exceeding 30 to 35 mm Hg may not lead to clinical evidence of pulmonary edema.

Diminished permeability of the capillary alveolar barrier is a second protective mechanism that might be operative in patients with *chronic* pulmonary venous hypertension in excess of 25 mm Hg. There is morphological evidence of thickening of the layer between the capillary lumen and the alveolar space.[102-105] A third mechanism operating in patients with chronic increased resistance to pulmonary venous drainage is the reactive constriction of small muscular pulmonary arteries and arterioles (Fig. 27–4). This constriction, which results in considerable elevation of pulmonary artery pressure, is usually associated with a significant decline in right ventricular output (and therefore pulmonary blood flow). The lower pulmonary blood flow tends to diminish the formation of pulmonary edema, since it results in substantially lower left atrial and pulmonary venous pressures at any given size of the mitral valve orifice[106] or for any given impairment of left ventricular function. Despite this protective effect of pulmonary vasoconstriction, pulmonary hypertension is often tolerated poorly in these patients, who commonly show prominent signs of right ventricular failure.

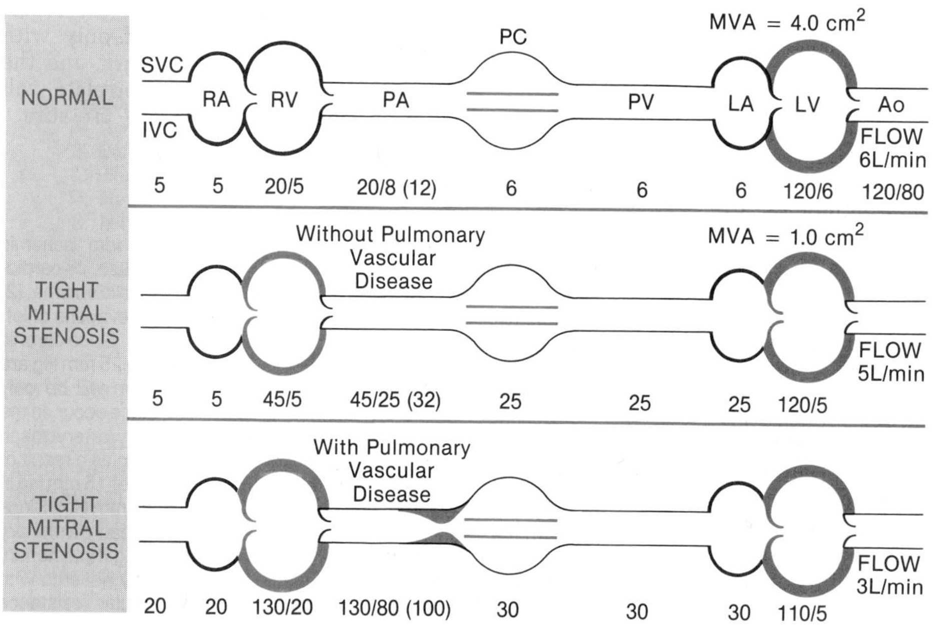

FIGURE 27–5. Schematic diagram of cardiopulmonary circulation in patients with tight mitral stenosis with and without pulmonary vascular disease. Pressures (in mm Hg) are listed for the superior and inferior venae cavae (SVC and IVC), right atrium (RA), right ventricle (RV), pulmonary arteries (PA), capillaries (PC), veins (PV), left atrium (LA), left ventricle (LV), and aorta (Ao) for the normal circulation (upper panel) and for the two types of mitral stenosis (middle and lower panels). Note that with pulmonary vascular disease (the "second stenosis") severe pulmonary hypertension occurs, and right ventricular failure develops. (Modified from the data of Dexter[93] and Schlant.[94])

Thus, the patient trades pulmonary for peripheral edema and dyspnea for the fatigue and lethargy of low cardiac output.

Effects of Surgery. After corrective surgery on the mitral valve, both pulmonary vascular resistance and pulmonary hypertension decline,[107,108] the major extent of which is noted within the first postoperative week. Mitral stenosis is now commonly treated with balloon dilatation (balloon valvuloplasty)[109–113] (pp. 931 and 1376) and this has provided the opportunity to observe the effects of relieving the mitral valve obstruction free from the obscuring effects of general anesthesia, intubation, and thoracotomy. Substantial reversibility of pulmonary hypertension and reduction of pulmonary vascular resistance has been observed following balloon valvuloplasty in patients with advanced mitral stenosis,[109,114] and the time course has generally followed that reported previously in patients undergoing mitral valve replacement.[107,108] As might be expected, the extent of reversal of pulmonary vascular obstruction has varied depending on the adequacy of the valvuloplasty procedure in producing an increase in mitral orifice area and whether the patient develops mitral valve restenosis in the months following balloon dilatation.[114] Factors involved in the improvement of pulmonary hypertension include reduction of reactive vasoconstriction resulting from (1) distention of the pulmonary vascular bed (i.e., from relief of myogenic vasoconstriction); (2) the resolution of edema within the walls of small arteries and arterioles; and (3) reversal of the morphological changes in Heath-Edwards Grades I to III (p. 800) seen commonly in mitral stenosis.

MITRAL REGURGITATION. Although pulmonary hypertension is widely recognized as developing in patients with left atrial hypertension due to mitral stenosis, it can also occur in patients with pure mitral regurgitation.[115] In one series, nearly half of a cohort of 41 patients with severe mitral regurgitation had pulmonary artery systolic pressures in excess of 50 mm Hg. In this subgroup of patients, pulmonary vascular resistance was three times normal and cardiac output was substantially depressed, compared with that in patients in whom severe mitral regurgitation was associated with only minimal pulmonary artery pressure elevation.[115] Presumably, the pulmonary hypertension in these patients is reversible, just as it is in mitral stenosis, although data on this point have not been reported.

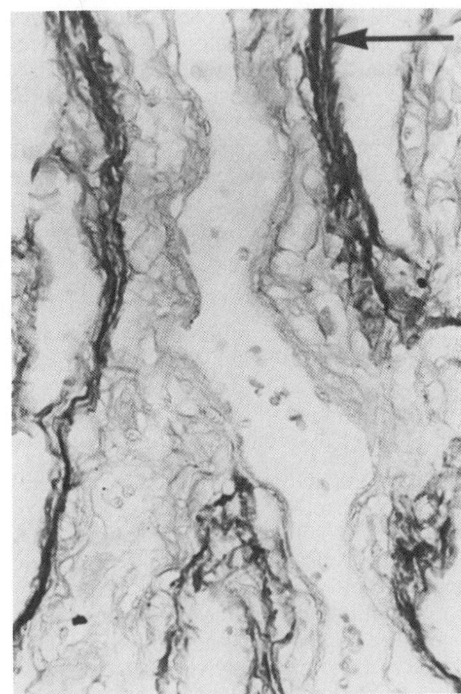

FIGURE 27–6. Longitudinal section of a small pulmonary vein, receiving two venules, from a girl of 16 years with pulmonary veno-occlusive disease. Both the vein and its tributaries show extensive blockage by loose, basophilic fibrous tissue. The remaining lumen, much reduced in size, passes through the vein and one of its tributaries. There is some "arterialization" of the venous media (arrow). (Elastic–van Gieson × 375.) (From Harris, P., and Heath, D.: The Human Pulmonary Circulation. 3rd ed. New York, Churchill Livingstone, 1986, p. 438.)

PULMONARY HYPERTENSION SECONDARY TO PULMONARY VENOUS OBSTRUCTION

Obstruction to pulmonary venous drainage also occurs in association with unusual conditions, such as cor triatriatum, stenosis of pulmonary veins, obstructive forms of anomalous pulmonary venous connection, and pulmonary veno-occlusive disease.

COR TRIATRIATUM (see also p. 929). This is a malformation in which partitioning of the left atrium creates two left atrial subchambers. The posterior subchamber receives the pulmonary venous inflow, which then drains through an opening in the partition into the anterior subchamber and thence through the mitral orifice into the left ventricle. When the opening in the partition separating the two left atrial subchambers is small, severe pulmonary venous and pulmonary arterial hypertension result.

PULMONARY VENO-OCCLUSIVE DISEASE. This is an uncommon condition characterized by progressive fibrotic obstruction of the veins and particularly the venules of both lungs.[5] Histological examination may reveal the veins to be blocked by loose fibrous tissue (Fig. 27–6). Later, there may be intimal fibrosis in many veins resembling organization of a thrombus, with a central luminal channel surrounded by a rim of collagenous tissue or with recanalization of a number of wide luminal channels, separated by septa. However, the histological picture in some cases demonstrates extensive blockage of pulmonary venules by basophilic fibrous tissue[5] and intimal proliferation[117] without any evidence of a thrombotic process. The lungs show pulmonary edema with congestion and areas of interstitial fibrosis and hemosiderosis. The involvement of veins and lungs may be diffuse, but in some instances the most severe lesions are focal and not equally distributed. The condition usually affects children or young adults and is characterized clinically by exertional dyspnea, orthopnea, and cyanosis. The pulmonary artery pressure is usually markedly elevated (frequently ≥ 70 mm Hg systolic); right ventricular failure may be present.

The pathogenesis of the obstructive changes is unknown, and it is debated whether this condition represents a distinct entity or a syndrome of various causes.[118] Since it has been observed that a febrile, influenza-like illness sometimes precedes pulmonary veno-occlusive disease,[5,117] it has been proposed that a viral infection may deplete the pulmonary venous endothelium of its plasminogen activator, thus leading to in situ thrombosis.[119] In pulmonary veno-occlusive disease, in contrast to primary pulmonary hypertension, the radiographic changes are suggestive of pulmonary venous hypertension with Kerley B lines and sometimes interstitial and alveolar pulmonary edema. However, in some cases there is no radiological evidence of increased pulmonary venous pressure. If the pulmonary veno-occlusive disease affects large veins, the wedge pressure will be elevated, and this measurement will then serve to distinguish this condition from primary pulmonary hypertension.[5] However, if the disease affects primarily the smaller veins, the wedge pressure may not reflect the level of the pressure within the pulmonary capillaries and may even be normal. The explanation for this discrepancy depends on the heterogeneity of pulmonary venular involvement; a theoretical explanation is presented by Harris and Heath.[5]

INCREASED RESISTANCE TO FLOW THROUGH THE PULMONARY VASCULAR BED

PULMONARY PARENCHYMAL DISEASE

Pulmonary hypertension is a common sequel to chronic bronchitis and emphysema (Chap. 49).[69] It had long been believed that the elevated pulmonary artery pressures in patients with emphysema resulted from destruction of the pulmonary vascular bed. Current views minimize this pathogenic pathway, because no direct correlation exists between the severity of the emphysema and the degree of right ventricular hypertrophy.[120,121]

PATHOPHYSIOLOGY. Hypoxia-induced vasoconstriction (p. 791) probably plays a major role in producing pulmonary hypertension in patients with chronic bronchitis and emphysema.[122-124] There is also evidence for a pulmonary vasoconstrictive action by hydrogen ions, particularly in the presence of hypoxia. In this regard, in patients with chronic obstructive lung disease pulmonary artery pressure correlates inversely with arterial oxygen saturation and directly with arterial Pco_2,[125-128] providing indirect evidence for a role for hypoxia and hypercapnia in the production of pulmonary hypertension. When patients with chronic bronchitis and emphysema inspire high concentrations of oxygen acutely, there is only a modest decrease in pulmonary artery pressure and vascular resistance,[126,129-131] both of which remain considerably elevated. This suggests that muscular hypertrophy of pulmonary arterioles may in itself be of importance in maintaining the hypoxic pulmonary hypertension.

TRIALS WITH OXYGEN THERAPY. The results of two large trials designed to assess the role of long-term oxygen therapy in cor pulmonale due to chronic bronchitis and emphysema have been disappointing.[132,133] Long-term domiciliary oxygen therapy in one study was associated with no change in mean pulmonary artery pressure after 500 days of oxygen treatment, compared with a 3-mm Hg increase in the control group.[132] In another study, nocturnal oxygen administration was associated with a 7 per cent increase in pulmonary vascular resistance after 6 months, as compared with an 11 per cent decrease in patients receiving continuous oxygen.[133] However, the efficacy of oxygen in prolonging life was greatest in patients with a low pulmonary vascular resistance, and the authors concluded that changes in pulmonary vascular resistance were not the cause of the lower mortality in patients on continuous oxygen therapy.[133] These findings and others[5] suggest that factors other than simple hypoxemic pulmonary hypertension are operative in producing the cor pulmonale of chronic bronchitis and emphysema.

Blood volume and red cell mass, in particular, increase during acute respiratory failure and may contribute to the development of elevated pulmonary arterial pressures. By increasing blood viscosity, increases in hematocrit to within the range commonly seen in chronic bronchitis and emphysema (i.e., 50 to 55 per cent) result in 30 to 50 per cent increases in the transpulmonary arteriovenous pressure gradient at constant blood flow.

SPECIFIC DISORDERS. In patients with *chronic obstructive lung disease,* the extent of destruction of alveoli and the accompanying reductions in alveolar surface area do not correlate closely with the degree of pulmonary hypertension. Thus, the decrease in the cross-sectional area of the pulmonary capillary bed in such patients plays a minor role in elevating pulmonary vascular resistance. A particular association exists between centrilobular (as opposed to panacinar) emphysema and pulmonary hypertension. Right ventricular hypertrophy may occur when only 10 to 15 per cent of the lung is involved in centrilobular emphysema, in contrast to 40 to 70 per cent involvement in patients with panacinar emphysema. This difference may reflect poorer gas exchange in the former circumstance. In patients with advanced bullous emphysema, physical compression of or enchroachment on pulmonary capillary beds may play a role, and reduction of pulmonary artery pressure following resection of bullae has been reported[134]; this may be related to reduced compression of the vessel and in part to the associated improvement of gas exchange.

Progressive interstitial pulmonary fibrosis may be associated with pulmonary hypertension. The latter occurs particularly in patients with *progressive systemic sclerosis* (p. 1736), in whom the fibrotic process leads to major reduction in the cross-sectional area of the pulmonary vascular bed due to obliteration of alveolar capillaries and narrowing and obliteration of many small arteries and arterioles.[2,5] Moreover, a marked elevation of pulmonary artery pressure (≥100 mm Hg systolic) and resistance (≥2000 dynes-sec-cm^{-5}) in patients with a variant of scleroderma, the *CREST syndrome* (calcinosis, Raynaud's phenomenon, esophageal dysmotility, sclerodactyly, and telangiectasia), has been reported[135] (p. 1736). In patients with the CREST form of *scleroderma,* marked right ventricular dysfunction may be present with right ventricular ejection fractions less than 30 per cent, presumably reflecting systolic overload of the right ventricle due to severe pulmonary vascular disease,[136,136a] and in some instances sclerodermatous narrowing of coronary arteries.

Fibrous obliteration of the pulmonary vascular bed and pulmonary hypertension have also been described in patients with various forms of pulmonary vasculitis (Table 27–2). These include isolated Raynaud's phenomenon,[137,138] dermatomyositis,[139] rheumatoid arthritis,[140] and systemic lupus erythematosus.[141,142] In the latter a *lupus anticoagulant* may be present in the IgG or IgM fractions of the serum; this may cause a paradoxical hypercoagulable state, intrapulmonary microthrombi, and pulmonary hypertension.[142] Pulmonary hypertension is an uncommon accompaniment of the Hamman-Rich syndrome,[143] desquamative interstitial pneumonia, idiopathic pulmonary hemosiderosis,[144] and sarcoidosis.[5,145] It is not clear whether significant pulmonary hypertension may result from pulmonary fibrosis due to radiation therapy.

Diffuse lymphatic spread of carcinoma may also cause pulmonary hypertension and right heart failure.[146] In many cases tumor microemboli and the attendant thrombotic and fibrotic reaction lead to vascular obstruction. Obstruction of the major pulmonary arteries by tumor (usually sarcoma) may be a cause of right ventricular and main pulmonary artery hypertension.[2,147] Congenital pulmonary aplasia or hypoplasia, the latter often observed in Down syndrome,[148] may be responsible for an elevation of pulmonary vascular resistance and pulmonary hypertension.

EISENMENGER SYNDROME

(See also pp. 763 and 810)

Decreased cross-sectional area of the pulmonary arteriolar bed with irreversible pulmonary hypertension characterizes

TABLE 27–2 PULMONARY VASCULITIDES

VASCULITIDES IN WHICH LUNG IS THE MAJOR ORGAN INVOLVED:
Wegener's granulomatosis
Lymphomatoid granulomatosis
Lymphocytic angiitis and granulomatosis
Churg-Strauss syndrome
Overlap vasculitis
Necrotizing sarcoid granulomatosis
VASCULITIDES IN WHICH LUNG MAY BE INVOLVED:
Henoch-Schönlein syndrome
Disseminated leukocytoclastic vasculitis
Cryoglobulinemia
Disseminated giant cell arteritis
Behçet's disease
Takayasu's disease
Polyarteritis nodosa
DISEASES IN WHICH PULMONARY VASCULITIS MAY BE PART OF THE SPECTRUM OF PATHOLOGY:
Collagen-vascular disorders
Rheumatoid arthritis
Systemic lupus erythematosus
Progressive systemic sclerosis
Eosinophilic pneumonias
Sarcoidosis
Immunoblastic lymphadenopathy
Organic dust diseases (hypersensitivity pneumonitides)
Bronchocentric granulomatosis
Ulcerative colitis
Ankylosing spondylitis
Hughes-Stovin syndrome

From Fulmer, J. D., and Kaltreider, H. B.: The pulmonary vasculitides. Chest *82*:615, 1982.

the so-called Eisenmenger syndrome. This term was used by Wood[149] to refer to patients with congenital cardiac lesions and severe pulmonary hypertension in whom reversal of a left-to-right shunt has occurred. Left-to-right shunts are due usually to congenital cardiovascular malformations[150-154] (e.g., atrial and ventricular septal defects, patent ductus arteriosus).

PATHOPHYSIOLOGY (p. 896). Pulmonary hypertension in congenital heart disease may occur simply because of increased pulmonary blood flow. When chronic, the increased pulmonary flow is often associated with a passive reduction in pulmonary resistance and little elevation of pulmonary vascular pressures. In a normal adult with a pulmonary blood flow (PBF) of 5 liters/min, a pulmonary vascular resistance (PVR) of 60 dynes-sec-cm^{-5}, and a mean left atrial pressure (LA) of 6 mm Hg, the pulmonary artery mean pressure (PA) may be calculated from the expression

$$\text{PVR} = \frac{(\text{PA} - \text{LA})80}{\text{PBF}} = \frac{(\text{PA} - 6)80}{5} = 60 \text{ dynes-sec-cm}^{-5}$$

$$\text{PA} = \frac{60 \times 5}{80} + 6 = 10 \text{ mm Hg}$$

If PBF is doubled, a reduction in PVR to 30 dynes-sec-cm^{-5} will maintain PA mean pressure at a normal level of 10 mm Hg. However, if PBF is increased four- to sixfold, the reserve capacity of the pulmonary vascular bed will be exceeded, and pulmonary artery pressure will rise. Thus, if the PVR is 30 dynes-sec-cm^{-5}, a PBF of 30 liters/min will be associated with a mean PA pressure that is only minimally elevated at 17 mm Hg, although the high right ventricular stroke volumes associated with the augmentation in pulmonary blood flow result in considerably higher values (40 to 45 mm Hg) for pulmonary artery and right ventricular systolic pressures. If the capacity of the pulmonary vascular bed to accommodate extra blood flow is diminished owing to mild parenchymal lung disease that results in a higher, albeit still normal, PVR of 90 dynes-sec-cm^{-5}, the mean PA pressure in the patient with a PBF of 30 liters/min will approximate 40 mm Hg; systolic PA and right ventricular systolic pressure will exceed 60 mm Hg. If no underlying arteriolar vascular disease exists, abolition of the shunt by corrective operation restores pulmonary blood flow and PA pressure to normal.

Commonly, an increase in pulmonary vascular resistance makes a variable contribution to the pulmonary hypertension associated with congenital heart disease. The increase in vascular resistance may have both a functional and a fixed component. The former—the "Bayliss" or myogenic theory—is thought to be related to pulmonary arteriolar vasoconstriction stimulated by distention of muscular pulmonary arteries and arterioles. According to this concept, distention of the vessel acts as a stimulus to vasoconstriction, which leads to increased work of the vascular smooth muscle and in turn to hypertrophy of the smooth muscle in the vessel wall.[5]

If a congenital cardiovascular defect causes pulmonary hypertension from the time of birth, the small, muscular arteries of the fetal lung may undergo delayed or only partial involution, resulting in persistently high levels of pulmonary vascular resistance (p. 791). This is true especially of those lesions in which a left-to-right shunt enters the right ventricle or pulmonary artery directly (i.e., a post-tricuspid valve shunt, such as ventricular septal defect or patent ductus arteriosus); these patients experience a higher incidence of severe and irreversible pulmonary vascular damage than those in whom the shunt is proximal to the tricuspid valve (pre-tricuspid shunts, as in atrial septal defect and partial anomalous pulmonary venous drainage). In the latter category, pulmonary hypertension may result from a large pre-tricuspid left-to-right shunt, which enhances the risk of pulmonary vascular damage.

PATHOLOGY (Table 27–3). The extent of reversibility of pulmonary vascular obstructive disease in the presence of congenital heart disease varies. From an anatomical point of view, reversible conditions are those in which the decreased pulmonary arteriolar cross-sectional area is the result of medial hypertrophy and vasoconstriction; irreversibility is associated with the presence of necrotizing arteritis and plexiform lesions in these small vessels.[150-154] The classification by Heath and Edwards[155] of six grades of structural change is widely employed to assess the potential reversibility of pulmonary vascular disease and is summarized as follows: *Grade I* is characterized by hypertrophy of the media of small muscular pulmonary arteries and arterioles. In *Grade II*, intimal cellular proliferation is added to the medial hypertrophy. *Grade IIII* is characterized by advanced medial thickening with hypertrophy and hyperplasia, together with progressive intimal proliferation and concentric fibrosis that results in obliteration of many arterioles and small arteries. In *Grade IV*, dilatation and so-called "plexiform lesions" of the muscular pulmonary arteries and arterioles are observed (Fig. 27–7). The latter consist of a plexiform net-

TABLE 27–3 HISTOPATHOLOGIC CLASSIFICATION OF PRIMARY PULMONARY VASCULAR DISEASE

PRESENT CLASSIFICATION	PREVIOUS CLASSIFICATION	CHARACTERISTIC HISTOPATHOLOGIC FEATURES*
Primary Pulmonary Arteriopathy With:		
Plexiform lesions with or without thrombotic lesions	Plexogenic pulmonary arteriopathy	Plexiform lesions; medial hypertrophy, eccentric or concentric-laminar intimal proliferation and fibrosis, fibrinoid degeneration, arteritis, dilatation lesions, and thrombotic lesions
Thrombotic lesions	Thromboembolic pulmonary arteriopathy	Thrombi (fresh, organizing, or organized, and recanalized-collander lesions); varying degrees of medial hypertrophy; no plexiform lesions
Isolated medial hypertrophy	Plexogenic pulmonary arteriopathy	Medial hypertrophy; increase of medial muscle, muscular arteries, muscularization of nonmuscularized intra-acinar arteries; no appreciable intimal or luminal obstructive lesions
Intimal fibrosis and medial hypertrophy	Plexogenic pulmonary arteriopathy	Eccentric or concentric-laminar proliferation and fibrosis; varying degrees of medial hypertrophy; no thrombotic or plexiform lesions
Isolated arteritis	Plexogenic pulmonary arteriopathy	Active or healed arteritis limited to pulmonary arteries; varying degrees of medial hypertrophy intimal fibrosis, and thrombotic lesions; no plexiform lesions
Pulmonary veno-occlusive disease	Pulmonary veno-occlusive disease	Intimal fibrosis and recanalized thrombi (collander lesions); pulmonary veins and venules; arterialized veins, capillary congestion, alveolar edema and siderophages, dilated lymphatics, pleural and septal edema and arterial medial hypertrophy, intimal fibrosis, and thrombotic lesions
Pulmonary capillary hemangiomatosis	—	Infiltrating thin-walled blood vessels widespread throughout pulmonary parenchyma, pleura, bronchi, and walls of pulmonary veins and arteries

* Medial hypertrophy may be accompanied by muscularization of arterioles.

From Pietra, G. G., Edwards, W. D., Kay, J. M. et al.: Histopathology of Primary Pulmonary Hypertension: A qualitative and quantitative study of pulmonary blood vessels from 58 patients in the National Heart, Lung and Blood Institute Primary Pulmonary Hypertension Registry. Circulation *80*:1198, 1989.

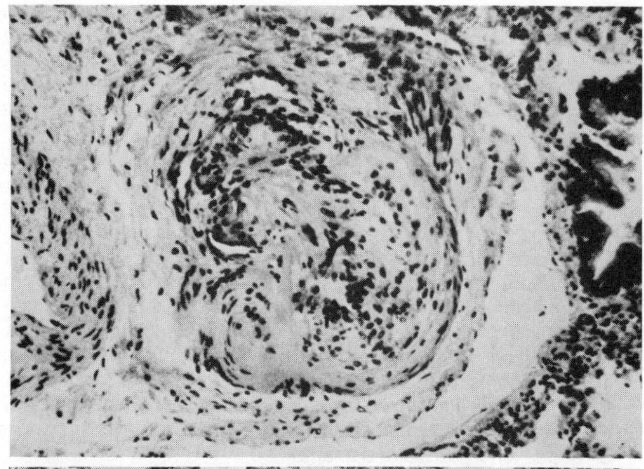

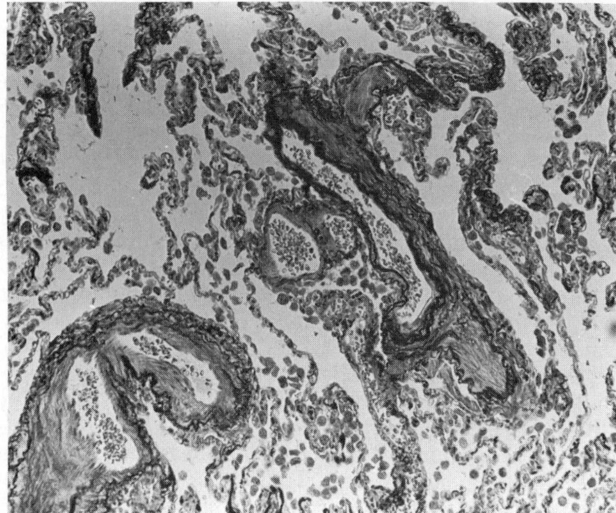

FIGURE 27–7. ***Top,*** **Histological section from the lung of a 3-year-old boy with a common atrioventricular canal and severe pulmonary hypertension. A muscular pulmonary artery with an early plexiform lesion is seen as well as fibrinoid necrosis of the media and active proliferation of intimal cells. (From Wagenvoort, C. A., and Wagenvoort, N.: Pathology of Pulmonary Hypertension. 2nd ed. New York, John Wiley and Sons, 1977.)** ***Bottom,*** **Photomicrograph of a lung biopsy specimen from a 35-year-old man with a patent ductus arteriosus and systemic pulmonary hypertension. A predominance of advanced changes is seen, including plexiform and dilatation lesions.**

work of capillary-like channels within a dilated segment of a muscular pulmonary artery. The channels are separated by proliferating endothelial cells, which often contain thrombi; indeed, the network of capillary channels may constitute recanalization of a thrombus. *Grade V* changes include complex plexiform, angiomatous, and cavernous lesions and hyalinization of intimal fibrosis (Fig. 27–8). Finally, *Grade VI* is characterized by the presence of necrotizing arteritis.

The Heath and Edwards classification implies that the morphological alterations are sequential, with Grade I being the earliest stage and Grade VI being the "end stage" of pulmonary vascular obliterative disease. That such an orderly progression may not in fact occur is suggested by the findings of Wagenvoort, which indicate that plexiform lesions develop gradually in areas affected by necrotizing arteritis. They have suggested that fibrinoid necrosis of a small segment of a pulmonary arterial branch leads to medial destruction and subsequent aneurysmal dilatation of the vessel as well as the formation of a fibrin clot in the lumen, often with admixture of platelets.[2,150] Organization of the fibrin clot by strands of intimal cells leads to formation of the plexus; the small capillary-like channels within the plexus (Fig. 27–7) provide continuity to the distal portion of the artery, which undergoes poststenotic dilatation. With time, the inflammatory component of the process subsides, fibrin disappears, and the strands of intimal cells become fibrotic. Wagenvoort's view is supported by animal experiments in which end-to-end systemic-pulmonary anastomoses resulted in arteritis and fibrinoid necrosis before the appearance of plexiform lesions.[156,157] Thus, although Heath-Edwards Grades I, II, and III may represent chronological progression, evidence exists that Grade VI (necrotizing arteritis) changes appear next, followed by Grades IV and V as end-stage alterations.

CLINICAL CONSIDERATIONS. As already mentioned, *Eisenmenger syndrome* is the term used by Wood to refer to patients with congenital central communications with severe pulmonary hypertension, in whom reversal of a left-to-right shunt has occurred across the pulmonary-systemic communication.[149] The patients described originally by Eisenmenger had ventricular septal defects, and the term *Eisenmenger complex* is applied to patients with severe pulmonary hypertension and right-to-left shunt through such a defect. The broader term *Eisenmenger syndrome* is applied to any anomalous circulatory communication that leads to obliterative pulmonary vascular disease, including pre- and post-tricuspid shunts. Heath-Edwards Grades IV to VI changes are usual in these patients; occasionally, lesser anatomical changes predominate and may be reversible after successful corrective operation.

When the pulmonary vascular resistance has increased so that it equals or exceeds systemic resistance, and the anatomical changes of the pulmonary vessels are predominantly those of Grades IV to VI, surgical closure of the anomalous circula-

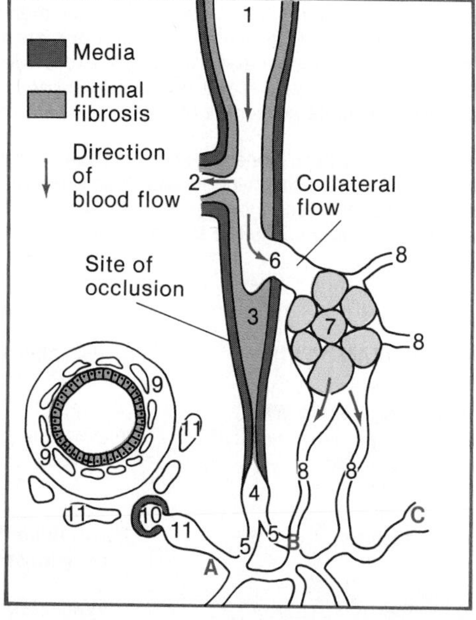

FIGURE 27–8. Diagram to show the origin and probable connections of small thin-walled blood vessels in the lung in grade 5 hypertensive pulmonary vascular disease. 1 = Dilated muscular pulmonary artery with thin media and intimal fibrosis: this is part of the generalized dilatation proximal to the site of vascular occlusion. 2 = Hypertrophied muscular pulmonary artery arising as a side branch of 1 with heaped-up intimal fibrous tissue at the site of origin. 3 = Terminal muscular pulmonary artery totally occluded by fibrous tissue: the media may be thick, as shown, or abnormally thin. 4 = Terminal dilated pulmonary arteriole. 5 = Capillaries in alveolar walls arising from pulmonary arteriole. 6 = Dilated, thin-walled, vein-like branch of hypertrophied parent muscular pulmonary artery. 7 = Localized "dilatation lesion": an angiomatoid lesion is shown. 8 = Capillaries in alveolar walls arising from dilatation lesions. 9 = Dilated thin-walled vessel in submucosa of small bronchus. 10 = Small bronchial artery in fibrous coat of small bronchus giving rise to thin-walled branches shown as 11. A = Bronchopulmonary anastomosis at capillary level. B = Anastomosis between capillaries arising from parent muscular pulmonary artery and from "dilatation lesions". C = Possible anastomosis between thin-walled vessels derived from pulmonary artery and those derived from pulmonary vein. (From Harris, P., and Heath, D.: The Human Pulmonary Circulation. 3rd ed. New York, Churchill Livingstone, 1986, p. 255.)

tory communication will be associated with a prohibitive immediate risk and if the patient survives will, in any case, fail to relieve pulmonary hypertension. Operation will, in fact, hasten death in most survivors who had either balanced shunts or predominant right-to-left shunts, since closure of the right-to-left communication merely increases the load on an already overburdened right ventricle. Structural changes in the pulmonary vascular bed are evident in pulmonary arteriograms, which reveal dilated central pulmonary arteries and narrowing of the peripheral branches (Fig. 27–9). These changes can be evaluated by means of quantitative analysis of the pulmonary wedge angiogram.[158] This technique has been employed successfully by Rabinovitch, Reid, and coworkers, who have demonstrated progressively more abrupt tapering of the pulmonary arteries in patients with increasingly abnormal hemodynamics and increasingly severe structural changes in lung biopsy tissue.[158]

OTHER CONDITIONS ASSOCIATED WITH DECREASED CROSS-SECTIONAL AREA OF THE PULMONARY VASCULAR BED

Primary Pulmonary Hypertension. This condition has been called "unexplained pulmonary hypertension" by a working committee of the World Health Organization[159] and is discussed in detail below.

Hepatic Cirrhosis and Portal Vein Thrombosis. These conditions have been occasionally associated with pulmonary hypertension and obliterative changes in the pulmonary arteriolar bed.[159–163,163a] Fishman has speculated that there is a common pathophysiological mechanism to these cases and others in which pulmonary hypertension is associated with ingestion of a variety of substances (*Crotalaria* alkaloids, aminorex[164]), and he has termed this "dietary pulmonary hypertension."[165] According to this concept, certain metabolites of ingested foods or drugs may induce pulmonary hypertension if they gain access to the pulmonary circulation or if, by damaging the liver, they lead to release of vasoactive substances that subsequently reach the lungs and injure pulmonary vessels. In at least one case of pulmonary hypertension complicated by portal hypertension, a high cardiac output was thought to play some role in the pathophysiology; treatment with a beta-adrenergic blocking agent, atenolol, resulted in a progressive reduction in pulmonary hypertension.[163]

Persistent Fetal Circulation in the Newborn (see also p. 893). This condition has been reported as a cause of severe pulmonary hypertension.[166–168] Affected infants exhibit cyanosis, tachypnea, acidemia, normal pulmonary parenchymal markings on chest x-ray, and anatomically normal hearts. Cyanosis is the result of right-to-left shunting across the foramen ovale and through a patent ductus arteriosus.[166] The condition may be due to persistence of extremely muscular small pulmonary arteries, a diminution in the absolute number of these resistance vessels, or a combination of the two.[168]

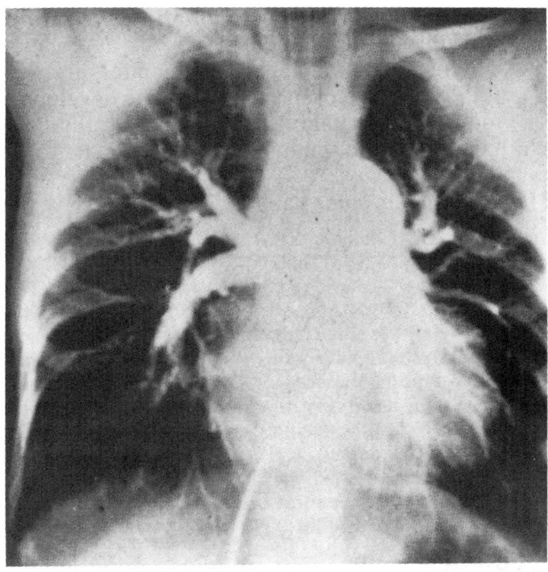

FIGURE 27–9. Pulmonary arteriogram of a boy aged 4 years with a ventricular septal defect and patent ductus arteriosus and reversed shunt. The narrowness of the peripheral branches of the pulmonary artery contrasts with the dilation of its main branches. Pulmonary arterial pressure, 90/60 mm Hg; wedge pressure, 4 mm Hg. Pulmonary blood flow, 1.6 L · min^{-1}; systemic flow 3.2 L · min^{-1}. (From Harris, P., and Heath, D.: The Human Pulmonary Circulation. 3rd ed. New York, Churchill Livingstone, 1986, p. 317.)

INCREASED RESISTANCE TO FLOW THROUGH LARGE PULMONARY ARTERIES

Pulmonary Thromboembolism (Chap. 48). This condition may cause pulmonary hypertension by impeding blood flow through the major pulmonary arteries and their branches. Generally, a single episode of pulmonary embolism resolves, and follow-up studies reveal normal pulmonary vasculature and pressure in the majority of patients.[169,170] In some patients, chronic pulmonary hypertension results when repeated, multiple emboli fail to resolve or trigger in-situ thrombosis.[171] Increasing numbers of these patients have been identified by the use of ventilation-perfusion lung scans, pulmonary angiography, and fiberoptic angioscopy.[172] It is important to make the diagnosis of pulmonary hypertension due to chronic pulmonary thromboembolism, since surgical treatment by thromboendarterectomy has been highly successful[171,173,174] (p. 810). Recently, balloon angioplasty has been used successfully in the treatment of pulmonary hypertension due to pulmonary embolism.[175]

Peripheral Pulmonic Stenosis. This is a congenital lesion that occurs particularly in association with supravalvular aortic stenosis or as a sequela of the rubella syndrome (p. 931). Hypertension in the proximal pulmonary arteries depends on the extent, location, and severity of the stenotic lesions.[2,176,177]

Unilateral Absence of Either the Right or the Left Pulmonary Artery. This is a rare congenital anomaly.[178] Often the condition is associated with a ventricular septal defect or patent ductus arteriosus, and the incidence of pulmonary hypertension is high. Pulmonary hypertension may also be observed in the absence of associated abnormalities, presumably because the thick-walled fetal pulmonary arterial bed is stimulated to constrict and undergo anatomical obliterative changes when the total cardiac output flows through only one lung from birth onward. The same mechanism may operate in patients with unilateral pulmonary artery stenosis in whom elevated pressure is observed in the main and uninvolved pulmonary arteries. Relief of the obstructive lesion by operation has been associated with marked improvement.[179]

HYPOVENTILATION

As discussed earlier (p. 791), conditions associated with hypoxia may cause pulmonary hypertension, particularly if there is associated acidemia.[32,33] A number of disorders that affect the upper airways, neuromuscular control, or pulmonary parenchyma lead to hypoventilation and (in the setting of a reactive pulmonary vascular bed) pulmonary hypertension.

The Obesity-Hypoventilation Syndrome[180,181] (see also p. 1593). Also called the pickwickian syndrome, this condition may lead to substantial pulmonary hypertension (mean pulmonary artery pressure ≥ 50 mm Hg), which correlates with the presence of hypoxemia and acidosis (Fig. 49–4, p. 1585). *Pharyngeal-tracheal obstruction* occurs in the presence of hypertrophied tonsils and adenoids[182,183] and may cause reversible pulmonary hypertension.

Neuromuscular Disorders. These include myasthenia gravis, poliomyelitis, and damage to the central respiratory center.[184] They may cause hypoventilation of sufficient severity to result in pulmonary hypertension (p. 1818). *Disorders of the chest wall* (kyphoscoliosis, pectus excavatum) may also cause hypoventilation and pulmonary hypertension (p. 1810).

The pulmonary hypertension in all of these conditions subsides with restoration of normal respiration and correction of the hypoxia. It should also be recognized that hypoxia may intensify pulmonary hypertension of other causes. For example, severe pulmonary hypertension occurring in children with a left-to-right shunt who reside at high altitude is often due to the combination of high pulmonary blood flow and superimposed hypoxic pulmonary vasoconstriction; pulmonary pressures may fall rapidly toward normal when residence is established at sea level.

OTHER CAUSES OF PULMONARY HYPERTENSION

High-Altitude Pulmonary Edema (see also p. 559). This entity is associated with reversible pulmonary hypertension. It is observed particularly in individuals acclimatized to high altitudes who, after a stay of some days or weeks at sea level, return to high altitude.[185] The finding of high-altitude pulmonary edema in four persons without a right pulmonary artery has been reported,[186] giving support to speculation concerning the combined role of hypoxia and hyperfusion in patients with this condition.[187]

Other Conditions. Severe pulmonary hypertension is an occasional but unusual finding in patients with *isolated partial anomalous pulmonary venous drainage.*[188] Speculation exists that the cause may be the increase in pulmonary blood flow associated perhaps with a reflex pulmonary arterial vasoconstriction secondary to distention of the right atrium.

plexogenic pulmonary arteriopathy,[198,202] suggesting a role for intense vasoconstriction with resultant fibrinoid necrosis of the muscular pulmonary arteries.

COLLAGEN-VASCULAR DISEASE (see also Chap. 56). The occurrence of arteritis and of fibrinoid necrosis in the walls of the smaller pulmonary arteries, and the frequent presence of Raynaud's phenomenon in patients with PPH, have raised the possibility that PPH may be a form of collagen-vascular or autoimmune disease. Since Raynaud's phenomenon is an expression of vasospasm in digital arteries, its presence in 10 per cent of patients with PPH[197] suggests that vasospasm in pulmonary arteries may be present as well. Interestingly, in families of patients with PPH, other members not affected by the disease may exhibit Raynaud's phenomenon. Pulmonary hypertension occurs frequently in patients with the so-called CREST syndrome[135,136] (p. 798), a variant of scleroderma. The histological changes in the pulmonary vessels in patients with this syndrome resemble those seen in patients with PPH and are similar to those seen in the pulmonary vessels of about 10 per cent of patients with the more usual forms of progressive systemic sclerosis.[135]

TAKAYASU'S (GIANT CELL) ARTERITIS (see also p. 1544). This frequently involves the pulmonary vessels (Fig. 27–10), but the pathological changes resemble those seen in systemic arteries. In the vast majority of these patients, the aorta and major arch vessels are involved as well. This condition can also be distinguished from PPH by the fact that the occlusive changes occur in the large and intermediate vessels rather than in the more distal vessels characteristic of PPH.[194,195]

OTHER ETIOLOGICAL FACTORS. A number of cases of PPH coexisting with postnecrotic *hepatic cirrhosis* have been reported, suggesting that a vasculitis might be responsible for the pulmonary hypertension.[160–163,211] *Polyarteritis nodosa* and *hypersensitivity* to a variety of *drugs,* including penicillin, chloramphenicol, and the sulfonamides, have also been suggested as etiologies for PPH,[214] although allergic vasculitis is unlikely to affect only the pulmonary vasculature. Occasionally a patient with PPH has been erroneously diagnosed as suffering from polyarteritis nodosa limited to the lungs.[2,215]

AMINOREX FUMARATE. Pulmonary hypertension has developed in a number of individuals in Europe who had ingested this anorexigenic drug, which has, of course, been removed from the market.[154,214–217] The clinical course of these patients was similar to that of patients with PPH, although in some instances regression of pulmonary hypertension upon withdrawal of the drug was reported.[219] Although causation has not been demonstrated definitively, the circumstantial evidence in favor of this relationship is impressive. Since only 0.2 per cent of individuals ingesting the drug developed pulmonary hypertension, some other factor such as a genetic predisposition or an idiosyncratic reaction must be involved.

MONOCROTALINE. Severe pulmonary hypertension can be produced in rats by the administration of *monocrotaline* or other pyrrolizidine alkaloids derived from the seeds of the plant *Crotalaria spectabillis* or of *fulvine,* an alkaloid derived from *Crotalaria fulva.*[220,221] Severe necrotizing pulmonary arteritis and luminal obstruction in small venules develops in these animals,[220,221] along with thickening of the main pulmonary artery.[232]

Monocrotaline-induced pulmonary vascular disease appears to follow activation of lung ornithine decarboxylase, an important enzyme in the biosynthesis of polyamines, such as spermidine and spermine.[223] A role for platelets in the production of pulmonary hypertension following monocrotaline lung injury has been suggested by a study[224] using antiplatelet antiserum to induce thrombocytopenia. When given 3 to 6 days after monocrotaline administration, the antiplatelet serum substantially blunted the development of pulmonary hypertension.[224] Although natives of the West Indies who ingest *Crotalaria fulva* in "bush tea" may develop veno-occlusive disease of the liver,[225] no instances of pulmonary hypertension in humans have been attributed to *Crotalaria.*

FEMALE HORMONES. The following observations suggest that *female hormones* may be involved in the genesis of PPH: (1) This condition occurs most frequently in young women, (2) there is a tendency for exacerbations to occur in the postpartum period, and (3) there may be an association between the use of oral contraceptives and the development of PPH.[226] The manner in which this endocrine effect may operate on the pulmonary vascular bed is obscure.

In most individual patients considered on clinical evidence to have PPH, there is no clear evidence that thromboembolism, congenital or immunological abnormalities, collagen-vascular disease, or drug ingestion were causes of the pulmonary hypertension. Although pulmonary hypertension can truly be said to be primary in such patients, some factors have been identified that may shed some light on the mechanisms underlying its development, even in these patients. It is well known that there is considerable variation among individuals in the reactivity of the pulmonary vascular bed. Vasoconstrictive stimuli, such as hypoxia or acidosis, can produce marked pulmonary hypertension in one person and be essentially without effect in another. The pulmonary arterial pressor response to hypoxia is particularly great in individuals with blood group A.[13,15] This variability in the responsivity of the pulmonary vascular bed undoubtedly accounts for the fact that only a minority of individuals develp pulmonary edema on exposure to high altitude (p. 793). Also, the severity of pulmonary hypertension and the level of pulmonary vascular resistance vary considerably among individuals with congenital heart disease and comparably sized ventricular septal defects. Presumably, there is a *genetic basis* for these differences in pulmonary vascular reactivity, just as there appears to be a genetic basis for the increased reactivity of the systemic vascular bed in essential systemic hypertension (p. 826).

The finding of increased pulmonary vascular reactivity and pulmonary vasoconstriction in patients with PPH suggests that a marked *vasospastic* or *constrictive* tendency underlies the development of PPH in predisposed individuals. The autonomic nervous system has been considered a factor in the development of PPH through stimulation of the pulmonary vascular bed by either neuronally released or circulating catecholamines. In some patients with PPH, the response to pulmonary vasodilators such as tolazoline, acetylcholine, or isoproterenol is a reduction in both pulmonary artery pressure and pulmonary vascular resistance,[54,227–229] supporting the notion of the importance of the autonomic nervous system in maintaining an elevated level of pulmonary vascular resistance. Other patients, however, are unresponsive to pulmonary vasodilating agents. Samet and Bernstein reported an interesting case of a patient with PPH who, when examined initially, exhibited marked pulmonary vasodilatation in response to an infusion of acetylcholine.[230] Three years later, on repeat catheterization, the pulmonary hypertension was more severe, and the patient did not respond to acetylcholine infusion. This observation suggests that patients with PPH initially may have increased pulmonary vasomotor tone. As the disease progresses, functional changes give way to fixed anatomical lesions unaffected by pharmacological intervention.

FAMILIAL PPH. Such cases have been reported with autosomal dominant inheritance[231–234]; other than from a positive family history, there is no way to distinguish these patients from those with the sporadic form of the disease. They may represent instances of the genetic transmission of extreme pulmonary vascular reactivity. The interplay between certain environmental factors such as hypoxia and a genetic predisposition for pulmonary vascular reactivity may also underlie the development of PPH. The reactivity of the pulmonary vascular bed of cattle to hypoxia has been shown clearly to be genetically determined.[2] In addition, it has been reported that the incidence of PPH increases at high altitude and that children with this condition improve when they move to lower altitudes[2]; conversely, the condition of patients with PPH may become worse if they ascend to higher altitudes.

PATHOLOGICAL FINDINGS AND ETIOLOGICAL CONSIDERATIONS

Several pathological findings (Tables 27–3 and 27–4) are common to almost all patients with PPH (Fig. 27–12): (1) intimal thickening of the smaller pulmonary arteries and arterioles with fibrosis, producing a characteristic "onionskin" configuration; (2) increased thickness of the media of muscular pulmonary arteries and muscularization of arterioles; (3) necrotizing arteritis in the walls of muscular pulmonary arteries with fibrinoid necrosis of the media of such vessels[203]; and (4) *plexiform lesions,* i.e., dilated, thin-walled side branches of muscular pulmonary arteries probably resulting from endothelial proliferation (Figs. 27–11 and 27–12). These lesions are responsible for the term *plexogenic pulmonary arteriopathy,* which is now frequently used to characterize the pathological changes in this condition. Although characteristic of PPH, these anatomical changes are not pathognomonic of the disease and are also found in patients with pulmonary hypertension secondary to cardiac shunts (p. 906).

The pathological diagnosis of PPH can be made when the aforementioned features—particularly the plexiform lesions—occur in the absence of congenital cardiac shunts. The pattern of elastic tissue of the pulmonary trunk is of the adult variety in PPH (p. 802), consistent with the belief that the pulmonary hypertension was acquired during adult life.[235] A number of pathological findings are *secondary* to the pulmonary hypertension itself, i.e., atherosclerosis of the major pulmonary arterial trunks and marked right ventricular hypertrophy.

Reid and coworkers examined the lungs of a number of patients with PPH using quantitative pathological techniques and electron microscopy.[207,236] These investigators noted thickening of the basement membranes and of the endothelial cells of small (<40 μm), nonmuscular pulmonary arterioles. The endothelial cells also contained increased numbers of organelles and pinocytotic vesicles, suggesting heightened metabolic activity; indeed, in some nonmuscular pulmonary arterioles, proliferation of endothelial cells obliterated the vascular lumen.[236] Quantitative analysis of the vessels in patients with PPH demonstrated a distinct reduction in the number of small, nonmuscular pulmonary arterioles. Residual, nonfunctioning "ghost vessels" seemed to remain in place of these small arterioles. At more proximal levels of the pulmonary vascular bed, there was considerable hypertrophy of smooth muscle of the media of small muscular pulmonary arteries.[207]

There has been much speculation recently concerning a possible role for pulmonary vascular endothelial dysfunction in the pathophysiology of PPH. The rapid proliferation of information about endothelial cell regulation of vascular smooth muscle contraction provides an attractive platform for a hypothesis about the genesis of PPH. Vascular endothelial cells can promote relaxation or contraction of adjacent smooth muscle cells via elaboration of EDRF (endothelial-derived relaxing factor) or endothelin, respectively.[20–23] The secretion of EDRF by vascular endothelium, which serves to dampen or counter many direct vasoconstrictor influences, is lost with endothelial dysfunction that may result from a variety of causes (e.g., shear stress[238]). Conversely, secretion of the potent vasoconstrictor peptide endothelin may be enhanced in the presence of hypoxia or in the setting of platelet aggregation. Endothelial denudation results in platelet adherence to exposed tissue collagen, with release of platelet derived smooth muscle mitogens which also have vasoconstrictor properties.[239] Another hypothesis for the development of pulmonary hypertension involves the disruption or activation of endothelial cells. This process in turn leads to an inflammatory response and thrombosis, thereby narrowing the lumen of the pulmonary vessels (Fig. 27–13). In a person who is susceptible—whether on a genetic or an acquired basis—stimuli for pulmonary vasoconstriction result in excessive responses and transient pulmonary hypertension. Frequent episodes of pulmonary vasoconstriction and the resultant

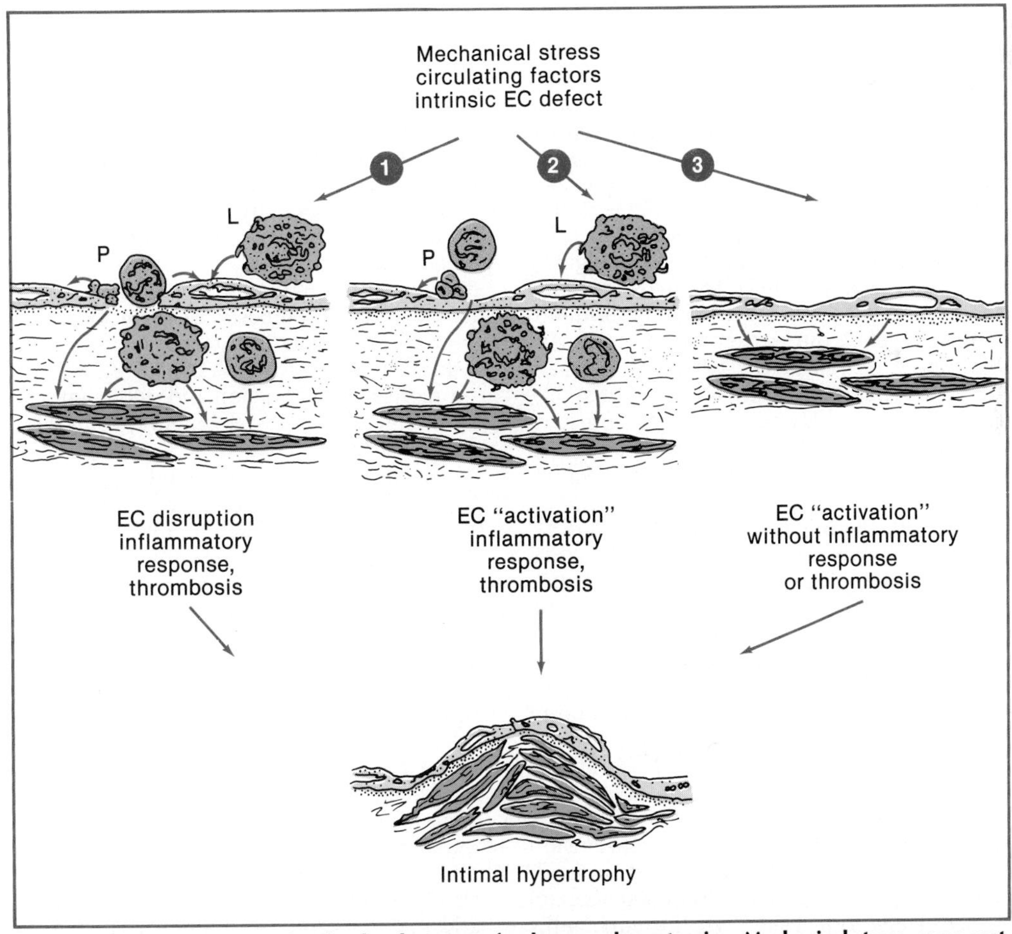

FIGURE 27–13. A hypothesis for the development of pulmonary hypertension. Mechanical stress, some sort of circulating factor, or an intrinsic endothelial cell defect begins the pathogenetic process. These perturbations can lead to endothelial cell (EC) and basement membrane (BM) disruption with subsequent adhesion of leukocytes (L) and platelets (P) (Pathway 1) or more subtle endothelial cell "activation." The activated endothelial cell either initiates a thrombotic and/or inflammatory response (Pathway 2) or releases growth factors without inflammation (Pathway 3). These growth factors stimulate the proliferation of EC and smooth muscle cells (SMC) ultimately leading to intimal hypertrophy. (From Albelda, SM: Role of growth factors in pulmonary hypertension. *In* Fishman, A. P. [ed.]: The Pulmonary Circulation: Normal and Abnormal. Philadelphia, University of Pennsylvania Press, 1990, p. 213.)

pulmonary hypertension eventually cause hypertrophy of the smooth muscle in the media of these vessels and perhaps damage and thicken the endothelial cells in the nonmuscular vessels, with subsequent failure of EDRF release. Intense vasoconstriction may lead to fibrinoid necrosis of the arteriolar wall, causing development of plexiform lesions. Ultimately, the vessels are reduced in number, and the residua of these destroyed vessels can be seen histologically as "ghost vessels." Destruction of large numbers of pulmonary arterioles reduces the cross-sectional area of the pulmonary vascular bed, thus producing a permanent increase in pulmonary vascular resistance and fixed pulmonary hypertension. The latter, in turn, damages other blood vessels and initiates a vicious circle, with progressively rising pulmonary arterial pressure.

CLINICAL FEATURES

NATURAL HISTORY AND SYMPTOMATOLOGY. One of the most extensive studies on the natural history of PPH was reported from the Mayo Clinic.[201] This study consisted of a long-term follow-up of 120 patients in whom PPH was diagnosed by clinical and hemodynamic criteria. Seventy-three per cent of the patients were female, and the mean age at diagnosis was 34 years (3 to 64 years). The median interval from initial clinical manifestation to the time of clinical and hemodynamic diagnosis was 1.9 years. The four most frequent clinical features at the time of diagnosis were exertional dyspnea (75 per cent), loud second heart sound (98 per cent), roentgenographic abnormalities (95 per cent) including cardiomegaly and prominent central pulmonary arteries, and electrocardiographic abnormalities (95 per cent) such as right ventricular hypertrophy, right axis deviation, and right atrial enlargement. Less frequent clinical features included exertional dizziness or syncope (30 per cent), exertional chest pain (8 per cent), and peripheral edema (8 per cent). Ten per cent of the study population had Raynaud's phenomenon, 7 (6 per cent) had chronic liver disease, and 5 (4 per cent) had a history of superficial thrombophlebitis. In two families, PPH affected two brothers. A national registry for PPH was begun in 1981, and a report[197] of baseline data on 187 patients in the registry appeared in 1987. The clinical profile in these 187 patients with PPH collected from 32 centers was remarkably similar to that in the Mayo Clinic series. In the registry report 63 per cent of patients were women, the mean age was 36 ± 15 years (range 1 to 81 years), the mean interval from onset of symptoms to diagnosis was 2 years, and the most common presenting symptoms were dyspnea (60 per cent), fatigue (19 per cent), syncope (or near-syncope) (13 per cent) and Raynaud's phenomenon (10 per cent).

The *prognosis* of PPH in the Mayo Clinic series[201] is illustrated in Figure 27–14. Survival is poor in patients with PPH, with only 21 per cent surviving to 5 years. However, patients who received anticoagulants clearly had a better survival rate than did those who did not receive anticoagulants. This was not a randomized study, and the choice to administer anticoagulants was determined by individual physicians using their clinical judgment for each case. However, the utilization of anticoagulant therapy in patients with a clinical and hemodynamic diagnosis of PPH is supported by the findings at autopsy in the Mayo Clinic series. Fifty-six patients underwent autopsy, and lung tissue in these patients revealed two major pathological types: thromboembolic pulmonary hypertension in 32 patients (57 per cent) and plexogenic pulmonary arteriopathy in 18 patients (32 per cent). Thus, thromboembolism without any evidence of plexiform lesions was the major pathological feature in more than half the patients autopsied. As a result of these findings, Fuster and coworkers[201] recommend anticoagulation as standard therapy for patients with a clinical and hemodynamic diagnosis of PPH. Prognosis in PPH has been strongly correlated with the presence and severity of pericardial effusion, as assessed by echocardiography.[240] Patients with moderate or large pericardial effusions had a very poor prognosis, possibly because the pericardial effusion served as an indicator of the presence of severe, sustained right heart failure.[240] Mean pulmonary artery pressure, mean right atrial pressure, and New York Heart Association Functional Class correlate inversely and cardiac index directly with survival in PPH[240,241] (Fig. 24–14), reflecting the importance of the severity of pulmonary vascular obstruction.

The mode of death in patients with PPH is variable, and in the Mayo Clinic series contributing factors included right heart failure (64 per cent), pneumonia (7 per cent), sudden death (7 per cent), death related to cardiac catheterization (5 per cent), pulmonary artery dissection with tamponade (1 per cent), and death during a minor operation (1 per cent). In 15 per cent of cases, the contributing factors or cause of death could not be determined.

Some patients with PPH, followed by means of serial catheterization over a number of years, exhibit some hemodynamic improvement if they are given pulmonary vasodilating agents when they are first seen.[227] During later stages of the disease, however, such drugs often have no effect on the pulmonary vascular bed.[227,230] Late in the course of the disease, patients develop right ventricular failure, and exertional syncope may occur, presumably because of a low fixed cardiac output and hypoxemia. PPH is a fatal disease in almost all instances; the duration of symptoms varies, but on the average death occurs approximately 3 years after the onset of symptoms. The course may be more precipitous in some patients, particularly in children. However, a few patients have lived for as long as 30 years after the onset of symptoms. In at least one reported case, PPH appeared to regress.[242]

Patients with PPH commonly complain of exertional dyspnea, syncope, precordial chest pain, weakness, and later, dyspnea at rest. These symptoms probably result from low cardiac output or hypoxemia or both. Precordial chest pain may also be secondary to ischemia of the right ventricular subendocardium or distention of the major pulmonary arteries or both.[243,244] The pain may radiate to the neck but not characteristically to the arms. Palpitations are also common and may be caused by ventricular tachyarrhythmias, which occur not infrequently in the late stages of PPH. Occasionally, cough and hemoptysis occur. These latter symptoms may be due to rupture of dilated plexiform lesions, to in situ pulmonary arterial thromboses, or to episodes of pulmonary embolism occurring late in the course of the disease.

PHYSICAL EXAMINATION. Findings are consistent with pulmonary hypertension and right ventricular pressure overload: a large *a* wave in the jugular venous pulse; a low-volume carotid arterial pulse with a normal upstroke; a left parasternal (right ventricular) heave; a systolic pulsation produced by a dilated, tense pulmonary artery in the second left interspace; an ejection click and flow murmur in the same area; a closely split second heart sound with a loud pulmonic component; and a fourth heart sound of right ventricular origin. Late in the course, signs of right ventricular failure (hepatomegaly, peripheral edema, and ascites) may be present. Patients with severe pulmonary hypertension may also have prominent *v* waves in the jugular venous pulse, owing to tricuspid regurgitation; a third heart sound of right ventricular origin; a high-pitched early diastolic murmur of pulmonic regurgitation; and a holosystolic murmur of tricuspid regurgitation. Cyanosis is a late finding in PPH and may be due to a patent foramen ovale with a right-to-left shunt occurring secondary to elevation of right atrial pressure. Other causes for cyanosis include a markedly reduced cardiac output with systemic vasoconstriction, intrapulmonary right-to-left shunting via vascular anastomoses, and ventilation-perfusion mismatches in the lung itself. Uncommonly, the left laryngeal nerve becomes paralyzed as a consequence of compression by a dilated pulmonary artery.[245]

LABORATORY FINDINGS

HEMATOLOGICAL AND CHEMICAL STUDIES. Results of these studies are usually normal in patients with PPH. If

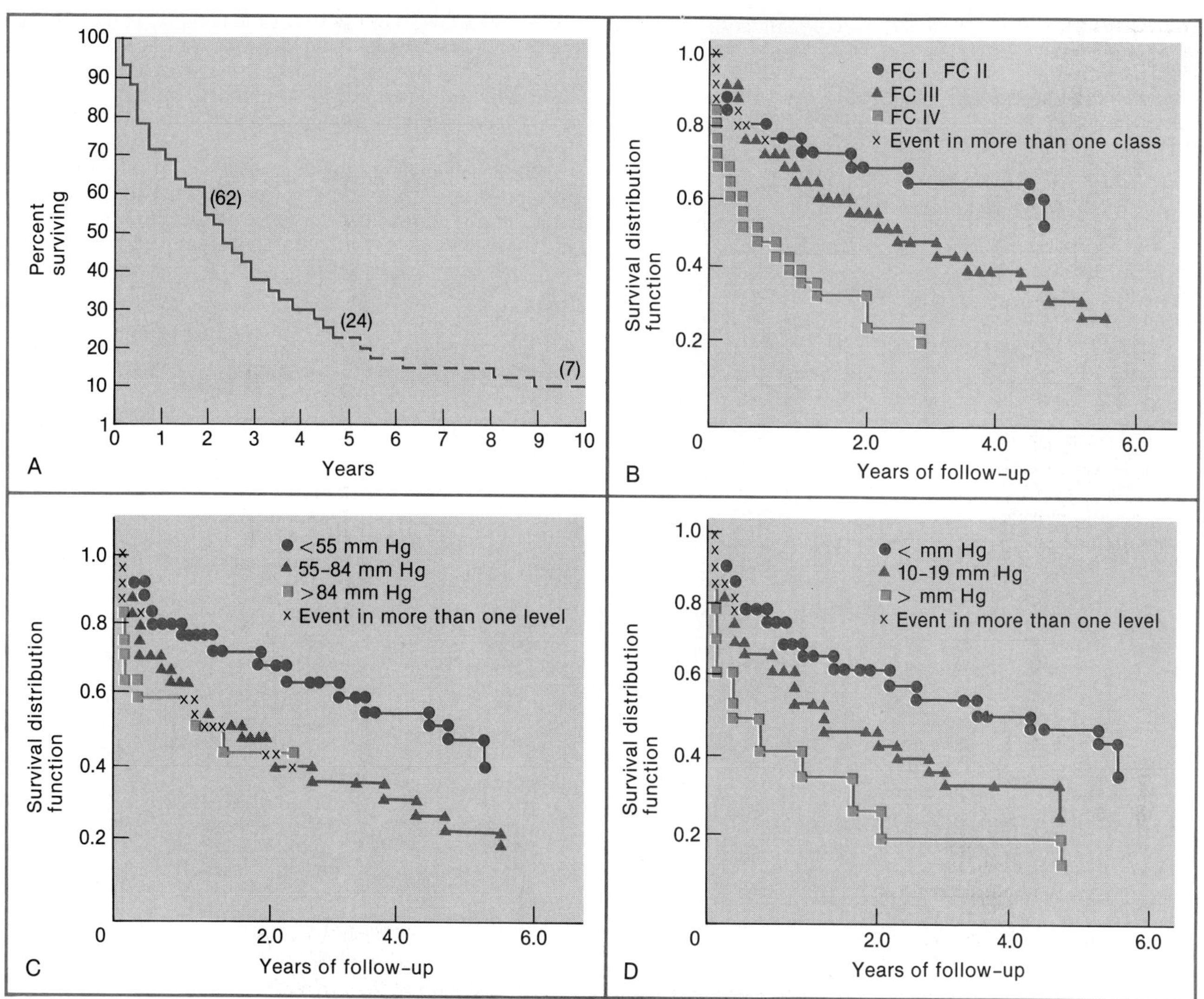

FIGURE 27–14. Prognosis in patients with a clinical and hemodynamic diagnosis of primary pulmonary hypertension. *Panel A,* the observed survival for the entire group (115 patients who survived diagnostic cardiac catheterization). (From Fuster, V., et al.: Primary pulmonary hypertension: Natural history and the importance of thrombosis. Circulation *70*:580, 1984, by permission of the American Heart Association, Inc.) *Panel B,* Survival time from baseline catheterization varied significantly ($p < 0.0001$) by New York Heart Association functional class with 4.9 years as the median survival time for functional classes I and II, 2.6 years and 0.5 years for functional classes III and IV, respectively. *Panel C,* Survival time from baseline catheterization varied significantly ($p < 0.0005$) by level of mean pulmonary artery pressure with 4 years as the median survival time for the <55 mm Hg group, and 1.8 years and 1 year for the 55–84 and >84 mm Hg groups, respectively. *Panel D,* Survival time from baseline catheterization varied significantly ($p < 0.0005$) by level of mean right atrial pressure with 3.8 years as the median survival time for the <10 mm Hg group, and 1.5 and 0.08 years for the 10–19 and >20 mm Hg groups, respectively. (*B* through *D,* from D'Alonzo, G. E., Barst, R. J., Levy, P. S. et al.: Survival in patients with primary pulmonary hypertension: Results of a national prospective registry. Ann. Intern. Med., *in press.*)

there is arterial oxygen desaturation, polycythemia may be present. A number of investigators have reported hypercoagulable states, abnormal platelet function, defects in fibrinolysis, and other abnormalities of coagulation in patients with PPH.[206,209] Abnormal liver function tests can indicate right ventricular failure with resultant systemic venous hypertension.

ELECTROCARDIOGRAPHY. The electrocardiogram in PPH usually exhibits right atrial and right ventricular enlargement. A direct correlation between the amplitude of the R in V_1, the R/S ratio in V_1 and the level of pulmonary arterial pressure has been reported.[246]

ROENTGENOGRAPHY. X-ray examination of the chest in patients with PPH shows enlargement of the main pulmonary artery and its major branches, with marked tapering of peripheral arteries.[247,248] The right ventricle and atrium may also be enlarged. Fluoroscopic examination may disclose exaggerated pulsations of secondary pulmonary arterial branches, reflecting an elevation in pulmonary arterial pulse pressure. However, in contrast to the plethoric peripheral lung fields in patients with left-to-right shunts, oligemia is noted in these lung regions in patients with PPH (Fig. 27–15). It has been suggested that survival in PPH correlates inversely with the size of the main pulmonary artery[248]—a reasonable suggestion, since the latter correlates with the height of the pulmonary arterial pressure. The diameter of the pulmonary artery may be determined from computed tomographic (CT) scans and used to estimate pulmonary artery pressures.[249]

PULMONARY FUNCTION TESTS. Pulmonary function tests may show mild restriction with a reduced diffusion capacity for carbon monoxide (DL_{CO}) and hypoxemia with hypocapnea. Some patients have increased residual volumes and reduced maximum voluntary ventilation.

ECHOCARDIOGRAPHY. This usually demonstrates enlargement of the right atrium and ventricle, normal or small left ventricular dimensions, and a thickened interventricular septum. The septal/posterior left ventricular wall ratio may be abnormally increased, as in hypertrophic obstructive car-

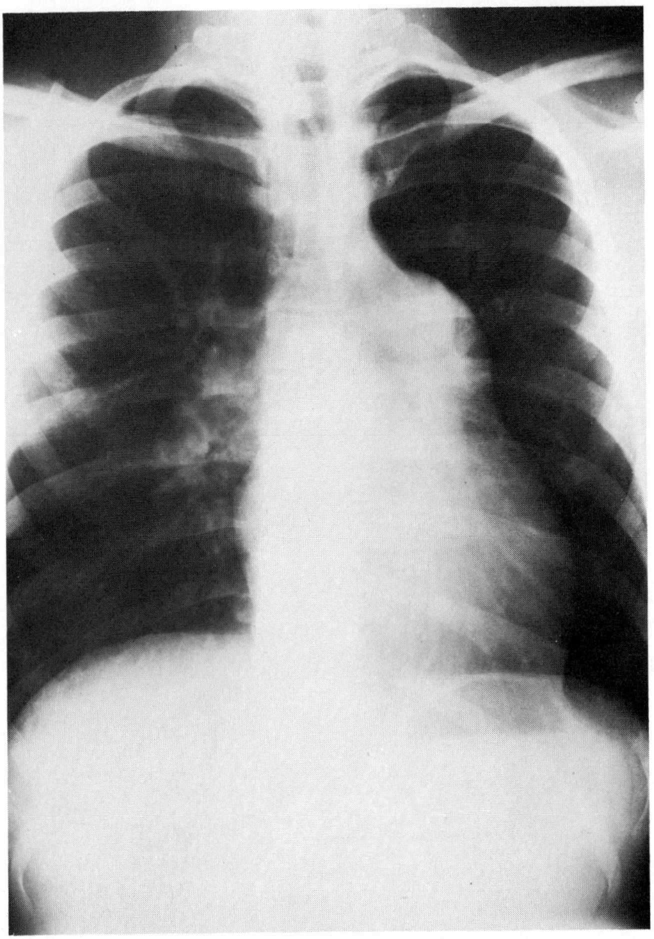

FIGURE 27–15. Frontal chest roentgenogram of a 15-year-old boy with PPH. Note the enlarged main pulmonary artery and the radiolucent lung fields.

diomyopathy (p. 1404), but the other echocardiographic signs characteristic of that condition are not present. Systolic prolapse of the mitral valve is frequently present, as is abnormal septal motion of the ventricular septum, presumably due to right ventricular dilatation or tricuspid and pulmonic regurgitation or both.[250] Doppler echocardiographic evidence of right ventricular systolic hypertension may be obtained by measuring the velocity of the tricuspid regurgitant jet and using the Bernouilli formula (p. 79). Doppler techniques have demonstrated a decrease in the velocity ratio of mitral early flow to atrial flow in patients with PPH, secondary to both a decrease in early and an increase in atrial flow velocities.[239,251]

LUNG SCINTIGRAPHY. Perfusion lung scans in patients with PPH are usually either normal or demonstrate small, nonspecific, subsegmental defects. Lung scanning may be hazardous late in the course of the disease because the macroaggregated albumin particles employed in scanning may significantly reduce the already critically narrowed cross-sectional area of the pulmonary vascular bed.[252]

CARDIAC CATHETERIZATION AND ANGIOGRAPHY (Table 27–5). The diagnosis of PPH cannot be confirmed without performing cardiac catheterization and pulmonary angiography. Some patients may be too ill for one or both of these procedures (see below), and in such individuals, the diagnosis must remain tentative and be based primarily on exclusion, following clinical evaluation and noninvasive tests. Right-heart catheterization reveals elevated pulmonary arterial and right-ventricular systolic pressures that may approach, equal, or sometimes even exceed systemic arterial levels; right artial pressure may also be increased. The calculated pulmonary vascular resistance is extremely high, approaching or sometimes even exceeding systemic vascular resistance. When tricuspid regurgitation is absent, the *a* wave in the right atrial pressure tracing is predominant; when it is present, the height of the *v* wave may equal or exceed that of the *a* wave. Left ventricular diastolic, left atrial, and pulmonary capillary wedge pressures are low or normal, but it is often difficult to record the pulmonary capillary wedge pressure. A patent foramen ovale with a right-to-left shunt may be present.

Pulmonary angiography demonstrates large central pulmonary arteries with marked peripheral tapering. Postmortem arteriograms demonstrate absence of "background haze" secondary to the loss of small, nonmuscular pulmonary arterioles

TABLE 27–5 APPLICATIONS OF CATHETERIZATION IN ESTABLISHING ETIOLOGIC DIAGNOSIS OF PULMONARY HYPERTENSION

CONDITION	TEST APPLIED	FINDING
Congenital heart disease	Step-up in O_2 saturation in right heart;	Left to right shunt and location of shunt
	Step-down in O_2 saturation in left heart	Right to left shunt and location of shunt
	Cardiac angiography	Anatomic definition
Peripheral pulmonary artery stenoses	Intrapulmonary arterial pressure	Intrapulmonary arterial pressure gradients
	Pulmonary angiogram	Pulmonary arterial branch stenoses
Major pulmonary arterial occlusion by clot, or tumor*	Continuous pressure recording from distal pulmonary artery to main pulmonary artery	Focal pressure gradient in a lobar or larger pulmonary artery, intravascular filling defect or narrowing
	Selective or main pulmonary angiography	
Mitral stenosis Cor triatriatum Supravalvular mitral ring	Simultaneous wedge and left ventricular pressure recording	An elevated wedge pressure and mean mitral valve diastolic pressure gradient >3 mm Hg at rest, both of which increase with exercise
Mitral regurgitation	Simultaneous wedge and left ventricular pressure recording Left ventriculogram	Large systolic pressure wave in wedge tracing. Regurgitation of contrast from left ventricular angiogram into the left atrium.
Left ventricular dysfunction or diastolic overload	Left ventricular pressure Left ventriculogram	Left ventricular end diastolic pressure >15 mm Hg Left ventricular contraction abnormality and/or ejection fraction <50%, or increased diastolic volume

* Ventilation and perfusion lung scans precede catheterization.

Modified from Reeves, J. T., and Groves, B. M.: Approach to the patient with pulmonary hypertension. In Weir, E. K., and Reeves, J. T.: Pulmonary Hypertension. Mt. Kisco, NY, Futura Publishing Co., 1984, p. 20.

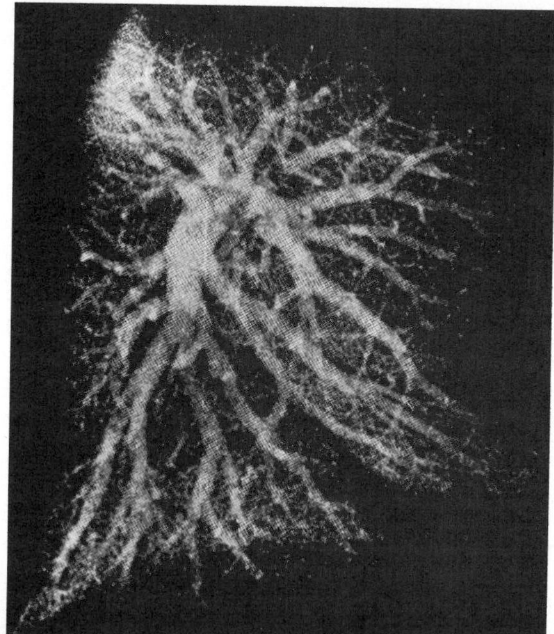

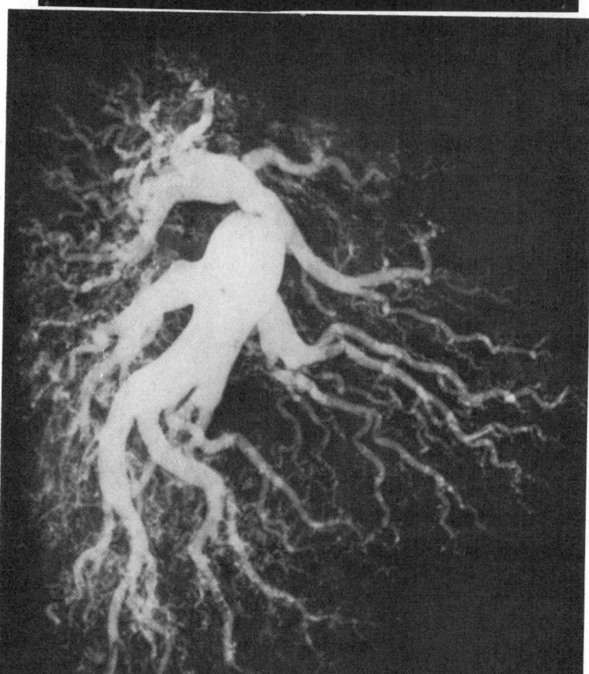

FIGURE 27–16. *A*, Postmortem pulmonary arteriogram of a normal lung in a 22-year-old man. The caliber of the pulmonary arteries tapers down gradually, and there is a rather dense background filling of vessels. *B*, Postmortem pulmonary arteriogram from an 18-year-old man with unexplained plexogenic pulmonary arteriopathy (primary pulmonary hypertension). The main branches are dilated. (From Wagenvoort, C. A., and Wagenvoort, N.: Pathology of Pulmonary Hypertension. New York, copyright 1977, reprinted by permission of John Wiley and Sons, Inc.)

(Fig. 27–16).[207] Right ventriculography usually demonstrates a thick-walled chamber, sometimes with delayed emptying, i.e., elevated right ventricular end-diastolic and end-systolic volumes and a reduced ejection fraction, a result of the markedly elevated pulmonary vascular resistance.

Cardiac catheterization and angiography carry an increased risk in patients with PPH. In the Mayo Clinic series,[201] five deaths were related to cardiac catheterization in the study cohort of 120 patients. Interestingly, pulmonary angiography had been performed in only one of these patients. Maintenance of adequate oxygenation by administration of supplemental oxygen and avoidance of vasovagal reactions (and rapid treatment of those that occur) should reduce the risk of invasive studies in this patient group. The risk of inducing atrial and/or ventricular arrhythmias can be minimized by the use of balloon flotation catheters and avoidance of prolonged attempts at catheterization by inexperienced operators. Pulmonary angiography can be performed safely using a segmental angiographic technique with hand injection of small amounts of radiographic contrast through the terminal lumen of a balloon-flotation catheter, while the balloon is inflated.[253] The new nonionic contrast agents appear to be better tolerated in these patients.

DIAGNOSIS

(Table 27–6)

It is essential that diagnostic efforts be pursued vigorously in patients with severe pulmonary hypertension in order to ensure that no patient with secondary pulmonary hyperten-

TABLE 27–6 DIAGNOSTIC STUDIES USEFUL FOR ELUCIDATING CAUSES OF PULMONARY HYPERTENSION

POTENTIAL CAUSE OF PULMONARY HYPERTENSION	POSSIBLE DIAGNOSTIC STUDIES
a) Pulmonary embolic disease	ventilation/perfusion scans and/or selective, lobar pulmonary angiography
b) Pulmonary venous thrombosis or obstruction	chest x-ray, angiography, lung biopsy
c) Congenital intra-cardiac shunts causing increased pulmonary blood flow	indicator dilution studies
d) Increased left atrial pressure; secondary to mitral or aortic valve disease, left ventricular dysfunction or systemic hypertension	pulmonary artery wedge pressure or left atrial pressure (via patent foramen ovale) (>15mm Hg)
e) Pulmonary airways disease (e.g., chronic bronchitis and emphysema)	respiratory function tests (FVC/FEV_1)
f) Hypoxic pulmonary hypertension associated with (i) impaired ventilation; either central (CNS) or peripheral (chest wall problems or upper airway obstruction); (ii) residence at high altitude	sleep apnea studies and respiratory tests
g) Interstitial lung disease, pneumoconioses and fibrosis (e.g., silicosis, rheumatoid disease and sarcoidosis)	chest x-ray, spirometry and carbon monoxide diffusion, rheumatoid factor, lymph node biopsy
h) Collagen disease (e.g., SLE, polyarteritis nodosa, scleroderma)	LE cells, skin, muscle, or other tissue biopsy, esophageal motility studies
i) Parasitic disease (schistosomiasis or filariasis)	rectal biopsy, complement fixation, skin tests, blood smears
j) Cirrhosis or portal vein thrombosis	liver function tests
k) Peripheral pulmonary artery stenosis (including Takayasu's disease and fibrosing mediastinitis)	selective pulmonary angiography, or pressure gradient at catheterization
l) Sickle cell disease	erythrocyte morphology, hemoglobin electrophoresis
m) Choriocarcinoma and hydatidiform mole	serum or urinary beta subunit of chorionic gonadotrophin
n) Intravenous injection of pulverized pills	lung biopsy

Modified from Weir, E. K.: Diagnosis and management of primary pulmonary hypertension. *In* Weir, E. K., and Reeves, J. T.: Pulmonary Hypertension. Mt. Kisco, NY, Futura Publishing Co., 1984, p. 141.

sion is erroneously classified as having PPH. Secondary pulmonary hypertension is often treatable in that the cause can be attacked directly; even when it cannot, the prognosis may not be as grave as it is in PPH. Patients with PPH may tolerate diagnostic procedures poorly. These individuals can experience sudden cardiovascular collapse and even death during or shortly after the induction of general anesthesia for surgical procedures, during cardiac catheterization and angiography, and even following radioisotopic lung scanning.[252] Although the mechanisms responsible for cardiovascular collapse and sudden death have not been defined clearly, it may be presumed that these interventions act as stimuli to further constriction of the already narrowed pulmonary vascular bed, followed by the sudden development or exacerbation of right heart failure or arrhythmias or both.

The *differential diagnosis* of PPH includes a number of well-defined causes of secondary pulmonary hypertension. Exclusion of mitral stenosis, congenital cardiac defects (including cor triatriatum), pulmonary embolism, and pulmonary venous obstruction by means of catheterization and angiography is imperative. "Silent" mitral stenosis, i.e., without the characteristic diastolic murmur, can be excluded by means of echocardiographic visualization of the motion of the mitral valve and the absence of a transvalvular pressure gradient (Chap. 34). *Congenital heart defects* with Eisenmenger syndrome can usually be ruled out if significant left-to-right or right-to-left shunts are absent, although occasional patients with equal pulmonary and systemic vascular resistances may have no detectable shunt at rest. The use of indicator-dilution curves and angiography may be quite helpful in this regard. *Cor triatriatum* (p. 929) is recognized by appropriate hemodynamic studies and angiographic visualization of the left atrial membrane. This entity presents a characteristic left atrial echocardiogram with normal mitral valve motion. Cardiac catheterization reveals a hemodynamic pattern similar in some ways to mitral stenosis, i.e., a diastolic pressure gradient between the left ventricle and the pulmonary capillary bed. *Pulmonary embolism* (Chap. 48) can be excluded by means of balloon-occlusion segmented pulmonary angiography,[253] and *sickle cell disease with in situ pulmonary vascular thrombosis* (Chap. 57) can be evaluated by hemoglobin electrophoresis. The presence of severe *pulmonary parenchymal disease* can be recognized by the characteristic physical findings, chest roentgenogram, and pulmonary function tests (Chap. 49). *Collagen vascular disease* is suggested by the involvement of other organ systems or the presence of abnormal immunological phenomena, such as antinuclear antibodies and LE cells (Chap. 56). *Pulmonary veno-occlusive disease* (p. 797) is characterized by progressive narrowing of nearly all small pulmonary veins and venules, many of which exhibit complete occlusion by fibrous tissue. It is suggested clinically by the finding of a normal or elevated[6] pulmonary artery "wedge" pressure together with chest x-ray evidence of Kerley B lines and pulmonary edema.

Treatment of Pulmonary Hypertension

Treatment of pulmonary hypertension (Table 27–7) is most successful when the inciting cause is identified and removed before the pulmonary vasculature has been irreversibly damaged. Thus, closure of central circulatory shunts while they are still predominantly left-to-right, and before extensive plexiform and angiomatoid lesions have developed in the lungs, will usually correct pulmonary hypertension in the setting of congenital heart disease with central left-to-right shunt. Patients with hypoventilation secondary to hypertrophied tonsils and adenoids will experience cure of associated pulmonary hypertension with tonsillectomy.[182,183]

In patients in whom removal of the inciting cause is not possible (or in whom the cause is unknown, as in PPH), therapy for pulmonary hypertension is directed at decreasing resistance to pulmonary blood flow and improving the cardiocirculatory response to right ventricular pressure overload.

Decreasing resistance to pulmonary blood flow can be accomplished only when the site of the increased resistance (Table 27–1) is identified. Thus, when left ventricular failure with secondary left atrial hypertension is the cause of increased resistance to pulmonary blood flow, relief of left ventricular failure (Chap. 17) will lower pulmonary artery pressure. When decreased cross-sectional area of the pulmonary vascular bed is responsible for pulmonary hypertension, *pulmonary vasodilators* may be tried; it is likely that they will be effective only in cases in which active vasoconstriction of small muscular arteries or arterioles is contributing significantly to the pulmonary hypertension.

The use of pulmonary vasodilators as chronic therapy for PPH[38–43,198,254–285] is based on the observation that muscular hypertrophy, rather than intimal hyperplasia, is the earliest finding in these patients. Because of the difficulty in predicting or interpreting the results of vasodilator therapy in patients with unexplained pulmonary hypertension, lung biopsy has been recommended whenever possible before

TABLE 27–7 TREATMENT OF PULMONARY HYPERTENSION

I. REMOVE INCITING CAUSE (when possible)
Examples: Surgical correction of mitral stenosis[107,108] or cor triatriatum,[116] closure of anatomical site of predominant left-to-right shunt, removal of massively hypertrophied tonsils and adenoids,[182] avoidance of offending drug or agent (aminorex, *Crotalaria* alkaloids, intravenous drug abuse)

II. DECREASE RESISTANCE TO PULMONARY BLOOD FLOW
- **A. Lower left atrial or left ventricular diastolic pressure, when these are elevated**
- **B. Pulmonary vasodilators**
  1. **Oxygen[70,123,124,278]**
  2. **Hydralazine[258,260,270]**
  3. **Phentolamine[272,285]**
  4. **Isoproterenol[273,283]**
  5. **Diazoxide[275–277]**
  6. **Nifedipine[26,256–259,261–263,280–282]**
  7. **Prostaglandins[39–43,279]**
  8. **Tolazoline[38,55]**
  9. **Verapamil[263–266]**
  10. **Nitroglycerin[267,268]**
  11. **Captopril[269]**
- **C. Anticoagulation: recurrent pulmonary embolism,[169] pulmonary veno-occlusive disease, PPH[201,291]**
- **D. Heart-lung transplantation[287–290]**

III. IMPROVE CARDIOCIRCULATORY RESPONSE TO RIGHT VENTRICULAR PRESSURE OVERLOAD
- **A. Appropriate pulmonary toilet to maximize alveolar ventilation and oxygenation**
- **B. Prophylaxis (vaccines) for influenza and pneumonia; prompt, vigorous treatment of any pulmonary infection**
- **C. Diuretics (spironolactone and furosemide or a thiazide) with low-salt diet**
- **D. Pulmonary vasodilators (see IIB)**
- **E. Inotropic agents (digitalis glycosides, newer oral beta agonists, etc.)**

starting pulmonary vasodilator therapy.[159] There is much to recommend this approach, including the possibility of uncovering a specific but unexpected cause of the pulmonary hypertension, such as pulmonary thromboembolism or a collagen-vascular disorder, as well as assessing the reversibility or irreversibility of the vascular changes prior to treatment. This latter point is all the more important, since vasodilator therapy may be hazardous in some patients with advanced pulmonary hypertension.[38,254,255,258,263,264,267]

VASODILATORS. These agents that have been used for either the acute or the chronic treatment of pulmonary hypertension include oxygen,[70,123,124,278] hydralazine,[258,260,270,271] phentolamine,[272,285] sublingual isoproterenol,[273,283] diazoxide,[275-277] nifedipine,[26,256-259,261-263,280-282] prostacyclin,[39-43,260,279] tolazoline,[38,54] verapamil,[263-266] nitroglycerin,[267,268] and captopril.[269] Effectiveness of these agents has been quite variable. In one report of 10 women with PPH, only sublingual isoproterenol (alone or combined with isosorbide dinitrate) produced a fall in pulmonary vascular resistance: diazoxide, hydralazine, phentolamine, and tolazoline were ineffective.[38] In contrast, hydralazine was found to be effective in each of 4 patients with PPH by one group[270] and in 6 of 12 patients by a second group.[271] Similar conflicting results have been reported for diazoxide.[38,275-277]

Prostacyclin (PGI_2) has been reported to reverse completely the pulmonary vasoconstriction in a neonate with persistent fetal circulation.[279] The hemodynamic effects of prostacyclin on the pulmonary circulation have been reported to resemble those of hydralazine, and the suggestion has been made that acute effects of prostacyclin admininstration may predict the response to hydralazine.[260] Treatment of PPH with chronic intravenous infusion of prostacyclin (PGI_2, epoprostenol) has been reported.[42] In a randomized multicenter trial, 23 patients with PPH were randomized to chronic intravenous PGI_2 via a permanent intravenous catheter and a portable syringe pump (11 patients) or conventional treatment (12 patients), which included oral vasodilators, supplemental O_2, and digoxin as deemed indicated by the investigator. All patients were anticoagulated. After 2 months, cardiac output had increased and pulmonary resistance had decreased significantly in the PGI_2 group but not in the control group. Hemodynamic and symptomatic benefit persisted with continued PGI_2 infusion up to 18 months in some patients, although dose requirements increased.

Nifedipine has been reported to prevent the acute pulmonary vasoconstriction associated with hypoxia,[26] and several reports suggest that nifedipine and diltiazem may have therapeutic value in pulmonary hypertension of various etiologies.[256-259,261,262] In particular, the use of high dosages of the calcium antagonists nifedipine or diltiazem has been reported to produce substantial reductions in pulmonary arterial pressure and pulmonary vascular resistance in patients with PPH[256] (Fig. 27-17). Thirteen patients received an initial test dose of either 60 mg diltiazem or 20 mg nifedipine followed by consecutive hourly doses until a 50 per cent fall in pulmonary vascular resistance (PVR) and a 33 per cent fall in pulmonary artery pressure was achieved, or until untoward side effects developed. Although little hemodynamic change was seen after the first dose, in 8 of 13 patients continued hourly doses led to a fall in mean pulmonary artery pressure of 48 per cent (61 mm Hg to 35 mm Hg) and in PVR of 60 per cent (15 to 6 units). Subsequent chronic treatment with high-dosage nifedipine (up to 240 mg/day) or diltiazem up to 720 mg/day) was undertaken in the eight patients who showed a favorable hemodynamic response. In five patients restudied at one year, sustained reductions in pulmonary artery pressure and PVR were present in four while the one patient in whom dosage had been reduced to conventional levels had a return of pressure and PVR to previous levels.[256] It should be noted that some patients with PPH (5/13 in this report[256]) failed to respond even to these massive dosages of nifedipine or diltiazem.

Variable results are not surprising, since most institutions have been able to study only small numbers of patients, and the underlying pathological condition (reversible vs. irreversible pulmonary vascular changes) has been unknown for the majority of patients in nearly all published reports on vasodilation therapy for pulmonary hypertension. Despite these shortcomings, there is some evidence that the findings on acute drug testing predict long-term results of treatment for individual patients.[256,257,261,265,268,270-272,278] Accordingly, it seems reasonable to assess the acute hemodynamic response to a variety of agents in the patient with severe pulmonary hypertension and to use the results of this assessment to design chronic therapy. As already mentioned, it is essential to determine the underlying cause of the patient's pulmonary hypertension whenever possible, since this may affect therapy in a fundamental way. An aggressive diagnostic approach, including lung biopsy, may be necessary in many cases.

HEART-LUNG TRANSPLANTATION (Ch. 18). This procedure has been performed as therapy for advanced, otherwise untreatable pulmonary vascular disease.[286-290] The largest experience with combined heart and lung transplantation is at Stanford University, where 70 such transplants were performed between March 9, 1981 and June 1990.[289,290] Indications for operation have included PPH (approximately 45 per cent of patients), Eisenmenger syndrome (45 per cent of patients) and miscellaneous causes (e.g., cystic fibrosis).[287] Recently, five single lung transplants have been performed, two of which were in patients with Eisenmenger syndrome due to atrial septal defect and included surgical closure of the septal defect.[290] Immunosuppression therapy has most recently consisted of cyclosporine, prednisone, and azathioprine, and management has included routine bronchoscopic surveillance for earlier detection of rejection and infection. With these approaches, survival at 1, 2, and 3 years has been 73 per cent, 73 per cent, and 65 per cent.[289] Problems with proliferative coronary atherosclerosis and obliterative bronchiolitis remain major long-term obstacles. Thus, although progress has been made in improving the results of combined heart and lung transplantation, major problems still exist. With advances in immunosuppressive therapy and surgical technique, it is likely that additional numbers of patients will be treated with lung or combined heart-lung transplantation.

ANTICOAGULATION. This is clearly indicated in pulmonary hypertension associated with recurrent pulmonary emboli. Its role in other forms of pulmonary hypertension (e.g., veno-occlusive disease) is conjectural and rests on postmor-

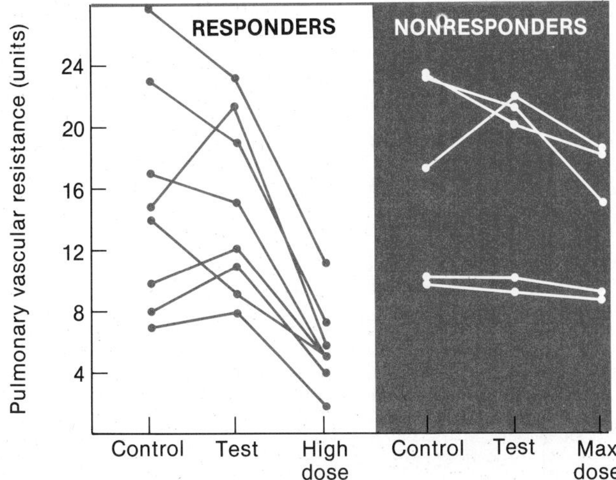

FIGURE 27-17. The effect of high-dose calcium antagonist treatment on pulmonary vascular resistance in patients with primary pulmonary hypertension. The patients are divided as responders and nonresponders. In the responders all but one had a reduction in pulmonary vascular resistance to 7 Wood units or less with high-dose therapy. (From Rich, S., and Brundage, B. H.: High dose calcium channel-blocking therapy for primary pulmonary hypertension: Evidence for long-term reduction in pulmonary arterial pressure and regression of right ventricular hypertrophy. Circulation 76:135, 1987).

tem or biopsy studies showing thrombi in large and small pulmonary veins or arteries.[2,5,117,171,198,201,202,291] However, the Mayo Clinic group[201,291] has reported clinical evidence that anticoagulants may improve the prognosis in at least some patients with severe PPH.

Even when pulmonary hypertension can be neither cured nor improved, the cardiocirculatory response to right ventricular pressure overload can often be improved with amelioration of right heart failure and an increase in forward cardiac output. The elements of a program designed to accomplish these goals are given in Table 27–7, III, A to E.

REFERENCES

NORMAL PULMONARY CIRCULATION

1. Comroe, J. H., Jr.: The main functions of the pulmonary circulation. Circulation *33*:146, 1966.
2. Wagenvoort, C. A., and Wagenvoort, N.: Pathology of Pulmonary Hypertension. 2nd ed. New York, John Wiley and Sons, 1977.
3. Fritts, H. W., Harris, P., Chidsey, C. A. et al: Estimation of flow rate through bronchial-pulmonary vascular anastomoses with use of T-1824 dye. Circulation *23*:390, 1961.
4. Barratt-Boyes, B. G., and Wood, E. H.: Cardiac output and related measurements and pressure values in the right heart and associated vessels, together with an analysis of the hemodynamic response to the inhalation of high oxygen mixtures in healthy subjects. J. Lab. Clin. Med. *51*:72, 1958.
5. Harris, P., and Heath, D.: The Human Pulmonary Circulation. 3rd ed. New York, Churchill Livingstone, 1986, 702 pp.
6. Harris, P., Segel, N., and Bishop, J. M.: The relation between pressure and flow in the pulmonary circulation in normal subjects and in patients with chronic bronchitis and mitral stenosis. Cardiovasc. Res. *1*:73, 1968.
7. Nihill, M. R., McNamara, D. G., and Vick, R. L.: The effects of increased blood viscosity on pulmonary vascular resistance. Am. Heart J. *92*:65, 1976.
8. Dawes, G. S., Mott, J. C., Widdicombe, J. G., and Wyatt, D. G.: Changes in the lungs of the newborn lamb. J. Physiol. *121*:141, 1953.
9. Adams, F. H., and Lind, J.: Physiologic studies on the cardiovascular status of normal newborn infants. Pediatrics *19*:431, 1957.
10. Rudolph, A. M.: The changes in the circulation after birth. Their importance in congenital heart disease. Circulation *41*:343, 1970.
11. Friedman, W. F., Molony, D. A., and Kirkpatrick, S. E.: Prostaglandins: Physiological and clinical correlations. Adv. Pediatr. *25*:151, 1978.
12. Naeye, R. L.: Arterial changes during the perinatal period. Arch. Pathol. *71*:121, 1961.
13. Fishman, A. P.: Hypoxia on the pulmonary circulation: How and where it acts. Circ. Res. *38*:221, 1976.
14. Von Euler, U. S., and Liljestrand, G.: Observations on the pulmonary arterial blood pressure in the cat. Acta Physiol. Scand. *12*:301, 1946.
15. Silove, E. D., Inoue, T., and Grover, R. F.: Comparison of hypoxia, pH, and sympathomimetic drugs on bovine pulmonary vasculature. J. Appl. Physiol. *24*:355, 1968.
16. Haneda, T., Nakajima, T., Shirato, K. et al.: Effects of oxygen breathing on pulmonary vascular input impedance in patients with pulmonary hypertension. Chest 83:520, 1983.
17. Grover, R. F., Vogel, J.H.K., Averill, K. H., and Blount, S. G.: Pulmonary hypertension. Individual and species variability relative to vascular reactivity. Am. Heart J. *66*:1, 1963.
18. Weir, E. K., Tucker, A., Reeves, J. T., and Will, D. H.: Pulmonary hypertension in cattle at high altitude. Cardiovasc. Res. *8*:745, 1975.
19. Fishman, A. P.: The enigma of hypoxic pulmonary vasoconstriction. *In* Fishman, A. P. (ed): The Pulmonary Circulation: Normal and Abnormal. Philadelphia, University of Pennsylvania Press, 1990, pp. 109–129.
20. Furchgott, R. F., and Zawadzki, J. W.: The obligatory role of endothelial cells in the relaxation of arterial smooth muscle by acetylcholine. Nature *288*:373, 1980.
21. Griffith, T. M., Edwards, D. H., Davies, R. L., et al.: EDRF coordinates the behaviour of vascular resistance vessels. Nature *329*:442, 1987.
22. Hickey, K. A., Rubanyi, G., Paul, R. J., and Highsmith, R. F.: Characterization of a coronary vasoconstrictor produced by cultured endothelial cells. Am. J. Physiol. *248*:C550, 1985.
23. Yanagisawa, M., Kurihara, H., Kimura, S., et al.: A novel potent vasoconstrictor peptide produced by vascular endothelial cells. Nature *332*:411, 1988.
23a. Stewart, D. J., Levy, R. D., Cernacek, P., and Langleben, D.: Increased plasma endothelin-1 in pulmonary hypertension: Marker or mediator of disease? Ann. Intern. Med. *114*:464, 1991.
24. Kotlikoff, M. I., and Fishman, A. P.: Endothelin: Mediator of hypoxic vasoconstriction? *In* Fishman, A. P. (ed): The Pulmonary Circulation: Normal and Abnormal. Philadelphia, University of Pennsylvania Press, 1990, pp. 85–89.
25. McMurty, I. F., Davidson, A. B., Reeves, J. T., and Grover, R. F.: Inhibition of hypoxic pulmonary vasoconstriction by calcium antagonist in isolated rat lungs. Circ. Res. *38*:99, 1976.
26. Simonneau, G., Escourron, P., Duroux, P., and Lockhart, A.: Inhibition of hypoxic pulmonary vasoconstriction by nifedipine. N. Engl. J. Med. *304*:1582, 1981.
27. Rabinovitch, M., Gamble, W., Nadas, A. S., et al.: Rat pulmonary circulation after chronic hypoxia: Hemodynamic and structural features. Am. J. Physiol. *236*:H818, 1979.
28. Rabinovitch, M., Gamble W. J., Miettinen, O. S., and Reid, L.: Age and sex influence on pulmonary hypertension of chronic hypoxia and on recovery. Am. J. Physiol. *240*:H62, 1981.
29. Glazier, J. B., and Murray, J. F.: Sites of pulmonary vasomotor reactivity in the dog during alveolar hypoxia and serotonin and histamine infusion. J. Clin. Invest. *50*:2550, 1971.
30. Bergofsky, E. H.: Mechanisms underlying vasomotor regulation of regional pulmonary blood flow in normal and disease states. Am. J. Med. *57*:378, 1974.
31. Hauge, A.: Hypoxia and pulmonary vascular resistance: The relative effects of pulmonary arterial and alveolar Po_2. Acta Physiol. Scand. *76*:121, 1969.
32. Enson, Y., Giuntini, C., Lewis, M. L., et al.: The influence of hydrogen ion concentration and hypoxia on the pulmonary circulation. J. Clin. Invest. *43*:1146, 1964.
33. Vogel, J.G.K., and Blount, G., Jr.: The role of hydrogen ion concentration in the regulation of pulmonary arterial pressure: Observations in a patient with hypoventilation and obesity. Circulation *32*:788, 1965.
34. Kadowitz, P. J., Joiner, P. D., and Hyman, A. L.: Effect of sympathetic nerve stimulation on pulmonary vascular resistance in the intact spontaneously breathing dog. Proc. Soc. Exp. Biol. Med. *147*:68, 1974.
35. Fritts, H. W., Harris, P., Clauss, R. H., et al.: The effect of acetylcholine on the human pulmonary circulation under normal and hypoxic conditions. J. Clin. Invest. *37*:99, 1958.
36. Wood, P., Besterman, E. M., Towers, M. K., and McIlroy, M. B.: The effect of acetylcholine on pulmonary vascular resistance and left atrial pressure in mitral stenosis. Br. Heart J. *19*:279, 1957.
37. Kadowitz, P. J., and Hyman, A. L.: Differential effects of prostaglandins A_1 and A_2 on pulmonary vascular resistance in the dog. Proc. Soc. Exp. Biol. Med. *149*:282, 1975.
38. Hermiller, J. B., Bambach, D., Thompson, M. J., et al.: Vasodilators and prostaglandin inhibitors in primary pulmonary hypertension. Ann. Intern. Med. *97*:480, 1982.
38a. Meyrick, B., Niedermeyer, M. E., Ogletree, M. L., and Brigham, K. L. Pulmonary hypertension and increased vasoreactivity caused by repeated indomethacin treatment in sheep. J. Appl. Physiol. *59*:443, 1985.
39. Jones, D. K., Whigenbottam, T. W., and Wallwork, J.: Treatment of primary pulmonary hypertension with intravenous epoprostenol (prostacyclin). Br. Heart J. *57*:270, 1987.
40. Guadagni, D. N., Ikram, H., and Maslowski, A. H.: Haemodynamic effects of prostacyclin (PGI_2) in pulmonary hypertension. Br. Heart J. *45*:385, 1981.
41. Rubin, L. J., Groves, B. M., Reeves, J. T., et al.: Prostacyclin-induced acute pulmonary vasodilation in primary pulmonary hypertension. Circulation *66*:334, 1982.
42. Rubin, L. J., Mendoza, J., Hood, M., et al.: Treatment of primary pulmonary hypertension with continuous intravenous prostacyclin (epoprostenol). Ann. Intern. Med. *112*:485, 1990.
43. Barst, R. J.: Pharmacologically induced pulmonary vasodilatation in children and young adults with primary hypertension. Chest *89*:497, 1986.
44. Kay, J. M., Waymire, J. C., and Grover, R. F.: Lung mast cell hyperplasia and pulmonary histamine forming capacity in hypoxic rats. Am. J. Physiol. *226*:178, 1974.
45. Haas, F., and Bergofsky, E. H.: Role of the mast cell in the pulmonary pressor response to hypoxia. J. Clin. Invest. *51*:3154, 1972.
46. Hauge, A.: Role of histamine in hypoxic pulmonary hypertension in the rat. I. Blockade or potentiation of endogenous amines, kinins, and ATP. Circ. Res. *22*:371, 1968.
47. Hauge, A., and Melmon, K. L.: Rise of histamine in hypoxic pulmonary hypertension in the rat. II. Depletion of histamine, serotonin, and catecholamines. Circ. Res. *22*:385, 1968.
48. Susmano, A., and Carleton, R. A.: Prevention of hypoxic pulmonary hypertension by chlorpheniramine. J. Appl. Physiol. *31*:531, 1971.
49. Salvaterra, C. G., and Rubin, L. J.: Cardiovascular effects of pulmonary hypertension. Trends Cardiovasc. Med. *1*:65, 1991.
50. Goldring, R. M., Turino, G. M., Cohen, G., et al.: The catecholamines in the pulmonary arterial pressor response to acute hypoxia. J. Clin. Invest. *41*:1211, 1962.
51. Patel, D. J., Lange, R. L., and Hecht, H. H.: Some evidence for active constriction in the human pulmonary vascular bed. Circulation *18*:19, 1958.
52. Long, W. A., and Brown, D. L.: Central neural regulation of the pulmonary circulation. *In* Fishman, A. P. (ed): The Pulmonary Circulation: Normal and Abnormal. University of Pennsylvania Press, Philadelphia, 1990, pp 131–149.
53. Sanders, J., Miller, D. D., and Patil, P. N.: Alpha adrenergic and histaminergic effects of tolazoline-like imidazolines. J. Pharmacol. Exp. Ther. *195*:362, 1975.
54. Rudolph, A. M., Paul, M. H., Sommer, L. S., and Nadas, A. S.: Effects of tolazoline hydrochloride (Priscoline) on circulatory dynamics of patients with pulmonary hypertension. Am. Heart J. *55*:424, 1958.
55. Vogel, J.H.K., Grover, R. F., Jamieson, G., and Blount, S. G., Jr.: Long-term physiologic observations in patients with ventricular septal defect and increased pulmonary vascular resistance. Adv. Cardiol. *11*:108, 1974.
56. Tucker, A., Hoffman, E. A., and Weir, E. K.: Histamine receptor antago-

nism does not inhibit hypoxic pulmonary vasoconstriction in dogs. Chest *71*(Suppl):261, 1977.
57. Okpako, D. T.: A dual action of histamine on guinea pig lung vessels. Br. J. Pharmacol. *45*:311, 1972.
58. Tucker, A., Weir, E. K., Reeves, J. T., and Grover, F.: Histamine H_1 and H_2 receptors in pulmonary and systemic vasculature of the dog. Am. J. Physiol. *229*:1008, 1975.
59. Shepherd, J. T., Donald, D. E., Linder, E., and Swan, H.J.C.: Effect of small doses of 5-hydroxytryptamine (serotonin) on pulmonary circulation in the closed chest dog. Am. J. Physiol. *197*:963, 1959.
60. Harris, P., Fritts, H. W., and Cournand, A.: Some circulatory effects of 5-hydroxytryptamine in man. Circulation *21*:1134, 1960.
61. Moret, P., Covarrubias, E., Coudert, J., and Duchosall, F.: Cardiocirculatory adaptation to chronic hypoxia. Acta Cardiol. (Brux.) *27*:596, 1972.
62. Penazola, D., Sime, F., Banchero, N., et al.: Pulmonary hypertension in healthy men born and living at high altitudes. Am. J. Cardiol. *11*:150, 1963.
63. Hecht, H. H., and McClement, J. H.: A case of chronic mountain sickness in the United States: Clinical, physiologic, and electrocardiographic observations. Am. J. Med. *25*:470, 1968.
64. Penazola, D., Sime, F., Banchero, N., and Gamboa, R.: Pulmonary hypertension in healthy men born and living at high altitudes. Med. Thorac. *19*:449, 1962.
65. Vogel, J.H.K., Weaver, W. F., Rose, R. L., et al.: Pulmonary hypertension on exertion in normal men living at 10,150 feet (Leadville, Colorado). Med. Thorac. *19*:461, 1962.
66. Niewoehner, D. E., Kleinerman, J., and Rice, D. B.: Pathologic changes in the peripheral airways of young cigarette smokers. N. Engl. J. Med. *291*:755, 1974.
67. United States Department of Health, Education, and Welfare: The health consequences of smoking: A report of the Surgeon General, 1972. DHEW publication No. v72 (HSM) 72-7516. Washington, D.C., U.S. Government Printing Office, 1972.
68. Spain, D. M., Siegel, H., and Bradess, V. A.: Emphysema in apparently healthy adults: smoking, age, and sex. J.A.M.A. *224*:322, 1973.
69. Burrow, B., Kettel, L. J., Niden, A. H., et al.: Patterns of cardiovascular dysfunction in chronic obstructive lung disease. N. Engl. J. Med. *286*:912, 1972.
70. Neff, T. A., and Petty, T. L.: Long-term continuous oxygen therapy in chronic airway obstruction. Ann. Intern. Med. *72*:621, 1970.

SECONDARY PULMONARY HYPERTENSION

70a. Turley, K.: The challenge of pulmonary hypertension. Chest *99*:6, 1991.
71. Brooks, H. L., Kirk, E. S., Vokonas, P. S., et al.: Performance of the right ventricle under stress. J. Clin. Invest. *50*:2176, 1971.
72. Berman, J. L., Green, L. G., and Grossman, W.: Right ventricular diastolic pressure in coronary artery disease. Am. J. Cardiol. *44*:1263, 1979.
73. Lorell, B. H., Leinbach, R. C., Pohost, G. M., et al.: Right ventricular infarction. Am. J. Cardiol. *43*:463, 1979.
74. Vasco, J. S., Elkins, R. C., Fogarty, T. J., and Morrow, A. G.: The experimental production of chronic mitral valvular obstruction. J. Thorac. Cardiovasc. Surg. *53*:875, 1967.
75. Haddy, F. J., Ferrin, A. L., Hannon, D. W., et al.: Cardiac function in experimental mitral stenosis. Circ. Res. *1*:219, 1953.
76. Silove, E. D., Tavernor, W. D., and Berry, C. L.: Reactive pulmonary arterial hypertension after pulmonary venous constriction in the calf. Cardiovasc. Res. *6*:36, 1972.
77. Charms, B. L., Brofman, B. L., and Adicoff, A.: Differential pulmonary artery occlusion in patients with chronic pulmonary disease. Am. J. Med. *26*:527, 1959.
78. Soderholm, B., and Werko, L.: Acetylcholine and the pulmonary circulation in mitral valvular disease. Br. Heart J. *21*:1, 1959.
79. Kay, J. M., and Edwards, F. R.: Ultrastructure of the alveolar-capillary wall in mitral stenosis. J. Pathol. *111*:239, 1973.
80. Szidon, J. P., Pietra, G. G., and Fishman, A. P.: The alveolar-capillary membrane and pulmonary edema. N. Engl. J. Med. *286*:1200, 1972.
81. Hicks, J. D.: Acute arterial necrosis in the lungs. J. Pathol. Bacteriol. *65*:333, 1953.
82. Whitaker, W., Black, A., and Warrack, A.J.N.: Pulmonary ossification in patients with mitral stenosis. J. Fac. Radiol. (Lond.) *7*:29, 1955.
83. Jordan, S. C., Hicken, P., Watson, D. A., et al.: Pathology of the lungs in mitral stenosis in relation to respiratory function and pulmonary haemodynamics. Br. Heart J. *28*:101, 1966.
84. Grossman, W., and Lorell, B. H.: Diastolic Relaxation of the Heart. Boston, Martinus Nijhoff, 1988.
85. Lorell, B. H., and Grossman, W.: Cardiac hypertrophy: The consequences for diastole. J. Am. Coll. Cardiol. *9*:1189, 1987.
86. Grossman, W.: Diastolic dysfunction and congestive heart failure. Circulation *81*(Suppl. III):1, 1990.
87. Dodek, A., Kassebaum, D. G., and Bristow, J. D.: Pulmonary edema in coronary artery disease without cardiomegaly: Paradox of the stiff heart. N. Engl. J. Med. *286*:1347, 1972.
88. Benotti, J. R., Grossman, W., and Cohn, P. F.: The clinical profile of restrictive cardiomyopathy. Circulation *61*:1206, 1980.
89. Kern, M. J., Lorell, B. H., and Grossman, W.: Cardiac amyloidosis masquerading as constrictive pericarditis. Cathet. Cardiovasc. Diagn. *8*:629, 1982.
90. Lorell, B. H., and Grossman, W.: Profiles in constrictive pericarditis, restrictive cardiomyopathy and cardiac tamponade. *In* Grossman, W. and Baim, D. S. (eds.): Cardiac Catheterization, Angiography and Intervention. 4th ed. Philadelphia, Lea and Febiger, 1991.
91. Sawyer, C. G., Burwell, C. S., Dexter, L., et al.: Chronic constrictive pericarditis: Further consideration of the pathologic physiology of the disease. Am. Heart J. *44*:207, 1952.
92. Grossman, W.: Profiles in valvular heart disease. *In* Grossman, W. and Baim, D. S., (eds.): Cardiac Catheterization, Angiography and Intervention. 4th ed. Philadelphia, Lea and Febiger, 1991.
93. Dexter, L.: Physiologic changes in mitral stenosis. N. Engl. J. Med. *254*:829, 1956.
94. Schlant, R. C.: Altered cardiovascular function of rheumatic heart disease and other acquired valvular disease. *In* Hurst, J. L., and Logue, R. B. (eds.): The Heart. 4th ed. New York, McGraw-Hill Book Co., 1978, p. 971.
95. Wood, P.: An appreciation of mitral stenosis. I. Clinical features; II. Investigation and results. Br. Med. J. *1*:1051 and 1131, 1954.
96. Araujo, J., and Lukas, D. S.: Interrelationships among pulmonary capillary pressure, blood flow and valve size in mitral stenosis: Limited regulatory effects of the pulmonary vascular resistance. J. Clin. Invest. *31*:1082, 1952.
97. Wood, P.: Pulmonary hypertension with special reference to the vasoconstrictive factor. Br. Heart J. *20*:557, 1958.
98. Davies, L. G., Goodwin, J. F., and VanLeuven, B. D.: The nature of pulmonary hypertension in mitral stenosis. Br. Heart J. *16*:440, 1954.
99. Robin, E. R., and Meyer, E. C.: Cardiopulmonary effects of pulmonary venous hypertension with special reference to pulmonary lymphatic flow. Circ. Res. *8*:324, 1960.
100. Uhley, H. N., Leeds, S. E., Sampson, J. J., and Friedman, M.: Role of pulmonary lymphatics in chronic pulmonary edema. Circ. Res. *11*:966, 1962.
101. Parker, F., and Hicken, P.: The relation between left atrial hypertension and lymphatic distention in lung biopsies. Thorax *15*:54, 1960.
102. Parker, F., and Weiss, S.: The nature and significance of the structural changes in the lungs in mitral stenosis. Am. J. Pathol. *12*:573, 1936.
103. Coalson, J. J., Jacques, W. E., Campbell, G. S., and Thompson, W. M.: Ultrastructure of the alveolar capillary membrane in congenital and acquired heart disease. Arch. Pathol. *83*:377, 1967.
104. Kay, J. M., and Edwards, F. R.: Ultrastructure of the alveolar capillary wall in mitral stenosis. J. Pathol. *111*:239, 1973.
105. Heath, D., and Edwards, J. E.: Histological changes in the lung in diseases associated with pulmonary venous hypertension. Br. J. Dis. Chest *53*:8, 1959.
106. Carabello, B. A., and Grossman, W.: Calculation of stenotic valve orifice area. *In* Grossman, W., and Baim, D. S. (eds.): Cardiac Catheterization, Angiography, and Intervention. 4th ed. Philadelphia, Lea and Febiger, 1991.
107. Braunwald, E., Braunwald, N. S., Ross, J., Jr., and Morrow, A. G.: Effects of mitral valve replacement on pulmonary vascular dynamics of patients with pulmonary hypertension. N. Engl. J. Med. *273*:509, 1965.
108. Dalen, J. E., Matloff, J. M., Evans, G. L., et al.: Early reduction of pulmonary vascular resistance after mitral valve replacement. N. Engl. J. Med. *277*:387, 1967.
109. McKay, R. G., Lock, J. E., Keane, J. F., et al.: Percutaneous mitral valvuloplasty in an adult patient with calcific rheumatic mitral stenosis. J. Am. Coll. Cardiol. *7*:1410, 1986.
110. Palacios, I. F., Lock, J. E., Keane, J. F., and Block, P. C.: Percutaneous transvenous balloon valvotomy in a patient with severe calcific mitral stenosis. J. Am. Coll. Cardiol. *7*:1416, 1986.
111. McKay, C. R., Kawanishi, D. T., and Rahimtoola, S. H.: Catheter balloon valvuloplasty of the mitral valve in adults using a double balloon technique: Early hemodynamic results. J.A.M.A. *257*:1753, 1987.
112. Lock, J. E., Khalilullah, M., Shrivastava, S., et al.: Percutaneous catheter commissurotomy in rheumatic mitral stenosis. N. Engl. J. Med. *313*:1515, 1985.
113. Inoue, K., Owaki, T., Nakamura, T., et al.: Clinical application of transvenous mitral commissurotomy by a new balloon catheter. J. Thorac. Cardiovasc. Surg. *87*:394, 1984.
114. Levine, M. J., Weinstein, J. S., Diver, D. J., et al.: Progressive improvement in pulmonary vascular resistance following percutaneous mitral valvuloplasty. Circulation *79*:1061, 1989.
115. Alexopoulos, D., Lazzam, C., Borrica, S., et al.: Isolated chronic mitral regurgitation with preserved systolic left ventricular function and severe pulmonary hypertension. J. Am. Coll. Cardiol. *14*:319, 1989.
116. Magidson, A.: Cor triatriatum. Severe pulmonary arterial hypertension and pulmonary venous hypertension in a child. Am. J. Cardiol. *9*:603, 1962.
117. Stoler, M. H., Anderson, N. M., and Stuard, I. D.: A case of pulmonary veno-occlusive disease in infancy. Arch. Pathol. Lab. Med. *106*:645, 1982.
118. Wagenvoort, C. A.: Pulmonary veno-occlusive disease: Entity or syndrome. Chest *69*:82, 1976.
119. Liebow, A. A., McAdam, A. J., Carrington, C. B., and Vigmonte, M.: Intrapulmonary veno-obstructive disease. Circulation *36*(Suppl. II):172, 1967.
120. Cromie, J. B.: Correlation of anatomic pulmonary emphysema and right ventricular hypertrophy. Am. Rev. Respir. Dis. *84*:657, 1961.
121. Hicken, P., Heath, D., and Brewer, D.: The relation between the weight of the right ventricle and the percentage of abnormal air space in the lung in emphysema. J. Pathol. Bacteriol. *92*:519, 1966.
122. Harvey, R. M., Ferrer, M. I., Richards, D. W., and Cournand, A.: Influence of chronic pulmonary disease on the heart and circulation. Am. J. Med. *10*:719, 1951.

123. Abraham, A. S., Cole, R. B., Green, I. D., et al.: Factors contributing to the reversible pulmonary hypertension in patients with acute respiratory failure studied by serial observation during recovery. Circ. Res. *24*:51, 1969.

124. Abraham, A. S., Cole, R. B., and Bishop, J.: Effects of prolonged oxygen administration on the pulmonary hypertension of patients with chronic bronchitis. Circ. Res. *23*:147, 1968.

125. Segel, N., and Bishop, J. M.: The circulation in patients with chronic bronchitis and emphysema at rest and during exercise with special reference to the influence of changes in blood viscosity and blood volumes on the pulmonary circulation. J. Clin. Invest. *45*:1555, 1966.

126. Horsfield, K., Segel, N., and Bishop, J. M.: The pulmonary circulation in chronic bronchitis at rest and during exercise breathing air and 80% oxygen. Clin. Sci. *34*:473, 1968.

127. Harvey, R. M., Ferrer, M. I., Richards, D. W., Jr., and Cournand, A.: Influence of chronic pulmonary disease on the heart and circulation. Am. J. Med. *10*:719, 1951.

128. Yu, P. N., Lovejoy, F. W., Joos, H. A., et al.: Studies of pulmonary hypertension. I. Pulmonary circulatory dynamics in patients with pulmonary emphysema at rest. J. Clin. Invest. *32*:130, 1953.

129. Kitchin, A. H., Lowther, C. P., and Matthews, M. B.: The effect of exercise and of breathing oxygen-enriched air on the pulmonary circulation in emphysema. Clin. Sci. *21*:93, 1961.

130. Wilson, R. H., Hoseth, W., and Dempsey, M. E.: The effects of breathing 99.6% oxygen on pulmonary vascular resistance and cardiac output in patients with pulmonary emphysema and chronic hypoxia. Ann. Intern. Med. *42*:629, 1955.

131. Aber, G. M., Harris, A. M., and Bishop, J. M.: The effect of acute changes in inspired oxygen concentration of cardiac, respiratory and renal function in patients with chronic obstructive airways disease. Clin. Sci. *26*:133, 1964.

132. Stuart-Harris, C., Bishop, J. M., Clark, T.J.H., et al.: Long-term domiciliary oxygen therapy in chronic hypoxic cor pulmonale complicating chronic bronchitis and emphysema. Lancet *1*:681, 1981.

133. Nocturnal Oxygen Therapy Trial Group: Continuous or nocturnal oxygen therapy in hypoxic chronic obstructive airways disease? Ann. Intern. Med. *93*:391, 1980.

134. Foreman, S., Weill, H., Duke, R., et al.: Bullous disease of the lung: Physiologic improvement after surgery. Ann. Intern. Med. *69*:757, 1968.

135. Salerni, R., Rodnan, G. P., Leon, D. F., and Shaver, J. A.: Pulmonary hypertension in the CREST syndrome variant of progressive systemic sclerosis (scleroderma). Ann. Intern. Med. *86*:394, 1977.

136. Follansbee, W. P., Curtiss, E. I., Medsger, T. A., et al.: Myocardial function and perfusion in the CREST syndrome variant of progressive systemic sclerosis. Am. J. Med. *77*:489, 1984.

136a. Morgan, J. M., Griffiths, M., du Bois, R. M., and Evans, T. W.: Hypoxic pulmonary vasoconstriction in systemic sclerosis and primary pulmonary hypertension. Chest *99*:551, 1991.

137. Seldin, D. W., Ziff, M., and DeGraff, A. V., Jr.: Raynaud's phenomenon associated with pulmonary hypertension. Tex. State J. Med. *58*:654, 1962.

138. Winters, W. L., Jr., Joseph, R. R., and Lerner, N.: "Primary" pulmonary hypertension and Raynaud's phenomenon. Arch. Intern. Med. *114*:821, 1964.

139. Caldwell, I. W., and Aitchison, J. D.: Pulmonary hypertension in dermatomyositis. Br. Heart J. *18*:273, 1956.

140. Walker, W. C., and Wright, V.: Pulmonary lesions and rheumatoid arthritis. Medicine *47*:501, 1968.

141. Santini, D., Fox, D., Kloner, R. A., et al.: Pulmonary hypertension in systemic lupus erythematosus: Hemodynamics and effects of vasodilator therapy. Clin. Cardiol. *3*:406, 1980.

142. Asherson, R. A., Mackworth-Young, C. G., Boey, M. L., et al.: Pulmonary hypertension in systemic lupus erythematosus. Br. Med. J. *287*:1024, 1983.

143. Muschenheim, C.: Some observations on the Hamman-Rich disease. Am. J. Med. Sci. *241*:279, 1961.

144. Soergel, K. H., and Sommers, S. C.: Idiopathic pulmonary hemosiderosis and related syndromes. Am. J. Med. *32*:499, 1962.

145. Manglo, A., Fisher, J., Libby, D. M., and Saddekni, S.: Sarcoidosis, pulmonary hypertension, and acquired peripheral pulmonary artery stenosis. Cathet. Cardiovasc. Diagn. *11*:69, 1985.

146. Kane, R. D., Hawkins, H. K., Miller, J. A., and Noce, P. S.: Microscopic pulmonary tumor emboli associated with dyspnea. Cancer *36*:1473, 1975.

147. Jacques, J. E., and Barclay, R.: The solid sarcomatous pulmonary artery. Br. J. Dis. Chest *11*:123, 1974.

148. Cooney, T. P., and Thurlbeck, W. M.: Pulmonary hypoplasia in Down's syndrome. N. Engl. J. Med. *307*:1170, 1982.

149. Wood, P.: The Eisenmenger syndrome, or pulmonary hypertension with reversed central shunt. Br. Med. J. *2*:755, 1958.

150. Yamaki, S., and Wagenvoort, C. A.: Comparison of primary plexogenic arteriopathy in adults and children. A morphometric study in 40 patients. Br. Heart J. *54*:428, 1985.

151. Haworth, S. G.: Pulmonary vascular disease in different types of congenital heart disease. Implications for interpretation of lung biopsy findings in early childhood. Br. Heart J. *52*:557, 1984.

152. Rabinovitch, M., Keane, J. F., Norwood, W. I., et al.: Vascular structure in lung tissue obtained at biopsy correlated with pulmonary hemodynamic findings after repair of congenital heart defects. Circulation *69*:655, 1984.

153. Davies, N.J.H., Shinebourne, E. A., Scallan, M. J., et al.: Pulmonary vascular resistance in children with congenital heart disease. Thorax *39*:895, 1984.

154. Takahashi, T., Wagenvoort, C. A.: Density of muscularized arteries in the lung. Arch. Pathol. Lab. Med. *107*:23, 1983.

155. Heath, D., and Edwards, J. E.: The pathology of hypertensive pulmonary vascular disease. A description of six grades of structural changes in the pulmonary arteries with special references to congenital cardiac septal defects. Circulation *18*:533, 1958.

156. Harley, R. A., Friedman, P. J., Saldana, M., et al.: Sequential development of lesions in experimental extreme pulmonary hypertension. Am. J. Pathol. *52*:52A, 1968.

157. Saldana, M. E., Harley, R. A., Liebow, A. A., and Carrington, C. B.: Extreme experimental pulmonary hypertension in relation to polycythemia. Am. J. Pathol. *52*:935, 1968.

158. Rabinovitch, M., Keane, J. F., Fellows, K. E., et al.: Quantitative analysis of the pulmonary wedge angiogram in congenital heart defects. Circulation *63*:152, 1981.

159. Fishman, A. P.: Unexplained pulmonary hypertension. Circulation *65*:651, 1982.

160. Senior, R. M., Britton, R. C., Turino, G. M., et al.: Pulmonary hypertension associated with cirrhosis of the liver and portacaval shunts. Circulation *37*:88, 1968.

161. Segel, N., Kay, J. M., Bayley, T. J., and Paton, A.: Pulmonary hypertension with hepatic cirrhosis. Br. Heart J. *30*:575, 1968.

162. Edwards, B. S., Weir, E. K., Edwards, W. D., et al.: Coexistent pulmonary and portal hypertension: Morphologic and clinical features. J. Am. Coll. Cardiol. *10*:1233, 1987.

163. Boot, H., Visser, F. C., Thijs, J. C., and Meuwissen, S.G.M.: Pulmonary hypertension complicating portal hypertension: A case report with suggestions for a different therapeutic approach. Eur. Heart. J. *8*:656, 1987.

163a. Robalino, B. D., and Moodie, D. S.: Association between primary pulmonary hypertension and portal hypertension: Analysis of its pathophysiology and clinical, laboratory and hemodynamic manifestations. J. Am. Coll. Cardiol. *17*:492, 1991.

164. Kay, J. M., Smith, P., and Heath, D.: Aminorex and the pulmonary circulation. Thorax *26*:262, 1971.

165. Fishman, A. P.: Dietary pulmonary hypertension. Circ. Res. *35*:657, 1974.

166. Levin, D. E., Heymann, M. A., Kitterman, J. A., et al.: Persistent pulmonary hypertension of the newborn infant. J. Pediatr. *89*:626, 1976.

167. Finn, M. C., Williams, L. C., and King, T. D.: Persistent fetal circulation in the newborn. J. La. State Med. Soc. *129*:169, 1977.

168. Haworth, S. G., and Reid, L.: Persistent fetal circulation: Newly recognized structural features. J. Pediatr. *88*:614, 1976.

169. Paraskos, J. A., Adelstein, S. J., Smith, R. E., et al.: Late prognosis of acute pulmonary embolism. N. Engl. J. Med. *289*:55, 1973.

170. Dalen, J. E., Banas, J. S., Jr., Brooks, H. L., and Dexter, L.: Resolution rate of acute pulmonary embolism in man. N. Engl. J. Med. *280*:1194, 1969.

171. Rich, S., Levitsky, S., and Brundage, B. H.: Pulmonary hypertension from chronic pulmonary thromboembolism. Ann. Intern. Med. *108*:425, 1988.

172. Shure, D., Gregoratos, G., and Moser, K. M.: Fiberoptic angioscopy: Role in diagnosis of chronic pulmonary arterial obstruction. Ann. Intern. Med. *103*:844, 1985.

173. Moser, K. M., Daily, P. O., Peterson, K., et al.: Thromboembolic pulmonary hypertension. Ann. Intern. Med. *107*:560, 1987.

174. Chitwood, W. R., Sabiston, D. C., and Wechsler, A. S.: Surgical treatment of chronic unresolved pulmonary embolism. Clin. Chest Med. *5*:507, 1984.

175. Voorburg, J.A.I., Cats, V. M., Buis, B., and Bruschke, A.V.G.: Balloon angioplasty in the treatment of pulmonary hypertension caused by pulmonary embolism. Chest *94*:1249, 1988.

176. Delaney, T. B., and Nadas, A. S.: Peripheral pulmonic stenosis. Am. J. Cardiol. *13*:451, 1964.

177. McCue, C. M., Robertson, L. W., Lester, R. G., and Mauck, H. P.: Pulmonary artery coarctations. J. Pediatr. *67*:222, 1965.

178. Pool, P. E., Vogel, J.H.K., and Blount, S. G., Jr.: Congenital unilateral absence of a pulmonary artery. Am. J. Cardiol. *10*:706, 1962.

179. Cohn, L. H., Sanders, J. H., Jr., and Collins, J. J., Jr.: Surgical treatment of congenital unilateral pulmonary arterial stenosis with contralateral pulmonary hypertension. Am. J. Cardiol. *38*:257, 1976.

180. Burwell, C. S., Robin, E. D., Whaley, R. D., and Bickelmann, A. G.: Extreme obesity associated with alveolar hypoventilation. Am. J. Med. *21*:811, 1956.

181. James, T. N., Frame, B., and Coates, E. D.: De subitaneis mortibus. III. Pickwickian syndrome. Circulation *48*:1311, 1973.

182. Noonan, A. J.: Reversible cor pulmonale due to hypertrophied tonsils and adenoids: Studies in two cases. Circulation *32*(Suppl. II):164, 1965.

183. Menashe, V. D., Farrchi, C., and Miller, M.: Hypoventilation and cor pulmonale due to chronic upper airway obstruction. J. Pediatr. *57*:198, 1965.

184. Naeye, R. L.: Alveolar hypoventilation and cor pulmonale secondary to damage to the respiratory center. Am. J. Cardiol. *8*:416, 1961.

185. Hultgren, H. N., Lopez, C. E., Lundberg, E., and Miller, H.: Physiologic studies of pulmonary edema at high altitude. Circulation *29*:393, 1964.

186. Hackett, P. H., Creagh, C. E., Grover, R. F., et al.: High altitude pulmonary edema in persons without the right pulmonary artery. N. Engl. J. Med. *302*:1070, 1980.

187. Staub, N. C.: Pulmonary edema—Hypoxia and overperfusion. N. Engl. J. Med. *302*:1085, 1980.

188. Saaluke, M. G., Shapiro, S. R., Perry, L. W., and Scott, L. P.: Isolated partial anomalous pulmonary venous drainage associated with pulmonary vascular obstructive disease. Am. J. Cardiol. *39*:439, 1977.
189. Heath, D., DuShane, J. W., Wood, E. H., and Edwards, J. E.: The etiology of pulmonary thrombosis in cyanotic congenital heart disease with pulmonary stenosis. Thorax *13*:213, 1958.
190. Durant, J. R., and Cortes, F. M.: Occlusive pulmonary vascular disease associated with hemoglobin SC disease. Am. Heart J. *71*:100, 1966.
191. Rowley, P. T., and Enlander, D.: Hemoglobin SC disease presenting as acute cor pulmonale. Am. Rev. Respir. Dis. *98*:494, 1968.
192. Houck, R. J., Bailey, G. L., Daroca, P. J., et al.: Pentazocine abuse: Report of a case with pulmonary arterial cellulose granulomas and pulmonary hypertension. Chest *77*:2, 1980.
193. Oliva, P. B., and Vogel, J.H.K.: Reactive pulmonary hypertension in alveolar proteinosis. Chest *58*:167, 1970.
194. Kawai, C., Ishikawa, K., Kato, M., et al.: Pulmonary pulseless disease: Pulmonary involvement in so-called Takayasu's disease. Chest *73*:651, 1978.
195. Lande, A., and Bard, R.: Takayasu's arteritis: An unrecognized cause of pulmonary hypertension. Angiography *27*:114, 1976.
196. Rose, A. G., Halper, J., and Factor, S. M.: Primary arteriopathy in Takayasu's disease. Arch. Pathol. Lab. Med. *108*:644, 1984.

PRIMARY PULMONARY HYPERTENSION

197. Rich, S., Dantzker, D. R., Ayres, S. M., et al.: Primary pulmonary hypertension. A national prospective study. Ann. Intern. Med. *107*:216, 1987.
198. Palevsky, H. I., Schloo, B. L., Pietra, G. G., et al.: Primary pulmonary hypertension. Vascular structure, morphometry and responsiveness to vasodilator agents. Circulation *80*:1207, 1989.
199. Newman, J. H., and Ross, J. C.: Primary pulmonary hypertension: A look at the future. J. Am. Coll. Cardiol. *14*:551, 1989.
200. Rich, S., and Brundage, B. H.: Pulmonary hypertension: A cellular basis for understanding the pathophysiology and treatment. J. Am. Coll. Cardiol. *14*:545, 1989.
201. Fuster, V., Steele, P. M., Edwards, W. D., et al.: Primary pulmonary hypertension: Natural history and the importance of thrombosis. Circulation *70*:580, 1984.
202. Pietra, G. G., Edwards, W. D., Kay, J. M., et al.: Histopathology of primary pulmonary hypertension. A qualitative and quantitative study of pulmonary blood vessels from 58 patients in the National Heart, Lung, and Blood Institute, Primary Pulmonary Hypertension Registry. Circulation *80*:1198, 1989.
203. Edwards, W. D., and Edwards, J. E.: Clinical primary pulmonary hypertension—three pathological types. Circulation *56*:884, 1977.
204. Harrison, C. V.: Experimental pulmonary arteriosclerosis. J. Pathol. Bacteriol. *60*:289, 1948.
205. Bernard, P. J.: Pulmonary arteriosclerosis and cor pulmonale due to recurrent-thromboembolism. Circulation *10*:343, 1954.
206. Inglesby, T. V., Singer, J. W., and Gordon, D. S.: Abnormal fibrinolysis in familal pulmonary hypertension. Am. J. Med. *55*:5, 1973.
207. Anderson, E. G., Simon, G., and Reid, L.: Primary and thrombo-embolic pulmonary hypertension: a quantitative pathological study. J. Pathol. *110*:273, 1973.
208. Stuard, I. D., Heusinkveld, R. S., and Moss, A. J.: Microangiopathic hemolytic anemia and thrombocytopenia in primary pulmonary hypertension. N. Engl. J. Med. *287*:869, 1972.
209. Franz, R. C., Ziady, F., Coetzee, W.J.C., and Hugo, N.: A possible causal relationship between defective fibrinolysis and pulmonary hypertension. S. Afr. Med. J. *55*:170, 1979.
210. Tubbs, R. R., Levin, R. D., Shirey, E. K., and Hoffman, G. C.: Fibrinolysis in familial pulmonary hypertension. Am. J. Clin. Pathol. *71*:384, 1979.
211. Naeye, R. L.: "Primary" pulmonary hypertension with coexisting portal hypertension. A retrospective study of six cases. Circulation *22*:376, 1960.
212. Segel, N., Kay, J. M., Bayley, T. J., and Paton, A.: Pulmonary hypertension with hepatic cirrhosis. Br. Heart J. *30*:575, 1968.
213. Senior, R. M., Britton, R. C., Turino, G. M., et al.: Pulmonary hypertension associated with cirrhosis of the liver and with portacaval shunts. Circulation *37*:88, 1968.
214. Barnard, P. J., and Davel, J.G.A.: Primary pulmonary vascular disease with cor pulmonale: Report of three cases in children, one with congenital hypertension and two siblings with allergic vasculitis and disorders of skeletal epiphyses. Am. J. Dis. Child. *92*:115, 1956.
215. Braunstein, H.: Periarteritis nodosa limited to the pulmonary circulation. Am. J. Pathol. *31*:837, 1955.
216. Gurtner, H. P., Gertsch, M., Salzmann, C., et al.: Häufen sich die primär vaskulären Forem des Cor Pulmonale? Schweiz. Med. Woenschr. *98*:1579, and 1695; 1968.
217. Gahl, von K., Fabel, H., Freiser, E., et al.: Primäre vaskuläre pulmonale Hypertonie. Z. Kreislaufforsch. *59*:868, 1970.
218. Gurtner, H. P.: Pulmonary hypertension, "plexogenic pulmonary arteriopathy" and the appetite depressant drug aminorex: Post or propter? Bull. Eur. Physiopathol. Resp. *15*:897, 1979.
219. Gertsch, M., and Stucki, P.: Weitgehend reversibele primär vaskuläre pulmonale Hypertonie bei einem Patienten mit Menocil-Einnahme. Z. Kreislaufforsch. *59*:902, 1970.
220. Meyrick, B., and Reid, L.: Development of pulmonary arterial changes in rats fed *Crotalaria spectabilis*. Am. J. Pathol. *94*:37, 1979.
221. Wagenvoort, C. A., Wagenvoort, N., and Dijk, H. J.: Effect of fulvine on pulmonary arteries and veins of the rat. Thorax *29*:522, 1974.
222. Guzowski, D. E., and Salgado, E. D.: Changes in the main pulmonary artery of rats with monocrotaline-induced pulmonary hypertension. Arch. Pathol. Lab. Med. *111*:741, 1987.
223. Olson, J. W., Hacker, A. D., Altiere, R. J., and Gillespie, M. N.: Polyamines and the development of monocrotaline-induced pulmonary hypertension. Am. J. Physiol. *247*:H682, 1984.
224. Hilliker, K. S., Bell, T. G., Lorimer, D., and Roth, R. A.: Effects of thrombocytopenia on monocrotaline pyrrole-induced pulmonary hypertension. Am. J. Physiol. *246*:H747, 1984.
225. Stuart, K. L., and Bras, G.: Veno-occlusive disease of the liver. Q. J. Med. *26*:291, 1957.
226. Kleiger, R. E., Boxer, M., Ingham, R. E., and Harrison, D. C.: Pulmonary hypertension in patients using oral contraceptives. A report of six cases. Chest *69*:143, 1976.
227. Daoud, F. S., Reeves, J. T., and Kelly, D. B.: Isoproterenol as a potential pulmonary vasodilator in primary pulmonary hypertension. Am. J. Cardiol. *42*:817, 1978.
228. Shepherd, J. T., Edwards, J. E., Burchell, H. B., et al.: Clinical, physiological and pathological considerations in patients with idiopathic pulmonary hypertension. Br. Heart J. *19*:70, 1957.
229. Marshall, R. J., Helmholz, H. F., and Shepherd, J. T.: Effect of acetylcholine on pulmonary vascular resistance in a patient with idiopathic pulmonary hypertension. Circulation *20*:391, 1959.
230. Samet, P. and Bernstein, W. H.: Loss of reactivity of the pulmonary vascular bed in primary pulmonary hypertension. Am. Heart J. *66*:197, 1963.
231. Robertson, B., Rosenhamer, G., and Lindberg, J.: Idiopathic pulmonary hypertension in two siblings. Acta Med. Scand. *186*:569, 1969.
232. Melmon, K. L., and Braunwald, E.: Familial pulmonary hypertension. N. Engl. J. Med. *269*:770, 1963.
233. Rogge, J. D., Mishkin, M. E., and Genovese, P. D.: The familial occurrence of primary pulmonary hypertension. Ann. Intern. Med. *65*:672, 1966.
234. Kingdon, H. S., Cohen, L. S., Roberts, W. C., and Braunwald, E.: Familial occurrence of primary pulmonary hypertension. Arch. Intern. Med. *118*:422, 1966.
235. Heath, D., Edwards, J. E.: Configuration of elastic tissue of pulmonary trunk in idiopathic pulmonary hypertension. Circulation *21*:59, 1960.
236. Meyrick, B., Clarke, S. W., Symons, C., et al.: Primary pulmonary hypertension—A case report including electron microscopic study. Br. J. Dis. Chest *68*:11, 1974.
237. Suarez, L. D., Sciandro, E. E., Llera, J. J., and Perosio, A. M.: Long-term followup in primary pulmonary hypertension. Br. Heart J. *41*:702, 1979.
238. Miller, V. M., Aarhus, L. L., and Vanhoutte, P. M.: Mediation of endothelium dependent responses by chronic alterations of blood flow. Am. J. Physiol. *251*:H520, 1986.
239. Morgan, K. G., DeFeo, T. T., Wenc, K., and Weinstein, R.: Alterations of excitation-contraction coupling by platelet-derived growth factor in enzymatically isolated and cultured vascular smooth muscle cells. Pfluegers Archiv. *405*:77, 1985.
240. Eysmann, S. B., Palevsky, H. I., Reichek, N., et al.: Two-dimension and Doppler-echocardiographic and cardiac catheterization correlates of survival in primary pulmonary hypertension. Circulation *80*:353, 1989.
241. Kanemoto, N., and Sasamoto, H.: Pulmonary hemodynamics in primary pulmonary hypertension. Jpn. Heart J. *20*:395, 1979.
242. Bourdillon, P.D.V., and Oakley, C. M.: Regression of primary pulmonary hypertension. Br. Heart J. *38*:264, 1976.
243. Ross, R. S.: Right ventricular hypertension as a cause of precordial pain. Am. Heart J. *61*:134, 1961.
244. Viar, W. N., and Harrison, T. R.: Chest pain in association with pulmonary hypertension; its similarity to the pain of coronary disease. Circulation *5*:1, 1952.
245. Wilmhurst, P. T., Webb-Peploe, M. M., and Corker, R. J.: Left recurrent laryngeal nerve palsy associated with primary pulmonary hypertension and recurrent pulmonary embolism. Br. Heart J. *49*:141, 1983.
246. Kanemoto, N.: Electrocardiographic and hemodynamic correlations in primary pulmonary hypertension. Angiology *39*:781, 1988.
247. Kanemoto, N., Furuya, H., Etoh, T., Sasamoto, H., and Matsuyama, S.: Chest roentgenograms in primary pulmonary hypertension. Chest *76*:45, 1979.
248. Anderson, G., Reid, L., and Simon, G.: The radiographic appearances in primary and in thromboembolic pulmonary hypertension. Clin. Radiol. *24*:113, 1973.
249. Kuriyama, K., Gamsu, G., Stern, R. G., et al.: CT-determined pulmonary artery diameters in predicting pulmonary hypertension. Invest. Radiol. *19*:16, 1984.
250. Goodman, D. J., Harrison, D. C., and Popp, R. L.: Echocardiographic features of primary pulmonary hypertension. Am. J. Cardiol. *33*:438, 1974.
251. Louie, E. K., Rich, S., and Brundage, B. H.: Doppler echocardiographic assessment of impaired left ventricular filling with right ventricular pressure overload due to primary pulmonary hypertension. J. Am. Coll. Cardiol. *8*:1298, 1986.
252. Child, J. S., Wolfe, J. D., Tashkin, D., and Nakano, F.: Fatal lung scan in a case of pulmonary hypertension due to obliterative pulmonary vascular disease. Chest *67*:308, 1975.
253. Benotti, J. R., and Grossman, W.: Pulmonary angiography. In Grossman, W., and Baim, D. S. (eds.): Cardiac Catheterization, Angiography and Intervention. 4th ed. Philadelphia, Lea and Febiger, 1991.
254. Oakley, C. M.: Management of primary pulmonary hypertension. Br. Heart J. *53*:1, 1985.

255. Packer, M.: Vasodilator therapy for primary pulmonary hypertension. Limitations and Hazards. Ann. Intern. Med. *103*:258, 1985.
256. Rich, S., and Brundage, B. H.: High-dose calcium channel-blocking therapy for primary pulmonary hypertension: Evidence of long-term reduction in pulmonary arterial pressure and regression of right ventricular hypertrophy. Circulation *76*:135, 1987.
257. Rubin, L. J., Nicod, P., Hillis, L. D., and Firth, B. G.: Treatment of primary pulmonary hypertension with nifedipine. A hemodynamic and scintigraphic evaluation. Ann. Intern. Med. *99*:433, 1983.
258. Fisher, J., Borer, J. S., Moses, J. W., et al.: Hemodynamic effects of nifedipine versus hydralazine in primary pulmonary hypertension. Am. J. Cardiol. *54*:646, 1984.
259. Ocken, S., Reinitz, E., and Strom, J.: Nifedipine treatment of pulmonary hypertension in a patient with systemic sclerosis. Arthritis Rheum. *86*:794, 1983.
260. Groves, B. M., Rubin, L. J., Frosolono, M. F., et al: A comparison of the acute hemodynamic effects of prostacyclin and hydralazine in primary pulmonary hypertension. Am. Heart J. *110*:1200, 1985.
261. Lunde, P., and Rasmussen, K.: Long-term beneficial effect of nifedipine in primary pulmonary hypertension. Am. Heart J. *108*:415, 1984.
262. Salto, D., Haraoka, S., Yoshida, H., et al: Primary pulmonary hypertension improved by long-term oral administration of nifedipine. Am. Heart J. *105*:1041, 1983.
263. Packer, M., Medine, N., and Yushak, M.: Adverse hemodynamic and clinical effects of calcium channel blockade in pulmonary hypertension secondary to obliterative pulmonary vascular disease. J. Am. Coll. Cardiol. *4*:890, 1984.
264. Packer, M., Medina, N., Yushak, M., and Wiener, I.: Detrimental effects of verapamil in patients with primary hypertension. Br. Heart J. *52*:106, 1984.
265. Malcic, I., and Richter, D.: Verapamil in primary pulmonary hypertension. Br. Heart J. *53*:345, 1985.
266. O'Brien, J. T., Hill, J. A., and Pepine, C. J.: Sustained benefit of verapamil in pulmonary hypertension with progressive systemic sclerosis. Am. Heart J. *109*:380, 1985.
267. Hoit, B., Gregoratos, G., and Shabetai, R.: Paradoxical pulmonary vasoconstriction induced by nitroglycerin in idiopathic pulmonary hypertension. J. Am. Coll. Cardiol. *6*:490, 1985.
268. Pearl, R. G., Rosenthal, M. H., Schroeder, J. S., and Ashton, J.P.A.: Acute hemodynamic effects of nitroglycerin in pulmonary hypertension. Ann. Intern. Med. *99*:9, 1983.
269. Niarchos, A. P., Whitman, H. H., Goldstein, J. E., and Laragh, J. H.: Hemodynamic effects of captopril in pulmonary hypertension of collagen vascular disease. Am. Heart J. *104*:834, 1982.
270. Rubin, L. J., and Peter, R. H.: Oral hydralazine therapy for primary pulmonary hypertension. N. Engl. J. Med. *302*:69, 1980.
271. Lupi-Herrera, E., Sandoval, J., Seoane, M., and Bialostozky, D.: The role of hydralazine therapy for pulmonary arterial hypertension of unknown cause. Circulation *65*:645, 1982.
272. Ruskin, J. N., and Hutter, A. M.: Primary pulmonary hypertension treated with oral phentolamine. Ann. Intern. Med. *90*:772, 1979.
273. Shettigar, U. R. Hultgren, H. N., Specter, M., et al.: Primary pulmonary hypertension: favorable effect of isoproterenol. N. Engl. J. Med. *295*:1414, 1978.
274. Rozkovec, A., Stradling, J. R., Shepherd, G., et al.: Prediction of favourable responses to long term vasodilator treatment of pulmonary hypertension by short-term administration of epoprostenol (prostacyclin) or nifedipine. Br. Heart J. *59*:696, 1988.
275. Wang, S.W.S., Pohl, J.E.F., Rowlands, D. J., and Wade, E. G.: Diazoxide in the treatment of primary pulmonary hypertension. Br. Heart J. *40*:572, 1978.
276. Klinke, W. P., and Gilbert, J.A.L.: Diazoxide in primary pulmonary hypertension. N. Engl. J. Med. *302*:91, 1980.
277. Buch, J., and Wennevold, A.: Hazards of diazoxide in pulmonary hypertension. Br. Heart J. *46*:401, 1981.
278. Nagasaka, Y., Akuisu, H., Lee, Y. S., et al.: Long-term favorable effects of oxygen administration on a patient with primary pulmonary hypertension. Chest *74*:299, 1978.
279. Lock, J. E., Olley, P. M., Coceani, P. M., et al.: Use of prostacyclin in persistent fetal circulation. Lancet *1*:1343, 1979.
280. DeFeyter, P. J., Kerkkamp, H.J.J., and deJong, J. P.: Sustained beneficial effect of nifedipine in primary pulmonary hypertension. Am. Heart J. *105*:333, 1983.
281. Melot, C., Naejie, R., Mols, P., et al.: Effects of nifedipine on ventilation/perfusion matching in primary pulmonary hypertension. Chest *83*:203, 1983.
282. Olivari, M. T., Cohn, J. N., Carlyle, P., and Levine, T. B.: Beneficial hemodynamic and exercise response to nifedipine in primary pulmonary hypertension. J. Am. Coll. Cardiol. *1*:735, 1983.
283. Lupi-Herrera, E., Bialostozky, D., and Sobrino, A.: The role of isoproterenol in pulmonary artery hypertension of unknown etiology (primary). Chest *79*:292, 1981.
284. Fyler, D. C.: Can vasodilators ameliorate pulmonary hypertension? J. Cardiovasc. Med. *8*:237, 1983.
285. Cohen, M. L., and Kronzon, I.: Adverse hemodynamic effects of phentolamine in primary pulmonary hypertension. Ann. Intern. Med. *95*:591, 1981.
286. Jamieson, S. W., Stinson, E. B., Oyer, P. E., et al.: Heart and lung transplantation for pulmonary hypertension. Am. J. Surg. *147*:740, 1984.
287. Dawkins, K. D., Jamieson, S. W., Hunt, S. A., et al.: Long-term results, hemodynamics, and complications after combined heart and lung transplantation. Circulation *71*:919, 1985.
288. Dawkins, K. D., Haverich, A., Derby, G. C., et al.: Long-term hemodynamics following combined heart and lung transplantation in primates. J. Thorac. Cardiovasc. Surg. *89*:55, 1985.
289. McCarthy, P. M., Starnes, V. A., Theodore, J., et al.: Improved survival after heart-lung transplantation. J. Thorac. Cardiovasc. Surg. *99*:54, 1990.
290. Shumway, N. E.: Current status of cardiac transplantation. Proceedings of the Annual Meeting of the New England Cardiovascular Society, Newton, MA, June 6, 1990.
291. Cohen, M., Edwards, W. D., and Fuster, V.: Regression in thromboembolic type of primary pulmonary hypertension during 2½ years of antithrombotic therapy. J. Am. Coll. Cardiol. *7*:172, 1986.

Systemic Hypertension: Mechanisms and Diagnosis

by NORMAN M. KAPLAN, M.D.

Definitions, Prevalence, and Consequences of Hypertension

Hypertension is the major risk factor for coronary, cerebral, and renal vascular diseases, which cause over half of all deaths in the United States. In the Framingham cohort, the risk of developing coronary disease rose progressively with increasing systolic or diastolic pressure, both in the middle-aged and the elderly[1] (Fig. 28–1). The number of persons identified as having hypertension continues to increase. On the basis of data from the 1976–1980 National Health and Examination Survey, the number of hypertensive persons in the United States in 1983 was estimated to be 57.7 million[2]—more than double the estimate made in 1960–1962. This rise reflects both the greater population at risk (including more elderly persons) and the use of a lower level of blood pressure as a criterion for diagnosis (i.e., 140/90 rather than 160/95 mm Hg). Lowering this criterion has been justified because of the increased risk for eventual cardiovascular disease associated with systolic blood pressure levels above 140 mm Hg and diastolic levels above 90.[3] However, because these numbers are based on only one set of readings, the number of persons whose blood pressure is persistently elevated may be overestimated by as much as one-third.[4]

The greater awareness of the dangers of elevated blood pressure along with the availability of safer and more effective antihypertensive agents has led to a therapeutic explosion. *In*

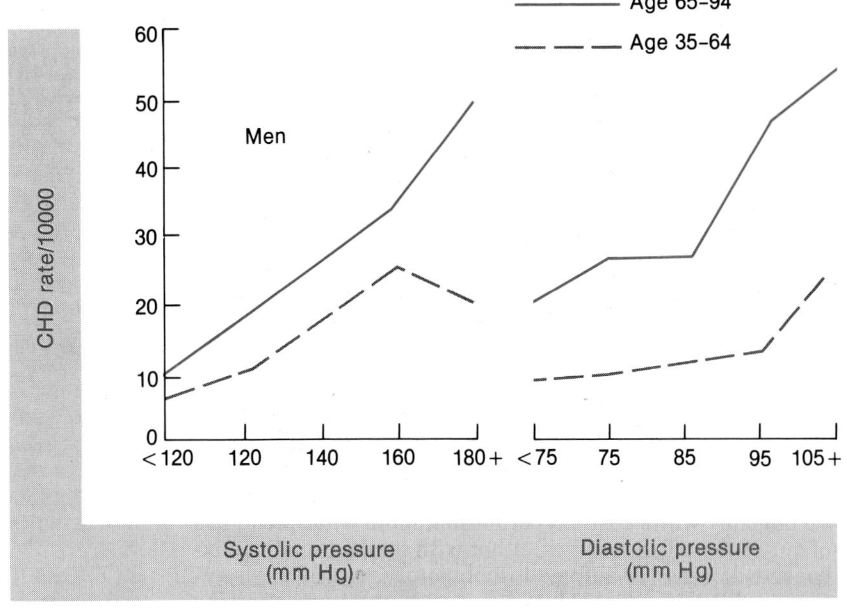

FIGURE 28–1. Biennial rate of coronary heart disease (CHD) according to blood pressure in Framingham men. (From Levy, D., Wilson, P. W. F., Anderson, K. M., and Castelli, W. P.: Stratifying the patient at risk from coronary disease: New insights from the Framingham Heart Study. Am. Heart J. *119:*712, 1990.)

TABLE 28–6 FEATURES OF "INAPPROPRIATE" HYPERTENSION

1. Onset before age 20 or after age 50
2. Level of blood pressure > 180/110 mm Hg
3. Organ damage
   a. Funduscopic findings of Grade 2 or higher
   b. Serum creatinine > 1.5 mg/100 ml
   c. Cardiomegaly (on x-ray) or left ventricular hypertrophy (on electrocardiogram)
4. Features indicative of secondary causes
   a. Unprovoked hypokalemia
   b. Abdominal bruit
   c. Variable pressures with tachycardia, sweating, tremor
   d. Family history of renal disease
5. Poor response to therapy that is usually effective

per cent greater *relative* risk of having a major coronary event over an 8.6-year period than did those with diastolic pressures below 80. However, this large increased *relative* risk translates to an *absolute* excess risk of only 3.5 men per 100 over the 8.6-year interval. Obviously the majority of those with even higher diastolic pressures did not suffer a major coronary event.

Nonetheless, because there are so many persons with hypertension, the fact that even a minority of them will suffer a premature cardiovascular event in the course of their disease makes hypertension a major societal problem. In fact, when the death rates for various levels of diastolic blood pressure are multiplied by the proportion of people in the population who have these various levels, the majority of excess deaths attributable to hypertension are found to occur among those with minimally elevated pressures.[38]

As the public and the medical profession have become aware of the overall societal consequences of even mild hypertension, enthusiasm for its early recognition and aggressive treatment has continued to mount. A closer look at the issue of deciding upon the need for therapy is provided in Chapter 29. However, further consideration of the natural course of hypertension, as it applies to the individual patient, is needed in order to answer a basic question: Are the blood pressure and the consequent risk high enough to justify medical intervention? Unless the risk is high enough to mandate some form of intervention, there seems to be no need to identify and label the person as hypertensive, since psychological and socioeconomic burdens accompany this label; unless risks clearly outweigh these burdens, caution is obviously advised. A cogent view of this issue has been offered by Rose:[39]

> As doctors we are trained to feel responsible for patients—that is, to care for the sick; and from that position accepting responsibility for those with major risk factors is not too difficult a transition. They are almost patients. A general practitioner, say, makes a routine measurement of a man's blood pressure and finds it raised. Thereafter both the man and the doctor will say that he 'suffers' from high blood pressure. He walked in a healthy man but he walks out a patient, and his newfound status is confirmed by the giving and receiving of tablets. An inappropriate label has been accepted because both public and professional felt that if the man were not a patient the doctor would have no business treating him. In reality the care of the symptomless hypertensive person is preventive medicine, not therapeutics.

Rose would certainly not deny the benefits of preventive medicine but goes on to emphasize the need for great caution is applying preventive measures to large groups of people:

> If a preventive measure exposes many people to a small risk, the harm it does may readily . . . outweigh the benefits, since these are received by relatively few. . . . We may thus be unable to identify that small level of harm to individuals from long-term intervention that would be sufficient to make that line of prevention unprofitable or even harmful. Consequently we cannot accept long-term mass preventive medication.

We are thus left with a dilemma: For hypertensive individuals as a group, even those with the least elevated pressures, risk is increased; for the individual hypertensive, the risk may not justify the labeling or treatment of the condition.

ASSESSMENT OF INDIVIDUAL RISK

Guidelines are available to help practitioners resolve this dilemma in dealing with the individual patient. These guidelines are based upon the overall assessment of cardiovascular risk and the biological aggressiveness of the hypertension. They are intended to apply only to those with *mild* hypertension, as defined in the Hypertension Detection and Follow-up Program as diastolic pressure between 90 and 104 mm Hg; those with diastolic levels persistently above 105 mm Hg have been shown to be at high enough risk from the hypertension per se to justify immediate intervention.

OVERALL CARDIOVASCULAR RISK. The Framingham Study and other epidemiological surveys have clearly defined certain risk factors for premature cardiovascular disease in addition to hypertension (see Ch. 37). For varying levels of blood pressure, the Framingham data (available in the Coronary and Stroke Risk Handbooks published by the American Heart Association) show the increasing likelihood of a vascular event over the next eight years for both men and women at various ages as more and more risk factors are added. For example, a 40-year-old man with a systolic blood pressure of 195 mm Hg who is otherwise at low risk would have a 4.6 per cent chance of a vascular event in the next eight years. A man of the same age with the same pressure but with all the additional risk factors (elevated serum cholesterol, cigarette smoking, glucose intolerance, and left ventricular hypertrophy on the electrocardiogram) has a 70.8 per cent chance. Obviously the higher the overall risk, the more intensive the interventions should be.

An interesting—and disturbing—connection between untreated hypertension and *hypercholesterolemia* has been noted in multiple populations.[40] This connection may be mediated through insulin resistance and hyperinsulinemia, anticipated in those with upper body obesity[41] but also found in nonobese hypertensives[42] (p. 828). Clearly, through this association, hypertensives are often burdened with an even greater risk than imposed by their blood pressure alone.

TARGET ORGAN DAMAGE. The biological aggressiveness of a given level of hypertension varies among individuals. This inherent propensity to induce vascular damage can be ascertained best by examination of the eyes, heart, and kidney.

Funduscopic Examination. As described by Keith et al. in 1939, vascular changes in the fundus reflect both hypertensive retinopathy and arteriosclerotic retinopathy.[43] The two processes first induce narrowing of the arteriolar lumen (Grade 1) and then sclerosis of the adventitia and/or thickening of the arteriolar wall, visible as arteriovenous nicking (Grade 2). Progressive hypertension induces rupture of small vessels, seen as hemorrhages and exudates (Grade 3) and eventually papilledema (Grade 4). Although the Grade 3 and 4 changes are clearly indicative of an accelerated-malignant form of hypertension, lesser changes have not been found to be of much prognostic value.[44]

Cardiac Involvement. Hypertension places increased tension on the left ventricular myocardium causing it to hypertrophy, and accelerates the development of atherosclerosis within the coronary vessels. The combination of increased demand and lessened supply increases the likelihood of myocardial ischemia, leading to higher incidences of myocardial infarction, sudden death, arrhythmias, and congestive failure in hypertensives (Fig. 28–1).

1. *Left ventricular hypertrophy (LVH).* Hypertrophy as a response to the increased afterload of an elevated systemic vascular resistance can be viewed as necessary and protective up to a certain point. Beyond that point, a variety of dysfunctions accompany LVH.

In the past, LVH was recognized by electrocardiography, based on increased voltage of QRS complexes, intrinsicoid deflection over leads V_5 or V_6 greater than 0.06 sec, and ST-segment depression greater than 0.5 mm (p. 125). Increasingly, echocardiography is being used (p. 70), because it is much more sensitive in recognizing early cardiac involvement. By echocardiography left ventricular mass is shown to progressively increase with increases in blood pressure[45,45a] (Fig. 28–5). LVH may be noted by echocardiography even before blood pressures become overtly abnormal in young offspring of hypertensive parents[46] and larger left ven-

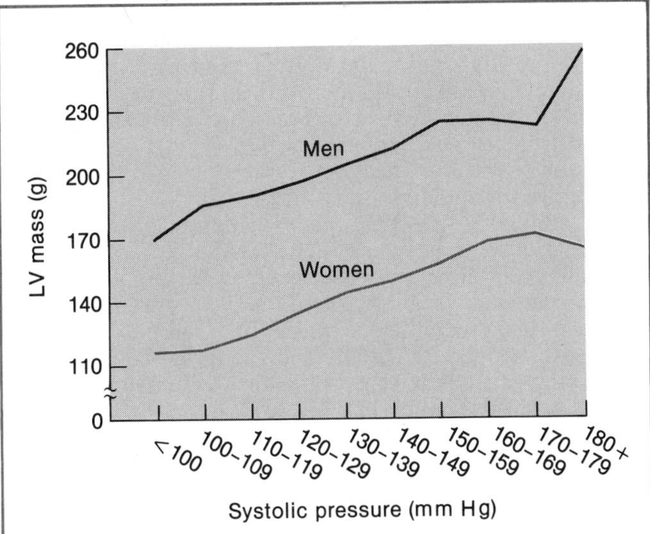

FIGURE 28–5. Mean left ventricular mass by sex and by systolic pressure, including participants taking antihypertensive medications, aged 17 to 90 years. Those data were obtained by M-mode echocardiograms taken on 2226 men and 2746 women in the Framingham Study, cohort examination 16 and offspring cycle 2, 1979 to 1983. (From Savage, D. D., Levy, D., Danneberg, A. L., et al.: Association of echocardiographic left ventricular mass with body size, blood pressure and physical activity [the Framingham Study]. Am. J. Cardiol. *65*:371, 1990.)

tricular mass by echocardiography may identify subjects at risk of developing hypertension.[47] Left ventricular mass is greater in those whose pressure does not fall during sleep, reflecting a more persistent pressure load.[48]

The pathogenesis of LVH involves a number of variables other than the pressure load. One of these is hemodynamic volume load, as measured by two-dimensional (2-D) echo-derived left ventricular end-diastolic volume.[49] Other determinants are obesity, levels of sympathetic nervous system and renin-angiotensin activity, and whole blood viscosity, presumably by way of its influence on peripheral resistance.[50] The correlation is much closer between LVH and pressures taken during the stresses of work by ambulatory monitoring than between LVH and casual pressures.[50] Moreover, left ventricular mass index was independently correlated with "job strain," as was diastolic blood pressure measured at the workplace.[51]

The basic signals that initiate and maintain myocardial hypertrophy probably include a number of growth factors whose effects may be transmitted via the alpha$_1$-adrenergic receptor to activate intracellular transducing proteins and ribonucleic acid (RNA) transcription factors.[52]

Different patterns of hypertrophy may evolve.[53] The pattern of LVH may have important prognostic implications.[53a] In a 10-year follow-up of 250 hypertensives, all-cause mortality was higher and cardiovascular events were most frequent in those with *concentric* LVH.[54] The degree of increased muscle mass is a strong and independent risk factor for cardiac mortality over and above the extent of coronary artery disease.[55] In addition, the risk of ventricular arrhythmias is increased at least twofold in the presence of LVH.[56]

Since the presence of LVH may connote a number of deleterious effects of hypertension on cardiac function, a great deal of effort has been expended in showing that treatment of hypertension will cause LVH to regress. Treatment with all antihypertensive drugs except those that further activate sympathetic nervous system activity, e.g., diuretics and direct vasodilators such as hydralazine when used alone, has been shown to cause LVH regression.[57] With regression, left ventricular function usually improves.[58]

2. *Abnormalities in left ventricular function.* Even before LVH and its attendant complications develop, changes in both systolic and diastolic function may be seen. Those with minimally increased left ventricular muscle mass may have supernormal contractility reflecting an increased inotropic state with a high percentage of fractional shortening and increased wall stress.[59] The earliest functional cardiac changes in hypertension are in left ventricular diastolic function with prolongation and incoordination of isovolumic relaxation, reduced rate of rapid filling, and increase in the relative amplitude of the *a* wave, probably caused by increased passive stiffness.

With increasing hemodynamic load, either systolic or diastolic dysfunction may evolve, progressing to different forms of congestive heart failure[60] (Fig. 28–6). The syndrome of severe concentric hypertrophy with a small ventricular cavity leading to dyspnea and pulmonary congestion has been most frequently reported in black hypertensive women.[61] In addition, impaired coronary flow reserve and thallium perfusion defects may be observed in hypertensives without obstructive coronary disease.[62]

3. *Features of coronary artery disease.* As detailed elsewhere (p. 1175), hypertension is a major risk factor for myocardial ischemia and infarction.[62a] Moreover, in the Framingham cohort, the prevalence of silent myocardial infarction was significantly increased in hypertensive subjects.[17] Hypertensive persons are thus at an increased risk for both the sustaining of myocardial infarction and the nonrecognition thereof. They are also more susceptible to silent ischemia[63] and sudden death.[17] Beyond these multiple additional risks associated with hypertension, a higher incidence of coronary events has been recognized when elevated diastolic blood pressures are reduced with either diuretic or beta-blocker–based therapies to levels below 85 to 90 mm Hg.[64] This J-shaped curve in the incidence of coronary disease probably reflects a reduction in perfusion pressure through coronary vessels either narrowed or having impaired vasodilatory reserve in the presence of an hypertrophied myocardium.

4. *Renal function.* Renal dysfunction, too subtle to be recognized, may be responsible for the development of most cases of essential hypertension. As discussed on p. 828, increased renal retention of salt and water may be a mechanism initiating primary hypertension, but the retention is so small that it escapes detection. With detailed study, both structural damage and functional derangements reflecting intraglomerular hypertension can be found in almost all hypertensive persons and even in some normotensive children of hypertensive parents.[65] In patients with longstanding hypertension, a loss of concentrating ability may be manifested by nocturia, decreased creatinine clearance, and albuminuria. As hypertension-induced nephrosclerosis proceeds, the plasma creatinine level begins to rise, and eventually renal insufficiency with uremia develops in 10 to 20 per cent of patients, making hy-

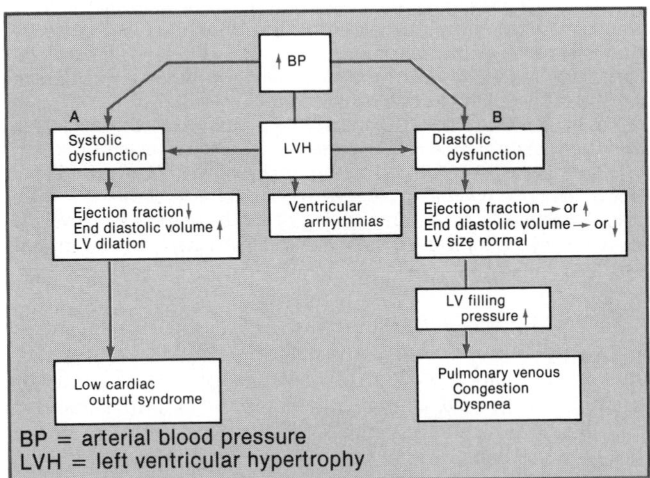

FIGURE 28–6. Consequences of systolic and diastolic dysfunction related to hypertension. *A*, Systolic dysfunction and congestive heart failure may occur late in the evolution of hypertensive heart disease, because of impaired ventricular contraction. *B*, Diastolic dysfunction is the most common manifestation of the effect of hypertension on cardiac function and also can lead to congestive heart failure due to increased filling pressures. LV = left ventricular. (From Shepherd, R. F. J., Zachariah, P. K., Shub, C.: Hypertension and left ventricular diastolic function. Mayo Clin. Proc. *64*:1521, 1989.)

pertension the leading cause for end-stage renal disease.[66] Prognosis is closely related to the degree of renal damage.[67]

5. *Cerebral involvement.* Hypertension, particularly systolic, is a major risk factor for stroke and for transient ischemic attacks caused by extracranial atherosclerosis.[68] As with the coronary circulation, the hemodynamic reserve in the cerebral circulation may be reduced, predisposing hypertensives to cerebral ischemia when blood pressure is lowered quickly and markedly.[69]

PLASMA RENIN ACTIVITY AS A PROGNOSTIC GUIDE. In 1972, Brunner et al. published data showing that a group of hypertensives with low levels of plasma renin activity (PRA) had a more benign course, with no heart attacks or strokes uncovered on retrospective analysis.[70] Subsequently, many investigators have examined the relationship between renin levels and cardiovascular complications and found that, with few exceptions,[71] patients with low PRA do *not* have a more benign course than do those with normal PRA.

On the basis of the aforementioned assessments of overall cardiovascular risk and severity of hypertension, it should be possible to determine the approximate risk status and prognosis for individual patients. This can most easily be accomplished with the Framingham data, as described on page 822.

SHORT-TERM COURSE OF LOW-RISK HYPERTENSION. Data on the four-year experiences of over 1600 "low-risk" hypertensives who served as controls in the Australian Therapeutic Trial document the validity of this assessment.[72] To enter this placebo-versus-drug trial, the patients had to be free of all identifiable cardiovascular disease, with the second set of diastolic pressures between 95 and 109 mm Hg. Thus, they could be considered "low-risk" hypertensives. Over the next four years, in the majority of these patients, who were given placebo tablets but neither nondrug nor drug therapy, blood pressures *dropped progressively,* from an average of 157/102 to 144/91 mm Hg. Diastolic pressure was below 95 mm Hg in 47.5 per cent at the end of the trial. The fall in blood pressure was not related to any recognizable change in the patients' status; similar decreases occurred independent of changes in or stability of body weight. Of great interest was the lack of excess morbidity or mortality among those whose diastolic pressures remained below 100 mm Hg.

These results support strongly the view that certain patients can be characterized as being at relatively low risk and can therefore safely do without drug therapy long enough for the clinician to monitor both their blood pressure levels over time and the effectiveness of nondrug measures, if indicated. The large number of patients whose pressures fell and the high average degree of fall may seem surprising, but none of these patients started with any identifiable cardiovascular disease or complications due to hypertension. Moreover, placebo may be more effective than no therapy.

Similar results were observed in the even larger Medical Research Council (MRC) trial in England, in which over 18,000 patients with pretreatment diastolic pressures between 95 and 109 mm Hg were randomly assigned to antihypertensive drugs or placebo.[73] At the end of five years, these pressures had dropped to below 90 mm Hg in 43 per cent of the men and 50 per cent of the women on placebo.

THE POTENTIAL FOR PROGRESSION. Although these data reflect the benign nature of "low-risk" hypertension over the short term, it should be noted that the diastolic blood pressure rose above 110 mm Hg in 12 per cent of the nondrug-treated patients in both the Australian and English trials. Therefore, continued monitoring of the blood pressure levels is obviously needed for all patients with even the mildest "low-risk" hypertension.

A SYNTHESIS OF RISK. In the MRC trial, older age, male sex, hypercholesterolemia, and cigarette smoking, along with the level of systolic blood pressure at entry, were related significantly to the subsequent development of cardiovascular complications.[73] Although the ability to discriminate between those who did and did not suffer a coronary or cerebrovascular event in this five-year trial was not precise, the degree of risk from hypertension can be categorized with reasonable accuracy, taking into account (1) the level of blood pressure; (2) the biological nature of the hypertension, based on target organ function; and (3) the coexistence of other risks. Although risk is increased for the hypertensive population as a whole, problems are more likely in those with higher levels of pressure (diastolic above 100 mm Hg), considerable target organ damage (retinopathy, cardiomegaly, renal damage), and other risk factors (hypercholesterolemia, cigarette smoking, diabetes). For them, immediate and effective reduction of pressure appears to be indicated. But for the majority, who are at relatively low risk, the more reasonable approach would be to continue to monitor the blood pressure while encouraging healthful habits, such as weight control, moderate sodium restriction, isotonic exercise, and relaxation, in hopes of slowing progression of the disease (Ch. 29).

This approach, involving the screening of *all* adults and identification of *all* persons with elevated blood pressure, has been shown to have cost-effectiveness comparable to other cardiovascular interventions[74] (p. 1694). Because there is no certain way to predict the course of the blood pressure, even hypertensives who are not treated should be followed, and recognition of their hypertension should motivate them to follow good health habits. In this way, no harm should be done and the potential benefit may be considerable if progression of the disease can be slowed by nondrug methods.

COMPLICATIONS OF HYPERTENSION

The higher the level of blood pressure, the more likely that various cardiovascular diseases will develop prematurely through acceleration of atherosclerosis, the pathological hallmark of uncontrolled hypertension. If untreated, about 50 per cent of hypertensive patients die of coronary heart disease or congestive failure, about 33 per cent of stroke, and 10 to 15 per cent of renal failure. Those with rapidly accelerating hypertension die more frequently of renal failure, as do those who are diabetic, once proteinuria or other evidence of nephropathy develops.[75] It is easy to underestimate the role of hypertension in producing the underlying vascular damage that leads to these cardiovascular catastrophes. Death is usually attributed to stroke or myocardial infarction instead of to the hypertension that was largely responsible. Moreover, hypertension may not persist after a myocardial infarction or stroke.

In general, the vascular complications of hypertension can be considered as either "hypertensive" or "atherosclerotic" (Table 28–7). The former are more directly caused by the increased blood pressure per se and can be prevented by lowering this level; the latter have more multiple causations (Ch. 37). Although hypertension may represent the most significant of the known risk factors of atherosclerosis in quantitative terms, lowering blood pressure may not by itself halt the atherosclerotic process.

The path from hypertension to vascular disease likely involves three interrelated processes: *pulsatile flow, endothelial cell dysfunction,* and *smooth muscle cell hypertrophy.* Higher systolic pressures are probably more responsible for these changes than are lower diastolic levels, providing an explanation for the closer approximation of cardiovascular risk to systolic pressure.

PULSATILE FLOW. The role of pulsatile flow has been summarized by O'Rourke as follows:[76]

TABLE 28–7 VASCULAR COMPLICATIONS OF HYPERTENSION

HYPERTENSIVE	ATHEROSCLEROTIC
Accelerated-malignant phase	Coronary heart disease
Hemorrhagic stroke	Sudden death
Congestive heart failure	Other arrhythmias
Nephrosclerosis	Atherothrombotic stroke
Aortic dissection	Peripheral vascular disease

Adapted from Smith, W. M.: Treatment of mild hypertension. Results of a ten-year intervention trial. Circ. Res. 25(Suppl. I):98, 1977, by permission of the American Heart Association, Inc.

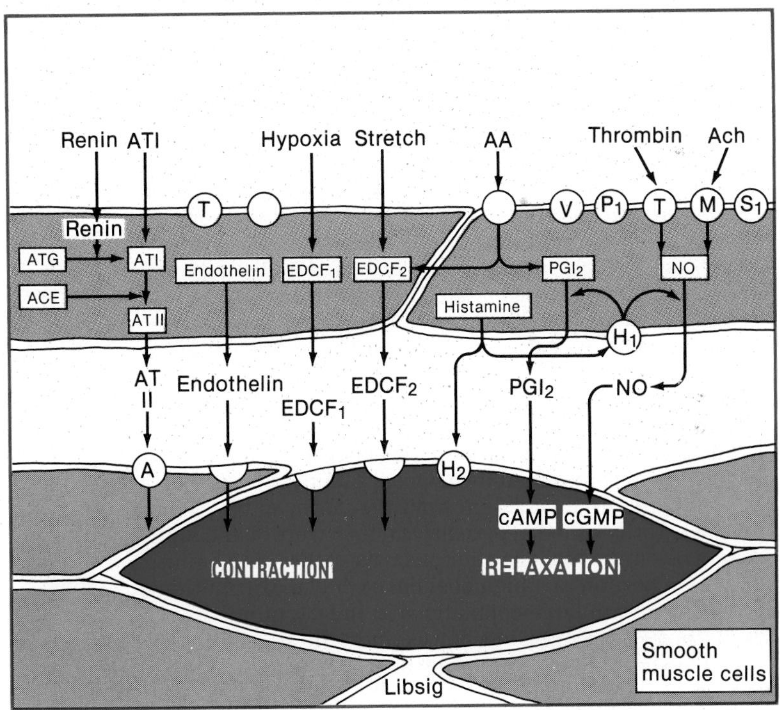

FIGURE 28–7. Endothelium-derived vasoactive substances. AA = arachidonic acid; ACE = angiotensin converting enzyme; ATG = angiotensinogen; ACh = acetylcholine; ATI/II = angiotensin I/II; cAMP/cGMP = cyclic adenosine/guanosine monophosphate; EDCF = endothelium-derived constricting factor(s); NO = nitric oxide; PGI_2 = prostacyclin. (From Lüscher, T. F., Yang, Z., Diederich D., and Bühle, F. R.: Endothelium-derived vasoactive substances: Potential role in hypertension, atherosclerosis, and vascular occlusion. J. Cardiovasc. Pharmacol. *14*(Suppl. 6):S63, 1989.)

Changes in the arterial pressure wave appear to have a deleterious effect on the arteries themselves and predispose to their further degeneration. There is a higher peak pressure, a higher pulse pressure, and a higher rate of change of pressure. All these factors might be expected, on the basis of principles of material fatigue, to lead inextricably on to fatigue and fracture of elastic fibers, and thence to dilation, thinning, and ultimately rupture of the arterial wall.

ENDOTHELIAL CELL DYSFUNCTION. The endothelial cell is probably both a victim of and an active participant in the vascular damage that is caused by hypertension. Rather than serving as the simple lining of a passive conduit, endothelial cells are now known to be the source of multiple relaxing and constricting substances, most having a paracrine influence on the underlying smooth muscle cells[77] (Fig. 28–7). Of these, two that appear to be particularly active are the endothelium-derived relaxing factor (EDRF) now characterized as nitric oxide or its precursor,[78] and the endothelins, which are long-acting vasoconstrictors.[79] They and other endothelium-derived substances may play a major role in both the causation of hypertension and the development of vascular damage. Their production may be altered by lipoproteins,[80] thereby providing another link between hyperlipidemia, hypertension, and arterial dysfunction.[81]

SMOOTH MUSCLE HYPERTROPHY. The third mechanism for vascular damage is an extension of what will be described as an apparent primary mechanism for the induction and persistence of hypertension, vascular smooth muscle cell hypertrophy (see p. 827). While hyperplasia of these cells is more typical of atherosclerosis, the two processes are almost certainly intertwined.[82]

Taken together, these three interrelated processes are probably responsible for the arteriolar and arterial sclerosis that is the usual consequence of longstanding hypertension leading to the target organ damages described earlier in this chapter as the features to be included in overall assessment of hypertension risks. Beyond the damage to eyes, heart, brain, and kidney, the large vessels such as the aorta may be directly affected, leading to aneurysms and dissection.[83]

RISK OF HYPERTENSION IN SPECIAL GROUPS

BLACKS. Although on the average blood pressure in blacks is not higher than that in whites during adolescence,[26] adult blacks have hypertension more frequently, producing higher rates of morbidity and mortality. In particular, they suffer more renal damage, leading to a significantly greater prevalence of end-stage disease requiring chronic dialysis.[84] Hypertension in blacks has been characterized as having a relatively greater component of fluid volume excess, including a higher prevalence of low plasma renin activity and a greater responsiveness to diuretic therapy.[85] These and other features suggestive of volume excess may reflect larger degrees of one or more of the abnormalities in sodium transport across cell membranes that are described on p. 828.[86]

Perhaps blacks evolved the physiological machinery that would offer protection in their ancestral habitat, i.e., hot, arid climates in which avid sodium conservation was necessary for survival because the diet was relatively low in sodium.[87] When they migrate to areas where sodium intake is excessive, they are then more susceptible to "sodium overload." In addition to susceptibility to exposure to excess sodium, it has been theorized that blacks may also be more susceptible to hypertension because they tend to ingest less potassium.[88]

WOMEN. In general, women suffer less cardiovascular morbidity and mortality than men for any degree of hypertension (Fig. 28–1). Moreover, before menopause, hypertension is less common in women than in men (Fig. 28–3). Perhaps the lower frequency and severity of hypertension reflect the lower blood volume afforded women by their monthly menses.

Mechanisms of Primary (Essential) Hypertension

No single or specific cause is known for most hypertension, referred to as *primary* in preference to *essential*. Since persistent hypertension can develop only in response to an increase in cardiac output or a rise in peripheral resistance, defects may be present in one or more of the multiple factors that affect these two forces (Fig. 28–8). The interplay of various derangements in factors affecting cardiac output and peripheral resistance may precipitate the disease, and these may differ in both type and degree in different patients. Looking for a single defect in all patients with essential hypertension may be a mistake.[89]

The search for such defects to unravel the pathogenesis of primary hypertension may be misguided for another reason —it may not be a *distinct* disease caused by *specific* abnormalities. Pickering advocated the concept that hypertension was only a quantitative deviation from the norm, so that people were arbitrarily called *hypertensive* if they were on the higher portion of a unimodal distribution curve rather than being on a separate portion of a biomodal curve.[90] The distribution of blood pressure in large populations is, in fact, unimodal (Fig. 28–2), but such curves do not exclude the possibility that those who become hypertensive have certain qualitative differences.

HEMODYNAMIC PATTERNS

Before presenting a specific hypothesis that includes such qualitative differences in the various factors shown in Figure 28–8 to affect the basic quation BP = CO × PR, the hemodynamic patterns that have been measured in patients with hypertension may be considered. One cautionary factor should be kept in mind: The pathogenesis of the disease is probably a slow and gradual process. By the time blood pressure becomes elevated, the initiating factors may no longer be apparent, since they may have been "normalized" by the compensatory interactions already alluded to. Nonetheless, when a group of untreated young hypertensive patients was initially studied, cardiac output was normal or slightly increased and peripheral resistance was normal.[91] Over the next 20 years, cardiac output fell progressively while peripheral resistance rose. Although this pattern may be common, it may not occur invariably. In a few patients a high-output state may persist.[92]

Regardless of how hypertension begins, the eventual primacy of increased resistance can be shown even in models of hypertension that feature an initial increase in fluid volume and cardiac output.[93] For example, patients with primary aldosteronism whose disease was completely controlled with the aldosterone antagonist spironolactone were followed after this drug was discontinued and the syndrome was allowed to recur in its natural manner.[94] Initially, plasma volume was expanded; however, it returned toward normal as peripheral resistance rose progressively.

GENETIC PREDISPOSITION

As seen in Figure 28–8, genetic alterations may initiate the cascade to permanent hypertension. Clearly, heredity plays a role, although no discriminatory gene markers are currently available.[95] In studies of twins and family members in which the degree of familial aggregation of blood pressure levels is compared with the closeness of genetic sharing, the genetic contributions have been estimated to range from 30 to 60 per cent.[96] Unquestionably, environment plays some role: the significant correlation between blood pressures of spouses has no other recognizable explanation.[97] Moreover, the considerable regional variations in blood pressure in British men were strongly influenced by where they had lived for most of their adult lives rather than by where they were born and brought up, suggesting greater roles for factors acting in adult life than for those acting early in life such as genetic inheritance and intrauterine environment.[98]

Although the debate concerning the roles of heredity and environment may be largely academic, it could have important practical implications. First, children and siblings of hypertensives should be more carefully screened. Second, they should be vigorously advised to avoid environmental factors known to aggravate hypertension and increase cardiovascular risk (e.g., smoking, inactivity, and sodium).

THE INHERITED DEFECT. If heredity does indeed play a role, what is inherited? A number of possibilities have been suggested, including a heightened sympathetic nervous response to stress,[95a] a defect in renal excretion of sodium, and a defect in the transport of sodium across cell membranes.[96]

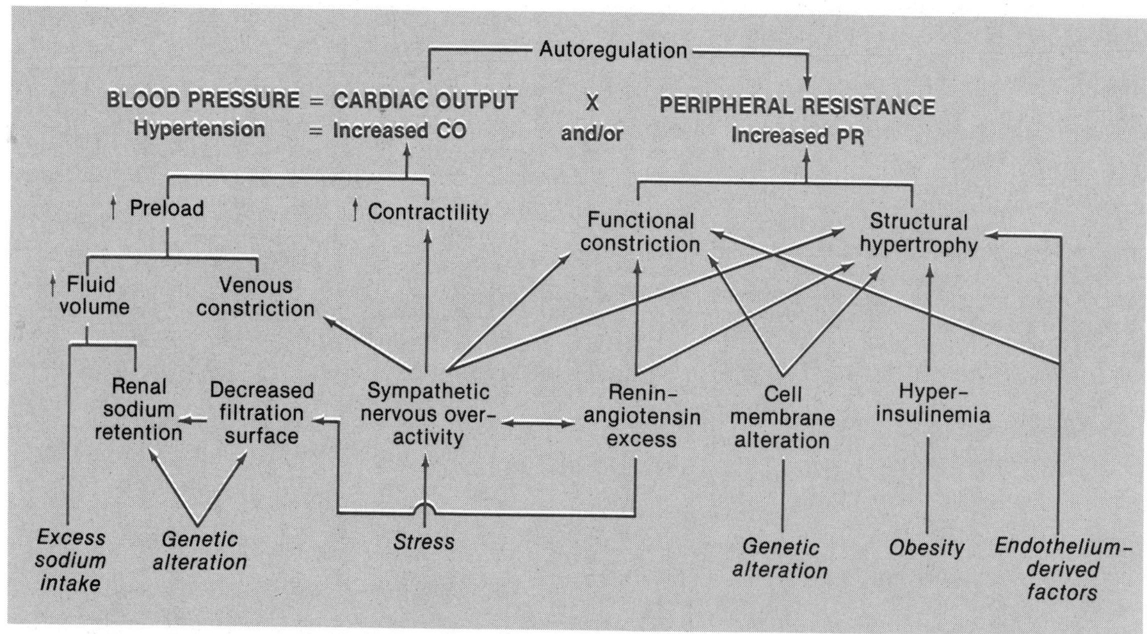

FIGURE 28–8. Some of the factors involved in the control of blood pressure that affect the basic equation: Blood pressure = cardiac output × peripheral resistance. Cellular hyperplasia may be seen along with hypertrophy. (From Kaplan, N. M.: Clinical Hypertension, 5th ed. Baltimore, © by Williams and Wilkins, 1990, p. 57.)

These may be interrelated: When two groups of normotensive young men underwent an hour of mental stress, nine of the 13 whose parents were hypertensive (the high-risk group) showed a fall in sodium excretion, whereas sodium excretion rose slightly among those with normotensive parents (the low-risk group).[99] The fall in sodium excretion was greater in those whose heart rate increased during the mental stress (the high reactors), suggesting a common pathway of the genetic influence on renal sodium excretion through the sympathetic nerves.

VASCULAR HYPERTROPHY

With the knowledge that an increased peripheral resistance is both necessary and sufficient to perpetuate hypertension even if it starts with an increased cardiac output, we will focus on those factors known to increase this resistance (Fig. 28–8). Although functional constriction of vascular smooth muscle is portrayed as a possible mechanism, it appears that the high peripheral resistance in hypertension is mainly determined by structural hypertrophy which, in turn, gives rise to a generalized increase in contractility of vascular smooth muscle. Small resistance vessels from subcutaneous tissue from untreated hypertensive subjects had on average a 29 per cent increase in the ratio of media thickness to lumen diameter compared with vessels from normotensive persons.[100] The in vitro responses of these vessels to various pressor agents were either unchanged or depressed, indicating that the increased contractility induced by pressor agents in vivo is caused by the increased muscle mass.

On the other hand, similar studies by the same investigators on resistance vessels from young normotensive offspring of hypertensive parents found no morphological changes but rather an increased sensitivity to norepinephrine, suggesting an alteration in sympathetic nervous activity before hypertension is established.[101] Such data from human subjects support the hypothesis proposed by Folkow[102] of a "positive-feedback interaction" wherein even mild functional pressor influences, if repeatedly exerted, may lead to structural hypertrophy which, in turn, reinforces and perpetuates the elevated pressure. Lever[103] has added two hypotheses to Folkow's first: A reinforcement of the hypertropic response to stimuli that initially raise the pressure, e.g., defects in the vascular cell membrane, and the action of various trophic mechanisms that may cause vascular hypertrophy directly and that Lever refers to as the "slow pressor mechanism."

The simple scheme shown by Lever contains, then, both a fast pressor mechanism and a slow hypertrophic effect, which can be induced by a number of pressor-growth promoters.[104] Lever uses renovascular hypertension as one model in which hypertension is initiated by a fast-acting pressor (angiotensin II) and maintained by the trophic action of the hormone to induce vascular hypertrophy. The evidence for the model derives, first, from the fact that the direct, immediate pressor actions of angiotensin II are less than the degree of chronic hypertension that occurs with equal concentrations of the hormone, suggesting an additional contribution of a "slow mechanism." Second, lower concentrations of angiotensin II are needed to maintain hypertension than to initiate it. Third, angiotensin II is a known growth stimulant for vascular smooth muscle.

Whereas the immediate pressor effect is mediated by increased free intracellular calcium, the slowly developing vascular hypertrophy is postulated to involve phosphatidylinositol metabolism in the cell membrane[105] (Fig. 28–9). The binding of angiotensin II to its receptor activates the enzyme phospholipase C, which hydrolyzes the membrane phosphatidylinositol 4,5-biphosphate (PIP_2) and releases inositol triphosphate (IP_3) into the cytosol and diacylglycerol (DG) in the plane of the membrane. The cytosolic IP_3 mobilizes calcium from its intracellular stores and causes an immediate contraction. The DG in the membrane activates protein kinase C which increases the activity of an amiloride-sensitive Na^+/H^+

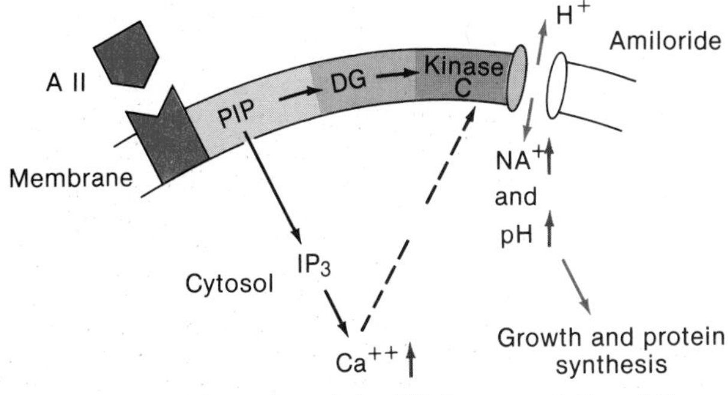

FIGURE 28–9. Schematic and simplified representation of the main events in a signalling system activated by growth factors. For example, angiotensin II (AII) occupies a membrane receptor; phosphatidylinositol bisphosphate (PIP) is hydrolyzed by phosphodiesterase in the membrane releasing inositol triphosphate (IP_3) into the cytosol and diacygly-cerol (DG) in the plane of the membrane. The latter activates kinase C linked to an amiloride-sensitive Na^+/H^+ exchanger whose activity increases. Sodium enters the cell down an electrochemical gradient and protons are extruded. The increased cell alkalinity which results is believed to promote growth and protein synthesis. (From Lever, A. F.: Slow pressor mechanisms in hypertension: A role for hypertrophy of resistance vessels? J. Hypertens. 4:515, 1986.)

exchanger. Thereby, sodium enters the cell down an electrochemical gradient and protons are extruded so that the cell becomes more alkaline. Increased cell alkalinity is believed to initiate DNA synthesis and thereby promote cell hypertrophy.

This scheme to explain the immediate pressor action and the slow hypertrophic effect of angiotensin II is thought to be common to the action of pressor-growth promoters.[106] When present in high concentrations over long periods, as with angiotensin II in renal artery stenosis, each of these pressor-growth promoters causes hypertension. Moreover, when the source of the excess pressor-growth promoter is removed, hypertension may recede slowly, presumably reflecting the time needed to reverse vascular hypertrophy.

No marked excess of any known pressor hormones is identi-

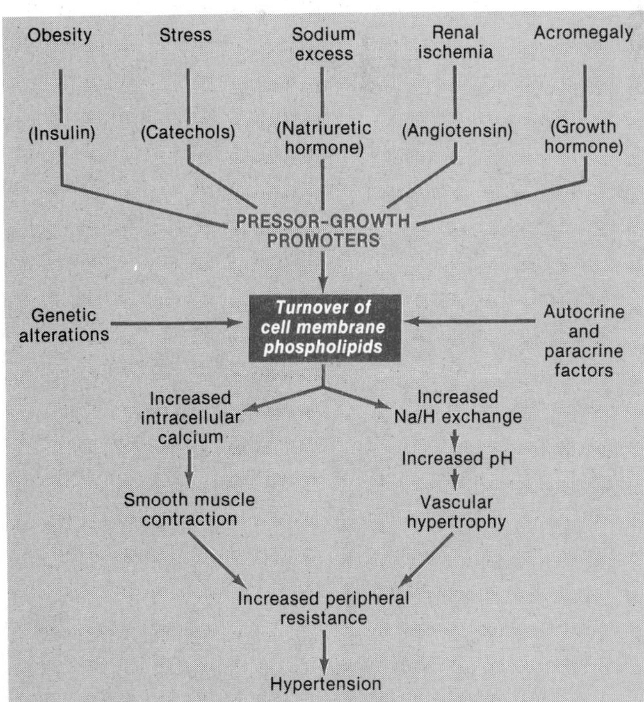

FIGURE 28–10. Scheme for the induction of hypertension by numerous pressor hormones that act as vascular growth promoters. (From Kaplan, N. M.: Clinical Hypertension, 5th ed. Baltimore, © by Williams and Wilkins, 1990, p. 93.)

fiable in the majority of hypertensive patients. Nonetheless, a lesser excess of one or more may have been responsible for initiation of a process sustained by the positive feedback postulated by Folkow[102] and the trophic effects emphasized by Lever.[103] This sequence encompasses a variety of specific initiating mechanisms that accentuate and maintain the hypertension by a nonspecific feedback-trophic mechanism (Fig. 28–10). If this double process is fundamental to the pathogenesis of primary hypertension, the difficulty in recognizing the initiating causal factor is easily explained. As formulated by Lever (103):

> The primary cause of hypertension will be most apparent in the early stages; in the later stages, the cause will be concealed by an increasing contribution from hypertrophy. . . . A particular form of hypertension may wrongly be judged to have "no known cause" because each mechanism considered is insufficiently abnormal by itself to have produced the hypertension. The cause of essential hypertension may have been considered already but rejected for this reason.

HYPERINSULINEMIA

A large number of circulating hormones and locally acting substances, some shown in Figure 28–7, may be involved. It is theorized that one hormone that is a prime candidate for a major role is insulin. This belief comes in part from the knowledge that hypertension is more common in the obese and that hyperinsulinemia is a hallmark of obesity. The associations are most striking in people with upper body obesity,[41] who have the highest prevalence of hypertension and the most pronounced hyperinsulinemia.[107]

The high levels of insulin in subjects with upper body obesity arise both from increased secretion of insulin, common to all forms of obesity, and from decreased hepatic removal and degradation of insulin, which appear to be related to the high rate of lipolysis of intra-abdominal fat.[108,109] (Fig. 28–11). The excessive quantity of free fatty acids coming from this fat are believed to be responsible for both the hyperinsulinemia and the hypertriglyceridemia and low HDL-cholesterol levels common in upper body obesity.[110]

Insulin is a potent trophic hormone, and insulin receptors are present on endothelial and arterial smooth muscle cells.[111] Insulin activates the amiloride-sensitive Na^+/H^+ exchanger[112] noted earlier to be the putative switch for protein synthesis and hypertrophy. In addition to its trophic action, insulin can raise the blood pressure by at least two other mechanisms: increase in circulating catecholamines[113] and stimulation of renal sodium reabsorption.[114]

The presence of hyperinsulinemia in obesity and its potential causal role in the hypertension of upper body obesity is rather obvious (Fig. 28–11). Less obvious but of even greater possible importance is the fact that hyperinsulinemia is also common in *nonobese* patients with primary hypertension.[115] Their hyperinsulinemia is attributable to peripheral insulin resistance,[115,116] but the reason for this resistance is unknown. It could reflect a simple inability of insulin to reach the skeletal muscle cells wherein its major peripheral actions on glucose metabolism occur.[117,118] Another possible explanation for the peripheral insulin resistance and resultant hyperinsulinemia in hypertension is a genetic or acquired increase in the proportion of type IIB muscle fibers, fibers that are fast twitch, glycolytic, and less sensitive to the action of insulin.[119] Marked interindividual variations in the proportion of these fibers are seen in normal persons,[120] and hypertensives have been found to have a greater proportion of fast-twitch fibers.[121] Moreover, the proportion of type IIB fibers is reduced after extensive isotonic exercise,[122] which is known to improve insulin sensitivity while it lowers blood pressure.

Regardless of how it occurs, insulin resistance with resultant hyperinsulinemia is likely to be a pressor-growth promotor involved in the pathogenesis of primary hypertension, both in the obese and the nonobese.

In addition to the overall pathogenetic mechanism shown in Figure 28–10, at least two other hypotheses that do not involve the entire scheme shown in Figure 28–10 continue to receive experimental support. The first involves defects in the transport of sodium across and the binding of calcium to cell membranes. The second implicates disturbances in the renin-angiotensin system.

DEFECTS IN CELL TRANSPORT OR BINDING

Considerable circumstantial evidence supports a causal role for sodium in the genesis of hypertension (Table 28–8). This evidence includes an increase in intracellular sodium in hypertensive animals and people, an increase that extends even to the normotensive children of hypertensive parents.[123] In addition, the higher intracellular sodium concentration has been linked to an increase in intracellular calcium in cells from hypertensives.[124] De Wardener and coworkers proposed that an increased fluid volume stimulates the secretion of a digitalis-like natriuretic hormone, presumably of hypothalamic origin, that inhibits the Na^+, K^+-ATPase pump.[125] Inhibition of the sodium pump would increase renal sodium excretion and restore vascular volume while at the same time

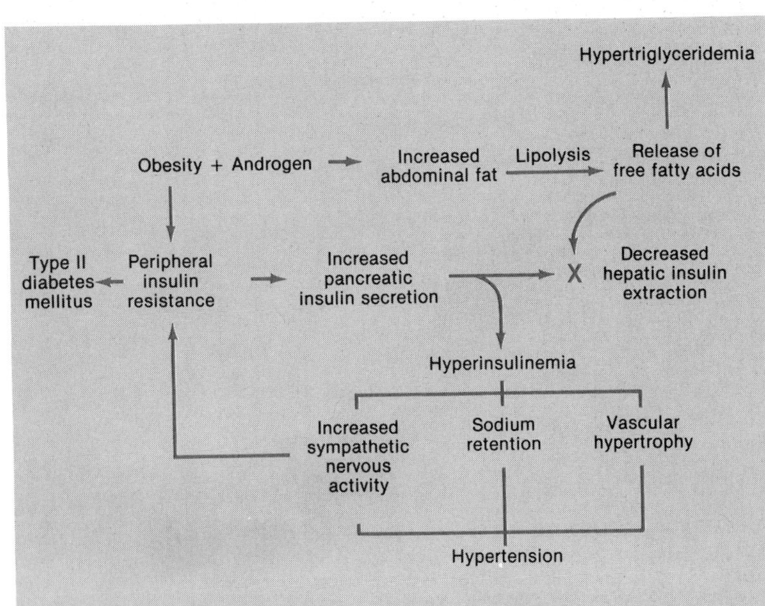

FIGURE 28–11. An overall scheme for the mechanism by which upper-body obesity could promote glucose intolerance, hypertriglyceridemia, and hypertension via hyperinsulinemia. (From Kaplan, N. M.: The deadly quartet: Upper body obesity, glucose intolerance, hypertriglyceridemia and hypertension. Arch. Intern. Med. 149:1514, 1989. Copyright 1989, American Medical Association.)

TABLE 28-8 EVIDENCE FOR A ROLE OF SODIUM IN PRIMARY (ESSENTIAL) HYPERTENSION

1. **In multiple populations, the rise in blood pressure with age is directly correlated with increasing levels of sodium intake.**
2. **Multiple, scattered groups who consume little sodium (less than 50 mmol/day) have little or no hypertension. When they consume more sodium, hypertension appears.**
3. **Animals given sodium loads, if genetically predisposed, develop hypertension.**
4. **Some people, when given large sodium loads over short periods, develop an increase in vascular resistance and blood pressure.**
5. **An increased concentration of sodium is present in the vascular tissue and blood cells of most hypertensives.**
6. **Sodium restriction, to a level of 60 to 90 mmol per day will lower blood pressure in most people. The antihypertensive action of diuretics requires an initial natriuresis.**

leading to hypertension by increasing intracellular sodium content (Fig. 28–12). A major problem with this hypothesis has been the difficulty in isolating the putative digitalis-like hormone, but this may have been overcome.[126]

While the search for the putative pressor natriuretic hormone has been widely pursued, a natriuretic hormone from the cardiac atria has been identified and widely studied. Atrial natriuretic peptide (ANP) is vasodilatory[127] and appears to be involved in the normal regulation of body fluid volume[128] (p. 1858). ANP appears to be involved in the pressure-natriuresis that occurs with acute volume expansion[129]; however, its concentration may be *decreased* in patients with established hypertension.[130] If present and persistent, such a deficiency could be responsible for the initial reduced renal sodium excretion and hypervolemia (Fig. 28–12).

Beyond the postulated role of a hypothalamic inhibitor of the sodium pump, the transport of sodium may be altered directly, for example by an inherited defect in the structure of the cell membrane. An increased activity of the Na^+/H^+ antiporter[131] could be involved in the amplification of the capacity of various stimuli to produce vascular smooth muscle cell contraction and hypertrophy (Fig. 28–10). Moreover, the activity of the Na^+/H^+ antiporter was found to be increased in fibroblasts of normotensive blacks compared with those from normotensive whites, which could help explain the higher prevalence of hypertension in blacks.[132]

Third, a primary defect in calcium binding to the inner aspect of the cell membrane could increase the free cytosolic calcium concentration.[133] At this time, a number of ion transport defects have been identified and a great deal of speculation offered as to their role in the pathogenesis of hypertension. We are left intrigued but uncertain.[134] Since transport mechanisms may be affected by vasoactive substances such as endothelin,[135] it is likely that these transport mechanisms may play an intermediate role, helping translate systemic influences into cellular actions.

THE RENIN-ANGIOTENSIN SYSTEM

Both as a direct pressor and as a growth promoter, the renin-angiotensin mechanism may also be involved in the pathogenesis of hypertension. All functions of renin are mediated through the synthesis of angiotensin II. This system is the primary stimulus for the secretion of aldosterone and hence mediates the mineralocorticoid responses to varying sodium intakes and volume loads. When sodium intake is reduced or effective plasma volume shrinks, the increase in renin-angiotensin II stimulates aldosterone secretion, and this, in turn, is responsible for a portion of the enhanced renal retention of sodium and water (Fig. 28–13).

In addition to this primary role in the preservation of normal fluid volume, the renin-angiotensin system participates in the control of the blood pressure under circumstances of sodium depletion or volume contraction. When fluid volume is normal, blockade of the renin-angiotensin system does little to the blood pressure, but during volume contraction the increased levels of renin-angiotensin play an important role in maintaining the integrity of the circulation.

As will be described, hypertension may develop either in the face of renin levels that are suppressed by an adrenal adenoma that causes mineralocorticoid excess or when renin levels are elevated from a kidney made ischemic by renovascular stenosis. The fact that renin levels may be either low or high in patients with primary hypertension (Fig. 28–14) has led some to believe that an excess of mineralocorticoid activity on the one hand or a more subtle, diffuse intrarenal ischemia on the other may be involved in the pathogenesis of primary hypertension.

LOW-RENIN HYPERTENSION. Excess mineralocorticoid

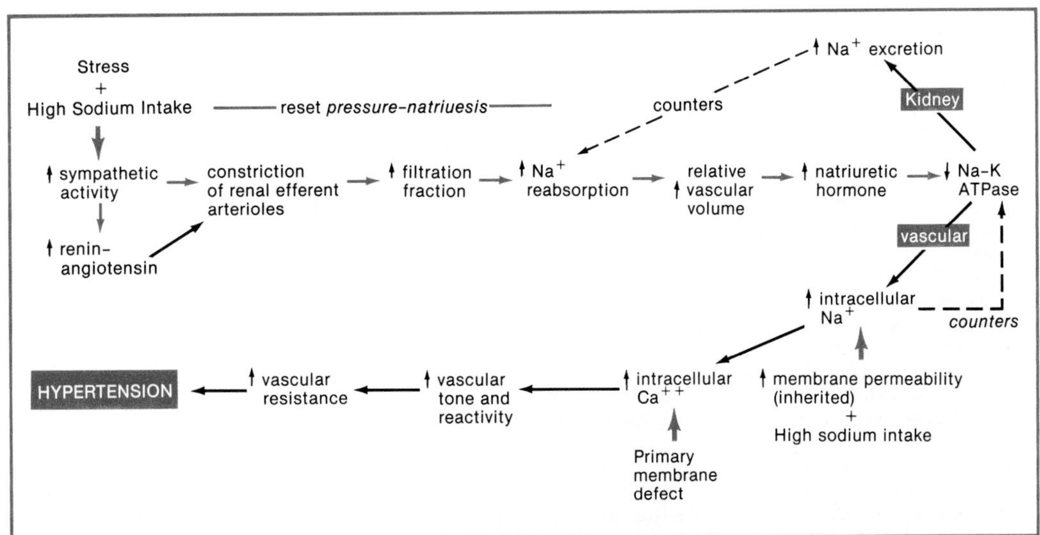

FIGURE 28–12. Hypothesis for the pathogenesis of primary (essential) hypertension, starting from three points, shown as heavy arrows. One, starting, on the top left, is the combination of stress and high sodium intake, which induces an increase in natriuretic hormone and thereby inhibits sodium transport. The second, starting at the bottom right, invokes an inherited defect in sodium transport plus a high sodium intake to induce an increase in intracellular sodium. The third invokes a primary defect in the binding of calcium to cell membranes.

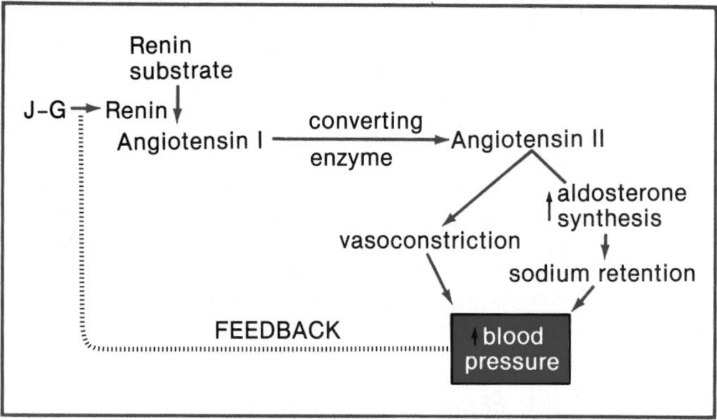

FIGURE 28-13. Overall scheme of the renin-angiotensin mechanism.

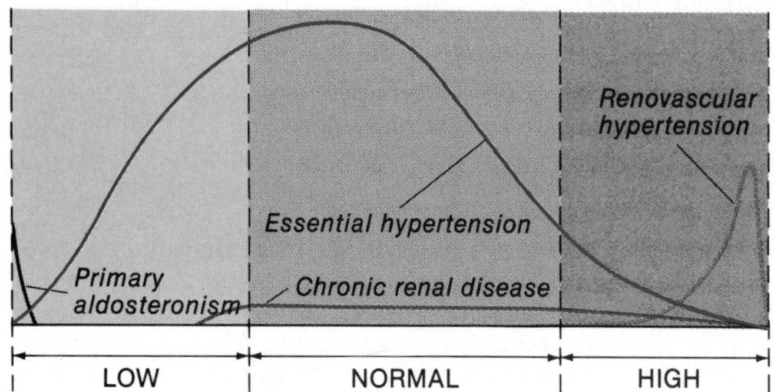

FIGURE 28-14. Schematic representation of plasma renin activity in various hypertensive diseases. The expected number of patients with each type of hypertension is indicated along with their proportion of low, normal, or high renin levels. (From Kaplan, N. M.: Renin profiles: The unfulfilled promises. J.A.M.A. *238:*611, 1977. Copyright 1977, American Medical Association.)

suppresses renin secretion via the negative feedback seen in Figure 28-13 by causing volume expansion and an elevated blood pressure. Therefore, an excess level of mineralocorticoid has been sought among the 30 per cent of hypertensive patients with low or suppressed levels of plasma renin activity. Although elevated levels of deoxycorticosterone and 19-nor-deoxycorticosterone have been reported, no such elevations were found in a systematic, prospective study of 46 low-renin hypertensives.[136]

While the still-fruitless search for increased levels of mineralocorticoid has proceeded, a syndrome of *apparent mineralocorticoid excess* with hypertension and hypokalemia but extremely low aldosterone levels has been identified.[137] Although these patients exhibited flagrant evidences of mineralocorticoid excess, more subtle forms may be more widely recognized in the future and could explain some cases of low-renin hypertension. The abnormality is caused by a deficiency of the 11-beta-hydroxysteroid dehydrogenase (11β-OHSD) responsible for conversion of cortisol to cortisone in the kidney. Cortisol is capable of acting as a mineralocorticoid by interacting with mineralocorticoid receptors; however, in the normal state, the conversion of cortisol to cortisone by 11β-OHSD prevents this from happening. In the absence of 11β-OHSD, cortisol exerts a profound mineralocorticoid effect. Of further interest, the mineralocorticoid action of licorice has been shown to result from its inhibition of 11β-OHSD.[138] Licorice is added to some brands of chewing tobacco as a flavoring agent in quantities sufficient to induce hypertension.[139]

The absence of significant volume expansion and hypokalemia argue further against a role of mineralocorticoid excess in the pathogenesis of ordinary low-renin hypertension. Subjects with low renin hypertension, in fact, may have a more normal renin mechanism than patients with higher renin levels, since an elevated blood pressure should diminish renin release by interaction with renal baroreceptors. Therefore, it is likely that the separation of a segment of hypertensives into a low renin category is largely artifactual. Renin levels in essential hypertension follow a continuum with a skewing toward low levels likely because a disproportionate number of hypertensives are elderly and black, two groups whose renin levels tend to be low whether or not they are hypertensive. The renin levels in both groups are lower probably because they have fewer functioning renal juxtaglomerular cells—in the elderly because of the progressive loss of functioning nephrons with age and in blacks as a consequence of nephrosclerosis.

A more direct causal relation between a reduced number of functioning glomeruli and low-renin hypertension has been postulated by Brenner and colleagues.[140] They propose that "a major renal abnormality that initiates essential hypertension is a decreased filtration surface area (FSA), due to a reduced number of nephrons and/or a decrease in FSA per glomerulus. Just as alterations in renal hemodynamics, reduced ability to excrete sodium, and raised blood pressure characterize the adaptive response to an acquired decrease in the number of functioning nephrons, inborn deficiencies may enhance susceptibility to essential hypertension. As schematized (in Fig. 28-15), this hypothesis suggests that a decrease in FSA may contribute to renal sodium retention, and thus to systemic (low-renin) hypertension. Systemic hypertension then leads to glomerular capillary hypertension and eventual glomerular sclerosis, which in turn further decreases FSA, perpetuating a vicious circle."[140]

The scheme shown in Figure 28-15 could explain the presence of low renin levels and the vicious circle of increasing loss of renal function once the process begins, as in diabetic nephropathy. Whether an inborn deficiency is responsible for most low-renin hypertension is uncertain. Those relatively rare low renin hypertensive states in which volume expansion, usually mediated by mineralocorticoid excess, is known to be responsible are considered in subsequent portions of this chapter.

NORMAL AND HIGH RENIN HYPERTENSION. As previously noted, renin levels should be suppressed in the presence of hypertension, assuming that the high systemic pressure reaches the juxtaglomerular cells. Therefore, the presence of normal renin levels may be inappropriate and may play a role in sustaining the hypertension. Even more ominous is the presence of higher than usual levels of plasma renin activity in 10 to 20 per cent of those with essential hypertension (Fig. 28-14).

A number of explanations have been offered for these "inappropriately normal" or high levels, beyond the proportion expected in a normal gaussian distribution curve. One of the more attractive is the concept of "nephron heterogeneity" described by Sealey et al.,[141] which assumes a mixture of ischemic nephrons, caused by afferent arteriolar narrowing, and normal nephrons in patients with essential hypertension. Excess renin from the ischemic nephrons could raise the total blood renin level to varying degrees and cause some persons to have normal or high renin hypertension.

This hypothesis is similar to that proposed by Goldblatt, who believed that "the primary cause of essential hypertension in man is intrarenal obliterative vascular disease, from any cause, usually arterial and arteriolar sclerosis, or any other condition which brings about the same disturbance of intrarenal hemodynamics".[142] When Goldblatt placed the clamp on the main renal arteries in canine studies, he was trying to explain the pathogenesis of primary (essential) hypertension rather than what he ended up explaining: the pathogenesis of renovascular hypertension. Nonetheless, his experimental concept is the basis for the more modern model of Sealey et al. The elevated renin from the ischemic population of

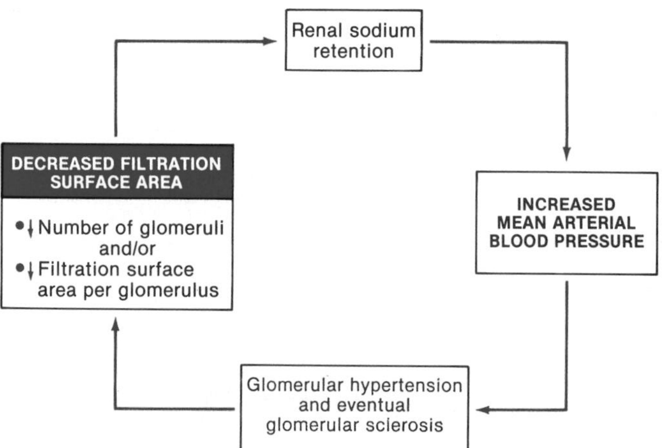

FIGURE 28-15. Relationship between decreased filtration surface area (FSA) and mean arterial pressure. Decreased FSA, due to decreased nephron number and/or FSA per glomerulus, leads to renal sodium retention, and thereby to increased mean arterial pressure. Systemic hypertension in turn promotes glomerular hypertension and eventual sclerosis further decreasing the functioning filtration surface area. (From Brenner, B. M., Garcia, D. L., and Anderson, S.: Glomeruli and blood pressure: Less of one, more the other? Am. J. Hypertens. 1:335, 1988.)

nephrons, although diluted in the systemic circulation, provides the "normal" renin levels that are usual in patients with primary hypertension in whom would otherwise be expected to shut down renin secretion and in whom levels would be low. These diluted levels are still high enough to impair sodium excretion in the nonischemic hyperfiltering nephrons but are too low to support efferent tone in the ischemic nephrons, thereby reducing sodium excretion in them as well.

Sealey and associates' concept of nephron heterogeneity differs from Brenner and associates' concept of nephron scarcity. Nevertheless Sealey et al. agree that "a reduction in nephron number related to either age or ischemia could amplify the impaired sodium excretion and promote hypertension."[141]

In further support of their hypothesis, Sealey et al. invoke the findings of Hollenberg and Williams in hypertensive patients with normal renin levels[143] in this manner: "These investigators have classified patients with essential hypertension as either nonmodulators or modulators according to their renal hemodynamic responses to saline and angiotensin II infusions. Nonmodulators have impaired plasma renin suppression, renal blood flow, and natriuresis during saline infusion. The latter responses are corrected by converting enzyme inhibition therapy, suggesting that inappropriate renin secretion, perhaps from an ischemic subpopulation of nephrons, is an important contributing factor in these patients. In contrast, the modulator group of hypertensive patients responds to saline infusion with an exaggerated natriuresis, and converting enzyme inhibition does not alter the associated renal hemodynamic responses."[141]

These nonmodulating hypertensives are sodium-sensitive, and the two groups probably overlap considerably. Although "inappropriate renin secretion from an ischemic subpopulation of nephrons" as suggested by Sealey et al. could be involved in the pathogenesis of the nonmodulating normal renin hypertensive state, Williams and Hollenberg offer this explanation: "These patients have an abnormality related to locally produced AII or the AII receptor which prevents them from changing their target tissue responsiveness to exogenous AII when sodium intake is modified, thus reducing their ability to excrete a sodium load. Paradoxically, converting enzyme inhibitors, which theoretically should be ineffective in these patients, are more effective than they are in the nonsalt-sensitive subgroups. Finally, preliminary data strongly suggest that the nonmodulating trait is inherited."

The renin-angiotensin system is probably active in multiple individual organs, probably from in situ synthesis of various components rather than by transport from renal J-G cells through the circulation. The complete system has been found, among other places, in endothelial cells,[144] the brain,[145] and adrenal cortex,[146] broadening the potential roles of this mechanism far beyond its previously accepted boundaries. Moreover, the role of prorenin, which comprises 90 per cent of the circulating plasma renin activity, remains totally unknown.[147]

OTHER MECHANISMS OF HYPERTENSION

Along with insulin, angiotensin, and natriuretic hormone, catecholamines arising in response to stress are shown in Figure 28–10 to be pressor-growth promoters. Increased sympathetic nervous activity could raise blood pressure in a number of ways—either alone or in concert with stimulation of renin release by catecholamines—by causing arteriolar and venous constriction, by increasing cardiac output, or by altering the normal renal pressure-volume relationship. In addition to cardiac stimulation by sympathetic activity, vagal inhibitory responses to baroreceptor and other stimuli may also be important. In humans with denervated transplanted hearts, both pulse and blood pressures fail to display the usual nocturnal fall, and hypertension is frequent.[148] The transient increase in epinephrine during stress reactions may invoke a more prolonged pressor response by facilitating the release of norepinephrine from sympathetic neurons.[149]

Although other hormones that have pressor actions are known, their possible role in human primary hypertension remains unknown. These include vasopressin[150] and serotonin.[151] Similarly, a number of vasodepressor hormones are known but their function, too, remains uncertain. These include kallikrein[152] and medullipin, a renomedullary lipid.[153]

The foregoing does not exhaust the list of suggested mechanisms underlying primary hypertension. Excesses of various minerals, particularly lead,[154] and changing ratios among dietary sodium, potassium, calcium, and magnesium have also been postulated.[155] Support for these and other postulated mechanisms is meager, and the overall schemes involving intracellular sodium and calcium and the pressor-growth promotor mechanisms for vascular hypertrophy seem more than adequate to explain the pathogenesis of primary hypertension. However, a number of associations between hypertension and other conditions have been noted and may offer additional insights into the potential causes and possible prevention of the disease. For example, when associations among 35 anthropometric, biochemical, and life style characteristics and nine different blood pressure measurements in 618 adults were examined by multiple regression analysis, certain correlations were found to be significant: body size and psychological stress were associated with higher systolic blood pressure, while obesity, smoking, ethanol consumption, and plasma sodium were associated with diastolic blood pressure.[156] Urine sodium and potassium excretion could not be correlated with any blood pressure measure. Although such correlations do not prove causality, they do suggest that those features associated with hypertension may be involved in its pathogenesis.

ASSOCIATION OF HYPERTENSION WITH OTHER CONDITIONS

OBESITY. Hypertension is more common among obese individuals and probably adds to their increased risk of developing ischemic heart disease. In the Framingham offspring study, adiposity, as measured by subscapular skinfold thickness, was the major controllable contributor to hypertension.[157] This finding corroborates the critical importance of the *distribution* of body fat, since blood pressure as well as blood lipids and glucose levels tend to be highest in those with central or upper body obesity.[107] As noted previously, these may all be interconnected via insulin resistance and hyperinsulinemia (Fig. 28–11). Children seem particularly vulnerable to the hypertensive effects of weight gain.[26] Therefore, avoidance of childhood obesity with the hope of avoiding subsequent hypertension seems important. The evidence that weight reduction will lower established hypertension is discussed on p. 856.

SLEEP APNEA. One of the contributors to the hypertension in obese people is sleep apnea. Snoring and sleep apnea are clearly associated with hypertension, and this, in turn, may be induced by increased sympathetic activity in response to hypoxemia during apnea.[158]

PHYSICAL INACTIVITY. Physical fitness may help prevent hypertension, and persons who are already hypertensive may lower their blood pressure by means of regular isotonic exercise.[159] Preventing hypertension may be one of the ways that exercise seems to protect against the development of cardiovascular disease.[160] Among 16,936 Harvard male alumni followed for 16 to 50 years, those who did not engage in vigorous sports play were at 35 per cent greater risk for developing hypertension, whether or not they had higher blood pressures while at Harvard, a family history of hypertension, or obesity—factors that also increased the risk of hypertension.[161]

ALCOHOL INTAKE. The role of alcohol in amounts consumed by a large segment of the population deserves special emphasis. Even in small quantities alcohol may raise blood pressure; in larger quantities alcohol may be responsible for a significant number of cases of hypertension. In all studies of this problem, the relationship between alcohol and blood pressure has been found to be independent of other known variables. Some have found a linear, progressively increasing level of blood pressure with increasing consumption of alcohol[162]; most report a threshold effect,[163] whereas some find lower levels of blood pressure among those who drink 1 to 2 ounces of ethanol a day than among those who drink none at all.[164] The latter pattern more clearly parallels the association with total and coronary mortality[165] as well as ischemic stroke.[166] The reduction in coronary disease in persons who ingest small amounts of alcohol, beyond any effect on blood pressure, may reflect a greater mobilization of tissue-free cholesterol for hepatic removal and excretion.[167]

The pressor effect of alcohol primarily reflects an increase in cardiac output and heart rate, possibly a consequence of increased sympathetic nerve activity.[168] Alcohol in vitro reduces sodium influx into leukocytes[169] so the specific cellular mechanism involved in this pressor response remains uncertain.

SMOKING (see also p. 759). Cigarette smoking raises blood pressure, probably through the nicotine-induced release of norepinephrine from adrenergic nerve endings. The increased risk of stroke among cigarette smokers probably involves an acute fall in cerebral blood flow.[170] When smokers quit, a trivial rise in blood pressure may occur, probably reflecting a gain in weight.

DIABETES MELLITUS (see also p. 1842). Hypertension is present in about two-thirds of patients with longstanding diabetes who have the associated intercapillary glomerulosclerosis described by Kimmelstiel and Wilson, and the prevalence of hypertension in the overall diabetic population is increased.[171] The coexistence of diabetes and hypertension almost redoubles the already high rate of cardiovascular mortality seen in nondiabetic hypertensives.[172]

When they are hypertensive, patients with diabetes mellitus may confront some interesting problems. With progressive renal insufficiency and automatic neuropathy, they may have few functional juxtaglomerular cells and a reduced ability to stimulate the release of renin. As a result, very low renin levels are often observed, with a tendency toward development of the syndrome of hyporeninemic hypoaldosteronism. If hypoglycemia develops because of too much insulin or other drugs, severe hypertension may occur as a result of stimulated sympathetic nervous activity.

Diabetics are also susceptible to special problems associated with antihypertensive therapy. Diuretics may exacerbate the carbohydrate intolerance, probably by inducing potassium deficiency. Those in whom the condition is brittle and who are prone to hypoglycemia may have difficulties with beta-adrenoceptor blocking agents, since these drugs blunt their protective catecholamine response, and severe hypoglycemia may develop with sweating as the only warning. On the other hand, successful reduction of their blood pressure may protect them from the otherwise inexorable progress of diabetic nephropathy. Angiotensin-converting enzyme inhibitors may be especially effective in reducing the high intraglomerular pressures that are probably responsible for the progressive glomerulosclerosis of diabetes.[173]

POLYCYTHEMIA (see also p. 1750). Polycythemia vera is frequently associated with hypertension. More common is a "pseudo-" or "stress" polycythemia with a high hematocrit and increased blood viscosity but contracted plasma volume as well as normal red cell mass and serum erythropoietin levels. Such patients may also have elevated plasma fibrinogen levels.[174]

GOUT. Hyperuricemia is present in 25 to 50 per cent of individuals with untreated primary hypertension, about five times the frequency found in normotensive persons. Hyperuricemia likely reflects decreased renal blood flow, presumably a reflection of nephrosclerosis.[175] When diuretics are used, the uric acid level rises further; however, even after prolonged exposure, patients with diuretic-induced hyperuricemia do not seem to develop urate deposition.[176] Nonetheless, gout may be precipitated by diuretic-induced hyperuricemia in those who are genetically susceptible.[177]

In addition to these conditions which are often associated with hypertension, several diseases actually induce hypertension, i.e., cause secondary hypertension.

Secondary Forms of Hypertension

(See Tables 28-4 and 28-5, pp. 820 and 821)

ORAL CONTRACEPTIVE USE

The use of estrogen-containing oral contraceptive pills is probably the most common cause of secondary hypertension in women. Most women who take them experience a slight rise in blood pressure, and about 5 per cent develop hypertension (i.e., blood pressure above 140/90 mm Hg) within 5 years of oral contraceptive use. This is more than twice the incidence seen among women of the same age who do not use these agents.[178] Although the hypertension is usually mild, it may persist after the oral contraceptive is discontinued, it may be severe, and it is almost certainly a factor in the increased cardiovascular mortality seen among young women who take these agents.[179] Despite these facts, these drugs have provided effective and safe birth control for millions of women and the need for oral contraceptives remains.

The dangers of oral contraceptives should be kept in proper perspective. While it is true that use of these drugs is associated with increased morbidity and mortality, the absolute numbers are quite small and overall mortality from cardiovascular disease has been progressively declining among women in the United States at a rate equal to that noted among American men. Moreover, the risks appear to have been lessened by more careful selection of users and lower doses of hormones. Data accumulated through 1987 reveal a relative risk for cardiovascular mortality among oral contraceptive users 1.5 times greater than that seen among women using other forms of birth control, whereas data reported in 1981 reveal a 4.2 relative risk.[180] The 1.5 relative risk translates to 13.4 deaths per 100,000 women years of use. Most of these deaths occurred in women who smoked and had other cardiovascular risk factors and who were taking formulations with more than 50 μg of estrogen. Thus, the currently used low-estrogen and progesterone forms seem quite safe for the purposes of temporary birth control.

INCIDENCE. The best data on the incidence of oral contraceptive-induced hypertension came from a large study of the Royal College of General Practitioners. The incidence of hypertension was 2.6 times greater among 23,000 pill users compared with 23,000 nonusers, resulting in a 5 per cent incidence over 5 years of oral contraceptive use.[178] In addition, this incidence increased with long duration of pill use, being only slightly higher than that among controls during the first year but rising to almost three times higher by the fifth year. In a much smaller but more carefully performed prospective study of 186 Scottish women, systolic pressure rose in 164 (by more than 25 mm Hg in eight) and diastolic pressure rose in 150 (by more than 20 mm Hg in two) during the first two years of oral contraceptive use. After three years, the mean rise in 83 of these women was 9.2 mm Hg.[181] The current use of smaller amounts of estrogen (20 to 35 μg) than the 50 μg taken by most of these women may induce less hypertension.[182]

CLINICAL FEATURES. The likelihood of developing hypertension among women using oral contraceptives is much greater among those who are over age 35 or obese or who drink large quantities of alcohol.[183] The presence of hypertension during a prior pregnancy increases this likelihood but not enough to preclude pill use in such women who require contraception. In most women, the hypertension is mild; however, in some it may accelerate rapidly and cause severe renal damage.[184] When the pill is discontinued, blood pressure falls to normal within three to six months in about half the patients. Whether the pill caused permanent hypertension in the other half or just uncovered primary hypertension at an earlier time is not clear.

MECHANISMS OF HYPERTENSION. Oral contraceptive use probably causes hypertension by renin-aldosterone-mediated volume expansion. Estrogens and the synthetic progestogens used in oral contraceptive pills both cause sodium retention.[185] This probably results from the following sequence of events (Fig. 28–16): (1) Estrogens increase the hepatic synthesis of renin substrate. (2) In the presence of increased substrate, more angiotensin is generated from whatever level of renin is present in the circulation. As a result of the increased level of angiotensin II, renin release is partially inhibited, so that its concentration in peripheral blood is lowered back to normal.[186] (3) The increased levels of angiotensin stimulate adre-

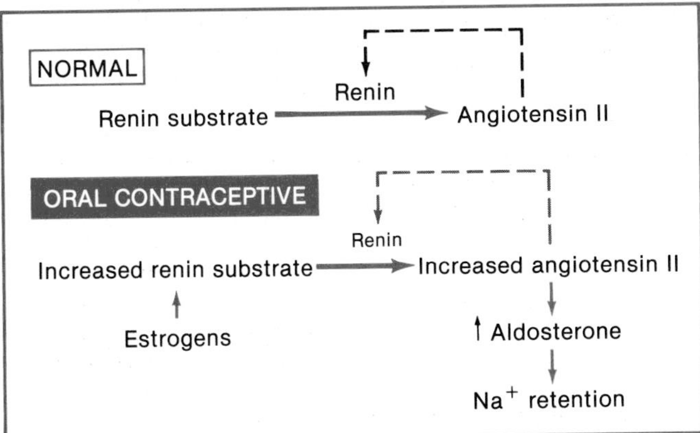

FIGURE 28-16. Schematic representation of the changes in the renin-angiotensin system induced by oral contraceptives containing estrogen. The dotted lines show the feedback inhibition of renin release by angiotensin II. (From Kaplan, N. M.: Clinical Hypertension, 5th ed. Baltimore, © by Williams and Wilkins, 1990, p. 346.)

nal synthesis of aldosterone, which causes sodium retention. The amount of progestogen may also be important; more vascular disease has been noted with the use of 250 μg of levonorgestrel than with 150 μg of this progestogen.[187]

In keeping with the probable role of hyperinsulinemia in other hypertensive states (see p. 828) this may be involved in oral contraceptive-induced hypertension as well because plasma insulin levels are increased for at least six months after start of oral contraceptive use, reflecting peripheral insulin resistance.[188]

MANAGEMENT. The use of estrogen-containing oral contraceptives should be restricted in women over age 35, particularly if they also smoke or are hypertensive or obese. Women given the pill should be properly monitored as follows: (1) the supply should be limited initially to three months and thereafter to six months; (2) they should be required to return for a blood pressure check before an additional supply is provided; and (3) if blood pressure has risen, an alternative contraceptive should be offered. If the pill remains the only acceptable contraceptive, the elevated blood pressure can be reduced with appropriate therapy. In view of the probable role of aldosterone, use of a diuretic-spironolactone combination seems appropriate. In those who stop taking oral contraceptives, evaluation for secondary hypertensive diseases should be postponed for at least three months to allow the changes in the renin-angiotensin-aldosterone system to remit. If the hypertension does not recede, additional workup and therapy may be needed.

POSTMENOPAUSAL ESTROGEN USE. Millions of women use estrogen for its potential benefits after menopause. It does not appear to induce hypertension, even though it does induce various changes in the renin-angiotensin-aldosterone system seen with oral contraceptive use.[189] Moreover, the majority of case-control studies have shown a significantly *lower* mortality rate from coronary artery disease among postmenopausal estrogen users than nonusers.[190]

RENAL PARENCHYMAL DISEASE

(See also Ch. 62)

After oral contraceptive use, renal parenchymal disease is the most common cause of secondary hypertension, responsible for 2 to 5 per cent of cases seen in unselected adult populations (Table 28-5). As chronic glomerulonephritis becomes less common, hypertensive nephrosclerosis and diabetic nephropathy have become the most common causes of end-stage renal disease (ESRD).[84] The hypertension that is usual in diabetic nephropathy contributes significantly to the progression of renal damage.[191] The higher prevalence of hypertension among United States blacks is probably responsible for their significantly higher rate of ESRD, with hypertension as the underlying cause in as many as one-half of these patients.[84]

Not only does hypertension cause renal failure and renal failure cause hypertension but also more subtle renal dysfunction may be involved in patients with primary hypertension. As discussed earlier (p. 829), the kidneys may initiate the hemodynamic cascade eventuating in primary hypertension. As that disease progresses, some renal dysfunction is demonstrable in most patients; progressive renal damage is the end result and is the cause of death in at least 10 per cent of hypertensives. Since early treatment of hypertension will likely protect against nephrosclerosis, there is hope that improved control of hypertension will slow the progression and reduce the frequency of ESRD.

In hypertension with renal parenchymal disease the sequence of progressively worsening renal damage is: (1) acute renal diseases that are often reversible; (2) unilateral and bilateral diseases without renal insufficiency; (3) chronic renal disease with renal insufficiency; and (4) hypertension in the anephric state and after renal transplantation.

ACUTE RENAL DISEASES. Hypertension may appear with any sudden, severe insult to the kidneys that either markedly impairs the excretion of salt and water, which leads to volume expansion, or reduces renal blood flow, which sets off the renin-angiotensin-aldosterone mechanism. Bilateral ureteral obstruction is an example of the former; sudden bilateral renal artery occlusion, as by emboli, is an example of the latter. Relief of either may dramatically reverse severe hypertension. This has been particularly striking in men with high-pressure chronic retention of urine, who may manifest both renal failure and severe hypertension, both of which may be relieved by prostatic resection.[192] Some of the collagen diseases may also produce rapidly progressive renal damage. The more common acute processes are glomerulonephritis and oliguric renal failure.

Acute Glomerulonephritis. Although the classic syndrome of type-specific poststreptococcal nephritis appearing after pharyngitis has become much less common, glomerular lesions of various types may be associated with hypertension. Moreover, although the epidemic poststreptococcal disease is usually self-limited, the disease in some patients follows a progressive, smoldering course that may lead to renal insufficiency.[193] Typically, hypertension accompanies the oliguria and fluid retention of acute renal injury. The presence of renal damage in acute glomerulonephritis is usually obvious, with abnormalities of the urinary sediment; however, these may be minimal, and severe hypertension may be the presenting feature.

Hypertension is best relieved by sodium and fluid restriction and by appropriate doses of potent diuretics such as furosemide. Dialysis and parenteral antihypertensive drugs may be needed if encephalopathy supervenes. In milder cases, the hypertension recedes as the edema is relieved. However, some patients have a rapidly progressive course, often with prolonged anuria.

Acute Oliguric Renal Failure. Acute renal failure occurs after shock develops, particularly in patients in whom renin levels are already high, such as those with cirrhosis and ascites or at the end of pregnancy. The release of even more renin by decreased blood pressure and effective circulating blood volume may flood the renal vasculature and cause such intense renal vasoconstriction that renal function shuts down.[194] Hypertension in this setting is usually not an important problem and can be controlled by preventing volume overload. High doses of furosemide may be helpful, but dialysis is often needed. When acute renal failure occurs in the setting of accelerated or malignant hypertension, aggressive therapy (including dialysis) may be followed by sustained recovery of renal function.[195]

Vasculitis. Rapidly progressive renal deterioration with severe hypertension occurs not infrequently during the course of scleroderma and other forms of vasculitis (p. 798). Therapy with antihypertensives, particularly angiotensin-converting enzyme inhibitors, may reverse the process.[196]

Extracorporeal Shock Wave Lithotripsy. As this procedure has been utilized increasingly to treat nephrolithiasis, some patients have been found to develop hypertension subsequently. In a prospective study of 731 patients followed for at least 1 year after the procedure, the prevalence of hyperten-

TABLE 28-10 CLASSIFICATION OF FIBROMUSCULAR DYSPLASIA OF THE RENAL ARTERIES

	INTIMA	MEDIA			ADVENTITIA
	Intimal Fibroplasia	Medial Fibroplasia	Perimedial Fibroplasia	Medial Hyperplasia	Periarterial Fibroplasia
Frequency	5%	70%	20%	5%	1%
Angiographic appearance	Single smooth lesion	String of beads	Smaller beads	Single smooth lesion	Single lesion
Progressive	Yes	1/3	Yes	Yes	?
Occlusion of artery	Yes	No	Yes	Yes	?
Comments	Children	Also extrarenal	Young women	Teenagers	?

From Pickering, T. G.: Renovascular hypertension: Etiology and pathophysiology. Semin. Nucl. Med. *19*:79, 1989.

collateral flow will become available to preserve the viability of the kidney. In this way, the seemingly nonfunctioning kidney may be responsible for continued renin secretion and hypertension. If recognized, such totally occluded vessels can sometimes be repaired, with return of renal function and relief of hypertension.[230]

Renovascular stenosis is often bilateral, although usually one side is clearly predominant. In the Cooperative Study on Renovascular Hypertension, 25 per cent of the subjects had bilateral atherosclerotic or fibroplastic disease.[231] In eight young women with one small kidney that was initially thought to be the cause of their hypertension, fibroplastic disease in the renal artery of the contralateral kidney was found to be responsible.[232] The possibility of bilateral disease should be suspected in those with renal insufficiency, particularly if rapidly progressive oliguric renal failure develops without evidence of obstructive uropathy and, even more so, if it develops after start of ACE inhibitor therapy.[233]

MECHANISMS. Since Goldblatt produced renovascular hypertension in the dog in 1934, the pathophysiology of this disease has been studied extensively. Confusion has arisen because of the use of one-kidney models, which are more appropriate to the study of renal parenchymal hypertension. The sequence of changes in the two-kidney (one-clip) model and in patients with renovascular hypertension almost certainly starts with the release of increased amounts of renin when sufficient ischemia is induced to diminish pulse pressure in the renal afferent arterioles. A reduction of renal perfusion pressure by 50 per cent leads to an immediate and persistent increase in renin secretion from the ischemic kidney, with suppression of secretion from the contralateral one. With time, renin levels fall (but not to the low levels expected based on the elevated blood pressure), accompanied by an expanded body fluid volume and increased cardiac output.[226]

In patients with proved renovascular hypertension of many years' duration, excess renin secretion persists, so that the experimental data are confirmed clinically. However, when renovascular hypertension induces extensive nephrosclerosis in the contralateral kidney, a different picture may evolve. Relief of the stenosis may not relieve the hypertension; rather the contralateral kidney becomes the culprit, with the stenotic kidney's vessels having been protected from the high pressure. With removal of the contralateral kidney, the hypertension may recede.[234]

DIAGNOSIS. The presence of certain clinical features indicates the need for a screening test for renovascular hypertension in perhaps 10 per cent of all hypertensives (Table 28-9). A positive screening test, or very strong clinical features, calls for more definitive confirmatory tests.

The differing clinical picture of the two major forms of renovascular disease was clearly delineated by the Cooperative Study on Renovascular Hypertension.[235] According to the Study, patients with atherosclerotic lesions were older, had a higher systolic blood pressure and more frequent arterial disease in areas outside the kidney, and were more likely to develop target-organ damage than were patients with essential hypertension. In contrast, patients with fibromuscular hyperplasia were young, predominantly female, more likely to have no family history of hypertension, and less prone to develop cardiomegaly.

Some patients have renovascular hypertension but may have none of the clinical features just described and in Table 28-9, clinically resembling patients with mild primary hypertension. Nonetheless, these features should be used to exclude the majority of hypertensives from additional workup and to identify the 10 per cent or so who should undergo a complete evaluation. In the past, routine performance in all hypertensives of intravenous pyelography or other screening tests with a high percentage of false-positive findings resulted in more false-positive than true-positive results, mandating even more unnecessary examinations, with their attendant costs and risks. Results with the *oral captopril challenge test,* described below, look very promising. This may be a screening test that can be applied to a larger population to find the disease in those who do not have the more classic clinical features.

Those who manifest the features shown in Table 28-9 should be strongly suspected of having this condition. Features of particular importance include the onset of severe hypertension after age 60 and the presence of hypokalemia indicative of secondary aldosteronism from the high renin levels,[236] recurrent episodes of acute pulmonary edema,[237] and acute loin pain in the absence of ureteric obstruction.[238]

Among blacks, less atherosclerosis develops in the main renal arteries, and the incidence of renovascular hypertension is lower.[239] Among diabetic hypertensive persons, despite their greater propensity for vascular disease, the incidence of atherosclerotic renal artery stenosis is not increased.[225]

Diagnostic Tests. Until recently, various screening tests were advocated for those with suspicious clinical features, including intravenous pyelography, isotopic renography, and peripheral plasma renin activity assays. However, each of these is relatively nonspecific and not highly sensitive, so that many false-positive and false-negative results were obtained. Increasingly, the diagnostic approach has become more direct: Arteriography is recommended as the first and definitive test when renovascular hypertension is strongly suspected.

However, as shown in Figure 28-18, isotopic renography and plasma renin measurements after an oral captopril challenge may be a reasonable initial test in those with suggestive clinical features, to be followed by renal arteriography and then renal vein renin assays. The latter procedure may not be needed if isotopic renography after captopril indicates significant renal ischemia in the kidney with renal artery disease by arteriography.

Even though arteriography is increasingly available and relatively safe, it cannot be used as a screening test except in those who seem very likely to have the disease, such as a young woman with recent onset of severe hypertension and a diastolic bruit over one kidney. For screening among populations with an expected prevalence of perhaps 5 per cent (taking only those with clinical features suggestive of renovascu-

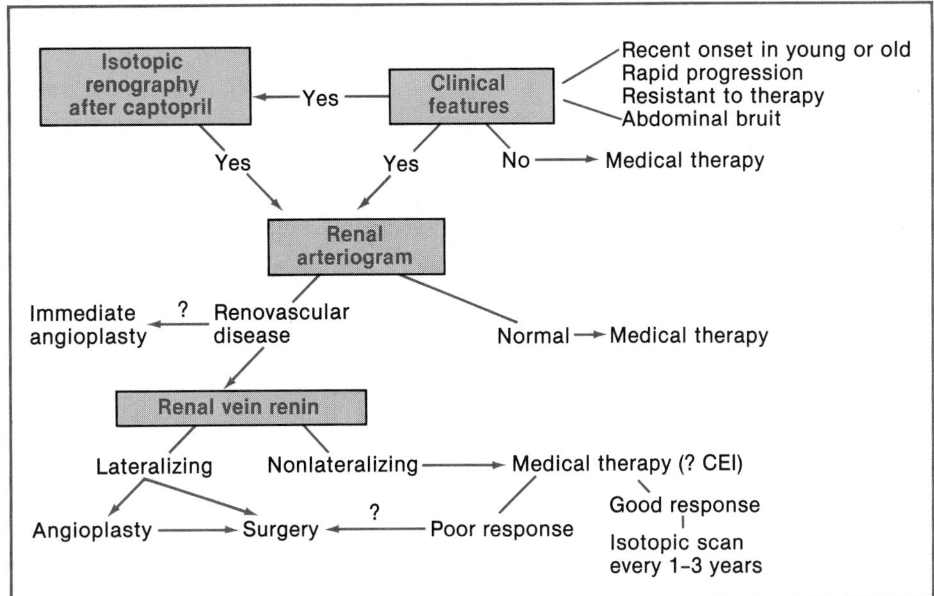

FIGURE 28-18. Scheme for the evaluation and management of renal vascular hypertension. (From Kaplan, N. M.: Clinical Hypertension. 5th ed. Baltimore, © by Williams and Wilkins, 1990, p. 312.)

lar hypertension), an easy and safe procedure that results in few false-negatives is needed. A certain number of false-positive results must be expected; considering that about 20 per cent of all adults will have primary hypertension, at least 20 per cent of patients with renovascular hypertension would be expected to have positive screening tests but would not be cured through repair of the stenosis. Therefore these results would be classified as "false-positives."

Initial experience with measurement of peripheral blood renin activity (PRA) before and one hour after a single 50-mg dose of the angiotensin-converting enzyme inhibitor captopril suggests that this approach may provide an easy, noninvasive way to establish the functional significance of a lesion, either after or preferably before arteriography[240] (Fig. 28-19). The procedure requires only that the patient be on normal sodium dietary intake and off diuretics and ACE inhibitors; if possible, other antihypertensive medications should be withdrawn for three weeks, although the test was almost equally valid among those examined while on therapy. After the patient sits for 30 minutes, venous blood is obtained for basal PRA, and 50 mg of captopril is given orally. At 60 minutes, another blood sample for stimulated PRA is obtained. The criteria for a positive test for renovascular hypertension are (1) a stimulated PRA of 12 ng/ml/hr or more, (20) an absolute increase in PRA of 10 ng/ml/hr or more, and (3) a 150 per cent or greater increase in PRA or, if baseline PRA is below 3 ng/ml/hr, a 400 per cent increase. Among the 112 patients with essential hypertension tested, only two showed false-positive results; among the 40 with renovascular hypertension, there were no false-negative results.

The test was accurate in patients with good renal function, but it gave both false-positive and false-negative results in a considerable portion of those with impaired renal function. This procedure may prove to be generally useful as a screening test for renovascular disease. The authors recommend it was a way to identify the process in many patients who would not otherwise be screened. This seems increasingly to be a good idea, since relief of renovascular hypertension by either angioplasty or surgery is being reported in a larger proportion of patients, including many who would not have been candidates for repair only a few years ago. At the same time, problems with the most effective form of medical therapy, ACE inhibitors, have surfaced. Others have found the test to be of excellent sensitivity and acceptable sensitivity.[241] Poor results have been noted when the test was modified and different diagnostic criteria used.[242]

Combination of isotopic renography with plasma renin measurement one hour after the oral captopril dose provides additional diagnostic information. Either labeled hippurate, a measure of renal blood flow, or diethylenetriaminepentaacetic acid (DTPA), a measure of glomerular filtration rate, may be used.[243] If the postcaptopril test shows a significant difference, the procedure should be repeated without captopril to document the ischemic origin of the differences in blood flow or GFR. With advances in renal artery duplex ultrasonography, this may become a useful screening procedure, although

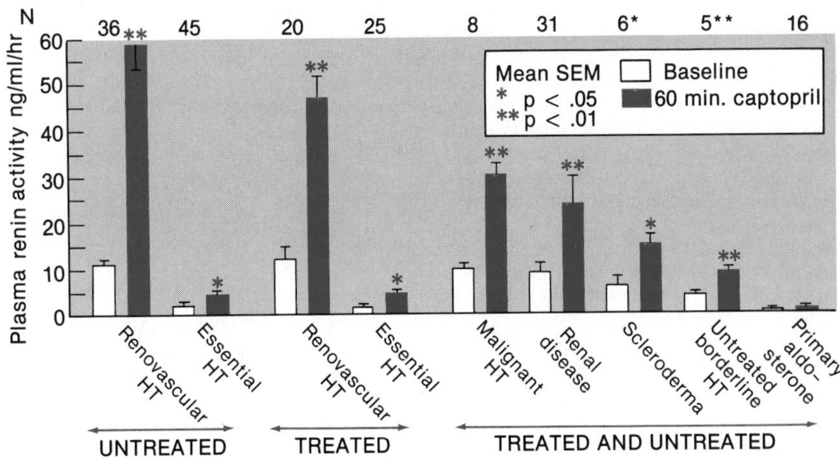

FIGURE 28-19. Seated blood pressure and plasma renin response 60 minutes after an oral dose of captopril in groups of various types of treated and untreated hypertensive patients. N = number in each group. (From Muller, F. B., Sealey, J. E., Case, D. B., et al.: The captopril test for identifying renovascular disease in hypertensive patients. Am. J. Med. *80*:633, 1986.)

currently it is mainly of value in following patients after intervention.[244]

MANAGEMENT. Little is known about the natural history of untreated renovascular disease so it is difficult to assess the results of therapy. Advances in medical therapy have made it easier to control the hypertension, and the availability of transluminal angioplasty offers another "curative" approach. However, current evidence supports surgical repair as being more likely to provide relief of hypertension and preserve renal function.

The availability of ACE inhibitors (p. 496) may be considered a two-edged sword; one edge provides better control of renovascular hypertension than may be possible with other antihypertensive medications,[245] while the other edge exposes the already ischemic kidney to a further loss of blood flow by removing the high levels of angiotensin II that were supporting its circulation.[246] Although ACE inhibitors may be effective and safe (particularly in concert with angioplasty[247]), their use has the potential to make the already ischemic kidney more ischemic, with an increased possibility of complete occlusion of the stenotic artery.[248] Calcium entry blockers and other antihypertensive drugs may be almost as effective as ACE inhibitors and considerably safer.[249]

Angioplasty. As experience builds with angioplasty, it has been shown to improve 60 to 70 per cent of patients, more with fibromuscular disease than with atherosclerosis, as is also the case for surgery.[250] It will probably be performed more and more frequently as the initial procedure, particularly in patients who are poor candidates for major surgery, even in the presence of severe stenoses.[230]

Surgery. Despite the availability of better medical therapy and angioplasty, surgical repair is being shown to relieve renovascular hypertension in an increasing number of patients, including the elderly[251] and those with renal insufficiency.[252] Most agree that surgery is indicated in patients whose hypertension is not well controlled or whose renal function deteriorates on medical therapy as well as in those with only a transient response to angioplasty or when lesions are not amenable to that procedure.

RENIN-SECRETING TUMORS

Made up of juxtaglomerular cells or hemangiopericytomas, these tumors have been found mostly in young patients with severe hypertension, very high renin levels in both peripheral blood and the kidney harboring the tumor, and secondary aldosteronism manifested by hypokalemia.[253] The tumor can usually be recognized by selective renal angiography, usually performed for suspected renovascular hypertension, although a few are extrarenal.[254] More commonly, children with Wilms' tumors may have hypertension and high renin levels that revert to normal after nephrectomy.[255]

ADRENAL CAUSES OF HYPERTENSION (see Ch. 61)

Three adrenal causes of hypertension are considered here—primary excesses of aldosterone, cortisol, and catecholamines—along with congenital adrenal hyperplasia. Together these constitute the causes of less than 1 per cent of all hypertensive diseases. Each can usually be recognized with relative ease, and patients suspected of having these disorders can be screened by means of readily available tests. More of a problem than the diagnosis of these adrenal disorders is the need to exclude their presence because of the increasing identification of incidental adrenal masses when abdominal computed tomography (CT) is done to diagnose intraabdominal pathology. Unsuspected adrenal tumors have been found in from 1 to 10 per cent of abdominal CT scans obtained for reasons unrelated to the adrenal gland.[256,257] As known from prior autopsy studies, most of these adrenal tumors are nonfunctioning. The threat of malignancy can probably be best excluded by adrenal scintigraphy with the radioiodinated derivative of cholesterol, NP-59.[258] Benign lesions almost always take up the isotope, while malignant ones almost always do not.

Primary Aldosteronism (see also p. 1837)

This disease is relatively rare in unselected populations (Table 28–5), although it may be found in the majority of hypertensive patients with unprovoked hypokalemia.[259]

PATHOPHYSIOLOGY. Primary aldosterone excess usually arises from solitary benign adenomas. As diagnostic tests have improved and become more readily available, larger numbers of patients with minimal features have been recognized. Many of these patients have been found to have bilateral adrenal hyperplasia, the number averaging about one-third of all cases of aldosteronism. Other variants of primary aldosterone excess include familial glucocorticoid-suppressible hyperaldosteronism[260] and rare extraadrenal tumors which hypersecrete aldosterone.[261] Glycyrrhizic acid in licorice in candy, liquor, or chewing tobacco may cause apparent mineralocorticoid excess[138] (see p. 830).

Whatever the source, excess aldosterone causes hypertension and hypokalemia, here defined as a plasma potassium level below 3.2 mEq/liter. Very rarely, the syndrome has been recognized in normotensive persons.[262] Not so rarely, hypokalemia may be absent or only intermittent, but in most patients with adenomas, persistent hypokalemia is observed.[259]

The hypertension begins as a volume overload but soon converts, as do apparently all forms of hypertension, to increased peripheral resistance.[94] Hypertension may be severe, with a mean pressure in one group of 136 patients of 205/123 mm Hg and four of the patients showing histological evidence of malignant hypertension on renal biopsy.[263] Furthermore, 23 per cent of these patients had a serious vascular complication such as stroke or myocardial infarction. In association with the increased pressure and expanded blood volume, renin secretion is suppressed. Although this finding has been almost invariable with hyperaldosteronism, the overwhelming majority of hypertensive patients with suppressed renin do not have this syndrome (see p. 830).

Hypokalemia results from the aldosterone-mediated increase in renal potassium excretion. Although hypokalemia may not be recognized until diuretics or salt loads are ingested, the effects may be striking, with muscular weakness, polyuria, metabolic alkalosis, impaired carbohydrate tolerance, blunting of circulating reflexes, and the development of multiple renal cysts.[264]

DIAGNOSIS. Serious consideration should be given to the diagnosis of primary aldosteronism when hypertension and hypokalemia coexist. If the rare normokalemic patient with the disease is thereby missed, little will be lost as long as the patient is protected by appropriate treatment of the hypertension. Since this is likely to include a diuretic, significant hypokalemia will soon become manifested, making the diagnosis obvious.

A high plasma aldosterone-to-renin ratio in plasma is a useful screening test that can be performed immediately upon recognition of hypokalemia in a hypertensive patient, without special conditions or preparation.[259]

Potassium Wasting. The next step in evaluating the hypokalemic hypertensive should be to determine potassium excretion in a 24-hour urine sample collected while the patient is hypokalemic, receiving no supplemental potassium or diuretic, and ingesting a normal sodium intake (i.e., urinary sodium excretion is above 100 mEq/day) (Fig. 28–20). If, under these circumstances, urinary potassium is less than 30 mEq/day, mineralocorticoid excess is highly unlikely, and the workup can be ended; if the value is greater than this, further evaluation is warranted. In most hypertensive patients hypokalemia is caused by the prior use of diuretics. Losses may be large and may require prolonged potassium supplementation. On the other hand, severe hypokalemia appearing soon after the initiation of diuretic therapy may presage primary aldosteronism.

Renin Suppression. If urinary potassium-wasting has been documented, the patient should receive potassium supplementation for long enough, often weeks to months, to bring the plasma potassium level within the normal range and maintain it, so that subsequent studies will be unaffected by hypokalemia. One or another mild stimulus to renin secretion may be applied to demonstrate suppression.

Aldosterone Excess. Increased levels of aldosterone can be found in urine or blood. When urine is analyzed, the 24-hour collection should contain over 100 mEq of sodium to ensure that high aldosterone levels are not simply secondary to sodium restriction. Various techniques to suppress endogenous aldosterone secretion have been used to ensure further that the aldosterone excess is primary. These include high-sodium diets, infusions of saline, injections of deoxycorticosterone acetate (DOCA), and oral administration of fludrocortisone

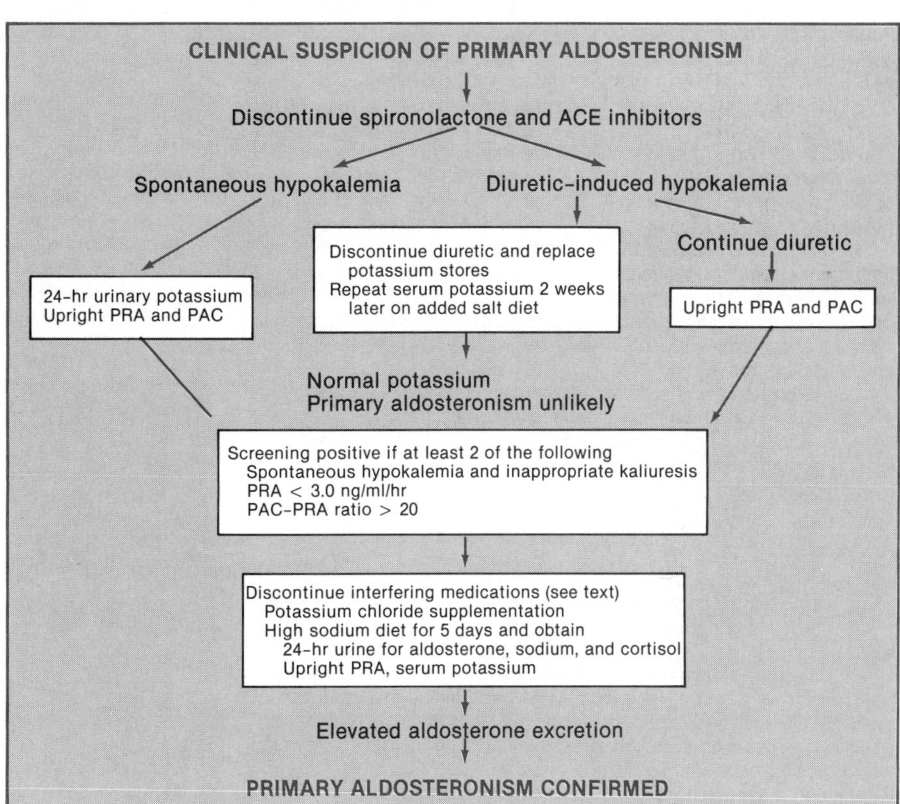

FIGURE 28-20. Algorithm for screening and diagnostic confirmation of primary aldosteronism. ACE = angiotensin-converting enzyme; PAC = plasma aldosterone concentration; PRA = plasma renin activity. (From Young, W. F. Jr., Hogan, M. J., Klee, G. G., et al.: Primary aldosteronism: Diagnosis and treatment. Mayo Clin. Proc. *65*:96, 1990.)

(Florinef). Reliable documentation of high and nonsuppressible aldosterone levels can be obtained with the saline suppression test of plasma aldosterone, in which two liters of normal saline are infused over a four-hour interval.[265] The plasma aldosterone level remains elevated in patients with primary aldosteronism but is suppressed to below 10 ng/dl in patients with essential hypertension or secondary aldosteronism. Patients with bilateral hyperplasia often exhibit intermediate levels (between 5 and 10 ng/dl).

Once the diagnosis of primary aldosteronism is made, the type of adrenal pathology should be determined and only those patients with a tumor should be subjected to operation, since it may not be possible to determine the type of pathology at operation without removing both adrenal glands.

Bilateral Adrenal Hyperplasia. Various maneuvers are available to differentiate patients with apparent aldosterone excess due to bilateral adrenal hyperplasia from those with an adrenal adenoma.[266] Basal levels of plasma 18-hydroxycorticosterone (18-OHB) and changes in plasma aldosterone levels after four hours of upright posture from 8 AM to 12 noon often have been found to distinguish patients with adenomas (who usually have basal 18-OHB levels above 100 ng/dl and falls in upright plasma aldosterone) from those with bilateral hyperplasia (who usually have basal 18-OHB levels below 50 ng/dl and postural rises in plasma aldosterone presumably invoked by their supersensitivity to posture-mediated rises in renin-angiotensin).[259] However, the best initial test to identify the type of adrenal disease is CT, which is capable of identifying adrenal lesions as small as 1.0 cm. If CT fails to define an adrenal adenoma when the clinical situation is strongly suggestive, either magnetic resonance imaging of the adrenals[267] or an adrenal scintillation scan with an iodinated cholesterol derivative[268] should be tried. If these are nondiagnostic, bilateral adrenal vein catheterization with venography and analysis of venous steroid levels may be utilized.[269] Rather than false-negative tests, there will probably be more problems with false-positive CT scans, i.e., finding nonfunctioning adrenal tumors, which are present in a considerable number of both normotensive and hypertensive persons.[256,257]

THERAPY. Once the diagnosis of primary aldosteronism is made and the type of adrenal disorder has been established, the choice of therapy is fairly easy: Patients with a solitary adenoma require resection of the tumor; those with bilateral hyperplasia should be treated with spironolactone (p. 1838) and a thiazide diuretic (p. 860).[259] Fortunately, the doses of spironolactone required for chronic therapy are usually low enough to avoid bothersome side effects. Other potassium-sparers will also control the disease if spironolactone is poorly tolerated. Other antihypertensive agents may be needed for some patients with bilateral hyperplasia. When an adenoma is resected, about 75 per cent of patients will become normotensive, while the other 25 per cent remain hypertensive, either from preexisting primary hypertension or from renal damage due to prolonged secondary hypertension.

CUSHING'S SYNDROME (see also p. 1837)

Hypertension occurs in about 80 per cent of patients with Cushing's syndrome. If left untreated, it can cause congestive heart failure and death.[270] As with hypertension of other endocrine causes, the longer it is present, the less likely it is to disappear when the underlying cause is relieved.

MECHANISM OF HYPERTENSION. Blood pressure may increase for a number of reasons.[271] The secretion of a mineralocorticoid, DOC or aldosterone, or another hypertension-producing steroid may also be increased along with cortisol. The excess cortisol exerts a sufficient intrinsic salt-retaining effect to expand volume and lead to hypertension. Cortisol stimulates the synthesis of renin substrate, which in turn causes more angiotensin to be generated. Vascular reactivity to pressor substances, including norepinephrine, increases.

DIAGNOSIS. The syndrome should be suspected in patients with central obesity, thin skin, muscle weakness, and osteoporosis. If clinical features are suggestive, the diagnosis can be either ruled out or virtually assured by the measurement of free cortisol in a 24-hour urine or the simple overnight *dexamethasone suppression test*.[272] In normal subjects, the level of plasma cortisol in a sample drawn at 8 AM after a bedtime dose of 1 mg of dexamethasone should be below 7 μg/100 mg. If the level is higher, additional workup is in order to establish both the diagnosis of cortisol excess and the pathological type. Measurement of urine free cortisol levels is almost as good a screening test: Most patients who do not have Cushing's syndrome excrete less than 100 μg/24 hours.

If screening tests are abnormal, a longer dexamethasone suppression test should be done, using 0.5 mg every six hours and then 2.0 mg every six hours, each for two days. Urinary free cortisol excretion and plasma cortisol levels should be measured on the second day of each dose.

Patients with Cushing's syndrome fail to suppress urine free cortisol to below 25 μg/day on the 0.5 mg dose; if Cushing's syndrome is caused by excess pituitary ACTH drive with bilateral adrenal hyperplasia, urinary free cortisol will be suppressed to below 40 per cent of the control value on the 2.0 mg dose. As plasma ACTH assays become more reliable, they will provide an additional means of differentiating pituitary and ectopic ACTH excess from adrenal tumors with ACTH suppression. The response to corticotropin-releasing hormone (CRH) and inferior petrosal sinus sampling may help identify the pituitary cause for the syndrome.[272]

THERAPY. In about two-thirds of patients with Cushing's syndrome, the process begins with overproduction of ACTH by the pituitary, which leads to bilateral adrenal hyperplasia. Although pituitary hyperfunction may reflect a hypothalamic disorder, the majority of patients have discrete pituitary adenomas that can usually be resected by selective transsphenoidal microsurgery.[273]

If an adrenal tumor is present, it should be surgically removed. With earlier diagnosis and more selective surgical therapy, it is hoped that more patients with Cushing's syndrome will be cured without the need for lifelong glucocorticoid replacement therapy and with permanent relief of their hypertension.

PHEOCHROMOCYTOMA (see also p. 1839)

The wild fluctuations in blood pressure and dramatic symptoms of pheochromocytoma usually alert both the patient and the physician to the possibility of this diagnosis. However, such fluctuations may be missed or, as occurs in half of the patients, the hypertension may be persistent. The symptoms may be incorrectly ascribed to psychoneurosis by practitioners not sensitized to "spells," which usually represent menopausal hot flushes or anxiety-induced hyperventilation. Unfortunately, if the diagnosis is missed, severe complications may arise from exceedingly high blood pressure and damage to the heart by catecholamines (p. 1436). Stroke and hypertensive crises with encephalopathy and retinal hemorrhages may occur, probably because blood pressure levels soar in vessels unprepared by a chronic hypertensive condition. Fortunately, a simple and inexpensive test will detect the disease with virtual certainty, so that diagnostic indecision may be minimized.

PATHOPHYSIOLOGY. Pheochromocytomas may arise wherever the sympathetic ganglia from the primitive neural crest come to lie. These cells differentiate into ganglion cells, neuroblasts, and chromaffin cells. Tumors develop from each of these cell types; ganglioneuromas and neuroblastomas usually occur in children and are recognized by the presence of large quantities of the precursor of catecholamines, dihydroxyphenylalanine.[274] Paragangliomas may arise in chemoreceptor tissue, where they are called *chemodectomas,* at multiple sites along the sympathetic chain, including the organ of Zuckerkandl, and in the urinary bladder.[275] Pheochromocytomas are often found in patients with neurofibromatosis and hypertension.[276]

About 90 per cent of pheochromocytomas arise in the adrenal medulla; 10 per cent are bilateral and another 10 per cent are malignant. Multiple adrenal tumors are particularly common in patients with simple familial pheochromocytoma and multiple endocrine neoplasia Type II in association with medullary carcinoma of the thyroid (Sipple's syndrome) or with mucosal ganglioneuromas in addition (Type IIB or III). Diffuse medullary hyperplasia may precede the development of tumors, and the tumors may, in fact, reflect extreme degrees of nodular hyperplasia.[277] Adrenal pheochromocytomas have been found to produce a number of hypothalamic and pituitary-like hormones, e.g., ACTH and somatostatin, whereas these hormones were not found in five extraadrenal pheochromocytomas.[278] Measurement of plasma levels of these immunoreactive hormones may prove useful in establishing the location of the catecholamine-secreting tumor.

Secretion from nonfamilial pheochromocytomas varies considerably, with small tumors tending to secrete larger proportions of active catecholamines. If the predominant secretion is epinephrine, which is formed primarily in the adrenal medulla, the symptoms reflect its effects—mainly systolic hypertension due to increased cardiac output, tachycardia, sweating, flushing, and apprehension. If norepinephrine is predominantly secreted, as from some of the adrenal tumors and from almost all the extraadrenal tumors, the symptoms include both systolic and diastolic hypertension from peripheral vasoconstriction but less tachycardia, palpitations, and anxiety. The hemodynamic features of 24 untreated patients with surgically proven pheochromocytomas were quite similar to those found in 24 untreated patients of similar sex, age, weight, and blood pressure with primary hypertension, with increased total peripheral resistance as the primary fault in both groups.[279]

TABLE 28–11 FEATURES SUGGESTIVE OF PHEOCHROMOCYTOMA

Hypertension: Persistent or paroxysmal
- Markedly variable blood pressures (± orthostatic hypotension)
- Sudden paroxysms (± subsequent hypertension) in relation to:
  - Stress: anesthesia, angiography, parturition
  - Pharmacological provocation: histamine, nicotine, caffeine, beta blockers, glucocorticoids, tricyclic antidepressants
  - Manipulation of tumors: abdominal palpation, urination
- Rare patients persistently normotensive
- Unusual settings
  - Childhood, pregnancy, familial
  - Multiple endocrine adenomas: medullary carcinoma of thyroid (MEN-2), mucosal neuromas (MEN-2b)
  - Neurocutaneous lesions: Neurofibromatosis

Associated Symptoms:
- Sudden spells with headache, sweating, palpitations, nervousness, nausea, and vomiting
- Pain in chest or abdomen

Associated Signs:
- Sweating, tachycardia, arrhythmia, pallor, weight loss

From Kaplan, N. M.: Clinical Hypertension. 4th ed. Baltimore, © by Williams and Wilkins, 1986, p. 386.

DIAGNOSIS. Many more hypertensive patients have variable blood pressures and "spells" than the 0.1 per cent or so who harbor a pheochromocytoma. Spells with paroxysmal hypertension may occur with a number of stresses, and a large number of conditions may involve transient catecholamine release. A pheochromocytoma should be suspected in patients with hypertension that is either paroxysmal or persistent and accompanied by the symptoms and signs listed in Table 28–11. In addition, children and patients with rapidly accelerating hypertension should be screened. Those whose tumors secrete predominantly epinephrine are prone to postural hypotension from a contracted blood volume and blunted sympathetic reflex tone. Suspicion should heightened if activities such as bending over, exercise, palpation of the abdomen, smoking, or dipping snuff cause repetitive spells that begin abruptly, advance rapidly, and subside within minutes.

High levels of catecholamines may induce myocarditis (Ch. 43), which may progress to cardiomyopathy and left ventricular failure.[280] Electrocardiographic changes of ischemia may also be seen.[281] Beta-blockers given to such patients may raise the pressure and induce coronary spasm through blockade of beta-mediated vasodilation.[282]

LABORATORY CONFIRMATION. The easiest and best procedure is either a 24-hour or spot urine assay for total metanephrine. This catecholamine metabolite is least affected by various interfering substances including antihypertensive drugs.[283] The ranges and sensitivities for the three urinary tests reported in multiple series are shown in Table 28–12, showing the superiority of the metanephrine assay.[284] Urinary metanephrine excretion will be increased if patients are taking sympathomimetic drugs, monoamine oxidase inhibitors, or the alpha- and beta-adrenoceptor blocker labetalol.[285] Interference with the measurement of metanephrine may occur for the next few days after use of x-ray contrast media

TABLE 28–12 URINARY TESTS FOR PHEOCHROMOCYTOMA

COMPOUND	URINARY EXCRETION (mg/day or μg/mg creatinine)		NO. OF PATIENTS WITH TUMOR	% PATIENTS WITH TUMOR CORRECTLY IDENTIFIED
	Normal Adults	Pheochromocytoma		
Free catecholamines	< 0.1	0.1 to 10.0	179	85
Metanephrine + normetanephrine	< 1.2	1.0 to 100.0	282	96
Vanillylmandelic acid	< 6.5	5 to 600	294	84

From Manu, P., and Runge, L. A.: Biocemical screening for pheochromocytoma: Superiority of urinary metanephrines measurements. Am. J. Epidemiol. *120*:788, 1984.

containing methylglucamine (e.g., Renografin, Hypaque) leading to a falsely low value. Therefore, the urine should be collected before an intravenous pyelogram or other such procedure is done.

If urine assays are equivocal, measurement of a plasma norepinephrine level three hours after a single 0.3 mg oral dose of the adrenergic inhibitor clonidine has been shown to separate the nonpheochromocytoma patients, whose levels are suppressed, from those with disease, whose levels are not suppressed.[286]

LOCALIZATION OF THE TUMOR. Once the diagnosis has been made, medical therapy should be started and tumor localized by CT scan, which usually demonstrates these typically large tumors with ease. Radioisotopes that localize in chromaffin tissue are available and are of additional help in the few patients in whom localization is not possible by CT.[283]

THERAPY. Once diagnosed and localized, pheochromocytomas should be resected. Great care should be taken in preparing patients for operation and managing them through the procedure.[287] The most important part of their preoperative management is adrenoceptor blockade sufficient to overcome vasoconstriction and allow the reduced blood volume to reexpand. If the tumor is unresectable, chronic medical therapy with the alpha blocker phenoxybenzamine (Dibenzyline) or the inhibitor of catechol synthesis α-methyl-tyrosine (Demser) can be used.

CONGENITAL ADRENAL HYPERPLASIA

Two distinct enzymatic defects may induce hypertension: (1) *11-hydroxylase deficiency,* which leads to virilization (from excessive androgens) and hypertension with hypokalemia (from excessive DOC). A partial deficiency has been recognized in 15 patients with what appeared to be ordinary primary hypertension[288] and in women with only hirsutism or menstrual irregularities.[289] (2) *17-Hydroxylase deficiency,* which also causes hypertension from excess DOC, but, in addition, causes failure of secondary sexual development because sex hormones are also deficient.[290] Affected children are hypertensive, but the defect in sex hormone synthesis may not become obvious until after puberty. Thereafter, affected males display ambiguity of sexual development and fail to mature.

OTHER CAUSES OF HYPERTENSION

A host of other causes of hypertension are known (Table 28–4). One that is likely becoming more common is ingestion of various drugs—prescribed (e.g., cyclosporine[291] and erythropoietin[292]), over the counter (e.g., phenylpropanolamine[293]), and illicit (e.g., cocaine).

COARCTATION OF THE AORTA (see pp. 920 and 967)

Congenital narrowing of the aorta may occur at any level of the thoracic or abdominal aorta. It is usually found just beyond the origin of the left subclavian artery or distal to the insertion of the ligamentum arteriosum. The coarctation may be localized or more diffuse. Other cardiac anomalies usually accompany the latter, giving rise to considerable mortality during the first year of life, although operative treatment of both the coarctation and associated anomalies may reduce this mortality rate. With less severe postductal lesions, damage is more insidious, and symptoms may not appear until the teenage years or later.

Hypertension in the arms and weak or absent femoral pulses are the classic features of coarctation. The pathogenesis of the hypertension may be more complicated than simple mechanical obstruction; a generalized vasoconstrictor mechanism is likely to be involved, which may be either renin-angiotensin or sympathetic nervous activity.[294] The lesion may be detected by two-dimensional echocardiography (Fig. 31–28, p. 920), and aortography proves the diagnosis (Fig. 31–29, p. 920). To diminish the development of congestive heart failure, endocarditis, and stroke, the obstruction should be corrected in early childhood.[295] Immediately after surgical repair, the blood pressure may transiently rise even further, and mesenteric arteritis may develop. These changes may reflect very high levels of renin-angiotensin and catecholamines and can be prevented by the prophylactic use of beta blockers.[296]

HYPERPARATHYROIDISM (see p. 1841)

As noted earlier, calcium may be intimately involved in the pathogenesis of primary hypertension, and increased levels of parathyroid hormone may be present as a response to a urinary calcium leak. In addition, hypertension occurs in over one-half of patients with hyperparathyroidism[297] and is found commonly in patients with other hypercalcemic states. As more patients are found to be hypertensive and undergo routine testing of serum calcium, asymptomatic hypercalcemia associated with hyperparathyroidism is not infrequently recognized. Moreover, thiazide diuretics—the most frequently used drug in the treatment of hypertension—may accentuate previously borderline hypercalcemia.

The mechanism by which hypercalcemia elevates blood pressure probably involves a direct increase in the contractility of vascular smooth muscle and activation of the sympathetic nervous system.[298] After surgical correction of hyperparathyroidism, hypertension usually persists.[297,298]

HYPERTENSION AFTER HEART SURGERY

(See also p. 1677)

Transient hypertension may develop postoperatively for various reasons: pain, physical and emotional excitement, hypoxia, hypercapnia, and excessive volume loads.[299] More severe hypertension has been noted to follow a number of cardiovascular surgical procedures:

1. *Coronary bypass surgery.* The incidence, exceeding 33 per cent, is far higher than after other major cardiac or noncardiac surgery. The problem appears more commonly on the background of preexisting hypertension, greater than 50 per cent obstruction of the left main coronary artery, or the preoperative use of beta blockers. The hemodynamic pattern of increased peripheral resistance can be explained by the markedly elevated plasma catecholamine levels measured in such patients in the presence of renin-angiotensin levels that are not increased.[300] In those patients who had previously received beta blocker therapy, the postoperative hypertension may also reflect a rebound phenomenon. Therefore, continuation of beta blocker therapy through the perioperative period is likely to reduce the frequency of the problem. If it occurs, therapy is often required: intravenous nitroprusside, labetalol,[301] and the calcium antagonists nifedipine or nicardipine[302] are all effective.
2. *Aortic valve replacement.* Transient hypertension may give way to more permanent hypertension. In one series, 53 per cent of 116 patients were hypertensive five years after surgery, and hypertension was a major determinant of late failure of the homograft valve.
3. *Closure of an atrial septal defect.*
4. *Cardiac transplantation.* With current immunosuppression using cyclosporine and high doses of adrenal steroids, hypertension is almost invariable and can be resistant to intensive therapy.[303] Fortunately, with effective antihypertensive therapy, left ventricular hypertrophy may be prevented.[304]

Special Topics in Hypertension

HYPERTENSION DURING PREGNANCY

Hypertension appearing during the latter third of pregnancy or immediately after delivery in a previously normotensive nonproteinuric woman, previously called preeclampsia or pregnancy-induced hypertension, is now termed *gestational hypertension.*[305] This disorder should be distinguished from chronic hypertension and renal disease. Both may progress into eclampsia, defined as the occurrence of convulsions. Gestational hypertension is of unknown cause but occurs more frequently in primigravid women with a positive family history of the syndrome[306] and in women with trisomy 13,[307] suggesting a genetic mechanism. Immunologic incompatibility between mother and fetus and a higher incidence of racial dissimilarity of the parents may play a role.[308] Additional predisposing factors include increased age, black race, multiple gestations, concomitant heart or renal disease, and chronic hypertension.[309] In the population in which these factors were identified, diabetes mellitus did not play a significant independent role as a predisposing factor.

TABLE 28–13 DIFFERENCES BETWEEN PREECLAMPSIA AND CHRONIC HYPERTENSION

	PREECLAMPSIA	CHRONIC HYPERTENSION
Age	Young (< 20)	Older (> 30)
Parity	Primigravida	Multipara
Onset	After 20 weeks of pregnancy	Before 20 weeks of pregnancy
Weight gain and edema	Sudden	Gradual
Systolic blood pressure	< 160	> 160
Funduscopic findings	Spasm, edema	Arteriovenous nicking, exudates
Proteinuria	Present	Absent
Plasma uric acid	Increased	Normal
Blood pressure after delivery	Normal	Elevated

CLINICAL FEATURES. The features shown in Table 28–13 should help distinguish gestational hypertension from chronic, primary hypertension. The distinction should be made since management and prognosis are different: Gestational hypertension is self-limited and rarely recurs in subsequent pregnancies, whereas chronic hypertension progresses and usually complicates all pregnancies. The separation may be difficult because of a lack of knowledge of pre-pregnancy blood pressure and because of the usual tendency for high pressures to fall considerably during the middle trimester, so that hypertension present before pregnancy may not be recognized.

In gestational hypertension, the blood pressure usually rises only late in pregnancy. Among 84 patients with the onset of hypertension before 37 weeks gestation, 55 had renal disease documented by kidney biopsy six months postpartum when morphological changes due solely to gestational hypertension should have subsided.[310] Gestational hypertension was the diagnosis in only 10 per cent of primiparous women with onset of hypertension before 37 weeks, whereas it was the diagnosis in three-fourths of primigravid women with onset of hypertension after 37 weeks.

The hemodynamic features of gestational hypertension are a further rise in cardiac output than that usually seen in normal pregnancy accompanied by an inappropriately high peripheral resistance.[311] The mother may be particularly vulnerable to encephalopathy because of her previously normal blood pressure. As is described in more detail on p. 844, cerebral blood flow is normally maintained constant over a fairly narrow range of mean arterial pressure, roughly between 60 and 100 mm Hg in normotensive individuals. In a previously normotensive young woman, an acute rise in blood pressure to 150/100 mm Hg may exceed the upper limit of autoregulation, resulting in a "breakthrough" of cerebral blood flow (acute dilation) that leads to cerebral edema, convulsions, and all of the clinical manifestations of eclampsia.[312, 313] Other findings may help predict gestational hypertension, including the blood pressure response to the roll-over test,[306] plasma concentrations of fibronectin derived from endothelial cells,[314] and the urine calcium/creatinine ratio.[306]

PATHOGENESIS. The common factor that predisposes to development of gestational hypertension is *reduced uteroplacental perfusion.* Although disturbances in the renin-angiotensin system may be involved,[315] increasing attention has been directed toward the possible role of disturbed prostaglandin relationships, either as the cause of or as a consequence of uteroplacental hypoperfusion.[316] Either increased activity of the lipoxygenase pathway or decreased production of prostacyclin by the fetal-placental unit could lead to the various clinical manifestations of the syndrome (Fig. 28–21). Decreased synthesis of prostacyclin may precede the appearance of hypertension.[317] Inhibition of prostacyclin production could be induced by the higher concentrations of progesterone in placentas of women with gestational hypertension.[318]

Whether or not this scheme explains the pathogenesis, small doses of aspirin, in the range of 40 to 100 mg/d, which reduce thromboxane but have little effect on prostacyclin,[319] prevent development of gestational hypertension in women at high risk for the syndrome.[320,321] Ingestion of aspirin during the first trimester of pregnancy was not associated with an increased risk of congenital heart defects,[322] and the low doses of aspirin (40 to 100 mg per day) being used maintain hemostatic competence in the fetus;[320] therefore, larger trials of low-dose aspirin are clearly indicated. At present, however, the FDA has advised women in the last trimester to avoid all aspirin-containing products to prevent excessive bleeding during delivery.

Other physiological abnormalities may be involved in the pathogenesis of gestational hypertension. In keeping with its probable role in other hypertensive states (see p. 828), hyperinsulinemia is present in half of women with hypertension during the third trimester.[323] Plasma levels of atrial natriuretic peptide (ANP, p. 829) are higher during normal pregnancy but no higher in those with gestational hypertension.[324] A reduction of the Na^+,K^+-ATPase pump in red blood cells of pregnant women with gestational hypertension and an increase in intracellular sodium that would be expected to accompany inhibition of the pump have been reported.[325] Possibly related to this, platelet intracellular free calcium concentrations are higher in primigravid women with gestational hypertension.[326]

TREATMENT

GESTATIONAL HYPERTENSION. Women with gestational hypertension and their fetuses can be protected from excessive morbidity and mortality by maneuvers that lower the blood pressure without impairing uteroplacental perfusion.[327] These maneuvers include modified bed rest, a nutritious diet with normal amounts of sodium, and antihypertensive agents when diastolic blood pressure above 100 mm Hg indicates impairment of renal function and predisposition to overt eclampsia. Low-dose aspirin will probably be used increasingly.

The traditional drug therapy of gestational hypertension remote from term has been methyldopa and, if a parenteral agent is needed closer to the time of delivery, hydralazine. Equally good or better experience has been reported with beta-blockers,[328] the alpha-blocker prazosin,[329] the combined alpha- and beta-blocker labetalol,[330] and the calcium antago-

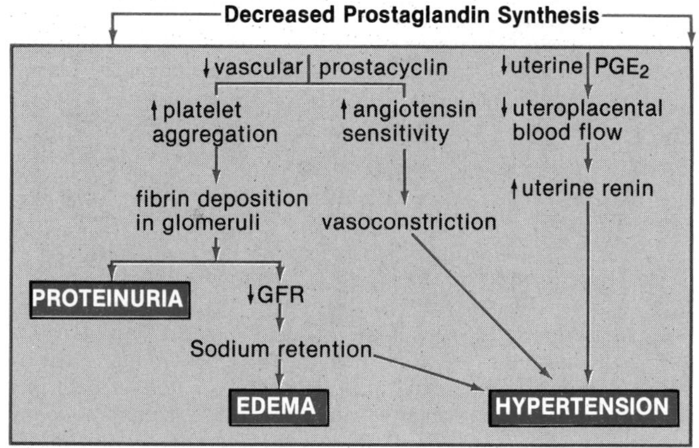

FIGURE 28–21. A scheme for the pathogenesis of gestational hypertension with proteinuria and edema based upon decreased prostaglandin synthesis.

nist nifedipine.[331] Caution remains necessary with the use of angiotensin-converting enzyme inhibitors.[332] In addition, the use of atenolol has been associated with intrauterine growth retardation.[332a]

Despite these generally favorable reports, caution is advised in the use of drugs for mild gestational hypertension. In one of the few controlled studies comparing modified bed rest versus antihypertensive drug therapy, half of 200 primigravid women with relatively mild hypertension at 26 to 35 weeks gestation were given labetalol and the other half were monitored while in the hospital.[333] Those given labetalol had a significant fall in blood pressure whereas the controls did not, but those in both groups had some worsening of renal function. However, the number of small-for-gestational age infants was higher in the labetalol group (19 versus 9 per cent). Thus, drug treatment of maternal blood pressure did not improve perinatal outcome and was associated with fetal growth retardation.

CHRONIC HYPERTENSION. If pregnancy begins while a woman is on antihypertensive drug therapy, the medications, including diuretics, are usually continued, on the basis of the belief that the mother should be protected and that the fetus will not suffer from any sudden hemodynamic shifts such as occur when therapy is first begun. Among women with chronic hypertension who were not undergoing treatment, therapy with either hydralazine or methyldopa significantly reduced the incidence of gestational hypertension when compared with that in a placebo-treated group.[334] However, despite treatment with drugs, the incidence of fetal growth retardation remains higher in patients with chronic hypertension.[335]

MANAGEMENT OF ECLAMPSIA. With appropriate care of gestational hypertension, eclampsia hardly ever supervenes; when it does, however, maternal and fetal mortality remain very high.[336] Although excellent results have been reported with the use of magnesium sulfate,[337] the English recommend intravenous diazepam to control convulsions.[336] Patients with severe eclampsia who have persistent oliguria after a fluid challenge should undergo hemodynamic monitoring, since management may require additional volume or a reduction in preload or afterload.[338]

CONSEQUENCES OF PREGNANCY-RELATED HYPERTENSION. The long-term prognosis of women with gestational hypertension is excellent. When 200 women with the most severe form, eclampsia, were followed for up to 44 years, the distribution of blood pressure was identical to that in the general population.[339] Chesley concludes that "eclampsia neither is a sign of latent essential hypertension nor causes hypertension." The long-term mortality rate in black women having eclampsia and of white women having eclampsia as multiparas is increased, probably because they had underlying but previously unrecognized chronic hypertension or renal disease.

After delivery, women may develop transient or persistent hypertension. In many, early primary hypertension may have been masked by the hemodynamic changes of pregnancy. Some women develop postpartum heart failure that may be an idiopathic cardiomyopathy but is usually related to hypertension, preexisting heart disease, or complications of pregnancy.[340] A small number develop rapidly progressive acute oliguric renal failure associated with severe hypertension.

HYPERTENSION IN CHILDREN AND ADOLESCENTS

(See also Ch. 33)

The linkage between hypertension in children and adolescents and that in adults is being strengthened, but long-term tracking studies are not available to document the natural history of the process. As an example, taken from the description of abnormal sodium transport in the pathogenesis of primary hypertension earlier in this chapter (p. 826), half the normotensive children of hypertensive parents have the abnormality,[96] but it will take another 30 or more years to determine whether the abnormality presages the development of hypertension.

TABLE 28–14 EPIDEMIOLOGIC FACTORS RELATED TO BLOOD PRESSURE LEVELS IN CHILDREN AND ADOLESCENTS

Factors
Genetic
Parental and sibling blood pressure levels
Erythrocyte sodium flux
Urinary kallikrein level
Haptoglobin phenotype 1-1
Environmental
Socioeconomic status
Rural vs. urban residence
Migration from developing area
Pulse rate
Small for gestational age (SGA)
Mixed genetic and environmental
Height
Weight
Muscle mass
Sodium/potassium excretion
Stress
Skinfold thickness

From Lieberman, E.: *In* Kaplan, N. M. (ed.): Clinical Hypertension. 5th ed. Baltimore, © by Williams and Wilkins, 1990, p. 414.

As in adults, care is needed in establishing the presence of persistently elevated blood pressures in children using the upper limits of normal shown in Table 28–3. Recall that only 38 per cent of 10- to 14-year-olds initially in the upper quartile remained in the upper quartile 4 years later.[27] Children who have the highest pressures tend to be larger and more mature, with higher levels of adrenal androgen secretion.[341] Obesity is associated with higher levels of pressure,[342] although children who are thin and in the upper range of blood pressure levels tend to remain at that high level, more than do those who are obese.[27] Additional factors related to blood pressure levels are listed in Table 28–14. Interestingly, blood pressures among healthy black children are not higher—and may be lower—than those seen among white children.[343] Thus, the reason for the greater incidence of hypertension in black adults must be sought among factors that are active mainly beyond adolescence or that have a long "incubation."

PRIMARY (ESSENTIAL) HYPERTENSION. When asymptomatic children with persistently elevated pressures are studied, most are found to have no recognizable secondary cause. In the Muscatine survey, 23 of the 41 with high pressures were obese; of the 18 lean subjects, 13 had primary hypertension.[344] The *hemodynamic profile* in children with primary hypertension is similar to that of adults in that an elevated peripheral vascular resistance is the major finding.[345] Thus, hypertension in children does not usually fit a "hyperdynamic" pattern, with high cardiac output and fast pulse rates. Nonetheless, normotensive children of hypertensive parents, who are thereby more likely to develop hypertension, often show a greater cardiovascular response to mental and other types of stress than do normotensive children of normotensive parents.[99]

Cardiac effects of even relatively small elevations in blood pressure may be found by echocardiography: Heart size and contractile functions are significantly increased in comparison to findings in normotensive subjects of the same age.[345] Abnormal patterns of left ventricular filling have been noted on pulsed Doppler examinations in children with only mildly elevated blood pressures.[345] Whether these changes are a cause or an effect of the elevated pressures remains uncertain, as does their relationship to the subjects' subsequent cardiovascular status.

SECONDARY HYPERTENSION IN CHILDREN. As more experience is gained, the need for extensive laboratory workup for the majority of postpubertal children with relatively mild hypertension continues to be deemphasized.[26] Only those with moderate or severe hypertension (i.e., 10 mm Hg or more above the 95th percentile for their age and sex) or an abnormality on initial laboratory screening studies (i.e., elevated serum creatinine) need to undergo additional testing. Most instances of hypertension in children have no apparent cause, but when diastolic pressure exceeds 120 mm Hg, approximately 95 per cent will have secondary hypertension. Thus, it seems appropriate to investigate more thoroughly only those hypertensive children with abnormalities on the physical examination or on urinalysis and those with a blood pressure level 10 mm Hg or more above the 95th percentile.[346]

The proper therapy for children with hypertension remains uncertain.[347] In general, the guidelines for treatment of adult hypertension provided in the next chapter are appropriate for the young, although a longer trial of weight reduction and sodium restriction seems indicated before drug treatment is begun.[26] The long-term effects of various antihypertensive agents need to be more carefully assessed.

HYPERTENSION IN THE ELDERLY

As more people live longer, more predominantly systolic and combined systolic and diastolic hypertension will be seen. Earlier, we noted the high frequency and risks of systolic hypertension among the elderly.[347a,347b] To a large extent, the progressive rise in systolic pressure reflects a loss of compliance within the major arteries due to permanent sclerosis; therapy may be either ineffectual, since vasodilation may not be possible, or poorly tolerated, since a shrinkage of fluid volume or decrease in cardiac output may diminish blood flow to the brain. Baroreceptor sensitivity often decreases with age, so that the buffering effect of this reflex with changes in posture and the like may be lost; elderly people may experience a greater fall in blood pressure upon standing as well as a propensity for postprandial hypotension.[19] In elderly patients with significant hypertension of recent onset, chronic renal disease or atherosclerotic renovascular disease may be a cause of the elevated blood pressure. The elderly present a number of special therapeutic challenges which will be covered in the next chapter.

HYPERTENSIVE CRISES

DEFINITIONS. A number of clinical circumstances may require rapid reduction of the blood pressure (Table 28–15). These may be separated into *emergencies*, which require immediate reduction of blood pressure (within one hour) and *urgencies*, which can be treated more slowly. A persistent diastolic pressure exceeding 130 mm Hg is often associated with acute vascular damage; some patients may suffer vascular damage from lower levels of pressure, while others manage to withstand even higher levels without apparent harm. As discussed below, the rapidity of the rise may be more important than the absolute level in producing acute vascular damage. Therefore, in practice, all patients with diastolic blood pressures above 130 mm Hg should be treated, some more rapidly with parenteral drugs, others more slowly with oral agents, as described on p. 870.

When the rise in pressure causes acute damage to retinal vessels, the term *accelerated-malignant hypertension* is used. The separation has been based upon the presence of retinal hemorrhages or exudates (accelerated) and papilledema (malignant). The clinical features and survival rates of those with or without papilledema are so similar that there is no reason to separate the two.[348]

Hypertensive encephalopathy is characterized by headache, irritability, alterations in consciousness, and other manifestations of central nervous dysfunction with sudden and marked elevations in blood pressure. Symptoms can be reversed by a reduction in the pressure.

TABLE 28–15 CIRCUMSTANCES REQUIRING RAPID TREATMENT OF HYPERTENSION

***Hypertensive Emergencies*:**
- **Cerebrovascular**
  - **Hypertensive encephalopathy (any cause)**
  - **Intracerebral hemorrhage**
  - **Subarachnoid hemorrhage**
  - **Atherothrombotic brain infarction with severe hypertension**
  - **Malignant hypertension (some cases)**
- **Cardiac**
  - **Acute aortic dissection**
  - **Acute left ventricular failure**
  - **Acute coronary insufficiency**
  - **After coronary bypass surgery**
- **Others**
  - **Excessive circulating catecholamines:**
    - **Pheochromocytoma crisis**
    - **Food or drug interactions with monoamine oxidase inhibitors**
  - **Head injury**
  - **Postoperative bleeding from vascular suture lines**
  - **Severe epistaxis**

***Hypertensive Urgencies*:**
- **Accelerated and malignant hypertension**
- **Rebound hypertension after sudden cessation of antihypertensive drugs**
- **Surgical**
  - **Severe hypertension in patients requiring immediate surgery**
  - **Postoperative hypertension**
  - **Severe hypertension after kidney transplantation**
- **Severe body burns**

From Kaplan, N. M.: Clinical Hypertension. 4th ed. Baltimore, © by Williams and Wilkins, 1986, p. 386.

INCIDENCE. In about 1 per cent of patients with primary hypertension, the disease progresses to an accelerated-malignant phase. Presumably, if the condition were left untreated, many more patients would follow this pattern, since the incidence was higher before effective therapies became available and seems to be decreasing steadily.[349]

Any hypertensive disease can initiate a crisis. Some, including pheochromocytoma and renovascular hypertension, do so at a higher rate than does primary hypertension. However, since hypertension is of unknown cause in over 90 per cent of all patients, most hypertensive crises appear in the setting of preexisting primary hypertension.[349]

PATHOPHYSIOLOGY. Whenever blood pressure rises and remains above a critical level, various processes set off a series of local and systemic effects that cause further rises in pressure and vascular damage (Fig. 28–22). Two distinct but usually concurrent processes are involved in the pathogenesis of hypertensive encephalopathy. One is *functional*, i.e., dilatation of cerebral arterioles, allowing excessive cerebral blood flow that leads to hypertensive encephalopathy.[350] The other is *structural*, i.e., acute damage to the arteriolar wall, resulting in increased permeability. Both processes are most likely the consequences of high blood pressure and may develop without apparent involvement of the renin-angiotensin-aldosterone or other hormonal mechanisms.

Studies in animals and humans by Strandgaard and associates have elucidated the mechanism of encephalopathy.[350] First, they directly measured the caliber of pial arterioles over the cerebral cortex in cats whose blood pressure was varied over a wide range by infusion of vasodilators or angiotensin II. As the pressure fell, the arterioles became dilated; as the pressure rose, they become constricted. Thus, a constant cerebral blood flow was maintained by means of autoregulation, which is dependent upon the cerebral sympathetic nerves. However, when mean arterial pressure rose above 180 mm Hg, the tightly constricted vessels could no longer withstand the pressure and suddenly dilated. This began in an irregular manner, first in areas with less muscle tone and then diffusely, producing generalized vasodilatation. This "breakthrough" of cerebral blood flow hyperperfuses the brain under high pressure, causing leakage of fluid into the perivascular tissue and resulting in cerebral edema and the syndrome of hypertensive encephalopathy. The vessel walls, in reaction to this excessive pressure, probably contribute to the injury by generating toxic superoxide anion radicals from accelerated arachidonate metabolism.[351]

In human subjects, cerebral blood flow was measured repetitively by an isotopic technique while blood pressure was lowered or raised with vasodilators or vasoconstrictors in a manner similar to that employed in the animal studies.[350] Curves depicting cerebral blood flow as a function of arterial pressure demonstrated autoregulation with a constancy of flow over mean pressures in normotensive persons from about 60 to 120 mm Hg and in hypertensive patients from about 110 to 180 mm Hg. This "shift to the right" in hypertensive patients is the result of structural thickening of the arterioles as an adaptation to the chronically elevated pressures. When pressures were raised beyond the upper limit of autoregulation, the same "breakthrough" with hyperperfusion occurred as was seen in the animal studies. In previously normotensive persons whose vessels have not been altered by prior exposure to high pressure, breakthrough occurred at a mean arterial pressure of about 120 mm Hg; in hypertensive patients, the breakthrough occurred at about 180 mm Hg.

These studies confirm clinical observations. In previously normotensive persons, severe encephalopathy occurs with relatively little hypertension. In children with acute glomerulonephritis and in women with eclampsia, convulsions may occur owing to hypertensive encephalopathy with blood pressures as low as 150/100 mm Hg. Obviously, chronically hypertensive patients withstand such pressures without difficulty; however, when pressures increase significantly, they too may develop encephalopathy.

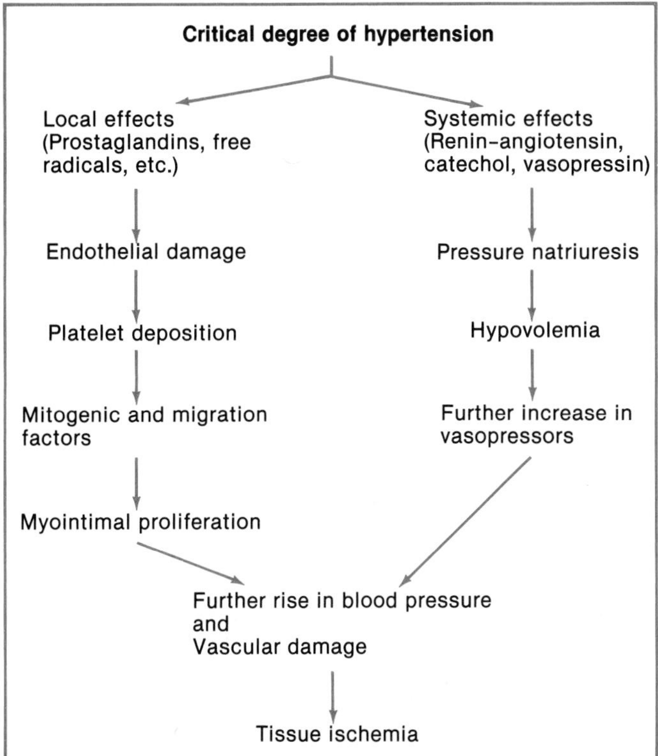

FIGURE 28-22. A scheme for the initiation and progression of malignant hypertension. (From Kaplan, N. M.: Clinical Hypertension. 5th ed. Baltimore, © by Williams and Wilkins, 1990, p. 269.)

TABLE 28-16 CLINICAL CHARACTERISTICS OF HYPERTENSIVE CRISIS

Blood pressure: Usually > 140 mm Hg diastolic
Funduscopic findings: Hemorrhages, exudates, papilledema
Neurological status: Headache, confusion, somnolence, stupor, visual loss, focal deficits, seizures, coma
Cardiac findings: Prominent apical impulse, cardiac enlargement, congestive failure
Renal: Oliguria, azotemia
Gastrointestinal: Nausea, vomiting

From Kaplan, N. M.: Clinical Hypertension. 5th ed. Baltimore, © by Williams and Wilkins, 1990, p. 269.

MANIFESTATIONS AND COURSE. The symptoms and signs of hypertensive crises are usually dramatic (Table 28-16). However, some patients may be relatively asymptomatic, despite markedly elevated pressures and extensive organ damage. Young black men are particularly prone to hypertensive crisis with severe renal insufficiency but little obvious prior distress. When the blood pressure is so high as to induce encephalopathy or accelerated-malignant hypertension, the following clinical features are frequently present:

1. Renal insufficiency with protein and red cells in the urine and azotemia; acute oliguric renal failure may also develop.
2. Elevated levels of plasma renin from the diffuse intrarenal ischemia, resulting in secondary aldosteronism, often manifested by hypokalemia. Although not causal, the secondarily elevated renin and aldosterone levels most likely exacerbate the hypertensive process.
3. Microangiopathic hemolytic anemia with red cell fragmentation and intravascular coagulation.
4. Cardiac size and function may *not* be abnormal in those who suddenly develop malignant hypertension.[352]

If left untreated, patients die quickly from brain damage or more gradually from renal damage. Before effective therapy was available, less than 25 per cent of patients with malignant hypertension survived one year and only 1 per cent survived five years. With therapy including renal dialysis, over 90 per cent survive one year and about 80 per cent survive five years.[353] Death in patients with severe hypertension is usually from stroke or renal failure if it occurs in the first few years

TABLE 28-17 DISEASES TO BE DIFFERENTIATED FROM A HYPERTENSIVE CRISIS

Acute left ventricular failure
Uremia from any cause, particularly with volume overload
Cerebral vascular accident
Subarachnoid hemorrhage
Brain tumor
Head injury
Epilepsy (postictal)
Collagen diseases, particularly lupus, with cerebral vasculitis
Encephalitis
Overdose and withdrawal from narcotics, amphetamines, and so on
Hypercalcemia
Acute anxiety with hyperventilation syndrome

after onset. If therapy keeps patients alive for longer than five years, death will usually be due to coronary artery disease, in which factors other than the high pressure per se are probably also involved.

DIFFERENTIAL DIAGNOSIS. The presence of hypertensive encephalopathy or accelerated-malignant hypertension demands immediate, aggressive therapy to lower blood pressure effectively. Except in pregnancy or in catecholamine excess, therapy may be instituted before the specific cause is known. However, certain serious diseases as well as psychogenic problems, i.e., acute anxiety with hyperventilation or panic attacks,[354] can mimic a hypertensive crisis (Table 28–17), and management of these conditions obviously requires different diagnostic and therapeutic approaches. In particular, blood pressure should not be lowered too abruptly in a patient with a stroke.[355] Specific therapy of hypertensive crises is described on p. 870.

REFERENCES

DEFINITIONS, PREVALENCE, AND CONSEQUENCES OF HYPERTENSION

1. Levy, D., Wilson, P. W. F., Anderson, K. M., and Castelli W. P.: Stratifying the patient at risk from coronary disease: New insights from the Framingham Heart Study. Am. Heart J. *119*:712, 1990.
2. Subcommittee on Definition and Prevalence of the 1984 Joint National Committee: Hypertension prevalence and the status of awareness, treatment, and control in the United States. Hypertension *7*:457, 1985.
3. Working Group on Risk and High Blood Pressure: An epidemiological approach to describing risk associated with blood pressure levels. Hypertension *7*:641, 1985.
4. Kaplan, N. M.: Clinical Hypertension, 5th ed. Baltimore, Williams and Wilkins, 1990.
5. Gross, T. P., Wise, R. P., and Knapp, D. E.: Antihypertensive drug use: Trends in the United States from 1973 to 1985. Hypertension *13*(Suppl. I):I, 1989.
6. Bonita, R., and Beaglehole, R.: Increased treatment of hypertension does not explain the decline in stroke mortality in the United States, 1970–1980. Hypertension 13:(Suppl I):I, 1989.
7. Pickering, T. G.: The clinical significance of diurnal blood pressure variations: Dippers and nondippers. Circulation *81*:700, 1990.
8. Irvine, M. J., Garner, D. M., Olmsted, M. P., and Logan, A. G.: Personality differences between hypertensive and normotensive individuals: Influence of knowledge of hypertension status. Psychosom. Med. *51*:537, 1989.
9. Pickering, T. G., James, G. D., Boddie, C., et al: How common is white coat hypertension? JAMA *259*:225, 1988.
10. Evans, C. E., Haynes, R. B., Goldsmith, C. H., and Hewson, S. A.: Home blood pressure-measuring devices: A comparative study of accuracy. J. Hypertens. *7*:133, 1989.
11. Prisant L. M., and Carr, A. A.: Ambulatory blood pressure monitoring and echocardiographic left ventricular wall thickness and mass. Am J. Hypertens. *3*:81, 1990.
12. Mejia, A. D., Egan, B. M., Schork, N. J., and Zweifler, A. J.: Artefacts in measurement of blood pressure and lack of target organ involvement in the assessment of patients with treatment-resistant hypertension. Ann. Intern. Med. *11*:270, 1990.
13. Saito, I., Takeshita, E., Hayashi, S., et al.: Comparison of clinic and home blood pressure levels and the role of the sympathetic nervous system in clinic-home differences. Am. J. Hypertens. *3*:219, 1990.
14. Muller, J. E., Tofler, G. H., and Stone, P. H.: Circadian variation and triggers of onset of acute cardiovascular disease. Circulation *79*:733, 1989.
15. Froom, P., Bar-David, M., Ribak, J., et al.: Predictive value of systolic blood pressure in young men for elevated systolic blood pressure 12 to 15 years later. Circulation *68*:467, 1983.
16. Menotti, A., Seccareccia, F., Giampaoli, S., and Giuli, B.: The predictive role of systolic, diastolic and mean blood pressures on cardiovascular and all causes of death. J. Hypertens. *7*:595, 1989.
17. Kannel, W. B.: Contribution of the Framingham Study to preventive cardiology. J. Am. Coll. Cardiol. *15*:206, 1990.
18. Tjoa, H. I., and Kaplan, N. M.: Treatment of hypertension in the elderly. JAMA *264*:1015, 1990.
19. Lye, M., Vargas, E., Faragher, E. B., et al: Haemodynamic and neurohumoral responses in elderly patients with postural hypotension. Eur. J. Clin. Invest. *20*:90, 1990.
20. 1988 Joint National Committee: The 1988 Report of the Joint National Committee on Detection, Evaluation, and Treatment of High Blood Pressure. Arch. Intern. Med. *148*:1023, 1988.
21. The Pooling Project Research Group: Relationship of blood pressure, serum cholesterol, smoking habit, relative weight and ECG abnormalities to incidence of major coronary events: Final report of the pooling project. J. Chronic Dis. *31*:201, 1978.
22. McClellan, W., Neel, J., and Owen, S.: Correlates of drug therapy of diastolic blood pressure between 80–89 mm Hg by physicians in the community. Am. J. Hypertens. *2*:869, 1989.
23. Report of the British Hypertension Society working party: Treating mild hypertension. Agreement from the large trials. Br. Med. J. *298*:694, 1989.
24. WHO/ISH: 1989 guidelines for the management of mild hypertension: Memorandum from a WHO/ISH meeting. J. Hypertens. *7*:689, 1989.
25. Hypertension Detection and Follow-up Program Cooperative Group: Blood pressure studies in 14 communities. A two-stage screen for hypertension. JAMA *237*:2385, 1977.
26. Lieberman, E.: Hypertension in childhood and adolescence. *In* Kaplan, N. M. (ed.): Clinical Hypertension, 5th ed. Baltimore, Williams and Wilkins, 1990, p. 407.
27. Burke, G. L., Freedman, D. S., Webber, L. S., and Berenson, G. S.: Persistence of high diastolic blood pressure in thin children: The Bogalusa heart study. Hypertension *8*:24, 1986.
28. National Center for Health Statistics, Rowland, W., and Roberts, J. (eds.): Blood Pressure Levels and Hypertension in Persons Aged 6–74 Years: United States, 1976–80. Advance Data From Vital and Health Statistics, No. 84, DHHS Pub. No. (PHS)82–1250. Hyattsville, MD, Public Health Service, October 8, 1982.
29. Otten, M. W., Jr., Teutsch, S. M., Williamson, D. F., and Marks, J. S.: The effect of known risk factors on the excess mortality of black adults in the United States. JAMA *263*:845, 1990.
30. Rudnick, K. V., Sackett, D. L., Hirst, S., and Holmes, C.: Hypertension in family practice. Can. Med. Assoc. J. *3*:492, 1977.
31. Danielson, M., and Dammstrom, B.: The prevalence of secondary and curable hypertension. Acta Med. Scand. *209*:451, 1981.
32. Sinclair, A. M., Isles, C. G., Brown, I., et al: Secondary hypertension in a blood pressure clinic. Arch. Intern. Med. *147*:1289, 1987.
33. Balla, J. I., Elstein, A. S., and Christensen, C.: Obstacles to acceptance of clinical decision analysis. Br. Med. J. *298*:579, 1989.
34. MacMahon, S., Peto, R., Cutler, J., et al.: Blood pressure, stroke, and coronary heart disease. Part I. Prolonged differences in blood pressure: Prospective observational studies corrected for the regression dilution bias. Lancet *335*:765, 1990.
35. Weiss, N. S.: Relation of high blood pressure to headache, epistaxis, and selected other symptoms. N. Engl. J. Med. *287*:631, 1972.
36. Cooper, W. D., Glover, D. R., Hormbrey, J. M., and Kimber, G. R.: Headache and blood pressure: Evidence of a close relationship. J. Hum. Hypertens. *3*:41, 1989.
37. Bulpitt, C. J., Dollery, C. T., and Carne, S.: Change in symptoms of hypertensive patients after referral to hospital clinic. Br. Heart J. *38*:121, 1976.
38. Hypertension Detection and Follow-Up Program Cooperative Group: The Hypertension Detection and Follow-Up Program. A progress report. Circ. Res. *40*:1, 1977.
39. Rose, G.: Strategy of prevention: Lessons from cardiovascular disease. Br. Med. J. *282*:1847, 1981.
40. Williams, R. R., Hunt, S. C., Hopkins, P. N., et al.: Familial dyslipidemic hypertension. Evidence from 58 Utah families for a syndrome present in approximately 1% of patients with essential hypertension. JAMA *259*:3579, 1988.
41. Kaplan, N. M.: The deadly quartet. Upper-body obesity, glucose intolerance, hypertriglyceridemia, and hypertension. Arch. Intern. Med. *149*:1514, 1989.
42. Pollare, T., Lithell, H., and Berne, C.: Insulin resistance is a characteristic feature of primary hypertension independent of obesity. Metabolism *39*:167, 1990.
43. Sapira, J. D.: An internist looks at the fundus oculi. Dis. Mon. *30*:1, 1984.
44. Dimmitt, S. B., Eames, S. M., Gosling, P., et al.: Usefulness of ophthalmoscopy in mild to moderate hypertension. Lancet *1*:1103, 1989.
45. Savage, D. D., Levy, D., Dannenberg, A. L., et al.: Association of echocardiographic left ventricular mass with body size, blood pressure and physical activity (the Framingham Study). Am. J. Cardiol. *65*:371, 1990.
45a. de Simone, G., Devereux, R. B., Roman, M. J., et al.: Echocardiographic left ventricular mass and electrolyte intake predict arterial hypertension. Ann. Intern. Med. *114*:202, 1991.
46. Nielsen, J. R., Oxhøj, H., and Fabricius, J.: Left ventricular structural changes in young men at increased risk of developing essential hypertension. Assessment by echocardiography. Am. J. Hypertens. *2*:885, 1989.
47. de Simone, G., Devereux, R. B., Schlussel, C. Y., et al.: Echocardiographic left ventricular mass predicts risk of developing subsequent borderline hypertension. J. Am. Coll. Cardiol. *15*:211A, 1990.
48. Verdecchia, P., Schillaci, G., Guerrieri, M., et al.: Circadian blood pressure changes and left ventricular hypertrophy in essential hypertension. Circulation *81*:528, 1990.
49. Ganau, A., Devereux, R. B., Pickering, T. G., et al.: Relation of left ventricular hemodynamic load and contractile performance to left ventricular mass in hypertension. Circulation *81*:25, 1990.
50. Devereux, R. B.: Does increased blood pressure cause left ventricular hypertrophy or vice versa? Ann. Intern. Med. *112*:157, 1990.
51. Schnall, P. L., Pieper, C., Schwartz, J. E., et al.: The relationship between "job strain," workplace diastolic blood pressure, and left ventricular mass index. JAMA *263*:1929, 1990.
52. Long, C. S., Ordahl, C. P., and Simpson, P. C.: α_1-Adrenergic receptor stimulation of sarcomeric actin isogene transcription in hypertrophy of cultured rat heart muscle cells. J. Clin. Invest. *83*:1078, 1989.
53. Nielsen, I.: Can dilated cardiomyopathy be an expression of hypertensive heart disease? Scand. J. Clin. Lab. Invest. *49*(Suppl 1):16, 1989.

53a. Koren, M. J., Devereux, R. B., Casale, P. N., et al.: Relation of left ventricular mass and geometry to morbidity and mortality in uncomplicated essential hypertension. Ann. Intern. Med. *114*:345, 1991.
54. Koren, M. J., Casale, P. N., Savage, D. D., and Laragh, J. H.: Left ventricular geometry and cardiac risk factors define high and low risk subgroups among essential hypertensives. J. Am. Coll. Cardiol. *15*:111A, 1990.
55. Cooper, R. S., Simmons, B. E., Castaner, A., et al.: Left ventricular hypertrophy is associated with worse survival independent of ventricular function and number of coronary arteries severely narrowed. Am. J. Cardiol. *65*:441, 1990.
56. Siegel, D., Cheitlin, M. D., Black, D. M., et al.: Risk of ventricular arrhythmias in hypertensive men with left ventricular hypertrophy. Am. J. Cardiol. *65*:742, 1990.
57. Agabiti-Rosei, E., Muiesan, M. L., and Muiesan, G.: Regression of structural alterations in hypertension. Am. J. Hypertens. *2*:70S, 1989.
58. Schmieder, R. E., Messerli, F. H., Sturgil, D., et al.: Cardiac performance after reduction of myocardial hypertrophy. Am. J. Med. *87*:22, 1989.
59. de Simone, G., Di Lorenzo, L., Costantino, G., et al.: Supernormal contractility in primary hypertension without left ventricular hypertrophy. Hypertension *11*:457, 1988.
60. Shepherd, R. F. J., Zachariah, P. K., and Shub, C.: Hypertension and left ventricular diastolic function. Mayo Clin. Proc. *64*:1521, 1989.
61. Karam, R., Lever, H. M., and Healy, B. P.: Hypertensive hypertrophic cardiomyopathy or hypertrophic cardiomyopathy with hypertension? A study of 78 patients. J. Am. Coll. Cardiol. *13*:580, 1989.
62. Houghton, J. L., Frank, M. J., Carr, A. A., et al.: Relations among impaired coronary flow reserve, left ventricular hypertrophy and thallium perfusion defects in hypertensive patients without obstructive coronary artery disease. J. Am. Coll. Cardiol. *15*:43, 1990.
62a. Gorlin, R.: Hypertension and ischemic heart disease: The challenge of the 1990's. Am. Heart J. *121*:658, 1991.
63. O'Kelly, B. F., Tubau, J. F., Szlachcic, J., et al.: Incidence and correlates of thallium defects in asymptomatic hypertensive patients. Circulation *80*(Suppl II):II-536, 1989.
64. Cruickshank, J. M.: Coronary flow reserve and the J curve relation between diastolic blood pressure and myocardial infarction. Br. Med. J. *297*:1227, 1988.
65. Grunfeld, B., Perelstein, E., Simsolo, R., et al.: Renal functional reserve and microalbuminuria in offspring of hypertensive parents. Hypertension *15*:257, 1990.
66. Ordonez, J. D., Hiatt, R. A., and Quesenberry, C. P. Epidemiologic features of treated end-stage renal disease in a large prepaid health plan. Am. J. Public Health *80*:47, 1990.
67. Shulman, N. B., Ford, C. E., Hall, W. D., et al.: Prognostic value of serum creatinine and effect of treatment of hypertension on renal function. Results from the Hypertension Detection and Follow-up Program. Hypertension *13*(Suppl. I):I–80, 1989.
68. Harmsen, P., Rosengren, A., Tsipogianni, A., and Wilhelmsen, L.: Risk factors for stroke in middle-aged men in Göteborg, Sweden. Stroke *21*:223, 1990.
69. Fujii, K., Sadoshima, S., Okada, Y., et al.: Cerebral blood flow and metabolism in normotensive and hypertensive patients with transient neurologic deficits. Stroke *21*:283, 1990.
70. Brunner, H. R., Laragh, J. H., Baer, L., et al.: Essential hypertension: Renin and aldosterone, heart attack and stroke. N. Engl. J. Med. *286*:441, 1972.
71. Alderman, M., Madhavan, S., Ooi, W. L., et al.: High renin/sodium pheontype predicts myocardial infarction (MI): Renin hypothesis confirmed. Circulation *80*(Suppl. II):II, 1989.
72. Management Committee: Untreated mild hypertension. Lancet *1*:185, 1982.
73. Medical Research Council Working Party: MRC trial of treatment of mild hypertension: Principal results. Br. Med. J. *291*:97, 1985.
74. Littenberg, B., Garber, A. M., and Sox, H. C., Jr.: Screening for hypertension. Ann. Intern. Med. *112*:192, 1990.
75. Chase, H. P., Garg, S., K., Harris, S., et al.: High-normal blood pressure and early diabetic nephropathy. Arch. Intern. Med. *150*:639, 1990.
76. O'Rourke, M.: Arterial stiffness, systolic blood pressure, and logical treatment of arterial hypertension. Hypertension *15*:339, 1990.
77. Lüscher, T. F., Yang, Z., Diederich, D., and Bühler, F. R.: Endothelium-derived vasoactive substances: Potential role in hypertension, atherosclerosis, and vascular occlusion. J. Cardiovasc. Pharmacol. *14*(Suppl. 6):S63, 1989.
78. Dusting, G. J., Macdonald, P. S., Higgs, E. A., and Moncada, S.: The endogenous nitrovasodilator produced by the vascular endothelium. Aust. N.Z. J. Med. *19*:493, 1989.
79. Inoue, A., Yanagisawa, M., Kimura, S., et al.: The human endothelin family: Three structurally and pharmacologically distinct isopeptides predicted by three separate genes. Proc. Natl. Acad. Sci. USA *86*:2863, 1989.
80. Takahashi, M., Yui, Y., Yasumoto, H., et al.: Lipoproteins are inhibitors of endothelium-dependent relaxation of rabbit aorta. Am. J. Physiol. *258*:H1, 1990.
81. Henry, P. D.: Hyperlipidemic arterial dysfunction. Circulation *81*:697, 1990.
82. Owens, G. K.: Control of hypertrophic versus hyperplastic growth of vascular smooth muscle cells. Am J. Physiol. *257*:H1755, 1989.
83. Lederle, F. A., Walker, J. M., and Reinke, D. B.: Selective screening for abdominal aortic aneurysms with physical examination and ultrasound. Arch. Intern. Med. *148*:1753, 1988.
84. Whelton, P. K., and Klag, M. J.: Hypertension as a risk factor for renal disease. Review of clinical and epidemiological evidence. Hypertension *13*(Suppl. I):I, 1989.
85. Falkner, B., and Kushner, H.: Effect of chronic sodium loading on cardiovascular response in young blacks and whites. Hypertension *15*:36, 1990.
86. Aviv, A., and Gardner, J.: Racial differences in ion regulation and their possible links to hypertension in blacks. Hypertension *14*:584, 1989.
87. Wilson, T.W.: History of salt supplies in West Africa and blood pressure today. Lancet *1*:784, 1986.
88. Barlow, R. J., Connel, M. A., and Milne, F. J.: A study of 48-hour faecal and urinary electrolyte excretion in normotensive black and white South African males. J. Hypertens. *401*:197, 1986.

MECHANISMS OF PRIMARY (ESSENTIAL) HYPERTENSION

89. Editorial: Catecholamines in essential hypertension. Lancet *1*:1088, 1977.
90. Pickering G.: Hypertension: Definitions, natural histories and consequences. Am. J. Med. *52*:570, 1972.
91. Lund-Johansen, P.: Central haemodynamics in essential hypertension at rest and during exercise: A 20-year follow-up study. J. Hypertens. *7*(Suppl 6):S52, 1989.
92. Andersson, O. K., Beckman-Suurküla, M., Sannerstedt, R., et al.: Does hyperkinetic circulation constitute a pre-hypertensive stage? A 5-year follow-up of haemodynamics in young men with mild blood pressure elevation. J. Intern. Med. *226*:401, 1989.
93. Julius, S., Mejia, A. D., Schork, N. J., and Krause, L. C.: Neurogenic hyperkinetic borderline hypertension (BHT) in Tecumseh, Michigan. Circulation *81*:16:1990.
94. Wenting, G. J., Man In'T Veld, A. J., and Schalekamp, M. A. D. H.: Time-course of vascular resistance changes in mineralocorticoid hypertension of man. Clinc. Sci. *61*:97, 1981.
95. Williams, R. R.: Will gene markers predict hypertension? Hypertension *14*:610, 1989.
95a. Julius S.: Autonomic nervous system dysregulation in human hypertension. Am. J. Cardiol. *67*:3B, 1991.
96. Williams, R. R., Hunt, S. C., Hasstedt, S. J., et al.: Current knowledge regarding the genetics of human hypertension. J. Hypertens. *7*(Suppl 6):S8, 1989.
97. Speers, M. A., Kasl, S. V., Freeman, D. H., and Ostfeld, A. M.: Blood pressure concordance between spouses. Am. J. Epidemiol. *123*:818, 1986.
98. Elford, J., Phillips, A., Thomson, A. G., and Shaper, A. G.: Migration and geographic variations in blood pressure in Britain. Br. Med. J. *300*:291:1990.
99. Light, K. C., Koepke, J. P., Obrist, P. A., and Willis, P. W.: Psychological stress induces sodium and fluid retention in men at high risk for hypertension. Science *220*:429, 1983.
100. Aalkjaer, C., Heagerty, A. M., Petersen, K. K., et al.: Evidence for increased media thickness, increased neuronal amine uptake, and depressed excitation-contraction coupling in isolated resistance vessels from essential hypertensives. Circ. Res. *61*:181, 1987.
101. Aalkjaer, C., Heagerty, A. M., Bailey, I., et al.: Studies of isolated resistance vessels from offspring of essential hypertensive patients. Hypertension *9*(Suppl III):III–155, 1987.
102. Folkow, B.: Structure and function of the arteries in hypertension. Am. Heart J. *114*:938, 1987.
103. Lever, A. F.: Slow pressor mechanisms in hypertension: A role for hypertrophy of resistance vessels? J. Hypertens. *4*:515, 1986.
104. Heagerty, A. M., Izzard, A. S., Ollerenshaw, J. D., and Bund, S. J.: Blood vessels and human essential hypertension. Int. J. Cardiol. *20*:15, 1988.
105. Griendling, K. K., Berk, B. C., Ganz, P., et al.: Angiotensin II stimulation of vascular smooth muscle phosphoinositide metabolism. Hypertension *9*(Suppl III)III–181, 1987.
106. Berridge, M. J.: The Croonian Lecture, 1988. Inositol lipids and calcium signalling. Proc. R. Soc. Lond. *B234*:359, 1988.
107. Björntorp, P.: Classification of obese patients and complications related to the distribution of surplus fat. Nutrition 6:131, 1990.
108. Peiris, A. N., Mueller, R. A., Smith, G. A., et al.: Splanchnic insulin metabolism in obesity: Influence of body fat distribution. J. Clin. Invest. *78*:1648, 1986.
109. Stromblad, G., and Bjorntorp, P.: Reduced hepatic insulin clearance in rats with dietary-induced obesity. Metabolism *35*:323, 1986.
110. Ostlund, R. E., Jr., Staten, M., Kohrt, W. M., et al.: The ratio of waist-to-hip circumference, plasma insulin level, and glucose intolerance as independent predictors of the HDL_2 cholesterol level in older adults. N. Engl. J. Med. *322*:229, 1990.
111. Banskota, N. K., Taub, R., Zellner, K., et al.: Characterization of induction of protooncogene-c-myc and cellular growth in human vascular smooth muscle cells by insulin and IGF-1. Diabetes *38*:123, 1989.
112. Rosic, N. K., Standaert, M. L., and Pollet, R. J.: The mechanism of insulin stimulation of (Na^+,K^+)-ATPase transport activity in muscle. J. Biol. Chem. *260*:6206, 1985.
113. Rowe, J. W., Yound, J. B., Minaker, K. L., et al.: Effect of insulin and glucose infusions on sympathetic nervous system activity in normal man. Diabetes *30*:219, 1981.
114. Baum, M.: Insulin stimulates volume absorption in the rabbit proximal convoluted tubule. J. Clin. Invest. *79*:1104, 1987.
115. Ferrannini, E., Buzzigoli, G., Bonadonna, R., et al.: Insulin resistance in essential hypertension. N. Engl. J. Med. *317*:350, 1987.
116. Swislocki, A. L. M., Hoffman, B. B., and Reaven, G. M.: Insulin resistance, glucose intolerance and hyperinsulinemia in patients with hypertension. Am. J. Hypertens. *2*:419, 1989.
117. Henrich, H. A., Romen, W., Heimgärtner, W., et al.: Capillary rarefaction

characteristics of the skeletal muscle of hypertensive patients. Klin. Wochenschr. 66:54, 1988.
118. Yang, Y. J., Hope, I. D., Ader, M., and Bergman, R. N.: Insulin transport across capillaries is rate limiting for insulin action in dogs. J. Clin. Invest. 84:1620, 1989.
119. Lillioja, S., Young, A. A., Culter, C. L., et al.: Skeletal muscle capillary density and fiber type are possible determinants of in vivo insulin resistance in man. J. Clin. Invest. 80:415, 1987.
120. Simoneau, J.- A., and Bouchard, C.: Human variation in skeletal muscle fiber-type proportion and enzyme activities. Am. J. Physiol. 257:E567, 1989.
121. Frisk-Holmberg, M., Essén, B., Fredrikson, M., et al.: Muscle fiber composition in relation to blood pressure response to isometric exercise in normotensive and hypertensive subjects. Acta Med. Scand. 213:21, 1983.
122. Larsson, L., and Ansved, T.: Effects of long-term physical training and detraining on enzyme histochemical and functional skeletal muscle characteristics in man. Muscle Nerve 8:714, 1985.
123. Pedersen, K. E., Nielsen, J., R., Klitgaard, N. A., and Johansen, T.: Sodium content and sodium efflux of mononuclear leucocytes from young subjects at increased risk of developing essential hypertension. Am. J. Hypertens. 3:182, 1990.
124. Blaustein, M. P.: Sodium/calcium exchange and the control of contractility in cardiac muscle and vascular smooth muscle. J. Cardiovasc. Pharmacol. 12(Suppl. 5):S56, 1988.
125. DeWardener, H. E., and Clarkson, E. M.: Concept of natriuretic hormone. Physiol. Rev. 65:658, 1985.
126. Bova, S., Blaustein, M. P., Harris, D. W., et al.: Effects of an endogenous digitalis-like factor (EDLF) on heart and aorta. Hypertension 16:316, 1990.
127. Jespersen, B., Eiskjaer, H., and Pedersen, E. B.: Effect of atrial natriuretic peptide on blood pressure, guanosine 3′:5′-cyclic monophosphate release and blood volume in uraemic patients. Clin. Sci. 78:67, 1990.
128. Clinkingbeard, C., Sessions, C., and Shenker, Y.: The physiological role of atrial natriuretic hormone in the regulation of aldosterone and salt and water metabolism. J. Clin. Endocrinol. Metab. 70:582, 1990.
129. Mizelle, H. L., Hall, J. E., and Hildebrandt, D. A.: Atrial natriuretic peptide and pressure natriuresis: Interactions with the renin-angiotensin system. Am. J. Physiol. 257:R1169, 1989.
130. Talartschik, J., Eisenhauer, T., Schrader, J., et al.: Low atrial natriuretic peptide plasma concentrations in 100 patients with essential hypertension. Am. J. Hypertens. 3:45, 1990.
131. Semplicini, A., Canessa, M., Mozzato, M. G., et al: Red blood cell Na^+/H^+ and Li^+/Na^+ exchange in patients with essential hypertension. Am. J. Hypertens. 2:903, 1989.
132. Hatori, N., Gardner, J. P., Tomonari, H., et al.: Na^+-H^+ antiport activity in skin fibroblasts from blacks to whites. Hypertension 15:140, 1990.
133. Postnov, Y. V.: An approach to the explanation of cell membrane alteration in primary hypertension. Hypertension 15:332, 1990.
134. Ives, H. E.: Ion transport defects and hypertension. Where is the link? Hypertension 14:590, 1989.
135. Rosati, C., Jeanclos, E., Nazaret, C., et al.: Stimulation of Na^+-H^+ exchange, the Na^+-K^+ pump and Na^+, K^+, Cl^- cotransport by endothelin-1 in cultured vascular smooth muscle cells. J. Hypertens. 7(Suppl 6):S138, 1989.
136. Gomez-Sanchez, C. E., Holland, O. B., and Upcavage R.: Urinary free 19-nor-deoxycorticosterone and deoxycorticosterone in human hypertension. J. Clin. Endocrinol. Metab. 60:234, 1985.
137. Stewart, P. M., Corrie, J. E. T., Shackleton, C. H. L., and Edwards, C. R. W.: Syndrome of apparent mineralocorticoid excess. J. Clin. Invest. 82:340, 1988.
138. Stewart, P. M., Wallace, A. M., Atherden, S. M. et al.: Mineralocorticoid activity of carbenoxolone: Contrasting effects of carbenoxolone and liquorice on 11β-hydroxysteroid dehydrogenase activity in man. Clin. Sci. 78:49, 1990.
139. Morris, D. J., Davis, E., and Latif, S. A.: Licorice, tobacco chewing, and hypertension. N. Engl. J. Med. 322:849, 1990.
140. Brenner, B. M., Garcia, D. L., and Anderson, S.: Glomeruli and blood pressure: Less of one, more the other? Am. J. Hypertens. 1:335, 1988.
141. Sealey, J. E., Blumenfeld, J. D., Bell, G. M., et al.: On the renal basis for essential hypertension: Nephron heterogeneity with discordant renin secretion and sodium excretion causing a hypertensive vasoconstriction-volume relationship. J. Hypertens 6:763, 1988.
142. Goldblatt, H.: Reflections. Urol. Clin. North Am. 2:219, 1975.
143. Williams, G. H., and Hollenberg, N. K.: Non-modulating hypertension: A subset of the sodium sensitive essential hypertension population. Hypertension (In press).
144. Tang, S.- S., Stevenson, L., and Dzau, V. J.: Endothelial renin-angiotensin pathway. Adrenergic regulation of angiotensin secretion. Circ. Res. 66:103, 1990.
145. Ferrario, C. M., Barnes, K. L., Block, C. H., et al.: Pathways of angiotensin formation and function in the brain. Hypertension 15(Suppl I):I, 1990.
146. Horiba, N., Nomura, K., and Shizume, K.: Exogenous and locally synthesized angiotensin II and glomerulosa cell functions. Hypertension 15:190, 1990.
147. Hare, G. M. T., and Osmond, D. H.: New renin-angiotensin from plasma prorenin? Am. J. Hypertens. 3:196, 1990.
148. Reeves, R. A., Shapiro, A. P., Thompson, M. E., and Johnsen, A.- M.: Loss of nocturnal decline in blood pressure after cardiac transplantation. Circulation 73:401, 1986.
149. Vincent, H. H., Boomsma, F., Man in'T Veld, A. J., and Schalekamp, M. A. D. H.: Stress levels of adrenaline amplify the blood pressure response to sympathetic stimulation. J. Hypertens. 4:255, 1986.
150. Goldsmith, S. R.: Vasopressin as vasopressor. Am. J. Med. 82:1213, 1987.
151. Robertson, J. I. S.: Serotonin and vascular disease: A survey. Cardiovasc. Drugs Ther. 4:137, 1990.
152. Oza, N. B., Schwartz, J. H., Goud, H. D., and Levinsky, N. G.: Rat aortic smooth muscle cells in culture express kallikrein, kininogen, and bradykininase activity. J. Clin. Invest. 85:597, 1990.
153. Muirhead, E. E.: Discovery of the renomedullary system of blood pressure control and its hormones. Hypertension 15:114, 1990.
154. Maheswaran, R., and Beevers, D. G.: Lead and blood pressure. J. Hypertens. 7(Suppl. 6):S381, 1989.
155. Witteman J. C. M., Willett, W. C., Stampfer, M. J., et al.: A prospective study of nutritional factors and hypertension among. U.S. women. Circulation 80:1320, 1989.
156. Jorde, L. B., Williams, R. R., and Kuida, H.: Factor analysis suggesting contrasting determinants for different blood pressure measurements. Hypertension 8:243, 1986.

ASSOCIATION WITH OTHER CONDITIONS

157. Sonne-Holm, S., Sørensen, T. I. A., Jensen, G., and Schnohr, P: Independent effects of weight change and attained body weight on prevalence of arterial hypertension in obese and non-obese men. Br. Med. J. 299:767, 1989.
158. Eisenberg, E., Zimlichman, R., and Lavie, P.: Plasma norepinephrine levels in patients with sleep apnea syndrome. N. Engl. J. Med. 322:932, 1990.
159. Jennings, G. L., Deakin, G., Dewar, E., et al.: Exercise, cardiovascular disease and blood pressure. Clin. Exper. Hypertens. A11:1035, 1989.
160. Blair, S. N., Kohl, H. W., III., Paffenbarger, R. S., Jr., et al.: Physical fitness and all-cause mortality. A prospective study of healthy men and women. JAMA 262:2395, 1989.
161. Paffenbarger, R. S., Jr.: Contributions of epidemiology to exercise science and cardiovascular health. Med. Sci. Sports Exerc. 20:426, 1988.
162. MacMahon, S.: Alcohol consumption and hypertension. Hypertension 9:111, 1987.
163. Criqui, M. H., Langer, R. D., and Reed, D. M.: Dietary alcohol, calcium, and potassium. Circulation 80:609, 1989.
164. Witteman, J. C. M., Willett, W. C., Stampfer, M. J., et al.: Relation of moderate alcohol consumption and risk of systemic hypertension in women. Am. J. Cardiol. 65:633, 1990.
165. Klatsky, A. L., Armstrong, M. A., and Friedman, G. D.: Alcohol and cardiovascular deaths. Circulation 80(Suppl. II):II614, 1989.
166. Camargo C. A., Jr.: Moderate alcohol consumption and stroke. The epidemiologic evidence. Stroke 20:1611, 1989.
167. Karsenty, C., Baraona, E., Savolainen, M. J., and Lieber, C. S.: Effects of chronic ethanol intake on mobilization and excretion of cholesterol in baboons. J. Clin. Invest. 75:976, 1985.
168. Grassi, G. M., Somers, V. K., Renk, W. S., et al.: Effects of oral alcohol intake on blood pressure and sympathetic nerve activity in normotensive humans: A preliminary report. J. Hypertens. 7(Suppl. 6):S20, 1989.
169. Main, J., and Thomas, T.: Ethanol predominantly alters sodium influx in human leucocytes. Clin. Sci. 78:235, 1990.
170. Cruickshank, J. M., Neil-Dwyer, G., Dorrance, D. E., et al.: Acute effects of smoking on blood pressure and cerebral blood flow. J. Hum. Hypertens. 3:443, 1989.
171. Jarrett, R. J.: Cardiovascular disease and hypertension in diabetes mellitus. Diabetes Metab. Rev. 5:547, 1989.
172. Aromaa, A., Reunanen, A., and Pyorala, K.: Hypertension and mortality in diabetic and non-diabetic Finnish men. J. Hypertens. 2(Suppl 3):205, 1984.
173. Anderson, S., and Brenner, B. M.: Progressive renal disease: A disorder of adaptation. Q. J. Med. 70:185, 1989.
174. Letcher, R. L., Chien, S., Pickering, T. G., et al.: Direct relationship between blood pressure and blood viscosity in normal and hypertensive subjects. Role of fibrinogen concentration. Am. J. Med. 70:1195, 1981.
175. Messerli, F. H., Frohlich, E. D., Dreslinski, G. R., et al.: Serum uric acid in essential hypertension: An indicator of renal vascular involvement. Ann. Intern. Med. 93:817, 1980.
176. Dykman, D., Simon, E. E., and Avioli, L. V.: Hyperuricemia and uric acid nephropathy. Arch. Intern. Med. 147:1341, 1987.
177. Campion, E. W., Glynn, R. J., and DeLabry, L. O.: Asymptomatic hyperuricemia. Am. J. Med. 82:421, 1987.

SECONDARY FORMS OF HYPERTENSION

178. Woods, J. W.: Oral contraceptives and hypertension. Hypertension 11(Suppl II):II, 1988.
179. Croft, P., and Hannaford, P. C.: Risk factors for acute myocardial infarction in women: Evidence from the Royal College of General Practitioners' Oral Contraception Study. Br. Med. J. 298:165, 1989.
180. Vessey, M. P., Villard-Mackintosh, L., McPherson, K., and Yeates, D.: Mortality among oral contraceptive users: 20-year follow-up of women in a cohort study. Br. Med. J. 299:1487, 1989.
181. Weir, R. J.: Effect on blood pressure of changing from high to low dose steroid preparation in women with oral contraceptive induced hypertension. Scott. Med. J. 27:212, 1982.
182. Malatino, L. S., Glen, L., Wilson, E. S. B., et al.: The effects of low-dose estrogen-progestogen oral contraceptives on blood pressure and the renin-angiotensin system. Curr. Ther. Res. 43:743, 1988.
183. Wallace, R. B., Barrett-Connor, E., Criqui, M., et al.: Alteration in blood

pressures associated with combined alcohol and oral contraceptive use —The Lipid Research Clinics Prevalence Study. J. Chronic Dis. *35*:251, 1982.

184. Lim, K. G., Isles, C. G., Hodsman, G. P., et al.: Malignant hypertension in women of childbearing age and its relation to the contraceptive pill. Br. Med. J. *294*:1057, 1987.

185. McAreavey, D., Cumming, A. M. M., Boddy, K., et al.: The renin-angiotensin system and total body sodium and potassium in hypertensive women taking oestrogen-progestagen oral contraceptives. Clin. Endocrinol. *18*:111, 1983.

186. Derkx, F. H. M., Stuenkel, C., Schalekamp, M. P. A., et al.: Immunoreactive renin, prorenin, and enzymatically active renin in plasma during pregnancy and in women taking oral contraceptives. J. Clin. Endocrinol. Metab. *63*:1008, 1986.

187. Kay, C. R.: Progestogens and arterial disease—Evidence from the Royal College of General Practitioners' study. Am. J. Obstet. Gynecol. *141*:762, 1982.

188. Kasdorf, G., and Kalkhoff, R. K.: Prospective studies of insulin sensitivity in normal women receiving oral contraceptive agents. J. Clin. Endocrinol. Metab. *66*:846, 1988.

189. Hassager, C., Riis, B. J., Strom, V., et al.: The long-term effect of oral and percutaneous estradiol on plasma renin substrate and blood pressure. Circulation *76*:753, 1987.

190. Knopp, R. H.: The effects of postmenopausal estrogen therapy on the incidence of arteriosclerotic vascular disease. Obstet. Gynecol. *72*:23S, 1988.

191. Reddi, A. S., and Camerini-Davalos, R. A.: Diabetic nephropathy. An update. Arch. Intern. Med. *150*:31, 1990.

192. Ghose, R. R., and Harindra, V.: Unrecognized high pressure chronic retention of urine presenting with systemic arterial hypertension. Br. Med. J. *298*:1626, 1989.

193. Garcia, R., Rubio, L., and Rodriguez-Iturbe, B.: Long-term prognosis of epidemic poststreptococcal glomerulonephritis in Maracaibo: Follow-up studies 11 to 12 years after the acute episode. Clin. Nephrol. 15:291, 1981.

194. Oken, D. E.: On the differential diagnosis of acute renal failure. Am. J. Med. *71*:916, 1981.

195. Bakir, A. A., Bazilinski, N., and Dunea, G.: Transient and sustained recovery from renal shutdown in accelerated hypertension. Am. J. Med. *80*:172, 1986.

196. Eknoyan, G., and Suki, W. N.: Renal vascular phenomena in systemic sclerosis (scleroderma). Semin. Nephrol. *5*:34, 1985.

197. Lingeman, J. E., Woods, J. R., and Toth, P. D.: Blood pressure changes following extracorporeal shock wave lithotripsy and other forms of treatment for nephrolithiasis. JAMA *263*:1789, 1990.

198. Strandgaard, S., Kamper, A., Skaarup, P., et al.: Changes in glomerular filtration rate, lithium clearance and plasma protein clearances in the early phase after unilateral nephrectomy in living healthy renal transplant donors. Clin. Sci. *75*:655, 1988.

199. Smith, H. W.: Unilateral nephrectomy in hypertensive disease. J. Urol. *76*:685, 1956.

200. Lüscher, T. F., Wanner, C., Hauri, D., et al.: Curable renal parenchymatous hypertension. Current diagnosis and management. Cardiology *72*(Suppl. 1):33, 1985.

201. Calabrese, G., Vageli, G., Cristofano, C., and Barsotti, G.: Behaviour of arterial pressure in different stages of polycystic kidney disease. Nephron *32*:207, 1982.

202. Siamopoulos, K., Sellars, L., Mishra, S. C., et al.: Experience in the management of hypertension with unilateral chronic pyelonephritis: Results of nephrectomy in selected patients. Q. J. Med. *207*:34, 1983.

203. Baumgart, P., Walger, P., Gerke, M, et al.: Nocturnal hypertension in renal failure, haemodialysis and after renal transplantation. J. Hypertens. *7*(Suppl. 6):S70, 1989.

204. Parving, H.- H., Hommel, E., Nielsen, M. D., and Giese, J.: Effect of captopril on blood pressure and kidney function in normotensive insulin dependent diabetics with nephropathy. Br. Med. J. *299*:533, 1989.

205. Koomans, H. A., Roos, J. C., Boer, P., et al.: Salt sensitivity of blood pressure in chronic renal failure. Evidence of renal control of body fluid distribution in man. Hypertension *4*:190, 1982.

206. Swaminathan, R., Glegg, G., Cumberbatch, M., et al.: Erythrocyte sodium transport in chronic renal failure. Clin. Sci. *62*:489, 1982.

207. Brunner, H. R., Wauters, J., McKinstry, D., et al.: Inappropriate renin secretion unmasked by captopril (SQ14 225) in hypertension of chronic renal failure. Lancet *2*:704, 1978.

208. Henrich, W. L., Mitchell, H., Anderson, S, et al.: Effect of antihypertensive therapy on plasma catecholamines in renal failure patients. Clin. Nephrol. *16*:131, 1981.

209. Jacobson, H. R.: Ischemic renal disease: An overlooked clinical entity? Kidney Int. *34*:729, 1988.

210. Ying, C. Y., Tifft, C. P., Gavras, H., and Chobanian, A. V.: Renal revascularization in the azotemic hypertensive patients resistant to therapy. N. Engl. J. Med. *311*:1070, 1984.

211. Parving, H.- H., Andersen, A. R., Smidt, U. M., et al.: Effect of antihypertensive treatment on kidney function in diabetic nephropathy. Br. Med. J. *294*:1443, 1987.

212. Iwasaki, R., Kigoshi, T., Uchida, K., and Morimoto, S.: Plasma 18-hydroxycorticosterone and aldosterone responses to angiotensin II and corticotropin in diabetic patients with hyporeninemic and normoreninemic hypoaldosteronism. Acta Endocrinol. (Copenh.) *121*:83, 1989.

213. Nadler, J. L., Lee, F. O., Hsueh, W., and Horton, R.: Evidence of prostacyclin deficiency in the syndrome of hyporeninemic hypoaldosteronism. N. Engl. J. Med. *314*:1015, 1986.

214. Stillman, M. T., and Schlesinger, P. A.: Nonsteroidal anti-inflammatory drug nephrotoxicity. Should we be concerned? Arch. Intern. Med. *150*:268, 1990.

215. Sandler, D. P., Smith, J. C., Weinberg, C. R., et al.: Analgesic use and chronic renal disease. N. Engl. J. Med. *320*:1238, 1989.

216. Muther, R. S., Potter, D. M., and Bennett, W. M.: Aspirin-induced depression of glomerular filtration rate in normal humans: Role of sodium balance. Ann. Intern. Med. *94*:317, 1981.

217. Henrich, W. L.: Hemodynamic instability during hemodialysis. Kidney Int. *30*:605, 1986.

218. Curtis, J. J., Luke, R. G., Dustan, H. P., et al.: Remission of essential hypertension after renal transplantation. N. Engl. J. Med. *309*:1009, 1983.

219. Cheigh, J. S., Haschemeyer, R. H., Wang, J. C. L., et al.: Hypertension in kidney transplant recipients. Effect on long-term renal allograft survival. Am. J. Hypertens. *2*:341, 1989.

220. Ribstein, J., Mourad, G., Mion, C., and Mimran, A.: Chronic angiotensin converting enzyme inhibition as an alternative to native kidneys removal in post-transplant hypertension. J. Hypertens. *4*(Suppl. 5):S255, 1986.

221. Guidi, E., Bianchi, G., Rivolta, E., et al.: Hypertension in man with a kidney transplant: Role of familial versus other factors. Nephron *41*:14, 1985.

222. Strandgaard, S., and Hansen, U.: Hypertension in renal allograft recipients may be conveyed by cadaveric kidneys from donors with subarachnoid hemorrhage. Br. Med. J. *292*:1041, 1986.

223. Working Group on Renovascular Hypertension: Detection, evaluation, and treatment of renovascular hypertension. Final Report. Arch. Intern. Med. *147*:820, 1987.

224. Vetrovec, G. W., Landwehr, D. M., and Edwards, V. L.: Incidence of renal artery stenosis in hypertensive patients undergoing coronary angiography. J. Interven. Cardiol. *2*:2, 1989.

225. Olin, J. W., Melia, M., Young, J. R., et al.: Prevalence of atherosclerotic renal artery stenosis in patients with atherosclerosis elsewhere. Am. J. Med. *88*:1–46N, 1990.

226. Pickering, T. G.: Renovascular hypertension: Etiology and pathophysiology. Semin. Nucl. Med. *19*:79, 1989.

227. Sang, C. N., Whelton, P. K., Hamper, U. M., et al.: Etiologic factors in renovascular fibromuscular dysplasia. A case-control study. Hypertension *14*:472, 1989.

228. Lüscher, T. F., Lie, J. T., Stanson, A. W., et al.: Arterial fibromuscular dysplasia. Mayo Clin. Proc. *62*:931, 1987.

229. Bookstein, J. J.: Segmental renal artery stenosis in renovascular hypertension. Radiology *90*:1073, 1968.

230. Geyskes, G. G., Klinge, O. J., Kooiker, C. J., et al.: Renovascular hypertension: The small kidney updated. Q. J. Med. *66*:203, 1988.

231. Bookstein, J. J., Abrams, H. L., Buenger, R. E., et al.: Radiologic aspects of renovascular hypertension. Part 3. Appraisal of arteriography. JAMA *21*:368, 1972.

232. de Jong, P. E., van Bockel, J. H., and de Zeeuw, D.: Unilateral renal parenchymal disease with contralateral renal artery stenosis of the fibrodysplasia type. Ann. Intern. Med. *110*:437, 1989.

233. Scoble, J. E., Maher, E. R., Hamilton, G., et al.: Atherosclerotic renovascular disease causing renal impairment—A case for treatment. Clin. Nephrol. *31*:119, 1989.

234. Thal, A. P., Grage, T. B., and Vernier, R. L.: Function of the contralateral kidney in renal hypertension due to renal artery stenosis. Circulation *27*:36, 1963.

235. Simon, N., Franklin, S. S., Bleifer, K. W., and Maxwell, M. H. P.: Clinical characteristics of renovascular hypertension. J.A.M.A. *220*:1209, 1972.

236. Anderson, G. H., Jr., Blakeman, N., and Streeten, D. H. P.: Prediction of renovascular hypertension: Comparison of clinical diagnostic indices. Am. J. Hypertens. *1*:301, 1988.

237. Pickering, T. G., Devereux, R. B., James, G. D., et al.: Recurrent pulmonary oedema in hypertension due to bilateral renal artery stenosis: Treatment by angioplasty or surgical revascularisation. Lancet *2*:551, 1988.

238. Stinchcombe, S. J., Manhire, A. R., Bishop, M. C., and Gregson, R. H. S.: Fibromuscular dysplasia of renal arteries: A neglected cause of acute loin pain. Br. Med. J. *300*:183, 1990.

239. Keith, T. A., III: Renovascular hypertension in black patients. Hypertension *4*:438, 1982.

240. Muller, F. B., Sealey, J. E., Case, D. B., et al.: The captopril test for identifying renovascular disease in hypertensive patients. Am. J. Med. *80*:633, 1986.

241. Frederickson, E. D., Wilcox, C. S., Bucci, C. M., et al.: A prospective evaluation of a simplified captopril test for the detection of renovascular hypertension. Arch. Intern. Med. *150*:569, 1990.

242. Postma, C. T., van der Steen, P. H. M., Hoefnagels, W. H. L., et al.: The captopril test in the detection of renovascular disease in hypertensive patients. Arch. Intern. Med. *150*:625, 1990.

243. Geyskes, G. G., Oei, H. Y., Puylaert, C. B. A. J., and Dorhout Mees, E. J.: Renovascular hypertension identified by captopril-induced changes in the renogram. Hypertension *9*:451, 1987.

244. Hawkins, P. G., McKnoulty, L. M., Gordon, R. D., et al.: Non-invasive renal artery duplex ultrasound and computerized nuclear renography to screen for and follow progress in renal artery stenosis. J. Hypertens. *7*(Suppl 6):S184, 1989.

245. Hollenberg, N. K.: Medical therapy for renovascular hypertension: A review. Am. J. Hypertens. *1*:338S, 1988.

246. Hricik, D. E.: Angiotensin-converting enzyme inhibition in renovascular hypertension: The narrowing gap between functional renal failure and progressive renal atrophy. J. Lab. Clin. Med. *115*:8, 1990.

247. Kumagai, H., Suzuki, H., Matsukawa, S., et al.: Captopril therapy follow-

ing percutaneous transluminal angioplasty for bilateral renal artery stenosis. Arch. Intern. Med. *149*:1973, 1989.
248. Postma, C. T., Hoefnagels, W. H. L., Barentsz, J. O., et al.: Occlusion of unilateral stenosed renal arteries—Relation to medical treatment. J. Hum. Hypertens. *3*:185, 1989.
249. Fiorentini, C., Galli, C., Tamborini, G., et al.: Hemodynamic and renin responses to nifedipine in renovascular hypertension. Am. Heart J. *119*:353, 1990.
250. Ramsay, L. E., and Waller, P. C.: Blood pressure response to percutaneous transluminal angioplasty for renovascular hypertension: An overview of published series. Br. Med. J. *300*:569, 1990.
251. Hansen, K. J., Ditesheim, J. A., Metropol, S. H., et al.: Management of renovascular hypertension in the elderly population. J. Vasc. Surg. *10*:266, 1989.
252. Kaylor, W. M., Novick, A. C., Ziegelbaum, M., and Vidt, D. G.: Reversal of end stage renal failure with surgical revascularization in patients with atherosclerotic renal artery occlusion. J. Urol. *141*:486, 1989.
253. Duprez, D., De Smet, H., Roels, H., and Clement, D.: Hypertension due to a renal renin-secreting tumour. J. Hum. Hypertens. *4*:59, 1990.
254. Geddy, P. M., and Main, J.: Renin-secreting retroperitoneal leiomyosarcoma: An unusual cause of hypertension. J. Hum. Hypertens. *4*:57, 1990.
255. Leckie, B. J., McIntyre, G. D., Millan, W. D., et al.: Renin and inactive (prorenin) in the plasma of patients with malignant renal tumors. Clin. Exp. Hypertens. *A9*:1325, 1987.
256. Copeland, P. M.: The incidentally discovered adrenal mass. Ann. Intern. Med. *98*:940, 1983.
257. Belldegrun, A., Hussain, S., Seltzer, S. E., et al.: Incidentally discovered mass of the adrenal gland. Surg. Gynecol. Obstet. *163*:203, 1986.
258. Gross, M. D., Shapiro, B., Gouffard, J. A., et al.: Distinguishing benign from malignant euadrenal masses. Ann. Intern. Med *109*:613, 1988.
259. Young, W. F., Jr., Hogan, M. J., Klee, G. G., et al.: Primary aldosteronism: Diagnosis and treatment. Mayo Clin. Proc. *65*:96, 1990.
260. O'Mahony, S., Burns, A., and Murnaghan, D. J.: Dexamethasone-suppressible hyperaldosteronism: A large new kindred. J. Hum. Hypertens. *3*:255, 1989.
261. Jackson, B., Valentine, R., and Wagner, G.: Primary aldosteronism due to a malignant ovarian tumor. Aust. N.Z. J. Med. *16*:69, 1986.
262. Matsunaga, M., Hara, A., Song, T. S., et al.: Asymptomatic normotensive primary aldosteronism. Case report. Hypertension *5*:240, 1983.
263. Ferriss, J. B., Beevers, D. G., Brown, J. J., et al.: Clinical, biochemical and pathological features of low renin ("primary") hyperaldosteronism. Am. Heart J. *95*:375, 1978.
264. Torres, V. E., Young, W. F., Jr., Offord, K. P., and Hattery, R. R.: Association of hypokalemia, aldosteronism, and renal cysts. N. Engl. J. Med. *322*:345, 1990.
265. Holland, O. B., Brown, H., Kuhnert, L. V., et al.: Further evaluation of saline infusion for the diagnosis of primary aldosteronism. Hypertension *6*:717, 1984.
266. McLeod, M. K., Thompson, N. W., Gross, M. D., and Grekin, R. J.: Idiopathic aldosteronism masquerading as discrete aldosterone-secreting adrenal cortical neoplasms among patients with primary aldosteronism. Surgery *106*:1161, 1989.
267. Spapen, H. D. M., Achten, E., De Geeter, F., et al.: Magnetic resonance imaging of the adrenal glands in the diagnosis of primary hyperaldosteronism. J. Intern. Med. *226*:463, 1989.
268. Gross, M. D., and Shapiro, B.: Scintigraphic studies in adrenal hypertension. Semin. Nucl. Med. *19*:122, 1989.
269. Vaughan, N. J. A., Jowett, T. P., Slater, J. D. H., et al.: The diagnosis of primary hyperaldosteronism. Lancet *1*:120, 1981.
270. Ross, E. J., and Linch, D. C.: The clinical response to treatment in adult Cushing's syndrome following remission of hypercortisolaemia. Postgrad. Med. J. *61*:205, 1985.
271. Sudhir, K., Jenning, G. L., Esler, M. D., et al.: Hydrocortisone-induced hypertension in humans: Pressor responsiveness and sympathetic function. Hypertension *13*:416, 1989.
272. Kaye, T. B., and Crapo, L.: The Cushing syndrome: An update on diagnostic tests. Ann. Intern. Med. *112*:434, 1990.
273. Mampalam, T. J., Tyrrell, J. B., and Wilson, C. B.: Transsphenoidal microsurgery for Cushing disease; A report of 216 cases. Ann. Intern. Med. *109*:487, 1988.
274. Goldstein, D. S., Stull, R., Eisenhofer, G., et al.: Plasma dihydroxyphenylalanine in neuroblastoma and pheochromocytoma. Ann. Intern. Med. *105*:887, 1986.
275. Goldfarb, D. A., Novick, A. C., Bravo, E. L., et al.: Experience with extra-adrenal pheochromocytoma. J. Urol. *142*:931, 1989.
276. DeAngelis, L. M., Kelleher, M. B., Post, K. D., and Fetell, M. R.: Multiple paragangliomas in neurofibromatosis: A new neuroendocrine neoplasia. Neurology *37*:129, 1987.
277. Gagel, R. F., Tashjian, A. H., Jr., Cummings, T., et al.: The clinical outcome of prospective screening for multiple endocrine neoplasia type 2a. An 18-year experience. N. Engl. J. Med. *318*:478, 1988.
278. Sasaki, A., Yumita, S., Kimura, S., et al.: Immunoreactive corticotropin-releasing hormone, growth hormone-releasing hormone, somatostatin, and peptide histidine methionine are present in adrenal pheochromocytomas, but not in extra-adrenal pheochromocytoma. J. Clin. Endocrinol. Metab. *70*:996, 1990.
279. Bravo, E., Fouad-Tarazi, F., Rossi, G., et al.: A reevaluation of the hemodynamics of pheochromocytoma. Hypertension *15*(Suppl I):I–128, 1990.
280. Scott, I., Parkes, R., and Cameron, D. P.: Phaeochromocytoma and cardiomyopathy. Med. J. Aust. *148*:94, 1988.
281. Haas, G. J., Tzagournis, M., and Boudoulas, H.: Pheochromocytoma: Catecholamine-mediated electrocardiographic changes mimicking ischemia. Am. Heart J. *116*:1363, 1988.
282. Goldbaum, T. S., Henochowicz, S., Mustafa, M., et al.: Pheochromocytoma presenting with Prinzmetal's angina. Am. J. Med. *81*:921, 1986.
283. Sheps, S. G., Jiang, N.- S., Klee, G. G., and van Heerden, J. A.: Recent developments in the diagnosis and treatment of pheochromocytoma. Mayo Clin. Proc. *65*:88, 1990.
284. Manu, P., and Runge, L. A.: Biochemical screening for pheochromocytoma: Superiority of urinary metanephrines measurements. Am. J. Epidemiol. *120*:788, 1984.
285. Feldman, J. M.: Falsely elevated urinary excretion of catecholamines and metanephrines in patients receiving labetalol therapy. J. Clin. Pharmacol. *27*:288, 1987.
286. Sheps, S. G., Jiang, N.- S., and Klee, G. G.: Diagnostic evaluation of pheochromocytoma. Endocrinol. Metab. Clin. North. Am. *17*:397, 1988.
287. Shapiro, B., and Fig, L. M.: Management of pheochromocytoma. Endocrinol. Metab. Clin. North. Am. *18*:443, 1989.
288. de Simone, G., Tommaselli, A. P., Rossi, R., et al.: Partial deficiency of adrenal 11-hydroxylase. A possible cause of primary hypertension. Hypertension *7*:204, 1985.
289. Lucky, A. W., Rosenfield, R. L., McGuire, J., et al.: Adrenal androgen hyperresponsiveness to adrenocorticotropin in women with acne and/or hirsutism: Adrenal enzyme defects and exaggerated adrenarche. J. Clin. Endocrinol. Metab. *62*:840, 1986.
290. D'Alberton, A., Reschini, E., Motta, T., and Catania, A.: Male pseudohermaphroditism due to 17-hydroxylase deficiency. J. Endocrinol. Invest. *12*:193, 1989.
291. Porter, G. A., Bennett, W. M., and Sheps, S. G.: Cyclosporine-associated hypertension. Arch. Intern. Med. *150*:280, 1990.
292. Eschbach, J. W., Kelly, M. R., Haley, N. R., et al.: Treatment of the anemia of progressive renal failure with recombinant human erythropoietin. N. Engl. J. Med. *321*:158, 1989.
293. Blackburn, G. L., Morgan, J. P., Lavin, P. T., et al.: Determinants of the pressor effect of phenylpropanolamine in healthy subjects. JAMA *261*:3267, 1989.
294. Murphy, A. M., Blades, M., Daniels, S., and James, F. W.: Blood pressure and cardiac output during exercise: A longitudinal study of children undergoing repair of coarctation. Am. Heart J. *117*:1327, 1989.
295. Cohen, M., Fuster, V., Steele, P. M., et al.: Coarctation of the aorta: Long-term follow-up and prediction of outcome after surgical correction. Circulation *80*:840, 1989.
296. Gidding, S. S., Rocchini, A. P., Beekman, R., et al.: Therapeutic effect of propranolol on paradoxical hypertension after repair of coarctation of the aorta. N. Engl. J. Med *312*:1224, 1985.
297. Maheswaran, R., and Beevers, D. G.: Clinical correlates in parathyroid hypertension. J. Hypertens. *7*(Suppl 6):S190, 1989.
298. Dominiczak, A. F., Lyall, F., Morton, J. J., et al.: Blood pressure, left ventricular mass and intracellular calcium in primary hyperparathyroidism. Clin. Sci. *78*:127, 1990.
299. Heuser, D., Guggenberger, H., and Fretschner, R.: Acute blood pressure increase during the perioperative period. Am. J. Cardiol. *63*:26C, 1989.
300. Weinstein, G. S., Zabetakis, P. M., Clavel, A., et al.: The renin-angiotensin system is not responsible for hypertension following coronary artery bypass grafting. Ann. Thorac. Surg. *43*:74, 1987.
301. Cruise, C. J., Skrobik, Y., Webster, R. E., et al.: Intravenous labetalol versus sodium nitroprusside for treatment of hypertension postcoronary bypass surgery. Anesthesiology *71*:835, 1989.
302. Kaplan, J. A.: Clinical considerations for the use of intravenous nicardipine in the treatment of postoperative hypertension. Am. Heart J. *119*:443, 1990.
303. Starling, R. C., and Cody, R. J.: Cardiac transplant hypertension. Am. J. Cardiol. *65*:106, 1990.
304. Angermann, C. E., Spes, C., Willems, S., et al.: Regression and prevention of left ventricular hypertrophy are possible in hypertensive heart transplant recipients. J. Am. Coll. Cardiol. *15*:223A, 1990.

SPECIAL TOPICS

305. Davey, D. A., and MacGillivray, I.: Semantic changes suggested in hypertension disorders. Am. J. Obstet. Gynecol. *161*:1422, 1989.
306. O'Brien, W. F.: Predicting preeclampsia. Obstet. Gynecol. *75*:445, 1990.
307. Boyd, P., Lindenbaum, R. H., and Redman, C.: Pre-eclampsia and trisomy 13: A possible association. Lancet *2*:425, 1987.
308. Alderman, B. W., Sperling, R. S., and Daling, J. R.: An epidemiological study of the immunogenetic aetiology of pre-eclampsia. Br. Med. J. *292*:372, 1986.
309. Guzick, D. S., Klein, V. R., Tyson, J. E., et al.: Risk factors for the occurrence of pregnancy-induced hypertension. Clin. Exp. Hypertens. *B6*:281, 1987.
310. Ihle, B. U., Long, P., and Oats, J.: Early onset pre-eclampsia: Recognition of underlying renal disease. Br. Med. J. *294*:79, 1987.
311. Mabie, W. C., Ratts, T. E., and Sibai, B. M.: The central hemodynamics of severe preeclampsia. Am. J. Obstet. Gynecol. *161*:1443, 1989.
312. Moutquin, J. M., Raiville, C., Giroux, L., et al.: A prospective study of blood pressure in pregnancy: Prediction of preeclampsia. Am. J. Obstet. Gynecol. *151*:191, 1985.
313. Chesley, L. C., and Sibai, B. M.: Clinical significance of elevated mean arterial pressure in the second trimester. Am. J. Obstet. Gynecol. *159*:275, 1988.
314. Lockwood, C. J., and Peters, J. H.: Increased plasma levels of ED1$^+$ cellular

fibronectin precede the clinical signs of preeclampsia. Am. J. Obstet. Gynecol. *162*:358, 1990.
315. Loquet, P. H.., Broughton Pipkin, F., Symonds, E. M., and Rubin, P. C.: Influence of raising maternal blood pressure with angiotensin II on utero-placental and feto-placental blood velocity indices in the human. Clin. Sci. *78*:95, 1990.
316. Woods, L. L.: Importance of prostaglandins in hypertension during reduced uteroplacental perfusion pressure. Am. J. Physiol. *257*:R1558, 1989.
317. Fitzgerald D. J., Entman, S. S., Mulloy, K., and Fitzgerald, G. A.: Decreased prostacyclin biosynthesis preceding the clinical manifestation of pregnancy-induced hypertension. Circulation *75*:956, 1987.
318. Walsh, S. W., and Coulter, S.: Increased placental progesterone may cause decreased placental prostacyclin production in preeclampsia. Am. J. Obstet. Gynecol. *161*:1586, 1989.
319. Nelson, D. M., and Walsh, S. W.: Aspirin differentially affects thromboxane and prostacyclin production by trophoblast and villous core compartments of human placental villi. Am. J. Obstet. Gynecol. 161:1593, 1989.
320. Benigni, A., Grergorini, G., Frusca, T., et al.: Effect of low-dose aspirin on fetal and maternal generation of thromboxane by platelets in women at risk for pregnancy-induced hypertension. N. Engl. J. Med. *321*:357, 1989.
321. Schiff, E., Peleg, E., Goldenberg, M., et al.: The use of aspirin to prevent pregnancy-induced hypertension and lower the ratio of thromboxane A_2 to prostacyclin in relatively high-risk pregnancies. N. Engl. J. Med. *321*:351, 1989.
322. Werler, M. M., Mitchell, A. A., and Shapiro, S.: The relation of aspirin use during the first trimester of pregnancy to congenital cardiac defects. N. Engl. J. Med. *321*:1639, 1989.
323. Bauman, W. A., Maimen, M., and Langer, O.: An association between hyperinsulinemia and hypertension during the third trimester of pregnancy. Am. J. Obstet. Gynecol. *159*:446, 1988.
324. McCance, D. R., McKnight, J. A., Traub, A. I., et al.: Plasma atrial natriuretic factor levels during normal pregnancy and pregnancy complicated by diabetes mellitus and hypertension. J. Hum. Hypertens. *4*:31, 1990.
325. Testa, I., Rabini, R. A., Danieli, G., et al.: Abnormal membrane cation transport in pregnancy-induced hypertension. Scand. J. Clin. Lab. Invest. *48*:7, 1988.
326. Kilby, M. D., Broughton Pipkin, F., Cockbill, S., et al.: A cross-sectional study of basal platelet intracellular free calcium concentration in normotensive and hypertensive primigravid pregnancies. Clin. Sci. *78*:75, 1990.
327. Rasmussen, K.: Fetal haemodynamics before and after treatment of maternal hypertension in pregnancy. Dan. Med. Bull. *34*:170, 1987.
328. Plouin, P.- F., Breart, G., Llado, J., et al.: A randomized comparison of early with conservative use of antihypertensive drugs in the management of pregnancy-induced hypertension. Br. J. Obstet. Gynaecol. *97*:134, 1990.
329. Lubbe, W. F.: Hypertension in pregnancy: Whom and how to treat. Br. J. Clin. Pharmacol. *24*:15S, 1987.
330. Pickles, C. J., Symonds, E. M., and Broughton Pipkin, F.: The fetal outcome in a randomized double-blind controlled trial of labetalol versus placebo in pregnancy-induced hypertension. Br. J. Obstet. Gynaecol. *96*:38, 1989.
331. Greer, I. A., Walker, J. J., Bjornsson, S., and Calder, A. A.: Second line therapy with nifedipine in severe pregnancy induced hypertension. Clin. Exp. Hypertens. Pregnancy *B8*:277, 1989.
332. Rose, F. W., Bosco, L. A., Graham, C. F., et al.: Neonatal anuria with maternal angiotensin-converting enzyme inhibition. Obstet. Gynecol. *74*:371, 1989.
332a. Butters, L., Kennedy, S., and Rubin, P. C.: Atenolol in essential hypertension during pregnancy. Br. Med. J. *301*: 587, 1990.
333. Sibai, B. M., Gonzalez, A. R., Mabie, W. C., and Moretti, M.: A comparison of labetalol plus hospitalization verus hospitalization alone in the management of preeclampsia remote from term. Obstet. Gynecol. *70*:323, 1987.
334. Welt, S. I., Dorminy, J. H., Jelovsek, F. R., et al.: The effect of prophylactic management and therapeutics on hypertension disease in pregnancy: Preliminary studies. Obstet. Gynecol. *57*:557, 1981.
335. Mabie, W. C., Pernoll, M. L., and Biswas, M. K.: Chronic hypertension in pregnancy. Obstet. Gynecol. *67*:197, 1986.
336. Moodley, J.: Treatment of eclampsia. Br. J. Obstet. Gynaecol. *97*:99, 1990.
337. Pritchard, J. A., Cunningham, F. G., and Pritchard, S. A.: The Parkland Memorial Hospital protocol for treatment of eclampsia. Evaluation of 245 cases. Am. J. Obstet. Gynecol. *148*:951, 1984.
338. Clark, S. L., Greenspoon, J. S., Aldahl, D., and Phelan, J. P.: Severe preeclampsia with persistent oliguria: Management of hemodynamic subsets. Am. J. Obstet. Gynecol. *154*:490, 1986.
339. Chesley, L. C.: Hypertension in pregnancy: Definitions, familial factor, and remote prognosis. Kidney Int. *18*:234, 1980.
340. Cunningham, F. G., Pritchard, J. A., Hankins, G. D. V., et al.: Peripartum heart failure: Idiopathic cardiomyopathy or compounding cardiovascular events? Obstet. Gynecol. *67*:157, 1986.
341. Katz, S. H., Hediger, M. L., Zemel, B. S., and Parks, J. S.: Blood pressure, body fat, and dehydroepiandrosterone sulfate variation in adolescence. Hypertension *8*:277, 1986.
342. Mahoney, L. T., and Lauer, R. M.: Consistency of blood pressure levels in children. Semin. Nephrol. *9*:230, 1989.
343. Baron, A. E., Freyer, B., and Fixler, D. E.: Longitudinal blood pressures in blacks, whites, and Mexican Americans during adolescence and early adulthood. Am. J. Epidemiol. *123*:809, 1986.
344. Lauer, R. M., Anderson, A. R., Beaglehole, R., and Burns, T. L.: Factors relating to tracking of blood pressure in children: U. S. National Center for Health Statistics Health Examination Surveys Cycles II and III. Hypertension *6*:307, 1984.
345. Berenson, G. S., Lawrence, M., and Soto, L.: The heart and hypertension in childhood. Semin. Nephrol. *9*:236, 1989.
346. De Santo, N. G., Trevisan, M., and Capasso, G.: Introduction. Semin. Nephrol. *9*:207, 1989.
347. Kotchen, J. M., Holley, J., and Kotchen, T. A.: Treatment of high blood pressure in the young. Semin. Nephrol. *9*:296, 1989.
347a. Pearson, A. C., Gudipati, C., Nagelhout, D., et al.: Echocardiographic evaluation of cardiac structure and function in elderly subjects with isolated systolic hypertension. J. Am. Coll. Cardiol. *17*:422, 1991.
347b. Joosens, J. V., and Kesteloot, H.: Trends in systolic blood pressure, 24-hour sodium excretion, and stroke mortality in the elderly in Belgium. Am. J. Med. *90*(Suppl. A):3A, 1991.
348. Ahmed, M. E. K., Walker, J. M., Beevers, D. G., and Beevers, M.: Lack of difference between malignant and accelerated hypertension. Br. Med. J. *292*:235, 1986.
349. Bennett, N. M., and Shea, S.: Hypertensive emergency: Case criteria, sociodemographic profile, and previous case of 100 cases. Am. J. Public Health *78*:636, 1988.
350. Strandgaard, S., and Paulson, O. B.: Cerebral blood flow and its pathophysiology in hypertension. Am. J. Hypertens. *2*:486, 1989.
351. Kontos, H. A.: Oxygen radicals in cerebral vascular injury. Circ. Res. *57*:508, 1985.
352. Shapiro, L. M., and Beevers, D. G.: Malignant hypertension: Cardiac structure and function at presentation and during therapy. Br. Heart J. *49*:477, 1983.
353. Kawazoe, N., Eto, T., Abe, I., et al.: Long-term prognosis of malignant hypertension: Difference between underlying diseases such as essential hypertension and chronic glomerulonephritis. Clin. Nephrol. *29*:53, 1988.
354. White, W. B., and Baker, L. H.: Episodic hypertension secondary to panic disorder. Arch. Intern. Med. *146*:1129, 1986.
355. Brott, T., and Reed, R. L.: Intensive care for acute stroke in the community hospital setting. The first 24 hours. Storke *24*:1, 1989.

29

Systemic Hypertension: Therapy

by NORMAN M. KAPLAN, M.D.

INDICATIONS FOR THERAPY

The treatment of most patients with hypertension is usually not difficult. Current therapy reduces the blood pressure in the majority of patients with hypertension, most of whom start with only minimally elevated pressure (Fig. 28–2, p. 818). Only a small percentage, likely less than 5 per cent of patients, are resistant to therapy.[1] The active drug therapy of patients with *mild* hypertension, defined as diastolic blood pressure (DBP) between 90 and 104 mm Hg, has expanded markedly in the past few years as a result of the confluence of three events: (1) even minimally elevated pressures have been shown to increase the overall risk for premature cardiovascular disease; (2) trials have shown that progression of hypertension, strokes, and probably heart failure can be reduced by drug therapy; and (3) medications that are easier to take have become available and intensively marketed.

Because of these factors and the inherent desire for patients and physicians to take direct action against perceived dangers, millions of asymptomatic persons are now being treated with antihypertensive drugs. The number of people worldwide now being *continuously* treated for hypertension represents the largest use of long-term drug therapy. The use of such therapy is more "aggressive" in the United States than anywhere else; indeed, treatment of hypertension is now the most common reason for patient visits to doctors and the most common indication for prescribing drugs. These statistics reflect the practice of more than two-thirds of United States physicians to institute drug therapy at levels of DBP between 90 and 100 mm Hg in asymptomatic patients[2] and for as many as 20 per cent to treat patients with DBP below 90.[3] In Canada, England, and elsewhere, most physicians institute drug therapy only at DBP levels above 100 mm Hg.[4]

Such aggressive therapy has been vigorously defended and credited with at least some of the reduction in coronary and stroke mortality seen in the United States since 1968.[5] Others question the wisdom of such therapeutic activism. In the words of an English practitioner: "In the U.S., the threshold for diagnosis is the threshold for treatment. The question 'to treat or not to treat' need no longer be asked. A free-fire zone has been created above diastolic 90, in which we simply shoot everything that moves."[6]

Even in the United States the aggressive treatment of hypertension is now being seriously questioned for numerous reasons, including: (1) the awareness that the risks of relatively mild hypertension, although apparent for the aggregate, are not shared by all[7]; (2) the failure to show clear protection against coronary mortality by drug therapy in nine clinical trials involving more than 41,000 patients (Table 29–1) (Fig. 29–1).[8–17] As a result of this apparent inability to protect against coronary disease, concerns have arisen about biochemical changes induced by the drugs used in these trials, changes that may have, at the same time they reduced risk by lowering blood pressure, increased risk in various ways, such as by lowering potassium levels, raising lipid levels, or altering

TABLE 29-1 RANDOMIZED DRUG TREATMENT TRIALS IN LESS-SEVERE HYPERTENSION: DESIGN FEATURES AND PROTOCOL IMPLEMENTATION

STUDY, YEAR REPORTED	NO. OF PARTICIPANTS	STUDY POPULATION Age (yr)	STUDY POPULATION Entry DBP (mm Hg)	LENGTH OF FOLLOW-UP (yr)	DESIGN-CONTROLS	STEP 1 DRUG(S)	DBP EFFECT (mm Hg) Baseline	DBP EFFECT (mm Hg) Net Change
VA, 1970	380	Mean, 52	90–114	3.8	DB-placebo	HCTZ + RES + HDRZ	104	−19
PHS, 1977	389	21–55	90–114	6.5–9.0	DB-placebo	CTZ	99	−10
VA-NHLBI, 1978	1012	21–50	85–105	1.5	DB-placebo	CTLD	93	−7
Oslo, 1980	785	40–49	95–109	5.5	Open-untreated	HCTZ	97	−10
ANBP, 1980	3427	30–69	95–109	4.0	SB-placebo	CTZ	100	−6
EWPHE, 1985	840	Mean, 72	90–119	4.7	SB-placebo	HCTZ + TMTR	101	−10
MRC, 1985	17,354	35–64	90–109	5.5	SB-placebo	BDFZ or PROP	98	−6
HDFP, 1979	10,940	30–69	90+	5.0	Open-referred care	CLTD	101	−5
MRFIT, 1982 (hypertensive subjects)	8012	35–57	90–114	7.0	Open-usual care	CLTD or HCTZ	96	−4

DBP, diastolic blood pressure; VA, Veterans Administration; PHS, US Public Health Service Hospitals Cooperative Study; VA-NHLBI, VA National Heart, Lung, and Blood Institute Feasibility Study; Oslo, Oslo study; ANBP, Australian National Blood Pressure Study; EWPHE, European Working Party on Hypertension in the Elderly; MRC, British Medical Research Council trial; HDFP, Hypertension Detection and Follow-up Program; MRFIT, Multiple Risk Factor Intervention Trial; DB, double-blind; SB, single-blind; HCTZ, hydrochlorothiazide; RES, reserpine; HDRZ, hydralazine; CTZ, chlorothiazide; CTLD, chlorthalidone; TMTR, triamterene; BDFZ, bendrofluazide; and PROP, propranolol.

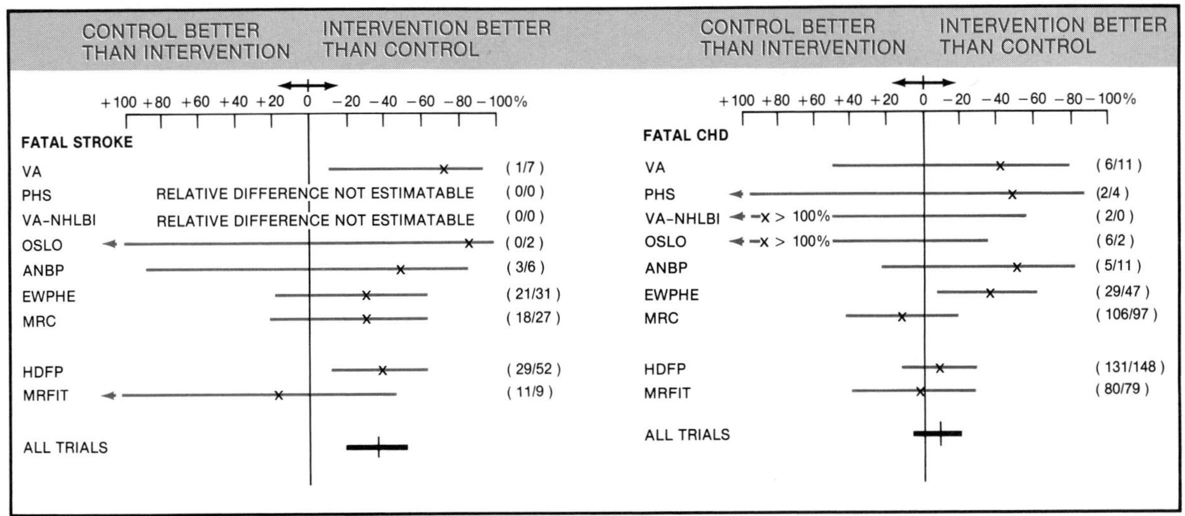

FIGURE 29-1. Bar graph showing estimates (X) with approximate 95 per cent confidence intervals (−) of the relative difference in fatal coronary heart disease (CHD) and nonfatal myocardial infarction (MI) between intervention and control groups. The numbers in parentheses are the numbers of events (intervention/control). (Note that the data from the EWPHE trial are reported only for total cardiac mortality.) See the legend to Table 29-1 for explanation of the abbreviations. (From Culter, J. A., MacMahon, S. W., and Furberg, C. D.: Controlled clinical trials of drug treatment for hypertension. A review. Hypertension *13*[Suppl I]:I-36, 1989.)

glucose tolerance; (3) concerns about the adverse effects of therapy, not only upon such biochemical markers but also upon the quality of life[18] and the potential for too much of a reduction in blood pressure to induce additional coronary ischemia[19]; and (4) the recognition by cost-to-benefit analysis[20] that the financial cost of protecting the relatively few who benefit (out of the much larger number who are treated without benefit) is much larger than anticipated.[21]

RESULTS OF CLINICAL TRIALS

The inability to show clear protection against coronary disease by reduction of the blood pressure in the nine controlled clinical trials which compared active therapy with placebo (Table 29-1) may not reflect a failure of the therapy, but a misguided attempt. Nonetheless, in some of these seven placebo-controlled trials and in the two large trials (HDFP and MRFIT) wherein therapy was given to all, but more to one half than to the other half, a greater reduction of the blood pressure did protect some of the participants[16,17] (Table 29-2). In both of these large trials, those patients who had *normal* electrocardiograms at entry were protected by more intensive therapy, whereas those with *abnormal* entry electrocardiograms suffered higher coronary mortality with more therapy. These data go along with those from many other less well-controlled studies that have shown a hazard for increasing myocardial ischemia when pressures are lowered below a critical level, i.e., a *J shaped* relating blood pressure on the abscissa to risk of coronary events on the ordinate with a threshold of 85 to 90 mm Hg diastolic.[19,22] In light of the potential importance of the

TABLE 29-2 CORONARY MORTALITY RATES PER 1000 PERSON-YEARS IN PATIENTS WITH OR WITHOUT ECG ABNORMALITIES AT ENTRY

TRIAL (REFERENCE)	NO. OF SUBJECTS	CORONARY HEART DISEASE RATE PER 1000 PERSON-YEARS		
		Less Therapy	More Therapy	Difference (%)
HDFP[16]*				
Normal ECG	3210	3.1	2.0	−35
Abnormal ECG	1963	3.5	4.3	+23
MRFIT[14]				
Normal ECG	5593	3.4	2.6	−24
Abnormal ECG	2418	2.9	4.9	+70

* The HDFP (Hypertension and Follow-up Program) patients were those men with diastolic blood pressure of between 90 and 104 mm Hg not on antihypertensive therapy at baseline, who were therefore similar to those in the MRFIT (Multiple Risk Factor Intervention Trial) population.

J-curve, particularly in hypertensives with preexisting coronary disease, it is described on p. 855.

Whatever the reasons, antihypertensive therapy, *as used in these nine trials,* has not been found clearly to protect against coronary disease, the major cause of morbidity and mortality among hypertensive patients. Since a diuretic, often in relatively high doses, was the first and often the only drug in all of the trials except for half of the treated patients in the Medical Research Council (MRC) trial, the presence of diuretic-induced biochemical derangements has been offered as a potential explanation of the lack of coronary protection. A different approach, specifically the use of a beta blocker as first drug, was used in the other half of the treated patients in the MRC trials. However, it too, failed to provide overall protection against coronary disease, other than in those men who did not smoke. Two other trials[23,24] have compared beta-blockers against diuretics and they too failed to demonstrate any clear advantage of either drug.[25]

The failure to show protection against coronary disease by drug treatment of mild hypertension may not reflect a fault of reduction of the blood pressure, but a fault of the manner by which it was lowered. Unfortunately, there are no data on coronary protection with any other drugs than diuretics and beta-blockers but, as indicted below, there is a strong likelihood that they will be more protective. In the meantime, it should be noted that reduction of the blood pressure in these trials did significantly reduce stroke mortality (Fig. 29-1) and almost completely prevented progression of the elevated pressures to more dangerous levels of hypertension.

GUIDELINES FOR TREATMENT

The sum of current evidence, then, supports the view that the risks of mild hypertension are not so great and the benefits of active therapy are not so large as to mandate that *all* mildly hypertensive persons be treated. A more aggressive course could be justified if there were *no* risks or problems associated with active therapy but, in all trials, 20 per cent to 40 per cent of patients given drug therapy experienced some adverse effects, seldom life-threatening but often enough to interfere with the quality of life.[26] Perhaps this percentage will be reduced with newer antihypertensive agents.

In view of the legitimate concerns arising from the evidence now available, a reconsideration of the common practice of treating *all* mild hypertension seems appropriate. The need for active drug therapy for those with moderate or severe hypertension, i.e., DBP above 105 mm Hg, is incontrovertible. Nonetheless, there is a need to ensure that their pressure is *persistently* elevated: Even among the patients enrolled in the Australian trial whose DBP was between 105 and 109 after two sets of readings four weeks apart, 11 per cent of those given only placebo pills had DBP persistently below 90 mm Hg for the next four years. Their blood pressure fell mostly during the first four months. Therefore, unless there is an obvious need for the more immediate institution of drug therapy, such as progressive target organ damage or blood pressures so high as to threaten immediate danger, all patients should be given the opportunity to achieve a spontaneous reduction of their initially high pressures over a four- to six-month interval. During that time they should have their pressures carefully monitored, since if it goes up—as it did in 10 to 15 per cent of the placebo-treated patients in the trials shown in Table 29-1—immediate institution of drug therapy may be indicated.

As noted in the preceding chapter, the monitoring logically can be done at home and, for some, with ambulatory 24-hour monitoring, which may provide, in a condensed manner, better prognostic evidence than multiple blood pressure measurements taken in the office. While the blood pressure is being monitored, the use of appropriate nondrug therapies may help lower the pressure even more, without risk and with relatively little inconvenience. Such nondrug therapies may not only lower the blood pressure but also reduce overall cardiovascular risk by amelioration of such conditions as hyperlipidemia, glucose intolerance, and alcohol abuse.

THE LEVEL OF BLOOD PRESSURE TO TREAT

Despite the uncertainty as to the ability of drug therapy *as it has been provided* to protect against coronary disease in those with mild hypertension, successful reduction of elevated blood pressure will protect against progression of hypertension, stroke, and probably congestive heart failure and renal damage. Therefore, drug therapy is indicated in essentially *all* patients with DBP persistently above 100 mm Hg, in *many* with DBP above 95 mm Hg, and in *some* with DBP above 90 mm Hg or an even lower level.

The risk associated with elevations of systolic pressure has been shown to be even more linear and equally strong than with elevations of diastolic pressure (p. 817). Unfortunately, most trials have mainly considered DBP levels, so that there is less evidence concerning the levels of systolic blood pressure that mandate therapy. This is particularly true among the large segment of elderly people with predominant or pure systolic hypertension. A trial to determine whether therapy will protect them has been begun,[27] but it will be sometime in 1991 before the results are known. Meantime, elevations of systolic pressure above 170 mm Hg, at any age, deserve gradual reduction by appropriate nondrug and drug therapies.

Rationale for Use of Different Levels

The benefit of treating essentially all patients with persistent DBP above 100 mm Hg seems well established on the basis

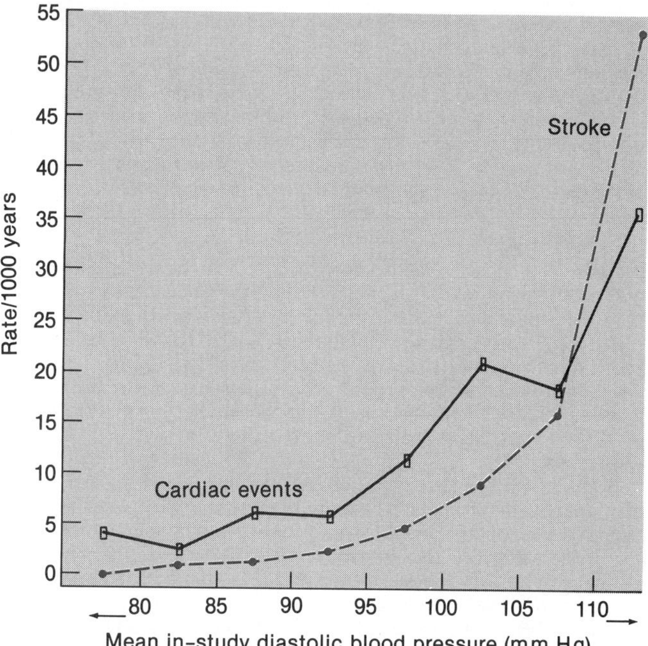

FIGURE 29-2. Absolute rate of cardiac events and stroke related to diastolic blood pressure during antihypertensive treatment. The extremes of the diastolic pressure scale include all values at or below 80 and above 110 mm Hg. Square = cardiac events, Circle = stroke. (From IPPPSH Collaborative Group: Cardiovascular risk and risk factors in a randomized trial of treatment based on the beta-blocker oxprenolol: The International Prospective Primary Prevention Study in Hypertension [IPPPSH]. J. Hypertens. 3:388, 1985.)

of the clinical trials shown in Table 29-1. The evidence for benefit of those with DBP above 95 mm Hg is less certain but reasonably strong (Fig. 29-2). These curves[23] show progressive falls in both cardiac events and stroke when blood pressures were reduced from above 110 to below 95 mm Hg. Below 95 mm Hg, no significant falls in the already quite low event rates were observed. Similar protection in those whose initial readings were above 95 mm Hg was demonstrated in the Australian[13] and the MRC trials.[15]

Those with DBP between 90 and 95 mm Hg, who constitute 40 per cent of the entire hypertensive population, have not been found to benefit from drug therapy in the controlled trials shown in Table 29-1. Part of this failure may reflect the finding that many of the patients in these trials were not, in fact, hypertensive: None of the trials required more than a two-month run-in period before randomization to active or placebo therapy, and it has been shown that readings in as many as one-third to one-half of patients with DBP above 95 mm Hg will be persistently below 90 mm Hg after four to six months *on no therapy*.

In addition, the risks are relatively small at such low levels of elevated blood pressure, and the trials, despite their size and duration, may not have been adequate to show protection with so little preexisting risk. Moreover, the trials mainly involved low-risk, otherwise healthy patients, unlike many seen in clinical practice. In the Hypertension Detection and Follow-up Program (HDFP) trial, those patients with initial DBP between 90 and 95 mm Hg whose pressures were lowered more aggressively (the stepped-care group) had fewer cardiovascular events than did those whose pressures were lowered less. However, the more intensively treated (Special Intervention) half of the patients in the Multiple Risk Factor Intervention trial (MRFIT) whose initial DBP was between 90 and 94 mm Hg had a *higher* total and coronary death rate than did those given less therapy (Usual Care), so the evidence from the two large nonplacebo-controlled trials done in the United States remains contradictory.

In hopes of documenting further the benefits of antihypertensive therapy for the millions with mild to moderate hypertension, additional analysis of the subsequent mortality among MRFIT participants[28] and meta-analysis of trials involving more severe hypertensives[25] have been performed. Unfortunately, they have shed little light on the issue of coronary protection for mild-to-moderate hypertension.

Therefore, there is legitimate cause for the disagreement as to the level at which to institute drug therapy, some believing that drug therapy should be given to all with DBP above 90 mm Hg, others believing that it should be given only to those with DBP above 100 mm Hg. The disagreement is not only of academic interest. As many as 40 million persons in the United States alone are in that 90 to 100 mm Hg range, so obviously the issue has great clinical and economic relevance.

On the basis of available data, the position adopted by a conference sponsored by the World Health Organization and the International Society of Hypertension seems to be an appropriate compromise (Fig. 29-3).[29] In substance, it states that after three to six months of observation, 95 mm Hg DBP should be used as the level for institution of active drug therapy. Some patients who are at high overall risk of developing coronary artery disease should probably be treated even if they have lower levels of DBP. Included in this group are patients with known coronary artery disease, patients with a history of hypercholesterolemia, cigarette smoking, and a family history of premature coronary artery disease, and diabetics with mild hypertension who have early evidence of glomerulosclerosis that is likely to progress if untreated. For such patients, active drug therapy may even be indicated at DBP levels below 90 mm Hg. More clinical trials are needed among such patients, but those at high risk may need the benefits potentially available from lower blood pressure, despite the risks attendant to the therapy used to achieve the lower pressure.

Although it has not been possible to predict with certainty which patients will develop complications, the larger the

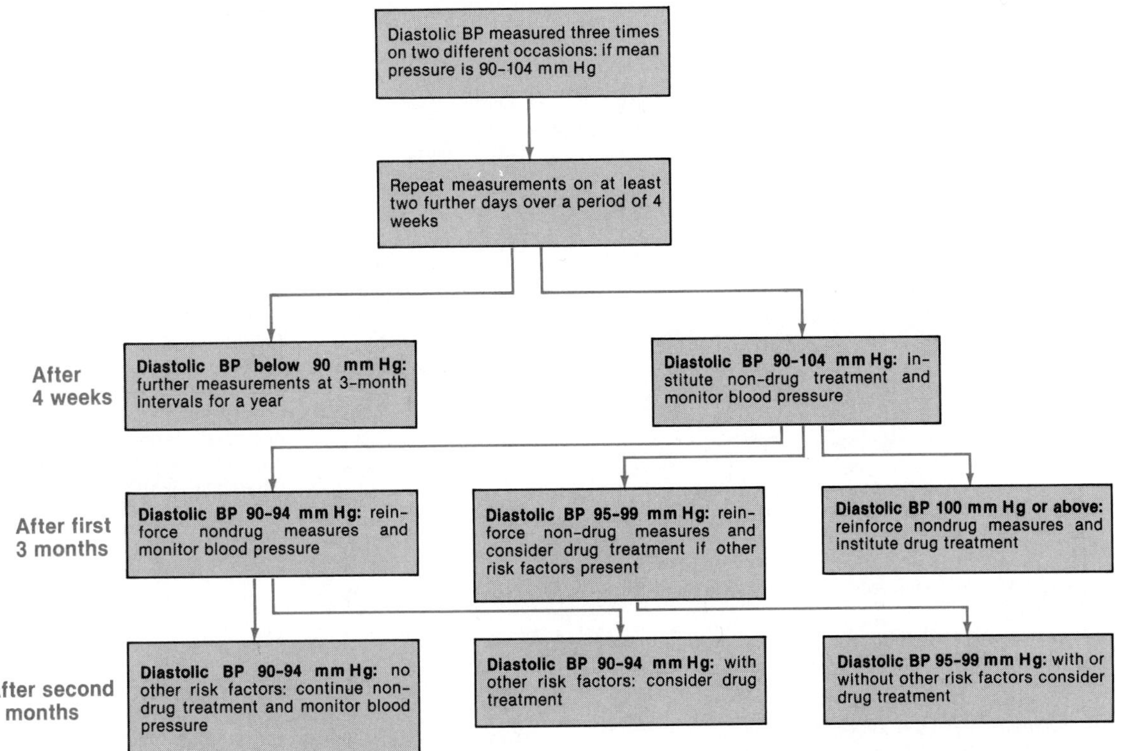

FIGURE 29–3. Definition, blood pressure (BP) measurement, and management of hypertension. (From WHO/ISH Mild Hypertension Liaison Committee. 1989 guidelines for the management of mild hypertension: Memorandum from WHO/ISH meeting. J. Hypertens. *7*:689, 1989.)

number of other cardiovascular risk factors present, the larger the number of complications observed and the greater the potential for protection by the amelioration of these other risk as well.[30] The importance of cessation of cigarette smoking has been particularly emphasized.[15] Because of their relatively lower degree of risk at every level of pressure, women are relatively less in need of therapy than are men. The level for instituting therapy in most women may appropriately be a DBP of 100 mm Hg, rather than the level of 95 for most men.

THE LEVEL OF BLOOD PRESSURE TO REACH

Once having decided to treat, the clinician must consider the goal of therapy. Until recently, most assumed that the effects of reduction of blood pressure on cardiovascular risk would fit a straight line downward (line A in Fig. 29–4),[31] justifying the opinion "the lower, the better." However, data from large trials indicated a more gradual decline in risk when pressures were reduced to moderate levels (line B in Fig. 29–4), around 95 mm Hg in the IPPPSH trial (Fig. 29–2).[23] Subsequently, Cruickshank[19] has called attention to a J-curve (line C in Fig. 29–4), reflecting a progressive fall in risk as pressure is lowered, but only to a certain level; below that level, the risk for coronary ischemic events goes back up. Cruickshank recalled the warning of Stewart in 1979[32] and added data of his own[33] to that of five other studies,[24,34–37] all indicating a rise in coronary events when treatment reduced DBP levels below a J-point that was usually between 85 and 90 mm Hg (Fig. 29–5). More recently, Alderman et al.[22] have provided additional confirmation, with a rise in coronary events when DBP was lowered, on average, to below 85 mm Hg. Recall, too, the data from HDFP and MRFIT (Table 29–2) showing higher coronary mortality rates among mild hypertensives with baseline ECG abnormalities if they were given more intensive therapy.[38,39] The apparent propensity to induce myocardial ischemia when pressures lowered below a certain critical threshold may not apply to other vital organs. Therefore, maximal protection against stroke or renal damage may require greater

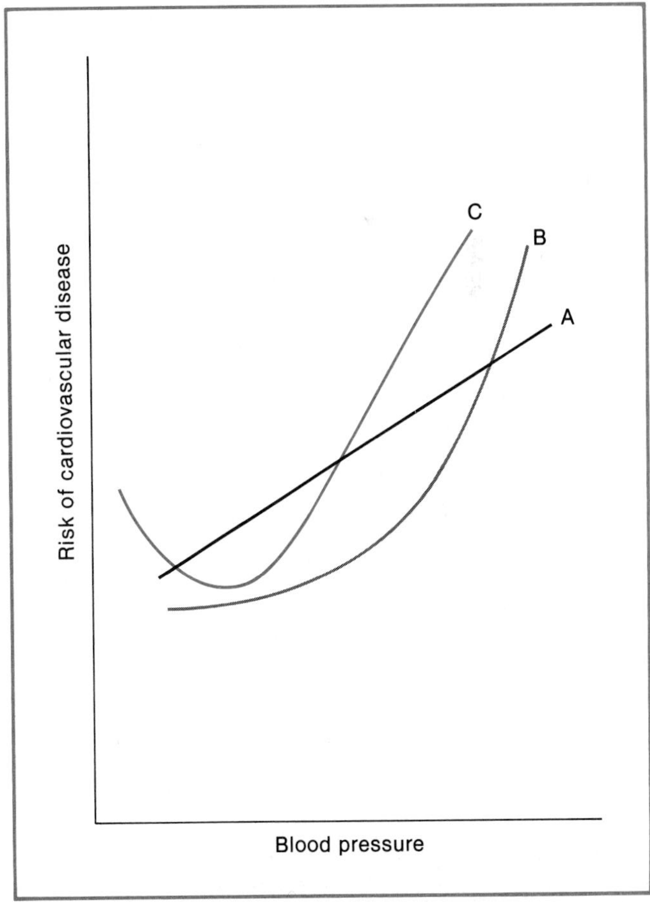

FIGURE 29–4. Three models representing hypothetical relationships between levels of blood pressure and risk of cardiovascular disease. (From Epstein, F. H.: Proceedings of the XVth International Congress of Therapeutics, September 5–9, 1979. Brussels, Excerpta Medica, 1980.)

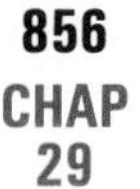

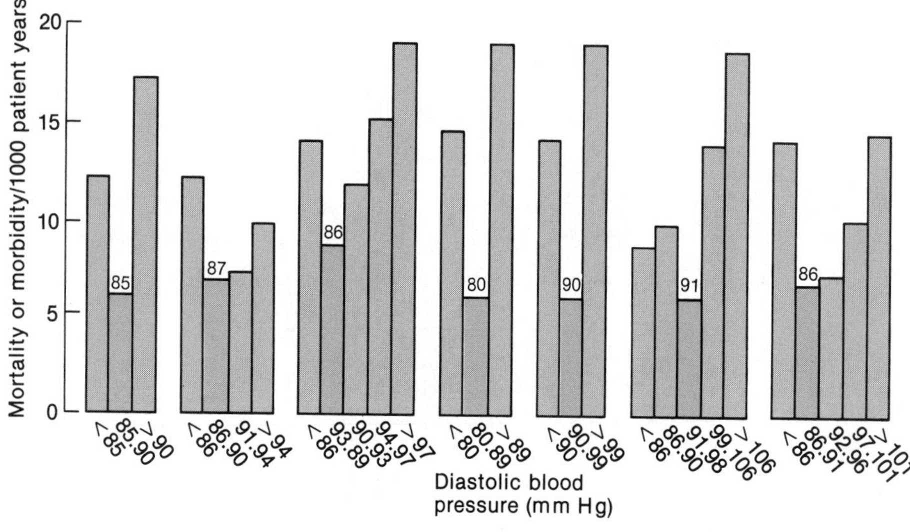

FIGURE 29-5. Relation of diastolic blood pressure (phase V) during treatment to mortality or morbidity from coronary heart disease. The six studies included 14,536 patients. Information from the Heart Attack Primary Prevention in Hypertension trial (HAPPHY) is by personal communication (Wilhelmsen, L.). The numbers on top of the histograms indicate diastolic blood pressure in millimeters of mercury at which J point (lowest incidence of myocardial infarction) occurred. (From Cruickshank, J. M.: Coronary flow reserve and the J curve relation between diastolic blood pressure and myocardial infarction. Br. Med. J. *297*:1227, 1988.)

falls in pressure than the coronary circulation can safely handle.

Why the special vulnerability of the coronary circulation in the presence of hypertension? Multiple explanations are available, including (1) the myocardium is usually hypertrophied, requiring even more nutrients; (2) oxygen delivery to the myocardium is near maximal even in nonhypertrophied hearts so that little more can be extracted when perfusion pressure is lowered; (3) coronary arteries do not autoregulate as well as cerebral arteries, particularly if they are sclerotic[40]; and (4) coronary vascular reserve is limited, so that a fall in perfusion pressure may not be tolerated.[41]

The presence of a *J*-curve has been stoutly defended and almost as aggressively denied.[42] Some deny that it occurs except as an "irregularity" of small sets of data in a particularly vulnerable group of patients.[43] On the other hand, the denial of a *J*-curve based on the absence of a lower threshold of risk in long-term observations on normotensive and mildly hypertensive people free of coronary artery disease and given no antihypertensive therapy[43] should be given no credence as evidence against the presence of such a threshold in more significantly hypertensive patients, often with preexisting coronary artery disease, who are given antihypertensive therapy and whose pressures are thereby "artificially" lowered. This is all the more valid when therapy involves drugs that have the propensity to worsen other coronary risks as they lower the pressure. The prudent course is to accept the considerable evidence that a *J*-curve does exist and hope to avoid it by careful, gradual reduction in pressure with agents that do not simultaneously incite other risks. This is particularly important in the elderly who display a *J*-curve even if on no therapy, presumably reflecting deteriorating general health.[44]

Once good control of blood pressure in a patient has been achieved, it may be possible to reduce or withdraw drug therapy. Perhaps one-fourth of patients with initially mild hypertension who achieve good control with therapy will remain normotensive for at least one year after their therapy is stopped.[45] However, such patients need to remain under observation.

There is no simple or single answer to the questions of whom to treat with drugs for mild hypertension and how low the pressure should be reduced. Each patient must be considered separately, taking various factors into account. The foregoing discussion should indicate the wisdom of withholding drug therapy from any of these patients, at least until the effects of time and nondrug therapies have been given a chance, and avoiding too fast and too great falls in pressure.

NONDRUG THERAPY

Interest in the use of various nondrug therapies for the treatment of hypertension—particularly diet and exercise—has risen markedly in the past few years. Yet many practitioners either do not use them or use them in a casual, perfunctory manner. This hesitant attitude can be attributed both to the sparseness of firm evidence indicating that these therapies succeed and to the difficulty many have faced in convincing patients to adhere to them. This situation is likely to change: Evidence for the effectiveness of these approaches is growing,[46-48] techniques for improving adherence are being popularized, and patients seem increasingly willing to adopt changes in life style. These changes come at a propitious time, when many more people are being identified as hypertensive and are considered in need of lowering of their blood pressure. Although most have turned first to drugs, the evidence presented in the previous section suggests that these can be safely withheld from many hypertensives to allow nondrug therapies a chance to be effective.

In part, the underuse of nondrug therapies is due to excitement over newly available drugs and the massive advertising campaigns to promote their use. Without commercial advocates, nondrug therapies have been unable to compete. Moreover, when physicians decide to treat a condition, they expect almost immediate results with virtual certainty. Such expectations were clearly justified when the majority of patients had fairly severe hypertension; however, as the large number of patients with mild hypertension enter the picture, a more gradual approach to their management seems more appropriate.

Data from long-term controlled studies of a nondrug therapy document a relatively small but significant reduction in blood pressure both in normotensives who are especially prone to develop hypertension[49,50] and in hypertensives whose therapy has been stopped.[46-48] Of equal, if not greater, benefit is the concomitant reduction in other risk factors even if the pressure fall is less than provided by drug therapy.[51]

Just as the increased awareness of the problem of patients' frequent poor adherence to drug therapy has led to attempts to improve the situation,[52] similar attention toward adherence to nondrug therapies will probably improve their effectiveness. These measures should be introduced gradually and gently. Too many and too drastic changes in life style may discourage patients from accepting needed care. Eventually, however, all hypertensive patients should benefit from mild restriction of dietary salt, reduction of excess body weight, and moderation of alcohol intake.[53] Although high blood lipid levels and cigarette smoking have little, if any, direct effect on blood pressure, patients with hypertension should be encouraged to eliminate these and other reversible risk factors that predispose to cardiovascular disease (see Chap. 37).

WEIGHT REDUCTION. In most published studies, weight loss has been shown to reduce blood pressure (Fig. 29-6).[54] In a review of adequately controlled intervention studies published through 1985, a 1.0 kilogram decrease in body weight was accompanied by an average reduction of 1.6/1.3 mm Hg in blood pressure. There may be a threshold, around 4 kg, to observe an effect[55] and a floor below which further weight loss may not be accompanied by further falls in blood pressure.[56] Use of a very low calorie supplement may achieve faster weight loss and marked falls in blood pressure[57] while improving exercise endurance.[58] Moreover, weight loss may reduce the sensitivity of blood pressure to sodium,[59] improving further the response to nondrug therapy. Although the rate of recidivism among obese people may be high, an attempt at weight reduction in all obese hypertensive patients should be made, using whatever level of caloric restriction the patient is able to maintain.

DIETARY SODIUM RESTRICTION. On page 828 evidence was presented incriminating the typically high sodium content of the diet of people living in developed, industrial-

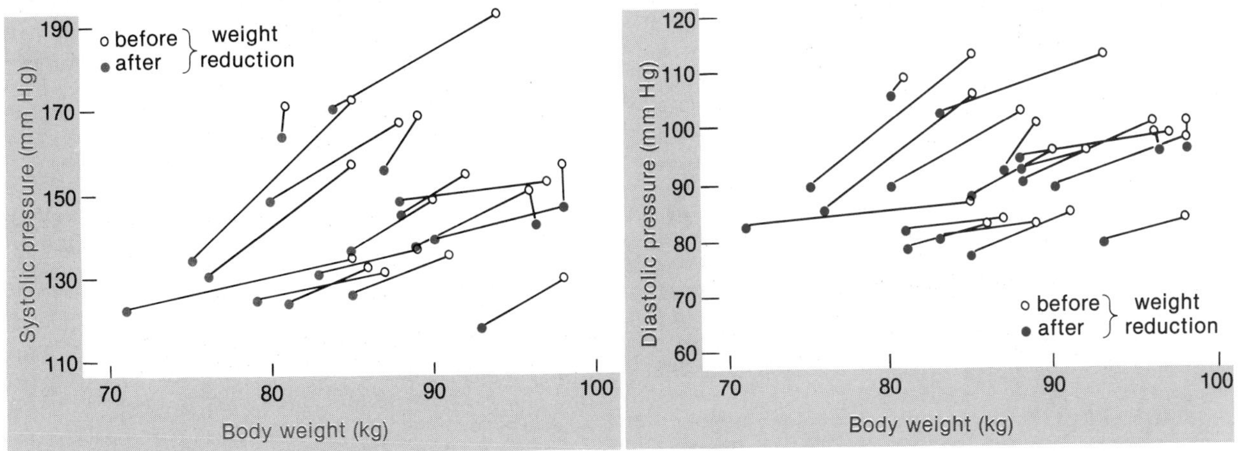

FIGURE 29–6. Systolic and diastolic blood pressure before and after body weight reduction. (From Staessen, J., Fagard, R., Lijnen, P., and Amery, A.: Body weight, sodium intake and blood pressure. J. Hypertens. *7*(Suppl 1):S19, 1989.)

ized societies as a cause of hypertension. Once hypertension is present, modest salt restriction may help lower the blood pressure. In the review by Staessen et al. of 24 intervention studies,[54] an average reduction in sodium intake of 100 mmol per day produced a decrease in blood pressure of 5.4/6.5 mm Hg. Two additional large-scale studies published subsequent to the Staessen et al. review confirm the effectiveness and feasibility of moderate sodium restriction in treating hypertension.[60,61] In a smaller but more controlled study, the fall in blood pressure was shown to be greater at a daily sodium intake of 50 mmol than at 100 mmol per day.[62]

However, rigid degrees of sodium restriction are not only difficult for patients to achieve but may also be counterproductive. The marked stimulation of renin-aldosterone that accompanies rigid sodium restriction may prevent the blood pressure from falling and increase the amount of potassium wastage if diuretics are concomitantly used.[63] Not all hypertensives will respond to a moderate degree of sodium restriction to a level of 70 to 100 mmol sodium, or approximately 2 gm per day. Blacks tend to be more sodium sensitive,[64] and elderly patients may be particularly responsive to sodium restriction, perhaps because of their usually lower renin responsiveness.[65]

Even if the blood pressure does not fall with moderate degrees of sodium restriction, the patient may still benefit: Improved beta-adrenergic responsiveness,[66] increased antihypertensive effectiveness of other drugs (with the possible exception of calcium antagonists[67]), and less diuretic-induced potassium wastage[63] have all been reported among patients on moderate sodium restriction. Although there is no assurance that moderate sodium restriction will help, there is no evidence that it will hurt. For example, neither the intake of other vital nutrients[68] nor exercise tolerance in a hot environment[69] are reduced by a lower sodium intake. Therefore, I consider it to be useful for all persons, as a preventive measure in those who are normotensive, and, more certainly, as partial therapy in those who are hypertensive. Population-wide reductions may be possible[70] with a considerable potential thereby to reduce cardiovascular mortality.[71]

The easiest way to accomplish moderate sodium restriction is to substitute natural foods for processed foods, since natural foods are low in sodium and high in potassium, whereas most processed foods have had sodium added and potassium removed. Additional guidelines include the following:

1. Add no sodium chloride to food during cooking or at the table.
2. If a salty taste is desired, use a half sodium and half potassium chloride preparation (such as Lite Salt), or a pure potassium chloride substitute.
3. Avoid or minimize the use of "fast" foods, many of which have high sodium content.
4. Recognize the sodium content of some antacids and proprietary medications. (For example, Alka-Seltzer contains more than 500 mg of sodium; Rolaids are virtually sodium free.)

POTASSIUM SUPPLEMENTATION. Some of the advantages of a lower sodium intake may relate to its tendency to increase body potassium content, both by a coincidental increase in dietary potassium intake and by a decrease in potassium wastage if diuretics are being used. Although potassium deficiency clearly exerts multiple effects that may increase blood pressure,[72] evidence that correction of hypokalemia[73] or addition of dietary potassium to normokalemics will lower the blood pressure is skimpy.[74] Nonetheless, diuretic-induced hypokalemia may be more of a danger than many suspect, so that, for various reasons, hypertensive patients should be protected from potassium depletion. Moreover, certainly in experimental animals[75] and perhaps in humans as well,[76] extra-dietary potassium intake protects against vascular damage and strokes.

MAGNESIUM SUPPLEMENTATION. In controlled trials little effect on blood pressure is seen with magnesium supplements.[77] However, those who are magnesium depleted may not be able to replete concomitant potassium deficiency.[78]

CALCIUM SUPPLEMENTATION. As noted on page 827, an increase in free calcium concentration in vascular smooth muscle cells may be a final step in the pathogenesis of primary hypertension. Nonetheless, some hypertensive patients have a lower calcium intake and higher urinary calcium excretion than do normotensives.[79] In 22 mostly short-term studies, about one-third of hypertensives given 1 to 2 gm of supplemental calcium per day have a fall in blood pressure.[80] Because others given calcium supplements have a rise in blood pressure, the best course is to ensure that calcium intake is not inadvertently reduced by reduction of milk and cheese consumption in an attempt to reduce saturated fat and sodium intake while not giving supplemental calcium.

OTHER DIETARY CHANGES. Some lowering of the blood pressure has been noted in studies of a lacto-ovo-vegetarian diet[81] and high doses of polyunsaturated fish oil.[82] No additional effect of 6 gm daily supplements of fish oil was found in those who regularly ate fish three or more times a week.[83] Neither decreases in total dietary fat[84] nor increases in dietary fiber[85] seem to alter blood pressure. In the attempt to reduce calories and overall coronary risk, substitution of carbohydrate for fat may aggravate further the hyperinsulinemia often present in primary hypertension and therefore be counterproductive.[86]

When consumed by noncoffee drinkers, caffeine equivalent to the amount in two cups of coffee will raise the blood pressure, probably by activation of the sympathetic nervous system.[87] However, chronic caffeine ingestion is *not* associated with significant rises in blood pressure because of tolerance to the hemodynamic effects.

MODERATION OF ALCOHOL. Moderate alcohol consumption, less than 1 oz of ethanol per day, does not increase the prevalence of hypertension. Heavier drinking clearly exerts a pressor effect that makes *alcohol abuse the most common cause of reversible hypertension*.[88] One to two portions of alcohol-containing beverages a day, containing 0.5 to 1.0 oz of ethanol, need not be prohibited, particularly since fewer coronary events have been noted in those who consume that amount.[89]

ISOTONIC EXERCISE. Isometric exercise, such as weightlifting, pushing, and pulling, may be harmful to the hypertensive patient. During an isometric contraction, blood pressure rises often to high levels reflexly.[90] On the other hand, in well-controlled studies, regular isotonic exercise results in a 5 to 10 mm Hg reduction in blood pressure, accompanied by, and probably related to, a fall in sympathetic nervous activity.[91] Beta-blockers may diminish the ability to perform exercise whereas most other antihypertensive drugs do not.[92]

RELAXATION TECHNIQUES. Various forms of relaxation—transcendental meditation, yoga, biofeedback, psychotherapy—have reduced the blood pressure of some hypertensive persons.[93] Responders tend to be those with overt signs of sympathetic nervous overactivity.[94]

THE POTENTIAL OF NONDRUG THERAPY

Part of the antihypertensive effect reported with these and other nondrug therapies may be attributable to the nonspecific fall in blood pressure so often seen when repeated readings are taken. Such decreases may reflect a statistical regression toward the mean, a placebo effect, or a relief of anxiety and stress with time. The same phenomenon is probably also responsible for much of the initial response to drug therapy, so that success may be attributed to both drugs and nondrugs when it is deserved by neither.

As noted, increasingly long and strong evidence from controlled studies attests to the efficacy of multifaceted nondrug programs to reduce the blood pressure. Whether such success can be achieved by individual practitioners is uncertain. However, because help is available, including various educational materials for patients, professional assistants such as dietitians and psychologists, and groups organized for weight reduction, exercise, and relaxation therapies, the effort seems both increasingly easy and likely to be successful in lowering blood pressure.

Antihypertensive Drug Therapy

If the nondrug therapies just described are not followed or prove to be ineffective, or if the level of hypertension at the onset is so high that immediate drug therapy is deemed necessary, the general guidelines listed in Table 29–3 should be helpful in improving patient adherence to lifelong treatment.

GENERAL GUIDELINES

Although most of the points listed in Table 29–3 are rather obvious, a few deserve additional comment. Item 5E, "Use the fewest daily doses needed," actually has not been found to influence adherence significantly,[95] but patients prefer to take medications less frequently. At present, most antihypertensive medications can be taken by most patients either once or twice a day. Although a few patients may have better control with more frequent doses, even patients with end-organ damage and resistant hypertension can often be managed by once-a-day therapy. In 55 such patients, a once-a-day regimen of diuretic, minoxidil, and nadolol controlled 46 for almost a year, although six had intolerable side effects.[96]

PHARMACOLOGICAL PRINCIPLES. Item 6b in Table 29–3 suggests starting with small doses of medication, aiming for a reduction of 5 to 10 mm Hg in blood pressure at each step. Some physicians, by nature and training, desire to control a patient's hypertension rapidly and completely. Regardless of which drugs are used, this approach often leads to easy fatigability, weakness, and postural dizziness, which many patients find intolerable, particularly when they felt well before therapy was begun. Although hypokalemia and other electrolyte abnormalities may be responsible for some of these symptoms, a more likely explanation has been provided by the studies of Strandgaard and Haunsø.[97] As shown in Figure 29–7, they reconfirmed the constancy of cerebral blood flow by autoregulation over a range of mean arterial pressures from about 60 to 120 mm Hg in normal subjects and from 110 to 180 mm Hg in patients with hypertension. This shift to the right protects the hypertensive patient from a surge of blood flow, which could cause cerebral edema. However, the shift also predisposes the

TABLE 29-3 GENERAL GUIDELINES TO IMPROVE PATIENT ADHERENCE TO ANTIHYPERTENSIVE THERAPY

1. **Be aware of the problem of nonadherence and be alert to signs of patient nonadherence.**
2. **Establish the goal of therapy: to reduce blood pressure to normotensive levels with minimal or no side effects.**
3. **Educate the patient about the disease and its treatment.**
   a. **Involve the patient in decision making.**
   b. **Encourage family support.**
4. **Maintain contact with the patient.**
   a. **Encourage visits and calls to allied health personnel.**
   b. **Allow the pharmacist to monitor therapy.**
   c. **Give feedback to the patient via home BP readings.**
   d. **Make contact with patients who do not return.**
5. **Keep care inexpensive and simple.**
   a. **Do the least work-up needed to rule out secondary causes.**
   b. **Obtain follow-up laboratory data only yearly unless indicated more often.**
   c. **Use home blood pressure readings.**
   d. **Use nondrug, no-cost therapies.**
   e. **Use the fewest daily doses of drugs needed.**
   f. **If appropriate, use combination tablets.**
   g. **Tailor medication to daily routines.**
6. **Prescribe according to pharmacological principles.**
   a. **Add one drug at a time.**
   b. **Start with small doses, aiming for 5 to 10 mm Hg reductions at each step.**
   c. **Prevent volume overload with adequate diuretic and sodium restriction.**
   d. **Be willing to stop unsuccessful therapy and try a different approach.**
   e. **Anticipate side effects.**
   f. **Adjust therapy to ameliorate side effects that do not spontaneously disappear.**
   g. **Continue to add effective and tolerated drugs, stepwise, in sufficient doses to achieve the goal of therapy.**

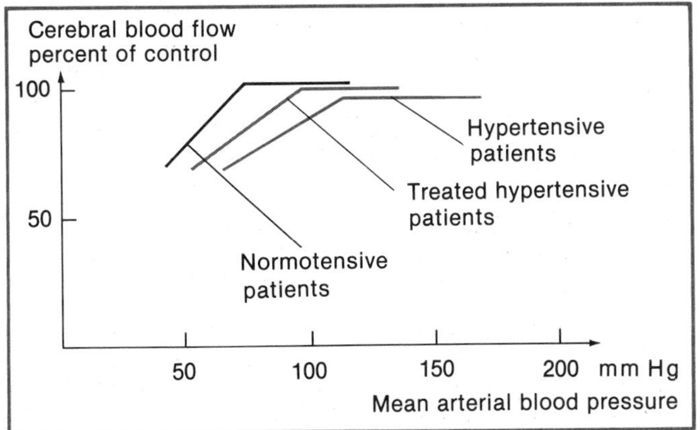

FIGURE 29–7. Mean cerebral blood flow autoregulation curves from normotensive, severely hypertensive, and effectively treated hypertensive patients are shown. Modified from Strandgaard (Circulation 53:720, 1976). (From Strandgaaard, S., Haunsø, S.: Why does antihypertensive treatment prevent stroke but not myocardial infarction? Lancet *2*:658, 1987.)

hypertensive patient to cerebral ischemia when blood pressure is lowered.

The lower limit of autoregulation necessary to preserve a constant cerebral blood flow in hypertensive patients is a mean of about 110 mm Hg. Thus acutely lowering the pressure from 160/110 (mean = 127) to 140/85 (mean = 102) may induce cerebral hypoperfusion, although hypotension in the accepted sense has not been produced. This provides an explanation for what many patients experience at the start of antihypertensive therapy, i.e., manifestations of cerebral hypoperfusion, even though blood pressure levels do not seem inordinately low.

Thus, there should be a gradual approach to antihypertensive therapy in order to avoid symptoms related to overly aggressive blood pressure reduction. Fortunately, as shown in the middle of Figure 29–7, if therapy is continued for a period of time, the curve of cerebral autoregulation shifts back toward normal, allowing patients to tolerate greater reductions in blood pressure without experiencing symptoms. There appear to be differences in the effects of various types of antihypertensive drugs on cerebral autoregulation and blood flow: Direct vasodilators such as hydralazine may cause autoregulation to be lost; alpha-adrenergic blockers help to preserve cerebral blood flow at low pressure; angiotensin-converting enzyme (ACE) inhibitors cause a resetting of the autoregulatory curve to lower levels, which probably explains why patients with congestive heart failure can tolerate such low systemic pressures when given these drugs.[98]

TABLE 29-4 CO-MORBID CONDITIONS AMONG 2706 HYPERTENSIVE PATIENTS

Diabetes	18.1%
Arthritis	36.1%
Back problems	4.4%
Chronic lung disease	7.4%
Angina	8.0%
Myocardial infarction	2.2%
Congestive heart failure	5.9%
None	37.3%

From Stewart, A. L., Greenfield, S., Hays, R. D., et al.: Functional status and well-being of patients with chronic conditions. Results from the Medical Outcomes study. JAMA *262*:907, 1989. Copyright 1989, the American Medical Association.

INDIVIDUALIZED THERAPY. Item 6g in Table 29–3 refers to the addition of drugs, stepwise, in sufficient doses to achieve the goal of therapy. Over the past 30 years the purely empirical basis for the use of antihypertensive drugs was replaced by a stepped-care approach, which involves use of a diuretic or a beta-adrenergic blocking drug first and stepwise addition of other drugs as needed.

Over the last few years, a more rational basis for selecting the initial drug has been recommended, an approach that more closely fits a patient's individual needs and demographics.[53] Individualized therapy involves three considerations: the patient's race (blacks responding less well to beta blockers and perhaps to ACE inhibitors), the patient's age (the elderly responding slightly better to diuretics and calcium antagonists), and the patient's concomitant conditions as enumerated in a recent survey (Table 29–4).[99] Some of the comorbid conditions point toward a choice, e.g., use of a calcium antagonist or beta blocker in a patient with angina; other conditions point away from certain choices, e.g., avoiding use of a beta-blocker in a patient with bronchospastic lung disease.

Even with a careful attempt to choose an appropriate drug for an individual patient, the choice may be either ineffectual in perhaps a third or unacceptable because of side effects in another 10 to 20 per cent of all patients. Therefore, the physi-

TABLE 29-5 THE CHOICE OF INITIAL THERAPY

	DIURETICS	CENTRALLY ACTING AGENTS	α-BLOCKERS	β-BLOCKERS	CONVERTING ENZYME INHIBITORS	CALCIUM ANTAGONISTS
HEMODYNAMIC EFFECT	Initial volume shrinkage	Reduce cardiac output	Peripheral vasodilation	Reduce cardiac output	Peripheral vasodilation	Peripheral vasodilation
SIDE EFFECTS OVERT	Weakness Palpitations	Sedation Dry mouth	Postural dizziness	Bronchospasm Fatigue Delay recovery Hypoglycemia	Cough Taste disturbance Rash	Flushing Local edema Constipation (verapamil)
HIDDEN	Hypokalemia Hypercholesterolemia Glucose intolerance Hyperuricemia	Withdrawal syndrome Autoimmune syndromes (methyldopa)		Glucose intolerance Hypertriglyceridemia Decrease HDL-cholesterol	Leukopenia Proteinuria	A-V conduction (verapamil, diltiazem)
CONTRAINDICATIONS	Preexisting volume contraction	Orthostatic hypotension Liver disease (methyldopa)	Orthostatic hypotension	Asthma Heartblock	Pregnancy	
CAUTIONS	Diabetes mellitus Gout Digitalis toxicity			Peripheral vascular disease Insulin-requiring diabetes Allergy Coronary spasm Withdrawal angina	Renal insufficiency Renovascular disease	Heart failure
SPECIAL ADVANTAGES	Effective in blacks, elderly Enhance effectiveness of all other agents	No alteration in blood lipids No fluid retention (guanabenz)	No decrease in cardiac output No alteration in blood lipids No sedation	Reduce recurrences of coronary disease Reduce manifestations of anxiety, Coexisting angina, migrane, glaucoma	No CNS side effects Unload congestive heart failure No coronary vasoconstriction Possible renal protection	Effective in blacks, elderly No CNS side effects Coronary vasodilation

From Kaplan, N. M.: Clinical Hypertension. 5th ed. Baltimore, © by Williams & Wilkins, 1990, p. 249.

cian must be willing to discontinue the initial choice and try a drug from another category. A more structured trial and error approach has been described in which each patient is put through multiple double-blind, randomized crossover trials against placebos to determine the best drug.[100] However, this approach probably is too much trouble for most physicians and patients. Other approaches have been recommended, including one based on the renin profile[101] and another on multiple hemodynamic features.[102] The general principles shown in Table 29–5 should serve well to ensure that each patient receives a drug likely to provide good control and few side effects.

For patients with more severe hypertension, in whom the first choice can be expected to be only partially effective, the stepped-care approach appears more logical. A diuretic will enhance the effectiveness of most other drugs used, preventing the "pseudotolerance" that develops because of the fluid retention that frequently follows the use of some adrenergic blocking drugs and vasodilators.[103] Increasingly, an ACE inhibitor or calcium antagonist is being chosen as the second or third drug when triple therapy is needed.

DIURETICS

(See also pp. 469 to 479)

Diuretics useful in the treatment of hypertension may be divided into four major groups by their primary site of action within the tubule, starting in the proximal portion and moving to the collecting duct: (1) agents acting on the proximal tubule, such as carbonic anhydrase inhibitors, which have limited antihypertensive efficacy; (2) loop diuretics; (3) thiazides and related sulfonamide compounds; and (4) potassium-sparing agents (Fig. 17–6, p. 474). A thiazide is the usual choice, often in combination with a potassium-sparing agent. Loop diuretics should be reserved for those patients with renal insufficiency or resistant hypertension.

MECHANISM OF ACTION. All diuretics initially lower the blood pressure by increasing urinary sodium excretion and by reducing plasma volume, extracellular fluid volume, and cardiac output. Within six to eight weeks the lowered plasma, extracellular fluid volume, and cardiac output return toward normal. At this point and beyond, the lower blood pressure is related to a fall in peripheral resistance, thereby improving the underlying hemodynamic defect of hypertension. The mechanism responsible for the lowered peripheral resistance is unknown, but there is a need for an initial diuresis, since diuretics fail to lower the blood pressure when the excreted sodium is returned or when given to chronic dialysis patients with nonfunctioning kidneys. With the shrinkage in blood volume and lower blood pressure, increased secretion of renin and aldosterone retard the continued sodium diuresis. Both renin-induced vasoconstriction and aldosterone-induced sodium retention prevent continued diminution of body fluids and progressive fall in blood pressure while diuretic therapy is continued.

CLINICAL EFFECTS. With continuous diuretic therapy, blood pressure usually falls about 10 mm Hg, although the degree depends on various factors, including the initial height of the pressure, the quantity of sodium ingested, the adequacy of renal function, and the intensity of the counterregulatory renin-aldosterone response. The antihypertensive effect of the diuretic persists indefinitely, although it may be overwhelmed by dietary sodium intake above 8 gm per day.

If other antihypertensive drugs are used, a diuretic may also be needed. Without a concomitant diuretic, antihypertensive drugs that do not block the renin-aldosterone mechanism may cause sodium retention. This mechanism probably reflects the success of the drugs in lowering the blood pressure and may involve the abnormal renal pressure-natriuresis relationship that is presumably present in primary hypertension. Just as it takes more pressure to excrete a given load of sodium in the hypertensive individual, so does a lowering of pressure toward normal incite sodium retention.

The critical need for adequate diuretic therapy to keep intravascular volume diminished has been repeatedly documented.[103] Therefore, diuretics are likely to continue to be widely used in antihypertensive therapy. Drugs that inhibit the renin-aldosterone mechanism, such as ACE inhibitors, or which induce some natriuresis themselves, such as calcium antagonists, may continue to work without the need for concomitant diuretics. However, a diuretic will enhance the effectiveness of all other types of drugs, including calcium antagonists.[104]

DOSAGE AND CHOICE OF AGENT. Most patients with mild to moderate hypertension and serum creatinine concentrations below 2.0 mg/dl will respond to the lower doses of the various diuretics listed in Table 29–6. An amount equivalent to 12.5 mg of hydrochlorothiazide is usually adequate; larger doses will have some additional antihypertensive effect but at the price of additional potassium wastage.[105] For uncomplicated hypertension, a moderately long-acting thiazide is a logical choice and a single morning dose of hydrochlorothiazide will provide a 24-hour antihypertensive effect. The nonthiazide agent indapamide has special properties that make it an attractive choice: It seldom disturbs lipid or glucose levels[106] and it may exert an additional vasodilatory action by increasing prostacyclin generation in vascular smooth muscle cells.[107] With renal failure, manifested by a serum creatinine level above 2.0 mg/dl or creatinine clearance below 25 ml/min, thiazides are usually not effective, and multiple doses of furosemide or a single dose of metolazone will be needed.[108]

SIDE EFFECTS. A number of biochemical changes often accompany successful diuresis, including a decrease in plasma potassium and increases in glucose, insulin, and cholesterol (Fig. 29–8).

Hypokalemia. Serum potassium falls an average of 0.67 mmol/liter after institution of continuous, daily diuretic therapy for hypertension.[109] Among 158 hypertensives given diuretics for two years, plasma potassium levels fell to between

TABLE 29-6 DIURETICS AND POTASSIUM-SPARING AGENTS

	DAILY DOSAGE (MG)	DURATION OF ACTION (HR)
THIAZIDES		
Bendroflumethiazide (Naturetin)	2.5–5.0	More than 18
Benzthiazide (Aquatag, Exna)	12.5–50	12–18
Chlorothiazide (Diuril)	125–500	6–12
Cyclothiazide (Anhydron)	0.5–2	18–24
Hydrochlorothiazide (Esidrix, HydroDIURIL, Oretic)	12.5–50	12–18
Hydroflumethiazide (Saluron)	12.5–50	18–24
Methyclothiazide (Enduron)	2.5–5.0	More than 24
Polythiazide (Renese)	1–4	24–48
Trichlormethiazide (Metahydrin, Naqua)	1–4	More than 24
RELATED SULFONAMIDE COMPOUNDS		
Chlorthalidone (Hygroton)	12.5–50	24–72
Indapamide (Lozol)	2.5	24
Metolazone (Zaroxolyn, Diulo)	1–10	24
Quinethazone (Hydromox)	25–100	18–24
LOOP DIURETICS		
Bumetanide (Bumex)	0.5–5	4–6
Ethacrynic acid (Edecrin)	25–100	12
Furosemide (Lasix)	40–480	4–6
POTASSIUM-SPARING AGENTS		
Amiloride (Midamor)	5–10	24
Spironolactone (Aldactone)	25–100	8–12
Triamterene (Dyrenium)	50–100	12

From Kaplan, N. M.: Clinical Hypertension. 5th ed. Baltimore, © by Williams & Wilkins, 1990, p. 190.

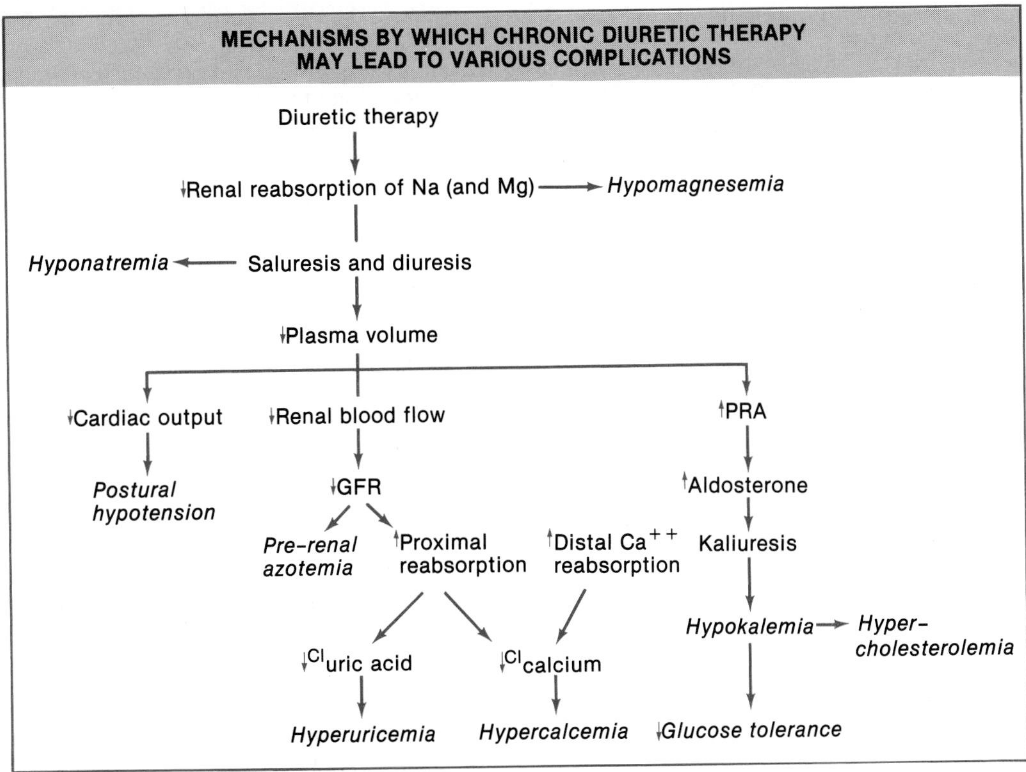

FIGURE 29–8. The mechanisms by which chronic diuretic therapy may lead to various complications. The mechanism for hypercholesterolemia remains in question, although it is shown as arising via hypokalemia. (From Kaplan, N. M.: Clinical Hypertension. 5th ed. Baltimore, © by Williams & Wilkins, 1990, p. 194.)

3.0 and 3.3 mmol/liter in 29 per cent and to between 2.6 and 2.9 mmol/liter in 7 per cent.[110] This fall in serum concentration may not reflect a significant decrease in total body potassium nor may it progress after the initial decline.[111] Nevertheless, it may precipitate potentially hazardous ventricular ectopic activity, even in patients not known to be susceptible because of concomitant digitalis therapy or myocardial irritability.[112] The arrhythmogenic effect of diuretic-induced hypokalemia may become manifested only at times of stress, when catecholamines may lower the plasma potassium level another 0.5 to 1.0 mmol/liter or when beta-adrenergic agonists are used as bronchodilators.[113] Although not all investigators find that patients with diuretic-induced hypokalemia have an increased propensity to cardiac arrhythmias,[114] increased frequencies of ventricular ectopic activity have been documented in hypokalemic patients with ischemic heart disease[115] or after an acute myocardial infarction.[116]

Most patients are unaware of mild diuretic-induced hypokalemia, although it may contribute to leg cramps, polyuria, and muscle weakness. But subtle interference with antihypertensive therapy may accompany even mild hypokalemia, and correction of hypokalemia may result in a fall in blood pressure.[73] In addition to increasing the propensity to ventricular ectopic activity, hypokalemia may be responsible for the loss of carbohydrate tolerance and the rise in plasma lipids seen with diuretic use.

Prevention of hypokalemia is preferable to correction of potassium deficiency. The following maneuvers should help prevent diuretic-induced hypokalemia:

- Use the smallest dose of diuretic needed.
- Use a moderately long-acting (12- to 18-hour) diuretic, such as hydrocholorothiazide, since longer-acting drugs (e.g., chlorthalidone) may increase potassium loss.
- Restrict sodium intake to less than 100 mmol per day (i.e., 2 gm sodium).
- Increase dietary potassium intake.
- Restrict concomitant use of laxatives.
- Use a combination of a thiazide with a potassium-sparing agent. If the latter is prescribed, avoid supplemental potassium, since dangerous hyperkalemia may supervene if these drugs are given together.
- The concomitant use of a beta blocker or an ACE inhibitor may diminish potassium loss, presumably by blunting the diuretic-induced rise in renin-aldosterone.

If hypokalemia is to be treated, these principles should be followed, along with some form of supplemental potassium. Potassium chloride is preferred for correction of the associated alkalosis. Despite the occasional appearance of mucosal lesions in the stomach after large doses, slow-release formulations of potassium chloride are both safe and effective, and most patients prefer them to liquid preparations. If tolerated, granular potassium chloride can be given as a salt substitute; thereby, extra potassium will be provided while sodium intake is reduced. Caution is necessary when supplemental potassium chloride is given to older patients with borderline renal function in whom hyperkalemia may be induced.

HYPOMAGNESEMIA. In some patients concomitant diuretic-induced magnesium deficiency will prevent the restoration of intracellular deficits of potassium,[78] so that hypomagnesemia should be corrected. Magnesium deficiency may also be responsible for some of the arrhythmias ascribed to hypokalemia.[117]

HYPERURICEMIA. The serum uric acid level is elevated in as many as one-third of untreated hypertensive patients. With chronic diuretic therapy, hyperuricemia appears in another third of patients, probably as a consequence of increased proximal tubular reabsorption accompanying volume contraction. Diuretic-induced hyperuricemia precipitates acute gout, most frequently in those who are obese and consume large amounts of alcohol.[118] Since asymptomatic hyperuricemia does not cause urate deposition, most researchers agree that it need not be treated. If therapy is used, a uricosuric drug such as probenecid should be given. Although allopurinol is often used, it is more likely to cause side effects and is a less rational choice, since the problem is a failure to excrete uric acid and not its overproduction.

HYPERLIPIDEMIA. Serum cholesterol levels often rise after diuretic therapy.[119] Although the rise in lipids can be prevented by a diet low in saturated fat, the propensity toward worsening of the lipid profile may inhibit the potential for diuretic therapy to reduce the incidence of coronary disease while it lowers blood pressure.

HYPERGLYCEMIA AND INSULIN RESISTANCE. Diuretics may impair glucose tolerance and rarely may precipitate diabetes mellitus. Perhaps of even greater concern, diuretics are associated with additional insulin resistance and hyperinsulinemia.[120] The manner by which diuretics reduce insulin sensitivity is uncertain but, in view of the multiple potential pressor actions of hyperinsulinemia (p. 828), this could be a significant problem.

HYPERCALCEMIA. A slight rise in serum calcium, less than 0.5 mg/dl, is frequently seen with thiazide diuretic therapy, at least in part because increased calcium reabsorption accompanies the increased sodium reabsorption in the proximal tubule induced by contraction of extracellular fluid volume.[121] The rise is of little concern except in patients with previously unrecognized hyperparathyroidism, who may experience a much more marked rise. On the other hand, the diuretic-induced positive calcium balance is associated with a reduction in the incidence of hip fractures in the elderly.[122]

OTHER PROBLEMS. A high incidence of impotence (22.6 per cent) was found among men taking 10 mg of bendroflumethiazide per day, compared with a rate of 10.1 per cent among those on placebo and 13.2 per cent among those on propranolol in the large MRC trial.[123] This high rate may reflect the rather large dose of the diuretic and perhaps the resultant hypokalemia.

Nonsteroidal antiinflammatory drugs (NSAID's) may inhibit the antihypertensive effects of both thiazides and loop diuretics, presumably by inhibiting the synthesis of vasodilatory prostaglandins in the kidney.[124]

OTHER DIURETICS

LOOP DIURETICS. Loop diuretics are usually needed in the treatment of hypertensive patients with renal failure defined here as a serum creatinine exceeding approximately 2.0 mg/dl. Furosemide has been most widely used, although metolazone may be as effective and requires only a single daily dose. Many physicians use furosemide in the management of uncomplicated hypertension, but as noted earlier, this drug seems to provide a less effective antihypertensive action when given once or twice a day than do longer-acting diuretics.

POTASSIUM-SPARING AGENTS. These drugs are normally used in combination with a diuretic. Of the three currently available, one (spironolactone) is an aldosterone antagonist, while the other two (triamterene and amiloride) are direct inhibitors of potassium secretion. In combination with a thiazide diuretic, they will diminish the amount of potassium wasting. Although they are more expensive than thiazides alone, they may decrease the total cost of therapy by reducing the need to monitor and treat potassium depletion.

AN OVERVIEW OF DIURETICS IN HYPERTENSION

Diuretics have been effective for the treatment of millions of hypertensive patients during the past 30 years. They reduce DBP and maintain it below 90 mm Hg in about half of all hypertensive patients, providing the same degree of effectiveness as most other antihypertensive drugs.[104] In two groups that constitute a rather large portion of the hypertensive population, the elderly[125] and blacks,[126] diuretics may be particularly effective. One diuretic tablet per day is usually all that is needed, minimizing cost and maximizing adherence to therapy.

The side effects of diuretic therapy are usually not overtly bothersome, but the hypokalemia, hypercholesterolemia, hyperinsulinemia, and worsening of glucose tolerance that often accompany prolonged diuretic therapy have given rise to increasing concerns about their long-term benignity. This concern has been fueled by the failure of diuretic-based therapy to reduce coronary mortality in the major trials of the therapy of mild hypertension (Table 29–1). Therefore, the author believes that the use of diuretics will continue to diminish in the future. When they are used, they will be given in smaller doses and more care will be taken to monitor and prevent the various biochemical changes that they may induce.

ADRENERGIC RECEPTOR BLOCKING DRUGS

A number of adrenergic receptor blocking drugs are available, including some that act centrally on vasomotor center activity, peripherally on neuronal catecholamine discharge, or by blocking alpha- and/or beta-adrenergic receptors (Table 29–7); some act at multiple sites. Figure 29–9, a schematic view of the ending of an adrenergic nerve and the effector cell with its receptors, depicts how some of these drugs act. When the nerve is stimulated, norepinephrine, which is synthesized intraneuronally and stored in granules, is released into the synaptic cleft. It binds to postsynaptic alpha- and beta-adrenergic receptors and thereby initiates various intracellular processes. In vascular smooth muscle, alpha stimulation causes constriction and beta stimulation causes relaxation. In the central vasomotor centers, sympathetic outflow is inhibited by alpha stimulation; the effect of central beta stimulation is unknown.

An important aspect of sympathetic activity involves the feedback of norepinephrine to alpha- and beta-adrenergic receptors located on the neuronal surface, i.e., *presynaptic* receptors.[127] Presynaptic alpha-adrenergic receptor activation inhibits release, whereas presynaptic beta activation stimulates further norepinephrine release. The presynaptic receptors probably play a role in the action of some of the drugs to be discussed.

Elucidation and quantitation of the various actions of these drugs remain incomplete. The listing in Table 29–7 is based on the predominant site of action according to currently available data. The action of beta-adrenergic receptor blockers probably depends on a peripheral effect but they almost certainly also act on central vasomotor mechanisms.

DRUGS THAT ACT WITHIN THE NEURON

Reserpine, guanethidine, and related compounds act to inhibit the release of norepinephrine from peripheral adrenergic neurons, each in a different manner.

TABLE 29-7 ADRENERGIC INHIBITORS USED IN TREATMENT OF HYPERTENSION

1. **PERIPHERAL NEURONAL INHIBITORS**
   a. Reserpine
   b. Guanethidine (Ismelin)
   c. Guanadrel (Hylorel)
   d. Bethanidine (Tenathan)
2. **CENTRAL ADRENERGIC INHIBITORS**
   a. Methyldopa (Aldomet)
   b. Clonidine (Catapres)
   c. Guanabenz (Wytensin)
   d. Guanfacine (Tenex)
3. **α-RECEPTOR BLOCKERS**
   b. α_1- and α_2-receptor
      (1) Phenoxybenzamine (Dibenzyline)
      (2) Phentolamine (Regitine)
   b. α_1-receptor
      (1) Doxazosin (Cardura)
      (2) Prazosin (Minipress)
      (3) Terazosin (Hytrin)
4. **β-RECEPTOR BLOCKERS**
   a. Acebutolol (Sectral)
   b. Atenolol (Tenormin)
   c. Betaxolol (Kerlone)
   d. Carteolol (Cartrol)
   e. Metoprolol (Lopressor)
   f. Nadolol (Corgard)
   g. Penbutolol (Levatol)
   h. Pindolol (Visken)
   i. Propranolol (Inderal)
   j. Timolol (Blocadren)
5. **α- AND β-RECEPTOR BLOCKER:** Labetalol (Normodyne, Trandate)

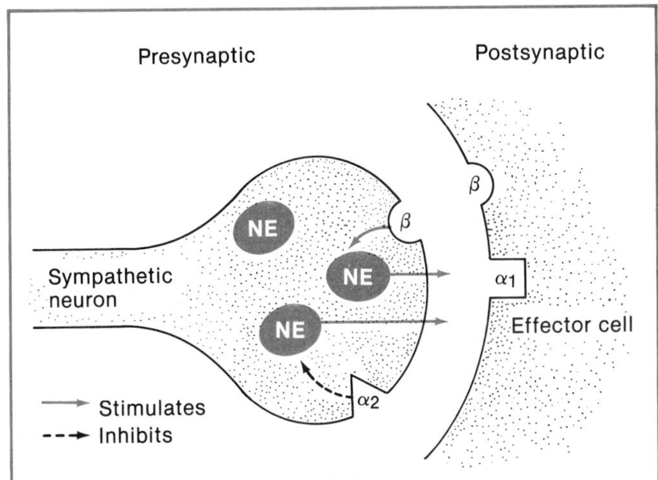

FIGURE 29-9. Simplified schematic view of the adrenergic nerve ending showing that norepinephrine (NE) is released from its storage granules when the nerve is stimulated and enters the synaptic cleft to bind to alpha$_1$ and beta receptors on the effector cell (postsynaptic). In addition, a short feedback loop exists, in which NE binds to alpha$_2$ and beta receptors on the neuron (presynaptic), to inhibit or to stimulate further release, respectively.

RESERPINE. Reserpine, the most active and widely used of the derivatives of the rauwolfia alkaloids, depletes the postganglionic adrenergic neurons of norepinephrine by inhibiting its uptake into storage vesicles, exposing it to degradation by cytoplasmic monoamine oxidase. The peripheral effect is predominant, although the drug enters the brain and depletes central catecholamine stores as well. This probably accounts for the sedation and depression seen with reserpine use. The drug has certain advantages: Only one dose a day is needed; in combination with a diuretic, the antihypertensive effect is significant, greater than that noted with propranolol in one comparative study[128]; little postural hypotension is noted; and many patients experience no side effects. The drug has a relatively flat dose-response curve, so that a dose of only 0.05 mg per day will give almost as much antihypertensive effect as 0.125 or 0.25 mg per day but fewer side effects.[129] However, the psychological depression that occurs in perhaps 2 per cent of patients may be severe but difficult to recognize and treat. The possible risk of breast cancer associated with reserpine use raised in 1974 has not been substantiated.[130] Although it remains popular in some places, the use of reserpine has declined progressively.

GUANETHIDINE. This agent and a series of related guanidine compounds, including guanadrel, bethanidine, and debrisoquine, act by inhibiting the release of norepinephrine from the adrenergic neurons, perhaps by a local anesthetic-like effect on the neuronal membrane. In order to act, the drug must be transported actively into the nerve through an amine pump. Various drugs, in particular tricyclic antidepressants, amphetamines, and ephedrine, competitively block the uptake of guanethidine into the nerves and thereby antagonize its effects.

Their low lipid solubility prevents these drugs from entering the brain, so that sedation, depression, and other side effects involving the central nervous system are not seen. Initially, the predominant hemodynamic effect is to decrease cardiac output; after continued use, peripheral resistance declines. Blood pressure is reduced further when the patient is upright, owing to gravitational pooling of blood in the legs, since compensatory sympathetic nervous system–mediated vasoconstriction is blocked. This results in the most common side effect, postural hypotension. Patients should be advised to arise slowly, sleep with the head of the bed elevated, and wear elastic hose to minimize this potential problem. Unlike reserpine, guanethidine has a steep dose-response curve, so that it can be successfully used in treating hypertension of any degree in daily doses of 10 to 300 mg. Like reserpine, it has a long biological half-life and may be given once daily. As other drugs have become available, guanethidine has been mainly relegated to the treatment of severe hypertension unresponsive to all other agents; often it is added to other agents.

Guanadrel, bethanidine, and *debrisoquin* are similar to guanethidine but have a shorter duration of action and perhaps fewer side effects.[131]

DRUGS THAT ACT UPON RECEPTORS

Predominantly Central Alpha Agonists

From the late 1960's until recently, methyldopa was the most widely used of the adrenergic receptor blockers, but its use has fallen off as beta blockers and other drugs have become more popular. In addition, three other drugs—clonidine, guanabenz, and guanfacine—which act similarly to methyldopa but have fewer serious side effects have become available.

METHYLDOPA. The primary site of action of methyldopa is within the central nervous system, where alpha-methylnorepinephrine, derived from methyldopa, is released from adrenergic neurons and stimulates central alpha adrenergic receptors, reducing the sympathetic outflow from the central nervous system.[132] The blood pressure mainly falls as a result of a decrease in peripheral resistance with little effect on cardiac output. However, as is true with all adrenergic receptor blockers, patients with borderline cardiac function may develop congestive failure by removal of adrenergic receptor support. On the other hand, methyldopa, probably in concert with other antihypertensive agents that decrease sympathetic activity, may reduce the degree of left ventricular hypertrophy as noted by echocardiography.[133] Renal blood flow is well maintained, and significant postural hypotension is unusual. Therefore, the drug has been widely used in hypertensive patients with renal failure or cerebrovascular disease.

Methyldopa need be given no more than twice daily. The dosage range is from 250 to 3,000 mg per day, with most patients responding to 750 to 1,500 mg. Smaller doses are needed in the presence of renal insufficiency. As in the case of the other adrenergic receptor blockers and peripheral vasodilators that may cause reactive fluid retention, methyldopa is best used in combination with a diuretic.

Side effects include some that are common to centrally acting drugs that reduce sympathetic outflow: sedation, dry mouth, orthostatic hypotension, impotence, and galactorrhea. However, methyldopa causes some unique side effects that are probably of an autoimmune nature, since a positive antinuclear antibody test is seen in about 10 per cent of patients who take the drug, and red cell autoantibodies occur in about 20 per cent. Clinically apparent hemolytic anemia is quite rare, probably because methyldopa also impairs reticuloendothelial function so that antibody-sensitized cells are not removed from the circulation and hemolyzed.[134] Inflammatory disorders in various organs have been reported, most commonly involving the liver (with diffuse parenchymal injury similar to viral hepatitis).[135]

CLONIDINE. Although of different structure, clonidine shares many features with methyldopa: It probably acts at the same central sites, has similar antihypertensive efficacy, and causes many of the same bothersome but less serious side effects (e.g., sedation, dry mouth). It does not, however, induce the autoimmune and inflammatory side effects.

As an alpha-adrenergic receptor agonist, the drug also acts on presynaptic alpha receptors and inhibits norepinephrine release (Fig. 29–9), and plasma catecholamine levels fall.[132] The drug has a fairly short biological half-life, so that when it is discontinued, the inhibition of norepinephrine release disappears within about 12 to 18 hours, and plasma catecholamine levels rise. This is probably responsible for the rapid rebound of the blood pressure to pretreatment levels and the occasional appearance of withdrawal symptoms, including tachycardia, restlessness, and sweating. Rarely, the blood pressure increases beyond the pretreatment level. Similar "overshoots" have been reported less commonly after the discontinuation of a variety of other antihypertensives.[136] If the rebound requires treatment, clonidine may be reintroduced or alpha adrenergic receptor antagonists given. By itself, clonidine often induces fluid retention, so that it should generally be used with a diuretic. After control has been achieved with two daily doses of clonidine and a diuretic, it may be maintained with a single bedtime dose.

Clonidine is available in a *transdermal* preparation, which may provide smoother blood pressure control for as long as seven days with fewer side effects. However, bothersome skin rashes preclude its use in perhaps one-fourth of patients.[137]

Clonidine has been used to treat severe hypertension with

hourly doses of 0.1 and 0.2 mg.[138] In addition, it may suppress withdrawal symptoms from opiates and nicotine and may have wider use in various psychiatric disorders.[139]

GUANABENZ. This drug differs in structure but shares many characteristics with both methyldopa and clonidine, acting primarily as a central alpha agonist. It may differ, however, in not causing fluid retention,[140] so that it may turn out to be effective without the need for a concomitant diuretic. Moreover, unlike diuretics, the use of guanabenz has been found to reduce serum cholesterol.[141]

GUANFACINE. This drug is also similar to clonidine but is longer acting, which enables once-a-day dosing and minimizes rebound hypertension.[142]

Alpha-Adrenergic Receptor Antagonists

Before 1977 the only alpha blockers used to treat hypertension were phenoxybenzamine (Dibenzyline) and phentolamine (Regitine). These drugs are effective in acutely lowering blood pressure, but their effects are offset by an accompanying increase in cardiac output, and side effects are frequent and bothersome. Their limited efficacy may reflect their blockade of presynaptic alpha-adrenergic receptors, which interferes with the feedback inhibition of norepinephrine release (Fig. 29–9). Increased catecholamine release would then blunt the action of postsynaptic alpha-adrenergic receptors. Their use has largely been limited to the treatment of patients with pheochromocytomas.

PRAZOSIN. This is the first of a group of selective antagonists of the postsynaptic $alpha_1$ receptors. Although prazosin was introduced as a peripheral vasodilator, subsequent study has clearly shown that primary effect of this group of drugs to be that of a postsynaptic alpha blocker.[143] By blocking alpha-mediated vasoconstriction, prazosin induces a fall in peripheral resistance with both venous and arteriolar dilation. Because the presynaptic alpha adrenergic receptor is left unblocked, the feedback loop for the inhibition of norepinephrine release is intact, an action which is also certainly responsible for the greater antihypertensive effect of the drug and the absence of concomitant tachycardia, tolerance, and renin release.

The inhibition of norepinephrine release may also account for the propensity toward greater first-dose falls in blood pressure. In a careful study of concentration-effect relationships, the first dose of 1 mg provided a greater effect (11.5 mm Hg fall in systolic blood pressure per nanogram of drug per milliliter of plasma) than seen after continued intake of 1 mg twice a day (8.7 mm Hg per ng/ml).[144] There was no long-term attenuation of the antihypertensive effect over the next three months. The problem of greater first-dose effects can be mitigated by limiting the first dose to 1 mg and withholding diuretic therapy for a few days before the start of prazosin.

Prazosin is as effective as other first-line antihypertensives and is similarly aided by concomitant use of a diuretic. When given to patients whose condition is poorly controlled on standard triple therapy (diuretic, beta blocker, and vasodilator), prazosin may reduce blood pressure even more than anticipated.[145] It can be safely and effectively used in patients with renal failure. The favorable hemodynamic changes—a fall in peripheral resistance with maintenance of cardiac output—make prazosin an attractive choice for patients who wish to remain physically active. Patients who may have trouble with beta blockers, including those with asthma or peripheral vascular disease, should be able to tolerate alpha blockade. In addition, blood lipids are not adversely altered and may actually improve with alpha blockers, unlike the adverse effects observed with diuretics and beta blockers.[146] Moreover, improved insulin sensitivity with lesser rises in plasma glucose and insulin levels after a glucose load has been observed with prazosin.[147]

Side effects, beyond first-dose postural hypotension, include the nonspecific effects of lower blood pressure, such as dizziness, weakness, fatigue, and headaches. Most patients, however, find the drug easy to take, with little sedation, dry mouth, or impotence.

OTHER ALPHA BLOCKERS. Two other alpha blockers, terazosin[148] and doxazosin,[149] are available. Beyond longer duration of action, they appear to differ little from prazosin.

Beta-Adrenergic Receptor Antagonists

(See also p. 644)

In the 1980's, beta-adrenergic receptor blockers became the most popular form of antihypertensive therapy after diuretics. Their popularity reflects their relative effectiveness and freedom from many bothersome side effects. However, they are no more effective in lowering blood pressure than are other antiadrenergic receptor agents, such as reserpine,[128] and side effects occur in a significant number of patients, including a variety of central nervous system-related dysfunctions.[150] Some of these side effects, including fatigue, brochospasm, peripheral vasospasm, and depression, may be quite bothersome. For the majority of patients who do not develop such side effects, beta blockers are usually easy to take, since somnolence, dry mouth, and impotence are seldom encountered. Because beta blockers have been found to reduce mortality if taken either before or after acute myocardial infarction,[151] i.e., secondary prevention, it was assumed that they might offer special protection against initial coronary events, i.e., primary prevention. In three large clinical trials (p. 853), a beta-blocker provided no more protection than did a diuretic. In the continuation of the HAPPHY trial, the group who remained on metoprolol experienced a lower eventual coronary mortality rate than did the one who continued on a diuretic.[152]

THE VARIETY OF BETA BLOCKERS. Some beta blockers now available in the United States are listed in Table 40–3, (p. 1308), and others are available in other countries. A number of agents with additional vasodilatory effects will probably soon be approved for use in the United States, and they may be free of many of the unfavorable hemodynamic and adverse effects of currently available agents.[153] Pharmacologically, those now available differ considerably from one another with respect to degree of absorption, protein binding, and bioavailability. However, the three most important differences affecting their clinical use are cardioselectivity, intrinsic sympathomimetic activity, and lipid solubility. Despite these differences, they all seem to be about equally as effective as are antihypertensives.

Cardioselectivity. As seen in Figure 29–10, beta blockers can be classified by their degree of cardioselectivity relative to their blocking effect on the $beta_1$ adrenergic receptors in the heart compared with that on the $beta_2$ receptor in the bronchi, peripheral blood vessels, and elsewhere.[154] Such cardioselec-

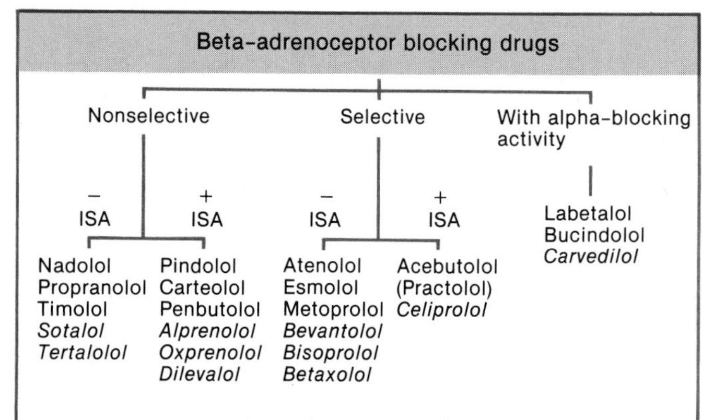

FIGURE 29–10. Classification of beta-adrenergic receptor blockers based on cardioselectivity and intrinsic sympathomimetic activity (ISA). Those not approved for use in the United States are in italics. (From Kaplan, N. M.: Clinical Hypertension. 5th ed. Baltimore, © by Williams & Wilkins, 1990, p. 215).

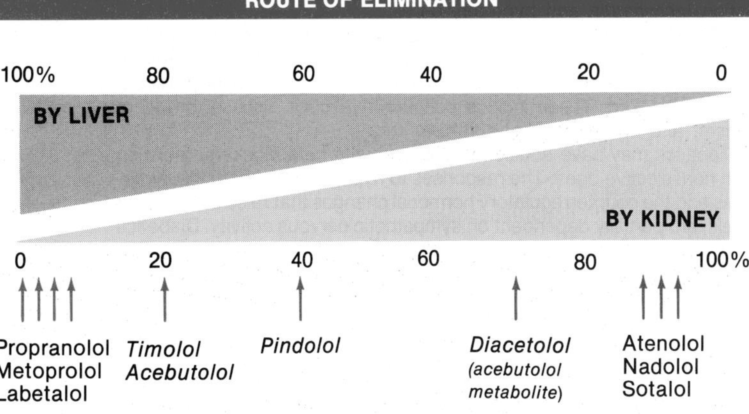

FIGURE 29–11. The relative degree of clearance by hepatic uptake and metabolism (liver) and renal excretion (kidney) of 10 beta-adrenoceptor blocking agents. The differences largely reflect differences in lipid solubility, which progressively diminishes from left to right. (Modified from Meier, J.: Beta-adrenoceptor-blocking agents: Pharmacokinetic differences and their clinical implications illustrated on pindolol. Cardiology *64*[Suppl 1]:1, 1979.)

tivity can be easily shown using small doses in acute studies; with the rather high doses used to treat hypertension, much of this effect is lost.

Intrinsic Sympathomimetic Activity (ISA). Some of these drugs have ISA, interacting with beta receptors to cause a measurable agonist response but at the same time blocking the greater agonist effects of endogenous catecholamines. As a result, while in usual doses they lower the blood pressure about the same degree as do other beta blockers, they cause a smaller decline in heart rate, cardiac output, and renin levels. A drug with ISA may prove useful when a beta blockers is needed for patients in whom bradycardia or peripheral vascular disease is a problem. During exercise the influence of ISA is reduced, so that similar hemodynamic effects are noted as with non-ISA beta blockers.[155] As noted under Side Effects, ISA may blunt the adverse effects on lipid metabolism seen with non-ISA beta blockers.[156]

Lipid Solubility. Atenolol and nadolol are among the least lipid-soluble of the beta blockers. This could translate into two clinically important advantages. First, because they escape hepatic inactivation and are excreted virtually unchanged through the kidneys (Fig. 29–11), they remain as active drugs in the plasma much longer, allowing once-a-day dosage. However, with the relatively large doses used to treat hypertension, once-a-day administration actually is effective with most, if not all, beta blockers. Second, because they do not enter the brain as readily, they may cause fewer central nervous system side effects.[150] In view of the reported high rate of such side effects, this could be a major advantage of less lipid-soluble agents.[157]

Mode of Action. Despite these and other differences, the various beta blockers now available are approximately equipotent as antihypertensive agents. How they lower the blood pressure remains uncertain, although a number of possible mechanisms are likely to be involved. In those without ISA, cardiac output falls 15 to 20 per cent and renin release is reduced about 60 per cent. Central nervous beta-adrenergic receptor blockade may reduce sympathetic discharge, but similar antihypertensive effects are seen with those drugs that are more lipid soluble, and therefore in high concentration within the central nervous system, and those that are less lipid soluble. Recall, too, that blockade of presynaptic beta adrenergic receptor should inhibit catecholamine release (Fig. 29–9).

At the same time that beta blockers lower blood pressure through various means, their blockade of peripheral beta adrenergic receptor inhibits vasodilation, leaving alpha receptors open to catecholamine-mediated vasoconstriction.[158] However, over time, vascular resistance tends to return to normal, which presumably preserves the antihypertensive effect of a reduced cardiac output. As seen in Figure 29–14, the eventual level of vascular resistance differs and some vasoconstriction may persist with agents such as timolol and atenolol.[159] A decrease in peripheral blood flow is a common problem with beta blocker therapy in cold climates.

Clinical Effects. Even in small doses, beta blockers begin to lower the blood pressure within a few hours, although their maximal effect may not be noted for some weeks. Even though progressively higher doses have usually been given, careful study has shown a near-maximal effect from smaller doses: In a double-blind crossover study involving 24 patients, 40 mg of propranolol twice a day provided the same antihypertensive effects as 80, 160, or 240 mg twice a day.[160] The degree of blood pressure reduction is at least comparable to that noted with other antihypertensive drugs. By itself, a beta blocker will lower the diastolic pressure to below 90 mm Hg in about half of patients with mild to moderate hypertension; when it is combined with a diuretic, the percentage rises to about 80.[128] Duration of action is well beyond the drugs' plasma half-life so that most can be used once daily. One of the attractions of these drugs is the constancy of their antihypertensive action, altered little by changes in activity, posture, or temperature. Because the sympathetic nervous system is blocked, the hemodynamic responses to stress are reduced, probably enough to interfere with athletic performance.[155]

Beta blockers have been proposed as initial monotherapy.[53] This approach may be effective for some younger hypertensives with a hyperdynamic circulation but may not be suitable for many older or black patients. Both blacks[126] and patients over age 50[161,162] have been found to respond less well to beta blocker monotherapy.

SPECIAL USES FOR BETA BLOCKERS

COEXISTING ISCHEMIC HEART DISEASE. Even without evidence that beta blockers protect patients from initial coronary events, the antiarrhythmic and antianginal effects of these drugs make them especially valuable in the hypertensive patients with coexisting coronary disease.

PATIENTS NEEDING ANTIHYPERTENSIVE VASODILATOR THERAPY. If a diuretic and an adrenergic receptor blocker are inadequate to control blood pressure, the addition of a vasodilator is a logical third step. When used alone, direct vasodilators induce reflex sympathetic stimulation of the heart. The simultaneous use of beta blockers prevents this undesirable increase in cardiac output, which not only bothers the patient but also dampens the antihypertensive effect of the vasodilator.

PATIENTS WITH HYPERKINETIC HYPERTENSION. Some hypertensive patients have increased cardiac output that may persist for many years. Beta blockers are particularly effective in such patients, but a reduction in exercise capacity may necessitate restriction of their use in young athletes.

PATIENTS WITH MARKED ANXIETY. The somatic manifestations of anxiety—tremor, sweating, and tachycardia—can be helped, without the undesirable effects of methods commonly used to control anxiety, such as alcohol and tranquilizers.

PERIOPERATIVE STRESS. The ultra-short-acting cardioselective in-

ACE inhibitors may find wider use if the inability to modulate adrenal and renal responses to different levels of sodium intake, ascribed to fixed high angiotensin II levels, is found to be a common defect in normal and high-renin hypertensives (p. 829). The defect appears to be corrected by ACE inhibitor therapy, holding the promise for a more specific form of therapy for a large portion of the hypertensive population.

These drugs have been a mixed blessing for patients with renovascular hypertension. On the one hand, the response of plasma renin to a single dose of captopril may provide a simple diagnostic test for the disease (p. 837). More importantly, they usually control the blood pressure effectively.[195] On the other hand, the removal of the high levels of angiotensin II that they produce may deprive the stenotic kidney of the hormonal drive to its blood flow, thereby causing a marked fall of renal perfusion. With these drugs, patients with solitary kidneys or bilateral disease may develop renal failure.[196]

Patients with intraglomerular hypertension, specifically those with diabetic nephropathy or reduced renal functional mass, may benefit especially from the reduction in efferent arteriolar resistance that follows reduction in angiotensin II. The experimental evidence for this protection is strong.[197] The clinical evidence, although limited as of this writing, is supportive.[198]

SIDE EFFECTS. Most patients who take an ACE inhibitor experience no side effects. In most studies patients have significantly fewer adverse effects from an ACE inhibitor than from other agents.[199] The major advantages are related to the absence of effects intimately involved in the sites of action of other drugs: no central nervous system side effects, no reduction in cardiac output, no interference with sympathetic activity. Beyond the decrease in bothersome overt side effects, ACE inhibitor therapy does not produce biochemical changes that may be of even more concern even though they are not so obvious: neither rises in lipids, glucose, or uric acid nor falls in potassium levels are seen, and insulin sensitivity may improve.[120]

To be sure, ACE inhibitors may cause both specific and nonspecific adverse effects. Among the specific ones are rash, loss of taste, glomerulopathy manifested by proteinuria, and leukopenia. In addition, these drugs may cause a hypersensitivity reaction with angioneurotic edema[200] or a cough which, although often persistent, is not associated with pulmonary dysfunction.[201] There is at least a potential problem for those patients taking an ACE inhibitor who coincidentally develop volume depletion, as from gastroenteritis, since they may be unable to marshal the compensatory homeostatic responses that involve increased angiotensin II and aldosterone. Lastly, patients on potassium supplements or sparing agents may not be able to excrete potassium loads and therefore may develop hyperkalemia.[202]

AN OVERVIEW OF ACE INHIBITOR THERAPY. These drugs are widely used for all degrees and forms of hypertension. Their use will increase further if their particular ability to decrease intrarenal hypertension experimentally is translated into greater protection from progressive renal damage clinically. Moreover, their increasing use as unloaders in patients with congestive heart failure may be accompanied by their use in patients after myocardial infarction if the preliminary evidence of their attenuating the development of left ventricular enlargement is confirmed.[188]

OTHER DRUGS. A variety of other forms of antihypertensive therapy are under investigation.[203] One that has been widely studied is the serotonin S_2-receptor blocker *ketanserin*, which has been found to reduce HMG CoA reductase activity in cultured skin fibroblasts; this may explain the fall in LDL cholesterol levels reported with its use.[204] A fascinating observation that a single injection of interleukin-2 controlled the blood pressure in SHR rats for at least 6 months[205] is likely to provoke clinical study of this and other immune reactants.

SPECIAL CONSIDERATIONS IN THERAPY

CHOICE OF DRUGS. Increasingly, the rigid, diuretic-first stepped-care approach has been broadened to include other classes of drugs for initial monotherapy following the overall individualized approach.[53] Excluding only direct vasodilators that are seldom tolerated when used alone, a drug from any other class can be chosen. There is little overall difference in their effectiveness, but black patients tend to respond less well to beta blockers and ACE inhibitors, whereas older persons may respond particularly well to calcium antagonists and diuretics. The choice is then logically made on the basis of the favorable or unfavorable effects of the drugs on concomitant conditions (Table 29–4). Certain tradeoffs may be required: Reserpine or a thiazide may be given in only one dose per day at little cost, but the side effects may be excessive; methyldopa, despite its efficacy, may cause some unique and serious problems and is no longer an acceptable choice; if poor patient compliance is likely, clonidine should be avoided; alpha blockers may provide more "physiological" control of the blood pressure but may cause bothersome postural hypotension; beta blockers are acceptable for many patients but may cause fatigue, inability to exercise as strenuously, central nervous system problems, and rarely serious side effects, even after careful exclusion of patients known to be susceptible. ACE inhibitors and calcium antagonists—particularly now that they are available for once-daily use—will be increasingly chosen. In general, vasodilators that reduce peripheral resistance are preferable to those that reduce cardiac output (Fig. 29–13). The logical process is to substitute a drug from another class if the first choice is not effective and to choose drugs of different classes if more than one is needed. For a second drug, a diuretic may be used, if it was not the first choice. If a third drug is needed, a vasodilator usually is added. In the past, this was usually hydralazine; increasingly it will be a calcium antagonist or an ACE inhibitor.

REASONS FOR INADEQUATE RESPONSES. Often patients do not respond well because they do not take their medications. On the other hand, what appears to be a poor response based on office readings of blood pressure may turn out to be an adequate response when home readings are used.[206] However, a number of factors may be responsible for a poor response even if the appropriate medication is taken regularly (Table 29–10). Most common is volume overload owing either to inadequate diuretic or excessive dietary sodium intake. Larger doses or more potent diuretics often bring resistant hypertension under control. On the other hand, there are a few patients whose blood pressure is resistant to therapy because of overly vigorous diuresis, which contracts vascular volume and activates both renin and catecholamines. This is most likely to occur in patients with obligatory salt-wasting resulting from interstitial renal disease.

ANESTHESIA IN HYPERTENSIVE PATIENTS. In the absence of significant cardiac dysfunction, hypertension does

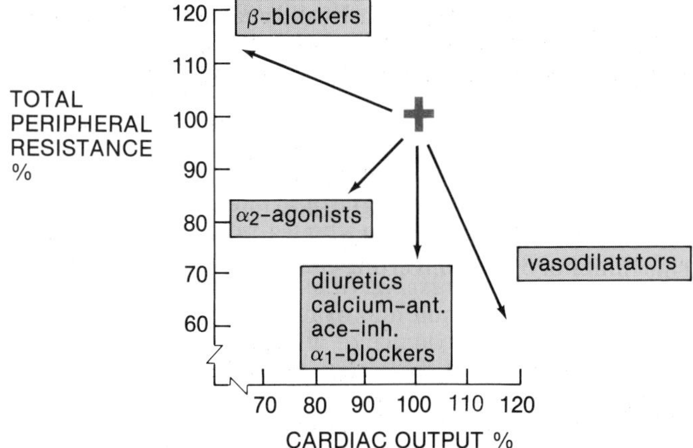

FIGURE 29–13. Relative effects of different categories of antihypertensive agents on cardiac output and total peripheral resistance in hypertension. The black cross indicates the situation before treatment. (From Man in't Veld, A. J., Van den Meiracker, A. H., and Schalemkamp, M. A.: Do beta-blockers really increase peripheral vascular resistance? Review of the literature and new observations under basal conditions. Am. J. Hypertens. *1*:91, 1988.)

TABLE 29-10 CAUSES OF POOR RESPONSE TO ANTIHYPERTENSIVE DRUGS

1. **Inadequate drugs**
   a. Doses too low
   b. Inappropriate combinations, e.g., two centrally acting adrenergic inhibitors
   c. Rapid inactivation, e.g., hydralazine
   d. Incomplete absorption related to food intake
   e. Antagonism from other drugs
      (1) Sympathomimetics
      (2) Antidepressants
      (3) Adrenal steroids
      (4) Nonsteroidal antiinflammatory drugs
2. **Associated conditions**
   a. Alcohol intake above 2 oz/day
   b. Renal insufficiency
   c. Renovascular hypertension
   d. Pheochromocytoma
3. **Volume overload**
   a. Inadequate diuretic
   b. Excessive sodium intake
   c. Fluid retention from reduction of blood pressure
   d. Progressive renal damage
4. **Volume depletion → increased renin → vasoconstriction**
   a. Renal salt-wasting
   b. Overly aggressive diuretic therapy

not add to the cardiovascular risks of surgery.[207] Most anesthesiologists suggest that hypertension should be well controlled by means of medications before anesthesia and surgery. Caution is needed in discontinuing beta blockers[165] and clonidine[136]; intravenous or patch preparations may be used to see the patient through surgery. The very short-acting beta-blocker esmolol has been successful in preventing surges in blood pressure during intubation.[163] Patients receiving calcium antagonists may occasionally manifest adverse effects when inhalation agents such as halothane, enflurane, and isoflurane are used, either because the cardiovascular effects of these agents are similar to or because they may increase the plasma levels of the calcium antagonists.[208]

Hypertension is often observed during and immediately after coronary bypass surgery (p. 841); various intravenous agents have been successfully used to lower the pressure. Nitroprusside has been the usual choice during the postoperative period, but toxicity, often in the form of loss of consciousness and cyanide or thiocyanate toxicity, may develop in those who are critically ill and given the drug for prolonged periods.[209] Moreover, its tendency to raise intracranial pressure[210] and to reduce cardiac output[211] detracts further from its usefulness.

HYPERTENSIVE CHILDREN (see also p. 999). Almost nothing is known about the effects of various antihypertensive medications given to children over long periods. Because most of the anti-adrenergic drugs act on the central nervous system, their effects on growth hormone, gonadotropins, and other hormones involved in maturation and growth should be ascertained. However, in the absence of adequate data, an approach similar to that advocated for adults is advised.[212] The dosages of drugs are shown in Table 33–3, p. 1002. Emphasis should be placed on weight reduction in hypertensive children who are obese, in the hope of attempting to control hypertension without the need for drug therapy.[213]

HYPERTENSION DURING PREGNANCY. This topic is discussed in Chapter 59.

THE ELDERLY WITH SYSTOLIC HYPERTENSION. Here again, almost no long-term controlled data are available as to the indications for therapy and the appropriate choice of drugs. If both systolic and diastolic pressures are elevated, elderly patients should be treated in a manner similar to that for younger persons[214]; they seem to respond as well and have no more problems with medications.[215] In view of the reduced effectiveness of the baroreceptor reflex[216] and the failure of peripheral resistance to rise appropriately with standing,[217] drugs with a propensity to cause postural hypotension should be avoided, and all drugs should be given in slowly increasing doses to prevent excessive lowering of the pressure. Thereby, the occasional episodes of serious cerebral ischemia and stroke related to antihypertensive therapy[218] should be avoidable. The elderly may have many features that contribute to an increased risk of therapy (Table 29–11); beyond all else, medications should be given in gradual progression to avoid serious adverse reactions.[219]

Patients with acute stroke are particularly vulnerable to immediate reductions in systemic blood pressure because there is often a transient rise in this pressure in an attempt to maintain adequate perfusion to the ischemic brain.[220]

Isolated systolic hypertension in the elderly presents a risk, particularly for strokes.[221] It is likely that judicious lowering of the pressure will protect against and not precipitate cardiovascular catastrophes. Admittedly, most isolated elevations of systolic pressure are due to structural hardening of the arterial walls, and the vessels may not be able to dilate as well as the functionally constricted, more pliant vessels of young people. The goals of therapy should not be rigid; a systolic pressure of 160 mm Hg seems reasonable for people over 60 years of age. It is hoped that data on the effectiveness of therapy for isolated systolic hypertension will be forthcoming from the Systolic Hypertension in the Elderly Program (SHEP) trial.[27] The preliminary data from this trial show that the systolic pressures of most will respond to small dosages of a diuretic, without inordinate side effects.[222]

As noted on page 844, some elderly persons may have high blood pressure as measured by the sphygmomanometer but may have less or no hypertension when direct intraarterial readings are made. Presumably their pseudohypertension is related to the failure of the sphygmomanometer cuff to collapse the rigid artery beneath the cuff. For those patients with vessels that feel rigid and who have few retinal or cardiac findings of hypertension, as would be expected with high sphygmomanometer readings, direct intraarterial measurements should be made before therapy is begun in order to avoid inordinate lowering of blood pressures which are not, in fact, elevated.

HYPERTENSION WITH RENAL FAILURE (see also pp. 833 and 1863). In the presence of renal failure, hypertension is usually predominantly caused by volume excess, and most patients can be successfully treated with sodium restriction and diuretics. When serum creatinine exceeds 2.0 mg/dl, thiazides are usually ineffective, and either metolazone or high doses of furosemide are required.[223] A few patients with chronic renal disease have a more resistant form of hypertension, usually associated with—and perhaps caused by—high levels of plasma renin activity. Medical therapy has been increasingly effective, not only in controlling the hypertension

TABLE 29-11 FACTORS THAT MIGHT CONTRIBUTE TO INCREASED RISK OF PHARMACOLOGICAL TREATMENT OF HYPERTENSION IN THE ELDERLY

FACTORS	POTENTIAL COMPLICATIONS
Diminished baroreceptor activity	Orthostatic hypotension
Decreased intravascular volume	Orthostatic hypotension, dehydration
Sensitivity to hypokalemia	Arrhythmia, muscular weakness
Decreased renal and hepatic function	Drug accumulation
Polypharmacy	Drug interaction
CNS changes	Depression, confusion

but also in halting the deterioration of renal function.[224] With appropriate therapy, which may include hemodialysis for some time, hypertension can be controlled in most patients and the deterioration of renal function slowed. Although experimental evidence suggests that ACE inhibitors may be even more effective in preserving residual renal function, particularly when diabetic nephropathy is responsible,[198] clinical evidence suggests that calcium antagonists may do as well.[225]

HYPERTENSION WITH CONGESTIVE HEART FAILURE. Cardiac output may fall so markedly in hypertensive patients who are in heart failure that their blood pressure is reduced, obscuring the degree of hypertension; often, however, the diastolic pressure is raised by intense vasoconstriction while the systolic pressure falls as a result of the reduced stroke volume. Lowering the blood pressure may, by itself, relieve the heart failure. Chronic unloading has been most efficiently accomplished with ACE inhibitors[188] (p. 867). Antihypertensive drugs that primarily decrease cardiac output, particularly beta blockers, which remove the heart's needed sympathetic support, may be dangerous in the presence of heart failure.

HYPERTENSION WITH ISCHEMIC HEART DISEASE. The coexistence of ischemic heart disease makes antihypertensive therapy even more essential, since relief of the hypertension may ameliorate the coronary disease. Beta blockers and calcium antagonists are particularly useful if angina or arrhythmias are present. Caution is needed to avoid decreased coronary perfusion that is likely responsible for the *J*-curve seen in multiple trials[19,22] (see p. 853).

The often markedly high levels of blood pressure during the early phase of an acute myocardial infarction may reflect sympathetic nervous hyperreactivity to pain. Cautious use of antihypertensive drugs that do not decrease cardiac output may be useful in the immediate postinfarction period, whereas beta-blockers have been shown to provide long-term benefit, and ACE inhibitors may turn out to prevent myocardial dysfunction.[226]

HYPERTENSION WITH DIABETES MELLITUS (see also p. 832). Diuretics may worsen diabetic control, probably because they induce potassium depletion. Brittle diabetics on insulin should not be given nonselective beta blockers, since these drugs may prevent the outpouring of catecholamines that counteracts a precipitous fall in blood sugar levels, thereby preventing the recognition of impending hypoglycemia and delaying the rebound rise in the blood sugar. In keeping with the multiple potential pressor effects of hyperinsulinemia (p. 828), reduction of the dose of exogenous insulin may help control the blood pressure.[227]

Impotence, although not infrequently observed in any hypertensive patient treated too fast and too vigorously so that penile blood flow is further reduced, is an even more common problem among diabetics. External negative pressure devices may provide excellent relief and avoid the need for surgical implants and intrapenile injections of vasodilators.[228]

HYPERTENSION WITH PSYCHIATRIC ILLNESS. Patients who are anxious and emotionally labile may benefit from the calming effects of beta blockers on the somatic manifestations of anxiety. However, caution is advised in using beta blockers, particularly the lipid-soluble ones,[157] which may induce depression, insomnia, and nightmares. If antidepressant or antipsychotic medications are needed, they will not blunt the effects of beta blockers, ACE inhibitors, or calcium entry blockers, as they may those of guanethidine, methyldopa, or clonidine.

THERAPY FOR HYPERTENSIVE CRISES

When diastolic blood pressure exceeds 140 mm Hg, rapidly progressive damage to the arterial vasculature is demonstrable experimentally, and a surge of cerebral blood flow may rapidly lead to encephalopathy (p. 844). If such high pressures persist or if there are any signs of encephalopathy, the pressures should be lowered using parenteral agents in those patients considered to be in immediate danger or with oral agents in those who are alert and in no other acute distress.

TABLE 29-12 PARENTERAL DRUGS FOR TREATMENT OF HYPERTENSIVE EMERGENCY (IN ORDER OF RAPIDITY OF ACTION)

DRUG	DOSAGE	ONSET OF ACTION	ADVERSE EFFECTS
VASODILATORS			
Nitroprusside (Nipride, Nitropress)	0.25–10 μg/kg/min as I.V. infusion	Instantaneous	Nausea, vomiting, muscle twitching, sweating, thiocyanate intoxication
Nitroglycerin	5–100 μg/min as I.V. infusion	2–5 min	Tachycardia, flushing, headache, vomiting, methemoglobinemia
Diazoxide (Hyperstat)	50–100 mg/IV bolus, repeated or 15–30 mg/min by I.V. infusion	2–4 min	Nausea, hypotension, flushing, tachycardia, chest pain
Hydralazine (Apresoline)	10–20 mg I.V. 10–50 mg I.M.	10–20 min 20–30 min	Tachycardia, flushing, headache, vomiting, aggravation of angina
Enalapril (Vasotec IV)	1.25–5 mg q 6 hr	15 min	Precipitous fall in BP in high renin states; response variable
Nicardipine	5–10 mg/hr I.V.	10 min	Tachycardia, headache, flushing, local phlebitis
ADRENERGIC INHIBITORS			
Phentolamine (Regitine)	5–15 mg I.V.	1–2 min	Tachycardia, flushing
Trimethaphan (Arfonad)	0.5–5 mg/min as I.V. infusion	1–5 min	Paresis of bowel and bladder, orthostatic hypotension, blurred vision, dry mouth
Esmolol (Brevibloc)	500 μg/kg/min for 4 min, then 150–300 μg/kg/min I.V.	1–2 min	Hypotension
Propranolol (Inderal)	1–10 mg load; 3 ng/hr	1–2 min	Beta blocker side effects, e.g., bronchospasm, decreased cardiac output
Labetalol (Normodyne, Trandate)	20–80 mg I.V. bolus every 10 min 2 mg/min I.V. infusion	5–10 min	Vomiting, scalp tingling, burning in throat, postural hypotension, dizziness, nausea

A number of drugs for this purpose currently are available (Table 29–12). If diastolic pressure exceeds 140 mm Hg and the patient has any complications, such as an aortic dissection, a constant infusion of nitroprusside is most effective and will almost always lower the pressure to the desired level. Constant monitoring, preferably with an intra-arterial line, is mandatory because a slightly excessive dose may lower the pressure abruptly to levels that will induce shock. The potency and rapidity of action of nitroprusside have made it the treatment of choice for life-threatening hypertension. However, nitroprusside acts as a venous and arteriolar dilator, so that venous return and cardiac output are lowered[211] and intracranial pressures may increase.[210] Therefore, other parenteral agents are being more widely used. These include labetalol[170] and the calcium antagonist nicardipine.[229]

With any of these agents, intravenous furosemide is often needed to lower the blood pressure further and prevent retention of salt and water. Diuretics should not be given if volume depletion is initially present. As the experimental evidence of different effects of various antihypertensive drugs on cerebral blood flow and autoregulation[230] becomes translated into clinical practice, more changes in the management of patients with severe hypertension probably will be dictated.

For patients in less immediate danger, oral therapy may be used. Almost every drug has been used and most will, with repeated doses, reduce high pressures. While clonidine, 0.1 to 0.2 mg every hour, has been successfully used, the current preference of many is nifedipine, 10 mg by mouth or sublingually repeated in 30 minutes if needed.[186] The sublingual route provides a slower route and probably, therefore, a safer one. The pressure almost always falls about 25 per cent within the first 30 minutes. Rarely, and not unexpectedly, a few patients may suffer tissue ischemia with such rapid and marked falls in pressure.[231] A safer course for some patients, particularly if their current high pressures are simply a reflection of stopping previously effective oral medication, is simply to restart that medication and monitor their response closely. if their nonadherence to therapy was caused by side effects, appropriate changes should be made.

Fortunately, fewer patients in hypertensive crisis are being seen, presumably because more hypertension in more patients is being recognized and treated before the disease enters this malignant course. It is hoped that the continued successful treatment of many more hypertensive persons will lead to similar increases in prevention of the other subtler but more frequent long-range sequelae of hypertension.

REFERENCES

INDICATIONS FOR THERAPY

1. Kaplan, N. M.: Clinical Hypertension, 5th ed. Baltimore, Williams & Wilkins, 1990, p. 252.
2. Cloher, T. P., and Whelton, P. K.: Physician approach to the recognition and initial management of hypertension. Arch. Intern. Med. *146*:529, 1986.
3. McClellan, W., Neel, J., and Owen, S.: Correlates of drug therapy of diastolic blood pressure between 80–89 mm Hg by physicians in the community. Am. J. Hypertens. *2*:869, 1989.
4. Report of the British Hypertension Society working party: Treating mild hypertension. Agreement from the large trials. Br. Med. J. *298*:694, 1989.
5. Bonita, R., and Beaglehole, R.: Increased treatment of hypertension does not explain the decline in stroke mortality in the United States, 1970–1980. Hypertension *13*(Suppl I):1–69, 1989.
6. Hart, J. T.: The practitioner's view. *In* Gross, F., and Strasser, T. (eds.): Mild Hypertension: Recent Advances. New York, Raven Press, 1983, p. 365.
7. Berglund, G.: Goals of antihypertensive therapy. Is there a point beyond which pressure reduction is dangerous? Am. J. Hypertens. *2*:586, 1989.
8. Cutler, J. A., MacMahon, S. W., and Furberg, C. D.: Controlled clinical trials of drug treatment for hypertension. A review. Hypertension *13*(Suppl I):1–36, 1989.
9. Veterans Administration Cooperative Study Group on Antihypertensive Agents: Effects of treatment on morbidity in hypertension. II. Results in patients with diastolic blood pressure averaging 90 through 114 mm Hg. JAMA *213*:1143, 1970.
10. U. S. Public Health Service Hospitals Cooperative Study Group, Smith, W. M.: Treatment of mild hypertension. Results of a ten-year intervention trial. Circ. Res. *40*(Suppl I):I–98, 1977.
11. Perry, H. M., Goldman, A. I., Lavin, M. A., et al.: Evaluation of drug treatment in mild hypertension: VA-NHLBI feasibility trial. Ann. NY Acad. Sci. *304*:267, 1978.
12. Helgeland, A.: Treatment of mild hypertension: A five year controlled drug trial. The Oslo Study. Am. J. Med. *69*:725, 1980.
13. Management Committee: The Australian therapeutic trial in mild hypertension. Lancet *1*:1261, 1980.
14. Amery, A., Birkenhager, W., Brixko, P. et al.: Mortality and morbidity results from the European Working Party on high blood pressure in the elderly trial. Lancet *1*:1349, 1985.
15. Medical Research Council Working Party: MRC trial of treatment of mild hypertension: Principal results. Br. Med. J. *291*:97, 1985.
16. Hypertension Detection and Follow-up Program Cooperative Research Group: The effect of antihypertensive drug treatment on mortality in the presence of resting electrocardiographic abnormalities at baseline: The HDFP experience. Circulation *70*:996, 1984.
17. Multiple Risk Factor Intervention Trial Research Group: Baseline rest electrocardiographic abnormalities, antihypertensive treatment, and mortality in the Multiple Risk Factor Intervention Trial. Am. J. Cardiol. *55*:1, 1985.
18. Bulpitt, C. J., and Fletcher, A. E.: Importance of well-being to hypertensive patients. Am. J. Med. *84*(Suppl 1B):40, 1988.
19. Cruickshank, J. M.: Coronary flow reserve and the J curve relation between diastolic blood pressure and myocardial infarction. Br. Med. J. *297*:1227, 1988.
20. Littenberg, B., Garber, A. M., and Sox, H. C. Jr.: Screening for hypertension. Ann. Intern. Med. *112*:192, 1990.
21. Ménard, J.: Hypertension costs: Source, evolution and impact of cost-containment measures in various health-care systems. Clin. Exp. Hypertens. *A11*:1149, 1989.
22. Alderman, M. H., Ooi, W. L., Madhavan, S., and Cohen, H.: Treatment-induced blood pressure reduction and the risk of myocardial infarction. JAMA 262:920, 1989.
23. IPPPSH Collaborative Group: Cardiovascular risk and risk factors in a randomized trial of treatment based on the beta-blocker oxprenolol: The International Prospective Primary Prevention Study in Hypertension (IPPPSH). J. Hypertens. *3*:379, 1985.
24. Wilhelmsen, L., Berglund, G., Elmfeldt, D. et al.: Beta-blockers versus diuretics in hypertensive men: Main results from the HAPPHY trial. J. Hypertens. 5:561, 1987.
25. Collins, R., Peto, R., MacMahon, S., et al.: Blood pressure, stroke and coronary heart disease. Part II, short-term reductions in blood pressure: Overview of randomised drug trials in their epidemiological context. Lancet 335:827, 1990.

GUIDELINES FOR TREATMENT

26. Curb, J. D., Schneider, K., Taylor, J. O., et al.: Antihypertensive drug side effects in the hypertension detection and follow-up program. Hypertension *11*(Suppl II):II–51, 1988.
27. Perry, H. M. Jr., Smith, W. M., McDonald, R. H., et al.: Morbidity and mortality in the Systolic Hypertension in the Elderly Program (SHEP) pilot study. Stroke *20*:4, 1989.
28. Multiple Risk Factor Intervention Trial Research Group. Mortality rates after 10.5 years for participants in the multiple risk factor intervention trial. Findings related to a priori hypotheses of the trial. JAMA *263*:1795, 1990.
29. WHO/ISH Mild Hypertension Liaison Committee. 1989 guidelines for the management of mild hypertension: Memorandum from a WHO/ISH meeting. J. Hypertens. *7*:689, 1989.
30. Samuelsson, O.: Experiences from hypertension trials. Impact of other risk factors. Drugs *36*(Suppl 3):9, 1988.
31. Epstein, F. H.: Proceedings of the XVth International Congress of Therapeutics, Sept. 5–9, 1979. Brussels: Excerpta Medica, 1980.
32. Stewart, I. M. G.: Relation of reduction in pressure to first myocardial infarction in patients receiving treatment for severe hypertension. Lancet *1*:861, 1979.
33. Cruickshank, J. M., Thorp, J. M., and Zacharias, F. J.: Benefits and potential harm of lowering high blood pressure. Lancet *1*:581, 1987.
34. Samuelsson, O., Wilhemlsen, L., Andersson, O. K., et al.: Cardiovascular morbidity in relation to change in blood pressure and serum cholesterol levels in treated hypertension. Results from the Primary Prevention Trial in Göteborg, Sweden. JAMA *258*:1768, 1987.
35. Cooper, J., Warrender, T. S.: Randomised trial of treatment of hypertension in elderly patients in primary care. Br. Med. J. *293*:1145, 1986.
36. Waller, P. C., Isles, C. G., Lever, A. F., et al.: Does therapeutic reduction of diastolic blood pressure cause death from coronary heart disease? J. Hum. Hypertens. *2*:7, 1988.
37. Fletcher, A. E., Beevers, D. G., Bulpitt, C. J., et al.: The relationship between a low treated blood pressure and IHD mortality: A report from the DHSS Hypertension Care Computing Project (DHCCP). J. Hum. Hypertens. *2*:11, 1988.
38. Kuller, L. H., Hulley, S. B., Cohen, J. D., and Neaton, J.: Unexpected effects of treating hypertension in men with electrocardiographic abnormalities: A critical analysis. Circulation *73*:114, 1986.
39. Cooper, S. P., Hardy, R. J., Labarthe, D. R., et al.: The relation between degree of blood pressure reduction and mortality among hypertensives in the hypertension detection and follow-up program. Am. J. Epidemiol. *127*:387, 1988.
40. Berglund, G.: Goals of antihypertensive therapy. Is there a point beyond which pressure reduction is dangerous? Am. J. Hypertens. *2*:586, 1989.

41. Pepi, M., Alimento, M., Maltagliati, A., and Guazzi, M. D.: Cardiac hypertrophy in hypertension. Repolarization abnormalities elicited by rapid lowering of pressure. Hypertension *11*:84, 1988.
42. Amery, A., Berglund, G., Cruickshank, J. M., et al.: How much should blood pressure be lowered? The problem of the J-shaped curve. J. Hypertens. *7(Suppl 6)*:S338, 1989.
43. MacMahon, S., Peto, R., Cutler, J., et al.: Blood pressure, stroke and coronary heart disease: Part I. Prolonged differences in blood pressure: Prospective observational studies corrected for the regression dilution bias. Lancet *335*:765, 1990.
44. Staessen, J., Bulpitt, C., Clement, D., et al.: Relation between mortality and treated blood pressure in elderly patients with hypertension: Report of the European Working Party on High Blood Pressure in the Elderly. Br. Med. J. *298*:1552, 1989.
45. Alderman, M. H., and Lamport, B.: Withdrawal of drug therapy in the treatment of hypertension. *In* Kaplan, N. M., Brenner, B. M., and Laragh, J. H. (eds.): New Therapeutic Strategies in Hypertension. New York, Raven Press, 1989, p. 171.

NONDRUG THERAPY

46. Stamler, R., Stamler, J., Grimm, R., et al.: Nutritional therapy for high blood pressure. Final report of four-year randomized controlled trial—The Hypertension Control Program. JAMA *257*:1484, 1987.
47. Oberman, A., Wassertheil-Smoller, S., Langford, H. G., et al.: Pharmacologic and nutritional treatment of mild hypertension: Changes in cardiovascular risk status. Ann. Intern. Med. *112*: 89, 1990.
48. Aberg, H., and Tibblin, G.: Addition of non-pharmacological methods of treatment in patients on antihypertensive drugs: Results of previous medication, laboratory tests and life quality. J. Intern. Med. *226*:39, 1989.
49. Stamler, R., Stamler, J., Gosch, F. C., et al.: Primary prevention of hypertension by nutritional-hygienic means. Final report of a randomized, controlled trial. JAMA *262*:1801, 1989.
50. Hypertension Prevention Trial Research Group: The Hypertension Prevention Trial: Three-year effects of dietary changes on blood pressure. Arch. Intern. Med. *150*:153, 1990.
51. Berglund, A., Andersson, O. K., Berglund, G., and Fagerberg, B.: Antihypertensive effect of diet compared with drug treatment in obese men with mild hypertension. Br. Med. J. *299*:480, 1989.
52. Lüscher, T. F., and Vetter, W.: Adherence to medication. J. Hum. Hypertens. *4*(Suppl 1):43, 1990.
53. 1988 Joint National Committee. The 1988 report of the Joint National Committee on detection, evaluation, and treatment of high blood pressure. Arch. Intern. Med. *148*:1023, 1988.
54. Staessen, J., Fagard, R., Lijnen, P., and Amery, A.: Body weight, sodium intake and blood pressure. J. Hypertens. *7(Suppl 1)*:S19, 1989.
55. Smoller, S. W., Blaufox, M. D., Oberman, A., et al.: TAIM Study: Adequate weight loss as effective as drug therapy for mild hypertension. Circulation *81*:4, 1990.
56. Cohen, N., and Flamenbaum, W.: Obesity and hypertension. Demonstration of a "floor effect. Am. J. Med. *80*:177, 1986.
57. Vertes, V., Frolkis, J. P., and Martin, P. J.: Clinical utility of nondrug therapy for hypertension. Mt. Sinai J. Med. *55*:296, 1988.
58. Krotiewski, M., Grimby, G., Holm, G., and Szczepanik, J.: Increased muscle dynamic endurance associated with weight reduction on a very-low-calorie diet. Am. J. Clin. Nutr. *51*:321, 1990.
59. Rocchini, A. P., Key, J., Bondie, D., et al.: The effect of weight loss on the sensitivity of blood pressure to sodium in obese adolescents. N. Engl. J. Med. *321*:580, 1989.
60. Weinberger, M., Cohen, S. J., Miller, J. Z., et al.: Dietary sodium restriction as adjunctive treatment of hypertension. JAMA *259*:2561, 1988.
61. Australian National Health and Medical Research Council Dietary Salt Study Management Committee. Fall in blood pressure with modest reduction in dietary salt intake in mild hypertension. Lancet *1*:399, 1989.
62. MacGregor, G. A., Markandu, N. D., Sagnella, G. A., et al.: Double-blind study of three sodium intakes and long-term effects of sodium restriction in essential hypertension. Lancet *2*:1244, 1989.
63. Ram, C. V. S., Garrett, B. N., and Kaplan, N. M.: Moderate sodium restriction and various diuretics in the treatment of hypertension. Arch. Intern. Med. *141*:1015, 1981.
64. Falkner, B., and Kushner, H.: Effect of chronic sodium loading on cardiovascular response in young blacks and whites. Hypertension *15*:36, 1990.
65. Niarchos, A. P., Weinstein, D. L., Laragh, J. H.: Comparison of the effects of diuretic therapy and low sodium intake in isolated systolic hypertension. Am. J. Med. *77*:1061, 1984.
66. Feldman, R. D.: Defective venous beta-adrenergic response in borderline hypertensive subjects is corrected by a low sodium diet. J. Clin. Invest. *85*:647, 1990.
67. Luft, F. C., and Weinberger, M. H.: Review of salt restriction and the response to antihypertensive drugs. Satellite symposium on calcium antagonists. Hypertension *11*(Suppl I):I–229, 1988.
68. Nowson, C. A., and Morgan, T. O.: Change in blood pressure in relation to change in nutrients effected by manipulation of dietary sodium and potassium. Clin. Exp. Pharmacol. Physiol. *15*:225, 1988.
69. Hargreaves, M., Morgan, T. O., Snow, R., and Guerin, M.: Exercise tolerance in the heat on low and normal salt intakes. Clin. Sci. *76*:553, 1989.
70. Forte, J. G., Pereira Miguel, J. M., Pereira Miguel, M. J., et al.: Salt and blood pressure: A community trial. J. Hum. Hypertens. *3*:179, 1989.
71. Stamler, J., Rose, G., Stamler, R., et al.: INTERSALT study findings. Public health and medical care implications. Hypertension *14*:570, 1989.
72. Krishna, G., Miller, E., and Kapoor, S.: Increased blood pressure during potassium depletion in normotensive men. N. Engl. J. Med. *320*:1177, 1989.
73. Kaplan, N. M., Carnegie, A., Raskin, P., et al.: Potassium supplementation in hypertensive patients with diuretic-induced hypokalemia. N. Engl. J. Med. *312*:746, 1985.
74. Grimm, R. H. Jr., Neaton, J. D., Elmer, P. J., et al.: The influence of oral potassium chloride on blood pressure in hypertensive men on a low-sodium diet. N. Engl. J. Med *322*:569, 1990.
75. Tobian, L., Jahner, T. M., and Johnson, M. A.: High K diets markedly reduce atherosclerotic cholesterol ester deposition in aortas of rats with hypercholesterolemia and hypertension. Am. J. Hypertens. *3*:133, 1990.
76. Khaw, K.T., and Barrett-Connor, E.: Dietary potassium and stroke-associated mortality. A 12-year prospective population study. N. Engl. J. Med. *316*:235, 1987.
77. Whelton, P. K., and Klag, M. J.: Magnesium and blood pressure: Review of the epidemologic and clinical trial experience. Am. J. Cardiol. *63*:26G, 1989.
78. Whang, R., Flink, E. B., Dyckner, T., et al.: Magnesium depletion as a cause of refactory potassium repletion. Arch. Intern. Med. *145*:1686, 1985.
79. Zoccali, C., Mallamaci, F., Cuzzola, F. et al.: Mechanisms of hypercalciuria in essential hypertension. J. Hypertens. *7(Suppl 6)*:S406, 1989.
80. Grobbe, D. E., and Waal-Manning, H. J.: The role of calcium supplementation in the treatment of hypertension. Current evidence. Drugs *39*:7, 1990.
81. Rouse, I. L., Beilin, L. J., Mahoney, D. P., et al.: Nutrient intake, blood pressure, serum and urinary prostaglandins and serum thromboxane B_2 in a controlled trial with a lacto-ovo-vegetarian diet. J. Hypertens. *4*:241, 1986.
82. Knapp, H. R., and FitzGerald, G. A.: The antihypertensive effects of fish oil. A controlled study of polyunsaturated fatty acid supplements in essential hypertension. N. Engl. J. Med. *320*:1037, 1989.
83. Bønaa, K. H., Bjerve, K. S., Straume, B., et al.: Effect of eicosapentaenoic and docosahexaenoic acids on blood pressure in hypertension. A population-based intervention trial from the Tromsø study. N. Engl. J. Med. *322*:795, 1990.
84. Sacks, F. M.: Dietary fats and blood pressure: A critical review of the evidence. Nutr. Rev. *47*:291, 1989.
85. Swain, J. F., Rouse, I. L., Curley, C. B., and Sacks, F. M.: Comparison of the effects of oat bran and low-fiber wheat on serum lipoprotein levels and blood pressure. N. Engl. J. Med. *322*:147, 1990.
86. Parillo, M., Coulston, A., Hollenbeck, C., and Reaven, G.: Effect of a low fat diet on carbohydrate metabolism in patients with hypertension. Hypertension *11*:244, 1988.
87. Sharp, D. S., and Benowitz, N. L.: Pharmacoepidemiology of the effect of caffeine on blood pressure. Clin. Pharmacol. Ther. *47*:57, 1990.
88. Moore, R. D., Levine, D. M., Southard, J., et al.: Alcohol consumption and blood pressure in the 1982 Maryland hypertension survey. Am. J. Hypertens. *3*:1, 1990.
89. Jackson, R., Scragg, R., and Beaglehole, R.: CHD risk associated with regular and acute consumption of alcohol. Circulation *81*:9, 1990.
90. Grossman, E., Oren, S., Garavaglia, G. E., et al.: Disparate hemodynamic and sympathoadrenergic responses to isometric and mental stress in essential hypertension. Am. J. Cardiol. *64*:42, 1989.
91. Hagberg, J. M., Montain, S. J., Martin, W. H. III, and Ehsani, A. A.: Effect of exercise training in 60- to 69-year-old persons with essential hypertension. Am. J. Cardiol. *64*:348, 1989.
92. Thompson, P. D., Cullinane, E. M., Nugent, A. M., et al.: Effect of atenolol or prazosin on maximal exercise performance in hypertensive joggers. Am. J. Med. *86*(Suppl 1B):104, 1989.
93. Patel, C., and Marmot, M.: Can general practitioners use training in relaxation and management of stress to reduce mild hypertension? Br. Med. J. *296*:21, 1988.
94. McGrady, A., and Higgins, J. T., Jr.: Prediction of response to biofeedback-assisted relaxation in hypertensives: Development of a hypertensive predictor profile (HYPP). Psychosomatic Med. *51*:277, 1989.
95. Cramer, J. A., Mattson, R. H., Prevey, M. L., et al.: How often is medication taken as prescribed? A novel assessment technqiue. JAMA *261*:3273, 1989.

ANTIHYPERTENSIVE DRUG THERAPY

96. Spitalewitz, S., Porush, J. G., and Reiser, I. W.: Minoxidil, nadolol, and a diuretic. Once-a-day therapy for resistant hypertension. Arch. Intern. Med. *146*:882, 1986.
97. Strandgaard, S., and Haunsø, S.: Why does antihypertensive treatment prevent stroke but not myocardial infarction? Lancet *2*:658, 1987.
98. Barry, D. I.: Cerebrovascular aspects of antihypertensive treatment. Am. J. Cardiol. *63*:14C, 1989.
99. Stewart, A. L., Greenfield, S., Hays, R. D., et al.: Functional status and well-being of patients with chronic conditions. Results from the Medical Outcomes study. JAMA *262*:907, 1989.
100. Guyatt, G. H., Keller, J. L., Jaeschke, R., et al.: The n-of-1 randomized controlled trial: Clinical usefulness. Our three-year experience. Ann. Intern. Med. *112*:293, 1990.
101. Laragh, J. H.: Perspectives in choosing therapy for hypertension. *In* Kaplan, N. M., Brenner, B. M., and Laragh, J. H. (eds.): New Therapeutic Strategies in Hypertension. New York, Raven Press, 1989, p. 141.
102. Bravo, E. L.: Rational drug therapy based on understanding the pathophysiology of hypertension. Cleve. Clin. J. Med. *56*:362, 1989.

103. Graves, J. W., Bloomfield, R. L., and Buckalew, V. M. Jr.: Plasma volume in resistant hypertension: Guide to pathophysiology and therapy. Am. J. Med. Sci. *298*:361, 1989.
104. Burris, J. F., Weir, M. R., Oparil, S., et al.: An assessment of diltiazem and hydrochlorothiazide in hypertension. JAMA *263*:1507, 1990.
105. McVeigh, G., Galloway, D., and Johnston, D.: The case for low dose diuretics in hypertension: Comparison of low and conventional doses of cyclopenthiazide. Br. Med. J. *297*:95, 1988.
106. Prisant, L. M., Beall, S. P., Nichoalds, G. E., et al.: Biochemical, endocrine, and mineral effects of indapamide in black women. J. Clin. Pharmacol. *30*:121, 1990.
107. Uehara, Y., Shirahase, H., Nagata, T., et al.: Radical scavengers of indapamide in prostacyclin synthesis in rat smooth muscle cell. Hypertension *15*:216, 1990.
108. Brater, D. C.: Use of diuretics in chronic renal insufficiency and nephrotic syndrome. Semin. Nephrol. *8*:333, 1988.
109. Morgan, D. G., and Davidson, C.: Hypokalemia and diuretics: An analysis of publications. Br. Med. J. *280*:905, 1980.
110. Sandor, F. F., Pickens, P. T., and Crallan, J.: Variations of plasma potassium concentrations during long-term treatment of hypertension with diuretics without potassium supplements. Br. Med. J. *284*:711, 1982.
111. Velazquez, H., and Wright, F. S.: Control by drugs of renal potassium handling. Annu. Rev. Pharmacol. Toxicol. *26*:293, 1986.
112. Holland, O. B., Kuhnert, L., Pollard, J., et al.: Ventricular ectopic activity with diuretic therapy. Am. J. Hypertens. *1*:380, 1988.
113. Lipworth, B. J., McDevitt, D. G., and Struthers, A. D.: Electrocardiographic changes induced by inhaled salbutamol after treatment with bendrofluazide: Effects of replacement therapy with potassium, magnesium and triamterene. Clin. Sci. *78*:255, 1990.
114. Myers, M. G.: Diuretic therapy and ventricular arrhythmias in persons 65 years of age and older. Am. J. Cardiol. *65*;599, 1990.
115. Schulman, M., and Narins, R. G.: Hypokalemia and cardiovascular disease. Am. J. Cardiol. *65*:4E, 1990.
116. Clausen, T. G., Brocks, K., and Ibsen, H.: Hypokalemia and ventricular arrhythmias in acute myocardial infarction. Acta Med. Scand. *224*:531, 1988.
117. Abraham, A. S., Rosenmann, D., Kramer, M., et al.: Magnesium in the prevention of lethal arrhythmias in acute myocardial infarction. Arch. Intern. Med. *147*:753, 1987.
118. Waller, P. C., and Ramsay, L. E.: Predicting acute gout in diuretic-treated hypertensive patients. J. Hum. Hyperten. *3*:457, 1989.
119. Lardinois, C. K., and Neuman, S. L.: The effects of antihypertensive agents on serum lipids and lipoproteins. Arch. Intern. Med. *148*:1280, 1988.
120. Pollare, T., Lithell, H., and Berne, C.: A comparison of the effects of hydrochlorothiazide and captopril on glucose and lipid metabolism in patients with hypertension. N. Engl. J. Med. *321*:868, 1989.
121. Stier, C. T. Jr., and Itskovitz, H. D.: Renal calcium metabolism and diuretics. Annu. Rev. Pharmacol. Toxicol. *26*:101, 1986.
122. LaCroix, A. Z., Wienpahl, J., White, L. R., et al.: Thiazide diuretic agents and the incidence of hip fracture. N. Engl. J. Med. *322*:286, 1990.
123. Medical Research Council Working Party on Mild to Moderate Hypertension: Adverse reactions to bendrofluazide and propranolol for the treatment of mild hypertension. Lancet *2*:539, 1981.
124. Wright, J. T., McKinney, J. M., Lehany, A. M., et al.: The effect of high-dose short-term ibuprofen on antihypertensive control with hydrochlorothiazide. Clin. Pharmacol. Ther. *45*:440, 1989.
125. Materson, B. J., Cushman, W. C., Goldstein, G., et al.: Treatment of hypertension in the Elderly: I. Blood pressure and clinical changes. Results of a Department of Veterans Affairs Cooperative Study. Hypertension *15*:348, 1990.
126. Veterans Administration Cooperative Study Group on Antihypertensive Agents: Comparison of propranolol and hydrochlorothiazide for the initial treatment of hypertension. I. Results of short-term titration with emphasis on racial difference in response. JAMA *248*:1996, 1982.
127. van Zwieten, P. A.: Basic pharmacology of alpha-adrenoceptor antagonists and hybrid drugs. J. Hypertens. *6(Suppl 2)*:S3, 1988.
128. Veterans Administration Cooperative Study Group on Antihypertensive Agents: Propranolol in the treatment of essential hypertension. JAMA *237*:2303, 1977.
129. Participating Veterans Administration Medical Centers: Low dose vs. standard dose of reserpine. JAMA *248*:2471, 1982.
130. Horwitz, R. I., and Feinstein, A. R.: Exclusion bias and the false relationship of reserpine and breast cancer. Arch. Intern. Med. *145*:1873, 1985.
131. Owens, S. D., and Dunn, M. I.: Efficacy and safety of guanadrel in elderly hypertensive patients. Arch. Intern. Med. *148*:1515, 1988.
132. Struthers, A. D., Brown, M. J., Adams, E. F., and Dollery, C. T.: The plasma noradrenaline and growth hormone response to α-methyldopa and clonidine in hypertensive subjects. Br. J. Clin. Pharmacol. *19*:311, 1985.
133. Fouad, F. M., Nakashima, Y., Tarazi, R. C., and Salcedo, E. E.: Reversal of left ventricular hypertrophy in hypertensive patients treated with methyldopa. Am. J. Cardiol. *49*:795, 1982.
134. Kelton, J. G.: Impaired reticuloendothelial function in patients treated with methyldopa. Am. J. Cardiol. *49*:795, 1982.
135. Kaplowitz, N., Aw, T. Y., Simon, F. R., and Stolz, A.: Drug-induced hepatotoxicity. Ann. Intern. Med. *104*:826, 1986.
136. Houston, M. C.: Abrupt cessation of treatment in hypertension: Consideration of clinical features, mechanisms, prevention and management of the discontinuation syndrome. Am. Heart J. *102*:415, 1981.
137. Schmidt, G. R., Schuna, A. A., and Goodfriend, T. L.: Transdermal clonidine compared with hydrochlorothiazide as monotherapy in elderly hypertensive males. J. Clin. Pharmacol. *29*:133, 1989.
138. Zeller, K. R., Kuhnert, L. V., and Matthews, C.: Rapid reduction of severe asymptomatic hypertension. A prospective, controlled trial. Arch. Intern. Med. *149*:2186, 1989.
139. Franks, P., Harp, J., and Bell, B.: Randomized, controlled trial of clonidine for smoking cessation in a primary care setting. JAMA *262*:3011, 1989.
140. Gehr, M., MacCarthy, E. P., and Goldberg, M.: Guanabenz: A centrally acting, natriurtic antihypertensive drug. Kidney Int. *29*:1203, 1986.
141. Kaplan, N. M., and Grundy, S.: Comparison of the effects of guanabenz and hydrochlorothiazide on plasma lipids. Clin. Pharmacol. Ther. *44*:297, 1988.
142. Wilson, M. F., Haring, O., Lewin, A., et al.: Comparison of guanfacine versus clonidine for efficacy, safety and occurrence of withdrawal syndrome in step-2 treatment of mild to moderate essential hypertension. Am. J. Cardiol. *57*:43E, 1986.
143. Cubeddu, L. X.: New alpha$_1$-adrenergic receptor antagonists for the treatment of hypertension: Role of vascular alpha receptors in the control of peripheral resistance. Am. Heart J. *116*:133, 1988.
144. Elliott, H. L., Donnelly, R., Meredith, P. A., and Reid, J. L.: Predictability of antihypertensive responsiveness and α-adrenoceptor antagonism during prazosin treatment. Clin. Pharmacol. Ther. *46*:576, 1989.
145. Heagerty, A. M., Russell, G. I., Bing, R. F., et al.: The addition of prazosin to standard triple therapy in the treatment of severe hypertension. Br. J. Clin. Pharmacol. *13*:539, 1982.
146. Grimm, R. H., Jr.: α_1-Antagonists in the treatment of hypertension. Hypertension *13*(Suppl I):I–131, 1989.
147. Pollare, T., Lithell, H., Selinus, I., and Berne, C.: Application of prazosin is associated with an increase of insulin sensitivity in obese patients with hypertension. Diabetologia *31*:415, 1988.
148. Yasumoto, K., Takata, M., Yoshida, K., et al.: Reversal of left ventricular hypertrophy by terazosin in hypertensive patients. J. Hum. Hypertens. *4*:13, 1990.
149. Donnelly, R., Elliott, H. L., Meredith, P. A., and Reid, J. L.: Concentration-effect relationships and individual responses to doxazosin in essential hypertension. Br. J. Clin. Pharmacol. *28*:517, 1989.
150. Dahlöf, C., and Dimenäs, E.: Side effects of β-blocker treatments as related to the central nervous system. Am. J. Med. Sci. *299*:236, 1990.
151. Nidorf, S. M., Parsons, R. W., Thompson, P. L., et al.: Reduced risk of death at 28 days in patients taking a β blocker before admission to hospital with myocardial infarction. Br. Med. J. *300*:71, 1990.
152. Wilkstrand, J., Warnold, I., Olsson, G., et al.: Primary prevention with metoprolol in patients with hypertension. Mortality results from the MAPHY study. JAMA *259*:1976, 1988.
153. Parati, G., Ravogli, A., Bragato, R., et al.: Clinical and hemodynamic effects of celiprolol in essential hypertension. J. Cardiovasc. Pharmacol. *14(Suppl 7)*:S14, 1989.
154. Pringle, T. H., and Riddell, J. G.: The cardioselectivity of beta adrenoceptor antagonists. Pharmacol. Ther. *45*:39, 1990.
155. Duncan, J. J., Vaandrager, H., Farr, J. E., et al.: Effect of intrinsic sympathomimetic activity on the ability of hypertensive patients to derive a cardiorespiratory training effect during chronic β-blockade. Am. J. Hypertens. *3*:302, 1990.
156. Fogari, R., Zoppi, A., Pasotti, C., et al.: Plasma lipids during chronic antihypertensive therapy with different β-blockers. J. Cardiovasc. Pharmacol. *14(Suppl 7)*:S28, 1989.
157. Conant, J., Engler, R., Janowsky, D., et al.: Central nervous system side effects of β-adrenergic blocking agents with high and low lipid solubility. J. Cardiovasc. Pharmacol. *13*:656, 1989.
158. Man in't Veld, A. J., Van Den Meiracker, A. H., and Schalekamp, M. A.: Do beta-blockers really increase peripheral vascular resistance? Review of the literature and new observations under basal conditions. Am. J. Hypertens. *1*:91, 1988.
159. Merli, I. P., Levenson, J., Filitti, V., and Simon, A.: Comparative long-term vasoactive effects of atenolol and carteolol on the properties of the small and large arteries of the upper extremities in human essential hypertension. Clin. Pharmacol. Ther. *46*:686, 1989.
160. Serlin, M. M., Orme, M. L'E., Baber, N. A., et al.: Propranolol in the control of blood pressure: A dose-response study. Clin. Pharmacol. Ther. *27*:586, 1980.
161. Buhler, F.: Antihypertensive treatment according to age, plasma renin, and race. Drugs *35*:495, 1988.
162. Kaplan, N. M.: Critical comments on recent literature. Age and the response to antihypertensive drugs. Am. J. Hypertens. *2*:213, 1989.
163. Oxorn, D., Knox, J. W. D., and Hill, J.: Bolus doses of esmolol for the prevention of perioperative hypertension and tachycardia. Can. J. Anaesth. *37*:206, 1990.
164. Pollare, T., Lithell, H., Selinus, I., and Berne, C.: Sensitivity to insulin during treatment with atenolol and metoprolol: A randomised, double blind study of effects on carbohydrate and lipoprotein metabolism in hypertensive patients. Br. Med. J. *298*:1152, 1989.
165. Psaty, B. M., Koepsell, T. D., Wagner, E. H., et al.: The relative risk of incident coronary heart disease associated with recently stopping the use of β-blockers. JAMA *263*:1653, 1990.
166. Koch, G., Fransson, L., Karlegärd, L., and Kothari, P.: Responses of glomerular filtration, renal blood flow and salt-water handling to acute cardioselective and non-selective β-adrenoceptor blockade in essential hypertension. Eur. J. Clin. Pharmacol. *36*:343, 1989.
167. Butters, L., Kennedy, S., and Rubin, P. C.: Atenolol in essential hypertension during pregnancy. Br. Med. J. *301*:587, 1990.
168. Bacon, P. J., Brazier, D. J., Smith, R., and Smith, S. E.: Cardiovascular responses to metipranolol and timolol eyedrops in healthy volunteers. Br. J. Clin. Pharmac. *27*:1, 1989.

169. Goa, K. L., Benfield, P., and Sorkin, E. M.: Labetalol. A reappraisal of its pharmacology, pharmacokinetics and therapeutic use in hypertension and ischaemic heart disease. Drugs *37*:583, 1989.
170. Huey, J., Thomas, J. P., Hendricks, D. R., et al.: Clinical evaluation of intravenous labetalol for the treatment of hypertensive urgency. Am. J. Hypertens. *1*:284S, 1988.
171. Wallin, J. D., Cook, E., Fletcher, E., et al.: Dilevalol in severe hypertension. A multicenter trial of bolus intravenous dosing. Arch. Intern. Med. *149*:2655, 1989.
172. Shepherd, A. M. M., and Irving, N. A.: Differential hemodynamic and sympathoadrenal effects of sodium nitroprusside and hydralazine in hypertensive subjects. J. Cardiovasc. Pharmacol. *8*:527, 1986.
173. Cinquegrani, M. P., and Liang, C.: Indomethacin attenuates the hypotensive action of hydralazine. Clin. Pharmacol. Ther. *39*:564, 1986.
174. Halstenson, C. E., Opsahl, J. A., Wright, E., et al.: Disposition of minoxidil in patients with various degrees of renal function. J. Clin. Pharmacol. *29*:798, 1989.
175. Sanz, E., Lopez Novoa, J. M., Linares, M. et al.: Intravascular and interstitial fluid dynamics in rats treated with minoxidil. J. Cardiovasc. Pharmacol. *15*:485, 1990.
176. Houston, M. C., McChesney, J. A., and Chatterjee, K.: Pericardial effusion associated with minoxidil therapy. Arch. Intern. Med. *131*:69, 1981.
177. Kaplan, N. M.: Calcium entry blockers in the treatment of hypertension. Current status and future prospects. JAMA *262*:817, 1989.
178. Holzgreve H., Distler, A., Michaelis, J., et al.: Verapamil versus hydrochlorothiazide in the treatment of hypertension: Results of long term double blind comparative trial. Br. Med. J. *299*:881, 1989.
179. Nikkilä, M. T., Inkovaara, J. A., Heikkinen, J. T., and Olsson, S.-O. R.: Antihypertensive effect of diltiazem in a slow-release formulation for mild to moderate essential hypertension. Am. J. Cardiol. *63*:1227, 1989.
180. Soro, S., Cocca, A., Pasanisi, F., et al.: The effects of nicardipine on sodium and calcium metabolism in hypertensive patients: A chronic study. J. Clin. Pharmacol. *30*:133, 1990.
181. Wei, J. Y.: Use of calcium entry blockers in elderly patients. Special considerations. Circulation *80*(Suppl IV):IV–171, 1989.
182. Weinberger, M. H.: The role of age, race, and plasma renin activity in influencing the blood pressure response to nitrendipine or hydrochlorothiazide. J. Cardiovasc. Pharmacol. *9*(Suppl 4):S272, 1987.
183. Pollare, T., Lithell, H., Mörlin, C., et al.: Metabolic effects of diltiazem and atenolol: Results from a randomized, double-blind study with parallel groups. J. Hypertens. *7*:551, 1989.
184. Marone, C., Luisoli, S., Bomio, F., et al.: Body sodium-blood volume state, aldosterone, and cardiovascular responsiveness after calcium entry blockade with nifedipine. Kidney Int. *28*:658, 1985.
185. Messerli, F. H., Nunez, B. D., Nunez, M. M., et al.: Hypertension and sudden death. Disparate effects of calcium entry blocker and diuretic therapy on cardiac dysrhythmias. Arch. Intern. Med. *149*:1263, 1989.
186. Jaker, M., Atkin, S., Soto, M., et al.: Oral nifedipine vs oral clonidine in the treatment of urgent hypertension. Arch. Intern. Med. *149*:260, 1989.
187. Bursztyn, M., Garvas, I., Tifft, C. P., et al.: Effects of a novel renin inhibitor in patients with essential hypertension. J. Cardiovasc. Pharmacol. *15*:493, 1990.
188. Gavras, H.: Angiotensin converting enzyme inhibition and its impact on cardiovascular disease. Circulation *81*:381, 1990.
189. Perry, I. J., and Beevers, D. G.: ACE inhibitors compared with thiazide diuretics as first-step antihypertensive therapy. Cardiovasc. Drugs Ther. *3*:815, 1989.
190. Waeber, B., Nussberger, J., Juillerat, L., and Brunner, H. R.: Angiotensin converting enzyme inhibition: Discrepancy between antihypertensive effect and suppression of enzyme activity. J. Cardiovasc. Pharmacol. *14*(Suppl 4):S53, 1989.
191. Zimmerman, B. G., Raich, P. C., Vavrek, R. J., and Stewart, J. M.: Bradykinin contribution to renal blood flow effect of angiotensin converting enzyme inhibitor in the conscious sodium-restricted dog. Circ. Res. *66*:242, 1990.
192. Ajayi, A. A., and Reid, J. L.: The effect of enalapril on baroreceptor mediated reflex function in normotensive subjects. Br. J. Clin. Pharmacol. *21*:338, 1986.
193. Herrick, A. L., Waller, P. C., Berkin, K. E., et al.: Comparison of enalapril and atenolol in mild to moderate hypertension. Am. J. Med. *86*:421, 1989.
194. Weinberger, M. H.: Blood pressure and metabolic responses to hydrochlorothiazide, captopril, and the combination in black and white mild-to-moderate hypertensive patients. J. Cardiovasc. Pharmacol. *7*:S52, 1985.
195. Hollenberg, N. K.: The treatment of renovascular hypertension: Surgery, angioplasty, and medical therapy with converting-enzyme inhibitors. Am. J. Kidney Dis. *10*(Suppl 1):52, 1987.
196. Wenting, G. J., Derkx, F. H. M., Tan-Tjiong, L., et al.: Risks of angiotensin converting enzyme inhibition in renal artery stenosis. Kidney Int. *31*(Suppl 20):S–180, 1987.
197. Remuzzi, A., Puntorieri, S., Battaglia, C., et al.: Angiotensin converting enzyme inhibition ameliorates glomerular filtration of macromolecules and water and lessens glomerular injury in the rat. J. Clin. Invest. *85*:541, 1990.
198. Keane, W. F., Anderson, S., Aurell, M., et al.: Angiotensin converting enzyme inhibitor and progressive renal insufficiency. Current experience and future directions. Ann. Intern. Med. *111*:503, 1989.
199. Schoenberger, J. A., Testa, M., Ross, A. D., et al.: Efficacy, safety, and quality-of-life assessment of captopril antihypertensive therapy in clinical practice. Arch. Intern. Med. *150*:301, 1990.
200. Chin, H. L., and Buchaan, D. A.: Severe angioedema after long-term use of an angiotensin-converting enzyme inhibitor. Ann. Intern. Med. *112*:312, 1990.
201. Boulet, L.- P., Milot, J., Lampron, N., and Lacourcière, Y.: Pulmonary function and airway responsiveness during long-term therapy with captopril. JAMA *261*, 413, 1989.
202. Katzman, P. L., Henningsen, N. C., Fagher, B., et al.: Renal and endocrine effects of long-term converting enzyme inhibition as compared with calcium antagonism in essential hypertension. J. Cardiovasc. Pharmacol. *15*:360, 1990.
203. Taylor, D. G., and Kaplan, H. R.: New antihypertensive drugs. *In* Kaplan, N. M., Brenner, B. M., and Laragh, J. H. (eds.): New Therapeutic Strategies in Hypertension. New York, Raven Press, 1989, p. 125.
204. Suzukawa, M., and Nakamura, H.: Effects of ketanserin tartrate on 3-hydroxy, 3-methylglutaryl coenzyme A reductase activity in cultured human skin fibroblasts. Cardiovasc. Drugs Ther. *4*:69, 1990.
205. Tuttle, R. S., and Boppana, D. P.: Antihypertensive effect of interleukin-2. Hypertension *15*:89, 1990.

SPECIAL CONSIDERATIONS IN THERAPY

206. Mejia, A. D., Egan, B. M., Schork, N. J., and Zwiefler, A. J.: Artefacts in measurement of blood pressure and lack of target organ involvement in the assessment of patients with treatment-resistant hypertension. Ann. Intern. Med. *112*:270, 1990.
207. Estafanous, F. G.: Hypertension in the surgical patient: Management of blood pressure and anesthesia. Cleve. Clin. J. Med. *56*:385, 1989.
208. Haworth, R. A., Goknur, A. B., and Berkoff, H. A.: Inhibition of Na-Ca exchange by general anesthetics. Circ. Res. *65*:1021, 1989.
209. Patel, C. B., Laboy, V., Venus, B., et al.: Use of sodium nitroprusside in post-coronary bypass surgery. A plea for conservatism. Chest *80*:663, 1986.
210. Cottrell, J. E., Patel, K., Turndorf, H., and Ransohoff, J.: Intracranial pressure changes induced by sodium nitroprusside in patients with intracranial mass lesions. J. Neurosurg. *48*:329, 1978.
211. Brush, J. E., Jr., Udelson, J. E., Bacharach, S. L., et al.: Comparative effects of verapamil and nitroprusside on left ventricular function in patients with hypertension. J. Am. Coll. Cardiol. *14*515, 1989.
212. Lieberman, E.: Hypertension in childhood and adolescence. *In* Kaplan, N. M. (ed.): Clinical Hypertension, 5th ed. Baltimore, Williams & Wilkins, 1990, p. 407.
213. Berenson, G. S., Shear, C. L., Chiang, Y. K., et al.: Combined low-dose medication and primary intervention over a 30-month period for sustained high blood pressure in childhood. Am. J. Med. Sci. *299*:79, 1990.
214. Potter, J. F., and Haigh, R. A.: Benefits of antihypertensive therapy in the elderly. Br. Med. Bull. *46*:77, 1990.
215. Goldstein, G., Materson, B. J., Cushman, W. C., et al.: Treatment of hypertension in the elderly: II. Cognitive and behavioral function. Results of a Department of Veterans Affairs Cooperative Study. Hypertension *15*:361, 1990.
216. Kawamoto, A., Shimada, K., Matsubayashi, K., et al.: Cardiovascular regulatory functions in elderly patients with hypertension. Hypertension *13*:401, 1989.
217. Lye, M., Vargas, E., Faragher, E. B., et al.: Haemodynamic and neurohumoral responses in elderly patients with postural hypotension. Eur. J. Clin. Invest. *20*:90, 1990.
218. Jansen, P. A. F., Schulte, B. P. M., and Gribnau, F. W. J.: Cerebral ischaemia and stroke as side effects of antihypertensive treatment: Special danger in the elderly. A review of the cases reported in the literature. Neth. J. Med. *30*:193, 1987.
219. Col, N., Fanale, J. E., and Kronholm, P.: The role of medication noncompliance and adverse drug reactions in hospitalizations of the elderly. Arch. Intern. Med. *150*:841, 1990.
220. Lavin, P.: Management of cerebral infarction or transient ischemic attacks. Arch. Intern. Med. *150*:692, 1990.
221. Applegate, W. B.: Hypertension in elderly patients. Ann. Intern. Med. *110*:901, 1989.
222. Hulley, S. B., Furberg, C. D., Gurland, B., et al.: Systolic hypertension in the elderly program (SHEP): Antihypertensive efficacy of chlorthalidone. Am. J. Cardiol. *56*:913, 1985.
223. Brater, D. C.: Use of diuretics in chronic renal insufficiency and nephrotic syndrome. Semin. Nephrol. *8*:333, 1988.
224. Heyka, R. J., and Vidt, D. G.: Control of hypertension in patients with chronic renal failure. Cleve. Clin. J. Med. *56*:65, 1989.
225. Stornello, M., Valvo, E. F., and Scapellato, L.: Hemodynamic, renal, and humoral effects of the calcium entry blockers nicardipine and converting enzyme inhibitor captopril in hypertensive type II diabetic patients with nephropathy. J. Cardiovasc. Pharmacol. *14*:851, 1989.
226. Wilhelmsen, L.: Practical guidelines for drug therapy after myocardial infarction. Drugs *38*:1000, 1989.
227. Tedde, R., Sechi, L. A., Marigliano, A., et al.: Antihypertensive effect of insulin reduction in diabetic-hypertensive patients. Am. J. Hypertens. *2*:163, 1989.
228. Moul, J. W., and McLeod, D. G.: Negative pressure devices in the explanted penile prosthesis population. J. Urol. *142*:729, 1989.
229. Wallin, J. D.: Intravenous nicardipine hydrochloride: Treatment of patients with severe hypertension. Am. Heart J. *119*:434, 1990.
230. Barry, D. I.: Cerebrovascular aspects of antihypertensive treatment. Am. J. Cardiol. *63*:14C, 1989.
231. Schwartz, M., Naschitz, J. E., Yeshurun, D., and Sharf, B.: Oral nifedipine in the treatment of hypertensive urgency: Cerebrovascular accident following a single dose. Arch. Intern. Med. *150*:686, 1990.

tation may be initiated by high intraventricular pressure acting on ventricular baroreceptors which may blunt the carotid and aortic baroreceptor-mediated compensatory reflexes. Other rare causes of syncope in valvular aortic stenosis include ventricular tachyarrhythmias, paroxysmal AV block, and atrial fibrillation with loss of the "atrial kick." Syncope is prognostically important in aortic stenosis, with an average survival of 2 to 3 years in affected patients after its onset in the absence of valve replacement.

Similar pathophysiological processes may be responsible for syncope in *hypertrophic cardiomyopathy* (HCM, p. 1404). Syncope is reported in as many as 30 per cent of patients with this condition. Left ventricular outflow obstruction is dynamic and intensifies by an increase in contractibility, a decrease in left ventricular volume, or a decrease in afterload and distending pressure. Thus, the Valsalva maneuver, severe coughing paroxysm, or specific drugs (e.g., digitalis) may precipitate hypotension and syncope. Ventricular tachycardia is reported in approximately 25 per cent of adult patients with HCM and is associated with an increased risk of sudden death. Thus, ventricular arrhythmias constitute an important cause of syncope in HCM.[30,31]

Effort syncope commonly occurs in *pulmonary hypertension* (p. 790) (in up to 30 per cent of patients with primary pulmonary hypertension). The limitations to right ventricular outflow may lead to diminished capacity to increase cardiac output. Exertional syncope may also occur with severe *pulmonic stenosis* on the basis of a similar mechanism. Patients with congenital heart disease (e.g., tetralogy of Fallot, patent ductus arteriosus, and interventricular or interatrial septal defects) can with effort or crying experience syncope due to sudden reversal of a left-to-right shunt and a fall in arterial oxygen saturation.

Atrial myxomas may result in obstruction of the mitral or tricuspid valve, leading to symptoms of cardiac failure and rarely syncope (p. 1452). Syncope, dyspnea, and cardiac murmurs that change with body position are particularly suggestive of myxoma.[32] Mitral stenosis may rarely lead to syncope which may be due to severe obstruction to outflow, atrial fibrillation with rapid ventricular response, pulmonary hypertension, or a cerebral embolic event.

Syncope may occasionally be the presenting symptom of a *myocardial infarction.* Five to 12 per cent of elderly patients with acute myocardial infarction present with syncope rather than chest pain. Mechanisms responsible for syncope include (1) sudden pump failure producing a decrease in perfusion pressure of the brain, and (2) rhythm disturbances, which include both ventricular tachyarrhythmias and bradyarrhythmias. Bradycardia secondary to vagal influences is reported in up to 17 per cent of patients with acute myocardial infarction and occurs most commonly in patients with inferior or posterior myocardial infarction due to vascular occlusion of branches that supply the sinus or AV node. Unstable angina and coronary artery spasm also have been rarely associated with syncope.[33]

Syncope occurs in 5 per cent of patients with aortic dissection. Loss of consciousness may be due to stroke or related to rupture into the pericardial space, resulting in sudden cardiac tamponade.[34] Syncope is reported in 10 to 15 per cent of patients with *pulmonary embolism* (p. 1558) and is more likely to occur with massive embolism (>50 per cent obstruction of the pulmonary vascular bed). Massive pulmonary embolism results in acute right ventricular failure, which leads to increased right ventricular filling pressure and reduced stroke volume. Subsequent decreased cardiac output and hypotension lead to loss of consciousness. Consciousness is regained if the embolus migrates distally in the pulmonary artery. Transient sinus bradycardia and AV block, possibly due to a parasympathetic reflex in patients with recurrent pulmonary embolism and chronic cor pulmonale, are reported as well as syncope due to right atrial thromboembolism.

ARRHYTHMIAS. Bradycardia leads to a prolonged ventricular filling period resulting in increased stroke volume to maintain cardiac output. Marked bradycardia (<30/min) may result in an inadequate compensatory increase in stroke volume and lead to syncope. Mild to moderate tachycardias increase cardiac output, but very rapid heart rates lead to a decrease in diastolic filling and cardiac output resulting in hypotension and syncope. *Sinus bradycardia* may result from excessive vagal tone, decreased sympathetic tone, or sinus node disease. Sinus bradycardia in healthy young athletes is generally attributed to increased vagal tone and decreased sympathetic activity. This bradycardia may be occasionally exaggerated, resulting in postexertional syncope in trained athletes.[35,36] Sinus bradycardia also occurs with ophthalmological surgery, myxedema, intracranial and mediastinal tumors, and with use of a large number of parasympathomimetic, sympatholytic, beta blocker, and other drugs. Conjunctival instillation of beta blockers may also cause symptomatic bradycardia.

Syncope is reported in 25 to 70 per cent of patients with the *sick sinus syndrome.* This syndrome is characterized by disturbances of sinoatrial impulse formation or conduction (p. 677). Electrocardiographic manifestations include sinus bradycardia, pauses, arrest, or exit block. Supraventricular tachycardia or atrial fibrillation may also occur in association with bradycardia or atrial fibrillation with slow ventricular response (tachycardia-bradycardia syndrome).[37] *Ventricular tachycardia* (p. 651) is an important cause of syncope and usually occurs in the setting of known organic heart disease. Severity of symptoms is related to its rate, duration, and myocardial pump function. Torsades de pointes and syncope occur in the setting of syndromes of congenital prolongation of Q-T interval (with or without deafness) as well as acquired long Q-T syndromes (p. 708) that occur with drugs, electrolyte abnormalities, and central nervous system disorders.[38] Antiarrhythmic drugs are the most common cause of torsades de pointes which occurs with quinidine (quinidine syncope), procainamide, disopyramide, flecanide, encainide, amiodarone, and satolol.[39,40] Other tachyarrhythmias that may cause syncope include atrial fibrillation or flutter with rapid ventricular response, AV nodal reentrant tachycardia, and supraventricular tachycardia in patients with Wolff-Parkinson-White syndrome.[41]

DIAGNOSTIC EVALUATION

The results of diagnostic testing in recent studies[1,42–47] are shown in Table 30–3. In those patients in whom an etiology could be determined, the history and physical examination identified a potential cause in 50 to 85 per cent. Furthermore, many of the cardiac and noncardiac causes (e.g., aortic stenosis, hypertrophic cardiomyopathy, pulmonary embolism, subclavian steal) would be suspected on the basis of the history, physical examination, and electrocardiogram. These entities often need selective confirmatory tests. In one study, suggestive findings were helpful in assigning the ultimate cause of syncope in 8 per cent of the patients.[47] In the remaining patients, arrhythmia detection, upright tilt testing, and psychiatric evaluation were of decisive value.

HISTORY. A detailed account of the syncopal episode, the events surrounding the loss of consciousness, and associated symptoms provides valuable information for diagnosing many of the entities. For example, in vasovagal syncope, precipitating factors, in conjunction with autonomic symptoms, indicate the diagnosis. Syncope during or immediately after micturition, cough, defecation, and swallowing is easily diagnosed by history but may require a search for an underlying organic disorder. Syncope associated with symptoms of brain stem ischemia suggests neurological causes such as transient ischemic attacks, basilar artery migraines, and subclavian steal syndrome; loss of consciousness with glossopharyngeal or trigeminal neuralgia is due to bradyarrhythmias or a vasodepressor response. A detailed drug history is important, and a drug challenge (such as with nitroglycerin) in a controlled

TABLE 30-3 SOME STUDIES OF DIAGNOSTIC TESTING IN SYNCOPE

AUTHOR	TYPE OF PATIENT	NO. OF PATIENTS	NO. WITH DIAGNOSIS		Diagnosis by (n)					
			n	%	H&P	ECG	PEM	EPS	EEG/CT	OTHERS§
Kapoor[42]*	Admitted SUO	121	13	—	—	—	7	3	—	3
Day[1]	ED	198	173	87	147	4	4	—	18	—
Silverstein[45]	MICU	108	57	53	42†	—	8	—	—	7‡
Kapoor[43]	All	433	254	59	140	30	54	7	2	21
Eagle[44]	Admitted	100	61	61	52†	—	3	—	2	4
Martin[46]	ER	170	106	62	90‖	2	5	—	9	—

Modified from Kapoor, W. N., et al.: Diagnostic and prognostic implications of recurrences in patients with syncope. Am. J. Cardiol. *63*:730, 1989; and Kapoor, W. N.: Diagnostic evaluation of syncope. Am. J. Med. *90*:91, 1991.

* Excluded patients in whom a diagnosis was made by H&P and ECG.

† On admission examination (may exclude ECG).

‡ 7 or 8 (data unclear).

§ Variety of tests including cardiac catheterization, echocardiogram, cardiac enzymes, stress test, noninvasive cerebrovascular studies, radionuclide brain scan, cerebral angiography, ventilation/perfusion scan.

‖ Calculated; exact number not given in the article.

SUO = Syncope of unknown origin
ED = Emergency department
MICU = Medical intensive care unit
H&P = History and physical
PEM = Prolonged electrocardiographic monitoring
EPS = Electrophysiological studies
EEG/CT = Electroencephalogram/Brain CT scan

setting can occasionally provide valuable diagnostic information.

There are specific clinical associations that may suggest various causes of syncope. Examples include syncope with arm exercise suggesting subclavian steal syndrome, loss of consciousness with head rotation or extension suggesting carotid sinus syncope, syncope in a deaf child with effort or emotional distress suggesting prolonged Q-T syndromes, and fainting with flushing and itching suggesting mastocytosis. Detailed accounts of such associations have been summarized elsewhere.[19]

PHYSICAL EXAMINATION. The physical examination may help diagnose specific entities and exclude others. Orthostatic hypotension, cardiovascular signs, and neurological examination are particularly important. However, since orthostatic hypotension is common, this finding in itself is a difficult one to use for attributing syncope to orthostatic hypotension. Development of symptoms similar to spontaneous episodes or severe hypotension (systolic blood pressure <90 mm Hg) during standing implicates orthostatic hypotension as a cause of syncope in the absence of another explanation. Several cardiovascular findings serve as clues to specific entities. Differences in the pulse intensity and blood pressure (generally >20 mm Hg) in the arms suggest aortic dissection or subclavian steal syndrome. Special attention to the cardiovascular examination for aortic stenosis, hypertrophic cardiomyopathy, pulmonary hypertension, myxomas, and aortic dissection is needed for consideration of these entities.

LABORATORY TESTS. Routine blood tests are rarely abnormal, nor do they yield diagnostically helpful information in patients with syncope. In studies of patients with syncope which included patients with seizure, 2 to 3 per cent had hypoglycemia, hyponatremia or hypocalcemia, or renal insufficiency.[1,43,47] These tests confirmed clinical suspicion of these problems, and in one report only one unexpected finding (hyponatremia) was noted, occurring in a patient with seizure rather than syncope.[1] Bleeding was diagnosed clinically rather than on the basis of a complete blood count. A glucose tolerance test did not delineate the cause of syncope in any of the patients undergoing this test.[42]

CAROTID MASSAGE. The technique of carotid massage is not standardized. Commonly, massage is done in the supine position, and occasionally repeated in the sitting and standing positions if the vasodepressor type is suspected and the supine test is negative. Electrocardiographic and blood pressure monitoring are necessary. Mixed cardioinhibitory and vasodepressor response is diagnosed when carotid sinus massage is performed after the cardioinhibitory response is abolished with atropine or atrioventricular sequential pacing. While the duration of massage has varied from 5 sec to 40 sec, recent recommendations suggest a limit of 5 sec.[18] Simultaneous bilateral massage should *never* be done. At least 15 seconds should be allowed between massage from one side to the other. Complications of carotid sinus massage include prolonged asystole, ventricular fibrillation, transient or permanent neurological deficit, and sudden death. Complication rates are not available but are considered extremely low; however, in patients with cerebrovascular disease the test should be done only if all other diagnostic modalities are exhausted and the pretest probability of carotid sinus syncope remains high.

Carotid sinus syncope is diagnosed in patients who are found to have carotid sinus hypersensitivity if they have (1) episodes related to activities that press or stretch the carotid sinus or (2) recurrent syncope with a negative work-up. Symptom reproduction during carotid sinus massage is helpful but not mandatory.[18]

Diagnosis of Arrhythmias

Ascribing syncope to arrhythmias is often difficult because in most patients symptoms have resolved by the time of testing; thus a causal inference is often made on the basis of arrhythmias detected during asymptomatic periods. This can result in uncertainty—as of this writing there are no validated criteria for attributing syncope to arrhythmias by the use of electrocardiographic abnormalities during asymptomatic periods. It has not been possible to develop a "gold standard" test (a test used to establish the patient's true disease status) to determine the value of ambulatory monitoring or electrophysiological testing in syncope. In attributing syncope to arrhythmias, index tests (i.e., tests in which performance is being measured, such as ECG, ambulatory monitoring, and electrophysiological studies) have been used as elements in the global diagnosis of arrhythmic syncope. Because gold standard tests have not been independent of index tests, it is not possible to estimate the sensitivity and specificity of various tests for arrhythmias. Each of the tests used for arrhythmia detection will be described.

ELECTROCARDIOGRAM. In one study, an abnormal electrocardiogram was reported in 50 per cent of patients presenting with syncope.[47] The most common abnormalities were bifascicular block, old myocardial infarction, and left ventricular hypertrophy. In recent syncope studies, 2 to 11 per cent of patients had an etiology assigned by means of ECG.[1,43-47] In one study, 30 of 433 patients had a cause of syncope assigned by means of an electrocardiogram or rhythm strip (20 per cent by paramedics in the field, 20 per cent on a rhythm strip in the emergency department or in the hospital with recurrence of syncope, and 60 per cent by 12-lead electrocardiogram).[47] This constituted 30 per cent of arrhythmias diagnosed in this study. While the most commonly assigned diagnoses included ventricular tachycardia and bradyarrhythmias, a possible acute myocardial infarction was found in five patients with syncope.

Exercise treadmill testing can be used to provoke syncope with exercise and to search for tachyarrhythmias or bradyarrhythmias occurring during or after abrupt termination of exercise.[35,36] In a study of exercise testing in syncope, complex ventricular dysrhythmias or supraventricular tachycardia were found in only 3 of 119 patients.[48]

PROLONGED ELECTROCARDIOGRAPHIC MONITORING (p. 615). The central problem in attributing syncope to arrhythmias is that the vast majority of detected arrhythmias in patients with syncope are brief and result in no symptoms.[49-52] On the other hand, arrhythmias are commonly reported in normal or ambulatory asymptomatic individuals. For example, ambulatory monitoring in asymptomatic individuals has shown sinus bradycardia (<40 beats/min during sleep) in up to 24 per cent of subjects, brief episodes of supraventricular tachycardia in up to 50 per cent of subjects, PACs or PVCs in 50 to 75 per cent, and frequent, multiform, or paired PVCs in up to 15 per cent of subjects. Some electrocardiographic abnormalities, however, are rarely reported in asymptomatic individuals. These include sinus pauses >2 sec (occurring in approximately 2 per cent of subjects) and brief runs of unsustained ventricular tachycardia (mostly less than 5 beat runs) in up to 4 per cent of asymptomatic persons. Mobitz II and complete AV block are even more rare.

One method of assessing the impact of ambulatory monitoring in syncope is to determine the presence or absence of arrhythmias in patients who develop symptoms during monitoring. Table 30–4 shows the incidence of symptomatic arrhythmias in studies on monitoring that met the following criteria: the patient population included those with syncope or presyncope; data on the presence or absence of symptoms during monitoring were reported; and monitoring duration was ≥12 hours.[47,51,53-56] Only 4 per cent of patients had symptomatic correlation of symptoms with an arrhythmia. In approximately 17 per cent of patients, arrhythmias were not associated with symptoms, thus potentially excluding rhythm disturbance as an etiology for the syncope. In approximately 80 per cent of patients, no symptoms induced by arrhythmias were found. The causal relation between these arrhythmias and syncope therefore is uncertain.

Extending the duration of monitoring to longer than 24 hours does not seem to resolve the problem of interpretation of abnormalities on monitoring. Experience with patients undergoing three 24-hour periods of Holter monitoring showed arrhythmias by specific criteria in 14.7 per cent during the first day, an additional 11.1 per cent the second day, and an additional 4.2 per cent the third day.[51] However, only one of 95 patients had arrhythmias associated with symptoms, and these occurred during the first 24 hours. Thus, there was no increased yield of symptom-producing arrhythmias when monitoring was extended beyond 24 hours.

Correlating arrhythmias detected on monitoring with mortality and sudden death in follow-up also does not help clarify the role of these arrhythmias in syncope. Frequent or repetitive ventricular ectopy in patients with syncope is an independent predictor of mortality and sudden death (3.7 fold increased risk of death and 14.9 fold increased risk of sudden death).[49] Sinus pauses were also associated with a 3.3 fold increased risk of death in patients with syncope,[49] although other studies have shown no increase in mortality in patients with sick sinus syndrome. The increased mortality is probably a manifestation of underlying heart disease, and inferences regarding the cause of syncope are difficult to draw from such outcome data.

Patient-activated transtelephonic electrocardiographic recording without a memory loop[57-59] is generally more useful for the evaluation of dizziness, presyncope, chest pain, and pacemaker failure, and in patients with a prolonged prodrome to their loss of consciousness, an unusual situation for most patients with arrhythmic syncope. Patient-activated intermittent loop recorders are more likely to capture the rhythm during syncope after the patient has regained consciousness, since several minutes of retrograde electrocardiographic recording can be obtained. In a study of 39 patients with a history of frequent syncope or presyncope, 35 per cent had symptoms during monitoring (mean duration of monitoring 28 days, range 3 to 140 days). During these symptoms, only three patients had arrhythmias while 11 had "normal" cardiac rhythm.[59] This type of device is more likely to capture an event in patients who have relatively frequent symptoms (at least one per month). A study of syncope recurrence has shown that only 5 per cent have recurrent fainting at one month, 11 per cent by 3 months, and 16 per cent by 6 months.[60] Thus, loop monitoring is likely to be useful for capturing a symptomatic period in a very small subset of patients with a negative initial work-up.

TABLE 30–4 PROLONGED ELECTROCARDIOGRAPHIC MONITORING IN SYNCOPE

STUDY	NO. OF PATIENTS	PRESENTING SYMPTOM	SYMPTOMS DURING MONITORING		NO SYMPTOMS DURING MONITORING	
			Arrhythmia	No Arrhythmia	Arrhythmia	No Arrhythmia
			%			
Jonas[53]	358*	Dizziness or syncope	4	—	16	80
Boudoulas[48]	119	Dizziness or syncope	26	13	27	34
Clark[54]	98	Dizziness or syncope	3	39	41	17
Zeldis[55]	74†	Syncope or near syncope	14	24	—	—
Kala[56]	107	Dizziness or syncope	7	7	16	69
Gibson[50]	1512	Dizziness or presyncope	2	15	10	79
Bass[51]‡	95	Syncope	1	20	26	53
Kapoor[47]§	249	Syncope	6	22	17	55
TOTAL‖ (Pooled)	2612		4	17	13	69

From Kapoor, W. N.: Diagnostic evaluation of syncope. Am. J. Med. *90*:91, 1991.
* 12 hours (in 102 patients) or 24 hours (in 256 patients) of monitoring.
† Total study included 371 with several symptoms (chest pain, palpitations, dizziness and syncope). Only patients with syncope or near syncope are included here.
‡ Prospective study of 72 hours of monitoring.
§ Includes 39 (11%) patients who underwent telemetry only.
‖ Total does not add up to 100% because of missing information from two studies.

ELECTROPHYSIOLOGICAL STUDIES. The indications for electrophysiological studies in patients with syncope have not been systematically defined, but they are more likely to be "positive" in patients with known heart disease who have abnormal ventricular function, electrocardiogram, or ambulatory monitoring.[61-67] These tests are also more likely to be positive in patients with bundle branch block, helping to identify isolated conduction disease or ventricular tachyarrhythmias.[68,69] Predictors of a *negative* electrophysiological study in patients with syncope include the absence of heart disease, an ejection fraction >40 per cent, normal 12-lead electrocardiogram and 24-hour ambulatory (Holter) electrocardiogram, absence of injury during syncope, and multiple or prolonged (>5 min) episodes of syncope.[65]

In studies of patients with syncope undergoing electrophysiological testing, the proportion with positive findings has ranged between 18 and 75 per cent (mean of 60 per cent).[61] Approximately 35 per cent (range 0 to 80) had inducible ventricular tachycardia, 20 per cent (0 to 60) supraventricular tachycardia, 35 per cent (range 11 to 60) conduction disturbance (abnormal sinus node, atrioventricular node, or His-Purkinje function), and 10 per cent (range 0 to 24) other abnormalities (including hypervagotonia and carotid hypersensitivity). Studies of special groups such as the elderly,[70] those with bundle branch block,[68,69] carotid sinus hypersensitivity,[71,72] excess vagal tone,[73] and electrophysiological studies with upright tilt have also been reported.[74] Several issues need to be considered in using electrophysiological studies in the evaluation of syncope:[61]

1. In most instances, arrhythmias during electrophysiological evaluation do not produce syncope in the laboratory. Thus, a causal relationship often has to be inferred.

2. The clinical significance of some of the electrophysiological abnormalities may be difficult to determine. The sensitivity and specificity of abnormal electrophysiologic findings will be reviewed briefly to develop a perspective on the use of these tests for the management of syncope.

The finding of prolonged sinus node recovery time (p. 617) has a relatively low sensitivity for diagnosis of sinus node dysfunction (18 to 69 per cent), although it is reported to have high specificity (88 to 100 per cent)[75,76] when electrophysiological results are compared with ambulatory monitoring. The performance of other tests of sinus node function (e.g., sinoatrial conduction time) is also controversial.[66,67] Tests for atrioventricular nodal conduction and refractoriness are also difficult to interpret and vary considerably with autonomic tone. A prolonged H-V interval and block between H and V with atrial pacing is a marker of significant conduction system disease that may have resulted in bradyarrhythmias and syncope; however, cutpoints for the length of H-V interval have varied widely when attributing syncope to conduction system disease. (Criteria have ranged from >55 msec to >100 msec.) However, the finding of an H-V interval >100 msec is quite uncommon in patients with syncope. Supraventricular tachycardia and atrial fibrillation or flutter may occasionally be initiated during electrophysiological studies, especially if aggressive induction procedures are used. The significance of these induced arrhythmias is uncertain unless they reproduce the patient's spontaneous symptoms.[66,67]

Patients with structural heart disease have higher rates of inducible ventricular tachycardia as compared with those without cardiac disease (approximately 55 to 70 per cent vs. <20 per cent). The finding of *sustained monomorphic* ventricular tachycardia has a high sensitivity and specificity for the presence of spontaneous ventricular tachycardia. However, induction of *polymorphic* or nonsustained ventricular tachycardia may frequently represent a nonspecific response to an aggressive ventricular stimulation protocol.[66,67]

In *summary*, the following electrophysiological findings are potentially important in attributing syncope to arrhythmias: sustained monomorphic ventricular tachycardia, sinus node recovery time ≥3.0 sec, and pacing-induced infranodal block; H-V interval >100 msec; and paroxysmal supraventricular tachycardia, which produces symptoms similar to spontaneous syncope.

3. The proportion of patients with positive findings has varied in reports of electrophysiological testing in syncope for the following reasons: first, the cases of patients studied have not been clinically uniform. Some studies have included only patients with recurrent syncope, while in others those with one episode or with presyncope only were evaluated. Furthermore, most studies have included patients with a wide variety of underlying heart conditions and some have reported on patients without clinical heart disease. Second, the extent of noninvasive evaluation before electrophysiological tests has varied and probably has affected the yield of these studies, since more thorough noninvasive evaluation may identify some of the arrhythmias found on electrophysiological studies. Finally, the protocol and criteria for abnormal results have differed in various laboratories. The variations have included performing left ventricular (in addition to right ventricular) stimulation, the use of isoproterenol, and the number of extrastimuli for induction procedures. The criteria for attributing syncope to abnormalities have also varied, and multiple abnormalities are found in some patients, making it difficult to determine to which of these syncope should be attributed.

4. There are problems in interpreting patient outcome after therapy based on testing. In previous reports on electrophysiological testing in syncope, recurrence on follow-up is used as the treatment endpoint. In patients with normal studies, recurrence rates averaging 35 per cent have been reported, while recurrence rates in those with abnormal testing have averaged 15 per cent.[61] Length of follow-up has ranged from 11 to 36 months. The interpretation of the rate of recurrence is complicated, however, because it may be caused by many different mechanisms: side effects of drugs, noncompliance, inadequate treatment, and the results of an incorrect initial diagnosis. Furthermore, recurrences are sporadic and thus analysis of their rate over time may be difficult.

The incidence of sudden death in patients undergoing electrophysiological testing has received less attention. In one study, the incidence was markedly higher in patients having positive studies than in those with negative studies (48 per cent vs. 9 per cent at 3 years).[62] In other studies a low rate of overall mortality and of sudden death has been noted in patients with negative studies, thus defining a low-risk group of patients with syncope.[77]

What is the current role of electrophysiological studies in syncope? A thorough clinical and noninvasive evaluation using a careful history and physical examination, an electrocardiogram, ambulatory monitoring, and other noninvasive or directed tests should ordinarily be carried out before electrophysiological study is considered. Because of spontaneous resolution of syncope in most patients, a single episode with a negative noninvasive evaluation *may not* justify an invasive work-up. Upright tilt testing and neuropsychiatric evaluation may be utilized before electrophysiological testing in patients with unexplained syncope, especially in those with more than five episodes in the last year who do not have evidence of organic heart disease. In patients with recurrent unexplained syncope and organic heart disease (moderate or marked left ventricular dysfunction and/or severe coronary artery disease, valvular heart disease, or hypertrophic cardiomyopathy), electrophysiological testing may help define potential arrhythmias and select specific therapy.

Upright Tilt Testing

This refers to maintaining the patient in a head-up position for a brief period to provoke syncope, bradycardia, or hypotension. Upright posture is associated with gravitational pooling of blood that results in a decline in central venous pressure, stroke volume, and blood pressure. These effects lead to the activation of arterial and cardiopulmonary baroreceptor reflexes as well as activation of the renin-angiotensin system and the release of vasopressin, which leads to vasoconstriction, tachycardia, and fluid retention. However, in individuals susceptible to vasovagal syncope, intense activation of cardiopulmonary mechanoreceptors may occur, leading to reversal of these normal compensatory responses, thereby resulting in bradycardia and hypotension. This type of syncope has also been termed *neurally mediated syncope.*

Urinary concentrations of epinephrine and norepinephrine in patients before vasovagal syncope have been reported to be higher than those in control subjects, and circulating catecholamine levels measured immediately before the syncopal episode have also occasionally been reported to be higher.[78] These findings suggest that enhanced adrenergic activity may play a role in vasovagal syncope. It has been postulated that catecholamine release could paradoxically enhance susceptibility to bradycardia and hypotension resulting in syncope by activation of cardiac mechanoreceptors. These considerations have led to the use of the intravenous infusion of catecholamines (such as isoproterenol) to induce syncope. Since upright posture is also a provocative stimulus for vasovagal syncope, use of upright tilt testing in conjunction with isoproterenol may result in higher rates of provocation of vasovagal syncope. Upright tilt testing has been used primarily to investigate patients with syncope of unknown cause after electrophysiological testing. In patients with negative electrophysiological studies, rates of provocation of hypotension on upright tilt testing (without isoproterenol) of 27 to 67 per cent are reported as compared to approximately 10 per cent in controls (without syncope).[79-84] A study using intravenous infusion of isoproterenol during upright tilt testing showed that 87 per cent of patients who had prior negative electrophysiological testing had a positive test as compared to 11 per cent in patients who had positive electrophysiological testing and 11 per cent in control patients.[82]

Although it is not possible to generalize these results to all patients with syncope of unknown cause, it is likely that a large proportion of patients with unexplained syncope have vasovagal reactions that are difficult to diagnose clinically. Upright tilt testing can suggest the diagnosis in these patients. Effective therapy for this disorder has not been determined, although preliminary studies suggest that beta blockers, disopyramide, anticholinergic agents, and fludrocortisone plus salt may be promising.[85]

Other Cardiovascular Testing

Echocardiogram, stress testing, ventricular function studies, and cardiac catheterization are generally needed for clarification or further evaluation of specific findings on the history and physical examination.[47] These tests are valuable when used in a selective manner to define the type, extent, or severity of cardiac diseases. Similarly, aortography and cerebrovascular flow studies are used in specific situations directed by the clinical presentation. There are no data available to justify the routine use of any of these diagnostic tests.

SIGNAL-AVERAGED ECG. Detection of low amplitude signals (late potentials) (p. 620) has a sensitivity of 73 to 89 per cent and a specificity of 89 to 100 per cent for prediction of inducible sustained ventricular tachycardia in patients with syncope.[86-88] The overall usefulness of this technique in managing patients presenting with syncope is still not totally clear, and further studies will be needed. Some centers have used signal-averaged electrocardiography as a screening test for ventricular tachycardia in selecting patients for electrophysiological studies. However, complete electrophysiological studies are generally needed to evaluate syncope when the decision is made to perform this test, since other abnormalities (e.g., sinus node dysfunction, other conduction system disease, induced supraventricular tachycardia) as well as multiple abnormalities cannot be excluded by this test.

Autonomic Function Studies

Clinical data with a focus on autonomic symptoms, diseases causing orthostatic hypotension, and drugs frequently provide clues to the etiology of orthostatic hypotension, and there is often little need for additional diagnostic testing.[12] Many of the illnesses listed in Table 30–2 are clinically diagnosable,

TABLE 30–5 USEFUL CLINICAL TESTS OF AUTONOMIC FAILURE

A. CARDIOVASCULAR REFLEXES

Tests Performed and Responses

1. Change of posture: BP and pulse rate monitored while subject is supine and then repeated measurements are made at 60° head-up tilt position: test of total baroreflex pathway. Pulse rate and plasma noradrenalin responses to standing. Lower-body negative pressure is an alternative to tilt or standing.
2. Deep breathing: presence or absence of sinus arrhythmia; test of vagal efferent pathway.
3. Carotid massage: right and left sides, in turn monitoring cardiac rate and blood pressure; test of vagal efferent pathway.
4. Hyperventilation: for 30 seconds, causing hypocapnia and fall in blood pressure; response suggests afferent lesion, if baroreflex block.
5. Inspiratory gasp: causing reflex vasoconstriction of hands; spinal cord reflex.
6. Stress: causing hypertension and tachycardia; tests of sympathetic efferent pathway.
   (a) Handgrip, submaximal sustained for 90 sec.
   (b) Sudden cortical arousal by unexpected noise.
   (c) Mental arithmetic (rapid serial subtraction of 7 from 100).
   (d) Cold pressor test–hand immersed in water at 4°C for 90 sec.
7. Breath holding: Test of central breathing control; prolonged if vagal afferent dysfunction.
8. Valsalva maneuver: After a deep inspiration the patient performs a forced expiration for 12 sec through a tube connected to a mercury manometer. Most subjects can maintain a pressure of 30 mm Hg. In normal subjects there is an increased tachycardia for the 10 sec of sustained forced expiration. Blood pressure falls initially but should cease to fall after the first few seconds if peripheral sympathetic vasoconstriction is normal. On release from blowing there is normally a BP overshoot and a compensatory reflex bradycardia.
9. Pharmacological and biochemical tests:
   (a) Plasma noradrenalin at rest and after 5 to 10 minutes standing or tilt.
   (b) Pressor response and cardiac slowing to infusion of noradrenalin; test of baroreflex sensitivity.
   (c) Pressor response and noradrenalin response to infusion of tyramine; test of cytoplasmic stores of noradrenalin.
   (d) Cardiac rate response to isoprenaline infusion; test of β-receptor cardiac function.
   (e) Cardiac response to atropine; test of vagal function.

B. SWEATING

1. Response to body heating in order to cause a rise of 1°C oral or rectal temperature in the course of 90 min. Record sweating and measure hand blood flow. Test of sympathetic pathway from hypothalamus to periphery.
2. Response to brief trunk heating with electric lamp source for 90 sec; a reflex response, without involving change of blood temperature, utilizing same efferent pathway as response to body heating.
3. Responses to intramuscular pilocarpine; acts directly on sweat glands.
4. Pilomotor and sudomotor response to intradermal methacholine; absent with complete postganglionic lesion.

C. PUPILLARY RESPONSES

1. Instillation of 1:1000 adrenalin. Response: dilatation after sympathetic postganglionic denervation; no effect on normal pupil.
2. Instillation of 4% cocaine. Response: dilatation of normal pupil; no effect after sympathetic denervation.
3. Instillation of fresh 2.5% methacholine. Response: constriction after parasympathetic denervation; no effect on normal pupil.

Adapted from Bannister, S. R. (ed.): Autonomic Failure. 2nd ed. Oxford, Oxford University Press, 1988, pp. 291–292.

and management decisions can be readily carried out. Specific tests of autonomic function are occasionally used when no clear reason for orthostasis is apparent to define further the cause of neurological diseases responsible for postural hypotension.[89] Table 30–5 lists some examples of the tests available for this purpose.[89]

ELECTROENCEPHALOGRAPHY AND BRAIN CT SCAN. EEG and CT scan are occasionally helpful in determining a cause of syncope (Table 30–3). These tests have been useful in evaluating patients who have focal neurological symptoms in association with syncope or when a convulsive disorder is suspected clinically in a patient with syncope.[1,47] Nonselective use of EEG and brain CT scans has not been rewarding.

PROGNOSIS

The one-year mortality of patients with a cardiac cause of syncope is consistently high in all recent studies, ranging between 18 and 33 per cent.[1,42–46,49] These rates have been higher than those in patients with a noncardiac cause (0 to 12 per cent) or in patients with unknown cause (6 per cent). The incidence of sudden death in patients with a cardiac cause was also markedly higher as compared with the other two groups (Fig. 30–1).[49] Even when adjustments for differences in baseline rate of heart and other diseases were made, cardiac syncope was still an independent predictor of mortality and sudden death.

It is not known whether syncope predisposes to increased risk of mortality independent of underlying diseases. In the Framingham study, patients less than 60 years of age experiencing syncope who did not have cardiovascular or neurological diseases had rates of mortality, sudden death, stroke, and myocardial infarction similar to patients without syncope.[90] However, such information is not available in patients with underlying cardiac or noncardiac diseases.

Recurrence of syncope often leads to concerns regarding morbidity and mortality. Recurrence rates of 12 to 15 per cent per year are reported in follow-up, and the rates were not significantly different in patients with cardiac causes as compared with the other groups.[60] In approximately 5 per cent of patients, new causes were assigned on evaluation of recurrent syncope. Although recurrences were associated with fractures and soft tissue injury in 12 per cent of patients, they did not predict an increased risk of mortality or sudden death.[60]

APPROACH TO DIAGNOSTIC EVALUATION

Using the recent studies on the evaluation of syncope discussed above, a diagnostic approach can be suggested (Fig. 30–2). A detailed history and physical examination will identify the vast majority of causes. Furthermore, the history and physical examination may reveal findings suggestive of specific entities as possible causes (e.g., findings of aortic stenosis or neurological signs and symptoms suggestive of a seizure disorder) that may require further noninvasive or invasive tests for establishing a diagnosis and initiating treatment. An electrocardiogram is generally needed for the evaluation of patients with syncope, the cause of which is not evident from the history and physical examination. Although the diagnostic yield is low (e.g., for arrhythmias), abnormalities can be treated quickly if found. Furthermore, patients with a normal electrocardiogram have a low likelihood of arrhythmias as a cause of syncope and are at low risk of sudden death.[65,91,92] Thus, the electrocardiogram can offer both diagnostic and prognostic information which may have an important role in further evaluation and management.

In patients in whom a cause of syncope is not determined by the history and physical examination and initial electrocardiogram, further diagnostic testing can be approached by classifying patients into those with and without heart disease. If the presence or absence of heart disease cannot be determined clinically, specific tests such as echocardiogram, stress test, and ventricular function studies may be needed. In patients with coronary artery disease, congestive heart failure, valvular heart disease, hypertrophic cardiomyopathy, and bundle branch block or bifascicular block, prolonged electrocardiographic monitoring forms the first step in evaluation. If prolonged monitoring is not diagnostic, these patients may be candidates for electrophysiological studies because these tests are more likely to be positive in patients with heart disease. The findings of electrophysiological studies can form the basis for potential therapy.

Patients with negative electrophysiological studies have a favorable prognosis; empiric therapy with a pacemaker or antiarrhythmics is not justified. Because a large proportion of patients with negative electrophysiological studies and recurrent unexplained syncope have been reported through upright tilt testing to have neurally mediated syncope, this test may help define a potential cause for syncope in this group of patients. Therapy of this entity can be attempted in patients who have frequent symptoms.

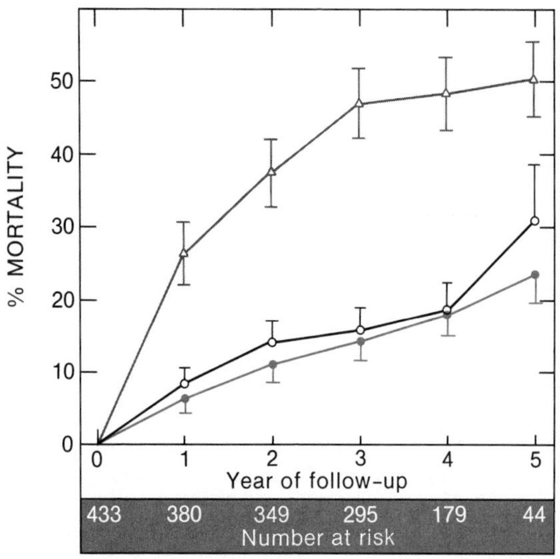

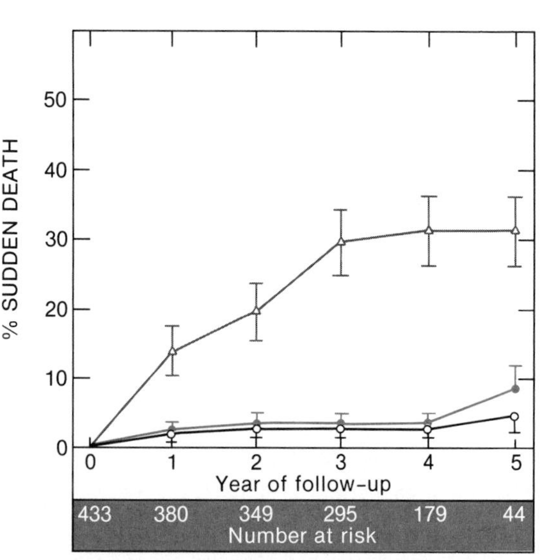

FIGURE 30–1. Actuarial mortality and sudden death incidences of patients with cardiac cause of syncope (triangles), noncardiac cause of syncope (open circles), and syncope of unknown cause (solid circles). The mortality and sudden death of patients with a cardiac cause of syncope were significantly higher than in patients with noncardiac cause ($p < 0.00001$) or patients with syncope of unknown cause ($p < 0.00001$).

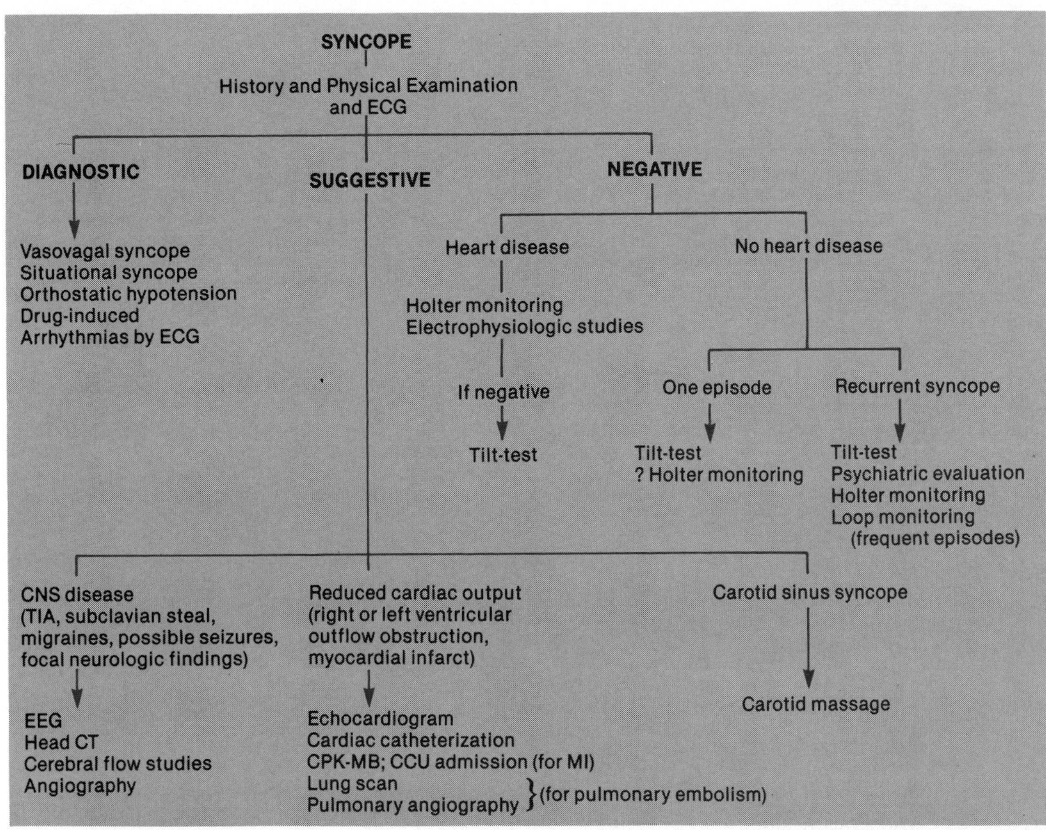

FIGURE 30-2. Flow diagram showing the approach to the evaluation of syncope.

Younger patients (less than 60 years of age) with syncope and without heart disease have an excellent prognosis.[93] Furthermore, in patients with a normal electrocardiogram, the likelihood of arrhythmias is low, and prolonged electrocardiographic monitoring rarely leads to a specific diagnosis.[91,92] Because the yield of electrophysiological studies in patients without heart disease is low, such studies are not justified in most of these patients. A large proportion of these patients (especially those with recurrent syncope) probably have vasovagal syncope or psychiatric disorders that should be investigated. Similar conclusions probably apply to older patients without heart disease, but further studies are needed to define better the role of prolonged electrocardiographic monitoring and other tests in these patients.

Patients with recurrent syncope constitute a difficult management challenge. Patients with multiple episodes are less likely to have arrhythmias[65] and are more likely to have psychiatric illnesses.[23] The extent of initial evaluation of these patients is guided by the presence or absence of heart disease (as already noted). In patients with frequent recurrent syncope in whom there is a high index of suspicion of arrhythmias from the history, patient-activated intermittent electrocardiographic loop recorders are especially attractive if a cause is not established by other means. Using this approach, a cause of syncope can be assigned to more than 60 per cent of patients presenting with this symptom. Patients without a diagnosis have a favorable prognosis regarding mortality and sudden death, but need to be followed closely and reevaluated upon recurrence, since a potential cause may become apparent in a small proportion of patients after repeated episodes.

REFERENCES

1. Day, S. C., Cook, E. F., Funkenstein, H., and Goldman, L.: Evaluation and outcome of emergency room patients with transient loss of consciousness. Am. J. Med. *73*:15, 1982.
2. Lipsitz, L. A., Pluchino, F. C., Wei, J. Y., and Rowe, J. W.: Syncope in institutionalized elderly: The impact of multiple pathological conditions and situational stress. J. Chron. Dis. *39*:619, 1986.
3. Syncope. *In* Fowler, N. O.: Diagnosis of Heart Disease. New York, Springer-Verlag, 1991, pp. 400–409.
4. Engel, G. L.: Psychologic stress, vasodepressor (vasovagal) syncope, and sudden death. Ann. Intern. Med. *89*:403, 1978.
5. Schraeder, P. L., Pontzer, R., and Engel, T. R.: A case of being scared to death. Arch. Intern. Med. *143*:1793, 1983.
6. Kapoor, W. N., Peterson, J. R., and Karpf, M.: Micturition syncope. J.A.M.A. *253*:796, 1985.
7. Kapoor, W., Peterson, J., and Karpf, M.: Defecation syncope. A symptom with multiple etiologies. Arch. Intern. Med. *146*:2377, 1986.
8. Kollef, M. H., and Schachter, D. T.: Defecation syncope caused by pulmonary embolism (Letter). Ann. Intern. Med. *113*:86, 1990.
9. Levin, B., and Posner, J. B.: Swallow syncope. Report of a case and review of the literature. Neurology *22*:1086, 1972.
10. Kunis, R. L., Garfein, O. B., Pepe, A. J., et al.: Deglutition syncope and atrioventricular block selectively induced by hot food and liquid. Am. J. Cardiol. *55*:613, 1985.
11. Kadish, A. H., Wesler, L., and Marchlinski, F. E.: Swallowing syncope: Observations in the absence of conduction system or esophageal disease. Am. J. Med. *81*:1098, 1986.
12. Lipsitz, L.: Orthostatic hypotension in the elderly. N. Engl. J. Med. *321*:952, 1989.
13. Atkins, D., Sefcik, T., and Kapoor, W.: Orthostatic hypotension and syncope. Clin. Res. *38*:701A, 1990.
14. Bannister, S. R. (ed.): Autonomic Failure: A Textbook of Clinical Disorders of the Autonomic Nervous System. 2nd ed. Oxford Medical Publishers, 1988, pp. 1–20.
15. Ausman, J. I., Shrontz, C. E., Pearce, J. E., et al.: Veterbrovasilar insufficiency. A review. Arch. Neurol. *42*:803, 1985.
16. Fields, W. S., and Lemak, N. A.: Joint study of extracranial arterial occlusion. VII. Subclavian steal—a review of 168 cases. JAMA *222*:1139, 1972.
17. Sacquegna, T., Cortelli, P., Baldrati, A., et al.: Impairment of consciousness and memory in migraine: A review. Headache *27*:30, 1987.
18. Strasberg, B., Sagie, A., Erdman, S., et al.: Carotid sinus hypersensitivity and the carotid sinus syndrome. Prog. Cardiovasc. Dis. *5*:379, 1989.
19. Ross, R. T.: Syncope. Philadelphia, W. B. Saunders Company, 1988, pp. 113–117.
20. St. John, J. N.: Glossopharyngeal neuralgia associated with syncope and seizures. Neurosurgery *10*:380, 1982.
21. Kapoor, W. N., and Jannetta, P. J.: Trigeminal neuralgia associated with seizure and syncope. J. Neurosurg. *61*:594, 1984.
22. Jacome, D. E.: Temporal lobe syncope: Clinical variants. Clin. Electroencephal. *20*:58, 1989.
23. Kapoor, W., Fortunato, M., Sefcik, T., and Schulberg, H.: Psychiatric illnesses in patients with syncope (Abstract). Clin. Res. *37*(2):316A, 1989.
24. Katon, W.: Panic disorder and somatization. Review of 55 cases. Am. J. Med. *77*:101, 1984.
25. Cregler, L. L., and Mark, H.: Cardiovascular dangers of cocaine abuse. Am. J. Cardiol. *57*:1185, 1986.
26. Lowenstein, D. H., Massa, S. M., Rowbotham, M. C., et al.: Acute neurologic and psychiatric complications associated with cocaine abuse. Am. J. Med. *83*:841, 1987.

27. Johnson, R. H.: Autonomic failure in alcoholics. *In* Bannister, R. (ed.): Autonomic Failure. A Textbook of Clinical Disorders of the Autonomic Nervous System. 2nd ed. Oxford Medical Publishers, 1988, pp. 690–714.
28. Linzer, M., Felder, A., Hackel, A., et al.: Psychiatric syncope. Psychosom. Med. *31*:181, 1990.
29. Grech, E. D., and Ramsdale, D. R.: Exertional syncope in aortic stenosis. Am. Heart J. *121*:603, 1991.
30. Kowey, P. R., Eisenberg, R., and Engel, T. R.: Sustained arrhythmias in hypertrophic obstructive cardiomyopathy. N. Engl. J. Med. *310*:1566, 1984.
31. Fananapazir, L., Tracy, C. M., Leon, M. B., et al.: Electrophysiologic abnormalities in patients with hypertrophic cardiomyopathy. Circulation *80*:1259, 1989.
32. Markel, M. L., Waller, B. F., and Armstrong, W. F.: Cardiac myxoma. A review. Medicine *66*:114, 1987.
33. Igarashi, Y., Yamazoe, M., Suzuki, K., et al.: A possible role of coronary artery spasm in unexplained syncope. Am. J. Cardiol. *65*:713, 1990.
34. DeSanctis, R. W., Doroghazi, R. M., Austen, W. G., and Buckley, M. J.: Aortic dissection. N. Engl. J. Med. *317*:1060, 1987.
35. Kapoor, W.: Syncope with abrupt termination of exercise. Am. J. Med. *67*:597, 1989.
36. Hirata, T., Yano, K., Okui, T., et al.: Asystole with syncope following strenuous exercise in a man without organic heart disease. J. Electrocardiol. *20*:280, 1987.
37. Rosenqvist, M., Vallin, H., Edhag, O.: Clinical and electrophysiological course of sinus node disease: Five-year follow-up study. Am. Heart J. *109*:513, 1985.
38. Jackman, W. M., Friday, K. J., Anderson, J. L., et al.: The long QT syndromes: A critical review, new clinical observations and a unifying hypothesis. Prog. Cardiovasc. Dis. *31*:115, 1988.
39. Laakso, M., Aberg, A., Savola, J., et al.: Diseases and drugs causing prolongation of the QT interval. Am. J. Cardiol. *59*:862, 1987.
40. Bigger, J. T., Jr., and Sahar, D. I.: Clinical types of proarrhythmic response to antiarrhythmic drugs. Am. J. Cardiol. *59*:2E, 1987.
41. Paul, T., Guccione, P., and Garson, A.: Relation of syncope in young patients with Wolff-Parkinson-White syndrome to rapid ventricular response during atrial fibrillation. Am. J. Cardiol. *65*:318, 1990.

DIAGNOSTIC EVALUATION

42. Kapoor, W., Karpf, M., Maher, Y., et al.: Syncope of unknown origin: The need for a more cost-effective approach to its diagnostic evaluation. J.A.M.A. *247*:2687, 1982.
43. Kapoor, W., Karpf, M., Wieand, S., et al.: A prospective evaluation and follow-up of patients with syncope. N. Engl. J. Med. *309*:197, 1983.
44. Eagle, K. A., and Black, H. R.: The impact of diagnostic tests in evaluating patients with syncope. Yale J. Biol. Med. *56*:1, 1983.
45. Silverstein, M. D., Singer, D. E., Mulley, A., et al.: Patients with syncope admitted to medical intensive care units. JAMA *248*:1185, 1982.
46. Martin, G. J., Adams, S. L., Martin, H. G., et al.: Prospective evaluation of syncope. Ann. Emerg. Med. *13*:499, 1984.
47. Kapoor, W.: Evaluation and outcome of patients with syncope. Medicine *69*:160, 1990.
48. Boudoulas, H., Schaael, S. F., Lewis, R. P., and Robinson, J. L.: Superiority of 24-hour outpatient monitoring over multi-stage exercise testing for the evaluation of syncope. J. Electrocardiol. *12*:103, 1979.
49. Kapoor, W., Cha, R., Peterson, J., et al.: Prolonged electrocardiographic monitoring in patients with syncope: The importance of frequent or repetitive ventricular ectopy. Am. J. Med. *82*:20, 1987.
50. Gibson, T. C., and Heitzman, M. R.: Diagnostic efficacy of 24-hour electrocardiographic monitoring for syncope. Am. J. Cardiol. *53*:1013, 1984.
51. Bass, E. B., Curtiss, E. I., Arena, V. C., et al.: The duration of Holter monitoring in patients with syncope: Is 24 hours enough? Arch. Intern. Med. *150*:1073, 1990.
52. DiMarco, J. P., and Philbrick, J. T.: Use of ambulatory electrocardiographic (Holter) monitoring. Ann. Intern. Med. *113*:53, 1990.
53. Moazez, F., Peter, T., Simonson, J., et al.: Syncope of unknown origin. Am. Heart J. *121*:81, 1991.
54. Clark, P. I., Glasser, S. P., and Spoto, E.: Arrhythmias detected by ambulatory monitoring: Lack of correlation with symptoms of dizziness and syncope. Chest *77*:722, 1980.
55. Zeldis, S. M., Levine, B. J., Michelson, E. L., and Morganroth, J.: Cardiovascular complaints: Correlation with cardiac arrhythmias on 24-hour electrocardiographic monitoring. Chest *78*:456, 1980.
56. Kala, R., Viitasalo, M. T., Tiovenon, L., and Eisalo, A.: Ambulatory ECG recording in patients referred because of syncope or dizziness. Acta Med. Scand. *668*(Suppl):13, 1982.
57. Linzer, M., Prystowsky, E. N., Brunetti, L. L., et al.: Recurrent syncope of unknown origin diagnosed by ambulatory continuous loop ECG recording. Am. Heart. J. *6*:1632, 1988.
58. Brown, A. P., Dawkins, K. D., and Davies, J. G.: Detection of arrhythmias: Use of a patient-activated ambulatory electrocardiogram device with a solid-state memory loop. Br. Heart J. *58*:251, 1987.
59. Cumbee, S. R., Pryor, R. E., and Linzer, M.: Cardiac loop ECG recording: A new noninvasive diagnostic test in recurrent syncope. South. Med. J. *83*:39, 1990.
60. Kapoor, W., Peterson, J., Wieand, H. S., and Karpf, M.: Diagnostic and prognostic implications of recurrences in patients with syncope. Am. J. Med. *83*:700, 1987.
61. Kapoor, W. N., Hammill, S. C., and Gersh, B. J.: Diagnosis and natural history of syncope and the role of invasive electrophysiologic testing. Am. J. Cardiol. *63*:730, 1989.
62. Bass, E. B., Elson, J. J., Fogoros, R. N., et al.: Long-term prognosis of patients undergoing electrophysiologic studies for syncope of unknown origin. Am. J. Cardiol. *62*:1186, 1988.
63. Olshansky, B., Mazuz, M., and Martins, J. B.: Significance of inducible tachycardia in patients with syncope of unknown origin: A long-term follow-up. Am. J. Cardiol. *5*:216, 1985.
64. Doherty, J. U., Pembrook-Rogers, D., Grogan, E. W., et al.: Electrophysiologic evaluation and follow-up characteristics of patients with recurrent unexplained syncope and presyncope. Am. J. Cardiol. *55*:703, 1985.
65. Krol, R. B., Morady, F., Flaker, G. C., et al.: Electrophysiologic testing in patients with unexplained syncope: Clinical and noninvasive predictors of outcome. J. Am. Coll. Cardiol. *10*:358, 1987.
66. DiMarco, J. P.: Electrophysiologic studies in patients with unexplained syncope. Circulation *75*(Suppl III):140, 1987.
67. McAnulty, J. H.: Syncope of unknown origin: The role of electrophysiologic studies. Circulation *75*(Suppl III):144, 1987.
68. Twidale, N., Heddle, W. G., Ayres, B. F., et al.: Clinical implications of electrophysiology study findings in patients with chronic bifascicular block and syncope. Aust. N. Z. J. Med. *18*:841, 1988.
69. Click, R. L., Gersh, B. J., Sugrue, D. D., et al.: Role of invasive electrophysiologic testing in patients with symptomatic bundle branch block. Am. J. Cardiol. *59*:817, 1987.
70. Sugrue, D. D., Holmes, D. R., Gersh, B. J., et al.: Impact of intracardiac electrophysiologic testing on the management of elderly patients with recurrent syncope or near syncope. J. Am. Geriatr. Soc. *35*:1079, 1987.
71. Sugrue, D. D., Gersh, B. J., Holmes, D. R., et al.: Symptomatic "isolated" carotid sinus hypersensitivity: Natural history and results of treatment with anticholinergic drugs or pacemaker. J. Am. Coll. Cardiol. *7*:158, 1986.
72. Nelson, S. D., Kou, W. H., DeBuitleir, M., et al.: Value of programmed ventricular stimulation in presumed carotid sinus syndrome. Am. J. Cardiol. *60*:1073, 1987.
73. McLaran, C. J., Gersh, B. J., Osborn, M. J., et al.: Increased vagal tone as an isolated finding in patients undergoing electrophysiologic testing for recurrent syncope: Response to long-term anticholinergic agents. Br. Heart J. *55*:53, 1986.
74. Hammill, S. C., Holmes, D. R., Wood, D. L., et al.: Electrophysiologic testing in the upright position: Improved evaluation of patients with rhythm disturbances using a tilt table. J. Am. Coll. Cardiol. *4*:65, 1984.
75. Crossen, K. J., and Cain, M. E.: Assessment and management of sinus node dysfunction. Mod. Concepts Cardiovasc. Dis. *55*:43, 1986.
76. Fujimura, O., Yee, R., Klein, G. J., et al.: The diagnostic sensitivity of electrophysiologic testing in patients with syncope caused by transient bradycardia. N. Engl. J. Med. *321*:1703, 1989.
77. Kushner, J. A., Kou, W. H., Kadish, A. H., and Morady, F.: Natural history of patients with unexplained syncope and a nondiagnostic electrophysiologic study. J. Am. Coll. Cardiol. *14*:391, 1989.
78. Vingerhoets, A.J.J.M.: Biochemical changes in two subjects succumbing to syncope. Psychosom. Med. *46*:95, 1984.
79. Calkins, H., Kadish, A., Souza, J., et al.: Comparison of responses to isoproterenol and epinephrine during head-up tilt in suspected vasodepressor syncope. Am. J. Cardiol. *67*:207, 1991.
80. Grubb, B. P., Temesy-Armos, P., Hahn, H., and Elliott L.: Utility of upright tilt-table testing in the evaluation and management of syncope of unknown origin. Am. J. Med. *90*:6, 1991.
81. Strasberg, B., Rechavia, E., Sagie, A., et al.: The head-up tilt table test in patients with syncope of unknown origin. Am. Heart J. *118*(5 Pt 1):923, 1989.
82. Almquist, A., Goldenberg, I. F., Milstein, S., et al.: Provocation of bradycardia and hypotension by isoproterenol and upright posture in patients with unexplained syncope. N. Engl. J. Med. *320*:346, 1989.
83. Waxman, M. B., Yao, L., Cameron, D. A., et al.: Isoproterenol induction of vasodepressor-type reaction in vasodepressor-prone patients. Am. J. Cardiol. *63*:58, 1989.
84. Raviele, A., Gasparini, G., DiPede, F., et al.: Usefulness of head-up tilt test in evaluating patients with syncope of unknown origin and negative electrophysiologic study. Am. J. Cardiol. *65*:1322, 1990.
85. Milstein, S., Buetikofer, J., Dunnigan, A., et al.: Usefulness of disopyramide for prevention of upright tilt-induced hypotension-bradycardia. Am. J. Cardiol. *65*:1339, 1990.
86. Kuchar, D. L., Thorburn, C. W., and Sammel, N. L.: Signal-averaged electrocardiogram for evaluation of recurrent syncope. Am. J. Cardiol. *58*:949, 1986.
87. Gang, E. S., Peter, T., Rosenthal, M. E., et al.: Detection of late potentials on the surface electrocardiogram in unexplained syncope. Am. J. Cardiol. *58*:1014, 1986.
88. Winters, S. L., Stewart, D., and Gomes, J. A.: Signal averaging of the surface QRS complex predicts inducibility of ventricular tachycardia in patients with syncope of unknown origin: A prospective study. J. Am. Coll. Cardiol. *10*:775, 1987.
89. Bannister, R.: Testing autonomic reflexes. *In* Bannister, R. (ed.): Autonomic Failure: A textbook of clinical disorders of the autonomic nervous system. 2nd ed. Oxford University Press, 1988, pp. 289–307.
90. Savage, D. D., Corwin, L., McGee, D. L., et al.: Epidemiologic features of isolated syncope: The Framingham Study. Stroke *16*:626, 1985.
91. Kapoor, W., Peterson, J., and Karpf, M.: A rapid identification of low risk patients with syncope. Implications regarding hospitalization and cost (Abstract). Clin. Res. *34*:823A, 1986.
92. Kapoor, W., Peterson, J., and Karpf, M.: The usefulness of initial electrocardiogram in evaluating patients with syncope (Abstract). Clin. Res. *35*:762A, 1987.
93. Kapoor, W., Snustad, D., Peterson, J., et al.: Syncope in the elderly. Am. J. Med. *80*:419, 1980.

PART III

DISEASES OF THE HEART, PERICARDIUM, AORTA, AND PULMONARY VASCULAR BED

31

Congenital Heart Disease in Infancy and Childhood

by WILLIAM F. FRIEDMAN, M.D.

General Considerations

DEFINITION

Congenital cardiovascular disease is defined as an *abnormality in cardiocirculatory structure or function that is present at birth, even if it is discovered much later.* Congenital cardiovascular malformations usually result from altered embryonic development of a normal structure or failure of such a structure to progress beyond an early stage of embryonic or fetal development. The aberrant patterns of flow created by an anatomical defect may, in turn, significantly influence the structural and functional development of the remainder of the circulation. For instance, the presence in utero of mitral atresia may prohibit normal development of the left ventricle, aortic valve, and ascending aorta. Similarly, constriction of the fetal ductus arteriosus may result directly in right ventricular dilatation and tricuspid regurgitation in the fetus and newborn, contribute importantly to the development of pulmonary arterial aneurysms in the presence of ventricular septal defect and absent pulmonic valve, or, further, result in an alteration in the number and caliber of fetal and newborn pulmonary vascular resistance vessels. In this same regard, postnatal events may markedly influence the clinical presentation of a specific "isolated" malformation. The infant with Ebstein's malformation of the tricuspid valve may improve dramatically as the magnitude of tricuspid regurgitation diminishes with normal fall in pulmonary vascular resistance after birth; the infant with hypoplastic left heart syndrome or interrupted aortic arch may not exhibit circulatory collapse, and the baby with pulmonic atresia or severe stenosis may not become cyanotic until normal spontaneous closure of a patent ductus arteriosus occurs. Ductal constriction many days after birth also may be a central factor in some infants in the development of coarctation of the aorta. Still later in life the patient with a ventricular septal defect may experience spontaneous closure of the abnormal communication, or develop right ventricular outflow tract obstruction and/or aortic regurgitation, or pulmonary vascular obstructive disease. These selected examples serve to emphasize that anatomical and physiological changes in the heart and circulation may continue indefinitely from prenatal life in association with any specific congenital cardiocirculatory lesion.

Certain congenital defects are not apparent on gross inspection of the heart or circulation. Examples include the electrophysiological pathways for ventricular preexcitation or interruptions in the cardiac conduction system giving rise to paroxysmal supraventricular tachycardia or congenital complete heart block, respectively. Similarly, abnormalities in the development of myocardial autonomic innervation or in the ultrastructure of myocardial cells may ultimately prove to contribute to asymmetrical septal hypertrophy and left ventricular outflow tract obstruction. These examples make clear that occasional difficulties arise in distinguishing between congenital anomalies that are readily apparent at or shortly after birth and lesions that may have as their basis a subtle or undetectable abnormality that is present at birth.

INCIDENCE. The true incidence of congenital cardiovascular malformations is difficult to determine accurately, partly because of the difficulties in definition discussed above. About 0.8 per cent of live births are complicated by a cardiovascular malformation.[1] This figure does not take into account what may be the two most common cardiac anomalies: the congenital, nonstenotic bicuspid aortic valve[2] and the leaflet abnormality associated with mitral valve prolapse.[3] Moreover, the widely quoted 0.8 per cent incidence figure fails to include small preterm infants, almost all of whom have persistent patent ductus arteriosus. Further, if the calculations were to include stillbirths and abortuses, the incidence would be greatly increased. Cardiac malformations occur 10 times more often in stillborn than in liveborn babies, and many early spontaneous abortions are associated with chromosomal defects (see Chap. 51).[1] Thus, it is clear that past statistical analyses have seriously *underestimated* the incidence of congenital heart disease.

Precise data concerning frequency of individual congenital lesions also are lacking, and the results of many analyses differ, depending on the source (living or dead) and the selection of the study population. Table 31–1 is a compilation from both clinical and pathological studies that approximates the frequency of occurrence of specific cardiovascular malformations.[4,5]

Taken *in toto*, children with congenital heart disease are predominantly male. Moreover, specific defects may show a definite sex preponderance; patent ductus arteriosus and atrial septal defect are more common in *females*, whereas valvular aortic stenosis, congenital aneurysm of the sinus of Valsalva, coarctation of the aorta, tetralogy of Fallot, and transposition of the great arteries are more common in *males*.

Extracardiac anomalies occur in about 25 per cent of infants with significant cardiac disease,[6] and their presence may significantly increase mortality. The extracardiac anomalies often are multiple, in part involving the musculoskeletal system; one third of infants with both cardiac and extracardiac anomalies have some established syndrome.

TABLE 31–1 FREQUENCY OF OCCURRENCE OF CARDIAC MALFORMATIONS AT BIRTH

DISEASE	PERCENTAGE
Ventricular septal defect	30.5
Atrial septal defect	9.8
Patent ductus arteriosus	9.7
Pulmonic stenosis	6.9
Coarctation of the aorta	6.8
Aortic stenosis	6.1
Tetralogy of Fallot	5.8
Complete transposition of the great arteries	4.2
Persistent truncus arteriosus	2.2
Tricuspid atresia	1.3
All others	16.5

Data based on 2310 cases.

ETIOLOGY

Malformations appear to result from an interaction between multifactorial genetic and environmental systems too complex to allow a single specification of cause;[7,7a] in most instances, a causal factor cannot be identified. Maternal rubella, ingestion of thalidomide early during gestation, and chronic maternal alcohol abuse are environmental insults known to interfere with normal cardiogenesis in humans.[8–10] *Rubella syndrome* consists of cataracts, deafness, microcephaly, and, either singly or in combination, patent ductus arteriosus, pulmonic valvular and/or arterial stenosis, and atrial septal defect. *Thalidomide* exposure is associated with major limb deformities and, occasionally, with cardiac malformations without predilection for a specific lesion. Tricuspid valve anomalies are associated with the ingestion of *lithium* during pregnancy. The *fetal alcohol syndrome* consists of microcephaly, micrognathia, microphthalmia, prenatal growth retardation, developmental delay, and cardiac defects. The latter—often defects of the ventricular septum—occur in about 45 per cent of affected infants. *Maternal lupus erythematosus* during pregnancy has been linked to congenital complete heart block (p. 714). Animal experiments have incriminated hypoxia, deficiency or excess of several vitamins, intake of several categories of drugs, and ionizing irradiation as teratogens capable of causing cardiac malformations. The precise relation of these animal teratogens to human malformations is not clear.

The genetic aspects of congenital heart disease are discussed extensively in Chap. 51. A single gene mutation may be causative in the familial forms of atrial septal defect with prolonged AV conduction, mitral valve prolapse, ventricular septal defect, congenital heart block, situs inversus, pulmonary hypertension, the combination of supravalvular aortic stenosis and peripheral pulmonary arterial stenosis, and the syndromes of Noonan, LEOPARD, Holt-Oram, Ellis–van Creveld, and Kartagener. Table 31–2 provides a partial list of syndromes in which cardiovascular anomalies may be manifestations of the pleiotropic effects of single genes or examples of gross chromosomal defects.[10a] Less than 10 per cent of all cardiac malformations can be accounted for by chromosomal aberrations or genetic mutations or transmission.

The finding that, with some exceptions, only one of a pair of monozygotic twins is affected by congenital heart disease indicates that the vast majority of cardiovascular malformations are not inherited in a simple manner.[11] Family studies indicate a twofold to tenfold increase in the incidence of congenital heart disease in siblings of affected patients or in the offspring of an affected parent. Malformations often are concordant or partially concordant within families.[12] Because the incidence of congenital heart disease in the offspring or siblings of an index patient is only 2 to 10 per cent, it is seldom wise to discourage the parents of one affected child from having additional children if either parent is free of a cardiovascular anomaly.[1] Moreover, the low recurrence rate and the increasing possibilities for effective treatment for nearly all cardiac lesions usually justify a positive approach to family counseling. When two or more members of the family are affected, the recurrence risk may be quite high, and a pedigree should be obtained before further counseling. If a dominant or recessive mendelian pattern is established, the mendelian laws apply, and the risk of recurrence in each pregnancy is equal.

TABLE 31-2 SYNDROMES WITH ASSOCIATED CARDIOVASCULAR INVOLVEMENT

SYNDROME	MAJOR CARDIOVASCULAR MANIFESTATIONS	MAJOR NONCARDIAC ABNORMALITIES
	Heritable and Possibly Heritable	
Ellis-van Creveld	Single atrium or atrial septal defect	Chondrodystrophic dwarfism, nail dysplasia, polydactyly
TAR (thrombocytopenia-absent radius)	Atrial septal defect, tetralogy of Fallot	Radial aplasia or hypoplasia, thrombocytopenia
Holt-Oram	Atrial septal defect (other defects common)	Skeletal upper limb defect, hypoplasia of clavicles
Kartagener	Dextrocardia	Situs inversus, sinusitis, bronchiectasis
Laurence-Moon-Biedl-Bardet	Variable defects	Retinal pigmentation, obesity, polydactyly
Noonan	Pulmonic valve dysplasia, cardiomyopathy (usually hypertrophic)	Webbed neck, pectus excavatum, cryptorchidism
Tuberous sclerosis	Rhabdomyoma, cardiomyopathy	Phakomatosis, bone lesions, hamartomatous skin lesions
Multiple lentigines (LEOPARD)	Pulmonic stenosis	Basal cell nevi, broad facies, rib anomalies
Rubinstein-Taybi	Patent ductus arteriosus (others)	Broad thumbs and toes, hypoplastic maxilla, slanted palpebral fissures
Familial deafness	Arrhythmias, sudden death	Sensorineural deafness
Weber-Osler-Rendu	Arteriovenous fistulas (lung, liver, mucous membranes)	Multiple telangiectasias
Apert	Ventricular septal defect	Craniosynostosis, midfacial hypoplasia, syndactyly
Incontinentia pigmenti	Patent ductus arteriosus	Irregular pigmented skin lesions, patchy alopecia, hypodontia
Alagille (arteriohepatic dysplasia)	Peripheral pulmonic stenosis, pulmonic stenosis	Biliary hypoplasia, vertebral anomalies, prominent forehead, deep-set eyes
DiGeorge	Interrupted aortic arch, tetralogy of Fallot, truncus arteriosus	Thymic hypoplasia or aplasia, parathyroid aplasia or hypoplasia, ear anomalies
Friedreich's ataxia	Cardiomyopathy and conduction defects	Ataxia, speech defect, degeneration of spinal cord dorsal columns
Muscular dystrophy	Cardiomyopathy	Pseudohypertrophy of calf muscles, weakness of trunk and proximal limb muscles
Cystic fibrosis	Cor pulmonale	Pancreatic insufficiency, malabsorption, chronic lung disease
Sickle cell anemia	Cardiomyopathy, mitral regurgitation	Hemoglobin SS
Conradi-Hünermann	Ventricular septal defect, patent ductus arteriosus	Asymmetrical limb shortness, early punctate mineralization, large skin pores
Cockayne	Accelerated atherosclerosis	Cachectic dwarfism, retinal pigment abnormalities, photosensitivity dermatitis
Progeria	Accelerated atherosclerosis	Premature aging, alopecia, atrophy of subcutaneous fat, skeletal hypoplasia
	Connective Tissue Disorders	
Cutis laxa	Peripheral pulmonic stenosis	Generalized disruption of elastic fibers, diminished skin resilience, hernias
Ehlers-Danlos	Arterial dilatation and rupture, mitral regurgitation	Hyperextensible joints, hyperelastic and friable skin
Marfan	Aortic dilatation, aortic and mitral incompetence	Gracile habitus, arachnodactyly with hyperextensibility, lens subluxation
Osteogenesis imperfecta	Aortic incompetence	Fragile bones, blue sclerae
Pseudoxanthoma elasticum	Peripheral and coronary arterial disease	Degeneration of elastic fibers in skin, retinal angioid streaks
	Inborn Errors of Metabolism	
Pompe disease	Glycogen storage disease of heart	Acid maltase deficiency, muscular weakness
Homocystinuria	Aortic and pulmonary artery dilatation, intravascular thrombosis	Cystathionine synthetase deficiency, lens subluxation, osteoporosis
Mucopolysaccharidoses: Hurler; Hunter	Multivalvular and coronary and great artery disease, cardiomyopathy	Hurler: Deficiency of α-L-iduronidase, corneal clouding, coarse features, growth and mental retardation Hunter: Deficiency of L-idurano-sulfate sulfatase, coarse facies, clear cornea, growth and mental retardation

Table continued on following page

TABLE 31–2 SYNDROMES WITH ASSOCIATED CARDIOVASCULAR INVOLVEMENT *Continued*

SYNDROME	MAJOR CARDIOVASCULAR MANIFESTATIONS	MAJOR NONCARDIAC ABNORMALITIES
Morquio; Scheie; Maroteaux-Lamy	Aortic regurgitation	Morquio: Deficiency of *N*-acetylhexosamine sulfate sulfatase, cloudy cornea, severe bone changes involving vertebrae and epiphyses Scheie: Deficiency of α-L-iduronidase, cloudy cornea, normal intelligence, peculiar facies Maroteaux-Lamy: Deficiency of arylsulfatase B, cloudy cornea, osseous changes
	Chromosomal Abnormalities	
Trisomy 21 (Down syndrome)	Endocardial cushion defect, atrial or ventricular septal defect, tetralogy of Fallot	Hypotonia, hyperextensible joints, mongoloid facies, mental retardation
Trisomy 13 (D)	Ventricular septal defect, right ventricle patent ductus arteriosus, double-outlet right ventricle	Single midline intracerebral ventricle with midfacial defects, polydactyly, nail changes, mental retardation
Trisomy 18 (E)	Congenital polyvalvular dysplasia, ventricular septal defect, patent ductus	Clenched hand, short sternum, low arch dermal ridge pattern on fingertips, mental retardation
Cri du chat (short-arm deletion-5)	Ventricular septal defect	Cat cry, microcephaly, antimongoloid slant of palpebral fissures, mental retardation
XO (Turner)	Coarctation of aorta, biscuspid aortic valve, aortic dilatation	Short female, broad chest, lymphedema, webbed neck
XXXY and XXXXX	Patent ductus arteriosus	XXXY: Hypogenitalism, mental retardation, radial-ulnar synostosis XXXXX: Small hands, incurving of fifth fingers, mental retardation
	Sporadic Disorders	
VATER association	Ventricular septal defect	Vertebral anomalies, anal atresia, tracheo-esophageal fistula, radial and renal anomalies
CHARGE association	Tetralogy of Fallot (other defects common)	Colobomas, choanal atresia, mental and growth deficiency, genital and ear anomalies
Williams	Supravalvular aortic stenosis, peripheral pulmonic stenosis	Mental deficiency, elfin facies, loquacious personality, hoarse voice
Cornelia de Lange	Ventricular septal defect	Micromelia, synophrys, mental and growth deficiency
Shprintzen (velocardiofacial)	Ventricular septal defect, tetralogy of Fallot, right aortic arch	Cleft palate, prominent nose, slender hands, learning disability
	Teratogenic Disorders	
Rubella	Patent ductus arteriosus, pulmonic valvular and/or arterial stenosis, atrial septal defect	Cataracts, deafness, microcephaly
Alcohol	Ventricular septal defect (other defects)	Microcephaly, growth and mental deficiency, short palpebral fissures, smooth philtrum, thin upper lip
Dilantin	Pulmonic stenosis, aortic stenosis, coarctation, patent ductus arteriosus	Hypertelorism, growth and mental deficiency, short phalanges, bowed upper lip
Thalidomide	Variable	Phocomelia
Lithium	Ebstein's anomaly, tricuspid atresia	None

Modified from Friedman, W. F.: Congenital heart disease. *In* Wilson, J. D., et al. (eds): Harrison's Principles of Internal Medicine. 12th ed. New York, McGraw-Hill Book Co., 1991, p. 924.

PREVENTION

The feasibility of preventive programs depends on what is learned in the future about the 90 per cent or more of cardiovascular anomalies for which no cause currently is known. Strict testing in animals of new drugs that may be teratogenic when taken during pregnancy may be expected to reduce the chances of another thalidomide tragedy. In this regard, the dictum cannot be emphasized too strongly that no medication should be taken during pregnancy without prior consultation with a physician. Physicians who deal with pregnant women should be aware of known teratogens as well as drugs that may have a functional rather than a structural damaging influence on the fetal and newborn heart and circulation, and should recognize that drugs abound for which there is inadequate information concerning their teratogenic potential. Similarly, appropriate radiological equipment and techniques for reducing gonadal and fetal radiation exposure should always be used to reduce the potential hazards of this likely cause of birth defects.

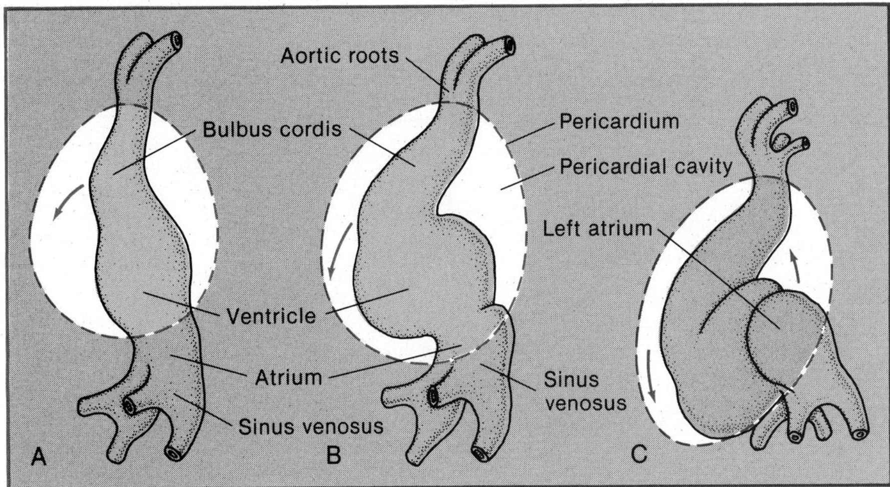

FIGURE 31-1. Formation of the cardiac loop as seen from the left side at *(A)* 32 days, *(B)* 34 days and *(C)* 38 days. Dashed line indicates parietal pericardium. The atrium gradually assumes an intrapericardial position. (From Clark, E. B., and Van Mierop, L. H. S.: Development of the cardiovascular system. *In* Moss' Heart Disease in Infants, Children, and Adolescents. Baltimore, Williams and Wilkins, 1989.)

Detection of abnormal chromosomes in fetal cells obtained from amniotic fluid or chorionic villus biopsy (Chap. 51) may predict cardiac malformation as one component of the multisystem involvement that may exist in such syndromes as Down, Turner, or trisomy 13-15 (D1) or 16-18 (E). Similarly, identification in such cells of the enzyme disorders observed in the mucopolysaccharidoses, homocystinuria, or type II glycogen storage disease may allow one to predict the ultimate presence of cardiac disease. Finally, immunization of children with rubella vaccine will avoid the effects of maternal rubella and its cardiac consequences.

EMBRYOLOGY

NORMAL CARDIAC DEVELOPMENT. Correlation of anatomical features of malformed hearts and embryonic cardiac morphology allows a developmental analysis of various anomalies. Detailed accounts of the normal development of the cardiovascular system are provided elsewhere.[13-15] In brief, during the first month of gestation the primitive, straight cardiac tube is formed, comprising the sinuatrium, the primitive ventricle, the bulbus cordis, and the truncus arteriosus in series (Fig. 31-1). In the second month of gestation this tube doubles over on itself to form two parallel pumping systems, each with two chambers and a great artery. The two atria develop from the sinuatrium; the atrioventricular canal is divided by the endocardial cushions into tricuspid and mitral orifices; and the right and left ventricles develop from the primitive ventricle and bulbus cordis. Differential growth of myocardial cells causes the straight cardiac tube to bear to the right, and the bulboventricular portion of the tube doubles over on itself, bringing the ventricles side by side (Fig. 31-2). Migration of the atrioventricular canal to the right and of the ventricular septum to the left serves to align each ventricle with its appropriate atrioventricular valve. At the distal end of the cardiac tube the bulbus cordis divides into a subaortic muscular conus and a subpulmonic muscular conus; the subpulmonic conus elongates and the subaortic conus resorbs, allowing the aorta to move posteriorly and connect with the left ventricle.

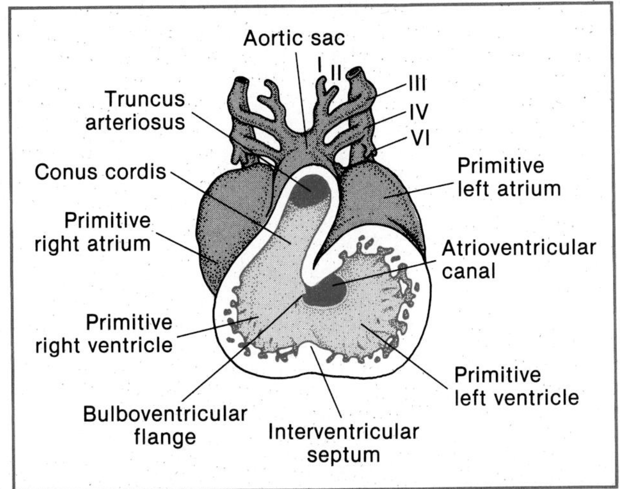

FIGURE 31-2. Frontal section through the heart of a 5-mm embryo showing the side-by-side primitive ventricles and the single opening of the atrium into the ventricles. (From Clark, E. B., and Van Mierop, L.H.S.: Development of the cardiovascular system. *In* Moss' Heart Disease in Infants, Children, and Adolescents. Baltimore, Williams and Wilkins, 1989.)

ABNORMAL DEVELOPMENT. A host of anomalies may result from defects in this basic developmental pattern. Thus, double-inlet left ventricle (p. 953) is observed if the tricuspid orifice does not align over the right ventricle. The various types of persistent truncus arteriosus (p. 915) result from failure of the truncus to divide into main pulmonary artery and aorta. Double-outlet anomalies of the right ventricle (p. 953) are produced by failure of either the subpulmonic or subaortic conus to resorb, whereas resorption of the subpulmonic instead of the subaortic conus may be central to transposition of the great arteries (p. 941).

THE ATRIA. The primitive sinuatrium is separated into right and left atria by the downgrowth from its roof of the septum primum toward the atrioventricular canal, thereby creating an inferior intraatrial ostium primum opening (Fig. 31-3). Multiple perforations form in the anterosuperior portion of the septum primum as the septum secundum begins to develop to the right of the former. The coalescence of these perforations forms the ostium secundum. The septum secundum completely separates the atrial chambers except for a central opening—the fossa ovalis—which is covered by tissue of the septum primum, forming the valve of the foramen ovale. Fusion of the endocardial cushions anteriorly and posteriorly divides the atrioventricular canal into tricuspid and mitral inlets (Fig. 31-4). The inferior portion of the atrial septum, the superior portion of the ventricular septum, and portions of the septal leaflets of both the tricuspid and mitral valves are formed from the endocardial cushions. The integrity of the atrial septum depends on growth of the septum primum and septum secundum and proper fusion of the endocardial cushions. Atrial septal defects (p. 906) and varying degrees of endocardial cushion defect (p. 92) are the result of developmental deficiencies of this process.

THE VENTRICLES. Partitioning of the ventricles occurs as cephalic growth of the main ventricular septum results in its fusion with the endocardial cushions and the infundibular or conus septum. Defects in the ventricular septum may occur owing to a deficiency of septal substance; malalignment of septal components in different planes, preventing their fusion; or an overly long conus, keeping the septal components apart. Isolated defects probably result from the first mechanism, whereas the latter two appear to generate the ventricular defects seen in tetralogy of Fallot (p. 935) and transposition complexes (p. 941).

THE LUNGS. These structures arise from the primitive foregut and are drained early in embryogenesis by channels from the splanchnic plexus to the cardinal and umbilicovitelline veins. An outpouching from the posterior left atrium forms the common pulmonary vein, which communicates with the splanchnic plexus, establishing pulmonary venous drainage to the left atrium. The umbilicovitelline and anterior cardinal vein communications atrophy as the common pulmonary vein is incorporated into the left atrium. Anomalous pulmonary venous connections (p. 951) to the umbilicovitelline (portal) venous system or to the cardinal system (superior vena cava) result from failure of the common pulmonary vein to develop or establish communications to the splanchnic plexus. Cor triatriatum (p. 929) results from a narrowing of the common pulmonary vein-left atrial junction.

THE GREAT ARTERIES. The truncus arteriosus is connected to the dorsal aorta in the embryo by six pairs of aortic arches. Partition of the truncus arteriosus into two great arteries is a result of the fusion of tissue arising from the back wall of the vessel and the truncus septum. Rotation of the truncus coils the aorticopulmonary septum and creates the normal

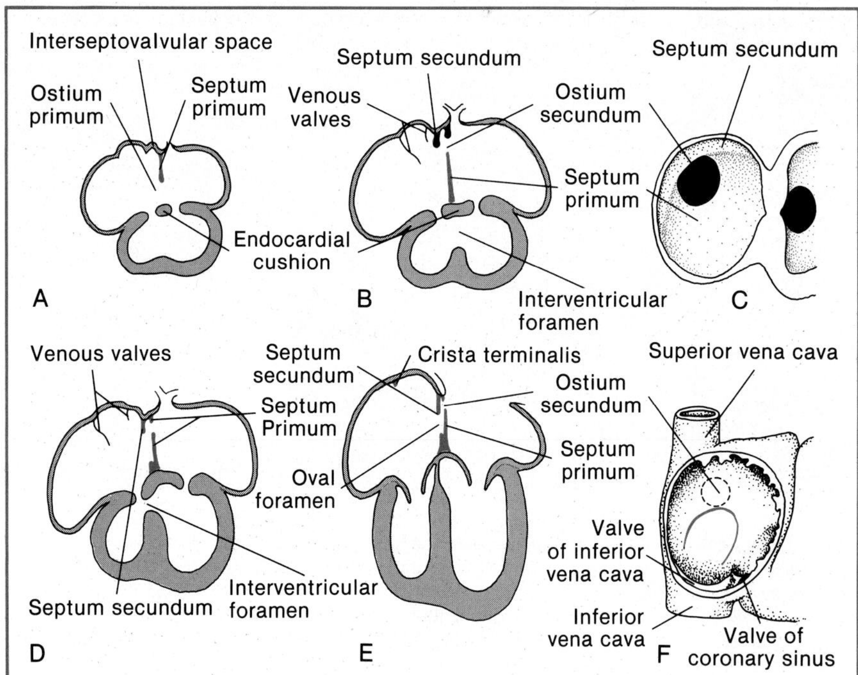

FIGURE 31–3. Diagrammatic representation of the atrial septa at 30 days *(A)*, at 33 days *(B)*, at 33 days (seen from the right side) *(C)*, at 37 days *(D)*, and in the newborn *(E)*; the newborn atrial septum viewed from the right *(F)*. (From Clark, E. B., and Van Mierop, L.H.S.: Development of the cardiovascular system. *In* Moss' Heart Disease in Infants, Children, and Adolescents. Baltimore, Williams and Wilkins, 1989.)

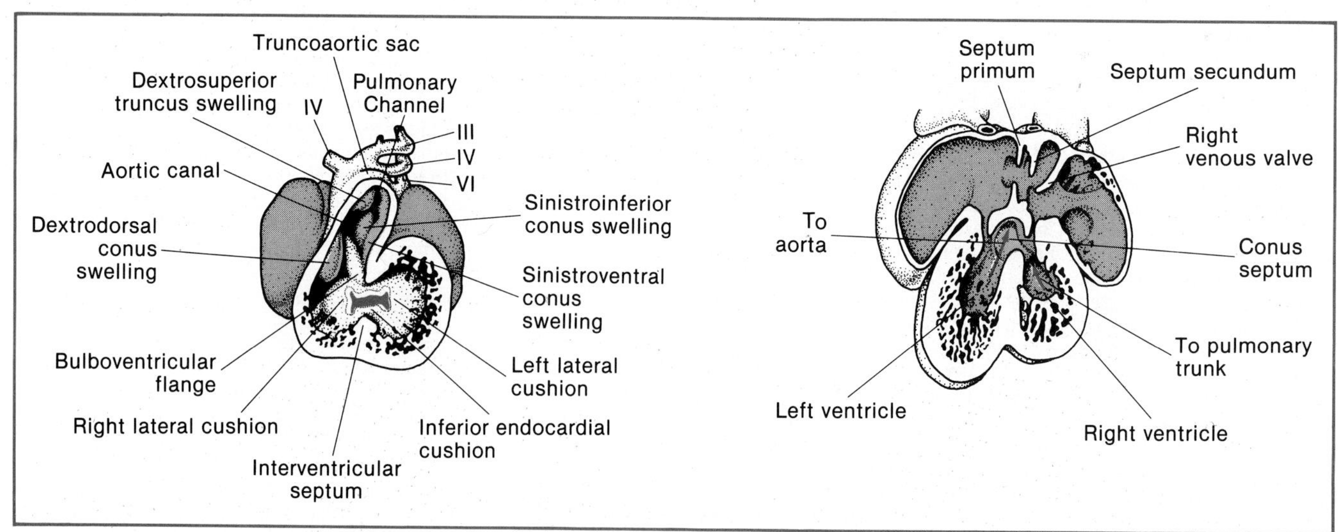

FIGURE 31–4. Frontal section through the heart of a 9-mm embryo (left panel) and 15-mm embryo (right panel). At 9 mm, development is noted of the cushions in the atrioventricular canal, and the truncus and conus swellings are visible. At 15 mm, the conus septum is completed; note the septation in the atrial region. (From Clark, E. B., and Van Mierop, L.H.S.: Development of the cardiovascular system. *In* Moss' Heart Disease in Infants, Children, and Adolescents. Baltimore, Williams and Wilkins, 1989.)

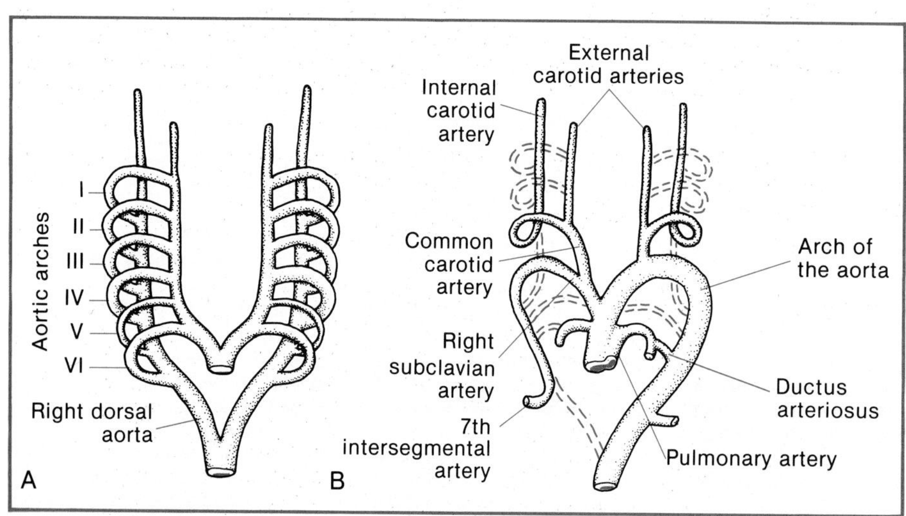

FIGURE 31–5. *A*, Aortic arches and dorsal aortas before transformation into the definitive vascular pattern. *B*, Aortic arches and dorsal aortas after transformation. The obliterated components are indicated by broken lines. (From Clark, E. B., and Van Mierop, L.H.S.: Development of the cardiovascular system. *In* Moss' Heart Disease in Infants, Children, and Adolescents. Baltimore, Williams and Wilkins, 1989.)

spiral relation between aorta and pulmonary artery. Semilunar valves and their related sinuses are created by absorption and hollowing out of tissue at the distal side of the truncus ridges. Aorticopulmonary septal defect (p. 915) and persistent truncus arteriosus (p. 915) represent varying degrees of partitioning failure.

Although the six aortic arches appear sequentially, portions of the arch system and dorsal aorta disappear at different times during embryogenesis (Fig. 31-5). The first, second, and fifth sets of paired arches regress completely. The proximal portions of the sixth arches become the right and left pulmonary arteries and the distal left sixth arch becomes the ductus arteriosus. The third aortic arch forms the connection between internal and external carotid arteries, while the left fourth arch becomes the arterial segment between left carotid and subclavian arteries; the proximal portion of the right subclavian artery forms from the right fourth arch. An abnormality in regression of the arch system in a number of sites can produce a wide variety of arch anomalies, whereas a failure of regression usually results in a double aortic arch malformation.

FETAL AND TRANSITIONAL CIRCULATIONS

Although the illness created by the presence of a cardiac malformation is almost always recognized only after an affected baby is born, important effects on the circulation have existed from early in pregnancy until the time of delivery. Thus knowledge of the changes in cardiocirculatory structure, function, and metabolism that accompany development is central to a systematic comprehension of congenital heart disease.

FETAL CIRCULATORY PATHWAYS. Dynamic alterations occur in the circulation during the transition from fetal to neonatal life when the lungs take over the function of gas exchange from the placenta. The single fetal circulation consists of parallel pulmonary and systemic pathways (Fig. 31-6) in contrast to the two-circuit system in the newborn and adult, in whom the pulmonary vasculature exists in series with the systemic circulation. Prenatal survival is not endangered by major cardiac anomalies as long as one side of the heart can drive blood from the great veins to the aorta; in the fetus, blood can bypass the nonfunctioning lungs both proximal and distal to the heart. Oxygenated blood returns from the placenta through the umbilical vein and enters the portal venous system. A variable amount of this stream bypasses the hepatic microcirculation and enters the inferior vena cava by way of the ductus venosus. Inferior vena caval blood is composed of flow from the ductus venosus, hepatic vein, and lower body venous drainage, which is summarily deflected to a significant extent across the foramen ovale into the left atrium. Almost all superior vena caval blood passes directly through the tricuspid valve entering the right ventricle. Most of the blood that reaches the right ventricle bypasses the high-resistance, unexpanded lungs and passes through the ductus arteriosus into the descending aorta. The right ventricle contributes about 55 per cent and the left 45 per cent to the total fetal cardiac output. The major portion of blood ejected from the left ventricle supplies the brain and upper body, with lesser flow to the coronary arteries; the balance passes across the aortic isthmus to the descending aorta, where it joins with the large stream from the ductus arteriosus before flowing to the lower body and placenta.

FETAL PULMONARY CIRCULATION. In fetal life, pulmonary arteries and arterioles are surrounded by a fluid medium, have relatively thick walls and small lumina, and resemble comparable arteries in the systemic circulation. The low pulmonary blood flow in the fetus (7 to 10 per cent of the total cardiac output) is the result of high pulmonary vascular resistance. Fetal pulmonary vessels are highly reactive to changes in oxygen tension or in the pH of blood perfusing them as well as to a number of other physiological and pharmacological influences.

EFFECTS OF CARDIAC MALFORMATIONS ON THE FETUS. Although fetal somatic growth may be unimpaired, the hemodynamic effects in utero of many cardiac malformations may alter the development and structure of the fetal heart and circulation.[16] Thus, total anomalous pulmonary venous connection in utero may result in underdevelopment of the left atrium and left ventricle (p. 949), and premature closure of the foramen ovale may result in hypoplasia of the left ventricle. Moreover, postnatally, the caliber of the aortic isthmus may be reduced (p. 922) in the presence of lesions in utero that create left ventricular hypertrophy and impede filling because of reduced compliance of that chamber. It may also

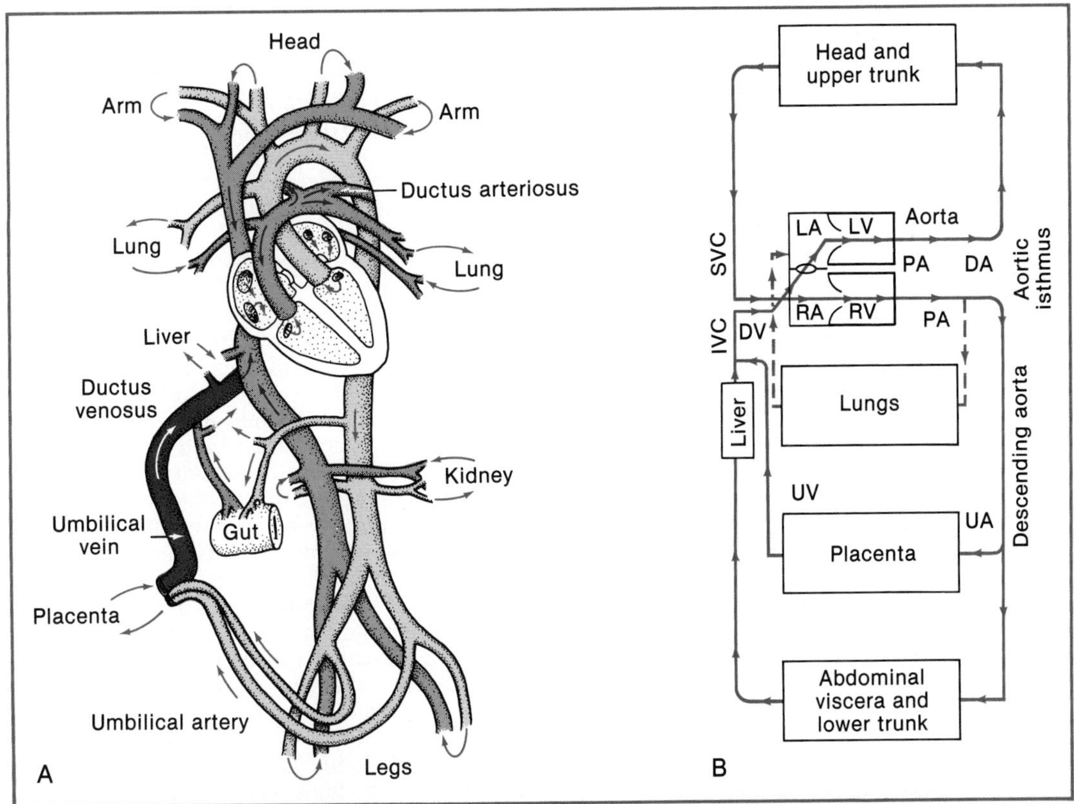

FIGURE 31-6. *A*, The fetal circulation. Shading shows the relative oxygenation of the blood, and arrows indicate its direction of flow. *B*, Prenatally, a fraction of umbilical venous (UV) blood enters the ductus venosus (DV) and bypasses the liver. This relatively well-oxygenated blood flows across the foramen ovale to the left heart, preferentially perfusing the coronary arteries, head, and upper trunk. Superior vena caval (SVC) blood is ejected by the right heart into the pulmonary artery (PA) and ductus arteriosus (DA). This stream circulates to the placenta as well as to the abdominal viscera and lower trunk. Dashed lines indicate diminished blood flow to and from the lungs and across the aortic isthmus. IVC = inferior vena cava, RA = right atrium, LA = left atrium, RV = right ventricle, LV = left ventricle, PA = pulmonary artery. (From Kaplan, S.: Congenital heart disease. *In* Vaughan, V. C., and McKay, R. J. [eds.]: Nelson Textbook of Pediatrics. 10th ed. Philadelphia, W. B. Saunders Company, 1975.)

be reduced in the presence of a lesion that interferes with left ventricular filling directly (e.g., mitral stenosis) or indirectly by diverting a proportion of left ventricular output away from the ascending aorta while increasing right ventricular output and ductus arteriosus flow (e.g., atrioventricular septal defect with left ventricular–right atrial shunt or aortic or subaortic stenosis with ventricular septal defect). Similarly, obstruction in utero to right ventricular outflow is associated with an increase in proximal aortic flow and diameter and almost never with aortic coarctation (p. 967). In these and other examples it is important to recognize that malformations compatible with fetal survival may nonetheless result in abnormal development of the circulation in utero and also affect circulatory adjustments after birth.

FUNCTION OF THE FETAL HEART. Compared with the adult heart, the fetal and newborn heart is unique with respect to its ultrastructural appearance,[17] its mechanical and biochemical properties,[17–20] and its autonomic innervation.[19–22] During late fetal and early neonatal development there is maturation of the excitation-contraction coupling process[23,24] and the biochemical composition of the heart's energy-utilizing myofibrillar proteins and of adenosine triphosphate and creatine phosphate energy-producing proteins.[20] Moreover, fetal and neonatal myocardial cells are small in diameter and reduced in density, so that the young heart contains relatively more noncontractile mass (primarily mitochondria, nuclei, and surface membranes) than later in postnatal life. As a result, force generation and the extent and velocity of shortening are decreased, and stiffness and water content of ventricular myocardium are increased in the fetal and early newborn periods. The diminished function of the young heart is reflected in its limited ability to increase cardiac output in the presence of either a volume load or a lesion that increases resistance to emptying.[25] Although functional integrity exists of efferent and afferent cardiac autonomic pathways early in life, fetal and newborn myocardium lacks the complete development of sympathetic but not cholinergic innervation. Thus, adaptation to cardiocirculatory stress in fetal or early newborn life may be less effective than in adulthood.

CHANGES AT BIRTH. The fundamental change that normally occurs at birth is a division of the single parallel fetal circulation into separate, independent circulations. Inflation of the lungs at the first inspiration produces a marked reduction in pulmonary vascular resistance owing partly to the sudden suspension in air of fetal pulmonary vessels previously supported by fluid media. The reduced extravascular pressure assists new vessels to open and already patent vessels to enlarge. The rapid decrease in pulmonary vascular resistance is related more importantly to vasodilatation owing to the increase in oxygen tension to which pulmonary vessels are exposed than to physical expansion of alveoli with gas. Pulmonary arterial pressure falls, and pulmonary blood flow increases greatly. Systemic vascular resistance rises when clamping of the umbilical cord removes the low-resistance placental circulation. Increased pulmonary blood flow increases the return of blood to the left atrium and raises left atrial pressure, which in turn closes the foramen ovale. The shift in oxygen dependence from the placenta to the lungs produces a sudden increase in arterial blood oxygen tension, which, in concert with alterations in the local prostaglandin milieu, initiates constriction of the ductus arteriosus.[26] Pulmonary pressure falls further as the ductus constricts. In healthy mature infants the ductus arteriosus is profoundly constricted at 10 to 15 hours and is closed functionally by 72 hours, with total anatomical closure following within a few weeks by a process of thrombosis, intimal proliferation, and fibrosis. A high incidence exists in preterm infants of persistent patency of the ductus arteriosus because of an immaturity of those mechanisms responsible for constriction (p. 913). In surviving preterm infants the ductus arteriosus spontaneously closes within 4 to 12 months of birth.

The ductus venosus, ductus arteriosus, and foramen ovale remain potential channels for blood flow after birth. Thus persistent patency of the ductus venosus may mask the most marked signs of pulmonary venous obstruction in infants with total anomalous pulmonary venous connection below the diaphragm (p. 949). Similarly, lesions producing right or left atrial volume or pressure overload may stretch the foramen ovale and render incompetent the flap valve mechanism for its closure. Anomalies that depend on patency of the ductus arteriosus for preserving pulmonary or systemic blood flow remain latent until the ductus arteriosus constricts. A common example is the sudden intensification of cyanosis observed in the infant with tetralogy of Fallot when the magnitude of pulmonary hypoperfusion is unmasked by spontaneous closure of the ductus arteriosus. Moreover, there is increasing evidence that ductal constriction is a key factor in the postnatal development of coarctation of the aorta (p. 967). Lastly, it should be recognized that because the ductus arteriosus is potentially patent after birth and the pulmonary resistance vessels are hyperreactive, hypoxic pulmonary vasoconstriction of diverse causes may result in a right-to-left shunt through the ductus.

TABLE 31–3 FEATURES OF HEART FAILURE IN INFANTS

Poor feeding and failure to thrive
Respiratory distress—mainly tachypnea
Rapid heart rate (160 to 180 beats/min)
Pulmonary rales or wheezing
Cardiomegaly and pulmonary edema on x-ray
Hepatomegaly (peripheral edema unusual)
Gallop sounds
Color—ashen pale or faintly cyanotic
Excessive perspiration
Diminished urine output

PATHOLOGICAL CONSEQUENCES OF CONGENITAL CARDIAC LESIONS

CONGESTIVE HEART FAILURE

(See also p. 446)

Although the basic mechanisms of cardiac failure, as outlined in Chap. 14, are similar for all ages, the pediatric cardiologist should clearly recognize that the common causes, time of onset, and often the approach to treatment vary with age.[27–29] The development of fetal echocardiography has allowed the diagnosis of intrauterine cardiac failure.[30,31] The cardinal findings of fetal heart failure are scalp edema, ascites, pericardial effusion, and decreased fetal movements. Although abnormalities in several organ systems may result in nonimmunological fetal hydrops, cardiac causes include a host of structural, functional, rhythm, and metabolic disturbances of the heart. Infants under 1 year of age with cardiac malformations account for 80 to 90 percent of pediatric patients who develop congestive failure. Moreover, cardiac decompensation in the infant is a medical emergency necessitating immediate treatment if the patient is to be saved.

In the preterm infant, especially under 1500 gm birthweight, persistent patency of the ductus arteriosus is the most common cause of cardiac decompensation, and other forms of structural heart disease are rare.[32] In the full-term newborn the earliest important causes of heart failure are the hypoplastic left heart and coarctation of the aorta syndromes, paroxysmal atrial tachycardia, cerebral or hepatic arteriovenous fistula, and myocarditis. Among the lesions commonly producing heart failure beyond age 1 to 2 weeks, when diminished pulmonary vascular resistance allows substantial left-to-right shunting, are ventricular septal and atrioventricular septal defects, transposition of the great arteries, truncus arteriosus, and total anomalous pulmonary venous connection, often with pulmonary venous obstruction. Although heart failure usually is the result of a structural defect or of myocardial disease, it should be recognized that the newborn myocardium may be severely depressed by such abnormalities as hypoxemia and acidemia, anemia, septicemia, marked hypoglycemia, hypocalcemia, and polycythemia. In the older child, heart failure often is due to acquired disease (Chap. 33) or is a complication of open-heart surgical procedures. In the acquired category are rheumatic and endomyocardial diseases, infective endocarditis, hematological and nutritional disorders, and severe cardiac arrhythmias.

CLINICAL MANIFESTATIONS IN THE INFANT. The clinical expression of cardiac decompensation in the infant consists of distinctive signs of pulmonary and systemic venous congestion and altered cardiocirculatory performance that resemble, but often are not identical to, those of the older child or adult (Table 31–3).[33] These reflect the interplay between the hemodynamic burden and adaptive responses. Common symptoms and signs are feeding difficulties and failure to gain weight and grow, tachypnea, tachycardia, pulmonary rales and rhonchi, liver enlargement, and cardiomegaly. Less frequent manifestations include peripheral edema, ascites, pulsus alternans, gallop rhythm, and inappropriate sweating. Pleural and pericardial effusions are exceedingly rare. The distinction between left and right heart failure is less obvious in the infant than in the older child or adult, since most lesions that create a left ventricular pressure or volume overload also result in left-to-right shunting of blood through the foramen ovale and/or patent ductus arteriosus as well as pulmonary hypertension owing to elevated pulmonary venous pressures. Conversely, augmented filling or elevated pressure of the right ventricle in the infant reduces left ventricular compliance disproportionately when compared with the older child or adult and gives rise to signs of both systemic and pulmonary venous congestion.[19]

Fatigue and dyspnea on exertion express themselves as a feeding problem in the infant. Characteristically, the respiratory rate in heart failure is rapid (50 to 100 breaths/min). In the presence of left ventricular failure, interstitial pulmonary edema reduces pulmonary compliance and results in tachypnea and retractions. Excessive pulmonary blood flow by way of significant left-to-right shunts may further decrease lung compliance. Moreover, upper airway obstruction may be produced by selective enlargement of cardiovascular structures. In patients with large left-to-right shunts and left atrial and main pulmonary artery enlargement, the left main stem bronchus may be compressed, resulting in emphysematous expansion of the left upper or lower lobe or left lower lobe collapse.[34] Respiratory distress with grunting, flaring of the alae nasi, and intercostal retractions is observed when failure is severe and especially when pulmonary infection precipitates cardiac decompensation, which often is the case. Under these circumstances pulmonary rales may be due to the infection or failure, or both. A resting heart rate with little variability is characteristic of heart failure. Hepatomegaly is regularly seen in infants in failure, although liver tenderness is uncommon. Cardiomegaly may be assessed roentgenographically, but it must be recognized that in the normal newborn infant, the cardiac diameter may be as much as 60 per cent of the thoracic diameter, and the large thymus gland in infants occasionally interferes with evaluation of heart size. Two-dimensional and Doppler echocardiography provide a good estimate of cardiac performance and chamber dimensions, and values may be compared with data derived from normal infants.[35-39]

Cardiac decompensation may progress with extreme rapidity in the first hours and days of life, producing a clinical picture of advanced cardiogenic shock and a profoundly obtunded infant. The presence of marked hepatomegaly and gross cardiomegaly usually allows distinction from noncardiac causes of diminished systemic perfusion.

CYANOSIS

(See also page 7)

Cyanosis is produced by reduced hemoglobin in cutaneous vessels in excess of approximately 3 gm/dl. Peripheral cyanosis usually reflects an abnormally great extraction of oxygen from normally saturated arterial blood, commonly the result of peripheral cutaneous vasoconstriction. Central cyanosis is a result of arterial blood oxygen unsaturation, most often in patients with congenital heart disease caused by shunting of systemic venous blood into the arterial circuit. Infants especially (as compared with adults) may appear cyanotic when in heart failure because of both peripheral and central factors; the latter may include severe impairment of pulmonary function that commonly exists with alveolar hypoventilation, ventilation-perfusion inequality, or impaired oxygen diffusion. In patients with central cyanosis owing to arterial oxygen unsaturation, the degree of cutaneous discoloration depends on the absolute amount of reduced hemoglobin, the magnitude of the right-to-left shunt relative to systemic flow, and the oxyhemoglobin saturation of venous blood. The last of these depends in turn on the tissue extraction of oxygen. Commonly, cyanosis appears or intensifies with physical activity or exercise as the saturation of systemic venous blood declines concurrent with an increase in right-to-left shunting across a defect as peripheral vascular resistance decreases. Oxygen transfer to the tissues is affected by shifts in the oxygen hemoglobin dissociation relation, which may be altered by blood pH and levels of red blood cell 2,3-diphosphoglycerate concentration.

CLUBBING AND POLYCYTHEMIA. Prominent accompaniments of arterial hypoxemia are polycythemia and clubbing of the digits. The latter is associated with an increased number of capillaries with increased blood flow through extensive arteriovenous aneurysms and an increase of connective tissue in the terminal phalanges of the fingers and toes. Polycythemia is a physiological response to chronic hypoxemia that stimulates erythrocytosis. The extremely high hematocrits observed in patients with arterial oxygen unsaturation cause a progressive increase in blood viscosity, especially beyond packed red blood cell volumes of 60 per cent. Both the hematocrit and the circulating whole blood volume are increased in polycythemia accompanying cyanotic congenital heart disease; the hypervolemia is the result of an increase in red cell volume. The augmented red blood cell volume provoked by hypoxemia provides an increased oxygen-carrying capacity and enhanced oxygen supply to the tissues. The compensatory polycythemia often is of such severity that it becomes a liability and produces adverse physiological effects such as thrombotic lesions in diverse organs and a hemorrhagic diathesis.[41] In this regard, oral steroid contraceptives are contraindicated in the adolescent cyanotic female because of the enhanced risk of cerebral thrombosis.

MANAGEMENT. Red cell volume reduction and replacement with plasma or albumin (erythrophoresis) lowers blood viscosity and increases systemic blood flow and systemic oxygen transport, and thus may be helpful in the management of patients with severe hypoxic polycythemia (hematocrit ≥ 65 per cent). A final hematocrit of 55 to 63 per cent should be achieved; the higher level is necessary in patients with low initial oxygen saturation to avoid a severe reduction in arterial oxygen content. Acute phlebotomy without fluid replacement is contraindicated.

CEREBRAL AND PULMONARY COMPLICATIONS. Cerebrovascular accidents and brain abscesses occur particularly in cyanotic patients with substantial arterial desaturation.[42-44] *Cerebral thrombosis* is most common under age 2 years in severely cyanotic children, even in the presence of relatively low hematocrits, and occurs especially in a clinical setting in which oxygen requirements are raised by fever or, if blood viscosity is increased, dehydration.

Brain abscess is an important complication of cyanotic heart disease.[43,44] Such abscesses are rare under 18 months of age and commonly are of insidious onset marked by headache, low-grade fever, vomiting, and a change in personality. Seizures or paralysis less frequently heralds the onset of a brain abscess. Abscess must be suspected in any cyanotic child with focal neurological signs. Morbidity and mortality are related inversely to oxygen saturation levels. Brain abscess is thought to occur in about 2 per cent of the population with cyanotic congenital heart disease; a mortality rate of 30 to 40 per cent often is related to delay in diagnosis and treatment.

Paradoxical embolus is a rare complication of cyanotic heart disease, usually observed only at necropsy.[45] Emboli arising in systemic veins may pass directly to the systemic circulation, since right-to-left intracardiac shunts allow venous blood to bypass the normal filtering action of the lungs.

Retinopathy, consisting of dilated tortuous vessels progressing to papilledema, and retinal edema occasionally are observed in cyanotic patients, and appear to be related to decreased arterial oxygen saturation and/or to erythrocytosis but not to hypercapnia.

Hemoptysis is an uncommon but major complication in cyanotic patients with congenital heart disease, and occurs most often in the presence of pulmonary vascular obstructive disease or in patients with an extensive bronchial collateral circulation or pulmonary venous congestion.[46] Massive hemoptysis almost always represents rupture of a dilated bronchial artery.

SQUATTING. After exertion, patients with cyanotic heart disease, especially tetralogy of Fallot, typically assume a squatting posture to obtain relief from breathlessness.[47] Squatting appears to improve arterial oxygen saturation by increasing systemic vascular resistance, thereby diminishing the right-to-left shunt, and also by the pooling of markedly desaturated blood in the lower extremities. In addition, systemic venous return, and therefore pulmonary blood flow, may increase.

HYPOXIC SPELLS. Hypercyanotic or hypoxemic spells commonly complicate the clinical course in younger children with certain types of cyanotic heart disease, especially tetralogy of Fallot (p. 935).[47] The spells are characterized by anxiety, hyperpnea, and a sudden marked increase in cyanosis; they are the result of an abrupt reduction in pulmonary blood flow. Unless terminated, the hypercyanotic episodes may lead to convulsions and may even be fatal. The sudden reduction in pulmonary blood flow may be precipitated by fluctuations in arterial pCO_2 and pH, a sudden fall in systemic or increase in pulmonary vascular resistance, or an acute increase in the severity of right ventricular outflow tract obstruction either by augmented contraction of the hypertrophied muscle in the right ventricular outflow tract or by a decrease in right ventricular cavity volume owing to tachycardia.

Treatment. This consists of oxygen administration, placing the child in the knee-chest position, and administration of morphine sulfate. Additional medications that may prove of value include the intravenous administration of sodium bicarbonate to correct the accompanying acidemia, alpha-adrenoceptor stimulants such as phenylephrine hydrochloride (Neo-Synephrine) or methoxamine to raise peripheral resistance and diminish right-to-left shunting, and beta-adrenoceptor blocking agents, which reduce cardiac sympathetic tone and depress cardiac contractility directly, and which increase ventricular volume by reducing heart rate.

ACID-BASE IMBALANCE

Disturbances in blood gas and acid-base equilibrium are noted particularly in infants with either congestive heart failure or cyanosis.[48] Large-volume left-to-right shunts, especially with pulmonary edema, may be associated with moderate respiratory acidemia and a lowering of arterial oxygen tensions, reflecting an increase in the alveolar-arterial oxygen tension gradient and ventilation-perfusion imbalance. Interference with carbon dioxide transport implies moderate to severe failure in these infants. Lesions associated with a reduced systemic cardiac output, such as severe coarctation of the aorta or critical aortic stenosis in infancy, often present as cardiac failure complicated by a severe metabolic acidemia and relatively high values of arterial oxygen tension. The latter finding, even in the presence of right-to-left shunting across a patent ductus arteriosus, is a result of diminished systemic perfusion and an elevated pulmonary-systemic blood flow ratio. Respiratory acidemia and depressed levels of oxygen tension are observed in infants with obstruction to pulmonary venous return and right-to-left atrial shunting. Many infants with severe hypoxemia caused by lesions such as transposition of the great arteries or pulmonic atresia show metabolic acidemia and marked reductions in carbon dioxide tension secondary to hyperventilation, resulting from hypoxic stimulation of peripheral chemoreceptors.

IMPAIRED GROWTH

Impaired growth and physical development and delayed onset of adolescence are common features of many cyanotic and, to a lesser extent, acyanotic forms of congenital heart disease.[49] Mental development seldom is affected. The severity of growth disturbance depends on the anatomical lesion and its functional effect. Most children with mild defects grow normally. Weight gain is commonly slower than linear growth in acyanotic patients with large left-to-right shunts, whereas in cyanotic congenital heart disease, height and weight usually parallel each other. Boys appear to be more retarded in growth than girls, especially in the second decade. Skeletal maturity (i.e., bone age) is delayed in cyanotic children in relation to the severity of hypoxemia.

In some children, prenatal factors such as intrauterine infection and chromosomal or other hereditary and nonhereditary syndromes are responsible for growth retardation. In other patients, extracardiac malformations may contribute to poor weight gain and linear growth. Additional explanations for the mechanisms of growth interference have implicated malnutrition as a result of anorexia and inadequate nutrient and caloric intake, hypermetabolic state, acidemia and cation imbalance, tissue hypoxemia, diminished peripheral blood flow, chronic cardiac decompensation, malabsorption or protein loss, recurrent respiratory infections, and endocrine or genetic factors. In some instances, the underdevelopment is influenced little by operative correction of the underlying cardiac anomaly. Among factors that may be responsible for persistent growth retardation postoperatively are age at operation, hemodynamically significant residual lesions, and sequelae or complications of operation. As a general rule, it is unwise preoperatively to guarantee to the parents of a child with heart disease that surgery will result in accelerated growth and development.

PULMONARY HYPERTENSION

(See also Chap. 27)

Pulmonary hypertension is a common accompaniment of many congenital cardiac lesions, and the status of the pulmonary vascular bed often is the principal determinant of the clinical manifestations, the course, and whether surgical treatment is feasible.[50] Increases in pulmonary arterial pressure result from elevations of pulmonary blood flow and/or resistance, the latter sometimes caused by an increase in vascular tone, but usually the result of underdevelopment and/or obstructive, obliterative structural changes within the pulmonary vascular bed.[51-53]

Pulmonary vascular resistance normally falls rapidly immediately after birth, owing to onset of ventilation and subsequent release of hypoxic pulmonary vasoconstriction. Subsequently the medial smooth muscle of pulmonary arterial resistance vessels thins gradually.[54] This latter process often is delayed by several months in infants with large aorticopulmonary or ventricular communications, at which time levels of pulmonary vascular resistance are still somewhat elevated. In patients with high pulmonary arterial pressure from birth, failure of normal growth of the pulmonary circulation may occur, and anatomical changes in the pulmonary vessels in the form of proliferation of intimal cells and intimal and medial thickening often progress, so that in the older child or adult vascular resistance ultimately may become fixed by obliterative changes in the pulmonary vascular bed. The causes of pulmonary vascular obstructive disease remain unknown, although increased pulmonary blood flow, increased pulmonary arterial blood pressure, elevated pulmonary venous pressure, polycythemia, systemic hypoxia, acidemia, and the nature of the bronchial circulation have all been implicated. There are many patients with pulmonary vascular obstruction whose cardiac anomaly places them at particular risk quite early in life, precluding survival to adulthood. Patients at particularly high risk for the development of significant pulmonary vascular obstruction are those with certain forms of cyanotic congenital heart disease, such as complete transposition of the great arteries with or without ventricular septal defect or patent ductus arteriosus, single ventricle without pulmonary stenosis, double-outlet right ventricle, and truncus arteriosus. Other conditions in which pulmonary vascular obstruction appears to progress rapidly include large ventricular septal defect, as well as the less common conditions of unilateral pulmonary artery absence, congenital left-to-right shunts in an environment of high altitude or in association with the Down syndrome of trisomy 21, and complete atrioventricular canal defects, even those unassociated with a chromosomal anomaly.

MECHANISMS OF DEVELOPMENT OF PULMONARY HYPERTENSION. Intimal damage appears to be related to shear stresses, since endothelial cell damage occurs at high-flow shear rates. A reduction in pulmonary arteriolar lumen size due to either thickened medial muscle or vasoconstriction increases the velocity of flow. Shear stress also increases as blood viscosity rises; therefore, infants with hypoxemia and high hematocrits as well as increased pulmonary blood flow are at increased risk of developing pulmonary vascular disease. In patients with left-to-right shunts, pulmonary arterial hypertension, if not present in infancy or childhood, may never occur or may not develop until the third or fourth decade or later. Once developed, intimal proliferative changes with hyalinization and fibrosis are not reversible by repair of the underlying cardiac defect. In severe pulmonary vascular obstructive disease, arteriovenous malformations may develop and predispose to massive hemoptysis.

Most vexing is the variability among patients with the same or similar cardiac lesions in both the time of appearance and rate of progression of their pulmonary vascular obstructive process. Although genetic influences may be operative (an example is the apparent acceleration of pulmonary vascular disease in patients with congenital heart disease and trisomy 21), evidence is now accumulating for important prenatal and postnatal modifiers of the pulmonary vascular bed that appear, at least in part, to be lesion-dependent. Thus a quantitative variability exists in the pulmonary vascular bed related to the *number,* not just the size and wall structure, of arterial vessels within the pulmonary circulation.[55,56] Modeling of the blood vessels occurs proximal to and within terminal bronchioles (preacinar and intraacinar vessels, respectively) continuously from before birth. The intraacinar vessels, in particular, increase in size and number from late fetal life throughout childhood with minimal muscularization of their walls. The ensuing increase in the cross-sectional area of the pulmonary arterial circulation allows the cardiac output to rise substantially without an increase in pulmonary arterial pressure. If, however, the presence of a cardiac lesion interferes with the normal growth and multiplication of these most peripheral arteries, the resulting elevation of pulmonary vascular resistance may first be related to failure of the intraacinar pulmonary circulation to develop fully, and then secondarily to the morphological changes of obliterative vascular disease—medial thickening, intimal proliferation, hyalinization and fibrosis, angiomatoid and plexiform lesions, and ultimately, arterial necrosis.[53]

In essence, the morphometric framework adds an important dimension, that of growth and development of the pulmonary circulation, to the traditional view of pulmonary vascular obstructive disease occurring primarily as a result of anatomical changes in the individual pulmonary arterioles. Research attention currently focuses on the cell biology of the vessel wall and abnormalities in endothelial cell–smooth muscle interactions in pulmonary hypertension.[51,56]

ASSESSMENT OF THE PATIENT WITH PULMONARY HYPERTENSION. It is important to understand the difficulties that exist with standard methods of assessing the severity of pulmonary vascular obstructive disease. Clinical, electrocardiographic, and echocardiographic observations do not distinguish between reversible and irreversible elevations in pulmonary vascular resistance. Hemodynamic measurements at cardiac catheterization are the mainstay in assessing the pulmonary vascular bed, especially its reactivity. The premium on accuracy is high because the presence, degree, and reactivity of pulmonary vascular obstruction determine the feasibility and long-term outcome of operation. Surgery must not be offered to patients with severe, fixed pulmonary vascular obstruction, even when the cardiac defect is anatomically correctable. Such patients either do not survive operation or, if they do, are not benefited and more often than not are harmed.

The aims of hemodynamic study are to quantify and compare the pulmonary and systemic flows and resistances and to determine the reactivity of the pulmonary vascular bed in patients with pulmonary hypertension. Because resistance to pulmonary blood flow cannot be measured directly, it is calculated from the ratio of pressure gradient to flow across the pulmonary bed according to Poiseuille's equation, which refers to steady flow of a newtonian fluid through straight, rigid tubes. There are potential errors in applying the equation and errors inherent in the methods of measurement. Furthermore, it is not possible in every patient to catheterize the pulmonary artery; when this is the case pulmonary venous wedge pressures may be used, but they are not always reliable indicators of pulmonary artery pressure, and the moment of hemodynamic evaluation may not be representative of potentially variable states of the pulmonary circulation. Nonetheless, a practical index of pulmonary vascular resistance can be established from measurements of pulmonary and systemic arterial pressures and calculated flows. One can then determine whether administration of drugs or oxygen reduces the pulmonary vascular resistance, implying that the resistance is not fixed and therefore may decrease or at least not progress after successful operation. A reduction in calculated pulmonary vascular resistance in response to oxygen inhalation or pharmacological intervention does not exclude coexisting anatomical pulmonary vascular disease, but does imply that there is a component of potentially reversible vasoconstriction contributing to the high resistance.

Other Diagnostic Methods. Because of the aforementioned shortcomings, additional methods have been developed to study the morphology of the small pulmonary arteries in patients with pulmonary hypertension. An example is the use of high-resolution magnification for *pulmonary wedge angiography* to determine the presence and extent of obstructive pulmonary vascular changes.[57] Pulmonary wedge angiograms, assessed quantitatively, appear to correlate well with both hemodynamic findings and histological observations of the structural state of the pulmonary vascular bed. Of additional interest is the current practical application of morphometric structural analyses that attempt to identify for operation patients whose postoperative pulmonary hemodynamics might be expected to improve, if not normalize.[58] Thus, *lung biopsy* at surgery has been proposed in patients with equivocal hemodynamic data to aid in determining whether to proceed with operation in reasonable anticipation of postoperative regression of elevated pulmonary vascular resistance.

THE MORPHOMETRIC APPROACH. Decisions on optimal timing of operations often are difficult because of the varying rates of development of pulmonary vascular disease in different patients with the same anomaly and because the evaluation of pulmonary vascular resistance and reactivity in the catheterization laboratory is a less than perfect science. Preoperative lung biopsy using the Heath-Edwards criteria has enjoyed little popularity, especially because sampling errors may result from the scatter of different grades of lesions in different parts of the lung. Accordingly, it is attractive to seek an alternative method that would obviate these problems. In this regard, application of a morphometric approach holds promise because the described changes in pulmonary vessel morphological characteristics are more uniformly distributed throughout the lung and, importantly, lend themselves to quantification.

Three abnormalities have been identified as anatomical markers of elevated pulmonary vascular resistance: (1) an excessive and premature extension of vascular smooth muscle into intraacinar pulmonary arteries, (2) failure of preacinar arterial wall thickness to regress normally, and (3) failure of pulmonary arteries to grow and proliferate normally during postnatal development. Frozen-section lung biopsy provides a firmer basis for judgment of whether reparative or palliative operation should proceed. The technique has proved useful in patients with univentricular hearts or tricuspid atresia in determining the feasibility of a Fontan procedure (p. 975) and in patients with lesions known to exhibit early and rapidly progressive pulmonary vascular disease, such as complete transposition of the great arteries, complete atrioventricular canal defect, and nonrestrictive ventricular septal defect.

CLINICAL MANIFESTATIONS OF PULMONARY HYPERTENSION. When this condition is associated with a large left-to-right shunt, the clinical manifestations reflect the specific malformation responsible. When pulmonary vascular resistance is elevated and a significant right-to-left shunt exists, the patient is cyanotic, and polycythemia and clubbing are noted. A dominant *a* wave in the jugular venous pulse may be seen, reflecting vigorous right atrial contraction caused by diminished compliance of the right ventricle. In some instances there are large systolic *c-v* waves, which suggest tricuspid regurgitation. A prominent right ventricular parasternal lift and palpable systolic expansion of the pulmonary artery are present. A soft pulmonary systolic ejection murmur preceded by an ejection sound and followed by a markedly accentuated pulmonic component of the second heart sound often is audible on auscultation; an early diastolic decrescendo blowing murmur of pulmonary regurgitation may be heard. If right ventricular failure and dilatation supervene, the systolic murmur of tricuspid regurgitation may be audible at the lower left sternal border. Right ventricular enlargement may be evident on the chest roentgenogram and electrocardiogram. The former examination also reveals a conspicuously enlarged pulmonary artery, prominent hilar pulmonary vascular markings, and attenuated peripheral vessels. The presence of pulmonary hypertension is suggested by analysis of Doppler waveforms of right and left ventricular ejection.[59,60] The site of the underlying defect may be localized by means of two-dimensional and Doppler echocardiography and/or cardiac catheterization and angiocardiography. Pressures in the right side of the heart are essentially identical to systemic pressures in cyanotic patients if the shunt is at the ventricular or aorticopulmonary levels, but they usually are lower than systemic pressures in patients with an intraatrial shunt. No specific treatment has proved beneficial for obstructive pulmonary vascular disease.

This fact underscores the importance of efforts to define the optimal age at operation to provide the highest probability of postoperative normalization of the pulmonary vascular bed. It is important to emphasize that almost all congenital cardiovascular defects are amenable to surgical repair in infancy, and it is likely that the surgical art will progress to the point that virtually all patients with lesions associated with pulmonary hypertension will be operated on within the first 3 to 18 months of life. When this goal is reached without increased operative mortality, the incidence of postoperative pulmonary vascular obstruction may well achieve the status of a bygone concern.

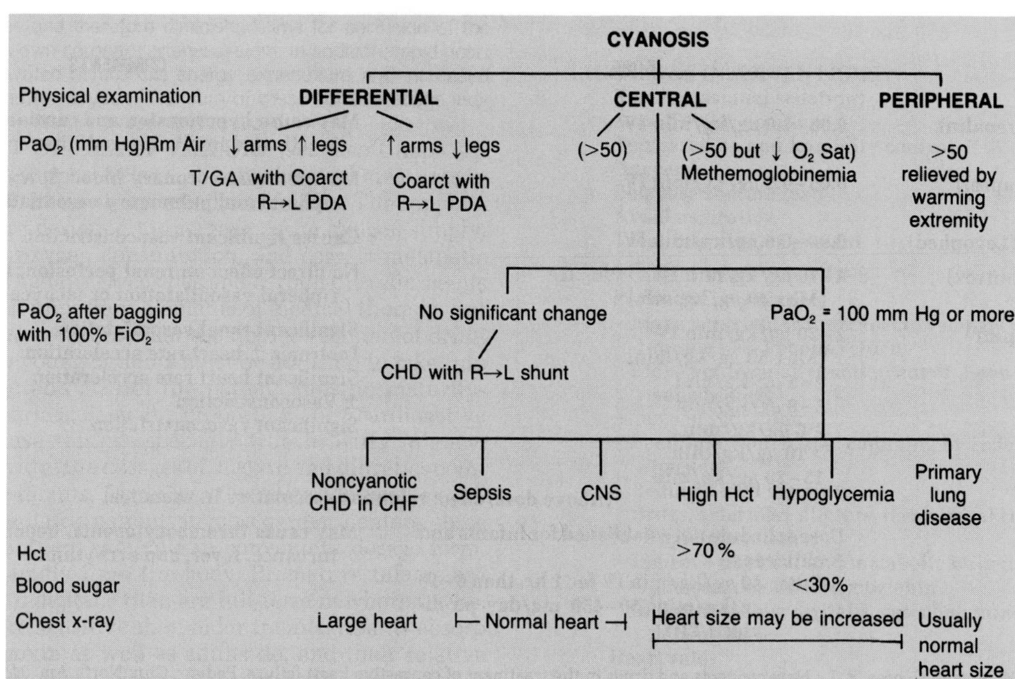

FIGURE 31–8. Flow chart for the evaluation of cyanotic infants. Tests to be done are listed at the left. The response to each of these tests leads along the line to the proper diagnostic category. CHD = congenital heart disease, CHF = congestive heart failure, CNS = central nervous system, Hct = hematocrit, PDA = patent ductus arteriosus, T/GA = transposition of great arteries. (From Kirkpatrick, S. E., et al.: Differential diagnosis of congenital heart disease in the newborn–University of California, San Diego, School of Medicine, and University Hospital, San Diego [Specialty Conference]. West. J. Med. *128*:127, 1978.)

cular resistance to dilate the pulmonary blood vessels and thus reduce the magnitude of the venoarterial shunt. Central cyanosis also may be due to the replacement of normal by abnormal hemoglobin, as in methemoglobinemia.

Several factors influence the oxygen saturation produced at any given arterial pO_2. These include temperature, pH, ratio of fetal to adult hemoglobin, and erythrocyte concentration of 2,3-diphosphoglycerate. For example, fetal hemoglobin has a higher affinity for oxygen than does adult hemoglobin and therefore would be more highly saturated at any given pO_2. Thus, determination of the systemic arterial oxygen tension may provide a more accurate picture of the underlying pathophysiology than simply measuring the oxygen saturation.[76]

DIFFERENTIAL CYANOSIS. Differential cyanosis virtually always indicates the presence of congenital heart disease, often with patency of the ductus arteriosus and coarctation of the aorta as components of the abnormal anatomical complex. If the upper part of the body is pink and the lower part of the body blue, coarctation of the aorta or interruption of the aortic arch is probable, with oxygenated blood supplying the upper body and desaturated blood supplying the lower body by way of right-to-left flow through the ductus arteriosus. The latter also occurs in patients with patent ductus arteriosus and markedly elevated pulmonary vascular resistance. A patient with transposition of the great arteries and coarctation of the aorta with retrograde flow through a patent ductus arteriosus demonstrates the reverse situation, i.e., the lower part of the body is pink and the upper part blue. Simultaneous determinations of oxygen saturation in the temporal or right brachial artery and the femoral artery are helpful in confirming the presence of differential cyanosis.

CENTRAL NERVOUS SYSTEM AND HEMATOLOGICAL CAUSES OF CYANOSIS. Irregular, shallow breathing secondary to central nervous system depression results in reduced alveolar ventilation and an abnormally low alveolar oxygen tension. Alveolar arterial pCO_2 becomes elevated, and arterial pO_2 is reduced. Sedatives and hypnotics administered to the mother during labor cause central nervous system depression in the newborn and intracranial hemorrhage secondary to birth trauma, accounting for most cases.

Methemoglobinemia, either congenital or acquired, is a rare cause of cyanosis in the newborn, with recognizable cyanosis occurring in affected babies when 15 per cent or more of the total hemoglobin is replaced by methemoglobin. Venous blood exposed to room air normally becomes pink but remains dark in infants with methemoglobinemia. Arterial blood with a normal partial pressure of oxygen but a low oxygen saturation should suggest the diagnosis, which may be established conclusively by spectrophotometry.

Differentiating Between Pulmonary and Cardiac Causes of Cyanosis

The distinction between respiratory signs and symptoms arising from cyanotic cardiac disease and those associated with a primary pulmonary disorder is an important challenge to the cardiologist.[33] Upper airway obstruction precipitates cyanosis by producing alveolar hypoventilation owing to reduced pulmonary ventilation. Mechanical obstruction may occur from the nares to the carina, and the important diagnostic possibilities among congenital abnormalities are choanal atresia, vascular ring, laryngeal web, and tracheomalacia. Acquired causes include vocal cord paresis, obstetrical injury to the cricothyroid cartilage, and foreign body. Structural abnormalities in the lungs resulting from intrapulmonary disease are more frequently a basis for cyanosis among newborns than is upper airway obstruction. Hyaline membrane disease, atelectasis, or pneumonitis causing inflammation, collapse, and fluid accumulation in the alveoli results in reduction of the oxygenation of blood reaching the systemic circulation.

Successfully distinguishing between these various causes of cyanosis depends on interpretation of the respiratory pattern, the cardiac physical examination, evaluation of arterial blood gases (Table 31–9), and interpretation of the electrocardiogram, chest x-ray, and echocardiogram.

RESPIRATORY PATTERNS. The key to differential diagnosis at the bedside commonly is the proper evaluation of the pattern of respiration. Term infants normally exhibit a progressive reduction in respiratory rate during the first day of life from 60 to 70 per minute to 35 to 55 per minute. Moreover, mild intercostal retractions and minimal expiratory grunting disappear within several hours of birth. An increased depth of respiration in the presence of cyanosis, but without other signs of respiratory distress, often is associated with congenital cardiac disease in which inadequate pulmonary blood flow is the most important functional component.

The most important variations from normal respiratory patterns are apnea and bradypnea, and tachypnea. Intermittent apneic episodes are common in premature infants with central nervous system immaturity or disease. In addition, higher

TABLE 31–9 ARTERIAL BLOOD GAS PATTERNS IN VARIOUS DISORDERS CAUSING CYANOSIS IN INFANTS

PATTERN	pH	pO_2	pCO_2	RESPONSE TO O_2	VENOUS pH	SUGGESTED CONDITION
1	↓	↓↓	↑	↑↑	↓	Hyaline membrane or other pulmonary parenchymal disease
2	↓	↓	↑↑↑	↑	↓	Hypoventilation
3	—	↓	—	↑	—	Venous admixture
4	↓	↓↓	—	—	↓	Decreased or ineffective pulmonary blood flow
5	↓↓↓	↓	—↑	—↑	↓↓↓↓	Systemic hypoperfusion

— = no effect.

centers may be depressed as a result of severe hypoxemia, acidemia, or the administration of pharmacological agents to mother or baby. The association of apneic episodes, lethargy, hypotonicity, and a reduction in spontaneous movements most often points to intracranial disease as an underlying cause.

Diverse conditions result in tachypnea in the newborn period. Tachypnea in the presence of intrinsic pulmonary disease with upper or lower airway obstruction usually is accompanied by flaring of the alae nasi, chest-wall retractions, and grunting. In contrast, tachypnea associated with intense cyanosis in the absence of obvious respiratory distress suggests the presence of cyanotic congenital heart disease. In general, highest respiratory rates (80 to 110/min) are seen in association with primary lung, and not heart, disease. An initial chest x-ray frequently is diagnostic, especially if the problem is aspiration, mucous plug, adenomatoid malformation, lobar emphysema, diaphragmatic hernia, pneumothorax, lung agenesis, pulmonary hemorrhage, or an abnormal thoracic cage configuration. Choanal atresia may be excluded by passing a feeding tube through the nares, and the more common types of esophageal atresia and tracheoesophageal fistula may be excluded by passing the tube farther into the stomach.

CARDIAC EXAMINATION. Specific findings on cardiovascular examination may direct attention to a cardiac cause for cyanosis. Peripheral perfusion is poor in the presence of severe primary myocardial disease or the hypoplastic left heart syndrome. In contrast, peripheral pulses are bounding and the dorsalis pedis and palmar pulses are easily palpable in infants with patent ductus arteriosus, truncus arteriosus, or aorticopulmonary window. A marked discrepancy between upper- and lower-extremity blood pressures helps to identify the infant with coarctation of the aorta. Inspection and palpation of the precordium allow an overall estimate of cardiac activity. A suprasternal notch and precordial thrill occasionally may be felt in the infant with patent ductus arteriosus, critical aortic stenosis, or coarctation of the aorta. Characterization of the second heart sound may be of help, since it often is single in infants with a hypoplastic left heart complex, pulmonary atresia with or without an intact ventricular septum, or truncus arteriosus. Wide splitting of the second heart sound may occur in infants with total anomalous pulmonary venous return. Ejection sounds often are detectable in infants with persistent truncus arteriosus and occasionally with critical aortic or pulmonic stenosis. The presence of a third heart sound is normal, but a gallop rhythm may provide a clue to myocardial failure. Wide splitting of the first and second heart sounds and prominent third and fourth heart sounds may produce the characteristically rhythmic auscultatory cadence of Ebstein's anomaly of the tricuspid valve (p. 940). The presence of a cardiac murmur may point clearly to underlying cardiac disease, but the absence of a murmur does not exclude the presence of a cardiac malformation. Moreover, cardiac murmurs of specific anomalies often are atypical in the newborn period. However, certain cardiac murmurs such as the decrescendo holosystolic murmur of tricuspid regurgitation in Ebstein's anomaly or the transient tricuspid regurgitation of infancy may point clearly to an accurate diagnosis. Auscultation of the head and abdomen may detect the murmur of an arteriovenous malformation at those sites in infants who present with findings of severe heart failure.

BLOOD GAS AND pH PATTERNS. Arterial blood gas analysis may be a reliable method of evaluating cyanosis, suggesting the type of altered physiology, and assessing responses to therapeutic maneuvers.[48] Specimens for blood gas analysis should be obtained in room air and in 100 per cent oxygen. Stick capillary samples from the patient's warmed heel may be used, although determinations obtained by arterial puncture are preferable for evaluation of oxygenation, since they are less susceptible to alterations in regional blood flow in the critically ill infant. Sampling of right radial or temporal arterial blood is preferable, since these sites are proximal to flow through a ductus arteriosus and do not reflect right-to-left ductal shunting, as would a sample from the descending aorta obtained by means of an umbilical artery catheter. A trial of continuous positive airway pressure may improve oxygenation in infants with either hyaline membrane disease or pulmonary edema. Arterial blood gas patterns in various pathophysiological conditions are listed in Table 31–9. Pattern 1 typically is observed in infants with ventilation-perfusion abnormalities resulting from primary respiratory disease, often associated with elevated pulmonary vascular resistance and venoarterial shunting across a patent foramen ovale or patent ductus arteriosus. Pulmonary hypoventilation with CO_2 retention produces pattern 2. In the presence of a lesion causing obligatory venous admixture, such as total anomalous pulmonary venous connection (pattern 3), the response to oxygen may reflect an increase in pulmonary venous return secondary to a fall in pulmonary vascular resistance. Pattern 4 typically is seen in infants with a cardiac malformation that results in reduced pulmonary blood flow. Oxygen administration in these infants does not alter the arterial pO_2. The alterations of pattern 5 are observed when systemic hypoperfusion is the principal hemodynamic problem. In these babies the arteriovenous oxygen difference is high, and the acidemia may be progressive and unrelenting.

ELECTROCARDIOGRAM. This is less helpful in suggesting a diagnosis of heart disease in the premature and newborn infant than in the older child. Right ventricular hypertrophy is a normal finding in the neonate, and the range of normal voltages is wide. However, specific observations may offer major clues to the presence of a cardiovascular anomaly. A counterclockwise, superiorly oriented frontal QRS loop with absent or reduced right ventricular forces suggests the diagnosis of tricuspid atresia (p. 938). In contrast, when the QRS axis is normal but left ventricular forces predominate, the diagnosis of pulmonic atresia must be considered (p. 933). The counterclockwise, superior QRS orientation also is observed in infants with an endocardial cushion defect (p. 92) and in some with double-outlet right ventricle (p. 948); right ventricular forces in these babies are increased. The initial septal vector should be assessed from the electrocardiogram. Often Q waves are not clearly seen in the lateral precordial leads in the first 72 hours of life. A leftward, posteriorly directed septal vector giving rise to Q waves in the right precordial leads is abnormal, and suggests the presence of marked right ventricular hypertrophy, single ventricle (p. 953), or inversion of the ventricles. T-wave alterations may be seen in a normal neonatal electrocardiogram and may be of no particular consequence. However, by 72 hours of age the T waves should be inverted in V_3 and V_1 and upright in the lateral precordium; persistently upright T waves in the right precordial leads are a sign of right ventricular hypertrophy. Depressed or flattened T waves in the lateral precordium may suggest subendocardial ischemia and a left heart outflow tract obstructive lesion, electrolyte disturbance, acidosis, or hypoxemia. An electrocardiographic pattern of myocardial infarction suggests a diagnosis of anomalous pulmonary origin of the coronary artery (p. 918). Finally, rhythm disturbances such as complete heart block or supraventricular tachycardia can be detected readily by electrocardiography.

RADIOGRAPHIC EXAMINATION (see also p. 228). The chest x-ray often is the single most useful part of the examination in differentiating between respiratory and cardiac causes of cyanosis in the newborn period. Determination of a normal cardiac and abdominal situs aids in ruling out several kinds of complex cyanotic cardiac malformations associated with asplenia or polysplenia with abdominal heterotaxy and dextrocardia (p. 969). The distinct appearance of pulmonary parenchymal disease, such as the classic reticulogranular pattern of hyaline membrane disease, may allow a specific radiological diagnosis. In those premature infants with a large ductus arteriosus the x-ray appearance often evolves from the typical findings of hyaline membrane disease to increased pulmonary vascular markings and finally to perihilar and generalized pulmonary edema. Most important, the pediatric cardiologist depends heavily on the evaluation of pulmonary vascular markings to categorize congenital cardiac malformations in the newborn infant according to function. In the presence of cyanosis, diminished pulmonary vascular markings call attention to the group of anomalies that includes tetralogy of Fallot, pulmonic stenosis with intact ventricular septum, pulmonic atresia, tricuspid atresia, and Ebstein's malformation of the tricuspid valve. Reduced pulmonary blood flow is responsible for the systemic arterial desaturation in these babies. Increased pulmonary vascular markings in the cyanotic infant are associated with lesions in which an obligatory admixture of systemic venous and pulmonary venous blood occurs. The more common anomalies in this category include transposition of the great arteries, hypoplastic left heart syndrome, truncus arteriosus, and total anomalous pulmonary venous drainage.

As mentioned earlier, overall heart size in the normal newborn infant is greater than in the older child, and cardiothoracic ratios up to 0.60 are within normal limits. The thymus shadow occasionally obscures the cardiac silhouette and prohibits accurate estimation of heart size. An enlarged heart on x-ray examination suggests a cardiac disorder. However, in the presence of severe respiratory difficulties with an increase in carbon dioxide tension and a decrease in both pH and arterial oxygen tension, cardiomegaly may be only moderate. A right aortic arch suggests the presence of either tetralogy of Fallot or persistent truncus arteriosus. An ovoid heart with a narrow base associated with increased pulmonary vascular marking is typical of transposition of the great arteries. A boot-shaped heart with concavity of the pulmonary outflow tract suggests tetralogy of Fallot, pulmonic atresia, or tricuspid atresia.

FETAL ECHOCARDIOGRAPHY (see also pp. 89 to 92). Ultrasound technology now allows examination of human fetal cardiac development and function in utero.[30,31] Diagnostic-quality images of the fetal heart in utero can be obtained as early as 16 weeks of gestation. Cardiac structures are imaged primarily by cross-sectional echocardiography and augmented by a combination of rangegated pulse Doppler ultrasonography and M-mode echocardiography.[77-79] The analysis of the structure and function of the fetal heart during the second and third trimesters of pregnancy has allowed cardiologists to counsel prospective parents, and in a number of instances to formulate management plans for pregnancy, delivery, and the immediate postnatal period. Using fetal echocardiography, major forms of congenital heart disease have been diagnosed in utero, and cardiac rhythm abnormalities have been detected, permitting direct efforts at transplacental therapy. In particular, it has been established that a high incidence exists

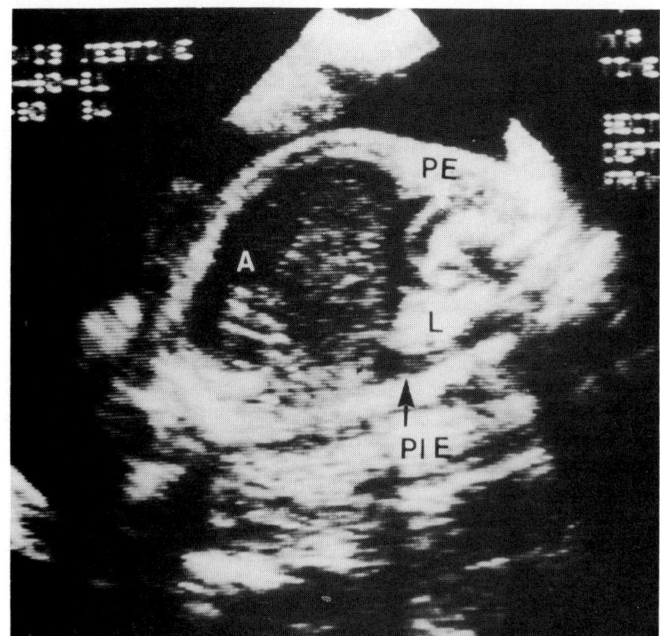

FIGURE 31-9. Abdominal ultrasound examination of a 28-week fetus with nonimmunological hydrops fetalis. A = ascites, PE = pericardial effusion, L = lung, PIE = pleural effusion. The fetal heart is to the right and inferior of the white arrow showing the pericardial effusion.

of cardiac pathology in the presence of nonimmune fetal hydrops. It appears clear that hydrops fetalis often represents end-stage fetal cardiac decompensation (Fig. 31-9). Atrioventricular valve insufficiency often causes fetal right ventricular volume overload and systemic venous hypertension leading to hydrops fetalis.

Pulsed Doppler ultrasound examination of the fetus importantly supplements the echocardiographic findings in identifying the responsible defects, such as Ebstein's malformation of the tricuspid valve, atrial isomerism with atrioventricular septal defects, and the absent pulmonary valve and hypoplastic left heart syndromes.

Fetal cardiac ultrasound is of especial importance in analyzing disturbances of fetal cardiac rhythm, which usually are first suspected on the basis of auscultatory findings. Transabdominal electrocardiography cannot identify atrial depolarization, and is of limited value in the analysis of cardiac arrhythmias in utero. However, M-mode recordings of cardiac motion versus time allow conclusions regarding electrical events in the fetal heart, as they are reflected by the mechanical responses that are recorded echocardiographically. Supraventricular tachyarrhythmias are a common cause of nonimmune fetal hydrops (Fig. 31-10). Detection is of practical use in the management of these patients because the arrhythmia is treatable with use of various antiarrhythmic drugs, such as digoxin, procainamide, propranolol, and verapamil, administered to the mother and reaching the fetus transplacentally or, rarely, under sonographic guidance, by means of injection of drugs, such as amiodarone, into the umbilical vein.[80]

ECHOCARDIOGRAPHY IN THE NEONATE. Echocardiography is of immense value in distinguishing heart disease from lung disease in the newborn.[81] Echocardiographic diagnoses that often can be made with certainty include hypoplastic left heart syndrome, aortic valve stenosis, membranous and fibromuscular subvalvular aortic stenosis, aortic coarctation, hypertrophic cardiomyopathy, cor triatriatum, atrial septal defect, tricuspid atresia, Ebstein's anomaly of the tricuspid valve, valvular pulmonic stenosis, atrioventricular septal defect, single ventricle, double-outlet right ventricle, transposition of the great arteries, and patent ductus arteriosus. The echocardiogram provides suggestive and occasionally conclusive evidence for tetralogy of Fallot, truncus

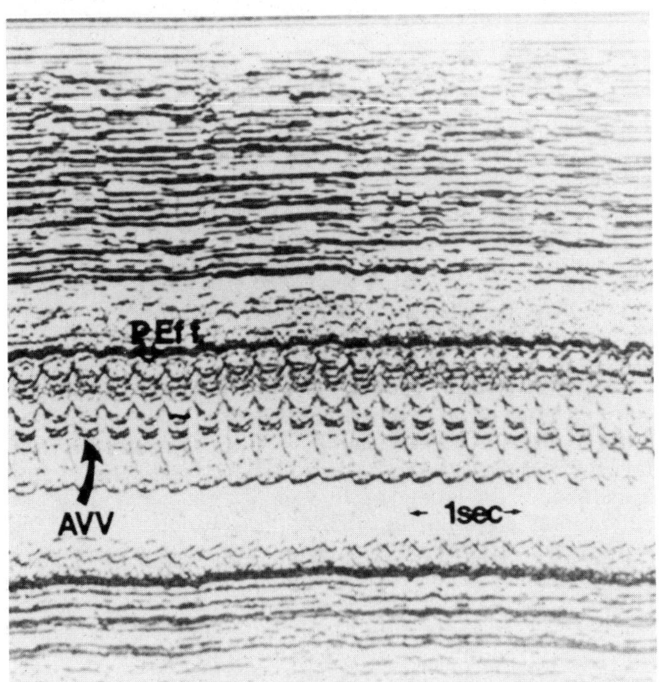

FIGURE 31-10. M-mode echocardiogram at 35 weeks' gestation, showing fetal supraventricular tachycardia and pericardial effusion (PEff). The tracing, taken at the midventricular level, allows the heart rate to be calculated from atrioventricular valve (AVV) motion (250 beats/min). (Courtesy of Charles Kleinman, M.D.)

arteriosus, total anomalous pulmonary venous connection, and pulmonary atresia with an intact ventricular septum.

Doppler ultrasonography (p. 67) has supplemented the two-dimensional echocardiographic examination by its ability to quantify valve gradients, cardiac output, blood flow patterns in the cardiac chambers and great arteries, and often shunt size.[81-84] For example, the pulmonary-systemic blood flow ratio can be calculated by multiplying the square of the ratio of the great vessel diameters by the ratio of the peak systolic flow velocities, the pulmonary variable being the numerator in each ratio.[82] The coupling of Doppler ultrasonographic techniques with the two-dimensional echocardiogram, and the representation in color of abnormalities in flow, volume, and direction (p. 68), greatly improves diagnostic accuracy.

CARDIAC CATHETERIZATION (see also Chap. 7). If a cardiac anomaly is identified by noninvasive studies or if a clear-cut differentiation cannot be made between cardiac and pulmonary disease, heart catheterization and angiocardiography often are necessary to define the underlying state precisely. However, fewer cardiac catheterizations are being performed in infants and children of all ages since the beginning of aggressive pursuit of preoperative diagnoses by noninvasive imaging modalities, particularly two-dimensional–Doppler flow echocardiography.[84] Hemodynamic study of the newborn infant carries a small but distinct risk.[85] As a general rule, cardiac catheterization is not performed unless the information sought is central to the management of the infant. Most infants with serious heart disease require therapeutic intervention, and thus catheterization should be performed only when surgical support is readily available. Cardiac catheterization usually is indicated in most newborns who experience congestive heart failure in the first days after birth if the cause is an anatomical abnormality rather than an arrhythmia or a metabolic disturbance. Preferably, medical measures will have been instituted to stabilize the clinical state before a hemodynamic study is performed.

It is generally agreed that many newborns with cyanotic congenital heart disease require prompt cardiac catheterization, since there is considerable risk of rapid deterioration.[16] Under these circumstances hemodynamic and angiographic study may not only provide the anatomical diagnosis required before emergency operation but also allow the opportunity for therapeutic maneuvers such as balloon atrial septostomy to facilitate intercirculatory mixing in patients with complete transposition of the great arteries or to augment interatrial shunting in patients with a restrictive patent foramen ovale and either tricuspid, pulmonic, or mitral atresia, or total anomalous pulmonary venous connection. The selective infusion of low doses of prostaglandin E_1 (0.05–0.1 μg/kg/min) intravenously has been used before and at cardiac catheterization for the emergency palliation of ductus-dependent cardiac lesions such as pulmonary atresia, aortic coarctation, and interruption of the aortic arch.[71] Because a patent ductus arteriosus maintains pulmonary and systemic blood flow, respectively, in these infants, dilatation of the ductus with vasodilatory prostaglandins may retard their clinical deterioration. Thus, prostaglandin E_1 infusion has been shown to be an effective short-term measure to correct hypoxemia and acidemia and to improve the preoperative and intraoperative status of infants who require surgical relief of the congenital cardiac lesion that is causing pulmonary or systemic hypoperfusion.

Therapeutic Catheterization (see also Chap. 41). Balloon atrial septostomy was the first catheter intervention that proved useful to treat congenital heart disease, and remains the standard initial palliation in infants with complete transposition of the great arteries.[86] Recently, additional transcatheter techniques have been used successfully to treat congenital heart disease.[87-92] These include knife blade atrial septostomy, umbrella closure of patent ductus arteriosus and atrial septal defect, and balloon and coil embolization of large systemic pulmonary artery collateral vessels and arteriovenous fistulas. Other procedures that have expanded the role of the cardiac catheter from a diagnostic tool to a therapeutic instrument include transvenous or transarterial pacemaker insertion and retrieval of foreign bodies from the cardiovascular system. Transluminal balloon angioplasty currently is used principally in pediatrics for dilation of pulmonic valve stenosis, recoarctation of the aorta, and peripheral pulmonary artery stenosis. Unresolved questions exist about transluminal angioplasty in native coarctation and congenital aortic, subaortic, and mitral stenosis. Also investigational is the use of vascular stents, particularly after recurrence of vessel stenoses after balloon dilatation.

Electrophysiological Studies (see also Chap. 22). The cardiac catheterization laboratory also is being used with increasing frequency to define the anatomical and physiological diagnoses of arrhythmias, thus facilitating an accurate prognosis and providing a rational basis for pharmacological or surgical treatment.[93-96] The invasive electrophysiological approach provides unique information that cannot be obtained noninvasively. These include determination of conduction times of individual components of the conducting system and measurement of refractory periods for structures such as the atrioventricular node, His bundle, and bundle branches. In addition, one can determine the initiating features, sustaining mechanisms, and possible perturbations that terminate the arrhythmia. This last maneuver is particularly important, because it may enable the planning of effective drug treatment. It also may determine the advisability of catheter ablation, pacemaker control, or surgical treatment of the rhythm disturbance.

Specific Cardiac Defects

Many classifications of congenital cardiovascular lesions have been proposed on the basis of hemodynamic, anatomical, and radiographic factors. Although there is overlapping between groups, the following arrangement of cardiac anomalies is used in this chapter: (1) communications between the systemic and pulmonary circulations without cyanosis (left-to-right shunts), (2) obstructing valvular and vascular lesions with or without associated right-to-left shunt, (3) abnormalities in the origins of the great arteries and veins (the transposition complexes), (4) malpositions of the heart and cardiac apex, and (5) miscellaneous anomalies.

LEFT-TO-RIGHT SHUNTS

ATRIAL SEPTAL DEFECT

(See also p. 1632)

MORPHOLOGY. Atrial septal defect is one of the most commonly recognized congenital cardiac anomalies in adults but is very rarely diagnosed and even less commonly results in disability in infants.[97] The anatomical sites of interatrial defects are shown in Figure 31–11. Defects of the sinus venosus type are high in the atrial septum near the entry of the superior vena cava and are frequently associated with and may be a consequence of anomalous connection of pulmonary veins from the right lung to the junction of the superior vena cava and right atrium.[98] Most often the atrial septal defect involves the fossa ovalis, is midseptal in location, and is of the ostium secundum type. This type of defect is a true deficiency of the atrial septum and should not be confused with a patent foramen ovale. Embryologically the left side of the atrial septum is derived from the septum primum, which possesses an opening—the interatrial ostium secundum (Fig. 31–3). The ostium secundum lies forward and superior to the position of the foramen ovale. The latter is formed by the septum secundum and occupies the right side of the atrial septum. Tissue of the septum primum lying to the left of the foramen ovale serves as a flap valve that usually becomes fused postnatally with the side of the foramen ovale, yielding an anatomically closed or sealed foramen. "Probe patency," or an incomplete seal of the foramen ovale, occurs in about 25 per cent of adults. A widely patent foramen ovale may be considered an acquired form of atrial septal defect that occurs especially when a disproportion exists between the size of the foramen ovale and the effective length of its valve. Enlargement of the foramen ovale per se is commonly associated with obstructive lesions of the right side of the heart, whereas a short valve relative to the size of the foramen often is seen in large-volume left-to-right shunts in which left atrial dilatation is prominent.

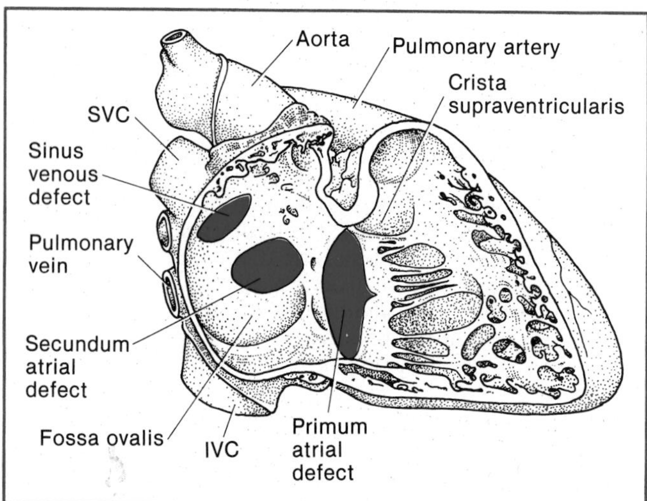

FIGURE 31–11. Composite locations of atrial defects. S.V.C. = superior vena cava, I.V.C. = inferior vena cava.

Ostium primum atrial septal anomalies are a form of atrioventricular septal defect and will be dealt with in the next section. Lutembacher's syndrome is a designation applied to the rare combination of atrial septal defect and mitral stenosis, which is almost invariably the result of acquired rheumatic valvulitis.[99] Ten to 20 per cent of patients with ostium secundum atrial septal defect also have prolapse of the mitral valve as an associated anomaly.[100]

HEMODYNAMICS. The magnitude of the left-to-right shunt through an atrial septal defect depends on the size of the defect and the relative compliance of the ventricles, and the relative resistance in both the pulmonary and the systemic circulation.[101] In patients with a small atrial septal defect or patent foramen ovale, the left atrial pressure may exceed the right by several millimeters of mercury, whereas the mean pressures in both atria are nearly identical when the defect is large. Left-to-right shunting occurs predominantly in late ventricular systole and early diastole with some augmentation during atrial contraction. The shunt results in diastolic overloading of the right ventricle and increased pulmonary blood flow. During the first few days and weeks of life pulmonary resistance falls and systemic resistance rises, facilitating right ventricular emptying and impeding left ventricular emptying; the left-to-right shunt rises. Early in infancy left-to-right flow through even a large interatrial communication commonly is limited by both the reduced chamber compliance of the thick neonatal right ventricle and the elevated pulmonary and reduced systemic vascular resistance of the neonate. The pulmonary vascular resistance commonly is normal or low in the older infant or child with atrial septal defect, and the volume load usually is well tolerated, even though pulmonary blood flow may be two to five times greater than systemic. A transient and small right-to-left shunt occurring with the onset of left ventricular contraction and especially during respiratory periods of decreasing intrathoracic pressure is common in patients with ostium secundum defect, even in the absence of pulmonary hypertension.

CLINICAL FINDINGS. Patients with atrial septal defect usually are asymptomatic early in life, although occasional reports exist of congestive heart failure and recurrent pneumonia in infancy.[97] Children with atrial septal defect may experience easy fatigability and exertional dyspnea. They tend to be somewhat underdeveloped physically and prone to respiratory infection. Atrial arrhythmias, pulmonary arterial hypertension, development of pulmonary vascular obstruction, and heart failure are exceedingly uncommon in the pediatric age range, in contrast to their common appearance in adults with atrial septal defect. In the former group, diagnosis often is entertained after detection of a heart murmur on routine physical examination prompts a more extensive cardiac evaluation.

Common findings on *physical examination* include a prominent right ventricular cardiac impulse and palpable pulmonary artery pulsation. The first heart sound is normal or split, with accentuation of the tricuspid valve closure sound. Increased flow across the pulmonic valve is responsible for a midsystolic pulmonary ejection murmur. After the normal postnatal drop in pulmonary vascular resistance, the second heart sound is split widely and is relatively fixed in relation to respiration in patients with normal pulmonary pressures and low pulmonary vascular impedance because of a delay in pulmonic valve closure. With pulmonary hypertension the splitting interval is a function of the electromechanical intervals of each ventricle; wide splitting occurs with shortening of the left and/or lengthening of the right ventricular electromechanical interval.[102] If the shunt is large, increased blood flow across the tricuspid valve is responsible for a middiastolic rumbling murmur at the lower left sternal border. In patients with associated prolapse of the mitral valve an apical holosystolic or late systolic murmur radiating to the axilla often is heard, but a midsystolic click may be difficult to discern. Moreover, left ventricular precordial overactivity usually is absent because mitral regurgitation is mild in most patients.

In the teenage patient, the physical findings may be altered when an increase in pulmonary vascular resistance results in diminution of the left-to-right shunt. Both the pulmonary and the tricuspid murmurs decrease in intensity, whereas the pulmonic component of the second heart sound becomes accentuated and the two components of the second heart sound may fuse; a diastolic murmur of pulmonic incompetence appears. Cyanosis and clubbing accompany development of a right-to-left shunt.

The *electrocardiogram* in patients with an ostium secundum defect usually shows right-axis deviation, right ventricular hypertrophy, and rSR′ or rsR′ pattern in the right precordial leads with a normal QRS duration (Fig. 31-12 and Fig. 30, p. 159). It is not clear whether the delay in right ventricular activation is a manifestation of right ventricular volume overload or a true conduction delay in the right bundle branch and peripheral Purkinje system.[103] Left-axis deviation of the P wave in the frontal plane (manifested by a negative P wave in lead III) suggests the presence of a sinus venosus rather than an ostium secundum type of atrial septal defect. Left-axis deviation and superior orientation and counterclockwise rotation of the QRS loop in the frontal plane suggests the presence of either an ostium primum defect or a secundum atrial septal defect in association with mitral valve prolapse. Prolongation of the P-R interval may be seen with all types of atrial septal defects; the prolonged internodal conduction time may be related to both the increased size of the atrium and the increased distance for internodal conduction produced by the defect itself.[103] *Chest roentgenograms* (Figs. 8-41*A*, p. 229, and 32-4, p. 969) reveal enlargement of the right atrium and ventricle, dilatation of the pulmonary artery and its branches, and increased pulmonary vascular markings. Dilatation of the proximal portion of the superior vena cava occasionally is noted in patients with a sinus venosus defect. Left atrial dilatation is

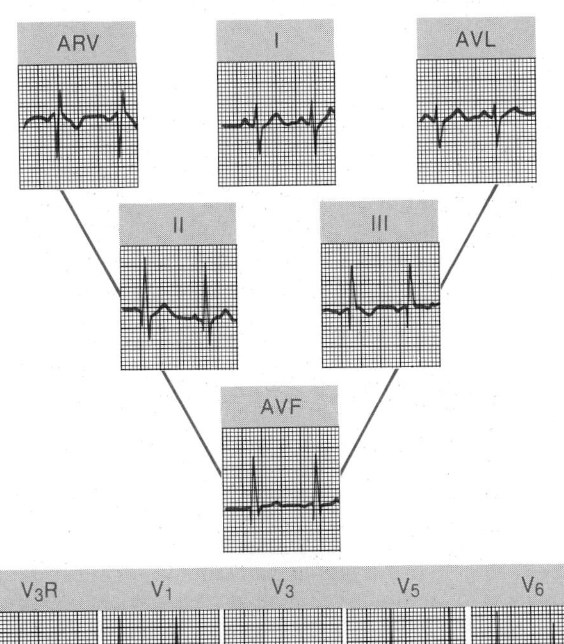

FIGURE 31-12. Typical electrocardiographic tracing in secundum atrial septal defect showing right axis deviation, rSR′ in the right precordial leads, and right ventricular hypertrophy. (Courtesy of Delores A. Danilowicz, M.D.)

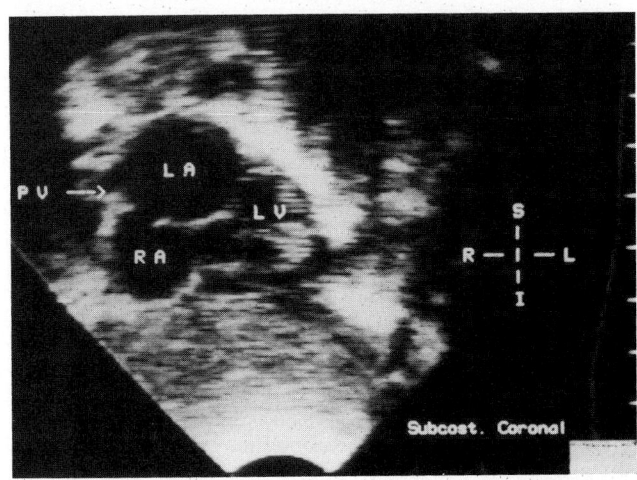

FIGURE 31-13. Subcostal coronal view showing a secundum atrial septal defect between the left atrium (LA) and the right atrium (RA). The right upper pulmonary vein (PV) is seen entering the left atrium. This view is posterior to the major portion of the ventricles; the left ventricle (LV) is seen, but only a small portion of the right ventricle (unlabeled) is apparent. I = inferior, L = left, R = right, S = superior. (Courtesy of Norman Silverman, M.D.)

extremely rare but may be observed when significant mitral regurgitation exists. Echocardiographic features include pulmonary arterial and right ventricular dilatation and anterior systolic (paradoxical) or "flat" interventricular septal motion if significant right ventricular volume overload is present.[81] The defect may be visualized directly by two-dimensional echo imaging, particularly from a subcostal view of the interatrial septum[36] (Fig. 31-13; also see Fig. 4-76, p. 93). Transesophageal color-coded Doppler echocardiography provides excellent visualization of defects of the atrial septum.[104] Associated mitral valve prolapse also may be identified by echocardiographic examination (Figs. 4-50 and 4-51, p. 84). Findings on ultrafast computed tomographic scanning are illustrated in Figure 11-12, p. 319.

In most institutions, two-dimensional echocardiography, supplemented by conventional or color-coded Doppler flow and/or contrast echocardiography, has supplanted cardiac catheterization as the confirmatory test for atrial septal defect.[105,106] Cardiac catheterization is then used if inconsistencies exist in the clinical data or if significant pulmonary hypertension is suspected.

Diagnosis may be readily confirmed at *cardiac catheterization* by passage of the catheter across the atrial defect. The site at which the catheter crosses, if high in the cardiac silhouette, may suggest a sinus venosus defect; if midseptal, a patent foramen ovale or ostium secundum defect; or, if low, a primum defect.[107] Serial determinations of the oxygen saturation or indicator dilution curve techniques may be used to estimate the magnitude of the shunt. In young patients, pressures on the right side of the heart often are normal, despite a large shunt. When a high oxygen saturation is found in the superior vena cava or when the catheter enters pulmonary veins directly from the right atrium, a sinus venosus defect is likely, and indicator dilution curves and selective angiography will aid in identifying the number and location of the anomalous veins. Partial anomalous pulmonary venous connection, although usually associated with sinus venosus defect, may accompany secundum defects. Selective left ventricular angiography will identify prolapse of the mitral valve and allow assessment of the magnitude of mitral regurgitation that may be present in such patients.

In contrast to adults, children with sinus venosus or secundum types of atrial septal defect seldom require treatment for heart failure or antiarrhythmic medications for atrial fibrillation or supraventricular tachycardia. Respiratory tract infections should be treated promptly. Although the risk of infective endocarditis is low, antibiotics should be administered prophylactically before dental procedures.

MANAGEMENT. *Operative repair* (ideally in those 2 to 4 years of age) should be advised for all patients with uncomplicated atrial septal defects in whom there is evidence of significant left-to-right shunting, i.e., with pulmonary-systemic flow ratios exceeding about 1.5:1.0. Rarely, an atrial septal aneurysm is seen in association with a secundum-type atrial septal defect.[108] Such patients may experience spontaneous closure, and may be followed more conservatively until an older age before advising operation. The defect is closed by suture or with a patch of prosthetic material with the patient on cardiopulmonary bypass. Earlier surgical repair is definitive treatment for the small number of infants and young children with significant symptoms or congestive failure. The surgical mortality rate is less than 1 per cent, and results usually are excellent. Although the mitral valve may be examined directly at operation, it seldom is necessary in childhood to attempt plication or replacement of a ballooning or prolapsing mitral valve. Operation should not be carried out in patients with small defects and trivial left-to-right shunts (pulmonary-systemic flow ratio ≤1.5:1.0) or in those with severe pulmonary vascular disease (pulmonary-systemic resistance ratio ≥0.7:1.0) without a significant left-to-right shunt.[109] Still investigational is the use of transcatheter closure by way of a clamshell-configuration double umbrella using fluoroscopic or transesophageal echocardiographic imaging guidance.[89]

Subtle evidence of left ventricular dysfunction may be observed preoperatively at cardiac catheterization in children with isolated large atrial septal defects but without overt left or right ventricular failure.[110] Thus decreased left ventricular stroke volume and cardiac output have been observed in children with both low and normal left ventricular end-diastolic volumes. In routine catheterization studies carried out on patients whose atrial septal defects were closed during preadolescence or later, a residual reduced cardiac output response to intense upright exercise in the absence of residual shunts, arrhythmias, or pulmonary arterial hypertension has been observed.[110,111] Normal myocardial function is preserved in patients in whom the defects were closed in early childhood.

Intracardiac electrophysiological studies reveal a high incidence of intrinsic dysfunction of the sinoatrial and atrioventricular nodes, which persists after surgical repair. These intrinsic nodal abnormalities are more common in sinus venosus than in ostium secundum defects,[112,113] but occur in both varieties. There also is evidence that the type of venous cannulation at the time of operative repair may contribute to the incidence and severity of arrhythmias observed at long-term follow-up.[114]

ATRIOVENTRICULAR (AV) SEPTAL DEFECT

AV septal defects comprise a range of malformations characterized by varying degrees of incomplete development of the inferior portion of the atrial septum, the inflow portion of the ventricular septum, and the AV valves (Fig. 31–3). These anomalies also have been called endocardial cushion defects and AV septal defects. The basic defect is a deficiency of the AV septum which separates the left ventricular inlet from the right atrium; it causes anomalies which range in severity from a small ostium primum atrial septal defect to a complete AV septum, which also involves defects in the interventricular septum and the mitral and tricuspid valves. The latter often are abnormal to varying degrees, with five or six leaflets present of variable size, and variability also in the completeness of their commissures. Often AV septal defects are encountered in association with other congenital abnormalities, such as asplenia or polysplenia syndromes, trisomy 21 (Down syndrome), and Ellis–van Creveld syndrome of ectodermal dysplasia and polydactyly.

OSTIUM PRIMUM DEFECT (PARTIAL AV CANAL). Ostium primum atrial septal defects lie immediately adjacent to the AV valves, either of which may be deformed and incompetent. Most often only the anterior or septal leaflet of the mitral valve is displaced, and it commonly is cleft; the tricuspid valve usually is not involved. A cleft often is considered to be present in the mitral valve, although it is likely that the valve is in fact a trileaflet structure, with the cleft representing an abnormal commissure. The interatrial defect often is large, and the size of the left-to-right interatrial shunt in these patients is controlled by the same factors that exist in patients with ostium secundum atrial septal defect. Moreover, the clinical features are quite similar, and principally consist of right ventricular precordial hyperactivity, a wide and persistently split second heart sound, a right ventricular outflow tract systolic ejection murmur, and a middiastolic tricuspid flow rumble. The murmurs of AV valve regurgitation may be audible if either valve is significantly abnormal; however, serious AV valve regurgitation usually is absent. In the occasional patient, mitral regurgitation is substantial and creates prominent signs of left ventricular overload.

Chest roentgenography usually reveals right atrial and ventricular cardiomegaly, prominence of the right ventricular outflow tract, and increased pulmonary vascular markings. The *electrocardiogram* is characteristic, and shows a right ventricular conduction defect accompanied by left anterior division block, left-axis deviation, and superior orientation and counterclockwise rotation of the QRS loop in the frontal plane (Fig. 5–21, p. 131).[115] Hemodynamic factors do not appear to be important in producing the characteristic electrocardiogram. Rather, the superior QRS vector in patients with a shortened H-V interval appears to be related to early activation of the posterobasal left ventricular wall; in other patients with a normal conduction time between the bundle of His and the ventricles, the counterclockwise superior inscription of the frontal plane vector appears to be related to late activation of the anterolateral left ventricular wall.[116,117] A prolonged P-R interval is observed in many patients with an ostium primum atrial septal defect; prolonged internodal conduction may be related to displacement of the AV node in a posteroinferior direction in some patients or to the enlarged right atrium, or both.[118]

Echocardiographic features (Fig. 4–77, p. 93) include enlargement of both the right ventricle and the pulmonary artery, systolic anterior ventricular septal motion, prolonged mitral-septal apposition in diastole, and various abnormalities in mitral valve motion.[119,120] The defect is easily visualized from the precordial apical and subxiphoid positions, with the latter views best demonstrating the relation between the atrial defect, AV valves, and the interventricular septum (Figs. 31–14 and 4–77, p. 93, color plate No. 4). Interatrial septal tissue is absent in the region of the crest of the interventricular septum; the trileaflet configuration of the mitral valve also may be identified. The subxiphoid long-axis view of the left ventricular outflow tract exhibits the "gooseneck" deformity in a manner similar to that with a right anterior oblique left ventricular angiogram (see Fig. 31–16). Echocardiography is particularly useful for detecting and characterizing double-orifice mitral valve, an association in about 3 per cent of patients with ostium primum atrial defect. It also allows detection of single left ventricular papillary muscle, hypoplasia of the left ventricle, and coarctation of the aorta, seen especially in symptomatic infants with an ostium primum atrial defect but without trisomy 21.[121] The *angiographic features* resemble those in the complete form of AV septal defect and are discussed below.

COMPLETE AV SEPTAL DEFECT. The complete form of the AV septal defect includes, in addition to the ostium primum atrial septal defect, a ventricular septal defect in the posterior basal inlet portion of the ventricular septum and a common AV orifice. The common AV valve usually has six leaflets: left superior and inferior, left and right lateral, and right superior and inferior. The left and right superior leaflets together often are referred to as the "anterior" bridging leaflet. No attachment exists between the left superior and inferior leaflets and the right superior and inferior leaflets. The left superior leaflet may cross the crest of the ventricular septum to reside partially on the right ventricular side. A classifica-

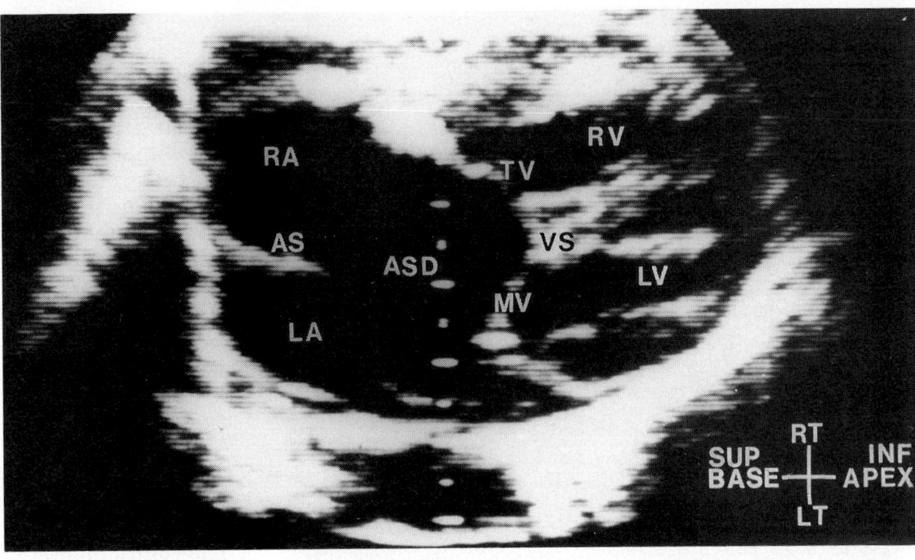

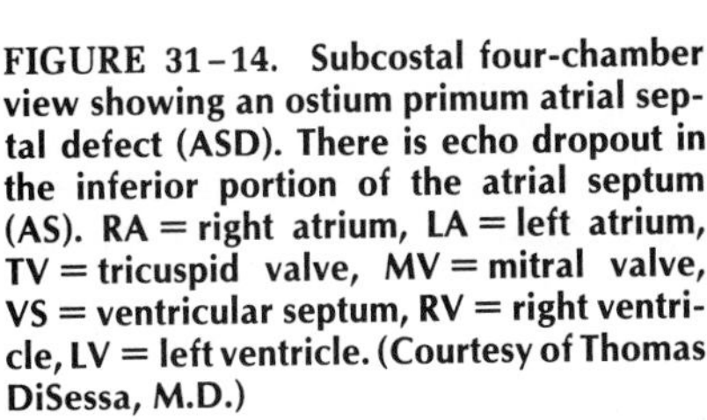

FIGURE 31-14. Subcostal four-chamber view showing an ostium primum atrial septal defect (ASD). There is echo dropout in the inferior portion of the atrial septum (AS). RA = right atrium, LA = left atrium, TV = tricuspid valve, MV = mitral valve, VS = ventricular septum, RV = right ventricle, LV = left ventricle. (Courtesy of Thomas DiSessa, M.D.)

tion of complete AV canal defect into types A, B, and C reflects the variability and the degree of left superior leaflet bridging of the ventricular septum. Thus in type A the left superior leaflet is entirely over the left ventricle, and together with the right superior leaflet is attached by chordae tendineae to the crest of the ventricular septum. In type C there is marked rightward displacement of the left superior leaflet, which floats freely over the crest of the ventricular septum and is not attached to it by chordae tendineae. In type B chordal attachments extend medially to an anomalous papillary muscle adjacent to the septum in the right ventricle.

A high incidence (about 35 per cent) of additional cardiovascular lesions exists in patients with common AV canal. Principal among these are tetralogy of Fallot, double-outlet right ventricle, transposition of the great arteries, total anomalous pulmonary venous connection, variable sites of left ventricular outflow tract obstruction, pulmonic stenosis, and persistent left superior vena cava. Moreover, the complete AV septal anomaly commonly is seen in patients with Down syndrome.

Diagnosis. Patients with common AV septal defects present clinically under age 1 year with a history of frequent respiratory infections and poor weight gain. Heart failure in infancy is extremely common. The *physical findings* are similar to those observed in patients with ostium primum atrial septal defect but may include as well the holosystolic, lower left sternal border murmur of an interventricular communication and/or the decrescendo, holosystolic apical murmur of mitral regurgitation. The *electrocardiographic features* of complete AV canal defects resemble those in the partial ostium primum variety of AV septal anomalies (Fig. 31-12, p. 907). *Radiographically*, the usual findings are generalized cardiomegaly and engorged pulmonary vessels. Two-dimensional echocardiography is diagnostic (Figs. 31-15 and 4-78, p. 94).[119,120] The atrial defect appears as a dropout of echoes from the leftmost portion of the interatrial septum immediately above the AV valves. AV leaflet morphology is best seen from the parasternal and subxiphoid short-axis views, with simultaneously visualized superior and inferior leaflets. The ventricular defect lies beneath the AV valve leaflets. On *hemodynamic study*, patients with persistent common AV canal invariably have elevated pulmonary arterial pressures; beyond age 2 years a significant number of these patients have progressively severe pulmonary vascular obstructive disease.

Diagnosis also is reliably established by selective left ventricular *angiocardiography* using rapid injection of relatively large quantities of contrast material. The findings include an absence of the AV septum and a deficiency of the inlet portion of the ventricular septum, with elongation of the left ventricular outflow tract in relation to the inflow tract. The leaflets of the left AV valve often may be visualized to determine the location and magnitude of valvar incompetence. The aortic valve is elevated and displaced anteriorly relative to the AV valves, changing the relation between the anterior components of the left AV valve and the aorta, which produces a pathognomonic "gooseneck" deformity seen angiographically in diastole (Fig. 31-16). Additional findings include a jet of

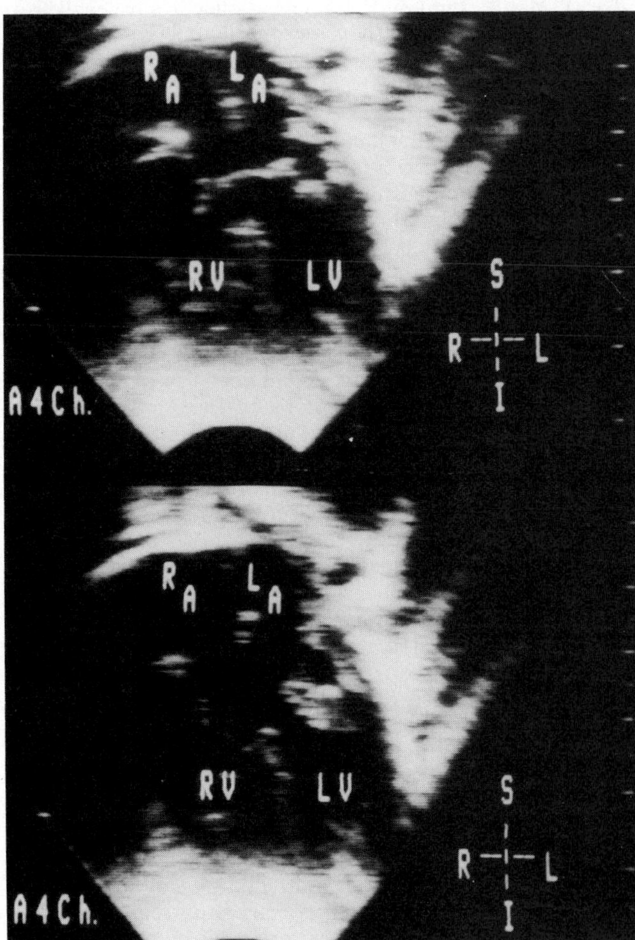

FIGURE 31-15. Apical four-chamber views of a common atrioventricular septal defect. The images are oriented anatomically. In systole, shown in the top panel, the atrioventricular valve leaflet is closed, with no apparent attachment of the atrioventricular valve to the ventricular septum. The interatrial and interventricular septal defects are represented by echo dropout above and below the common AV valve. In diastole, shown in the bottom panel, the AV valve is open, showing the valve resting on the crest of the ventricular septum and the entire defect allowing communication between all four cardiac chambers. RA = right atrium, LA = left atrium, RV = right ventricle, LV = left ventricle. (Courtesy of Norman Silverman, M.D.)

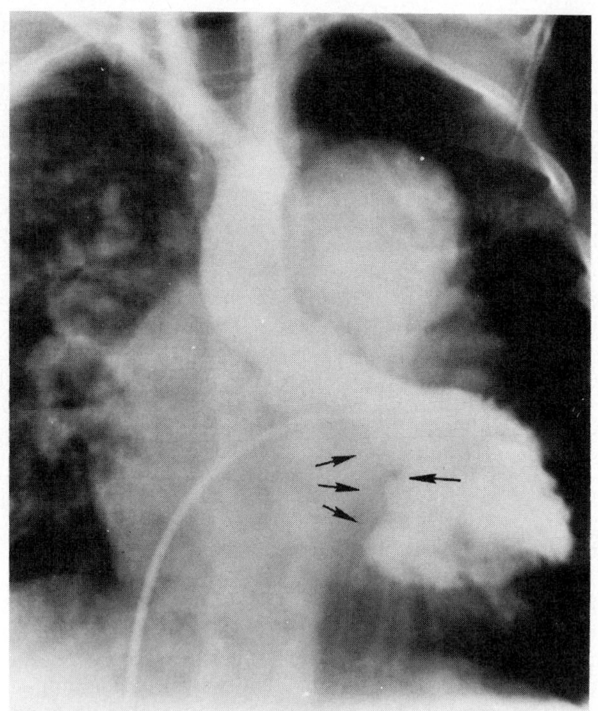

FIGURE 31–16. Left ventriculogram in systole in a patient with an endocardial cushion defect. The concavity of the right border of the left ventricle (left arrows) is caused by the abnormal position of the mitral orifice.

contrast material from left ventricle directly to right atrium or by way of mitral regurgitation and left-to-right atrial shunting. Conventional anteroposterior and lateral left ventricular angiographic views may not always differentiate between the partial and complete types of AV septal defects because all have the characteristic "gooseneck" left ventricular outflow tract deformity and because mitral regurgitation into the right atrium may obscure the presence or absence of a defect in the ventricular septum. Axial cine angiography, however, permits a more accurate distinction between types of AV septal defects, since the hepatoclavicular view helps greatly in separating a left ventricular–right atrial communication and shunt from left ventricular–left atrial regurgitation with subsequent left-to-right atrial shunt. In addition, the long axial oblique view portrays the AV portion of the ventricular septum.[122]

Management. In patients with complete AV canal, cardiac decompensation should be controlled initially. If an adequate response to medical therapy occurs early in life, hemodynamic study is indicated at about age 3 to 6 months to determine the level of pulmonary vascular resistance, since infants with the complete form of the AV septal defect are at high risk of obstructive pulmonary vascular disease. The level of major shunting should be determined during the initial hemodynamic and angiographic study, since if it is mainly at the ventricular level, pulmonary artery banding occasionally may be advised for intractable heart failure and failure to thrive. Often, however, there is a significant left ventricular–right atrial shunt either directly or indirectly by way of mitral regurgitation and left-to-right interatrial shunting, which will be unaffected by pulmonary artery banding and requires complete surgical correction. In most centers primary repair in patients who have intractable heart failure, growth failure, or severe pulmonary hypertension is the preferred approach at any age.[123–126] Mild to moderate regurgitation often persists after surgical repair, particularly if significant AV valve incompetence existed preoperatively.[127] Rarely, if left AV leaflet tissue is remarkably deficient or deformed, mitral valve replacement may be required. Recent advances in the surgical approach to complex forms of AV septal defects have greatly improved the outlook for patients born with this malformation.[127a] These include a more precise preoperative detection of such anatomical features as additional muscular ventricular septal defects, malalignment of the complete AV septum, and left ventricular hypoplasia.[126] Operative improvement is primarily related to a clearer understanding of the anatomy of this complex lesion and to the ability to reconstruct the left AV valve, often by splitting of papillary muscles and shortening of chordae tendineae, with or without annuloplasty. Many surgeons prefer to close the septal defects with a single patch rather than separating ventricular and atrial patches. Suture placement is avoided in the region of the AV node and the bundle of His.

VENTRICULAR SEPTAL DEFECT

(See also p. 944)

Among the most prevalent of cardiac malformations, defects of the ventricular septum occur commonly, both as isolated anomalies and in combination with other anomalies. The ventricular septum is made up of four compartments: the membranous septum, the inlet septum, the trabecular septum, and the outlet, or infundibular, septum. Defects result from a deficiency of growth or a failure of alignment or fusion of component parts. Defects most commonly are classified as occurring in or adjacent to one or more of the septal components (Fig. 31–17).[127–130]

The most common defects occur in the region of the membranous septum, and are referred to as paramembranous or perimembranous defects because they are larger than the membranous septum itself, and are associated with a muscular defect at a portion of their perimeter. They also are known as infracristal, subaortic, or conoventricular defects. These perimembranous defects also can be defined by their adjacent

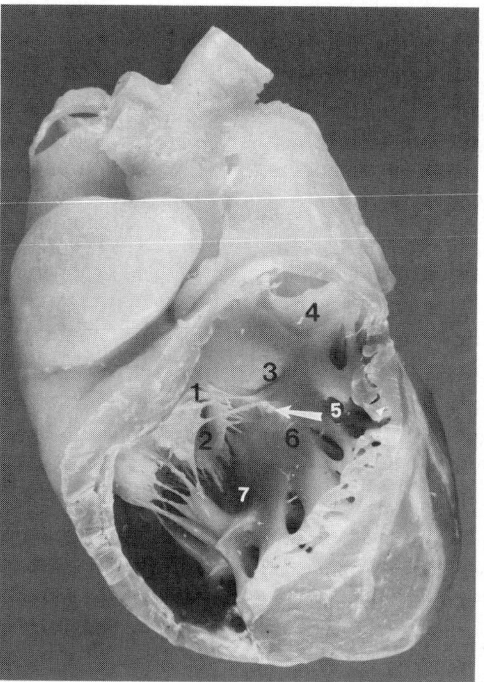

FIGURE 31–17. Heart specimen with right ventricular free wall removed to expose the locations of the various sites of ventricular septal defects. Perimembranous defects (1) lie at the right superior margin of the tricuspid valve. Inlet or atrioventricular septal defects (2) lie beneath the septal leaf of the tricuspid valve and may extend to the tricuspid annulus. Malalignment subaortic outflow or conoseptal defects (3) lie superior to the attachment of the septal tricuspid leaflet to the papillary muscle of the conus (arrow). The subpulmonary defect (4) is to the left of malalignment defects, and also is referred to as doubly committed subarterial. Muscular defects lie within the trabecular septum and may be located in the anterior (5), middle (6), or posterior (7) muscular septum. (Courtesy of Roberta G. Williams, M.D.)

areas as inlet, trabecular, or outlet. A second type of defect is one with an entirely muscular rim. Such muscular defects also can be defined as inlet, trabecular, outlet, or various combinations, and vary greatly in size, shape, and number. A third type of defect occurs when the outlet septum is deficient, and commonly is referred to as supracristal, subpulmonary, outlet, infundibular, or conoseptal. Because the aortic and pulmonary valves are in fibrous continuity, this type of defect also may be referred to as doubly committed subarterial. A septal deficiency of the site of the atrioventricular septum characterizes defects called atrioventricular septal, atrioventricular canal, or inlet septal defects.

The other feature of any defect may be a malalignment of the septal components. Either the inlet or the outlet septum can be malaligned. Malalignment of the inlet septum produces either mitral or tricuspid valve override and/or straddle. Malalignment of the outlet septum can be to the right or the left of the trabecular septum; when to the left of the trabecular septum, the ventricular septal defect is characteristic of tetralogy of Fallot, double-outlet ventricle, truncus arteriosus, and, in some cases, transposition of the great arteries.

TWO-DIMENSIONAL ECHOCARDIOGRAPHY. This technique identifies the type of defect in the ventricular septum.[131-134] Perimembranous ventricular septal defects are identified by septal dropout in the area behind the septal leaflet of the tricuspid valve and below the right border of the aortic annulus. The subaortic or anterior malalignment type of ventricular septal defect appears just below the posterior semilunar valve cusps, entirely superior to the tricuspid valve. The subpulmonary ventricular septal defect appears as echo dropout within the outflow septum, which extends to the pulmonary annulus. One or two of the aortic cusps may be visualized protruding through the defect into the right ventricular outflow tract. The inlet atrioventricular septal–type of ventricular septal defect extends from the fibrous annulus of the tricuspid valve into the muscular septum, and often is entirely beneath the septal tricuspid leaflet. Muscular defects may appear anywhere throughout the ventricular septum, and may be either single and large, or small and multiple. Anatomical localization of all ventricular septal defects is facilitated by coupling two-dimensional ultrasound images (Fig. 4–80, p. 94) with a Doppler system, and also by superimposing a color-coded direction and velocity of blood flow on the real-time images.[135-138]

PATHOPHYSIOLOGY. In general, the functional disturbance caused by a ventricular septal defect depends primarily on its size and the status of the pulmonary vascular bed rather than on the location of the defect. A small ventricular septal defect with high resistance to flow permits only a small left-to-right shunt. A large interventricular communication allows a large left-to-right shunt only if there is no pulmonic stenosis or high pulmonary vascular resistance, since these factors also determine shunt flow. Resistance to left ventricular emptying also affects shunt flow because it is an important factor in determining left ventricular pressure. Large defects allow both ventricles to function hemodynamically as a single pumping chamber with two outlets, equalizing the pressure in the systemic and pulmonary circulations. In such patients the magnitude of the left-to-right shunt varies inversely with pulmonary vascular resistance.

A wide spectrum exists in the natural history of ventricular septal defects, ranging from spontaneous closure to congestive cardiac failure and death in early infancy. Within this spectrum are possible development of pulmonary vascular obstruction, right ventricular outflow tract obstruction, aortic regurgitation, and infective endocarditis.[137-146]

INFANCY. It is unusual for a ventricular septal defect to cause difficulties in the immediate postnatal period, although congestive heart failure during the first 6 months of life is a frequent occurrence. Early diagnosis is helpful to insure more careful observation of the affected infant.[143] The examining physician usually suspects the diagnosis because of a harsh systolic murmur at the lower left sternal border. The electrocardiogram and chest roentgenogram are within normal limits in the immediate neonatal period because appreciable left-to-right shunting occurs only after the pulmonary vascular resistance decreases as the pulmonary vessels lose their fetal characteristics. It is desirable to follow these infants closely. A ventricular septal defect that either decreases in size or closes completely during the first year of life presents no problems to the practicing physician. Spontaneous closure occurs by age 3 years in about 45 per cent of patients born with ventricular septal defect; occasional patients, however, do not experience spontaneous closure until age 8 to 10 years.[141] Closure is more common in patients born with a small ventricular septal defect; nonetheless, about 7 per cent of infants with a large defect and congestive heart failure early in life also may experience spontaneous closure. Partial rather than complete closure is common in patients with both large and small ventricular septal defects. Anatomically, reduction of the ventricular septal defect often is based on adherence of the tricuspid valve to the defect, hypertrophy of septal muscle, or ingrowth of fibrous tissue. Rarely, closure of the ventricular septal defect is the result of prolapse of an aortic cusp[145] or infective endocarditis.[144] Some defects close when an aneurysm forms in the ventricular septum.[142] On auscultation a click may be heard in early systole as the aneurysm tenses toward the right; the septal aneurysm may be detected by echocardiography as an anterior systolic bulge in the right ventricular outflow tract. A persistent minute ventricular septal defect is not life-threatening unless infective endocarditis develops. With proper precautions the incidence of this complication is less than 1 per cent.

If a moderate or large defect maintains its size after birth, the net left-to-right shunt increases during the first month of life as pulmonary vascular resistance falls. *Physical examination* during this time usually reveals a thrill along the lower left sternal border, and the holosystolic murmur of flow across the interventricular defect is accompanied by a low-pitched diastolic rumble at the apex, reflecting increased flow across the mitral valve. *Chest roentgenograms* reveal increased pulmonary vascular markings; evidence of left or biventricular hypertrophy may be observed on the electrocardiogram. Infants with a large left-to-right shunt tend to do poorly, with recurrent upper and lower respiratory tract infections, failure to gain weight, and congestive heart failure. Congestive heart failure may be severe and intractable despite intensive medical management.

Management. We currently recommend primary intracardiac repair of the ventricular septal defect rather than surgical banding of the pulmonary artery[147] to reduce pulmonary blood flow and alleviate heart failure. An exception is made for the rare infant with multiple ventricular septal defects and a sievelike septum, who is at higher risk for complications following operative repair. Operation usually is deferred, along with debanding of the pulmonary artery, until the child reaches 3 to 5 years. Primary closure of the ventricular septal defect, preferably through the right atrium, may be performed in infancy using cardiopulmonary bypass, profound hypothermia and cardiocirculatory arrest, or a combination of the two techniques. Mortality is less than 10 per cent if the defect is isolated and uncomplicated but approaches 25 per cent if multiple anomalies are present.[148]

Fortunately, medical treatment often is successful in controlling congestive heart failure. Nevertheless, these infants should be referred for cardiac catheterization to evaluate pulmonary vascular resistance and to detect associated defects that may require operation, such as patent ductus arteriosus and coarctation of the aorta.

It is of utmost importance to identify patients who may develop irreversible pulmonary vascular obstructive disease (the Eisenmenger reaction).[146,149,150] Retrospective analyses of children who develop this complication indicate that infants with systemic or near systemic pressures in the pulmonary artery at the time of initial hemodynamic study are most at risk. If early primary closure is not recommended, recatheterization before age 18 months and a second determination of pulmonary vascular resistance should be performed in these patients to decide whether surgical intervention is obligatory to prevent development of fixed obliterative changes in the pulmonary vessels. It is likely that multiple factors are involved in the development of pulmonary vascular disease (Chap. 27 and p. 896).[50-56] The anatomically large ventricular septal defect allows some or all of the systemic pressure to be transmitted to the pulmonary arteries, thereby retarding regression of their muscular media. Medial hypertrophy in the first months of life is responsible for higher pulmonary vascular resistance than would be anticipated for the amount of pulmonary blood flow. The shearing forces created by the high velocity of flow through narrowed pulmonary arterioles cause endothelial damage that is progressive. Although an elevation in left atrial pressure may contribute to the rise in pulmonary vascular resistance, it is not an essential factor, since pulmonary venous pressures can be low in patients who later develop pulmonary vascular disease. Nonetheless, pulmonary venous hypertension also may contribute to pulmonary arterial vasoconstriction and thus to increased shear forces. In this same regard, pulmonary vasoconstriction enhancing the risk of pulmonary vascular obstruction also may be caused by hypoxia caused by either high altitude or lung disease. At high altitudes, large ventricular septal defects have higher pulmonary vascular resistances and smaller shunts than at low altitudes.

CHILDHOOD. Beyond the first year of life a variable clinical picture emerges in children with ventricular septal defect.[139-147] If a small defect is present, the child usually is asymptomatic, the electrocardiogram usually is normal, and the chest roentgenogram shows normal or only a mild increase in pulmonary vascular markings. Effort intolerance and fatigue are associated with moderate left-to-right shunts. These children exhibit cardiomegaly with a forceful left ventricular impulse and a prominent systolic thrill along the lower left sternal border. The second heart sound normally is split, with moderate accentuation of the pulmonic component; a third heart sound and rumbling diastolic murmur that reflects increased flow across the mitral valve are audible at the cardiac apex. The characteristic murmur resulting from flow across the defect is harsh and holosystolic, is best heard along the third and fourth interspaces to the left of the sternum, and is widely transmitted over the precordium. A basal midsystolic ejection murmur due to increased flow across the pulmonic valve also may be heard. The electrocardiogram reveals left or combined ventricular hypertrophy (Fig. 31, p. 159), and the chest roentgenogram and CT scan (Fig. 8-41C, p. 229) show cardiomegaly, left atrial enlargement, and vascular engorgement (Fig. 11-13, p. 319).

RIGHT VENTRICULAR OUTFLOW TRACT OBSTRUCTION. With time, the clinical picture changes in 5 to 10 per cent of patients with ventricular septal defect and a moderate to large left-to-right shunt early in life. It begins to resemble more closely the tetralogy of Fallot (p. 935), i.e., subvalvular right ventricular outflow tract obstruction develops owing to progressive hypertrophy of the crista supraventricularis. Depending on the severity of the latter process, it ultimately may result in reduced blood flow and a right-to-left shunt across the ventricular septal defect. As right ventricular outflow tract obstruction develops, the holosystolic murmur is replaced by the crescendo-decrescendo ejection systolic murmur of pulmonic stenosis, and the pulmonary closure sound becomes softer. Right ventricular hypertrophy is evident on the electrocardiogram, and the chest roentgenogram shows a reduction in pulmonary vascular markings and a smaller heart size with a right ventricular configuration. Infundibular hypertrophy may progress quite rapidly within the first year of life, but the typical evolution to a clinical picture of cyanotic tetralogy of Fallot often takes 1 to 4 years. In those infants who develop right ventricular outflow obstruction the incidence of spontaneous closure or reduction in size of a ventricular septal defect is low.

AORTIC REGURGITATION. This well-described complication of ventricular septal defect occurs in about 5 per cent of patients.[151-153] It usually is noted after age 5 years when a physician detects the early diastolic blowing murmur and wide pulse pressure of aortic regurgitation while following a patient with a ventricular septal defect. The diagnosis is readily confirmed by Doppler echocardiography. In such patients aortic regurgitation may become the predominant hemodynamic abnormality. It is of interest that ventricular septal defect with aortic regurgitation is rare in Europe and the United States, with an incidence of about 4 per cent of all cases of isolated ventricular septal defect, whereas in Japan the incidence is substantially higher (about 10 per cent). In the Japanese, in particular, aortic regurgitation is the result of herniation of an aortic leaflet (usually the right coronary) through a subpulmonic supracristal ventricular septal defect. In these patients, closure of the ventricular septal defect may be all that is required to relieve aortic regurgitation. In many patients, however, especially in the Western world, the ventricular septal defect is below the infundibular septum (crista supraventricularis). Although aortic leaflet herniation, especially of the right or noncoronary cusp, may occur in some of these patients, quite often aortic regurgitation results from a primary abnormality of the valve, usually one defective commissure. In the latter situation, plication of the elongated leaflet may lessen, but not abolish, the aortic regurgitation; in some patients prosthetic aortic valve replacement may be necessary to provide hemodynamic relief. In most patients with ventricular septal defect and aortic regurgitation, the ventricular septal defect is small to moderate in size, and mild right ventricular outflow tract obstruction exists. The latter is caused by either subpulmonic infundibular stenosis or projection of the herniated aortic cusp into the right ventricular outflow tract. The distinction between types of ventricular septal defect with aortic regurgitation usually can be made by two-dimensional and Doppler echocardiography and by selective left ventricular angiocardiography to define the site of the interventricular communication in combination with retrograde aortography to assess the anatomy and competence of the aortic valve (Fig. 31-18).[152,153]

Management. Treatment of the patient with ventricular septal defect and aortic regurgitation is controversial. In patients with a large, hemodynamically significant left-to-right shunt, repair of the ventricular septal defect is indicated, but aortic regurgitation is repaired only if at least moderate aortic regurgitation exists. If a supracristal ventricular septal defect without aortic regurgitation is identified at cardiac catheterization in early childhood, a sensible argument for prophylactic closure of the ventricular septal defect can be put forth to prevent the potential complication of aortic valve incompetence. In the presence of moderate or severe aortic regurgitation, valvuloplasty is preferred to valve replacement, in recognition of the fact that the severity of aortic regurgitation may increase in subsequent years and that reoperation with valve replacement may be necessary. Operation should probably be deferred in asymptomatic patients with a subcristal ventricular septal defect and an insignificant left-to-right shunt in whom aortic regurgitation is not severe. If the defect is

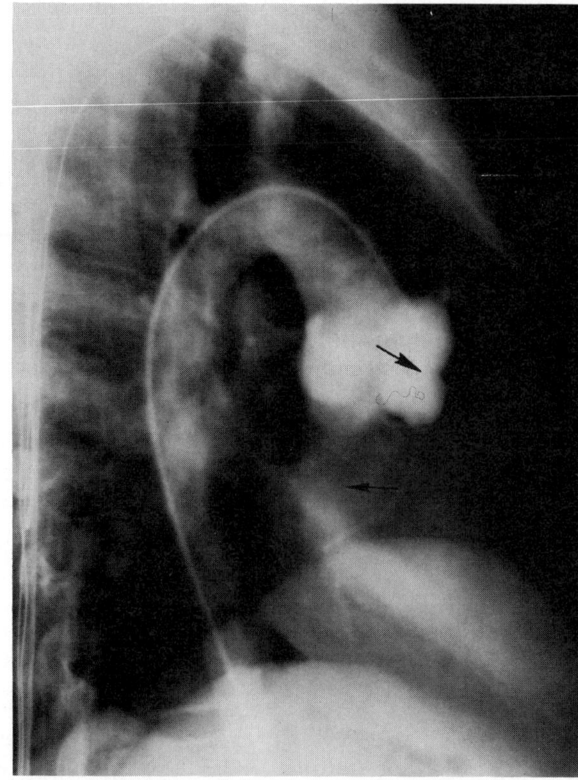

FIGURE 31-18. Retrograde aortogram showing herniation of the right coronary cusp through a supracristal ventricular septal defect (upper arrow) and the jet of aortic regurgitation (lower arrow). (Courtesy of Robert White, M.D.)

supracristal in the same clinical setting, its closure may not alleviate the mild degree of aortic incompetence but may retard its progression.

PULMONARY VASCULAR OBSTRUCTION. If a child who previously had a loud murmur and thrill associated with poor growth suddenly has a growth spurt, fewer respiratory infections, and a diminution of the intensity of the cardiac murmur and disappearance of the thrill, he or she may be developing severe obliterative changes in the pulmonary vascular bed. An increase in intensity of the pulmonic component of the second heart sound, a reduction in heart size on the chest roentgenogram (Fig. 32–9, p. 971), and more pronounced right ventricular hypertrophy on the electrocardiogram also are noted. These changes occur because the increased pulmonary vascular resistance causes a decrease in the left-to-right shunt. If these changes are suspected, cardiac catheterization should be repeated; if they are confirmed, prompt surgical repair is indicated before an inoperable predominant right-to-left shunt ensues. If operation is performed under age 2 years, pulmonary vascular resistance may be expected to fall to normal levels.[150] In older patients the degree to which pulmonary vascular resistance is elevated before operation is a critical factor determining prognosis. If the pulmonary vascular resistance is one-third or less of the systemic value, progressive pulmonary vascular disease after operation is unusual. However, if a moderate-to-severe increase in pulmonary vascular resistance exists preoperatively, either no change or progression of pulmonary vascular disease is common postoperatively. Moreover, the presence of increased pulmonary vascular resistance results in a higher immediate postoperative mortality rate for surgical closure of ventricular septal defect. These observations make it clear that a large ventricular septal defect should be approached surgically very early in life when pulmonary vascular disease is still reversible or has not yet developed.

OTHER FORMS OF VENTRICULAR DEFECT. Unusual forms of ventricular septal defect include multiple muscular defects and left ventricular–right atrial communications. Defects in the muscular ventricular septum frequently are multiple small fenestrations that produce a large net left-to-right shunt.[139] Their recognition is a necessary preliminary to successful operation, since incomplete repair may result in postoperative cardiac failure and death. A shunt from the left ventricle to right atrium may occur with a ventricular septal defect in the most superior portion of the ventricular septum, since the tricuspid valve is lower than the mitral valve. The clinical, electrocardiographic, and radiological findings in these patients do not differ appreciably from those in patients with a simple ventricular septal defect, although right atrial enlargement may provide a clue to correct diagnosis of left ventricular–right atrial communication.[155] The pathophysiology of single or common ventricle (p. 953) may resemble that of a large ventricular septal defect, although these defects are dissimilar embryologically. The single chamber frequently is the morphological left ventricle; malposition of the great arteries is quite common. There may be no detectable cyanosis if selective streaming and increased pulmonary blood flow rather than complete mixing occurs. Pulmonary hypertension invariably is present unless pulmonic stenosis exists. It is imperative to differentiate a single ventricle from a large ventricular septal defect by echocardiography[134] and angiography[122] because the operative approaches to the former malformation require a complex septation technique or the atriopulmonary Fontan connection.

MANAGEMENT OF VENTRICULAR SEPTAL DEFECT. It is rarely necessary to restrict the activities of a child with an isolated ventricular septal defect. Infective bacterial endocarditis is always a threat, and antibiotic prophylaxis for dental procedures and minor surgery is indicated (Table 31–4).[156] Respiratory infections require prompt evaluation and treatment. These children should be seen at least once or twice yearly to detect changes in the clinical picture that suggest the development of pulmonary vascular obliterative changes.

When clinical findings suggest a moderate shunt but no pulmonary hypertension, elective hemodynamic evaluation should be advised between ages 3 and 6 years. Of prime importance in the hemodynamic evaluation is a determination of pressure and blood flow in the pulmonary artery.[157] Surgical treatment is not recommended for children who have normal pulmonary arterial pressures with small shunts (pulmonary-systemic flow ratios of less than 1.5 to 2.0 : 1). In such patients the remaining risk of infective endocarditis[156] does not exceed the risk of operation. Moreover, although the inherent risk of operation is small, the possibility of postoperative heart block, infection, or other complications of operation and cardiopulmonary bypass dictates a conservative approach when the cardiac defect may be well tolerated for life.

With larger shunts, elective operation may be advised before the child enters school, thus minimizing any subsequent distinction of these patients from their normal classmates. A total assessment of the psychosocial dynamics of the family and child is helpful in determining the proper age for elective operation in each patient.

Under investigation is transcatheter closure by umbrella or clamshell occluder devices (p. 915) inserted by crossing the ventricular defect by way of the left ventricle to guide a venous catheter through a long sheath, and, ultimately, placing the device across the ventricular septum from the right ventricular side.[158]

Complete heart block is the most significant surgically induced conduction system abnormality, occurring immediately after surgery in fewer than 1 per cent of patients. Late-onset complete heart block occasionally is a problem, especially in the 10 to 25 per cent of patients whose postoperative electrocardiographic findings show complete right bundle branch block with left anterior hemiblock.[159] When the latter electrocardiographic pattern is observed in patients with transient complete heart block in the early postoperative period, electrophysiological studies should be conducted at postoperative cardiac catheterization. It would appear that patients presenting postoperatively with right bundle block and left anterior hemiblock fall into two populations, defined by either peripheral damage to the conduction system or damage to the bundle of His or its proximal branches.[160] The former has not been associated with transient postoperative complete heart block, and these patients usually have a benign course. Trifascicular damage may be demonstrated in the latter population by a prolonged H-V interval, which implies a higher risk of complete heart block later in life. Although the prophylactic use of permanent pacemakers in asymptomatic patients with evidence of trifascicular damage is not currently recommended, this group certainly requires careful follow-up and continued study.

Treadmill exercise studies in patients who preoperatively had normal or only moderately elevated pulmonary vascular resistance and essentially normal postoperative cardiac catheterization data may uncover late abnormalities in circulatory function.[161,162] Despite normal cardiac output at rest, an impaired cardiac output response to exercise is noted in some. Moreover, despite a normal pulmonary arterial pressure at rest, markedly abnormal increases in pulmonary arterial pressure may be noted during exercise. These findings may be related to abnormal left ventricular function after closure of the ventricular septal defect and/or to persistent pathological changes in the pulmonary arterioles or to abnormal pulmonary vascular reactivity.[163] A direct relation exists between age at operation and the magnitude of the pulmonary arterial pressure response to intense exercise, suggesting that early operation may prevent permanent impairment of the functional capacity of the myocardium and pulmonary vascular bed.

Occasionally a child may come to medical attention who has already developed pulmonary vascular obstruction and a net right-to-left shunt across the ventricular septal defect. Symptoms may consist of exertional dyspnea, chest pain, syncope, and hemoptysis; the right-to-left shunt leads to cyanosis, clubbing, and polycythemia. There currently is little to offer this group of patients other than continuing support to the patient and family.

PATENT DUCTUS ARTERIOSUS

(See also p. 974)

The ductus arteriosus normally exists in the fetus as a widely patent vessel connecting the pulmonary trunk and the descending aorta just distal to the left subclavian artery (Fig. 31–5). In the fetus most of the output of the right ventricle bypasses the unexpanded lungs by way of the ductus arteriosus and enters the descending aorta, where it travels to the placenta, the fetal organ of oxygenation. Until recently it was assumed that during fetal life the ductus arteriosus was a pas-

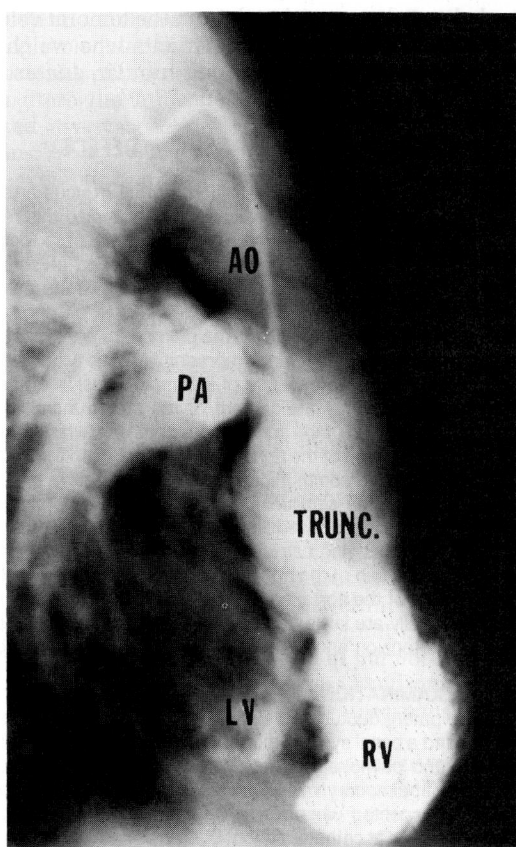

FIGURE 31–21. Right ventriculogram in the lateral view in a patient with type I truncus arteriosus. The contrast agent enters the left ventricle (LV) across a ventricular septal defect. The pulmonary artery (PA) arises directly from the persistent truncus arteriosus (TRUNC). AO = aorta, RV = right ventricle. (Courtesy of Robert White, M.D.)

teries.[191] The defect results from failure of septation of the embryonic truncus by the infundibular truncal ridges (Fig. 31–4). It is always accompanied by a ventricular septal defect, frequently with a right-sided aortic arch. The ventricular septal defect is due to the absence or underdevelopment of the distal portion of the pulmonary infundibulum. The truncal valve usually is tricuspid but is quadricuspid in about one-third of patients and rarely can be bicuspid. Truncal valve regurgitation and truncal valve stenosis are each seen in 10 to 15 per cent of patients. There may be a single coronary artery, displacement of the coronary ostia (usually the left ostium posteriorly), or a single posterior descending coronary artery arising from the right coronary or, less often, from the left circumflex artery, especially in patients with a single coronary artery.[192,193]

Truncus malformations may be classified either anatomically according to the mode of origin of pulmonary vessels from the common trunk or from a functional point of view, based on the magnitude of blood flow to the lungs.[194] In the common type (type I) of truncus arteriosus malformation a partially separate pulmonary trunk of variable length exists because of the presence of an incompletely formed aorticopulmonary septum (Fig. 31–21). The pulmonary trunk usually is very short and gives rise to left and right pulmonary arteries. When the aorticopulmonary septum is absent, there is no discrete main pulmonary artery component, and both pulmonary artery branches arise directly from the truncus. In type II, each pulmonary artery arises separately but close to the other from the posterior aspect of the truncus. In type III, each pulmonary artery arises from the lateral aspect of the truncus. Less commonly, one pulmonary artery branch may be absent, with collateral arteries supplying the lung that does not receive a pulmonary artery branch from the truncus. Truncus arteriosus malformation should not be confused with "pseudotruncus arteriosus," which is the severe form of tetralogy of Fallot with pulmonary atresia in which the single aorta arises from the heart accompanied by a remnant of atretic pulmonary artery (p. 935).

Pulmonary blood flow is governed by the size of the pulmonary arteries and the pulmonary vascular resistance. In infancy, pulmonary blood flow is usually excessive, since pulmonary vascular resistance is not greatly increased. Thus, despite an obligatory admixture of systemic and pulmonary venous blood in the common trunk, only minimal cyanosis is present. Rarely, pulmonary blood flow is restricted by hypoplastic or stenotic pulmonary arteries arising from the truncus. Pulmonary vascular obstruction usually does not restrict pulmonary blood flow before 1 year of age.[195] Hence, the infant with truncus arteriosus usually presents with mild cyanosis coexisting with the cardiac findings of a large left-to-right shunt. Symptoms of heart failure and poor physical development usually appear in the first weeks or months of life. The most frequent physical findings include cardiomegaly, a systolic ejection sound accompanied by a thrill, a loud single second heart sound, a harsh systolic murmur, and a low-pitched middiastolic rumbling murmur and bounding pulses. Truncus arteriosus often is a feature of the *DiGeorge syndrome* (Table 31–2); thus facial dysmorphism, a high incidence of extracardiac malformations (particularly of the limbs, kidneys, and intestines), atrophy or absence of the thymus gland, T-lymphocyte deficiency, and predilection to infection also may be features of the clinical presentation.[196] Recent evidence suggests that embryonic abnormalities in the cardiac neural crest play a major role in the creation of the cardiovascular malformation as well as the other components of the syndrome.[196a]

Truncal valve incompetence is suggested by the presence of a diastolic decrescendo murmur at the base of the heart.[197] The physical findings are quite different if pulmonary blood flow is restricted by either high pulmonary vascular resistance or pulmonary arterial stenosis: cyanosis is prominent, congestive failure is rare, and only a short systolic ejection may be audible occasionally accompanied by continuous murmurs posteriorly of bronchial collateral flow. Left ventricular hypertrophy alone or in combination with right ventricular hypertrophy is present electrocardiographically when a prominent left-to-right shunt exists; right ventricular hypertrophy is observed in patients with restricted pulmonary blood flow. The radiographic findings depend on the hemodynamic circumstances. Gross cardiomegaly with left or combined ventricular enlargement, left atrial enlargement, and a small or absent main pulmonary artery segment with pulmonary vascular engorgement are the usual radiographic features. A right aortic arch is common (25 to 30 per cent of patients). When pulmonary blood flow is reduced, both heart size and pulmonary vascular markings are less prominent.

The *echocardiographic* features of truncus arteriosus (Fig. 31–22) include the detection of a large truncal root overriding the ventricular septum, truncal valve abnormalities, an in-

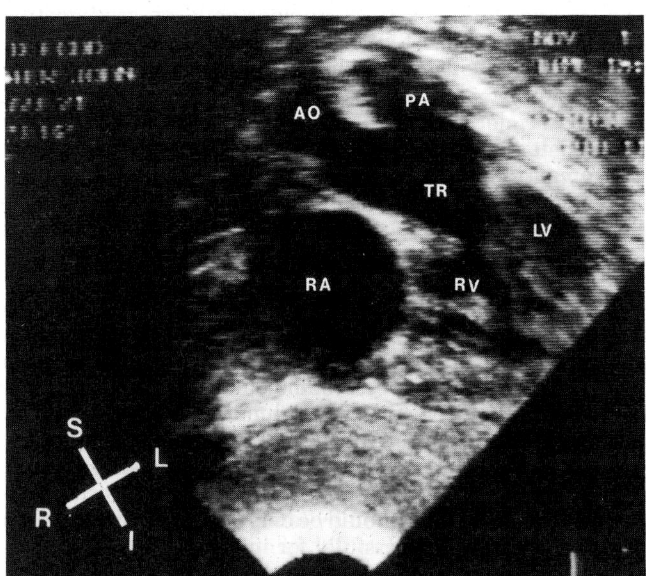

FIGURE 31–22. Truncus arteriosus, shown by a subcostal view with superior angulation of the transducer to image the truncal root (TR). The tricuspid valve is closed in ventricular systole. The truncal root sits above both the right ventricle (RV) and left ventricle (LV). The pulmonary artery (PA) arises directly from the truncus. AO = aorta, RA = right atrium.

crease in the right ventricular dimension, and mitral valve–truncal root continuity. The dimension of the left atrium determined echocardiographically provides a good index of pulmonary flow. Differentiation between truncus arteriosus and tetralogy of Fallot by ultrasound may be difficult unless either the separate origin of the pulmonary arteries or a single trunk from the ascending portion of a single arterial root can be identified. Diagnosis should be suspected at cardiac catheterization if the catheter fails to enter the central pulmonary arteries from the right ventricle. Selective angiocardiography and retrograde aortography are necessary to establish a precise diagnosis and to reveal the common trunk arising from the heart and the origin of the pulmonary arteries from the truncus.[198]

The early fatal course as well as early development of pulmonary vascular obstructive disease in patients surviving infancy is responsible for the poor prognosis associated with truncus arteriosus. In infants and young children with large left-to-right shunts, surgical banding of one or both pulmonary arteries to reduce pulmonary flow has been used with little success. Corrective operation is preferred before age 3 months to avoid the development of severe pulmonary vascular obstructive disease.[199]

SURGICAL TREATMENT. Operation consists of closure of the ventricular septal defect, leaving the aorta arising from the left ventricle; the pulmonary arteries are excised from their truncus origin and a valve-containing prosthetic conduit or aortic homograft valve conduit is used to establish continuity between the right ventricle and the pulmonary arteries (Fig. 31–23). Truncal valve regurgitation significantly enhances the risk of corrective surgery, since valve replacement is associated with significantly increased surgical mortality. Patients with only one pulmonary artery are especially prone to early development of severe pulmonary vascular disease but otherwise are not at increased risk from surgery. With truncus arteriosus defects, the possible inequalities of pressure and flow between the two pulmonary arteries often make precise calculation of pulmonary resistance difficult. Corrective operation may be performed in patients with at least one adequate pulmonary artery having low distal pressure or arteriolar resistance. Conversely, significant systemic arterial desaturation in a patient with two pulmonary arteries and with neither pulmonary artery stenosis nor a previous pulmonary artery band signifies that high pulmonary vascular resistance exists and that the condition is probably inoperable. It is not yet clear how often and at what age the conduit between the right ventricle and pulmonary artery must be replaced with a larger prosthesis because of either growth of the patient, in whom a small conduit causes eventual obstruction, heterograft valve degeneration, or obstruction created by neointimal proliferation within a prosthetic conduit. When operation is carried out with a conduit in the first year of life, conduit replacement often is required within 3 to 5 years.

CORONARY ARTERIOVENOUS FISTULA

(See also p. 970)

Coronary arteriovenous fistula is an unusual anomaly that consists of a communication between one of the coronary arteries and a cardiac chamber or vein. The right coronary artery, or its branches, is the site of the fistula in about 55 per cent of cases; the left coronary artery is involved in about 35 per cent, and both coronary arteries in 5 per cent. Connections between the coronary system and a cardiac chamber appear to represent persistence of embryonic intertrabecular spaces and sinusoids. Most of these fistulas drain into the right ventricle, right atrium, or coronary sinus; fistulous communication to the pulmonary artery, left atrium, or left ventricle is much less frequent. Most often the shunt through the fistula is of small magnitude, and myocardial blood flow is not compromised.[199] Potential complications include pulmonary hypertension and congestive heart failure if a large left-to-right shunt exists, bacterial endocarditis, rupture or thrombosis of the fistula or an associated arterial aneurysm, and myocardial ischemia distal to the fistula due to decreased coronary blood flow.

Most patients are asymptomatic and are referred because of a cardiac murmur that is loud, superficial, and continuous at the lower or midsternal border. The site of maximal intensity of the murmur is related to the site of drainage and usually is different from the second left intercostal space—the classic site of the continuous murmur of persistent ductus arteriosus—except when the fistula drains into the pulmonary artery or right ventricle. In the latter situation the murmur is louder in diastole than in systole because of compression of the fistula by contracting myocardium. The electrocardiogram and chest roentgenogram quite often are normal and seldom show selective chamber enlargement or myocardial ischemia. Significantly enlarged coronary arteries may be detected by two-dimensional echocardiography, and the actual diagnosis of an arteriovenous fistula occasionally can be made by combining two-dimensional echocardiography and Doppler techniques to detect the entrance site of the shunt, which is characterized by a continuous turbulent systolic and diastolic flow pattern.[200,201] (Fig. 32–7, p. 970)

Retrograde thoracic aortography or coronary arteriography can be used reliably to identify the size and anatomical features of the fistulous tract, which can be closed by suture obliteration in most cases.[202] In the presence of a large left-to-right shunt and symptoms of heart failure, the decision to

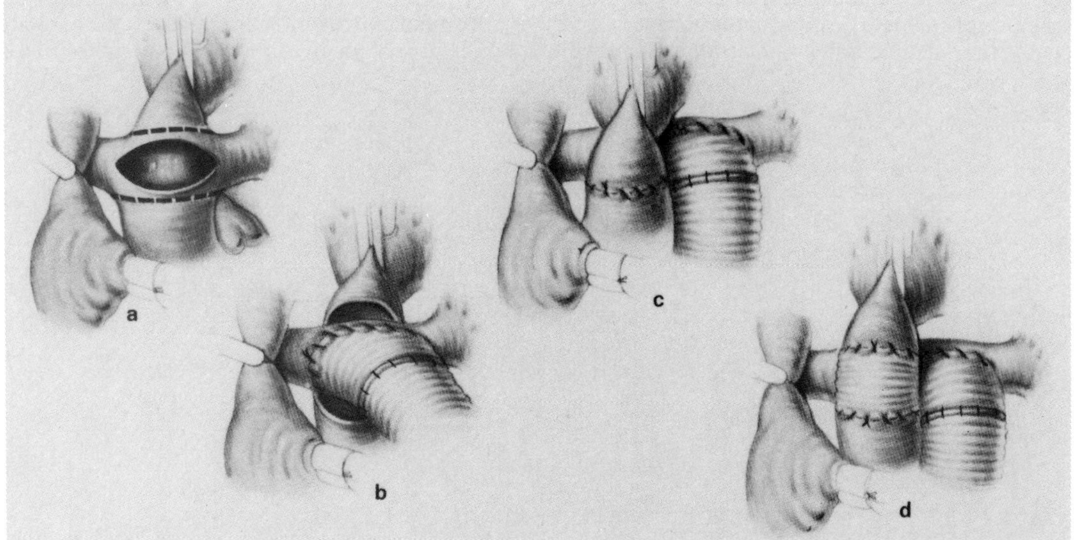

FIGURE 31–23. **Operative correction of truncus arteriosus, type III. The pulmonary arteries arise separately from the truncus. An anterior incision is made and a segment of aorta containing the orifices of both pulmonary arteries is excised from the truncus (a). The cuff of tissue containing the two pulmonary arteries is anastomosed to an extracardiac valved conduit (b). Aortic continuity is restored by direct suture (c), or by interposing a preclotted graft (d). The diagram does not show closure of the ventricular septal defect. (From Stark, J., and DeLaval, M.: Surgery for Congenital Heart Defects. New York, Grune and Stratton, 1983, p. 420.)**

operate is clearly justified. Most often the fistula is closed in asymptomatic patients to prevent future symptoms or complications, such as infective endocarditis. The prognosis after successful closure of a coronary artery–cardiac chamber fistula is excellent.

ANOMALOUS PULMONARY ORIGIN OF THE CORONARY ARTERY

This rare malformation occurs in about 0.4 per cent of patients with congenital cardiac anomalies. In almost all patients the left coronary artery originates from the posterior sinus of the pulmonary artery.[203]

Unusual cases have been reported in which the right coronary artery, or the entire coronary artery system, originates from the main pulmonary trunk. Embryologically the distal coronary artery system is formed by 9 weeks from solid angioblastic buds that extend throughout the epicardium to form the major coronary artery branches. Proximally the coronary network forms a ring around the truncus arteriosus, joining with coronary buds from the primitive aortic sinuses as the truncus partitions to form the great arteries. The varieties of anomalous pulmonary origin of the coronary artery are the result of displacement in this proximal process.

During fetal life pulmonary artery pressure is slightly greater than aortic pressure, and perfusion of the left coronary artery is antegrade. After birth, when pulmonary artery pressure falls below aortic pressure, perfusion of the left coronary artery from the pulmonary artery ceases, and the direction of flow in the anomalous vessel reverses. Blood flows from the aorta to the right coronary artery, then through collateral channels to the left coronary artery, and finally to the pulmonary artery. In effect, the left coronary artery behaves as a fistulous communication between the aorta and pulmonary artery. If adequate collateral channels exist or develop between the two coronary artery circulations, total myocardial perfusion through the right coronary artery increases. In 10 to 15 per cent of patients myocardial ischemia never develops because extensive intercoronary collaterals allow survival to adolescence or adulthood. In fact, if collateral blood flow is considerable, the patient may develop the clinical manifestations of a large arteriovenous shunt and a continuous or diastolic murmur. Older children or adults usually present with a continuous murmur or with mitral regurgitation resulting from dysfunction of ischemic or infarcted papillary muscles. In some instances the coronary anomaly is unsuspected until a previously well adolescent or adult experiences angina, heart failure, or sudden death.

By far the most common clinical presentation is that of the infant who suffers a myocardial infarction and develops congestive heart failure.[204,205] The infant syndrome usually becomes manifested at age 2 to 4 months with angina-like symptoms that may be misinterpreted as colic. Feeding and defecation often are accompanied by dyspnea, irritability and crying, pallor, diaphoresis, and occasional loss of consciousness. The diagnosis of anomalous origin of the coronary artery is supported by the electrocardiographic demonstration of deep Q waves in association with ST-segment alterations and T-wave inversions in leads I, aV_L, V_5, and V_6 (Fig. 31–24). Chest roentgenograms show moderate to severe enlargement of the left atrium and ventricle. The origin of the anomalous left coronary artery occasionally may be visualized echocardiographically from long- or short-axis views of the pulmonary artery.[206,207] Absence of the left coronary artery from its usual origin in the left sinus of Valsalva does not distinguish this lesion from single coronary artery. Color-flow Doppler examination reveals diastolic turbulent flow in the pulmonary artery near the coronary orifice, and also may disclose associated mitral regurgitation. Contrast echocardiography from a radial artery injection demonstrates even small left-to-right shunts from the right coronary artery system, through the anomalous left coronary artery, into the pulmonary artery.[207] Ischemia or infarction is suggested by the echocardiographic findings of segmental wall motion abnormalities, particularly involving the anterolateral free wall of the left ventricle. Stress thallium scintigraphy shows a characteristic defect of the anterolateral wall of the left ventricle.

Aortography or coronary angiography is the definitive diagnostic procedure, and demonstrates the retrograde drainage of the coronary vessel into the pulmonary artery (Fig. 31–25). It should be recognized that ventricular arrhythmias may complicate the course of hemodynamic study. Management of these infants depends, in part, on the magnitude of shunting into the pulmonary artery, which may be determined by oximetry, indicator dilution curves, or angiography.

MANAGEMENT. *Medical treatment* is indicated in infants with myocardial infarction for congestive heart failure, arrhythmias, and cardiogenic shock. In patients with a small left-to-right shunt or no shunt at all, the prognosis is exceedingly poor with conservative management, justifying an attempt to reestablish a two–coronary artery system. The *operations* that have been used include reimplanting the left coronary artery into the aortic root, surgically creating an aortopulmonary window and a tunnel to convey blood from the window across the back of the pulmonary trunk to the origin of the anomalous left coronary artery, with reconstruction of the anterior wall of the pulmonary trunk, or anastomosis of the left coronary artery with the subclavian artery or with the aorta by means of a graft.[208,209] If clinical deterioration occurs in infants in whom a sizable left-to-right shunt into the pulmonary artery exists, simple ligation of the left coronary artery at its origin prevents retrograde flow and allows perfusion of the left ventricle with blood supplied through anastomoses with the right coronary artery. If medical management stabilizes the infant with significant intercoronary collaterals, operation may be postponed to allow the patient to grow, since increased

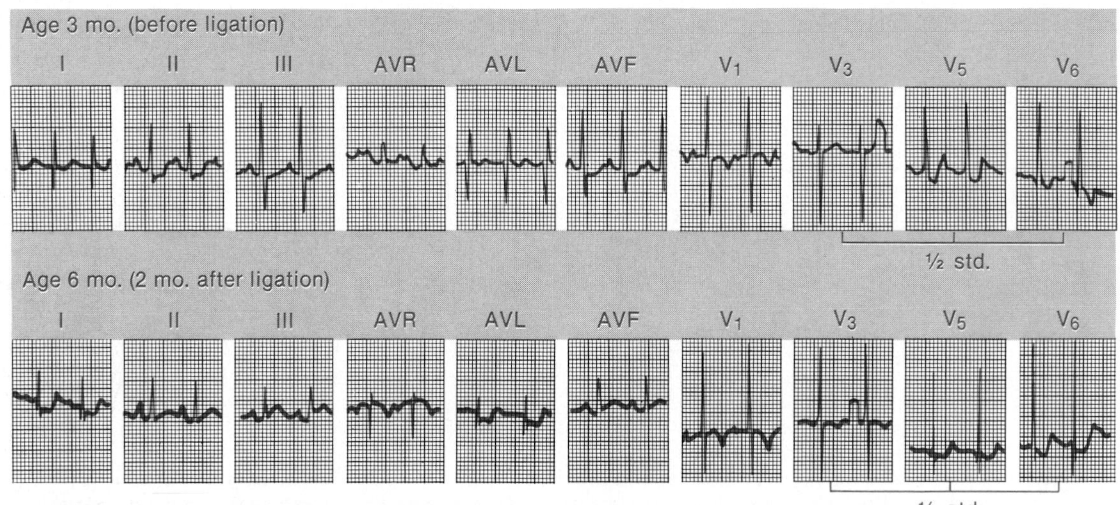

FIGURE 31–24. Typical electrocardiogram of an infant with anomalous left coronary artery before *(above)* and after *(below)* ligation of the anomalous left coronary artery. Arrows point to the abnormal Q waves. (Courtesy of Delores A. Danilowicz, M.D.)

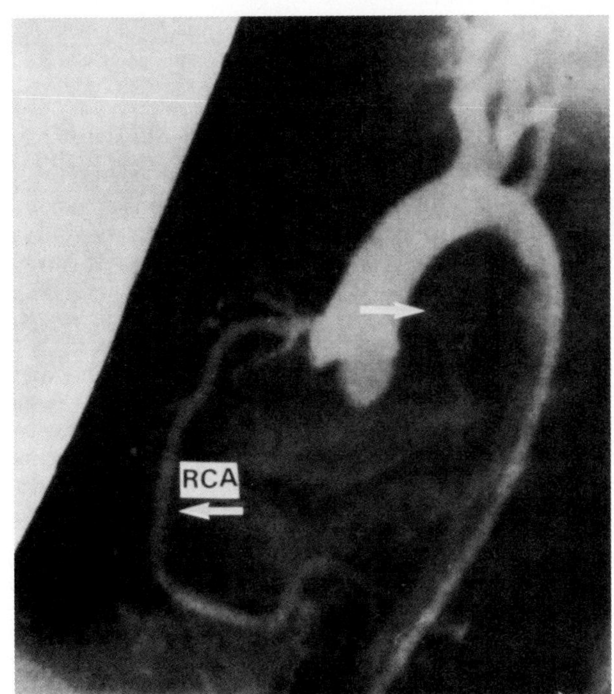

FIGURE 31-25. Lateral view of anomalous left coronary artery. Retrograde aortogram fills the right (RCA) and then the left coronary artery through collateral channels. The left coronary artery enters the main pulmonary artery (upper arrow). (Courtesy of Robert Freedom, M.D.)

size of the vessels enhances the likelihood of successful reimplantation or coronary arterial bypass surgery. The outcome of surgery and ultimate prognosis are significantly influenced by the degree of myocardial damage suffered preoperatively. Uncommonly, it is necessary to consider aneurysmectomy or mitral valve replacement.

AORTIC SINUS ANEURYSM AND FISTULA

(See also p. 970)

Congenital aneurysm of an aortic sinus of Valsalva, particularly the right coronary sinus, is an uncommon anomaly that occurs more often in males than in females. The malformation consists of a separation, or lack of fusion, between the media of the aorta and the annulus fibrosis of the aortic valve.[210] The receiving chamber of the aorticocardiac fistula usually is the right ventricle, but occasionally, when the noncoronary cusp is involved, the fistula drains into the right atrium.

Five to 15 per cent of aneurysms originate in the posterior or noncoronary sinus; seldom is the left aortic sinus involved. Associated anomalies are common and include bicuspid aortic valve, ventricular septal defect, and coarctation of the aorta.

It is not clear whether the aneurysm itself is present at birth, although the deficiency in the aortic media would appear to be congenital. Reports in children are infrequent, since progressive aneurysmal dilatation of the weakened area develops but may not be recognized until the third or fourth decade of life, when rupture into a cardiac chamber occurs.

The *unruptured aneurysm* usually does not produce a hemodynamic abnormality, although pressure on the intracardiac conduction system by an unruptured aneurysm may be a rare cause of complete atrioventricular block; rarely, myocardial ischemia may be caused by coronary arterial compression. Rupture often is of abrupt onset, causes chest pain, and creates continuous arteriovenous shunting and volume loading of both right and left heart chambers, which results in heart failure. An additional complication is bacterial endocarditis, which may originate either on the edges of the aneurysm or on those areas in the right side of the heart that are traumatized by the jet-like stream of blood flowing through the fistula.

The presence of this anomaly should be suspected in a patient with a history of chest pain or recent onset, symptoms of diminished cardiac reserve, bounding pulses, and a loud superficial continuous murmur accentuated in diastole when the fistula opens into the right ventricle, as well as a thrill along the right or left lower parasternal border. The *physical findings* may be difficult to distinguish from those produced by a coronary arteriovenous fistula. *Electrocardiography* shows biventricular hypertrophy, and chest roentgenography demonstrates generalized cardiomegaly. Two-dimensional and pulsed Doppler *echocardiographic* studies may detect the walls of the aneurym and disturbed flow within the aneurysm or at the site of perforation, respectively.[211] *Cardiac catheterization* reveals a left-to-right shunt at the ventricular or, less commonly, the atrial level; the diagnosis may be established definitively by retrograde thoracic aortography (Fig. 31-26). Preoperative medical management consists of measures to relieve cardiac failure and to treat coexistent arrhythmias or endocarditis, if present. At operation the aneurysm is closed and amputated, and the aortic wall is reunited with the heart, either by direct suture or with a prosthesis.[212] Every effort should be made to preserve the aortic valve in children, since patch closure of the defect combined with prosthetic valve replacement greatly enhances the risk of operation in small patients.

VALVULAR AND VASCULAR LESIONS WITH OR WITHOUT RIGHT-TO-LEFT SHUNT

AORTIC ARCH OBSTRUCTION

The conventional anatomical and clinical divisions into preductal and postductal coarctation or infantile and adult types, respectively, is misleading, since the anatomical localization is inaccurate and the age-dependency of clinical presentation does not hold true (i.e., the adult type often is seen in the first weeks of life). A spectrum of anatomical lesions exists, causing obstruction of the aortic arch or proximal portion of the descending aorta. These range from a localized coarctation or constriction of the lumen, most commonly located just distal to the origin of the left subclavian artery and closely related to the attachment of the ductus arteriosus with the aorta, to diffuse narrowing or interruption of a portion of the aortic arch. In this chapter, aortic arch obstruction is divided into three types: (1) localized juxtaductal coarctation, (2) hypoplasia of the aortic isthmus, and (3) aortic arch interruption. *Pseudocoarctation* is used synonymously with "kinking," or

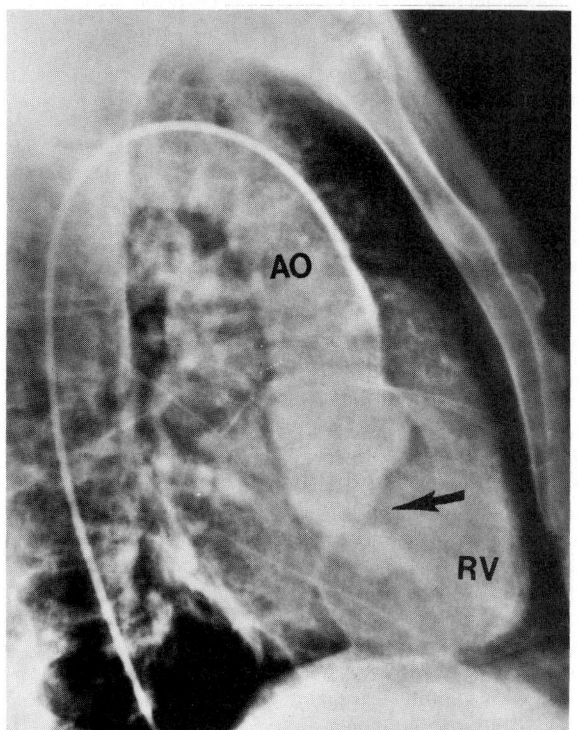

FIGURE 31-26. A retrograde aortogram shows the fistulous connection between the noncoronary sinus of Valsalva and the right ventricle (RV) (arrow). AO = aorta. (Courtesy of Robert White, M.D.)

"buckling," of the aorta, which is a subclinical form of localized juxtaductal coarctation of the aorta.[213]

LOCALIZED JUXTADUCTAL COARCTATION

(See also p. 967)

MORPHOLOGY. This lesion consists of a localized shelf-like thickening and infolding of the media of the posterolateral aortic wall opposite the ductus arteriosus; the wall of the aorta into which the ductus or ligamentum arteriosum inserts is not involved.[214] Juxtaductal coarctation occurs two to five times more commonly in males than in females, and there is a high degree of association with gonadal dysgenesis (Turner syndrome) and bicuspid aortic valve. Other common associated anomalies include ventricular septal defect and mitral stenosis or regurgitation. The most important extracardiac anomaly is aneurysm of the circle of Willis.

PATHOGENESIS. Juxtaductal coarctation is probably related to an abnormality in the pattern of ductus arteriosus blood flow in utero, which, in turn, may be the result of associated intracardiac anomalies.[214,215] Thus, in fetal life, blood flow through the aortic isthmus constitutes only 12 to 17 per cent of the total cardiac output, while blood flow through the ductus arteriosus exceeds that across the aortic valve. The dorsal aortic wall directly opposite the ductus arteriosus will resemble morphologically the apex of a normal branch point of the aorta if ductal flow pathways in utero diverge, with some flow directed cephalad into the aortic isthmus and the remainder proceeding into the descending aorta. The aortic branch point is identical histologically to the posterior shelf of juxtaductal aortic coarctation. A divergence of ductal flow is fostered by the presence of lesions in the fetus that create an imbalance between left and right ventricular outputs, with right-sided flow predominating (e.g., bicuspid aortic valve, mitral valve anomaly). In the absence of an anomaly fostering augmented ductal flow, a branch point may be created by an alteration in the angle at which the ductus arteriosus meets the aorta, pointing the ductal stream directly against the posterior aortic wall rather than obliquely down into the descending aorta. Cardiac anomalies that cause augmented ascending aortic blood flow (e.g., pulmonic atresia or stenosis, tetralogy of Fallot) prevent development of a branch point and indeed are almost never seen in association with juxtaductal coarctation of the aorta.

During fetal life the posterior aortic shelf is not obstructive, since blood may pass readily from the ascending aorta to the descending aorta by traversing the anterior aortic segment and the aortic end of the ductus arteriosus. Postnatally, however, when the ductus undergoes obliteration at its aortic end, the shelf-like projection of the posterior aortic wall unmasks the obstruction to aortic flow (Fig. 31-27). After pharmacological interventions that dilate the ductus arteriosus (prostaglandin E_1 infusion) the pressure difference may be obliterated across the site of coarctation, since the fetal flow pattern is reestablished.[71,216]

The pathogenesis of juxtaductal coarctation already described explains the prevalence of associated intracardiac anomalies that foster reduced ascending aortic flow and augmented ductus arteriosus flow in utero, and the absence of associated intracardiac anomalies in which the converse flow conditions exist in utero. The dependence of aortic obstruction on constriction of the ductus arteriosus postnatally explains the variable onset after birth of the clinical manifestations of coarctation, as well as the dramatic alleviation of obstruction produced pharmacologically by dilatation of the ductus arteriosus.

CLINICAL FINDINGS. The manifestations of juxtaductal coarctation of the aorta depend on the prominence of the posterolateral aortic shelf, which determines the intensity of obstruction, and on the rapidity with which obstruction develops. Rapid, severe obstruction in infancy is a prominent cause of left ventricular failure and systemic hypoperfusion. Substantial left-to-right shunting across a patent foramen ovale and pulmonary venous hypertension secondary to heart failure cause pulmonary arterial hypertension. Because little or no aortic obstruction existed during fetal life, the collateral circulation in the newborn period is often poorly developed. Characteristically in these infants, peripheral pulses are weak throughout the body until left ventricular function is improved with medical management; a significant pressure difference then develops between the arms and the legs, allowing detection of a pulse discrepancy. Cardiac murmurs are nonspecific in infancy and commonly are derived from associated lesions. The electrocardiogram shows right-axis deviation and right ventricular hypertrophy; the chest x-ray shows generalized cardiomegaly and pulmonary arterial and venous engorgement. Hemodynamic study allows delineation of the site and extent of aortic obstruction and the detection of associated cardiac malformations. Most infants with early-onset severe heart failure respond poorly to medical management, and balloon angioplasty,[217] surgical excision of the coarctation, or a subclavian flap angioplasty[218] often is required.

Aortic obstruction may develop slowly in infants in whom the posterolateral aortic shelf is not prominent at birth and in whom ductus arteriosus constriction is gradual. In these babies compensatory myocardial hypertrophy and an extensive collateral circulation have time to develop. If the obstruc-

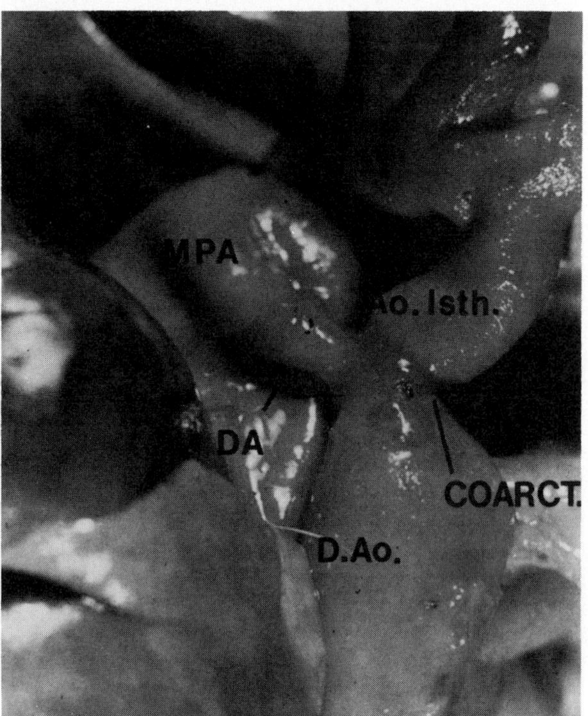

FIGURE 31-27. **Juxtaductal coarctation (COARCT) unmasked by constriction of the ductus arteriosus (DA). MPA = main pulmonary artery, D.Ao. = descending aorta, Ao.Isth. = aortic isthmus. (Courtesy of Norman Talner, M.D.)**

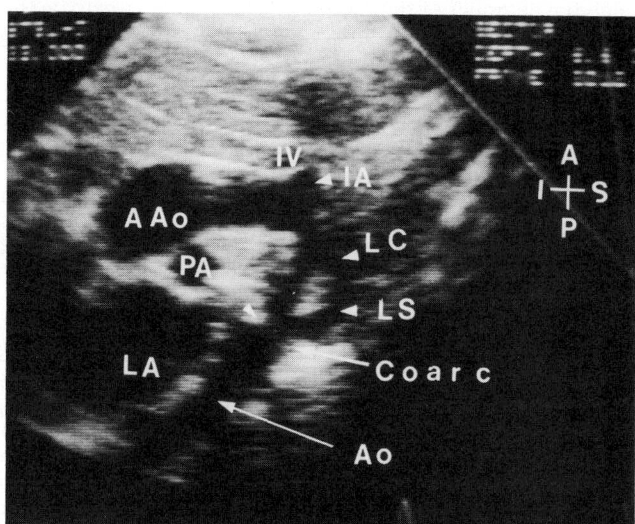

FIGURE 31-28. **Aortic coarctation (Coarc) is visualized from the suprasternal notch. The aorta (Ao) can be traced from the ascending aorta (AAo). The aortic arch is somewhat narrowed and the relationship of the left subclavian artery (LS) to the coarctation is identified clearly. LA = left atrium, PA = pulmonary artery, IA = innominate artery, LC = left carotid artery. (Courtesy of Norman Silverman, M.D.)**

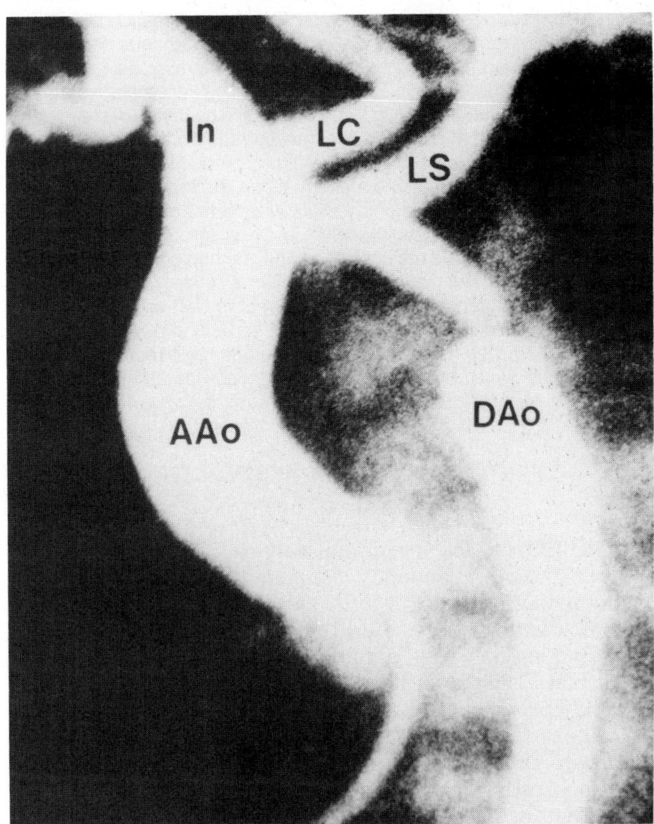

FIGURE 31–29. Retrograde aortogram demonstrates the discrete site of coarctation of the aorta, hypoplasia of the aortic isthmus, and poststenotic dilation of the descending aorta (DAo). AAo = ascending aorta, In = innominate artery, LC = left common carotid artery, LS = left subclavian artery.

tion does not intensify and cardiac failure does not occur by age 6 to 9 months, circulatory compensation is likely until adult life.

Most children with isolated juxtaductal coarctation are asymptomatic. Complaints of headache, cold extremities, and claudication with exercise may be noted, although attention usually is directed to the cardiovascular system by detection of a heart murmur or upper-extremity hypertension on routine physical examination. Mechanical factors rather than those of renal origin play the primary role in the production of hypertension. Absent, markedly diminished, or delayed pulsations in the femoral arteries and a low or unobtainable arterial pressure in the lower extremities with hypertension in the arms are the basic clues to the diagnosis.[219] A midsystolic murmur over the anterior chest, back, and spinous processes is most frequent, becoming continuous if the lumen is sufficiently narrowed to result in a high-velocity jet across the lesion throughout the cardiac cycle. Additional systolic and continuous murmurs over the lateral thoracic wall may reflect increased flow through dilated and tortuous collateral vessels. *Electrocardiography* reveals left ventricular hypertrophy of varying degrees, depending on the height of arterial pressure above the obstruction and the patient's age. Combined with right ventricular hypertrophy, this usually implies a complicated lesion. *Chest roentgenograms* (Fig. 8–40, p. 229) may show a dilated left subclavian artery high on the left mediastinal border and a dilated ascending aorta. Indentation of the aorta at the site of coarctation and prestenotic and poststenotic dilatation (the "3" sign) along the left paramediastinal shadow is almost pathognomonic. Poststenotic dilation also may be detected by indentation of the barium-filled esophagus. Notching of the ribs, an important radiographic sign, is due to erosion by dilated collateral vessels, increases with age, and usually becomes apparent between the 4th and 12th years of life. The aortic coarctation may be visualized directly by two-dimensional echocardiography from high parasternal or suprasternal notch views with short focused transducers, and from the subxiphoid window with extended focal range transducers (Fig. 31–28). Doppler examination reveals a flow disturbance and high-velocity jet at the site of obstruction and provides a reasonable estimate of the transcoarctation pressure gradient.[220,221] Computed tomography,[222] magnetic resonance imaging (Fig. 11–39, p. 331), or cardiac catheterization and aortography (Fig. 31–29) are usually indicated to accurately localize the site of obstruction, determine the length of the coarctation, and, particularly, identify associated malformations.[223] Preoperative catheterization may be avoided for selected patients with typical clinical and two-dimensional and Doppler echocardiographic findings.[224]

MANAGEMENT. Controversy exists concerning the role of balloon angioplasty (p. 1365) in the treatment of native coarctation.[217] Concerns exist about residual pressure gradients and aneurysm formation, especially late after angioplasty. It is clear that angioplasty can effectively reduce obstruction in many patients, albeit with an unpredictable late outcome.

Subclavian flap aortoplasty (Fig. 31–30), particularly in neonates and infants, or surgical resection and end-to-end anastomosis of uncomplicated juxtaductal coarctation of the aorta can be accomplished with excellent results in most patients[218,225]; some surgeons prefer an on-lay patch across the site of obstruction.[226] In children who are asymptomatic it is preferable to delay surgery until age 4 to 6 years, at which time coarctation seldom recurs.[227] Paradoxical hypertension of short duration often is noted in the immediate postoperative period. A resetting of carotid baroreceptors and increased catecholamine secretion appear to be responsible for the initial phase of systemic hypertension with a later, second phase of prolonged elevation of systolic and particularly diastolic blood

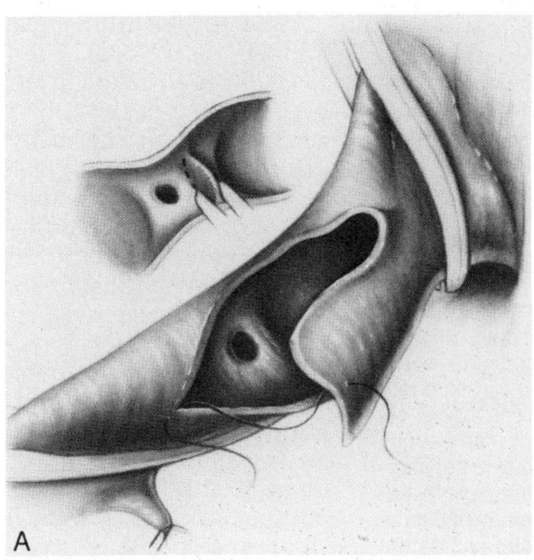

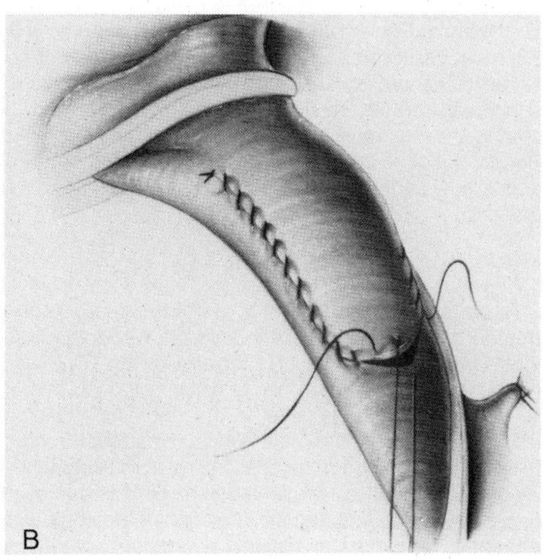

FIGURE 31–30. Subclavian flap aortoplasty repair of aortic coarctation. *A*, The left subclavian artery has been ligated and divided; the aorta is incised from below the coarctation ridge of tissue, which is carefully excised. *B*, The distal end of the subclavian artery forms a flap, which is sutured to the aortotomy. (From Stark, J., and DeLaval, M.: Surgery for Congenital Heart Defects. New York, Grune and Stratton, 1983, p. 216.)

pressure related to activation of the renin-angiotensin system.[228,230] A necrotizing panarteritis of the small vessels of the gastrointestinal tract of uncertain cause occasionally complicates the course of recovery.

A 5 to 10 per cent risk of recurrent narrowing exists after repair of coarctation in infancy.[231] This problem is treated most effectively by transcutaneous balloon angioplasty,[232] which may be expected to markedly reduce, but not abolish entirely, the pressure differences across the site of recoarctation.

In those patients who survive the first 2 years of life, complications of juxtaductal coarctation are uncommon before the second or third decade. The chief hazards to patients with coarctation result from severe hypertension, and include the development of cerebral aneurysms and hemorrhage, hypertensive encephalopathy, rupture of the aorta, left ventricular failure, and infective endocarditis. Systemic hypertension in the absence of residual coarctation has been observed in resting or exercise-stressed patients postoperatively and appears to be related to the duration of preoperative hypertension.[233,234] Lifelong observation is desirable because of the late onset of hypertension in some postoperative patients.

HYPOPLASIA OF THE AORTIC ARCH

The aortic isthmus, the portion of aorta between the left subclavian artery and the ductus arteriosus, normally is narrowed in the fetus and newborn. The lumen of the aortic isthmus is about two-thirds that of the ascending and descending portions of the aorta until age 6 to 9 months, when the physiological narrowing disappears.[235] Pathological tubular hypoplasia of the aortic arch usually is noted in the aortic isthmus and often is referred to as preductal or infantile coarctation of the aorta.[236] Associated major cardiac malformations occur in virtually all such infants and include large ventricular septal defect, atrioventricular septal defect, transposition of the great arteries, the Taussig-Bing type of anomaly, and double-outlet right ventricle. The ventricular septal defect most often is subpulmonary, lying within the substance of the infundibular septum. Thus, muscle persists between the aortic and pulmonary valve leaflets, which, when displaced leftward, produces subaortic stenosis. Persistent patency of the ductus arteriosus commonly coexists, and right-to-left flow across the ductus arteriosus usually provides filling of the descending aorta. The adequacy of blood flow to the lower body depends on the degree of aortic hypoplasia, the caliber of the ductus arteriosus, and the relationship between pulmonary and systemic vascular resistance. Substantial right-to-left shunting through a wide-open ductus arteriosus minimizes the arterial blood pressure difference between the upper and lower body. Differential cyanosis of the toes and feet with normal color of the fingers and hands may be difficult to discern because intracardiac left-to-right shunting and pulmonary edema attenuate the differences in oxygen saturation in the ascending and descending aorta. Clinical deterioration is associated with ductal constriction or a fall in pulmonary vascular resistance. Moreover, the clinical presentation often is dictated by the hemodynamic effects of complex associated intracardiac malformations. Infants most often present with findings of a large left-to-right intracardiac shunt, pulmonary hypertension, and marked cardiac decompensation. Although tubular hypoplasia is detectable by two-dimensional echocardiography, cardiac catheterization often is required to evaluate the full extent of intracardiac and extracardiac lesions.[237] Surgical repair of aortic arch hypoplasia usually must be accompanied by operative palliation or correction of associated intracardiac lesions. Aortic angioplasty incorporating the subclavian–aortic anastomosis, and a tubular prosthetic conduit are among the operative approaches to correct long segment narrowing. Recoarctation is common and often necessitates transcatheter balloon aortoplasty and/or a second operation later in life to relieve anastomotic stenosis.

AORTIC ARCH INTERRUPTION

Aortic arch interruption is a rare and usually lethal anomaly; unless treated surgically almost all infants die within the first month of life.[238] Interruptions distal to the left subclavian artery (Type A) occur with almost equal frequency to interruptions distal to the left common carotid artery (Type B); interruptions distal to the innominate artery (Type C) are extremely uncommon. The right subclavian artery often is of variable origin, frequently arising from the descending aortic segment distal to the interruption.[239] The clinical presentation resembles that seen in tubular hypoplasia or severe juxtaductal coarctation of the aorta with a patent ductus arteriosus. In almost all patients a ventricular septal defect and patent ductus arteriosus coexist with the arch interruption. Because the ductus arteriosus provides lower-body blood flow, its spontaneous constriction results in profound clinical deterioration. The latter may be temporarily ameliorated by prostaglandin E_1 infusion.[71,216] The ventricular septal defect most often is subpulmonary, lying within the substance of the infundibular septum. Thus, muscle persists between the aortic and pulmonary valve leaflets, which, when displaced leftward, produces subaortic stenosis. Other complex intracardiac malformations, such as transposition of the great arteries, aortopulmonary window, and truncus arteriosus, are common.[240] An association is frequent with DiGeorge syndrome of thymic hypoplasia or aplasia and the accompanying immunological and hypocalcemia problems.[241] The major clinical problem is severe congestive heart failure as a consequence of volume overload of the left ventricle resulting from an associated intracardiac left-to-right shunt and of pressure overload imposed by systemic hypertension. Operation by direct anastomosis seldom is possible, and reconstitution usually necessitates interposition of a tubular synthetic graft or a direct anastomosis between the aorta and one of its major brachiocephalic vessels.[238,239]

CONGENITAL VALVULAR AORTIC STENOSIS

(See also p. 1035)

MORPHOLOGY. Congenital valvular aortic stenosis is a relatively common anomaly, estimated to occur in 3 to 6 per cent of patients with congenital cardiovascular defects. However, it must be appreciated that the true incidence of the malformation is probably grossly underestimated because the congenital bicuspid aortic valve may be undetected in early life, and becomes stenotic and of clinical significance only in adult life, at a time when it may be indistinguishable from the acquired forms of aortic stenosis (Fig. 32–1, p. 967). Congenital valvular aortic stenosis occurs much more frequently in males than in females, with the sex ratio approximating 4:1. Associated cardiovascular anomalies have been noted in as many as 20 per cent of patients.[241] Patent ductus arteriosus and coarctation of the aorta occur most frequently with valvular aortic stenosis; all three of these lesions may coexist.

The basic malformation consists of thickening of valve tissue with varying degrees of commissural fusion. The valve most commonly is bicuspid with a single fused commissure and an eccentrically placed orifice. Sometimes a third commissure, incomplete or rudimentary, is apparent. Less commonly, the valve has three fused cusps with a stenotic central orifice. In some patients the stenotic aortic valve is unicuspid and dome-shaped with no or one lateral attachment to the aorta at the level of the orifice. In infants and young children with severe aortic stenosis the aortic valve ring may be relatively underdeveloped. This lesion forms a continuum with the hypoplastic left heart syndrome and the aortic atresia and hypoplasia complexes. Secondary calcification of the valve is extremely rare in childhood, but the dynamics of blood flow associated with the congenitally deformed aortic valve ultimately lead to thickening of the cusps and calcification in adult life. When the obstruction is hemodynamically significant, concentric hypertrophy of the left ventricular wall and dilatation of the ascending aorta occur.

HEMODYNAMICS (see also Figs. 4–55, p. 86; 7–9, p. 188; and 34–25, p. 1036). The hemodynamic abnormalities produced by obstruction to left ventricular outflow are discussed on p. 1036. A peak systolic gradient exceeding 75 mm Hg in association with a normal cardiac output or an effective aortic orifice less than 0.5 cm^2/m^2 body surface area is considered to reflect critical obstruction to left ventricular outflow.[241,242] The normal outflow orifice approximates 2.0 cm^2/m^2 body surface area; areas of 0.5 to 0.8 cm^2/m^2 signify moderate obstruction. When the area is larger than 0.8 cm^2/m^2, the obstruction is considered to be mild; when less than 0.4 cm^2/m^2, it is severe.

The resting cardiac output and stroke volume usually are within normal limits. During exercise, most children with critical stenosis show an elevation of the cardiac output and an associated elevation in the transvalvular pressure gradient.[243,244] When left ventricular failure occurs, the cardiac output decreases, and the left atrial, left ventricular end-diastolic, and pulmonary vascular pressures increase.

The blood supply to the myocardium may be significantly compromised in infants and children with aortic stenosis, despite normal patency of the coronary arteries.[245] Coronary blood flow and arterial oxygen content are critical determinants of oxygen supply to the myocardium. Because intramyocardial compressive forces are greatest in the subendocardium, blood flow to that region of left ventricle is entirely diastolic in the presence of elevated left ventricular systolic pressure. In patients with left ventricular outflow tract obstruction, coronary vasodilatation may give an inadequate response to an increase in the demands of the myocardium for oxygen at rest or with exercise. When subendocardial vessels are maximally dilated, the coronary artery driving pressure and the duration of diastole determine the magnitude of subendocardial flow. When the duration of systolic ejection lengthens across the stenotic orifice, diastole is shortened, especially at high heart rates. Moreover, a reduction occurs in coronary driving pressure if left ventricular end-diastolic pressure is high or if aortic diastolic pressure is low, e.g., with aortic regurgitation or heart failure. In patients with severe aortic stenosis the redistribution of flow away from the subendocardium and the ischemia that results in that portion of ventricular muscle may be estimated by relating the diastolic pressure–time index (DPTI) (i.e., the area between the aortic and left ventricular pressures in diastole) to the systolic pressure–time index (SPTI) (a measure of myocardial oxygen demands). Inadequate subendocardial oxygen delivery has been shown to exist when the ratio [DPTI × arterial oxygen content/SPTI] falls below 10.[245]

INFANCY. Special comment concerning this malformation as it is seen in infants is warranted, in view of the unique problems presented by patients in this age group.[246–250] Fortunately isolated aortic valvular stenosis seldom causes symptoms in infancy. This lesion, however, occasionally may be responsible for profound and intractable heart failure. Despite normal coronary arterial anatomy, infarction of left ventricular papillary muscles may occur, resulting in an acquired form of mitral valvular regurgitation that intensifies the heart failure state. In addition, endocardial fibroelastosis may result from limited subendocardial oxygen delivery and myocardial degeneration may be significant.[250] The symptomatic infant with isolated valvular aortic stenosis is irritable, pale, and hypotensive, and presents with tachycardia, cardiomegaly, and pulmonary congestion manifested by dyspnea, tachypnea, subcostal retractions, and diffuse rales. Cyanosis may be observed secondary to pulmonary venous desaturation. The systolic murmur in infants often is atypical; it is best heard at the apex or along the lower left sternal border and may be confused with that caused by a ventricular septal defect. In infants with heart failure the murmur occasionally may be absent or extremely soft, becoming louder when myocardial contractility is improved with digitalis and other medical measures. The response to medical management of the infant with heart failure is frequently poor.

The electrocardiographic findings may not be characteristic; left ventricular hypertrophy and/or strain as well as right atrial enlargement and right ventricular hypertrophy may be detected shortly after birth.[246] The latter signs of right heart involvement result from both pulmonary hypertension secondary to elevated left ventricular diastolic and left atrial pressures and from volume loading of the right ventricle caused by left-to-right shunting across the foramen ovale. Survival past the early neonatal period does not preclude subsequent difficulties, and clinical deterioration may recur with the onset of physiological anemia.

Congenital aortic stenosis must be considered a medical emergency in the seriously ill newborn, and echocardiography, and sometimes cardiac catheterization and angiocardiography, may be indicated in the first 24 hours of life. Two-dimensional echocardiographic long-axis views of the left ventricular outflow tract demonstrate doming of the aortic valve. The parasternal short-axis view bisects the face of the valve, demonstrating the anatomy of the commissures.[251,252] M-mode recordings best demonstrate wall thickness and motion. Doppler echocardiography provides an accurate estimate of the pressure gradient across the site of obstruction (Fig. 4–54, p. 85).[253–255] Hemodynamic findings commonly include left-to-right shunting at the atrial level, elevated left atrial and left ventricular end-diastolic pressures, and a small pressure drop across the aortic valve as a result of a markedly reduced cardiac output. Occasionally, right-to-left shunting across a patent ductus arteriosus is encountered. The presence of a normal or enlarged left ventricular cavity and normal or dilated ascending aorta allows distinction of aortic stenosis from the hypoplastic left heart syndrome angiographically. Because prolonged periods of stabilization are uncommon with medical therapy, early and definitive establishment of the diagnosis and prompt balloon valvuloplasty or valvulotomy usually are justified.[256–258] Poor myocardial performance resulting from endocardial fibroelastosis, subendocardial ischemia, or reduced left ventricular compliance, and inadequate relief of obstruction with or without significant aortic regurgitation are among the factors accounting for high operative mortality and morbidity. Open repair under direct vision is the preferred type of operation.[257,258,258a]

CHILDHOOD. Congenital aortic stenosis may be responsible for severe obstruction to left ventricular outflow in the absence of the clinical symptoms of diminished cardiac reserve that are so frequent in other forms of congenital heart disease. Most children with congenital aortic stenosis grow and develop normally and are asymptomatic. Attention usually is called to these children when a murmur is detected on routine examination. When symptoms occur, those noted most commonly are fatigability, exertional dyspnea, angina pectoris, and syncope. Less often described are abdominal pain, profuse sweating, and epistaxis. The symptomatic child usually has critical stenosis. There is a distinct threat of sudden death in patients with severe obstruction[242] (p. 899). Although the precise cause is poorly understood, ventricular arrhythmias, perhaps initiated by acute myocardial ischemia, are probably the most common inciting event. It has been speculated that an abrupt rise in intracavity left ventricular systolic pressure elicits a reflex hypotensive syncope that promotes acute ischemia and ventricular fibrillation.[260] Bacterial endocarditis occurs in about 4 per cent of patients with congenital valvular aortic stenosis.

DIAGNOSIS. Physical Findings. When the magnitude of obstruction is significant, a left ventricular lift usually is palpable, and a precordial systolic thrill often is palpated over the base of the heart with transmission to the jugular notch and along the carotid arteries; presystolic expansion often is palpable. The obstruction usually is mild if neither a left ventricular lift nor a thrill is present.

Opening of the aortic valve produces a systolic aortic ejection sound that typically is present at the cardiac apex when the valve is mobile, particularly in patients with mild to moderate stenosis. A delay in closure of the stenotic aortic valve leads to a single or a closely split second heart sound, and paradoxical splitting may be present. A fourth heart sound normally is associated with severe obstruction. A loud, harsh, rhomboid-shaped systolic murmur starts after completion of left ventricular isometric contraction and is best heard at the base of the heart. The murmur, like the thrill, radiates to the suprasternal notch and carotid vessels as well as to the apex. An early diastolic blowing murmur of aortic regurgitation is present in some patients, but unless the valve leaflets have been eroded by bacterial endocarditis, the regurgitation usually is not hemodynamically significant; uncommonly, in patients with a congenitally bicuspid valve, aortic regurgitation may be severe and may predominate.

Electrocardiography. There is a tendency for electrocardiographic signs of left ventricular hypertrophy to vary with the severity of obstruction, although a normal or near-normal electrocardiogram does not exclude severe aortic stenosis.[261] The presence of a left ventricular "strain pattern," consisting of left ventricular hypertrophy combined with ST-segment

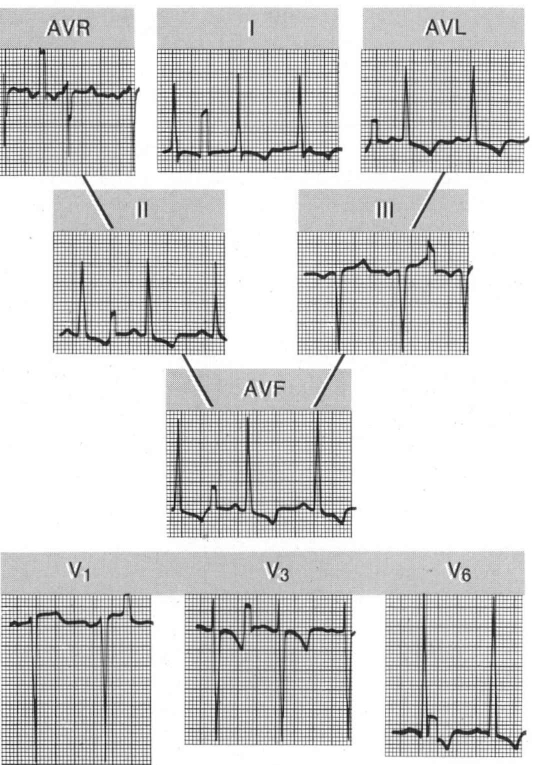

FIGURE 31-31. Electrocardiogram in congenital aortic stenosis. This tracing shows left ventricular hypertrophy and the typical left ventricular "strain" pattern (V_6, arrow). (Courtesy of Delores A. Danilowicz, M.D.)

depressions and T-wave inversion in the left precordial leads, usually indicates that severe aortic stenosis is present (Fig. 31-31).

In patients under 10 years of age the electrocardiogram is a more reliable guide in indicating the severity of the stenosis than it is in older patients.[259] Findings in the younger age group that often accompany severe obstruction are T-wave vectors in the frontal plane to the left of −40 degrees, widening of the angle between the mean QRS and T forces in the frontal plane in excess of 100 degrees, an S wave in V_1 greater than 16 mm, and an R wave in V_5 exceeding 20 mm. Nonetheless, it is important to recognize that these voltages may be excessive in patients who do not have severe stenosis. A good relation appears to exist between exercise-induced electrocardiographic changes and the severity of obstruction; ischemic ST-segment changes have been observed in patients with normal resting cardiac indices and transvalvular pressure differences in excess of 50 mm Hg or an abnormal left ventricular oxygen supply-demand ratio.[243]

Roentgenography. Overall heart size is normal or the degree of enlargement is slight in most children with congenital valvular aortic stenosis. Concentric left ventricular hypertrophy accompanies moderate or severe obstruction and is manifested by rounding of the cardiac apex in the frontal projection and posterior displacement in the lateral view.

Echocardiography. The M-mode echocardiographic findings that may suggest a diagnosis of aortic valve stenosis include multiple diastolic closure lines, or a single eccentrically placed diastolic closure line in the aortic lumen; left ventricular posterior wall and septal thickening; reduced separation of thickened aortic valve leaflets; and aortic root dilation. Two-dimensional echocardiography demonstrates a bicuspid aortic valve, impaired mobility of cusp tissue, altered phasic movement of the aortic valve with increased superior and reduced lateral excursions of valve echoes, and an increase in the internal aortic root dimension distal to the level of the valve annulus.[241] The parasternal short-axis view of the valve demonstrates the leaflet anatomy (Fig. 31-32).

The most accurate noninvasive approach to quantify the severity of obstruction combines continuous-wave Doppler flow analysis with the two-dimensional echocardiographic determination of the area of the orifice.[253-255] A simple estimate of the transvalvular gradient (in millimeters of mercury) may be calculated as four times the square of the peak Doppler velocity (meters per second).

The Doppler-derived aortic valve area, calculated by the continuity equation, correlates well with the catheterization-derived aortic valve area, calculated by the Gorlin equation, when either the time-velocity integral ratio or the peak flow velocity ratio between the left ventricular outflow tract and the aortic valve is used in the equation as follows:

$$\text{AVA} = (\text{area})_{\text{LVOT}} \times \frac{(\text{TVI})_{\text{LVOT}}}{(\text{TVI})_{\text{AV}}}$$

where AV = aortic valve, AVA = aortic valve area, LVOT = left ventricular outflow tract, and TVI = time-velocity integral. The simplified continuity equation uses peak velocity ratio instead of time-velocity integral:

$$\text{AVA} = (\text{area})_{\text{LVOT}} \times \frac{(\text{V})_{\text{LVOT}}}{(\text{V})_{\text{AV}}}$$

where V = peak flow velocity.[253]

Cardiac catheterization is more important for establishing the site and severity than for detecting the presence of aortic stenosis, since the malformation usually is readily diagnosed by clinical examination. Catheterization is indicated in any child with a clinical diagnosis of aortic stenosis in whom the clinical examination, roentgenogram, resting or exercise electrocardiogram, or echocardiogram suggests the possibility of severe obstruction.[242] Even in the absence of such findings, hemodynamic study should be performed if symptoms exist that might be related to aortic stenosis.

The site and severity of obstruction are established at car-

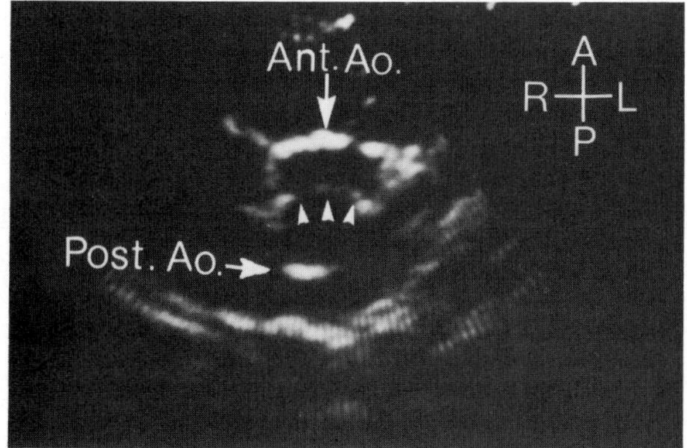

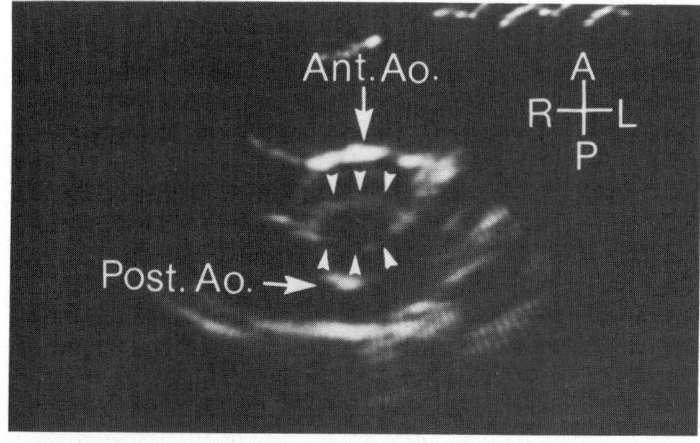

FIGURE 31-32. Short-axis view at the base of the heart of a bicuspid aortic valve. In the left panel the valve is imaged as a single diastolic echo (arrows) in the aortic root. In systole (right panel), the valve opens (arrows) with a typical fish-mouth appearance. Ant.Ao. = anterior aorta, Post.Ao. = posterior aorta. (From DiSessa, T. G., and Friedman, W. F.: Cardiovascular Clinics. Fowler, N. [ed.], Philadelphia, F. A. Davis Co., 1983.)

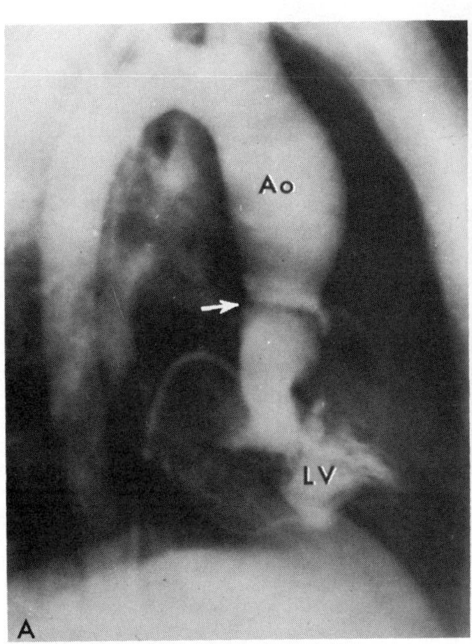

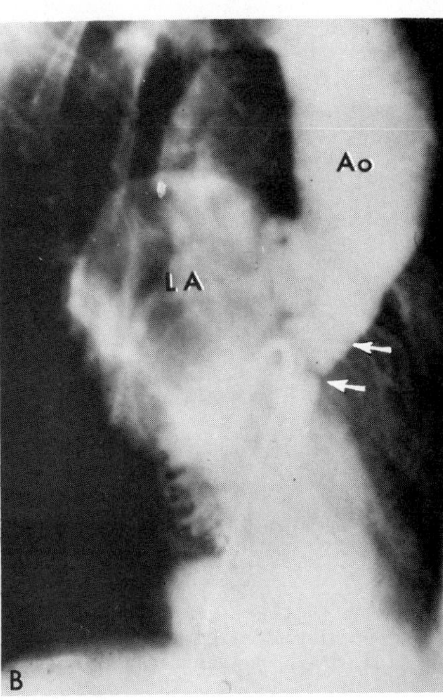

FIGURE 31-33. *A*, Left ventricular angiocardiogram obtained by the transseptal method in a patient with congenital valvular aortic stenosis. Ao = post-stenotic dilatation of the aorta; LV = left ventricle. Arrow denotes the thickened valve cusp. *B*, Selective angiocardiogram in a patient with discrete subvalvular stenosis (bottom arrow). Associated mitral regurgitation is evident from the reflux of contrast into an enlarged left atrium (LA). The aortic valve (top arrow) is normal, and the right coronary artery is visualized. (From Friedman, W. F., and Kirkpatrick, S. E.: Congenital aortic stenosis. *In* Moss, A. J., Adams, F. H., and Emmanouilides, G. C. [eds.]: Heart Disease in Infants, Children and Adolescents. 2nd ed. Baltimore, Williams and Wilkins, 1977.)

diac catheterization, and associated malformations are identified. Typically, the angiocardiographic features of valvular stenosis are thickening of the aortic cusps and of the left ventricular wall with slight or no dilatation of the left ventricular cavity, poststenotic dilatation of the ascending aorta, and occasionally a jet of contrast material entering the ascending aorta through a narrowed valve orifice that is central or eccentric (Fig. 31-33). The leaflets of the bicuspid valve are domed in systole; a central jet corresponds to the orifice of the stenotic valve. In contrast, the stenotic orifice of the unicommissural valve may be visualized by the systolic jet in contact with the posterior wall of the aorta, with leaflet tissue and valve motion seen only anteriorly.

Congenital aortic stenosis frequently is a progressive disorder, even early in life, in a significant fraction of patients presenting initially with mild obstruction.[262-265] Thus, clinical deterioration may be anticipated because of an intensification in the severity of stenosis rather than the development of significant aortic regurgitation. Progression of obstruction usually is the result of the increase in cardiac output that occurs concurrent with increased body growth. Less often, a decrease in the area of the orifice is an added factor in the intensification of obstruction. The onset of symptoms or changes in the phonocardiogram or graphic pulse tracings, chest roentgenograms, electrocardiograms, or vectorcardiograms cannot be depended on to indicate progressive obstruction in the individual patient; Doppler echocardiography is most reliable.

MANAGEMENT. The malformed aortic valve is a potential site of bacterial infection; antibiotic prophylaxis is recommended for all patients, regardless of the severity of obstruction. Strict avoidance of strenuous physical activity is advised if severe aortic stenosis is present. Participation in competitive sports also should probably be restricted in patients with milder degrees of obstruction. Digitalis should be administered to patients who have symptoms of diminished cardiac reserve and also should be considered in patients with left ventricular hypertrophy, even if they are not in heart failure.

The most important decision concerns the advisability of *surgical treatment*. Among the factors influencing the indications, techniques, and results of operation are the patient's age, the nature of the valvular deformity, and the experience of the surgical team.[242] The recommendation that operation is indicated depends more often on the presence of severe obstruction than on the symptoms described by the patient. Operation currently is advised for any child with critical stenosis (i.e., a peak systolic pressure gradient exceeding 75 mm Hg, measured in the basal state when the cardiac output is normal) or a calculated effective orifice less than 0.5 cm^2/m^2 body surface area. In the presence of clinical symptoms, a left ventricular strain pattern on the electrocardiogram, or an abnormal exercise electrocardiogram, operation may be recommended with less rigid regard to the hemodynamic assessment of the severity of stenosis. After severe stenosis has been established hemodynamically, the potential hazard of sudden death dictates that surgical treatment not be postponed unnecessarily. Operation is carried out under direct vision after institution of cardiopulmonary bypass; judicious incision of the fused commissures enlarges the valve orifice and does not result in significant aortic regurgitation. A mortality rate less than 2 per cent can be expected when operation is performed by an experienced surgeon. Substantial relief of obstruction occurs in most patients unless the valve ring is hypoplastic. Balloon aortic valvuloplasty (p. 1043) currently is an experimental procedure for unoperated congenital valvular aortic stenosis. Preliminary data suggest that percutaneous valvuloplasty provides effective acute relief of valvular aortic stenosis. Significant complications have included death, aortic regurgitation, and femoral artery thrombosis or damage. Follow-up data are required before the percutaneous approach can be established as a treatment of choice for infants or children with this anomaly.[256,266]

Long-term follow-up studies have provided evidence that aortic valvulotomy is a safe and effective means of treatment with excellent relief of symptoms that were present preoperatively.[267-269] In some patients, aortic regurgitation may be progressive and require prosthetic valve replacement. Moreover, after commissurotomy the valve leaflets remain somewhat deformed, and it is quite possible that further degenerative changes, including calcification, will lead to significant stenosis later in life.[269-271] Thus, prosthetic valve replacement is required in about 35 per cent of patients within 15 to 20 years of the original operation. Because the valves are not rendered anatomically normal, antibiotic prophylaxis is indicated in all patients postoperatively, even if the systolic pressure gradient has been completely abolished.

DISCRETE SUBAORTIC STENOSIS

This malformation accounts for 8 to 10 per cent of all cases of congenital aortic stenosis and occurs twice as frequently in males as in females. The lesion consists of a membranous diaphragm or fibromuscular ring encircling the left ventricular outflow tract just beneath the base of the aortic valve.

Distinction of subvalvular from valvular aortic stenosis is

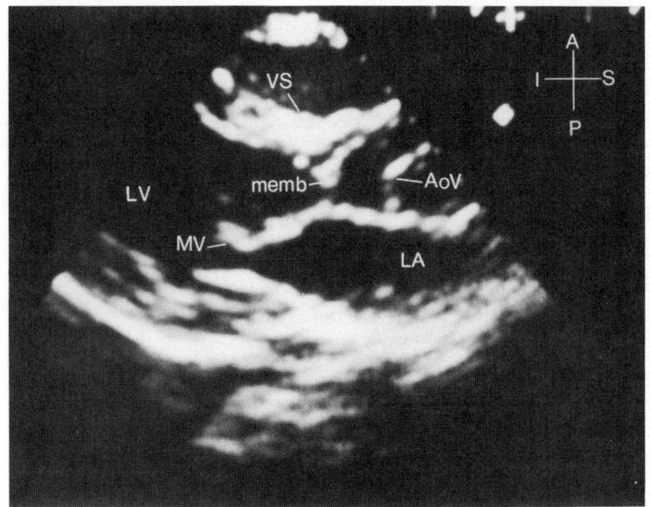

FIGURE 31-34. Long-axis view of discrete membranous subaortic stenosis. A discrete membrane (memb) is imaged in the left ventricular (LV) outflow tract beneath and parallel to the aortic valve (AoV), extending from the ventricular septum (VS) to the anterior leaflet of the mitral valve (MV). LA = left atrium.

extremely difficult by means of clinical findings alone.[241] Rarely, systolic ejection sound is heard, and the diastolic murmur of aortic regurgitation is more common than it is in valvular aortic stenosis. Dilatation of the ascending aorta is common, but valvular calcification is not observed.

Echocardiography is useful in the differentiation between valvular and subvalvular stenosis (Figs. 4-71 and 4-72, p. 92).[272,273] Two-dimensional echocardiographic studies from the apical two-chamber and left parasternal and subxiphoid long-axis views demonstrate persistent, prominent echoes in the subaortic left ventricle in both systole and diastole (Fig. 31-34). Doppler sampling proximal to the aortic valve shows increased flow velocity.[274] Most important, echocardiography also can identify hypertrophic subaortic stenosis when it coexists with fixed subaortic stenosis and can differentiate between the two forms of obstruction.

Definitive distinction between valvular and subvalvular obstruction is provided by transesophageal Doppler echocardiography[275] and by recording pressure tracings as a catheter is withdrawn across the outflow tract and valve, or by localizing the site of obstruction with selective left ventricular angiocardiography (Fig. 31-33).

Mild degrees of aortic valvular regurgitation commonly are observed in patients with discrete subaortic stenosis and appear to be caused by thickening of the valve and impaired mobility of the cusps secondary to the trauma created by the high-velocity jet passing through the subaortic diaphragm. Further deformation of these abnormal valve cusps by the vegetations of bacterial endocarditis often results in severe aortic regurgitation.

Because of the likelihood of both progressive obstruction and aortic regurgitation, the presence of even mild or moderate subaortic stenosis warrants consideration of elective operation.[276,277] The risks of operation in patients with discrete subaortic stenosis and valvular aortic stenosis are essentially the same. Surgical correction is accomplished by excising the membrane or fibrous ridge. Operation may be expected to improve the hemodynamic state substantially; it frequently is totally curative.[278-280] In a small number of patients, secondary muscular hypertrophy of the outflow tract and a pressure gradient may persist after the operative relief of valvular or discrete subvalvular aortic stenosis. Balloon dilatation also has been reported to be a successful mode of therapy, but is still considered experimental.[281]

UNCOMMON FORMS OF SUBAORTIC STENOSIS

In some patients, valvular and subvalvular aortic stenosis coexist, with hypoplasia of the aortic valve ring and thickened valve leaflets, producing a tunnel-like narrowing of the left ventricular outflow tract.[282] Additional findings often include a small ascending aorta. The subvalvular fibrous process usually extends onto the aortic valve cusps and almost always makes contact with the ventricular aspect of the anterior mitral leaflet at its base. The presence of "tunnel stenosis" may be suspected echocardiographically and angiographically from the appearance of the outflow tract and the aortic root. Operative treatment often is complicated by the necessity for prosthetic or homograft replacement of the aortic valve as well as for enlarging the aortic annulus, proximal aorta, and left ventricular outlet tract (the Konno operation). Operation is controversial, utilizing a prosthetic, valve-containing conduit between the left ventricular apex and descending aorta.[283]

Various anatomical lesions other than a discrete membrane or ridge may produce subaortic stenosis.[277,284] Among these are abnormal adherence of the anterior leaflet of the mitral valve to the left septal surface, and the presence in the left ventricular outflow tract of accessory endocardial cushion tissue. In some patients with atrioventricular canal, the part of the ventricular septum that contributes to the wall of the left ventricular outflow tract is deficient, and the ventricular aspect of the anterior leaflet of the common atrioventricular valve is adherent to the posterior edge of the deficient septum, resulting in a narrow left ventricular outflow tract. Malalignment of the conoventricular septum, resulting in an inferior ventricular septal defect, produces a leftward superior deviation and insertion of the conal septum, obstructing left ventricular outflow.[284] In patients with a single ventricle and an outflow chamber, the bulboventricular foramen serves as a potential site of aortic outflow obstruction. Additional, rarer causes of subaortic stenosis include redundant dysplastic left atrioventricular valve tissue in patients with congenitally corrected transposition of the great arteries and anomalous muscle bundles of the left ventricular outflow tract. A muscular type of subaortic stenosis may result from a convergence of all the mitral chordae into one or two fused papillary muscles; a "parachute" deformity of the mitral valve is produced that often is seen in association with supravalvular stenosis of the left atrium and coarctation of the aorta. In some of these patients, discrete membranous subvalvular aortic obstruction also has been noted.

In patients with ventricular septal defect, muscular subaortic stenosis has been shown to develop after surgical banding of the pulmonary artery, possibly as a result of hypertrophy of the conal septum or crista supraventricularis encroaching on the left ventricular outflow tract above the septal defect.

Subaortic muscular hypetrophy secondary to diffuse involvement of the myocardium by glycogen storage disease (Pompe's disease) is an extremely rare cause of obstruction to left ventricular outflow. A positive family history, symptoms of muscle weakness, heart failure in infancy, and the characteristic electrocardiographic findings of a short PR interval, high-voltage QRS and T waves, and left ventricular hypertrophy warrant skeletal muscle biopsy or fibroblast culture, permitting an antemortem diagnosis.

The last, relatively uncommon form of subaortic stenosis to be mentioned occurs infrequently in patients with congenitally corrected transposition of the great arteries in whom an anomalous muscle bundle in the subaortic area of the arterial ventricle obstructs outflow.

SUPRAVALVULAR AORTIC STENOSIS

Supravalvular aortic stenosis is a congenital narrowing of the ascending aorta that may be localized or diffuse, originating at the superior margin of the sinuses of Valsalva just above the levels of the coronary arteries.

The clinical picture of supravalvular obstruction usually differs in major respects from that observed in the other forms of aortic stenosis. Chief among these differences is the association of supravalvular aortic stenosis with idiopathic infantile hypercalcemia, a disease that may be related to deranged vitamin D metabolism.[285-288]

The designation supravalvular aortic stenosis syndrome, or Williams' syndrome, is applied to the distinctive clinical picture produced by coexistence of the cardiac and multisystem disorder. Additional manifestations of this syndrome include a peculiar elfin facies (Fig. 31-35), mental retardation, auditory hyperacusis, narrowing of peripheral systemic and pulmonary arteries, inguinal hernia, strabismus, and abnormalities of dental development.[289] In some patients, moderate thickening of the aortic cusps and valvular pulmonary stenosis may occur in association with peripheral pulmonary artery stenosis. Rarely, patients have mitral valve abnormalities with prolapse and mitral regurgitation.

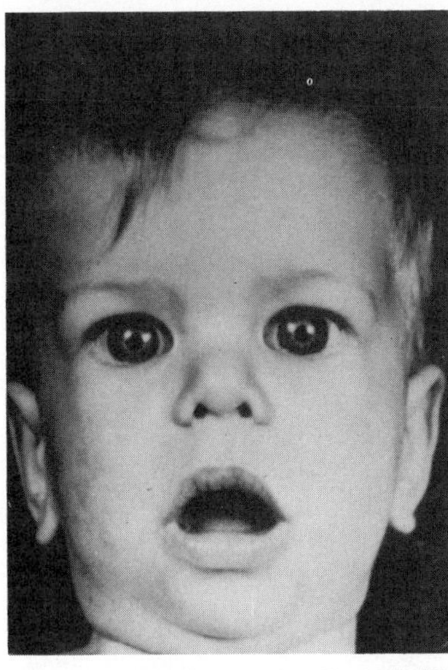
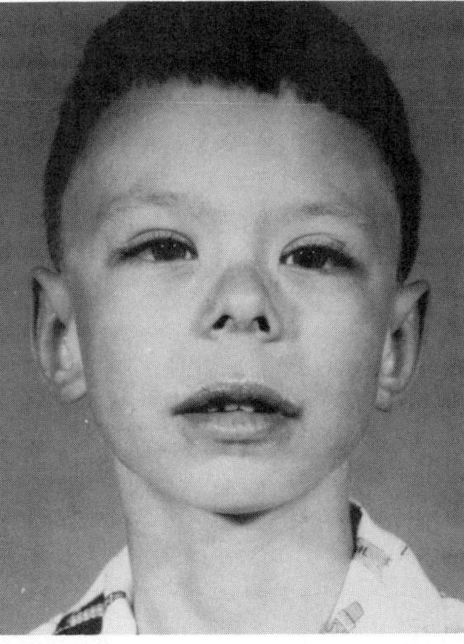
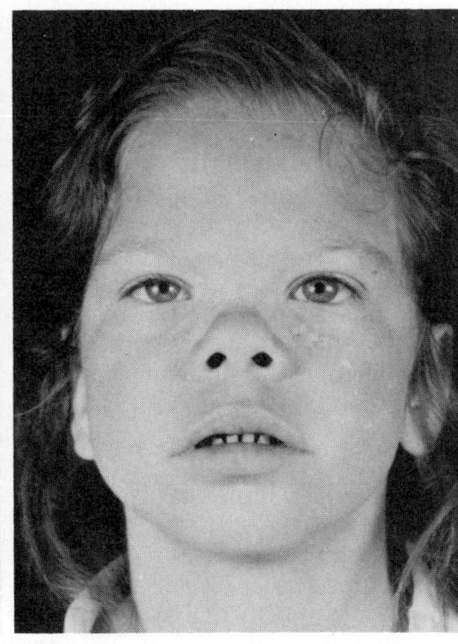

FIGURE 31-35. Typical elfin facies in three patients with supravalvular aortic stenosis. (From Friedman, W. F., and Kirkpatrick, S. E.: Congenital aortic stenosis. *In* Moss, A. J., Adams, F. H., and Emmanouilides, G. C. [eds.]: Heart Disease in Infants, Children and Adolescents. 2nd ed. Baltimore, Williams and Wilkins, 1977.)

Experimental hypervitaminosis D produced in the pregnant rabbit has caused craniofacial abnormalities and malformations resembling those of supravalvular aortic stenosis in the offspring.[285,286] In patients the metabolism of vitamin D is abnormal.[290] In humans, with one exception, chromosomal studies have consistently revealed normal karyotypes. Supravalvular aortic stenosis most often is a feature of the distinctive syndrome described above. Peripheral pulmonary artery stenosis and the aortic anomaly also are seen, however, in familial and sporadic forms unassociated with the other features of the syndrome.[291] Genetic studies suggest that the familial anomaly is transmitted as an autosomal dominant with variable expression. Some family members may have supravalvular pulmonic stenosis either as an isolated lesion or in combination with the supravalvular aortic anomaly. Unlike with the other forms of aortic stenosis, there appears to be no sex predilection.

Three anatomical types of supravalvular aortic stenosis are recognized, although some patients may have findings of more than one type. Most common is the hourglass type, in which marked thickening and disorganization of the aortic media produce a constricting annular ridge at the superior margin of the sinuses of Valsalva. The membranous type is the result of fibrous or fibromuscular semicircular diaphragm with a small central opening stretched across the lumen of the aorta. Uniform hypoplasia of the ascending aorta characterizes the hypoplastic type.

Because the coronary arteries arise proximal to the site of outflow obstruction in supravalvular aortic stenosis, they are subjected to the elevated pressure that exists within the left ventricle. These vessels often are dilated and tortuous, and premature coronary arteriosclerosis has been observed. Moreover, if the free edges of some or all of the aortic cusps adhere to the site of supravalvular stenosis, coronary artery inflow may be reduced. The formation of thoracic aortic aneurysms has been described in several patients.

Most patients with supravalvular aortic stenosis syndrome are mentally retarded and resemble one another in their facial features. The typical appearance is similar to that of the elfin facies observed in the severe form of idiopathic infantile hypercalcemia and is characerized by a high prominent forehead, epicanthal folds, underdeveloped bridge of the nose and mandible, overhanging upper lip, strabismus, and anomalies of dentition (Fig. 31-35). Recognition of this distinctive appearance, even in infancy, should alert the physician to the possibility of underlying multisystem disease. In addition, a positive family history in a patient with a normal appearance and clinical signs suggesting left ventricular outflow obstruction should lead to the suspicion of either supravalvular aortic stenosis or hypertrophic obstructive cardiomyopathy.[291] Patients with supravalvular aortic obstruction appear to be subject to the same risks of unexpected sudden death and infective endocarditis as those with valvular aortic stenosis.

With few exceptions, the major *physical findings* resemble those observed in patients with valvular aortic stenosis. Among these exceptions are accentuation of aortic valve closure due to elevated pressure in the aorta proximal to the stenosis, an infrequent systolic ejection sound, and the especially prominent transmission of a thrill and murmur into the jugular notch and along the carotid vessels. Uncommonly, there is an early diastolic, decrescendo, blowing murmur of aortic regurgitation caused by the fusion of one or more cusps to the area of stenosis. The narrowing of the peripheral pulmonary arteries that often coexists in these patients frequently produces a late systolic or continuous murmur that may help to distinguish this anomaly from valvular aortic stenosis. This differentiation is reinforced by the frequent finding of a significant disparity between the arterial pressures in the upper extremities in supravalvular aortic stenosis; the systolic pressure in the right arm tends to be the higher of the two and occasionally exceeds that in the femoral arteries. The disparity in pulses may relate to the tendency of a jet stream to adhere to a vessel wall (Coanda effect) and selective streaming of blood into the innominate artery.[292,293]

Electrocardiography usually reveals left ventricular hypertrophy when obstruction is severe. Biventricular, or even right ventricular, hypertrophy may be found if significant narrowing of peripheral pulmonary arteries coexists. Radiographically, in contrast to valvular and discrete subvalvular

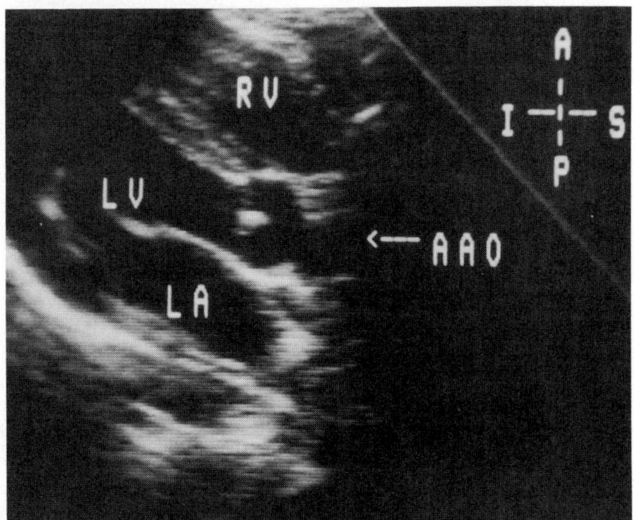

FIGURE 31-36. Supravalvar aortic stenosis is seen in a parasternal long-axis view. The constriction is distal to the sinuses of Valsalva in the ascending aorta (AAO). RV = right ventricle, LV = left ventricle, LA = left atrium. (Courtesy of Norman Silverman, M.D.)

aortic stenosis, poststenotic dilation of the ascending aorta seldom is seen. The sinuses of Valsalva usually are dilated, and the ascending aorta and aortic arch are of normal size or appear small.

Echocardiography is the most valuable technique for localizing the site of obstruction to the supravalvular area (Fig. 31–36), and Doppler examination and retrograde aortic catheterization can determine the degree of hemodynamic abnormality.[294]

The supravalvular aortic lumen may be widened by the insertion of an oval- or diamond-shaped fabric patch in those patients with a normal ascending aorta.[295,296] If the aorta is markedly hypoplastic, this operation merely displaces the pressure gradient distally without abolishing the obstruction. Under these circumstances, repair may require replacement or widening of the entire hypoplastic aorta with an appropriate prosthesis. Operation may be recommended when relatively little hypoplasia of the ascending aorta and arch exists and when the obstruction is discrete and significant, i.e., with a systolic gradient exceeding 50 mm Hg.

HYPOPLASTIC LEFT HEART SYNDROME

This designation is used to describe a group of closely related cardiac anomalies characterized by underdevelopment of the left cardiac chambers, atresia or stenosis of the aortic and/or the mitral orifices, and hypoplasia of the aorta.[297] These anomalies are an especially common cause of heart failure in the first week of life. The left atrium and ventricle often exhibit *endocardial fibroelastosis.* Pulmonary venous blood traverses a patent foramen ovale, and a dilated and hypertrophied right ventricle acts as the systemic, as well as the pulmonary, ventricle; the systemic circulation receives blood by way of a patent ductus arteriosus (Fig. 31–37). The diagnosis should be considered in infants, particularly males, with the sudden onset of heart failure, systemic hypoperfusion, and nonspecific murmur. Electrocardiography frequently reveals right axis deviation, right atrial and ventricular enlargement, and ST and T-wave abnormalities in the left precordial leads. Chest roentgenography may show only slight enlargement shortly after birth, but with clinical deterioration there are marked cardiomegaly and increased pulmonary venous and arterial vascular markings.

The *echocardiographic* findings usually are diagnostic (Fig. 31–38), and include a diminutive aortic root and left ventricular cavity and absence or poor visualization of aortic and mitral valve echoes, which, when seen, are of diminished amplitude and mobility.[298] Retrograde aortography shows hypoplasia of the ascending aorta (Fig. 31–39).

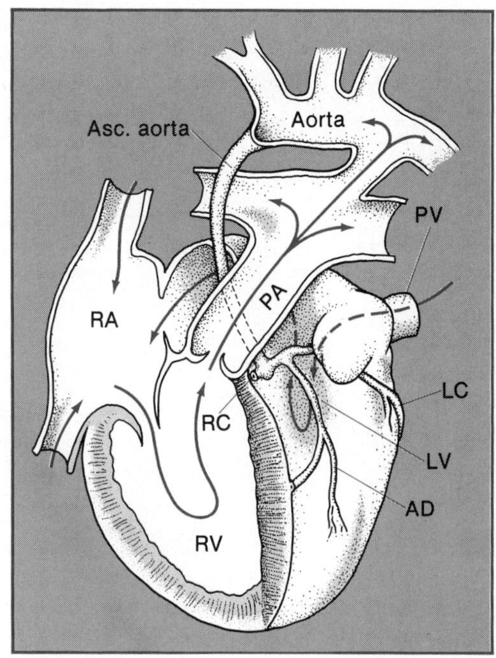

FIGURE 31–37. Hypoplastic left heart with aortic hypoplasia, aortic valve atresia, and a hypoplastic mitral valve and left ventricle. R.A. = right atrium, R.V. = right ventricle, R.C. = right coronary artery, P.A. = pulmonary artery, P.V. = pulmonary vein, L.C. = left coronary artery, L.V. = left ventricle, A.D. = anterior descending coronary artery. (From Neufeld, H. N., et al.: Diagnosis of aortic atresia by retrograde aortography. Circulation *25*:278, 1962, by permission of the American Heart Association, Inc.)

MANAGEMENT. Medical therapy directed at cardiac decompensation, hypoxemia, and metabolic acidemia seldom prolongs survival beyond the first days of life. Constriction of the patent ductus arteriosus and limited flow through a re-

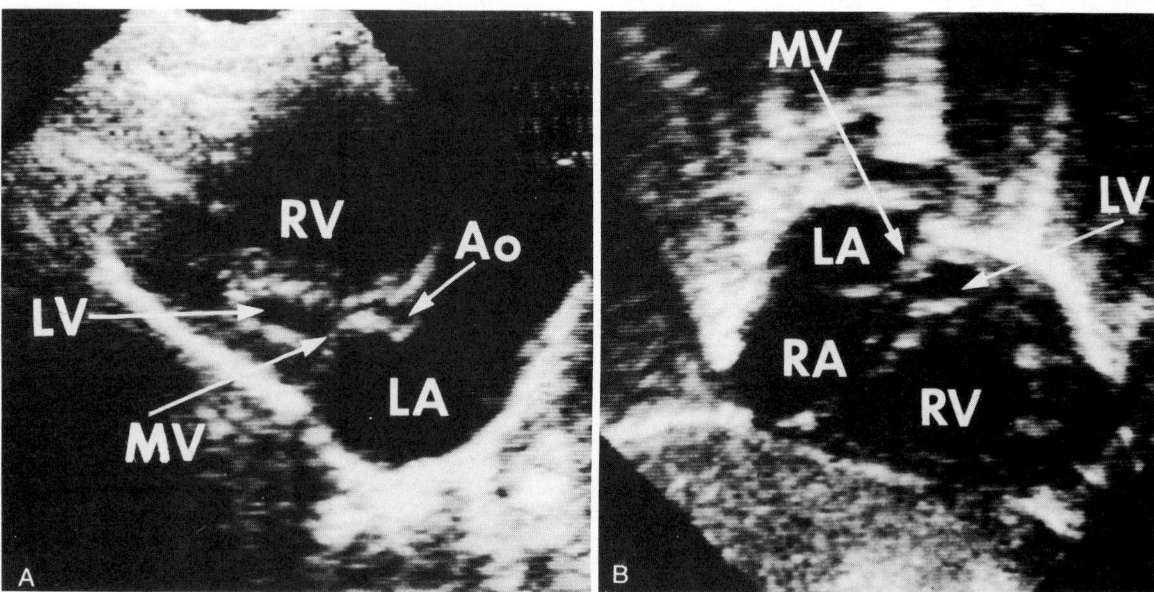

FIGURE 31–38. ***A,*** **Hypoplastic left heart in a parasternal long-axis view in a newborn with aortic atresia, intact ventricular septum, and patent but hypoplastic mitral valve (MV). The left ventricular (LV) cavity is diminutive and the ascending aorta (Ao) is hypoplastic. Right ventricular (RV) dilation is noted.** ***B,*** **In the subcostal four-chamber view dilatation of the right atrium (RA) and right ventricle (RV) is noted. The endocardial echoes are very bright owing to fibroelastosis. (From Perloff, J.: The Clinical Recognition of Congenital Heart Disease. 3rd ed. Philadelphia, W. B. Saunders Company, 1986.)**

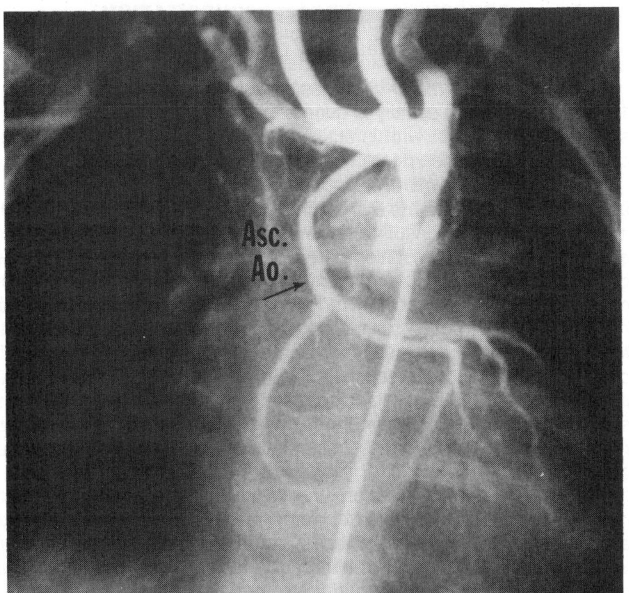

FIGURE 31–39. Retrograde aortogram showing marked hypoplasia of the ascending aorta (asc. Ao.) (arrow) in an infant with hypoplastic left heart syndrome. (From Freedom, R. M., et al.: Aortic atresia with normal left ventricle: Distinctive angiocardiographic findings. Cath. Cardiovasc. Diag. *3*:283, 1977.)

strictive patent foramen ovale are the principal factors responsible for early death. Prostaglandin E_1 infusion is effective in maintaining ductal patency. Some centers are attempting staged surgical management in an effort to provide long-term palliation.[297,299–302] The first stage, often referred to as the Norwood procedure, consists of creating an unobstructed communication between the right ventricle and aorta, and enlargement of the ascending aorta. The right ventricular–aortic connection has been accomplished with homograft or prosthetic conduits from the right ventricle or pulmonary trunk to the descending aorta, or by direct connection between the proximal pulmonary trunk and ascending aorta, which also enlarges the ascending aorta. Pulmonary blood flow and pressure are controlled by a tubed interposition systemic-pulmonary shunt to the distal pulmonary artery. The patent ductus arteriosus is ligated. A large interatrial communication also must be assured in stage 1 to allow free access of pulmonary venous blood to the tricuspid valve. In stage 2 an interatrial baffle is created to provide continuity between left atrium and tricuspid valve; the pulmonary arterial circulation is provided by direct anastomosis of the right atrium to the pulmonary arteries (the Fontan connection). Some surgeons prefer to perform a modified superior vena cava–pulmonary artery shunt (the Glenn operation) as an intermediate step before the Fontan procedure. In some centers, the preferred operation is human cardiac transplantation.[303]

CONGENITAL AORTIC REGURGITATION

Congenital aortic valve regurgitation is a rare isolated congenital cardiac lesion.[304] Aortic regurgitation most often occurs in association with congenital valvular aortic stenosis in which the valve commissures are fused, inhibiting cusp mobility, subvalvular aortic stenosis in which the aortic ring is dilated and the valve cusps are deformed, coarctation of the aorta when the aortic ring is dilated and the aortic valve is bicuspid, ventricular septal defect (p. 910), and endocardial fibroelastosis. Aortic valve regurgitation also may accompany aortic sinus aneurysm or be secondary to dilatation of the ascending aorta in patients with Marfan syndrome, Turner syndrome, cystic medial necrosis, or osteogenesis imperfecta, in which the aortic lesions are manifestations of the underlying connective tissue disorder.

Severe aortic regurgitation also may occur through channels other than the aortic valve.[305,306] Thus aortico–left ventricular tunnel is a rare anomaly that must be distinguished from congenital aortic valve regurgitation, since the approach to management of the former usually does not include consideration for prosthetic valve replacement. The aortico–left ventricular tunnel is an abnormal channel beginning in the ascending aorta above the right coronary orifice and ending in the left ventricle below the right aortic cusp. The channel usually passes behind the right ventricular infundibulum and through the ventricular septum.

Echocardiography, Doppler studies, and aortography combine to establish a precise diagnosis. Exercise testing is useful to assess the severity of the lesion.[307] In infants and children with congenital aortic regurgitation the severity of regurgitation increases with time, and valve replacement, rather than plication, is almost always necessary to correct the lesion. Operation should be deferred until symptoms, signs, and noninvasive assessment dictate its necessity. Conversely, closure of an aortic–left ventricular communication is advisable before progressive dilation of the aortic annulus creates secondary changes in the aortic valve itself which may necessitate aortic valve replacement.

PULMONARY VEIN ATRESIA AND STENOSIS

Pulmonary vein atresia is a rare anomaly in which the pulmonary veins do not connect with the heart or with a major systemic vein.[308] The lesion is incompatible with life, but infants may survive for days, probably because communications exist between the pulmonary veins and the bronchial or esophageal veins that allow limited egress for pulmonary venous blood. Pulmonary vein stenosis may occur as a focal stenosis at the atrial junction or generalized hypoplasia or one or more pulmonary veins. There is an extremely high incidence of associated cardiac malformations, including atrial septal defect, tetralogy of Fallot, tricuspid and mitral atresia, and endocardial cushion defect. The severe pulmonary vein obstruction imposed by pulmonary vein abnormalities causes severe cyanosis, congestive cardiac failure, and early death. Focal stenosis of one or more pulmonary veins at the atrial junction, recognized by two-dimensional echocardiography or angiography, may be relieved surgically.[309] Results of transcutaneous balloon angioplasty have been disappointing.

COR TRIATRIATUM

In this malformation failure of resorption of the common pulmonary vein results in a left atrium divided by an abnormal fibromuscular diaphragm into a posterosuperior chamber receiving the pulmonary veins and an anteroinferior chamber giving rise to the left atrial appendage and leading to the mitral orifice.[310] The communication between the divided atrial chambers may be large, small, or absent, depending on the size of the opening in the subdividing diaphragm, which determines the degree of obstruction to pulmonary venous return. Elevations of both pulmonary venous pressure and pulmonary vascular resistance result in severe pulmonary artery hypertension.

The diagnosis is established by two-dimensional echocardiography; cardiac catheterization and angiography are necessary only if major associated cardiac anomalies are suspected.[311,312] The obstructive membrane is visualized in the parasternal long- and short-axis and four-chamber (Fig. 31–40) views and can be distinguished from a supravalvular mitral ring by its position superior to the left atrial appendage, which forms part of the distal chamber. Also present are diastolic fluttering of the mitral leaflets and high-velocity flow detected by Doppler examination in the distal atrial chamber and at the mitral orifice.

The diagnosis should be suspected at cardiac catheterization if the pulmonary arterial wedge pressure is higher than a simultaneous left atrial pressure. The diagnosis also may be established by visualizing the obstructing lesion angiographically. Although rare, it is important to recognize the malformation because it may be easily correctable at operation.[313]

CONGENITAL MITRAL STENOSIS

Anatomical types of mitral stenosis include the parachute deformity of the valve, in which shortened chordae tendineae converge and insert into a single large papillary muscle; thickened leaflets with shortening and fusion of the chordae tendinase; an anomalous arcade of obstructing papillary muscles; accessory mitral valve tissue; and a supravalvular circumferential ridge of connective tissue arising at the base of the atrial

feed both the left and right coronary systems, or they may be via a single, dilated vessel. The proximal coronary arteries in some patients may be atrophic, proximal to a communication between the sinusoids and the distal coronary artery, particularly in hearts with severe hypoplasia of the right ventricle. In these circumstances, the distal coronary vessels are supplied by communications with the right ventricle, and the coronary circulation is, therefore, right ventricule-dependent. In this group, decompression of the right ventricle by a surgical procedure would be associated with a high risk of myocardial ischemia and death.

Because the pulmonic valve is imperforate and completely obstructed, systemic venous blood returning to the heart bypasses the right ventricle through an interatrial communication. Right ventricular output does not contribute to the effective cardiac output and is proportional to the magnitude of tricuspid regurgitation and the size and extent of the sinusoidal communications with the coronary arterial tree. The blood supply to the lungs is derived from the bronchial circulation and from flow through a persistently patent ductus arteriosus. The size and patency of the ductus arteriosus are critical determinants in postnatal survival; ductus closure results in death. Reduced pulmonary blood flow by way of a partially constricted ductus arteriosus results in profound hypoxemia, tissue hypoxia, and metabolic acidemia.

CLINICAL FEATURES. The diagnosis is suggested by roentgenographic findings of pulmonary hypoperfusion and the electrocardiographic observation of a normal QRS axis, absent or diminished right ventricular forces, and/or dominant left ventricular forces. In the minority of infants with marked tricuspid regurgitation, the right ventricle and right atrium are massively enlarged. The echocardiogram in the usual infant shows a small right ventricular cavity and diminutive or absent pulmonic valve echoes.[353,354] Doppler examination shows continuous retrograde flow to the pulmonary artery and/or its branches through a patent ductus arteriosus which usually is narrow and tortuous. Only if tricuspid valve echoes are imaged by ultrasound examination can tricuspid atresia be distinguished from pulmonic atresia. Contrast echocardiography showing filling of the right ventricle across the tricuspid valve in diastole may clarify the latter distinction.

Cardiac catheterization usually is performed on an emergency basis. Because survival depends on patency of the ductus arteriosus, infusion of prostaglandin E_1 (0.05–0.1 μg/kg/min) intravenously may dramatically reverse clinical deterioration and improve arterial blood gases and pH.[71] The usual hemodynamic findings are right atrial and right ventricular hypertension, with right ventricular pressure often greater than systemic pressure, and a massive right-to-left interatrial shunt. Selective angiocardiography establishes the

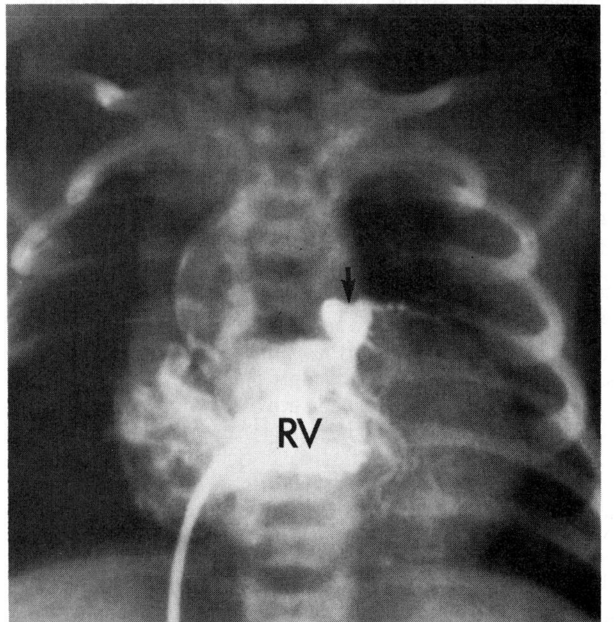

FIGURE 31–45. Right ventricular angiocardiogram in the frontal projection in a 1-day-old infant with an atretic pulmonic valve (arrow). The cavity of the right ventricle (RV) is small and eccentrically shaped. (Courtesy of Robert Freedom, M.D.)

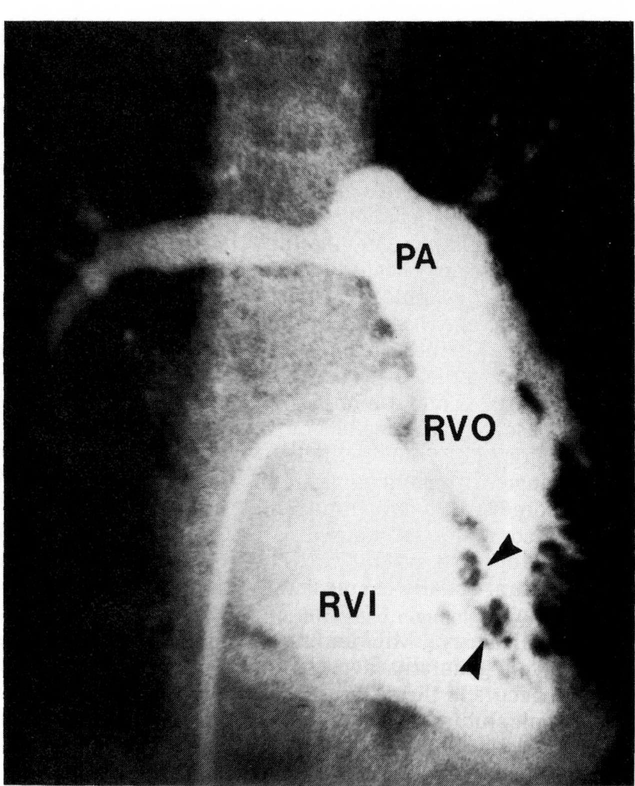

FIGURE 31–46. Intraventricular right ventricular obstruction. The right ventricular inflow (RVI) and outflow (RVO) tracts are separated by bands (arrows), creating intraventricular right ventricular obstruction. PA = pulmonary artery.

diagnosis and allows evaluation of the degree of separation between the right ventricular infundibular and pulmonary trunk, the size of the right ventricular cavity and of the pulmonary arteries (Fig. 31–45), the anatomy and function of the tricuspid valve, and the anatomical and functional details of the coronary circulation.

MANAGEMENT. In the majority of infants with a diminutive right ventricle, balloon atrial septostomy followed by a systemic-pulmonary artery shunt provides palliation. Infants with moderate right ventricular hypoplasia most often require a surgical pulmonary valvotomy and a systemic-pulmonary artery shunt, whereas in infants with only mild right ventricular hypoplasia, often valvotomy alone is necessary. The ultimate prognosis is poor unless continuity can be established between the right ventricle and the pulmonary arteries by pulmonary valvotomy or prosthetic conduit at initial or second operation.[349,355] Decompression of the right ventricle permits that chamber to grow and both the tricuspid and the pulmonary orifices to enlarge. In other patients who are unsuitable candidates for a one- or two-stage approach to biventricular repair, the Fontan right atrium–pulmonary anastomosis may be effective several years after shunt pallliation in the newborn period.[349]

INTRAVENTRICULAR RIGHT VENTRICULAR OBSTRUCTION

Infundibular pulmonic stenosis with an intact ventricular septum and the presence of anomalous muscle bundles are the two principal causes of intraventricular right ventricular obstruction (Fig. 31–46).[356]

SUBPULMONIC INFUNDIBULAR STENOSIS. This anomaly usually occurs at the proximal portion of the infundibulum and consists of a fibrous band at the junction of the right ventricular cavity and outflow tract. The clinical manifestations, course, and prognosis of patients with infundibular stenosis are similar to those of patients with valvular stenosis, although the former diagnosis is suggested by the absence of a systolic ejection sound and a systolic murmur lower along the left sternal border. Doppler echocardiography, withdrawal pressure tracings, and selective right ventricular angiocardiography permit localization of the site of obstruction and assessment of its extent and severity. Surgical treatment consists of resection of the fibrotic narrowed area and hypertrophied muscle. Occasionally it may be necessary to widen the outflow tract with a pericardial or prosthetic patch.

ANOMALOUS MUSCLE BUNDLES. A two-chambered right ventricle is formed by right ventricular obstruction due to anomalous muscle bundles; most of the patients have an associated malalignment or perimembranous ventricular septal defect, and about 5 per cent have subaortic stenosis.[356] Aberrant hypertrophied muscle bands traverse the right ventricular cavity, extending from its anterior wall to the crista supraventricularis and/or the portion of the adjacent interventricular septum. The anomalous pyramid-shaped muscle mass obstructs blood flow through the body of the right ventricle and produces a proximal high-pressure inflow chamber and a distal low-pressure chamber. Thus this type of obstruction is distinguishable from that in tetralogy of Fallot, in which hypertrophied infundibular muscle protrudes into but does not cross the cavity of the right ventricle.

The clinical, electrocardiographic, and chest roentgenographic findings resemble those observed in pulmonic valvular or subvalvular infundibular obstruction, although the systolic thrill and murmur may be displaced lower along the left sternal border. Progressive obstruction occurs in some patients. The diagnosis may be established by two-dimensional echocardiography. Selective right ventricular angiocardiography is necessary for most accurate diagnosis and reveals a filling defect in the midportion of the right ventricle which often does not change significantly with systole and diastole.

Management. The treatment for anomalous muscle bundles consists of surgical removal.[357,358] In the absence of preoperative recognition of the anomaly, the surgeon should be alerted to the correct diagnosis by the presence of a dimple on the ordinarily smooth anterior surface of the right ventricle and/or the inability to view the tricuspid valve through a longitudinal ventriculotomy because of the presence of the abnormal muscle mass.

TETRALOGY OF FALLOT

(See also p. 971)

DEFINITION. The overall incidence of this anomaly approaches 10 per cent of all forms of congenital heart disease, and it is the most common cardiac malformation responsible for cyanosis after 1 year of age.[359,360] The four components of this malformation are (1) ventricular septal defect, (2) obstruction to right ventricular outflow, (3) overriding of the aorta, and (4) right ventricular hypertrophy. The basic anomaly is the result of an anterior deviation of the septal insertion of the infundibular ventricular septum from its usual location in the normal heart between the limbs of the trabecular septum. The malalignment interventricular defect usually is large, approximating the aortic orifice in size, and is located high in the septum just below the right cusp of the aortic valve, separated from the pulmonic valve by the crista supraventricularis. The aortic root may be displaced anteriorly and straddle or override the septal defect, but, as in the normal heart, it lies to the right of the origin of the pulmonary artery. In most cases no dextroposition of the aorta exists; overriding of the aorta is a phenomenon secondary to the subaortic location of the ventricular septal defect.

HEMODYNAMICS. The degree of obstruction to pulmonary blood flow is the principal determinant of the clinical presentation. The site of obstruction is variable[361]; infundibular stenosis is the only major obstruction in about 50 per cent of patients and coexists with valvular obstruction in another 20 to 25 per cent (Fig. 31–47). Supravalvular and peripheral pulmonary arterial narrowing may be observed, and unilateral absence of a pulmonary artery (usually the left) is found in a small number of patients. Circulation to the abnormal lung is accomplished by bronchial and other collateral arteries.[362–365] Atresia of the pulmonic valve, infundibulum, or main pulmonary artery occasionally is referred to as "pseudotruncus arteriosus." True truncus arteriosus with absent pulmonary arteries (Type 4) differs from Fallot's tetralogy, in which pulmonary artery branches are present but are fed by a patent ductus arteriosus and/or bronchial arteries (see Fig. 31–50).[363] A right-sided aortic knob, aortic arch, and descending aorta occur in about 25 per cent of patients with tetralogy of Fallot. The coronary arteries may have surgically important variations[366–368]: the anterior descending artery may originate from the right coronary artery; a single right coronary artery may give off a left branch that courses anterior to the pulmonary trunk; a single left coronary artery may give off a right branch that crosses the infundibulum of the right ventricle. Enlargement of the infundibular branch of the right coronary artery often presents a problem with respect to a right ventriculotomy. Associated cardiac anomalies exist in about 40 per cent of patients. Major associated cardiac anomalies include patent ductus arteriosus, multiple (usually muscular) ventricular septal defects, and complete atrioventricular septal defects. Localized single or multiple peripheral pulmonary arterial stenotic lesions are common; rarely, the right or left pulmonary artery may arise anomalously from the ascending aorta. Infrequently, aortic valve regurgitation results from aortic cusp prolapse. Associated extracardiac anomalies are present in 20 to 30 per cent of patients.

The relation between the resistance to blood flow from the ventricles into the aorta and into the pulmonary vessels plays a major role in determining the hemodynamic and clinical picture.[359] Thus, the severity of obstruction to right ventricular outflow is of fundamental significance. When right ventricular outflow tract obstruction is severe, the pulmonary blood flow is markedly reduced, and a large volume of unsaturated systemic venous blood is shunted from right to left across the ventricular septal defect. Severe cyanosis and polycythemia occur, and symptoms and sequelae of systemic hypoxemia are prominent. At the opposite end of the spectrum, the term "acyanotic" or "pink" tetralogy of Fallot often is used to describe an interventricular communication and a milder degree of obstruction to right ventricular outflow with little or no venoarterial shunting. In many infants and children the obstruction to right ventricular outflow is mild but progres-

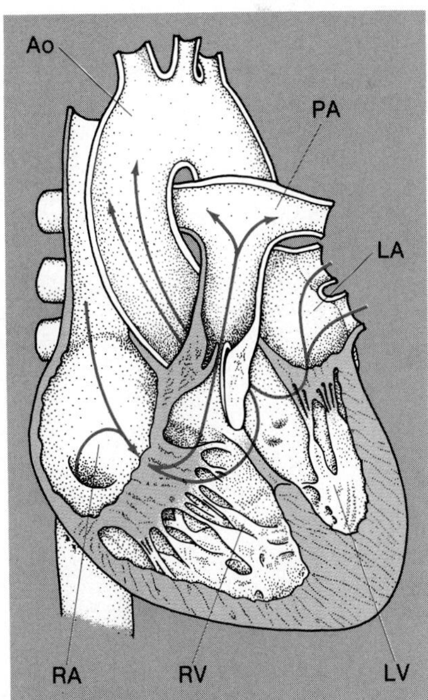

FIGURE 31–47. Tetralogy of Fallot with infundibular and valvular pulmonic stenosis. The arrows indicate direction of blood flow. A substantial right-to-left shunt exists across the ventricular septal defect. RA = right atrium; LA = left atrium; RV = right ventricle; LV = left ventricle; Ao = aorta; PA = pulmonary artery.

sive, so that early in life pulmonary exceeds systemic blood flow, and the symptoms resemble those produced by a simple ventricular septal defect.

CLINICAL MANIFESTATIONS. Few children with tetralogy of Fallot remain asymptomatic or acyanotic. Most are cyanotic from birth or develop cyanosis before age 1 year. In general, the earlier the onset of systemic hypoxemia, the more likely the possibility that severe pulmonary outflow tract stenosis or atresia exists. Dyspnea with exertion, clubbing, and polycythemia is common. When resting after exertion, children with tetralogy characteristically assume a squatting posture. The latter may be obvious even in infancy; many cyanotic infants prefer to lie in a knee-chest position. Spells of intense cyanosis related to a sudden increase in venoarterial shunting and a reduction in pulmonary blood flow most often have their onset between 2 and 9 months of age and constitute an important threat to survival.[369,370] The attacks are not restricted to patients with severe cyanosis; they are characterized by hyperpnea and increasing cyanosis that progresses to limpness and syncope and occasionally terminates in convulsions, a cerebrovascular accident, and death.

Physical Examination. This reveals variable degrees of underdevelopment and cyanosis. Clubbing of the terminal digits may be prominent after the first year of life. The heart is not hyperactive or enlarged; a right ventricular impulse and systolic thrill often are palpable along the left sternal border. An early systolic ejection sound that is aortic in origin may be heard at the lower left sternal border and apex; the second heart sound is single, the pulmonic component rarely being audible. A systolic ejection murmur is produced by flow across the narrowed right ventricular infundibulum or pulmonic valve. The intensity and duration of the murmur vary inversely with the severity of obstruction—the opposite of the relation that exists in patients with pulmonic stenosis and an intact ventricular septum. Polycythemia, decreased systemic vascular resistance, and increased obstruction to right ventricular outflow may all be responsible for a decrease in intensity of the murmur; with extreme outflow tract stenosis or pulmonic atresia and during an attack of paroxysmal hypoxemia, there may be no or only a very short, faint murmur. A continuous murmur faintly audible over the anterior or posterior chest reflects flow through enlarged bronchial collateral vessels. A loud continuous murmur of flow through a patent ductus arteriosus occasionally may be heard at the upper left sternal border.

LABORATORY EXAMINATIONS. The *electrocardiogram* ordinarily shows right ventricular and, less frequently, right atrial hypertrophy. In a patient with acyanotic tetralogy, combined ventricular hypertrophy may be noted initially, progressing to right ventricular hypertrophy as cyanosis develops. *Roentgenographic* examination (Fig. 32–14, p. 974) characteristically reveals a normal-sized, boot-shaped heart (coeur en sabot) with prominence of the right ventricle and a concavity in the region of the underdeveloped right ventricular outflow tract and main pulmonary artery. The pulmonary vascular markings typically are diminished, and the aortic arch and knob may be on the right side; the ascending aorta usually is large. A uniform, diffuse, fine reticular pattern of vascular markings is noted in the presence of prominent collateral vessels.

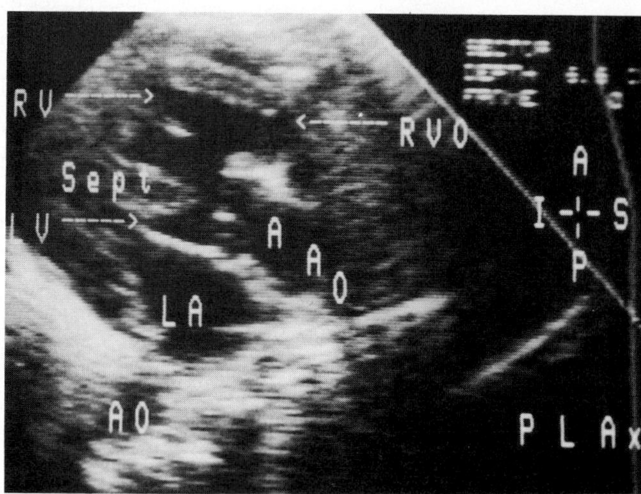

FIGURE 31–48. **Tetralogy of Fallot in a parasternal long-axis (PLAx) view, which demonstrates the aorta overriding the ventricular septum (Sept). RV = right ventricle, RVO = right ventricular outflow tract, LV = left ventricle, LA = left atrium, AO = ascending aorta. (Courtesy of Norman Silverman, M.D.)**

Echocardiographic findings include aortic enlargement, aortic–septal discontinuity, and aortic overriding of the ventricular septum.[371] Two-dimensional echocardiography (Fig. 4–82, p. 94) shows the right ventricular outflow tract to be narrowed and in a more horizontal orientation than normal. The main pulmonary artery and its branches are mildly to severely hypoplastic. The usual malalignment ventricular septal defect lies superior to the tricuspid valve and immediately below the aortic valve cusps. These findings are best displayed in views of the long axis of the right ventricular outflow tract, which are the subxiphoid short axis and the high transverse parasternal echo windows. Echo views which show the anteroposterior coordinates best indicate the overriding of the aorta; these are the parasternal long-axis, apical two-chamber, and subxiphoid views (Fig. 31–48). The echocardiographic examination also reveals the origin of the main pulmonary artery from the right ventricle, and continuity of the main pulmonary artery with its right and left branches,

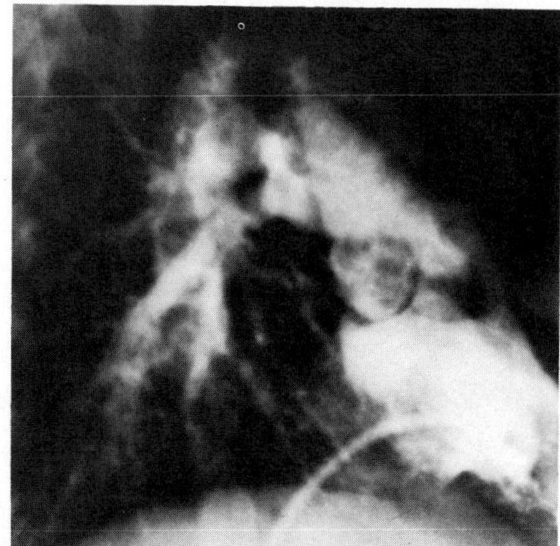

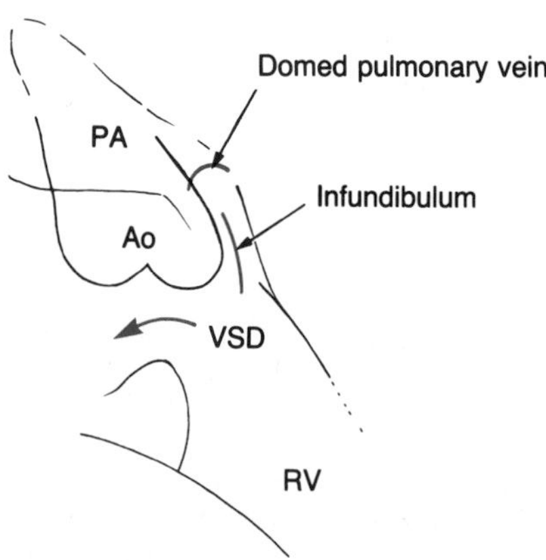

FIGURE 31–49. **Lateral view of a right ventriculogram in a child with tetralogy of Fallot showing simultaneous opacification of the pulmonary artery (P.A.) and aorta (Ao.). P.V. = pulmonic valve; V.S.D. = ventricular septal defect; R.V. = right ventricle.**

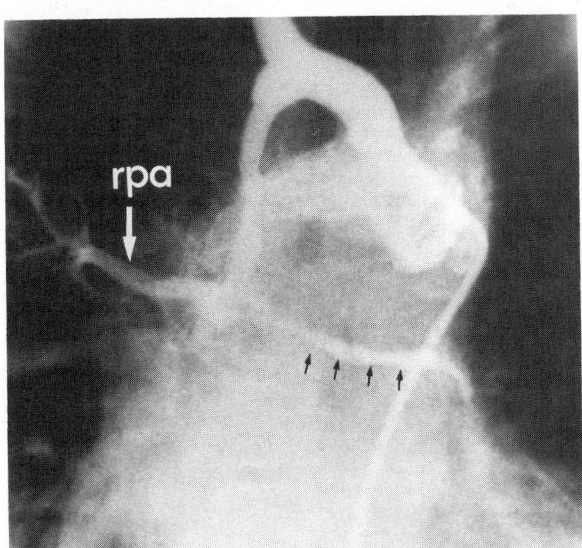

FIGURE 31–50. Selective systemic collateral bronchial arteriogram demonstrates "gull-wing" configuration of the hypoplastic right pulmonary artery (rpa) and left pulmonary artery (arrows) in a patient with tetralogy of Fallot and pulmonic atresia. (Courtesy of Robert Freedom, M.D.)

and is accurate for diagnosing coronary abnormalities.[367,368] The demonstration of mitral–semilunar valve continuity helps to distinguish tetralogy from double-outlet right ventricle with pulmonic stenosis, in which discontinuity of the mitral valve echo and the aortic cusp echo is a critical feature.

Cardiac Catheterization and Angiocardiography (Fig. 31–49). These are necessary to confirm the diagnosis; assess the magnitude of right-to-left shunting; provide details of additional muscular ventricular septal defects, if present; evaluate the architecture of the right ventricular outflow tract, pulmonic valve, and annulus and the morphology and caliber of the main branches of the pulmonary arteries; and analyze the anatomy of the coronary arteries. *Axial cineangiography*, utilizing the sitting-up projection, greatly facilitates evaluation of the pulmonary outflow tract and arteries.[122,361,365] The preoperative assessment of tetralogy with pulmonic atresia must include delineation of the arterial supply to both lungs by selective catheterization and visualization of bronchial collateral arteries with late serial filming; pulmonary arteries may be opacified only after the bronchial collateral arteries have cleared of contrast material (Fig. 31–50).[361,363] A patient with pulmonic atresia should not be ruled out as a candidate for surgical correction unless an inadequate pulmonary arterial supply to the lungs is clearly demonstrated.[362] Rarely, injection of contrast through a catheter in the pulmonary venous capillary wedge position is required to assess the possibility that anatomical pulmonary arteries are present.[364] Computer-assisted axial tomography may visualize central pulmonary arteries when conventional angiography cannot.

MANAGEMENT. Among the factors that may complicate the management of patients with tetralogy are iron deficiency anemia, infective endocarditis, paradoxical embolism, polycythemia, coagulation disorders, and cerebral infarction or abscess. Paroxysmal hypercyanotic spells may respond quickly to oxygen, placing the child in the knee-chest position, and morphine. If the spell persists, metabolic acidosis will develop from prolonged anaerobic metabolism, and infusion of sodium bicarbonate may be necessary to interrupt the attack. Vasopressors, beta-adrenoceptor redundant blockade, or general anesthesia occasionally may be necessary.[370]

Total Surgical Correction. This operation is advisable ultimately for almost all patients with tetralogy of Fallot.[367a–369a] Early definitive repair, even in infancy, currently is advocated in most centers that are experienced in intracardiac surgery in infants. Successful early correction appears to prevent the consequences of progressive infundibular obstruction and acquired pulmonic atresia, delayed growth and development, and complications secondary to hypoxemia and polycythemia with bleeding tendencies. The size of the pulmonary arteries, rather than the age or size of the infant or child, is the most important determinant in assessing candidacy for primary repair; marked hypoplasia of the pulmonary arteries is a relative contraindication for early corrective operation.

Palliative Surgery. When marked hypoplasia of the pulmonary arteries exists, a palliative operation designed to increase pulmonary blood flow is recommended and usually consists in the smallest infants of a systemic-pulmonary arterial anastomosis.[370a] A transventricular infundibulectomy or valvulotomy is an alternative palliative procedure that may be considered. Balloon dilatation of the pulmonary valve may afford palliation in selected infants.[372] Total correction can then be carried out at a lower risk later in childhood or adolescence. The palliative procedures relieve hypoxemia caused by diminished pulmonary blood flow and reduce the stimulus to polycythemia. Because pulmonary venous return is augmented, the left atrium and ventricle are stimulated to enlarge their capacity in anticipation of total correction. In the most severe forms of tetralogy of Fallot with pulmonic atresia, the goals of operation include establishment of nonstenotic continuity between the right ventricle and pulmonary arteries, closure of the intracardiac shunt, and interruption of surgically created shunts or major collateral arteries to the lungs.[360,371a] When atresia is confined to the infundibulum or pulmonic valve, repair may be accomplished by infundibular resection and reconstruction of the outflow tract with a pericardial patch. If a long segment of pulmonary arterial atresia exists, a valve-containing conduit is inserted from the right ventricle to the distal pulmonary artery. The presence of a single pulmonary artery in the hilus of either lung is a prerequisite for repair of pulmonic atresia. A conduit also may be necessary in less severe forms of right ventricular outflow tract obstruction when an anomalous coronary artery crosses the right ventricular outflow tract.

A variety of complications are common in the postoperative period after palliative or corrective operation. Mild-to-moderate left ventricular decompensation may be secondary to the sudden increase in pulmonary venous return; varying degrees of pulmonic valvular regurgitation increase right ventricular cavity size further.[373] Bleeding problems frequently are seen, especially in older polycythemic patients. Complete right bundle branch block or the pattern of left anterior hemiblock often is seen, but disabling dysrhythmias are infrequent.[374,376] Restricted pulmonary arterial flow is the greatest cause for early and late mortality and poor late results.[359] After convalescence from intracardiac repair, symptoms of hypoxemia and severe exercise intolerance are relieved even in the presence of some residual right ventricular outflow tract obstruction, pulmonic valve incompetence, and/or cardiomegaly.[371,377] However, cardiovascular performance at rest or during exercise may remain below normal,[378,379] and major complications, such as trifascicular block, complete heart block, ventricular arrhythmias, and sudden death, may rarely occur many years after surgical treatment.

CONGENITAL ABSENCE OF THE PULMONIC VALVE

PATHOLOGY AND PATHOGENESIS. In the majority of cases of this rare malformation the lesion is associated with a ventricular septal defect, a narrowed obstructive annulus of the pulmonic valve, and marked aneurysmal dilatation of the pulmonary arteries. The combination of anomalies often is referred to as tetralogy of Fallot with absent pulmonic valve. The obstructing lesion principally consists of underdeveloped, primitive valve tissue within a hypoplastic annulus; infundibular obstruction and the ventricular septal defect do not differ from classic tetralogy of Fallot. The massively dilated pulmonary arteries often are the major determinant of the clinical course, since they frequently result in upper airway obstruction and severe respiratory distress in infancy.[380] Poststenotic pulmonary artery aneurysms develop in utero, and their size and location appear to be related to the magnitude of pulmonic regurgitation in fetal life, the orienta-

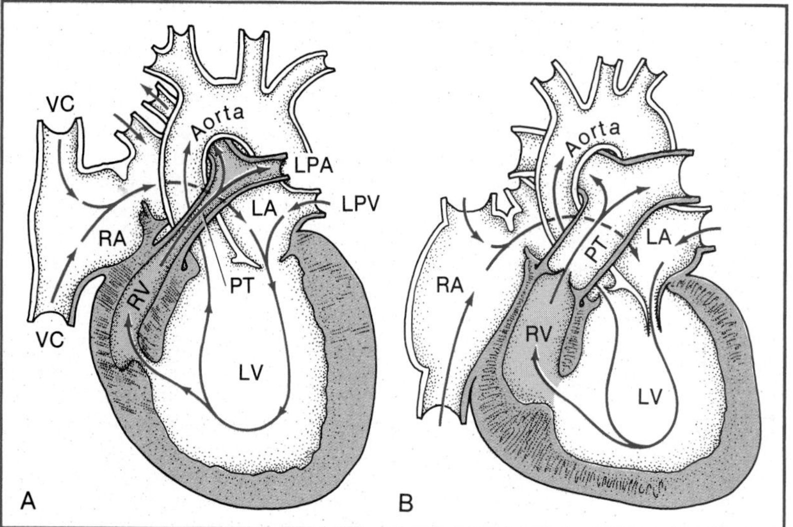

FIGURE 31-51. *A,* Tricuspid atresia with normally related great arteries, a small ventricular septal defect, diminutive right ventricular chamber, and narrowed outflow tract. *B,* An example of tricuspid atresia and complete transposition of the great arteries in which the left ventricular chamber is essentially a common ventricle, with the aorta arising from an infundibular component (R.V.) of the common ventricle. V.C. = vena cava; R.A. = right atrium; L.A. = left atrium; R.V. = right ventricle; L.V. = left ventricle; L.P.V. = left pulmonary vein; L.P.A. = left pulmonary artery. (Modified from Edwards, J. E., and Burchell, H. B.: Congenital tricuspid atresia: Classification. Med. Clin. North Am. *33*:1177, 1949.)

tion of the right ventricular infundibulum to the right or left, and the size of the ductus arteriosus.[381] It has been suggested that the aneurysmal dilatation is related pathogenetically to agenesis of the ductus arteriosus.[382]

CLINICAL AND LABORATORY FINDINGS. The *clinical features* often are distinctive, with an early onset of severe respiratory distress caused by tracheobronchial compression accompanied by a systolic ejection and a widely transmitted low-pitched, decrescendo diastolic murmur at the upper left sternal border. In the absence of pulmonary complications cyanosis is commonly mild. *Roentgenographically* the heart is moderately enlarged; hyperinflated lung fields are observed with large hilar densities representing the aneurysmally dilated pulmonary arteries. The *echocardiographic* features are similar to those seen in classic tetralogy of Fallot, in addition to massive dilatation of the main pulmonary artery and branch pulmonary arteries. Remnants of pulmonary cusps may be visible. Right ventricular dilatation is produced by significant pulmonary regurgitation; the latter is identified by retrograde diastolic flow in the pulmonary arteries and right ventricle at Doppler examination. Definitive diagnosis is established by cardiac catheterization and selective angiocardiography.

Prognosis is related to the intensity of upper airway obstruction; pulmonary complications are the usual cause of death in infancy. If survival beyond infancy is accomplished, the respiratory symptoms usually diminish, probably because of maturational changes in the structure of the tracheobronchial tree. The surgical approach in infancy often is unsatisfactory; a variety of procedures have been attempted, ranging from aneurysmorrhaphy to pulmonary artery suspension to transection and reanastomosis of pulmonary artery segments to homograft insertion.[383,384] Also suggested are ligation of the main pulmonary artery and creation of a systemic-pulmonary shunt, and primary repair of the ventricular septal defect with pulmonary arterial plication. In older patients the stenotic anulus may be widened with a patch and the ventricular septal defect closed. It seldom is necessary to replace the pulmonic valve.

TRICUSPID ATRESIA

MORPHOLOGY. This anomaly is characterized by absence of the tricuspid orifice, an interatrial communication, hypoplasia of the right ventricle, and the presence of a communication between the systemic and pulmonary circulations, usually a ventricular septal defect.[385,386] Thus there is a univentricular atrioventricular connection, consisting of a left-sided mitral valve between the morphological left atrium and left ventricle. Unequal division of the atrioventricular canal by fusion of the right-sided endocardial cushions has been proposed as the embryological fault. Patients may be subdivided into those with normally related great arteries (60 to 70 per cent of cases) and those with D-transposition of the great arteries; further classification depends on the presence of pulmonic stenosis or atresia and the absence or size of the ventricular septal defect (Fig. 31-51). Additional cardiovascular malformations often are present, especially in patients with D-transposition of the great arteries, and include persistent left superior vena cava, patent ductus arteriosus, coarctation of the aorta, and juxtaposition of the atrial appendages.

PATHOPHYSIOLOGY. The association with other cardiac malformations determines whether or not pulmonary blood flow is decreased, normal, or increased and therefore the degree of systemic hypoxemia.[387] The clinical picture usually is dominated by symptoms resulting from greatly diminished pulmonary blood flow with severe cyanosis. Cyanosis results from an obligatory admixture of systemic and pulmonary venous blood in the left atrium, and its intensity primarily depends on the magnitude of pulmonary blood flow. Heart failure, rather than cyanosis, is the predominant problem in infants with torrential pulmonary blood flow, which results when D-transposition of the great arteries, a ventricular septal defect, and an unobstructed pulmonary outflow tract coexist. If the latter patients survive infancy, they are candidates for pulmonary vascular obstructive disease; a favorable response to pulmonary arterial banding is common early in life.

CLINICAL FEATURES. The diagnosis is easily established in the vast majority of infants with tricuspid atresia and pulmonary hypoperfusion. The *electrocardiographic* findings of left-axis deviation, right atrial enlargement, and left ventricular hypertrophy in a cyanotic infant strongly suggest tricuspid atresia.[387] *Echocardiography* reveals a small or absent right ventricle, large left ventricle, and absent tricuspid valve echoes (Figs. 31-52 and 4-70, p. 91); further, it may demonstrate the relation of the great arteries unless pulmonic atresia is present. Contrast cross-sectional echocardiography reveals the abnormal flow patterns; apical and subxiphoid cross-sectional views best reveal the atretic tricuspid orifice. *Roentgenographically,* there are diminished pulmonary vascular markings and a concavity in the region of the cardiac silhouette usually occupied by the main pulmonary artery. The

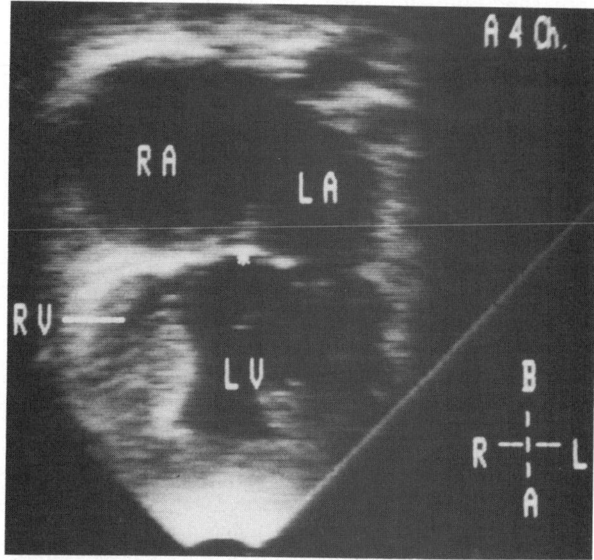

FIGURE 31-52. Tricuspid atresia is seen in an apical four-chamber view. The bright horizontal echoes arise from the AV sulcus tissue preventing communication between the right atrium (RA) and right ventricle (RV). The RV is small and communicates with the left ventricle (LV) via a small ventricular septal defect. (Courtesy of Norman Silverman, M.D.)

right atrial shadow may be prominent unless left-sided juxtaposition of the atrial appendages exists, which produces a straight and flattened right heart border.

CARDIAC CATHETERIZATION AND ANGIOGRAPHY. The right ventricle cannot be entered directly from the right atrium. When the great arteries are related normally, pulmonary blood flow is found to be derived from shunting through a ventricular septal defect or by way of a patent ductus arteriosus; the latter and the bronchial collaterals are the source of pulmonary flow if the ventricular septum is intact. In complete transposition the pulmonary artery fills directly from the left ventricle and the aorta indirectly through a ventricular septal defect and the hypoplastic right ventricle. Because complete admixture exists in the left atrium of pulmonary and systemic venous return, the degree of systemic arterial hypoxemia depends on the pulmonary-systemic flow ratio. Right atrial angiography does not opacify the right ventricle unless by way of a ventricular septal defect (Fig. 31-53). Selective left ventricular *angiography* permits identification of the hypoplastic right ventricle, the size and location of the ventricular septal defect, the type of pulmonary obstruction, the relation between the great arteries, and the size of the distal pulmonary arterial tree.

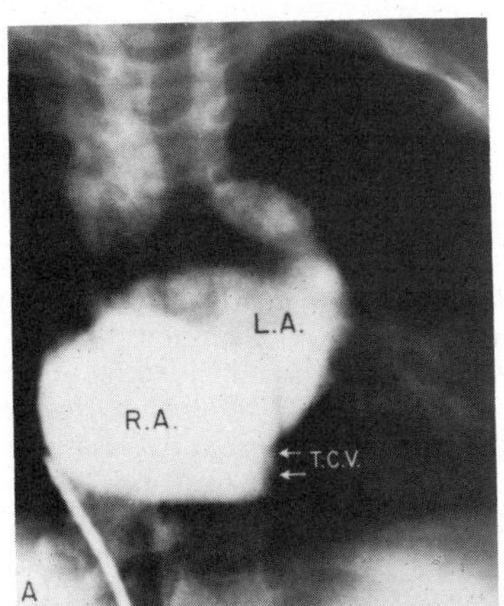

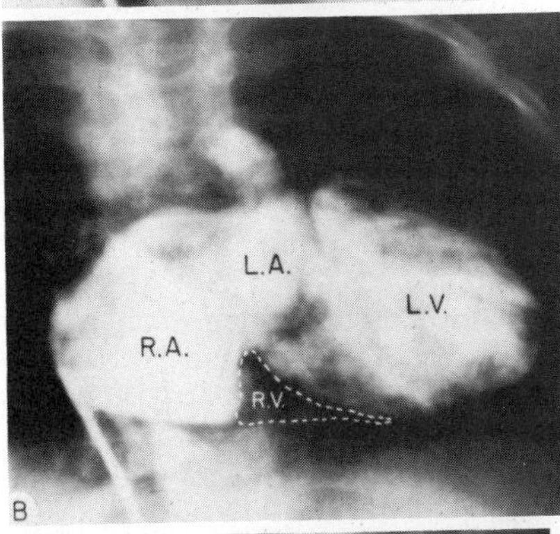

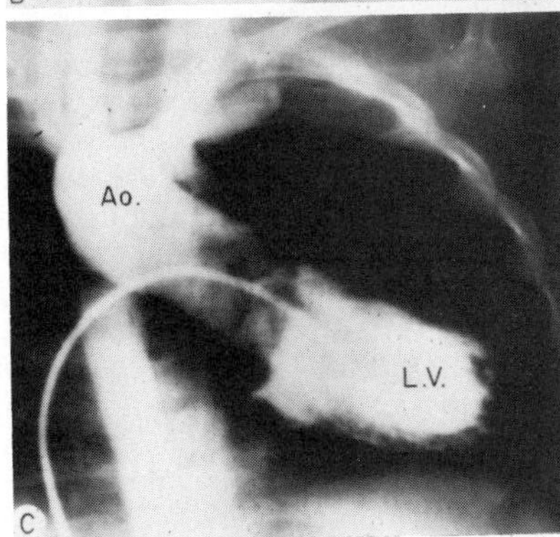

FIGURE 31-53. Right atrial angiogram in an infant with tricuspid atresia shows flow of contrast material from right atrium (R.A.) to left atrium *(A)*, and then to left ventricle (L.V.) *(B)* and aorta (Ao.) *(C)*. The tricuspid valve (T.C.V.) is atretic, and a radiolucency exists in the region of the right ventricle (R.V.).

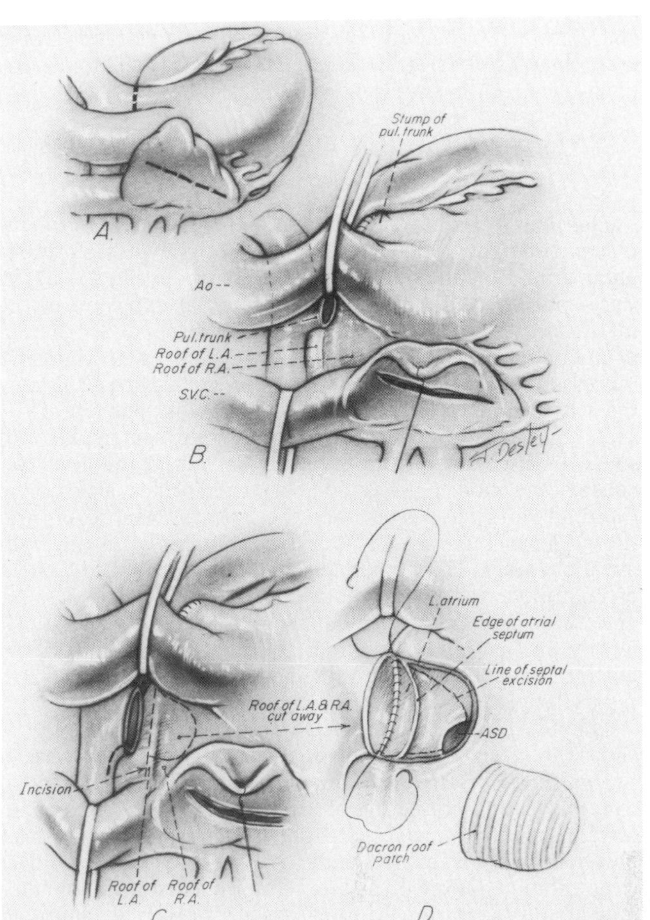

FIGURE 31-54. The Fontan operation with direct right atrial-pulmonary artery connection. *A*, The right atrium is opened through an oblique incision and the pulmonary artery transsected above the pulmonary valve. *B*, The proximal pulmonary trunk is closed and the distal end brought toward the right atrium beneath the aorta. *C*, The pulmonary artery is enlarged if a complex atrial septal baffle is required, the atrial septum is excised, and a circular button of atrial roof is removed. *D*, The posterior wall of the openings into the pulmonary artery and the atria are anastomosed; if the anterior wall of the right atrium and the pulmonary artery cannot easily be brought together for direct anastomoses, a convex Dacron roof patch is employed. AO = aorta, RA = right atrium, LA = left atrium, ASD = atrial septal defect. (From Kirklin, J. W., and Barratt-Boyes, B. G.: Cardiac Surgery. New York, John Wiley & Sons, 1986, p. 873.)

MANAGEMENT. *Balloon atrial septostomy* in those infants with a restrictive interatrial communication and palliative operations designed to increase pulmonary blood flow (systemic arterial- or venous-pulmonary artery anastomosis) are capable of producing clinical improvement of significant duration in patients with diminished blood flow.[387,388]

Functional correction of the anomaly has been accomplished by direct anastomosis or insertion of a nonvalved prosthetic conduit between the right atrium and pulmonary artery and closure of the interatrial communication (Fontan procedure) (Fig. 31-54).[389,390,390a,390b] If the right ventricle is not markedly hypoplastic, it may be utilized in the correction to generate forward flow into the pulmonary vascular bed. Also, if the right ventricle is not too hypoplastic, it may be used as a pumping chamber by anastomosis of the right atrial appendage to the right ventricle with the aid of a pericardial patch, leaving the outflow tract and pulmonic valve intact.[387] A previously existing systemic artery-to-pulmonary artery anastomosis must be closed, but a systemic vein-to-pulmonary artery anastomosis may be left in place. Candidates for these corrective procedures must have normal pulmonary vascular resistance and a mean pulmonary artery pressure less than 20 mm Hg, pulmonary arteries of adequate size, and good left ventricular function.[389,391] The postoperative period usually is characterized transiently by a superior vena cava syndrome with right heart failure, edema, ascites, and hepatomegaly. Long-term results have been good.[392-397]

EBSTEIN'S ANOMALY OF THE TRICUSPID VALVE

(See also p. 970)

This malformation is characterized by a downward displacement of the tricuspid valve into the right ventricle due to anomalous attachment of the tricuspid leaflets (Fig. 31-55).[398] Case-control studies suggest that maternal exposure in the first trimester to lithium carbonate, used in the management of manic-depressive psychosis, is associated with a greatly increased risk of this anomaly in exposed offspring.[399] Tricuspid valve tissue is dysplastic, and a variable portion of the septal and inferior cusps adhere to the right ventricular wall some distance away from the atrioventricular junction. Because of the abnormally situated tricuspid orifice, a portion of the right ventricle lies between the atrioventricular ring and the origin of the valve, which is continuous with the right atrial chamber. This proximal segment is "atrialized," and a distal, functionally small ventricular chamber exists. The degree of impairment of right ventricular function depends primarily on the extent to which the right ventricular inflow portion is atrialized and on the magnitude of tricuspid valve regurgitation.

CLINICAL MANIFESTATIONS. These are variable because the spectrum of pathology varies widely and because of the presence of associated malformations.[400] An interatrial communication consisting of a patent foramen ovale or an ostium secundum atrial septal defect is present in more than half the cases. The most common important associated defect is pulmonic stenosis or atresia. Other coexistent anomalies may include an ostium primum type of atrial septal defect and ventricular septal defect alone or in combination with other lesions. The Ebstein's lesion commonly is observed in association with congenitally corrected transposition of the great arteries, in which the tricuspid valve is in the left atrioventricular orifice (p. 946). The usual manifestations in infancy are cyanosis, a cardiac murmur, and severe congestive heart failure. The magnitude of tricuspid regurgitation in the neonate is enhanced because the pulmonary vascular resistance is normally high early in life.[401] In this regard it may be difficult in some newborn infants with Ebstein's anomaly and massive tricuspid regurgitation to distinguish between organic pulmonic atresia and the presence of elevated perinatal pulmonary vascular resistance.[402] In such infants retrograde aortography is quite likely to fill the pulmonary root and allow visualization of the pulmonic valve by way of a patent ductus arteriosus, serving to differentiate a normal from an abnormal pulmonary outflow tract.[403] The tricuspid regurgitation in infants with Ebstein's anomaly may lessen substantially, and cyanosis may disappear early in life as pulmonary vascular resistance falls, only to recur at a later age when right ventricular dysfunction and/or paroxysmal arrhythmias develop. In some infants with Ebstein's malformation, cyanosis is suddenly intensified as the degree of pulmonary hypoperfusion is unmasked by spontaneous closure of a patent ductus arteriosus.

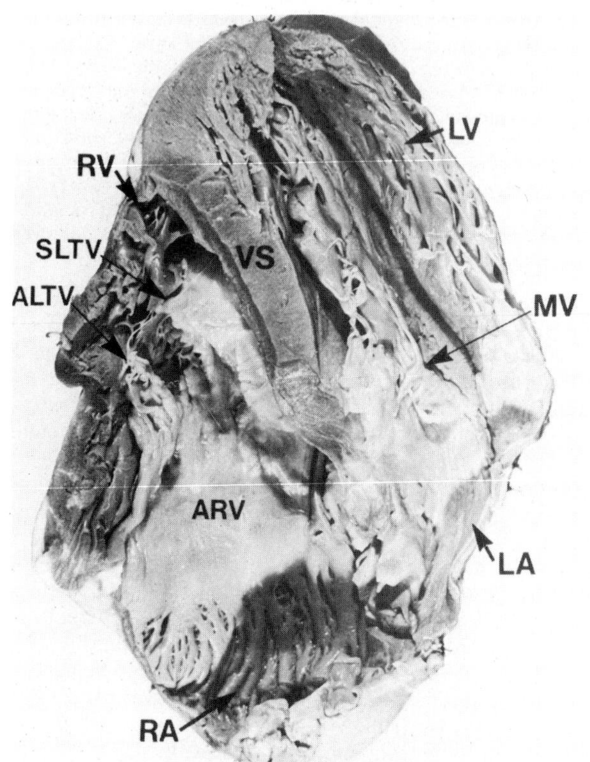

FIGURE 31-55. Anatomical specimen of Ebstein's anomaly of the tricuspid valve, cut in the same plane as an apical four-chamber echocardiographic view (Fig. 31-56). The septal and anterior leaflets of the tricuspid valve (SLTV, ALTV) are displaced into the right ventricle (RV), producing a large atrialized right ventricle (ARV). VS = ventricular septum, RA = right atrium, LA = left atrium, MV = mitral valve, LV = left ventricle. (Courtesy of Thomas DiSessa, M.D.)

Beyond infancy the onset of symptoms is insidious; the most common complaints are exertional dyspnea, fatigue, and cyanosis. About 25 per cent of patients suffer episodes of paroxysmal atrial tachycardia. A prominent systolic pulsation of the liver and a large *v* wave in the jugular venous pulse accompany the systolic thrill and murmur of tricuspid regurgitation. Wide splitting of the first and second heart sounds and prominent third and fourth heart sounds may produce a characteristically rhythmic auscultatory cadence with a triple, quadruple, or quintuple combination of sounds.

LABORATORY FINDINGS. The *electrocardiographic abnormalities* commonly fall into two categories: those with a right bundle branch block pattern and those with the Wolff-Parkinson-White syndrome (Fig. 32-10, p. 972). The pattern in the latter is almost always type B, resembling left bundle branch block with predominant S waves in the right precordial leads. The presence of the Wolff-Parkinson-White pattern increases the risk of supraventricular paroxysmal tachycardia.[404] The electrocardiogram most often shows giant P waves, a prolonged P-R interval, and prolonged terminal QRS depolarization, producing variable degrees of right bundle branch block. These distinctive findings help to distinguish Ebstein's anomaly from other forms of right ventricular dysplasia whose presenting problem often is an arrhythmia. *Roentgenographic* (Figs. 8-42C, p. 230, and 32-6, p. 970) and fluoroscopic studies usually demonstrate an enlarged right atrium, a small right ventricle, and a pulmonary artery with reduced pulsations; the pulmonary vascularity may be reduced if a large right-to-left shunt is present.

The principal *echocardiographic findings* observed in patients with this anomaly, as well as in those with other forms of right ventricular volume overload, are an increase in right ventricular dimension, paradoxical ventricular septal motion, an increase in tricuspid valve excursion, and an abnormal closing velocity of the tricuspid valve. More specific findings for Ebstein's anomaly include a delay in tricuspid valve closure relative to mitral closure and a decrease in the E-F slope of the tricuspid valve, an abnormal anterior position of the tricuspid valve during diastole, and the detection of tricuspid valve echoes with more lateral placement of the transducer than usual.[405] Two-dimensional echocardiographic techniques are superior for observation of the inferior and leftward displacement of the tricuspid valve and simultaneously demonstrate the abnormal positional relation between the tricuspid and mitral valves (Figs. 31-56 and 4-69, p. 91).[402,405] Moreover, the boundaries of the atrialized right ventricle may be defined. Specific diagnosis requires identification, usually from an apical four-chamber view, of displacement of the septal tricuspid leaflet.[406] Tricuspid regurgitation, if present, is detected by Doppler examination.

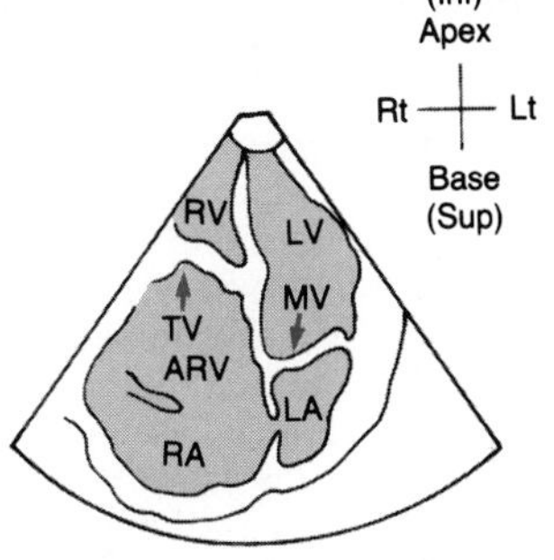

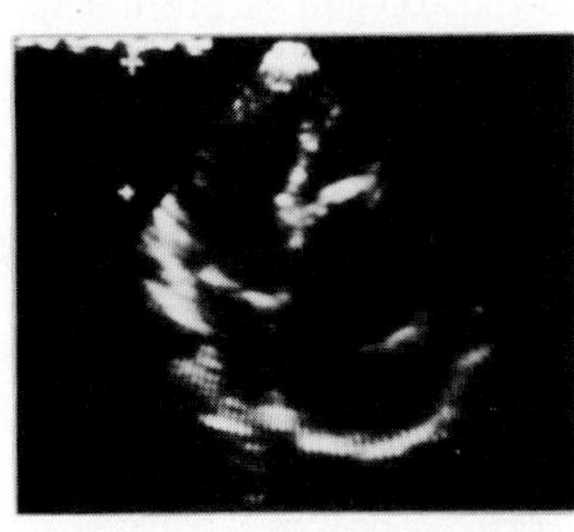

FIGURE 31-56. Apical four-chamber view of Ebstein's anomaly, corresponding to the anatomical specimen in Figure 31-55. RA = right atrium, LA = left atrium, MV = mitral valve, LV = left ventricle, TV = tricuspid valve, ARV = atrialized right ventricle, RV = right ventricle. (Courtesy of Thomas DiSessa, M.D.)

At *cardiac catheterization* the intracavitary electrocardiogram recorded just proximal to the tricuspid valve shows a right ventricular type of complex, while the pressure recorded is that of the right atrium (Fig. 31-57). A right-to-left atrial shunt normally is present. The hemodynamic findings depend on the degree of tricuspid regurgitation. The cardiac muscle is unusually irritable, and a high incidence of significant arrhythmias during catheterization has been noted. Selective right ventricular *angiocardiography* shows the position of the displaced tricuspid valve, the size of the right ventricle, and the configuration of the outflow portion of the right ventricle.

MANAGEMENT. Ebstein's anomaly may be compatible with a relatively long and active life, with most patients surviving into the third decade.[400,407] In some disabled patients moderate improvement has resulted from anastomosis of the superior vena cava to the right pulmonary artery (the Glenn procedure) to divert systemic venous return from the right atrium and to increase pulmonary blood flow. Benefit has resulted in older patients from replacement or repair of the tricuspid valve and closure of the atrial defect with or without ligation and marsupialization of the thin atrialized portion of the right ventricle.[408,409,409a] In patients with a preexcitation syndrome (p. 693) that is producing life-threatening rhythm disturbances the accessory conduction pathways should be divided. It should be recognized, however, that patients with Ebstein's anomaly are poor surgical risks at all ages.

The term *transposition* identifies a group of malformations that have in common abnormal relation between the cardiac chambers and great arteries. In this chapter the term is used to include both anomalous insertion of the pulmonary veins and cardiac malpositions.

COMPLETE TRANSPOSITION OF THE GREAT ARTERIES

(See also p. 946)

MORPHOLOGY. This is a common and potentially lethal form of heart disease in newborns and infants.[410] The malformation consists of the origin of the aorta arising from the morphological right ventricle and that of the pulmonary artery from the morphological left ventricle. With rare exceptions there is no fibrous continuity between the aortic and mitral valves. The origin of the aorta usually is to the right and anterior to, but may be lateral to, the main pulmonary artery. Thus, dextro- or D-transposition is a term often used interchangeably with complete transposition. The embryogenesis of complete transposition of the great arteries is controversial. There is consensus that the ventricular origins of the great arteries are reversed after development of a straight rather than a spiral infundibulotruncal septum. Transposition appears to result from a transfer of the pulmonary artery, instead of the aorta, from the heart tube's outlet zone to the left ventricle.[410a] The latter may result from maldevelopment of the infundibulum, or a combination of both infundibulum maldevelopment and truncal malseptation; the former results if the subpulmonary, rather than the subaortic, infundibulum is absorbed.

The anatomical arrangement results in two separate and parallel circulations. Some communication between the two circulations must exist after birth to sustain life; otherwise, unoxygenated systemic venous blood is directed inappropriately to the systemic circulation and oxygenated pulmonary venous blood is directed to the pulmonary circulation. Almost all patients have an interatrial communication (Fig. 31-58). Two-thirds have a patent ductus arteriosus, and about one-third have an associated ventricular septal defect. Complete transposition occurs more frequently in the offspring of diabetic mothers and more often in males than in females. Without treatment, about 30 per cent of these infants die within the first week of life, 50 per cent within the first month, 70 per cent within 6 months, and 90 per cent within the first year.[410] Those who live beyond infancy have, as a general rule, either

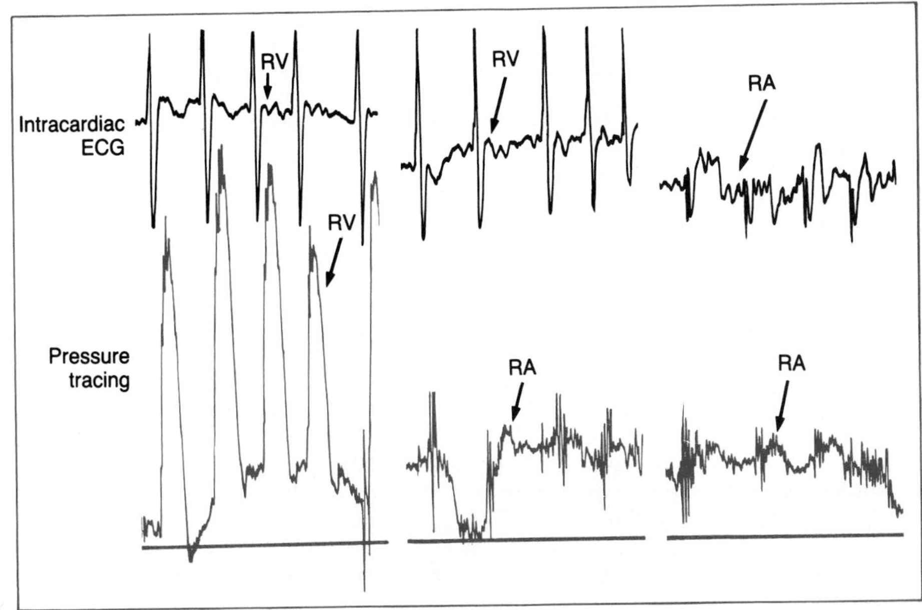

FIGURE 31-57. With a catheter in the "atrialized" portion of the right ventricle (RV), the intracardiac electrocardiogram in a patient with Ebstein's anomaly continues to show a ventricular complex, while right atrial pressure (RA) is recorded at the same site. (Courtesy of Delores A. Danilowicz, M.D.)

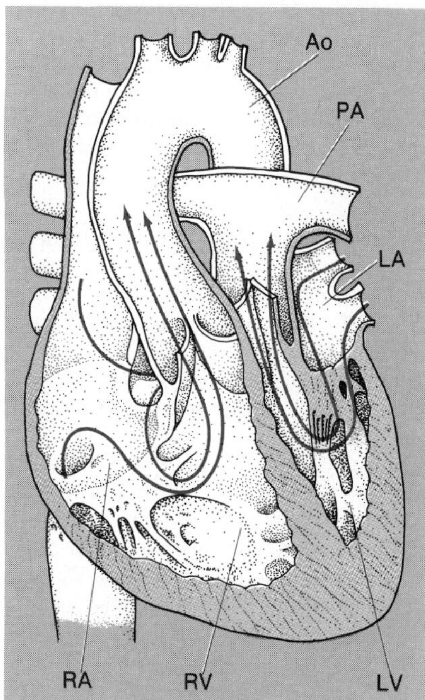

FIGURE 31–58. Complete transposition of the great arteries. Intercirculatory mixing occurs only at the atrial level. RA = right atrium; LA = left atrium; RV = right ventricle; LV = left ventricle; Ao = aorta; PA = pulmonary artery.

an isolated large atrial septal defect or a single ventricle, or ventricular septal defect and pulmonic stenosis. Current aggressive medical and surgical approaches to this group of patients have transformed the prognosis for an infant with this malformation from hopeless to hopeful.

The *clinical course* is determined by the degree of tissue hypoxia, the ability of each ventricle to sustain an increased workload in the presence of reduced coronary arterial oxygenation, the nature of the associated cardiovascular anomalies, and the anatomical and functional status of the pulmonary vascular bed.[411] A bidirectional shunt is always present because continuous unidirectional shunting would result in a progressive depletion of the circulating volume in either the pulmonary or the systemic vascular bed.

HEMODYNAMICS. A major determinant of the systemic arterial oxygen saturation is the amount of blood exchanged between the two circulations by intercirculatory shunts. The net volume of blood passing left to right from the pulmonary to the systemic circulation represents the anatomical left-to-right shunt and is in fact the effective systemic blood flow (i.e., the amount of oxygenated pulmonary venous return reaching the systemic capillary bed). Conversely, the volume of blood passing right to left from the systemic to the pulmonary circulation constitutes the anatomical right-to-left shunt and is in fact the effective pulmonary blood flow (i.e., the net volume of unsaturated systemic venous return perfusing the pulmonary capillary bed). The net volume exchange between the two circulations per unit time is equal. The magnitude of the intercirculatory mixing volume is modified by the number of intercirculatory communications that exist, the presence of associated obstructive intracardiac and extracardiac anomalies, the extent of the bronchopulmonary circulation, and the relation between pulmonary and systemic vascular resistance. For example, in the newborn with an intact ventricular septum and a constricted or closed patent ductus arteriosus, inadequate mixing through a small patent foramen ovale often is the cause of severe hypoxemia. If a large interatrial communication or a ventricular septal defect exists, systemic arterial oxygen saturation is influenced more importantly by the pulmonary–systemic blood flow relation than by the adequacy of mixing; augmented pulmonary blood flow produces a higher systemic arterial saturation if the left ventricle can sustain a high-output state without the intervention of congestive heart failure and pulmonary edema. The systemic arterial oxygen saturation will be quite low, despite adequate intercirculatory mixing sites, if pulmonary blood flow is reduced by left ventricular outflow tract obstruction or increased pulmonary vascular resistance.

Infants with complete transposition of the great arteries are particularly susceptible to the early development of *pulmonary vascular obstructive disease*.[52,412] Severe morphological alterations develop in the pulmonary vascular bed by the age of 1 or 2 years in almost all patients with an associated large ventricular septal defect or large patent ductus arteriosus in the absence of obstruction to left ventricular outflow. Advanced pulmonary vascular disease also is seen within this same time frame in 5 to 10 per cent of patients without a patent ductus arteriosus and with an intact ventricular septum. Systemic arterial hypoxemia, increased pulmonary blood flow, and pulmonary hypertension contribute to the development of pulmonary vascular obstruction in these patients as they do in other forms of congenital heart disease. Among the additional factors implicated in the accelerated and more widespread pulmonary vascular obstruction found in patients with complete transposition is the presence of extensive bronchopulmonary anastomotic channels, which enter the pulmonary vascular bed proximal to the pulmonary capillary bed; thus, oxygen tension is reduced at the precapillary level, causing pulmonary vasoconstriction.[413] Beyond the early neonatal period many patients have an abnormal distribution pattern of pulmonary blood flow, with preferential flow to the right lung.[414] The asymmetrical distribution of pulmonary blood flow in these individuals results from an abnormal rightward inclination of the main pulmonary artery in the transposition malformation that favors flow from the main to the right pulmonary artery. Persistently increased pulmonary blood flow to the right lung would be expected to contribute to pulmonary vascular obstructive changes within the lung; in the left pulmonary vascular bed, thrombotic changes may occur because of the combination of reduced flow and polycythemia. Finally, it should be recognized that a prenatal alteration in pulmonary vascular smooth muscle may exist, since blood perfusing the fetal lungs in complete transposition of great arteries has a higher than normal pO_2 and may serve to dilate pulmonary vessels in utero. Postnatally such vessels may have an enhanced capacity to constrict in response to vasoactive stimuli and suffer anatomical, obliterative changes.

CLINICAL FINDINGS. Average birthweight and size of infants born with complete transposition of the great arteries are greater than normal. The usual clinical manifestations are dyspnea and cyanosis from birth, progressive hypoxemia, and congestive heart failure. Early in postnatal life the clinical manifestations and course are influenced principally by the magnitude of intercirculatory mixing. The most severe cyanosis and hypoxemia are observed in infants with only a small patent foramen ovale or ductus arteriosus and an intact ventricular septum in whom mixing is inadequate, or in those infants with relatively reduced pulmonary blood flow because of left ventricular outflow tract obstruction.[415,416] With a large persistent patent ductus arteriosus or a large ventricular septal defect, cyanosis may be minimal and heart failure is the usual dominant problem after the first few weeks of life.[410] It should be recognized that a patent ductus arteriosus is present in about half of newborn infants with transposition, although it closes functionally and anatomically soon after birth in almost all cases. If the ductus arteriosus remains open, better mixing of the venous and arterial circulations usually is at the expense of pulmonary artery hypertension.[417]

Cardiac murmurs are of little diagnostic significance and are absent or insignificant in about 30 to 50 per cent of infants with complete transposition of the great arteries and an intact ventricular septum. In infants with a large persistent patent ductus arteriosus, fewer than half exhibit physical signs typical of ductus arteriosus, such as continuous murmur, bounding pulses, or a prominent middiastolic rumble. Moreover, *differential cyanosis* caused by reversed pulmonary-to-sys-

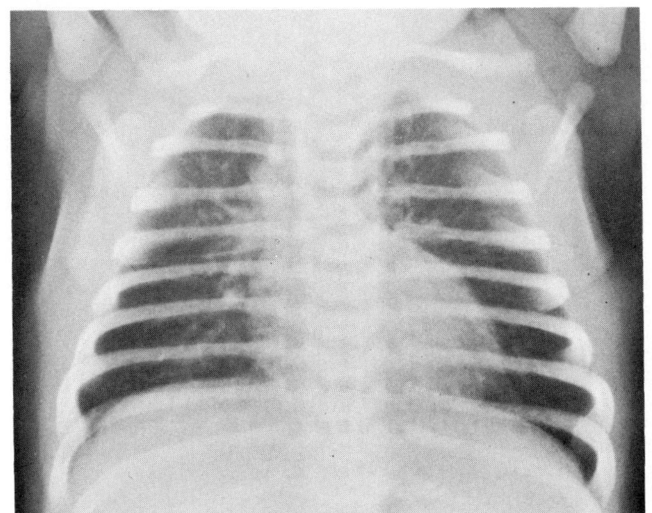

FIGURE 31–59. **Chest roentgenogram in a 4-day-old infant with complete transposition of the great arteries showing an oval-shaped heart with a narrow base and increased pulmonary vascular markings.**

temic shunting across the ductus arteriosus is difficult to detect because of generalized arterial desaturation. In those infants with a large ventricular septal defect, a pansystolic murmur usually emerges within the first 7 to 10 days of life. In newborns with transposition and severe pulmonic stenosis or atresia, the clinical findings are similar to those in the infant with tetralogy of Fallot.

The most usual *electrocardiographic findings* include right-axis deviation, right atrial enlargement, and right ventricular hypertrophy, reflecting that the right ventricle is the systemic pumping chamber. Combined ventricular hypertrophy may be present in those patients with a large ventricular septal defect and elevated pulmonary blood flow. Isolated left ventricular hypertrophy is encountered rarely in patients with a ventricular septal defect and a hypoplastic right ventricle, in many of whom the tricuspid valve is displaced abnormally and straddles a ventricular septal defect. In the first days of life the chest x-ray may appear normal, particularly in infants with an intact ventricular septum. Thereafter, roentgenographic findings often are highly suggestive of the diagnosis,[418] and consist of (1) progressive cardiac enlargement in early infancy; (2) a characteristic oval or egg-shaped cardiac configuration in the anteroposterior view, and a narrow vascular pedicle created by superimposition of the aortic and pulmonary artery segments; and (3) increased pulmonary vascular markings (Fig. 31–59). A right aortic arch is seen in about 4 per cent of infants with an intact ventricular septum and 11 per cent of infants with a ventricular septal defect.

CT scanning (Fig. 11–17, p. 321) and MR imaging (Fig. 11–38, p. 331) may be helpful in diagnosis as well.

ECHOCARDIOGRAPHY. Two-dimensional echocardiography is extremely useful in the diagnosis of complete transposition of the great arteries.[419–422,422a] In sagittal cross sections the aorta is observed to ascend retrosternally in contrast to the normal posterior sweep of the pulmonary artery. With transverse short-axis cross-sectional imaging, the diagnosis is confirmed by demonstrating that the anterior great artery (the aorta) is to the right of the posterior great artery (pulmonary) or that the two arteries are visualized side by side (Fig. 31–60). Moreover, from this plane the course of the two great arteries may be traced to delineate their ventricle of origin, demonstrating that the anterior rightward vessel (aorta) originates from the right ventricle and the posterior leftward vessel (pulmonary artery) originates from the left ventricle (Fig. 31–61). Echocardiography also may assist in identifying associated defects. Ventricular septal defects may be localized to the membranous, atrioventricular, and trabecular muscular septa, and malalignment types of ventricular septal defects may be identified if the infundibular septum is shifted either anteriorly or posteriorly. A subaortic obstruction may be created by anterior shifting of the infundibular septum, whereas a posterior shift may narrow the subpulmonary area. The nature of left ventricular outflow tract obstruction may be further identified as a fixed obstruction caused by a fibromuscular ridge or as a dynamic obstruction caused by deviation of the interventricular septum toward the left ventricular cavity and the apposition between a thickened interventricular septum and systolic anterior motion of the mitral valve.[422,423]

CARDIAC CATHETERIZATION AND ANGIOCARDIOGRAPHY. Infants with simple, complete transposition of the great arteries who present in the first few weeks of life to a center prepared to correct the anomaly by the arterial switch operation (see below) often are taken to the operating room shortly after two-dimensional echocardiography and Doppler examination are performed.[422a] In these cases, transcatheter balloon atrial septostomy is not performed unless a delay is expected in taking the patient to the operating room. In essentially all other patients, cardiac catheterization and angiography are components of the initial evaluation of the patient.

The diagnostic portion of the cardiac catheterization allows confirmation of the anatomical derangement of the great ar-

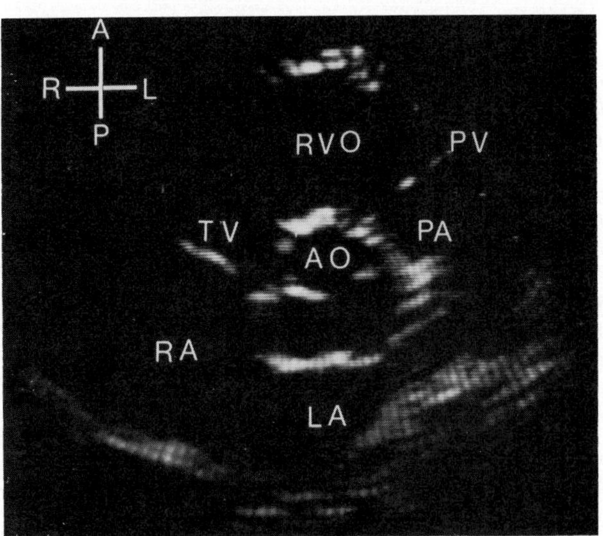

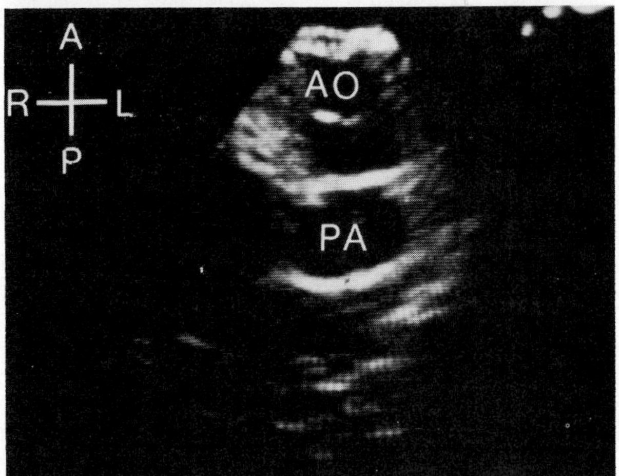

FIGURE 31–60. ***Top,*** **A two-dimensional echocardiographic short-axis scan demonstrates normal great artery relations. The right ventricular outflow tract (RVO) wraps around the aorta (AO) in a clockwise manner. The pulmonic valve (PV) is to the left of the aortic valve.** ***Bottom,*** **Short-axis scan shows the abnormal great artery relations in an infant with transposition of the great arteries. The aorta (AO) is directly anterior and slightly to the right of the pulmonary artery (PA). The clockwise partial encirclement of the aorta by the right ventricular outflow tract is no longer observed. A = anterior, L = left, P = posterior, R = right, LA = left atrium, RA = right atrium, TV = tricuspid valve.**

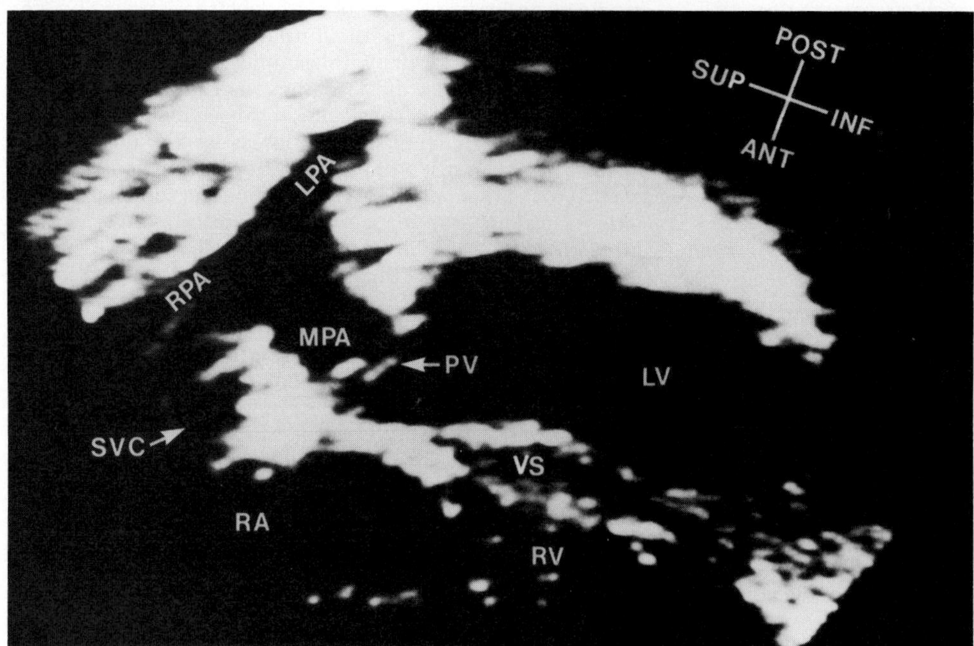

FIGURE 31-61. Complete transposition of the great arteries in a subcostal long-axis view with anterior transducer tilt. The main pulmonary artery (MPA) is seen exiting the left ventricle (LV) and bifurcating into its right and left branches (RPA, LPA). SVC = superior vena cava, RA = right atrium, RV = right ventricle, VS = ventricular septum, PV = pulmonary valve. (Courtesy of Thomas DiSessa, M.D.)

teries and establishes the presence of associated lesions; in the newborn, unless prompt arterial switch repair is planned, as discussed above, it should always be accompanied by a palliative balloon atrial septostomy, which serves to enlarge the interatrial communication and improve oxygenation. In the older neonate, usually beyond age 3 weeks, thickening of the atrial septum may preclude satisfactory balloon septostomy. In these instances, transcatheter blade septostomy is the preferred approach to palliation. Two-dimensional echocardiography, with or without fluoroscopy, may be used as the imaging mode for both balloon and blade creation of an atrial septal defect.[424] Subcostal four-chamber and sagittal views image cardiac anatomy and catheter position during the procedure, substantially reducing radiation dosage.

Both the diagnostic and the palliative procedures can be performed by percutaneous entry into the femoral vein, umbilical vein catheterization, or direct cutdown into the femoral or saphenous vein. The catheter passes easily across the foramen ovale into the left atrium and left ventricle and may be manipulated into the pulmonary artery by means of a flow-directed balloon-guided catheter or by manipulation of a standard catheter bent in the form of a J loop within the left ventricle, with the tip pointed posteriorly to the pulmonary artery. When a large ventricular septal defect is present, a catheter often can be manipulated directly across it from the right ventricle into the pulmonary artery.

The major abnormal hemodynamic findings include right ventricular pressure at systemic levels and either a high or low left ventricular pressure, depending on pulmonary blood flow, pulmonary vascular resistance, and the presence or absence of left ventricular outflow tract obstructive lesions. Oxygen saturation in the aorta is lower than that in the pulmonary artery. Application of the Fick principle to the calculation of pulmonary and systemic blood flow rates in these patients is an important source of error. Assumed values of oxygen consumption are unreliable in the severely hypoxemic infant. Moreover, because systemic and particularly pulmonary arteriovenous oxygen differences may be quite reduced, small errors in oxygen saturation values result in large errors in flow calculations. Furthermore, because bronchial collaterals enter the pulmonary circuit at the precapillary level, a true mixed pulmonary artery saturation cannot be sampled; pulmonary blood flow is therefore overestimated when one uses a sample from the central pulmonary artery, and pulmonary vascular resistance values often are underestimated.

Selective Ventricular Angiography. This is diagnostic and demonstrates that the anteriorly placed aorta arises from the right ventricle and that the posteriorly placed pulmonary artery in continuity with the mitral valve arises from the left ventricle. The status of the ductus arteriosus and the site and size of a ventricular septal defect can be well visualized by angiography (Fig. 31-62). Interventricular defects posterior and inferior to the crista supraventricularis occur in about

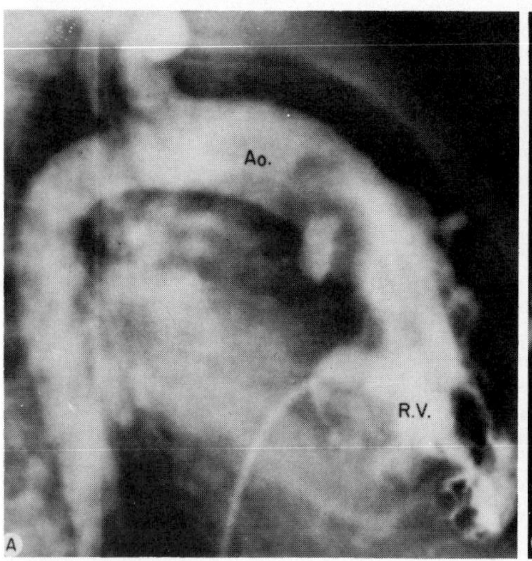

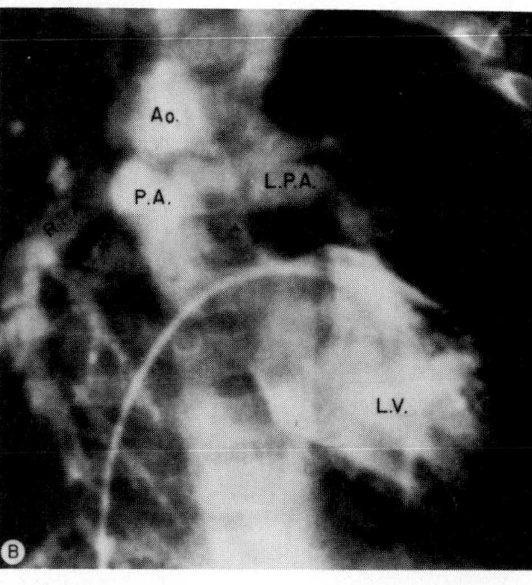

FIGURE 31-62. Lateral *(A)* and frontal *(B)* views of selective ventriculograms in a child with complete transposition of the great arteries and a ventricular septal defect (V.S.D.). Ao. = aorta, R.V. = right ventricle, P.A. = pulmonary artery, L.V. = left ventricle, R.P.A. = right pulmonary artery, L.P.A. = left pulmonary artery. (Courtesy of Delores A. Danilowicz, M.D.)

half of these patients; less often the defects are anterior and superior to the crista supraventricularis or are of the atrioventricular septal type.[425] A variety of lesions may be identified as the cause of left ventricular outflow tract obstruction, including ventricular septal hypertrophy with systolic anterior movement of the mitral valve, discrete or tunnel fibromuscular subpulmonic stenosis, valvular and supravalvular stenosis, and, rarely, an aneurysm of the membranous ventricular septum or redundant tricuspid valve tissue protruding through a ventricular septal defect.

A number of coronary arterial patterns are seen in patients with complete transposition of the great arteries.[426,427] In the majority, the left coronary artery originates in the left sinus and the right coronary artery originates in the posterior sinus, with single ostium above both the left and the posterior sinus. In almost 20 per cent of patients the left circumflex artery arises as a branch of the right coronary artery; a single coronary artery is present in about 6 per cent; in 3 to 4 per cent of patients either the right coronary and anterior descending arteries originate in the left sinus, with the left circumflex originating in the posterior sinus, or two ostia are present above one sinus, one giving rise to the right and the other to the left coronary artery.

MANAGEMENT. Medical treatment often is of limited help but should be vigorous since both functional and anatomical corrections of the malformation achieve good results. Conservative measures include the use of oxygen, digitalis, diuretics, iron (if an associated iron-deficiency anemia is present), and intravenous sodium bicarbonate for severe hypoxemic metabolic acidosis. Dilatation of the ductus arteriosus by prostaglandin E_1 in the early neonatal period both augments pulmonary blood flow and enhances intercirculatory mixing.[71] The creation or enlargement of an interatrial communication is the simplest procedure for providing increased intracardiac mixing of systemic and pulmonary venous blood; preferably this is achieved by rupturing the valve of the foramen ovale by balloon catheter during transseptal catheterization of the left side of the heart (Rashkind's procedure), or by blade septostomy. Surgical atrial septectomy seldom is required. The balloon should be inflated to a diameter of about 15 mm before pullback to the right atrium. Salutary results consist of a fall in left atrial pressure, equalization of mean left and right atrial pressures, and an increase in the systemic arterial oxygen saturation. When the foramen ovale is stretched by the balloon without accomplishing rupture of the septum primum valve of the fossa ovalis, the improvement in oxygenation is short-lived. Infusion or reinfusion intravenously of prostaglandin E_1 (0.05 to 0.1 mg/kg/min) has been shown to improve systemic oxygenation temporarily in the latter situation, by dilating the ductus arteriosus and thereby facilitating intercirculatory mixing.[71] Although balloon atrial septotomy usually is successful in stabilizing the infant's condition and allowing survival in the neonatal period, the initial rise in systemic arterial oxygen saturation to 65 to 75 per cent often is not sustained beyond 6 to 9 months of age.

Surgical Treatment. The development of *corrective operations* for infants born with transposition of the great arteries has greatly improved prognosis.[428,428a] Intraatrial correction by the *Mustard* technique is accomplished by excision of the interatrial septum and creation of a new interatrial septum with a pericardial baffle diverting the systemic venous return into the left ventricle through the mitral valve and thence to the left ventricle and pulmonary artery, while the pulmonary venous blood is diverted through the tricuspid valve and right ventricle to the aorta.[428b] The *Senning* procedure is based on a similar principle and consists of diversion of left pulmonary venous blood by a coronary sinus flap and rerouting of caval flow by the use of an atrial wall flap.[428c] In medical centers in which the venous switch approach is preferred, the intraatrial corrective operation is performed at any age in patients with an intact ventricular septum who do not improve after balloon atrial septotomy. If palliative septotomy provides adequate relief of hypoxemia, the atrial rerouting operation is performed routinely in most infants with transposition of the great arteries and intact ventricular septum by 3 to 9 months of age, with a surgical mortality less than 5 per cent.[428] Clinical improvement usually is quite dramatic. In some patients postoperative complications are observed that are directly related to the intraatrial repair (shunts across the intraatrial patch and obstruction to either systemic or pulmonary venous return or both).[429] There is a high incidence of early and late postoperative dysrhythmias that are more likely to have their basis in injury to the sinoatrial node and/or its arterial supply than in disruption of internodal tracts or damage to the atrioventricular node.[430,431,431a] Tricuspid regurgitation is a less common complication of operation and may be related in some patients to a preexisting abnormality of the tricuspid valve, whereas in most it is related to right ventricular dysfunction.[432] Although the assessment of right ventricular contractility is difficult, it would appear that the right ventricular pump function is impaired before Mustard operation and does not return to normal after successful surgery.[433-438] It seems unlikely that the right ventricle can perform as a systemic pumping chamber for the duration of a normal life span.

A one-stage anatomical correction is now the approach of choice in major centers that care for infants with congenital heart disease.[428,439-443,443a] In this operation both coronary arteries are transposed to the posterior artery; the aorta and pulmonary arteries are transsected, contraposed, and anastomosed (Jatene operation) (Fig. 31–63). The arterial switch anatomical correction may be complicated by coronary ostial stenosis, acquired supravalvular aortic and/or pulmonary stenosis, and pulmonic and/or aortic incompetence. The major advantages of the arterial switch procedure, when com-

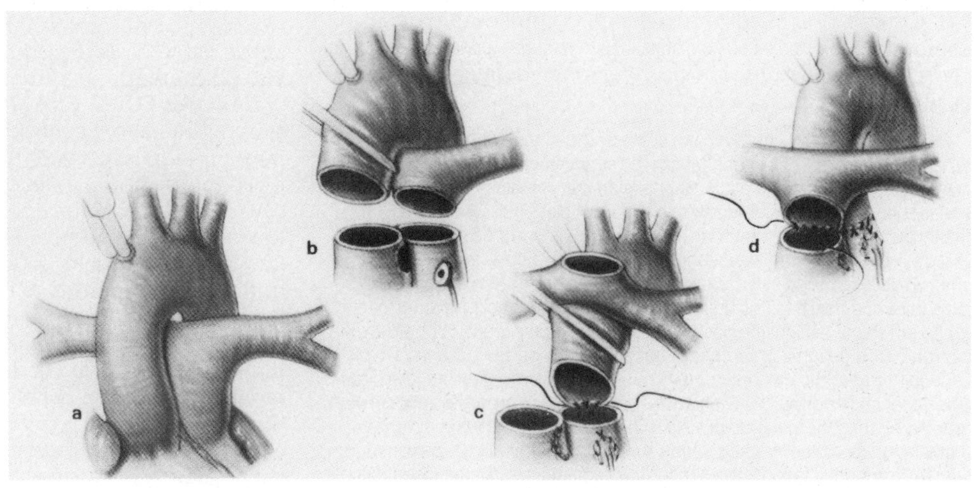

FIGURE 31–63. Complete transposition of the great arteries, corrected by a modified arterial switch operation. The aorta and pulmonary artery are transected and the orifices of the coronary arteries are excised with a rim of adjacent aortic wall (b). The aorta is brought under the bifurcation of the pulmonary artery, and the proximal pulmonary artery and the aorta are anastomosed without necessitating graft interposition. The coronary arteries are transferred to the pulmonary artery (c). The mobilized pulmonary artery is directly anastomosed to the proximal aortic stump (d). (From Stark, J., and DeLaval, M.: Surgery for Congenital Heart Defects. New York, Grune and Stratton, 1983, p. 379.)

pared with the atrial switch procedure, are the restoration of the left ventricle as the systemic pump and the potential for long-term maintenance of sinus rhythm.[444-450,450a]

Within the first month of life the arterial switch operation may be performed as a single-stage repair. In such patients, the origin and branching patterns of the coronary arteries are defined reliably preoperatively by two-dimensional echocardiography.[426] In older infants it appears necessary to prepare the left ventricle to withstand the systemic pressure which is produced after switching the great arteries, since, if the ventricular septum is intact, left ventricular pressure and left ventricular wall thickness diminish normally in relation to the postnatal reduction in pulmonary artery pressure. In these infants a two-stage approach is used, the first of which consists of banding the pulmonary artery; the arterial switch is performed soon thereafter, in some centers as early as 1 to 2 weeks later.[451]

In the unusual infant with an intact ventricular septum and a significant patent ductus arteriosus, an early intraatrial corrective operation with closure of the ductus is indicated at 4 to 6 months of age to prevent the likely progression of pulmonary vascular disease. Debate exists concerning the optimal management of patients with a large ventricular septal defect.[428] In some centers pulmonary artery banding is advocated early in life, followed by definitive intracardiac repair at 1 to 2 years of age. Others favor a one-stage intraatrial repair with patch closure of the ventricular septal defect before age 3 to 6 months. Still others perform an arterial switch anatomical correction within the first 3 to 4 months of age, unless the coronary arterial anatomy is considered unfavorable at operation.[440-442] Infants with transposition of the great arteries plus a ventricular septal defect and left ventricular outflow tract obstruction may require a systemic–pulmonary artery anastomosis when a pronounced diminution in pulmonary blood flow exists. A later corrective procedure for these patients bypasses the left ventricular outflow obstruction and uses an intracardiac ventricular baffle connecting the left ventricle to the aorta and an extracardiac prosthetic conduit between the right ventricle and the distal end of a divided pulmonary artery (Rastelli procedure).[440] In patients with significant pulmonary vascular obstructive disease the risk associated with definitive repair (anatomical correction or intraatrial baffle and closure of the ventricular septal defect) is great. In this group of patients a "palliative" Mustard or Senning procedure leaving the ventricular septal defect open often provides good, short-term, symptomatic improvement by increasing arterial oxygen tension and reducing the stimulus to progressive polycythemia.[452]

CONGENITALLY CORRECTED TRANSPOSITION OF THE GREAT ARTERIES

(See also p. 941)

This term is applied to two distinctly different anomalies: anatomically corrected transposition or malposition of the great arteries and physiologically corrected, levo- or L-transposition of the great arteries.

MORPHOLOGY. Anatomically corrected malposition of the great arteries is a rare form of congenital heart disease in which the great arteries are abnormally related to each other and to the ventricles but arise, nonetheless, above the anatomically correct ventricles.[453,454] Because of this, the term *malposition*, rather than *transposition*, is preferable. The anomaly results from either leftward looping of the ventricular segment of the embryonic heart tube in the situs solitus heart, or rightward looping in the situs inversus heart. In this unusual malformation the aorta is anterior and to the left (levo- or L-malposition) and the pulmonary artery is posteromedial and to the right, presumably because of a subaortic conus which causes mitral-aortic discontinuity. When no other defect exists, the circulation proceeds normally. When an associated lesion prompts echocardiographic examination, the diagnosis is indicated by the finding of atrioventricular concordance in association with wide mitral-aortic discontinuity with an anteriorly placed aorta. At cardiac catheterization, the diagnosis of the abnormal relation between the great arteries may be made by biplane angiocardiography. Anomalies commonly associated with anatomically corrected malposition of the great arteries include ventricular septal defect, left juxtaposition of the atrial appendages, tricuspid atresia or stenosis, and valvular and subvalvular pulmonic stenosis.

DEFINITION. Invariably, the term *congenitally corrected transposition* is applied to the heart in which a functional correction of the circulation exists by virtue of the relation between the ventricles and great arteries.[455,456] Corrected or L-transposition occurs when the primitive cardiac tube loops to the left, instead of to the right, during embryogenesis.[457] The anatomical right ventricle comes to lie on the left and receives oxygenated blood from the left atrium; this blood is ejected into an anteriorly placed, left-sided aorta. The anatomical left ventricle lies to the right and connects the right atrium to a posteriorly placed pulmonary artery. Thus, there are both ventriculoarterial and atrioventricular discordant connections, with ventricular inversion. This arrangement of the great arteries and ventricles (in contrast to the uncorrected, complete, or D-transposition) permits functional correction, so that systemic venous blood passes into the pulmonary trunk while arterialized pulmonary venous blood flows into the aorta. In the heart with congenitally corrected transposition, the venae cavae and coronary sinus drain into a right atrium that is normal in position and structure.

Venous blood flows from the right atrium, designated as the "venous atrium," across an atrioventricular valve that has the structure of a normal mitral valve and into the right-sided "venous ventricle." The venous ventricle, however, has the morphological characteristics of a normal left ventricle, i.e., its interior lining is trabeculated, it has no crista supraventricularis, and the atrioventricular valve is in continuity with the posteriorly placed semilunar valve. It ejects blood into the pulmonary trunk, which arises posterior to the ascending aorta. Oxygenated blood returns from the lungs to the left atrium, which is normal in position and structure; from here it flows into the left-sided "arterial ventricle" across an atrioventricular valve that has the structure of a normal tricuspid valve. The interior lining of the arterial ventricle has the morphological characteristics of a normal right ventricle (i.e., it has coarse trabeculations and a crista supraventricularis), and the tricuspid atrioventricular valve is not in continuity with the anteriorly placed semilunar valve. The arterial ventricle ejects blood into the aorta, which arises anterior to the pulmonary trunk. In addition to inversion of the cardiac ventricles, there is inversion of the conduction system and coronary arteries. Commonly associated anatomical lesions include atrial and ventricular septal defects, often accompanied by valvular or subvalvular pulmonary stenosis; single ventricle with an outlet chamber with or without pulmonic stenosis; left atrioventricular valve regurgitation, usually because of an Ebstein's malformation of the left-sided tricuspid valve; and abnormalities of visceral and atrial situs.[458]

CLINICAL MANIFESTATIONS. The clinical presentation, course, and prognosis of patients with congenital functionally corrected transposition vary, depending on the nature and severity of the complicating intracardiac anomalies.[458,459] Patients in whom corrected transposition exists as an isolated anomaly present no functional alterations and have no symptoms. Asymptomatic children with an increase in the size of the systemic ventricle, due to significant left-to-right shunting or tricuspid regurgitation, usually develop symptoms of systemic ventricular dysfunction by the third or fourth decade.[458-461]

The *physical findings* in congenitally corrected transposition are those of the associated lesions with two exceptions: (1) a single accentuated second heart sound usually is present in the second left intercostal space, representing closure of the aortic valve lying lateral and anterior to the pulmonic valve; and (2) there is a high incidence of cardiac dysrhythmias

LABORATORY EXAMINATION. Because of the inversion of the heart's conduction system, the *electrocardiogram* may provide important clues in the diagnosis. An abnormal direction of initial (septal) depolarization from right to left causes leftward, anterior, and superior orientation of the initial QRS forces and reversal of the precordial Q-wave pattern (Q waves are present in the right precordial leads and absent in the left). In addition to inversion of the conduction system, the His bundle is elongated because of the greater distance between the atrioventricular node and the base of the ventricular septum.[462] The His bundle is located beneath the pulmonic valve in the position of mitral pulmonary continuity; thus, it is subject to significant excursions during mitral valve closure. This arrangement may be a causal factor in the arrhythmias and atrioventricular conduction disturbances commonly observed in these patients. First-degree atrioventricular (AV) block occurs in about 50 per cent, and complete AV block occurs in 10 to 15 per cent of patients. Other degrees of AV dissociation may be observed as well as paroxysmal supraventricular tachycardia and ventricular extrasystoles. In some patients, Kent bundle connections provide the anatomical substrate for preexcitation.[463]

Roentgenographic examination characteristically reveals absence of the normal pulmonary artery segment and a smooth convexity of the left supracardiac border produced by the displaced ascending aorta (Fig. 8–42*B*, p. 230). The latter may be visualized by radionuclide scintillation scans of the central circulation. The main pulmonary trunk is medially displaced and absent from the cardiac silhouette; the right pulmonary hilus often is prominent and elevated compared with the left, producing a right-sided "waterfall" appearance.

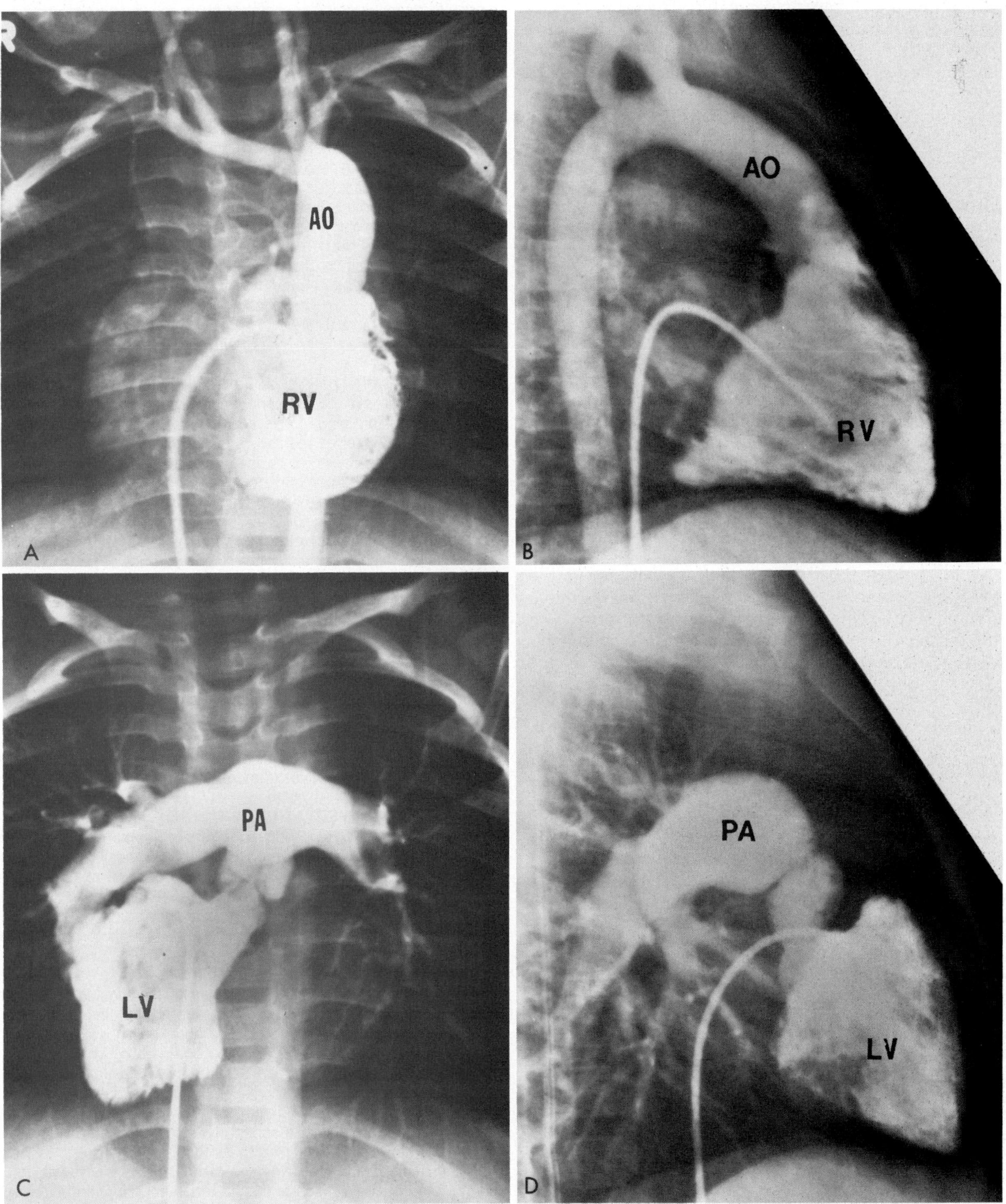

FIGURE 31–64. Congenitally corrected (levo-)transposition of the great arteries in a 4-year-old boy. *A*, Anteroposterior ventriculogram in left-sided ventricle with mesocardia. The morphological right ventricle (RV) is left-sided, indicating an L-ventricular loop (inverted ventricles in situs solitus). The aorta (AO) originates above the morphological right ventricle and is thus transposed and in the classic levo-transposition position. *B*, Lateral ventriculogram is left-sided ventricle (same frame as *A*). The aorta originates anteriorly above the morphological right ventricle (RV). *C*, Anteroposterior ventriculogram in right-sided morphological left ventricle (LV). The transposed pulmonary artery (PA) arises from this ventricle, and the ventricular septum appears intact. Pulmonic valve thickening is also evident. The aorta *(A)* is to the left of the pulmonary artery. Note that the ventricular septum in the L-ventricular loop is visualized best in the anteroposterior views. *D*, Lateral ventriculogram in right-sided ventricle (same frame as *C*). The pulmonary artery is posterior to the aorta, and supravalvular pulmonic narrowing is seen. (From Freedom, R. M., et al.: The differential diagnosis of levo-transposed or malposed aorta. An angiocardiographic study. Circulation *50*:1040, 1974, by permission of the American Heart Association, Inc.)

Two-dimensional echocardiography seeks to identify the morphology of each ventricle by defining the characteristics of the inflow and outflow tracts and papillary and trabecular muscle morphology, ventricular shape, and great artery position.[464] By tracing the great arteries back to their ventricles of origin in subxiphoid and parasternal short-axis planes, one would find that the anterior leftward great artery (the aorta) arises from the left-sided ventricle and is not in continuity with the left-sided atrioventricular valve. The great arteries exit the heart in parallel fashion; the position, origin, and branching pattern of the great arteries are observed in subxiphoid and suprasternal views, while the anteroposterior and right-left positions of the great arteries can be seen from the parasternal short-axis view. Because the ventricular septum lies in the anteroposterior plane parallel to the echo beam, it may not be visualized from a left parasternal view. In apical-basal or subxiphoid, four-chamber echocardiographic views, the right and left ventricular morphology and the inverted position of the atrioventricular valves may be ascertained correctly. The latter views also demonstrate the level of attachment of the atrioventricular valves and allow detection of inferior displacement of the left-sided tricuspid valve when Ebstein's anomaly coexists.

At *cardiac catheterization* the diagnosis should be suspected when the venous catheter enters a posterior and midline main pulmonary trunk. Retrograde arterial catheter passage establishes the typical position of the ascending aorta at the upper left cardiac border. Hemodynamic abnormalities depend on the lesions associated with corrected transposition. Selective *angiocardiography* allows visualization of the transposed great arteries and morphological differentiation of the two ventricles (Fig. 31–64). The ventricles usually lie side by side, with the ventricular septum oriented in an anteroposterior direction. Selective aortography demonstrates the inverted coronary arterial pattern that is invariably present in corrected transposition. The competence of the left atrioventricular valve may be determined by injection of contrast material into the arterial ventricle.[465] When a left-sided Ebstein's malformation exists, the leaflets are displaced distal to the true valve annulus. The level of the annulus may be determined by visualization of the circumflex branch of the left coronary artery, which courses posteriorly in the AV groove.

Specific problems have attended operative repair of the lesions associated with congenitally corrected transposition, owing primarily to the course of the atrioventricular conduction system and the coronary arterial pattern.[466,467] Intraoperative electrophysiological mapping of the course of the conduction system has been proposed to reduce, but not abolish, the risk of surgically induced heart block. The AV bundle is located anteriorly and in relation to the anterolateral quadrant of the pulmonary outflow tract. Thus, when a ventricular septal defect is present, the bundle usually is related to the anterior and superior margins of the defect and lies beneath the pulmonic valve. In corrected transposition, the coronary arteries have a course appropriate to their ventricles, i.e., the anterior descending and circumflex arteries supply the morphological left ventricle, and the right coronary artery supplies the morphological right ventricle. However, because the great arteries are transposed, the noncoronary sinus is the anterior sinus of the aortic valve.

The inversion of the coronary arterial system occasionally may limit and preclude an incision into the venous ventricle, thereby interfering with exposure of intracardiac defects in the usual manner. The disadvantage in approaching intracardiac anomalies using an incision in the morphological right ventricle is that this is the systemic ventricle. When significant pulmonary stenosis exists with a ventricular septal defect, a valved extracardiac conduit often is a required part of the surgical repair. Surgical risks are especially high in patients in whom significant regurgitation exists from the arterial ventricle to the arterial atrium. In these patients, annuloplasty, or more usually valve replacement, is required. In all operative approaches, if complete heart block has been present intermittently or permanently preoperatively or intraoperatively, permanent epicardial atrial and ventricular pacemaker leads are implanted.

DOUBLE-OUTLET RIGHT VENTRICLE

MORPHOLOGY. Other designations applied to this lesion include origin of both great arteries from the right ventricle, partial transposition, complete transposition of the aorta and levo-position of the pulmonary artery, complete dextroposition of the aorta, and the Taussig-Bing complex. This is an extremely heterogeneous category of malformations in which an abnormal relation exists between the aorta and the pulmonary trunk, which arise wholly or in large part from the right ventricle.[468,470]

A uniform definition or classification of double-outlet right ventricle does not exist.[469] To some, double-outlet right ventricle means origin of one great artery and at least 50 per cent of the other over the right ventricle; others require the presence of bilateral conus muscle between both great arteries and the atrioventricular annulus. One or both great arteries may arise from an infundibular chamber; there may be considerable variability in the amount of subarterial conus muscle. Thus, the semilunar valves may lie side by side, or with the pulmonary valve more anterior and superior, or with a more anterior and superior aortic valve. A malalignment type of ventricular septal defect is almost always present in double-outlet right ventricle because the infundibular septum is positioned abnormally. When the amount of conus muscle beneath the two great arteries varies, the ventricular septal defect commonly is positioned beneath the more posterior semilunar valve, which in fact usually overrides the interventricular septum through this ventricular septal defect. The amount of conus muscle underneath the valve determines the position of the semilunar root in relation to the ventricles below. Thus double-outlet right ventricle resides within the spectrum of conotruncal abnormalities ranging from tetralogy of Fallot to transposition of the great arteries. The ventricular septal defect occasionally, extends beneath both great arteries and is referred to as doubly committed. In some instances, the ventricular septal defect is remote to both great arteries, or is considered uncommitted, in which case the defect often lies in the inlet or muscular portion of the interventricular septum.

More than half of patients with double-outlet right ventricle have associated anomalies of the atrioventricular valves.[471] Mitral atresia associated with a hypoplastic left ventricle is common; less often observed are tricuspid stenosis, Ebstein's anomaly of the tricuspid valve, complete atrioventricular septal defect, and overriding or straddling of either atrioventricular valve. Aortic coarctation may be associated with double-outlet right ventricle, particularly when the subaortic area is narrowed by malalignment of the infundibular septum. Double-outlet right ventricle also may be a component of the multiple cardiovascular anomalies of the splenic dysgenesis or heterotaxy syndromes. An increased incidence of the anomaly occurs in infants with the trisomy 18 syndrome.

The pathological features in most patients include side-by-side pulmonic and aortic valves and discontinuity between the mitral and aortic valves. The latter exists because muscular infundibulum is usual beneath both semilunar valves. The ventricular septal defect may be remote from or closely related to one or both semilunar valves (Fig. 31–65).[471] When the interventricular defect is subpulmonic, with or without a straddling pulmonary trunk, the complex is designated "Taussig-Bing." In most patients the interventricular septal defect is below the crista supraventricularis and is subaortic in location. Least often the defect either is remote from both semilunar valves ("uncommitted") or underlies both ("doubly committed").

CLINICAL MANIFESTATIONS. The clinical and physiological picture is determined by the size and location of the ventricular septal defect and the presence or absence of pulmonic stenosis. In the Taussig-Bing form of double-outlet right ventricle, the malformation resembles physiologically and clinically complete transposition with ventricular septal defect and pulmonary hypertension. When the ventricular septal defect is subaortic, the stream of blood from the left ventricle is directed preferentially to the aorta. Thus, there may be little or no detectable cyanosis, and these patients usually clinically resemble those with an isolated, large ventricular septal defect and pulmonary hypertension. The most important determinant of the natural history in both these types of double-outlet right ventricle is the progression of pulmonary vascular obstruction. In contrast, when there is pulmonary outflow tract obstruction, which often is severe and found commonly in those patients in whom the ventricular septal defect is subaortic, clinical findings are similar to those of cyanotic tetralogy of Fallot. In some patients, especially without pulmonic stenosis, the electrocardiogram shows a superiorly oriented counterclockwise frontal plane QRS loop in addition to right ventricular hypertrophy.[472] The pattern appears to result from relative hypoplasia of the anterosuperior left bundle and preferential activation of the posteroinferior left ventricular wall. The presence of the latter electrocardiographic pattern in patients with double-outlet right ventricle should raise the possibility of a coexistent atrioventricular septal defect or abnormality of the mitral valve.[471]

DIAGNOSIS. Two-dimensional *echocardiography* may reliably distinguish double-outlet right ventricle from other lesions causing cyanosis, such as tetralogy of Fallot and transposition of the great arteries.[469,473] The relative anteroposterior positions of the great arteries can be determined from the parasternal short-axis view. The parasternal long-axis view shows the position of the more posterior semilunar root relative to the interventricular septum and anterior mitral leaflet, and is the best view for demonstrating the presence of subarterial conus muscle. Subxiphoid

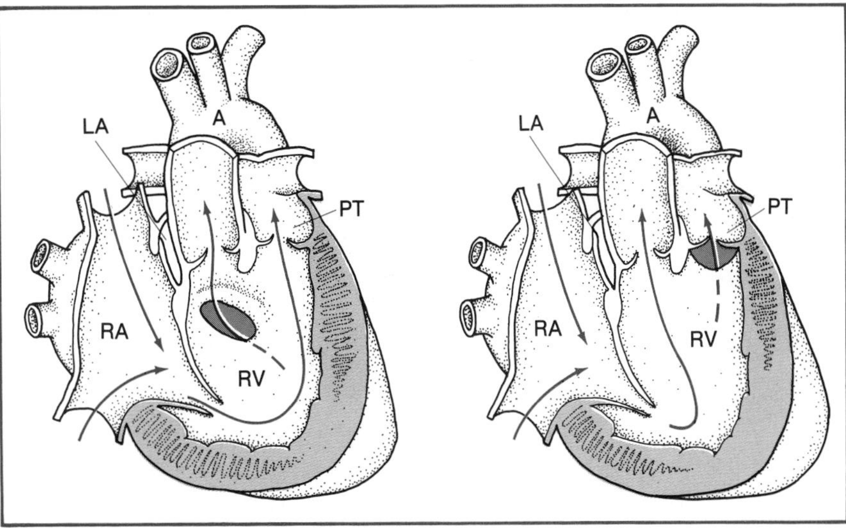

FIGURE 31-65. Double-outlet right ventricle (RV) with side-by-side relation of great arteries is illustrated in both panels. A subaortic ventricular septal defect (VSD) below the crista supraventricularis *(left)* favors delivery of left ventricular blood to the aorta (A). Location of the VSD above the crista *(right)* favors streaming to the pulmonary trunk (PT). LA = left atrium; RA = right atrium; PT = pulmonary trunk. (From Sridaromont, S., et al.: Double outlet right ventricle: Hemodynamic and anatomic correlations. Am. J. Cardiol. *38*:85, 1976.)

views best demonstrate the position of both great arteries over the ventricles. Each great artery is displayed on long- and short-axis subxiphoid sweeps. In reporting echocardiographic results, it is imperative to state each component anatomical feature, i.e., the position of both great arteries, the presence and amount of infundibulum under each semilunar valve, the anatomy of both subpulmonary and subaortic outflow tracts, the position and size of the associated ventricular septal defect, and the presence of all other associated lesions, particularly atrioventricular valve anomalies and coarctation of the aorta.

In each of the different types of double-outlet right ventricle, precise delineation of the malformation also depends on careful angiocardiographic analysis. The diagnosis can be established with confidence when the angiographic findings include simultaneous opacification of both great vessels from the right ventricle, aortic and pulmonic valves at the same transverse level, and separation of the aortic valve from the aortic leaflet of the mitral valve by the crista supraventricularis (Fig. 31-66).[474] The position of the ventricular septal defect and the relation between the great arteries must be defined to plan surgical procedures appropriately.

SURGICAL TREATMENT. In double-outlet right ventricle with subaortic ventricular septal defect, repair is accomplished by creating an intraventricular baffle that conducts left ventricular blood to the aorta.[475,476] When the ventricular septal defect is subpulmonic, repair is accomplished by use of one of three procedures: by creating an intraventricular conduit that conducts left ventricular blood to the pulmonary arteries and performing the Mustard or Senning procedure, by creating an intraventricular baffle directing left ventricular blood to the aorta and connecting the right ventricle to the pulmonary artery by use of a valve-containing conduit, or by closure of the ventricular septal defect and arterial switch.[477-479] When the ventricular septal defect is doubly committed, i.e., both subaortic and subpulmonic, operation consists of creating an intraventricular baffle that conducts left ventricular blood to the aorta. The type of double-outlet right ventricle in which the ventricular septal defect is remote and uncommitted to either semilunar orifice may be approached by a venous switch operation, permitting the right ventricle to eject into the aorta, followed by placement of a conduit between the left ventricle and the pulmonary trunk. Alternatively, some patients may be candidates for a modified Fontan procedure (p. 939), particularly if additional findings include a common atrioventricular orifice, hypoplastic ventricles, a straddling tricuspid valve, or a straddling mitral valve.[477]

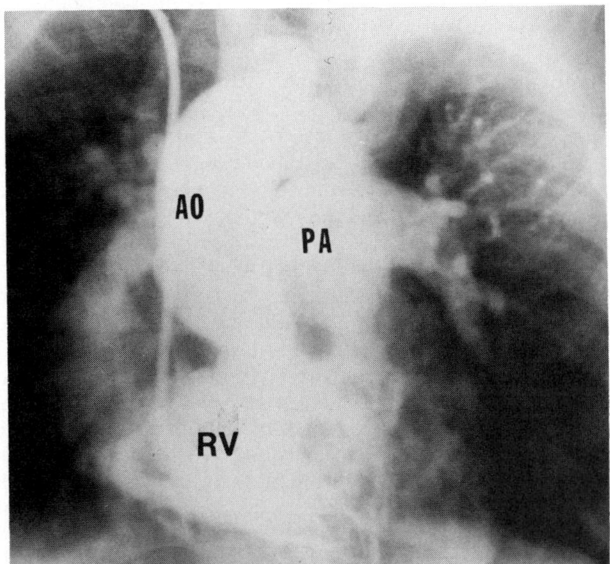

FIGURE 31-66. Simultaneous opacification of both great arteries from a right ventricular injection of contrast material in a patient with double-outlet right ventricle (RV). The aortic and pulmonic valves are at the same transverse level. AO = aorta, PA = pulmonary artery. (Courtesy of Robert White, M.D.)

DOUBLE-OUTLET LEFT VENTRICLE

One of the rarest cardiac anomalies consists of the origin of both great arteries from the morphological left ventricle. Conal musculature or an infundibulum usually is absent or deficient beneath the orifices of both semilunar valves.[480] A broad spectrum of associated malformations exists. A ventricular septal defect and valvular or subvalvular pulmonic stenosis have been present in most patients. Angiocardiographic assessment of the spatial relations of the origins of the great arteries is essential to an accurate diagnosis and to evaluating the possibility of operative repair.[481]

TOTAL ANOMALOUS PULMONARY VENOUS CONNECTION

This anomaly has been estimated to account for 1 to 3 per cent of all cases of congenital heart disease and 2 per cent of deaths therefrom in the first year of life.[308,482] The anomaly is the result of persistence during embryogenesis of communications between the pulmonary portion of the foregut plexus and the cardinal or umbilicovitelline system of veins, resulting in the connection of all the pulmonary veins either to the right atrium directly or to the systemic veins and their tributaries. Because all venous blood returns to the right atrium, an interatrial communication is an integral part of this malformation. Additional major cardiac malformations occur in about 30 per cent of patients.[308] Among these are common atrium, single ventricle, truncus arteriosus, and anomalies of the systemic veins. Extracardiac malformations, particularly of the alimentary, endocrine, and genitourinary systems, are present in 25 to 30 per cent of cases.

MORPHOLOGY. The anatomical varieties of total anomalous pulmonary venous connection may be subdivided, depending on the level of the abnormal drainage (Fig. 31-67). Table 31-10 provides average figures of the distribution of the sites of anomalous connection.[308] The anomalous connection usually is supradiaphragmatic and to the left brachiocephalic vein, right atrium, coronary sinus, or superior vena cava. In about 13 per cent, particularly in males, the distal site of connection is below the diaphragm. In this situation a common trunk originates from the confluence of pulmonary veins and descends in front of the esophagus, penetrating the diaphragm through the esophageal hiatus. The anomalous trunk then connects into the portal vein or one of its tributaries, the ductus venosus, or, rarely, to one of the hepatic veins. In rare cases various combinations of anomalous connection occur in which drainage is to multiple levels.

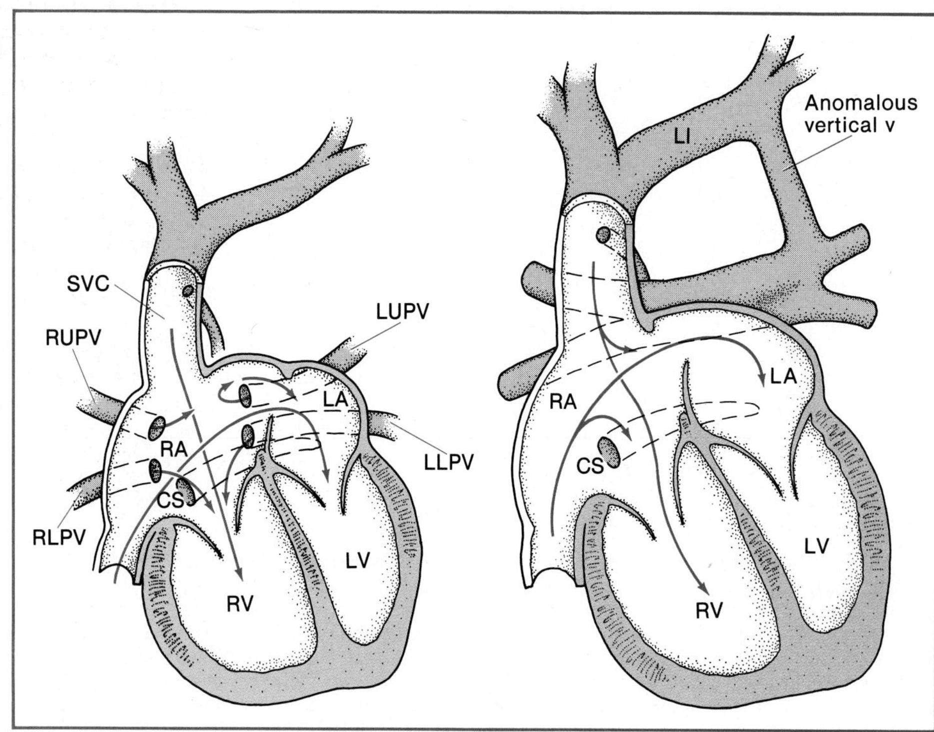

FIGURE 31-67. Two common types of total anomalous pulmonary venous connection are illustrated. These are connections to the right atrium *(left)* and to the left innominate vein *(right).* S.V.C. = superior vena cava; I.V.C. = inferior vena cava; R.A. = right atrium; L.A. = left atrium; C.S. = coronary sinus; R.V. = right ventricle; L.V. = left ventricle; R.U.P.V. = right upper pulmonary veins; L.U.P.V. = left upper pulmonary veins; R.L.P.V. = right lower pulmonary veins; L.L.P.V. = left lower pulmonary veins; R.H. = right hepatic vein; L.H. = left hepatic vein; L.P.V. = left portal vein; R.P.V. = right portal vein; L.I. = left innominate vein. (From Wagenvoort, C. A., et al.: Pathology of the Pulmonary Vasculature. Springfield, Ill., Charles C Thomas, 1964.)

HEMODYNAMICS. The physiological consequences and, accordingly, the clinical picture depend on the size of the interatrial communication and on the magnitude of the pulmonary vascular resistance.[482] When the interatrial communication is small, systemic blood flow is markedly limited.[483] Right atrial and systemic venous pressures are elevated, and hepatic enlargement and peripheral edema are present. The size of the interatrial communication also is an important determinant in the development in utero and postnatally of the left atrium and left ventricle. Left atrial cavity size usually is somewhat reduced, whereas left ventricular volumes may be reduced or normal. The magnitude of pulmonary blood flow and therefore the ratio of oxygenated to unoxygenated blood that returns to the right atrium are a function of pulmonary vascular resistance. The arterial oxygen saturation, which ranges from markedly reduced to normal values, is inversely related to the pulmonary vascular resistance. In this regard, in most patients the principal determinant of pulmonary pressures and resistance is related less to augmented pulmonary blood flow and pulmonary arteriolar vascular obstruction than to the presence and intensity of pulmonary venous obstruction.[484-486] Obstruction to pulmonary venous return and pulmonary venous hypertension are invariably present in patients with infradiaphragmatic anomalous pulmonary venous connection and in many with a supradiaphragmatic pathway. In the former type, pulmonary venous obstruction results from the length and narrowness of the common pulmonary venous trunk, compression at the esophageal hiatus of the diaphragm, constriction at the subdiaphragmatic site of insertion, or pulmonary venous return that must pass first through the portal-hepatic circulation before returning to the right atrium. When venous obstruction occurs in supradiaphragmatic types of drainage, constriction may exist at the entrance site of the anomalous veins into the systemic venous circulation, and/or the anomalous venous channel may be kinked or situated abnormally and compressed between the left pulmonary artery and left bronchus.[484,487] The presence of a small, restrictive patent foramen ovale occasionally results in pulmonary venous obstruction. Pulmonary vascular obstructive disease is rare during infancy, although exceptions have been reported.[488] In patients without pulmonary venous obstruction the risk of developing the Eisenmenger reaction is comparable to that in patients with an atrial septal defect.

TABLE 31-10 SITE OF CONNECTION IN TOTAL ANOMALOUS PULMONARY VENOUS CONNECTION

1. Connection to right atrium	**15%**
2. Connection to common cardinal system	
a. (Right) superior vena cava	**11%**
b. Azygos vein	**1%**
3. Connection to left common cardinal system	
a. Left innominate vein	**36%**
b. Coronary sinus	**16%**
4. Connection to umbilicovitelline system	
a. Portal vein	**6%**
b. Ductus venosus	**4%**
c. Inferior vena cava	**2%**
d. Hepatic vein	**1%**
5. Multiple sites	**7%**
6. Unknown	**1%**

CLINICAL MANIFESTATIONS. The majority of patients with total anomalous pulmonary venous connection have symptoms during the first year of life, and 80 per cent will die before age 1 year if left untreated.[482] The few who remain asymptomatic have a relatively good prognosis; once the condition is detected, operation may be elected later in childhood. Symptomatic infants with total anomalous pulmonary venous connection present with signs of heart failure and/or cyanosis. Infants with pulmonary venous obstruction present with the early onset of severe dyspnea, pulmonary edema, cyanosis, and right heart failure. Cardiac murmurs often are not prominent. In the unobstructed forms of total anomalous pulmonary venous connection the characteristic physical findings include right ventricular precordial overactivity and minimal cyanosis unless congestive heart failure intervenes. Multiple heart sounds often are audible, consisting of a first heart sound followed by an ejection sound; a fixed, widely split second heart sound with an accentuated pulmonic component; and a third and often a fourth heart sound. A soft systolic ejection murmur is usual along the left sternal border, and a middiastolic murmur of flow across the tricuspid valve commonly is audible at the lower left sternal border.

LABORATORY FINDINGS. The *electrocardiogram* shows right-axis deviation and right atrial and right ventricular hypertrophy. *Roentgenograms* of the chest reveal increased pulmonary blood flow; the right atrium and ventricle are dilated and hypertrophied, and the pulmonary artery segment is enlarged (Fig. 31–68).[489] In addition, the specific site of anomalous connection may cause a characteristic appearance of the cardiac silhouette. Thus, in patients with total anomalous pulmonary venous connection to the left brachiocephalic vein, the superior vena cava on the right, left brachiocephalic vein superiorly, and vertical vein on the left produce a cardiac shadow that resembles a snowman or figure of eight. The upper right cardiac border may be prominent when the anomalous connection is to the right superior vena cava.

Echocardiography demonstrates marked enlargement of the right ventricle and a small left atrium.[490,491] An echo-free space representing the common pulmonary venous chamber occasionally may be seen to lie behind the left atrium on ultrasound examination. Diagnostic echocardiographic findings include an absence of pulmonary vein connections to a small left atrium in the presence of right to left bulging of the septum primum at the foramen ovale. Positive diagnosis is made by identifying pulmonary venous connection to the systemic veins, coronary sinus, or right atrium, rather than to the left atrium. All four pulmonary veins and their connections must be identified to diagnose mixed types accurately.[491] There is no standard echocardiographic method for tracing pulmonary venous pathways because of their diverse anatomical positions.

At *cardiac catheterization* those patients found to have systemic arterial saturations below 70 per cent and with pulmonary artery pressure at or above systemic levels are likely to have pulmonary venous obstruction. Variations in oxygen saturation in the systemic venous circulation may be helpful. In the subdiaphragmatic type, a step-up may not be apparent in inferior vena caval oxygen saturations obtained by way of femoral vein cannulation because of the contribution of highly oxygenated renal venous blood to the caval stream. In contrast, sampling of the hepatic or portal vein by way of a catheter inserted through the umbilical vein will yield diagnostically higher oxygen saturations, indicating anomalous return to those vessels. Selective pulmonary arteriography and *indicator dilution* studies at cardiac catheterization are especially helpful in determining the drainage pathways of the pulmonary veins. Indicator dye injected into the right ventricle or pulmonary artery takes longer to reach the peripheral arterial sampling site than does dye injected into the vena cava or right atrium. The contours of dilution curves obtained from a peripheral artery after injection into both the right atrium and a pulmonary vein are identical and show a large right-to-left shunt, while the left atrial curve is normal. If the cardiac catheter can be manipulated directly into the anomalous trunk through its site of connection, selective injection of contrast material into the common channel provides anatomical definition of the pulmonary venous tree. If the pulmonary veins cannot be entered directly, selective right and left main pulmonary artery injection of contrast material often is more helpful than is injection into a main pulmonary artery, since many infants have a persistent patent ductus arteriosus through which the contrast agent flows right to left. Moreover, the drainage from both lungs must be outlined clearly to exclude a mixed type of anomalous venous drainage. Pulmonary venous obstruction may be detected by noting a pressure difference between the pulmonary artery wedge pressure and the right atrium.

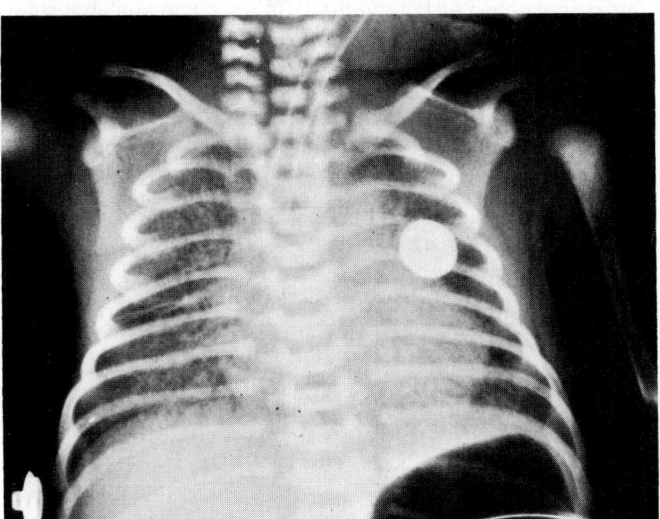

FIGURE 31–68. Chest roentgenogram in an infant with total anomalous pulmonary venous connection below the diaphragm shows normal overall heart size but diffuse pattern of pulmonary venous hypertension in both lung fields.

MANAGEMENT. Balloon atrial septotomy may provide dramatic palliation for the infant in whom the small size of an interatrial communication limits the amount of blood reaching the left side of the heart and systemic circulation.[483] Unless pulmonary vascular disease is present, results of operation for total anomalous pulmonary venous connection in patients beyond infancy are generally good.[491–493] The procedure consists of creating an anastomosis between the common pulmonary venous channel and left atrium and closing the atrial defect and the anomalous venous pathway. Improved results of operation in infancy require that postoperative pulmonary venous hypertension be averted by construction of a generally large anastomosis with or without enlargement of the left atrium. Normal hemodynamics and cardiac function have been demonstrated after surgical correction.[494]

PARTIAL ANOMALOUS PULMONARY VENOUS CONNECTION

(See also p. 949)

In this condition one or more of the pulmonary veins, but not all, are connected to the right atrium or to one or more of its venous tributaries. An atrial septal defect, particularly one of the sinus venosus type, commonly accompanies this anomaly; the usual connection involves the veins of the right upper and middle lobes and the superior vena cava.[308] Exclusive of atrial septal defects, major additional cardiac malformations occur in about 20 per cent of patients; these include ventricular septal defect, tetralogy of Fallot, and a variety of complex anomalies.

In the absence of associated anomalies the physiological disturbance is determined by the number of anomalous veins and their site of connection, the presence and size of an atrial septal defect, and the state of the pulmonary vascular bed.[495] In the usual patient with isolated partial pulmonary venous connection the hemodynamic state and physical findings are similar to those in atrial septal defect. Rarely, venous drainage of the right lung is into the inferior vena cava. This condition often is associated with hypoplasia of the right lung, dextroposition of the heart, pulmonary parenchymal abnormalities, and anomalous systemic supply to the lower lobe of the right lung from the abdominal aorta or its main branches.[496] This complex has been designated the "scimitar syndrome" because of the characteristic roentgenographic finding of a crescent-like shadow in the right lower lung field that is produced by the anomalous venous channel.

At *cardiac catheterization*, partial anomalous pulmonary venous connection to the coronary sinus, azygos vein, or superior vena cava may be identified by careful and frequent oximetry sampling. Oximetry is of limited value when the anomalous connection is to the inferior vena cava because of both reduced flow through the right lung and the contribution to the vena caval stream of highly oxygenated blood from the renal veins. Selective angiography is most helpful in cases in which the anomalous veins connect far away from the right atrium. Surgical repair offers definitive therapy at low risk if pulmonary vascular obliterative disease has not yet developed.

MALPOSITIONS OF THE HEART AND CARDIAC APEX

Positional anomalies of the heart are conditions in which the cardiac apex is located in the right side of the chest (dextrocardia) or is centrally located (mesocardia) or in which there is a normal location of the heart in the left side of the chest but abnormal position of the viscera (isolated levocardia). Such hearts commonly are abnormal with respect to chamber localization and great artery attachments; associated complex intracardiac and extracardiac lesions are common.

Problems of terminology abound in the literature describing these complex cardiac anomalies, although sensible and uniform systems of classification are available.[497,498]

ANATOMICAL FEATURES. Defining the cardiac anatomy in instances of cardiac malposition requires a description of three cardiac segments—the visceroatrial situs, the ventricular loop, and the conotruncus (the atria, ventricles, and great arteries, respectively). In addition to defining positional interrelation, the description of the malposed heart also must include the connections of the ventricles to the atria and great arteries as well as chamber identification, both morphologically and functionally.

To accomplish accurate diagnosis often requires a synthesis of findings from noninvasive tests such as two-dimensional echocardiography, computed tomography, and magnetic resonance imaging (when available), as well as hemodynamic and cineangiographic findings obtained at cardiac catheterization.[499,500]

In general, the determination of the body situs indicates the position of the atria. The visceral situs usually can be determined by the location of the stomach bubble and liver on a routine roentgenogram and of the inferior vena cava by means of echocardiography or the position of a cardiac catheter, or by means of a computed axial tomogram or venous or radioisotope angiocardiogram. Atrial anatomy is best investigated noninvasively by using subxiphoid long- and short-axis and apical four-chamber echocardiographic views. Venous contrast injections may be useful to define systemic venous connections.

Situs solitus is the normal arrangement of viscera and atria, with the right atrium right-sided and the left atrium left-sided. Situs solitus is further characterized by a trilobed right lung and eparterial bronchus (i.e., the right upper lobe bronchus passes above the right pulmonary artery), a bilobed left lung and hyparterial bronchus (i.e., the left bronchus passes below the left pulmonary artery), the major lobe of the liver on the right, a left-sided stomach and spleen, and right-sided venae cavae. Situs inversus is a mirror image of normal. Situs ambiguus or visceral heterotaxy refers to an anatomically uncertain or indeterminate body configuration. The latter often is seen in association with congenital asplenia, which resembles bilateral right-sidedness, and congenital polysplenia, which resembles bilateral left-sidedness.[501-503]

ASPLENIA. Cardiac anomalies associated commonly with asplenia include anomalous systemic venous connection, atrial septal or complete endocardial cushion defect, common ventricle, transposition of the great arteries, severe pulmonic stenosis or atresia, and anomalous pulmonary venous connection. Polysplenia commonly is associated with absence of the hepatic portion of the inferior vena cava with azygos continuation, bilateral superior venae cavae, anomalous pulmonary venous connection, and atrial septal defect (either ostium secundum or endocardial cushion). Pulmonic stenosis and double-outlet right ventricle are each observed in about 25 per cent of cases. It is important to recognize these complex syndromes to distinguish them from forms of cyanotic heart disease that may be more amenable to corrective surgical therapy. Diagnosis is suggested by a symmetrical liver shadow roentgenographically and, in asplenia, by the presence of Howell-Jolly and Heinz bodies in red blood cells demonstrated on blood smear, and it is confirmed by a negative or abnormal radioactive spleen scan.

Once the type of visceral situs is defined, it is necessary to describe the bulboventricular loop. The primitive cardiac tube normally bends to the right (D-loop), which brings the anatomical right ventricle to the right of the anatomical left ventricle. An L-loop brings the morphological right ventricle left-sided relative to the morphological left ventricle. The L-loop is normal in the presence of situs inversus, but in situs solitus it is synonymous with inverted ventricles.

VENTRICULAR MORPHOLOGY. The number, morphology, and size of the ventricle can be ascertained by using a variety of echocardiographic views. The morphological features of each ventricle also can be identified angiographically. The anatomical right ventricle is equipped with a tricuspid valve, is highly trabeculated, and contains the septal band of the single papillary muscle; its infundibulum lies anterior to and superiorly beyond the outlet of the left ventricle. The anatomical right ventricle usually connects with whichever of the two great arteries is the more anterior. The anatomical left ventricle is smooth-walled and contains an outlet that lies posterior to the right ventricular infundibulum; its entrance is guarded by a bicuspid mitral valve, the anterior leaflet of which is normally in continuity with elements of the semilunar valve at its outlet.

GREAT ARTERIES. The great arteries are described in terms of their positional interrelations and their ventricular connections. Each outflow tract and semilunar valve should be examined in both long- and short-axis echocardiographic views.[500] The ventriculoarterial alignments may be determined by direct visualization from the subxiphoid window. The relation between the great arteries can best be demonstrated noninvasively using parasternal short-axis echocardiographic views, which display the semilunar roots. The aortic arch and brachiocephalic arteries are seen well using suprasternal notch views. The pulmonary artery is seen from high parasternal or suprasternal notch short-axis sections. The ventricular attachments may be normal or may form the anomalies of double-outlet right or left ventricle or transposition. The arterial interrelations are described as D (dextro), in which the ascending aorta sweeps toward the right and lies to the right of the main pulmonary artery; L (levo), in which the ascending aorta sweeps toward the left and lies to the left of the main pulmonary artery; or A (antero), which is the rare situation in which the aorta lies directly in front of the pulmonary artery. The D, L, and A descriptions of the aorticopulmonary artery interrelations should not be confused with the D- or L-loop designation of the ventricular interrelations.[498]

Using segmental sets composed of descriptive units of visceroatrial situs/ventricular loop/great artery relations greatly simplifies expression of the type of cardiac anatomy present in cardiac malposition. For example, the normal heart in a patient with situs inversus and dextrocardia is referred to as inversus/L loop/L normal; complete transposition of the great arteries in a patient with situs inversus is referred to as inversus/L loop/L transposition; functionally corrected transposition in a patient with situs solitus is referred to as solitus/L loop/L transposition; dextrocardia and functionally corrected transposition is designated solitus/D loop/D transposition with dextrocardia.

After the cardiac chambers are diagnosed functionally (arterial and venous), the positional and morphological relations are understood, and the presence of associated anomalies has been established, the principles of medical and surgical treatment apply to these cardiac malpositions as they do to normally located hearts.

OTHER CONDITIONS

Congenital Pericardial Defects

(See also p. 1506)

Isolated pericardial defects are rare. They most commonly occur in males and usually are left-sided, although they may be right-sided, diaphragmatic, or total.[504] The anomaly is produced by deficient formation of the pleuropericardial membrane, or, if diaphragmatic, defective formation of the septum transversum. Associated congenital anomalies of the heart and lungs occur in about 30 per cent of cases. Most patients with the isolated defect are asymptomatic. Nonspecific anterior chest pain may be the result of torsion of the great arteries due to absence of the stabilizing forces of the left pericardium.[505]

With complete absence of the left pericardium a conspicuous apical impulse may be noted shifted leftward to the anterior or midaxillary line. Electrocardiographic changes may be related to levo-position of the heart; a leftward displacement of the QRS transition in the precordial leads and vertical or right-axis deviation are usual. The diagnosis may be suggested by chest roentgenograms.[506] With complete left pericardial absence, the heart is levo-posed, and the aortic knob, pulmonary artery, and ventricles form three prominent left heart border convexities.

A partial left pericardial defect may be suspected on the basis of varying degrees of prominence of the pulmonary artery and/or the left atrial appendage. Echocardiographic findings often mimic those observed in patients with right ventricular volume overload (enlarged right ventricle and abnormal ventricular septal motion), probably owing to the altered cardiac position and motion within the thorax.[507,508] Other echocardiographic clues include lateral extension of the left atrial appendage as it herniates through the pericardial defect; this is best seen in short-axis views. The anomaly can be definitively diagnosed by computed tomography, magnetic resonance imaging, or angiocardiography, or by inducing a left pneumothorax and observing air under the right pericardium when the patient is placed in the right lateral decubitus position.[509]

Complete absence of the left pericardium requires no treatment. However, partial defects may impose serious risks, including herniation and strangulation of the ventricles or left atrial appendage with left-sided defects, or the possibility of a superior vena cava obstructive syndrome with right-sided defects.[510] In the diaphragmatic type, cardiac compression by abdominal contents requires surgical repair.[511] Partial left or right defects may be closed with a patch of mediastinal pleura.

Single Atrium

Single or common atrium is a rare, isolated detect. The anomaly consists of an absent atrial septum, usually with a cleft in the anteromedial leaflet of the mitral valve and, occasionally, with a cleft tricuspid valve as well. The lesion may be seen as one component of the Ellis–van Creveld syndrome (Table 31–2) or of the complex cardiac anomalies seen in patients with asplenia or polysplenia.

Single atrium may be suspected clinically by the presence of cardiac murmurs of an atrial septal defect and mitral regurgitation associated with mild cyanosis, roentgenographic evidence of cardiac enlargement and increased pulmonary blood flow, and electrocardiographic features of atrioventricular septal defect.[512] An absence of echoes from any part of the atrial septum is the essential feature of two-dimensional echocardiographic examination, which also may show a cleft anterior mitral leaflet, increased right ventricular end-diastolic dimension, paradoxical ventricular septal motion, and dilated, pulsatile pulmonary trunk. Angiographically, the absence of the atrial septum produces a large, globe-shaped single atrial structure. Selective left ventricular angiocardiography shows the characteristic gooseneck appearance seen in the various forms of atrioventricular septal defect. In the absence of pulmonary vascular obstructive disease surgical correction is indicated by means of a prosthetic patch.

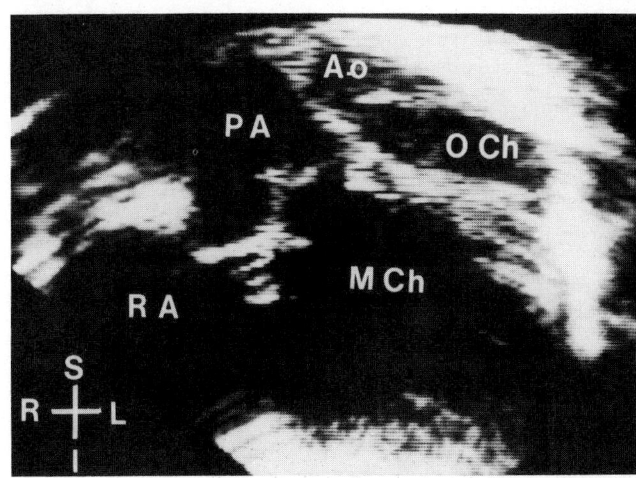

FIGURE 31–69. Single ventricle imaged in a subcostal coronal view. The pulmonary artery (PA) arises from a main chamber (MCh) of left ventricular type. The right atrioventricular valve is seen in part between the main chamber and the right atrium (RA). The ascending aorta (AO) arises anteriorly from a small outlet chamber (OCh). The bulboventricular foramen or ventricular septal defect is not identified in this plane. (Courtesy of Norman Silverman, M.D.)

Univentricular Atrioventricular Connection (Single Ventricle)

Hearts with univentricular atrioventricular connection constitute a family of complex lesions in which both atrioventricular valves, or a common atrioventricular valve, open into a single ventricular chamber.[513] Terminology is varied, and the anomaly often is referred to as single or common ventricle, which is imprecise but useful shorthand for the entity. The definition excludes examples of tricuspid or mitral atresia. Single ventricle is almost always accompanied by abnormal great artery positional relations; the incidence of L-malposition of the great arteries is about equal to that of D-malposition.[514] Associated anomalies are common, and include, in particular, pulmonic valvular or subvalvular stenosis, subaortic stenosis, total or partial anomalous pulmonary venous connection, and coarctation of the aorta.

MORPHOLOGY. In about 80 per cent of patients the single ventricle morphologically resembles a left ventricular chamber that is separated from an infundibular outlet chamber by a bulboventricular septum.[515] The opening is variously called the bulboventricular foramen and ventricular septal defect. The infundibular chamber is considered to represent developmentally the outflow tract of the right ventricle. When the great arteries are malposed the infundibulum lying anterior at the basal position of the single ventricle communicates with the aorta and may be in one of two positions: noninverted (D-malposition), when it is situated at the right basal aspect of the heart, or inverted (L-malposition), when it is located at the left base of the heart. In the unusual situation in which the great arteries normally are related, the infundibulum communicates with the pulmonary trunk.[514] *Double-inlet left ventricle* is a term used synonymously to describe the most frequently encountered single ventricular chamber that has the anatomical characteristics of the left ventricle. Less commonly the single ventricular chamber resembles a right ventricle (double-inlet right ventricle) or contains features suggestive of both ventricles or neither one; the latter two situations occasionally have been designated common ventricle and single ventricle of the primitive type, respectively.[514]

CLINICAL FINDINGS. Depending on the associated anomalies, the clinical presentation of single ventricle mimics other conditions in which cyanosis and decreased or increased pulmonary blood flow coexist, e.g., tetralogy of Fallot or tricuspid atresia in the former instance or complete transposition of the great arteries and double-outlet right ventricle in the latter. The *electrocardiogram in* double-inlet left ventricle without inversion of the infundibulum (D-malposition) usually shows features of left ventricular hypertrophy. With infundibular inversion (L-malposition) the electrical forces are directed anteriorly and rightward, as they are in ventricular inversion without associated defects. In patients with the more primitive types of common or single ventricle there is a repetitious rS pattern in all the precordial electrocardiographic leads. *Chest roentgenographic* findings resemble those observed in patients with complete (dextro-) transposition of the great arteries or functionally corrected (levo-) transposition of the great arteries without features distinctive for single ventricle.

In those patients in whom two separate atrioventricular valves communicate with the single ventricular chamber, *echocardiography* (Fig. 4–83, p. 95) suggests the correct diagnosis when echoes are visualized from the two valves without an intervening interventricular septum.[515,516] In the absence of ventricular septal echoes when the two valves are not visualized simultaneously, they may be identified separately with a careful long-axis sweep of the ventricle. It is possible to detect the presence of a small outflow chamber anterior to the atrioventricular valves by using subxiphoid or parasternal short-axis views, and a plane orthogonal to the long-axis plane (Fig. 31–69). The single ventricle with a single atrioventricular valve is suspected when the excursion of echoes from the single valve located posteriorly in the ventricular chamber is of large amplitude. Enhanced assessment of the atrioventricular valve in patients with single

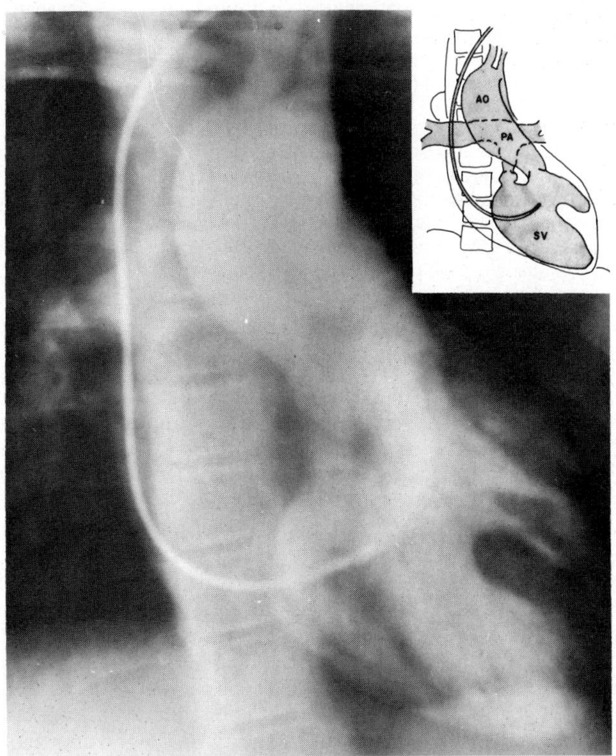

FIGURE 31–70. Selective ventriculogram in a child with single ventricle (SV). There is levo-malposition of the great arteries with the aorta (AO) communicating with a small outflow chamber. The pulmonary artery (PA) arises from a single ventricular chamber, which has the anatomical characteristics of a left ventricle. There is moderate pulmonic stenosis.

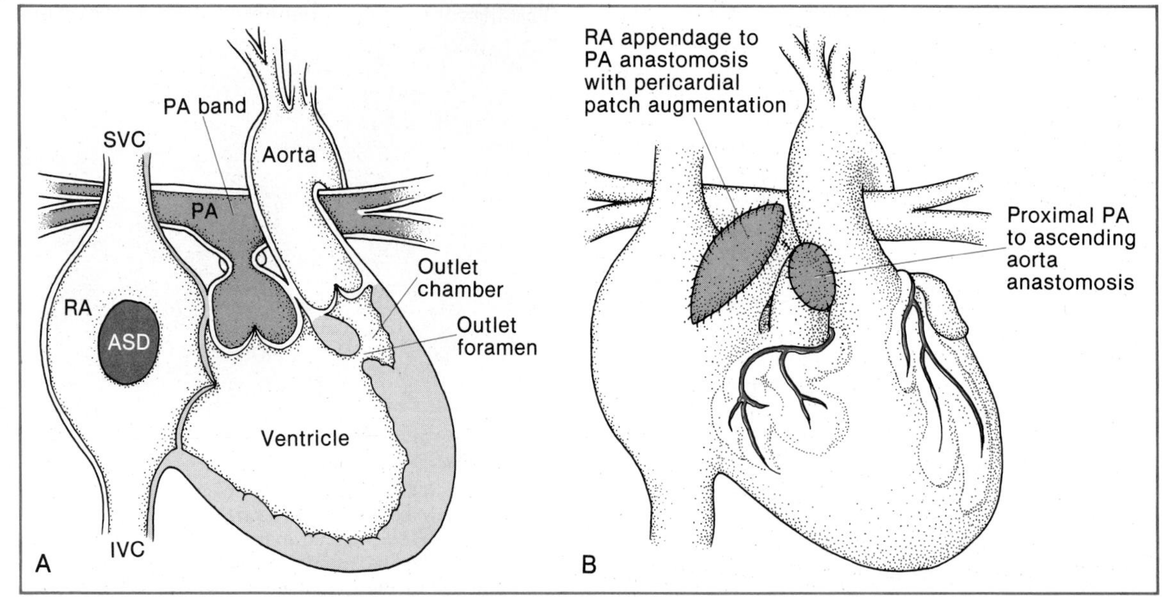

FIGURE 31-71. ***A,*** **The preoperative anatomy of a univentricular heart of the left ventricular type with left anterior subaortic outlet chamber, ventricular arterial discordance, left atrioventricular valve atresia, atrial septal defect (ASD), and subaortic stenosis caused by a restrictive bulboventricular outlet foramen.** ***B,*** **The physiologic operative repair. The proximal pulmonary artery (PA) anastomosed to the ascending aorta (augmented by a prosthetic patch) and a modified Fontan procedure created (right atrial to the pulmonary artery anastomosis). Not shown is the interatrial baffle committing the pulmonary venous return to the right atrioventricular valve. (From Lin, A. E., et al.: Subaortic obstruction in complex heart disease. Reprinted with permission from the American College of Cardiology. J. Am. Coll. Cardiol.** ***7:*****617, 1986.)**

ventricle is provided by Doppler echocardiography.[517] Selective ventriculography is necessary to delineate with certainty the anatomical type of single ventricle and to diagnose the associated great artery interrelations and the presence or absence of additional lesions (Fig. 31-70).[518,519]

SURGICAL TREATMENT. Attempts to partition the single ventricle with a Dacron or Teflon prosthetic patch have met with modest success as well as a high incidence of postoperative complete heart block.[520,521] The septation operation is best performed in patients with double-inlet left ventricle, a rudimentary right ventricular outflow chamber which is anterior and leftward, and a discordant ventriculoarterial connection, with either absent or mild pulmonary stenosis. Creation of an atriopulmonary conduit (the Fontan procedure) and closure of the tricuspid orifice is a technique best applied to patients with severe pulmonary stenosis or previous pulmonary artery banding procedure (Fig. 31-71).[522] In these patients, subaortic obstruction caused by a restricted bulboventricular foramen requires a pulmonary artery-to-ascending aorta anastomosis.[523,524] Palliative procedures designed to either increase pulmonary blood flow (systemic-pulmonary anastomosis) or limit pulmonary blood flow (pulmonary artery banding) often allow survival to adolescence in patients with a single ventricle.

VASCULAR RINGS

MORPHOLOGY. The normal development of the aortic arch system is described on page 1528 (Fig. 31-5). The term *vascular ring* is used for those aortic arch or pulmonary artery malformations that exhibit an abnormal relation with the esophagus and trachea, causing compression, dysphagia, and/or respiratory symptoms.[524a] The most common and serious vascular ring is produced by a double aortic arch in which both the right and left fourth embryonic aortic arches persist. In the most common type of double aortic arch there is a left ligamentum arteriosum or ductus arteriosus, and both arches are patent, the right being larger than the left. A right aortic arch with a left ductus or ligamentum arteriosum connecting the left pulmonary artery and the upper part of the descending aorta and with an anomalous right subclavian artery arising from the left descending aorta are additional important vascular ring arrangements.[525] The latter anomaly frequently exists in cases of tetralogy of Fallot and otherwise uncomplicated coarctation of the aorta. An unusual cause of tracheal compression is the "vascular sling" created by an anomalous left pulmonary artery that arises from a rightward, elongated pulmonary trunk and courses between the trachea and esophagus before it branches normally within the left lung.[526] This arrangement commonly is associated with other cardiac and extracardiac anomalies.

CLINICAL FINDINGS. The symptoms produced by vascular rings depend on the tightness of anatomical constriction of the trachea and esophagus and consist principally of respiratory difficulties, cyanosis (associated especially with feeding), stridor, and dysphagia. The electrocardiogram is normal unless associated cardiovascular anomalies are present. The barium esophagogram is a useful screening procedure. Prominent posterior indentation of the esophagus is observed in the common vascular ring arrangements, although the pulmonary artery "vascular sling" produces an anterior indentation. Unusual and rare aortic arch anomalies may create rings that impinge on the trachea but do not compress the esophagus and that will be detected not by this simple radiographic procedure but rather by bronchoscopy. Computed tomography examination is helpful in the diagnosis of this malformation. Selective contrast angiography usually is required to delineate the anatomy of the aorta and its branches or the course of the main pulmonary arteries. Computed axial tomography and magnetic resonance imaging offer excellent imaging alternatives.[527,528]

MANAGEMENT. The severity of symptoms and the anatomy of the malformation are the most important factors in determining treatment. Patients, particularly infants, with respiratory obstruction require prompt surgical intervention. Operative repair of the double aortic arch requires division of the minor arch (usually the left).[529] A reported 20 to 30 per cent operative mortality is related, in part, to problems in postoperative respiratory care, especially when there is coexistent residual anatomical tracheal narrowing. Patients with a right aortic arch and a left ductus or ligamentum arteriosum require division of the ductus or ligamentum and/or ligation and division of the left subclavian artery, which is the posterior component of the ring. Operation seldom is indicated for patients with an aberrant right subclavian artery derived from a left aortic arch and left descending aorta. In patients with a pulmonary artery vascular sling, operation consists of detachment of the left pulmonary artery at its origin and anastomosis to the main pulmonary artery directly or by way of a conduit of its proximal end brought anterior to the trachea.[529]

CONGENITAL ARRHYTHMIAS

This classification refers to arrhythmias that are present in infancy, whose causes, when known, relate to a structural malformation or defect of the conduction system or to an acquired prenatal condition such as myocarditis, hypoxia, acidosis, or transplacental passage of a drug or substance from mother to fetus. In these latter examples, the substrate for the postnatal expression of the rhythm disturbance existed before birth and the arrhythmia is therefore designated "congenital." Complete heart block and supraventricular and ventricular tachycardias are the most common important congenital arrhythmias.[530] The electrophysiological and electrocardiographic features of these arrhythmias are discussed elsewhere in the text (Chaps. 24 and 25).

CONGENITAL COMPLETE HEART BLOCK

(See also p. 969)

The atrioventricular node and the His bundle originate during fetal development as separate structures and later join together. Anatomical studies have shown the basic lesion in congenital complete heart block to consist of discontinuity between the atrial musculature and the AV node or the His bundle, if the AV node is absent. The anatomical interruption occasionally may be situated between the AV node and the main His bundle, or within the bundle itself.[531,532] No known cause exists for the vast majority of cases of congenital heart block in infants, who usually have otherwise anatomically normal hearts. However, fetal myocarditis, idiopathic hemorrhage and necrosis involving conduction tissue, and degeneration and fibrosis related in some instances to the transplacental passage of anti–Ro antibody and other immune complexes from mothers with systemic lupus erythematosus are all entities capable of causing congenital heart block.[533–535] Less often, congenital heart block may be associated with various forms of congenital heart disease, the most common malformation being congenitally corrected transposition of the great arteries.

Detection of consistent fetal bradycardia (heart rate 40 to 80 beats/min) by auscultation, fetal echocardiography (Fig. 31–72), or electronic monitoring allows anticipation of the correct diagnosis.[536] The newborn, especially with a ventricular rate less than 50 beats/min and atrial rate in excess of 150 beats/min, is at highest risk; the presence of an associated cardiovascular anomaly greatly lessens the chances of survival. Treatment is not required for the asymptomatic infant. Digitalization is recommended for the baby in congestive heart failure, irrespective of complete heart block. Isoproterenol and other sympathomimetic drugs and atropine do not have permanent or beneficial effects. Congestive heart failure and Stokes-Adams attacks require pacemaker treatment at any age.[530,537,540] Initial management of the child in whom permanent epicardial pacemaker insertion is indicated usually involves preoperative insertion of a transvenous intracardiac electrode into the right ventricle to protect the patient from serious arrhythmias during the induction of anesthesia.[538] A variety of problems may be anticipated after pacemaker implantation related to growth of the patient, which stresses the electrical lead system; the fragility of the lead system in a physically active young patient; and the limited life span of the pulse generator. Patients with congenital complete heart block who survive infancy usually remain asymptomatic until late in childhood or adolescence.[539]

SUPRAVENTRICULAR TACHYCARDIA

Paroxysmal tachycardia of supraventricular origin may have its origin in utero or in the immediate postnatal period.[30,541,542] The most frequent arrhythmias producing symptoms are paroxysmal atrial tachycardia with or without ventricular preexcitation, atrial flutter, and junctional tachycardia. The arrhythmia may cause intrauterine cardiac failure; its detection and persistence prenatally should prompt consideration of administration of digitalis, or if that fails, of propranolol or quinidine, to the mother if amniocentesis indicates surfactant deficiency and fetal lung immaturity, since early delivery is not indicated if the baby will have hyaline membrane disease. Cesarean delivery or induced labor may be indicated if the fetus is close to term. No recognizable cause exists for the disorder in the vast majority of infants. The transplacental passage of long-acting thyroid-stimulating (LATS) and immune gamma 2 globulin from hyperthyroid mothers, hypoglycemia, and Ebstein's anomaly of the tricuspid valve occasionally are causative.[543] Wolff-Parkinson-White syndrome (p. 693) is present in 10 to 50 per cent of infants with supraventricular tachycardia.[544] Symptoms produced by the tachyarrhythmia after birth are subtle and often go undetected until signs of heart failure have been present for 24 to 36 hours. Conversion to normal sinus rhythm usually is accomplished by administration of digitalis, direct-current cardioversion, transesophageal atrial pacing, or eliciting a diving reflex by covering the face with an ice-cold wet washcloth for 4 to 5 seconds.[545–548] Conversion should be fol-

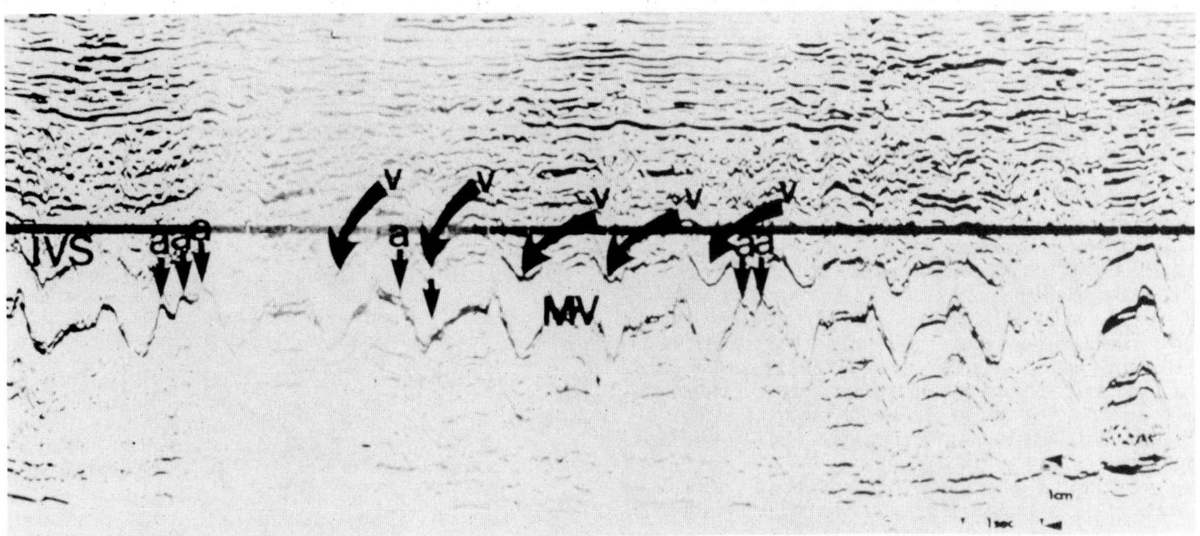

FIGURE 31–72. Fetal M-mode echocardiogram of complete heart block at 28 weeks' gestation. A slow ventricular rate of 45 to 50 beats/min is seen by the undulations (v, curved arrows) of the interventricular septum (IVS). Atrial contractions (a, straight vertical arrows) cause regular undulations of the mitral valve (MV) at a rate of 120–130 beats/min. The atrial activity has no fixed relationship to the idioventricular rhythm. (Courtesy of Charles Kleinman, M.D.)

lowed by digitalization on a prophylactic basis. Common practice consists of digitalis treatment for 9 to 12 recurrence-free months followed by its abrupt cessation. Recurrence of tachycardia, particularly in those infants with ventricular preexcitation, is not uncommon; maintenance of normal rhythm may require the administration, alone or in combination, of digitalis, phenytoin sodium, verapamil, and propranolol.[546a] The rate of recurrence falls substantially between ages 2 and 10 years, with a slight rise during adolescence. In general, the prognosis is excellent.[549]

ELECTROPHYSIOLOGICAL STUDIES. Beyond infancy, patients whose condition is refractory to medical treatment are candidates for electrophysiological catheter evaluation, which facilitates differentiation of a causative ectopic anatomical focus within the atria from accessory conduction pathways.[530,550] Endocardial mapping is performed to specifically localize the site of earliest activation in the atrium, or to identify multiple foci of ectopic impulses. Electrophysiological studies should include measurement of resting intervals and sinus and atrioventricular node function, including recovery times, effective refractory period, and Wenckebach conduction. Premature atrial stimulation may be used to interrupt tachycardia. Premature ventricular stimulation is used to measure retrograde conduction and localize the site of earliest atrial activation, and to assess the effective refractory period of the accessory pathway. Coronary sinus and right atrial catheters provide localization of the site of earliest atrial activation during tachycardia, and allow measurement of the antegrade effective refractory period of the accessory pathway.

If the tachyarrhythmia is refractory to pharmacological therapy or catheter ablative techniques, it may be treated definitively with intraoperative mapping and a variety of operative maneuvers, including cryoablation, surgical division of accessory conduction pathways, subendocardial excision of the ectopic focus, and atrial disconnection.[551,552]

ATRIAL FLUTTER. Uncommonly, atrial flutter is the cause of supraventricular tachycardia,[546] especially in the setting of newborn infants with hydrops fetalis, whose intrauterine tachyarrhythmia is an alternation between supraventricular tachycardia with Wolff-Parkinson-White syndrome and atrial flutter. Another common clinical setting for atrial flutter is in the infant under age 6 months with an otherwise normal heart, who shows frequent premature atrial contractions. In infants, classic flutter waves may not be present on a surface electrocardiogram or rhythm strip; detection may require recordings of transesophageal atrial electrograms. Acute treatment with electrical conversion or overdrive pacing, either through the esophagus or with an intracardiac atrial catheter, effectively terminates the rhythm disturbance.[546,547] If synchronized direct-current electrocardioversion is used, standby pacing should be available; if overdrive pacing is utilized, the same pacing catheter can be used to pace the heart in the event of a systole. Uncommonly, chronic drug treatment with digitalis, digitalis plus quinidine, or amiodarone may be required.

Junctional automatic tachycardia is characterized by a narrow QRS complex and AV dissociation, with the ventricular rate faster than the normal atrial rate. Ventricular dysfunction and congestive heart failure occur early, and the rhythm disturbance usually is not convertible to sinus rhythm by any medical treatment.[530] Because sudden death commonly occurs, pacemaker implantation is recommended with a subsequent effort at either catheter or surgical ablation.

VENTRICULAR TACHYCARDIA. Ventricular tachycardia is defined as three or more consecutive premature ventricular contractions. The definition, however, fails to identify a high-risk group. Infants or children who meet this criterion but seldom require treatment and seem to be at little risk have no symptoms and no evidence of anatomical heart disease. Potentially serious ventricular tachycardia in the newborn is associated with Q-T prolongation, mitral valve prolapse, and Marfan syndrome. In these settings the tachycardia is potentially life-threatening and always merits treatment.[530]

The cause of long Q-T syndrome (p. 708) is unknown; proposed are regional abnormalities of ventricular repolarization on the basis of an imbalance of right and left sympathetic innervation of the heart. The two most effective treatments are beta blockade and high thoracic left sympathectomy, which reduce the incidence of syncope and sudden death without affecting the Q-T interval.

The treatment of ventricular tachycardia (p. 651) consists of intravenous administration of lidocaine, followed by direct-current electrical cardioversion. In the absence of Q-T prolongation, but in the presence of mitral prolapse or other cardiac abnormalities, chronic treatment should be undertaken of multiform premature ventricular contractions, couplets, or ventricular tachycardia. In infants and children unresponsive to conventional or investigational antiarrhythmic drugs, surgical treatment—by either cryoablation or excision—may be lifesaving.[553]

REFERENCES

1. Hoffman, J.I.E.: Congenital heart disease. Ped. Clin. North Am. *37*:45, 1990.
2. Roberts, W. C.: Anatomically isolated aortic valvular disease: The case against its being of rheumatic etiology. Am. J. Cardiol. *49*:151, 1970.
3. Warth, D. C., King, M. E., Cohen, J. M., et al.: Prevalence of mitral valve prolapse in normal children. J. Am. Coll. Cardiol. *5*:1173, 1985.
4. Fontana, R. S., and Edwards, J. E.: Congenital Cardiac Disease: A Review of 357 Cases Studied Pathologically. Philadelphia, W. B. Saunders Company, 1962.
5. Bankl, H.: Congenital Malformations of the Heart and Great Vessels: Synopsis of Pathology, Embryology and Natural History. Baltimore-Munich, Urban and Schwarzenberg, 1977.
6. Greenwood, R. D.: Cardiovascular malformations associated with extracardiac anomalies and malformation syndromes. Clin. Pediatr. *23*:145, 1984.
7. Nora, J. J., and Nora, A. H.: Maternal transmission of congenital heart diseases: New recurrence risk figures and the questions of cytoplasmic inheritance and vulnerability to teratogens. Am. J. Cardiol. *59*:459, 1987.
7a. Kirby, M. L., and Waldo, K. L.: Role of neural crest in congenital heart disease. Circulation *82*:332, 1990.
8. de la Cruz, M. V., Munoz-Castellanos, L., and Nadal-Ginard, S.: Extrinsic factors in the genesis of congenital heart disease. Br. Heart J. *33*:203, 1971.
9. Ruttenberg, H. D.: Concerning the etiology of congenital cardiac disease. Am. Heart J. *84*:437, 1972.
10. Ouelette, E. M., Rossett, H. L., Rossman, M. P., and Wiener, L.: Adverse effects on offspring of maternal alcohol abuse during pregnancy. N. Engl. J. Med. *297*:528, 1977.
10a. Stevens, C. A., Carey, J. C., and Shigeoka, A. O.: DiGeorge anomaly and velocardiofacial syndrome. Pediatrics *85*:526, 1990.
11. Noonan, J.: Twins, conjoined twins, and cardiac defects. Am. J. Dis. Child. *132*:17, 1978.
12. Corone, P., Bonaiti, C., Feingold, J., et al.: Familial congenital heart disease: How are the various types related? Am. J. Cardiol. *51*:942, 1983.
13. Anderson, R. H., and Ashley, G. T.: Anatomic development of the cardiovascular system. *In* Davies, J., and Dobbing, J. (eds.): Scientific Foundations of Paediatrics. London, Heinemann, 1974, p. 165.
14. Langman, J., and van Mierop, L.H.S.: Development of the cardiovascular system. *In* Moss, A. J., and Adams, F. H. (eds.): Heart Disease in Infants, Children and Adolescents. Baltimore, Williams and Wilkins, 1968, p. 3.
15. Los, J. A.: Embryology. *In* Watson, H. (ed.): Paediatric Cardiology. London, Lloyd Luke Ltd., 1968, p. 1.
16. Rudolph, A. M.: Congenital Diseases of the Heart. Chicago, Year Book Medical Publishers, 1974.
17. Sheldon, C. A., Friedman, W. F., and Sybers, H. D.: Scanning electron microscopy of fetal and neonatal lamb cardiac cells. J. Molec. Cell. Cardiol. *8*:853, 1976.
18. McPherson, R. A., Kramer, M. F., Covell, J. W., and Friedman, W. F.: A comparison of the active stiffness of fetal and adult cardiac muscle. Pediatr. Res. *10*:660, 1976.
19. Friedman, W. F.: The intrinsic physiologic properties of the developing heart. Prog. Cardiovasc. Dis. *15*:87, 1972.
20. Ingwall, J. S., Kramer, M. F., Woodman, D., and Friedman, W. F.: Maturation of energy metabolism in the lamb: Changes in myosin ATPase and creatine kinase activities. Pediatr. Res. *15*:1128, 1981.
21. Friedman, W. F.: Physiological properties of the developing heart. Paediatric Cardiology. Vol. 6. New York, Churchill Livingstone, 1987, p. 3.
22. Geis, W. P., Tatooles, C. J., Priola, D. V., and Friedman, W. F.: Factors influencing neurohumoral control of the heart and newborn. Am. J. Physiol. *228*:1685, 1975.
23. Klitzner, T. S., and Friedman, W. F.: Excitation contraction coupling in developing mammalian myocardium. Pediatr. Res. *23*:428, 1988.
24. Klitzner, T. S., and Friedman, W. F.: A diminished role for the sarcoplasmic reticulum in newborn myocardial contraction. Pediatr. Res. *26*:98, 1989.
25. Romero, T. E., and Friedman, W. F.: Limited left ventricular response to volume overload in the neonatal period. Pediatr. Res. *13*:910, 1979.
26. Friedman, W. F., Printz, M. P., Kirkpatrick, S. E., and Hoskins, E. J.: The vasoactivity of the fetal lamb ductus arteriosus studied in utero. Pediatr. Res. *17*:331, 1983.

PATHOLOGICAL CONSEQUENCES

27. Friedman, W. F., and George, B. L.: Medical progress—Treatment of congestive heart failure by altering loading conditions of the heart. J. Pediatr. *106*:697, 1985.
28. Friedman, W. F., and George, B. L.: Treatment of cardiac failure in infants. Compr. Ther. *12*:8, 1986.

29. Artman, M., Parrish, M. D., and Graham, T. P., Jr.: Congestive heart failure in childhood and adolescence: Recognition and management. Am. Heart J. *105*:471, 1983.
30. Schmidt, K. G., Araujo, L., and Silverman, N. H.: Evaluation of structural and functional abnormalities of the fetal heart by echocardiography. Am. J. Cardiol. Imag. *2*:57, 1988.
31. Schmidt, K. G., Silverman, N. H., Van Hare, G. F., et al.: Two-dimensional echocardiographic determination of ventricular volumes in the fetal heart. Circulation *81*:325, 1990.
32. Milne, M. J., Sung, R.Y.T., Fok, T. F., and Crozier, I. G.: Doppler echocardiographic assessment of shunting via the ductus arteriosus in newborn infants. Am. J. Cardiol. *64*:102, 1989.
33. Sahn, D. J., and Friedman, W. F.: Difficulties in distinguishing cardiac from pulmonary disease in the neonate. Pediatr. Clin. North Am. *20*:293, 1973.
34. Stanger, P., Lucas, R. V., Jr., and Edwards, J. E.: Anatomic factors causing respiratory distress in acyanotic congenital cardiac disease: Special reference to bronchial obstruction. Pediatrics *43*:760, 1969.
35. DiSessa, T. G., and Friedman, W. F.: Echocardiographic evaluation of cardiac performance. Cardiol. Clin. *1*:487, 1983.
36. DiSessa, T. G., and Friedman, W. F.: Echocardiographic evaluation of cardiac performance. *In* Friedman, W. F., and Higgins, C. B. (eds.): Pediatric Cardiac Imaging. Philadelphia, W. B. Saunders Company, 1984, p. 219.
37. Mercier, J. C., DiSessa, T. G., Jarmakani, J., and Friedman, W. F.: Two dimensional echocardiographic assessment of left ventricular volumes and ejection fraction. Circulation *65*:962, 1982.
38. Hanseus, K., Bjorkhem, G., and Lundstrom, N. R.: Dimensions of cardiac chambers and great vessels by cross-sectional echocardiography in infants and children. Pediatr. Cardiol. *9*:7, 1988.
39. Riggs, T. W., Rodriguez, R., Snider, A. R., and Batton, D.: Doppler echocardiographic evaluation of right and left diastolic function in normal neonates. J. Am. Coll. Cardiol. *13*:700, 1989.
40. Teitel, D., and Rudolph, A. M.: Perinatal oxygen delivery and cardiac function. Adv. Pediatr. *32*:321, 1985.
41. Rosenthal, A., Nathan, D. G., Marty, A. T., et al.: Acute hemodynamic effects of red cell volume reduction, polycythemia of cyanotic congenital heart disease. Circulation *42*:297, 1970.
42. Voigt, G. C., and Wright, J. R.: Cyanotic congenital heart disease and sudden death. Am. Heart J. *87*:773, 1974.
43. Fischbein, C. A., Rosenthal, A., Fischer, E. G., et al.: Risk factors for brain abscess in patients with congenital heart disease. Am. J. Cardiol. *34*:97, 1974.
44. Shaher, R. M., and Deuchard, D. C.: Hematogenous brain abscess in cyanotic congenital heart disease. Am. J. Med. *52*:349, 1972.
45. Corrin, C.: Paradoxical embolism. Br. Heart J. *26*:549, 1964.
46. Haroutunian, L. M., and Neill, C. A.: Pulmonary complications of congenital heart disease: Hemoptysis. Am. Heart J. *84*:540, 1972.
47. Guntheroth, W. G., Morgan, B. C., and Mullens, G. L.: Physiologic studies of paroxysmal hyperpnea in cyanotic congenital heart disease. Circulation *31*:70, 1965.
48. Talmer, N. S.: Congestive heart failure in the infant. Pediatr. Clin. North Am. *18*:1011, 1971.
49. Rosenthal, A., and Castaneda, A. R.: Growth and development after cardiovascular surgery in infants and children. *In* Rosenthal, A., Sonnenblick, E. H., and Lesch, M. (eds.): Postoperative Congenital Heart Disease. New York, Grune and Stratton, 1975, p. 110.
50. Friedman, W. F., Heiferman, M. F., and Perloff, J. K.: Late postoperative pulmonary vascular disease—Clinical concerns. *In* Engle, M. A., and Perloff, J. K. (eds.): Congenital Heart Disease After Surgery. New York, Yorke Medical Publishers, 1983, p. 151.
51. Rabinovitch, M.: Structure and function of the pulmonary vascular bed: An update. Cardiol. Clin. *7*:227, 1989.
52. Rabinovitch, M., Keane, J. F., and Norwood, W. I.: Vascular structure and lung biopsy tissue correlated with pulmonary hemodynamic findings after repair of congenital heart defects. Circulation *69*:655, 1984.
53. Heath, D., and Edwards, J. E.: The pathology of hypertensive pulmonary vascular disease. Circulation *18*:533, 1958.
54. Levin, D. L., Rudolph. A. M., Heymann, M. A., and Phibbs, R. H.: Morphological development of the pulmonary vascular bed in the fetal lamb. Circulation *53*:144, 1976.
55. Rabinovitch, M., and Reid, L. M.: Quantitative structural analysis of the pulmonary vascular bed in congenital heart defects. *In* Engle, M. A. (ed.): Pediatric Cardiovascular Disease. Philadelphia, F. A. Davis, 1981, p. 149.
56. Friedman, W. F.: Proceedings of the National Heart, Lung and Blood Institute Pediatric Cardiology Workshop: Pulmonary Hypertension. Pediatr. Res. *20*:8, 1986.
57. Rabinovitch, M., Keane, J. F., Fellows, K. E., et al.: Quantitative analysis of the pulmonary wedge angiogram in congenital heart defects. Circulation *63*:152, 1981.
58. Rabinovitch, M., Castaneda, A. R., and Reid, L.: Lung biopsy with frozen section as a diagnostic aid in patients with congenital heart defects. Am. J. Cardiol. *47*:77, 1981.
59. Zeller, S. T., and Gutgesell, H. P.: Noninvasive estimation of pulmonary artery pressure. J. Pediatr. *114*:735, 1989.
60. Morera, J., Hoadley, S. D., Roland, J. M., et al.: Estimation of the ratio of pulmonary to systemic pressures by pulsewave Doppler echocardiography for assessment of pulmonary artery pressures. Am. J. Cardiol. *63*:862, 1989.
61. Van Hare, G. F., Ben-Shachar, G., Liebman, J., et al.: Infective endocarditis in infants and children during the past 10 years: A decade of change. Am. Heart J. *107*:1235, 1984.
62. Dajani, A. S.: Prevention of bacterial endocarditis. Pediatr. Infect. Dis. *4*:349, 1985.
62a. Dajani, A. S., Bisno, A. L., Chung, K. J., et al.: Prevention of bacterial endocarditis. Recommendations by the American Heart Association. JAMA *264*:2919, 1990.
63. Selbst, S. M., Ruddy, R. M., Clark, B. J., et al.: Pediatric chest pain: A prospective study. Pediatrics *82*:319, 1988.
64. Graham, T. P., Gessner, I. H., Friedman, W. F., et al.: Recommendations for use of laboratory studies for pediatric patients with suspected or proven heart disease: A statement of the Committee on Congenital Cardiac Defects of the Council on Cardiovascular Disease in the Young of the AHA. Circulation *74*:443a, 1986
65. Driscoll, D. J., and Edwards, W. D.: Sudden unexpected death in children and adolescents. J. Am. Coll. Cardiol. *5*:118B, 1985.
66. Denfield, S. W., and Garson, A., Jr.: Sudden death in children and young adults. Ped. Clin. North Am. *37*:215, 1990.

APPROACH TO THE HIGH-RISK INFANT

67. Friedman, W. F., and George, B. L.: New concepts and drugs in the treatment of congestive heart failure. Pediatr. Clin. North Am. *31*:1197, 1984.
68. Anderson, P.A.W.: Maturation in cardiac contractility. Cardiol. Clin. *7*:209, 1989.
69. Talner, N. S., and Lister, G.: Perioperative care of the infant with congenital heart disease. Cardiol. Clin. *7*:419, 1989.
70. Park, M. K.: Use of digoxin in infants and children, with specific emphasis on dosage. J. Pediatr. *108*:871, 1986.
71. Freed, M. D., Hegmann, M. A., Lewis, A. B., et al.: Prostaglandin E_1 in infants with ductus arteriosus dependent congenital heart disease. Circulation *64*:899, 1981.
72. Lewis, A. B., Freed, M. D., Hegmann, M. A., et al.: Side effects of therapy with prostaglandin E_1 in infants with critical congenital heart disease. Circulation *64*:893, 1981.
73. Friedman, W. F., Kurlinski, J., Jacob, J., et al.: Inhibition of prostaglandin and prostacyclin synthesis in clinical management of PDA. Semin. Perinatol. *4*:125, 1980.
74. Friedman, W. F.: Patent ductus arteriosus in respiratory distress syndrome. Pediatr. Cardiol. *4*(Suppl 2):3, 1983.
75. Montigny, M., Davignon, A., Fouron, J. C., et al.: Captopril in infants for congestive heart failure secondary to a large ventricular to right shunt. Am J. Cardiol. *63*:631, 1989.
76. Snyder, J. V.: Assessment of systemic oxygen transport. In Snyder, J. V. (ed.): Oxygen Transport in the Clinically Ill. Chicago, Year Book Medical Publishing Co., 1987, p. 179.
77. Kleinman, C. S., and Donnerstein, R. L.: Ultrasonic assessment of cardiac function in the intact human fetus. J. Am. Coll. Cardiol. *5*:84S, 1985.
78. Silverman, N. H., Kleinman, C. S., Rudolph, A. M., et al.: Fetal atrioventricular valve insufficiency associated with nonimmune hydrops: A two-dimensional echocardiographic and pulsed Doppler ultrasound study. Circulation *72*:825, 1985.
79. Reed, K. L., Appelton, C. P., Anderson, C. F., et al.: Doppler studies of venacaval flows in human fetuses. Circulation *81*:498, 1990.
80. Gembruch, U., Manz, M., Bald, R., et al.: Repeated intravascular treatment with amiodarone in a fetus with refractory supraventricular tachycardia and hydrops fetalis. Am. Heart J. *118*:1335, 1989.
81. Silverman, N. H., and Schmidt, K. G.: The current role of Doppler echocardiography in the diagnosis of heart disease in children. Cardiol. Clin. *7*:265, 1989.
82. Cloez, J. L., Schmidt, K. G., Birk, E., and Silverman, N. H.: Determination of pulmonary systemic blood flow ratio in children by simplified Doppler echocardiographic method. J. Am. Coll. Cardiol. *11*:825, 1988.
83. Sahn, D. J.: Applications of color flow mapping in pediatric cardiology. Cardiol. Clin. *7*:255, 1989.
84. Krabill, K. A., Ring, W. S., Foker, J. E., et al.: Echocardiographic versus cardiac catheterization diagnosis of infants with congenital heart disease requiring cardiac surgery. Am. J. Cardiol. *60*:351, 1987.
85. Stanger, P., Heymann, M. A., Tarnoff, H., et al.: Complications of cardiac catheterization of neonates, infants and children. Circulation *50*:595, 1974.
86. Rashkind, W. J., Tait, M.A.S., and Gibson, R. J., Jr.: Interventional cardiac catheterization in congenital heart disease. Int. J. Cardiol. *7*:1, 1985.
87. Lock, J. E., Keane, J. F., and Fellows, K. E.: The use of catheter intervention procedures for congenital heart disease. J. Am. Coll. Cardiol. *7*:1420, 1986.
88. Mullins, C. E., Latson, L. A., Neches, W. H. et al.: Balloon dilation of miscellaneous lesions: Results of valvuloplasty and angioplasty of congenital anomalies registry. Am. J. Cardiol. *65*:802, 1990.
89. Mullins, C. E.: Pediatric and congenital therapeutic cardiac catheterization. Circulation *79*:1153, 1989.
90. Beckman, R. H., Rocchini, A. P., and Rosenthal, A.: Therapeutic cardiac catheterization for pulmonary valve and pulmonary artery stenosis. Cardiol. Clin. *7*:331, 1989.
91. Perry, S. B., Zeevi, B., Keane, J. F., and Lock, J. E.: Interventional catheterization of left heart lesions, including aortic and mitral valve stenosis and coarctation of the aorta. Cardiol. Clin. *7*:341, 1989.
92. Hellenbrand, W. E., and Mullins, C. E.: Catheter closure of congenital heart defects. Cardiol. Clin. *7*:351, 1989.
93. Zipes, D. P., Akthar, M., Denes, P., et al.: Guidelines for clinical intracar-

diac electrophysiologic studies. A report of the American College of Cardiology/AHA Task Force on assessment of diagnostic and therapeutic cardiovascular procedures. J. Am. Coll. Cardiol. *14*:1827, 1989.

94. Perry, J. C., and Garson, A., Jr.: Diagnosis and treatment of arrhythmias. Adv. Pediatr. *36*:177, 1989.
95. Case, C. L., Crawford, F. A., and Gillette, P. C.: Surgical treatment of dysrhythmias in infants and children. Ped. Clin. North Am. *37*:79, 1990.
96. Kugler, J. D., Bansal, A. M., Cheatham, J. P., et al.: Drug-electrophysiology studies in infants, children and adolescents. Am. Heart J. *110*:144, 1985.

SPECIFIC CARDIAC DEFECTS

97. Hunt, C. E., and Lucas, R. V., Jr.: Symptomatic atrial septal defect in infancy. Circulation *42*:1042, 1973.
98. Davea, J. E., Cheitlin, M. D., and Bedynek, J. L.: Sinus venosus atrial septal defect. Am. Heart J. *85*:177, 1973.
99. Bashi, V. V., Ravikumar, E., Jairaj, P. S., et al.: Coexistent mitral valve disease with left-to-right shunt at the atrial level: Clinical profile, hemodynamics, and surgical considerations in 67 consecutive patients. Am. Heart J. *114*:1406, 1987.
100. Leachman, R. D., Cokkinos, D. V., and Cooley, D. A.: Association of ostium secundum atrial septal defects with mitral valve prolapse. Am. J. Cardiol. *38*:167, 1976.
101. Levin, A. R., Spach, M. S., Boineau, J. P., et al.: Atrial pressure flow dynamics and atrial septal defects (secundum type). Circulation *37*:476, 1968.
102. O'Toole, J. D., Reddy, I., Curtiss, E. I., and Shaver, J. A.: The mechanism of splitting of the second heart sound in atrial septal defect. Circulation *41*:1047, 1977.
103. Clark, E. B., and Kugler, J. D.: Preoperative secundum atrial septal defect with coexisting sinus node and atrioventricular node dysfunction. Circulation *65*:976, 1982.
104. Mugge, A., Daniel, W. G., Klopper, J. W., and Lichtlen, P. R.: Visualization of patent foramen ovale by transesophageal color-coded Doppler echocardiography. Am. J. Cardiol. *62*:837, 1988.
105. Shub, C., Tajik, A. J., Seward, J. B., et al.: Surgical repair of uncomplicated atrial septal defect without "routine" preoperative cardiac catheterization. J. Am. Coll. Cardiol. *6*:49, 1985.
106. Freed, M. D., Nadas, A. S., Norwood, W. I., and Castaneda, A. R.: Is routine preoperative cardiac catheterization necessary before repair of secundum and sinus venosus atrial septal defects? J. Am. Coll. Cardiol. *4*:333, 1984.
107. Taketa, R. M., Sahn, D. J., Simon, A. L., et al.: Catheter positions in congenital cardiac malformations. Circulation *51*:749, 1975.
108. Brand, A., Keren, A., Branski, D., et al.: Natural course of atrial septal aneurysm in children and the potential for spontaneous closure of associated septal defect. Am. J. Cardiol. *64*:996, 1989.
109. Steele, P. M., Fuster, V., Cohen, M., et al.: Isolated atrial septal defect with pulmonary vascular obstructive disease—long term follow up and prediction of outcome after surgical correction. Circulation *76*:1037, 1987.
110. Levin, A. R., Liebson, P. R., Ehlers, K. H., and Daimant, B.: Assessment of left ventricular function in atrial septal defect. Pediatr. Res. *9*:894, 1975.
111. Epstein, S. E., Beiser, G. D., Goldstein, R. E., et al.: Hemodynamic abnormalities in response to mild and intense upright exercise following operative correction of an atrial septal defect or tetralogy of Fallot. Circulation *42*:1065, 1973.
112. Karpawich, P. P., Antillon, J. R., Cappola, P. R., and Agarwal, K. C.: Pre- and postoperative electrophysiologic assessment of children with secundum atrial septal defect. Am. J. Cardiol. *55*:519, 1985.
113. Bink-Boelkens, M.T.E., Bergstra, A., and Landsman, M.L.J.: Functional abnormalities of the conduction system in children with an atrial septal defect. Int. J. Cardiol. *20*:263, 1988.
114. Bink-Boelkens, M.T.E., Meuzelaar, K. J., and Eygelaar, A.: Arrhythmias after repair of secundum atrial septal defect: The influence of surgical modification. Am. Heart J. *115*:629, 1988.
115. Borkon, A. M., Pieroni, D. R., Varghese, P. J., et al.: The superior QRS axis in ostium primum ASD. Am. Heart J. *92*:15, 1975.
116. Goodman, D. J., Harrison, D. C., and Cannom, D. S.: Atrioventricular conduction in patients with incomplete endocardial cushion defect. Circulation *49*:630, 1974.
117. Jacobsen, J. R., Gillette, P. C., Corbett, B. N., et al.: Intracardiac electrography in endocardial cushion defects. Circulation *54*:599, 1976.
118. Waldo, A. L., Kaiser, G. A., Bowman, F. O., Jr., and Malm, J. R.: Etiology of prolongation of the PR interval in patients with an endocardial cushion defect. Circulation *43*:19, 1973.
119. Smallhorn, J. F., Tommasini, G., and Anderson, R. H.: Assessment of atrioventricular septal defects by two-dimensional echocardiography. Br. Heart J. *47*:109, 1982.
120. Lipshultz, S. E., Sanders, S. P., Mayer, J. E., et al.: Are routine preoperative cardiac catheterization angiography necessary before repair of ostium primum atrial septal defect? J. Am. Coll. Cardiol. *11*:373, 1988.
121. DeBia, S.E.L., DiCommo, V., Ballerini, L., et al.: Prevalence of left-sided obstructive lesions in patients with atrial ventricular canal without Down's syndrome. J. Thorac. Cardiovasc. Surg. *91*:467, 1986.
122. Elliott, L. P., Bargeron, L. M., Jr., and Green, C. E.: Angled angiography: General approach and findings. *In* Friedman, W. F., and Higgins, C. B. (eds.): Pediatric Cardiac Imaging. Philadelphia, W. B. Saunders Company, 1984, p. 1.
123. Castaneda, A. R., Mayer, J. E., and Jonas, R. A.: Repair of complete atrioventricular canal in infancy. World J. Surg. *9*:590, 1985.
124. Santos, A., Boucek, M., Ruttenberg, H., et al.: Repair of atrioventricular septal defects in infancy. J. Thorac. Cardiovasc. Surg. *91*:505, 1986.
125. Clapp, S. K., Perry, B. L., Farooki, Z. Q., et al.: Surgical and medical results of complete atrioventricular canal: A ten-year review. Am. J. Cardiol. *59*:454, 1987.
126. Pacifico, A. D.: Surgical treatment of complex atrial ventricular septal defects. Cardiol. Clin. *7*:399, 1989.
127. Ceithaml, E. L., Midgley, F. M., and Perry, L. W.: Long term results after surgical repair of incomplete endocardial cushion defects. Am. Thorac. Surg. *48*:413, 1989.
127a. Soto, B., Ceballos, R., and Kirklin, J. W.: Ventricular septal defects: A surgical viewpoint. J. Am. Coll. Cardiol. *14*:1291, 1989.
128. Van Praagh, R., Geva, T., and Kreutzer, J.: Ventricular septal defects: How shall we describe, name and classify them? J. Am. Coll. Cardiol. *14*:1298, 1989.
129. Hagler, D. J., Edwards, W. D., Seward, J. B., and Tajik, A. J.: Standardized nomenclature of the ventricular septum and ventricular septal defects, with applications for two-dimensional echocardiography. Mayo Clin. Proc. *60*:741, 1985.
130. Baker, E. J., Leung, M. P., Anderson, R. H., et al.: The cross-sectional anatomy of ventricular septal defects: A reappraisal. Br. Heart J. *69*:339, 1988.
131. Helmcke, F., Souza, A., Nanda, N. C., et al.: Two-dimensional and color Doppler assessment of ventricular septal defect of congenital origin. Am. J. Cardiol. *63*:1112, 1989.
132. Sharif, D. S., Huhta, J. C., Marantz, P., et al.: Two-dimensional echocardiographic determination of ventricular septal defect size: Correlation of autopsy. Am. Heart J. *117*:1333, 1989.
133. Beerman, L. B., Park, S. C., Fischer, D. R., et al.: Ventricular septal defect associated with aneurysm of the membranous septum. J. Am. Coll. Cardiol. *5*:118, 1985.
134. Ortiz, E., Robinson, P. J., Deanfield, J. E., et al.: Localisation of ventricular septal defects by simultaneous display of superimposed colour Doppler and cross sectional echocardiographic images. Br. Heart J. *54*:53, 1985.
135. Murphy, D. J., Ludomirsky, A., and Huhta, J. C.: Continuous-wave Doppler in children with ventricular septal defect: Noninvasive estimation of interventricular pressure gradient. Am. J. Cardiol. *57*:428, 1986.
136. Kurokawa, S., Takahashi, M., Katoh, Y., et al.: Noninvasive evaluation of the ratio of pulmonary to systemic flow in ventricular septal defect by means of Doppler two-dimensional echocardiography. Am. Heart J. *116*:1033, 1988.
137. Williams, R. G.: Doppler color-flow mapping and prediction of ventricular defect outcome. J. Am. Coll. Cardiol. *13*:1119, 1989.
138. Hornberger, L. K., Sahn, D. J., Krabill, K. A., et al.: Elucidation of the natural history of ventricular septal defects by serial Doppler color-flow mapping studies. J. Am. Coll. Cardiol. *13*:1111, 1989.
139. Friedman, W. F., Mehrizi, A., and Pusch, A. L.: Multiple muscular ventricular septal defects. Circulation *32*:35, 1964.
140. Dickinson, D. F., Arnold, R., and Wilkinson, J. L.: Ventricular septal defects in children born in Liverpool. Evaluation of natural course and surgical implications in an unselected population. Br. Heart J. *46*:47, 1981.
141. Weidman, W. H., Blount, S. G., Jr., DuShane, J. W., et al.: Clinical course in ventricular septal defect. Natural history study. Circulation *56*(Suppl.):I-56, 1977.
142. Ramaciotti, C., Keren, A., and Silverman, N. H.: Importance of (perimembranous) ventricular septal aneurysm in the natural history of isolated perimembranous ventricular septal defect. Am. J. Cardiol. *57*:268, 1986.
143. Friedman, W. F., and Pitlick, P. T.: Ventricular septal defect in infancy—University of California, San Diego (Specialty Conference). West. J. Med. *120*:295, 1974.
144. Blumenthal, S., Griffiths, S. P., and Morgan, B. C.: Bacterial endocarditis in children with heart disease. (A review based on the literature and experience with 58 cases.) Pediatrics *26*:993, 1960.
145. Moe, D. J., and Guntheroth, W. G.: Spontaneous closure of uncomplicated ventricular septal defect. Am. J. Cardiol. *60*:674, 1987.
146. Neutze, J. M., Ishikawa, T., Clarkson, P. M., et al.: Assessment and follow up of patients with ventricular septal defect and elevated pulmonary vascular resistance. Am. J. Cardiol. *63*:327, 1989.
147. Yeager, S. B., Freed, M. D., Keane, J. F., et al.: Primary surgical closure of ventricular septal defect in the first year of life: results in 128 infants. J. Am. Coll. Cardiol. *3*:1269, 1984.
148. McDaniel, N., Gutgesell, H. P., Nolan, S. P., and Kron, I. L.: Repair of large musclar ventricular septal defects in infants employing left ventriculotomy. Ann. Thorac. Surg. *47*:593, 1989.
149. Hislop, A., Haworth, S. G., Shinebourne, E. A., and Reid, L.: Quantitative structural analysis of pulmonary vessels in isolated ventricular septal defect in infancy. Br. Heart J. *37*:1014, 1975.
150. DuShane, J. W., and Kirklin, J. W.: Late results of the repair of ventricular septal defect on pulmonary vascular disease. *In* Kirklin, J. W. (ed.): Advances in Cardiovascular Surgery. New York, Grune and Stratton, 1973, p. 9.
151. Rhodes, L. A., Keane, J. F., Keane, J. P., et al.: Long-term follow up (up to 43 years) of ventricular septal defect with audible aortic regurgitation. Am. J. Cardiol. *66*:340, 1990.
152. Griffin, M. L., Sullivan, I. D., Anderson, R. H., and Macartney, F. J.: Doubly committed subarterial ventricular septal defect: New morphological criteria with echocardiographic and angiocardiographic correlation. Br. Heart J. *59*:474, 1988.
153. Schmidt, K. G., Cassidy, S. C., Silverman, N. H., and Stanger, P.: Doubly

committed subarterial ventricular septal defects: Echocardiographic features and surgical implications. J. Am. Coll. Cardiol. *12*:1538, 1988.
154. Okita, Y., Miki, S., Kusuhara, K., et al.: Long-term results of aortic valvuloplasty for aortic regurgitation associated with ventricular septal defect. J. Thorac. Cardiovasc. Surg. *96*:769, 1988.
155. Leung, M. P., Mok, C. K., Lo, R.N.S., and Lau, K. C.: An echocardiographic study of perimembranous ventricular septal defect with left ventricular to right atrial shunting. Br. Heart J. *55*:45, 1986.
156. Gersony, W. M., and Hayes, C. J.: Bacterial endocarditis in patients with pulmonary stenosis, aortic stenosis, or ventricular septal defect. Natural history study. Circulation *56*(Suppl.):I-84, 1977.
157. deLeval, M.: Ventricular septal defects. *In* Stark, J., and deLeval, M. (eds.): Surgery for Congenital Heart Defects. New York, Grune and Stratton, Inc., 1983, p. 271.
158. Lock, J. E., Block, P. C., McKay, R. G., et al.: Transcatheter closure of ventricular septal defects. Circulation *78*:361, 1988.
159. Godman, M. J., Roberts, N. K., and Izukawa, T.: Late postoperative conduction disturbances after repair of ventricular septal defect in tetralogy of Fallot. Circulation *49*:214, 1974.
160. Okarama, E. O., Guller, B., Molony, J. D., and Weidman, W. H.: Etiology of right bundle-branch block pattern after surgical closure of ventricular-septal defects. Am. Heart J. *90*:14, 1975.
161. Otterstad, J. E., Simonsen, S., and Erikssen, J.: Hemodynamic findings at rest and during mild supine exercise in adults with isolated uncomplicated ventricular septal defects. Circulation *71*:650, 1985.
162. Maron, B. J., Redwood, D. R., Hirschfield, J. W., Jr., et al.: Postoperative assessment of patients with ventricular septal defect and pulmonary hypertension. Response to intense upright exercise. Circulation *48*:864, 1973.
163. Graham, T. P., Jr., Atwood, G. F., Boucek, R. J., Jr., et al.: Right ventricular volume characteristics in ventricular septal defect. Circulation *54*:800, 1976.
164. Heymann, M. A., and Rudolph, A. M.: Control of the ductus arteriosus. Physiol. Rev. *55*:62, 1975.
165. Friedman, W. F., Printz, M. P., Kirkpatrick, S. E., and Hoskins, E. J.: The vasoactivity of the fetal lamb ductus arteriosus studied in utero. Pediatr. Res. *17*:331, 1983.
166. Skidgel, R. A., Friedman, W. F., and Printz, M. P.: Prostaglandin biosynthetic activities of the fetal lamb ductus arteriosus, other blood vessels and fetal lung. Pediatr. Res. *18*:12, 1984.
167. Printz, M. P., Skidgel, R. A., and Friedman, W. F.: Studies of pulmonary prostaglandin biosynthetic and catabolic enzymes as factors in ductus arteriosus patency and closure: Evidence for a shift in products with gestational age. Pediatr. Res. *18*:19, 1984.
168. Gittenberger-DeGroot, A. C.: Persistent ductus arteriosus: Most probably a primary congenital malformation. Br. Heart J. *39*:610, 1977.
169. Friedman, W. F., Hirschklau, M. J., Printz, M. P., et al.: Pharmacologic closure of patent ductus arteriosus in the premature infant. N. Engl. J. Med. *295*:526, 1976.
170. Douidar, S. M., Richardson, J., and Snodgrass, W. R.: Use of indomethacin in ductus closure: An update evaluation. Dev. Pharmacol. Ther. *11*:196, 1988.
171. Sahn, D. J., Vaucher, Y., Williams, D. E., et al.: Echocardiographic detection of large left to right shunts and cardiomyopathies in infants and children. Am. J. Cardiol. *38*:73, 1976.
172. Liao, P. K., Su, W. J., and Hung, J. S.: Doppler echocardiographic flow characteristics of isolated patent ductus arteriosus: Better delineation by Doppler color-flow mapping. J. Am. Coll. Cardiol. *12*:1285, 1988.
173. Hiraishi, S., Horiguchi, Y., Misawa, H., et al.: Noninvasive Doppler echocardiographic evaluation of shunt flow dynamics of the ductus arteriosus. Circulation *75*:1146, 1987.
174. Cloez, J. L., Issaz, K., and Pernot, C.: Pulsed Doppler flow characteristics of ductus arteriosus in infants with associated congenital anomalies of the heart or great arteries. Am. J. Cardiol. *57*:845, 1986.
175. Yeh, T. F., Achanti, B., Patel, H., and Pildes, R. S.: Indomethacin therapy in premature infants with patent ductus arteriosus—determination of therapeutic plasma levels. Dev. Pharmacol. Ther. *12*:169, 1989.
176. Jacob, J., Gluck, L., DiSessa, T. G., et al.: The contribution of PDA in the neonate with severe RDS. J. Pediatr. *96*:79, 1980.
177. Merritt, T. A., Harris, J. P., and Roghmann, K.: Early closure of the patent ductus arteriosus in very low birth weight infants: A controlled trial. J. Pediatr. *99*:281, 1981.
178. Gersony, W. M., Peckham, G. J., Ellison, R. C., et al.: Effects of indomethacin in premature infants with patent ductus arteriosus: Results of a national collaborative study. J. Pediatr. *102*:895, 1983.
179. Cassady, G., Crouse, D. T., Kirklin, J. W., et al.: A randomized control trial of very early prophylactic ligation of the ductus arteriosus in babies who weighed 1000 g or less at birth. N. Engl. J. Med. *320*:1511, 1989.
180. Wagner, H. R., Ellison, R. C., Zierler, S., et al.: Surgical closure of patent ductus arteriosus in 268 preterm infants. J. Thorac. Cardiovasc. Surg. *87*:870, 1984.
181. Jarmakani, M. M., Graham, T. P., Jr., Canent, R. V., Jr., et al.: Effect of site of shunt on left heart volume characteristics in children with ventricular septal defect and patent ductus arteriosus. Circulation *40*:411, 1969.
182. Bessenger, F. B., Jr., Blieden, L. C., and Edwards, J. E.: Hypertensive pulmonary vascular disease associated with patent ductus arteriosus. Circulation *52*:157, 1975.
183. Latson, L. A., Hofschire, P. J., Kugler, J. D., et al.: Transcatheter closure of patent ductus arteriosus in pediatric patients. J. Pediatr. *115*:549, 1989.
184. Krichenko, A., Benson, L. N., Burrows, P., et al.: Angiographic classification of the isolated, persistently patent ductus arteriosus and implications for percutaneous catheter closure. Am. J. Cardiol. *63*:877, 1989.
185. Musewe, N. N., Benson, L. N., Smallhorn, J. F., and Freedom, R. M.: Two-dimensional echocardiographic and color-flow Dopper evaluation of ductal occlusion with the Rashkind prothesis. Circulation *80*:1706, 1989.
186. Ali Khan, M. A., Mullins, C. E., Nihill, M. R., et al.: Percutaneous catheter closure of the ductus arteriosus in children and young adults. Am. J. Cardiol. *64*:218, 1989.
187. Hellenbrand, W. E., and Mullins, C. E.: Catheter closure of congenital cardiac defects. Cardiol. Clin. *7*:351, 1989.
188. Kutsche, L. M., and Van Mierop, L.H.S.: Anatomy and pathogenesis of aorticopulmonary septal defect. Am. J. Cardiol. *59*:443, 1987.
189. Tiraboschi, R., Salomone, G., Crupi, G., et al.: Aorto-pulmonary window in the first year of life: Report on 11 surgical cases. Ann. Thorac. Surg. *46*:438, 1988.
190. Prasad, T. R., Valiathan, M. S., Chyamakrishnan, K. G., et al.: Surgical management of aortopulmonary septal defect. Ann. Thorac. Surg. *47*:877, 1989.
191. Crupi, G., Macartney, F. J., and Anderson, R. H.: Persistent truncus arteriosus: A study of 66 autopsy cases with special reference to definition and morphogenesis. Am. J. Cardiol. *40*:569, 1977.
192. Shrivastava, F., and Edwards, J. E.: Coronary arterial origin and persistent truncus arteriosus. Circulation *55*:551, 1977.
193. Suzuki, A., Ho, S. Y., Anderson, R. H., and Deanfield, J. E.: Coronary arterial and sinusal anatomy in hearts with a common arterial trunk. Ann. Thorac. Surg. *48*:792, 1989.
194. Calder, L., Van Praagh, R., Sears, W. P., et al.: Truncus arteriosus communis. Am. Heart J. *92*:23, 1976.
195. Juaneda, E., and Haworth, S. G.: Pulmonary vascular disease in children with truncus arteriosus. Am. J. Cardiol. *54*:1314, 1984.
196. Radford, D. J., Perkins, L., Lachman, R., and Thong, Y. H.: Spectrum of DiGeorge syndrome in patients with truncus arteriosus: Expanded DiGeorge syndrome. Pediatr. Cardiol. *9*:95, 1988.
196a. Kirby, M. L., and Waldo, K. L.: Role of neural crest in congenital heart disease. Circulation *82*:332, 1990.
197. Gelband, H., Van Meter, S., and Gersony, W. M.: Truncal valve abnormalities in infants with persistent truncus arteriosus. Circulation *45*:397, 1972.
198. Yoshizato, T., and Julsrud, P. R.: Truncus arteriosus revisited: An angiographic demonstration. Pediatr. Cardiol. *11*:36, 1990.
199. Bove, E. L., Beekman, R. H., Snider, A. R., et al.: Repair of truncus arteriosus in the neonate and young infant. Ann. Thorac. Surg. *47*:499, 1989.
200. Cooper, M. J., Bernstein, D., and Silverman, N. H.: Recognition of left coronary artery fistula to the left and right ventricles by contrast echocardiography. J. Am. Coll. Cardiol. *6*:923, 1985.
201. Miyatake, K., Okamoto, M., Kinoshita, N., et al.: Doppler echocardiographic features of coronary arteriovenous fistula. Complementary roles of cross sectional echocardiography and the Doppler technique. Br. Heart J. *51*:508, 1984.
202. Ruttenhouse, E. A., Doty, D. B., and Ehrenhaft, J. L.: Congenital coronary artery-cardiac chamber fistula. Review of operative management. Ann. Thorac. Surg. *20*:468, 1975.
203. Angelini, P.: Normal and anomalous coronary arteries: Definitions and classification. Am. Heart J. *117*:418, 1989.
204. Hurwitz, R. A., Caldwell, R. L., Girod, D. A., et al.: Clinical and hemodynamic course of infants and children with anomalous left coronary artery. Am. Heart J. *118*:1176, 1989.
205. Menahem, S., and Venables, A. W.: Anomalous left coronary artery from the pulmonary artery: A 15-year sample. Br. Heart J. *58*:378, 1987.
206. Vaksmann, G., Mauran, P., Ray, C., et al.: Visualization of anomalous origin of the left main coronary artery from the pulmonary trunk by pulsed and color Doppler echocardiography. Am. Heart J. *116*:181, 1988.
207. Schmidt, K. G., Cooper, M. J., Silverman, N. H., and Stanger, P.: Pulmonary artery origin of the left coronary artery: Diagnosis by two-dimensional echocardiography, pulsed Doppler ultrasound and color-flow mapping. J. Am. Coll. Cardiol. *11*:396, 1988.
208. Rein, A.J.J.T., Colan, S. D., Parness, I. A., and Sanders, S. P.: Regional and global left ventricular function in infants with anomalous origin of the left coronary artery from the pulmonary trunk: Preoperative and postoperative assessment. Circulation *75*:115, 1987.
209. Guikahue, M. K., Sidi, D., Kachaner, J., et al.: Anomalous left coronary artery arising from the pulmonary artery in infancy: Is early operation better? Br. Heart J. *60*:522, 1988.
210. Boutefeu, J. M., Morat, P. R., Hahn, C., and Hauf, E.: Aneurysms of the sinus of Valsalva. Report of seven cases in review of the literature. Am. J. Med. *65*:18, 1978.
211. Engle, P. J., Held, J. S., Bel-Kahn, J.V.D., and Spitz, H.: Echocardiographic diagnosis of congenital sinus of Valsalva aneurysm. Circulation *63*:705, 1981.
212. Barragry, T. P., Ring, W. S., Moller, J. H., and Lillehei, C. W.: 15 to 30 year follow up of patients undergoing repair of ruptured congenital aneurysms of the sinus of Valsalva. Ann. Thorac. Surg. *46*:515, 1988.
213. Smyth, P. T., and Edwards, J. E.: Pseudocoarctation, kinking or buckling of the aorta. Circulation *46*:1027, 1972.
214. Hutchins, G. M.: Coarctation of the aorta explained as a branch point of the ductus arteriosus. Am. J. Pathol. *63*:203, 1971.
215. Talner, N. S., and Berman, M. A.: Postnatal development of obstruction in coarctation of the aorta: Role of the ductus arteriosus. Pediatrics *56*:562, 1975.
216. Heymann, M. A., Berman, W., Jr., Rudolph, A. M., and Whitman, V.:

Dilatation of the ductus arteriosus by prostaglandin E_1 in aortic arch abnormalities. Circulation *59*:169, 1979.
217. Tynan, M., Finley, J. P., Fontes, V., et al.: Balloon angioplasty for the treatment of native coarctation: Results of valvuloplasty and angioplasty of congenital anomalies registry. Am. J. Cardiol. *65*:790, 1990.
218. Kopf, G. S., Hellenbrand, W., Kleinman, C., et al.: Repair of aortic coarctation in the first three months of life: Immediate and long-term results. Ann. Thorac. Surg. *41*:425, 1986.
219. Van Son, J.A.M., Skotnicki, S. H., Van Asten, W. N., et al.: Quantitative assessment of coarctation in infancy by Doppler spectral analysis. Am. J. Cardiol. *63*:1282, 1989.
220. Shaddy, R. E., Snider, A. R., Silverman, N. H., and Lutin, W.: Pulsed Doppler findings in patients with coarctation of the aorta. Circulation *73*:82, 1986.
221. Rao, P. S., and Carey, P.: Doppler ultrasound in the prediction of pressure gradients across aortic coarctation. Am. Heart J. *118*:299, 1989.
222. Godwin, G. D., Herfkens, R. L., Brundage, D. H., and Lipton, N. J.: Evaluation of coarctation of the aorta by computed tomography. J. Comput. Assist. Tomogr. *5*:153, 1981.
223. Graham, T. P., Jr., Burger, J., Boucek, R. J., Jr., et al.: Absence of left ventricular volume loading in infants with coarctation of the aorta and a large ventricular septal defect. J. Am. Coll. Cardiol. *14*:1545, 1989.
224. George, B., DiSessa, T. G., Williams, R. G., et al.: Coarctation repair without cardiac catheterization in infants. Am. Heart J. *114*:1421, 1987.
225. Cohen, M., Fuster, V., Steele, P. M., et al.: Coarctation of the aorta: Long-term follow up and prediction of outcome after surgical correction. Circulation *80*:840, 1989.
226. Bromberg, B. I., Beekman, R. H., Rocchini, A. P., et al.: Aortic aneurysm after patch aortoplasty repair of coarctation: A prospective analysis of prevalence, screening tests and risks. J. Am. Coll. Cardiol. *14*:734, 1989.
227. Beekman, R. H., Rocchini, A. P., Behrendt, D. M., and Rosenthal, A.: Reoperation for coarctation of the aorta. Am. J. Cardiol. *48*:1108, 1981.
228. Igler, F. O., Boerboom, L. E., Werner, P. H., et al.: Coarctation of the aorta and narrow receptor resetting. Circulation Res. *48*:365, 1981.
229. Gidding, S. S., Rocchini, A. P., Beekman, R., et al.: Therapeutic effect of propranolol on paradoxical hypertension after repair of coarctation of the aorta. N. Engl. J. Med. *312*:1224, 1985.
230. Choy, M., Rocchini, A. P., Beekman, R. H., et al.: Paradoxical hypertension after repair of coarctation of the aorta in children: Balloon angioplasty versus surgical repair. Circulation *75*:1186, 1987.
231. Johnson, R. G., Williams, G. R., Razook, J. D., et al.: Reoperation in congenital aortic stenosis. Ann. Thorac. Surg. *40*:156, 1985.
232. Hellenbrand, W. E., Allen, H. D., Golinko, R. J., et al.: Balloon angioplasty for aortic re-coarctation: Results of valvuloplasty and angioplasty of congenital anomalies registry. Am. J. Cardiol. *65*:793, 1990.
233. Murphy, A. M., Blades, M., Daniels, S., and James, F. W.: Blood pressure in cardiac output during exercise: A longitudinal study of children undergoing repair of coarctation. Am. Heart J. *117*:1327, 1989.
234. Maron, B. J., Humphries, J., Rowe, R. D., and Mellits, E. D.: Prognosis of surgically corrected coarctation of the aorta. Circulation *47*:119, 1973.
235. Van Woezik, E.V.M., Kline, H. W., and Krediet, P.: Normal internal calibers of ostia, great arteries and aortic isthmus in children. Br. Heart J. *39*:860, 1977.
236. Bharati, S., and Lev, M.: The surgical anatomy of the heart in tubular hypoplasia of the transverse aorta (preductal coarctation). J. Thorac. Cardiovasc. Surg. *91*:79, 1986.
237. Graham, T. P., Jr., Atwood, G. F., Boerth, R. C., et al.: Right and left heart size and function in infants with symptomatic coarctation. Circulation *56*:641, 1977.
238. Hammon, J. W., Jr., Merrill, W. H., Prager, R. L., et al.: Repair of interrupted aortic arch and associated malformations in infancy: Indications for complete or partial repair. Ann. Thorac. Surg. *42*:17, 1986.
239. Sell, J. E., Jonas, R. A., Mayer, J. E., et al.: The results of a surgical program for interrupted aortic arch. J. Thorac. Cardiovasc. Surg. *96*:864, 1988.
240. Dekker, A. O., Gittenberger-DeGroot, A. C., and Roozendaal, H.: The ductus arteriosus and associated cardiac anomalies in interruption of the aortic arch. Pediatr. Cardiol. *2*:185, 1982.
241. Friedman, W. F.: Congenital aortic stenosis. *In* Adams, F. H., and Emmanouilides, G. C. (eds.): Moss' Heart Disease in Infants, Children and Adolescents. 4th ed. Baltimore, Williams and Wilkins, 1989.
241a. Stevens, C. A., Carey, J. C., and Shigeoka, A. O.: DiGeorge anomaly and velocardiofacial syndrome. Pediatrics *85*:526, 1990.
242. Friedman, W. F., and Pappelbaum, S. J.: Indications for hemodynamic evaluation and surgery in congenital aortic stenosis. Pediatr. Clin. North Am. *18*:1207, 1971.
243. Kveselis, D. A., Rocchini, A. P., Rosenthal, A., et al.: Hemodynamic determinants of exercise-induced ST-segment depression in children with valvar aortic stenosis. Am. J. Cardiol. *55*:1133, 1985.
244. Cyran, S. E., James, F. W., Daniels, S., et al.: Comparison of the cardiac output and stroke volume response to upright exercise in children with valvular and subvalvular aortic stenosis. J. Am. Coll. Cardiol. *11*:651, 1988.
245. Lewis, A. L., Heymann, M. A., Stanger, P., et al.: Evaluation of subendocardial ischemia in valvar aortic stenosis in children. Circulation *49*:978, 1974.
246. Lakier, J. B., Lewis, A. B., Heymann, M. A., et al.: Isolated aortic stenosis of the neonate: Natural history and hemodynamic considerations. Circulation *50*:801, 1974.
247. Balaji, S., Keeton, B. R., Sutherland, G., et al.: Aortic valvotomy for critical aortic stenosis in neonates and infants aged less than one year. Br. Heart J. *61*:358, 1989.
248. Karl, T. R., Sano, S., Brawn, W. J., and Mee, R.B.B.: Critical aortic stenosis in the first month of life: Surgical results in 26 infants. Ann. Thorac. Surg. *50*:105, 1990.
249. Sink, J. D., Smallhorn, J. F., Macartney, F. J.: Mangement of critical aortic stenosis in infancy. J. Thorac. Cardiovasc. Surg. *87*:82, 1984.
250. Broderick, T. W., Higgins, C. B., and Friedman, W. F.: Critical aortic stenosis in neonates. Radiology *129*:393, 1978.
251. Skjaerpe, T., Hegrenaes, L., and Hatle, L.: Noninvasive estimation of valve area in patients with arotic stenosis by Doppler ultrasound anad two-dimensional echocardiography. Circulation *72*:810, 1985.
252. Ohlsson, J., and Wranne, B.: Noninvasive assessment of valve area in patients with aortic stenosis. J. Am. Coll. Cardiol. *7*:501, 1986.
253. Oh, J. K., Taliercio, C. P., Holmes, D. R., et al.: Prediction of the severity of aortic stenosis by Doppler aortic valve area determination: Prospective Doppler-catheterization correlation in 100 patients. J. Am. Coll. Cardiol. *11*:1227, 1988.
254. Bengur, A. R., Snider, A. R., Serwer, G. A., et al.: Usefulness of the Doppler mean gradient in evaluation of children with aortic valve stenosis in comparison to gradient at catheterization. Am. J. Cardiol. *64*:756, 1989.
255. Meliones, J. N., Snider, R., Serwer, G. A., et al.: Pulsed Doppler assessment of left ventricular diastolic filling in children with left ventricular outflow obstruction before and after balloon angioplasty. Am. J. Cardiol. *63*:231, 1989.
256. Kasten-Sportes, C. H., Piechaud, J. F., Sidi, D., and Kachaner, J.: Percutaneous balloon valvuloplasty in neonates with critical aortic stensis. J. Am. Coll. Cardiol. *13*:1101, 1989.
257. Wheller, J. J., Hosier, D. M., Teske, D. W., et al.: Results of operation for aortic valve stenosis in infants, children and adolescents. J. Thorac. Cardiovasc. Surg. *96*:474, 1988.
258. Karl, T. R., Sano, S., Brown, W. J., and Mee, R.B.B.: Critical aortic stenosis in the first month of life: Surgical results in 26 infants. Ann. Thorac. Surg. *50*:105, 1990.
259. Braunwald, E., Goldblatt, A., Aygen, M. M., et al.: Congenital aortic stenosis. I. Clinical and hemodynamic findings in 100 patients. Circulation *27*:426, 1963.
260. Johnson, A. M.: Aortic stenosis, sudden death, and the left ventricular baroreceptors. Br. Heart J. *33*:1, 1971.
261. Wagner, H. R., Weidman, W. H., Ellison, R. C., and Miettinen, O. S.: Indirect assessment of severity in aortic stenosis. Natural history study. Circulation *56*(Suppl.):I-20, 1977.
262. El-Said, G., Gallioto, F. J., Mullens, C. E., and McNamara, D. G.: Natural hemodynamic history of congenital aortic stenosis in childhood. Am. J. Cardiol. *30*:6, 1972.
263. Hurwitz, R. A.: Aortic valve stenosis in childhood: Clinical and hemodynamic history. J. Pediatr. *82*:228, 1973.
264. Friedman, W. F., Modlinger, J., and Morgan, J.: Serial hemodynamic observations in asymptomatic children with valvar aortic stenosis. Circulation *43*:91, 1971.
265. Cohen, L. S., Friedman, W. F., and Braunwald, E.: Natural history of mild congenital aortic stenosis elucidated by serial hemodynamic studies. Am. J. Cardiol. *30*:1, 1972.
266. Rocchini, A. P., Beekman, R. H., Ben Shachar, G., et al.: Balloon aortic valvuloplasty: Results of the valvuloplasty and angioplasty of congenital anomalies registry. Am. J. Cardiol. *65*:784, 1990.
267. Bisset, G. S., III, Meyer, R. A., Hirschfeld, S. S., et al.: Aortic valve replacement in childhood: Evaluation of left ventricular function by electrocardiography, echocardiography and graded exercise testing. Am. J. Cardiol. *52*:568, 1983.
268. Dorn, G. W., Donner, R., Assey, M. E., et al.: Alterations in left ventricular geometry, wall stress, and ejection performance after correction of congenital aortic stenosis. Circulation *78*,:1358, 1988.
269. DeBoer, B. A., Robbins, R. C., Maron, B. J., et al.: Late results of aortic valvotomy for congenital valvular aortic stenosis. Ann. Thorac. Surg. *50*:69, 1990.
270. DeBoer, D. A., Robbins, R. C., Maron, B. J., et al.: Late results of aortic valvotomy for congenital valvar aortic stenosis. Ann. Thorac. Surg. *50*:69, 1990.
271. Friedman, W. F., Novak, V., and Johnson, A. D.: Congenital aortic stenosis in adults. *In* Roberts, W. C. (ed.): Congenital Heart Disease in Adults. Philadelphia, F. A. Davis, 1979, p. 235.
272. DiSessa, T. G., Hagan, A. D., Isabel-Jones, J. B., and Friedman, W. F.: Two-dimensional echocardiograpic evaluation of discrete subaortic stenosis from the apical long axis view. Am. Heart J. *101*:774, 1981.
273. Pierli, C., Marino, B., Picardo, S., et al.: Discrete subaortic stenosis: Surgery in children based on two-dimensional and Doppler echocardiography. Chest *96*:325, 1989.
274. Kinney, E. L., Machado, H., Cortada, X., and Galbut, D. L.: Diagnosis of discrete subaortic stenosis by pulsed and continuous wave echocardiography. Am. Heart J. *110*:1069, 1985.
275. Mugge, A., Daniel, W. G., Wolpers, H. G., et al. Improved visualization of discrete subvalvular aortic stenosis by transesophageal color-coded Doppler echocardiography. Am. Heart J. *117*:474, 1989.
276. Newfeld, E. A., Muster, A. J., Paul, M. H., et al.: Discrete subvalvular aortic stenosis in childhood. Am. J. Cardiol. *38*:53, 1976.
277. Douville, E. C., Sade, R. M., Crawford, F. A., Jr., and Wiles, H. B.: Subvalvar aortic stenosis: timing of operation. Ann. Thorac. Surg. *50*:29, 1990.
278. Brown, J., Stevens, L., Lynch, L., et al.: Surgery for discrete subvalvular aortic stenosis: Actuarial survival, hemodynamic results, and acquired aortic regurgitation. Ann. Thorac. Surg. *40*:151, 1985.
279. Moses, R. D., Barnhart, G. R., and Jones, M.: The late prognosis after

localized resection for fixed (discrete and tunnel) left ventricular outflow tract observation. J. Thorac. Cardiovasc. Surg. *87*:410, 1984.

280. Ivert, T., Astudillo, R., Birdon, L., and Wranne, B.: Late results after a section of fixed subaortic stenosis. Scand. J. Thorac. Cardiovasc. Surg. *23*:211, 1989.
281. Lababidi, Z., Weinhaus, L., Stoeckle, H., Jr., and Walls, J. T.: Transluminal balllоon dilatation for discrete subaortic stenosis. Am. J. Cardiol. *59*:423, 1987.
282. Maron, B. J., Redwood, D. R., Roberts, W. C., et al.: Tunnel subaortic stenosis. Circulation *54*:404, 1976.
283. Ergin, M. A., Cooper, R., LaCourte, M., et al.: Experience with left ventricular apicoaortic conduits for complicated left ventricular outflow obstruction in children and young adults. Ann. Thorac. Surg. *32*:369, 1981.
284. Waldman, J. D., Schneeweiss, A., Edwards, W. D., et al.: The obstructive subaortic conus. Circulation *70*:339, 1984.
285. Friedman, W. G., and Roberts, W. C.: Vitamin D and the supravalvular aortic stenosis syndrome: The transplacental effects of vitamin D on the aorta of the rabbit. Circulation *34*:77, 1966.
286. Friedman, W. F.: Vitamin D embryopathy. Adv. Teratol. *3*:85, 1968.
287. Friedman, W. F., and Mills, L. F.: The relationship between vitamin D and the craniofacial and dental anomalies of the supraventricular aortic stenosis syndrome. Pediatrics *43*:12, 1969.
288. Garcia, R. C., Friedman, W. F., Kaback , M. M., and Rowe, R. D.: Idiopathic hypercalcemia and supravalvular aortic stenosis: Documentation of a new syndrome. N. Engl. J. Med. *271*:117, 1964.
289. Morris, C. A., Demsey, S. A., Leonard, C. O., et al.: Natural history of Williams syndrome: Physical characteristics. J. Pediatr. *113*:318, 1988.
290. Taylor, A. B., Stern, P. H., and Bell, N. H.: Abnormal regulation of circulating 25-hydroxy vitamin D in the Williams syndrome. N. Engl. J. Med. *306*:972, 1982.
291. Kahler, R. L., Braunwald, E., Plauth, W. H., Jr., and Morrow, A. G.: Familial congenital heart disease. Am. J. Med. *40*:384, 1966.
292. French, J. W., and Guntheroth, W. G.: An explanation of asymmetric upper extremity blood pressure in supravalvular aortic stenosis: The Coanda effect. Circulation *42*:31, 1970.
293. Goldstein, R. E., and Epstein, S. E.: Mechanism of elevated innominate artery pressures in supravalvular aortic stenosis. Circulation *42*:23, 1970.
294. Brand, A., Keren, A., Reifen, R. M., et al.: Echocardiographic and Doppler findings in the Williams syndrome. Am. J. Cardiol. *63*:633, 1989.
295. Stewart, S., Alexson, C., and Manning, J.: Extended aortoplasty to relieve supravalvular aortic stenosis. Ann. Thorac. Surg. *46*:427, 1988.
296. Flaker, G., Teske, D., Kilman, J. et al.: Supravalvular aortic stenosis. A 20-year clinical perspective and experience with patch aortoplasty. Am. J. Cardiol. *15*:256, 1983.
297. Sade, R. M., Crawford, F. A., Jr., and Fyfe, D. A.: Symposium on hypoplastic left heart syndrome. J. Thorac. Cardiovasc. Surg. *91*:937, 1986.
298. Bash, S. E., Huhta, J. C., Vick, G. W., III, et al.: Hypoplastic left heart syndrome: Is echocardiography accurate enough to guide surgical palliation? J. Am. Coll. Cardiol. *7*:610, 1986.
299. Norwood, W. I., Lang, P., and Hansen, D. D.: Physiologic repair of aortic atresia-hypoplastic left heart syndrome. N. Engl. J. Med. *308*:23, 1983.
300. Norwood, W. I.: Hypoplastic left heart syndrome. Cardiol. Clin. *7*:377, 1989.
301. Gustafson, R. A., Murray, G. F., Warden, H. E., et al.: Stage I palliation of hypoplastic left heart syndrome: The importance of neoaorta construction. Ann. Thorac. Surg. *48*:43, 1989.
302. Pigott, J. D., Murphy, J. D., Barber, G., and Norwood, W. I.: Palliative reconstructive surgery for hypoplastic left heart syndrome. Ann. Thorac. Surg. *45*:122, 1988.
303. Bailey, L. L., and Gundry, S. R.: Hypoplastic left heart syndrome. Pediatr. Clin. North Am. *37*:137, 1990.
304. Frahm, C. J., Braunwald, E., and Morrow, A. G.: Congenital aortic regurgitation. Am. J. Med. *31*:63, 1961.
305. Tuna, I. C., and Edwards, J. E.: Aortico-left ventricular tunnel and aortic insufficiency. Ann. Thorac. Surg. *45*:5, 1988.
306. Hovaguimian, H., Cobanoglu, A., and Starr, A.: Aortico-left ventricular tunnel: A clinical review and new surgical classification. Ann. Thorac. Surg. *45*:106, 1988.
307. Goforth, D., James, F. W., Kaplan, S., and Donner, R.: Maximal exercise in children with aortic regurgitation: An adjunct to noninvasive assessment of disease severity. Am. Heart J. *108*:1306, 1984.
308. Lucas R. V., Jr.: Anomalous venous connection, pulmonary and systemic. *In* Adams, F. H., and Emmanouilides, G. C. (eds.): Moss' Heart Disease in Infants, Children and Adolescents. 4th ed. Baltimore, Williams and Wilkins, 1989, p. 580.
309. Pacifico, A. D., Mandke, N. V., McGrath, L. B., et al.: Repair of congenital pulmonary venous thrombosis with living autologous atrial tissue. J. Thorac. Cardiovasc. Surg. *89*:604, 1985.
310. Marin-Garcia, J., Tandon, R., Lucas, R. V., Jr., and Edwards, J. E.: Cor triatriatum: Study of 20 cases. Am. J. Cardiol. *35*:59, 1975.
311. Burton, D. A., Chin, A., Weinberg, P. M., Pigott, J. D.: Identification of cor triatriatum dexter by two-dimensional echocardiography. Am. J. Cardiol. *59*:409, 1987.
312. Smith, I. O., Silverman, N. H., Oldershaw, P., et al.: Cor triatriatum sinistrum: Diagnostic features on cross-sectional echocardiography. Br. Heart J. *51*:211, 1984.
313. Oglietti, J., Cooley, D. A., Izquierdo, J. P., et al.: Cor triatriatum: Operative results in 25 patients. Ann. Thorac. Surg. *35*:415, 1983.
314. Ruckman, R. N., and Van Praagh, R.: Anatomic types of congenital mitral stenosis: Report of 49 autopsy cases with consideration of diagnosis and surgical implications. Am. J. Cardiol. *42*:592, 1978.
315. Parr, G. V. S., Fripp, R. A., Whitman, V., et al.: Anomalous mitral arcade: Echocardiographic and angiographic reception. Pediatr. Cardiol. *4*:163, 1983.
316. Brandi-Pifano, S., Palacios, I. F., Block, P. C., et al.: Echophonocardiography in patients undergoing percutaneous mitral balloon valvotomy (PMV): The learning curve of PMV. Am. Heart J. *117*:25, 1989.
317. Ortiz, E., and Somerville, J.: Assessment by cross-sectional echocardiography of surgical mitral valve disease in children and adolescents. Br. Heart J. *56*:267, 1986.
318. Mazzera, E., Corno, A., Di Donato, R., et al.: Surgical bypass of the systemic atrioventricular valve in children by means of a valve conduit. J. Thorac. Cardiovasc. Surg. *96*:321, 1988.
319. Stellin, G., Mazzucco, A., Bortolotti, U., et al.: Repair of congenital malformations of the mitral valve in children. Tex. Heart Inst. J. *16*:102, 1989.
320. Zweng, T. N., Bluett, M. K., Mosca, R., et al.: Mitral valve replacement in the first 5 years of life. Ann. Thorac. Surg. *47*:720, 1989.
321. Alday, L. E., and Juaneda, E.: Percutaneous balloon dilation in congenital mitral stenosis. Br. Heart J. *57*:479, 1987.
322. Perloff, J. K.: Evolving concepts of mitral valve prolapse. N. Engl. J. Med. *307*:369, 1982.
323. Carpentier, A.: Congenital malformations of the mitral valve. *In* Stark, J., and deLeval, M. (eds.): Surgery for Congenital Heart Defects. New York, Grune and Stratton, Inc., 1983, p. 467.
324. Carpentier, A., Branchini, B., Cour, J. C., et al.: Congenital malformations of the mitral valve in children: Pathology and surgical treatment. J. Thorac. Cardiovasc. Surg. *72*:854, 1976.
325. Lamberti, J. J., Gensen, T. S., Grehl, T. M., et al.: Late reoperation for systemic atrioventricular valve regurgitation after repair of congenital heart defects. Ann. Thorac. Surg. *47*:517, 1989.
326. White, R. I., Jr., Mitchell, S. E., Barth, K. H., et al.: Angioarchitecture of pulmonary arteriovenous malformations: An important consideration before embolotherapy. Am. J. Radiol. *140*:681, 1983.
327. Gonzalez, V. R., Pieper, W. M., and Kap-herr, S. H.: Pulmonary arteriovenous fistula in childhood. Z. Kinderchir. *40*:101, 1985.
328. Gomes, A. S., Busuttil, R. W., Baker, J. D., et al.: Congenital arteriovenous malformations: The role of transcatheter arterial embolization. Arch. Surg. *118*:817, 1983.
329. D'Cruz, I. A., Agustssou, M. M., Bicoff, J. P., et al.: Stenotic lesions of the pulmonary arteries. Clinical hemodynamic findings in 84 cases. Am. J. Cardiol. *13*:441, 1964.
330. Venables, A. W.: The syndrome of pulmonary stenosis complicating maternal rubella. Br. Heart J. *27*:49, 1965.
331. Danilowicz, D. A., Rudolph, A. M., Hoffman, J. I. E., and Heymann, M. A.: Physiologic pressure differences between main and branch pulmonary arteries in infants. Circulation *45*:410, 1972.
332. Eldredge, W. J., Tingelstad, J. B., Robertson, L. W., et al.: Observations on the natural history of pulmonary artery coarctation. Circulation *45*:404, 1972.
333. Kan, J. S., Marvin, W. J., Jr., Bass, J. L., et al.: Balloon angioplasty-branch pulmonary artery stenosis: Results from the valvuloplasty and angioplasty of congenital anomalies registry. Am. J. Cardiol. *65*:798, 1990.
334. Mullins, C. E., O'Laughlin, M. P., Vick, W., III, et al.: Implantation of balloon-expandable intravascular grafts by catheterization in pulmonary arteries and systemic veins. Circulation *77*:188, 1988.
335. Koretzky, E., Moller, J. H., Korns, M. E., et al.: Congenital pulmonary stenosis resulting from dysplasia of valve. Circulation *40*:43, 1969.
336. Aldousany, A. W., DiSessa, T. G., Dubois, R., et al.: Doppler estimation of pressure gradient in pulmonary stenosis: Maximal instantaneous vs peak-to-peak, vs mean catheter gradient. Pediatr. Cardiol. *10*:145, 1989.
337. Frantz, E. G., and Silverman, N. H.: Doppler ultrasound evaluation of valvular pulmonary stenosis from multiple transducer positions in children requiring pulmonary valvuloplasty. Am. J. Cardiol. *61*:844, 1988.
338. Srinivasan, V., Konyer, A., Broda, J. J., and Subramanian, S.: Critical pulmonary stenosis in infants less than three months of age: A reappraisal of closed transventricular pulmonary valvotomy. Ann. Thorac. Surg. *34*:46, 1982.
339. Rao, P. S.: Balloon pulmonary valvuloplasty: A review. Clin. Cardiol. *12*:55, 1989.
340. Radtke, W., and Lock, J.: Balloon dilation. Pediatr. Clin. North Am. *37*:193, 1990.
341. Stanger, P., Cassidy, S. C., Girod, D. A., et al.: Balloon pulmonary valvuloplasty: Results of the valvuloplasty and angioplasty of congenital anomalies registry. Am. J. Cardiol. *65*:775, 1990.
342. Marantz, P. M., Huhta, J. C., Mullins, C. E., et al.: Results of balloon valvuloplasty in typical and dysplastic pulmonary valve stenosis: Doppler echocardiographic follow up. J. Am. Coll. Cardiol. *12*:476, 1988.
343. Lange, P. E., Onnasch, G. W., and Heintzen, P. H.: Valvular pulmonary stenosis. Natural history and right ventricular function in infants and children. Eur. Heart J. *6*:706, 1985.
344. Mody, M. R.: The natural history of uncomplicated valvular pulmonary stenosis. Am. Heart J. *90*:317, 1975.
345. Ellison, R. C., and Miettinen, O. S.: Interpretation of rSR′ in pulmonic stenosis. Am. Heart J. *88*:7, 1974.
346. Krabill, K. A., Wang, Y., Einzig, S., and Moller, J. H.: Rest and exercise hemodynamics in pulmonary stenosis: Comparison of children and adults. Am. J. Cardiol. *56*:360, 1985.
347. Danilowicz, D., Hoffman, J. I. E., and Rudolph, A. M.: Serial studies of pulmonary stenosis in infancy and childhood. Br. Heart J. *37*:808, 1975.

348. Wennevold, A., and Jacobsen, J. R.: Natural history of valvular pulmonary stenosis in children below the age of two years: Long-term follow-up with serial heart catheterizations. Eur. J. Cardiol. *8*:371, 1978.
349. Kopecky, S. L., Gersh, B. J., McGoon, M. D., et al.: Long-term outcome of patients undergoing surgical repair of isolated pulmonary valve stenosis: Follow up at 20–30 years. Circulation *78*:1150, 1988.
349a. Laks, H., and Billingsley, A. M.: Advances in the treatment of pulmonary atresia with intact ventricular septum: Palliative and definitive repair. Cardiol. Clin. *7*:387, 1989.
350. Freedom, R. M., Wilson, G., Trusler, G., et al.: Pulmonary atresia and intact ventricular septum: A review of the anatomy, myocardium and factors influencing right ventricular growth and guidelines for surgical intervention. Scand. J. Thorac. Cardiovasc. Surg. *17*:1, 1983.
351. Van de Wal, H.J.C.M., Smith, A., Becker, A. E., et al.: Morphology of pulmonary atresia with intact ventricular septum with patients dying after operation. Ann. Thorac. Surg. *50*:98, 1990.
352. O'Connor, W. N., Stahr, B. J., Cottrill, C. M., et al.: Ventriculocoronary connections in hypoplastic right heart syndrome: Autopsy serial section study of six cases. J. Am. Coll. Cardiol. *11*:1061, 1988.
353. Trowitzsch, E., Colan, S. D., and Sanders, S. P.: Two-dimensional echocardiographic evaluation of right ventricular size and function in newborns with severe right ventricular outflow tract obstruction. J. Am. Coll. Cardiol. *6*:388, 1985.
354. Leung, M. P., Mok, C. K., and Hui, P. W.: Echocardiographic assessment of neonates with pulmonary atresia and intact ventricular septum. J. Am. Coll. Cardiol. *12*:719, 1988.
355. Milliken, J. C., Laks, H., Hellenbrand, W., et al.: Early and late results in the treatment of patients with pulmonary atresia and intact ventricular septum. Circulation *72*:II-61, 1985.
356. Danilowicz, D., and Ishmael, R.: Anomalous right ventricular muscle bundle: Clinical pitfalls and extracardiac anomalies. Clin. Cardiol. *4*:146, 1981.
357. Kveselis, D., Rosenthal, A., Ferguson, P., et al.: Long-term prognosis after repair of double-chamber right ventricle with ventricular septal defect. Am. J. Cardiol. *54*:1292, 1984.
358. Ford, D. K., Bollaboy, C. A., Derkac, W. M., et al.: Transatrial repair of double-chambered right ventricle. Ann. Thorac. Surg. *46*:412, 1988.
359. Pinsky, W. W., and Arciniegas, E.: Tetralogy of Fallot. Pediatr. Clin. North Am. *37*:179, 1990.
360. Perloff, J. K., Friedman, W. F., Laks, H., and Child, J. S.: From the cyanotic infant to the acyanotic adult—the odyssey of the blue baby. UCLA School of Medicine Interdisciplinary Conference. West. J. Med. *139*:673, 1983.
361. Soto, B., and McConnell, M. E.: Tetralogy of Fallot: Angiographic and pathological correlation. Semin. Thorac. Cardiovasc. Surg. *2*:12, 1990.
362. Barbero-Marcial, M., and Jatene, A. D.: Surgical management of the anomalies of the pulmonary arteries in the tetralogy of Fallot with pulmonary atresia. Semin. Thorac. Cardiovasc. Surg. *2*:93, 1990.
363. Liao, P. K., Edwards, W. D., Julsrud, P. R., et al.: Pulmonary blood supply in patients with pulmonary atresia and ventricular septal defect. J. Am. Coll. Cardiol. *6*:1343, 1985.
364. Johnson, R. J., Sauer, U., Buhlmeyer, K., and Haworth, S. G.: Hypoplasia of the intrapulmonary arteries in children with right ventricular overflow tract obstruction, ventricular septal defect, and major aortopulmonary collateral arteries. Pediatr. Cardiol. *6*:137, 1985.
365. Smyllie, J. H., Sutherland, G. R., and Keeton, B. R.: The value of Doppler color-flow mapping in determining pulmonary blood supply in infants with pulmonary atresia with ventricular septal defect. J. Am. Coll. Cardiol. *14*:1759, 1989.
366. Fellows, K. E., Freed, M. D., Keane, J. F., et al.: Results of routine preoperative coronary angiography and tetralogy of Fallot. Circulation *51*:561, 1977.
366a. Kirklin, J. K., Kirklin, J. W., and Pacifico, A. D.: Transannular outflow tract patching for tetralogy: Indications and results. Semin. Thorac. Cardiovasc. Surg. *2*:61, 1990.
367. Jureidini, S. B., Appleton, R. S., and Nouri, S.: Detection of coronary artery abnormalities in tetralogy of Fallot by two-dimensional echocardiography. J. Am. Coll. Cardiol. *14*:960, 1989.
367a. Castaneda, A. R.: Classical repair of tetralogy of Fallot: Timing, technique, and results. Semin. Thorac. Cardiovasc. Surg. *2*:70, 1990.
368. Pacifico, A. D., Kirklin, J. K., Colvin, E. V., et al.: Transatrial-transpulmonary repair of tetralogy of Fallot. Semin. Thorac. Cardiovasc. Surg. *2*:76, 1990.
369. Morgan, B. C., Guntheroth, W. G., Blume, R. S., and Fyler, D. C.: A clinical profile of paroxysmal hyperpnea in cyanotic congenital heart disease. Circulation *31*:66, 1965.
369a. Hammon, J. W., Jr., Henry, C. L., Jr., Merrill, W. H., et al.: Tetralogy of Fallot: Selective surgical management to minimize operative mortality. Ann. Thorac. Surg. *40*:280, 1985.
370. Shaddy, R. E., Viney, J., Judd, V. E., and McGough, E. C.: Continuous intravenous phenylephrine infusion for treatment of hypoxemic spells in tetralogy of Fallot. J. Pediatr. *114*:468, 1989.
370a. Rosankranz, E. R.: Modified Blalock-Taussig shunts in the treatment of tetralogy of Fallot. Semin. Thorac. Cardiovasc. Surg. *2*:27, 1990.
371. McConnell, M. E.: Echocardiography in classical tetralogy of Fallot. Semin. Thorac. Cardiovasc. Surg. *2*:2, 1990.
371a. Pacifico, A. D., Kirklin, J. K., Colvin, E. V., et al.: Tetralogy of Fallot: Late results and reoperations. Semin. Thorac. Cardiovasc. Surg. *2*:108, 1990.
372. Qureshi, S. A., Kirk, C. R., Lamb, R. K., et al.: Balloon dilatation of the pulmonary valve in the first year of life in patients with tetralogy of Fallot: A preliminary study. Br. Heart J. *60*:232, 1988.
373. Naito, Y., Fujita, T., Yagihara, T., et al.: Usefulness of left ventricular volume in assessing tetralogy of Fallot for total correction. Am. J. Cardiol. *56*:356, 1985.
374. Garson, A., Jr., Randall, D. C., Gillette, P. C., et al.: Prevention of sudden death after repair of tetralogy of Fallot: Treatment of ventricular arrhythmias. J. Am. Coll. Cardiol. *6*:221, 1985.
375. Zahka, K. G., Horneffer, P. J., Rowe, S. A., et al.: Long-term valvular function after total repair of tetralogy of Fallot: Relation to ventricular arrhythmias. Circulation *78*(Suppl. III):14, 1988.
376. Chandar, J. S., Wolff, G. S., Garson, A., Jr., et al.: Ventricular arrhythmias in postoperative tetralogy of Fallot. Am. J. Cardiol. *65*:655, 1990.
376a. Vaksmann, G., Fournier, A., Davignon, A., et al.: Frequency and prognosis of arrhythmias after operative "correction" of tetralogy of Fallot. Am. J. Cardiol. *66*:346, 1990.
377. Oku, H., Shirotani, H., Sunakawa, A., and Yokoyama, T.: Postoperative long-term results in total correction of tetralogy of Fallot: Hemodynamics and cardiac function. Ann. Thorac. Surg. *41*:413, 1986.
378. Rosenthal, A., Behrendt, D., Sloan, H., et al.: Long-term prognosis (15 to 26 years) after repair of tetralogy of Fallot: I. Survival and symptomatic status. Ann. Thorac. Surg. *38*:151, 1984.
379. Sandor, G.G.S., Patterson, M.W.H., Tipple, M., et al.: Left ventricular systolic and diastolic function after total correction of tetralogy of Fallot. Am. J. Cardiol. *60*:1148, 1987.
380. Ilbawi, M. N., Fedorchik, J., Muster, A. J., et al.: Surgical approach to severely symptomatic newborn infants with tetralogy of Fallot and absent pulmonary valve. J. Thorac. Cardiovasc. Surg. *91*:584, 1986.
381. Fischer, D. R., Neches, W. H., Beerman, L. B., et al.: Tetralogy of Fallot with absent pulmonic valve: Analysis of 17 patients. Am. J. Cardiol. *53*:1433, 1984.
382. Emmanouilides, G. C., Thanopoulos, B., Siassi, B., and Fishbein, M: Agenesis of ductus arteriosus associated with the syndrome of tetralogy of Fallot and absent pulmonary valve. Am. J. Cardiol. *37*:403, 1976.
383. Dunnigan, A., Oldham, H. N., and Benson, D. W.: Absent pulmonary valve syndrome in infancy: Surgery reconsidered. Am. J. Cardiol. *48*:117, 1981.
384. Kron, I. L., Johnson, A. M., Carpenter, M. A., et al.: Treatment of absent pulmonary valve syndrome with homograft. Ann. Thorac. Surg. *46*:579, 1988.
385. Rigby, M. L., Carvalho, J. S., Anderson, R. H., and Redington, A.: The investigation and diagnosis of tricuspid atresia. Int. J. Cardiol. *27*:1, 1990.
386. Wenink, A.C.J., and Ottenkamp, J.: Tricuspid atresia. Microscopic findings in relation to "absence" of the atrioventriculaar connection. Int. J. Cardiol. *16*:57, 1987.
387. Sade, R. M., and Fyfe, D. A.: Tricuspid atresia: Current concepts in diagnosis and treatment. Pediatr. Clin. North Am. *7*:151, 1990.
388. Fesslova, V., Hunter, S., Stark, J., and Taylor, J.F.N.: Long-term clinical outcome of patients with tricuspid atresia. I. "Natural history." J. Cardiovasc. Surg. *30*:262, 1989.
389. Fontan, F., Deville, C., Quaegebeur, J., et al.: Repair of tricuspid atresia in 100 patients. J. Thorac. Cardiovasc. Surg. *85*:647, 1983.
390. Fontan, F., Kirklin, J. W., Fernandez, G., et al.: Outcome after a "perfect" Fontan operation. Circulation 81:1520, 1990.
390a. Nakazawa, M., Katayama, H., Imai, Y., et al.: A quantitative analysis of hemodynamic effects of the right ventricle included in the circulation of the Fontan procedure. Circulation *83*:822, 1991.
390b. Mayer, J. E., Jr., Bridges, N. D., Lock, J. E., et al.: Factors associated with improved survival after modified Fontan operations. J. Am. Coll. Cardiol. *17*:33a, 1991.
391. Weber, H. S., Hellenbrand, W. E., Kleinman, C. S., et al.: Predictors of rhythm disturbances and subsequent morbidity after the Fontan operation. Am. J. Cardiol. *64*:762, 1989.
392. Mair, D. D., Hagler, D. J., Puga, F. J., et al.: Fontan operation in 176 patients with tricuspid atresia. Circulation *82*(Suppl. IV): 164, 1990.
393. Sampson, C., Martinez, J., Rees, S., et al.: Evaluation of Fontan's operation by magnetic resonance imaging. Am. J. Cardiol. *65*:819, 1990.
394. Matsushita, T., Matsuda, H., Ogawa, M., and Yabuuchi, H.: Assessment of the intrapulmonary ventilation-perfusion distribution after the Fontan procedure for complex cardiac anomalies: Relation to pulmonary hemodynamics. J. Am. Coll. Cardiol. *15*:842, 1990.
395. Fernandez, G., Costa, F., Fontan, F., et al.: Prevalence of reoperation for pathway obstruction after Fontan operation. Ann. Thorac. Surg. *48*:654, 1989.
396. Zellers, T. M., Driscoll, D. J., Mottram, C. D., et al.: Exercise tolerance and cardiorespiratory response to exercise before and after the Fontan operation. Mayo Clin. Proc. *64*:1489, 1989.
397. Rhodes, J., Garofano, R. P., Bowman, F. O., Jr., et al.: Effect of right ventricular anatomy on the cardiopulmonary response to exercise. Implications for the Fontan procedure. Circulation *81*:1811, 1990.
398. Gussenhoven, E. J., Stewart, P. A., Becker, A. E., et al.: "Offsetting" of the septal tricuspid leaflet in normal hearts and in hearts with Ebstein's anomaly. Am. J. Cardiol. *53*:172, 1984.
399. Zalzstein, E., Koran, G., Einarson, T., and Freedom, R. M.: A case control study on the association between first trimester exposure to lithium and Ebstein's anomaly. Am. J. Cardiol. *65*:817, 1990.
400. Guiliani, E. R., Fuster, V., Brandenberg, R. O., and Mair, D. D.: Ebstein's anomaly; The clinical features and natural history of Ebstein's anomaly of the tricuspid valve. Mayo Clin. Proc. *54*:163, 1979.
401. Boucek, R. J., Jr., Graham, T. P., Jr., Morgan J. P., et al.: Spontaneous resolution of massive congenital tricuspid insufficiency. Circulation *54*:795, 1976.

402. Roberson, D. A., and Silverman, N. H.: Ebstein's anomaly: Echocardiographic and clinical features in the fetus and neonate. J. Am. Coll. Cardiol. *14*:1300, 1989.
403. Freedom, R. M., Culham, J.A.G., Olley, P. M., et al.: The differentiation of functional from organic pulmonary atresia: The role of aortography. Am. J. Cardiol. *41*:914, 1978.
404. Kastor, J. A., Goldreier, B. N., Josephson, M. E., et al.: Electrophysiologic characteristics of Ebstein's anomaly of the tricuspid valve. Circulation *52*:987, 1975.
405. Gussenhoven, W. J., Spitaels, S.E.C., Bom, N., and Becker, A. E.: Echocardiographic criteria for Ebstein's anomaly of tricuspid valve. Br. Heart J. *43*:31, 1980.
406. Hirschklau, M. J., Sahn, D. J., Hagan, A. D., et al.: Cross-sectional echocardiographic features of Ebstein's anomaly of the tricuspid valve. Am. J. Cardiol. *40*:400, 1977.
407. Driscoll, D. J., Mottram, C. D., and Danielson, G. K.: Spectrum of exercise intolerance in 45 patients with Ebstein's anomaly and observations on exercise tolerance in 11 patients after surgical repair. J. Am. Coll. Cardiol. *11*:831, 1988.
408. Pasque, M., Williams, W. G., Coles, G. J., et al.: Tricuspid valve replacement in children. Ann. Thorac. Surg. *44*:164, 1987.
409. Carpentier, A., Chauvaud, S., Mace, L., et al.: A new reconstructive operation for Ebstein's anomaly of the tricuspid valve. J. Thorac. Cardiovasc. Surg. *96*:92, 1988.
409a. Quaegebeur, J. M., Sreeram, N., Fraser, A. G., et al.: Surgery for Ebstein's Anomaly: The clinical and echocardiographic evaluation of a new technique. J. Am. Coll. Cardiol. *17*:722, 1991.
410. Paul, M. H.: D-Transposition of great arteries. *In* Adams, F. H., and Emmanouilides, G. C. (eds.): Moss' Heart Disease in Infants, Children and Adolescents, 4th ed. Baltimore, Williams and Wilkins, 1989, p. 371.
410a. Anderson, R. H., Henry, G. W., and Becker, A. E.: Morphologic aspects of complete transposition. Cardiol. Young *1*:41, 1991.
411. Mair, D. D., and Ritter, D. G.: Factors influencing systemic arterial oxygen saturation in complete transposition of the great arteries. Am. J. Cardiol. *31*:742, 1973.
412. Lakier, J. B., Stanger, P., Heymann, M. A., et al.: Early onset of pulmonary vascular obstruction in patients with aortopulmonary transposition and intact ventricular septum. Circulation *51*:875, 1975.
413. Aziz, K. U., Paul, M. H., and Rowe, R. D.: Bronchopulmonary circulation in D-transposition of the great arteries: Possible role and genesis of accelerated pulmonary vascular disease. Am. J. Cardiol. *39*:432, 1977.
414. Muster, A. J., Paul, M. H., Van Grondell, E. A., and Conway, J. J.: Asymmetric distribution of the pulmonary blood flow between the right and left lungs in D-transposition of the great arteries. Am. J. Cardiol. *38*:352, 1976.
415. Sansa, M., Tonkin, I. L., Bargeron, L. M., and Elliott, L. P.: Left ventricular outflow tract obstruction in transposition of the great arteries. Am. J. Cardiol. *44*:88, 1979.
416. Chiu, I., Anderson, R. H., Macartney, F. J., et al.: Morphologic features of an intact ventricular septum susceptible to subpulmonary obstruction in complete transposition. Am. J. Cardiol. *53*:1633, 1984.
417. Waldman, J. D., Paul, M. H., Newfeld, E. A., et al.: Transposition of the great arteries with intact ventricular septum and patent ductus arteriosus. Am. J. Cardiol. *39*:232, 1977.
418. Tonkin, I. L., Kelley, M. J., Bream, P. R., and Elliott, L. P.: The frontal chest film as a method of suspecting transposition complexes. Circulation *53*:1016, 1976.
419. Chin, A. J., Yeager, S. B., Sanders, S. P., et al.: Accuracy of prospective two-dimensional echocardiographic evaluation of left ventricular outflow tract in complete transposition of the great arteries. Am. J. Cardiol. *55*:759, 1985.
420. Deal, B. J., Chin, A. J., Sanders, S. P., et al.: Subxiphoid two-dimensional echocardiographic identification of tricuspid valve abnormalities in transposition of the great arteries with ventricular septal defect. Am. J. Cardiol. *55*:1146, 1985.
421. Marino, B., de Simone, G., Pasquini, L., et al.: Complete transposition of the great arteries: Visualization of left and right outflow tract obstruction by oblique subcostal two-dimensional echocardiography. Am. J. Cardiol. *55*:1140, 1985.
422. Chin, A. J., Yeager, S. B., Sanders, S. P., et al.: Accuracy of prospective two-dimensional echocardiographic evaluation of left ventricular outflow tract in complete transposition of the great arteries. Am. J. Cardiol. *55*:759, 1985.
422a. Rigby, M. L., and Chan, K-Y: The diagnostic evaluation of patients with complete transposition. Cardiol. Young *1*:26, 1991.
423. DiSessa, T. G., Childs, W., Ti, C. C., and Friedman, W. F.: Systolic anterior motion of the mitral valve in a one day old infant with transposition of the great vessels. J. Clin. Ultrasound *6*:186, 1978.
424. Lin, A. E., Di Sessa, T. G., Williams, R. G., et al.: Balloon and blade atrial septostomy facilitated by two-dimensional echocardiography. Am. J. Cardiol. *57*:273, 1986.
425. Moene, R. J., Oppenheimer-Dekker, A., Wenink, A.C.G., et al.: Morphology of ventricular septal defect in complete transposition of the great arteries. Am. J. Cardiol. *55*:1566, 1985.
426. Pasquini, L., Sanders, S. P., Parness, I. A., and Colan, S. D.: Diagnosis of coronary artery anatomy by two-dimensional echocardiography in patients with transposition of the great arteries. Circulation *75*:557, 1987.
427. Oberhoffer, R. M., Ho, S. Y., and Anderson, R. H.: Coronary artery diameters in the heart with complete transposition of the great vessels. J. Am. Coll. Cardiol. *15*:1433, 1990.
428. Kirklin, J. W., Colvin, E. V., McConnell, M. E., and Bargeron, L. M.: Complete transposition of the great arteries: Treatment in the current era. Pediatr. Clin. North Am. *37*:171, 1990.
428a. Kirklin, J. W.: The surgical repair for complete transposition. Cardiol. Young *1*:13, 1991.
428b. Oelert, H.: Modification of the Mustard operation for surgical treatment of complete transposition by creating a confluence of the caval veins. Cardiol. Young *1*:71, 1991.
428c. Merrill, W. H., Stewart, J. R., Hammon, J. W., Jr., et al: The Senning operation for complete transposition: Mid-term physiologic, electrophysiologic, and functional results. Cardiol. Young *1*:80, 1991.
429. Wong, K. Y., Venables, A. W., Kelly, M. J., and Kalff, V.: Longitudinal study of ventricular function after the Mustard operation for transposition of the great arteries: A long-term follow up. Br. Heart J. *60*:316, 1988.
430. Vetter, V. L., Tanner, C. S., and Horowitz, L. N.: Inducible atrial flutter after the Mustard repair of complete transposition of the great arteries. Am. J. Cardiol. *61*:428, 1988.
431. Duster, M. C., Bink-Boelkens, M.T.E., Wampler, D., et al.: Long-term follow-up of dysrhythmias following the Mustard procedure. Am. Heart J. *109*:1323, 1985.
431a. Deanfield, J. E., Cullen, S., and Gewillig, M.: Arrhythmias after surgery for complete transposition: Do they matter? Cardiol. Young *1*:91, 1991.
432. Kato, H., Nakano, S., Matsuda, H., et al.: Right ventricular myocardial function after atrial switch operation for transposition of the great arteries. Am. J. Cardiol. *63*:226, 1989.
433. George, B. L., Laks, H., Klitzner, T. S., et al.: Results of the Senning procedure in infants with simple and complex transposition of the great arteries. Am. J. Cardiol. *59*:426, 1987.
434. Reybrouck, T., Dumoulin, M., and Van Der Hauwaert, L. G.: Cardiorespiratory exercise testing after venous switch operation in children with complete transposition of great arteries. Am. J. Cardiol. *61*:861, 1988.
435. Ensing, G. J., Heise, C. T., and Driscoll, D. J.: Cardiovascular response to exercise after the Mustard operation for simple and complex transposition of great arteries. Am. J. Cardiol. *62*:617, 1988.
436. Musewe, N. N., Reisman, J., Benson, L. M., et al.: Cardiopulmonary adaptation at rest and during exercise 10 years after Mustard atrial repair for transposition of the great arteries. Circulation *77*:1055, 1988.
437. Turina, M. I., Siebenmann, R., Von Segesser, L., et al.: Late functional deterioration after atrial correction for transposition of the great arteries. Circulation *80*(Suppl. I):162, 1989.
438. Benson, L. N., Bonet, J., Olley, P. M., et al.: Assessment of right ventricular function during supine bicycle exercise after Mustard's operation. Circulation *65*:1052, 1982.
439. Danford, D. A.: Factors influencing choice of procedure in transposition of the great arteries: A decision-analysis approach. J. Am. Coll. Cardiol. *16*:471, 1990.
440. Corno, A., George, B., Pearl, J., and Laks, H.: Surgical options for complex transposition of the great arteries. J. Am. Coll. Cardiol. *14*:742, 1989.
441. Bove, E. L., Beekman, R. H., Snider, A. R., et al.: Arterial repair for transposition of the great arteries and large ventricular septal defect in early infancy. Circulation *78*(Suppl. III):26, 1988.
442. Di Donato, R. M., Wernofsky, G., Walsh, E. P., et al.: Results of the arterial switch operation for transposition of the great arteries with ventricular septal defect. Surgical considerations and mid-term follow up data. Circulation *80*:1689, 1989.
443. Castaneda, A. R., Mayer, J. E., Jonas, R. A., et al.: Transposition of the great arteries: The arterial switch operation. Cardiol. Clin. *7*:369, 1989.
443a. Planche, C., Serraf, A., Lacour-Gayet, F., et al.: Anatomic correction of complete transposition with ventricular septal defect in neonates: Experience with 42 consecutive cases. Cardiol Young *1*:101, 1991.
444. Colan, S. D., Trowitz, S.C.H.E., Wernvosky, G., et al.: Myocardial performance after arterial switch operation for transposition of the great arteries with intact ventricular septum. Circulation *78*:132, 1988.
445. Sandor, G.S.S., Freedom, R. M., Williams, W. G., et al.: Left ventricular systolic and diastolic function after two-stage anatomic correction of transposition of the great arteries. Am. Heart J. *115*:1257, 1988.
446. Gleason, M. M., Chin, A., Andrews, B. A., et al.: Two-dimensional and Doppler echocardiographic assessment of neonatal arterial repair for transposition of the great arteries. J. Am. Coll. Cardiol. *13*:1320, 1989.
447. Martin, M. M., Snider, R., Bove, E. L., et al.: Two-dimensional and Doppler echocardiographic evaluation after arterial switch repair in infancy for complete transposition of the great arteries. Am. J. Cardiol. *63*:332, 1989.
448. Wernovsky, G., Hougen, T. J., Walsh, E. P., et al.: Mid-term results after the arterial switch operation for transposition of the great arteries with intact ventricular septum: Clinical, hemodynamic, echocardiographic, and electrophysiologic data. Circulation *77*:1333, 1988.
449. Villafane, J., White, S., Elbl, F., et al.: An electrocardiographic mid-term follow up study after anatomic repair of transposition of the great arteries. Am. J. Cardiol. *66*:350, 1990.
450. Martin, R. P., Ettedgui, J. A., Qureshi, S. A., et al.: A quantitative evaluation of aortic regurgitation after anatomic correction of transposition of the great arteries. J. Am. Coll. Cardiol. *12*:1281, 1988.
450a. Redington, A. N.: Functional assessment of the heart after corrective surgery for complete transposition. Cardiol. Young *1*:84, 1991.
451. Jonas, R. A., Giglia, T. M., Sanders, S. P., et al.: Rapid, two-stage arterial switch for transposition of the great arteries and intact ventricular septum beyond the neonatal period. Circulation *80*(Suppl. I):203, 1989.
452. Corno, A. F., Parisi, F., Marino, B., et al.: Palliative Mustard operation: An expanded horizon. Eur. J. Cardiothorac. Surg. *1*:144, 1987.

453. Colli, A. M., De Leval, M., and Somerville, J.: Anatomically corrected malposition of the great arteries. Am. J. Cardiol. *55*:1367, 1985.
454. Kirklin, J. W., Pacifico, A. D., Bargeron, L. M., Jr., and Soto, B.: Cardiac repair and anatomically corrected malposition of the great arteries. Circulation *48*:153, 1973.
455. Berry, W. B., Roberts, W. C., Morrow, A. G., and Braunwald, E.: Corrected transposition of the aorta and pulmonary trunk: Clinical, hemodynamic, and pathologic findings. Am. J. Med. *36*:35, 1964.
456. Freedberg, D. Z., and Nadas, A. S.: Clinical profile of patients with congenital corrected transposition of the great arteries. N. Engl. J. Med. *282*:1053, 1970.
457. Allwork, S. P., Bentall, H. H., Becker, A. E., et al.: Congenitally corrected transposition of the great arteries. Morphologic study of 32 cases. Am. J. Cardiol. *38*:910, 1976.
458. Bjarke, B. B., and Kidd, B.S.L.: Congenitally corrected transposition of the great arteries: A clinical study of 101 cases. Acta Paediatr. Scand. *65*:153, 1976.
459. Huhta, J. C., Danielson, G. K., Ritter, D. G., and Ilstrup, D. M.: Survival in atrioventricular discordance. Pediatr. Cardiol. *6*:57, 1985.
459a. Dimas, A. P., Moodie, D. S., Strba, R., and Gill, C. C.: Long-term function of the morphologic right ventricle in adult patients with corrected transposition of the great arteries. Am. Heart J. *118*:526, 1989.
460. Peterson, R. J., Franch, R. H., Fajman, W. A., and Jones, R. H.: Comparison of cardiac function in surgically corrected and congenitally corrected transposition of the great arteries. J. Thorac. Cardiovasc. Surg. *96*:227, 1988.
461. Benson, L. N., Burns, R., Schwaiger, M., et al.: Radionuclide angiographic evaluation of ventricular function in isolated congenitally corrected transposition of the great arteries. Am. J. Cardiol. *58*:319, 1986.
462. Waldo, A. L., Pacifico, A. D., Bargeron, L. M., Jr., et al.: Electrophysiological delineation of specialized AV conduction system in patients with corrected transposition of the great vessels and ventricular septal defect. Circulation *52*:435, 1975.
463. Bharati, B., Rosen, K., Steinfield, L., et al.: The anatomic substrate for pre-excitation in corrected transposition. Circulation *62*:831, 1980.
464. Meissner, M. D., Panidis, I. P., Eshaghpour, E., et al.: Corrected transposition of the great arteries: Evaluation by two-dimensional and Doppler echocardiography. Am. Heart J. *111*:599, 1986.
465. Freedom, R. M., Harrington, D. P., and White, R. I., Jr.: The differential diagnosis of levotransposed or malposed aorta: An angiocardiographic study. Circulation *50*:1040, 1974.
466. Russo, P., Danielson, G. K., and Driscoll, D. J.: Transaortic closure of ventricular septal defect in patients with corrected transposition with pulmonary stenosis or atresia. Circulation *76*(Suppl. III):88, 1987.
467. McGrath, L. B., Kirklin, J. W., Blackstone, E. H., et al.: Death and other events after cardiac repair in discordant atrioventricular connection. J. Thorac. Cardiovasc. Surg. *90*:711, 1985.
468. Piccoli, G., Pacifico, A. D., Kirklin, J. W., et al.: Changing results and concepts in the surgical treatment of double-outlet right ventricle: Analysis of 137 operations in 126 patients. Am. J. Cardiol. *52*:549, 1983.
469. Hagler, D. J., Ritter, D. G., and Puga, F. J.: Double-outlet right ventricle. *In* Adams, F. H., and Emmanoulides, G. C. (eds.): Moss' Heart Disease in Infants, Children and Adolescents. 4th ed. Baltimore, Williams and Wilkins, 1989, p. 442.
470. Bostrom, M.P.G., and Hutchins, G. M.: Arrested rotation of the outflow tract may explain double-outlet right ventricle. Circulation *77*:1258, 1988.
471. Sondheimer, H. M., Freedom, R. M., and Olley, P. M.: Double outlet right ventricle: Clinical spectrum and prognosis. Am. J. Cardiol. *39*:709, 1977.
472. Goitein, K. J., Neches, W. H., Park, S. C., et al.: Electrocardiogram in double chamber right ventricle. Am. J. Cardiol. *45*:604, 1980.
473. Macartney, F. J., Rigby, M. L., Anderson, R. H., et al.: Double outlet right ventricle. Cross-sectional echocardiographic findings, their anatomical explanation and surgical relevance. Br. Heart J. *52*:164, 1984.
474. Sridaromont, S., Ritter, D. G., Feldt, R. H., et al.: Double outlet right ventricle: Anatomic and angiocardiographic correlations. Mayo Clin. Proc. *53*:555, 1978.
475. Kirklin, J. W., Pacifico, A. D., Blackstone, E. H., et al.: Current risks and protocols for surgery for double outlet right ventricle: Derivation from an 18-year experience. J. Thorac. Cardiovasc. Surg. *92*:913, 1986.
476. Musumeci, F., Shumway, S., Lincoln, C., and Anderson, R. H.: Surgical treatment for double-outlet right ventricle at the Brompton Hospital, 1973 to 1986. J. Thorac. Cardiovasc. Surg. *96*:278, 1988.
477. Russo, P., Danielson, G. K., Puga, F. J., et al.: Modified Fontan procedure for biventricular hearts with complex forms of double-outlet right ventricle. Circulation *78*(Suppl. III):20, 1988.
478. Shen, W. K., Holmes, D. R., Jr., Porter, C. J., et al.: Sudden death after repair of double-outlet right ventricle. Circulation *81*:128, 1990.
479. Kanter, K., Anderson, R., Lincoln, C., et al.: Anatomic correction of double-outlet right ventricle and subpulmonary ventricular septal defect (the "Taussig-Bing" anomaly). Ann. Thorac. Surg. *41*:287, 1986.
480. Van Praagh, R., and Weinberg, P. M.: Double outlet left ventricle. *In* Adams, F. H., and Emmanouilides, G. C. (eds.): Moss' Heart Disease in Infants, Children and Adolescents. 3rd ed. Baltimore, Williams and Wilkins, 1983, p. 370.
481. Murphy, E. A., Gillis, D. A., and Sridhara, K. S.: Intraventricular repair of double outlet left ventricle. Ann. Thorac. Surg. *31*:364, 1981.
482. Gathman, G. E., and Nadas, A. S.: Total anomalous pulmonary venous connection: Clinical and physiologic observations in 75 pediatric patients. Circulation *42*:143, 1970.
483. Ward, K. E., Mullins, C. E., Huhta, J. C., et al.: Restrictive interatrial communication in total anomalous pulmonary venous connection. Am. J. Cardiol. *57*:1131, 1986.
484. Lucas, R. V., Jr., Lock, J. E., Tandon, R., and Edwards, J. E.: Gross and histologic anatomy of total anomalous pulmonary venous connections. Am. J. Cardiol. *62*:292, 1988.
485. Jonas, R. A., Smolinsky, A., Mayer, J. E., and Castaneda, A. R.: Obstructed pulmonary venous drainage with total anomalous pulmonary venous connection to the coronary sinus. Am. J. Cardiol. *59*:431, 1987.
486. Lincoln, C. R., Rigby, M. L., Marcanti, C., et al.: Surgical risk factors in total anomalous pulmonary venous connection. Am. J. Cardiol. *61*:608, 1988.
487. Elliott, L. P., and Edwards, J. E.: The problem of pulmonary venous obstruction in total anomalous pulmonary venous connection to the left innominate vein. Circulation *25*:913, 1962.
488. Newfeld, E. A., Wilson, A., Paul, M. H., and Reisch, J. S.: Pulmonary vascular disease in total anomalous pulmonary venous drainage. Circulation *61*:103, 1980.
489. Haworth, S. G., Reid, L., and Simon, G.: Radiological features of the heart and lungs in total anomalous pulmonary venous return in early infancy. Clin. Radiol. *28*:561, 1977.
490. Smallhorn, J. F., and Freedom, R. M.: Pulsed Doppler echocardiography in the preoperative evaluation of total anomalous pulmonary venous connection. J. Am. Coll. Cardiol. *8*:1413, 1986.
491. Chin, A. J., Sanders, S. P., Sherman, F., et al.: Accuracy of subcostal two-dimensional echocardiography in prospective diagnosis of total anomalous pulmonary venous connection. Am. Heart J. *113*:1153, 1987.
491a. Lamb, R. K., Qureshi, S. A., Wilkinson, J. L., et al.: Total anomalous pulmonary venous drainage. 17-year surgical experience. J. Thorac. Cardiovasc. Surg. *96*:368, 1988.
492. Corno, A., Giamberti, A., Carotti, A., et al.: Total anomalous pulmonary venous connection: Surgical repair with a double-patch technique. Ann. Thorac. Surg. *49*:492, 1990.
493. Phillips, S. J., Kongtahworn, C., Zeff, R. H., et al.: Correction of total anomalous pulmonary venous connection below the diaphragm. Ann. Thorac. Surg. *49*:734, 1990.
494. Matthew, R., Thilenius, O. G., Replogle, R. L., and Arcilla, R. A.: Cardiac function in total anomalous pulmonary venous return before and after surgery. Circulation *55*:361, 1977.
495. Van Meter, C., Jr., LeBlanc, J. G., Culpepper, W. S., III, and Ochsner, J. L.: Partial anomalous pulmonary venous return. Circulation *82*(Suppl. IV): 195, 1990.
496. Gikonyo, D. K., Tandon, R., Lucas, R. V., Jr., and Edwards, J. E.: Scimitar syndrome in neonates: Report of four cases and review of the literature. Pediatr. Cardiol. *6*:193, 1986.
497. Stanger, P., Rudolph, A. M., and Edwards, J. E.: Cardiac malpositions: An overview based on a study of 65 necropsy specimens. Circulation *56*:159, 1977.
498. Van Praagh, R.: Diagnosis of complex congenital heart disease: Morphologic-anatomic method and terminology. Cardiovasc. Intervent. Radiol. *7*:115, 1984.
499. Tonkin, I.L.D.: The definition of cardiac malpositions with echocardiography and computed tomography. *In* Friedman, W. F., and Higgins, C. B. (eds.): Pediatric Cardiac Imaging. Philadelphia, W. B. Saunders Company, 1984, p. 157.
500. Silverman, N. H.: An ultrasonic approach to the diagnosis of cardiac situs, connections, and malposition. *In* Friedman, W. F., and Higgins, C. B. (eds.): Pediatric Cardiac Imaging. Philadelphia, W. B. Saunders Company, 1984, p. 188.
501. Anderson, C., Devine, W. A., Anderson, R. H., et al.: Abnormalities of the spleen in relation to congenital malformations of the heart: Survey of necropsy findings in children. Br. Heart J. *63*:122, 1990.
502. Peoples, W. M., Moller, J. H., and Edwards, J. E.: Polysplenia: A review of 146 cases. Pediatr. Cardiol. *4*:129, 1983.
503. Momma, K., Takao, A., and Shibata, T.: Characteristics and natural history of abnormal atrial rhythms in left isomerism. Am. J. Cardiol. *65*:231, 1990.
504. Nasser, W. K.: Congenital absence of the left pericardium. Am. J. Cardiol. *26*:466, 1970.
505. Morgan, J. R., Rogers, A. K., and Forker, A. D.: Congenital absence of the left pericardium: Clinical findings. Ann. Intern. Med. *74*:370, 1971.
506. Pernot, C., Hoeffel, J. C., and Henry, M.: Radiologic patterns of congenital malformation of the pericardium. Radiol. Clin. (Basel) *44*:505, 1975.
507. Nicolosi, G. L., Borgioni, L., Alberti, E., et al.: M-mode and two-dimensional echocardiography in congenital absence of the pericardium. Chest *81*:610, 1982.
508. Rowland, T. W., Twible, E. A., Norwood, W. I., Jr., and Keane, J. F.: Partial absence of the left pericardium: Diagnosis by two-dimensional echocardiography. Am. J. Dis. Child. *136*:628, 1982.
509. Schiavone, W. A., and O'Donnell, J. K.: Congenital absence of the left portion of parietal pericardium demonstrated by nuclear magnetic resonance imaging. Am. J. Cardiol. *55*:1439, 1985.
510. Jones, J. W., and McManus, B. M.: Fatal cardiac strangulation by congenital partial pericardial defect. Am. Heart J. *107*:183, 1984.
511. Rowland, T. W., Twible, E. A., Norwood, W. J., Jr., and Keane, J. F.: Partial absence of the left pericardium. Am. J. Dis. Child. *136*:628, 1982.
512. Rastelli, G., Kirklin, J. W., and Titus, J. L.: Anatomic observations on complete form of persistent common atrioventricular canal with special reference to atrioventricular valves. Mayo Clin. Proc. *41*:296, 1966.
513. Anderson, R. H., Macartney, F. J., Tynan, M., et al.: Univentricular atrioventricular connection: The single ventricle trap unsprung. Pediatr. Cardiol. *4*:273, 1983.
514. Thies, W. R., Soto, B., Diethelm, E., et al.: Angiographic anatomy of hearts

with one ventricular chamber: The true single ventricle. Am. J. Cardiol. *55*:1363, 1985.

515. Huhta, J. C., Seward, J. B., Tajik, A. J., et al.: Two-dimensional echocardiographic spectrum of univentricular atrioventricular connection. J. Am. Coll. Cardiol. *5*:149, 1985.

516. DiSessa, T. G., Isabel-Jones, J. G., Heins, H., et al.: Two dimensional echocardiographic features of the univentricular heart. Cardiovasc. Ultrason. *3*:89, 1984.

517. Moak, J. P., and Gersony, W. M.: Progressive atrioventricular valvular regurgitation in single ventricle. Am. J. Cardiol. *59*:656, 1987.

518. Sano, T., Ogawa, M., Taniguchi, T., and Kawashima, Y.: Assessment of ventricular contractile state and function in patients with univentricular heart. Circulation *79*:1247, 1989.

519. Sano, T., Ogawa, M., Yabuuchi, H., and Kawashima, Y.: Quantitative cineangiographic analysis of ventricular volume and mass in patients with single ventricle: Relation to ventricular morphologies. Circulation *77*:62, 1988.

520. Stefanelli, G., Kirklin, J. W., Naftel, D. C., et al.: Early and intermediate-term (10-year) results of surgery for univentricular atrioventricular connection ("single ventricle"). Am. J. Cardiol. *54*:811, 1984.

521. Pacifico, A. D., Kirklin, J. K., and Kirklin, J. W.: Surgical management of double inlet ventricle. World J. Surg. *9*:579, 1985.

522. Laks, H., Milliken, J. C., Perloff, J. K., et al.: Experience with the Fontan procedure. J. Thorac. Cardiovasc. Surg. *88*:939, 1984.

523. Rothman, A., Lang, P., Lock, J. E., et al.: Surgical management of subaortic obstruction in single left ventricle and tricuspid atresia. J. Am. Coll. Cardiol. *10*:421, 1987.

524. Lin, A. E., Laks, H., Barber, G., et al.: Subaortic obstruction in complex congenital heart disease: Management by proximal pulmonary artery to ascending aorta end-to-side anastomosis. J. Am. Coll. Cardiol. *7*:617, 1986.

524a. Stevenson, O., Soderlund, S., Thoren, C., and Wallgren, G.: Arterial anomalies causing compression of the trachea and/or the esophagus. Acta Paediatr. Scand. *60*:81, 1971.

525. Park, C. D., Waldhausen, J. A., Friedman, S., et al.: Tracheal compression by the great arteries in the mediastinum: Report of 39 cases. Arch. Surg. *103*:626, 1971.

526. Gikonyo, B. M., Jue, K. L., and Edwards, J. E.: Pulmonary vascular sling: Report of seven cases and review of the literature. Pediatr. Cardiol. *10*:81, 1989.

527. Baron, R. L., Gutierrez, F. R., and McKnight, R. C.: Computed tomographic evaluation of the great arteries and aortic arch malformations. *In* Friedman, W. F., and Higgins, C. B. (eds.): Pediatric Cardiac Imaging. Philadelphia, W. B. Saunders Company, 1983, p. 135.

528. Biancaniello, T. M., and Heneghan, M. A.: Cardiac imaging with nuclear magnetic resonance: Technical considerations and potential clinical application. *In* Friedman, W. F., and Higgins, C. B. (eds): Pediatric Cardiac Imaging. Philadelphia, W. B. Saunders Company, 1983, p. 270.

529. deLeval, M.: Vascular rings. *In* Stark, J., and deLeval, M. (eds.): Surgery for Congenital Heart Defects. New York, Grune and Stratton, Inc., 1983, p. 227.

530. Perry, J. C., and Garson, A., Jr.: Diagnosis and treatment of arrhythmias. Adv. Pediatr. *36*:177, 1989.

531. Anderson, R. H., Wenick, A.C.G., Losekoot, T. G., and Becker, A. E.: Congenitally complete heart block. Circulation *56*:90, 1977.

532. Ho, S. Y., Esscher, E., Anderson, R. H., and Michaelsson, M.: Anatomy of congenital complete heart block and relation to maternal anti–ro antibodies. Am. J. Cardiol. *58*:291, 1986.

533. Ross, B. A.: Congenital complete atrioventricular block. Pediatr. Clin. North Am. *37*:69, 1990.

534. Sholler, G. F., and Walsh, E. P.: Congenital complete heart block in patients without anatomic cardiac defects. Am. Heart J. *118*:1193, 1989.

535. Beyon, J. P., Ben-Chetrit, E., Karp, S., et al.: Acquired congenital heart block. Pattern of maternal antibody response to biochemically defined antigens in neonatal lupus. J. Clin. Invest. *84*:627, 1989.

536. Steinfeld, L., Rappaport, H. L., Rossback, H. C., and Martinez, E.: Diagnosis of fetal arrhythmias using echocardiographic and Doppler techniques. J. Am. Coll. Cardiol. *8*:1425, 1986.

537. Mahoney, L. T., Marvin, W. J., Jr., Atkins, D. L., et al.: Pacemaker management for acute onset of heart block in childhood. J. Pediatr. *107*:207, 1985.

538. Epstein, M. L., Knauf, D. G., and Alexander, J. A.: Long-term follow-up of transvenous cardiac pacing in children. Am. J. Cardiol. *57*:889, 1986.

539. Michaelsson, M., and Engle, M. A.: Congenital complete heart block: An international study of the natural history. Cardiovasc. Clin. *4*:85, 1982.

540. Kugler, J. D., and Danford, D. A.: Pacemakers in children: An update. Am. Heart J. *117*:665, 1989.

541. Zales, V. R., Dunnigan, A., and Benson, D. W., Jr.: Clinical and electrophysiologic features of fetal and neonatal paroxysmal atrial tachycardia resulting in congestive heart failure. Am. J. Cardiol. *62*:225, 1988.

542. Kleinman, C. S., Donnerstein, R. L., DeVore, G. R., et al.: Fetal echocardiography for evaluation of in utero congestive heart failure. N. Engl. J. Med. *306*:568, 1982.

543. Radford, D. J., Izukawa, T., and Rowe, R. D.: Congenital paroxysmal atrial tachycardia. Arch. Dis. Child. *51*:613, 1976.

544. Deal, B. J., Keane, J. F., Gillette, P. C., and Gardon, A., Jr.: Wolff-Parkinson-White syndrome and supraventricular tachycardia during infancy: Management and follow-up. J. Am. Coll. Cardiol. *5*:130, 1985.

545. Benson, D. W., Jr., Dunnigan, A., Benditt, D. G., et al.: Prediction of digoxin treatment failure in infants with supraventricular tachycardia: Role of transesophageal pacing. Pediatrics *75*:288, 1985.

546. Klitzner, T. S., and Friedman, W. F.: Cardiac arrhythmias: The role of pharmacologic intervention. Cardiol. Clin. *7*:299, 1989.

546a. Garson, A., Jr., Bink-Boelkens, M., Hesslein, P. S., et al.: Atrial flutter in the young: A collaborative study of 380 cases. J. Am. Coll. Cardiol. *6*:871, 1985.

547. Dunnigan, A., Benson, W., Jr., and Benditt, D. G.: Atrial flutter in infancy: Diagnosis, clinical features and treatment. Pediatrics *75*:725, 1985.

547a. Trippel, D. L., and Gillette, P. C.: Atenolol in children with supraventricular tachycardia. Am. J. Cardiol. *64*:233, 1989.

548. Dick, M., Scott, W. A., Serwer, G. S., et al.: Acute termination of supraventricular tachyarrhythmias in children by transesophageal atrial pacing. Am. J. Cardiol. *61*:925, 1988.

549. Benson, D. W., Jr., Dunnigan, A., and Benditt, D. G.: Follow-up evaluation of infant paroxysmal atrial tachycardia: Transesophageal study. Circulation *75*:542, 1987.

550. Zipes, D. P., et al.: Guidelines for clinical intracardiac electrophysiologic studies. A report of the American College of Cardiology/American Heart Association Task Force on Assessment of Diagnostic and Therapeutic Cardiovascular Procedures. J. Am. Coll. Cardiol. *14*:1827, 1989.

551. Case, C. L., Crawford, F. A., and Gillette, P. C.: Surgical treatment of dysrhythmias. Pediatr. Clin. North Am. *37*:79, 1990.

552. Garson, A., Jr., Moak, J. P., Friedman, R. A., et al.: Surgical treatment of arrhythmias in children. Cardiol. Clin. *7*:319, 1989.

553. Garson, A., Jr., Gillette, P. C., Titus, J. L., et al.: Surgical treatment of ventricular tachycardia in infants. N. Engl. J. Med. *310*:1443, 1984.

32

Congenital Heart Disease in Adults

by JOSEPH K. PERLOFF

Congenital heart disease in adults has emerged as a special area of cardiovascular interest.[1,1a] The patient population includes those who have never undergone cardiac surgery, those who have undergone cardiac surgery and require no further operation, those who have had palliation with or without anticipation of reparative surgery, and those who are inoperable apart from organ transplantation. The number of adults with congenital heart disease is steadily increasing, and the trend promises to continue. This chapter begins with a brief historical perspective and then focuses on the multidisciplinary facilities for comprehensive care, the survival patterns (natural and postoperative), medical considerations, surgical considerations, and postoperative residua and sequelae.

HISTORICAL PERSPECTIVES

Congenital heart disease is, by definition, present at birth, but survival patterns vary widely. In 1888, Etienne-Louis Arthur Fallot wrote: "We have seen from our observations that cyanosis, especially in the adult, is the result of a small number of cardiac malformations well determined."[2] Fallot was referring to the tetralogy that still bears his name.

In the first half of the twentieth century, the untiring work of Maude Abbott culminated in her remarkable *Atlas of Congenital Heart Disease,* which was based on 1000 pathology specimens personally studied.[3] The atlas was not only a landmark in the orderly classification of the anomalies but also provided invaluable information on natural survival patterns. The seminal contributions of Gross, Blalock, Taussig, and Crafoord materially modified those survival patterns, and the sense of despair that had surrounded congenital cardiac anomalies—those "hopeless futilities"—began to dissipate.

In 1939, Robert Gross, a pediatric surgeon at Harvard, ligated a patent ductus in a 7½-year-old girl.[4] A few years later, Helen Brooke Taussig, a pediatric cardiologist in Baltimore, conceived the idea of "creating" a patent ductus arteriosus in cyanotic children suffering from deficient pulmonary blood flow. In 1945, Alfred Blalock, a vascular surgeon at Johns Hopkins, sutured the end of a subclavian artery to the side of a pulmonary artery in a patient with Fallot's tetralogy, establishing the Blalock-Taussig anastomosis.[5] Previously, "a blue baby with a malformed heart was considered beyond the reach of surgical aid." In the early 1940s, Clarence Crafoord of the Karolinska Institute, while operating on patients with patent ductus arteriosus, "began to wonder whether it might not also be possible to treat coarctation of the aortic isthmus by surgical means."[6] The postwar introduction of cardiac catheterization, for which Andre F. Cournand, Dickinson W. Richards, and Werner Forssman received the Nobel prize in 1956, was a major step forward. The development of extra-corporeal circulation in the early to mid-1950's was destined to make virtually all congenital malformations of the heart accessible to the skills of cardiac surgeons. The stage was set for "accurate visualization of structures within the heart for a period sufficient to permit precise corrective measures."[7]

The culmination of these historical landmarks resulted in one of the most successful diagnostic and therapeutic programs that medicine has witnessed. Formidable technical resources are at our disposal, permitting remarkably accurate anatomical and physiological cardiac diagnoses and astonishing feats of reparative surgery. Survival patterns have been affected, often profoundly. Accordingly, congenital heart disease should be considered not only in terms of its age of onset but also in terms of the age range that survival now permits—an uninterrupted continuum from fetal life to senescence. Although long-term management remains concerned with natural survival, it is increasingly involved with the growing numbers of postoperative patients who continue to need medical surveillance. The quality of care provided by pediatric cardiologists to patients from birth to maturity must be matched with care of equal quality during adulthood.

Congenital heart disease in adults is represented by natural survival and postoperative survival patterns. *Unoperated* adults experience improved longevity and well-being owing to refinements in the medical management of hematological disorders, renal function, urate metabolism, pulmonary physiology, infective endocarditis, electrophysiological abnormalities, pregnancy, and noncardiac surgery. Proper care of patients *after* operation requires knowledge of the preoperative congenital cardiac malformation, the nature and effects of surgical intervention, and the presence, type, and extent of postoperative residua and sequelae. The ideal objective of complete cure is rarely achieved, so operations necessarily leave behind a broad range of residua and sequelae that require prolonged, if not indefinite, medical attention. Uninterrupted, long-term continuity care is essential if the concerns inherent in this new and increasing patient population are to be addressed.[8-10]

A MULTIDISCIPLINARY CENTER FOR CARE OF ADULTS WITH CONGENITAL HEART DISEASE

The UCLA Adult Congenital Heart Disease Center is a university hospital facility for congenital heart disease in adults.[1] The staff consists of a medical cardiologist, a pediatric cardiologist, a cardiologist with appointments in medicine and pediatrics, two cardiac surgeons, and a clinical cardiovascular nurse specialist. The cardiologists have a thorough understanding of the diagnostic modalities, the reparative and palliative surgical techniques, and the cardiovascular and general medical illnesses that adults with congenital heart disease may acquire during the course of aging. Dedication to task is a collaborative effort, especially in the setting of a university hospital in which intellectual interchange, teaching, and research are as paramount as optimal patient care.

Patients qualify for entry into the center when they reach age 18 years, or when they are judged to have achieved appropriate psychological and physical maturity. The transition from pediatric to adult care is simplest for 18-year-olds who consider themselves young adults. Conversely, patients in their 20's may be physically small, emotionally immature, and all too dependent on the familiar pediatric setting that has provided a sense of security for so many years. Every effort should be made to avoid reinforcing this dependency. Adult care is best provided in an adult setting, whether outpatient or inpatient. Referrals are from pediatric cardiology in the same institution, and from internists, family practitioners, pediatricians, or cardiologists within or outside the immediate geographical area. Patients are referred either directly to the Adult Congenital Heart Disease Center or to a colleague in the Division of Cardiothoracic Surgery.

The outpatient clinic is an important aspect of the center. Appointments are made through a single group of secretaries with whom the patients become familiar. The same outpatient rooms and the same nurses are used for each clinic session to provide the patients with a sense of familiarity. The outpatient laboratory serving the clinic gives priority to the processing of blood counts. The clinical nurse specialist arranges for phlebotomy during the outpatient visit as soon as its necessity is determined. Medical and pediatric cardiac fellows are assigned to the clinic together with medical and pediatric residents. Initial patient assessment is by a fellow or resident, who then confers with a staff cardiologist. When time permits, these presentations are made to the group as a whole, unless the problem is judged to be relatively routine. All follow-up and consultation reports are dictated by the staff cardiologists because the reports are designed to provide educational as well as practical information for referring physicians and to serve as reliable data sources. Inpatients include elective admissions for cardiac or noncardiac surgery, admissions for labor and delivery, admissions to the cardiac intensive care unit, usually for arrhythmias, and admissions for medical management. Other inpatients are referred directly to a cardiac surgeon and are routinely seen in hospital by a staff cardiologist. Before discharge, follow-up arrangements are made in collaboration with the surgeon and the referring physician. The clinical nurse specialist coordinates the inpatient-outpatient interface.

The noninvasive, catheterization, and angiographic laboratories must offer the same diagnostic quality for adults with congenital heart disease as that offered by the pediatric laboratories for infants and children. Adults with congenital heart disease are best studied in laboratories that are designed for adults, provided the quality of the investigations equals that achieved in pediatric laboratories. Results will be less than optimal unless the cardiologists and technologists in the adult laboratories have training, expertise, and experience in the complex problems of congenital heart disease, a goal that can be reached when there is a sufficient volume and variety of patients.

Noncardiac consultants formally incorporated into the Adult Congenital Heart Disease Center include those in hematology, renal function, urate metabolism, pulmonary medicine, cardiac surgery, electrophysiology, insurability and vocational counseling, genetics and epidemiology, gynecology and obstetrics, psychiatry, anesthesiology, and pathology. The objective is to have ready access to specialists who have gained experience in the specific problems associated with congenital heart disease in adults.

The center assumes a major role in the training and education of fellows, residents, and nurse specialists who will become the next generation of responsible professionals. Implicit in the educational mission is the idea that pediatric cardiologists should have an understanding of cardiovascular disease in adults, and medical cardiologists should have an understanding of heart disease in children.[11]

The center is a lively area of clinical research, which is prompted by a desire to address unresolved questions posed by the patient population under surveillance. Investigations usually require collaboration with colleagues in a number of other disciplines, thus stimulating valuable interdisciplinary interchange.

SURVIVAL PATTERNS

NATURAL SURVIVAL

Natural survival includes malformations that do not require operation, malformations that remain amenable to operation in adulthood, and malformations that are inoperable except for organ transplantation. Management of adults with congenital heart disease must take into account acquired disorders of the heart and circulation that may coexist and modify the physiological expressions of the basic congenital malformation. This discussion deals chiefly with common or uncommon defects in which survival to adulthood is expected, and with some common defects in which adult survival is exceptional, but does not deal with uncommon defects in which adult survival is exceptional.

Common Defects in Which Survival to Adulthood Is Expected

BICUSPID AORTIC VALVE (see also p. 922 and Figs. 4–66, p. 90; 31–31, p. 924; 31–32, p. 924; 31–33, p. 925). This disorder is the most frequent congenital anomaly to which that structure is subject and is one of the most common gross morphological congenital anomalies of the heart or great arteries.[12,13] Bicuspid aortic valves that are functionally normal at birth undergo one of several patterns of evolution.[12,13] The valve can remain functionally normal throughout a normal life span or can develop gradual obstruction caused by fibrocalcific thickening, a substrate that accounts for about one-half of surgical cases of calcific aortic stenosis in adults (Fig. 32–1).[14] The natural history of bicuspid aortic valves occasionally is punctuated by dissecting aortic aneurysms, which sometimes become manifested years after otherwise successful valve replacement. The relationship between aortic root disease and a congenitally bicuspid aortic valve is more than casual.[15] A bicuspid aortic valve may develop progressive regurgitation with or without the impetus of infective endocarditis and is an important cause of anatomically isolated valvular aortic regurgitation—mild to severe, chronic or acute—in adults.[16]

COARCTATION OF THE AORTA (see also p. 920 and Figs. 11–39, p. 331; 8–40, p. 229; 31–29, p. 921, 31–30, p. 921). This anomaly may not cause significant symptoms until after 20 to 30 years of age.[17] Most patients who survive infancy reach adulthood. Sporadic examples of exceptional longevity (Fig. 32–2) should not obscure the inherent risks that significantly shorten life span. On an average, death occurs in the mid-30's.[13] The oldest recorded survivor was Raynaud's patient (1828), a 92-year-old man.[18]

Longevity and morbidity in adults with coarctation of the aorta are influenced by coexisting congenital and acquired cardiac and vascular diseases. The most common associated congenital malformation is the bicuspid aortic valve,[13] the natural history of which was just described. Less common, but potentially lethal, is a congenital aneurysm of the circle of Willis, which typically announces itself by sudden rupture.[19] Aortic dissection or rupture is a dramatic complication, with peak incidence in the third and fourth decades.[20] Ruptures originate either in the proximal ascending aorta (the most common site) or in a post-coarctation aneurysm (distal compartment). Left ventricular failure in unoperated coarctation

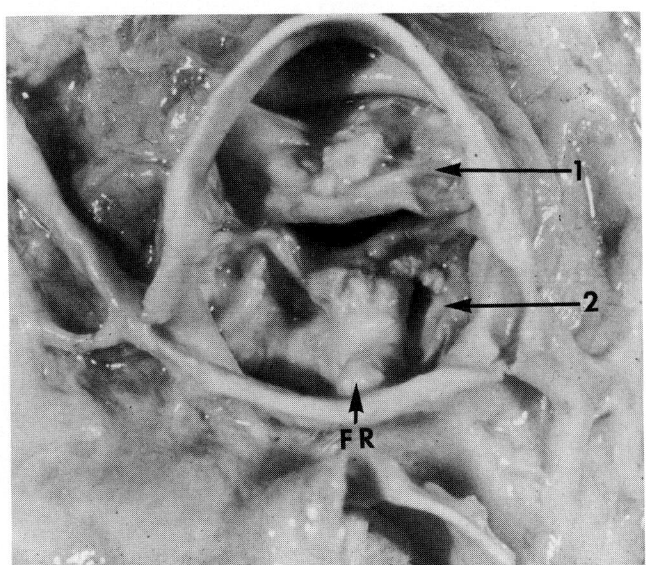

FIGURE 32–1. Necropsy specimen from an adult with bicuspid aortic stenosis. The first arrow points to one calcified leaflet, the second arrow points to a second calcified leaflet, and the vertical arrow points to calcium in the false raphe (FR). (Courtesy of Dr. William C. Roberts, National Heart Lung and Blood Institute, Bethesda, MD.)

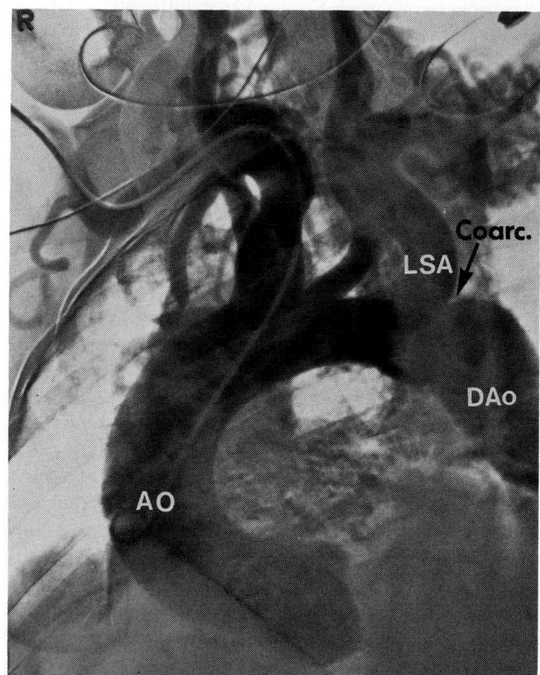

FIGURE 32–2. Lateral aortogram from a 62-year-old woman with coarctation (Coarc) of the aorta just distal to the left subclavian artery (LSA). There is poststenotic dilatation of the descending aorta (DAo). Arterial collaterals are conspicuous.

of the aorta occurs in patients who are either younger than 1 year of age or older than age 40 years, but seldom in between.[13] Hypertension predisposes to premature coronary artery disease.[21]

PULMONARY VALVE STENOSIS (see also p. 972, and Figs. 4–67 and 4–68, p. 90; 8–42*A*, p. 230; Fig. 7, p. 156; Fig. 31–42, p. 932; 31–43, p. 933). Represented by a pliant conical or dome-shaped valve with a narrow outlet at its apex, pulmonary valve stenosis typically occurs as an isolated congenital anomaly and is the most common variety of congenital obstruction to right ventricular outflow.[13] With the exception of pinpoint pulmonary valve stenosis in neonates, survival into adolescence and adulthood is the rule. Longevity depends chiefly on three variables: (1) the initial severity of obstruction, (2) whether a given degree of obstruction remains constant or progresses, and (3) the functional adequacy of the pressure-overloaded right ventricle.[13] Patients with typical isolated pulmonary stenosis usually experience an increase in valve orifice with age, although the development of secondary hypertrophic subpulmonary stenosis (Fig. 32–3*A*) or fibrocalcific thickening may augment the degree of obstruction. While subjective complaints become more prevalent as years go by, equivalent degrees of stenosis may handicap one patient in childhood yet leave another relatively unencumbered as an adult. Right ventricular failure is the most common mode of death, usually occurring after the fourth decade.[22–25] Infective endocarditis is a risk (except perhaps in mild pulmonary valve stenosis), with a reported incidence of 2 to 7 per cent.

OSTIUM SECUNDUM ATRIAL SEPTAL DEFECT (see also p. 906 and Figs. 4–76, p. 92; 8–41*A*, p. 229; Fig. 30, p. 159; 31–11, p. 906; 31–12, p. 907; 31–13, p. 907). *This anomaly is among the most common congenital cardiac malformations in adults* (Fig. 32–4), accounting for 30 to 40 per cent in patients age 40 years or older.[13,26,27] The malformation often goes unrecognized for decades because symptoms may be absent and physical signs are subtle. Although life expectancy is not normal, survival into adulthood of patients who are not operated on is the rule, and many patients live to advanced ages.[26–31] Natural survival beyond age 40 to 50 years is, however, less than 50 per cent, with an attrition rate after age 40 years of about 6 per cent per annum.[13] One of the author's patients died at age 87 years with atrial fibrillation and right ventricular failure, and another lived relatively comfortably until 3 months before his 95th birthday.[32]

Virtually all patients with ostium secundum atrial septal defects who survive beyond the sixth decade are symptomatic. Older patients deteriorate chiefly on three counts. First, an age-related decrease in left ventricular distensibility augments the left-to-right shunt. Second, atrial arrhythmias, especially fibrillation but also atrial flutter or paroxysmal atrial tachycardia, increase in frequency after the fourth decade and precipitate right ventricular failure. Third, the majority of symptomatic adults older than age 40 have mild to moderate pulmonary hypertension in the presence of a persistent large left-to-right shunt, so the aging right ventricle is doubly beset by both pressure and volume overload.[13] If advanced pulmonary vascular disease occurs at all, it seldom does so before the third decade. Even so, the patient's life span often stretches into the fourth decade.[13,33]

The incidence, extent, and degree of mitral valve disease in patients with ostium secundum atrial septal defect increases with age, and significant mitral regurgitation occurs in about

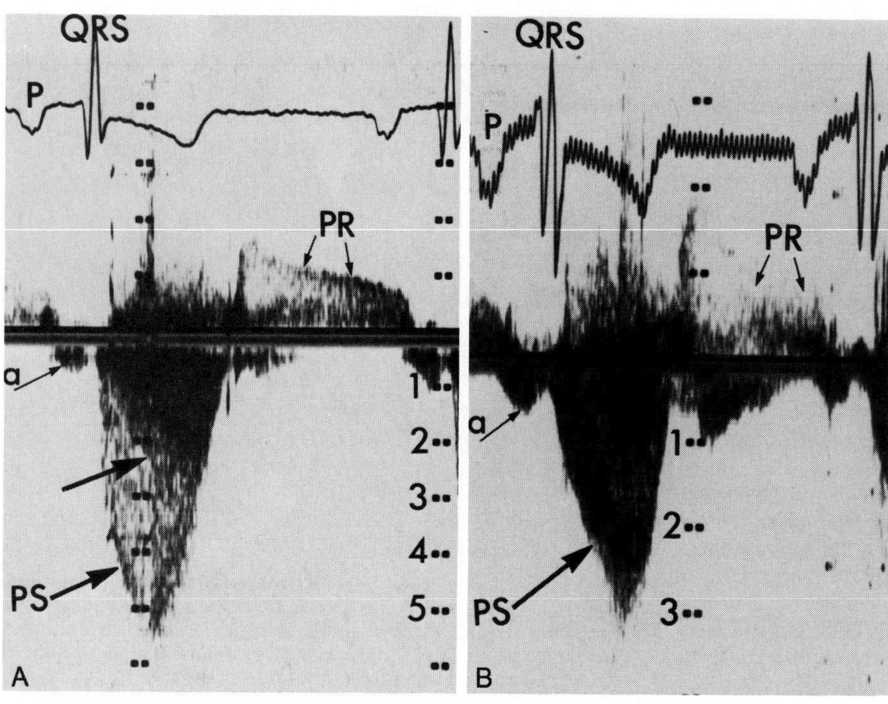

FIGURE 32–3. *A,* Continuous wave Doppler across the right ventricular outflow tract of a 33-year-old male with severe pulmonary valve stenosis (PS) and secondary hypertrophic subpulmonary stenosis. The peak instantaneous gradient across the valve was 120 mm Hg. Within the major symmetric flow disturbance envelope, there is an asymmetric, lower-velocity pattern (upper unmarked arrow) caused by the hypertrophic subpulmonary stenosis. a = presystolic flow in response to an increased force of right atrial contractions; PR = pulmonary regurgitation. *B,* After balloon dilatation, the gradient at valve level was virtually abolished, leaving only the subpulmonary (PS) gradient.

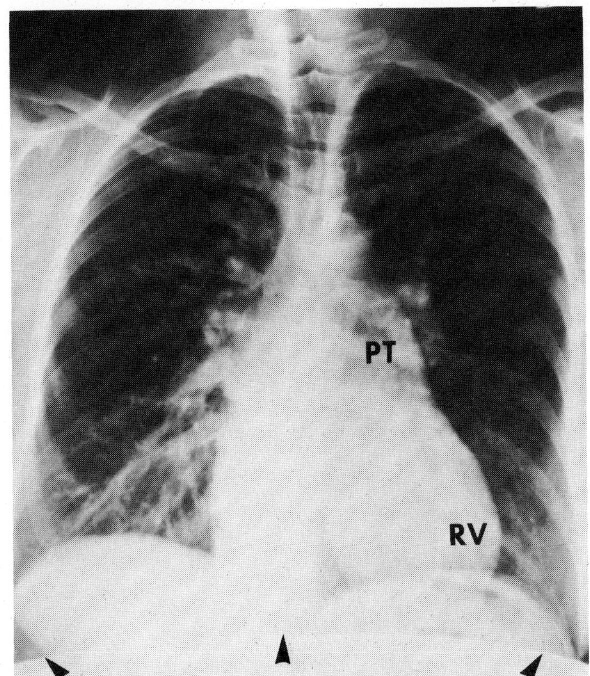

FIGURE 32-4. Chest radiograph from a 32-year-old woman with an uncomplicated ostium secundum atrial septal defect. She was in the third trimester of her ninth pregnancy. Note the lead shield (arrowheads) over the abdomen. The pulmonary trunk (PT) is dilated. An enlarged right ventricle (RV) occupies the apex.

15 per cent.[34-36] Mitral valve abnormalities have been attributed chiefly to the effects on the mitral apparatus of left ventricular cavity deformity (size as well as shape).[37,38] The female-male ratio is about two to one. Because the natural history of ostium secundum atrial septal defect extends into adulthood, it is the rule for women to reach childbearing age (Fig. 32-4) (see pp. 977 and 978).

PATENT DUCTUS ARTERIOSUS (see also p. 913 and Fig. 8-41*B*, p. 229). This congenital vascular anomaly permits asymptomatic survival in most patients, at least after the first year of life.[39-43] At the beginning of the second decade, the risk of infective endarteritis exceeds the risk of heart failure.[13] Beginning in the third decade (occasionally earlier), more and more patients with sizable left-to-right shunts develop cardiac failure, whereas those with small shunts (restrictive ductus) remain asymptomatic. One of the author's patients was an 84-year-old woman with a small patent ductus arteriosus of little or no physiological significance, and another 84-year-old patient had a moderately restrictive ductus with atrial fibrillation and congestive heart failure (Fig. 32-5). There is a significant cumulative risk of infective endocarditis, especially if the patent ductus is restrictive (see later). Patients with patent ductus arteriosus and large shunts (nonrestrictive ductus) seldom reach adulthood unless a rise in pulmonary vascular resistance relieves the left ventricle of excessive volume overload.[42] Differential cyanosis is a distinctive feature of the reversed shunt.

Uncommon Defects in Which Survival to Adulthood Is Expected

SITUS INVERSUS WITH DEXTROCARDIA (p. 984). Patients with this anomaly, which usually occurs with a structurally normal heart,[13] experience normal longevity but are susceptible to *acquired* cardiac and noncardiac diseases. Symptoms so related may lead to the discovery of the hitherto unsuspected cardiac malposition. Angina pectoris or myocardial infarction in adults with complete situs inversus is associated with pain in the *right* anterior chest with radiation to the *right* shoulder and *right* arm. The pain of appendicitis is referred to the *left* lower quadrant, and biliary colic presents in the *left* upper quadrant, owing to the mirror image positions of the abdominal viscera. When situs inversus with dextrocardia coexists with congenital malformations of the heart, longevity is determined by the associated anomalies.

SITUS SOLITUS WITH DEXTROCARDIA. This malformation occasionally occurs with a structurally normal heart, which not only permits adult survival but usually delays clinical recognition.[13] A routine chest radiograph may provide the first evidence of the malposition. Coexisting congenital cardiac malformations, which normally are present, determine longevity.

CONGENITAL COMPLETE HEART BLOCK (see also pp. 955 and 984). This disorder usually permits survival into adulthood.[13,44-46] The key determinants of longevity are the ventricular rate, the presence of intrinsically normal ventricular myocardium, and the hemodynamic adjustments at rest and with exercise. Despite the frequency of asymptomatic survival into adulthood, optimism is dampened by the ultimate fate of large numbers of adolescents and adults with congenital complete heart block; nor is mortality in childhood negligible.[13,44]

UNCOMPLICATED CONGENITALLY CORRECTED TRANSPOSITION OF THE GREAT ARTERIES (see also p. 946 and Figs. 8-42A, p. 230; 31-65, p. 949). This malformation permits good but not normal longevity because of the functional inadequacy of a morphologic right ventricle in the systemic location.[47-50] More often than not the natural history is influenced by the presence and degree of the congenital cardiac malformations that commonly coexist.[13] Survival into the sixth decade is uncommon, with only a few patients reaching the seventh decade, and only one reaching age 73 years.[51] Incompetence of the inverted left atrioventricular valve (Ebstein-like anomaly) may go unrecognized until late childhood or early adulthood, prompting the mistaken diagnosis of acquired mitral regurgitation. The risk of complete atrioventricular block accrues at a rate of about 2 per cent per year.[13] Complete heart block may announce itself with a Stokes-Adams attack or sudden death.

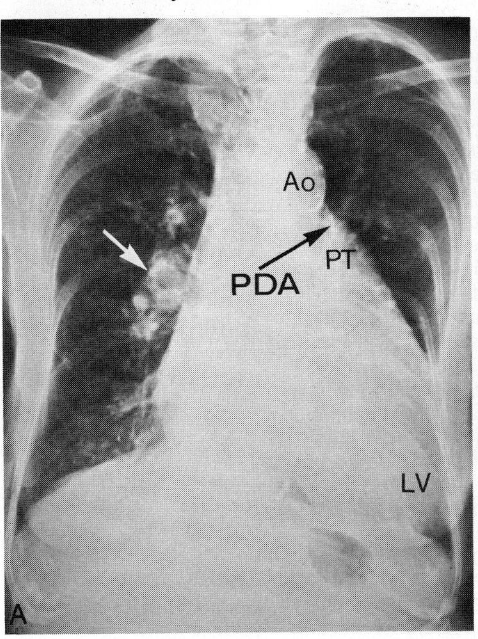

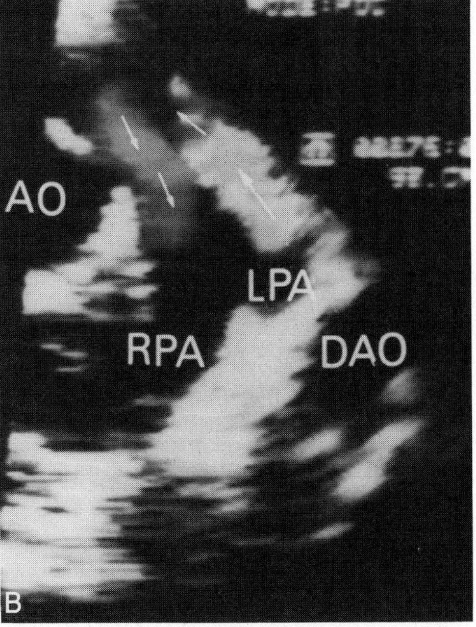

FIGURE 32-5. *A,* Radiograph from an 84-year-old woman with a moderately restrictive calcified patent ductus arteriosus (PDA). The pulmonary trunk (PT) and its right branch (unmarked white arrow) are dilated. Pulmonary arterial pressure was 90/40 mm Hg. The enlarged left ventricle (LV) occupies the apex. The aortic knuckle (Ao) is calcified. *B,* Black and white print of a color-flow image (parasternal short axis). Arrows trace the direction of ductal flow, moving first down the left lateral wall of the pulmonary trunk and then up the opposite wall. LPA = left pulmonary artery; RPA = right pulmonary artery; DAo = descending aorta.

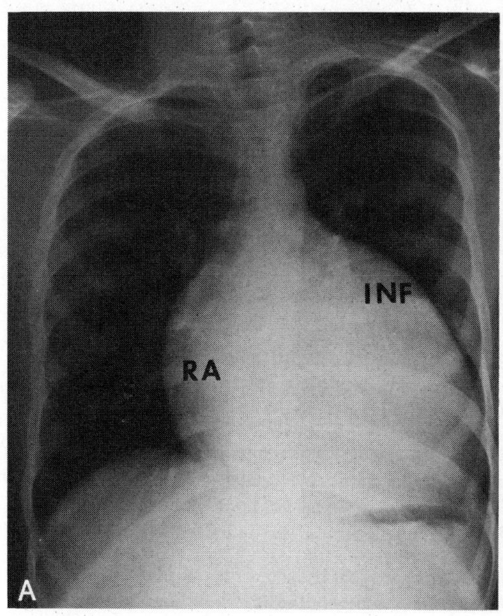

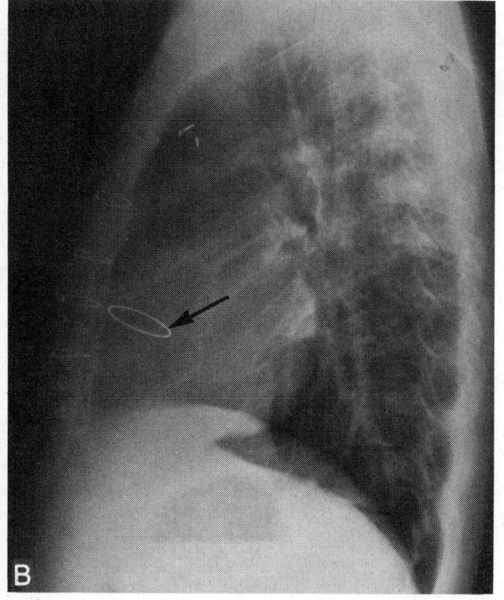

FIGURE 32–6. *A,* Preoperative chest radiograph from a 22-year-old man with cyanotic Ebstein's anomaly, Wolff-Parkinson-White bypass tracts, and syncope induced by atrial flutter with 1:1 antegrade conduction. There is a large right atrium (RA) and a hump-shaped infundibulum (INF). *B,* Lateral chest radiograph after tricuspid valve reconstruction and atrioventricular dissociation. Arrow identifies the Carpentier ring.

CONGENITAL MITRAL REGURGITATION (see also p. 930). Sometimes this lesion occurs as the only clinically overt component of an endocardial cushion defect.[13] Adult survival depends on the degree of regurgitation and the adaptive response of the volume-overloaded left ventricle. The mistaken diagnosis of acquired mitral regurgitation is not uncommon.

EBSTEIN'S ANOMALY OF THE TRICUSPID VALVE (see also p. 940 and Figs. 4–69, p. 91; 8–42C, p. 230). This lesion permits longevity into adulthood, depending on the physiological state of the malformed right ventricle, the presence of an interatrial communication (right-to-left shunt), and the presence and severity of atrial tachyarrhythmias, especially when accompanied by accelerated conduction through Wolff-Parkinson-White bypass tracts. The natural history ranges from neonatal death to relatively asymptomatic survival into adulthood, even to advanced age.[52–60,60a] For patients who survive the first year of life, a cumulative mortality of 12.4 per cent is distributed about evenly through childhood and adolescence.[13] Paroxysmal supraventricular tachycardia occurs in about 25 to 30 per cent of patients with Ebstein's anomaly.[13] Syncope heightens suspicion of accelerated bypass conduction (rapid atrial fibrillation or one-to-one atrial flutter). A rapid ventricular response by way of a bypass tract is held responsible for sudden death. Despite the aforementioned qualifications, there are accounts of astonishing longevity, with survivals into the eighth decade.[56,57] The oldest recorded patient with Ebstein's anomaly lived to age 85 years and had no cardiac symptoms until age 79.[13]

CONGENITAL PULMONARY VALVE REGURGITATION (see also p. 1059). This malformation typically permits adult survival. Longevity depends on the degree of regurgitant flow and on the adaptive response of the right ventricle to volume overload.[61,62] Because the regurgitation is seldom more than moderate, and because the right ventricle readily adapts to low pressure volume overload, most patients tolerate the anomaly through middle age and occasionally into the sixth or even eighth decade of life.[13,63] Right heart failure may occur in older adults after decades of stability because of the additive effects of a rise in pulmonary arterial pressure caused by acquired bronchopulmonary disease or because of the passive elevation of pulmonary arterial pressure that accompanies left ventricular failure.[13] The risk of infective endocarditis is relatively low.

LUTEMBACHER'S SYNDROME. This syndrome consists of an atrial septal defect that coexists with *acquired* mitral stenosis.[13] Longevity depends on the degree of mitral valve obstruction and the size of the interatrial communication. Mitral stenosis augments the left-to-right interatrial shunt, but the atrial septal defect decompresses the left atrium, reducing the gradient across the stenotic mitral valve. Lutembacher's original patient was a 61-year-old woman who had been pregnant 7 times,[68] and Firket's patient was a 74-year-old woman who had experienced 11 pregnancies.[69] The oldest reported patient was an 81-year-old woman who experienced no symptoms related to her heart until her 75th year.[70]

ANEURYSM OF A SINUS OF VALSALVA (see also p. 106). This defect typically begins as a blind pouch or diverticulum that takes origin from a localized site in one aortic sinus. The substantial majority of ruptures develop well after puberty but before age 30 years, usually in males ranging in age from 11 to 67 years.[71,72] The physiological consequences depend on the rapidity with which the rupture develops, the amount of blood flowing through the abnormal communication, and the chamber (site) that receives the shunt. Death usually is within a year after an unrelieved acute large perforation. A small perforation that progresses gradually may at first go unnoticed; small chronic perforations are susceptible to infective endocarditis. About 20 per cent of congenital sinus of Valsalva aneurysms are unperforated and are discovered at necropsy or cardiac surgery.[13] In one of our patients, an 85-year-old man, the diagnosis of a previously unsuspected aortic sinus aneurysm was made by echocardiography with Doppler interrogation and color-flow imaging.

CORONARY ARTERIOVENOUS FISTULAS (see also p. 917). This anomaly represents one of the most common major congenital malformations of the coronary circulation that permit adult survival.[13,73] Both coronary arteries arise from the aorta, but a fistulous branch of one or more arteries communicates directly with a cardiac chamber or with the pulmonary trunk, coronary sinus, vena cava, or a pulmonary vein (Fig. 32–7). Longevity depends on the amount of blood flowing through the communication, the chamber or vessel into which the fistula drains, and myocardial ischemia that may result from the fistulous bypass (coronary steal). Adult survival is expected, although life span is not normal. Survivals have been recorded in the seventh to the ninth decades, with the oldest patient living to age 85 years.[13]

CONGENITAL PULMONARY ARTERIOVENOUS FISTULAS (see also p. 930). These fistulas typically occur without coexisting congenital heart

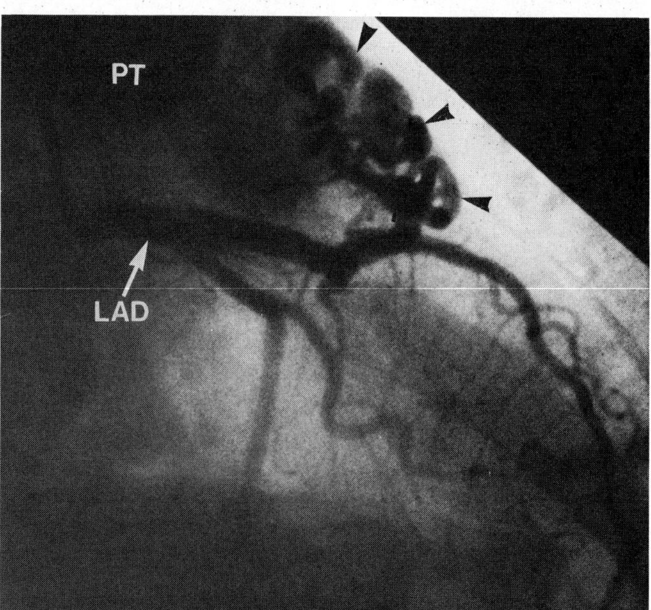

FIGURE 32–7. Selective left coronary arteriogram from an asymptomatic 63-year-old woman who had a continuous murmur beneath her left clavicle. Arrows at the right point to a congenital coronary arteriovenous fistula arising from a branch of the left anterior descending (LAD) coronary artery. PT = pulmonary trunk.

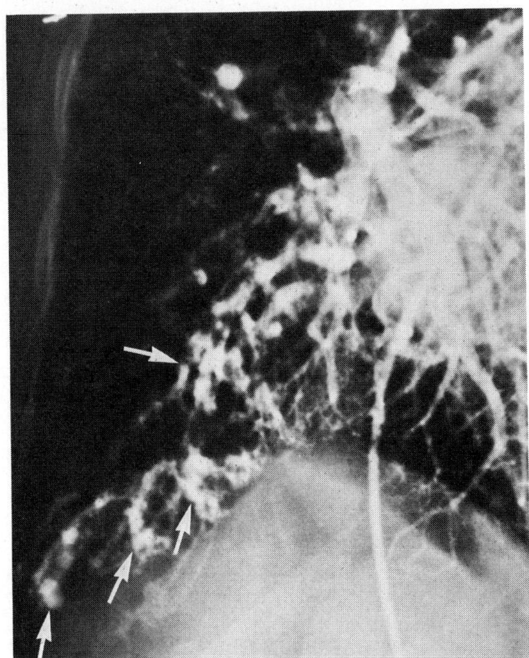

FIGURE 32-8. Selective right pulmonary arteriogram from a 71-year-old man with congenital bilateral pulmonary arteriovenous fistulae (arrows). His 73-year-old sister was similarly afflicted. Neither had telangiectasia.

disease but usually are associated with hereditary telangiectasia.[74] A substantial majority of the fistulas go unrecognized until adult life. In one large series, the mean patient age was 39 years (range 3 to 73 years), with the distinct minority younger than age 20 years.[13] Two of the author's patients without telangiectasia are siblings age 71 and 73 years (Fig. 32-8).[75]

Common Defects in Which Adult Survival Is Exceptional

VENTRICULAR SEPTAL DEFECT (see also p. 910, and Figs. 4-74, p. 93; Fig. 31, p. 159; 8-41C, p. 229; 11-13, p. 319). These are among the most common congenital cardiac malformations at birth but are seldom found in adults.[76-80] In his remarks on adult survival in congenital heart disease, Paul Wood asked, "Where's the maladie de Roger? Assuming it does not provide immortality, it must either close spontaneously in middle life or have long since run its mortal course."[81] Patients who survive into adulthood comprise two main groups: (1) those with small or moderately restrictive perimembranous or muscular defects that have closed spontaneously or that have decreased in size so that they are clinically inapparent, and (2) patients with nonrestrictive ventricular septal defects but with elevated pulmonary vascular resistance that relieves the left ventricle of excessive volume overload while imposing no increase in afterload on the right ventricle (Eisenmenger's complex).

The chief reason for adult survival of patients born with ventricular septal defects is spontaneous closure.[82] The long-term fate of perimembranous ventricular septal defects that have closed by aneurysm formation is unknown, but there is cautious optimism.[83] The occasional adult survivor with persistent patency of a small perimembranous ventricular septal defect confronts a cumulative risk of infective endocarditis.[84] It is not uncommon for patients with Eisenmenger's complex to reach adulthood (p. 763). The author's oldest patient died of noncardiac causes at age 69 years (Fig. 32-9). Longevity in Eisenmenger's complex has improved significantly because of meticulous hematological management (see later).

FALLOT'S TETRALOGY (see also p. 935 and Fig. 4-82, p. 94). This is the cyanotic malformation that most frequently permits survival to adulthood.[2,13] Individual reports describe survivals from the fifth to the seventh decades of life.[13,85,86] Nevertheless, survival patterns based on an analysis of more than 500 necropsy cases disclosed that two-thirds of patients born with the tetralogy reached their first birthday, 50 per cent reached age 3 years, about 25 per cent completed the first decade of life, and thereafter the attrition rate was 6.4 per cent per year.[13] But differently, 11 per cent of patients are alive at age 20 years, 6 per cent at age 30 years, and 3 per cent at age 40. Systemic hypertension in adult survivors with the tetralogy is a special problem because the increased afterload is imposed on both the left *and* right ventricles (biventricular aorta).[13] The rise in right ventricular systolic pressure augments pulmonary blood flow and reduces cyanosis, but at the price of right ventricular (or biventricular) failure. Infective endocarditis on an incompetent biventricular aortic valve in Fallot's tetralogy may result in catastrophic acute severe regurgitation into both right and left ventricles.

SURVIVAL AFTER CARDIAC SURGERY OR INTERVENTIONAL CATHETERIZATION

An understanding of prognosis after cardiac surgery or interventional catheterization requires knowledge of the preoperative congenital malformation, the nature and effects of the therapeutic intervention, and the postoperative residua and sequelae.[1,87] Success is measured by the length of survival, the quality of life, and the need for reoperation. It is axiomatic that techniques have evolved and will continue to do so. Patients who underwent cardiac surgery two to three decades ago benefited from the anatomical repairs but often suffered from the deleterious effects of what would now be considered inadequate myocardial protection. Prosthetic materials—valves, patches, and conduits—that were state of the art at that time have been superseded by many generations of improved devices and materials. This discussion is concerned with late survival after surgery or interventional catheterization involving cardiac valves, intraatrial or intraventricular repairs, central arterial procedures, and creation of a complete or partial vena caval or atrial-dependent pulmonary circulation.

Congenitally Malformed Cardiac Valves

Congenitally stenotic or incompetent semilunar or atrioventricular valves are treated by cardiac surgery or, if ste-

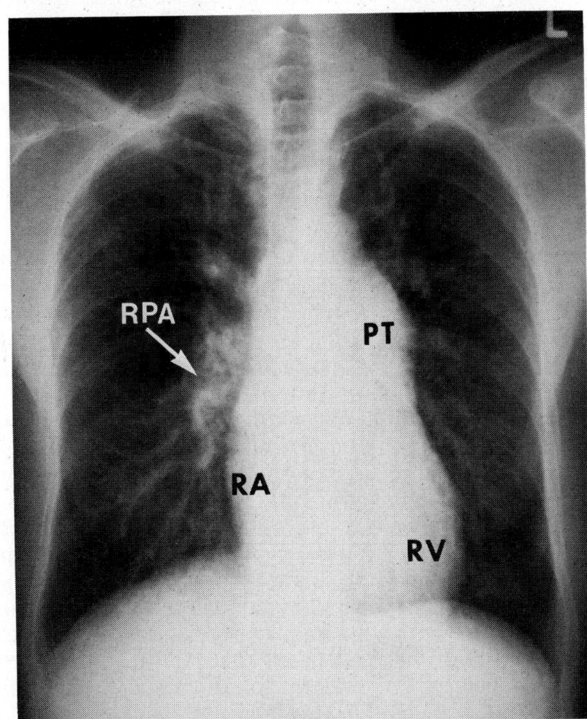

FIGURE 32-9. Radiograph from a 67-year-old man with Eisenmenger's complex; he died at age 69 of Legionnaire's disease. The pulmonary trunk (PT) and its branches (RPA = right pulmonary artery) are conspicuously dilated but the heart size is virtually normal.

notic, interventional catheterization. Surgery involves reconstruction or replacement of the malformed valve, either alone or with repair of coexisting defects. Long-term results are colored by these variables.

ISOLATED PULMONARY VALVE STENOSIS (see also p. 968). This anomaly lends itself to surgical repair with excellent results. Postoperative valvular residua are relatively minor, and residual poststenotic dilatation of the pulmonary arterial trunk is of no clinical significance, even when marked. These exemplary results are qualified by the age of the patient at operation and the severity of the preoperative gradient. If marked to severe pulmonary stenosis is relieved surgically during childhood, long-term survival patterns are similar to age- and sex-matched controls.[1] Adults who undergo surgical valvotomy after age 21 years also have excellent results, but the more severe the preoperative stenosis and the longer that the right ventricle has confronted the increased afterload, the less optimal are the long-term results, including late death from right ventricular failure. These conclusions support the current practice of relieving hemodynamically significant pulmonary stenosis during childhood and underscore the desirability of surveillance through adulthood.

Balloon dilatation has largely replaced surgical repair of typical isolated congenital pulmonary valve stenosis (Fig. 32–3).[88–91] Refinements in techniques have resulted in relief of gradients comparable to the results achieved at surgery. Long-term results are not yet available, but balloon valvuloplasty promises to be as effective as surgical valvotomy.

CONGENITAL AORTIC STENOSIS (see also p. 922). When caused by a bicuspid aortic valve, this malformation is amenable to direct repair in young patients or valve replacement in older patients.[92–95] Surgical valvotomy or balloon valvuloplasty presupposes that there is a pliant, noncalcified bicuspid valve with obstruction caused by congenital fusion (nonseparation) of the commissures. The best that valvotomy can achieve is a functionally normal bicuspid aortic valve with minor degrees of regurgitation. Valvotomy of a congenitally stenotic bicuspid aortic valve in childhood or adolescence provides temporary relief of obstruction, but the valve has the same, if not a greater, tendency than does a native, functionally normal bicuspid aortic valve to thicken, calcify, and become stenotic with the passage of time. Significant postvalvotomy aortic regurgitation tends to develop gradually, but infective endocarditis can cause sudden, severe incompetence that requires urgent valve replacement. The risk of infective endocarditis is not reduced by valvotomy, even if there is complete relief of bicuspid aortic stenosis. The longer the interval after operation, the greater the need for reoperation.[93–95]

Balloon dilatation in young patients with congenital bicuspid aortic stenosis is associated with considerable variability and unpredictability of results.[96,97] This procedure does not permit the meticulous relief of commissural fusion that is possible under direct vision. The best that can be achieved by ideal balloon separation of fused commissures is an outlook that approximates that just described for open operation.

Surgically important *congenital aortic regurgitation* may occur during the natural history of a bicuspid aortic valve or after valvotomy for bicuspid aortic stenosis. Prime objectives of operation (valve replacement) for aortic regurgitation are the removal of left ventricular volume overload and the preservation or restoration of satisfactory left ventricular function. Even if these objectives are achieved, a minority of patients succumb late after operation, not because of heart failure but because of what is presumed to be a disturbance in ventricular rhythm (sudden death). The fate of the aortic prosthesis and the need for anticoagulants are important determinants of late postoperative outcome.

EBSTEIN'S ANOMALY (see also pp. 940 and 970). This malformation is the most common cause of surgically important congenital tricuspid regurgitation. Operation relieves the right ventricular volume overload and improves right ventricular function.[98–100] Closure of the interatrial communication removes the risk of paradoxical emboli, and interruption of right atrioventricular bypass tracts eliminates the risk of a rapid ventricular response to atrial flutter or fibrillation (Fig. 32–10). Supraventricular arrhythmias may recur postoperatively, but if the accessory pathways are divided, the ventricular response is not accelerated, and the arrhythmias respond to conventional pharmacological management.

Every attempt should be made to reconstruct rather than replace the tricuspid valve (Fig. 32–6), even though there are obligatory residual abnormalities following use of the large anterior leaflet to create a unicuspid valve. Replacement of the valve carries a late mortality of 10 to 15 per cent.[101] Tissue valves are preferred; a mechanical prosthesis poses the risk of pulmonary embolization even with anticoagulation. Abnormal left ventricular geometry and function have been identified in patients with Ebstein's anomaly,[53,60a] but the long-term postoperative effects are unknown.

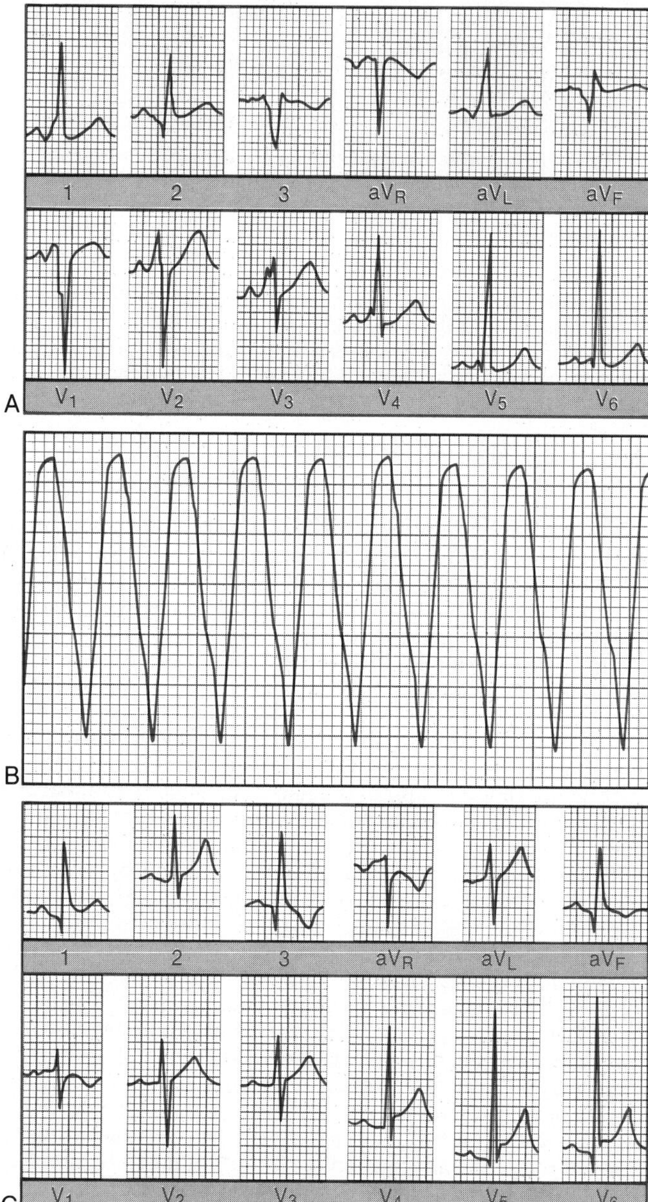

FIGURE 32–10. *A,* Twelve-lead electrocardiogram from a patient with Ebstein's anomaly of the tricuspid valve. There are typical fusion beats due to a right atrioventricular bypass tract. The delta wave is directed to the left, superior and posterior. *B,* Lead V_1 showing antegrade wide QRS tachycardia via the right bypass tract. *C,* Twelve-lead electrocardiogram after tricuspid valve reconstruction with interruption of the bypass tract by surgical dissociation between right atrium and right ventricle. The delta wave is absent.

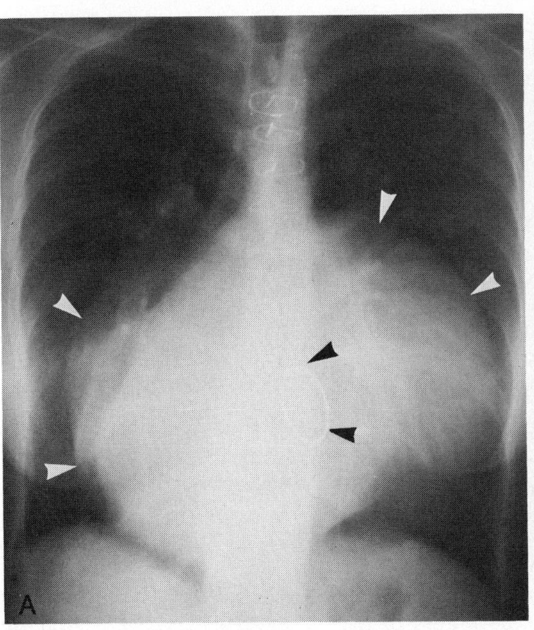

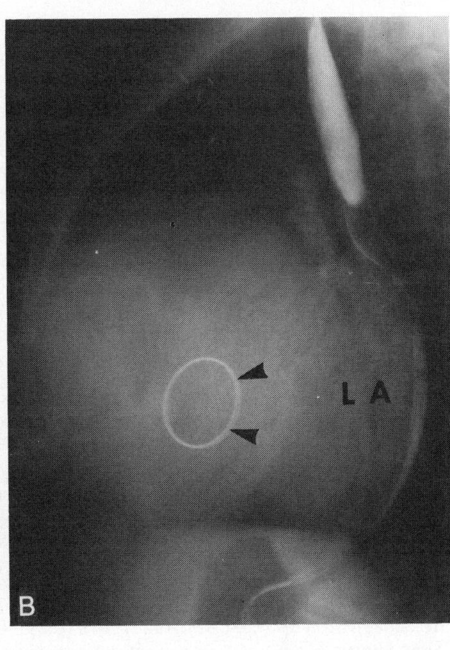

FIGURE 32-11. Chest radiographs from a 24-year-old woman with congenitally corrected transposition of the great arteries 5 years after replacement of an incompetent left atrioventricular valve with a tissue valve (arrowheads). *A,* The cardiac silhouette shown here is identical with the preoperative silhouette, resembling a huge ball consisting almost entirely of a massive left atrium (white arrowheads) that appears to be suspended from a narrow vascular pedicle. Neither great artery is border-forming. *B,* Lateral projection showing the prosthetic ring (black arrowheads) and the huge left atrium (LA).

ISOLATED INCOMPETENCE OF A LEFT-SIDED ATRIOVENTRICULAR VALVE IN CONGENITALLY CORRECTED TRANSPOSITION OF THE GREAT ARTERIES. This lesion is caused by an Ebstein-like anomaly of a tricuspid valve in the systemic (inverted) position.[102] When surgical relief is indicated, the valve almost always requires replacement (Fig. 32-11). Long-term outcome is determined chiefly by the chronicity of preoperative regurgitation, by the functional adequacy (or inadequacy) of a morphological right ventricle in the systemic location, and by a 2 per cent per year accrued incidence of high-degree intranodal heart block.[13]

Intraatrial Surgery

ATRIAL SEPTAL DEFECT (OSTIUM SECUNDUM) (see also p. 906). This malformation lends itself to surgical closure with excellent long-term results. Operation before 24 years of age resulted in a 30-year actuarial survival that was the same as age- and sex-matched controls (98 per cent and 97 per cent).[103] When operation was performed on patients who were 24 to 40 years of age and whose preoperative pulmonary arterial pressures were normal, survival also approximated that of the control group. When pulmonary arterial systolic pressure exceeded 40 mm Hg, late survival was one-half of that of the control group, although life expectancy in the surgically treated older patients was better than with medical treatment. Even patients who were 60 years of age or older at the time of operation benefited, at least in the short term, regardless of pulmonary arterial pressure or functional class as long as the left-to-right shunt through the atrial septal defect remained large.[104]

After operation in childhood, right ventricular dimensions decrease, often strikingly,[105] but when adults undergo surgery, right ventricular dimensions remain abnormal in about 80 per cent of cases. If there is preoperative right ventricular failure and tricuspid regurgitation, late postoperative right atrial and right ventricular dilatation are the rule, and right ventricular ejection fraction seldom normalizes. These patients improve but usually remain symptomatic, and long-term outcome is influenced by preoperative pulmonary vascular resistance.[106]

A minority of patients who undergo surgical closure of an ostium secundum atrial septal defect during childhood experience the late onset of supraventricular arrhythmias believed to be related to patchy fibrosis of the right atrium secondary to dilatation, and perhaps to sinus node dysfunction.[107,108] In adults, chronic preoperative atrial fibrillation usually persists after surgical repair, but cardioversion followed by antiarrhythmic therapy may be efficacious. When operation is performed on patients older than age 40 years, about one-half of those in preoperative sinus rhythm experience late postoperative development of atrial fibrillation.

Intraatrial Surgery for Complex Cyanotic Congenital Heart Disease

COMPLETE TRANSPOSITION OF THE GREAT ARTERIES (p. 941). This malformation has been managed until recently by a Rashkind balloon atrial septostomy performed on the neonate followed by intraatrial redirection of venous return (Mustard or Senning venous switch operation) during the first 6 months of life.[1] These procedures have given way to the *arterial switch operation,* but there are large numbers of patients, including many young adults, who underwent intraatrial redirection of venous return 5 to 25 years ago.[109,110] Twenty-year survival after *atrial* switch operations has been reported at 80 to 90 per cent, but complications are the rule. Apart from postoperative electrophysiological sequelae (Fig. 32-12), an issue of fundamental importance is the long-term

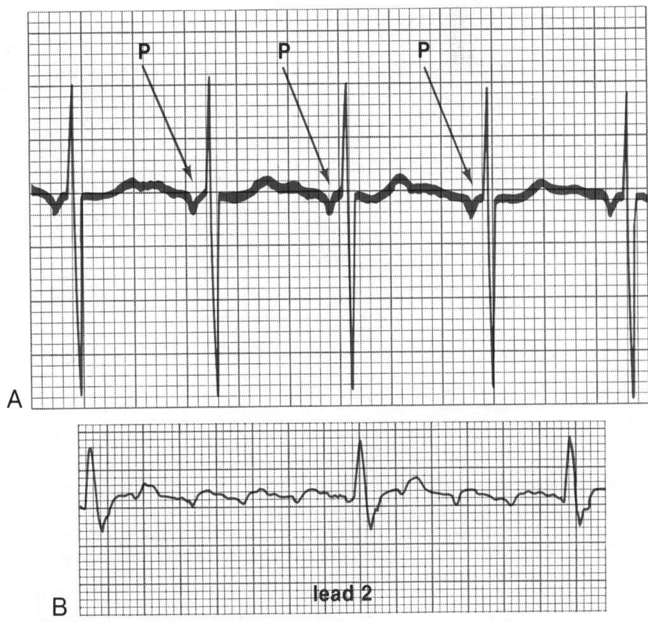

FIGURE 32-12. *A,* Junctional ectopic rhythm early after a Mustard repair for complete transposition of the great arteries. *B,* Late-onset atrial flutter with a slow ventricular response (impaired atrioventricular conduction) in a 25-year-old man who had a Mustard repair in infancy. The patient developed sinus node dysfunction in addition to atrial tachyarrhythmias.

adequacy of a morphological right ventricle in the systemic location.[111-113] The postoperative right ventricle normally does not increase its ejection fraction in response to exercise, and there is a high incidence of coexisting left ventricular dysfunction.

Intraventricular Surgery

Intraventricular surgery is performed through a right atrial incision or through a ventriculotomy in the morphological right ventricle. Long-term survival depends on a number of variables, including patient age at operation, the degree of relief of the loading conditions imposed on ventricular myocardium, myocardial protection during operation, electrophysiological sequelae, and the durability of prosthetic materials.

FALLOT'S TETRALOGY. This malformation is a case in point. When intraventricular repair is performed during infancy, long-term survival is good, but about 15 per cent of patients require reoperation.[114-117] The incidence of bifascicular block or high-degree heart block (Fig. 32–13) has decreased significantly with current operative techniques. Patients who had undergone early palliative shunts followed by intracardiac repair at about 2 years of age experienced 87 per cent survival 10 to 20 years after operation; all but a minority were free from significant cardiac or vascular symptoms and for all practical purposes were leading normal lives. Some patients who reach adulthood after having undergone Blalock-Taussig shunts in infancy or early childhood maintain symptomatic improvement for decades after operation, and benefit from intracardiac repair as adults (Fig. 32–14). However, patients who are 40 years or older at the time of intraventricular repair have a late mortality of about 15 per cent.[118,119] Late postoperative *left* ventricular function is related to age at the time of intracardiac repair and to previous shunt procedures (Fig. 32–14). Patients with severe cyanotic Fallot's tetralogy have reductions in left ventricular volume and ejection fraction related to decreased pulmonary arterial blood flow. If intracardiac repair is undertaken after 2 years of age, volumes of the left side of the heart increase but left ventricular function remains subnormal.[120,121]

Central Arterial Surgery

PATENT DUCTUS ARTERIOSUS (p. 913). Division of an isolated restrictive (small) patent ductus arteriosus in childhood represents one of the few categoric cures of congenital malformations of the heart and circulation. Transcatheter ductal occlusion must compete with this record, which is ideal except for the thoracotomy. After operation, patients are normal in the literal sense. When the ductus is moderately restrictive or nonrestrictive (large), division in childhood usually results in regression of left atrial and left ventricular enlargement, and in normalization of pulmonary arterial and right ventricular systolic pressures. If a relatively large (nonrestrictive) ductus remains undivided until after childhood, long-term outcome depends on the preoperative pulmonary

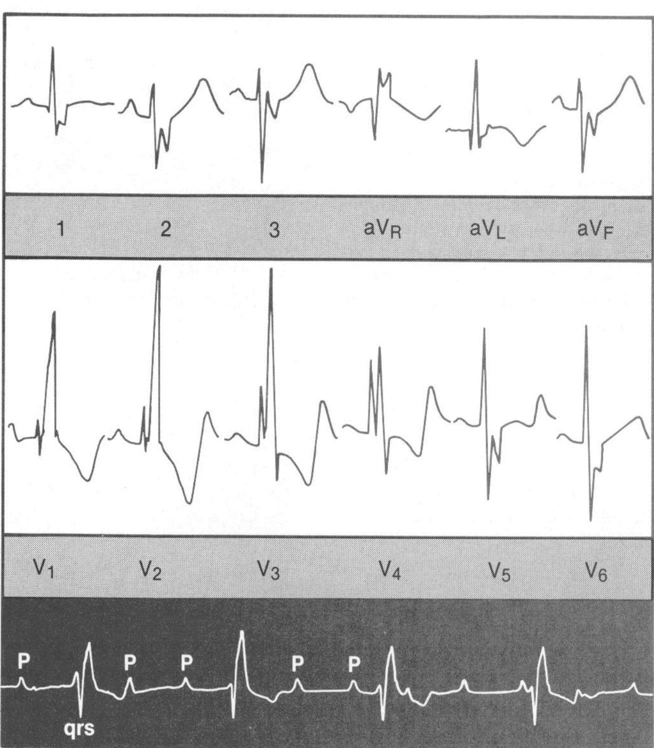

FIGURE 32–13. Twelve-lead electrocardiogram (top panel) and single channel electrocardiogram from a patient with Fallot's tetralogy after intracardiac repair. Bifascicular block (right bundle branch block with left anterior fascicular block) *(top)* progressed to complete atrioventricular block *(bottom)*.

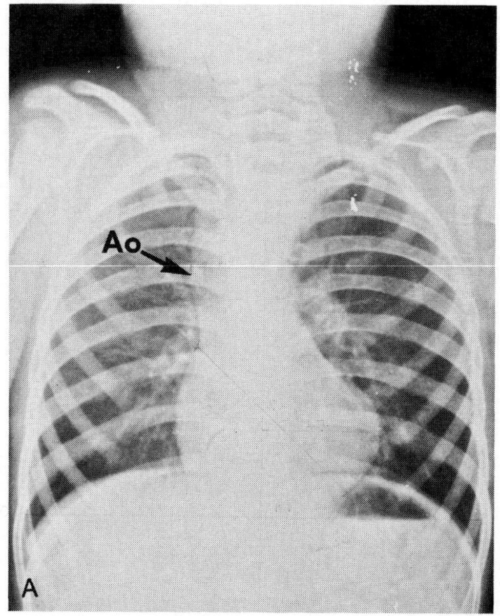

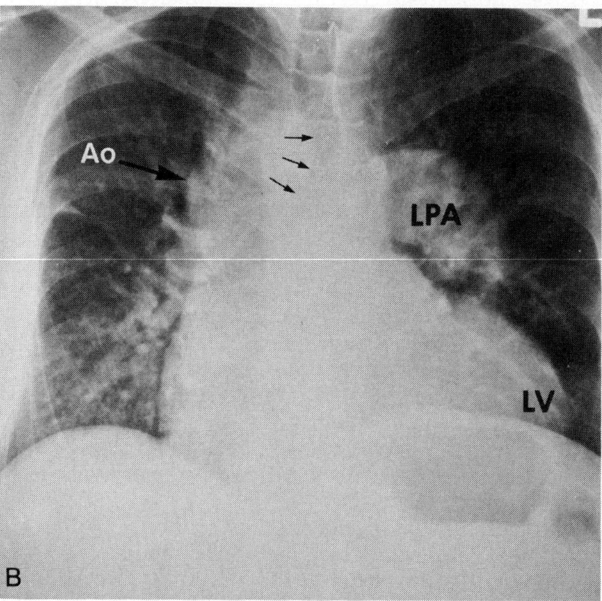

FIGURE 32–14. *A,* Radiograph before a left Blalock-Taussig shunt in a 4-year-old boy with cyanotic Fallot's tetralogy and a right aortic arch (Ao). *B,* Same patient at age 50 years. Pulmonary vascularity is increased. The left pulmonary artery (LPA) is aneurysmal. The large right ascending aorta (Ao) indents the trachea (small arrows), and an enlarged left ventricle (LV) occupies the apex. The patient underwent intracardiac repair with revision of the shunt.

vascular resistance and the effects of chronic left ventricular volume overload (Fig. 32–5).[122]

COARCTATION OF THE AORTA. After surgical repair, residual, sequelae, and complications are frequent and require indefinite follow-up.[123–127] There are three principal concerns: residual systolic hypertension despite absence of coarctation gradients, a bicuspid aortic valve, and recoarctation. The major predisposing factor for hypertension after coarctation repair is the duration of preoperative hypertension that results in baroreceptor abnormalities and changes in compliance of the walls of the major arteries.[124,128] The natural history of a coexisting functionally normal bicuspid aortic valve after coarctation repair is the same as that of an isolated congenitally bicuspid aortic valve, including the risk of infective endocarditis. Recurrence of coarctation after reparative surgery is related to the technique used for the initial operation.[129] After infancy, end-to-end anastomosis has the lowest incidence of recoarctation. Complications of premature coronary atherosclerosis, including myocardial infarction and congestive heart failure, were major causes of death in 12 per cent of patients 11 to 25 years after coarctectomy.[123] Cerebrovascular accidents owing to rupture of an aneurysm of the circle of Willis have been reported in normotensive patients long after successful coarctation repair.[126] Abnormalities of the mitral apparatus occur in 26 to 58 per cent of patients with coarctation of the aorta and vary from clinically occult and functionally benign to grossly overt stenosis or incompetence of the orifice.[130]

CONGENITAL SINUS OF VALSALVA ANEURYSMS. These typically rupture well after puberty but before age 30 years (see earlier discussion).[13] Surgical mortality is low, and when aortic regurgitation is not present preoperatively, late results of repair are excellent.

Caval to Pulmonary Arterial Circulations

THE FONTAN PROCEDURE[131] (see p. 954). This operation has undergone a number of modifications, the most recent of which is total caval-to-pulmonary arterial connection.[132] The Fontan and modified Fontan procedures are applied chiefly to tricuspid atresia or single ventricle with pulmonary stenosis but now include physiologically analogous complex cyanotic malformations in which biventricular repair is not feasible because of an underdeveloped ventricle. Late results depend principally on ventricular function and on maintenance of sinus rhythm.[133] Atrial fibrillation or flutter adversely elevates mean right atrial pressure chiefly because of the effect of the atrial arrhythmia on left ventricular filling pressure, a rise that results in an increase in right atrial and caval mean pressures. Ventricular function is better in the presence of a morphological *left* ventricle, as in tricuspid atresia or univentricular hearts of the left ventricular type.[134] Long-term function is, as a rule, not as good when a Fontan procedure is performed on patients with univentricular hearts of the *right* ventricular type.[134] Patients who are carefully selected for operation have fared well and often are New York Heart Association functional class I or II as late as 15 years after surgery. Operation in patients 18 years or older also has been successful, sometimes achieving remarkable degrees of rehabilitation. Ninety-three per cent of these adult patients are in New York Heart Association functional class I or II.[135–137]

MEDICAL MANAGEMENT OF CONGENITAL HEART DISEASE IN THE ADULT

CYANOTIC CONGENITAL HEART DISEASE: HEMATOLOGICAL MANAGEMENT, RENAL FUNCTION, AND URATE METABOLISM

In response to tissue hypoxia, erythropoietin is produced by specialized sensor cells in the kidneys, resulting in an increase in the number of circulating red blood cells and in an expanded blood volume.[138,139] If an increase in erythrocyte mass is sufficient to raise the tissue oxygen concentration above the threshold for release of erythropoietin by the renal oxygen sensors, a new equilibrium is established at a higher hematocrit. However, erythrocytosis may exceed the range at which blood viscosity becomes a limiting factor in tissue oxygen delivery. An equilibrium is not achieved, and increased erythropoietin secretion and expansion of the erythrocyte mass proceed despite the detrimental effects of the further increase in hematocrit.[140] Iron deficiency significantly affects blood viscosity and shortens erythrocyte survival time.[141,142] Iron-deficient microcytic red cells are relatively rigid and resist deformation at high shear rates and in the microcirculation; accordingly, whole blood viscosity is increased. Phlebotomy-induced iron deficiency results in microcytosis, which leads to a reduction in the oxygen-carrying capacity of the erythrocytes and to an increase in viscosity that may offset potential benefits of hematocrit reduction. The erythrocytosis of cyanotic congenital heart disease is fundamentally different from polycythemia vera (primary polycythemia, p. 1749), an idiopathic clonal disorder of the bone marrow that results in an autonomous overproduction of red cells and is accompanied by thrombocytosis, leukocytosis, and basophilia.

Cyanotic patients with erythrocytosis fall into two categories: compensated and decompensated.[140,143] Those with *compensated* erythrocytosis establish equilibrium hematocrits in an iron replete state. Symptoms attributable to hyperviscosity usually are mild or absent when hematocrit levels are less than 65 per cent, and absent, mild, or moderate even at higher hematocrit levels, occasionally 70 per cent or more. Phlebotomy for relief of hyperviscosity symptoms is required rarely, if at all. Patients with *decompensated* erythrocytosis fail to establish equilibrium conditions and manifest unstable, rising hematocrit levels and recurrent, moderate to severe symptoms attributable to hyperviscosity. Erythrocyte production is not controlled, and negative feedback inhibition does not occur. Symptomatic hyperviscosity is common, prompting therapeutic phlebotomy that depletes iron stores. The pathophysiological mechanisms responsible for symptoms in patients with decompensated erythrocytosis are complex but are believed to be related to tissue hypoxia, iron deficiency, and hyperviscosity.

The risk of *cerebrovascular accidents* (stroke) in patients with cyanotic congenital heart disease is greatest in children younger than age 4 years with iron deficiency.[143,144] Dehydration is an important aggravating cause in these young patients in whom the cerebrovascular accidents are due to thromboses of intracranial veins and sinuses. By contrast, adults with cyanotic congenital heart disease do not appear to be at increased risk of stroke, even if the hematocrit level is above 65 per cent and the erythrocytosis is decompensated (iron deficient).[140,143] Cerebrovascular accidents in cyanotic adults usually are associated with excessive, injudicious phlebotomies or with use of aspirin or anticoagulants that reinforce the intrinsic hemostatic defects (see later) and cause intracranial bleeding.[143]

Phlebotomy is not recommended for adult patients with compensated erythrocytosis, including those with hematocrit levels in the range of 70 per cent, as long as symptoms attributed to hyperviscosity are mild or absent. Phlebotomy is recommended in patients with significant hyperviscosity symptoms and with hematocrit levels of 65 per cent or greater, provided dehydration is not the cause. Dehydration is treated by volume replacement, not phlebotomy. A comparatively simple, safe outpatient method for phlebotomy in adults involves the removal of 500 ml of blood over 30 to 45 minutes while quantitative volume replacement with isotonic saline or salt-free dextran is carried out.

Symptoms of iron deficiency usually are indistinguishable from those of hyperviscosity, but in adults with cyanotic heart disease, symptomatic hyperviscosity in an *iron replete state* seldom occurs with hematocrit levels of less than 65 per cent.[143] Symptoms in patients with hematocrit levels lower than 65 per cent are almost always due to iron deficiency, so phlebotomy aggravates rather than alleviates the symptoms.

Cyanotic congenital heart disease patients, especially those with decompensated erythrocytosis, should be cautioned to avoid over-the-counter preparations that contain iron. When iron is administered therapeutically in symptomatic iron-deficient patients with inappropriately low hematocrit levels, the dose should be small (325 mg of ferrous sulfate per day). Hematocrit levels rise quickly, so erythrocyte response should be closely monitored. Significant erythrocytosis can lead to inaccuracies in laboratory determinations. Hematocrits must be based on automated blood counts because microhematocrit centrifugation methods result in plasma trapping and falsely elevated hematocrit levels.[143]

Home oxygen therapy is sometimes advised, especially during sleep.[145] From both the hematological and respiratory points of view, there is little evidence that home oxygen is useful in adults with cyanotic congenital heart disease, and the drying effect on nasal mucous membranes tends to increase the risk of epistaxes.

HEMOSTASIS (see also p. 1767). Coagulation is abnormal in cyanotic congenital heart disease.[143,146-149] For the most part, bleeding tendencies are mild and characterized by easy bruising, petechial hemorrhages in the skin and mucous membranes, epistaxes, gingival bleeding, and hemoptysis.[143] Platelet counts usually are in the low range of normal, but when the increased blood volume is taken into account, the total circulating platelet mass is closer to normal than platelet concentrations indicate. Inherent abnormalities in platelet function[150] are reinforced by aspirin and other nonsteroidal antiinflammatory agents. Aspirin, oral anticoagulants, and heparin are ill-advised because the inherent risk of stroke is low and because these drugs have no demonstrated efficacy in reducing that negligible risk and instead may significantly aggravate the existing hemostatic defects and increase the risk of bleeding. Abnormalities of the intrinsic and extrinsic coagulation systems, with elevations of the prothrombin time and activated partial thromboplastin time, respectively, and specific deficiencies of several coagulation factors have been reported.[146] Failure to adjust the citrate concentration for the hematocrit level during blood collection may lead to spurious test results for the prothrombin time and activated partial thromboplastin time.

Serious bleeding may occur during surgery or accidental trauma.[151] Phlebotomy has been shown to temporarily improve hemostasis in some erythrocytotic patients, so preoperative phlebotomy is selectively used to reduce the hematocrit level to just below 65 per cent. The activated partial thromboplastin time is a useful estimate of the overall response of the intrinsic coagulation system to preoperative phlebotomy. Phlebotomized units are reserved for potential autologous transfusions.

RENAL FUNCTION AND URATE METABOLISM. These variables often are abnormal in adults with cyanotic congenital heart disease and erythrocytosis.[152,153] High plasma uric acid levels are secondary to inappropriately low fractional uric acid excretion by the kidney rather than to urate overproduction.[152] Enhanced urate reabsorption is believed to result from renal hypoperfusion reinforced by a high filtration fraction. Accordingly, hyperuricemia serves as a marker of abnormal intrauterine hemodynamics.[153] Renal histopathology is characterized by enlarged, hypercellular glomeruli, basement membrane thickening, focal interstitial fibrosis, tubular atrophy, and hyalinization of afferent and efferent arterioles.[154]

Arthralgias are relatively common in erythrocytotic adults with cyanotic congenital heart disease, but acute gouty arthritis is relatively uncommon, despite elevated uric acid levels, an observation similar to that in other forms of secondary hyperuricemia.[155] If colchicine is used to treat acute gouty arthritis, special care must be taken to avoid the dehydrating effects of vomiting and diarrhea. Nonsteroidal antiinflammatory agents may then be considered but should be used cautiously in patients with potential hemostatic defects. Whereas uricosuric agents are not routinely advised, they can be efficacious in patients with hyperuricemia and recurrences of gouty arthritis. Intraarticular steroid injections are sometimes required. Overt tophaceous deposits of urate are exceptional, even in patients with considerable chronic hyperuricemia (Fig. 32–15).[152]

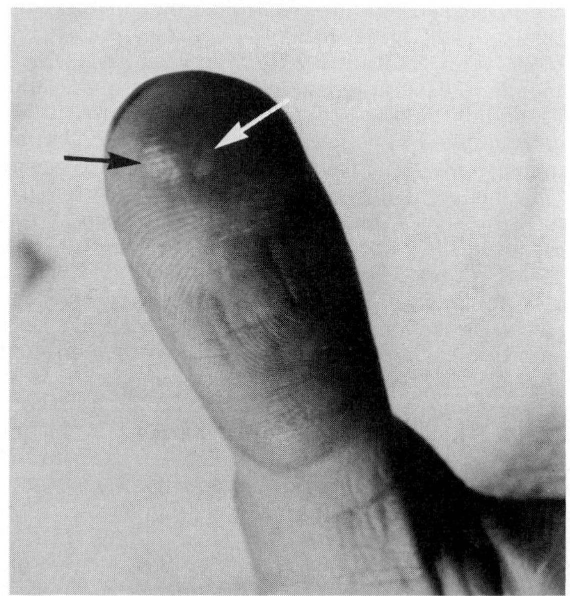

FIGURE 32–15. **Urate deposit (arrows) on the pad of the thumb of a 24-year-old man with complex cyanotic congenital heart disease.**

CYANOTIC CONGENITAL HEART DISEASE: DYNAMICS OF OXYGEN UPTAKE AND CONTROL OF VENTILATION

Diversion of systemic venous blood from the pulmonary circulation into the systemic arterial circulation is a basic pathological fault in patients with cyanotic congenital heart disease. Exercise tends to increase significantly the degree of venoarterial shunting and materially influences the dynamics of oxygen uptake (VO_2) and ventilation. Patients with cyanotic congenital heart disease have markedly abnormal responses in achieving a new steady state for VO_2 after the onset of exercise.[156] The prolonged onset and recovery VO_2 kinetics result in large oxygen deficits and hypoxemia, even with low levels of exercise, and suggest that patients with significant right-to-left shunts may rely on an unusual degree of anaerobic metabolism to perform exercise. Patients with right-to-left

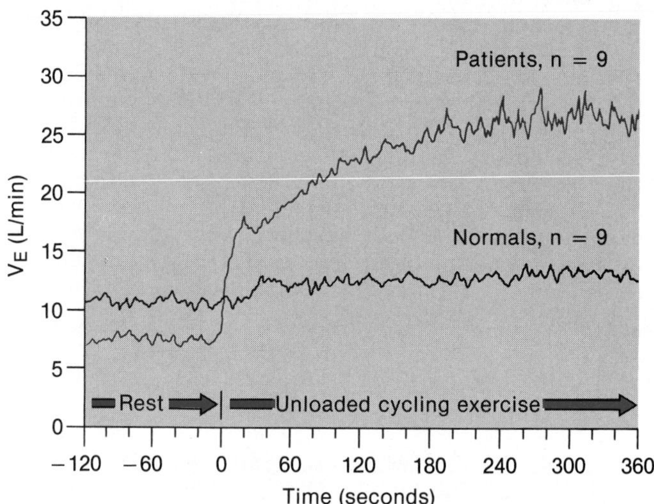

FIGURE 32–16. **The increase in ventilation in response to unloaded cycle ergometric exercise in nine adults with right-to-left shunts, and in nine normal subjects. The patients had higher minute ventilation both at rest and in response to exercise. (From Sietsema, K. E., et al.: Control of ventilation during exercise in patients with central venous to systemic arterial shunts. J. Appl. Physiol. *64*:234, 1988.)**

shunts also have greater increases in ventilation during exercise than do normal subjects; dyspnea on exertion may be a prominent clinical complaint.[157] Unlike the prolonged kinetics of VO_2, cyanotic patients exhibit large increases in ventilation in phase I, and in contrast to normal subjects, ventilation increases more rapidly than VO_2 in phase II (Fig. 32–16).[157] Ventilatory stimuli that are potentially augmented by exercise in patients with right-to-left shunts include hypoxemia, metabolic acidosis, and shunting of carbon dioxide into the systemic arterial circulation.

INFECTIVE ENDOCARDITIS: RISKS AND PROPHYLAXIS

(See also Chap. 35)

With the advent of intracardiac surgery and of prosthetic devices, the clinical and bacteriological profile of infective endocarditis changed significantly.[1,158] Certain operations (ligation of a patent ductus arteriosus) eliminate the risk, whereas others (shunts, prosthetic valves, or conduits) materially increase the risk. However, certain general principles still prevail, namely, that there are two major predisposing causes of infective endocarditis: a susceptible cardiac or vascular substrate, and the presence of bacteremia. Susceptible lesions include those associated with high-velocity flow, jet impact, and focal increases in the rate of shear. Portals of entry include the oral cavity, the genitourinary tract in males, the upper and lower gastrointestinal tract, the airways and respiratory tract, obstetrical and gynecological procedures, and certain types of noncardiac surgery. Prophylaxis for infective endocarditis comprises nonchemotherapeutic and chemotherapeutic (antimicrobial) measures.

The risk of infective endocarditis in congenital heart disease has been classified as low-risk unoperated anomalies, low- or no-risk postoperative, intermediate-risk unoperated, intermediate-risk postoperative, and high-risk postoperative.[1] Examples of low-risk unoperated anomalies include ostium secundum atrial septal defect and mild pulmonary valve stenosis. A no-risk postoperative lesion is typified by division of a patent ductus arteriosus. Intermediate-risk unoperated lesions are represented by functionally normal bicuspid aortic valve, aortic regurgitation, restrictive ventricular septal defect, or patent ductus arteriosus. Intermediate-risk postoperative lesions are represented by bicuspid aortic stenosis, and residual left atrioventricular valve or aortic regurgitation. High-risk postoperative substrates include rigid prosthetic valves, especially left-sided, external valved conduits, and aortopulmonary shunts.

Chemotherapeutic prophylaxis is based on the cardiac lesion, the source of potential bacteremia, and the absence or presence of a history of antibiotic sensitivity. The American Heart Association recommendations (p. 1098) have been incorporated into convenient wallet-sized instructions that can be given to patients and referring physicians.

Nonchemotherapeutic prophylaxis includes day-to-day oral hygiene, skin care, nail care, and avoidance of certain female contraceptive devices.[1] The spongy, fragile gums of some patients with cyanotic congenital heart disease are of special concern, necessitating twice-yearly teeth and gum prophylaxis. Meticulous skin care is important, especially in adolescents and young adults with acne, which may be distributed beyond the face. Biting or picking of fingernails risks injury to contiguous skin and predisposes to paronychial infection with staphylococci. Intrauterine devices are best avoided because of the risk of bacteremia.

PREGNANCY AND CONGENITAL HEART DISEASE

(See p. 1793)

Central to this topic is the interplay between maternal circulatory and respiratory physiology and maternal congenital heart disease, and the effects of this interplay on the fetus, which is exposed to immediate risks that threaten its viability and to remote risks that express themselves as developmental defects or transmitted congenital anomalies.

THE UNOPERATED PATIENT

In a practical sense, the most important category of unoperated patients are those with common congenital cardiac anomalies that are likely to be found in adult women.

OSTIUM SECUNDUM ATRIAL SEPTAL DEFECT (see also p. 1794). Because the natural history of this defect spans the reproductive years, and because the majority of affected patients are female, the malformation is of special importance. Young women with uncomplicated ostium secundum atrial septal defects usually tolerate pregnancy—even multiple pregnancies—with no tangible ill effects (Fig. 32–4). After the fourth decade, however, patients with otherwise uncomplicated secundum defects experience an increased incidence of supraventricular arrhythmia that may cause right ventricular failure and peripheral edema and, accordingly, serve to increase the probability of venous stasis and thrombophlebitis.

An important concern is the risk of paradoxical embolization from leg veins because emboli tend to course from the inferior vena cava through the atrial septal defect into the systemic circulation.[13,160,161] Meticulous leg care is advised to minimize venous stasis. Also important but less well known are potentially hazardous effects of acute blood loss in patients with unoperated ostium secundum atrial septal defects.[1] Hemorrhage during delivery results in a rise in systemic vascular resistance and a fall in systemic venous return, a combination that augments the left-to-right shunt, sometimes appreciably. Pulmonary hypertension is uncommon in young women with ostium secundum atrial septal defects, but its presence, even in the absence of a reversed shunt, increases the risk of pregnancy.

PATENT DUCTUS ARTERIOSUS (see also p. 1794). This anomaly occurs predominantly in females but is becoming less important as a complication of pregnancy because the clinical diagnosis is simple and surgical or bioprosthetic closure is routine and curative in childhood (see earlier). Asymptomatic young women with a small or moderate-sized ductus and normal pulmonary arterial pressure can anticipate an uncomplicated pregnancy, apart from the risk of infective endocarditis during delivery. One of the author's patients, a 57-year-old woman with a moderately restrictive patent ductus, endured 20 pregnancies with 12 live births (Fig. 32–17). The gestational fall in systemic vascular resistance tends to decrease ductal flow, but if the shunt is large, that benefit is not likely to compensate for the hemodynamic burden of pregnancy. At highest risk is the patient with a nonrestrictive patent ductus and a reversed shunt. The hazard of pulmonary vascular disease is again underscored, and the low oxygen saturation in the descending aorta puts the fetus at risk.

ISOLATED PULMONARY VALVE STENOSIS (see also p. 1795). Fifty per cent of patients are female[13]; survival to adulthood is usual, even if there is significant obstruction to right ventricular outflow. Mild to moderate pulmonary stenosis poses little or no threat to the mother, and occasionally even severe pulmonary stenosis is well tolerated despite the gestational volume overload imposed on an already pressure-overloaded

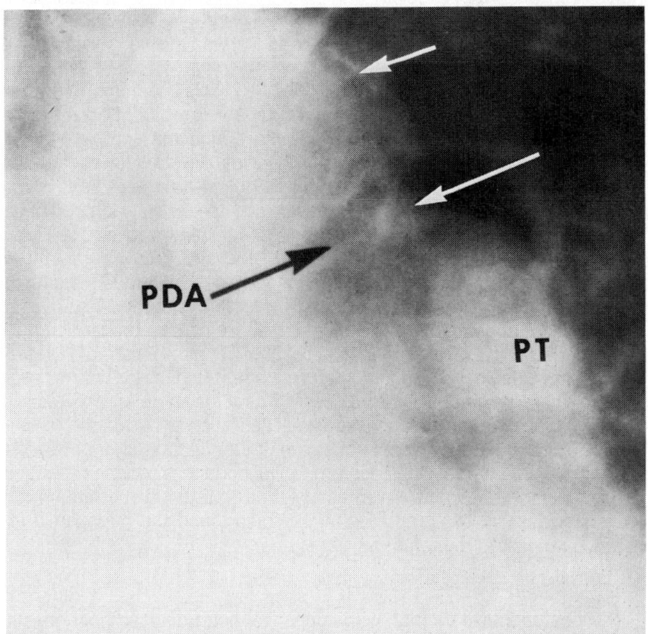

FIGURE 32–17. Chest radiograph (closeup) from a 57-year-old woman with a calcified patent ductus arteriosus (PDA, paired arrows) that was moderately restrictive. She had had 20 pregnancies with 12 live births. The pulmonary trunk (PT) is dilated. The aorta (Ao) also contains calcium (unmarked large white arrow).

right ventricle. Infective endocarditis prophylaxis is called for during delivery, although the risk in patients with mild pulmonary stenosis is negligible, if not absent.

COARCTATION OF THE AORTA (see also p. 1794). This lesion occurs chiefly in males but is dealt with here because maternal morbidity is high.[13] Pregnancy increases the risk of aortic rupture or dissection and of cerebral hemorrhage from rupture of an aneurysm of the circle of Willis.[13,160] Blood pressure variations of pregnant women with aortic coarctation are similar in direction but occur from a higher initial level than in normal pregnancy. The incidence of toxemia is much less with the hypertension of coarctation than in pregnant women with other forms of hypertension. Left ventricular failure is exceptional despite the increased gestational blood volume that is added to the pressure-overloaded left ventricle. The risk of infective endocarditis is significantly higher on a coexisting bicuspid aortic valve than at the site of coarctation (see earlier).

BICUSPID AORTIC VALVE. An isolated functionally normal bicuspid aortic valve is likely to go unrecognized in young women. The clinical index of suspicion is low because the malformation occurs predominantly in males and the auscultatory signs are subtle. Because of the high susceptibility of the bicuspid aortic valve to infective endocarditis, the anomaly may become evident after delivery because of fever or the development of acute severe aortic regurgitation.[16]

CHRONIC BICUSPID AORTIC REGURGITATION. When moderate or even severe, this lesion usually is well tolerated during pregnancy, provided that the adaptive response of the left ventricle permits normal function, which normally is the case. The gestational fall in systemic vascular resistance coupled with a more rapid heart rate (shorter diastole) results in a decrease in regurgitant flow. The risk of infective endocarditis is high, and prophylaxis is required during delivery.

In the occasional young woman with congenital *bicuspid aortic stenosis,* the increased cardiac output of pregnancy is imposed on a pressure-overloaded left ventricle. Most asymptomatic women entering pregnancy with mild-to-moderate aortic stenosis do well, but if obstruction is marked to severe, circulatory reserve is limited. Dyspnea, angina pectoris, or cerebral symptoms that precede conception or that appear during early gestation predict serious sequelae. The stenotic valve is at risk of infective endocarditis.

FALLOT'S TETRALOGY (see also p. 1795). This is the most common cyanotic malformation that permits natural survival to reproductive age, and the sex distribution is nearly equal.[13] A paucity of symptoms and the presence of mild cyanosis before conception do not assure a smooth course. The gestational fall in systemic vascular resistance, coupled with the augmented cardiac output and increased venous return to an obstructed right ventricle, results in an augmentation of the right-to-left shunt and a fall in systemic arterial oxygen saturation. Cyanosis deepens, but the hematocrit level may rise less than anticipated because of the gestational increase in plasma volume. Labile hemodynamics during labor, delivery, and the puerperium incurs additional risks.[160] A sudden fall in systemic resistance may precipitate intense cyanosis, syncope, and death. Conversely, bearing down during labor may abruptly and dangerously reduce systemic blood flow. Infective endocarditis during delivery is an additional concern.

CONGENITAL COMPLETE HEART BLOCK. This uncommon disorder permits survival into childbearing age, and about one-half of patients are female. Asymptomatic young women with congenital complete heart block usually experience uneventful pregnancies, provided the duration of the QRS complex is not prolonged.[162-164] Stokes-Adams attacks occasionally occur during gestation, however, and the heart and circulation may not respond adequately to the volatile demands of labor and delivery.

EBSTEIN'S ANOMALY OF THE TRICUSPID VALVE. About 50 per cent of patients are female, and the majority reach adulthood.[13] The functionally inadequate right ventricle, already volume-overloaded by tricuspid regurgitation, copes poorly with the gestational increase in cardiac output.[165] Paroxysmal atrial arrhythmias occur in about one-third of nongravid patients with Ebstein's anomaly and are potential hazards during pregnancy. Wolff-Parkinson-White bypass tracts set the stage for excessively rapid ventricular rates in response to atrial fibrillation or flutter; the consequences can be catastrophic. Cyanosis in Ebstein's anomaly (right-to-left shunt at atrial level) may first become manifest during pregnancy because of a rise in right ventricular filling pressure. The right-to-left interatrial shunt increases the risk of paradoxical embolization, and the hypoxemia increases the risk to the fetus.

THE POSTOPERATIVE PATIENT

The postoperative woman with congenital heart disease now constitutes one of the most important categories of pregnancy and heart disease and represents a growing patient population. A prime objective of reparative surgery is to increase the safety and success of pregnancy and to preserve the subsequent health of mother and child. Operations should, therefore, be anticipatory. With few exceptions, cardiac surgery or interventional catheterization is not curative; the risk of pregnancy to the mother is then determined chiefly by the presence, type, and degree of cardiac and vascular residua and sequelae. There is a consensus, however, that successful operation before gestation can be pivotal in reducing maternal risk. Operation has no bearing on genetic transmission of maternal congenital heart disease.

An asymptomatic woman of childbearing age who has undergone closure of an *ostium secundum atrial septal defect* as a child or young adult can anticipate pregnancy devoid of maternal risk.[160] Successful closure of the defect also eliminates the risk of paradoxical embolization. There are few or no significant postoperative residua or sequelae except for occasional atrial tachyarrhythmias years after successful repair. When a small *patent ductus arteriosus* has been closed in childhood, pregnancy is tolerated normally. More circumspect is the response to gestation after closure of a moderately restrictive or nonrestrictive ductus. Postoperative pulmonary vascular disease and depressed left ventricular function are important residua, depending on the degree. In any case, there is no risk of endocarditis. When surgical repair or balloon dilatation of *congenital pulmonary valve stenosis* leaves behind little or no gradient, the mother can anticipate a normal pregnancy except for a low, if not absent, risk of infective endocarditis. Mild-to-moderate low-pressure pulmonary regurgitation is not an important sequel.

Complete relief of *coarctation of the aorta,* especially in early childhood, materially increases the probability of long-term normalization of blood pressure and decreases the risk of gestational aortic dissection or rupture by removing the zone of aortic cystic medial necrosis.[166] Balloon dilatation of native (unoperated) coarctation may significantly reduce the intraaortic pressure gradient, but the risk of aortic rupture or dissection during pregnancy can be no less (and may be greater) than in mild native coarctation. Susceptibility to infective endocarditis at the site of successful coarctation repair is, for all practical purposes, absent, but the risk of infection on a coexisting bicuspid aortic valve is unaffected. To what extent successful correction of aortic coarctation diminishes the hazard of gestational rupture of an aneurysm of the circle of Willis is open to question, but the incidence of death resulting from intracranial hemorrhage is reassuringly low.[167]

In congenital *aortic valve stenosis,* surgical relief of gradients of 50 mm Hg or more appreciably lowers the risk of pregnancy except for susceptibility to infective endocarditis. Risk during pregnancy is lowest when postoperative left ventricular function is normal or nearly so. Aortic valve replacement should be avoided, especially with a rigid prosthesis that requires anticoagulants.

A woman with moderate to marked *aortic regurgitation* who wants to become pregnant is best advised to do so before aortic valve replacement. If a prosthetic valve is required in a female of reproductive age, there are persuasive arguments for the use of a tissue valve (no need for anticoagulants, with their adverse effects during pregnancy, p. 1797).

Pregnancy after successful intracardiac repair of *Fallot's tetralogy* is accompanied by justifiable optimism, especially in women with little or no outflow gradient and no more than mild postoperative low-pressure pulmonary regurgitation. Surgical relief of cyanosis increases the likelihood of successful conception and substantially improves the stability of the pregnancy and the prospect of normal growth and development of the fetus. However, electrophysiological sequelae of intracardiac repair—bifascicular block, high-degree heart block, or right ventricular electrical instability (Figs. 32–13 and 32–18)—cannot be ignored.

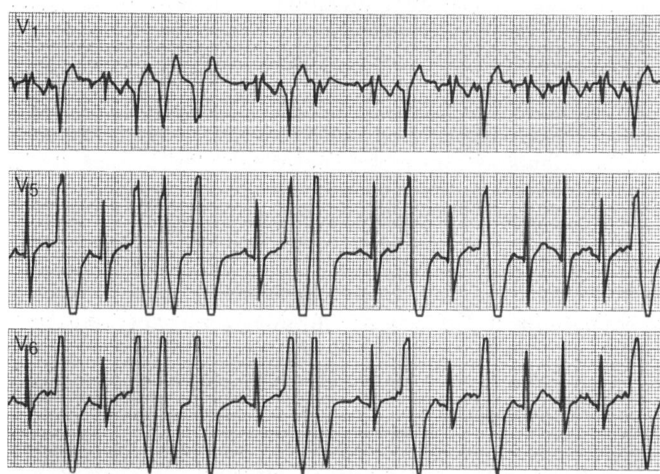

FIGURE 32–18. Rhythm response to isotonic exercise in a 41-year-old patient 5 years after intracardiac repair of Fallot's tetralogy. There are short runs of nonsustained ventricular tachycardia (From James, F. W., et al.: Response to exercise in patients after total correction of tetralogy of Fallot. Circulation *54*:671, 1976.)

Congenital complete heart block in young women occasionally requires insertion of a pacemaker, but even so, relative confidence that pregnancy can proceed is justified. If ventricular function is normal, which usually is the case, an artificial fixed-rate pacemaker appears to provide satisfactory physiological support.

Surgical repair of *Ebstein's anomaly of the tricuspid valve* ideally takes the form of reconstruction into a relatively competent unicuspid atrioventricular valve. Dissociation of right atrium from right ventricle eliminates active or potential bypass tracts (Fig. 32–10). The risk of pregnancy to the mother, including susceptibility to infective endocarditis, is then appreciably reduced but not eliminated.

Pregnancy after repair of certain forms of *complex cyanotic congenital heart disease* is now a practical objective. After a Fontan operation for single ventricle or tricuspid atresia with pulmonary stenosis, patients can achieve a two-fold increment in cardiac index in response to isotonic exercise.[135] The implication is that women who have undergone successful Fontan repairs and have normal systemic ventricular function confront the physiological burden of pregnancy with circulations that potentially possess adequate hemodynamic reserve.[133]

MEDICAL MANAGEMENT OF THE PREGNANT WOMAN

The expectant mother's cardiac reserve is reduced by the hemodynamic burden of pregnancy, but the reduction can almost always be countered by addressing the factors that encroach on circulatory reserve. There is little or no convincing evidence that oxygen administration benefits cyanotic pregnant women.

Maternal mortality usually varies directly with functional class, but in the presence of certain congenital cardiac malformations, childbearing imposes such a formidable threat to maternal survival that pregnancy is proscribed or should be interrupted irrespective of functional class. The cardiac symptoms on which the New York Heart Association functional classes were originally based are more relevant to acquired than to congenital heart disease. In cyanotic patients, for example, what is subjectively reported as effort dyspnea is less likely to result from heart failure than from stimulation of the respiratory center by the changes in blood gas composition and pH in response to the increased right-to-left shunt induced by exercise. Effort fatigue may be due to the effect of iron deficiency on exercise performance (see p. 1791).

The two major maternal cardiac risks are pulmonary vascular disease and pulmonary edema. Pulmonary vascular disease limits or precludes appropriate adaptive responses to the circulatory changes of pregnancy and to the volatile changes during labor, delivery, and the puerperium. Primary pulmonary hypertension epitomizes this risk, and Eisenmenger's complex combines the maternal risk of pulmonary vascular disease with the fetal risk of cyanosis. A sudden fall in systemic vascular resistance in Eisenmenger's complex may precipitate intense cyanosis, and a sudden rise in systemic resistance associated with bearing down during labor may abruptly depress cardiac output and provoke fatal syncope. Pulmonary edema (p. 551) is less common in congenital heart disease than in acquired heart disease, but the functional adequacy of the ventricle that serves the systemic circulation—before or after operation—is central to this concern.

In women with functionally mild unoperated lesions and in patients after successful intracardiac repairs, management of labor and delivery is essentially the same as for normal women except for the selective risk of infective endocarditis (see Chap. 35). In high-risk patients, a flotation catheter offers the security of meticulous hemodynamic surveillance during labor and delivery and in the immediate postpartum period, but individual judgments are required. In Eisenmenger's complex, for example, the risks involved with use of a Swan-Ganz catheter outweigh the benefits.[168] Oxygen often is administered during labor, especially in cyanotic women, although the efficacy of so doing is unproved.

After expulsion of the placenta, bleeding can be reduced by uterine massage or intravenous oxytocin. Blood loss should be minimized, especially in patients with pulmonary vascular disease or Fallot's tetralogy. The risk of sudden hemorrhage in women with ostium secundum atrial septal defect was pointed out earlier.

The probability of thromboembolism increases during the postpartum period, and patients with lesions susceptible to paradoxical embolization are at particular risk (see earlier). Meticulous leg care, use of elastic support stockings, and early ambulation are important preventive measures.

Prophylaxis for infective endocarditis during labor and delivery is dealt with in Chapter 35.

MEDICAL MANAGEMENT OF THE FETUS

Maternal congenital heart disease exposes the fetus to immediate risks that threaten its intrauterine viability and to remote risks that are evidenced as congenital and developmental malformations. Immediate risks are determined chiefly by the functional class of the mother, maternal cyanosis, and anticoagulants. Extracorporeal circulation is associated with a high incidence of fetal wastage, but cardiac surgery seldom is required during pregnancy, especially in patients with congenital heart disease. The hypertension of coarctation of the aorta does not threaten the fetus as do other hypertensive disorders. Remote risks to the fetus take the form of genetic parental transmission, teratogenic effects of certain cardiac drugs, and the harmful effects of certain environmental toxins and environmental exposures.

Maternal cyanosis threatens the growth, development, and viability of the fetus, and materially increases fetal wastage.[160,169] Infants born to cyanotic mothers are typically dysmature (small for gestational age) or premature (gestation less than 37 weeks). There is little or no evidence that maternal oxygen administration favorably affects the growth-retarded fetus, despite the fact that high levels of inspired oxygen may raise arterial saturation even in the presence of a right-to-left shunt. The rate of spontaneous abortion is high and increases approximately in parallel to the mother's hypoxemia. Even when cyanosis is initially mild, the risk of fetal wastage is not low because a right-to-left shunt often increases during the course of pregnancy in response to the anticipated fall in systemic vascular resistance. Surgical correction of congenital heart disease eliminates cyanosis and improves maternal functional class, underscoring the desirability of anticipatory operative intervention.

The use of *anticoagulants* involves risks to the fetus that cannot be satisfactorily resolved. An attempt should be made to minimize the need for anticoagulants, and their use should be judicious. There is no consensus regarding the best method for administering anticoagulants to pregnant women. The options are discussed on pages 1805 and 1806.

GENETICS, EPIDEMIOLOGY, COUNSELING, AND PREVENTION

(See also Chap. 51)

There is substantial evidence that the presence of a congenital heart lesion in a first-degree relative is a risk factor to the fetus, even in the absence of a known genetic disorder.[170] There also is evidence that *maternal* congenital heart disease

TABLE 32–1 CHARACTERISTICS OF CYTOPLASMIC INHERITANCE

INHERITANCE OF MITOCHONDRIAL GENOMES						
Parental genotypes	Maternal Cc	×	Paternal CC	Maternal CC	×	Paternal Cc
Offspring genotypes		Cc			CC	

CC = normal mitochondrial genomes
Cc = some normal, some mutated mitochondrial genomes

CHARACTERISTICS OF INHERITANCE

Many mitochondrial gene copies are inherited. Inheritance is through the maternal lineage only. Offspring show variable phenotypes due to ratio of C:c mitochondrial DNAs caused by random segregation. Affected phenotypes are not manifested until a certain proportion of mutated mitochondrial DNAs is reached—a threshold effect.

is a greater fetal risk than congenital heart disease in other relatives, including the father. Possible reasons for this maternal effect include nonmendelian inheritance (cytoplasmic transmission [Table 32–1] and parental imprinting) and an effect of the maternal environment on the developing embryo.[170] If the mother has congenital heart disease, the recurrence risk in her offspring is 6.7 per cent (range 2.5 to 18 per cent), but if the father is affected, the risk is only 2.1 per cent (range 1.5 to 3 per cent). Potential parents with congenital heart disease—male or female—should be provided with genetic counseling regarding the recurrence risk in offspring.

Potential teratogenic or developmental fetal injury associated with cardiac or noncardiac drugs used during pregnancy is discussed on page 1803. In the first trimester, particularly before the 9th week, the risk of exposure is teratogenicity. In the second and third trimesters, the risks are represented by adverse effects on fetal growth and development, especially the central nervous system, which continues to develop throughout gestation.

In brief, congenital cardiovascular malformations cannot, as a rule, be assigned to specific antecedent causes, although malformations can result from heredity, from environmental exposures that require little or no apparent genetic predisposition, or from genetic-environmental interactions. Many cases of inherited malformations remain unexplained by classical genetics. Recent work has focused on cytoplasmic inheritance or parental imprinting to explain the observed risks.

EXERCISE AND ATHLETICS BEFORE AND AFTER SURGERY OR INTERVENTIONAL CATHETERIZATION

Patients with certain types of congenital disorders of the heart or circulation are at greater risk of complications or sudden death if they expose themselves to the stress of strenuous exercise or competitive sports.[171] Apart from the somewhat arbitrary distinction between competitive and recreational athletics, a number of other points are relevant. Consideration must be given to (1) the type, intensity, and duration of exercise; (2) the risk of body collision inherent in a given type of athletic activity, especially in patients receiving anticoagulants; (3) the training program (conditioning) required for a given sport; (4) the emotional response (stress) that the athlete experiences in anticipation of or during a particular sport event; and (5) the risk of injury either to the athlete or to spectators if the athletic activity induces loss of consciousness.[172]

Two general types of exercise are recognized: isotonic (dynamic) and isometric (static). *Isotonic exercise* is associated with changes in muscle length and with rhythmic muscle contractions that develop comparatively little force. A steady state can be achieved. *Isometric exercise* results in sudden development of a comparatively large force with little or no change in muscle length; a steady state cannot be achieved, even temporarily. There often is a continuum between the two types, with most physical activity incorporating both isotonic and isometric components. After certain types of reparative surgery, conditioning improves physical performance and permits activities at normal or near-normal levels. However, the risk entailed by conditioning (training) for a specific competitive athletic activity may exceed the risk of the competitive event itself. The heightened emotional response of an athlete before or during a sporting event may trigger a disturbance in cardiac rhythm and a loss of consciousness, putting the athlete, as well as participants and bystanders, at risk of injury. At issue in the following discussion are the type and severity of a given congenital malformation, whether surgery was undertaken and, if so, its type and success.

Sometimes patients with *congenital complete heart block* perform optimally,[13] but prolonged, high-intensity isotonic exercise is ill-advised, and strenuous isometric exercise is unwise, although often tolerated. If a pacemaker is required, patients are allowed isotonic or isometric exercise that falls within the limits of sensible moderation.

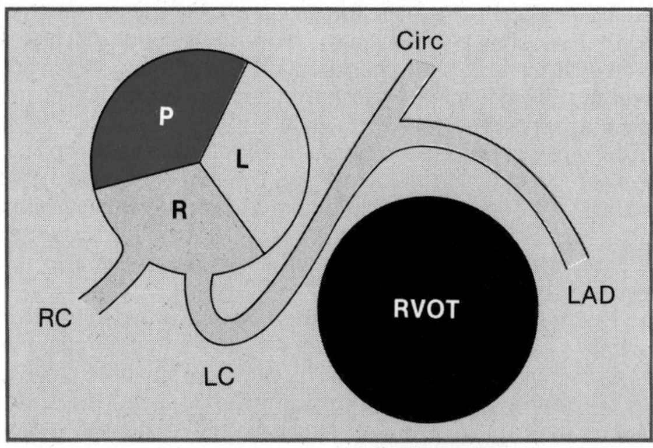

FIGURE 32–19. **Illustration of the left coronary artery (LC) arising from a right aortic sinus (R) and coursing between the aorta and the right ventricular outflow tract (RVOT). P = posterior aortic sinus; L = left aortic sinus; RC = right coronary artery; Circ = circumflex coronary artery; and LAD = left anterior descending artery.**

An aberrant coronary artery coursing between the aorta and right ventricular outflow tract can cause angina pectoris, myocardial infarction, and sudden death.[173] The risk is greatest when the *left* coronary artery arises from the right aortic sinus and passes between the aorta and the right ventricular outflow tract (Fig. 32–19), especially in males. Most cases of sudden death occur during or immediately after relatively strenuous physical effort. The mechanism is believed to be coronary arterial compression in response to exercise-induced dilatation of the great arteries in the setting of preexisting acute angulation of the proximal course of the aberrant coronary, causing intrinsic narrowing of its lumen.[174,175] If the anomaly is identified and surgically corrected, subsequent athletic activity need not be restricted, provided that coronary flow is unobstructed and myocardial ischemia absent.

In *coarctation of the aorta*, the distensibility characteristics of the proximal aorta, the sensitivity or "set" of carotid sinus baroreceptors, and the efferent sympathetic activity play important roles in systemic hypertension (see earlier).[13] The aorta proximal to the coarctation is less distensible than is the postcoarctation aorta, accounting in part for the disproportionate rise in systolic blood pressure in the proximal compartment. The excessive rise in systolic blood pressure during isotonic exercise represents an exaggeration of the disproportionate systolic hypertension in the resting state. After successful repair of coarctation, the excessive rise in exercise-induced systolic hypertension is in large part related to the patient's age at the time of repair. Patients without recoarctation but with postoperative hypertension may experience abnormal increases in blood pressure (especially systolic) during exercise.

Unoperated patients with mild congenital *aortic valve stenosis* (resting gradient of 20 mm Hg or less) are not restricted in athletic activity, provided that the electrocardiogram is normal, the response to exercise stress testing is normal, left ventricular function is normal or supernormal, and there are no significant disturbances in rhythm as measured by 24-hour ambulatory electrocardiography. Patients with *moderate* congenital aortic stenosis (resting gradients higher than 20 but less than 50 mm Hg), especially those at the upper range, are advised to confine their athletics to low-intensity isotonic exercise. Isometric exercise, by increasing the aortic root systolic pressure, may reduce the gradient, but in so doing increases an already elevated left ventricular afterload. In patients with *marked* to *severe* aortic stenosis (peak systolic gradients in excess of 50 mm Hg), high-intensity isotonic or isometric exercise or competitive sports should be avoided.

A legitimate concern in advising exercise limitations in patients with aortic stenosis is the perceived risk of sudden death. The syncope that precedes sudden death is believed to be initiated by left ventricular baroreceptors activated by an exercise-induced increase in left ventricular pressure or stretch, which causes vasodilatation in skeletal muscle followed by systemic hypotension.[176] Malignant ventricular arrhythmias seldom *initiate* syncope but are believed to be the chief cause of death *after* a faint. Syncope-induced hypotension is much more likely to provoke electrical ventricular instability in adults with coexisting coronary artery disease than in younger patients with normal coronary arteries and no myocardial ischemia.

Recommendations based on the criteria above do not necessarily apply to exercise in patients after valvotomy or valvuloplasty for congenital aortic stenosis. Even if the postoperative pressure gradient is 20 mm Hg or less, athletic activity should be limited to low or moderate intensity when left ventricular internal dimensions at end-diastole are increased, when aortic regurgitation is more than mild, when the scalar electrocardiogram shows residual abnormalities of repolarization at rest or with exercise, or when important disturbances in ventricular rhythm are present at rest, with exercise, or on 24-hour ambulatory electrocardiogram. These recommendations are valid even if left ventricular systolic function is within normal range as measured by two-dimensional echocardiography or radionuclide imaging.

Patients with mild *pulmonary valve stenosis* (peak systolic gradient < 25 mm Hg) are allowed unrestricted athletic activity. When obstruction is moderate (gradient between 25 and 50 mm Hg) high-intensity competitive sports may be tolerated but are unwise because right ventricular systolic pressure rises appreciably in response to strenuous isotonic exercise. Most such patients have some degree of electrocardiographic evidence of right ventricular hypertrophy. When the resting peak systolic gradient exceeds 50 mm Hg, especially if there is echocardiographic or radionuclide evidence of impaired right ventricular function, isotonic exercise should be limited to mild intensity and short duration. After successful balloon dilatation or valvotomy, most patients need few restrictions and, as a rule, may participate in high-intensity competitive athletics. If residual obstruction to right ventricular outflow after surgery or balloon valvuloplasty is moderate or greater, athletic activity should be limited to noncompetitive low- to moderate-intensity exercise, especially if right ventricular internal dimensions are increased and systolic function is less than normal.

Most patients with uncomplicated *ostium secundum atrial septal defects* who escape early detection are asymptomatic and usually experience normal tolerance to high-intensity exercise. As long as the pulmonary vascular resistance is normal (which usually is the case), these young adults should not be restricted, although elective repair is advisable. When surgery abolishes the shunt in early childhood, long-term outlook is excellent and athletic activity is unrestricted, provided that the pulmonary vascular resistance is normal, the sinus node function and atrioventricular conduction are normal, and the right atrial and the right ventricular volumes are normal or nearly so.

A small *ventricular septal defect* with a functionally normal heart imposes no limitations on physical activity. Such patients can safely participate in competitive sports without restriction, but it is uncommon to find adult patients in this category. An important variation on the theme is the adult who had a moderately restrictive perimembranous ventricular septal defect that decreased in size or closed spontaneously in infancy. There is a consensus that such patients are physiologically normal and should be permitted unrestricted physical activity. Two-dimensional echocardiographic studies with Doppler interrogation and color-flow imaging should be performed to determine whether the defect closed by formation of a "septal aneurysm" and whether a trivial residual shunt persists. Although there is no evidence that strenuous athletic activity risks rupturing a septal aneurysm, it is prudent to be aware of the morphological substrate.

After surgical closure of a moderate to large ventricular septal defect, recommendations regarding levels of physical activity and competitive sports depend on the postoperative pulmonary arterial pressure; the absence of significant disturbances in ventricular rhythm during maximal exercise stress testing and during 24-hour ambulatory electrocardiography; and two-dimensional echocardiographic evidence of an intact ventricular septum together with normalization of left ventricular and left atrial size and left ventricular function. It also is desirable for the 12-lead scalar electrocardiogram to exhibit little or no evidence of left ventricular volume overload or right ventricular pressure overload. If the aforementioned criteria are met, patients are permitted unrestricted isotonic or isometric exercise. Persistent postoperative elevation of pulmonary arterial pressure, especially if accompanied by exercise-induced right ventricular ectopic rhythms, requires that patients limit physical activity to low intensity and short duration.

A small *patent ductus arteriosus* is of little or no physiological significance, and patients are allowed normal physical activity. Similarly, there are no postoperative restrictions on athletic activity after division of an isolated restrictive patent ductus arteriosus in childhood. Recommendations for patients who have undergone division of a moderately restrictive or nonrestrictive patent ductus with large left-to-right shunt and variable elevations of pulmonary arterial pressure depend on the guidelines set forth earlier for postoperative moderately restrictive to nonrestrictive ventricular septal defect.

Pulmonary vascular disease is an important situation in which strenuous exercise should be avoided. In patients with suprasystemic pulmonary vascular resistance and right-to-left shunts (p. 919), even low levels of isotonic exercise tend to be accompanied by marked decrements in systemic arterial oxygen content and in the development of tissue lactic acidosis. The exercise-induced increase in right-to-left shunt poses a special problem in the elimination of metabolically produced carbon dioxide, resulting in high ventilatory requirements and subjective dyspnea (Fig. 32–16) and, occasionally, in respiratory acidosis. In nonrestrictive patent ductus arteriosus with suprasystemic pulmonary vascular resistance and reversed shunt, certain symptoms are related to selective flow of poorly oxygenated blood to the *lower* extremities (reversed shunt). Exercise may cause leg fatigue but comparatively little dyspnea because the ventilatory stimuli of hypoxemia, hypercapnia, and acidemia circumvent the respiratory center (venous blood is delivered to the lower body but not to the vital centers of the head and neck).[13]

In *Fallot's tetralogy*, isotonic exercise results in a fall in systemic resistance together with augmented venous return to a right ventricle with fixed obstruction to outflow, so the right-to-left shunt is increased. The subjective sensation of breathlessness is caused chiefly by the response of the respiratory center to the sudden change and blood gas composition and pH. The relief of effort-induced dyspnea by squatting, a time-honored hallmark of Fallot's tetralogy in children, is seldom witnessed in adults.[13] Squatting exerts its salutory effect by countering the exercise-induced fall in systemic vascular resistance and by decreasing the amount of low oxygen content inferior vena caval blood that is received by the right ventricle and shunted into the aorta during exercise. High-intensity *isometric* exercise in Fallot's tetralogy abruptly reduces flow from the right ventricle into the aorta in the face of fixed obstruction to right ventricular outflow, so systemic flow suddenly falls, precipitating syncope and, occasionally, sudden death. All but low-intensity isometric exercise is proscribed.

After intracardiac repair of Fallot's tetralogy, recommendations regarding the level of physical activity and participation in athletics depend on the patient's age at operation and the presence and degree of postoperative residua and sequelae.[177,178] Postoperative patients with Fallot's tetralogy should undergo two-dimensional echocardiography with Doppler interrogation and color-flow imaging, exercise stress testing, and 24-hour ambulatory electrocardiography. If obstruction to right ventricular outflow is mild or absent, if the shunt is absent or trivial, if low-pressure pulmonary valve regurgitation is no more than mild or moderate, if there are no detectable disturbances in ventricular rhythm, and if right ventricular size and function are normal, no limitations are imposed on athletic activity, either isotonic or isometric.[177,178] Of particular concern is a residual right ventricular outflow gradient that increases significantly with exercise and is accompanied by right ventricular electrical instability believed to originate at the site of the ventriculotomy scar (Fig. 32–18). Postoperative bifascicular block, uncommon with current operative techniques, is a potential electrophysiological risk (Fig. 32–13). Occurrence of bifascicular block in isolation (without the aforementioned residua or sequelae) does not in itself preclude unrestricted physical activity, provided the 24-hour ambulatory electrocardiogram records no additional evidence of impaired atrioventricular conduction.

In *complete transposition of the great arteries* (p. 944) data are derived chiefly from patients who have undergone atrial switch operations in early life. With few exceptions, obligatory and important postoperative residua and sequelae require that physical activity be restricted to mild or moderate intensity and limited duration. Recommendations regarding athletic activity for patients after undergoing the *arterial* switch operation cannot be made as of this writing. However, it is believed that uncomplicated arterial switch repairs may circumvent the electrophysiological sequelae after atrial switch operations (Fig. 32–12), while permitting the morphological left ventricle to serve as the systemic pump.

The *Fontan operation* (p. 975) permits study of the human circulation in which total right atrial or total caval flow is channeled directly into the pulmonary artery or into a small right ventricle that serves only as a conduit. The principal congenital malformations amenable to the Fontan repair are tricuspid atresia and single ventricle with pulmonary stenosis. Exercise performance improves but remains subnormal,[135,179] and cardiac index increases but seldom more than twofold. Patients with optimal repairs are permitted moderate-intensity isotonic and isometric exercise if the following criteria are met: (1) a satisfactory working capacity as judged by exercise stress testing; (2) stable sinus rhythm with no significant disturbances in atrial or ventricular rhythm in response to exercise or on 24-hour ambulatory electrocardiography; (3) normal ventricular function as determined by two-dimensional echocardiography or radionuclide imaging; and (4) normal systemic arterial oxygen saturation.

INSURABILITY, EMPLOYABILITY, AND PSYCHOSOCIAL CONSIDERATIONS

Most young adults who have undergone surgical repair of congenital heart lesions are eligible for *health insurance* and *life insurance.* As newer and more successful therapeutic modalities are applied, and as the long-term benefits of these therapeutic advances are realized, patients are likely to enjoy greater access to insurance. Life insurance ratings and premiums are based on known mortality rates over periods of 10 to 20 years, calculated from the age of the person at the time of application.[180,181] *Group life insurance* is a form of term life insurance that provides death benefits for applicants who are members of a specific group. The larger the group, the lower the premiums, as a rule. Comparatively less medical information is required for group term life insurance applications, so the probability of denial is significantly lower than for other types of life insurance. Term insurance is a relatively inexpensive solution for young parents who desire death benefits only, and policies are available to most young adults with congenital heart disease if purchased through a large group. Companies willing to consider applications for *whole life insurance* from patients with congenital heart disease may not insure a child, but might approve an adolescent (over age 15) with the same congenital malformation. These positions reflect the insurance companies' theory that by adolescence, a sufficient amount will be known about a patient's prognosis to provide a basis for judgment. *The Medical Information Bureau* pools medical information from life insurance applications. That information is available for review by referring physicians and patients.

The future of *health insurance* systems is uncertain, as reflected by major changes during the past 20 years. Options include fee-for-service insurance, health maintenance organizations, independent practice associations, Medicare, and Medicaid. An appreciable number of young adults who have had repair of congenital cardiac defects can anticipate a normal or near-normal life span and lifestyle, but the constraints imposed by fee-for-service health insurance plans (no coverage for preexisting conditions or for ambulatory services) make these plans least attractive. This is especially true for patients who anticipate further surgery or catheterization or for those who require frequent ambulatory evaluation or diagnostic testing.

EMPLOYABILITY. The opportunities for employment of adults with congenital cardiac defects are influenced by education, type of cardiac lesion, job discrimination, and cardiac surgery.[181] Legislation has been enacted to protect the rights of patients and to provide them with assistance in seeking employment. Overprotective attitudes by parents and teachers combined with absence of discipline may seriously reduce the patient's competitive spirit and curtail educational achievements. Job discrimination is one of the most important factors affecting employment opportunities for patients with congenital heart disease. The smaller the company to which the application is made, the greater the reluctance of employers to hire anyone with a thoracotomy scar or a preexisting cardiac disorder.

In selected occupations (bus drivers and airline pilots, for example), the safety of others is in the hands of a single person. To make rational recommendations about medical fitness for these occupations, the patient's risk of incapacity or sudden death must be clearly defined. The National Rehabilitation Act of 1973 prevents job discrimination against the disabled by almost all employers with 10 or more employees. The Vocational Rehabilitation Act of 1920, strengthened by amendments, offers a wide range of services, including medical evaluation and treatment, guidance and counseling, training for the right job, living expenses during rehabilitation, and follow-up to ascertain the satisfaction of the employee and employer. These services are significantly underutilized, especially by cardiac patients.

PSYCHOSOCIAL CONSIDERATIONS. There are special, if not unique, psychological problems of patients who have experienced dramatic and sometimes traumatic diagnostic and therapeutic interventions during key developmental phases of their lives. The trend toward earlier diagnosis and reparative surgery in congenital heart disease has made it difficult to generalize from results of studies done 10 to 20 years ago. Despite methodological difficulties and a number of constraints, some understanding has been achieved by critical assessment of available data combined with clinical experience. Most patients with congenital heart disease function psychologically within normal range, although sometimes low self-esteem, insecurity, and feelings of vulnerability are matters of concern.[182] Parental knowledge, understanding, and attitude largely determine patients' and parents' perceptions of the congenital heart disease and significantly affect psychological adjustments. Difficulty in accepting illness may be manifested by denial and potentially self-destructive behavior, especially in adolescents. The adult with congenital heart disease faces tangible problems in the workforce, in dating, in marriage, and in parenthood. Cyanosis impairs intellectual function, although the degree of impairment is usually mild and may be overestimated in IQ tests that depend on gross motor function at a young age.[183] Early surgery in patients with cyanotic congenital heart disease appears to improve intellectual and psychological development.[184,185] Circulatory arrest with profound hypothermia results in no major detrimental sequelae but may have subtle adverse effects on intellectual function, especially if the circulatory arrest and hypothermia are prolonged.[186] Longitudinal studies of the psychosocial aspects of congenital heart disease promise to improve our understanding of the expanding population of adolescents and adults with these disorders.

CARDIAC SURGICAL CONSIDERATIONS IN ADULTS WITH CONGENITAL HEART DISEASE

OPERATION AND REOPERATION

Operation or reoperation in adults with congenital heart disease often involves special surgical considerations peculiar to older patients.[1] These considerations must take into account the congenital cardiac malformation per se (previously operated or unoperated) together with acquired cardiac and noncardiac diseases of adulthood. Certain general considerations apply to adult congenital heart disease patients who have not had surgery and to those who have had palliative or reparative surgery. In cyanotic adults undergoing their initial operation, aortopulmonary collateral and hematological disorders are matters of concern. In patients who have had palliative procedures, the general concerns at the time of reoperation are shunts and bands. In adults who have undergone reparative surgery, the chief concerns at the time of reoperation are prosthetic materials such as conduits and valves. Concerns that apply to both unoperated patients and patients undergoing reoperation include pulmonary vascular disease, ventricular function, myocardial protection (cardioplegia), blood salvage techniques, the risk of infective endocarditis, the residua and sequelae of previous cardiac surgery, as well as coexisting acquired heart disease, the incidence of which varies with patient age.

Perioperative management of hemostatic defects in adult patients with cyanotic congenital heart disease is outlined on p. 1714. When preoperative phlebotomy is required to improve hemostasis, the blood should be stored for potential autologous transfusion. Reoperation after palliative procedures include revision of Blalock-Taussig shunts (Fig. 32–14), Glenn shunts, Potts or Waterston shunts, and pulmonary arterial bands. The most significant considerations regarding reoperation of patients who have had prior reparative surgery are related to native valve reconstruction and to prosthetic materials, either conduits or valves. Operative planning requires knowledge of the basic congenital malformation, knowledge of the initial surgical procedure, and knowledge of the postoperative residua, sequelae, and complications. Perhaps the most important variable that precludes reparative or palliative surgery or reoperation is pulmonary vascular disease. Ventricular function is the second major determinant of operability or reoperability. Volume and pressure overload, myocardial ischemia, and ventricular morphology are important variables that influence ventricular function and require meticulous preoperative assessment.

Certain general principles apply intraoperatively, such as myocardial protection and cardioplegia, and systemic hypothermia. Intraoperative salvage of red blood cells and platelet-rich plasma before cardiopulmonary bypass has greatly diminished the need for nonautologous blood and blood products. Minimizing blood and blood product usage is even more important at reoperation than at initial operation because of the greater risk of bleeding and the need for transfusions at reoperation. The sternotomy incision at reoperation is a technical concern. There is a significant risk of bleeding when an enlarged right ventricle is apposed to the sternum and when right ventricular outflow conduits adhere to the sternum. The risk of reopening the sternum can be materially reduced if reoperation is anticipated at the initial repair, with placement of an anterior patch of synthetic pericardium.

The selection, use, and long-term effects of prosthetic materials are additional major considerations. There are three categories of prostheses: patches, valves, and conduits. The devices or materials selected must achieve an immediately successful technical result, while the long-term postoperative effects of the prosthetic materials on morbidity and mortality are taken into account (Figs. 32–20 and 32–21). The choice of materials is based on the patient's age and size, the nature of the congenital malformation, the type of repair undertaken, whether or not subsequent repairs are anticipated, the availability of various synthetic and biological materials and devices, complications of long-term anticoagulation, and the risk of infection.

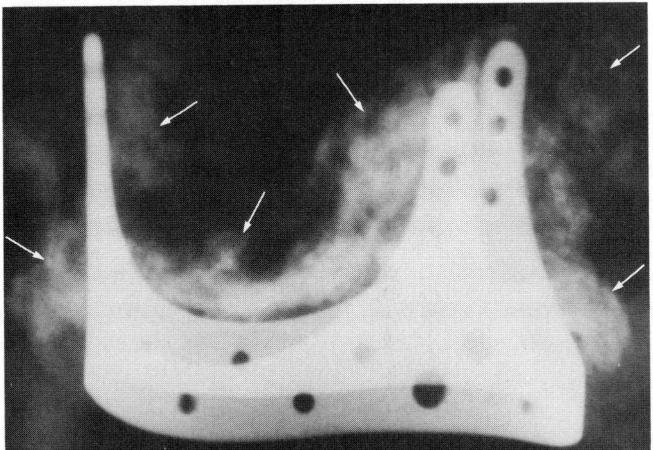

FIGURE 32–20. Lateral radiograph of an Ionescu-Shiley pericardial bioprosthetic valve removed from a 19-year-old male 4 years after insertion. The specimen shows extensive calcification (arrows).

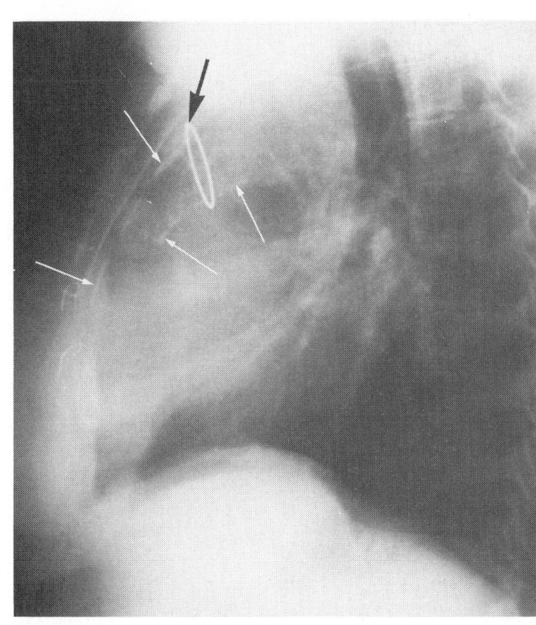

FIGURE 32–21. Lateral chest radiograph from a 19-year-old woman who, at age 8, underwent intracardiac repair for Fallot's tetralogy. An external valve conduit (porcine valve) was inserted because an anomalous coronary artery coursed across the right ventricular outflow tract. The radiograph shows calcification of the conduit (small arrows) above and below the porcine valve (large arrow).

CARDIAC CATHETERIZATION AS A THERAPEUTIC INTERVENTION

(See also Chap. 41)

Interventional cardiac catheterization is now the preferred primary treatment or an adjunct to the surgical treatment of increasing numbers of pediatric and adult patients with congenital malformations of the heart and circulation (see also p. 202).[90,91] *Corrective or reparative* interventional catheterization procedures apply to pulmonary valve stenosis, recoarctation of the aorta, patent ductus arteriosus, and potentially to selected patients with atrial septal defect or ventricular septal defect. *Palliative* interventions can be either instead of surgery or as adjuncts to surgery. Procedures performed in lieu of surgery are applied to lesions such as aortic valve stenosis, postoperative systemic or pulmonary venous obstruction, previously unoperated coarctation of the aorta, obstructed bioprosthetic valves, and congenital pulmonary arteriovenous fistulas (Fig. 32–22). Palliative procedures that are adjuncts to surgery apply to patients with systemic-to-pulmonary arterial collateral circulation, systemic-to-pulmonary arterial surgical shunts, pulmonary or systemic venous obstruction, certain intraatrial communications, and selected patients with peripheral pulmonary artery stenosis. Therapeutic cardiac catheterization, like cardiac surgery, has three principal objectives: (1) preservation of or improvement in cardiac function, (2) increase in longevity, and (3) maintenance of or improvement in quality of life. When the catheterization technique achieves these ends, surgical morbidity and mortality are circumvented.

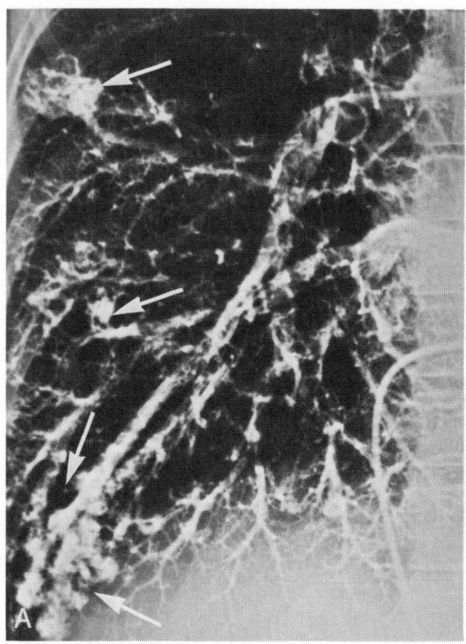

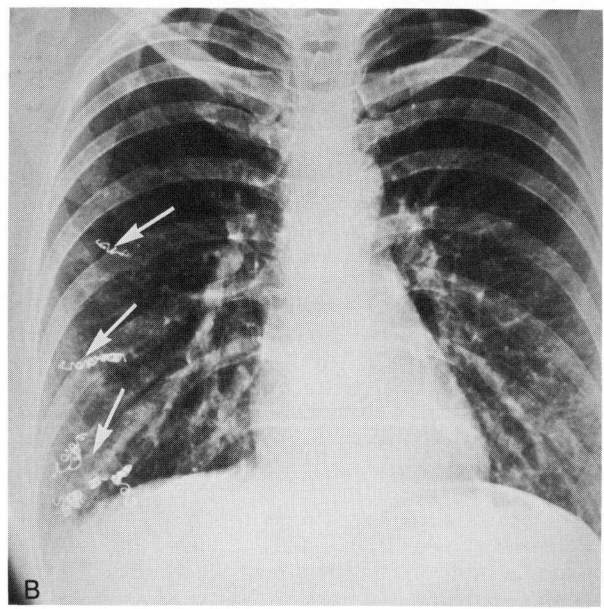

FIGURE 32–22. *A,* **Pulmonary arteriogram showing congenital pulmonary arteriovenous fistulas in the right middle and lower lobes of a 50-year-old woman with hereditary hemorrhagic telangiectasia (Rendu-Osler-Weber syndrome). Arrows point to the larger fistula that was subjected to coil occlusion.**

NONCARDIAC SURGERY IN ADULTS WITH CONGENITAL HEART DISEASE

(See also Chap. 55)

When adults with congenital heart disease require noncardiac surgery, perioperative risks can be reduced, often appreciably, when problems inherent in this patient population are anticipated. The author discusses patients with cyanotic or acyanotic congenital heart disease who have *not* undergone cardiac surgery and patients who have undergone reparative cardiac surgery.

SITUS INVERSUS WITH DEXTROCARDIA (p. 969). This arrangement usually occurs in people with structurally and functionally normal hearts and may go unrecognized until an illness that requires surgery brings an adult patient to attention. Accompanying symptoms are likely to be misconstrued and diagnostic conclusions incorrect unless the mirror image visceral positions are known. In acute appendicitis the abdominal pain is present in the *left* lower quadrant, and with biliary colic the pain is in the *left* upper quadrant. The risk of noncardiac surgery is the same in the presence of situs inversus as in patients with normal situs, provided no congenital malformations coexist in the mirror image heart.

CONGENITAL COMPLETE HEART BLOCK (p. 955). Patients with this condition who undergo noncardiac surgery should have electrocardiographic monitoring during and immediately after operation. Intraoperative vagotonic stimuli at ophthalmic or gastrointestinal surgery should be minimized and treated with intravenous atropine expectantly or if there is a sudden decrease in heart rate. If the preoperative scalar electrocardiogram shows wide QRS complexes and a relatively slow ventricular response, especially if the patient has a history of syncope or near syncope, a temporary right ventricular pacemaker should be inserted.

BICUSPID AORTIC VALVE. Noncardiac surgery in an adult with a functionally normal or mildly stenotic or incompetent bicuspid aortic valve imposes the risk of infective endocarditis. Fibrocalcific obstruction of a congenital bicuspid aortic valve accounts for about one-half the cases of surgically important pure aortic stenosis in adults.[14] The immediate risks of noncardiac surgery are determined by the degree of obstruction, the functional adequacy of the afterloaded left ventricle, and the presence of acquired coronary artery disease. When emergency noncardiac surgery is required in an adult with severe calcific bicuspid aortic stenosis and marginal left ventricular function, hemodynamic monitoring with a flotation catheter is obligatory. If surgery is elective, consideration should be given to aortic valve replacement. Balloon valvuloplasty in this setting is less successful if the stenosis is due to calcification of a congenitally *bicuspid* aortic valve than if the stenosis results from calcification of a previously normal *trileaflet* aortic valve. Coronary angiography helps to determine whether angina pectoris is caused by coexisting coronary artery disease or to augmented oxygen demands of the increased left ventricular mass. If the former is the case, the margin of safety during noncardiac surgery might be increased by preoperative coronary angioplasty. Intraoperative monitoring of systemic blood pressure is important because a sudden fall in systemic vascular resistance may not be compensated by an increase in stroke volume, owing to fixed obstruction to left ventricular outflow. An attempt to correct hypotension with rapid infusion of intravenous fluids may cause pulmonary edema. Pharmacological support of systemic resistance is safer than intravenous infusion and just as efficacious.

CONGENITAL BICUSPID AORTIC REGURGITATION. Patients with hemodynamically significant congenital bicuspid aortic regurgitation face noncardiac surgery with risks determined by left ventricular function and susceptibility to infective endocarditis. If left ventricular function is normal, noncardiac surgery is well tolerated. Moderate intraoperative anesthetic hypotension is not a hazard, serving instead to decrease regurgitant flow and reduce the volume overload on the left ventricle. If left ventricular function is depressed, elective noncardiac surgery raises the question of preemptive replacement of the aortic valve. A tissue valve is preferred to avoid anticoagulants in patients who anticipate subsequent noncardiac surgery. Emergency noncardiac operation in the presence of depressed left ventricular function calls for hemodynamic monitoring with a flotation catheter and postoperative pharmacological afterload reduction. Infective endocarditis is a risk; meticulous prophylaxis is mandatory.

EBSTEIN'S ANOMALY OF THE TRICUSPID VALVE (p. 940). Patients with acyanotic Ebstein's anomaly who require, noncardiac surgery confront four risks: (1) the functionally inadequate right ventricle, (2) atrial tachyarrhythmias with or without accessory pathways, (3) paradoxical embolism through an intraatrial communication, and (4) infective endocarditis on the malformed tricuspid valve. Right ventricular failure is less a perioperative risk than the sudden occurrence of atrial flutter or fibrillation, especially with rapid antegrade conduction by way of right bypass tracts. Patients with histories of rapid heart action or with fusion beats (type B Wolff-Parkinson-White) on scalar electrocardiogram (Fig. 32–10*A*) require electrocardiographic monitoring. Postoperative thrombophlebitis and the attendant risk of paradoxical embolization are minimized by the use of support hose and early ambulation.

OSTIUM SECUNDUM ATRIAL SEPTAL DEFECT (p. 906). In asymptomatic young adults with this malformation normal pulmonary arterial pressure imposes comparatively little risk during noncardiac surgery, but there are two caveats. In response to hemorrhage, systemic resistance rises and venous return diminishes, a combination that augments the left-to-right intraatrial shunt, sometimes considerably. An additional concern is the risk of paradoxical emboli from leg veins because thrombi carried by the inferior vena cava tend to stream across the atrial septal defect into the systemic circulation. Meticulous leg care and early ambulation minimize venous stasis.

CYANOTIC CONGENITAL HEART DISEASE. In patients with these malformations both general and specific concerns apply. Cyanotic adults have an increased incidence of acute cholecystitis caused by *calcium bilirubinate stones* (Fig. 32–23). Accordingly, cholecystectomy is a surgical procedure that such patients may anticipate. Sometimes biliary colic becomes evident years after intracardiac surgery has eliminated the cyanosis. Perioperative improvement in *hemostasis* in cyanotic patients can be addressed if surgery is elective. Phlebotomized units are stored for potential autologous transfusion. *Oxygen inhalation* would seem to be desirable in cyanotic patients during and immediately after noncardiac surgery, and there are no ill effects from so doing. Administration of high levels of inspired oxygen may significantly raise arterial oxygen saturation even in the presence of right-to-left shunts, but there is little or no evidence that its routine perioperative use is beneficial. *Intravenous lines, infusions, and drugs* must be managed with special care in cyanotic patients. The introduction of air into peripheral veins risks delivery of the air into the systemic circulation because of the right-to-left shunt. Use of an air filter obviates the risk.

Fallot's tetralogy represents a large category of adults with uncorrected cyanotic congenital heart disease. Older patients with this malformation may, therefore, come to noncardiac surgery without intracardiac repair or with only a shunt created in infancy or childhood. Meticulous perioperative monitoring of oxygen saturation (pulse oximeter) and blood pressure is important because a sudden fall in systemic resistance may precipitate intense cyanosis and occasionally death, or a sudden rise in systemic resistance may abruptly and dangerously depress systemic blood flow. The risk of postoperative postural hypotension is mentioned later. Susceptibility to infective endocarditis requires prophylaxis.

Cyanotic patients with *elevated pulmonary vascular resistance* face noncardiac surgery with risks inherent in the cyanosis per se, in addition to the formidable risks of pulmonary vascular disease. Fixed pulmonary resistance precludes rapid adaptive responses to potentially labile intraoperative or postoperative hemodynamic changes. In Eisenmenger's complex or physiologically analogous lesions, a sudden fall or a sudden rise in systemic vascular resistance precipitates responses similar to those already described in Fallot's tetralogy. Every effort should be made to minimize the postural hypotension that tends to occur during early convalescence in patients having general anesthesia. Because the attendant drop in systemic vascular resistance suddenly augments the right-to-left shunt, convalescent cyanotic patients with pulmonary vascular disease should change positions slowly until the risk of postoperative postural hypotension has abated.

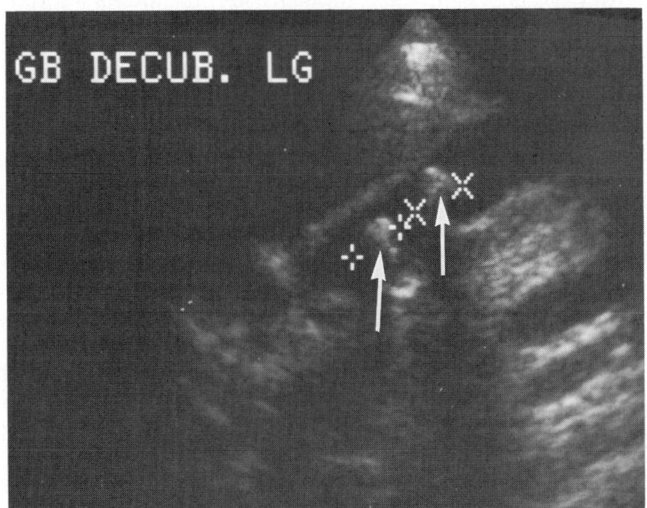

FIGURE 32–23. Abdominal ultrasound in a cyanotic 31-year-old woman with a univentricular heart and pulmonary vascular disease. She developed biliary colic due to calcium bilirubinate stones (arrows).

The Postoperative Patient

Adults with congenital heart disease who have undergone *reparative surgery* comprise an increasing percentage of patients who require subsequent noncardiac operations. If the cardiac surgery is curative, as it is after division of a small patent ductus arteriosus in childhood, there is no added risk of a noncardiac surgical procedure. Early uncomplicated correction of simple pulmonary valve stenosis also is close to a cure, and subsequent noncardiac surgery imposes little or no risk, including, in all probability, susceptibility to infective endocarditis. Closure of an ostium secundum atrial septal defect in childhood is close to a cure.

Valvular residua and sequelae after cardiac surgery or therapeutic catheterization are relevant to medical management when patients undergo noncardiac surgery in adulthood. Successful repair of coarctation of the aorta may leave behind a functionally normal bicuspid aortic valve susceptible to infective endocarditis. Direct repair of congenital bicuspid aortic stenosis at best creates a functionally normal bicuspid aortic valve that remains at risk of infective endocarditis. After complete relief of congenital pulmonary valve stenosis by direct repair or balloon dilatation, the risk of infective endocarditis is low, if not absent. The functional adequacy of the right ventricle is an important perioperative variable. In Fallot's tetralogy, reconstruction of the right ventricular outflow tract may largely or entirely abolish the pressure gradient, and if the functional adequacy of the right ventricle is satisfactory, the risk of noncardiac surgery is low. It is advisable to use prophylaxis for infective endocarditis, even though susceptibility is relatively low.

After surgical repair of *Ebstein's anomaly of the tricuspid valve* (tricuspid reconstruction and division of active or potential bypass tracts), atrial arrhythmias remain a consideration during medical management of noncardiac surgery, but without the fear of accelerated conduction (Fig. 32–10). Closure of the intraatrial communication eliminates cyanosis, so the hematological derangements are no longer concerns, and the risk of paradoxic embolization is eliminated. The postoperative right ventricle is not functionally normal, but the hemodynamic risk during subsequent noncardiac surgery is small. If residual tricuspid regurgitation is more than mild, prophylaxis for infective endocarditis is advisable.

PROSTHETIC MECHANICAL VALVES. These devices complicate the management of subsequent noncardiac surgery. The immediate intraoperative and perioperative concern is anticoagulation, in addition to and apart from the risk of infective endocarditis. If noncardiac surgery is elective, and if the prosthesis carries a high thromboembolic risk, warfarin should be replaced with an in-hospital continuous infusion of heparin, which is discontinued 4 to 6 hours before elective operation, restarted within 48 hours after operation, and then replaced by warfarin. For a lower-risk prosthetic valve in the aortic location, it is considered relatively safe to discontinue warfarin 2 to 3 days before noncardiac surgery and resume the drug 2 to 3 days postoperatively. Emergency noncardiac surgery in an anticoagulated patient with a mechanical prosthesis is managed differently. Cessation of warfarin and administration of vitamin K do not achieve immediate reversal of the anticoagulant effects, which persist for 24 hours or longer. Rapid reversal of the hemostatic defects before emergency noncardiac surgery requires infusion of fresh frozen plasma. If vitamin K is used preoperatively, the response to readministration of warfarin after operation is blunted.

ELECTROPHYSIOLOGICAL SEQUELAE. After reparative surgery for congenital heart disease, electrophysiological sequelae are important concerns in the management of subsequent noncardiac surgery. The most diverse and complex of these sequelae are after intraatrial repairs (Mustard or Senning operations) for complete transposition of the great arteries (Fig. 32-12) and require monitoring during noncardiac surgery. Intraventricular surgery, as in Fallot's tetralogy, may result in electrophysiological sequelae that are potentially important concerns during noncardiac surgery (Figs. 32-13 and 32-18). Awareness of the presence or potential presence of these sequelae serves to decrease perioperative risk.

After repair of coarctation of the aorta, *systemic hypertension* may persist to some degree or recur even if the obstruction has been completely relieved, but the incidence is declining because of the success of early operation. Nevertheless, pharmacological control of perioperative systemic hypertension is sometimes necessary during noncardiac surgery. The longer the duration of systemic hypertension before repair of coarctation, the greater the incidence of premature coronary artery disease, a point to be considered in subsequent perioperative management.

VENTRICULAR FUNCTION. This is an important variable in the long-term management of patients after operation for congenital heart disease. The adequacy of ventricular function (left, right, or single ventricle) is a major determinant of risk during noncardiac surgery in adulthood. Excessive perioperative intravenous fluids should be avoided, and hemodynamic monitoring should be used when the morphological substrate permits.

Adults with congenital heart disease have not only the preoperative or postoperative malformation with which they were born but also *cardiovascular and noncardiac diseases that are acquired with age.* Medical management during noncardiac surgery must take into account acquired diseases of the heart and circulation, especially coronary artery disease and systemic hypertension, and noncardiac acquired medical disorders.

POSTOPERATIVE RESIDUA AND SEQUELAE

Residua

These are represented by cardiac, vascular, or noncardiovascular disorders that are intentionally left behind at the time of reparative heart surgery (Table 32-2). With few exceptions, the residua are obligatory, that is, do not result from the operation having fallen short of its goal, at least in a technical sense.[186] By contrast, *sequelae* are alterations or disorders that are intentionally incurred—occasionally or invariably—at the time of reparative surgery and are looked on as necessary and acceptable consequences of operation (Table 32-3). *Complications* are unintentional aftermaths of reparative surgery that range in severity from inconsequential to fatal; complications and sequelae may imperceptibly merge. Surgery is considered curative if no residua, sequelae, or complications of the heart or circulation are present after operation. This definition implies that normal cardiovascular function is achieved and maintained, life expectancy is normal, and further medical or surgical treatment for the congenital heart disease is unnecessary. These ideals seldom are realized, and even curative cardiac surgery does not preclude noncardiac residua.

Residua after reparative surgery for congenital heart disease are listed in Table 32-2. Electrophysiological abnormalities are, with some exceptions, inherent components of certain congenital cardiac malformations. These abnormalities often are evident in the standard preoperative 12-lead electrocardiogram, and they persist—sometimes harmlessly, sometimes not so harmlessly—after reparative surgery. Electrophysiological residua include: (1) axis deviation, especially left; (2) conduction defects, especially atrioventricular; (3) disorders of impulse formation, especially of the sinus node; and (4) arrhythmias, especially atrial.

TABLE 32-2 RESIDUA AFTER REPARATIVE SURGERY FOR CONGENITAL HEART DISEASE

1. **Electrophysiological**
2. **Valvular**
3. **Ventricular**
   a. **Chamber morphology**
   b. **Chamber mass**
   c. **Chamber function**
   d. **Myocardial connective tissue**
4. **Vascular**
   a. **Anatomical (morphological) vascular anomalies or defects**
   b. **Elevated resistance and/or pressure—systemic, pulmonic**
5. **Noncardiovascular residua**
   a. **Developmental abnormalities**
   b. **Somatic defects**
   c. **Medical disorders**

TABLE 32-3 SEQUELAE OF REPARATIVE SURGERY FOR CONGENITAL HEART DISEASE

A. **Electrophysiological**
   1. **Atriotomy**
      a. **Intraatrial repair**
      b. **Intraventricular repair**
   2. **Ventriculotomy**
      a. **The incision site**
      b. **The intracardiac repair**
B. **Native valves**
   1. **Left ventricular or right ventricular *outflow* repair**
   2. **Left ventricular or right ventricular *inflow* repair**
C. **Prosthetic materials**
   1. **Patches**
   2. **Valves**
   3. **Conduits**
D. **Myocardial and endocardial sequelae**

RESIDUAL ABNORMALITIES OF CARDIAC VALVES. These abnormalities after reparative surgery for congenital heart disease fall into three general categories: (1) congenitally malformed cardiac valves that are functionally normal and do not require attention during reparative surgery; (2) intrinsically normal cardiac valves that are rendered incompetent because of the physiological stress imposed by the congenital malformation that prompted surgical repair; and (3) residually incompetent or stenotic congenitally malformed cardiac valves that do not lend themselves to complete repair. Aortic valve abnormalities that represent functionally unimportant residua include a bicuspid aortic valve with coarctation of the aorta, and mild aortic regurgitation that may accompany Fallot's tetralogy, perimembranous ventricular septal defect, or truncus arteriosus. Congenital mitral valve abnormalities that represent functionally unimportant residua include the "cleft" but competent anterior mitral leaflet of an endocardial cushion defect (p. 92) and a reduction in interpapillary muscle distance associated with coarctation of the aorta. Postoperative residual incompetence of intrinsically normal pulmonary or tricuspid valves usually is in response to pulmonary hypertension or right ventricular hypertension (obstruction to outflow) which is intrinsic to the basic congenital malformation that warranted surgery.

RESIDUAL VENTRICULAR ABNORMALITIES. After reparative surgery, certain ventricular abnormalities are permanent, such as the intrinsic morphology of a chamber, or may change with the passage of time, as in the case of alterations in chamber mass and function. In patients undergoing either atrial switch operations for complete transposition of the great arteries or operations for congenitally corrected transposition of the great arteries, an important postoperative residuum is the presence of a morphological right ventricle in the systemic location. A pivotal question is whether a morphological right ventricle that is perfused by a right coronary artery can, in the long run, perform as a systemic chamber as well as an anatomical left ventricle perfused by a left coronary artery.

The development of increased ventricular mass and its regression after reparative surgery are important properties of ventricular myocardium (Chap. 14).[187,188] An increase in ventricular mass in excess of the process of normal growth is determined by the nature of the inciting stimulus (hemodynamic or hypoxic), the duration and type of the hemodynamic stimulus (pressure or volume overload), myocardial age (maturity) at the time the stimulus is imposed, and the type of cell involved.[188-190] The response of a given cell type at the time of a hemodynamic or hypoxic stimulus depends chiefly on myocardial maturity. If overload or hypoxia is imposed on the immature heart, the cellular response is characterized by replication (hyperplasia) of myocytes and fibroblasts.[191] If the stimuli continue beyond immaturity, myocytes then respond by hypertrophy (enlargement) and fibroblasts by hyperplasia (replication).[189] Of concern is the cellular basis for the decrease in mass after surgical removal of ventricular overload or hypoxia[37,38] (Figs. 32–24 and 32–25). Regression of hypertrophy at the cellular level means a decrease in size of enlarged myocytes, but the fate of myocytes that had replicated in excess of their otherwise genetically regulated numbers is not clear.[192] A postoperative reduction in ventricular mass in the setting of hyperplasia implies, at least in part, that the numerically excessive myocytes become smaller in size, not fewer in number. If this contention is valid, its long-term functional significance is unknown. The response of preoperative hyperplasia of connective tissue cells to operative removal of the overload or hypoxic stimulus is also unknown, although there is evidence that connective tissue cells do not regress as readily as myocytes.[193]

VASCULAR RESIDUA. After primary repair of congenital cardiac malformations, vascular residua consist of anatomical anomalies or defects, or elevated resistance and/or pressure in the systemic or pulmonary circulation (Table 32–2). A more than casual relation exists between aortic root disease and bicuspid or unicuspid unicommissural aortic valves, and on rare occasions, bicuspid or unicuspid aortic stenosis is dramatically complicated by a dissecting aneurysm.[14] The aortic root defect—if present before operation—remains as a postoperative risk. Rupture of an aneurysm of the circle of Willis is a cerebral complication of coarctation of the aorta. The predisposition is likely to persist after surgery, and rupture may occur in normotensive patients long after successful coarctation repair.[194]

Congenital anomalies of the coronary arteries occur in a number of congenital malformations of the heart; an example is Fallot's tetralogy, in which a coronary arterial anomaly is

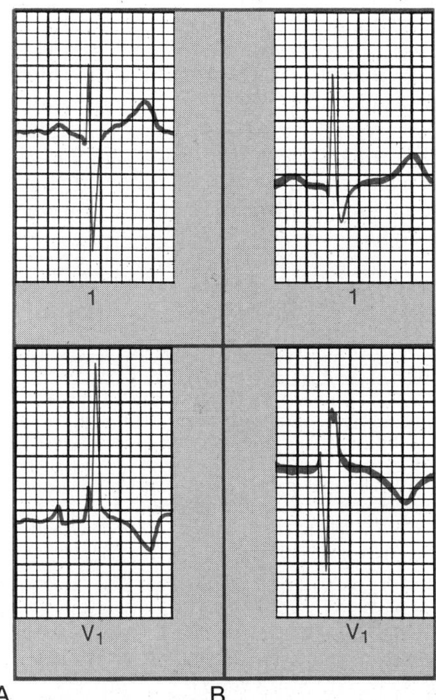

FIGURE 32–24. ***A,*** **Leads 1 and V_1 from a 2-year-old boy with severe pulmonary valve stenosis.** ***B,*** **Leads 1 and V_1 7 years after surgical pulmonary valvotomy. Right axis deviation has resolved and the rR′ in lead V_1 has been replaced with an rSr′. These are electrocardiographic features of regression of right ventricular hypertrophy.**

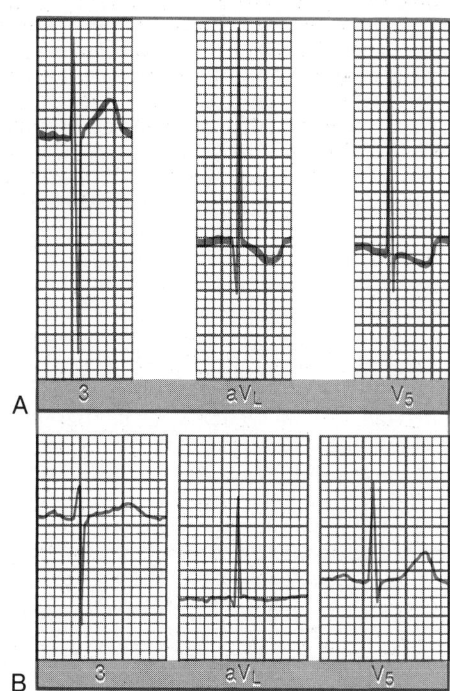

FIGURE 32–25. **Electrocardiographic leads 3, aVl, and V_5 before and after ligation of an anomalous left coronary artery that arose from the pulmonary trunk.** ***A,*** **Before operation (age 4 months) there was left axis deviation with voltage and repolarization criteria for left ventricular hypertrophy in leads aVl and V_5. Lead aVl exhibits a deep but narrow Q wave.** ***B,*** **Five years after operation the left axis deviation persists, but left ventricular hypertrophy and the deep Q wave in lead aVl have disappeared.**

present in 2 to 10 per cent of patients.[13] Although these anomalous arteries are functionally unimportant, they may be injured during operation. Not unimportant, however, is the residual coronary artery disease (intimal proliferation, medial thickening, premature atherosclerosis) initiated by the hypertension of coarctation of the aorta and that may become clinically overt after successful repair.

The younger the patient is at the time of successful coarctation repair, the more probable the long-term normalization of postoperative blood pressure.[195] Even if the resting blood pressure is normal after operation, systemic *systolic* pressure may rise disproportionately during exercise, implying a residual decrease in compliance of major proximal systemic arterial walls.

The preoperative status of the *pulmonary vascular bed,* especially the resistance vessels, is a major determinant of the presence and degree of residual postoperative pulmonary vascular disease. Early operation sets the stage for normal development of the pulmonary vascular bed, and reduces the probability that preoperative alterations will result in increased muscularity of small pulmonary arteries, intimal hyperplasia, and a reduction in the number of intraacinar vessels.[196] Refinements and safety of surgical repair within the first 6 to 12 months of life make it likely that postoperative pulmonary vascular disease will diminish in importance.

Noncardiac residua can be important long-term concerns after reparative surgery (Table 32–2). Developmental abnormalities such as the mental deficiency of Down syndrome or the physical deficiencies of Turner or the Ellis–van Creveld syndrome are examples. Specific residual somatic defects include dysmorphism and limb abnormalities. Spinal cord injuries during repair of coarctation of the aorta[197] are more properly considered complications rather than residua as defined earlier. Preoperative medical or psychosocial disorders may remain as important postoperative residua, and a healed brain abscess can serve as a focus of a seizure disorder. Cataracts and deafness persist as medical residua after division of the patent ductus in children with the rubella syndrome.[13]

After reparative surgery for congenital heart disease, sequelae may involve electrophysiological mechanisms, native cardiac valves, prosthetic materials, myocardium, and endocardium (Table 32–3). *Electrophysiological sequelae* of intraatrial repair become overtly manifest as disturbances in rhythm and conduction, including sinoatrial dysfunction, junctional rhythm, atrial fibrillation, atrial flutter, and impaired atrioventricular conduction varying from P-R interval prolongation to complete atrioventricular block. Electrophysiological sequelae of intraventricular repair by way of a right atrial incision result from injury to internodal conduction pathways, the proximal right bundle branch alone or in combination with the left anterior fascicle (left anterior hemiblock with right bundle branch block or bifascicular block). A right ventriculotomy is responsible for two electrophysiological sequelae: an alteration in the sequence of ventricular activation, and electrical instability of the incised right ventricle (Fig. 32–18).[198] The surface electrocardiogram is useful in determining the site of origin of abnormal right ventricular activation when a right bundle branch block pattern coexists with left anterior fascicular block. Bifascicular block sets the stage for postoperative complete heart block, which is a hazardous electrophysiological sequel (Fig. 32–13).

Sequelae involving native cardiac valves occur after left ventricular or right ventricular outflow repairs, or left ventricular or right ventricular inflow repairs. Postoperative aortic regurgitation as a sequel of repair of congenital bicuspid aortic stenosis is an example. Direct repair or balloon dilatation of simple congenital pulmonary valve stenosis is commonly followed by mild postinterventional pulmonary regurgitation (Fig. 32–26), a physiologically minor and therefore acceptable sequel. Repair of complex obstruction to right ventricular outflow, as in Fallot's tetralogy, usually induces pulmonary regurgitation. The importance of this sequel depends on the degree of regurgitant flow and the functional state of the recipient ventricle.

Sequelae associated with left ventricular inflow repair accompany operations for congenital mitral regurgitation or congenital obstruction to left ventricular inflow. Assuming complete relief of the mitral regurgitation of an endocardial cushion defect, the morphological abnormalities intrinsic to the congenitally malformed valve leave the left ventricular inflow guarded by an abnormal mitral apparatus. How these repaired valves will function decades after operation is not yet clear. Reconstruction of the tricuspid valve in Ebstein's anomaly is somewhat analogous. Repair is necessarily followed by sequelae intrinsic to the basic tricuspid valve malformation, even if competence is established.

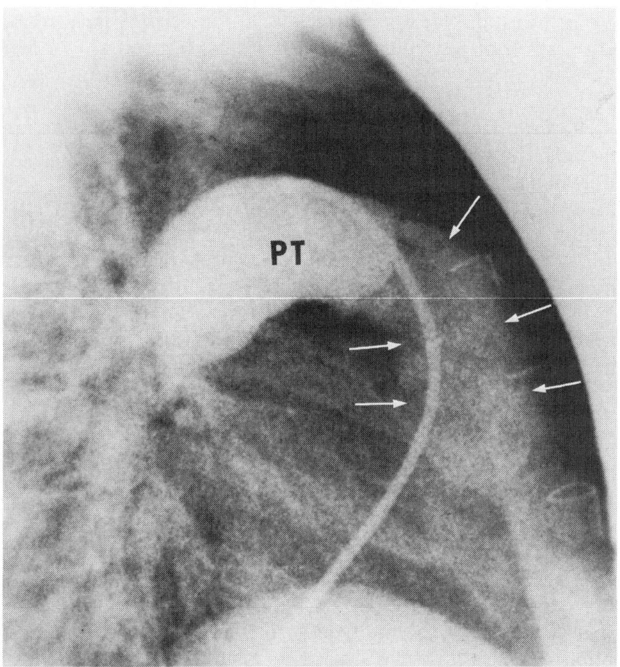

FIGURE 32–26. Pulmonary regurgitation (arrows) after open valvotomy for typical congenital pulmonary valve stenosis. PT = pulmonary trunk.

PROSTHETIC MATERIALS. Insertion of these materials represents a special category of sequelae after reparative surgery for congenital heart disease. Patches often are devoid of sequelae, such as an endogenous pericardial patch for closure of an ostium secundum atrial septal defect. However, a patch can set the stage for undesirable sequelae, as when an ostium primum atrial septal defect is closed with synthetic material that is struck by a jet of mitral regurgitation, which causes hemolytic anemia. Valve replacement results in sequelae that vary in signficance according to the physical and hemodynamic characteristics of the prosthetic device (bioprosthetic or synthetic), the site of insertion, and patient age at the time of insertion. Sequelae and complications imperceptibly merge. Reoperation is required when an infant or child outgrows the original valve prosthesis. Bioprosthetic valves degenerate at rates determined chiefly by the patient's age at the time of insertion (p. 1065) and by the tissue characteristics of the device (endogenous or exogenous materials, homografts or xenografts) (Fig. 32–20). Susceptibility to infective endocarditis varies from negligible with aortic homografts to high with mechanical valvular prostheses. The incidence of thromboembolic complications is low with aortic homografts and high with rigid prostheses. Anticoagulants reduce but do not eliminate thromboembolic risks and carry inherent risks of anticoagulant-induced bleeding and the risks of teratogenicity during pregnancy (see earlier).

Conduits can be nonvalved (usually synthetic) or valved (bioprosthetic or mechanical valves). In addition to the risks of degeneration (Fig. 32–21), thrombogenicity, anticoagulation, and infective endocarditis, conduits—especially valved conduits—are subject to pseudointimal proliferation (peel). Conduit obstruction can therefore result from both nongrowth and pseudointimal proliferation.

MYOCARDIAL SEQUELAE. These originate at the site of the ventriculotomy or atriotomy incision. Morphological or mechanical sequelae at these sites usually are negligible or absent, unless there is aneurysm formation, which is more properly considered a complication. Electrophysiological sequelae were discussed earlier. *Endocardial sequelae* after intraventricular repair have been called "surgical fibroelastosis."[199,200] The cause and functional significance of these endocardial lesions, which are not necessarily confined to the chamber in which the intracardiac repair was done, have not been established.

REFERENCES

1. Perloff, J. K., and Child, J. S.: Congenital Heart Disease in Adults. Philadelphia, W. B. Saunders Company, 1991.
2. Fallot, A.: Contribution a l'anatomie pathologique de la maladie bleue (cyanose cardiaque). Marseilleméd. *25*:418, 1888.
3. Abbott, M. E.: Atlas of Congenital Heart Disease. New York, American Heart Association, 1936.
4. Gross, R. E., and Hubbard, J. P.: Surgical ligation of a patent ductus arteriosus: Report of first successful case. JAMA *112*:729, 1939.
5. Blalock, A., and Taussig, H. B.: Surgical treatment of malformations of the heart in which there is pulmonary stenosis or pulmonary atresia. JAMA *128*:189, 1945.
6. Crafoord, C., and Nylin, G.: Congenital coarctation of the aorta and its surgical treatment. J. Thorac. Surg. *14*:347, 1945.
7. Kirklin, J. W., DuShane, J. W., Patrick, R. T., et al.: Intracardiac surgery with the aid of a mechanical pump-oxygenator system (Gibbon type): Report of eight cases. Proc. Staff Meet. Mayo Clin. *30*:201, 1955.
8. Perloff, J. K.: Pediatric congenital cardiac becomes a postoperative adult. The changing population of congenital heart disease. Circulation *47*:606, 1973.
9. Somerville, J.: Congenital heart disease in adults and adolescents. Br. Heart J. *56*:395, 1986.
10. Engle, M. A., Adams, F. H., Betson, C., et al.: Resources for long-term care of congenital heart disease. Circulation *44*:A-205, 1971.

11. Garson, A.: The science and practice of pediatric cardiology in the next decade. Am. Heart J. *114*:462, 1987.

SURVIVAL PATTERNS

12. Roberts, W. C.: The congenitally bicuspid aortic valve: A study of 85 autopsy cases. Am. J. Cardiol. *26*:72, 1970.
13. Perloff, J. K.: The Clinical Recognition of Congenital Heart Disease. 3rd ed. Philadelphia, W. B. Saunders Company, 1987.
14. Subramanian, R., Olson, L. J., and Edwards, W. D.: Surgical pathology of pure aortic stenosis: A study of 374 cases. Mayo Clin. Proc. *59*:683, 1984.
15. Larson, E. W., and Edwards, W. D.: Risk factors for aortic dissection. A necropsy study of 161 cases. Am. J. Cardiol. *53*:849, 1984.
16. Morganroth, J., Perloff, J. K., Zeldes, S. M., and Dunkman, W. B.: Acute severe aortic regurgitation. Ann. Intern. Med. *87*:223, 1977.
17. Campbell, M.: Natural history of coarctation of the aorta. Br. Heart J. *32*:633, 1970.
18. Jarcho, S.: Coarctation of the aorta (Reynaud, 1828). Am. J. Cardiol. *9*:591, 1962.
19. Hodes, H. L., Steinfeld, L., and Blumenthal, S.: Congenital cerebral aneurysms and coarctation of the aorta. Arch. Pediatr. *76*:28, 1959.
20. Edwards, J. E.: Aneurysms of the thoracic aorta complicating coarctation. Circulation *48*:195, 1973.
21. Vladover, Z., and Neufeld, H. N.: Coronary arteries in coarctation of the aorta. Circulation *37*:449, 1968.
22. Campbell, M.: The natural history of congenital pulmonic stenosis. Br. Heart J. *31*:394, 1969.
23. Nugent, E. W., Freedom, R. M., Nora, J. J., et al.: Clinical course in pulmonary stenosis. Circulation *56*(Suppl I):38, 1977.
24. Moller, J. H., and Adams, P., Jr.: Natural history of pulmonary valvular stenosis: Serial cardiac catheterization in 21 children. Am. J. Cardiol. *16*:654, 1965.
25. Kaplan, S., and Adolph, R. J.: Pulmonic valve stenosis in adults. Cardiovasc. Clin. *10*:328, 1979.
26. Sanders, C., Bittner, V., Nath, P. H., et al.: Atrial septal defect in older adults: Atypical radiographic appearances. Radiology *167*:123, 1988.
27. Campbell, M.: Natural history of atrial septal defect. Br. Heart J. *32*:820, 1970.
28. Rodstein, M., Zeman, F. D., and Gerber, I. E.: Atrial septal defect in the aged. Circulation *23*:665, 1961.
29. Colmers, R. E.: Atrial septal defects in elderly patients: Report of three patients aged 68, 72, and 78. Am. J. Cardiol. *1*:768, 1958.
30. Craig, R. J., and Selzer, A.: Natural history and prognosis of atrial septal defect. Circulation *37*:805, 1968.
31. Markman, P. G., Horvitt, E. G., and Wade, E. G.: Atrial septal defect in the middle-aged and elderly. Q. J. Med. *34*:409, 1965.
32. Perloff, J. K.: Ostium secundum atrial septal defect—survival for 87 and 94 years. Am. J. Cardiol. *53*:388, 1984.
33. Wood, P.: The Eisenmenger syndrome or pulmonary hypertension with reversed central shunt. Br. Med. J. *2*:701, 1958.
34. Nagata, S., Yasuharu, N., Sakakibara, H., et al.: Mitral valve lesion associated with secundum atrial septal defect. Br. Heart J. *49*:51, 1983.
35. Davies, M. J.: Mitral valve in secundum atrial septal defect. Br. Heart J. *46*:126, 1981.
36. Boucher, C. A., Liberthson, R. R., and Buckley, M. J.: Secundum atrial septal defect and significant mitral regurgitation: Incidence, management and morphologic basis. Chest *75*:697, 1979.
37. Popio, K. A., Gorlin, R., Teichholz, L., et al.: Abnormalities of left ventricular function and geometry in adults with an atrial septal defect. Am. J. Cardiol. *36*:302, 1975.
38. Wanderman, K. L., Ovsyheer, I., and Gueron, M.: Left ventricular performance in patients with atrial septal defect: Evaluation with noninvasive methods. Am. J. Cardiol. *41*:487, 1978.
39. Campbell, M.: Natural history of persistent ductus arteriosus. Br. Heart J. *30*:4, 1968.
40. Marquis, R. M., Miller, H. C., McCormack, R.J.M., et al.: Persistence of ductus arteriosus with left to right shunt in the older patient. Br. Heart J. *48*:469, 1982.
41. White, P. D., Maxurkie, S. J., and Boschetti, A. E.: Patency of the ductus arteriosus at 90. N Engl. J. Med. *280*:146, 1969.
42. Fishman, L.: Patent ductus arteriosus in a patient surviving to seventy-four years. Am. J. Cardiol. *6*:685, 1960.
43. Bain, C.W.C.: Longevity in patent ductus arteriosus. Br. Heart J. *19*:574, 1957.

UNCOMMON DEFECTS WITH EXPECTED ADULT SURVIVAL

44. McHenry, M. M.: Factors influencing longevity in adults with congenital complete heart block. Am. J. Cardiol. *29*:416, 1972.
45. Reybrouck, T., Vanden Eynde, B. B., Dumoulin, M., and Van der Hauwaert, L. G.: Cardiorespiratory response to exercise in congenital complete atrioventricular block. Am. J. Cardiol. *64*:896, 1989.
46. Dewey, R. C., Capeless, M. A., and Levy, A. M.: Use of ambulatory electrocardiographic monitoring to identify high-risk patients with congenital complete heart block. N. Engl. J. Med. *316*:835, 1987.
47. Bjarke, B. B., and Kidd, B.S.L.: Congenitally corrected transposition of the great arteries: A clinical study of 101 cases. Acta Paediatr. Scand. *65*:153, 1976.
48. Cumming, G. R.: Congenital corrected transposition of the great vessels without associated intracardiac anomalies. Am. J. Cardiol. *10*:605, 1962.
49. Nagle, J. P., Cheitlin, M. D., and McCarty, R. J.: Corrected transposition of the great vessels without associated anomalies. Chest *60*:363, 1971.
50. Schiebler, G. L., Edwards, J. E., Burchell, H. B., et al.: Congenital corrected transposition of the great vessels. Pediatrics *27*:851, 1961.
51. Lieberson, A. D., Schumacker, R., and Childress, D.: Corrected transposition of the great vessels in a 73 year old man. Circulation *39*:96, 1969.
52. Anderson, K. R., Zuberbuhler, J. R., Anderson, R. H., et al.: Morphologic spectrum of Ebstein's anomaly of the heart. Mayo Clin. Proc. *54*:174, 1979.
53. Benson, L. N., Child, J. S., Schwaiger, M., et al.: Left ventricular geometry and function in adults with Ebstein's anomaly of the tricuspid valve. Circulation *75*:353, 1987.
54. Watson, H.: Natural history of Ebstein's anomaly of tricuspid valve in childhood and adolescence: An international cooperative study of 505 cases. Br. Heart J. *36*:417, 1974.
55. Radford, D. J., Graff, R. F., and Neilson, G. H.: Diagnosis and natural history of Ebstein's anomaly. Br. Heart J. *54*:517, 1985.
56. Makous, N., and Vander Veer, J. B.: Ebstein's anomaly and life expectancy: Report of a survival to over seventy-nine. Am. J. Cardiol. *18*:100, 1966.
57. Adams, J.C.L., and Hudson, R.: Case of Ebstein's anomaly surviving to age 79. Br. Heart J. *18*:129, 1956.
58. Giuliani, E. R., Fuster, V., Brandenburg, R. O., and Mair, D. D.: Ebstein's anomaly: The clinical features and natural history of Ebstein's anomaly of the tricuspid valve. Mayo Clin. Proc. *54*:163, 1979.
59. Seward, J. B., Tajik, A. J., Feist, D. J., and Smith, H. C.: Ebstein's anomaly in an 85 year old man. May Clin. Proc. *54*:193, 1979.
60. Leung, M. P., Baker, E. J., Anderson, R. H., and Zuberbuhler, J. R.: Cineangiographic spectrum of Ebstein's malformations: Its relevance to clinical presentation and outcome. J. Am. Coll. Cardiol. *11*:154, 1988.
60a. Saxena, A., Fong, L. V., and Tristam, M., et al: Left ventricular function in patients > 20 years of age with Ebstein's anomaly of the tricuspid valve. Am. J. Cardiol. *67*:217, 1991.
61. Collins, N. P., Braunwald, E., and Morrow, A. G.: Isolated congenital pulmonary valvular regurgitation. Am. J. Med. *28*:159, 1960.
62. Cortes, F. M., and Jacoby, W. J.: Isolated congenital pulmonary valvular insufficiency. Am. J. Cardiol. *10*:287, 1962.
63. Pouget, J. M., Kelly, C. E., and Pilz, C. G.: Congenital absence of the pulmonic valve: Report of a case in a 73 year old man. Am. J. Cardiol. *19*:732, 1967.
64. Rich, S., and Brundage, B. H.: Pulmonary hypertension: A cellular basis for understanding the pathophysiology and treatment. J. Am. Coll. Cardiol. *14*:545, 1989.
65. McGoon, M. D., and Edwards, W. D.: Primary pulmonary hypertension: Current status. Mod. Conc. Cardiovasc. Dis. *54*:29, 1985.
66. Fuster, V., Steele, P. M., Edwards, W. D., et al.: Primary pulmonary hypertension: Natural history and the importance of thrombosis. Circulation *70*:580, 1984.
67. Bjornsson, J., and Edwards, W. D.: Primary pulmonary hypertension: A histopathologic study of 80 cases. Mayo Clin. Proc. *60*:16, 1985.
68. Lutembacher, R.: De la stenose mitrale avec communication interauriculaire. Arch. Mal. Coeur *9*:237, 1916.
69. Firkett, C. H.: Examen anatomique d'un cas de persistence du trou ovale de botal, avec lésions valvulaires considérables du couer gauche, chez une femme de 74 ans. Ann. Soc. Med. Chir. Liege. *19*:188, 1880.
70. Rosenthal, L.: Atrial septal defect with mitral stenosis (Lutembacher's syndrome) in a woman of 81. Br. Med. J. *2*:1351, 1956.
71. Botefeu, J. M., Moret, P. R., Hahn, C., and Hauf, E.: Aneurysms of the sinus of Valsalva: Report of seven cases and review of the literature. Am. J. Med. *65*:18, 1983.
72. Mayer, E. D., Ruffman, K., Saggau, W., et al.: Ruptured aneurysms of the sinus of Valsalva. Ann. Thorac. Surg. *42*:81, 1986.
73. Liberthson, R. R., Sagar, K., Berkoben, J. P., et al.: Congenital coronary arteriovenous fistula: Report of 13 patients, review of the literature and delineation of management. Circulation *59*:849, 1979.
74. Dines, D. E., Seward, J. B., and Bernatz, P. E.: Pulmonary arteriovenous fistula. Mayo Clin. Proc. *58*:176, 1983.
75. Wong, L. B., and Perloff, J. K.: Familial occurrence of congenital pulmonary arteriovenous fistulae in octogenarian siblings. Am. J. Cardiol. *62*:1149, 1988.
76. Campbell, M.: Natural history of ventricular septal defect. Br Heart J. *33*:246, 1971.
77. Corone, P., Doyon, F., Gaudeau, S., et al.: Natural history of ventricular septal defect: A study involving 790 cases. Circulation *55*:908, 1977.
78. Weidman, W. H., DuShane, J. W., and Ellison, R. C.: Clinical course in adults with ventricular septal defect. Circulation *56*:I-78, 1977.
79. Ellis, J. H. IV, Moodie, D. S., Sterba, R., and Gill, C. C.: Ventricular septal defect in the adult: Natural and unnatural history. Am. Heart J. *114*:115, 1987.
80. Otterstad, J. E., Nitter-Hauge, S., and Myhre, E.: Isolated ventricular septal defect in adults: Clinical and haemodynamic findings. Br. Heart J. *50*:343, 1983.
81. Wood, P.: Foreword. *In* Bedford, E. D., and Caird, F. L.: Valvular Diseases of the Heart in Old Age. Boston, Little, Brown, and Company, 1960.
82. Moe, D. G., and Guntheroth, W. G.: Spontaneous closure of uncomplicated ventricular septal defect. Am. J. Cardiol. *60*:674, 1987.
83. Ramaciotti, C., Keren, A., and Silverman, N. H.: Importance of (perimembranous) ventricular septal aneurysm in the natural history of isolated perimembranous ventricular septal defect. Am. J. Cardiol. *57*:268, 1986.

84. Shah, P., Singh, W.S.A., Rose, V., and Keith, J. D.: Incidence of bacterial endocarditis in ventricular septal defects. Circulation *34*:127, 1966.
85. Abraham, K. A., Cherian, G., Rao, V. D., et al.: Tetralogy of Fallot in adults: A report on 147 patients. Am. J. Med. *66*:811, 1979.
86. Bertranou, E. G., Blackstone, E. H., Hazelrig, J. B., et al.: Life expectancy without surgery in tetralogy of Fallot. Am. J. Cardiol. *42*:458, 1978.
87. Perloff, J. K.: Late postoperative concerns in adults with congenital heart disease. Cardiovasc. Clin. *11*:431, 1980.
88. Kan, J. S., White, R. I., Jr., Mitchell, S. E., and Gardner, T. S.: Percutaneous balloon valvuloplasty: A new method for treating congenital pulmonary valve stenosis. N Engl. J. Med. *307*:540, 1982.
89. Mullins, C. E.: Pediatric and congenital therapeutic cardiac catheterization. Circulation *79*:1153, 1989.
90. Stanger, P., Cassidy, S. C., Girod, D. A., et al.: Balloon pulmonary angioplasty: Results of the valvuloplasty and angioplasty of congenital anomalies registry. Am. J. Cardiol. *65*:775, 1990.
91. Nishimura, R. A., Holmes, D. R., and Reeder, G. S.: Percutaneous balloon valvuloplasty. Mayo Clin. Proc. *65*:198, 1990.
92. Sandor, G.G.S., Olley, P. M., Trusler, G. A., et al.: Long-term follow-up of patients after valvotomy for congenital valvular aortic stenosis in children. J. Thorac. Cardiovasc. Surg. *80*:171, 1980.
93. Presbitero, P., Sommerville, J., Revel-Chion, R., and Ross, D.: Open aortic valvulotomy for congenital aortic stenosis: Late results. Br. Heart J. *47*:26, 1982.
94. Hsieh, K., Keane, J. F., Nadas, A. S., et al.: Long-term follow-up of valvulotomy before 1968 for congenital aortic stenosis. Am. J. Cardiol. *58*:338, 1986.
95. Jones, M., Barnhart, G. R., and Morrow, A. G.: Late results after operation for left ventricular outflow tract obstruction. Am. J. Cardiol. *50*:569, 1982.
96. Choy, M., Beekman, R. H., Rocchini, A. P., et al.: Percutaneous balloon valvuloplasty for valvar aortic stenosis in infants and children. Am. J. Cardiol. *59*:1010, 1987.
97. Helgason, H., Keane, J. F., Fellow, K. E., et al.: Balloon dilatation of the aortic valve: Studies in normal lambs and in children with aortic stenoses. J. Am. Coll. Cardiol. *9*:816, 1987.
98. Danielson, G. K., and Fuster, V.: Surgical repair of Ebstein's anomaly. Ann. Surg. *196*:499, 1982.
99. Westaby, S., Karp, R. B., Kirklin, J. W., et al.: Surgical treatment in Ebstein's malformation. Ann. Thorac. Surg. *34*:388, 1982.
100. Driscoll, D. J., Mottram, C. D., and Danielson, G. K.: Spectrum of exercise intolerance in 45 patients with Ebstein's anomaly and observations on exercise tolerance in 11 patients after surgical repair. J. Am. Coll. Cardiol. *11*:831, 1988.
101. Behz, P. R., and Bleslovsky, A.: Ebstein's anomaly: Sixteen years' experience with valve replacement without plication of the right ventricle. Thorax *39*:8, 1984.
102. Hwang, B., Bowman, F., Malm, J., and Krongrad, E.: Surgical repair of congenitally corrected transposition of the great arteries: Results and follow-up. Am. J. Cardiol. *50*:781, 1982.
103. Murphy, J. G., Gersh, B. J., McGoon, M. D., et al.: Long-term outcome of patients undergoing surgical repair of isolated atrial septal defect: Follow-up at 28-32 years. (In press.)
104. St. John Sutton, M. G., Tajik, A. J., and McGoon, D. C.: Atrial septal defect in patients 60 years or older: operative results and long-term postoperative follow-up. Circulation *64*:402, 1981.
105. Meyer, R. A., Korfhagen, J. C., Covitz, W., and Kaplan, S.: Long-term follow-up study after closure of secundum atrial septal defect in children: An echocardiography study. Am. J. Cardiol. *50*:143, 1982.
106. Steele, P. M., Fuster, V., Cohen, M., et al.: Isolated atrial septal defect with pulmonary vascular obstructive disease—long-term follow-up and prediction of outcome after surgical correction. Circulation *76*:1037, 1987.
107. Bink-Boelkens, M. T., Velvis, H., Van der Heide, J. J., et al.: Dysrhythmias after atrial surgery in children. Am. Heart J. *106*:125, 1983.
108. Bolens, M., and Friedli, B.: Sinus node function and conduction system before and after surgery for secundum atrial septal defect: an electrophysiologic study. Am. J. Cardiol. *53*:1415, 1984.
109. Williams, W. G., Trusler, G. A., Kirklin, J. W., et al.: Early and late results of a protocol for simple transposition leading to an atrial switch (Mustard) repair. J Thorac. Cardiovasc. Surg. *45*:717, 1988.
110. Turina, M., Siebenmann, R., Nussbaumer, P., and Senning, A.: Long-term outlook after atrial correction of transposition of the great arteries. J. Thorac. Cardiovasc. Surg. *95*:828, 1988.
111. Musewe, N. N., Reisman, J., Benson, L. N., et al.: Cardiopulmonary adaptation at rest and during exercise ten years after Mustard atrial repair for transposition of the great arteries. Circulation *77*:1055, 1988.
112. Parrish, M. D., Graham, T. P., Bender, H. W., et al.: Radionuclide angiographic evaluation of right and left ventricular function during exercise after repair of transposition of the great arteries. Circulation *67*:178, 1983.
113. Ramsay, J. M., Venables, A. W., Kelly, M. J., and Kalff, V.: Right and left ventricular function at rest and with exercise after the Mustard operation for transposition of the great arteries. Br. Heart J. *51*:364, 1984.
114. Katz, N. M., Blackstone, E. H., Kirklin, J. W., et al.: Late survival and symptoms after repair of tetralogy of Fallot. Circulation *65*:403, 1982.
115. Fuster, V., McGoon, D. C., Kennedy, M. A., et al.: Long-term evaluation (12 to 22 years) of open heart surgery for tetralogy of Fallot. Am. J. Cardiol. *46*:635, 1980.
116. Abe, T., Asai, Y., Sugiki, K., and Komatsu, S.: Reoperation after initial correction of tetralogy of Fallot. J. Cardiovasc. Surg. *26*:568, 1985.
117. Zhao, H., Miller, D. C., Reitz, B. A., and Shumway, N. E.: Surgical repair of tetralogy of Fallot: Long-term follow-up with particular emphasis on late death and reoperation. J. Thorac. Cardiovasc. Surg. *89*:204, 1985.
118. Hu, D.C.K., Seward, J. B., Puga, F. J., et al.: Total correction of tetralogy of Fallot at age 40 years or older: long-term follow-up. J. Am. Coll. Cardiol. *5*:40, 1985.
119. Hughes, C. F., Lim, Y. C., Cartmill, T. B., et al.: Total intracardiac repair for tetralogy of Fallot in adults. Ann. Thorac. Surg. *43*:634, 1987.
120. Jarmakani, J. M., Graham, T. P., and Canent, R. V.: Left heart function in children with tetralogy of Fallot before and after palliative or corrective surgery. Circulation *46*:478, 1972.
121. Borow, K. M., Green, L. H., Castenada, A. R., and Keane, J. F.: Left ventricular function after repair of tetralogy of Fallot and its relationship to age of surgery. Circulation *61*:1150, 1980.
122. Fisher, R. G., Moodie, D. S., Sterba, R., and Gill, C. G.: Patent ductus arteriosus in adults—long-term follow-up: Nonsurgical versus surgical treatment. J. Am. Coll. Cardiol. *8*:280, 1986.
123. Koller, M., Rothlin, M., and Senning, A.: Coarctation of the aorta: Review of 362 operated patients. Long-term follow-up and assessment of prognostic variables. Eur. Heart J. *8*:670, 1987.
124. Daniels, S. R., James, F. W., Loggie, J.M.H., and Kaplan, S.: Correlates of resting and maximal exercise systolic blood pressure after repair of coarctation of the aorta: A multivariate analysis. Am. Heart J. *113*:349, 1987.
125. Presbitero, P., Demarie, D., Villani, M., et al.: Long-term results (15 to 30 years) of surgical repair of aortic coarctation. Br. Heart J. *57*:462, 1987.
126. Liberthson, R. L., Pennington, D. G., Jacobs, M. L., and Daggett, W. M.: Coarctation of the aorta: Review of 234 patients and clarification of management problems. Am. J. Cardiol. *43*:835, 1979.
127. Cohen, M., Fuster, V., Steele, P. M., et al.: Coarctation of the aorta: Long-term follow-up and prediction of outcome after surgical correction. Circulation *80*:840, 1989.
128. Clarkson, P. M., Nicholson, M. R., Barratt-Boyes, B. G., et al.: Results after repair of coarctation of the aorta beyond infancy: A 10 to 28 year follow-up with particular reference to late systemic hypertension. Am. J. Cardiol. *51*:1481, 1983.
129. Hesslein, P. S., McNamara, D. G., Morriss, M.J.H., et al.: Comparison of resection versus patch aortoplasty for repair of coarctation in infants and children. Circulation *64*:164, 1981.
130. Celano, V., Pieroni, D. R., Morera, J. A., et al.: Two-dimensional echocardiographic examination of mitral valve abnormalities associated with coarctation of the aorta. Circulation *69*:924, 1984.
131. Fontan, F., and Baudet, E.: Surgical repair of tricuspid atresia. Thorax *26*:240, 1971.
132. de Leval, M. R., Kilner, P., Gewillig, M., and Bull, C.: Total cavopulmonary connection: A logical alternative to atriopulmonary connection for complex Fontan operations. Experimental studies and early clinical experience. J. Thorac. Cardiovasc. Surg. *96*:682, 1988.
133. Girod, D. A., Fontan, F., Deville, C., et al.: Long-term results after the Fontan operation for tricuspid atresia. Circulation *75*:605, 1987.
134. Matsuda, H., Kawashima, Y., Kishimoto, H., et al.: Problems with the modified Fontan operation for univentricular heart of the right ventricular type. Circulation *76*(suppl II):1, 1987.
135. Barber, G., DiSessa, T., Child, J. S., et al.: Hemodynamic responses to isolated increments in heart rate by atrial pacing after a Fontan procedure. Am. Heart J. *115*:837, 1988.
136. Humes, R. A., Mair, D. D., Porter, C. J., et al.: Results of the modified Fontan operation in adults. Am. J. Cardiol. *61*:602, 1988.
137. Laks, H., Milliken, J. C., Perloff, J. K., et al.: Experience with the Fontan procedure. J. Thorac. Cardiovasc. Surg. *88*:939, 1984.

MEDICAL MANAGEMENT OF CONGENITAL HEART DISEASE IN THE ADULT

138. Berman, W., Jr., Wood, S. C., Yabek, S. M., et al.: Systemic oxygen transport in patients with congenital heart disease. Circulation *75*:360, 1987.
139. Tyndall, M. R., Teitel, D. F., Lutin, W. A., et al.: Serum erythropoietin levels in patients with congenital heart disease. J. Pediatr. *110*:538, 1987.
140. Rosove, M. H., Perloff, J. K., Hocking, W. G., et al.: Chronic hypoxaemia and decompensated erythrocytosis in cyanotic congenital heart disease. Lancet *2*:313, 1986.
141. Linderkamp, O., Klose, H. J., Betke, K., et al.: Increased blood viscosity in patients with cyanotic congenital heart disease and iron deficiency. J. Pediatrics *95*:567, 1979.
142. Giddings, S. S., and Stockman, J. A.: Effect of iron deficiency on tissue oxygen delivery in cyanotic congenital heart disease. Am. J. Cardiol. *61*:605, 1988.
143. Perloff, J. K., Rosove, M. H., Child, J. S., and Wright, G. B.: Adults with cyanotic congenital heart disease: Hematologic management. Ann. Intern. Med. *109*:406, 1988.
144. Cottrill, C. M., and Kaplan, S.: Cerebral vascular accidents in cyanotic congenital heart disease. Am. J. Dis. Child. *125*:484, 1973.
145. Bowyer, J. J., Busst, C. M., Denison, D. M., and Shinebourne, E. A.: Effect of long term oxygen treatment at home in children with pulmonary vascular disease. Br. Heart J. *55*:385, 1986.
146. Suarez, C. R., Menendez, C. E., Griffin, A. J., et al.: Cyanotic congenital heart disease in children: Hemostatic disorders and relevance of molecular markers of hemostasis. Semin. Thromb. Hemost. *10*:285, 1984.
147. Rosove, M. H., Hocking, W. G., Harwig, S. S., and Perloff, J. K.: Studies of beta-thromboglobulin, platelet factor 4, and fibrinopeptide A in eryth-

rocytosis due to cyanotic congenital heart disease. Thromb. Res. *29*:225, 1983.

148. Gill, J. C., Wilson, A. D., Endres-Brooks, J., and Montgomery, R. R.: Loss of the largest von Willebrand factor multimers from the plasma of patients with congenital cardiac defects. Blood *67*:758, 1986.
149. Henriksson, P., Vårendh, G., and Lundström, N. R.: Haemostatic defects in cyanotic congenital heart disease. Br. Heart J. *41*:23, 1979.
150. Ware, J. A., Reaves, W. H., Horak, J. K., and Solis, R. T.: Defective platelet aggregation in patients undergoing surgical repair of cyanotic congenital heart disease. Ann. Thorac. Surg. *36*:289, 1983.
151. Ekert, H., Gilchrist, G. S., Stanton, R., and Hammond, D.: Hemostasis in cyanotic congenital heart disease. J. Pediatr. *76*:221, 1970.
152. Ross, E. A., Perloff, J. K., Danovitch, G. M., et al.: Renal function and urate metabolism in late survivors with cyanotic congenital heart disease. Circulation *73*:396, 1986.
153. Young, D.: Hyperuricemia in cyanotic congenital heart disease. Am. J. Dis. Child. *134*:902, 1980.
154. Spear, G. S.: The glomerular lesion of cyanotic congenital heart disease. Bull. Johns Hopkins Hosp. *140*:185, 1977.
155. German, D. C., and Holmes, E. W.: Hyperuricemia and gout. Med. Clin. North Am. *70*:419, 1986.
156. Sietsema, K. E., Cooper, D. M., Perloff, J. K., et al.: Dynamics of oxygen uptake during exercise in adults with cyanotic congenital heart disease. Circulation *73*:1137, 1986.
157. Sietsema, K. E., Cooper, D. M., Perloff, J. K., et al.: Control of ventilation during exercise in patients with central venous-to-systemic arterial shunts. J. Appl. Physiol. *64*:234, 1988.
158. Carvalho, J. S., Belcher, P., and Knight, W. B.: Infection of modified Blalock shunts. Br. Heart. J. *58*:287, 1987.
159. Watanakunakorn, C.: Changing epidemiology and newer aspects of infective endocarditis. Adv. Intern. Med. *22*:21, 1977.
160. Pitkin, R. M., Perloff, J. K., Koos, B. J., and Beall, M. H.: Pregnancy and congenital heart disease. Ann. Intern. Med. *112*:445, 1990.
161. Loscalzo, J.: Paradoxical embolization: Clinical presentation, diagnostic strategies, and therapeutic options. Am. Heart J. *112*:141, 1986.
162. Esscher, E. B.: Congenital complete heart block in adolescence and adult life: A follow-up study. Eur. Heart J. *2*:281, 1981.
163. Esscher, E. B.: Congenital complete heart block (review). Acta Paediatr. Scand. *70*:131, 1981.
164. Michaelson, M., and Engle, M. A.: Congenital complete heart block: An internal study of the natural history. Cardiovasc. Clin. *4*:85, 1972.
165. Waickman, L. A., Skorton, D. J., Varner, M. W., et al.: Ebstein's anomaly and pregnancy. Am. J. Cardiol. *53*:357, 1984.
166. Isner, J. M., Donaldson, R. F., Fulton, D., et al.: Cystic medial necrosis in coarctation of the aorta. Circulation *75*:689, 1987.
167. Steele, P. M., Fuster, V., Ritter, D. G., and McGoon, D. C.: Isolated coarctation of the aorta—long term operative results. *In* Engle, M. A., and Perloff, J. K. (eds.): Congenital Heart Disease After Surgery. New York, Yorke Medical Books, 1983.
168. Devitt, J. H., Noble, W. H., and Byrick, R. J.: A Swan-Ganz catheter related complication in a patient with Eisenmenger's syndrome. Anesthesiology *57*:335, 1982.
169. Shime, J., Mocarski, E. J., Hastings, D., et al.: Congenital heart disease in pregnancy: Short- and long-term implications. Am. J. Obstet. Gynecol. *156*:313, 1987.
170. Nora, J. J., and Nora, A. H.: Maternal transmissions of congenital heart diseases: New recurrence risk figures and the questions of cytoplasmic inheritance and vulnerability to teratogens. Am. J. Cardiol. *59*:459, 1987.
171. Maron, B. J., Epstein, S. E., and Mitchell, J. H.: Sixteenth Bethesda Conference: Cardiovascular abnormalities in the athlete: Recommendations regarding eligibility for competition. J. Am. Coll. Cardiol. *6*:1189, 1985.
172. Mitchell, J. H., Blomqvist, G., Haskell, W. L., et al.: Classification of sports. Am. J. Coll. Cardiol. *6*:1189, 1985.
173. Barth, C. W., and Roberts, W. C.: Left main coronary artery originating from the right sinus of Valsalva and coursing between the aorta and pulmonary trunk. J. Am. Coll. Cardiol. *7*:366, 1986.
174. Cheitlin, M. D., De Castro, C. M., and McAllister, H. A.: Sudden death as a complication of anomalous left coronary origin from the anterior sinus of Valsalva, a not so minor congenital anomaly. Circulation *50*:780, 1974.
175. Maron, B. J., Roberts, W. C., McAllister, H. A., et al.: Sudden death in young athletes. Circulation *62*:218, 1980.
176. Mark, A. L., Abboud, F. M., Schmidt, P. G., and Heistad, D. D.: Reflex vascular responses to left ventricular outflow obstruction and activation of ventricular baroreceptors in dogs. J. Clin. Invest. *52*:1147, 1982.
177. James, F. W., Kaplan, S., Schwartz, D. C., et al.: Response to exercise in patients after total correction of tetralogy of Fallot. Circulation *54*:671, 1976.
178. Garson, A., Gillette, P. C., Gutgesell, H. P., and McNamara, D. G.: Stress-induced ventricular arrhythmias after repair of tetralogy of Fallot. Am. J. Cardiol. *46*:1006, 1980.
179. Driscoll, D. J., Danielson, O. K., Puga, F. J., et al.: Exercise tolerance and cardiorespiratory response to exercise after the Fontan operation for tricuspid atresia or functional single ventricle. J. Am. Coll. Cardiol. *7*:1087, 1986.
180. Truesdell, S. C., Skorton, D. J., and Lauer, R. M.: Life insurance for children with cardiovascular disease. Pediatrics *77*:687, 1986.
181. Manning, J. A.: Insurability and employability of young cardiac patients. *In* Engle, M. A. (ed.): Pediatric Cardiovascular Disease. Philadelphia, F. A. Davis Co., 1981.
182. Sillanpaa, M.: Social adjustment and functioning of chronically ill and impaired children and adolescents. Acta Paediatr. Scand. [Suppl] *340*:1, 1987.
183. Rasof, B., Linde, L. M., and Dunn, O. J.: Intellectual development in children with congenital heart disease. Child. Dev. *38*:1043, 1967.
184. Finly, K. H., Buse, S. T., Popper, R. W., et al.: Intellectual functioning of children with tetralogy of Fallot: Influence of open heart surgery and earlier palliative operations. J. Pediatr. *85*:318, 1974.
185. Baer, P. E., Freedman, D. A., and Garson, A.: Longterm psychological follow-up of patients after corrective surgery for tetralogy of Fallot. J. Am. Acad. Child. Psychiatry *5*:622, 1984.
186. Dickinson, D. F., and Sambrooks, J. E.: Intellectual performance in children after circulatory arrest with profound hypothermia in infancy. Arch. Dis. Child. *54*:1, 1979.
186. Stark, J.: Do we really correct congenital heart defects? J. Thorac. Cardiovasc. Surg. *97*:1, 1989.

CARDIAC SURGICAL CONSIDERATIONS IN ADULTS WITH CONGENITAL HEART DISEASE

187. Grossman, W.: Cardiac hypertrophy: Useful adaptation or pathologic process? Am. J. Med. *69*:576, 1980.
188. Zak, R., Kizu, A., and Bugaisay, L.: Cardiac hypertrophy: its characteristics as a growth process. Am. J. Cardiol. *44*:941, 1979.
189. Zak, R.: Cell proliferation during cardiac growth. Am. J. Cardiol. *31*:211, 1973.
190. Anversa, P., Ricci, R., and Olivetti, G.: Quantitative structural analysis of the myocardium during physiologic growth and induced cardiac hypertrophy: A review. J. Am. Coll. Cardiol. *7*:1140, 1986.
191. Ghani, Q. P., and Hollenberg, M.: Poly-adenosine biphosphate ribose metabolism and regulation of myocardial cell growth by oxygen. Biochem. J. *170*:378, 1978.
192. Hathaway, D. R., and March, K. L.: Molecular cardiology: New avenues for the diagnosis and treatment of cardiovascular disease. J. Am. Coll. Cardiol. *13*:265, 1989.
193. Cutilleta, A. F., Bowell, R. T., Rudnik, M., et al.: Regression of myocardial hypertrophy: I. Experimental model, changes in heart weight, nucleic acids and collagen. J. Mol. Cell. Cardiol. *7*:67, 1975.
194. Simon, A. B., and Zloto, A. E.: Coarctation of the aorta: Longitudinal assessment of operated patients. Circulation *50*:456, 1974.
195. Nanton, M. A., and Olley, P. M.: Residual hypertension after coarctectomy in children. Am. J. Cardiol. *37*:769, 1976.
196. Hislop, A., and Reid, L. M.: Intrapulmonary arterial development during fetal life—branching pattern and structure. J. Anat. *113*:35, 1972.
197. Pollock, J. C., Jamieson, M. P., and McWilliams, R.: Somatosensory evoked potentials in the detection of spinal chord ischemia in aortic coarctation repair. Ann. Thorac. Surg. *41*:251, 1986.
198. Horowitz, L. N., Alexander, J. A., and Edmunds, L. H.: Postoperative right bundle branch block: Identification of three levels of block. Circulation *62*:319, 1980.
199. Bharati, S., and Lev, M.: Sequelae of atriotomy on the endocardium, conduction system and coronary arteries. *In* Engle, M. A., and Perloff, J. K. (eds.): Congenital Heart Disease After Surgery, New York, Yorke Medical Books, 1983.
200. Miller, A. J., Pick, R., and Katz, L. N.: Ventricular endomyocardial change after impairment of cardiac lymph flow in dogs. Br. Heart. J. *25*:182, 1963.

Acquired Heart Disease in Infancy and Childhood

by WILLIAM F. FRIEDMAN, M.D.

Because many of the topics discussed in this chapter are given more substantial coverage elsewhere in this text, the emphasis herein is placed on features of acquired heart disease that are relatively unique to or common in infancy and childhood, although the disease processes per se may not recognize age-related boundaries. Acute rheumatic fever and rheumatic heart disease are discussed in Chapter 56. The hyperlipidemias are discussed in Chapter 37.

NONRHEUMATIC INFLAMMATORY DISEASE

INFECTIVE MYOCARDITIS

(See also Chap. 43)

Infectious processes that cause inflammatory disease of the heart may occur at any age, including fetal life. Causative agents include viruses, rickettsiae, bacteria, spirochetes, fungi, protozoa, and helminths. As a general rule, few of the generalized illnesses caused by these agents feature significant involvement of the heart. Myocardial involvement may be demonstrated histologically, but in most cases little or no expression of cardiac inflammation is detected clinically. Important exceptions are infections caused by certain viruses, diphtheria, and trypanosomes; these are discussed individually below.

VIRAL MYOCARDITIS. Coxsackie B and rubella viruses are the most common causative agents in infective myocarditis of the newborn. The rubella embryopathy and its associated cardiovascular malformations are discussed on page 888. Active *rubella myocarditis* occurs in utero, and may cause varying degrees of myocardial damage.[1] Invariably, however, other cardiovascular manifestations of the rubella syndrome dominate the clinical picture.

Coxsackie B typically causes outbreaks of epidemic myocarditis but may occur in the isolated infant in the newborn nursery, commonly with a fatal outcome.[2,3] The illness is of sudden onset, and is characterized by fever, tachycardia, signs of systemic hypoperfusion, cyanosis, and, occasionally, cardiac failure. In some infants signs and symptoms of encephalomyelitis and hepatitis predominate. The diagnosis is suggested by electrocardiographic findings of atrial and/or ventricular arrhythmias, generalized ST-segment and T-wave changes, and low-voltage QRS complexes, accompanied by the appearance of marked generalized cardiomegaly and pulmonary vascular congestion on the chest roentgenogram. Echocardiography reveals dilatation of both ventricles and depressed indices of cardiac performance. Echocardiography is especially helpful in excluding congenital cardiac structural anomalies. The diagnosis is strongly suggested or confirmed when the virus can be isolated from pericardial fluid, pharyngeal secretions, or feces, and when elevations occur in type-specific–neutralizing, hemagglutination-inhibiting, or complement-fixing antibody.[4] Digitalis, diuretics, and general supportive measures are of limited benefit. Although increased sensitivity to the toxic effects of the glycosides is common, digitalis should be administered cautiously and continued until heart size is normal, since cardiac failure may recur when the drug is discontinued.

Numerous viral agents have been identified as a cause of myocarditis in childhood beyond infancy.[5–7] The most common are Coxsackie A and B (Fig. 33–1), influenza, adenovirus, and ECHO virus. Moreover, myocarditis, usually of mild degree, may be associated with the common viral infectious diseases of childhood, including mumps, measles, infectious mononucleosis, varicella, and variola. Although the diagnosis usually is one of exclusion, it may be suggested by the presence of sustained tachycardia out of proportion to fever, cardiomegaly without significant murmurs, poor-quality heart sounds, a gallop rhythm, an unexplained arrhythmia, and the electrocardiographic findings already mentioned. Radionuclide gallium-67 scanning of the heart, showing a dense gallium uptake, provides suggestive evidence of active myocarditis.[8] Although endomyocardial biopsy is a reasonably safe procedure in infants, children, and adolescents, a poor correlation exists between clinical and endomyocardial biopsy diagnoses of acute myocarditis in these age-groups.[9–11a] Important differential diagnostic possibilities include endocardial fibroelastosis, glycogen storage disease with cardiac involvement, anomalous pulmonary origin of a coronary artery, critical aortic stenosis in infancy, and coarctation of the aorta or hypoplastic left heart syndromes.

The vast majority of these children recover from the acute episode of myocarditis with few or no sequelae. The results of treating patients with antiviral therapy or with immunosuppresants and antiinflammatory drugs have been disappointing.[11,12,12a] Some patients may retain a permanent conduction defect or mild cardiac enlargement as a result of the acute illness. Moreover, a child may progress from the acute episode to a chronic dilated cardiomyopathy, characterized by signs of left ventricular dysfunction and mitral valve insufficiency. Unfortunately there are no predictive criteria to identify the latter situation.[13] Cardiac transplantation has been successful in some of these children with cardiomyopathy and a chronic, relentless, and refractory course of heart failure. However, cardiac transplantation in children, especially in infants or very young children, is complicated by growth suppression related to the required corticosteriod doses, and the complex-

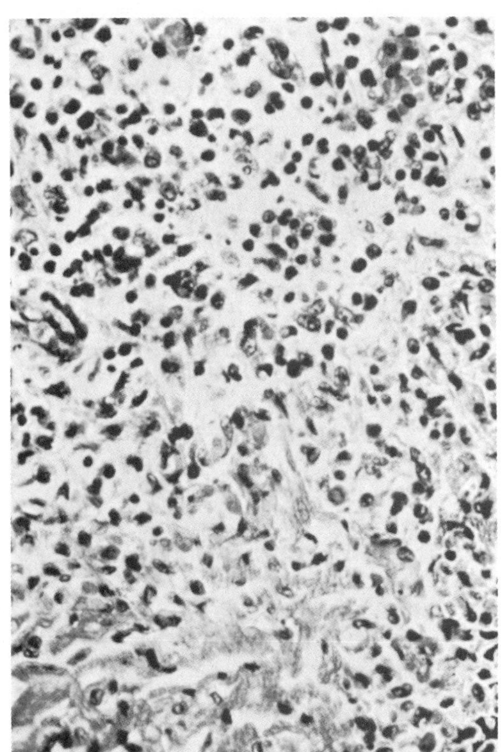

FIGURE 33-1. Photomicrograph of Coxsackie B_2 viral myocarditis. The major features are myocardial necrosis, edema, and heavy infiltrate of lymphocytes and large mononuclear cells. (×400.)(From Gore, I., and Kline, I. K.: Pericarditis and myocarditis. *In* Gould, S. E. (ed.): Pathology of the Heart and Blood Vessels. 3rd ed. Springfield, Ill., Charles C Thomas, 1968, p. 740.)

ity and severity of the immunosuppression in these infection-prone age groups.

DIPHTHERITIC CARDIOMYOPATHY. Diphtheria usually occurs in unimmunized children, especially in the western United States. Cardiac involvement is the result of the bacterial endotoxin rather than cardiac invasion by the bacillus.[14] Cardiac dysfunction appears to be related to abnormal fat metabolism, since diphtheria toxin causes marked depletion of myocardial carnitine, a cofactor required for the beta-oxidation of fats.[15] Thus, what was formerly designated a form of myocarditis is now considered an acute metabolic cardiomyopathy. The pathology includes extensive intracellular fat vacuolization and glycogen depletion. Plasma carnitine deficiences have also been found in children with other forms of dilated cardiomyopathy.[16]

Cardiac involvement occurs in about 10 per cent of affected patients and is the most common cause of death from this disease. Heart disease is most reliably indicated by electrocardiographic changes, which range from ST-segment and T-wave changes to arrhythmias and conduction disturbances, including complete heart block.[17] Occasionally, the electrocardiographic pattern of myocardial infarction may emerge. The electrocardiogram is a fair indicator of the extent of myocardial involvement and of prognosis. The latter usually is favorable if only ST-segment and T-wave changes are observed in the absence of conduction system disturbances. Right or left bundle branch block and complete atrioventricular block are associated with mortality rates of 50 to 80 per cent. The electrocardiographic findings may be accompanied by evidence of myocardial dysfunction and ventricular chamber dilatation on cardiac ultrasound.

Treatment of diphtheritic cardiomyopathy usually is unsatisfactory. All patients should receive diphtheria antitoxin and intravenous penicillin after appropriate skin testing. Although corticosteroids have been used in the treatment of the myocardial problem, their value is debatable. Digitalis, diuretics, and antiarrhythmic medications usually are indicated. Parenteral adminstration of carnitine has been found to partially reverse diphtheritic cardiac dysfunction and reduce the risk of cardiac death.[18] This observation requires confirmation. If the child recovers from the acute episode of diphtheritic cardiomyopathy, the prognosis is quite good.

MYOCARDITIS CAUSED BY TRYPANOSOMAL INFECTION. Chagas' disease (p. 1432) is a chronic parasitosis caused by *Trypanosoma cruzi*, transmitted to humans by the bite of insects in the reduviid family. In the United States the disease is seen mostly in the southern states; endemic infection occurs in Latin America. Its most important clinical manifestation is a late-developing, chronic myocarditis and, much less frequently, an early acute myocarditis that is fatal in up to 10 per cent of cases.[19] In patients who survive the acute stage, cardiomyopathy may occur after an interval of 10 to 30 years.[20] Diagnosis of the acute illness is supported by findings of edema and adenitis in the region of the insect bite, associated with low-grade intermittent fever, sweating, muscle pain, and, at times, diarrhea and vomiting; weeks or months later cardiomegaly, gallop rhythm, and conduction disturbances may be noted. Xenodiagnosis (examination of the excreta of laboratory-bred insects fed on the patient) or complement-fixation tests provide confirmation. Endomyocardial biopsy reveals mitochondrial, nuclear, and cell membrane abnormalities early in the myocardial degenerative process. Late stages are characterized by severe myofibrillar lysis and variable amounts of fibrous tissue and cellular infiltrates.[21] There is no satisfactory treatment. Prophylaxis consists of control of the carrier of the parasites, reduviid bugs, by benzene hexachloride. A nitrofuran compound, nifurtinox, appears effective in the acute stage of infection, but not during the intracellular parasitic infection period.[22]

Trypanosoma rhodesiense, which causes African sleeping sickness, may also produce myocardial hemorrhage, interstitial edema, mononuclear infiltration, and myocardial degeneration.[23] Cardiac involvement is usually relatively mild, and the clinical picture is dominated by evidence of encephalitis.

MYOCARDITIS CAUSED BY HUMAN IMMUNODEFICIENCY VIRUS (see also p. 1427). In infants and children, the cardiac complications of the acquired immunodeficiency syndrome (AIDS) range from incidental microscopic inflammatory findings at necropsy to clinically significant, extensive, and chronic cardiac dysfunction.[24,25] In most patients infected with the human immunodeficiency virus (HIV), the virus appears to have been transmitted from mother to child; other routes of transmission include contaminated blood products. Older children or adolescents also can be infected by routes more commonly associated with adults, such as sharing needles used for the injection of drugs, and sexual activity.

Cardiovascular abnormalities have been observed in as many as 65 per cent of infants or children with AIDS, whether induced by opportunistic infection or by the HIV infection itself.[25] As the prevalence of AIDS escalates, it is predictable that the cardiac involvement in infants and children with this disease will become better defined. Ventricular dysfunction, pericardial effusion, dilated cardiomyopathy, and rhythm disturbances (including high-grade atrial and ventricular ectopy and sudden death) provide evidence that HIV infection may have multiple direct or indirect effects on the heart. The latter may be due to infection with a variety of opportunistic organisms as well as to toxins, drugs, and autoimmunity. Other possible contributors to the cardiomyopathy include the myocardial depressant action of overwhelming noncardiac infection, the hypoxic and ischemic influence of severe lung disease, renal failure, autonomic dysfunction, chronic anemia, malnutrition, elevated endogenous catecholamines, vasoactive substances related to stress, and therapeutic interventions, including the use of steroids. Serial noninvasive assessment of this patient population, particularly by echocardiography, will, it is hoped, enable early or even anticipatory medical therapy, improving the cardiovascular status of children with HIV infection.

INFECTIVE PERICARDITIS (see also p. 1484)

Numerous infectious agents may be responsible for infective pericarditis. Viral and tuberculous inflammatory pericardial disease are discussed in detail in Chap. 45. Of special concern in infancy and childhood is disease caused by pyogenic bacteria.[26,27] Purulent pericarditis occurs most often in the first two decades of life, and is especially common in children under 6 years of age. Acute bacterial pericarditis usually is fatal if misdiagnosed or incorrectly treated. The most common pathogens are *Staphylococcus aureus, Streptococcus pneumoniae, Haemophilus influenzae,* and *Neisseria meningitides.* Unusual organisms that cause purulent pericarditis include *Escherichia coli, Pseudomonas, Salmonella, Klebisella, Proteus,* and *Bacteroides. H. influenzae,* in particular, affects infants and young children, usually in association either with upper respiratory tract infection and croup, with lower respiratory tract pneumonia, bronchitis, or, occasionally, with meningitis.

Presenting clinical signs and symptoms vary, depending on the age of the patient, the responsible organism, and the site(s) of associated infection. The latter two require identification if therapy is to be effective. Fever, tachycardia, dyspnea, and chest pain are invariably present. Pericardial exudate resulting from the acute suppurative process commonly produces signs of life-threatening cardiac tamponade. Physical findings suggestive of purulent pericarditis include neck vein distention and hepatomegaly, pulsus paradoxus, and/or systemic hypotension with a narrow pulse pressure, muffled and distant heart sounds, marked cardiomegaly, and a point of maximal cardiac impulse well within the area of percussed dullness. Although the presence of a pericardial friction rub clearly points to pericardial involvement, this sign occurs infrequently.

An enlarged, globular cardiac configuration on chest x-ray and electrocardiographic findings of diminished QRS amplitude and abnormalities of the ST segment (usually elevated) and T waves (often inverted) usually focus attention on the pericardium. Echocardiographic evaluation (p. 102) is reliable for establishing the diagnosis of significant pericardial effusion and for directing and guiding pericardiocentesis.[28] Culture and examination of pericardial fluid obtained by pericardiocentesis are essential for diagnosis and treatment. Unless effective surgical drainage is combined with antibiotic treatment, the mortality rate is high. Operation should consist of creation of a subxiphoid pericardial window with placement of a drainage tube, or anterior pericardiectomy with tube drainage.[29] Early aggressive diagnosis and treatment reduce the risk of death substantially (10 to 20 per cent). Pericardial constriction is uncommon, but all patients should be followed carefully for this complication.

POSTPERICARDIOTOMY SYNDROME (see also p. 1688)

In the first year after cardiac operation in which the pericardium is opened, and seldom in the second or third postoperative year, a febrile illness may occur, consisting of a pericardial and pleural inflammatory reaction with effusion and often with pulmonary parenchymal involvement. The illness occurs in about 35 per cent of children undergoing pericardiotomy and usually is self-limiting; infants undergoing open-heart surgery are seldom affected. It is characterized by fever; chest, neck, or shoulder pain that becomes worse with inspiration; anorexia; and laboratory findings of leukocytosis and an elevated erythrocyte sedimentation rate.[30] Recurrences are uncommon and usually mild. Physical, electrocardiographic, and roentgenographic signs of pericardial involvement vary with the magnitude of the effusion. Echocardiographic detection of the effusion is common between 4 and 10 days postoperatively.[31] Cardiac tamponade, although not usual, occurs with sufficient frequency to warrant careful observation of the patient.

Viral infection and an autoimmune reaction have been implicated in the pathogenesis. Serum antibodies and a rise in titer frequently are found against adenovirus, Coxsackie virus, and cytomegalovirus. Elevations in levels of heart-reactive antibody are common.

An association recently has been shown between antinuclear antibodies, which are immunoglobulins directed toward antigenic nuclear material, and postpericardiotomy syndrome.[32]

The syndrome must be distinguished from infective endocarditis and the postperfusion syndrome of atypical lymphocytosis and hepatosplenomegaly, which occurs about 3 to 6 weeks after extracorporeal circulation and is caused by cytomegalovirus infection.[33]

Treatment of the postpericardiotomy syndrome depends on the degree of patient discomfort and the magnitude of pericardial and/or pleural effusion. In some patients signs of cardiac tamponade will require pericardiocentesis. Bed rest and salicylates or indomethacin lessen patient discomfort and diminish the production of pleural or pericardial fluid. Corticosteroids are indicated for severe illness and promptly relieve fever and symptoms. Antibiotics are not useful in the treatment. Prolonged therapy is seldom necessary because of the self-limited nature of this postoperative complication. Late or recurrent tamponade, although rare, may require reinstitution of treatment.[34]

PRIMARY CARDIOMYOPATHIES

(See also Chap. 43)

The important *nonobstructive* cardiomyopathies, of special concern in infants and children, are the familial forms of endocardial fibroelastosis,[35–40] which afflict many of the patients also designated as having *dilated (congestive) cardiomyopathy.*[41–44] By definition, this diagnostic term excludes patients whose myocardial dysfunction is caused by infection, a congenital cardiac anomaly, or increased preload or afterload.[46] Dilated (congestive) cardiomyopathy often is a disease of infants, with most cases becoming manifested before the age of 1 year, with a history of respiratory or diarrheal illness preceding the onset of cardiac symptoms. Most severely ill patients probably have endocardial fibroelastosis, although the latter can be confirmed definitely only after myocardial biopsy or autopsy. Beyond age 2 years, dilated cardiomyopathy, like the condition in adults, is characterized by an unobstructed, dilated, and poorly contracting left ventricle. For this group of children, debate also exists as to whether endocardial fibroelastosis should be categorized as a separate entity under dilated or congestive cardiomyopathy, and whether it is an end stage of dilated cardiomyopathy of *any* cause.[45] In children with the clinical picture of dilated cardiomyopathy, a poor outcome is anticipated by a reduced left ventricular shortening fraction, a familial incidence of cardiomyopathy, and the presence of endocardial fibroelastosis. The overall mortality of dilated cardiomyopathy exceeds 30 per cent, the vast majority of fatal cases occurring during the first episode of cardiac failure.

ENDOCARDIAL FIBROELASTOSIS (EFE). Various designations have been applied to this condition, including endocardial sclerosis, fetal endocarditis, fetal endomyocardial fibrosis, and elastic tissue hyperplasia.[35] In recent years familial cases have been encountered more commonly than has the isolated form. The data provided by family studies fit neither an autosomal recessive nor a multifactorial mode of inheritance. Although the reasons are obscure, a marked reduction has been observed in the past decade of isolated, nonfamilial EFE. No definite cause for this condition has been established, although a host of theories have been proposed; inadequate subendocardial blood flow and/or prenatal or postnatal inflammation or infection currently are considered the most likely pathogenetic pathways.[37,45]

A distinction has been made between primary EFE, in which there is no cardiac malformation, and EFE secondary to congenital malformations of the heart.[38] In the *secondary* variety, focal areas of opaque fibroelastotic thickening of the mural endocardium or cardiac valves are observed in association with cardiac malformations. Underlying cardiovascular anomalies are almost always obstructive lesions, particularly of the left side of the heart, and these create cardiac hypertrophy and an imbalance in the myocardial oxygen supply-demand relation. Thus, secondary EFE quite commonly occurs in aortic stenosis, coarctation of the aorta, and hypoplastic left heart syndrome.

This discussion focuses on the *primary* form of EFE, which invariably involves the left ventricle and mitral and aortic valves without significant associated cardiac defects.

Although the use of the term "primary" implies that this form of EFE is a specific disease entitity, most would agree that it is the end result of many different diseases.[45,46] Further, as already discussed, no clear separation exists clinically between primary EFE and dilated cardiomyopathy. Primary EFE commonly produces a marked dilatation of the left ventricle; rarely, a "contracted" type of primary EFE is observed, in which the left ventricle is relatively hypoplastic or normal in size. In the latter situation the right and left atria and the right ventricle are markedly enlarged and hypertrophied, with minimal or no endocardial sclerosis. In the common, dilated type of primary EFE, microthrombi may be found adherent to the endocardium. The diffuse endocardial hyperplasia may be several millimeters thick (Fig. 33–2). The aortic

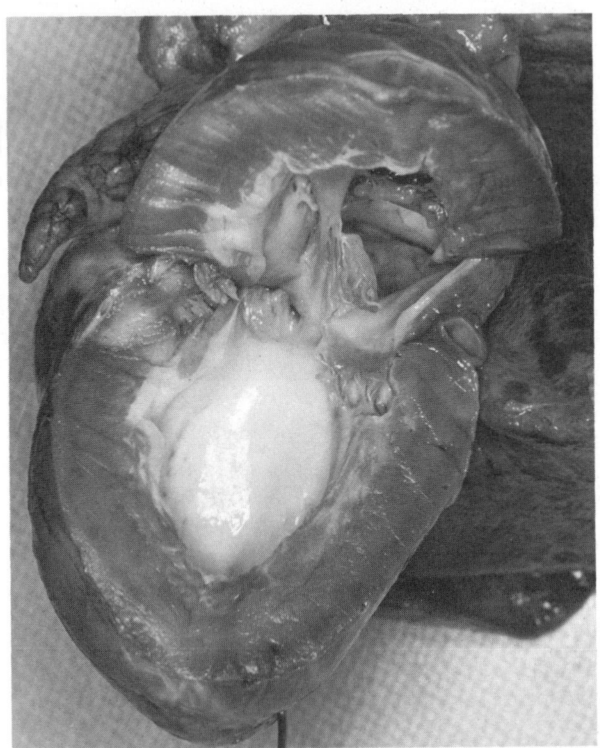

FIGURE 33-2. Diffuse left ventricular endocardial fibroelastosis. There is myocardial hypertrophy and obliteration of the papillary muscles as well as encroachment of the sclerotic subendocardial process onto the base of the aortic cusps. (From Tingelstaad, J. B., et al.: The electrocardiogram in the contracted type of primary endocardial fibroelastosis. Am. J. Cardiol. *27*:304, 1971.)

and mitral valve leaflets are thickened and distorted; mitral regurgitation is especially common. The papillary muscles and chordae tendineae are involved in the fibroelastic process and are shortened and distorted.

Primary EFE is a disease of infancy; symptoms usually develop between 2 and 12 months of age, although rarely they may be present shortly after birth. Clinical features reflect left ventricular dysfunction and congestive heart failure.[47,48] Noted initially are fatigue and breathlessness during feeding, failure to thrive, irritability, pallor, increased sweating, peripheral cyanosis, cough, wheezing, or grunting. Symptoms usually are rapidly progressive. Examination of the infant reveals tachycardia, cardiomegaly, a gallop rhythm, and hepatosplenomegaly. Cardiac murmurs may be absent; about 40 per cent of infants have the characteristic apical systolic murmur of mitral regurgitation.

Chest roentgenography reveals marked, generalized cardiomegaly with normal or congested pulmonary vascular markings. A typical electrocardiographic finding is left ventricular hypertrophy with inverted T waves in the left precordial leads; less common are tracings suggestive of myocardial infarction, varying degrees of atrioventricular block, and arrhythmias. Echocardiographic features include an increase in left atrial and left ventricular dimensions, reduced left ventricular septal and posterior wall motion, reduced ejection fraction, and abnormal mitral valve motion.[46,49] Dense echoes along the endocardium of the left ventricle are a diagnostic clue.

The *diagnosis* of primary EFE usually is made easily by the characteristic clinical findings but is, nonetheless, one of exclusion. Differential diagnosis includes anomalous pulmonary origin of the left coronary artery, myocarditis, hypertrophic obstructive cardiomyopathy, anomalies that cause left ventricular outflow tract obstruction, and glycogen storage disease of the heart. The first four of these entities differ appreciably from fibroelastosis in their electrocardiographic or echocardiographic features; the skeletal muscle biopsy in glycogen storage disease is diagnostic.

Hemodynamic studies reveal evidence of left ventricular dysfunction.[46a] This includes elevations in left ventricular end-diastolic and left atrial pressures, moderate pulmonary hypertension, widened arteriovenous oxygen differences, and reduced left ventricular stroke volume and cardiac output. Angiography usually demonstrates a markedly dilated left ventricle, a reduced ejection fraction, and varying degrees of mitral regurgitation. The configuration of the left ventricular chamber usually is globular or spherical; dyskinetic or akinetic patterns of contraction are uncommon. Endomyocardial biopsy shows a diagnostic invasion of the endocardium and subendocardium by fibroelastic tissue.[9-11,11a,50,51] The *contracted form* of primary EFE produces a clinical picture of left-sided obstructive disease, particularly if the mitral valve is small. Left atrial pressure is elevated, with pulmonary artery pressures at or near systemic arterial levels.

The optimal management of patients with primary EFE consists of early and prolonged treatment with digitalis. Glycoside therapy should be continued for many years after the disappearance of symptoms, since cessation of the drug may result in acute cardiac failure, even when the heart size has returned to normal. The results of pericardial poudrage and mitral valve replacement in seriously afflicted infants have been disappointing. Cardiac transplantation may be recommended, although the survival data for this approach have not been impressive for infants and children with cardiomyopathies.[44]

SECONDARY CARDIOMYOPATHIES

The designation "secondary" cardiomyopathy refers to intrinsic myocardial disease that is secondary to or associated with systemic disease or diseases of other organs or in other systems. Myocardial diseases coexisting with collagen vascular disorders (Chap. 56), neuromuscular disorders (Chap. 60), neoplasms (Chap. 57), acute glomerulonephritis (Chap. 62), and thalassemia (Chap. 57) are discussed elsewhere in this text. Additional secondary cardiomyopathies of special interest to those caring for infants and children are those seen in infants of diabetic mothers, and associated with glycogen storage disease, neonatal thyrotoxicosis, infantile beriberi, protein-calorie malnutrition, tropical endomyocardial fibrosis, anthracycline toxicity, and the mucocutaneous lymph node syndrome. Attention is directed to each of these latter disorders.

CARDIOMYOPATHY IN INFANTS OF DIABETIC MOTHERS

Infants born of diabetic mothers are exposed to chronic hyperinsulinism in utero and to reactive hypoglycemia after birth. Such infants occasionally display two basic forms of cardiomyopathy, both of which usually are transient.[52-55] Evidence exists that suboptimal metabolic control of maternal diabetes during pregnancy increases the incidence of these abnormalities.[55] In some of these infants, hypertrophy and hyperplasia of myocardial cells constitute a diffuse process, producing reversible signs and symptoms that resemble those of congestive cardiomyopathy. In other infants, the clinical findings are indistinguishable from those of hypertrophic obstructive cardiomyopathy.[56] The natural history in this latter group has been one of gradual spontaneous regression within 1 to 12 months of obstructive murmurs, cardiomegaly, and electrocardiographic and echocardiographic abnormalities typical of hypertrophic obstructive cardiomyopathy.

GLYCOGEN STORAGE DISEASE

Glycogen storage disease is the result of a deficiency of one or more of the enzymes involved in the biosynthesis and degradation of glycogen. The heart is importantly involved in type II (Pompe's disease), which results from a deficiency of alpha-1, 4-glucosidase (acid maltase), a lysosomal enzyme that hydrolyzes glycogen into glucose.[57] This disease is a heredi-

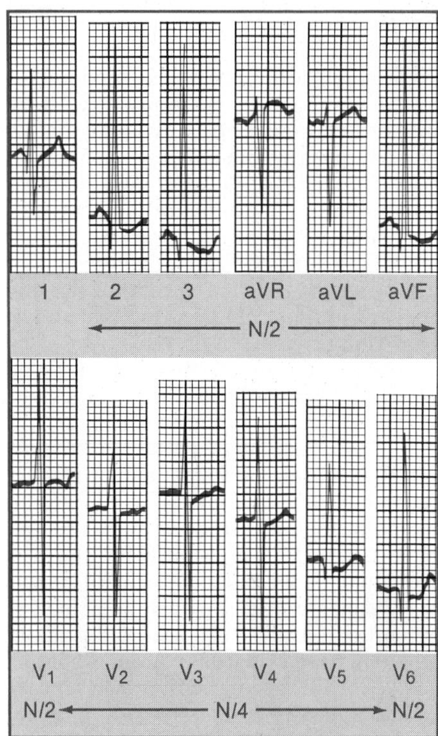

FIGURE 33-3. Electrocardiogram of an infant with glycogen storage disease showing a short PR interval and left ventricular hypertrophy.

tary error of metabolism transmitted through a single recessive gene. Generalized glycogenesis takes place, occurring especially in the heart, the skeletal muscles, and the liver. The glycogen within cardiac muscle cells is biochemically normal but is present in excessive amounts, both within lysosomes and free in the cytoplasm.[57] As a result, the heart enlarges, often to a marked degree, and congestive heart failure supervenes. Glycogen deposition within the myocardium usually is uniform, although occasionally the interventricular septum is especially involved, producing subpulmonic obstruction or a constellation of features indistinguishable from hypertrophic obstructive cardiomyopathy. Selective angiography has revealed a distinctive trabeculation of the left ventricle in some infants.[58]

Clinical signs of type II glycogen storage disease usually become prominent in the early neonatal period.[59,59a] Characteristic symptoms include failure to thrive, progressive hypotonia, lethargy, and a weak cry. Prominent early features include nonspecific cardiac murmurs, cardiomegaly, signs of congestive heart failure, macroglossia, poor skeletal muscle tone, and weakness. The electrocardiogram shows extremely tall, broad QRS complexes with a short P-R interval (commonly less than 0.09 sec) (Fig. 33-3).

The short P-R interval may be the result of facilitated atrioventricular conduction owing to myocardial glycogen deposition. Less often, deep Q waves are observed over the mid or left precordium as well as T-wave inversion and ST-segment elevation. Chest roentgenograms show an enlarged globular heart associated with pulmonary vascular congestion (Fig. 33-4). In rare patients with cardiac glycogenosis the cardiac murmur suggests left ventricular outflow tract obstruction and/or mitral regurgitation; the echocardiographic, hemodynamic, and angiographic features in this subgroup are indistinguishable from those in infants with hypertrophic obstructive cardiomyopathy. Diagnosis is confirmed by demonstrating the enzymatic deficiency in lymphocytes, skeletal muscle, or liver. Skeletal muscle biopsy reveals histological and histochemical evidence of glycogen deposition.

Cardiac glycogenosis may be confused with other entities that cause cardiac failure in the early months of life, including endocardial fibroelastosis, anomalous pulmonary origin of the left coronary artery, fixed and dynamic forms of left ventricular outflow tract obstruction, coarctation of the aorta, and myocarditis. The short P-R interval and the skeletal muscle hypotonia in glycogen storage disease help to distinguish this disorder from *endocardial fibroelastosis.* Infants with an anomalous pulmonary origin of the *left coronary artery* usually have a distinctive electrocardiographic pattern of anterolateral myocardial infarction. In infants with *coarctation of the aorta* the pulse and blood pressure discrepancies between the upper and lower extremities point to the proper diagnosis (p. 967). *Myocarditis* usually is of abrupt onset in a previously healthy child and is not associated with marked hypotonia; the generally low-voltage electrocardiogram does not show the short P-R interval. The skeletal muscle hypotonia and the macroglossia in infants with glycogen storage disease occasionally raise the possibilities of amyotonia congenita and cretinism or mongolism, respectively.

Cardiac glycogenosis leads to progressive impairment of myocardial function; Pompe's disease is uniformly fatal, usually within the first year of life. Death quite often is the result of either cardiac failure or complications of respiratory management such as pneumonia or aspiration.

NEONATAL THYROTOXICOSIS

Thyroid-stimulating immunoglobulin traverses the placental barrier and stimulates the fetal thyroid gland when maternal hyperthyroidism exists.[60] Many infants are born prematurely or are small for gestational age. Jitteriness and irritability are noted early. Cardiac findings include tachycardia, bounding pulses, systolic hypertension, and a precordial systolic murmur. Congestive heart failure frequently is present, and the presenting finding occasionally is an episode of paroxysmal atrial tachycardia. A neonatal goiter may be observed, especially if the mother received iodine therapy during pregnancy.

Diagnosis should be anticipated whenever a history of hyperthyroidism exists in the mother. Neonatal thyrotoxicosis occurs in the offspring of about 1 to 2 per cent of these women. A maternal level of thyroid-stimulating immunoglobulin should be obtained before delivery in anticipation of the problem arising in the newborn infant, since high levels often are observed in both mother and offspring. The serum levels of thyroxine are increased in the newborn.

The infant who has heart failure may be treated with digitalis and propylthiouracil or carbamizole. The latter two drugs will not be completely effective for many weeks; a beta blocker usually is helpful in addition to these agents. Supportive measures such as sedation and minimal stimulation may be helpful. Exchange transfusion or corticosteroid treatment is of no proven benefit.

Infants usually improve between the second and third month of life, although lack of attention to the problem or inadequate therapy may result in a fatal outcome.

INFANTILE BERIBERI (see also p. 461)

Thiamine (vitamin B_1) deficiency mainly occurs in regions of Southeast Asia, India, Brazil, and Africa, in which the dietary staple is polished rice or

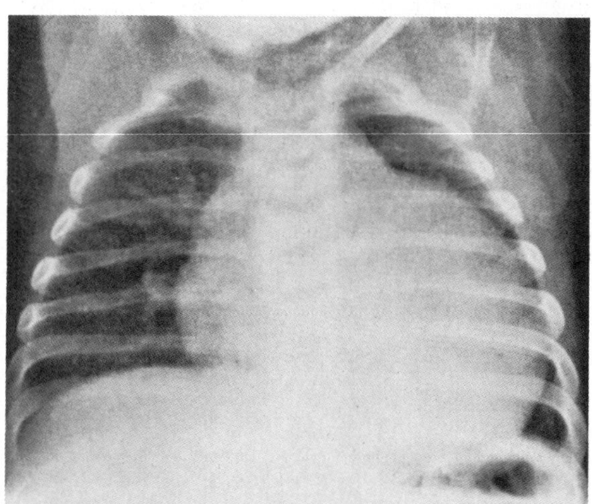

FIGURE 33-4. Chest roentgenogram of an infant with glycogen storage disease showing massive cardiomegaly and pulmonary edema. (From Taussig, H.: Congenital Malformations of the Heart. Vol. 2. 2nd ed. Boston, Commonwealth Fund, Harvard University, 1960, p. 901.)

cassava. Thiamine functions as a coenzyme in decarboxylation of alpha-keto acids and in the utilization of pentose in the hexose monophosphate shunt. A reduction in myocardial energy production causes symptoms in the infant, usually between 1 and 4 months of age, who is breastfed by a thiamine-deficient mother.[61] Such infants usually are edematous, irritable, pale, and anorectic. Hoarseness or aphonia is common, owing to involvement of the recurrent laryngeal nerve; blepharoptosis occurs in one-third of infants. Typically, cardiac involvement manifests as dilation of the right ventricle and prominent signs of systemic venous congestion. Electrocardiographic findings are nonspecific, and radiological findings principally consist of right ventricular dilatation. Infantile beriberi may be rapidly fatal but responds quickly and well to administration of thiamine (25 to 50 mg intravenously initially, with reduction of the dose to 10 mg/day for several days, and then orally for several weeks). Dramatic amelioration occurs within a few days of the cardiac findings. Cure is complete with no known sequelae.

PROTEIN-CALORIE MALNUTRITION (see also p. 1848)

This is a major public health problem in underdeveloped areas of the tropics.[62,63] In infants inadequate diet results in a state of emaciation termed "marasmus"; "kwashiorkor" is a designation applied to this syndrome in children beyond 1 year of age. The disease results from a deficiency of protein relative to calories, although the latter and other essential nutrients often are lacking as well. General muscle wasting, loss of subcutaneous fat, and atrophy of most organs, including the heart, are typical in marasmic infants. In both marasmus and kwashiorkor, thinning and atrophy of cardiac muscle fibers and interstitial edema or vacuolization of the myocardial fibers are noted.[64] As the condition progresses, listlessness becomes prominent. Cardiovascular collapse is easily precipitated in these infants by the stress of infection.

In both infancy and childhood the principal physical findings reflect systemic hypoperfusion and principally consist of hypothermia, hypotension, tachycardia, and low-amplitude peripheral arterial pulsations. Peripheral usually nonpitting edema is prominent, as are wasting of the skeletal musculature, exfoliative dermatitis, and gray or red discoloration of the hair. Changes seen on electrocardiogram and on radiographic examination are nonspecific.

Treatment should be directed at correction of fluid and electrolyte imbalance, eradication of infection, and management of such associated problems as anemia and parasitic infestation. Care is required in the correction of dehydration or severe anemia, since volume overload of the heart is easily produced. Supplements of potassium and magnesium often are required, and because of deficiences in these elements, digitalis should probably be avoided or used with extreme caution. If the infant or child survives the initial phase, a well-balanced diet will effect an impressive recovery over several months' duration.

TROPICAL ENDOMYOCARDIAL FIBROSIS (see also p. 1422)

Endomyocardial fibrosis is a rare, acquired, progressive disease, usually involving children and young adults from Africa, Southeast Asia, and South America. This cardiomyopathy of unknown cause is characterized by focal endocardial fibrosis of one or, rarely, both ventricles.[65] Controversy exists as to whether or not endomyocardial fibrosis, which is not associated with eosinophilia, and Löffler's endocarditis with eosinophilia (Chap. 43) are the same disorder described from temperate climates.[66] Endocardial fibrosis is located almost exclusively in the inflow tracts of the ventricles, and commonly involves one or the other atrioventricular valve. Partial obliteration of either cardiac chamber results in reduced ventricular compliance with impairment of filling. The fibrotic process often involves the chordae tendineae, resulting in mitral and/or tricuspid regurgitation. Plaques of heaped-up fibrous tissue without elastic fibers are especially common within the left ventricle. Endomyocardial fibrosis involving the right ventricle may have to be differentiated from Ebstein's anomaly of the tricuspid valve (p. 940), and endomyocardial fibrosis involving the left ventricle may have to be differentiated from rheumatic mitral regurgitation.

When left ventricular disease predominates, the clinical findings often resemble those of mitral stenosis or regurgitation. When endocardial involvement of the right ventricle is more severe than that of the left ventricle, the patient usually presents with findings of markedly elevated systemic venous pressure and tricuspid regurgitation.

Treatment is supportive. Survival usually depends on the extent of endocardial and valvular involvement and is better when right ventricular disease predominates.[67] Mean survival after the onset of symptoms is about 24 months. Specific treatment does not exist, and corticosteroid therapy has not proved efficacious. Surgical excision (decortication) of affected tissue with prosthetic valve replacement has been associated with clinical improvement.[68] However, children most severely affected by this disease commonly reside in regions of the tropics and subtropics where cardiac surgery is not readily available.

MUCOCUTANEOUS LYMPH NODE SYNDROME (KAWASAKI DISEASE)

The mucocutaneous lymph node syndrome in infancy (Kawasaki disease) was first described in Japan in 1967. Many thousands of cases from Japan have been reported, and the disorder is being recognized with increasing frequency in North America and Europe.[69]

The syndrome presents as a febrile illness in children that occurs before the age of 10 and usually before the age of 2 years. They commonly have fever and ocular and oral manifestations followed in 5 days by a rash and indurative edema of the hands and feet, with palmar and plantar erythema. Finally, after about 2 weeks, cutaneous desquamation occurs. Diagnostic criteria include (1) a fever lasting for 5 or more days that is unresponsive to antibiotics; (2) bilateral congestion of the ocular conjunctiva; (3) peripheral limb changes that include an indurative peripheral edema and erythema of the palms and feet, followed later in the course of the illness by a membranous desquamation of the fingertips; (4) changes in the lips and mouth, including dry, erythematous, and fissured lips, injected oropharyngeal mucosa, and a strawberry tongue; and (5) a polymorphous exanthema of the trunk without crusts or vesicles. Diagnosis is accepted when the first criterion and at least three of the remainder are present.

In addition to the mucous membrane and cutaneous effects, multiple organ system involvement has been noted. Noncardiovascular complications of the illness include arthritis, cerebrospinal fluid pleocytosis, pulmonary infiltrates, and hydrops of the gallbladder. The illness often is accompanied by cervical adenopathy, diarrhea, leukocytosis with a predominance of neutrophils, thrombocytosis, sterile pyuria and proteinuria, elevated liver transaminases, an elevation in the erythrocyte sedimentation rate and alpha$_2$-globulin, and a positive C-reactive protein.

An extensive search for the cause of Kawasaki disease has been unproductive. Multiple immunoregulatory abnormalities have been suggested to be involved in the pathogenesis of the illness.[70] Abnormalities include a T-cell lymphocytopenia, a decrease in CD^{8+} T cells, increased numbers of activated CD^{4+} lymphocytes, B-cell hyperactivity, and increased endothelial cell proliferation. Some hypothesize that a retrovirus with tropism for endothelial and lymphoid cells may be associated with the acute disease,[70] whereas others question the role of toxin-producing bacteria in pathogenesis, particularly streptococcal erythrogenic toxins.[71] Tumor necrosis factor, a polypeptide mediator secreted by activated macrophages and T lymphocytes, also has been viewed as a potential mediator of inflammation in this illness.[72]

On the basis of pathological data, progression of the disease may be divided into four stages.[73,74] In stage I, lasting for 1 to 9 days, acute perivasculitis of the small arteries is evident and involves the vasa vasorum of the major coronary arteries. Pericarditis, interstitial myocarditis, and endocardial inflammation also are seen; these changes chiefly consist of neutrophilic, eosinophilic, and lymphocytic infiltrations. In stage II, of 12 to 25 days' duration, panvasculitis involves the major coronary arteries. It affects the intima, media, and adventitia and results in aneurysm and thrombus formation. In stage III, of 28 to 31 days' duration, granulating thrombi and marked intimal thickening cause partial or total occlusion of the major coronary arteries. Stage IV follows and may be of many years' duration, during which healing occurs, consisting of scarring, calcification, and recanalization of occluded arteries.

The syndrome has an associated acute mortality of 1 to 3 per cent, secondary to complications from coronary artery involvement, myocarditis, or pericarditis, with a majority of deaths occurring in the third or fourth week of illness.[75] Other children may die later in life as a result of myocardial infarction.[76] Autopsy examination has almost uniformly demonstrated coronary arterial aneurysms, with occlusion caused by

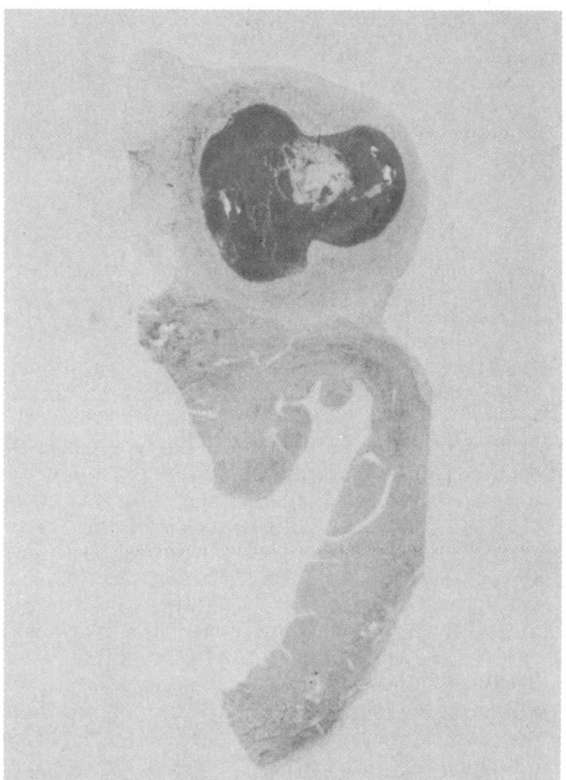

FIGURE 33–5. Low-power photomicrograph of a coronary artery aneurysm with recent occlusive thrombosis in a patient with mucocutaneous lymph node syndrome. (From Landing, B. H., and Larson, E. J.: Are infantile periarteritis nodosa with coronary artery involvement and fatal mucocutaneous lymph node syndrome the same? Comparison of 20 patients from North America with patients from Hawaii and Japan. Pediatrics *59*:651, 1977. Copyright American Academy of Pediatrics, 1977.)

thromboendarteritis (Fig. 33–5). The spectrum of cardiovascular involvement is outlined in Table 33–1.

The disease often has been misdiagnosed in the United States as scarlet fever, Stevens-Johnson syndrome, Rocky Mountain spotted fever, rheumatoid arthritis, scleroderma, or lupus erythematosus.

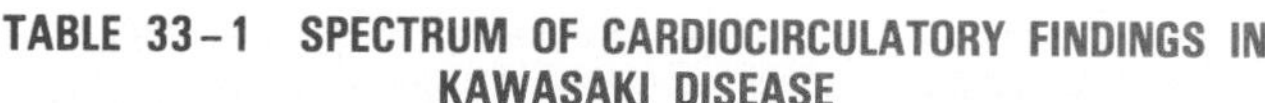

TABLE 33–1 SPECTRUM OF CARDIOCIRCULATORY FINDINGS IN KAWASAKI DISEASE

- CARDITIS (myocarditis, pericarditis)
  - Congestive heart failure
  - Arrhythmias
- CORONARY ANGIITIS
  - Thromboendarteritis—aneurysms
    - Regression
    - Thrombosis—recanalization
    - Obstruction—stenosis
    - Collaterals
    - Rupture
  - Myocardial ischemia or infarction
    - Ventricular aneurysm
    - Papillary muscle of dysfunction—mitral regurgitation
- ARTERIAL INVOLVEMENT
  - Pulmonary/renal angitis—pulmonary/renal hypertension
  - Arteritis, aneurysms: femoral, iliac, brachial, cerebral, hepatic, etc.

Infants and children with this syndrome should be closely watched for signs of cardiac involvement. A significant number of patients show evidence of myocarditis or pericarditis, or both, in the early phases of the disease.[77] Electrocardiographic evidence of myocarditis with low voltage and nonspecific ST-T wave changes is seen in 45 per cent of patients, echocardiographic evidence of poor left ventricular function in 25 per cent, pericardial effusion in 9 per cent, cardiomegaly on chest radiographs in 25 per cent, pericardial effusion in 9 per cent, and a gallop rhythm in 12 per cent. Aneurysms of the coronary arteries with narrowing, tortuosity, and obstruction are almost invariably present on aortography and coronary angiography (Fig. 33–6).[78–82a] Success has been achieved in visualizing aneurysmal coronary lesions with two-dimensional cross-sectional echocardiography (Fig. 33–7).[83–85] About half of the children with coronary aneurysms diagnosed shortly after the acute phase of the disease subsides have normal-appearing vessels by angiography 1 or 2 years later.[86–89a] In those patients with residual cardiac abnormalities after recovery from the acute illness phase, a variety of findings have been described. These include impairment of left ventricular function secondary to the coronary arterial involvement, papillary muscle dysfunction with mitral regurgitation,[89b] impaired left

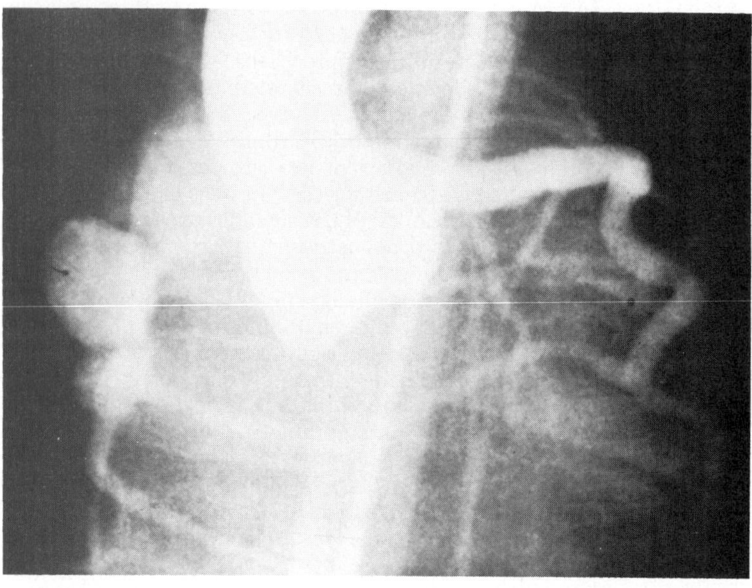

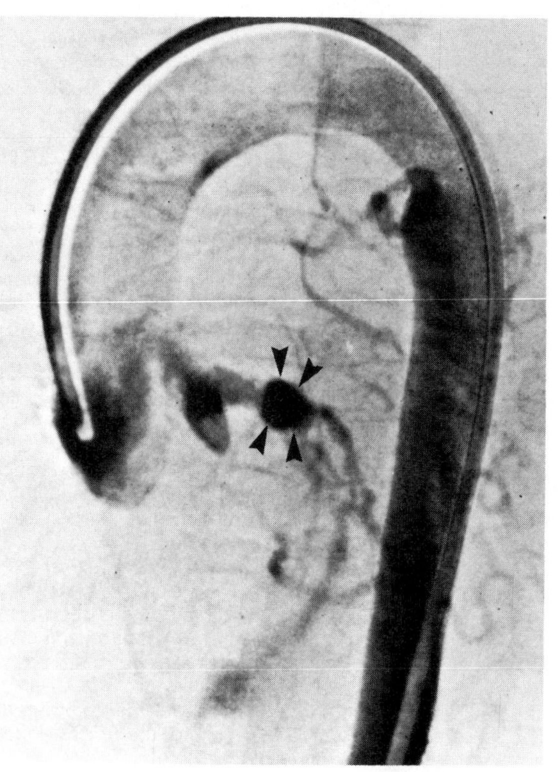

FIGURE 33–6. Aortic root cineangiograms from two patients with mucocutaneous lymph node syndrome. In the left panel, a dilated proximal left coronary artery is observed with collateral circulation and retrograde filling of the right coronary system, and three aneurysms of the right coronary artery. In the right panel, subtraction technique shows an aneurysm of the left coronary artery (arrowheads). (Courtesy of Thomas G. DiSessa, M. D.)

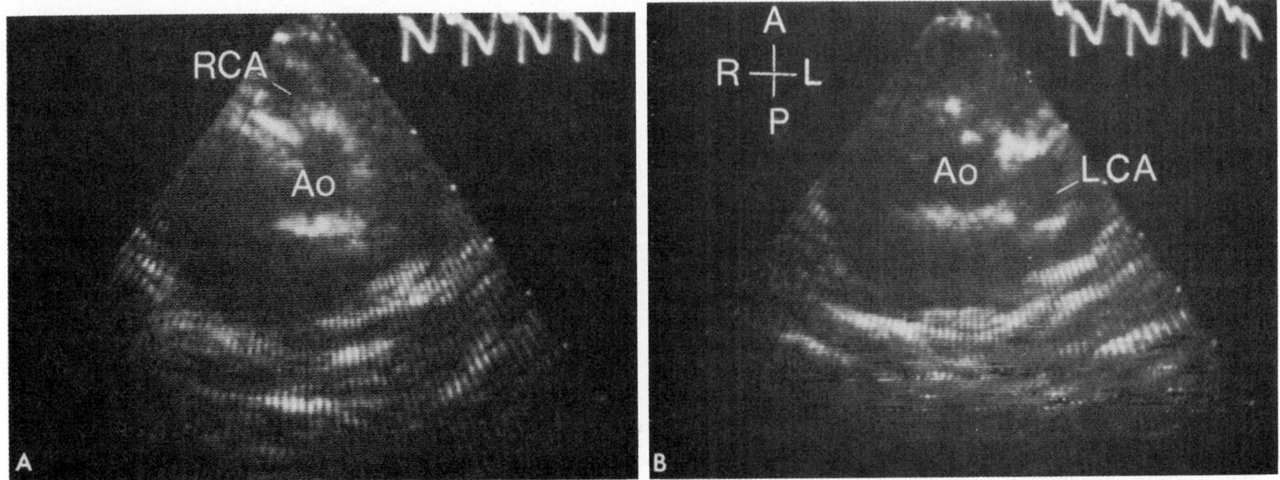

FIGURE 33-7. Short-axis cross-sectional echocardiographic views of aneurysms of the proximal right coronary artery (RCA) (*A*) and proximal left coronary artery (LCA) (*B*) in a 3-year-old boy with mucocutaneous lymph node syndrome. The right ventricular outflow tract is anterior (A) to the aorta (Ao) and the left atrium is posterior (P). R = right; L = left.

ventricular function,[89c] and abnormalities of the distensibility of the coronary arteries (even after aneurysms have disappeared and no morphological abnormalities are recognized by coronary arteriography).[90-94]

To date, no treatment has proved effective to prevent the formation of coronary artery aneurysms. It appears that corticosteroid therapy is *detrimental* during the acute illness. High-dose salicylate treatment (50 to 100 mg/kg/day) is advisable for all patients in the acute phase of the illness, and later in low doses (3-5 mg/kg/day) to inhibit platelet aggregation in the hope of preventing subsequent thrombus formation and occlusion of the coronary arteries. In many children with Kawasaki disease, there is failure to achieve therapeutic serum concentrations of salicylate despite high oral doses because of impaired gastrointestinal absorption of salicylate.[95] Therefore, regular monitoring of serum salicylate levels is advisable. In children who have no evidence of coronary artery disease and in whom the platelet count has returned to normal, the aspirin may be discontinued after 2 to 6 months. In patients who develop coronary arterial involvement, aspirin therapy should be maintained indefinitely (3 to 5 mg/kg/day). High-dose intravenous gamma globulin therapy has been demonstrated to be safe and effective in reducing the prevalence of coronary artery abnormalities when administered early in the course of Kawasaki disease.[96,97] The suggested dosage of intravenous gamma globulin has been 400 mg/kg/day for 4 days, although it is likely that a single large dose of intravenous gamma globulin (2 gm/kg), infused over 10 hours, is as safe and effective as the 4-day regimen.[98,99]

Two-dimensional echocardiography is indicated in all children with a diagnosis of Kawasaki disease, with or without evidence of significant cardiac involvement. Coronary angiography is recommended for those patients with severe symptoms of cardiovascular involvement, persistence of cardiomegaly or heart failure, ischemic ST-T wave changes or an electrocardiographic pattern of myocardial infarction, signs of mitral insufficiency, or cardiac calcification by chest x-ray. The prognosis for children with vascular involvement should be guarded;[100,101] some will be candidates for coronary arterial bypass surgery.[102]

Anthracycline Toxicity

(See also p. 1756)

Anthracycline drugs such as doxorubicin and daunomycin, used as cancer chemotherapeutic agents, cause a dose-related cardiomyopathy.[103] The risk of cardiac involvement increases significantly with doses in excess of 400 mg/m^2.[104] The onset of cardiac symptoms often is delayed, occurring 2 to 3 months after the anthracycline dose. Cardiac dysfunction usually presents first as unexplained tachycardia, progressing to dyspnea, congestive heart failure, hepatomegaly, and, often, death. The cardiomyopathy most often is reversible only in its early stages. Later, it usually is poorly responsive to digitalis, diuretics, and afterload reducing agents. Quite often patients are in remission from their neoplasm when the drug's cardiotoxicity proves lethal. Long-term followup has disclosed elevated levels of left ventricular wall stress and impairment of diastolic function in children without overt cardiomyopathy.[105] Further, there are occasional reports of late-onset heart failure in previously asymptomatic children, many years after their cancer chemotherapy.[106]

SYSTEMIC HYPERTENSION

(See also p. 843)

Unfortunately, many physicians consider hypertension a disease of adults and not children. Thus, all too frequently, blood pressure is not recorded during the pediatric physical examination. It should be emphasized that elevations in systemic blood pressure may occur in as many as 2 per cent of children, and it has been well documented that undetected or untreated hypertension may lead to unfortunate consequences.[107] Three points in particular require recognition:[108]

1. Causes of hypertension in infants and children differ markedly from those in adults. Most children have secondary rather than essential forms of hypertension (Table 33-2); therefore, it is important to search for a remedial cause.
2. Offspring of hypertensive parents are known to have an increased susceptibility to blood pressure elevation.
3. Children with elevated blood pressure require the same surveillance and treatment as adults.

Accurate blood pressure measurements require cuffs of different sizes because of the variation in arm size from infancy through adolescence. To measure blood pressure correctly, the inner rubber bag should be wide enough to cover two-thirds of the length and three-fourths of the circumference of the upper arm or thigh while leaving the antecubital or popliteal fossa free. A cuff that is too small is likely to produce spuriously high readings. In infants under age 2 years the flush technique may be used, although a Doppler instrument is preferred.[109,110] Because disappearance of the Korotkoff sound may cause underestimation of the diastolic pressure, both muffling (the fourth phase of the Korotkoff sound) and disap-

TABLE 33–2 CONDITIONS AND DRUGS ASSOCIATED WITH HYPERTENSION IN INFANTS AND CHILDREN

CONGENITAL
- Coarctation of the aorta
- Gonadal dysgenesis (Turner syndrome)
- Rubella syndrome
- Pseudoxanthoma elasticum (Ehlers-Danlos syndrome)
- Ask-Upmark syndrome (segmental renal artery dysplasia)
- Renal arterial abnormalities
- Multiple systemic and pulmonary artery stenoses
- Solitary renal cyst
- Hydronephrosis

GENETIC
- Diabetes mellitus
- Neurofibromatosis (von Recklinghausen's disease)
- Adrenogenital syndrome
- Pheochromocytoma
- Polycystic kidney disease (infantile and adult forms)
- Familial nephritis (Alport syndrome)
- Little syndrome
- Fabry's disease (angiokeratoma corporis diffusum)
- Familial dysautonomia (Riley-Day syndrome)
- Essential hypertension
- Tuberous sclerosis with angiolipomas
- Primary hyperparathyroidism
- Porphyria

PHARMACOLOGICAL
- Sympathomimetics: ephedrine, epinephrine, isoproterenol
- Adrenal steroids
- Heavy metals: mercury, lead
- Licorice

ACQUIRED, RENAL
- Unilateral hydronephrosis
- Unilateral pyelonephritis
- Renal trauma
- Renal tumors
- Unilateral multicystic kidney
- Unilateral ureteral occlusion
- Renal artery stenosis
- Renal arteritis
- Fibromuscular dysplasia of the renal artery
- Renal fistula
- Renal artery aneurysm
- Chronic pyelonephritis superimposed on abnormal kidneys
- Nephritis: shunt nephritis, acute poststreptococcal disease, anaphylactoid purpura, disseminated lupus erythematosus
- Renal tuberculosis
- Renal cortical necrosis: hemolytic uremic syndrome; sepsis
- Renal vein thrombosis
- Radiation nephritis
- Postrenal transplantation

ACQUIRED, OTHER THAN RENAL
- Hyperthyroidism
- Retrosternal goiter
- Guillain-Barré syndrome or poliomyelitis
- Cerebral edema
- Stevens-Johnson syndrome
- Neuroblastoma
- Hypercalcemia or hypernatremia
- Adrenal adenoma or hyperplasia: primary aldosteronism or Cushing's syndrome
- Hyperuricemic nephropathy
- Burns

Modified from Lieberman, E.: Diagnostic evaluation of hypertensive children. Pediatr. Ann. *6*:390, 1977.

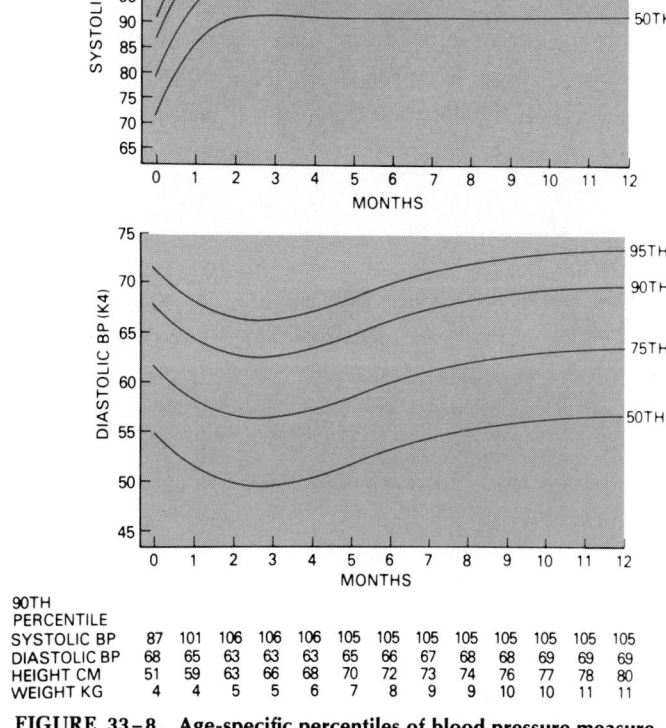

pearance (fifth phase) should be recorded. The fourth phase is the more accurate measure of diastolic pressure in most prepubertal children; beyond adolescence the fifth phase sound more closely reflects diastolic pressure.[110,111]

The normal ranges of blood pressure relative to age are shown in Figures 33–8 through 33–13 and serve as a guide in judging unsafe levels. Because considerable variation exists in most children's pressures, it should be recognized that a single blood pressure recording at or higher than the 90th percentile at a single point in time may not be an abnormal finding. In an apparently healthy child measurements should be repeated serially; further investigation is warranted if the blood pressure persists at or above the 90th percentile.[112,113] In contrast, definite or severe hypertension (i.e., pressures repeatedly well beyond the broad limits of normal) requires prompt investigation and treatment.[114,115] Particularly urgent attention must be paid to those children whose systolic and diastolic pressures are remarkably high (i.e., equal to or greater than 180 and 110 mm Hg, respectively). Other findings identifying the patient at acute risk include localized neurological signs and/or generalized seizures; blurred vision or such eye ground changes as retinal hemorrhage, exudate, papilledema, or retinal arterial constriction; renal or abdominal pain; evidence of left ventricular hypertrophy or cardiac decompensation; renal

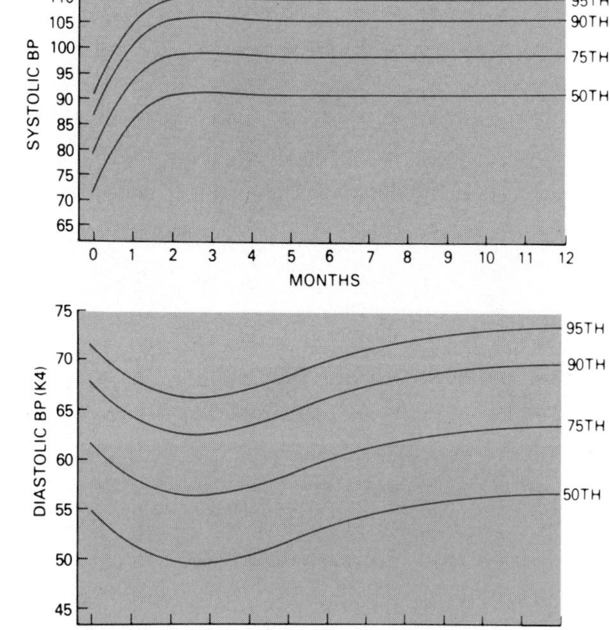

90TH PERCENTILE													
SYSTOLIC BP	87	101	106	106	106	105	105	105	105	105	105	105	105
DIASTOLIC BP	68	65	63	63	63	65	66	67	68	68	69	69	69
HEIGHT CM	51	59	63	66	68	70	72	73	74	76	77	78	80
WEIGHT KG	4	4	5	5	6	7	8	9	9	10	10	11	11

FIGURE 33–8. Age-specific percentiles of blood pressure measurements in boys—birth to 12 months of age. Korotkoff phase IV used for diastolic blood pressure. (From Horan, M. J., et al.: Report of the second task force on blood pressure control in children—1987. Pediatrics *79*:1, 1987. Copyright American Academy of Pediatrics, 1987.)

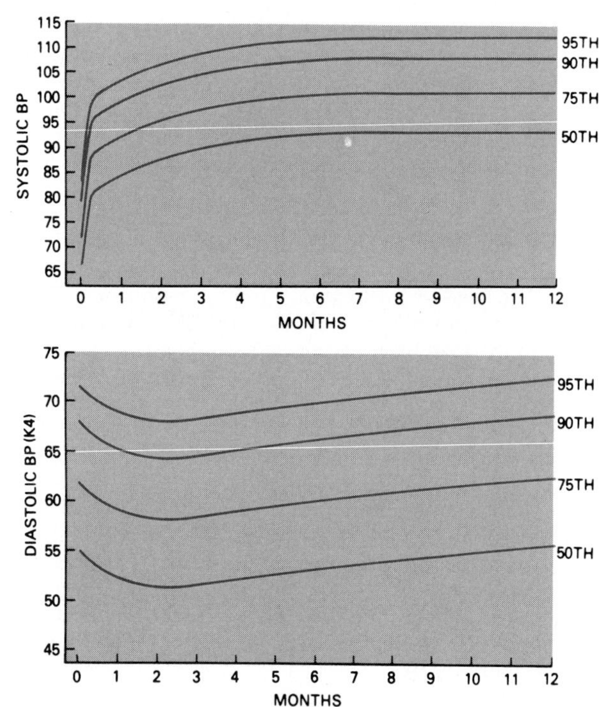

90TH PERCENTILE													
SYSTOLIC BP	76	98	101	104	105	106	106	106	106	106	106	105	105
DIASTOLIC BP	68	65	64	64	65	65	66	66	66	67	67	67	67
HEIGHT CM	54	55	56	58	61	63	66	68	70	72	74	75	77
WEIGHT KG	4	4	4	5	5	6	7	8	9	9	10	10	11

FIGURE 33–9. Age-specific percentiles of blood pressure measurements in girls—birth to 12 months of age. Korotkoff phase IV used for diastolic blood pressure. (From Horan, M. J., et al.: Report of the second task force on blood pressure control in children—1987. Pediatrics *79*:1, 1987. Copyright American Academy of Pediatrics, 1987.)

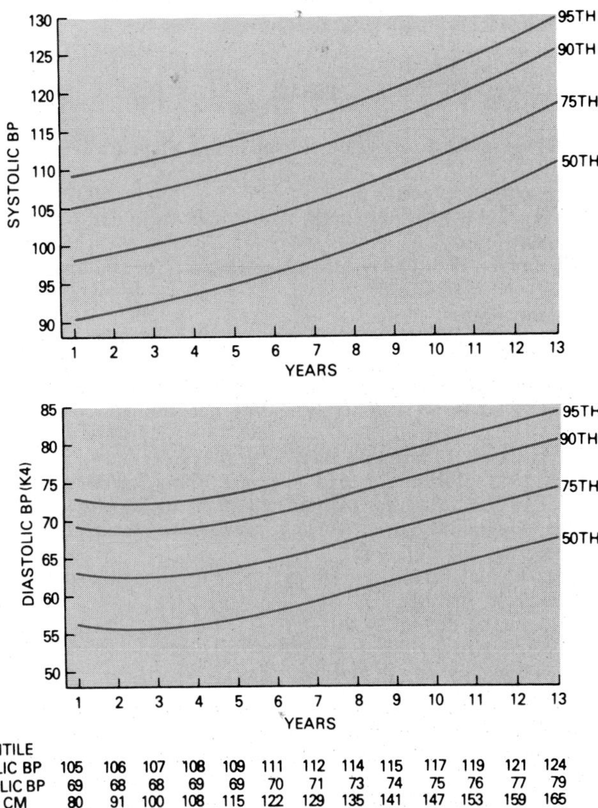

90TH PERCENTILE	1	2	3	4	5	6	7	8	9	10	11	12	13
SYSTOLIC BP	105	106	107	108	109	111	112	114	115	117	119	121	124
DIASTOLIC BP	69	68	68	69	69	70	71	73	74	75	76	77	79
HEIGHT CM	80	91	100	108	115	122	129	135	141	147	153	159	165
WEIGHT KG	11	14	16	18	22	25	29	34	39	44	50	55	62

FIGURE 33–10. Age-specific percentiles of blood pressure measurements in boys—1 to 13 years of age. Korotkoff phase IV used for diastolic blood pressure. (From Horan, M. J., et al.: Report of the second task force on blood pressure control in children—1987. Pediatrics *79*:1, 1987. Copyright American Academy of Pediatrics, 1987.)

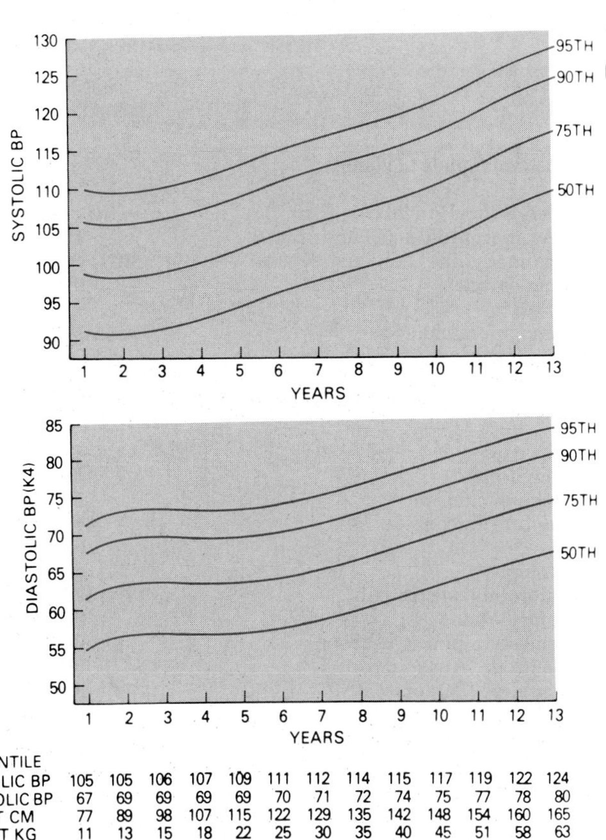

90TH PERCENTILE	1	2	3	4	5	6	7	8	9	10	11	12	13
SYSTOLIC BP	105	105	106	107	109	111	112	114	115	117	119	122	124
DIASTOLIC BP	67	69	69	69	69	70	71	72	74	75	77	78	80
HEIGHT CM	77	89	98	107	115	122	129	135	142	148	154	160	165
WEIGHT KG	11	13	15	18	22	25	30	35	40	45	51	58	63

FIGURE 33–11. Age-specific percentiles of blood pressure measurements in girls—1 to 13 years of age. Korotkoff phase IV used for diastolic blood pressure. (From Horan, M. J., et al.: Report of the second task force on blood pressure control in children—1987. Pediatrics *79*:1, 1987. Copyright American Academy of Pediatrics, 1987.)

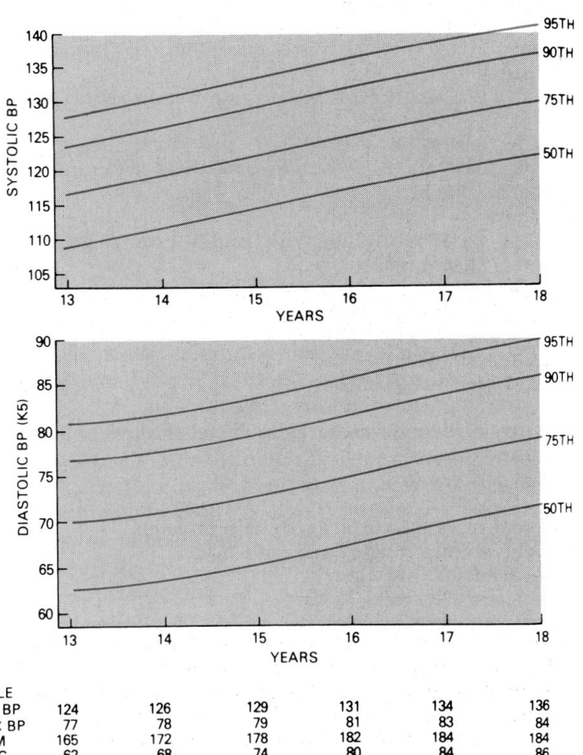

90TH PERCENTILE	13	14	15	16	17	18
SYSTOLIC BP	124	126	129	131	134	136
DIASTOLIC BP	77	78	79	81	83	84
HEIGHT CM	165	172	178	182	184	184
WEIGHT KG	62	68	74	80	84	86

FIGURE 33–12. Age-specific percentiles of blood pressure measurements in boys—13 to 18 years of age. Korotkoff phase V used for diastolic blood pressure. (From Horan, M. J., et al.: Report of the second task force on blood pressure control in children—1987. Pediatrics *79*:1, 1987. Copyright American Academy of Pediatrics, 1987.)

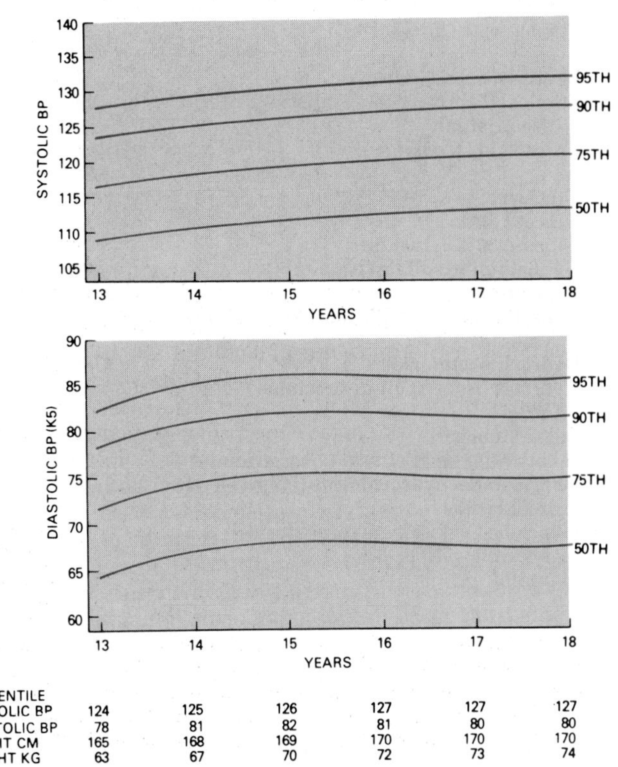

90TH PERCENTILE	13	14	15	16	17	18
SYSTOLIC BP	124	125	126	127	127	127
DIASTOLIC BP	78	81	82	81	80	80
HEIGHT CM	165	168	169	170	170	170
WEIGHT KG	63	67	70	72	73	74

FIGURE 33–13. Age-specific percentiles of blood pressure measurements in girls—13 to 18 years of age. Korotkoff phase V used for diastolic blood pressure. (From Horan, M. J., et al.: Report of the second task force on blood pressure control in children—1987. Pediatrics *79*:1, 1987. Copyright American Academy of Pediatrics, 1987.)

and the higher the blood pressure elevation, the more vigorous should be the laboratory evaluation. It should be recognized that although essential hypertension often is a diagnosis by exclusion in prepubertal children, it is a viable diagnosis, particularly in adolescents.[116,117] In the author's opinion the need for extensive laboratory investigations has been overemphasized in children or adolescents with mild sustained elevations in blood pressure.

Asymptomatic children and adolescents with borderline or only mildly elevated blood pressure (<5 to 10 mm Hg beyond the 90th percentile values for age) may not require antihypertensive pharmacological agents but should receive counseling regarding weight control, salt abuse, and avoidance of agents with pressor effects (e.g., caffeine, some bronchoconstrictors, nicotine). These patients should be encouraged to be physically active, especially in exercises improving cardiovascular fitness. Isometric or static exercise such as wrestling and weight lifting should be avoided, especially in children with evidence of left ventricular hypertrophy. If the latter exists or if these conservative measures do not result in normalization of blood pressure, treatment with antihypertensive drugs is indicated.

Drug therapy (Table 33–3) is aimed at prescribing the least complex regimen with the fewest side effects (see also Chap. 29). Pharmacological management is usually undertaken if diastolic blood pressure is greater than 85 mm Hg in children less than age 12 years, and greater than 90 mm Hg in children older than 12 years. If left ventricular hypertrophy is evident by echocardiogram, drug treatment is advisable at lower diastolic pressures. An oral thiazide diuretic usually is the initial drug of choice and may be combined with a potassium-sparing drug or with a dietary regimen that provides adequate potassium. If blood pressure control is not achieved, a beta-adrenergic blocking agent such as atenolol may be added to the regimen. Occasionally it is necessary to use an angiotensin enzyme blocker or a central sympathetic inhibitor such as clonidine. Of the calcium-antagonists, nifedipine has been used most often, but a broad experience in pediatric patients is lacking.

Acute, life-threatening episodes of hypertension occur rarely and in a variety of clinical situations.[118] Encephalopathy is the most severe complication of an acute hypertensive crisis; its presence demands immediate lowering of the systemic arterial blood pressure. Diazoxide is the agent of choice as a first drug for the patient with encephalopathy. If diazoxide is ineffective, catecholamine-producing tumors must be suspected and consideration given to using alpha-adrenergic blocking agents such as phentolamine or phenoxybenzamine. Sodium nitroprusside usually is considered the agent to be administered when all others have failed. If a cause for sustained hypertension has been detected, medical and/or surgical treatment should be directed at the underlying disease process.

HYPERLIPIDEMIAS

(See also Chap. 37)

The importance of prevention of arteriosclerosis in childhood is now generally accepted.[119–121] Hyperlipidemic children are at high risk of becoming hyperlipidemic adults and are therefore at greater risk of future atherosclerotic disease.[123–125] Although opinions vary about the feasibility of maintaining low serum lipid levels in normal children by dietary modification, a consensus exists that children whose serum cholesterol or triglyceride levels are beyond the 95th percentile for their age and sex should be treated. Guidelines for abnormal levels in the first two decades of life are provided in Table 33–4.

In the author's opinion, as part of routine pediatric practice, all children should have a random nonfasting cholesterol test performed. If the cholesterol level exceeds 200 mg/dl, a lipid profile should be obtained and, if the LDL cholesterol exceeds

TABLE 33–4 FASTING LIPID AND LIPOPROTEIN LEVELS (mg/dl) IN CHILDREN BY AGE

	MALES			FEMALES		
	5%	50%	95%	5%	50%	95%
Cholesterol						
0–4 yr	114	155	203	112	156	200
5–9 yr	121	160	203	126	164	205
10–14 yr	119	158	202	124	160	201
15–19 yr	113	150	197	120	158	203
Triglycerides						
0–4 yr	29	56	98	34	64	112
5–9 yr	30	56	101	32	60	105
10–14 yr	32	66	125	37	75	131
15–19 yr	37	78	148	39	75	132
HDL Cholesterol						
5–9 yr	38	56	74	36	53	73
10–14 yr	37	55	74	37	52	70
15–19 yr	30	46	63	35	52	74
LDL Cholesterol						
5–9 yr	63	93	129	68	100	140
10–14 yr	64	100	140	68	97	132
15–19 yr	62	94	130	59	96	137

Data from Lipid Research Clinics: Population Studies Data Book. Dept. of Health and Human Services (NIH) 80-1527, Vol. I: The Prevalence Study.

130 mg/dl, appropriate therapy should be instituted. Serum lipid levels should be analyzed at regular intervals in all children from families with hyperlipidemia or with histories that include hypertension, myocardial infarction, stroke, or peripheral vascular disease among parents or grandparents before age 50.[119,126–128] Differentiation is necessary between acquired hyperlipidemia and one of the familial, and presumably genetic, hyperlipidemias.[124]

Homozygous familial hypercholesterolemia causes severe atherosclerosis of the coronary arteries and myocardial infarction in childhood; rarely it causes atherosclerosis of the aortic valve, leading to critical aortic stenosis that requires surgical treatment.[128]

REFERENCES

NONRHEUMATIC INFLAMMATORY DISEASE

1. Ainger, L. E., Lawyer, N. G., and Fitch, C. W.: Neonatal rubella myocarditis. Br. Heart J. *28*:691, 1966.
2. Ayuthya, T.S.N., Jayavasu, J., and Pongpanich, B.: Coxsackie group B virus in primary myocardial disease in infants and children. Am. Heart J. *88*:311, 1974.
3. Suckling, P. V., and Vogelpoel, L.: Coxsackie myocarditis of the newborn. Lancet *2*:421, 1970.
4. Lerner, A. M., and Wilson, F. M.: Virus myocardiopathy. Progr. Med. Virol. *15*:63, 1973.
5. Oda, T., Hamamoto, K. and Morinaga, H.: Clinical aspects of non-rheumatic myocarditis in children. Jpn. Circ. J. *43*:443, 1979.
6. Wink, K., and Schmitz, H.: Cytomegalovirus myocarditis. Am. Heart J. *100*:667, 1980.
7. Arita, M., Ueno, Y., and Masuyama, Y.: Complete heart block in mumps myocarditis. Br. Heart J. *46*:342, 1981.
8. O'Connell, J. B.: Gallium-67 imaging in patients with dilated cardiomyopathy and biopsy proven myocarditis. Circulation *70*:58, 1984.
9. Leatherbury, L., Chandra, R. S., Shapiro, S. R., and Perry, L. W.: Value of endomyocardial biopsy of infants, children and adolescents with dilated or hypertrophic cardiomyopathy and myocarditis. J. Am. Coll. Cardiol. *12*:1547, 1988.
10. Schmaltz, A. A., Apitz, J., Hort, W., and Maisch, B.: Endomyocardial biopsy in infants and children: Experience in 60 patients. Pediatr. Cardiol. *11*:15, 1990.
11. Fisher, L. L., and Fisher, B. A.: Recognition and treatment of viral myocarditis. Primary Cardiol. *16*:46, 1990.
11a. Yoshizato, T., Edwards, W. D., Alboliras, E. T., et al: Safety and utility of endomyocardial biopsy in infants, children and adolescents: Our view of 66 procedures in 53 patients. J. Am. Coll. Cardiol. *15*:436, 1990.
12. Rezkalla, S. H., and Kolner, R. A.: Management strategies in viral myocarditis. Am. Heart J. *117*:706, 1989.
12a. Chan, K. Y., Iwahara, M., Benson, L. N., et al.: Immunosuppressive therapy in the management of acute myocarditis in children: A clinical trial. J. Am. Coll. Cardiol. *17*:458, 1991.

13. Taliercio, C. P., Seward, J. B., Driscoll, D. J., et al.: Idiopathic dilated cardiomyopathy in the young: Clinical profile and natural history. J. Am. Coll. Cardiol. *6*:1126, 1985.
14. Wittels, B., and Bressler, R. J.: Biochemical lesions of diphtheria toxin in the heart. J. Clin. Invest. *43*:630, 1964.
15. Challoner, D. R., and Prols, H. G.: Free fatty acid oxidation and carnitine levels in diphtheritic guinea pig myocardium. J. Clin. Invest. *51*:2071, 1972.
16. Ino, T., Sherwood, W. G., Benson, L. N. et al.: Cardiac manifestations and disorders of fat and carnitine metabolism in infancy. J. Am. Coll. Cardiol. *11*:1301, 1988.
17. Srivastava, S. C., Puri, D. S., and Lumba, S. T.: An electrocardiographic study of myocarditis and diphtheria. J. Assoc. Phys. India *14*:365, 1966.
18. Ramos, A., Elias, P., Barrucand, L., and DaSilva, J.: The protective effect of carnitine in human diphtheritic myocarditis. Pediatr. Res. *18*:815, 1984.
19. Prata, A.: Chagas' heart disease. Cardiologia *52*:79, 1968.
20. Rosenbaum, M. B.: Chagasic myocardiopathy. Progr. Cardiovasc. Dis. *7*:199, 1964.
21. Guerra, H. A. C., Palacios-Prue, E., Scorza, C. D., et al.: Clinical, histochemical, and ultrastructural correlation in septal endomyocardial biopsies from chronic chagasic patients: Detection of early myocardial damage. Am. Heart J. *113*:716, 1987.
22. Drugs for parasitic infections. *In* Abramowicz, M. (ed.): The Medical Letter of Drugs and Therapeutics, Vol. 28 (Issue 706). The Medical Letter, Inc., New Rochelle, January 1986.
23. Koten, J. W., and DeRaadt, P.: Myocarditis and *Trypanosoma rhodesiense* infections. Trans. R. Soc. Trop. Med. Hyg. *63*:485, 1969.
24. Stewart, J. M., Kaul, A., Gromisch, D. S., et al.: Symptomatic cardiac dysfunction in children with immunodeficiency virus infection. Am. Heart J. *117*:140, 1989.
25. Lipshultz, S. E., Chanock, S., Sanders, S. P., et al.: Cardiovascular manifestations of human immunodeficiency virus infection in infants and children. Am. J. Cardiol. *63*:1489, 1989.
26. Okoroma, E. O., Terry, L. W., and Scott, L. T.: Acute bacterial pericarditis in children: Report of 25 cases. Am. Heart J. *90*:709, 1975.
27. VanReken, D., Strauss, A., Hernandez, A., and Feigin, R. D.: Infectious pericarditis in children. J. Pediatr. *85*:165, 1974.
28. Callahan, J. A., Seward, J. B., Nishimura, R. A., et al.: Two dimensional echocardiographically guided pericardiocentesis: Experience in 117 consecutive patients. Am. J. Cardiol. *55*:476, 1985.
29. Lajos, T. Z., Black, H. E., Cooper, R. G., and Wanka, J.: Pericardial decompression. Ann. Thorac. Surg. *19*:47, 1975.
30. Engle, M. A., Ehlers, K. H., O'Laughlin, J. E., et al.: The post-pericardiotomy syndrome: Iatrogenic illness with immunologic and virologic components. *In* Engle, M. A. (ed.): Pediatric Cardiovascular Disease. Philadelphia, F. A. Davis Co., 1981, p. 381.
31. Clapp, S. K., Garson, J., Jr., Gutgesell, H. P., et al.: Postoperaive pericardial effusion and its relation to post-pericardiotomy syndrome. Pediatrics *66*:585, 1980.
32. Mason, T. G., Neal, W. A., and DiBartolomeo, A. G.: Elevated antinuclear antibody titers and the postpericardiotomy syndrome. J. Pediatr. *116*:403, 1990.
33. Paloheimo, J. A., Van Essen, R., Klemola, E., et al.: Sub-clinical cytomegalovirus infections and cytomegalovirus mononucleosis after open heart surgery. Am. J. Cardiol. *22*:624, 1968.
34. Kron, I. L., Rheuban, K., and Nolan, S. P.: Late cardiac tamponade in children. Ann. Surg. *199*:173, 1984.

PRIMARY CARDIOMYOPATHIES

35. Greenwood, R. D., Nadas, A. S., and Flyler, D. C.: The clinical course of primary myocardial disease in infants and children. Am. Heart J. *92*:549, 1976.
36. Goodwin, J. F.: The frontiers of cardiomyopathy. Br. Heart J. *48*:1, 1982.
37. Schryer, M. J. P., and Karnauchow, P. N.: Endocardial firboelastosis: Etiologic and pathogenic considerations in children. Am. Heart J. *88*:557, 1974.
38. Moller, J. N., Lucas, R. V., Adams, P., et al.: Endocardial fibroelastosis. A clinical and anatomic study of 47 patients with emphasis on its relationship to mitral insufficiency. Circulation *30*:759, 1964.
39. Taliercio, C. P., Seward, J. B., Driscoll, D. J., et al.: Idiopathic dilated cardiomyopathy in the young: Clinical profile and natural history. J. Am. Coll. Cardiol. *6*:1126, 1985.
40. Hanukoglu, A., Fried, D., and Somekh, E.: Inheritance of familial primary endocardial fibroelastosis. Clin. Pediatr. *25*:272, 1986.
41. Tripp, M. E.: Congestive cardiomyopathy of childhood. *In* Barness, L. A., (ed.): Advances in Pediatrics. Chicago, Year Book Medical Publishers, 1984, pp. 179–203.
42. Guntheroth, W. G.: Congestive cardiomyopathy in children. J. Am. Coll. Cardiol. *15*:194, 1990.
43. Chen, S., Nouri, S., Balfour, I., et al.: Clinical profile of congestive cardiomyopathy in children. J. Am. Coll. Cardiol. *15*:189, 1990.
44. Griffin, M. L., Hernandez, A., Martin, T. C., et al.: Dilated cardiomyopathy in infants and children. J. Am. Coll. Cardiol. *11*:139, 1988.
45. Lurie, P. R.: Endocardial fibroeleastosis is not a disease. Am. J. Cardiol. *62*:468, 1988.
46. Brandenburg, R. O.: Report of the WHO/ISFC Task Force on definition and classification of cardiomyopathy. Circulation *64*:437a, 1971.
46a. Ino, T., Benson, L. N., Freedom, R. M., and Rowe, R. D.: Endocardial fibroelastosis: Natural history and prognostic risk factors. Am. J. Cardiol. *62*:431, 1988.
47. Lambert, E. C., and Vlad, P.: Primary endomyocardial disease. Pediatr. Clin. North Am. *5*:1057, 1958.
48. Sellers, F. J., Keith, J. D., and Manning, J. A.: The diagnosis of primary endocardial fibroelastosis. Circulation *29*:49, 1964.
49. Akiba, T., Yoshikawa, M., Kinoda, M., et al.: Assessment of cardiac performance by first-pass radionuclide angiocardiography in infants and children with normal heart and endocardial fibroelastosis. Tohoku J. Exp. Med. *148*:15, 1986.
50. Neustein, H. B., Lurie, P. R., and Fugita, M.: Endocardial fibroelastosis found on transvascular endomyocardial biopsy in children. Arch. Pathol. Lab. Med. *103*:214, 1979.
51. Billingham, M. E.: The safety and utility of endomyocardial biopsy in infants, children and adolescents. J. Am. Coll. Cardiol. *15*:443, 1990.

SECONDARY CARDIOMYOPATHIES

52. Gutgesell, H. P., Speer, M. E., and Rosenberg, H. S.: Characterization of the cardiomyopathy in infants with diabetic mothers. Circulation *51*:441, 1980.
53. Trowitzsch, E, Bigalke, U., Gisbertz, R., and Kallfelz, H. C.: Echocardiographic profile of infants of diabetic mothers. Eur. J. Pediatr. *140*:311, 1983.
54. Walther, F. J., Siassi, B., King, J., and Wu, P. Y-K.: Cardiac output in infants of insulin-dependent diabetic mothers. J. Pediatr. *107*:109, 1985.
55. Miller, E., Hare, J. W., Cloherty, J. P., et al.: Elevated maternal hemoglobin A_{1C} in early pregnancy and major congenital anomalies in infants of diabetic mothers. N. Engl. J. Med. *304*:1331, 1981.
56. Deorari, A. K., Saxena, A., Singh, M., and Shrivastava, S.: Echocardiographic assessment of infants born to diabetic mothers. Arch. Dis. Child *64*:721, 1989.
57. Bordiuk, J. N., Logato, M. J., Lovelace, R. E., and Blumenthal, S: Pompe's disease: Electron myographic, electron microscopic and cardiovascular aspects. Arch. Neurol. (Chicago) *23*:113, 1970,
58. Dickenson, E. F., Houlsby, W. T., and Wilkinson, J. L.: Unusual angiographic appearance of the left ventricle in two cases of Pompe's disease (glycogenosis type 2.) Br. Heart J. *41*:238, 1979.
59. Hwang, G., Meng, C. C., Lin, C. Y., and Hsu, H. C.: Clinical analysis of five infants with glycogen storage disease of the heart—Pompe's disease. Jpn. Heart J. *27*:25, 1986.
59a. DeDominicis, E., Finocchi, G., Vincenzi, M., et al.: Echocardiographic and pulsed Doppler features in glycogen storage disease type II of the heart (Pompe's disease). Acta Cardiologica *XLVI*:107, 1991.
60. Caddell, J. L.: Metabolic and nutritional disease. *In* Adams, F. H., and Emmanouilides, G. C. (eds.): Moss' Heart Disease in Infants, Children and Adolescents. 4th ed. Baltimore, Williams and Wilkins Co., 1989, pp. 750–777.
61. Sanstead, H. H.: Clinical manifestations of certain vitamin deficienceis. *In* Goodhart, M. S., and Shils, M. E. (eds.): Modern Nutrition in Health and Disease. 5th ed. Philadelphia, Lea and Febiger, 1973, p. 593.
62. Sanstead, H. H.: Mineral metabolism and protein malnutrition. *In* Olson, R. E. (ed.): Protein Calorie Malnutrition. New York, Academic Press, 1975, p. 213.
63. Cadell, J. L.: Diseases of the cardiovascular system. *In* Jelliffe, B. B. (ed.): Diseases of Children in the Subtropics and Tropics. London, Edward Arnold, Ltd., 1970, p. 398.
64. Nutter, D. O., Murray, T. G., Heymsfield, S. B., and Fuller, E. O.: The effect of chronic protein-calorie undernutrition in the rate on myocardial function and cardiac function. Circ. Res. *45*:144, 1979.
65. Roberts, W. C., and Ferrans, V. J.: Pathological aspects of certain cardiomyopathies. Circ. Res. *34*(Suppl. II):II–128, 1974.
66. Roberts, W. C., Buja, L. M., and Ferrans, V. J.: Löffler's fibroplastic parietal endocarditis, eosinophilic leukemia, and Davies' endomyocardial fibrosis: The same disease at different stages? Pathol. Microbiol. (Basel) *35*:90, 1970.
67. Barretto, A. C. P., DaLuz, T. L., Oliveira, S. A, et al.: Determinants of survival in endomyocardial fibrosis. Circulation *80*(Suppl. I):177, 1989.
68. Valithan, M. S., Balkrishnan, K. G., Sankarkumar, R., and Kartha, C. C.: Surgical treatment of endomyocardial fibrosis. Ann. Thorac. Surg. *43*:68, 1987.
69. DiSessa, T. G., Klitzner, T., Hiraishi, S., et al.: Cardiovascular effects of Kawasaki's disease. J. Cardiovasc. Med. *6*:1159, 1981.
70. Burns, J. C., Huang, A. S., Newburger, J. W., et al.: Characterization of the polymerase activity associated with cultured peripheral blood mononuclear cells from patients with Kawasaki disease. Pediatr. Res. *27*:109, 1990.
71. Abe, Y., Nakano, S., Nakahara, T., et al.: Detection of serum antibody by the antimitogen assay against streptococcal erythrogenic toxins. Age distribution in children and the relation to Kawasaki disease. Pediatr. Res. *27*:11, 1990.
72. Lang, B. A., Silverman, E. D., Laxer, R. M., and Lau, A. S.: Spontaneous tumor necrosis factor production in Kawasaki disease. J. Pediatr. *115*:939, 1989.
73. Hiraishi, S., Yashiro, K., Oguchi, K., and Nakazawa, K.: Clinical course of cardiovascular involvement in the mucocutaneous lymph node syndrome. Am. J. Cardiol. *47*:323, 1981.
74. Fujiwara, T., Fujiwara, H., and Hamashima, Y.: Frequency and size of coronary arterial aneurysm at necropsy in Kawasaki disease. Am. J. Cardiol. *59*:808, 1987.
75. Nakano, H., Saito, A., Ueda, K., and Nojima, K.: Clinical characteristics of myocardial infarction following Kawasaki disease: Report of 11 cases. J. Pediatr. *108*:198, 1986.

76. Kato, H., Ichinose, E., and Kawasaki, T.: Myocardial infarction in Kawasaki disease: Clinical analyses in 195 cases. J. Pediatr. *108*:923, 1986.
77. Meade, R. H., and Brandt, L.: Manifestation of Kawasaki disease in New England outbreak of 1980. J. Pediatr. *100*:558, 1982.
78. Onouchi, Z., Shimazu, S., Takamatsu, T., and Hamaoka, K.: Aneurysms of the coronary arteries in Kawasaki disease: An angiographic study of 30 cases. Circulation *66*:6,1982.
79. Nakanishi, T., Takao, A., Nakazawa, M., et al.: Mucocutaneous lymph node syndrome: Clinical, hemodynamic, and angiographic features of coronary obstructive disease. Am. J. Cardiol. *55*:6662, 1985.
80. Chung, K., Brandt, L., Fulton, D. R., and Kreidberg, M. B.: Cardiac and coronary arterial involvement in infants and children with mucocutaneous lymph node syndrome. Am. J. Cardiol. *50*:136, 1982.
81. Yoshida, H., Maeda, T., and Taniguchi, N.: Subcostal two-dimensional echocardiographic imaging of peripheral right coronary artery in Kawasaki disease. Circulation *65*:956, 1982.
82. Koren, G., Lavi, S., Rose, V., and Rowe, R.: Kawasaki disease. Review of risk factors for coronary aneurysms. J. Pediatr. *108*:388, 1986.
82a. Tatara, K., Kusakawa, S., Itoh, K., et al.: Collateral circulation in Kawasaki disease with coronary occlusion or severe stenosis. Am. Heart J. *121*:797, 1991.
83. Anderson, T. M., Meyer, R. A., and Kaplan, S.: Long-term echocardiographic evaluation of cardiac size and function in patients with Kawasaki's disease. Am. Heart J. *110*:107, 1985.
84. Ichida, F., Fatica, N. S., O'Loughlin, J. E., et al.: Correlation of electrocardiographic and echocardiographic changes in Kawasaki disease. Am. Heart J. *116*:812, 1988.
85. Fujiwara, T., Fujiwara, H., Ueda, T., et al.: Comparison of macroscopic, postmortem, angiographic and two-dimensional echocardiographic findings of coronary aneurysms in children with Kawasaki disease. Am. J. Cardiol. *6*:199, 1986.
86. Grenadier, E., Allen, H.D., Goldberg, S. J., et al.: Left ventricular wall motion abnormalities in Kawasaki's disease. J. Am. Coll. Cardiol. *1*:714, 1983.
87. Kato, H., Ichinose, E., Matsunaga, S., et al.: Fate of coronary aneurysms in Kawasaki disease: Serial coronary angiography and long-term follow-up study. Am. J. Cardiol. *49*:1758, 1982.
88. Anderson, T., Meyer, R. A., and Kaplan, S.: Long term evaluation of cardiac size and function in patients with Kawasaki disease. J. Am. Coll. Cardiol. *1*:714, 1983.
89. Suma, K., Takeuchi, Y., Shiroma, K., et al.: Early and late postoperative studies in coronary arterial lesions resulting from Kawasaki's disease in children. J. Thorac. Cardiovasc. Surg. *84*:224, 1982.
89a. Suzuki, A., Kamiya, T., Yasuo, O., and Kuroe, K.: Extended long-term follow-up study of coronary arterial lesions in Kawasaki disease. J. Am. Coll. Cardiol. *17*:33A, 1991.
89b. Akagi, T., Kato, H., Inoue, O., et al.: Valvular heart disease in Kawasaki syndrome: Incidence and natural history. Am. Heart J. *120*:366, 1990.
89c. Paridon, S. M., Ross, R. D., Kuhns, L. R., and Pinsky, W.W.: Myocardial performance and perfusion during exercise in patients with coronary artery disease caused by Kawasaki disease. J. Pediatr. *116*:52, 1990.
90. Takahashi, M., Mason, W., and Lewis, A. B.: Regression of coronary aneurysms in patients with Kawasaki syndrome. Circulation *75*:387, 1987.
91. Gidding, S. S., Shulman, S. T., Ilbawi, M., et al.: Mucocutaneous lymph node syndrome (Kawasaki's disease): delayed aortic and mitral insufficiency secondary to active valvulitis. J. Am. Coll. Cardiol. *7*:894, 1986.
92. Newburger, J. W., Sanders, S. P., Burns, J. C., et al.: Left ventricular contractility and function in Kawasaki syndrome: Effect of intravenous gamma globulin. Circulation *79*:1237, 1989.
93. Paridon, S. M., Ross, R. D., Kuhns, M. R., and Pinsky, W. W.: Myocardial performance and perfusion during exercise in patients with coronary-artery disease caused by Kawasaki disease. J. Pediatr. *116*:52, 1990.
94. Kurisu, Y., Azumi, T., Sugahara, T., et al.: Variation in coronary arterial dimension (distensible abnormality) after disappearing aneurysm in Kawasaki disease. Am. Heart J. *114*:532, 1987.
95. Koren, G., and MacLaod, S. M.: Difficulty in achieving therapeutic serum concentrations of salicylate in Kawasaki's disease. J. Pediatr. *105*:991, 1984.
96. Newburger, J. W., Takahasi, M., Burns, J. C., et al.: The treatment of Kawasaki syndrome with intravenous gamma globulin. N. Engl. J. Med. *315*:341, 1986.
97. Glode, M. P., Joffe, L. S., Wiggins, J., Jr., et al.: Effect of intravenous immune globulin on the coagulopathy of Kawasaki syndrome. J. Pediatr. *115*:469, 1989.
98. Engle, M. A., Fatica, N. S., Bussel, J. B., et al.: Clinical trial of single-dose intravenous gamma globulin in acute Kawasaki disease. Am. J. Dis. Child. *143*:1300, 1989.
99. Newburger, J. W., Takahashi, M., Beiser, A. S., et al.: A single intravenous infusion of gamma globulin as compared with four infusions in the treatment of acute Kawasaki syndrome. N. Engl. J. Med. *324*:1633, 1991.
99a. Shackelford, P. G., and Strauss, A. W.: Kawasaki syndrome. N. Engl. J. Med. *324*:1664, 1991.
100. Ohyagi, A., Hirose, K., Tsujimoto, S. et al.: Kawasaki's disease complicated by acute myocardial infarction nine years after onset. Am. Heart J. *110*:670, 1985.
101. Kohr, R. M.: Progressive asymptomatic coronary artery disease as a late fatal sequelae of Kawasaki's disease. J. Pediatr. *108*:256, 1986.
102. Suzuki, A., Kamiya, T., Ono, Y., et al.: Aorto-coronary bypass surgery for coronary arterial lesions resulting from Kawasaki disease. J. Pediatr. *116*:567, 1990.
103. Seraydarian, M. W., Artaza, L., and Yang, J. J.: Metablic involvement and adriamycin cardiotoxicity. *In* Tajaddin, M., Bhatrab, B., and Siddegue, H. H. (eds.): Advances in Myocardiology, Vol. 2. Baltimore, University Park Press, 1980.
104. Legha, S. S., Benjamin, R. S., and MacKay, H. J.: Reduction of doxorubicin cardiotoxicity by prolonged continuous intravenous infusion. Ann. Intern. Med. *96*:133, 1982.
105. Hausdorf, G., Morf, G., Beron, G., et al.: Long term doxorubicin cardiotoxicity in childhood: Noninvasive evaluation of the contractile state and diastolic filling. Br. Heart J. *60*:309, 1988.
106. Goorin, A. M., Chauvenet, A. R., Perez-Atayde, A. R., et al.: Initial congestive heart failure, six to 10 years after doxorubicin chemotherapy for childhood cancer. J. Pediatr. *116*:144, 1990.

SYSTEMIC HYPERTENSION

107. New, M. I., and Levine, L. S.: Hypertension in childhood and adolescence. Cardiovasc. Rev. *3*:115, 1982.
108. Lieberman, E.: Diagnostic evaluation of hypertensive children. Pediatr. Ann. *6*:390, 1977.
109. Colan, S. D., Fujii, A, Borow, K. M., et al.: Noninvasive determination of systolic, diastolic and end-systolic blood pressure in neonates, infants, and young children: Comparison with central aortic measurements. Am. J. Cardiol. *52*:867, 1983.
110. Horan, M. J., et al.: Report of the second task force on blood pressure control in children—1987. Pediatrics *79*:1, 1987.
111. Berenson, G. S., Webber, L. S., and Voors, A. W.: Diagnosing hypertension in children. J. Cardiovasc. Med. *6*:273, 1982.
112. Mehta, S. K.: Pediatric hypertension: A challenge for pediatrics. Am. J. Dis. Child. *141*:893, 1987.
113. Lauer, R. M., Burns, T. L., and Clarke, W. R.: Assessing children's blood pressure—considerations of age and body size: The Muscatine study. Pediatrics *75*:1081, 1985.
114. Rocchini, A. P.: Childhood hypertension: Etiology, diagnosis, and treatment. Pediatr. Clin. North Am. *31*:1259, 1984.
115. Balfe, J. W., Levin, L., Tsuru, N., and Chan, J. C. M.: Hypertension in childhood. Adv. Pediatr. *36*:201, 1989.
116. Lauer, R. M., and Clarke, W. R.: Childhood risk factors for high adult blood pressure: The Muscatine study. Pediatrics *84*:633, 1989.
117. Rocchini, A. P., Katch, V., Anderson, J. et al.: Blood pressure in obese adolescents: Effect of weight loss. Pediatrics *82*:16, 1988.
118. Fleischmann, L. E.: Management of hypertensive crises in children. Pediatr. Ann. *6*:410, 1977.

HYPERLIPIDEMIAS

119. Schieken, R. M.: The management of the family at high risk for coronary heart disease. *In* Friedman, W. F., and Talner, N. S. (eds.): Cardiology Clinics: Update in Pediatric Cardiology. Philadelphia, W. B. Saunders Company, Vol. 7, No. 2, 1989, pp. 467–477.
120. Garcia, R. E., and Moodie, D. S.: Routine cholesterol surveillance in childhood. Pediatrics *84*:751, 1989.
121. Jacobson, M. S., and Lillienfeld, D. E.: The pediatrician's role in atherosclerosis prevention. J. Pediatr. *112*:836, 1988.
122. Lauer, R. M., Lee, J., and Clarke, W. R.: Factors affecting the relationship between childhood and adult cholesterol levels: The Muscatine study. Pediatrics *82*:309, 1988.
123. Nader, P. R., Taras, H. L., Sallis, J. F., and Patterson, T. L.: Adult heart disease prevention in childhood: A national survey of pediatricians, practices and attitudes. Pediatrics *79*:843, 1987.
124. Breslow, J. L.: Genetic basis of lipoprotein disorders. J. Clin. Invest. *84*:373, 1989.
125. Leaf, A.: Management of hypercholesterolemia. Are preventive interventions advisable? N. Engl. J. Med. *321*:680, 1989.
126. Schaefer, E. J., and Levy, R. I.: Pathogenesis and management of lipoprotein disorders. N. Engl. J. Med. *312*:1300, 1985.
127. Neill, C. A., Ose, L., and Kwiterovich, P. O., Jr.: Hyperlipidemia: Clinical clues in the first two decades of life. Johns Hopkins Med. J. *140*:171, 1977.
128. Forman, M. B., Kinsley, R. M., DuPlessis, J. P. , et al.: Surgical correction of combined supravalvular and valvular aotic stenosis in homozygous familial hypercholesterolemia. SA Med. J. *1*:579, 1982.

Valvular Heart Disease

by EUGENE BRAUNWALD, M.D.

Mitral Stenosis

ETIOLOGY AND PATHOLOGY

The predominant cause of mitral stenosis (MS) is rheumatic fever[1,2] (p. 1721). Far less frequently, MS is congenital in etiology,[3] and this form is observed almost exclusively in infants and young children (p. 929). Rarely, mitral stenosis is a complication of malignant carcinoid (p. 1424), systemic lupus erythematosus, rheumatoid arthritis,[4] and the mucopolysaccharidoses of the Hunter-Hurley phenotype.[5] Amyloid deposits may occur on rheumatic valves and contribute to the obstruction to left atrial emptying.[6] Methysergide therapy is an unusual but documented cause of MS.[7] MS, generally of rheumatic origin, may be associated with atrial septal defect in Lutembacher syndrome (p. 970). Left atrial tumor, particularly myxoma (p. 1454); ball-valve thrombus in the left atrium (usually associated with MS)[8]; and a congenital membrane in the left atrium, i.e., cor triatriatum (p. 929), may also obstruct left atrial outflow and therefore simulate MS. Although calcification of the mitral annulus usually causes mitral regurgitation (MR), when subvalvular or intravalvular extension is extensive, MS may result.[9] Approximately 25 per cent of all patients with rheumatic heart disease have pure MS, and an additional 40 per cent have combined MS and MR.[10] Two-thirds of all patients with rheumatic MS are female.

Rheumatic fever results in four forms of fusion of the mitral valve apparatus leading to stenosis: (1) commissural, (2) cuspal, (3) chordal, and (4) combined.[11] Thickening of the commissures alone occurs in 30 per cent, of the cusps alone in 15 per cent, and of the chordae alone in 10 per cent; in the remainder, thickening of more than one of these structures is involved. Characteristically, mitral valve cusps fuse at their edges, and fusion of the chordae results in thickening and shortening of these structures. The stenotic mitral valve is typically funnel-shaped, and the orifice is frequently shaped like a "fish mouth" or buttonhole, with calcium deposits in the valve leaflets sometimes extending to involve the valve ring, which may become quite thick[11] (Figs. 34–1 and 56–6, p. 1726). The thickened leaflets may be so adherent and rigid that they cannot open or shut, reducing or rarely even abolishing the first heart sound (S_1) and leading to combined MS and MR.[12] There is a rough correlation between the severity of calcification and the transvalvular gradient.[13] When rheumatic fever results exclusively or predominantly in contraction and fusion of the chordae tendineae, with little fusion of the valvular commissures, dominant MR results.[14]

It probably takes a minimum of 2 years after the onset of acute rheumatic fever for severe MS to develop, and most patients in temperate climates remain asymptomatic for at least a decade more.[1,15] Symptoms commence most commonly in the third or fourth decade, although mild MS in the aged is becoming a more frequent finding.[16,17] In the tropics, particularly in underdeveloped areas, the disease advances more rapidly, and severe MS may be present in early adolescence.[18] The debate continues about whether the anatomical changes in severe MS result from a smoldering rheumatic process or whether once the valve has been deformed by the initial episode, the constant trauma produced by the turbulent blood flow leads to progressive fibrosis, thickening, and calcification of the valve apparatus.[19]

Enlargement of the left atrium and resultant elevation of the left main stem bronchus, calcification of the left atrial wall, the development of mural thrombi, and obliterative changes in the pulmonary vascular bed (p. 796) may all result from chronic MS.

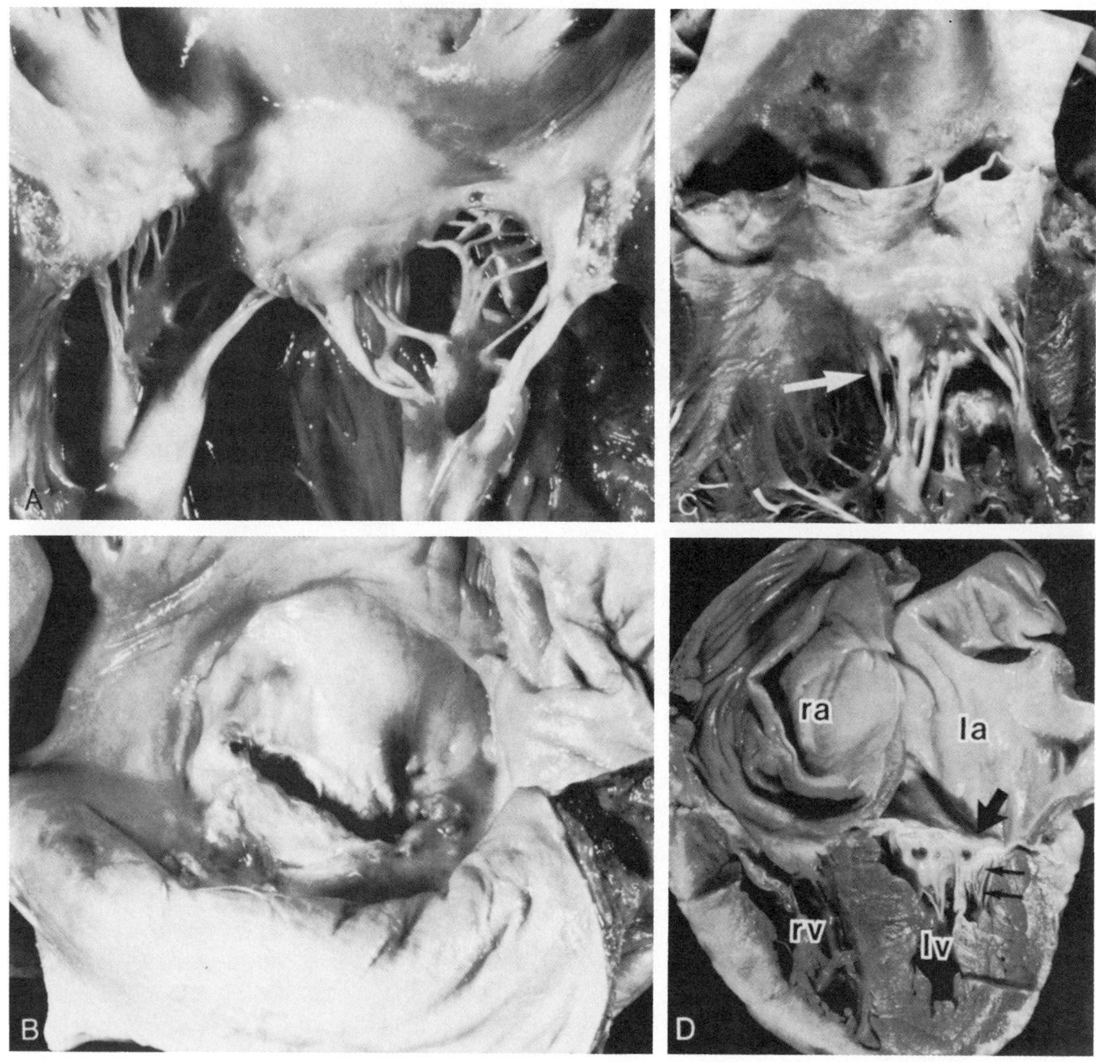

FIGURE 34–1. Rheumatic mitral stenosis. *A*, Moderate valvular changes including diffuse leaflet fibrosis, commissural fusion, and chordal thickening and fusion. In another case, atrial view (*B*) and subvalvular and aortic aspects (*C*) show prominent subvalvular involvement; severe subvalvular distortion is evident (arrow). *D*, Severe rheumatic mitral stenosis with specimen shown in apical four-chamber echocardiographic view, demonstrating small left ventricle (lv) and enlarged left atrium (la), right ventricle (rv), and right atrium (ra). Note the calcified stenotic valve (arrow) and prominent subvalvular changes (double arrows). (*A* and *D* from Schoen, F. J., and St. John Sutton, M.: Contemporary issues in the pathology of valvular heart disease. Hum. Pathol. *18*:568, 1987.)

PATHOPHYSIOLOGY

In normal adults the cross-sectional area of the mitral valve orifice is 4 to 6 cm². When the orifice is reduced to approximately 2 cm², which is considered to represent mild MS, blood can flow from the left atrium to the left ventricle only if propelled by an abnormal, though small, pressure gradient. When the mitral valve opening is reduced to 1 cm², which is considered to represent critical MS, a left atrioventricular pressure gradient of approximately 20 mm Hg (and therefore, in the presence of a normal left ventricular diastolic pressure, a mean left atrial pressure of approximately 25 mm Hg) is required to maintain normal cardiac output at rest (Figs. 34–2 and 34–3 and 7–10, p. 189). The elevated left atrial pressure in turn raises pulmonary venous and capillary pressures, resulting in exertional dyspnea (p. 449). The first bouts of dyspnea in patients with MS are usually precipitated by exercise, emotional stress, sexual intercourse, infection, or atrial fibrillation, all of which increase the rate of blood flow across the mitral orifice and result in further elevation of the left atrial pressure.[20,21]

In order to assess the severity of obstruction of the mitral valve (and, for that matter, of any valve), it is essential to measure both the transvalvular pressure gradient and the flow rate. The latter depends not only on cardiac output but on heart rate as well. An increase in heart rate shortens diastole proportionately more than systole and diminishes the time available for flow across the mitral valve. Therefore, at any given level of cardiac output, tachycardia augments the transmitral valvular pressure gradient and elevates left atrial pressures further.[22,23] This explains the sudden development of dyspnea and pulmonary edema in previously asymptomatic patients with MS who experience atrial fibrillation with a rapid ventricular rate[24]; it also accounts for the equally rapid improvement in these patients when the ventricular rate is slowed by means of cardiac glycosides and/or beta-adrenoceptor blocking agents, even when the cardiac output per minute remains constant. Hydraulic considerations dictate that at any given orifice size the transvalvular gradient is a function of the square of the transvalvular flow rate (p. 194 and Fig. 34–3).[25] Thus, a doubling of flow rate will quadruple the pressure gradient, so that a stress such as exercise in patients with moderate or severe MS will cause marked elevation of left atrial pressure.[26]

Atrial contraction augments the presystolic transmitral valvular gradient by approximately 30 per cent in patients with MS (Fig. 7–10, p. 189). Withdrawal of atrial transport when atrial fibrillation develops decreases cardiac output by about 20 per cent. The more rapid ventricular rate that occurs in atrial fibrillation until it is pharmacologically controlled raises the transvalvular pressure gradient. Thus, hemody-

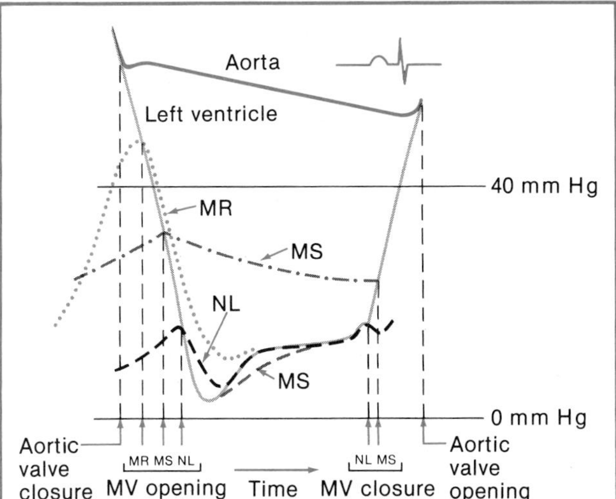

FIGURE 34–2. Schematic relationship of left ventricular (————), aortic (▬▬▬), and pulmonary atrial wedge (PAW) pressures. Note that the higher the left atrial *v* wave, the earlier the pressure crossover, and the earlier the mitral valve (MV) opening. The higher left atrial end-diastolic pressure with severe mitral stenosis (MS) also results in later closure of the mitral valve. PAW pressures in severe mitral regurgitation (MR) (• • • • • • •), mitral stenosis (— • — • — •), and normal (— — — —). The LV diastolic pressure in mitral stenosis (– – – – – –) rises slowly, denoting the absence of a rapid filling wave. (From Braunwald, E., and Turi, Z. G.: Pathophysiology of mitral valve disease. *In* Ionescu, M. I., and Cohn, L. H. [eds.]: Mitral Valve Disease. London, Butterworths, 1985, p. 3.)

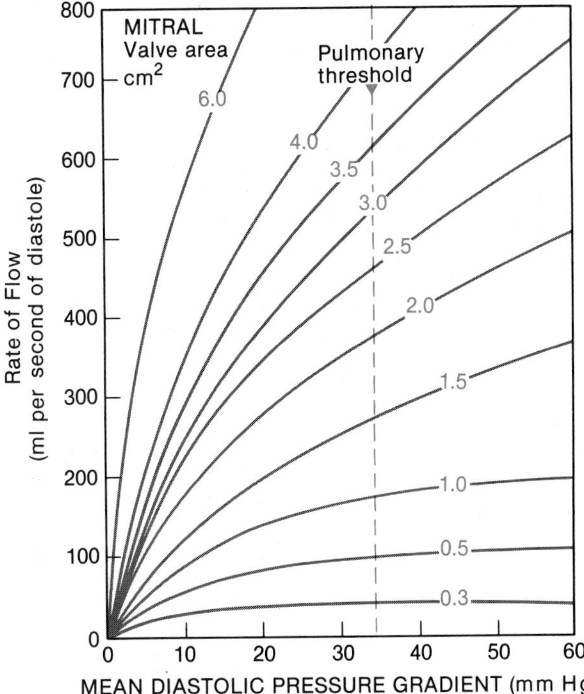

FIGURE 34–3. Graph illustrating the relation between mean diastolic gradient across the mitral valve and rate of flow across the mitral valve per second of diastole, as predicted by the Gorlin formula. Note that when the mitral valve area is 1.0 cm² or less, very little additional flow can be achieved by an increased pressure gradient. (From Wallace, A. G.: Pathophysiology of cardiovascular disease. *In* Smith, L. H., Jr., and Thier, S. O. [eds.]: Pathophysiology: The Biological Principles of Disease. The International Textbook of Medicine. Vol. 1. Philadelphia, W. B. Saunders Company, 1981, p. 1192.)

namic considerations indicate the desirability of maintaining sinus rhythm in patients with MS.[27]

INTRACARDIAC AND INTRAVASCULAR PRESSURES

Left ventricular diastolic pressure is normal in patients with pure MS; coexisting MR, aortic valve lesions, systemic hypertension, ischemic heart disease, and cardiomyopathy may all be responsible for elevations of left ventricular diastolic pressure. In approximately 85 per cent of patients with pure MS, the end-diastolic volume is within the normal range, whereas it is reduced in the remainder.[28] In approximately one-fourth of patients with pure MS the ejection fraction and other ejection indices of systolic performance (p. 426) are below normal, most likely resulting from chronic reduction in preload and elevated afterload caused by reduced left ventricular thickness.[29] Regional hypokinesis is common,[30] perhaps caused by extension of the scarring process from the mitral valve into the adjacent posterior basal myocardium[31] or by associated ischemic heart disease. The left ventricular mass is normal or slightly reduced.[28] It has long been postulated that persistent myocardial dysfunction, perhaps caused by smoldering rheumatic myocarditis, may be responsible for the poor results following surgical treatment of some patients with pure MS.[32] The bulk of available evidence suggests that myocardial *contractility* (as opposed to systolic performance) is normal or slightly impaired in the majority of patients.[33,34] Associated ischemic heart disease may be responsible for myocardial dysfunction.[35] Most patients with MS show a normal elevation of ejection fraction and reduction of end-systolic volume during exercise.[36]

In MS and sinus rhythm, the *left atrial pressure pulse* generally exhibits a prominent atrial contraction (*a*) wave (Fig. 7–10, p. 189) and a gradual pressure decline after mitral valve opening (*y* descent); the mean left atrial pressure is elevated. In patients with mild to moderate MS without elevation of pulmonary vascular resistance, pulmonary arterial pressure may be normal or only slightly elevated at rest and may rise only during exercise. However, in patients with severe MS and/or those in whom the pulmonary vascular resistance is significantly increased, pulmonary arterial pressure is elevated when the patient is at rest, and in rare cases of extreme elevation of the pulmonary vascular resistance it may exceed the systemic arterial pressure. Further elevations of left atrial and pulmonary vascular pressures occur during exercise (Fig. 7–10, p. 189) or tachycardia or both. With moderate elevation of pulmonary artery pressure, right ventricular performance is maintained.[37] However, an elevation of pulmonary arterial systolic pressure exceeding 70 mm Hg represents a serious impedance to emptying of the right ventricle and causes right ventricular failure with elevations of the right ventricular end-diastolic and right atrial pressures. During exercise, patients with MS and pulmonary hypertension commonly fail to exhibit normal elevation of right ventricular ejection fraction.[36]

The *clinical and hemodynamic features* of MS of any given severity are dictated largely by the levels of cardiac output and pulmonary vascular resistance. The response to a given degree of mitral obstruction may be characterized at one end of the hemodynamic spectrum by a normal cardiac output and a high left atrioventricular pressure gradient or, at the opposite end of the spectrum, by a markedly reduced cardiac output and low transvalvular pressure gradient. In some patients with moderately severe stenosis (mitral valve area = 1.0 to 1.5 cm²) cardiac output at rest may be normal and it rises normally during exertion as well. In these patients, marked elevation of left atrial and pulmonary capillary pressures and the high transvalvular pressure gradient together lead to severe pulmonary congestion during exertion. However, in the majority of patients with severe MS, cardiac output rises subnormally during exertion, thus reducing the pulmonary venous pressure and the severity of symptoms of pulmonary conges-

the murmur is a guide to the severity of mitral narrowing. In patients with combined MS and MR, a long diastolic murmur always signifies the presence of significant stenosis and, in general, persists for as long as the gradient across the mitral valve exceeds approximately 3 mm Hg. The murmur usually commences immediately after the mitral OS. In mild MS, the early diastolic murmur is brief but resumes in presystole. In severe stenosis, the murmur is holodiastolic, with presystolic accentuation in patients with sinus rhythm.

Although a *presystolic murmur* is usually present in patients with sinus rhythm in whom transvalvular blood flow is accelerated by atrial contraction, such a murmur may also occur in patients with atrial fibrillation, in whom it results from the increased velocity of blood flow across a mitral valve orifice that begins to narrow after the onset of left ventricular contraction.[62] Since, in patients with atrial fibrillation, this murmur results from motion of the mitral valve leaflets, a flexible mitral valve is required for its generation; its absence in a patient with moderate or severe obstruction suggests a rigid calcified valve or a markedly reduced cardiac output or both.

The *diastolic rumbling murmur* of MS may be masked by the presence of obesity, pulmonary emphysema, and a low cardiac output with a low flow rate across the mitral valve. The rumble may be sharply localized and thus missed unless palpation is used to detect the apex of the left ventricle and to pinpoint the area at which auscultation should be carried out. In so-called "silent" MS, there is usually marked right ventricular enlargement, so that the right ventricle occupies the cardiac apex, and cardiac output is reduced, so that the murmur either is not audible at all or can be heard only in the mid- or posterior axillary line.[63] Auscultation of the murmur is facilitated by placing the patient in the left lateral position and auscultating during expiration after a few sit-ups or other maneuvers described later.

Dynamic Auscultation. The diastolic murmur and OS of MS are often reduced during inspiration and augmented during expiration[53,54,64]—the opposite of what occurs when these findings are secondary to tricuspid stenosis (p. 1053). During inspiration the A_2-OS interval widens, and three sequential sounds (A_2, P_2, and OS) are frequently audible. Sudden standing and the resultant reduction of venous return lower left atrial pressure and widen the A_2-OS interval[65]; this maneuver is useful in distinguishing an A_2-OS combination from a split S_2, which narrows on standing. In contrast, A_2-OS is significantly narrowed during exercise as left atrial pressure rises. The diastolic rumbling murmur of MS is reduced during the strain of a Valsalva maneuver and in any condition in which transmitral valve flow rate declines. Amyl nitrite, coughing, isometric or isotonic exercise, and sudden squatting are all useful in accentuating a faint or equivocal murmur of MS. Progressive narrowing of A_2-OS on serial examinations suggests an increase in the severity of stenosis, whereas widening of A_2-OS after mitral commissurotomy indicates that the severity of stenosis has been reduced significantly.

DIFFERENTIAL DIAGNOSIS. It is important to recognize that a variety of conditions other than MS may exhibit auscultatory findings that can be confused with MS, and these are summarized in Table 34-2. In addition to the findings listed in the table, the *Carey-Coombs murmur* of acute rheumatic fever (p. 1727) is a sign of active mitral valvulitis and can be confused with the murmur of MS. It is a soft, early diastolic murmur, usually varies from day to day, and is higher pitched than the diastolic rumbling murmur of established MS. In pure, severe MR—indeed, in any condition in which there is increased flow across a nonstenotic mitral valve—there may also be a short, diastolic murmur following an S_3. *Left atrial myxoma* may produce auscultatory findings similar to those in rheumatic valvular MS (p. 1452). A high-frequency early systolic murmur is audible along the lower left sternal border in one-third of patients with MS.[66] This should be distinguished from the apical (often holosystolic or late systolic) murmur of MR. In addition, a *pansystolic murmur of tricuspid regurgitation* and an S_3 originating from the right ventricle may be audible in the fourth intercostal space in the left parasternal region in patients with severe mitral stenosis. These signs, secondary to pulmonary hypertension, may be confused with the findings of MR.[67] However, the inspiratory augmentation of the murmur and of the S_3 and the prominent *v* wave in the jugular venous pulse aid in establishing that the mur-

TABLE 34-2 CONDITIONS IN WHICH AUSCULTATORY FINDINGS MAY SIMULATE THOSE IN MITRAL STENOSIS

AUSCULTATORY EVENT	CONDITION OTHER THAN MITRAL STENOSIS	EXPLANATION OF EVENT
Loud and snapping first sound	Hyperkinetic states	High left ventricular dP/dt at time of mitral closure
Early diastolic opening snap	Myxoma of left atrium	Tumor movement into ventricle Abrupt checking of tumor (tumor plop)
	Constrictive pericarditis	Checking of ventricular filling by pericardium
	Tricuspid stenosis	Stenotic valve
Diastolic rumbling murmur	Aortic regurgitation (Austin Flint murmur)	Preclosure of mitral valve (?) Regurgitant stream (?) Fluttering of mitral valve
	Dilated ventricle Myocarditis Cardiomyopathy	Preclosure of mitral valve (?) Centrifugal displacement of papillary muscles
	Hypertrophic, restrictive ventricle Hypertrophic obstructive cardiomyopathy Aortic valve disease	Impaired filling of left ventricle (?) Impaired opening of mitral valve
	Tricuspid stenosis	Narrow orifice
	Myxoma of left atrium	Narrow orifice
	Augmented atrioventricular flow Mitral regurgitation Left-to-right shunts	Preclosure of valve (?) Centrifugal displacement of papillary muscles
Crescendo presystolic murmur	Aortic regurgitation (Austin Flint murmur)	Preclosure of mitral valve opposing atrial systole
	Hypertrophic, restrictive ventricle	Summation of S_4 and S_1 may simulate presystolic murmur
	Tricuspid stenosis	Narrow orifice
	Myxoma of left atrium	Narrow orifice

Modified from Criley, J. M., et al.: Departures from the expected auscultatory events in mitral stenosis. *In* Likoff, W. (ed.): Cardiovascular Clinics, Vol. 5, No. 2, Valvular Heart Disease. Philadelphia, F. A. Davis, 1973, p. 213.

mur originates from the tricuspid valve. A decrescendo diastolic murmur along the left sternal border in patients with MS and pulmonary hypertension is usually due to aortic regurgitation and rarely represents a Graham Steell murmur of pulmonary regurgitation[68] (p. 56); the latter, when present, characteristically increases during inspiration.

LABORATORY EXAMINATION

ELECTROCARDIOGRAPHY. The ECG and vectorcardiogram are relatively insensitive techniques for the detection of mild MS, but they do show characteristic changes in moderate or severe obstruction[69,70] (Fig. 34–4). Left atrial enlargement (P-wave duration in lead II > 0.12 sec, terminal negative P force in lead $V_1 > 0.003$ mV/sec, P-wave axis between +45 and −30 degrees) is a principal electrocardiographic feature of MS (Fig. 5–10, p. 124) and is found in 90 per cent of patients with significant MS and sinus rhythm.[71] The ECG signs of left atrial enlargement correlate more closely with left atrial volume than with left atrial pressure[72] and often regress following successful valvulotomy.[21] When atrial fibrillation is present, the fibrillatory waves are coarse, i.e., greater than 0.1 mV in amplitude in V_1, also suggesting the presence of atrial enlargement.[73] The development of atrial fibrillation correlates with the preexistent ECG diagnosis of left atrial enlargement and is related to the size and the extent of fibrosis of the left atrial myocardium,[39–41] the duration of atriomegaly, and the age of the patient.[74]

Whether or not there is ECG evidence of right ventricular hypertrophy depends largely on the height of right ventricular systolic pressure; it is infrequent in patients with right ventricular systolic pressures less than 70 mm Hg.[71] However, approximately half of all patients with right ventricular systolic pressures between 70 and 100 mm Hg manifest the electrocardiographic criteria for right ventricular hypertrophy, including both a mean QRS axis that is greater than 80 degrees in the frontal plane and an R : S ratio greater than 1.0 in V_1.[75] In other patients with this degree of pulmonary hypertension there is no frank evidence of right ventricular hypertrophy, but the R : S ratio fails to increase from right to midprecordial leads. When right ventricular systolic pressures exceed 100 mm Hg, electrocardiographic evidence of right ventricular hypertrophy is found quite consistently. The mean QRS axis averages +150 degrees, and there is a Q-R morphology in the right precordial leads, accompanied by inverted or biphasic T waves.[76]

The *QRS axis in the frontal plane* often correlates with the severity of valve obstruction and with the level of pulmonary vascular resistance in pure MS; thus, a mean frontal axis between 0 and +60 degrees suggests that the mitral valve area exceeds 1.3 cm^2, whereas an axis greater than 60 degrees suggests that the valve area is less than 1.3 cm^2. In patients in whom pulmonary vascular resistance is greater than 650 dynes·sec·cm^{-5}, the mean axis usually exceeds +110 degrees.[75]

VECTORCARDIOGRAPHY. The characteristic *vectorcardiographic finding* in MS is right ventricular hypertrophy Type C (Fig. 5–15, p. 128) characterized by counterclockwise rotation in the horizontal plane and a terminal deflection directed to the right, posteriorly, and superiorly.[71,75–77] In other patients with MS without frank right ventricular hypertrophy, QRS loops with posterior and rightward terminal appendages are evident without conduction delays.[71,75] There is vectorcardiographic evidence of right ventricular hypertrophy Type A (Fig. 5–15, p. 128) in only 10 per cent of patients with MS, but when present it indicates that both the hypertrophy and the stenosis are severe. Vectorcardiograms showing right ventricular hypertrophy Type B (Fig. 5–15) are infrequent in MS.

Rotation of the P loop in the frontal plane, with superior orientation of the terminal P forces and a wide angle between the initial and terminal P vectors, occurs in about one-fourth of patients with pure mitral stenosis and may be the only evidence of left atrial enlargement.[78] The terminal portion of the P loop is usually directed posteriorly and inferiorly, and the T loop is often directed leftward and posterosuperiorly and is discordant with respect to the QRS loop, resulting in a diphasic T wave with initial negativity and terminal positivity in lead V_1.

RADIOLOGICAL FINDINGS (see also p. 223). Although the cardiac silhouette may be normal in the frontal projection, with the exception of an enlarged atrial appendage (Fig. 8–35, p. 224) in patients with hemodynamically significant MS, left atrial enlargement is almost invariably evident on the lateral and left anterior oblique views.[79,80] The size of the left atrium does *not* correlate with the severity of obstruction. However, extreme left atrial enlargement rarely occurs in pure MS; when it is present, MR is usually severe. Enlargement of the pulmonary artery, right ventricle, and right atrium (as well as the left atrium) is commonly seen in severe MS (Fig. 8–34, p. 224). Occasionally, calcification of the mitral valve is evident on the chest roentgenogram (Fig. 8–30, p. 221), but, more commonly, fluoroscopy is required to detect valvular calcification.

Radiological changes in the lung fields (Fig. 8–34, p. 224) are useful in estimating the height of pulmonary venous pressure and thereby the severity of MS. Interstitial edema, an indication of severe obstruction, is manifested as Kerley B lines (dense, short, horizontal lines most commonly seen in the costophrenic angles).[81] This finding is present in 30 per cent of patients with resting pulmonary artery wedge pressures below 20 mm Hg and in 70 per cent of patients with pressures exceeding 20 mm Hg. Severe, longstanding mitral obstruction often results in Kerley A lines (straight, dense lines up to 4 cm in length and running toward the hilum) as well as the findings of pulmonary hemosiderosis[82] (Fig. 8–34*B*, p. 224) and rarely of parenchymal ossification.

Angiography. Angiograms exposed in the right and left anterior oblique projections afford the best views of the mitral valve.[83] Although ideally contrast medium should be injected into the left atrium, it is often possible to achieve good visualization of the left side of the heart by injecting a large volume of contrast medium into the main pulmonary artery. Such angiograms provide an assessment of left atrial size, may demonstrate thickening and reduced motion of the valve leaflets, and may outline large intraluminal thrombi.[84] Left cine ventriculography is useful in the assessment of mitral valve motion. Although this technique allows visualization of only the ventricular aspect of the leaflet in patients with pure MS, it makes possible simultaneous assessment of left ventricular contractile function and of the subvalvular mitral apparatus.

ECHOCARDIOGRAPHY (see also p. 81). MS can ordinarily be readily diagnosed by M-mode echocardiography (Fig. 4–44, p. 82), but this technique does not allow a precise determination of its severity. Echocardiograms of a thickened, calcified stenotic rheumatic valve demonstrate increased acoustic impedance and fusion of the mitral valve leaflets and poor leaflet separation in diastole.[85,86] The leaflets fail to close in mid-diastole and may not reopen widely during atrial contraction. Normally, the posterior leaflet of the mitral valve moves posteriorly during early diastole, but in more than 90 per cent of patients with MS, both leaflets move anteriorly at this time (Fig. 34–5, *top*) and there is inadequate separation of the leaflets. The E–F slope is reduced,[87] but this finding is not

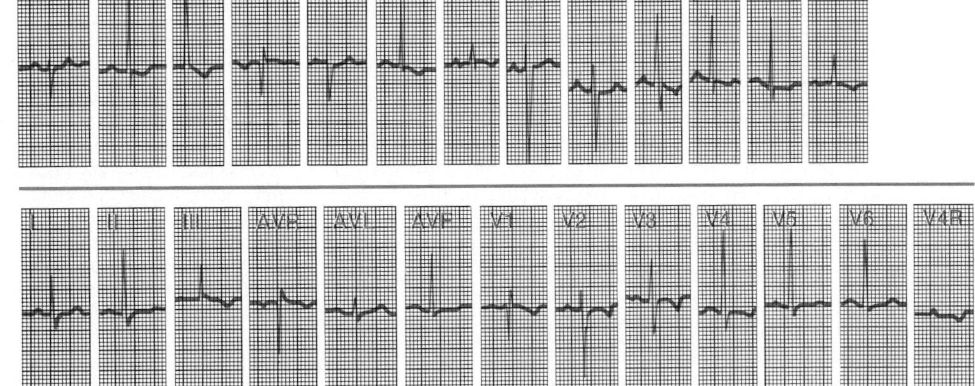

FIGURE 34–4. ***Upper tracing,*** **ECG of a patient with tight mitral stenosis, pulmonary hypertension, right atrial enlargement, right axis deviation, and right ventricular hypertrophy.** ***Lower tracing,*** **Six months after commissurotomy, the signs of right ventricular hypertrophy have regressed. (From Barlow, J. B.: Perspectives on the Mitral Valve. Philadelphia, F. A. Davis, 1987, p. 169.)**

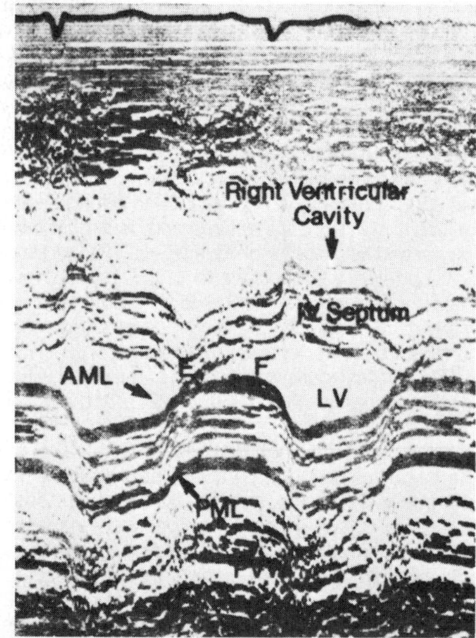

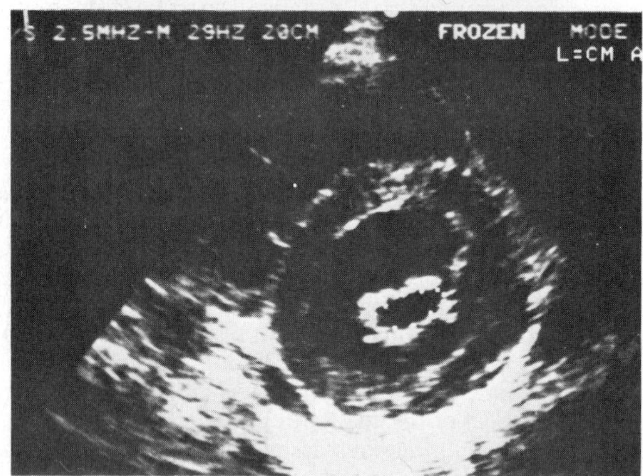

FIGURE 34–5. *Top,* M-mode echocardiogram of a patient with mitral stenosis. Note the decreased E-F slope, absence of the A wave, and thickened leaflets. The posterior mitral leaflet (PML) moves in an anterior direction with the anterior mitral leaflet (AML) during diastole. IV = interventricular septum, LV = left ventricle, PVW = posterior ventricular wall. (From Dalen, J. E.: Mitral stenosis. *In* Dalen, J. E., and Alpert, J. S. [eds.]: Valvular Heart Disease. 2nd ed. Boston, Little, Brown and Company, 1987, p. 73.) *Bottom,* Two-dimensional parasternal short-axis view of the mitral valve orifice during diastole, demonstrating the echocardiographic method of mitral valve area calculation. The innermost border of the mitral orifice was planimetered with the use of a light-pen system to obtain the area (in cm^2). (From Smith, M. D., et al.: Comparative accuracy of two-dimensional echocardiography and Doppler pressure half-time methods in assessing severity of mitral stenosis in patients with and without prior commissurotomy. Circulation *73*:100, 1986, by permission of the American Heart Association, Inc.)

pathognomonic of MS, since it may occur in other conditions in which left ventricular compliance and the velocity of left ventricular filling are reduced. However, in these other conditions the posterior leaflet of the mitral valve moves normally. The maximal diastolic separation of the anterior and posterior leaflets,[88] their rate of diastolic apposition, and the slope of motion of the left ventricular posterior wall during diastole appear to correlate more closely with the mitral valve area.[87,88] Two-dimensional echocardiography (Fig. 34–5, *bottom*, and Fig. 4–45, p. 82) is more accurate than M-mode echocardiography in determining mitral orifice size.[89–91] It reveals restricted motion and doming of the valve leaflets. The orifice can often be imaged directly and measured. This technique also provides information on the pliability and extent of calcification of the valve and its suitability for balloon mitral valvuloplasty (p. 1017).

Other important echocardiographic findings in patients with pulmonary hypertension and MS include a small or absent *a* wave in the pulmonic valve echogram (Fig. 4–42, p. 81). The left atrium is usually enlarged, and in isolated MS the left ventricular cavity is normal or reduced in size. Echocardiography is also useful in detecting mitral annular calcification, which may accompany MS and in which a band of dense echoes is present in the region of the mitral annulus, in contrast to the thin and delicate echoes recorded from the normal mitral annulus. The technique is helpful in the estimation of pulmonary artery pressure. Two-dimensional echocardiography may be helpful in the preoperative recognition of left atrial thrombus[92] in assessing mitral valve calcification and left ventricular contractility.

Doppler echocardiography is especially useful in quantifying the severity of MS[91,93] (Fig. 4–46, p. 82). The peak velocity of transmitral flow is increased, and the rate of decline of flow during early diastole is reduced. The time required for peak velocity to reach half its initial level correlates with the size of the mitral orifice. Doppler color flow imaging can be used to enhance the accuracy of the Doppler data by guiding the position of the beam[94] and to determine whether mitral regurgitation and other valvular abnormalities coexist. A detailed echocardiographic examination in a patient with MS can frequently provide sufficient information to allow development of a therapeutic plan without the need for invasive cardiac catheterization.

MANAGEMENT

MEDICAL TREATMENT

Patients with rheumatic heart disease should receive penicillin prophylaxis for beta-hemolytic streptococcal infections and prophylaxis for infective endocarditis (p. 1090). Anemia and infections should be treated promptly and aggressively in patients with valvular heart disease. Adolescents and young adults with serious valvular heart disease should be advised to avoid entering occupations requiring strenuous exertion.

In symptomatic patients with mitral valve disease, considerable improvement occurs with oral diuretics and the restriction of sodium intake. Digitalis glycosides do not alter the hemodynamics and usually do not benefit patients with MS and sinus rhythm[86,95] but are of great value in slowing the ventricular rate in patients with atrial fibrillation and in the treatment of right-sided heart failure. Measures designed to reduce pulmonary venous pressure, including sedation, assumption of the upright posture, and aggressive diuresis, are used to treat hemoptysis. Beta blockers may increase exercise capacity by reducing heart rate, even in patients with sinus rhythm.[96]

In patients with rheumatic heart disease and heart failure and/or atrial fibrillation, anticoagulant therapy is helpful in preventing venous thrombosis and pulmonary embolism in those who have experienced one or more previous embolic episodes, in those who are at high risk of embolization, i.e., with atrial fibrillation, and in those with mechanical prosthetic heart valves. However, no firm evidence exists that anticoagulant therapy reduces the incidence of pulmonary or systemic embolism in patients in sinus rhythm in whom such episodes have not previously occurred.

TREATMENT OF ARRHYTHMIAS. Frequent premature atrial contractions often presage atrial fibrillation, and the administration of antiarrhythmic drugs, as outlined on page 628, may be effective in preventing this complication. However, once atrial fibrillation has developed, these agents may be ineffective in restoring sinus rhythm or even in maintaining sinus rhythm following electrical cardioversion, because of the pathological changes that occur in the atrium secondary to the arrhythmia itself. After electrical cardioversion, sinus rhythm can often be maintained with antiarrhythmic drugs in young patients with mild MS without marked left atrial enlargement who have been in atrial fibrillation less than 6 months and who are maintained by adequate doses of quinidine. In any event, if elective cardioversion (pharmacological or electrical) is to be attempted in the patient with MS and atrial fibrillation, a preparatory three-week course of anticoagulation should be given to minimize the risk of systemic embolism when sinus rhythm resumes. Immediate treatment of atrial fibrillation should be directed toward reducing the ventricular rate by means of digitalis and, if possible, toward reestablishing sinus rhythm by a combination of pharmacological treatment and cardioversion. However, it must be appreciated that in 1 to 2 per cent of patients with MS, systemic embolism develops following electrical or pharmacological cardioversion. Paroxysmal atrial fibrillation and repeated conversions, spontaneous or induced, carry the risk of embolization.[97] In patients who cannot be converted or maintained in sinus rhythm, the ventricular rate at rest should be maintained at approximately 60 to 65 beats/min with digitalis. If this is not possible, small doses of a beta blocker, such as atenolol (25 mg daily), may be added. Multiple repeat cardioversions are not indicated if the patient has not sustained sinus rhythm while on adequate doses of quinidine.

NATURAL HISTORY

The development of effective surgical treatment has obscured our understanding of the natural history of MS (Fig. 34-6) and, for that matter, of all valvular lesions.[98] Although few meaningful data are available, it appears that in temperate zones such as the United States and Europe, after an asymptomatic period of 20 to 25 years following an attack of rheumatic fever, it takes approximately 5 years for most patients to progress from mild disability (i.e., early Class II) to severe disability (i.e., Class III or IV). The progression is much more rapid in patients in subtropical areas such as Pakistan, the Middle East, Central America, and the Philippines.[99] Polynesians, as well as Eskimos in Alaska and blacks in Alabama, also show an accelerated course. Economic conditions as well as genetic ones may play a role. In the presurgical era, Olesen found 62 per cent 5-year and 38 per cent 10-year survival rates among patients in New York Heart Association functional Class III but only 15 per cent 5-year survival rate in patients in Class IV.[100] Among asymptomatic patients (Class I) with MS treated medically, 40 per cent had a worsened course or had died within 10 years. Among mildly symptomatic patients (Class II), the comparable number was 80 per cent.[101] In medically treated patients with MS or with combined MS and MR, Munoz et al. found a 45 per cent 5-year survival rate.[44] In a comparable group of patients subjected to mitral commissurotomy, the 5-year survival rate was substantially better. In an unselected mix of patients with MS of varying severity, 80 per cent were alive after 5 years and 60 per cent after 10 years of medical treatment.[102]

SURGICAL TREATMENT

INDICATIONS FOR OPERATION. Patients with MS who are asymptomatic or minimally symptomatic frequently re-

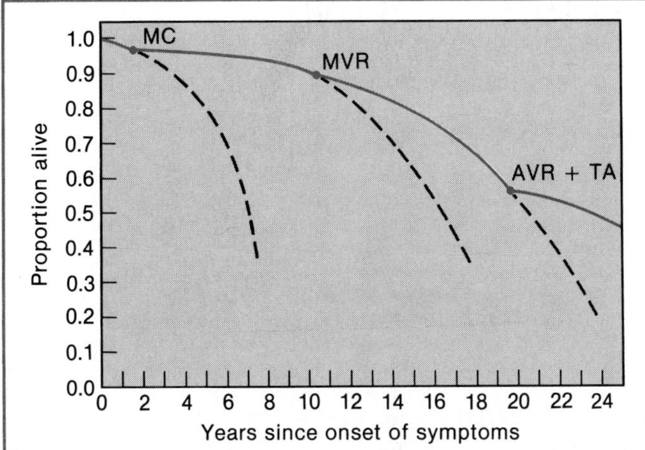

FIGURE 34-6. Schematic representation of the subsequent life history after the initial development of symptoms in a large group of patients with mitral stenosis. The red solid circles and red lines indicate a surgical procedure. The dashed lines represent estimated survival of patients not receiving the surgical procedure. MC = mitral commissurotomy, MVR = mitral valve replacement, TA = tricuspid annuloplasty, AVR = aortic valve replacement. (From Kirklin, J. W., and Barratt-Boyes, B. G.: Cardiac Surgery. New York, John Wiley and Sons, 1986, p. 328.)

main so for years. However, once severe symptoms develop, if the stenosis is not relieved mechanically, the disease may progress relatively rapidly, as already discussed. Operation (or balloon valvuloplasty) should therefore be carried out in symptomatic patients with moderate to severe MS (i.e., a mitral valve orifice size less than approximately 1.0 cm^2/m^2 body surface area [BSA]).

There has been considerable debate concerning the need for routine cardiac catheterization in determining whether operation is indicated.[103-105] A careful clinical evaluation and noninvasive assessment, particularly using two-dimensional and Doppler echocardiography, can provide sufficient information to permit an informed decision in the majority of patients. However, the consequences of valvular surgery, particularly valve replacement, are so profound that I recommend preoperative catheterization and angiography in the following groups of patients with MS: (1) patients with heart murmurs and other findings suggesting the presence of valve lesions in addition to MS, (2) patients with associated chronic obstructive pulmonary disease, (3) patients in whom left atrial myxoma should be excluded, and (4) patients who have angina or angina-like chest pain or who have risk factors for coronary artery disease in whom associated coronary artery disease must be excluded. Critical narrowing of one or more coronary vessels occurs in approximately one-fourth of all adults with severe MS. It is more common in men over 45 years who have angina and risk factors for coronary artery disease.[35,106,107] I believe that preoperative catheterization can be omitted in the young (<40 years) patient without angina who has typical symptoms and classic findings of pure, severe MS on physical examination and by noninvasive tests, including two-dimensional and Doppler echocardiography.

Care of mildly symptomatic patients (Class II) must be individualized. It is necessary to consider and balance three important factors: (1) the size of the mitral orifice, (2) the degree to which the patient's life style is impaired by the mitral obstruction, (3) the risk of the procedure (operation or balloon valvuloplasty), and (4) the history of complications, particularly systemic embolism. If there are no obvious contraindications to one of these procedures, left heart catheterization should be performed to determine the size of the valve orifice. In general, mechanical relief of obstruction can be deferred in patients with mild symptoms and mild stenosis (i.e., mitral valve orifice size > approximately 1.0 cm^2/m^2 BSA), whereas it should be recommended for those with mild symptoms and more severe stenosis (i.e., mitral valve orifice size < approximately 1.0 cm^2/m^2 BSA). However, this plan is subject to qualification. For instance, mechanical relief of obstruction might well be deferred in a retired, sedentary woman in her seventies and a mitral valve orifice of 0.8 cm^2/m^2 BSA. On the other hand, a 25-year-old laborer whose family's economic well-being depends on his continued physical exertion might be an excellent candidate for mechanical relief of obstruction, although his mitral valve orifice size is 1.2 cm^2/m^2 BSA.

Because of the high rate of recurrence, operation is also indicated in patients with MS in whom systemic embolism has previously occurred, even if they are otherwise asymptomatic and even though there is no definitive evidence that the incidence of recurrent emboli will be significantly reduced. Anticoagulants should be administered up to the time of operation. Although the risk of operation is higher in patients with advanced disease characterized by severe pulmonary hypertension and right-sided heart failure, surviving patients nearly always show striking clinical and hemodynamic improvement, with a marked reduction in pulmonary vascular pressures. In the pregnant patient with MS, operative treatment should be carried out only if serious pulmonary congestion occurs despite intensive medical treatment including bed rest (p. 1796).

There is no evidence that surgical treatment improves the prognosis of patients with no or only slight functional impairment. Therefore, valvulotomy is *not* indicated in patients who are entirely asymptomatic, except in unusual circumstances.

For example, some years ago I saw a 33-year-old woman with MS who had had hemoptysis and pulmonary edema during the second trimester of a pregnancy 2 years previously. She then became asymptomatic but wished to have another child. Hemodynamic study showed a pulmonary wedge pressure of 17 mm Hg and a mitral orifice area of 1.7 cm^2/m^2 BSA. Prophylactic mitral commissurotomy was undertaken in this patient, since it was virtually certain that another pregnancy would have resulted in serious heart failure. At present I would recommend balloon mitral valvuloplasty (p. 1376) for such a patient.

SURGICAL TECHNIQUES. Three basically different operative approaches are available for the treatment of rheumatic MS (Fig. 34–7): (1) closed mitral valvotomy[108,109]; (2) open commissurotomy, i.e., commissurotomy carried out under direct vision with the aid of cardiopulmonary bypass; and (3) mitral valve replacement.[110] *Closed mitral commissurotomy*, performed with the aid of a transventricular dilator, is generally preferred to simple transatrial finger fracture.[108–110] It is an effective operation, provided that MR, atrial thrombosis, or valvular calcification is not serious and that chordal fusion and shortening are not severe. Unfortunately, few patients satisfy all these criteria, and they are difficult to identify preoperatively. In one large series,[108] hospital mortality was 1.5 per cent and 0.3 per cent of patients developed severe MR. Marked symptomatic improvement occurred in 86 per cent of survivors. Actuarial survival rate was 89.5 per cent after 18 years. Closed valvotomy for restenosis was carried out with a 6.7 per cent mortality. Long-term follow-up has shown that the results are best if the operation is carried out before chronic atrial fibrillation and/or heart failure have occurred.[109] Therefore, if possible, closed mitral commissurotomy should be carried out with "pump standby"; if the surgeon is unable to achieve a satisfactory result, the patient can be placed on cardiopulmonary bypass, and the commissurotomy carried out under direct vision. Closed mitral commissurotomy is rarely used in the United States today, but is more popular in developing nations, where the expense of open-heart surgery is a more important factor and where patients with mitral valve disease are younger. In any event, echocardiography is useful in selecting suitable candidates for closed mitral valvulotomy by identifying patients without valvular calcification or dense fibrosis.[111]

Most surgeons in the United States, Canada, and Western Europe now prefer to carry out *direct-vision* or *open commissurotomy*.[110–115] Cardiopulmonary bypass is established, and in order to obtain a dry, quiet heart, body temperature is usually lowered, the heart is arrested, and the aorta is occluded intermittently. Thrombi are removed from the left atrium and its appendage, and the latter is often amputated in order to remove a potential source of postoperative emboli. The commissures are incised, and when necessary fused chordae are separated, the underlying papillary muscle is split, and the valves are debrided of calcium; mild or even moderate mitral regurgitation may be corrected with suture plication or annuloplasty. Left atrial and ventricular pressures are measured after bypass has been discontinued to confirm that the commissurotomy has in fact been effective. In patients with atrial fibrillation, conversion to sinus rhythm is carried out at the completion of the operation. In a series of open mitral valve reconstructive procedures for MS at Brigham and Women's Hospital, the actuarial probability of survival at 10 years was 95 per cent; thromboemboli occurred in 9 of 120 patients. The annual reoperation rate was 1.7 per cent.[116]

The mortality rate after mitral commissurotomy, whether open or closed, ranges from 1 to 3 per cent, depending on the condition of the patient and the skill and experience of the surgical team.[113–116] In general, open commissurotomy provides better hemodynamic relief of mitral valve obstruction than does the closed procedure,[115,117] and the risk of dislodging thrombi from the atrium or calcium from the mitral valve is also less.[113,116] Left atrial size, the need for mitral or tricuspid annuloplasty, and the presence of left atrial thrombus are all "risk factors" for a less than optimal outcome.[117] However, it must be recognized that mitral commissurotomy, whether open or closed, is a *palliative* rather than a curative operation, and even when successful, it merely "turns the clock back." (The generally more effective open valvulotomy turns the clock farther backward than does the closed valvulotomy or balloon mitral valvuloplasty.) Thus, valvulotomy does not result in a normal mitral valve but, at best, results in one resembling the valve as it existed perhaps a decade earlier. Since the valve is not normal postoperatively, turbulent flow usually persists in the paravalvular region, and the resultant trauma may well play a role in restenosis. These changes are analogous to the gradual development of obstruction in a congenitally bicuspid aortic valve (p. 967) and are not usually the result of recurrent rheumatic fever.

Mitral valve replacement is discussed on pages 1027 and 1042.

Although a contemporary control series of medically and surgically treated patients is not available (nor is it likely that it ever will be), appropriate surgical treatment appears to prolong survival substantially in patients with MS (Fig. 34–6).

Mitral Restenosis. This condition can be diagnosed with certainty only on the basis of three satisfactory hemodynamic or echocardiographic investigations: a preoperative study, a second study following a satisfactory operation in which an increase in the size of the valvular orifice can be demonstrated, and a third after the reappearance of symptoms, when a reduction in size relative to the earlier postoperative study is noted. On clinical grounds alone, the incidence of "restenosis" has been estimated to range widely, from 2 to 60 per cent[118]; approximately 10 per cent of patients who have undergone mitral commissurotomy require reoperation within 5

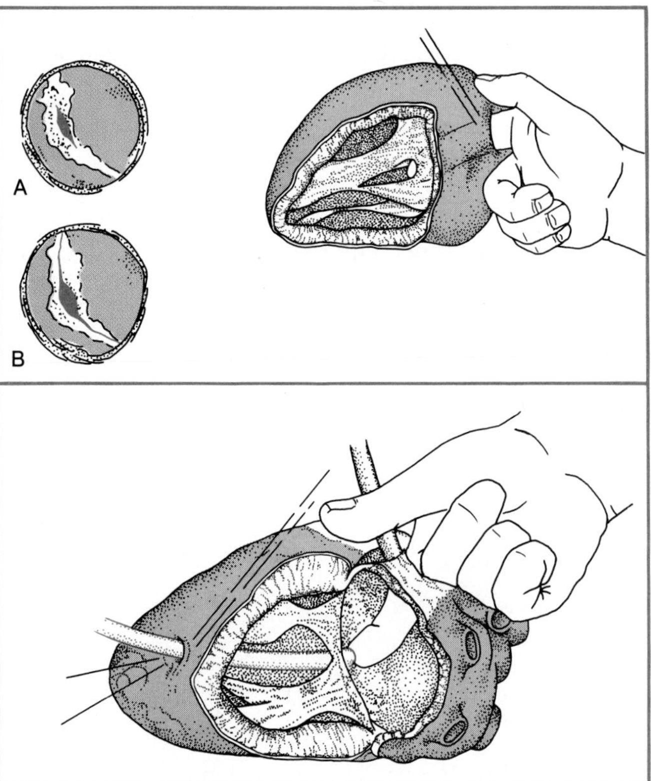

FIGURE 34–7. *Top*, Closed digital mitral commissurotomy. Mitral valve before (A) and after (B) valvotomy. *Bottom*, Transventricular closed mitral commissurotomy. Finger of the surgeon's right hand in the left atrium. Tubbs dilator through the apex of the left ventricle in the ostium of the mitral valve. (From deVivie, E. R., and Hellberg, K.: Closed transventricular mitral commissurotomy. *In* Ionescu, M. I., and Cohn, L. H. [eds.]: Mitral Valve Disease: Diagnosis and Treatment. London, Butterworths, 1985, pp. 140–141.)

years, but that fraction increases to 60 per cent by 10 years.[119] The recurrence of symptoms is *not necessarily* due to restenosis. Recurrent symptoms may be due to one of four other conditions: (1) an inadequate first operation with residual stenosis; (2) the presence or development of MR, either at operation or as a consequence of infective endocarditis; (3) the progression of aortic valve disease; and (4) the development of ischemic heart disease. In a study in which the size of the mitral valve orifice was estimated using two-dimensional echocardiography in 18 patients who had undergone successful mitral commissurotomy, no change in the mitral valve area occurred over a 10- to 14-year period in 13 patients, whereas in 5 (28 per cent) true restenosis developed.[119] Approximately 10 per cent of patients returning to the hospital with persistent or recurrent symptoms 6 years after operation have true restenosis.[120]

Thus, in properly selected patients, mitral commissurotomy results in a significant increase in the size of the mitral orifice and, at a low risk, favorably alters the clinical course of an otherwise progressive disease. Pulmonary artery pressure falls promptly and decisively when mitral obstruction is effectively relieved.[121-124] Some patients maintain clinical improvement for many (10 to 15) years of follow-up. When a second operation is required because of symptomatic deterioration, the valve is usually calcified and more seriously deformed than at the time of the first operation, and adequate reconstruction is not always possible. Accordingly, mitral valve replacement is often necessary.[125] Also, in patients with combined MS and MR, and in those with extensive calcification involving the commissures of the valve, mitral replacement rather than commissurotomy is often required. The operative mortality following mitral valve replacement ranges from 3 to 8 per cent in most hospitals. As described below (p. 1062), the long-term fate of the prosthetic valves is not yet clear; also, the hazards of lifelong anticoagulant treatment in patients with mechanical prostheses cannot be neglected. Therefore, in patients in whom preoperative evaluation suggests that valve replacement may be required, the threshold for operation should be higher than in patients believed to require commissurotomy alone. If possible, a second conservative procedure, i.e., open commissurotomy, should be performed; in some instances this has led to excellent outcome.[126]

BALLOON MITRAL VALVULOPLASTY

(See also Chap. 41)

This procedure represents an alternative to surgical treatment of MS. The technique consists of advancing a small balloon flotation catheter across the interatrial septum (after transseptal puncture), enlarging the opening and advancing one large (23 to 25 mm) or two smaller (12 to 18 mm) balloons across the mitral orifice, and inflating them within the orifice[86,127-133] (Fig. 41-19, p. 1376). Commissural separation and fracture of nodular calcium appear to be the mechanisms responsible for improvement in valvular function. In several series the hemodynamic results have been quite favorable (Fig. 34-8), with reduction of the gradient from an average of approximately 18 to 6 mm Hg, a small (average 20 per cent) increase in cardiac output, and, on the average, a 50 to 100 per cent increase in the calculated mitral valve area. The reported mortality ranges from 0 to 4 per cent. Complications include embolic events (despite absence of detectable thrombus on two-dimensional echocardiography), cardiac perforation in 0 to 4 per cent, and the development of mitral regurgitation severe enough to require operation in another 2 per cent (approximately one-third of patients develop milder degrees of regurgitation). Results are especially impressive in younger patients without valvular thickening or calcification.[133a] Improvement in exercise tolerance has paralleled the favorable hemodynamic changes (Fig. 34-9).

Approximately 35 per cent of patients are left with a small residual atrial septal defect, but this closes or decreases in size in the majority. Rarely, the defect is large enough to cause right heart failure.[129,129a] Elevated pulmonary vascular resistance declines rapidly (but usually not completely) following mitral balloon valvuloplasty,[130,132] and pulmonary function improves as well.[131] In follow-up studies over 1 to 2 years, hemodynamic benefit has been maintained in the majority of patients, and they have not required surgical treatment, i.e., with commissurotomy or mitral valve replacement. Approximately 10 per cent have developed restenosis.

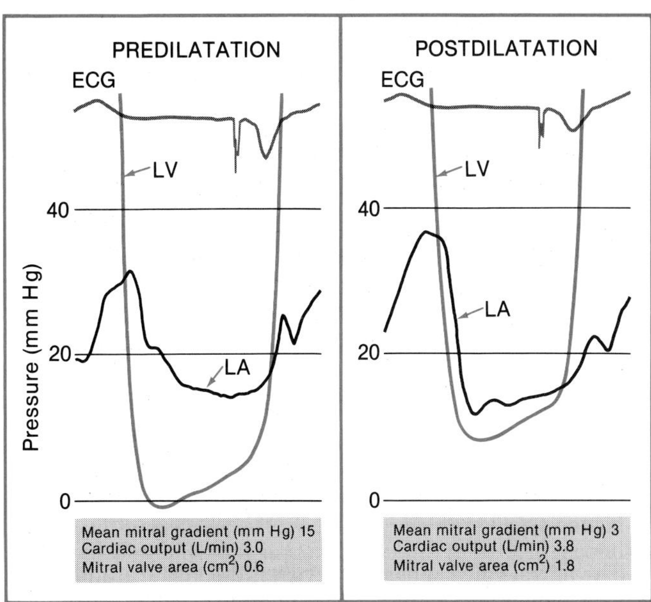

FIGURE 34-8. Simultaneous left atrial (LA) and left ventricular (LV) pressure before and after balloon valvuloplasty of the mitral valve in a patient with severe mitral stenosis. (Courtesy of Raymond G. McKay, M.D.)

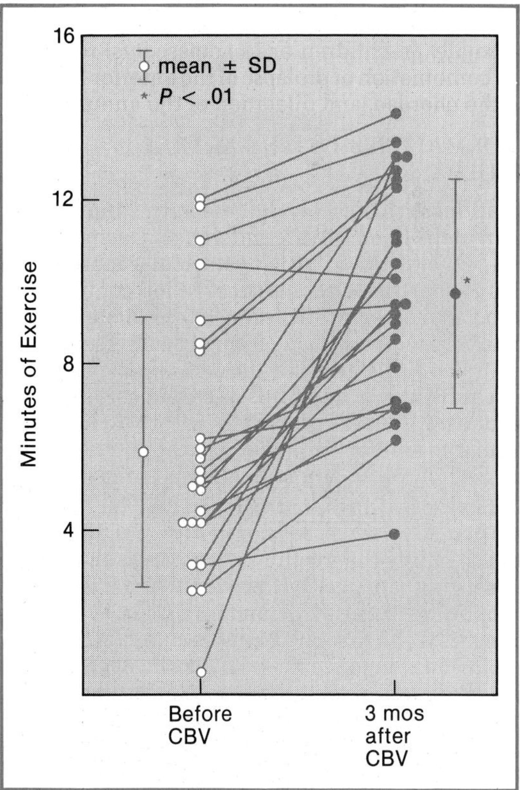

FIGURE 34-9. Exercise treadmill time (Bruce protocol) before and 3 months after catheter balloon valvuloplasty (CBV) in patients with mitral stenosis. (From McKay, C. R., et al.: Improvement in exercise capacity and exercise hemodynamics 3 months after double-balloon, catheter balloon valvuloplasty treatment of patients with symptomatic mitral stenosis. Circulation *77*:1013, 1988, by permission of the American Heart Association, Inc.)

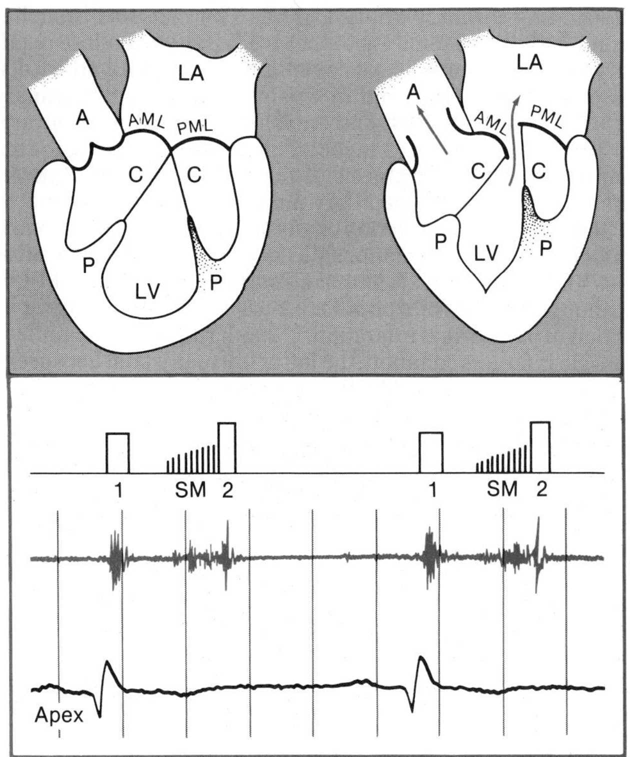

FIGURE 34–11. *Top,* Mitral regurgitation due to papillary muscle dysfunction. At the onset of systole (left), the anterior and posterior mitral valve leaflets (AML and PML) approximate. Later in systole (right), the anterior papillary muscle (P, nonhatched) contracts while the posterior papillary muscle (P, hatched) fails to contract because of ischemia or infarction. Part of the posterior leaflet is allowed to prolapse into the left atrium (LA) during systole, producing regurgitation. This process may involve either papillary muscle. C = chordae tendineae, LV = left ventricle, A = aorta. *Bottom,* Late systolic murmur (SM) that developed in a patient following an inferior myocardial infarction and is probably due to weakening of the posterior papillary muscle with prolapse of the mitral leaflet into the atrium during late systole. (From Ravin, A., et al.: Auscultation of the Heart. 3rd ed. Chicago, Year Book Medical Publishers, 1977, p. 99. Copyright © 1977 by Year Book Medical Publishers, Inc., Chicago.)

domyocardial fibrosis,[163] trauma affecting the leaflets[164] and/or papillary muscles[165] (p. 1523), Kawasaki disease (p. 997),[166] left atrial myxoma (p. 1454), a variety of congenital anomalies including cleft anterior leaflet,[167] and ostium secundum atrial septal defect.[168]

PATHOPHYSIOLOGY

Since the regurgitant mitral orifice is in parallel with the aortic valve, the impedance to ventricular emptying is reduced in MR. Consequently, as the left ventricle decompresses into the left atrium—both during isometric contraction and early during ejection—the left ventricular volume declines. Almost half of the regurgitant volume is ejected into the left atrium before the aortic valve opens.[169] The volume of MR is dependent on the impedance to left ventricular emptying and is increased by aortic stenosis.

The volume of mitral regurgitant flow depends on a combination of the instantaneous size of the regurgitant orifice and the pressure gradient between the left ventricle and left atrium[170–174]; both of these factors—orifice size and pressure

TABLE 34-4 HELPFUL POINTS IN DIFFERENTIAL DIAGNOSIS OF MITRAL REGURGITATION, VENTRICULAR SEPTAL DEFECT, TRICUSPID REGURGITATION, AND AORTIC STENOSIS

PHYSICAL, ROENTGENOGRAPHIC, OR ELECTROCARDIOGRAPHIC FEATURE	MITRAL REGURGITATION	VENTRICULAR SEPTAL DEFECT	TRICUSPID REGURGITATION	AORTIC STENOSIS
Systolic murmur	Harsh and pansystolic	Harsh and pansystolic	Pansystolic	Ejection, crescendo-decrescendo
Primary location of murmur	Apex	Left sternal border	Left sternal border	Base of heart; occasionally apical
Radiation of murmur	Axilla; occasionally base and neck	Left precordium	Little	Carotids
Thrill	Occasionally present at apex	Usually present at left sternal border	Rare	Occasionally present at base
Murmur with inspiration	No change	No change	Increases	No change
Valsalva maneuver	May increase	Increases or no change	No change	Decreases
Venous pressure	Often normal	Slightly elevated with prominent A and V waves	Elevated, with very prominent V waves	Usually normal
Pulsatile liver	No	No	Yes	No
Pulmonary component of S_2	Normal; occasionally increased	Normal or loud; usually delayed	Usually increased	Normal
Apical impulse	Hyperkinetic; occasional heaving	Hyperkinetic	Weak or normal	Forceful and sustained
ECG	Left ventricular hypertrophy; left atrial hypertrophy	Biventricular hypertrophy (Katz-Wachtel phenomenonon)	Right ventricular hypertrophy, occasional right atrial hypertrophy	Left ventricular hypertrophy with associated ST-T changes
Chest roentgenogram	Moderately enlarged heart, marked left atrial enlargement	Enlarged left and right ventricle	Enlarged right ventricle	Often normal heart size or left ventricular hypertrophy

From Haffajee, C. I.: Chronic mitral regurgitation. *In* Dalen, J. E., and Alpert, J. S.: Valvular Heart Disease. 2nd ed. Boston, Little, Brown and Company, 1987, p. 141.

gradient—are labile. Left ventricular systolic pressure and therefore the left ventricular–left atrial gradient are dependent on systemic vascular resistance and forward stroke volume,[170] and in patients in whom the mitral annulus is not calcific or rigid, the cross-sectional area of the mitral annulus may be altered by many interventions. Thus, increases of both preload and afterload and depressions of contractility increase left ventricular size and enlarge the mitral annulus and thereby the regurgitant orifice.[174] In MR caused by conditions in which the mitral valve apparatus is not rigid, such as ventricular dilatation due to ischemic heart disease, hypertensive heart disease or cardiomyopathy, dysfunction of papillary muscles, and rupture of chordae tendineae, the volume of regurgitant flow is influenced significantly by left ventricular dimensions, which in turn affect the regurgitant orifice. When ventricular size is reduced by treatment with positive inotropic agents, diuretics, and particularly vasodilators, the volume of regurgitant flow may become diminished, as reflected in the height of the *v* wave in the left atrial pressure pulse and in the intensity and duration of the systolic murmur. Conversely, left ventricular dilatation may increase MR.

In experiments in which the acute effects of equally severe MR and aortic regurgitation (AR) on the left ventricle were compared, left ventricular end-diastolic pressure, volume, and radius rose with both lesions, but far *less* so with MR.[175,176] Peak left ventricular wall tension rose markedly when AR was induced but either did not change greatly or actually declined with MR. According to Laplace's law (p. 377), myocardial wall tension is related to the product of intraventricular pressure and ventricular radius. Since acute MR reduces both late systolic ventricular pressure and radius, left ventricular wall tension declines markedly (and proportionately to a greater extent than left ventricular pressure), permitting the velocity of myocardial fiber shortening to increase. The ratio of wall thickness (h) to ventricular radius (r) is lower and the fractional shortening of myocardium greater in patients with MR than AR.[177,178]

At any given left ventricular end-diastolic and aortic systolic pressures, *acute* MR enhances early diastolic filling of the left ventricle[179] and reduces the tension developed by the left ventricular myocardium. The reduced load on the ventricle allows a greater proportion of the contractile energy of the myocardium to be expended in shortening than in tension development and explains how the left ventricle can adapt to the load imposed by MR. Thus, the reduction in left ventricular tension in *acute* MR may allow the left ventricle to increase its total output. Although the left ventricle initially compensates for the development of acute MR (in part by emptying more completely),[176,177] as regurgitation persists, the left ventricular end-diastolic volume increases. This may increase wall tension to normal or supranormal levels.[179,180] Then, an increase in left ventricular volume and mitral annulus diameter may create a vicious circle in which "MR begets more MR."[181]

A large volume of MR induced experimentally produces only slightly increased myocardial oxygen consumption,[182] because myocardial fiber shortening, which is elevated in MR, is not one of the principal determinants of myocardial oxygen consumption.[183] One of these, mean left ventricular wall tension, may actually be reduced in MR whereas the other two, contractility and heart rate, are little affected. In addition, the duration of left ventricular systolic tension is reduced in MR. These experimental observations correlate with the low incidence of clinical manifestations of myocardial ischemia in patients with severe MR compared with that occurring in aortic stenosis or aortic regurgitation, conditions in which myocardial oxygen demands are augmented.

In patients with chronic MR, both left ventricular end-diastolic volume and mass are increased; i.e., typical volume overload (eccentric) hypertrophy develops. The degree of hypertrophy is appropriate to the left ventricular dilatation, so that the ratio of left ventricular mass to end-diastolic volume is normal. In acute MR the left ventricle at first dilates rapidly. Before the myocardium becomes hypertrophied, the ratio of left ventricular mass to end-diastolic volume is reduced; i.e., the left ventricle is thin-walled. A shift to the right occurs in the left ventricular diastolic pressure-volume curve with chronic MR (Fig. 34–12).[183a]

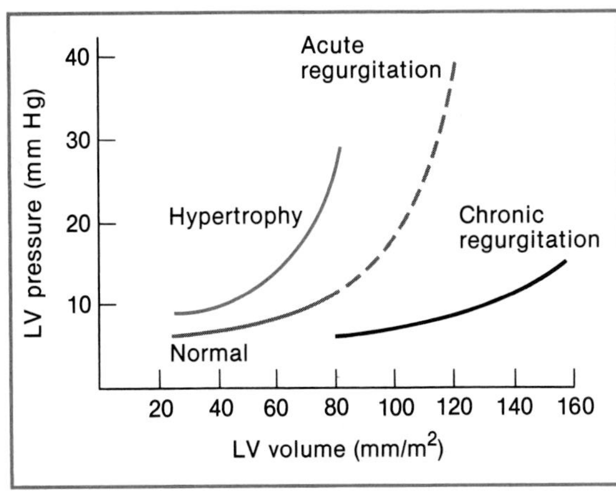

FIGURE 34–12. Diagrammatic representation of the changes in the diastolic pressure-volume relationship that occur in valve disease. Hypertrophy without significant ventricular dilatation (e.g., in aortic stenosis) produces a somewhat steeper curve than normal. Acute regurgitation produces a sudden volume load on the ventricle without time for other changes to occur and the ventricle operates at the upper (steep) end of the normal curve (broken line). Chronic aortic and mitral regurgitation with volume overload produces a flattened curve so that large volumes are accommodated without the large rise in end-diastolic pressure which occurs in acute regurgitation. (From Hall, R. J., and Julian, D. G.: Diseases of the Cardiac Valves. New York, Churchill Livingstone, 1989, p. 291.)

ASSESSMENT OF MYOCARDIAL CONTRACTILITY IN MITRAL REGURGITATION (see also p. 434)

Patients with severe MR often exhibit small elevations in ejection phase indices of myocardial contractility, such as ejection fraction (EF), fractional fiber shortening (FS), and velocity of circumferential fiber shortening (VCF) when they are in the compensated state as a consequence of reduced afterload.[184] However, by the time patients become seriously symptomatic, EF, FS, and mean VCF have usually declined to *normal* levels. As MR persists, the tendency for a low impedance leak, which usually increases myocardial shortening, is counteracted by the impairment of myocardial function characteristic of severe chronic diastolic overload. However, even in patients with overt heart failure secondary to MR, the EF and FS may be only slightly reduced.[179,180,184] Ejection phase indices of myocardial contractility are exquisitely sensitive to afterload, and wall tension (afterload) is dependent on preload (end-diastolic ventricular volume).[185,186] Therefore, *normal* values for the ejection phase indices of myocardial performance in patients with acute MR may actually reflect impaired myocardial function, whereas moderately reduced values (e.g., an ejection fraction of 40 to 50 per cent) generally signify severe, not moderate, impairment of contractility. An ejection fraction under 40 per cent in patients with severe MR usually represents advanced myocardial

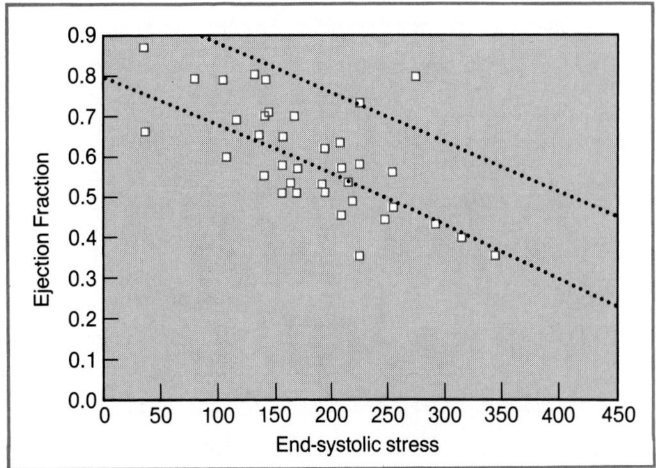

FIGURE 34–13. Ejection fraction–end-systolic stress (σ_{es}) relationships in 27 patients with MR (data points) versus the normal 95 per cent prediction (dashed lines). (From Wisenbach, T.: Does normal pump function belie muscle dysfunction in patients with chronic severe mitral regurgitation? Circulation *77*:515, 1988, by permission of the American Heart Association, Inc.)

dysfunction; such patients are high operative risks and may not experience marked improvement following mitral valve replacement.[187] Reduction of ejection fraction at any level of end-systolic stress is often found in MR and reflects impaired contractility (Fig. 34–13).

END-SYSTOLIC VOLUME. Preoperative myocardial contractility is an important determinant of the risk of operative death and of cardiac failure in the perioperative period and of the level of left ventricular function postoperatively. Therefore, it is not surprising that the end-systolic pressure (or stress/dimension) relation has emerged as a useful index for evaluating left ventricular function in patients with valvular regurgitation (p. 428).[188–190] Indeed, the simple measurement of end-systolic volume has been found to be more useful as a predictor of outcome than the ejection fraction, end-diastolic volume, or end-diastolic pressure.[191–193] Patients with severe MR with a normal preoperative end-systolic volume (<30 ml/m^2) retained normal left ventricular function postoperatively, whereas marked enlargement of the end-systolic volume (>90 ml/m^2) signified a high perioperative mortality and residual left ventricular dysfunction. Patients with MR and modest enlargement of end-systolic volume (between 30 and 90 ml/m^2) usually tolerate operation satisfactorily but may have reduced left ventricular function postoperatively. For any level of end-systolic volume, patients with MR have more severe left ventricular dysfunction than do patients with aortic regurgitation.[189] This finding reflects the lower afterload in MR and correlates with the clinical observation that patients with MR have a less favorable response to surgical intervention than do those with aortic regurgitation.[191]

HEMODYNAMICS. Effective (forward) *cardiac output* is usually depressed in seriously symptomatic patients, whereas total left ventricular output (the sum of forward and regurgitant flow, which can be measured by radionuclide ventriculography)[192] is usually elevated until quite late in the patient's course. The atrial contraction (*a*) wave in the left atrial pressure pulse is usually not as prominent in MR as in MS, but the *v* wave is often much taller[173] (Figs. 7–15, p. 196 and 7–17*A*, p. 201), since it is inscribed during ventricular systole, when the left atrium is filled with blood from the pulmonary veins as well as from the left ventricle (Fig. 34–14). Indeed, backward transmission of the tall *v* wave into the pulmonary arterial bed may result in an early diastolic "pulmonary arterial *v* wave."[194] In patients with pure MR, during early diastole, as the distended left atrium suddenly empties, the *y* descent is particularly rapid. However, in patients with combined MS and MR, the *y* descent is gradual. Although a left atrioventricular pressure gradient persisting throughout diastole signifies the presence of significant associated MS, a brief early diastolic gradient may occur in patients with pure severe regurgitation as a result of the torrential flow of blood across a normal-sized mitral orifice (Fig. 34–2).

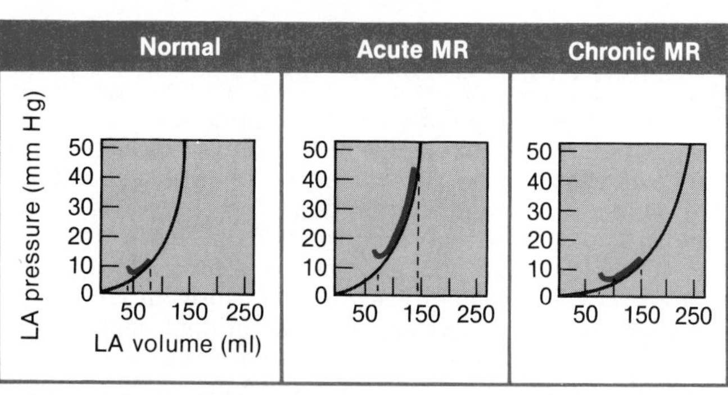

FIGURE 34–15. Schematic left atrial pressure-volume curves in a normal individual *(left),* a patient with acute mitral regurgitation *(center),* and a patient with chronic mitral regurgitation *(right).* The phasic increase in left atrial pressure and volume during left ventricular systole is indicated by the heavy trace superimposed on the left atrial pressure-volume curve. In the normal subject, there is an LA volume increase of 40 ml, due to return of blood from the pulmonary veins, during the period of time when the mitral valve is closed. This causes a peak *v* wave of 10 mm Hg. This valve acutely becomes insufficient *(center),* and the increase in LA volume during LV systole increases (in this example to 80 ml) because of the combination of the regurgitant volume and the pulmonary venous return, resulting in *v* waves to 45 mm Hg. In the same patient one year later *(right)* left atrial enlargement had occurred, so that the same degree of mitral regurgitation caused a much-reduced *v* wave because of increased left atrial compliance. (From Barry, W. H.: Invasive investigations for the diagnosis of mitral valve disease. *In* Ionescu, M. I., and Cohn, L. H. [eds.]: Mitral Valve Disease: Diagnosis and Treatment. London, Butterworths, 1985, p. 92.)

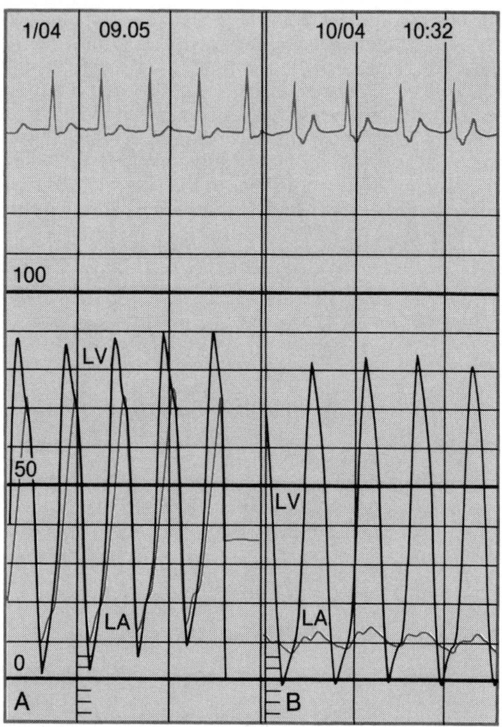

FIGURE 34–14. Intraoperative simultaneous left ventricular (LV) and left atrial (LA) pressures (mm Hg) before *(A)* and after *(B)* mitral valvuloplasty for correction of severe acute mitral regurgitation. Note the height of the *v* wave in the preoperative tracing. (From Barlow, J. B.: Perspectives on the Mitral Valve. Philadelphia, F. A. Davis, 1987, p. 257.)

LEFT ATRIAL COMPLIANCE. The compliance of the left atrium (and pulmonary venous bed) is an important determinant of the hemodynamic[193] and clinical picture in MR. Three major subgroups of patients with severe MR based on left atrial compliance have been identified[176,195,196] (Figs. 34–15 and 34–16) and are characterized as follows:

1. Normal or Reduced Compliance. There is little enlargement of the left atrium but marked elevation of the mean left atrial pressure, particularly of the *v* wave,[197–200] and pulmonary congestion is a prominent symptom. In most cases, severe MR has developed suddenly, as occurs with rupture of chordae tendineae, infarction of one of the heads of a papillary muscle, or perforation of a mitral leaflet as a consequence of trauma or endocarditis. Initially in acute MR the left atrium operates on the steep portion of the pressure-volume curve. Sinus rhythm is usually present; with the passage of weeks or a few months the left atrial wall frequently exhibits striking hypertrophy, is capable of contracting vigorously, and facilitates left ventricular filling.[193] Thickening of the walls of the pulmonary veins and proliferative changes in the pulmonary arteries as well as marked elevation of pulmonary vascular resistance usually develop over the course of 6 to 12 months.

2. Markedly Increased Compliance. At the opposite end of the spectrum from patients in the first group are those with severe, longstanding MR with massive enlargement of the left atrium and normal or only slightly elevated left atrial pressure. The atrial wall contains only a small remnant of muscle surrounded by a great deal of fibrous tissue. Longstanding MR in these patients has altered the physical properties of the left atrial wall and thereby displaced the atrial pressure-volume curve, allowing a normal or almost normal pressure to exist in a greatly enlarged left atrium. (This shift in the left atrial pressure-volume curve with persistent MR has been documented in animal experiments.[193]) Pulmonary artery pressure and

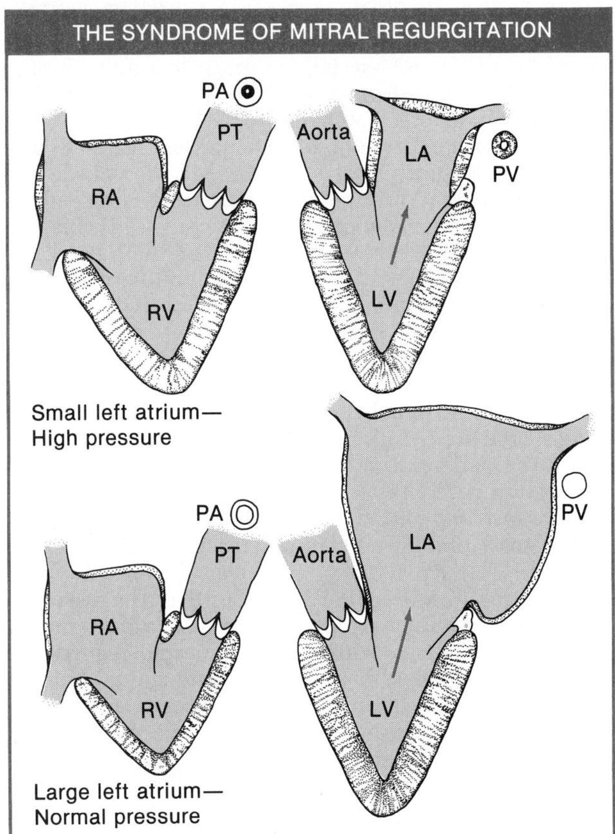

FIGURE 34-16. Diagram depicting the two extremes of the spectrum in pure mitral regurgitation. When severe mitral regurgitation appears suddenly in individuals with previously normal or near-normal hearts (*top*), the left atrium (LA) is relatively small and the high pressure within it is reflected back into the pulmonary vessels and right ventricle (RV). The anatomical indicator of this latter physiological event is severe hypertrophy of the left atrial and right ventricular walls and marked intimal proliferation and medial hypertrophy of the pulmonary arteries (PA), arterioles, and veins (PV). At the other extreme with severe chronic mitral regurgitation (*bottom*), the left atrial cavity is of giant size and its wall is thin. It is thus able to "absorb" the left ventricular (LV) pressure without reflecting it back into the pulmonary vessels or right ventricle. As a consequence, pulmonary vessels remain normal, and the right ventricular wall does not thicken. PT = pulmonary trunk; RA = right atrium. (From Roberts, W. C., et al.: Nonrheumatic valvular cardiac disease. A clinicopathologic survey of 27 different conditions causing valvular dysfunction. *In* Likoff, W. [ed.]: Cardiovascular Clinics. Vol. 5, No. 2, Valvular Heart Disease. Philadelphia, F. A. Davis, 1973, p. 403.)

pulmonary vascular resistance are normal or only slightly elevated at rest. Atrial fibrillation and a low cardiac output are almost invariably present.[195]

3. Moderately Increased Compliance. This, the most common subgroup, consists of patients between the ends of the spectrum represented by groups 1 and 2; these patients have severe chronic MR and exhibit variable degrees of enlargement of the left atrium, associated with significant elevation of the left atrial pressure.

CLINICAL MANIFESTATIONS

(See Table 34-1, p. 1010)

HISTORY

The nature and severity of the symptoms of patients with chronic MR are a function of the severity of regurgitation, its rate of progression, the level of pulmonary artery pressure, and the presence of associated valvular, myocardial, or coronary artery disease. Since symptoms usually do not develop in patients with chronic MR until the left ventricle fails, the time interval between the initial attack of rheumatic fever (when one has occurred) and the development of symptoms tends to be longer in MR than in MS and often exceeds 2 decades. Acute pulmonary edema occurs less frequently in chronic MR than in MS, presumably because sudden surges in left atrial pressure are less common.[20] Similarly, although hemoptysis and systemic embolization do occur in MR, they are less common than in MS. On the other hand, chronic weakness and fatigue secondary to a low cardiac output are more prominent features in MR.

Patients with mild MR may remain asymptomatic for their entire lives.[64] The majority of patients with MR of rheumatic origin have only mild disability, unless regurgitation progresses as a result of chronic rheumatic activity, infective endocarditis, or rupture of chordae tendineae.[196] The development of atrial fibrillation affects the course adversely but perhaps not as dramatically as it does in MS. The course in patients with chronic MR tends to be less dramatic and is punctuated with fewer acute complications than in patients with MS. However, this more indolent course may, in fact, be deceptive. By the time that symptoms secondary to a reduced cardiac output and/or pulmonary congestion become apparent, serious and sometimes even irreversible left ventricular dysfunction may have developed. In contrast, patients with MS have the benefit of an "early warning system," i.e., symptoms of pulmonary congestion with frequent, sudden elevations of left atrial pressure.

In patients with severe chronic MR with a greatly enlarged left atrium and with relatively mild left atrial hypertension (group 2 with increased left atrial compliance, already described), pulmonary vascular resistance does not usually rise appreciably. Instead, the major symptoms, fatigue and exhaustion, are related to a low cardiac output. However, right heart failure, characterized by congestive hepatomegaly, ankle edema, and ascites, is observed both in patients with longstanding severe MR and in patients with acute MR and elevated pulmonary vascular resistance. Angina pectoris is rare unless coronary artery disease coexists.

NATURAL HISTORY. This is variable and depends on a combination of the volume of regurgitation, the state of the myocardium, and the cause of the underlying disorder. The condition in asymptomatic patients with mild MR usually remains stable for many years[197]; severe regurgitation develops in only a small percentage of these, in some cases because of intervening infective endocarditis[196] or rupture of chordae tendineae or both. Regurgitation tends to progress more rapidly in patients with connective tissue diseases, such as Marfan syndrome, than in those with chronic MR on a rheumatic basis. Because the natural history of severe MR has been altered greatly by surgical intervention, it is difficult now to predict the course of patients on medical therapy alone. However, in an unselected group of patients with MR who were treated medically before surgical treatment of severe MR became commonplace, approximately 80 per cent survived 5 years after the diagnosis and almost 60 per cent survived 10 years.[102] Patients with combined MS and MR had a poorer prognosis, with only 67 per cent surviving 5 years and 30 per cent surviving 10 years after diagnosis. Munoz et al., in studying a group of patients with greater disability, found that medically treated patients with severe MR had a 5-year survival rate of only 45 per cent.[44] Among medically treated patients with MR, the arteriovenous oxygen difference and ventricular end-diastolic volume were significant (inverse) predictors of survival.[197]

PHYSICAL EXAMINATION

Palpation of the arterial pulse is helpful in differentiating aortic stenosis from MR; both may produce a prominent systolic murmur at the base of the heart. The carotid arterial upstroke is sharp in mitral regurgitation[201] and delayed in aortic stenosis; the volume of the pulse may be normal in both conditions or reduced in the presence of heart failure.

The cardiac impulse is brisk, hyperdynamic, and displaced to the left[20] (Table 2-1, p. 26; Fig. 2-18, p. 28), and a prominent left ventricular filling wave is frequently palpable in early diastole. Systolic expansion of the enlarged left atrium may result in a late systolic thrust in the parasternal region, which may be confused with right ventricular enlargement.[202]

AUSCULTATION.[203] With severe, chronic MR due to defective valve cusps, S_1, produced by valve closure, is usually diminished.[204] Wide splitting of S_2 is common and results from the shortening of left ventricular ejection and an earlier A_2 as a consequence of reduced resistance to left ventricular outflow. When pulmonary hypertension is present, P_2 is louder than A_2. The abnormal increase in the flow rate across the mitral orifice during the rapid filling phase is usually associated with an S_3, the auscultatory counterpart of a palpable rapid filling wave. A left ventricular S_3, i.e., one that is not augmented by inspiration, excludes predominant MS (unless aortic regurgitation, ischemic heart disease, or another cause of an S_3 is present).

The *systolic murmur* is the most prominent physical finding in MR; it must be differentiated from the systolic murmur heard in aortic stenosis, tricuspid regurgitation, ventricular septal defect, and sometimes MS (Table 34–4). In most cases of severe MR the systolic murmur commences immediately after the soft S_1 and continues beyond and may obscure A_2 because of the persistence of the pressure difference between the left ventricle and left atrium (Figs. 3–20 and 3–21, p. 53). The holosystolic murmur of chronic MR is usually constant in intensity, blowing, high-pitched, and loudest at the apex with radiation to the axilla and left infrascapular area; however, radiation toward the sternum or the aortic area may ocur with abnormalities of the posterior leaflet. The murmur shows little change even in the presence of large beat-to-beat variations of left ventricular stroke volume, as occur in atrial fibrillation, in contrast to most midsystolic (ejection) murmurs, such as in aortic stenosis, which vary greatly in intensity with stroke volume and therefore with the duration of diastole.[205] There is little correlation between the intensity of the systolic murmur and the severity of MR. Indeed, in patients with severe MR due to left ventricular dilatation, acute myocardial infarction, or paraprosthetic valvular regurgitation or in those who have marked emphysema, obesity, chest deformity, or a prosthetic heart valve, the systolic murmur may be barely audible or even absent, a condition referred to as "silent MR."

Pansystolic and late systolic murmurs (and pansystolic murmurs with late systolic accentuation) are characteristic of MR. When the murmur is confined to late systole, the regurgitation is usually mild and may be secondary to prolapse of the mitral valve or papillary muscle dysfunction, conditions that cause late systolic regurgitation. These causes of MR are frequently associated with a normal S_1 because initial closure of the mitral valve cusps may be unimpaired. The systolic murmur is usually of no more than Grade 3/6 intensity and is a mid- to late diamond-shaped murmur, or exhibits late systolic accentuation and radiates more frequently to the lower left sternal border than to the axilla.[155] The murmur of papillary muscle dysfunction is particularly variable; it may become accentuated or holosystolic during acute myocardial ischemia and often disappears when ischemia is relieved.[206] The response of a mid- to late-systolic murmur to a number of maneuvers, as described on page 1024, helps to establish the diagnosis of prolapse of the mitral valve.

Dynamic Auscultation (Table 2–8, p. 38; Fig. 2–20, p. 40). The holosystolic murmur of rheumatic MR shows little variation during respiration. However, sudden standing and amyl nitrite inhalation usually diminish the murmur (Table 34–5; Fig. 3–39, p. 62) whereas squatting and methoxamine or phenylephrine augment it. The murmur is reduced during the strain of the Valsalva maneuver and shows a left-sided response, i.e., a transient overshoot, six to eight beats following release. The murmur is usually intensified by isometric exercise, differentiating it from the systolic murmurs of valvular aortic stenosis and hypertrophic obstructive cardiomyopathy, both of which are reduced by this intervention. The murmur of MR due to left ventricular dilatation *decreases* in intensity and duration with effective therapy with cardiac glycosides, diuretics, rest, and particularly vasodilators.

The holosystolic murmur of MR resembles that produced by a ventricular septal defect. However, the latter is usually loudest at the left sternal border rather than the apex and is often accompanied by a parasternal thrill. The murmur of MR may also be confused with that of tricuspid regurgitation, which is usually heard best along the left sternal border, is augmented during inspiration, and is accompanied by a prominent *v* wave and *y* descent in the jugular venous pulse.

When the chordae tendineae to the posterior leaflet of the mitral valve rupture, the regurgitant jet is often directed anteriorly, so that it impinges on the atrial septum adacent to the aortic root and causes a systolic murmur most prominent at the base of the heart, which can be confused with that of aortic stenosis. The acoustic energy derived from the mitral regurgitant jet may be transmitted to the aorta by the impact of the jet on the portion of the left atrial wall adjacent to the aortic root.[207] On the other hand, when the chordae to the anterior leaflet rupture, the jet is usually directed to the posterior wall of the left atrium, and the murmur may be transmitted to the spine or even to the top of the head.[208]

Differential Diagnosis. Patients with rheumatic disease of the mitral valve exhibit a spectrum of abnormalities, ranging from pure MS to pure MR. The presence of an S_3, a rapid left ventricular filling wave and left ventricular impulse on palpation, and a soft S_1 all favor predominant MR, whereas an accentuated S_1, a prominent OS with a short A_2-OS interval, and a soft short systolic murmur all point to predominant MS. Elucidation of the predominant valvular lesion may be complicated by the presence of a holosystolic murmur of tricuspid regurgitation in patients with pure MS and pulmonary hypertension; this murmur, as has already been noted, may sometimes be heard at the apex when the right ventricle is greatly enlarged and may therefore be mistaken for the murmur of MR. Many patients with severe tricuspid regurgitation have a low cardiac output and an inaudible or barely audible dia-

TABLE 34-5 EFFECT OF VARIOUS INTERVENTIONS ON SYSTOLIC MURMURS

INTERVENTION	HYPERTROPHIC OBSTRUCTIVE CARDIOMYOPATHY	AORTIC STENOSIS	MITRAL REGURGITATION	MITRAL PROLAPSE
Valsalva	↑	↓	↓	↑ or ↓
Standing	↑	↑ or unchanged	↓	↑
Handgrip or squatting	↓	↓ or unchanged	↑	↓
Supine position with legs elevated	↓	↑ or unchanged	Unchanged	↓
Exercise	↑	↑ or unchanged	↓	↑
Amyl nitrite	↑↑	↑	↓	↑
Isoproterenol	↑↑	↑	↓	↑

↑↑ = Markedly increased.

Modified from Paraskos, J. A.: Combined valvular disease. *In* Dalen, J. E., and Alpert, J. S. (eds.): Valvular Heart Disease. Boston, Little, Brown and Company, 1987, p. 365.

stolic murmur of MS, further complicating the clinical diagnosis. An S_3 originating from the right ventricle in patients with MS and pulmonary hypertension may falsely suggest the presence of MR. On the other hand, systolic expansion of the left atrium, as occurs in severe MR, often produces a late systolic parasternal expansion that may be confused with right ventricular hypertrophy and falsely attributed to mitral stenosis.

LABORATORY EXAMINATION

(Table 34–6)

ELECTROCARDIOGRAPHY. The principal *electrocardiographic* findings in patients with MR are left atrial enlargement and atrial fibrillation.[71,203,209] Electrocardiographic evidence of left ventricular enlargement occurs in about one-third of patients with severe MR. Approximately 15 per cent exhibit electrocardiographic evidence of right ventricular hypertrophy, a change which reflects the presence of pulmonary hypertension of sufficient severity to counterbalance even the hypertrophied left ventricle of MR.

RADIOLOGICAL FINDINGS (see also p. 224). Cardiomegaly with left ventricular and particularly with left atrial enlargement is a common finding in patients with chronic severe MR.[83,210] However, there is little correlation between left atrial size and pressure. Changes in the lung fields are less prominent in MR than in MS, but interstitial edema with Kerley B lines is frequently seen with acute regurgitation or with progressive left ventricular failure.

In patients with combined MS and MR, overall cardiac enlargement and particularly left atrial dilatation are prominent findings. However, it is often difficult to determine which lesion is predominant from the plain chest roentgenogram, since it may be difficult to distinguish between right and left ventricular enlargement. Predominant MS is suggested by relatively mild cardiomegaly, principally straightening of the left cardiac border with significant changes in the lung fields, whereas predominant MR is more likely when the heart is greatly enlarged and the changes in the lungs are relatively inconspicuous. When the left atrium is aneurysmally dilated chronic MR is almost always the dominant lesion. Calcification of the mitral valve occurs in patients with stenosis, regurgitation, or mixed lesions.

Calcification of the mitral annulus, an important cause of MR in the elderly, is most prominent in the posterior third of the cardiac silhouette[83] and is best visualized on films exposed in the lateral or right anterior oblique projection, in which it appears as a dense, coarse, C-shaped opacity (Fig. 8–29, p. 221).

The diagnosis of MR can be established definitively by means of left ventricular angiocardiography:[211] the prompt appearance of contrast material in the left atrium following its injection into the left ventricle indicates the presence of MR. The injection should be rapid enough to permit left ventricular opacification but slow enough to avoid the development of premature ventricular contractions, which can induce spurious regurgitation.

The regurgitant volume can be determined from the difference between the total left ventricular stroke volume, estimated angiocardiographically, and the simultaneous measurement of the effective forward stroke volume by Fick's method (p. 189). The results of such studies suggest that in patients with severe regurgitation, the regurgitant volume may approach and in rare instances may even exceed the effective forward stroke volume.

Qualitative but clinically useful estimates of the severity of MR may be made by cineangiographic observation of the degree of opacification of the left atrium and pulmonary veins following the injection of contrast material into the left ventricle. MR secondary to rheumatic heart disease is characterized angiographically by a central regurgitant jet and by thickened leaflets that exhibit reduced motion, whereas in regurgitation due to other causes, particularly dilatation or calcification of the mitral annulus or ruptured chordae and papillary muscles, the systolic jet may be eccentric, and the valves consist of thin filaments that display excessive motion. The etiology of the regurgitation, e.g., prolapse of the mitral valve, and a flail leaflet are often distinguishable angiographically.

ECHOCARDIOGRAPHY (see also p. 83). Two-dimensional echocardiography is more useful in determining the etiology and hemodynamic consequences of than in estimating the severity of MR.[212] Severe MR results in enlargement of the left atrium and left ventricle, with increased systolic motion of both of these chambers. The underlying cause of the regurgitation—e.g., rupture of chordae tendineae,[213] mitral valve prolapse (Figs. 4–50 and 4–51, p. 84), a flail leaflet[213a] (Fig. 4–52, p. 84), and vegetation (Fig. 35–2, p. 1035)—can often be determined, and the echocardiogram may also show calcification of the mitral annulus as a band of dense echoes between the mitral apparatus and the posterior wall of the heart.[144,214] This technique is also useful for estimating the hemodynamic consequences of MR; with left ventricular dysfunction, end-diastolic and end-systolic volumes are increased.

Doppler echocardiography in MR reveals a high-velocity jet in the left atrium during systole. The severity of the regurgitation is a function of the distance from the valve that the jet can

TABLE 34-6 NONINVASIVE ASSESSMENT OF MITRAL REGURGITATION: COMPARISON OF FINDINGS IN ACUTE AND CHRONIC FORMS

ACUTE MITRAL REGURGITATION	CHRONIC MITRAL REGURGITATION
ECG	
Commonly normal unless acute ischemia is the cause of regurgitation	Left atrial enlargement (P mitrale) Atrial fibrillation common Left ventricular hypertrophy common with severe regurgitation
Radiology and Fluoroscopy	
Heart size usually normal If regurgitation is severe there may be pulmonary congestion and interstitial edema	Cardiomegaly common, mainly due to left ventricular enlargement Left atrial enlargement, especially with rheumatic mitral disease Fluoroscopy may demonstrate calcium in rheumatic mitral disease
Phonocardiography and Pulse Tracings	
Systolic murmur frequently terminates before S_2 S_3 common Apex cardiogram shows marked systolic impulse	Systolic murmur usually holosystolic S_3 occurs with more severe regurgitation Systolic impulse less marked than with acute severe mitral regurgitation
M-Mode Echocardiography	
Left atrium usually of normal size Left ventricle usually of normal size, may be vigorously hypercontractile Cause of acute regurgitation may be demonstrated; flail mitral leaflet, ruptured chordae or vegetations in infective endocarditis, etc.	Left atrium usually enlarged Left ventricle frequently dilated, with signs of volume overload Cause of chronic regurgitation may be defined; rheumatic disease, mitral valve prolapse, etc.
Two-Dimensional Echocardiography	
In both acute and chronic regurgitation more clearly defines severity of left ventricular volume overload and enhances assessment of left ventricular function. In majority of cases can define etiology of regurgitation, and is especially useful in elucidating difficult diagnostic problems in M-mode echocardiography	
Doppler Ultrasound	
Facilitates detection of mitral regurgitation by identifying turbulent flow within left atrium in systole Aids quantification of degree of mitral regurgitation	
Nuclear Cardiology	
Principal use is in quantitative assessment of ventricular performance, e.g., ejection fraction (EF). Quantification of the degree of mitral regurgitation can be achieved by comparing left and right ventricular stroke volumes. In acute regurgitation the EF is usually normal if increased. A decreased EF implies pre-existing regurgitation or severe ischemic damage to the left ventricle. In chronic regurgitation the EF is usually normal and may be decreased if long-standing volume overload leads to left ventricular dysfunction	

From Bloomfield, P., et al.: Noninvasive investigations for the diagnosis of mitral valve disease. *In* Ionescu, M. I., and Cohn, L. H. (eds.): Mitral Valve Disease: Diagnosis and Treatment. London, Butterworths, 1985, p. 63.

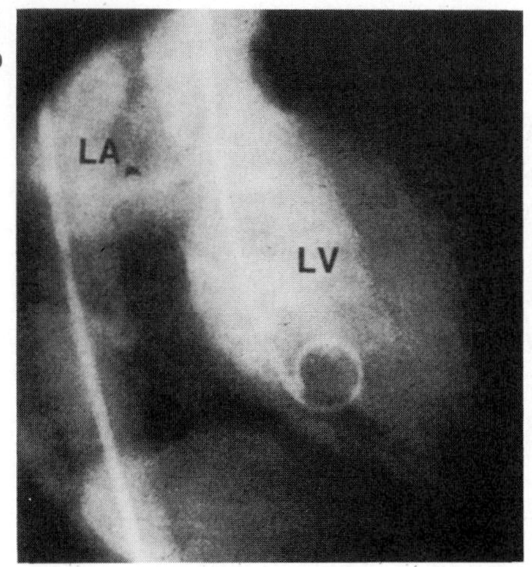

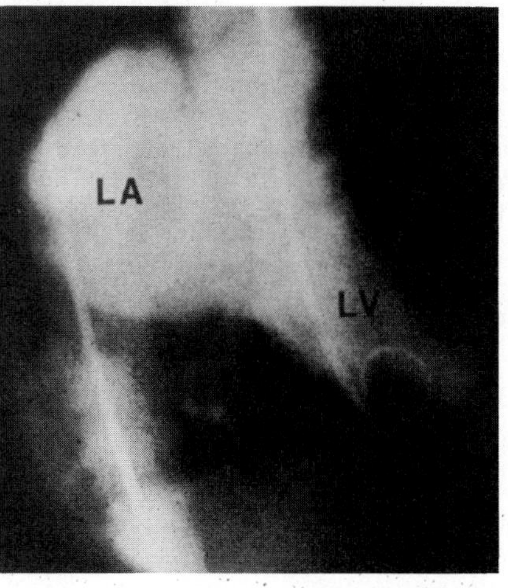

FIGURE 34–17. Diastolic *(left)* and systolic *(right)* frames of a left ventricular cineangiogram from a patient with severe mitral regurgitation. Dense opacification of the left atrium is seen in the first systolic frame. Left ventricular contraction is excellent. (From Hall, R. J., and Julian, D. G.: Diseases of the Cardiac Valves. New York, Churchill Livingstone, 1989, p. 66.)

be detected (Fig. 4–47, p. 83) and the size of the left atrium. Both color flow Doppler (Fig. 4–48, color plate No. 2, and Fig. 4–49, color plate No. 2) and pulsed techniques[215] have been found to correlate well with angiographic methods in estimating the severity of MR. Other methods of assessing the severity of MR include measurement of the absolute mitral jet (>8 cm^2 specifies severe MR[216]) and evaluation of the difference between left ventricular inflow and aortic outflow.[217]

ANGIOGRAPHY. Contrast left ventriculography shows systolic opacification of the left atrium (Fig. 34–17).

Gated pool imaging or first-pass angiography may reveal an increased end-diastolic volume; the regurgitant fraction can be estimated from the ratio of left ventricular to right ventricular stroke volume[192,218]; in patients with mitral regurgitation and impaired left ventricular function, ejection fraction fails to rise normally during exercise.[219] Radionuclide angiograms are useful for interval follow-up of patients. Progressive increases in ventricular end-diastolic or end-systolic volume often suggest that surgical treatment is necessary (discussed later).

ACUTE MITRAL REGURGITATION

The causes of acute MR are shown in Table 34–3 (*bottom*). They are diverse and represent acute manifestations of disease processes that may, under other circumstances, cause chronic MR. Especially important causes of acute MR are infective endocarditis with disruption of valve leaflets or rupture of chordae tendineae, ischemic dysfunction or rupture of a papillary muscle, and malfunction of a prosthetic valve.

One major hemodynamic difference between acute and chronic MR derives from the differences in the compliance of the left atrium, as discussed on page 1022 and as illustrated in Figures 34–15 and 34–16. As shown in Table 34–7 (*top*), acute severe MR causes a marked reduction of forward stroke volume, a slight reduction of end-systolic volume, a rise in end-diastolic volume. The differences in the clinical features between acute and chronic MR are summarized in Table 34–7 (*bottom*). In patients with acute MR with a normal-sized left atrium (group 1 with normal or reduced left atrial compliance, p. 1022) the left atrial pressure rises abruptly, possibly leading to pulmonary edema, marked elevation of pulmonary vascular resistance, and right-sided heart failure. Because the *v* wave is markedly elevated in acute MR, the pressure gradient between the left ventricle and atrium declines at the end of systole (Fig. 34–13*A*), and the murmur may not be holosystolic but decrescendo, ending well before A_2. It is usually lower-pitched and softer than the murmur of chronic MR. A left-sided S_4 is common.[197] Pulmonary hypertension, common in acute MR, may increase the intensity of P_2 and the mur-

TABLE 34-7 CHARACTERISTICS OF ACUTE AND CHRONIC REGURGITATION

	LV End Diastolic Volume	LV End Systolic Volume	Forward Stroke Volume	Ejection Fraction	Left Atrial Compliance	Left Atrial Pressure	LV Muscle Function
Acute MR	↑	↓	↓↓	↑	n	↑↑↑	n
Compensated chronic MR	↑↑↑	↓	n	↑	↑	n or ↑	n
Decompensated chronic MR	↑↑↑↑	↑↑	n or ↓	n or ↓	↑	↑↑	↓↓↓

CLINICAL FEATURE	CHRONIC MITRAL REGURGITATION	ACUTE MITRAL REGURGITATION
Systolic murmur	Harsh, pansystolic	Softer, low pitched, descrescendo, ends before A_2
Primary location of murmur	Apex	Base of heart
Radiation of murmur	Axilla	Neck, spine, top of head
Thrill	Apex	Absent
Venous pressure	Normal	Increased with large V waves
Apical impulse	Hyperkinetic, heaving	Hyperkinetic, heaving until LV failure occurs
ECG	LVH, LAE	Normal or infarct pattern
Chest x-ray	Cardiomegaly, marked LA enlargement, Kerley B lines	Normal size heart, may show pulmonary edema

n = normal, LA = left atrial, LAE = left atrial enlargement, LVH = left ventricular hypertrophy, MR = mitral regurgitation.

Data from Kusiak, V., and Brest, A. N.: Acute mitral regurgitation: Pathophysiology and management. *In* Frankl, W. S., and Brest, A. N. (eds.): Cardiovascular Clinics. Valvular Heart Disease: Comprehensive Evaluation and Management. Philadelphia, F. A. Davis, 1986, p. 273 (top portion); and from Carabello, B. A., and Grossman, W.: Effects of acute and chronic mitral regurgitation on left ventricular mechanics and contractile muscle function. *In* Duran, C., et al. (eds.): Recent Progress in Mitral Valve Disease. London, Butterworths, 1984, p. 188 (bottom portion).

murs of pulmonary and tricuspid regurgitation, and a right-sided S_4 may also develop. Rarely in patients with severe acute MR, a *v* wave (late systolic pressure rise) in the pulmonary artery pressure pulse may cause premature closure of the pulmonary valve, early P_2, and paradoxical splitting of S_2.[203] Acute MR, even if severe, often does not increase overall cardiac size on the chest roentgenogram and may produce only mild left atrial enlargement despite marked elevation of left atrial pressure. With acute MR, there may be little increase in the internal diameter of either of these chambers on the echocardiogram, but increased systolic motion of the ventricle is prominent.

ACUTE VS. CHRONIC MITRAL REGURGITATION

(See Table 34–7)

MANAGEMENT

MEDICAL TREATMENT

This includes all the measures used in the treatment of heart failure, as outlined in Chapter 17. Afterload reduction is of particular benefit in the management of MR—both the acute and the chronic forms.[220,221] By reducing the impedance to ejection into the aorta, the volume of blood regurgitating into the left atrium is reduced. In addition, decreasing left ventricular volume reduces the diameter of the mitral annulus and thereby the regurgitant orifice.[222] Mean left atrial pressure and, in particular, the elevated *v* wave, declines. Thus in the management of MR, vasodilator therapy is actually directed at relieving the physiological abnormality rather than simply dealing with its consequences. Afterload reduction with intravenous nitroprusside may be life-saving in acute MR due to rupture of the head of a papillary muscle occurring in the course of an acute myocardial infarction. It may permit stabilization of the patient's condition and thereby allow coronary arteriography and operation to be carred out with the patient in optimal condition. When surgical treatment is contraindicated, chronic afterload reduction with an angiotensin inhibitor or oral hydralazine may improve the clinical state for months or even years in patients with severe, chronic MR. Digitalis glycosides play a more important role in the management of MR than of MS. Like diuretics, they are indicated in patients with MR, cardiomegaly, and sinus rhythm. Cardiac glycosides are particularly helpful in patients with established atrial fibrillation.

Appropriate prophylaxis to prevent infective endocarditis (p. 1099) is indicated in MR as in all valvular lesions.

Left-sided cardiac catheterization, selective left ventricular angiocardiography, and coronary arteriography are indicated in patients with functional disability despite optimal medical management. The objectives of these studies are to (1) confirm the presence of regurgitation and estimate its severity; (2) aid in the identification of patients with primary myocardial disease and relatively mild, functional MR secondary to ventricular dilatation who are not likely to benefit greatly from operation and in whom the operative risk is relatively high; (3) detect and assess the severity of any associated valve lesions; and (4) determine the presence and assess the extent of coronary artery disease. Because of the additional risks when surgical treatment is carried out in patients with left ventricular dysfunction, definitive diagnosis and characterization of left ventricular function and consideration of surgical treatment should not be deferred until after the patient has developed severe heart failure.

SURGICAL TREATMENT

When operative treatment is under consideration, the chronic, often slowly progressive nature of MR must be weighed against the immediate risks and long-term uncertainties attendant upon surgery. Surgical mortality depends on the patient's hemodynamic and clinical state (particularly the function of the left ventricle) and on the presence of associated conditions such as renal, hepatic, or pulmonary disease, as well as on the skill and experience of the surgical team.[222a] The decision to replace or reconstruct the valve is of critical importance, since surgical mortality associated with mitral valve reconstruction appears to be lower than that associated with replacement (Fig. 34–18), although the patients selected for the two procedures differ. Surgical mortality does not depend significantly on *which* of the currently widely used tissue or mechanical valve prostheses is employed (pp. 1061 to 1062).

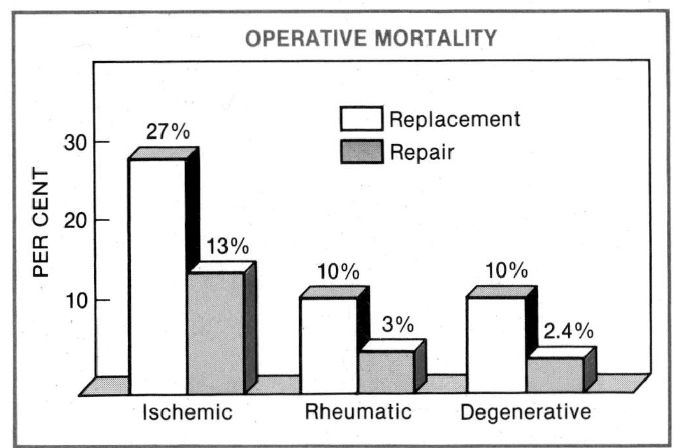

FIGURE 34–18. The operative mortality for mitral valve repair has been lower than for valve replacement regardless of the etiology. (From Cosgrove, D. M., and Stewart, W. J.: Mitral valvuloplasty. Curr. Prob. Cardiol. *14*:359, 1989.)

The reconstructive procedure consists of annuloplasty, often with use of a rigid prosthetic ring (Carpentier ring) or a flexible ring (Duran ring) (Fig. 34–19) or resection and repair of the valve (Fig. 34–20). Replacement,[223] reimplantation, elongation, or shortening of chordae tendineae has been successful in selected patients with pure or predominant MR. Reconstructive procedures have been useful in patients who have severe noncalcific MR with pliable valves, a dilated mitral annulus, MR secondary to ruptured chordae to the posterior leaflet, or perforation of a mitral leaflet due to infective endocarditis, in the absence of severe subvalvular chordal thickening and major loss of leaflet substance.[151,224–232] The results of these "plastic" operations have, in general, been more favorable in children and adolescents with pliable valves and in patients with MR secondary to mitral valve prolapse, annular dilatation, papillary muscle secondary to ischemia, dysfunction or rupture, or chordal rupture than they have been in older patients with the rigid, calcified deformed valves of rheumatic heart disease. Many of these patients still require mitral valve replacement, which is also usually the procedure of choice in patients with badly scarred mitral valves who have previously undergone mitral commissurotomy.

Although mitral valve replacement—with mechanical or bioprostheses—has been used successfully in the treatment of MR for 3 decades, there has been some dissatisfaction with the results of this operation. First, left ventricular function often deteriorates following this procedure, contributing to early and late mortality and late disability. The increase in afterload consequent to abolition of the low impedance leak was first believed to be responsible, but now it is clear that the loss of annular-chordal-papillary muscle continuity interferes with left ventricular function in patients who have undergone mitral valve replacement. This does not occur after mitral valve reconstruction.[233] Indeed, animal experiments have shown convincingly that the normal function of the mitral valve apparatus "primes" the left ventricle for normal contraction and that this is prevented when operation causes discontinuity of this apparatus.

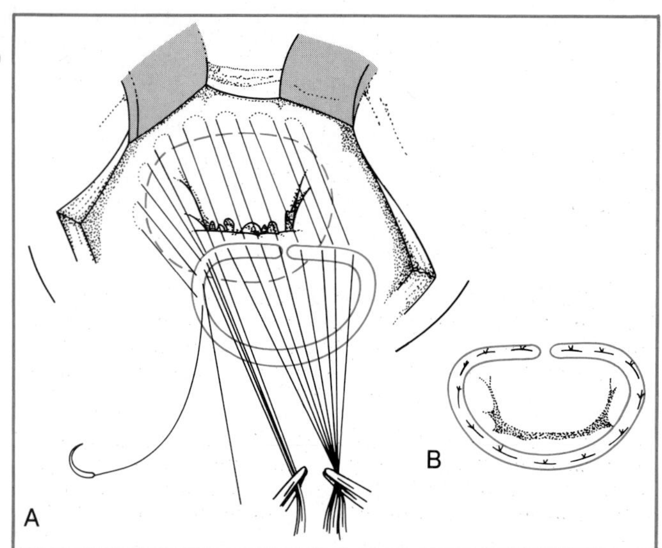

FIGURE 34-19. Illustration of insertion of annuloplasty ring. (From Galloway, A. C., Colvin, S. B., Baumann, F. G., et al.: Current concepts of mitral valve reconstruction for mitral insufficiency. Circulation *78*:1087, 1988, by permission of the American Heart Association, Inc.)

A second disadvantage of prosthetic mitral valve replacement results from the prosthesis itself: thromboembolism or hemorrhage in the case of mechanical prostheses, late mechanical dysfunction of bioprostheses, and the hazard of infective endocarditis with all prostheses. For these reasons, increasing efforts are being made to reconstruct the mitral valve whenever possible, especially in patients with pure and predominant regurgitation. Indeed, these procedures, widely employed in Europe since the early 1960's, are now frequently used by U.S. surgeons as well. In many centers in the United States, approximately half of all patients requiring operation for pure or predominant MR receive reconstructive procedures and the other half valve replacement.

Intraoperative Doppler color flow mapping is extremely useful in assessing the adequacy of the reconstruction. In the minority of patients with persistent severe MR in whom the results are unsatisfactory, the problem can usually be corrected before the chest is closed.[234,235] Occasionally, the rigid Carpentier ring, placed in the mitral annulus with mitral valve reconstruction, causes serious left ventricular outflow tract obstruction.[236]

Progressive reduction in the prevalence of rheumatic heart disease—in which damaged valves often are not suitable for reconstructive surgery—with a simultaneous rise in degenerative causes of MR (including mitral valve prolapse and rupture of chordae tendineae) as well as in ischemic causes is producing an increase in the proportion of patients in whom reconstruction is carried out.

The potential advantages of repair of MR (as opposed to replacement with a prosthetic valve) are many; chronic anticoagulation and the hazards of bleeding and thromboembolism attendant upon implantation of a mechanical prosthesis are largely eliminated, as are the risks of late failure of a bioprosthesis. However, there is a distinct learning curve for mitral reconstructive procedures.[229] Furthermore, many regurgitant valves, particularly those which are thickened, severely deformed, calcified, and partly stenotic, do not lend themselves to reconstruction; mitral valve replacement is necessary. When severe MR is caused by myxomatous degeneration—especially when there is severe associated chordal disease—mitral valve replacement is usually required.[228]

RESULTS. Mortality rates of 1 to 4 per cent in patients with predominant MS and of 2 to 7 per cent in patients with pure or predominant MR in functional Class II or III who undergo elective isolated mitral valve replacement are now common in many centers.[151,237-239] Operative mortality tends to be lower (1 to 4 per cent) in patients undergoing reconstructive surgery. Age per se is no barrier to successful surgery; mitral valve replacement can be carried out in patients older than 70 years with the same or only slightly higher risk as in younger patients, if their general health status is adequate. Surgical treatment substantially improves survival in patients with symptomatic MR. Factors such as an age of less than 60 years, a preoperative New York Heart Association functional Class of II, a cardiac index exceeding 2.0 liters/min/m^2, a left ventricular end-diastolic pressure less than 12 mm Hg, and a normal ejection fraction and end-systolic volume all correlate with improved immediate as well as long-term survival rates. Patients with moderate impairment of the ejection fraction (40 to 50 per cent) exhibit improved survival rates following surgical compared with medical treatment. In other series, only age and preoperative ejection fraction predicted long-term survival following mitral valve replacement.[240]

In most patients with MR, the clinical state and the quality of life improve following valve replacement. Severe pulmonary hypertension is relieved almost uniformly,[121,122] and left

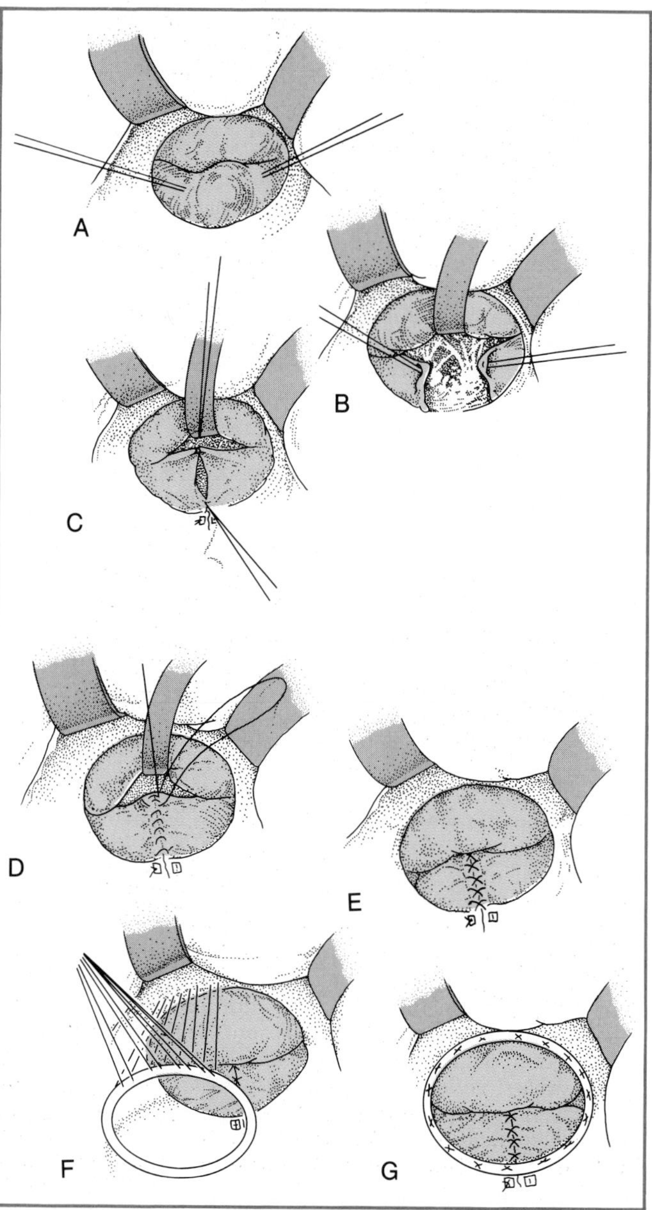

FIGURE 34-20. Valve repair techniques for quadrilateral resection of posterior leaflet of mitral valve. (From Cohn, L. H., DiSesa, V. J., Couper, G. S., et al.: Mitral valve repair for myxomatous degeneration and prolapse of the mitral valve. J. Thorac. Cardiovasc. Surg. *98*:987, 1989.)

ventricular end-diastolic volume and mass are reduced. Depressed contractile function due to mitral regurgitation improves after mitral valve replacement.[240a] However, some patients with MR who had marked left ventricular dysfunction preoperatively sometimes remain symptomatic with a depressed ejection fraction[241] after a technically satisfactory operation, especially mitral valve replacement. Furthermore, long-term survival in patients with predominant MR who undergo mitral valve replacement may be poorer than in those with pure stenosis or mixed stenotic and regurgitant lesions, presumably because left ventricular dysfunction may be quite advanced and largely irreversible by the time patients with pure regurgitation become seriously symptomatic.[242–247] However, even though it is clearly desirable to operate on patients with MR before they develop marked left ventricular dysfunction, and despite these limitations of the results of surgical treatment in patients with severe left ventricular failure, operation is still indicated in the majority of these patients, since conservative therapy has little to offer.

The cause of the MR also plays an important role in the outcome following surgical treatment. In patients in whom mitral dysfunction is secondary to ischemic heart disease, the 5-year survival rate is about 30 per cent, whereas in rheumatic mitral regurgitation it is much better, approximately 70 per cent. Furthermore, occlusive coronary artery disease coexisting with, but not the primary cause of, mitral dysfunction is associated with decreased perioperative and long-term postoperative survival as well.[248] However, some improvement from mitral valve replacement can be expected even in patients with MR secondary to ischemic heart disease who are medically unresponsive and in congestive heart failure, as long as the cardiac index and ejection fraction exceed 1.5 liters/min/m^2 and 0.35, respectively. When left ventricular dysfunction is more severe, however, the risk of perioperative death becomes prohibitive.[249,250]

Surgical Treatment of Acute Mitral Regurgitation. Emergency surgical treatment of acute left ventricular failure caused by acute MR due to myocardial infarction and rupture of the head of a papillary muscle, by trauma to the mitral valve, or by endocarditis is associated with higher mortality rate than is the elective surgical treatment of chronic MR. However, unless such patients with acute, severe MR and heart failure are treated aggressively, a fatal outcome is almost certain. If the condition of patients with MR secondary to acute infarction can be stabilized by medical treatment, it is preferable to defer operation until 4 to 6 weeks after infarction. Vasodilator treatment may be useful during this period. However, medical management should not be prolonged if multisystem (renal or pulmonary or both) failure occurs. Surgical mortality is also higher in patients with refractory heart failure (functional Class IV), in those in whom a previously implanted prosthetic valve must be replaced because of thromboembolism or valve dysfunction, and in those with active infective endocarditis (of a natural or prosthetic valve). Despite the higher surgical risks, the efficacy of early operation has been established in patients with infective endocarditis complicated by medically uncontrollable congestive heart failure, recurrent emboli, or both[244] (p. 1096). Since fungal endocarditis responds poorly to medical management, it is now the practice to recommend valve replacement in these cases *before* the onset of heart failure or embolization.

INDICATIONS FOR OPERATION. In view of advanced surgical techniques, reductions in operative mortality, and improvements in mitral reconstructive procedures and in artificial valves, as well as poor long-term results in many patients whose MR is corrected after a long history of heart failure, a more aggressive stance concerning the desirability of operation is in order. Only a few years ago I, along with many cardiologists, recommended operation for patients with chronic severe MR only if they were in functional Class III or IV,[251] i.e., with symptoms at rest or on ordinary activity despite intensive medical treatment. However, it is now my policy to recommend operation also for patients with severe MR who are in Class II, i.e., who become distinctly symptomatic only on heavy exertion, particularly if cardiomegaly and an elevated left ventricular end-systolic volume ($>$30 ml/m^2 BSA) persist despite aggressive medical therapy.

The asymptomatic patient with severe MR presents a particularly challenging problem. Careful history and performance of an exercise test often reveal that these patients are not, in fact, truly asymptomatic. If that is the case, they may be considered for surgical treatment, as already discussed. However, patients with severe MR who are truly asymptomatic or only mildly symptomatic and have normal ventricular function (ejection fraction $>$ 70 per cent) are followed. In asymptomatic patients with ejection fractions between 55 and 70 per cent it is useful to follow the end-systolic wall stress/end-systolic volume index ratio using noninvasive techniques and to time operation when these indices have begun to fall but before the patient becomes severely symptomatic. If valve replacement is likely to be necessary, a somewhat higher threshold for clinical and hemodynamic impairment is employed than if valvular reconstruction is contemplated.

The following preoperative hemodynamic indices are predictive of a favorable surgical outcome: EF $>$ 0.70 and an end-systolic volume index $<$50 ml/m^2, while predictors of poor outcome are an EF of $<$0.55 and an end-systolic volume index of $>$75 ml/m^2. Crawford et al. have reported that preoperative pulmonary hypertension (mean pulmonary artery pressure $>$20 mm Hg) correlates with persistent postoperative left ventricular dilatation and that surgery should be considered in patients with MR before the ejection fraction decreases to 0.50 and before the end-systolic volume index exceeds 50 ml/m^2.[190]

The Mitral Valve Prolapse Syndrome

ETIOLOGY AND PATHOLOGY

(Fig. 34–21)

The mitral valve prolapse (MVP) syndrome has been given many names, including the systolic click–murmur syndrome, Barlow syndrome, billowing mitral valve syndrome, ballooning mitral cusp syndrome, floppy valve syndrome, and redundant cusp syndrome.[253–258] It is a common but variable clinical syndrome resulting from diverse pathogenic mechanisms of the mitral valve apparatus. The MVP syndrome has become recognized as one of the most prevalent cardiac valvular abnormalities, affecting as much as 5 to 10 per cent of the population.[256,259,260] It had been thought for many years that midsystolic clicks and late systolic murmurs, the auscultatory hallmarks of this syndrome, were of extracardiac origin. However, in 1963 Barlow et al. demonstrated that these auscultatory findings are frequently associated with prolapse of the mitral valve, often with regurgitation.[261] Barlow and collaborators have distinguished between "billowing" and "prolapse" of the mitral valve.[261] Normally, the mitral valve billows slightly into the left atrium and an exaggeration should be termed "billowing mitral valve." A "floppy valve" is regarded as an extreme form of billowing. MVP occurs when the leaflet edges of the valve do not coapt, causing MR. With chordal rupture, the prolapsed mitral valve is "flail." Obviously, these conditions blend into one another, and it is often difficult to separate them sharply.

it is likely that more rigorous criteria for diagnosis based on two-dimensional echocardiography will indicate a much lower prevalence.[254] In one series, about 20 per cent of patients who underwent mitral valve replacement had myxomatous proliferation of the valve on histopathological examination.[310] Indeed, MVP is now the most common cause of isolated regurgitation requiring mitral valve replacement.[311] Echocardiographic evidence of MVP has been found in more than 90 per cent of patients with Marfan syndrome[312] and in many of their first-degree relatives.

HISTORY

The overwhelming majority of patients with MVP are asymptomatic[313] (Fig. 34–21). In many cases, otherwise asymptomatic patients with MVP suffer from undue anxiety, perhaps precipitated by their having been informed of the presence of heart disease. Boudoulas et al. have called attention to a "MVP syndrome" with a characteristic nonejection click and a variety of nonspecific symptoms, such as fatigability, palpitations, postural orthostasis, and neuropsychiatric symptoms, as well as symptoms of autonomic dysfunction.[313] Patients may complain of palpitations, chest discomfort, and, when MR is severe, symptoms of diminished cardiac reserve. Chest discomfort may be typical of angina but most often is atypical in that it is prolonged, not clearly related to exertion, and punctuated by brief attacks of severe stabbing pain at the apex. The discomfort may be secondary to tension on papillary muscles and may be associated with abnormalities of wall motion or indentations of the wall of the left ventricle at the base of these muscles on angiography. It may be difficult to differentiate this discomfort from angina because of the coexistence of the MVP syndrome and true angina pectoris secondary to coronary artery disease.

Since MVP is sometimes associated with another form of heart disease, e.g., atrial septal defect, symptoms produced by the latter may predominate. It has been suggested that many of the symptoms are related to dysfunction of the autonomic nervous system, which occurs frequently in the MVP syndrome.[314–316] Some patients with MVP exhibit increased excretion and circulating concentrations of epinephrine and norepinephrine, presumably secondary to increased adrenergic tone, which may be responsible for many of the symptoms of the syndrome. Some exhibit excessive vasoconstriction, others striking orthostatic tachycardia.[315] Although many of the symptoms of MVP resemble those of neurocirculatory asthenia, the two conditions appear to be distinct and unrelated.[317] Patients with MVP also have an unusually high incidence of migraine.[313]

PHYSICAL EXAMINATION

Palpation of the chest and of the carotid pulses confirms the presence of MR, which may range from nonexistent to severe. The physical findings unique to the MVP syndrome are detected by auscultation and can be corroborated by phonocardiography.[253,258] The most important is a systolic click at least 0.14 sec after S_1 (Figs. 3–7 and 3–8, p. 46). This can be differentiated from a systolic ejection click, since it occurs distinctly *after* the beginning of the upstroke of the carotid pulse. Occasionally multiple mid- and late-systolic clicks are audible most readily along the lower left sternal border and are believed to be produced by sudden tensing of the elongated chordae tendineae and of the prolapsing leaflets. The click is often, although not invariably, followed by a mid- to late-crescendo systolic murmur that continues to A_2. This murmur is similar to that produced by papillary muscle dysfunction (Fig. 2–20, p. 40), which is readily understandable, since both result from mid- to late-systolic MR. In general, the duration of the murmur is a function of the severity of the regurgitation, and when the murmur is confined to the latter portion of systole, regurgitation usually is not severe. However, as regurgitation becomes more severe, the murmur commences earlier and becomes holosystolic.

It is important to emphasize the variability of the physical findings in the MVP syndrome. Some patients exhibit both a midsystolic click and a mid- to late-systolic murmur; others present with one or the other of these two findings; still others have only a click on one occasion and only a murmur on another, both on a third examination, and no abnormality at all on a fourth. MVP may also cause an early diastolic sound or murmur, best heard at the apex or left sternal border 70 to 110 msec following A_2, at a time when the prolapsed posterior leaflet descends into the left ventricle.[318] Conditions other than MVP cause midsystolic clicks; these include tricuspid valve clicks, extracardiac causes, and atrial septal aneurysms.[319]

DYNAMIC AUSCULTATION. The auscultatory and phonocardiographic findings are exquisitely sensitive to physiological and pharmacological interventions, and recognition of the changes induced by these interventions is of great value in the diagnosis of the MVP syndrome (Fig. 2–20, p. 40) (Table 34–5).[253,258] The mitral valve begins to prolapse when the reduction of left ventricular volume during systole reaches a critical point at which the mitral valve leaflets no longer coapt; at that instant, the click occurs and the murmur commences. Any maneuver that decreases left ventricular volume, such as a reduction of impedance to left ventricular outflow, a reduction in venous return, or an augmentation of contractility, results in an earlier occurrence of prolapse during systole. As a consequence, the click and onset of the murmur move closer to S_1. When prolapse is severe or left ventricular size is markedly reduced or both, prolapse may begin with the onset of systole, and as a consequence, the click may not be audible and the murmur may be holosystolic. On the other hand, when left ventricular volume is augmented by an increase in venous return, a reduction of myocardial contractility, bradycardia, or an increase in the impedance to left ventricular emptying, both the click and the onset of the murmur will be delayed. Indeed, if the left ventricle becomes extremely large, prolapse may not occur at all, and the abnormal auscultatory features may disappear entirely.

During the straining phase of the Valsalva maneuver, upon sudden standing, and early during the inhalation of amyl nitrite, cardiac size decreases, and both the click and the onset of the murmur occur earlier in systole. In contrast, a sudden change from the standing to the prone position, leg-raising, squatting, maximal isometric exercise, and, to a lesser extent, expiration will delay the click and the onset of the murmur (Fig. 3–8, p. 46). During the overshoot phase of the Valsalva maneuver (i.e., six to eight cycles following release) and with prolongation of the R-R interval either following a premature contraction or in atrial fibrillation, the click and onset of the murmur are usually delayed, and the intensity of the murmur is reduced.

In general, when the onset of the murmur is delayed, both its duration and its intensity are diminished, reflecting a reduction in the severity of MR. With some maneuvers, however, there is a discrepancy between changes in the intensity and duration of the murmur. Following amyl nitrite inhalation, for example, the reduced left ventricular size results in an earlier click and longer murmur, but the lower left ventricular systolic pressure diminishes the severity of regurgitation and the intensity of the murmur. Conversely, phenylephrine and methoxamine delay the click and the onset of the murmur, but the larger volume of regurgitation consequent to the elevated left ventricular systolic pressure increases regurgitation and the intensity of the murmur. Emotional stress may increase the intensity of the click and exacerbate arrhythmias in MVP,[320] a finding that might explain the intermittency of the auscultatory findings and arrhythmias in these patients. In the diagnosis of the MVP syndrome, it is generally more helpful to determine the effect of interventions on the *timing of the click* and murmur than on the *intensity of the murmur*.

There may be confusion between the systolic murmurs of

hypertrophic cardiomyopathy (HCM) and of MVP, particularly because midsystolic clicks and a late systolic murmur have been reported in HCM and because the murmur may increase in intensity and duration with standing and decrease with squatting in both conditions (p. 1408). However, the response to several interventions may be helpful in differentiating these two conditions. During the strain of the Valsalva maneuver, the murmur of HCM increases in intensity[321] in contrast to that in the syndrome, which becomes longer but usually not louder. The murmur of HCM becomes louder after amyl nitrite inhalation, whereas that of MVP does not. Following a premature beat, the murmur of HCM increases in intensity and duration, whereas that due to MVP usually remains unchanged or decreases.

LABORATORY EXAMINATION

ELECTROCARDIOGRAPHY

Most commonly, the electrocardiogram is within normal limits in asymptomatic patients with typical auscultatory and echocardiographic findings. In a minority of asymptomatic patients and in many symptomatic patients, the electrocardiogram shows inverted or biphasic T waves and nonspecific ST-segment changes in leads II, III, and aV_f and occasionally in the anterolateral leads as well.[253] The ST- and T-wave changes may become exaggerated during amyl nitrite inhalation and exercise. These electrocardiographic findings may be related to ischemia of the papillary muscles, or of the left ventricle at their bases, resulting from increased tension on these structures produced by the prolapsing valve. Alternatively, it is possible that the electrocardiographic abnormality reflects an underlying cardiomyopathy.

ARRHYTHMIAS. A spectrum of arrhythmias, including atrial and ventricular premature contractions and supraventricular and ventricular tachyarrhythmias[322–328] as well as bradyarrhythmias due to sinus node dysfunction or varying degrees of atrioventricular block,[329] have been observed in the MVP syndrome. Indeed, this syndrome should be considered patients with otherwise unexplained arrhythmias. The mechanism of the arrhythmias is not clear. Diastolic depolarization of muscle fibers in the anterior mitral leaflet in response to stretch has been demonstrated experimentally,[330] and the abnormal stretch of the prolapsed leaflet may be of pathogenetic significance. Wit et al. have shown that mitral valve leaflets contain atrium-like muscle fibers in continuity with left atrial myocardium. It is possible that mechanical stimulation of these fibers generates slow-response action potentials and sustained rhythmic action that penetrates the cardiac chambers.[331] Although most of these arrhythmias are of litle clinical importance, recurrent ventricular tachycardia, refractory to the usual agents, and even ventricular fibrillation have been reported. These serious ventricular arrhythmias are significantly more frequent in patients with ST-segment and T-wave abnormalities on the resting electrocardiogram.[332]

Paroxysmal supraventricular tachycardia is the most common sustained tachyarrhythmia in patients with the MVP syndrome and may be related to the high incidence of atrioventricular bypass tracts in this condition.[322] These bypass tracts are always left-sided and may be associated with the mitral valve abnormality. In the general population only 20 per cent of patients with paroxysmal supraventricular tachycardia have such bypass tracts, whereas the incidence in patients with MVP is three times as great. Conversely, there is evidence that there is high incidence of MVP among patients with the Wolff-Parkinson-White syndrome.[333] However, the absence of electrocardiographic evidence of the Wolff-Parkinson-White syndrome should not be taken as evidence against the existence of bypass tracts in patients with the MVP syndrome who suffer attacks of supraventricular tachycardia. These considerations suggest that patients with the MVP syndrome who develop paroxysmal supraventricular tachycardia should be subjected to electrophysiological investigation. The outcome of such studies may be important, since digitalis or propranolol, which may be useful in reentry tachycardias, may be hazardous in the presence of antegrade conduction over an atrioventricular bypass tract. There is also an increased association between MVP and prolongation of the Q-T interval, and this association may play a role in the genesis of ventricular arrhythmias.[316,334]

MVP AND SUDDEN DEATH. The relation between the MVP syndrome and sudden death is not clear. Jeresaty collected 25 patients with MVP who died suddenly,[335] and Pocock et al. reviewed 17 patients.[336] But these are "numerators without denominators," and when the high incidence of both conditions is considered, it is difficult to interpret the coincidence. Considering the frequency of both conditions, these numbers are not very impressive. It is not clear how many, indeed if any, of these instances of sudden death were in fact caused by or related to the MVP syndrome. The immediate cause of the sudden, unexpected death is probably an episode of tachyarrhythmia,[337] although complete heart block with prolonged asystole has also been reported in this syndrome and cannot be excluded.[338]

Kligfield et al. have identified the following as potential risks for sudden death in MVP: the presence of significant MR, complex ventricular arrhythmias, prolongation of the Q-T interval, and a history of syncope and palpitations.[323,324] Boudoulas et al. identified nine patients with MVP who had experienced cardiac arrest. Ventricular fibrillation was documented in eight; seven were successfully resuscitated. Six living survivors have been followed for 3 to 14 years.[329]

ECHOCARDIOGRAPHY (see also p. 83). Echocardiography plays a key role in the diagnosis of MVP and has been most useful in the delineation of this syndrome[339] (Figs. 3–7, p. 46, 4–50 and 4–51, p. 84). The most common echocardiographic finding on M-mode echocardiography is abrupt posterior movement of the posterior leaflet or of both mitral leaflets in midsystole. A second finding is pansystolic posterior prolapse of one or both leaflets, giving rise to a U- or hammock-shaped configuration in the C-D segment (Fig. 4–50, p. 84) (the opposite of what is seen in hypertrophic obstructive cardiomyopathy, in which the anterior leaflet of the mitral valve moves toward the ventricular septum in midsystole). Holosystolic "hammocking" of less than 5 mm is not specific for MVP. Rarely, there is a sudden posterior collapse of the anterior mitral leaflet as it approaches the prolapsing posterior leaflet in early systole.[340] All three of these echocardiographic patterns have in common the motion of the mitral valve posterior to the C-point. Although the systolic click usually occurs at the time of the abrupt posterior movement, there is considerable variability in the relationship between the auscultatory and echocardiographic events.

In some patients, M-mode echocardiography has missed MVP that was detected by two-dimensional echocardiography.[341,342] The echocardiogram is helpful in the identification of patients at significant risk of developing severe MR or infective endocarditis; in addition to systolic displacement of one or both leaflets into the left atrium, the leaflets are distinctly thickened[263] or redundant[263] in these patients (Fig. 34–23). Doppler echocardiography frequently reveals mild MR that is not always associated with an audible murmur. Color flow Doppler is useful in identifying the location and severity of the regurgitant jets.[344] Moderate or severe MR is found in 10 per cent of patients, usually in men over the age of 50.[344]

The echocardiographic findings of MVP have been reported to occur in a large number of first-degree relatives of patients with established MVP,[345] but the variability in physical findings in this syndrome, already commented upon, extends to the echocardiogram.[346] Thus, some patients have a systolic click with or without a murmur and show no evidence of MVP on the echocardiogram. Conversely, the echocardiographic findings of MVP may be observed in patients without the click or murmur. Others have both the typical echocardiographic and auscultatory features.

Two-dimensional echocardiography has also revealed prolapse of the tricuspid and aortic valves in approximately one-fifth of patients with MVP.[347] Conversely, however, prolapse of the tricuspid and aortic valves[348] occurs *uncommonly* in patients without prolapse of the mitral valve; the latter echocardiographic finding is usually not associated with any aortic regurgitation.

STRESS SCINTIGRAPHY

The differential diagnosis between two common conditions—MVP associated with atypical chest pain and electrocardiographic abnormalities, and primary coronary artery disease associated with MVP—may be aided by exercise electrocardiography,[224] but myocardial scintigraphy using thallium-201 during exercise (p. 287) is probably more specific in this disorder. When findings are normal, i.e., when there is no evidence of exercise-induced regional myocardial ischemia, the diagnosis of MVP unrelated to ischemic heart disease is favored.[349] However, the reverse is not always the case, since patients having MVP with or without associated coronary artery disease may exhibit myocardial perfusion defects—

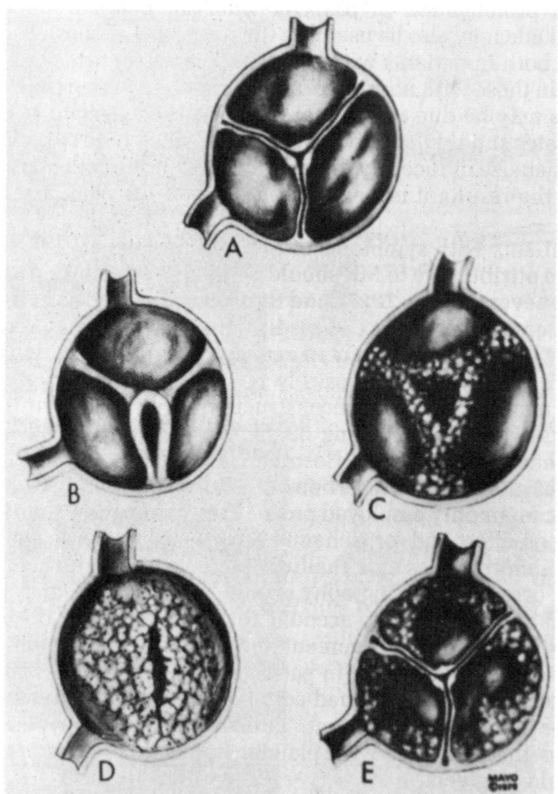

FIGURE 34–24. Types of aortic valve stenosis. *A*, Normal aortic valve. *B*, Congenital aortic stenosis. *C*, Rheumatic aortic stenosis. *D*, Calcific aortic stenosis. *E*, Calcific senile aortic stenosis. (From Brandenburg, R. O., et al.: Valvular heart disease—When should the patient be referred? Pract. Cardiol. *5*:50, 1979.)

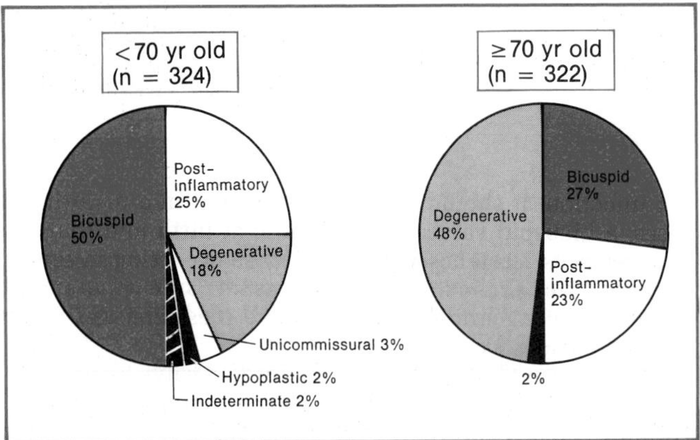

FIGURE 34–25. Causes of aortic stenosis, shown for two age groups. Among patients younger than 70 years (*left*), calcification of congenitally bicuspid valves accounted for half of the surgical cases. In contrast, in those 70 years of age or older (*right*), degenerative calcification accounted for almost half of the cases. (From Passik, C. S., et al.: Temporal changes in the causes of aortic stenosis: A surgical pathologic study of 646 cases. Mayo Clin. Proc. *62*:119, 1987.)

may extend in the direction of the cusps, no commissural fusion is present. Degenerative "wear and tear" appears to be the most likely cause of this form of AS, which is commonly accompanied by calcifications of the mitral annulus and coronary arteries but rarely by aortic regurgitation. Both diabetes mellitus and hypercholesterolemia are risk factors for the development of this lesion.[375,376] The stenosis is produced by the calcific deposits that prevent the cusps from opening normally during systole (Fig. 34–26).

In atherosclerotic aortic valvular stenosis, severe atherosclerosis involves the aorta and other major arteries; this form of AS occurs most frequently in patients with severe hypercholesterolemia and is observed in children with homozygous type II hyperlipoproteinemia (p. 1137). Calcific aortic stenosis is observed in Paget's disease of bone[377] as well as in end-stage renal disease.[378,379] *Rheumatoid involvement* of the valve is a rare cause of AS and results in nodular thickening of the valve leaflets and involvement of the proximal part of the aorta (p. 1732). *Ochronosis* is another rare cause of aortic stenosis.[380]

Roberts studied hearts with AS obtained from patients between 15 and 65 years of age and found that almost 40 per cent were tricuspid. Since there were thickening of the mitral valve and a history of acute rheumatic fever in half of these cases, it is likely that the AS was rheumatic in etiology; in the remainder it was either congenital or degenerative in origin. In 90 per cent of hearts of patients with AS who were older than 65 years and who were examined at autopsy, the valves were tricuspid, with nodular calcific deposits on the aortic aspects of the cusps, but without commissural fusion.[368]

Hemodynamically significant AS leads to severe concentric left ventricular hypertrophy,[381] with heart weights as great as 1000 gm. The interventricular septum often bulges into and encroaches on the right ventricular cavity. When left ventricular failure supervenes, the left ventricle dilates,[381] the left atrium enlarges, and changes secondary to backward failure occur in the pulmonary vascular bed, right side of the heart, and systemic venous bed.

PATHOPHYSIOLOGY

The left ventricle responds to the *sudden* production of severe obstruction to outflow by dilatation and reduction of stroke volume. However, in adults with AS, the obstruction usually develops and increases gradually over a prolonged period. In infants and children with congenital AS, the valve orifice shows little change as the child grows, thereby also intensifying the relative obstruction quite gradually. Left ventricular function can be well maintained in experimentally produced, chronic, gradually developing subcoronary AS.[382] Left ventricular ouput is maintained by the presence of left ventricular hypertrophy, which may sustain a large pressure gradient across the aortic valve for many years without a reduction in cardiac output, left ventricular dilatation, or the development of symptoms. A peak systolic pressure gradient exceeding 50 mm Hg in the presence of a normal cardiac output or an effective aortic orifice less than about 0.75 cm^2 in an average-sized adult, i.e., 0.4 cm^2/m^2 of body surface area (less than approximately one-fourth of the normal orifice) is generally considered to represent critical obstruction to left ventricular outflow.[383]

As contraction of the left ventricle becomes progressively more isometric, the left ventricular pressure pulse exhibits a rounded, rather than flattened, summit. The elevated left ventricular end-diastolic pressure, which is characteristic of severe AS, does not necessarily signify the presence of left ventricular dilatation or failure but often reflects diminished compliance of the hypertrophied left ventricular wall; usually it results from both processes.[384–386]

In patients with severe AS, large *a* waves usually appear in the left atrial pressure pulse because of the combination of enhanced contraction of a hypertrophied left atrium and diminished left ventricular compliance. Atrial contraction plays a particularly important role in filling of the left ventricle in AS.[27] It raises left ventricular end-diastolic pressure without producing a concomitant elevation of mean left atrial pressure.[387] This "booster pump" function of the left atrium prevents the pulmonary venous and capillary pressures from rising to levels that would produce pulmonary congestion, while at the same time maintaining left ventricular end-diastolic pressure at the elevated level necessary for effective left ventricular contraction. Loss of appropriately timed, vigorous atrial contraction, as occurs in atrial fibrillation or atrioventricular dissociation, may result in rapid clinical deterioration in patients with severe AS.

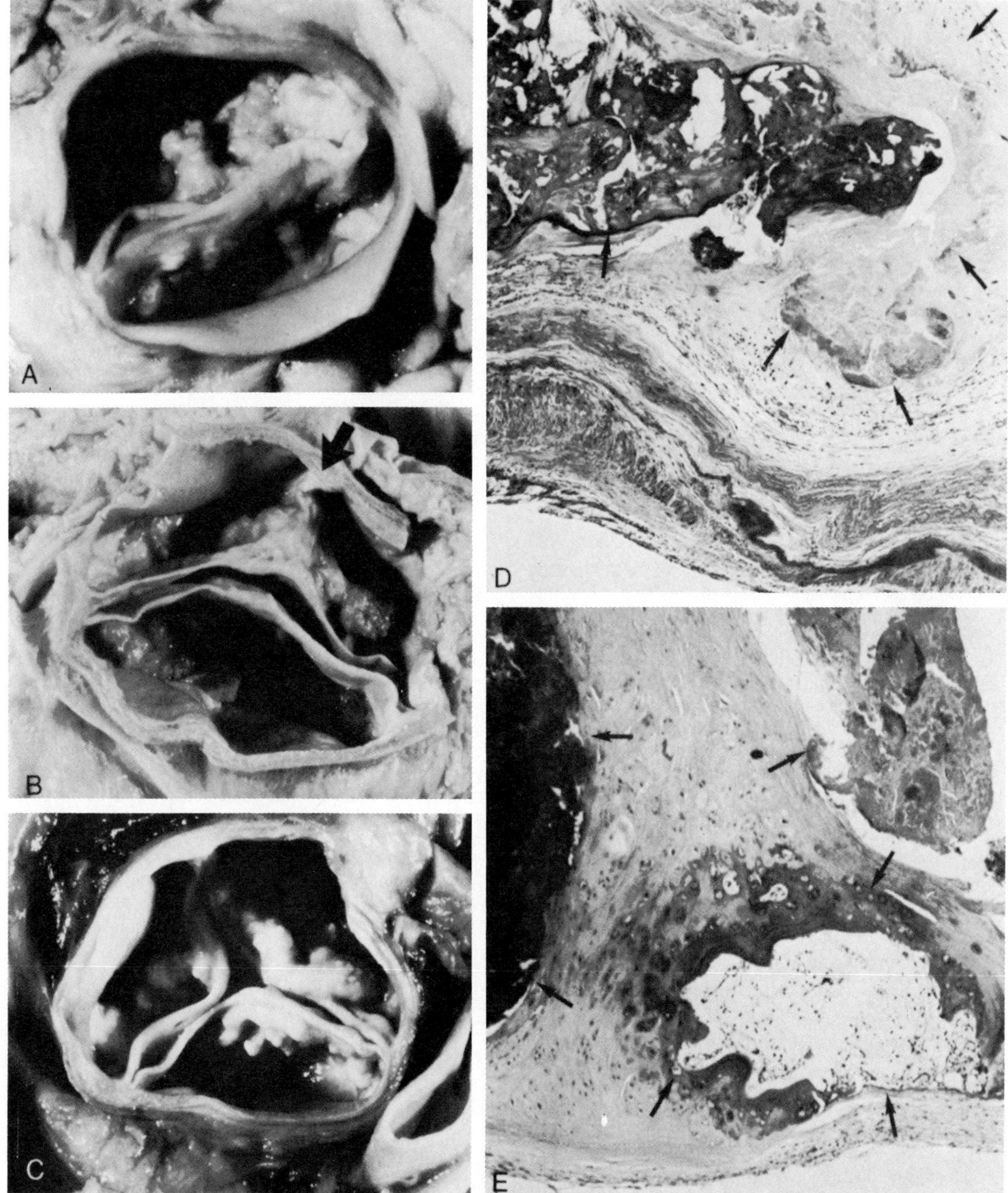

FIGURE 34–26. **Calcific aortic stenosis. *A*, Congenitally bicuspid aortic valve, characterized by two equal cusps with basal mineralization. *B*, Congenitally bicuspid aortic valve having two unequal cusps, the larger with a central raphe (arrow). *C*, Otherwise anatomically normal tricuspid aortic valve in an elderly patient, characterized by isolated cusps with calcification localized to basilar aspect; cuspal free edges are not involved. *D* and *E*, Photomicrographs of calcific deposits in calcific aortic stenosis; deposits are rimmed by arrows (hematoxylin and eosin, 15×). *D*, Shows deposits with underlying cusp largely intact; transmural calcific deposits are shown in *E*. (*A* and *C*, from Schoen, F. J., St. John Sutton, M.: Contemporary issues in the pathology of valvular heart disease. Hum. Pathol. *18*:568, 1987.)**

Although the *cardiac output* at rest is within normal limits in the majority of patients with severe AS,[383] it often fails to rise normally during exertion. Late in the course of the disease the cardiac output, stroke volume, and therefore the left ventricular–aortic pressure gradient all decline, whereas the mean left atrial, pulmonary capillary, pulmonary arterial, right ventricular systolic and diastolic, and right atrial pressures rise, often sequentially. AS intensifies the severity of any existing mitral regurgitation by increasing the pressure gradient responsible for driving blood from the left ventricle to the left atrium. In addition, the dilatation of the left ventricle, which occurs late in the course of some patients with aortic valve disease, may produce mitral regurgitation, superimposing the hemodynamic changes associated with this lesion on those produced by AS. Also, as a consequence of pulmonary hypertension or bulging of the hypertrophied septum into the right ventricular cavity or both, the *a* wave in the right atrial pressure pulse becomes prominent.

Left ventricular end-diastolic volume usually remains normal until quite late in the course of the disease, but left ventricular mass increases in response to the chronic pressure overload, resulting in an increase in the mass/volume ratio. However, the increase in mass may not be as great as that seen with aortic regurgitation (AR) or combined AS and AR.

MYOCARDIAL FUNCTION IN AORTIC STENOSIS

In experimental animals, when the aorta is suddenly constricted, left ventricular pressure rises, and there is a large increase in wall stress, whereas both extent and velocity of shortening decline. As pointed out in Chapter 14, the development of ventricular hypertrophy is one of the principal mechanisms by which the heart adapts to such an increased

TABLE 34-10 EFFECT OF AORTIC VALVE DISEASE ON MYOCARDIAL OXYGEN SUPPLY AND DEMAND

$M\dot{V}O_2$					
AS	AR	DETERMINANTS OF SUPPLY	DETERMINANTS OF DEMAND	AS	AR
−↑	↓↓↓	**Diastolic BP**	**LV systolic pressure**	↑↑↑	↑
↓	↓	**Diastolic filling time**	**LV volume**	—	↑↑↑
↓*	↓	**Epicardial coronary arteries**	**Systolic ejection time**	↑	↑
↓↓↓	↓	**Coronary vascular resistance**	**Heart rate**	—	—
		Humoral	**Contractility**	—	—
		Autonomic nervous system			
		Catecholamines	**LV mass**	↑↑↑	↑↑↑
		Compression by LV			
↓↓	↓↓	**LV filling pressure**			
		(effect on intramural coronary veins)			
—	—	**RV filling pressure**			

AS, aortic stenosis; AR, aortic regurgitation; BP, blood pressure; LV, left ventricular; $M\dot{V}O_2$, myocardial oxygen consumption. Arrows refer to effect on supply or demand. Number of arrows indicates magnitude of effect. ↑ indicates increased demand; ↓, decreased demand; and —, no effect.

*If coronary disease present.

From Cheitlin, M. D.: The timing of surgery in mitral and aortic valve disease. Curr. Prob. Cardiol. *12*:115, 1987.

hemodynamic burden.[388,389] The increased systolic wall stress induced by AS apparently leads to parallel replication of sarcomeres and concentric hypertrophy (Fig. 14–8, p. 400), and the increase in left ventricular wall thickness is often sufficient to counterbalance the increased pressure so that peak systolic wall tension returns to normal or remains so if the obstruction develops slowly[390–392] (Fig. 14–9, p. 401). An inverse correlation between wall stress and ejection fraction exists in patients with AS.[392] This suggests that the depressed ejection fraction and velocity of fiber shortening that occur in *some* patients are a consequence of inadequate wall thickening,[393] resulting in "afterload mismatch."[394] Patients having AS with compensated pressure overload as well as some with depressed left ventricular ejection fractions and overt congestive failure may have normal values for the rate of intraventricular stress ($d\sigma/dt$) and pressure (dP/dt) development.[395,396] In others, the lower ejection fraction is secondary to a depression of contractility; in the latter, the effectiveness of surgical treatment is reduced.[397] Thus, both altered contractility and increased afterload are operative in depressing left ventricular performance.[398]

From these considerations it is clear that in order to evaluate myocardial function in patients with AS, it is critical to relate the ejection phase indices to the existing wall tension (p. 422). Wall thickness is a critical determinant of ventricular performance in patients with AS; inadequate hypertrophy, an intrinsic depression of myocardial contractility, or a combination of these two defects may lead to a depression of ventricular performance.

DIASTOLIC STIFFNESS (see p. 402). Although ventricular hypertrophy is a key adaptive mechanism to the pressure load imposed by AS, it results in an adverse pathophysiological consequence, i.e., an increase in diastolic stiffness (Fig. 34–12, p. 1021). As a result, greater intracavitary pressure is required for ventricular filling. Some patients with AS manifest an increase in chamber stiffness due simply to an increase in muscle mass but with no alteration in muscle stiffness; others exhibit increases in muscle stiffness as well as in chamber stiffness, both of which contribute to the elevation of ventricular diastolic filling pressure at any level of ventricular diastolic volume.[384–386,399,400] Chamber stiffness may revert toward normal as hypertrophy regresses following relief of AS,[386] and at least in some patients muscle stiffness may also revert to normal. Whether this occurs in all patients is not clear. It is expected that this regression of stiffness would not occur in patients with extensive myocardial fibrosis. Indeed, in some patients stiffness increases postoperatively as ventricular hypertrophy regresses, while interstitial fibrosis remains unchanged.[385] The rate of ventricular thinning in diastole is slowed in AS (Fig. 15–25, p. 439).

STRUCTURE. A variety of changes in the myocardial ultrastructure have been documented in patients with severe AS. These include unusually large nuclei, loss of myofibrils, accumulation of mitochondria, large cytoplasmic areas devoid of contractile material, and proliferation of fibroblasts and collagen fibers in the interstitial space.[401] The depression of cardiac function that occurs late in the course of the disease may well be related to these morphological alterations. In adults with AS, both myocardial cellular hypertrophy and relative and absolute increases in connective tissue occur.[402–404] An inverse correlation between left ventricular ejection fraction and myocardial fiber diameter has been reported.[404]

ISCHEMIA (Table 34–10). In AS, coronary blood flow at rest is elevated in absolute terms but is normal when corrected for myocardial mass.[402] There may be inadequate myocardial oxygenation in severe AS, even in the absence of coronary artery disease. The hypertrophied left ventricular muscle mass, the increased systolic pressure, and the prolongation of ejection all elevate myocardial oxygen consumption,[405] and the abnormally heightened pressure compressing the coronary arteries exceeds the coronary perfusion pressure, thereby interfering with coronary blood flow.[406,407] Myocardial perfusion is also impaired by the relative decrease in myocardial capillary density and by the elevation of left ventricular end-diastolic pressure, which lowers the aortic–left ventricular pressure gradient in diastole, i.e., the coronary perfusion pressure gradient. Therefore, the subendocardium in severe AS is susceptible to ischemia, and this underperfusion may be responsible for the development of myocardial ischemia.[406] Marcus et al. have demonstrated a reduction in the velocity of coronary blood flow during reactive hyperemia at the time of operation in patients with severe AS,[408] and this may be responsible for the angina commonly observed in these patients. Metabolic evidence of myocardial ischemia, i.e., lactate production, can be demonstrated when myocardial oxygen needs are stimulated by exercise or isoproterenol in patients with AS, in both the presence and the absence of coronary arterial narrowing.

CLINICAL MANIFESTATIONS

HISTORY

In the natural history of adults with AS, a long latent period exists during which there is gradually increasing obstruction and an increase in the pressure load on the myocardium while the patient remains asymptomatic. The cardinal manifestations of AS, which commence most commonly in the sixth decade of life, are angina pectoris, syncope, and heart failure.[409] In patients in whom the obstruction remains unrelieved, once these symptoms become manifested, the prognosis is poor; survival curves show that the interval from the onset of symptoms to the time of death is approximately 2 years in patients with heart failure, 3 years in those with syncope, and 5 years in those with angina.[410,411] *Dyspnea* is the most common initial complaint.[412] *Angina* occurs in approximately two-thirds of patients with critical AS (about half of whom have significant coronary artery obstruction)[413] and usually resembles that observed in patients with coronary artery disease, in that it is commonly precipitated by exertion and relieved by rest. It results from the combination of increased oxygen needs by the hypertrophied myocardium and reduction of oxygen delivery secondary to the excessive compression of coronary vessels[402,408,414] (see Ischemia, above). Rarely, it results from calcium emboli to the coronary vascular bed.[415] Angina may, of course, also result from coexisting coronary artery disease, but the absence of angina in a patient with severe AS does not exclude serious obstructive coronary artery disease.[416,417]

Syncope is often orthostatic and is most commonly due to the reduced cerebral perfusion that occurs during exertion when arterial pressure declines consequent to systemic vasodilatation in the presence of a fixed cardiac output. This may be related to an inappropriate left ventricular baroreceptor response.[418]It may also be caused by arrhythmias[419]; premonitory symptoms are common. Exertional hypotension may also be manifested as "graying out" spells or giddiness on effort.[420] Syncope at rest may be due to transient ventricular fibrillation, from which the patient recovers spontaneously; transient atrial fibrillation with loss of the "atrial kick" and a precipitous decline in cardiac output; or transient atrioventricular block due to extension of the calcification of the valve into the conduction system. Syncope has also been attributed to malfunction of the baroreceptor mechanism.[373] Exertional dyspnea with orthopnea, paroxysmal nocturnal dyspnea, and pulmonary edema reflect varying degrees of pulmonary venous hypertension. These are late symptoms in AS, and their presence for more than 5 years should suggest the possibility of associated mitral valvular disease. *Gastrointestinal bleeding*, idiopathic or due to angiodysplasia (most commonly of the right colon) or other vascular malformations, occurs more often than expected in patients with calcific AS; it may cease after aortic valve replacement.[421,422] Infective endocarditis is a greater risk in younger patients with milder valvular deformity than in older patients with rocklike calcific aortic deformities. Cerebral emboli resulting in stroke or transient ischemic attacks may result from microthrombi on thickened bicuspid valves.[423] Calcific AS may cause embolization of calcium to a variety of organs, including the heart, kidney, and brain. Abrupt loss of vision has been reported when calcific emboli occluded the central retinal artery.[424]

Since cardiac output is usually well maintained for many years in patients with severe AS, marked fatigability, debilitation, peripheral cyanosis, and other manifestations of a low cardiac output are usually not prominent until quite late in the natural history of the disease. Atrial fibrillation, pulmonary hypertension, and systemic venous hypertension in patients with isolated AS are often preterminal findings. Although AS may be responsible for sudden death (p. 763), this usually occurs in patients who had previously been symptomatic.

PHYSICAL EXAMINATION

The arterial pulse characteristically rises slowly and is small and sustained (pulsus parvus et tardus) (Fig. 2–12, p. 23).[425,426] In the advanced stage, systolic and pulse pressures are both reduced. However, in patients with mild stenosis with associated regurgitation and in older patients with an inelastic arterial bed, both systolic and pulse pressures may be normal or even increased. A systolic pressure exceeding 200 mm Hg is rare in patients with critical AS.[425] The anacrotic notch and coarse systolic vibrations are felt most readily in the carotid arterial pulse, producing the so-called carotid shudder. Simultaneous palpation of the apex and carotid arteries reveals a distinct lag in the latter in patients with severe AS.[427] Although pulsus alternans occurs commonly in AS with left ventricular dysfunction,[428] obstruction of the aortic valve may prevent its being recognized by examination of the peripheral arterial pulse. The jugular venous pulse usually shows prominent *a* waves, reflecting reduced right ventricular compliance consequent to hypertrophy of the ventricular septum.[429] With pulmonary hypertension and secondary right ventricular failure and tricuspid regurgitation, *v* or *c-v* waves may be prominent.

The cardiac impulse is sustained with left ventricular failure; it becomes displaced inferiorly and laterally (Table 2–1, p. 26). Presystolic distention of the left ventricle, i.e., a prominent precordial *a* wave, is often both visible and palpable. A hyperdynamic left ventricle suggests concomitant aortic or MR. A systolic thrill is usually best appreciated when the patient leans forward in full expiration. It is felt most readily in the second left intercostal space on either side of the sternum or in the suprasternal notch and is frequently transmitted along the carotid arteries.

Rarely, right ventricular failure with systemic venous congestion, hepatomegaly, and edema precedes left ventricular failure. Probably this is caused by the so-called Bernheim effect, which results from the hypertrophied ventricular septum's bulging into and encroaching on the right ventricular cavity and leads to impairment of right ventricular filling. In such cases, the jugular venous pressure is elevated and the *a* wave is prominent.

AUSCULTATION (Tables 34–4, p. 1020, and 34–11). S_1 is normal or soft and S_4 is prominent, presumably because atrial contraction is vigorous and the mitral valve is partially closed

TABLE 34-11 DIFFERENTIAL DIAGNOSIS OF AORTIC STENOSIS: PHYSICAL FINDINGS

TYPE OF STENOSIS	MAXIMUM MURMUR AND THRILL	AORTIC EJECTION SOUND	AORTIC COMPONENT OF SECOND SOUND	REGURGITANT DIASTOLIC MURMUR	ARTERIAL PULSE
Acquired nonrheumatic or rheumatic	Second right sternal border to neck; may be at apex in the aged	Uncommon	Decreased or absent	Common	Delayed upstroke; anacrotic notch; ± small amplitude
Hypertrophic subaortic	Fourth left sternal border to apex (± regurgitant systolic murmur at apex)	Rare	Normal or decreased	Very rare	Brisk upstroke, sometimes bisferiens
Congenital valvular	Second right sternal border to neck (along left sternal border in some infants)	Very common in children, disappearing with decrease in valve mobility with age	Normal or increased in childhood; decreased with decrease in valve mobility with age	Uncommon in child; not uncommon in adult	Delayed upstroke; anacrotic notch; ± small amplitude
Congenital subvalvular	Discrete: like valvular; tunnel: left sternal border	Rare	Not helpful (normal, increased, decreased or absent)	Almost all	(Delayed upstroke; anacrotic notch; ± small amplitude)
Congenital supravalvular	First right sternal border to neck and sometimes to medial aspect of right arm; occasionally greater in neck than in chest	Rare	Normal or decreased	Uncommon	Rapid upstroke in right carotid, delayed in left carotid; right arm pulse pressure greater than left

From Levinson, G. E.: Aortic stenosis. *In* Dalen, J. E., and Alpert, J. S.: Valvular Heart Disease. 2nd ed. Boston, Little, Brown and Company, 1987, p. 202.

during presystole.[430,431] S_2 may be single because calcification and immobility of the aortic valve make A_2 inaudible, because P_2 is buried in the prolonged aortic ejection murmur, or because prolongation of left ventricular systole makes A_2 coincide with P_2. Paradoxical splitting of S_2, which suggests associated left ventricular dysfunction, may also occur (Fig. 2–21, p. 31). With left ventricular failure and secondary pulmonary hypertension, P_2 may become accentuated. When the valve is rigid, A_2 may be inaudible, but when the valve is flexible, A_2 may be snapping and accentuated.

An aortic ejection sound (p. 44) occurs simultaneously with the halting upward movement of the aortic valve (Fig. 3–3, p. 45). It is dependent on mobility of the valve cusps and disappears when they become severely calcified. Thus, it is common in children with congenital AS but is rare in elderly adults with acquired calcific AS and rigid valves. This sound occurs approximately 0.06 sec after the onset of S_1, has a frequency similar to that of S_1, and is heard most readily with the diaphragm of the stethoscope along the left sternal border, although it is often well transmitted to the apex, where it may be confused with S_1 (and the S_1 may be mistaken for an S_4). In contrast to a pulmonic ejection sound, aortic ejection sounds usually do not vary with respiration.

The *systolic murmur* of AS is heard best at the base of the heart but is often well transmitted along the carotid vessels and to the apex (Fig. 3–16, p. 51). Cessation of the murmur before A_2 is usually helpful in differentiating it from a pansystolic mitral murmur, but it may be falsely considered to be a pansystolic murmur because it may end with S_2, which represents pulmonic valve closure, A_2 being soft or even inaudible. In patients with calcified aortic valves, the murmur is harsh and rasping at the base, but high-frequency components selectively radiate to the apex (the so-called Gallavardin phenomenon [Fig. 3–17, p. 51]), where it may actually be more prominent and where it may be mistaken for the murmur of MR. Frequently, there is a "quiet area" between the base and apex where the murmur is diminished in intensity, supporting the erroneous impression that the apical and basal murmurs have different origins. In general, the more severe the stenosis, the longer the duration of the murmur[432] and the more likely that it peaks in mid-systole.[433]

In patients with degenerative or atherosclerotic AS, there may be heavy valvular calcification, but obstruction may not be severe because the commissural fusion characteristic of congenital and rheumatic AS is absent. The nonfused calcified cusps vibrate freely, resulting in a softer, more musical murmur, more prominent at the apex than the murmur of congenital or rheumatic AS.[432] High-pitched decrescendo diastolic murmurs secondary to aortic regurgitation are common in many patients with dominant AS.

In hypertrophic cardiomyopathy (HCM), the murmur is delayed in onset and may continue up to A_2; the carotid artery characteristically rises sharply and is bisferiens. Palpation of the carotid pulse is also extremely helpful in differentiating between valvular AS on the one hand and HCM and MR on the other, because the arterial pulse generally rises slowly in AS but sharply in the other two conditions. However, confusion can arise in the young patient with congenital AS, in whom sudden upward displacement ("doming") of the pliant aortic leaflet or leaflets with ventricular systole may result in a brisk initial upstroke in the carotid pulse, coincident with the systolic ejection click.

When the left ventricle fails in AS and the cardiac output falls, the murmur becomes softer or disappears altogether, and the slowly rising pulse is more difficult to recognize. Stated simply, the clinical picture changes to that of severe left ventricular failure with a low cardiac output. Thus, occult AS may be a cause of intractable heart failure, and critical AS should be actively sought in patients with severe heart failure of unknown cause, since operative treatment may be life-saving and may result in substantial clinical improvement.[434,435]

Dynamic Auscultation (Table 34–5). The murmur of valvular AS is augmented by the inhalation of amyl nitrite and with squatting or lying flat and is reduced in intensity during the Valsalva strain, which increases the murmur of HCM or that produced with vasopressors, moderate isometric exercise, or standing.[436] It varies in intensity from beat to beat when the duration of diastolic filling varies, as in atrial fibrillation or following a premature contraction, and this characteristic is helpful in differentiating AS from MR, in which the murmur is usually unaffected. An aortic diastolic murmur is frequently present in patients with valvular AS.

LABORATORY EXAMINATION

ELECTROCARDIOGRAPHY

The principal electrocardiographic change is left ventricular hypertrophy, which is found in approximately 85 per cent of patients with severe AS. The absence of left ventricular hypertrophy does not exclude the presence of critical AS, and the correlation between the absolute voltages in precordial leads and the severity of obstruction, which is quite good in children with congenital AS, is not as good in adults. However, a good correlation has been reported between the sum of the QRS amplitudes in 12 leads and the height of the left ventricular systolic pressure.[437] T-wave inversion and ST-segment depressions in leads having upright QRS complexes are common. ST-segment depressions greater than 0.3 mV in patients with AS (left ventricular "strain") suggest that severe ventricular hypertrophy is present. The progressive development of ST-segment and T-wave abnormalities suggests that hypertrophy has progressed. Occasionally, a "pseudoinfarction" pattern is present, characterized by a loss of *r* waves in the right precordial leads and an early vector directed posteriorly in the horizontal plane of the vectorcardiogram, simulating anteroseptal infarction. There is evidence of left atrial enlargement in more than 80 per cent of patients with severe isolated AS[438]; the principal manifestation is prominent late negativity of the P wave in V_1 rather than an increased duration in lead II, suggesting that hypertrophy rather than dilatation is present. Atrial fibrillation is an uncommon and late sign of pure AS, and, when present in a patient who is not greatly disabled, should suggest the possibility of mitral valvular disease or ischemic heart disease.

The extension of calcific infiltrates from the aortic valve into the conduction system may cause various forms and degrees of atrioventricular and intraventricular block in 5 per cent of patients with calcific AS.[439–441] Conduction defects are more common in patients who also have mitral annular calcium.[441] Almost 10 per cent of all instances of left anterior hemiblock are secondary to aortic valvular disease.[442] Ambulatory electrocardiography frequently shows complex ventricular arrhythmias,[443] particularly in patients with myocardial dysfunction.[444]

VECTORCARDIOGRAPHY

In patients with severe AS, the vectorcardiogram usually shows an increase in the maximal spatial voltage and counterclock inscription of the loop in the transverse plane, with the major forces in the left posterior quadrant. In the left sagittal plane, the QRS loop is usually directed posteriorly and superiorly.[445]

GRAPHIC RECORDINGS

The indirect carotid, jugular, and apical pulse tracings and the phonocardiographic findings in AS are discussed in Chapters 2 and 3.

RADIOLOGICAL FINDINGS

Routine radiological examination may be entirely normal despite the presence of critical AS. The heart is usually of normal size or slightly enlarged, with a rounding of the left ventricular border and apex (Fig. 8–8*A*, p. 208), unless regurgitation or left ventricular failure is present and causes substantial cardiomegaly. Poststenotic dilatation of the ascending aorta is a common finding. Calcification of the aortic valve is found in almost all adults with hemodynamically significant AS[446,447] (Fig. 8–28, p. 220); it may have to be sought on fluoroscopy (or the echocardiogram) rather than on the roentgenogram. This is an important finding. Indeed, the *absence* of calcium in the region of the aortic valve on careful fluoroscopic examination in a patient older than 35 essentially rules out severe valvular AS. The converse is not true, however, and in patients over the age of 60, severe calcification of the aortic valve may occur with only mild obstruction. The left atrium may be slightly enlarged, and there may be radiological signs of pulmonary venous hypertension. However, when left atrial enlargement is marked, particularly if the atrial appendage is prominent, the presence of associated mitral valvular disease should be suspected.

Angiographic studies of the aortic valve are best performed by injecting contrast medium into the left ventricle and filming in the 30-degree right anterior oblique and 60-degree left anterior oblique projections. These examinations often make it possible to ascertain the number of cusps of the stenotic valve and to demonstrate doming of a thickened valve and a systolic jet. There is some hazard associated with the rapid injection of a large volume of contrast material into a high-pressure left ventricle, and this is ordinarily not indicated in patients with AS, critical obstruction, and/or left ventricular failure.

ECHOCARDIOGRAPHY (see also p. 85). The normal range of opening of the aortic valve is 1.6 to 2.6 cm, and normally the aortic valve leaflets are barely visible in systole. In patients with severe AS, thickened leaflets and a barely discernible aortic orifice in systole can often be recognized on the M-mode echocardiogram. However, a reduced aortic valve opening may also be seen in other conditions, such as heart failure, in which there is decreased blood flow across the aortic valve. In patients with a bicuspid aortic valve, the valve cusps are asymmetrical, resulting in their eccentric position within the aortic root. Dense, multiple echoes within the aortic root in the area of the aortic leaflets suggest valvular calcification and support the diagnosis of AS. Systolic vibrations of the interventricular septum are common in congenital AS.[448] Two-dimensional echocardiography may also be helpful in determining the severity of the stenosis, by imaging the orifice (Fig. 4-53, p. 85). Doppler echocardiography allows calculation of the left ventricular-aortic pressure gradient[449-452] using a modified Bernouilli equation (Fig. 4-54, p. 85). The noninvasively determined gradients correlate well with those determined by left heart catheterization.

MANAGEMENT

MEDICAL TREATMENT

Patients who are asymptomatic should be advised to report promptly to their physician the development of *any* symptoms possibly related to AS. Noninvasive assessment of the severity of obstruction by Doppler echocardiography should be carried out. In patients with mild obstruction, this measurement should be repeated every 2 years in asymptomatic patients because obstruction tends to become more severe over time.[453-456] There is a close correlation between the left ventricular-aortic systolic pressure gradient determined by echocardiography and left heart catheterization. Those with known or suspected critical obstruction should be cautioned to avoid vigorous athletic and physical activity. However, such restrictions do not apply to patients with mild obstruction. Because there is a tendency for the obstruction to become progressively more severe in patients with AS, asymptomatic patients with AS should be followed carefully; on follow-up examinations, it is essential to look for signs of possible progression.[457] Repeated clinical examinations and electrocardiographic and echocardiographic studies at intervals of 6 to 12 months are indicated in asymptomatic patients with severe AS. The necessity for endocarditis prophylaxis should be explained (p. 1097).

There is no need to use digitalis glycosides unless evidence exists of an increase in ventricular volume or a reduced ejection fraction. Although diuretics are beneficial when there is abnormal accumulation of fluid, they must be used with caution, because hypovelemia may reduce the elevated left ventricular end-diastolic pressure, lower cardiac output, and produce orthostatic hypotension. Beta-adrenoceptor blockers can depress myocardial function and induce left ventricular failure and should be used only with great caution, if at all, in patients with AS.

Atrial arrhythmias occur in fewer than 10 per cent of patients with severe AS, perhaps because of the late occurrence of left atrial enlargement in this condition. When such an arrhythmia is observed in a patient with AS, the possibility of associated mitral valve disease should be considered. In light of the adverse hemodynamic effects of loss of atrial booster pump function with atrial fibrillation in patients with AS,[387] an effort should be made to prevent the development of this arrhythmia by prophylaxis with an antiarrhythmic agent when premature atrial contractions are frequent. When atrial fibrillation does occur, the rapid ventricular rate may cause angina or electrocardiographic evidence of myocardial ischemia or both; in some cases, loss of the "atrial kick" and a sudden fall in cardiac ouput may cause serious hypotension. Therefore, this arrhythmia should be treated promptly (p. 683), and a search for previously unrecognized mitral valve disease should be undertaken.

Adults considered to have severe AS should undergo catheterization if any symptoms develop. The purpose of catheterization in patients with AS is to localize the site and document the severity of the obstruction, to determine the state of left ventricular function, and to ascertain the presence or absence of associated valvular disease and coronary artery disease.

NATURAL HISTORY

In contrast to MS, which leads to symptoms almost immediately after its development, patients with severe AS may be asymptomatic for many years despite the presence of severe obstruction. The systolic pressure gradient can exceed 150 mm Hg, and the peak left ventricular systolic pressure can reach approximately 300 mm Hg with relatively little increase in overall heart size on radiographic examination and with normal left ventricular end-diastolic and end-systolic volumes. Patients with severe chronic AS tend to be free of cardiovascular symptoms until relatively late in the course of the disease. In Rapaport's series, 40 per cent of patients treated medically survived for 5 years and 20 per cent for 10 years after diagnosis.[102] In another series of patients with hemodynamically significant valvular AS treated medically, the 5-year survival rate was 64 per cent. However, once patients with AS become symptomatic with angina or syncope, the average survival is 2 to 3 years, whereas with congestive heart failure it is 1½ years[413] (Fig. 34-27). Sudden death, like syncope, in patients with severe AS may be due to cerebral hypoperfusion followed by arrhythmia. Among symptomatic patients with moderate or severe AS not subjected to operation, mortality rates from onset of symptoms were approximately 25 per cent at 1 year and 50 per cent at 2 years; more than half

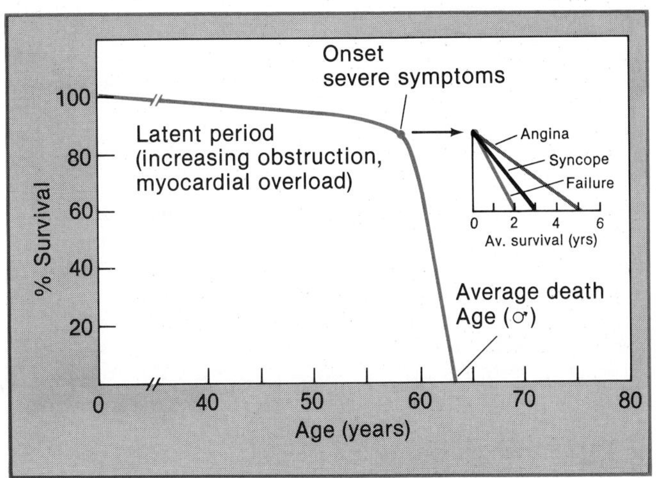

FIGURE 34-27. Natural history of aortic stenosis without operative treatment. (From Ross, J., Jr., and Braunwald, E.: Aortic stenosis. Circulation *38*[Suppl. V]:61, 1968, by permission of the American Heart Association, Inc.)

of the deaths were sudden. Asymptomatic patients have an excellent prognosis insofar as survival is concerned[458]; only about 4 per cent of the deaths in AS occur suddenly in asymptomatic patients. While severe AS is a potentially lethal disease, death, even when sudden, usually occurs in symptomatic patients. A number of authors have followed asymptomatic patients with critical AS,[459-462] and sudden death is extremely rare. Pellika et al. followed 113 asymptomatic patients; symptoms developed in 38 per cent within 2 years. No sudden deaths occurred during 118 patient-years of follow-up.[462] The obstruction tends to progress more rapidly in patients with degenerative calcific disease than in those with congenital or rheumatic disease.[463]

SURGICAL TREATMENT

INDICATIONS FOR OPERATION. The most critical decision in the management of patients with AS—indeed, of all patients with valvular heart disease—concerns the advisability and timing of surgical treatment.[464] The indications for surgery as well as the techniques and results of operation depend on the patient's age and the nature of the valvular deformity. In children and adolescents with noncalcific congenital AS, who most commonly have bicuspid aortic valves, simple commissural incision under direct vision usually leads to substantial hemodynamic improvement at a low risk, i.e., a mortality rate of less than 1 per cent (p. 925).[465] Therefore, this procedure (or aortic balloon valvuloplasty) is indicated not only in symptomatic patients but also in asymptomatic children and adolescents with critical aortic stenosis, i.e., a calculated effective orifice less than 0.75 cm^2/m^2 BSA. Despite the salutary hemodynamic results following this procedure, the valve is not rendered entirely normal anatomically, and the turbulent blood flow through it may lead to further deformation, calcification, the development of regurgitation, and restenosis after 10 to 20 years, probably requiring reoperation and valve replacement later.

In most adults with calcific AS, satisfactory valvular function cannot be restored, even by deliberate sculpturing procedures carried out under direct vision, and valve replacement is the surgical treatment of choice.[466] Ultrasonic decalcification and other repairs may be effective immediately in a fraction of patients but even in them restenosis is a serious problem.[467-470] The aortic valve should, in general, be replaced in patients who have hemodynamic evidence of severe obstruction (aortic valve orifice < 0.75 cm^2 or < 0.4 cm^2/m^2 BSA) as well as symptoms believed to result from AS. (Prosthetic valves are discussed on pp. 1061 to 1064.) Surgical treatment should also be carried out in asymptomatic patients with serious left ventricular dysfunction and progressive cardiomegaly. Although a prospective randomized controlled study has not been done, the long-term mortality in patients undergoing operation in the latter group appears to be lower than that in medically treated patients without operation.[471] As artificial valves and surgical skills continue to improve, it is likely that patients with severe AS will become candidates for operation at progressively earlier stages in the natural history of their disease. At the present time, I do not recommend prophylactic replacement of a critically narrow calcific aortic valve in *asymptomatic* adults unless they exhibit progressive left ventricular dysfunction.

RESULTS. Successful replacement of the aortic valve results in substantial clinical and hemodynamic improvement in patients with AS, AR, or combined lesions[466-475] including many patients in their 70's and 80's.[468,469] In patients without frank left ventricular failure, the operative risk ranges from 2 to 8 per cent in most centers. Risk factors for higher mortality include high New York Heart Association (NYHA) class, impairment of left ventricular function, age, and the presence of associated aortic regurgitation.[466] The 5-year actuarial survival rate of hospital survivors is approximately 85 per cent. Risk factors for late death include preoperative NYHA class, left ventricular function, preoperative ventricular arrhythmias, associated significant aortic regurgitation, older age, and concomitant untreated coronary artery disease.[466] Symptoms secondary to elevations of left atrial pressure and myocardial ischemia are relieved in almost every patient. Hemodynamic results are equally impressive; elevated end-diastolic and end-systolic volumes show significant reductions. Ventricular performance often returns to normal more frequently in patients with AS than in those with AR.[476] However, the finding that the strongest predictor of postoperative left ventricular dysfunction is preoperative dysfunction[471,477] suggests that patients should, if possible, be operated on before left ventricular function becomes seriously impaired. The increased left ventricular mass is reduced toward (but not to) normal within 18 months after aortic valve replacement in patients with AS.[399,478] When restudied 5 years postoperatively, left ventricular mass had returned to normal.[479] Myocyte hypertrophy regresses before fibrous tissue is resorbed.

When operation is carried out in patients with frank left ventricular failure or a depressed ejection fraction, the operative risk is higher, and the mortality ranges from 10 to 25 per cent, depending on the skill of the surgical team and the severity of depression of left ventricular function.[480] A depressed relation between ejection fraction and wall stress is a poor prognostic index, as is a depressed level of dP/dt max at any given left ventricular end-diastolic pressure.[472] Obviously, it is desirable to perform surgery before the development of heart failure, but emergency operation is sometimes lifesaving even in the most desperate situations, such as cardiac arrest or pulmonary edema from AS. Certainly, in view of the extremely poor prognosis of such patients when they are treated medically, there is usually little choice but to advise immediate mechanical relief of obstruction, i.e., balloon angioplasty (see later discussion) or emergency surgery.[481] Many symptomatic patients with calcific AS are elderly, and particular attention must be directed to the adequacy of their hepatic, renal, and pulmonary function. However, the results of aortic valve replacement are satisfactory in patients older than 70[468] or even 80.[469] If the patient's general condition permits, age, per se, while adding to the risk, should not be considered a contraindication to operation.[482]

In patients with AS and obstructive coronary artery disease (a relatively common combination), aortic valve replacement and myocardial revascularization should be performed together.[417] Although the risk of aortic valve surgery is in-

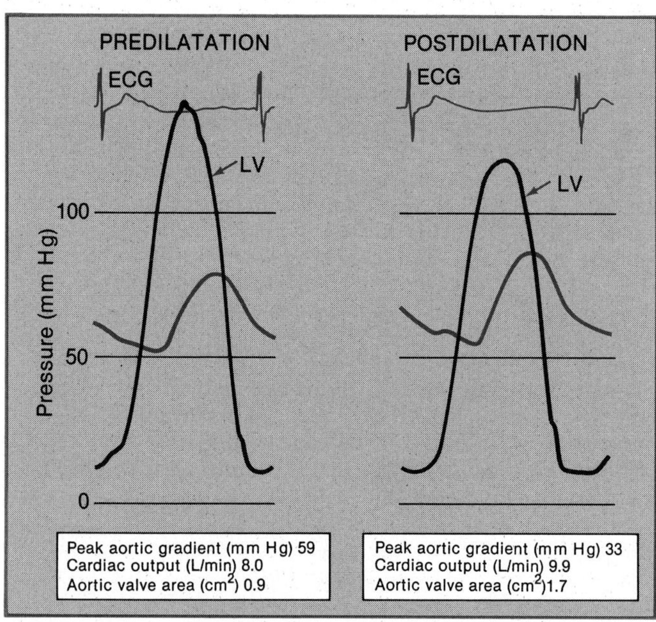

FIGURE 34-28. Simultaneous left ventricular (LV) and arterial pressure tracings recorded before and after balloon valvuloplasty in a patient with severe aortic stenosis. (Courtesy of Raymond G. McKay, M.D.)

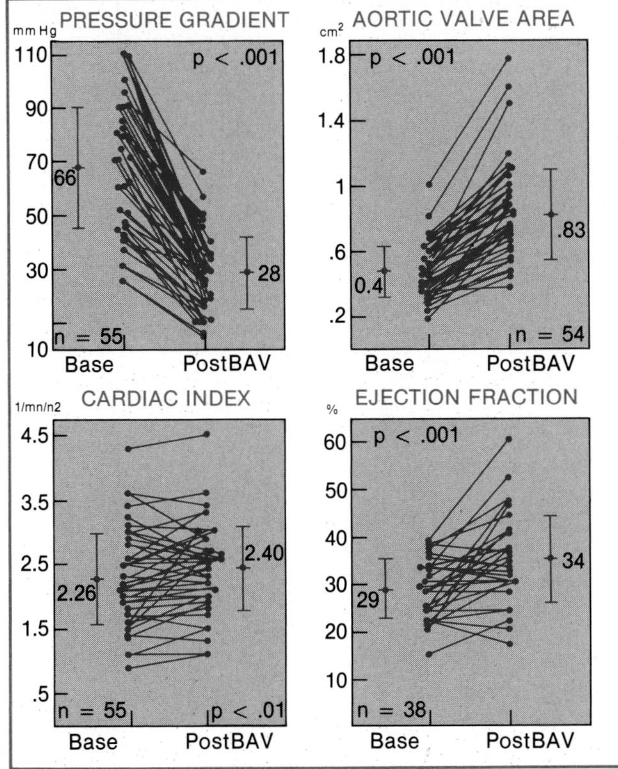

FIGURE 34-29. Plots of changes in pressure gradient, valve area, cardiac index, and ejection fraction at baseline (Base) after balloon aortic valvuloplasty (BAV). (From Berland, J., et al.: Percutaneous balloon valvuloplasty in patients with severe aortic stenosis and low ejection fraction. Circulation *79*:1189, 1989, by permission of the American Heart Association, Inc.)

creased by the association of coronary artery disease, the operative mortality in patients undergoing the combined procedure is not necessarily higher than that of isolated aortic valve replacement in this group.[466] Indeed, the surgical risk rises if severe coronary artery disease is left untreated. The ability to avoid serious myocardial ischemia in the perioperative period is a major factor that has served to reduce operative mortality. After the patient has been placed on cardiopulmonary bypass, the heart is protected by means of hypothermic cardiac arrest alone or combined with cardioplegia. The calcified valve must be removed with great care to avoid embolization of calcified fragments into the systemic circulation.

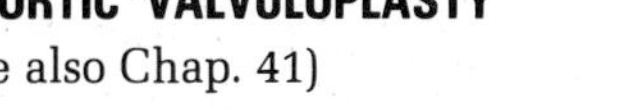

BALLOON AORTIC VALVULOPLASTY

(See also Chap. 41)

This technique (Fig. 41-20, p. 1377) represents an increasingly attractive alternative to aortic valvotomy in children and adolescents with congenital AS (p. 1035), but its value is limited in adults with calcific AS. A series of balloon dilatation catheters are advanced along a guidewire positioned at the left ventricular apex. In balloon dilatation of calcified stenotic aortic valves carried out on postmortem specimens and in the operating room, fracture of calcified nodules and/or separation of fused commissures were found to be responsible for the relief of obstruction[483]; stretching of the aortic valve ring is probably also involved.[484] There is considerable variation in patient response. However, this technique results initially in relief of obstruction in most patients[485,486,486a] (Fig. 34-28). On the average, valve area initially increases by about 60 per cent, from 0.50 to 0.80 cm,^{2} and the mean gradient declines from approximately 60 to 30 mm Hg. Left ventricular ejection fraction tends to rise in patients with depressed left ventricular function. A major problem is restenosis, which occurs in about half of the patients within 6 months. Symptoms lessen in severity in the majority of patients but recur in approximately 30 per cent by 6 months. In most series, patients have been elderly, with heart failure, and were considered poor operative risks. One-year mortality is approximately 25 per cent. Independent correlates of event-free survival were a prevalvuloplasty left ventricular systolic pressure ≥130 mm Hg, a pulmonary capillary wedge pressure ≤15 mm Hg, an aortic valve area ≥0.8 cm^2, and a reduction in the transvalvular gradient >15 mm Hg.[487,487a]

In critically ill patients, the mortality from the procedure is 3 to 7 per cent, and another 6 per cent develop serious complications such as myocardial perforation, myocardial infarction, and severe aortic regurgitation.[484-490] While the overall intermediate-term (6 to 12 months) results of balloon aortic valvuloplasty have been disappointing, largely because of restenosis, the procedure does have a role in the management of severe calcific AS in patients who are not surgical candidates. This includes patients with cardiogenic shock due to critical AS,[484] patients with critical AS who require an urgent noncardiac operation, as a "bridge" to aortic valve replacement in patients with severe heart failure who are at extremely high operative risk, and in pregnant women with critical AS.[490a] In the adult, balloon aortic valvuloplasty is *not* a substitute for surgery (as balloon mitral valvuloplasty may be [p. 1017]).

Balloon aortic valvuloplasty appears to be useful in patients with critical AS who refuse surgical treatment or in whom surgical intervention is not advised because of an extremely high expected mortality. The procedure is also effective in young patients with noncalcific congenital AS.

Aortic Regurgitation

ETIOLOGY AND PATHOLOGY

Aortic regurgitation (AR) may be caused by primary disease of either the aortic valve leaflets or the wall of the aortic root or both (Table 34-12 and Fig. 34-30). Among patients with pure AR coming to valve replacement, the percentage with aortic root disease has been increasing steadily during the past few decades and now accounts for more than one-third of the patients.[491]

VALVULAR DISEASE

Rheumatic fever is a common cause of primary disease of the valve leading to regurgitation.[11,491,492] The cusps become infiltrated with fibrous tissues and retract, a process that prevents cusp apposition during diastole and that usually leads to regurgitation into the left ventricle through a defect in the center of the valve. Often the associated fusion of the commissures may also restrict the opening of the valve, resulting in combined AS and AR (Fig. 34-31B); some associated mitral valve involvement is common. Other primary valvular causes of AR include *infective endocarditis* (Chap. 35), in which the infection may destroy the valve or cause perforation of a leaflet, or the vegetations may interfere with proper coaptation of the cusps. *Trauma* (Fig. 46-8, p. 1524) resulting in a tear of the ascending aorta and loss of commissural support can cause prolapse of an aortic cusp. Although the most common complication of a congenitally *bicuspid valve* is stenosis in adult life, incomplete closure and/or prolapse of the larger of the two cusps of a *bicuspid valve* may cause regurgitation in childhood.[493] More commonly, progressive regurgitation of a

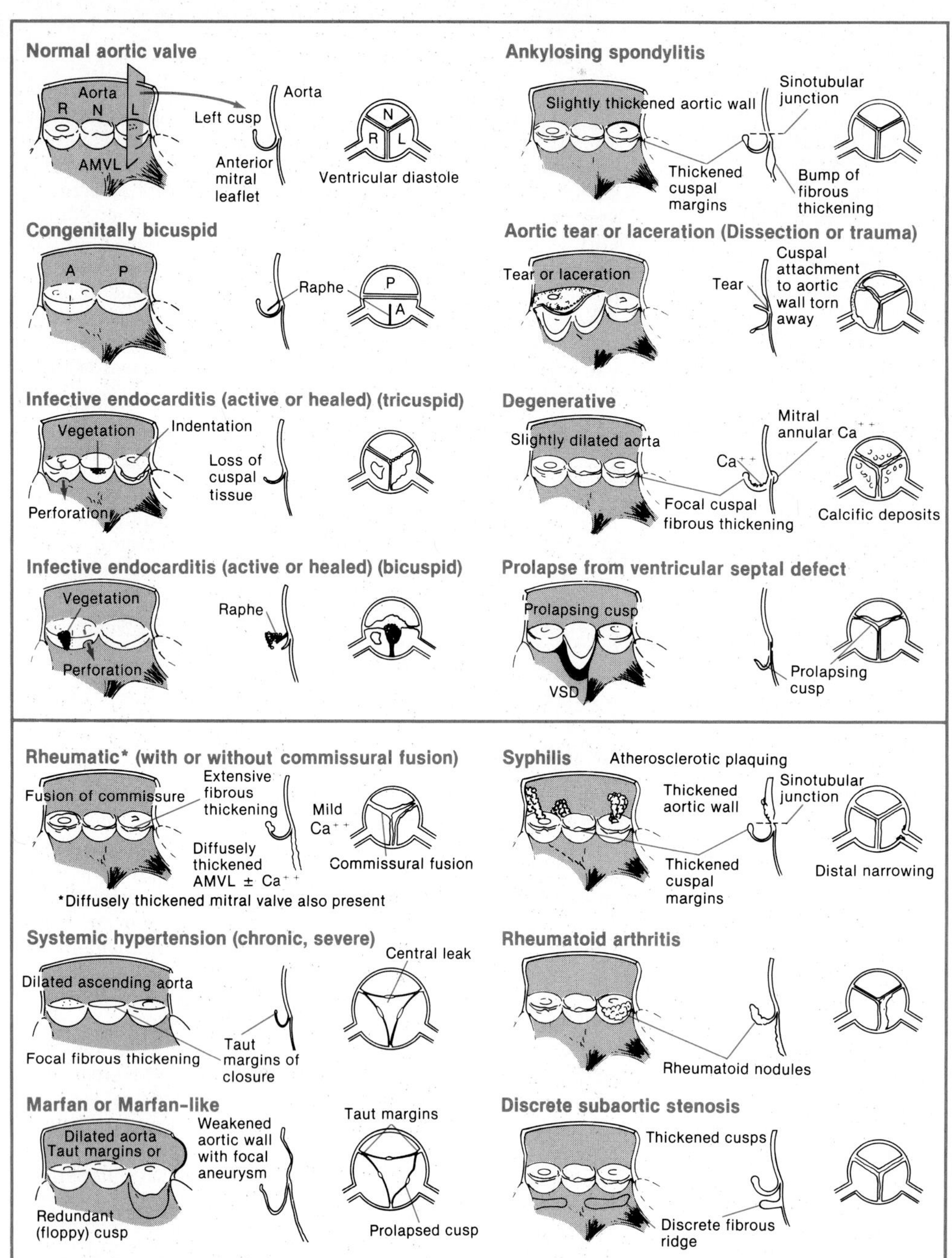

FIGURE 34–30. Diagram of various causes of pure aortic regurgitation. (From Waller, B. F.: Rheumatic and nonrheumatic conditions producing valvular heart disease. *In* Frankl, W. S., and Brest, A. N. [eds.]: Cardiovascular Clinics. Valvular Heart Disease: Comprehensive Evaluation and Management. Philadelphia, F. A. Davis, 1986, pp. 30–31.)

congenitally bicuspid valve develops in the third and fourth decades.[494,495] Progressive regurgitation may also occur in patients with Marfan syndrome, Ehlers-Danlos syndrome, cystic medionecrosis of the aorta, myxomatous proliferation of the aortic valve,[496] and related diseases of connective tissue. Less common causes of AR include a variety of forms of congenital AR; rupture of a congenitally fenestrated valve,[497] particularly in the presence of hypertension[498]; AR in association with systemic lupus erythematosus[499]; rheumatoid arthritis[500]; ankylosing spondylitis[501]; Jaccoud's arthropathy[502]; Whipple's disease[503]; and Crohn's disease in the absence of ankylosing spondylitis.[504] Isolated congenital AR is an uncommon lesion on necropsy studies, but when present, it is usually associated with a bicuspid valve.[505]

AORTIC ROOT DISEASE

(See also Chap. 47)

A variety of diseases produce aortic regurgitation by causing marked dilatation of the ascending aorta (Fig. 34–31C). These conditions include annuloaortic ectasia, cystic medionecrosis of the aorta (either isolated or associated with classic Marfan syndrome), osteogenesis imperfecta, syphilitic aortitis, ankylosing spondylitis, Behçet syndrome,[506] psoriatic arthritis, arthritis associated with ulcerative colitis, relapsing polychondritis, Reiter syndrome, giant cell arteritis, osteogenesis imperfecta, and systemic hypertension.[498,507–512]

Table 34–13 presents a comparison of the findings in four important conditions in which dilation of the aorta causes AR. In each of these, the aortic annulus may become greatly dilated, the aortic leaflets separate, and AR may ensue. Dissection of the diseased aortic wall may occur and may aggravate the AR. Dilatation of the aortic root may also have secondary effects on the aortic valve, since it results in tension and bowing of the individual cusps, which may thicken, retract, and become too short to close the aortic orifice. This leads to intensification of the AR, which increases left ventricular stroke volume, further dilating the ascending aorta and thus leading to a vicious circle in which "regurgitation begets regurgitation."

AR, regardless of its etiology, produces dilatation and hypertrophy of the left ventricle, dilatation of the mitral valve ring, and sometimes hypertrophy and dilatation of the left atrium. Endocardial pockets frequently develop in the left ventricular cavity at sites of impact of the regurgitant jet.

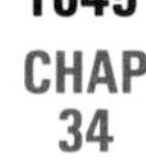

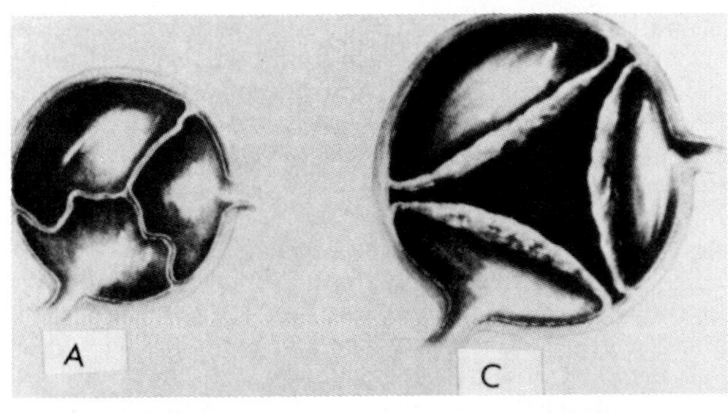

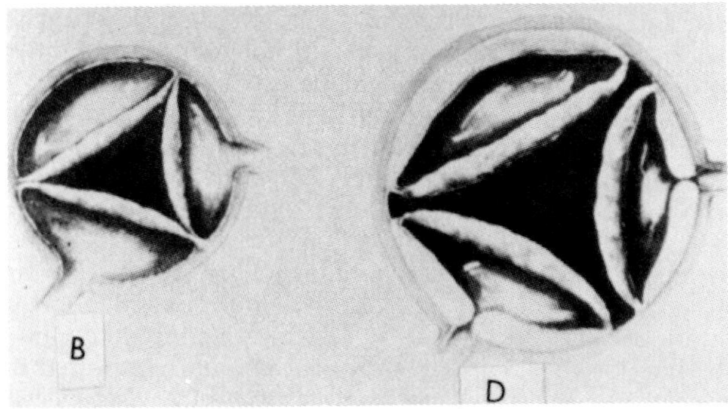

FIGURE 34-31. Variations in the aortic valve. *A*, The normal valve. *B*, Shortening of the cusps characteristic of rheumatic aortic regurgitation. The caliber of the aorta is normal. *C*, Dilatation of the aorta, as occurs in syphilitic aortitis and other conditions in which dilatation is responsible for aortic regurgitation. The main feature results from bowing of the leaflets. Commissural separation is illustrated and may also be present. *D*, In addition to the features shown in *C*, there is atherosclerosis of the aorta, as occurs in syphilitic aortitis, with consequent coronary ostial narrowing. (From Roberts, W. C.: Valvular, subvalvular and supravalvular aortic stenosis: Morphologic features. *In* Edwards, J. E. [ed.]: Clinical-Pathologic Correlations #2. Philadelphia, F. A. Davis, 1973, p. 133.)

TABLE 34-12 MECHANISMS OF AORTIC REGURGITATION

1. Cusp abnormality	Perforation Reduction in area of cusps	Bacterial endocarditis Rheumatic disease Rheumatoid disease
2. Aortic root distortion (aortitis)		Ankylosing spondylitis Nonspecific urethritis Nonspecific aortitis Rheumatoid disease Syphilis Fallot-type VSD
3. Loss of commissural support		Dissection tears of aorta
4. Aortic root dilatation	Aortitis (inflammatory) "Aortopathy" (noninflammatory)	Syphilis All other aortitis Marfan syndrome Familial Idiopathic Ehlers-Danlos Pseudoxanthoma elasticum

From Davies, M. J.: Pathology of Cardiac Valves. London, Butterworths, 1980.

PATHOPHYSIOLOGY

In contrast to MR, in which a fraction of the left ventricular stroke volume is ejected into the low-pressure left atrium, in AR the entire left ventricular stroke volume is ejected into a high-pressure chamber, i.e., the aorta (although the low aortic diastolic pressure does facilitate ventricular emptying during early systole). Whereas in MR the reduction of wall tension (i.e., reduced afterload) allows more complete systolic emptying, in AR the increase in left ventricular end-diastolic volume provides major hemodynamic compensation.[513-517]

Severe AR may occur with a normal effective forward stroke volume and a normal ejection fraction (total [forward plus regurgitant] stroke volume/end-diastolic volume), together with an elevated preload, i.e., left ventricular end-diastolic volume pressure and stress[518a] (Figs. 34-32 and 34-33). In accord with Laplace's law, left ventricular dilatation also increases the left ventricular systolic tension required to develop any level of systolic pressure. The increased end-diastolic wall stress leads to volume overload (eccentric) hypertrophy, with replication of sarcomeres in series, elongation of fibers, and sufficient wall thickening to maintain or return end-diastolic wall stress to normal levels the ratio of ventricular wall thickness to cavity radius (h/R) remains normal.[519]

TABLE 34-13 CARDIOVASCULAR MANIFESTATIONS OF CONDITIONS CAUSING AORTIC REGURGITATION

	SYPHILIS	AKYLOSING SPONDYLITIS	RHEUMATOID ARTHRITIS	MARFAN SYNDROME
Average age	50	45	70	30
Predominant sex	Men	Men	Women	Men
Aortic regurgitation	++++	++++	+	++++
Mitral regurgitation	0	++	+	+++
Conduction disturbances	+	++++	++	+
Serology (STS)	+	0	0	0
Morphology of aorta				
Thickened adventitia	++++	++++	+	+
Degenerated media	+++	+++	0	++++
Intimal proliferation	+++	+++	0	+
Vasa vasorum abnormal	++++	++++	0	0
Calcium	++	+	0	0
Aneurysms	+++	0	0	+++
Rupture	+	0	0	+
Dissection	0	0	0	+
Limited to sinuses	0	+	0	0
Morphology of aortic valve				
Cusp thickening				
Diffuse	0	+	0	0
Focal	+	0	+	+
Cusp calcification	0	0	0	0
Shortening	0	+	0	0
Commissural abnormality	+	+	0	0

From Roberts, W. C., et al.: Nonrheumatic valvular cardiac disease: A clinicopathologic survey of 27 different conditions causing valvular dysfunction. *In* Likoff, W. (ed.): Cardiovascular Clinics. Vol. 5, No. 2, Valvular Heart Disease. Philadelphia, F. A. Davis, 1973, p. 424.

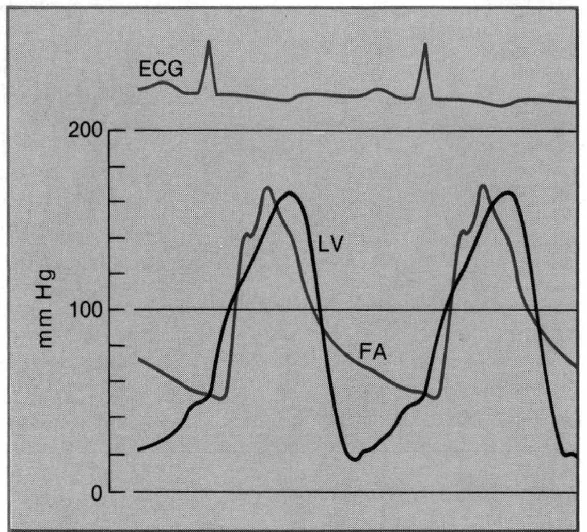

FIGURE 34–32. Pressure curves obtained from a 63-year-old man with symptoms of left ventricular failure and a loud decrescendo diastolic murmur. The femoral arterial (FA) pressure tracing demonstrates a widened pulse pressure of 115 mm Hg and equalization with left ventricular (LV) pressure late in diastole. The LV pressure curve exhibits a steady pressure increase throughout diastole, culminating in a markedly elevated end-diastolic pressure of 45 mm Hg. These findings are indicative of severe aortic regurgitation.

This contrasts with the events in AS, in which there is pressure overload (concentric) hypertrophy with replication of sarcomeres in parallel (p. 399) and an increased h/R (p. 402). In AR, left ventricular mass is usually greatly elevated, often to levels even higher than in isolated AS[381] and sometimes exceeding 1000 gm.

Patients with severe chronic AR have the largest end-diastolic volumes of those with any form of heart disease (resulting in so-called *cor bovinum*). However, end-diastolic pressure is not uniformly elevated (i.e., left ventricular compliance often becomes increased [Fig. 14–5, p. 398 and Fig. 34–12, p. 1021]), and there is a wide scatter in the relationship between end-diastolic volume and end-diastolic pressure.[381] In the more severe cases of AR, the regurgitant flow may exceed 20 liters/min, so that the total left ventricular output approaches 25 liters/min, a level that can be achieved only by a trained endurance runner during maximal exercise. Thus, the adaptive response to chronic and gradually increasing AR permits the ventricle to function as an effective high-compliance pump, handling large end-diastolic and stroke volumes, often with little increase in filling pressure (Fig. 34–33C). During exercise, peripheral vascular resistance declines, and with an increase in heart rate, diastole shortens and the regurgitation per beat decreases,[520–522] facilitating an increment in effective forward cardiac output without substantial increases in end-diastolic volume and pressure. The ejection fraction and related ejection phase indices (p. 426) are often within normal limits, both at rest and during exercise when

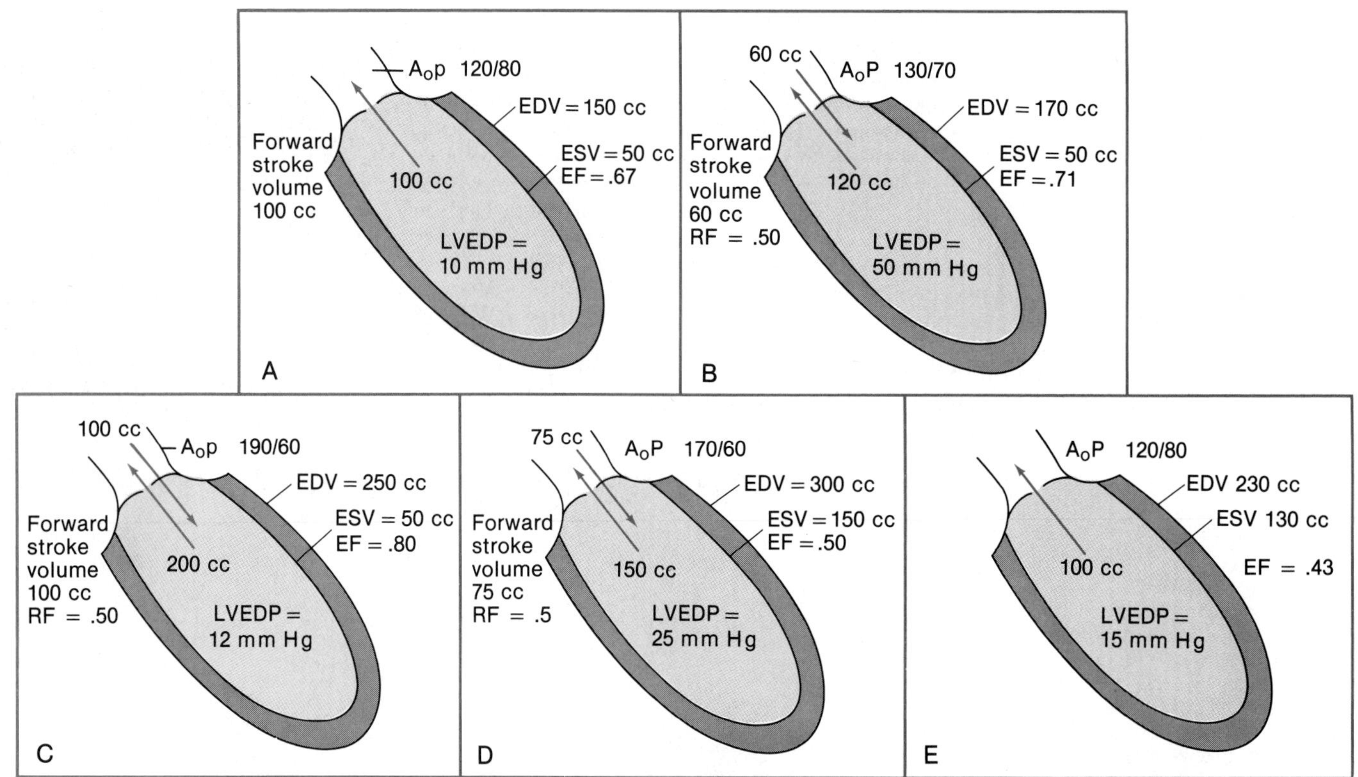

FIGURE 34–33. Hemodynamics of aortic regurgitation. *A*, Normal conditions. *B*, The hemodynamic changes that occur in severe acute aortic regurgitation. Although total stroke volume is increased, forward stroke volume is reduced. Left ventricular end-diastolic pressure rises dramatically. *C*, Hemodynamic changes occurring in chronic compensated aortic regurgitation are shown. Eccentric hypertrophy produces increased end-diastolic volume, which permits an increase in total as well as forward stroke volume. The volume overload is accommodated and left ventricular filling pressure is normalized. Ventricular emptying and end-systolic volume remain normal. *D*, In chronic decompensated aortic regurgitation, impaired left ventricular emptying produces an increase in end-systolic volume and a fall in ejection fraction, total stroke volume, and forward stroke volume. There is further cardiac dilatation and reelevation of left ventricular filling pressure. *E*, Immediately following valve replacement, preload estimated by end-diastolic volume decreases, as does filling pressure. End-systolic volume also is decreased but to a lesser extent. The result is an initial fall in ejection fraction. Despite these changes, elimination of regurgitation leads to an increase in forward stroke volume. AoP = aortic pressure; EDV = end-diastolic volume; ESV = end-systolic volume; EF = ejection fraction; LVEDP = left ventricular end-diastolic pressure; RF = regurgitant fraction. (From Carabello, B. A.: Aortic regurgitation: Hemodynamic determinants of prognosis. *In* Cohn, L. H., and DiSesa, V. J. [eds.]: Aortic Regurgitation: Medical and Surgical Management. New York, Marcel Dekker, Inc., 1986.)

myocardial function, as reflected in the slope of the end-systolic pressure-volume relation, is depressed.[523-525] Therefore, the latter is a more sensitive index of contractility than the former (p. 429).

As left ventricular function deteriorates, the left ventricle dilates (Fig. 34-33*D*). Ventricular end-diastolic volume increases without further elevation of the aortic regurgitant volume; left ventricular end-diastolic h/R declines,[526] systolic wall tension rises, and afterload mismatch occurs[527] so that ejection fraction declines with any additional stress.[528] Ultimately the ejection fraction and forward stroke volume decline at rest, and ventricular emptying is impaired; i.e., end-systolic volume increases. Many of these changes precede the development of symptoms. In advanced stages there may be considerable elevation of the left atrial, pulmonary artery wedge, pulmonary arterial, right ventricular, and right atrial pressures and lowering of the effective cardiac output, first during the stress of exercise[522] and then even at rest.

As is the case in MR (p. 1022), the end-systolic volume provides a useful overall index of myocardial function in patients with AR and correlates with operative mortality and postoperative left ventricular dysfunction.[191] Both the immediate and the long-term results are excellent in patients with normal left ventricular end-systolic volumes (<30 ml/m^2), poor in patients in whom this index is elevated (>90 ml/m^2), and variable in patients with intermediate values. In general, however, for any given preoperative level of impairment of left ventricular function, the outlook for left ventricular function in the postoperative period is somewhat better in patients with AR than with MR.

When *acute* AR is induced experimentally, preload, wall tension, and myocardial oxygen consumption all rise substantially,[182,514] a situation contrasting with that produced by *acutely* induced MR. In patients with chronic severe AR, total myocardial oxygen requirements are also augmented by the increase in left ventricular mass. Since the major portion of coronary blood flow occurs during diastole, when arterial pressure is lower than normal, coronary perfusion pressure is reduced.[529] The result—a combination of increased oxygen demand and reduced supply—sets the stage for the development of myocardial ischemia, especially during exercise.[530] Indeed, patients with severe AR exhibit a reduction of coronary reserve,[531] which may be responsible for myocardial ischemia, which in turn may play a role in the deterioration of left ventricular function. The heightened activity of the adrenergic nervous system as a compensatory mechanism in patients with chronic AR is reflected in an abnormal increase in plasma catecholamine content during exercise, accompanied by a reduction in cardiac norepinephrine stores.[532]

Symptomatic patients with severe chronic AR generally exhibit a depression of the relations between end-systolic pressure (or wall stress) and end-systolic volume. This depression of myocardial function, combined with the increased demands placed on the left ventricle, augments left ventricular end-diastolic volume and ultimately pressure, causing symptoms of pulmonary congestion. These patients also demonstrate a failure of the normal decline in end-systolic volume or rise in ejection fraction during exercise, as determined by radionuclide angiography.[533] However, abnormal left ventricular function can be discerned even in subgroups of asymptomatic patients with normal ejection fractions; this dysfunction is reflected in failure of the normal increase in ejection fraction during exercise[534,535] or a depressed end-systolic pressure-volume relation.[535] Radionuclide ventriculography is of value in the identification of those patients with severe chronic AR, who, although asymptomatic or almost so, are at greater risk of developing left ventricular failure and therefore are candidates for consideration of surgical treatment.

ACUTE AORTIC REGURGITATION

In contrast to the pathophysiological events in chronic AR described above, in which the left ventricle has had the opportunity to adapt to the increased load, in *acute* regurgitation (caused most commonly by infective endocarditis, aortic dissection, and trauma) the regurgitant blood fills a ventricle of normal size that cannot accommodate the combined large regurgitant volume and inflow from the left atrium.[536,537] Since

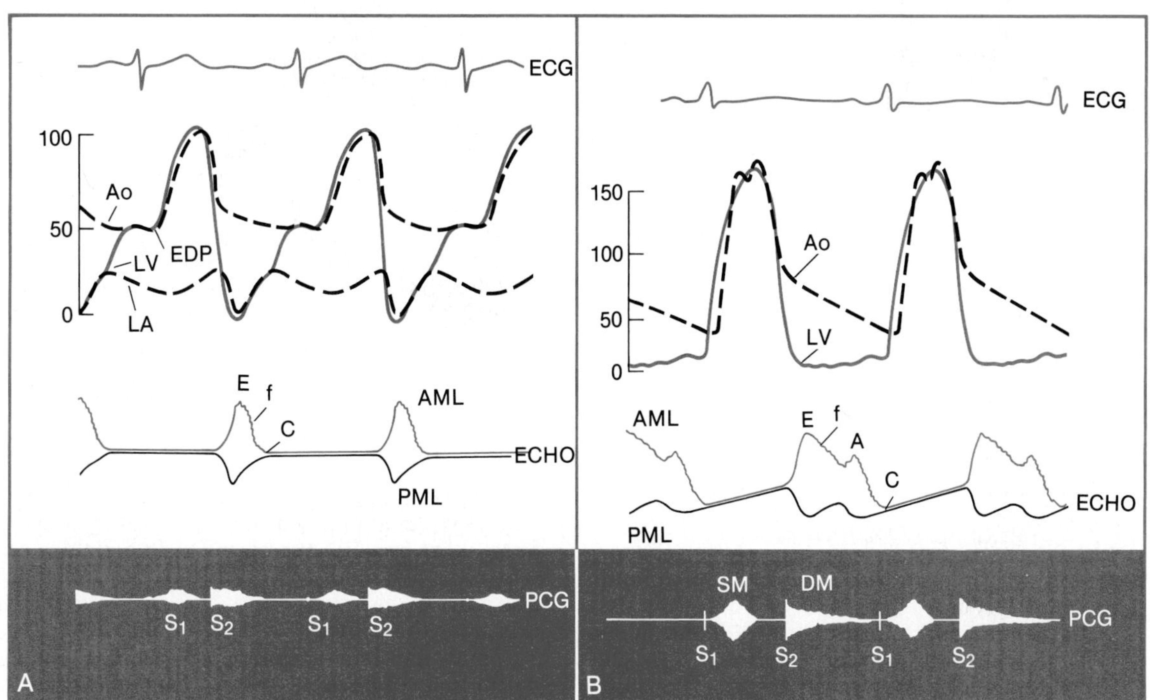

FIGURE 34-34. Schematic representations contrasting the hemodynamic, echocardiographic (ECHO), and phonocardiographic (PCG) manifestations of acute severe *(A)* and chronic severe *(B)* aortic regurgitation. Ao = aorta; LV = left ventricle; LA = left atrium; EDP = end-diastolic pressure; f = flutter of anterior mitral valve leaflet; AML = anterior mitral valve leaflet; PML = posterior mitral valve leaflet; SM = systolic murmur; DM = diastolic murmur; C = closure point of mitral valve. (From Morganroth, J., et al.: Acute severe aortic regurgitation. Ann. Intern. Med. *87*:225, 1977.)

total stroke volume cannot rise a great deal acutely, *forward* stroke volume declines, left ventricular diastolic pressure rises rapidly to high levels,[513] and the left ventricle operates on a steep portion of its pressure-volume curve (Fig. 34–14).[514]

The hemodynamic findings in acute AR contrast with those in chronic AR.[538] For a similar severe degree of AR, the patient with acute regurgitation has a much smaller aortic pulse pressure and effective forward cardiac output, a smaller left ventricular volume throughout the cardiac cycle, and a higher heart rate than the patient with chronic AR. In addition, as left ventricular pressure rises rapidly above left atrial pressure during early diastole, the mitral valve closes prematurely in diastole (Fig. 34–34).[539] Preclosure of the mitral valve is accompanied by diastolic mitral regurgitation.[539] This protects the pulmonary venous bed from backward transmission of the greatly elevated end-diastolic pressure. Premature closure of the mitral valve, together with the tachycardia that shortens diastole, reduces the time interval during which the mitral valve is open. Left ventricular and aortic systolic pressures exhibit little change. Since aortic diastolic pressure cannot decline below the elevated left ventricular end-diastolic pressure, the systemic arterial pulse pressure widens relatively little.

CLINICAL MANIFESTATIONS

HISTORY

CHRONIC AORTIC REGURGITATION. In patients with chronic, severe AR, the left ventricle gradually undergoes enlargement while the patient remains asymptomatic or almost so.[492,540] Symptoms of reduced cardiac reserve or myocardial ischemia develop, most often in the fourth or fifth decade and usually only after considerable cardiomegaly and myocardial dysfunction have occurred. When symptoms do develop, exertional dyspnea, orthopnea, and paroxysmal nocturnal dyspnea are the principal complaints. Syncope is rare, and although angina pectoris is less frequent than it is in patients with AS, nocturnal angina, often accompanied by diaphoresis, which occurs when the heart rate slows and arterial diastolic pressure falls to extremely low levels, may be particularly troublesome. These episodes are occasionally accompanied by abdominal discomfort, presumably caused by splanchnic ischemia. Patients with severe AR often complain of an uncomfortable awareness of the heartbeat, especially on lying down, and disagreeable thoracic pain due to pounding of the heart against the chest wall. Tachycardia, occurring with emotional stress or exertion, may produce palpitations and head pounding; premature ventricular contractions are particularly distressing because of the great heave of the volume-loaded left ventricle during the postpremature beat. These complaints may be present for many years before symptoms of overt left ventricular dysfunction develop.

ACUTE AORTIC REGURGITATION. In light of the limited ability of the left ventricle to tolerate AR, patients with this valvular lesion often develop sudden clinical manifestations of cardiovascular collapse, with weakness, severe dyspnea, and hypotension; angina is uncommon.[538,541]

PHYSICAL EXAMINATION

In patients with chronic severe AR, the head frequently bobs with each heartbeat (*de Musset's sign*),[542] and the pulses are of the water-hammer or collapsing type with abrupt distention and quick collapse (*Corrigan's pulse*, p. 23). This pulse is readily visible in the carotid arteries and can be best appreciated by palpation of the radial artery with the patient's arm elevated. A *bisferiens pulse* may be present (Fig. 2–13, p. 24) and is more readily recognized in the brachial and femoral than in the carotid arteries. A variety of auscultatory findings provide confirmation of a wide pulse pressure. *Traube's sign* (also known as "pistol shot sounds"[542a]) refers to booming systolic and diastolic sounds heard over the femoral artery, *Müller's sign* consists of systolic pulsations of the uvula, and *Duroziez's sign* consists of a systolic murmur heard over the femoral artery when it is compressed proximally and a diastolic murmur when it is compressed distally. Capillary pulsations, i.e., *Quincke's sign*, can be detected by pressing a glass slide on the patient's lip or by transmitting a light through the patient's fingertips.

Systolic arterial pressure is elevated, and diastolic pressure is abnormally low. *Hill's sign* refers to popliteal cuff systolic pressure exceeding brachial cuff pressure by more than 60 mm Hg. Korotkoff sounds often persist to zero even though intraarterial pressure rarely falls below 30 mm Hg. The point of change in intensity of the Korotkoff sounds, i.e., the muffling of these sounds in phase IV, correlates with the diastolic pressure. As heart failure develops, peripheral vasoconstriction may occur and arterial diastolic pressure may rise. However, this finding should not be interpreted as a reduction in the severity of the AR.

The apical impulse is diffuse and hyperdynamic and is displaced laterally and inferiorly; there may be systolic retraction over the parasternal region. A rapid ventricular filling wave is often palpable at the apex, as is a systolic thrill at the base of the heart or suprasternal notch and over the carotid arteries, resulting from the augmented stroke volume. In many patients, a carotid shudder is palpable or may be recorded.[543]

AUSCULTATION. In *chronic* severe AR, a soft S_1 and prolongation of the P-R interval frequently are present. A_2 is soft or absent, and P_2 may be obscured by the early diastolic murmur.[544,544a] Thus, S_2 is variable; it may be absent or single or exhibit narrow or paradoxical splitting. A systolic ejection sound, presumably related to abrupt distention of the aorta by the augmented stroke volume, is frequently audible. An S_3 gallop correlates with an increased left ventricular end-systolic volume and has been suggested as a sign useful in considering patients with severe regurgitation for surgical treatment.[545]

The aortic regurgitant murmur is one of high frequency that begins immediately after A_2 (Figs. 2–24*E*, p. 35 and 3–31, p. 58). It may be distinguished from the murmur of pulmonic regurgitation (p. 1059) by its earlier onset, i.e., immediately after A_2 rather than after P_2, and often by the presence of a widened pulse pressure. The murmur is heard best through the diaphragm of the stethoscope while the patient is sitting up and leaning forward, with the breath held in deep expiration. In severe AR, the murmur reaches an early peak and then has a dominant decrescendo pattern throughout diastole.

The severity of the regurgitation correlates better with the *duration* than with the *intensity* of the murmur. In mild AR, the murmur may be limited to the early phase of diastole and is typically high-pitched; in moderately severe and severe regurgitation, the murmur is holodiastolic and may have a rough quality. When the murmur is musical ("cooing dove" murmur), it usually signifies eversion or perforation of an aortic cusp. In severe AR and left ventricular decompensation, equilibration of aortic and left ventricular pressures in late diastole (Fig. 34–32) abolishes this component of the regurgitant murmur. The diastolic murmur is best heard along the left sternal border in the third and fourth intercostal spaces when regurgitation is due to primary valvular disease, but it is often more readily audible along the right sternal border when it is due mainly to dilatation of the ascending aorta.[546] Murmurs in the latter position may be overlooked if auscultation along the right sternal border is not carried out routinely.

A mid- and late-diastolic apical rumble, the *Austin Flint murmur*, is common in severe AR and may occur in the presence of a normal mitral valve (Figs. 3–31 and 3–32, p. 58). This murmur appears to be created by rapid antegrade flow across a mitral orifice[520] that may be being narrowed by the rapidly rising left ventricular diastolic pressure caused by severe aortic reflux.[547] The Austin Flint murmur may be difficult to differentiate from that due to MS, but the presence of an opening snap and a loud S_1 in MS and the absence of these findings in AR are helpful clues (Table 34–14). As the left ventricular end-diastolic pressure rises, the Austin Flint murmur commences and terminates earlier, and in acute AR with premature diastolic closure of the mitral valve, the presystolic portion of the Austin Flint murmur is eliminated. A short, midsystolic murmur, grades 1 to 4/6, related to the increased ejection rate and stroke volume, may be audible at the base of the heart and transmitted to the carotid vessels. It may be higher pitched and less rasping than the murmur of aortic stenosis but is often accompanied by a systolic thrill.

Dynamic Auscultation. The diastolic murmur of AR may be accentuated when the patient sits up and leans forward or by any intervention that raises the arterial pressure, such as infusion of a vasopressor drug, squatting, or isometric exercise. It is reduced by interventions that lower the systolic pressure, such as amyl nitrite inhalation and the strain of the Valsalva maneuver.[548] The Austin Flint murmur, like that of AR, is augmented by isometric exercise and vasopressors and is reduced by amyl nitrite inhalation (Fig. 3–32, p. 58).[548]

ACUTE AORTIC REGURGITATION. These patients often appear gravely ill, with tachycardia, severe peripheral vasoconstriction and cyanosis, and sometimes pulmonary congestion and edema (Table 34–15).[536,538,541] The peripheral signs of AR are often not impressive and certainly not as dramatic as in patients with chronic AR.[539] Duroziez's murmur, pistol shot sounds over the peripheral arteries, and bisferiens pulses are usually absent in acute AR. The normal pulse pressure may lead to serious underestimation of the severity of the valvular lesion. The left ventricular impulse is normal or nearly so, and the rocking motion of the chest characteristic of chronic AR is not apparent. S_1 may be soft or absent because of premature closure of the mitral valve.[549] Instead, the sound of mitral valve closure is heard occasionally in mid-diastole. However, closure of the mitral valve may be incomplete, and diastolic mitral regurgitation may occur.[550] Evidence of pulmonary hypertension, with an accentuated P_2 and an S_3 and S_4, is frequently present. The early diastolic murmur of acute AR is lower pitched and shorter than that of chronic AR, because as left ventricular end-diastolic pressure rises, the pressure gradient between the aorta and the left ventricle is rapidly reduced. The Austin Flint murmur, if present, is brief and ceases when left ventricular pressure exceeds left atrial pressure in diastole.

TABLE 34-14 CHARACTERISTICS DISTINGUISHING THE MURMUR OF MITRAL STENOSIS FROM THE AUSTIN FLINT MURMUR

CLINICAL OR LABORATORY FINDING	MITRAL STENOSIS	AUSTIN FLINT MURMUR
Opening snap present	+	–
S_1 increased	+	–
S_3 present	–	+
Left ventricular enlargement and/or hypertrophy (physical examination, ECG, chest roentgenogram)	–	+
Right ventricular enlargement and/or hypertrophy (physical examination, ECG, chest roentgenogram)	+	–
Murmur decreases with amyl nitrite	–	+
Echocardiographic evidence of organic mitral stenosis	+	–
Presence of atrial fibrillation	+	–

From Alpert, J. S.: Chronic aortic regurgitation. *In* Dalen, J. E., and Alpert, J. S. (eds.): Valvular Heart Disease. 2nd ed. Boston, Little, Brown and Company, 1987, p. 291.

TABLE 34-15 MANIFESTATIONS OF SEVERE AORTIC REGURGITATION

	ACUTE	CHRONIC
CLINICAL FINDING		
Congestive heart failure	Early and sudden	Late and insidious
Arterial pulse		
Rate per minute	Increased	Normal
Rate of rise	Not increased	Increased
Systolic pressure	Normal to decreased	Increased
Diastolic pressure	Normal to decreased	Decreased
Pulse pressure	Near-normal	Increased
Contour of peak	Single	Bisferiens
Pulsus alternans	Common	Uncommon
Left ventricular impulse	Near-normal to laterally displaced; not hyperdynamic	Laterally displaced, hyperdynamic
Auscultation		
First heart sound	Soft to absent	Normal
Aortic component S_2	Soft	Normal or decreased
Pulmonic component of S_2	Normal or increased	Normal
Fourth heart sound	Consistently absent	Usually absent
Third heart sound	Common	Uncommon
Aortic systolic murmur	Grade 3 or less	Grade 3 or more
Aortic regurgitant murmur	Short, medium-pitched	Long, high-pitched
Austin Flint murmur	Mid-diastolic	Presystolic, mid-diastolic, or both
Peripheral arterial auscultatory signs	Absent	Present
LABORATORY FINDING		
ECG	Normal left ventricular voltage with minor repolarization abnormalities	Increased left ventricular voltage with major repolarization abnormalities
Chest roentgenogram		
Left ventricle	Normal to moderately increased	Markedly increased
Aortic root	Usually normal	Prominent
Pulmonary venous pattern	Redistributed to upper lobes	Normal
ECHOCARDIOGRAPHIC VARIABLE		
Mitral valve		
Closure	Early	Normal
Opening	Late	Normal
Anterior leaflet E-F slope	Reduced	Normal
Diastolic fluttering	Yes	Yes
Septal wall motion	Normal	Hyperkinetic
Posterior wall motion	Normal	Hyperkinetic
End-diastolic dimension	Normal	Increased
End-systolic dimension	Normal	Normal
Shortening fraction	Normal	Increased

Modified from Benotti, J. R.: Acute aortic insufficiency. *In* Dalen, J. E., and Alpert, J. S. (eds.): Valvular Heart Disease. 2nd ed. Boston, Little, Brown and Company, 1987, pp. 331 and 337.

LABORATORY EXAMINATION

ELECTROCARDIOGRAM. *Chronic* AR results in left axis deviation and a pattern of left ventricular diastolic volume overload, characterized by an increase in initial forces (prominent Q waves in leads I, aV_l, and V_3 to V_6) and a relatively small *r* wave in V_1 (Fig. 34–35). With the passage of time, these initial forces diminish, but the total QRS amplitude increases. The T waves may be tall and upright in left precordial leads early in the course, but more commonly they are inverted, with ST-segment depressions.[551] Left intraventricular conduction defects occur late in the course and are usually associated with left ventricular dysfunction. When AR is caused by

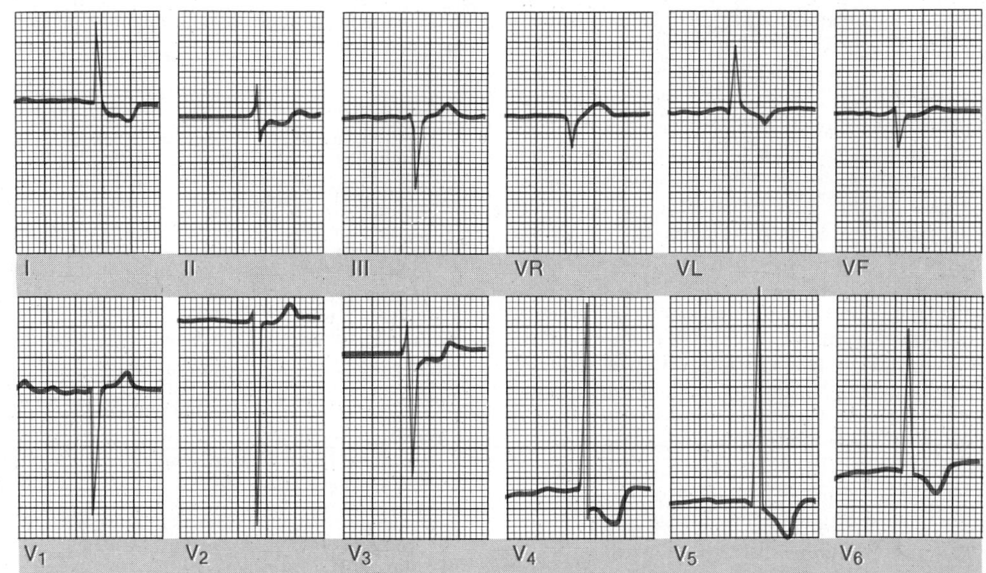

FIGURE 34–35. Atrial fibrillation and left ventricular hypertrophy. The most prominent features are the gross increase in precordial voltage (RV5 + SV2 = 70 mm) and the marked anterolateral ST/T wave changes (leads I, aVL, and V4-6). The patient had aortic regurgitation and normal coronary arteries and was not taking digitalis. (Normal standardization, i.e., 1 mV = 10 mm.) (From Hall, R. J., and Julian, D. G.: Diseases of the Cardiac Valves. New York, Churchill Livingstone, 1989, p. 39.)

an inflammatory process, P-R prolongation may result.[552] However, the electrocardiogram is not an accurate predictor of the severity of AR or cardiac weight.[552] In *acute* AR, the electrocardiogram may or may not show left ventricular hypertrophy, despite the presence of left ventricular failure, depending upon the severity and duration of the regurgitation. However, nonspecific ST-segment and T-wave changes are common.

RADIOLOGICAL FINDINGS (see also p. 223). Cardiac size is a function of the duration and severity of regurgitation and the state of left ventricular function. In acute AR, there may be little cardiac enlargement, but marked enlargement is a common finding in chronic AR. Typically, the left ventricle enlarges in an inferior and leftward direction, causing a significant increase in the long axis (Figs. 8–3, p. 207, 8–8*B*, p. 208, and 8–33, p. 223) but sometimes little or no increase in the transverse diameter of the heart. Calcification of the aortic valve is uncommon in patients with pure AR but is often present in patients with combined AS and AR. As in the case with AS, the presence of distinct left atrial enlargement in the absence of heart failure should suggest the possibility of mitral valve disease. Dilatation of the ascending aorta is usually more marked than in AS and may involve the entire aortic arch, including the aortic knob. Severe, aneurysmal dilatation of the aorta should suggest that aortic root disease (e.g., Marfan syndrome, cystic medionecrosis, or annuloaortic ectasia) is responsible for the AR. Linear calcifications in the wall of the ascending aorta are seen in syphilitic aortitis but are nonspecific and are observed in degenerative disease as well.

For angiographic assessment of AR, contrast material should be injected rapidly (i.e., 25 to 35 ml/sec) into the aortic root, and filming should be carried out in the right and left anterior oblique projections. Opacification may be improved by filming during a Valsalva maneuver. In acute AR, there is only a slight increase in ventricular end-diastolic volume, but with the passage of time both the end-diastolic volume and the thickness of the ventricular wall increase, usually in parallel.

ECHOCARDIOGRAPHY (p. 86). The severity of regurgitation is reflected in increased motion of the septum and posterior wall, as recorded by M-mode echocardiography. In chronic AR, the left ventricular end-diastolic diameter and extent of systolic shortening are both augmented (Fig. 34–36*A*). There is increased motion of the interventricular septum and posterior left ventricular wall in compensated patients, but shortening is normal or reduced in patients with left ventricular failure. Serial studies, particularly with two-dimensional echocardiography, may detect early changes in left ventricular function, as reflected in increased end-diastolic and end-systolic diameters and reduced fractional shortening, which may be of assistance in selecting the optimal time for surgical intervention. Echocardiography is helpful in identifying the cause of AR. It may show thickening of the valve cusps, prolapse of the valve, a flail leaflet (Fig. 34–

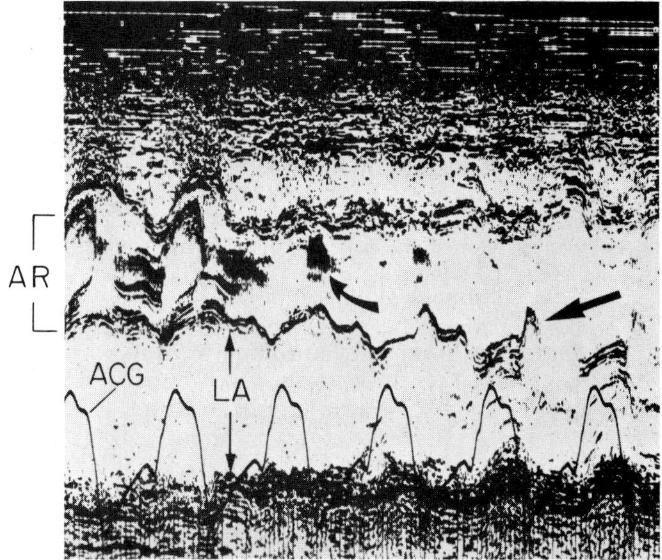

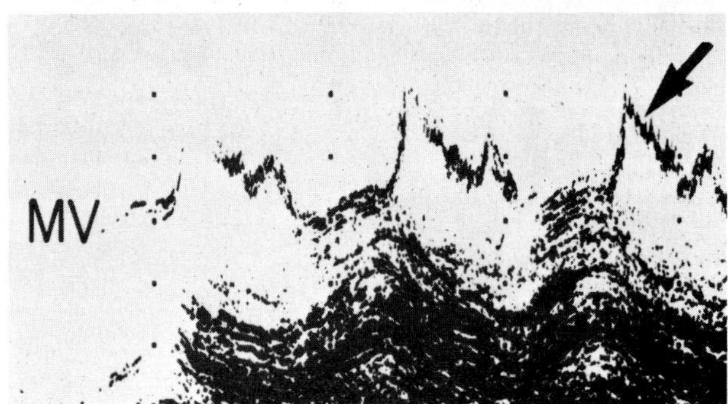

FIGURE 34–36. ***Top,*** **M-mode electrocardiogram in severe aortic regurgitation. A markedly dilated aortic root (AR) is apparent on the left, appearing anterior to a slightly enlarged left atrium (LA). The left ventricle (at the right of the tracing) is dilated and demonstrates vigorous symmetrical contractile motion of the posterior wall and interventricular septum. Projecting anterior to the mitral valve is an abnormal diastolic echo (curved arrow) suggestive of a partially disrupted aortic valve cusp prolapsing into the left ventricular outflow tract. ACG = apexcardiogram.** ***Bottom,*** **Echocardiogram in aortic regurgitation. High-frequency diastolic vibrations (arrow) of the anterior mitral valve leaflet (MV) are typical of aortic regurgitation.**

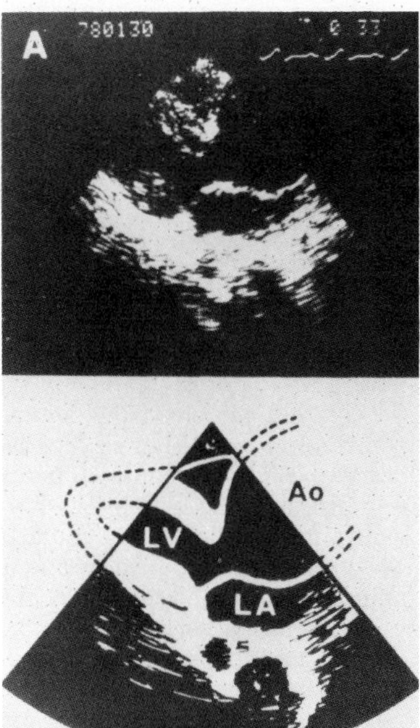

FIGURE 34-37. *A, B,* Long-axis view and schematic of the aortic root in end systole by two-dimensional echocardiography. The unusually dilated aortic root is visualized. (From Imaizumi, T., et al.: Utility of two-dimensional echocardiography in the differential diagnosis of the etiology of aortic regurgitation. Am. Heart J. *103*:887, 1982.)

36*A*), vegetations, or dilatation of the aortic root[553] (Fig. 34-37).

In *acute AR* (Table 34-14 and Fig. 34-34) the echocardiogram reveals a reduction in amplitude of the opening movement of the mitral valve, premature closure and delayed opening of the mitral valve,[554] and a reduction in the E-F slope, indicating that the left ventricle is operating on the steep portion of its pressure-volume curve. Left ventricular end-diastolic dimensions are not markedly increased, and fractional shortening is normal. This contrasts with the findings in chronic AR, in which end-diastolic dimensions and wall motion are increased. Occasionally, with equilibration of aortic and left ventricular pressures in diastole, premature opening of the aortic valve may be detected.[555]

High-frequency, diastolic fluttering of the anterior leaflet of the mitral valve during diastole[556] (Fig. 34-36*B*) is an important echocardiographic finding in both acute and chronic AR; it does not occur, however, when the mitral valve is rigid. This sign, which, unlike the Austin Flint rumble, occurs even in mild AR, results from the movement imparted to the anterior leaflet of the mitral valve by the jet of blood regurgitating from the aorta.

Doppler echocardiography (Figs. 4-56, p. 86, 4-57, p. 87, and 4-58, p. 87) is the most sensitive and accurate noninvasive technique in the detection of AR and is superior to the M-mode and two-dimensional techniques in this regard.[557] It readily detects mild degrees of AR that may be inaudible. In addition, it provides an approach to the measurement of the regurgitation flow and the regurgitant orifice.[558,559]

RADIONUCLIDE TECHNIQUES. Radionuclide angiography, by allowing determination of the regurgitant fraction and of the left ventricular/right ventricular stroke volume ratio, provides an accurate noninvasive assessment of AR.[560,561] This technique is nonspecific, because the ratio will be increased by associated MR and reduced by tricuspid or pulmonary regurgitation. However, in the absence of these complicating lesions, a left ventricular/right ventricular stroke volume ratio of 2.5 or more denotes severe AR. As indicated earlier, these techniques are of value in the assessment of left ventricular function in patients with AR.[533-535] Serial measurements are of value in the early detection of deterioration of left ventricular function.

MANAGEMENT

ACUTE AORTIC REGURGITATION. Since early death due to left ventricular failure is frequent in patients with *severe acute* AR despite intensive medical management, prompt surgical intervention is indicated. Even a normal ventricle cannot sustain the burden of acute severe volume overload; therefore, the risk of *acute* AR is much greater than that of chronic AR.[536,538,541] While the patient is being prepared for surgery, intravenous treatment with a positive inotropic agent (dopamine or dobutamine) and/or vasodilator (nitroprusside) may be necessary. The agent and dosage should be selected on the basis of arterial pressure (Chap. 17). In patients with acute AR secondary to active infective endocarditis who are stable hemodynamically, operation may be deferred to allow 7 to 10 days of intensive antibiotic therapy if the patient remains stable.[541] However, aortic valve replacement should be undertaken at the earliest sign of hemodynamic instability, if there is echocardiographic evidence of diastolic closure of the mitral valve,[562] or immediately upon completion of a 10-day course of antibiotics when acute, severe regurgitation has developed (p. 1091). The cautious use of vasodilators may be helpful in stabilizing the patient's condition but is no substitute for prompt surgery in the patients with pulmonary edema, severe pulmonary congestion, and/or an obvious low forward cardiac output state.

NATURAL HISTORY OF CHRONIC AORTIC REGURGITATION. Management must take into account the natural history of the lesion.[563] Moderately severe or even severe chronic AR is associated with a generally favorable prognosis for many years. Approximately 75 per cent of patients survive for 5 years and 50 per cent for 10 years after diagnosis.[102] However, as is the case for AS, once the patient becomes symptomatic, the condition often deteriorates rapidly, and sudden death may occur, usually in previously symptomatic patients. Without surgical treatment, death usually occurs within 4 years after the development of angina and within 2 years after the onset of heart failure. Even during the asymptomatic period gradual deterioration of left ventricular function may occur; it is important, therefore, to intervene surgically before these changes have become irreversible.

MEDICAL TREATMENT

Patients with mild or moderate AR who are asymptomatic with normal or only minimally increased cardiac size require no therapy but should be followed clinically and with echocardiography and with antibiotic prophylaxis for endocarditis. Patients with limitations of cardiac reserve and/or left ventricular dysfunction secondary to AR should not engage in vigorous sports or heavy exertion.[564] Cardiac glycosides should be employed in patients with severe AR, left ventricular dilatation, and sinus rhythm, even in the absence of symptoms. If present, systemic arterial diastolic hypertension should be treated, since it increases the regurgitant flow; however, drugs that impair left ventricular function, such as propranolol, should be avoided. Atrial fibrillation and bradyarrhythmias are poorly tolerated and should be prevented if possible. Since these and other cardiac arrhythmias and infections are poorly tolerated in patients with severe AR, such complications must be treated promptly and vigorously. Even though nitroglycerin and other nitrates are not as helpful in relieving anginal pain in patients with AR as they are in patients with coronary artery disease or AS, they are worth a trial. Patients with AR secondary to syphilitic aortitis (p. 1548) should receive a full course of penicillin therapy. Although patients with left ventricular failure secondary to AR require surgical treatment, they also respond, at least temporarily, to treatment with digitalis glycosides, salt restriction, and diuretics. The response to vasodilator therapy is often impressive. Hemodynamic studies have shown beneficial effects of intravenous hydralazine,[565,566] sublingual nifedipine,[567] and oral prazosin.[568] This form of therapy may be particularly helpful in stabilizing patients with acute lesions or those with decompensated chronic AR who are awaiting operation. Long-term administration of hydralazine[569–571] and nifedipine[572] appears to improve systolic function; either drug combined with digitalis glycosides[573] may be useful for the long-term management of the asymptomatic patient with severe AR.

Asymptomatic patients with severe *chronic* AR and normal left ventricular function should be examined at intervals of approximately 3 to 6 months. In addition to clinical examination, x-ray, and electrocardiogram, serial noninvasive assessments of left ventricular size and performance at rest and during exercise should be carried out using echocardiography or radionuclide angiography or both.

SURGICAL TREATMENT

INDICATIONS FOR OPERATION. There is general agreement that operative correction is *not* indicated in patients with severe chronic AR who are asymptomatic, have good exercise tolerance, and have normal left ventricular function. Similarly, there is a consensus that in the absence of contraindications surgical treatment is advisable in patients with severe AR who are symptomatic as a result of this lesion and who have impaired left ventricular function. Between these two ends of the clinical-hemodynamic spectrum are many patients in whom it may be quite difficult to balance the immediate risks of operation and the continuing risks of an implanted prosthetic valve on the one hand against the hazards of allowing a severe volume overload to damage the left ventricle on the other.[574–580]

Irreversible changes in left ventricular function can develop in some patients with AR so that even after successful correction of AR, this subset of patients may have persistent cardiomegaly and depressed left ventricular function.[581–585] Symptoms of impaired left ventricular function present preoperatively may persist and occasionally even get worse despite successful valve replacements. While it is best to operate on patients before irreversible left ventricular changes have occurred, most of the patients in the latter category are, in fact, also benefited, and do even worse with continued medical management. Patients whose ventricular function does not return to normal after aortic valve replacement often exhibit histological changes in the left ventricle, including massive fiber hypertrophy and increased interstitial fibrous tissue.[586] On the other hand, postoperative left ventricular function is usually excellent in patients who have normal systolic function preoperatively.[584]

In order to minimize the risk of postoperative left ventricular dysfunction, every effort should be made to operate on patients *before* serious left ventricular dysfunction occurs. Although quantitative biplane ventriculography is the most precise method for assessing left ventricular performance, it cannot be readily employed in serial fashion. Instead, serial echocardiograms or radionuclide ventriculograms should be obtained to detect changes in left ventricular size and function. These examinations can provide valuable information concerning progressive deterioration in left ventricular function at rest. Radionuclide angiography, in particular (p. 168), is a safe, simple, and noninvasive method that allows repeated evaluation of ejection fraction and end-systolic volume both at rest and during exercise. However, it is impaired ventricular function at *rest* that becomes the basis for selection of patients for operation; failure of a normal ejection fraction to respond normally to *exercise* portends impaired function at rest.

Since AR has complex effects on both preload and afterload, the selection of appropriate indices of ventricular contractility is a challenge.[587] Simple left ventricular end-diastolic volume and the ejection phase indices such as ejection fraction and ventricular fraction shortening are too strongly influenced by loading to be accurate indicators of ventricular contractility but may be useful empirical predictors of postoperative function.[477] Preoperative left ventricular end-systolic volume and dimensions are largely preload dependent and are good predictors of postoperative left ventricular function.[588,589] The relationship between end-systolic wall stress and ejection fraction or per cent[590] fractional shortening may be even more useful. However, in the absence of such measurements *serial* changes in ventricular end-diastolic and/or ejection phase indices can be employed to detect *relative* deterioration of ventricular function.

Patients with severely impaired left ventricular systolic function preoperatively are at high risk of developing irreversible left ventricular dysfunction and, indeed, of dying of congestive heart failure postoperatively. Other patients with impaired left ventricular function preoperatively, improve postoperatively—both symptomatically and insofar as left ventricular function is concerned. Bonow et al. have reported that, after valve replacement, survival was excellent in patients with normal resting ejection fractions preoperatively. However, patients with subnormal ejection fraction and only a brief (<1 year) duration of left ventricular dysfunction also did well postoperatively and maintained their preoperative levels of exercise tolerance. On the other hand, patients with subnormal ejection fraction and impaired exercise tolerance and/or prolonged left ventricular dysfunction exhibited poor postoperative survival.[575,586]

In *conclusion*, the decision to recommend aortic valve replacement in some patients with severe AR remains difficult. Operation should be deferred in asymptomatic patients with normal left ventricular function and should be recommended in symptomatic patients regardless of the status of their left ventricular function. Asymptomatic patients with impaired left ventricular function must be treated individually, taking into account associated medical conditions and coronary artery disease that may add to the surgical risk, as well as the experience level of the surgical team. A decision should be based not on a single abnormal measurement of impaired left ventricular function but rather on several observations of depressed performance and impaired exercise tolerance, carried out at intervals of 4 to 6 months. If abnormalities are shown consistently and if any trend to deterioration is noted, operation should be carried out forthwith. If evidence of left ventricular dysfunction is borderline or is not consistent, the patient may be followed closely.

OPERATIVE PROCEDURES. The surgical treatment of AR and of combined AS and AR is valve replacement. (Prosthetic valves are discussed on pp. 1061–1064.) Since the aortic annulus in patients with severe AR is usually not as narrow as it is in patients with AS, a larger artificial valve can be inserted, and mild postoperative obstruction to left ventricular outflow is less of a problem than it is in some patients with AS. Occasionally, when a leaflet has been torn from its attachments to the aortic annulus by trauma, surgical repair without valve replacement may be possible. In patients in whom AR is due to aneurysmal dilatation of the aortic annulus (Chap. 47) and the ascending aorta, regurgitation may occasionally be reduced or eliminated by narrowing the annulus or by excising a portion of the aorta. More often, effective treatment in these patients requires replacement of the aortic valve and excision of the aneurysmal portion of the aorta and its replacement with a graft, sometimes with reimplantation of the coronary arteries. This more extensive procedure is associated with a higher operative risk than is aortic valve replacement alone.

Aortic valve replacement is discussed on page 1042. In general, results in patients with AR are similar to those in patients with AS, with a large percentage of patients exhibiting striking clinical improvement. Reductions in heart size and in left ventricular diastolic volume and mass occur in the majority of patients.[466,591] However, as already indicated, the extent of

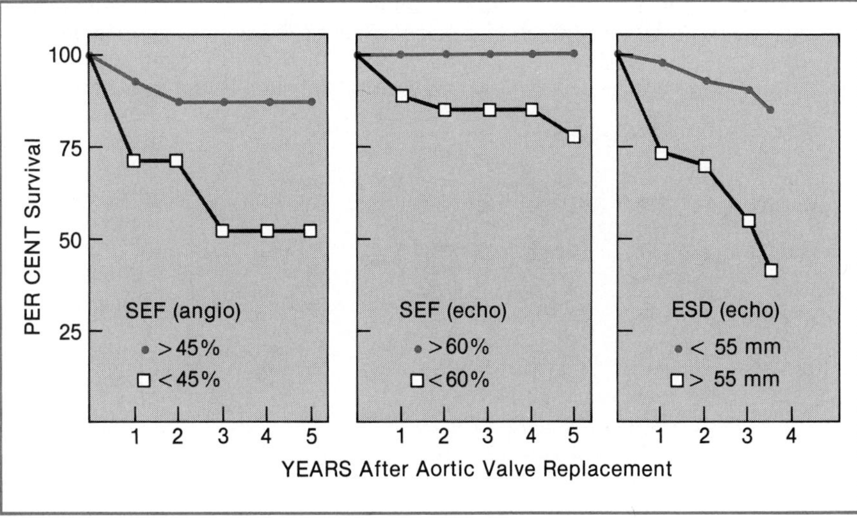

FIGURE 34-38. Relation of preoperative ventricular function to postoperative survival. Data of Greves et al. *(left)* and those of Bonow et al. *(right)* show remarkable agreement: both groups incorporated limits clearly in abnormal range. Cunha et al *(center)* selected a limit that was well within normal range. These and other published data indicate that preoperative ventricular function is an important determinant of postoperative survival. SEF indicates systolic ejection fraction; ESD = echocardiographically measured dimension at end-systole; angio = angiography; echo = echocardiography. (From Errichetti, A., et al.: Is valve replacement indicated in asymptomatic patients with aortic stenosis or aortic regurgitation? *In* Cheitlin, M. [ed.]: Dilemmas in Clinical Cardiology. Philadelphia, F. A. Davis Co., 1990, p. 204.)

improvement in left ventricular function may not be as salutary as in patients with aortic stenosis, perhaps because the ventricular dysfunction is more advanced and less reversible in patients with volume overload by the time they become symptomatic and are referred for surgical treatment[592-593] than it is in patients with pressure overload. As is the case for AS, the operative risk of aortic valve replacement in patients with AR depends on the general condition of the patient, the state of left ventricular function, and the skill and experience of the surgical team; the mortality rate ranges from 3 to 8 per cent in most medical centers. A late mortality of approximately 5 to 10 per cent per year is observed in survivors in whom cardiac enlargement was marked and prolonged left ventricular dysfunction was present preoperatively (Fig. 34–38). Follow-up studies have shown both early rapid and then slower long-term reductions of ventricular mass, ejection fraction,[495] myocyte hypertrophy, and ventricular fibrous content.[404,479] By extending the indications for operation to symptomatic patients with normal left ventricular function as well as to asymptomatic patients with early left ventricular dysfunction, both early and late results are improving.[575,576,586] It is likely that with the continued improvement of surgical techniques and results, it will become possible to extend the recommendation for operative treatment to asymptomatic patients with severe regurgitation and normal or nearly normal cardiac function. However, given the risks of operation and the long-term complications of artificial valves, I believe that the time for such a policy has not yet arrived.

Tricuspid, Pulmonic, and Multivalvular Disease

TRICUSPID STENOSIS

ETIOLOGY AND PATHOLOGY

Tricuspid stenosis (TS) is almost always rheumatic in origin.[594] Other causes of obstruction to right atrial emptying are unusual and include congenital tricuspid atresia (p. 938), right atrial tumors (which may produce a clinical picture suggesting rapidly progressive TS [p. 1453]), and the carcinoid syndrome (which more frequently produces tricuspid regurgitation [TR] [p. 1056] but which may occasionally produce TS). Rarely, obstruction to right ventricular inflow can be due to pericardial constriction, extracardiac tumors, and vegetations.

Rheumatic TS *almost* never occurs as an isolated lesion but generally accompanies mitral valve disease[595-600]; in many patients the aortic valve is also involved. TS is present at autopsy in about 15 per cent of patients with rheumatic heart disease but is of clinical significance in only about 5 per cent.[601]

Organic tricuspid valve disease is more common in India than in North America or Western Europe; it has been reported to occur in the hearts of more than one-third of patients with rheumatic heart disease studied at autopsy on the subcontinent.[602] The anatomical changes of rheumatic TS resemble those of MS, with fusion and shortening of the chordae tendineae and fusion of the leaflets at their edges producing a diaphragm with a fixed central aperture.[11] As is the case for MS, TS is more common in women and, in the United States, TS is seen most commonly in persons between the ages of 20 and 60. Again, as in mitral valve disease, stenosis, regurgitation, or some combination of the two may exist.

The right atrium is often greatly dilated, and its walls are thickened. There may be evidence of severe passive congestion, with enlargement of the liver and spleen.

PATHOPHYSIOLOGY

A diastolic pressure gradient between the right atrium and ventricle—the hemodynamic expression of TS—is augmented when the transvalvular blood flow increases during exercise or inspiration and is reduced when flow declines during expiration. A mean diastolic pressure gradient exceeding 5 mm Hg is usually sufficient to elevate mean right atrial pressure to levels that result in systemic venous congestion and, unless sodium intake has been restricted or diuretics have been given, is associated with jugular venous distention, ascites, and edema.

In patients with sinus rhythm, the right atrial *a* wave may be extremely tall (Fig. 34–39) and may even approach the level of the right ventricular systolic pressure. Resting cardiac output is usually markedly reduced and fails to rise during exercise, accounting for the normal or only slightly elevated left atrial, pulmonary arterial, and right ventricular systolic pressures, despite the presence of accompanying mitral valve disease.

A *mean* diastolic pressure gradient across the tricuspid valve as low as 2 mm Hg is sufficient to establish the diagnosis

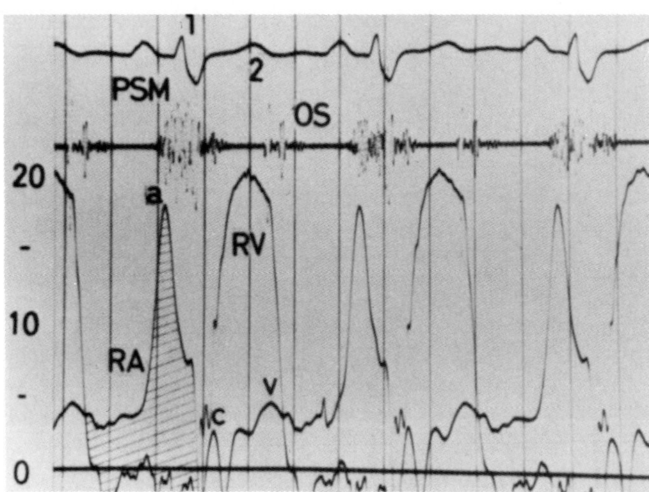

FIGURE 34-39. Phonocardiogram and right heart pressures in a patient with tricuspid stenosis. The giant right atrial *a* wave (a) nearly equals right ventricular (RV) systolic pressure and produces a large diastolic gradient (shaded area). A presystolic murmur (PSM), loud first heart sound (1), and early diastolic opening snap (OS) simulate the findings in mitral stenosis. (Time lines = 0.2 sec.) (From Criley, J. M., et al.: Departures from the expected auscultatory events in mitral stenosis. *In* Likoff, W. [ed.]: Valvular Heart Disease. Philadelphia, F. A. Davis, 1973, p. 214.)

of TS. However, exercise, deep inspiration, and the rapid infusion of fluid or the administration of atropine may enhance greatly a borderline gradient in the presence of TS.[596] Therefore, whenever this diagnosis is suspected, right atrial and ventricular pressures should be recorded simultaneously, using two catheters or a single catheter with a double lumen, with one lumen opening on either side of the tricuspid valve. The effects of respiration on any pressure difference should be examined.

CLINICAL MANIFESTATIONS

(Table 34-16)

HISTORY. The low cardiac output characteristic of TS causes fatigue, and patients often complain of discomfort due to hepatomegaly, swelling of the abdomen, and anasarca.[602a] The severity of these symptoms, which are secondary to an elevated systemic venous pressure, is out of proportion to the degree of dyspnea.[597] Some patients complain of a fluttering discomfort in the neck, caused by giant *a* waves in the jugular venous pulse. Despite the coexistence of MS, the symptoms characteristic of this valve lesion, i.e., hemoptysis, paroxysmal nocturnal dyspnea, and acute pulmonary edema, are usually absent in the presence of severe TS. Indeed, the *absence* of the symptoms of pulmonary congestion in a patient with obvious MS should suggest the possibility of TS.

PHYSICAL EXAMINATION. Because of the high frequency with which MS occurs in patients with TS, the diagnosis of the latter is commonly overlooked, since the physical findings are mistakenly attributed to MS, which is, of course, more common and may be more obvious. Therefore, a high index of suspicion is required to detect the tricuspid valve lesion. In the presence of sinus rhythm (which is surprisingly common), the *a* wave in the jugular venous pulse is tall, sharp, and flicking and on first impression may be confused with an arterial pulsation; a presystolic hepatic pulsation is often palpable. The *y* descent is slow and barely appreciable, indicating the absence of normal rapid, early right ventricular filling. The lung fields are clear, and despite engorgement of the neck veins and the presence of ascites and anasarca, the patient may be comfortable while lying flat. A parasternal (right ventricular) lift is inconspicuous, and pulmonic valve closure is not palpable, but occasionally the pulsations of a greatly enlarged right atrium may be felt to the right of the sternum. Thus, on inspection and palpation the combination of a prominent *a* wave in the jugular venous pulse in a patient with MS without the clinical signs of pulmonary hypertension or right ventricular enlargement should suggest the diagnosis of TS. This suspicion is strengthened when a diastolic thrill is felt at the lower left sternal edge, particularly if it appears or becomes more prominent during inspiration.[20]

The auscultatory findings of the accompanying MS are usually prominent and often overshadow the more subtle signs of TS. A tricuspid valvular opening snap (OS) may be audible but is often difficult to distinguish from a mitral OS. However, the tricuspid OS usually follows the mitral OS, and is localized to the lower left sternal border, whereas the mitral OS is usually most prominent at the apex and radiates more widely. The diastolic murmur of TS is commonly heard best along the lower left parasternal border in the fourth intercostal space and is usually softer, higher pitched, and shorter in duration than the murmur of MS. The presystolic component has a scratchy quality, commences earlier (0.06 sec after the P wave in TS compared with 0.12 in MS), and has a crescendo-decrescendo configuration, diminishing before S_1.[598] The diastolic murmur and OS of TS are both augmented by inspiration (Fig. 3-34, p. 58), the Mueller maneuver, assumption of the right lateral decubitus position, leg-raising, inhalation of amyl nitrite, squatting, and both isotonic and isometric exercise. They are reduced during expiration or the strain of the Valsalva maneuver and return to control levels immediately (i.e., within two to three beats) after Valsalva release.

LABORATORY EXAMINATION

ELECTROCARDIOGRAM

In a patient with valvular heart disease in the absence of atrial fibrillation, TS is suggested by the presence of ECG evidence of right atrial enlargement disproportionate to the degree of right ventricular hypertrophy. The P-wave amplitude in leads II and V_1 exceeds 0.25 mV (p. 124), and there may be depression of the P-R segment resulting from increased magnitude of the atrial T wave. Since most patients with TS have mitral valve

TABLE 34-16 CLINICAL AND LABORATORY FEATURES OF RHEUMATIC TRICUSPID STENOSIS

HISTORY
- Long history
- Progressive fatigue, edema, anorexia
- Minimal orthopnea, paroxysmal nocturnal dyspnea
- Rheumatic fever in two-thirds of patients
- Female preponderance
- Orthopnea and paroxysmal nocturnal dyspnea are unusual
- Pulmonary edema and hemoptysis are rare

PHYSICAL FINDINGS
- Signs of multivalvular involvement
- Wasting
- Peripheral cyanosis
- Neck vein distension, with prominent V waves
- Right ventricular lift
- Associated murmurs of mitral and aortic valve disease
- Holosystolic murmur maximal at left lower sternal border, accentuating with inspiration
- Hepatic pulsation
- Ascites, peripheral edema

LABORATORY FINDINGS
- Normal sinus rhythm is frequently present with large A waves in the neck veins
- Absent right ventricular lift
- Auscultation reveals a diastolic rumble at lower left sternal edge, increasing in intensity with inspiration
- Electrocardiogram shows tall right atrial P waves and no right ventricular hypertrophy
- Roentgenogram shows a dilated right atrium without an enlarged pulmonary artery segment

Modified from Ockene, I. S.: Tricuspid valve disease. *In* Dalen, J. E., and Alpert, J. S. (eds.): Valvular Heart Disease. 2nd ed. Boston, Little, Brown and Company, 1987, pp. 356 and 390.

disease, the ECG signs of biatrial enlargement (p. 125) with abnormally tall, broad P waves in leads II, III, and aV_f and prominent positive and negative deflections in V_f are commonly found. Right atrial dilatation may rotate the ventricular septum and affect QRS morphology in a manner so that the large volume of the right atrium between the exploring electrode and the ventricles reduces the amplitude of the QRS complex in lead V_1 (which often has a Q wave), whereas the QRS complex is much taller in V_2.

RADIOLOGICAL FINDINGS

The key radiological findings in TS are marked cardiomegaly, with conspicuous enlargement of the right atrium (i.e., prominence of the right heart border), which extends into a dilated superior vena cava and azygos vein, but without dilatation of the pulmonary artery. The vascular changes in the lungs characteristic of mitral valve disease may be masked, with little or no interstitial edema or vascular redistribution.

Angiography carried out following injection of contrast material into the right atrium and filming in the 30-degree right anterior oblique projection is useful for evaluating the appearance of the tricuspid valve. Thickening and decreased mobility of the leaflets, a jet through the constricted orifice, and thickening of the right atrial wall are characteristic findings.

ECHOCARDIOGRAM (see also p. 87). Although the motion of the normal tricuspid valve is similar to that of the normal mitral valve, it is more difficult to image. Not surprisingly, the changes in the echocardiogram of the tricuspid valve in TS resemble those observed in the mitral valve in MS (p. 1013). The M-mode echocardiogram usually shows thickening of the leaflets, a reduction in the E-F slope of the anterior leaflet, and paradoxical motion of the septal leaflet in diastole.[603,604] Calcification and thickening of the tricuspid valve often results in multiple and disorganized echoes. Two-dimensional echocardiography is more useful in the diagnosis of TS.[605] It characteristically shows diastolic doming of the leaflets, thickening and restriction of excision of the other leaflets, and reduced separation of the tips of the leaflets[606,607] (Fig. 34–40). Doppler echocardiography shows a prolonged slope of antegrade flow[608] and compares well with cardiac catheterization in the quantification of TS and in the assessment of associated tricuspid regurgitation.[608]

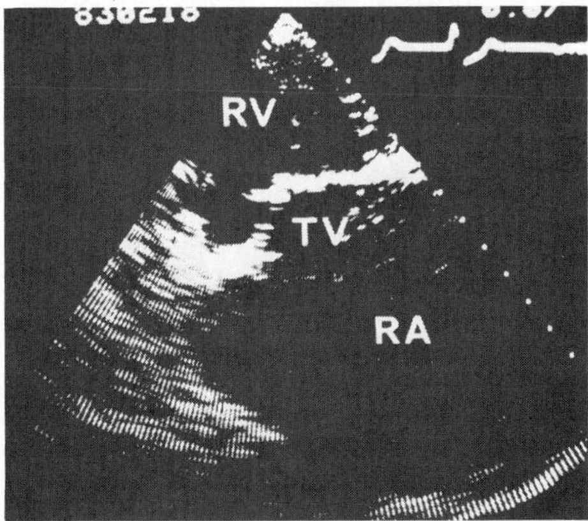

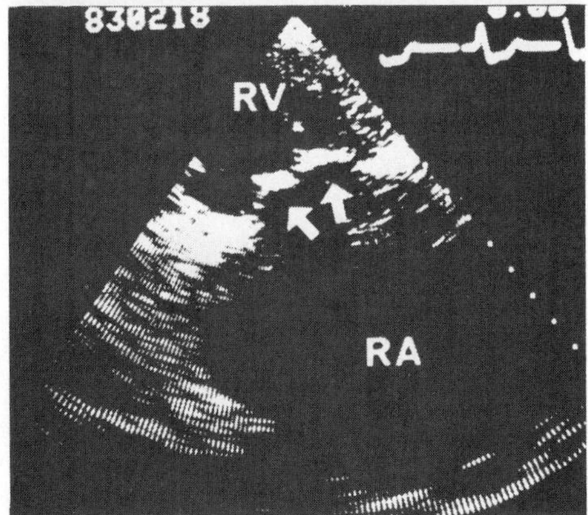

FIGURE 34–40. Two-dimensional echocardiograms in the long-axis view in a patient with tricuspid stenosis. *Top,* Systolic frame. *Bottom,* Diastolic frame that shows doming of both leaflets of the tricuspid valve (TV) (arrows). RA = right atrium; RV = right ventricle. (From Shimada, R., et al.: Diagnosis of tricuspid stenosis by M-mode and two-dimensional echocardiography. Am. J. Cardiol. *53*:164, 1984.)

MANAGEMENT

Although the fundamental approach to the management of severe TS is surgical treatment, intensive sodium restriction and diuretic therapy may diminish the symptoms secondary to the accumulation of excess salt and water. A prolonged preparatory period of diuresis may diminish hepatic congestive and thereby improve hepatic function sufficiently to diminish the risks of subsequent operation.

Surgical treatment of TS should be carried out at the time of mitral commissurotomy or valve replacement in patients with TS in whom mean diastolic pressure gradients exceed 5 mm Hg and tricuspid orifices are less than approximately 2.0 cm². Most patients with TS have coexisting valvular disease that requires surgery. The final decision concerning surgical treatment is made at the operating table. Since TS is almost always accompanied by some TR, simple finger fracture commissurotomy often does not result in significant hemodynamic improvement but may merely substitute severe regurgitation for stenosis. However, open valvulotomy in which the stenotic tricuspid valve is converted into a functionally bicuspid one may result in substantial improvement. The commissures between the anterior and septal leaflets and between the posterior and septal leaflets are opened; it is not advisable to open the commissure between the anterior and posterior leaflets for fear of producing severe regurgitation. If open commissurotomy does not restore reasonable normal valve function, the tricuspid valve may have to be replaced.[609,610] A tissue valve (p. 1062) is preferred to a mechanical prosthesis in the tricuspid position because of the high risk of thrombosis of the latter[611,612] (p. 1062) and the long-term durability of bioprostheses in the tricuspid position.[613] The feasibility of tricuspid balloon valvuloplasty has been demonstrated,[614] but it is not clear how this procedure will be used most effectively.

TRICUSPID REGURGITATION

ETIOLOGY AND PATHOLOGY

(Table 34–17)

The most common cause of tricuspid regurgitation (TR) is not intrinsic involvement of the valve itself but *dilatation of the right ventricle* and of the tricuspid annulus, which may be complications of right ventricular failure of any cause (Fig. 34–41). Functional TR is observed in patients with right ventricular hypertension secondary to any form of cardiac and pulmonary vascular disease, most commonly mitral valve disease,[613-617] right ventricular infarction[618] (p. 1205), congenital heart disease (e.g., pulmonic stenosis and pulmonary hypertension secondary to Eisenmenger syndrome), primary pulmonary hypertension, and rarely in cor pulmonale. Severe TR has been reported to be the presenting manifestation in thyrotoxicosis.[619] In infants, TR may complicate right ventricular failure secondary to neonatal pulmonary diseases and pulmonary hypertension with persistence of the fetal pulmonary circulation.[620] In all of these cases, TR reflects the presence of, and in turn aggravates, severe right ventricular failure. TR results from dilatation of the tricuspid annulus, reduction of the narrowing of the annulus during systole, and resultant failure of systolic valve coaptation of the tricuspid valve leaflets.[621-623] Functional regurgitation may diminish or disappear as the right ventricle decreases in size with the treatment of heart failure. TR can also occur as a consequence of dilatation of the annulus in Marfan syndrome, in which it is not associated with right ventricular dilatation secondary to pulmonary hypertension.

A variety of disease processes can affect the tricuspid valve

TABLE 34-17 CAUSES AND MECHANISMS OF PURE TRICUSPID REGURGITATION

CAUSES

I. Anatomically ABNORMAL valve
   A. Rheumatic
   B. Nonrheumatic
      1. Infective endocarditis
      2. Ebstein's anomaly
      3. Floppy (prolapse)
      4. Congenital (non-Ebstein's)
      5. Carcinoid
      6. Papillary muscle dysfunction
      7. Trauma
      8. Connective tissue disorders (Marfan)
      9. Rheumatoid arthritis
      10. Radiation injury
II. Anatomically NORMAL valve (functional)
   A. Elevated right ventricular systolic pressure (dilated annulus)

MECHANISMS

Condition	Leaflet Area	Annular Circumference	Leaflet Insertion
1. Floppy	↑	↑	Normal
2. Ebstein's anomaly	↑	↑	Abnormal
3. Pulmonary/right ventricular systolic hypertension	Normal	↑	Normal
4. Papillary muscle dysfunction	Normal	Normal	Normal
5. Carcinoid	↓/Normal	Normal	Normal
6. Rheumatic	↓/Normal	Normal	Normal
7. Infective endocarditis	↓/Normal	Normal	Normal

Modified from Waller, B. F.: Rheumatic and nonrheumatic conditions producing valvular heart disease. *In* Frankel, W. S., and Brest, A. N. (eds.): Cardiovascular Clinics. Valvular Heart Disease: Comprehensive Evaluation and Management. Philadelphia, F. A. Davis, 1986, pp. 35 and 95.

apparatus *directly* and lead to regurgitation. Thus, organic TR may occur on a congenital basis, as part of Ebstein's anomaly, (p. 940), in atrioventricular canal, and when the tricuspid valve is involved in the formation of an aneurysm of the ventricular septum,[624] or it may occur as an isolated congenital lesion.[625] Rheumatic fever may attack the tricuspid valve directly,[613] and when it does so, it usually leads to both regurgitation and stenosis (Fig. 34–41*B*). Infarction, rupture, or ischemia of the papillary muscles of the right ventricle in coronary artery disease[618] and in perinatal asphyxia is an important cause of TR. TR may result from prolapse of the tricuspid valve caused by myxomatous changes in the valve and chordae tendineae; this condition usually, but not always, accompanies prolapse of the mitral valve[626–628] and may be associated with atrial septal defect.[629] Other causes include trauma,[630] dilated cardiomyopathy[631] infective endocarditis,[632] particularly staphylococcal endocarditis in drug addicts, and surgical excision that has been necessary in patients with infective endocarditis unresponsive to medical management.[633]

TR can occur in the *carcinoid syndrome*[634] (Fig. 34–42, p. 1057), which leads to focal or diffuse deposits of fibrous tissue on the endocardium of the valvular cusps and cardiac chambers and on the intima of the great veins and coronary sinus. The white, fibrous carcinoid plaques are most extensive on the right side of the heart, where they are usually deposited on the ventricular surfaces of the tricuspid valve and cause the cusps to adhere to the underlying right ventricular wall, thereby producing tricuspid regurgitation.[635,636] Less common causes of tricuspid regurgitation include cardiac tumors, particularly right atrial myxoma; endomyocardial fibrosis; methysergide-induced valvular disease[637]; and systemic lupus erythematosus involving the tricuspid valve.[638]

CLINICAL MANIFESTATIONS

HISTORY. In the absence of pulmonary hypertension, TR is generally well tolerated. However, when pulmonary hypertension and TR coexist, cardiac output declines, and the manifestations of right-sided heart failure become intensified. Thus, the symptoms of TR result from a reduced cardiac output and from ascites, painful congestive hepatomegaly, and massive edema. Occasionally, patients complain of throbbing pulsations in the neck due to jugular venous distention, which intensify on effort,[20] and systolic pulsations of the eyeballs are sometimes noted.[639] In the many patients with TR who have mitral valve disease, the symptoms of the latter usually predominate. Symptoms of pulmonary congestion may abate as TR develops, but they are replaced by weakness, fatigue, and other manifestations of a depressed cardiac output.

PHYSICAL EXAMINATION (Figs. 2–7, p. 19, and 16–3, p. 453). Evidence of weight loss and cachexia, cyanosis, and jaundice is often present on inspection. Atrial fibrillation is common. There is jugular venous distention,[640] the normal *x* and *x′* descents disappear, and a prominent systolic ("s") wave, i.e., a *c-v* wave, is apparent. The descent of this wave, the *y* descent, is sharp and becomes the most prominent event in the venous pulse (unless there is coexisting TS, in which case it is slowed). The *s* waves and *y* descents become more prominent during inspiration.[641] A venous systolic thrill and murmur in the neck may be present in severe TR.[642] The right ventricular impulse is hyperdynamic and thrusting in quality. Rarely, a right atrial systolic impulse may be observed or palpated along the right lower sternal edge.[20] In patients with combined mitral valve disease and TR, a relatively quiet zone may be present between the apex and the left sternal edge.

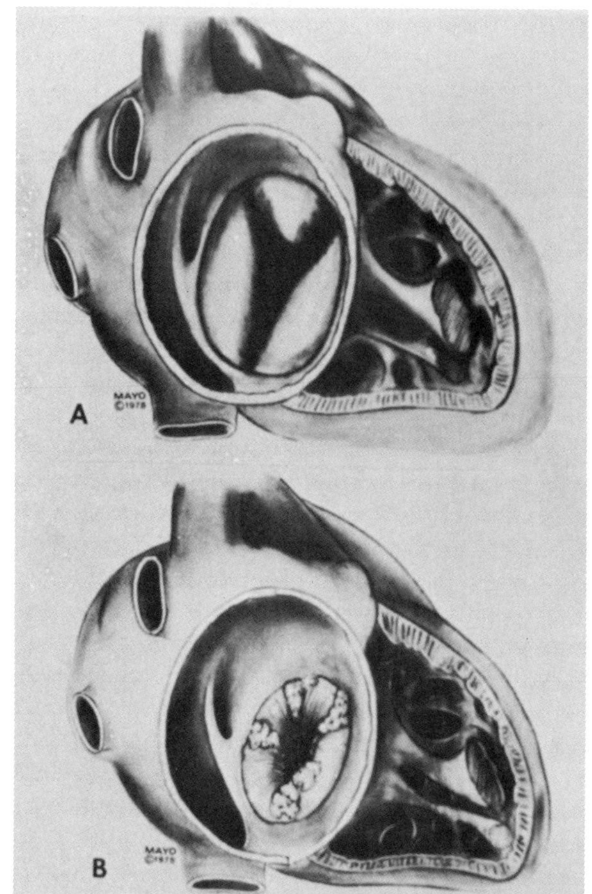

FIGURE 34–41. Types of tricuspid incompetence. *A*, Functional tricuspid incompetence secondary to dilatation of the right ventricle. *B*, Organic rheumatic tricuspid incompetence. (From Brandenburg, R. O., et al.: Valvular heart disease—When should the patient be referred? Pract. Cardiol. *5*:50, 1979.)

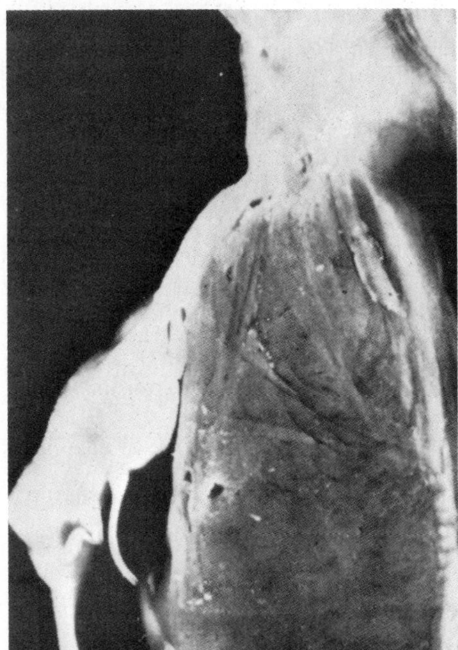

FIGURE 34-42. Septal tricuspid leaflet thickened by carcinoid plaques and fused to underlying ventricular septum. (From Callahan, J. A., et al.: Echocardiographic features of carcinoid heart disease. Am. J. Cardiol. *50*:766, 1982.)

Systolic pulsations of an enlarged tender liver are commonly present initially, but in chronic TR with congestive cirrhosis, the liver may be firm and nontender. Ascites and edema are frequent.

Auscultation (Table 34-4, p. 1020). This usually reveals an S_3 originating from the right ventricle, i.e., one which is accentuated by inspiration; when TR is associated with pulmonary hypertension, P_2 is accentuated as well. The murmur of TR is usually high-pitched, pansystolic, and loudest in the fourth intercostal space in the parasternal region but occasionally in the subxiphoid area. When TR is mild, the murmur may be short. With acute TR due to infective endocarditis or trauma, the murmur is usually of low intensity and limited to the first half of systole. When the right ventricle is greatly dilated and occupies the anterior surface of the heart, the murmur may be most prominent at the apex and difficult to distinguish from that produced by MR.

The response of the murmur to respiration and other maneuvers is of considerable aid in establishing the diagnosis of tricuspid regurgitation (Table 2-8, p. 38). It is usually augmented during inspiration[20,643,644] (Rivero-Carvello's sign, p. 53). However, when the failing ventricle can no longer increase its stroke volume, the inspiratory augmentation is lost. Under these circumstances, respiratory variation may be elicited by standing and thereby reducing venous return. The murmur also increases during inspiration, the Mueller maneuver (forced inspiration against a closed glottis), exercise, leg-raising, hepatic compression, and amyl nitrite inhalation as well as after a prolonged diastole. It demonstrates an immediate overshoot after release of the Valsalva strain. It is reduced in intensity and duration in the standing position and during the strain of the Valsalva maneuver. Rarely, TR is silent except for the selective appearance of a soft systolic murmur during inspiration.[645]

Increased atrioventricular flow may cause a short early diastolic flow rumble in the left parasternal region following S_3.

LABORATORY EXAMINATION

ELECTROCARDIOGRAM. This is usually nonspecific and characteristic of the lesion causing TR. Incomplete right bundle branch block, Q waves in lead V_1, and atrial fibrillation are commonly found.

RADIOLOGICAL FINDINGS. Marked cardiomegaly secondary to the condition responsible for the dilatation of the right ventricle is usually evident. The right atrium is prominent.[641] Evidence of elevated right atrial pressure may include distention of the azygos vein and the presence of pleural effusion. Ascites with upward displacement of the diaphragm may be present. Rarely, with prolonged elevation of right ventricular pressure, the tricuspid ring may calcify. The findings of pulmonary arterial and venous hypertension are common. Fluoroscopy may reveal systolic pulsations of the right atrium.

ECHOCARDIOGRAM (see also p. 87). In patients with TR secondary to dilation of the tricuspid annulus, the right atrium, right ventricle, and tricuspid annulus are usually dilated.[621-623] There is evidence of right ventricular diastolic overload, with paradoxical motion of the ventricular septum similar to that in atrial septal defect. Exaggerated motion and delayed closure of the tricuspid valve are evident in patients with Ebstein's anomaly. In patients with TR secondary to right ventricular dilatation and pulmonary hypertension, the pulmonic valve echogram shows a diminished or absent *a* deflection. *Prolapse of the tricuspid valve* due to myxomatous degeneration may be evident on M-mode and two-dimensional echocardiography[625,646] (Fig. 4-59, p. 87). Simultaneous echocardiographic studies of the tricuspid valve and phonocardiography may reveal a nonejection systolic click originating from the right side of the heart that occurs at the onset of prolapse. Echocardiographic indications of tricuspid valve abnormalities, especially TR by Doppler examination, can be detected in the majority of patients with carcinoid heart disease.[634]

Contrast echocardiography involving rapid injection of saline or indocyanine green dye into an antecubital vein made while a two-dimensional echocardiogram is being recorded (p. 69) is both sensitive and specific for TR.[647] The injection produces microcavities that are readily visible on echocardiography and normally travel as a bolus through the circulation. In TR, these microcavities can be seen to travel back and forth across the tricuspid orifice and to pass into the inferior vena cava and hepatic veins during systole.[648] TR secondary to carcinoid heart disease shows thickened, retracted valve leaflets, fixed in a semiopen position throughout the cardiac cycle[647,649] whereas that due to endocarditis may reveal vegetations on the valve, or a flail valve.

Pulsed Doppler echocardiography revealing systolic flow from right ventricle to right atrium is an exquisitely sensitive technique for detecting TR.[650] A semiquantitative assessment can be made by measuring reverse velocity in the inferior vena cava[651] and hepatic veins.[652] The peak velocity of TR flow is useful in the noninvasive estimation of right ventricular (and pulmonary artery) systolic pressure.[654] Real-time two-dimensional color-coded Doppler imaging is an extremely accurate, sensitive, and specific method for assessing TR[655] and is helpful in selecting patients for surgical treatment[656] and in assessing postoperative results.[657] The velocity of TR flow is useful in the noninvasive estimation of right ventricular (and pulmonary artery) systolic pressure.

HEMODYNAMIC AND ANGIOGRAPHIC FINDINGS. The right atrial and right ventricular end-diastolic pressures are characteristically elevated in TR, whether the condition is due to organic disease of the tricuspid valve or is secondary to right ventricular systolic overload (e.g., pulmonary hypertension and pulmonic stenosis). The right atrial pressure tracing reveals absence of the x descent and a prominent *v* or *c-v* wave ("ventricularization" of the atrial pressure). Therefore, as the severity of tricuspid regurgitation increases, the right atrial pressure pulse increasingly resembles the right ventricular pressure pulse (Fig. 34-43).[598] A rise or no change in right atrial pressure on deep inspiration, rather than the usual fall, is characteristic.[641,658] Pulmonary artery (or right ventricular) systolic pressure may offer a rough guide as to whether the TR

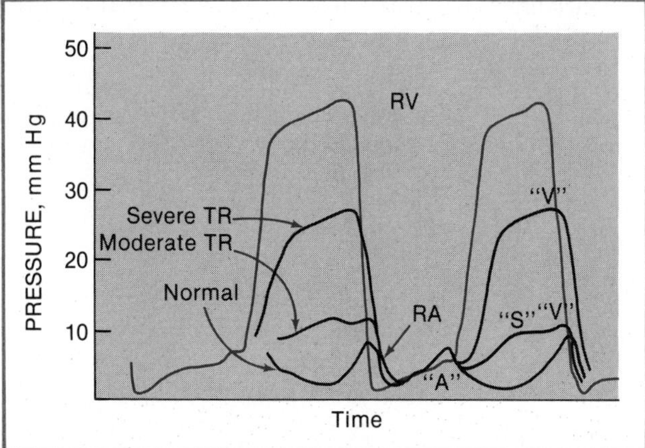

FIGURE 34–43. Appearance of right atrial (RA) pressure contour in patients with severe tricuspid regurgitation (TR), moderate TR, and no TR (normal). Note the regurgitant systolic ("S") wave that blends with the normal filling ("V") wave in severe TR. The resultant RA pressure waveform resembles a right ventricular (RV) pressure recording. (From Grossman, W. [ed.]: Cardiac Catheterization and Angiography. 3rd ed. Philadelphia, Lea and Febiger, 1986, p. 378.)

is primary (i.e., due to disease of the valve or its supporting structures) or secondary to right ventricular dilatation. A pulmonary artery or right ventricular systolic pressure less than 40 mm Hg favors a primary etiology, whereas a pressure greater than 60 mm Hg suggests that TR is secondary.

Diagnosis and quantitative assessment of TR can be aided in many instances by right ventriculography, but the fact that the catheter must be positioned across the tricuspid valve cannot exclude the possibility of a false-positive diagnosis of TR.[659] Modifications of previous angiographic techniques have been introduced in which a special, preformed catheter is positioned in the right ventricle, and angiography is carried out at low injection rates[660]; or a special balloon catheter is employed to minimize the induction of extrasystoles, which can also cause spurious regurgitation.[661]

MANAGEMENT

TR in the absence of pulmonary hypertension usually does not require surgical treatment. Indeed, both patients and experimental animals tolerate total excision of the tricuspid valve, as long as right ventricular systolic pressure is normal.[662] In some patients dilatation of the right side of the heart occurs months or years after tricuspid valvectomy (usually carried out for acute infective endocarditis), and insertion of a prosthetic valve can then be carried out after adequate sterilization of the valve ring.[662] *Surgical treatment* of acquired regurgitation secondary to annular dilatation was greatly improved when Carpentier introduced the concept of suturing the annulus to a right prosthetic ring of appropriate dimensions.[657,663] Annuloplasty without insertion of a prosthetic ring (so-called DeVega annuloplasty) has also been found to be effective in patients with annular dilatation. This technique is now widely employed.[664-666]

In patients with TR associated with mitral valve disease and pulmonary hypertension, the severity of the regurgitation should be assessed by palpation of the valve at the time of mitral commissurotomy or valve replacement. Patients with mild TR usually do not require surgical treatment[667]; pulmonary vascular pressures decline following successful mitral valve surgery, and the mild TR tends to disappear. Excellent results have been reported in patients with moderate TR with the use of tricuspid annuloplasty,[663] often utilizing a Carpentier ring[664,668,669] (Fig. 34–44). However, management of severe TR is more controversial. It is not clear whether severe TR should be treated by annuloplasty or valve replacement, but most surgeons prefer the former approach. If it does not provide a good functional result at the operating table, they resort to valve replacement.[670]

Organic disease of the tricuspid valve responsible for TR, as in Ebstein's anomaly[671,672] or carcinoid heart disease,[673] when severe enough to require surgery, usually requires valve replacement. The risk of thrombosis of valvular prostheses is greater in the tricuspid than in the mitral position, presumably because pressure and flow rates are lower in the right side of the heart. For this reason, the artificial valve of choice for the tricuspid position in adults at present is a large porcine heterograft. Anticoagulants are not required, and a durability of more than 10 years has been established.

In treating the difficult problem of tricuspid endocarditis in heroin addicts, it has been noted that total excision of the tricuspid valve *without immediate replacement* can be tolerated by these patients, who usually do not have associated pulmonary hypertension. However, surgery should be carried out in patients with resistant or relapsing infection after optimal antibiotic therapy.[661] When antibiotic therapy is unsuccessful, valvular replacement frequently results in reinfection or continued infection. Diseased valvular tissue should be excised to eradicate the endocarditis, and antibiotic treatment can be continued. Most patients tolerate loss of the tricuspid valve without great difficulty. However, if medical management does not control the tricuspid regurgitation and the infection has been controlled, an artificial valve can be inserted later.[662]

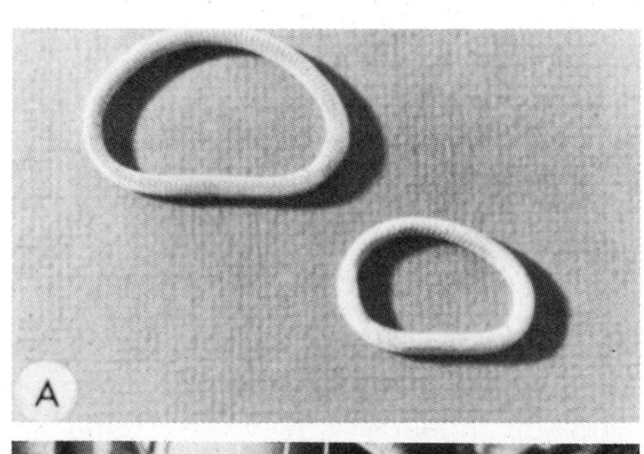

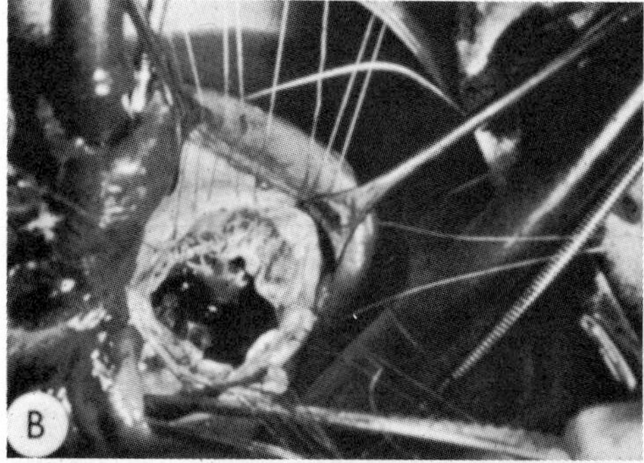

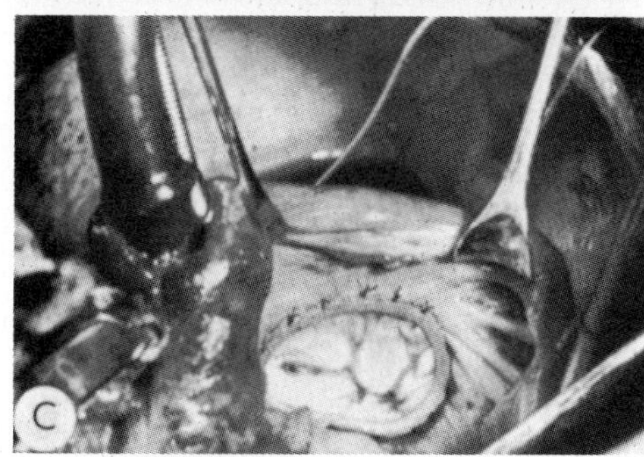

FIGURE 34–44. *A*, Carpentier rings. *B*, Ring being sutured into place. *C*, Completion of Carpentier ring annuloplasty. (From Starr, A.: Acquired disease of the tricuspid valve. *In* Sabiston, D. C., Jr., and Spencer, F. C. [eds.]: Gibbon's Surgery of the Chest. Philadelphia, W. B. Saunders Company, 1976, p. 1182.)

PULMONIC VALVE DISEASE

ETIOLOGY AND PATHOLOGY

The congenital form is the most common cause of *pulmonic stenosis* (PS).[674] Its manifestations in children are discussed on page 931 and in adults on page 968. *Rheumatic* inflammation of the pulmonic valve is very uncommon, is usually associated with involvement of other valves, and rarely leads to serious deformity. However, a high incidence of significant pulmonic valve involvement secondary to rheumatic fever has been reported in Mexico City, perhaps related to the pulmonary hypertension that occurs at high altitudes and the resultant greater stress on the pulmonic valve.[675] *Carcinoid* plaques, similar to those involving the tricuspid valve, are often present in the outflow tract of the right ventricle in patients with malignant carcinoid and result in constriction of the pulmonic valve ring, retraction and fusion of the valve cusps, and either PS or the combination of PS and pulmonic regurgitation (PR) (Fig. 34–45).[676] Obstruction in the region of the pulmonic valve may be extrinsic to the valve apparatus and may be produced by cardiac tumors or aneurysm of the sinus Valsalva.[677]

By far the most common cause of PR is dilatation of the valve ring secondary to pulmonary hypertension (of any etiology) or to dilatation of the pulmonary artery, either idiopathic[678,679] or consequent to a connective tissue disorder such as Marfan syndrome.[680] The second most common cause is infective endocarditis.[676,681–683] Less frequently, it is iatrogenic and is induced at the time of surgical treatment of congenital PS or tetralogy of Fallot. It may also result from a variety of lesions directly affecting the pulmonic valve. These include congenital malformations, such as absent, malformed, fenestrated, or supernumerary leaflets.[11] These anomalies may occur as isolated lesions[684] but more often are associated with other congenital anomalies, particularly tetralogy of Fallot, ventricular septal defect, and pulmonic valvular stenosis. Less common causes include carcinoid syndrome,[676] rheumatic involvement,[685] injury produced by a pulmonary artery flow-directed catheter,[686] syphilis,[629] and chest trauma.[683]

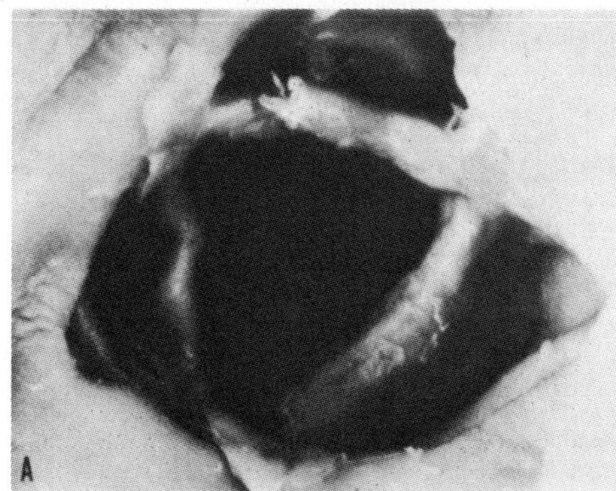

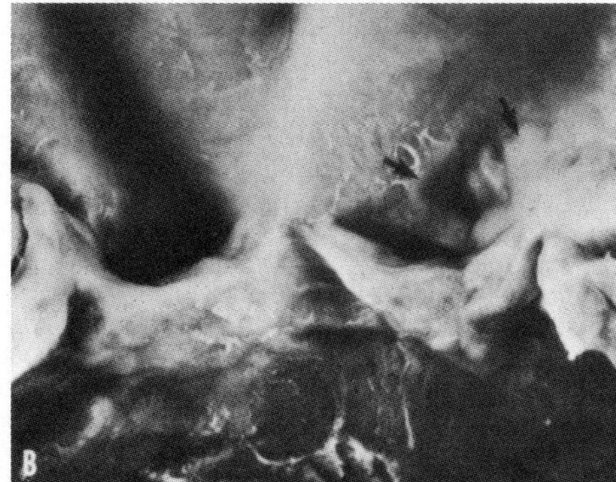

FIGURE 34–45. Carcinoid heart disease; pulmonary valve viewed from above (*A*) and opened (*B*). The thickened and retracted cusps result in valvular incompetence. The constricted annulus results in valvular stenosis. Carcinoid plaques (arrows) extend onto the pulmonary trunk. (From Callahan, J. A., et al.: Echocardiographic features of carcinoid heart disease. Am. J. Cardiol. *50*:767, 1982.)

CLINICAL MANIFESTATIONS

Like TR, isolated PR causes right ventricular volume overload and may be tolerated for many years without difficulty unless it complicates or is complicated by pulmonary hypertension, in which case it is usually accompanied by and aggravates right ventricular failure. Patients with PR caused by infective endocarditis who develop septic pulmonary emboli and pulmonary hypertension often exhibit severe right ventricular failure.[683] In most patients the clinical manifestations of the primary disease are severe and usually overshadow the PR, which often results only in incidental auscultatory findings. *Physical examination* reveals a hyperdynamic right ventricle, producing palpable systolic pulsations in the left parasternal area and an enlarged pulmonary artery that often results in palpable systolic pulsations in the second left intercostal space; sometimes systolic and diastolic thrills are felt in the same area. A tap reflecting pulmonic valve closure is usually easily palpable in the second intercostal space in patients with pulmonary hypertension and secondary PR.

AUSCULTATION. In patients with congenital absence of the pulmonic valve, P_2 is not audible, but this sound is accentuated in patients with PR secondary to pulmonary hypertension, particularly when the dilated pulmonary artery is near the chest wall. There may be wide splitting of S_2 due to prolongation of right ventricular ejection accompanying the augmented stroke volume.[685] A nonvalvular systolic ejection click due to the sudden expansion of the pulmonary artery by the augmented right ventricular stroke volume frequently initiates a midsystolic ejection murmur, most prominent in the second left intercostal space. An S_3 and S_4 originating from the right ventricle are often audible, most readily in the fourth intercostal space at the left parasternal area, and are augmented by inspiration.

In the absence of pulmonary hypertension, the diastolic murmur of PR is low-pitched and is usually heard best at the third and fourth left intercostal spaces adjacent to the sternum (Fig. 3–32, p. 58). The murmur commences when pressures in the pulmonary artery and right ventricle diverge, approximately 0.04 sec after P_2. It is diamond-shaped in configuration and brief, reaching a peak intensity when the gradient between these pressures is maximal and ending with equilibration of the pressures.[687] The murmur becomes louder during inspiration[688] and following inhalation of amyl nitrite.

When pulmonary artery systolic pressure exceeds approximately 60 mm Hg, dilatation of the pulmonic annulus results in a regurgitant jet of high velocity that is responsible for the so-called Graham Steell murmur of PR. (Doppler ultrasound reveals pulmonary regurgitation at much lower pulmonary arterial pressures.[689]) The Graham Steell murmur is a high-pitched, blowing decrescendo murmur beginning immediately after P_2 and is most prominent in the left parasternal region in the second to fourth intercostal spaces. Thus, although it resembles the murmur of AR, it is usually accompanied by the findings of severe pulmonary hypertension, i.e., an accentuated P_2 or fused S_2, an ejection sound, and a systolic murmur of tricuspid regurgitation. Sometimes a low-frequency presystolic murmur is present, i.e., a right-sided Austin Flint murmur originating from the tricuspid valve that is analogous to the more common left-sided Austin Flint murmur originating from the mitral valve.[690]

The Graham Steell murmur of PR secondary to pulmonary hypertension usually increases in intensity with inspiration, exhibits little change after amyl nitrite inhalation or vasopressors, is diminished during the Valsalva strain, and returns to baseline intensity almost immediately after release of the Valsalva strain. This murmur resembles and may be confused with the diastolic blowing murmur of AR. However, indicator dilution studies[691] and aortography have established that a diastolic blowing murmur along the left sternal border in patients with rheumatic heart disease and pulmonary hypertension—even in the absence of peripheral signs of AR—is usually due to AR and not PR.

LABORATORY EXAMINATION

ELECTROCARDIOGRAM. In the absence of pulmonary hypertension, PR often results in an ECG that reflects right ventricular diastolic overload, i.e., an rSr′ (or rsR′) configuration in the right precordial leads. PR secondary to pulmonary hypertension is usually associated with ECG evidence of right ventricular hypertrophy.

RADIOLOGICAL FINDINGS. Both the pulmonary artery and the right ventricle are usually enlarged,[692] but these signs are nonspecific. Fluoros-

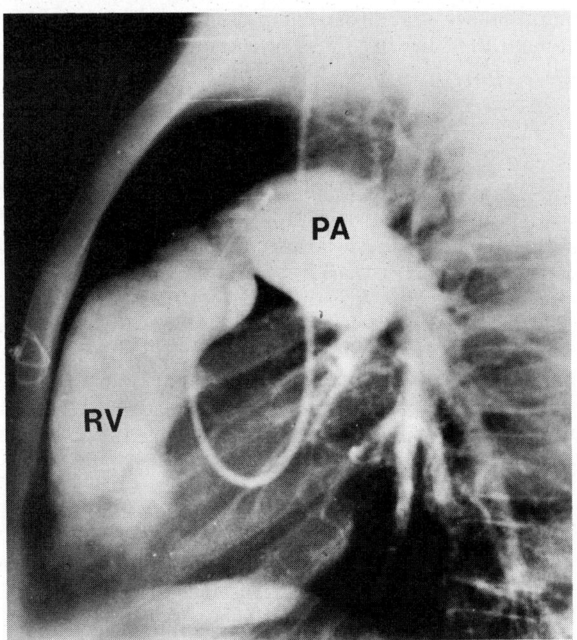

FIGURE 34-46. Pulmonic valvular regurgitation. Contrast medium has been injected into the main pulmonary artery (PA) and regurgitates back into an enlarged right ventricle (RV). (From Carlsson, E., et al.: The radiological diagnosis of cardiac valvular insufficiency. Circulation *55*:921, 1977, by permission of the American Heart Association, Inc.)

copy may demonstrate pronounced pulsation of the main pulmonary artery. PR can be diagnosed by observing opacification of the right ventricle following injection of contrast material into the main pulmonary artery (Fig. 34-46). The diagnosis is supported by noting superimposition of the pulmonary artery and right ventricular pressure curves during mid and late diastole. Indicator dilution techniques with injections into the pulmonary artery and sampling from the right ventricle,[693] as well as intracardiac phonocardiography,[629] can also be helpful in establishing the diagnosis in mild cases.

ECHOCARDIOGRAM. This shows right ventricular dilatation and, in patients with pulmonary hypertension, right ventricular hypertrophy as well. Diastolic fluttering of the tricuspid valve leaflets, similar to that of the mitral valve leaflets in AR, is often noted. Abnormal motion of the septum characteristic of volume overload of the right ventricle in diastole and/or septal flutter[694] may be evident. The motion of the pulmonic valve may point to the etiology of the pulmonic regurgitation.[695] Absence of *a* waves and systolic notching of the posterior leaflet suggest pulmonary hypertension; large *a* waves indicate pulmonic stenosis. PR can be detected by contrast echocardiography.[696] The pulsed Doppler technique is extremely accurate in detecting PR. Abnormal Doppler signals in the right ventricular outflow tract whose velocity is sustained throughout diastole are generally observed in patients in whom dilatation of the valve ring (functional regurgitation) is the cause. When the velocity falls during diastole, the pulmonary artery pressure is usually normal, and the regurgitation is caused by an abnormality of the valve itself.[695]

MANAGEMENT. PR per se is seldom severe enough to require specific treatment. Cardiac glycosides are useful in the management of right ventricular dilatation or failure. Treatment of the primary condition such as infective endocarditis or of the lesion responsible for the pulmonary hypertension, such as surgical treatment of mitral valvular disease, often ameliorates the PR. Surgical treatment of primary PR directed specifically at the pulmonic valve is required only occasionally because of intractable right heart failure, and under such circumstances valve replacement may be carried out.[697]

MULTIVALVULAR DISEASE

Multivalvular involvement is common, particularly in patients with rheumatic heart disease, and a variety of clinical and hemodynamic syndromes can be produced by different combinations of valvular abnormalities. Development of PR and TR secondary to dilatation of the pulmonic valve ring and tricuspid annulus, respectively, as a consequence of pulmonary hypertension secondary to disease involving the mitral or aortic valve or both, has already been discussed (pp. 1055 and 1060), as has the combination of *organic* rheumatic tricuspid and mitral valvular disease. In patients with multivalvular disease, the clinical manifestations depend on the relative severities of each of the lesions.[698] When the valvular abnormalities are of approximately equal severity, as a general rule, clinical manifestations produced by the more proximal (upstream) of two valvular lesions, i.e., the mitral valve in patients with combined mitral and aortic valvular disease and the tricuspid valve in patients with combined tricuspid and mitral valvular disease, are more prominent than those produced by the distal lesion.

It is important to recognize multivalvular involvement preoperatively, since failure to correct all significant valvular disease at the time of operation increases mortality considerably. In patients with multivalvular disease, the relative severity of each lesion may be difficult to estimate by clinical examination and noninvasive techniques, because one lesion may mask the manifestations of the other. For this reason, patients suspected of multivalvular involvement and in whom surgical treatment is under consideration should undergo (in addition to careful clinical examination and noninvasive workup, with emphasis on two-dimensional and Doppler echocardiography), right- and left-sided cardiac catheterization and angiography. If there is any question concerning the presence of significant AS in patients undergoing an operation on the mitral valve, the aortic valve should be inspected, since overlooking this condition can lead to a high perioperative mortality. Similarly, it is useful to palpate the tricuspid valve at the time of operation on the mitral valve.

Mitral Stenosis and Aortic Regurgitation

Approximately two-thirds of patients with severe MS have an early blowing diastolic murmur along the left sternal border with a normal pulse pressure; in 90 per cent of these the murmur is due to AR and is usually of little clinical importance. However, approximately 10 per cent of patients with MS have severe rheumatic AR,[699] which can usually be recognized by the peripheral signs of a widened pulse pressure, left ventricular dilatation and increased wall motion on echocardiography, and signs of left ventricular enlargement on radiological and electrocardiographic examinations.

In keeping with the general observation that a proximal lesion may mask a distal lesion, significant AR may be missed in patients with severe MS. The widened pulse pressure, in particular, may be absent in the latter. On clinical examination of patients with obvious AR, errors may be made in that MS may be missed or, conversely, may be falsely diagnosed. An accentuated S_1 and an opening snap in a patient with AR should suggest the possibility of mitral valvular disease. On the other hand, an Austin Flint murmur is often inappropriately considered to be the diastolic rumbling murmur of MS (Table 34-14). These two murmurs may be distinguished at the bedside by means of amyl nitrite inhalation, which diminishes the Austin Flint murmur (Fig. 3-32, p. 58) but augments the murmur of MS; isometric handgrip and squatting augment both the diastolic murmur of AR and the Austin Flint murmur. Echocardiography, particularly pulsed Doppler echocardiography, is of decisive value in the detection of both lesions. Diastolic fluttering of the anterior leaflet of the mitral valve and of the ventricular spectrum is an important clue to the presence of AR in a patient with MS. Evidence of rapid left ventricular filling in diastole by echocardiography should suggest the presence of associated AR.

Hemodynamic analysis reveals that MS reduces the left ventricular volume overload characteristic of AR.[607] This combination is relatively uncommon.

Mitral Stenosis and Aortic Stenosis

When severe MS and AS coexist, the former masks many of the manifestations of the latter.[701] The cardiac output tends to be reduced further than in patients with isolated AS, and the atrial booster pump mechanism, so important in filling the ventricle in AS (p. 1035), has little impact when MS is present. The reduction in cardiac output lowers both the transaortic valvular pressure gradient and the left ventricular systolic pressure, diminishes the incidence of angina, and retards the development of aortic calcification and left ventricular hypertrophy.[702] On the other hand, clinical manifestations associated with MS, such as pulmonary congestion and hemoptysis, atrial fibrillation, and systemic embolization, occur more frequently than in patients with isolated AS. On physical examination, presystolic distention of the left ventricle and an S_4, common in pure AS, are usually not present. The midsystolic murmur characteristic of AS may be reduced in intensity and duration because of the reduced stroke volume. The *electrocardiogram* may fail to demonstrate left ventricular hypertrophy, but left atrial enlargement is common in patients in sinus rhythm. The *chest roentgenogram* is usually typical of MS except that calcium may be present in the region of the aortic valve. The two-dimensional and Doppler *echocardiograms* are of the greatest value because stenosis of both valves may be evident. However, the low cardiac output characteristic of the combination of lesions may reduce the transvalvular gradients estimated by Doppler echocardiography. The indirect *carotid pulse* tracing reveals a delayed upstroke.

It is vital to recognize the presence of hemodynamically significant aortic valvular disease (stenosis and/or regurgitation) preoperatively in patients who are to undergo surgical correction of MS, since isolated mitral valvulotomy may be hazardous in such patients; this operation can impose a sudden hemodynamic load on the left ventricle that may lead to acute pulmonary edema.

Aortic Stenosis and Mitral Regurgitation

The combination of severe AS and MR is a hazardous one, but fortunately it is relatively uncommon. Obstruction to left ventricular outflow augments the volume of MR flow,[170] whereas the presence of MR diminishes the ventricular preload necessary for maintenance of the left ventricular stroke volume in AS. The result is a reduced forward cardiac output and marked left atrial and pulmonary venous hypertension. The physical findings may be confusing because the delayed arterial pulse of AS may be counteracted by the sharp upstroke of MR, and it may be difficult to recognize two distinct systolic murmurs. Amyl nitrite tends to increase the intensity of the murmur of AS and to reduce that of MR. On echocardiography and roentgenography the left atrium and ventricle are usually larger than in isolated AS. Usually both valves must be treated surgically in patients with severe AS and MR.

Aortic Regurgitation and Mitral Regurgitation

This relatively frequent combination of lesions[703] may be caused by rheumatic heart disease or by prolapse of both valves due to myxomatous degeneration,[704] or dilatation of both annuli in connective tissue disorders. The clinical features of AR usually predominate, and it sometimes is difficult to determine whether the MR is due to organic involvement of this valve or dilatation of the mitral valve ring secondary to left ventricular enlargement. When both valvular leaks are severe, this combination of lesions is poorly tolerated. The normal mitral valve ordinarily serves as a "backup" to the aortic valve, and premature (diastolic) closure of the mitral valve limits the volume of reflux that occurs in patients with acute AR.[513] With combined regurgitant lesions, regardless of the etiology of the mitral lesion, blood may reflux from the aorta through both chambers of the left side of the heart into the pulmonary veins. Physical and laboratory examination will usually show evidence of both lesions. Both lesions are frequently associated with an S_3 and a brisk arterial pulse. The relative severity of each lesion can be assessed best by contrast angiography.

When MR occurs in patients with AR secondary to left ventricular dilatation, it often regresses following aortic valve replacement. If severe, it may be corrected by annuloplasty at the time of aortic valve replacement. Replacement of an intrinsically normal mitral valve that is regurgitant due to a dilated annulus is neither necessary nor advisable.

Surgical Treatment of Multivalvular Disease

Combined aortic and mitral valve replacement is usually associated with a higher risk and poorer survival than is replacement of either of the two valves alone.[705] Kirklin reported a 5-year survival rate of 70 per cent after double-valve replacement compared to 80 per cent for single-valve replacement.[706] The long-term survival is strongly dependent on the functional status preoperatively.[707] Also, patients operated on for the combination of AR and MR fared worse than did patients receiving double-valve replacement for any of the other combinations.[706] The operative risk of double valve replacement is about twice as high as it is for single valve replacement, and like the latter has been slowly but steadily declining.[708]

Hemodynamically significant disease involving the mitral, aortic, and tricuspid valves is uncommon. Patients with these lesions often present in advanced heart failure with marked cardiomegaly, and surgical correction of all three valvular lesions is imperative. Attempts to shorten the duration of operation by leaving one severely impaired valve in place after a double valve replacement are usually unsatisfactory. However, triple valve replacement is a long and complex operation. In one early series, the mortality rate was 18 per cent in patients in functional Class III and 40 per cent in Class IV.[709] In a more recent one it was only 5 per cent.[710,711] However, even this high risk must often be accepted because of the otherwise dismal prognosis in these patients. An alternative is to replace the mitral and aortic valves and carry out a tricuspid valvuloplasty.[710,711]

Patients who survive triple-valve replacement usually show substantial clinical improvement in the early postoperative period,[712–714] and postoperative catheterization studies show marked reductions in pulmonary arterial and capillary pressures.[715] However, some patients succumb to arrhythmias[714] or congestive heart failure in the late postoperative period despite normally functioning prostheses. The cause of cardiac failure in this situation is not known, but it may be related to intraoperative myocardial ischemia, microemboli from the multiple prostheses, or continued subclinical episodes of rheumatic myocarditis.

When multiple prosthetic valves must be inserted, it is logical to select either two (or three) bioprostheses or mechanical prostheses for the left side of the heart. If the patient is to be exposed to the hazards of anticoagulants for one mechanical prosthesis, it seems unreasonable to add the potential risks of early failure of a bioprosthesis. However, the use of a bioprosthesis in the tricuspid position is suggested.[710]

Prosthetic Cardiac Valves

The first successful replacements of cardiac valves in the human were accomplished by Nina Braunwald,[715] Harken et al.,[716] and Starr[717] in 1960. Two major groups of artificial (prosthetic) valves are currently available in models designed for both the atrioventricular (mitral and tricuspid) and the aortic positions: mechanical prostheses and bioprostheses (tissue valves).

MECHANICAL PROSTHESES

(Table 34–18)

Mechanical prosthetic valves are classified into two major groups: caged-ball and tilting-disc valves. The *Starr-Edwards* caged-ball valve (Figs. 34–47*A* and 34–48) is still widely used in both the aortic and mitral positions.[718,719] It has the longest record of predictable performance of any artificial valve. A disadvantage is its bulky cage design. It is therefore not suitable in patients with a small left ventricular cavity or a small aortic annulus or in a valve–aortic arch composite graft. In a small number of patients it induces hemolysis, which may be greatly exaggerated and become of clinical importance if a perivalvular leak develops.

Several types of tilting-disc valves are widely employed; these are less bulky and have a lower profile than the caged-ball valve. The *St. Jude* valve (Fig. 34–47*E*), constructed of pyrolytic carbon, has two semicircular discs that pivot between open and closed positions without the need for supporting struts (Fig. 34–48). It possesses favorable flow characteristics and causes a lower transvalvular gradient at any outer diameter and cardiac output than the caged-ball or tilting valves.[720,721] It is the most widely used mechanical prosthetic valve in the United States at the time of this writing. The St. Jude valve appears to have particularly favorable hemodynamic characteristics in the smaller sizes; therefore, it may be especially useful in children. Thrombogenicity in the mitral position *may* be less than for other prosthetic valves. As with other mechanical prostheses, permanent anticoagulation is needed—antiplatelet agents alone are not sufficient.[720] A variation of the St. Jude valve, the *Duromedics* prosthesis (Fig. 34–47*F*), is also a bileaflet valve with curved leaflets and a hinge design, which supposedly enhances central flow and hemodynamic performance. This valve appears to cause less regurgitation than other tilting-disc valves; the incidence of valve thrombosis and thromboembolism appears to be low.[722]

The *Lillehei-Kaster* pivoting-disc valve consists of a titanium valve housing with a Teflon fabric sewing ring in which a pyrolyte disc is suspended. In the open position, the disc swings to an angle of 80 degrees, providing a large central flow orifice. This is an excellent valve in larger sizes in the aortic position, but a relatively high incidence of thrombosis pre-

TABLE 34-18 RELATIVE RISK OF SPECIFIC PROSTHESIS-ASSOCIATED COMPLICATIONS WITH VARIOUS VALVE TYPES

	GENERIC VALVE TYPE/MODELS USED						
COMPLICATIONS	Caged-Ball (Bare-Cage)/ Starr-Edwards, Smerloff-Cutter	Caged-Ball (Cloth-Covered)/ Starr-Edwards, Braunwald-Cutter	Caged-Disc/ Beall	Tilting-Disc/ Björk-Shiley Hall-Medtronic Lillehei-Kaster	Bileaflet Tilting-Disc/ St. Jude/ Edwards-Duromedics	Porcine Bioprosthesis/ Hancock/ Carpentier-Edwards	Pericardial Bioprosthesis/ Ionescu-Shiley
Obstruction	++	++	+++	+	+	+	+
Hemolysis[a]	+	+	+	+	+	+	+
Paravalvular leak	++	++	++	++	++	++	++
Endocarditis	++	++	++	++	++	++	++
Thrombosis/thromboembolism	+++	+++	+++	+++	++	+	+
Extrinsic interference	+	++	++	++	+	+	+
Component fracture/ escape	+	++	+	+[b]	+	+	+
Ball (or disc) variance	+[c]	+	+	NA	+	NA	NA
Ball (or disc) abrasive wear	+	+[d]	+++[e]	+	+	NA	NA
Cloth wear	NA	++	NA	NA	NA	NA	NA
Leaflet tears	NA	NA	NA	NA	NA	+++	+++
Calcification	NA	NA	NA	NA	NA	+++	+++

NA = not applicable, + = rare, ++ = frequent, +++ = major problem; [a] = new onset or increasing hemolysis generally indicates dysfunctional valve; [b] = some Björk-Shiley valves are partially susceptible; [c] = lipid uptake unusual in valves fabricated since 1964; [d] = occurs only with cloth-covered valves with silicone ball; [e] = except in valves with pyrolytic carbon disc.

From Schoen, F. J.: Valvular heart disease. *In* Interventional and Surgical Cardiovascular Pathology. Philadelphia, W. B. Saunders Company, 1989, p. 156.

cludes its use in the mitral position.[723-725] Two adaptations of the Lillehei-Kaster tilting-disc valve, the *Omniscience*[724,726] (Fig. 34–47*C*) and the *Omnicarbon*[723] valves, have been introduced in an effort to improve hemodynamics and decrease thrombogenicity. Early reports suggest that both of these goals may have been achieved. A closely related valve is the *Medtronic-Hall* valve (Fig. 34–47*D*). Its pivoting disc has a central perforation that allows improved hemodynamics; thrombogenicity appears to be quite low, less than 1 episode per 100 patient-years in the aortic position and 1.5 per 100 patient-years in the mitral position[727,728]; mechanical performance is excellent over the long term. The *Björk-Shiley* valve[729-731] (Fig. 34–47*B*) consists of a low-profile cobalt base alloy covered with a Teflon fabric sewing ring; its design allows an excellent ratio between the diameter of the valve orifice and tissue annulus. It contains a suspended tilting-disc occluder made of pyrolytic carbon (pyrolyte). Two serious problems with this valve have been reported in a small number of patients: (1) sudden thrombosis and (2) strut fracture. Changes have been made to overcome the first of these problems, but in some models the incidence of strut fracture is prohibitive. Accordingly, this valve, previously very popular, is not being used in the United States at present.

DURABILITY AND THROMBOGENICITY. Most of these mechanical prosthetic valves have an excellent record of durability—up to 30 years in the case of the caged-ball valves. However, patients with any mechanical prosthesis, regardless of design or site of placement, require long-term anticoagulation because of the hazard of thromboembolism, which is greatest in the first postoperative year. Without anticoagulation, the incidence of thromboembolism is three- to sixfold higher than with proper doses.[731] Anticoagulation with sodium warfarin should begin about 2 days after operation, and a prothrombin time in the range of 1.5 times control should be achieved. This relatively conservative approach reduces the risk of anticoagulant hemorrhage yet does not appear to be associated with a greater frequency of thromboembolism than a prothrombin time of 2.0 to 2.5 times control. It must be recognized that (1) the administration of warfarin carries its own mortality and morbidity, estimated at 0.2 and 2.2 per 100 patient-years, respectively; and (2) despite treatment with anticoagulants, the incidence of thromboembolic complications with the best mechanical prostheses is still about 0.2 (fatal) and 1 to 2 (nonfatal) per 100 patient-years. This incidence tends to be slightly higher for prostheses in the mitral than in the aortic position; thrombosis of mechanical prostheses in the tricuspid position is quite high, and for this reason bioprostheses are preferred at this site. The incidence of embolization in patients who have experienced repeated emboli from a prosthetic valve despite anticoagulants may be reduced by replacement with a tissue valve.

TISSUE VALVES

Largely to overcome the risk of thromboembolism that is inherent in all mechanical prosthetic valves and the attendant hazards and inconvenience of permanent anticoagulant therapy just discussed, considerable effort has been devoted to the development of nonthrombogenic tissue valves.[732,733] The first of these to be widely used were chemically sterilized homografts. These exhibited a high incidence of breakdown within 3 years. Fresh antibiotic-treated cryopreserved frozen-irradiated homografts were then developed. These are more durable[734-737]; while they have many desirable properties, their use has been restricted by the problems inherent in their procurement.

PORCINE HETEROGRAFTS. To overcome this difficulty, porcine heterografts were developed and have been used clinically since 1965. Two porcine heterografts are widely used today[725,726,738-742]: (1) The *Hancock* valve is fixed with 0.2 per cent glutaraldehyde and is mounted on a Dacron cloth–covered flexible polypropylene strut. In the smaller aortic models, the right coronary cusp is replaced by a posterior cusp from another valve to reduce obstruction resulting from the septal shelf of the valve. (2) The *Carpentier-Edwards* valve[738] (Fig. 34–47*G*) is pressure-fixed with 0.625 per cent glutaraldehyde and is mounted on a Teflon-covered Eljiloy strut in a manner as to minimize the septal shelf. The hemodynamic profiles of the porcine heterografts are similar to those of comparably sized low-profile mechanical prostheses.[743,744] In contrast to the latter, however, the valve orifice is blood flow–dependent, with greater orifice size as transvalvular flow increases. The Hancock valve has been reported to have slightly better hemodynamics than the Carpentier-Edwards valve.[734,735]

During the first 3 postoperative months, while the sewing ring becomes endothelialized, the thromboembolic rate is high enough that anticoagulation is extremely desirable. Thereafter, anticoagulants are not required for porcine valves in the aortic position, and the thromboembolic rate is approxi-

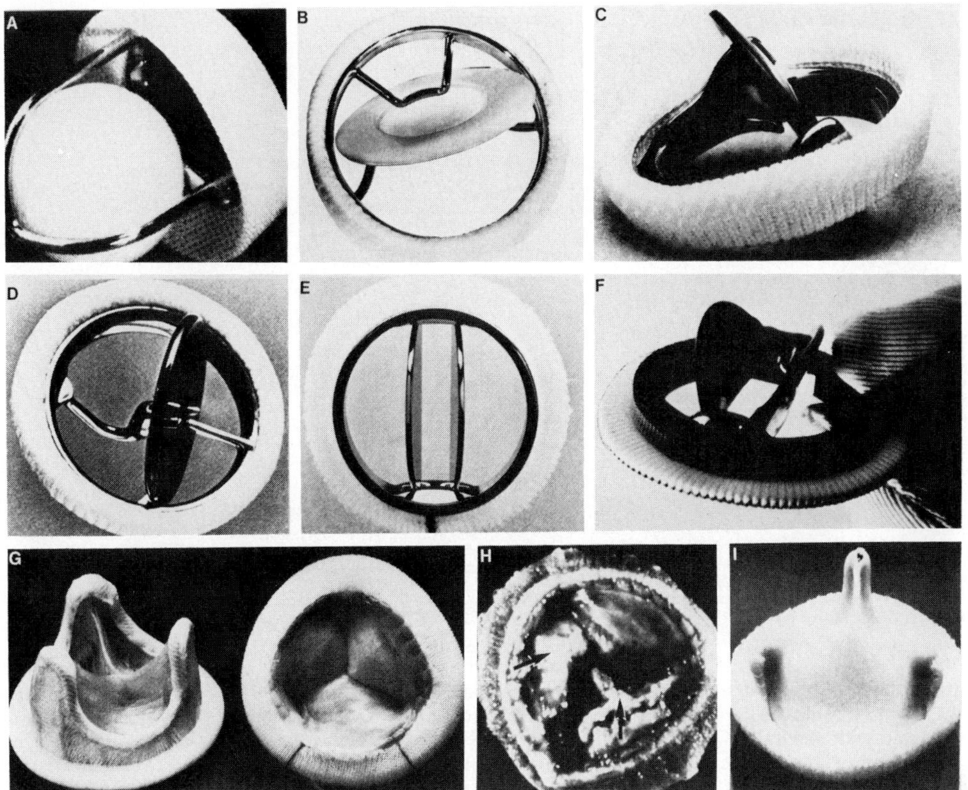

FIGURE 34–47. Prosthetic cardiac valves. *A*, Starr-Edwards caged-ball valve with cloth sewing ring and bare struts. *B*, Björk-Shiley tilting disc valve. *C*, Omniscience tilting disc valve. *D*, Medtronic-Hall tilting disc valve. *E*, St. Jude medical bileaflet valve as viewed end on. Note the large size of the effective orifice area compared with the potential orifice area and the minimal obstruction to flow by the leaflets. *F*, Duromedics bileaflet valve. *G*, Carpentier-Edwards prosthetic valve. *H*, Porcine valve removed several years following implantation because of primary valve failure; arrows point to areas of calcification and destruction of leaflets. *I*, Ionescu-Shiley pericardial valve. (*A* from Starek, P.J.K., and *F* from Clark, R. E., *in* Heart Valve Replacement and Reconstruction. Chicago, Year Book Medical Publishers, 1987, pp. 223 and 286. *B* from Björk, V.; C from Austin, E. H., III.; *E* and *I* from Crawford, F. A., Jr.; *G* and *H* from Magilligan, D. J., Jr., *in* Crawford, F. A. [ed.]: Cardiac Surgery: Current Heart Valve Prostheses, Vol. 1. Philadelphia, Hanley and Belfus, 1987, pp. 184, 204, 252, 270, 271, and 286. *D* from Cobanoglu, A., and Brockman, S. K., *in* Frankl, W. S., and Brest, A. N. [eds.]: Valvular Heart Disease: Comprehensive Evaluation and Management. Philadelphia, F. A. Davis, 1986, p. 404.)

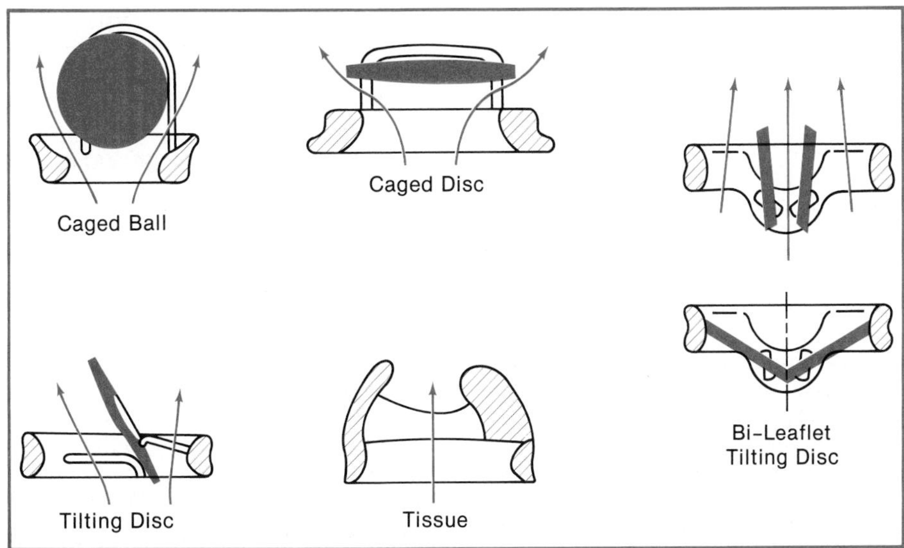

FIGURE 34–48. Designs and flow patterns of major categories of prosthetic heart valves: caged-ball, caged-disc, tilting-disc, bi-leaflet tilting-disc, and bioprosthetic (tissue) valves. While flow in mechanical valves must course along both sides of the occluder, bioprostheses have a central flow pattern. (Reproduced by permission from Schoen, F. J., et al.: Bioengineering aspects of heart valve replacement. Ann. Biomed. Eng. *10*:97, 1982. Copyright 1983, Pergamon Press Limited, 1983; and from Schoen, F. J.: Pathology of cardiac valve replacement. *In* Morse, D., Steiner, R. M., Fernandez, J. [eds.]: Guide to Prosthetic Cardiac Valves, p. 209. New York, Springer-Verlag, 1985. Copyright Springer-Verlag, Inc., 1985.)

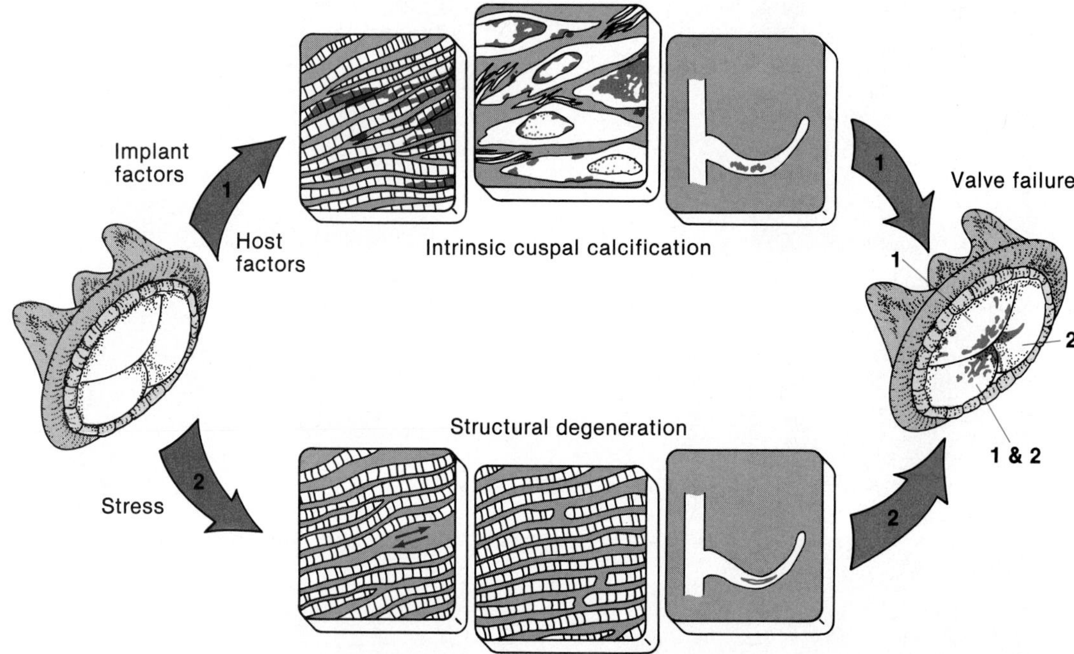

FIGURE 34–49. Unified model for bioprosthetic heart valve failure relating isolated tissue processes of mineralization (Pathway 1) and collagen degeneration (Pathway 2) to gross clinical failures. Such failures have calcification with cuspal stiffening (1), cuspal defects without calcific deposits (2), or cuspal tears associated with mineralization (1 and 2). These processes may occur independently or they may be synergistic. Specifically, implant and host factors interact to induce the collagen-oriented and cell-oriented calcific deposits noted ultrastructurally. The deposits predominate in the central portions of valve cusps, particularly at flexion points such as the commissures (Pathway 1). Stress causes shear between and fracture of collagen fibers, which may create gross cuspal defects (Pathway 2). Although dynamic mechanical activity is not a prerequisite for calcification, stress may promote (i.e., accelerate) this process through unknown mechanisms. (Amended from Schoen, F. J., and Levy, R. J.: Bioprosthetic heart valve failure: Pathology and pathogenesis. Cardiol. Clin. *2*:717, 1984.)

mately 1 to 2 episodes per 100 patient-years without these drugs.[733,739,742] When these valves have been placed in the mitral position in patients who are in sinus rhythm, anticoagulants are not needed (after the first 3 postoperative months), and the thromboembolic rate is also approximately 1 to 2 per 100 patient-years. This is comparable to that in patients with the St. Jude or other mechanical valves receiving anticoagulants and therefore subject to the risks of thrombosis. In patients undergoing mitral valve replacement who have experienced a previous embolus, in whom thrombus is found in the left atrium at operation or who remain in atrial fibrillation postoperatively (approximately one-third of all patients receiving mitral valve replacements), the hazard of thromboembolism persists. Indeed, in patients with atrial fibrillation the incidence of postoperative emboli following implantation of a porcine bioprosthesis into the mitral position is three times as high as in patients in sinus rhythm. Therefore, anticoagulants are required in those patients with these risk factors. This negates the principal advantage of the tissue valves. It is unlikely that any replacement of the mitral valve can be associated with a thromboembolic rate much below 0.5 per 100 patient-years, since some of the emboli in patients with longstanding mitral disease are derived from the left atrium rather than from the valve itself.[745]

The major problem with porcine bioprostheses is their limited durability (Fig. 34–49). Cuspal tears, degeneration, fibrin deposition, disruption of the fibrocollagenous structure, perforation, fibrosis, and calcification sufficiently severe to require reoperation (Fig. 34–47*H*) begin to appear in the fourth or fifth postoperative year, so that by 10 years the rate of primary tissue failure is approximately 20 per cent. It then accelerates,[733] and in one report in which a 15-year follow-up is described[734] the actuarial freedom from bioprosthetic primary tissue failure was only 45 per cent for valves in the mitral and 50 per cent for valves in the aortic position. It is likely that with the passage of time even more of these valves will fail, and essentially all valves implanted into patients aged less than 60 years will have to be replaced.[746] Fortunately, however, these valves usually do not fail suddenly (as is usually the case for failure of mechanical prostheses), and the second operation can often be carried out on an elective basis, with a surgical mortality in the range of 10 to 15 per cent.[742] Color Doppler echocardiography with two-dimensional transthoracic[743,744] or transesophageal imaging is extremely helpful in the early detection of bioprosthetic malfunction. The time after implantation at which tissue valves fail varies inversely with age; it is prohibitively rapid in children and young adults. Valve degeneration is extremely rare in patients older than 70 years at the time of implantation.[733,739] Bioprostheses also have extremely limited durability in patients with chronic renal failure and hypercalcemia related to secondary hyperparathyroidism.

PERICARDIAL XENOGRAFT. A second major type of bioprosthetic valve is the *Ionescu-Shiley pericardial xenograft* (Fig. 34–47*I*),[747,748] which consists of glutaraldehyde-treated bovine pericardium from which three leaflets are mounted on a Dacron velour–covered titanium frame. This valve has an unacceptable rate of failure[747,748] and therefore is no longer widely used.

HEMODYNAMICS OF VALVE REPLACEMENTS

All valve replacements—mechanical prostheses as well as tissue valves—have an effective in vitro orifice size that is *smaller* than the normal valve at the same site.[732,733,749] After implantation, tissue ingrowth and endothelialization reduce the size of the in vivo effective orifice further. Therefore, all prosthetic valves currently available must be considered to be mildly stenotic. However, postoperative hemodynamic measurements of the rigid prostheses show reasonably good function, with effective mitral valve orifice areas averaging 1.7 to 2.0 cm^2 and mitral valve gradients of 4 to 8 mm Hg at rest. Although definitive comparisons have not been carried out, the cloth-covered Starr-Edwards valve appears to be intrinsically slightly more stenotic than the tilting-disc valves. The St. Jude valve, in turn, may be slightly superior to the latter. In hemodynamic studies, the porcine mitral valves behave in a manner similar to that of an artificial prosthetic valve of the same diameter.[645a,650a] Serious hemodynamic obstruction of an artificial valve in the mitral position is quite uncommon, unless the valve is placed in a small left ventricular cavity or an unusually small mitral annulus or unless the prosthesis chosen is inappropriate in size.

The problem of intrinsic stenosis may be more serious in patients who undergo aortic valve replacements for AS. The annulus into which the prosthesis is inserted in these patients is usually smaller than it is in patients with AR, and the surgeon may be forced to select an artificial valve of relatively small size. As a consequence, aortic valve replacement may not abolish obstruction in AS but may merely convert severe obstruction to a mild or moderate type. When the smaller models of the porcine xenograft or mechanical prosthesis are placed into the aortic position, effective orifice areas of about 1.1 to 1.3 cm^2 are common. In such patients, peak transvalvular gradients as high as 40 mm Hg during exercise have been recorded. It is possible that the poor late results observed in a minority of patients undergoing replacement of stenotic aortic valves may be the delayed effects of moderate stenosis of the prosthesis. In patients with AS who do not exhibit clinical improvement postoperatively, it is important to evaluate the function of both the prosthetic valve and the left ventricle. Rarely, reoperation to correct a malfunctioning prosthesis may be necessary.

SELECTION OF AN ARTIFICIAL VALVE

Most comparisons of mechanical and bioprostheses indicate similar overall results, in terms of early and late mortality, prosthetic valve endocarditis and other complications, and the need for reoperation, at least for the first 5 years postoperatively. As indicated, there appear to be no significant differences insofar as hemodynamics are concerned, except that in patients with an unusually small left ventricular cavity or mitral or aortic annulus, the low-profile (tilting-disc) St. Jude or Edwards-Duromedics prosthesis or a tissue valve may perform better than other valves.[749–751]

The major task in selection of an artificial valve is to weigh the advantage of durability and the disadvantage of the risk of thromboembolism and of anticoagulant treatment inherent in mechanical prostheses on the one hand with the advantages of low thrombogenicity and the serious disadvantage of abbreviated durability of the bioprostheses on the other. Tissue valves are preferred over mechanical prostheses in patients in whom anticoagulation is difficult to control or in whom it is especially hazardous because they are prone to hemorrhage or are noncompliant. Because of the problems with the long-term durability of bioprostheses, I believe that a mechanical prosthetic valve should be employed in patients under the age of approximately 65 to 70 years who do not have any of the aforementioned contraindications to anticoagulants.[752] Thus, the following groups of patients should receive bioprostheses: (1) those with coexisting disease who are prone to hemorrhage; (2) those who are noncompliant insofar as permanent anticoagulant treatment is concerned, (3) those who are unwilling to take anticoagulants on a regular basis; and (4) those over the age of 65 to 70 years, in whom bioprosthetic valves deteriorate very slowly and who by reason of their age may be at greater risk of hemorrhage while taking anticoagulants.

Special Situations

Pregnancy (see also p. 1802). Women with artificial valves can tolerate the hemodynamic burden of pregnancy well, but the hypercoagulable state of pregnancy increases the risk of thromboembolism in such patients. Anticoagulation must not be interrupted, although an increased risk of fatal fetal hemorrhage is seen in those in whom it is continued. There is also a risk of fetal malformation caused by the probable teratogenic effect of warfarin. Although these problems represent arguments for the use of tissue valves in all women of childbearing age,[753–756] their limited durability in young adults makes their use unacceptable. Therefore, every effort should be made to defer valve replacement until after childbirth. In pregnant women with critical mitral or aortic stenosis, balloon valvuloplasty should be considered. Women of childbearing potential with a mechanical prosthesis should be counseled against pregnancy. When a woman in whom a mechanical prosthetic valve is already in place becomes pregnant, the risk to the fetus if the mother receives oral anticoagulants appears to be lower than the risk to the mother if anticoagulants are discontinued.[757] Therefore, coumarin derivatives should be continued until 2 weeks before expected delivery, when the patient should probably be given prophylactic heparin.[753,754,756] This approach appears to be safe for the mother but is associated with increased fetal wastage.

Noncardiac Surgery. When this is required in patients with prosthetic valves who are receiving anticoagulants, the risk is minimal when the drug regimen is stopped 1 to 3 days preoperatively and for a similar period postoperatively. It may be desirable, however, to protect the patient with low molecular weight dextran during the perioperative period.

Patients Who Are Destined to Receive Anticoagulants. Patients with earlier implantation of a mechanical prosthesis, chronic atrial fibrillation in the presence of an enlarged left atrium, a history of thromboembolism, or the presence of a thrombus in the left atrium at operation (and who therefore are destined to receive anticoagulants) should receive a mechanical prosthesis because the potential advantage of a tissue valve is negated.

Children and Patients Receiving Chronic Hemodialysis. The high incidence of bioprosthetic valve failure in children and adolescents[752,758–760] and in patients on chronic hemodialysis virtually prohibits their use in these groups. In young adults between the ages of 25 and 35, the failure of bioprosthetic valves is somewhat higher than it is in older adults; this serves as a relative, but not an absolute, contraindication to their use in this age group.

In children, a mechanical prosthesis (generally the St. Jude valve) with its favorable hemodynamics is preferred despite the disadvantages inherent in anticoagulants in this age group.[761] Similarly, mechanical prostheses should be used in patients with chronic renal failure and/or hypercalcemia.

Tricuspid Position. The risk of thrombosis for all valves is highest in the tricuspid position because of the lower pressures and velocity of blood flow; this complication appears to be highest for tilting-disc valves, intermediate for caged-ball valves, and lowest for the bioprostheses, which are the valves of choice as tricuspid replacements. In the tricuspid position bioprostheses exhibit a much slower rate of mechanical deterioration than in the mitral or aortic position.

DETECTION OF PROSTHETIC VALVE DYSFUNCTION. Artificial valves have distinctive auscultatory and phonocardiographic characteristics.[762] Transthoracic and transesophageal echocardiography, phonocardiography, and cineradiography are extremely useful in the identification of artificial valve dysfunction.[762–765] Two-dimensional and Doppler echocardiography are particularly useful in the follow-up of patients who demonstrate clinical deterioration in the postoperative period following porcine heterograft implantation. These techniques may prove capable of distinguishing between failure of a bioprosthesis (abnormal valve motion) and left ventricular dysfunction.

REFERENCES

MITRAL STENOSIS

1. Kinare, S. G., and Kulkarni, H. L.: Quantitative study of the mitral valve in chronic rheumatic heart disease. Int. J. Cardiol. 16:271, 1987.
2. Olson, L. J., Subramanian, R., and Ackermann, D. M.: Surgical pathology of the mitral valve: A study of 712 cases spanning 21 years. Mayo Clin. Proc. 62:22, 1987.
3. Ruckman, R. N., and Van Praagh, R.: Anatomic types of congenital mitral stenosis: Report of 49 autopsy cases with consideration of diagnostic and surgical implications. Am. J. Cardiol. 42:592, 1978.
4. Bortolotti, U., Valente, M., Agozzino, L., et al.: Rheumatoid mitral stenosis requiring valve replacement. Am. Heart J. 107:1049, 1984.
5. Johnson, G. L., Vine, D. L., Cottrill, C. M., and Noonan, J. A.: Echocardiographic mitral valve deformity in the mucopolysaccharidoses. Pediatrics 67:401, 1981.
6. Ladefoged, C., and Rohr, N.: Amyloid deposits in aortic and mitral valves. Virchows Arch. (A) 404:301, 1984.
7. Misch, K. A.: Development of heart valve lesions during methysergide therapy. Br. Med. J. 2:365, 1974.
8. Matagliati, A., Pepi, M., and Fiorentini, C.: Doppler and echocardio-

136. Davies, M. J.: Aetiology and pathology of the diseased mitral valve. *In* Ionescu, M. I., and Cohn, L. H. (eds.): Mitral Valve Disease: Diagnosis and Treatment. London, Butterworths, 1985, pp. 27–42.
137. Dajee, H., Hurley, E. J., and Szarnicki, R. J.: Cardiac valve replacement in systemic lupus erythematosus. A review. J. Thorac. Cardiovasc. Surg. *85*:718, 1983.
138. Marcus, R. H., Sareli, P., Pocock, W. A., et al.: Functional anatomy of severe mitral regurgitation in active rheumatic carditis. Am. J. Cardiol. *63*:577, 1989.
139. Boltwood, C. M., Tei, C., Wong, M., and Shah, P. M.: Quantitative echocardiography of the mitral complex in dilated cardiomyopathy: The mechanism of functional mitral regurgitation. Circulation *68*:498, 1983.
140. Keren, G., Sonnenblick, E. H., and LeJemtel, T. H.: Mitral annulus motion: Relation to pulmonary venous and transmitral flows in normal subjects and in patients with dilated cardiomyopathy. Circulation *78*:621, 1988.
141. Bloor, C. M.: Valvular heart disease in the elderly. J. Am. Geriatr. Soc. *30*:466, 1982.
142. Nestico, P. F., DePace, N. L., Kotler, M. N., et al.: Calcium phosphorus metabolism in dialysis patients with and without mitral anular calcium. Analysis of 30 patients. Am. J. Cardiol. *51*:497, 1983.
143. Ritschard, T., Blumberg, A., and Jenzer, H. R.: Mitralanulusverkalkungen bei Dialyse-Patienten. Schweiz. Med. Wschr. *117*:1363, 1987.
144. Zanolla, L., Marino, P., Nicolosi, G. L., et al.: Two-dimensional echocardiographic evaluation of mitral valve calcification. Sensitivity and specificity. Chest *82*:154, 1982.
145. Mellino, M., Salcedo, E. E., Lever, H. M., et al.: Echographic-quantified severity of mitral annulus calcification: Prognostic correlation to related hemodynamic, valvular, rhythm, and conduction abnormalities. Am. Heart J. *103*:222, 1982.
146. Labovitz, A. J., Nelson, J. G., Windhorst, D. M., et al.: Frequency of mitral valve dysfunction from mitral annular calcium as detected by Doppler echocardiography. Am. J. Cardiol. *55*:133, 1985.
147. Kaul, S., Pearlman, J. D., Touchstone, D. A., and Esquival, L.: Prevalence and mechanisms of mitral regurgitation in the absence of intrinsic abnormalities of the mitral leaflets. Am. Heart J. *118*:963, 1989.
148. Takamoto, T., and Popp, R. L.: Conduction disturbances related to the site and severity of mitral anular calcification: A two-dimensional echocardiographic and electrocardiographic correlative study. Am. J. Cardiol. *51*:1644, 1983.
149. Scott-Jupp, W., Barnett, N. L., Gallagher, P. J., et al.: Ultrastructural changes in spontaneous rupture of mitral chordae tendineae. J. Pathol. *133*:185, 1981.
150. Oliveira, D. B. G., Dawkins, K. D., Kay, P. H., and Paneth, M.: Chordal rupture I: Aetiology and natural history. Br. Heart J. *50*:312, 1983.
151. Oliveira, D. B. G., Dawkins, K. D., Kay, P. H., and Paneth, M.: Chordal rupture II: Comparison between repair and replacement. Br. Heart J. *50*:318, 1983.
152. Hickey, A. J., Wilcken, D. E. L., Wright, J. S., and Warren, B. A.: Primary (spontaneous) chordal rupture: Relation to myxomatous valve disease and mitral valve prolapse. J. Am. Coll. Cardiol. *5*:1341, 1985.
153. Godley, R. W., Wann, L. S., Rogers, E. W., et al.: Incomplete mitral leaflet closure in patients with papillary muscle dysfunction. Circulation *63*:565, 1981.
154. Gallagher, P. J., Caves, P. K., and Stinson, E. B.: Pathological changes in spontaneous rupture of chordae tendineae. Ann. Cir. Gynaecol. *66*:135, 1977.
155. Burch, G. E., DePasquale, N. P., and Phillips, J. H.: The syndrome of papillary muscle dysfunction. Am. Heart J. *75*:399, 1968.
156. Izumi, S., Miyatake, K., Beppu, S., et al.: Mechanism of mitral regurgitation in patients with myocardial infarction: A study using real-time two-dimensional Doppler flow imaging and echocardiography. Circulation *76*:777, 1987.
157. Hickey, M. St.J., Smith, L. R., Muhlbaier, L. H., et al.: Current prognosis of ischemic mitral regurgitation: Implications for future management. Circulation *78*(Suppl. I):I51, 1988.
158. Ballester, M., Jajoo, J., Rees, S., et al.: The mechanism of mitral regurgitation in dilated left ventricle. Clin. Cardiol. *6*:333, 1983.
159. Becker, A. E., and Anderson, R. H.: Mitral insufficiency complicating acute myocardial infarction. Eur. J. Cardiol. *2*:351, 1975.
160. Morrow, A. G., Cohen, L. S., Roberts, W. C., et al.: Severe mitral regurgitation following acute myocardial infarction and ruptured papillary muscle. Hemodynamic findings and results of operative treatment in four patients. Circulation *37*(Suppl. II):124, 1968.
161. Balu, V., Hershowitz, S., Masud, A. R. Z., et al.: Mitral regurgitation in coronary artery disease. Chest *81*:550, 1982.
162. Gottdiener, J. S., Maron, B. J., Schooley, R. T., et al.: Two-dimensional echocardiographic assessment of the idiopathic hypereosinophilic syndrome. Anatomic basis of mitral regurgitation and peripheral embolization. Circulation *67*:572, 1983.
163. Metras, D., Ouezzin-Coulibaly, A., Ouattara, K., et al.: Endomyocardial fibrosis masquerading as rheumatic mitral incompetence. A report of six surgical cases. J. Thorac. Cardiovasc. Surg. *86*:753, 1983.
164. Mazzucco, A., Rizzoli, G., Faggian, G., et al.: Acute mitral regurgitation after blunt chest trauma. Arch. Intern. Med. *143*:2326, 1983.
165. Jolly, D. T.: Traumatic rupture of a papillary muscle of the mitral valve due to blunt thoracic trauma. Can. Fam. Phys. *29*:1960, 1983.
166. Gidding, S. S., Shulman, S. T., Ibawi, M., et al.: Mucocutaneous lymph node syndrome (Kawasaki disease): Delayed aortic and mitral insufficiency secondary to active valvulitis. J. Am. Coll. Cardiol. *7*:894, 1986.
167. DiSegni, E., and Edwards, J. E.: Cleft anterior leaflet of the mitral valve with intact septa. A study of 20 cases. Am. J. Cardiol. *51*:919, 1983.
168. Nagata, S., Nimura, Y., Sakakibara, H., et al.: Mitral valve lesion associated with secundum atrial septal defect. Analysis of real-time two-dimensional echocardiography. Br. Heart J. *49*:151, 1983.
169. Eckberg, D. L., Gault, J. H., Bouchard, R. L., et al.: Mechanics of left ventricular contraction in chronic severe mitral regurgitation. Circulation *47*:1252, 1973.
170. Braunwald, E., Welch, G. H., Jr., and Sarnoff, S. J.: Hemodynamic effects of quantitatively varied experimental mitral regurgitation. Circ. Res. *5*:539, 1957.
171. Pierpont, G. L., and Talley, R. C.: Pathophysiology of valvar heart disease. Arch. Intern. Med. *142*:998, 1982.
172. Spratt, J. A., Olsen, C. O., Tyson, G. S., Jr., et al.: Experimental mitral regurgitation. Physiological effects of correction on left ventricular dynamics. J. Thorac. Cardiovasc. Surg. *86*:479, 1983.
173. Braunwald, E., and Turi, Z. G.: Pathophysiology of mitral valve disease. *In* Ionescu, M. I., and Cohn, L. H. (eds.): Mitral Valve Disease: Diagnosis and Treatment. London, Butterworths, 1985, pp. 3–10.
174. Yellin, E. L., Yoran, C., Frater, R. W. M., and Sonnenblick, E. H.: Dynamics of acute experimental mitral regurgitation. *In* Ionescu, M. I., and Cohn, L. H. (eds.): Mitral Valve Disease: Diagnosis and Treatment. London, Butterworths, 1985, pp. 11–26.
175. Urschel, C. W., Covell, J. W., Sonnenblick, E. H., et al.: Myocardial mechanics in aortic and mitral valvular regurgitation: The concept of instantaneous impedance as a determinant of the performance of the intact heart. J. Clin. Invest. *47*:867, 1968.
176. Braunwald, E.: Mitral regurgitation: Physiological, clinical and surgical considerations. N. Engl. J. Med. *281*:425, 1969.
177. Corin, W. J., Monrad, E. S., Murakami, T., et al.: The relationship of afterload to ejection performance in chronic mitral regurgitation. Circulation *76*:59, 1987.
178. Nwasokwa, O., Camesas, A., Weg, I., and Bodenheimer, M. M.: Differences in left ventricular adaptation to chronic mitral and aortic regurgitation. Chest *95*:106, 1989.
179. Katayama, K., Tajimi, T., Guth, B. D., et al.: Early diastolic filling dynamics during experimental mitral regurgitation in the conscious dog. Circulation *78*:390, 1988.
180. Knotos, G. J., Jr., Schaff, H. V., Gersh, B. J., and Bove, A. A.: Left ventricular function in subacute and chronic mitral regurgitation: Effect on function early postoperatively. J. Thorac. Cardiovasc. Surg. *98*:163, 1989.
181. Keren, G., Katz, S., Strom, J., et al.: Dynamic mitral regurgitation: An important determinant of the hemodynamic response to load alterations and inotropic therapy in severe heart failure. Circulation *80*:306, 1989.
182. Urschel, C. W., Covell, J. W., Graham, T. P., et al.: Effects of acute valvular regurgitation on the oxygen consumption of the canine heart. Circ. Res. *23*:33, 1968.
183. Braunwald, E.: Control of myocardial oxygen consumption: Physiologic and clinical considerations. Am. J. Cardiol. *27*:416, 1971.
183a. Corin, W. J., Murakami, T., Monrad, E. S., et al.: Left ventricular passive diastolic properties in chronic mitral regurgitation. Circulation *83*:797, 1991.
184. Ross, J., Jr.: Left ventricular function and the timing of surgical treatment in valvular heart disease. Ann. Intern. Med. *94*:498, 1981.
185. Mirsky, I., Corin, W. J., Murakami, T., et al.: Correction for preload in assessment of myocardial contractility in aortic and mitral valve disease: Application of the concept of systolic myocardial stiffness. Circulation *78*:68, 1988.
186. Wisenbach, T.: Does normal pump function belie muscle dysfunction in patients with chronic severe mitral regurgitation? Circulation *77*:515 1988.
187. Osbakken, M. D., Bove, A. A., and Spann, J. F.: Left ventricular regional wall motion and velocity of shortening in chronic mitral and aortic regurgitation. Am. J. Cardiol. *47*:1055, 1981.
188. Ramanthan, K. B., Knowles, J., Connor, M. J., et al.: Natural history of chronic mitral insufficiency: Relation of peak systolic pressure/end-systolic volume ratio to morbidity and mortality. J. Am. Coll. Cardiol. *3*:1412, 1984.
189. Wisenbaugh, T., Spann, J. F., and Carabello, B. A.: Differences in myocardial performance and load between patients with similar amounts of chronic aortic versus chronic mitral regurgitation. J. Am. Coll. Cardiol. *3*:913, 1984.
190. Crawford, M. H., Souchek, J., Oprian, C. A., et al.: Determinants of survival and left ventricular performance after mitral valve replacement. Circulation *81*:1173, 1990.
191. Borow, K., Green, L. H., Mann, T., et al.: End-systolic volume as a predictor of postoperative left ventricular performance in volume overload from valvular regurgitation. Am. J. Med. *68*:655, 1980.
192. Boucher, C. A., Bingham, J. B., Osbakken, M. D., et al.: Early changes in left ventricular size and function after correction of left ventricular volume overload. Am. J. Cardiol. *47*:991, 1981.
193. Kihara, Y., Sasayama, S., Miyazaki, S., et al.: Role of the left atrium in adaptation of the heart to chronic mitral regurgitation in conscious dogs. Circ. Res. *62*:543, 1988.
194. Grose, R., Strain, J., and Cohen, M. V.: Pulmonary arterial V waves in mitral regurgitation. Clinical and experimental observations. Circulation *69*:214, 1984.
195. Braunwald, E., and Awe, W. C.: The syndrome of severe mitral regurgitation with normal left atrial pressure. Circulation *27*:29, 1963.
196. Roberts, W. C., Braunwald, E., and Morrow, A. G.: Acute severe mitral

regurgitation secondary to ruptured chordae tendineae. Clinical, hemodynamic and pathologic considerations. Circulation *33*:58, 1966.
197. Cohen, L. S., Mason, D. T., and Braunwald, E.: Significance of an atrial gallop sound in mitral regurgitation: A clue to the diagnosis of ruptured chordae tendineae. Circulation *35*:112, 1966.
198. Gorlin, R.: Natural history, medical therapy and indications for surgery in mitral valve disease. *In* Ionescu, M. I., and Cohen, L. H. (eds.): Mitral Valve Disease: Diagnosis and Treatment. London, Butterworths, 1985, pp. 105–126.
199. Kusiak, V., and Brest, A. N.: Acute mitral regurgitation: Pathophysiology and management. *In* Frankl, W. S., and Brest, A. N. (eds.): Cardiovascular Clinics. Valvular Heart Disease: Comprehensive Evaluation and Management. Philadelphia, F. A. Davis, 1986, pp. 257–280.
200. Rippe, J. M., and Howe, J. P., III: Acute mitral regurgitation. *In* Dalen, J. E., and Alpert, J. S. (eds.): Valvular Heart Disease. 2nd ed. Boston, Little, Brown and Company, 1987, pp. 151–176.
201. Elkins, R. C., Morrow, A. G., Vasko, J. S., and Braunwald, E.: The effects of mitral regurgitation on the pattern of instantaneous aortic blood flow. Clinical and experimental observations. Circulation *36*:45, 1967.
202. Basta, L. L., Wolfson, P., Eckberg, D. L., and Abboud, F. M.: The value of left parasternal impulse recordings in the assessment of mitral regurgitation. Circulation *48*:1055, 1973.
203. Barlow, J. B.: Mitral regurgitation. *In* Perspectives on the Mitral Valve. Philadelphia, F. A. Davis, 1987, pp. 113–131.
204. Haffajee, C. I.: Chronic mitral regurgitation. *In* Dalen, J. E., and Alpert, J. S. (eds.): Valvular Heart Disease. 2nd ed. Boston, Little, Brown and Company, 1987, pp. 111–150.
205. Karliner, J. S., O'Rourke, R. A., Kearney, D. J., and Shabetai, R.: Haemodynamic explanation of why the murmur of mitral regurgitation is independent of cycle length. Br. Heart J. *35*:397, 1973.
206. Schreiber, T. L., Fisher, J., Mangla, A., and Miller, D.: Severe "silent" mitral regurgitation: A potentially reversible cause of refractory heart failure. Chest *96*:242, 1989.
207. Antman, E. M., Angoff, G. H., and Sloss, J. J.: Demonstration of the mechanism by which mitral regurgitation mimics aortic stenosis. Am. J. Cardiol. *42*:1044, 1978.
208. Merendino, K. A., and Hessel, E. A.: The murmur on top of the head in acquired mitral insufficiency. J.A.M.A. *199*:392, 1967.
209. Morris, J. J., Estes, E. H., Whalen, R. E., et al.: P wave analysis in valvular heart disease. Circulation *29*:242, 1964.
210. Priest, E. A., Finlayson, J. K., and Short, D. S.: The x-ray manifestations in the heart and lungs of mitral regurgitation. Prog. Cardiovasc. Dis. *5*:219, 1962.
211. Wexler, L., Silverman, J. F., DeBusk, R. F., and Harrison, D. C.: Angiographic features of rheumatic and nonrheumatic mitral regurgitation. Circulation *44*:1080, 1971.
212. Pizzarello, R. A., Turnier, J., Goldman, M. A., et al.: Clinical and echocardiographic features of isolated severe pure mitral regurgitation. Clin. Cardiol. *7*:565, 1984.
213. Sweatman, T., Selzer, A., Kamageki, M., and Cohn, K.: Echocardiographic diagnosis of mitral regurgitation due to ruptured chordae tendineae. Circulation *46*:580, 1972.
213a. Himelman, R. B., Kusumoto, F., Oken, K., et al.: The flail mitral valve: Echocardiographic findings by precordial and transesophageal imaging and Doppler color flow mapping. J. Am. Coll. Cardiol. *17*:272, 1991.
214. Nair, C. K., Aronow, W. S., Sketch, M. H., et al.: Clinical and echocardiographic characteristics of patients with mitral annular calcification. Am. J. Cardiol. *51*:992, 1983.
215. Helmcke, F., Nanda, N. C., Hsiung, M. C., et al.: Color doppler assessment of mitral regurgitation with orthogonal planes. Circulation *75*:175, 1987.
216. Cujec, B., David, T., Wilansky, S., and Pollick, C.: Color flow imaging in severe mitral and aortic regurgitation. Can. J. Cardiol. *4*:341, 1988.
217. Jenni, R., Ritter, M., Eberli, F., et al.: Quantification of mitral regurgitation with amplitude-weighted mean velocity from continuous wave Doppler spectra. Circulation *79*:1294, 1989.
218. Thompson, R., Ross, I., and Elmes, R.: Quantification of valvular regurgitation by cardiac gated pool imaging. Br. Heart J. *46*:629, 1981.
219. Boucher, C. A., Okada, R. D., and Pohost, G. M.: Current status of radionuclide imaging in valvular heart disease. Am. J. Cardiol. *46*:1153, 1980.
220. Chatterjee, K.: Vasodilator therapy for mitral regurgitation. *In* Duran, C., Angell, W. W., Johnson, A. D., and Oury, J. H. (eds.): Recent Progress in Mitral Valve Disease. London, Butterworths, 1984, pp. 138–148.
221. Hoit, B. D.: Medical treatment of valvular heart disease. Curr. Opin. Cardiol. *6*:207, 1991.
222. Yoran, C., Yellin, E. L., Becker, R. M., et al.: Mechanism of reduction of mitral regurgitation with vasodilator therapy. Am. J. Cardiol. *43*:773, 1979.
222a. Cohn, L. H.: Valvular surgery. Curr. Opin. Cardiol. *6*:235, 1991.
223. Frater, R.W.M., Vetter, O., Zussa, C., and Dahm, M.: Chordal replacement in mitral valve repair. Circulation *82*(Suppl. IV):125, 1990.
224. Craver, J. M., Cohen, C., and Weintraub, W. S.: Case-matched comparison of mitral valve replacement and repair. Ann. Thorac. Surg. *49*:964, 1990.
225. Tandon, A. P., Silverton, N. P., and Ionescu, M. I.: Mitral valve repair (the Woller annuloplasty). *In* Ionescu, M. I., and Cohn, L. H. (eds.): Mitral Valve Disease: Diagnosis and Treatment. London, Butterworths, 1985, pp. 171–178.
226. Rahko, P. S., and Berkoff, H. A.: Echocardiographic comparison of cardiac size and function before and after surgery for isolated MR: superiority of mitral valve repair vs replacement. Acta Cardiol. *45*:189, 1990.
227. Duran, C. G., Revuelta, J. M., Gaite, L., et al.: Stability of mitral reconstructive surgery at 10–12 years for predominantly rheumatic valvular disease. Circulation *78*(Suppl. I):I91, 1988.
228. Kirklin, J. W.: Mitral valve repair for mitral incompetence. Mod. Concepts Cardiovasc. Dis. *56*:7, 1987.
229. Rankin, J. S., Feneley, M. P., Hickey, M. St.J., et al.: A clinical comparison of mitral valve repair versus valve replacement in ischemic mitral regurgitation. J. Thorac. Cardiovasc. Surg. *95*:165, 1988.
230. Carpentier, A.: Mitral reconstruction in predominant mitral incompetence. *In* Duran, C., Angell, W. W., Johnson, A. D., and Oury, J. H. (eds.): Recent Progress in Mitral Valve Disease. London, Butterworths, 1984, pp. 265–276.
231. Galloway, A. C., Colvin, S. B., Baumann, F. G., et al.: Current concepts of mitral valve reconstruction for mitral insufficiency. Circulation *78*:1087, 1988.
232. Cohn, L. H.: Surgery for mitral regurgitation. JAMA *260*:2883, 1988.
233. Sarris, G. E., Cahill, P. D., Hansen, D. E., et al.: Restoration of left ventricular systolic performance after reattachment of the mitral chordae tendineae. J. Thorac. Cardiovasc. Surg. *95*:969, 1988.
234. Stewart, W. J., Currie, P. J., Salcedo, E. E., et al.: Intraoperative Doppler color flow mapping for decision-making in valve repair for mitral regurgitation. Circulation *81*:556, 1990.
235. Pitarys, C. J., III, Forman, M. B., Panayiotou, H., and Hansen, D. E.: Long-term effects of excision of the mitral apparatus on global and regional ventricular function in humans. J. Am. Coll. Cardiol. *15*:557, 1990.
236. Shiavone, W. A., Cosgrove, D. M., Lever, H. M., et al.: Long-term follow-up of patients with left ventricular outflow tract obstruction after Carpentier ring mitral valvuloplasty. Circulation *78*(Suppl. I):60, 1988.
237. Björk, V. O., Henze, A., and Lindblom, D.: The current status of prosthetic valves in the mitral position. *In* Duran, C., Angell, W. W., Johnson, A. D., and Oury, J. H. (eds.): Recent Progress in Mitral Valve Disease. London, Butterworths, 1984, pp. 201–210.
238. Gore, J. M.: Prosthetic heart valves. *In* Dalen, J. E., and Alpert, J. S. (eds.): Valvular Heart Disease. 2nd ed. Boston, Little, Brown and Company, 1987, pp. 509–528.
239. Lee, S.J.K., and Bay, K. S.: Mortality risk factors associated with mitral valve replacement: A survival analysis of 10 year follow-up data. Can. J. Cardiol. *7*:11, 1991.
240. Phillips, H. R., Levine, F. H., Carter, J. E., et al.: Mitral valve replacement for isolated mitral regurgitation: Analysis of clinical course and late postoperative left ventricular ejection fraction. Am. J. Cardiol. *48*:647, 1981.
240a. Nakano, K., Swindle, M. M., Spinale, F., et al.: Depressed contractile function due to canine mitral regurgitation improves after correction of the volume overload. J. Clin. Invest. *87*:2153, 1991.
241. Huikuri, H.: Effect of mitral valve replacement on left ventricular function in mitral regurgitation. Br. Heart J. *49*:328, 1983.
242. Schneider, R. M., and Helfant, R. H.: Timing of surgery in chronic mitral and aortic regurgitation. *In* Frankl, W. S., and Brest, A. N. (eds.): Cardiovascular Clinics. Valvular Heart Disease: Comprehensive Evaluation and Management. Philadelphia, F. A. Davis, 1986, pp. 361–374.
243. Carabello, B. A., and Grossman, W.: Effects of acute and chronic mitral regurgitation on left ventricular mechanics and contractile muscle function. *In* Duran, C., Angell, W. W., Johnson, A. D., and Oury, J. H. (eds.): Recent Progress in Mitral Valve Disease. London, Butterworths, 1984, pp. 181–192.
244. Smith, D. R.: Clinical diagnosis and evaluation of mitral valve disease. *In* Ionescu, M. I., and Cohn, L. H. (eds.): Mitral Valve Disease: Diagnosis and Treatment. London, Butterworths, 1985, pp. 43–52.
245. Cosgrove, D. M.: Valve reconstruction versus valve replacement. *In* Crawford, F. A. (ed.): Cardiac Surgery: Current Heart Valve Prostheses, Vol. 1. Hanley and Belfus, Philadelphia, 1987, pp. 143–158.
246. Peterson, K. L.: The timing of surgical intervention in chronic mitral regurgitation. Cathet. Cardiovasc. Diag. *9*:433, 1983.
247. Peterson, K. L., and Tajimi, T.: The timing of surgical intervention in mitral regurgitation. *In* Duran, C., Angell, W. W., Johnson, A. D., and Oury, J. H. (eds.): Recent Progress in Mitral Valve Disease. London, Butterworths, 1984, pp. 171–180.
248. Bonchek, L. I.: Current status of cardiac valve replacement: Selection of a prosthesis and indications for operation. Am. Heart J. *101*:96, 1981.
249. Pinson, C. W., Cobanoglu, A., Metzdorff, M. T., et al.: Late surgical results for ischemic mitral regurgitation. Role of wall motion score and severity of regurgitation. J. Thorac. Cardiovasc. Surg. *88*:663, 1984.
250. Connolly, M. W., Gelbfish, J. S., Jacobowitz, I. J., et al.: Surgical results for mitral regurgitation from coronary artery disease. J. Thorac. Cardiovasc. Surg. *91*:379, 1986.
251. Fowler, N. O., and van der Bel-Kahn, J. M.: Indications for surgical replacement of the mitral valve. With particular reference to common and uncommon causes of mitral regurgitation. Am. J. Cardiol. *44*:148, 1979.
252. Cohn, L. H., Kowalker, W., Bhatia, S., et al.: Comparative morbidity of mitral valve repair versus replacement for mitral regurgitation with and without coronary artery disease. Ann. Thorac. Surg. *45*:284, 1988.

THE MITRAL VALVE PROLAPSE SYNDROME

253. Pocock, W. A.: Mitral leaflet billowing and prolapse. *In* Barlow, J. B. (ed.): Perspectives on the Mitral Valve. Philadelphia, F. A. Davis, 1987, pp. 45–112.
254. Perloff, J. K., Child, J. S., and Edwards, J. E.: New guidelines for the clinical diagnosis of mitral valve prolapse. Am. J. Cardiol. *57*:1124, 1986.

255. Krivokapich, J., Child, J. S., Dadourian, B. J., and Perloff, J. K.: Reassessment of echocardiographic criteria for diagnosis of mitral valve prolapse. Am. J. Cardiol. *61*:131, 1988.
256. Savage, D. D., Garrison, R. J., Devereux, R. B., et al.: Mitral valve prolapse in the general population. I. Epidemiologic features: The Framingham Study. Am. Heart J. *106*:571, 1983.
257. Fontana, M. E., Sparks, E. A., Boudoulas, H., and Wooley, C. F.: Mitral valve prolapse and the mitral valve prolapse syndrone. Curr. Prob. Cardiol. *XVI*:311–375, 1991.
258. Mitral valve prolapse. *In* Fowler, N. O.: Diagnosis of Heart Disease. New York, Springer-Verlag, 1991, pp. 171–180.
259. Procacci, P. M., Savran, S. V., Schreiter, S. L., and Bryson, A. L.: Prevalence of clinical mitral valve prolapse in 1,169 young women. N. Engl. J. Med. *294*:1086, 1976.
260. Markiewicz, W., Stoner, J., London, E., et al.: Mitral valve prolapse in one hundred presumably healthy young females. Circulation *53*:464, 1976.
261. Barlow, J. B., Pocock, W. A., Marchand, P., and Denny, M.: The significance of the late systolic murmurs. Am. Heart J. *66*:443, 1963.
262. Wann, L. S., Grove, J. R., Hess, T. R., et al.: Prevalence of mitral prolapse by two-dimensional echocardiography in healthy young women. Br. Heart J. *49*:334, 1983.
263. Marks, A. R., Choong, C. Y., Sanfilippo, A. J., et al.: Identification of high-risk and low-risk subgroups of patients with mitral valve prolapse. N. Engl. J. Med. *320*:1031, 1989.
264. Levine, R. A., Handschumacher, M. D., Sanfilippo, A. J., et al.: Three-dimensional echocardiographic reconstruction of the mitral valve, with implications for the diagnosis of mitral valve prolapse. Circulation *80*:589, 1989.
265. Ballester, M., Presbitero, P., Foale, R., et al.: Prolapse of the mitral valve in secundum atrial septal defect: A functional mechanism. Eur. Heart J. *4*:472, 1983.
266. Goldhaber, S. Z., Rubin, I. L., Brown, W., et al.: Valvular heart disease (aortic regurgitation and mitral valve prolapse) among institutionalized adults with Down's syndrome. Am. J. Cardiol. *57*:278, 1986.
267. Goldhaber, S. Z., Brown, W. D., and St. John Sutton, M. G.: High frequency of mitral valve prolapse and aortic regurgitation among asymptomatic adults with Down's syndrome. JAMA *258*:1793, 1987.
268. Noah, M. S., Sulimani, R. A., Famuyiwa, F. O., et al.: Prolapse of the mitral valve in hyperthyroid patients in Saudi Arabia. Int. J. Cardiol. *19*:217, 1988.
269. Froom, P., Margulis, T., Grenadier, E., et al.: Von Willebrand factor and mitral valve prolapse. Thromb. Haemost. *60*:230, 1988.
270. Margaliot, S. Z., Barzilay, J., Bar-David, M., et al.: Spontaneous pneumothorax and mitral valve prolapse. Chest *89*:93, 1986.
271. Jackson, A. C.: Neurologic disorders associated with mitral valve prolapse. Can. J. Neurol. Sci. *13*:15, 1986.
272. Streib, E. W., Meyers, D. G., and Sun, S. F.: Mitral valve prolapse in myotonic dystrophy. Muscle Nerve *8*:650, 1985.
273. Whittaker, P., Boughner, D. R., Perkins, D. G., and Canham, P. B.: Quantitative structural analysis of collagen in chordae tendineae and its relation to floppy mitral valves and proteoglycan infiltration. Br. Heart J. *57*:264, 1987.
274. Johnson, G. L., Humphries, L. L., Shirley, P. B., et al.: Mitral valve prolapse in patients with anorexia nervosa and bulimia. Arch. Intern. Med. *146*:1525, 1986.
275. Liberthson, R., Sheehan, D. V., King, M. E., and Weyman, A. E.: The prevalence of mitral valve prolapse in patients with panic disorders. Am. J. Psychiatry *143*:511, 1986.
276. Waite, P., and McCallum, C. A.: Mitral valve prolapse in craniofacial skeletal deformities. Oral Surg. Oral Med. Oral Pathol. *61*:15, 1986.
277. Sakuraba, H., Yanagawa, Y., Igarashi, T., et al.: Cardiovascular manifestations of Fabry's disease. Clin. Genet. *29*:276, 1986.
278. Comens, S. M., Alpert, M. A., Sharp, G. C., et al.: Frequency of mitral valve prolapse in systemic lupus erythematosus, progressive systemic sclerosis and mixed connective tissue disease. Am. J. Cardiol. *63*:59, 1989.
279. Chan, F. L., Chen, W. W., Wong, P.H.C., and Chow, J.S.F.: Skeletal abnormalities in mitral valve prolapse. Clin. Radiol. *34*:207, 1983.
280. Chen, W. W., Chan, F. L., Wong, P.H.C., and Chow, J.S.F.: Familial occurrence of mitral valve prolapse: Is this related to the straight back syndrome? Br. Heart J. *50*:97, 1983.
281. Kalter, S., Fuentes, F., and Price, E.: Mitral and tricuspid valve prolapse in a patient with mixed connective tissue disease. South. Med. J. *786*:794, 1983.
282. Lu-Li, S., Guang-Gen, C., and Ru-Lian, L.: Valve prolapse in Behçet's disease. Br. Heart J. *54*:100, 1985.
283. Olsen, E.G.J., and Al-Rufaie, H. K.: The floppy mitral valve. Study on pathogenesis. Br. Heart J. *44*:674, 1980.
284. Pyeritz, R. E., and Wappel, M. A.: Mitral valve dysfunction in the Marfan syndrome. Am. J. Med. *74*:797, 1983.
285. Davies, M. J., Moore, B. P., and Braimbridge, M. V.: The floppy mitral valve. Study of incidence, pathology and complications in surgical, necropsy and forensic material. Br. Heart J. *40*:368, 1978.
286. Jaffe, A. S., Geltman, E. M., Rodey, G. E., and Uitto, J.: Mitral valve prolapse: A consistent manifestation of Type IV Ehlers-Danlos syndrome. The pathogenetic role of the abnormal production of Type III collagen. Circulation *64*:121, 1981.
287. King, B. D., Clark, M. A., Baba, N., et al.: "Myxomatous" mitral valves: Collagen dissolution as the primary defect. Circulation *66*:288, 1982.
288. Hammer, D., Leier, C. V., Baba, N., et al.: Altered collagen composition in a prolapsing mitral valve with ruptured chordae tendineae. Am. J. Med. *67*:863, 1979.
289. Tomaru, T., Uchida, Y., Mohri, N., et al.: Postinflammatory mitral and aortic valve prolapse: A clinical and pathological study. Circulation *76*:68, 1987.
290. Stein, P. D., Wang, C.-H, Riddle, J. M., et al.: Scanning electron microscopy of operatively excised severely regurgitant floppy mitral valves. Am. J. Cardiol. *64*:392, 1989.
291. Baker, P. B., Bansal, G., Boudoulas, H., et al.: Floppy mitral valve chordae tendineae: Histopathologic alterations. Hum. Pathol. *19*:507, 1988.
292. Hickey, A. J., and Wilcken, D.E.L.: Age and the clinical profile of idiopathic mitral valve prolapse. Br. Heart J. *55*:582, 1986.
293. Malcolm, A. D.: Mitral valve prolapse associated with other disorders. Causal coincidence, common link, or fundamental genetic disturbance? Br. Heart J. *53*:353, 1985.
294. Pader, E.: The familial incidence of mitral valve prolapse. A report of three generations in one family. N.Y. State J. Med. *84*:395, 1984.
295. Wordsworth, P., Ogilvie, D., Akhras, F., et al.: Genetic segregation analysis of familial mitral valve prolapse shows no linkage to fibrillar collagen genes. Br. Heart J. *61*:300, 1989.
296. Cabeen, W. R., Jr., Reza, M. J., Kovick, R. B., and Stern, M. S.: Mitral valve prolapse and conduction defects in Ehlers-Danlos syndrome. Arch. Intern. Med. *137*:1227, 1977.
297. Lebwohl, M. G., Distefano, D., Prioleau, P. G., et al.: Pseudoxanthoma elasticum and mitral valve prolapse. N. Engl. J. Med. *307*:228, 1982.
298. Sanyal, S. K., Johnson, W. W., Dische, M. R., et al.: Dystrophic degeneration of papillary muscle and ventricular myocardium. A basic for mitral valve prolapse in Duchenne's muscular dystrophy. Circulation *62*:430, 1980.
299. Mason, J. W., Koch, F. H., Billingham, M. E., and Winkle, R. A.: Cardiac biopsy evidence for a cardiomyopathy associated with symptomatic mitral valve prolapse. Am. J. Cardiol. *42*:557, 1978.
300. Beardsley, T. L., and Foulks, G. N.: An association of keratoconus and mitral valve prolapse. Ophthalmology *89*:35, 1982.
301. Rippe, J. M., Sloss, J. J., Angoff, G., and Alpert, J. S.: Mitral valve prolapse in adults with congenital heart disease. Am. Heart J. *97*:561, 1979.
302. Zema, M. J., Chiaramida, S., DeFilipp, G. J., et al.: Somatotype and idiopathic mitral valve prolapse. Cathet. Cardiovasc. Diagn. *8*:105, 1982.
303. Giesby, M. J., and Pyeritz, R. E.: Association of mitral valve prolapse and systemic abnormalities of connective tissue: A phenotypic continuum. JAMA *262*:523, 1989.
304. Gottdiener, J. S., Sherber, H. S., and Harvey, W. P.: Midsystolic click and mitral valve prolapse following mitral commissurotomy. Am. J. Med. *64*:295, 1978.
305. Barlow, J. B., Pocock, W. A., and Obel, I.W.P.: Mitral valve prolapse: Primary, secondary, both or neither? Am. Heart J. *102*:140, 1981.
306. Crawford, M. H.: Mitral valve prolapse due to coronary artery disease. Am. J. Med. *62*:447, 1977.
307. Imaizumi, T., Chandraratna, P.A.N., Whayne, T. F., Jr., et al.: Transmural myocardial infarction. With the prolapsing mitral-leaflet syndrome and normal coronary arteries. Arch. Intern. Med. *138*:1354, 1978.
308. Sakuma, T., Kakihana, M., Togo, T., et al.: Mitral valve prolapse syndrome with coronary artery spasm: A possible cause of recurrent ventricular tachyarrhythmia. Clin. Cardiol. *8*:306, 1985.
309. Devereux, R. B., Kramer-Fox, R., and Kligfield, P.: Mitral valve prolapse: Causes, clinical manifestations, and management. Arch. Intern. Med. *111*:305, 1989.
310. Tutassaura, H., Gerein, A. N., and Miyagishima, R. T.: Mucoid degeneration of the mitral valve. Clinical review, surgical management and results. Ann. J. Surg. *132*:276, 1976.
311. Guy, F. C., MacDonald, R.P.R., Fraser, D. B., and Smith, E. R.: Mitral valve prolapse as a cause of hemodynamically important mitral regurgitation. Can. J. Surg. *23*:166, 1980.
312. Pan, C. W., Chen, C. C., Wang, S. P., et al.: Echocardiographic study of cardiac abnormalities in families of patients with Marfan's syndrome. J. Am. Coll. Cardiol. *6*:1016, 1985.
313. Boudoulas, H., Kolibash, A. J., Jr., Baker, P., et al.: Mitral valve prolapse and the mitral valve prolapse syndrome: A diagnostic classification and pathogenesis of symptoms. Am. Heart J. *118*:796, 1989.
314. Davies, A. O., Mares, A., Pool, J. L., and Taylor, A. A.: Mitral valve prolapse with symptoms of beta-adrenergic hypersensitivity. Beta$_2$-adrenergic receptor supercoupling with desensitization on isoproterenol exposure. Am. J. Med. *82*:193, 1987.
315. Gaffney, F. A., Bastian, B. C., Lane, L. B., et al.: Abnormal cardiovascular regulation in the mitral valve prolapse syndrome. Am. J. Cardiol. *52*:316, 1983.
316. Puddu, P. E., Pasternac, A., Tubau, J. F., et al.: QT interval prolongation and increased plasma catecholamine levels in patients with mitral valve prolapse. Am. Heart J. *105*:422, 1983.
317. Leor, R., and Markiewicz, W.: Neurocirculatory asthenia and mitral valve prolapse—Two unrelated entities? Isr. J. Med. Sci. *17*:1137, 1981.
318. Wei, J. Y., and Fortuin, N. J.: Diastolic sounds and murmurs associated with mitral valve prolapse. Circulation *63*:559, 1981.
319. Alexander, M. D., Bloom, K. R., Hart, P., et al.: Atrial septal aneurysm: A cause of midsystolic click. Report of a case and review of the literature. Circulation *63*:1186, 1981.
320. Combs, R. L., Shah, P. M., Klorman, R. S., and Klorman, R.: Effects of induced psychological stress on click and rhythm in mitral valve prolapse. Am. Heart J. *99*:714, 1980.
321. Braunwald, E., Oldham, H. N., Jr., Ross, J., Jr., et al.: The circulatory response of patients with idiopathic hypertrophic stenosis to nitroglycerin and to the Valsalva maneuver. Circulation *29*:422, 1964.
322. Kligfield, P., Hochreiter, C., Kramer, H., et al.: Complex arrhythmias in mitral regurgitation with and without mitral valve prolapse: Contrast to

arrhythmias in mitral valve prolapse without mitral regurgitation. Am. J. Cardiol 55:1545, 1985.
323. Kligfield, P., Levy, D., Devereux, R. B., and Savage, D. D.: Arrhythmias and sudden death in mitral valve prolapse. Am. Heart J. 113:1298, 1987.
324. Kligfield, P., and Devereux, R. B.: Is the mitral valve prolapse patient at high risk of sudden death identifiable? *In* Cheitlin, M. D. (ed.): Dilemmas in Clinical Cardiology. Philadelphia, F. A. Davis, 1991, pp. 143–157.
325. Bharati, S., Granston, A. S., Liebson, P. R., et al.: The conduction system in mitral valve prolapse syndrome with sudden death. Am. Heart J. 101:667, 1981.
326. Ware, J. A., Magro, S. A., Luck, J. C., et al.: Conduction system abnormalities in symptomatic mitral valve prolapse: An electrophysiologic analysis of 60 patients. Am. J. Cardiol. 53:1075, 1984.
327. Kavey, R.-E.W., Blackman, M. S., Sondheimer, H. M., and Byrum, C. J.: Ventricular arrhythmias and mitral valve prolapse in childhood. J. Pediatrics 105:885, 1984.
328. Kramer, H. M., Devereux, R. B., Savage, D. D., and Kramer-Fox, R.: Arrhythmias in mitral valve prolapse. Arch. Intern. Med. 144:2360, 1984.
329. Boudoulas, H., Schaal, S. F., Stang, J. M., et al.: Mitral valve prolapse: Cardiac arrest with long-term survival. Int. J. Cardiol. 26:37, 1990.
330. Wit, A. L., Fenoglio, J. J., Wagner, B. M., and Bassett, A. L.: Electrophysiological properties of cardiac muscle in the anterior mitral valve leaflet and the adjacent atrium in the dog. Possible implications for the genesis of atrial dysrhythmias. Circ. Res. 32:731, 1973.
331. Wit, A. L., Fenoglio, J. J., Hordof, A. J., and Reemtsma, K.: Ultrastructure and transmembrane potentials of cardiac muscle in the human anterior mitral valve leaflet. Circulation 59:1283, 1979.
332. Campbell, R.W.F., Godman, M. G., Fiddler, G. I., et al.: Ventricular arrhythmias in syndrome of balloon deformity of mitral valve. Definition of possible high risk group. Br. Heart J. 38:1053, 1976.
333. Gallagher, J. J., Gilbert, M., and Svenson, R. H.: Wolff-Parkinson-White syndrome. The problem, evaluation and surgical correction. Circulation 57:767, 1975.
334. Bekheit, S. G., Ali, A. A., Deglin, S. M., and Jain, A. C.: Analysis of QT interval in patients with idiopathic mitral valve prolapse. Chest 81:620, 1982.
335. Jeresaty, R. M.: Mitral Valve Prolapse. New York, Raven Press, 1979, 251 pp.
336. Pocock, W. A., Bosman, C. K., Chesler, E., et al.: Sudden death in primary mitral valve prolapse. Am. Heart J. 107:378, 1984.
337. Chesler, E., King. R. A., and Edwards, J. E.: The myxomatous mitral valve and sudden death. Circulation 67:632, 1983.
338. Leichtman, D., Nelson, R., Gobel, F. L., et al.: Bradycardia with mitral valve prolapse: A potential mechanism of sudden death. Ann. Intern. Med. 85:453, 1976.
339. Hershman, W. Y., Moskowitz, M. A., Marton, K. I., and Balady, G. J.: Utility of echocardiography in patients with suspected mitral valve prolapse. Am. J. Med. 87:371, 1989.
340. Waller, B. F., Maron, B. J., DelNegro, A. A., et al.: Frequency and significance of M-mode echocardiographic evidence of mitral valve prolapse in clinically isolated pure mitral regurgitation: Analysis of 65 patients having mitral valve replacement. Am. J. Cardiol. 53:139, 1984.
341. Abbasi, A. S., DeCristofaro, D., Anabtawi, J., and Irwin, L.: Mitral valve prolapse: Comparative value of M-mode, two-dimensional and Doppler echocardiography. J. Am. Coll. Cardiol. 2:1219, 1983.
342. Alpert, M. A., Carney, R. J., Flaker, G. C., et al.: Sensitivity and specificity of two-dimensional echocardiographic signs of mitral valve prolapse. Am. J. Cardiol. 54:792, 1984.
343. Morganroth, J., Mardelli, T. J., Naito, M., and Chen, C. C.: Apical cross-sectional echocardiography. Standard for the diagnosis of idiopathic mitral valve prolapse syndrome. Chest 79:23, 1981.
344. Panidis, I. P., McAllister, M., Ross, J., and Mintz, G. S.: Prevalence and severity of mitral regurgitation in the mitral valve prolapse syndrome: A Doppler echocardiographic study of 80 patients. J. Am. Coll. Cardiol. 7:975, 1986.
345. Sahn, D. J., Wood, J., Allen, H. D., et al.: Echocardiographic spectrum of mitral valve motion in children with and without mitral valve prolapse: The nature of false-positive diagnosis. Am. J. Cardiol. 39:422, 1977.
346. Arvan, S., and Tunick, S.: Relationship between auscultatory events and structural abnormalities in mitral valve prolapse: A two-dimensional echocardiographic evaluation. Am. Heart J. 108:1298, 1984.
347. Ogawa, S., Hayashi, J., Sasaki, H., et al.: Evaluation of combined valvular prolapse syndrome of two-dimensional echocardiography. Circulation 65:174, 1982.
348. Rodger, J. C., and Morley, P.: Abnormal aortic valve echoes in mitral prolapse. Echocardiographic features of floppy aortic valve. Br. Heart J. 47:337, 1982.
349. Klein, G. J., Kostuk, W. J., Boughner, D. R., and Chamberlain, M. J.: Stress myocardial imaging in mitral leaflet prolapse syndrome. Am. J. Cardiol. 42:746, 1978.
350. Butman, S., Chandraratna, P. A. N., Milne, N., et al.: Stress myocardial imaging in patients with mitral valve prolapse: Evidence of a perfusion abnormality. Cathet. Cardiovasc. Diagn. 8:243, 1982.
351. Gottdiener, J. S., Borer, J. S., Bacharach, S. L., et al.: Left ventricular function in mitral valve prolapse: Assessment with radionuclide cineangiography. Am. J. Cardiol. 47:7, 1981.
352. Ranganathan, N., Silver, M. D., Robinson, T. I., and Wilson, J. K.: Idiopathic prolapse mitral leaflet syndrome. Angiographic-clinical correlations. Circulation 54:707, 1976.
353. Cohen, M. V., Shah, P. K., and Spindola-Franco, H.: Angiographic-echocardiographic correlation of mitral valve prolapse. Am. Heart J. 97:43, 1979.
354. Cipriano, P. R., Kline, S. A., and Baltaxe, H. A.: An angiographic assessment of left ventricular function in isolated mitral valvular prolapse. Invest. Radiol. 15:293, 1980.
355. Mills, P., Rose, J., Hollingsworth, J., et al.: Long-term prognosis of mitral valve prolapse. N. Engl. J. Med. 297:13, 1977.
356. Greenwood, R. D.: Mitral valve prolapse: Incidence and clinical course in a pediatric population. Clin. Pediatr. 23:318, 1984.
357. Chesler, E., and Gornick, C. C.: Maladies attributed to myxomatous mitral valve. Circulation 83:328, 1991.
358. Devereux, R. B., Hawkins, I., Kramer-Fox, R., et al.: Complications of mitral valve prolapse: Disproportionate occurrence in men and older patients. Am. J. Med. 81:751, 1986.
359. Hickey, A. J., MacMahon, S. W., and Wilcken, D.E.L.: Mitral valve prolapse and bacterial endocarditis: When is antibiotic prophylaxis necessary? Am. Heart J. 109:431, 1985.
360. MacMahon, S. W., Hickey, A. J., Wilcken, D.E.L., et al.: Risk of infective endocarditis in mitral valve prolapse with and without systolic murmurs. Am. J. Cardiol. 59:105, 1987.
361. Danchin, N., Briancon, S., Mathieu, P., et al.: Mitral valve prolapse as a risk factor for infective endocarditis. Lancet 1:743, 1989.
362. Schnee, M. A., and Bucal, A. A.: Fatal embolism in mitral valve prolapse. Chest 83:285, 1983.
363. Vared, Z., Oren, S., Rabinowitz, B., et al.: Mitral valve prolapse. Quantitative analysis and long-term followup. Isr. J. Med. Sci. 21:644, 1985.
364. Barletta, G. A., Gagliardi, R., Benvenuti, L., and Fantini, F.: Cerebral ischemic attacks as a complication of aortic and mitral valve prolapse. Stroke 16:219, 1985.
365. Makino, H., and Al-Sadir, J.: Myocardial infarction in patients with mitral valve prolapse and normal coronary arteries. J. Am. Coll. Cardiol. 1:661, 1983.
366. Winkle, R. A., and Harrison, D.: Propranolol for patients with mitral valve prolapse. Am. Heart J. 93:422, 1977.
367. Cohn, L. H., DiSesa, V. J., Couper, G. S., et al.: Mitral valve repair for myxomatous degeneration and prolapse of the mitral valve. J. Thorac. Cardiovasc. Surg. 98:987, 1989.

AORTIC STENOSIS

368. Roberts, W. C.: Valvular, subvalvular and supravalvular aortic stenosis. Morphologic features. Cardiovasc. Clin. 5:97, 1973.
369. Panidis, I. P., and Segal, B. L.: Aortic valve disease in the elderly. *In* Frankl, W. S., and Brest, A. N. (eds.): Cardiovascular Clinics. Valvular Heart Disease: Comprehensive Evaluation and Management. Philadelphia, F. A. Davis, 1986, pp. 289–312.
370. Levinson, G. E.: Aortic stenosis. *In* Dalen, J. E., and Alpert, J. S. (eds.): Valvular Heart Disease. 2nd ed. Boston, Little, Brown and Company, 1987, pp. 197–282.
371. Moller, J. H., Nakib, A., Elliott, R. S., and Edwards, J. E.: Symptomatic congenital aortic stenosis in the first year of life. J. Pediatr. 67:728, 1966.
372. Braunwald, E., Goldblatt, A., Aygen, M. M., et al.: Congenital aortic stenosis: Clinical and hemodynamic findings in 100 patients. Circulation 27:426, 1963.
373. Selzer, A.: Changing aspects of the natural history of valvular aortic stenosis. N. Engl. J. Med. 317:91, 1987.
374. Passik, C. S., Ackermann, D. M., Pluth, J. R., and Edwards, W. D.: Temporal changes in the causes of aortic stenosis: A surgical pathologic study of 646 cases. Mayo Clin. Proc. 62:119, 1987.
375. Narang, N. K., Andrew, A.M.R., Chaudhury, H. R., and Gaba, B. S.: Aortic stenosis due to familial hypercholesterolemic xanthomatosis. A case report with brief review of literature. Indian Heart J. 30:189, 1978.
376. Deutscher, S., Rockette, H. E., and Krishnaswami, V.: Diabetes and hypercholesterolemia among patients with calcific aortic stenosis. J. Chron. Dis. 37:407, 1984.
377. Strickberger, S. A., Schulman, S. P., and Hutchins, G. M.: Association of Paget's disease of bone with calcific aortic valve disease. Am. J. Med. 82:953, 1987.
378. Maher, E. R., Pazianas, M., and Curtis, J. R.: Calcific aortic stenosis: A complication of chronic uraemia. Nephron 47:119, 1987.
379. Maher, E. R., Young, G., Smyth-Walsh, B., et al.: Aortic and mitral valve calcification in patients with end stage renal diseases. Lancet I:875, 1987.
380. Dereymacker, L., Van Parijs, G., Bayart, M., et al.: Ochronosis and alkaptonuria: Report of a new case with calcified aortic valve stenosis. Acta Cardiol. 45:98, 1990.
381. Kennedy, J. W., Twiss, R. D., and Blackmon, J. R.: Quantitative angiography. III. Relationships of left ventricular pressure volume and mass in aortic valve disease. Circulation 38:838, 1968.
382. Carabello, B. A., Mee, R., Collins, J. J., Jr., et al.: Contractile function in chronic gradually developing subcoronary aortic stenosis. Am. J. Physiol. 240:H80, 1981.
383. Grossman, W.: Profiles in valvular heart disease. *In* Grossman, W., and Baim, D. (eds.): Cardiac Catheterization and Angiography. 4th ed. Philadelphia, Lea and Febiger, 1991.
384. Diver, D. J., Royal, H. D., Aroesty, J. M., et al.: Influence of left ventricular load on abnormal diastolic function in patients with aortic stenosis. J. Am. Coll. Cardiol. *(in press)*.
385. Hess, O. M., Ritter, M., Schneider, J., et al.: Diastolic stiffness and myocardial structure in aortic valve disease before and after replacement. Circulation 69:855, 1984.
386. Murakami, T., Hess, O. M., Gage, J. E., et al.: Diastolic filling dynamics in patients with aortic stenosis. Circulation 73:1162, 1986.

387. Braunwald, E., and Frahm, C. J.: Studies on Starling's law of the heart. IV. Observations on the hemodynamic functions of the left atrium in man. Circulation *24*:633, 1961.
388. Donner, R., Carabello, B. A., Black, I., and Spann, J. F.: Left ventricular wall stress in compensated aortic stenosis in children. Ann. J. Cardiol. *51*:946, 1983.
389. DePace, N. L., Ren, J-F., Iskandrian, A. S., et al.: Correlation of echocardiographic wall stress and left ventricular pressure and function in aortic stenosis. Circulation *67*:854, 1983.
390. Sasayama, S., Ross, J., Jr., Franklin, D., et al.: Adaptations of the left ventricle to chronic pressure overload. Circ. Res. *38*:172, 1976.
391. Spann, J. F., Bove, A. A., Natarajan, G., and Kreulens, T.: Ventricular performance, pump funcha, and compensatory mechanisms in patients with aortic stenosis. Circulation *62*:576, 1980.
391a. Brouwer, C. B., Verwers, F. A., Alpert, J. S., and Goldberg, R. J.: Isolated aortic stenosis: Analysis of clinical and hemodynamic subsets. J. Appl. Cardiol. *4*:565, 1989.
392. Krayenbuehl, H. P., Hess, O. M., Ritter, M., et al.: Left ventricular systolic function in aortic stenosis. Eur. Heart J. *9*(Suppl. E):19, 1988.
393. Gunther, S., and Grossman, W.: Determinants of ventricular function in pressure overload hypertrophy in man. Circulation *59*:679, 1979.
394. Ross, J., Jr.: Afterload mismatch and preload reserve: A conceptual framework for the analysis of ventricular function. Prog. Cardiovasc. Dis. *18*:255, 1976.
395. Fifer, M. A., Gunther, S., Grossman, W., et al.: Myocardial contractile function in aortic stenosis as determined from the rate of stress development during isovolumic systole. Am. J. Cardiol. *44*:1318, 1979.
396. Dineen, E., and Brent, B. N.: Aortic valve stenosis: Comparison of patients with to those without chronic congestive heart failure. Am. J. Cardiol. *57*:419, 1986.
397. Carabello, B. A., Green, L. H., Grossman, W., et al.: Hemodynamic determinants of prognosis of aortic valve replacement in critical aortic stenosis and advanced congestive heart failure. Circulation *62*:42, 1980.
398. Huber, D., Grimm, J., Koch, R., and Krayenbuehl, H. P.: Determinants of ejection performance in aortic stenosis. Circulation *64*:126, 1981.
399. Dineen, E., and Brent, B. N.: Aortic valve stenosis: Comparison of patients to those without chronic congestive heart failure. Am. J. Cardiol. *57*:419, 1986.
400. Fifer, M. A., Borow, K. M., Colan, S. D., and Lorell, B. H.: Early diastolic left ventricular function in children and adults with aortic stenosis. J. Am. Coll. Cardiol. *5*:1147, 1985.
401. Schwarz, F., Flameng, W., Schaper, J., et al.: Myocardial structure and function in patients with aortic valve disease and their relation to postoperative results. Am. J. Cardiol. *41*:661, 1978.
402. Bertrand, M. E., LaBlanche, J. M., Tilmant, P. Y., et al.: Coronary sinus blood flow at rest and during isometric exercise in patients with aortic valve disease. Mechanism of angina pectoris in presence of normal coronary arteries. Am. J. Cardiol. *47*:199, 1981.
403. Bonow, R. O.: Left ventricular structure and function in aortic valve disease. Circulation *79*:966, 1989.
404. Krayenbuehl, H. P., Hess, O. M., Monrad, E. S., et al.: Left ventricular myocardial structure in aortic valve disease before, intermediate, and later after aortic valve replacement. Circulation *79*:744, 1989.
405. Smucker, M. L., Tedesco, C. L., and Manning, S. B.: Demonstration of an imbalance between coronary perfusion and excessive load as a mechanism of ischemia during stress in patients with aortic stenosis. Circulation *78*:573, 1988.
406. Vinten-Johansen, J., and Weiss, H. R.: Oxygen consumption in subepicardial and subendocardial regions of the canine left ventricle—The effect of experimental acute valvular aortic stenosis. Circ. Res. *46*:139, 1980.
407. Matsuo, S., Tsuruta, M., Hayano, M., et al.: Phasic coronary artery flow velocity determined by Doppler flowmeter catheter in aortic stenosis and aortic regurgitation. Am. J. Cardiol. *62*:917, 1988.
408. Marcus, M. L., Dot, D. B., Hiratzka, L. F., et al.: Decreased coronary reserve. A mechanism for angina pectoris in patients with aortic stenosis and normal coronary arteries. N. Engl. J. Med. *307*:1362, 1982.
409. Kennedy, K. D., Nishimura, R. A., Holmes, D. R., et al.: Natural history of moderate aortic stenosis. J. Am. Coll. Cardiol. *17*:313, 1991.
410. Ross, J., Jr., and Braunwald, E.: The influence of corrective operations on the natural history of aortic stenosis. Circulation *37*(Suppl. V):61, 1968.
411. Frank, S., Johnson, A., and Ross, J., Jr.,: Natural history of valvular aortic stenosis. Br. Heart J. *35*:41, 1973.
412. Kelly, T. A., Rothbart, R. M., Cooper, M., et al.: Comparison of outcome of asymptomatic to symptomatic patients older than 20 years of age with valvular aortic stenosis. Am. J. Cardiol. *61*:123, 1988.
413. Hakki, A.-H., Kimbiris, D., Iskandrian, A. S., et al.: Angina pectoris and coronary artery disease in patients with severe aortic valvular disease. Am. Heart J. *100*:441, 1980.
414. Lombard, J. T., and Selzer, A.: Valvular aortic stenosis: A clinical and hemodynamic profile of patients. Ann. Intern. Med. *106*:292, 1987.
415. Holley, K. E., Bahn, R. C., McGoon, D. C., and Mankin, H. T.: Spontaneous calcific embolization associated with calcific aortic stenosis. Circulation *27*:197, 1963.
416. Vandeplas, A., Willems, J. L., Piessens, J., and DeGeest, H.: Frequency of angina pectoris and coronary artery disease in severe isolated valvular aortic stenosis: Am. J. Cardiol. *62*:117, 1988.
417. Mullany, C. J., Elveback, L. R., Frye, R. L., et al.: Coronary artery disease and its management: Influence on survival in patients undergoing aortic valve replacement. J. Am. Coll. Cardiol. *10*:66, 1987.
418. Grech, E. D., and Ramsdale, D. R.: Exertional syncope in aortic stenosis: Evidence to support inappropriate left ventricular baroreceptor response. Am. Heart J. *121*:603, 1991.
419. Schwartz, L. S., Goldfischer, J., Sprague, G. J., and Schwartz, S. P.: Syncope and sudden death in aortic stenosis. Am. J. Cardiol. *23*:647, 1969.
420. Kulbertus, H. E.: Ventricular arrhythmias, syncope and sudden death in aortic stenosis. Eur. Heart J. *9*(Suppl. E):51, 1988.
421. Shoenfeld, Y., Eldar, M., Bedazovsky, B., et al.: Aortic stenosis associated with gastrointestinal bleeding. A survey of 612 patients. Am. Heart J. *100*:179, 1980.
422. Love, J. W.: The syndrome of calcific aortic stenosis and gastrointestinal bleeding: Resolution following aortic valve replacement. J. Thorac. Cardiovasc. Surg. *83*:779, 1982.
423. Pleet, A. B., Massey, E. W., and Vengrow, M. E.: TIA, stroke, and the bicuspid aortic valve. Neurology *31*:1540, 1981.
424. Brockmeier, L. B., Adolph, R. J., Gustin, B. W., et al.: Calcium emboli to the retinal artery in calcific aortic stenosis. Am. Heart J. *101*:32, 1981.
425. Wood, P.: Aortic stenosis. Am. J. Cardiol. *1*:553, 1958.
426. Aortic stenosis. *In* Fowler, N.O.: Diagnosis of Heart Disease. New York, Springer-Verlag, 1991, pp. 134–145
427. Abrams, J.: Aortic stenosis. *In* Essentials of Cardiac Physical Diagnosis. Philadelphia, Lea and Febiger, 1987, pp. 205–224.
428. Cooper, T., Braunwald, E., and Morrow, A. G.: Pulsus alternans in aortic stenosis: Hemodynamic observations in 50 patients studied by left heart catheterization. Circulation *18*:64, 1958.
429. Perloff, J. K.: Clinical recognition of aortic stenosis. The physical signs and differential diagnosis of the various forms of obstruction to left ventricular outflow. Prog. Cardiovasc. Dis. *10*:323, 1968.
430. Goldblatt, A., Aygen, M. M., and Braunwald, E.: Hemodynamic-phonocardiographic correlations of the fourth heart sound in aortic stenosis. Circulation *26*:92, 1962.
431. Caulfield, W. H., deLeon, A. C., Perloff, J. K., and Steelman, R. B.: The clinical significance of the fourth heart sound in aortic stenosis. Am. J. Cardiol. *28*:179, 1971.
432. Morton, B. C.: Natural history and management of chronic aortic valve disease. Can. Med. Assoc. J. *126*:477, 1982.
433. Forssell, G., Jonasson, R., and Orinius, E.: Identifying severe aortic valvular stenosis by bedside examination. Acta Med. Scand. *218*:397, 1985.
434. Morgan, D.J.R., and Hall, R.J.C.: Occult aortic stenosis as cause of intractable heart failure. Br. Med. J. *1*:784, 1979.
435. Dymond, D. S., Wolf, F. G., and Schmidt, D. H.: Severe left ventricular dysfunction in critical aortic stenosis—reversal following aortic valve replacement. Postgrad. Med. J. *59*:781, 1983.
436. Delman, A. J., and Stein, E.: Valvular aortic stenosis. *In* Dynamic Cardiac Auscultation and Phonocardiography. Philadelphia, W. B. Saunders Company, 1979, p. 795.
437. Siegel, R. J., and Roberts, W. C.: Electrocardiographic observations in severe aortic valve stenosis: Correlative necropsy study of clinical, hemodynamic, and ECG variables demonstrating relation of 12-lead QRS amplitude to peak systolic transaortic pressure gradient. Am. Heart J. *103*:210, 1982.
438. Gooch, A. S., Calatayud, J. B., Rogers, P. A., and Garman, P. A.: Analysis of the P wave in severe aortic stenosis. Dis. Chest *49*:459, 1966.
439. Thompson, R., Mitchell, A., Ahmed, M., et al.: Conduction defects in aortic valve disease. Am. Heart J. *98*:3, 1979.
440. Rasmussen, K., Thomsen, P.E.B., and Bagger, J. P.: H-V interval in calcific aortic stenosis. Relation to left ventricular function and effect of valve replacement. Br. Heart J. *52*:82, 1984.
441. Nair, C. K., Aronow, W. S., Stokke, K., et al.: Cardiac conduction defects in patients older than 60 years with aortic stenosis and without mitral annular calcium. Am. J. Cardiol. *53*:169, 1984.
442. Rosenbaum, M., Elizari, M., and Lazari, J.: Los Hemibloques. Buenos Aires, Paidos, 1968, p. 363.
443. Klein, R. C.: Ventricular arrhythmias in aortic valve disease: Analysis of 102 patients. Am. J. Cardiol. *53*:1079, 1984.
444. Olshausen, K. V., Schwarz, F., Apfelbach, J., et al.: Determinants of the incidence and severity of ventricular arrhythmias in aortic valve disease. Am. J. Cardiol. *51*:1103, 1983.
445. Bell, H., Pugh, D., and Dunn, M.: Vectorcardiographic evolution of left ventricular hypertrophy. Br. Heart J. *30*:70, 1968.
446. Siegel, R. J., Maurer, G., Navatpumin, T., and Shah, P. K.: Accurate noninvasive assessment of critical aortic valve stenosis in the elderly. J. Am. Coll. Cardiol. *1*:639, 1983.
447. Szamosi, A., and Wassberg, B.: Radiologic detection of aortic stenosis. Acta Radiol. Diagn. *24*:201, 1983.
448. Vukas, M., Wallentin, I., and Hjalmarson, A.: Analysis of systolic vibrations of interventricular septum in patients with aortic valvular stenosis. Acta Med. Scand. *210*:397, 1981.
449. Galan, A., Zoghbi, W. A., and Quiñones, M. A.: Determination of severity of valvular aortic stenosis by Doppler echocardiography and relation of findings to clinical outcome and agreement with hemodynamic measurements determined at cardiac catheterization. Am. J. Cardiol. *67*:1007, 1991.
450. Agatston, A. S., Chengot, M., Rao, A., et al.: Doppler diagnosis of valvular aortic stenosis in patients over 60 years of age. Am. J. Cardiol. *56*:106, 1985.
451. Yeager, M., Yock, P. G., and Popp, R. L.: Comparison of Doppler-derived pressure gradient to that determined at cardiac catheterization in adults with aortic valve stenosis: Implications for management. Am. J. Cardiol. *57*:644, 1986.
452. Currie, P. J., Hagler, D. J., Seward, J. B., et al.: Instantaneous pressure gradient: A simultaneous Doppler and dual catheter correlative study. J. Am. Coll. Cardiol. *7*:800, 1986.
453. Jonasson, R., Jonsson, B., Nordlander, R., et al.: Rate of progression of severity of valvular aortic stenosis. Acta Med. Scand. *213*:51, 1983.

454. Nestico, P. F., DePace, N. L., Kimbiris, D., et al.: Progression of isolated aortic stenosis. Analysis of 29 patients having more than one cardiac catheterization. Am. J. Cardiol. *52*:1054, 1983.
455. Hoagland, P. M., Cook, E. F., Wynne, J., and Goldman, L.: Value of noninvasive testing in adults with suspected aortic stenosis. Am. J. Med. *80*:1041, 1986.
456. Cohen, L. S., Friedman, W. F., and Braunwald, E.: Natural history of mild congenital aortic stenosis elucidated by serial hemodynamic studies. Am. J. Cardiol. *30*:1, 1972.
457. Cheitlin, M. D., Gertz, E. W., Brundage, B. H., et al.: Rate of progression of severity of valvular aortic stenosis in the adult. Am. Heart J. *98*:689, 1979.
458. Chizner, M. A., Pearle, D. L., and deLeon, A. C., Jr.: The natural history of aortic stenosis in adults. Am. Heart J. *99*:419, 1980.
459. Braunwald, E.: On the natural history of severe aortic stenosis (editorial). J. Am. Coll. Cardiol. *15*:1018, 1990.
460. Turina, J., Hess, O., Sepulchri, F., and Krayenbuehl, H. P.: Spontaneous course of aortic valve disease. Eur. Heart J. *8*:471, 1987.
461. Kelly, T. A., Rothbart, R. M., Cooper, C. M., et al.: Comparison of outcome of asymptomatic patients older than 20 years with valvular aortic stenosis. Am. J. Cardiol. *61*:123, 1988.
462. Pellikka, P. A., Nishimura, R. A., Bailey, K. R., and Tajik, A. J.: The natural history of adults with asymptomatic hemodynamically significant aortic stenosis. J. Am. Coll. Cardiol. *15*:1012, 1990.
463. Wagner, S., and Selzer, A.: Patterns of progression of aortic stenosis: A longitudinal hemodynamic study. Circulation *65*:709, 1982.
464. Usher, B. W.: Valve surgery: Indications and long-term results. Curr. Opin. Cardiol. *6*:219, 1991.
465. Kirklin, J. W., and Barratt-Boyes, B. G.: Congenital valvular aortic stenosis. *In* Cardiac Surgery. New York, John Wiley and Sons, 1986, pp. 972–988.
466. Kirklin, J. W., and Barratt-Boyes, B. G.: Aortic valve disease. *In* Cardiac Surgery. New York, John Wiley and Sons, 1986, pp. 374–420.
467. McBride, L. R., Naunheim, K. S., Fiore, A. C., et al.: Aortic valve decalcification. J. Thorac. Cardiovasc. Surg. *100*:36, 1990.
468. Culliford, A. T., Galloway, A. C., Colvin, S. B., et al.: Aortic valve replacement for aortic stenosis in persons aged 80 years and over. Am. J. Cardiol. *67*:1256, 1991.
469. Shapira, N., Lemole, G. M., Fernandez, J., et al.: Aortic valve repair for aortic stenosis in adults. Ann. Thorac. Surg. *50*:110, 1990.
470. Levinson, J. R., Akins, C. W., Buckley, M. J., et al.: Octagenarians with aortic stenosis: Outcome after aortic valve replacement. Circulation *80*(Suppl. I):49, 1989.
471. Lund, O.: Preoperative risk evaluation and stratification of long-term survival after valve replacement for aortic stenosis. Circulation *82*:124, 1990.
472. Mirsky, I., Henschke, C., Hess, O. M., and Krayenbuehl, H. P.: Prediction of postoperative performance in aortic valve disease. Ann. J. Cardiol. *48*:295, 1981.
473. Acar. J., Ducimetiere, P., Cadilhac, M., et al.: Prognosis of surgically treated chronic aortic valve disease. Predictive indicators of early postoperative risk and long-term survival, based on 439 cases. J. Thorac. Cardiovasc. Surg. *82*:114, 1981.
474. St. John Sutton, M., Plappert, T., Spiegel, A., et al.: Early postoperative changes in left ventricular chamber size, architecture, and function in aortic stenosis and aortic regurgitation and their relation to intraoperative changes in afterload: A prospective two-dimensional echocardiographic study. Circulation *76*:77, 1987.
475. Monrad, E. S., Hess, O. M., Murakami, T., et al.: Abnormal exercise hemodynamics in patients with normal systolic function late after aortic valve replacement. Circulation *77*:613, 1988.
476. Pantely, G., Morton, M., and Rahimtoola, S. H.: Effects of successful, uncomplicated valve replacement on ventricular hypertrophy, volume and performance in aortic stenosis and in aortic incompetence. J. Thorac. Cardiovasc. Surg. *75*:383, 1978.
477. Hwang, M. H., Hammermeister, K. E., Oprian, C., et al.: Preoperative identification of patients likely to have left ventricular dysfunction after aortic valve replacement. Participants in the Veterans Administration Cooperative Study on Valvular Heart Disease. Circulation *80*(Suppl. I):165, 1989.
478. Kennedy, J. W., Doces, J., and Stewart, D. K.: Left ventricular function before and following aortic valve replacement. Circulation *56*:944, 1977.
479. Monrad, E. S., Hess, O. M., Murakami, T., et al.: Time course of regression of left ventricular hypertrophy after aortic valve replacement. Circulation *77*:1345, 1988.
480. O'Tolle, J. D., Geiser, E. A., Reddy, S., et al.: Effect of preoperative ejection fraction on survival and hemodynamic improvement following aortic valve replacement. Circulation *58*:1175, 1978.
481. Smith, N., McAnulty, J. H., and Rahimtoola, S. H.: Severe aortic stenosis with impaired left ventricular function and clinical heart failure: Results of valve replacement. Circulation *58*:255, 1978.
482. Kay, P. H., and Paneth, M.: Aortic valve replacement in the over seventy age group. J. Cardiovasc. Surg. *22*:312, 1981.
483. Safian, R. D., Mandell, V. S., Thurer, R. E., et al.: Postmortem and intraoperative balloon valvuloplasty of calcific aortic stenosis in elderly patients: Mechanisms of successful dilation. J. Am. Coll. Cardiol. *9*:655, 1987.
484. Beatt, K. J.: Balloon dilatation of the aortic valve in adults: a physician's view. Br. Heart J. *63*:207, 1990.
485. Kuntz, R. E., Tosteson, A. N. A., Berman, A. D., et al.: Predictors of event-free survival after balloon aortic valvuloplasty. N. Engl. J. Med. *325*:17, 1991.
486. Bashore, T. M., Davidson, C. J., and the Mansfield Scientific Aortic Valvuloplasty Registry Investigators: Follow-up recatheterization after balloon aortic valvuloplasty. J. Am. Coll. Cardiol. *17*:1188, 1991.
486a. Nishimura, R. A., Holmes, D. R., Jr., Michela, M. A., et al.: Follow-up of patients with low output, low gradient hemodynamics after percutaneous balloon aortic valvuloplasty: The Mansfield Scientific Aortic Valvuloplasty Registry. J. Am. Coll. Cardiol. *17*:828, 1991.
487. McKay, R. G.: The Mansfield Scientific Aortic Valvuloplasty Registry: Overview of acute hemodynamic results and procedural complications. J. Am. Coll. Cardiol. *17*:485, 1991.
488. Holmes, D. R., Jr., Nishimura, R. A., and Reeder, G. S.: In-hospital mortality after balloon aortic valvuloplasty: Frequency and associated factors. J. Am. Coll. Cardiol. *17*:189, 1991.
489. Cribier, A., and Letac, B.: Percutaneous balloon aortic valvuloplasty in adults with calcific aortic stenosis. Curr. Opin. Cardiol. *6*:212, 1991.
489a. Isner, J. A., and the Mansfield Scientific Aortic Valvuloplasty Registry Investigators: Acute catastrophic complications of balloon aortic valvuloplasty. J. Am. Coll. Cardiol. *17*:1436, 1991.
490. Berland, J., Cribier, A., Savin, T., et al.: Percutaneous balloon valvuloplasty in patients with severe aortic stenosis and low ejection fraction. Circulation *79*:1189, 1989.
490a. Angel, J. L., Chapman, C., and Knuppel, R. A.: Percutaneous balloon aortic valvuloplasty in pregnancy. Obstet. Gynecol. *72*:438, 1988.

AORTIC REGURGITATION

491. Olson, L. J., Subramanian, R., and Edwards, W. D.: Surgical pathology of pure aortic insufficiency: A study of 225 cases. Mayo Clin. Proc. *59*:835, 1984.
492. Alpert, J. S.: Chronic aortic regurgitation. *In* Dalen, J. E., and Alpert, J. S. (eds.): Valvular Heart Disease. 2nd ed. Boston, Little, Brown and Company, 1987, pp. 283–318.
493. Stewart, W. J., King, M. E., Gillam, L. D., et al.: Prevalence of aortic valve prolapse with bicuspid aortic valve and its relation to aortic regurgitation: A cross-sectional echocardiographic study. Am. J. Cardiol. *54*:1277, 1984.
494. Frahm, C. J., Braunwald, E., and Morrow, A. G.: Congenital aortic regurgitation. Clinical and hemodynamic findings in four patients. Am. J. Med. *31*:63, 1961.
495. Roberts, W. C., Morrow, A. G., McIntosh, C. L., et al.: Congenitally bicuspid aortic valve causing severe, pure aortic regurgitation without superimposed infective endocarditis. Am. J. Cardiol. *47*:206, 1981.
496. Tonnemacher, D., Reid, C., Kawanishi, D., et al.: Frequency of myxomatous degeneration of the aortic valve as a cause of isolated aortic regurgitation severe enough to warrant aortic valve replacement. Am. J. Cardiol. *60*:1194, 1987.
497. Morain, S. V., Casanegra, P., Maturana, G., and Dubernet, J.: Spontaneous rupture of a fenestrated aortic valve. Surgical treatment. J. Thorac. Cardiovasc. Surg. *73*:716, 1977.
498. Waller, B. F., Kishel, J. C., and Roberts, W. C.: Severe aortic regurgitation from systemic hypertension. Chest *82*:365, 1982.
499. Chartash, E. K., Lans, D. M., Paget, S. A., et al.: Aortic insufficiency and mitral regurgitation in patients with severe systemic lupus erythematosus and the antiphospholipid syndrome. Am. J. Med. *86*:407, 1989.
500. Kramer, P. H., Imboden, J. B., Jr., Waldman, F. M., et al.: Severe aortic insufficiency in juvenile chronic arthritis. Am. J. Med. *74*:1088, 1983.
501. Demoulin, J. C., Lespagnard, J., Bertholet, M., and Soumagne, D.: Acute fulminant aortic regurgitation in ankylosing spondylitis. Am. Heart J. *105*:859, 1983.
502. Tahakur, R., Gupta, L. C., Misra, M., et al.: Jaccoud's arthropathy—diagnostic and therapeutic implications. Postgrad. Med. J. *64*:809, 1988.
503. Bostwick, D. G., Bensch, K. G., Burke, J. S., et al.: Whipple's disease presenting as aortic insufficiency. N. Engl. J. Med. *305*:995, 1981.
504. Burdick, S., Tresch, D. D., and Komokowski, R. A.: Cardiac valvular dysfunction associated with Crohn's disease in the absence of ankylosing spondylitis. Am. Heart J. *118*:174, 1989.
505. Darvill, F. R., Jr.: Aortic insufficiency of unusual etiology. JAMA *184*:753, 1963.
506. Chikamori, T., Doi, Y. L., Yonezawa, Y., et al.: Aortic regurgitation secondary to Behçet's disease. A case report and review of the literature. Eur. Heart J. *11*:572, 1990.
507. Emanuel, R., Ng, R.A.L., Marcomichelakis, J., et al.: Formes frustes of Marfan's syndrome presenting with severe aortic regurgitation. Clinicogenetic study of 18 families. Br. Heart J. *39*:190, 1977.
508. Reid, G. D., Patterson, M.W.H., Patterson, A. C., and Cooperberg, P. L.: Aortic insufficiency in association with juvenile ankylosing spondylitis. J. Pediatr. *95*:78, 1979.
509. Paulus, H. E., Pearson, C. M., and Pitts, W., Jr.: Aortic insufficiency in five patients with Reiter's syndrome: A detailed clinical and pathologic study. Am. J. Med. *53*:464, 1972.
510. Hollingsworth, P., Hall, P. J., Knight, S. C., and Newman, R.: Lone aortic regurgitation, sacroiliitis, and HLA B27: Case history and frequency of association. Br. Heart J. *42*:229, 1979.
511. Heppner, R. L., Babitt, H. I., Blanchine, J. W., and Warbasse, J. R.: Aortic regurgitation and aneurysm of sinus of Valsalva associated with osteogenesis imperfecta. Am. J. Cardiol. *31*:654, 1973.
512. Esdah, J., Hawkins, D., Gold, P., et al.: Vascular involvement in relapsing polychondritis. Can. Med. Assoc. J. *116*:1019, 1977.
513. Welch, G. H., Jr., Braunwald, E., and Sarnoff, S. J.: Hemodynamic effects of quantitatively varied experimental aortic regurgitation. Circ. Res. *5*:546, 1957.
514. Belenkie, I., and Rademaker, A.: Acute and chronic changes after aortic valve damage in the intact dog. Am. J. Physiol. *241*:H95, 1981.

515. Iskandrian, A. S., Hakki, A-H., Manno, B., et al.: Left ventricular function in chronic aortic regurgitation. J. Am. Coll. Cardiol. *1*:1374, 1983.
516. Boucher, C. A., Wilson, R. A., Kanarek, D. J., et al.: Exercise testing in asymptomatic or minimally symptomatic aortic regurgitation: Relationship of left ventricular ejection fraction to left ventricular filling pressure during exercise. Circulation *67*:1091, 1983.
517. Johnson, L. L., Powers, E. R., Tzall, W. R., et al.: Left ventricular volume and ejection fraction response to exercise in aortic regurgitation. Am. J. Cardiol. *51*:1379, 1983.
518. Florenzano, F., and Glantz, S. A.: Left ventricular mechanical adaptation to chronic aortic regurgitation in intact dogs. Am. J. Physiol. *252*:H969, 1987.
518a. Borow, K. M., and Marcus, R. H.: Aortic regurgitation: The need for an integrated physiologic approach. J. Am. Coll. Cardiol. *17*:898, 1991.
519. Grossman, W., Jones, D., and McLaurin, L. P.: Wall stress and patterns of hypertrophy in the human left ventricle. J. Clin. Invest. *56*:56, 1975.
520. Laniado, S., Yellin, E. L., Yoran, C., et al.: Physiologic mechanism in aortic insufficiency. I. The effect of changing heart rate on flow dynamics. II. Determinants of Austin Flint murmur. Circulation *66*:226, 1982.
521. Kawanishi, D. T., McKay, C. R., Chandraratna, A. N., et al.: Cardiovascular response to dynamic exercise in patients with chronic symptomatic mild-to-moderate and severe aortic regurgitation. Circulation *73*:62, 1986.
522. Massie, B. M., Kramer, B. L., Loge, D., et al.: Ejection fraction response to supine exercise in asymptomatic aortic regurgitation: Relation to simultaneous hemodynamic measurements. J. Am. Coll. Cardiol. *5*:847, 1985.
523. Mehmel, H. C., Olshausen, K. V., Schuler, G., et al.: Estimation of left ventricular myocardial function by the ejection fraction in isolated, chronic, pure aortic regurgitation. Am. J. Cardiol. *54*:610, 1984.
524. Iskandrian, A. S., Hakki, A-H., and Kane-Marsch, S.: Left ventricular pressure/volume relationship in aortic regurgitation. Am. Heart J. *110*:1026, 1985.
525. Shen, W. F., Roubin, G. S., Choong, C.Y.-P., et al.: Evaluation of relationship between myocardial contractile state and left ventricular function in patients with aortic regurgitation. Circulation *71*:31, 1985.
526. Scognamiglio, R., Roelandt, J., Fasoli, G., et al.: Relation between myocardial contractility, hypertrophy and pump performance in patients with chronic aortic regurgitation: An echocardiographic study. Int. J. Cardiol. *6*:473, 1984.
527. Ricci, D. R.: Afterload mismatch and preload reserve in chronic aortic regurgitation. Circulation *66*:826, 1982.
528. Greenberg, B., Massie, B., Thomas, D., et al.: Association between the exercise ejection fraction response and systolic wall stress in patients with chronic aortic insufficiency. Circulation *71*:458, 1985.
529. Falsetti, H. L., Carroll, R. J., and Cramer, J. A.: Total and regional myocardial blood flow in aortic regurgitation. Am. Heart J. *97*:485, 1979.
530. Uhl, G. S., Boucher, C. A., Oliveros, R. A., and Murgo, J. P.: Exercise-induced myocardial oxygen supply-demand imbalance in asymptomatic or mildly symptomatic aortic regurgitation. Chest *80*:686, 1981.
531. Nitenberg, A., Foult, J-M., Antony, I., et al.: Coronary flow and resistance reserve in patients with chronic aortic regurgitation, angina pectoris, and normal coronary arteries. J. Am. Coll. Cardiol. *11*:478, 1988.
532. Maurer, W., Ablasser, A., Tschada, R., et al.: Myocardial catecholamine metabolism in patients with chronic aortic regurgitation. Circulation *66*(Suppl. I):139, 1982.
533. Dehmer, G. J., Firth, E. G., Hillis, L. D., et al.: Alterations in left ventricular volumes and ejection fraction at rest and during exercise in patients with aortic regurgitation. Am. J. Cardiol. *48*:17, 1981.
534. Lewis, S. M., Riba, A. L., Berger, H. J., et al.: Radionuclide angiographic exercise left ventricular performance in chronic aortic regurgitation: Relationship to resting echographic ventricular dimensions and systolic wall stress index. Am. Heart J. *103*:498, 1982.
535. Schuler, G., Olshausen, K. V., Schwarz, F., et al.: Noninvasive assessment of myocardial contractility in asymptomatic patients with severe aortic regurgitation and normal left ventricular ejection fraction at rest. Am. J. Cardiol. *50*:45, 1982.
536. Benotti, J. R.: Acute aortic insufficiency. *In* Dalen, J. E., and Alpert, J. S. (eds.): Valvular Heart Disease. 2nd ed. Boston, Little, Brown and Company, 1987, pp. 319–352.
537. Dervan, J., and Goldberg, S.: Acute aortic regurgitation: Pathophysiology and management. *In* Frankl, W. S., and Brest, A. N. (eds.): Cardiovascular Clinics. Valvular Heart Disease: Comprehensive Evaluation and Management. Philadelphia, F. A. Davis, 1986, pp. 281–288.
538. Perloff, J. K.: Acute severe aortic regurgitation: Recognition and management. J. Cardiovasc. Med. *8*:209, 1983.
539. Downes, T. R., Nomeir, A-M., Hackshaw, B. T., et al.: Diastolic mitral regurgitation in acute but not chronic aortic regurgitation: Implications regarding the mechanism of mitral closure. Am. Heart J. *117*:1106, 1989.
540. Spagnuolo, M., Kloth, H., Taranta, A., et al.: Natural history of rheumatic aortic regurgitation: Criteria predictive of death, congestive heart failure and angina in young patients. Circulation *44*:368, 1971.
541. Benotti, J. R., and Dalen, J. E.: Aortic valvular regurgitation: Natural history and medical treatment. *In* Cohn, L. H., and DiSesa, V. J. (eds.): Aortic Regurgitation: Medical and Surgical Management. New York, Marcel Dekker, 1986, pp. 1–54.
542. Sapira, J. D.: Quincke, DeMusset, Duroziez and Hill: Some aortic regurgitations. South. Med. J. *74*:459, 1981.
542a. Boudoulas, H., Triposkiadis, F., Dervenagas, et al.: Mechanisms of pistol shot sounds in aortic regurgitation. Acta Cardiol. *XLVI*:139, 1991.
543. Alpert, J. S., Veiweg, W.V.R., and Hagan, A. D.: Incidence and morphology of carotid shudders in aortic valve disease. Am. Heart J. *92*:435, 1976.
544. Sabbah, H. N., Khaja, F., Anbe, D. T., and Stein, P. D.: The aortic closure sound in pure aortic insufficiency. Circulation *56*:859, 1977.
544a. Aortic Insufficiency, *In* Fowler, N. O.: Diagnosis of Heart Disease. New York, Springer-Verlag, 1991, pp. 123–133.
545. Abdulla, A. M., Frank, M. J., Erdin, R. A., Jr., and Canedo, M. I.: Clinical significance and hemodynamic correlates of the third heart sound gallop in aortic regurgitation. A guide to optimal timing of cardiac catheterization. Circulation *64*:464, 1981.
546. Harvey, W., Corrado, M. A., and Perloff, J. K.: "Right-sided" murmurs of aortic insufficiency. Am. J. Med. Sci. *245*:53, 1963.
547. Fortuin, N. J., and Craige, E.: On the mechanism of the Austin Flint murmur. Circulation *45*:558, 1972.
548. Delman, A. J., and Stein, E.: Aortic regurgitation. *In* Dynamic Cardiac Auscultation and Phonocardiography. Philadelphia, W. B. Saunders Company, 1979, pp. 811–824.
549. Spring, D. A., Folts, J. D., Young, W. P., and Rowe, G. G.: Premature closure of the mitral and tricuspid valves. Circulation *45*:663, 1972.
550. Wong, M.: Diastolic mitral regurgitation. Hemodynamic and angiographic correlation. Br. Heart J. *31*:468, 1969.
551. Estes, E. H.: Left ventricular hypertrophy in acquired heart disease: A comparison of the vectorcardiogram in aortic stenosis and aortic insufficiency. *In* Hoffman, I. (ed.): Vectorcardiography. Amsterdam, North Holland Publishing Co., 1976.
552. Roberts, W. C., and Day, P. J.: Electrocardiographic observations in clinically isolated, pure, and chronic, severe aortic regurgitation: Analysis of 30 necropsy patients aged 19 to 65 years. Am. J. Cardiol. *55*:431, 1985.
553. DePace, N. L., Nestico, P. F., Kotler, M. N., et al.: Comparison of echocardiography and angiography in determining the cause of severe aortic regurgitation. Br. Heart J. *51*:36, 1984.
554. Meyer, T., Sareli, P., Pocock, W. A., et al.: Echocardiographic and hemodynamic correlates of diastolic closure of mitral valve and diastolic opening of aortic valve in severe aortic regurgitation. Am. J. Cardiol. *59*:1144, 1987.
555. Weaver, W. F., Wilson, C. S., Rourke, T., and Caudill, C. C.: Mid-diastolic aortic valve opening in severe acute aortic regurgitation. Circulation *55*:112, 1977.
556. Louie, E. K., Mason, T. J., Shah, R., et al.: Determinants of anterior mitral leaflet fluttering in pure aortic regurgitation from pulsed Doppler study of the early diastolic interaction between the regurgitant jet and mitral inflow. Am. J. Cardiol. *61*:1085, 1988.
557. Grayburn, P. A., Smith, M. D., Handshoe, R., et al.: Detection of aortic insufficiency by standard echocardiography, pulsed Doppler echocardiography and auscultation. Ann. Intern. Med. *104*:599, 1986.
558. Downes, T. R., Nomeir, A-D., Hackshaw, B. T., et al.: Diastolic mitral regurgitation in acute but not chronic aortic regurgitation: Implications regarding the mechanism of mitral closure. Am. Heart J. *117*:1106, 1989.
559. Masuyama, T., Kodama, K., Kitabatake, A., et al.: Noninvasive evaluation of aortic regurgitation by continuous-wave Doppler echocardiography. Circulation *73*:460, 1986.
560. Manyari, D. E., Nolewajka, A. J., and Kostuk, W. J.: Quantitative assessment of aortic valvular insufficiency by radionuclide angiography. Chest *81*:170, 1982.
561. Steingart, R. M., Yee, C., Weinstein, L., and Scheuer, J.: Radio-nuclide ventriculographic study of adaptations to exercise in aortic regurgitation. Am. J. Cardiol. *51*:483, 1983.
562. Sareli, P., Klein, H. O., Schamroth, C. L., et al.: Contribution of echocardiography and immediate surgery to the management of severe aortic regurgitation from active infective endocarditis. Am. J. Cardiol. *57*:413, 1986.
563. Goldschlager, N., Pfeifer, J., Cohn, K., et al.: The natural history of aortic regurgitation. A clinical and hemodynamic study. Am. J. Med. *54*:577, 1973.
564. Cheitlin, M. D., Bonow, R. O., Parmley, W. W., et al.: Task force II: Acquired valvular heart disease. J. Am. Coll. Cardiol. *6*:1209, 1985.
565. Greenberg, B. H., DeMots, H., Murphy, E., and Rahimtoola, S. H.: Mechanism for improved cardiac performance with arteriolar dilators in aortic insufficiency. Circulation *63*:263, 1981.
566. Elkayam, U., McKay, C. R., Weber, L., et al.: Favorable effects of hydralazine on the hemodynamic response to isometric exercise in chronic severe aortic regurgitation. Am. J. Cardiol. *54*:1603, 1984.
567. Fioretti, P., Benussi, B., Scardi, S., et al.: Afterload reduction with nifedipine in aortic insufficiency. Am. J. Cardiol. *49*:1728, 1982.
568. Jebavy, P., Koudelkova, E., and Henzlova, M.: Unloading effects of prazosin in patients with chronic aortic regurgitation. Am. Heart J. *105*:567, 1983.
569. Kleaveland, J. P., Reichek, N., McCarthy, D. M., et al.: Effects of six-month afterload reduction therapy with hydralazine in chronic aortic regurgitation. Am. J. Cardiol. *57*:1109, 1986.
570. Greenberg, B., Massie, B., Bristow, J. D., et al.: Long-term vasodilator therapy of chronic aortic insufficiency. Circulation *78*:92, 1988.
571. Dumesnil, J. G., Tran, K., and Dagenais, G. R.: Beneficial long-term effects of hydralazine in aortic regurgitation. Arch. Intern. Med. *150*:757, 1990.
572. Scognamiglio, R., Fasoli, G., Ponchia, A., and Dalla-Volta, S.: Long-term nifedipine unloading therapy in asymptomatic patients with chronic severe aortic regurgitation. J. Am. Coll. Cardiol. *16*:424, 1990.
573. Crawford, M. H., Wilson, R. S., O'Rourke, R. A., and Vittitoe, J. A.: Effect of digoxin and vasodilators on left ventricular function in aortic regurgitation. Int. J. Cardiol. *23*:385, 1989.
574. Hoshino, P. K., and Gaasch, W. H.: When to intervene in chronic aortic regurgitation. Arch. Intern. Med. *146*:346, 1986.
575. Bonow, R. O., Picone, A. L., McIntosh, C. L., et al.: Survival and functional results after valve replacement for aortic regurgitation from 1976 to

1983: Impact of preoperative left ventricular function. Circulation *72*:1244, 1985.

576. Turina, J., Turina, M., Rothlin, M., and Krayenbuehl, H. P.: Improved late survival in patients with chronic aortic regurgitation by earlier operation. Circulation *70*(Suppl. I):147, 1984.

577. Gee, D. S., Juni, J. E., Santinga, J. T., and Buda, A. J.: Prognostic significance of exercise-induced left ventricular dysfunction in chronic aortic regurgitation. Am. J. Cardiol. *56*:605, 1985.

578. Stone, P. H., Clark, R. D., Goldschlager, N., et al.: Determinants of prognosis of patients with aortic regurgitation who undergo aortic valve replacement. J. Am. Coll. Cardiol. *3*:1118, 1984.

579. Nishimura, R., McGoon, M. D., Schaff, H. V., and Giuliani, E. R.: Chronic aortic regurgitation: Indications for operation—1988. Mayo Clin. Proc. *63*:270, 1988.

580. Louagie, Y., Brohet, C., Robert, A., et al.: Factors influencing postoperative survival in aortic regurgitation. J. Thorac. Cardiovasc. Surg. *88*:225, 1984.

581. Borow, K. M., Surgical outcome in chronic aortic regurgitation: A physiologic framework for assessing preoperative predictors. J. Am. Coll. Cardiol. *10*:1165, 1987.

582. Taniguchi, K., Nakano, S., Matsuda, H., et al.: Depressed myocardial contractility and normal ejection performance after aortic valve replacement in patients with aortic regurgitation. J. Thorac. Cardiovasc. Surg. *98*:258, 1989.

583. Toussaint, C., Cribier, A., Cazor, J. L., et al.: Hemodynamic and angiographic evaluation of aortic regurgitation 8 and 27 months after aortic valve replacement. Circulation *64*:456, 1981.

584. Bonow, R. O., Rosing, D. R., Kent, K. M., and Epstein, S. E.: Timing of operation for chronic aortic regurgitation. Am. J. Cardiol. *50*:325, 1982.

585. Errichetti, A., Greenberg, J. M., and Gaasch, W. M.: Is valve replacement indicated in asymptomatic patients with aortic stenosis or aortic regurgitation? *In* Cheitlin, M. (ed.): Dilemmas in Clinical Cardiology. Philadelphia, F. A. Davis, 1991.

586. Bonow, R. O.: Noninvasive evaluation: Prognosis and timing of operation in symptomatic and asymptomatic patients with chronic aortic regurgitation. *In* Cohn, L. H., and DiSesa, V. J. (eds.): Aortic Regurgitation: Medical and Surgical Management. New York, Marcel Dekker, 1986, pp. 55–86.

587. Bonow, R. O., Dodd, J. T., Maron, B. J., et al.: Long-term serial changes in left ventricular function and reversal of ventricular dilatation after valve replacement for chronic aortic regurgitation. Circulation *78*:1108, 1988.

588. Carabello, B. A., Usher, B. W., Hedrik, G. H., et al.: Predictors of outcome for aortic valve replacement in patients with aortic regurgitation and left ventricular dysfunction: A change in the measuring stick. J. Am. Coll. Cardiol. *10*:991, 1987.

589. Taniguchi, K., Nakano, S., Hirose, H., et al.: Preoperative left ventricular function: Minimal requirement for successful late results of valve replacement for aortic regurgitation. J. Am. Coll. Cardiol. *10*:510, 1987.

590. Wisenbaugh, T., Booth, D., DeMaria, A., et al.: Relationship of contractile state to ejection performance in patients with chronic aortic valve disease. Circulation *73*:47, 1986.

591. Carroll, J. D., Gaasch, W. H., Naimi, S., and Levine, H. J.: Regression of myocardial hypertrophy: Electrocardiographic-echocardiographic correlations after aortic valve replacement in patients with chronic aortic regurgitation. Circulation *65*:980, 1982.

592. Carroll, J. D., Gaasch, W. H., Zile, M. R., and Levine, H. J.: Serial changes in left ventricular function after correction of chronic aortic regurgitation. Dependence on early changes in preload and subsequent regression of hypertrophy. Am. J. Cardiol. *51*:476, 1983.

593. Donaldson, R. M., Florio, R., Rickards, A. F., et al.: Irreversible morphological changes contributing to depressed cardiac function after surgery for chronic aortic regurgitation. Br. Heart J. *48*:589, 1982.

TRICUSPID, PULMONIC, AND MULTIVALVULAR DISEASE

594. Hauck, A. J., Freeman, D. P., Ackermann, D. M., et al.: Surgical pathology of the tricuspid valve: A study of 363 cases spanning 25 years. Mayo Clin. Proc. *63*:851, 1988.

595. Smith, J. A., and Levine, S. A.: Clinical features of tricuspid stenosis. Am. Heart J. *23*:739, 1942.

596. Ribeiro, P. A., Al Zaibag, M., Al Kasab, S., et al.: Provocation and amplification of the transvalvular pressure gradient in rheumatic tricuspid stenosis. Am. J. Cardiol. *61*:1307, 1988.

597. Perloff, J. K., and Harvey, W. P.: The clinical recognition of tricuspid stenosis. Circulation *22*:346, 1960.

598. Morgan, J. R., Forker, A. D., Coates, J. R., and Myers, W. S.: Isolated tricuspid stenosis. Circulation *44*:729, 1971.

599. Ockene, I. S.: Tricuspid valve disease. *In* Dalen, J. E., and Alpert, J. S. (eds.): Valvular Heart Disease. 2nd ed. Boston, Little, Brown and Company, 1987, pp. 353–402.

600. Wooley, C. F., Fontana, M. E., Kilman, J. W., and Ryan, J. M.: Tricuspid stenosis: Atrial systolic murmur, tricuspid opening snap and right atrial pressure pulse. Am. J. Med. *78*:375, 1985.

601. Kitchin, A., and Turner, R.: Diagnosis and treatment of tricuspid stenosis. Br. Heart J. *26*:354, 1964.

602. Mahapatra, R. K., Agarwal, J. B., and Wasir, H. S.: Rheumatic tricuspid stenosis. Indian Heart J. *30*:138, 1978.

602a. Tricuspid valve disease. *In* Fowler, N. O.: Diagnosis of Heart Disease. New York, Springer-Verlag, 1991, pp. 181–186.

603. Daniels, S. J., Mintz, G. S., and Kotler, M. N.: Rheumatic tricuspid valve disease. Two-dimensional echocardiographic, hemodynamic, and angiographic correlations. Am. J. Cardiol. *51*:492, 1983.

604. Pillai, M. G., Sharma, S., Munsi, S. C., Desai, A. G., and Panday, S. R.: Value of echocardiography in detecting rheumatic tricuspid stenosis. J. Cardiovasc. Ultrasonogr. *4*:185, 1985.

605. Ribeiro, P. A., Al Zaibag, M., and Sawyer, W.: A prospective study comparing the haemodynamic with the cross-sectional echocardiographic diagnosis of rheumatic tricuspid stenosis. Eur. Heart J. *10*:120, 1989.

606. Guyer, D. E., Gillam, L. D., Foale, R. A., et al.: Comparison of the echocardiographic and hemodynamic diagnosis of rheumatic tricuspid stenosis. J. Am. Coll. Cardiol. *3*:1135, 1984.

607. Shimada, R., Takeshita, A., Nakamura, M., et al.: Diagnosis of tricuspid stenosis by M-mode and two-dimensional echocardiography. Am. J. Cardiol. *53*:164, 1984.

608. Fawzy, M. E., Mercer, E. N., Dunn, B., et al.: Doppler echocardiography in the evaluation of tricuspid stenosis. Eur. Heart J. *10*:985, 1989.

609. Péterffy, A., Jonasson, R., and Henze, A.: Haemodynamic changes after tricuspid valve surgery. Scand. J. Thorac. Cardiovasc. Surg. *15*:161, 1981.

610. Throburn, C. W., Morgan, J. J., Shanahan, M. X., and Chang, V. P.: Long-term results of tricuspid valve replacement and the problem of prosthetic valve thrombosis. Am. J. Cardiol. *51*:1128, 1983.

611. Boskovic, D., Elezovic, I., Boskovic, D., et al.: Late thrombosis of the Björk-Shiley tilting disc valve in the tricuspid position. J. Thorac. Cardiovasc. Surg. *91*:1, 1986.

612. Cobanoglu, A., and Starr, A.: Tricuspid valve surgery: Indications, methods, and results. *In* Frankl, W. S., and Brest, A. N. (eds.): Cardiovascular Clinics. Valvular Heart Disease: Comprehensive Evaluation and Management. Philadelphia, F. A. Davis, 1986, pp. 375–388.

613. Guerra, F., Bortolotti, U., Thiene, G., et al.: Long-term performance of the Hancock porcine bioprosthesis in the tricuspid position. A review of 45 patients with 14-year follow-up. J. Thorac. Cardiovasc. Surg. *99*:838, 1990.

614. Goldenberg, I. F., Pedersen, W., Olson, J., et al.: Percutaneous double balloon valvuloplasty for severe tricuspid stenosis. Am. Heart J. *118*:417, 1989.

615. Shafie, M. Z., Hayat, N., and Majid, O. A.: Fate of tricuspid regurgitation after closed valvotomy for mitral stenosis. Chest *88*:870, 1985.

616. Cohen, S. R., Sell, J. E., McIntosh, C. L., and Clark, R. E.: Tricuspid regurgitation in patients with acquired, chronic, pure mitral regurgitation. 1. Prevalence, diagnosis, and comparison of preoperative clinical and hemodynamic features in patients with and without tricuspid regurgitation. J. Thorac. Cardiovasc. Surg. *94*:481, 1987.

617. Morrison, D. A., Ovitt, T., and Hammermeister, K. E.: Functional tricuspid regurgitation and right ventricular dysfunction in pulmonary hypertension. Am. J. Cardiol. *62*:108, 1988.

618. Vatterott, P. J., Nishimura, R. A., Gersh, B. J., and Smith, H. C.: Severe isolated tricuspid insufficiency in coronary artery disease. Int. J. Cardiol. *14*:295, 1987.

619. Dougherty, M. J., and Craige, E.: Apathetic hyperthyroidism presenting as tricuspid regurgitation. Chest *63*:767, 1973.

620. Scheck-Krejca, H., Zulstra, F., Roelandt, J., and Vletter-McGhie, J.: Diagnosis of tricuspid regurgitation: Comparison of jugular venous and liver pulse tracings with combined two-dimensional and Doppler echocardiography. Eur. Heart J. *7*:973, 1986.

621. Come, P. C., and Riley, M. F.: Tricuspid anular dilatation and failure of tricuspid leaflet coaptation in patients with tricuspid regurgitation. Am. J. Cardiol. *55*:599, 1985.

622. Tei, C., Pilgrim, J. P., Shah, P. M., et al.: The tricuspid valve annulus: Study of size and motion in normal subjects and in patients with tricuspid regurgitation. Circulation *66*:665, 1982.

623. Mikami, T., Kudo, T., Sakurai, N., et al.: Mechanisms for development of functional tricuspid regurgitation determined by pulsed Doppler and two-dimensional echocardiography. Am. J. Cardiol. *53*:160, 1984.

624. Esaghpour, E., Kawai, N., and Linhart, J. W.: Tricuspid insufficiency associated with aneurysm of the ventricular septum. Pediatrics *61*:586, 1978.

625. Sakai, K., Inoue, Y., and Osawa, M.: Congenital isolated tricuspid regurgitation in an adult. Am. Heart J. *110*:680, 1985.

626. Schlamowitz, R. A., Gross, S., Keating, E., et al.: Tricuspid valve prolapse: A common occurrence in the click-murmur syndrome. J. Clin. Ultrasound *10*:435, 1982.

627. Weinreich, D. J., Burke, J. F., Bharati, S., and Lev, M.: Isolated prolapse of the tricuspid valve. J. Am. Coll. Cardiol. *6*:475, 1985.

628. Jackson, D., Gibbs, H. R., and Zee-Cheng, C. S.: Isolated tricuspid valve prolapse diagnosed by echocardiography. Am. J. Med. *80*:281, 1986.

629. Chandraratna, P.A.N., Littman, B. B., and Wilson, D.: The association between atrial septal defect and prolapse of the tricuspid valve. An echocardiographic study. Chest *73*:839, 1978.

630. Gayet, C., Pierre, B., Delahaye, J-P., et al.: Traumatic tricuspid insufficiency: An underdiagnosed disease. Chest *92*:429, 1987.

631. Dickerman, S. A., and Rubler, S.: Mitral and tricuspid valve regurgitation in dilated cardiomyopathy. Am. J. Cardiol. *63*:629, 1989.

632. Ginzton, L. E., Siegel, R. J., and Criley, J. M.: Natural history of tricuspid valve endocarditis: A two-dimensional echocardiographic study. Am. J. Cardiol. *49*:1853, 1982.

633. Arbulu, A., and Asfaw, I.: Tricuspid valvulectomy without prosthetic replacement. Ten years of clinical experience. J. Thorac. Cardiovasc. Surg. *82*:684, 1981.

634. Lundin, L., Norheim, I., Landelius, J., et al.: Carcinoid heart disease: Relationship of circulating vasoactive substances to ultrasound-detectable cardiac abnormalities. Circulation *77*:264, 1988.

635. Callahan, J. A., Wroblewski, E. M., Reeder, G. S., et al.: Echocardiographic features of carcinoid heart disease. Am. J. Cardiol. *50*:762, 1982.
636. Gutman, J. M., and Schiller, N. B.: Carcinoid heart disease: Diagnostic usefulness of echocardiography. Primary Cardiol. *9*:130, 1983.
637. Mason, J. W., Billingham, M. E., and Friedman, J. P.: Methysergide-induced heart disease: A case of multivalvular and myocardial fibrosis. Circulation *56*:889, 1977.
638. Laufer, J., Frand, M., and Milo, S.: Valve replacement for severe tricuspid regurgitation caused by Libman-Sacks endocarditis. Br. Heart J. *48*:294, 1982.
639. Allen, S. J., and Naylor, D.: Pulsation of the eyeballs in tricuspid regurgitation. Can. Med. Assoc. J. *133*:119, 1985.
640. Abrams, J.: Tricuspid regurgitation. *In* Essentials of Cardiac Physical Diagnosis. Philadelphia, Lea and Febiger, 1987, pp. 375–400.
641. Cha, S. D., and Gooch, A. S.: Diagnosis of tricuspid regurgitation: Current status. Arch. Intern. Med. *143*:1763, 1983.
642. Amidi, M., Irwin, J. M., Salerni, R., et al.: Venous systolic thrill and murmur in the neck: A consequence of severe tricuspid insufficiency. J. Am. Coll. Cardiol. *7*:942, 1986.
643. Cha, S. D., Gooch, A. S., and Maranhao, V.: Intracardiac phonocardiography in tricuspid regurgitation: Relation to clinical and angiographic findings. Am. J. Cardiol. *48*:578, 1981.
644. Maisel, A. S., Atwood, J. E., and Goldberger, A. L.: Hepatojugular reflux: Useful in the bedside diagnosis of tricuspid regurgitation. Ann. Intern. Med. *101*:781, 1984.
645. Sepulveda, G., and Lukas, D. S.: The diagnosis of tricuspid insufficiency: Clinical features in 60 cases with associated mitral valve disease. Circulation *11*:552, 1955.
646. Hubbard, W. N., Westgate, C., Shapiro, L. M., and Donaldson, R. M.: Acquired abnormalities of the tricuspid valve—an ultrasonographic study. Int. J. Cardiol. *14*:311, 1987.
647. Meltzer, R. S., van Hoogenhuyze, D., Serruys, P. W., et al.: Diagnosis of tricuspid regurgitation by contrast echocardiography. Circulation *63*:1093, 1981.
648. Tei, C., Shah, P. M., and Ormiston, J. A.: Assessment of tricuspid regurgitation by directional analysis of right atrial systolic linear reflux echoes with contrast M-mode echocardiography. Am. Heart J. *103*:1025, 1982.
649. Forman, M. B., Byrd, B. F., Oates, J. A., and Robertson, R. M.: Two-dimensional echocardiography in the diagnosis of carcinoid heart disease. Am. Heart J. *107*:492, 1984.
650. Curtius, J. M., Thyssen, M., Breuer, H.W.M., and Loogen, F.: Doppler versus contrast echocardiography for diagnosis of tricuspid regurgitation. Am. J. Cardiol. *56*:333, 1985.
651. Diebold, B., Touati, R., Blanchard, D., et al.: Quantitative assessment of tricuspid regurgitation using pulsed Doppler echocardiography. Br. Heart J. *50*:443, 1983.
652. Pennestri, F., Loperfido, F., Salvatori, M. F., et al.: Assessment of tricuspid regurgitation by pulsed Doppler ultrasonography of the hepatic veins. Am. J. Cardiol. *54*:363, 1984.
653. Yock, P. G., and Popp, R. L.: Noninvasive estimation of right ventricular systolic pressure by Doppler ultrasound in patients with tricuspid regurgitation. Circulation *70*:657, 1984.
654. Skjaerpe, T., and Hatle, L.: Noninvasive estimation of systolic pressure in the right ventricle in patients with tricuspid regurgitation. Eur. Heart J. *7*:704, 1986.
655. Suzuki, Y., Kambara, H., Kadota, K., et al.: Detection and evaluation of tricuspid regurgitation using a real-time, two-dimensional, color-coded, Doppler flow imaging system: Comparison with contrast two-dimensional echocardiography and right ventriculography. Am. J. Cardiol. *57*:811, 1986.
656. Wong, M., Matsumara, M., Kutsuzawa, S., and Omoto, R.: The value of Doppler echocardiography in the treatment of tricuspid regurgitation in patients with mitral valve replacement. J. Thorac. Cardiovasc. Surg. *99*:1003, 1990.
657. Lambertz, H., Minale, C., Flachskampf, F. A., et al.: Long-term follow-up after Carpentier tricuspid valvuloplasty. Am. Heart J. *117*:615, 1989.
658. Lingameni, R., Cha, S. D., Maranhao, V., et al.: Tricuspid regurgitation: Clinical and angiographic assessment. Cathet. Cardiovasc. Diagn. *5*:7, 1979.
659. Pepino, C. J., Nichols, W. W., and Selby, J. H.: Diagnostic tests for tricuspid insufficiency: How good? Cathet. Cardiovasc. Diagn. *5*:1, 1979.
660. Lingameni, R., Cha, S. D., Maranhao, V., et al.: Tricuspid regurgitation: Clinical and angiographic assessment. Cathet. Cardiovasc. Diagn. *5*:7, 1979.
661. Ubago, J. L., Figueroa, A., Colman, T., et al.: Right ventriculography as a valid method for the diagnosis of tricuspid insufficiency. Cathet. Cardiovasc. Diagn. *7*:433, 1981.
662. Barbour, D. J., and Roberts, W. C.: Valve excision only versus valve excision plus replacement for active infective endocarditis involving the tricuspid valve. Am. J. Cardiol. *57*:475, 1986.
663. Carpentier, A., Deloche, A., and Dauptain, J.: A new reconstructive operation for correction of mitral and tricuspid insufficiency. J. Thorac. Cardiovasc. Surg. *61*:1, 1971.
664. Kirklin, J. W., and Barratt-Boyes, B. G.: Tricuspid valve disease. *In* Cardiac Surgery. New York, John Wiley and Sons, 1986, pp. 447–462.
665. Stolf, N.A.G., Moreira, L.F.P., Costa, R., et al.: The DeVega annuloplasty as surgical treatment for tricuspid incompetence. Int. J. Surg. *68*:201, 1983.
666. Cohen, S. R., Sell, J. E., McIntosh, C. L., and Clark, R. E.: Tricuspid regurgitation in patients with acquired, chronic, pure mitral regurgitation. II. Nonoperative management, tricuspid valve annuloplasty, and tricuspid valve replacement. J. Thorac. Cardiovasc. Surg. *94*:488, 1987.
667. Minale, C., Lambertz, H., Nikol, S., et al.: Selective annuloplasty of the tricuspid valve. Two years experience. J. Thorac. Cardiovasc. Surg. *99*:846, 1990.
668. Duran, C.M.G., Pomar, J. L., Colman, T., et al.: Is tricuspid valve repair necessary? J. Thorac. Cardiovasc. Surg. *80*:849, 1980.
669. Chidambaram, M., Abdulali, S. A., Baliga, B. G., and Ionescu, M. I.: Long-term results of DeVega tricuspid annuloplasty. Ann. Thorac. Surg. *43*:185, 1987.
670. Kratz, J. M., Crawford, F. A., Stroud, M. R., et al.: Trends and results in tricuspid valve surgery. Chest *88*:837, 1985.
671. Abe, T., and Komatsu, S.: Valve replacement for Ebstein's anomaly of the tricuspid valve. Chest *84*:414, 1983.
672. Silver, M. A., Cohen, S. R., McIntosh, C. L., et al.: Late (5 to 132 months) clinical and hemodynamic results after either tricuspid valve replacement of annuloplasty for Ebstein's anomaly of the tricuspid valve. Am. J. Cardiol. *54*:627, 1984.
673. Miller, B. R., Vohr, F. H., Christian, F. V., and Singh, A. K.: Cardiac valvular replacement in carcinoid heart disease. Am. J. Med. *75*:896, 1983.
674. Kirshenbaum, H. D.: Pulmonary valve disease. *In* Dalen, J. E., and Alpert, J. S. (eds.): Valvular Heart Disease. 2nd ed. Boston, Little, Brown and Company, 1987, pp. 403–438.
675. Vela, J. E., Conteras, R., and Sosa, F. R.: Rheumatic pulmonary valve disease. Am. J. Cardiol. *23*:12, 1969.
676. Altrichter, P. M., Olson, L. J., Edwards, W. D., et al.: Surgical pathology of the pulmonary valve: A study of 116 cases spanning 15 years. Mayo Clin. Proc. *64*:1352, 1989.
677. Seymour, J., Emanuel, R., and Patterson, N.: Acquired pulmonary stenosis. Br. Heart J. *30*:776, 1968.
678. Brayshaw, J. R., and Perloff, J. K.: Congenital pulmonary insufficiency complicating idiopathic dilatation of the pulmonary artery. Am. J. Cardiol. *10*:282, 1962.
679. Runco, V., and Levin, H. S.: The spectrum of pulmonic regurgitation. *In* Physiologic Principles of Heart Sounds and Murmurs. American Heart Association Monograph No. 46, 1975, p. 175.
680. Childers, R. W., and McCrea, P. C.: Absence of the pulmonary valve. A case occurring in the Marfan's syndrome. Circulation *29*:598, 1964.
681. Cassling, R. S., Rogler, W. C., and McManus, B. M.: Isolated pulmonic valve infective endocarditis: A diagnostically elusive entity. Am. Heart J. *109*:558, 1985.
682. Cremieux, A. C., Witchitz, S., Malergue, M. C., et al.: Clinical and echocardiographic observations in pulmonary valve endocarditis. Am. J. Cardiol. *56*:610, 1985.
683. DePace, N. L., Nestico, P. F., Iskandrian, A. S., and Morganroth, J.: Acute severe pulmonic valve regurgitation: Pathophysiology, diagnosis and treatment. Am. Heart J. *108*:567, 1984.
684. Collins, N. P., Braunwald, E., and Morrow, A. G.: Isolated congenital pulmonic valvular regurgitation. Am. J. Med. *28*:159, 1960.
685. Jacoby, W. J., Tucker, D. H., and Sumner, R. G.: The second heart sound in congenital pulmonary valvular insufficiency. Am. Heart J. *69*:603, 1965.
686. O'Toole, J. D., Wurtzbacher, J. J., Wearner, N. E., and Jain, A. C.: Pulmonary valve injury and insufficiency during pulmonary-artery catheterization. N. Engl. J. Med. *301*:1167, 1979.
687. Bousvaros, G. A., and Deuchar, D. C.: The murmur of pulmonary regurgitation which is not associated with pulmonary hypertension. Lancet *2*:962, 1961.
688. Enomoto, D., Fenster, P. E., Ewy, G. A., and Salomon, N.: Effect of mitral regurgitation on the murmur of pulmonic regurgitation. Chest *83*:822, 1983.
689. Masuyama, T., Kodama, K., Kitabatake, A., et al.: Continuous-wave Doppler echocardiographic detection of pulmonary regurgitation and its application to noninvasive estimation of pulmonary artery pressure. Circulation *74*:484, 1986.
690. Green, E. W., Agruss, N. S., and Adolph, R. J.: Right-sided Austin Flint murmur. Documentation by intracardiac phonocardiography, echocardiography and postmortem findings. Am. J. Cardiol. *32*:370, 1973.
691. Braunwald, E., and Morrow, A. G.: A method for detection and estimation of aortic regurgitant flow in man. Circulation *17*:505, 1958.
692. Pernot, C., Hoeffel, J. C., Henry, M., et al.: Radiological patterns of congenital absence of the pulmonary valve in infants. Radiology *102*:619, 1972.
693. Collins, N. P., Braunwald, E., and Morrow, A. G.: Detection of pulmonic and tricuspid valvular regurgitation by means of indicator solutions. Circulation *20*:561, 1959.
694. Van Meurs-Van Woezik, H., McGhie, J., and Roelandt, J.: Septal flutter in pulmonary insufficiency. J. Cardiovasc. Ultrasonogr. *3*:159, 1984.
695. Miyatake, K., Okamoto, M., Kinoshita, N., et al.: Pulmonary regurgitation studied with the ultrasonic pulsed Doppler technique. Circulation *65*:969, 1982.
696. Meltzer, R. S., Vered, Z., Hegesh, T., et al.: Diagnosis of pulmonic regurgitation by contrast echocardiography. Am. Heart J. *107*:102, 1984.
697. Emery, R. W., Landes, R. G., Moller, J. H., and Nicoloff, D. M.: Pulmonary valve replacement with a porcine aortic heterograft. Ann. Thorac. Surg. *27*:148, 1979.
698. Paraskos, J. A.: Combined valvular disease. *In* Dalen, J. E., and Alpert, J. S. (eds.): Valvular Heart Disease. 2nd ed. Boston, Little, Brown and Company, 1987, pp. 439–508.
699. Segal, J., Harvey, W. P., and Hufnagel, C. A.: Clinical study of one hundred cases of severe aortic insufficiency. Am. J. Med. *21*:200, 1956.
700. Gash, A. K., Carabello, B. A., Kent, R. L., et al.: Left ventricular performance in patients with coexistent mitral stenosis and aortic insufficiency. J. Am. Coll. Cardiol. *3*:703, 1984.
701. Zitnik, R. S.: The masking of aortic stenosis by mitral stenosis. Am. Heart J. *69*:22, 1965.
702. Schattenberg, T. T., Titus, J. L., and Parkin, T. W.: Clinical findings in

acquired aortic valve stenosis. Effect of disease of other valves. Am. Heart J. *73*:322, 1967.

703. Melvin, D. B., Tecklenberg, P. L., Hollingsworth, J. F., et al.: Computer-based analysis of preoperative and postoperative prognostic factors in 100 patients with combined aortic and mitral valve replacement. Circulation *48*(Suppl. III):58, 1973.
704. Rippe, J. M.: Multiple floppy valves. An echocardiographic syndrome. Am. J. Med. *66*:817, 1979.
705. Baxley, W. A., and Soto, B.: Hemodynamic evaluation of patients with combined mitral and aortic prostheses. Am. J. Cardiol. *45*:42, 1980.
706. Kirklin, J. W., and Barratt-Boyes, B. G.: Combined aortic and mitral valve disease with or without tricuspid valve disease. *In* Cardiac Surgery. New York, John Wiley and Sons, 1986, pp. 431–446.
707. Stephenson, L. W., Edie, R. N., Harken, A. H., and Edmunds, L. H.: Combined aortic and mitral valve replacement: Changes in practice and prognosis. Circulation *69*:640, 1984.
708. Nitter-Hauge, S., and Horstkotte, D.: Management of multivalvular heart disease. Eur. Heart J. *8*:643, 1987.
709. Stephenson, L. W., Kouchoukos, N. T., and Kirklin, J. W.: Triple valve replacement: An analysis of eight years' experience. Ann. Thorac. Surg. *23*:327, 1977.
710. Coll-Mazzei, J. V., Jegaden, O., Janody, P., et al.: Results of triple valve replacement: Perioperative mortality and long-term results. J. Cardiovasc. Surg. *28*:369, 1987.
711. Michel, P. L., Houdart, E., Ghanem, G., et al.: Combined aortic, mitral and tricuspid surgery: Results in 78 patients. Eur. Heart J. *8*:457, 1987.
712. MacManus, Q., Grunkemeier, G., and Starr, A.: Late results of triple valve replacement: A 14-year review. Ann. Thorac. Surg. *25*:402, 1978.
713. Péterffy, A., Jonasson, R., and Björk, V. O.: Ten years' experience of surgical management of triple valve disease. Early and late results in thirty-four consecutive cases. Scand. J. Thorac. Cardiovasc. Surg. *13*:191, 1979.
714. Vatterott, P. J., Gersh, B. J., Fuster, V., et al.: Long-term followup (2–20 years) of patients with triple valve replacement (abstr.). J. Am. Coll. Cardiol. *1*:586, 1983.

PROSTHETIC CARDIAC VALVES

715. Braunwald, N. S., Cooper, T. S., and Morrow, A. G.: Complete replacement of the mitral valve. J. Thorac. Cardiovasc. Surg. *40*:1, 1960.
716. Harken, D. E., Soroff, M. S., and Taylor, M. C.: Partial and complete prostheses in aortic insufficiency. J. Thorac. Cardiovasc. Surg. *40*:744, 1960.
717. Starr, A., and Edwards, M. L.: Mitral replacement: Clinical experience with a ball-valve prosthesis. Ann. Surg. *154*:726, 1961.
718. Pilegaard, H. K., Lund, O., Nielsen, T. T., et al.: Twenty-two-year experience with aortic valve replacement: Starr-Edwards ball valves versus disc valves. Texas Heart Inst. J. *18*:24, 1991.
719. Grunkemeier, G. L., and Starr, A.: Twenty-five year experience with Starr-Edwards heart valves: Follow-up methods and results. Can. J. Cardiol. *4*:381, 1988.
720. Nair, C., Mohiuddin, S. M., Hilleman, D. E., et al.: Ten-year results with the St. Jude medical prosthesis. Am. J. Cardiol. *65*:217, 1990.
721. Burckhardt, D., Streibel, D., Vogt, S., et al.: Heart valve replacement with St. Jude medical valve prosthesis: Long-term experience in 743 patients in Switzerland. Circulation *78*(Suppl. I):I18, 1988.
722. Austin, E. H., III: Other mechanical prostheses. *In* Crawford, F. A. (ed.): Cardiac Surgery: Current Heart Valve Prostheses. Vol. 1. Hanley and Belfus, Philadelphia, 1987, pp. 237–268.
723. Damle, A., Gelfand, E., and Callaghan, J.: Six years clinical experience with the Omniscience cardiac valve. Can. J. Cardiol *4*:372, 1988.
724. Stewart, S., Cianciotta, D., Hicks, G. L., and DeWeese, J. A.: The Lillehei-Kaster aortic valve prosthesis. J. Thorac. Cardiovasc. Surg. *95*:1023, 1988.
725. Cobanoglu, A., and Brockman, S. K.: Selection of a prosthetic heart valve. *In* Frankl, W. S., and Brest, A. N. (eds.): Cardiovascular Clinics. Valvular Heart Disease: Comprehensive Evaluation and Management. Philadelphia, F. A. Davis, 1986, pp. 399–414.
726. Starek, P.J.K., Beaudet, R. L., and Hall, K.-V.: The Medtronic-Hall valve: Development and clinical experience. *In* Crawford, F. A. (ed.): Cardiac Surgery: Current Heart Valve Prostheses. Vol. 1. Hanley and Belfus, Philadelphia, 1987, pp. 223–236.
727. Beaudet, R. L., Nakhle, G., Beaulieu, C. R., et al.: Medtronic-Hall prosthesis: Valve related deaths and complications. Can. J. Cardiol. *4*:376, 1988.
728. Lindblom, D., Rodriguez, L., and Björk, V. O.: Mechanical failure of the Björk-Shiley valve. J. Thorac. Cardiovasc. Surg. *97*:95, 1989.
729. Lindblom, D.: Long-term clinical results after mitral valve replacement with the Björk-Shiley prosthesis. J. Thorac. Cardiovasc. Surg. *95*:321, 1988.
730. Björk, V. O.: The Björk-Shiley tilting disc valve: Past, present, and future. *In* Crawford, F. A. (ed.): Cardiac Surgery: Current Heart Valve Prostheses. Vol. 1. Hanley and Belfus, Philadelphia, 1987, pp. 183–202.
731. Harker, L. A.: Antithrombotic therapy following mitral valve replacement. *In* Duran, C., et al. (eds.): Recent Progress in Mitral Valve Disease. London, Butterworths, 1984, pp. 340–348.
732. Alam, M., Rosman, H. S., Lakier, J. B., et al.: Doppler and echocardiographic features of normal and dysfunctioning bioprosthetic valves. J. Am. Coll. Cardiol. *10*:851, 1987.
733. Akins, C. W., Carroll, D. L., Buckley, M. J., et al.: Late results with Carpentier-Edwards porcine bioprosthesis. Circulation *82*(Suppl. IV):65, 1990.
734. Sugimoto, J. T., and Karp, R. B.: Homografts and cyropreserved valves. *In* Crawford, F. A. (ed.): Cardiac Surgery: Current Heart Valve Prostheses. Vol. 1. Hanley and Belfus, Philadelphia, 1987, pp. 295–316.
735. Khan, S. S., Mitchell, R. S., Derby, G. C., et al.: Differences in Hancock and Carpentier-Edwards porcine xenograft aortic valve hemodynamics: Effect of valve size. Circulation *82*(Suppl. IV):117, 1990.
736. Matsuki, O., Okita, Y., Almeida, R. S., et al.: Two decades experience with aortic valve replacement with pulmonary autograft. J. Thorac. Cardiovasc. Surg. *95*:705, 1988.
737. O'Brien, M. F., Stafford, E. G., Gardner, M. A. H., et al.: A comparison of aortic valve replacement with viable cryopreserved and fresh allograft valves, with a note on chromosomal studies. J. Thorac. Cardiovasc. Surg. *94*:812, 1987.
738. Carpentier, A., Lemaigre, G., and Robert, L.: Biological factors affecting long-term results of valvular heterografts. J. Thorac. Cardiovasc. Surg. *58*:467, 1969.
739. Cohn, L. H., Collins, J. J., DiSesa, V. J., et al.: Fifteen-year experience with 1678 Hancock porcine bioprosthetic heart valve replacements. Ann. Surg. *210*:435, 1989.
740. Bortolotti, U., Milano, A., Mazzucco, A., et al.: Results of reoperation for primary tissue failure of porcine bioprostheses. J. Thorac. Cardiovasc. Surg. *90*:564, 1985.
741. Fawzy, M. E., Halim, M., Ziady, G., et al.: Hemodynamic evaluation of porcine bioprostheses in the mitral position by Doppler echocardiography. Am. J. Cardiol. *59*:643, 1987.
742. Magilligan, D. J., Jr.: Porcine bioprostheses. *In* Crawford, F. A. (ed.): Cardiac Surgery: Current Heart Valve Prostheses. Vol. 1. Philadelphia, Hanley and Belfus, 1987, pp. 269–284.
743. Nellessen, U., Masuyama, T., Appleton, C. P., et al.: Mitral prosthesis malfunction: Comparative Doppler echocardiographic studies of mitral prostheses before and after replacement. Circulation *79*:330, 1989.
744. Khuri, S. F., Folland, E. D., Sethi, G. K., et al.: Six month postoperative hemodynamics of the Hancock heterograft and the Björk-Shiley prosthesis: Results of a Veteran's Administration cooperative prospective randomized trial. J. Am. Coll. Cardiol. *12*:8, 1988.
745. Janusz, M. T., Jamieson, W.R.E., Burr, L. H., et al.: Thromboembolism risks and role of anticoagulants in patients in chronic atrial fibrillation following mitral valve replacement with porcine bioprostheses. J. Am. Coll. Cardiol. *1*:587, 1983.
746. Jamieson, W. R. E., Tyers, G. F. O., Janusz, M. T., et al.: Age as a determinant for selection of porcine bioprostheses for cardiac valve replacement: Experience with Carpentier-Edwards standard bioprosthesis. Can. J. Cardiol. *7*:181, 1991.
747. Crawford, F. A.: The Ionescu-Shiley pericardial xenograft. *In* Crawford, F. A. (ed.): Cardiac Surgery: Current Heart Valve Prostheses. Vol. 1. Philadelphia, Hanley and Belfus, 1987, pp. 285–294.
748. Trowbridge, E. A., Lawford, P. V., Crofts, C. E., and Roberts, K. M.: Pericardiac heterografts: Why do these valves fail? J. Thorac. Cardiovasc. Surg. *95*:577, 1988.
749. Bloomfield, P., Wheatley, D. J., Prescott, R. J., and Miller, H. C.: Twelve-year comparison of a Björk-Shiley mechanical heart valve with porcine bioprostheses. N. Engl. J. Med. *324*:573, 1991.
750. Roberts, W. C.: Complications of cardiac valve replacement: Characteristic abnormalities of prostheses pertaining to any specific site. Am. Heart J. *103*:113, 1982.
751. Nashof, S.A.M., Sethia, B., Turner, M. A., et al.: Björk-Shiley and Carpentier-Edwards valves: A comparative analysis. J. Thorac. Cardiovasc. Surg., *93*:394, 1987.
752. Hammond, G. L., Geha, A. S., Klopf, G. S., and Hashim, S. W.: Biological versus mechanical valves. Analysis of 1116 valves inserted in 1012 adult patients with a 4818 patient-year and a 5327 valve-year followup. J. Thorac. Cardiovasc. Surg. *93*:182, 1987.
753. Oakley, C.: Valve prostheses and pregnancy. Br. Heart J. *58*:303, 1987.
754. Sareli, P., England, M. J., Berk, M. R., et al.: Maternal and fetal sequelae of anticoagulation during pregnancy in patients with mechanical heart valve prostheses. Am. J. Cardiol. *63*:1462, 1989.
755. Salazar, E., Zajarias, A., Gutierrez, N., and Iturbe, I.: The problem of cardiac valve prostheses, anticoagulants, and pregnancy. Circulation *70*(Suppl. I):169, 1984.
756. Iturbe-Alessio, I., Fonesca, M.D.C., Mutchinik, O., et al.: Risks of anticoagulant therapy in pregnant women with artificial heart valves. N. Engl. J. Med. *315*:1390, 1986.
757. Limet, R., and Grondin, C. M.: Cardiac valve prostheses, anticoagulation and pregnancy. Ann. Thorac. Surg. *23*:337, 1977.
758. John, S.: Valve replacement in the young patients with rheumatic heart disease: Review of a twenty year experience. J. Thorac. Cardiovasc. Surg. *99*:631, 1990.
759. Ilbawi, M. N., Idriss, F. S., DeLeon, S. Y., et al.: Valve replacement in children: Guidelines for selection of prosthesis and timing of surgical intervention. Ann. Thorac. Surg. *44*:398, 1987.
760. Selwyn, L., Rao, S., Mardin, M. K., et al.: Prosthetic valves in children and adolescents. Am. Heart J. *121*:557, 1991.
761. Gardner, T. J.: Anticoagulants for children requiring heart valve replacement. *In* Dunn, J. M. (ed.): Cardiac Valve Disease in Children. New York, Elsevier, 1988, p. 359
762. Smith, N. D., Raizada, V., and Abrams, J.: Auscultation of the normally functioning prosthetic valve. Ann. Intern. Med. *95*:594, 1981.
763. Radhakrishnan, S., Behl, V. K., Bajaj, R., et al.: Doppler echocardiographic evaluation of normal and thrombosed Björk-Shiley mitral prosthetic valves. Int. J. Cardiol *20*:387, 1988.
764. Klein, H. O., Schamroth, C. L., Marcus, B. D., et al.: Echo-phonocardiographic assessment of the Medtronic-Hall mitral valve prosthesis: Observations on normal and abnormal function. J. Cardiovasc. Ultrasonogr. *5*:115, 1986.
765. Alam, M., Serwin, J. B., Rosman, H. S., et al.: Transesophageal echocardiographic features of normal and dysfunctioning bioprosthetic valves. Am. Heart J. *121*:1149, 1991.

35

Infective Endocarditis

by OKSANA M. KORZENIOWSKI, M.D., and DONALD KAYE, M.D.

DEFINITION AND CLASSIFICATION

Infective endocarditis (IE) usually refers to bacterial or fungal infection within the heart, although chlamydial and rickettsial infections also occur; the role of viruses is unknown. Extracardiac endothelium also can be colonized by microorganisms, and the infection (more properly called endarteritis) produces a clinical syndrome indistinguishable from that of IE.[1]

Endocarditis historically has been classified as *acute* or *subacute* on the basis of the clinical course as observed before availability of antimicrobial therapy. *Acute* endocarditis denoted infection on a normal valve by virulent organisms such as *Staphylococcus aureus, Streptococcus pneumoniae, Neisseria gonorrhoeae, Streptococcus pyogenes,* and *Haemophilus influenzae,* which rapidly destroyed the heart valve and caused widespread metastatic foci. Death occurred in less than 6 weeks. *Subacute* endocarditis referred to infection on abnormal valves (usually rheumatic) with relatively avirulent organisms such as viridans streptococci or *Staphylococcus epidermidis.* The course was indolent (up to 2 years), and metastatic foci were uncommon. Such classic presentations of IE are now encountered less frequently. Currently, patients with prosthetic cardiac valves, users of illicit parenteral drugs, and patients with mitral valve prolapse or other nonrheumatic abnormalities, rather than patients with rheumatic heart disease, account for the majority of cases of endocarditis. The bacteriology in each population differs, and correlations between organism and course are variable. Current useful classifications refer to underlying anatomy (i.e., native valve intravenous (IV) drug abuser or prosthetic valve) and infecting organism, and serve as a basis for therapy and prognosis (e.g., viridans streptococcal endocarditis on a native valve).

NATIVE VALVE ENDOCARDITIS

Most people (60 to 80 per cent) with native valve endocarditis who do not use parenteral drugs have an identifiable predisposing cardiac lesion.[2] The nature of the predisposing lesion and, to some extent, the bacteriology of the infection are determined by the patient's age.

Demographic Characteristics

CHILDREN (see also Chap. 33). The incidence of IE in infancy and childhood is low. It has been reported as 0.34 cases per 100,000 children per year and as ~1 in 4500 pediatric hospital admissions.[3]

Rheumatic Heart Disease. In children infected after the neonatal period, 75 to 100 per cent have identifiable predisposing lesions (Table 35-1).[5,6] Early series implicated rheumatic carditis as the underlying lesion in about one-third of cases of pediatric endocarditis.[7,8] Over the past 20 years the incidence of rheumatic fever has been decreasing and, consequently, rheumatic heart disease has been implicated in fewer cases of endocarditis. In several series from the 1970's and 1980's, only 1.5 to 10 per cent of endocarditis cases were on valves damaged by rheumatic fever.[3,9,10] Most infections involved the mitral and aortic valves. A resurgence in rheumatic fever recently was documented in several metropolitan areas in the United States (p. 1721), and carditis developed in 50 to 90 per cent of the affected children.[11,12] If the trend continues, an increase in the incidence of endocarditis on rheumatic valves can be anticipated.

Congenital Heart Disease. The association between congenital heart disease (CHD) and endocarditis was firmly established by autopsy series in the preantibiotic era. Of 181 children with CHD autopsied, 16.5 per cent had evidence of endocarditis.[13] Ventricular septal defect, patent ductus arteriosus, and tetralogy of Fallot were the most common underlying lesions, but patients with cyanotic heart disease associated with shunts and stenotic valves were noted to be at particular risk. Aortic valve disease accounted for 9 per cent of pediatric patients with IE. Infection of the pulmonary valve is uncommon but most often occurs in conjunction with infection at other structurally abnormal sites, such as uncorrected ventricular septal defect and tetralogy of Fallot.[14] Early series examining the impact of palliative or corrective surgery on the incidence of IE in CHD established cardiac surgery as a risk factor for endocarditis, both directly by way of postsurgical infections, especially in patients with synthetic material in the circulation, and indirectly as a consequence of prolongation of life in such patients.[15] Ostium secundum atrial septal defects seldom become infected because the lesion results in a low-pressure shunt with low turbulence; however, endocarditis that involves the mitral valve has been documented in patients with ostium primum defects.

Viridans streptococci and group D streptococci cause 40 to 50 per cent of pediatric cases (Table 35-1).[5,10,16] The beta-hemolytic streptococci seldom cause endocarditis. Enterococci are responsible for 4 per cent and pneumococci for less than 3 per cent of cases. *S. aureus* is responsible for 25 per cent of pediatric cases of endocarditis, but the incidence appears to be increasing.

ADULTS. The spectrum of recognized cardiac lesions underlying IE in adults has been changing as a result of the decline in the incidence of rheumatic heart disease and improvement in cardiac diagnostic techniques.[2] In a recent series, the major categories of underlying lesions, in descending frequency, were mitral valve prolapse, no underlying disease, degenerative lesions of the aortic and mitral valves, CHD, and rheumatic heart disease (Table 35-1).[2]

In most recent series evaluating nonaddict patients with native valve endocarditis, mitral valve prolapse (p. 1029) has gained prominence as the most common underlying predisposing cardiac lesion.[2,17,18] Mitral valve prolapse with redundancy of the mitral valve is an extremely common condition, with prevalence estimates ranging from 2.5 to 5.0 per cent in the general healthy population and up to 20 per cent in young women.[19] In two series prevalence rates of mitral valve prolapse in patients with IE were 32 per cent (18/56) and 54 per cent (19/35).[2,17] Male gender, the presence of a systolic murmur, and age above 45 years characterize patients at highest risk for IE. The risk for IE with mitral valve prolapse but no murmur is 0.0046 per cent per year; the risk for IE with mitral valve prolapse and a systolic murmur is 0.0520 per cent per year; the incidence of IE in the general population 15 years and older is 0.004 per cent per year.[18,20]

TABLE 35–1 INCIDENCE OF PREDISPOSING VALVULAR LESIONS AND MICROBIAL ISOLATES IN PATIENTS WITH ENDOCARDITIS ON NATIVE VALVES

	CHILDREN (%)		ADULTS %			
	Neonates	Older	<60 yr.	>65 yr.	Pregnant	Addict*
Predisposing Lesion						
RHD	–	1.5–10	25–30	8	74**	–
CHD	28	75–100	10–20	2		10
MVP	–	–	20–50	10	–	–
DHD	–	–	–	30	–	–
Parenteral drug use	–	–	–	–	8	100*
Other	–	–	10–15	10	–	10
None	72	–	25–50	40	18	–
Organisms						
Streptococci	20	40–50	50–70	30	60	6–12
Enterococci	–	4	10	15	6	8
Staphylococci	60	30	25	45	18	60
S. aureus	(80)	(80)	(90)	(65)	(90)	(99)
S. epidermidis	(20)	(20)	(10)	(35)	(10)	(1)
GNB	10	5	<1	5	2	10
Fungi	10	1	<1	–	–	5
Diphtheroids	–	–	<1	–	–	2
Polymicrobial	4	–	–	–	4	5
Other	–	–	<1	–	6	–
Culture negative	4	0–15	5–10	5	4	4–10

RHD, rheumatic heart disease; CHD, congenital heart disease; MVP, mitral valve prolapse; DHD, degenerative heart disease; other, idiopathic hypertrophic subaortic stenosis, Marfan's syndrome, etc.; GNB, gram-negative bacilli.

* All patients are parenteral drug users.

** 74 percent includes RHD and CHD.

Rheumatic heart disease was the underlying lesion in 37 to 76 per cent of cases in the past.[2] It now accounts for about 30 per cent (21 to 42 per cent) of heart lesions in adults with endocarditis.[21] Most patients with rheumatic heart disease and endocarditis are middle-aged or older.[22] The mitral valve is the most commonly involved valve (>85 per cent), and women predominate (2:1) in series in which the mitral valve is solely involved. The aortic valve is the next most commonly affected site (50 per cent), and a male predominance (4:1) is seen with isolated lesions.[23] A tricuspid valve affected by rheumatic heart disease occasionally may be involved, but usually in association with involvement of either the mitral or aortic valve.

Congenital heart disease is the underlying lesion in 10 to 20 per cent of patients.[2] The most common predisposing lesions in adults include patent ductus arteriosus, ventricular septal defect, bicuspid aortic valve, coarctation of the aorta, and pulmonic stenosis. Isolated pulmonic valve endocarditis, in patients with CHD, in particular, atrial and ventricular septal defects, patent ductus arteriosus, and tetralogy of Fallot, is being increasingly recognized as improvements in echocardiographic technology have provided visual access to this site.[24] Bicuspid aortic valve is an important risk factor, especially in men over age 60. Hypertrophic obstructive cardiomyopathy (p. 1404) is a risk factor for endocarditis; about 5 per cent of patients with this condition develop IE.[25] Enhanced risk is conferred on people with a high peak systolic pressure gradient. Sites of involvement include the aortic valve, the mitral valve, and the subaortic endocardium, reflecting the hemodynamic abnormalities (i.e., mitral regurgitation caused by displacement of the anterior leaflet by the abnormal ventricular architecture and turbulence of the jet stream crossing the aortic valve distal to the intraventricular obstruction). Marfan syndrome, when associated with aortic insufficiency, has been involved in IE.[26] The vegetations are found primarily on the mitral valve. Luetic aortic valves are uncommon underlying lesions. Degenerative heart disease, particularly calcific aortic stenosis, is important in predisposing the elderly to endocarditis.

THE ELDERLY. There is a significant trend toward increased age among patients diagnosed with endocarditis.[27] In evaluating patients seen between 1976 and 1985, the percentage over age 60 ranged from 26 per cent of those treated in a veterans' hospital to 23 per cent treated in a university center to 60 per cent treated in a community hospital (the last institution having the lowest proportion of intravenous IV drug abusers).[28] The factors accounting for this shift in age distribution are a marked reduction in the frequency of rheumatic heart disease, longer survival as a result of modern medical and surgical therapy, of patients with CHD and those with valves damaged by rheumatic fever and aging of the population in general. The longer average life span is associated with an increased incidence of degenerative valve disease. The most common predisposing factor to endocarditis in those over age 65 is a prosthetic intravascular device. In elderly patients with native valve endocarditis, degenerative cardiac lesions (i.e., aortic sclerosis with or without a bicuspid aortic valve, calcified mitral annulus, postmyocardial infarction thrombi, atrial thrombi, and ventricular aneurysms) appear to be gaining prominence (Table 35–1).[29,30] Pomerance reported that of those with endocarditis, 33 per cent older than age 65 had no apparent underlying lesion at autopsy, compared with 22 per cent of those younger than 65 years.[31] It is likely that many of those older than 65 had minor degenerative cardiac lesions that were undetected at autopsy but were sufficient to serve as a nidus for initiation of endocarditis. Others may in fact have no structural defects but may have nosocomially acquired endocarditis related to intravenous catheters (23 per cent in one series) infected with a virulent organism such as *S. aureus*.[28] Overall, in the elderly, the mitral valve is involved more commonly than the aortic valve. However, gender difference exists—the aortic valve is involved in 61 per cent of male cases but in only 31 per cent of female cases.

DIABETES MELLITUS. Diabetes has been documented as an associated disease with IE in 15 per cent (8/53) of elderly patients.[28] Although not directly documented, metabolic, immunological, and vascular abnormalities in diabetes may have a significant impact on the susceptibility of patients to endocarditis.[32] Accelerated atherosclerosis results in a high incidence of calcific valvular nodular lesions.[33] Urinary tract infections and soft tissue infections are common in diabetes as a consequence of both poor perfusion and inhibition of leukocytic migration and phagocytosis by acidosis, and can serve as sources of bacteremia.[34] Furthermore, an increased incidence of colonization by *S. aureus* of the skin and nares has been documented in insulin-dependent diabetics.[35] A strong association of group B streptococcal infections with diabetes has been noted, and bacteremias and cases of endocarditis have been documented in diabetics.[36,37]

PREGNANCY (see also p. 1080). IE is an important but uncommon complication of pregnancy.[38] The calculated incidence of IE is 0.03 to 0.14 cases per 1000 deliveries and 5.5 to 9.0 cases per 1000 for patients with preexisting cardiac disease. These incidence rates, however, are based on earlier eras (1950's through 1970); the true incidence reflecting improved management of obstetric complications, legalization of abortion, falling incidence of rheumatic heart disease, and increasing use of IV drugs by women is unknown. Underlying cardiac disease was present in about 75 per cent of cases of IE in obstetric and gynecologic practice (Table 35–1).[39] Most cases were caused by streptococci—primarily viridans streptococci and S. aureus. In pregnancy, the most common portal of entry of bacteria was dental procedures. Puerperal endocarditis occurred after both vaginal delivery and cesarean delivery. Potential predisposing factors included premature labor, prolonged rupture of membranes, prolonged third stage of labor, and manual removal of the placenta.[39] Based on the number of abortions performed yearly in the United States, the incidence of endocarditis is believed to be below 1 per 1 million abortions.

MICROBIOLOGY

Streptococci (50 to 70 per cent), enterococci (10 per cent), and staphylococci (25 per cent) account for the majority of cases of endocarditis on native valves in nonintravenous drug abusers (Table 35–1).[2,18,27,28]

VIRIDANS STREPTOCOCCI. This organism is a normal inhabitant of the oropharynx, and accounts for more than half of all streptococcal infections.[40] These organisms usually are beta-hemolytic and nontypable by the Lancefield system. This group includes a variety of species, including *Streptococcus mitior* (25 per cent of cases of IE on native valves in non-drug abusers), *Streptococcus sanguis* (~20 per cent), *Streptococcus mutans* (~10%), *Streptococcus anginosus* (~5 per cent), and *Streptococcus salivarius* (~1 per cent).[40,41] Most are highly susceptible to penicillin and cause infections primarily on abnormal heart valves. The clinical course usually is indolent. *S. mutans* is fastidious on culture and frequently hydrolyzes bile-esculin; thus it may be confused with enterococci.[42] It grows best on horse blood agar in 5 to 10 per cent carbon dioxide on subculture, requires more than 3 days for primary isolation, and morphologically is quite pleomorphic. Nutritionally deficient variant streptococci, usually *S. mitior*, may be difficult to isolate.[43] Therapy for IE caused by nutritionally deficient variant streptococci tends to result in more frequent relapses than with other viridans species.[42]

ENTEROCOCCI. These organisms were classified as streptococci and recently reclassified as a separate genus. They include *Enterococcus faecalis, Enterococcus faecium,* and *Enterococcus durans.*[44] They are alpha-, beta-, or gamma-hemolytic, and normally inhabit the gastrointestinal tract and the anterior urethra. They grow well in sodium azide ("SF broth"), 40 per cent bile, 6.5 per cent sodium chloride, and 0.1 per cent methylene blue, and can survive at high temperatures (56°C) and high pH (9.6). Enterococci can attack normal or damaged heart valves.[45] Most patients are older men (60 years or older), many of whom give a recent history of genitourinary manipulation, trauma, or disease (cystoscopy, urethral catheterization, or prostatectomy), or, less commonly, young women (less than 40 years old) who have undergone abortion, pregnancy, or cesarean delivery.[46] Correct biochemical identification of enterococci is important because the organisms are relatively resistant to penicillin G and penicillin alone is not bactericidal. Thus, high doses of penicillin must be used and an aminoglycoside must be added to achieve a bactericidal effect on these organisms.[47] Recent identification of beta-lactamase–producing strains,[48] strains with high-level resistance to all aminoglycosides,[49] and vancomycin-resistant enterococci[50] has further increased the complexity of therapeutic regimens.

OTHER STREPTOCOCCI. *S. bovis* and *S. equinus* are group D streptococci. They differ biochemically from enterococci (which also type with group D typing serum) and can be separated from enterococci by determination of arginine or starch hydrolysis. They usually are readily killed by penicillin alone.[51] *S. bovis* endocarditis primarily occurs in the elderly (older than 60 years of age) and frequently is associated with the presence of colonic polyps (67 per cent versus 21 per cent of patients with enterococcal endocarditis) or colonic malignancy (18 per cent versus 2 per cent enterococcal endocarditis).[52,53]

Other Lancefield group streptococci account for less than 5 per cent of cases of endocarditis. Group A and group B streptococci can attack normal valves and produce distant metastases. Group B streptococci (*Streptococcus agalactiae*) are normal inhabitants of the mouth, vagina, anterior urethra, and gastrointestinal tract.[36] *S. agalactiae* has now been recognized as a significant pathogen in adults with diabetes mellitus, carcinoma, and hepatic failure as well as being a major pathogen in neonates and young pregnant women.[37] An association of *S. agalactiae* bacteremia with colonic villus adenomas recently has been noted.[54] More than 70 cases of *S. agalactiae* endocarditis have been reported since the 1940's. Most patients have fulminant disease with large, crumbling vegetations and systemic emboli, perhaps reflecting the absence of fibrinolysin production by the bacterium.[37] A similar clinical syndrome with high morbidity and mortality also has been reported as caused by group G streptococci.[55] Susceptibility to penicillin of the typable streptococci is variable, and an aminoglycoside may need to be added to achieve an adequate bactericidal effect.[55]

STREPTOCOCCUS PNEUMONIAE. This form of endocarditis occurred in 10 per cent of patients in series collected before the advent of penicillin. It now accounts for only 1 to 3 per cent of cases of IE, even though pneumococcal bacteremia remains common.[56–59] *S. pneumoniae* can infect normal valves, has a predilection for the aortic valve, and has an unusually high incidence of tricuspid valve involvement. Alcoholism is recognized as a risk factor for endocarditis (~40 per cent of patients), as are advanced age and diabetes. The course is fulminant with rapid valvular destruction, frequent perivalvular abscess formation, and purulent pericarditis. Sixty to 90 per cent of patients have concurrent meningitis. Most pneumococcal isolates remain sensitive to penicillin, but relatively resistant strains (minimal inhibitory concentration to penicillin $\geq$0.1 to $\leq$2.0 μg/ml) are being recognized with increasing frequency in the United States as well as in other countries.[60] Strains highly resistant to multiple antibiotics (but reliably susceptible to vancomycin), first recognized in South Africa, have been identified in Europe, the United States, and Canada.[61]

STAPHYLOCOCCI. These organisms cause 25 per cent of cases of native valve endocarditis.[62] Most are coagulase-positive (*S. aureus*). Coagulase-negative (*S. epidermidis*) species account for less than 10 per cent of isolates (1 to 3 per cent of cases of native valve endocarditis). The great majority of staphylococci, acquired either in the hospital or in the community, are highly resistant to penicillin G because of their ability to elaborate beta-lactamase.[63] *S. aureus* endocarditis usually is fulminant with multiple metastatic abscesses, and affected valves are rapidly destroyed.[64,65] *S. aureus* bacteremia commonly occurs in patients with soft tissue infections and as a nosocomial complication in patients with intravascular catheters. Because *S. aureus* can attack either normal or damaged valves, sometimes it is difficult to determine if a valve has been infected in patients with positive blood cultures for *S. aureus* but who have none of the characteristic clinical features of IE.

The percentage of patients with *S. aureus* bacteremia who have underlying IE is variable: 50 to 60 per cent of patients in populations with a high prevalence of underlying predisposing cardiac lesions, 15 to 25 per cent of patients in unselected populations, and 1 to 16 per cent of patients with a removable focus of infection (i.e., an IV catheter) but no underlying valvular disease.[66] Three clinical risk criteria—absent primary focus, community acquisition, and metastatic sequelae—that are strongly predictive (74 per cent) of IE in IV drug abusers (discussed below) are much less reliable (50 per cent predictive value) in non-addicts with *S. aureus* bacteremia.[66]

Community-acquired strains of *S. aureus* usually are susceptible to penicillinase-resistant beta-lactam antibiotics. The clinical significance of antibiotic tolerance (marked dissociation of minimal inhibitory concentration and minimal bactericidal concentration of cell wall–active antibiotics after 18 to 24 hours of incubation) has not been established.[67] Methicillin-resistant strains of *S. aureus* are becoming a major problem in nosocomially acquired infections.[62]

S. epidermidis. This organism causes an indolent infection on previously damaged valves.[62,68] Coagulase-negative staphylococci are common skin commensals, and the most common bacteria to contaminate blood cultures. A presumptive diagnosis of endocarditis caused by these organisms rests on repeated isolation of the same strain from multiple separate blood cultures. Determination of species, antibiogram analysis, phage typing, and plasmid profiles have been used with variable success to demonstrate strain identity.[62] Several reports have noted species other than *S. epidermidis* (*Staphylococcus warneri, Staphylococcus cohnii, Staphylococcus saprophyticus, Staphylococcus hemolyticus,* and *Staphylococcus hominis*) as causes of native valve endocarditis. In nosocomially acquired (i.e., catheter-related) coagulase-negative staphylococcal endocarditis, *S. epidermidis* predominated.[68] Most cases of coagulase-negative IE on native valves are community acquired, and the infecting strains are commonly susceptible to methicillin; nosocomial infections are caused by methicillin-resistant strains (frequently also gentamicin- and rifampin-resistant strains).[68] However, the association of antibiotic susceptibility and the location where endocarditis was acquired is not absolute. Thus, antibiotic susceptibility of isolates must be rigorously tested.[62]

OTHER ORGANISMS. Almost all species of bacteria occasionally are identified as causes of native valve endocarditis. Most commonly encountered are *N. gonorrhoeae*,[69,70] *Haemophilus* sp.,[71] and other closely related fastidious, slow-growing, gram-negative bacilli of the HACEK group (*Actinobacillus actinomycetemcomitans, Cardiobacterium hominis, Eikenella corrodens*, and *Kingella* sp.)[72-76]; *Pseudomonas*[77,77a]; *Listeria*[78]; and diphtheroids.[79] Clinical courses can be fulminant or indolent. Serum-susceptible gram-negative enteric organisms and anaerobic organisms are less capable of sustaining endocardial infection.[80,81] Spirochetes (e.g., *Spirillum minor*),[82] cell wall–deficient bacteria,[83] *Brucella*,[84] rickettsiae (*Coxiella burnetii*),[85] and chlamydiae[86] are rare causes of endocarditis.

Fungi. These organisms seldom cause native valve endocarditis in the absence of parenteral drug abuse. Factors that predispose to fungemia (i.e., severe underlying illness, corticosteroids, prolonged use of broad-spectrum antibiotics, and cytotoxic agents) can result in endocarditis in patients with IV catheters.[87] *Candida, Torulopsis*, and *Aspergillus* species usually are implicated. The course is indolent but grave; large vegetations frequently embolize to major vessels in the lower extremities.[87,88,88a]

ENDOCARDITIS IN INTRAVENOUS DRUG ABUSERS

The frequency of endocarditis in IV drug abusers is difficult to estimate.[89] There appear to be differences in relative risk for infection based on the drugs used (i.e., the risk with cocaine is lower than with heroin or amphetamines), the frequency of use, and the modes of drug preparation.[90] Such individuals with endocarditis usually are men (male-female ratio 3 : 1) and young (mean age 30 years).[64,91,92] Underlying cardiac disease is found in about 20 per cent, usually either congenital lesions or residua of previous endocarditis (Table 35–1).[93]

Recent echocardiographic studies have demonstrated mild degrees of tricuspid and pulmonic regurgitation in valves of IV drug abusers without a history of previous endocarditis (13/26 patients versus 1/13 controls).[94] This suggests that IV drug abuse is the human equivalent of stress-induced valvular abnormalities described in animals. These findings might explain the right-sided predilection of IE in drug users.[95] The sites of endocardial involvement based on clinical criteria are a tricuspid valve infected in about 54 per cent, aortic in 25 per cent, and mitral in 20 per cent.[64,91,93] The recent availability of Doppler echocardiography (p. 88) has led to the identification of vegetations that involve the pulmonic valve. In two series collectively describing 42 patients with isolated pulmonary valve endocarditis, 10 patients (24 per cent) were IV drug abusers.[14,96] Patients with pulmonic valve IE constitute 1.1 to 1.4 per cent of all patients with endocarditis. Mixed right- and left-sided endocarditis occurs in 6 per cent.

The sites of involvement as determined in a detailed autopsy series of 80 addicts dying during the first episode of endocarditis (59/80), recurrent endocarditis (10/80), or healed endocarditis (11/80) differ from clinically determined distributions, and reflect the increased mortality of IE in drug addicts when the left side of the heart is involved.[97] The first episode of IE involved a single right-sided cardiac valve in 30 per cent, both a right- and left-sided valve in 16 per cent, a single left-sided valve in 41 per cent, and both left-sided valves in 13 per cent—an average of 1.3 valves per patient. The tricuspid valve was infected in 44 per cent, the mitral in 43 per cent, aortic in 40 per cent, and pulmonic in 3 per cent. In 81 per cent of patients the infected valves were determined to have been anatomically normal before the onset of IE, and 71 per cent of patients had sufficient valvular damage to cause valvular dysfunction.

MICROBIOLOGY. The skin is the most frequent source of microorganisms responsible for endocarditis in IV drug abusers, although contamination of drugs and associated paraphernalia also contributes to bacteremias.[92,98] *S. aureus* is isolated from 60 per cent of cases of IE in these persons; various species of streptococci and enterococci from almost 20 per cent, gram-negative bacilli (predominantly *Pseudomonas* and *Serratia* sp.) from 10 per cent, and fungi (usually *Candida*) from 5 per cent. Anaerobic organisms are uncommon causes of IE, and diagnosis may be delayed because of difficulties in isolating such species from blood cultures.[99] Recent reports have identified *Streptococcus mitis* and group A streptococcus as causes of endocarditis among drug addicts.[100]

Five per cent of addict patients have more than a single microorganism isolated from the blood. In most cases of polymicrobial endocarditis, there are two or three isolates and rarely four or five pathogens.[101] Multiple organisms can either cause the primary infection or be acquired during the course of therapy. *S. aureus* is by far the most common organism isolated in tricuspid endocarditis, and accounts for 80 per cent of clinical isolates. Similarly, in 70 to 80 per cent of cases of *S. aureus* endocarditis in IV drug abusers only the tricuspid valve is involved.

The vast majority (70 to 100 per cent) of addicts with right-sided endocarditis are noted to have pneumonia or multiple septic emboli, but the murmur of tricuspid regurgitation frequently is not present, and that accompanying pulmonic valve endocarditis may be misinterpreted as a functional or flow murmur.[102] Moreover, patients with a syndrome compatible with tricuspid endocarditis may actually have an extracardiac site of endovascular infection (i.e., septic thrombophlebitis involving the subclavian or femoral venous system) rather than endocarditis.[103]

PROSTHETIC VALVE ENDOCARDITIS

Infections of prosthetic valves account for 5 to 15 per cent of all cases of endocarditis.[17,21] The overall incidence of endocarditis in patients with prosthetic valves is 1 to 4 per cent.[104-106,106a] Rutledge and coworkers retrospectively reviewed 1598 patients undergoing prosthetic valve replacement at the National Institutes of Health from 1961 to 1981, and performed an actuarial analysis of the risk of IE.[107] Overall, 43/1598 patients (2.7 per cent) developed endocarditis. The cumulative risk was 3 per cent at 5 years and 5 per cent at 10 years. The risk for prosthetic valve endocarditis (PVE) development peaked 15 days after operation at 45 episodes per 100,000 patient days; the risk then rapidly declined and from 150 days to 20 years remained stable at about 1 episode per 100,000 patient days. Using all patients and all episodes of PVE, the overall rate of infection was 5.9 episodes per 1000 patient years; if a patient survived 60 days without developing PVE, the subsequent rate was 3.7 episodes per 1000 patient years. These findings are consistent with results of others.[106,108]

By convention, PVE is termed "early" when symptoms appear within 60 days of valve insertion and "late" when symptoms occur after that time. The early and late groups differ in clinical features, microbial patterns, and mortality rates. Early PVE usually reflects contamination arising in the perioperative period. Most contamination probably occurs intraoperatively by way of direct wound inoculation or contamination of the bypass machine. Postoperative sources include IV catheters (particularly central lines), arterial lines, urethral catheters, cardiac pacing wires, and endotracheal tubes. The attack rate for early PVE before 1969 was 2.5 per cent of all patients undergoing valve replacement and subsequently has been 0.75 per cent of all such patients.[104-106]

Despite use of prophylactic antibiotics, staphylococcal infection accounts for 45 to 50 per cent of early PVE (Table 35–2). *S. epidermidis* is the most common organism isolated, with an average incidence of 25 to 30 per cent; *S. aureus* causes 20 to 25 per cent. The remainder of cases are caused by gram-negative aerobic organisms (about 20 per cent), fungi (particularly *Candida* and *Aspergillus*, 10 to 12 per cent), streptococci and enterococci (5 to 10 per cent), and diphtheroids (5 to 10 per cent). Occasional unusual causes of PVE include atypical mycobacteria,[109] *Legionella*,[110] mycoplasma,[111] unusual fungi,[112] and *Coxiella*.[113]

Late PVE occurs after valves have been endothelialized. The incidence depends on the length of follow-up. It has been estimated to occur at an overall incidence of 0.2 to 0.5 per cent per patient year. The source for infection is presumed to be seeding of the valve by transient bacteremia arising from dental, genitourinary, or gastrointestinal manipulation. Thus the bacteriology more closely resembles that of native valve endocarditis (Table 35–2). Viridans streptococci are the most

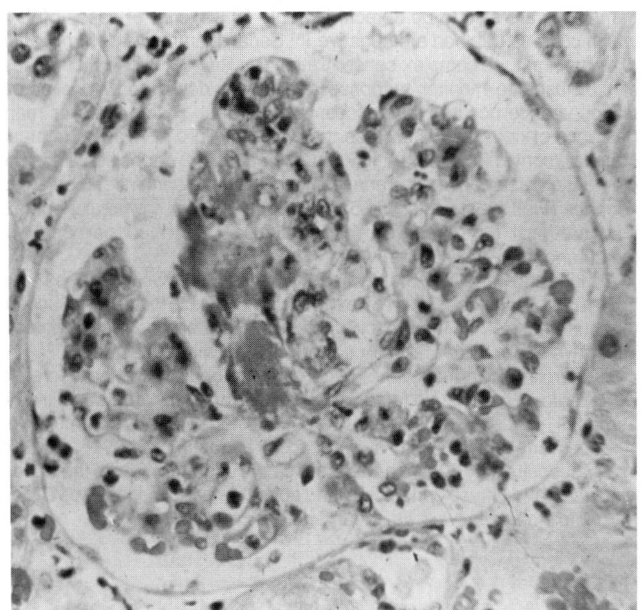

FIGURE 35-4. Microscopic section of glomerulus from patient with IE showing focal hypercellularity and focal necrosis (400×). (From Kaye, D.: Infective Endocarditis. Baltimore, University Park Press, 1976.)

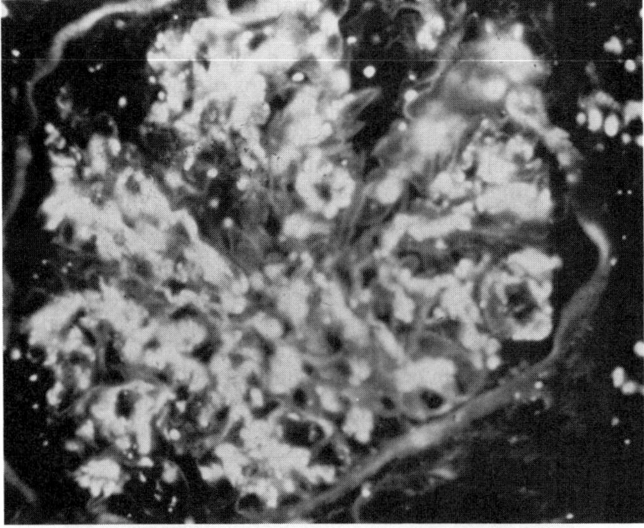

FIGURE 35-5. Microscopic section of glomerulus from patient with IE prepared with fluorescein-tagged antihuman globulin (bright areas). Granular immunoglobulin depositis are seen along the glomerular basement membrane and in the mesangium (400×). (From Kaye, D.: Infective Endocarditis. Baltimore, University Park Press, 1976.)

Heart murmurs are almost always present (>99 per cent of cases) except in acute infections or with right-sided or mural infection. The appearance of a new regurgitant murmur or true changes in a preexisting murmur (not changes in intensity owing to differences in heart rate or cardiac output) have been reported as uncommon (only 16.7 per cent of subacute cases in earlier series[170]), but when present, they suggest acute staphylococcal disease and correlate with development of congestive heart failure. Of interest, in two recent series of patients with IE based on strict clinical criteria, new or changing murmurs were found in 36 to 52 per cent of patients.[28] New or changing murmurs are less common in the elderly. The possibility of endocarditis must always be considered in a febrile patient with a known heart murmur.[28]

Splenomegaly (present in about 30 per cent of cases), *petechiae* (20 to 40 per cent), and *clubbing* of the fingers tend to occur in disease of long duration (greater than 6 weeks).[170,171] *Splenic enlargement* occurred in 80 to 90 per cent of cases in the preantibiotic era; enlargement is still common except in acute cases but less pronounced. *Splenic infarctions*[155a] have been reported in 44 per cent of autopsy cases but are seldom detected clinically. *Clubbing*, formerly present in 25 to 30 per cent of patients with subacute forms of endocarditis, now occurs in only 10 to 20 per cent of patients with disease of long duration.

Petechiae (Fig. 35-6) are most frequently found on the conjunctivae, palate, buccal mucosa, and skin above the clavicles; they may be embolic or vasculitic. Petechiae are not specific to endocarditis, because lesions develop in patients with hematological disorders, vasculitis, scurvy, or renal insufficiency and as a consequence of fat or cholesterol emboli. *Splinter hemorrhages* (subungual, linear, dark red streaks) are nonspecific (Fig. 35-7). They often are related to trauma. Lesions located proximally in the nailbed are more suggestive of endocarditis than are distal lesions. The number of fingers involved is variable; in some cases the toes may be involved. *Osler nodes* (small, tender nodules, usually on the finger or toe pads, that persist for hours to days) occur in 10 to 25 per cent of patients, but also in other diseases.[172] They also may be present on the dorsal surfaces of toes, soles, forearms, and ears; on occasion they become necrotic[173] (p. 18). Immune complexes have been demonstrated in dermal vessels of Osler nodes, but occasional recovery of bacteria after aspiration suggests that they also may result from septic emboli.[174] *Janeway lesions* (1- to 4-mm, nontender, hemorrhagic areas on the palms and soles) are due to septic emboli.[175] They are most commonly seen in acute endocarditis (Fig. 35-8). *Roth spots* (oval, retinal hemorrhages with a pale center located near the optic disk) occur in less than 5 per cent of patients with endocarditis, and also are found in patients with connective tissue disease and hematological disorders (Fig. 35-9).

Musculoskeletal complaints (arthralgias or arthritis) may mimic rheumatological disorders.[166] *Systemic emboli* may occur during or after therapy, and are recognized in about a third of patients. *Pulmonary emboli* are common in addicts with tricuspid valve endocarditis (70 to 100 per cent are noted to have pneumonia or septic pulmonary emboli) and can be seen in left-sided endocarditis with left-to-right cardiac shunts.[64,65]

Neurological manifestations are present in about one-third of patients with endocarditis.[177] Major cerebral emboli to the middle cerebral artery system account for 25 per cent and mycotic aneurysms for 2 to 10 per cent, but brain abscesses and purulent meningitis, cerebral arteritis, cranial nerve palsy, intracerebral bleeding, and encephalomalacia have been documented. The most common complaint is *headache*, and most patients show improvement with supportive care and antimicrobial therapy. *Mycotic aneurysms* account for 2.5 to 6.2 per cent of all intracranial aneurysms (Fig. 35-10).[154] In a Mayo Clinic series of 628 patients with IE treated between 1963 and 1979, 8 (1.3 per cent) were found to have cerebral mycotic aneurysms; all 8 complained of severe, unremitting, localized headache, a complaint that should strongly suggest the possibility of a mycotic aneurysm.[154] Many other reports suggest that most patients with intracranial mycotic aneurysms are asymptomatic.[148] The true incidence of mycotic aneurysms is unknown. The diagnosis usually is made after a sudden catastrophic hemorrhage.[159]

Congestive heart failure (CHF) is the most common complication of IE.[178] Contributing factors include valve destruction, myocarditis, coronary artery emboli with myocardial infarction, and myocardial abscesses. CHF with aortic valve infective endocarditis is associated with a higher mortality than is CHF with mitral valve infection.[179] *Renal disease* is present in most patients with endocarditis, and is due to glomerulonephritis (up to 80 per cent), infarction (50 per cent), or abscesses (uncommon).[165] Renal insufficiency may result. Metastatic infection (i.e., pyogenic meningitis, splenic abscess, pyelonephritis, osteomyelitis, discitis) occurs most frequently in endocarditis caused by *S. aureus*.[148,154] Persistence of fever, localized pain, persistently abnormal results of liver function tests, and "breakthrough bacteremia" after institution of ap-

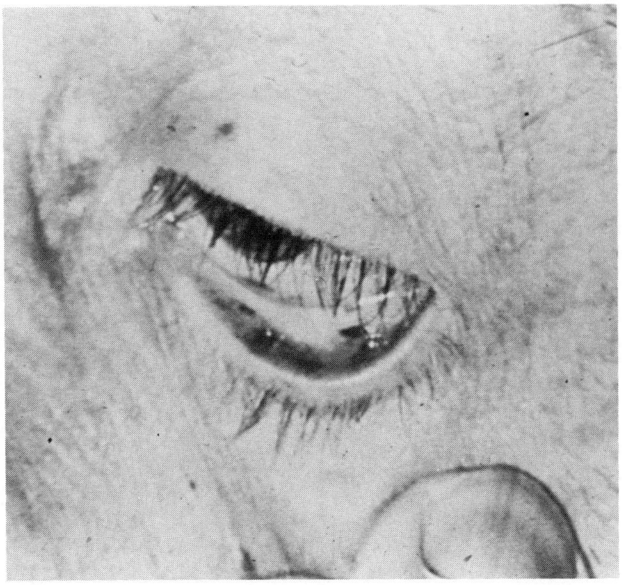

FIGURE 35-6. Conjunctival petechiae in a patient with IE. (From Kaye, D.: Infective Endocarditis. Baltimore, University Park Press, 1976.)

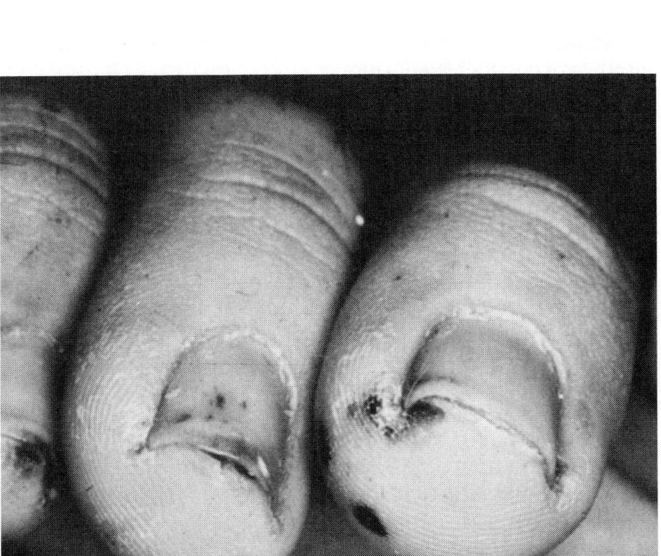

FIGURE 35-7. Subungual hemorrhages (splinter hemorrhages) and digital petechiae in a patient with IE.

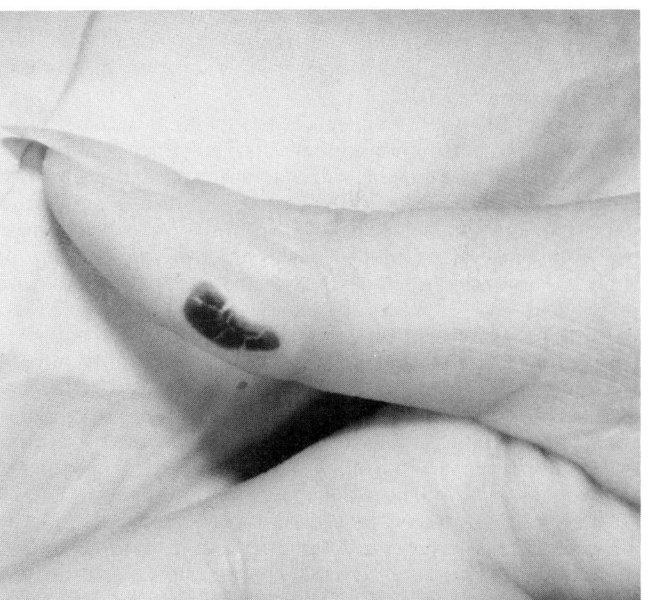

FIGURE 35-8. Janeway lesions on the thumb in a patient with endocarditis.

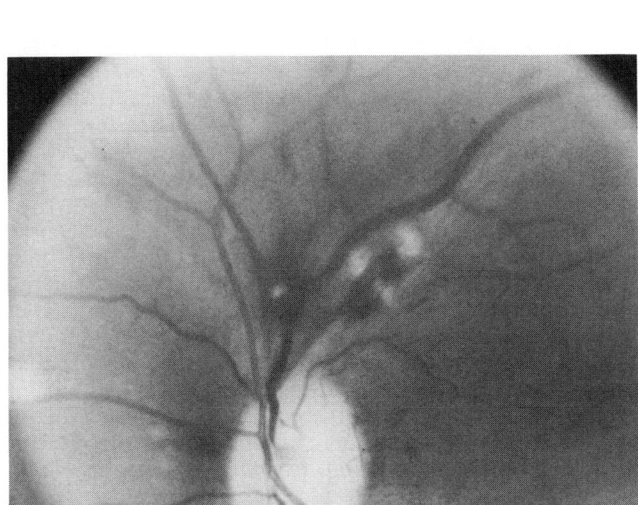

FIGURE 35-9. Roth spot (retinal hemorrhage with a clear center) in a patient with IE.

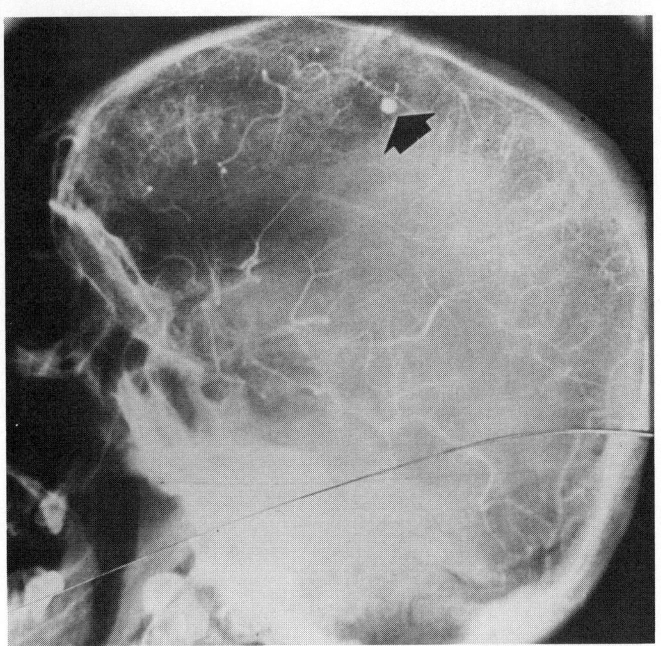

FIGURE 35-10. Angiographic demonstration of a large aneurysm (arrow) of cerebral artery in a patient with IE. (From Kaye, D.: Infective Endocarditis. Baltimore, University Park Press, 1976.)

propriate therapy suggest the diagnosis of metastatic abscess. Patients with metastatic infections are at high risk for relapse of IE.

DIFFERENTIAL DIAGNOSIS

The diagnosis of IE may be suspected either by clinical presentation or by results of blood cultures in the absence of a suggestive syndrome. Proof of endocarditis requires isolation of the infecting microorganism from blood, from an embolus, or from a vegetation or demonstration of infected vegetations at surgery or autopsy.[170]

Endocarditis should be suspected in a patient with a significant heart murmur when unexplained fever is present for at least 1 week or in a febrile IV drug abuser even in the absence of a murmur.[95,102] Endocarditis also should be suspected in a young person with a stroke[154,180] and in patients with a prosthetic valve who are febrile or who have valve dysfunction, such as a new murmur.[105,181] Even with a syndrome classic for endocarditis, a definitive diagnosis requires positive blood cultures or positive cultures of surgical or autopsy specimens (vegetation or emboli) because other diseases can duplicate the syndrome of endocarditis.[17,28a] For example, atrial myxoma, NBTE, acute rheumatic fever, systemic lupus erythematosus, other connective tissue diseases, thrombotic thrombocytopenic purpura, and sickle cell disease can produce a syndrome that is indistinguishable from that of IE.

After cardiac surgery, fever may be related to infection at other sites, to the postcardiotomy syndrome, or to a "post-pump syndrome" (such as with cytomegalovirus infection) rather than to endocarditis (Chap. 53)[182] Furthermore, any patient with an existing heart murmur can develop fever related to another occult illness or to drugs. Therefore, in the absence of postive blood cultures, a search must be made for other causes of fever.

Another setting in which endocarditis should be suspected is in the patient who is treated with antimicrobial agents with response of symptoms (e.g., fever, malaise) only to relapse when therapy is stopped. Some patients have multiple episodes of symptoms, treatment, and then relapse. Furthermore, the therapy is likely to temporarily suppress positive blood cultures, confusing the diagnosis.

Although a murmur may not be present at the time of diagnosis, it may become detectable during therapy or even after therapy is completed.[28,169] Development of a murmur *during therapy* is particularly prone to occur with acute endocarditis, most often caused by coagulase-positive staphylococci.[63-66] The appearance of a *new murmur* usually is related to perforation of the valve, rupture of chordae tendineae, or rupture of a papillary muscle. With prosthetic valve or tricuspid valve endocarditis, a murmur may never appear.[95,102,183]

Not uncommonly, febrile patients with or without a murmur have blood cultures performed as part of a diagnostic evaluation. When blood cultures are reported as positive, the possibility of endocarditis arises. Three factors must be considered in evaluating the significance of the microorganisms isolated from the blood. The first is whether the bacteremia is sustained or transient, as an intravascular infection such as endocarditis tends to produce sustained bacteremia[184]; in turn, sustained bacteremia must always raise the possibility of intravascular infection. We define sustained bacteremia as presence of the same microorganism in blood for at least 1 hour, as transient bacteremias are cleared in 30 minutes or less.[185] Isolation of an organism from blood cultures at only a single point in time may indicate contamination or transient bacteremia and does not constitute evidence for endocarditis.

The second major consideration is the identity of the microorganism. Certain bacteria, such as salmonellae, brucellae, meningococci, and enteric gram-negative bacilli, produce sustained bacteremia relatively frequently but are *rare causes of IE*. Other organisms, such as viridans streptococci and coagulase-negative staphylococci, seldom, if ever, produce sustained bacteremia without an intravascular focus. Coagulase-positive staphylococci and pneumococci often produce sustained bacteremia which may or may not be indicative of endocarditis.[66,186,187]

The third factor to consider is whether or not there is another explanation for the sustained bacteremia, such as infection at another site. Combinations of these factors often come into play. For example, sustained pneumococcal bacteremia in the absence of pneumonia strongly suggests endocarditis, but in the presence of pneumonia it may or may not indicate endocarditis. Sustained coagulase-negative staphylococcal bacteremia in the absence of an intravascular catheter is highly suggestive of endocarditis; in the presence of a catheter, endocarditis may or may not be present.

LABORATORY

BLOOD CULTURES

The critical diagnostic finding in IE is bacteremia or fungemia. In the absence of previous antimicrobial therapy, blood cultures are positive in more than 95 per cent of patients. The bacteremia is continuous; if any cultures are positive, all are likely to be positive.[184] For example, in one large series of 206 patients with blood culture–positive streptococcal endocarditis, 750 of 789 (95 per cent) blood cultures were positive for the causative organisms.[184] Intermittently positive and negative cultures were unusual. The first culture was positive in 95 per cent and the first or second in 98 per cent of the patients. Although constant, the bacteremia usually was low grade with less than 100 bacteria per milliliter of blood in more than 80 per cent of patients. Because the bacteremia of endocarditis is continuous, there is no advantage to obtaining cultures at any particular time or body temperature. Arterial blood offers *no* advantage over antecubital vein blood.[188]

In subacute disease, in the absence of previous therapy, three cultures should be obtained at least 1 hour apart. In those in whom the diagnosis seems likely, therapy should be started without waiting for a confirmatory positive culture. Blood cultures may be negative in as many as 25 per cent of patients who received recent outpatient antibiotic therapy,[189-191] and it is prudent, depending on the clinical status of the patient, to delay treatment to maximize the chance of obtaining positive blood cultures. In general, in acute disease, therapy should not be delayed for more than 2 to 3 hours while obtaining three blood cultures. Cultures should be spaced at least 30 minutes apart to allow proof that the bacteremia was continuous.

Only one culture should be obtained from each venipuncture site. At least 10 ml of blood should be obtained per culture and diluted tenfold in culture medium using both aerobic and anaerobic techniques. The yield of positive cultures is increased by observing them over 3 weeks and making periodic Gram stains and subcultures. Addition of pyridoxal hydrochloride to media will improve the chances of isolating nutritionally deficient variant streptococci.[43,192] Hypertonic media have been advocated to improve recovery of cell wall–deficient bacteria from previously treated patients. Their value, however, is controversial.[193]

Blood cultures may be negative in infections with fastidious organisms such as *H. parainfluenzae, Brucella* sp., or anaerobes. Prolonged incubation, up to 4 weeks, may increase recovery. Fifty per cent of patients with *Candida* endocarditis and almost all with *Aspergillus, Histoplasma, Coxiella burnetii,* or *Chlamydia psittaci* endocarditis have negative blood cultures.[85–88,194,195] With fungi, large peripheral emboli are common, necessitating embolectomy.[87,194] Histological examination and culture of the embolus may be diagnostic.

Although fastidious organisms are an occasional cause of negative blood cultures, administration of antimicrobial agents is a more common cause. The period of time required for the blood cultures to become positive again may be as short as 24 hours or as long as 2 weeks, depending on the activity of the antimicrobial agent against the infecting organism and the length of time the therapy was given. If therapy is given for only 2 to 3 days and then discontinued, cultures will probably rapidly revert to positive. With longer therapy, blood cultures will probably become positive by the time fever recurs.

Other obvious causes of negative blood cultures are incorrect diagnosis and improper blood culture techniques.

Other Laboratory Features[170,171,196]

In subacute IE a normochromic, normocytic *anemia* usually is present (70 to 90 per cent of cases) and worsens with duration of illness. The *white blood cell count* usually is normal, but the *differential count* may be slightly shifted to the left. In acute endocarditis (particularly staphylococcal), *leukocytosis* with a shift to the left often is present. *Thrombocytopenia* may occur. The *erythrocyte sedimentation rate* is almost always elevated except in patients with heart or kidney failure. A positive *rheumatoid factor* is present in 50 per cent of patients with endocarditis for 3 to 6 weeks.[167,197] Although circulating *immune complexes* are present in virtually all patients,[162,198] *hypergammaglobulinemia* is detected in only one-quarter. These tend to disappear with therapy.

High serum titers of *antibodies directed against teichoic acid* constituents of the cell wall of staphylococci suggest endocarditis or other deep-seated infection.[65,66,186] Unfortunately false-positive reactions and cross-reactions with other gram-positive bacteria limit their usefulness in diagnosis. Serologic tests for *C. burnetii, C. psittaci,* and *Brucella* are positive in endocarditis caused by these organisms but are not diagnostic of endocarditis.

Large mononuclear cells (earlobe histiocytes) occasionally can be seen on peripheral blood smears from patients with subacute endocarditis, but the yield is higher (25 per cent) if the first drop of blood obtained after earlobe massage and puncture is examined. These cells are not specific for endocarditis. *Intraleukocytic bacteria* can be seen in buffy coat preparations of blood in up to 50 per cent of patients.[199]

The urinalysis usually is abnormal, with *proteinuria, microscopic hematuria,* and/or *microscopic pyuria* in most patients. Reduction in *serum complement* parallels the incidence of abnormal renal function, especially that caused by diffuse glomerulonephritis.

IMAGING STUDIES

ECHOCARDIOGRAPHY (see also p. 88 and Figs. 4–60 to 4–62). This technique has assumed an increasingly important role in the assessment and management of patients with suspected IE.[14,125,200–206,206a] Two-dimensional echocardiograms can demonstrate the vegetation in up to 80 per cent of patients with native valve endocarditis, but the usual sensitivity reported is about 60 per cent (Fig. 4–60, p. 88). In the absence of a prosthetic valve, vegetations larger than 5 mm in diameter are reliably detected and those under 3 mm usually are missed. Transesophageal echocardiography has been reported to be more sensitive than transthoracic echocardiography.[202–206,206b,206c] M-mode echocardiograms are less sensitive than two-dimensional studies in detecting vegetations. Knowledge of which valve is involved in endocarditis is important for surgical management and determination of prognosis. In addition, echocardiography can provide valuable information about the degree of valvular destruction and its hemodynamic effects and whether myocardial or valve ring abscess or aneurysm of the sinus of Valsalva is present. Doppler ultrasound can help to quantitate the degree of valvular insufficiency. Serial echocardiographic findings can contribute to decisions for surgical intervention.

In addition to the lack of sensitivity in terms of at least a 20 per cent false-negative rate, echocardiography lacks specificity. Thickened valves, noninfected thrombi, nodules, tumors, and flail leaflets can be misinterpreted as vegetations.[207,208]

Vegetations often are not visualized during the first 2 weeks of endocarditis. Once visualized, they usually remain unchanged in size during therapy and may remain the same size for months after successful therapy.[125,209]

Some have reported that patients with vegetations visualized on echocardiography have an increased risk of developing emboli and CHF, and require valve replacement.[200–202] Others have not found these relationships. It seems likely that vegetations greater than or equal to 10 mm in size are associated with a greater risk of emboli.[203,210]

Recent technological developments using digital image processing of two-dimensional echocardiograms may permit differentiation between active and healed vegetations.[209] Echocardiography usually is not useful in nontissue PVE because of the production of intense interfering echoes by the metal.[211]

Nontissue PVE more commonly is evaluated by serial phonocardiography, cineradiography, and Doppler echocardiography.[212] Changes in the timing or the intensity of the prosthetic sounds detected by phonocardiography may suggest obstruction by a vegetation. Disappearance of an opening click or the sound produced by a closing valve suggests presence of a vegetation. Cineradiography of the valve shows abnormal motion with valve dehiscence (Fig. 35–11). Doppler echocardiography is a sensitive detector of new valvular insufficiency, which indicates valvular dysfunction.

RADIOISOTOPIC SCANNING. This may be carried out with gallium-67 and with indium-111–labeled white blood cells, and has been used to localize vegetations and myocardial abscesses in endocarditis.[213–215] Although these techniques have been found to be useful in selected patients, because of their low sensitivity they add little to the usual diagnosis and management of endocarditis.

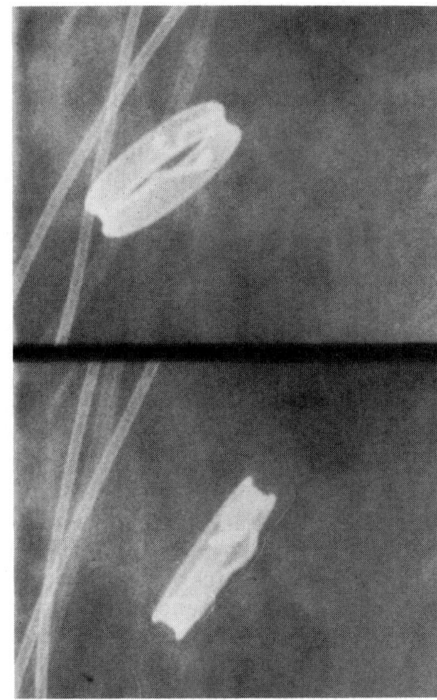

FIGURE 35–11. Fluoroscopic demonstration of the instability (rocking) of a prosthetic valve in a patient with IE.

function.[104,105,288] Patients with delayed-onset streptococcal PVE are most likely to be cured with antibiotics alone.

Although it is ideal to treat with optimal antimicrobial therapy long enough to sterilize blood cultures before surgery, when a definite indication for surgery is present, the procedure should not be delayed. Delay of surgery, especially in the presence of heart failure, may convert an elective procedure with a relatively low mortality rate to an emergency procedure with a high mortality rate. Persistence of infection with the same organism has been uncommon (probably <5 per cent) after valve replacement, even when only short courses of antimicrobial therapy have been given before surgery.[286,290-293a] Postoperative antimicrobial therapy should be continued long enough to eradicate metastatic foci of infection.

Myocardial or valve ring abscesses must be drained surgically. Myocardial invasion extending from the valve annulus is common in PVE. Prompt surgical intervention may be lifesaving. Surgery should be considered in patients with large vegetations demonstrated by echocardiography and recurrent major arterial emboli. Many consider emboli a major indication for surgery. However, it is difficult to decide when to operate in patients with recurrent emboli, as there are no data to indicate the likelihood of additional emboli.[148,294] Our approach is not to routinely recommend surgery after one major embolus. With two or more emboli, and perhaps even after one embolus in the presence of very large vegetations on echocardiography (i.e., ≥10 mm), surgery often is recommended. We do not use size of the vegetation alone as an indication for cardiac surgery.

Some have considered infection caused by *S. aureus* to be an indication for cardiac surgery.[295] The authors do not advocate cardiac surgery for *S. aureus* infection unless other indications also are present.

A recent approach to the surgical management of IE has been valvuloplasty with resection of the vegetation. This procedure is applicable only to patients in whom the valve is relatively intact.[296-299] In future years this may become the preferred approach for patients with endocarditis refractory to therapy or with emboli.

Endocarditis restricted to the tricuspid valve is most often seen in IV drug abusers. When it is caused by fungi or antibiotic-resistant gram-negative bacilli, one approach has been resection of the valve without replacement.[299,300] This approach is of particular potential importance in those persons who are likely to return to use of intravenous drugs after surgery and in whom valvuloplasty with resection of the vegetatin is not possible. Presence of a prosthetic valve in an active IV drug abuser would provide an extremely susceptible focus for subsequent episodes of endocarditis. Many patients tolerate absence of the tricuspid valve for long periods of time. If pulmonary artery hypertension begins to develop, a tricuspid prosthetic valve can be implanted.

Recently, a patient with *Mycoplasma hominis* endocarditis involving mitral and aortic valve prostheses was cured with heart transplantation.[301] Noncardiac surgical intervention may be required for drainage of abscesses. Large emboli often require vascular procedures to reopen major arteries.

ANTICOAGULATION

Anticoagulants are of no value in treatment of IE. They do not prevent embolization of parts of the vegetation and do not add to the effectiveness of appropriate antimicrobial agents in preventing growth of the vegetation. Anticoagulation also increases the potential hazard of bleeding from a mycotic aneurysm or from a cerebral embolus and infarction. However, anticoagulation may have to be used if indications for anticoagulation exist, such as presence of a prosthetic valve or pulmonary emboli from a source other than from a cardiac vegetation.[148,302] Careful control is important to keep the parameters of anticoagulation (e.g., prothrombin time) in low therapeutic ranges.

RESPONSE TO THERAPY

Most patients defervesce by 3 to 7 days after effective antimicrobial therapy has been started.[251,303] *Persistence or recurrence of fever* may be due to associated myocardial or metastatic abscesses, recurrent emboli, superinfection of the vegetation, or (most commonly with recurrence of fever) febrile reactions to antimicrobial agents.[154,304,305] Blood cultures should be obtained periodically during treatment, and they usually become negative after several days of therapy. Lack of response of bacteremia may be associated with myocardial or metastatic abscess formation (especially with *S. aureus*)[148,154,251] Some patients may have positive blood cultures for as long as 1 or occasionally 2 weeks while receiving curative therapy. This is most likely to occur with enterococcal and especially *S. aureus* endocarditis.

If a *rash* develops, therapy can be continued and antihistamines or even corticosteroids given to suppress the reaction. If the rash is severe, therapy should be altered. Weight gain, improvement in appetite, and a rise in hemoglobin may not be seen until weeks after therapy has been completed. Petechiae, Osler nodes, and emboli may occur during and for weeks after successful antimicrobial therapy.[148] Splenomegaly may take months to resolve. Changes in murmurs from destruction of the valve or from shrinkage or rupture may occur during or after therapy. Heart failure may result, and is the principal cause of death, particularly in patients with aortic valve endocarditis.[154]

Mycotic aneurysms may regress on drug therapy or may rupture on therapy weeks to years later.[148,306] Despite the fact that cerebral aneurysms may rupture without warning, with present knowledge it is not reasonable to submit all patients with endocarditis for evaluation for cerebral aneurysm. Symptoms of headache and/or transient or permanent neurological abnormalities (e.g., visual field defects) in a patient with endocarditis must raise the question of cerebral aneurysm[148,154,157,306] and suggests leakage or enlargement of an aneurysm. Although computed tomographic scans may be suggestive, cerebral angiography is necessary for diagnosis and should be pursued in patients with central nervous system symptoms.[154,306] When aneurysms are found in symptomatic patients, surgical intervention must be seriously considered.

Aneurysms in the chest or abdomen often are asymptomatic and unsuspected until they rupture, requiring emergency surgery.[159] In an extremity a pulsatile mass suggests an aneurysm and the need for surgery.[154,158]

Renal insufficiency from glomerulonephritis usually improves with therapy for the endocarditis.[154,165,307] Occasional patients do not improve with control of the endocarditis, and in some of these patients corticosteroids, plasma exchange, and/or cytotoxic chemotherapy has been reported to be effective.[307-309]

RELAPSES AND NEW EPISODES

The great majority of relapses of endocarditis occur within 2 months of stopping antimicrobial therapy, and most occur within 4 weeks.[310,311] Blood cultures 2 to 4 weeks after completion of therapy detect the majority of relapses. Although delayed relapses are unusual with bacterial endocarditis, they are not uncommon with fungal endocarditis and Q fever endocarditis.[312] Relapses caused by the same fungus have been reported as long as 2 years after replacement of a prosthetic valve for fungal endocarditis. In fact, a case of ours reported as a cure subsequently relapsed after 2 years.[194]

New episodes of endocarditis commonly occur in patients who have had IE. At least 6 per cent of patients with native valve endocarditis and who are not drug abusers will have one or more additional episodes of endocarditis.[313] We saw one patient who had seven distinct episodes over a period of 20 years. IV drug abusers are at particularly high risk for additional episodes.[93,97] The results of treatment of those with subsequent episodes of endocarditis on native valves are no worse than results of therapy for first episodes of endocarditis.[313]

PROGNOSIS

The prognosis of IE varies according to the infecting microorganisms, the type of cardiac valve (native versus prosthetic and aortic versus mitral versus tricuspid), the age of the patient, and the presence or absence of complications.

NATIVE VALVE ENDOCARDITIS

The cure rates for native valve endocarditis are greater than or equal to 90 per cent for streptococcal endocarditis, 75 to 90 per cent for enterococcal endocarditis, and 60 to 75 per cent for *S. aureus* endocarditis (some series report mortality rates as high as 70 per cent in *S. aureus* endocarditis).[47,224,252,253,314] Mortality from streptococcal or enterococcal endocarditis is seldom related to failure of antibiotic therapy. (This may change with the emergence of antibiotic-resistant enterococci.) The usual causes of death are heart failure, emboli, rupture of mycotic aneurysms, complications of cardiac surgery, and renal failure. Death from *S. aureus* endocarditis may be caused by overwhelming infection or by the complications listed above. Results have been poor in endocarditis caused by fungi, gram-negative enteric organisms, and *Pseudomonas* sp. because of resistance to antimicrobial agents.

In addition to the effect of the microorganism on prognosis, a *poorer prognosis* has been associated with the old and the very young, aortic versus mitral valve involvement, left-sided versus right-sided endocarditis, myocardial abscess, rupture of a mycotic aneurysm, emboli (especially coronary artery emboli), heart failure, renal insufficiency, and cardiac surgery in the presence of active versus inactive endocarditis.[47,224,252,253,314,315]

Other underlying diseases also increase the chance of mortality. Delay of diagnosis results in more complications and a worse prognosis. The striking effect of right-sided versus left-sided endocariditis can be illustrated by the fact that more than 90 per cent of IV drug abusers with *S. aureus* endocarditis localized to the tricuspid valve can be cured with antibiotic therapy alone, as contrasted with at least a 25 to 40 per cent mortality with left-sided *S. aureus* endocarditis.[62] The presence of large vegetations on echocardiogram may indicate a poorer prognosis than small or absent vegetations.[200-203,210]

After cure of endocarditis the risk of increased mortality remains. Most of the deaths that occur during therapy or after cure of endocarditis are related to heart failure, a major embolus, or rupture of a mycotic aneurysm. Cardiac surgery with valve replacement may be required during therapy for the episode of endocarditis or after bacteriological cure. In a recent series of patents with IE,[314] 25 per cent died in the hospital, 30 per cent had died by 1 year after discharge, and about 40 per cent by 5 years.

PROSTHETIC VALVE ENDOCARDITIS

The prognosis is clearly worse in PVE than in native valve endocarditis. Late PVE (>60 days after surgery) has a better prognosis, with a mortality rate of 19 to 50 per cent, than early PVE (<60 days postoperatively), with a mortality rate of 41 to 80 per cent.[104,181,288,316,317] The valve dysfunction and dehiscence and intracardiac abscesses, which are much more common with early disease, and the antibiotic-resistant organisms associated with early disease contribute to the higher mortality. Streptococcal PVE has the best prognosis, whereas PVE caused by fungi, coagulase-positive and coagulase-negative staphylococci, *Corynebacterium* sp., enteric gram-negative bacilli, and *Pseudomonas* has a much worse prognosis.[104,181,288,316-318]

In addition to infecting organism and time of onset, increased mortality has been associated with the clinical observations of persistent fever on antibiotic therapy, changing murmurs, new conduction abnormalities, and increasing heart failure.[288,316,319] These poor prognostic clinical features are probably in turn related to uncontrolled infection, myocardial abscesses, and/or valve dysfunction. It also has been observed that early valve replacement in PVE patients (who have indications for replacement) is associated with a lower mortality than when surgery is delayed.[288,320]

PREVENTION

In the pathogenesis of bacterial endocarditis the causative microorganisms usually gain access to the bloodstream from the oropharynx, but in IV drug abusers and occasionally others the portal of entry is the skin. The respiratory, genitourinary, or gastrointestinal tract or an intravascular catheter, suture, or infusion also can act as a portal of entry.

The optimal approach to prophylaxis of IE is prevention or correction of underlying cardiovascular defects which predispose to intravascular infection, and some progress toward this goal is being achieved through modern medicosurgical therapy. The other approach consists of use of antimicrobial agents to prevent bacterial invasion of the bloodstream and subsequent localization and multiplication at an intravascular site.

Antibiotic prophylaxis of IE can be applied only to events or procedures recognized as providing potential bacterial portals of entry and only in patients with a recognized predisposing cardiac lesion. Therefore, most cases of IE are not preventable, as only half of patients who develop endocarditis have a previously recognized predisposing cardiac lesion,[171,321] and an apparent portal of entry (other than in drug abusers) can be demonstrated in patients with IE in less than 25 per cent of cases.[169,321-326] In fact, it has been calculated that less than 10 per cent of cases of IE are theoretically preventable with prophylaxis.[322]

Viridans streptococci are the predominant organisms in the flora of the oral cavity, the most common bacterial species isolated from the blood after trauma to the tissues of the mouth, and the most common cause of IE. However, many other bacterial species can be detected in the mouth, are occasionally isolated from blood after dental trauma, and can cause IE (Table 35–3).[128] Prophylaxis of endocarditis after procedures in the mouth is aimed primarily at viridans streptococci. The frequency of bacteremia is related to the degree of disease of the gum and to the degree of trauma inflicted during the procedure (Table 35–3).[128] Procedures attended by bleeding are far more likely to cause bacteremia than those that are not.

Enterococci are responsible for a relatively large number of cases of IE that develop after urinary tract surgical procedures or delivery, abortion, pelvic inflammatory disease, and instrumentation of the female genitourinary tract.[45,46] Although *gram-negative enteric bacilli* are responsible for most of the cases of bacteremia after urinary tract manipulation, these organisms are unusual as causes of IE, and prophylaxis of endocarditis is directed at the enterococcus.

The *gastrointestinal tract* occasionally has been identified as a portal of entry for microorganisms in patients with IE. Although bacteremia occasionally occurs in association with instrumentation of the intestinal tract, such as sigmoidoscopy and colonoscopy, IE after these procedures is rare.[327,328] However, it appears advisable to administer antimicrobial agents to patients with valvular or congenital heart disease who undergo procedures on the lower gastrointestinal tract that are likely to be associated with considerable trauma to soft tissues (i.e., surgery).

Surgical procedures on the *gallbladder* also have occasionally been implicated as providing a portal of entry in IE; therefore, antimicrobial prophylaxis should be considered in connection with this type of surgery. Although the predominant bacterial flora of the gastrointestinal tract is anaerobic, anaerobes are rare causes of endocarditis. Gram-negative aerobic bacilli and enterococci also are found in large numbers in the intestinal tract, but, as the former organisms are rare causes of endocarditis, prophylaxis should be directed at the enterococcus. Endocarditis also may complicate localized infection

Antibiotic prophylaxis is to be used with procedures that are likely to cause bacteremia, as listed in Table 35–13, which also lists some procedures that infrequently cause bacteremia and for which prophylaxis is *not* recommended.

The regimens recommended for dental and other oral and upper respiratory tract procedures are aimed at viridans streptococci. The adult regimens are listed in Tables 35–14 and 35–15. The latter gives alternative regimens for patients who are unable to take oral medication. Although the oral regimen in Table 35–14 is appropriate for patients with all cardiovascular lesions, including those at high risk for IE (e.g., those with prosthetic valves), Table 35–15 outlines regimens for the physician who *elects* to use a parenteral regimen in high-risk patients.

When a series of dental procedures is anticipated, it is recommended to wait 7 days between procedures and to do multiple procedures at the same sitting. This may help to reduce the chances of emergence of antibiotic-resistant flora. If a patient is receiving continuous oral penicillin for prevention of rheumatic fever, mouth flora resistant to penicillin may develop. In such cases, erythromycin or another nonpenicillin regimen in Table 35–14 or 35–15 should be used.

Antibiotic prophylaxis is used with procedures that are likely to cause significant trauma to the large bowel, genitourinary tract, and the gallbladder and is directed at the enterococcus. Adult regimens are found in Table 35–16. Prophylaxis at the time of cardiac surgery with placement of foreign material (e.g., prosthetic valves) is directed primarily at staphylococci. An aminoglycoside often is added for activity against gram-negative bacilli in an attempt to prevent endocardial infection as well as infection at other sites, such as the sternum. Reasonable regimens are listed in Table 35–17.

REFERENCES

1. Johnson, F., Darling, R. C., Mundth, E. D., et al.: The management of infected arterial aneurysms. J. Cardiovasc. Surg. *18*:361, 1977.
1a. Infective endocarditis. *In* Fowler, N. O.: Diagnosis of Heart Disease. New York, Springer-Verlag, 1991, pp. 410–416.

NATIVE VALVE ENDOCARDITIS

2. McKinsey, D. S., Ratts, T. E., and Bisno, A. L.: Underlying cardiac lesions in adults with infective endocarditis: The changing spectrum. Am. J. Med. *82*:681, 1987.
3. Sholler, G. E., Hawker, R. E., and Celermajer, J. M.: Infective endocarditis in childhood. Pediatr. Cardiol. *6*:183, 1986.
4. Millard, D. D., and Shulman, S. T.: The changing spectrum of neonatal endocarditis. Clin. Perinatol *15*:587, 1988.
5. Saiman, L., and Prince, A.: Infections of the heart. Adv. Pediatr. Infect. Dis. *4*:139, 1989.
6. Johnson, C. M., and Rhodes, K. H.: Pediatric endocarditis. Mayo Clin. Proc. *57*:86, 1982.
7. Johnson, D. H., Rosenthal, A., and Nadas, A. S.: A forty-year review of bacterial endocarditis in infancy and childhood. Circulation *51*:581, 1975.
8. Zakrzewski, T., and Keith, J. D.: Bacterial endocarditis in infants and children. J. Pediatr. *67*:1179, 1965.
9. VanHare, G. F., Ben-Shachar, G., Liebman, J., et al.: Infective endocarditis in infants and children during the past 10 years: A decade of change. Am. Heart J. *107*:1235, 1984.
10. Schollin, J., Bjarke, B., and Wesstrom, G.: Infective endocarditis in Swedish children. I. Incidence, etiology, underlying factors and port of entry of infection; II. Location, major complications, laboratory findings, delay of treatment, treatment and outcome. Acta Paediatr. Scand. *75*:993, 1986; *75*:999, 1986.
11. Wald, E. R., Dashefsky, B., Feidt, C., et al.: Acute rheumatic fever in western Pennsylvania and the tri-state area. Pediatrics *80*:371, 1987.
12. Veasy, L. G., Weidmeier, S. E., Orsmond, G. S., et al.: Resurgence of acute rheumatic fever in the intermountain area of the United States. N. Engl. J. Med. *316*:421, 1987.
13. Cutler, J. G., Ongley, P. A., Shwachman, H., et al.: Bacterial endocarditis in children with heart disease. Pediatrics *22*:706, 1958.
14. Cremieux, A. C., Witchitz, S., Malergue, M. C., et al.: Clinical and echocardiographic observations in pulmonary valve endocarditis. Am. J. Cardiol. *56*:610, 1985.
15. Blumenthal, S., Griffiths, S. P. and Morgan, B. C.: Bacterial endocarditis in children with congenital heart disease. Pediatrics *26*:993, 1960.
16. Geva, T., and Frand, M.: Infective endocarditis in children with congenital heart disease: The changing spectrum 1965–1985. Eur. Heart J. *9*:1244, 1988.
17. Nagger, C. Z., and Forgacs, P.: Infective endocarditis: A challenging disease. Med. Clin. North Am. *70*:1279, 1986.
18. MacMahon, S. W., Roberts, J. K., Kramer-Fox, R., et al.: Mitral valve prolapse and infective endocarditis. Am. Heart J. *113*:1291, 1987.
19. Lavie, C. J., Khandheria, B. K., Seward, J. B., et al.: Factors associated with the recommendation for endocarditis prophylaxis in mitral valve prolapse. JAMA *262*:3308, 1989.
20. MacMahon, S. W., Hickey, A. J., Wilcken, D.E.L., et al.: Risk of infective endocarditis in mitral valve prolapse with and without precordial systolic murmurs. Am. J. Cardiol. *58*:105, 1986.
21. Griffin, M. R., Wilson, W. R., Edwards, W. D., et al.: Infective endocarditis—Olmstead County, Minnesota, 1950 through 1981. JAMA *254*:1199, 1985.
22. Weinberger, I., Rotenberg, Z., Zacharovitch, D., et al.: Native valve infective endocarditis in the 1970's versus the 1980's: Underlying cardiac lesions and infecting organisms. Clin. Cardiol. *13*:94, 1990.
23. Kaye, D.: Definitions and demographic characteristics. In: Kaye, D. (ed.): Infective endocarditis. Baltimore, University Park Press, 1976, pp. 1–10.
24. Sharma, S., Desai, A. G., Pillai, M. G., et al.: Clinical and diagnostic features of pulmonary valve endocarditis in the setting of congenital cardiac malformations. Int. J. Cardiol. *9*:457, 1985.
25. Stulz, P., Zimmerli, W., Mihatsch, J., and Gradel, E.: Recurrent infective endocarditis in idiopathic hypertrophic subaortic stenosis. Thorac. Cardiovasc. Surg. *37*(2):99, 1989.
26. Soman, V. R., Breton, G., Hershkowitz, M., and Mark, H.: Bacterial endocarditis of mitral valve in Marfan syndrome. Br. Heart J. *36*:1247, 1974.
27. Kaye, D.: Changing pattern of infective endocarditis. Am. J. Med. *78*(Suppl 6B):157, 1985.
28. Terpenning, M. S., Buggy, B. P., and Kauffman, C. A.: Infective endocarditis: Clinical features in young and elderly patients. Am. J. Med. *83*:626, 1987.
28a. von Reyn, C. E., Levy, B. S., Arbeit, N. O., et al.: Infective carditis: An analysis based on strict case definitions. Ann. Intern. Med. *94*:505, 1981.
29. Stekilber, J. M., Melton, L. J., IV, Ilstrup, D. M., et al.: Influence of referral bias on the apparent clinical spectrum of infective endocarditis. Am. J. Med. *88*:582, 1990.
30. Applefeld, M. M., and Hornick, R. B.: Infective endocarditis in patients over age 60. Am. Heart J. *88*:90, 1974.
31. Pomerance, A.: Cardiac pathology in the elderly. Cardiovasc. Clin. *12*:9, 1981.
32. Rayfield, E. J., Ault, M. J., Keusch, G. T., et al.: Infection and diabetes: The case for glucose control. Am. J. Med. *72*:439, 1982.
33. Seltzer, A.: Changing aspects of the natural history of valvular aortic stenosis. N. Engl. J. Med. *317*:91, 1987.
34. Cooper, G., and Platt, R.: *Staphylococcus aureus* bacteremia in diabetic patients. Endocarditis and mortality. Am. J. Med. *73*:658, 1982.
35. Tuazon, C. U., Perez, A., Kishaba, T., et al.: *Staphylococcus aureus* among insulin-injecting diabetic patients; an increased carrier risk. J.A.M.A. *231*:1272, 1975.
36. Casey, J. I., Maturlo, S., Albin, J., and Edberg, S. C.: Comparison of carriage rates of group B streptococcus in diabetic and non-diabetic persons. Am. J. Epidemiol. *116*:704, 1982.
37. Gallagher, P. G., and Watanakunakorn, C.: Group B streptococcal endocarditis: Report on seven cases and review of the literature, 1962–1985. Rev. Infect. Dis. *8*:175, 1986.
38. Seaworth, B. J., and Durack, D. T.: Infective endocarditis in obstetric and gynecologic practice. Am. J. Obstet. Gynecol. *54*:180, 1986.
39. Cox, S. M., Hankins, G. D., Leveno, K. S., and Cunningham, F. G.: Bacterial endocarditis: A serious pregnancy complication. J. Reprod. Med. *33*:671, 1988.
40. Roberts, R. B., Krieger, A. G., Schiller, N. L., et al.: Viridans streptococcal endocarditis: The role of various species including pyridoxal-dependent streptococci. Rev. Infect. Dis. *1*:955, 1979.
41. Coykendale, A. L.: Classification and identification of the viridans streptococci. Clin. Microbiol. Rev. *2*:315, 1989.
42. Harder, E. J., Wilkowske, C. J., Washington, J. A., et al.: *Streptococcus mutans* endocarditis. Ann. Intern. Med. *80*:364, 1974.
43. Stein, D. S., and Nelson, K. E.: Endocarditis due to nutritionally deficient streptococci: Therapeutic dilemma. Rev. Infect. Dis. *9*:908, 1987.
44. Facklam, R. R., and Carey, R. B.: Streptococci and aerococci. In: Lennete, E. H., Balows, A., Hausler, W. J., Jr., et al. (eds.): Manual of Clinical Microbiology. 4th ed. Washington, D.C., American Society of Microbiology, 1985, pp. 154–175.
45. Mandell, G. L., Kaye, D., Levison, M. E., et al.: Enterococcal endocarditis: An analysis of 38 patients observed at the New York Hospital—Cornell Medical Center. Arch. Intern. Med. *125*:258, 1970.
46. Maki, D. G., and Agger, W. A.: Enterococcal bacteremia: Clinical features, the risk of endocarditis and management. Medicine (Baltimore) *67*:248, 1988.
47. Bisno, A. L., Dismukes, W. E., Durack, D. T., et al.: Antimicrobial treatment of infective endocarditis due to viridans streptococci, enterococci and staphylococci. JAMA *261*:1471, 1989.
48. Ingerman, M., Pitsakis, P. G., Rosenberg, A., et al.: Beta-lactamase production in experimental endocarditis due to aminoglycoside-resistant *Streptococcus faecalis*. J. Infect. Dis. *155*:1226, 1987.
49. Zervos, M. J., Terpenning, M. S., Schaberg, D. R., et al.: High-level aminoglycoside-resistant enterococci colonization of nursing home and acute care hospital patients. Arch. Intern. Med. *147*:1591, 1987.
50. Uttley, A.H.C., Collins, C. H., Naidoo, J., and George, R. C.: Vancomycin-resistant enterococci. Lancet *1*:57, 1988.

51. Moellering, R. C., Watson, B. K., Kunz, L. J.: Endocarditis due to group D streptococci. Comparison of disease caused by *Streptococcus bovis* with that produced by enterococci. Am. J. Med. *57*:239, 1974.
52. Leport, C., Bure, A., Leport, J., and Vilde, J. L.: Incidence of colonic lesions in *Streptococcus bovis* and enterococcal endocarditis. Lancet *1*:748, 1987.
53. Emiliani, V. J., Chodos, J. E., Comer, G. M., et al.: *Streptococcus bovis* brain abscess associated with an occult colonic villous adenoma. Am. J. Gastroenterol. *85*:78, 1990.
54. Wiseman, A., René, P., and Crelinsten, G. L.: *Streptococcus agalactiae* endocarditis: An association with villous adenomas of the large intestine. Ann. Intern. Med. *103*:893, 1985.
55. Venezio, F. R., Gullberg, R. M., Westenfelder, G. O., et al.: Group G streptococcal endocarditis and bacteremia. Am. J. Med. *81*:29, 1986.
56. Ugolini, V., Pacifico, A., Smitherman, T. C., and Mackowiak, P. A.: Pneumococcal endocarditis update: Analysis of 10 cases diagnosed between 1974 and 1984. Am. Heart J. *112*:813, 1986.
57. Powderly, W. G., Stanley, S. L., Jr., and Medoff, G.: Pneumococcal endocarditis: Report of a series and review of the literature. Rev. Infect. Dis. *8*:786, 1986.
58. Sands, M., Brown, R. B., Ryczak, M., and Hamilton, W.: *Streptococcus pneumoniae* endocarditis. South Med. J. *80*:780, 1987.
59. Bruyn, G.A.W., Thompson, J., and van der Meer, J.W.M.: Pneumococcal endocarditis in adult patients. A report of five cases and review of the literature. Q. J. Med. *74*:33, 1990.
60. Editorial: Penicillin-resistant pneumococci. Lancet *1*:1142, 1988.
61. Klugman, K. P., and Koornof, H. J.: Drug resistance patterns and serogroups or serotypes of pneumococcal isolates from cerebrospinal fluid or blood, 1979–1986. J. Infect. Dis. *158*:956, 1988.
62. Karchmer, A. W.: Staphylococcal endocarditis, laboratory and clinical basis for antibiotic therapy. Am. J. Med. *78*:(Suppl 6B):116, 1985.
63. Eykyn, S. J.: Staphylococcal sepsis. The changing pattern of disease and therapy. Lancet *1*:100, 1988.
64. Chambers, H. F., Korzeniowski, O. M., Sande, M. A., et al.: *Staphylococcus aureus* endocarditis: Clinical manifestations in addicts and non-addicts. Medicine *62*:170, 1983.
65. Espersen, F., and Frimodt-Moller, N.: *Staphylococcus aureus* endocarditis. A review of 119 cases. Arch. Intern. Med. *146*:1118, 1986.
66. Bayer, A. S., Lam, K., Ginzton, L., et al.: *Staphylococcus aureus* bacteremia clinical, serologic, and echocardiographic findings in patients with and without endocarditis. Arch. Intern. Med. *147*:457, 1987.
67. Kaye, D.: The clinical significance of tolerance of *Staphylococcus aureus*. Ann. Intern. Med. *93*:924, 1980.
68. Caputo, G. M., Archer, G. L., Calderwood, S. B., et al.: Native valve endocarditis due to coagulase-negative staphylococci, clinical and microbiologic features. Am. J. Med. *83*:619, 1987.
69. Wall, T. C., Peyton, R. B., and Corey, G. R.: Gonococcal endocarditis: A new look at an old disease. Medicine (Baltimore) *68*:375, 1989.
70. Owens, J. E., and Kelchak, J. A.: Gonococcal endocarditis: Report of a case and review of the literature. J.S.C. Med. Assoc. *86*:93, 1990.
71. Lynn, D. J., Kane, J. G., and Parker, R. H.: *Haemophilus parainfluenzae* and *influenzae* endocarditis: A review of forty cases. Medicine (Baltimore) *56*:115, 1977.
72. Ellner, J. J., Rosenthal, M. S., Lerner, P. I., et al.: Infective endocarditis caused by slow-growing, fastidious, gram-negative bacteria. Medicine (Baltimore) *58*:145, 1979.
73. Schack, S. H., Smith, P. W., Penn, R. G., and Rapaport, J. M.: Endocarditis caused by *Actinobacillus actinomycetemcomitans*. J. Clin. Microbiol. *20*:579, 1984.
74. Lane, T., MacGregor, R. R., Wright, D., et al.: *Cardiobacterium hominis:* An elusive cause of endocardits. J. Infect. Dis. *6*:75, 1983.
75. Decker, M. D., Graham, B. S., Hunter, E. R., et al.: Endocarditis and infections of intravascular devices due to *Eikenella corrodens*. Am. J. Med. Sci. *292*:209, 1986.
76. Jenny, D. B., Letendre, P. W., and Iverson, G.: Endocarditis due to Kingella species. Rev. Infect. Dis. *10*:1065, 1988.
77. Cohen, P. S., Maguire, J. H., and Weinstein, L.: Infective endocarditis caused by gram-negative bacteria: A review of the literature. Prog. Cardiovasc. Dis. *22*:205, 1980.
77a. Komshian, S. V., Tablan, O. C., Palutke, W., and Reyes, M. P.: Characteristics of left-sided endocarditis due to *Pseudomonas aeruginosa* in the Detroit Medical Center. Rev. Infect. Dis. *12*:693, 1990.
78. Carvajal, A., and Frederiksen, W.: Fatal endocarditis due to *Listeria monocytogenes*. Rev. Infect. Dis. *10*:616, 1988.
79. Lindner, P. S., Hardy, D. J., and Murphy, T. E.: Endocarditis due to *Corynebacterium pseudodiphtheriticum*. N.Y. State J. Med. *86*:102, 1986.
80. Yersin, B., Glauser, M. P., Guze, P. A., et al.: Experimental *Escherichia coli* endocarditis in rats. Roles of serum bactericidal activity and duration of catheter placement. Infect. Immunol. *56*:1273, 1988.
81. Nord, C. E.: Anaerobic bacteria in septicemia and endocarditis. Scand. J. Infect. Dis. *31*(Suppl):95, 1982.
82. McIntosh, C. S., Vickers, P. J., and Isaacs, A. J.: Spirillum endocarditis. Postgrad. Med. J. *51*:645, 1975.
83. Popat, K., Barnardo, D., Webb-Peploe, M.: *Mycoplasma pneumoniae* endocarditis. Br. Heart J. *44*:111, 1980.
84. Al-Kasab, S., Fagih, M. R., Al-Yousef, S., et al.: *Brucella* infective endocarditis: Successful combined medical and surgical therapy. J. Thorac. Cardiovasc. Surg. *95*:862, 1988.
85. Shafer, R. W., and Braverman, E. R.: Q-fever endocarditis: Delay in diagnosis due to an apparent clinical response to corticosteroids. Am. J. Med. *86*:729, 1989.
86. Jones, R. B., Priest, J. B., and Kuo, C. C.: Subacute chlamydial endocarditis. JAMA *247*:655, 1982.
87. Rubinstein, E., Noriega, E.R., Simberkoff, M. S., et al.: Fungal endocarditis: Analysis of 24 cases and a review of the literature. Medicine *54*:331, 1975.
88. Woods, G. L., Wood, R. P., and Shaw, B. W., Jr.: *Aspergillus* endocarditis in patients without prior cardiovascular surgery: Report of a case in a liver transplant recipient and review. Rev. Infect. Dis. *11*:263, 1989.
88a. Johnston, P. G., Lee, J., Domanski, M., et al.: Late recurrent candida endocarditis. Chest *99*:1531, 1991.

ENDOCARDITIS IN INTRAVENOUS DRUG ABUSERS

89. Scheidegger, C., and Zimmerli, W.: Infectious complications in drug addicts: Seven-year review of 269 hospitalized narcotics abusers in Switzerland. Rev. Infect. Dis. *11*:486, 1989.
90. Chambers, H. F., Morris, D. L., Tauber, M. G., and Modin, G.: Cocaine use and the risk for endocarditis in intravenous drug users. Ann. Intern. Med. *106*:833, 1987.
91. Julander, I.: Staphylococcal septicemia and endocarditis in 80 drug addicts. Aspects on epidemiology, clinical and laboratory findings and prognosis. Scand. J. Infect. Dis. *41*(Suppl):49, 1983.
92. Levine, D. P., Crane, L. R., and Zervos, M. J.: Bacteremia in narcotic addicts at the Detroit Medical Center. II. Infectious endocarditis: A prospective comparative study. Rev. Infect. Dis. *8*:374, 1986.
93. Baddour, L. M.: Twelve year review of recurrent native valve infective endocarditis: A disease of the modern antibiotic era. Rev. Infect. Dis. *10*:1163, 1988.
94. Eichacker, P. Q., Miller, K., Robbins, M., et al.: Echocardiographic evaluation of heart valves in IV drug abusers without a previous history of endocarditis. Clin. Res. *32*:670A, 1984.
95. Robbins, M. J., Sveiro, R., Fishman, W. H., and Strom, J. A.: Right-sided valvular endocarditis: Etiology, diagnosis, and approach to therapy. Am. Heart J. *111*:128, 1986.
96. Cassling, R. S., Rogler, W. C., and McManus, B. M.: Isolated pulmonic valve infective endocarditis: A diagnostically elusive entity. Am. Heart J. *109*:558, 1985.
97. Dressler, F. A., and Roberts, W. C.: Infective endocarditis in opiate addicts: Analysis of 80 cases studied at necropsy. Am. J. Cardiol. *63*:1240, 1989.
98. Tuazon, C. W., and Sheagren, J. W.: Increased rate of carriage of *Staphylococcus aureus* among narcotic addicts. J. Infect. Dis. *129*:725, 1974.
99. Kolander, S. A., Cosgrove, E. M., and Molavi, A.: Clostridial endocarditis. Report of a case caused by *Clostridium bifermentans* and review of the literature. Arch. Intern. Med. *149*:455, 1989.
100. Rapeport, K. B., Girón, J. A., and Rosner, F.: *Streptococcus mitis* endocarditis. Report of 17 cases. Arch. Intern. Med. *146*:2361, 1986.
101. Saravolatz, L. D., Burch, K. H., and Quinn, E. L.: Polymicrobial infective endocarditis: An increasing clinical entity. Am. Heart J. *95*:163, 1978.
102. Burns, J.M.A., Hogg, K. J., Hillis, W. S., and Dunn, F. G.: Endocarditis in intravenous drug abusers with staphylococcal septicemia. Br. Heart J. *61*:356, 1980.
103. Barg, W. L., Supena, R. B., and Fekety, R.: Persistent staphylococcal bacteremia in an intravenous drug abuser. Antimicrob. Agents Chemother. *29*:209, 1986.

PROSTHETIC VALVE ENDOCARDITIS

104. Cowgill, L. D., Addonizio, V. P., Hopeman, A. R., and Harken, A. H.: Prosthetic valve endocarditis. Curr. Probl. Cardiol. *11*:617, 1986.
105. Heimburger, T. S., and Duma, R. J.: Infections of prosthetic heart valves and cardiac pacemakers. Infect. Dis. Clin. North Am. *3*:221, 1989.
106. Calderwood, S. B., Swinski, L. A., Waternaux, C. M., et al.: Risk factors for the development of prosthetic valve endocarditis. Circulation *72*:31, 1985.
106a. Chen, S. C., Sorrell, T. C., Dwyer, D. E., et al.: Endocarditis associated with prosthetic cardiac valves. Med. J. Aust. *152*:458, 1990.
107. Rutledge, R., Kim, J., and Applebaum, R. E.: Actuarial analysis of the risk of prosthetic valve endocarditis in 1,598 patients with mechanical and bioprosthetic valves. Arch. Surg. *120*:469, 1985.
108. Ivert, I.S.A., Dismukes, W. E., Cobbs, G., et al.: Prosthetic valve endocarditis. Circulation *69*:222, 1984.
109. Laskowski, L. F., Marr, J. J., Spernoga, J. F., et al.: Fastidious mycobacteria grown from porcine prosthetic heart valve cultures. N. Engl. J. Med. *297*:101, 1977.
110. Thompkins, L. S., Roessler, B. J., Redd, S. C., et al.: *Legionella* prosthetic valve endocarditis. N. Engl. J. Med. *318*:530, 1988.
111. Cohen, J. I., Sloss, L. J., Kundsin, R., and Golightly, L.: Prosthetic valve endocarditis caused by *Mycoplasma hominis*. Am. J. Med. *86*:819, 1989.
112. Svirbely, J. R., Ayers, L. W., and Briesching, W. J.: Filamentous *Histoplasma capsulatum* endocarditis involving mitral and aortic valve porcine bioprostheses. Arch. Pathol. Lab. Med. *109*:273, 1985.
113. Fernandez-Guerrero, M. L., Muelas, J. M., Aguado, J. M., et al.: Q-fever endocarditis on porcine bioprosthetic valves. Ann. Intern. Med. *108*:209, 1988.
114. Karchmer, A. W., Archer, G. L., and Dismukes, W. E.: *Staphylococcus epidermidis* causing prosthetic valve endocarditis: Microbiologic and clinical observations as guides to therapy. Ann. Intern. Med. *98*:447, 1983.

115. Rodgers, G. M., Greenberg, C. S., and Shuman, M. A.: Characterization of the effects of cultured vascular cells on the activation of blood coagulation. Blood *61*:1155, 1983.
116. Richardson, M., Kinlough-Rathbone, R. L., Groves, H. M., et al.: Ultrastructural changes in re-endothelialized and non-endothelialized rabbit aorta neo-intima following reinjury with a balloon catheter. Br. J. Exp. Pathol. *65*:597, 1984.
117. Ferguson, D.J.P., McColm, A. A., Savage, T. J., et al.: A morphologic study of experimental rabbit staphylococcal endocarditis and aortitis. I. Formation and effect of infected and uninfected vegetations on the aorta. Br. J. Exp. Pathol. *67*:667, 1986.
118. Ferguson, D.J.P., McColm, A. A., Savage, T. J., et al.: A morphologic study of experimental rabbit staphylococcal endocarditis and aortitis. II. Inter-relationship of bacteria, vegetation and cardiovasculature in established infections. Br. J. Exp. Pathol. *67*:679, 1986.
119. Rodbard, S.: Blood velocity and endocarditis. Circulation *27*:18, 1963.
120. Lepeschkin, E.: On the relation between the site of valvular involvement in endocarditis and the blood pressure resting on the valve. Am. J. Med. Sci. *224*:318, 1952.
121. Lopez, J. A., Ross, R. S., Fishbein, M. C., and Siegel, R. J.: Nonbacterial thrombotic endocarditis: A review. Am. Heart J. *113*:773, 1987.
122. Durack, D. T., and Beeson, P. B.: Experimental bacterial endocarditis. I. Colonization of a sterile vegetation. Br. J. Exp. Pathol. *53*:44, 1972.
123. Baddour, L. M., Christensen, G. D., Lowrance, J. H., and Simpson, W. A.: Pathogenesis of experimental endocarditis. Rev. Infect. Dis. *11*:452, 1989.
124. Baddour, L. M. Production and progress of the disease in rabbits. Br. J. Exp. Pathol. *54*:142, 1973.
125. Editorial: Vegetations, valves and echocardiography. Lancet *2*:1118, 1988.
126. Durack, D. T.: Experimental bacterial endocarditis. IV. Structure and evolution of early lesions. J. Pathol. *115*:81, 1975.
127. Roberts, W. C., and Buchbinder, N. A.: Healed left-sided infective endocarditis: A clinicopathologic study of 59 patients. Am. J. Cardiol. *40*:876, 1977.
128. Everett, E. D., and Hirschmann, J. V.: Transient bacteremia and endocarditis prophylaxis. A review. Medicine (Baltimore) *56*:61, 1977.
129. Sipes, J. N., Thompson, R. L., and Hook, E. W.: Prophylaxis of infective endocarditis: A re-evaluation. Ann. Rev. Med. *28*:371, 1977.
130. Baskin, G.: Prosthetic endocarditis after endoscopic variceal sclerotherapy: A failure of antibiotic prophylaxis. Am. J. Gastroenterol. *84*:311, 1989.
131. Rogosa, M., Hampp, E. G., Nevin, T. A., et al.: Blood sampling and cultural studies in the detection of post-operative bacteremia. J. Am. Dent. Assoc. *60*:171, 1960.
132. Durack, D. T.: Current issues in the prevention of infective endocarditis. Am. J. Med. *78*(Suppl B):149, 1985.
133. Hamill, R. J., Vann, J. M., and Proctor, R. A.: Phagocytosis of *Staphylococcus aureus* by cultured bovine aortic endothelial cells: Model for post-adherence events in endovascular infections. Infect. Immun. *54*:833, 1986.
134. Rotrosen, D., Edwards, J. E., Jr., Gibson, T. R., et al.: Adherence of *Candida* to cultured vascular endothelial cells: Mechanisms of attachment and endothelial cell penetration. J. Infect. Dis. *152*:1264, 1985.
135. Hamill, R. J.: Role of fibronectin in infective endocarditis. Rev. Infect. Dis. *9*(Suppl 4):5360, 1987.
136. Sage, M. D., Koelmeyer, T. D., Smeeton, W.M.I., and Galler, L. L.: Evolution of Swan-Ganz catheter-related pulmonary valve nonbacterial endocarditis. Am. J. Forensic Med. Pathol. *9*:112, 1988.
137. Gibbons, R. J., and Nygaard, M.: Synthesis of insoluble dextran and its significance in the formation of gelatinous depositis by plaque-forming streptococci. Arch. Oral Biol. *13*:1249, 1968.
138. Scheld, W. M., Valone, J. A., and Sande, M. A.: Bacterial adherence in the pathogenesis of endocarditis. J. Clin. Invest. *61*:1394, 1978.
139. Proctor, R. A., Mosher, D. F., and Olbrantz, P. J.: Fibronectin binding to *Staphylococcus aureus*. J. Biol. Chem. *257*:14788, 1982.
140. Kuusela, P., Vartio, T., Vuento, M., and Myhre, E. B.: Attachment of staphylococci and streptococci on firbonectin, fibronectin fragments, and fibrinogen bound to a solid phase. Infect. Immun. *50*:77, 1985.
141. Myhre, E. B., and Kuusela, P.: Binding of human fibronectin to groups A, C, and G streptococci. Infect. Immun. *40*:29, 1983.
142. Skerl, K. G., Calderone, R. A., Segal, E., et al.: *In vitro* binding of *Candida albicans* yeast cells to human fibronectin. Can. J. Microbiol. *30*:221, 1984.
143. Nealon, T. J., Beachey, E. H., Courtney, H. S., and Simpson, W. A.: Release of fibronectin-lipoteichoic acid complexes from group A streptococci with penicillin. Infect. Immun. *51*:529, 1986.
144. Korzeniowski, O. M., Scheld, W. M., Bithell, T. C., et al.: Bacterial-platelet interaction in staphylococcal endocarditis (E). Abstr. 239. Presented at the 18th Interscience Conference on Antimicrobial Agents and Chemotherapy. American Society for Microbiology, October 1978.
145. Sullam, P. M., Valone, F. H., and Mills, J.: Mechanisms of platelet aggregation by viridans group streptococci. Infect. Immun. *55*:1743, 1987.
146. Hendrix, H., Lindhou, T., Mertins, K., et al.: Activation of human prothrombin by stoichiometric levels of staphylocoagulase. J. Biol. Chem. *258*:3637, 1983.
147. Drake, T. A., Rodgers, G. M., and Sande, M. A.: Tissue factor is a major stimulus for vegetation formation in enterococcal endocarditis in rabbits. J. Clin. Invest. *73*:1750, 1984.
148. Weinstein, L.: Life-threatening complications of infective endocarditis and their management. Arch. Intern. Med. *146*:953, 1986.
149. Arnett, E. N., and Roberts, W. C.: Valve ring abscess in active endocarditis: Frequency, location and clues to clinical diagnosis from the study of 95 necropsy patients. Circulation *54*:140, 1976.
150. Sandler, M. A., Kotler, M. N., Bloom, R. D., and Jacobson, L.: Pericardial abscess extending from mitral vegetation: An unusual complication of infective endocarditis. Am. Heart J. *118*:857, 1989.
151. DiNubile, M. J., Calderwood, S. B., Steinhaus, D. M., and Karchmer, A. W.: Cardiac conduction abnormalities complicating native valve active infective endocarditis. Am. J. Cardiol. *58*:1213, 1986.
152. Bhatnagar, N. K., Dhasmana, J. P., Russell, G. A., and Jordan, S. C.: Aspergillus ball thrombus occluding a homograft conduit. Eur. J. Cardiothorac. Surg. *3*:270, 1989.
153. Roberts, W. C., Ewy, G. A., Glancy, D. L., et al.: Valvular stenosis produced by active infective endocarditis. Circulation *36*:449, 1967.
154. Wilson, W. R., Giulliani, E. R., Danielson, G. K., and Geraci, J. E.: Management of complications of infective endocarditis. Mayo Clin. Proc. *57*:162, 1982.
155. Dowling, G. P., and Buja, M. L.: Sudden death due to left coronary artery occlusion in infective endocarditis. Arch. Pathol. Lab. Med. *112*:932, 1988.
155a. Ting, W., Silverman, N. A., Arzouman, D. A., and Levitsky, S.: Splenic septic emboli in endocarditis. Circulation *82*(Suppl. IV):IV–105, 1990.
156. Nakayama, D. K., O'Neill, J. A., Jr., Wagner, H., et al.: Management of vascular complications of bacterial endocarditis. J. Pediatr. Surg. *21*:636, 1986.
157. Wilson, W. R., Lie, J. T., Houser, O. W., et al.: The management of patients with mycotic aneurysms. Curr. Clin. Top. Infect. Dis. *2*:151, 1981.
158. Mansur, A. J., Grinberg, M., Leao, P. P., et al.: Extracranial mycotic aneurysms in infective endocarditis. Clin. Cardiol. *9*:65, 1986.
159. Cosmo, L. Y., Risi, G., Nelson, S., et al.: Fatal hemoptysis in acute bacterial endocarditis. Am. Rev. Respir. Dis. *137*:1223, 1988.
160. Bayer, A. S., and Theofilopoulos, A. N.: Immunopathogenetic aspects of infective endocarditis. Chest *97*:204, 1990.
161. Maisch, B.: Autoreactive mechanisms in infective endocarditis. Springer Semin. Immunopathol. *11*:439, 1989.
162. Bayer, A. S., Theofilopoulos, P. N., Eisenberg, R., et al.: Circulating immune complexes in infective endocarditis. N. Engl. J. Med. *295*:1500, 1970.
163. McKenzie, P. E., Hawke, D., Woodroffe, A. J., et al.: Serum and tissue immune complexes in infective endocarditis. J. Clin. Lab. Immunol. *4*:125, 1980.
164. Maisch, B., Mayer, E., Schubert, U., et al.: Immune reactions in infective endocarditis. II. Relevance of circulating immune complexes, serum inhibition factors, lymphocytotoxic reactions, and antibody dependent cellular cytotoxicity against cardiac target cells. Am. Heart J. *106*:338, 1983.
165. Feinstein, E. I.: Renal complications of bacterial endocarditis. Am. J. Nephrol. *5*:457, 1985.
166. Churchill, M. A., Geraci, J. E., and Hunder, G. G.: Musculoskeletal manifestations of bacterial endocarditis. Ann. Intern. Med. *87*:754, 1977.
167. Williams, R. C.: Rheumatoid factors in subacute bacterial endocarditis and other infectious diseases. Scand. J. Rheumatol. *Suppl 75*:300, 1988.
168. Williams, R. C., Jr., and Kilpatrick, K.: Immunofluorescence studies of cardiac valves in infective endocarditis. Arch. Intern. Med. *145*:297, 1985.

CLINICAL MANIFESTATIONS

169. Starkenbaum, M., Durack, D., and Beeson, P.: The "incubation period" of subacute bacterial endocarditis. Yale J. Biol. Med. *50*:49, 1977.
170. Weinstein, L., and Schlesinger, J. J.: Pathoanatomic, pathophysiologic and clinical correlations in endocarditis. N. Engl. J. Med. *291*:832, 1974.
171. Weinstein, L., and Rubin, R. H.: Infective endocarditis—1973. Prog. Cardiovasc. Dis. *16*:239, 1973.
172. Yee, J., and McAllister, K.: The utility of Osler's nodes in the diagnosis of infective endocarditis. Chest *92*:751, 1987.
173. Watanakunakorn, C.: Osler's nodes on the dorsum of the foot. Chest *94*:1088, 1988.
174. Albeit, J. S., Krous, H. F., Dalen, J. E., et al.: Pathogenesis of Osler's nodes. Ann. Intern. Med. *85*:471, 1976.
175. Kerr, A., Jr., and Tan, J. S.: Biopsies of the Janeway lesion of infective endocarditis. J. Cutan. Pathol. *6*:124, 1979.
176. Silverberg, H. H.: Roth spots. Mt. Sinai J. Med. *37*:77, 1970.
177. Salgado, A. V., Furlan, A. J., Keys, T. F., et al.: Neurologic complications of endocarditis: A 12 year experience. Neurology *39*:173, 1989.
178. Varma, M.P.S., McCluskey, D. R., Khan, M. M., et al.: Heart failure associated with infective endocarditis. A review of 40 cases. Br. Heart J. *55*:191, 1986.
179. Mills, J., Utley, J., and Abbott, J.: Heart failure in infective endocarditis: Predisposing factors, course and treatment. Chest *66*:151, 1974.
180. Jones, H. R., and Siekert, R. G.: Neurological manifestations of infective endocarditis. Brain *112*:1295, 1989.
181. Brottier, E., Gin, H., Brottier, L., et al.: Prosthetic valve endocarditis: Diagnosis and prognosis. Eur. Heart J. *5*(Suppl C):123, 1984.
182. Armstrong, J. A., Tarr, G. C., Ho M., et al.: Cytomegalovirus infection in children undergoing open-heart surgery. Yale J. Biol. Med. *49*:83, 1976.

183. Rouveix, E., Witchitz, S., Bouvet, E., et al.: Tricuspid infective endocarditis: 56 cases. Eur. Heart J. 5(Suppl C):111, 1984.

LABORATORY

184. Werner, A. S., Cobbs, C. G., Kaye, D., et al.: Studies on the bacteremia of bacterial endocarditis. JAMA *202*:199, 1967.
185. Scheld, W. M.: Pathogenesis and pathophysiology of infective endocarditis. In: Sande, M. A., Kaye, D., and Root, R. K. (eds.): Endocarditis. New York, Churchill Livingstone, 1984, pp. 1–32.
186. Tuazon, C. U., Sheagren, J. N., Choa, M. S., et al.: *Staphylococcus aureus* bacteremia: Relationship between formation of antibodies to teichoic acid and development of metastatic abscesses. J. Infect. Dis. *137*:57, 1978.
187. Ehni, W. F., and Reller, B.: Short-course therapy for catheter-associated *Staphylococcus aureus* bacteremia. Arch. Intern. Med. *149*:533, 1989.
188. Hook, E. W.: Annotation. Yale J. Biol. Med. *38*:521, 1966.
189. Pesanti, E. L., and Smith, I. M.: Infective endocarditis with negative blood cultures. An analysis of 52 cases. Am. J. Med. *66*:43, 1979.
190. Van Scoy, R. E.: Culture-negative endocarditis. Mayo Clin. Proc. *57*:149, 1982.
191. Pazin, G. J., Saul, S., and Thompson, M. E.: Blood culture positivity. Suppression by outpatient antibiotic therapy in patients with bacterial endocarditis. Arch. Intern. Med. *142*:263, 1982.
192. Carey, R. B., Gross, K. C., and Roberts, R. B.: Vitamin-B_6-dependent *Streptococcus mitior (mitis)* isolated from patients with systemic infections. J. Infect. Dis. *131*:722, 1975.
193. Auckenthaler, R. W.: Laboratory diagnosis of infective endocarditis. Eur. Heart J. 5(Suppl C):49, 1984.
194. Carrizosa, J., Levison, M. E., Lawrence, T., et al.: Cure of *Aspergillus ustus* endocarditis of prosthetic valve. Arch. Intern. Med. *133*:486, 1974.
195. Pierce, M. A., Saag, M. S., Dismukes, W. E., et al.: Case report: Q fever endocarditis. Am. J. Med. Sci. *292*:104, 1986.
196. Mandell, G. L.: The laboratory in diagnosis and management. In: Kaye, D. (ed.): Infective endocarditis. Baltimore, University Park Press, 1976, pp. 155–166.
197. Williams, R. C., Jr., and Kunkel, H. G.: Rheumatoid factor, complement and conglutinin aberrations in patients with subacute bacterial endocarditis. J. Clin. Invest. *41*:666, 1962.
198. Mohammed, I., Ansell, B. M., Holborow, E. J., et al.: Circulating immune complexes in subacute endocarditis and poststreptococcal glomerulonephritis. J. Clin. Pathol. *30*:308, 1977.
199. Powers, D. L., and Mandell, G. L.: Intraleukocytic bacteria in endocarditis patients. J.A.M.A. *227*:312, 1974.
200. Buda, A. J., Zotz, R. J., Le Mire, M. S., et al.: Prognostic significance of vegetations detected by two-dimensional echocardiography in infective endocarditis. Am. Heart J. *112*:1291, 1986.
201. Bayer, A. S., Blomquist, I. K., Bello, E., et al.: Tricuspid valve endocarditis due to *Staphylococcus aureus*. Chest *93*:247, 1988.
202. Erbel, R., Rohmann, S., Drexler, M., et al.: Improved diagnostic value of echocardiography in patients with infective endocarditis by transoesophageal approach. A prospective study. Eur. Heart J. *9*:43, 1988.
203. Mugge, A., Daniel, W. G., Frank, G., et al.: Echocardiography in infective endocarditis: Reassessment of prognostic implications of vegetation size determined by the transthoracic and the transesophageal approach. J. Am. Coll. Cardiol. *14*:631, 1989.
204. Schwinger, M. E., Tunick, P. A., Freedberg, R. S., et al.: Vegetations on endocardial surface struck by regurgitant jets: Diagnosis by transesophageal echocardiography. Am. Heart J. *119*:1212, 1990.
205. Taams, M. A., Gussenhoven, E. J., Bos, E., et al.: Enhanced morphological diagnosis in infective endocarditis by transoesophageal echocardiography. Br. Heart J. *63*:109, 1990.
206. Klodas, E., Edwards, W. D., and Khandheria, B. K.: Use of echocardiography for improving detection of valvular vegetations in subacute bacterial endocarditis. J. Am. Soc. Echocardiogr. *2*:386, 1989.
206a. Steckelberg, J. M., Murphy, J. G., Ballard, D., et al.: Emboli in infective endocarditis: The prognostic value of echocardiography. Ann. Intern. Med. *114*:635, 1991.
206b. Tunick, P. A., Freedberg, R. S., Schrem, S. S., and Kronzon, I.: Unusual mitral annular vegetation diagnosed by transesophageal echocardiography. Am. Heart J. *120*:444, 1990.
206c. Daniel, W. G., Mugge, A., Martin, R. P., et al.: Improvement in the diagnosis of abscesses associated with endocarditis by transesophageal echocardiography. N. Engl J. Med. *324*:795, 1991.
207. Kinney, E. L., and Wright, R. J.: Aortic valve vegetations: Examples of overestimation and underestimation of disease by two-dimensional echocardiography. Am. Heart J. *113*:1248, 1987.
208. Gross, C. M., Prisant, M., Paolini, D., et al.: Echocardiographic appearance of a flail bioprosthetic mitral valve leaflet mimicking vegetation. Am. Heart J. *117*:953, 1989.
209. Tak, T., Rahimtoola, S. H., Kumar A., et al.: Value of digital image processing of two-dimensional echocardiograms in differentiating active from chronic vegetations of infective endocarditis. Circulation *78*:116, 1988.
210. Jaffe, W. M., Morgan, D. E., and Pearlman, A. S.: Infective endocarditis, 1983–1988: Echocardiographic findings and factors influencing morbidity and mortality. J. Am. Coll. Cardiol. *15*:1227, 1990.
211. Martin, R. P., French, J. W., and Popp, R. L.: Clinical utility of two-dimensional echocardiography in patients with bioprosthetic valves. Adv. Cardiol. *27*:294, 1980.
212. Panidis, I. P., Ross, J., and Mintz, G. S.: Normal and abnormal prosthetic valve function as assessed by Doppler echocardiography. J. Am. Coll. Cardiol. *8*:317, 1986.
213. Hardoff, R., Luder, A. S., and Lorber, A.: Early detection of infantile endocarditis by gallium-67 scintigraphy. Eur. J. Nucl. Med. *15*:219, 1989.
214. Cerqueira, M. D., and Jacobson, A. F.: Indium-111 leukocyte scintigraphic detection of myocardial abscess formation in patients with endocarditis. J. Nucl. Med. *30*:703, 1989.
215. Machac, J., Vallabhajosula, S., Goldman, M. E., et al.: Value of blood-pool subtraction in cardiac indium-111 labeled platelet imaging. J. Nucl. Med. *30*:1445, 1989.

ANTIMICROBIAL THERAPY

216. Durack, D. T., and Beeson, P. B.: Experimental bacterial endocarditis. II. Survival of bacteria in endocardial vegetations. Br. J. Exp. Pathol. *53*:50, 1972.
217. Cremieux, A. C., Maziere, B., and Vallois, J. M.: Evaluation of antibiotic diffusion into cardiac vegetations by quantitative autoradiography. J. Infect. Dis. *159*:938, 1989.
218. Bayer, A. S., Crowell, D., and Nast, C. C.: Intravegetation antimicrobial distribution in aortic endocarditis analyzed by computer-generated model. Chest *97*:611, 1990.
219. Washington, J. A.: In vitro testing of antimicrobial agents. Infect. Dis. Clin. North Am. *3*:375, 1989.
220. Mulligan, M. J., and Cobbs, C. G.: Bacteriostatic versus bactericidal activity. Infect. Dis. Clin. North Am. *3*:389, 1989.
221. Holloway, Y., Dankert, J., and Hess, J.: Penicillin tolerance and bacterial endocarditis. Lancet *1*:589, 1980.
222. Eliopoulos, G. M.: Synergism and antagonism. Infect. Dis. Clin. North Am. *3*:399, 1989.
223. Moellering, R. C.: Treatment of enterococcal endocarditis. In: Sande, M. A., Kaye, D., and Root, R. K. (eds.): Endocarditis. New York, Churchill Livingstone, 1984, pp. 113–133.
224. Wilson, W. R., and Geraci, J. E.: Treatment of streptococcal infective endocarditis. Am. J. Med. 78(Suppl 6B):128, 1985.
225. Meeson, J., McColm, A. A., and Acred, P.: Differential response to benzylpenicillin in vivo of tolerant and non-tolerant variants of *Streptococcus sanguis*. II. J. Antimicrob. Chemother. *25*:103, 1990.
226. Levison, M. E., and Bush, L. M.: Pharmacodynamics of antimicrobial agents, bactericidal and post antibiotic effects. Infect. Dis. Clin. North Am. *3*:415, 1989.
227. Weinstein, M. P., Stratton, C. W., Ackley, A., et al.: Multicenter collaborative evaluation of a standardized serum bactericidal test as a prognostic indicator in infective endocarditis. Am. J. Med. *78*:262, 1985.
228. Wolfson, J. S., and Swartz, M. N.: Serum bactericidal activity as a monitor of antibiotic therapy. N. Engl. J. Med. *312*:968, 1985.
229. Reller, L. B.: The serum bactericidal test. Rev. Infect. Dis. *8*:803, 1986.
230. Craig, W. A., and Ebert, S. C.: Protein binding and its significance in antibacterial therapy. Infect. Dis. Clin. North Am. *3*:407, 1989.
231. Poretz, D. M., Eron, L. J., Goldenberg, R. I., et al.: Intravenous antibiotic therapy in an outpatient setting. JAMA *248*:336, 1982.
232. Guntheroth, W. G., Cammarano, A. A., and Kirby, W.M.M.: Home treatment of infective endocarditis with oral amoxicillin. Am. J. Cardiol. *55*:1231, 1985.
233. Gayet, J. L., Etienne, J., Malquarti, V., et al.: Indices of effectiveness of medical and surgical treatment in 40 cases of prosthetic valve endocarditis. Eur. Heart J. *5*:(Suppl C):133, 1984.
234. Myers, J. P., and Linnemann, C. C.: Bacteremia due to methicillin-resistant *Staphylococcus aureus*. J. Infect. Dis. *145*:532, 1982.
235. Craven, D. E., Kollisch, N. R., Hsieh, C. R., et al.: Vancomycin treatment of bacteremia caused by oxacillin-resistant *Staphylococcus aureus*. J. Infect. Dis. *147*:137, 1983.
236. King, K., and Harkness, J. L.: Infective endocarditis in the 1980s. Treatment and management. Med. J. Aust. *144*:588, 1986.
237. Guzman, F., Gartmill, I., Holden, M. P., et al.: *Candida* endocarditis: Report of four cases. Int. J. Cardiol. *16*:131, 1987.
238. Handrick, W., Kohler, W., Spencker, F. B., et al.: Endocarditis due to nutritionally variant streptococci. Infection *16*:371, 1988.
239. DiNubile, M. J.: Treatment of endocarditis caused by relatively resistant nonenterococcal streptococci: Is penicillin enough? Rev. Infect. Dis. *12*:112, 1990.
240. Wilson, W. R., Wilkowske, C. J., Wright, A. J., et al.: Treatment of streptomycin-susceptible and streptomycin-resistant enterococcal endocarditis. Ann. Intern. Med. *100*:816, 1984.
241. Besnier, J. M., Leport, C., Bure, A., et al.: Vancomycin-aminoglycoside combinations in therapy of endocarditis caused by *Enterococcus* species and *Streptococcus bovis*. Eur. J. Clin. Microbiol. Infect. Dis. *9*:130, 1990.
242. Green, G. R., Peters, G. A., and Geraci, J. E.: Treatment of bacterial endocarditis in patients with penicillin hypersensitivity. Ann. Intern. Med. *67*:235, 1967.
243. Lipman, M. L., and Silva, J.: Endocarditis due to *Streptococcus faecalis* with high-level resistance to gentamicin. Rev. Infect. Dis. *11*:325, 1989.
244. Eliopoulos, G. M., Eliopoulos, C. T.: Therapy of enterococcal infections. Eur. J. Clin. Microbiol. Infect. Dis. *9*:118, 1990.
245. Patterson, J. E., Masecar, B. L., and Zervos, M. J.: Characterization and comparison of two penicillinase-producing strains of *Streptococcus (Enterococcus) faecalis*. Antimicrob. Ag. Chemother. *32*:122, 1988.

246. Bush, L. M., Calmon, J., Cherney, C. L., et al.: High-level penicillin-resistance among isolates of enterococci. Ann. Intern. Med. *110*:515, 1989.
247. Kaplan, A. H., Gilligan, P. H., and Facklam, R. R.: Recovery of resistant enterococci during vancomycin prophylaxis. J. Clin. Microbiol. *26*:1216, 1988.
248. Leclerq, R., Derlot, E., Duval, J., et al.: Plasmid-mediated resistance to vancomycin and teicoplanin in *Enterococcus faecium*. N. Engl. J. Med. *319*:157, 1988.
249. Sande, M. A., and Korzeniowski, O. M.: The antimicrobial therapy of infective endocarditis. New York, Grune & Stratton, 1981, pp. 113–122.
250. Watanakunakorn, C., and Baird, I. M.: Prognostic factors in *Straphylococcus aureus* endocarditis and results of therapy with a penicillin and gentamicin. Am. J. Med. Sci. *273*:133, 1977.
251. Korzeniowski, O., and Sande, M. A.: The National Collaborative Endocarditis Study Group: Combination antimicrobial therapy for *Staphylococcus aureus* endocarditis in patients addicted to parenteral drugs and in nonaddicts. A prospective study. Ann. Intern. Med. *97*:496, 1982.
252. Frimodt-Moller, N., Espersen, F., and Rosdahl, V. T.: Antibiotic treatment of *Staphylococcus aureus* endocarditis. A review of 119 cases. Acta Med. Scand. *222*:175, 1987.
253. Karchmer, A. W.: Antibiotic therapy of nonenterococcal streptococcal and staphylococcal endocarditis: Current regimens and some future considerations. J. Antimicrob. Chemother. *21*(Suppl C):91, 1988.
254. Faville, R. J., Zaske, D. E., Kaplan, E. L., et al.: *Staphylococcus aureus* endocarditis: Combined therapy with vancomycin and rifampin. JAMA *240*:1963, 1978.
255. Acar, J. F., Goldstein, F. W., and Duval, J.: Use of rifampin for the treatment of serious staphylococcal and gram-negative bacillary infections. Rev. Infect. Dis. *5*:S502, 1983.
256. Zak, O., Scheld, W. M., and Sande, M. A.: Rifampin in experimental endocarditis due to *Staphylococcus aureus* in rabbits. Rev. Infect. Dis. *5*:S481, 1983.
257. Chambers, H. F., Miller, R. T., and Newman, M. D.: Right-sided *Staphylococcus aureus* endocarditis in intravenous drug abusers: Two-week combination therapy. Ann. Intern. Med. *109*:619, 1988.
258. Chambers, H. F., and Sande, M. A.: Teicoplanin versus nafcillin and vancomycin in the treatment of experimental endocarditis caused by methicillin-susceptible or -resistant *Staphylococcus aureus*. Antimicrob. Ag. Chemother. *26*:61, 1984.
259. Martino, P., Venditti, M., Micozzi, A., et al.: Teicoplanin in the treatment of gram-positive bacterial endocarditis. Antimicrob. Ag. Chemother. *33*:1329, 1989.
260. Leport, C., Perronne, C., Massip, P., et al.: Evaluation of teicoplanin for treatment of endocarditis caused by gram-positive cocci in 20 patients. Antimicrob. Ag. Chemother. *33*:871, 1989.
261. Kaatz, G. W., Barriere, S. L., Schaberg, D. R., et al.: Ciprofloxacin versus vancomycin in the therapy of experimental methicillin-resistant *Staphylococcus aureus* endocarditis. Antimicrob. Ag. Chemother. *31*:527, 1987.
262. Rouse, M. S., Walcox, R. M., Henry, N. K., et al.: Ciprofloxacin therapy of experimental endocarditis caused by methicillin-resistant *Staphylococcus epidermidis*. Antimicrob. Ag. Chemother. *34*:273, 1990.
263. Dworkin, R. J., Lee, B. L., Sande, M. A., et al.: Treatment of right-sided *Staphylococcus aureus* endocarditis in intravenous drug users with ciprofloxacin and rifampicin. Lancet *2*:1071, 1989.
264. Humphreys, H., and Mulvihill, E.: Ciprofloxacin-resistant *Staphylococcus aureus*. Lancet *2*:383, 1985.
265. Kobasa, W. D., Kaye, K. L., Shapiro, T., et al.: Therapy for experimental endocarditis due to *Staphylococcus epidermidis*. Rev. Infect. Dis. *5*(Suppl 3):533, 1983.
266. Wilson, W. R., and Geraci, J. E.: Antibiotic treatment of infective endocarditis. Ann. Rev. Med. *34*:413, 1983.
267. Levison, M. E.: Therapy of endocarditis due to gram-negative bacteria and fungi. In: Sande, M. A., Kaye, D., and Root, R. K. (eds.): Endocarditis. New York, Churchill Livingstone, 1984, pp. 151–161.
268. Geraci, J. E., and Wilson, W. R.: Endocarditis due to gram-negative bacteria. Report of 56 cases. Mayo Clin. Proc. *52*:145, 1982.
269. Neu, H. C.: The quinolones. Infect. Dis. Clin. North Am. *3*:625, 1989.
270. Donowitz, G. R., and Mandell, G. L.: Beta-lactam antibiotics. N. Engl. J. Med. *318*:419, 1988.
271. Donowitz, G. R.: Third generation cephalosporins. Infect. Dis. Clin. North Am. *3*:595, 1989.
272. Sobel, J. D.: Imipenem and aztreonam. Infect. Dis. Clin. North Am. *3*:613, 1989.
273. Lipman, B., and Neu, H. C.: Imipenem: A new carbapenem antibiotic. Update on antibiotics. II. Med. Clin. North Am. *72*:567, 1988.
274. Diekson, G., Rodriguez, K., and Arcey, S.: Efficacy of imipenem/cilastatin in endocarditis. Am. J. Med. *78*:109, 1985.
275. Neu, H. C.: Aztreonam: The first monobactam. Med. Clin. North Am. *72*:555, 1988.
276. Bush, L. M., Calmon, J., and Johnson, C. C.: Newer penicillins and beta-lactamase inhibitors. Infect. Dis. Clin. North Am. *3*:571, 1989.
277. Reyes, M. P., and Lerner, A. M.: Current problems in the treatment of infective endocarditis due to *Pseudomonas aeruginosa*. Rev. Infect. Dis. *5*:314, 1983.
278. Maderazo, E. G., Hickingbotham, N., and Cooper, B.: *Aspergillus* endocarditis: Cure without surgical valve replacement. South. Med. J. *83*:351, 1990.
279. Haldane, E. V., Marrie, T. J., Faulkner, R. S., et al.: Endocarditis due to Q fever in Nova Scotia: Experience with five patients in 1981–1982. J. Infect. Dis. *148*:978, 1983.
280. Street, A. C., and Durack, D. T.: Experience with trimethoprim-sulfamethoxazole in treatment of infective endocarditis. Rev. Infect. Dis. *10*:915, 1988.
281. Brearley, B. F., and Hutchinson, D. N.: Endocarditis associated with *Chlamydia trachomatis* infection. Br. Heart J. *46*:220, 1981.
282. Daikos, G. L., Kathpalia, S. B., Lolans, V. T., et al.: Long-term oral ciprofloxacin: Experience in the treatment of incurable infective endocarditis. Am. J. Med. *84*:786, 1988.

SURGICAL MANAGEMENT

283. Abdelnoor, M., Nitter-Hauge, S., and Trettli, S.: Relative survival of patients after heart valve replacement. Eur. Heart J. *11*:23, 1990.
284. Teoh, K. H., Ivanov, J., Weisel, R. D., et al.: Determinants of survival and valve failure after mitral valve replacement. Ann. Thorac. Surg. *49*:643, 1990.
285. Jones, E. L., Weintraub, W. S., Craver, J. M., et al.: Ten-year experience with the porcine bioprosthetic valve: Interrelationship of valve survival and patient survival in 1,050 valve replacements. Ann. Thorac. Surg. *49*:370, 1990.
286. Alsip, S. G., Blackstone, E. H., Kirklin, J. W., et al.: Indications for cardiac surgery in patients with active infective endocarditis. Am. J. Med. *78*(Suppl 6B):138, 1985.
287. Karp, R. B.: Role of surgery in infective endocarditis. Cardiovasc. Clin. *17*(3):141, 1987.
288. Cowgill, L. D., Addonizio, P. Hopeman, A. R., et al.: A practical approach to prosthetic valve endocarditis. Ann. Thorac. Surg. *43*:450, 1987.
289. Griffin, F. M., Jr., Jones, G., and Cobbs, C. G.: Aortic insufficiency in bacterial endocarditis. Ann. Intern. Med. *76*:23, 1972.
290. Sweeney, M. S., Ott, D. A., and Livesay, J. J.: Comparison of bioprosthetic and mechanical valve replacement for active endocarditis. J. Thorac. Cardiovasc. Surg. *90*:676, 1985.
291. Mullany, C. J., McIsaacs, A. I., and Rowe, R. H.: The surgical treatment of infective endocarditis. World J. Surg. *13*:132, 1989.
292. Aslamaci, S., Dimitri, W. R., and Williams, B. T.: Operative considerations in active native valve infective endocarditis. J. Cardiovasc. Surg. *30*:328, 1989.
293. Tuna, I. C., Orszulak, T. A., Schaff, H. V., et al.: Results of homograft aortic valve replacement for active endocarditis. Ann. Thorac. Surg. *49*:619, 1990.
293a. Dreyfus, G., Serraf, A., Jebara, V. A., et al.: Valve repair in acute endocarditis. Ann. Thorac. Surg. *49*:706, 1990.
294. Cobbs, C. G., and Gnann, J. W.: Indications for surgery. In: Sande, M. A., Kaye, D., and Root, R. K. (eds.): Endocarditis. New York, Churchill Livingstone, 1984, pp. 201–212.
295. Richardson, J. V., Karp, R. B., Kirklin, J. W., et al.: Treatment of infective endocarditis: A 10-year comparative analysis. Circulation *58*:589, 1978.
296. Fleisher, A. G., David, I., Mogtader, A., et al.: Mitral valvuloplasty and repair for infective endocarditis. J. Thorac. Cardiovasc. Surg. *93*:311, 1987.
297. Evora, P.R.B., Brasil, J.C.F., and Elias, L. C.: Surgical excision of the vegetation: Treatment of tricuspid valve endocarditis. Cardiology *75*:287, 1988.
298. Yee, E. S., and Ullyot, D. J.: Reparative approach for right-sided endocarditis. J. Thorac. Cardiovasc. Surg. *96*:133, 1988.
299. Yee, E. S., and Khonsari, S.: Right-sided infective endocarditis: Valvuloplasty, valvectomy or replacement. J. Cardiovasc. Surg. *30*:744, 1989.
300. Barbour, D. J., and Roberts, W. C.: Valve excision only versus valve excision plus replacement for active infective endocarditis involving the tricuspid valve. Am. J. Cardiol. *57*:475, 1986.
301. DiSesa, V. J., Sloss, L. J., and Cohn, L. H.: Heart transplantation for intractable prosthetic valve endocarditis. J. Heart Transplant *9*:142, 1990.
302. Wilson, W. R., Geraci, J. E., Danielson, G. K., et al.: Anticoagulant therapy and central nervous system complications in patients with prosthetic valve endocarditis. Circulation *57*:1004, 1978.

RESPONSE TO THERAPY

303. Levison, M. E.: Response to therapy. In: Kaye, D. (ed.): Infective Endocarditis. Baltimore, University Park Press, 1976, pp. 185–199.
304. Douglas, A., Moore-Gillon, J. M., and Eykyn, S.: Fever during treatment of infective endocarditis. Lancet *1*:1342, 1986.
305. Zabalgoitia-Reyes, M., Mehlman, D. J., and Talano, J. V.: Persistent fever with aortic valve endocarditis. Arch. Intern. Med. *145*:327, 1985.
306. Brust, J.C.M., Dickinson, P.C.T., and Hughes, J.E.O.: The diagnosis and treatment of cerebral mycotic aneurysms. Ann. Neurol. *27*:238, 1990.
307. Neugarten, J., and Baldwin, D. S.: Glomerulonephritis in bacterial endocarditis. Am. J. Med. *77*:297, 1984.
308. Rovzar, M. A., Logan, J. L., Ogden, D. A., et al.: Immunosuppressive therapy and plasmapheresis in rapidly progressive glomerulonephritis associated with bacterial endocarditis. Am. J. Kidney Dis. *7*:428, 1986.
309. McKinsey, D. S., McMurray, T. I., and Flynn, J. M.: Immune complex glomerulonephritis associated with *Staphylococcus aureus* bacteremia: Response to corticosteroid therapy. Rev. Infect. Dis *12*:125, 1990.
310. Cates, J. E., and Christie, R. V.: Subacute bacterial endocarditis. Q. J. Med. *20*:93, 1951.
311. Wilson, W. R., Giuliani, E. R., Danielson, G. K., et al.: Symposium on

infective endocarditis. II. General considerations in the diagnosis and treatment of infective endocarditis. Mayo Clin. Proc. *57*:81, 1982.

312. Noseda, A., Liesnard, C., Goffin, Y., et al.: Q fever endocarditis: Relapse five years after successful valve replacement for a first unrecognized episode. J. Cardiovasc. Surg. *29*:360, 1988.
313. Levison, M. E., Kaye, D., Mandell, G. L., and Hook, E.: Characteristics of patients with multiple episodes of bacterial endocarditis. JAMA *211*:1355, 1970.
314. Malquarti, V., Saradarian, W., Etienne, J., et al.: Prognosis of native valve infective endocarditis: A review of 253 cases. Eur. Heart J. 5(Suppl C):11, 1984.
315. Julander, I.: Unfavorable prognostic factors in *Staphylococcus aureus* septicemia and endocarditis. Scand. J. Infect. Dis. *17*:179, 1985.
316. Leport, C., Vilde, J. L., and Bricaire, F.: Fifty cases of late prosthetic valve endocarditis: Improvement in prognosis over a 15 year period. Br. Heart J. *58*:66, 1987.
317. Dismukes, W. E.: Prosthetic valve endocarditis. Factors influencing outcome and recommendations for therapy. In: Bisno, A. L. (ed.) Treatment of Infective Endocarditis. New York, Grune & Stratton, 1981, pp. 167–191.
318. Wilson, W. R., Danielson, G. K., Giuliani, E. R., et al.: Prosthetic valve endocarditis. Mayo Clin. Proc. *57*:155, 1982.
319. Calderwood, S. B., Swinski, L. A., Karchmer, A. W., et al.: Prosthetic valve endocarditis: Analysis of factors affecting outcome of therapy. J. Thorac. Cardiovasc. Surg. *92*:776, 1986.
320. Cortina, J. M., Martinell, J., and Artiz, V.: Surgical treatment of active prosthetic valve endocarditis. J. Thorac. Cardiovasc. Surg. *35*:209, 1987.

PREVENTION

321. Bayliss, R., Clarke, C., Oakley, C., et al.: The teeth and infective endocarditis. Br. Heart J. *50*:506, 1983.
322. Kaye, D.: Prophylaxis against bacterial endocarditis: A dilemma. In: Kaplan, E. L., and Taranta, A. V. (eds.): Infective Endocarditis. Dallas, American Heart Association (AHA Monograph No. 52):67, 1977.
323. Pelletier, L. J., Jr., and Petersdorf, R. G.: Infective endocarditis: A review of 125 cases from the University of Washington hospitals, 1963–1972. Medicine (Baltimore) *56*:282, 1977.
324. Lowes, J. A., Hamer, J., Williams, G., et al.: 10 years of infective endocarditis at St. Bartholomew's Hospital: Analysis of clinical features and treatment in relation to prognosis and mortality. Lancet *1*:133, 1980.
325. Moulsdale, M. T., Eykyn, S. J., and Phillips, I.: Infective endocarditis, 1970–1979: A study of culture-positive cases in St. Thomas's Hospital. Q. J. Med. *49*:315, 1980.
326. Guntheroth, W. G.: How important are dental procedures as a cause of infective endocarditis? Am. J. Cardiol. *54*:797, 1984.
327. Meyer, G. W.: Endocarditis prophylaxis and gastrointestinal procedures. Am. J. Gastroenterol. *84*(12):1492, 1989.
328. Fleischer, D: Recommendations for antibiotic prophylaxis before endoscopy. Am. J. Gastroenterol. *84*(12):1489, 1989.
329. Kaye, D.: Prophylaxis of endocarditis. *In* Kaye, D. (ed.): Infective Endocarditis. Baltimore, University Park Press, 1976, pp. 245–265.
330. Lowy, F., and Steigbigel, N. H.: Infective endocarditis. Am. Heart J. *96*:689, 1978.
331. Goodman, J. S., Schaffner, W., Collins, H. A., et al.: Infection after cardiovascular surgery: Clinical study including examination of antimicrobial prophylaxis. N. Engl. J. Med. *287*:117, 1968.
332. Pallasch, T. J.: A critical appraisal of antibiotic prophylaxis. Int. Dent. J. *39*:183, 1989.
333. Fekete, T.: Controversies in the prevention of infective endocarditis related to dental procedures. Dent. Clin. North Am. *34*(1):79, 1990.
334. Lockhart, P. B., Crist, D., and Stone, P. H.: The reliability of the medical history in the identification of patients at risk for infective endocarditis. J. Am. Dent. Assoc. *119*:417, 1989.
335. Sadowsky, D., and Kunzel, C.: Recommendations for prevention of bacterial endocarditis: Compliance by dental general practitioners. Circulation *77*:1316, 1988.
336. Bender, I. B., Naidorf, I. J., and Garvey, G. J.: Bacterial endocarditis: A consideration for physician and dentist. J. Am. Dent. Assoc. *10*:415, 1984.
337. Durack, D. T., Bisno, A. L., and Kaplan, E. L.: Apparent failure of endocarditis prophylaxis. Analysis of 52 cases submitted to a national registry. JAMA *250*:2318, 1983.
338. Glauser, M. P., Bernard, J. P., Mareillon, P., and Francioli, P.: Successful single-dose amoxicillin prophylaxis against experimental streptococcal endocarditis: Evidence for two mechanisms of protection. J. Infect. Dis. *147*:568, 1983.
339. Francioli, P., Mareillon, P., and Glauser, M. P.: Comparison of single-doses of amoxicillin or of amoxicillin-gentamicin for the prevention of endocarditis caused by *Streptococcus faecalis* and by viridans streptococci. J. Infect. Dis. *152*:83, 1985.
340. Dajani, A. S., Bisno, A. L., Chung, K. J., et al.: Prevention of bacterial endocarditis. JAMA *264*:2919, 1990.
341. Devereux, R. B., Hawkins, J., Kramer-Fox, R., et al.: Complications of mitral valve prolapse: Disproportionate occurrence in men and older patients. Am. J. Med. *81*:751, 1986.
342. Hickey, A. J., MacMahon, S. W., and Wilcken, D.E.L.: Mitral valve prolapse and bacterial endocarditis: When is antibiotic prophylaxis necessary? Am. Heart J. *109*(3 pt 1):431, 1985.
343. Bor, D. H., and Himmelstein, D. U.: Endocarditis prophylaxis for patients with mitral valve prolapse: A quantitative analysis. Am. J. Med. *76*:711, 1984.
344. Clemens, J. D., and Ransohoff, D. F.: A quantitative assessment of predental antibiotic prophylaxis for patients with mitral valve prolapse. J. Chronic Dis. *37*:531, 1984.
345. Kaye, D.: Prophylaxis for infective endocarditis: An update. Ann. Intern. Med. *104*:419, 1986.

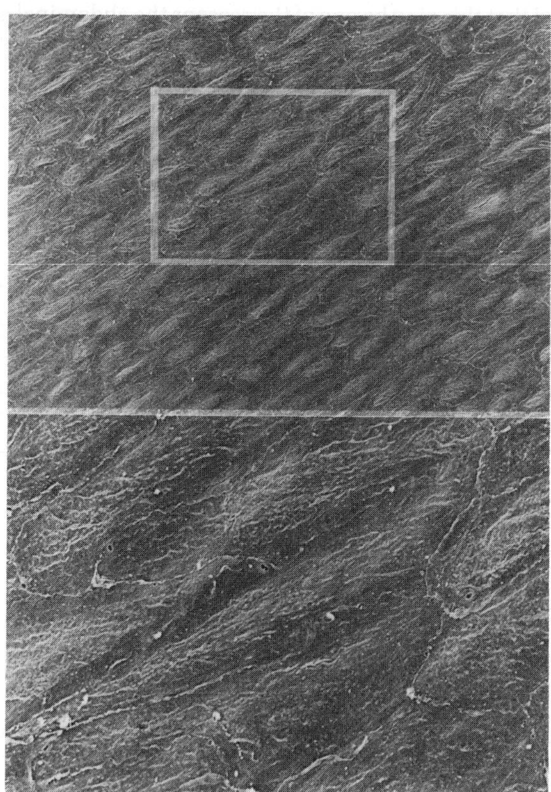

FIGURE 36–3. Scanning electron micrographs of the thoracic aorta endothelium from normal monkey *(Macaca nemestrina).* ×540. At somewhat higher magnification, the overlapping folds of the endothelial cells can be clearly visualized. The elongated and elliptical appearance of the endothelium can also be seen. The long axes of the cells appear to be diagonal and are oriented in the main direction of the flow of blood in the artery. ×2100. (From Ross, R.: Atherosclerosis: A problem of the biology of arterial wall cells and their interactions with blood components. Arteriosclerosis *1*:297, 1981, by permission of the American Heart Association.)

Although the endothelial cells, as seen en face by light and scanning electron microscopy (Fig. 36–3) and in cross section by light and transmission electron microscopy (Fig. 36–4), appear to be highly similar morphologically in different parts of the arterial tree, there may be functional differences in these lining cells in different anatomical sites. For example, capillary endothelial cells contain receptors on their surfaces for a potent growth-regulatory peptide, platelet-derived growth factor (PDGF), whereas these receptors are absent on arterial endothelium.[35] Other differences are likely to be found, not only between capillary and arterial endothelium, but among endothelial cells in different parts of the arterial tree itself. With these differences, one might anticipate that there might be differences in the way in which endothelial cells respond to injury after exposure to various injurious agents in different parts of the arterial tree. Endothelial cells are normally attached to each other by tight junctions and by gap junctions. They transport substances in both directions via the process of endocytosis, sometimes called *transcytosis.* Transendothelial channels have been observed in capillary endothelium; however, it is not clear whether they play a role in macromolecular transport in arterial tissue. It has also been suggested that the junctions between endothelial cells may serve as potential sites of increased endothelial transport, particularly when the endothelium has been injured.

Endothelial cells rest on a basement membrane that consists of a particular form of collagen (type IV collagen) intermixed with particular types of proteoglycan molecules. The endothelial cells are undoubtedly responsible for the synthesis of these connective tissue molecules.[33] The basement membrane probably also serves as a crude form of filter.

Endothelial cells have receptors for many different molecules on their surface, including receptors for low-density lipoprotein (LDL),[36] for growth factors, and probably for a number of pharmacological agents. A special capacity of endothelium that may be particularly important in atherogenesis is its ability to modify lipoproteins. LDLs appear to be "modified" by a process of low-level oxidation when they are bound to LDL receptors, internalized, and transported through the

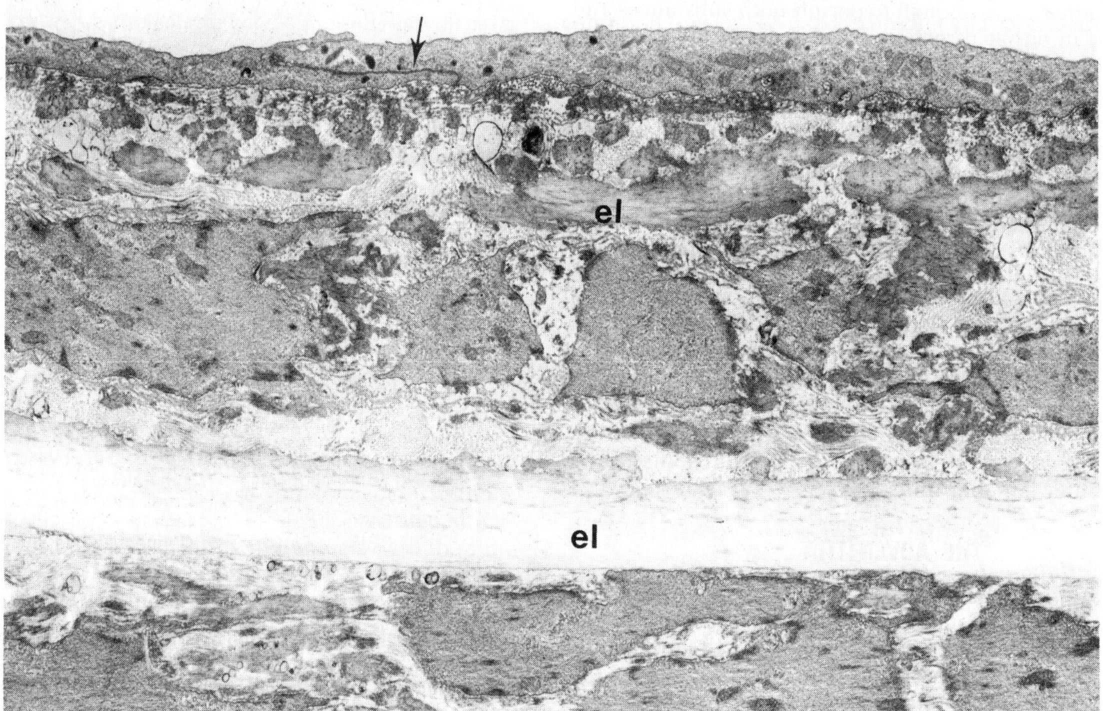

FIGURE 36–4. Transmission electron micrograph of a developing monkey aorta. Two endothelial cells can be seen at the lumen with a junction between them (arrow). Beneath the endothelial cells are newly forming elastic fibers (el) that are separated from the endothelium by basement membrane and collagen fibrils. Beneath the newly forming elastic fibers is a layer of smooth muscle cells separated from another layer by a well-formed elastica (el). No nuclei are apparent in the endothelial cells in this particular thin section.

endothelium. Such modified LDLs can bind to a specific type of receptor, termed a scavenger receptor, on the surface of macrophages, where they are ingested and contribute to the formation of foam cells. This activity is probably important in atherogenesis (see below). The endothelium normally provides a nonthrombogenic surface because of its capacity to form prostaglandin derivatives, particularly prostacyclin (PGI_2) (Chap. 59), a potent vasodilator that is an effective inhibitor of platelet aggregation,[29,32] and because of its surface coat of heparan sulfate. Endothelial cells also make the most potent vasodilator thus far discovered, endothelial-derived relaxing factor (EDRF), a thiolated form of nitric oxide. EDRF formation by endothelium may be critical in maintaining a balance between vasoconstriction and vasodilation in the process of arterial homeostasis.[37] Endothelial cells can also secrete agents that are effective in lysing fibrin clots, including plasminogen, as well as procoagulant materials such as von Willebrand factor.[34] They also secrete a number of vasoactive agents, such as endothelin,[38] angiotensin-converting enzyme, and platelet-derived growth factor, which may be important in vasoconstriction.

A particular characteristic of the endothelium that may be of great importance is the fact that endothelial cells grow in an obligate monolayer. Such growth is representative of cells that line most body surfaces, including epithelial surfaces, and is characterized by the fact that the endothelial cells cannot crawl over one another at sites of injury to facilitate repair of a surface that has been deendothelialized. In other words, only the cells at the margin of an injury can participate in the regenerative response. Thus if a particular anatomical site is repeatedly injured over a prolonged period, and if the endothelial cells that regenerate lose their replication capacity, cells distal to the site, capable of replicating, may not be able to participate simply because they cannot reach the site to do so.

Arterial endothelial cells are capable of synthesizing and secreting at least two mitogens, one of which is a form of PDGF.[39-41] PDGF is a growth factor for mesenchymally derived, connective tissue-forming cells such as fibroblasts and smooth muscle, but not for arterial endothelial cells. The capacity of endothelium, when it has been appropriately "activated," to form such growth factors may be important in atherogenesis. This will be discussed further in the section concerning the response-to-injury hypothesis of atherosclerosis (see p. 1113).

Thus, the endothelium forms an obligate monolayer that lines the entire arterial tree, is metabolically active, produces vasoactive substances, has a nonthrombogenic surface, and can form procoagulant materials. It also serves as the permeability barrier that controls the passage of molecules into the artery. All of these activities demonstrate the dynamic nature of the endothelial lining and how potentially important this cell layer is in the maintenance of arterial homeostasis.

SMOOTH MUSCLE

The cell that proliferates in the arterial intima to form the intermediate and advanced lesions of atherosclerosis, the smooth muscle cell, is originally derived from the media. In his early work, Wissler[42] described this cell as a "multifunctional medial mesenchymal cell." It is now widely accepted that proliferation of smooth muscle cells in the intima represents the sine qua non of the lesions of advanced atherosclerosis (Fig. 36–5).

Twenty years ago, the only functional capacity attributed to the smooth muscle cell was its ability to contract. In 1971, it became possible to maintain and propagate pure populations of smooth muscle cells in culture and to demonstrate that this cell, like the fibroblast, is one of the principal connective tissue-forming cells in the body.[43] It is capable of synthesizing and secreting several forms of collagen, both elastic fiber proteins and several different types of proteoglycans.[44] The principal role of the smooth muscle cell in the fully formed adult artery is presumably to maintain the tone of the arterial wall by its capacity to maintain the slow contractions peculiar to smooth muscle. The smooth muscle cell responds to numerous vasoactive agents, such as epinephrine and angiotensin, which induce contraction and vasoconstriction, and prostacyclin and EDRF, which can induce relaxation and vasodilation. Smooth muscle cells, like fibroblasts, contain specific high-affinity receptors for a number of ligands. These ligands include LDL[45] (see p. 1127) (which is the principal cholesterol-carrying plasma lipoprotein that participates in regulation of cholesterol metabolism), insulin (which is involved in glucose metabolism), and growth stimulators such as PDGF[46] and growth inhibitors such as transforming growth factor beta (TGF β) (which help to regulate cell multiplication). Arterial smooth muscle cells of the newborn rat, in contrast to adult rat smooth muscle, have been shown to be capable of synthesizing and secreting PDGF.[47] These observations suggest possible roles for smooth muscle in growth and development and possibly in atherosclerosis as well (to be discussed below).

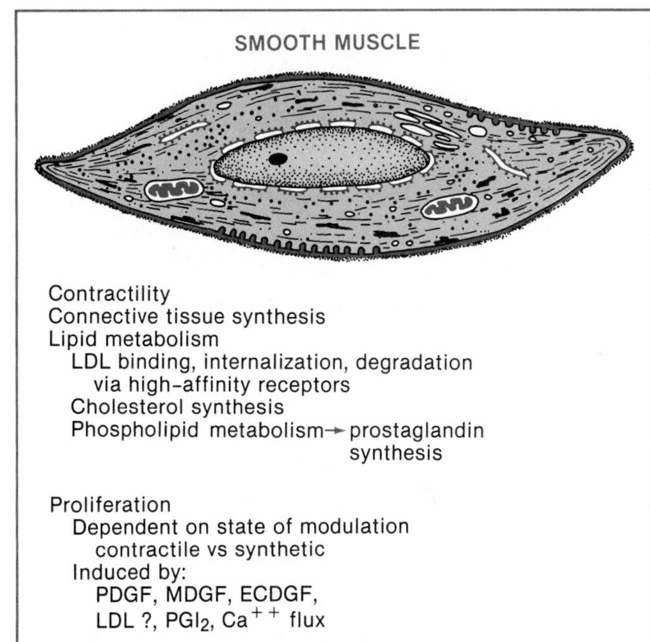

FIGURE 36–5. A smooth muscle cell showing many of the phenotypic characteristics of normal smooth muscle, as well as factors that can induce smooth muscle proliferation. (From Ross, R.: Atherosclerosis: A problem of the biology of arterial wall cells and their interactions with blood components. Arteriosclerosis *1*:304, 1981, by permission of the American Heart Association.)

Smooth muscle cells appear to be capable of presenting two different phenotypes in culture.[48,49] The first of these, the *contractile phenotype*, is generally thought to be associated with cell contractility because the cells contain extensive myofibrils throughout their cytoplasm consisting of actin and myosin filaments. These contractile filaments bind to one another and to the subplasmalemmal surface of the cell by dense bodies. Such cells do *not* appear to be capable of responding to mitogens such as PDGF. When a smooth muscle cell becomes appropriately stimulated, it loses its contractile phenotype and changes to a cell that has decreased content of myofilaments and that contains an extensively developed rough endoplasmic reticulum and Golgi complex. Such a cell has been described as being in a *synthetic phenotype*. Smooth muscle cells in the synthetic phenotype appear to be involved in the formation of numerous secretory proteins, including connective tissue matrix macromolecules. These two different smooth muscle phenotypes have been described in cell culture as well as in the artery wall.

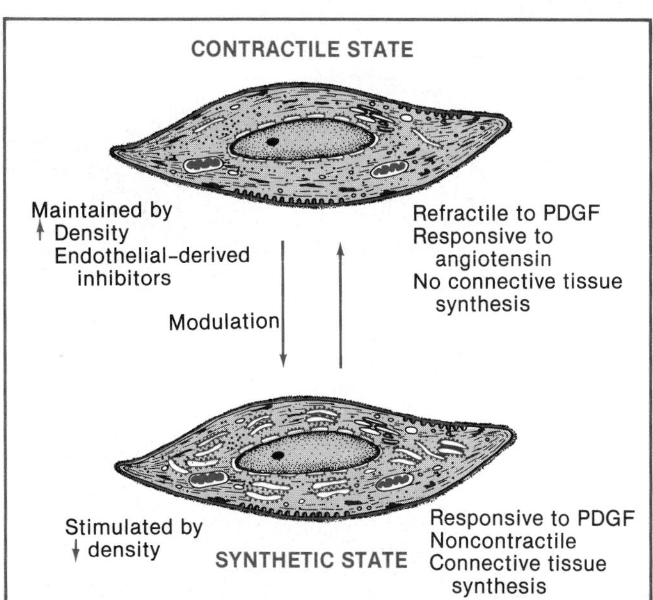

FIGURE 36-6. The state of modulation of smooth muscle cells in which the contractile versus the synthetic state is maintained by different sets of factors. (From Ross, R.: Atherosclerosis: A problem of the biology of arterial wall cells and their interactions with blood components. Arteriosclerosis *1*:305, 1981, by permission of the American Heart Association.)

It has been suggested that the phenotypic differentiation of the smooth muscle cell may be important in terms of its capacity to respond to mitogens such as PDGF, and thus to form the proliferative lesions of atherosclerosis. Smooth muscle cells in the contractile phenotype have been described as nonresponsive to mitogens, whereas those in the synthetic phenotype have been described as responsive.[48,49] For the lesions of atherosclerosis to form, the smooth muscle cells must, in most cases, migrate from the media into the intima, where they can respond mitogenically. Consequently, control of the phenotypic state of smooth muscle cells could be important in understanding and preventing atherogenesis (Fig. 36-6).

One characteristic feature of the smooth muscle cells found in the lesions of atherosclerosis is the accumulation of lipid that results in formation of vacuolated cells, or foam cells. Most of the lipids that are deposited in these cells are in the form of cholesteryl esters that result from increase in cholesterol synthesis and esterification, and also a decrease in degradation of cholesteryl esters in the lysosomes of the cell.

Although smooth muscle cells were originally conceived of as only the receiver of signals such as those derived from mitogens, it has now been demonstrated that they not only can respond to mitogens such as PDGF but that they can synthesize and secrete substances such as PDGF and other growth-regulatory molecules so that they may stimulate themselves and their neighbors. Thus, smooth muscle cells may respond in autocrine fashion to molecules they themselves form. For example, it is well known that a marked intimal smooth muscle proliferative lesion can be induced by passing an intraarterial balloon embolectomy catheter through an artery. The pressure exerted by the balloon is sufficient to strip off the lining endothelium, expand the artery, and damage many of the smooth muscle cells in the wall of the artery. The exposed subendothelial connective tissue attracts platelets to adhere and degranulate, and many of the injured subendothelial smooth muscle cells undergo a change and migrate from the media into the intima, where they proliferate and form a myointimal hyperplastic fibrotic lesion. If the smooth muscle cells are cultured from such a lesion and are compared with those cultured from a contralateral uninjured artery, the cells from the proliferative lesion secrete a form of PDGF (see section on Growth Factors), and thus may participate in further enlargement of the lesion by autocrine stimulation. Similarly, when smooth muscle cells derived from lesions of atherosclerosis are grown in culture, they secrete PDGF into the culture medium. Interestingly, there are data to suggest that smooth muscle cells derived from human occlusive fibrous plaques of the superficial femoral arteries have a limited capacity to divide in culture. When placed in culture, these cells respond less well to mitogens and act like senescent cells that have already undergone numerous cell doublings.[50] Although the cells may secrete mitogens in culture, it remains to be determined whether they are capable of secreting mitogens and responding to them in vivo.

Some data relevant to these observations have come from studies in nonhuman primates where Northern analyses of advanced lesions of atherosclerosis, using cDNA probes for different growth-regulatory peptides, have demonstrated increased messenger RNA for PDGF-B chain, and for both receptors of PDGF. Recent studies (see below), however, show that the principal source of the PDGF-B chain in these lesions is the macrophage. The smooth muscle cells appear to be the principal recipient of the growth regulatory peptides. Thus the regulation of smooth muscle cells via cellular interaction in the lesions of atherosclerosis needs to be further explored.

MACROPHAGES

Macrophages in all tissues, whether they are resident macrophages or cells that have entered the tissue during an inflammatory response, are derived at some point in their life span from circulating monocytes.[51] When the monocyte enters a tissue, it appears to take on characteristics peculiar to the host tissue. In most inflammatory sites, the macrophage acts as a scavenger cell to remove foreign substances by phagocytosis and intracellular hydrolysis and as a second line of defense after the neutrophil against microbial organisms.[52]

Macrophages are capable of secreting a large number of biologically important substances, including chemotactic agents such as leukotriene B4[53] and interleukin 1,[54] and oxygen metabolites such as superoxide anion,[55] which can be toxic to other cells. Macrophages have recently been shown to be capable of synthesizing and secreting at least six different growth factors.[56] These include (1) PDGF,[57] a growth factor for mesenchymal cells such as smooth muscle and fibroblasts; (2) interleukin 1, a cytokine that induces PDGF gene expression in fibroblasts[54,58]; (3) fibroblast growth factor (FGF),[59] a mitogen for endothelial cells and thus a potentially important angiogenic agent; (4) epidermal growth factor (EGF) and EGF-like molecules [e.g., transforming growth factor alpha (TGF α)], both of which bind to the same receptor and are capable of stimulating the growth of epithelial cells; (5) TGF β, a substance that participates in a synergistic way with some of the aforementioned growth factors in aiding the proliferation of many cells in different tissues and in many instances in inhibiting cell growth; and (6) M-CSF, a growth factor for monocyte macrophages[60] (Fig. 36-7).

As a result of its scavenging capacity and its ability to form and secrete growth factors, the macrophage is probably the key cell responsible for the promotion of connective tissue proliferation so commonly associated with chronic inflammatory responses. Macrophages, like smooth muscle, are a major source of foam cells in the lesions of atherosclerosis. In fact, they are the principal cells in the fatty streak, the initial lesion of atherosclerosis. They accumulate large amounts of lipid in the form of droplets that contain large amounts of cholesteryl ester. The role of the macrophage in atherogenesis will be discussed below.

PLATELETS

(see also Chap. 58)

Although they are probably uninvolved in the generation of many lesions, platelets are clearly implicated in the genesis of some of the lesions of atherosclerosis. (This will be discussed in greater detail below.) However, platelets are also important because they are regularly involved in one of the principal sequelae of atherosclerosis, thrombosis. It is usually a mural or occlusive thrombus or both that leads to infarction.

Platelets are amazing cells in that, although they are capable of little to no protein synthesis, they contain, sequestered in their granules, numerous prepacked extraordinarily potent molecules[61,62] (Fig. 36–8). Among these are a number of factors that participate in the coagulation cascade and, in addition, at least four extremely potent growth factors or mitogens. These are the same growth factors that can be formed by the activated macrophage, namely, PDGF,[63] FGF, EGF[64] or TGF α, and TGF β.[65] It appears that each of these growth factors is present in a class of granules, the alpha granules, which were originally thought to represent a single class on the basis of cell fractionation studies. They may, however, represent several different granules that are similar in morphological and flotation characteristics. Thus, when they are separated by cell fractionation and density gradient centrifugation, they appear to sequester into a single population.

When the platelet is exposed to substrates that induce platelet adherence, aggregation, and degranulation, each of these growth factors is potentially released and thus is capable of eliciting a proliferative response by essentially all of the resident cells in a particular tissue. In other words, platelets contain growth factors potentially stimulatory for each of the cell types present in any tissue in which platelet aggregation and release may occur. Thus, at sites of injury in which collagen exposure, thrombin and fibrin formation, or adenosine diphosphate release occur, platelet aggregation and thrombosis can occur, leading to release of the numerous vasoactive, stimulatory, and proliferative agents carried by the platelets. Each of these agents may play an important role in stimulating an early vasoconstrictive and proliferative response.[66] This early reparative response to injury may be important in the initiation of the lesions of atherosclerosis as well.

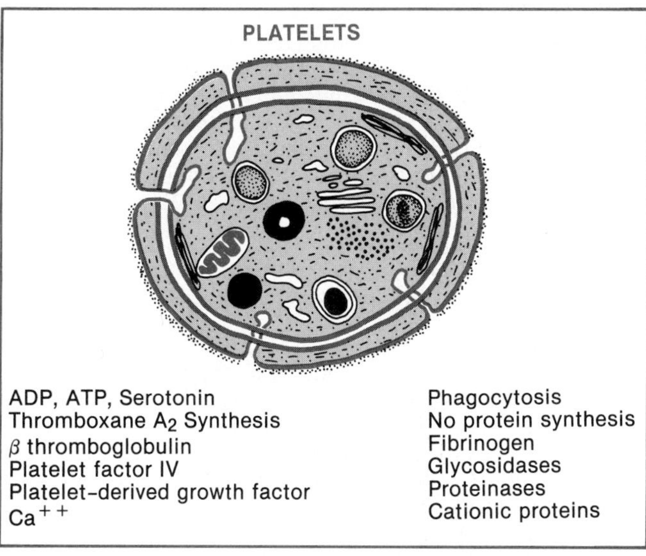

PLATELETS
ADP, ATP, Serotonin
Thromboxane A_2 Synthesis
β thromboglobulin
Platelet factor IV
Platelet-derived growth factor
Ca^{++}
Phagocytosis
No protein synthesis
Fibrinogen
Glycosidases
Proteinases
Cationic proteins

FIGURE 36–8. A platelet demonstrating the principal constituents of the platelet, which are listed beneath the figure. (From Ross, R.: Atherosclerosis: A problem of the biology of arterial wall cells and their interactions with blood components. Arteriosclerosis *1*:301, 1981, by permission of the American Heart Association.)

MONOCYTE/MACROPHAGE

Neutral proteases
Acid hydrolases
Complement
Enzyme inhibitors
Reactive metabolites of O_2
Bioactive lipids
Chemotactic factors
Growth factors
Factors inhibitory to replication of lymphocytes, viruses, and tumor cells
Modified LDL receptors

FIGURE 36–7. A monocyte/macrophage cell containing a large number of substances, many of which are not present in the circulating monocyte but are formed after the monocyte leaves the blood and enters a specific tissue. A few of the components that can be found in macrophages are listed beneath the diagram. (From Ross, R.: Atherosclerosis: A problem of the biology of arterial wall cells and their interactions with blood components. Arteriosclerosis *1*:302, 1981, by permission of the American Heart Association.)

T-LYMPHOCYTES

T-lymphocytes, both CD-8+ and CD-4+, have been observed in all phases of atherogenesis in humans and in nonhuman primates.[67–70] Their involvement in the lesions of atherosclerosis supports the notion that these lesions may develop, at least in part, as a result of an immune or possibly autoimmune response. Experimentally induced autoimmunity has been shown to induce rampant proliferative lesions of atherosclerosis in rabbits.[71] In humans, rejected cardiac transplants characteristically have extensive occlusive lesions of atherosclerosis in the coronary arteries. However, in contrast to the lesions observed in common atherosclerosis, the majority of which are eccentric lesions, those observed in the rejected hearts are concentric in appearance. The nature of the antigen(s) that may play a role in common atherosclerosis is unknown. However, interactions between T-lymphocytes and activated macrophages, both of which are prominent in the lesions, suggest that antigen presentation and the release of cytokines and growth factors between the activated macrophages and T cells may be important in this process.[72,73]

THE LESIONS OF ATHEROSCLEROSIS

Although atherosclerosis has been known for many centuries, its clinical effects are manifested principally in medium-sized muscular arteries, including the coronary, carotid, basilar, and vertebral arteries, as well as several arteries affecting the lower extremities, particularly the iliac and superficial femoral arteries. Larger arteries, such as the aorta and the iliac arteries, can also be involved, and the principal clinical sequelae in these large arteries is usually aneurysmal dilatation and its related effects.[74]

The earliest lesions of atherosclerosis can usually be found in young children and infants in the form of a lesion called the *fatty streak*, whereas the advanced lesion, the fibrous plaque, generally appears during early adulthood and progresses with age.[75–78] Until recently, most tissues that had been prepared for examination were derived from autopsy specimens and were sufficiently poorly preserved so that when the cells became laden with lipid and appeared as foam cells, it was virtually impossible to determine the origin of the cell. Advances in tissue fixation and embedding have permitted new modes of preservation. Furthermore, monoclonal antibodies have been developed that are specific for smooth muscle cells, for macrophages, and for lymphocytes. With the use of these antibodies and with improved preservation techniques, it has been possible to identify specifically the origin of the cells in the different lesions of atherosclerosis.

THE FATTY STREAK

Fatty streaks were observed by Stary[78] in his studies of a series of children and young adults. He demonstrated that by the age of 10 years, the fatty streaks consisted principally of lipid-laden macrophages, together with varying (but usually small) numbers of lipid-filled smooth muscle cells that accumulated beneath them as the lesions increased in size. Grossly, the fatty streak appears as an area of yellow discoloration due to the large amount of lipid deposited in the foam cells. The bulk of this lipid is in the form of cholesterol and cholesteryl ester, which probably enters the fatty streak by transport of lipoproteins from the plasma via the endothelial cells, after which it is taken up by macrophages and smooth muscle cells. The plasma lipids present in the intima are ingested by macrophages and are hydrolyzed and re-esterified once they have been taken up by these cells.

Stary also studied fatty streaks in the coronary arteries of a series of children and young adults and observed that they were localized at anatomical sites that were the same as the sites in other older individuals that were occupied by advanced fibromuscular lesions, or fibrous plaques. His data and that of others suggested that over a time, fatty streaks at particular sites are converted by a series of changes into the more advanced fibroproliferative lesions of atherosclerosis, whereas fatty streaks at other anatomical sites either remain the same or regress and disappear. McGill[79] has gone on to review data to demonstrate that with time, fatty streaks occupy increasing surface areas of the coronary arteries and that these sites also precede the formation of advanced lesions. Thus, although it is difficult to derive firm conclusions from these types of data, such observations suggest that the fatty streak in many instances, if not the large majority, is the precursor lesion that becomes converted into the advanced occlusive form of atherosclerosis.

Once foam cells have formed in fatty streaks and in advanced lesions, it may become extremely difficult to define the cell of origin. The cells become filled with lipid droplets that appear as empty vacuoles in paraffin-embedded tissues which are often surrounded by a very thin rim of cytoplasm (Fig. 36–9). Electron microscopic examination may permit identification of some of these cells; however, large numbers remain difficult if not impossible to identify using standard techniques of tissue staining.

Several monoclonal antibodies have been developed, at least two of which appear to be specific for cell type. Tsukada et al.[80] have developed monoclonal antibodies against smooth muscle–alpha actin and against a cytoplasmic antigen present in macrophages. Fortunately, these antigens resist some modes of fixation and embedding in paraffin. With these monoclonal antibodies, it has been possible to positively identify macrophages, T-lymphocytes, and smooth muscle cells in lesions of atherosclerosis. Thus it can be said definitively that the fatty streak consists principally of lipid-laden macrophages and T-lymphocytes, together with small and variable numbers of smooth muscle cells (Fig. 36–9).

DIFFUSE INTIMAL THICKENING

One form of lesion, described as a diffuse intimal thickening, consists of increased numbers of intimal smooth muscle cells surrounded by variable amounts of connective tissue. It is not entirely clear whether these sites of thickened intima represent developmental thickenings or whether such multilayered cushions of intimal smooth muscle cells are sites that formed because of increased stress on the artery wall, but which do not progress to advanced lesions of atherosclerosis. This is a somewhat poorly understood and controversial subject.

THE FIBROUS PLAQUE

The advanced lesion of atherosclerosis is generally called a fibrous plaque. When the fibrous plaque becomes involved with thrombosis, hemorrhage, and/or calcification, it is often called a *complicated lesion*.

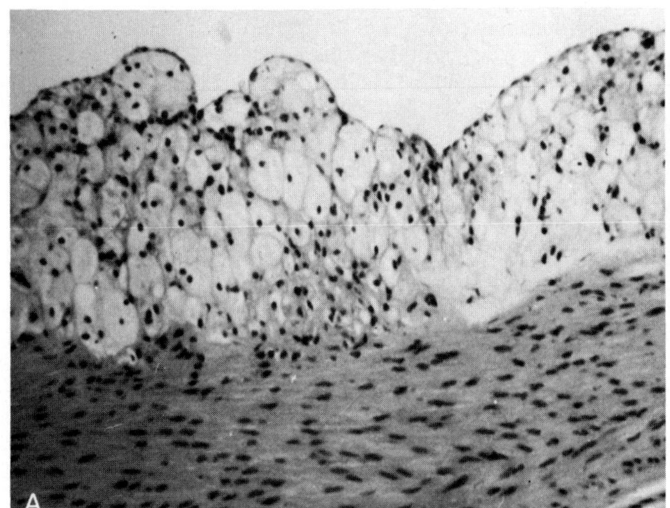

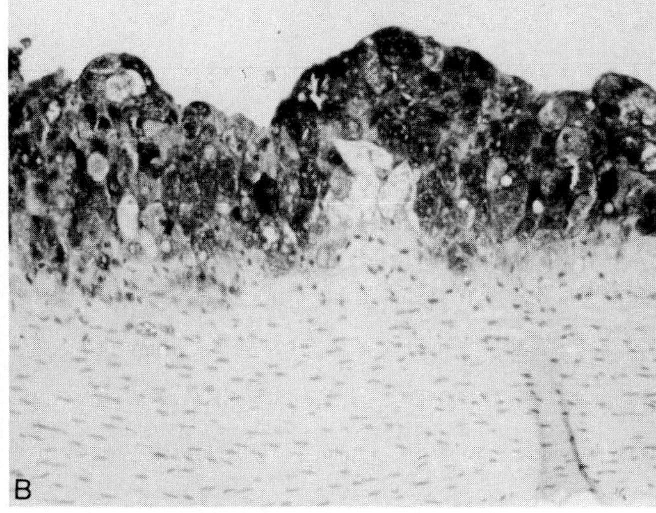

FIGURE 36–9. Light micrographs demonstrating portions of a fatty streak obtained from an aorta of a hypercholesterolemic monkey. This particular fatty streak contains several layers of macrophages. *A* is a routinely fixed and embedded paraffin section that has been stained with hematoxylin and eosin. The macrophage-rich areas are seen as clear, since they are lipid-containing and the lipid has been extracted during the process of dehydration and embedding. *B* demonstrates an adjacent section that has been stained with immunoperoxidase coupled to an antibody specific for a cytoplasmic antigen present within the macrophage. The macrophages stain densely black in this micrograph, demonstrating that the large majority of the lipid-rich cells in the fatty streak are macrophages. Such antibodies make it possible to recognize cell type, even after the cells have become distorted by inclusions.

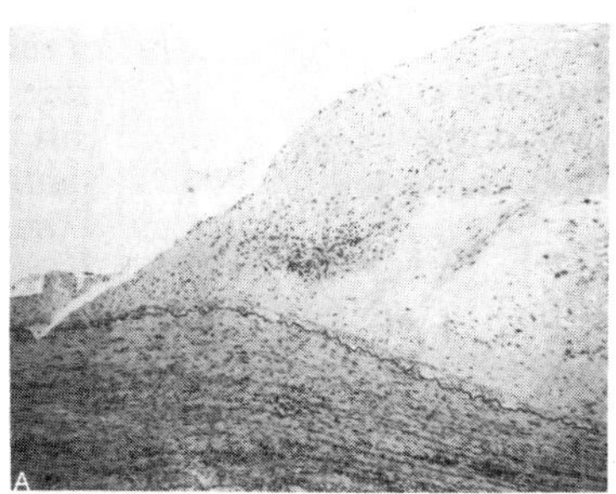

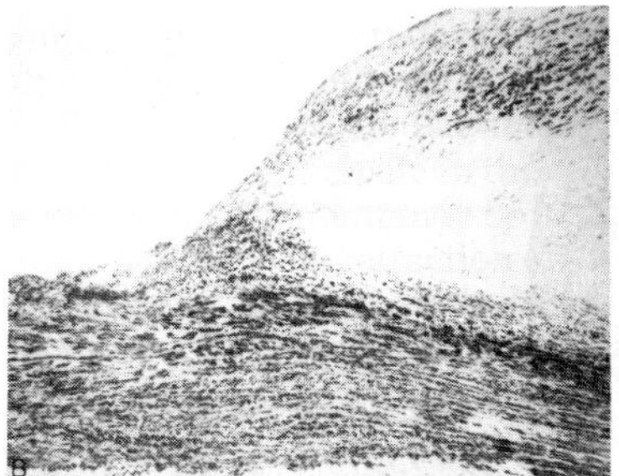

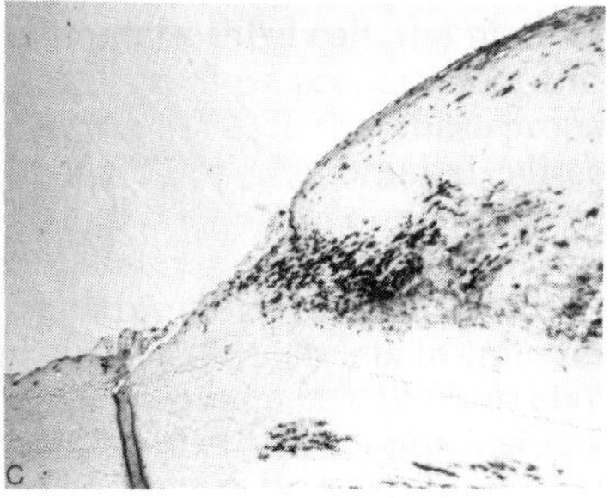

FIGURE 36–10. Three light micrographs demonstrating adjacent sections of a human fibrous plaque from a carotid endarterectomy specimen. *A* was stained with hematoxylin and eosin. In the elevated portion of the lesion, the area adjacent to the lumen consists of a fibrous cap of parallel layers of smooth muscle cells covering a mixture of cells. With H & E it is impossible to determine cell type. *B* is an adjacent section that has been stained using immunoperoxidase coupled to an anti–smooth muscle actin antibody. The smooth muscle cells in the fibrous cap, in the media underlying the lesion, and in patches and individual cells located throughout the lesion are stained black. *C* is an adjacent section stained with immunoperoxidase coupled to an anti-macrophage antibody. Individual macrophages can be seen dispersed among the smooth muscle cells in the fibrous cap, but are found principally in the area deep to the fibrous cap between the fibrous cap and the media, where most of the lipid-containing cells in this particular lesion can be found.

Fibrous plaques are grossly white in appearance and are usually elevated. In many cases they protrude into the lumen of the artery and, if sufficiently large, compromise the flow of blood. These lesions consist of large numbers of intimal smooth muscle cells, together with numerous macrophages and T-lymphocytes. When the macrophages and smooth muscle contain lipid, the lipid is primarily in the form of cholesterol and cholesteryl ester. The proliferated smooth muscle cells are surrounded by collagen and elastic fibers, by large amounts of proteoglycan, and, in individuals who are hypercholesterolemic, by varying amounts of lipid deposited in the cells and in the connective tissue. Fibrous plaques characteristically are covered by a fibrous cap.

In a study of a large series of male patients who had advanced occlusive lesions of the superficial femoral artery, we observed that the fibrous cap of each lesion consisted largely of a particular form of smooth muscle cell that is thin and pancake shaped and that is surrounded by numerous lamellae of basement membrane, proteoglycan, and large numbers of collagen fibrils. The connective tissue in the fibrous cap is exceedingly dense. Beneath the fibrous cap lies a mixture of smooth muscle cells, macrophages, and numerous lymphocytes, principally CD-8+ and some CD-4+ T cells. Using the monoclonal antibodies already described, as well as antibodies to lymphocytes, it has been possible to identify definitively each of these cell types in the advanced lesions of atherosclerosis. In this highly cellular portion of the fibrous plaque, there are also large amounts of connective tissue. Beneath the cell-rich region, there is often a zone of necrotic tissue and debris which may contain cholesterol crystals and regions of calcification as well as numerous enlarged foam cells (Fig. 36–10).

Some fibrous plaques are densely fibrous and contain relatively little lipid, whereas others are rich in lipid deposits. Such differences can be found in different arteries within a given individual but are often associated with different risk factors. For example, it is common that the fibrous plaques observed in the superficial femoral arteries of those who are heavy cigarette smokers are extremely fibrous and contain relatively little lipid. On the other hand, individuals who are hypercholesterolemic and have advanced lesions in the coronary arteries often have large amounts of lipid within the lesions.[50]

There appears to be a general pattern in the distribution of advanced lesions of atherosclerosis in humans. Generally, the abdominal aorta is more extensively involved than the thoracic aorta.[22] Lesions in the aorta are usually most prominent near the ostia of major branches that leave the aorta. Some arteries such as the renal arteries appear to be spared from atherosclerosis, except at their ostia.[81] The coronary arteries generally demonstrate the most intense involvement, with lesions of atherosclerosis located within the first 6 cm of the artery.[82] In hypertensive patients, lesions of the carotid, cerebral, and basilar arteries are more common. It has been suggested that the severity of lesion formation in a given artery may be related in part to the particular nature of the characteristics of the blood flow in the artery, and that rheological forces play a major role in determining the localization, extent, and severity of lesions in susceptible individuals.[83,84]

The principal clinical results of advanced lesions of atherosclerosis are derived either from the fact that they partially or totally occlude the lumen of the affected artery or because cracks and fissures develop in the lesions, leading to thrombosis and embolism or to aneurysmal dilatation (which usually occurs in large arteries such as the aorta).

HYPOTHESES OF ATHEROGENESIS

Current theories of the pathogenesis of the lesions of atherosclerosis relate back to early proposals made by Virchow,[85] Rokitansky,[86] and Duguid.[87] Virchow believed that a form of low-grade injury to the artery wall resulted in a type of inflammatory insudation, which in turn caused increased passage and accumulation of plasma constituents in the intima of the artery.[85] Rokitansky's belief, subsequently elaborated upon by Duguid, was that an encrustation of small mural thrombi existed at sites of arterial injury, that these thrombi went on to organize by the growth of smooth muscle cells into them, and they would become incorporated into the lesions and thus serve as sites where the lesions would progress.[86,87]

In 1973, these two notions about atherogenesis were combined with new knowledge of the cellular and molecular biology of the artery wall in a hypothesis termed the *response-to-injury hypothesis of atherosclerosis.*[2] This hypothesis has been modified as new data have come forth. It now takes into account many aspects of the behavior of arterial and blood cells described above, as well as the numerous risk factors that have been associated with atherogenesis, including hyperlipidemia, hormone dysfunction, altered rheological forces as may occur in hypertension, and alteration of the endothelial barrier by factors associated with cigarette smoking, diabetes, and so on.[3,6,88]

A second hypothesis that was also formulated in 1973, the *monoclonal hypothesis*, suggests that the lesions of atherosclerosis may represent some form of neoplasia.[14] Both of these are discussed below.

THE RESPONSE-TO-INJURY HYPOTHESIS

The response-to-injury hypothesis of atherosclerosis states that some form of "injury" may occur to the lining endothelial

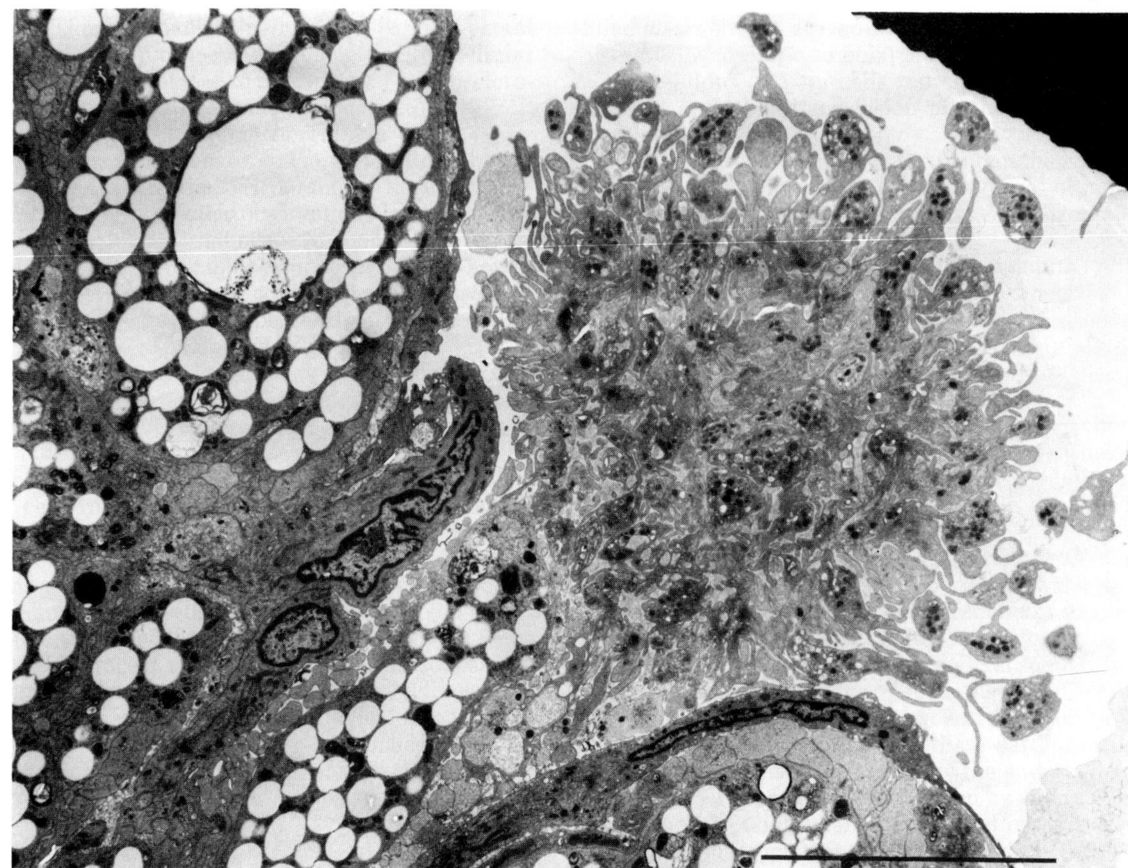

FIGURE 36–18. Transmission electron micrograph of platelets adherent to an exposed macrophage from a fatty streak in a fat-fed monkey that had been hypercholesterolemic for 6 months. The platelets in this thrombus are generally adherent to exposed foam cells and penetrate into the depth of a crevice in the fatty streak. Many of the platelets have undergone degranulation and have released their contents. Bar = 10 μ. (From Faggiotto, A., and Ross, R.: Studies of hypercholesterolemia in the nonhuman primate: II. Fatty streak conversion to fibrous plaque. Arteriosclerosis *4*:349, 1984, by permission of the American Heart Association.)

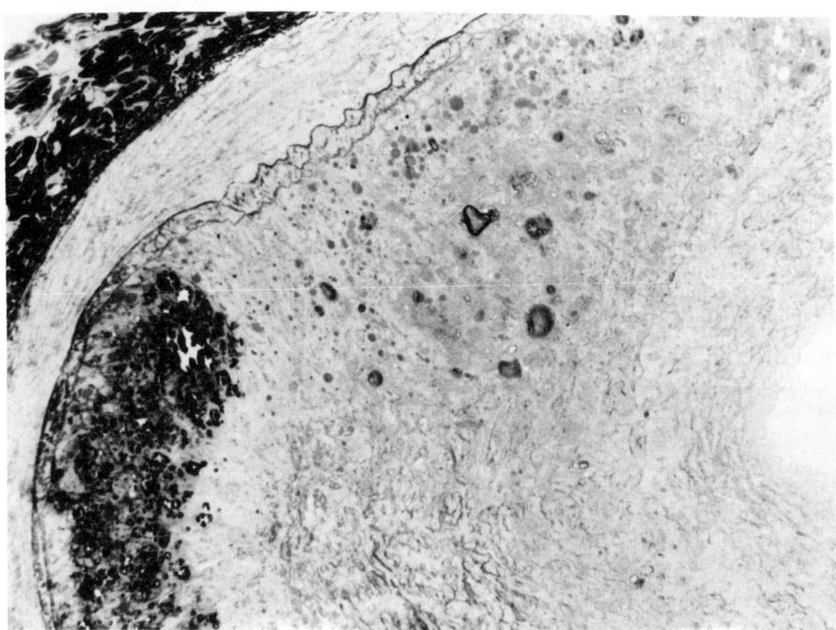

FIGURE 36–19. Light micrograph demonstrating an advanced fibrous plaque that formed in the internal iliac artery of a monkey that was hypercholesterolemic for 7 months. The lesion has occluded approximately 70 per cent of the arterial lumen and consists of numerous layers of smooth muscle cells surrounded by fibrous connective tissue. An area of lipid and necrotic tissue occupies the left side and upper portion of this lesion. (From Faggiotto, A., and Ross, R.: Studies of hypercholesterolemia in the nonhuman primate: II. Fatty streak conversion to fibrous plaque. Arteriosclerosis *4*:345, 1984, by permission of the American Heart Association.)

endothelium remains intact over preexisting lesions such as fatty streaks. This can undoubtedly be explained by the fact that both activated macrophages and endothelium can serve as sources of growth factors so that platelet interactions are not required for smooth muscle proliferation to occur.

This leads to the need to determine what constitutes endothelial injury. It also suggests that nondenuding forms of injury or endothelial dysfunction are more important than the denuding forms described above. Reidy and Schwartz[130,131] have indicated that one of the most common results of endothelial injury may be detachment of individual endothelial cells, which are rapidly replaced by neighboring cells so that endothelial continuity is maintained. Several markers have been developed that can be used to identify sites of endothelial injury. Hansson et al.[132] demonstrated that injured endothelial cells take up IgG whereas normal endothelium will not, and that such IgG uptake can be correlated with increased replication of the endothelium. Furthermore, Reidy and Schwartz[133] showed that a linear correlation exists between the extent of endothelial injury (the number of denuded cells) and the localization of indium-111-labeled platelets at these sites. Platelets would adhere because injured endothelium appears to have lost its nonthrombogenic properties.

Thus, there may be several different forms of endothelial injury and more subtle techniques may be necessary to uncover them. This raises the interesting question, as suggested earlier, whether one subtle form of endothelial injury may be the stimulation of these cells to synthesize and secrete growth factors, including PDGF, that could then play a critical role in the genesis of the events previously described. If this were the case, then endothelial disjunction, retraction, and subendothelial exposure are clearly not necessary for lesions of atherosclerosis to develop, since both activated endothelium and macrophages could be sufficient in themselves to provide a mitogenic stimulus for smooth muscle cells to form lesions of atherosclerosis.

REGRESSION OF ATHEROSCLEROSIS

ANIMAL STUDIES. A number of studies have demonstrated that lesions of experimentally induced atherosclerosis can in fact regress. When hypercholesterolemic swine and nonhuman primates that have developed severe lesions are fed a normocholesterolemic diet, these lesions can regress. Fatty streaks formed in the monkeys receiving the high-fat, high-cholesterol diet of Faggiotto et al.[122] were found to regress completely within 1 month after the animals resumed a normal diet. Most of the studies of regression of the advanced lesions of atherosclerosis have been performed in nonhuman primates, principally in different strains of macaques and in squirrel monkeys. The studies were performed by providing the monkeys with atherogenic diets that took them through stages of fatty streak development and on to fibrous plaque formation. When cholesterol was removed from the diet and plasma cholesterol concentrations returned to normal, Faggiotto et al.[122] observed that reasonably rapid regression of fatty streaks occurred. Of greater potential interest, significant reduction in the size of the smooth muscle proliferative lesions has been observed by several different investigators. Some of the earliest studies were performed by Armstrong et al.,[134] who demonstrated that coronary atherosclerosis could regress. These studies were subsequently confirmed by Wissler and Vesselinovitch.[135] Perhaps the largest number of studies have been performed by Clarkson and his colleagues.[136] They demonstrated the clear therapeutic benefit of lowering plasma cholesterol concentrations after having induced fibrous plaques in animals on hypercholesterolemic regimens for periods of 12 months and longer. Regression occurred principally in lesions in the abdominal aorta and in the coronary arteries, in contrast to those that formed at the carotid bifurcation, which appeared, on some occasions, to develop lesions relatively independently of plasma lipid concentrations. When regression occurs and plasma cholesterol levels return to baseline, the lesions of atherosclerosis become smaller, contain less lipid, and demonstrate marked decreases in their content of cholesterol and cholesteryl esters. Remodeling of connective tissue proteins also appears to take place, as shown by decreases in both collagen and elastic fiber proteins in these lesions. Thus it seems that, over a sufficiently long period, advanced lesions can in some cases also regress.

HUMAN STUDIES. It has been demonstrated that advanced, semiocclusive lesions of human coronary atherosclerosis also can regress. In a quantitative image analysis study of coronary angiograms from a series of patients being aggressively treated with lipid-lowering regimens of either niacin and colestipol or lovastatin and colestipol, Brown and colleagues[137] have demonstrated statistically significant regression in association with decreases in plasma cholesterol and LDL. This provides clear evidence that the lesions of atherosclerosis are able to regress at apparently all stages of lesion development.

A number of investigators have probed the capacity of fish oils, which contain large amounts of omega-3 fatty acids, to decrease plasma cholesterol levels and potentially to induce lesion regression when added to the diet of hypercholesterolemic individuals.[138] Not only do these diets lead to decrease in plasma cholesterol levels, but they also change the balance of prostaglandins that are formed by the cells. It is well known that platelets have the capacity to use arachidonic acid to form the prostaglandin derivative thromboxane A_2, a proaggregating factor for platelets. On the other hand, endothelial cells and smooth muscle use the same fatty acid to form, via cyclooxygenase, the prostaglandin metabolite prostacyclin (PGI_2), an extraordinarily potent antiaggregant and vasodilator. When the omega-3 fatty acids are fed to animals (and if they are particularly rich in eicosapentaenoic acid), they shift the balance because thromboxane A_3 derived from this fatty acid is inactive as a platelet aggregant, whereas PGI_3 is as active as PGI_2, thus favoring antiaggregant, vasodilator effects over effects that might lead to platelet aggregation and thrombosis.

THROMBOSIS

(see also Chapter 58)

As described at the beginning of this chapter, thrombosis was originally considered to be an important component in the initiation and progression of the lesions of atherosclerosis. It now appears that thrombosis may play several roles. One prominent and potentially important clinical role is that of thrombi which become incorporated into existing advanced lesions of atherosclerosis, rapidly resulting in lumen narrowing and increase in lesion dimensions. Perhaps one of the most persistent and common complications of atherosclerosis is the formation of cracks and fissures in the advanced lesions of atherosclerosis that can act as sites for platelet attachment and formation of mural and potentially occlusive thrombi, which could lead to unstable angina or myocardial infarction.

As discussed earlier, there is good evidence in nonhuman primates and in rabbits that mural thrombi can contribute to the initiation and development of lesions of atherosclerosis.[94-98] This has also been demonstrated in humans at the perianastomotic site of coronary bypass surgery, where new lesions of atherosclerosis form in approximately 30 per cent of all bypass grafts.[139] In monkeys or rabbits receiving a hyperlipemic diet, intraarterial balloon catheter deendothelialization can lead to intimal smooth muscle proliferative lesions that appear very much like those found in hypercholesterolemic patients.

Thrombi have been observed in the coronary arteries of the vast majority of individuals who die from transmural myocardial infarction. However, thrombi are much less common in individuals who die from subendothelial infarction. Thrombosis is even less common in individuals who die of sudden cardiac death, although both thrombosis and embolism are well recognized as complications of cerebrovascular disease as well as peripheral vascular disease.

The role of the endothelium in the process of thrombosis is not entirely clear since, as discussed earlier, endothelial cells have both nonthrombogenic and procoagulant activities. Endothelial cells produce von Willebrand factor as well as plasminogen activator and prostacyclin. The development of agents that can alter thromboxane formation and thus prevent platelet interaction, or alter prostacyclin formation and thus promote platelet interactions, should make it possible to obtain a clearer idea of the role of these agents as compared with others that can be produced by the endothelial cells in the process of thrombosis in general.

CONCLUSIONS

It is clear that knowledge in the field of atherosclerosis has exploded and is changing rapidly. The opportunity to use the tools of cell and molecular biology, as well as new noninvasive methods for examining individuals at the clinical level, has broadened our understanding of the roles of the cells in atherogenesis. Cell and molecular biology have rapidly increased our understanding of the principal cells involved in atherosclerosis: endothelium, smooth muscle, platelets, and monocyte/macrophages and T-lymphocytes. How the risk factors that are commonly associated with an increased incidence of atherosclerosis are related to these cellular interactions is beginning to be understood, particularly in relation to hypercholesterolemia. Unfortunately, there are no good animal models that permit us to study the questions related to cigarette smoking, hypertension, diabetes, or some of the other risk factors that are epidemiologically associated with atherosclerosis. Without these, it is difficult to know the nature of the cellular interactions that occur during the genesis of the disease process as it is associated with each of these important risk factors.

Perhaps the most critical aspect of this problem is the need to understand the basis of the genetic susceptibility of individuals to these risk factors and thus to circumstances that can lead to these increased cellular interactions. Once the genetic loci for the various apoproteins are identified, and once it is possible to demonstrate altered genetic loci for these and other factors important in atherogenesis in individuals who are at increased risk for heart attack and/or stroke, it should be possible to begin to probe this question using these new tools.

Acknowledgments

This work was supported in part by U.S. Public Health Service Grant HL-18645 and NIH grant RR-00166 to the Northwest Regional Primate Center. The author is particularly indebted to Elaine Raines, Agostino Faggiotto, Junichi Masuda, Michael Rosenfeld, Toyohiro Tsukada, Masakiyo Sasahara, Shogo Katsuda, Allen Gown, and to Daniel Bowen-Pope, with whom work reported from his laboratory was performed.

REFERENCES

RISK FACTORS

1. Report of the Working Group on Arteriosclerosis of the National Heart, Lung, and Blood Institute. Vol. 2. DHEW Publication No. (NIH) 82-2035, Washington D.C., U.S. Government Printing Office, 1981.
2. Ross, R., and Glomset, J.: Atherosclerosis and the arterial smooth muscle cell. Science *180*:1332, 1973.
3. Ross, R., and Glomset, J. A.: The pathogenesis of atherosclerosis. N. Engl. J. Med. *295*:369, 1976.
4. Ross, R., and Harker, L.: Hyperlipidemia and atherosclerosis. Science *193*:1094, 1976.
5. Wissler, R. W., Vesselinovitch, D., and Getz, G. J.: Abnormalities of the arterial wall and its metabolism in atherogenesis. Prog. Cardiovasc. Dis. *18*:341, 1976.
6. Dawber, T. R., Moore, F. E., and Mann, G. V.: Measuring the risk of coronary heart disease in adult population groups: II. Coronary heart disease in the Framingham study. Am. J. Public Health *47*:4, 1957.
7. Chapman, J. M., Goerke, L. S., Dixon, W., et al.: Measuring the risk of coronary heart disease in adult population groups: IV. The clinical status of a population group in Los Angeles under observation for two or three years. Am. J. Public Health *47*:33, 1957.
8. Doyle, J. T., Heslin, A. S., Hillboe, H. E., et al.: Measuring the risk of coronary heart disease in adult population groups: III. A prospective study of degenerative cardiovascular disease in Albany: Report of three years' experience: I. Ischemic heart disease. Am. J. Public Health *47*:25, 1957.
9. Drake, R. M., Buechley, R. W., and Breslow, L.: Measuring the risk of coronary heart disease in adult population groups: V. An epidemiological investigation of coronary heart disease in the California health survey population. Am J. Public Health *47*:43, 1957.
10. Report of Inter-Society Commission for Heart Disease Resources. Primary prevention of the atherosclerotic disease. Circulation *42*:55, 1970.
11. Stamler, J., Berkson, D. M., and Lindberg, H. A.: Risk factors: Their role in the etiology and pathogenesis of the atherosclerotic diseases. *In* Wissler, R. W., Geer, J. C., and Kaufman, N. (eds.): The Pathogenesis of Atherosclerosis. Baltimore, Williams and Wilkins, 1962, p. 41.
12. Kuller, L. H.: Epidemiology of cardiovascular disease: Current perspectives. Am. J. Epidemiol. *104*:425, 1976.
13. Ross, R.: The pathogenesis of atherosclerosis—an update. N. Engl. J. Med. *314*:488, 1986.
14. Benditt, E. P., and Benditt, J. M.: Evidence for a monoclonal origin of human atherosclerotic plaques. Proc. Natl. Acad. Sci. USA *70*:1753, 1973.
15. Inkeles, S., and Eisenberg, D.: Hyperlipidemia and coronary atherosclerosis: A review. Medicine *70*:110, 1981.
16. Lipid Research Clinics Program. The Lipid Research Clinics Coronary Primary Prevention Trial Results: I. Reduction in incidence of coronary heart disease. JAMA *251*:351, 1984.
17. Lipid Research Clinics Program. The Lipid Research Clinics Coronary Primary Prevention Trial Results: II. The relationship of reduction in incidence of coronary heart disease to cholesterol lowering. JAMA *251*:365, 1984.
18. Smoking and Health. Chap. 3. Criteria for Judgment. DHEW Publication No. (NIH) 1103, Washington, D.C., U.S. Government Printing Office, 1964.
19. The Pooling Project Research Group: Relationship of blood pressure, serum cholesterol, smoking habit, relative weight, and ECG abnormalities to incidence of major coronary events: Final report of the pooling project. J. Chronic Dis. *31*:201, 1978.
20. Oberman, A., Harlan, W. R., Smith, M., and Graybiel, A.: The cardiovascular risk associated with different levels and types of elevated blood pressure. Minn. Med. *52*:1283, 1969.

THE NORMAL ARTERY

21. Report of the Hypertension Task Force. Vol. 1. DHEW Publication No. (NIH) 79-1623, Washington, D.C., U.S. Government Printing Office, 1964.
22. Glagov, S.: Hemodynamic risk factors: Mechanical stress, mural architecture, medial nutrition and the vulnerability of arteries to atherosclerosis. *In* Wissler, R. W., and Geer, J. C. (eds.): The Pathogenesis of Atherosclerosis. Baltimore, Williams and Wilkins, 1972, p. 164.
23. Wolinsky, H., and Glagov, S.: Comparison of abdominal and thoracic aortic medial structure in mammals. Deviation of man from the usual pattern. Circ. Res. *25*:677, 1969.

CELLS OF THE ARTERY AND FROM THE BLOOD POTENTIALLY INVOLVED IN ATHEROGENESIS

24. Schwartz, S. M., and Benditt, E. P.: Clustering of replicating cells in aortic endothelium. Proc. Natl. Acad. Sci. USA *73*:651, 1976.
25. Schwartz, S. M., and Benditt, E. P.: Aortic endothelial cell replication. Effects of age and hypertension in the rat. Circ. Res. *41*:248, 1977.
26. Simionescu, N., Simionescu, M., and Palade, G. E.: Permeability of muscle capillaries to small heme-peptides. Evidence for the existence of patent transendothelial channels. J. Cell Biol. *64*:586, 1975.
27. Huttner, I., Boutet, M., and More, R. H.: Studies on protein passage through arterial endothelium. I. Structural correlates of permeability in rat arterial endothelium. Lab. Invest. *28*:672, 1973.
28. Renkin, E. M.: Multiple pathways of capillary permeability. Circ. Res. *41*:735, 1977.
29. Moncada, S., Herman, A. G., Higgs, E. A., and Vane, J. R.: Differential formation of prostacyclin (PGX or PGI_2) by layers of the arterial wall. An explanation for the antithrombotic properties of vascular endothelium. Thromb. Res. *11*:323, 1977.
30. Fielding, C. J.: Metabolism of cholesterol-rich chylomicrons. Mechanism of binding and uptake of cholesteryl esters by the vascular bed of the perfused rat heart. J. Clin. Invest. *62*:141, 1978.
31. Furchgott, R. F.: Role of endothelium in responses of vascular smooth muscle. Circ. Res. *53*:557, 1983.
32. Gimbrone, M. A. Jr., and Alexander, R. W.: Angiotensin II stimulation of prostaglandin production in cultured human vascular endothelium. Science *189*:219, 1975.

33. Jaffe, E. A., Minick, C. R., Adelman, B., et al.: Synthesis of basement membrane by cultured human endothelial cells. J. Exp. Med. *144*:209, 1976.
34. Jaffe, E. A., Hoyer, L. W., and Nachman, R. L.: Synthesis of antihemophilic factor antigen by cultured human endothelial cells. J. Clin. Invest. *52*:2757, 1973.
35. Rubin, K., Hansson, G. K. Ronnstrand, L. et al.: Induction of B-type receptors for platelet-derived growth factor in vascular inflammation: Possible implications for development of vascular proliferative lesions. Lancet *1*:1353, 1988.
36. Steinberg, D.: Lipoproteins and atherosclerosis. A look back and a look ahead. Arteriosclerosis *3*:283, 1983.
37. Yanagisawa, M., Kurihara, H., Kimura, S., et al.: A novel potent vasoconstrictor peptide produced by vascular endothelial cells. Nature *322*:411, 1988.
38. Furchgott, R. F.: Role of endothelium in responses of vascular smooth muscle. Circ. Res. *53*:557, 1983.
39. Gajdusek, C. M., DiCorleto, P. E., Ross, R., and Schwartz, S. M.: An endothelial cell-derived growth factor. J. Cell Biol. *85*:467, 1980.
40. DiCorleto, P. E., Gajdusek, C. M., Schwartz, S. M., and Ross, R.: Biochemical properties of the endothelium-derived growth factor: Comparison to other growth factors. J. Cell. Physiol. *114*:339, 1983.
41. DiCorleto, P. E., and Bowen-Pope, D. F.: Cultured endothelial cells produce a platelet-derived growth factor–like protein. Proc. Natl. Acad. Sci. USA *80*:1919, 1983.
42. Wissler, R. W.: The arterial medial cell, smooth muscle, or multifunctional mesenchyme? J. Atheroscler. Res. *8*:201, 1968.
43. Ross, R.: The smooth muscle cell: II. Growth of smooth muscle in culture and formation of elastic fibers. J. Cell Biol. *50*:172, 1971.
44. Burke, J. M., and Ross, R.: Synthesis of connective tissue macromolecules by smooth muscle. Int. Rev. Connect. Tissue Res. *8*:119, 1979.
45. Chait, A., Ross, R., Albers, J. J., and Bierman, E. L.: Platelet-derived growth factor stimulates activity of low density lipoprotein receptors. Proc. Natl. Acad. Sci. USA *77*:4084, 1980.
46. Bowen-Pope, D. F., Seifert, R. A., and Ross, R.: The platelet-derived growth factor receptor. *In* Boynton, A. L., and Leffert, H. L. (eds): Control of Animal Cell Proliferation: Recent Advances. Vol. 1. New York, Academic Press, 1985, p. 281.
47. Seifert, R. A., Schwartz, S. M., and Bowen-Pope, D. F.: Developmentally regulated production of platelet-derived growth factor–like molecules. Nature *311*:669, 1984.
48. Chamley-Campbell, J., Campbell, G., and Ross, R.: Phenotype-dependent response of cultured aortic smooth muscle to serum mitogens. J. Cell Biol. *89*:379, 1981.
49. Thyberg, J., Palmberg, L., Nilsson, J., et al.: Phenotype modulations in primary cultures of arterial smooth muscle cells. On the role of platelet-derived growth factor. Differentiation *25*:156, 1983.
50. Ross, R., Wight, T. N., Strandness, E., and Thiele, B.: Human atherosclerosis: I. Cell constitution and characteristics of advanced lesions of the superficial femoral artery. Am. J. Pathol. *114*:79, 1984.
51. Van Furth, R.: Current view on the mononuclear phagocyte system. Immunobiology *161*:178, 1982.
52. Nathan, C. F., Murray, H. W., and Cohn, Z. A.: Current concepts: The macrophage as an effector cell. N. Engl. J. Med. *303*:622, 1980.
53. Martin, T. R., Altman, L. C., Albert, R. K., and Henderson, W. R.: Leukotriene B4 production by human alveolar macrophage: A potential mechanism for amplifying inflammation in the lung. Am. Rev. Respir. Dis. *129*:106, 1984.
54. Bevilacqua, M. P., Pober, J. S., Cotran, R. S., and Gimbrone, M. A. Jr.: Interleukin 1 (IL1) acts upon vascular endothelium to stimulate procoagulant activity and leukocyte adhesion. J. Cell. Biochem. Suppl. *9A*:148, 1985.
55. Cathcart, M. K., Morel, D. W., and Chisolm, G., III.: Monocytes and neutrophils oxidize low-density lipoprotein making it cytotoxic. J. Leuk. Biol. *38*:341, 1985.
56. Ross, R., Raines, E. W., and Bowen-Pope, D. F.: The biology of platelet-derived growth factor. Cell *46*:155, 1986.
57. Shimokado, K., Raines, E. W., Madtes, D. K., et al.: A significant part of macrophage-derived growth factor consists of at least two forms of PDGF. Cell *43*:277, 1985.
58. Raines, E. W., Dower, S. K., and Ross, R.: IL-1 mitogenic activity for fibroblasts and smooth muscle cells is due to PDGF-AA. Science *243*:393, 1989.
59. Baird, A., Mormede, P., and Bohlen, P.: Immunoreactive fibroblast growth factor in cells of peritoneal exudate suggests its identity with macrophage-derived growth factor. Biochem. Biophys. Res. Commun. *126*:358, 1985.
60. Ralph, P.: Colony stimulating factors. *In* Zembala, M., and Asherson, G. (eds.): Human Monocytes. New York, Academic Press, 1989, p. 228.
61. Holmsen, H., and Weiss, H. J.: Secretable storage pools in platelets. Annu. Rev. Med. *30*:119, 1979.
62. Pepper, D. S.: Macromolecules released from platelet storage organelles. Thromb. Haemost. *42*:1667, 1980.
63. Ross, R., Glomset, J., Kariya, B., and Harker, L.: A platelet-dependent serum factor that stimulates the proliferation of arterial smooth muscle cells in vitro. Proc. Natl. Acad. Sci. USA *71*:1207, 1974.
64. Oka, Y., and Orth, D. N.: Human plasma epidermal growth factor/beta-urogastrone is associated with blood platelets. J. Clin. Invest. *72*:249, 1983.
65. Assoian, R. K., Komoriya, A., Meyers, C. A., et al.: Transforming growth factor-β in human platelets. Identification of a major storage site, purification, and characterization. J. Biol. Chem. *258*:7155, 1983.
66. Baumgartner, H. R.: Platelet-interaction with vascular structures. Thromb. Diath. Haemorrh. *51*(Suppl.):161, 1972.
67. Jonasson, L., Holm, J., Skalli, O., et al: Regional accumulations of T cells, macrophages, and smooth muscle cells in the human atherosclerotic plaque. Arteriosclerosis *6*:131, 1986.
68. Gown, A. M., Tsukada, T., and Ross, R.: Human atherosclerosis: II. Immunocytochemical analysis of the cellular composition of human atherosclerotic lesions. Am. J. Pathol. *125*:191, 1986.
69. Munro, J. M., van der Walt, J. D., Munro, C. S., et al.: An immunohistochemical analysis of human aortic fatty streaks. Hum. Pathol. *18*:375, 1987.
70. Emeson, E. E., and Robertson, A. L.: T lymphocytes in aortic and coronary intimas. Their potential role in atherogenesis. Am. J. Pathol. *130*:369, 1988.
71. Minick, C. R., and Murphy, G. E.: Experimental induction of atheroarteriosclerosis by the synergy of allergic injury to arteries and lipid-rich diet: II. Effect of repeated injections of horse serum in rabbits fed a lipid-rich, cholesterol-poor diet. Am. J. Pathol. *73*:265, 1973.
72. Hansson, G. K., Holm, J., and Jonasson, L.: Detection of activated T lymphocytes in the human atherosclerotic plaque. Am. J. Pathol. *135*:169, 1989.
73. Hansson, G. K., Jonasson, L., Holm, J., and Claesson-Welsh, L.: MHC antigen expression in the atherosclerotic plaque: Smooth muscle cells express HLA-DR, HLA-DQ, and the invariant gamma chain. Clin. Exp. Immunol. *64*:261, 1986.

THE LESIONS OF ATHEROSCLEROSIS

74. McGill, H. C., Jr. (ed.): The Geographic Pathology of Atherosclerosis. Baltimore, Williams and Wilkins, 1968.
75. Geer, J. C., McGill, H. C., Jr., and Strong, J. P.: The fine structure of human atherosclerotic lesions. Am. J. Pathol. *38*:263, 1961.
76. Geer, J. C.: Fine structure of human aortic intimal thickening and fatty streaks. Lab. Invest. *14*:1764, 1965.
77. Ghidoni, J. J., and O'Neal, R. M.: Recent advances in molecular pathology. A review: Ultrastructure of human atheroma. Exp. Mol. Pathol. *7*:378, 1967.
78. Stary, H. C.: Evolution of atherosclerotic plaques in the coronary arteries of young adults. Arteriosclerosis *3*:471a, 1983.
79. McGill, H. C., Jr.: Persistent problems in the pathogenesis of atherosclerosis. Arteriosclerosis *4*:443, 1984.
80. Tsukada, T., Rosenfeld, M., Ross, R., and Gown, A. M.: Immunocytochemical analysis of cellular components in atherosclerotic lesions. Use of monoclonal antibodies with the Watanabe and fat-fed rabbit. Arteriosclerosis. *6*:601, 1986.
81. Glagov, S., and Ozoa, A.: Significance of the relatively low incidence of atherosclerosis in the pulmonary, renal and mesenteric arteries. Ann. N.Y. Acad. Sci. *149*:940, 1968.
82. Strong, J. P., Eggen, D. A., and Oalmann, M. C.: The natural history, geographic pathology, and epidemiology of atherosclerosis. *In* Wissler, R. W., and Geer, J. C. (eds.): The Pathogenesis of Atherosclerosis. Baltimore, Williams and Wilkins, 1972, p. 20.
83. Glagov, S., Rowley, D. A., Cramer, D. B., and Page, R. G.: Heart rate during 24 hours of usual activity in 100 normal men. J. Appl. Physiol. *29*:799, 1970.
84. Wissler, R. W., and Vesselinovitch, D.: Atherosclerosis—relationship to coronary blood flow. Am. J. Cardiol. *52*(2):2A, 1983.

THE HYPOTHESES OF ATHEROGENESIS

85. Virchow, R.: Phlogose und thrombose in gefassystem, gesammelte abhandlungen zur wissenschaftlichen medicin. Frankfurt-am-Main, Meidinger Sohn and Co., 1856, p. 458.
86. von Rokitansky, C.: A Manual of Pathological Anatomy, translated by Day, G. E. Vol. 4. London, The Sydenham Society, 1852.
87. Duguid, J. B.: Thrombosis as a factor in the pathogenesis of coronary atherosclerosis. J. Pathol. Bacteriol. *58*:207, 1946.
88. Ross, R.: Atherosclerosis—a problem of the biology of arterial wall cells and their interaction with blood components. Arteriosclerosis *1*:293, 1981.
89. Leary, T.: The genesis of atherosclerosis. Arch. Pathol. *32*:507, 1941.
90. Parthasarathy, S., Quinn, M. T., Schwenke, D. C., et al.: Oxidative modification of beta-very low density lipoprotein. Potential role in monocyte recruitment and foam cell formation. Arteriosclerosis *9*:398, 1989.
91. Assoian, R. K., Grotendorst, G. R., Miller, D. M., and Sporn, M. B.: Cellular transformation by coordinated action of three peptide growth factors from human platelets. Nature *309*:804, 1984.
92. Sporn, M. B., Roberts, A. B., Wakefield, L. M., and de Crombrugghe, B.: Some recent advances in the chemistry and biology of transforming growth factor-beta. J. Cell Biol. *105*:1039, 1987.
93. Ross, R., Masuda, J., Raines, E. W., et al.: Localization of PDGF-B protein in macrophages in all phases of atherogenesis. Science *248*:1009, 1990.
94. Stemerman, M. B., and Ross, R.: Experimental arteriosclerosis: I. Fibrous plaque formation in primates, an electron microscope study. J. Exp. Med. *136*:769, 1972.
95. Sheppard, B. L., and French, J. E.: Platelet adhesion in the rabbit abdominal aorta following the removal of the endothelium: A scanning and

transmission electron microscopical study. Proc. R. Soc. Lond. (Biol.) *176*:427, 1971.

96. More, S.: Thromboatherosclerosis in normolipemic rabbits: A result of continued endothelial damage. Lab. Invest. *29*:478, 1973.
97. Friedman, R. J., Moore, S., and Singal, D. P.: Repeated endothelial injury and induction of atherosclerosis in normolipemic rabbits by human serum. Lab. Invest. *32*:404, 1975.
98. Harker, L. A., Ross, R., Slichter, S. J., and Scott, C. R.: Homocystine-induced arteriosclerosis: The role of endothelial cell injury and platelet response in genesis. J. Clin. Invest. *58*:731, 1976.
99. Libby, P., Warner, S. J. C., Salomon, R. N., and Birinyi, L. K.: Production of platelet-derived growth factor-like mitogen by smooth-muscle cells from human atheroma. N. Engl. J. Med. *318*:1493, 1988.
100. Lindner, D., and Gartler, S. M.: Glucose-6-phosphate dehydrogenase mosaicism: Utilization as a cell marker in the study of leiomyomas. Science *150*:67, 1965.
101. Hajjar, D. P. Fabricant, C. G., Minick, C. R., and Fabricant, J.: Virus-induced artherosclerosis: Herpesvirus infection alters aortic cholesterol metabolism and accumulation. Am. J. Pathol. *122*:62, 1986.
102. Fialkow, P. J.: Use of genetic markers to study cellular origin and development of tumor in human females. Adv. Cancer Res. *15*:191, 1972.

LIPIDS AND LIPOPROTEINS IN ATHEROSCLEROSIS

103. Jackson, R. L., and Gotto, A. M., Jr.: Hypothesis concerning membrane structure, cholesterol, and atherosclerosis. *In* Paoletti, R., and Gotto, A. M., Jr. (eds.): Atherosclerosis Reviews. Vol. 1. New York, Raven Press, 1976, p 1.
104. Carew, T., Schwenke, D. C., and Steinberg, D.: Antiatherogenic effect of probucol unrelated to its hypocholesterolemic effect: Evidence that the antioxidants in vivo can selectively inhibit low density lipoprotein degradation in macrophage-rich fatty streaks and slow the progression of atherosclerosis in the Watanabe heritable hyperlipidemic (WHHL) rabbit. Proc. Natl. Acad. Sci. USA *84*:7725, 1987.
105. Kita, T., Nagano, Y., Yokode, M., et al.: Probucol prevents the progression of atherosclerosis in Watanabe heritable hyperlipidemic rabbit, an animal model for familial hypercholestrolemia. Proc. Natl. Acad. Sci. USA *84*:5928, 1987.
106. Boyd, H. C., Gown, A. M., Wolfbauer, G., and Chait A.: Direct evidence for a protein recognized by a monoclonal antibody against oxidatively modified LDL in atherosclerotic lesions from a Watanabe heritable hyperlipidemic rabbit. Am. J. Pathol. *135*:815, 1989.

GROWTH FACTORS

107. Heldin, C.-H., Westermark, B., and Wasteson, A.: Platelet-derived growth factor: Purification and partial characterization. Proc. Natl. Acad. Sci. USA *76*:3722, 1979.
108. Antoniades, H. N.: Human platelet-derived growth factor (PDGF): Purification of PDGF-I and PDGF-II and separation of their reduced subunits. Proc. Natl. Acad. Sci. USA *78*:7314, 1981.
109. Raines, E. W., and Ross, R.: Platelet-derived growth factor: I. High yield purification and evidence for multiple forms. J. Biol. Chem. *257*:5154, 1982.
110. Huang, J. S., Huang, S. S., Kennedy, B., and Deuel, T. F.: Platelet-derived growth factor: Specific binding to target cells. J. Biol. Chem. *257*:8130, 1982.
111. Heldin, C.-H., Westermark, B., and Wasteson, A.: Specific receptors for platelet-derived growth factors on cells derived from connective tissue and glia. Proc. Natl. Acad. Sci. USA *78*:3664, 1981.
112. Bowen-Pope, D. F., and Ross, R.: Platelet-derived growth factor: II. Specific binding to cultured cells. J. Biol. Chem. *257*:5161, 1982.
113. Grotendorst, G., Seppa, H. E. J., Kleinman, H. K., and Martin, G.: Attachment of smooth muscle cells to collagen and their migration toward platelet-derived growth factor. Proc. Natl. Acad. Sci. USA *78*:3669, 1981.
114. Grotendorst, G. R., Chang, T., Seppa, H. E. J., et al.: Platelet-derived growth factor is a chemoattractant for vascular smooth muscle cells. J. Cell. Physiol. *113*:261, 1982.
115. Witte, L. D., and Cornicelli, J. A.: Platelet-derived growth factor stimulates low density lipoprotein receptor activity in cultured human fibroblasts. Proc. Natl. Acad. Sci. USA *77*:5962, 1980.
116. Bowen-Pope, D. F., Malpass, T. W., Foster, D. M., and Ross, R.: Platelet-derived growth factor in vivo: Levels, activity, and rate of clearance. Blood *46*:458, 1984.
117. Raines, E. W., Bowen-Pope, D. F., and Ross, R.: Plasma binding proteins for platelet-derived growth factor that inhibit its binding to cell-surface receptors. Proc. Natl. Acad. Sci. USA *81*:3424, 1984.
118. Doolittle, R. F., Hunkapiller, M. W., Hood, L. E., et al.: Simian sarcoma virus onc gene, v-sis, is derived from the gene (or genes) encoding a platelet-derived growth factor. Science *221*:275, 1983.
119. Waterfield, M. D., Scrace, G. T., Whittle, N., et al.: Platelet-derived growth factor is structurally related to the putative transforming protein P^{28sis} of simian sarcoma virus. Nature *304*:35, 1983.
120. Bowen-Pope, D. F., Vogel, A., and Ross, R.: Production of platelet-derived growth factor-like molecules and reduced expression of platelet-derived growth factor receptors accompany transformation by a wide spectrum of agents. Proc. Natl. Acad. Sci. USA *81*:2396, 1984.
121. Seifert, R. A., Hart, C. E., Phillips, P. E., et al.: Two different subunits associate to create isoform-specific platelet-derived growth factor receptors. J. Biol. Chem. *264*:8771, 1989.

CELLULAR EVENTS THAT OCCUR DURING ATHEROSCLEROSIS

122. Faggiotto, A., Ross, R., and Harker, L.: Studies of hypercholesterolemia in the nonhuman primate: I. Changes that lead to fatty streak formation. Arteriosclerosis *4*:323, 1984.
123. Faggiotto, A., and Ross, R.: Studies of hypercholesterolemia in the nonhuman primate: II. Fatty streak conversion to fibrous plaque. Arteriosclerosis *4*:341, 1984.
124. Masuda, J., and Ross, R.: Atherogenesis during low-level hypercholesterolemia in the nonhuman primate: I. Fatty streak formation. Arteriosclerosis *10*:164, 1990.
125. Masuda, J., and Ross, R.: Atherogenesis during low-level hypercholesterolemia in the nonhuman primate: II. Fatty streak conversion to fibrous plaque. Arteriosclerosis *10*:178, 1990.
126. Gerrity, R. G., Naito, H. K., Richardson, M., and Schwartz, C. J.: Dietary induced atherogenesis in swine: Morphology of the intima in prelesion stages. Am. J. Pathol. *95*:775, 1979.
127. Gerrity, R. G.: The role of the monocyte in atherogenesis: I. Transition of blood-borne monocytes into foam cells in fatty lesions. Am. J. Pathol. *103*:181, 1981.
128. Gerrity, R. G., Goss, J. A., and Soby, L.: Control of monocyte recruitment by chemotactic factor(s) in lesion-prone areas of swine aorta. Arteriosclerosis *5*:55, 1985.
129. Rosenfeld, M. E., Faggiotto, A., and Ross, R.: The role of the mononuclear phagocyte in primate and rabbit models of atherosclerosis. *In* Van Furth, R. (ed.): Mononuclear Phagocytes: Characteristics, Physiology, and Function. The Hague, Netherlands, Martinus Nijhoff, 1985, p. 795.
130. Reidy, M. A., and Schwartz, S. M.: Endothelial regeneration: III. Time course of intimal changes after small defined injury to rat aortic endothelium. Lab. Invest. *44*:301, 1981.
131. Reidy, M. A., and Schwartz, S. M.: Endothelial injury and regeneration: IV. Endotoxin: A nondenuding injury to aortic endothelium. Lab. Invest. *48*:25, 1983.
132. Hansson, G. K., Bondjers, G., Bylock, A., and Hjalmarsson, L: Ultrastructural studies on nonatherosclerotic rabbits. Exp. Mol. Pathol. *33*:301, 1980.
133. Reidy, M. A., and Schwartz, S. M.: Recent advances in molecular pathology: Arterial endothelium—assessment of in vivo injury. Exp. Mol. Pathol. *41*:419, 1984.

REGRESSION OF ATHEROSCLEROSIS

134. Armstrong, M. L., Warner, E. D., and Conner, W. E.: Regression of coronary atheromatosis in rhesus monkeys. Circ. Res. *27*:59, 1970.
135. Wissler, R. W., and Vesselinovitch, D.: Studies of regression of advanced atherosclerosis in experimental animals and man. Ann. N.Y. Acad. Sci. *275*:363, 1976.
136. Clarkson, T. B., Bond, M. G., Bullock, B. C., et al.: A study of atherosclerosis regression in Macaca mulatta: V. Changes in abdominal aorta and carotid and coronary arteries from animals with atherosclerosis induced for 38 months and then regressed for 24 or 48 months at plasma cholesterol concentrations of 300 or 200 mg/dl. Exp. Mol. Pathol. *41*:96, 1984.
137. Brown, B. G., Albers, J. J., Fisher, L. D., et al.: Familial atherosclerosis treatment study: A randomized trial demonstrating coronary disease regression and clinical benefit from lipid-altering therapy among men with high apolipoprotein-B. N. Engl. J. Med. in press.
138. Cannon, P. J.: Eicosanoids and the blood vessel wall. Circulation *70*:00, 1984.

THROMBOSIS

139. Chesebro, J. H., Clements, L. P., Fuster, V., et al.: A platelet-inhibitor-drug trial in coronary-artery bypass operations. Benefit of perioperative dipyridamole and aspirin therapy on early postoperative vein-graft patency. N. Engl. J. Med. *307*:73, 1982.

Risk Factors for Coronary Artery Disease

by JOHN A. FARMER, M.D., and ANTONIO M. GOTTO, Jr., M.D., D.Phil.

DECLINING MORTALITY

Great progress against specific aspects of coronary artery disease (CAD) has been made over the past 40 years. For example, in 1950, the United States age-adjusted mortality rate from myocardial infarction was 226.4 per 100,000 people. By 1987 that rate had dropped to 124.1 per 100,000. Over the same period, the age-adjusted mortality rates from strokes and hypertension per 100,000 fell from 88.8 and 56.0, respectively, to 30.7 and 6.6.[1] These declining mortality rates mask the fact that CAD remains the major cause of death among Americans. In 1988, cardiovascular disease claimed 982,579 American lives (45.3 per cent of all deaths in the United States), and 511,050 of those deaths were due to CAD.[1] Moreover, the CAD mortality rate remains higher in the United States than in other industrialized nations. According to the World Health Organization, 55 of every 100,000 Americans die of CAD each year. That compares with CAD mortality rates of 33 and 15 per 100,000 people in Switzerland and Japan, respectively. Further progress against CAD in the United States may depend in part on whether we can precisely identify the factors behind the declining CAD mortality rates recorded since the 1950's and on whether we can continue to affect these factors positively.

Between 1968 and 1976, the age-adjusted mortality from CAD in the United States progressively declined by 20 per cent.[2] Goldman and Cook in 1984 estimated that more than half of that decline was related to lifestyle changes, specifically to decreases in serum cholesterol and cigarette smoking.[2a] They attributed as much as 24 per cent of the CAD reduction to smoking cessation. Dietary changes would also appear to be crucial. Since the 1950's, Americans have been eating less saturated fat and red meat and fewer dairy products while eating more polyunsaturated fats. Public concern about "heart-healthy" eating has grown stronger with each recent decade. The U.S. antihypertension campaign of the 1970's also is cited as a possible explanation for the declining CAD mortality rates during recent years. The declining rate of fatal cerebrovascular events, in particular, apparently reflects the growing awareness of hypertension as a cardiovascular risk factor, as well as the improved availability and effectiveness of well-tolerated antihypertensive agents. However, these advances against hypertension have not translated into fewer deaths from CAD. Indeed, clinical studies have indicated that some of the widely used antihypertensives, although they successfully lower blood pressure, tend to increase serum cholesterol levels, a result that negates the expected benefits of lower blood pressure on CAD mortality.

Other factors that have had a beneficial effect on CAD mortality rates in the United States include improvements in prehospital care, greater availability of coronary care units, the introduction of thrombolytic therapy and percutaneous transluminal angioplasty, and refinements in surgical techniques. Diagnostic advances such as thallium scintigraphy, gated wall-motion stress tests, and positron-emission tomography probably have not yet had an important impact on CAD mortality. But these imaging techniques are expected to cause further reductions in CAD mortality, especially among patients with subclinical or clinically manifest coronary atherosclerosis. That coronary artery bypass surgery has become part of common medical practice also should reduce these rates.

Because no single factor can be cited as the sole catalyst for the declining CAD mortality rates in the past, it is logical to assume that no one factor will be totally responsible for any mortality reductions in the future. Indeed, our ability to collectively identify and manage CAD risk factors will profoundly affect our efforts to maintain the trend of declining CAD mortality rates well into the 21st century. With this in mind, our goal here is to identify the risk factors for CAD and to review the current guidelines for their diagnosis and effective management.

DYSLIPIDEMIA

Dyslipidemia is one of three major modifiable risk factors for CAD. Hypertension and smoking, the other two such factors, are discussed in a later section.

Dyslipidemia has numerous forms, from hypercholesterolemia to hypoalphalipoproteinemia. The term itself simply refers to an abnormal metabolism of plasma lipids. This abnormal metabolism can be caused by genetic, dietary, or secondary disease factors. The various types of dyslipidemia, their probable causes, and the suggested treatment regimens for each are discussed later in this section. The traditional definition of hyperlipoproteinemia has been based on plasma cholesterol levels exceeding the 95th percentile value for age and sex, in comparison with measurements in a comparable nonrestricted population. The Lipid Research Clinics data provide the most complete sets available (Table 37–1).

TABLE 37-1 REFERENCE VALUES FOR PLASMA CHOLESTEROL AND LIPOPROTEIN CHOLESTEROL

	mg/dl												
	PLASMA CHOLESTEROL					LDL CHOLESTEROL				HDL CHOLESTEROL			
PERCENTILE	5	50	75	90	95	5	50	75	95	5	10	50	95
AGE (YR)													
						Men							
5–19	115	155	170	185	200	65	95	105	130	35*	40*	55*	75*
20–24	125	165	185	205	220	65	105	120	145	30	30	45	65
25–29	135	180	200	225	245	70	115	140	165	30	30	45	65
30–34	140	190	215	240	255	80	125	145	185	30	30	45	60
35–39	145	200	225	250	270	80	135	155	190	30	30	45	60
40–44	150	205	230	250	270	85	135	155	185	25	30	45	65
45–69	160	215	235	260	275	90	145	165	205	30	30	50	70
70+	150	205	230	250	270	90	145	165	185	30	35	50	75
						Women							
5–19	120	160	175	190	200	65	100	110	140	35	40	55	70
20–24	125	170	190	215	230	55	105	120	160	35	35	55	80
25–34	130	175	195	220	235	70	110	125	160	35	40	55	80
35–39	140	185	205	230	245	75	120	140	170	35	40	55	80
40–44	145	195	215	235	255	75	125	145	175	35	40	60	90
45–49	150	205	225	250	270	80	130	150	185	35	40	60	85
50–54	165	220	240	265	285	90	140	160	200	35	40	60	90
55+	170	230	250	295	295	95	150	170	215	35	40	60	95

From the Lipid Research Clinics Population Studies Data Book. Vol. 1: The Prevalence Study, Washington, D.C., U.S. Government Printing Office, 1988. USDHHS/NIH pub. no. 88-1927.

* For HDL values for men aged 15–19 yr use values for age group 20–24 yr.

HDL = high-density lipoprotein; LDL = low-density lipoprotein.

PLASMA LIPOPROTEINS

The major classes of plasma lipids are cholesterol, cholesteryl ester, triglyceride, and phospholipid. Although lipids are vital components of many of the body's tissues, they are insoluble in water. To reach those tissues, lipids must be transported in the bloodstream by complex, water-soluble molecules called *lipoproteins.* Structurally, lipoproteins consist of a core of nonpolar cholesteryl ester and triglyceride covered by a polar surface monolayer made up of phospholipids, free cholesterol, and the protein or polypeptide moieties called apolipoproteins, or apoproteins (apos) (Table 37–2). Each of the plasma lipids has one or more apoproteins that perform specific functions essential to lipid transport and cellular uptake (Figs. 37–1 and 37–2).

The five principal lipoprotein classes are defined according to their density on ultracentrifugation and by their mobility on agarose gel electrophoresis. In addition, they can be classified on the basis of size and relative concentrations of cholesterol or triglyceride and by their apoprotein content. The major lipoprotein classes are chylomicrons, very-low-density lipoproteins (VLDLs), intermediate-density lipoproteins (IDLs), low-density lipoproteins (LDLs), and high-density lipoproteins (HDLs).

CHYLOMICRONS. Chylomicrons are the largest of the lipoproteins. Their primary function is to transport dietary, or exogenous, triglyceride and cholesterol from the intestinal lumen to sites of metabolism or storage. The chylomicrons are formed in the gastrointestinal (GI) tract. In the lumen of the GI tract, dietary fat is degraded into free fatty acids and monoglycerides. These substances enter the intestinal villi, where they are reconstructed into a triglyceride particle. Dietary cholesterol absorbed into the intestinal wall is then esterified to cholesteryl esters, mainly cholesteryl oleate, by the enzymatic reaction catalyzed by acyl:cholesterol acyltransferase. The triglyceride and cholesteryl esters are then combined with apos B-48, A-I, and A-IV within the intestinal wall to form chylomicron particles.

The nascent chylomicrons enter the systemic circulation by way of the lymphatics. Apos E and C are then added to the

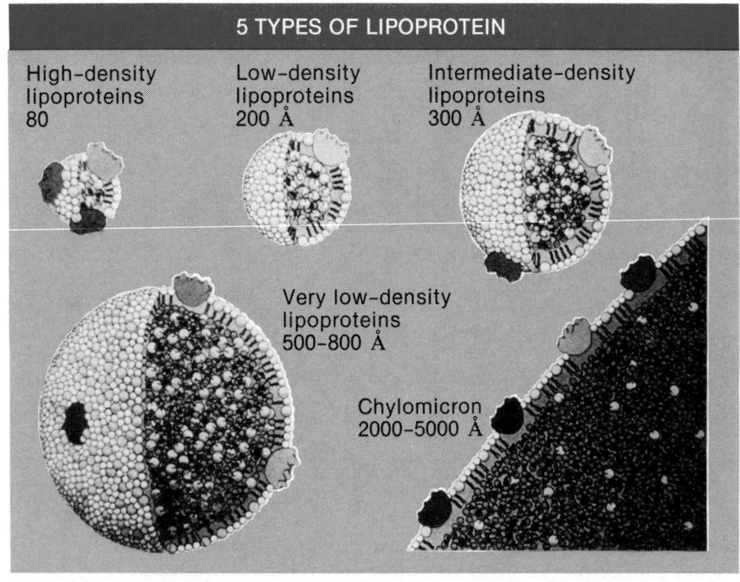

FIGURE 37–1. **The major categories of circulating lipoproteins differ as to size, relative lipid composition, electrophoretic mobility, and apoprotein content. Chylomicrons are large, triglyceride-rich particles that are formed in the wall of the intestine and carry dietary fat. Very low-density lipoproteins are smaller, triglyceride-rich particles of hepatic origin. Intermediate-density lipoproteins are formed from very low-density lipoprotein catabolism and are recognized by the apoprotein B/E receptor. The low-density lipoprotein particle has only apoprotein B-100 on its surface and is highly correlated with atherosclerosis risk. High-density lipoproteins are the smallest of the major lipoproteins and act in reverse cholesterol transport. (From Federman, D. D., and Rubenstein, E. (eds.): Scientific American Medicine, Section 9, Subsection II. © 1987 Scientific American, Inc., All rights reserved.)**

TABLE 37-2 COMPOSITION AND PROPERTIES OF HUMAN PLASMA LIPOPROTEINS

PROPERTIES	CHYLOMICRONS	VLDL	IDL	LDL	HDL
Density (gm/ml)	0.95	0.95–1.006	1.006–1.019	1.019–1.063	1.061–1.210
Electrophoretic mobility	Origin	Pre-Beta	Beta	Beta	Alpha
Major lipid constituents	Triglyceride (exogenous)	Triglyceride (endogenous), phospholipid	Esterified cholesterol, phospholipid	Triglyceride, esterified cholesterol	Phospho-lipid, cholesterol
Apoprotein constituents	Apo A-I Apo II Apo IV Apo B-48	Apo B-100 Apo C-I Apo C-II Apo C-III Apo E	Apo B-100 Apo E	Apo B-100	Apo A-I Apo A-II Apo C-II Apo E

From Beigel, Y., and Gotto, A.: Lipoproteins in Health and Disease: Diagnosis and Management. The Baylor College of Medicine Cardiology Series 9:6, No. 1., 1986. Used with permission, Associates in Medical Marketing Co., Inc.
HDL = high-density lipoprotein; IDL = intermediate-density lipoprotein; LDL = low-density lipoprotein; VLDL = very low-density lipoprotein.

particles. Normally, the chylomicrons are cleared rapidly from the blood and are virtually absent in the fasting state. The clearing of the chylomicrons is modulated by the enzyme lipoprotein lipase (LPL). LPL catalyzes hydrolysis of the triglyceride core of the chylomicron, leaving a remnant particle rich in cholesterol, apo C, apo E, and apo B-48. During this process, apoproteins, phospholipids, and cholesterol from the surface of the chylomicron are transferred to HDL particles. The chylomicron remnants are cleared rapidly from the circulation by receptors present on the surface of liver cells. These receptors recognize the apo E component of the remnant particle. Remnants that contain the apo E_2 moiety bind less well, and are thus removed less quickly, than remnants that contain either the apo E_3 or E_4 moiety. The chylomicron remnant receptor, possibly identical to the LDL receptor–related entity, does not appear to be down-regulated as remnant particles are taken up.

Chylomicron remnants are thought to be atherogenic, and an abnormal delay in their clearance is therefore undesirable. Delays in chylomicron clearance may be secondary to a genetically inherited deficiency of LPL or its activator, apo C-II. Interestingly, in the most severe forms of these conditions, which produce fasting hyperchylomicronemia syndromes, accelerated atherogenesis does not appear to be a clinical feature. Instead, it is partial degradation of the chylomicron to a remnant that renders the particle atherogenic. Delayed clearance of the remnant particles may damage the vascular endothelium, and thus predispose to atherosclerosis.

Hyperchylomicronemia also may be secondary to other acquired hypertriglyceridemic states, such as those seen with exogenous estrogen use, uncontrolled diabetes, and excessive alcohol intake. The presence of chylomicrons in the serum is necessary for the diagnosis of type I or V hyperlipoproteinemia in the Fredrickson and Lees classification system (see Typing of Hyperlipoproteinemia).

VERY LOW-DENSITY LIPOPROTEIN. VLDLs are intermediate in size between chylomicrons and IDLs. They are relatively large particles, with diameters ranging from 500 to 800 Å. VLDLs are produced in the liver. Their primary lipid component is triglyceride, but cholesterol, cholesteryl ester, and phospholipid are also present. Their surface components are apos B-100, C, and E and phospholipid. The synthesis of VLDL is increased by excess carbohydrate, alcohol, or caloric consumption. The function of VLDL is to transport endoge-

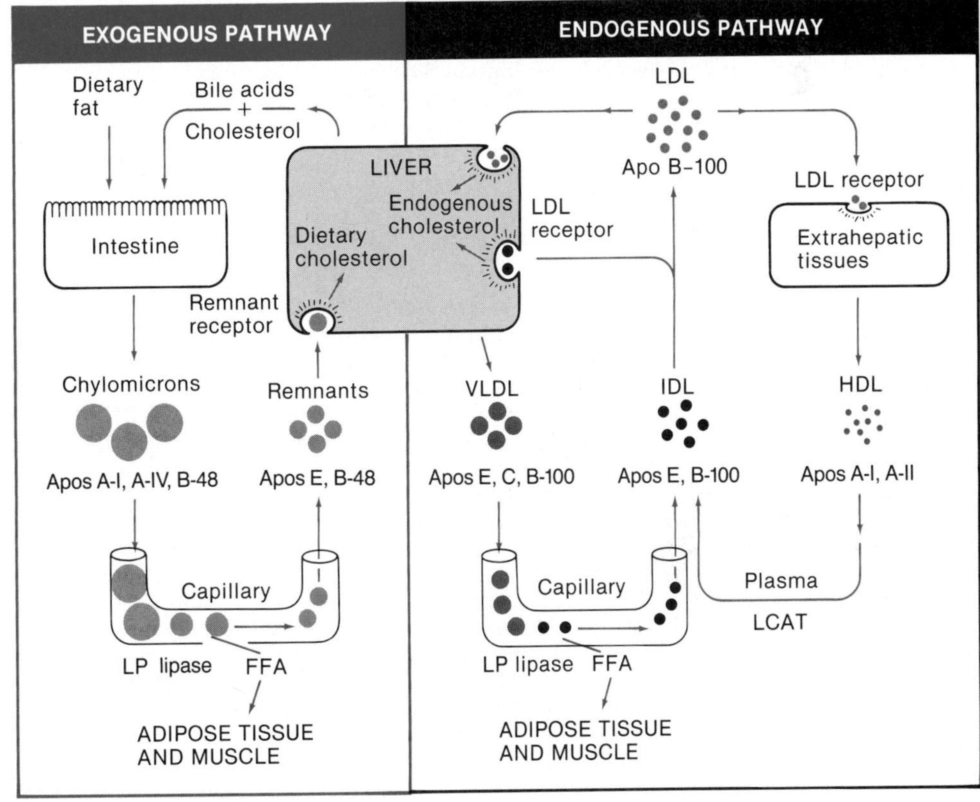

FIGURE 37–2. Model for plasma triglyceride and cholesterol transport in humans. VLDL, very low-density lipoprotein; IDL, intermediate-density lipoprotein; LDL, low-density lipoprotein; HDL, high-density lipoprotein; LCAT, lecithin:cholesterol acyltransferase; LP lipase, lipoprotein lipase; FFA, free fatty acids. The major apoprotein for each class of lipoproteins is shown. In HDL, apo E is a minor but crucial apoprotein. In chylomicrons, apo E and apo C-II are minor but crucial; they are added in the lymph or after the chylomicrons reach the circulation. (From Brown, M. S., and Goldstein, J. L.: The hyperlipoproteinemias and other disorders of lipid metabolism. *In* Wilson, J. E., et al. (eds.): Harrison's Principles of Internal Medicine. 12th ed. New York, McGraw-Hill, 1991, p. 1816.)

nously synthesized triglycerides and cholesterol into the peripheral tissues, where the lipids' fatty acids can be utilized for energy or stored as triglyceride.

When VLDL particles enter the systemic circulation, their triglyceride core is hydrolyzed by LPL. As the VLDL particle is degraded, most of its surface apoproteins, except for apo B-100, are transferred with other surface components to HDL. The remaining VLDL remnant is called IDL. Unlike the chylomicron remnant, IDL contains apo B-100 rather than apo B-48. The metabolism of VLDL is complex and not fully understood. Some of the larger particles appear to be directly removed from the circulation. The rest of the particles enter the cascade, in which they are converted to IDL and eventually to LDL, as discussed below.

INTERMEDIATE-DENSITY LIPOPROTEIN. IDLs, which carry both cholesterol and triglyceride, are the product of the enzymatic (LPL-mediated) breakdown of VLDL. After their formation, IDLs may be removed by the liver by means of the binding of apo E to the LDL, or B/E, receptor. The remainder are converted to LDL, a process thought to be mediated by hepatic triglyceride lipase. IDLs have a high cholesterol content and migrate in the beta region on electrophoresis. Elevations of IDLs are thought to predispose to premature CAD and peripheral artery disease. Accumulation of IDL is characteristic of dysbetalipoproteinemia, also called Fredrickson's type III hyperlipoproteinemia. This relatively uncommon form of hyperlipoproteinemia is associated with both triglyceride and cholesterol elevations (see Typing of Hyperlipoproteinemia, p. 1135).

LOW-DENSITY LIPOPROTEIN. LDL, which is 45 per cent cholesterol by weight, is the major carrier of cholesterol to the nerve tissues, cell membranes, and other cells that require the cholesterol for metabolic functions, including the synthesis of steroid hormones. LDLs have a density of 1.019 to 1.063 gm/ml, a diameter of 180 to 280 Å, and beta electrophoretic mobility. LDL usually is formed from VLDL breakdown. Direct synthesis has not been completely excluded. Increased LDL synthesis may occur by means of enhanced conversion of VLDL remnants or direct hepatic production of apo B–containing lipoproteins.

Apo B-100 is the only protein found in LDL, and makes up about 20 per cent of the LDL mass. Each particle is thought to contain 1 molecule of apo B-100, but the ratio of protein mass to total particle mass can vary from the large to the small particle range. LDL particles are heterogeneous, differing in their hydrated density and cholesteryl ester content. The content of cholesteryl ester in the LDL particle, for example, may vary up to 40 per cent by weight. Patients with greater concentrations of small, dense LDL have been reported to have a three-times greater risk for acute myocardial infarction (MI), regardless of weight or gender.[3] Small, dense LDL molecules are commonly associated with male gender, diabetes, depressed HDL levels, and familial combined hyperlipoproteinemia.

LDL particles are recognized by specific LDL, or apo B/E, receptors on the surfaces of hepatic and certain nonhepatic cells (Fig. 37–2). These receptors also recognize and bind some of the apo E–containing IDL particles, preventing their conversion into LDL. Bound LDL particles (and IDL particles) are then internalized into the cells.[4] About 75 per cent of the LDLs in the bloodstream are removed by this specific receptor-mediated binding. The remaining LDL particles are cleared by scavenger, or macrophage, receptors or by non-receptor-mediated mechanisms. The number of LDL receptors is not fixed, and can be modified by genetic defects, saturated fat and cholesterol intake, or certain pharmacological agents.

The prototype disease involving the LDL receptor is familial hypercholesterolemia. In this condition, heterozygotes have a 50 per cent reduction in LDL receptors, whereas homozygotes have little or no receptor activity. Familial hypercholesterolemia is fairly common, occurring in 1 in every 500 people. Familial combined hyperlipidemia (FCH) is even more common, possibly occurring in 1 in every 300 people. Clinically, FCH patients may be difficult to differentiate from those with familial hypercholesterolemia. In FCH, most patients lack tendon xanthomas and the hyperlipidemia does not present in childhood; most family studies show varying Fredrickson's phenotypes.

The characteristic defect in FCH is thought to be an overproduction of apo B-100 by the liver.[5,6] Also, FCH patients have a lower ratio of apo A-I to apo B-100. About 80 per cent of patients with an elevated LDL value do not have only one gene defect; the dyslipidemia is secondary to polygenic factors. Hence, elevations of LDL due to primary receptor defects are relatively uncommon.

HIGH-DENSITY LIPOPROTEIN. HDLs are produced by the liver and the GI tract and by the peripheral catabolism of chylomicrons and VLDLs. HDL particles carry cholesteryl ester as their major lipid and apos A-I and A-II as their major proteins. Much of the apoprotein component of HDL is transferred in the systemic circulation to VLDLs or chylomicrons. Apo C-II, an obligatory activator of LPL, is one of the apoproteins transferred by HDL. By weight, HDL particles are about 30 per cent cholesterol, 45 per cent protein, and 25 per cent phospholipid (predominantly phosphatidylcholine). Small amounts of triglycerides are present.

HDL particles exist in several subtypes. For clinical purposes, HDL_2 and HDL_3 are the major circulating subfractions. HDL_2, which migrates with alpha mobility, is the subfraction most closely associated with statistical protection against premature atherosclerosis. It has a density of 1.061 to 1.25 gm/ml and a diameter of 90 to 120 Å. HDL_3 is a smaller particle, with a density of 1.125 to 1.210 gm/ml and a diameter of 50 to 90 Å. Alcohol consumption increases both HDL subfractions, with a greater impact on HDL_3. Lower levels of both subfractions are associated with male gender; hypertriglyceridemia; diabetes mellitus; obesity; uremia; the use of androgens, progestins, or tobacco products; and diets rich in polyunsaturated fat but low in total fat content.

Several epidemiological studies have addressed whether there is a varying clinical impact on CAD depending on the relative levels of HDL_2 and HDL_3.[7] In males with CAD who have an associated low level of circulating HDL, both fractions of HDL are depressed with more of a decline in HDL_2. The initial National Cholesterol Education Program (NCEP) guidelines (see below) do not recommend routine screening of HDL levels. In the authors' opinion, however, a complete lipoprotein profile, including determination of HDL levels, should be obtained in any patient with established CAD. In their own practice, they measure HDL cholesterol in anyone with a total cholesterol value exceeding 200 mg/dl.

HDL particles are thought to participate in the reverse transport of free cholesterol from peripheral tissues by way of a putative HDL receptor. Oram and coworkers[8] report that apos A-I and A-II interact with this receptor. This receptor-mediated reverse transport could explain why patients with elevated HDL concentrations are less prone to CAD.

Another explanation for the inverse relation between HDL levels and CAD incidence may be related to the observation that most patients with low levels of HDL have elevated levels of the more cholesterol- and triglyceride-rich lipoproteins. In this case, low HDL levels may serve only as a marker for other, concurrent lipid abnormalities. Hence, the independent clinical impact of low HDL concentrations is difficult to determine.[9] Patients with certain variant forms of apo A-I, such as A-I Milano, may have decreased levels of HDL without evidence of accelerated atherosclerosis.

Just as low levels of HDL are statistically associated with atherosclerosis, HDL is increased on a genetic basis in *familial hyperapolipoproteinemia*. This condition has been described as being associated with longevity.

LIPOPROTEIN (a) (see also p. 1780). Lipoprotein (a), or Lp(a), has been established as an independent CAD risk factor. The structure of Lp(a) is similar to that of an LDL molecule whose apo B-100 is linked by a disulfide bridge to apoprotein (a). It has a density of 1.05 to 1.12 gm/ml and a size of about

TABLE 37-3 SUMMARY OF APOPROTEINS

NAME	LIPOPROTEIN	MOLECULAR WEIGHT	FUNCTION
apo A-I	HDL, chylomicrons*	28,000	Structural; activator of LCAT enzyme
apo A-II	HDL, chylomicrons	16,000	Structural
apo A-IV	HDL, chylomicrons,* VLDL	46,000	Unknown
apo B-100	LDL, VLDL	550,000	Structural; synthesis and secretion of VLDL; binds to LDL receptor (B/E)
apo B-48	Chylomicrons	250,000	Structural; synthesis and secretion from intestine
apo C-I	HDL, chylomicrons, VLDL	6,000	Activator of LCAT
apo C-II	HDL, chylomicrons, VLDL	7,000	Activator of lipoprotein lipase
apo C-III	HDL, chylomicrons, VLDL	7,000	Stabilizes surface; provides negative charge
apo D	HDL, chylomicrons*	21,000	Cholesteryl ester exchange
apo E	HDL, VLDL, chylomicrons*	34,000	Binds to receptor on cell membrane of liver (E and B/E) and macrophage

From Cholesterol & Coronary Disease . . . Reducing the Risk. Lecture Guide. New York, Science & Medicine, 1986.
* Only in nascent chylomicrons.
HDL = high-density lipoprotein; LDL = low-density lipoprotein; LCAT = lecithin:cholesterol acyltransferase; VLDL = very low-density lipoprotein.

250Å, and it migrates in the pre-beta region. Lp(a) levels range from 1 mg/dl to 200 mg/dl, with the largest number of values below 20 mg/dl. Thus, this lipoprotein does not have the normal, bell-shaped distribution of population serum values seen in the other lipoproteins.

Although Lp(a) is structurally similar to LDL, the former appears to be regulated independently and carries an independent relation to overall coronary risk. If serum levels of both LDL and Lp(a) are elevated, the risk of CAD is markedly increased.[10] Recent angiographic studies have documented a positive correlation between Lp(a) levels and the severity of coronary atherosclerosis.[11,11a,11b]

The mechanism by which high levels of Lp(a) are related to coronary atherosclerosis is unclear. It has been suggested that because of the structural similarities of Lp(a) to plasminogen,[12] high levels of Lp(a) may inhibit the thrombolytic activity of naturally occurring tissue plasminogen activity. Plasminogen is composed of five sequences of amino acids rich in cysteine (Fig. 37–3). Each sequence is called a kringle. Lp(a) lacks the first three kringles, but has a sequence that is highly homologous to the fourth kringle of plasminogen. There is no serine protease activity in Lp(a) and no thrombolytic activity. An alternative explanation for the association between elevated Lp(a) levels and atherosclerosis is that Lp(a) may somehow alter the LDL-mediated delivery of cholesterol to the atherosclerotic plaque. Lp(a) is highly polymorphic and contains variable quantities of carbohydrate as well as having a heterogeneity of kringles.

The control mechanisms of Lp(a) are unknown. Dietary changes that increase LDL levels do not affect Lp(a) levels. The effects of pharmacological agents are unclear, although Lp(a) has been reported to be decreased by niacin, neomycin, and stanozolol.[13,14]

APOPROTEINS

(See Table 37–3)

Apoproteins are key lipoprotein components that serve both as enzymatic cofactors and as recognition elements that bind to specific receptors on peripheral tissues, including the vascular endothelial cells. It is the apo E component of the chylomicron remnant, for example, that is recognized by receptors on the hepatocyte. The apoproteins are distinguished alphabetically and numerically as apo A-I through apo E.

A great deal of research has been conducted in the use of apoproteins as CAD markers. Some investigators have found that the concentrations of apo A-I and apo B-100 are better predictors of CAD than are measurements of total plasma lipids or lipoproteins. In one study, apo A-I was the best predictor of atherosclerotic risk in patients undergoing coronary arteriography.[15] In this study, higher levels of apo A-I were associated with a decreased prevalence of obstructive coronary lesions. Indeed, apo A-I was found to be a better CAD predictor than either total cholesterol or HDL. These observations have not been generally reproduced.

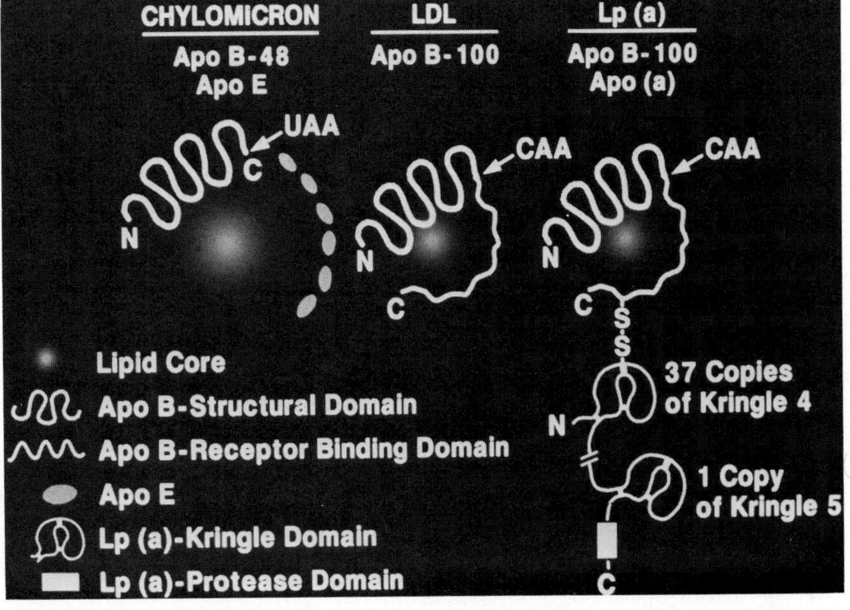

FIGURE 37–3. Chylomicrons are large, triglyceride-rich particles with several classes (A, B, C, E) of surface apoproteins. Apoprotein (apo) C-II activates lipoprotein lipase, which degrades the chylomicrons to remnant particles. The B class of apoproteins is apo B-48. Low-density lipoprotein (LDL) has only one apoprotein (B-100), which is recognized by the apo B/E receptor. Lipoprotein (a) [Lp(a)] has two major associated proteins—apo B-100 and apo(a), a unique protein. Lp(a) has structural similarity to plasminogen (one form has 7 repeating units of kringle 4) but lacks the serine protease activity. Arrow site at which codon 2,153 in the apo B gene is changed at the mRNA level from CAA (glutamine) to UAA (termination) in intestinal cells. (Adapted from Brown, M. S., and Goldstein, J. L.: Plasma lipoproteins: Teaching old dogmas new tricks. Nature *330*:113, 1987.)

APOPROTEIN A. Apo A-I, the prototype of apo A, is a major protein in HDL and also is seen in chylomicrons. It has a molecular weight of 28,000 and is synthesized in the GI tract and liver. Its specific regions called amphipathic helices are enriched with charged amino acids that form areas of polar and nonpolar residues.[16] Apo A-I functions as the activator of lecithin:cholesterol acyltransferase (LCAT), and also has been found as a degradation product in amyloid fibrils.[17]

Apo A-II is a minor constituent of HDL and does not appear to be present in all species. Human apo A-II is of hepatic origin and consists of two identical chains attached by a single disulfide linkage. Apo A-II may be an activator of hepatic triglyceride lipase, which hydrolyzes triglyceride and phospholipid while utilizing HDL_2 as its preferred substrate. Apo A-IV is synthesized in the gut, and is present in HDL, chylomicrons, and as a free protein. Its molecular weight is 46,000, and its structure is helical. Although its function is not known, it also may be an activator of LCAT.

Although levels of apo A-I are inversely related to CAD risk, there are several genetic conditions in which the relationship of apo A-I to the subsequent development of coronary atherosclerosis is less clear. Genetic deficiencies of apo A-I are associated with extremely low HDL levels. The genetic codes for apos A-I, A-IV, and C-III are close together on the long arm of chromosome 11.[18] Combined A-I/C-III deficiency is associated with severe premature atherosclerosis.[19] A kindred with apo A-II deficiency has been reported with no significant reduction in either the level of circulating HDL or evidence of atherosclerosis.

APOPROTEIN B. Apo B occurs in two forms. Apo B-48 is synthesized by the small intestine, and apo B-100 is secreted by the liver. Apo B-48 is present on the surfaces of chylomicrons and chylomicron remnants. Apo B-100 is found in VLDL, IDL, and LDL. Apo B-100 is the primary apoprotein of LDL, and accounts for 25 per cent of its weight. It also is the recognition site for the LDL, or apo B/E, receptor on cell surfaces. It has recently been determined that a single gene regulates the synthesis of both apo B-48 and apo B-100. The gene for apo B-100 has been localized to chromosome 2 and exists as a 40-kilobase structure.[20] The structure in the amino acid sequence of human apo B-100 and the corresponding cDNA messenger have recently been determined.[21] A unique editing mechanism introduces a stop codon into the mRNA for apo B by means of a single base change. This allows the biosynthesis of two proteins from a single gene and mRNA, with either apo B-100 or apo B-48 being synthesized.[22,23]

APOPROTEIN D. Apo D is a relatively minor constituent found in HDL and the chylomicron. Its molecular weight is 21,000. It has been reported to be involved in cholesteryl ester exchange but does not appear to be the exchange site itself. Apo D is not in the family of the other soluble apoproteins.

APOPROTEIN E. Most apo E is synthesized in the liver. However, other tissues, including the small bowel, kidney, adrenals, and the cells of the reticuloendothelial system, have the ability to synthesize this apoprotein. Apo E accounts for about 15 per cent of the protein content of VLDL, 7 per cent of the protein content of chylomicron remnants, and 2 per cent of the protein content of HDL. It can be recognized by the LDL, or apo B/E, receptor and by specific apo E receptors in the liver whose function appears to be the removal of chylomicron remnants. The ability of apo E to interact with the LDL receptor is thought to be the result of ligand recognition sites between residues 140 and 150. Apo E is polymorphic and contains three major alleles: apos E_2, E_3, and E_4. These respective alleles are present in about 10 per cent, 76 per cent, and 13 per cent of whites. Their various combination results in homozygotes for apos $E_{2/2}$, $E_{3/3}$, and $E_{4/4}$. Also, apos $E_{2/3}$, $E_{2/4}$, and $E_{3/4}$ exist in the heterozygous state. The polymorphism of apo E has been determined on a molecular basis and results from the substitution of an amino acid at residues 112 and 158 in the protein.[23]

About 90 per cent of patients with type III hyperlipoproteinemia (HLP) are homozygous for the $E_{2/2}$ phenotype. This disorder is characterized by hypercholesterolemia, hypertriglyceridemia, and IDL or VLDL particles abnormally enriched in cholesterol. These particles have beta electrophoretic mobility and are termed beta-VLDLs. Premature coronary and peripheral vascular disease is characteristically associated with type III HLP. Type III HLP is also characterized by the delayed clearance of chylomicron remnants in the serum due to impaired binding of these remnants to the lipoprotein receptors in isolated cells. Because the $E_{2/2}$ genotype occurs in 1 per cent of the population, and type III HLP is rare, a second abnormality must be present.

Apo E isoforms may account for as much as 15 per cent of the variability of cholesterol and LDL levels in the population.[24] Also, recent Finnish studies suggest that E_4 may be associated with increased cholesterol absorption in the GI tract.[25] In the Prospective Cardiovascular Muenster (PROCAM) study, E_2 was associated with lower cholesterol levels and E_3 or E_4 with higher levels of total cholesterol and LDL in populations with and without CAD.[26,27]

GENETIC VARIATION OF APOPROTEINS

Restriction fragment length polymorphism (RFLP) analysis is a powerful tool for studying the genetic variation of apoproteins. When the genomic DNA molecules from different individuals are digested with enzymes called restriction endonucleases, the pattern of gene fragments varies. Each restriction endonuclease is specific for a defined DNA recognition sequence. A change in the digestion pattern could represent simply a point mutation, or it could be due to a deletion, insertion, or rearrangement of the DNA. RFLP analysis was initially used with the enzyme *Eco*RI to detect the abnormality in the DNA of patients with familial deficiency of apo A-I and apo C-III.

The genes for apos A-I, C-III, and A-IV have been localized to chromosome 11, and several kindreds have been described with abnormalities at this locus (see below). These genes have been isolated and shown clinically to be associated with abnormalities of HDL regulation. The most extensively evaluated RFLP for this locus used *Sac*I.[28] This minor allele has been shown to be associated with elevated triglycerides and decreased HDL in certain racial groups. The RFLP may or may not be in the coding region of the protein. Association with elevations or decreases in serum lipid or lipoprotein levels could be due to a disequilibrium linkage with another gene.

Population screening has revealed at least 11 variants of apo A-I. The abnormal gene is associated with one normal gene in a heterozygous manner. It produces mutants that contain abnormal amino acid substitutions. Examples are apo A-I Milano and apo A-I Marburg. Both are associated with low HDL levels. Other apo A-I mutants (i.e., Giessen and Muenster) fail to activate LCAT. RFLP studies with apo A-II have revealed several alleles for the apo A-II gene.[29] A cDNA probe has revealed a minor allele of 3.7 kilobases. In patients homozygous for the minor allele, increased levels of apo A-II have been found.[29] Apo A-II has been reported to be an activator of hepatic triglyceride lipase.

RFLP analysis has been used to study the cluster of genes for apos A-I, C-III, and A-IV.[30] Two alleles have been identified in the apo C-III region: S1 and S2. They vary among racial groups; in addition, the S2 region has been associated with low HDL levels, MI survivors, and type V HLP. One of the most widely studied mutants is the *Xba*I polymorphism for apo B-100. Characteristic lipid changes are present in some populations but not in all. Unfortunately, this has been the case for most of the apoprotein polymorphism described, including that for apo A-I by Ordovas and associates.[31]

FAMILIAL APO C-II DEFICIENCY. The gene for apo C-II has been isolated, sequenced, and localized to chromosome 19.[32] The deficiency state involving apo C-II results in hyperchylomicronemia, but the disorder is highly complex and may involve a variety of potential defects. Several degradation steps occur before the final form of apo C-II is reached: pro-apo C-II and pre-pro-apo C-II isoforms undergo proteolysis and processing before the formation of the mature 73–amino acid sequence.[33] The deficiency of apo C-II on a familial basis has been well described. Its clinical presentation is similar to that of lipoprotein lipase deficiency. In one family, the apo C-II was nonfunctional and was characterized by an abnormal electrophoretic migration pattern due to an amino acid deletion.[34]

DEFECTS IN STRUCTURE AND SYNTHESIS OF APO B.[34a] The polymorphism of apo B has been observed in case-control studies of whites with and without CAD and in RFLP studies of the DNA coding sequence. So far, more than 60 variations have been reported.[35,36] The polymorphism is not associated with alterations in LDL content, although the X-2 allele with endonuclease *Xba*I and the B1 allele with *Eco*RI have been reported to occur with increased frequency in patients with CAD. There is great variability among populations.

Several genetic diseases have been described that result in decreased levels or the absence of apo B. Abetalipoproteinemia is characterized by the absence of LDL and by acanthocytosis. It appears to be transmitted as an autosomal recessive trait. On Southern blot analysis, the gene appears normal[37]; hence, the defect in abetalipoproteinemia appears to be a post-translational event. Homozygous hypobetalipoproteinemia has similar clinical manifestations; in this condition, however, the levels of apo B are reduced to one-half of normal. As a rule, CAD is not present, but the number of patients studied so far is small.

THE LIPID HYPOTHESIS OF ATHEROGENESIS

The lipid hypothesis states that dyslipidemia, as manifested by elevated LDL levels and/or decreased HDL levels, is central to the initiation and propagation of atherosclerotic plaque and CAD. It has been known since the nineteenth century that atherosclerotic plaques are laden with cholesterol. But the first scientific credence for the lipid hypothesis came in the early years of this century, when Anitschkow and his colleagues in czarist Russia experimentally induced atherosclerosis in rabbits by cholesterol feeding. Anitschkow reported that cholesterol was an essential ingredient in the development of atherosclerosis.

More recently, the lipid hypothesis has been supported by a large body of epidemiological studies that link the level of mean serum cholesterol to the incidence of coronary morbidity and mortality in many populations (Fig. 37–4). Indeed, virtually every major epidemiological study to date has shown a significant correlation between the level of serum cholesterol at the time of entry and the subsequent risk of CAD. The Seven Countries Study found that CAD was less common in Japan and Mediterranean countries (where the average diet is low in cholesterol and saturated fat) than in the United States, Finland, and The Netherlands (where the cholesterol and saturated fat content of the average diet is higher).[38] In the United States, the Framingham Heart Study and more recently the Multiple Risk Factor Intervention Trial (MRFIT) have shown that the incidence of CAD is positively associated with serum cholesterol levels in a continuous, graded, and progressive manner (Fig. 37–5).

Recent analyses of other epidemiological studies have also lent credence to the lipid hypothesis. Simons analyzed epidemiological data from 19 countries and found that in men, 45

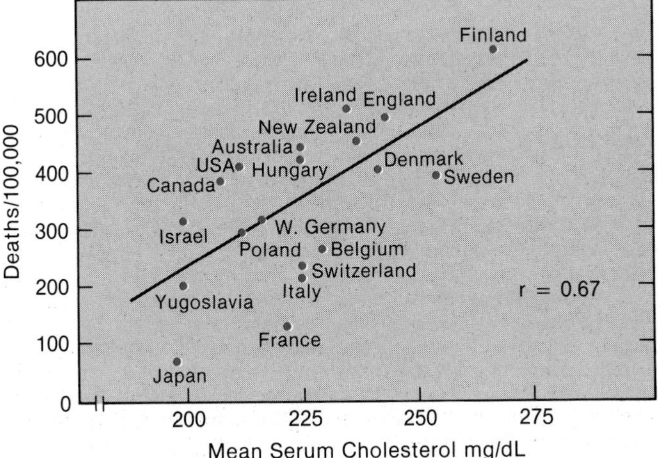

FIGURE 37–4. Coronary artery disease mortality rate versus serum cholesterol. (From Simons, L. A.: Interrelations of lipids and lipoproteins with coronary artery disease mortality in 19 countries. Am. J. Cardiol. *57*:5G, 1986.)

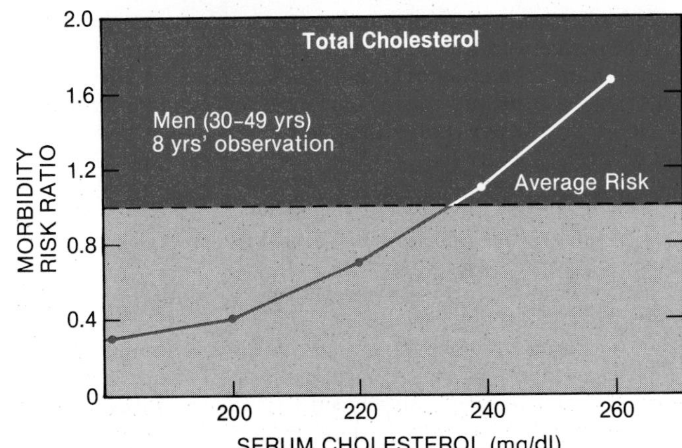

FIGURE 37–5. Various total cholesterol concentrations as related to coronary artery disease risk. Men in Framingham aged 30 to 49 were found to have significantly higher risk if their total cholesterol value exceeded 240 mg/dl.

per cent of the interpopulation differences in CAD mortality could be accounted for by the variation in serum cholesterol levels.[39] He noted that the variability in HDL levels could explain 32 per cent of the mortality differences, and the ratio of total serum cholesterol to HDL could account for 55 per cent. Meanwhile Peto, although unable to identify a level of cholesterol below which CAD is extremely rare, noted that in societies in which average cholesterol levels are under 150 mg/dl and low levels of total serum cholesterol are accompanied by low levels of LDL cholesterol, risks for atherosclerosis and CAD are greatly reduced (personal communication).

ATHEROSCLEROSIS PREVENTION STUDIES

Although the epidemiological data correlating the risk of CAD to levels of cholesterol are compelling, it does not necessarily follow that clinical benefits will accrue from dietary or pharmacological cholesterol lowering. Nonetheless, several controlled clinical trials of the lipid hypothesis have shown that reducing serum cholesterol will reduce overall CAD risk. This conclusion is substantiated by meta-analyses of the available trials. Yusuf and colleagues combined the results of 22 randomized trials involving more than 40,000 subjects.[40] In these trials, various means were used to alter serum cholesterol, including lowering total fat consumption, substituting polyunsaturated for saturated fat, and using pharmacological agents. The meta-analysis examined both primary prevention trials (for people with no clinical evidence of coronary atherosclerosis at the time of entry into the trial) and secondary prevention trials (for patients with documented atherosclerosis). The duration of these trials ranged from 1 to 7 years.

In the overall analysis, the treated subjects had 23 per cent fewer coronary events than the control subjects, a highly significant difference. It must be emphasized, however, that in the earlier trials, the degree of cholesterol lowering was relatively modest and the trials' durations were much shorter than the decades usually required for the buildup of atherosclerotic plaque. Nonetheless, in the 14 trials conducted for less than 4 years, a 10 per cent reduction in serum cholesterol level led to a 10 per cent reduction in coronary events. The reduction in CAD was double (lowering cholesterol 10 per cent leading to 20 per cent less CAD) in the eight trials that treated subjects for longer periods of time. Some of the more important prevention trials are summarized below.

Rossouw and colleagues performed a meta-analysis of the results of eight secondary prevention trials (post-MI, comprising 7837 participants) selected according to strict criteria. They found that across the eight trials, a 10 per cent mean reduction in serum cholesterol meant reductions of 19, 12, and 15 per cent in the number of nonfatal, fatal, and all MIs. Across four primary prevention trials selected by the same criteria, Rossouw and coworkers found respective reductions of 25, 12, and 22 per cent with a 10 per cent reduction in total cholesterol.[41]

SECONDARY PREVENTION TRIALS

Secondary prevention refers to the treatment of patients with established atherosclerotic disease in an attempt to prevent, postpone, or cause regression of the clinical or anatomical manifestations of atherosclerosis. The Veterans Administration Center in Los Angeles used a randomized trial design in 846 domiciled veterans. Patients with and without clinical evidence of coronary disease at the time of entry were included. The average patient age was 65 years. One group of patients was placed on a diet higher in unsaturated (versus saturated) fat content and somewhat lower in cholesterol content. By 8-year follow-up the group placed on the unsaturated fat diet had a 23 per cent reduced CAD incidence. Overall mortality was not different between the groups.[42]

The Coronary Drug Project was performed in post-MI patients and used high- or low-dose estrogens (allocation n = 2220) or clofibrate (n = 1103), niacin (n = 1119), dextrothyroxine (n = 1110), or placebo (n = 2789).[43] This trial was constituted as a randomized, double-blind clinical trial. The niacin, clofibrate, and placebo groups were on study for a mean 6.2 years; treatment in the other three arms was stopped early. No benefit was seen with clofibrate (1.8 gm per day), but niacin recipients (prescribed 3.0 mg/day) showed some improvement: average total serum cholesterol lowered from 253 to 227 mg/dl and average triglycerides lowered from 190 to 139 mg/dl at 1 year, with a 27 per cent lower incidence of nonfatal MI than placebo recipients at 5 years but without a significant difference in overall mortality. However, 9 years after the termination of the trial, total mortality was 11 per cent lower in the niacin group than in the placebo group, a highly significant difference.[44] The researchers estimated that nearly 30 per cent of the niacin recipients took less than 60 per cent of the protocol amount of drugs.[44]

The National Heart, Lung and Blood Institute (NHLBI) conducted a trial in patients with type II HLP and angiographic evidence of CAD.[45] Repeat angiography was performed in 116 of the 143 patients to determine CAD progression. Diet alone reduced the LDL cholesterol level 6 per cent in both the cholestyramine and placebo groups. After randomization, and averaged over the 5 years of treatment, LDL cholesterol was reduced another 26 per cent in the cholestyramine group (the drug allocated at 6 gm four times daily) and 5 per cent in the placebo group. HDL cholesterol increased 8 per cent in the drug group and 2 per cent in the placebo group over the 5 years. These lipid level modifications, in turn, greatly reduced the rate of progression of the angiographically demonstrated plaques.[45] Lack of progression correlated best with a favorable HDL–total cholesterol ratio.

The nonrandomized Leiden trial obtained similar results with a strict diet.[46] Other recent trials involving secondary prevention are discussed in the section on the progression of coronary atherosclerosis. These recent studies had adequate statistical power to analyze angiographic endpoints, in addition to the use of pharmacological agents, with a greater degree of lipid and lipoprotein modification.

PRIMARY PREVENTION STUDIES

The primary prevention studies reviewed in this section were designed to test whether modifying CAD risk factors, primarily hypercholesterolemia, would prevent the subsequent formation and progression of atherosclerotic plaque.

WORLD HEALTH ORGANIZATION TRIAL. In this trial, hypercholesterolemic European men were randomized in a double-blind manner and treated with a placebo or clofibrate (1.6 gm/daily). After 5 years of treatment,[47] the incidence of major ischemic heart disease was 20 per cent lower in the clofibrate group than in the control high-cholesterol group. Since the mortality from ischemic heart disease was essentially the same in the two groups, the difference lay in nonfatal MI (4.6 and 6.2 per thousand). Mean serum cholesterol was reduced 9 per cent from baseline levels in the clofibrate group. The overall mortality was increased in the group receiving the hypolipidemic agent; however, the excess mortality did not continue after the end of treatment.[48] This study had a number of flaws, but still raises a cautionary note about the risk of casual and relatively indiscriminate use of hypolipidemic drugs in a general population.

THE OSLO STUDY. This primary prevention trial used diet to lower cholesterol.[49] Because the study also incorporated programs to encourage smoking cessation, its results cannot be interpreted as a pure test of the lipid hypothesis. In the special-intervention group, 24 per cent of the control patients discontinued smoking, compared with 17 per cent in the placebo group. Also, the special-intervention group experienced a mean 13 per cent reduction in total cholesterol levels over the 5 years, compared with 3 per cent among controls. The smoking cessation and cholesterol lowering, in turn, resulted in 47 per cent fewer nonfatal and fatal MIs and sudden death for the special-intervention group and a 55 per cent reduction in CAD death. The statistical significance of this reduction could not be definitely determined because of the relatively small sample size. (N = 1232). More recent analysis of the Oslo Study, at a follow-up of 102 months, documented 19 deaths in the treated group versus 31 deaths in the control group, a difference approaching statistical significance.[50]

THE MULTIPLE RISK FACTOR INTERVENTION TRIAL. In the MRFIT, high-risk men either were referred to their own physicians for standard care or were enrolled in an intensive treatment program consisting of dietary treatment for lowering plasma cholesterol, counseling against cigarette smoking, and treatment of elevated blood pressure with diet and medication. This was not a placebo-controlled study; in fact, blood pressure and smoking cessation improved significantly in both groups. No significant difference in CAD or overall mortality was observed between the two groups after an average 7 years of follow-up.[51]

Special intervention led to a 49 per cent lower CAD mortality rate compared with usual care.[51] This was of particular interest because of the significant reductions in sudden coronary death and CAD incidence achieved by lipid-lowering dietary intervention and smoking cessation in the Oslo Study.[49] A negative aspect was the finding that patients with nonspecific ST-segment and T-wave changes on initial electrocardiograms who were treated with diuretics in the special-intervention group appeared to have a higher mortality rate. Whether these results were due to the lipid, insulin, or electrolyte effects of diuretic therapy is unclear.[51]

Recent MRFIT follow-up data have revealed a significant decrease in overall and CAD mortality in the special-intervention group at 10.5 years (an average 3.8 years after the end of intervention). The special-intervention patients had 11 per cent lower CAD mortality and 8 per cent lower all-causes mortality than the usual-care patients. The mortality differences were mainly due to a 24 per cent reduction in the death rate from acute MI in the special-intervention group compared with the usual-care groups.[52]

THE CORONARY PRIMARY PREVENTION TRIAL PERFORMED BY THE LIPID RESEARCH CLINICS (LRC-CPPT). This trial provided definitive proof of the lipid hypothesis.[53] This was a large-scale study carried out in 12 specialized lipid research clinics in North America. More than 3800 men were enrolled after meeting strict entry criteria: no clinical evidence of CAD, serum cholesterol in excess of 265 mg/dl and LDL elevation of 175 mg/dl or more even after dietary therapy, and without severe hypertension, hypertriglyceridemia, or diabetes. The men were randomized to receive either a placebo or the bile acid sequestrant cholestyramine. The prevalence of smoking was the same in both groups. The recommended dose of cholestyramine was 24 gm/day. Because of poor compliance, only a minority of patients took that much cholestyramine; the average actual dose was probably about 14 gm. Treatment was continued for 7 to 10 years (mean, 7.4 years), with definite endpoints of acute MI and CAD mortality tabulated.

Patients who received drug therapy lowered their total and LDL cholesterol levels 9 per cent and 13 per cent more than control patients. This degree of cholesterol lowering was associated with a graded effect on coronary endpoints (Fig. 37–6). The mean decrease in nonfatal MI and/or CAD death was 19 per cent. In patients who were randomized to cholestyramine but were unable to take the medication because of associated side effects, there was no reduction in cholesterol and no concomitant alteration in overall cardiac risk. However, those patients who daily took 20 gm or more of cholestyramine had a mean 19 per cent reduction in total cholesterol and a mean 28 per cent reduction in LDL cholesterol averaged over 7 years. Many cholestyramine recipients, especially those who took 20 gm or more daily, sustained total and LDL cholesterol levels at least 25

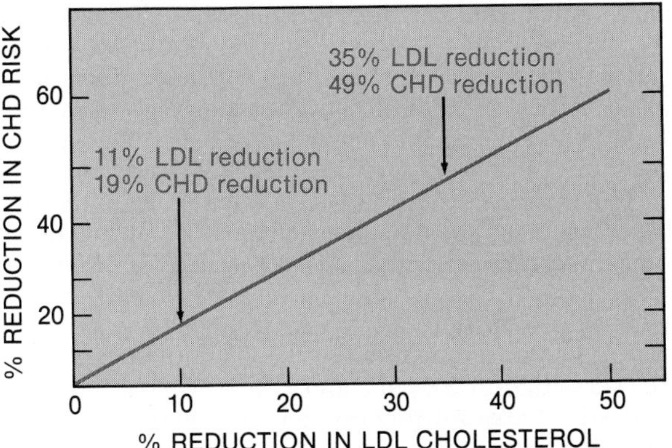

FIGURE 37-6. Relation of reduction in low-density lipoprotein (LDL) cholesterol to reduction in coronary heart disease (CHD) risk (Cox proportional hazards model) in the Lipid Research Clinics Coronary Primary Prevention Trial. When the cholestyramine-treated group was analyzed separately, a 19 per cent reduction in CHD was associated with each 11 per cent decrement in LDL cholesterol or 8 per cent decrement in total cholesterol.[44]

per cent and 35 per cent, respectively, below baseline. The proportional hazards model applied to the cholestyramine group predicted a 49 per cent reduction in CAD risk for a 35 per cent reduction in LDL cholesterol. As a rough rule of thumb, this study demonstrated that a 1 per cent reduction of total cholesterol results in a 2 per cent decrease in CAD risk.

Secondary cardiovascular endpoints were also lower in frequency in the cholestyramine-treatment group and on the order of the 19 per cent reduction of CAD risk. For example, there were reductions of 20, 25, and 21 per cent in the development of angina, new positive exercise test, and incidence of coronary bypass surgery, respectively, compared with those in the placebo group.

Total mortality was equivalent between the two groups, despite the decline in cardiovascular deaths. Apparently the treated group had a higher level of mortality from noncardiovascular causes, primarily motor vehicle accidents and other forms of violent death. These results have been extensively analyzed by the investigators, who perceive a statistical quirk unrelated to any pathological effect of cholestyramine or cholesterol lowering.

THE HELSINKI HEART STUDY. This primary prevention trial used gemfibrozil in the treatment of middle-aged men with dyslipidemia.[54] Like the LRC-CPPT, the Helsinki study was a randomized, double-blind trial of asymptomatic middle-aged men who ranged in age from 40 to 55 years and who had non-HDL cholesterol levels of 200 mg/dl or higher at entry. The total treatment group was 4081 men who were randomized to receive gemfibrozil 600 mg/twice daily or a placebo. Patients were followed for both cardiac death and MI for 5 years. By the end of the trial period, the treated group had experienced 34 per cent fewer coronary events. As in the LRC-CPPT, there was no decrease in overall mortality because of an increase in violent and other noncardiovascular deaths in the treatment group. There was no significant increase in serious drug-related side effects such as cholelithiasis, although GI side effects and the number of abdominal surgical procedures were increased in the gemfibrozil group.

Gemfibrozil has a powerful effect on hypertriglyceridemia, and when the effects on cardiovascular mortality in the Helsinki study were analyzed further, it became apparent that the largest benefit from the drug was seen in the patients with Fredrickson IIb HLP, a lipid disorder characterized by elevated cholesterol and triglycerides. The role of hypertriglyceridemia as a primary CAD risk factor remains controversial. However, there is an inverse relation between elevated triglycerides and low levels of HDL that may be reversed with gemfibrozil therapy. Although not definitely proved by the Helsinki Heart Study, it is attractive to speculate that the larger-than-expected improvement in mortality from a cholesterol lowering of 8 per cent was due to the combined effects on raising HDL and reducing LDL associated with gemfibrozil. On the basis of these findings, the Food and Drug Administration expanded its indication for gemfibrozil to subjects with elevated levels of LDL and triglycerides and low levels of HDL who have failed dietary therapy, resins, or nicotinic acid.

HYPERTRIGLYCERIDEMIA

Several genetic, epidemiological, and clinical studies have linked elevated triglycerides to an increased CAD risk. For example, in the remnant lipoprotein disorder (type II), dysbetalipoproteinemia (which in part is characterized by elevated triglyceride levels), premature atherosclerosis, including CAD and peripheral arterial disease, frequently occurs. Also, a number of studies have shown that depressed lipoprotein lipase activity and the subsequent extended postprandial lipemia lead to a decreased clearance of triglyceride-rich lipoprotein remnants, an increased triglyceride exchange between LDL and HDL, a greater concentration of atherogenic small, dense LDL lipoproteins, and presumably an increased risk for CAD.[55]

At least two epidemiological or clinical studies lend credence to the positive correlation between elevated triglycerides and CAD risk. Recent analysis of the Framingham data indicates that triglyceride elevation constitutes a CAD risk, which for women is independent of other CAD risk factors. The triglyceride value was an independent risk factor in a Swedish study.[56]

As mentioned above, the Helsinki Heart Study patients in whom the greatest drop in CAD mortality was seen were those with type IIb HLP, a condition manifested by elevated LDL and triglyceride levels and depressed HDL levels. Gemfibrozil treatment in this study lowered the patients' LDL and triglyceride concentrations, while raising their HDL concentrations. The precise effect of the triglycerides modification cannot be determined at this point, and an independent effect of triglycerides could not be statistically validated.

In the *Cholesterol-Lowering Atherosclerosis Study* (CLAS) conducted by Blankenhorn et al. (see below), the proportion of apo C-III in HDL was correlated with decreased progression of disease. This suggests that a rapid rate of metabolism of the triglyceride-rich lipoproteins is anti-atherogenic. In addition, multivariate analysis of the placebo group in this study indicated that the concentration of triglyceride-rich lipoproteins was a significant predictor of atherosclerotic progression.[57] Despite this evidence, it is not clear whether elevated triglycerides are an independent and causal factor in the development of atherosclerosis. Multivariate analyses in many studies have failed to show the independent relation of hypertriglyceridemia and atherosclerosis.

The link between elevated triglycerides and CAD risk may be secondary to other disorders.[58] Various disease entities that are associated with hypertriglyceridemia, such as diabetes mellitus and chronic renal failure, have a definite association with atherosclerosis risk. Certain genetic disorders, such as FCH, which presents with several Fredrickson phenotypes within the same family, confer increased risk for atherosclerosis. In this situation, the triglycerides may represent the presence of other lipoprotein abnormalities that are associated with CAD, such as decreased levels of apo A-I and elevated levels of apo B-100 or remnant particles. However, the causal role of elevated triglycerides on CAD development cannot be ruled out for at least two reasons. First, it is not clear that multivariate analysis is a proper statistical tool to determine causal relations between lipoproteins, since the lipoproteins are highly interrelated metabolically and have rapid kinetic turnover rates. Second, cross-sectional studies have shown an inverse relation between hypertriglyceridemia and HDL, which is presumably due to the interrelated formation of HDL cholesterol with the efficient breakdown of the triglyceride core of VLDL particles.[59] Our ability to delineate further subfractions of the various lipoproteins may better determine the role of triglycerides in atherosclerosis. For example, it has been demonstrated that subforms of VLDL, particularly when associated with high levels of apo E, are readily taken up by residual macrophages with subsequent conversion into the foam cells that are precursors for advanced atherosclerosis.[60]

Current treatment guidelines for hypertriglyceridemia are based on the recommendations of a National Institutes of Health–sponsored consensus conference convened in 1983.[61] This conference classified triglyceride levels under 250 mg/dl as normal, levels between 250 and 500 mg/dl as borderline risk for CAD, and levels above 500 mg/dl as high risk. The guidelines of the European Atherosclerosis Society are quite different, and include triglyceride levels above 200 mg/dl in the treatment algorithm. Patients with borderline hypertriglyceridemia should be examined for possible secondary causes, such as obesity, diabetes, excess alcohol consumption, or the administration of certain drugs, such as noncardioselective beta blockers. Patients with elevated triglyceride levels are also at high risk for pancreatitis, and thus should be placed on a low-fat diet and treated with a fibric acid derivative, such as gemfibrozil, if diet therapy is ineffective.

CAN THE PROGRESS OF ATHEROSCLEROSIS BE HALTED?

Data from the *Bogalusa Heart Study* show a stepwise correlation between LDL concentrations and the extent of fatty streaks in the aorta (Fig. 37–7). It is believed, on the basis of the Bogalusa data, that the presence of fatty streaks in young people is the precursor of advanced atherosclerotic lesions. In the Bogalusa study, the aortic fatty streaks strongly correlated with antemortem levels of LDL and total serum cholesterol and were inversely related to the HDL-LDL ratio.[62]

Cabin and Roberts studied the relation between the autopsy extent of coronary artery narrowing by atherosclerotic plaques and fasting levels determined during life.[63] They quantitatively analyzed multiple 5-mm segments of 160 epicardial coronary arteries in 40 patients. Total cholesterol correlated positively with the number of severely narrowed coronary arteries per subject but not with the degree of severe narrowing. However, there was a significant relationship between triglyceride level and the (percentage) degree of severe narrowing.

Several studies have correlated aggressive control of dyslipidemia with angiographic regression of established CAD. As already mentioned, in the NHLBI's type II HLP trial, cholestyramine treatment lowered LDL levels. Also, cholestyramine improved the HDL–total cholesterol ratio. These changes, in turn, were associated with a decrease in the rate of progression of atherosclerosis.[64] Thirty-two per cent of the patients in the treatment group experienced atherosclerotic progression, compared with 49 per cent of the patients in the placebo group.

Blankenhorn and colleagues in CLAS studied the effects of combination hypolipidemic therapy on coronary atherosclerosis in patients who had angiographically documented CAD and who had undergone coronary artery bypass. Patients were enrolled in the study if they demonstrated that they

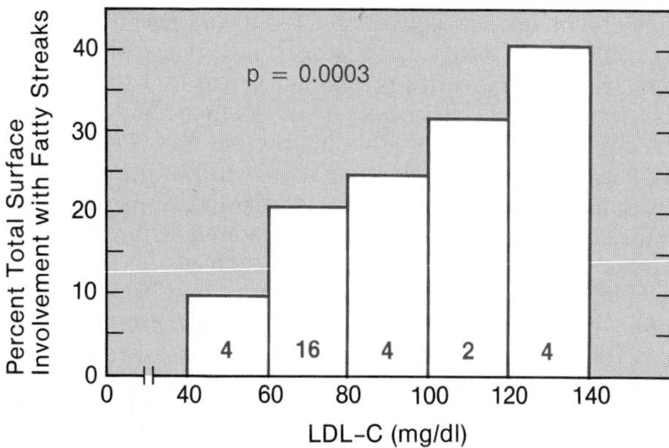

FIGURE 37–7. Atherosclerotic fatty streak involvement of the aorta related to levels of low-density lipoprotein cholesterol (LDL-C) in 30 young persons. Increasing LDL-C levels are significantly related to increasing amounts of aortic fatty streaks. (To convert values for cholesterol to millimoles per liter, multiply by 0.026.) (Reprinted by permission from Newman, W. P., Freedman, D. S., and Voors, A. W.: Relation of serum lipoprotein levels and systolic blood pressure to early atherosclerosis. The Bogalusa Heart Study. N. Engl. J. Med. *314*:138, 1986.)

could tolerate full-dose niacin and colestipol therapy. Angiography was performed at the beginning of and post-study. A global coronary score was assigned to the angiograms after qualitative interpretation of both the native vessels and bypass grafts by a panel of experts. The scores ranged from −3, representing maximum regression, to +3, representing maximum progression. After 2 years,[65] patients in the pharmacologically treated group had experienced a 26 per cent decrease in total cholesterol, a 43 per cent decrease in LDL, and a 37 per cent increase in HDL concentrations, when compared with the placebo group. Moreover, a total of 16.2 per cent of patients in the treated group had evidence of anatomical regression, compared with only 3.6 per cent in the placebo group. In addition, no atherosclerotic progression was noted in 45 per cent of the treated group, compared with 36.6 per cent of the placebo group. A subgroup of patients continued on the study, and the results at 4 years[66] confirmed the 2-year findings.

Although only a minority of the general population with dyslipidemia is able to tolerate maximum colestipol plus niacin therapy, this study unequivocally demonstrated that modifying patient lipid profiles can delay progression of angiographically established atherosclerosis. Another interesting finding of the study was that among patients on placebo, those who did not develop new lesions had an average fat intake of 27 per cent of total calories, versus 34 per cent in those who formed new lesions.

The *Familial Atherosclerosis Treatment Study* (FATS) evaluated changes in angiographically demonstrable coronary disease on aggressive lipid lowering.[67] The men in this study had apo B-100 levels over 125 mg/dl and a family history of premature atherosclerosis. Participants were required to have at least 50 per cent stenosis in one vessel or 30 per cent or greater in three. Unlike the CLAS patients, the FATS patients had not had bypass grafts. Also, quantitative coronary angiography was used, viewing nine defined proximal segments of the major coronary arteries. Patients were divided into three comparably sized groups, two on treatment and one receiving placebo. All received dietary counseling. Treatment was daily, either colestipol 30 gm plus niacin 4 gm or colestipol 30 gm plus lovastatin 40 mg. Patients assigned to the placebo group whose baseline LDL cholesterol level exceeded the 90th percentile for age were given colestipol instead of placebo. A subgroup of patients in the niacin group received 6 gm of niacin a day when the LDL reduction was deemed inadequate. The patients were followed for 2.5 years and then underwent repeat angiography.

The colestipol-niacin group achieved a 32 per cent reduction in LDL and a 43 per cent increase in HDL. The colestipol-lovastatin group achieved a 46 per cent reduction in LDL and a 15 per cent increase in HDL. The control group achieved only a 7 per cent reduction in LDL and a 5 per cent increase in HDL. Moreover, in the colestipol-niacin group, only 25 per cent had definite lesion progression without regression, whereas 39 per cent had regression as the only change, comparable to figures of 21 per cent and 32 per cent in the colestipol-lovastatin group but quite different from values of 46 per cent for progression and 11 per cent for regression in the conventional-therapy group. Examples of regression in treated patients are shown in Figure 37–8. The negative anatomical changes correlated with a worsened clinical outcome. Three patients in the colestipol-lovastatin group experienced cardiovascular events, compared with two in the colestipol-niacin group and 10 in the control group. This well-designed study further supported the lipid hypothesis, and demonstrated that anatomical regression and decrease in clinical events can be achieved with lipid-lowering therapy. The role that HDL elevation played in these results is unclear. It has been suggested, however, that pharmacological elevations of HDL may also play a role in anatomical regression.

Quantitative angiography also showed atherosclerotic lesion regression with treatment (diet with niacin, colestipol, and/or lovastatin) versus lesion progression in a control group (diet, in some cases with low-dose colestipol) in the University

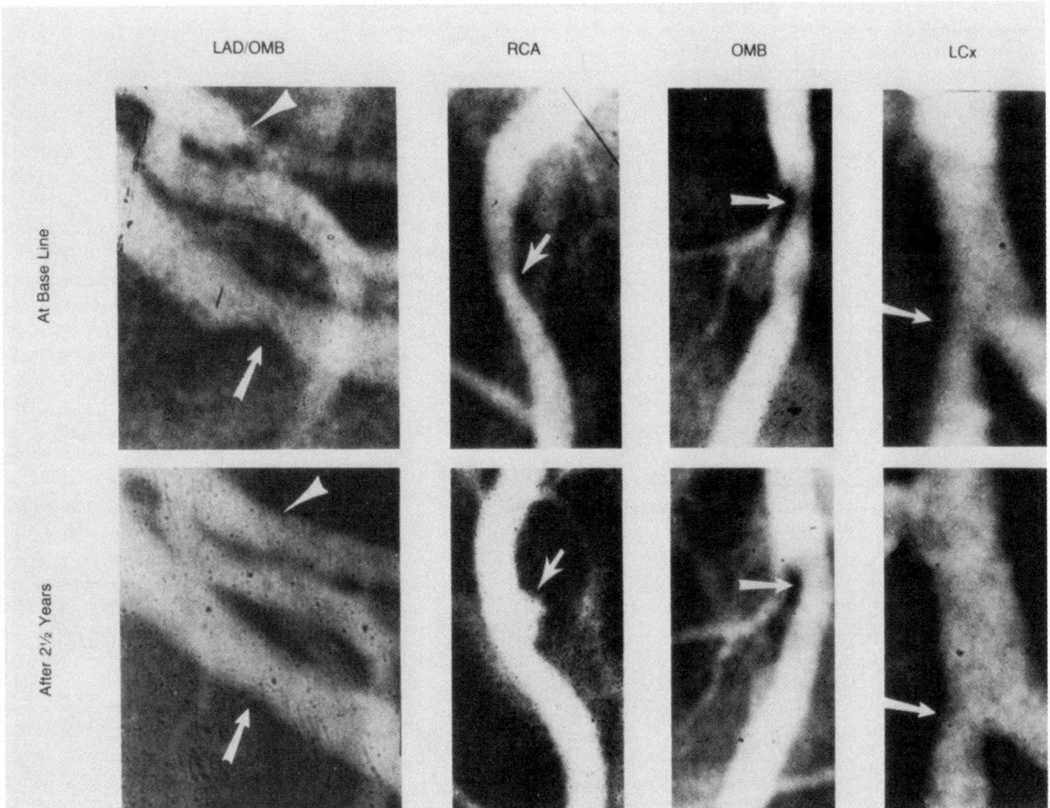

FIGURE 37–8. Examples of atherosclerotic lesion regression in patients treated intensively in the Familial Atherosclerosis Treatment Study. The top row shows images obtained at baseline; the bottom row, images obtained 2½ years later. LAD, left anterior descending artery; OMB, obtuse marginal branch; RCA, right coronary artery; LCx, left circumflex artery. Stenosis caused by the lesions in these vessels decreased as follows: LAD, from 100 to 28 per cent; OMB, from 39 to 18 per cent; RCA, from 48 to 30 per cent (note the plaque ulcer present at 2½ years); OMB, from 69 to 37 per cent; and LCx, from 44 to 30 per cent. (Reprinted by permission from Brown, G., Albers, J. J., Fisher, L. D., et al.: Regression of coronary artery disease as a result of intensive lipid-lowering therapy in men with high levels of apolipoprotein B. N. Engl. J. Med. *323*:1289, 1990.)

of California, San Francisco Arteriosclerosis Specialized Center of Research (SCOR) Intervention Trial.[68] All 72 patients in this randomized trial had heterozygous familial hypercholesterolemia, and the authors concluded that reduction of LDL cholesterol can induce lesion regression in CAD.

Gordon and associates in a meta-analysis of four major trials found that a 1 mg/dl increment in HDL cholesterol was associated with significant reductions in CAD risk: 2 per cent in men and 3 per cent in women.[69] They found HDL levels to be essentially unrelated to noncardiovascular disease mortality.

DIAGNOSIS OF HYPERLIPIDEMIA

Because of the frequent lack of overt physical findings or symptomatology in patients with dyslipidemia, the first step when HLP is suspected is to determine accurate plasma lipoprotein levels. However, the basic screening test currently recommended for all adults is that for serum cholesterol.

The traditional definition of HLP was levels of plasma cholesterol and triglycerides exceeding the 95th percentile for adjusted age and gender. This approach used a statistical variation from the median and included patients who were 2 standard deviations above and below the mean cholesterol for that group. In the United States and other countries where CAD incidence is high, these statistically derived guidelines were inadequate.

The National Cholesterol Education Program (NCEP) reported its findings after evaluating clinical risks from hypercholesterolemia and issued new screening recommendations based on three categories of cholesterol levels (Fig. 37–9).[70–72] According to the NCEP guidelines, less than 200 mg/dl cholesterol is desirable. Patients with these low cholesterol levels should merely be given education concerning the risks involved in the development of CAD, general dietary information, and instructions to repeat cholesterol testing within 5 years.

Borderline cholesterol levels in these guidelines are between 200 and 239 mg/dl in the absence of established CAD or other CAD risk factors (hypertension, smoking, diabetes mellitus, body weight over 30 per cent of ideal, HDL under 35 mg/dl, family history of CAD, and male gender). Patients with a cholesterol value in this range who do not have established CAD or two other risk factors should be given dietary information and instructions to repeat cholesterol testing within 1 year. Patients with these borderline cholesterol levels who have CAD or other CAD risk factors are considered at high risk, as are patients with total cholesterol 240 mg/dl or higher. High-risk patients should undergo a complete lipoprotein analysis with further therapeutic intervention based on the calculated LDL level.

From the fasting sample, total cholesterol, HDL, and triglycerides can be measured directly. LDL and its cholesterol content can be calculated mathematically. HDL is determined by measuring the cholesterol that is in solution after precipitating the apo B–containing lipoproteins. LDL can then be calculated by the following formula: LDL = total cholesterol − HDL − (triglycerides/5). The formula is not valid for triglyceride levels over 400 mg/dl or in type III HLP.

TYPING OF HYPERLIPOPROTEINEMIA

The Fredrickson and Lees classification of hyperlipoproteinemia (Table 37–4) remains a practical approach for the clinician.[73] This system is based on laboratory definitions as opposed to genetics and does not take into account underlying pathophysiology or HDL measurements.

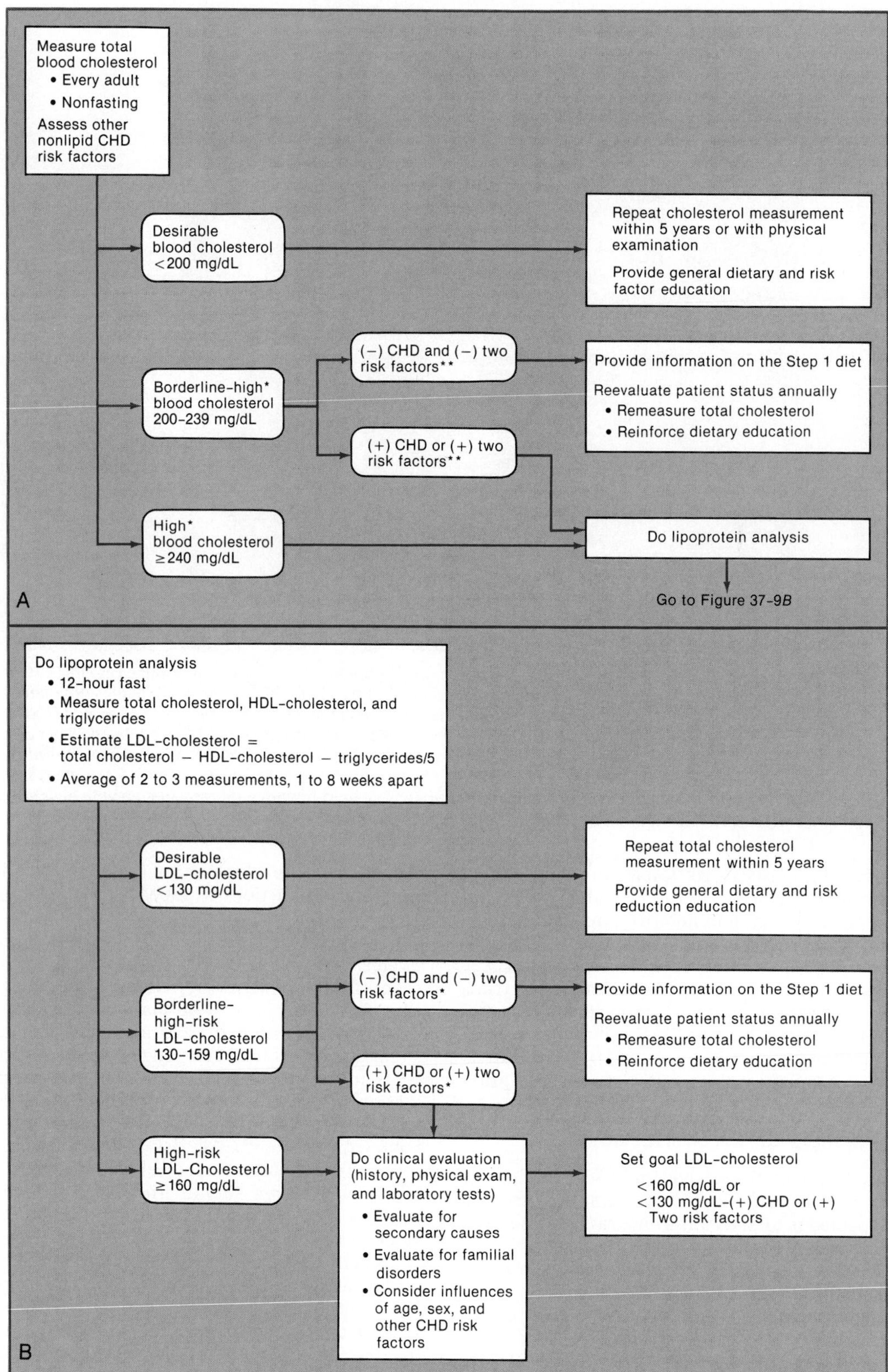

FIGURE 37–9. ***A***, **Initial classification based on total cholesterol. CHD indicates coronary heart disease; asterisk, must be confirmed by obtaining repeat measurements and then using the average value; double asterisks, one of which can be male sex. (From The Expert Panel: Report of the National Cholesterol Education Program Expert Panel on Detection, Evaluation and Treatment of High Blood Cholesterol in Adults. Arch. Intern. Med. *148*:36, 1988.)** ***B***, **Classification based on low-density lipoprotein (LDL)-cholesterol. Asterisk, one of which can be male sex. CHD, coronary heart disease; HDL, high-density lipoprotein. (From The Expert Panel: Report of the National Cholesterol Education Program Expert Panel on Detection, Evaluation and Treatment of High Blood Cholesterol in Adults. Arch. Intern. Med. *148*:36, 1988.)**

TABLE 37-4 HYPERLIPOPROTEINEMIA PHENOTYPE DEFINITIONS AND THEIR ASSOCIATION WITH GENETIC AND OTHER DISORDERS

FREDRICKSON AND LEES PHENOTYPE	LABORATORY DEFINITION	ASSOCIATED WITH GENETIC DISORDERS	CONDITIONS ASSOCIATED WITH SECONDARY HYPERLIPOPROTEINEMIA
Type I	Hyperchylomicronemia and absolute deficiency of LPL Cholesterol normal Triglycerides greatly increased	Familial LPL deficiency Apo C-II deficiency	Dysglobulinemia, pancreatitis, poorly controlled diabetes mellitus
Type IIa	LDL increased Cholesterol increased Triglycerides normal VLDL normal	Familial hypercholesterolemia LDL receptor abnormal Familial combined hyperlipidemia Polygenic hypercholesterolemia	Hypothyroidism, acute intermittent porphyria, nephrosis, idiopathic hypercalcemia, dysglobulinemia, anorexia nervosa
Type IIb	LDL increased VLDL increased Cholesterol increased Triglycerides increased	Familial hypercholesterolemia Familial combined hyperlipidemia	
Type III	Floating beta lipoproteins VLDL cholesterol/VLDL triglyceride >0.35 Apo E_2 homozygote on isoelectric focusing Cholesterol increased Triglycerides increased	Familial dysbetalipoproteinemia	Diabetes mellitus, hypothyroidism, dysglobulinemia (monoclonal gammopathy)
Type IV	VLDL increased Cholesterol normal or increased Triglycerides increased	Familial hypertriglyceridemia Familial combined hyperlipidemia	Glycogen storage disease, hypothyroidism, disseminated lupus erythematosus, diabetes mellitus, nephrotic syndrome, renal failure, ethanol abuse
Type V	Chylomicrons and VLDL increased LDL present but reduced Cholesterol increased Triglycerides greatly increased	Familial hypertriglyceridemia Familial multiple lipoprotein type hyperlipidemia	Poorly controlled diabetes mellitus, glycogen storage disease, hypothyroidism, nephrotic syndrome, dysglobulinemia, pregnancy, estrogen administration (either contraceptive or therapeutic) in women with familial hypertriglyceridemia

From Gotto, A. M.: Practical approach to phenotyping hyperlipoproteinemia. *In* Kligfield, P. D. (ed.): Cardiology Reference Book. New York, Co-Medica, Inc., 1984.

LDL = low-density lipoprotein; LPL = lipoprotein lipase; VLDL = very low density lipoprotein.

TYPE I HLP: FAMILIAL GENETIC DYSLIPIDEMIAS. The diagnosis of familial chylomicronemia, or type I HLP, requires the presence of chylomicrons in the fasting plasma above a clear supernatant. Type I HLP may be a primary genetic disorder, manifested chemically by the absence of apo C-II or lipoprotein lipase, or a condition secondary to poorly controlled diabetes mellitus, pancreatitis, or dysglobulinemia. The hyperchylomicronemic state of type I HLP is characterized by the appearance of extraordinarily large lipoprotein complexes. These macromolecular particles appear in normal people after consumption of a fatty meal. They usually are rapidly cleared from the plasma by means of activation of lipoprotein lipase by the apo C-II present on the surface of the chylomicrons. The diagnosis of type I HLP can be established by chemical determinations of the activity of lipoprotein lipase after heparin administration. The presence of an inhibitor to lipoprotein lipase can be determined by bioassay: there is a lack of activity when the patient's serum is added to a source that normally has enzyme activity. The primary genetic form of type I HLP—familial lipoprotein lipase deficiency—is not associated with complications of premature atherosclerosis, despite high levels of cholesterol and triglycerides. This disorder is clinically manifested in childhood by recurrent abdominal pain secondary to pancreatitis. The gene that governs the production of lipoprotein lipase has been mapped to chromosome 8.[74] The absence of lipoprotein lipase noted in some forms of HLP may be secondary to mutations of this gene and to the subsequent accumulation of triglycerides localized to chylomicron particles because of impaired degradation. A clinically similar condition can occur when there is a deficiency of the apo C-II activator for lipoprotein lipase. This deficiency is less common than that of lipoprotein lipase enzyme. RFLP studies to determine genetic variation indicate that the genetic defect of apo C-II deficiency is heterogeneous.[75] The diagnosis of apo C-II deficiency depends on the determination of absent or defective apo C-II by electrophoretic techniques or assays.[76]

Dietary treatment is similar in both of these conditions. The infusion of fresh plasma with normal amounts of apo C-II may activate lipoprotein lipase if a deficiency state exists.

TYPE II HLP. Type II HLP is defined as an elevation of total plasma cholesterol, predominantly in the LDL fraction. It may represent a primary genetic disorder or be secondary to underlying disease such as hypothyroidism, nephrotic syndrome, or dysglobulinemia. In type IIa HLP, triglycerides and VLDL are normal. In type IIb, both these fractions are elevated.

GENETIC FORMS OF HYPERCHOLESTEROLEMIA

POLYGENIC HYPERCHOLESTEROLEMIA. The most common cause of an isolated elevation of total cholesterol and LDL cholesterol is polygenic hypercholesterolemia, which may be the underlying disorder in as many as 80 per cent of the people found to be hypercholesterolemic by routine screening. However, the exact incidence of polygenic hypercholesterolemia in patients with the type II phenotype has not been definitely determined. Polygenic hypercholesterolemia is not well understood from a genetic standpoint, and no single gene disorder has been implicated. Presumably, exogenous factors interact with a poorly understood genetic predisposition to result in increased LDL production or decreased LDL catabolism. Dietary treatment significantly reduces cholesterol levels in these patients.

FAMILIAL HYPERCHOLESTEROLEMIA. Familial hypercholesterolemia (FH) has a strong association with premature atherosclerosis. In the rare homozygous form of FH (which occurs in roughly 1 in 1 million Americans), clinical evidence of atherosclerosis—including acute MI, severe coronary atherosclerosis, and aortic stenosis—may occur in the first decade of life. The primary genetic defect in FH is an autosomal dominant disorder caused by a mutation in the LDL-receptor gene. The gene frequency in the United States is 1 per 500 people. Higher frequencies have been noted in Lebanon and among Afrikaners; this heterozygosity perhaps occurs in 1 per cent of these populations. In FH, LDL production is increased, whereas the cells' ability to recognize the apo B surface component of LDL is decreased. Also, the production of LDL may be increased because of a decrease in IDL removal by the liver and enhanced conversion to LDL.

The LDL receptor is located in coated pits on the surface of hepatic and extrahepatic tissues as a glycoprotein of 839 amino acids. The LDL receptor protrudes from the coated pit, and has a highly complex structure consisting of a ligand-binding domain of 292 amino acids that recognizes apos B and E. A subsequent domain is composed of about 400 amino acids with a homology to the precursors of the epidermal growth factor. This latter domain is followed by a series of O-linked sugars in a membrane-spanning domain of 222 amino acids. The carboxy-terminal portion of the LDL receptor is located within the cytoplasm and is composed of 50 amino acids.[77] Patients with homozygous FH typically have no functioning LDL receptors, although some homozygotes, called receptor defective, exhibit up to 10 per cent of normal receptor activity. Patients with the heterozygous state have about half of the normal-functioning LDL receptors. Goldstein and Brown have described four classes of LDL-receptor mutations that affect respectively the receptor's formation, transport, LDL binding, and clustering in the coated pit.[78]

In a class I mutation, a null allele results in a total failure to produce the LDL receptor. In a class II mutation, the LDL-receptor protein is formed, but with a transport defect that alters its migration between the endoplasmic reticulum and the Golgi complex. The class III mutation is associated with normal synthesis and transport of the LDL-receptor protein, but with LDL receptors that cannot recognize apoproteins on the LDL particle. With a class IV mutation, the LDL receptor fails to internalize and cluster properly in the coated pits. Many mutations of the LDL gene have been identified, each resulting in the phenotypic clinical manifestations of FH.

There is a mechanism for the clearance of LDL that is independent of the presence of the LDL receptor (Fig. 37–2, p. 1127). In receptor-absent homozygous patients, LDL clearance occurs by means of a non-receptor–mediated mechanism. This form of clearance is referred to as the "scavenger pathway" and presumably occurs in macrophages of the reticuloendothelial system or by other poorly defined non-receptor–mediated pathways. Patients with a normal complement of LDL receptors clear about one-third of their LDL by the scavenger pathway.

Monocytes and macrophages are able to express receptors for LDL that have been altered by oxidation or chemically. Contact with the endothelial cell can induce LDL oxidation. This uptake was attributed to the presence of a specific receptor—called the acetyl LDL receptor, or scavenger receptor—which is distinct from the LDL receptor. In fact, this specific receptor does not recognize native LDL.[79]

Most patients with a type IIa phenotype do not have FH. The clinical hallmarks of the FH patient are a positive family history and tendinous xanthomas. Quantification of the number and function of the LDL receptors can only be done by specialized medical centers.[80,81]

FAMILIAL COMBINED HYPERLIPIDEMIA. FCH is relatively common in the United States, occurring in about 1 in 300 people. It is an autosomal dominant disease. The presentation may vary within families, with several Fredrickson phenotypes seen (IIa, IIb, IV). FCH is associated with an increased risk for premature atherosclerosis. Although the disease may clinically mimic FH, patients with FCH lack tendinous xanthomas. FCH may be heterogeneous. The underlying mechanism is thought to be an overproduction of apo B-100 by the liver. Small, dense LDL particles with an increased content of apo B-100 are seen. It is possible the FCH could represent the heterozygous state of LPL deficiency.

TYPE III HLP: FAMILIAL DYSBETALIPOPROTEINEMIA. Type III HLP, or broad-beta-lipoproteinemia or dysbetalipoproteinemia, occurs in about 1 in 10,000 people. The expression of this genetic condition seldom occurs before adulthood, and the $E_{2/2}$ phenotype is seen in more than 90 per cent of patients. Atherosclerosis is clinically manifested as peripheral vascular disease or CAD.[3]

The lipid profile in patients with type III HLP is roughly equal elevations of both cholesterol and triglycerides, which are derived from incomplete catabolism of chylomicrons and VLDL particles. Lipoprotein electrophoresis reveals an increase in VLDL and a second band that encompasses both VLDL and LDL fractions. This broad band contains remnant intermediates termed beta-VLDLs. In normal subjects, the ratio of VLDL cholesterol to total triglycerides usually is less than 0.2, whereas in type III HLP, the ratio exceeds 0.37.

Delineation of apo E subtypes is a useful diagnostic tool for type III HLP, but it is not widely available. In patients with type III HLP, the presence of apo E_2 leads to defective binding of apo E–containing lipoproteins and the accumulation of remnant particles. Other factors must play a role, because approximately 1 per cent of the U.S. population carries the apo $E_{2/2}$ phenotype but without demonstrable lipoprotein abnormality or associated vascular disease. It has been suggested that some unknown environmental influence interacts with the underlying apo $E_{2/2}$ phenotype to alter the lipid profile. Type III HLP is associated in rare cases with another disease such as hypothyroidism. Although physical examination may be normal, a characteristic palmar lesion—xanthoma striatum palmare, which consists of yellow streaks in the palmar creases—frequently is present (Fig. 37–10). Tuberoeruptive xanthomas may be present on the tibial tuberosities and the

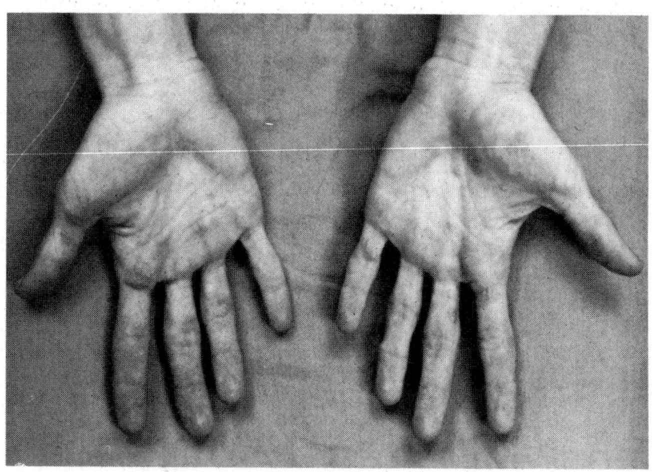

FIGURE 37–10. Palmar xanthomas.

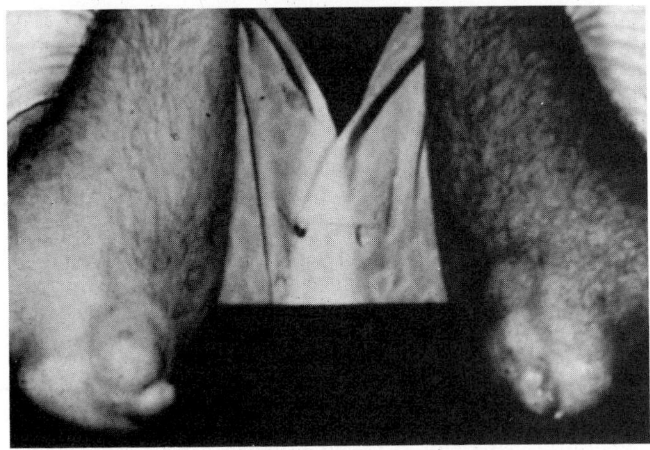

FIGURE 37–11. Tuberoeruptive xanthomas on the elbow.

elbows (Fig. 37–11). Tendinous xanthomas, which are common in type II, are rare in type III.[82]

GENETIC FORMS OF HYPERTRIGLYCERIDEMIA

Familial Combined Hyperlipoproteinemia

FAMILIAL DYSBETALIPOPROTEINEMIA. Hypertriglyceridemia's genetic forms have been described above.

TYPE IV HLP: FAMILIAL ENDOGENOUS HYPERTRIGLYCERIDEMIA. Type IV HLP is caused by an accumulation of VLDL in fasting plasma, which results in a cloudy or turbid appearance. Type IV HLP may be genetic in origin or secondary to another, underlying disease. Two main patterns with a genetic basis have been recognized. *Primary (familial) endogenous hypertriglyceridemia* is a relatively common autosomal dominant disorder. The incidence of its heterozygous form is 1 per cent in the general population. VLDL production is increased in this condition, whereas HDL levels are decreased.[83] The metabolic defect appears to be an oversynthesis of hepatic triglyceride and VLDL in which large triglyceride-rich particles are produced. Triglyceride levels usually are in the 200 to 500 mg/dl range.

FCH also may present as a type IV pattern. The physician should not be deterred by the overlap, since FCH patients also are predisposed to CAD. It should be noted, however, that the risk for patients with familial hypertriglyceridemia is less clearly delineated.[84] Premature CAD is common in some kindreds but not in others.

TYPE V HLP. Type V HLP is an uncommon dyslipidemia characterized by the presence of chylomicrons and VLDL in the fasting plasma. The phenotype occurs in about 2 of every 1000 men and is less frequent in women. Type V HLP usually is recognized in adults. Examination of fasting plasma reveals a creamy supernatant composed of chylomicrons overlying a turbid layer of VLDL-rich serum. The underlying causes are complex, and include genetic and secondary factors. Type V HLP does not have a clear pattern of inheritance, although elevations of chylomicrons usually are associated with a decreased activity of lipoprotein lipase. Type V HLP also can be associated with apo C-II deficiency. Other secondary causes include obesity (especially when associated with rapid weight gain), excessive alcohol intake, and administration of exogenous estrogens.[85,86]

A type V pattern may be seen in patients with genetic forms of hypertriglyceridemia. Effective treatment will decrease the chylomicron levels and cause the phenotype to revert to type IV or IIb. Type V HLP is difficult to differentiate from the frequently associated diabetes mellitus. The frequent presence of other risk factors for premature atherosclerosis, such as diabetes, hypertension, and obesity, clouds the primary contribution of type V HLP to CAD.[87,88]

Causes of secondary hypertriglyceridemia or of a type IV pattern are common and should be actively sought in any given patient. Diabetes mellitus frequently is associated with elevated triglycerides. There are several possible mechanisms for this association. For example, obese diabetics who are insensitive to the action of insulin require elevated levels of insulin to maintain a given level of plasma glucose. The increased insulin levels may, in turn, increase VLDL synthesis. In diabetics with insulin deficiency, the mechanism is more complex and relates to the prevention of triglyceride catabolism with lipoprotein lipase. The antilipolytic action of insulin prevents triglyceride breakdown and secondary free fatty acid release from adipocytes. The flux of unesterified fatty acids to the liver is thought to be a major factor driving VLDL synthesis. Insulin also is required to maintain adequate activity of lipoprotein lipase. As a result of absolute or relative insulin deficiency, remnant lipoproteins accumulate in the blood. Exogenous insulin restores lipoprotein lipase and prevents marked elevations of VLDL and chylomicrons.

Reduced lipoprotein lipase activity also occurs in myxedema and renal failure and may partially account for the commonly seen elevated triglyceride levels. If the nephrotic syndrome accompanies renal insufficiency, the associated hypoalbuminemia is thought to stimulate the VLDL production. Other causes of a type IV pattern are excessive alcohol intake and hepatocellular disease (glycogen or lipid storage abnormalities).

TREATMENT OF HYPERLIPOPROTEINEMIA

Before the initiation of therapy, a careful medical examination should be performed to determine if the hyperlipidemia is secondary to an underlying disease or has a genetic basis. Underlying conditions, such as diabetes, renal insufficiency, myxedema, biliary obstruction, nephrotic syndrome, and dysproteinemia, should be identified and treated. A careful dietary history also should be obtained to estimate caloric intake and the amounts of cholesterol, total fat, and saturated fat in the diet.

CONCURRENT MEDICATIONS. The concurrent use of medications should be documented and the need for continuation determined. Commonly used medications that alter lipid profiles include the diuretics and beta blockers. Estrogens tend to raise HDL, VLDL, and triglyceride levels while reducing LDL. Their effect on cardiac risk, especially in postmenopausal women, is the subject of current debate. Progesterone analogs decrease elevated levels of triglycerides but also decrease HDL.

The effect of antihypertensive agents on the blood lipids is complex. Noncardioselective beta blockers tend to increase VLDL levels, presumably because they also inhibit the adrenergic stimulation of lipoprotein lipase. It has been demonstrated that beta I and beta II agonists increase the lipase enzyme activity, whereas alpha agonists inhibit it. Despite their potential adverse effects on lipids, both cardioselective beta blockers (metoprolol) and nonselective beta blockers (propranolol, timolol) have been shown to reduce rates of MI and cardiac mortality.

Alpha-adrenergic blockers, such as prazosin, do not adversely affect lipids and may actually raise HDL. Whether this effect will translate into cardioprotection has not been determined. The calcium blockers, angiotensin-converting enzyme inhibitors, and centrally acting $alpha_2$ agonists tend to have a neutral effect on lipids. The role of the angiotensin-converting enzyme inhibitors is under investigation. There is increasing evidence that essential hypertension is associated with an insulin-resistant state. Captopril has been demonstrated to enhance, because of an increase in insulin sensitivity with its use, the insulin-mediated disposal of glucose when compared with hydrochlorothiazide.[89] The long-term clinical effects of this action have yet to be determined, but it may explain in part the lack of improvement in coronary mortality in hypertensive patients treated with thiazide derivatives.

LDL cholesterol below a level of 130 mg/dl is considered desirable (Fig. 37–9). LDL levels between 130 and 159 mg/dl are classified as borderline high risk if CAD or other CAD risk factors are absent. High-risk LDL elevations are values of 160 mg/dl or more, or between 130 and 159 mg/dl with existing CAD or two additional risk factors. The NCEP recommends dietary therapy for an LDL value of 160 mg/dl or higher if the patient is free of clinically evident coronary disease and does not have two of the established risk factors. The minimal goal is to lower the LDL cholesterol to under 160 mg/dl. If coronary disease is present or the patient has two or more of the established risk factors, the minimal goal for dietary therapy would be an LDL level below 130 mg/dl.

INDICATIONS FOR DRUG THERAPY. Drug therapy is recommended if a patient free of coronary disease and other risk factors has an LDL cholesterol value over 190 mg/dl after 3 to 6 months of dietary treatment. If the patient has coronary disease or the presence of two or more other risk factors, 160 mg/dl would be the threshold for the initiation of drug therapy after dietary therapy. Current NCEP treatment guidelines do not take into account for the LDL-HDL ratio.

As already stated, drug therapy should be considered only if patients still have high cholesterol levels despite at least 6 months of intensive dietary therapy. Drug therapy for patients who are at extreme risk for CAD or who have marked elevations of LDL might be considered at an earlier point. The treatment goal for LDL cholesterol should be to decrease the circulating LDL to less than 160 mg/dl if the patient is free of CAD and two of the established risk factors, or 130 mg/dl if these other factors are present. In the case of established atherosclerosis, the goal should not be limited to lowering the lipid value, but should include the anatomical regression of coronary disease. The threshold to achieve regression has not yet been determined but may be <100 mg/dl of LDL cholesterol. Drug therapy should be monitored by repeat cholesterol tests performed regularly every 4 to 6 weeks after the initiation of therapy. At the end of 12 weeks, the physician should check for any drug toxicity, altered liver function, or impairment of concomitant drug absorption due to binding in the GI tract.

DIETARY THERAPY

Dietary therapy should be the initial intervention in all forms of lipid disorders. Although there is considerable variability in individual response to a low-fat, low-cholesterol diet, alterations of diet can be expected to play a significant role in improving most lipid profiles.

Angiographic studies have demonstrated the benefit of dietary therapy in halting the progression of atherosclerosis. In the 2-year *Leiden Intervention Trial*, patients in whom angiography had shown at least one coronary vessel with 50 per cent obstruction were given a vegetarian diet that contained twice as much polyunsaturated as saturated fat. Less than 100 mg of cholesterol was consumed each day. By the end of the trial, body weight, systolic blood pressure, total cholesterol, and the ratio of total cholesterol to HDL had all been lowered. There also was an increase in the linoleic acid content of cholesteryl esters. Angiograms performed after 24 months of dietary intervention indicated that about half of the patients showed no progression of coronary atherosclerosis. Progression of disease was seen in patients who had total cholesterol-HDL ratios greater than 6.9 throughout the trial period.[46]

The CLAS data (p. 1134) showed that the appearance of new coronary lesions can be influenced by diet.[90] This study's dietary therapy mainly involved the substitution of low-fat meats as a protein source. Similar findings on the benefits of dietary therapy were recently reported by Ornish and colleagues, whose study combined a vegetarian diet with relaxation therapy and exercise.[91]

Dietary goals should be established and a concerted effort made to ensure patient compliance. The diet should be nutritious, balanced, and of high culinary standard. These steps enhance adherence while achieving a reduction in circulating total and LDL cholesterol levels.

The minimal goals of dietary therapy should be to reduce LDL cholesterol to under 160 mg/dl and to lower the total cholesterol to under 240 mg/dl in patients without CAD or two additional risk factors and to less than 130 mg/dl if any of these conditions apply. Some clinicians would hold that the serum cholesterol should be more aggressively treated. The NCEP has described a two-step dietary program which parallels the dietary recommendations of the American Heart Association (AHA).[70,92] The NCEP specifically recommends a progressive initiation of dietary therapy designed to decrease dietary consumption of saturated fatty acids, promote weight loss, and lower total cholesterol. Although the AHA's Step One Diet can be initiated by the physician, implementation of the AHA's Step Two Diet should involve the aid of a registered dietitian. If a patient is overweight, total caloric intake should be decreased, as should the intake of saturated fat and cholesterol. In the average American diet, about 15 per cent of the total caloric intake consists of saturated fat, but in some people this may be considerably higher. A high consumption of saturated fat may decrease the activity of hepatic LDL receptors. In general, the diet should be aimed at balancing total calories and decreasing total fat, saturated fat, and cholesterol intake to the prescribed levels.

In the AHA's Step One Diet (Table 37–5), the recommended daily intake of total fat is less than 30 per cent of calories, with less than 10 per cent of total caloric intake coming from saturated fat. The daily consumption of total cholesterol should be less than 300 mg. The patient should have adequate instruction from the physician or staff, and a trial of 6 weeks should be implemented before lipids are rechecked. Not all saturated fatty acids elevate serum cholesterol. Recent studies by Bonanome and Grundy, for example, have shown that some saturated fatty acids have a neutral effect on cholesterol and that palmitic acid exerts a significant cholesterol-raising effect.[93] Saturated fatty acid intake can be replaced by the consumption of monounsaturated or polyunsaturated acids. Polyunsaturated fats can be increased to 10 per cent of calories, but the advisability of increasing their intake beyond this level is questioned by many authorities. The consumption of polyunsaturated fats has been shown to be associated with a better

TABLE 37-5 AMERICAN HEART ASSOCIATION DIETARY THERAPY OF HIGH BLOOD CHOLESTEROL IN ADULTS

NUTRIENT	RECOMMENDED INTAKE	
	Step One Diet	**Step Two Diet**
Total fat	Less than 30% of total calories	Less than 30% of total calories
Saturated fatty acids	Less than 10% of total calories	Less than 7% of total calories
Polyunsaturated fatty acids	Up to 10% of total calories	Up to 10% of total calories
Monounsaturated fatty acids	10% to 15% of total calories	10% to 15% of total calories
Carbohydrates	50% to 60% of total calories	50% to 60% of total calories
Protein	10% to 20% of total calories	10% to 20% of total calories
Cholesterol	Less than 300 mg/d	Less than 200 mg/d
Total calories	To achieve and maintain desirable weight	To achieve and maintain desirable weight

risk factor profile, including benefits in the lipid profile and alterations of glucose tolerance and blood pressure. The NCEP has recommended that monounsaturated fats, mainly oleic acid, make up 10 per cent to 15 per cent of total calories. These fats are found in olive oil and canola oil.

In Mediterranean countries, the intake of monounsaturated fats is high, primarily representing the consumption of olive oil. The incidence of CAD is considerably lower in these countries.[94]

A high dietary intake of cholesterol has been documented to induce the process of atherosclerosis in a variety of laboratory animals, including nonhuman primates. In humans, response of circulating cholesterol levels to alterations in diet is highly variable. However, an excess intake of cholesterol can elevate LDL in susceptible individuals and may add to the presence of cholesterol-rich atherogenic particles in the postprandial state. Hence, dietary restriction of cholesterol may be justifiable, even when other dietary measurements to minimize cholesterol have been successfully instituted.

Protein intake should be between 10 per cent and 20 per cent of the total caloric intake. The total amount of carbohydrates should be about 50 to 60 per cent of total calories. As dietary fat is reduced, it is considered prudent to replace it with complex carbohydrates, including vegetable fiber. The precise action of dietary fiber is not known. Although recent studies have shown that an increased consumption of oat bran may have a hypolipidemic effect, much of this effect may be due to the substitution of complex carbohydrates as fiber for fat in the diet rather than to a direct action.[95,96] There is a 4 to 5 per cent independent effect of soluble fiber in the reduction of serum cholesterol. Fiber in the diet may have other health benefits, including reduced risk from colon cancers.

If the patient is above ideal body weight, caloric restriction should be implemented to achieve weight reduction. Certain patients will respond to alterations in body weight with profound changes in circulating LDL levels. Ethanol is calorie dense, and its restriction can play a role in weight reduction; moderate use of ethanol can increase HDL cholesterol,[9] but the clinical significance of this effect is unknown.

After initiation of the Step One Diet, the serum cholesterol should be retested at 6 and 12 weeks. Serum cholesterol can serve as a surrogate measure of LDL in most patients. If specific goals are not achieved, and the patient can adhere to a more restricted diet, the patient should be referred to a registered dietitian for further instruction and for institution of the Step Two Diet. In the Step Two Diet (Table 37–5), saturated fats are decreased to less than 7 per cent of total calories and cholesterol to less than 200 mg/day. The polyunsaturated and monounsaturated fatty acid contents of the diet should remain at 10 per cent and in the 10 to 15 per cent range, respectively. Carbohydrate and protein intake should represent 50 to 60 per cent and 10 to 20 per cent of total calories, respectively, as in Step One.

An inadequate response to diet has several possible explanations. Some patients appear to be biologically resistant to an impact of diet on LDL lowering, despite good adherence. Adherence is a major problem and requires a concerted effort at guidance by physicians and dietitians. In some cases, a prolonged period of dietary therapy may be needed to alter the pattern of eating. Adequate time should be allowed for the patient to institute the recommended dietary changes and required adaptations of lifestyle. In patients with severe hyperlipidemia, it is not necessary to wait the 6 months before beginning pharmacological therapy.

The NCEP has also provided recommendations for dietary therapy in special groups. During pregnancy, elevated levels of triglycerides and cholesterol occur in the third trimester. As a general rule, these elevations are not clinically significant. The elevated lipids usually return to the baseline range about 4 to 6 weeks after delivery.

It is prudent to follow lipid values in hypertriglyceridemic patients and in those who have conditions that might predispose to this disorder. Dietary therapy in elderly patients should be individualized on physiological rather than chronological age, and the value of diet modification should be weighed against the possibility of an inadequate nutritional state. For the severe primary lipid disorders, such as FH, the lipid levels usually do not improve with dietary therapy alone. Dietary therapy should be implemented, however, to minimize the doses of pharmacological agents used.

For most patients with borderline elevations of lipids, intensive dietary therapy (i.e., the Step Two Diet) is not required. The NCEP states that population-based approaches to altering levels of lipids—in the entire community—will have a significant impact. Special attention should be given to younger people who are believed to be at increased risk for long-term development of CAD. The role of diet modification is pivotal in the treatment of the dyslipidemic patient and that dietary therapy must be continued, even after the decision has been made to use a pharmacological agent.

OMEGA-3 UNSATURATED FATTY ACIDS

The role of the consumption of oils from cold-water fish to protect against coronary disease remains controversial. The rationale for the use of these agents stems from the recognition that Greenland Eskimos have a low incidence of atherosclerotic cardiovascular disease, although this association has not been definitely established by extensive epidemiological data. Inhibition of atherosclerosis has been documented in several animal models on fish oil feeding.[97]

Fish oils are rich in eicosapentaenoic acid, an omega-3 unsaturated fatty acid that replaces an arachidonic acid in the platelet membrane. This replacement alters platelet aggregation and secondarily increases bleeding time. Eicosapentaenoic acid and docosahexaenoic acid appear to be the most important omega-3 fatty acids in the cold-water fish. Fish that contain omega-3 fatty acids include salmon, mackerel, rainbow trout, sardines, sablefish, and albacore tuna. In addition to the antiplatelet effect, the consumption of fish oil supplements has been shown to affect thrombosis. Experiments are under way to test the effects of fish oil supplements on patients undergoing angioplasty. The specific mechanisms are unknown, but it has been shown that fish oils will decrease fibrinogen levels.[98]

Fish oils may have beneficial effects on blood pressure as well. Human studies have documented that the intake of cold-water fish at a dose level of 280 gm/day can result in a 12 per cent decrease in systolic blood pressure.[99] Similar results were recorded in a number of epidemiological studies, in which fish consumption correlated with lower blood pressure.[100]

Although the consumption of fish oils does not greatly affect circulating LDL levels, it has been shown to decrease triglyceride levels markedly by inhibiting hepatic VLDL secretion. The benefit from fish oil supplements is rapid, and maximal lipid lowering can occur within 1 month of therapy. The use of fish oil supplements is more effective in the Fredrickson phenotypes associated with hypertriglyceridemia (IIb, IV, and V). Although usually this measure is effective in lowering lipids, there have been reports that a rebound phenomenon may occur later in the treatment phase, resulting in a decreased efficacy of therapy.[101] Moreover, fish oil supplements may have adverse effects in diabetic patients because of altered secretion of insulin and increased hepatic output of glucose.[102] Despite the apparent benefits of fish oil consumption in clinical and epidemiological studies, we do not recommend the intake of fish oil supplements as of this writing. It does seem prudent, however, to incorporate cold-water fish that are rich in omega-3 fatty acids into the diet at least twice a week.

DRUG TREATMENT

(See Tables 37–6 and 37–7)

Drug treatment of lipid disorders should not be used until a precise diagnosis is firmly established and the presence of

TABLE 37-6 SUMMARY OF LIPID-LOWERING AGENTS

AGENTS	MECHANISM OF ACTION	BIOCHEMICAL SIDE EFFECTS	SYSTEMIC SIDE EFFECTS	DOSAGE RANGE (DAILY)
Bile acid resins Cholestyramine; Colestipol	Increases excretion of bile acids in the stool, increases LDL-receptor activity	May prevent absorption of fat-soluble vitamins	Constipation, bloating	12–24 gm (cholestyramine) 15–30 gm (colestipol)
Nicotinic acid	Decreases plasma levels of free fatty acids, possibly inhibits cholesterol synthesis, decreases hepatic VLDL synthesis	Altered liver function tests, increased uric acid, increased glucose intolerance	Cutaneous flushing, pruritus, gastrointestinal upset	3–6 gm
Probucol	Enhances scavenger pathway removal of LDL	Decreased HDL	Diarrhea, nausea, flatulence	500–1000 mg
Fibric acid derivatives Gemfibrozil Clofibrate	Decreases hepatic VLDL synthesis, increases lipoprotein lipase activity	Altered liver function tests, increased CPK, potentiation of warfarin	Increased incidence of cholelithiasis and perhaps of GI cancer; myositis, diarrhea, nausea, rash (rare)	600–1200 mg (gemfibrozil) 1–2 gm (clofibrate)
HMG CoA reductase inhibitors Lovastatin Pravastatin	Inhibits HMG CoA reductase, increases LDL-receptor activity	Elevated transaminase levels, increased CPK	Mild GI symptoms; myositis syndrome	Starting dose 20 mg; range 40–80 mg

CPK = creatine phosphokinase; GI = gastrointestinal; HDL = high-density lipoprotein; HMG-CoA = 3-hydroxy-3-methylglutaryl coenzyme A; LDL = low-density lipoprotein; VLDL = very low-density lipoprotein.

treatable secondary causes has been ruled out. Before the institution of pharmacological hypolipidemic therapy, maximum dietary efforts should be instituted. As noted earlier, diet should be considered the mainstay of therapy, and a strenuous effort should be made to lower elevated lipids by nonpharmacological means. Drug therapy should be considered only when dietary treatment and other nonpharmacological interventions have failed to improve the lipid profile adequately.

The NCEP has provided risk-stratification guidelines for patients with hyperlipidemia. A number of factors—including the patient's age, associated illnesses, presence of documented atherosclerosis, and renal or hepatic dysfunction—play a role and must be considered before a patient is committed to pharmacological intervention.

The role of drugs in the treatment of hypertriglyceridemia is controversial. For example, Hoeg and coworkers recommend dietary therapy for patients in whom the triglyceride value is between 200 and 500 mg/dl.[103] If the value exceeds 500 mg/dl and the patient is at increased risk for pancreatitis or has a strong personal history of coronary disease, pharmacological therapy in addition to dietary measures is recommended.[103] If the triglyceride value exceeds 1000 mg/dl and this parameter is uncontrolled, Hoeg and associates recommend referral to a specialized center for evaluation and treatment.[103] The NCEP recommends total and LDL cholesterol values as the keys to establishing treatment guidelines (see above). However, the importance of individualizing the therapy must be emphasized.

TABLE 37-7 DRUG TREATMENT FOR HYPERLIPIDEMIAS

PHENOTYPE	DRUG TREATMENT
Type I	None
Type IIa	LOV BAS NA and PRO
	BAS + NA
	BAS + LOV
	BAS + PRO
Type IIb	BAS + NA
	BAS + GEM
Type III	NA, GEM, Clo
Type IV	NA, GEM
Type V	NA (limited by glucose intolerance)
	GEM
	NA + GEM

BAS = bile-acid sequestrant (cholestyramine, colestipol); Clo = clofibrate; GEM = gemfibrozil; LOV = lovastatin; NA = nicotinic acid (niacin); Pro = probucol.

BILE ACID SEQUESTRANTS. Cholestyramine and colestipol are quaternary ammonium salts that act as anion-exchange resins and bind bile salts in the intestine. This binding leads to an interruption of the enterohepatic circulation of bile salts and causes an enhanced excretion of sterols in the stool. The number and function of LDL receptors also are increased, with a secondary rise in the plasma clearance of LDL.

Cholestyramine and colestipol are considered first-line agents by the NCEP for the treatment of type II HLP and are highly effective in decreasing LDL cholesterol.[104] They are efficacious if the cholesterol is moderately elevated, as in the sporadic, polygenic forms of hyperlipidemia, but usually are not sufficient as single agents if the cholesterol is severely elevated, as in heterozygous familial hypercholesterolemics. Cholestyramine and colestipol also are ineffective in the rare homozygous type II HLP.

The bile acid sequestrants are difficult to use because of their frequent side effects, which include nausea, abdominal discomfort, constipation, and indigestion, and their sandy, gritty texture and unpleasant taste. Systemic side effects are rare because of the drugs' lack of absorption. Sequestrants may interfere with the absorption of other agents, such as digitalis, phenobarbital, thiazides, Coumadin (warfarin), thyroxine, and tetracycline. GI side effects have been lessened with recent preparations that are less bulky and have decreased carbohydrate content.

The resins come as granulated preparations in 4- or 5-gm packets and should be mixed with fluids or taken with meals. Stool softeners and increased fluid intake also may minimize the side effects. The dose should be low initially (e.g., one packet per day before a meal) and gradually increased (by one packet per day). The drug should be given 1 hour before or 4 hours after other medications. For patients who tolerate these agents, the average dose is three to six packets per day, usually given in divided doses with meals. Although the maximum dose is difficult to attain because of poor compliance, a 20 to 25 per cent reduction in LDL levels may be attained.

The LRC-CPPT study used the bile acid sequestrant cholestyramine as a single agent.[53] As noted above, this study indicated that a 1 per cent drop in total cholesterol was associated with approximately a 2 per cent drop in CAD risk. However, only a 9 per cent reduction of cholesterol was achieved overall in this trial because of inadequate compliance in the use of the drug.

Colestipol was used in the recent CLAS[55,56] and FATS[67,105] studies in combination with nicotinic acid. This drug combination produced angiographic regression of coronary atherosclerosis among patients who had undergone coronary bypass surgery (CLAS) or who had elevated levels of apo B-100 (FATS).

NICOTINIC ACID. The B vitamin nicotinic acid (niacin) is applied pharmacologically in doses that far exceed the levels required for its action as a nutrient. At the maximum dose of 3 to 6 gm/day, nicotinic acid is effective in the pharmacological management of all types of HLP except type I. Nicotinic acid decreases LDL levels by about 25 per cent and VLDL levels by about 75 per cent. The mechanism of this agent is complex and involves a reduction in LDL production, secondary to a decreased hepatic VLDL synthesis.[106] Nicotinic acid also inhibits the release of fatty acids from adipose tissues and thus decreases the level of substrate available for synthesis of triglycerides. Nicotinic acid increases HDL levels by 20 to 40 per cent, also probably as a result of the decreased VLDL production. The subfraction of HDL increased with nicotinic acid therapy appears to be predominantly HDL_2.

Like bile acid resins, nicotinic acid has frequent side effects. Common problems include cutaneous flushing and GI symptoms. The flushing and pruritus usually occur within 1 hour of administration and can be minimized by taking the drug with meals along with aspirin prophylaxis. The flushing tends to decrease with time; its basis is a prostaglandin-mediated capillary dilation. The documented GI effects relate to the elevation of the liver enzymes and gastritis, which may predispose the patient to peptic ulcer disease. Increased pigmentation of the skin may occur as well. Liver function tests should be closely monitored. Because another potential side effect is impairment of glucose tolerance, the drug should be used with caution in diabetics. Hyperuricemia has been reported, particularly in patients with gout.

Initial doses of nicotinic acid should be low (e.g., 50 mg), given with each meal, and gradually advanced to 1 gm three times daily. Nicotinic acid can be used for aggressive LDL lowering when administered with bile acid sequestrants. In the Coronary Drug Project, nicotinic acid was shown to decrease coronary and total mortality 9 years after the trial was terminated.[44] An overall decrease in total mortality of 11 per cent was seen in the trial's long-term follow-up. In the CLAS study[65,66] nicotinic acid combined with colestipol markedly improved lipid profiles and produced angiographic coronary regression, when compared with dietary treatment. Entry into this study required that patients be able to tolerate full-dose niacin and colestipol. Anatomical coronary lesion regression was seen after 4 years in 18 per cent of the patients who underwent diet plus drug therapy, compared with 6 per cent of the group with dietary intervention alone.[66]

PROBUCOL. Probucol lowers both LDL and HDL fractions. LDL cholesterol reductions averaging about 20 per cent can be expected after a full therapeutic trial, although the magnitude of the effect varies considerably from patient to patient. Probucol's mechanism of action is complex, and does not require the presence of LDL receptors. Presumably, the effect on lipids is accomplished by a non-receptor–mediated or scavenger pathway–modulated removal of LDL. The decrease in HDL that occurs is of concern, but its clinical impact has not been determined. Probucol also may modify LDL in the Watanabe rabbit by protecting against LDL oxidation.[79,107] This effect has been correlated with an antiatherosclerotic effect in this animal. Native LDL is poorly taken up by the resident macrophages in foam cell genesis. However, oxidatively modified LDL is preferentially taken up by these scavenger receptors, thus providing a mechanism for foam cell formation.[107a,107b] Apparently, antioxidants such as probucol can slow the progression of atherosclerosis in the Watanabe heritable hyperlipidemic (WHHL) rabbit. Probucol also may produce antiatherosclerotic activity, independent of its effect on lowering cholesterol.[108]

This pharmaceutical has been reported to increase the activity of the cholesteryl ester transfer protein, or lipid transfer protein. This effect would be expected to decrease HDL concentrations because of an alteration in lipoprotein kinetics. Probucol has been demonstrated to enhance a cholesterol efflux from human fibroblasts in vitro.[109] Its demonstrated stimulation of the production of apo E may further enhance the clearance of lipoproteins by way of their recognition and removal by the LDL receptor.[110] Probucol has little effect on VLDL; hence, it is most efficacious in the treatment of patients with type II HLP. Probucol has been combined with bile acid sequestrants for an additional effect on LDL lowering. The addition of probucol to lovastatin resulted in no further LDL decrease beyond that produced by lovastatin alone. There also appeared to be no added hypolipidemic benefit with the use of probucol as a third agent.[111]

The major side effects of probucol are gastrointestinal and usually are mild when the drug is used as a single agent. Prolongation of the QT and QT-C electrocardiogram intervals has been demonstrated experimentally and in humans. However, the relation of this alteration of repolarization to polymorphic ventricular tachycardia (torsades de pointes) has not been established.

As seen by a variety of imaging techniques, probucol yielded regression of tendinous xanthomas in FH patients; however, whether this effect correlates with coronary artery regression or has an impact on mortality has not been determined. A large-scale arterial regression study, the Probucol Quantitative Regression Swedish Trial, is investigating the development of atherosclerosis in hyperlipidemic patients through femoral quantitative angiographic techniques.[112,113]

FIBRIC ACID DERIVATIVES. Gemfibrozil and clofibrate are the fibric acid derivatives currently available in the United States. In Europe, fenofibrate, bezafibrate, and ciprofibrate are also used. The fibric-acid derivatives are effective in lowering VLDL, IDL, and triglycerides. Their mechanism of action is complex; one effect is to increase lipoprotein lipase activity and thereby increase the clearance of VLDL particles.[114,114a] Cholesterol secretion into the bile also is enhanced. These agents are effective in lowering triglycerides in patients with hypertriglyceridemia. In some cases, they can lower triglyceride levels by as much as 50 per cent, while increasing HDL levels by 10 per cent to 20 per cent.

Clofibrate was the agent used in the World Health Organization trial that showed a decrease in nonfatal MIs.[115] However, an increase in overall mortality was noted. In this trial, the MI incidence was directly related to serum cholesterol levels and blood pressure, and to the incidence of cigarette smoking. The decrease in MI was most evident in the patients who were hypertensive and heavy smokers. Clofibrate also appeared to lower fibrinogen levels, an effect that may have contributed to the lower MI incidence.

Gemfibrozil has been shown to be effective in all types of dyslipidemia with the exception of type I HLP.[114a] However, its main effect is the alteration of triglyceride-rich lipoproteins. Gemfibrozil reduces LDL cholesterol by about 10 per cent to 20 per cent, with a subsequent decrease in apo B in patients with type IIa HLP. Patients with type IIb experience minimal changes in LDL levels, whereas those with type IV HLP may experience an *increase* in LDL levels. VLDL and triglycerides may be decreased by up to 60 per cent, with a subsequent rise in the HDL fraction.

The efficacy of gemfibrozil in decreasing coronary death rates was demonstrated in the Helsinki Heart Study[54] (see p. 1133). This trial resulted in a 34 per cent reduction in coronary incidents with improvements seen in all of the Fredrickson

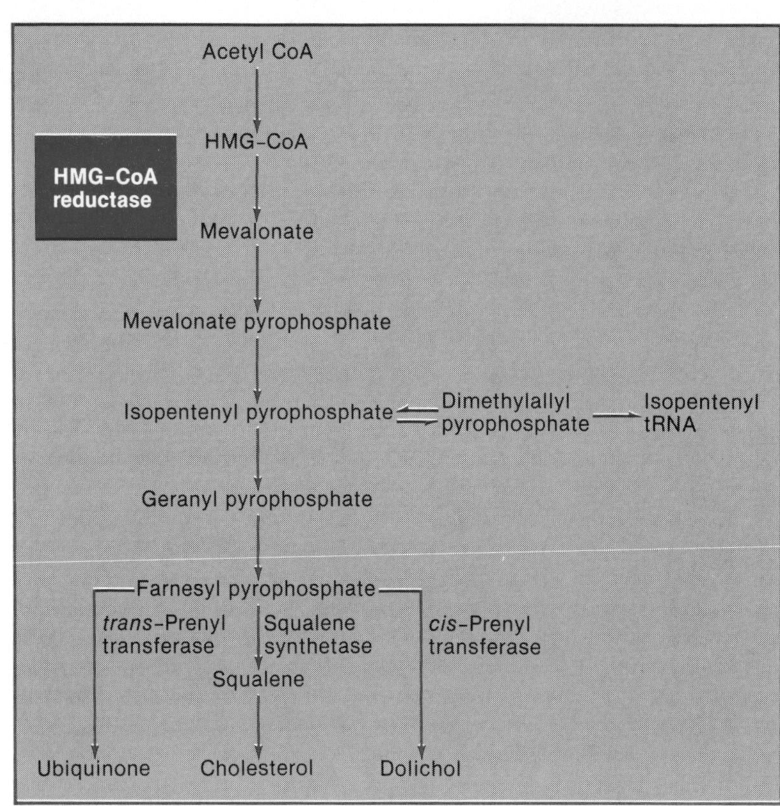

FIGURE 37-12. Cholesterol biosynthetic pathway. (From Alberts, A. W.: Effects of HMG CoA reductase inhibitors on cholesterol synthesis. Drug Invest. *2*(Suppl. 2):9, 1990.)

phenotypes in the study (IIa, IIb, and IV). The greatest benefit was experienced by patients with type IIb HLP.

Fibric-acid derivatives usually are well tolerated, with nausea and GI discomfort the major side effects. Myositis and glucose elevation have been reported but are relatively uncommon. Fibric acid derivatives may potentiate the effect of Coumadin.

HMG-CoA REDUCTASE INHIBITORS. Compactin, lovastatin, simvastatin, pravastatin, and fluvastatin are agents that inhibit 3-hydroxy-3-methylglutaryl coenzyme A HMG-CoA reductase, which is the rate-limiting enzyme in the cholesterol biosynthetic pathway (Fig. 37-12).[116] Their action is competition and partial blocking (Fig. 37-13), which occurs because the side chain in these agents has a structural resemblance to HMG-CoA. They decrease hepatic cholesterol synthesis and thus increase the number of LDL receptors expressed on the hepatic tissue surface. LDL-receptor activity can be determined by bioassay with culture of human fibroblasts, or by assay of the functional LDL-receptor activity on lymphocytes.[117,118]

The HMG-CoA reductase inhibitors represent a major advance in the treatment of hypercholesterolemic patients. Lovastatin and pravastatin are the only drugs of this class currently available in the United States. The prototype statin, compactin, was never marketed, presumably because of toxicity in animal experiments.

The main indication for the use of the HMG-CoA reductase inhibitors is in the treatment of patients with elevated levels of LDL cholesterol. In patients who also have mildly elevated triglycerides, lovastatin enhances clearance of postprandial lipoprotein levels, with a significant lowering of VLDL cholesterol and fasting triglycerides; hence its administration may benefit patients with type IIb HLP.[119] In patients with normal lipid profiles except for decreased levels of HDL, lovastatin has been shown to decrease LDL and apo B by about 25 per cent. In the large clinical trials in hypercholesterolemic subjects, reductase inhibitors have increased HDL cholesterol on average by 5 to 10 per cent.[120] The effects of reductase inhibitors on Lp(a) have not yet been well characterized. Lovastatin has reportedly decreased LDL cholesterol levels without a concomitant reduction in Lp(a). This suggests a different mechanism of clearance of Lp(a) from the circulation. There are some reports of an increase in Lp(a) levels with lovastatin therapy, although the data are quite limited.[121]

In addition to lowering plasma lipids, the reductase inhibitor *simvastatin* has been reported to decrease platelet aggregation and thromboxane B_2 formation induced by collagen.[122]

The reductase inhibitors may be combined with bile-acid sequestrants (Fig. 37-14) to produce dramatic decreases in

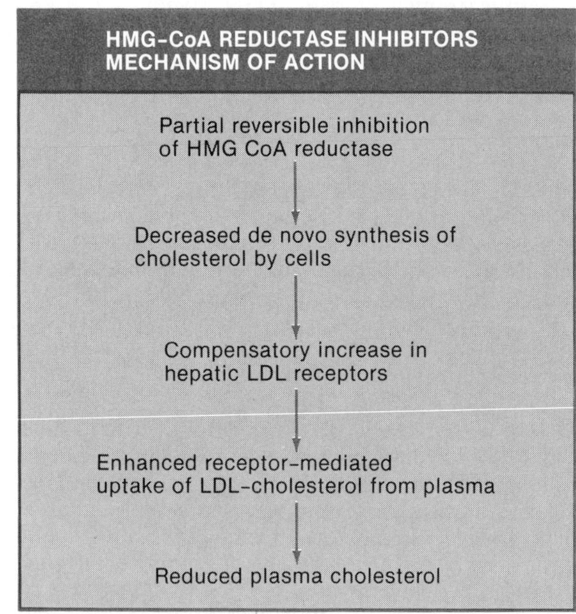

FIGURE 37-13. The mechanism of the 3-hydroxy-3-methylglutaryl-coenzyme A (HMG-CoA) reductase inhibitors involves partial inhibition of the rate-limiting enzyme in cholesterol synthesis that converts HMG-CoA to mevalonic acid. The subsequent decrease in intracellular cholesterol stimulates the synthesis of the low-density lipoprotein (LDL) or apoprotein B/E receptor, which allows increased recognition and plasma clearance of particles containing these apoproteins.

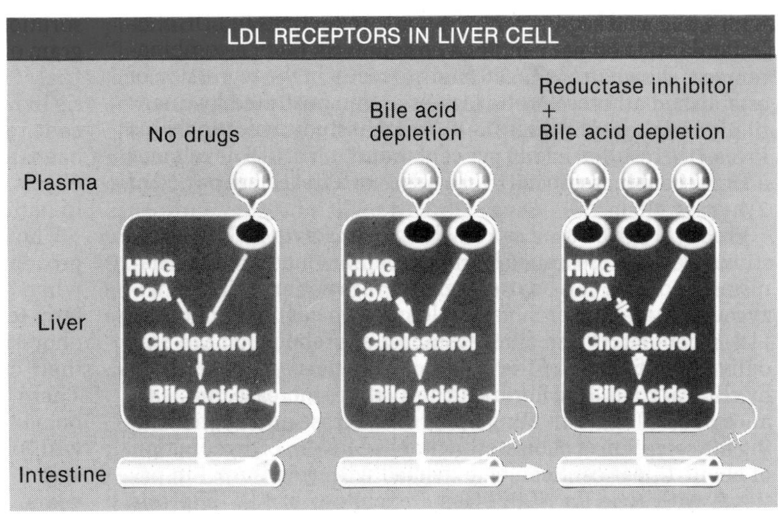

FIGURE 37–14. Rationale for the combination of a bile acid sequestrant and reductase inhibitor in the treatment of hypercholesterolemia. Bile acid sequestrants increase clearance of low-density lipoprotein (LDL) by increasing the number of apoprotein B/E receptors in addition to enhanced gastrointestinal loss via interception of the enterohepatic circulation. The compensatory increase in cholesterol synthesis may be blocked by addition of a reductase inhibitor that inhibits 3-hydroxy-3-methylglutaryl–coenzyme A (HMG-CoA) reductase–mediated cholesterol synthesis and further increases apoprotein B/E receptor activity. (From Brown, M. S., and Goldstein, J. L.: A receptor-mediated pathway for cholesterol homeostasis. Science *232*:34, 1986. Copyright 1986 by the American Association for the Advancement of Science.)

overall LDL levels. As already discussed, the bile-acid sequestrants increase LDL-receptor activity and sterol excretion in the GI tract. A compensatory increase in the activity of the HMG-CoA reductase enzyme system can be inhibited by the use of lovastatin, with reductions in LDL cholesterol of 50 per cent to 60 per cent reported.

The incidence of serious side effects with lovastatin is low. Nonetheless, the physician should be watchful for myositis, hepatocellular abnormalities, and lens opacities. Concerns about the potential for development of cataracts resulted from early experience with the drug MER-29, an agent that inhibited the penultimate step in the biosynthesis of cholesterol. This drug increased early cataract formation. Also, lovastatin at very high doses has been reported to cause cataracts in beagles, but this effect has not been encountered in other animals or in humans.

The inhibition of HMG-CoA reductase occurs early in the biosynthetic pathway of cholesterol (Fig. 37–12), and the fears concerning cataract formation have not been realized. Mild elevations of aspartate aminotransferase and alanine aminotransferase have been reported, requiring the discontinuation of therapy in about 0.6 per cent of outpatients. Myositis has been seen in transplant patients receiving concomitant cyclosporine therapy. The latter therapy raises blood levels of lovastatin and may result in marked elevation of creatinine phosphokinase and rhabdomyolysis. In patients not receiving cyclosporine, the incidence of myositis is probably 1 in 500. An increased incidence has been reported when the drug is given with gemfibrozil, nicotinic acid, or erythromycin. Available data on reductase inhibitors suggest that they are effectively removed in first-pass clearance by the liver and may be actively transported into hepatocytes. This highly effective first-pass clearance probably accounts for the relative efficacy and safety of the drugs as a class. Demonstrated differences in the uptake by nonhepatic tissues are potentially related to hydrophobicity and solubility in tissue. The clinical significance of these effects in humans is not established.

DEXTROTHYROXINE. Dextrothyroxine is the dextroisomer of the naturally occurring thyroid hormone levothyroxine and is used as a secondary drug in the treatment of type II HLP. Its mechanism of action is unclear, but it appears to increase the activity of LDL receptors in hypothyroid animals. Dextrothyroxine is approved by the Food and Drug Administration for use in patients with no evidence of CAD or cardiac arrhythmia. In the Coronary Drug Project, its use was associated with increased morbidity and mortality, leading to its early termination.[123] Dextrothyroxine should be reserved for selected young adults with primary hypercholesterolemia who are unable to take effective lipid-lowering drugs and who are free of CAD.

SPECIFIC TREATMENTS FOR HYPERLIPOPROTEINEMIA TYPES

(Table 37–7)

LIPOPROTEIN LIPASE AND APO C-II DEFICIENCY—TYPE I. Type I HLP is diagnosed in the pediatric age group as an autosomal recessive disorder of lipoprotein lipase.[124] A deficiency of apo C-II or a circulating inhibitor may cause a clinical presentation that is indistinguishable from other types of chylomicronemia. Therapy is initiated to decrease the risk of recurrent pancreatitis. Generally, if the triglyceride level can be kept under 1000 mg/dl, the development of pancreatitis is uncommon. Dietary fat should be restricted to 10 to 25 gm/day. Medium-chain triglycerides may be used to make the diet more palatable. These triglycerides are absorbed directly in the portal circulation and do not require lipoprotein lipase activation for metabolism. If there is documented apo C-II deficiency, the acute treatment of the abdominal pain associated with type I HLP can be specifically directed at replacement of the apoprotein. Apo C-II may be supplied by plasma infusions in a life-threatening situation. Drug therapy is ineffective in the three genetic defects that result in a type I phenotype. Hence, diet is the key to maintenance therapy of type I HLP.

POLYGENIC AND FAMILIAL HYPERCHOLESTEROLEMIA—TYPE II. Aggressive therapy is mandatory in patients with type II HLP because of the high incidence of premature coronary atherosclerosis and peripheral vascular disease. Therapy should be based on a careful genetic diagnosis, with secondary causes of elevated cholesterol diagnostically excluded. The patient should scrupulously follow the AHA Step One Diet and progress to the Step Two Diet before drug therapy is considered. Most patients with mild type II HLP have polygenic hypercholesterolemia and can be treated with diet alone. The NCEP recommends bile acid sequestrants (cholestyramine or colestipol) and niacin as primary therapeutic agents. Colestipol is given at 5 to 10 gm three times a day, cholestyramine at 4 to 8 gm three times a day. Nicotinic acid can be added in doses of 1.0 to 1.5 gm three times a day with meals and aspirin prophylaxis. The combination of colestipol and niacin has been shown to be associated with the regression of coronary atherosclerosis in both native circulation and coronary venous bypass grafts.[65] However, this combination often is hampered by poor compliance with therapy.

The advent of the HMG-CoA reductase inhibitors has markedly expanded the ability of the clinician to treat type II HLP successfully. These agents have been shown to be markedly effective in type II phenotypes, regardless of the underlying defect. Lovastatin in short-term use has been associated with a low incidence of serious side effects.[125] When it is combined

(see pp. 819 and 843)

A consensus report has been published to establish guidelines for the evaluation and treatment of pediatric patients as regards blood pressure.[166] This report stratifies blood pressure into three categories: (1) significant hypertension, in which the average confirmed systolic and diastolic pressures are above the 95th percentile for age and sex; (2) high normal, in which the average systolic and diastolic pressures are between the 90th and 95th percentiles for age and sex; and (3) normal, in which the average systolic and diastolic blood pressures are below the 90th percentile for age and sex.

The prevalence of significant hypertension is low in children. Markedly elevated blood pressure levels frequently are associated with a secondary cause (e.g., coarctation of the aorta, renal parenchymal anomalies, or reno-vascular disease), which should focus the investigation. A familial tendency for hypertension, hyperlipidemia, and increased insulin secretion, tentatively termed familial dyslipidemic hypertension, has been described in children and young adults, who often have truncal obesity. This may occur in 10 to 15 per cent of patients with presumed essential hypertension.[154,167] The urinary excretion of kallikrein has been reported to be inversely related to the level of high blood pressure and may be useful as a marker for some familial forms of hypertension.[168]

DIET AND HYPERTENSION

Although the exact relation of high sodium intake to hypertension has not been definitely established, an enormous amount of clinical evidence is available on this subject. The average U.S. consumption of salt is 10 to 15 gm/day, which exceeds the needs of the body. About two-thirds of the average dietary salt intake is obtained in processed food and one-third is added in cooking. NaCl has been shown to be more powerful in its pressor effect than other sodium salts.[169] Also, evaluation of 11 major clinical trials showed that an average decline in blood pressure of 6 mm Hg could be achieved by a 100-mmol/day decrease in sodium intake. A diet restricting sodium intake to a total of 2 gm, or 88 mmol, has been shown to be tolerable and efficacious.[170]

Although a vegetarian diet has been epidemiologically associated with lower blood pressure, these studies are fraught with potential methodological problems. Such a relation also is supported by experimental studies, although no precise mechanism has been described.[171,172] Daily consumption of more than 2 oz of alcohol is associated with an increased prevalence of hypertension.[173]

The role of dietary calcium in blood pressure remains controversial. Epidemiological studies suggest an inverse relationship.[174,175] The mechanism is unclear; the many explanations proferred include alteration of the vascular tone and the relationship of renin and angiotensin. Kaplan has hypothesized that volume expansion due to high dietary sodium intake will lead to hypercalciuria, secondary hyperparathyroidism, and subsequent hypertension. Increased dietary calcium intake would then restore parathormone levels to normal and thus reduce blood pressure.[176] Until the issue is clarified, dietary supplements of calcium for hypertension should not be routinely administered.

Decreased consumption of saturated fat has been correlated with lower blood pressure, as has increased intake of potassium.

EFFECTS OF TREATING HYPERTENSION

Meta-analysis of the major blood pressure–lowering trials has been performed by Yusuf and coworkers.[40] They reviewed the 14 major trials, which together involved 45,000 patients for an average of 5 years. In nine of the trials, a definite benefit was seen in stroke reduction. The impact on coronary disease was much less clear. The most important clinical trials are summarized below.

VETERANS ADMINISTRATION COOPERATIVE STUDY GROUP. The classic Veterans Administration trial demonstrated the efficacy of antihypertensive therapy in severe hypertension (> 114 mm Hg diastolic). The results in milder hypertension (90–104 mm Hg) were not statistically significant, although the numbers of patients were small.[177]

HYPERTENSION DETECTION AND FOLLOW-UP PROGRAM. More than 7800 patients with diastolic pressure between 90 and 104 mm Hg were enrolled in the Hypertension Detection and Follow-up Program (HDFP).[178] Half were referred to their usual source of medical care (referred care) and half received more intensive treatment under a stepped-care program (i.e., the study was not placebo controlled). The initial drug in the stepped-care approach was a diuretic, followed by addition of an adrenergic inhibitor and then hydralazine. After 5 years, the mean diastolic pressure was 83 mm Hg in the stepped-care group and 88 mm Hg in the referred-care group. The stepped-care group also had a 20 per cent lower overall mortality rate, including 45 per cent fewer deaths due to cerebrovascular disease, 46 per cent fewer deaths due to acute MI, and 20 per cent fewer deaths due to CAD. Across all the nearly 11,000 patients in the trial (including the 4000 with higher blood pressure at entry), total mortality was reduced 17 per cent with stepped care compared with referred care. On the basis of these findings, the second U.S. Joint National Committee recommended that the initial goal of antihypertensive therapy be to maintain diastolic pressure under 90 mm Hg.

AUSTRALIAN THERAPEUTIC TRIAL. The Australian Therapeutic Trial enrolled patients with diastolic blood pressure between 95 and 109 mm Hg who were free of CAD. Patients were randomly assigned to placebo or stepped-care therapy similar to that in the HDFP. The trial was stopped after a statistically significant difference of 30 per cent between the two groups was attained. The patients were treated for an average of 4 years. Interestingly, the blood pressure in the group treated with placebo also fell, and, at the end of the trial, only 22 per cent of the patients whose initial pressure was between 100 and 104 mm Hg failed to lower their blood pressure. The treated group's average blood pressure fell 12.2 mm Hg, compared with 6.6 mm Hg in the placebo group. Improvement in total CAD outcome was noted. An excess in complications was noted in the placebo-treated patients whose pressure remained over 100 mm Hg.[179]

MULTIPLE RISK FACTOR INTERVENTION TRIAL. The MRFIT studied not only hypertension intervention, but also the impact of smoking cessation and cholesterol lowering on CAD mortality.[51] The MRFIT enrolled 12,866 men and assigned them to usual care by their private physicians or to a specialized center for aggressive intervention to reduce cardiac risk. Although the special-intervention patients were able to reduce their major risk factors, there were no significant differences between this group and the usual-care group in CAD or total mortality. The reason for this failure is unclear but may relate to the use of thiazide diuretic therapy in the special-care group.[180] Long-term follow-up (10.5 years) has revealed a beneficial impact on risk reduction in the special-intervention group, emphasizing the fact that risk-factor reduction should be considered a lifelong commitment.[181]

MEDICAL RESEARCH COUNCIL TRIAL. The Medical Research Council (MRC) Trial[182] was a large drug trial in mild hypertension carried out in the United Kingdom. Diuretics were used as the first step after nonpharmacological means were used. The MRC compared diuretics or beta blockers to placebo in patients who had no prior treatment for high blood pressure and no history of MI, diabetes, or angina pectoris. By the trial's end, the rate of strokes was decreased in the treated group. There was no decrease in coronary events.

INTERNATIONAL PROSPECTIVE PRIMARY PREVENTION STUDY IN HYPERTENSION. The International Prospective Primary Prevention Study in Hypertension (IPPPSH)[183] was a large-scale trial (6357 patients) that examined the impact of a noncardioselective beta blocker with partial agonist activity (oxprenolol) versus placebo plus other agents with a treatment goal of a diastolic pressure not to exceed 95 mm Hg. With 3 to 5 years of follow-up, there were no statistically significant differences between the groups in stroke, MI, or sudden cardiac death.

METOPROLOL ATHEROSCLEROSIS PREVENTION IN HYPERTENSION. The previously mentioned MAPHY trial was in a large subgroup (3234 men) of the original Heart Attack Primary Prevention in Hypertensives Trial, and analyzed only the metoprolol versus diuretics results.[159] The drugs were administered in a nonblinded manner in this open trial. The metoprolol group had significant reductions in CAD, stroke, and overall mortality, as analyzed by the conservative intention-to-treat method. The benefit with metoprolol also was significant in the patients who used tobacco products. Despite some unanswered questions (e.g., study design, higher-than-expected mortality in the diuretics group), the MAPHY data suggest benefit from the use of a cardioselective beta blocker in hypertension.

REVIEW OF THE CLINICAL TRIALS. Diuretics and beta blockers are effective in reducing hypertension and subsequent morbidity and mortality from cardiovascular disease. Although they are well tolerated and effective in decreasing blood pressure, angiotensin-converting enzyme inhibitors and calcium antagonists have not been studied in placebo-controlled primary prevention trials. However, an impact on CAD is less clearly demonstrated. Care must be taken to correct induced metabolic abnormalities (e.g., hyperglycemia, hyperlipidemia, electrolyte abnormalities) and to avoid overzealous reduction of pressure to a point that jeopardizes coronary perfusion.

PHYSICAL ACTIVITY

(See also Chap. 42)

The role of physical activity in the prevention of CAD and in decreasing mortality after MI remains controversial. Recent epidemiological studies have shown an encouraging and beneficial trend in favor of this relatively low-cost and low-risk intervention (Fig. 37–15). Long-term physical activity is known to be important in maintaining ideal body weight and muscle mass. Exercise also may play an important role in

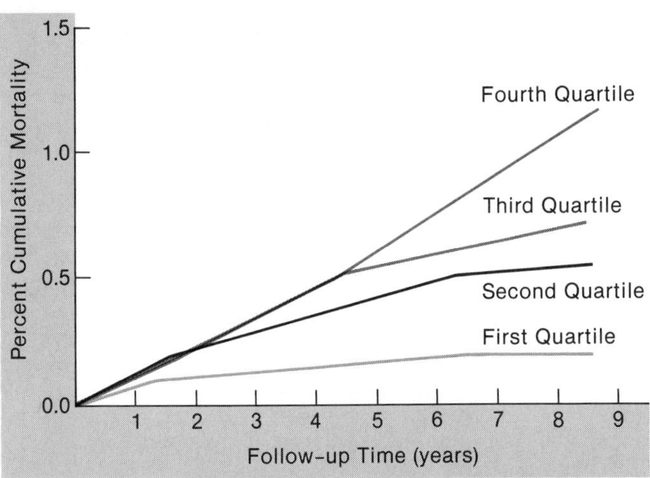

FIGURE 37-15. Life-table failure plots were computed from proportional hazards models that included age, smoking status, HDL level, LDL level, resting systolic blood pressure, and stage 2 exercise heart rate, with continuous variables set to mean values and smoking status to zero (yes = 1, no = 0). (Reprinted by permission from Ekelund, L.-G., Haskell, W. L., Johnson, J. L., et al.: Physical fitness as a predictor of cardiovascular mortality in asymptomatic North American men: The Lipid Research Clinics Mortality follow-up study. N. Engl. J. Med. *319*:1379, 1988, p. 1383.)

maintaining normal blood pressure and optimizing lipid values. Patients who exercise regularly have been reported to show a decreased incidence of sudden cardiac death (Chap. 26). In contrast, some people who have been sedentary may be at increased risk for malignant ventricular arrhythmia or acute MI when they begin to exercise. Thus, patients over age 40 are urged to undergo a thorough physical examination and exercise stress test before undertaking a program of vigorous physical activity.

Several epidemiological studies have shown a consistent inverse relationship between caloric intake per kilogram of body mass and CAD, probably because of the protective effect of increased physical activity. Multivariate analyses have revealed that people with high levels of physical fitness have lower rates of CAD and cancer. Conversely, decreased levels of physical fitness are associated with increased risk of atherosclerosis.[184] Several studies have shown that the relative risk for cardiovascular disease conferred by physical inactivity appears to parallel in magnitude that conferred by hypertension, dyslipidemia, or the use of tobacco products.[185] This impact of physical inactivity was documented in well-designed prospective studies with large numbers of patients, superseding the lack of benefit described by small-scale and poorly designed studies.

In addition to its possible role as a primary risk factor for the development of coronary disease, physical inactivity may affect the secondary association of other cardiac risk factors.[185a] The Framingham Offspring Study found that patients who participated in at least 1 hour of conditioning activities per week had an improved cardiac risk profile when HDL, heart rate, body mass index, and tobacco use were analyzed.[186] Decreased presence of associated risk factors in physically active people would be predicted to translate into altered CAD mortality. The U.S. Railroad Study, with 17 to 20 years of mortality follow-up, confirmed that the age-adjusted risk estimate for CAD death was increased to 1.39 for sedentary men who expended less than 40 kcal/week. The relationship of physical activity was independent and statistically significant when controlled in multivariate analysis.[187]

MECHANISMS OF POSSIBLE BENEFIT

The exact mechanism of the apparent protection afforded against atherosclerosis by physical activity is doubtless multifactorial. Regular aerobic exercise decreases both systolic and diastolic blood pressure levels, although the precise mechanism is not clear. Regular aerobic physical training has been shown to increase cardiac output and decrease systemic vascular resistance.[188] Exercise also may alter the renin-angiotensin-aldosterone axis, with subsequent decreases in circulating renin levels, although the changes in renin have not been documented uniformly. It does appear that the decrease in plasma renin correlates significantly with the subsequent increase in physical activity.[189] Prostacyclin activity also is increased with exercise, although the role that this plays in the regulation of blood pressure is unclear.[190] Meta-analysis of studies that evaluated changes in blood pressure of normotensive patients with exercise has revealed a mild but significant decrease in both systolic and diastolic pressures of about 4 mm Hg. In patients with initial hypertension, the decrease may be more significant and has resulted in an average decline of 11 mm Hg for systolic pressure and 6 mm Hg for diastolic pressure. This has been corroborated by 24-hour ambulatory recordings.[191]

Additional benefit may accrue to patients who undergo exercise training, by means of an alteration in the lipid profile. Special interest has been directed to the effect of physical exertion on HDL levels. An inverse relation between HDL and obesity has been documented.[192] The role of exercise in the alteration of lipid profiles has been well studied. In most of these studies, intense exercise is associated with decreased total and LDL cholesterol values and with increased HDL levels.[193] In addition to the increases in total HDL induced by exercise, an associated increase in apo A-I levels has been shown to be produced by physical training.[194] The relation between exercise and alcohol consumption in runners and inactive men has been studied. Exercise has a more profound positive impact on HDL levels than does alcohol in people who run 12 or more miles per week.

Another benefit from regular exercise is improved glucose tolerance, although it is not clear that the reduction of blood glucose alters CAD mortality. However, meta-analyses of studies evaluating the impact of physical activity on cardiac mortality have been performed to circumvent the statistical limitations of smaller studies. Isolated clinical trials using samples of up to 750 patients usually have shown a trend of improvement in mortality (about a 20 per cent change). In general, these changes have not reached statistical significance when populations undergoing exercise training were compared with nonexercising controls. However, a meta-analysis involving the 12 major exercise trials has shown a statistically significant benefit to an endurance exercise program.[195]

EXERCISE LEVELS. The level of exercise required to provide CAD protection has not been established. Sedentary patients may produce alterations in other risk factors, such as blood pressure, weight, lipids, HDL, and glucose tolerance, by means of a moderate exercise program. Whether more sustained exercise will increase the benefit has not been shown. Exercise energy expenditures of about 2000 kcal/week, or the equivalent of jogging 20 miles per week, have correlated with protection from the development of CAD.[196,197] A practical exercise prescription depends on the clinical status of the patient and on the existence of CAD and peripheral arteriosclerosis. Patients at increased risk for atherosclerosis, such as those with hypertension, dyslipidemia, or diabetes, and patients in whom coronary disease is suspected should be evaluated by an exercise treadmill test, clinical history, and physical examination. Treadmill testing is recommended in sedentary patients over age 40 who plan to begin an exercise program. If the patient has no evidence or history of ischemic heart disease, exercise programs may not need close monitoring because of the low risk involved.

RECOMMENDATIONS

The best available evidence indicates that regular and moderate physical activity is beneficial in the primary and secondary prevention of CAD. This conclusion is endorsed by the World Health Organization, which predicts that increased physical activity should result in decreased health care costs and lower mortality rates.[198] Exercise programs can be inexpensive, and they seem a prudent way to improve the general health and well-being of the population. To bring about a significant improvement in aerobic capacity, at least three sessions per week are required, each lasting between 20 and 30 minutes. Five sessions produce the maximum result, which is achieved after 4 to 6 weeks of training. Adherence to exercise programs is a major problem, and half of those who begin a regular program drop out. All patients with known CAD should undergo treadmill testing before beginning an exercise program. Patients treated for MI may undergo a submaximal treadmill test before discharge from the hospital. Prognosis may be estimated by ST shifts, exercise time, ectopy, and inappropriate blood pressure responses.[199] The role of the physician is pivotal in helping the patient establish attainable goals for an exercise program. A regular routine should be advocated, with flexibility as to the type of calorie expenditure. The physician should encourage and support the patient to maximize benefits and to minimize dropout.

OBESITY

The precise role of obesity as an independent cardiac risk factor remains unclear. Analysis of the Framingham data reveals an independent contribution to the risk of coronary disease by elevated blood cholesterol, blood pressure, glucose, and uric acid. Although all are increased with increasing body mass index, obesity still makes an independent contribution to the overall risk of coronary disease on multivariate analysis. Mortality rates also are increased with overall obesity and central obesity. In people in the highest quintile by body mass index, increased waist circumference and subscapular skin folds were associated with increased risk of coronary and cerebrovascular disease. The definition of obesity is arbitrary; this condition frequently is defined as an increase of 20 per cent above ideal body weight. Actuarial studies have defined ideal weight as that weight associated with the lowest mortality rates in people applying for life insurance. Body mass index has been advocated as the best approach to estimating obesity. The prevalence of obesity averages about 20 per cent for men between ages 45 to 54 and 15 per cent for women in the same age range. About 16 per cent of men are at least 20 per cent overweight, and 28 per cent of women are 20 per cent or more overweight.

A National Institutes of Health consensus conference on obesity concluded that obesity adversely affects both health and longevity.[200] Obesity has a direct relationship with all the coronary risk factors except smoking.[201] The number of cigarettes smoked per day shows an inverse trend when compared with body weight, possibly because of appetite suppression by smoking.[202,203] The strongest correlations with obesity are with blood pressure, hypertriglyceridemia, hyperinsulinemia (all positive correlations), and the concentration of HDL cholesterol (an inverse relationship).

Body mass index correlates positively with total serum cholesterol and inversely with HDL level.[204] Although the epidemiological association of hypertension and obesity is well established, the precise mechanism involved in the genesis of elevated blood pressure is not known. Obesity may alter peripheral vascular resistance, dietary salt intake, and neuroendocrine homeostasis.

The role that dietary salt plays in elevating blood pressure in obese patients is controversial. Some obese patients who are salt sensitive lower their blood pressure when they reduce their sodium intake.[205] Certain obese patients increase renal sodium reabsorption, secondary to autonomic nervous system alterations, and have a low-renin or salt-sensitive hypertensive state.

In obese patients, hyperinsulinemia may play a role in elevating blood pressure. Obese patients have resistance to the action of insulin because of decreased numbers of functioning receptors for insulin on the cell surface. Also, further decreases in insulin receptors occur when levels of circulating insulin are high. A relationship between insulin levels, diabetes, and hypertension has been determined epidemiologically.[206] Syndrome X has recently been defined as an underlying genetic disorder associated with insulin resistance, hyperinsulinemia, increased blood pressure, decreased HDL and HDL_2, increased VLDL triglyceride, and small, dense, apo B-rich LDL.[207] Postprandial lipemia may be part of this syndrome.[208] Familial dyslipidemic hypertension has been described as well.[209] Many of these characteristics are seen in familial combined hyperlipidemia. Possible suggested causes include the overproduction of hepatic apo B-100, heterozygous deficiency of lipoprotein lipase, and an increase in the activity of the cholesteryl ester transfer protein.[210]

FAT DISTRIBUTION

Studies carried out in several countries have shown the importance of the distribution of fat as a coronary risk factor. The difference in fat patterns between men and women implicates a hormonal basis for the variable degree of obesity in different anatomical areas. The waist-hip ratio (in women) has been positively correlated with the level of androgens.

The terms "overweight" and "obese" are not synonymous. Overweight refers to body mass index; obesity is estimated by the thickness of skin folds in various body regions. Upper values of body mass index and increased central obesity, as estimated by abdominal girth or waist-hip ratio, have been associated with increased relative risks of CAD.[211] Fat deposition in the abdomen has been associated both with hypertension and the risk of developing CAD complications (Fig. 37-16).[212] In men, CAD is correlated with the abdominal distribution of adiposity, which appears to be independent of obesity. The circumference of the waist compared with that of the hips has been associated with hypertension, hypercholesterolemia, elevated levels of fibrinogen, and hypertriglyceridemia. These variables have been epidemiologically correlated with CAD.[213]

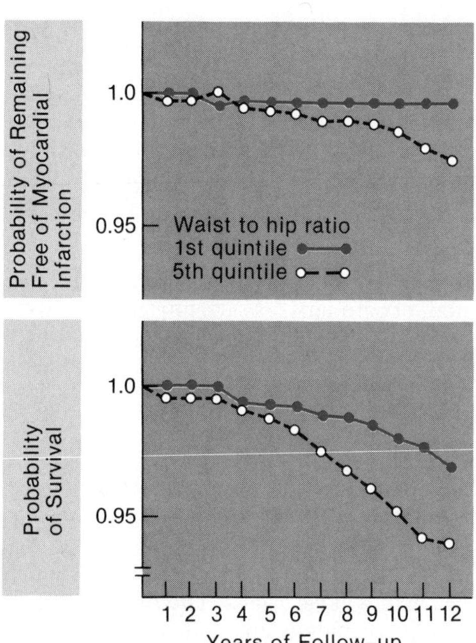

FIGURE 37-16. Probability of remaining free of myocardial infarction and dying of any cause for every year of a 12-year follow-up by highest and lowest quintiles of ratio of waist-to-hip circumference at entry. (From Lapidus, L., et al.: Distribution of adipose tissue and risk of cardiovascular disease and death: A 12-year follow-up of participants in the population study of women in Gothenburg, Sweden. Br. Med. J. *289*:1257, 1984.)

In women, the deposition of intraabdominal fat constitutes a greater risk for the development of CAD than obesity alone, when studied by a variety of anthropomorphic measurements: total body fat mass index, fat distribution (using waist-hip ratios), computed tomography, and subscapular-triceps skin fold ratios.[214] In women, body mass index and measurement of fasting levels of insulin are found to be strongly associated with CAD risk. The association is stronger for these variables than 2-hour postprandial glucose or insulin levels.[215] The positive association in women between the incidence of MI, angina, and stroke is linked to the waist-hip circumference ratio. This correlation is independent of age, smoking, serum cholesterol, systolic blood pressure, triglycerides, or body mass index.[211] Thus, a masculine distribution of adipose tissue increases CAD risk in both men and women. The waist-hip ratio appears to be a more significant predictor than the total degree of obesity. Although the role of obesity in the development of atherosclerotic complications is complex and remains controversial, obesity is associated with other cardiac risk factors and may increase the total risk in these patients. Hence, weight reduction should be encouraged in patients who have these additional risks. Dietary therapy should be aimed at weight reduction (to approach ideal body weight and to maintain the weight loss) as well as at any associated hyperlipidemia. Alteration of behavioral habits is a key element in the control of obesity. Exercise and other physical activities are adjuncts to weight control.

FAMILY HISTORY AND FAMILIAL AGGREGATION

A variety of studies, both case-control and prospective, point to familial aggregation of CAD. The aggregation of risk factors is well known and includes cholesterol, lipoproteins, blood pressure, diabetes, and obesity. Genetic and environmental influences on coronary risk may be difficult to distinguish.[216] A population predisposition to hypertension or hypercholesterolemia may be determined by its intake of salt, saturated fat, or calories overall. The family at high risk for the development of CAD usually has at least one member who has hyperlipidemia, low HDL, hypertension, a positive family history of coronary disease, or a positive family history of premature CAD. Familial-aggregation studies, genetic studies, and the tracking of blood pressure have yielded evidence that children born to families with a high prevalence of these risk factors also are at risk for development of CAD.[217] Preventive strategies are now available to the pediatrician.[218]

Familial-aggregation studies have included the evaluation of the siblings of patients with documented premature atherosclerosis. In the study by Becker and associates,[219] the siblings were apparently free of clinically evident coronary disease and were examined by questionnaire and interview. This wide-scale screening revealed that 48 per cent of the brothers and 41 per cent of the sisters were hypertensive, and that 45 per cent of the brothers and 22 per cent of the sisters had a lipid abnormality. There were high percentages of cigarette smoking and diabetes. Several risk factors frequently coexisted in the siblings; hence, there is a high degree of modifiable risk factors in first-degree relatives in families of a member affected by premature atherosclerosis. Despite the presence of classic risk factors in families, discriminant analyses evaluating the various risk factors have been unable to classify patients into exact risk groups. Hence, unknown risk variables must mediate the family history of coronary disease, and a positive family history for atherosclerosis should be considered an independent risk factor.[220]

Recent work by Austin and associates[221] has established a mendelian dominant inheritance for the atherogenic lipoprotein pattern associated with small, dense LDL. VLDL, IDL, and small, dense LDL are increased, whereas HDL and HDL_2 are decreased. Kindreds with this pattern may represent what has been called familial combined hyperlipidemia. This disorder may be caused by partial lipase deficiency or by an increase in cholesteryl ester transfer protein.

DIABETES MELLITUS

(See also p. 1842)

Diabetes mellitus is a well-established risk factor for coronary disease.[222] However, problems have arisen in establishing standardized criteria for the diagnosis of diabetes and in comparing the risk inherent in diabetics with that of patients who have glucose intolerance. Also, diabetes frequently coexists with other cardiac risk factors; dyslipidemia and hypertension are increased in prevalence in the diabetic population compared with normals. The definition of diabetes mellitus of the National Diabetes Data Group is given in Table 37-9. The mechanism of coronary events for patients with overt diabetes is multifactorial and may include such factors as increased platelet aggregation. Strict control of glucose intolerance in type II diabetics has been shown to exert a favorable effect on the concentration of adenosine diphosphate and on collagen-induced platelet aggregation. Strict control of diabetes also has been shown to be associated with decreased thromboxane A_2 synthesis, which may play a further role in platelet aggregation in the diabetic patient.[223] Hyperinsulinemia may pose an additional risk in the development of atherosclerosis in patients with both diabetes and glucose intolerance. A number of epidemiological and clinical studies implicate hyperinsulinemia and insulin resistance in an increased frequency of CAD.[224]

Insulin is a growth factor and may stimulate smooth muscle cell proliferation. It has been found to enhance the local synthesis of lipids and the uptake of lipid by smooth muscle cells and fibroblasts,[225] which could enhance the transformation of these cells into foam cells. Epidemiological studies have documented that elevated fasting insulin levels are a predictor for the development of coronary atherosclerosis in nondiabetic patients, independent of other CAD risk factors.[226,226a] In addition, postprandial elevations of circulating insulin also play a role in increased coronary risk. Hypertension and obesity also have been found to be associated with diabetes and glucose intolerance. The frequency of hypertension is about doubled in patients with altered glucose tolerance.[226b]

The Framingham Study found diabetes to be a major risk for CAD, on the basis of a fasting glucose over 120 mg/dl or a blood glucose greater than 160 mg/dl at 1 hour and of more than 110 mg/dl at 2 hours after an oral glucose load.[227] This rather liberal definition of glucose intolerance probably contributed to inconsistencies in reports of various international studies relating hyperglycemia to CAD. Frank diabetes occurs in 2 per cent to 6 per cent of the general population, and

TABLE 37-9 CRITERIA FOR DIABETES AND GLUCOSE INTOLERANCE IN NONPREGNANT ADULTS

DIABETES MELLITUS
(Type I = Insulin-dependent; Type II = Non-insulin-dependent)
Fasting plasma glucose ≥ 140 mg/dl
Sustained elevated plasma glucose levels during the OGTT
Two hour ≥ 200 mg/dl
One other value between 0 and 2 hours ≥ 200 mg/dl
Classic symptoms of diabetes with unequivocal elevation of plasma glucose
IMPAIRED GLUCOSE TOLERANCE (OGTT)
Fasting plasma glucose <140 mg/dl
One value between 0 and 2 hours ≥ 200 mg/dl
Two hour = 140-199 mg/dl

From Kaplan, N. M.: Diabetes and glucose intolerance. *In* Kaplan, N. M., and Stamler, J. (eds.): Prevention of Coronary Heart Disease: Practical Management of the Risk Factors. Philadelphia, W. B. Saunders Company, 1983, p. 114. Reproduced from the National Diabetes Data Group: Classification and diagnosis of diabetes mellitus and other categories of glucose intolerance. Diabetes 28:1039, 1979.

OGTT = Oral glucose tolerance test.

impaired glucose tolerance may occur in up to 20 per cent, depending on the level of glucose used for the diagnosis.[228] However, overt diabetes develops in less than 5 per cent of patients with moderate glucose intolerance, defined by plasma glucose of 140 to 199 mg/dl 2 hours after an oral glucose load. Hence, the use of more conservative criteria to diagnose apparent glucose intolerance may alter epidemiological findings.

In overt diabetes, the mortality associated with coronary atherosclerosis is definitely increased. In the First National Health and Nutrition Examination Survey (NAHANES I), the age-adjusted death rates for diabetic men and women were twice those seen in nondiabetics.[229] Seventy-five per cent of the excess mortality among diabetic men was due to CAD. However, the risk of ischemic heart disease in patients with asymptomatic impairment of glucose tolerance is not clear. In a multivariate analysis of 15 studies, the International Collaborative Group raised the issue of absolute asymptomatic hyperglycemia, especially in combination with other risk factors such as hypertension, smoking, and hypercholesterolemia.[230] The relation between CAD risk and hyperinsulinemia is a consistent finding. As further studies implicating a role for hyperinsulinemia accumulate, more sophisticated analysis may further establish the relationship of glucose intolerance, insulin resistance, and hypertension.

Control of hypertension is particularly important in protecting against microvascular diabetic complications in the eye and kidney. Formation of glycosylated LDL has been suggested as a potential predisposing factor to macrovascular disease.[231] We do not yet know whether maintaining normal glucose levels will reduce the macrovascular or atherosclerotic complications in diabetics. In type II diabetes, weight control has been shown to improve glucose control, lipid abnormalities, and other CAD risk factors. Weight loss with normalization of glucose enhances the activity of lipoprotein lipase, with reduction of VLDL and an increase in HDL levels. Weight loss also augments control of the glucose level in patients with impaired glucose tolerance.[232]

Smoking should be discontinued and hypertension controlled in the diabetic. Drugs that adversely affect glucose tolerance, such as diuretics in high doses, should be avoided. Captopril, a sulfhydryl-containing angiotensin-converting enzyme inhibitor, has recently been shown to alter favorably the insulin and glucose relation in the treatment of hypertension.[233] The value of strict control of blood glucose as regards long-term vascular complications in diabetes has been controversial. However, a consensus exists that microangiopathy affecting the retina and kidney is reduced by maintaining more normal levels of glucose. Patients receiving a diuretic have increased insulin resistance.[233,234] Insulin resistance decreases lipoprotein lipase levels, which leads to an increase in remnant lipoproteins. It also may lead to increased lipolysis in adipose tissue, increased free fatty acid flux to the liver, and enhanced triglycerides and VLDL secretion.

OTHER INFLUENCES

PSYCHOSOCIAL AND BEHAVIORAL FACTORS

Many investigators have hypothesized that psychosocial factors play an important role in the incidence of CAD in Western society. The mechanisms of many psychosocial factors, such as stress, are not well delineated. Six prospective and many case-control studies have assessed for any correlation of depression, anxiety, and neuroticism with CAD.[235] These studies report consistently that emotional distress precedes the development of the symptoms of CAD. However, it has been difficult to define a statistical relation between MI and stress. The largest prospective study, involving Swedish construction workers, showed a statistically significant relation between emotional factors and acute MI.[235]

The means by which chronic emotional distress would accelerate CAD have not been established, but mechanisms could include an imbalance between sympathetic- and parasympathetic-mediated release of catecholamines and acute increases in blood pressure. Several epidemiological studies have shown an inverse statistical relation of blood pressure and cigarette usage to educational level. There also appears to be, in general, an inverse correlation between educational level and both age-adjusted mortality from CAD and all-causes mortality, explained at least in part by shifts in exposure to (known) CAD risk factors as educational attainment increases.[236] Neither risk factor modification nor the decreases in the MI rates have been uniform across all socioeconomic groups. The higher the level of education and socioeconomic status, the greater the modification in life style, including adherence to a low-fat diet, and subsequent decline in the incidence of CAD.[237] Although such observations do not establish causality, the great challenge to the U.S. health care industry is to ensure that such changes are introduced in and adopted by all levels of society.

STRESS IN OCCUPATION. Job-related factors that appear to influence the induction or exacerbation of CAD include perceived job stress, role ambiguity, job autonomy, job change, unemployment, and retirement.[238] However, such causality is controversial, and several studies have revealed little statistical impact of occupational stress on cardiovascular morbidity and mortality. When stress was present, its demonstrable impact was believed to be weak.[239] The Honolulu Heart Study was unable to support the hypothesis that men in high-stress occupations have an enhanced risk of developing CAD. In this large-scale study involving more than 8000 men, there were no significant associations between the presence of CAD and individual job demands or low autonomy in the workplace.[240]

In a case-control study using death certificate verification derived from several geographical locations, the rates of acute MI and ischemic heart disease mortality were analyzed in police officers.[241] The authors proposed that the decreasing risk documented with increased age suggests that removal of stress at the time of retirement lowers the incidence of CAD. Various methodological problems exist in studies that attempt to correlate stress in the workplace and the development or exacerbation of CAD. This is especially pronounced in the assessment of the effect of blood pressure and its relation to job-induced stress. Random blood pressure measurements have a high potential for measurement error in addition to biological variability. This problem is compounded when a correlation is attempted with the assessment of stress. Blood pressure measurement has been improved with the availability of ambulatory monitoring, which increases the number of readings and minimizes interobserver variation. One study[242] weighed job-stimulated stress, as defined by high psychosocial demands associated with low decision latitude, against echocardiographically determined left ventricular mass and ambulatory blood pressure recordings. Multivariate analysis with control for age, race, body mass index, type A personality, 24-hour sodium excretion, education, alcohol consumption, and smoking showed a correlation between job strain and both hypertension and left ventricular mass index. Hence, job strain may predispose to left ventricular hypertrophy. Although not correlated with clinical events in this study, increased left ventricular mass has been linked in a number of epidemiological studies (e.g., Framingham Study[243]) to a variety of adverse cardiac outcomes, including stroke and CAD.

STRESS AND TYPE A PERSONALITY. The role of type A personality in the predisposition to CAD remains controversial. Type A people are characterized as highly competitive, ambitious, and in a constant struggle with their environment, in contradistinction to the type B personality, defined by greater passivity and less disturbance by environmental stress. The correlation of type A personality to CAD has been evaluated in several large studies, including the Framingham Study, in which type A behavior patterns were associated with a twofold increase in the development of angina pectoris.[244] However, there did not appear to be a translation into subsequent increases in fatal coronary events. The increased rate of stable angina among the subjects with type A personality traits could not be explained by the presence of other cardiac risk factors, such as diabetes, or by the presence of behavioral status, such as cigarette smoking or excessive alcohol intake. In addition, a high rate of silent MI occurs in type A subjects as assessed by exercise electrocardiography, with ST shifts as the basis for the diagnosis of total ischemic burden. Other studies have shown increased episodes of painful ischemia in type A people when compared with type B people with an equivalent ischemic burden.[245] More episodes of painful ischemia would seem to make seeking medical attention more likely, leading to treatment and thus introducing bias into a long-term study.

The Western Collaborative Group Study showed that type A men had more than twice the prevalence of CAD as type B men.[246] Interestingly, long-term survival data from this study revealed that the rate of sudden cardiac death did not relate to personality type (A versus B). However, among patients who survived at least 24 hours after a cardiac event, there appeared to be a protective benefit in the type A description: men with type A traits had a death rate of 19.1 per 1000 person-years (mean follow-up, 12.7 years), compared with 31.7 deaths per 1000 person-years in the type B group (mean follow-up, 11.5 years). This difference in mortality persisted after multivariate analysis for other cardiac risk factors.[247] Interpretation of the mortality data remains highly controversial, since other studies showed no effect or an inverse relation of type A personality to morbidity and mortality from CAD.[248,249]

The mechanism by which type A personality traits could influence atherogenesis is unclear. It is doubtless not a single mechanism. Stress may increase the risk imparted by traditional factors, and this process may be modulated by personal response. A rise in blood pressure might be expected to result from excess adrenergic output. Some studies have shown an increased adrenergic receptor density in the healthy offspring of parents with documented premature CAD and type A behavior. The pattern of receptor-density alteration was believed to be compatible with increased peripheral alpha-adrenergic receptor activity and potentially with increased coronary arterial vasoconstriction.[250] Lipid values are altered in people under stress, but this has not been conclusively shown to add to overall cardiac risk.[251] Type A people react differently even to nonstressful situations. Hence, although stress may play a role in the modification of risk factors, the effect of stress alone appears to be relatively minor and would not totally explain the epidemiologically documented risk.

Stress management has been advocated for primary and secondary prevention of CAD and has been shown to decrease reaction to anxiety-provoking situations. In particular, with an impetus from behavioral counseling, it may have a positive impact on the patient at risk for coronary disease.[252]

ESTROGENS AND GENDER

(See also p. 832)

The dictum that women have a lower incidence of CAD than men is a function of the age group examined. CAD is much less common in premenopausal women than in age-matched men, the difference most pronounced between ages 35 and 44. The purported protection of women from CAD becomes much less evident in their postmenopausal years, when the CAD rates for men and women begin to converge. The process of atherosclerosis does not appear to differ between men and women, and the risk factors correlated with the development of CAD appear to affect both sexes equally.

The presumption is that the differences in prevalence rates of coronary atherosclerosis between men and women are a function of the relative differences in estrogen and androgenic hormones. At puberty, circulating levels of testosterone increase in males and estrogen production increases in females. HDL levels are approximately equivalent in males and females until puberty, when they drop in the male as a result of the androgenic effect of testosterone. The greatest effect is in the HDL_2 fraction. According to the Framingham Study, the total cholesterol–HDL ratio estimates the net effect of the "two-way traffic" of cholesterol in and out of the tissues. When this ratio exceeds 7.5 in women, they have the same CAD risk as men. The Framingham data also implicate the triglyceride concentration as an independent risk factor in older women.[253]

Determining the causes of the changes in CAD rates in postmenopausal women is difficult because of the complexity of factors. The Framingham Study did not show an effect of change in life style, thus implicating an alteration in reproductive physiology.

Natural menopause has not been documented to alter glucose tolerance, insulin levels, or blood pressure. In women who undergo natural menopause, serum levels of HDL gradually decline and total serum cholesterol and LDL levels gradually rise; that is, the lipid profile changes in a way that would predispose to atherosclerosis.[254] These lipid changes are favorably altered by hormone-replacement therapy (estrogens). Postmenopausal women also have been shown to have increased levels of circulating small, dense LDL particles, which may further increase their risk for the development of atherosclerosis.[255] Case-control studies revealed a significant benefit as regards severity of angiographically demonstrable coronary atherosclerosis in women receiving estrogen in the postmenopausal period. This protective effect was independent of other variables.[256] The roles that hormone-replacement therapy and gender play in the subsequent development of coronary atherosclerosis remain controversial[257]; the bulk of evidence favors hormone replacement therapy in the form of estrogen in postmenopausal women.

The effect of oral contraceptives is more complex, since these prescriptions contain both estrogen and progesterone in varying quantities. Progesterone analogs decrease both triglyceride and HDL levels. The progestational agents were added to the estrogen therapy, both in oral contraceptives and in replacement therapy, to decrease the risk of endometrial and breast cancer. The effect of this addition on the development of CAD needs further clarification.[258,259] The estrogen and progesterone doses in oral contraceptive pills are generally low, and the impact on cardiac risk depends on their relative concentrations. The nontestosterone agents are especially potent in reducing HDL levels. However, as mentioned, estrogen increases HDL and triglycerides and decreases LDL levels. The study by Mann and colleagues[260] was one of the first to demonstrate an increased associated risk of acute MI with the use of oral contraceptives. The relative risk in oral contraceptive users was estimated to be 4.5 compared with nonusers. The impact on risk of the use of oral contraceptives appears to be increased by the concomitant use of tobacco products. However, recent studies have provided conflicting data on the risk of oral contraceptive agents and subsequent development of atherosclerosis. In the Nurses' Health Study, about 120,000 women, ages 30 to 55, were prospectively evaluated for cardiovascular disease for 8 years. There appeared to be no increased risk for cardiovascular disease according to past use of oral contraceptives, despite prolonged use among a few participants. Past use also did not correlate on multivariate analysis with any material increase in risk for atherosclerosis.[261,262]

Estrogen and progesterone use should be addressed on an individual basis. For women at risk of thromboembolic disease who have associated risk factors such as hypertension or tobacco use, hormone replacement therapy should be addressed in light of the potential risk–benefit ratio.

ALCOHOL

Excessive ingestion of alcohol is an established preventable cause of morbidity and mortality. The effects of alcohol on the

TABLE 37-10 CASE-CONTROL STUDIES OF ALCOHOL CONSUMPTION AND CORONARY ARTERY DISEASE

STUDY	SIZE OF POPULATION	LEVEL OF CONSUMPTION	RELATIVE RISK DRINKERS : NONDRINKERS
Klatsky et al. 1974	661 cases*	≤2 drinks/day	0.7
	661 controls	3–5 drinks/day	0.7
		6+ drinks/day	0.4
Stason et al. 1976	399 cases†	<6 drinks/day	1.0
	2486 controls	6+ drinks/day	0.6
Hennekens et al. 1978	568 cases‡	≤2 oz alcohol/day	0.4
		>2 oz alcohol/day	0.7
Petitti et al. 1979	Not given†	Any	0.3
Rosenberg et al. 1981	513 cases†	Any	0.7
	918 controls		

From Hennekens, C. H.: Alcohol. *In* Kaplan, N. M., and Stamler, J. (eds.): Prevention of Coronary Heart Disease: Practical Management of the Risk Factors. Philadelphia, W. B. Saunders Company, 1983, p. 132.

* Both fatal and nonfatal.
† Nonfatal.
‡ Fatal.

cardiovascular system are highly complex[262a]; alteration of cardiovascular function occurs by both primary and secondary mechanisms. Alcohol may be associated with a primary dilated cardiomyopathy in the absence of coronary atherosclerosis. The acute and chronic effects of ethanol on the cardiovascular system are variable, and epidemiological studies often are flawed by lack of control of other, coexisting risk factors. It is well established that excessive alcohol use is associated with high blood pressure.[263] However, it is not clear that alcohol intake of a moderate degree has a positive correlation with either total or CAD mortality. Multiple studies have demonstrated an inverse correlation between moderate alcohol consumption and subsequent cardiac events.[264]

The protective role that has been attributed to alcohol by some investigators has not been definitely established. Alcohol does raise HDL levels, although the specific subfraction (HDL_2, HDL_3, or a combined increase) involved has varied.[265] Low-dose alcohol (defined as one beverage per day) prospectively compared with abstention over an 8-week period increased apo A-I levels by 9 mg/dl and apo A-I–apo B ratios. But whether such lipid changes correlate with decreased prevalence or extent of CAD has not been established.

The epidemiological association between alcohol intake and CAD has been examined in a variety of large *case-control* studies (Table 37–10). There appears to be an inverse correlation between the daily consumption of small to moderate amounts of alcohol and coronary atherosclerosis. Of the five major *prospective* studies, four showed an inverse relationship to the incidence of CAD with mild to moderate alcohol use.[266] The Framingham Study assigned a relative risk of 0.7 to subjects consuming at least 30 oz of alcohol per month, the comparison with those drinking less.[267]

In other large epidemiological studies, light drinkers had a lower overall mortality rate than did heavy drinkers or nondrinkers. There remain many unanswered questions about the relationship of alcohol intake to coronary atherosclerosis. Overt CAD has been shown to be inversely related to moderate alcohol consumption, as has been the anatomical degree of atherosclerosis.[268–270] However, overt CAD correlated significantly with alcoholism. Also, heavy alcohol intake has been positively associated with prevalence of acute MI. This correlation was confirmed after control for tobacco usage and severity of underlying atherosclerosis, perhaps signifying a destabilizing effect by alcohol intake on the atherosclerotic plaque. Despite the inverse correlation of coronary mortality and moderate alcohol intake, other studies have shown associated problems of alcohol abuse to contribute to an increase in overall mortality. The authors currently do not recommend that patients consume alcohol as a preventive measure.

MINOR RISK FACTORS

A number of minor risk factors have also been implicated in the genesis of coronary atherosclerosis, notably certain trace elements, water hardness, hypercalcemia, hypercoagulability, vasectomy, coffee consumption, and hyperuricemia. In none of these categories is an effect fully documented or completely understood.

TRACE ELEMENTS. In the zinc/copper hypothesis, Klevay proposes that a deficiency of copper, or an excess of zinc, predisposes to secondary hypercholesterolemia, to result in coronary atherosclerosis.[271,272]

WATER HARDNESS. Both Leoni and coworkers[273] and Crawford and colleagues[274] in large studies found cardiovascular mortality to correlate inversely with water hardness. Unfortunately, in no such study has protection or risk clearly been linked to specific components in the water. Selenium and zinc have been described as protective, and lead and calcium as conferring increased risk, with magnesium variously placed in both categories. The inconsistency of the findings precludes any definite conclusions about CAD risk in relation to water hardness.

HYPERCALCEMIA. Calcium overload in the arterial wall may play a role in the pathogenesis of atherosclerosis. Intracellular calcium accumulation may increase vascular tone and enhance cholesterol accumulation and atherosclerotic plaque formation. The affinity of the arterial wall for calcium increases with age. Calcium antagonists such as verapamil, diltiazem, and nifedipine can inhibit experimental atherogenesis. Nifedipine has been reported in one clinical trial to decrease new coronary lesion formation.[275,276]

HYPERCOAGULABILITY[276a] (see also Chap. 58). Epidemiological studies, including the Framingham Study,[142] have shown a strong correlation between fibrinogen concentration and CAD risk.[277,277a] Indeed, this correlation is comparable in statistical strength to the classic CAD risk factors. Fibrinogen is positively associated with concentrations of cholesterol and triglycerides, and thus linked with hyperlipidemia. It correlates as well with smoking, obesity, and socioeconomic stress. Also, factor VII is positively correlated with hyperlipidemia, especially with elevated triglycerides. Because more than 90 per cent of patients with MI exhibit coronary thrombosis, one might expect high levels of fibrinogen to predispose to thrombotic events. But whether levels of fibrinogen and factor VII relate exclusively to the thrombotic process involved in coronary disease or play an accessory role in atherogenesis is not known. Fibrinogen has been statistically associated with the severity of angiographically determined CAD.[278] Fibrinogen remains significantly associated with the severity of coronary atherosclerosis in a progressive manner, even when adjustment is made for age, hypertension, dyslipidemia, cigarette smoking, and body mass index.[142,279]

Early on, researchers postulated that fibrin contributes to the growth of atherosclerotic plaque. The process may be by the incorporation of a mural thrombus into the intima of an artery. Fibrin can be diffusely or discretely deposited within an atherosclerotic plaque. Thus, it may be argued that the early proliferative plaque arises from a mural fibrin thrombus. All of the clotting factors are present in the intima. Prothrombin is present in the gelatinous atherosclerotic lesion, but the ratio of the antithrombin III inhibitor to prothrombin is 3 : 1.

Some studies have reported a reduction in the activity of antithrombin III with CAD, and many studies have described an apparent direct correlation between fibrinogen and cholesterol levels.[280] The relationship of the lipid profile to clotting mechanisms is complex. High levels of triglycerides have been shown to be associated with inhibitors of fibrinolysis, especially of alpha$_2$ antiplasmin.[281] With its close homology to plasminogen, Lp(a) at high concentrations might participate in the inhibition of thrombolysis, but this possibility remains to be explored. Split fibrin products have been demonstrated within the intima and exert potentially toxic effects, including chemotaxis and alteration of vascular permeability. Fibrin deposition in the vessel wall may be associated with the trapping of LDL. It has been shown that the intima contains not only extractable soluble LDL, but also an insoluble apo B-containing substance that remains in the tissues, some of which might be Lp(a).[282] This lighter substance can be released by pretreatment with plasminogen.

Platelet aggregation is believed to play a major role in atherogenesis. The role of antiplatelet therapy in the treatment of unstable angina and other acute ischemic syndromes has been well described (p. 1233).[283,284] Platelet aggregation is enhanced in patients with established coronary atherosclerosis.[285] The role of aspirin in the primary prevention of acute MI has recently been tested in the Physicians' Health Study,[286] in which the subjects were physicians. Aspirin prophylaxis (325 mg every other day) yielded a 44 per cent reduction in the risk of MI. The benefits of aspirin were significant for both fatal and nonfatal MI, and the MI benefit was apparent only in subjects 50 years of age or older. No reduction in overall mortality from cardiovasclar disease was established.

VASECTOMY. The subject of a correlation between vasectomy and nonfatal MI is controversial. In studies in nonhuman primates, vasectomy increased the severity of diet-induced atherosclerosis.[287] However, various investigators observed no excess risk for MI and no increase in the prevalence of hypertension or hypercholesterolemia in men who had undergone vasectomy. Moreover, epidemiological studies have shown no clear relation between vasectomy and coronary events. Finally, recent long-term studies have failed to indicate an association between the presence of sperm autoimmunization and the development of atherosclerosis.[288,289]

COFFEE CONSUMPTION. Epidemiological studies have not yet clarified whether coffee consumption is a risk factor for CAD. A recent Framingham multivariate analysis assessed survey data on coffee consumption in relation to age, systolic pressure, body mass index, and total cholesterol with regard to impact on CAD.[290] The analysis did not show an association between coffee consumption and the presence of atherosclerosis. Moreover, there was no demonstrable relationship between coffee intake and subsequent CAD events in patients with known CAD. The effects of coffee intake on lipids were gender dependent: an inverse correlation with total cholesterol and with LDL cholesterol in men, and a positive correlation with each of these lipid values in women.

HYPERURICEMIA. Several studies have shown a statistical association between elevated levels of uric acid and hypertriglyceridemia. The Framingham Study found that the concentration of uric acid also correlated with both systolic and diastolic blood pressure values.[291] Although uric acid was a predictor of MI in the Framingham cohort, on multivariate analysis—which included age, systolic blood pressure, relative weight, cigarette smoking, and serum cholesterol—serum uric acid was not an independent CAD predictor. Instead, hyperuricemia appeared to be a marker of metabolic disturbances that predispose to CAD.

ATHEROSCLEROSIS AFTER CARDIAC TRANSPLANTATION (see also p. 1352). For cardiac transplant patients, the advent of improved immunosuppressive agents has lowered the rates of morbidity and mortality due to acute rejection of the donor heart. However, accelerated atherosclerosis has emerged as a major problem affecting long-term post-transplant survival.[292] Chronic immune injury caused by the presence of cytotoxic B-cell antibodies and/or alterations of the lipid profile may play a role in transplant-associated atherosclerosis.[293] Cyclosporine has been shown to decrease LDL-receptor activity and thus to worsen the patient's lipid profile by increasing total and LDL cholesterol levels and by lowering HDL levels. Higher donor age and elevated plasma triglycerides also have been associated with atherosclerotic development in the donor heart.[294] Although logical on causative grounds, episodes of rejection or human leukocyte antigen mismatches have not been clearly shown to play a major role in transplant atherosclerosis. Moreover, several recent studies have shown no correlation of the level of maintenance steroids, the fasting blood sugar value, or the number of rejection episodes with the development of atherosclerosis in the donor heart.

REFERENCES

DECLINING MORTALITY OF CAD

1. American Heart Association. 1991 Heart and Stroke Facts. Dallas, American Heart Association, 1991.
2. Stern, M. P.: The recent decline in ischemic heart disease mortality. Ann. Intern. Med. *91*:630, 1979.

2a. Goldman, L., and Cook, E. F.: The decline in ischemic heart disease mortality rates: An analysis of the comparative effects of medical interventions and changes in lifestyle. Ann. Intern. Med. *101*:825, 1984.

DYSLIPIDEMIA

3. Austin, M. A., Breslow, J. L., Hennekens, C. H., et al.: Low-density lipoprotein subclass patterns and risk of myocardial infarction. JAMA *260*:1917, 1988.
4. Goldstein, J. L., and Brown, M. S.: Atherosclerosis: The low-density lipoprotein receptor hypothesis. Metabolism *26*:1257, 1977.
5. Teng, B., Sniderman, A. D., Soutar, A. K., and Thompson, G. R.: Metabolic basis of hyperapobetalipoproteinemia. Turnover of apolipoprotein B in low density lipoprotein and its precursors and subfractions compared with normal and familial hypercholesterolemia. J. Clin. Invest. *77*:663, 1986.
6. Kwiterovich, P. O., Jr., White, S., Forte, T., et al.: Hyperapobetalipoproteinemia in a kindred with familial combined hyperlipidemia and familial hypercholesterolemia. Arteriosclerosis *7*:211, 1987.
7. Miller, N. E.: Association of high density lipoprotein subclasses and apolipoprotein with ischemic heart disease and coronary atherosclerosis [Review]. Am. Heart J. *113*:589, 1987.
8. Oram, J. F., Brinton, E. A., and Bierman, E. L.: Regulation of high-density lipoprotein receptor activity in cultured human skin fibroblasts and human arterial smooth muscle cells. J. Clin. Invest. *72*:1611, 1983.
9. Gordon, D. J., and Rifkind, B. M.: High density lipoprotein. The clinical implication of recent studies [Review]. N. Engl. J. Med. *321*:1311, 1989.
10. Armstrong, V. W., Cremer, P., Eberle, P., et al.: The association between serum Lp(a) concentrations and angiography assessed coronary atherosclerosis: Dependence on serum LDL levels. Atherosclerosis *62*:249, 1986.
11. Dahlen, G. H., Guyton, J. R., Attar, M., et al.: Association of levels of Lp(a), plasma lipids, and other lipoproteins with coronary artery disease documented by angiography. Circulation *74*:758, 1986.

11a. Genest, J., Jr., Jenner, J. L., McNamara, J. R., et al.: Prevalence of lipoprotein (a) [Lp(a)] excess in coronary artery disease. Am. J. Cardiol. *67*:1039, 1991.

11b. Solymoss, B. C., Marcil, M., Lesperance, J., et al.: Lp(a) is related to complete obstruction of coronary arteries in men and to partial as well as complete obstruction in women. J. Am. Coll. Cardiol. *17*:62A, 1991.

12. Eaton, D. L., Fless, G. M., and Kohn, W. J.: Partial amino acid sequence of apolipoprotein(a) shows that it is homologous to plasminogen. Proc. Natl. Acad. Sci. USA *84*:3224, 1987.
13. Gurakar, A., Hoeg, J. M., Kostner, G., et al.: Levels of Lp(a) decline with neomycin and niacin treatment. Atherosclerosis *57*:293, 1985.
14. Albers, J. J., Taggart, H. M., Applebaum-Bowden, D., et al.: Reduction of lecithin-cholesterol acyltransferase, apolipoprotein D, and the Lp(a) lipoprotein with the anabolic steroid stanozolol. Biochim. Biophys. Acta *795*:293, 1984.
15. Kottke, B. A., Zinsmeister, A. R., Holmes, D. R., Jr., et al.: Apolipoproteins and coronary artery disease. Mayo Clin. Proc. *61*:313, 1986.
16. Gotto, A. M., Pownall, H. R., and Havel, R. J.: Introduction to the plasma lipoproteins: Methods [Review]. Methods Enzymol. *128*:3, 1986.
17. Michals, W. C., Duvulet, F. E., and Benson, M.: Apolipoprotein A-I in Iowa type hereditary amyloidosis. Clin. Res. *35*:595A, 1987.
18. Karathanasis, S. K., Ferris, E., and Haddad, I. A.: DNA inversion within the apolipoprotein A-I/C-III/A-IV encoding gene cluster of certain patients with premature atherosclerosis. Proc. Natl. Acad. Sci. USA *89*:7198, 1987.
19. Schaefer, E. J., Ordovas, J. M., Law, S. W., et al.: Familial apolipoprotein A-I and C-III deficiency, variant II. J. Lipid Res. *26*:1089, 1985.
20. Higuchi, K., Monge, J. C., Lee, N., et al.: The human apo B-100 gene: Apo B-100 is encoded by a single copy gene in the human genome. Biochem. Biophys. Res. Commun. *144*:1332, 1987.
21. Chen, S. H., Yang, C. Y., and Chen, P. F.: The completed cDNA and amino acid sequence of human apolipoprotein B-100. J. Biol. Chem. *261*:12918, 1986.
22. Higuchi, K., Hospattankar, I. V., Law, S. W., et al.: Human (apolipoprotein B) mRNA: Identification of two distinct apo B mRNAs, an mRNA with the apoB-100 mRNA containing a premature w-frame translational stop codon in both liver and intestine. Proc. Natl. Acad. Sci. USA *85*:1772, 1988.
23. Mahley, R. W.: Atherogenic lipoproteins and coronary artery disease: Concepts derived from recent advances in cellular and molecular biology. Circulation *72*:943, 1985.
24. Lenzen, H. J., Assmann, G., Buchwalsky, R., and Schulte, H.: Association of apolipoprotein E polymorphism, low-density lipoprotein cholesterol, and coronary artery disease. Clin. Chem. *32*:778, 1986.
25. Kesaniemi, Y. A., Ehnolm, C., and Miettinen, T. A.: Intestinal cholesterol absorption efficiency in man is related to apoprotein E phenotype. J. Clin. Invest. *80*:578, 1987.
26. Assmann, G., and Schulte, H.: PROCAM-Studie. Zuerich, Panscientia Verlag, 1986.
27. Assmann, G., Schulte, H., Oberwittler, W., and Hauss, W. H.: New aspects in the prediction of coronary heart disease. In: Fidge, N. H., and Nestel, P. J. (eds). The Prospective Cardiovascular Müenster Study. Atherosclerosis VII. Proceedings of the 7th International Atherosclerosis Symposium. Amsterdam, Elsevier Science Publishers, 1986, p. 19.
28. Kessling, A. M., Berg, K., Mockelby, E., and Humphries, S. E.: DNA polymorphisms around the apo A-I gene in normal and hyperlipidemic individuals selected for a twin study. Clin. Genet. *29*:485, 1986.

29. Scott, J., Knott, T. J., Priestley, L. M., et al.: High-density lipoprotein composition is altered by a common DNA polymorphism adjacent to apo A-II gene in man. Lancet *1*:771, 1985.
30. Seilhamer, J. J., Protter, A. A., Frossard, P., and Levy-Wilson, B.: Isolation and DNA sequence of full-length cDNA and of the entire gene for human apolipoprotein AI—discovery of a new genetic polymorphism in the apo AI gene. DNA *3*:309, 1984.
31. Ordovas, J. M., Schaefer, E. J., Salem, D., et al.: Apolipoprotein A-I gene polymorphism associated with premature coronary artery disease and familial hypoalphalipoproteinemia. N. Engl. J. Med. *314*:671, 1986.
32. Fojo, S. S., Law, S. W., and Brewer, H. B., Jr.: The human preproapoprotein C-II gene. Complete nucleic acid sequence and genomic organization. FEBS Lett. *213*:221, 1987.
33. Fojo, S. S., Taam, L., Fairwell, T., et al.: Human preproapolipoprotein C-II: Analysis of major plasma isoforms. J. Biol. Chem. *261*:9591, 1986.
34. Connelly, P. W., Maguire, G. F., Hoffmann, T., and Little, J. A.: Structure of apolipoprotein CII Toronto, a nonfunctional human apolipoprotein. Proc. Natl. Acad. Sci. USA *84*:270, 1987.
34a. Young, S. G., and Linton, M. F.: Genetic abnormalities in apolipoprotein B. Trends Cardiovasc. Med. *1*:59, 1991.
35. Blackhart, B. D., Ludwig, E. M., Pierotti, V. R., et al.: Structure of the human apolipoprotein B gene. J. Biol. Chem. *261*:15364, 1986.
36. Chan, L., Van Tuinen, P., and Gotto, A. M.: The human Apo B-100 gene: A highly polymorphic gene which maps to the short arm of chromosome 2. Biochem. Biophys. Res. Commun. *133*:248, 1985.
37. Lackner, K. J., Monge, J. C., Gregg, R. E., et al.: Analysis of the apolipoprotein B gene and messenger ribonucleic acid in abetalipoproteinemia. J. Clin. Invest. *78*:1707, 1986.

THE LIPID HYPOTHESIS OF ATHEROGENESIS

38. Keys, A. (ed.): Coronary heart disease in seven countries. Circulation *41*(Suppl. 1), 1970.
39. Simons, L. A.: Interrelations of lipids and lipoproteins with coronary artery disease mortality in 19 countries. Am. J. Cardiol. *57*:5G., 1986.
40. Yusuf, S., Wittes, J., and Friedman, L.: Overview of results of randomized clinical traits in heart disease. II. Unstable angina, heart failure, primary prevention with aspirin, and risk factor modification. JAMA *260*:2259, 1988.
41. Rossouw, J. E., Lewis, B., and Rifkind, B. M.: The value of lowering cholesterol after myocardial infarction. N. Engl. J. Med. *323*:1112, 1990.
42. Dayton, S., Pearce, M. L., Hashimoto, S., et al.: A controlled clinical trial of a diet high in unsaturated fat in preventing complications of atherosclerosis. Circulation *40*(Suppl II):1, 1969.
43. Coronary Drug Project Research group: Clofibrate and niacin in coronary heart disease. JAMA *231*:360, 1975.
44. Canner, P. L., Berge, K. G., Wenger, N. K., et al.: Fifteen year mortality in the Coronary Drug Project patients: Long-term benefit with niacin. J. Am. Coll. Cardiol. *8*:1245, 1986.
45. Brensike, J. F., Levy, R. I., and Kelsey, S. F.: Effects of therapy with cholestyramine on progression of coronary arteriosclerosis: Results of the NHLBI Type II Coronary Intervention Study. Circulation *69*:313, 1984.
46. Arntzenius, A. C., Kromhout, D., Barth, J. D., et al.: Diet, lipoproteins, and the progression of coronary atherosclerosis. The Leiden Intervention Trial. N. Engl. J. Med. *312*:805, 1985.
47. Committee of Principal Investigators: A cooperative trial in the primary prevention of ischemic heart disease using clofibrate. Br. Heart J. *40*:1069, 1978.
48. Committee of Principal Investigators: WHO cooperative trial on primary prevention of ischemic heart disease with clofibrate to lower serum cholesterol: Final mortality follow-up. Lancet *2*:600, 1984.
49. Hjermann, I., Velve-Byre, K., Holme, I., and Leren, P.: Effect of diet and smoking on the incidence of coronary heart disease: Report from the Oslo Study Group of a randomized trial in healthy men. Lancet *2*:1303, 1981.
50. Hjermann, I., Holme, I., and Leren, P.: Oslo Study, Diet and Antismoking Trial: Results after 102 months. Am. J. Med. *80*(Suppl 2A):7, 1986.
51. Multiple Risk Factor Intervention Trial Research Group: Multiple Risk Factor Intervention Trial: Risk factor changes and mortality results. JAMA *248*:1465, 1982.
52. Multiple Risk Factor Intervention Trial Research Group: Mortality rates after 10.5 years for participants in the Multiple Risk Factor Intervention Trial. Findings related to a priori hypotheses of the trial. JAMA *263*:1795, 1990.
53. Lipid Research Clinics Program: The Lipid Research Clinics' Coronary Primary Prevention Trial results. I. Reduction in incidence of coronary heart disease. II. The relationship of reduction in incidence of coronary heart disease to cholesterol lowering. JAMA *251*:351, 1984.
54. Manninen, V., Elo, M. O., and Frick, L.: Lipid alterations and decline in the incidence of coronary heart disease in the Helsinki Heart Study. JAMA *260*:641, 1988.
55. Austin, M. A.: Epidemiologic association between hypertriglyceridemia and coronary heart disease. Semin. Thromb. Haemost. *14*:137, 1988.
56. Carlson, L. A., and Bottiger, L. E.: Risk factors for ischemic heart disease in men and women. Results of the 19-year follow-up of the Stockholm Prospective Study. Acta Med. Scand. *218*:207, 1985.
57. Blankenhorn, D. H., Alaupovic, P., Wickham, E., et al.: Prediction of angiographic change in native human coronary arteries and aortocoronary bypass grafts. Lipid and nonlipid factors. Circulation *81*:470, 1990.
58. Kaplan, N. M.: The deadly quartet: upper body obesity, glucose intolerance, hypertriglyceridemia, and hypertension. Arch. Intern. Med. *149*:1514, 1989.
59. Phillips, N. R., Havel, R. J., and Kane, J. P.: Levels and interrelationships of serum and lipoprotein cholesterol and triglycerides. Arteriosclerosis *1*:13, 1981.
60. Havel, R. J.: Role of triglyceride-rich lipoproteins in progression of atherosclerosis. (comment). Circulation *81*:694, 1990.
61. Consensus Conference: Treatment of hypertriglyceridemia. JAMA *251*:1196, 1984.
62. Newman, W. P., III, Freedman, D. S., Voors, A. W., et al.: Relation of serum lipoprotein levels and systolic blood pressure to early atherosclerosis. The Bogalusa Heart Study. N. Engl. J. Med. *314*:138, 1986.
63. Cabin, H. S., and Roberts, W. C.: Relation of serum total cholesterol and triglyceride levels to the amount and extent of coronary arterial narrowing by atherosclerotic plaque in coronary heart disease. Quantitative analysis of 2,037 five mm segments of 160 major epicardial coronary arteries in 40 necropsy patients. Am. J. Med. *73*:227, 1982.
64. Levy, R. I., Brensike, J. F., Epstein, S. E., et al.: The influence of changes in lipid values induced by cholestyramine and diet on progression of coronary artery disease: Results of the NHLBI Type II Coronary Intervention Study. Circulation *69*:325, 1984.
65. Blankenhorn, D. H., Nessim, S. A., Johnson, R. L., et al.: Beneficial effects of combined colestipol-niacin therapy on coronary atherosclerosis and coronary venous bypass grafts. JAMA *257*:3233, 1987. (Published erratum appears in JAMA *259*:2698, 1988.)
66. Cashin-Hemphill, L., Mack, W. J., Pogoda, J. M., et al.: Beneficial effects of colestipol-niacin on coronary atherosclerosis: A 4-year follow-up. JAMA *264*:3013, 1990.
67. Brown, G., Albers, J. J., Fisher, L. D., et al.: Regression of coronary artery disease as a result of intensive lipid-lowering therapy in men with high levels of apolipoprotein B. N. Engl. J. Med. *323*:1289, 1990.
68. Kane, J. P., Malloy, M. J., Ports, T. A., et al.: Regression of coronary atherosclerosis during treatment of familial hypercholesterolemia with combined drug regimens. JAMA *264*:3007, 1990.
69. Gordon, D. J., Probstfield, J. L., Garrison, R. J., et al.: High-density lipoprotein cholesterol and cardiovascular disease: four prospective American studies. Circulation *79*:8, 1989.
70. The Expert Panel: Report of the National Cholesterol Education Program Expert Panel on detection, evaluation and treatment of high blood cholesterol in adults. Arch. Intern. Med. *148*:36, 1988.
71. National Cholesterol Education Program: Current status of blood cholesterol measurements in clinical laboratories in the U.S.: A report from the Laboratory Standardization Panel of the National Cholesterol Education Program. Clin. Chem. *80*:193, 1988.
72. Goodman, D. S., Bradford, R. H., Brewer, H. B., Jr., et al.: AHA Conference Report on Cholesterol. Diagnosis, evaluation and treatment: Current status and issues [Review]. Circulation *80*:735, 1989.
73. Fredrickson, D. S., and Lees, R. S.: System for phenotyping hyperlipoproteinemia. Circulation *31*:321, 1965.
74. Sparks, R. S., Zollner, S., Klisak, I., et al.: Mapping of loci for lipoprotein lipase to 8p22 and hepatic lipase to 15q21. Genomics *1*:138, 1987.
75. Hayden, M. R., Vergani, C., Humphries, S. E., et al.: The genetics and molecular biology of apolipoprotein C-II [Review]. Adv. Exp. Med. Biol. *201*:241, 1986.
76. Brunzell, J. D., Miller, N. E., Alaupovic, P., et al.: Familial chylomicronemia due to a circulating inhibitor of lipoprotein in lipase activity. J. Lipid Res. *24*:12, 1983.
77. Goldstein, J. L., Brown, M. S., Anderson, R. G., et al.: Receptor-mediated endocytosis: Concepts emerging from the LDL receptor system. Annu. Rev. Cell Biol. *1*:1, 1985.
78. Goldstein, J. L., and Brown, M. S.: Progress in understanding the LDL receptor and HMG-CoA reductase, two membrane proteins that regulated the plasma cholesterol [Review]. J. Lipid Res. *25*:1450, 1984.
79. Steinberg, D., Parthasarathy, S., Carew, T. E., et al.: Beyond cholesterol. Modifications of low-density lipoproteins that increase its atherogenicity [Review]. N. Engl. J. Med. *320*:915, 1989.
80. Cuthbert, J. A., East, C. A., Bilheimer, D. W., and Lipsky, P. E.: Detection of familial hypercholesterolemia by assaying functional low-density lipoprotein receptors on lymphocytes. N. Engl. J. Med. *314*:879, 1986.
81. Hobbs, H. H., Brown, M. S., Russel, D. W., et al.: Deletion in the gene for the low-density lipoprotein receptor in a majority of French Canadians with familial hypercholesterolemia. N. Engl. J. Med. *317*:734, 1987.
82. Morganroth, J., Levy, R. I., and Fredrickson, D. S.: The biochemical, clinical and genetic features of Type III hyperlipoproteinemia. Ann. Intern. Med. *82*:158, 1975.
83. Janus, E. D., Nicoll, A. M., Turner, P. R., et al.: Kinetic basis of the primary hyperlipidemias: Studies of apolipoprotein B turnover in genetically defined subjects. Eur. J. Clin. Invest. *10*:161, 1980.
84. Sniderman, A. D., Wolfson, C., Teng, B., et al.: Association of hyperapobetalipoproteinemia with endogenous hypertriglyceridemia and atherosclerosis. Ann. Intern. Med. *97*:833, 1982.
85. Chait, A., Mancini, M., February, A. W., and Lewis, B.: Clinical and metabolic study of alcoholic hyperlipidemia. Lancet *2*:62, 1972.
86. Sadbank, V., Bechan, M., and Bonnstein, B.: Hyperlipidemia neuropathy. Acta Neuropathol. Berl. *19*:290, 1971.
87. Fallat, R. W., and Glueck, C. J.: Familial and acquired Type V hyperlipoproteinemia. Atherosclerosis *23*:41, 1976.
88. Zilversmit, D. B.: Atherogenesis: A postprandial phenomenon. Circulation *60*:473, 1979.

89. Pollare, T., Lithell, H., and Berne, C.: A comparison of the effects of hydrochlorothiazide and captopril on glucose and lipid metabolism in patients with hypertension. N. Engl. J. Med. *321*:868, 1989.
90. Blankenhorn, D. H., Johnson, R. L., Mack, W. J., et al.: The influence of diet on the appearance of new lesions in human coronary arteries. JAMA *263*:1646, 1990.
91. Ornish, D., Brown, S. E., Scherwitz, L. W., et al.: Can lifestyle changes reverse coronary heart disease? The Lifestyle Heart Trial. Lancet *336*:129, 1990.
92. Gotto, A. M., Jr., Bierman, E. L., Connor, E., et al.: Recommendations for treatment of hyperlipidemia in adults. A joint statement of the Nutrition Committee and the Council on Arteriosclerosis. Circulation *69*:1065A, 1984.
93. Bonanome, A., and Grundy, S. M.: Effect of dietary stearic acid on plasma cholesterol and lipoprotein levels. N. Engl. J. Med. *318*:1244, 1988.
94. Trevisan, M., Krogh, V., Freudenheim, J., et al.: Consumption of olive oil, butter, and vegetable oils and coronary heart disease risk factors. The Research Group ATS-RF2 of the Italian National Research Council. JAMA *263*:688, 1990.
95. Swain, J. F., Rouse, I. L., Curley, C. B., and Sacks, F. M.: Comparison of the effects of oat bran and low-fiber wheat on serum lipoprotein levels and blood pressure. N. Engl. J. Med. *322*:147, 1990.
96. Connor, W. E.: Dietary fiber—nostrum or critical nutrient? N. Engl. J. Med. *322*:193, 1990.
97. Kim, D. N., Ho, H. T., Lawrence, D. A., et al.: Modification of lipoprotein patterns and retardation of atherogenesis by a fish oil supplement to a hyperlipidemic diet for swine. Atherosclerosis *76*:35, 1989.
98. Rogers, S., James, K. S., Butland, B. K., et al.: Effects of a fish oil supplement on serum lipids, blood pressure, bleeding time, hemostatic and rheological variables. A double blind randomized controlled trial in healthy volunteers. Atherosclerosis *63*:137, 1987.
99. Singer, P., Jaeger, W., Wirth, M., et al.: Lipid and blood pressure lowering effect of mackerel diet in man. Atherosclerosis *49*:99, 1983.
100. Zhu, B. Q., and Parmley, W. W. Modification of experimental and clinical atherosclerosis by dietary fish oil. Am. Heart. J. *119*:178, 1990.
101. Schectman, G., Kaul, S., Cherayil, G. D., et al.: Can the hypotriglyceridemic effect of fish oil concentrate be sustained? Ann. Intern. Med. *110*:346, 1989.
102. Glauber, H., Wallace, P., Griver, K., et al.: Adverse metabolic effect of omega-3 fatty acids in non-insulin-dependent diabetes mellitus. Ann. Intern. Med. *108*:663, 1988.
103. Hoeg, J. M., Gregg, R. E., and Brewer, H. B., Jr.: An approach to the management of hyperlipoproteinemia [Review]. JAMA *255*:512, 1986.
104. Levy, R. I.: Drugs used in the treatment of hyperlipoproteinemia. *In* Goodman, A. S., Gilman, A. S., and Gilman, A. (eds.): The Pharmacologic Basis of Therapeutics. New York, Macmillan, 1980, pp. 834–877.
105. Brown, B. G., Lin, J. T., Schaefer, C. A., et al.: Niacin or lovastatin combined with colestipol regress coronary atherosclerosis and prevent clinical events in men with elevated apolipoprotein. Circulation *80*(Suppl. II):II-266, 1989.
106. Grundy, S. M., Mok, H. Y., Zech, L., and Berman, M.: Influence of nicotinic acid on metabolism of cholesterol and triglycerides in man. J. Lipid Res. *22*:24, 1981.
107. Steinberg, D., Parthasarathy, S., and Carew, T. E.: In vivo inhibition of foam cell development by probucol in Watanabe rabbits. Am. J. Cardiol. *62*:6b, 1988.
107a. Tanner, F. C., Noll, G., Boulanger, C. M., and Luscher, T. F.: Oxidized low density lipoproteins inhibit relaxations of porcine coronary arteries. Role of scavenger receptor and endothelium-derived nitric oxide. Circulation *83*:2012, 1991.
107b. Rosenfield, M. E.: Oxidized LDL affects multiple atherogenic cellular responses. Circulation *83*:2137, 1991.
108. Carew, T., Schwenke, W., and Steinberg, D.: Antiatherogenic effect of probucol unrelated to its hypercholesterolemic effect: Evidence that antioxidants in vivo can selectively inhibit low density lipoprotein degradation in macrophage-rich fatty streaks and slow the progression of atherosclerosis in the Watanabe heritable hyperlipidemic rabbit. Proc. Natl. Acad. Sci. USA *84*:7725, 1987.
109. Goldberg, R., and Mendez, A.: Probucol enhances cholesterol efflux from cultured skin fibroblasts. Am. J. Cardiol. *62*:57B, 1988.
110. Aburatani, H., Matsumoto, A., Kodama, T., et al.: Increased levels of messenger ribonucleic acid for apolipoprotein E in the spleen of probucol-treated rabbits. Am. J. Cardiol. *62*:60B, 1988.
111. Witztum, J. L., Simmons, D., Steinberg, D., et al.: Intensive combination drug therapy of familial hypercholesterolemia with lovastatin, probucol and colestipol hydrochloride. Circulation *79*:16, 1989.
112. Erikson, U., Nilsson, S., and Stenport, G.: Probucol Quantitative Regression Swedish Trial: New angiographic technique to measure atheroma volume of the femoral artery. Am. J. Cardiol. *62*:44B, 1988.
113. Walldius, G., Carlson, L. A., Erickson, U., et al.: Development of femoral atherosclerosis in hypercholesterolemic patients during treatment with cholestyramine and probucol/placebo. Probucol Quantitative Regression Swedish Trial (PQRST): A status report. Am. J. Cardiol. *62*:37B, 1988.
114. Sitori, C. R., and Chiero, G.: Effects of lipid lowering agents and other treatment regimens on serum lipoprotein. Current Opinion in Lipidology *1*:262, 1990.
114a. Lupien, P. J., Brun, D., Gagné, C., et al.: Gemfibrozil therapy in primary type II hyperlipoproteinemia: Effects on lipids, lipoproteins and apolipoproteins. Can. J. Cardiol. *7*:27, 1991.
115. Committee of Principal Investigators: WHO cooperative trial of primary prevention of ischaemic heart disease with clofibrate to lower serum cholesterol: Final mortality follow-up. Lancet *2*:600, 184.
116. Mabuchi, H., Sakai, T., Sakai, Y., et al.: Reduction of serum cholesterol in heterozygous patients with familial hypercholesterolemia. Additive effects of compactin and cholestyramine. N. Engl. J. Med. *308*:609, 1983.
117. Bilheimer, D. W., Grundy, S. M., Brown, M. S., and Goldstein, J. L.: Mevinolin and colestipol stimulate receptor mediated clearance of low density lipoprotein from plasma in familial hypercholesterolemia heterozygotes. Proc. Natl. Acad. Sci. USA *80*:4124, 1983.
118. Cuthbert, J. A., and Lipsky, P. E.: Assessment of functional LDL receptor activity on lymphocytes of normal subjects and patients with mild hypercholesterolemia. Trans. Assoc. Am. Physicians *101*:1, 1988.
119. Weintraub, M. S., Eisenberg, S., and Breslow, J. L.: Lovastatin reduces postprandial lipoprotein levels in hypercholesterolemic patients with mild hypertriglycerides. Eur. J. Clin. Invest. *19*:480, 1989.
120. Vega, G. L., and Grundy, S. M.: Comparison of lovastatin and gemfibrozil in normolipidemic patients with hypoalphalipoproteinemia. JAMA *262*:3148, 1989.
121. Kostner, G. M., Gavish, D., Leopold, B., et al.: HMG-CoA reductase inhibitors lower LDL cholesterol without reducing Lp(a) levels. Circulation *80*:1313, 1989.
122. Davi, G., Averna, M., Novo, S., et al.: Effects of synvinolin on platelet aggregation and thromboxane B2 synthesis in type IIa hypercholesterolemic patients. Atherosclerosis *79*:79, 1989.
123. Coronary Drug Project Research Group: The Coronary Drug Project findings leading to further modifications of its protocol with respect to dextrothyroxine. JAMA *220*:996, 1972.
124. Eckel, R. H.: Lipoprotein lipase. A multifunctional enzyme relevant to common metabolic diseases [Review]. N. Engl. J. Med. *320*:1060, 1989.
125. Havel, R. J., Hunninghake, D. B., Illingworth, D. R., et al.: Lovastatin (mevinolin) in treatment of heterozygous familial hypercholesterolemia. Ann. Intern. Med. *107*:609, 1987.
126. Blum, C. B., and Levy, R. I.: Current therapy for hypercholesterolemia [Review]. JAMA *261*:3582, 1989.
127. Stuyt, P. M., Mol, M. J., Stalenhoef, A. F., et al.: Simvastatin in the effective reduction of plasma lipoprotein levels in familial dysbetalipoproteinemia (type III hyperlipoproteinemia). Am. J. Med. *88*:42N, 1990.
128. Leaf, D. A., Connor, W. E., Illingworth, D. R., et al.: The hypolipidemic effects of gemfibrozil in type V hyperlipidemia. A double-blind, crossover study. JAMA *262*:3154, 1989.
129. Buchwald, H., Varco, R. L., Matts, J. P., et al.: Effect of partial ileal bypass surgery on mortality and morbidity from coronary heart disease in patients with hypercholesterolemia. Report of the Program on the Surgical Control of the Hyperlipidemias (POSCH). N. Engl. J. Med. *323*:946, 1990.
130. Miettinen, T. A., and Lempinen, M.: Cholestyramine and ileal bypass in the treatment of familial hypercholesterolemia. Eur. J. Clin. Invest. *7*:509, 1977.
131. Starzl, T. E., Putnam, C. W., Chase, H. P., and Porter, K. A.: Portacaval shunt in hyperlipoproteinemia. Lancet *2*:940, 1973.
132. Forman, M. B., Baker, S. G., Mieny, C. J., et al.: Treatment of homozygous familial hypercholesterolemia with portacaval shunt. Atherosclerosis *41*:349, 1982.
133. Bilheimer, D. W., Goldstein, J. L., Grundy, S. C., et al.: Liver transplantation provides low density lipoprotein receptors and lowers plasma cholesterol in a child with homozygous familial hypercholesterolemia. N. Engl. J. Med. *311*:1658, 1984.
134. Lupien, P. J., Moorjani, S., Lou, M., et al.: Removal of cholesterol from blood by affinity binding to heparin-agarose: Evaluation on treatment in homozygous familial hypercholesterolemia. Pediatr. Res. *14*:113, 1980.
135. Thompson, G. R., Myant, N. B., Kilpatrick, D., et al.: Assessment of long-term plasma exchange for familial hypercholesterolemia. Br. Heart J. *43*:680, 1980.

TOBACCO USE

136. Migas, O. D.: The lipid effects of smoking. Am. Heart J. *115*:272, 1988.
137. Tiwari, A. K., Gode, J. D., and Dubey, G. P.: Effect of cigarette smoking on serum total cholesterol and HDL in normal subjects and coronary heart disease patients. Indian Heart J. *41*:92, 1989.
138. Trap-Jensen, J.: Effects of smoking on the heart and peripheral circulation [Review]. Am. Heart J. *115*:263, 1988.
139. Green, M. S., Jucha, E., and Luz, Y.: Blood pressure in smokers and nonsmokers: Epidemiologic findings. Am. Heart J. *111*:932, 1986.
140. Langford, H. G., Stamler, J., Wassertheil-Smoller, S., and Prineas, R. J.: All-cause mortality in the Hypertension Detection and Follow-up Program. Findings for the whole cohort and for persons with less severe hypertension with and without other traits related to risk of mortality. Prog. Cardiovasc. Dis. *29*:29, 1986.
141. Kannel, W. B., D'Agostino, R. B., and Belanger, A. J.: Fibrinogen, cigarette smoking, and the risk of cardiovascular disease: Insights from the Framingham Study. Am. Heart J. *113*:1006, 1987.
142. Kannel, W. B., Wolf, P. A., Castelli, W. P., and D'Agostino, R. B.: Fibrinogen and risk of cardiovascular disease. The Framingham Study. JAMA *258*:1183, 1987.

143. Meade, T. W., Imeson, J., and Stirling, Y.: Effects of changes in smoking and other characteristics on clotting factors and the risk of ischemic heart disease. Lancet *2*:986, 1987.
144. Nowak, J., Murray, J. J., Oates, J. A., and FitzGerald, G. A.: Biochemical evidence of a chronic abnormality in platelet and vascular function in healthy individuals who smoke cigarettes. Circulation *76*:6, 1987.
145. Winniford, M. D., Wheelan, K. R., Kremers, M. S., et al.: Smoking-induced coronary vasoconstriction in patients with atherosclerotic coronary artery disease: Evidence for adrenergically mediated alterations in coronary artery tone. Circulation *73*:662, 1986.
146. Deanfield, J. E., Shea, M. J., Wilson, R. A., et al.: Direct effects of smoking on the heart: Silent ischemic disturbances of coronary flow. Am. J. Cardiol. *57*:1005, 1986.
147. Kannel, W. B.: Hypertension, blood lipids, and cigarette smoking as co-risk factors for coronary heart disease. Ann. N.Y. Acad. Sci. *304*:128, 1978.
148. Cook, D. G., Shaper, A. G., Pocock, S. J., and Kussick, S. J.: Giving up smoking and the risk of heart attacks: A report from the British Regional Heart Study. Lancet *2*:1376, 1986.
149. Kaufman, D. W., Helmrich, S. P., Rosenberg, L., et al.: Nicotine and carbon monoxide content of cigarette smoke and the risk of myocardial infarction in young men. N. Engl. J. Med. *308*:409, 1983.
150. Allen, D. R., Browse, N. L., and Rutt, D. L.: Effects of cigarette smoke, carbon monoxide and nicotine on the uptake of fibrinogen by the canine arterial wall. Atherosclerosis *77*(1):83, 1989.
151. Palmer, J. R., Rosenberg, L., and Shapiro, S.: "Low yield" cigarettes and the risk of nonfatal myocardial infarction in women. N. Engl. J. Med. *320*:1569, 1989.
152. Svendsen, K. H., Kuller, L. H., Martin, M. J., and Ockene, J. K.: Effects of passive smoking in the Multiple Risk Factor Intervention Trial. Am. J. Epidemiol. *126*:783, 1987.

HYPERTENSION

153. Stamler, J., Stamler, R., and Liu, K.: High blood pressure. *In* Connor, W. E., and Bristow, J. D. (eds.): Coronary Heart Disease: Prevention, Complications, and Treatment. Philadelphia, J. B. Lippincott Company, 1985, pp. 85–109.
153a. Koren, M. J., Devereux, R. B., Casale, P. N., et al.: Relation of left ventricular mass and geometry to morbidity and mortality in uncomplicated essential hypertension. Ann. Intern. Med. *114*:345, 1991.
154. Williams, R. R., Hunt, S. C., and Hopkins, P. H.: Familial dyslipidemic hypertension. Evidence of 58 Utah families for a syndrome present in approximately 12% of patients with essential hypertension. JAMA *259*:3579, 1988.
155. Freis, E. D.: Critique of the clinical importance of diuretic induced hypokalemia and elevated cholesterol level. Arch. Intern. Med. *149*:2640, 1989.
156. Safar, M.: Therapeutic trials and large arteries in hypertension [Review]. Am. Heart J. *115*:702, 1988.
157. MacMahon, S. M., Cutler, J. A., Furburg, C. D., and Payne, G. H.: The effects of drug treatment for hypertension on morbidity and mortality from cardiovascular disease: A review of randomized controlled trials [Review]. Prog. Cardiovasc. Dis. *29*(3 Suppl. 1):99, 1986.
158. Subcommittee on Definition and Prevalence of the 1984 Joint National Committee: Hypertension prevalence and the status of awareness, treatment, and control in the United States: Final report. Hypertension *7*:457, 1985.
159. Wikstrand, J., Warnold, I., Olsson, G., et al.: Primary prevention with metoprolol in patients with hypertension. Mortality results from the MAPHY study. JAMA *259*:1976, 1988.
160. Kaplan, N. M.: Cardiovascular risk reduction: The role of antihypertensive treatment. Am. J. Med. *90*:19S, 1991.
161. Treating mild hypertension. Report of the British Hypertension Society Working Party. Recommendation for treatment of hypertension. Br. Med. J. [Clin. Res.] *298*:694, 1989.
162. Breckenridge, M. B., and Kostis, J. B.: Isolated systolic hypertension in the elderly: Results of a statewide survey of clinical practice in New Jersey. Am. J. Med. *86*:370, 1989.
163. Cloher, T. P., and Whelton, P. K.: Physician approach to the recognition and initial management of hypertension. Results of a statewide survey of Maryland physicians. Arch. Intern. Med. *146*:529, 1986.
164. Laragh, J. H.: Issues, goals and guidelines in selecting first line drug therapy for hypertension. Hypertension *13*:I103, 1989.
165. The 1988 Report of the Joint National Committee on Detection, Evaluation and Treatment of High Blood Pressure. Arch. Intern. Med. *148*:1023, 1988.
166. Report of the Second Task Force on Blood Pressure in Children, 1987. Task Force on Blood Pressure Control in Children. National Heart, Lung, and Blood Institute, Bethesda, Maryland. Pediatrics *79*:1, 1987.
167. Smoak, C. A., Burke, G. L., Webber, L. S., et al.: Relation of obesity to clustering of cardiovascular risk factors in children and young adults. The Bogalusa Heart Study. Am. J. Epidemiol. *125*:364, 1987.
168. Williams, R. R., Hunt, S. C., Hasstedt, S., et al.: Biological markers of genetically predisposed hypertension. *In* Hofman, A., Grobbee, D. E., Schalekamp, M.A.D.H. (eds.): The Early Pathogenesis of Primary Hypertension. Amsterdam, Excerpta Medica, *187*:208, 1987.
169. Weinberger, M. H.: Sodium chloride and blood pressure [Editorial]. N. Engl. J. Med. *317*:1084, 1987.
170. Weinberger, M. H., Cohen, S. J., Miller, J. Z., et al.: Dietary sodium restriction as adjunctive treatment of hypertension. JAMA *259*:2561, 1988.
171. Rouse, I. L., Beilin, L. J., and Mahoney, D. O.: Nutrient intake, blood pressure, serum and urinary prostaglandins and serum thromboxane B2 in a controlled trial with a lacto-ovo-vegetarian diet. J. Hypertens. *4*:241, 1986.
172. Margetts, B. M., Beilin, L. J., Vandongen, R., et al.: Vegetarian diet in mild hypertension. A randomized controlled trial. Br. Med. J. [Clin. Res.] *293*:1468, 1986.
173. Klatsky, A. L., Friedman, G. D., and Armstrong, M. A.: The relationships between alcoholic beverage use and other traits to blood pressure: A new Kaiser-Permanente study. Circulation *73*:628, 1986.
174. Kok, F. J., Vandenbroucke, J. P., Wessel, C., and Van der Heide, R. M.: Dietary sodium, calcium potassium and blood pressure. Am. J. Epidemiol. *123*:1043, 1986.
175. Trevisan, M., Krogh, V., Farinaro, E., et al.: Calcium-rich foods and blood pressure. Findings from the Italian National Research Council Study (the Nine Communities Study). Am. J. Epidemiol. *127*:1155, 1988.
176. Kaplan, N. M.: Calcium and potassium in the treatment of essential hypertension [Review]. Semin. Nephrol. *8*:176, 1988.
177. Veterans' Administration Co-operative Study Group on Antihypertensive Agents: Effects of treatment on morbidity in hypertension. JAMA *213*:1143, 1970.
178. Hypertension Detection and Follow-up Program Cooperative Group: Five year findings of the Hypertension Detection and Follow-up Program. I. Reduction in mortality of persons with high blood pressure, including mild hypertension. JAMA *242*:2562, 1979.
179. Management Committee: The Australian therapeutic trial in mild hypertension. Lancet *1*:1261, 1980.
180. Multiple Risk Factor Intervention Trial Research Group: Coronary heart disease, death, non-fatal acute myocardial infarction and other clinical outcomes in the Multiple Risk Factor Intervention Trial. Am. J. Cardiol. *58*:1, 1986.
181. Multiple Risk Factor Intervention Group: Mortality after 10.5 years for hypertensive patients in MRFIT. Circulation *82*:1616, 1990.
182. Paul, O.: The Medical Research Council Trial. Hypertension *8*:733, 1986.
183. The IPPPSH Collaborative Group: Cardiovascular risk and risk factors in a randomized trial of treatment based on the beta blocker oxprenolol: The International Prospective Primary Prevention Study in Hypertension (IPPPSH). J. Hypertens. *3*:379, 1985.

PHYSICAL ACTIVITY AND OBESITY

184. Blair, S. N., Kohl, H. W., Paffenberger, R. S., Jr., et al.: Physical fitness and all-cause mortality. A prospective study of healthy men and women. JAMA *262*:2395, 1989.
185. Powell, K. E., Thompson, P. D., Caspersen, C. J., and Kendrick, J. S.: Physical activity and the incidence of coronary heart disease [Review]. Annu. Rev. Public Health *8*:253, 1987.
185a. Caspersen, C. J., Bloemberg, B. P. M., Saris, W. H. M., et al.: The prevalence of selected physical activities and their relation with coronary heart disease risk factors in elderly men: The Zutphen study, 1985. Am. J. Epidemiol. *133*:1078, 1991.
186. Daneberg, A. L., Keller, J. B., Wilson, P. W., and Castelli, W. P.: Leisure time physical activity in the Framingham Offspring Study. Description, seasonal variation, and risk factor correlates. Am. J. Epidemiol. *129*:76, 1989.
187. Slattery, M. L., Jacobs, D. R., Jr., and Nichaman, M. Z.: Leisure time physical activity and coronary heart disease death. The US Railroad Study. Circulation *79*:304, 1989.
188. Jennings, G., Nelson, L., Nestel, P., et al.: The effects of changes in physical activity on major cardiovascular risk factors, hemodynamics, sympathetic function, and glucose utilization in man: A controlled study of four levels of activity. Circulation *73*:30, 1986.
189. Hespel, P., Lijnen, P., Van Hoof, R., et al.: Effects of physical endurance training on the plasma renin-angiotensin-aldosterone system in normal man. J. Endocrinol. *116*:443, 1988.
190. Fagard, R., Grauwels, R., Groeseneken, D., et al.: Plasma levels or renin, angiotensin II, and 6-keto-prostaglandin F1 alpha in endurance athletes. J. Appl. Physiol. *59*:947, 1985.
191. Fagard, R., Bielen, D., Hespel, P., et al.: Physical exercise in hypertension. *In* Laragh, J. H., and Brenner, B. M. (eds.): Hypertension: Pathophysiology, Diagnosis, and Management. Vol. 2. New York, Raven Press, 1990, pp. 1985–1997.
192. Gordon, T., Castelli, W. P., Hjortland, M. C., et al.: High-density lipoprotein as a protective factor against coronary heart disease. The Framingham Study. Am. J. Med. *62*:707, 1977.
193. Sellier, P., Corona, P., Audoin, P., et al.: Influence of training on blood lipids and coagulation. Eur. Heart J. *9*:32, 1988.
194. Hamalainen, E., Tikkanen, H., Harkonen, M., et al.: Serum lipoproteins, sex hormones and sex hormone binding globulin in middle-aged men of different physical fitness and risk of coronary heart disease. Atherosclerosis *67*:155, 1987.
195. Shepard, R. J.: Exercise in the tertiary prevention of ischemic heart disease: Experimental proof [Review]. Can. J. Sport Sci. *14*:74, 1989.
196. Paffenbarger, R. S., Jr., Wing, A. L., and Hyde, R. T.: Physical activity as an index of heart attack risk in college alumni. Am. J. Epidemiol. *108*:161, 1978.
197. Milvy, P., and Siegel, A. J.: Physical activity levels and altered mortality

from CHD with emphasis on marathon running: A critical review. Cardiovasc. Rev. Rep. *2*:233, 1981.

198. Briazgounor, I. P.: The role of physical activity in the prevention and treatment of noncommunicable diseases. World Health Stat. Q. *41*:242, 1988.

199. Froelicher, V. F., Perdue, S. T., Atwood, J. E., et al.: Exercise testing of patients recovering from myocardial infarction. Curr. Probl. Cardiol. *11*:369, 1986.

200. Burton, B. T., Foster, W. R., Hirsch, J., and Van Itallie, T. B.: Health implications of obesity: An NIH consensus development conference. Int. J. Obes. *9*:155, 1985 (Published erratum appears in Int. J. Obes. *10*:79, 1986).

201. Kannel, W. B., and Gordon, T.: Physiological and medical concomitants of obesity: The Framingham Study. *In* Bray, G. A. (ed.): Obesity in America. Washington, D.C., U.S. Department of Health, Education and Welfare, 1979, pp. 125–163. NIH publication no. 79–359.

202. Higgins, M., Kannel, W., Garrison, R., et al.: Hazards of obesity–The Framingham experience. Acta Med. Scand. [Suppl] *723*:23, 1988.

203. Jooste, P. L., Steenkamp, H. J., Benade, A. J., and Rossouw, J. E.: Prevalence of overweight and obesity and its relation to coronary heart disease in the CORIS Study. S. Afr. Med. J. *74*:101, 1988.

204. Knuiman, J. T., West, C. E., and Burema, J.: Serum total and high density lipoprotein cholesterol concentrations and body mass index in adult men from 13 countries. Am. J. Epidemiol. *116*:631, 1982.

205. Yamazi, I., Kobayakawa, H., and Komura, H.: Sympathetic nerve activity, plasma renin and water-sodium balance in obese patients with essential hypertension. Jpn. Circ. J. *50*:1155, 1986.

206. Modan, M., Halkin, H., Almog, S., et al.: Hyperinsulinemia: A link between hypertension, obesity and glucose intolerance. J. Clin. Invest. *75*:809, 1985.

207. Reaven, G. M., and Hoffman B. B.: Hypertension as a disease of carbohydrates and lipoprotein metabolism. Am. J. Med. *87*(Suppl. 6A):2S, 1989.

208. Patsch, J. R., Prasad, S., Gotto, A. M., Jr., and Patsch, W.: High density lipoprotein. Relationship of the plasma levels of this lipoprotein species to its composition, to the magnitude of postprandial lipemia, and to the activities of lipoprotein lipase and hepatic lipase. J. Clin. Invest. *80*:341, 1987.

209. Hunt, S. C., Wu, L. L., Hopkins, P. N., et al.: Apolipoprotein, low density lipoprotein subfraction, and insulin associations with familial combined hyperlipidemia. Study of Utah patients with familial dyslipidemic hypertension. Arteriosclerosis *9*:335, 1989.

210. Bjorntorp, P.: The associations between obesity, adipose tissue distribution and disease. Acta Med. Scand. Suppl. *723*:121, 1988.

211. Lapidus, L., Bentsson, C., and Larsson, B.: Distribution of adipose tissue and body fat and risk of cardiovascular disease. A 12-year follow-up of participants in the population study of women in Gothenburg, Sweden. Br. Med. J. [Clin. Res.] *289*:1257, 1984.

212. Larsson, B., and Svardsudd, K.: Distribution and the risk of cardiovascular disease. Br. Med. J. [Clin. Res.] *288*:1401, 1984.

213. Larsson, B., Seidell, J., Savardsudd, K., et al.: Obesity, adipose tissue distribution and health in men. The study of men born in 1913. Appetite *13*:37, 1989.

214. Peiris, A. N., Sothmann, M. S., Hoffmann, R. G., et al.: Adiposity, fat distribution and cardiovascular risk. Ann. Intern. Med. *110*:867, 1989.

215. Wing, R. R., Bunker, C. H., Kueller, L. H., et al.: Insulin, body mass index and cardiovascular risk factors in pre-menopausal women. Arteriosclerosis *9*:479, 1989.

FAMILY HISTORY AND DIABETES MELLITUS

216. Feinleib, M.: Genetics. *In* Kaplan, N. M., and Stamler, J. (eds.): Prevention of Coronary Heart Disease: Practical Management of the Risk Factors. Philadelphia, W. B. Saunders Company, 1983, pp. 120–129.

217. Sinaiko, A. R., and Wells, T. G.: Childhood hypertension. In: Laragh J. H., and Brenner, B. M. (eds.): Hypertension, vol. 2. Raven Press, New York, 1990, pp. 1855–1868.

218. Schieken, R. M.: The management of the family at high risk for coronary heart disease. Cardiol. Clin. *7*:467, 1989.

219. Becker, D. M., Becker, L. C., and Pearson, T. A.: Risk factors in siblings of people with premature coronary heart disease. J. Am. Coll. Cardiol. *12*:1273, 1988.

220. Jorde, L. B., and Williams, R. R.: Relation between family history of coronary artery disease and coronary risk variables. Am. J. Cardiol. *62*:708, 1988.

221. Austin, M. A., King, M. C., Vranizan, K. M., and Krauss, R. M.: Atherogenic lipoprotein phenotype. A proposed genetic marker for coronary heart disease risk. Circulation *82*:495, 1990.

222. Garcia, M. J., McNamara, P. M., Gordon, T., and Kannel, W. B.: Sixteen year follow-up study. Morbidity and mortality in diabetics in the Framingham population. Diabetes *23*:105, 1976.

223. Davi, G., Averna, M., Catalano, I., et al.: Platelet function in patients with Type II diabetes mellitus. The effect of glycemic control. Diabetes Res. *10*:7, 1988.

224. Stolar, M. W.: Atherosclerosis in diabetes. The role of hyperinsulinemia. Metabolism. *37*(Suppl. 1):J1, 1988.

225. Dzau, V. J.: Atherosclerosis and hypertension: Mechanisms and interrelationships. J. Cardiovasc. Pharmacol. *15*(Suppl. 5):S59, 1990.

226. Black, H. R.: The coronary artery disease paradox: The role of hyperinsulinemia and insulin resistance and implications for therapy. J. Cardiovasc. Pharmacol. *15*(Suppl. 5):S26, 1990.

226a. Kannel, W. B., and Ross, S. A.: States of insulin resistance: the interaction between hypertension, glucose intolerance, and coronary heart disease. Am. Heart J. *121*:1267, 1990.

226b. Reaven, G. M.: Insulin resistance and compensatory hyperinsulinemia: Role in hypertension, dyslipidemia, and coronary heart disease. Am. Heart J. *121*:1283, 1991.

227. Kannel, W. B., D'Agostino, R. B., Wilson, P. W., et al.: Diabetes, fibrinogen and risk of cardiovascular disease. The Framingham Experience. Am. Heart J. *120*:672, 1990.

228. West, K. M.: Epidemiology of Diabetes and Its Vascular Lesions. New York, Elsevier, 1978.

229. Kleinman, J. C., Donahue, R. P., Harris, M. I., et al.: Mortality among diabetics in a national health sample. Am. J. Epidemiol. *128*:389, 1988.

230. Joint Discussion: The International Collaborative Group. J. Chron. Dis. *32*:829, 1979.

231. Ishii, H., Umeda, F., Kunisaki, M., et al.: Modification of prostaglandin synthesis in washed human platelets and cultured bovine aortic endothelial cells by glycosylated low density lipoprotein. Diabetes Res. *12*:177, 1989.

232. Howard, B. V.: Lipoprotein metabolism in diabetes mellitus. J. Lipid Res. *28*:613, 1987.

233. Pollare, T., Lithell, H., and Berne, C.: A comparison of the effects of captopril and hydrochlorothiazide on glucose and lipid metabolism in patients with hypertension. N. Engl. J. Med. *321*:868, 1989.

234. Ferrannini, E., Buzzigoli, G., Bonadonna, R.: Insulin resistance in essential hypertension. N. Engl. J. Med. *317*:350, 1987.

235. Jenkins, C. D.: Psychosocial and behavioral factors. *In*: Kaplan, N. M., and Stamler, J. (eds.): Prevention of Coronary Heart Disease: Practical Management of the Risk Factors. Philadelphia, W. B. Saunders Company, 1983, p. 99.

236. Liu, K., Cedres, L. B., and Stamler, J.: Relationship of education to major risk factors and death from coronary heart disease, cardiovascular diseases and all causes. Findings of three Chicago epidemiologic studies. Circulation *66*:1308, 1982.

237. Colbourn, A. W.: The decline in coronary heart disease mortality: The DuPont experience. Part 2 (editorial). Del. Med. J. *58*:351, 1986.

238. Davidson, D. M.: Cardiovascular disease and occupation. Cardiovasc. Rev. Rep. *5*:503, 1984.

239. Aro, S., and Hasan, J.: Occupational class, psychosocial stress and morbidity. Ann. Clin. Dis. *19*:62, 1987.

240. Reed, D. M., LaCroix, A. Z., Karasek, R. A., et al.: Occupational strain and the incidence of coronary heart disease. Am. J. Epidemiol. *129*:495, 1989.

241. Dubrow, R., Burnett, C. A., Gute, D. M., and Brockert, J. E.: Ischemic heart disease and acute myocardial infarction among police officers. J. Occup. Med. *30*:650, 1988.

242. Schnall, P. L., Pieper, C., Schwartz, J. E., et al.: The relationship between job strain, workplace diastolic blood pressure, and left ventricular mass index. Results of a case-control study. JAMA *263*:1929, 1990.

243. Levy, D., Savage, D. D., Garrison, R. J., et al.: Echocardiographic criteria for left ventricular hypertrophy: The Framingham Heart Study. Am. J. Cardiol. *59*:956, 1987.

244. Eaker, E. D., Abbott, R. D., and Kannel, W. B.: Frequency of uncomplicated angina pectoris in Type A compared with Type B persons. The Framingham Study. Am. J. Cardiol. *63*:1042, 1989.

245. Siegel, W. C., Mark, D. B., Hlatky, M. A., et al.: Clinical correlates and prognostic significance of Type A behavior and silent myocardial ischemia on the treadmill. Am. J. Cardiol. *64*:1280, 1989.

246. Rosenman, R. H., Friedman, M., Straus, R., et al.: A predictive study of coronary heart disease. The Western Collaborative Group Study. JAMA *189*:15, 1964.

247. Ragland, D. R., and Brand, R. J.: Type A behavior and mortality from coronary heart disease. N. Engl. J. Med. *318*:65, 1988.

248. Shekelle, R. B., Gale, M., and Norusis, M.: Type A score (Jenkins Activity Survey) and risk of recurrent heart disease in the Aspirin Myocardial Infarction Study. Am. J. Cardiol. *56*:221, 1985.

249. Case, R. B., Heller, S. S., Case, N. B., et al.: Type A behavior and survival after acute myocardial infarction. N. Engl. J. Med. *312*:737, 1985.

250. Kahn, J. P., Perumal, A. S., Gully, R. J., et al.: Correlations of Type A behaviour with adrenergic receptor density: Implications for coronary artery disease pathogenesis. Lancet *2*:937, 1987.

251. Friedman, M., Rossenman, R. H., and Carroll, V.: Changes in serum cholesterol and blood clotting time in men subject to cycle variations of occupations stress. Circulation *17*:852, 1980.

252. Friedman, M.: Type A behavior: Its diagnosis, cardiovascular relation and the effect of its modification or recurrence of coronary artery disease. Am. J. Cardiol. *64*:12c, 1989.

253. Kannel, W. B.: Metabolic risk factors for coronary heart disease in women: Perspective from the Framingham Study. Am. Heart J. *114*:413, 1987.

254. Matthews, K. A., Meilahn, E., Kuller, L. H., et al.: Menopause and risk factors for coronary artery disease. N. Engl. J. Med. *321*:641, 1989.

255. Campos, H., McNamara, J. R., Wilson, P. W., et al.: Differences in low density lipoprotein subfractions and apolipoproteins in premenopausal and postmenopausal women. J. Clin. Endocrinol. Metab. *67*:30, 1988.

256. Sullivan, J. M., Vander-Zwag, R., Lemp, G. F., et al.: Postmenopausal estrogen use and coronary atherosclerosis. Ann. Intern. Med. *108*:358, 1988.

257. Godsland, I. F., Wynn, V., Crook, D., and Miller, N. E.: Sex, plasma, lipo-

proteins and atherosclerosis prevailing assumption and questions. Am. Heart J. *114*:1467, 1987.

258. Ernster, V. L., Bush, T. L., and Huggins, G. R.: Benefits and risks of menopausal estrogens and progestin hormone use. Prev. Med. *17*:201, 1988.
259. Stampfer, M. J., Willett, W. C., and Coldity, G. A.: A prospective study of this past use of oral contraceptive agents and risk of cardiovascular disease. N. Engl. J. Med. *319*:1313, 1988.
260. Mann, J. I., Vessey, M. P., Thorogood, M., and Doll, R.: Myocardial infarction in young women with special reference to oral contraceptive practice. Br. Med. J. [Clin. Res.] *2*:241, 1975.
261. Stampfer, M. J., Willett, W. C., Colditz, G. A., et al.: A prospective study of past use of oral contraceptive agents and risk of cardiovascular disease. N. Engl. J. Med. *319*:1313, 1988.
262. Stampfer, M. J., Willett, W. C., Colditz, G. A., et al.: Past use of oral contraceptives and cardiovascular disease: A meta-analysis in the context of the Nurses' Health Study. Am. J. Obstet. Gynecol. *163*:285, 1990.
262a. Steinberg, D., Pearson, T. A., and Kuller, L. H.: Alcohol and atherosclerosis. Ann. Intern. Med. *114*:967, 1991.
263. Regan, T. J.: Alcohol and the cardiovascular system. JAMA *264*:377, 1990.
264. Handa, K., Sasaki, J., and Saku, K.: Alcohol consumption, serum lipids and severity of angiographically determined coronary artery disease. Am. J. Cardiol. *65*:287, 1990.
265. Hartung, G. H., Reeves, R. S., Krock, L. P., et al.: Effect of alcohol and exercise on plasma HDL cholesterol subfractions and apolipoprotein A-I(APOA-I) in middle-aged men. Circulation *72*(Suppl. III):452, 1985.
266. Hennekens, C. H.: Alcohol. *In* Kaplan, N. M., and Stamler, J. (eds.): Prevention of Coronary Heart Disease: Practical Management of the Risk Factors. Philadelphia, W. B. Saunders Company, 1983, pp. 130–138.
267. Stason, W. B., Neff, R. K., Miettinen, O. S., and Jick, H.: Alcohol consumption and nonfatal myocardial infarction. Am. J. Epidemiol. *104*:603, 1976.
268. Anderson, A. J., Barboriak, J. J., and Rimm, A. A.: Risk factors and angiographically determined coronary occlusion. Am. J. Epidemiol. *107*:8, 1978.
269. Barboriak, J. J., Rimm, A. A., and Anderson, A. J.: Coronary artery occlusion and alcohol intake. Br. Heart J. *39*:289, 1977.
270. Barboriak, J. J., Anderson, A. J., and Hoffman, R. G.: Interrelationships between coronary artery occlusion, high-density lipoprotein cholesterol and alcohol intake. J. Lab. Clin. Med. *94*:348, 1979.
271. Klevay, L. M.: The role of copper, zinc and other chemical elements in ischemic heart disease. *In*: Rennert, O. M., and Chan, W. Y. (eds.): Metabolism of Trace Metals in Man, vol. 1. Boca Raton, FL, CRC Press, 1984, pp. 129–158.
272. Klevay, L. M.: Copper and ischemic heart disease. Bio-Trace Element Res. *5*:245, 1983.
273. Leoni, V., Fabiani, L., and Ticchiarelli, L.: Water hardness and cardiovascular mortality rate in Abruzzo, Italy. Arch. Environ. Health *40*:274, 1985.
274. Crawford, M. D., Clayton, D. G., Stanley, F., and Shaper, A. G.: An epidemiological study of sudden death in hard and soft water areas. J. Chronic Dis. *30*:69, 1977.
275. Chobanian, A. V.: Effects of calcium channel antagonists and other antihypertensives on atherogenesis. J. Hypertens. *5*(Suppl. 4):S543, 1987.
276. Weinstein, D. B., and Heiden, J. G.: Antiatherogenic effects of calcium channel blockers. Am. J. Med. *84*:102, 1988.
276a. Broze, G. J., Jr.: Endothelial injury, coagulation, and atherosclerosis. Coronary Artery. Dis. *2*:131, 1991.
277. Meade, T. W., Mellows, S., Brozovic, M., et al.: Haemostatic function and ischemic heart diseases. Principal results of the Northwich Park Heart Study. Lancet *2*:533, 1986.
277a. Yarnell, J. W. G., Baker, I. A., Sweetnam, P. M., et al.: Fibrinogen, viscosity, and white blood cell count are major risk factors for ischemic heart disease. The Caerphilly and Speedwell collaborative heart disease studies. Circulation *83*:836, 1991.
278. Lipinska, I., Gurewich, V., and Meriam, C. M.: Lipids, lipoproteins, fibrinogen and fibrinolytic activity in angiographically assessed coronary heart disease. Artery *15*:44, 1987.
279. Handa, K., Kono, S., and Saku, K.: Plasma fibrinogen levels as an independent indicator of the severity of coronary atherosclerosis. Atherosclerosis *77*:209, 1989.
280. Lobo, R. A.: Lipids, clotting factors and diabetes. Endogenous risks for cardiovascular disease. Am. J. Obstet. Gynecol. *158*:1584, 1988.
281. Small, M., Lowe, G. D., Beattie, J. M., et al.: Severity of coronary artery disease and basal fibrinolysis. Haemostasis *17*:305, 1987.
282. Smith, E. B., Massie, I. B., and Alexander, K. M.: The release of an immobilized lipoprotein fraction from atherosclerotic lesions by incubation with plasmin. Atherosclerosis *25*:71, 1976.
283. Cairns, J. A., Gent, M., Singer, J., et al.: Aspirin, sulfinpyrazone or both to treat in unstable angina. N. Engl. J. Med. *313*:1369, 1985.
284. Theroux, P., Ouimet, H., McCans, J., et al.: Aspirin, heparin, or both treat acute unstable angina. N. Engl. J. Med. *319*:1105, 1988.
285. Jaschonek, K., Karsch, K. R., Weisenberger, H., et al.: Platelet prostacyclin binding in coronary artery disease. J. Am. Coll. Cardiol. *8*:259, 1986.
286. Steering Committee of the Physicians' Health Study Group: Final report on the aspirin component of the ongoing physicians' health study. N. Engl. J. Med. *321*:129, 1989.
287. Alexander, N. J., and Clarkson, T. B.: Vasectomy increases the severity of diet-induced atherosclerosis in *Macaca fascicularis*. Science *201*:538, 1978.
288. Walker, A. M., Jick, H., Hunter, J. R., and McEvoy, J.: Vasectomy and nonfatal myocardial infarction: Continued observations indicate no elevation of risk. J. Urol. *130*:936, 1983.
289. Liu, S. C., and Fang, G. H.: Serum autoimmunity in vasectomyed men and its relation to atherosclerotic coronary artery disease? Clin. Reprod. Fertil. *3*:343, 1985.
290. Wilson, P. W., Garrison, R. J., Kannel, W. B., et al.: Is coffee consumption a contribution to cardiovascular disease? Insights from the Framingham Study. Arch. Intern. Med. *149*:1169, 1989.
291. Brand, F. N., McGee, D. L., Kannel, W. B., et al.: Hyperuricemia as a risk factor of coronary heart disease: The Framingham Study. Am. J. Epidemiol. *121*:11, 1985.
292. Billingham, M. E.: Cardiac transplant atherosclerosis. Transplant Proc. *19*:19, 1987.
293. Hess, M. L., Hastillo, A., Mohanakumar, T., et al.: Accelerated atherosclerosis in cardiac transplantation: Role of cytoxic B-cell antibodies and hyperlipidemia. Circulation *68*(Suppl. 2):94, 1983.
294. Gao, S. Z., Schroeder, J. S., Alderman, E. L., and Hunt, S. A.: Clinical and laboratory correlates of accelerated coronary disease in the cardiac transplant patient. Circulation *76*(Suppl. 5):56, 1987.

38

Coronary Blood Flow and Myocardial Ischemia

by EUGENE BRAUNWALD, M.D., and BURTON E. SOBEL, M.D.

Hypoxia, or *hypoxemia*, is a state of reduced oxygen supply to tissue despite adequate perfusion; *anoxia* is the absence of oxygen supply despite adequate perfusion. These conditions should be distinguished from *ischemia*, which is a condition of oxygen deprivation accompanied by inadequate removal of metabolites consequent to reduced perfusion. Although clinical manifestations of coronary insufficiency generally reflect the effects of ischemia, under selected experimental and clinical conditions, deprivation of oxygen can be separated from reduced washout of metabolites.[1] For example, in isolated hearts perfused at high flow rates with media equilibrated with a gas mixture poor in oxygen, anoxia without ischemia results, since washout of metabolites is not hindered. An analogous situation occurs in patients with cyanotic congenital heart disease, as well as in those with cor pulmonale, severe anemia, asphyxiation, and carbon monoxide poisoning.

Neither ischemia nor hypoxia can be defined in absolute terms, since the blood flow and quantity of oxygen required to support myocardium under one set of conditions will not necessarily pertain under another. In humans, blood flow of 60 to 90 ml/min per 100 gm of myocardium is generally required under basal physiological conditions. On the other hand, when the mechanical activity of the heart and its metabolic requirements are markedly reduced, myocardial viability may be maintained by perfusion at much lower rates, approximately 10 to 20 ml/min per 100 gm, or even with complete interruption of perfusion for periods of up to 100 minutes. Examples of conditions that reduce oxygen needs markedly include hypothermia with ventricular fibrillation or asystole, techniques widely used in cardiovascular surgery. Other examples of lowered cardiac oxygen needs, though less drastic, occur following the administration of nitroglycerin and of other nitrates, which reduce the preload and afterload, and of beta-adrenoceptor blockers, which lower heart rate and contractility. This reduction of oxygen needs is perhaps the *principal* mechanism by which these agents relieve anginal pain (p. 1307).

The importance of defining ischemia in *relative* rather than absolute terms is underscored by the use of a variety of stress tests to detect or assess the severity of coronary artery disease. During relative ischemia an imbalance occurs between myocardial oxygen demands and supply (Fig. 38–1). Whether the ischemia is manifested as anginal discomfort, deviation of the ST segment on the electrocardiogram (Chap. 5), relative dimi-

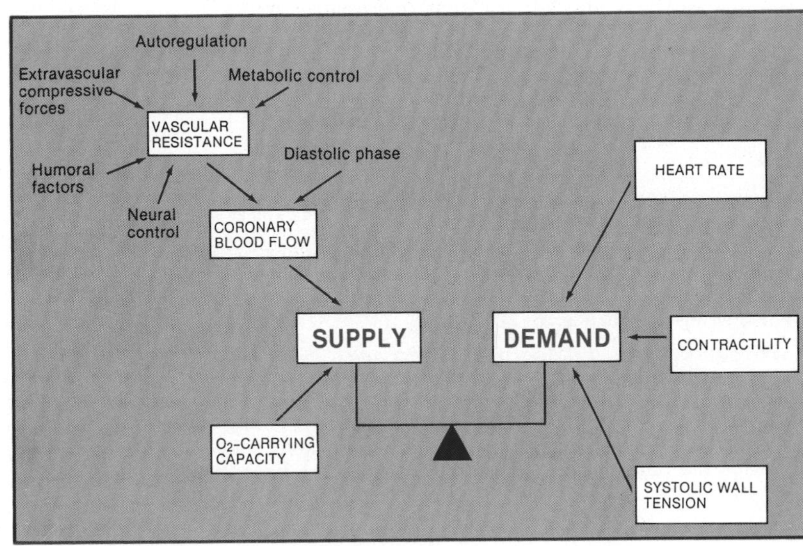

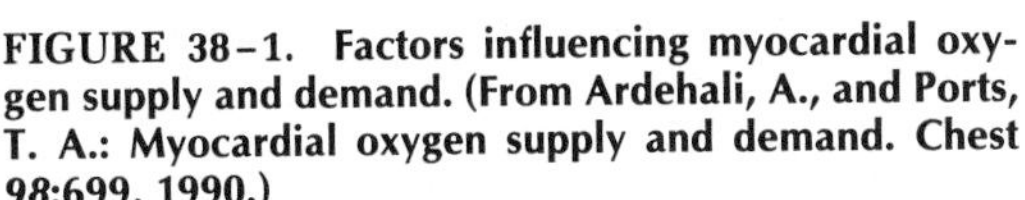
FIGURE 38–1. Factors influencing myocardial oxygen supply and demand. (From Ardehali, A., and Ports, T. A.: Myocardial oxygen supply and demand. Chest *98*:699, 1990.)

nution of accumulation of ^{201}Tl in myocardial "perfusion images," regional wall motion disorders, or diminution of ejection fraction detectable with gated blood pool images (Chap. 10), the underlying principle is the same. Induction of stress by isotonic exercise, atrial pacing, handgrip, or any other means leads to a transitory disparity in the balance between oxygen supply and demand. Although this balance may be adequate under conditions of rest, the disparity becomes apparent when the increased oxygen demands cannot be satisfied by an adequate augmentation of myocardial delivery. An additional cause of imbalance is a reduction of oxygen supply secondary to increased coronary vascular tone.

In this chapter we consider first the control of the balance between myocardial oxygen supply and demand and then the hemodynamic, biochemical, and electrophysiological consequences of ischemia.

DETERMINANTS OF MYOCARDIAL OXYGEN CONSUMPTION

(Table 38–1)

The heart is an aerobic organ; that is, it relies almost exclusively on the oxidation of substrates for the generation of energy, and it can develop only a small oxygen debt. Therefore, in a steady state, determination of the rate of myocardial oxygen consumption ($M\dot{V}O_2$) provides an accurate measure of its total metabolism. It has been known for many years that the total metabolism of the arrested, quiescent heart is only a small fraction of that of the working organ. The $M\dot{V}O_2$ of the beating canine heart ranges from 8 to 15 ml/min per 100 gm, while the oxygen of the noncontracting heart is approximately 1.5 ml/min per 100 gm.[2–4] This quantity of oxygen is required for those physiological processes not directly associated with contraction. Increases in the frequency of depolarization of the *noncontracting* heart are accompanied by only small increases of $M\dot{V}O_2$. Oxygen cost of electrical depolarization is trivial compared to the cost of contractile activity.[5]

MYOCARDIAL TENSION. As early as 1915 Evans and Matsuoka concluded from studies on the Starling heart-lung preparation that "there is a relation between the tension set up on contraction and the metabolism of the contractile tissue."[6] In 1955, in a systematic investigation of the relative effects of aortic pressure, stroke volume, and heart rate on $M\dot{V}O_2$, it became apparent that the energy needs of the myocardium do not correlate simply with the external work produced by the heart when work is calculated in the classic manner as the product of developed pressure and stroke volume. As a corollary, it was shown that myocardial efficiency, i.e., the ratio of the work performed to the oxygen consumed, varies widely according to the hemodynamic conditions.[7,8] These investigations suggested that the tension-time index, i.e. the area under the left ventricular pressure curve, is an important determinant of the $M\dot{V}O_2$. Subsequently, it was emphasized that the myocardial wall tension time integral is a

TABLE 38–1 MYOCARDIAL O_2 CONSUMPTION COMPONENTS

Total: 6–8 cc/min/100 gm			
Distribution			
Basal	20%	Volume work	15%
Electrical	1%	Pressure work	64%
Effects on $M\dot{V}O_2$ of 50% increases in			
Wall stress	25%	Heart rate	50%
Contractility	45%	Volume work	4%
Pressure work	50%		

The table demonstrates the dominant contribution to $M\dot{V}O_2$ made by pressure work and prominent effects of increasing pressure work and heart rate on $M\dot{V}O_2$.

From Gould, K. L.: Coronary Artery Stenosis. New York, Elsevier, 1991, p. 8.

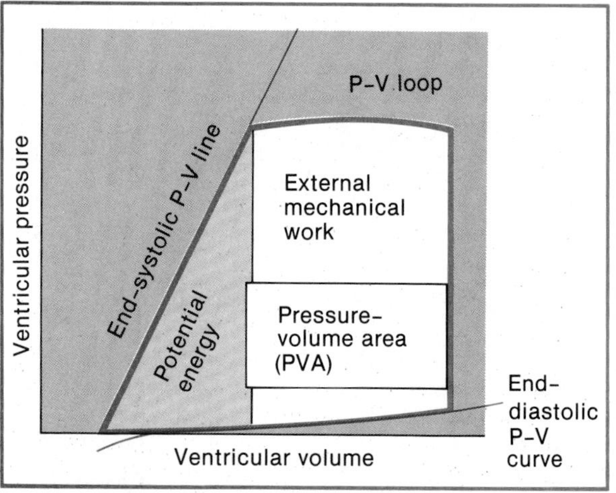

FIGURE 38–2. Schematic illustration of systolic pressure-volume area and its two components, external mechanical work (the P-V loop) and potential energy. End-systole is the time at which the P-V loop touches the end-systolic P-V relation line. The systolic segment of the P-V loop consists of the segments for the isovolumic contraction phase and the ejection phase. The diastolic segment of the P-V loop consists of the segments for the isovolumic relaxation phase and the filling phase. (From Suga, H., Goto, Y., Yamada, O., and Igarashi, Y.: Independence of myocardial oxygen consumption from pressure-volume trajectory during diastole in canine left ventricle. Circ. Res. *55*:735, 1984, by permission of the American Heart Association, Inc.)

more definitive determinant of myocardial energy utilization than is the developed pressure.[9,10] Later studies demonstrated that velocity of myocardial contraction—a reflection of the heart's contractility—is an additional important determinant of $M\dot{V}O_2$ (Fig. 38–1).[11]

Recent reexamination of the determinants of $M\dot{V}O_2$ has emphasized that they correlate closely with the left ventricular systolic pressure-volume area, which consists of the sum of the area within the systolic pressure-volume loop, i.e., the external mechanical work, and the end-systolic elastic potential energy in the ventricular wall, i.e., the area enclosed by the systolic pressure-volume trajectory and the E_{max} line[12–17a] (Fig. 38–2). The pressure-volume area varies linearly with $M\dot{V}O_2$ regardless of loading conditions. It has been demonstrated in isolated muscle as well as in the intact ventricle[18,19] that the pressure-volume area appears to be superior to the force-time integral as a correlate of $M\dot{V}O_2$.[13] Mechanical events during myocardial relaxation do *not* appear to affect $M\dot{V}O_2$ importantly.[4,12–15,20]

Rooke and Feigl have provided evidence that $M\dot{V}O_2$ is influenced by stroke volume, although less so than by pressure development.[3] They have also provided an experimental basis for the use of the systolic pressure–rate product (plus an estimate of the oxygen requirements of the noncontracting heart) as a clinically useful index of $M\dot{V}O_2$. These observations are consistent with Fenn's classic observations on skeletal muscle, which showed that the energy release (a variable related to oxygen consumption) is proportional to the sum of tension development and external work of the muscle.[21,22] Thus, both skeletal muscle and myocardium adjust their energy costs to external conditions imposed after stimulation (Fig. 38–3).[10]

MYOCARDIAL CONTRACTILITY. The net effect of positive inotropic stimuli (such as Ca^{++}, cardiac glycosides, and catecholamines) on $M\dot{V}O_2$ is the end result of their influence on two of its major determinants of that change in opposite directions in the intact heart. These are *wall tension*, which declines as a consequence of a reduction in heart size, and *myocardial contractility*, which, by definition, is augmented. In the failing, dilated ventricle, the increased contractility reduces the left ventricular end-diastolic pressure and volume. On the basis of the Laplace relation (p. 377), this reduction in ventricular volume leads to a decline in intramyocardial tension, which reduces $M\dot{V}O_2$. However, the decrease in $M\dot{V}O_2$

that might be expected to result from falling tension in the ventricular wall is opposed by the increase in contractility, which tends to augment $M\dot{V}O_2$. The net result of these opposing effects is to produce no change, a slight increase, or a small decrease in $M\dot{V}O_2$. Thus, the change in $M\dot{V}O_2$ that follows the stimulation of contractility depends on the extent to which intramyocardial tension is reduced in relation to the extent to which contractility is augmented.[10] In general, in the absence of heart failure, drugs that stimulate myocardial contractility elevate $M\dot{V}O_2$, because heart size and therefore wall tension are not reduced substantially and do not offset the effect on metabolism of the stimulation of contractility. The importance of contractility as an independent predictor of $M\dot{V}O_2$ is reflected in its displacement of the relation between the pressure-volume area and $M\dot{V}O_2$.[15,23] The conclusion that myocardial contractility is an important determinant of $M\dot{V}O_2$ is also supported by observations on the effects of reducing contractility. Thus, in animal experiments reductions in contractility and in the velocity of contraction produced by cardiac depressant drugs, including propranolol and procainamide, were shown to lower $M\dot{V}O_2$ when wall tension was held constant or almost so.[24] Also, reductions of $M\dot{V}O_2$ are sometimes seen in the presence of heart failure with its reduced contractility.

In experiments in which the relative effects on $M\dot{V}O_2$ of changes in tension development and in myocardial contractility were assessed in the same heart, it was concluded that the quantitative effects on $M\dot{V}O_2$ of changes in contractility and tension development are both substantial and of the same order of magnitude.[24] In these experiments heart rate was purposely held constant, since heart rate itself is an important determinant of $M\dot{V}O_2$. An augmentation of heart rate elevates the $M\dot{V}O_2$ by increasing the frequency of tension development per unit of time, as well as by increasing contractility.[7,25] Systolic wall tension, contractility, and heart rate thus have emerged as the three principal determinants of $M\dot{V}O_2$[26] (Fig. 38–1).

Although the precise energy costs of the *maintenance* of the active state of the myocardium have not yet been clearly defined, they are likely to be relatively low. In studies on isolated papillary muscles, $M\dot{V}O_2$ was found to be a function of the tension that is developed and the velocity of shortening of the unloaded muscle. Shortening against a load requires oxygen above and beyond that required for the development of tension. It has been suggested by Suga et al. that almost the entire increase in $M\dot{V}O_2$ produced by the administration of positive inotropic agents such as Ca^{++} and epinephrine results from the energy costs of enhanced excitation-contraction coupling. Specifically the increased energy costs result from the greater and more rapid Ca^{++} uptake by the sarcoplasmic reticulum[27] as well as from the increased contractile activity, rather than from a direct stimulating effect of positive inotropic agents on basal myocardial metabolism. It has been suggested that when all other parameters affecting $M\dot{V}O_2$ are held constant, severe valvular regurgitation does not increase $M\dot{V}O_2$ significantly because of the relatively low O_2 cost of the additional myocardial shortening associated with valvular regurgitation[7,16,17,28] (Table 38–2).

$M\dot{V}O_2$ is also influenced by the substrate utilized. Specifically, it varies directly with the fraction of energy derived from the metabolism of fatty acids, which in turn varies directly with the arterial concentration of fatty acids and inversely with that of glucose and insulin.[29]

TABLE 38–2 DETERMINANTS OF MYOCARDIAL OXYGEN CONSUMPTION

1. **Tension development**
2. **Contractile state**
3. **Heart rate**
4. **Shortening against a load (Fenn effect)**
5. **Maintenance of cell viability in basal state**
6. **Depolarization**
7. **Activation**
8. **Maintenance of active state**
9. **Direct metabolic effect of catecholamines**
10. **Fatty acid uptake**

Alterations in contractile performance sometimes affect $M\dot{V}O_2$ profoundly. For example, the spontaneously hypertensive rat exhibits reduced $M\dot{V}O_2$ (per gm of myocardium) compared with the normal rat at comparable mechanical activity. This improved mechanical efficiency appears to be related to the shift from V_1 to V_3 myosin isoforms.[31] Similar changes have been described in nonischemic, nonworking hearts.[32] On the other hand, the acutely reduced mechanical activity of the postischemic (stunned) heart (p. 1329) is *not* associated with any reduction of $M\dot{V}O_2$.[33] Presumably, abnormalities in energy utilization, in electromechanical coupling, or in the shunting of energy supplies to cellular repair processes might be responsible for the unexpectedly high $M\dot{V}O_2$ (and the low efficiency) of stunned myocardium.[33]

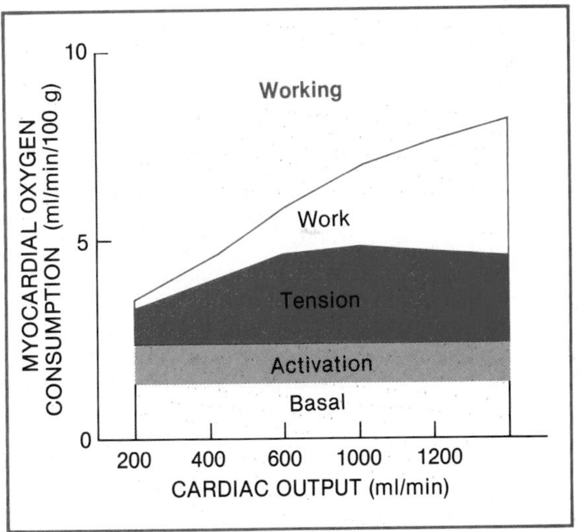

FIGURE 38–3. Basal metabolism, activation energy, tension-related energy, and energy for external work as components of myocardial oxygen consumption at various levels of cardiac output. (From Ando, H., Nakano, E., Ueno, Y., and Tokunaga, K.: New technique for analysis of cardiac energetics using a modified Fenn equation. J. Thorac. Cardiovasc. Surg. *97*:565, 1989.)

Regulation of Coronary Blood Flow

ANATOMICAL FACTORS. Coronary blood flow is influenced by anatomical, hydraulic, mechanical, and metabolic factors.[34–37] During diastole, when the aortic valve is closed, aortic diastolic pressure is transmitted without impediment through the dilated sinuses of Valsalva to the coronary ostia. The aortic arch and sinuses then act as a miniature reservoir, facilitating maintenance of relatively uniform coronary inflow through diastole. Both the left and right coronary arteries course across the epicardial surface of the heart. The major vessels and their principal branches serve as conductance vessels and normally offer little resistance to coronary blood flow. The epicardial conductance vessels can constrict

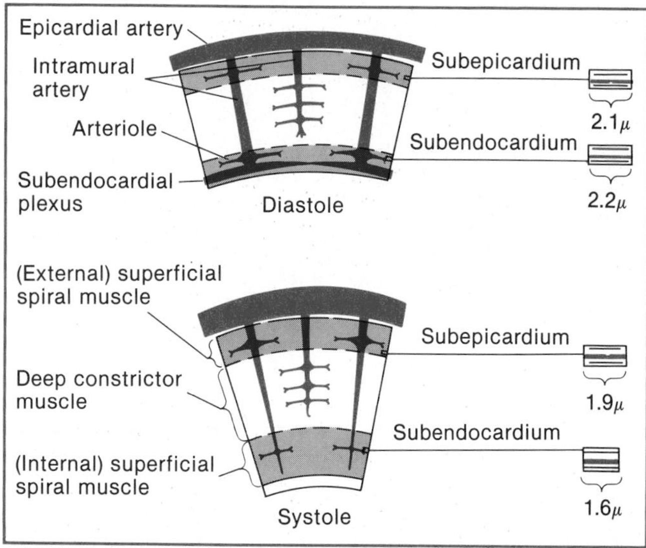

FIGURE 38-4. Cross-section of the left ventricular wall in diastole and systole. Factors involved in the susceptibility of the subendocardium to the development of ischemia include the greater dependence of this region on diastolic perfusion and the greater degree of shortening, and therefore of energy expenditure, of this region during systole. (From Bell, J. R., and Fox, A. C.: Pathogenesis of subendocardial ischemia. Am. J. Med. Sci. *268*:2, 1974.)

in response to alpha-adrenergic stimuli and dilate to nitroglycerin.[38] These vessels give rise to smaller penetrating vessels approximately at right angles (Fig. 38-4). A large pressure drop occurs in these intramural vessels and in the coronary arterioles, hence their designation as "resistance vessels." The dense capillary network of about 4000 capillaries/mm^2 cross-section of the normal heart is not uniformly patent, because precapillary sphincters appear to serve a regulatory function,[39] depending on the flow needs of the myocardium. This capillary density is reduced in the presence of ventricular hypertrophy.

COLLATERALS. Anastomotic connections without an intervening capillary bed exist between portions of the same coronary artery and between different coronary arteries. The distribution and extent of these collateral vessels differ markedly between species, as well as among different individuals of the same species. In canine or guinea pig hearts, an extensive epicardial network of collateral vessels is common, but epicardial collateral vessels are not prominent in porcine or primate hearts. In human hearts, the distribution and extent of collateral vessels are quite variable. Under physiological conditions, such vessels are generally less than 40 μ in diameter and appear to have little or no functional role. When myocardial perfusion is compromised by obstructions affecting major vessels, these collateral vessels enlarge and blood flow through them increases.[40] Exercise,[41,42] severe anemia,[43] and gradual (rather than abrupt) coronary occlusion[44] appear to enhance the development of collaterals. However, in experimental animals[44a] exercise does not reduce mortality resulting from subsequent coronary occlusion.[45] Perfusion via collaterals in the presence of total coronary occlusion may equal perfusion through a vessel with 90 per cent obstruction of the luminal diameter.[46] Positron emission tomographic imaging is a noninvasive technique for detecting coronary collaterals in humans.

Repeated brief (2 min) but not transient (15 sec) episodes of ischemia can serve as stimuli for collateral vessel formation.[47-49] With sustained coronary occlusion, collateral blood flow to salvaged tissue commences early, i.e., between 5 and 10 min following occlusion, and then rises progressively for 24 hours; this reflects the gradual recruitment of collateral vessels.[50]

Although debate continues concerning the functional significance of collaterals, two facts are clear: (1) collaterals become visible angiographically only when coronary occlusion is complete or virtually so, and (2) the presence of collaterals occasionally can prevent the development of a myocardial infarction in the presence of a total coronary occlusion. However, even when collaterals prevent myocardial infarction in the presence of coronary occlusion, they provide perfusion just sufficient to maintain myocardial viability; an increase in M$\dot{V}O_2$ induced by electrical pacing results in a deterioration of myocardial function.[51] Some studies have shown that the presence of collaterals appears to reduce the frequency of wall motion disorders in the face of coronary obstruction,[46] while others have not confirmed this.[47-49] In any event, when cardiac muscle is supplied entirely or largely by collateral vessels, it often becomes ischemic if its oxygen demands increase above basal levels.

PERFUSION PRESSURE. As in any vascular bed, blood flow in the coronary bed depends on the driving pressure and the resistance offered by this bed. However, the coronary circulation differs from other circulations in that the resistance offered by the bed is influenced importantly by phasic systolic compression of the coronary vessels coursing through the myocardium. The perfusion or effective coronary driving pressure is the pressure gradient between the coronary arteries and the pressure in either the right atrium or the left ventricle in diastole, since coronary flow drains primarily into these two chambers. However, effective perfusion pressure is not constant throughout the cardiac cycle. When the aortic valve is open and ejected blood flows rapidly past the coronary ostia, perfusion pressure is reduced slightly below aortic pressure because of the Venturi effect. In addition, phasic changes in right atrial pressure occurring during the cardiac cycle and in the left ventricle during diastole modify the effective perfusion pressure gradient, albeit only slightly, except in the presence of a tall right atrial *v* wave, as in tricuspid regurgitation.

FACTORS EXTRINSIC TO THE VASCULAR BED. Coronary vascular resistance is influenced both by factors *extrinsic* to the bed, particularly compressive forces within the myocardium (intramyocardial forces acting on the intramyocardial vessels), and by metabolic, neural, and humoral factors *intrinsic* to the bed causing changes in the cross-sectional area of coronary resistance vessels. Intramyocardial wall tension varies throughout the cardiac cycle and is dependent on both load and contractility.[51,52] Because ventricular wall tension is much higher in systole than it is in diastole, forces compressing intramyocardial vessels are much greater during this phase of the cardiac cycle. Therefore, most of the coronary blood flow to the left ventricle occurs during diastole. Sometimes there is even some backflow in the major coronary arteries during systole. This "throttling" effect of systole on myocardial perfusion[34] is particularly important when systolic intraventricular pressure is elevated but coronary perfusion pressure is not, as is the case with obstruction to left ventricular outflow by valvular or subvalvular aortic stenosis, or with severe aortic regurgitation. Since an increase in heart rate diminishes the total amount of diastolic time per minute while myocardial oxygen demand is augmented, tachycardia may cause myocardial ischemia.

Extravascular Compressive Forces. The important resistance to coronary blood flow caused by left ventricular compression can be demonstrated experimentally in a beating heart perfused at constant pressure in which asystole is induced transiently by vagal stimulation. At this time, coronary blood flow suddenly increases by approximately 50 per cent because of relief of the compressive effect.[35] Because compressive forces exerted by the right ventricle are ordinarily far less than those of the left ventricle, perfusion of the right ventricle is not interrupted during systole.

The calculation of coronary vascular resistance is complicated by the observation that under normal conditions coronary blood flow ceases when coronary driving pressure reaches levels of approximately 40 mm Hg, the so-called P_{zf} (pressure at zero flow). Although there is no question concerning the existence of a P_{zf} substantially above coronary venous pressure, considerable debate continues about the responsible mechanism.[53,54] Extravascular compressive forces in humans are reflected in the phasic coronary artery flow velocity determined by Doppler flow meter catheters. Patients with aortic stenosis exhibit a reduction of the fraction of forward flow in systole.[55,56]

Susceptibility of the Subendocardium to Ischemia. Extravascular compressive forces during systole are greater in subendocardial zones of the heart than in subepicardial ones (Fig. 38–3). Therefore, systolic flow is greatly reduced in this area.

Under physiological conditions, marked transitory disparities exist between endocardial and epicardial wall stresses and, correspondingly, between endocardial and epicardial flow throughout the cardiac cycle. Nevertheless, under physiological conditions, in conscious dogs the ratio of endocardial to epicardial flow averaged throughout the cardiac cycle is approximately 1.25 : 1 as a consequence of preferential dilatation of the subendocardial vessel,[57] which appears to be secondary to the increased wall stress and oxygen consumption in this region. Interventions that reduce the perfusion pressure gradient during diastole (as occurs with coronary obstruction, elevation of ventricular diastolic pressure, and tachycardia) lower the ratio of subendocardial to subepicardial flow and may cause the subendocardium to become ischemic.

The combination of a greater wall stress, and hence greater resistance to flow, and higher metabolic demands results in lower coronary vascular tone in the subendocardium than in the subepicardium. As a consequence, the reserve for vasodilatation is also less in the subendocardium than in the subepicardium, and as perfusion is reduced the deeper layers of myocardium become ischemic before the more superficial ones. This phenomenon is manifested by reduced intracellular oxygen tension and contractility and increased production of lactate in the inner layers of the ventricular wall as the heart becomes ischemic[58,59] (see Fig. 38–31, p. 1182).

The preferential susceptibility of the subendocardium to ischemia by the combination of limited reserve for vasodilatation, extrinsic compression from the higher wall stress to which it is subjected,[60] and the resultant high metabolic demands accounts for the electrocardiographic ST-segment depression characteristically associated with episodes of transient ischemia (Fig. 5–30, p. 137). Injury currents from the subendocardium, resulting in ST-segment depression, accompany the maldistribution of transmural flow and metabolic impairment of subendocardial tissue under these circumstances, even though net transmural flow may remain near normal[61] (Fig. 38–5). These considerations provide the basis for the recognition of myocardial ischemia by ST-segment depression during exercise stress testing (Chap. 6). When coronary flow is restricted, the adaptive changes in the subendocardium include its greater potential for glycolytic metabolism[62] due to higher glycolytic enzyme activity and, consequently, higher lactate production rates.[63] However, even though the glycogen content of subendocardium is higher than that of the subepicardium under aerobic conditions, concentrations of high-energy phosphate compounds are generally lower in the subendocardium than in other portions of the ventricular wall when coronary flow is restricted, because of the inability of the anaerobic metabolism of glucose to fulfill energy requirements completely.

PREDICTION OF SUBENDOCARDIAL ISCHEMIA. Griggs, Hoffman, Buckberg, Brazier and their collaborators have developed indexes for the evaluation of transmural blood flow and the prediction of subendocardial ischemia in the absence of coronary artery obstruction.[57,61–64] They reasoned that the delivery of oxygen to the subendocardium represents the product of arterial oxygen content and the driving force for subendocardial blood flow, which in turn depend on the integrated pressure difference between the aorta and left ventricle during diastole, termed the *diastolic pressure–time index* (DPTI). The demand for blood flow, i.e., MVO_2, is closely related to the area beneath the systolic portion of the ventricular pressure curve, i.e., the *systolic pressure–time index* (SPTI). The ratio DPTI × oxygen content/SPTI has been used as an index of the relation between subendocardial oxygen supply and demand. This ratio can be reduced by (1) opening an arteriovenous fistula or patent ductus arteriosus or inducing aortic regurgitation to diminish aortic diastolic pressure and thereby reducing DPTI; (2) increasing preload or afterload, causing left ventricular dysfunction, or reducing left ventricular compliance; these maneuvers all raise left ventricular diastolic pressure and also reduce DPTI; (3) inducing tachycardia to shorten diastole[65]; and (4) causing severe anemia or hypoxemia to reduce arterial oxygen content. With reduction of the DPTI × oxygen content/SPTI below a critical value of approximately 10, the endocardial/epicardial blood flow ratio also decreased.

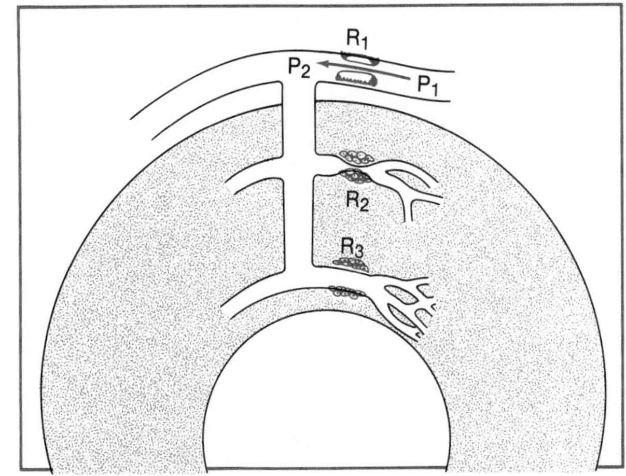

FIGURE 38–5. Effects of a stenosis in an epicardial vessel (R_1) on endocardial and epicardial flow. Endocardial vessels (R_3) are maximally dilated, whereas epicardial vessels (R_2) are not. A vasodilator stimulus resulting (for example, from an increase in heart rate) will augment transmural flow owing to dilation of subepicardial vessels. Increase in flow will cause a greater pressure drop across the stenosis (P_1-P_2) and the coronary driving pressure (P_2) will drop.

As long as the fall in resistance in subepicardial vessels (R_2) is greater than the resulting fall in driving pressure, flow will increase in the subepicardial region. However, because subendocardial vessels are already maximally dilated, the fall in coronary driving pressure will not be accompanied by a fall in resistance. Hence, flow to subendocardial vessels will fall. (From Epstein, S. E., Cannon, R. O., III, and Talbot, T. L.: Hemodynamic principles in the control of coronary blood flow. Am. J. Cardiol. *56*:8E, 1985.)

Although it is recognized that this index provides only an approximation of the oxygen supply-to-demand relationship,[51] it can explain a number of clinical findings, such as the development of angina and the electrocardiographic and biochemical evidence of ischemia caused by tachycardia in patients with aortic stenosis; in this situation DPTI falls and SPTI rises. Myocardial lactate production has been observed to occur during beta-adrenoceptor stimulation with isoproterenol in patients with aortic stenosis,[66] when left ventricular systolic pressure, contractility, heart rate, and therefore, MVO_2 rise while DPTI does not. When adrenergic stimulation was carried out in dogs with experimentally produced aortic stenosis, the myocardial lactate concentration and the lactate-pyruvate ratio rose while the reduction of ATP stores was more prominent in the inner than the outer half of the ventricle.[58,59] This indicates that the subendocardium is more vulnerable to ischemia and therefore becomes dependent on anaerobic metabolism more readily than does the subepicardium.

In experimentally produced aortic regurgitation, diastolic coronary blood flow falls but systolic flow rises, so that total coronary flow does not change.[67] However, with severe reductions in aortic diastolic pressure, DPTI declines and the subendocardial region exhibits biochemical evidence of anaerobic metabolism. As the DPTI × oxygen content/SPTI declines, the subendocardial lactate-pyruvate ratio rises, evidence of anaerobic metabolism in this region of myocardium. These observations are clinically relevant considering that angina pectoris occurs in a significant number of patients with severe aortic stenosis and/or regurgitation in the absence of coronary artery disease (Chap. 34). Other conditions in which subendocardial ischemia occurs include marked systemic hypotension, regardless of etiology (Chap. 21), and pulmonary embolism, particularly when complicated by fever, tachycardia, and anemia. In these conditions the ischemia results from a combination of lowered coronary perfusion

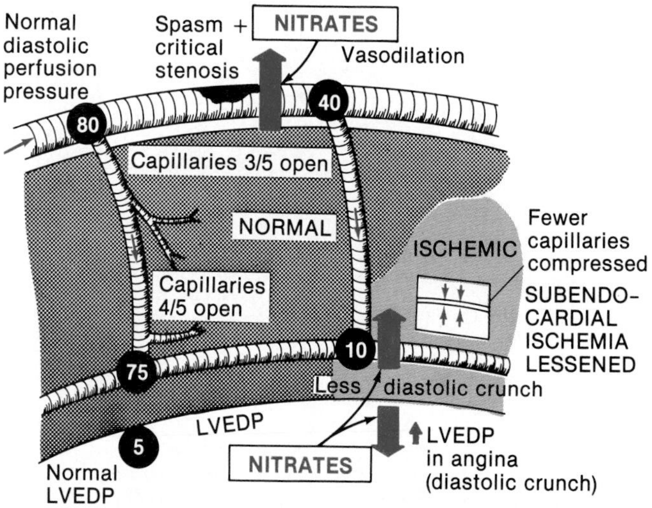

FIGURE 38-6. **Effects of a critical stenosis in an epicardial vessel and of nitrates on myocardial perfusion and function. When a patient with a critical stenosis exercises, subendocardial ischemia and an increase in left ventricular end-diastolic pressure (LVEDP) occur; this is accompanied by compression of subendocardial vessels. Alternatively, angina at rest can develop if there is superimposed coronary spasm. Nitrates bring relief by increasing the diameter of large coronary arteries, by relaxing spasm, by reducing LVEDP, and by decreasing diastolic compression. (Adapted from Parratt, J. R., Marshall, R. J., and Ledingham, M. C. A.: J. Physiol. [Paris]** ***76*****:791, 1980.)**

pressure, tachycardia, and increased subendocardial tension secondary to sympathetic stimulation of myocardial contractility. Since coronary blood flow ceases at a pressure higher than ventricular diastolic pressure (see discussion of P_{zf} above), as arterial pressure declines with systemic hypotension or aortic regurgitation, the coronary perfusion pressure declines to quite low levels.

In the presence of coronary obstruction the *effective* pressure perfusing the subendocardial region is determined by the gradient between the diastolic coronary pressure *distal* to the obstruction and the left ventricular end-diastolic pressure; hence the DPTI no longer reflects or even approximates the driving force for subendocardial blood flow. When left ventricular diastolic pressure is elevated in the ischemic ventricle, the endocardial/epicardial flow ratio declines, further reducing subendocardial blood flow.[68] The development of subendocardial ischemia can raise ventricular diastolic pressure further, largely by interfering with the ventricle's diastolic properties, thereby causing a vicious circle.

Since maldistribution of transmural blood flow compromises the subendocardial tissue, antianginal drugs may be effective if they improve the ratio of subendocardial to subepicardial flow even if they do not augment net transmural perfusion. Analysis of the washout of ^{86}Rb and fractional uptake of radioactive-labeled microspheres has shown that both nitroglycerin and beta-adrenoceptor blockers redistribute blood flow to the subendocardium.[69,70] This phenomenon may, in the case of nitroglycerin, reflect in part the direct effects of the drugs on the coronary vascular bed as well as the reduction of extravascular compressive forces induced by a lowering of ventricular diastolic pressure resulting from a reduction of preload (Fig. 38-6). Beta blockers reduce MVO_2 and thereby ischemia, which is most prominent in the subendocardium; the relief of ischemia in turn reduces diastolic wall tension (primarily in the subendocardium) and improves myocardial perfusion.

CONTROL OF CORONARY VASCULAR RESISTANCE

Coronary vascular resistance is influenced markedly by changes in the tone of the vascular bed, changes that are mediated by neural, metabolic, pharmacological, and myogenic factors, as well as by vasodilator and vasoconstrictor substances released by the endothelium.

NEURAL FACTORS. The coronary arteries are richly innervated by adrenergic and parasympathetic nerves,[35,38] and their activation can exert an important influence on coronary vasomotor tone. Both $alpha_1$ and $alpha_2$ adrenoceptors are present in the coronary arteries,[71] and when activated by neuronally released or circulating norepinephrine both cause coronary vasoconstriction[72-74] (Fig. 38-7), which appears to be mediated ultimately by an increased concentration of calcium in coronary vascular smooth muscle.[73-76] When inotropic and chronotropic effects are blocked[77] (to prevent the development of metabolic vasodilator stimuli), stimulation of cardiac nerves causes coronary vasoconstriction. The activation of $alpha_1$ receptors induced by the infusion of methoxamine has been demonstrated to reduce the diameter of coronary arteries while increasing intraluminal pressure.[38,78] Activation of the carotid chemoreceptor reflex causes marked coronary constriction, which can be blocked by surgical denervation or by the alpha blocker phentolamine.[78] On the other hand, $beta_1$ and $beta_2$ adrenoceptors in the large and small coronary arteries mediate vasodilation.[38,79,80] Beta blockade induces coronary constriction, but this effect appears *not* to be a direct action on the coronary arteries. Rather it results from blockade of beta-adrenoreceptor–mediated increases in $M\dot{V}O_2$.[81] The extent of cholinergic regulation of large coronary arteries is controversial,[82] although parasympathetic stimulation appears to dilate small coronary arteries.[38]

Intravenous administration of norepinephrine induces a brief fall, followed by a sustained rise, in coronary vascular resistance, accompanied by a decline in coronary sinus pO_2 (Fig. 38-7).[83] The early vasodilatation can be eliminated by beta-adrenoceptor blockade and presumably results from the augmented myocardial oxygen needs consequent to stimulation of myocardial beta receptors. The later increase in coronary vascular resistance can be prevented by alpha-adrenoceptor blockade and presumably results from stimulation by norepinephrine of alpha receptors in the coronary vascular bed. Blockade of $alpha_1$ receptors in patients with coronary artery disease attenuates the coronary vasoconstrictor response to the cold pressor test[84] and cigarette smoking,[85,86] indicating that both responses are mediated by stimulation of these receptors. Baroreceptor activity affects coronary vascular resistance reflexly. In the dog with sectioned vagal nerves, occlusion of the carotid arteries to produce baroreceptor hypotension induces an increase in heart rate and blood pressure, accompanied by a reduction in coronary vascular

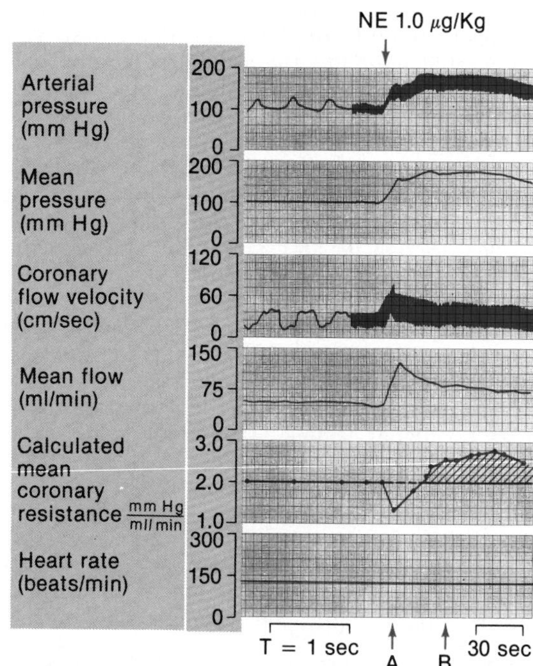

FIGURE 38-7. **Effects of intravenously administered norepinephrine (NE) in the intact unanesthetized dog with heart rate held constant. Coronary vascular resistance fell initially (*A*) and then showed a sustained increase (*B*). (From Vatner, S. F., Higgins, C. B., and Braunwald, E.: Effects of norepinephrine on coronary circulation and left ventricular dynamics in the conscious dog. Circ. Res.** ***34*****:812, 1974, by permission of the American Heart Association, Inc.)**

resistance.[87] When the reflex tachycardia and myocardial contractility (which would be expected to increase $M\dot{V}O_2$ and thereby lower coronary vascular resistance) are blocked with propranolol, an *increase* in coronary vascular resistance is observed, which can be prevented by cardiac sympathectomy. It may be concluded that with intact adrenergic nerves and beta receptors, the coronary dilatation consequent to carotid occlusion is due to heightened cardiac metabolic activity induced reflexly by baroreceptor hypotension. When this augmentation of myocardial beta-receptor–mediated activity is prevented by beta blockade, reflex coronary *vasoconstriction* secondary to carotid hypotension is unmasked.[88] Stimulation of the distal ends of the vagi produces coronary vasodilatation,[88,89] an effect that is mediated by the release of acetylcholine from vagal nerve endings and that can be blocked by atropine.[35]

Evidence also exists for *tonic* coronary constriction mediated by adrenergic nerves.[90] Acute surgical denervation of the heart produces a fall in coronary vascular resistance with a reduction in arteriovenous oxygen extraction and a rise in coronary venous O_2 content (primary vasodilatation).[91] Coronary vascular resistance in patients as well as in dogs[92] with innervated hearts declines by almost 25 per cent in response to alpha-adrenoceptor blockade, suggesting that basal coronary constrictor tone mediated by alpha receptors is released. However, coronary vascular resistance does *not* diminish when patients with cardiac transplants receive alpha-adrenoceptor blockade. This indicates that cardiac denervation had previously abolished the coronary constrictor tone.

In the conscious dog, stimulation of the carotid sinus nerves results in a substantial reduction in coronary vascular resistance.[90] This effect can be prevented by alpha-receptor blockade; therefore, it would appear that adrenergic coronary constrictor tone is present in the resting conscious dog and that coronary vasodilation attendant upon electrical stimulation of the carotid sinus nerves results from a reduction in this resting vasoconstrictor tone. Coronary vasodilation resulting from stimulation of the carotid sinus nerves occurs also during exercise. Apparently, alpha-receptor-mediated constrictor tone persists in the coronary vascular bed during exercise, despite the coexisting metabolic vasodilation. This conclusion is supported by studies using alpha-adrenoceptor blocking drugs which have shown that the increase in coronary blood flow and oxygen delivery to the myocardium during normal exercise is limited by alpha-adrenergic vasoconstriction.[93] $Alpha_1$ adrenoceptor stimulation of *ischemic* myocardium is capable of causing epicardial vasoconstriction and thereby influencing favorably the transmural distribution of blood flow[94–96] during exercise. Thus, alpha-adrenergic–mediated coronary constriction distal to the flow-limiting stenosis redistributes blood flow to the subendocardium.[97,98]

Efferent neural influences on the coronary vascular bed may also be activated reflexly by cardiopulmonary parasympathetic receptors. Stimulation of parasympathetic receptors leads to reflex systemic and coronary vasodilation,[99] while stimulation of somatic afferent fibers increases coronary resistance through alpha-adrenergically mediated vasoconstriction.[100] Chemoreceptor activation initially causes coronary dilation, a reflex that is mediated by the vagi and can be abolished by atropine.[35] As already noted, the late response is coronary vasoconstriction.[78] Intracoronary injection of veratrum alkaloids, as well as other metabolically active substances, induces reflex bradycardia and hypotension (the Bezold-Jarisch reflex),[101] the afferent limb of which involves the vagus nerves. The effects of efferent vagus nerve activity causing *coronary* vasodilation[102] have been documented, indicating that the Bezold-Jarisch reflex involves coronary efferent as well as afferent parasympathetic components.[99] Neurally controlled and alpha-adrenoceptor–mediated constriction of stenotic lesions of the coronary vascular bed in humans has been observed on coronary arteriograms[98] demonstrating the vasoconstrictor effects of handgrip.[103]

An increase in adrenergic outflow does *not* appear to be responsible for the episodes of coronary spasm in patients with Prinzmetal's (variant) angina[104] (p. 1342) or in the genesis of ischemia in so-called syndrome X (p. 1346).[105,105a] However, it has been reported that alpha-adrenoceptor stimulation can induce coronary spasm that can be prevented by phenoxybenzamine or prazosin in some patients.[98] The finding that administration of alpha receptor blockers can reduce exercise-induced ST-segment depression and angina[98,106,106a,107] indicates that alpha receptor–mediated coronary vasoconstriction plays some role in angina on effort. It has also been shown that cocaine is a potent coronary vasoconstrictor in humans and dogs,[107a] and since this effect can be prevented by an alpha receptor blocker, phentolamine, it appears to be mediated through alpha-adrenergic stimulation.[108]

AUTOREGULATION OF CORONARY BLOOD FLOW

When sudden alterations in perfusion pressure are imposed in many vascular beds, the abrupt changes in blood flow are only transitory, with flow promptly returning toward the previous steady-state level.[109] This phenomenon, called *autoregulation* (Fig. 38–8), applies also to the coronary vascular bed and tends to maintain myocardial perfusion within a relatively narrow range, regardless of transitory changes in perfusion pressure between approximately 60 and 130 mm Hg.[52] Demonstration of autoregulation is difficult in intact animals because modification of coronary perfusion pressure also changes both $M\dot{V}O_2$ and the extrinsic compression of the coronary vessels. However, under experimental conditions in which perfusion pressure is altered but ventricular pressure, cardiac contractility, and heart rate—the principal determinants of $M\dot{V}O_2$—are maintained constant, autoregulation is clearly evident. Autoregulation is more prominent in the subepicardial than in the subendocardial layers of the left ventricle. Drugs that cause relaxation of coronary vascular smooth muscle diminish autoregulation.[51]

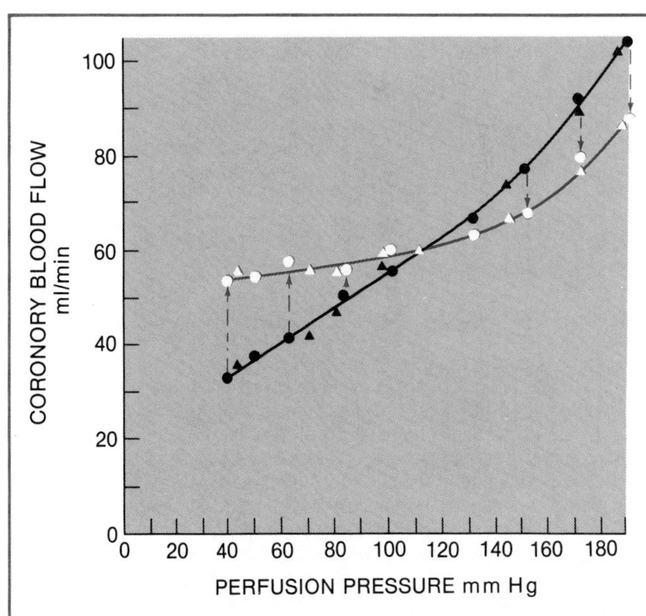

FIGURE 38–8. Autoregulation of coronary blood flow in the beating dog heart. The point where the curves cross represents the control steady-state pressure and flow. A sudden, sustained change in perfusion pressure caused an abrupt change in flow represented by the filled symbols and black line (transient flow). The open symbols and red line represent the steady-state flows obtained at each perfusion pressure. The points represented by triangles were obtained after blockade of cardiac prostaglandin synthesis with indomethacin. (Reproduced by permission from Rubio, K., and Berne, K. M.: Regulation of coronary blood flow. Prog. Cardiovasc. Dis. *18*:105, 1975.)

Autoregulation in the bed distal to a coronary obstruction may be compromised because the bed is already maximally dilated in the basal state. As a consequence, perfusion of this distal bed becomes dependent entirely on perfusion pressure (Fig. 38–5). Under these circumstances, augmentation of cardiac oxygen requirements, as occurs during exercise and *without* an increase in perfusion pressure, results in or intensifies ischemia. Since blood flow to regions supplied by normal vessels can be increased (because regional vasodilatation in these regions is possible), while blood flow to the compromised zone cannot (because its vessels are already maximally dilated), disparities in regional perfusion can become intensified. This explains exercise-induced regional dysfunction in the presence of subcritical coronary stenosis.[110] In addition, vasodilatation in the normal zones may reduce perfusion pressure to the ischemic area and deprive it further of blood flow, a phenomenon sometimes termed *coronary steal.* It has been observed that when coronary perfusion pressure falls to below the critical levels of 60 to 70 mm Hg, the coronary vessels become maximally dilated and flow becomes pressure-dependent, i.e., autoregulation is lost (Fig. 38–8). This observation underlines the importance of maintaining coronary perfusion pressure in patients with hypotension of any cause, including acute myocardial infarction.

When obstructive coronary artery disease is present, coronary perfusion pressure is lower than aortic pressure. A small reduction of the latter could then lower perfusion pressure below critical levels, thereby depressing myocardial perfusion, intensifying myocardial ischemia, and increasing left ventricular filling pressure, which decreases the perfusion pressure gradient further and may cause a vicious circle. In patients with cardiogenic shock, the reduction of perfusion pressure below the critical level at which autoregulation is lost lowers coronary blood flow even through nonobstructed vessels and may reduce collateral blood flow to the periinfarction zone, thereby enlarging the infarct (Fig. 39–11, p. 1210).

Several mechanisms have been implicated in the autoregulation of coronary blood flow, including myogenic and metabolic factors, vasoactive substances released by the endothelium, as well as extravascular compressive forces.[34,35]

MYOGENIC FACTORS. Stretch of vascular smooth muscle resulting from an increase in perfusion pressure stimulates the muscle to contract.[111] The consequent augmentation of resistance tends to return blood flow toward normal despite the higher perfusion pressure. Although this myogenic mechanism, sometimes called the *Bayliss effect* (after its discoverer, a collaborator of Ernest Starling), appears to be a general characteristic of vascular smooth muscle,[112] its role in the regulation of coronary blood flow has not been explicitly defined and is probably a modest one.[35]

METABOLIC CONTROL OF CORONARY BLOOD FLOW. It is likely that changes in regional myocardial metabolism are important determinants of autoregulation (and therefore coronary blood flow). Several mediators have been implicated, including oxygen, carbon dioxide, and vasodilator metabolites such as adenosine, that accumulate in hypoperfused regions of myocardium. There is a tight coupling between $M\dot{V}O_2$ and coronary blood flow.[52] It has been suggested that with increased energy expenditure by the heart there is a proportionally increased production of vasodilator metabolites, which in turn reduces coronary vascular resistance and raises coronary blood flow so that only small changes in myocardial oxygen extraction occur. This form of coronary vasodilatation is known as *secondary* dilatation, in contrast to the *primary* dilatation that occurs with denervation of the heart already described.

A marked reduction in coronary arterial perfusion pressure (while $M\dot{V}O_2$ is held constant) causes an immediate decrease in coronary flow. This would be expected to cause increased myocardial O_2 extraction and a reduced myocardial oxygen tension; the resultant hypoxia and accompanying accumulation of vasodilator metabolites then would be responsible for the ensuing (secondary) coronary vasodilatation.[113] It is possible that oxygen acts on vascular smooth muscle directly, possibly by altering the electrochemical potential of the muscle cells. Direct vasodilating effects of diminished oxygen tension have been demonstrated in the coronary, femoral, and other vessels.[114] Molecular oxygen diffusing across the walls of the vessels appears to be a primary determinant of constrictor tone of precapillary sphincters under physiological conditions.[115] Thus, diminution of oxygen tension increases the number of capillaries perfused within a predefined region of myocardium, presumably by relaxation of these sphincters.[116] In this manner, coronary blood flow would be expected to remain constant (or almost so) despite a reduction of coronary perfusion pressure. Transitory augmentation of the concentration of potassium in extracellular fluid, an early consequence of myocardial ischemia, may also modify the transmembrane potential of vascular smooth muscle cells, causing their relaxation and thus producing coronary vasodilatation.

Role of Adenosine (Fig. 38–9). Degradation of adenine nucleotides under conditions in which ATP utilization exceeds the capacity of myocardial cells to resynthesize high-energy phosphate compounds (a process dependent on oxidative phosphorylation in mitochondria) results in the production of adenosine monophosphate (AMP). The enzyme 5′-nucleotidase is responsible for the formation of adenosine.[117] Accordingly, adenosine and its metabolites, inosine and hypoxanthine, appear in interstitial fluid and in the coronary sinus venous effluent. *Adenosine* is a powerful vasodilator[118] that is considered to be an important, perhaps *the critical, mediator* linking metabolically induced vasodilatation to diminished coronary perfusion (Fig. 38–9). There is substantial evidence that an imbalance (a reduction) in the supply-to-demand ratio for oxygen is the primary determinant of adenosine formation.[117,119]

Concentrations of adenosine in the venous effluent are much lower than those in interstitial fluid, in part because capillary endothelium rapidly converts adenosine to inosine and hypoxanthine.[120] However, when the enzyme responsible for this conversion, adenosine deaminase, is inhibited by the administration of 8-azaguanine, marked increases in the concentration of adenosine in the effluent are unmasked.[121] If, at a constant level of myocardial metabolism, adenosine were being released at a constant rate, an elevation of coronary perfusion pressure and the resultant increase in coronary blood flow would augment the washout of adenosine, reduce its concentration, and thus increase coronary vascular resistance. Such a mechanism could provide a feedback to account for autoregulation of coronary blood flow. More important, it could also explain the close correlation between the energy expenditure of the heart and the level of coronary blood flow.[121,122] According to this concept, as the former rises, the ratio of oxygen supply to demand declines, and more ATP is degraded to AMP, which becomes available for and enhances adenosine formation. The latter causes coronary relaxation, thereby increasing coronary blood flow to a level appropriate to the $M\dot{V}O_2$.

It appears that adenosine acts on the surface of vascular smooth muscle cells, apparently on adenosine receptors on the cell membrane; presumably activation of these receptors blocks entry of Ca^{++} into these cells and thereby causes vasodilatation.[35] In addition to its potent vasodilating action, adenosine exerts a generally depressant activity on cardiac automaticity and atrioventricular conduction and attenuates the effects of adrenergic influences on myocardial contractility.[123]

Despite its importance, adenosine is almost certainly not the only metabolic factor involved, and its role in mediating the increase in coronary blood flow has been questioned. It is possible that adenosine does not act alone but interacts with other agents in response to hypoxia in causing coronary relaxation.[124] Prostaglandins, kinins, acetate, K^+, and a number of metabolites alter coronary vascular resistance profoundly and may play a role in mediating vasodilatation in response to hypoxia. The infusion of at least two prostaglandins synthesized in the heart (PGI_2 and PGE_2) can cause coronary vasodilatation,[125] and the inhibition of prostaglandin synthesis with indomethacin causes an increase in coronary vascular resistance in humans.[126]

ENDOTHELIAL CONTROL OF CORONARY VASCULAR TONE

The adult human possesses approximately 10^{12} vascular endothelial cells, which occupy an area exceeding 1000 m^2. It has long been appreciated that the endothelial cells serve as a nonthrombogenic diffusion barrier to the migration of substances out of and into the bloodstream and as a site for exchange of nutrients and metabolites between the capillaries and cells. However, during the past 15 years it has been appreciated that the endothelium is also the largest and most active paracrine organ in the body, producing potent vasoactive, anticoagulant, procoagulant, and fibrinolytic substances (Table 38–3).[126a] Abnormalities in the structure and function of the

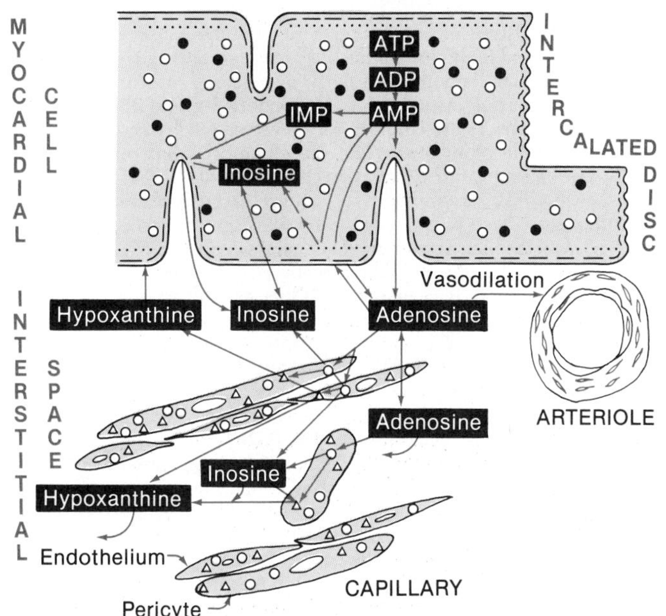

FIGURE 38-9. Schematic drawing depicting a myocardial interstitial space, an arteriole, and a capillary with the localization of enzymes involved in the formation and fate of adenosine. Adenosine formed by 5′-nucleotidase from AMP (which in turn arises from ATP) can enter the interstitial space. There it can induce arteriolar dilation and reenter the myocardial cell, where it is either phosphorylated to AMP by adenosine kinase or deaminated to inosine by adenosine deaminase, or it can enter the capillaries and leave the tissue. A large fraction of adenosine that crosses the capillary wall is deaminated to inosine, which in turn is split to hypoxanthine and ribose-1-PO_4 by nucleoside phosphorylase located in the endothelial cells, pericytes, and erythrocytes. Most of the adenosine is taken up by the myocardial cells, and that escaping into the circulation is largely in the form of inosine and hypoxanthine. Since adenylic acid deaminase (which deaminates AMP to IMP) is in low concentration in heart muscle, the major degradative pathway from AMP is via dephosphorylation to adenosine. ○, Adenosine deaminase; ●, adenylic acid deaminase; △, nucleoside phosphorylase; (---), 5′-nucleotidase; (···), adenosine kinase. (From Berne, R. M., and Rubio, R.: Coronary circulation. *In* Berne, R. M., Sperelakis, N., and Geiger, S. R. [eds.]: Handbook of Physiology, Section 2. The Cardiovascular System. Bethesda, Md., American Physiological Society, 1979, p. 924.)

endothelium are now believed to play important roles in the pathogenesis of many vascular (including coronary vascular) diseases.[127,128]

Among the many important vasoactive substances synthesized by endothelial cells is prostacyclin (PGI_2), an arachidonic acid metabolite whose release is stimulated by a variety of physiological stimuli (tissue hypoxia, hemodynamic stress, high-density lipoproteins, ATP, and leukotrienes) and pharmacological substances (calcium ionophores). Prostacyclin elevates intracellular concentrations of cyclic AMP and thereby serves as a potent relaxant of vascular smooth muscle and inhibitor of platelet aggregation.

ENDOTHELIUM-DERIVED RELAXING FACTOR. Endothelium also synthesizes *endothelium-derived relaxing factor* (EDRF),[129–131] which is, or acts like, nitric oxide (NO).[131a] It is derived from the amino acid L-arginine (through an as-yet unidentified biosynthetic pathway[132]) and is metabolized to inactive nitrite; the synthesis of EDRF can be inhibited by the L-arginine analog N^G monomethyl L-arginine.[133] The principal target organs of EDRF are, on one side, the subadjacent vascular smooth muscle cells and on the other side, circulating platelets (Fig. 38–10).

EDRF is released from normal endothelial cells by a broad array of stimulants, including acetylcholine,[134] thrombin, bradykinin, thromboxane A_2, histamine, and aggregating platelets, and by catecholamines acting on $alpha_2$ receptors on endothelial cells.[129] Receptors on normal endothelium that cause the release of EDRF when stimulated include muscarinic receptors (for acetylcholine), thrombin receptors, histaminergic receptors, vasopressin(ergic) and oxytocin(ergic) receptors, $alpha_2$-adrenoceptors (for circulating catecholamines), purinergic and serotonergic receptors stimulated by aggregating platelets, ADP, and serotonin (Fig. 38–11). In contrast to prostacyclin (which acts by increasing intracellular

TABLE 38-3 IMPORTANT SUBSTANCES PRODUCED BY OR ACTING THROUGH VASCULAR ENDOTHELIUM

VASODILATOR	VASOCONSTRICTOR	ANTICOAGULANT/ ANTITHROMBOTIC/ ANTIPLATELET	PROCOAGULANT
Produced by endothelium			
Adenosine	? Endothelin	Adenosine	Collagen
EDRF	Peptidoleukotrienes	EDRF	FVIII-VWF complex
EDHF		Glycosaminoglycans	Fibronectin
Peptidoleukotrienes		Plasminogen activator	Plasminogen inhibitors
PGE_2		PGE_1, PGE_2	
$PGF_{1\alpha}$		PGI_2	
PGI_2		Thrombomodulin	
		Tissue factor	
Acts through endothelium			
Acetylcholine	Angiotensin	Heparin	
ADP	Vasopressin		
Bradykinin			
Catecholamines			
Histamine			
Peptidoleukotrienes			
Serotonin			

ADP = adenosine diphosphate; EDHF = endothelium-derived hyperpolarizing factor; EDRF = endothelium-derived relaxing factor; FVIII = coagulation factor VIII; PG = prostaglandin; VWF = von Willebrand factor.

From Dinerman, J. L., and Mehta, J. L.: Endothelial, platelet and leukocyte interactions in ischemic heart disease: Insights into potential mechanisms and their clinical relevance. Reprinted by permission of the American College of Cardiology. J. Am. Coll. Cardiol. *16*:207, 1990.

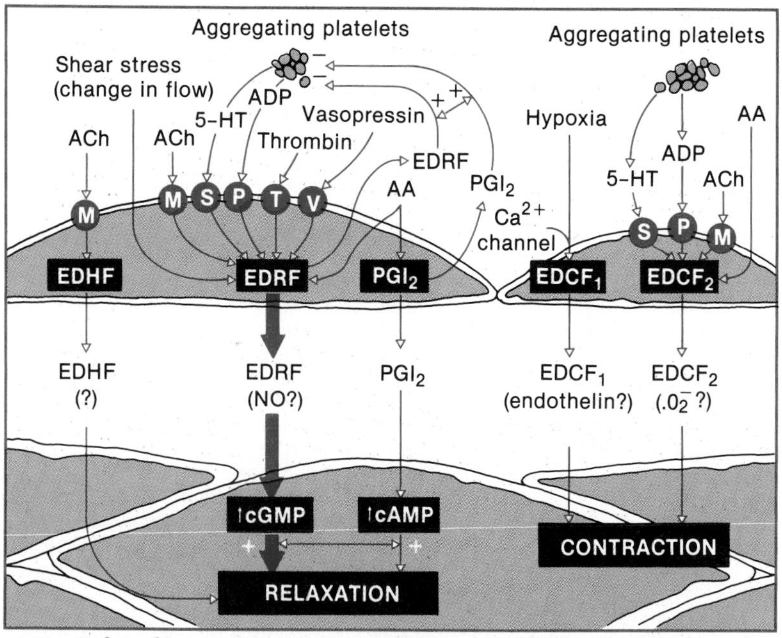

FIGURE 38-10. **Current concepts of endothelium-derived factors and their modulation of vascular smooth muscle contraction. Endothelium-derived relaxing factor (EDRF), a powerful vasodilator of the underlying smooth muscle, increases cyclic GMP (cGMP) levels through activation of soluble guanylate cyclase. The chemical nature of EDRF may be simply nitric oxide or a complex containing it. Prostacyclin (PGI_2) is another vasodilator released from the endothelium whose effects depend on elevation of cyclic AMP (cAMP) through activation of adenylate cyclase. EDRF and prostacyclin could act synergistically in terms of relaxing vascular smooth muscle and inhibiting platelet aggregation. The endothelial cells also secrete a hyperpolarizing factor (EDHF). The exact nature of EDHF is unknown; is most likely is a metabolite of arachidonic acid, presumably an epoxide or lipoxide.**

At least two endothelium-derived contracting factors exist; one is indomethacin-insensitive ($EDCF_1$) and the other is indomethacin-sensitive ($EDCF_2$). Recent data suggest that $EDCF_1$ may be endothelin, and $EDCF_2$ may be superoxide anions, although this remains to be proved. EDHF has a vasodilator effect and may contribute in part to the initial portion of endothelium-dependent relaxations. ACh, acetylcholine; 5-HT, 5-hydroxytryptamine, serotonin; ADP, adenosine diphosphate; AA, arachidonic acid; +, synergism or facilitation; −, inhibition; ?, exact nature unknown; M, muscarinic receptor; S, serotonergic receptor; P, purinergic receptor; T, thrombin receptor; V, vasopressinergic receptor. (From Vanhoutte, P. M., and Shimokawa, H.: Endothelium-derived relaxing factor and coronary vasospasm. Circulation *80*:1, 1989, by permission of the American Heart Association, Inc.)

cyclic AMP), EDRF acts on a receptor that is probably the heme moiety of soluble guanylate cyclase.[132] The resultant stimulation of guanylate cyclase increases vascular smooth muscle cell cyclic guanine monophosphate (GMP), which activates a cyclic GMP–dependent protein kinase. This in turn inhibits release of Ca^{++} from endoplasmic reticulum and other storage sites, causing relaxation of vascular smooth muscle. These biochemical actions of EDRF are shared by a number of nitrosodilators, such as nitroglycerin and nitroprusside, which act by generating NO. However, these substances do not require an intact endothelium for their vasodilator action, as do acetylcholine, thrombin, aggregating platelets, and the like. Thus, EDRF might be considered to be an "endogenous nitrate," while, conversely, nitroglycerin might be considered to be an "exogenous EDRF." N-Acetylcysteine, a reduced thiol, potentiates the inhibition of platelets by EDRF, an effect associated with increasing platelet cyclic GMP concentrations.[135]

The formation of EDRF in the basal state plays a significant role in setting resting arterial tone.[131] The endothelial response to shear stress plays an important physiological role in the control of vascular (including coronary vascular) tone. As blood flow through an artery increases, the shear stress on the endothelium rises. This in turn increases the release of EDRF and causes vasodilation, which enhances blood flow further. Absence of EDRF or damage to the endothelium abolishes this response to shear stress. Inflammatory mediators, such as bradykinin, histamine, and substance P, also augment local blood flow by increasing release of EDRF.

The two vasoactive and platelet-active products of normal endothelium, prostacyclin and EDRF, act in concert to inhibit platelet adhesion and aggregation and to relax vascular smooth muscle. Normal endothelium also opposes a variety of vasoconstrictor stimuli, including catecholamines, serotonin, and vasopressin, and enhances the vasorelaxant effects of dilators, such as histamine and adenosine nucleotides.[136] Vascular endothelium is normally the principal source of locally produced plasminogen activator, and by this action too it enhances the fluidity of the blood. Indeed, prostacyclin, EDRF, and t-PA act synergistically in this manner. In the absence of

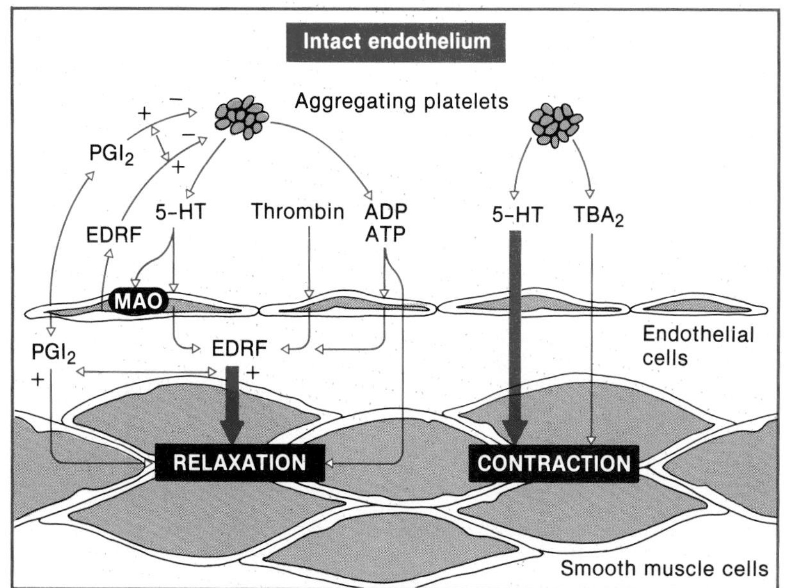

FIGURE 38-11. **Illustration of several effects of endothelium-derived relaxing factor (EDRF) during platelet aggregation; inhibition of platelet adhesion and aggregation and of platelet-induced contraction. Endothelium-dependent relaxations to aggregating platelets are achieved mainly by adenine nucleotides (ADP and ATP) and serotonin (5-HT), whereas direct, endothelium-independent contractions are achieved mainly by serotonin (5-HT) and thromboxanes (TBA_2), depending on the species and vascular beds tested. Under normal conditions in the presence of intact endothelium, those relaxations and contractions may be well balanced. EDRF and prostacyclin could act synergistically (arrowheads) against platelet aggregation and platelet-induced contractions. +, facilitation; −, inhibition. MAO, monoamine oxidase; PGI_2, prostacyclin. (From Vanhoutte, P. M., and Shimokawa, H.: Endothelium-derived relaxing factor and coronary vasospasm. Circulation *80*:1, 1989, by permission of the American Heart Association, Inc.)**

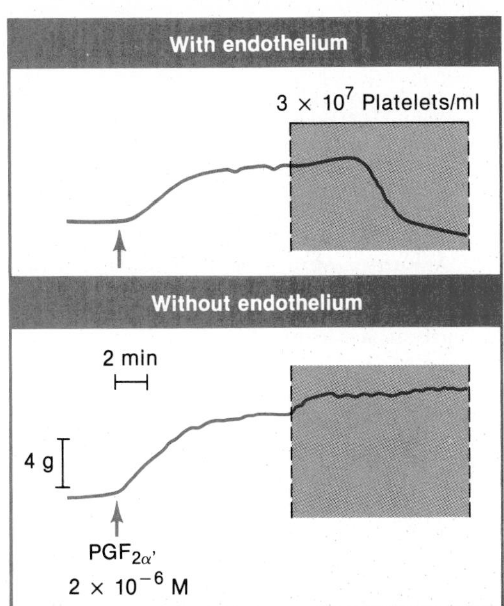

FIGURE 38-12. Example of the response of left circumflex artery rings with and without endothelium during contraction to prostaglandin $F_{2\alpha}$ ($PGF_{2\alpha}$) upon addition of platelet suspensions. The size of the contraction in response to $PGF_{2\alpha}$ was not significantly different in rings with or without endothelium. (From Cohen, R. A., Shepherd, J. T., and Vanhoutte, P. M.: Endothelial alpha receptors in canine pulmonary and systemic blood vessels. Eur. J. Pharmacol. *118*:123, 1985.)

an intact endothelium, platelets are potent vasoconstrictors, but in the presence of an intact endothelium, platelets actually exert an indirect vasodilating effect by effecting the release of EDRF (Fig. 38-12). Vascular endothelial cells also perform a variety of metabolic functions including the conversion of angiotensin I to II as well as the uptake of circulating norepinephrine and serotonin.[127]

In the face of thrombogenic vasoconstrictor stimuli, such as may be supplied by thrombin and platelets, the products of endothelial cells, i.e., prostacyclin and EDRF, oppose normal thrombogenesis and cause vascular dilatation. In contrast, in vessels with atherosclerotic plaques and in other conditions in which the endothelium has been damaged, the response to a thrombus is vascular contraction and further platelet aggregation, thereby resulting in interference with blood flow. A variety of disease processes interfere with the normal function of the endothelium. For example, disruption of the endothelium by atheromatous plaques can activate platelets and lead to thrombogenesis. Sites of endothelial damage in the coronary vascular bed can be responsible for localized regions of coronary spasm (Fig. 38-13). Indeed, the coronary spasm that frequently follows PTCA suggests that disruption of the endothelium may tip the balance of forces acting on the coronary artery diameter in favor of contraction.

There is experimental evidence that both hypertension and hypercholesterolemia also impair release of EDRF. Thus, endothelium-dependent relaxation in response to thrombin, ADP, and acetylcholine is reduced or absent in aortic rings from genetically hypertensive rats. Hypercholesterolemia in cynomolgus monkeys and swine[137a] impairs endothelium-dependent vascular relaxation.[137] Normal young adult human subjects exhibit coronary vasodilatation in response to the intracoronary artery infusion of acetylcholine, presumably as a consequence of the release of EDRF. In contrast, atherosclerotic coronary arteries, coronary vessels with minor irregularities, the apparently *uninvolved* vessels of patients with known coronary vascular disease,[138] vessels of patients after cardiac transplantation, and even apparently normal coronary arteries in older subjects all may display a constrictor effect to intracoronary acetylcholine, suggesting the presence of abnormally functioning endothelium.[139] The endothelial dysfunction characteristic of early atherosclerosis may, by impairing vasodilator function, cause abnormal coronary vasomotion during exercise.[140] In patients with ischemic heart disease, the combination of atherosclerotic plaques that encroach on the vascular lumen and the presence of vasoconstrictor stimuli, such as norepinephrine and angiotensin II, with the additional factor of endothelial dysfunction, may produce vascular obstruction.[141]

Oxygen-derived free radicals, frequently produced during postischemic reperfusion (p. 1239), inhibit endothelial dependent dilation and can thereby impede recovery of ischemically damaged myocardium.[142,143] In contrast, relaxation of coronary arteries to acetylcholine can be restored by dietary treatment of arteriosclerosis (Fig. 38-14). It is possible (through not proved) that the eicosapentaenoic acid in cod liver oil, by changing the fluidity of the membranes of endothelial cells, enhances synthesis and/or release of EDRF.[144]

ENDOTHELIN. Endothelial cells may also cause contraction of vascular smooth muscle cells (Fig. 38-15). Yanagisawa et al.[145] have cloned the precursor of a contractile factor produced by endothelial cells, a 21-residue vasoconstrictor polypeptide called *endothelin* (Fig. 38-16). Endothelin was ini-

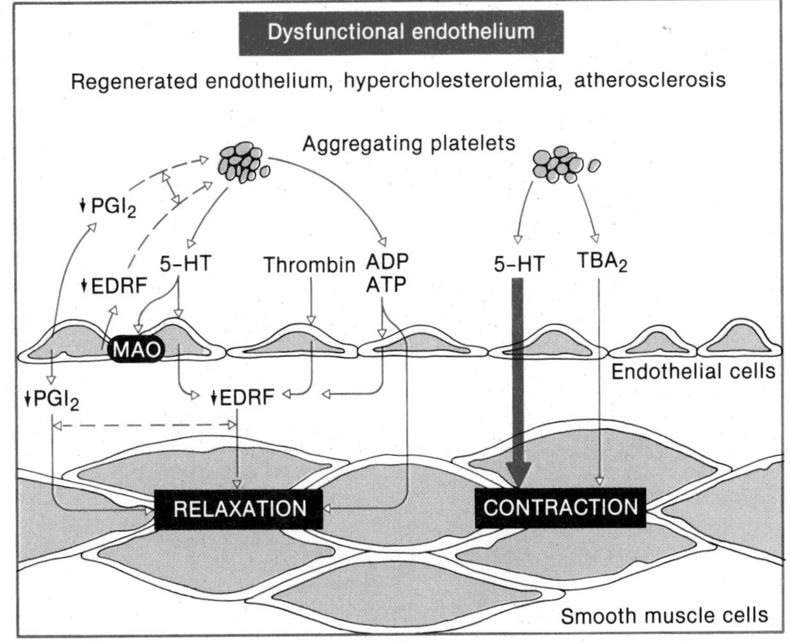

FIGURE 38-13. Illustration of endothelium-dependent responses under pathological conditions. The endothelium is dysfunctional in a regenerated state, hypercholesterolemia and atherosclerosis, releasing less endothelium-derived relaxing factor (EDRF), whereas the ability of the smooth muscle to contract is unaltered. As a result, the contractions predominate. In atherosclerosis, the production of both EDRF and prostacyclin (PGI_2) is reduced, and their synergistic actions against aggregating platelets may not occur. 5-HT, 5-hydroxytryptamine, serotonin; ADP, adenosine diphosphate; ATP, adenosine triphosphate; TBA_2, thromboxane A_2; MAO, monoamine oxidase; −, inhibition; +, synergism. (From Vanhoutte, P. M., and Shimokawa, H.: Endothelium-derived relaxing factor and coronary vasospasm. Circulation *80*:6, 1989, by permission of the American Heart Association, Inc.)

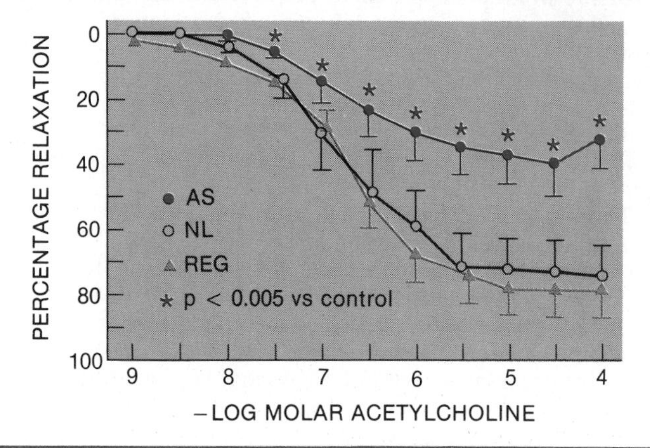

FIGURE 38–14. Responses to acetylcholine of iliac arteries of normal (NL), atherosclerotic (AS), and atherosclerosis regression (REG) monkeys. Atherosclerosis was induced by cholesterol feeding, while regression was achieved by withdrawal of the high cholesterol diet. *$p < 0.05$ vs. atherosclerotic. Responses to acetylcholine were reduced by approximately one-half in atherosclerotic vessels, and were restored to normal by dietary treatment of atherosclerosis. (Reproduced from Harrison, D. G., Armstrong, M. L., Freiman, P. C., and Heistad, D. D.: Restoration of endothelium-dependent relaxation by dietary treatment of atherosclerosis. J. Clin. Invest. *80*:1808, 1987, by copyright permission of the American Society for Clinical Investigation.)

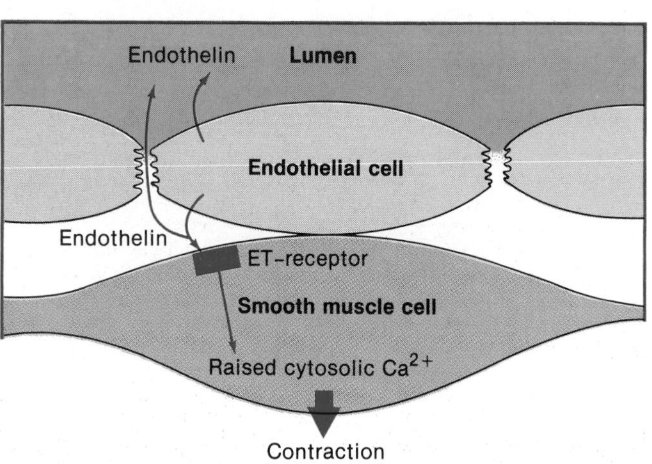

FIGURE 38–15. Schematic representation of the "spill-over" of endothelin into the circulation. The target site for the released endothelin is the endothelin (ET) receptor on the smooth muscle cell. Activation of this receptor results in a sustained rise in cytosolic Ca^{++}, and hence constriction. (From Naylor, W. G.: The Endothelins. Berlin, Springer-Verlag, 1990, p. 91.)

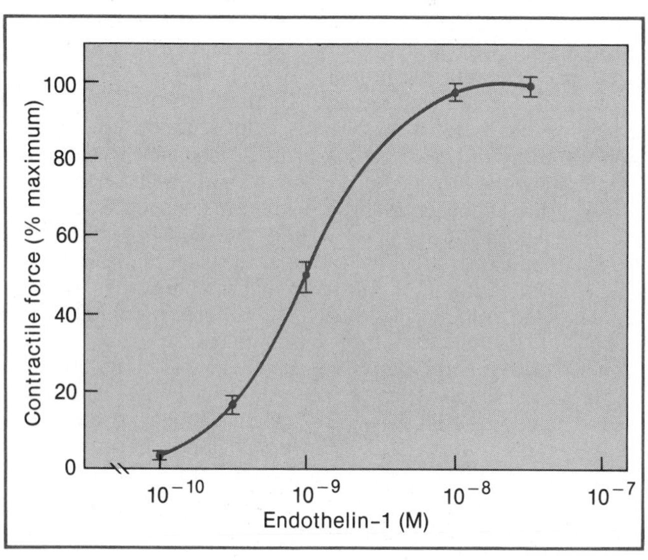

FIGURE 38–16. Dose-dependent constrictor effect of endothelin-1 on human left anterior descending coronary arteries. (From Naylor, W. G.: The Endothelins. Berlin, Springer-Verlag, 1990, p. 117, based on data from Chester, A. H., et al.: Influence of endothelin on human coronary arteries and localization of its binding sites. Am. J. Cardiol. *63*:1395, 1989.)

tially isolated from cultured endothelial cells, but it is also synthesized in a number of tissues, including the kidneys. Shear stress acting on endothelial cells apparently causes downregulation of the preendothelin gene, thereby contributing to flow-induced vasodilation.[146] Threshold concentrations of endothelin I also amplify the contractions of human arteries caused by norepinephrine and serotonin.[147] Endothelin has a potent, prolonged coronary vasoconstrictor action[148,149] (Fig. 38–16). Like EDRF, it may be a long-term modulator of coronary tone. Endothelin's action is not affected by calcium antagonists, but it is opposed by adenosine, substance P, and glyceryl trinitrate.[150] Many diverse tissues contain high-affinity binding sites for endothelin, including blood vessels, heart (especially the atria), lung, brain, and kidneys. Endothelin may also function as a neurotransmitter.[146]

PHARMACOLOGICAL AGENTS

As already pointed out, alpha$_1$-adrenoceptor agonists can cause constriction both of coronary conductance vessels, i.e., the large epicardial arteries, and coronary resistance vessels, i.e., the small intramural arteries and arterioles[38] (Figs. 38–7 and 38–8). This effect is opposed by the passive distention of these vessels consequent to an elevation of intravascular pressure as well as by the metabolically-induced coronary vasodilatation resulting from the increase in $M\dot{V}O_2$ accompanying the arterial hypertension induced by these drugs. Directly acting coronary vasodilators, such as nitroglycerin and isosorbide dinitrate,[151–153] augment perfusion of ischemic zones, as reflected by the increased rate of clearance of ^{133}Xe injected into the coronary arteries of patients with coronary artery disease.[154] These drugs have been shown to dilate coronary conductance vessels, coronary collaterals, and even atherosclerotic stenoses[155–157] (Fig. 40–4, p. 1305) as well as to reduce ventricular diastolic tension, which tends to limit flow to the subendocardium. Nitrates have a lesser effect on coronary resistance vessels[158] (Fig. 38–6).

Papaverine and calcium antagonists exert a *direct* action on the large epicardial conductance vessels as well as on the resistance vessels.[157] These agents increase blood flow to normal as well as ischemic myocardium.[159] Dipyridamole dilates the distal (resistance) vessels.[151,160] Because these are acted upon also by the endogenous vasodilator (adenosine), dipyridamole is of little or no value in the treatment of acute myocardial ischemia. Prostacyclin, which is produced by endothelial cells and which inhibits platelet aggregation, also is a potent coronary vasodilator,[124] whereas thromboxane A_2, which is produced by and aggregates platelets, is a potent coronary vasoconstrictor. Dazoxiben, a thromboxane A_2 synthetase inhibitor, can prevent cyclic increases in coronary vascular resistance in stenotic coronary arteries.[161] Serotonin is an extremely potent coronary vasoconstrictor that acts on serotonergic receptors.[38,162] It can be blocked by serotonergic antagonists such as methysergide and ketanserin. Ergonovine and related ergot alkaloids are used diagnostically to provoke coronary spasm in patients suspected of having Prinzmetal's (variant) angina (p. 1342); these compounds cause coronary constriction by acting on both alpha-adrenergic and serotonergic receptors.[38] Atrial natriuretic peptide (p. 412) is a potent dilator of coronary arteries and collaterals in experimental animals and humans.[163,164]

REACTIVE HYPEREMIA AND CORONARY FLOW RESERVE

Ischemia caused by transient coronary arterial occlusion is followed by an increase in blood flow above control levels, a response called *reactive hyperemia* (Fig. 38–17). The flow debt (although not the oxygen debt) is overpaid by the marked vasodilation that characterizes reactive hyperemia; this overpayment is probably related to the accumulation of vasodilator metabolites, especially adenosine.[51,165] The difference between basal coronary blood flow and peak flow during reactive hyperemia represents the *coronary flow reserve*, which has been measured in experimental animals[166–168] and estimated in patients.[169] The coronary reserve is reduced, even absent, in patients with severe obstructive coronary artery disease, and it can be restored to normal by bypass grafting. The coronary flow reserve in the left ventricles of patients with severe left ventricular hypertrophy secondary to aortic stenosis is reduced,[170,171] perhaps because of failure of the coronary circulation to grow apace with the increase in ventricular mass[170] as well as by compression of the intramural coronary vascular bed by the hypertrophied myocardium. Regression of experimentally produced hypertrophy has been found to restore impaired coronary flow reserve toward normal.[172–174]

Coronary flow reserve can be estimated noninvasively by positron emission tomographic imaging (to measure cardiac perfusion) both in the basal state and under the influence of a powerful vasodilator stress—the combination of intravenous dipyridamole and handgrip stress. Patients with left ventricular hypertrophy exhibited a reduction of the stress-to-rest perfusion ratio to 1.06 from normal values of 1.41.[175] Good correlations also have been reported between the severity of coronary stenosis determined by quantitative coronary arteriography and myocardial perfusion determined by positron emission tomography.[176] Coronary flow reserve has been estimated in a wide variety of conditions. A reduction of the coronary blood flow response to the vasodilating actions of dipyridamole has been demonstrated in patients with essential hypertension.[177] Using electrical pacing of the heart to evoke a vasodilator response, Cannon and associates described an abnormally reduced coronary flow reserve in patients with hypertrophic cardiomyopathy, in whom elevation of left ventricular filling pressure, probably related to an ischemia-induced reduction in ventricular compliance during tachycardia, was associated with a decline in coronary blood flow.[178] Similar reductions in vasodilator reserve were demonstrated in patients undergoing rejection of the transplanted heart.[179]

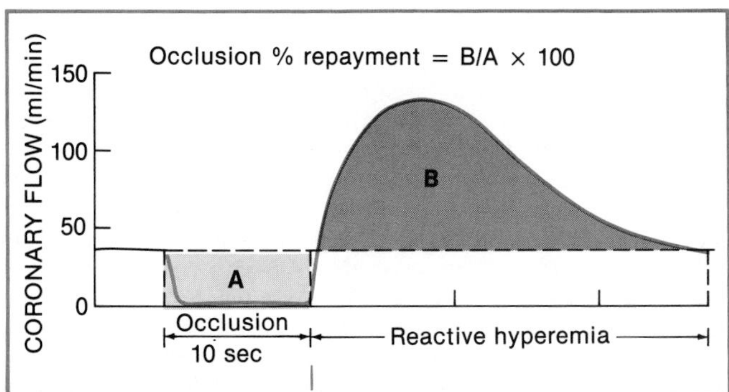

FIGURE 38–17. **Mean coronary flow prior to, during, and following coronary occlusion. Arrow indicates the release of occlusion. Area A represents the flow debt, and area B its repayment. (From Gould, K. L.: Coronary Artery Stenosis. New York, Elsevier, 1991, p. 13.)**

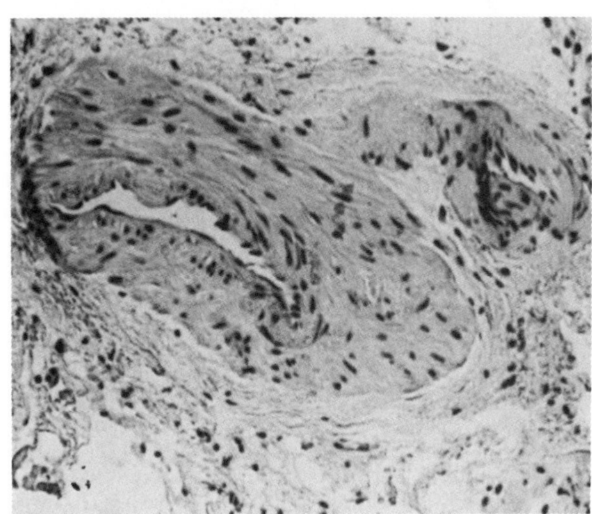

FIGURE 38–18. **Light micrograph from patient 2, showing markedly thickened small coronary arteries (hematoxylin and eosin ×320). (From Mosseri, M., Yarom, R., Gotsman, M. S., and Hasin, Y.: Histologic evidence for small-vessel coronary artery disease in patients with angina pectoris and patent large coronary arteries. Circulation *74*:964, 1986, by permission of the American Heart Association, Inc.)**

Patients with dilated cardiomyopathy, anginal chest pain, and angiographically normal coronary arteries have exhibited impaired vasodilator response to a metabolic stimulus (cardiac pacing) and a pharmacological stimulus (dipyridamole) and increased sensitivity to a vasoconstrictor stimulus (ergonovine).[180]

An inadequate flow reserve secondary to a vascular or extravascular abnormality that prevents normal coronary arterial dilatation in the face of ischemia represents a cause of myocardial ischemia that is being recognized with increasing frequency. Indeed, among patients with angina pectoris and patent large coronary arteries, a reduced flow of angiographic contrast medium has been reported, and right ventricular endomyocardial biopsy specimens have shown fibromuscular hyperplasia, hypertrophy of the media, and endothelial degeneration[181] (Fig. 38–18). Many of these patients with so-called microvascular angina[181a] also demonstrate an abnormally reduced dilator capacity to dipyridamole with a paradoxical vasoconstrictor response to bicycle exercise.[182] At autopsy intramyocardial small arteries uniformly showed a reduction in the ratio of vessel lumen to wall thickness.[183]

FACTORS LIMITING CORONARY PERFUSION

The normal intramyocardial coronary vascular bed has the capacity to reduce its resistance to approximately 15 to 20 per cent of basal levels during the stress of maximal exercise, i.e., a five- to sixfold increase in coronary blood flow, which is generally accompanied by an increase in arterial pressure and marked tachycardia, can occur during maximal exercise. It is then not surprising that when the diameter of a normal proximal coronary artery can be reduced by up to 80 per cent, sufficient dilatation of the intramyocardial coronary resistance vessels will occur so that the *total* coronary vascular resistance in series remains constant (Fig. 38–19).[184] However, when maximal dilatation of the resistance vessels has occurred in the presence of such a critical obstruction in a proximal artery, coronary blood flow cannot rise; any stimulus that increases $M\dot{V}O_2$, such as exercise- or pacing-induced tachycardia, will of necessity elicit ischemia. When obstruction of a proximal coronary artery reduces the lumen by more than approximately 90 to 95 per cent of normal, ischemia will be present even in the basal state, despite maximal dilatation of the resistance vessels, unless the myocardium distal to the obstructed vessel is perfused by collateral vessels or unless mechanical activity of the myocardium is reduced. Transient severe obstruction, as may occur with coronary spasm, will result in brief periods of ischemia, chest pain, electrocardiographic changes, and myocardial dysfunction. When severe ischemia persists, myocardial necrosis usually ensues. With lesser degrees of obstruction of an epicardial artery (e.g., 40 to 80 per cent of the control diameter lumen) the distal bed is *not* maximally dilated in the basal state, and although the capacity for further dilatation exists, this capacity is subnormal and ischemia may develop if myocardial oxygen demands are sufficiently augmented. With less than 40 per cent diameter stenosis, maximum flow during exercise is usually normal.

Basic considerations of fluid mechanics indicate that the pressure drop across a stenosis varies directly with the length of the stenosis and inversely with the fourth power of the radius (Bernoulli's theorem), emphasizing the greater importance of changes in the latter compared with the former.[185,186] Stenosis resistance changes relatively little with mild degrees of vascular narrowing but rises progressively and precipitously with severe obstruction; indeed, resistance almost triples as stenosis severity increases from 80 to 90 per cent.[187] As a consequence, with even a slight increase in the severity of stenosis—as might occur when platelets aggregate on a critically narrowed plaque or when the pressure distending the narrowed coronary artery declines, as occurs with a rise in blood flow during exercise or following administration of dipyridamole—the perfusion pressure distal to the obstruction may become reduced and subendocardial perfusion impaired.[185] Vascular resistance is not fixed even in the presence of an atherosclerotic plaque. As flow across such a lesion rises, substantial energy losses due to turbulence occur that are proportional to the flow squared. As a result, there is an exponential rise in the pressure gradient across the stenosis. As the transstenotic pressure drop increases, the pressure distending the artery declines. This may result in passive collapse[188] (Fig. 38–20), causing further damage.

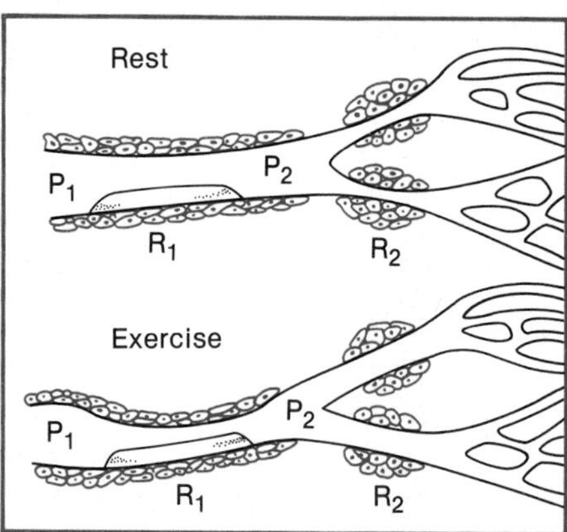

FIGURE 38–20. Diagrammatic representation of vessel collapse when myocardial flow increases. Under baseline conditions (Rest, *top*), flow across the stenosis (R_1) is modest and a large pressure gradient (P_1-P_2) does not develop. With a vasodilator intervention such as exercise *(bottom)*, the pressure gradient across the stenosis (P_1-P_2) increases. The resulting fall in intraluminal pressure may lead to collapse of the vessel at the level of the obstruction, thereby increasing the degree of stenosis. This leads to dilatation of the distal vessels (R_2). (From Epstein, S. E., Cannon, R. O., III, and Talbot, T. L.: Hemodynamic principles in the control of coronary blood flow. Am. J. Cardiol. *56*:9E, 1985.)

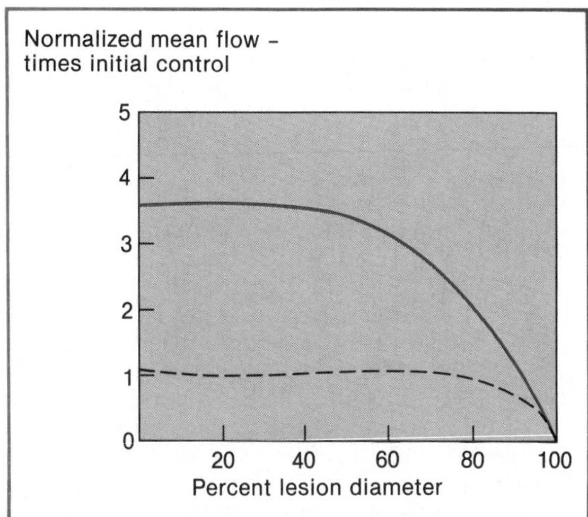

FIGURE 38–19. Relationship between resting *(dashed line)* and maximal coronary blood flow *(solid line)* and percentage of diameter stenosis in a dog. Progressive coronary stenosis was achieved by progressively narrowing a short segment of a proximal coronary artery. Resting coronary blood flow did not change until coronary diameter stenosis exceeded 80 percent. Maximal coronary blood flow began to decrease when percent diameter stenosis exceeded 50 percent. (From Marcus, M. L.: The Coronary Circulation in Health and Disease. New York, McGraw-Hill, 1983, and modified from Gould, K. L., Lipscomb, K.: Effects of coronary stenoses on coronary flow reserve and resistance. Am. J. Cardiol. *34*:50, 1974.)

FIXED AND DYNAMIC OBSTRUCTION

Myocardial ischemia and its consequences may occur as a result of fixed atherosclerotic lesions or may be secondary to transitory reduction of myocardial blood flow caused by coronary spasm and/or platelet aggregation.[189,190] The clinical sequelae of myocardial ischemia, whether produced by an increase in $M\dot{V}O_2$ in the face of fixed obstruction, by a reduction in myocardial oxygen supply, or by a combination of these factors, may be manifested clinically as angina pectoris, electrical instability, characteristic electrocardiographic changes, or depression of myocardial function, alone or in combination.

Maseri has clarified the interrelation between fixed and dynamic (variable) obstruction to blood flow.[189] Normal subjects can carry out maximal exercise, develop a 15- to 20-fold increase in body $\dot{V}O_2$ above resting levels, and yet not develop myocardial ischemia because they operate within their normal coronary reserve. Figure 38–21 shows the effects of fixed coronary obstruction that allows a fourfold increase in coronary blood flow. Ischemia occurs whenever $M\dot{V}O_2$ rises to a level that cannot be met by this coronary flow reserve. It is clear that transient reductions of coronary reserve below this level will occur in many patients with coronary atherosclerosis. In these patients, the anginal threshold will be quite variable (Fig. 38–21 II), a condition referred to a *mixed angina*.[191]

PLATE 5

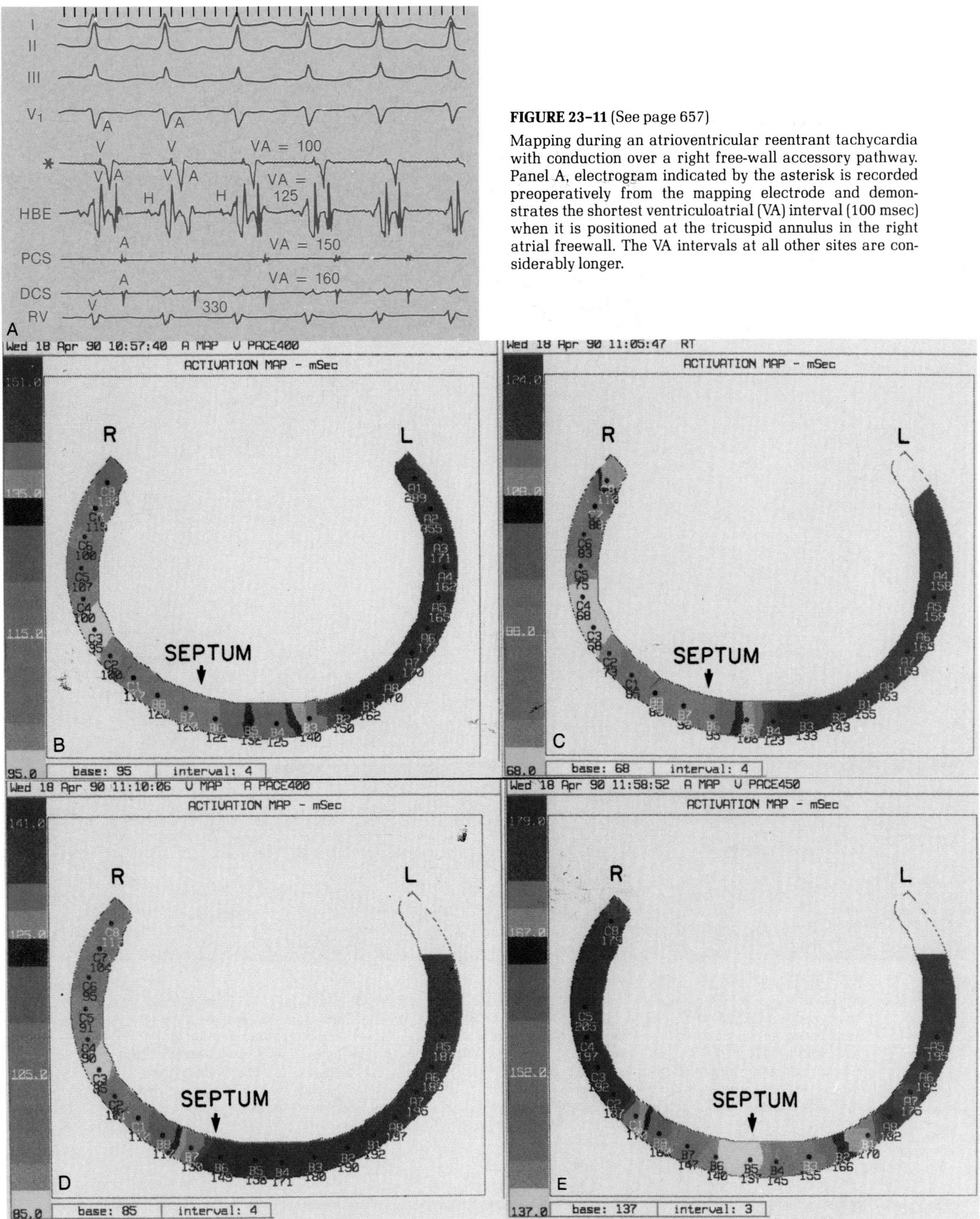

FIGURE 23–11 (See page 657)

Mapping during an atrioventricular reentrant tachycardia with conduction over a right free-wall accessory pathway. Panel A, electrogram indicated by the asterisk is recorded preoperatively from the mapping electrode and demonstrates the shortest ventriculoatrial (VA) interval (100 msec) when it is positioned at the tricuspid annulus in the right atrial freewall. The VA intervals at all other sites are considerably longer.

Panel B demonstrates the computerized isopotential map (Bard Systems) recorded at the atrial side of the annulus intraoperatively during ventricular pacing at a CL of 400 msec. The VA interval at site C3 is 95 msec (yellow). (The VA interval at site C6 registers 100 msec while at C5 it is 107 msec, probably due to slightly inappropriate electrode positioning.) The activation map during atrioventricular reentrant tachycardia confirms the location of the earliest atrial activation to be at C3 and C4 (panel C). During atrial pacing, the ventricle is similarly activated anterogradely early at the same site (panel D). Following surgical interruption of the accessory pathway, ventricular pacing results in earliest activation of the atrium concentrically, just to the right of the interventricular septum (panel E).

PLATE 6

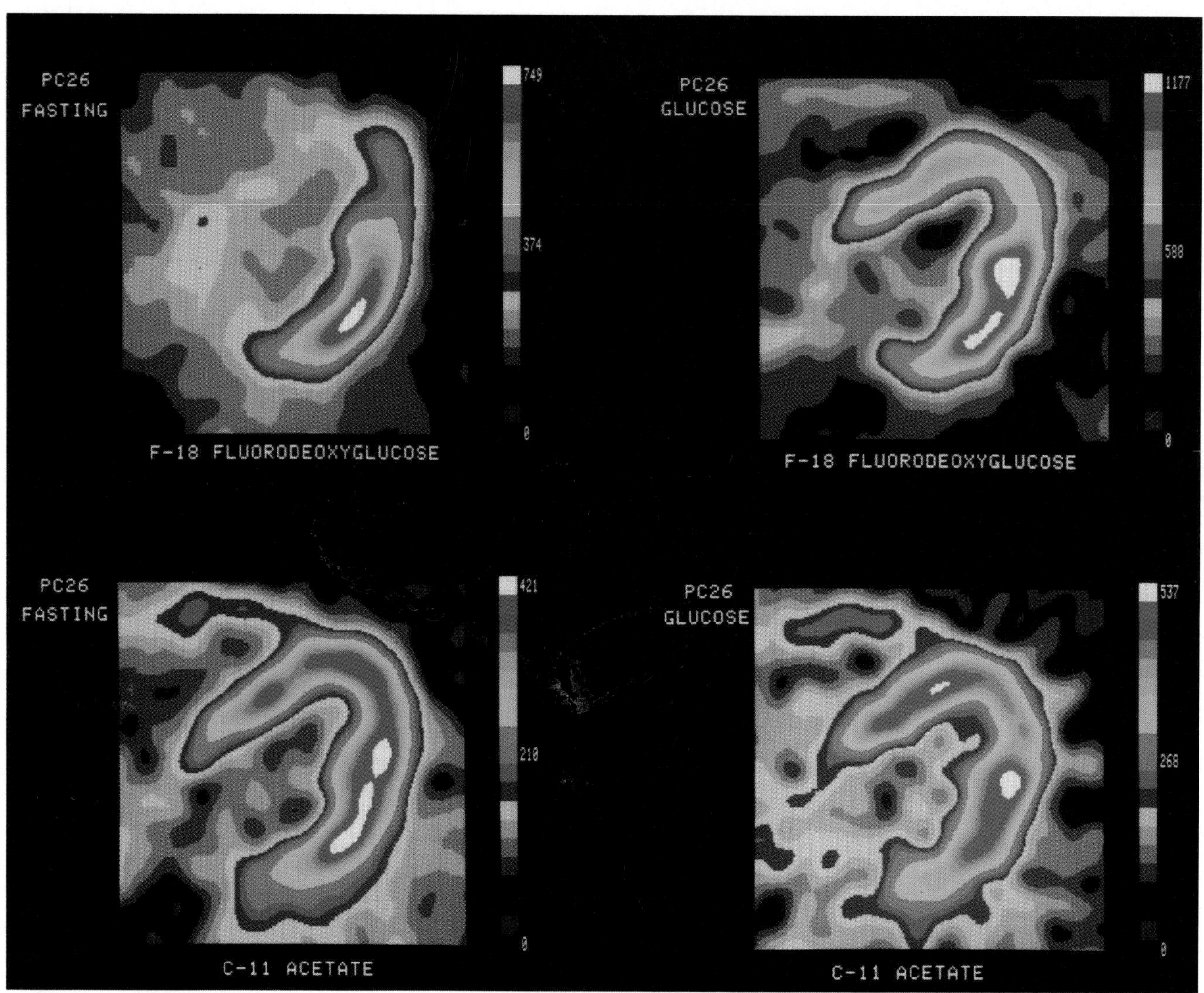

FIGURE 38–34 (See page 1184)

Midventricular positron-emission tomographic reconstructions are shown from a single normal subject. The tomograms depicted in the upper panels were performed after the intravenous administration of ^{18}F-fluorodeoxyglucose and those in the bottom panels after the intravenous administration of ^{11}C-acetate. The left-hand panels were acquired after a 5- to 8-hour fast; those in the right-hand panels were acquired after glucose administration. ^{11}C-acetate accumulation and clearance were homogenous during fasting and after feeding. (Reproduced, with permission, from Gropler, R., Siegel, B.A., Lee, K.J. et al.: Nonuniformity in myocardial accumulation of F-18 fluorodeoxyglucose in normal fasted humans. J. Nucl. Med. [in press].)

PLATE 7

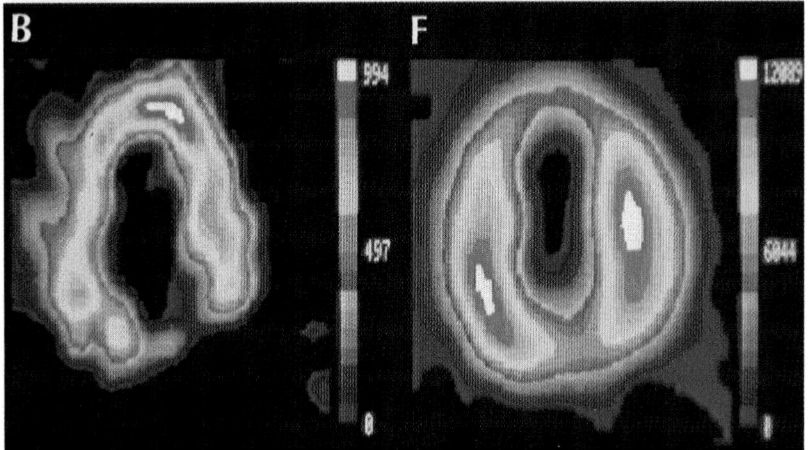

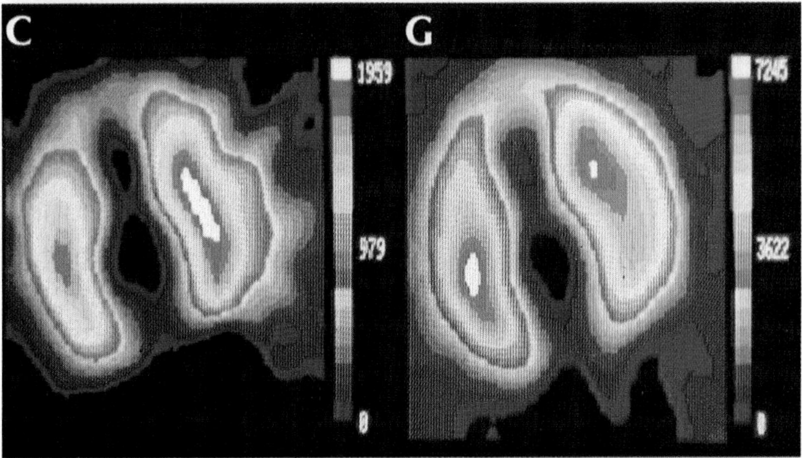

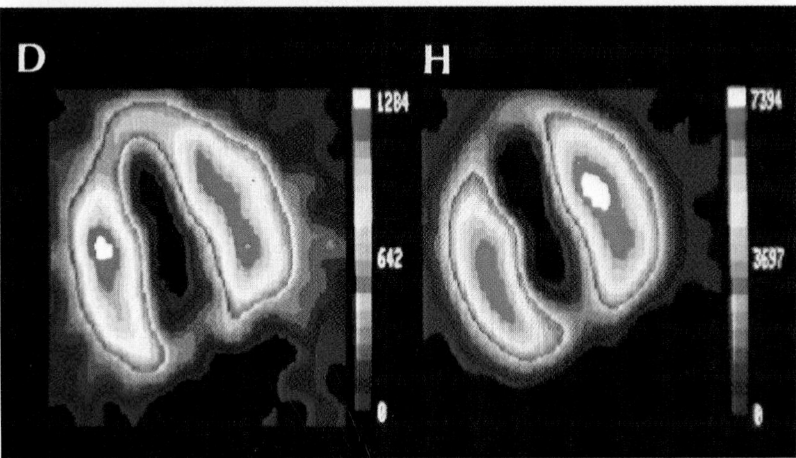

FIGURE 38–35 (See page 1184)

Transverse reconstructed tomograms from a single plane through the middle of the left ventricle of a dog given recombinant tissue-type plasminogen activator after 2 hours of coronary occlusion. Images have been corrected for vascular activity with the use of blood-pool images obtained prior to each flow determination after inhalation of ^{15}O-labeled carbon monoxide. Anterior myocardium is at the top of each image, with the lateral wall on the left, interventricular septum on the right, and the posterior region of the mitral valve at the bottom. Panels A through D represent myocardial perfusion and were obtained after intravenous injection of ^{15}O-labeled water. Panels E through H represent myocardial fatty acid uptake after intravenous injection of ^{11}C-labeled palmitate. Images A and E were obtained 90 minutes after occlusion of the left anterior descending coronary artery.

Note the large ischemic area in the anterior region, which partially resolves 1 hour after reperfusion (panels B and F). Panels C and G were obtained after 24 hours and show the late diminution in flow and metabolism in the reperfused zone. After 4 weeks of reperfusion, flow (panel D) has increased in the anterior region, but palmitate uptake (panel H) has recovered only minimally. (Reproduced, with permission, from Knabb, R.M., Bergmann, S.R., Fox, K.A.A., Sobel, B.E.: The temporal pattern of recovery of myocardial perfusion and metabolism delineated by positron emission tomography after coronary thrombolysis. J. Nucl. Med 28:1563, 1987.)

PLATE 8

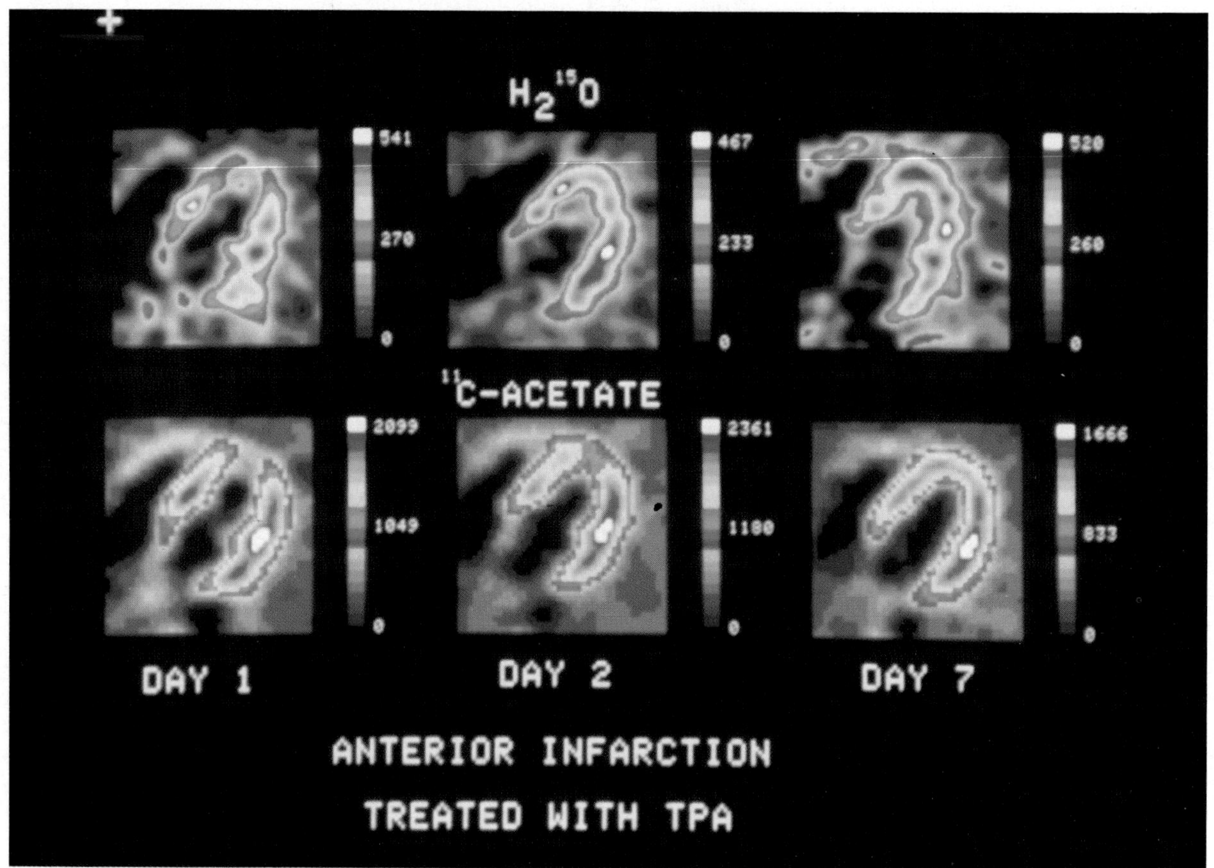

FIGURE 38-40 (See page 1190)

Midventricular positron-emission tomographic reconstructions from a patient with anterior myocardial infarction after treatment with t-PA are depicted at the intervals indicated. The top row of images represents relative perfusion. The bottom row of images illustrates the myocardial accumulation of ^{11}C-acetate reconstructed from data collected 3 to 8 minutes after administration of ^{11}C-acetate. The top of each image corresponds to the anterior and the left of each to the patient's right. Areas in white and red have the highest relative perfusion or content of tracer. Zones in blue and purple have the lowest. The discontinuity visible posteriorly is attributable to the mitral valve apparatus and atria, in which uptake is below the spatial resolution of the instrument.

A slight reduction in relative perfusion is observed in the anterior wall on the initial study, with normalization by 48 hours. A defect in accumulation of ^{11}C-acetate is evident in the initial study, with gradual improvement over the subsequent interval of observation. (Reproduced, with permission, from Henes, C.G., et al.: The time course of restoration of nutritive perfusion, myocardial oxygen consumption, and regional function after coronary thrombolysis. Coronary Artery Dis. 1:687,1990.)

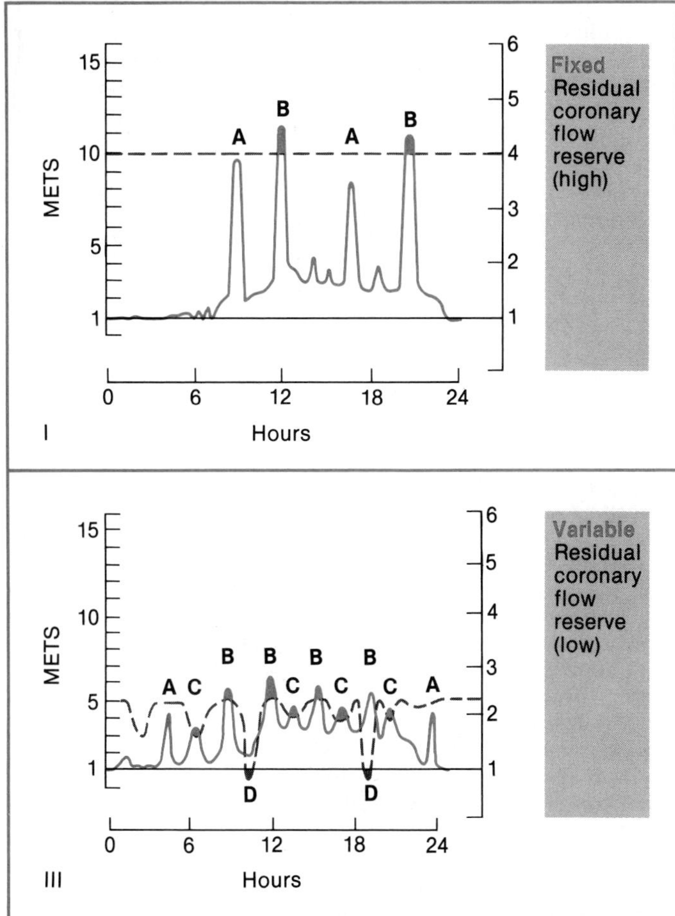

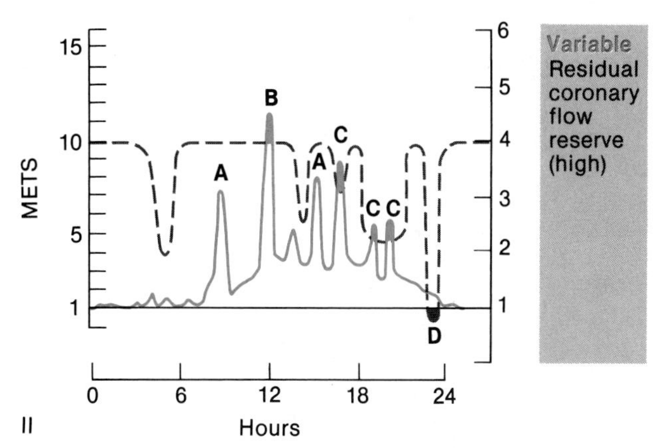

FIGURE 38-21. Schematic illustration of the relation between physical activity (during 24 hours) expressed as METS (multiple of basal metabolic oxygen consumption) and coronary flow reserve. Normally, during resting conditions, coronary flow reserve exactly matches the metabolic demand. However, when metabolic demands increase to a maximum of 16 METS, coronary flow reserve increases up to six times the resting value to match the increased demand for flow by the myocardium so that no ischemia occurs.

I. In this situation, a patient has a moderately severe fixed coronary artery obstruction that reduces coronary flow reserve to four times the resting value. *A*, the patient can exercise up to approximately 10 METS without developing ischemia; *B*, however, if he exercises above approximately 10 METS, he will consistently develop ischemia.

II. In this situation, the patient has a moderately severe stenosis that fixes the coronary reserve at four times resting levels as in I. In addition, he has a variable stenosis. Therefore, residual coronary flow reserve has an upper limit that is fixed but that can decrease because of the presence of the mechanisms that transiently interfere with coronary blood flow. Thus, the residual coronary flow reserve can vary throughout the day. Under these conditions, if the patient exercises beyond the maximal residual coronary flow reserve, he will always develop ischemia (*B*). However, he may also develop ischemia on other occasions after smaller degrees of exercise, when residual coronary flow reserve is decreased by these functional factors (*C*). Occasionally, coronary flow reserve decreases so that resting flow is impaired and ischemia occurs at rest (*D*). At other times of the day, this patient can exercise below the level of his maximal residual coronary flow reserve without experiencing ischemia (*A*).

III. In this situation, the patient has a very severe fixed stenosis and also variable stenosis. Maximal residual coronary flow reserve is reduced to little more than two times the resting value of coronary flow, thus allowing the patient to exercise up to a level of about 5 METS in the absence of any transient impairment of coronary flow. The combination of markedly reduced coronary flow reserve and of transient impairment of coronary flow results in frequent occurrences of ischemic episodes caused by excessive increase of demand above the maximal residual coronary flow (*B*) or by transient impairment of flow during exertion (*C*) or at rest (*D*). However, in the absence of transient impairment of flow, the patient can tolerate activities below 5 METS (*A*). (Modified from Maseri, A., Chierchia, S., and Kaski, J. C.: Mixed angina pectoris. Am. J. Cardiol., *56*:31E and 32E, 1985.)

Myocardial Ischemia and Ischemic Injury

EFFECTS OF ISCHEMIA ON MYOCARDIAL FUNCTION

In 1935 Tennant and Wiggers demonstrated that after ligation of a coronary artery the contraction of cardiac muscle supplied by this vessel ceases almost immediately and the affected area appears cyanotic, dilated, and bulging.[192] In the basal state there is no reserve in blood flow; any reduction in flow, even one as small as 10 to 20 per cent, results in an approximately similar percentage reduction of myocardial segment shortening.[193] Myocardial ischemia is generally associated with elimination of the normal contractile performance of a *localized area* of myocardium, resulting in an asynergic contraction.[194] Figure 38-22 shows the immediate regional myocardial functional responses to acute coronary occlusion: there is paradoxical motion (systolic bulging or dyskinesis) in the central ischemic zone, reduced contraction (akinesis or hypokinesis) in the adjacent area, and compensatory hyperfunction of the uninvolved normal myocardium, the latter mediated in part by adrenergic stimulation and the operation of the Frank-Starling mechanism.[195,196] A reduction of blood flow of 80 per cent below control results in akinesis, while a 95 per cent reduction causes dyskinesis. Animals and patients with a previous myocardial infarction exhibit impaired regional left ventricular function, although, if the damage is limited, hyperfunction of the residual myocardium will maintain global left ventricular function (Fig. 39-12, p. 1211). In the isolated heart, *global* ischemia causes a depression of myocardial contractility reflected in a decrease in the slope of the end-systolic pressure-volume relation (E_{max}) (p. 428). On the other hand, *regional* ischemia shifts the relationship

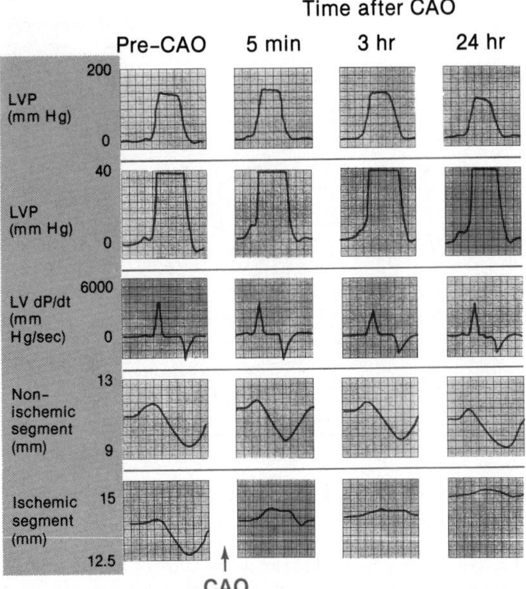

FIGURE 38–22. Phasic recordings are shown for left ventricular (LV) systolic (1st trace) and end-diastolic (2nd trace) pressures, LV dP/dt, and segment shortening in nonischemic and ischemic zones in a normal dog, before coronary artery occlusion (CAO), at 5 minutes and 3 and 24 hours after CAO. (From Amano, J., Thomas, J. X., Jr., Lavallee, M., Mirsky, I., Glover, D., Manders, W. T., Randall, W. C., and Vatner, S. F.: Effects of myocardial ischemia on regional function and stiffness in conscious dogs. Am. J. Physiol. *252*:H113, 1987.)

rightward, without affecting E_{max}. The shift reflects the behavior of the noncontractile ischemic segment of the ventricle, while the normal slope results from the compensatory hyperfunction of the nonischemic segment.[197]

Myocardial Stunning and Hibernation

For approximately 4 decades following Tennant and Wiggers' classic observations on the effects of coronary occlusion on myocardial contraction,[192] it was thought that following severe ischemia myocardium either became irreversibly injured, i.e., infarction developed, or promptly recovered. However, in the 1970's it became clear that after a *brief* episode of *severe* ischemia, prolonged dysfunction with gradual return of contractile activity occurred, a condition termed *myocardial stunning*[198–200] (Figs. 38–23 and 38–24). It then became evident in both experimental animals and patients that myocardial function could also be chronically depressed consequent to severe, chronic ischemia; this myocardial dysfunction could be ameliorated promptly by relief of the ischemia. This condition has been termed *myocardial hibernation*[201,202] (Figs. 38–25 and 38–26).

Those two conditions, myocardial stunning and hibernation, occur frequently, both in the experimental laboratory and in the clinic (Fig. 38–27). Since stunned myocardium occurs adjacent to necrotic tissue after prolonged coronary occlusion, many myocardial infarcts may be a mixture of necrotic and stunned tissue. Stunning may occur with demand-induced ischemia[203] with coronary spasm,[203a] and may be limited to the subendocardium.[204] It occurs in diastole as well as in systole[200,205] and can occur in the globally as well as in the regionally ischemic heart. Clinically, myocardial stunning probably occurs most frequently in the hearts of patients who have undergone ischemic cardiac arrest during cardiopulmonary bypass[206]; such hearts may not recover normal function for hours or days. Similarly, it occurs following thrombolytic therapy in patients having acute myocardial infarction[207] and in those with severe ischemia due to coronary vasospasm (Prinzmetal's angina) or unstable angina, or following coronary occlusion during balloon angioplasty. Myocardial hibernation is as common as stunning (p. 1329) and is manifested clinically as the improvement in ventricular function that is frequently seen after myocardial revascularization in patients with ischemic heart disease[208,209] (Fig. 38–25).

MECHANISM OF STUNNING. The mechanism responsible for stunning has not been elucidated definitively.[209a,209b] Studies with NMR spectroscopy demonstrate that changes in the ratio of phosphocreatine to inorganic phosphate correlate closely with reductions of nutritive perfusion and consequent changes in myocardial function.[210] Results implicate accumulation of inorganic phosphate or hydrogen ion or both as potential inhibitors of myocardial contractility. They are supported by studies with magnetic resonance imaging (MRI) in dogs subjected to coronary occlusion in which increased signal intensity with proton MRI was found to be a specific criterion of irreversible ischemic injury in contrast to stunning of myocardium.[211]

Stunned myocardium has been differentiated from irreversibly injured tissue by ultrasonic tissue characterization with

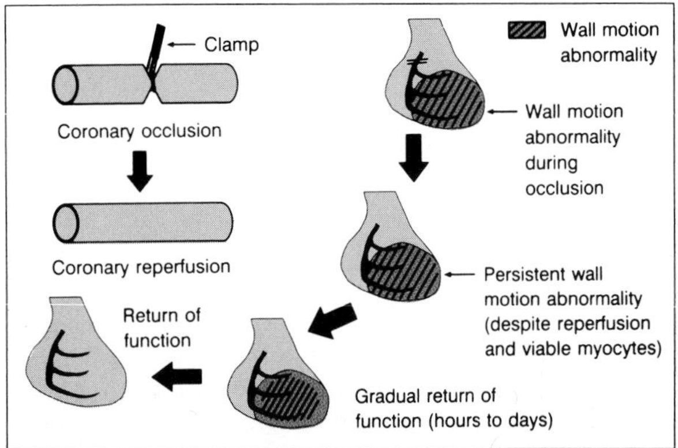

FIGURE 38–23. Schematic diagram of stunned myocardium. During coronary occlusion, a wall motion abnormality of the left ventricle is present in the region supplied by the occluded artery. With relief of ischemia and re-establishment of coronary blood flow, there is a persistent wall motion abnormality despite reperfusion and viable myocytes. There is then gradual improvement in function that requires hours to days for recovery. (From Kloner, R. A., Przyklenk, K., and Patel, B.: Altered myocardial states: The stunned and hibernating myocardium. Am. J. Med. *86*(Suppl. 1A):14, 1986.)

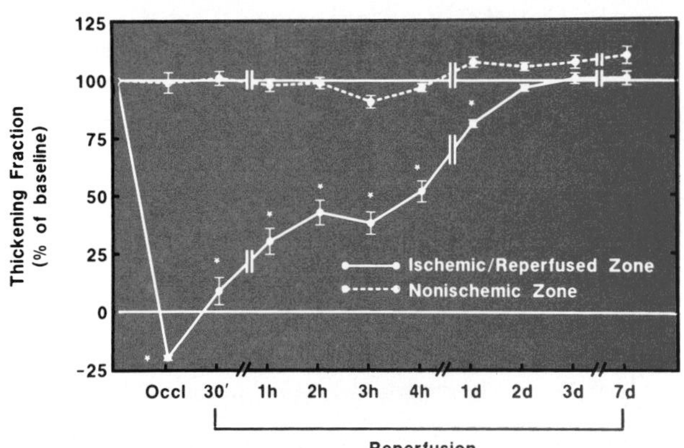

FIGURE 38–24. Changes in systolic thickening fraction during coronary occlusion (Occl) and at selected times after reperfusion in the nonischemic region and in the ischemic-reperfused region. Thickening fraction is expressed as percentage of preocclusion (baseline) values. It is an excellent indicator of local myocardial function. Data are mean values ± SEM (n = 10). Systolic function in the reperfused myocardium recovered slowly; on the average, thickening fraction was still significantly depressed at 24 hours, and returned to baseline at 48 hours after reflow. *p < 0.001 versus baseline. (From Charlat, M. L. et al.: Prolonged abnormalities of left ventricular diastolic wall thinning in the "stunned" myocardium in conscious dogs: Time course and relation to systolic function. Reprinted by permission of the American College of Cardiology. J. Am. Coll. Cardiol. *13*:185, 1989.)

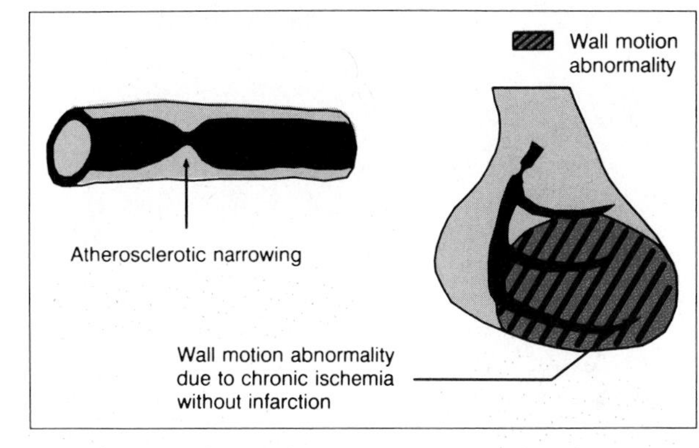

FIGURE 38–25. Schematic diagram of hibernating myocardium. Chronic ischemia without infarction results in a persistent regional wall motion abnormality. There is enough blood flow through the severe stenosis to allow for myocyte viability, but not enough to allow for normal contraction. The wall motion abnormality may be a protective mechanism whereby the left ventricle tries to reduce its oxygen demand in the setting of reduced oxygen supply. (From Kloner, R. A., Przyklenk, K., and Patel, B.: Altered myocardial states: The stunned and hibernating myocardium. Am. J. Med. *86*(Suppl. 1A):14, 1986.)

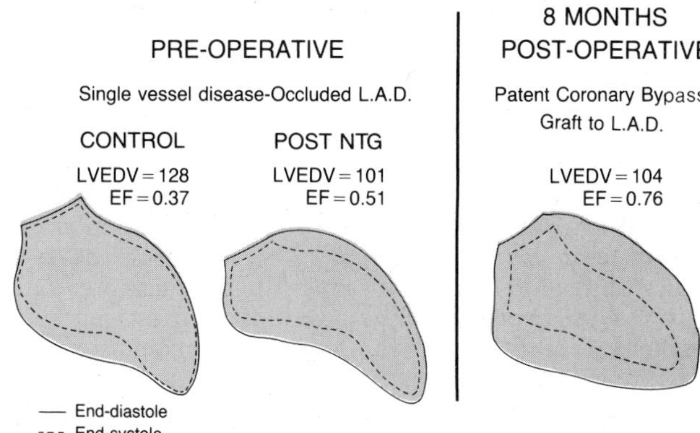

FIGURE 38–26. End-diastolic and end-systolic silhouettes of the left ventricle from the right anterior oblique contrast ventriculogram. In the preoperative studies, the ejection fraction (EF) in the control state was 0.37 and there was a large akinetic area involving the anteroapical wall. After nitroglycerin (NTG), there was an improvement of wall motion of the akinetic zone, and EF improved to 0.51. The patient had no history of myocardial infarction. Coronary arteriography showed one-vessel disease with a totally occluded left anterior descending coronary artery (LAD). The distal LAD was filled by collaterals from the circumflex coronary artery and the posterior descending coronary artery. Eight months postoperatively on routine study, the graft was fully patent and there was good filling of the LAD. The patient now shows normal left ventricular wall motion function and a normal ejection fraction of 0.76. LVEDV, Left ventricular end-diastolic volume. (From Rahimtoola, S. H.: Coronary bypass surgery for chronic angina—1981. Circulation *65*:225, 1982 by permission of the American Heart Association, Inc.)

integrated backscatter. Cardiac cycle–dependent variation of backscatter is depressed persistently in zones of infarction, whereas it is at least partially restored in stunned myocardium even before recovery of wall thickening is detectable echocardiographically.[212]

As judged from results of studies in patients with infarction treated with thrombolytic agents, in patients with angina, and in patients recovering from cardiopulmonary bypass, the duration of stunning is generally proportional to the duration of the preceding ischemia that is responsible.[213] In addition to local acidosis and accumulation of inorganic phosphate, increased intracellular sodium giving rise to excessive calcium uptake in myocardium subjected to ischemia has been implicated.[214] As judged from studies of sarcoplasmic reticulum isolated from stunned tissue from hearts of dogs subjected to transitory coronary occlusion and reflow, impaired calcium uptake may contribute as well.[215] Inhibition of calcium influx into cells and competition for calcium binding sites appear to protect against stunning, as judged from results of laboratory studies with isolated perfused hearts.[216]

Metabolic abnormalities have been detected in stunned myocardium and implicated in its pathogenesis (Fig. 38–28). Although accumulation of oxygen-derived free radicals may occur through the xanthine-oxidase system in the hearts of experimental animals,[217] the absence of this system in human myocardium implicates other sources of free radicals in

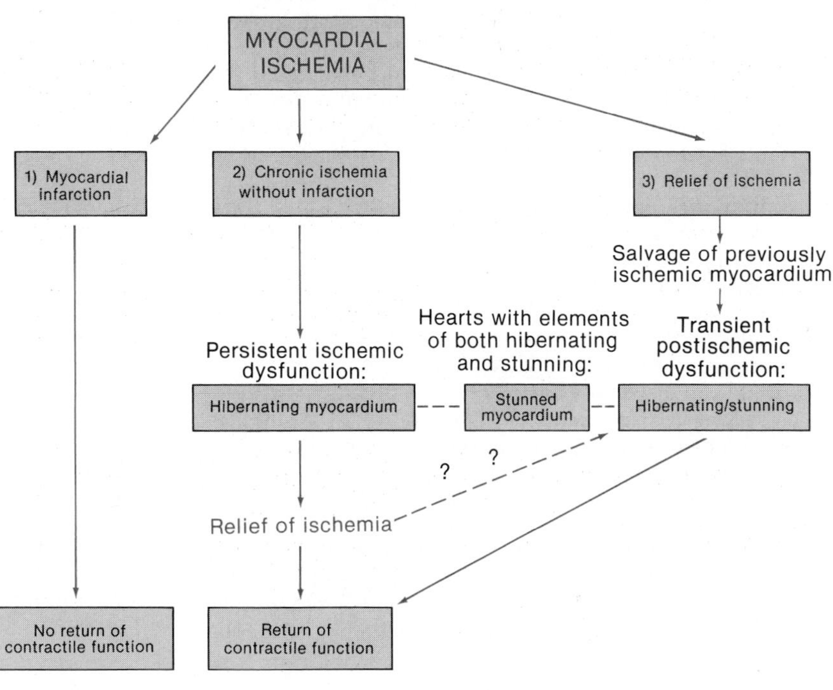

FIGURE 38–27. The three possible outcomes of myocardial ischemia. (From Kloner, R., et al.: Myocardial stunning and hibernation: Mechanisms and clinical implications. *In* Braunwald, E. (ed.): Heart Disease: A Textbook of Cardiovascular Medicine, 3rd ed. Philadelphia, W. B. Saunders Company. Update No. 11, p. 253, 1990.)

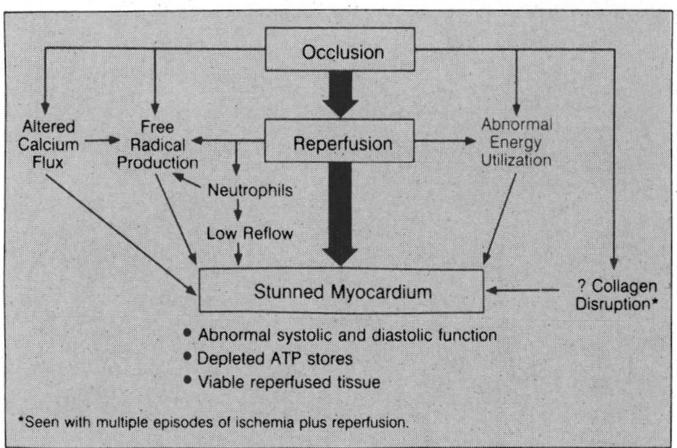

FIGURE 38-28. Potential mechanisms of stunned myocardium. (From Kloner, R. A., Przyklenk, K., and Patel, B.: Altered myocardial states: The stunned and hibernating myocardium. Am. J. Med. *86*(Suppl. 1A):14, 1986.)

human hearts. Infiltration of neutrophils into ischemic myocardium and consequent bombardment of the tissues with free radicals from activated white cells may be responsible for extending myocardial damage, in view of the diminution of apparent infarct size in dog hearts by prostacyclin analogs that inhibit neutrophil activation[218] and by free-radical scavengers.[219-223] Accumulating free radicals may contribute to stunning by direct attack on myocyte membranes resulting from lipid peroxidation, as judged from the protective effects of agents such as diltiazem that inhibit peroxidation without attenuating free-radical production in isolated perfused rabbit hearts.[224] Proarrhythmic effects that are manifested as reperfusion arrhythmias,[225] attenuation of vasodilator reserve,[226] and stunning may all be manifestations of free radical–induced injury accompanying ischemia. These effects may be attenuated by free-radical scavengers such as dimethylurea,[227] enzymes mediating catabolism of free radicals such as superoxide dismutase (SOD) and catalase,[228] and inhibitors of free-radical production.[229]

The contractility of stunned but viable myocardium can be stimulated by infused sympathomimetics.[230,231] However, it does not respond to sympathetic nerve stimulation.[232]

CLINICAL IMPLICATIONS OF STUNNING. The clinical importance of differentiating stunned from irreversibly injured myocardium cannot be overemphasized. If impaired ventricular performance is caused primarily by stunned myocardium, aggressive interventions designed to induce revascularization, including thrombolysis, angioplasty, and surgery, may be beneficial. Appropriate selection of patients for angiography and invasive intervention after attempted pharmacological thrombolysis rests in part on delineation of the extent of myocardium still in jeopardy but potentially salvageable. Several approaches are under development to facilitate differentiation of stunned from necrotic myocardium, including ultrasonic tissue characterization[212] and positron-emission tomography.[233-236] The latter approaches are based on the principle that persistent intermediary metabolism is a hallmark of persistent viability. Thus, in tomographic studies with nitrogen-13 ammonia ($^{13}NH_3$) (to estimate regional myocardial blood flow) and fluorine-18-deoxyglucose (^{18}FDG) (to measure glucose uptake and hence metabolism), wall motion abnormalities are reversible in areas in which glucose uptake is preserved before coronary bypass grafting.[233] In addition, residual glucose utilization detectable tomographically is often present despite fixed or only partially resolving stress thallium defects, underscoring the discordance between persistence of intermediary metabolism and apparent diminution of perfusion. Tomography is helpful in recognizing persistent aerobic oxidative metabolism with the use of tracers such as carbon-11–labeled acetate that may avoid ambiguities seen with tracers of aerobic and anaerobic metabolism combined, such as ^{18}FDG. In dogs with reperfusion after 15 minutes of myocardial ischemia, preservation of regional oxidative metabolism is detectable tomographically, as is oxidative metabolic reserve in stunned myocardium.

HEMODYNAMIC CONSEQUENCES OF ISCHEMIA

If sufficiently widespread, regional loss of myocardial contractile activity (whether sustained or transient) depresses overall left ventricular function, producing reductions of stroke volume, stroke work, cardiac output, and ejection fraction, while elevating ventricular of end-diastolic volume and pressure. Clinical evidence of heart failure occurs when regional asynergy is so severe and extensive that the uninvolved myocardium cannot sustain the excess load. Hemodynamic evidence of left ventricular failure develops when contraction ceases in 20 to 25 per cent of the left ventricle; with loss of 40 per cent or more of the left ventricular myocardium, severe pump failure ensues, and, if this loss is acute, fatal or near-fatal cardiogenic shock usually develops.

In patients with wall motion abnormalities secondary to coronary artery disease, maintenance of nearly normal regional myocardial oxygen consumption is a powerful predictor of subsequent resolution of regional wall motion abnormalities after revascularization, whereas preservation of glucose utilization before bypass grafting is of less predictive value.[235] The insensitivity of glucose utilization as a marker of persistent viability reflects the primary dependence of myocardial oxidative metabolism on fatty acid utilization[237] and the confounding effects of variable patterns of substrate utilization on the interpretation of tomographic images when labeled metabolites of carbohydrate utilization are used, as opposed to tracers of overall oxidative metabolism.[238-241]

Since the heart has virtually no stores of oxygen, its high rate of energy expenditure results in a sudden, striking decline of myocardial oxygen tension within seconds of coronary occlusion, coincident with the loss of contractility. During ischemia there is both a rightward shift and a reduction in the slope of the left ventricular end-diastolic pressure-volume relation.[242,243] The marginal zone contracts weakly, whereas the nonischemic myocardium exhibits a compensatory increase in its force of contraction. The rapid decline in contractility induced by ischemia cannot be attributed to alterations in excitability. Although the early stages of ischemia do not produce major changes in the amplitude and upstroke velocity of the action potential, the duration of the plateau phase of the action potential is shortened, which may signify a reduction in the slow inward current, carried largely by Ca^{++}.

Mechanism of Ischemic Impairment of Ventricular Contraction

The precise mechanism by which ischemia impairs left ventricular systolic function has not been defined. It is possible that ischemia reduces the release of Ca^{++} from the sarcolemma or the sarcoplasmic reticulum (SR)[244] or both and thereby interferes with the interaction of Ca^{++} with the contractile proteins. However, ischemic failure of cardiac contraction can occur despite normal or even elevated[245] intracellular Ca^{++} concentrations, and therefore ischemia must in some manner interfere with the ability of Ca^{++} to generate force in the myocardial cell.[246] During severe hypoxia the intracellular $[Ca^{++}]$ declines as contractility fails. In contrast, during ischemia $[Ca^{++}]$ usually rises, implying a reduced sensitivity to Ca^{++}.[247] One theory holds that the high intracellular $[H^+]$ induced by ischemia may compete with Ca^{++} for the receptors on the troponin molecules. Thus, the actin-myosin interaction is impaired, and it has been postulated that as a result of two processes, i.e., reduction of the sensitivity of the SR to any given concentration of Ca^{++} and competition between H^+ and Ca^{++} for the troponin receptor sites, contractility is reduced.[248] This idea is supported by the observations that the functional changes induced by primary acidosis in the face of adequate myocardial oxygenation are similar to those produced by ischemia[249] and that the reversal of acidosis by the administration of alkali improves contractile performance. In addition to the role played by intracellular [H^+], minor reductions of ATP may be important. It is possible that the concentrations of high-energy phosphate compounds in critical locations—such as the SR or the sarcolemma (where ion fluxes and cell volume may be affected)—are reduced by ischemia even when the overall intracellular concentration of these compounds is still normal or near normal.

ISCHEMIA AND HIGH-ENERGY PHOSPHATE DEPLETION. Despite the fact that prolonged ischemia depletes ATP from myocardium, impairment of function after transitory ischemia is not closely correlated with depression of overall ATP content at the end of the ischemic interval. "Buffering" of ATP stores by phosphocreatine is one factor responsible for the disparity.[250] Results from studies of isolated perfused hearts with nuclear magnetic resonance (NMR) magnetization transfer indicate that despite reduction of the creatine kinase reaction velocity, high-energy phosphate transfer does not limit availability of high-energy phosphate for contraction.[251] In fact, impairment of mechanical function and diminution of the rate of oxidative metabolism are parallel even though tissue ATP content is sustained by dephosphorylation of phosphocreatine.[252] Thus, limitation of oxidative metabolic reserve is not responsible for depression of contractility in ischemic or stunned myocardium, as judged from the persistence of close coupling between contractile performance and oxidative metabolism.[252] However, when cells are subjected to profound or prolonged ischemia, or when profound ischemic injury is complicated by reperfusion and flooding of cellular organelles with calcium, postischemic oxidative capacity may be reduced and may limit the maximal postischemic mechanical performance obtainable.[253]

Effects of ischemia on myocardium lead within seconds to the loss of the capacity for development of tension. Phosphocreatine content also declines rapidly and may be marked within a few minutes; ATP content declines more slowly and is associated with progressive intracellular hypoxia and acidosis; and accumulation of intracellular sodium, calcium, and hydrogen ion is striking and associated with impaired compartmentalization of activator calcium available for initiation of contraction. Accumulation of amphipathic metabolites such as long-chain acyl carnitine and lysophospholipids, strongly implicated in the genesis of malignant arrhythmias, may impair mechanical performance as well. Excitation-contraction coupling can be affected adversely by oxygen-derived free radicals elaborated within myocardium or by neutrophils infiltrating ischemic zones.[254]

EFFECTS OF ISCHEMIA ON VENTRICULAR DIASTOLIC PROPERTIES. Myocardial ischemia and infarction alter not only the contractile properties of the heart but also the diastolic pressure-volume relations of the left ventricle. Myocardial ischemia impairs ventricular relaxation[255-256a] as evidenced by a decreased rate of left ventricular pressure decline (negative dP/dt) and ventricular wall thinning, and it prolongs the isovolumetric relaxation period.[255,256] The globally ischemic ventricle is less compliant than normal[255,257-258a] (Fig. 38–29). In the presence of regional ischemia, the reduction of compliance involves the ischemic region, while the behavior of the nonischemic region conforms to that described by a higher and steeper portion of the pressure-volume curve. These changes are exaggerated when ischemia is induced in hearts with pressure overload hypertrophy.[259] In turn, the ischemia-induced changes in diastolic properties increase the resistance to ventricular filling and together with the reduced systolic properties of the ventricle contribute to the elevation of left ventricular diastolic pressure during ischemia. The mechanism responsible for the ischemia-induced impairment of myocardial relaxation has not been fully

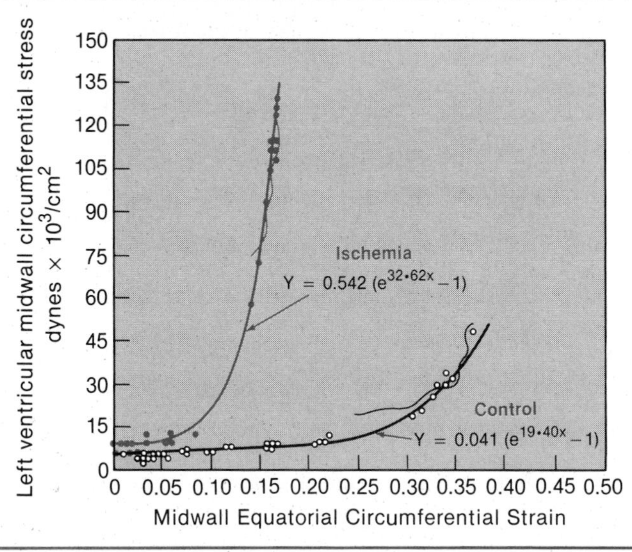

FIGURE 38–29. Diastolic pressure-strain and stress-strain relationships constructed from observations during control period and during ischemia. (From Visner, M. S., Arentzen, C. E., Parrish, D. G., Larson, E. V., O'Connor, M. J., Crumbley, A. J., III, Bache, R. J., and Anderson, R. W.: Effects of global ischemia on the diastolic properties of the left ventricle in the conscious dog. Circulation *71*:616, 1985, by permission of the American Heart Association, Inc.)

elucidated, but it has been proposed that reductions of myocardial high-energy stores impair the rate of uptake of Ca^{++} from the vicinity of the myofilaments into the SR, thus prolonging contraction.[260] Ca^{++} channel blockade will antagonize this process and by diminishing Ca^{++} influx into the cell will lower cytosolic [Ca^{++}], restoring rapid relaxation. On the other hand, caffeine, an agent known to prolong Ca^{++} availability, potentiates the ischemia-induced impairment of ventricular relaxation. In addition to increases in myocardial stiffness induced by ischemia, alterations in ventricular diastolic properties may reflect protraction of systolic events locally with regionally delayed onset of relaxation (postsystolic contraction), passively decreased segmental lengthening corresponding to a decrease in segmental shortening preceding it, regionally nonuniform loading conditions, and changes in coronary vascular pressure and chamber geometry.[261-264]

Ischemia thus causes impairment of cardiac contraction and incomplete ventricular emptying (systolic failure). In addition, it impairs ventricular relaxation and shifts the diastolic pressure-volume curve upward (diastolic failure). The combination of systolic and diastolic failure leads to elevated ventricular filling pressures, ultimately causing symptoms of pulmonary congestion.

ELECTROPHYSIOLOGICAL CONSEQUENCES OF ISCHEMIA

ST-SEGMENT CHANGES IN THE DETECTION OF ISCHEMIA. It has been known for more than a half century that ST-segment elevation is an electrocardiographic sign of coronary artery occlusion. Within 30 to 60 seconds after occlusion in dogs with open chests, epicardial leads from within the area of cyanosis show ST-segment elevation, reaching a maximum 5 to 7 minutes after occlusion. ST-segment elevation in the central area of cyanosis is usually more marked than at the periphery. With the use of small intracavitary electrodes, simultaneous ST-segment elevation is also noted on the endocardial surface, although it is less marked than that recorded on the epicardium.

The electrophysiological basis of ST-segment changes in myocardial ischemia is discussed on page 137; altered ion transport across the myocardial cell membrane apparently is the underlying cause. In the nonischemic myocardium, cell volume is regulated within narrow limits by the sarcolemmal "sodium pump" (p. 592). This active, metabolically dependent pump maintains a high extracellular [Na^+] as well as high intracellular [K^+] and colloids, thus stabilizing cell volume. It has been postulated that with ischemia the availability of energy necessary for this pumping is reduced. According to this concept Na^+, accompanied by Cl^- and H_2O, accumulates intracellularly and K^+ begins to leak into the extracellular space. The reduction in intracellular [K^+] or the accumulation of extracellular [K^+] or both are critical in the generation of the elevated ST segment, since small changes in the ratio of intracellular to extracellular [K^+] have a marked effect on the polarity of cellular membranes.

Interpretation of ST-Segment Elevations. The magnitude of epicardial ST-segment elevation generally correlates with the decrease in blood flow, lactate accumulation, and depletion of high-energy phosphate compounds in the underlying myocardium. In addition, ST-segment elevation is associated with a reduction in oxygen tension in the affected tissue below 65 per cent of control,[265] and the magnitude of the elevation correlates with intramyocardial oxygen tension. Measurements with a mass spectrometer have shown that intramyocardial ST-segment elevations are correlated with changes in myocardial gas tensions. Also, epicardial ST-segment elevations shortly after coronary artery occlusion correlate closely with subsequent depletion of myocardial creatine phosphokinase (CK) activity and with histological evidence of necrosis in the subjacent myocardium.[266] It is now clear that the distribution of *epicardial* ST-segment elevation provides an approximation of the extent of myocardial ischemia, but that the *intramyocardial* ST segment is a more sensitive index than the epicardial. However, it must be appreciated that ST-segment elevation, wherever measured, is not specific for myocardial ischemia, since the ST segment is also affected by changes in temperature, by drugs (including the digitalis glycosides and quinidine), by sympathetic stimulation of the heart, by epicardial injury due to pericarditis, and by localized intraventricular conduction defects.[267]

ALTERATIONS IN CELLULAR ELECTROPHYSIOLOGY INDUCED BY ISCHEMIA

The effects of ischemia on the electrophysiological properties of cardiac muscle are numerous and complex. Ischemia-induced ventricular tachyarrhythmias can be caused by increased automaticity (p. 603), triggered activity (p. 604), and reentry (p. 607). The early electrophysiological hallmarks of ischemia include a marked diminution in resting membrane potential, action potential amplitude, rate of upstroke of phase 0, and action potential duration. Activation of ATP-sensitive K^+ channels appears to be responsible for the latter. Within 10 minutes of ischemia, action potential alterations in amplitude and duration (2 : 1 alternans) become prominent, with subsequent diminution of excitability and conduction block. Although excitability may return transiently, it is generally persistently absent after 30 minutes of ischemia. Initially, the refractory period of cells in ischemic zones decreases, but with ischemia lasting for several minutes it lengthens and exceeds the duration of refractoriness in nonischemic tissue. Consequently, heterogeneity of refractoriness and postrepolarization refractoriness are prominent. These phenomena may account for continuous electrical activity spanning the interval between a normal sinus beat and a ventricular ectopic beat.[254] Although conduction velocity may increase transiently early after the onset of ischemia, it declines within 3 to 5 minutes as a result of hypoxia, acidosis, and increased intracellular calcium.[254] Initially, changes in passive membrane properties may contribute to the electrophysiologic effects induced first by ischemia increasing extracellular longitudinal resistance reflecting volume shifts and subsequently by increased intracellular longitudinal resistance with irreversible uncoupling of cells.[269]

REENTRY ARRHYTHMIAS (see also p. 609). The development of conduction delay contributes to spatial inhomogeneity of electrophysiological alterations along with disparities in refractory period duration. These alterations predispose to development of arrhythmias reflecting reentry caused by slow conduction and unidirectional block combined with delayed activation and inhomogeneous recovery of excitability.

ABNORMAL AUTOMATICITY (see also p. 603). Ventricular arrhythmias associated with ischemia may reflect nonreentrant mechanisms as well,[270] such as abnormal automaticity favored by diminished negativity of resting membrane potentials and triggered activity precipitated by early or delayed afterdepolarizations. The rapid reversibility of both types of electrophysiological alterations by prompt restoration of perfusion and the lack of concomitant morphological manifestations of myocyte injury under such circumstances suggest that subtle biochemical derangements accompanying brief ischemia are responsible. Accumulation of specific metabolites and ions has been implicated. Thus, electrophysiological derangements underlying malignant arrhythmias induced by ischemia appear to depend on the accumulation of toxic metabolites as well as on lack of oxygen for energy production itself.[271]

EFFECTS OF ISCHEMIA ON THE SARCOLEMMA. The function of the sarcolemma is exquisitely dependent on its structural integrity. Disruption of sarcolemma secondary to ischemia appears to reflect altered lipid metabolism. The generation of amphipathic metabolites such as long-chain acyl carnitine and lysophosphatidyl choline (LPC) as a result of impairment of beta-oxidation of fatty acids, the activation of phospholipases, and the inhibition of enzymes that catalyze catabolism of LPC appear to be responsible.[271] Such metabolites are toxic because their combined hydrophobic and hydrophilic (amphiphilic) properties endow them with detergent-like properties. Their presence, in even minute concentrations in the sarcolemma, alters the behavior of ion channels, the activity of membrane-associated receptors, and thereby the electrophysiological properties of the sarcolemma.[270] Thus, exposure of normoxic myocytes to amphiphiles induces electrophysiological derangements comparable to those induced by ischemia. Induction of ventricular fibrillation early after the onset of ischemia can be prevented by pharmacological inhibition of accumulation of amphiphiles in hearts of experimental animals.[272]

Arrhythmias occur in three phases in dogs with coronary occlusion.[158,159]

THE EARLY PERIOD. This phase begins almost immediately after coronary ligation, frequently culminates in ventricular fibrillation within 3 to 6 minutes, and usually lasts less than 30 minutes. Within minutes after coronary occlusion, marked alterations occur in the electrophysiological properties of ventricular myocardial cells, with shortening of action potential duration and refractoriness, decreased amplitude, upstroke velocity, and resting potential. Extracellular recordings from the epicardial surface of the ischemic zone show marked loss of amplitude and delay and fractionation of recorded electrograms, suggesting that activation in the myocardium is irregular and that the effects of ischemia are heterogeneous.

Initially after coronary occlusion, conduction velocity increases presumably related to the increase in extracellular K^+ (which may also contribute to the abbreviation of the action potential). Subsequently, conduction velocity slows. Available evidence suggests that inhomogeneities in the conduction velocity and in the shortening of the refractory period create the conditions necessary for reentry, which in turn is responsible for ventricular tachycardia and ventricular fibrillation early during ischemia.[272a] The cause of ventricular premature beats is less clear but may be related to the triggering of automatic activity by the current of injury.

This early arrhythmic phase observed in experimental animals could be related to the "prehospital" phase of arrhythmias observed in patients, which is also marked by a high incidence of ventricular fibrillation and sudden death. The arrhythmias of the early phase are intimately rate-related. Thus, vagally induced cardiac slowing can avert or abort ectopic ventricular rhythms. Conversely, ectopic ventricular rhythm can be induced by cardiac pacing.

Regional myocardial sympathetic stimulation appears to contribute to early malignant ventricular arrhythmia. During ischemia, beta-adrenoceptors are redistributed from intracellular vesicles to the sarcolemma. This may enhance the response of the ischemic myocardium to sympathomimetics, causing arrhythmia, increase of MVO_2, and extension of the ischemic zone. Sympathectomy and beta-adrenoceptor blockade mitigate both the regional augmentation of cyclic AMP and the frequency and severity of the early phase of ventricular arrhythmias.[273] On the other hand, the effectiveness of antiarrhythmic drugs such as quinidine and lidocaine during the early phase has been questioned.

THE INTERMEDIATE PERIOD IN THE DOG. After a period of quiescence, a delayed arrhythmic phase begins at about 6 to 9 hours following coronary occlusion in the dog and lasts for 24 to 72 hours. During this period spontaneous polymorphic ventricular rhythms occur, but ventricular fibrillation is uncommon. Multiple electrophysiological mechanisms are probably involved in the delayed arrhythmic phase, particularly abnormal automaticity of subendocardial Purkinje fibers. This phase may correspond to ventricular tachycardia and "accelerated idioventricular rhythms" (p. 706) commonly seen on the second and third days following infarction in humans. Antiarrhythmic drugs such as quinidine, procainamide, lidocaine, and disopyramide suppress these arrhythmias by reducing automaticity.

THE LATE PHASE. By 72 hours after coronary ligation in the dog, the spontaneous polymorphic ventricular rhythms have nearly subsided, but the heart is still prone to ventricular tachyarrhythmias and, occasionally, ventricular fibrillation.[274] These arrhythmias may be easily induced by rapid cardiac pacing or programmed premature stimulation[275] and may be the result of reentrant circuits in the subepicardial layer of the infarction, including the boundary zone between the infarction and surrounding viable myocardium. This late phase of ventricular vulnerability may correspond to the "post-coronary care unit" ventricular arrhythmias and late in-hospital ventricular fibrillation. Antiarrhythmic drugs, such as lidocaine or procainamide, appear to abolish these late reentrant arrhythmias by further depression or block of the already slowed conduction in the reentrant circuit. Electrophysiological abnormalities persist for long periods after myocardial infarction. These may be responsible, in part, for the prolonged increased risk of sudden death in such patients.

REPERFUSION ARRHYTHMIAS. There has been considerable interest in the mechanism of ventricular arrhythmias that occur with release of coronary occlusion and reperfusion (whether induced or spontaneous). Ventricular fibrillation is likely to occur abruptly without warning following reperfusion, whereas it is often heralded by ventricular ectopic beats with increasing frequency after occlusion. Chemical and electrical gradients caused by washout of metabolites and electrolytes that have accumulated in the ischemic zone are probably responsible for the electrophysiological derangement responsible for reperfusion arrhythmias.[276] Reperfusion is accompanied by changes in regional concentrations of K^+, Ca^{++}, H^+, catecholamines, and lysophosphoglycerides; the last are derived from degradation of membrane phospholipids in cells undergoing infarction.[277] Since the free-radical scavenger superoxide dismutase can protect the heart from reperfusion arrhythmias, these substances may also be important in its generation.[278] Reperfusion arrhythmias are more common in experimental animals such as the dog and pig. However, while they are less common in patients, the occasional abrupt onset of ventricular fibrillation in those with coronary occlusion and myocardial infarction who are undergoing thrombolytic, mechanical, or spontaneous reperfusion and in those with Prinzmetal's angina at the termination of an episode of coronary spasm is a clinical example of reocclusion arrhythmia.

BIOCHEMICAL MECHANISMS OF ELECTROPHYSIOLOGICAL DERANGEMENTS INDUCED BY ISCHEMIA. Physiological changes have not been identified with certainty. Ischemia depresses the energy-dependent sarcolemmal Na pump, which leads to a gain in intracellular Na^+ and loss of intracellular K^+ with consequent elevation of extracellular K^+ concentration in the vicinity of the sarcolemma, and augmented intracellular Ca^{++} secondary to increased Na/Ca exchange.[279] As a result of anaerobic metabolism, intracellular pH declines. Ischemia also results in release of norepinephrine from adrenergic nerve endings and an increase of tissue levels of cyclic AMP. Although it has been postulated that in the ischemic zone high concentrations of extracellular K^+ may depolarize the cells to the extent that the rapid Na^+ channel is inactivated, and high concentrations of catecholamines may stimulate the slow current carried principally by Ca^{++}, resulting in slow response action potentials, slowed conduction and reentrant ventricular arrhythmias associated with ischemia are more likely to reflect depression of the rapid Na inward current.[254]

It is less likely that slow response action potentials are responsible for ischemia-induced electrophysiological disturbances in the later stage of myocardial infarction. The extracellular $[K^+]$ is probably not as high as in the early stage of ischemia. Besides, total catecholamines in the ischemic region decline to a very low level on the day after coronary occlusion. However, ischemic myocardium still shows markedly depressed action potentials, slow conduction, and a high propensity for reentrant rhythms. In the later stage of ischemia, ischemic myocardial cells have been found to be exquisitely sensitive to the depressant effect of tetrodotoxin, a specific blocker of the fast Na^+ channel, and not to verapamil and D600, which are blockers of the slow Ca^{++} channel. These observations suggest that poor membrane responses of ischemic myocardial cells are related to depression of the fast Na^+ channel. The clinical relevance of studies of ischemia-induced ionic conductance changes relates to the choice of ideal antiarrhythmic therapy following ischemia. Thus, the antiarrhythmic effect of lidocaine on ischemia-induced reentrant ventricular arrhythmias (pp. 633 and 639) may be due to selective depression of ischemic myocardial cells forming part of the reentrant pathway. The finding that the effect of lidocaine on depressed ischemic cells is similar to that of tetrodotoxin suggests that lidocaine acts by further depressing the Na^+ channel in ischemic cells.

EFFECTS OF ISCHEMIA ON MYOCARDIAL METABOLISM

HIGH-ENERGY PHOSPHATE METABOLISM. During the first minutes of severe ischemia, the production of high-energy phosphates (the sum of ATP and creatine phosphate [CP]) declines and is greatly exceeded by their utilization (Figs. 38–30 and 38–31). Therefore, tissue stores decline progressively, with CP stores falling more rapidly than ATP stores. CP is depleted by transfer of high-energy phosphate to ADP as oxidative synthesis of ATP declines. In the absence of normal oxidative phosphorylation, ADP is converted to AMP (in the myokinase reaction), which in turn is broken down to adenosine and ultimately to inosine, hypoxanthine, and xanthine (Fig. 38–9, p. 1169).[280] When ATP content is reduced below 20 per cent of control values, cells become unable to regenerate high-energy phosphate, to maintain physiological ionic gradients, and to control their volume. The combination of reduced myocardial high-energy phosphate stores, cell swelling, and sarcolemmal damage (attributable potentially to oxygen-derived free radical attack with lipid peroxidation and the effects of accumulating amphipathic metabolites) appears to play a key role in cell death with ischemia or reperfusion (Fig. 38–32). When tissue is only *reversibly* injured by ischemia (i.e., when its viability can still be maintained by reperfusion), ATP stores are usually greater than 60 per cent of control and electronmicroscopy may reveal only glycogen loss, nuclear chromatin clumping, intermyofibrillar edema, and mitochondrial swelling but no sarcolemmal damage or accumulation of amorphous dense bodies in the mitochondria. Reduction of ATP below 30 per cent is usually associated with visible sarcolemmal damage and irreversible injury (i.e., the tissue is not viable despite reperfusion).

Phosphorus-31 NMR spectroscopy permits multiple sequential assessments of the same tissue and correlation of high-energy phosphate stores with mechanical activity. Both the magnitude of intracellular acidosis and associated increase in inorganic phosphate have been shown to correlate inversely with postischemic recovery of function; ATP but not CP content has been shown to correlate with return of contractile function after reperfusion.[281]

INTERMEDIARY METABOLISM IN ISCHEMIA (Fig. 38–33)

Under physiological conditions, myocardium derives most of its energy from oxidative phosphorylation, a process localized to the mitochondria. Oxidation of fatty acids predominates. When oxygen availability is limited, the rate of ATP synthesis declines, regeneration of ATP from ADP and phosphocreatine decreases, and ultimately, high-energy phosphate stores decline. Results of NMR spectroscopic studies indicate that the ratio of phosphocreatine to creatine is an index of energy reserve[282] and that energy production and consumption remain balanced when contractile reserve is taxed.[283] The diminution of contractility induced by ischemia reflects a limited turnover of high-energy phosphate stores[284,285] rather than reduction of total cellular content of ATP itself, until and unless ischemia is profound and sustained.[286] However, even intermittent ischemia depletes the mitochondria of adenine nucleotides[287] and may therefore limit oxidative metabolic reserve. After intense, transitory ischemia, the depletion of adenine nucleotides may persist for hours to days, in part

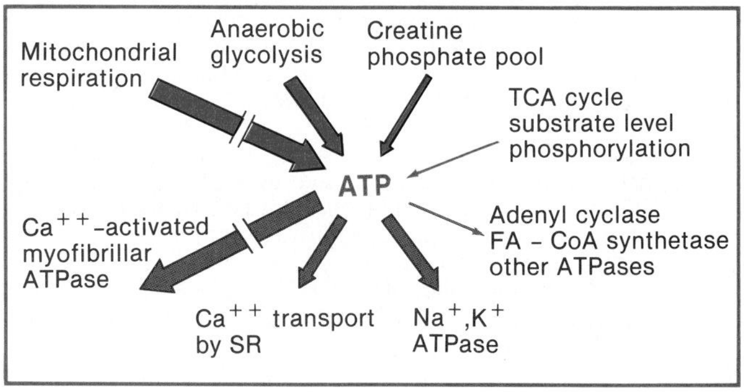

FIGURE 38-30. Principal reactions producing and utilizing high-energy phosphates (HEP) in ischemic tissue. The width of the arrows indicates the estimated quantitative importance of the various reactions. In severe ischemia, aerobic respiration is abolished. The preexisting stores of HEP, in the form of creatine phosphate (CP) or ATP, are relatively small. Thus, anaerobic glycolysis becomes the principal source of energy, producing 80 to 90 per cent of the HEP bonds that can be utilized by severely ischemic tissue. Substrate-level phosphorylation of α-ketoglutarate in the mitochondria does not require oxygen, but the tissue content of substrates that can be shuttled to α-ketoglutarate is small. Energy utilized also is markedly reduced during ischemia. Cardiac contraction, which is mediated by Ca^{++} activated myofibrillar ATPase, consumes much of the ATP produced in aerobic myocardium. However, contraction is abolished or severely depressed in areas of severe ischemia. Nevertheless, ATP continues to be required to remove Na^{+} from the cell, to keep Ca^{++} sequestered in the sarcoplasmic reticulum, and for a variety of other cellular processes that may continue to compete for the remaining ATP. (From Jennings, R. B., and Reimer, K. A.: Lethal myocardial ischemic injury. Am. J. Pathol. *102*:241, 1981.)

because of the limited capacity of myocardium for de novo purine synthesis. Depletion of adenine nucleotides may *contribute* to (but does not appear to be the cause of) stunning of myocardium, because recovery of segmental function with reperfusion is associated with restoration of high-energy phosphate stores.[287]

CARBOHYDRATE METABOLISM. During hypoxia, glycolytic flux increases, as does the uptake of glucose. There is evidence for functional compartmentalization of anaerobic glycolytic versus oxidative metabolism. Energy from glycolysis preferentially supports sarcolemmal function, whereas oxidative phosphorylation preferentially supports contractile function.[288] However, anaerobic glycolysis alone can meet myocardial energy requirements only transiently, even though augmentation of glycolytic flux by provision of glucose or prior augmentation of glycogen stores confers some resistance to the deterioration of function induced by anoxia or ischemia.[289] The persistence of anaerobic glycolytic flux may account for observations made with positron-emission tomography of patients in which metabolism/flow mismatches (persistence of uptake of ^{18}FDG despite diminished accumulation of $^{13}NH_3$ reflecting decreased perfusion) were seen in ischemic but presumably still viable myocardium[290,291,291a,291b] (p. 1301). However, tomographic documentation of viability may be provided more definitively by delineation of persistent oxidative metabolism, ascertainable by positron tomography with carbon-11-labeled acetate, which presages recovery of regional wall motion with reperfusion[235,238-241] (Fig. 38-34).

THE ROLE OF LACTATE. Lactate accumulates during ischemia, because oxidation of pyruvate is precluded by the inhibition of the tricarboxylic acid cycle, and washout of metabolites is reduced because of the limited perfusion. The initial burst of glycolytic activity accompanying hypoxia with or without ischemia appears to depend on allosteric effects of adenine nucleotides and other regulators of enzymes such as phosphorylase b, hexokinase, and phosphofructokinase.[292] However, under conditions of limited perfusion sufficient to induce hypoxia, the rapidly increasing concentration of lactic acid within the cell, the decline of pH, and the accumulation of other metabolites inhibit glycolytic flux at the phosphofructokinase and glyceraldehyde-3-phosphate dehydrogenase[292] steps, among others (Fig. 38-33).

In isolated perfused hearts, lactate exerts a deleterious effect on glycolytic flux independent of pH[190] by inhibiting the glyceraldehyde-phosphate dehydrogenase reaction, which is responsible for conversion of glyceraldehyde-3-phosphate to 1,2-diphosphoglyceric acid. On the other hand, acidosis itself inhibits glycolytic flux and the malate-aspartate cycle.[293] Persistent or prolonged ischemia results in inhibition of this and other shuttle reactions because of accumulation of reducing equivalents in the

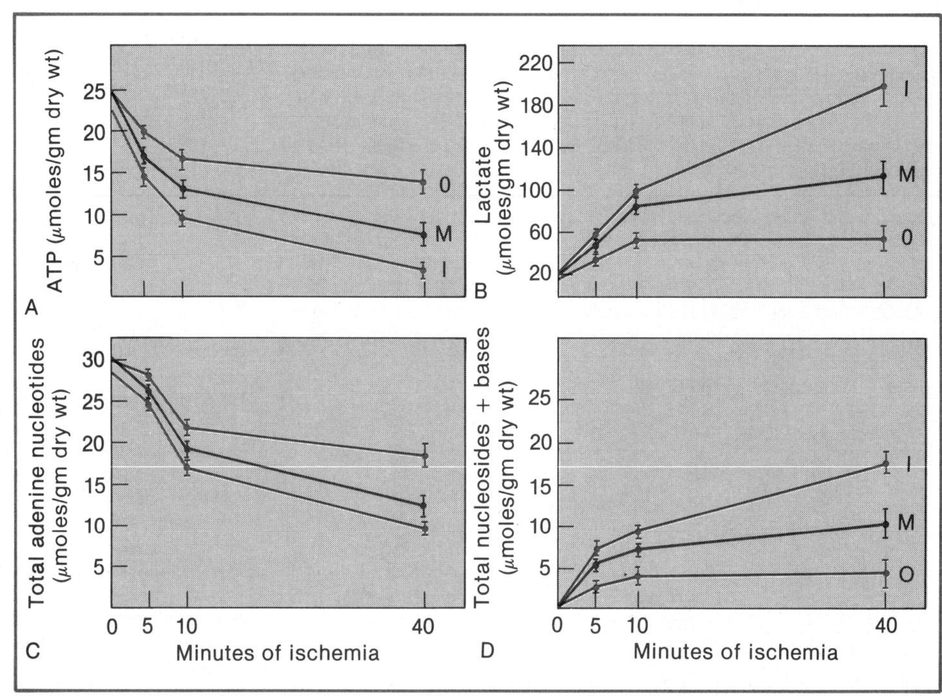

FIGURE 38-31. Time course of metabolic changes during myocardial ischemia plotted by transmural layer (I = inner, subendocardial; M = middle; O = outer, subepicardial). Ischemia was induced by circumflex occlusion in anesthetized dogs. Data for different times are based on different groups of dogs; $N = 4$ to 6; brackets indicate plus or minus one standard error of the mean. *A*, More rapid depletion of ATP in the inner layer, highly significant after 5 min of ischemia ($p < 0.01$). *B*, Tissue lactate accumulation, with the most rapid accumulation in the subendocardium. For all layers there was a progressive increase in lactate content during the first 10 min of ischemia. Between 10 and 40 min there was continued lactate accumulation in the inner and middle layers, but not in the outer layer. *C*, Total adenine nucleotide content (ATP + ADP + AMP). Adenine nucleotide degradation was most rapid in the subendocardium. Note the time lag between ATP depletion (graph A) and adenine nucleotide breakdown. *D*, Total nucleosides and bases, which are the products of adenine nucleotide degradation. Accumulation was fastest in the subendocardium. As with lactate (graph B), nucleoside and base content in the outer layer was maximal by 10 minutes and was not further increased at 40 minutes, even though adenine nucleotide breakdown in this layer continued (graph C). (From Reimer, K. A., and Jennings, R. B.: Myocardial ischemia, hypoxia and infarction. *In* Fozzard, H. A., Jennings, R. B., Haber, E., Katz, A. M., and Morgan, H. E. [eds.]: The Heart and Cardiovascular System. New York, Raven Press, 1986, p. 1144. From the studies of Murry, C. E. et al.: Collateral blood flow and transmural location: Independent determinants of ATP in ischemic canine myocardium. Fed. Proc. *44*:823, 1985.)

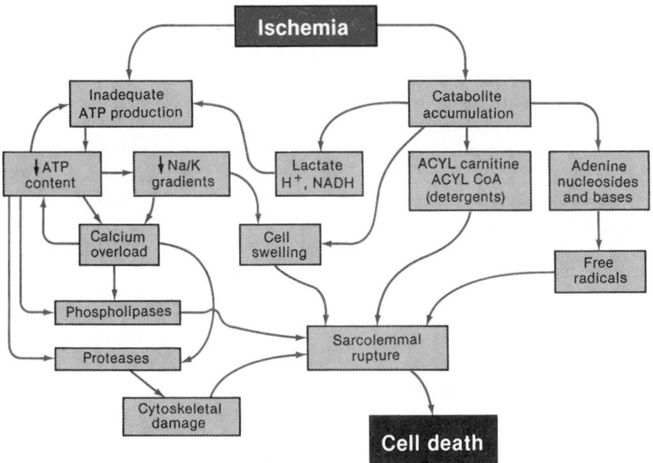

FIGURE 38–32. Some potential pathways leading to sarcolemmal damage, which form the basis for various hypotheses of events leading to irreversible ischemic cell injury. Two major facets of ischemia are the inadequate production of ATP and the accumulation of potentially noxious catabolites. Declining ATP content could have many adverse consequences including loss of sodium and potassium gradients, calcium overload, and activation of endogenous phospholipases or proteases. The latter could damage the sarcolemma and/or its cytoskeletal supports. Accumulation of catabolites such as lactate, H^-, and NADH inhibits anaerobic glycolysis and thereby inhibits ATP production in ischemia. Products of lipid degradation may act as detergents and damage cell membranes. Adenine nucleosides and bases accumulate and might be a major source of free radicals via the xanthine oxidase reaction. In addition, accumulating catabolites are an intracellular osmotic load that may accentuate cell swelling and facilitate the rupture of already weakened membranes. The relative importance of these various pathways in the pathogenesis of ischemic cell death has not been established. Moreover, many reactions occur in ischemic myocardium which have been less well studied and are not included on this diagram; it is not even certain that the most important assays are illustrated. (From Reimer, K. A., and Jennings, R. B.: Myocardial ischemia, hypoxia and infarction. *In* Fozzard, H. A., Jennings, R. B., Haber, E., Katz, A. M., and Morgan, H. E. [eds.]: The Heart and Cardiovascular System. New York, Raven Press, 1986, p. 1163.)

mitochondria (due to the lack of oxygen as a terminal electron and hydrogen receptor), with consequent acidosis and accumulation of metabolites that inhibit glycolytic flux. When flux is sufficiently inhibited, ischemic contracture results.[289]

The relationship between lactate production and the severity of impaired perfusion can be exploited diagnostically. Under physiological aerobic conditions, myocardium extracts lactate from the arterial blood with extraction fractions in the range of 20 per cent. In normal subjects, extraction persists despite acceleration of ventricular rate by pacing. However, when myocardial ischemia is present at rest or develops in response to stress induced by pacing or other physiological stimuli, lactate extraction declines or is replaced by net lactate production. Dual carbon-labeled isotopic experiments have demonstrated that in patients with coronary artery disease simultaneous lactate production and extraction can occur. During a pacing stress test, significant lactate release occurs even in the presence of net lactate extraction. Unfortunately, relationships between the concentrations of lactate in coronary sinus blood and in extracellular fluid, cytosol, and mitochondrial compartments are complex and are influenced by nonspecific factors such as acid-base balance, adrenergic stimulation of the heart, substrate availability, permeability of cell membranes to lactate and pyruvate, concomitant disorders such as diabetes mellitus, and prevailing levels of plasma free fatty acids. Thus, net lactate extraction is a relatively insensitive index of changes occurring in localized regions of the heart.

DIFFERENCES BETWEEN ISCHEMIA AND ANOXIA

A number of important differences exist between anoxia and ischemia.[1] Not only is oxidative metabolism reduced during ischemia, as it is in anoxia, but the anaerobic production of ATP also proceeds at less than maximal capacity. In the ischemic working heart the concentration of lactic acid rises and the intracellular pH falls rapidly as the acid products of glycolysis accumulate. In contrast, in the anoxic heart perfusion results in the washout of the acid products of glycolysis, thereby retarding the rate of development of intracellular acidosis. The increased lactate production is not sustained by the ischemic heart, which has a glycolytic rate about one-fourth that of the anoxic heart in a steady state. This is unrelated to a reduction of substrate availability. Thus, the addition of insulin and glucose to the perfusion medium fails to stimulate glycolysis to the extent observed in anoxia or under normal aerobic conditions. While insulin and elevated glucose in the perfusate are able to increase glucose transport and augment the intracellular glucose concentration, they do not prevent ischemia from inhibiting glucose utilization.

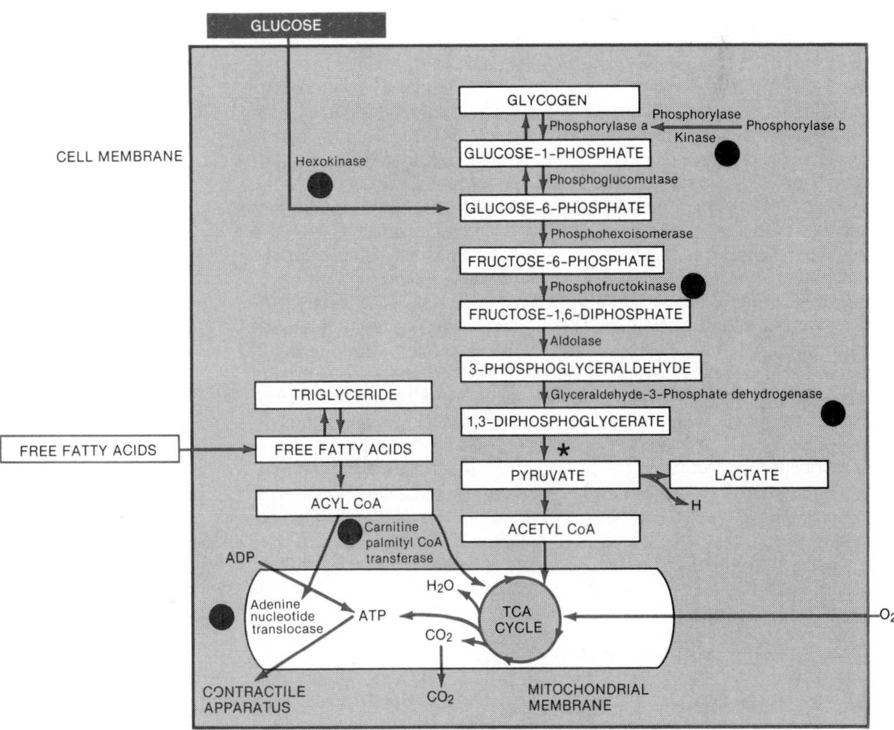

FIGURE 38–33. Effects of ischemia on glycolysis and free fatty acid metabolism. Ischemia increases intracellular lactate concentration; this accumulation inhibits several enzymes in the glycolytic pathway: Phosphofructokinase (*A*); hexokinase (*B*); and phosphorylase kinase (*C*), which prevents activation of phosphorylase b to phosphorylase a and therefore suppresses conversion of glycogen to glucose-1-phosphate. Glyceraldehyde-3-phosphate dehydrogenase (*D*) is suppressed by an elevation of intracellular lactate. (* denotes that the glycolytic pathway has been condensed at this point.) Ischemia increases the intracellular concentration of acyl CoA esters, in part because the intracellular accumulation of lactate inhibits carnitine palmityl coenzyme A transferase (*E*), the enzyme that catalyzes the transfer of acyl CoA from the cell cytoplasm to the mitochondria. Acyl CoA esters inhibit the effective exchange of ADP and ATP between the cytoplasm of the cell and the mitochondria by suppressing the activity of adenine nucleotide translocase (*F*). The antilipolytic agents are effective because they prevent a build-up of acyl CoA esters within the cytoplasm, and 1-carnitine exerts a salutary effect on ischemic myocardium by reversing the inhibition of adenine nucleotide translocase, thus allowing continued movement of ADP and ATP between the cell cytoplasm and the mitochondria. (TCA = tricarboxylic acid.) (Reproduced with permission from Hillis, L. D., and Braunwald, E.: Myocardial ischemia. N. Engl. J. Med. *296*:971, 1034, and 1093; 1977.)

Figure 38-34. See color plate 6

The lower glycolytic flux in the ischemic as compared with the anoxic heart probably results in part from the inhibition by intracellular acidosis of PFK (Fig. 38-33), a key enzyme in the glycolytic chain. The importance of intracellular pH is further supported by the observation that pretreatment of rat myocardium to an alkaline pH of 7.9 maintains tension during a subsequent period of hypoxia.

In ischemic as opposed to anoxi perfused myocardium, accumulation of metabolites other than hydrogen ion, such as long-chain acyl carnitine (due to inhibition of β-oxidation of fatty acids) and lysophospholipids (due to activation of phospholipases and inhibition of enzymes responsible for lysophospholipid metabolism,[294-296] is likely to contribute not only to electrophysiological impairment and arrhythmogenesis but also to depression of mechanical performance and progression of injury in ischemic myocardium.

FATTY ACID METABOLISM IN ISCHEMIA

Under normal aerobic conditions, 60 to 90 per cent of myocardial energy requirements is met by oxidation of free fatty acids (FFA),[297] which are trapped in cells in the form of fatty (acyl) esters containing coenzyme A (acyl-CoA). The preferential utilization of FFA by myocardium appears to depend on the high activity of several enzyme systems, including the acyl-CoA-carnitine transferase systems that facilitate continuing transport of acyl-CoA from the cytosol to the mitochondria in a series of steps in which acyl-CoA and acyl-carnitine are interconverted.

After fatty acids are taken up by myocardial cells and undergo esterification with CoA, the acyl-CoA intermediates generally remain trapped in the cell. Acyl-CoA may be incorporated into triglycerides in the cytosol or oxidized after transport through the mitochondrial membrane. Under aerobic conditions, oxidation predominates since the products formed (two carbon moieties called acetyl groups) are readily incorporated as intermediates into the citric acid cycle and oxidized to carbon dioxide and water. Oxidation of fatty acids inhibits glucose uptake, glycolytic flux, and glycogenolysis. The increased production of acetyl-CoA accompanying fatty acid oxidation inhibits pyruvate dehydrogenase, thereby limiting the flow of carbohydrate metabolism through the citric acid cycle. Accumulation of glucose-6-phosphate inhibits hexokinase, decreasing phosphorylation of glucose. The decreased phosphorylation, coupled with direct inhibition of membrane transport of glucose mediated by fatty acids, contributes to the overall reduction of carbohydrate metabolism when fatty acid availability is high and oxygenation adequate.

Striking changes in fatty acid metabolism result from myocardial ischemia. The limited supply of oxygen inhibits beta-oxidation—as do the increased ratio of NADH/NAD and the reduced concentration of flavoproteins.[292] With more prolonged ischemia, oxidation of fatty acids is inhibited by another mechanism: inhibition or loss of long-chain acyl-carnitine transferase enzyme activity, necessary for transport of cytosolic acyl-CoA to the mitochondria before oxidation.[297] Accordingly, intracellular concentrations of acyl-CoA increase and acetyl-CoA content declines.[298] The increased acyl-CoA accompanied by increased production of glycerol, a byproduct of the enhanced glycolytic flux induced by ischemia, leads to increased synthesis of triglycerides, which accumulate in the ischemic myocardium.

INTRAMYOCARDIAL ACCUMULATION OF ACYL-COA IN ISCHEMIA. Accumulation of acyl-CoA may be deleterious because it inhibits further formation of CoA esters of fatty acids. Thus, fatty acids entering the cell cannot be esterified and trapped and are therefore prone to egress promptly. Furthermore, oxidation of fatty acids entering the cell cannot proceed without initial esterification with CoA. Accordingly, accumulation of fatty acid labeled with carbon-11, which can be monitored externally in vivo by positron tomography (p. 1347) or with other tracers,[299] is diminished in ischemic or hypoxic zones. Restored metabolism accompanying reperfusion implemented promptly enough to maintain cell viability is reflected by a return of myocardial accumulation of fatty acid toward normal,[300] although the return of recovery may sometimes be prolonged. In working hearts subjected to ischemia followed by reperfusion, recovery of function cannot be sustained by the metabolism of glucose alone but, in fact, appears to depend on restoration of metabolism of fatty acids. When fatty acid metabolism is inhibited with oxfenicine, an inhibitor of long-chain acyl carnitine transferase activity,[301] ischemia followed by reperfusion results in profound stunning with concordant reduction of myocardial oxygen consumption despite increased oxidation of glucose. These results are consistent with the known coupling between diminished fatty acid oxidation and decreased function in ischemic myocardium.[299]

ISCHEMIA-INDUCED DEFECTS IN FATTY ACID METABOLISM. Detection of altered fatty acid metabolism is the basis for recognition of ischemic myocardium in experimental animals and patients after intravenous administration of cyclotron-produced, positron-emitting, ^{11}C-labeled fatty acids. In isolated perfused hearts, transitory diminution of perfusion leads to a reversible reduction of ^{11}C-palmitate accumulation, reflecting decreased uptake and oxidation of fatty acids in the perfusate. The uptake of tracer is independent of flow per se, as long as metabolic activity of the myocardium remains constant. In patients with myocardial infarction, diminished accumulation of ^{11}C-palmitate is evident in computer-reconstructed images obtained by positron emission tomography. Because this technique permits quantitative delineation of the distribution of the tracer in multiple cross-sections of the heart after intravenous administration, the diminution of ^{11}C-palmitate uptake detectable tomographically corresponds quantitatively to biochemical and morphometric criteria of infarction.[302] During physical exercise patients with ischemic heart disease exhibited reduced myocardial free fatty acid extraction.[303]

Reduced flow alone does not diminish uptake of a substrate if intermediary metabolism is not altered, since the extraction fraction increases. Thus, transitory ischemia without reduction of either myocardial oxygen consumption or fatty acid utilization would not be manifested tomographically by decreased ^{11}C-palmitate uptake.[304] However, prolonged ischemia, with impairment of oxidative metabolism but without necrosis, would give rise to a zone of decreased accumulation of the tracer evident by tomography. The two conditions (prolonged ischemia without necrosis and infarction per se) can be readily differentiated with the use of serial studies. Prolonged and persistent diminution of oxidative metabolism and hence persistently impaired regional uptake of ^{11}C-palmitate detectable tomographically are tantamount to necrosis in view of the well-established irreversibility of injury sustained by myocardium rendered ischemic for 2 hours or more.

In contrast to the regional variation of accumulation of ^{18}FDG in hearts of normal human subjects under conditions such as fasting,[305] accumulation of radiolabeled fatty acids is homogeneous.[306] Nevertheless, externally detectable clearance of radiolabeled tracers of fatty acid from myocardium does not provide a direct index of myocardial fatty acid metabolism because of sometimes pronounced and often variable efflux of nonmetabolized radiolabeled fatty acid.[307] Furthermore, variable contributions to overall energy production of diverse substrates, including glucose, palmitate, ketones, and lactate, preclude estimations of regional energy metabolism in ischemic or reperfused myocardium by analysis of uptake or clearance of a single tracer of any one metabolic pathway.[308,308a]

Uptake of Fatty Acids. Despite the limitations of estimation of fatty acid utilization (because of efflux) and the diversity of contributions of different pathways of intermediary metabolism to overall oxidative metabolism, uptake of palmitate quantifiable tomographically 1 hour after reperfusion is a powerful predictor of maintenance of myocardial viability evident 4 weeks later in the hearts of dogs subjected to coronary occlusion and reperfusion[240] (Fig. 38-35). Definitive assessments of overall myocardial oxygen utilization (and hence viability) can be made in normal, ischemic, and reperfused myocardium with the use of dynamic positron-emission tomography and radiolabeled acetate—a tracer entering essentially only one pathway of metabolism, namely mitochondrial oxidative phosphorylation.[239,241,254]

Figure 38-35. See color plate 7

PROTEIN AND NUCLEIC ACID METABOLISM IN ISCHEMIA

Characteristic changes in synthesis and degradation of myocardial proteins accompany ischemia. Synthesis decreases because of inhibition of peptide chain initiation and elongation. Efflux of alanine reflects not only its diminished utilization in protein synthesis but also augmented synthesis by transamination of pyruvate, a precursor accumulating because of impaired carbohydrate exudation. Thus, alanine release from the ischemic heart is analogous to lactate production, just as release of inosine (a product of degradation of adenine nucleotides) is analogous to lactate production.

Release of another amino acid, phenylalanine, has been employed in experimental preparations in which reincorporation into protein is prevented by pretreatment with cycloheximide (an inhibitor of protein synthesis) to provide an index of protein degradation under a variety of conditions, including normal oxygenation, anoxia, and simulated ischemia. The process of protein degradation requires energy derived from oxidative metabolism under physiological conditions based on observations with such preparations, since the rate of protein degradation declines by as much as 80 per cent in isolated hearts subjected to severe ischemia.[309] Although proteolysis mediated by lysosomal hydrolases has been implicated as a factor leading to irreversible injury in myocardium undergoing ischemic injury, increases in free and total lysosomal hydrolase activity do not occur until several hours after the onset of ischemia. Accordingly, it appears likely that the early loss of functional sarcolemmal integrity accompanied by electrophysiological manifestations, subsequent impairment of cell volume regulation, and leakage of cytoplasmic constituents reflects primary damage to the cell membrane itself. Only later during the evolution of ischemic injury do activation and liberation of lysosomal enzymes or activation of proteases appear to be prominent. It has been postulated that a Ca^{++}- activated neutral protease degrades subunits of troponin within the first few hours of severe ischemia. These and related observations suggest that the irreversible nature of injury sustained by ischemic myocardium is not due to proteolysis, even though activation of these enzymes may account for the release of relatively late markers of cell death and result in protein degradation late in the evolution of necrosis. Nevertheless, provision of branched chain amino acids along with glucose in oxygenated crystalloid solutions to energy-depleted ischemic rat hearts enhances protection of myocardium and recovery of function with reperfusion.[310]

Under physiological conditions, the myocardium extracts glutamic acid from arterial blood and produces ammonia and glutamine, which appear in the coronary venous effluent. When ischemia supervenes, ammonia derived from amino acids that cannot be incorporated into protein under these conditions is incorporated into alanine and glutamine with a consequent increase in their concentrations in the coronary sinus effluent. The increased production of alanine has been viewed as analogous to the increased production of lactate. Both are markers of ischemia. In the case of alanine, transamination of pyruvate serves as a sink for ammonia that would otherwise accumulate. In the case of lactate, the pyruvate serves as a sink for hydrogen ions.

EFFECTS OF ISCHEMIA ON GENETIC EXPRESSION OF SPECIFIC PROTEINS

As already outlined, the consequences of myocardial ischemia are prompt and are undoubtedly mediated initially by altered intermediary metabolism. Later or more sustained effects may reflect abnormalities in the synthesis of particular proteins mediated by changes in their genetic expression. In many tissues, "stress" such as hyperthermia or hypoxia induces the appearance of so-called heat shock or stress proteins with diverse effects. Recently, increased steady-state concentrations of a messenger RNA (mRNA) coding for one such protein in myocardium have been demonstrated after the induction of ischemia.[311] Proteins coded by the specific mRNA showed an increase in concentration despite a lack of overall change in the concentration of myosin and a decrease in the concentration of the predominant subunit of creatine kinase. Thus, myocardial ischemia induces specific alterations in steady-state concentrations of mRNAs coding for proteins with disparate functional properties in heart muscle cells.[311] These observations indicate that relatively long-term consequences of ischemia may reflect altered genetic expression leading to abnormal concentrations of specific intracellular proteins.[312]

Stimulation of hearts by heat shock, which induces expression of heat-shock proteins and acquisition of thermotolerance in other systems, can protect the stressed cells from injury induced by subsequent ischemia followed by reperfusion. Thus, when rats are rendered hyperthermic at 40°C for 15 minutes, hearts isolated and perfused later under conditions of low flow followed by reperfusion recover contractility within 5 minutes of reperfusion, in contrast to the case with hearts from control animals in which no recovery is evident at corresponding intervals. Release of creatine kinase induced by ischemia is markedly diminished, and ultrastructural integrity is better maintained as well.[312] The potential impact of altered genetic expression of specific proteins in mediating cardiac dysfunction is suggested by the relationship between slow relaxation and decreased relative expression of the calcium-ATPase gene with consequently diminished density of intracellular calcium pumps in rat hearts rendered hypertrophic.[313]

The importance of oxidative phosphorylation, i.e., the coupling of ATP synthesis to aerobic respiration, for the metabolic integrity of myocardium is underscored by some simple quantitative considerations. Complete oxidation of one mole of glucose gives rise to the net production of 36 moles of ATP. In contrast, only 2 moles of ATP are produced from complete anaerobic metabolism of 1 mole of glucose. Thus, even if the profound derangements in intermediary metabolism associated with increased production of reducing equivalents accompanying anaerobic glycolysis could be corrected, an 18-fold increase in glycolytic flux would be required for myocardium to synthesize comparable quantities of ATP via anaerobic compared to aerobic metabolism. The failure of energy production to keep pace with demand in ischemic cells is manifested by a prompt decline in the concentration of creatine phosphate, a major constituent of myocardial high-energy phosphate stores.

The dependence of myocardial viability on the availability of oxygen has stimulated careful assessment of the gradients of oxygen present within ischemic zones of the heart, based on analysis of the oxidation-reduction state of specific components of the electron transport chain and different spectra reflecting changes in the oxygenation of myoglobin.[314,315] Results obtained with optical techniques applied to the infarcted heart in vitro suggest that individual cells, and possibly individual mitochondria, are either fully aerobic or fully anaerobic in regions of myocardium subjected to ischemia. Thus, at any given instant, borders between anoxic and oxygenated tissue are very sharp. This phenomenon is in part a reflection of the very high affinity of mitochondria for oxygen. In response to ischemia, the mitochondria remain oxidized, despite very low levels of tissue oxygen tension, and become reduced only when virtually the last remaining oxygen has been utilized within a region. Thus, there appears to be a sharp, anatomically definable border between regions in which mitochondria are aerobic and anaerobic. However, this border is not static. As ischemia persists, there is expansion of the mass of severely ischemic tissue judging from morphological observations in canine hearts subjected to coronary occlusion. Early in the course of severe ischemia there is a potentially large mass of jeopardized but not yet irreversibly injured ischemic myocardium, susceptible to favorable influence by selected interventions.

THE "WAVEFRONT" OF ISCHEMIC NECROSIS. The percentage of transmural necrosis ultimately developing within a zone of myocardium rendered ischemic by coronary occlusion maintained for 40 minutes, 3 hours, 6 hours, and 24

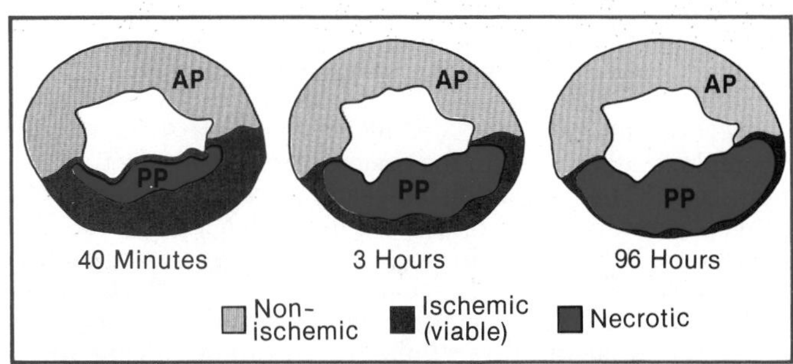

FIGURE 38-36. Progression of cell death versus time after circumflex coronary occlusion in dogs. Necrosis occurs first in the subendocardial myocardium. With longer occlusions, a wavefront of cell death moves from the subendocardial zone across the wall to involve progressively more of the transmural thickness of the ischemic zone. In contrast, the lateral margins in the subendocardial region of the infarct are established as early as 40 minutes after occlusion and are sharply defined by the anatomic boundaries of the ischemic bed. AP = anterior papillary muscle; PP = posterior papillary muscle. (From Reimer, K. A., Hill, M. L., and Jennings, R. B.: Prolonged depletion of ATP and of the adenine nucleotide pool due to delayed resynthesis of adenine nucleotides following reversible myocardial ischemic injury in dogs. J. Mol. Cell. Cardiol. *13*:229, 1981.)

hours, followed by reperfusion for 2 to 4 days, varies from 38 to 85 per cent with a "wavefront" of necrosis progressing from subendocardial to epicardial tissue,[1] presumably because the subendocardium has a greater oxygen demand and smaller oxygen supply than the epicardium (Fig. 38–36). Metabolic studies have shown greater and more rapid reductions of ATP and total adenosine nucleotides and greater and more rapid accumulation of lactate and nucleotides and bases, i.e., the products of degradation of adenine nucleotides in the subendocardium (Fig. 38–31). A cell in the subendocardium may be able to tolerate severe ischemia for a brief interval although it will become necrotic after 20 minutes. A cell with similar energy requirements in the subepicardium will be able to tolerate the milder degree of ischemia to which it is exposed following coronary occlusion for a longer period before becoming necrotic. As a consequence, when ischemic myocardium is reperfused 20 minutes to 5 hours after coronary occlusion, a progressively smaller epicardial zone of myocardium survives.[316]

ACTIVATION OF LYSOSOMAL ENZYMES AND COMPLEMENT

Most tissues contain latent lysosomal hydrolases capable of mediating proteolysis under certain conditions. Lysosomal hydrolases are activated by an acid pH, although mammalian cells contain neutral proteases as well. Relatively late reparative processes in myocardium undergoing infarction are accompanied by consistent increases in lysosomal hydrolase activity in tissue extracts as well as in the circulation, suggesting that activation of proteases with dissolution of cellular debris is a component to the response to irreversible injury. However, the extent to which activation of lysosomal hydrolase contributes to early manifestations of ischemia or irreversibility remains controversial. What is clear is that much of the lysosomal activity in the heart undergoing infarction comes from cells participating in the response to inflammation, such as polymorphonuclear leukocytes rather than myocardial cells per se.

In addition to degradation by activated lysosomal enzymes, ischemic injury may reflect the impact of activated complement either directly[317] or indirectly[318] by diminution of neutrophil activation. Complement may be activated by constituents of mitochondria released when heart muscle is subjected to ischemia.[317] Depletion of complement diminishes ischemic injury even when it is induced only after the onset of ischemia.[318] Salutary effects of depletion of complement appear to be greater than those seen with reduction of neutrophil activation and infiltration alone by nonsteroidal antiinflammatory agents such as ibuprofen.[318]

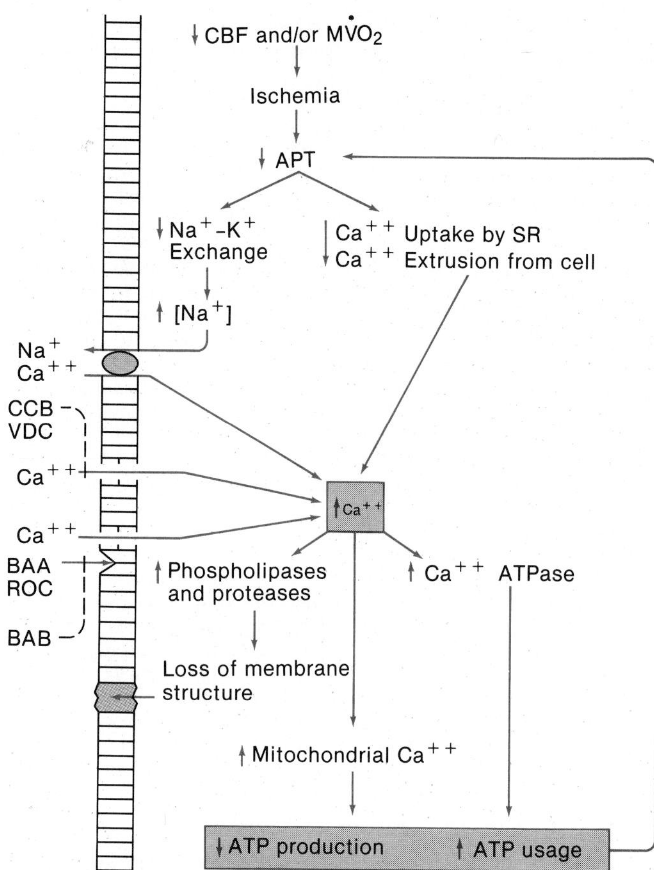

FIGURE 38–37. **Interactions between myocardial ischemia and $[Ca^{++}]$. A reduction of coronary blood flow (CBF), sometimes accompanied by an increase in myocardial oxygen requirements ($M\dot{V}O_2$), causes myocardial ischemia, which in turn reduces cellular ATP stores. This reduction interferes with the transsarcolemmal $Na^{+}-K^{+}$ exchange, which elevates intracellular $[Na^{+}]$, raising intracellular $[Ca^{++}]$ through an enhanced $Na^{+}-Ca^{++}$ exchange. Lowered ATP stores also reduce Ca^{++} uptake by the sarcoplasmic reticulum (SR) and reduce extrusion of Ca^{++} from cells. The resultant augmented intracellular $[Ca^{++}]$ causes mitochondrial Ca^{++} overload, which depresses ATP production further; activation of intracellular Ca^{++} ATPases, which augment ATP usage; and activation of sarcolemmal phospholipases and proteases, which impair the integrity of the cell membrane. Calcium-channel blockers (CCB) interfere with Ca^{++} influx through voltage-dependent channels (VDA). Beta-adrenoceptor agonists (BAA) recruit additional receptor-operated channels (ROC). Beta-adrenoceptor blockers (BAB) reduce Ca^{++} influx by interfering with the recruitment of ROC. (Reproduced with permission from Braunwald, E.: Mechanism of action of calcium channel blocking agents. N. Engl. J. Med. *307*:1618, 1982.)**

ROLE OF CALCIUM IN ISCHEMIC INJURY

Myocardial injury induced by ischemia is associated with complexes of calcium in the tissue detectable by electron microscopy.[1] The interaction between myocardial ischemia and myoplasmic $[Ca^{++}]$ is complex, as illustrated in Figure 38–37. Ischemia, however produced, is characterized by a reduction of myocardial ATP stores, which interferes with the transsarcolemmal $Na^{+}-K^{+}$ exchange, which in turn elevates intracellular $[Na^{+}]$, raising intracellular $[Ca^{++}]$ through an enhanced $Na^{+}-Ca^{++}$ exchange. Lowered ATP stores also reduce Ca^{++} uptake by the sarcoplasmic reticulum and reduce extrusion of Ca^{++} from cells. The resultant augmented intracellular $[Ca^{++}]$[319,320] causes mitochondrial Ca^{++} overload, which depresses ATP production further. Activation of intracellular Ca^{++} ATPases augments ATP usage and activates sarcolemmal phospholipases, which release membrane phospholipid degradation products whose detergent properties impair the integrity of the cell membrane.[321,322] Calcium antagonists interfere with Ca^{++} influx through voltage-dependent channels. Beta-adrenoceptor agonists recruit additional receptor-operated channels, and beta-adrenoceptor blockers reduce Ca^{++} influx by interfering with this recruitment of receptor-operated channels. Thus, one would expect beta blockers and Ca^{++} antagonists to have similar effects in the treatment of ischemia. Indeed, both groups of compounds delay ischemia-induced necrosis and, particularly when combined with reperfusion, reduce the extent of myocardial necrosis.[323–327]

The hypothesis that the entry of Ca^{++} into ischemic cells may be harmful is based on the observation that after a period of myocardial ischemia and subsequent reperfusion the accumulation of excess Ca^{++} in the mitochondria may interfere with their capacity to generate ATP. The destructive chain of metabolic events provoked by increased intracellular $[Ca^{++}]$ appears to be responsible, at least in part, for the death of cells in the ischemic myocardium. Henry and associates[328] found that during one hour of severe ischemia, the left ventricle undergoes progressive ischemic contracture, with the development of an elevated ventricular diastolic pressure and a fourfold increase in mitochondrial Ca^{++}. With subsequent reperfusion, both myocardial systolic function and relaxation remain abnormal, and a further marked increase in Ca^{++} accumulation occurs. Administration of nifedipine prevents ischemic contracture and permits recovery of systolic contractile function and of myocardial relaxation. These favorable hemodynamic changes are accompanied by a marked reduction in the accumulation of Ca^{++} in the mitochondria.

Ca^{++} antagonists have also been shown to reduce ATP depletion and myocardial damage during coronary occlusion, and particularly during reperfusion,[327-331] and nifedipine preserved left ventricular function in dogs with cardiopulmonary bypass that were subjected to prolonged total ischemia. These experiments demonstrate that in a setting analogous to the clinical practice of cardiac surgery, Ca^{++} antagonists protect myocardium, which is at first ischemic and is then reperfused. Thus, Ca^{++} antagonists may be valuable in protecting the myocardium from the Ca^{++}-associated ischemic injury occurring during open heart surgery. However, Ca^{++} antagonists do *not* appear to inhibit Ca^{++} influx into irreversibly injured myocardium. Instead, their protective action depends on an antiischemic effect resulting from a reduction of $M\dot{V}O_2$.

The accumulation of Ca^{++} in myocardium undergoing ischemic injury has important diagnostic and therapeutic implications. Myocardial infarct scintigraphy with agents such as ^{99m}Tc-stannous pyrophosphate permits detection and localization of infarction after intravenous injection of tracer. The tissue's avidity for the tracer appears to depend on the accumulation of Ca^{++} (p. 291).

Reduction of accumulation of intracellular Ca^{++} in jeopardized ischemic myocardium that has not yet undergone necrosis appears to protect the tissue and enhance salvage induced by reperfusion, as judged from studies in dogs with induced thrombotic coronary occlusion followed by clot lysis with intravenous streptokinase.[332] Effects of intravenous diltiazem given 30 minutes before administration of steptokinase were evident on positron-emission tomograms with $H_2{}^{15}O$ (to characterize perfusion) and carbon-11–labeled palmitate (to characterize intermediary metabolism). The extent of infarction expressed as the percentage of risk region was reduced by reperfusion alone but was even more markedly reduced by reperfusion coupled with cardiac protection conferred by diltiazem. These results were confirmed by direct analysis of myocardial creatine kinase content, which demonstrated less depletion of the enzyme in hearts subjected to reperfusion and concomitant calcium blockage compared with depletion in hearts subjected to reperfusion alone.

PHOSPHOINOSITIDES AND CALCIUM. The effects of many agonists on diverse cells are transduced by their interactions with surface receptors that are coupled to specific intracellular second messengers. One familiar example is beta-adrenergic stimulation of cardiac myocytes (p. 363). Stimulation is transduced by activation of cell surface receptors coupled to specific G proteins (p. 363) (named because of their interaction with GTP) that modulate activity of adenylate cyclase, increased synthesis of cyclic AMP, and cyclic AMP–dependent phosphorylation of proteins, one of which alters calcium channel function and increases calcium influx. Another particularly important bifurcating signal pathway responds to activation of other surface receptors coupled to other G proteins in response to agonists such as alpha-adrenergic agents. Activation of this system in cardiac myocytes gives rise to inositol 1,4,5-triphosphate (IP_3) (or a cyclic compound, inositol 1:2-cyclic 4,5-triphosphate) and diacylglycerol—both of which are products of Ca^{++}-dependent phospholipase-catalyzed hydrolysis of phosphatidylinositol 4,5-biphosphate. IP_3 releases Ca^{++} from the sarcoplasmic reticulum, and diacylglycerol activates protein kinase C. Both components of this signaling pathway (IP_3 and diacylglycerol) influence intracellular Ca^{++}-dependent responses.[333]

Increases in intracellular concentrations of phosphoinositides may mediate the positive inotropic effects of alpha-adrenergic agonists and contribute to Ca^{++} overload and alpha-adrenergic receptor–mediated arrhythmogenesis in ischemic and reperfused myocardium.[334] Amphiphiles accumulating with ischemia and reperfusion augment alpha-receptor density and Ca^{++} influx. Thus, it is not surprising that reperfusion appears to increase turnover of phosphoinositides.[335] Catecholamines increase intracellular Ca^{++} by beta-adrenergic cyclic AMP-mediated increased influx and by alpha-adrenergic IP_3-mediated effects on the sarcoplasmic reticulum, and increased adrenergic stimulation is a hallmark of ischemic and reperfused myocardium. Accordingly, attenuation of receptor-mediated activation of both the cyclic AMP and IP_3-diacylglycerol second messenger systems, inhibition of activation of phospholipase C, or inhibition of activated protein kinase C may retard the progression of ischemic injury and attenuate its manifestations, particularly when coupled with other measures designed to inhibit calcium overload secondary to ischemia or reperfusion.[336,337]

OXYGEN-DERIVED FREE RADICALS IN ISCHEMIC TISSUE INJURY

There is substantial evidence that ischemic tissue generates oxygen-derived free radicals (oxygen radicals), i.e., oxygen molecules containing an odd number of electrons, making them chemically reactive, and often leading to chain reactions.[338] There are three principal oxygen radicals: the superoxide anion ($\cdot O_2^-$), hydrogen peroxide (H_2O_2), and the hydroxyl radical ($\cdot OH$). Acute, severe ischemia appears to increase the production of oxygen radicals by several mechanisms: (1) dissociation of intramitochondrial electron transport; (2) ischemia-induced Ca^{++} influx activates phospholipase, which enhances arachidonic acid metabolism, which in turn may produce oxygen radicals; (3) ischemia converts the normal myocardial enzyme xanthine dehydrogenase to xanthine oxidase in some species, which in the presence of xanthine produces oxygen radicals; and/or (4) complement is activated in ischemic tissue and this enhances the accumulation of neutrophils, which in turn release oxygen radicals.[338]

The oxygen radicals, in turn, can contribute to ischemic damage or postischemic damage caused by reperfusion.[339] These moieties react with almost any biological molecule in their vicinity. It has been proposed that by causing perioxidation of cell membranes, oxygen radicals damage cell membranes and contribute to cell death. It has also been postulated that they can contribute to the development of irreversible injury by acting on the mitochondria and sarcoplasmic reticulum. This postulate is based largely on the observation that free radical scavengers such as superoxide dismutase and catalase prevent the ischemia-induced loss of Ca^{++} sequestration by the sarcoplasmic reticulum and preserve mitochondrial function.

Despite the demonstrable toxicity of oxygen-derived free radicals to cell membranes and the apparently protective effects of free radical scavengers in studies of experimental animals[225-228,340] and inhibitors of their production,[229,229a] salvage of myocardium by interventions attenuating free-radical production and persistence has not been observed consistently. High molecular weight "scavengers" such as catalase and superoxide dismutase may not penetrate the source of free radicals rapidly enough, and even brief exposure of vulnerable organelles to oxygen-derived free radicals may be sufficient to obviate their protective effects. Strategies focusing on attenuation of oxygen-derived free radical accumulation diminish stunning in ischemic myocardium subjected to reperfusion, and accordingly, these radicals have been implicated in its pathogenesis.[226,341-344] Neutrophil depletion during reperfusion reduces myocardial infarct size, presumably by reducing production of oxygen-derived free radicals.[345] Preservation of high concentrations of intracellular reducing agents such as glutathione that may attenuate otherwise increased concentrations of active oxygen radicals appears to confer protection as judged from preservation of both systolic and diastolic function in hearts subjected to ischemia and reperfusion.[346] In addition, agents such as diltiazem that inhibit lipid peroxidation inducible by oxygen-derived free radicals may be beneficial.[224]

RELEASE OF MYOCARDIAL ENZYMES IN DETECTION OF ACUTE MYOCARDIAL INFARCTION

(see also p. 1218)

Since biochemical markers of ischemic injury have become important clinical tools, some considerations required for their proper interpretation merit particular attention. Loss of functional integrity of the sarcolemma is a primary common denominator underlying liberation of cytoplasmic constituents into the circulation, such as transaminase (SGOT, AST), lactic dehydrogenase (LDH), and creatine kinase (CK).[347] Species of lower molecular weight, such as myoglobin, are liberated, but elevated concentrations persist in the circulation only briefly because of rapid renal clearance. Furthermore, myoglobin released from hypoperfused skeletal muscle may cloud interpretation of elevated values in plasma.

Accurate assessment of myocardial infarction based on analysis of plasma enzyme time-activity curves has been facilitated by the demonstration that one isoenzyme of creatine kinase, CK-MB, is localized primarily in the heart in humans.[347] Under carefully defined conditions in experimental animals, depletion of myocardial CK activity correlates with infarct size estimated independently by morphometric techniques or with the use of radioactively labeled microspheres. The corollary of these observations, namely, that increases in plasma enzyme activity reflect infarct size, has been recognized for many years.

On the basis of many clinical studies and observations in conscious experimental animals,[347,348] it has become clear that release of myocardial cytosolic enzymes into the circulation is tantamount to cell death when the cause of enzyme release is myocardial ischemia. Accordingly, infarct size has been estimated from analysis of plasma enzyme CK time-activity curves,[349–351] and from curves obtained by quantitative assay of plasma samples for CK-MB activity. Despite obvious imperfections, enzymatic estimates of infarct size have correlated with biochemical and morphological analyses of infarction in hearts of experimental animals, morbidity and mortality in patients, histochemical assessment of necrosis among patients who succumb to acute myocardial infarction,[352] early and late ventricular arrhythmia, and impairment of ventricular function. Time-activity curves are influenced by regional myocardial perfusion, local degradation of enzyme in the heart, the ratio of enzyme released compared with that destroyed,[353] inactivation of enzyme in lymph,[354] exchange of enzyme between vascular and extravascular compartments,[350] and potential variation in the rate of inactivation and removal of enzyme once it has reached the circulation.[354] Thus, the pattern of enzyme release and its overall magnitude may be influenced by interventions resulting in early reperfusion and accelerated washout. Nevertheless, analysis of plasma time-activity curves of CK-MB and other biochemical markers of ischemic injury has proved useful in quantitative assessment of the progress and extent of myocardial infarction in the clinical setting.

Because the rate of appearance of macromolecules such as CK in plasma is accelerated when myocardium is subjected to reperfusion (reflecting an increased rate of washout), the utility of enzymatic estimation of the extent of infarction in the setting of reperfusion has been questioned. However, recent studies in dogs in which estimates based on plasma enzyme time-activity curves were correlated with the actual extent of infarction as judged from direct measurements of infarct size in excised hearts demonstrated that enzymatic estimates remained valid when CK release was measured during the first 60 minutes after the onset of reperfusion. Analogous results were obtained in patients with myocardial infarction who had undergone early reperfusion and in whom enzymatic estimates were correlated with estimates of infarct size based on positron-emission tomography 1 to 2 weeks after the index episode.[355]

Despite their usefulness, results of assays of plasma enzymes and other macromolecules must be interpreted cautiously. An apparent lack of elevation may occur in the setting of unequivocal acute myocardial infarction if the extent of injury sustained is minimal, the frequency of sampling insufficient, or the extent of the peak elevation modest and difficult to define in terms of the "normal" range reflecting a distribution of values in the population. The biological implications of severe myocardial ischemia without infarction may be as great for patients with unstable angina as they are for patients with incipient or early evolving infarction or infarction of minimal extent. Accordingly, it is inappropriate to deprive patients of continued medical surveillance if the index of suspicion of coronary insufficiency is high, even when statistically definable elevations of plasma enzymes and other macromolecular markers of ischemic injury are not present in initially obtained plasma samples.

CREATINE KINASE ISOFORMS. Subforms of individual isoenzymes of CK-MM (isoforms), which may be distinguished by differences in isoelectric points (PI), exist in the plasma soon after myocardial infarction (Fig. 38–38). When CK-MM is released into the bloodstream it is in the MM_3 isoform; this evolves in the plasma sequentially and in a time-dependent manner with cleavage of carboxyterminal lysines on each of the M subunits by carboxypeptidase N[356] into two other isoforms, MM_2 and MM_1, having lower isoelectric points. Both in experimental animals and in patients with coronary occlusion, within one hour after occlusion the percentage of total circulating MM comprised by the MM_3 isoform rises, with a reciprocal reduction of MM_2. No conversion of isoforms appears to occur in normal, ischemic, or necrotic myocardium.[357] It appears possible to use a single blood sample, available at the time of initial presentation, in which relative distribution of CK-MM isoforms is estimated both to diagnose (with a sensitivity of 94 per cent)[358] and to time the onset of myocardial infarction. The isoform profile may be distinctly abnormal in the face of normal total CK or CK-MB.[359] However, since the MM_3 isoform is present in tissues other than the

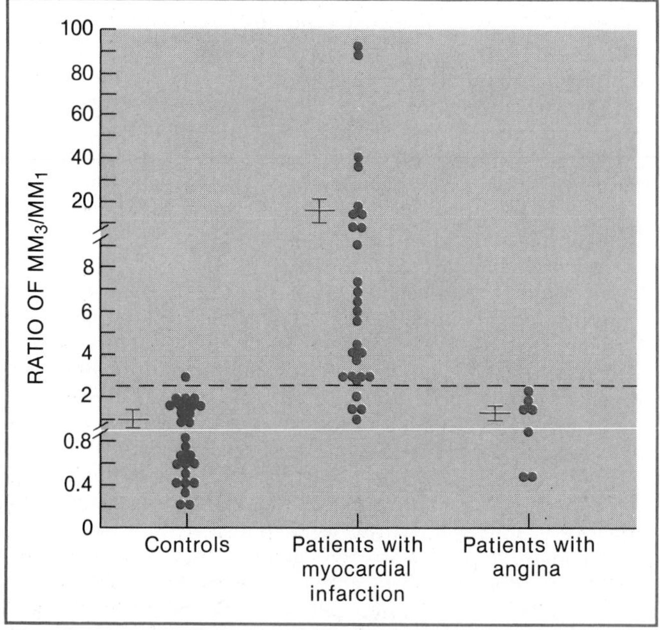

FIGURE 38–38. Comparison of the ratios of MM_3 to MM_1 in plasma from normal control subjects, patients with acute myocardial infarction, and patients with angina. (From Jaffe, A. S., Serota, H., Grace, A., and Sobel, B. E.: Diagnostic changes in plasma creatine kinase isoforms early after the onset of acute myocardial infarction. Circulation *74*:105, 1986, by permission of the American Heart Association, Inc.)

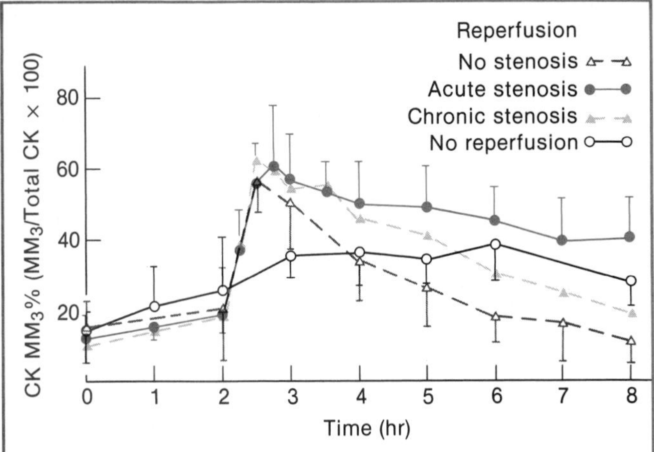

FIGURE 38–39. Plasma profiles of percent of creatine kinase activity composed of MM_3 in dogs subjected to coronary occlusion and release after 2 hours in the absence of coronary stenosis (n = 10) or with stenosis induced for 1 week (chronic, n = 5) or before occlusion (acute, n = 5), and in dogs subjected to persistent coronary occlusion (no reperfusion, n = 10). Data are presented as mean vaues ± 1 SD. (From Nohora, R., Myears, D. W., Sobel, B. E., and Abendschein, D. R.: Optimal criteria for rapid detection of myocardial reperfusion by creatine kinase MM isoforms in the presence of residual high grade coronary stenosis. Reprinted with permission from the American College of Cardiology. J. Am. Coll. Cardiol. *14*:1067, 1989.)

heart, the isoform profile in plasma is less specific for myocardial damage than is the CK-MB. The isoform profile (the percentage of concentrations of total CK activity in plasma comprised by MM_3) changes rapidly following myocardial reperfusion and appears to provide a prompt, reliable, and noninvasive index of the presence of myocardial reperfusion,[360,361] even in the presence of residual high-grade stenosis with the potential to attenuate washout of MM_3 into the circulation[362] (Fig. 38–39).

OTHER MACROMOLECULAR MARKERS. In addition to isoforms of CK-MM, isoforms of CK-MB have been recognized.[363] Three MB isoforms exist, but most assay systems detect only a tissue form and a second form that can comprise both converted products comigrating or copurifying under specific conditions. Alternatively, one of the two converted forms may be present only transiently in the circulation.[364,365] Despite the promise of analysis of CK-MB isoform profiles for early detection of reperfusion because of potentially greater specificity with MB- as opposed to MM-CK,[366] isoform analysis of MM is likely to afford more sensitivity and less ambiguity in view of the resolution of all three theoretically possible isoforms.

The pattern of release of many other macromolecular markers of ischemic injury into the circulation is qualitatively similar to that of individual isoenzymes of CK. Myoglobin has been used for early detection of reperfusion[367] because of its rapid clearance from the circulation as a result of glomerular filtration. In experimental animals, its pattern of release into the circulation with reperfusion is "staccato-like." [368] In patients, abrupt increases in the concentration of myoglobin in plasma are evident during the first 2 hours after coronary revascularization with myocardial infarction in progress.[369]

Myosin light chains have been assayed in plasma to detect irreversible ischemic injury. In dogs, the extent of infarction estimated from calculated myosin light-chain II release correlates closely with morphological estimates of infarct size whether or not reperfusion is induced within 3 or 6 hours after coronary occlusion.[370]

It appears likely that rapid, noninvasive estimation of the extent of infarction and accurate delineation of the time of occurrence of reperfusion based on assay of macromolecular markers will play an increasing role in decision making for management of patients with evolving myocardial infarction treated with thrombolytic agents in whom angioplasty or emergency surgery may be required because of failure of initial recanalization or demonstrably successful recanalization with subsequent early reocclusion.

MODIFICATION OF ISCHEMIC INJURY

A variety of interventions have been shown in animal experiments to modify the severity of ischemic injury, and in some instances parallel changes in infarct size have been observed. The theoretical basis for these interventions and the experimental results are discussed below. The clinical application of these observations is discussed on page 1227. The potency of any intervention designed to limit ischemic injury is inversely related to the interval between the onset of the ischemic stimulus and the time the intervention is applied. In the normothermic working dog heart no intervention can be expected to exert a significant beneficial effect if it is initiated more than 4 to 6 hours after the onset of severe ischemia, because by this time all tissue in the distribution of the occluded vessel is likely to have become irreversibly injured.

INTERVENTIONS THAT INCREASE MYOCARDIAL INJURY AFTER CORONARY ARTERY OCCLUSION

(Table 38–4)

Certain interventions known to increase $M\dot{V}O_2$ also increase the severity and extent of myocardial injury in the presence of residual, albeit restricted coronary blood flow. In the dog without heart failure, isoproterenol, digitalis (in the absence of heart failure), and amrinone[371] have a deleterious effect on ischemic myocardium. Exercise can precipitate ischemia in the presence of obstruction not severe enough to cause ischemia at rest. Also, pacing-induced tachycardia increases ischemic damage,[372] and a similar observation in patients has been reported. Hypoxemia,[373] anemia, and hypotension, regardless of how produced,[374] increase myocardial ischemic injury after coronary occlusion, since in all of these conditions the delivery of oxygen to the ischemic tissue is reduced; similarly, hypoglycemia augments ischemic injury.[375] Hyperthermia impairs mechanical performance of the ischemic myocardium; through its direct stimulation of $M\dot{V}O_2$ and heart rate, it exerts an adverse effect on myocardial oxygen balance.

The positive inotropic and chronotropic effects of isoproterenol improve the function of normal myocardium and elevate $M\dot{V}O_2$. When isoproterenol is administered in the presence of global myocardial ischemia, however, myocardial function deteriorates rapidly because of the intensification of ischemia.[376] The effects of isoproterenol on myocardial function in

TABLE 38–4 INTERVENTIONS THAT INCREASE MYOCARDIAL INJURY AFTER CORONARY ARTERY OCCLUSION

Increase Myocardial Oxygen Requirements
Isoproterenol
Digitalis and amrinone (in the absence of heart failure)
Tachycardia
Hyperthermia
Decrease Myocardial Oxygen Supply
Directly
Hypoxemia
Anemia
Through collateral vessels, reducing coronary perfusion pressure
Hemorrhage
Sodium nitroprusside
Other vasodilators (including isoproterenol)
Coronary vasoconstriction (indomethacin)
Decrease substrate availability
Hypoglycemia

the presence of regional ischemia are more complex. In the conscious dog with regional myocardial ischemia, isoproterenol elicits a spectrum of reactions in areas with different degrees of ischemia.[377] Severely ischemic sites exhibit no increase in blood flow, and a deterioration of function occurs during infusion of isoproterenol, as a result of an increase in $M\dot{V}O_2$, whereas normal or moderately ischemic areas show an improvement of both myocardial function and regional blood flow. The positive chronotropic and inotropic actions of isoproterenol cause an increase in infarct size in anesthetized dogs, and myocardial lactate production increases when isoproterenol is administered to patients with acute myocardial infarction.

An increase in the concentration of circulating fatty acids also aggravates ischemia following coronary occlusion. They augment $M\dot{V}O_2$ in the presence of limited oxygen supply; this intensifies ischemia, depresses myocardial contractility, and probably precipitates arrhythmias.

INTERVENTIONS THAT REDUCE MYOCARDIAL INJURY AFTER CORONARY ARTERY OCCLUSION

(Table 38–5)

THE PRIMACY OF REPERFUSION FOR SALVAGE OF ISCHEMIC MYOCARDIUM. As discussed on page 1230, coronary thrombolysis has become a cornerstone of early treatment of acute myocardial infarction precipitated by coronary thrombosis. Results of numerous laboratory and clinical investigations[378] have demonstrated that (1) myocardial infarction is a dynamic process that can be interrupted by interventions restoring nutritive perfusion, limiting myocardial oxygen requirements, supporting myocardial metabolism, and inducing favorable ventricular loading conditions; (2) damage to ischemic myocardium can be limited by prompt and sustained recanalization of infarct-affected arteries; (3) most acute transmural infarcts and many non-Q-wave infarcts result from acute coronary thrombosis that can be documented biochemically, angiographically, or morphologically; (4) mortality attributable to acute myocardial infarction is directly related to the extent of damage sustained by heart muscle rendered ischemic, which is also reflected by impairment of regional ventricular function; and (5) preservation of myocardial viability, restoration of regional wall motion in jeopardized ischemic zones, and reduction of mortality are inversely related to the duration of ischemia preceding induction and persistence of reperfusion.

TABLE 38–5 INTERVENTIONS THAT REDUCE EXPERIMENTAL MYOCARDIAL INJURY FOLLOWING CORONARY OCCLUSION

- **Increasing myocardial oxygen supply**
  - **Directly**
    - **Coronary artery reperfusion (surgery, PTCA, thrombolysis)**
    - **Elevating arterial pO_2, hyperbaric oxygenation**
    - **Fluorocarbons**
  - **Through collateral vessels**
    - **Elevation of coronary perfusion pressure (e.g., methoxamine, neosynephrine)**
    - **Intraaortic balloon counterpulsation**
  - **Coronary vasodilatation (calcium antagonists, nitroglycerin, prostacyclin)**
  - **Coronary venous retroperfusion**
- **Decreasing myocardial O_2 demand**
  - **Beta-adrenoceptor blockers**
  - **Cardiac glycoside in the failing heart**
  - **Intraaortic balloon in counterpulsation**
  - **Decreasing afterload in hypertensive individuals**
  - **Decreasing preload (nitroglycerin)**
  - **Inhibiting calcium influx (Ca^{++} antagonists)**
  - **Hypothermia**
- **Preventing myocardial edema**
  - **Increasing plasma osmolality (mannitol, hypertonic glucose)**
- **Augmenting anaerobic metabolism**
  - **Glucose-insulin-potassium, fructose diphosphate, ribose hypertonic glucose**
- **Enhancing transport to the ischemic zone of substrate utilized in energy production (presumed)**
  - **Hyaluronidase**
- **Prevention of injury by oxygen-free radicals (e.g., superoxide dismutase, allopurinol)**
- **Reduction of catabolism**
  - **Inhibition of adenine nucleotide catabolism (allopurinol)**
  - **Inhibition of lipolysis (β-pyridilcarbinol)**
- **Prevention of cell swelling**
  - **Osmotic agents (mannitol), Ca^{++} antagonists**
- **Reduction of inflammatory response**
  - **Glucocorticosteroids**
  - **Nonsteroidal antiinflammatory drugs (e.g., ibuprofen)**
- **Reduction of microvascular damage**
  - **Prevention of injury of vessels by free radicals**
  - **Prevention of platelet aggregation**
  - **Prevention of endothelial swelling (hypertonic agents)**

Myocardial ischemia in patients should be relieved by prompt and sustained recanalization of thrombotically occluded infarct-related arteries, generally accomplished with intravenous administration of activators of plasminogen.[379] The efficacy of coronary thrombolysis can be enhanced pharmacologically in two ways: with adjunctive agents and with conjunctive agents.[380]

Adjunctive Agents. Treatment with adjunctive agents is directed toward increasing the interval during which jeopardized ischemic myocardium remains salvageable as has been accomplished in experimental animals with calcium antagonists[332]; diminishing deleterious effects of neutrophil activation[381] or of oxygen-centered free radicals regardless of their origin[382–384]; diminishing calcium overload potentially exacerbated by reperfusion[385,386]; reducing oxygen requirements in jeopardized ischemic or reperfused myocardium with beta-adrenergic-blocking agents[387]; or preserving myocardial viability with combinations of protective measures.[388]

Treatment with conjunctive agents is directed toward accelerating thrombolysis or sustaining recanalization to prevent early thrombotic reocclusion or both on the basis of compelling evidence indicating that the efficacy of coronary thrombolysis depends on attenuation of ongoing thrombosis potentially exacerbated by procoagulant effects of plasminogen activators or plasmin[389–391] and by activation of platelets[392–395] as well as on fibrinolysis itself.[380,396] Conjunctive agents include PGE_1,[397,398] thromboxane receptor antagonists,[399] thromboxane synthetase inhibitors,[400] prostacyclin analogs,[401] $alpha_2$-antiplasmin,[402] heparin,[403] aspirin,[404] and hirudin.[405] Thus, even though protection of ischemic myocardium is best accomplished by prompt restoration of nutritive perfusion[406] and perfusion reserve[407] (as shown by positron-emission tomography with $H_2{}^{15}O$ before and after revascularization [Fig. 38–40]), the net impact of recanalization reflects the interplay of diverse factors that can affect myocardial viability.

Figure 38–40. See color plate 8

Several studies in animals have shown that early reperfusion results in smaller infarction than if the occlusion is sustained. As might be expected, the extent of salvage depends on the duration of occlusion.[1,315,408,409] Reperfusion after less than 15 to 20 minutes of coronary occlusion salvages essentially all of the ischemic tissue.[1] With longer periods of ischemia, a wavefront of necrosis beginning in the subendocardium and moving progressively outward, i.e., to the epicardium and laterally, occurs[410] (Fig. 38–36). When reperfusion is implemented after 6 hours of coronary occlusion, most of the jeopardized myocardium becomes necrotic and no tissue is salvaged.

OTHER INTERVENTIONS

The inhalation of an *oxygen-rich gas mixture* exerts a slight beneficial effect on the ischemic myocardium, presumably by enhancing delivery of oxygen to ischemic tissue through collaterals.[411] This may be greatly enhanced by combining inhalation of 100 per cent oxygen with fluorocarbon mixtures, i.e., so-called artificial blood, which greatly augments delivery.[412-415]

Intraaortic balloon counterpulsation (p. 580) reduces the severity of ischemic injury, presumably by reducing MVO_2, as a consequence of lowering systolic wall tension, while simultaneously augmenting oxygen delivery by increasing aortic diastolic (coronary perfusion) pressure. In experimental animals, *beta-adrenoceptor blockers* appear to prolong the survival of severely ischemic tissue, judging from changes in ST segments, QRS complexes, myocardial creatine kinase activity, and electron-microscopic, histochemical, and histological criteria.[416] In addition, these drugs appear to improve the ratio of subendocardial to subepicardial blood flow in both ischemic and normal areas of myocardium in dogs with coronary occlusion. Beta-adrenoceptor blockade appears to be more useful in *delaying* than preventing cell death and is especially effective in limiting infarct size in animals subjected to coronary occlusion and reperfusion.[325] Calcium antagonists have similar actions.[417] Ca^{++} antagonists may be beneficial when they are administered prophylactically, i.e., before the development of ischemia or early in its course.[323,326-331,418-420]

A number of *metabolic interventions* may also improve the energy balance of ischemic myocardium. As fatty acid oxidation is impaired by ischemia, glucose becomes the principal source of energy. In the ischemic dog heart, oxidative phosphorylation and cardiac function are enhanced by the infusion of glucose-insulin-potassium (GIK).[421] In the anoxic, isolated heart, both electrical and mechanical function improve and recovery occurs more rapidly when glucose is added to the perfusate,[422] and analogous effects have been observed in laboratory and some clinical studies in vivo.[423-425]

A number of agents that limit the inflammatory response reduce myocardial ischemic injury in the laboratory animal, and some have been tested in limited numbers of patients. *Cobra venom factor,* a protein that enzymatically cleaves C3 and prevents the effects of the complement system, reduces myocardial injury,[426] presumably by diminishing leukotaxis. The kallikrein system enhances leukotactic activity, capillary permeability, interstitial edema, and proteolytic activity, and *aprotinin,* an inhibitor of this system, diminishes ischemic injury.[427] Large doses of a *glucocorticosteroid* reduce myocardial infarct size in the dog with coronary occlusion.[428] However, they may inhibit healing of the infarct, increasing the risk of ventricular rupture or aneurysm formation.[429] Ibuprofen, a nonsteroidal antiinflammatory compound, reduces infarct size in experimental animals but interferes with infarct healing and scar formation.[430]

Mannitol reduces the extent of ischemic injury and improves the function of the ischemic myocardium, presumably by reducing cell swelling and improving collateral blood flow.[431]

Hyaluronidase, which depolymerizes mucopolysaccharides in extracellular matrix, has also been shown to reduce myocardial necrosis in the dog and rabbit, possibly by increasing the access of nutrients to myocytes or increasing washout of toxic metabolites. However, its clinical impact is modest, and it appears to be beneficial only to patients with infarction associated with early, spontaneous reperfusion.[432] In the dog, intravenous nitroglycerin, administered at a rate sufficient to cause a mild diminution in systemic arterial pressure, reduces the magnitude and extent of ischemic injury, particularly when reflex tachycardia secondary to hypertension is prevented. In addition, the administration of nitroglycerin shortly after coronary artery occlusion partially reverses the ventricular fibrillation threshold, whereas nitroglycerin and phenylephrine in combination restore this threshold to normal. Nitroglycerin is presumed to act by augmenting perfusion of the border of the ischemic zone by dilating collaterals and by reducing myocardial demands by lowering preload and afterload (Fig. 38-6).[433]

The idea that oxygen-derived free radicals may play a role in myocardial injury due to ischemia and reperfusion is discussed on page 1187). A variety of scavengers of oxygen radicals have been shown to reduce the size of myocardial infarction in some[338] but certainly not all experiments.[434,435] These agents include superoxide dismutase, catalase, their combination, *N*-2-mercaptopropionyl glycine, and allopurinol, an inhibitor of xanthine oxidase.[436] Neutrophils accumulate rapidly in ischemic tissue, and the injury they cause is mediated largely through release of oxygen radicals. Neutrophil depletion also limits infarct size[437]; however, beneficial effects of free radical scavengers have been seen even in animals depleted of neutrophils.

When myocardium is "preconditioned" by repeated brief episodes of ischemia, it appears to be protected from the deleterious effects of subsequent prolonged ischemia. It had been suggested that preconditioning reduces myocardial energy demand during subsequent ischemia.[438-440]

Despite the unequivocal utility of reperfusion in limiting cell death in the presence of severe ischemia, reperfusion can elicit a number of adverse reactions that may limit its beneficial actions[437a,437b].

ACCELERATION OF MYOCYTE NECROSIS. After reperfusion, ischemic cells often suddenly develop ultrastructural changes indicative of cell death, including "explosive swelling" and widespread architectural disruption. Nevertheless, it is likely that most—perhaps all—of the myocytes in which necrosis is accelerated by reperfusion were already irreversibly injured by the time reperfusion occurred and that reperfusion merely hastened the death of cells already destined not to recover. If reperfusion does cause necrosis of *reversibly* injured myocardium, the quantity of tissue so affected is likely to be small.

ISCHEMIC CELL SWELLING. This causes compression of myocardial capillaries interfering further with myocardial perfusion. Reperfusion intensifies this process and thereby contributes to necrosis of some reversibly injured cells.[441]

THE "NO-REFLOW" PHENOMENON. This refers to the failure to achieve sustained reperfusion after a prolonged period of ischemia. The areas of reduced or absent reflow often appear to result from ischemia-induced microvascular damage and myocardial contracture. The no-reflow phenomenon does *not* appear to augment myocyte death, because the zone of reflow is contained within areas in which myocytes were already necrotic at the time of the onset of reperfusion (Fig. 38-41).

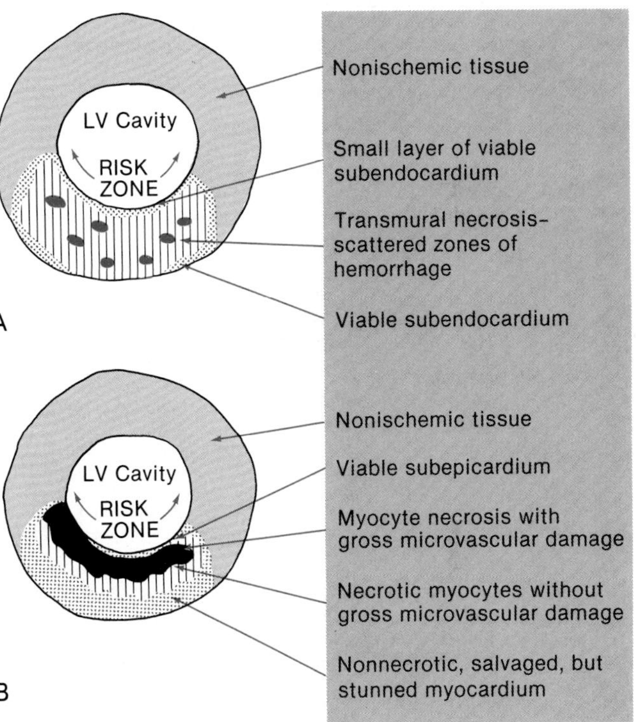

FIGURE 38-41. *A*, Schematic diagram showing a transverse section through a canine left ventricle subjected to a permanent coronary occlusion without reperfusion. The white area represents nonischemic myocardium supplied by the nonoccluded vessel. The infarct (hatched area) is transmural or near-transmural. There are scattered zones of hemorrhage (solid black). A small layer of viable subendocardium is present, which derives its oxygen directly from the ventricular cavity. Where collateral flow is high, there may be a small rim of surviving subepicardium (stippled areas). *B*, Schematic diagram showing a transverse section through a canine left ventricle subjected to coronary occlusion followed within 1 or 2 hours by coronary reperfusion. The hatched and solid black areas represent the infarct that is confined to the inner half of the myocardium. The solid black area represents the zone of gross microvascular damage including the zones of no-reflow and hemorrhage. It is smaller than and contained within the total infarct. The remainder of the infarct without severe microvascular damage is represented by the hatched area and is located in the midmyocardium. The epicardial portion of the ischemic zone (stippled area) has been salvaged by coronary reperfusion. It is nonnecrotic but stunned (postischemic ventricular dysfunction) for hours to days following coronary reperfusion. (From Braunwald, E., and Kloner, R. A.: Myocardial reperfusion: A double-edge sword? J. Clin. Invest. *76*:1715, 1985.)

REPERFUSION-INDUCED HEMORRHAGE. Reperfused infarcts frequently contain hemorrhagic areas.[442] Reperfusion-induced hemorrhage, like the "no-reflow" phenomenon, is caused largely by microvascular damage. It is generally contained within areas of myocardium already necrotic at the time of reperfusion.[443]

THE CALCIUM PARADOX AND THE OXYGEN PARADOX. The reintroduction of Ca^{++} and/or of oxygen to hearts previously perfused with Ca^{++}-free hypoxic media causes marked damage to the sarcolemma and entry of large quantities of Ca^{++} into the ischemic cells. These phenomena have been termed the *calcium paradox* and the *oxygen paradox,* respectively. Perfusion of ischemic cells with Ca^{++}-free solution occurs clinically only in the special circumstances when cardioplegia is produced during cardiac surgery by means of a Ca^{++}-free solution. However, the oxygen paradox may have clinical relevance. It may be mediated by oxygen-derived free radicals and potentially can be limited by free-radical scavengers of these substances.

REFERENCES

CONTROL OF MYOCARDIAL OXYGEN CONSUMPTION

1. Reimer, K. A., and Jennings, R. B.: Myocardial ischemia, hypoxia and infarction. *In* Fozzard, H. A., Jennings, R. B., Haber, E., Katz, A. M., and Morgan, H. E. (eds.): The Heart and Cardiovascular System. New York, Raven Press, 1986, pp. 1133–1202.
2. McKeever, W. P., Gregg, D. E., and Canney, P. C.: Oxygen uptake of the nonworking left ventricle. Circ. Res. *6*:612, 1958.
3. Rooke, G. A., and Feigl, E. O.: Work as a correlate of canine left ventricular oxygen consumption, and the problem of catecholamine oxygen wasting. Circ. Res. *50*:273, 1982.
4. Suga, H., Goto, Y., Yamada, O., and Igarashi, Y.: Independence of myocardial oxygen consumption from pressure-volume trajectory during diastole in canine left ventricle. Circ. Res. *55*:734, 1984
5. Klocke, F. J., Braunwald, E., and Ross, J., Jr.: Oxygen cost of electrical activation of the heart. Circ. Res. *18*:357, 1966.
6. Evans, C. L., and Matsuoka, Y.: The effect of various mechanical conditions on the gaseous metabolism and efficiency of the mammalian heart. J. Physiol. *49*:378, 1915.
7. Sarnoff, S. J., Braunwald, E., Welch, G. H. Jr., et al.: Hemodynamic determinants of oxygen consumption of the heart with special reference to the tension-time index. Am. J. Physiol. *192*:148, 1958.
8. Braunwald, E., Sarnoff, S. J., Case, R. B., et al.: Hemodynamic determinants of coronary flow: Effect of changes in aortic pressure and cardiac output on the relationship between myocardial oxygen consumption and coronary flow. Am. J. Physiol. *192*:157, 1958.
9. Rodbard, S., Williams, C. B., and Rodbard, D.: Myocardial tension and oxygen uptake. Circ. Res. *14*:139, 1964.
10. Teplick, R., Haas, G. S., Trautman, E., et al.: Time dependence of the oxygen cost of force development during systole in the canine left ventricle. Circ. Res. *59*:27, 1986.
11. Sonnenblick, E. H., Ross, J., Jr., Covell, J. W., and Braunwald, E.: Velocity of contraction as a determinant of myocardial oxygen consumption. Am. J. Physiol. *209*:919, 1965.
12. Starling, M. R., Mancini, J., Montgomery, D. G., and Gross, M. D.: Relation between maximum time-varying elastance pressure-volume areas and myocardial oxygen consumption in dogs. Circulation *83*:304, 1991.
13. Suga, H., Nozawa, T., Yasumura, Y., et al.: Force-time integral does not improve predictability of cardiac O_2 consumption from pressure-volume area (PVA) in dog left ventricle. Heart Vessels *5*:152, 1990.
14. Suga, H., Goto, Y., Igarashi, Y., et al.: Cardiac cooling increases E_{max} without affecting relation between O_2 consumption and systolic pressure-volume area in dog left ventricle. Circ. Res. *63*:61, 1988.
15. Schike, J. D., Burkhoff, D., Kass, D. A., et al.: Hemodynamic dependence of myocardial oxygen consumption indexes. Am. J. Physical. *258*:H1281, 1990.
16. Yasumura, Y., Nozawa, T., Futaki, S., et al.: Time-invariant oxygen cost of mechanical energy in dog left ventricle: Consistency and inconsistency of time-varying elastance model with myocardial energetics. Circulation *64*:764, 1989.
17. Ando, H., Nakano, E., Ueno, Y., and Tokunaga, K.: New technique for analysis of cardiac energetics using a modified Fenn equation. J. Thorac. Cardiovasc. Surg. *97*:565, 1989.

17a. Hasenfuss, G., Mulieri, L. A., Blanchard, E. M., et al.: Energetics of isometric force development in control and volume-overloaded human myocardium: Comparison with animal species. Circ. Res. *68*:836, 1991.

18. Hisano, R., and Cooper, G. IV: Correlation of force-length area with oxygen consumption in ferret papillary muscle. Circ. Res. *61*:318, 1987.
19. Mast, F., and Elzinga, G.: Heat released during relaxation equals force-length area in isometric contractions of rabbit papillary muscle. Circ. Res. *67*:893, 1990.
20. Duwel, C.M.B., and Westerhof, N.: Feline left ventricular oxygen consumption is not affected by volume expansion, ejection or redevelopment of pressure during relaxation. Pflugers Arch. *412*:409, 1988.
21. Fenn, W. O.: A quantitative comparison between the energy liberated and the work performed by the isolated sartorius muscle of the frog. J. Physiol. (Lond.) *58*:175, 1923.
22. Rall, J. A.: Sense and nonsense about the Fenn effect. Am. J. Physiol. *242*(Heart Circ. Physiol. 11):H1, 1982.
23. Suga, H., Futaki, S., Tanaka, N., et al.: Paired pulse pacing increases cardiac O_2 consumption for activation without changing efficiency of contractile machinery in canine left ventricle. Heart Vessels *4*:79, 1988.
24. Graham, T. P., Jr., Covell, J. W., Sonnenblick, E. H., et al.: Control of myocardial oxygen consumption: Relative influence of contractile state and tension development. J. Clin. Invest. *47*:375, 1968.
25. Boerth, R. C., Covell, J. W., Pool, P. E., and Ross, J., Jr.: Increased myocardial oxygen consumption and contractile state associated with increased heart rate in dogs. Circ. Res. *24*:725, 1969.
26. Ardehali, A., and Ports, T. A.: Myocardial oxygen supply and demand. Chest *98*:699, 1990.
27. Suga, H., Hisano, R., Goto, Y., Yamada, O., and Igarashi, Y.: Effect of positive inotropic agents on the relation between oxygen consumption and systolic pressure volume area in canine left ventricle. Circ. Res. *53*:306, 1983.
28. Urschel, C. W., Covell, J. W., Graham, T. P., et al.: Effects of acute valvular regurgitation on the oxygen consumption of the canine heart. Circ. Res. *23*:33, 1968.
29. Vik-Mo, H., and Mjos, O. E.: Influence of free fatty acids on myocardial oxygen consumption and ischemic injury. Am. J. Cardiol. *48*:361, 1981.
30. Loiselle, D. S.: Cardiac basal and activation metabolism. *In* Jacob, R., Just, H. J., and Holubarsch, C. H. (eds.): Cardiac Energetics: Basic Mechanisms and Clinical Implications. New York, Springer-Verlag, 1987, pp. 37–50.
31. Tubau, J. F., Wikman-Coffelt, J., Massie, B. M., et al.: Improved myocardial efficiency in the working perfused heart of the spontaneously hypertensive rat. Hypertension *10*:396, 1987.
32. Hornby, L., Hamilton, N., Marshall, D., et al.: Role of cardiac work in regulating myocardial biochemical characteristics. Am. J. Physiol. *258*:H1482, 1990.
33. Laxson, D. D., Homans, D. C., Dai, X., et al.: Oxygen consumption and coronary reactivity in postischemic myocardium. Circ. Res. *64*:9, 1989.

REGULATION OF CORONARY BLOOD FLOW

34. Braunwald, E., Ross, J., Jr., and Sonnenblick, E. H.: Regulation of coronary blood flow. *In* Mechanisms of Contraction of the Normal and Failing Heart. 2nd ed. Boston, Little, Brown, 1976, p. 200.
35. Berne, R. M., and Rubio, R.: Coronary circulation. *In* Berne, R. M., Sperelakis, N., and Geiger, S. R. (eds.): Handbook of Physiology; Section 2, The Cardiovascular System. Bethesda, American Physiological Society, 1979, p. 897.
36. Feigl, E. O.: Coronary physiology. Physiol. Rev. *63*:1, 1983.
37. Marcus, M. L., and Harrison, D. G.: Physiologic basis for myocardial perfusion imaging. *In* Marcus, M. L.,, et al. (eds.): Cardiac Imaging. Philadelphia, W. B. Saunders Company, 1991, pp. 8–23.
38. Young, M. A., and Vatner, S. F.: Regulation of large coronary arteries. Circ. Res. *59*:579, 1986.
39. Provenza, D. V., and Scherlis, S.: Coronary circulation in dog's heart: Demonstration of muscle sphincters in capillaries. Circ. Res. *7*:318, 1959.
40. Habib, G. B., Heibig, J., Forman, S. A., et al.: Influence of coronary collateral vessels on myocardial infarct size in humans: Results of Phase I thrombolysis in myocardial infarction (TIMI) trial. Circulation *83*:739, 1991.
41. Cohen, M. V., Yipintsoi, T., and Scheuer, J.: Coronary collateral stimulation by exercise in dogs with stenotic coronary arteries. J. Appl. Physiol. *52*:664, 1982.
42. Bloor, C. M., White, F. C., and Sanders, M.: Effects of exercise on collateral development in myocardial ischemia in pigs. J. Appl. Physiol. *56*:656, 1984.
43. Scheel, K. W., and Williams, S. E.: Hypertrophy and coronary and collateral vascularity in dogs with severe chronic anemia. Am. J. Physiol. *249*:H1031, 1985.
44. Patterson, R. E., Jones-Collins, B. A., Aamodt, R., and Ro, Y. M.: Differences in collateral myocardial blood flow following gradual vs. abrupt coronary occlusion. Cardiovasc. Res. *17*:207, 1983.

44a. Sabri, M. N., DiSciascio, G., Cowley, M. J., et al.: Coronary collateral recruitment: Functional significance and relation to rate of vessel closure. Am. Heart J. *121*:876, 1991.

45. Schaper, W.: Influence of physical exercise on coronary collateral blood flow in chronic experimental two-vessel occlusion. Circulation *65*:905, 1982.
46. Verani, M. S.: The functional significance of coronary collateral vessels: Anecdote confronts science. Cathet. Cardiovasc. Diagn. *9*:333, 1983.
47. Elayda, M. A., Mathur, V. S., Hall, R. J., et al.: Collateral circulation in coronary artery disease. Am. J. Cardiol. *55*:58, 1985.
48. Demer, L. L., Gould, K. L., Goldstein, R. A., and Kirkeeide, R. L.: Noninvasive assessment of coronary collaterals in man by PET perfusion imaging. J. Nucl. Med. *31*:259, 1990.
49. Mohri, M., Tomoike, H., Noma, M., et al.: Duration of ischemia is vital for collateral development: Repeated brief coronary artery occlusions in conscious dogs. Circ. Res. *64*:287, 1989.
50. Shen, Y., Knight, D. R., Canfield, D. R., et al.: Progressive change in collateral blood flow after coronary occlusion in conscious dogs. Am. J. Physiol. *256*:H478, 1989.
51. Marcus, M. L.: The Coronary Circulation in Health and Disease. New York, McGraw-Hill and Company, 1983, 465 pp.

52. Olsson, R. A., and Bugni, W. J.: Coronary circulation. *In* Fozzard, H. A., et al. (eds.): The Heart and Cardiovascular System. New York, Raven Press, 1986, pp. 987–1038.
53. Klocke, F. J., Mates, R. E., Canty, J. M., Jr., and Ellis, A. K.: Coronary pressure-flow relationships. Controversial issues and probable implications. Circ. Res. *56*:311, 1985.
54. Spnan, J.A.E.: Coronary diastolic pressure-flow relation and zero flow pressure explained on the basis of intramyocardial compliance. Circ. Res. *56*:293, 1985.
55. Matsuo, S., Tsuruta, M., Hayano, M., et al.: Phasic coronary artery flow velocity determined by Doppler flowmeter catheter in aortic stenosis and aortic regurgitation. Am. J. Cardiol. *62*:917, 1988.
56. Cole, J. S., and Hartley, C. J.: The pulsed Doppler artery catheter. Circulation *56*:18, 1977.
57. Klocke, F. J.: Coronary blood flow in man. Prog. Cardiovasc. Dis. *19*:117, 1976.
58. Griggs, D. M., Jr., Chen, C. C., and Tchokoev, V. V.: Subendocardial metabolism in experimental aortic stenosis. Am. J. Physiol. *224*:607, 1973.
59. Klocke, F. J.: Measurements of coronary flow reserve: Defining pathophysiology versus making decisions about patient care. Circulation *76*:1183, 1987.
60. Sabbah, H. N., and Stein, P. D.: Effect of acute regional ischemia on pressure in the subepicardium and subendocardium. Am. J. Physiol. *242*(Heart Circ. Physiol. 11):H240, 1982.
61. Brazier, J., Cooper, N., and Buckberg, G.: The adequacy of subendocardial oxygen delivery: The interaction of determinants of flow, arterial oxygen content and myocardial oxygen need. Circulation *49*:968, 1974.
62. Lundsgaard-Hansen, P., Meyer, C., and Riedwyl, H.: Transmural gradients of glycolytic enzyme activities in left ventricular myocardium. I. The normal state. Pfluegers Arch. *297*:89, 1967.
63. Buckberg, G. D., Fixler, D. E., Archie, J. P., and Hoffman, J.I.E.: Experimental subendocardial ischemia in dogs with normal coronary arteries. Circ. Res. *30*:67, 1972.
64. Hoffman, J.I.E.: Determinants of prediction of transmural myocardial perfusion. Circulation *58*:381, 1978.
65. Boudoulas, H.: Diastolic time: The forgotten dynamic factor. Implications for myocardial perfusion. Acta Cardiologica *XLVI*:61, 1991.
66. Fallen, E. L., Elliott, W. C., and Gorlin, R.: Mechanisms of angina in aortic stenosis. Circulation *36*:480, 1967.
67. Griggs, D. M., Jr., and Chen, C. C.: Coronary hemodynamics and regional myocardial metabolism in experimental aortic insufficiency. J. Clin. Invest. *53*:1599, 1974.
68. Dunn, R. B., and Griggs, D. M., Jr.: Ventricular filling pressure as a determinant of coronary blood flow during ischemia. Am. J. Physiol. *244*:H429, 1983.
69. Becker, L. C., Fortuin, N. J., and Pitt, B.: Effect of ischemia and antianginal drugs on the distribution of radioactive microspheres in the canine left ventricle. Circ. Res. *28*:263, 1971.
70. Mathes, P., and Rival, J.: Effect of nitroglycerin on total and regional coronary blood flow in the normal and ischaemic canine myocardium. Cardiovasc. Res. *5*:54, 1971.
71. Vatner, S. F.: Alpha-adrenergic tone in the coronary circulation of the conscious dog. Fed. Proc. *43*:2867, 1984.
72. Woodman, O. L., and Vatner, S. F.: Coronary vasoconstriction mediated by $alpha_1$ and $alpha_2$ adrenoceptors in the conscious dog. Am. J. Physiol. *253*:H388, 1987.
73. Young, M. A., Vatner, D. E., Knight, D. R., et al.: Alpha-adrenergic vasoconstriction and receptor subtypes in large coronary arteries of calves. Am. J. Physiol. *255*:H1452, 1988.
74. Morgan, K. G.: Role of calcium ion in maintenance of vascular smooth muscle tone. Am. J. Cardiol. *59*:24A, 1987.
75. Johns, A., Leijten, P., Yamamoto, H., Hwang, K., and van Breemen, C.: Calcium regulation in vascular smooth muscle contractility. Am. J. Cardiol. *59*:18A, 1987.
76. Adelstein, R. S., and Sellers, J. R.: Effects of calcium on vascular smooth muscle contraction. Am. J. Cardiol. *59*:4B, 1987.
77. Rinkema, L. E., Thomas, J. X., Jr., and Randall, W. C.: Regional coronary vasoconstriction in response to stimulation of stellate ganglia. Am. J. Physiol. *243*:H410, 1982.
78. Murray, P. A., Lavall, M., and Vatner, S. F.: Alpha-adrenergic-mediated reduction in coronary blood flow secondary to carotid chemoreceptor reflex activation in conscious dogs. Circ. Res. *54*:96, 1984.
79. Vatner, D. E., Knight, D. R., Homcy, C. J., et al.: Subtypes of beta-adrenergic receptors in bovine coronary arteries. Circ. Res. *59*:463, 1986.
80. Feldman, R. D., Christy, J. P., Paul, S. T., and Harrison, D. G.: Beta-adrenergic receptors on canine coronary collateral vessels: Characterization and function. Am. J. Physiol. *257*:H1634, 1989.
81. Vatner, S. F., and Hintze, T. H.: Mechanism of constriction of large coronary arteries by beta-adrenergic receptor blockade. Circ. Res. *53*:389, 1983.
82. Cox, D. A., Hintze, T. H., and Vatner, S. F.: Effects of acetylcholine on large and small coronary arteries in conscious dogs. J. Pharmacol. Exp. Ther. *225*:764, 1983.
83. Vatner, S. F., Higgins, C. B., and Braunwald, E.: Effects of norepinephrine on coronary circulation and left ventricular dynamics in the conscious dog. Circ. Res. *34*:812, 1974.
84. Kern, M. J., Horowitz, J. D., Ganz, P., et al.: Attenuation of coronary vascular resistance by selective $alpha_1$-adrenergic blockade in patients with coronary artery disease. J. Am. Coll. Cardiol. *5*:840, 1985.
85. Winniford, M. D., Wheelan, K. R., Kremers, M. S., et al.: Smoking-induced coronary vasoconstriction in patients with atherosclerotic coronary artery disease: Evidence for adrenergically mediated alterations in coronary artery tone. Circulation *74*:662, 1986.
86. Winniford, M. D., Jansen, D. E., Reynolds, G. A., et al.: Cigarette smoking-induced coronary vasoconstriction in atherosclerotic coronary artery disease and prevention by calcium antagonists and nitroglycerin. Am. J. Cardiol. *59*:203, 1987.
87. Szentivanyi, M., and Juhasz-Nagy, N.: Physiological role of the coronary constrictor fibers. Q. J. Exp. Physiol. *48*:93, 1963.
88. Hackett, J. G., Abboud, F. M., Mark, A. L., et al.: Coronary vascular responses to stimulation of chemoreceptors and baroreceptors. Circ. Res. *21*:8, 1972.
89. Higgins, C. B., Vatner, S. F., and Braunwald, E.: Parasympathetic control of the heart. Pharmacol. Rev. *25*:119, 1973.
90. Vatner, S. F., Franklin, D., VanCitters, R. L., and Braunwald, E.: Effects of carotid sinus nerve stimulation on the coronary circulation of the conscious dog. Circ. Res. *27*:11, 1970.
91. Brachfeld, N., Monroe, R. G., and Gorlin, R.: Effects of pericoronary denervation on coronary hemodynamics. Am. J. Physiol. *199*:174, 1960.
92. Macho, P., and Vatner, S. F.: Effects of prazosin on coronary and left ventricular dynamics in conscious dogs. Circulation *65*:1186, 1982.
93. Heyndrickx, G. R., Muylaert, P., and Pannier, J. L.: Alpha-adrenergic control of oxygen delivery to myocardium during exercise in conscious dog. Am. J. Physiol. *242*(Heart Circ. Physiol. 11):H805, 1982.
94. Laxson, D. D., Dai, X., Homans, D. C., and Bache, R. J.: The role of $alpha_1$- and $alpha_2$-adrenergic receptors in mediation of coronary vasoconstriction in hypoperfused ischemic myocardium during exercise. Circ. Res. *65*:1688, 1989.
95. Feigl, E. O.: The paradox of adrenergic coronary vasoconstriction. Circulation *76*:737, 1987.
96. Huang, A. H., and Feigl, E. O.: Adrenergic coronary vasoconstriction helps maintain uniform transmural blood flow distribution during exercise. Circ. Res. *62*:286, 1988.
97. Chilian, W. M., and Ackell, P. H.: Transmural differences in sympathetic coronary constriction during exercise in the presence of coronary stenosis. Circ. Res. *62*:216, 1988.
98. Heusch, G.: Alpha-adrenergic mechanisms in myocardial ischemia. Circulation *81*:1, 1990.
99. Feigl, E. O.: Reflex parasympathetic coronary vasodilation elicited from cardiac receptors in the dog. Circ. Res. *37*:175, 1975.
100. Pitetti, K. H., Iwamoto, G. A., Mitchell, J. H., and Ordway, G. A.: Stimulating somatic afferent fibers alters coronary arterial resistance. Am. J. Physiol. *256*:R1331, 1989.
101. Jarisch, A., and Zotterman, Y.: Depressor reflexes from the heart. Acta Physiol. Scand. *16*:31, 1948.
102. Feigl, E. O.: Parasympathetic control of coronary blood flow in dogs. Circ. Res. *25*:509, 1969.
103. Brown, B. G., Lee, A. B., Bolson, E. L., and Dodge, H. T.: Reflex constriction of significant coronary stenosis as a mechanism contributing to ischemic left ventricular dysfunction during isometric exercise. Circulation *70*:18, 1984.
104. Chierchia, S., Davies, G., Berkenboom, B., et al.: Alpha-adrenergic receptors and coronary spasm: An elusive link. Circulation *69*:8, 1984.
105. Galassi, A. R., Kaski, J. C., Pupita, G., et al.: Lack of evidence for alpha-adrenergic receptor–mediated mechanisms in the genesis of ischemia in syndrome X. Am. J. Cardiol. *64*:264, 1989.
105a. Cannon, R. O., III, Bonow, R. O., Bacharach, S. L., et al.: Left ventricular dysfunction in patients with angina pectoris, normal epicardial coronary arteries, and abnormal vasodilator reserve. Circulation *71*:218, 1985.
106. Gould, L., Reddy, G. V., and Gombrecht, R. F.: Oral phentolamine in angina pectoris. Jpn. Heart J. *14*:393, 1973.
106a. Cannon, R. O., III, Leon, M. B., Watson, R. M., et al.: Chest pain and "normal" coronary arteries—Role of small coronary arteries. Am. J. Cardiol. *55*:50B, 1985.
107. Berkenboom, G. M., Abramowicz, M., Vandermoten, P., and Degre, S. G.: Role of alpha adrenergic coronary tone in exercise-induced angina pectoris. Am. J. Cardiol. *57*:195, 1986.
107a. Hayes, S. N., Moyer, T. P., Morley, D., and Bove, A. A.: Intravenous cocaine causes epicardial coronary vasoconstriction in the intact dog. Am. Heart J. *121*:1639, 1991.
108. Lange, R. A., Cigarra, R. G., Yancy, C. W., et al.: Cocaine-induced coronary-artery vasoconstriction. N. Engl. J. Med. *321*:1557, 1989.
109. Johnson, P. C.: Autoregulation of blood flow. Circ. Res. *58*:483, 1986.
110. Lee, J.-D., Tajimi, T., Guth, B., et al.: Exercise-induced regional dysfunction with subcritical coronary stenosis. Circulation *73*:596, 1986.
111. Oien, A. H., and Aukland, K.: A mathematical analysis of the myogenic hypothesis with special reference to autoregulation of renal blood flow. Circ. Res. *52*:241, 1983.
112. Bayliss, W. M.: On the local reaction of the arterial wall to changes in arterial pressure. J. Physiol. (Lond.) *28*:220, 1902.
113. Coffman, J. D., and Gregg, D. E.: Oxygen metabolism and oxygen debt repayment after myocardial ischemia. Am. J. Physiol. *201*:881, 1961.
114. Detar, R., and Bohr, D. F.: Oxygen and vascular smooth muscle contraction. Am. J. Physiol. *214*:241, 1968.
115. Duling, B. R.: Microvascular responses to alterations in oxygen tension. Circ. Res. *31*:481, 1972.
116. Martini, J., and Honig, C. R.: Direct measurement of intercapillary distance in beating rat heart in situ under various conditions of O_2 supply. Microvasc. Res. *1*:244, 1969.
117. Sparks, H. V., Jr., and Bardenheuer, H.: Regulation of adenosine formation by the heart. Circ. Res. *58*:193, 1986.

Clinical and experimental difference between ischemia with S-T elevation and ischemia with S-T depression, Am. J. Cardiol. *7*:412, 1961.

233. Tillisch, J., Brunken, R., Marshall, R., et al.: Reversibility of cardiac wall-motion abnormalities predicted by positron tomography. N. Engl. J. Med. *314*:884, 1986.
234. Brunken, R., Schwaiger, M., Grover-McKay, M., et al.: Positron emission tomography detects tissue metabolic activity in myocardial segments with persistent thallium perfusion defects. J. Am. Coll. Cardiol. *10*:557. 1987.
235. Gropler, R. J., Siegel, B. A., Perez, J. E., et al.: Functional recovery after myocardial revascularization is characterized by improved glucose and oxidative metabolism. J. Nucl. Med. *31*:773, 1990.
236. Bergmann, S. R., Shelton, M. E., Weinheimer, C. J., et al.: Persistence of perfusion, metabolic, and functional reserve capacity in stunned myocardium. J. Nucl. Med. *31*:794, 1990.
237. Renstrom, B., Nellis, S. H., and Liedtke, A. J.: Metabolic oxidation of glucose during early myocardial reperfusion. Circ. Res. *65*:1094, 1989.
238. Myears, D. W., Sobel, B. E., and Bergmann, S. R.: Substrate utilization in ischemic and reperfused canine myocardium: quantitative considerations. Am. J. Physiol. *253*:H107, 1987.
239. Brown, M. A., Marshall, D. R., Sobel, B.E., and Bergmann, S. R.: Delineation of myocardial oxygen utilization with carbon-11-labeled acetate. Circulation. *76*:687, 1987.
240. Knabb, R. M., Bergmann, S. R., Fox, K.A.A., and Sobel, B. E.: The temporal pattern of recovery of myocardial perfusion and metabolism delineated by positron emission tomography after coronary thrombolysis. J. Nucl. Med. *28*:1563, 1987.
241. Walsh, M. N., Geltman, E. M., Brown, M. A., et al.: Noninvasive estimation of regional myocardial oxygen consumption by positron emission tomography with carbon-11 acetate in patients with myocardial infarction. J. Nucl. Med. *30*:1798, 1989.
242. Kass, D. A., Marino, P., Maughan, W. L., and Sagawa, K.: Determinants of end-systolic pressure-volume relations during acute regional ischemia in situ. Circulation *80*:1783, 1989.
243. Jennings, R. B., Murry, C. E., Steenbergen, C. Jr., and Reimer, K. A.: Development of cell injury in sustained acute ischemia. Circulation *82*:(Suppl. II):2, 1990.
244. Stern, M. D., Silverman, H. S., Houser, S. R., et al.: Anoxic contractile failure in rat heart myocytes is caused by failure of intracellular calcium release due to alteration of the action potential. Proc. Natl. Acad. Sci. USA *85*:6954, 1988.
245. Marban, E., Kitikaze, M., Kusuoka, H., et al.: Intracellular free calcium concentration measured with ^{19}F NMR spectroscopy in intact ferret hearts. Proc. Natl. Acad. Sci. USA *84*:6005, 1987.
246. Barry, W. H.: Mechanical dysfunction of the heart during and after ischemia. Circulation *82*:652, 1990.
247. Kihara, Y. Grossman, W., and Morgan, J. P.: Direct measurement of changes in intracellular calcium transients during hypoxia, ischemia, and reperfusion of the intact mammalian heart. Circ. Res. *65*:1029, 1989.
248. Braunwald, E., Ross, J., Jr., and Sonnenblick, E. H.: Mechanisms of Contractions in the Normal and Failing Heart. 2nd Ed. Boston, Little, Brown and Company, 1976, p. 357.
249. Williamson, J. R., Schaffer, S. W., Ford, C., and Safer, B.: Contribution of tissue acidosis to ischemic injury in the perfused rat heart. Circulation *53*(Suppl. I):3, 1976.
250. Gard, J. K., Kichura, G. M., Ackerman, J. J. H., et al.: Quantitative ^{31}P NMR analysis of metabolite concentrations in Langendorff-perfused rabbit hearts. Biophys. J. *48*:803, 1985.
251. Neubauer, S., Hamman, B. L., Perry, S., B., et al. Velocity of the creatine kinase reaction decreases in postischemic myocardium: A^{31}P-NMR magnetization transfer study of the isolated ferret heart. Circ. Res. *63*:1, 1988.
252. Marshall, R. C.: Correlation of contractile dysfunction with oxidative energy production and tissue high energy phosphate stores during partial coronary flow disruption in rabbit heart. J. Clin. Invest. *82*:86, 1988.
253. Zimmer, S. D., Ugurbil, K., Michurski, S. P., et al.: Alterations in oxidative function and respiratory regulation in the post-ischemic myocardium. J. Biol. Chem. *264*:12402, 1989.
254. Pogwizd, S. M., and Corr, P. B.: Electrophysiologic and biochemical mechanisms underlying malignant ventricular arrhythmias during early myocardial ischemia. *In* Heusch, G. (ed.): Pathophysiology and Rational Pharmacotherapy of Myocardial Ischemia. Darmstadt, Germany, Steinkopff Verlag Darmstadt, 1990, p. 137.
255. Visner, M. S., Arentzen, C. E., Parrish, G. D., et al.: Effects of global ischemia on the diastolic properties of the left ventricle in the conscious dog. Circulation *71*:610, 1985.
256. Momomura, S-I, Ferguson, J. J., Miller, M. J., et al.: Regional myocardial blood flow and left ventricular diastolic properties in pacing-induced ischemia. J. Am. Coll. Cardiol. *17*:781, 1991.

256a. Miyazaki, S., Guth, B. D., Miura, T., et al.: Changes of left ventricular diastolic function in exercising dogs without and with ischemia. Circulation *81*:1058, 1990.

257. Kass, D. A., Midei, M., Brinker, J., and Maughan, W. L.: Influence of coronary occlusion during PTCA on end-systolic and end-diastolic pressure volume relations in humans. Circulation *81*:447, 1990.
258. Wexler, L. F., Weinberg, E. O., Ingwall, J. S., and Apstein, C. S.: Acute alterations in diastolic left ventricular chamber distensibility: Mechanistic differences between hypoxia and ischemia in isolated perfused rabbit and rat hearts. Circ. Res. *59*:515, 1986.

258a. Takahashi, T., Levine, M. J., and Grossman, W.: Regional diastolic mechanics of ischemic and nonischemic myocardium in the pig heart. J. Am. Coll. Cardiol. *17*:1203, 1991.

259. Gaasch, W. H., Zile, M. R., Hoshino, P. K., et al.: Tolerance of the hypertrophic heart to ischemia: studies in compensated and failing dog hearts with pressure overload hypertrophy. Circulation *81*:164, 1990.
260. Imai, K., Wang, T., Millard, R. W., et al.: Ischemia-induced changes in canine cardiac sarcoplasmic reticulum. Cardiovasc. Res. *17*:696, 1983.
261. Krayenbuehl, H. P., Hess, O. M., and Nonogi, H.: On whether there is a true increase in myocardial stiffness during myocardial islchemia. Am. J. Cardiol. *63*:78E, 1989.
262. Nakamura, Y., Sasayama, S., Nonogi, H., et al.: Alterations in left ventricular relaxation, early diastolic filling and passive viscoelastic properties during postpacing ischemia. Am. J. Cardiol. *63*:72E, 1989.
263. Ross, J., Jr.: Is there a true increase in myocardial stiffness with acute ischemia? Am. J. Cardiol. *63*:87E, 1989.
264. Sys, S. U., and Brutsaert, D. L.: Is stiffness increased during ischemia? Am. J. Cardiol. *63*:83E, 1989.

ELECTROPHYSIOLOGICAL CONSEQUENCES OF ISCHEMIA

265. Sayen, J. J., Peirce, G., Katcher, A. H., and Sheldon, W. F.: Correlation of intramyocardial electrocardiograms with polarographic oxygen and contractility in the nonischemic and regional ischemic left ventricle. Circ. Res. *9*:1268, 1961.
266. Maroko, P. R., Kjekshus, J. K., Sobel, B. E., et al.: Factors influencing infarct size following experimental coronary artery occlusions. Circulation *43*:67, 1971.

266a. Carroll, J. D., Hess, O. M., Hirzel, H. O., and Krayenbuehl, H. P.: Exercise-induced ischemia: The influence of altered relaxation on early diastolic pressures. Circulation *67*:521, 1983.

267. Muller, J. E., Maroko, P. R., and Braunwald, E.: Evaluation of precordial electrocardiographic mapping as a means of assessing changes in myocardial ischemic injury. Circulation *52*:16, 1975.
268. Wilde, A.A.M., Escande, D., Schumacher, C. A., et al.: Potassium accumulation in the globally ischemic mammalian heart: A role for the ATP-sensitive potassium channel. Circ. Res. *67*:835, 1990.

268a. Sasayama, S., Nonogi, H., Miyazaki, S., Sakurai, T., Kawai, C., Eiho, S., and Kuwahara, M.: Changes in diastolic properties of the regional myocardium during pacing-induced ischemia in human subjects. J. Am. Coll. Cardiol. *5*:599, 1985.

269. Kleber, A. G., Riegger, C. B., and Janse, M. J.: Electrical uncoupling and increase of extracellular resistance after induction of ischemia in isolated, arterially perfused rabbit papillary muscle. Circ. Res. *61*:271, 1987.
270. Creer, M. H., Dobmeyer, D. J., and Corr, P. B.: Amphipathic lipid metabolites and arrhythmias during myocardial ischemia. *In* Zipes, D., and Jalife, J. (eds.): Cardiac Electrophysiology. Philadelphia, W. B. Saunders, 1990, pp. 417–432.
271. Corr, P. B., Saffitz, J. E., and Sobel, B. E.: What is the contribution of altered lipid metabolism to arrhythmogenesis in the ischemic heart? *In* Hearse, D. J., Manning, A. S., and Janse M. (eds.): Life-Threatening Arrhythmias During Ischemia and Infarction. New York, Raven Press, 1987, pp. 91–114.
272. Corr, P. B., Creer, M. H., Yamada, K. A., et al.: Prophylaxis of early ventricular fibrillation by inhibition of acylcarnitine accumulation. J. Clin. Invest. *83*:927, 1989.

272a. Mehra, R., Zeiler, R. H. Gough, W. B., and El-Sherif, N.: Reentrant ventricular arrhythmias in the late myocardial infarction period. 9. Electrophysiologic-anatomic correlation of reentrant circuits. Circulation *67*:11, 1983.

273. Corr, P. B., Witkowski, F. X., and Sobel, B. E.: Mechanisms contributing to malignant dysrhythmias induced by ischemia in the cat. J. Clin. Invest. *61*:109, 1978.
274. Kimura, S., Basset, A. L., Kohya, T., et al.: Automaticity, triggered activity, and responses to adrenergic stimulation in cat subendocardial Purkinje fibers after healing of myocardial infarction. Circulation *75*:651, 1987.
275. El-Sherif, N., Hope, R. R., Scherlag, B. J., and Lazzara, R.: Re-entrant ventricular arrhythmias in the late myocardial infarction period. 2. Patterns of initiation and termination of reentry. Circulation *55*:702, 1977.
276. Sobel, B. E., Corr, P. B., Robinson, A. K., et al.: Accumulation of lysophosphoglycerides with arrhythmogenic properties in ischemic myocardium. J. Clin. Invest. *61*:109, 1978.
277. Corr, P. B., Cain, M. E., Witkowski, F. X., et al.: Potential arrhythmogenic electrophysiological derangements in canine Purkinje fibers induced by lysophosphoglycerides. Circ. Res. *44*:822, 1979.
278. Bernier, M., Manning, A. S., and Hearse, D. J.: Reperfusion arrhythmias: Dose-related protection by anti-free radical interventions. Am. J. Physiol. *256*:H1344, 1989.
279. Tani, M., and Neely, J. R.: Intermittent perfusion of ischemic myocardium. Possible mechanisms of protective effects on mechanical function in isolated rat heart. Circulation *82*:536, 1990.

EFFECTS OF ISCHEMIA ON MYOCARDIAL METABOLISM

280. Jennings, R. B., Reimer, K. A., Hill, M. L., and Mayer, S. E.: Total ischemia in dog hearts in vitro. I. Comparison of high energy phosphate production, utilization and depletion, and of adenine nucleotide catabolism in total ischemia in vitro vs. severe ischemia in vivo. Circ. Res. *49*:892, 1981.

281. Flaherty, J. T., Weisfeldt, M. L., Bulkley, B. H., et al.: Mechanisms of ischemic myocardial cell damage assessed by phosphorus-31 nuclear magnetic resonance. Circulation 65:561, 1982.
282. Schaefer, S., Camacho, S. A., Gober, J., et al.: Response of myocardial metabolites to graded regional ischemia: ^{31}P NMR spectroscopy of porcine myocardium in vivo. Circ. Res. 64:968, 1989.
283. Marshall, R. C., Nash, W. W., Bersohn, M. M., and Wong, G. A.: Myocardial energy production and consumption remain balanced during positive inotropic stimulation when coronary flow is restricted to basal rates in rabbit heart. J. Clin. Invest. 80:1165, 1987.
284. Bittl, J. A., Balschi, J. A., and Ingwall, J. S.: Effects of norepinephrine infusion on myocardial high-energy phosphate content and turnover in the living rat. J. Clin. Invest. 79:1852, 1987.
285. Bittl, J. A., Balschi, J. A., and Ingwall, J. S.: Contractile failure and high-energy phosphate turnover during hypoxia: ^{31}P-NMR surface coil studies in living rat. Circ. Res. 60:871, 1987.
286. Asimakis, G. K., Sandhu, G. S., Conti, V. R., et al.: Intermittent ischemia produces a cumulative depletion of mitochondrial adenine nucleotides in the isolated perfused rat heart. Circ. Res. 66:302, 1990.
287. Guth, B. D., Martin, J. F., Heusch, G., and Ross, J., Jr.: Regional myocardial blood flow, function and metabolism using phosphorus-31 nuclear magnetic resonance spectroscopy during ischemia and reperfusion in dogs. J. Am. Coll. Cardiol. 10:673, 1987.
288. Mazer, C. D., Stanley, W. C., Hickey, R. F., et al.: Myocardial metabolism during hypoxia: Maintained lactate oxidation during increased glycolysis. Metabolism 39:913, 1990.
289. Owen, P., Dennis, S., and Opie, L. H.: Glucose flux rate regulates onset of ischemic contracture in globally underperfused rat hearts. Circ. Res. 66:344, 1990.
290. Mody, F. V., Brunken, R. C., Stevenson, L. W., et al.: Differentiating cardiomyopathy of coronary artery disease from nonischemic dilated cardiomyopathy utilizing positron emission tomography. J. Am. Coll. Cardiol. 17:373, 1991.
291. Fudo, T., Kambara, H., Hashimoto, T., et al.: F-18 deoxyglucose and stress N-13 ammonia positron emission tomography in anterior wall healed myocardial infarction. Am. J. Cardiol. 61:1191, 1988.
291a. Bonow, R. O., Dilsizian, V., Cuocolo, A., and Bacharach, S. L.: Identification of viable myocardium in patients with chronic coronary artery disease and left ventricular dysfunction. Circulation 83:26, 1991.
291b. Bonow, R. O., Dilsizian, V., Cuocolo, A., and Bacharach, S. L.: Identification of viable myocardium in patients with chronic coronary artery disease and left ventricular function. Circulation 83:26, 1991.
292. Rovetto, M. J., Lamberton, W. F., and Neely, J. R.: Mechanisms of glycolytic inhibition in ischemic rat hearts. Circ. Res. 37:742, 1975.
293. Williamson, J. R., Schaffer, S. W., Ford, C., and Safer, B.: Contribution of tissue acidosis to ischemic injury in the perfused rat heart. Circulation 53(Suppl. I):3, 1976.
294. Corr, P. B., Saffitz, J. E., and Sobel, B. E.: Lysophospholipids, long chain acylcarnitines, and membrane dysfunction in the ischemic heart. In Lipid Metabolism in the Normoxic and Ischaemic Heart. New York, Springer-Verlag, 1987, p. 199.
295. Miyazaki, Y., Gross, R. W., Sobel, B. E., and Saffitz, J. E.: Selective turnover of sarcolemmal phospholipids with lethal injury. Am. J. Physiol., 259:C325, 1990.
296. Knabb, M. T., Saffitz, J. E., Corr, P. B., and Sobel, B. E.: The dependence of electrophysiologic derangements on accumulation of endogenous long-chain acyl carnitine in hypoxic neonatal rat myocytes. Circ. Res. 58:230, 1986.
297. Camici, P., Marraccini, P., Lorenzoni, R.: Metabolic markers of stress-induced myocardial ischemia. Circulation 83(Suppl. III)III8, 1991.
298. Neely, J. R., Rovetto, M. J., Whitmer, J. T., and Morgan, H. E.: Effects of ischemia on ventricular function and metabolism in the isolated working rat heart. Am. J. Physiol. 225:651, 1973.
299. Vyska, K., Machulla, H. J., Stremmel, W., et al.: Regional myocardial free fatty acid extraction in normal and ischemic myocardium. Circulation 78:1218, 1988.
300. Bergmann, S. R., Lerch, R. A., Fox, K. A. A., et al.: Temporal dependence of beneficial effects of coronary thrombolysis characterized by positron tomography. Am. J. Med. 73:573, 1982.
301. Renstrom, B., Nellis, S. H., and Liedtke, A. J.: Metabolic oxidation of glucose during early myocardial reperfusion. Circ. Res. 65:1094, 1989.
302. Weiss, E. S., Ahmed, S. A., Welch, M. J., et al.: Quantification of infarction in cross sections of canine myocardium in vivo with positron emission transaxial tomography and ^{11}C-palmitate. Circulation 55:66, 1977.
303. Kimihara, S., Yokota, M., Iwase, M., et al.: Early detection of myocardial ischemia by myocardial free fatty acid extraction in patients with exercise-induced angina pectoris. Am. J. Cardiol. 64:180–185, 1989.
304. Fox, K. A. A., Nomura, H., Sobel, B. E., and Bergmann, S. R.: Consistent substrate utilization despite reduced flow in hearts with maintained work. Am. J. Physiol. 244:H799, 1983.
305. Gropler, R. J., Siegel, B. A., Lee, K. J., et al.: Nonuniformity in myocardial accumulation of ^{18}F-fluorodeoxyglucose in normal fasted humans. J. Nucl. Med., 31:1749, 1990.
306. Eisenberg, J. D., Sobel, B. E., and Geltman, E. M.: Differentiation of ischemic from nonischemic cardiomyopathy with positron emission tomography. Am. J. Cardiol. 59:1410, 1987.
307. Rosamond, T. L., Abendschein, D. R., Sobel, B. E., et al.: Metabolic fate of radiolabeled palmitate in ischemic canine myocardium: Implications for positron emission tomography. J. Nucl. Med. 28:1322, 1987.
308. Myears, D. W., Sobel, B. E., and Bergmann, S. R.: Substrate use in ischemic and reperfused canine myocardium: Quantitative considerations. Am. J. Physiol. 253:H107, 1987.
308a. Henes, C. G., Bergmann, S. R., Walsh, M. N., et al.: Assessment of myocardial oxidative metabolic reserve with positron emission tomography and carbon-11 acetate. J. Nucl. Med. 30:1489, 1989.
309. Rannels, D. E., McKee, E. E., and Morgan, H. E.: Regulation of protein synthesis and degradation in heart and skeletal muscle. In Litwack, G. (ed.): Biochemical Actions of Hormones. New York, Academic Press, 1976.
310. Schwalb, H., Izhar, U., Yaroslavsky, E., et al.: The effect of amino acids on the ischemic heart: Improvement of oxygenated crystalloid cardioplegic solution by an enriched branched chain amino acid formulation. J. Thorac. Cardiovasc. Surg. 98:551, 1989.
311. Mehta, H. B., Popovich, B. K., and Dillmann, W. H.: Ischemia induces changes in the level of mRNAs coding for stress protein 71 and creatine kinase M. Circ. Res. 63:512, 1988.
312. Currie, R. W., Karmazyn, M., Kloc, M., and Mailer, K.: Heat-shock response is associated with enhanced postischemic ventricular recovery. Circ. Res. 63:543, 1988.
313. de la Bastie, D., Levitsky, D., Rappaport, L., et al.: Function of the sarcoplasmic reticulum and expression of its Ca^{+}-ATPase gene in pressure overload-induced cardiac hypertrophy in the rat. Circ. Res. 66:554, 1990.
314. Chance, B.: Discussion. Circ. Res. 38(Suppl. I):69, 1976.
315. Reimer, K. A., Lowe, J. E., Rasmussen, M. M., and Jennings, R. B.: The wavefront phenomenon of ischemic cell death. I. Myocardial infarct size vs duration of coronary occlusion in dogs. Circulation 56:786, 1977.
316. Lavellee, M., Cox, D., Patrick, T. A., and Vatner, S. F.: Salvage of myocardial function by coronary artery reperfusion 1, 2, and 3 hours after occlusion in conscious dogs. Circ. Res. 53:235, 1983.
317. Kagiyama, A., Savage, H. E., Michael, L. H., et al.: Molecular basis of complement activation in ischemic myocardium: Identification of specific molecules of mitochondrial origin that bind human C1q and fix complement. Circ. Res. 64:607, 1989.
318. Crawford, M. H., Grover, F. L., Kolb, W. P., et al.: Complement and neutrophil activation in the pathogenesis of ischemic myocardial injury. Circulation 78:1449, 1988.
319. Steenbergen, C., Murphy, E., Levy, L., and London, R. E.: Elevation of cytosolic free calcium concentration early in myocardial ischemia in perfused rat heart. Circ. Res. 60:700, 1987.
320. Marban, E., Koretsume, Y., Corretti, M., et al.: Calcium and its role in myocardial cell injury during ischemia and reperfusion. Circulation 80(Suppl. IV):4, 1989.
321. Corr, P. B., Gross, R. W., and Sobel, B. E.: Arrhythmogenic amphiphilic lipids and the myocardial cell membrane. J. Mol. Cell. Cardiol. 14:619, 1982.
322. Sedlis, S. P., Corr, P. B., Sobel, B. E., and Ahumada, G. G.: Lysophosphatidyl choline potentiates Ca^{++} accumulation in rat cardiac myocytes. Am. J. Physiol. 13:H32, 1983.
323. Kloner, R. A., DeBoer, L.W.V., Carlson, N., and Braunwald, E.: The effect of verapamil on myocardial ultrastructure during and following release of coronary artery occlusion. Exp. Mol. Pathol. 36:277, 1982.
324. Braunwald, E., Muller, J. E., Kloner, R. A., and Maroko, P. R.: Role of beta-adrenergic blockade in the therapy of patients with myocardial infarction. Am. J. Med. 784:113, 1983.
325. Hammerman, H., Kloner, R. A., Briggs, L. L., and Braunwald, E.: Enhancement of salvage of reperfused myocardium by early beta-adrenergic blockade. J. Am. Coll. Cardiol. 3:1438, 1984.
326. Lo, H. M., Kloner, R. A., and Braunwald, E.: Effect of intracoronary verapamil on infarct size in the ischemic, reperfused canine heart: Critical importance of the timing of treatment. Am. J. Cardiol. 56:672, 1985.
327. Campbell, C. A., Kloner, R. A., Alker, K. J., and Braunwald, E.: Effect of verapamil on infarct size in dogs subjected to coronary artery occlusion with transient reperfusion. J. Am. Coll. Cardiol. 8:1169, 1986.
328. Henry, P. D., Shuchleib, R., Davis, J., et al.: Myocardial contracture and accumulation of mitochondrial calcium in ischemic rabbit heart. Am. J. Physiol. (Heart Circ. Physiol.) 2:H677, 1977.
329. DeBoer, L.W.V., Strauss, H. W., Kloner, R. A., et al.: Autoradiographic method for measuring the ischemic myocardium at risk: Effects of verapamil on infarct size after experimental coronary artery occlusion. Proc. Natl. Acad. Sci. 77:6119, 1980.
330. Nayler, W. G., Panagiotopoulos, S., Elz, J. S., and Sturrock, W. J.: Fundamental mechanisms of action of calcium antagonist in myocardial ischemia. Am. J. Cardiol. 59:75B, 1987.
331. Kloner, R. A., and Braunwald, E.: Effects of calcium antagonists on infarcting myocardium. Am. J. Cardiol. 59:84B, 1987.
332. Knabb, R. M., Rosamond, T. L., Fox, K.A.A., et al.: Enhancement of salvage of reperfused ischemic myocardium by diltiazem. J. Am. Coll. Cardiol. 8:861, 1986.
333. Berridge, M. J.: Inositol trisphosphate and diacylglycerol: Two interacting second messengers. Annu. Rev. Biochem. 56:159, 1987.
334. Kohl, C., Schmitz, W., Scholz, H., and Scholz, J.: Evidence for the existence of inositol tetrakisphosphate in mammalian heart: Effect of α_1-adrenoceptor stimulation. Circ. Res. 66:580, 1990.
335. Otani, H., Prasad, R., Engelman, R. M., et al.: Enhanced phosphodiesteratic breakdown and turnover of phosphoinositides during reperfusion of ischemic rat heart. Circ. Res. 63:930, 1988.
336. Heathers, G. P., Yamada, K. A., Kanter, E. M., and Corr, P. B.: Long-chain acylcarnitines mediate the hypoxia-induced increase in α_1-adrenergic receptors on adult canine myocytes. Circ. Res. 61:735, 1987.
337. Heathers, G. P., Yamada, K. A., Pogwizd, S. M., and Corr, P. B.: The

contribution of α- and β-adrenergic mechanisms in the genesis of arrhythmias during myocardial ischemia and reperfusion. *In* Kulbertus, H. E., and Frank, G. (eds.): Neurocardiology. Mount Kisco, Futura, 1988, pp. 143–178.

338. Ambrosio, G., Weisfeldt, M. L., Jacobus, W. E., and Flaherty, J. T.: Evidence for a reversible oxygen radical-mediated component of reperfusion injury: reduction by recombinant human superoxide dismutase administered at the time of reflow. Circulation *75*:282, 1987.
339. Rossen, R. D., Swain, J. L., Michael, L. H., et al.: Selective accumulation of the first component of complement and leukocytes in ischemic canine heart muscle. Circ. Res. *57*:119, 1985.
340. Naslund, U., Haggmark, S., Johansson, G., et al.: Limitation of myocardial infarct size by superoxide dismutase as an adjunct to reperfusion after different durations of coronary occlusion in the pig. Circ. Res. *66*:1294, 1990.
341. Kloner, R. A., Przyklenk, K., and Whittaker, P.: Deleterious effects of oxygen radicals in ischemia/reperfusion: Resolved and unresolved issues. Circulation *80*:1115, 1989.
342. Cohen, M. V.: Free radicals in ischemic and reperfusion myocardial injury: It is the time for clinical trials? Ann. Intern. Med. *111*:918, 1989.
343. Kaneko, M., Beamish, R. E., and Dhalla, N. S.: Depression of heart sarcolemmal Ca^{2+}-pump activity by oxygen free radicals. Am. J. Physiol. *256*:H368, 1989.
344. van der Kraaij, A. M. M., van Eijk, H. G., and Koster, J. F.: Prevention of postischemic cardiac injury by the orally active iron chelator 1,2-dimethyl-3-hydroxy-4-pyridone (L1) and the antioxidant (+)-cyanidanol-3. Circulation *80*:158, 1989.
345. Litt, M. R., Jeremy, R. W., Weisman, H. F., et al.: Neutrophil depletion limited to reperfusion reduces myocardial infarct size after 90 minutes of ischemia: Evidence for neutrophil-mediated reperfusion injury. Circulation *80*:1816, 1989.
346. Blaustein, A., Deneke, S. M., Stolz, R. I., et al.: Myocardial glutathione depletion impairs recovery after short periods of ischemia. Circulation *80*:1449, 1989.
347. Ahumada, G., Roberts, R., and Sobel, B. E.: Evaluation of myocardial infarction with enzymatic indices. Prog. Cardiovasc. Dis. *18*:405, 1976.
348. Ahmed, S. A., Williamson, J. R., Roberts, R., et al.: The association of increased plasma MB CPK activity and irreversible ischemic myocardial injury in the dog. Circulation *54*:187, 1976.
349. Shell, W. E., Kjekshus, J. K., and Sobel, B. E.: Quantitative assessment of the extent of myocardial infarction in the conscious dog by means of analysis of serial changes in serum creatine phosphokinase activity. J. Clin. Invest. *50*:2614, 1971.
350. Sobel, B. E., Markam, J., Karlsberg, R. P., and Roberts, R.: The nature of disappearance of creatine kinase from the circulation and its influence on enzymatic estimation of infarct size. Circ. Res. *41*:836, 1977.
351. Geltman, E. M., Ehsani, A. A., Campbell, M. K., et al.: The influence of location and extent of myocardial infarction on long-term ventricular dysrhythmia and mortality. Circulation *60*:805, 1979.
352. Hackel, D. B., Reimer, K. A., Ideker, R. E., et al.: Comparison of enzymatic and anatomic estimates of myocardial infarct size in man. Circulation *70*:824, 1984.
353. Vatner, S. F., Baig, H., Manders, W. T., and Maroko, P. R.: Effects of coronary artery reperfusion on myocardial infarct size calculated from creatine kinase. J. Clin. Invest. *61*:1048, 1978.
354. Clark, G. L., Robison, A. K., Gnepp, D. R., et al.: Effects of lymphatic transport of enzyme on plasma CK time-activity curves after myocardial infarction. Circ. Res. *43*:162, 1978.
355. Devries, S. R., Jaffe, A. S., Geltman, E. M., et al.: Enzymatic estimation of the extent of irreversible myocardial injury early after reperfusion. Am. Heart J. *117*:31, 1989.
356. Abendschein, D. R., Serota, H., Plummer, T. H., Jr., et al.: Conversion of MM creatine kinase isoforms in human plasma by carboxypeptidase N. J. Lab. Clin. Med. *110*:798, 1987.
357. Hashimoto, H., Abendschein, D. R., Strauss, A. W., and Sobel, B. E.: Early detection of myocardial infarction in conscious dogs by analysis of plasma MM creatine kinase isoforms. Circulation *71*:363, 1985.
358. Abendschein, D., Seacord, L. M., Nohara, R., et al.: Prompt detection of myocardial injury by assay of creatine kinase isoforms in initial plasma samples. Clin. Cardiol. *11*:661, 1988.
359. Jaffe, A. S., Serota, H., Grace, A., and Sobel, B. E.: Diagnostic changes in plasma creatine kinase isoforms early after the onset of acute myocardial infarction. Circulation *74*:105, 1986.
360. Devries, S. R., Sobel, B. E., and Abendschein, D. R.: Early detection of myocardial reperfusion by assay of plasma MM-creatine kinase isoforms in dogs. Circulation *74*:567, 1986.
361. Rude, R. E., Muller, J. E., and Braunwald, E.: Efforts to limit the size of myocardial infarcts. Ann. Intern. Med. *95*:736, 1981.
362. Nohara, R., Myears, D. W., Sobel, B. E., and Abendschein, D. R.: Optimal criteria for rapid detection of myocardial reperfusion by creatine kinase MM isoforms in the presence of residual high-grade coronary stenosis. J. Am. Coll. Cardiol. *14*:1067, 1989.
363. Wu, A.H.B.: Creatine kinase isoforms in ischemic heart disease. Clin. Chem. *35*:7, 1989.
364. Puleo, P. R., Guadagno, P. A., Roberts, R., and Perryman, M. B.: Sensitive, rapid assay of subforms of creatine kinase MB in plasma. Clin. Chem. *35*:1452, 1989.
365. Christenson, R. H., Ohman, E. M., Clemmensen, P., et al.: Characteristics of creatine kinase-MB and MB isoforms in serum after reperfusion in acute myocardial infarction. Clin Chem. *35*:2179, 1989.
366. Garabedian, H. D., Gold, H. K., Yasuda, T., et al.: Detection of coronary artery reperfusion with creatine kinase-MB determinations during thrombolytic therapy: Correlation with acute angiography. J. Am. Coll. Cardiol. *11*:729, 1988.
367. Katus, H. A., Diederich, K. W., Scheffold, T., et al.: Noninvasive assessment of infarct reperfusion: The predictive power of the time to peak value of myoglobin, CK MB, and CK in serum. Eur. Heart J. *9*:619, 1988.
368. Ellis, A. K., and Saran, B. R.: Kinetics of myoglobin release and prediction of myocardial myoglobin depletion after coronary artery reperfusion. Circulation *80*:676, 1989.
369. Ellis, A. K., Little, T., Zaki Masud, A. R., et al.: Early noninvasive detection of successful reperfusion in patients with acute myocardial infarction. Circulation *78*:1352, 1988.

MODIFICATION OF ISCHEMIC INJURY

370. Isobe, M., Nagai, R., Yamaoki, K., et al.: Quantification of myocardial infarct size after coronary reperfusion by serum cardiac myosin light chain II in conscious dogs. Circ. Res. *65*:684, 1989.
371. Maroko, P. R., Kjekshus, J. K., Sobel, B. E., et al: Factors influencing infarct size following experimental coronary artery occlusion. Circulation *43*:67, 1971.
372. Shell, W. E., and Sobel, B. E.: Deleterious effects of increased heart rate on infarct size in the conscious dog. Am. J. Cardiol. *31*:474, 1973.
373. Radvany, P., Maroko, P. R., and Braunwald, E.: Effect of hypoxemia on the extent of myocardial necrosis after experimental coronary occlusion. Am. J. Cardiol. *35*:795, 1975.
374. DeBoer, L.W.V., Rude, R. E., Davis, R. F., et al.: Extension of myocardial necrosis into normal epicardium following hypotension during experimental coronary occlusion. Cardiovasc. Res. *16*:423, 1982.
375. Libby, P., Maroko, P. R., and Braunwald, E.: The effect of hypoglycemia on myocardial ischemic injury during acute experiment coronary artery occlusion. Circulation *51*:621, 1975.
376. Davidson, S., Maroko, P. R., and Braunwald, E.: Effects of isoproterenol on contractile function of the ischemic and anoxic heart. Am. J. Physiol. *227*:439, 1974.
377. Vatner, S. F., Millard, R. W., Patrick, T. A., and Heyndrickx, G. R.: Effects of isoproterenol on regional myocardial function, electrogram, and blood flow in conscious dogs with myocardial ischemia. J. Clin. Invest. *57*:1261, 1976.
378. Fry, E. T. A., and Sobel, B. E.: Coronary thrombolysis. *In* Zipes, D. P., and Rowlands, D. J. (eds.): Progress in Cardiology. Philadelphia, Lea and Febiger, 1990, p. 199.
379. Tiefenbrunn, A. J., and Sobel, B. E.: Thrombolysis and myocardial infarction. Fibrinolysis, *5*:1, 1991.
380. Sobel, B. E.: Coronary thrombolysis. Coronary Artery Dis. *1*:3, 1990.
381. Simpson, P. J., Fantone, J. C., Mickelson, J. K., et al.: Identification of a time window for therapy to reduce experimental canine myocardial injury: Suppression of neutrophil activation during 72 hours of reperfusion. Circ. Res. *63*:1070, 1988.
382. Przyklenk, K., and Kloner, R. A.: "Reperfusion injury" by oxygen-derived free radicals? Effect of superoxide dismutase plus catalase, given at the time of reperfusion, on myocardial infarct size, contractile function, coronary microvasculature, and regional myocardial blood flow. Circ. Res. *64*:86, 1989.
383. Engler, R. L.: Free radical and granulocyte-mediated injury during myocardial ischemia and reperfusion. Am. J. Cardiol. *63*:19E, 1989.
384. Engler, R., and Covell, J. W.: Granulocytes cause reperfusion ventricular dysfunction after 15-minute ischemia in the dog. Circ. Res. *61*:20, 1987.
385. Opie, L. H.: Reperfusion injury and its pharmacologic modification. Circulation *80*:1049, 1989.
386. Klein, H. H., Pich, S., Lindert, S., et al.: Treatment of reperfusion injury with intracoronary calcium channel antagonists and reduced coronary free calcium concentration in regionally ischemic, reperfused porcine hearts. J. Am. Coll. Cardiol. *13*:1395, 1989.
387. Jang, I.-K., Van de Werf, F., Vanhaecke, J., and De Geest, H.: Coronary reperfusion by thrombolysis and early beta-adrenergic blockade in acute experimental myocardial infarction. J. Am. Coll. Cardiol. *14*:1816, 1989.
388. Torr, S., Drake-Holland, A. J., Main, M., et al.: Effects on infarct size of reperfusion and pretreatment with β-blockade and calcium antagonists. Basic Res. Cardiol. *84*:564, 1989.
389. Eisenberg, P. R., Sherman, L., Rich, M., et al.: Importance of continued activation of thrombin reflected by fibrinopeptide A to the efficacy of thrombolysis. J. Am. Coll. Cardiol. *7*:1255, 1986.
390. Eisenberg, P. R., Miletich, J. P., Sobel, B. E., and Jaffe, A. S.: Differential effects of activation of prothrombin by streptokinase compared with urokinase and tissue-type plasminogen activator (t-PA). Thromb. Res. *50*:707, 1988.
391. Eisenberg, P. R., and Miletich, J. P.: Induction of marked thrombin activity by pharmacologic concentrations of plasminogen activators in nonanticoagulated whole blood. Thromb. Res. *55*:635, 1989.
392. Sobel, B. E.: Coronary thrombolysis and the new biology. J. Am. Coll. Cardiol. *14*:850, 1989.
393. Fry, E.T.A., Grace, A., and Sobel, B. E.: Interactions between pharmacologic concentrations of plasminogen activators and platelets. Fibrinolysis *3*:127, 1989.
394. Fujii, S., and Sobel, B. E.: Induction of plasminogen activator inhibitor by products released from platelets. Circulation, *82*:1485, 1990.
395. Torr, S. R., Winters, K. J., Santoro, S. A., and Sobel, B. E.: The nature of interactions between tissue-type plasminogen activator and platelets. Thromb. Res., *59*:279, 1990.

396. Eisenberg, P. R., Miletich, J. P., and Sobel, B. E.: Factors responsible for differential procoagulation effects of diverse plasminogen activators in plasma. Blood, *in press.*
397. Terres, W., Beythien, C., Kupper, W., and Bleifeld, W.: Effects of aspirin and prostaglandin E_1 on in vitro thrombolysis with urokinase: Evidence for a possible role of inhibiting platelet activity in thrombolysis. Circulation *79*:1309, 1989.
398. Vaughan, D. E., Plavin, S. R., Schafer, A. I., and Loscalzo, J.: PGE_1 accelerates thrombolysis by tissue plasminogen activator. Blood *73*:1213, 1989.
399. Schumacher, W. A., and Grover, G. J.: The thromboxane receptor antagonist SQ 30,741 reduces myocardial infarct size in monkeys when given during reperfusion at a threshold dose for improving reflow during thrombolysis. J. Am. Coll. Cardiol. *15*:883, 1990.
400. Lefer, A. M., Mentley, R., and Sun, J-Z.: Potentiation of myocardial salvage by tissue type plasminogen activator in combination with a thromboxane synthetase inhibitor in ischemic cat myocardium. Circ. Res. *63*:621, 1988.
401. Nicolini, F. A., Mehta, J. L., Nichols, W. W., et al.: Prostacyclin analogue iloprost decreases thrombolytic potential of tissue-type plasminogen activator in canine coronary thrombosis. Circulation *81*:1115, 1990.
402. Reed, G. L., III, Matsueda, G. R., and Haber, E.: Inhibition of clot-bound α_2-antiplasmin enhances in vivo thrombolysis. Circulation *82*:164, 1990.
403. Hsia, J., Hamilton, W. P., Kleiman, N., et al.: The Heparin-Aspirin Reperfusion Trial (HART): A randomized trial of heparin versus aspirin adjunctive to tissue plasminogen activator-induced thrombolysis in acute myocardial infarction. N. Engl. J. Med., *in press.*
404. Thompson, P. L., Aylward, P. E., Federman, J., et al.: A randomized comparison of intravenous heparin versus oral aspirin and dipyridamole commenced at 24 hours after recombinant tissue plasminogen activator for acute myocardial infarction. Circulation, *in press.*
405. Haskel, E. J., Sobel, B. E., and Abendschein, D. R.: The relative efficacy of antithrombin compared with antiplatelet agents in accelerating coronary thrombolysis and preventing early reocclusion. Circulation, *83*:1048, 1991.
406. Walsh, M. N., Geltman, E. M., Steele, R. L., et al.: Augmented myocardial perfusion reserve after coronary angioplasty quantified by positron emission tomography with $H_2^{15}O$. J. Am. Coll. Cardiol. *15*:119, 1990.
407. Geltman, E. M., Henes, C. G., Senneff, M. J., et al.: Increased myocardial perfusion at rest and diminished perfusion reserve in patients with angina and angiographically normal coronary arteries. J. Am. Coll. Cardiol., *16*:586, 1990.
408. Schaper, J., and Schaper, W.: Reperfusion of ischemic myocardium: Ultrastructural and histochemical aspects. J. Am. Coll. Cardiol. *1*:1037, 1983.
409. Ellis, S. G., Henschke, C. I., Sandor, T., et al.: Time course of functional and biochemical recovery of myocardium salvaged by reperfusion. J. Am. Coll. Cardiol. *1*:1047, 1983.
410. Lavallee, M., Cox, D. A., and Vatner, S. F.: Effects of coronary artery reperfusion on recovery of regional myocardial function in conscious dogs. Eur. Heart J. *6*:109, 1985.
411. Maroko, P. R., Radvany, P., Braunwald, E., and Hale, S. L.: Reduction of infarct size by oxygen inhalation following acute coronary occlusion. Circulation *52*:360, 1975.
412. Glogar, D. H., Kloner, R. A., Muller, J., et al.: Fluorocarbons reduce myocardial ischemic damage after coronary occlusion. Science *211*:1439, 1981.
413. Tokioka, H., Miyazaki, A., Fung, P., et al.: Effects of intracoronary infusion of arterial blood or Fluosol-DA 20% on regional myocardial metabolism and function during brief coronary artery occlusions. Circulation *75*:473, 1987.
414. Schaer, G. L., Karas, S. P., Santoian, E. C., et al.: Reduction in reperfusion injury by blood-free reperfusion after experimental myocardial infarction. J. Am. Coll. Cardiol. *15*:1385, 1990.
415. Bajaj, A. K., Cobb, M. A., Virmani, R., et al.: Limitation of myocardial reperfusion injury by intravenous perfluorochemicals. Role of neutrophil activation. Circulation *79*:645, 1989.
416. Braunwald, E., Muller, J. E., Kloner, R. A., and Maroko, P. R.: Role of beta-adrenergic blockade in the therapy of patients with myocardial infarction. Am. J. Med. *74*:113, 1983.
417. Nayler, W. G., Panagiotopoulos, S., Elz, J. S., and Sturrock, W. J.: Fundamental mechanisms of action of calcium antagonists in myocardial ischemia. Am. J. Cardiol. *59*:75B, 1987.
418. Kloner, R. A., and Braunwald, E.: Effects of calcium antagonists on infarcting myocardium. Am. J. Cardiol. *59*:84B, 1987.
419. Henry, P. R., Shuchleib, R., Borda, L. J., et al.: Effects of nifedipine on myocardial perfusion and ischemic injury in dogs. Circ. Res. *43*:372, 1978.
420. Drury, J. K., Haendchen, R. V., Meerbaum, S., et al.: Diltiazem improves function and reduces infarct size after acute coronary occlusion. J. Am. Coll. Cardiol. *1*:692, 1983.
421. Calva, E., Mujica, A., Bisteni, A., and Sodi-Pallares, D.: Oxidative phosphorylation in cardiac infarct: Effect of glucose-KCl-insulin solution. Am. J. Physiol. *209*:371, 1965.
422. Henry, P. D., Sobel, B. E., and Braunwald, E.: Protection of hypoxic guinea pig hearts with glucose and insulin. Am. J. Physiol. *226*:390, 1974.
423. Maroko, P. R., Libby, P., Sobel, B. E., et al.: Effect of glucose-insulin-potassium infusion on myocardial infarction following experimental coronary artery occlusion. Circulation *45*:1160, 1972.
424. Mjøs, O. D.: Effect of reduction of myocardial free fatty acid metabolism relative to that of glucose on the ischemic injury during experimental coronary artery occlusion in dogs. *In* Hjalmarson, A., and Werko, L. (eds.): Experimental and Clinical Aspects on Preservation of the Ischemic Myocardium. Sweden, Molndal, 1976, p. 29.
425. Coleman, G. M., Gradinac, S., Taegtmeyer, H., et al.: Efficacy of metabolic support with glucose-insulin-potassium for left ventricular pump failure after aortocoronary bypass surgery. Circulation *80*(Suppl. I):91, 1989.
426. Maroko, P. R., Carpenter, C. B., Chiariello, M., et al.: Reduction by cobra venom factor of myocardial necrosis following coronary artery occlusion. J. Clin. Invest. *61*:661, 1978.
427. Diaz, P. E., Fishbein, M. C., Davis, M. A., et al.: Effect of kallikrein inhibitor aprotinin on myocardial ischemic injury following coronary artery occlusion in the dog. Am. J. Cardiol. *40*:541, 1977.
428. Libby, P., Maroko, P. R., Bloor, C. M., et al.: Reduction of experimental myocardial infarct size by corticosteroid administration. J. Clin. Invest. *52*:599, 1973.
429. Hammerman, H., Kloner, R. A., Hale, S., et al.: Dose-dependent effects of short-term methylprednisolone on myocardial infarct extent, scar formation, and ventricular function. Circulation *68*:446, 1983.
430. Brown, E. J., Kloner, R. A., Schoen, F. J., et al.: Scar thinning due to ibuprofen administration following experimental myocardial infarction. Am. J. Cardiol. *51*:877, 1983.
431. Willerson, J. T., Watson, J. T., and Platt, M. R.: Effect of hypertonic mannitol and intraaortic counterpulsation on regional myocardial blood flow and ventricular performance in dogs during myocardial ischemia. Am. J. Cardiol. *37*:514, 1976.
432. Roberts, R., Braunwald, E., Muller, J. E., et al.: Effect of hyaluronidase on mortality and morbidity in patients with early peaking of plasma creatine kinase MB and non-transmural ischaemia. Br. Heart J. *60*:290, 1988.
433. Flaherty, J. T.: Intravenous nitroglycerin in acute myocardial infarction. Cardiovasc. Rev. Rep. 46, June 1990.
434. Gallagher, K. P., Buda, A. J., Pace, D., et al.: Failure of superoxide dismutase and catalase to alter size of infarction in conscious dogs after three hours of occlusion followed by reperfusion. Circulation *73*:1065, 1986.
435. Uraizee, A., Reiner, K. A., Murry, C. E., and Jennings, R. B.: Failure of superoxide dismutase to limit size of myocardial infarction after 40 minutes of ischemia and four days of reperfusion in dogs. Circulation *75*:1237, 1987.
436. Werns, S. W., Shea, M. J., Mitsos, S. E., et al.: Reduction of the size of infarction by allopurinol in the ischemic-reperfused canine heart. Circulation *73*:518, 1986.
437. Braunwald, E., and Kloner, R. A.: Myocardial reperfusion: A double-edged sword? J. Clin. Invest. *76*:1713, 1985.
437a. Forman, M. B., Virmani, R., and Puett, D. W.: Mechanisms and therapy of myocardial reperfusion injury. Circulation *81*(Suppl. IV)69, 1990.
437b. Lefer, A. M., Tsao, P. S., Lefer, D. J., and Ma, X-L.: Role of endothelial dysfunction in the pathogenesis of reperfusion injury after myocardial ischemia. FASEB J *5*:2029, 1991.
438. Murry, C. E., Richard, V. J., Reimer, K. A., and Jennings, R. B.: Ischemic preconditioning slows energy metabolism and delays ultrastructural damage during a sustained ischemic episode. Circ. Res. *66*:913, 1990.
439. Li, G. C., Vasquez, J. A., Gallagher, K. P., and Lucchesi, B. R.: Myocardial protection with preconditioning. Circulation *82*:609, 1990.
440. Schott, R. J., Rohmann, S., Braun, E. R., and Schaper, W.: Ischemic preconditioning reduces infarct size in swine myocardium. Circ. Res. *66*:1133, 1990.
441. Jennings, R. B., Schaper, J., Hill, M. L., et al.: Effect of reperfusion late in the phase of reversible ischemic injury: Changes in cell volume, electrolytes, metabolites, and ultrastructure. Circ. Res. *56*:262, 1985.
442. Kloner, R. A., Ellis, S. G., Lange, R., and Braunwald, E.: Studies of experimental coronary artery reperfusion: Effects on infarct size, myocardial function, biochemistry, ultrastructure, and microvascular damage. Circulation *68*(Suppl. I):8, 1983.
443. Kloner, R. A., Ellis, S. G., Carlson, N. V., and Braunwald, E.: Coronary reperfusion for the treatment of acute myocardial infarction. Postischemic ventricular dysfunction. Cardiology *70*:233, 1983.

39

Acute Myocardial Infarction

by RICHARD C. PASTERNAK, M.D., EUGENE BRAUNWALD, M.D., and BURTON E. SOBEL, M.D.

In the United States nearly 1,500,000 patients suffer from acute myocardial infarction (AMI) annually and approximately one-fourth of all deaths are due to AMI.[1] More than 60 per cent of the deaths associated with AMI occur within one hour of the event and are attributable to arrhythmias, most often ventricular fibrillation (Chap. 26). Approximately 1.7 million patients with suspected AMI are admitted yearly to coronary care units in the United States; in about one-third of the patients, the diagnosis of MI is confirmed.[2]

In 1980, before the introduction of thrombolytic therapy, the mortality rates during hospitalization and the year following infarction were approximately 10 per cent each. However, there is considerable variation in prognosis depending on a wide variety of clinical factors, as discussed later, and several recent large-scale trials have suggested a far lower mortality when newer therapeutic modalities are used.[3,4] In the United States, the yearly economic burden of coronary artery disease is in excess of $100 billion.[5] Perhaps as much as half of this cost is related to myocardial infarction (MI) and its prevention and treatment. The average 5-year cost of an AMI has recently been estimated at over $50,000 per patient[6]; these costs appear to be increasing despite shorter average lengths of hospital stay.[7]

DIMINISHING MORTALITY IN MYOCARDIAL INFARCTION. In the United States, the decline in death rate from coronary artery disease (p. 1292) has been accompanied by diminished mortality from AMI. This fall in the mortality appears to be caused by two factors: a fall in the incidence of AMI by 25 per cent or more[8] and a similarly marked fall in the case fatality rate once a myocardial infarction has occurred.[8-11] The reasons for this decline in mortality undoubtedly are multifactorial. According to some estimates,[12,13] about 40 per cent of the fall in mortality is caused by such medical interventions as coronary care units, prehospital resuscitation, and newer mechanical and medical treatments of coronary artery disease. A marked overall decline in the incidence of sudden cardiac death suggests the effectiveness of both preventive measures and early treatment.[14]

There is no doubt that careful monitoring of cardiac rhythm and prompt treatment of *primary* arrhythmias have reduced sharply the incidence of in-hospital deaths from AMI. Accordingly, most deaths among patients with this condition who reach the hospital are now attributable to left ventricular failure and shock, and occur within the 3 or 4 days after the onset of infarction.[15,16] Only a minority of in-hospital deaths now result from *primary* arrhythmias and most of these occur in

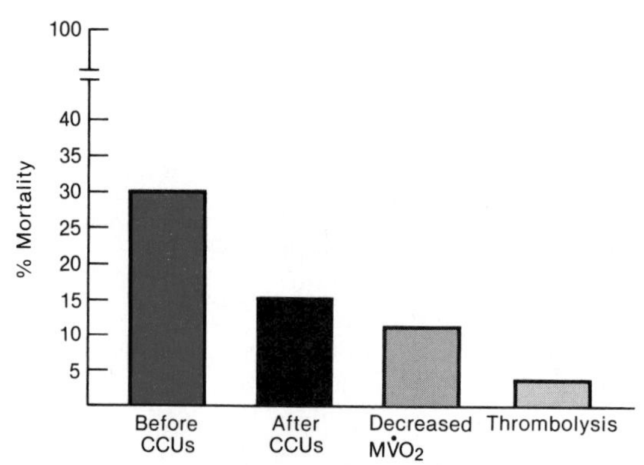

FIGURE 39-1. The mortality rates for patients with AMI managed in the era before use of defibrillation in coronary care units, after widespread utilization of defibrillation, and during the period in which reduction of myocardial oxygen requirements ($M\dot{V}O_2$) was a major focus of cardiovascular care, and presently for patients treated with thrombolysis. (From Sobel, B. E.: Coronary thrombolysis and the new biology. Reprinted with permission of the American College of Cardiology. J. Am. Coll. Cardiol. *14*:858, 1989.)

settings in which monitoring and/or treatment is inadequate. Nevertheless, arrhythmias occurring in the setting of extensive infarction and left ventricular failure (*secondary* arrhythmias) represent a relatively common cause of death.[17]

Before the advent of coronary care units, treatment of AMI was directed almost exclusively toward allowing healing of the infarct, preventing cardiac rupture and other complications such as pulmonary and systemic embolism, and sustaining arterial pressure and urine output. Subsequently, the major emphasis was on the prevention and aggressive treatment of arrhythmias. The concept that infarct size is an important determinant of prognosis and that its ultimate extent might be modified favorably by early implementation of selected physiological and pharmacological interventions has directed attention to the protection of jeopardized myocardium by attempts to decrease myocardial oxygen demand as well as by restoration of perfusion to ischemic tissue.[17,18] There have been recent dramatic strides, particularly in the area of thrombolytic therapy for AMI.[16,19,20] These developments are responsible for an ever-decreasing mortality from AMI, a decrease of over 80 per cent in the past 3 decades (Fig. 39–1).

For several years now we have been in an era in which the management of AMI may be characterized as "aggressive,"[21] in which there is wide recognition of the dynamic nature of the infarction process, and in which technological advances are occurring rapidly. This chapter addresses the underlying pathophysiology of AMI and the resulting clinical manifestations. Rapidly evolving management strategies are discussed in this pathophysiological context.

Pathology of Acute Myocardial Infarction

Almost all myocardial infarctions result from atherosclerosis of the coronary arteries, generally with superimposed coronary thrombosis. Nonatherogenic forms of coronary artery disease are discussed on p. 1352. The genesis of the coronary atherosclerotic lesion is a complex and controversial issue (see Chap. 36), and a number of risk factors have been associated with the development of atherosclerosis (see Chap. 37). However, regardless of the etiology and pathogenesis of the atherosclerotic process, the end result is plaques that cause luminal narrowing of the coronary arterial tree and, in many instances, a thrombus that causes further narrowing and often total occlusion. Below a certain critical level of blood flow, myocardial cells develop ischemic injury, a process described in detail in Chapter 38. When severe ischemia is prolonged, irreversible damage, i.e., MI, occurs.

Since the coronary luminal narrowing affects the major coronary arteries and their various branches to a different extent, MI usually occurs focally in specific regions of the heart. The location and size of a particular infarction depend on a number of different factors including (1) the location and severity of the atherosclerotic narrowings in the coronary arterial tree; (2) the size of the vascular bed perfused by the narrowed vessel(s); (3) the oxygen needs of the poorly perfused myocardium; (4) the extent of development of collateral blood vessels; (5) the presence, site, and severity of coronary arterial spasm; (6) the presence of tissue factors capable of modifying the necrotic process; and (7) the activity and effect of endogenously released thrombotic and thrombolytic substances.

GROSS PATHOLOGICAL CHANGES

Myocardial infarctions may be divided into two major types: *transmural infarcts*, in which myocardial necrosis involves the full thickness of the ventricular wall, and *subendocardial (nontransmural) infarcts*, in which the necrosis involves the subendocardium, the intramural myocardium, or both without extending all the way through the ventricular wall to the epicardium (Fig. 39–2).

Acute coronary thrombosis appears to be far more common when the infarction is transmural.[21a,22] Furthermore, the histological pattern of necrosis may differ, with contraction band injury (see below) occurring almost twice as often in nontransmural as in transmural infarction.[21a] Transmural infarcts are more frequently localized to the zone of distribution of a single coronary artery. Nontransmural infarctions, however, frequently occur in the setting of severely narrowed but still patent coronary arteries,[23] often in patients with pulmonary embolism, hypertension, hypotension, anemia, aortic stenosis, operative procedures, or cerebrovascular accidents. In the presence of severe atherosclerotic narrowing of the coronary arteries, these and other conditions associated with increased myocardial metabolic demands or decreased myocardial oxygen delivery or both are capable of producing patchy nontransmural myocardial necrosis, which tends to involve the subendocardium. In other instances, nontransmural infarcts appear to result from a total thrombotic occlusion that undergoes early spontaneous thrombolysis. Paradoxically, before their infarction, patients with nontransmural infarcts have, on average, a more severe stenosis in the infarct-related coronary artery than do patients suffering from transmural infarcts.[24] This finding suggests that a more severe lesion occurring before infarction protects against the development of transmural infarction, perhaps by fostering the development of supportive collateral circulation.

Myocardial infarction most commonly involves the left ventricle and interventricular septum; however, depending upon the criteria used, approximately one-third to two-thirds of patients with inferior infarction have some involvement of the right ventricle.[25,26] Among these patients, right ventricular infarction occurs exclusively in those with transmural infarction of the inferior posterior wall and the posterior portion of the septum. Patients with preexisting right ventricular hypertrophy are predisposed to develop right ventricular infarction with acute inferior MI.[27] Although right ventricular infarction almost invariably develops in association with infarction of the adjacent septum and left ventricular myocardium, *isolated* infarction of the right ventricle is seen in 3 to 5 per cent of autopsy-proven cases of myocardial infarction, usually in patients with chronic lung disease and right ventricular hypertrophy.[28]

ATRIAL INFARCTION. This occurs in 7 to 17 per cent of autopsy-proven cases of MI,[29] is often seen in conjunction with left ventricular infarction, and can result in rupture of the atrial wall. This type of infarct is more common on the right than the left side and occurs more frequently in the atrial appendages than in the lateral or posterior walls of the atrium. These differences in incidence might be explained by the considerably higher oxygen content of left atrial blood. Since right atrial infarction is usually associated with obstructive disease of the sinus node artery, it is accompanied frequently by atrial arrhythmias.

Gross changes (Fig. 39–3) do not appear in the myocardium until 6 hours after the onset of MI.[30] Initially, the myocardium in the affected region appears pale, bluish, and slightly swollen. Eighteen to 36 hours after the onset of the infarct, the

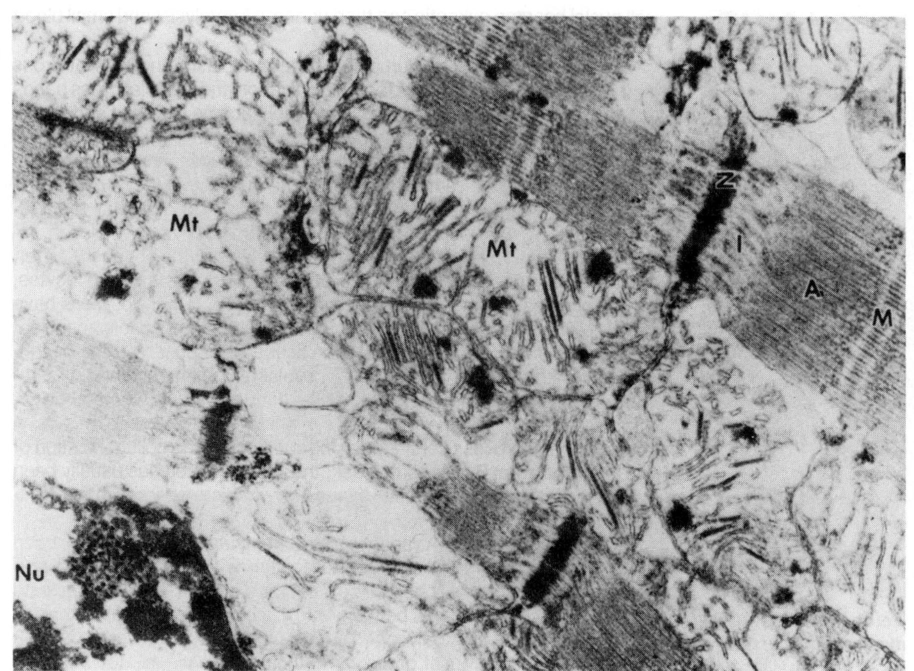

FIGURE 39-6. Electron micrograph of a muscle cell from the center of an infarct produced by permanent coronary occlusion in the dog. The myofibrils are fixed in a relaxed state and exhibit I, A, M, and Z bands. There is slight edema and no glycogen. (The clusters of granules resembling glycogen probably are ribosomes.) The mitochondria (Mt) are swollen and have linear densities and amorphous matrix (flocculent) densities. The nucleus (Nu) has clumped chromatin along the nuclear membrane and large lucent areas. (Tissue fixed with glutaraldehyde and osmium. Epoxy section stained with uranyl acetate and lead citrate, × 19,500.) (From Willerson, J. T., Hillis, L. D., and Buja, L. M. [eds.]: Pathogenesis and pathology of ischemic heart disease. *In* Ischemic Heart Disease. Clinical and Pathophysiological Aspects. New York, Raven Press, 1982, p. 47.)

ing and distortion of the transverse tubular system, the sarcoplasmic reticulum, and the mitochondria (Fig. 39-6).[36-38] When these changes are relatively mild, they are compatible with reversible ischemic injury. Changes after 60 minutes of occlusion include myocardial cell swelling, mitochondrial abnormalities such as swelling and internal disruption, aggregation and margination of nuclear chromatin, and relaxation of myofibrils. After 20 minutes to 2 hours of ischemia, changes in some cells become irreversible, and there is progression of these alterations; additional changes include indistinct, tight junctions at the intercalated discs, swollen sacs of the sarcoplasmic reticulum at the level of the A band, greatly enlarged mitochondria with few cristae, thinning and fractionation of myofilaments, disappearance of the heterochromatin, rarefaction of the euchromatin and peripheral aggregation of chromatin in the nucleus, disorientation of myofibrils, and clumping of mitochondria. Cells irreversibly damaged by ischemia are usually swollen, with an enlarged sarcoplasmic space; the sarcolemma may peel off the cells, defects in the plasma membrane may appear, and the mitochrondria are fragmented.

The swollen mitochondria obtained from ischemic myocardium contain deposits of calcium phosphate and amorphous matrix densities[39]; many of these changes become more intense when blood flow is restored.[40] However, it appears unlikely that the structural and functional deterioration of mitochondria—the hallmark of ischemic injury—is the primary mediator of myocardial cell death. In experimental infarction, reflow into an area rendered ischemic for 40 to 60 minutes results in violent cell swelling with vacuolization of myocardial cell cytoplasm and marked swelling of mitochondria. Cell membranes are lifted off the myofibrils, and subsarcolemmal blebs appear. The speed with which these morphological changes occur early after ischemic reflow suggests that ischemia produces a defect of volume regulation in myocardial cells.

PATTERNS OF MYOCARDIAL NECROSIS

COAGULATION NECROSIS. This results from severe, persistent ischemia and is usually present in the central region of infarcts, which results in the arrest of muscle cells[44] in the relaxed state and the passive stretching of ischemic muscle cells. On light microscopy the myofibrils are stretched, many with unclear pyknosis, with vascular congestion and healing by phagocytosis of necrotic muscle cells. There is evidence of mitochondrial damage with prominent amorphous (flocculent) densities but no calcification.

COAGULATIVE MYOCYTOLYSIS.[34,42] This form of myocardial necrosis, also termed *contraction band necrosis,*[43] results primarily from severe ischemia followed by reflow.[36] It is caused by increased Ca^{++} influx into dying cells, resulting in the arrest of cells in the contracted state. It is seen in the periphery of large infarcts and is present to a greater extent in nontransmural infarcts than in transmural ones.[21a] The entire infarct may show this form of necrosis when reperfusion occurs experimentally[44] or by surgery.[43] While patches of contraction band necrosis are found after successful reperfusion by thrombolytic therapy,[45] its presence in a large segment of some infarcts suggests that reperfusion through spontaneous thrombolysis or the release of spasm or both have occurred. It is characterized by hypercontracted myofibrils with contraction bands and mitochondrial damage, frequently with calcification, marked vascular congestion, and healing by lysis of muscle cells.

MYOCYTOLYSIS. This results from prolonged moderate ischemia and, like coagulative myocytolysis, is also frequently seen at the borders of an infarct as well as in patchy areas of infarction in patients with chronic ischemic heart disease. It is characterized by edema and cell swelling, early lysis of myofibrils, late lysis of nuclei, no neutrophilic response, and healing by lysis and phagocytosis of necrotic myocytes.[32,42]

CORONARY ARTERY ANATOMY AND PATHOLOGICAL ANATOMY

HISTORY. The importance of coronary artery obstruction has been the subject of much controversy since 1912, when Herrick proposed that AMI was due to occlusion of an epicardial coronary artery.[46] In the 3 decades following Herrick's description of the condition, the clinical manifestations of myocardial infarction were believed to stem from sudden coronary arterial occlusion, usually due to thrombosis; hence the terms *coronary thrombosis* and *acute myocardial infarction* became almost synonymous. One weakness of this concept was shown by Blumgart and colleagues, who demonstrated that *coronary occlusion could occur in the absence of infarction,* when the collateral circulation was adequate to maintain myocardial nutrition.[47] Equally important, Friedberg and Horn observed that *infarction could occur in the absence of coronary occlusion.*[48] The patients whom they described had severe coronary arterial narrowing. The areas of patchy, subendocardial infarction that occurred were thought to have developed secondary to relative insufficiency of coronary blood flow. Miller et al. then expanded on these observations, demonstrating that predominantly subendocardial infarcts were rarely associated with coronary occlusion, whereas transmural infarctions were frequently so.[23]

In over 75 per cent of patients with MI who come to autopsy, more than one coronary artery is severely narrowed.[32,49] One-third to two-thirds of patients with AMI have critical obstruction (to less than 25 per cent of luminal area) of all three coronary arteries, whereas the remainder are equally divided between those having one-vessel disease and those having two-vessel disease.[49,50] (Coronary arteriographic studies in surviving patients show that a higher percentage have one-vessel disease.) Most transmural infarcts occur distal to a totally occluded coronary artery. However, the converse is not the case, in that total occlusion of a coronary artery is not always associated with myocardial infarction. Collateral blood flow and other factors—such as the level of myocardial metabolism, the presence and location of stenoses in other coronary arteries, the rate of development of the obstruction, and the quantity of myocardium supplied by the obstructed vessel—all influence the viability of myocardial cells distal to the occlusion. In many series of patients studied at necropsy or by coronary arteriography, a small number (<5 per cent) of patients with MI are found to have normal coronary vessels.[32,50] In these patients, an embolus that has lysed or a prolonged episode of severe coronary spasm may have been responsible for the reduction in coronary flow.

Obstruction of the left anterior descending coronary artery usually causes infarction or threatens the viability of the anterior and apical regions of the left ventricle; portions of the septum, anterolateral wall, papillary muscles, and inferoapical wall of the left ventricle may also be involved. Obstruction of the left circumflex artery can cause infarction of the lateral or inferoposterior wall of the left ventricle. Occlusion of the right coronary artery usually results in infarction of the inferoposterior wall of the left ventricle, the inferior portions of the septum, posteromedial papillary muscle, and portions of the right ventricle. The size of the infarction and its location depend in part on the distribution of the obstructed coronary vessels. Thus, with occlusion of a dominant right coronary artery that supplies the posterior descending artery and posterior left ventricular wall, the inferoposterior wall of the left ventricle becomes infarcted, whereas the same region of the myocardium becomes involved with occlusion of the left circumflex coronary artery in the presence of a dominant left coronary artery.

Studies of patients who ultimately develop MI after having undergone coronary angiography at some time before its occurrence have been helpful in clarifying coronary anatomy before infarction. While high-grade stenoses, when present,[51,52] more frequently lead to MI than do less severe lesions, the majority of infarctions actually occur in areas supplied by a coronary artery with a previously identified stenosis of less than 50 per cent on angiograms performed months to years earlier.[53] This supports the concept (see below) that MI ultimately occurs secondary to recent destabilization of an atherosclerotic plaque. Certain angiographic characteristics, such as roughness of the luminal surface and lesion length, correlate with the risk of future infarction, further supporting this idea.[52]

RIGHT VENTRICULAR INFARCTION. Regardless of whether or not it is combined with involvement of the left ventricle, right ventricular infarction is generally associated with obstructive lesions of the right coronary artery. However, right ventricular infarction occurs less commonly than would be anticipated from the frequency of atherosclerotic lesions involving the right coronary artery.[54] This discrepancy probably can be explained by the lower oxygen demands of the right ventricle, since right ventricular infarcts occur more commonly in conditions such as pulmonary hypertension and right ventricular hypertrophy that are associated with increased right ventricular oxygen needs.[27,28] Moreover, the intercoronary collateral system of the right ventricle is richer than that of the left, and the thinness of the right ventricular wall allows the chamber to derive some nutrition from the blood within the right ventricular cavity.

Rather frequently, when an area of the ventricle is perfused by collateral vessels, an infarct occurs at a distance from a coronary occlusion. For example, following the gradual obliteration of the lumen of the right coronary artery, the inferior wall of the left ventricle may be maintained viable by collateral vessels arising from the left anterior descending coronary artery. In this circumstance, an occlusion of the left anterior descending artery may cause an infarct of the diaphragmatic wall.

CORONARY ARTERY THROMBOSIS

Conclusions drawn from autopsy studies of the coronary arteries following AMI are limited both by the selection bias (obviously only patients who die can be studied), and by post-

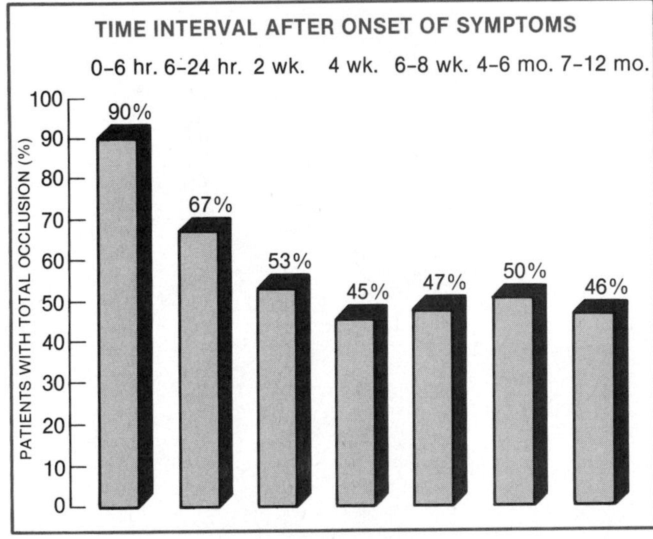

FIGURE 39-7. Percentage of patients with total coronary occlusion at different time intervals after the onset of symptoms of AMI. (Adapted from deFeyter, P. J., van den Brand, M., Serruys, P. W., and Wijns, W.: Early angiography after myocardial infarction: What have we learned? Am. Heart J. *109*:194, 1985.)

mortem events, including lysis of clots that were present premortem. For many years coronary angiography was avoided in the acute phases of MI because of potential complications.[55] Experience of the last decade, however, has shown that angiography is safe even during the acute phase of MI.[55,56] Angiographic studies performed in the earliest hours of transmural MI have revealed an approximate 90 per cent incidence of total occlusion in the infarct-related vessel.[56-58] Recanalization from spontaneous thrombolysis[58,59] as well as attrition due to some mortality among those patients with total occlusion results in a diminishing incidence of totally occluded vessels found in the period following myocardial infarction (Fig. 39-7).[50,56,59a]

Occlusion of a coronary artery leading to MI appears to be the final common pathway resulting from a complex and dynamic interaction among coronary atherosclerosis, vasospasm, plaque rupture, and platelet activation, ultimately leading to coronary artery thrombosis.[60-62]

CORONARY ATHEROSCLEROSIS IN MYOCARDIAL INFARCTION

At autopsy, the atherosclerotic plaque of patients who died of MI is primarily composed of fibrous tissue of varying density and cellularity.[63] Calcium, lipid-laden foam cells, and extracellular lipid each constitutes 5 to 10 per cent of the remaining area.[63] Roberts et al. have quantified the extent and severity of atherosclerosis in autopsied patients with a history of MI.[49,64] The entire length of the epicardial coronary tree was examined by dividing each coronary artery into 5-mm segments and assessing a cross-sectional area of each segment. The extent of severe narrowing (76 to 100 per cent) was largely unpredictable from clinical factors and varied between approximately 20 and 45 per cent of all coronary artery segments. Of the remaining segments without severe stenosis, about two-thirds showed moderate stenoses (51 to 75 per cent) and one-third, mild stenoses (26 to 50 per cent). Fewer than 6 per cent of segments examined were 25 per cent narrowed or less. Thus, the atherosclerotic processes were almost ubiquitous in most patients with MI. At autopsy, however, less advanced atherosclerosis may be present in survivors of MI.

The atherosclerotic plaques that are associated with thrombosis and a total occlusion, located in infarct-related vessels, are generally more complex and irregular than those in vessels not associated with MI.[65] Histological studies of these lesions often reveal plaque rupture or fissuring[66-69] (Fig. 39-8). Angiographic morphology suggestive of plaque rupture has been identified in the majority of stenoses associated with AMI or abrupt onset of unstable angina.[70] This finding is rare in the noninfarct-related vessels of AMI patients and in the vessels of patients with chronic stable angina pectoris.[70] While controversy exists regarding the exact role that plaque rupture plays in the sequence of events leading to coronary artery occlusion, it is probable that hemorrhage into an atherosclerotic plaque

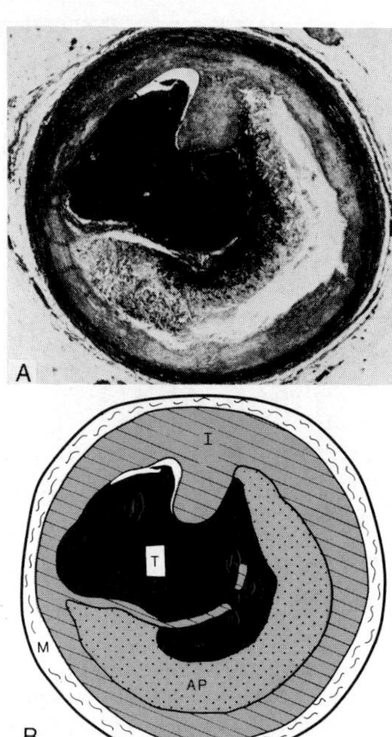

FIGURE 39-8. Histological cross section of a major plaque rupture *(A)* and accompanying diagram *(B)*. The plaque (AP) has a large defect in the fibrous cap, through which a dumb-bell mass of thrombus (T) has formed, part being within the plaque and part virtually occluding the lumen. AP = atherosclerotic plaque; I = intima; M = media. (From Davies, M. J., and Thomas, A. C.: Plaque fissuring—the cause of acute myocardial infarction, sudden ischemic death, and crescendo angina. Br. Heart J. *53*:363, 1985.)

can initiate a chain of events leading to coronary artery thrombus in MI.[61,62,66,68,69]

Platelet-rich thrombi are often associated with the surface of the most advanced atherosclerotic lesions, called *complicated plaques,* which are characterized by fibrocalcific degeneration, deposition of lipid, calcium, fibrous tissue, necrotic debris, extravasated blood, and a fibrous cap (Fig. 39-9). Impaired endothelial cell function associated with atherogenesis may predispose to platelet adhesion and activation. Conversely, platelet activation in association with such lesions may contribute to atherogenesis through release of growth factors. Luminal narrowing may potentiate platelet activation through augmentation of shear forces.

While it is now clear that transmural MI usually is caused by coronary thrombosis, the incidence of coronary thrombosis in subendocardial infarction is less clear, because angiographic studies provide only indirect evidence of thrombosis. The results of postmortem studies are difficult to interpret because thrombi can undergo organization or recanalization, which makes their pathological characteristics indistinguishable from nonocclusive atherosclerotic plaques.[66] Angiographic studies have suggested a wide variability in the frequency of coronary thrombosis with nontransmural infarction ranging from 20 to nearly 90 per cent.[22,71] The increasingly persuasive evidence that thrombosis plays a major role in patients with unstable ischemic syndromes[69-71] suggests that previous estimates of the incidence of thrombosis in nontransmural MI may have been less than the true frequency.

Rarely, coronary thrombosis may cause multifocal or circumferential infarction. However, the latter is more often the consequence of a severe imbalance between myocardial oxygen supply and demand when multiple high-grade fixed atherosclerotic lesions exist and myocardial oxygen demand is increased by such causes as tachycardia, increased ventricular wall tension, or increased myocardial contractility.

The rapidity with which thrombosis develops and the extent of coronary collaterals can determine whether acute coronary occlusion causes a transmural infarct, a subendocardial infarct, or no infarct.[36]

COMPOSITION OF THROMBI. At autopsy, coronary arterial thrombi, which are approximately 1 cm in length in most cases,[23] adhere to the luminal surface of an artery and are composed of platelets, fibrin, erythrocytes, and leukocytes. The composition of the thrombus may vary at different levels: A white thrombus is composed of platelets, fibrin, or both distally, and a red thrombus is composed of erythrocytes, fibrin, platelets, and leukocytes proximally. Early thrombi are usually small and nonocclusive and are composed almost exclusively of platelets.

In patients with MI, coronary thrombi are usually superimposed on or adjacent to atherosclerotic plaques (Fig. 39-8).[69] As already pointed out, the culprit plaques are often less than nearly occlusive. It has been suggested that degenerative changes in the atherosclerotic intima damage supportive perivascular tissue with resultant rupture of a plaque, sometimes accompanied by intramural hemorrhage.[36] This process may enlarge the volume of the plaque so that it occludes the arterial lumen without the occurrence of thrombosis, or the fissuring may disrupt the intima covering the plaque, thereby exposing collagen to flowing blood, a strong stimulus for thrombus formation.[67,68,72]

THE UNSTABLE PLAQUE. Pre- and postmortem angiographic studies have suggested that ulceration and plaque fissuring can be characterized radiographically as stenoses showing irregular borders (Fig. 8-35, p. 224) and intraluminal lucencies.[65,69] (The latter may be due to thrombus associated with the atherosclerotic lesion.) It has also been theorized that an angiographic pattern suggesting disruption of the atherosclerotic plaque is associated with histopathological evidence of coronary thrombosis as well as with the clinical syndromes of unstable angina (p. 1334) and AMI.[65,68-70]

ROLES OF PLATELETS AND COAGULATION FACTORS. While it is clear that platelets play an important role in the pathogenesis of atherosclerosis (Chap. 36), their precise *causal* role in MI remains controversial (p. 1110). It is quite likely that they are involved in the pathogenesis of coronary thrombosis.[60,62] Radiolabeled platelets incorporated into coronary thrombi have been identified scintigraphically in patients with AMI.[73] When atherosclerotic plaques undergo the changes noted earlier, exposed collagen leads to prompt platelet adhesion followed by formation of platelet aggregates, release of platelet granular constituents, and possible microembolization. The platelet in AMI has been characterized as hyperaggregable, and the degree of platelet hyperreactivity even appears to be a useful marker for future coronary events.[74] The phenomenon of hyperreactivity is probably related to the production, by aggregating platelets, of increased

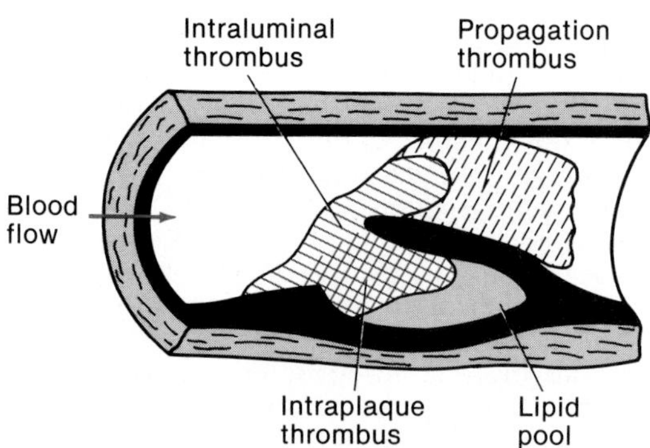

FIGURE 39-9. Representation of a longitudinal reconstruction of a coronary artery showing the histological components of an occluding thrombus. Much of the thrombus at the site of occlusion is contained within the plaque and compresses the lumen from outside. Intraluminal thrombus develops adjacent to a plaque fissure then propagates downstream. A plug of lipid has extruded into the lumen. (From Davies, M. J.: A macro and micro view of coronary vascular insult in ischemic heart disease. Circulation *82*[Suppl. II]:38, 1990, by permission of the American Heart Association, Inc.)

amounts of thromboxane A_2 (a potent platelet-aggregating prostaglandin that is also a powerful vasoconstrictor).[60,75,76]

An imbalance in the clotting system between prothrombotic activity and the fibrinolytic system may also be related to the development of AMI. A hypercoagulable state may lead to MI in some patients who do not have atherosclerotic lesions (see below). A reduced fibrinolytic capacity due to the presence of a plasma inhibitor of tissue plasminogen activator (PAI-1) may be important in the pathogenesis of AMI in certain patients.[77] Elevated levels of urinary fibrinopeptide A in AMI patients provide evidence of activation of the clotting system, specifically of recent production of fibrin by the action of thrombin on fibrinogen.[78]

TEMPORAL CORRELATIONS. In order to define the precise relationship between coronary thrombosis and AMI, it is important to understand the time course of thrombus formation in relation to the onset of infarction. Unfortunately, estimates of the age of coronary thrombi and myocardial infarction by histological criteria may be quite imprecise,[79] but several lines of evidence suggest that a thrombus is present acutely. The findings of elevated levels of markers that indicate active coagulation[76,78,80] is considered circumstantial evidence. As already noted, studies in which coronary arteriography performed on patients within the first few hours after the onset of AMI have demonstrated that the coronary artery supplying the area of evolving infarction is totally occluded in the majority of these patients.[56,57,81,82] If fibrinolytic agents are infused into the occluded artery (or intravenously in large doses) patency is achieved in a high percentage of cases. Angiography performed after fibrinolytic therapy usually demonstrates residual stenotic lesions at the site where coronary arterial occlusion had existed. Fresh thrombi have been recovered from the majority of patients with acute myocardial infarction undergoing emergency coronary bypass surgery,[56] and have been directly visualized through coronary angioscopy in the setting of unstable angina, a condition that frequently precedes the development of AMI.[83]

CORONARY ARTERY SPASM

(See also p. 1338)

In addition to causing AMI in rare patients with normal coronary arteries (see below), coronary artery spasm may also play a broader role in patients with atherosclerotic coronary artery disease.[84] It has been postulated that spasm may cause intimal damage that can initiate formation of an atherosclerotic plaque.[85,86] Epicardial coronary artery spasm has been identified in patients with fixed atherosclerotic coronary artery stenosis before, during, and after AMI.[86-88] An association between coronary artery spasm and coronary artery thrombosis has also been documented clinically.[89]

In the setting of AMI, there is evidence of increased production of vasodilating and vasoconstricting prostaglandins,[75,90] but it appears that the vasoconstricting activity of thromboxane A_2 predominates.[60,75] Thus, the presence of thromboxane A_2 and other vasoconstricting substances released by the aggregating platelets at the site of a coronary artery stenosis has the potential to initiate or maintain coronary artery constriction. It may be responsible for some observed cases of coronary artery spasm occurring with and perhaps contributing to the pathogenesis of AMI.

COLLATERAL CIRCULATION

(See also p. 1164)

Normal hearts contain an extensive network of interarterial anastomotic blood vessels, greater than 60 μm in diameter, involving epicardial, intramyocardial, and subendocardial connections. This collateral circulation exists at birth and apparently grows in size along with the rest of the coronary circulation but is beyond the limit of resolution of coronary arteriographic techniques and is not seen in living subjects without disease. In patients with coronary artery disease, these preexisting channels progressively enlarge, presumably as a consequence of the release of local vasodilators; flow through the collaterals will occur when pressure differences exist across these channels.[91] The coronary collateral circulation is particularly well developed in patients with (1) coronary occlusive disease, especially when it is severe, with the reduction of the luminal cross-sectional area by more than 75 per cent in one or more major vessels; (2) chronic hypoxia, as occurs in severe anemia, chronic obstructive pulmonary disease, and cyanotic congenital heart disease; and (3) left ventricular hypertrophy, which intensifies coronary collaterals. There is considerable variability in the development of collateral channels in patients with comparable degrees of obstructive coronary artery disease.

CORONARY COLLATERALS IN ACUTE MYOCARDIAL INFARCTION

Early angiography in patients with AMI and the performance of serial catheterizations for trials on the effects of reperfusion in these patients have allowed the careful study of the angiographic appearance of collaterals. Although well-developed collaterals are not the rule at the time of infarction, some collaterals are seen in nearly 40 per cent of patients with an acute total occlusion,[92] and more begin to appear soon after the total occlusion occurs.[22,93] The incidence of collaterals 1 to 2 weeks following AMI varies considerably and may be as high as 75 to 100 per cent in patients with persistent total occlusion of the infarct vessel, or as low as 17 to 42 per cent in patients with subtotal occlusion.[22,93-95,99a]

That the appearance of collaterals is closely related to the presence of a totally occluded vessel has been shown by studies at the time of coronary angioplasty. These studies have allowed for the demonstration that filling of collaterals improves within 1 to 2 minutes of a sudden temporary coronary artery occlusion induced by an angioplasty balloon.[96] Likewise, a total occlusion induced by transient coronary artery spasm may allow for the visualization of collaterals not seen before the spasm.[97] It is likely that the presence of a high-grade stenosis (> 90 per cent), possibly with periods of intermittent total occlusion, permits the development of collaterals that remain only as *potential* conduits until a total occlusion occurs or recurs. The latter event then brings these channels into full operation.

Supporting the argument in favor of a functional role for coronary collateral vessels is the finding that in patients with coronary occlusion and collaterals the area of myocardial necrosis is frequently smaller than the area supplied by an occluded coronary artery when collaterals are not present.[94,95,98,98a] Indeed, it is rather common for patients with abundant collaterals to have totally occluded coronary arteries without evidence of infarction in the distribution of that coronary vessel; thus, the survival of the myocardium distal to such occlusions must be dependent on collateral blood flow.

NONATHEROSCLEROTIC CAUSES OF ACUTE MYOCARDIAL INFARCTION

Numerous pathological processes other than atherosclerosis can, on occasion, involve the coronary arteries (p. 1213) and result in myocardial infarction (Table 39-1).[99,100] For example, coronary arterial occlusions can be the result of embolization of a coronary artery. Emboli most frequently lodge in the distribution of the left anterior descending coronary artery, commonly in the distal epicardial and intramural branches.[23] The causes of coronary embolism are numerous: infective and marantic endocarditis (Chap. 35), mural thrombi, prosthetic valves,[101] neoplasms,[102] air that is introduced at the time of cardiac surgery,[103] and calcium deposits from manipulation of calcified valves at operation. In situ thrombosis of coronary arteries can occur secondary to chest-wall trauma (Chap. 46). Oral contraceptive use probably is associated with AMI in healthy women,[104] although this point remains controversial.[105] The mechanism of this association may operate through an increased tendency for thrombosis.

A variety of inflammatory processes can be responsible for coronary artery abnormalities, some of which mimic athero-

TABLE 39-1 CAUSES OF MYOCARDIAL INFARCTION WITHOUT CORONARY ATHEROSCLEROSIS

CORONARY ARTERY DISEASE OTHER THAN ATHEROSCLEROSIS

Arteritis
- Luetic
- Granulomatous (Takayasu disease)
- Polyarteritis nodosa
- Mucocutaneous lymph node (Kawasaki) syndrome
- Disseminated lupus erythematosus
- Rheumatoid arthritis
- Ankylosing spondylitis

Trauma to coronary arteries
- Laceration
- Thrombosis
- Iatrogenic
- Radiation (radiotherapy for neoplasia)

Coronary mural thickening with metabolic disease or intimal proliferative disease
- Mucopolysaccharidoses (Hurler disease)
- Homocystinuria
- Fabry disease
- Amyloidosis
- Juvenile intimal sclerosis (idiopathic arterial calcification of infancy)
- Intimal hyperplasia associated with contraceptive steroids or with the postpartum period
- Pseudoxanthoma elasticum
- Coronary fibrosis caused by radiation therapy

Luminal narrowing by other mechanisms
- Spasm of coronary arteries (Prinzmetal's angina with normal coronary arteries)
- Spasm after nitroglycerin withdrawal
- Dissection of the aorta
- Dissection of the coronary artery

EMBOLI TO CORONARY ARTERIES

Infective endocarditis
Nonbacterial thrombotic endocarditis
Prolapse of mitral valve
Mural thrombus from left atrium, left ventricle, or pulmonary veins
Prosthetic valve emboli
Cardiac myxoma
Associated with cardiopulmonary bypass surgery and coronary arteriography
Paradoxical emboli
Papillary fibroelastoma of the aortic valve ("fixed embolus")
Thrombi from intracardiac catheters or guide wires

CONGENITAL CORONARY ARTERY ANOMALIES

Anomalous origin of left coronary from pulmonary artery
Left coronary artery from anterior sinus of Valsalva
Coronary arteriovenous and arteriocameral fistulas
Coronary artery aneurysms

MYOCARDIAL OXYGEN DEMAND-SUPPLY DISPROPORTION

Aortic stenosis, all forms
Incomplete differentiation of the aortic valve
Aortic insufficiency
Carbon monoxide poisoning
Thyrotoxicosis
Prolonged hypotension

HEMATOLOGICAL (IN SITU THROMBOSIS)

Polycythemia vera
Thrombocytosis
Disseminated intravascular coagulation
Hypercoagulability, thrombosis, thrombocytopenic purpura

MISCELLANEOUS

Cocaine abuse
Myocardial contusion
Myocardial infarction with normal coronary arteries
Complication of cardiac catheterization

Modified from Cheitlin, M., et al.: Myocardial infarction without atherosclerosis. J.A.M.A. *231*:951, 1975. Copyright 1975, American Medical Association.

sclerotic disease and may predispose to true atherosclerosis.[106] There is suggestive epidemiological evidence that viral infections, particularly with coxsackie B, may be an uncommon cause of MI.[107] Viral illnesses precede AMI occasionally in young persons who are later shown to have normal coronary arteries.[107,108]

Syphilitic aortitis may produce marked narrowing or occlusion of one or both coronary ostia,[109] whereas Takayasu's arteritis may result in obstruction of the coronary arteries (Chap. 47).[110] Necrotizing arteritis, polyarteritis nodosa,[111] mucocutaneous lymph node syndrome (Kawasaki disease) (p. 997),[112] systemic lupus erythematosus (p. 1234) and giant cell arteritis[114] (Chap. 56) can cause coronary occlusion. Therapeutic levels of mediastinal radiation can cause thickening and hyalinization of the walls of coronary arteries, with subsequent infarction.[115,116] MI may also be the result of coronary arterial involvement in amyloidosis (p. 1753), Hurler syndrome, pseudoxanthoma elasticum,[117] and homocystinuria (Chap. 51).

Involvement of the small coronary arteries (0.1 to 1.0 mm in diameter) by a number of disease processes may produce intimal and medial hyperplasia, necrosis, dissection, and thrombosis,[118] resulting in occlusions that produce *focal* areas of infarction and ultimately of fibrosis. Depending on the location and extent of the fibrotic reaction, arrhythmias, conduction defects, heart block, and heart failure can occur.

As *cocaine abuse* has become more common, reports of AMI following the use of cocaine have appeared with increasing frequency. Cocaine may cause AMI in patients with normal coronary arteries,[119-121] preexisting MI,[122] documented coronary artery disease,[121-123] or known coronary artery spasm.[125] Recurrent MI after further cocaine abuse has been reported as well.[119,124] Cocaine may cause MI by at least three mechanisms: (1) increasing myocardial oxygen demand via increases in heart rate and blood pressure, (2) diminishing coronary artery flow resulting from either coronary vasospasm and/or thrombosis,[119,121] and (3) active myocarditis (either hypersensitivity or toxic). Contraction band necrosis is the rule, and its extent appears to be related to the level of cocaine found in the blood or urine at autopsy.[126,128] In very high doses, cocaine appears to have a direct toxic effect on heart muscle that may produce cardiac failure and sudden death[127,129] with extensive myocyte necrosis.[126,127]

MYOCARDIAL INFARCTION WITH ANGIOGRAPHICALLY NORMAL CORONARY VESSELS

Approximately 6 per cent of all patients with AMI and perhaps four times that percentage of patients with this diagnosis under the age of 35 years do not have coronary atherosclerosis demonstrated by coronary arteriography or at autopsy.[50,59] Perhaps half the patients of this group, in turn, have a variety of other lesions involving the coronary vessels or myocardium (Table 39-1), whereas the others have no detectable coronary obstructive lesions.[130,131] Patients with AMI and normal coronary arteries tend to be young and to have relatively few coronary risk factors, except that they often have a history of cigarette smoking.[132-135] Usually they have no history of angina pectoris prior to the infarction.[136] The infarction in these patients is usually not preceded by any prodrome, but the clinical, laboratory, and electrocardiographic features of AMI are otherwise distinguishable from those present in the overwhelming majority of patients with AMI who have classic obstructive atherosclerotic coronary artery disease. In patients without coronary obstruction, the prognosis for survival of the acute event is usually excellent, but a few fatalities have occurred; therefore, it has been possible to document the presence of this syndrome at autopsy.[137] In 10 such patients, infarcts ranged from 5 to 33 per cent (mean of 18 per cent) of the left ventricle.[137] No thromboembolic material was seen in the coronary arterial tree despite the fact that the infarcts were only 2 days old in five patients and 3 or 4 days old in three others.

In patients who recover, areas of localized dyskinesis and hypokinesis can often be demonstrated by left ventricular angiography. Patients have been described as having both occlusion of the infarct-related artery during the acute phase of MI and normal coronary arteries during the convalescent phase.[138] In most cases, the initial total occlusion appears to have been due to thrombosis as thrombolytic therapy was used to produce complete recanalization.

POSSIBLE MECHANISMS

CORONARY SPASM. Numerous theories have been proposed to explain the occurrence of AMI in patients with normal coronary arteriograms. Patients with vasospastic angina are clearly at risk for MI: coronary spasm has been shown to cause MI in some patients with normal coronary arteries.[88,89] The administration of agents that provoke coronary artery spasm has been reported to cause MI in patients with normal coronary arteries,[139,140] and withdrawal of chronic nitrate vasodilation is presumably responsible for MI in others.[141] However, spasm may be induced in only a minority of patients with MI and normal coronary arteries.[132,133,138,142] Intracoronary vasodilators often have no effect when administered acutely in MI, even when patients are later (after thrombolysis) shown to have normal coronary arteries. It is attractive to hypothesize that many of these cases are caused by combined coronary artery spasm and thrombosis, perhaps with underlying endothelial irregularities or small plaques that are not apparent on coronary angiography.[89,138,143]

OTHER CAUSES. Additional suggested causes include (1) coronary emboli (perhaps from a small mural thrombus, a prolapsed mitral valve,[144] or a myxoma); (2) coronary artery disease in vessels too small to be visualized by coronary arteriography or coronary arterial thrombosis with subsequent recanalization (Table 39–1); (3) a variety of hematological disorders causing in situ thrombosis in the presence of normal coronary arteries (polycythemia vera, cyanotic heart disease with polycythemia,[145] sickle cell anemia,[146] disseminated intravascular coagulation, thrombocytosis, and thrombotic thrombocytopenic purpura); (4) augmented oxygen needs (thyrotoxicosis,[147] amphetamine use[148]); (5) hypotension secondary to sepsis, blood loss, or pharmacological agents, and (6) anatomical variations such as anomalous origin of a coronary artery (p. 254), coronary arteriovenous fistula (p. 970), or a myocardial bridge.[149]

PROGNOSIS. The long-term outlook for patients who have survived an AMI with normal coronary vessels on arteriography appears to be substantially better than for patients with MI and obstructive coronary artery disease.[130–134,137] Following recovery from the initial infarct, recurrent infarction, heart failure, and death are unusual in patients with normal coronary arteries.[134,135] Indeed, most of these patients have normal exercise electrocardiograms[150] and only a minority develop angina pectoris.

Pathophysiology of Acute Myocardial Infarction

SYSTOLIC FUNCTION

The fundamental pathological alteration underlying left ventricular dysfunction in AMI is loss of functioning myocardium. Depression of cardiac function in myocardial infarction is directly related to the extent of left ventricular damage.[151] Cessation of blood flow to a region of myocardium produces four sequential abnormal contraction patterns[152]: (1) *dyssynchrony*, dissociation in the time course of contraction of adjacent segments of myocardial segments; (2) *hypokinesis*, reduction in the extent of shortening; (3) *akinesis*, cessation of shortening; and (4) *dyskinesis*, paradoxical expansion, systolic bulging.[153,154] Accompanying dysfunction of the infarcting segment is initial *hyperkinesis* of the remaining normal myocardium in the intact ventricle.[155] This increased motion of the noninfarcted region subsides within 2 weeks of infarction, during which time some degree of recovery can be seen in the infarct region as well, particularly if reperfusion (p. 1229) of the infarcted area occurs.[156] It is thought to be the result of acute compensatory mechanisms including the Frank-Starling mechanism and increased levels of circulating catecholamines.[155] If a sufficient amount of myocardium undergoes ischemic injury, left ventricular pump function becomes depressed, and cardiac output, stroke volume, blood pressure, and peak dP/dt are reduced,[151,154] and end-systolic volume is increased. In fact, the degree to which end-systolic volume increases is perhaps the most powerful predictor of mortality following AMI.[157] The paradoxical systolic expansion of an area of ventricular myocardium decreases the stroke output of the left ventricle. With the passage of time, edema and cellular infiltration and ultimately fibrosis increase the stiffness of the infarcted myocardium back to and beyond control values.[158] Increasing stiffness in the infarcted zone of myocardium improves left ventricular function, since it prevents systolic paradoxical wall motion.

Areas with reduced and absent wall motion are universally seen in patients with transmural AMI. Rackley and collaborators have demonstrated a linear relationship between specific parameters of left ventricular function and clinical symptoms.[159] The earliest abnormality is a reduction in diastolic compliance, which can be observed with infarcts that involve only 8 per cent of the total left ventricle on angiographic examination. When the abnormally contracting segment exceeds 15 per cent, the ejection fraction may be reduced and elevations of left ventricular end-diastolic pressure and volume occur. Clinical heart failure accompanies areas of abnormal contraction exceeding 25 per cent, and cardiogenic shock, often fatal, accompanies loss of more than 40 per cent of the left ventricular myocardium.[159]

Unless extension of the infarct occurs, some improvement in wall motion takes place during the healing phase, as recovery of function occurs in initially reversibly injured myocardium. Regardless of the age of the infarct, patients who continue to demonstrate abnormal wall motion of 20 to 25 per cent of the left ventricle manifest hemodynamic signs of left ventricular failure.[160] Physical signs and symptoms of left ventricular failure also increase proportionally to increasing areas of abnormal left ventricular wall motion.[154] These findings are of interest in view of the experimental work of Pfeffer et al., who produced infarcts of varying sizes and studied left ventricular performance 3 weeks later.[151] Rats with relatively small infarcts (<30 per cent of the left ventricle) had no detectable impairment of function; those with moderate-sized infarcts (31 to 46 per cent) exhibited normal baseline measurements but inadequate responses to hemodynamic stresses; rats with large infarcts (>46 per cent) uniformly exhibited left ventricular failure.

Patients with AMI often also show reduced myocardial contractile function in noninfarcted zones of myocardium.[161] This may result from obstruction of the coronary artery supplying this region of the ventricle, which is perfused by collaterals from the vessel that becomes occluded, a condition that has been termed *ischemia at a distance*.[162] Conversely, the presence of collaterals developing before MI may allow for greater preservation of regional systolic function in an area of distribution of the occluded artery and improvement in left ventricular ejection fraction early after infarction.[94,163]

DIASTOLIC FUNCTION

As pointed out on page 1178, myocardial ischemia alters not only the systolic performance but also the diastolic characteristics of the left ventricle, ultimately raising its diastolic pressure at any given volume.[158,164,165] Left ventricular diastolic properties are altered in infarcted and ischemic myocardium, leading initially to an increase but later to a reduction in left ventricular compliance. These changes are associated with an initial rise in left ventricular end-diastolic pressure. Over a period of 2 weeks, this pressure begins to fall toward normal, as there is a compensatory increase in end-diastolic volume.[166] As with impairment of systolic function, the magnitude of the diastolic abnormality appears to be related to the size of the initial infarct. Patients who have recovered from AMI frequently continue to manifest decreased left ventricular compliance secondary to the fibrous scar that remains in the left ventricle.

CIRCULATORY REGULATION IN ACUTE MYOCARDIAL INFARCTION

The abnormality in circulatory regulation that is present in AMI is diagrammed in Figure 39–10. The process begins with an anatomical or functional obstruction in the coronary vascular bed, which results in regional myocardial ischemia and, if the ischemia persists, in infarction. If the infarct is of sufficient size, it depresses overall left ventricular function so that left ventricular stroke volume falls and filling pressures rise. The hemodynamic deterioration is more severe if an atrioventricular conduction disturbance develops or if a mechanical complication such as mitral regurgitation or ventricular septal rupture occurs. A marked depression of left ventricular stroke volume ultimately lowers aortic pressure and reduces coronary perfusion pressure; this condition may intensify myocardial ischemia and thereby initiate a vicious circle (Fig. 39–11). The inability of the left ventricle to empty also leads to an increased preload—that is, it dilates the well-perfused, normally functioning portion of the left ventricle. This compensatory mechanism tends to restore stroke volume to normal levels, but at the expense of a reduced ejection fraction. However, the dilatation of the left ventricle also elevates ventricular afterload, because Laplace's law (p. 377) dictates that at any given arterial pressure the dilated ventricle must develop a higher wall tension. This increased afterload not only depresses left ventricular stroke volume but also elevates myocardial oxygen consumption, which in turn intensifies regional myocardial ischemia. When regional myocardial dysfunction is limited and the function of the remainder of the left ventricle is normal, compensatory mechanisms will sustain overall left ventricular function. If a large portion of the left ventricle becomes necrotic, pump failure occurs; i.e., overall left ventricular function becomes so depressed that the circulation cannot be sustained despite the dilatation of the remaining viable portion of the ventricle.

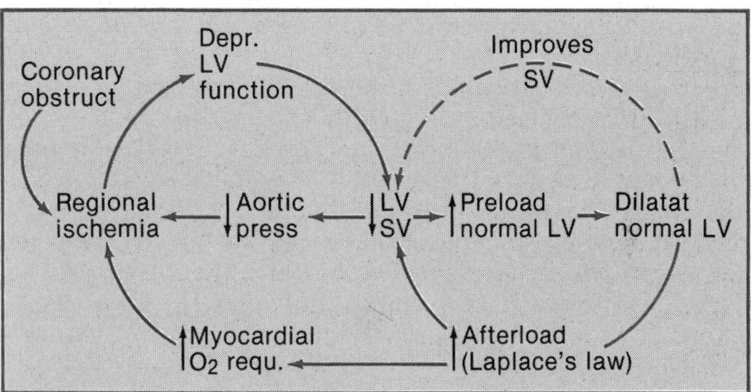

FIGURE 39–10. Changes in circulatory regulation in ischemic heart disease. DEPR. LV FUNCT., depressed left ventricular function; SV, stroke volume; DILATAT., dilatation; O_2 REQU., oxygen requirements. Solid lines indicate that the effect is produced or intensified; broken lines indicate that it is diminished. (Reprinted by permission from Braunwald, E.: Regulation of the circulation. N. Engl. J. Med. *290*:1420, 1974.)

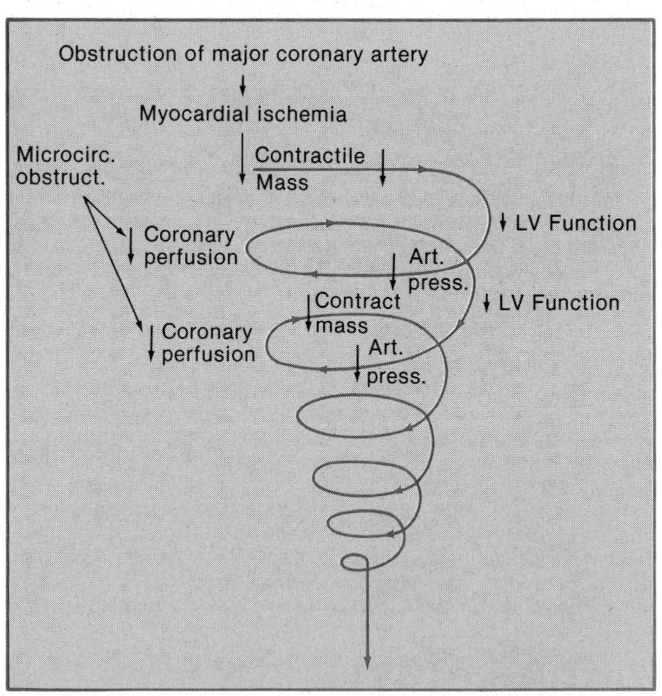

FIGURE 39–11. The sequence of events in the vicious circle in which coronary artery obstruction leads to cardiogenic shock and progressive circulatory deterioration. (From Pasternak, R. C., and Braunwald, E.: Acute myocardial infarction. *In* Wilson, J. D., et al. [eds.]: Harrison's Principles of Internal Medicine. New York, McGraw-Hill Book Co., 1991.)

EFFECTS OF TREATMENT. Some of the consequences of treating pump failure, discussed on page 1252, should be considered. The favorable effect of raising a depressed arterial pressure results from the increased coronary perfusion pressure and the subsequent augmented blood flow across the stenotic areas and through the collateral vessels. This improvement of coronary blood flow may limit the size of the infarction by improving oxygen delivery to the periinfarction zone. In this manner, myocardial fiber shortening may be augmented, thereby increasing stroke volume and cardiac output and elevating arterial pressure.

However, there are also some unfavorable effects of increasing arterial pressure because this intervention usually necessitates an elevation of left ventricular intracavitary pressure (unless it is achieved by a circulatory assist device, such as an intraaortic balloon). The increased afterload causes cardiac dilatation; intramyocardial tension rises, not only because of the higher intraventricular pressure but also because of the cardiac dilatation (p. 376). The increased wall tension augments myocardial oxygen needs and reduces myocardial fiber shortening (p. 425). These changes can cause further ischemia of the marginally viable myocardium adjacent to that supplied exclusively by the occluded vessel, and the area of infarction may be enlarged. Thus, cardiac function may deteriorate further.

It is obvious that the circulation is delicately balanced in patients with AMI. Unless the loss of viable myocardium is so extensive that it precludes survival, or is so small that the patient's survival is not threatened, the outcome may well depend on the clinician's appreciation of the interaction of the many factors that influence circulatory performance and their judicious manipulation.

VENTRICULAR REMODELING

As a consequence of MI, changes in left ventricular size, shape, and thickness involving both the infarcted and the noninfarcted segments of the ventricle often occur. These

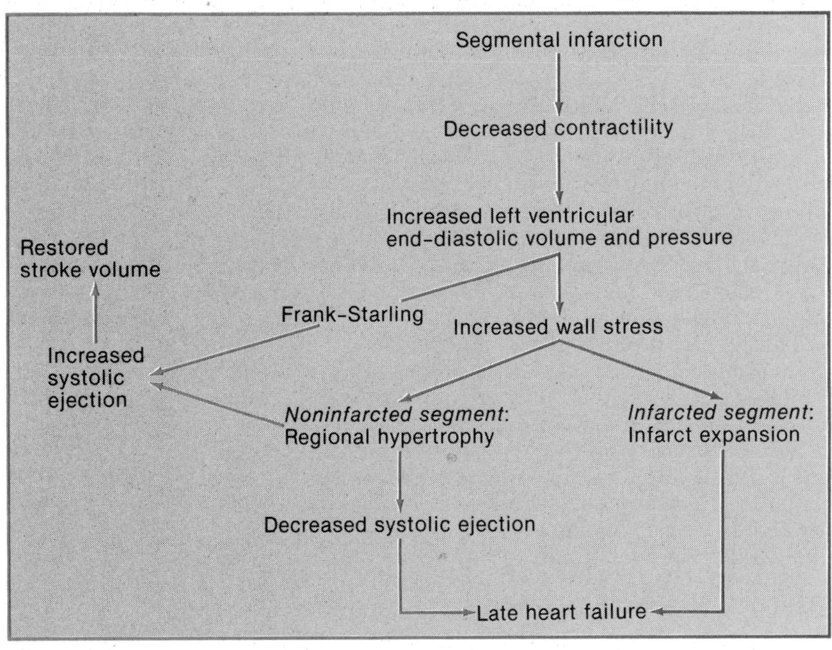

FIGURE 39-12. Hypothesis proposed to account for the mechanisms of left ventricular remodeling. (From McKay, R. G., et al.: Left ventricular remodeling after myocardial infarction: A corollary to infarct expansion. Circulation *74*:693, 1986, by permission of the American Heart Association, Inc.)

changes are referred to as "ventricular remodeling," a process that in turn can influence ventricular function and prognosis.[167]

INFARCT EXPANSION. An increase in the size of the infarcted segment, known as *infarct expansion*, is defined as "acute dilatation and thinning of the area of infarction not explained by additional myocardial necrosis."[168] Infarct expansion appears to be caused by (1) a combination of slippage between muscle bundles, reducing the number of myocytes across the infarct wall; (2) disruption of the normal myocardial cells; and (3) tissue loss within the necrotic zone.[163,169,170] At autopsy, more than one-fourth of hearts of patients succumbing to AMI have severe infarct expansion and wall thinning.[168,171] Infarct expansion occurs almost exclusively in transmural infarcts, is far more common with anterior-apical than with other infarcts, and correlates directly with infarct size.[168,171] The degree of infarct expansion also appears to be related to the preinfarction wall thickness, with existing hypertrophy possibly protecting against infarct thinning.[171] Infarct expansion is associated with both a higher mortality and a higher incidence of nonfatal complications such as heart failure and ventricular aneurysm.[172] Rupture of the ventricle may be considered to be a consequence of extreme infarct expansion.[171,173] Infarct expansion can be recognized echocardiographically as elongation of the noncontractile region of the ventricle.[174]

VENTRICULAR DILATATION. While infarct expansion plays an important role in the ventricular remodeling that occurs in the early weeks following myocardial infarction, remodeling is also caused by dilatation of the viable portion of the ventricle, which commences immediately following AMI, but may progress for months thereafter.[166,175,176,176a] This dilatation may be accompanied by a shift to the right of the pressure-volume curve of the left ventricle, resulting in a larger left ventricular volume at any given diastolic pressure. This dilatation of the noninfarct zone may be viewed as a compensatory mechanism that maintains stroke volume in the face of a large infarction (Fig. 39-12). Following AMI, an extra burden is placed on the residual functioning myocardium,[160] a burden that presumably is responsible for the hypertrophy.[177] This adaptive hypertrophy could help to compensate for the functional impairment caused by the infarct and may be responsible for some of the initial hemodynamic improvement seen in the weeks after infarction in some patients.[178] However, as illustrated in Figure 39-12, adaptive hypertrophy may undergo a transition, with ultimate impairment of contractile function of the viable myocardium in the presence of a large infarction, leading to further cardiac dilatation, loss of global function, and ultimately heart failure.[166]

In *summary*, ventricular remodeling occurs to an increasing extent with larger infarcts. It is a complex process that is not limited to areas of infarction. It begins at the time of AMI and probably continues for months to years, until either a stable hemodynamic state is achieved or progressively severe cardiac decompensation occurs, leading to death from congestive heart failure.

Ventricular remodeling after AMI can be affected by three independent factors, the first of which is infarct size. Acute reperfusion and other measures to restrict the extent of myocardial necrosis limit the increase in ventricular volume following AMI,[178a-180] and there is suggestive evidence that an open infarct artery per se also attenuates ventricular enlargement.[181,182,182a] The second factor is scar formation in the infarct. Glucocorticosteroids and nonsteroidal anti-inflammatory agents given early after MI can cause scar thinning and greater infarct expansion.[183,184] Third is the left ventricular distending pressures in the early post MI period; reduction of this pressure with nitroglycerin[185,186] or an angiotensin-converting enzyme inhibitor[187,187a] attenuates ventricular enlargement (p. 496).

PATHOPHYSIOLOGY OF OTHER ORGAN SYSTEMS IN ACUTE MYOCARDIAL INFARCTION

Alterations in Pulmonary Function

Changes in pulmonary gas exchange, ventilation, and distribution of perfusion all occur with AMI. Hypoxemia is a frequent consequence, with a severity, in general, proportional to that of left ventricular failure. Thus, there is an inverse relation between arterial oxygen tension and pulmonary artery diastolic pressure in patients with AMI. This suggests that increased pulmonary capillary hydrostatic pressure leads to interstitial edema, which results in arteriolar and bronchiolar compression that ultimately causes perfusion of poorly ventilated alveoli with resultant hypoxemia.[188] In addition to hypoxemia, there is a fall in diffusing capacity of carbon monoxide.[189] Hyperventilation often occurs in patients with AMI and may cause hypocapnia and respiratory alkalosis, particularly in restless, anxious patients with pain. Intrapulmonary shunting of blood has been noted in patients in whom left ventricular failure complicates AMI. With reversal of heart failure, hypoxemia and intrapulmonary shunting diminish.

INCREASE IN INTERSTITIAL WATER. A positive correlation has been demonstrated between pulmonary extravascular (interstitial) water content, left ventricular filling pressure, and the clinical signs and symptoms of left ventricular failure.[188] Over a period of 2 to 4 days following AMI, both the pulmonary extravascular water content and the wedge pressure decline. Presumably the increased pulmonary extravascular water represents a transudate secondary to increased pulmonary capillary pressure.

The increase in pulmonary extravascular water may also be responsible for the alterations in pulmonary mechanics observed in patients with AMI, i.e., reduction of airway conductance, pulmonary compliance, forced expiratory volume and midexpiratory flow rate, and an increase in closing volume—the last presumably related to the widespread closure of small, dependent airways during the first 3 days following AMI.[190] Ultimately, severe increases in extravascular water may lead to pulmonary edema (Chap. 20). Recovery of left ventricular function or diuresis reduces abnormally elevated values for closing volumes to normal. Presumably, competition for space between arteries and small airways in the bronchovascular sheath accounts for some of the elevation in airway resistance, particularly at left atrial pressures under 15 mm Hg. Higher left atrial pressures produce increases in airway resistance secondary to interstitial, alveolar, and peribronchial edema.

The "closing volume," i.e., the lung volume at which airway closure commences, can encroach on and sometimes exceed functional residual volume. This can lead to arterial hypoxemia by the shunting of blood through alveoli that are not well ventilated.

REDUCTION OF VITAL CAPACITY. For over 70 years it has been recognized that a fall in vital capacity is related to shortened life expectancy for the cardiac patient. It is now clear that virtually all indices of lung volume—total lung capacity, functional residual capacity, and residual volume, as well as vital capacity—fall in the setting of AMI.[191] These reductions correlate with the elevations of left-sided filling pressure and are most probably due to increases in pulmonary extravascular water. Lung volumes, oxygenation, and airway resistance all return toward normal by the time of discharge for most patients.[191]

Increased pulmonary venous pressure also results in redistribution of pulmonary blood flow from the bases to the apices of the lung in patients with AMI,[192] altering the relationship between ventilation and perfusion. However, at follow-up examination 3 to 25 weeks after MI, the ventilation/perfusion relationship has usually returned to normal or almost so.

REDUCTION OF AFFINITY OF HEMOGLOBIN FOR OXYGEN. In patients with MI, particularly when complicated by left ventricular failure or cardiogenic shock, the affinity of hemoglobin for oxygen is reduced, i.e., the P_{50} is increased.[193] The increase in P_{50} results from increased levels of erythrocyte 2,3-diphosphoglycerate (2,3-DPG), is maximal after 24 hours, and constitutes an important compensatory mechanism, responsible for an estimated 18 per cent increase in oxygen release from oxyhemoglobin in patients with cardiogenic shock.[193]

Alterations in Endocrine Function

PANCREAS. Hyperglycemia and impaired glucose tolerance are common in patients with AMI. Although the absolute levels of blood insulin are often in the normal range in patients with uncomplicated AMI, they are usually inappropriately low for the level of blood sugar elevation, and there may be relative insulin resistance as well.[194] Patients with cardiogenic shock often demonstrate marked hyperglycemia and depressed levels of circulating insulin, often with complete suppression of insulin secretion in response to tolbutamide.[195] These abnormalities in insulin secretion and the resultant impaired glucose tolerance appear to be secondary to a reduction in pancreatic blood flow as a consequence of splanchnic vasoconstriction, which accompanies severe left ventricular failure. In addition, increased activity of the sympathetic nervous system with augmented circulating catecholamines[196] inhibits insulin secretion[197] and augments glycogenolysis, also contributing to the elevation of blood sugar.[198] In fact, hyperglycemia, even without prior diabetes mellitus, is associated with an increased incidence of heart failure following AMI and a high mortality.[199]

Since hypoxic heart muscle derives a considerable portion of its energy from the metabolism of glucose (Chap. 38), and since insulin is essential for the uptake of glucose by the myocardium as well as for myocardial protein synthesis and inhibition of lysosomal activity, the deleterious effects of insulin deficiency are clear.[200]

ADRENAL MEDULLA. Excessive secretion of catecholamines produces many of the characteristic signs and symptoms of AMI. The plasma and urinary catecholamine levels are highest during the first 24 hours after the onset of chest pain,[198] with the greatest rise in plasma catecholamine secretion occurring during the first hour after the onset of MI.[201,201a] These high levels of circulating catecholamines in patients with AMI correlate with the occurrence of serious arrhythmias[197] and result in an increase in myocardial oxygen consumption, both directly and indirectly, as a consequence of catecholamine-induced elevation of circulating free fatty acids.[201] As might be anticipated, the concentration of circulating catecholamines correlates with extent of myocardial damage, incidence of cardiogenic shock, as well as both early and late mortality rates.[197,202]

It is not clear, however, whether the elevation in plasma catecholamines plays some role in determining the amount of myocardium that becomes necrotic or whether this elevation is a consequence of the myocardial damage, i.e., whether it is cause or effect or both. The time course of sympathetic activation, which begins extremely early before extensive myocardial necrosis is present, suggests at least a potential role for these circulating hormones in extending myocardial damage and certainly in the genesis of arrhythmias.[202] Circulating catecholamines enhance platelet aggregation; when this occurs in the coronary microcirculation, the release of the potent vasoconstrictor thromboxane A_2 may further impair cardiac perfusion.[75]

ADRENAL CORTEX. Plasma and urinary 17-hydroxycorticosteroids and ketosteroids, as well as aldosterone, are also markedly elevated in patients with AMI.[198] Their concentrations correlate directly with the peak level of serum glutamic oxaloacetic transaminase and serum creatine kinase,[202] implying that the stress imposed by larger infarcts is associated with greater secretion of adrenal steroids. Glucocorticosteroids also contribute to the impairment of glucose tolerance. Although it has been suggested that the secretion of glucocorticoids is increased, it is inadequate to meet the demands for the stress imposed by a massive AMI, particularly if it is accompanied by cardiogenic shock.[198]

THYROID GLAND. Although patients with AMI are generally euthyroid, there is evidence for a significant transient decrease in serum T_3 levels, a fall that is most marked on about the third day after the infarct.[203,204] This fall in T_3 is usually accompanied by a rise in reverse T_3 with variable changes or no change in T_4 and TSH levels. The alteration in peripheral thyroxin metabolism appears to correlate with infarct size[203] and may be mediated by the rise in endogenous levels of cortisol that accompanies AMI.[204]

Hematological Function

ALTERATIONS IN PLATELETS. AMI generally occurs in the presence of extensive coronary and systemic atherosclerotic plaques, which may serve as the site for the formation of platelet aggregates, a sequence that has been suggested as the initial step in the process of coronary thrombosis, coronary occlusion, and subsequent MI. Circulating platelets are hyperaggregable in patients with AMI.[76] Approximately one-third of these patients demonstrate shortened platelet survival times.[205] Types III and IV hyperlipoproteinemia, frequently present in patients with AMI, can also be responsible for shortening platelet survival. Findings suggestive of a hypercoagulable state as a risk factor for AMI are discussed on page 1779, and the role of platelets in AMI is discussed on page 1206. A wide variety of platelet abnormalities have been described, including, most recently, an increase in thromboxane A_2 receptors on platelets from AMI patients.[206]

COAGULATION TESTS. Elevated levels of serum fibrinogen degradation products, an end product of thrombosis[207]—as well as release of distinctive proteins when platelets are activated, i.e., platelet factor 4[208] and beta thromboglobulin[209]—have been reported in some patients with AMI. Fibrinopeptide A, a protein released from fibrin by thrombin, is a marker of ongoing thrombosis and is elevated during the early hours of AMI.[210,211] In fact, markedly elevated levels of fibrinopeptide A may be a marker for coronary reocclusion after initially successful thrombolytic therapy.[211-213] The interpretation of the coagulation tests in patients with AMI may be complicated by elevated blood levels of catecholamines, concomitant shock, and/or pulmonary embolism, conditions which are all capable of altering various tests of platelet and coagulation function.[214] Thus, it is not yet clear whether the aforementioned changes are the causes or consequences of AMI.

LEUKOCYTES. AMI is usually accompanied by leukocytosis that is thought to be related both to the necrotic process and its magnitude, in which leukocytes play an active role, and to their stimulation by elevated glucocorticoids that occur with infarction. It is now recognized that leukocytes also participate in the thrombotic process.[215] Activation of neutrophils may produce important intermediates, such as leukotriene B_4 and oxygen free radicals,[216,217] that have important microcirculatory effects.[215]

BLOOD VISCOSITY. An increase in blood viscosity also occurs in patients with AMI. During the first few days after infarction, this is mainly attributable to hemoconcentration, but later the increases in plasma viscosity and red cell aggregation correlate with elevated serum concentrations of alpha$_2$ globulin and fibrinogen, which are nonspecific reactions to tissue necrosis and which are also responsible for the elevated sedimentation rate characteristic of AMI.[218] The high values of blood viscosity indices are observed most frequently in patients with complications such as left ventricular failure, cardiogenic shock, and thromboembolism.

OTHER BIOCHEMICAL TESTS. Over the years, many isolated abnormal blood chemistries have been reported in patients with AMI. Many have not led to further understanding of the pathophysiology of AMI or have not been confirmed in subsequent studies. New abnormalities are regularly reported— recent examples include decreased selenium[219] and pyridoxal 5′-phosphate (a metabolite of vitamin B6) levels.[220] The importance of both is unknown at present.

ALTERATIONS IN RENAL FUNCTION

Both prerenal azotemia and acute renal failure can complicate the marked reduction of cardiac output that occurs in cardiogenic shock. A physiological compensation for this occurs with the increase in atrial natriuretic peptide seen following AMI, an increase that is correlated with the degree of left ventricular failure present.[221] An increase in atrial natriuretic peptide is also found when right ventricular infarction accompanies inferior wall infarction, suggesting that this neurohumoral abnormality may play a role in the hemodynamic disturbances of the right ventricular infarction syndrome (p. 412).[222]

Clinical Features of Acute Myocardial Infarction

PRECIPITATING FACTORS

In about one-half of patients with AMI, no precipitating factor can be identified.[217a] An early study noted the following patient activities at the onset of AMI: heavy physical exertion, 13 per cent; modest or usual exertion, 18 per cent; surgical procedure, 6 per cent; rest, 51 per cent; and sleep, 8 per cent.[223] A more recent study has confirmed the importance of physical activity and pointed to emotional stress (in about 18 per cent of patients) as another important trigger of AMI.[224] Others, too, have reported that a significant number of AMIs occur within a few hours of severe physical exertion.[225,226] It has been pointed out that the *severe exertion* that preceded an infarction was often performed at times when the patient was unduly fatigued or emotionally stressed.[227] Exertion before infarction is somewhat more common among patients without preexisting angina than in patients who have had a history of angina.[228] Thus, although adequate control studies have not been carried out, there is *suggestive* evidence that heavy exercise may play a precipitating role in some patients. Such infarctions could be the result of marked increases in myocardial oxygen consumption in the presence of severe coronary arterial narrowing. Alternatively, exertion or mental stress may trigger plaque disruption, initiating a cascade of events leading to AMI. Such a scenario has been proposed by Muller[62] and is illustrated in Figure 39–13.

Surgical procedures associated with acute blood loss have also been noted as precursors of AMI (p. 1711). Reduced myocardial perfusion secondary to hypotension and increased myocardial oxygen demands secondary to fever, tachycardia, and agitation are presumably responsible for the myocardial necrosis. Other factors reported as predisposing to AMI include respiratory infections, hypoxemia of any cause, pulmonary embolism, hypoglycemia, administration of ergot preparations, serum sickness, allergy, and wasp stings.[229,230] In patients with Prinzmetal's angina (p. 1342), AMI may develop in the territory of the coronary artery, which repeatedly undergoes spasm.[231] Rarely, munition workers exposed to high concentrations of nitroglycerin may develop myocardial infarction when they are withdrawn from this exposure, suggesting that it is caused by vasospasm.[141] Accelerating angina and rest angina, two forms of unstable angina, may culminate as infarction of the myocardium, again in the distribution of the affected vessel.[231]

Considerable evidence has accumulated that *emotional stresses* may be a precipitating factor in the initiation of AMI.[224,232] A number of reports have documented that upsetting life events occur commonly in patients who subsequently suffer an MI.[233] Such events have been quantified and scored as *Life Change Units*. Rahe and coworkers noted, on retrospective analysis, a significant buildup of Life Change Units in patients who subsequently suffered myocardial infarction or died suddenly.[233]

Trauma may precipitate an AMI in one of two ways. Myocardial contusion and hemorrhage into the myocardium may actually cause cell necrosis, or the injury may involve a coronary artery, causing occlusion of that vessel with resultant MI (Chap. 46). *Neurological disturbances* (transient ischemic attacks or strokes) may also precipitate AMI.[234]

CIRCADIAN PERIODICITY. An analysis of a large number of patients hospitalized with myocardial infarction, studied as part of the Multicenter Investigation of Limitation of Infarct Size (MILIS), has revealed a pronounced circadian periodicity for the time of onset of AMI.[235] In this retrospective review, a peak incidence of onset at about 9 AM was found when timing was estimated from either the occurrence of symptoms or from the first elevation of plasma creatine kinase MB (Fig. 39–14, *top*). This has been confirmed by other studies[236,237] such as a large World Health Organization report.[238] This early morning peak in MI parallels the onset of other related phenomena including sudden cardiac death,[239] thrombotic stroke,[240] and transient myocardial ischemia[241,242] (p. 1294) (Fig. 39–14, *bottom 3 panels*). Circadian rhythms affect many physiological and biochemical parameters; the

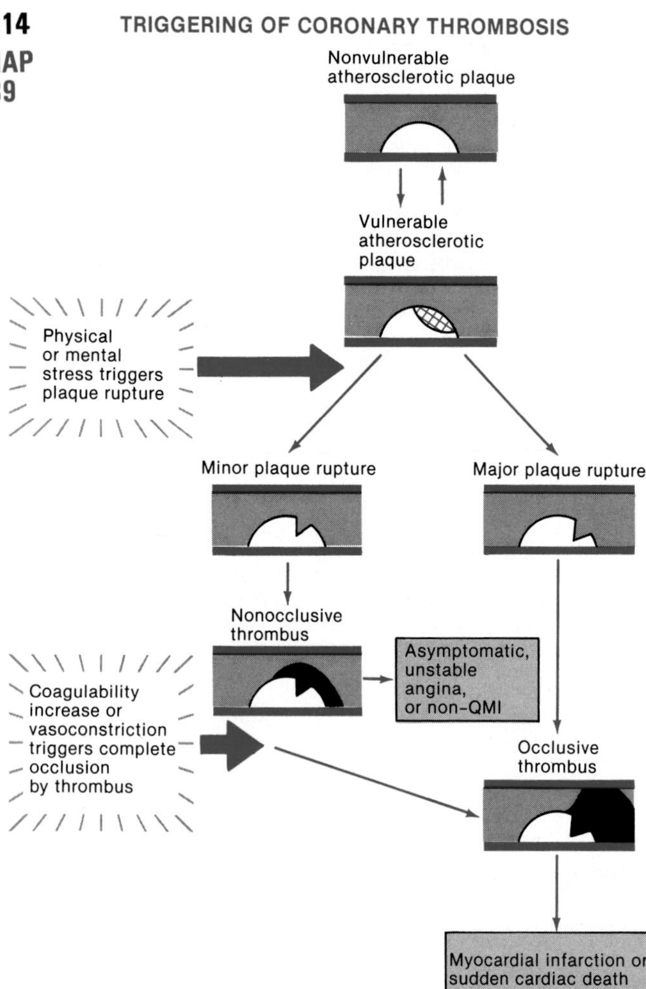

FIGURE 39–13. Schematic illustration of a hypothetical method by which daily activities may *trigger* coronary thrombosis. Three triggering mechanisms, (1) physical or mental stress producing hemodynamic changes leading to plaque rupture, (2) activities causing a coagulability increase, and (3) stimuli leading to vasoconstriction, have been added to the scheme depicting the role of coronary thrombosis in unstable angina, myocardial infarction, and sudden cardiac death. (From Muller, J. E., et al.: Circadian variation and triggers of onset of acute cardiovascular disease. Circulation *79*:733, 1989, by permission of the American Heart Association, Inc.)

early morning hours are associated with rises in plasma catecholamines and cortisol and increases in platelet aggregability. Interestingly, the characteristic circadian peak was *absent* in patients receiving beta blocker or aspirin therapy before their presentation with AMI.[243,244] In addition to beta blockade and aspirin, previous heart failure or MI, history of smoking or diabetes, and non-Q-wave infarction have all been identified as blunting this circadian variability in AMI.[245] Nevertheless, it appears possible that some cyclical aspects of combined vasospastic and prothrombotic factors, in the setting of preexisting atherosclerosis, can lead to AMI. The apparent relationship between a patient's biological rhythm and the onset of AMI appears to be of both pathophysiological and clinical importance.

CLINICAL HISTORY

PRODROMAL SYMPTOMS. Despite recent advances in the laboratory detection of AMI, the history remains of substantial value in establishing a diagnosis. A prodromal history can be elicited in 20 to 60 per cent of patients with AMI.[246,247] The prodrome is usually characterized by chest discomfort, resembling classic angina pectoris (described on pp. 4 and 1215), but it occurs at rest or with less activity than usual and can therefore be classified as unstable angina. However, the latter is often not disturbing enough to induce patients to seek medical attention, and if they do, they may not be hospitalized. Among patients who are hospitalized for unstable an-

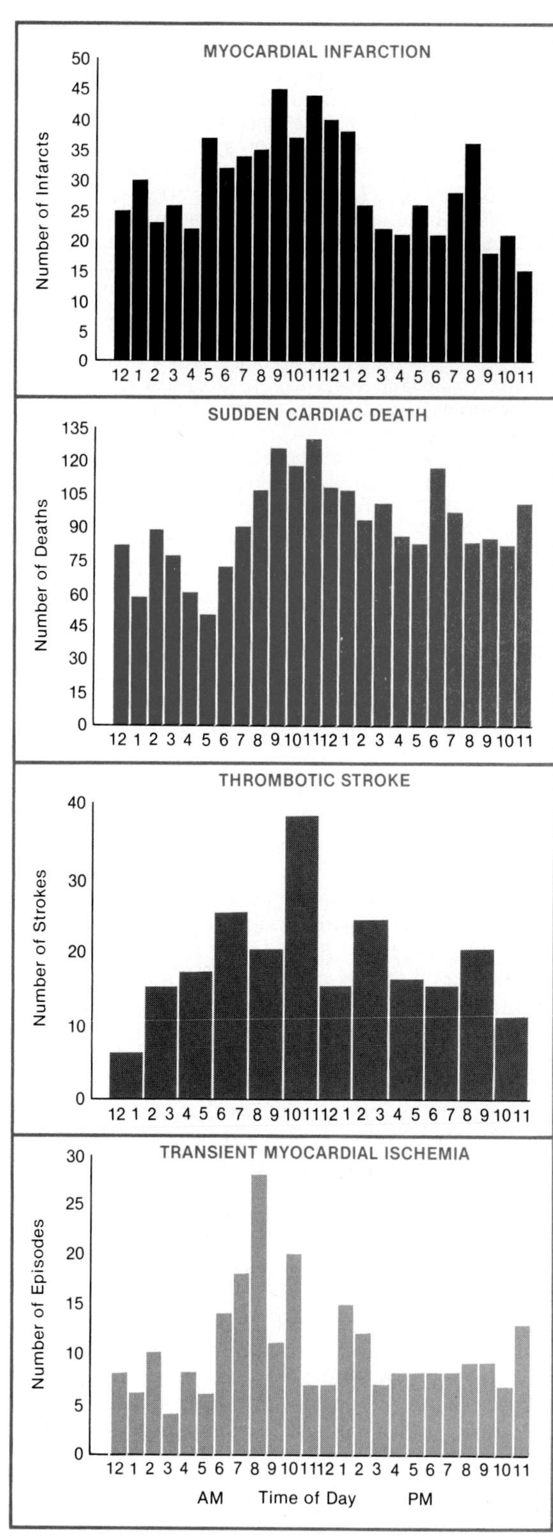

FIGURE 39–14. Bar graphs of time of day of onset of myocardial infarction, sudden cardiac death, stroke, and transient myocardial ischemia in four different groups of patients. The number of events is shown on the y axis and the hour of the day on the x axis. Note that each of the disorders exhibits a prominent increase in frequency of onset in the period from 6 AM to noon. (From Muller, J. E., et al.: Circadian variation and triggers of onset of acute cardiovascular disease. Circulation *79*:733, 1989, by permission of the American Heart Association, Inc.)

gina, fewer than 15 per cent develop AMI (p. 1341). Of the patients with AMI presenting with prodromal symptoms of unstable angina, approximately one-third have had symptoms from 1 to 4 weeks before hospitalization; in the remaining two-thirds, symptoms predated admission by a week or less, with one-third of these patients (20 per cent of all with prodromes) having had symptoms for 24 hours or less.[248]

NATURE OF THE PAIN. The pain of AMI is variable in intensity; in most patients it is severe and, in some instances, intolerable. The pain is prolonged, usually lasting for more than 30 minutes and frequently for a number of hours. The discomfort is described as constricting, crushing, oppressing, or compressing; often the patient complains of something sitting on or squeezing the chest. Although usually described as a squeezing, choking, viselike, or heavy pain, it may also be characterized as a stabbing, knifelike, boring, or burning discomfort. The pain is usually retrosternal in location, spreading frequently to both sides of the anterior chest, with predilection for the left side. Often the pain radiates down the ulnar aspect of the left arm, producing a tingling sensation in the left wrist, hand, and even fingers. Some patients note only a dull ache or numbness of the wrists in association with severe substernal or precordial discomfort. In some instances, the pain of AMI may begin in the epigastrium and simulate a variety of abdominal disorders, a fact which often causes MI to be misdiagnosed as "indigestion." In other patients the discomfort of AMI radiates to the shoulders, upper extremities, neck, jaw, and interscapular region, again usually favoring the left side. In patients with preexisting angina pectoris, the pain of infarction usually resembles that of angina with respect to quality and location. However, it is generally much more severe, lasts longer, and is not relieved by rest and nitroglycerin.

What follows is a lucid, personal, published description of the pain of AMI, provided by a distinguished, experienced physician:

> During the first 15 to 20 minutes when the pain was waxing and waning, I was pretending it was esophageal and popping a few Tums and drinking a glass of milk. After this, the pain certainly told me just what it seems to have told other patients. I felt I must sit down very, very quietly. Although I did so, the pain became a steadily expanding, deep, penetrating ache spreading from beneath mid-breast bone, around the sides of my chest, up my neck into my lower jaw, and down the inner aspect of my left arm into my fourth and fifth fingers. It cycled a bit. Sometimes it seemed most dreadful in my chest—then in my jaw and lower teeth—then in my left arm. But it conveyed one clear message. What I thought from the outset and continued to think through about 2 hours of what seemed absolutely intolerable pain was that if I remained *absolutely* immobile, not moving even an eyelash, perhaps it would let go of me. I would guess it took about 10 to 12 minutes to build to maximal intensity and there it stayed. During the entire period I sat absolutely still with my eyes closed, conscious of the fact that I was sweating profusely and that I probably looked very pale and lousy. Although my wife was bustling cheerfully about in the kitchen not 15 feet away, I said absolutely nothing, feeling that even moving my tongue or vocal chords was simply too much. There was no inclination to groan or cry out.
>
> There was another aspect of the pain frequently alluded to by others. There was absolutely no doubt in my mind that I was about to die. As the pain remained, I simply wished exodus would go ahead and happen. . . . The quality of the pain is as difficult for me to describe as it seems to have been for other observers over the last 70 plus years. It was not the bright or burning or well-localized pain one feels with a cut, a puncture, or a burn, from which one instinctively and swiftly retreats. A very difficult set of nerve endings is involved. It was a dreadful, deep, nauseating ache. If you would try multiplying a hundredfold the kind of ache you experience after working too long trying to screw a recalcitrant light bulb into a ceiling socket that's a little too high over your head to reach decently, you would be close. . . .
>
> As to intensity, I keep wanting to use the word *unbearable*. Obviously, this word is not really appropriate, as I did manage somehow to bear the pain. But it was an absolutely monstrous, awful sensation, and it was totally untouched by 20 or 30 or 40 milligrams of morphine administered to me over the next 2 hours. That morphine gave so little relief has made me empathize deeply with the hundreds of patients with the same disease I've treated with this drug over the years.[249]

In some patients, particularly the elderly, AMI is manifested clinically not by chest pain but rather by symptoms of acute left ventricular failure and chest tightness or by overwhelming weakness, accompanied by diaphoresis, nausea, vomiting, and diarrhea.[234] The pain of AMI may have disappeared by the time the physician first encounters the patient (or the patient reaches the hospital), or it may persist for many hours. Opiates—in particular, morphine—usually relieve the pain, although a persistent soreness, pressure, or dull ache may remain for several hours or more despite intensive treatment with analgesics. The longer a patient requires analgesic administration after hospital admission for ischemic pain, the more likely that MI will be confirmed in that patient.[250] Both angina pectoris and the pain of AMI are thought to arise from nerve endings in ischemic or injured, but not necrotic, myocardium.[251] Thus, in MI, stimulation of nerve fibers in an ischemic zone of myocardium surrounding the necrotic central area of infarction probably gives rise to the pain.

It has been suggested that the phenomenon of referred pain is modulated by the spatial and temporal patterns of excitation of these afferent sympathetic fibers as well as a variable contribution of vagal afferent fibers.[252] Experience with patients undergoing procedures to reperfuse myocardium in the setting of AMI suggests that pain often disappears suddenly and completely once blood flow to the infarct territory is restored.[253] In patients in whom reocclusion occurs after thrombolysis, pain recurs if the initial reperfusion has left viable myocardium. Thus, what has previously been thought of as the "pain of infarction," sometimes lasting for many hours, probably represents pain caused by ongoing ischemia. The recognition that pain implies ischemia and not inevitable infarction has important clinical ramifications and heightens the importance of seeking ways to relieve the ischemia, for which the pain is a marker. This finding suggests that the clinician should not be complacent about ongoing cardiac pain under any circumstances.

OTHER SYMPTOMS. Nausea and vomiting occur in more than 50 per cent of patients with transmural MI and severe chest pain,[254] presumably owing to activation of vagal reflex or to stimulation of left ventricular receptors as part of the Bezold-Jarisch reflex (p. 1167).[255] These symptoms occur more commonly in patients with inferior MI than in those with anterior MI. Occasionally a patient complains of diarrhea or a violent urge to evacuate the bowels during the acute phase of MI. Moreover, nausea and vomiting are common side effects of opiates. When the pain of AMI is epigastric in location and is associated with nausea and vomiting, the clinical picture may easily be confused with that of acute cholecystitis, gastritis, or peptic ulcer. Other symptoms include feelings of profound weakness, dizziness, palpitations, cold perspiration, and a sense of impending doom. On occasion, symptoms arising from an episode of cerebral embolism or other systemic arterial embolism are the first signs of an AMI. Rarely, patients with inferior infarction report intractable hiccupping, a finding which has been attributed to diaphragmatic irritation by the infarct. The aforementioned symptoms may or may not be accompanied by chest pain.[256] Finally, the feeling of general malaise or frank exhaustion often accompanies other symptoms preceding AMI.[257]

DIFFERENTIAL DIAGNOSIS. The pain of AMI may simulate the pain of *acute pericarditis* (p. 1469), which is usually associated with some pleuritic features, i.e., it is aggravated by respiratory movements and coughing and often involves the shoulder, ridge of the trapezius, and neck. *Pleural pain* is usually sharp, knifelike, and aggravated by each breath, which distinguishes it from the deep, dull, steady pain of AMI. *Pulmonary embolism* (Chap. 48) generally produces pain laterally in the chest, is often pleuritic in nature, and may be associated with hemoptysis. The pain due to *acute dissection of the aorta* (p. 1535) is usually localized in the center of the chest, is extremely severe, persists for many hours, and often radiates to the back and sometimes into the legs. Often one or more major arterial pulses are absent. Pain arising from the *costochondral and chondrosternal articulations* may be associated with localized swelling and redness; it is usually sharp and "darting" and is characterized by marked localized tenderness.

SILENT MI AND ATYPICAL PRESENTATION. Population studies suggest that between 20 and 60 per cent of nonfatal MIs are unrecognized by the patient and are discovered only on subsequent routine electrocardiographic[258,259] or postmortem examinations. Of these unrecognized infarctions, approximately half are truly silent, with the patients unable to recall any symptoms whatsoever referable to the infarction. The other half of patients with so-called silent infarction can recall an event characterized by symptoms compatible with acute infarction when leading questions are posed after the electrocardiographic abnormalities are discovered. Unrecognized or silent infarction occurs more commonly in patients without antecedent angina pectoris and is more common in patients with diabetes and hypertension,[258] although the association with diabetes is controversial. Silent MI is often followed by silent ischemia (p. 1347).

In an analysis of atypical presentations of AMI, Bean[260] lists the following: (1) congestive heart failure—beginning de novo or worsening of established failure; (2) classic angina pectoris without a particularly severe or prolonged attack; (3) atypical location of the pain; (4) central nervous system manifestations, resembling those of stroke, secondary to a sharp reduction in cardiac output in a patient with cerebral arteriosclerosis; (5) apprehension and nervousness; (6) sudden mania or psychosis; (7) syncope; (8) overwhelming weakness; (9) acute indigestion; and (10) peripheral embolism.

PHYSICAL EXAMINATION

GENERAL APPEARANCE. Patients suffering an AMI often appear anxious and in considerable distress. An anguished facial expression is common, and—in contrast to patients with angina pectoris, who often lie, sit, or stand quite still, realizing that all forms of activity increase the discomfort—patients suffering an AMI may be restless and move about in an effort to find a comfortable position. Others, like the physician who described his own symptoms (p. 1215), prefer to sit still. They often massage or clutch their chests and frequently describe their pain with a clenched fist held against the sternum. In patients with left ventricular failure and sympathetic stimulation, cold perspiration and skin pallor may be evident; they usually sit or are propped up in bed, gasping for breath. Between breaths, they may complain of chest discomfort or a feeling of suffocation. Cough production of frothy, pink, or blood-streaked sputum is common.

Patients in cardiogenic shock often lie listlessly, making few if any spontaneous movements. The skin is cool and clammy, with a bluish or mottled color over the extremities, and there is marked facial pallor with severe cyanosis of the lips and nailbeds. Depending on the degree of cerebral perfusion, the patient in shock may converse normally or may evidence confusion and disorientation. The patient is often anxious and frightened but may profess interest in only minimal communication.

VITAL SIGNS. The heart rate may vary from a marked bradycardia to rapid regular or irregular tachycardia, depending on the underlying rhythm and the degree of left ventricular failure. Most commonly, the pulse is rapid and regular initially (sinus tachycardia at 100 to 110 beats/min), slowing as the patient's pain and anxiety are relieved; premature ventricular beats are common, occurring in more than 95 per cent of patients evaluated early after the onset of symptoms.

Blood Pressure. The majority of patients with uncomplicated AMI are normotensive, although the reduced stroke volume accompanying the tachycardia may cause declines in systolic and pulse pressures and elevation of diastolic pressure. Among previously normotensive patients, a hypertensive response occasionally is seen, with the arterial pressure exceeding 160/90 mm Hg, presumably as a consequence of adrenergic discharge secondary to pain and agitation. It is rather common for previously hypertensive patients to become normotensive without treatment following AMI, although approximately two-thirds of these previously hypertensive patients eventually regain their elevated levels of blood pressure, generally 3 to 6 months after infarction. In patients with massive infarcts, arterial pressure falls acutely, owing to left ventricular dysfunction and venous pooling secondary to administration of morphine or nitrates or both; as recovery occurs, the arterial pressure tends to return to preinfarction levels. Patients in cardiogenic shock (p. 579), by definition, have systolic pressures below 90 mm Hg. However, hypotension does not necessarily signify cardiogenic shock, since some patients with inferior infarction, in whom the Bezold-Jarisch reflex is activated, may also have systolic blood pressure below 90 mm Hg.[261] Their prognosis is generally good and their hypotension eventually resolves spontaneously, although this resolution can be accelerated by atropine and assumption of the reverse Trendelenburg position. Other patients who are initially only slightly hypotensive may demonstrate gradually falling blood pressures with progressive reduction in cardiac output over several hours or days as they gradually develop cardiogenic shock as a consequence of increasing ischemia and extension of infarction (Fig. 38–11). Evidence of autonomic hyperactivity is common, varying in type with the location of the infarction. At some time in their initial presentation, more than half of patients with inferior MI have evidence of excess parasympathetic stimulation, with hypotension, bradycardia, or both, while about half of patients with anterior MI show signs of sympathetic excess, having hypertension, tachycardia, or both.[262]

Temperature and Respiration. Most patients with AMI develop *fever*, a nonspecific response to tissue necrosis, within 24 to 48 hours of the onset of infarction. Body temperature often begins to rise within 4 to 8 hours after the onset of infarction, and rectal temperature often reaches 101 to 102°F. Fever usually resolves by the seventh or eighth day following infarction.

The *respiratory rate* may be slightly elevated soon after the development of an AMI; in patients without heart failure, it results from anxiety and pain, since it returns to normal with treatment of physical and psychological discomfort. In patients with left ventricular failure, the respiratory rate correlates with the severity of failure; patients with pulmonary edema may have respiratory rates exceeding 40 per minute. However, the respiratory rate is not necessarily elevated in patients with cardiogenic shock. Cheyne-Stokes (periodic) respiration (p. 454) may occur in elderly individuals with cardiogenic shock and heart failure, particularly after opiate therapy and in the presence of cerebrovascular disease.

JUGULAR VENOUS PULSE. The height and contour of the jugular venous pulse reflect right atrial and right ventricular diastolic pressures (p. 18). Since these pressures are usually normal or only slightly elevated in patients with AMI (even in the presence of mild to moderate left ventricular failure), it is not surprising that usually the jugular venous pulse does not appear to be abnormal. The *a* wave may be prominent in patients with pulmonary hypertension secondary to left ventricular failure or reduced compliance. In contrast, right ventricular infarction (whether or not it accompanies left ventricular infarction) often results in marked jugular venous distention and, when it is complicated by necrosis or ischemia of right ventricular papillary muscles, tall *v* waves of tricuspid regurgitation are evident. In patients with AMI and cardiogenic shock, the jugular venous pressure is usually elevated. In patients with AMI, hypotension, and hypoperfusion, whose signs may specifically resemble those of patients with cardiogenic shock but who have flat neck veins, it is likely that the depression of left ventricular performance may be related, at least in part, to hypovolemia, but the differentiation can be made only by assessing left ventricular performance.

CAROTID PULSE. Palpation of the carotid arterial pulse provides a clue to the left ventricular stroke volume; a small pulse suggests a reduced stroke volume, whereas a sharp, brief upstroke is often observed in patients with mitral regurgitation or ruptured ventricular septum with a left-to-right shunt. Pulsus alternans reflects severe left ventricular dysfunction.

THE CHEST. Moist rales are audible in patients who develop left ventricular failure and/or a reduction of left ventricular compliance with AMI. Diffuse wheezing may be present in patients with severe left ventricular failure. Cough with hemoptysis, suggesting pulmonary embolism with infarction, may also occur. In 1967 Killip proposed a prognostic classification scheme based on the presence and severity of rales detected in patients presenting with AMI. Class I patients are free of rales and a third heart sound. Class II patients have rales but to only a mild-moderate degree (<50 per cent of lung fields) and may or may not have an S_3. Patients in Class III have rales in more than half of each lung field and frequently have pulmonary edema. Finally, Class IV patients are in cardiogenic shock. Despite overall improvement in mortality in each class, this classification remains useful today as evidenced by data from a recent large MI trial.[263]

CARDIAC EXAMINATION. Despite severe symptoms and extensive myocardial damage, the findings on examination of the heart may be surprisingly unremarkable in patients with AMI.[264] Palpation of the precordium may yield normal findings but more commonly reveals (in patients with sinus rhythm) a presystolic pulsation, synchronous with an audible fourth heart sound, reflecting a vigorous left atrial contraction filling a ventricle with reduced compliance. In the presence of left ventricular systolic dysfunction, an outward movement of the left ventricle may be palpated in early diastole, coincident with a third heart sound. When the anterior or lateral portion of the ventricle is dyskinetic, an abnormal systolic pulsation is present in the third, fourth, or fifth interspace to the left of the sternum. In some patients, this abnormal paradoxical precordial impulse is clearly separable from the point of maximal impulse, which is more lateral and to the left. In other patients, the abnormal impulse is a diffuse, rippling, precordial movement, approximately 5 to 10 cm in diameter, not clearly separable from the point of maximal impulse. Patients with longstanding hypertension or previous infarction with left ventricular hypertrophy often demonstrate a laterally displaced, sustained apical impulse.

Auscultation. The heart sounds, particularly the first sound, are frequently muffled and occasionally inaudible immediately after the infarct, and their intensity increases as healing occurs. A soft first sound may also reflect prolongation of the P-R interval. Patients with marked ventricular dysfunction and/or left bundle branch block may have paradoxical splitting of the second heart sound (p. 47). Individuals with postinfarction angina also may develop transient, paradoxically split second heart sounds during anginal episodes because of prolongation of the left ventricular preejection period.

A *fourth heart sound* is almost universally present in patients in sinus rhythm with AMI and is usually best heard between the left sternal border and the apex. This sound reflects atrial contraction and a reduction in left ventricular compliance (p. 50) and is associated with an elevation of left ventricular end-diastolic pressure, even in the absence of left ventricular systolic dysfunction. It is of little diagnostic value, since it is commonly audible in most patients with chronic ischemic heart disease and is recordable, although not often audible, in many normal subjects older than 45 years.

A *third heart sound* in AMI usually reflects extensive left ventricular dysfunction. It is usually heard in patients with large infarctions. This sound is heard best at the apex, with the patient in the left lateral recumbent position, and is more common in patients with transmural anterior infarctions than in those with inferior or nontransmural infarctions.[265] Patients with a third heart sound often have elevated left ventricular filling pressure. The mortality of patients who manifest a third heart sound during the acute phase of MI is higher than that of patients without such a sound.[265] A third sound may be caused not only by left ventricular failure but also by increased inflow into the left ventricle, as occurs when mitral regurgitation or ventricular septal defect complicates AMI. Third and fourth heart sounds emanating from the left ventricle are heard best at the apex; in patients with right ventricular infarcts, these sounds may be heard along the left sternal border and are intensified by inspiration.

Systolic murmurs, transient or persistent, are commonly audible in patients with AMI and generally result from mitral regurgitation secondary to papillary muscle dysfunction or left ventricular dilatation. A new, prominent holosystolic murmur at the apex, accompanied by a thrill, may represent rupture of a head of a papillary muscle (p. 1259). The findings in rupture of the interventricular septum are similar, although the murmur and thrill are usually most prominent along the left sternal border while being audible at the right sternal border as well. The systolic murmur of tricuspid regurgitation (caused by right ventricular failure due to pulmonary hypertension and/or right ventricular infarction or by infarction of a right ventricular papillary muscle) is also heard along the left sternal border but is characteristically intensified by inspiration and is accompanied by a prominent *v* wave in the jugular venous pulse. A *continuous murmur* is an unusual finding in AMI that may occur as a result of a variety of congenital abnormalities including a coronary artery arteriovenous fistula, an extremely rare cause of myocardial ischemia or infarction.[266]

Pericardial friction rubs are audible in 7 to 20 per cent of all patients with AMI and in a higher percentage of patients with transmural infarcts.[267] Rubs are notorious for their evanescence and, hence, are probably even more common than reported; frequent auscultation in patients with transmural infarction often results in the discovery of a rub which might otherwise have gone unnoticed. Although friction rubs may be heard by 24 hours or as late as 2 weeks after the onset of infarction, most commonly they are noted on the second or third day.[267] Occasionally, in patients with extensive infarction, a loud rub may be heard for many days. About 40 per cent of patients with a friction rub in the setting of AMI have a pericardial effusion on echocardiographic study[268] but only rarely are the classic electrocardiographic changes of pericarditis (p. 158) seen.[267] Delayed onset of the rub and the associated discomfort of pericarditis (as late as 3 months postinfarction) are characteristic of the postmyocardial infarction (Dressler) syndrome (p. 1263).[268–270]

Pericardial rubs are most readily audible along the left sternal border or just inside the point of maximal impulse and occur after either anterior or inferoposterior transmural infarction. Loud rubs may be audible over the entire precordium and even over the back. Occasionally, only the systolic portion of a rub is heard; it may be confused with a systolic murmur, and the diagnosis of rupture of the ventricular septum or mitral regurgitation may be considered. The presence of a pericardial friction rub does not exclude the presence of a significant pericardial effusion.

THE FUNDI. Hypertension, diabetes, and generalized atherosclerosis commonly accompany AMI, and since these conditions may produce characteristic changes in the fundus, a careful funduscopic examination may provide information concerning the underlying vascular status; this is particularly useful in patients unable to provide a detailed history.

THE ABDOMEN. As already noted, in patients with AMI (particularly inferior infarcts) with diaphragmatic irritation, the pain may localize in the epigastrium or the right upper quadrant. Pain in the abdomen associated with nausea, vomiting, restlessness, and even abdominal distention is often interpreted by patients as a sign of "indigestion,"[260] resulting in self-medication with antacids, and it may suggest an acute abdominal process to the physician. A normal abdominal examination aids in ruling this out and in pointing to the correct diagnosis. Right heart failure, characterized by hepatomegaly and a positive abdomino-jugular reflux, is unusual in patients with acute left ventricular infarction but does occur in patients with severe and usually prolonged left ventricular failure or right ventricular infarction.

THE EXTREMITIES. Coronary atherosclerosis is often associated with systemic atherosclerosis, and it is therefore common for patients with AMI to have a history of intermittent claudication and to demonstrate physical findings of peripheral vascular disease. Thus, diminished peripheral arterial pulses, loss of hair, and atrophic skin in the lower extremities are noted frequently in patients with coronary artery disease. Peripheral edema is a manifestation of right ventricular failure and, like congestive hepatomegaly, is unusual in patients with acute left ventricular infarction. Cyanosis of the nailbeds is common in patients with severe left ventricular failure and is particularly striking in patients with cardiogenic shock.

NEUROPSYCHIATRIC FINDINGS. Except for the altered mental status that occurs in patients with AMI who have a markedly reduced cardiac output and cerebral hypoperfusion, the neurological examination is normal unless the patient has suffered cerebral embolism secondary to a mural thrombus. Indeed, an underlying MI is common in patients with cerebral embolic stroke. There is an increased coincidence of cerebrovascular accidents and AMI. In a prospective study of patients with cerebrovascular accidents admitted to the hospital within 72 hours of the onset, 12.7 per cent have an associated AMI; in contrast, in a series of patients with AMI, only 1.7 per cent suffered a stroke. The coincidence was confined to patients with large myocardial infarcts as reflected in markedly elevated serum creatine kinase concentrations.[271] The coincidence between these two conditions may be explained by systemic hypotension due to MI precipitating a cerebral infarction and the converse, as well as by mural emboli from the heart causing cerebral emboli.

Patients with AMI often exhibit alterations of the emotional state, including intense anxiety, denial, and depression.

LABORATORY EXAMINATIONS

ENZYMES

Irreversibly injured myocardial cells release a number of enzymes into the circulation (Fig. 39–15), where they can be measured by specific chemical reactions (p. 1188).[272] Increased activities of many enzymes have been found in the serum or plasma of patients with AMI.[273] Following experimental MI, a small but significant myocardial venoarterial difference of enzyme activity can be measured, and elevated plasma levels of enzymes correlate with corresponding depletion of these same enzymes from infarcted tissue.[274] Determinations of serum activity of creatine kinase (CK), preferably its MB isoenzyme, and of lactic dehydrogenase (LDH) are frequently used in the laboratory diagnosis of AMI.

LACTIC DEHYDROGENASE (LDH). The activity of this enzyme exceeds the normal range by 24 to 48 hours after the onset of AMI, reaches a peak 3 to 6 days after the onset of pain, and returns to normal levels 8 to 14 days after the infarction. The total LDH, while sensitive, is not specific; false-positive elevations occur in patients with hemolysis, megaloblastic anemia, leukemia, liver disease, hepatic congestion, renal disease, a variety of neoplasms, pulmonary embolism, myocarditis, skeletal muscle disease, and shock.[272,273]

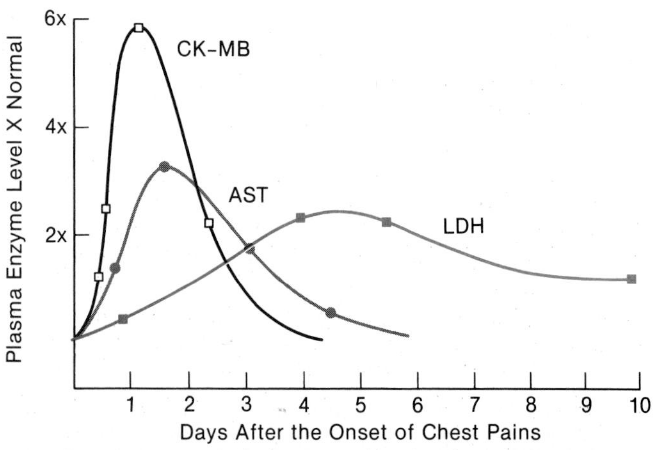

FIGURE 39–15. Typical plasma profiles for the MB isoenzyme of creatine kinase (CK-MB), aspartate amino transferase (AST), and lactate dehydrogenase (LDH) activities following onset of acute myocardial infarction. (Adapted from Hearse, D. J.: Myocardial enzyme leakage. J. Molec. Med. 2:185, 1977.)

LDH comprises five isoenzymes, which are numbered in the order of the rapidity of their migration toward the anode of an electrophoretic field. LDH_1 moves most rapidly, whereas LDH_5 is the slowest. Fractionation of serum LDH into its five isoenzymes increases diagnostic accuracy, since the heart contains principally LDH_1, whereas liver and skeletal muscle contain primarily LDH_4 and LDH_5. Thus, LDH_5 is commonly elevated in patients with congestive hepatomegaly. Most conditions causing elevated serum total LDH activity, such as liver or skeletal muscle disease or injury, are readily distinguished from AMI by analysis of LDH isoenzymes. Increased serum LDH_1 activity precedes elevation of serum total LDH and usually occurs within 8 to 24 hours after infarction.[275] Elevations of LDH and in the ratio of LDH_1 to total LDH occur in more than 95 per cent of patients with AMI.[272,276] Since hemolysis also raises serum LDH_1 activity, particular care must be taken in the withdrawal and handling of the blood specimens.

Many laboratories report the ratio of LDH_1 to LDH_2, which is elevated in MI. An LDH_1/LDH_2 ratio greater than 1.0 is commonly used as a cutoff defining abnormality in most series[273]; however, even a ratio as low as 0.76 has been reported to be more than 90 per cent sensitive and specific for the diagnosis of AMI.[275] LDH or LDH isoenzyme analysis for the diagnosis of AMI should be reserved for cases in which the CK has already fallen to normal—that is, when infarction is suspected to have occurred 2 to 4 days earlier. Although LDH isoenzyme testing may be useful, as already indicated, like aspartate aminotransferase (AST), the *routine* use of LDH and LDH isoenzyme determination is not justified and accounts for a considerable waste of resources.[277,278]

ASPARTATE AMINOTRANSFERASE (AST). For many years the activity of serum glutamic oxaloacetic acid transferase (SGOT)—now generally referred to as aspartate aminotransferase (AST)—was monitored for the diagnosis of AMI. Levels rise above normal 8 to 12 hours after the onset of chest pain, peak at 18 to 36 hours, and generally fall to normal within 3 to 4 days. However, because false-positive elevations occur frequently (with most hepatic or skeletal muscle diseases, following intramuscular injections or pulmonary embolism, and with shock), and because the time course of elevation and fall of AST is intermediate between that of CK and LDH, its incremental benefit for the diagnosis of AMI is negligible, and it is no longer routinely used.[277]

CREATINE KINASE (CK). Serum CK activity exceeds the normal range within 4 to 8 hours following the onset of AMI and declines to normal within 3 to 4 days after the onset of chest pain. The time of peak serum CK activity varies considerably, occurring as early as 8 hours after the onset of pain to as long as 58 hours later.[279] While the mean peak CK for AMI occurs at about 24 hours, peak levels occur earlier in patients who have had reperfusion as a result of the administration of thrombolytic therapy or mechanical recanalization (as well as in patients with early spontaneous thrombolysis), with peak CK occurring at about 12 hours after infarction in such cases.[273,280] With reperfusion, enzyme is released into the circulation more rapidly than for an infarct of comparable size without reperfusion.[281] Thus, reperfusion renders estimation of infarct size by enzyme analysis less accurate. Because the time-activity curve of serum CK is influenced by reperfusion, and because reperfusion itself influences infarct size, it has been suggested that the time to peak CK activity should be incorporated into enzymatic estimates of infarct size.[282]

Although elevation of the serum CK is the most sensitive enzymatic detector of AMI that can be used routinely,[272,273,283]

15 per cent false-positive results will occur in patients with muscle disease, alcohol intoxication, diabetes mellitus, skeletal muscle trauma, vigorous exercise, convulsions, intramuscular injections, thoracic outlet syndrome, and pulmonary embolism.[272,284] However, serum CK activity is normal in patients with heart failure and hepatic disease. CK values in women are normally about two-thirds of those in men.

CK ISOENZYMES. Three isoenzymes of CK (MM, BB, and MB) have been identified by electrophoresis. Extracts of brain and kidney contain predominantly the BB isoenzyme, skeletal muscle contains principally MM, and both MM and MB isoenzymes are present in cardiac muscle. The MB isoenzymes of CK may also be present in minor quantities in the small intestine, tongue, diaphragm, uterus, and prostate.[283,285] Strenuous exercise, particularly in trained long-distance runners or professional athletes, may cause elevation of both total CK and CK-MB.[286,287] For some athletes, both the percentage of MB released and the characteristic rise and fall of CK-MB may be similar to the changes seen after MI. The possibility has been raised that isoenzyme production is at least partially dynamic, with the relative portion of MB isoenzyme in cardiac muscle perhaps depending on maturation, preexisting coronary artery disease, or left ventricular hypertrophy.[288] Despite these issues and the fact that small amounts of CK-MB isoenzyme are found in tissues other than heart, elevated serum activity of CK-MB may be considered, for practical purposes, to be the result of AMI (except in the case of trauma or surgery on the aforementioned organs, which contain small quantities of the enzyme).

Isoforms of the MM and MB *isoenzymes* have been identified[289-291] (p. 1188). Certain isoforms appear to be released into the blood quite rapidly—perhaps as soon as 1 hour—after the onset of infarction. An assay of these isoforms may permit early identification of patients with AMI and early detection of successful reperfusion with AMI,[292] with or without residual high-grade stenosis[293,294] (Fig. 38–38, p. 1188).

Nevertheless, measurement of serum CK-MB isoenzyme continues to be the most useful and widely available test for myocardial necrosis.[273,295,296] The development of radioimmunoassay for the measurement of serum CK-MB has been helpful in increasing the accuracy, sensitivity, and specificity of this test,[297] although agarose gel electrophoresis is used routinely in most laboratories. A newer solid-phase immunoradiometric assay may further improve sensitivity.[298] In addition to AMI secondary to coronary obstruction, other forms of injury to cardiac muscle—such as those resulting from myocarditis, trauma, cardiac catheterization, shock,[299] and cardiac surgery—may also produce elevated serum CK-MB activity.[299-301] These latter causes of elevation of serum CK-MB values can usually be readily distinguished from AMI by the clinical setting. In approximately 15 per cent of patients with apparent AMI, the CK-MB may be elevated despite a normal total CK.[302,303] The importance of this finding is unclear. In an animal model, it has been shown that CK-MB may be released into the blood by transient severe ischemia without myocardial necrosis[304]; thus, minor elevation of CK-MB may not be diagnostic of AMI. Patients with minimally elevated CK-MB and normal CK, however, do have a prognosis that is generally worse than patients with suspected MI and no CK-MB elevation.[298,303,305] Thus, whether or not such elevations represent true "microinfarctions" may be less important than the prognostic connotations of this isolated elevation. Therefore, total CK is not a sensitive adequate screening test. On the basis of a careful analysis of factors affecting serum enzyme assays and a rational approach to minimizing resource consumption without adversely affecting diagnostic accuracy, Lee and Goldman[273] have proposed the series of recommendations on the use of serum enzyme assays for the diagnosis of AMI, shown in Table 39–2.

Serial measurement of CK-MB and application of the methods devised by Sobel and Shell (p. 1189)[272] allow prediction of infarct size determined at necropsy[306]; infarct size estimated by this method varies inversely with ejection fraction[307] and with survival.[308] Coronary artery reperfusion influences infarct size estimates by CK-MB as it does total CK-derived estimates. Thus, further refinements in the estimation of infarct size from CK-MB will depend on the incorporation of the effect of acute reperfusion into such estimates.[309]

TABLE 39–2 RECOMMENDATIONS ON THE USE OF SERUM ENZYME ASSAYS IN THE DIAGNOSIS OF ACUTE MYOCARDIAL INFARCTION

1. A single set of cardiac enzyme values in the emergency room is not sufficiently sensitive to exclude myocardial infarction. Although a single, markedly positive CK-MB value will greatly increase the probability of acute infarction, data are insufficient to support or reject a policy whereby low-risk patients, who otherwise would be sent home, would be observed until one or more CK-MB values are obtained.

2. If myocardial infarction is suspected, then samples of total CK and CK-MB levels should be measured on admission and about 12 and 24 hours later, although condensed versions of this strategy may ultimately prove to be equally efficacious and more cost effective. If myocardial infarction may have occurred more than 24 hours before admission, and if CK and CK-MB levels are not diagnostic, a total LDH level should be ordered. If the total LDH level is elevated, an assay of LDH isoenzymes should be obtained. If the first LDH1/LDH2 ratio is only slightly less than 1.0, a second assay is probably indicated.

3. If chest pain recurs after admission, CK and CK-MB assays should be done at 0, 12, and 24 hours. "Surveillance" enzyme assays are not recommended in asymptomatic patients without electrocardiographic changes.

4. Routine use of enzyme assays other than those for CK, CK-MB, and LDH isoenzymes is not recommended.

5. If more than 2 hours may pass before CK isoenzymes will be assayed, the serum sample should be preserved on ice.

6. Strategies including CK-MB assays can be used to diagnose myocardial infarction in the setting of noncardiac surgery and cardiac catheterization and after electrical countershock.

7. In the setting of cardiac surgery, myocardial infarction should be diagnosed if any two of the following are present: CK-MB elevation persisting more than 12 hours; new Q waves on an electrocardiogram; or regional defects on technetium pyrophosphate scintigraphy.

8. False-positive elevations of CK-MB can be minimized by diluting samples with marked elevations of total CK; detecting isoenzyme variants that masquerade as CK-MB on column chromatography assays by retesting the sample on an electrophoretic assay if the clinical presentation is atypical for myocardial infarction; or consideration of other sources of CK-MB (for example, myocarditis, renal failure, neuromuscular diseases, trauma) if a true elevation of CK-MB levels is found in the absence of a typical rise and fall of CK and CK-MB levels and other evidence for myocardial infarction.

From Lee, T., and Goldman, L.: Serum enzyme assays in the diagnosis of acute myocardial infarction. Recommendations based on a quantitative analysis. Ann. Intern. Med. *102*:221, 1986.

Other Laboratory Measurements

Numerous nonspecific manifestations may be recognized in patients with AMI. Although they are not generally employed in establishing the diagnosis, awareness of their coexistence with infarction is important in order to avoid misinterpretation or erroneous diagnosis of other disorders.

BLOOD SUGAR. Hyperglycemia occurs frequently following AMI, not only in diabetic patients, in whom ketoacidosis may be precipitated, but also (with a lower frequency) in nondiabetics, in whom several weeks may elapse before carbohydrate tolerance returns to normal[198,310] (p. 1212). The plasma urea and creatinine concentrations are normal, except in patients with severe left ventricular failure, in whom reduced renal perfusion and glomerular filtration may result in azotemia.

Hypokalemic alkalosis may be present in patients who develop an AMI while receiving thiazide or loop diuretics for antecedent hypertension or heart failure.

SERUM LIPIDS. These are often determined in patients with AMI.

However, the results may be misleading, since numerous factors that can alter the values are operating at the time of the patient's admission to the hospital; for example, stress increases serum cholesterol, whereas recumbency decreases it.[311] Serum triglycerides are affected by caloric intake, intravenous glucose, and recumbency.[311]

During the first 24 to 48 hours after admission, total cholesterol and HDL cholesterol remain at or near baseline values but generally fall precipitously after that.[312,313] The fall in HDL cholesterol after AMI is greater than the fall in total cholesterol; thus, the ratio of total cholesterol to HDL cholesterol is no longer useful for risk assessment early after MI.[314] Therefore, unless values are obtained very early in patients admitted for AMI, it is best to defer determinations of serum lipid levels until at least 8 weeks after the infarction has occurred.

MYOGLOBIN. This protein is released into the circulation from injured myocardial cells and can be demonstrated within a few hours after the onset of infarction; myoglobinemia is common in patients with AMI.[315] Peak levels of serum myoglobin are reached considerably earlier (3 to 20 hours) than peak values of serum CK.[316] However, the time of earlier appearance of myoglobin in the serum, its peak level, and the duration of detectable myoglobin release do *not* correlate well with these same parameters for serum CK and with clinical estimates of the severity of infarction. In contrast to CK, myoglobin (which has a molecular weight of only 17,000) is readily excreted into the urine. A more rapid rise in serum myoglobin has been observed following reperfusion, and its measurement has even been suggested as a useful index of successful reperfusion.[317] However, the clinical value of serial determinations of myoglobin in AMI is limited because of the brief duration of its elevation and the lack of specificity resulting from the fact that myoglobin is a constituent of skeletal muscle and is readily detected in the serum following damage to skeletal muscle.

HEMATOLOGICAL MANIFESTATIONS. An increase in the *white blood count* occurs frequently following AMI; it may be a response to tissue necrosis or increased secretion of adrenal glucocorticoids or both. The elevation of the white count usually develops within 2 hours after the onset of chest pain, reaches a peak 2 to 4 days following infarction, and returns to normal in 1 week; the peak white blood cell count usually ranges between 12 and 15 $\times 10^3$ per cubic millimeter but occasionally rises to as high as 20 $\times 10^3$ per cubic millimeter. Often there is an increase in the percentage of polymorphonuclear leukocytes and a shift of the differential count to band forms. The *erythrocyte sedimentation rate* (ESR) is usually normal during the first day or two after infarction, even though fever and leukocytosis may be present. It then rises to a peak on the fourth or fifth day and may remain elevated for several weeks. The increase in the ESR is secondary to elevated plasma alpha$_2$ globulin and fibrinogen,[318] but the peak does not correlate well with the size of the infarction or with the prognosis. The *hematocrit* often increases during the first few days following infarction as a consequence of hemoconcentration.[218]

ELECTROCARDIOGRAPHIC FINDINGS

(See also p. 136)

In the majority of patients with AMI, some change can be documented when serial electrocardiograms (ECGs) are compared. However, many factors limit the ability of the ECG to diagnose and localize MI: the extent of myocardial injury, the age of the infarct, its location, the presence of conduction defects, the presence of previous infarcts or acute pericarditis, changes in electrolyte concentrations, and the administration of cardioactive drugs. Nevertheless, serial standard 12-lead ECGs remain a clinically useful method for the detection and localization of MI.[296,319]

Although there is general agreement of electrocardiographic and vectorcardiographic criteria for the recognition of infarction of the anterior and inferior myocardial walls (Table 5–5, p. 144), there is less agreement on criteria for lateral and posterior infarcts[320]; here even the terminology may be confusing.[321] Although most patients continue to demonstrate the ECG changes from an infarction, particularly if they evolve Q waves for the rest of their lives, in a substantial minority the typical changes disappear, Q waves can regress,[322,323] and the ECG can even return to normal after a number of months or, more commonly, years.[324] Under many circumstances Q wave patterns may simulate MI.[325] Conditions that may mimic the electrocardiographic features of MI by producing a pattern of "pseudoinfarction" are listed in Table 39–3.

TABLE 39–3 CONDITIONS SIMULATING INFARCTION ON ECG

Ventricular hypertrophy
Right ventricular (cor pulmonale)
Left ventricular
Conduction disturbances
Left bundle branch block
Left anterior fascicular block
Wolff-Parkinson-White syndrome
Primary myocardial disease
Myocarditis
Dilated cardiomyopathy
Hypertrophic cardiomyopathy (both obstructive and nonobstructive)
Friedreich's ataxia
Muscular dystrophy
Pneumothorax
Pulmonary embolus
Amyloid heart disease
Primary and metastatic tumors of the heart
Traumatic heart disease
Intracranial hemorrhage
Hyperkalemia
Pericarditis
Early repolarization
Sarcoidosis involving the heart

From Taussig, A. S., et al.: Misleading ECGs: Patterns of infarction. J. Cardiovasc. Med. *9*:1147, 1983.

Q-WAVE AND NON-Q-WAVE INFARCTION. In the past an AMI (by enzyme or other clinical criteria) in which Q waves failed to develop on the ECG was referred to as a "subendocardial" or "nontransmural" MI. However, the presence or absence of Q waves on the surface ECG does not reliably predict the distinction between transmural and nontransmural or subendocardial MI.[326] True pathological subendocardial MI, as recognized at autopsy, is seen with ST-segment depression and/or T wave changes only about 50 per cent of the time.[327] Nevertheless, for the prognostic importance of identifying two different populations, a distinction should be made between AMI with and without Q waves.[328,329] Changes in the ST segment and T wave are quite nonspecific and may occur in a variety of conditions, including stable and unstable angina pectoris, ventricular hypertrophy, acute and chronic pericarditis, myocarditis, early repolarization, electrolyte imbalance, shock, metabolic disorders, and following the administration of digitalis (Ch. 17).[320] Serial ECGs may be of considerable aid in differentiating these conditions from non-Q-wave infarction.[330] Transient changes favor angina or electrolyte disturbances, whereas persistent changes argue for infarction if other causes such as shock, administration of glycoside, and persistent metabolic disorders can be eliminated. In the final analysis, the diagnosis of nontransmural infarction rests more on the combination of clinical findings and the elevation of serum enzymes than on the ECG.

ISCHEMIA AT A DISTANCE. Patients with new Q waves and ST-segment elevation diagnostic for MI in one territory often have ST-segment depression in other territories. These additional ST-segment changes may be caused by ischemia in a territory other than the area of infarction, termed "ischemia at a distance,"[162,331] or by reciprocal electrical phenomena.[332] A good deal of attention has been directed to associated ST-segment depression in the anterior leads, which occurs in the majority of patients with acute inferior MI.[333,334] However, despite the clinical importance of differentiation among causes of anterior ST-segment depression in such patients—including anterior ischemia, posterior wall infarction, and true reciprocal changes—such a differentiation cannot be made reliably by electrocardiographic or even vectorcardiographic[334] techniques. Although precordial ST-segment depression is more commonly associated with extensive infarction of the posterior, lateral, or inferior septal segments—rather than anterior wall subendocardial ischemia[335-336]—ancillary scintigraphic or angiographic techniques are necessary to document this. Regardless of whether the anterior ST-segment changes reflect anterior wall ischemia or are reciprocal to changes

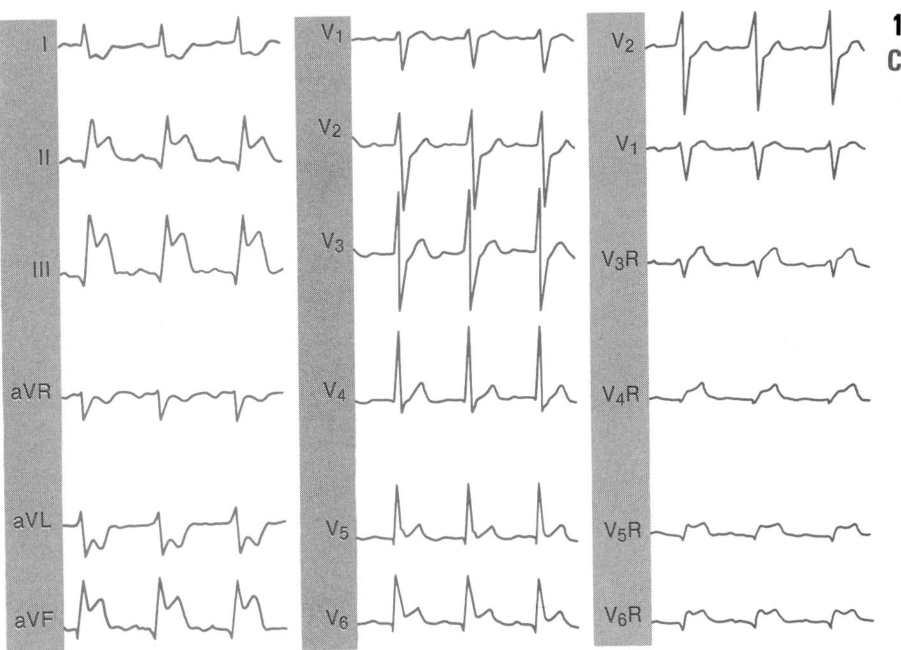

FIGURE 39-16. Leads I, II, III, aVR, aVL, aVF, leads V_1, V_2, V_3, V_4, V_5, and V_6, and right precordial leads V_2, V_1, V_3R, V_4R, V_5R, and V_6R recorded simultaneously. The ECG shows acute inferoposterior wall myocardial infarction. The right precordial leads show ST-segment elevation in leads V_3R, V_4R, V_5R, and V_6R, indicating right ventricular infarction as well. (From Brant, S. H.: Value of electrocardiography in diagnosing right ventricular involvement patients with an acute inferior wall myocardial infarction. Br. Heart J. *49*:368, 1983.)

elsewhere, this finding, as with ischemia at a distance, implies a poorer prognosis than is the case if such changes are not present.[331,334]

RIGHT VENTRICULAR INFARCTION. This is difficult to diagnose by the electrocardiogram, presumably because the right ventricular myocardial mass is small in comparison with the left. However, ST-segment elevation in right precordial leads (V_1, V_3R-V_6R) has been noted to be a relatively sensitive and specific sign of right ventricular infarction[337-340] (Fig. 39-16). Occasionally ST-segment elevation in the usual precordial leads (particularly V_2 and V_3) may be due to acute right ventricular infarction; this appears to occur only when the injury to the left ventricular inferior wall is minimal.[341] Usually, the concurrent inferior wall injury suppresses this anterior ST-segment elevation resulting from right ventricular injury. Likewise, right ventricular infarction itself appears to reduce the anterior ST-segment depression often seen with inferior wall myocardial infarction.[342] A QS or QR pattern in leads V_3R and/or V_4R also suggest right ventricular myocardial necrosis but have less predictive accuracy than ST-segment elevation in these leads.[339,340]

ATRIAL INFARCTION. This can be suspected occasionally from the ECG[343,344]; the most common electrocardiographic patterns are depression or elevation of the PQ segment, alterations in the contour of the P wave, and abnormal atrial rhythms, including atrial flutter, atrial fibrillation, wandering atrial pacemaker, and AV nodal rhythm.[322]

IMAGING IN ACUTE MYOCARDIAL INFARCTION

ROENTGENOGRAPHY

(See also p. 224)

The initial chest roentgenogram in patients with AMI is almost invariably a portable film obtained in the emergency room or the coronary care unit. Two findings are common: signs of left ventricular failure and cardiomegaly. Although the pulmonary vascular markings on the roentgenogram generally reflect the left ventricular end-diastolic pressure, significant discrepancies may occur because of what have been termed *diagnostic lags* and *post-therapeutic lags*. In the former, patients may have elevated left ventricular filling pressure and normal chest roentgenogram, and, because of the time required for pulmonary edema to accumulate after left ventricular filling pressure has become elevated, 12 hours may elapse before the radiographic findings reflect the hemodynamic status. The post-therapeutic phase lag represents the longer time interval, generally 1 or 2 days, required for pulmonary edema to resorb and the radiographic signs of pulmonary congestion to clear after left ventricular filling pressure has returned toward normal.[345]

Cardiomegaly in a patient with AMI usually signifies prior infarction or another form of antecedent cardiovascular disease such as chronic hypertension with subsequent left ventricular dilatation, and it is usually associated with impaired left ventricular function.[346] Since the chest film (especially the portable film in the A-P projection) is not a sensitive indicator of ventricular size, the converse is not true, in that patients may have increased end-diastolic volume and still demonstrate a normal-sized heart on roentgenographic examination. The degree of congestion and the size of the left side of the heart on the chest film are highly useful predictors for defining groups of patients with AMI who are at increased risk of dying after the acute event.[347]

Computed tomography (CT) (p. 315) can provide useful cross-sectional information in patients with MI. In addition to the assessment of cavity dimensions and wall thickness, left ventricular aneurysms may be detected, and, of particular importance in AMI, intracardiac thrombi can be identified. Although cardiac CT is a less convenient technique, it probably is more sensitive for thrombus detection than echocardiography.[348] Infarct sizing is possible with CT scanning but for this purpose remains a research tool rather than a clinical one[349] (Fig. 11-4, p. 314).

Radioisotopic Studies

(See Chap. 10)

All major forms of nuclear cardiac imaging—radionuclide angiography, perfusion scintigraphy, infarct-avid scintigraphy, and positron-emission tomography—are useful in detecting AMI, in assessing infarct size and jeopardized myocardium, in determining the effects of the infarct on ventricular function, and in establishing prognosis. The application of these techniques is discussed in Chapter 11.[296,350-353]

A new radiopharmaceutical agent, ^{99m}Tc hexakis 2-methoxy-2-isobutyl isonitrile (^{99m} Sesta MIBI), has been developed for myocardial perfusion imaging[354] (p. 277). This agent has already proved useful for the measurement of the area of myocardium at risk in AMI[355] and the recognition of salvaged myocardium following thrombolytic therapy.[356] Its use is likely to increase in the next several years.

Magnetic Resonance Imaging

(See Figs. 11-22, 11-23, and 11-25, pp. 325-326)

Cardiac imaging with magnetic resonance imaging (MRI) has been employed in experimental and clinical studies of

AMI.[357] In addition to localizing and sizing the area of infarction,[358] MRI techniques are capable of early recognition of MI[359] and of providing an assessment of the severity of the ischemic insult.[360] While imaging with this technique presents practical problems for routine studies in coronary care unit patients because patients must be transported to the MRI facility, this safe, noninvasive modality holds much promise. Potential capabilities of MRI are likely to include not only the ability to detect, localize, and size AMI but also to assess perfusion of infarcted and noninfarcted tissue as well as of reperfused myocardium; to identify areas of jeopardized but not infarcted myocardium; to identify myocardial edema, fibrosis, wall thinning, and hypertrophy; to assess ventricular chamber size and segmental wall motion; and to identify the temporal transition between ischemia and infarction and eventually to assess coronary anatomy and flow.[359,361,362]

Echocardiography

(See also p. 97)

As major technical improvements have been made, echocardiography has emerged as an extremely important imaging modality in all cardiac patients. The relative portability of echocardiographic equipment makes this technique ideal for the assessment of patients with AMI hospitalized in the critical care setting[363] or even in the emergency department before admission. In patients with chest pain compatible with AMI, but with a nondiagnostic ECG, the finding on echocardiography of a distinct region of disordered contraction can be helpful diagnostically.

M-MODE ECHOCARDIOGRAPHY. This sensitive technique for examining regional left ventricular wall motion[364] is limited to the imaging of small segments of the interventricular septum and posterior and anterior left ventricular walls. Abnormalities of left ventricular wall motion, usually corresponding to the electrocardiographic site of infarction, may be recognized in the majority of patients with transmural infarction, and hyperkinetic motion can be found in noninfarcted areas in approximately one-third of patients.[365] M-mode echocardiography is also useful in detecting small pericardial effusions in patients with postinfarction pericarditis.[366]

TWO-DIMENSIONAL ECHOCARDIOGRAPHY (see Figs. 4–90, p. 98; 4–93, 4–94, p. 99). This technique can provide both longitudinal and transverse views of the left ventricle. Also, a much larger fraction of the ventricular wall—including significant portions of the left ventricular apical, anterior, septal, inferior, and posterior walls—can be imaged[363] by this method than by the M-mode technique. Areas of abnormal regional wall motion are observed almost universally in patients with AMI.[367] Abnormal wall motion is less often noted echocardiographically when the infarction is nontransmural; however, abnormalities are still present in more than two-thirds of patients.[368] Left ventricular function, estimated from two-dimensional echocardiograms,[368] correlates well with estimates for angiographic studies and may be useful in establishing prognosis.[369,370]

It has recently been shown that two-dimensional echocardiography is diagnostically useful and cost-effective in the emergency department setting.[367,370,371] In patients who arrive with chest pain, echocardiography may be utilized rapidly to identify regional wall motion abnormalities, which are nearly universally present in patients with AMI. The rapid application of this technique can then aid in admission decisions and in selecting among other important therapeutic options such as whether or not to use thrombolytic therapy (p. 1230). Furthermore, the *early* use of echocardiography can aid in the early detection of mechanical complications of AMI and in the early assessment of right and left ventricular function, as already noted.

In addition to the abnormal wall motion seen following AMI, myocardium in the area of infarction is usually much thinner than noninfarcted myocardium. Ultrasonic tissue characterization techniques, which take advantage of the known increase in echo intensity from myocardial scar, appear to aid in the differentiation between ischemic and infarcted myocardium.[372] Motion within the originally defined area of dyssynergy may improve during the recovery phase of AMI, suggesting a beneficial effect of reperfusion therapy.[373] While reliably detecting and localizing an AMI, two-dimensional echocardiography has been less useful for quantifying the area of infarction because of difficulties in distinguishing between ischemic and infarcted tissue. Both fail to contract normally; in such assessments the area of actual tissue necrosis usually is overestimated.[374]

Two-dimensional echocardiography is extremely useful for the detection of most mechanical complications of AMI. Left ventricular aneurysms[375] and pseudoaneurysms[376] usually are easily and reliably identified. In addition, in patients with AMI who develop a loud systolic murmur, this type of echocardiography can be used to detect and localize a ventricular septal defect, as well as detect mitral regurgitation, and elucidate its cause.[377] Myocardial rupture, pericardial effusion, and left ventricular thrombus formation, all of which occur with AMI, may also be detected by this method.[363,378]

DOPPLER ECHOCARDIOGRAPHY. This technique (p. 97) allows for assessment of blood flow in the cardiac chambers and across cardiac valves.[379] Used in conjunction with two-dimensional echocardiography, it is of benefit in detecting and assessing the severity of mitral[380] or tricuspid regurgitation following AMI. Identification of the site of acute ventricular septal rupture, as well as quantification of shunt flow across the resulting defect, is also possible.[380,381] Reliable estimation of cardiac output has been made by combining Doppler echocardiographic measurements of flow with two-dimensional echocardiographic measurements of ascending aortic cross-sectional area through which blood flows.[382]

Estimation of Infarct Size

ELECTROCARDIOGRAPHY. Interest in limiting infarct size, in large part because of the recognition that the quantity of myocardium infarcted has important prognostic implications, has focused attention on the accurate determination of MI size. The ECG initially received greatest attention. Early studies by Maroko and others demonstrated that the sum of ST-segment elevations measured from many precordial leads was useful for assessing the extent of myocardial injury in patients with anterior MI.[383] While this technique is practical and easily utilized, it is applicable only to anterior infarctions. It is limited by the inability to distinguish between reversibly and irreversibly ischemic tissue, and it depends on the influence of myocardial geometry.[384] QRS scoring systems with planar[385,386] or vectorcardiographic[387] techniques to estimate infarct size have been developed. While demonstrating good correlations with infarct size at autopsy and with enzymatic estimates, these ECG techniques are also subject to major limitations. These include the effects of ventricular geometry[384] as well as the inability to size infarcts in patients with conduction defects, nontransmural MI, and multiple infarctions.

ENZYMATIC METHODS. Serial measurements of enzymes released by necrotic myocardium, particularly creatine kinase (CK) and its MB isoenzyme, are helpful in determining AMI size. Clinically, the peak CK or CK-MB is useful for a rough estimate of infarct size and is widely used prognostically. However, coronary artery recanalization—spontaneous or pharmacologically or mechanically achieved—dramatically changes the wash-out kinetics of CK from myocardium, resulting in early and exaggerated peak enzyme levels.[280,281] Nevertheless, accuracy can be attained with appropriate modification of enzymatic estimates of impact size.[388] Quantification of the cumulative release of CK[399] or CK-MB[306,389,390] has been closely correlated with other techniques for estimating infarct size and with the area of necrosis at autopsy. This quantitative approach has proved useful for determining, in clinical trials on groups of patients, the effects (if any) of different forms of therapy for AMI and for prognostic assessment. However, accurate quantitation by this method is not available early enough to be useful for the clinician caring for patients with AMI.

NONINVASIVE IMAGING TECHNIQUES. Echocardiography (Chap. 4, p. 97), radionuclide scintigraphy (Chap. 10, p. 277), CT scanning (Chap. 11, p. 315), and magnetic resonance imaging (Chap. 11, p. 337) have all been utilized for the clinical and experimental assessment of infarct size. Contrast enhancement[391] may improve upon the tendency of two-dimensional echocardiography to overestimate infarct size.[392] Infarct-avid scintigraphy and the myocardial perfusion and wall motion types all have been used experimentally to quantify infarct size, but are limited by the inability to detect small infarcts, by ventricular geometry, and again by difficulty in distinguishing ischemic from infarcted myocardium. Tomography has improved on techniques employing technetium-99m pyrophosphate to image AMI.[393] Imaging of radiolabeled myosin-specific antibodies, which bind to myosin exposed by the loss of plasma membrane in early myocardial necrosis, is the newest scintigraphic technique and holds promise for highly accurate quantification of infarct size.[351,394]

A comprehensive method of infarct size estimation has been proposed incorporating enzymatic (CK-MB) and electrocardiographic indices and two-dimensional echocardiography.[395] While proving accurate in one prospective study, the proposed formula requires further validation.

Management of Acute Myocardial Infarction

Many options are available for the treatment of AMI. These include the use of pharmacological agents to dissolve occlusive thrombi and to prevent or delay necrosis of jeopardized myocardium and mechanical procedures to recanalize occluded coronary arteries. While such approaches have been termed "aggressive,"[21] they are clearly warranted in increasing numbers of patients. Nevertheless, the sound management of patients with AMI still depends on a variety of conventional management measures that have come into use in the decades since Herrick's original description of the condition at the beginning of this century. These measures, which consist of bed rest, oxygen, treatment of arrhythmias, and prevention of complications, will be considered in this section before the more aggressive therapies are discussed.

Physician practices have changed dramatically as newer approaches to the care of the AMI patient have become available.[395a,396] Virtually all physicians in the U.S. have intensive care facilities available for their patients with AMI. In 1970, such facilities were *unavailable* to almost 20 per cent of family physicians and general practitioners. The use of antiarrhythmic agents has increased markedly, while the regular prescription of long-term anticoagulant therapy and cardiac glycosides has fallen by 50 per cent or more. Nitrates and/or beta blockers, rarely prescribed in 1970, are now given to the majority of patients. Average hospital stay is less than one-half of what it was in 1970. Invasive and/or noninvasive procedures to evaluate prognosis and the need for further therapy are now used in most post-MI patients, whereas only a small percentage of patients had such procedures performed in the early 1970's.[397] Finally, thrombolytic therapy, available but unused in 1970, is now standard care in suitable patients.

PREHOSPITAL CARE

Most deaths associated with AMI occur within the first hour after its onset, and death usually is due to ventricular fibrillation (Chap. 26).[398] Accordingly, the importance of the immediate implementation of definitive resuscitative efforts and of rapidly transporting the patient to a hospital cannot be overemphasized.[398a] First and foremost, patients must be educated to seek immediate medical attention should they develop manifestations of MI. In patients with previous infarcts or in those with chronic stable angina, these manifestations are not difficult to describe—severe chest pain resembling that with the first infarct or more severe and prolonged than with ordinary angina. The task is more difficult in patients in whom the AMI is the first clinical manifestation of coronary artery disease.

Public campaigns must inform the susceptible population (most adults) about the clinical manifestations of AMI. In fact, it has been shown that a media campaign in Göteborg, Sweden, shortened significantly (from 3 to 2 hours) the median delay time for the onset of symptoms to hospital arrival.[399] People must be educated concerning the benefits of seeking immediate medical help if they are suffering an AMI, both in terms of prevention and treatment of potentially fatal arrhythmias as well as salvage of jeopardized myocardium by reperfusion, for which time is particularly crucial. In fact, when thrombolytic therapy is employed, prompt hospital arrival following the onset of symptoms (within 2 hours) is associated with a lower mortality rate.[263,400] It has been suggested that primary care physicians need to become familiar with newer strategies to help facilitate early treatment.[401] Well-equipped ambulances and helicopters staffed by personnel trained in the acute care of the infarction victim allow definitive therapy to commence while the patient is being transported to the hospital.[402,403] These specially equipped and staffed ambulances have been termed *mobile coronary care units;* to be used effectively, they must be placed strategically within a community and excellent radio communication systems must be available. They should be equipped with battery-operated monitoring equipment and direct writing electrocardiograph, a battery-operated DC defibrillator, oxygen, endotracheal tubes and suction apparatus, and commonly used cardiovascular drugs. A radiotelemetry system that allows transmission of the ECG to the hospital is desirable but not essential. The effectiveness of such a system depends upon the competency of paramedics, transmission distances, and the availability of expert consultation on the receiving end.[404]

The effectiveness of these systems in Belfast, Ireland,[402] Seattle, Washington,[405] and Columbus, Ohio[406] has been amply documented. The rapid initiation of prehospital cardiopulmonary resuscitation facilitated by mobile coronary care units and trained paramedical personnel results in initially successful resuscitation in approximately two-thirds of patients. It has been demonstrated that the frequency of death *during* transportation can be diminished from 22 to 9 per cent when defibrillation equipment and trained paramedical personnel are available,[407] although reduced overall mortality has not been shown.[403] In addition to prompt defibrillation, the efficacy of prehospital care appears to depend on several factors, including early relief of pain with its deleterious physiological sequelae, reduction of excessive activity of the autonomic nervous system, and abolition of prelethal arrhythmias, such as ventricular tachycardia. However, these efforts must not inhibit rapid transfer to the hospital, as recently the application of such therapies has been found actually to delay hospital arrival, possibly diminishing the benefit of such an approach.[403]

Communication systems capable of transmitting the ECG over regular telephone lines are now available for the home. The prehospital use of such a system has been shown to reduce morbidity and mortality in a high-risk subset of patients supplied with the device.[408] Mobile intensive care and prehospital monitoring systems have also facilitated the acquisition of data about the earliest signs and symptoms of AMI, both for the understanding of early complications of AMI and for identifying patient subgroups with differing risks.[409] Observations of simple variables such as heart rate and blood pressure permit initial classification to high- or low-risk subgroups because patients initially presenting with hypotension have a mortality in excess of 50 per cent, whereas patients with isolated sinus bradycardia (and a normal or elevated blood pressure) appear to have a mortality that approaches zero.[409]

Recently the possibility that the prehospital use of thrombolytic therapy might be of benefit has been addressed,[410,411] and several pilot studies have been carried out.[412–415] It is estimated that approximately one-quarter of patients presenting with AMI would be candidates for such early treatment[416] and that an organized paramedic-based treatment system could allow for thrombolytic therapy to be given, on average, about 70 minutes earlier.[416]

CORONARY CARE UNITS

During the past two and a half decades the mortality of patients with AMI treated in coronary care units has declined significantly from what it had been before the introduction of these units.[8,10,417] Reduction in mortality has resulted in large part from the elimination of *primary* arrhythmias as a cause of death. Actually, most instances of primary arrhythmias occur *before* the patient reaches the hospital, and only about 5 per cent of patients develop a primary ventricular arrhythmia *after* they reach the hospital, an average of 5 to 6 hours after the onset of the attack in most series. Deaths from primary ventricular fibrillation have been prevented because the coronary care unit allows continuous monitoring of cardiac rhythm by highly trained nurses with the authority to administer immediate treatment and prophylaxis of arrhythmias in the absence of physicians, and because of the specialized equipment (defibrillators, pacemakers) and drugs available for instantaneous use.[417] Although all of these benefits can certainly be achieved for patients scattered throughout the hospital, the clustering of patients with AMI in the coronary (or cardiac) care unit has greatly improved the efficient use of the trained personnel, facilities, and equipment. In recent years, with increasing emphasis on hemodynamic monitoring and treatment of the serious complications of AMI with such modalities as thrombolytic therapy, afterload reduction, and intraaortic balloon counter pulsation, the coronary care unit has assumed even greater importance.[417] As interventional strategies including thrombolytic therapy and acute coronary angioplasty are used more routinely in AMI patients, facilities in which patients may undergo diagnostic and therapeutic angiographic procedures are being integrated into the coronary care unit structure.

ROLE OF THE CORONARY CARE UNIT IN UNCOMPLICATED AMI PATIENTS. At the same time, the value of coronary care units for patients with *uncomplicated AMI* has been questioned and restudied.[418] In one widely publicized randomized trial, carried out in England, patients with suspected infarction were evaluated initially at home; after a 2-hour observation interval they were divided at random into home-management and hospital-management groups.[419] Although the 6-week mortality rates among patients with infarction in the two groups were similar (13 per cent and 11 per cent, respectively), such relatively low overall mortality rates make detection of small although real differences difficult (i.e., a high Type II error). Furthermore, hospital care was provided for all high-risk patients. Under the general conditions of medical practice in the United States, it is difficult to provide the same immediate intensive care at home for all patients with suspected infarction that was made available in this study. Since prediction of the occurrence of early complications is imperfect, it appears that the observation and prompt treatment possible in a well-staffed coronary care unit continue to justify the reliance placed upon this setting as the primary one for early management of patients with suspected or confirmed AMI. Unfortunately, patient delay in seeking medical attention and the medical system's delay in responding reduce the potential impact of the coronary care unit because the patients do not reach the unit until the maximum danger has passed. Therefore, education of the public, of patients at high risk of AMI, and of those members of the medical profession involved in responding to the initial complaints of these patients is likely to be rewarded by further reductions of mortality.[401]

SELECTION OF PATIENTS FOR THE CCU. With increasing attention directed to the limitation of resources and to the economic impact of intensive care, there have been efforts to identify patients for whom hospitalization in a coronary care unit would likely be of benefit (p. 1702).[417] A single set of cardiac enzyme measurements obtained in the emergency department is not of sufficient sensitivity to rule out an AMI. On the other hand, the ECG, particularly in conjunction with a general clinical assessment, can be useful both for predicting which patients will have the diagnosis of AMI confirmed and identifying low-risk patients who may require less intensive care.[420] Of patients with a classic history of chest pain but with a normal ECG in the emergency department, less than 20 per cent will ultimately have an AMI on that admission, and less than 1 per cent will develop any significant complication.[421] Thus, a patient with a normal ECG may not require admission to a full-fledged coronary care unit. Careful analysis of the quality of pain may help identify such low-risk patients as well. Patients without a history of angina pectoris or MI presenting with pain that is sharp or stabbing and pleuritic, positional, or reproduced by palpation of the chest wall are extremely unlikely to have an AMI.[422]

More complex decision protocols, which have been utilized with the aid of simple computer programs accessible to the emergency department staff, have been successfully tested and found capable of accurately predicting which patients with acute chest pain are having an MI[423] and which have acute ischemic heart disease (including unstable angina).[424] These instruments, which incorporate clinical variables including ECG changes, the quality of pain and other symptoms, and the patient's age, have not yet achieved widespread use. As pressures increase to eliminate inappropriate coronary care unit admissions, emergency department clinicians may find it important to take advantage of such tools.

For patients with a low probability of MI, the clinician should consider admission to an intermediate care facility equipped with simple ECG monitoring and resuscitation equipment. This strategy has been shown to be cost-effective.[425] It may be preferable for many such patients who stand to gain little benefit from the high staffing, intense activity, and elaborate technology available to current coronary care units (with their attendant high costs) and who may be disturbed by that activity and equipment. Use of a nonintensive care facility for low-risk patients may reduce coronary care unit utilization by one-third, shorten hospital stays, and have no deleterious effect on patients' recovery.

RECOMMENDATIONS. While there is both a lack of direct evidence, in terms of improved patient survival, for the value of coronary care units and a lack of consensus concerning general admission policies and therapeutic strategies for these units,[426] several common principles and guidelines may be proposed: (1) Most patients with clear-cut AMI should be admitted to an intensive (coronary) care unit. Patients with hemodynamic instability, other serious medical problems, or continuing symptoms also should be admitted, even if the diagnosis of AMI is uncertain. Most patients with unstable angina (p. 1334), particularly if episodes of chest pain are occurring at rest, should also be admitted to the coronary care unit. (2) Once an AMI is ruled out, which may be as early as 24 hours after admission,[417,427] and symptoms are controlled with oral or topical pharmacological agents, discharge from the coronary care unit should be considered.[428] (3) In AMI patients with *uncomplicated* status, stays in the unit need be no longer than 2 days. (4) In patients with complicated AMI, the duration of the coronary care unit stay should depend on the need for "intensive" care—that is, hemodynamic monitoring, close nursing supervision, intravenous vasoactive drugs, and frequent changes in the medical regimen.

GENERAL MEASURES

General care measures should include (1) a liquid diet for 24 hours, because of the risk of nausea and vomiting or cardiac arrest early after infarction and the need to reduce the risk of aspiration. This should be followed by a 1500 calorie soft diet, with no added salt, divided into multiple small feedings for several days. Then, in the absence of heart failure, a regular diet, low in cholesterol and saturated fats, is appropriate. Caffeine-rich beverages should be avoided because of their possible arrhythmogenic effects. (2) Dioctyl sodium sulfosuccinate, 100 mg daily, or another stool softener should be used to prevent constipation and straining. (3) The emotional impact of an AMI and of hospitalization in a coronary care unit should be offset by thoughtful explanations of the nature of the illness, the function of the equipment, and the purpose of the procedures. A deliberate effort should be made to maintain the atmosphere in the coronary care unit as quiet and restful as possible. Oxazepam, 15 to 30 mg orally four times a day, is useful to allay the anxiety that is so common in this setting. Temazepam, 15 to 30 mg, or an equivalent may be given for sleep. (4) Derangements potentially contributing to arrhythmias, such as hypoxemia, hypovolemia, disturbances of acid-base balance or of electrolytes, and drug toxicity, should be identified and corrected.

CONTROL OF CARDIAC PAIN

The alleviation or reduction of pain is a critical factor in the care of patients with AMI.[429] Since the pain associated with MI is related to ongoing ischemia (p. 1201), many interventions that act to improve the oxygen supply-demand relationship (by either increasing supply or decreasing demand) may lessen the pain associated with AMI.

NITRATES. As long as hypotension (systolic pressure <100 mm Hg or a decline of >25 mm Hg from the patient's normal pressure) is not present, careful administration of nitrates may lessen pain. Once it is ascertained that hypotension is not present, a sublingual nitroglycerin tablet should be administered and the patient observed carefully for improvement in symptoms or change in hemodynamics. If an initial dose is well tolerated and appears to be of benefit, further nitrates should be administered, with careful monitoring of the vital signs. However, long-acting nitrate preparations should be avoided in the very early course of AMI. In patients with a prolonged period of waxing and waning chest pain, intravenous nitroglycerin may be of benefit in controlling symptoms and correcting ischemia, but careful monitoring of blood pressure is required.[430] Nitrates should be used cautiously in patients with inferior wall infarction because even small doses may produce sudden hypotension and bradycardia; a reaction that can be life-threatening can usually be easily reversed with intravenous atropine if it is recognized quickly.[431] In patients with suspected right ventricular myocardial infarction, nitrates should be used with *extreme caution*, if at all, since these patients may be particularly sensitive to the venodilating effects of the drug, with sudden hypotension resulting from inadequate right ventricular filling.[432]

ANALGESICS. Although a wide variety of analgesic agents has been used to treat the pain associated with MI, including meperidine, pentazocine, and morphine,[429] the last-named agent remains the drug of choice except in patients with well-documented morphine hypersensitivity. Four to 8 mg should be administered intravenously and doses of 2 to 8 mg repeated at intervals of 5 to 15 minutes until the pain is relieved or evident toxicity—i.e., hypotension, depression of respiration, or severe vomiting—precludes further administration of the drug. In some patients, remarkably large cumulative doses of morphine (2 to 3 mg/kg) may be required and are usually tolerated.

The reduction of anxiety resulting from morphine diminishes the patient's restlessness and the activity of the autonomic nervous system, with a consequent reduction of the heart's metabolic demands. The beneficial effect of morphine in patients with pulmonary edema is unequivocal (p. 563) and may relate to several factors, including peripheral arterial and venous dilatation (particularly among patients with excessive sympathoadrenal activity), reduction of the work of breathing, and slowing of heart rate secondary to combined withdrawal of sympathetic tone and augmentation of vagal tone.[433]

Hypotension following the administration of morphine can be minimized by maintaining the patient in a supine position and elevating the lower extremities if systolic arterial pressure declines below 100 mm Hg. Obviously, such positioning is undesirable in the presence of pulmonary edema, but morphine rarely produces hypotension under these circumstances. The concomitant administration of atropine in doses of 0.5 to 1.5 mg intravenously may be helpful in reducing the excessive vagomimetic effects of morphine, particularly when hypotension and bradycardia are present before it is administered. Respiratory depression is an unusual complication of morphine in the presence of severe pain or pulmonary edema, but as the patient's cardiovascular status improves, impairment of ventilation may supervene and should be watched for. It can be treated with naloxone, in doses of 0.1 to 0.2 mg intravenously initially, repeated after 15 minutes if necessary. Nausea and vomiting may be troublesome side effects of large doses of morphine and may be treated with a phenothiazine to avoid marked stress on the circulation.

Other analgesics such as meperidine are less effective than is morphine but equally likely to produce side effects and prone to augment ventricular rate.

OXYGEN. Hypoxemia is common in patients with AMI and is usually secondary to ventilation-perfusion abnormalities[434] that are sequelae of left ventricular failure; pneumonia and intrinsic pulmonary disease are additional causes of hypoxemia. It is common practice to treat all patients hospitalized with AMI with oxygen for 24 to 48 hours, based on the common occurrence of arterial hypoxemia and clinical[435] evidence that increased oxygen in the inspired air may protect ischemic myocardium. However, augmentation of the fraction of oxygen in the inspired air does not elevate oxygen delivery significantly in patients who are not hypoxemic. Furthermore, it may increase systemic vascular resistance and arterial pressure and thereby lower cardiac output slightly.

In view of these considerations, arterial oxygen tension may be estimated or measured at the time of the patient's admission to the coronary care unit; oxygen therapy may be omitted if it is normal. On the other hand, oxygen should be administered to patients with AMI when arterial hypoxemia is clinically evident or can be documented by measurement. In these patients, serial arterial blood gas measurements may be employed to follow the efficacy of oxygen therapy. Although patients with AMI may exhibit a reduction in precordial ST-segment elevation during 100 per cent oxygen breathing, no long-term effect on survival or on the development of complications has been documented.[435]

In general, the delivery of 2 to 4 liters/min of 100 per cent oxygen by mask or nasal prongs for 2 to 3 days is satisfactory for most patients with mild hypoxemia. If arterial oxygenation is still depressed on this regimen, the flow rate may have to be increased, and other causes for hypoxemia should be sought. In patients with pulmonary edema, endotracheal intubation and positive-pressure controlled ventilation may be necessary.

BETA-ADRENOCEPTOR BLOCKERS. Beta blocking agents have been used in the early hours of AMI in attempts to limit the size of the infarct (p. 1236). In the course of these studies, it has been recognized that beta blockers relieve pain and reduce the need for analgesics in many patients, presumably by reducing ischemia.[436] Patients most suited for the use of beta blockers early in the course of AMI are those who also have sinus tachycardia and hypertension, since beta blockers will improve the heart rate and blood pressure, thereby lowering myocardial oxygen demand. A popular and relatively safe protocol for the use of a beta blocker in this situation is as follows: (1) Patients with heart failure, hypotension, bradycardia, or heart block are first excluded. (2) Metoprolol is given in three 5-mg boluses. (3) Patients are observed for *2 to 5 minutes* after each bolus and if heart rate falls below 60 beats per minute, or systolic blood pressure falls below 100 mm Hg, no further drug is given; a total of three intravenous doses (15 mg) are administered. (4) If hemodynamic stability continues, 6 to 8 hours later the patient is begun on oral metoprolol 50 mg for one day, then advanced to 100 mg twice daily if the lower dose is well tolerated. An extremely short-acting beta blocker, esmolol, may also be useful and even safer than other currently available drugs.[436]

Unlike beta blockers, calcium antagonists are of little if any value in AMI and may be hazardous.[436a]

PHYSICAL ACTIVITY. In the absence of all complications, patients with AMI need not be confined to bed for more than 24 to 36 hours and, unless they are hemodynamically compromised, they may use a bedside commode from the time of admission. Progression of activity regimens should be individualized depending upon patients' clinical status, age, and physical capacity. A typical patient may sit in a chair for two half-hour periods on the second and for two one-hour periods or more on the third day. If arrhythmia, heart failure, and other significant complications have not occurred or if they are controlled, the patient may be transferred out of the coronary care unit after 2 to 3 days. Monitoring for at least an additional two days, and usually more, in an intermediate care unit is desirable.

In patients without hemodynamic compromise, early ambulation—including dangling feet on the side of the bed, sitting in a chair, standing, and walking around the bed—does not cause important changes in heart rate, blood pressure, or pulmonary wedge pressure.[437] While heart rate increases slightly (usually by less than 10 per cent), pulmonary wedge pressures fall slightly as the patient assumes the upright posture for activities. Early ambulatory activities are only rarely associated with any symptoms, and when symptoms do occur, they generally are related to hypotension. Thus, when Levine and Lown proposed the "armchair" treatment of AMI in the 1950's, they were undoubtedly correct that stress to the myocardium is less in the upright position.[438] As long as blood pressure and heart rate are monitored carefully, early ambulation offers considerable psychological and physical benefit without any clear medical risk.

HEMODYNAMIC ASSESSMENT

Major advances in the management of AMI have resulted from the hemodynamic monitoring that has become widespread in coronary care units.[439,440] This often consists of both an intraarterial catheter and a pulmonary artery catheter. The former is usually inserted into the radial artery for continuous monitoring of systemic pressure and for sampling for blood gas determination. Pulmonary artery catheterization is accomplished with a balloon-tipped flotation catheter, often advanced, with fluoroscopic guidance, from a peripheral or internal jugular vein through the right heart and into the pulmonary artery. Judicious positioning of the catheter allows recording of the pulmonary capillary wedge pressure when the balloon is inflated.[439] Blood may be sampled from the tip of the catheter in the pulmonary artery and, in some catheters, from a second lumen opening into the right atrium. Pulmonary artery balloon catheters with a thermistor near the tip for recording thermodilution measurements of cardiac output are used frequently.[441] Thus, a single catheter in the right heart can yield the following information: saturation of blood in the pulmonary artery and right atrium, pressures in the pulmonary artery, pulmonary wedge position, and right atrium and cardiac output. A good correlation exists between pulmonary artery wedge pressure (which is equal to pulmonary capillary pressure) and left ventricular diastolic pressure in patients with AMI.

Balloon-tipped catheters are now available with a fiberoptic bundle for transmission of light. By connecting this catheter to an oximeter, continuous pulmonary artery venous blood oxygen saturation can be monitored.[442]

In the past, central venous or right atrial pressure was used to gauge the degree of *left* ventricular failure in patients with AMI. However, this technique is fraught with error, since central venous pressure actually reflects *right* rather than left ventricular function. Right ventricular function, and therefore systemic venous pressure, may be normal or nearly so in patients with significant left ventricular failure.[440] Conversely, patients with right ventricular failure due to right ventricular infarction or pulmonary embolism may exhibit elevated right atrial and central venous pressures despite normal left ventricular function.[443] Low values for right atrial and central venous pressures imply hypovolemia, whereas elevated right atrial pressures usually result from right ventricular failure secondary to left ventricular failure, pulmonary hypertension, or right ventricular infarction, or less commonly from tricuspid regurgitation or pericardial tamponade.

The prognosis and the clinical status are related to both the cardiac output and the pulmonary artery wedge pressure. Patients with normal cardiac output after AMI have an extremely low expected mortality; prognosis worsens as cardiac output declines. Patients with cardiac indices in the range of 2.7 to 4.3 liters/min/sq meter usually have no clinical signs of impaired perfusion, whereas patients with cardiac indices ranging from 1.8 to 2.2 liters/min/sq meter demonstrate early signs of hypoperfusion (cool skin and decreasing urine output and mental acuity). Patients whose cardiac index is less than 1.8 liters/min/sq meter are usually in shock. The pulmonary artery wedge pressure reflects the state of left ventricular filling, its compliance, and its ability to empty. As pulmonary pressure rises, progressive increases in pulmonary congestion occur. Mortality is greater for patients with elevated pulmonary wedge pressures.[444]

Patients with intraventricular conduction defects or AV block or both after *anterior* infarction have lower cardiac indices and higher pulmonary capillary wedge pressures than do patients without these conduction disturbances. On the other hand, patients with these conduction defects and *inferior* myocardial infarction usually do not demonstrate such hemodynamic abnormalities.

PULMONARY ARTERY CATHETERIZATION (Table 39–4). Before inserting a pulmonary artery catheter into a patient with an AMI, the physician must decide that the potential benefit of the information to be obtained outweighs any potential risks. Complications from pulmonary artery catheters are relatively rare, but severe problems can occur, including sepsis, pulmonary infarction, and pulmonary artery rupture. By minimization of the duration of catheterization and by adherence to careful sterile techniques, risk can be diminished.[445] Accurate determination of hemodynamics by clinical assessment is difficult in critically ill patients. The use of a pulmonary artery catheter often leads to important changes in therapy that would not have occurred if the hemodynamic information had not been available.[446] Some believe, however, that the pulmonary artery catheter is often overused. It has been suggested that until clinical trials assessing its benefit are performed, the use of this technique should be curbed.[447,448] (At least one such trial has suggested that complications and mortality are actually higher in patients who received pulmonary artery catheterization,[449] although such patients might have been at higher risk initially.) This view emphasizes the importance of careful patient selection, meticulous technique, and correct interpretation of the data obtained.

TABLE 39–4 INDICATIONS FOR HEMODYNAMIC MONITORING OF AMI

Management of complicated AMI
- **Hypovolemia vs. cardiogenic shock**
- **Ventricular septal rupture vs. acute mitral regurgitation**
- **Severe left ventricular failure**
- **Right ventricular failure**

Refractory ventricular tachycardia

Differentiating severe pulmonary disease from left ventricular failure

Assessment of cardiac tamponade

Assessment of therapy in *selected* individuals
- **Afterload reduction in patients with severe left ventricular failure**
- **Inotropic agents**
- **Beta blockers**
- **Temporary pacing (ventricular vs. atrioventricular)**
- **Intraaortic balloon counterpulsation**
- **Mechanical ventilation**

From Gore, J. M., and Zwernet, P. L.: Hemodynamic monitoring of acute myocardial infarction. *In* Francis, G. S., and Alpert, J. S. (eds.): Modern Coronary Care. Boston, Little, Brown & Co., 1990, p. 138.

Patients most likely to benefit from pulmonary artery catheter monitoring include those whose AMI is complicated by: (1) hypotension that is not easily corrected by fluid administration; (2) hypotension in the presence of congestive heart failure; (3) hemodynamic compromise severe enough to require intravenous vasopressors or vasodilators or intraaortic balloon counterpulsation; and (4) mechanical lesions (or suspected ones) such as cardiac tamponade, severe mitral regurgitation, and a ruptured ventricular septum.[445]

THE INTERMEDIATE CORONARY CARE UNIT

Since the hazard of *primary* ventricular fibrillation is essentially over in 24 to 36 hours, there is little need for patients with entirely *uncomplicated* infarction to remain in a coronary care unit for more than 1 to 2 days. Obviously, patients with complicated infarction, particularly those with arrhythmias, pump failure, and recurrent ischemia, require continued care in such a unit. Patients who have undergone reperfusion and may be at risk of recurrent infarction also may require an extra day or so in the intensive cardiac care unit. There is an increased risk of ventricular tachycardia and ventricular fibrillation in the late MI period, particularly among patients with impaired left ventricular function or anterior infarction, accounting for between 10 and 30 per cent of total hospital deaths.[450] Recurrent ischemia or infarction also places such patients at increased risk.[451] In view of this significant in-hospital mortality after discharge from the coronary care unit, continued surveillance in intermediate coronary care units (also called step-down units) is justifiable. In fact, patients at an extremely low risk for complications should be considered as candidates for initial direct admission to such a facility.[425]

Risk factors for mortality in the hospital *after* discharge from the coronary care unit include intraventricular conduction defects,[452] sinus tachycardia persisting for more than 2 days, extensive anterior infarction, episodes of ventricular fibrillation and of atrial flutter or fibrillation occurring while the patient is in the coronary care unit, early recurrent angina and marked electrocardiographic ST-segment abnormalities induced by low levels of activity.[453,454] It is possible that a reduction in late hospital mortality can be achieved with the use of intermediate coronary care units, which permit prolonged continuous monitoring of the electrocardiogram and prompt, effective treatment of ventricular fibrillation and other serious arrhythmias. The availability of these units may be useful also in helping to identify those patients who remain free from complications for a minimum of one week, since early discharge from the hospital appears to be feasible for this subset.[455]

EARLY REHABILITATION (see p. 1263 and Chap. 42). Following myocardial infarction, patients are often eager for information, in need of reassurance, confused by misinformation and prior impressions, capable of counterproductive denial, and simply frightened. Cardiac rehabilitation should be carefully structured and often requires a considerable period of time, optimally beginning as early as possible once the patient is no longer in extreme danger. Intermediate care facilities provide ideal settings and ample opportunities to begin the rehabilitation process. Although intermediate care units were introduced for the purpose of decreasing mortality after coronary care unit discharge, studies have not shown any conclusive benefit in that regard.[456,457] Nevertheless, the capacity for the early detection of problems following AMI and the social and educational benefits of grouping such patients together strongly argue for continued utilization of the concept of intermediate coronary care. Furthermore, the economic advantage of grouping such patients together for sharing of resources, in terms of improving utilization of coronary care units and possibly for facilitating early discharge, outweighs any questions raised by the lack of a clear consensus regarding reduced mortality. An additional potential advantage that should not be underestimated is facilitation of patient education in a group setting with formal lectures and various types of audiovisual programs.

LIMITATION OF INFARCT SIZE

Infarct size is an important determinant of prognosis in patients with AMI.[458] Patients who succumb from cardiogenic shock generally exhibit massive infarcts.[459,460] Early impairment of ventricular function, presaging a poor prognosis, is correlated with extensive infarcts.[460,461] Survivors with large infarcts frequently exhibit late impairment of ventricular function, and the long-term mortality rate is higher than that for survivors with small infarcts (Fig. 39–17), who tend not to develop cardiac decompensation.[461-463] The occurrence of various manifestations and complications of AMI as well as the need for special treatments is also related to infarct size.[458] The influence of infarct size on mortality is most apparent during the patient's hospital course and in the first few months after infarction. The hospital mortality in patients with large infarcts, as estimated by technetium pyrophosphate scanning, is several times greater than it is in patients with small infarcts.[462] However, the importance of infarct size declines somewhat with time after the initial episode[463]; after recovery from an AMI it is the quantity of remaining myocardium whose viability is threatened because it is perfused by obstructed coronary vessels that becomes crucial to the prognosis.

In view of the prognostic importance of infarct size, the concept that modification of infarct size is possible has attracted a great deal of experimental and clinical attention over the past 2 decades.[17,18,464-466] Efforts to limit the size of the infarct have been divided among three different (sometimes overlapping) approaches: early reperfusion, reduction of myocardial energy demands, and stimulation of anaerobic energy production.[467] Before these areas are considered in more detail, issues concerning the infarction process and general clinical measures are discussed.

THE DYNAMIC NATURE OF INFARCTION. AMI is a dynamic process that often does not occur instantaneously but sometimes evolves relatively slowly, i.e., over a matter of hours (Fig. 39–18). As has been pointed out (p. 1190), in experimental animals the fate of jeopardized, ischemic tissue may be affected favorably by interventions that restore perfusion, reduce myocardial oxygen requirements, inhibit accumula-

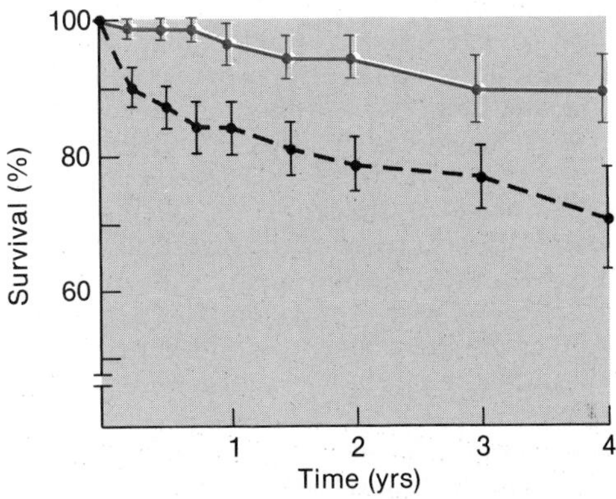

FIGURE 39–17. **The influence of the extent of initial myocardial infarction on survival. Survival is shown after initial myocardial infarction in a total of 173 patients with infarct size index (expressed in terms of CK-gram-equivalents/m^2) of <15 (solid line) vs. ≥ 15 (interrupted line). Brackets indicate standard errors. The graph depicts survival curves for all patients who survived for at least 24 hours after the onset of an initial myocardial infarction. Survival was significantly greater for patients with small compared with large infarcts ($P < 0.05$). (From Geltman, E. M., et al.: The influence of location and extent of myocardial infarction on long-term ventricular dysrhythmia and mortality. Circulation *60*:805, 1979, by permission of the American Heart Association, Inc.)**

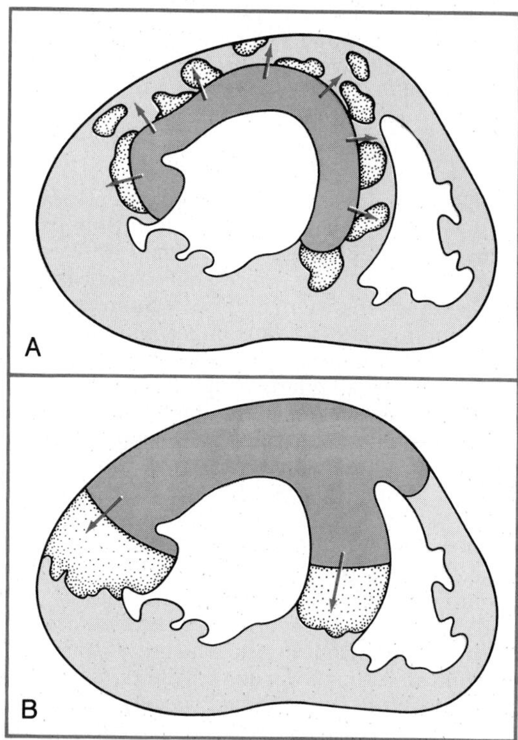

FIGURE 39-18. **Two types of extension of myocardial infarction. Type A (*A*) was observed at the edges of an infarct, usually subepicardially. Type B (*B*) occurred at the lateral margins. (From Alonso, D. R., et al.: Pathophysiology of cardiogenic shock: Quantification of myocardial necrosis, clinical, pathological and electrocardiographic correlation. Circulation *48*:588, 1973, by permission of the American Heart Association, Inc.)**

tion or facilitate washout of noxious metabolites, augment the availability of substrate for anaerobic metabolism,[17,18,464,465,467] or blunt the effects of mediators of injury such as calcium or oxygen free radicals,[468-470,470a] metabolites, and constituents of cell membranes.[471,472]

The perfusion of the myocardium associated with AMI appears to be reduced maximally immediately following coronary occlusion. In experimental animals, increases in blood flow to the peripheral portions of the ischemic zones become evident within 24 hours of acute coronary occlusion,[472] suggesting that dynamic factors contribute to the early limitation of perfusion. These may include the efflux of potassium from injured myocardial cells as well as the release of catecholamines as a consequence of ischemia of adrenergic neurons (and the resultant vasospasm). Spasm of coronary vessels has been implicated not only in Prinzmetal's variant angina (p. 1342) but also in association with the more common forms of MI involving atherosclerosis,[473,474] as well as in patients experiencing postinfarction angina at rest.[475] While spasm may play a contributory role in enhancing infarct size, other than in patients with Prinzmetal's angina it is unlikely to be the *principal* cause. While coronary spasm might play a role at the inception of coronary occlusion, by the time an angiogram is performed intracoronary nitroglycerin very rarely results in reperfusion.

Relatively prompt, *partial* restoration of reduced blood flow to the ischemic zone may result from spontaneous thrombolysis, from relief of coronary spasm (see above), or from improved systemic hemodynamics; the last factor includes augmented coronary perfusion pressure and reduced left ventricular end-diastolic pressure. Subsequently, perfusion of the jeopardized zone may be enhanced by the development of collateral circulation.[476] The prompt implementation of measures designed to protect ischemic myocardium and support myocardial perfusion may provide sufficient time for the development of anatomical and physiological compensatory mechanisms that limit the ultimate extent of infarction.

AMI in hospitalized patients may be complicated by extension of infarction or early reinfarction (p. 1262). Depending on the criteria utilized for detection, the incidence of these complications ranges from 8 to 30 per cent.[477] It is possible that interventions designed to protect ischemic myocardium during the initial event may also reduce the incidence of extension of infarction or early reinfarction. On the other hand, it has been suggested that preservation of ischemic myocardium could lead to persistent survival of cells in regions subjected to repetitive episodes of severe ischemia, leading to the development of arrhythmias. The relatively poor *late* prognosis of patients with non-Q-wave infarction[478,479] is consistent with this possibility. However, despite these hazards, there is no evidence that the implementation of interventions designed to protect ischemic myocardium results in any late deleterious effects. Furthermore, it has been reported that preservation of ischemic myocardium by trimethaphan in hypertensive patients with evolving infarction,[480] by intravenous nitroglycerin in normotensive patients,[481] and by the early administration of beta-adrenoceptor blocking agents[482-484] is actually associated with a reduced rather than an increased mortality.

Proof of the clinical efficacy of specific interventions has been difficult to acquire, in part because of the wide variations in the size of infarcts and their rate of evolution, in part because of the difficulties involved in measuring infarct size, and in part because it is difficult to predict what size any given infarct would have attained had the intervention under study not taken place.

ROUTINE MEASURES FOR INFARCT SIZE LIMITATION

Recognition that the ultimate size of a myocardial infarct does not depend solely on the pathological anatomy of the coronary vascular bed (which supplies oxygen) but also is affected by a variety of physiological variables (which determine the heart's demands for oxygen) suggests emphasis on a number of principles to be considered in the routine care of AMI. It is mandatory to maintain an optimal balance between myocardial oxygen supply and demand so that as much of the jeopardized zone of the myocardium surrounding the most profoundly ischemic zones of the infarct can be salvaged. During the period before irreversible injury has occurred, myocardial oxygen consumption should be minimized by maintaining the patient at rest, physically and emotionally, and by utilizing mild sedation and a quiet atmosphere that may lower heart rate, a major determinant of myocardial oxygen consumption. If the patient was receiving a beta-adrenoceptor blocking agent at the time the clinical manifestations of the infarction commenced, the drug should not be discontinued unless a specific contraindication develops, such as left ventricular systolic failure or bradyarrhythmia. Marked sinus bradycardia (heart rate less than approximately 50 beats/min) and the frequently coexisting hypotension should be treated with postural maneuvers (the reverse Trendelenburg position) to increase central blood volume and atropine or electrical pacing, but *not* with isoproterenol. On the other hand, the *routine* administration of atropine, with the resultant increase in heart rate, to patients without serious bradycardia is contraindicated. All forms of tachyarrhythmias require prompt and direct treatment, since they increase myocardial oxygen needs.

Diuretics are the first line of drugs indicated in the treatment of congestive heart failure. If they prove insufficient, vasodilators should be added,[485] unless the patient is already hypotensive. Inotropic agents such as cardioactive sympathomimetics or the phosphodiesterase inhibitor amrinone (p. 503) should be added only if there is evidence of persistent and severe ventricular failure despite diuretics and vasodilators; these agents should *not* be given prophylactically. Of the various sympathomimetic amines available, isoproterenol with its chronotropic and vasodilator effects is the most hazardous.

Dobutamine (or small doses of dopamine) (p. 502), which has less effect on heart rate and systemic vascular resistance than does norepinephrine, epinephrine, or isoproterenol, is the drug of choice when cardiac contractility *must* be augmented.

Particular attention must be paid to preserving arterial oxygenation in patients with hypoxemia, such as occurs in patients with chronic pulmonary disease, pneumonia, or left ventricular failure. Oxygen-enriched air should be administered to patients with hypoxemia, and bronchodilators and expectorants should be used when indicated. Severe anemia, which can also extend the area of ischemic injury, should be corrected by the cautious administration of packed red cells, accompanied by a diuretic if there is any evidence of left ventricular failure. Associated conditions, particularly infections and the accompanying tachycardia, fever, and elevated myocardial oxygen needs, require immediate attention.

Systolic arterial pressure should not be allowed to deviate by more than approximately 25 to 30 mm Hg from the patient's usual level, unless marked hypertension had been present before the AMI. It is likely that each patient has an optimum level of arterial pressure; as coronary perfusion pressure deviates from this level, the unfavorable balance between oxygen supply (which is related to coronary perfusion pressure) and myocardial oxygen demand (which is related to ventricular wall tension) that ensues will increase the extent of ischemic injury.

Rather than simply maintaining the patient's vital signs, the physician's attention should be directed toward controlling ischemia and preserving the myocardium as well as maintaining perfusion of peripheral organs. However, these two objects may sometimes conflict. In the first 4 hours after the onset of the clinical event, when the ultimate size of the infarct may not yet have been established definitively, myocardial preservation should ordinarily be given the highest priority. This may mean foregoing the stimulation of cardiac contractility by inotropic agents. Later, once the size of the infarct is fixed and if heart failure supervenes, it may be appropriate to stimulate the heart with positive inotropic agents, i.e., to employ an intervention that might have increased infarct size if given at an earlier time.

In some patients, particularly those with cardiogenic shock, tissue damage occurs in a "stuttering" manner with persistent release of CK into the bloodstream rather than abruptly, a condition that might more properly be termed *subacute infarction*.[460] This concept of the dynamic nature of the infarction process as well as the observation that the incidence of complications of AMI in both the early and late postinfarction periods is a function of infarct size[458,463] greatly expands the horizon for what can *potentially* be accomplished by techniques to limit myocardial necrosis.

REPERFUSION OF MYOCARDIAL INFARCTION

One of the two most important developments in the treatment of patients with AMI since Herrick's description of the syndrome 80 years ago[46] consists of establishing reperfusion of ischemic heart muscle in the early hours of myocardial infarction.[486] (The second is the prevention and treatment of life-threatening arrhythmias.) While reperfusion occurs spontaneously in some patients,[280] this may not occur early enough to salvage ischemic myocardium, and in any event it is now well recognized that a persistent thrombotic occlusion is present in the majority of patients with AMI while the myocardium is undergoing necrosis.[56] Efforts to recanalize an occluded coronary artery by pharmacological and/or mechanical means have been increasingly successful. Timely reperfusion of jeopardized myocardium clearly represents the most effective way of restoring the balance between myocardial oxygen supply and demand. When carried out within the first several hours after coronary occlusion in several species of experimental animals, reperfusion improves hemodynamics and decreases infarct size, as assessed by both indirect techniques (epicardial ST-segment recordings, precordial QRS maps, myocardial CK depletion, and positron-emission tomography) and direct techniques (morphology).[487–490] The extent of protection appears to be directly related to the rapidity with which reperfusion is implemented after the onset of coronary occlusion.[491]

While surgical reperfusion by coronary artery bypass grafting has been undertaken with variable success since the early 1970's,[492] the current era of nonsurgical reperfusion was launched by the pioneering effects of Chazov[493] and Rentrop[494] and their collaborators. These investigators demonstrated successful reperfusion of an occluded coronary artery by the intracoronary infusion of a thrombolytic agent, sometimes in conjunction with recanalization by means of a guidewire. Many different therapeutic approaches are now available to the clinician.[21] Much clinical research is currently directed at deciding on optimal reperfusion strategies and at understanding ancillary clinical issues such as patient selection, follow-up noninvasive testing, and the need for additional secondary preventive measures involving anticoagulants, antiplatelet agents, and revascularization.[495]

PATHOPHYSIOLOGY OF MYOCARDIAL REPERFUSION

By delivering oxygen to ischemic muscle, reperfusion has the potential to relieve ischemia. Prevention of cell death by the restoration of blood flow depends on the severity and duration of preexisting ischemia. Substantial experimental evidence for this concept[496] is supported by clinical studies showing that recovery of left ventricular systolic function,[497–499] improvement in diastolic function,[500] and reduction in overall mortality[466,501,502] are more favorably influenced, the earlier that blood flow is restored. Collateral coronary vessels also appear to play a role in the successful restoration of left ventricular function following reperfusion.[503] Collaterals are probably of greater importance in patients having reperfusion later than with reperfusion 1 to 2 hours after coronary artery occlusion; they provide sufficient perfusion of the myocardium to retard cell death.

REPERFUSION INJURY (see p. 1191). A specific form of reperfusion injury has been described as cell death that occurs following reperfusion in tissue that previously had been ischemic but not necessarily irreversibly damaged.[469,504,504a] Thus reperfusion may be a "double-edged sword."[505] On the one hand, blood flow must be restored to salvage ischemic myocardium, but it is possible, although not yet unequivocally established, that the process of restoring flow may damage cells not yet irreversibly injured. Reperfusion does increase the cell swelling that occurs with ischemia,[469,506] and this alone or with the condition known as the "no-reflow" phenomenon (impingement of swollen cells on the restoring of flow at the microvascular level[506]) could potentially lead to cellular injury. Available evidence indicates that, while reperfusion may accelerate necrosis of irreversibly injured myocytes, it does not add substantially to the area of myocardium ultimately damaged, for such cells are already destined to die.[507] Reperfusion of myocardium in which the microvasculature is damaged leads to the creation of a hemorrhagic infarct.[496,508] Reperfusion by means of thrombolytic therapy appears more likely to produce hemorrhagic infarction than reperfusion by mechanical means.[508] While concern has been raised that this hemorrhage may lead to extension of the infarct, this does not appear to be the case.[505,509] Histological study of patients not surviving in spite of successful reperfusion has revealed hemorrhagic infarcts, but this hemorrhage usually does *not* extend beyond the area of necrosis.[508–510] Necrosis in reperfused myocardium generally is of the contraction band type rather than the coagulation necrosis type seen after AMI.[510]

The sudden exposure of severely ischemic cells to both calcium and oxygen with the restoration of flow has been observed to affect the severity of ischemic damage.[504,505,510a] Toxicity from oxygen-derived free radicals, mediated at least in part by stimulated leukocytes, has attracted considerable attention[469,505,511] for its possible role in extending myocardial injury. Although unsupported by clinical evidence as of this writing, future therapy, likely to be carried out with reperfusion, may well include administration of agents that reduce leukocyte activation and scavenge oxygen free radicals. In addition, drugs such as beta-adrenoceptor blockers and verapamil, which *delay* the death of ischemic cells, may, if administered prophylactically to patients at high risk of occlusion (or reocclusion) or in the earliest phases of the development of an AMI, enhance the quantity of myocardium salvaged by early reperfusion.[512,513]

Reperfusion frequently causes changes in the cardiac rhythm. Transient sinus bradycardia occurs in many patients with inferior infarcts at the time of acute reperfusion; it is most often accompanied by some degree of hypotension. This combination of hypotension and bradycardia with a sudden increase in coronary flow has been ascribed to the Bezold-Jarisch reflex.[514] Premature ventricular contractions are the most common arrhythmia noted at the time of reperfusion, but these are frequent in all patients with AMI and it is not clear whether or not reperfusion actually increases their incidence. An accelerated idioventricular rhythm and ventricular tachycardia are more common acutely after successful reperfusion than after failed therapy.[515] When present, these rhythm disturbances may actually be a marker of successful restoration of coronary flow.[516] In general, clinical features are poor markers of reperfusion, with no single clinical finding or constellation of findings being reliably predictive of angiographically demonstrated coronary artery patency.[517] Nevertheless, the need for treatment of arrhythmias should be anticipated in any patient receiving therapy designed to recanalize a totally occluded coronary artery in the setting of AMI. Occasionally, reperfusion may actually lessen the severity of ventricular arrhythmias due to ongoing ischemia, or of heart block associated with an AMI.[518]

It has been suggested that improved survival and ventricular function after successful reperfusion are not due to limitation of infarct size alone.[181,495,519–521,521a] In addition to the possibility that early reperfusion may actually *prevent* AMI[519] and probably improves the electrical stability of the heart as noted earlier,[521b] the benefit of a patent artery may include a favorable effect on ventricular remodeling (p. 1210), improved diastolic function,[500] a lower incidence of cardiac rupture,[486,509] provision of collateral flow,[486,520] and later improvement in systolic left ventricular function.[521,522] Further support of this theory comes from information suggesting improved survival even when reperfusion occurs *after* the time period in which myocardial salvage could be anticipated. Therefore, it is reasonable to reexamine the width of the "time window"[490,491] previously thought to limit the benefit of reperfusion, but it is inappropriate to conclude that anything but maximum efforts should be applied to reducing the time interval between onset of clinical manifestations of AMI and institution of reperfusion therapy.[520]

CORONARY THROMBOLYSIS

Many years elapsed between the first report of intracoronary clot lysis in an experimental animal[524] and the widespread use of thrombolytic agents in AMI, even though the feasibility of such an approach was demonstrated as early as 1958.[525] It was not until relatively recently that the knowledge that coronary thrombosis is responsible for the initiation and/or the perpetuation of myocardial infarction (p. 1780) *and* the discovery that in most cases administration of thrombolytic agents restores angiographic patency to coronary vessels[57,81,493,526–528] sparked interest in the potential value of clot lysis in salvaging jeopardized tissue and limiting the extent of injury sustained in patients with evolving myocardial infarction. A large European trial in the late 1970's demonstrated that intravenous streptokinase reduced mortality at 6 months if given within 12 hours of AMI.[529] By the early 1980's reports of the use of thrombolytic agents in AMI became frequent. With publication of the first GISSI trial of over 11,000 patients in 1986,[512] in which intravenous streptokinase resulted in a significant reduction in mortality in patients treated within 6 hours of the onset of symptoms, the routine use of thrombolytic therapy in AMI was established. It is now clear that thrombolysis recanalizes thrombotic occlusion associated with the majority of cases, restoration of coronary flow improves myocardial function, and mortality is reduced.[530]

INTRACORONARY THROMBOLYSIS

Clinical investigation in the area of pharmacological reperfusion of ischemic myocardium initially focused on the use of *intracoronary* thrombolysis in the early hours of AMI (Fig. 39–19).[57,81,526,527] The fact that viability could be maintained in a portion of the successfully reperfused myocardium was reflected in studies showing the restoration of contractile activity.[155,498,507,528] On the basis of results of several successful trials, the Food and Drug Administration initially approved the use of *intracoronary* streptokinase and urokinase for the treatment of myocardial infarction.[507] Many factors affect the usefulness of this technique, which is dependent on the availability of a skilled catheterization team and well-equipped catheterization facility. Most reported experience with intracoronary thrombolysis has not been in both randomized and controlled trials, largely because it has been thought difficult to withhold thrombolytic therapy once a thrombotic coronary artery occlusion has been visualized angiographically, and it has not been considered ethical to catheterize patients if randomization to no thrombolytic therapy were possible for a portion of the patients. Because of the delay involved in catheterizing patients with AMI, current consensus is that intracoronary administration

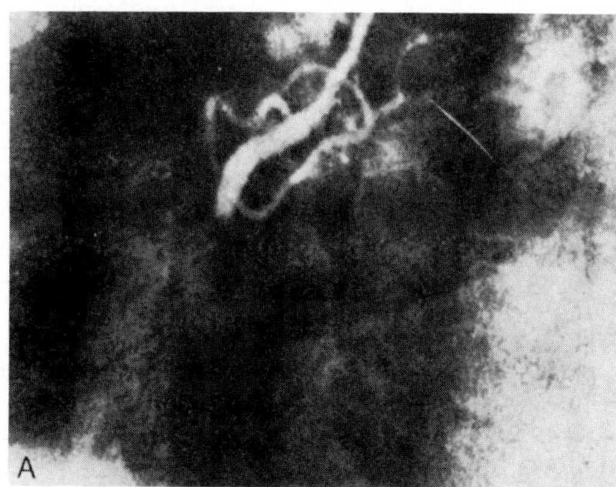

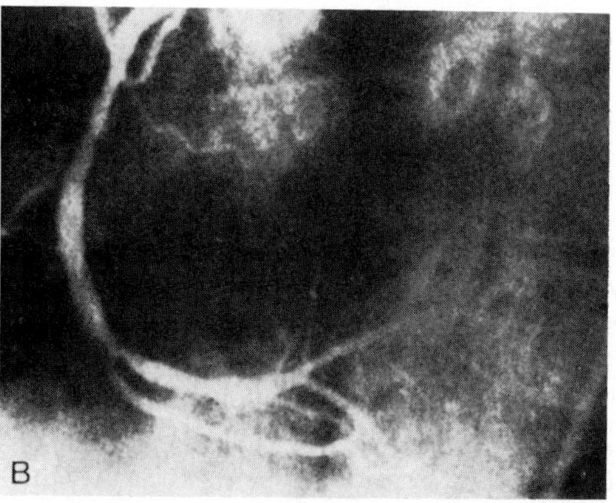

FIGURE 39–19. ***A,*** **Complete occlusion of the right coronary artery in a 38-year-old man with evolving inferoposterolateral myocardial infarction.** ***B,*** **The artery was patent after 20 minutes of intracoronary streptokinase infusion. This arteriogram was taken after an additional infusion of streptokinase for 60 minutes, which further improved patency. (From Ganz, W., et al.: Intracoronary thrombolysis in evolving myocardial infarction. Am. Heart J.** ***101:*****4, 1981.)**

TABLE 39-5 OVERALL COMPARISON OF INTRAVENOUSLY ADMINISTERED STREPTOKINASE, RECOMBINANT TISSUE-TYPE PLASMINOGEN ACTIVATOR (rt-PA), AND ANISOYLATED PLASMINOGEN ACTIVATOR COMPLEX (APSAC)

FACTOR	STREPTOKINASE	rt-PA	APSAC
Usual dose	1.5 million U in 30-60 min	60 mg for first hour, 40 mg during hrs 2-3	30 mg in 5 min
Clot selectivity	None	Relative	Minor
Patency of infarct-related artery	50-60%	75-85%	60%
Time dependency	High; <30% after 4 h	None	?
Reocclusion	5-20%	10-20%	10-20%
Improvement of left ventricular function	Yes	Yes	Yes
Improvement of survival	Yes, in numerous trials	Yes, in two small trials	Yes
Hypotension	Severe in <5%	None	None
Half-life	Long	Short	Long
Allergic reactions	Yes	No	Yes
Fibrinogenolysis	Severe	Moderate	Severe
Periaccess bleeding	Common	Common	Common
Intracranial bleeding	<0.5%	<0.5%	<0.5%
Repeat dosing possible	No, because of antibodies	Yes	No
Patient cost/dose	$125	$2,800	$1,800

Data from references 486, 540, 573.
APSAC = anisoylated plasminogen streptokinase activator complex (Eminase).

of thrombolytic therapy should be reserved for patients who develop coronary thrombosis during the course of an angiographic procedure and in whom either a coronary catheter is already in place or such placement is easily and rapidly achieved.

Intravenous Thrombolysis

This form of thrombolytic therapy has several important advantages over intracoronary use. Since only the placement of a peripheral intravenous line is required, therapy may be initiated early, in a variety of locations (emergency room, ambulance, helicopter, or home[411,413]) and at relatively low cost. In fact, as already noted, intravenous streptokinase has been used in the treatment of AMI for decades, preceding our recent definitive knowledge that thrombosis is the focal event in initiating AMI. This subject has perhaps been one of the most rapidly evolving in the management of patients with AMI.

CHOICE OF AGENTS. Three thrombolytic agents, streptokinase, recombinant tissue-type plasminogen activator (rt-PA), and anisoylated plasminogen streptokinase activator complex (APSAC), are currently approved by the Food and Drug Administration for intravenous use in patients with AMI (Chap. 58) (Table 39-5). By far the greatest international experience has been accumulated with streptokinase, in part owing to its low cost and demonstrated efficacy in reducing mortality in very large trials.[466,502] The usual dose is 1.5 million units given over 1 hour. APSAC was developed in part to provide an agent with kinetics more favorable to sustain a thrombolytic effect, as the approved dose of 30 mg can be given over 2 to 5 minutes.[531] The initial hope that APSAC would be more fibrin clot-selective than streptokinase has not been borne out.[486,532] It appears to induce recanalization at a rate approaching that seen with *intracoronary* streptokinase.[531,533] It possesses the distinct advantage of allowing administration as a single bolus injection compared with continued intravenous infusion (for streptokinase or rt-PA).

Tissue plasminogen activator is an endogenously produced enzyme released from vascular endothelium as part of the body's defense against in vivo thrombosis (p. 1571).[533a,533b] Its isolation from a melanoma cell line led to later production by recombinant DNA techniques. Although the agent is expensive, it has received much attention as an "elegant product of the molecular biology revolution."[534] The currently approved dose is 100 mg, given as 60 mg in the first hour (of this, 6 to 10 mg is given as an initial bolus), followed by 20 mg per hour for the next 2 hours. Currently, different dosing strategies are being explored for improved efficacy and safety, as discussed below. Four relatively small trials have compared intravenous streptokinase with rt-PA.[535-538] In the three trials employing early angiography, patency rate of the infarct-related artery was higher with rt-PA.[536-539] Although none of these studies showed reduced mortality with rt-PA, an analysis of pooled results suggests that mortality with streptokinase was 50 per cent greater than with rt-PA.[528,534] Additionally, pooled data from angiographic trials (of which there have been many) of streptokinase and rt-PA alone suggest a higher early patency rate with rt-PA.[540] However, the ultimate proof of superior efficacy depends on mortality trials that necessarily require many more patients. The results of one such trial (the International t-PA/SK Mortality Trial/GISSI 2) have recently been published.[263] Another (ISIS 3) has been presented[540a]; and one other large comparative trial (GUSTO) is under way. Both ISIS 3 and the International t-PA/SK Mortality Trial showed no significant difference in mortaity rates between the two agents.[263] However, in these trials, intravenous heparin was not administered early as it has been in most other trials with rt-PA, and this might have led to a lower early patency rate (as discussed below), thus diminishing its efficacy.

EFFECT ON MORTALITY. There is no doubt that early intravenous therapy with thrombolytic drugs improves survival in patients with AMI (Fig. 39-20). In fact, 30-day and 1-year mortality rates in some of the controlled trials are impressive, with survival in one treated group as high as 93.1 per cent at 12 months.[541] Mortality varies considerably depending on patients included for study and adjunctive therapies employed.[528] The benefit of thrombolytic therapy appears to be greatest when agents are administered as early as possible, with incremental benefit demonstrated if drug is administered less than 4 to 6 hours after the onset of pain, and even better results are seen when drug is given less than 1 to 2 hours after symptoms begin.[486,528] The impact of early treatment was first clearly shown in the initial GISSI trial[501] and confirmed in ISIS 2.[502] Although an analysis of patients treated 7 to 24 hours after symptom onset suggests a therapeutic benefit of thrombolysis as well, firm conclusions about the efficacy of such late therapy await the results of several ongoing placebo-controlled trials addressing this issue.

There has been debate about the relative benefit of thrombolytic therapy in inferior versus anterior myocardial infarction,[542] because, for example, initial results from the first GISSI trial showed no improvement in survival for inferior MI.[501] However, more careful analysis of data has subsequently shown that infarct *size* rather than *location* is the key variable, with no significant benefit in the smallest of infarcts, while the benefit (in terms of survival) increases with progressively larger infarcts.[501,543]

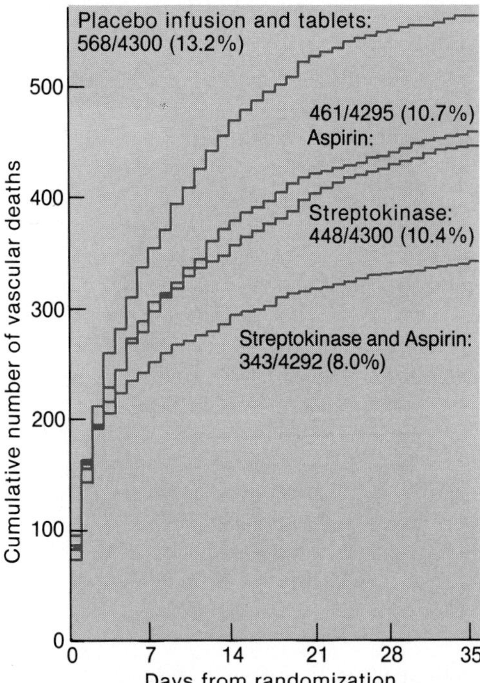

FIGURE 39-20. Cumulative vascular mortality (deaths from cardiac, cerebral, hemorrhagic, or other known vascular disease) in days 0–35 of the Second International Study of Infarct Survival (ISIS-2). The four curves describe mortality for patients allocated (i) active streptokinase only, (ii) active aspirin only, (iii) both active treatments, and (iv) neither. Note that individually, aspirin and streptokinase have a favorable effect of similar magnitudes, and that together the benefits appear additive. (From ISIS-2 [Second International Study of Infarct Survival] Collaborative Group: Randomized trial of intravenous streptokinase, oral aspirin, both, or neither among 17,187 cases of suspected acute myocardial infarction: ISIS-2. Lancet *2*:349, 1988.)

A wide variety of other clinical benefits appear to accrue to patients treated with thrombolytic agents, including a reduction in ventricular arrhythmias,[486] asystole,[544] and cardiac arrest,[502] as well as a significantly lower incidence of cardiogenic shock.[544] Longer-term follow-up is now available from early trials.[545,546] Results indicate that the early favorable results of thrombolytic therapy are sustained over time, with one study showing that the benefit of a lower mortality is maintained over the 5-year follow-up.[546]

EFFECT ON LEFT VENTRICULAR FUNCTION. While precise measurements of infarct size would be an ideal endpoint for clinical reperfusion studies, such measures have been found to be impracticable. Trials have used the myocardial sparing as indirectly reflected in the preservation of left ventricular function as an important endpoint—one that is also well known to be prognostically important as well. As with survival, improvement in global left ventricular function is related to the time of thrombolytic treatment, with greatest improvement occurring with earliest therapy.[486,528,547] Improvement in left ventricular function is apparently greater with anterior than with inferior infarcts.[486] Trials have failed to demonstrate any difference in global left ventricular function when streptokinase and rt-PA were compared.[538,548,549] However, global ejection fraction is an imprecise measurement of ventricular function because hyperkinesis of noninvolved myocardium may prevent the reduction that would result from akinesis of the involved muscle. Regional left ventricular function of the ischemic myocardium has been shown to improve with streptokinase,[550] with APSAC,[551] and with rt-PA.[552] When regional wall motion was analyzed in a streptokinase versus rt-PA study, the latter appeared to be of greater benefit.[548] Reperfusion with either streptokinase or rt-PA appears to prevent some degree of late ventricular dilatation following AMI.[175,553] In many studies, the survival benefit appears to exceed measured improvements in ventricular function.[547] This may reflect the impact on group data of survivors with markedly improved left ventricular function who would have died had they not been treated with a thrombolytic drug. In general, studies employing ventricular function as an endpoint have been much smaller than the survival trials and have at times included patients without Q-wave infarction in whom the benefit of thrombolytic therapy may well be produced by different mechanisms. Furthermore, as discussed on page 1267, long-term survival may be enhanced by long-term patency of the coronary artery as well as by diminished infarct size.

PATIENT SELECTION FOR THROMBOLYTIC THERAPY. In view of the established benefit of thrombolytic therapy, it is unfortunate that not more patients with AMI are being treated. Among patients presenting to emergency departments with MI, it has been estimated that 15 to 37 per cent are appropriate candidates for thrombolysis.[554–557] Firm recommendations cannot be made for the selection of patients in some instances. Most studies have excluded patients older than 70 to 75 years, yet among those that have included more elderly patients, thrombolytic therapy appears to be of benefit as judged from subgroup analysis.[501,502,558,559] In careful reviews of this subject, it was concluded that it is the elderly patient who may actually benefit most from thrombolytic therapy.[560,561] Patients with inferior, small, or prior infarcts have not been shown conclusively to benefit from thrombolytic therapy. Therapy should probably be reserved for those with at least a moderate amount of myocardium in jeopardy or otherwise at high risk (Table 39–6). The potential benefit of thrombolytic therapy in non-Q-wave MI is not yet clear but is currently under investigation. Finally, as already noted, the outside time limit for benefit is incompletely defined, and late therapy, while likely not to be universally helpful, should be considered for patients with clear evidence of ongoing ischemia.[561]

ADJUNCTIVE TREATMENT. Anticoagulants and antiplatelet therapy may play an important role in establishing and maintaining the success achieved by the use of thrombolytic drugs.[562a] The Second International Trial of Intravenous

TABLE 39-6

A) MORTALITY 6 WEEKS FOLLOWING THROMBOLYTIC THERAPY FOR EACH OF EIGHT RISK FACTORS IN 3261 PATIENTS*

RISK FACTOR	NO. OF PATIENTS WITH RISK FACTOR (%)	NO. OF DEATHS IN 6 WEEKS (%)
Age ≥70 years	374 (11.5)	42 (11.2)
Previous infarction	456 (13.7)	36 (7.9)
Anterior infarction	1681 (51.5)	94 (5.6)
Atrial fibrillation	66 (2.0)	7 (10.6)
Rales in more than one third of lung fields	105 (3.2)	13 (12.4)
Hypotension and sinus tachycardia	158 (4.8)	16 (10.1)
Female gender	577 (17.7)	41 (7.1)
Diabetes mellitus	425 (13.0)	36 (8.5)

B) MORTALITY 6 WEEKS FOLLOWING THROMBOLYTIC THERAPY ACCORDING TO NUMBER OF RISK FACTORS† PRESENT INITIALLY

NO. OF RISK FACTORS	NO. OF PATIENTS	NO. OF DEATHS WITHIN 6 WEEKS	MORTALITY RATE (%)
0	864	13	1.5
1	1384	32	2.3
2	689	48	7.0
3	231	30	13.0
≥4	93	16	17.2

* Seventy-eight patients with cardiogenic shock or pulmonary edema were excluded.

† Possible risk factors listed in A.

Data from analysis of patients enrolled in Phase II of the Thrombolysis in Myocardial Infarction (TIMI) trial. Hillis, L. D., Foreman, S., and Braunwald, E.: Risk stratification before thrombolytic therapy in patients with acute myocardial infarction. Reprinted by permission of the American College of Cardiology. J. Am. Coll. Cardiol. *16*:313, 1990.

TABLE 39-7 EARLY MORTALITY (≤42 DAYS) IN PATIENTS TREATED WITH INTRAVENOUS THROMBOLYTIC DRUGS WITH AND WITHOUT HEPARIN

	PLACEBO GROUPS			TREATMENT GROUPS		
	No. of	MORTALITY		No. of	MORTALITY	
RESULTS*	Patients	%	No.	Patients	%	No.
With intravenous heparin	**3025**	**9.3**	**280**	**8716**	**5.6**	**491**
Without intravenous heparin	**16,331**	**13.1**	**2144**	**34,581**	**9.3**	**3226**

From Tiefenbrunn, A. J., and Sobel, B. E.: Thrombolysis and myocardial infarction. Fibrinolysis 5:1, 1991

* Trials included are:

With heparin: ASSET, initial European Cooperative Study Group Trial (ECSG), ECSG IV, ECSG V, HART, ISIS II patients treated with streptokinase for whom intention to treat with intravenous heparin was noted, New Zealand I, New Zealand II, SCATI, TIMI II, TIMI IIB.

Without heparin: GISSI I, GISSI II, ISIS II, HART (patients from the nonheparin arm of the trial), SCATI (patients from the nonheparin arm of the trial).

(See references for further details of individual studies.)

Streptokinase[502,562a] demonstrated a clear benefit when aspirin was added to streptokinase (Fig. 39-20). Concurrent therapy with aspirin is now widely recommended with use of all thrombolytic agents, although optimal initial dose (80 to 325 mg) and ideal starting time (0 to 24 hours) have not been firmly established. Newer and potentially more potent antiplatelet drugs (p. 1266) are being actively studied and may well be of benefit in the future.[542]

The importance of interactions between heparin (and antiplatelet and other antithrombotic agents) and fibrinolytic drugs cannot be overemphasized. The clinical efficacy of thrombolysis appears to depend on a favorable balance between dissolution of clot and retardation or prevention of concomitant continuing thrombosis.[562,563] Unopposed, persistent thrombosis reflected by elevation of concentrations in plasma of fibrinopeptide A may compromise coronary thrombolysis by delaying recanalization or predisposing to early reocclusion or both. Results of laboratory studies demonstrate the efficacy of antithrombin agents in potentiating thrombolysis,[564] and a favorable impact of heparin on outcome in trials of thrombolytic agents is strongly suggested by comparison of recent results (Table 39-7).

In the absence of adequate anticoagulation, early patency induced by thrombolytic drugs may not be sustained.[565,566] Accordingly, apparent failure of thrombolysis may occur more often. Impairment of a treatment effect may be more prominent with rt-PA than with streptokinase because of the relative lack of generation of high concentrations of fibrin degradation products with rt-PA.

From a pathophysiological point of view, it should be recognized that fibrinolytic agents appear to exert clinically occult procoagulant effects even when lysis is successful. The presence of such effects underscores the importance of adequate concomitant anticoagulation.[567] While the use of heparin has been well studied, important questions remain. With rt-PA, intravenous heparin does not appear to be necessary in the first 90 minutes[568] or after 24 to 48 hours.[569] Likewise, subcutaneous heparin at 12 hours does not reduce mortality.[263] However, in the period immediately following discontinuation of intravenous rt-PA, heparin may be crucial in maintaining the high early patency rate of this agent,[565,566] for, without it, angiographic patency rates at 1 to 3 days are compromised by as much as 50 per cent. While the role of early intravenous heparin with streptokinase and APSAC has not been well studied, theoretically it may be of less importance in view of the prolonged half-lives of these agents. However, the results of one small trial suggest a benefit of early intravenous heparin with streptokinase.[570]

Many other potential adjunctive therapies have been or are being considered. Beta-adrenoceptor blockers appear to be useful for preventing recurrent ischemic episodes and reinfarction,[3,513] while no such benefit has been demonstrated for calcium antagonists.[571] While the early use of nitrates may improve coronary patency in some patients,[572] such concurrent therapy has not been tested in controlled prospective trials. Finally, the possibility has been raised that agents which scavenge damaging oxygen-derived free radicals may reduce ischemic injury when given with thrombolytic agents[542] (p. 1187), and studies are being carried out to test this hypothesis.

COMPLICATIONS OF THROMBOLYTIC THERAPY. Recent (<1 year) exposure to streptococci or streptokinase produces some degree of antibody-mediated resistance to streptokinase (and APSAC) in most patients, but this is of clinical consequence only rarely. In the International tPA/SK Mortality Trial, allergic reactions were seen in 1.7 per cent of patients given streptokinase. Hypotension can be expected in 4 to 10 per cent.[263,502] Bleeding complications are, of course, most common and potentially the most serious.[573] Most bleeding is relatively minor with all agents, with more serious episodes occurring in patients requiring invasive procedures. Overall, 70 per cent of bleeding episodes occur at the site of vascular punctures.[573] Intracranial hemorrhage is the most serious complication of thrombolytic therapy[573a]; its frequency of about 0.5 per cent (as judged from results of numerous trials[486]) appears to be only slightly increased over that seen with anticoagulants alone.[592] The incremental incidence of intracranial hemorrhage with thrombolysis appears to be at least partially offset by a lower frequency of thrombotic strokes, so that the overall incidence of stroke is usually not much higher in patients receiving thrombolytic therapy compared with control patients. (However, the more devastating nature of hemorrhagic strokes as compared with the thrombotic type must be considered.) In addition to the risks introduced by invasive procedures, the following all appear to confer an increased risk of bleeding: female gender, lesser body weight, hypertension, older age, fibrinogen depletion, and a prolonged bleeding time at baseline.[573-575] Reports of more unusual complications such as splenic rupture[576] or aortic dissection[577] and cholesterol embolization[578] are beginning to appear as well.

DOSES. Most trials employing intravenous streptokinase have used 1.5 million units over 1 hour as a standard dose. The clinical acceptance of this dose was not preceded by the usual dose-response trials, however. Surprisingly, few studies have tried different doses until very recently. Although smaller doses have been found to be nearly as effective as the standard dose, trials testing these doses have not been of sufficient power to confirm this with a high degree of certainty.[579,580] One recent multicenter trial compared two smaller doses (200,000 units and 500,000 units) with the standard dose (1.5 million units) and one larger dose (3 million units).[581] Patency rates of the infarct-related artery were 38, 75, 60, and 82 per cent, respectively, with the lowest and highest doses each differing significantly from the middle two doses. Complications were low and similar in all groups. The implications of this preliminary trial are important: namely, that at twice the standard dose streptokinase may achieve patency rates comparable with those routinely seen with rt-PA and intravenous heparin together.

Alternative dosing strategies has been more extensively studied with rt-PA. Of the various regimens differing from the standard recommended doses that have been studied, two important newer strategies have clinical relevance. The first is that of so-called "front-loading."[582] Various regimens employing a larger *initial* bolus have shown a high patency rate.[583,584] The specific scheme proposed and tested by Neuhaus[585] appears most promising as it has produced the highest recanalization rate—92 per cent—yet reported for rt-PA: 15 mg intravenous bolus, 50 mg intravenous over 30 minutes, followed by 35 mg over the following 60 minutes (total dose 100 mg over 90 minutes). The improved efficacy of this regimen does not appear to be associated with a higher reocclusion rate, and the regimen does not seem to produce more frequent side effects. If these results are confirmed, current dosing recommendations for rt-PA should be modified to conform to this approach. The second important consideration is that of selection of optimal *total* dosage. It is widely recognized that bleeding complications increase with higher dosages and lesser patient body weights.[574] Accordingly, dosing on the basis of weight has been considered.[552,586,587] There are not sufficient data on which to base recommendations at present, although a total dosage of 2.0 mg/kg does appear to produce a higher incidence of intracranial bleeding (as was already recognized when 150 mg rather than 100 mg total dosage was given in the early phase of the TIMI II study[3]). It seems probable that an ideal regimen will eventually incorporate both front loading and dosing based on body weight.

Repeat dosing with rt-PA has been successfully employed in patients with acute reinfarction after initially successful thrombolysis with either rt-PA or streptokinase.[588] There does not appear to be an increased risk of bleeding, even when a full dosage of rt-PA is employed.[588] Because of antigenicity, repeat infusion of streptokinase or APSAC should be avoided.

INVESTIGATIONAL AGENTS AND COMBINATIONS. Urokinase (p. 1773), a thrombolytic agent that has been available for many years but is not approved for *intravenous* use in AMI, remains investigational in the United States. While probably as effective as streptokinase,[589] given its high cost, it appears to offer no advantage when used as the sole agent. *Single-chain urokinase-type plasminogen activator* (p. 1572) (scuPA or prourokinase) has been studied alone[590,591] and in combination with urokinase[592] and rt-PA.[593] Synergism has been suggested for these combinations, allowing for lower drug doses with higher clot specificity and less frequent bleeding complications. Combinations of urokinase and rt-PA[594] and streptokinase and rt-PA[595,595a] have also been tried for similar reasons. As yet, none of the newer agents or combinations have proved clearly to be of additional benefit, however. In the future, "protein engineering" may lead to molecular alterations of plasminogen activators that will improve both efficacy and safety.[596-598]

CORONARY ANGIOPLASTY IN AMI

It is now established that reperfusion *can* be achieved by emergency percutaneous transluminal coronary angioplasty (PTCA).[599-602] Using a guidewire and balloon catheter, it is technically easier to cross a total occlusion consisting of a fresh thrombus than to cross a longstanding occlusion of a coronary artery. Thus, wire-guided balloon angioplasty can be useful to achieve prompt reperfusion in two quite different situations: (1) in lieu of thrombolytic therapy, or (2) when thrombolysis has failed or when a severe stenosis remains after successful thrombolysis.

PRIMARY ANGIOPLASTY IN AMI. Although PTCA can be performed quickly and relatively safely after the onset of ischemia,[602,602a] the majority of patients with AMI do not have ready access to facilities in which this procedure can be performed. Emergency PTCA requires the ready availability of considerable resources but, despite the difficulty in mustering such resources, several centers have reported relatively extensive experiences with primary PTCA in AMI.[603-606] In these centers, outcome is generally quite favorable, with high primary success rates (78 to 94 per cent successful angioplasties), reocclusion rates of 10 to 15 per cent, improvement in global ejection fraction, and in-hospital mortality as low as 1 per cent in patients with single-vessel coronary artery disease,[607] but considerably higher (12 per cent) in patients with multivessel disease.[608] Small trials comparing thrombolytic therapy with PTCA directly suggest that the latter may result in less subsequent ischemia,[609,610,611a] presumably based on significantly less severe residual coronary artery stenosis produced by PTCA. While in-hospital mortality has generally been higher in patients with cardiogenic shock,[604,605] emergency PTCA in this setting (with or without prior thrombolytic therapy) can often be life-saving.[607,611] Despite the impressive results, the strategy of primary PTCA has not achieved widespread acceptance both because of the tremendous effort and resources (human and physical) required on a continuous standby basis and because, on a comparative basis, it has not been shown to be superior to an initial attempt at reperfusion with thrombolytic therapy.[612]

ANGIOPLASTY AS AN ADJUNCT TO THROMBOLYSIS. Immediate PTCA following thrombolytic therapy has the theoretical benefit of further opening of a stenosed coronary artery to increase flow, perhaps enhancing myocardial recovery and diminishing the possibility of reocclusion. However, in three separate trials of early emergency PTCA, it has been shown that this strategy actually increases the possibility of abrupt reclosure of the coronary artery and increases complications, including the need for urgent coronary artery bypass surgery, while providing no benefit in terms of overall mortality or recovery of ventricular function.[613-615] In the TIMI II study, the strategy of elective catheterization and PTCA, if suitable anatomy was found, within the first 2 days was compared with a strategy of catheterization and PTCA *only* if ischemia developed later in the hospital course or at predischarge exercise stress testing.[3] Here again, the more invasive course with early catheterization failed to provide any benefit in terms of either survival (Fig. 39–21) or improved ventricular function. As a result of this large trial as well as earlier key trials,[613-615] PTCA can be considered elective in most patients receiving thrombolytic therapy after AMI, with "watchful waiting" for ischemia at rest or during a prehospital discharge exercise test and a careful decision based on the clinical picture rather than routine catheterization and angioplasty.[616,617] Patients in whom thrombolytic therapy fails to achieve reperfusion represent candidates for PTCA (rescue angioplasty), and in such patients PTCA can usually be safe and effective (greater than 75 per cent success rates).[618-620] Unfortunately, it is difficult to know in advance of administering thrombolytic therapy which patients will require angioplasty, as *early* PTCA (as already noted) is *not* a practical technique to be used

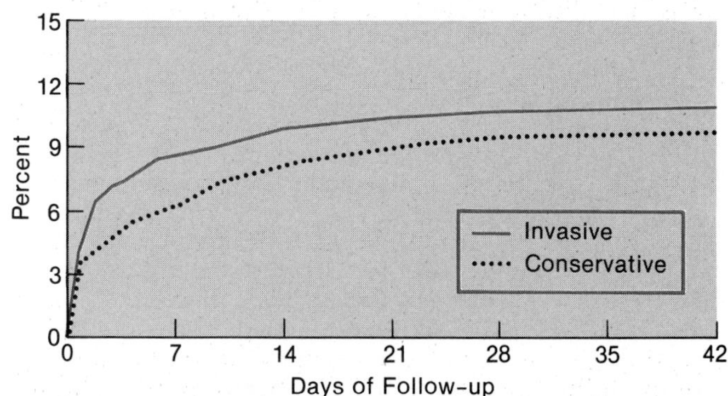

FIGURE 39–21. Cumulative percentage of patients in the invasive strategy and conservative strategy groups of the Thrombolysis in Myocardial Infarction (TIMI) Phase II trial who died or had confirmed nonfatal myocardial infarction (MI) during the 42 days after randomization. Invasive = coronary angiography and infarct-related artery coronary angioplasty (if vessel suitable) within 18–48 hours of thrombolytic therapy; Conservative = coronary angiography and angioplasty only if recurrent ischemia developed. (Reprinted by permission from the TIMI Study Group: Comparison of invasive and conservative strategies after treatment with intravenous tissue plasminogen activator in acute myocardial infarction. Results of the Thrombolysis in Myocardial Infarction [TIMI] Phase II Trial. N. Engl. J. Med. *320*:618, 1989.)

on a *routine* basis. Until there are better ways to recognize patients who might benefit from "rescue angioplasty," the question of optimal treatment of thrombolytic failure remains unresolved.[620] One approach employed in many centers is to perform emergency coronary arteriography on patients with AMI treated with thrombolytic therapy whose condition becomes or remains unstable followed by mechanical revascularization (PTCA or coronary bypass surgery) on those with persistently occluded infarct-related coronary arteries.

Either with or without previous thrombolytic therapy, certain clinical and angiographic features have been identified that can aid the clinician in selecting patients with AMI for PTCA. The most favorable outcome can be anticipated, not surprisingly, in younger patients with single-vessel disease and preserved ventricular function.[618,621] Emergency PTCA should probably be avoided in patients who have an open vessel if a clear-cut residual thrombus is present because abrupt closure appears to be relatively frequent in this situation. Emergency angioplasty also carries considerable more risk in patients with multilesion, multivessel disease and in those with severe hemodynamic compromise.[618,621] As already noted, however, in certain of the latter group, PTCA can be of substantial benefit albeit accompanied by high risk.[619]

Recommendations for Thrombolytic Therapy

On the basis of these considerations and of information from existing studies, as well as the authors' personal experience in the TIMI trials, and recognizing fully that this field is in rapid evolution, the following reperfusion strategy is recommended as of this writing.

1. Intravenous streptokinase (1.5 million units) administered over 1 hour, tissue plasminogen activator (t-PA) (a 6 mg bolus, a total of 60 mg during the first hour, 20 mg during the second hour and the third hour for a total of 100 mg), or Anistreplase (APSAC) (30 mg) given as a bolus should be given intravenously to all patients with impending or evolving transmural infarction (characteristic ischemic pain for ≥30 min, clear-cut new ST-segment elevation), if the drug can be administered within 4 to 6 hours of the onset of symptoms and if contraindications to the administration of this drug are not present (see below).

While as already stated there is still lively debate regarding the optimal thrombolytic agent(s), at this writing all three available thrombolytic agents appear to be effective in opening thrombolytically occluded coronary arteries and are approximately equally effective in reducing mortality. Cost considerations (SK is considerably less expensive than the other two agents) must sometimes influence the selection. This economic advantage must be considered in the light of the apparent greater effectiveness of rt-PA over SK in opening occluded coronary arteries SK and the concern that the large comparison trials of rt-PA and SK[263,540a] may not have used a heparin regimen optimal for rt-PA. This concern is being addressed in the ongoing GUSTO trial.

Patients who have received earlier treatment with either SK or APSAC should not receive these agents a second time because of the development of anti-SK antibodies. Finally, patients who are hypotensive or otherwise hemodynamically unstable should probably receive rt-PA because SK and APSAC may intensify the hypotension.

2. If symptoms have been present for more than 4 to 6 hours, thrombolytic therapy should be employed only if there is clinical evidence of ongoing ischemia, including continuing or recurrent chest pain and/or continuing elevation of electrocardiographic ST segments.

3. *Absolute* contraindications (Table 39–8) to thrombolytic therapy include active internal bleeding, recent prolonged or traumatic cardiopulmonary resuscitation, recent head trauma or known intracranial neoplasm, suspected or possible aortic dissection, suspected pregnancy, recorded blood pressure of greater than 200/110, previous allergic reaction to a thrombolytic agent (with streptokinase or APSAC only), and

TABLE 39–8 CONTRAINDICATIONS TO THROMBOLYTIC TREATMENT (GUIDELINES)

RISK OF BLEEDING
Recent trauma, major surgery, or head injury (within 6 weeks)
Gastrointestinal hemorrhage
Symptoms of proven peptic ulceration (within 3 months)
Bleeding diathesis or chronic liver disease with portal hypertension
Allergy (streptokinase or anistreplase)
Previous treatment with streptokinase or anistreplase
Stroke (residual disability), transient ischemic attack within 6 months, cerebrovascular hemorrhage (ever)
Pregnancy
RELATIVE CONTRAINDICATIONS
Serious organic disease associated with increased risk of bleeding or embolization
Uncontrolled hypertension
Systolic pressure >200 mm Hg or diastolic pressure >110 mm Hg
Noncompressible arterial puncture within 14 days
Dental extraction within 14 days
Active menstruation or lactation
Prolonged cardiopulmonary resuscitation
Diabetic proliferative retinopathy

From Verstraete, M.: Thrombolytic treatment in acute myocardial infarction. Circulation *82*(Suppl.II):96, 1990, by permission of the American Heart Association.

presence of any condition that readily leads to hemorrhage (e.g., diabetic hemorrhagic retinopathy). *Relative* contraindications include history of a cerebrovascular accident, known bleeding diathesis, recent trauma or major surgery (within 6 weeks), history of severe recently uncontrolled hypertension, significant liver dysfunction, and prior exposure to streptokinase or APSAC (if either of those agents is to be given). Either rt-PA or urokinase can be used repeatedly or after streptokinase. Finally, thrombolytic therapy should be used with great caution in the elderly (over 80 years), and in any patient who is agitated, lethargic, or confused.

4. Before the institution of thrombolytic therapy, consideration should be given to the patient's need for intravascular catheterization, as would be required for the placement of an arterial pressure monitoring line, a pulmonary artery catheter for hemodynamic monitoring, or a temporary transvenous pacemaker. If any of these are required, ideally they should be placed, as expeditiously as possible, *before* infusion of the thrombolytic agent is begun. If such procedures will require an additional delay of more than 30 minutes, they should be deferred for as long as possible after thrombolytic therapy is begun. In the early hours *after* institution of thrombolytic therapy, such catheterization should be performed only if crucial to survival, and then sites where excessive bleeding can be controlled should be chosen (e.g., subclavian vein catheterization should be avoided).

5. With infusion of rt-PA, intravenous heparin should be employed initially given as a bolus of 5000 units intravenously, followed by a continuous infusion. It should be begun at the rate of 1000 units/hr and adjusted to keep the activated partial thromboplastin time at $1\frac{1}{2}$ to 2 times control value. Aspirin (160 to 325 mg) should be administered within 24 hours of thrombolytic therapy regardless of the agent chosen. It should be continued indefinitely.

6. Emergency PTCA should be reserved for those patients who have access to a skilled cardiac catheterization team that is highly experienced in the performance of coronary angioplasty and readily available. Angioplasty should be employed on an emergency basis if thrombolytic therapy is contraindicated or if attempts at myocardial salvage have apparently failed after thrombolytic therapy, particularly if cardiac function is severely impaired and/or if there is clinical evidence of widespread ongoing ischemia. Primary PTCA may also be employed (without antecedent thrombolytic treatment or contraindications thereto) in the earliest (4) hours of an infarct in

patients with extensive ischemia and with the immediate availability of a skilled team and laboratory.

7. Elective PTCA should be reserved for patients who develop recurrent ischemia at any point during hospitalization, including during the predischarge exercise stress test. When a patient develops one of these indications and if a qualified catheterization team and well-equipped laboratory are not available in the facility in which the patient is located, the patient should be transferred promptly to a tertiary care center.

8. If recurrent ischemia develops and does not readily resolve, and if immediate catheterization with angioplasty backup is unavailable, retreatment with rt-PA should be considered. If prior therapy was within 12 hours (for rt-PA) or 24 hours (for streptokinase), the dose should be reduced by 25 to 50 per cent; otherwise a full dose can be administered, albeit cautiously.

9. Additional medical therapy with beta blockers, nitrates, and/or calcium antagonists should be routinely employed, as required, just as they are for other patients with AMI or for those undergoing coronary angioplasty.

SURGICAL REPERFUSION IN ACUTE MYOCARDIAL INFARCTION

There have been extensive improvements in intraoperative myocardial preservation with cardioplegia and hypothermia and in surgical techniques. These have allowed surgical reperfusion in coronary patients with AMI to be carried out at quite low short- and long-term mortality rates—approximately 2 per cent in-hospital and 25 per cent 10-year mortality rates in selected centers. This has kept alive the concept of emergency coronary revascularization as a possible measure to protect jeopardized myocardium in patients suffering AMI.[622–625] As appears to be the case for all methods designed to limit infarct size, this therapy can be successful only if it is applied within the first 4 to 6 hours (preferably the first 2 hours) of the onset of the acute event. In the usual patient who develops an AMI outside of the hospital, it is logistically difficult to bring the patient to the hospital, carry out a clinical evaluation, outline the coronary anatomy by arteriography, assemble the surgical team, commence operation, and place the patient on cardiopulmonary bypass in less than 4 hours after the onset of the event. It is therefore unlikely that surgical reperfusion can or will be widely applied on a regular basis in the routine treatment of AMI. Indeed, the operation is contraindicated in patients with uncomplicated transmural infarcts more than 6 hours after the onset of the event. When carried out at this time, surgical reperfusion appears to produce marked hemorrhage into the area of infarction.[626]

However, in some patients with AMI, including some with cardiogenic shock, infarction appears to occur in a stuttering manner over an interval of several days.[627] Theoretically, revascularization carried out more than 6 hours after the onset of the event might be of benefit in this group, but this has yet to be established firmly. Also, coronary bypass surgery can be carried out promptly in patients who develop coronary occlusion during cardiac catheterization, coronary arteriography, and PTCA, as well as in patients whose coronary anatomy has been assessed recently by coronary arteriography and who develop an infarction in the hospital while awaiting operation.

Patients undergoing successful thrombolysis but with important residual stenoses, who on anatomical grounds are more suitable for surgical revascularization than for PTCA, have undergone coronary artery bypass surgery with quite low mortality and morbidity.[628–630] Although postoperative chest tube drainage with relatively minor bleeding occurs more commonly than after elective bypass surgery, this problem is not of major concern.[628] PTCA is preferable in patients suitable for this procedure, whereas surgery should be reserved for those in whom PTCA has not been successful or could not be performed, or for patients with left main or extensive multivessel coronary artery disease for whom coronary artery bypass graft surgery would be recommended even in the absence of AMI. Thus, it is in this group of patients with AMI, i.e., those who have undergone or who are undergoing thrombolytic therapy with continued severe ischemic and hemodynamic instability, that a small subgroup can be identified who are likely to benefit from emergency revascularization. In this group, bypass of noninfarct-related coronary artery obstructions can be expected to produce additional benefit.

Elective coronary artery bypass surgery has been carried out soon after AMI for much the same reasons as just outlined (see #6 above). If recurrent ischemia occurs in multivessel or left main coronary disease, that is, if the patient has coronary anatomy unsuitable for PTCA, coronary artery bypass grafting is a reasonable alternative and should be used—particularly in patients with easily provoked ischemia or impaired left ventricular function. Large series of patients operated on within 30 days of AMI have been reported with excellent long-term survival.[631,632] However, when surgery is performed under urgent conditions with active and ongoing ischemia or cardiogenic shock, operative mortality rises steeply.[631,632] At autopsy, such patients have extensive myocardial necrosis that is often hemorrhagic.[633]

PHARMACOLOGICAL THERAPY OF ACUTE MYOCARDIAL INFARCTION

BETA-ADRENOCEPTOR BLOCKADE

(See also p. 1225)

The immediate administration of beta-adrenoceptor blockers reduces cardiac index, heart rate, blood pressure, and tension-time index levels. The next effect of these drugs is a reduction in myocardial oxygen consumption per minute and per beat. Favorable effects of beta-adrenoceptor blockade on the balance of myocardial oxygen supply and demand are reflected in the reduction of myocardial lactate production and diminution of ventricular arrhythmias.[634] Since beta-adrenoceptor blockade diminishes circulating levels of free fatty acids by antagonizing the lipolytic effects of catecholamines, and since elevated levels of fatty acids augment myocardial oxygen consumption and probably increase the incidence of arrhythmias, these metabolic actions of beta-blocking agents may also be beneficial to the ischemic heart.[634] The effects of beta blockers on AMI can be divided into those that are immediate (when the drug is given very early in the course of infarction) and long-term (secondary prevention), when the drug is initiated sometime after infarction. The former type, which is part of the acute management of AMI, is considered this section; the latter, on p. 1254.

Objective evidence of beneficial effects of beta blockers in acute myocardial ischemia has been reported by several investigators using various modifications of the precordial ST-segment mapping technique.[635,636] For example, Gold et al.[635] found that the likelihood of a beneficial clinical and electrocardiographic response increased in the presence of residual antegrade or collateral blood flow to the infarct zone, as determined by coronary arteriography. Peter et al.[637] found that patients treated within 4 hours of onset of symptoms of uncomplicated MI had significantly lower peak serum creatine kinase levels and less cumulative creatine kinase release into plasma than did patients without specific therapy. The same group[638] also found that patients with suspected MI, treated with propranolol within 4 hours of the onset of symptoms, had a significantly lower incidence of infarction. This suggests that threatened infarction might actually be prevented by early beta blockade. Similarly, Yusuf et al. have reported that intravenous atenolol, given a median of 4 hours following onset of symptoms of AMI, decreased the incidence of AMI, CK-MB release, the electrocardiographic evolution of infarction, and the severity of ischemic pain.[639] Alprenolol[640] and metoprolol[641] begun early in the course of infarction have been shown to limit enzymatically estimated infarct size.

RESULTS OF MULTICENTER TRIALS. At least 27 randomized beta blocker trials involving over 27,000 patients have been undertaken.[16] Of these, there have been four large trials designed to test the effects of early beta blockade in myocardial infarction. In the *Multicenter Investigation for the Limitation of Infarct Size* (MILIS) study, propranolol adminis-

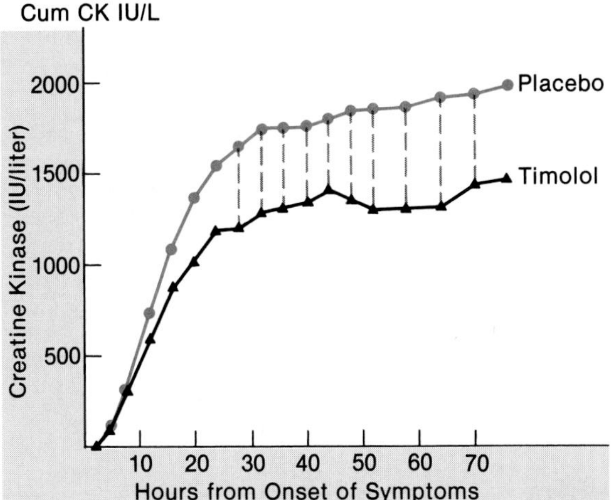

FIGURE 39–22. Mean cumulative release of creatine kinase during the evolution of acute myocardial infarction. Time zero denotes onset of symptoms. Significant differences between the two groups are indicated by vertical dashed lines. (Reprinted by permission from The International Collaborative Study Group: Reduction of infarct size with the early use of timolol in acute myocardial infarction. N. Engl. J. Med. *310*:9, 1984.)

tered an average of 8.5 hours after the onset of symptoms, when compared to control, failed to reduce infarct size.[642] More favorable results were reported by the *International Collaborative Study Group*, which reported on the use of intravenous timolol in the early phase of AMI.[643] In this study, patients were treated a mean of 3.4 hours after the onset of symptoms, and infarct size was smaller in timolol-treated patients as assessed by cumulative release of CK (Fig. 39–22) and by electrocardiographic indices.

In a large randomized trial using intravenous metoprolol (the *MIAMI Trial*),[644] infarct size was found to be smaller by enzymatic criteria (maximum serum activity of aspartate aminotransferase [AST]) in the metoprolol group but only in patients treated within 7 hours. All these studies are consistent with experimental and other clinical evidence that ischemic myocardium can be spared from irreversible injury only if treated early enough in the infarction process. For most patients, the outside time limit for salvaging viable myocardium is probably in the range of 4 to 6 hours. Benefit is highly variable if treatment is begun between 6 and 12 hours.

In an additional large multicenter trial *(ISIS 1)* involving over 16,000 patients, investigators reported a significant reduction in mortality among the patients randomized to intravenous atenolol when compared to placebo-treated patients.[645] Patients were treated at a mean of 5 hours after the onset of suspected AMI. Mortality was reduced by 15 per cent at one week and this difference was maintained for the first year of follow-up. The study further suggests that treatment of approximately 200 patients would result in avoidance of one reinfarction, one cardiac arrest, and one death in the first week after onset of an AMI.[645]

In the TIMI II trial the addition of a beta blocker (metoprolol) to thrombolytic therapy was studied.[3] While recurrent ischemia and reinfarction were reduced by metoprolol, mortality was not reduced nor was ventricular function improved. Thus, beta blockade may not enhance salvage of myocardium in the setting of early reperfusion but may confer clinical benefit by means of its antiischemic effect.[513]

Given the overall favorable effects of beta blockade in the aforementioned clinical trials, patients in a hyperdynamic state (sinus tachycardia, hypertension, no evidence of heart failure or bronchospasm) as well as patients seen in the first 4 hours would appear to be good candidates for this therapy, regardless of whether thrombolytic therapy is employed. Unless there are contraindications, beta blockade probably should be continued in patients who develop AMI. In addition, beta blockers are indicated in patients in whom infarction is complicated by persistent or recurrent ischemic pain, progressive or repetitive serum enzyme elevations suggestive of infarct extension, or tachyarrhythmias refractory to lidocaine and procainamide early after the onset of infarction. If adverse effects of beta blockers develop, or if patients present with complications of infarction that are contraindications to beta blockade such as heart failure or heart block, the beta blocker should be withheld or can be discontinued safely.[646]

RECOMMENDATIONS. In patients with AMI who have not received beta blockers in the preceding 24 hours, this therapy may be administered as metoprolol 15 mg intravenously, divided into three equal doses given at 2- to 5-minute intervals. During this period, heart rate and arterial pressure should be determined, and an electrocardiographic strip should be recorded after each injection. Intravenous beta blockade should not be administered in patients with a history of bronchial asthma, and administration should be halted if any of the following events are present or develop:

1. Second- or third-degree AV block or lengthening of the P-R interval beyond 0.24 sec.
2. Rales extending more than one-third of the way up the lung fields, or wheezes detected on auscultation.
3. Heart rate below 50 per minute.
4. Systolic arterial pressure below 90 to 95 mm Hg.
5. Pulmonary artery wedge pressure above 20 to 24 mm Hg. (While it is useful to monitor this pressure in patients in whom a beta blocker will be administered, it is by no means essential.)

The intravenous administration of metoprolol is followed 6 to 8 hours later by oral metoprolol given first as 50 mg twice daily for the first day and then advanced to 100 mg twice daily, if the lower dose is tolerated. Ideally, the dose should keep the heart rate between 50 to 65 beats/min and the systolic pressure above 95 mm Hg in the absence of heart failure, wheezing, or advanced AV block.

Selection of Beta Blocker. At the time of this writing, only metoprolol has been approved for intravenous use in AMI by the Food and Drug Administration. However, favorable effects have also been reported with atenolol, timolol, and alprenolol; these benefits probably occur with propranolol and esmolol, an ultrashort-acting agent, as well.

In the absence of any favorable evidence supporting the benefit of agents with intrinsic sympathomimetic activity (ISA) such as pindolol and oxprenolol, and with some unfavorable evidence for any benefit of these agents in secondary prevention,[647] beta blockers with ISA probably should not be chosen for treatment of AMI. Occasionally the clinician may wish to proceed with beta blocker therapy even in the presence of *relative* contraindications, such as a history of mild asthma, mild bradycardia, mild heart failure, or first-degree heart block. In this situation, a trial of the very short-acting beta blocker esmolol (p. 1304) may help determine whether the patient can tolerate beta blockade.[648,649] Since the hemodynamic effects of this drug, with a half-life of 9 minutes, disappear in less than 30 minutes, it offers considerable advantage over longer-acting agents when the risk of a beta blocker complication is relatively high.

Although antagonism of sympathetic stimulation to the heart might be expected to exacerbate pulmonary edema in patients with occult heart failure, usually only small changes in pulmonary capillary wedge pressure occur when the drug is used in patients with AMI.[634]

NITRATES

(See also p. 1304)

Intravenous nitroglycerin has been reported to reduce infarct size in AMI patients.[650,651] The early use of intravenous nitroglycerin appears to diminish the frequency of mechanical complications of AMI and improves postinfarction ventricular remodeling.[651] Furthermore, in patients with heart failure, mortality and serious ventricular arrhythmias appeared to be reduced in the nitroglycerin-treated group.[650,651] Bussmann and associates[652] found significantly lower values of peak serum CK, lower rates of CK release, and smaller calculated infarct sizes in nitroglycerin-treated patients. Flaherty and colleagues[653] have shown in a prospective, randomized trial that treatment with intravenous nitroglycerin for 48 hours followed by nitroglycerin ointment therapy for 72 hours enhanced postinfarction improvement of myocardial perfusion measured with ^{201}Tl scintigraphy.

As with other interventions to spare ischemic myocardium in AMI, intravenous nitroglycerin appears to be of greatest benefit in patients treated earliest.[651,653] Patients with inferior wall infarction are particularly sensitive to an excessive fall in preload, particularly if concurrent right ventricular infarction is present.[432] In such cases nitrate-induced venodilatation could impair cardiac output and reduce coronary blood flow, thus worsening myocardial oxygenation rather than improving it.[654]

HEMODYNAMIC EFFECTS. In patients with AMI, the administration of nitroglycerin and other nitrates such as isosorbide dinitrate diminishes pulmonary capillary wedge pressure and systemic arterial pressure as well as left ventricular end-systolic and end-diastolic volumes. It also reduces ventricular asynergy, to the extent that the local impairment of left ventricular function is due to reversibly injured, depressed myocardium rather than to zones of completed infarction or scar.[655] When systemic arterial and pulmonary capillary wedge pressures are normal or low prior to the administration of nitroglycerin, reflex tachycardia may result from the further reduction of ventricular filling and arterial pressures.

MODE OF ADMINISTRATION. Intravenous nitroglycerin can be administered safely to patients with evolving MI as long as the dose is titrated carefully to avoid induction of reflex tachycardia or systemic arterial hypotension (systolic blood pressure ≤ 95 mm Hg).[485] One useful regimen employs an initial infusion rate of 10 μg/min with stepwise increases of 10 μg/min until the mean arterial blood pressure is reduced by 10 per cent of its baseline level. Alternatively, it may be administered sublingually at doses of 0.3 to 0.6 mg. This route may be more hazardous, since the rate of absorption is difficult to control and arterial pressure may decline precipitously. Nitroglycerin is often useful for the relief of persistent pain and as a vasodilator in patients with infarction associated with left ventricular failure.

When continuous infusion of intravenous nitroglycerin is used, two important potential complications must be considered. First, most commercially available nitroglycerin for intravenous use is prepared in a solution with ethanol as a diluent. When high infusion rates are continued for several days, signs and symptoms of alcohol intoxication may occur.[656] Second, clinically significant methemoglobinemia has been reported to occur during administration of intravenous nitroglycerin.[657] Although uncommon, this problem is seen when unusually large doses of nitrates are administered. It is important not only for its potential to cause symptoms of lethargy and headache but also because elevated methemoglobin levels can impair the oxygen-carrying capacity of blood, potentially exacerbating ischemia.

Tolerance to intravenous nitroglycerin (as manifested by increasing nitrate requirements) develops in many patients, often as soon as 12 hours after the infusion is started.[658] Despite the theoretical and demonstrated benefit of sulfhydryl agents in diminishing tolerance, their use has not become widespread.[659,660]

ACTIONS. According to all of the available evidence, nitroglycerin very rarely opens previously occluded coronary arteries. Nevertheless, one or two 0.3 mg tablets of nitroglycerin should be given when a patient presents with acute chest pain, particularly if the diagnosis of AMI is not clear. Patients in whom the pain is caused by unstable angina often respond with prompt relief of chest pain. Despite the evidence of a favorable effect of nitroglycerin on infarct size as already discussed, *routine* use of this drug is not recommended in patients with established AMI. However, in patients with pump failure, pulmonary edema, or continuing ischemia, intravenous nitroglycerin may be useful for lowering preload and afterload, and for improving flow to ischemic myocardium. It is contraindicated in the presence of hypotension.

OTHER POTENTIALLY USEFUL APPROACHES TO PROTECTION OF ISCHEMIC MYOCARDIUM

The experimental observations indicating the potential usefulness of the interventions described below are summarized on pages 1190 to 1192.

CALCIUM ANTAGONISTS

Nifedipine. In multiple trials involving a total of over 5000 patients, nifedipine has not shown any benefit in infarct size reduction, prevention of progression to infarction, control of recurrent ischemia, or lowering of mortality.[661] Furthermore, several trials suggest a detrimental effect of early nifedipine.[662–665] Nifedipine does not appear to be helpful in conjunction with either thrombolytic therapy[664] or beta blockade.[662,665]

VERAPAMIL AND DILTIAZEM. Verapamil, although less well studied, has not had any demonstrated favorable effect on infarct size or other important endpoints in patients with AMI, with the exception of control of supraventricular arrhythmias.[661] Both verapamil and diltiazem have apparently reduced mortality in subgroups of patients free of heart failure.[666,667] While diltiazem has been shown to diminish myocardial oxygen requirements,[668] it has failed convincingly to reduce infarct size, improve ventricular function, and reduce ischemia.[661] Thus far, the promising effects of calcium antagonists in studies of animals with infarction[669] have not been widely translated to clinical benefit in patients with AMI.[436a,670]

GLUCOSE-INSULIN-POTASSIUM. Administration of a solution of glucose-insulin-potassium (300 gm of glucose, 50 units of insulin, and 80 mEq of KCl in 1000 ml of water administered at a rate of 1.5 ml/kg/hr) lowers the concentration of plasma free fatty acids and improves ventricular performance, as reflected in systolic arterial pressure, cardiac output, and stroke work at any level of left ventricular filling pressure[671]; also the frequency of ventricular premature beats decreases.[672] In a nonrandomized study, mortality appeared to be reduced,[673] hemodynamics improved, global ejection fraction increased, and both asynergy in the ischemic zone and pulmonary artery diastolic pressure reduced.[672] However, no definitive effect on enzymatically estimated infarct size or long-term mortality has been described in a prospective, controlled, randomized trial.

INTRAAORTIC BALLOON COUNTERPULSATION. From a theoretical standpoint, intraaortic balloon counterpulsation might be expected to limit infarct size for several reasons. In experimental animals, intraaortic balloon counterpulsation decreases afterload and myocardial oxygen consumption,[630] decreases preload, increases coronary blood flow, and improves cardiac performance.[674] No definitive information is available indicating that intraaortic balloon counterpulsation alters the prognosis in patients with relatively uncomplicated infarction. Leinbach et al., however, have reported an immediate, persistent fall in ST-segment elevation. This occurred in patients with anterior MI who had preservation of precordial R waves and good ventricular function,[675] in whom the left anterior descend-

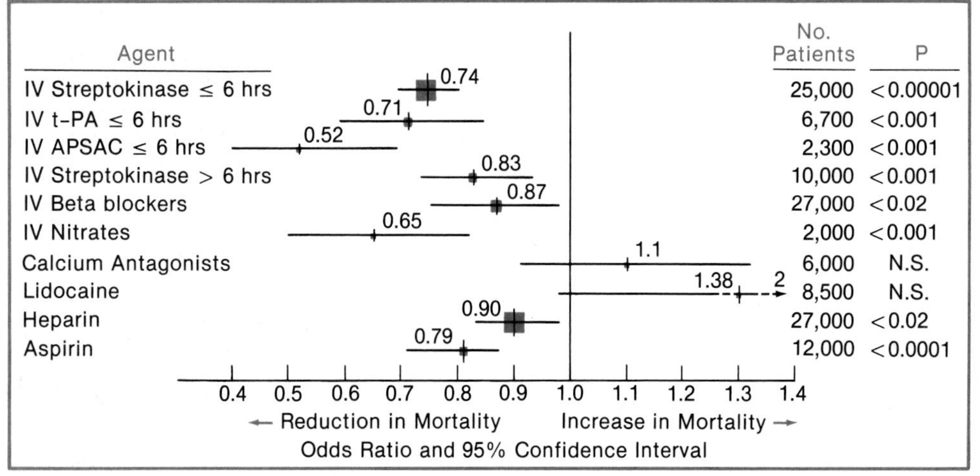

FIGURE 39–23. Summary of effects of various treatments on mortality in AMI. Odds ratios and their 95 per cent confidence intervals are plotted. The size of each square is related to the variance of the data. Larger squares reflect more data, and a narrower confidence interval indicates more precise estimates of treatment effect. IV, intravenous; t-PA, tissue plasminogen activator; APSAC, anisoylated plasminogen-streptokinase activator complex; NS, not significant. (From Yusuf, S., et al.: Routine medical management of acute myocardial infarction. Lessons from overviews of recent randomized controlled trials. Circulation *82*[Suppl II]:117, 1990, by permission of the American Heart Association, Inc.)

ing coronary artery was not totally occluded and who underwent intraaortic balloon pumping within 6 hours.

In a relatively small prospective trial intraaortic balloon pumping with intravenous nitroglycerin appeared to preserve function only in noninfarcted segments.[676] Given the relatively frequent rate of complications[677] after intraaortic balloon insertion and the absence of convincing data for infarct size reduction, intraaortic balloon pumping should be reserved for hemodynamically compromised patients and for those with refractory ischemia, for whom the benefit of this approach has been demonstrated.

OTHER AGENTS. Oxygen-derived free radicals are abundant in ischemic tissue and may contribute to myocardial injury, particularly following reperfusion (p. 1187). Evidence from studies in animals suggests that the extent of myocardial necrosis can be affected favorably by treatment with oxygen free radical scavengers such as superoxide dismutase.[678] Additionally, myocardial function is improved by the enhanced recovery induced by oxygen free radical scavengers after severe ischemia.[679] Studies in humans are under way to test the efficacy of this type of therapy for sparing injured myocardium.

The suggestion that magnesium metabolism is disturbed in AMI has led to several recent trials with intravenous magnesium. One such trial suggests that in-hospital mortality is reduced following a 48-hour magnesium infusion.[680] This improvement does not appear to be based solely on an antiarrhythmic effect.

Dozens of careful clinical trials carried out around the world by hundreds of collaborating investigators have made it possible to summarize and compare the results of different pharmacological therapies by the technique of meta-analysis. Such a comparison is shown in Figure 39–23.

Arrhythmias in Acute Myocardial Infarction

The genesis and diagnosis of arrhythmias are presented in Chapters 22 and 24 and their treatment in Chapters 23 and 25. The role of arrhythmias in complicating the course of patients with AMI and the prevention and treatment of these arrhythmias in this setting are discussed here and summarized in Table 39–9.

Some abnormality of cardiac rhythm has been noted in 72 to 96 per cent of patients with AMI treated in coronary care units.[234,681] The incidence of arrhythmias is higher in those patients seen earlier after the onset of symptoms. Moreover, many arrhythmias occur before hospitalization, before the patient is monitored.[682] Thus, the overall incidence of rhythm disturbance in AMI may actually be as high as 100 per cent. However, these data are difficult to interpret, since ambulatory electrocardiographic monitoring has also disclosed arrhythmias in a high percentage of asymptomatic, apparently healthy middle-aged men.[683]

Arrhythmias occurring in patients with AMI require vigorous treatment when they (1) impair hemodynamics; (2) compromise myocardial viability by augmenting myocardial oxygen requirements; or (3) predispose to malignant ventricular arrhythmias, i.e., ventricular tachycardia, ventricular fibril-

TABLE 39–9 CARDIAC ARRHYTHMIAS AND THEIR MANAGEMENT DURING ACUTE MYOCARDIAL INFARCTION

CATEGORY	ARRHYTHMIA	OBJECTIVE OF TREATMENT	THERAPEUTIC OPTIONS
I. *Electrical instability*	Ventricular premature beats	Prophylaxis against ventricular fibrillation	Antiarrhythmic agents (lidocaine, procainamide, beta blocker)
	Ventricular tachycardia	Prophylaxis against ventricular fibrillation, restoration of hemodynamic stability	Antiarrhythmic agents; cardioversion/defibrillation
	Ventricular fibrillation	Urgent reversion to sinus rhythm	Defibrillation; bretylium tosylate
	Accelerated idioventricular rhythm	Observation unless hemodynamic function is compromised	Increase sinus rate (atropine, atrial pacing); antiarrhythmic agents
	Nonparoxysmal AV junctional tachycardia	Search for precipitating causes (e.g., digitalis intoxication); suppress arrhythmia only if hemodynamic function is compromised	Atrial overdrive pacing; antiarrhythmic agents; cardioversion relatively contraindicated if digitalis intoxication present
II. *Pump failure/ Excessive sympathetic stimulation*	Sinus tachycardia	Reduce heart rate to diminish myocardial oxygen demands	Antipyretics; analgesics; consider beta blocker unless CHF present; treat latter if present with anticongestive measures (diuretics, afterload reduction)
	Atrial fibrillation and/or atrial flutter	Reduce ventricular rate; restore sinus rhythm	Verapamil, digitalis glycosides; anticongestive measures (diuretics, afterload reduction); cardioversion; rapid atrial pacing (for atrial flutter)
	Paroxysmal supraventricular tachycardia	Reduce ventricular rate; restore sinus rhythm	Vagal maneuvers; verapamil, cardiac glycosides, beta-adrenergic blockers; cardioversion; rapid atrial pacing
III. *Bradyarrhythmias and conduction disturbances*	Sinus bradycardia	Acceleration of heart rate only if hemodynamic function is compromised	Atropine; atrial pacing
	Junctional escape rhythm	Acceleration of sinus rate only if loss of atrial "kick" causes hemodynamic compromise	Atropine; atrial pacing
	Atrioventricular block and intraventricular block		Insertion of pacemaker

Modified from Antman, E. M., and Rutherford, J. D. (eds.): Coronary Care Medicine: A Practical Approach. Boston, Martinus Nijhoff Publishing, 1986, p. 78.

lation, or asystole. There is evidence that both the diminished threshold to ventricular fibrillation[684] and the incidence of malignant ventricular arrhythmias associated with infarction[463] are affected by the extent of the underlying infarction.[685]

When patients are seen *very early* during the course of MI they almost invariably exhibit evidence of increased activity of the autonomic nervous system. Thus sinus bradycardia, sometimes associated with AV block, and hypotension reflect the augmented vagal activity. Hypotension, regardless of cause, is hazardous in patients with AMI, since it impairs perfusion of marginally ischemic zones, intensifies ischemia, and may initiate or perpetuate the vicious circle illustrated in Figure 39–11 (p. 1210).

Activation of receptors within atrial and ventricular myocardium by necrotic tissue may cause enhanced efferent sympathetic activity, increased concentrations of circulating catecholamines, and local release of catecholamines from nerve endings within the heart. The last phenomenon may also result from direct ischemic damage of adrenergic neurons. In addition, ischemic myocardium may be hyperreactive to the arrhythmogenic effects of norepinephrine,[686] which may vary strikingly in concentration in different portions of the ischemic heart.[687] Sympathetic stimulation of the heart may also enhance the automaticity of ischemic Purkinje fibers. Furthermore, catecholamines facilitate propagation of slow current responses mediated by calcium, and stimulation of ischemic myocardium by catecholamines may exacerbate arrhythmias dependent on such currents.[686] Finally, it has been demonstrated that transmural infarction can interrupt both afferent and efferent limbs of the sympathetic nervous system innervating myocardium distal to the area of infarction (but still viable).[687] In addition to the potential for modifying a variety of cardiovascular reflexes, this creation of autonomic imbalance may promote the development of arrhythmias.[687] This explains why beta-adrenoceptor blocking agents may also be helpful in the treatment of ventricular arrhythmias, particularly when the latter are associated with other signs of heightened adrenergic activity.

The treatment of tachyarrhythmias involves not only the use of antiarrhythmic drugs but also correction of abnormalities of plasma electrolyte concentrations, acid-base balance disturbances, hypoxemia, anemia, and digitalis intoxication. In addition, it is essential to treat pericarditis, pulmonary emboli, and pneumonia or other infections, which may give rise to sinus tachycardia or other supraventricular tachyarrhythmias.

HEMODYNAMIC CONSEQUENCES OF CARDIAC ARRHYTHMIAS. Patients with significant left ventricular dysfunction have a relatively fixed stroke volume and depend on changes in heart rate to alter cardiac output. However, there is a narrow range over which the cardiac output is maximal, with significant reductions occurring at both faster and slower rates. Thus, all forms of bradycardia and tachycardia may depress the cardiac output in patients with AMI. Although the optimal rate insofar as cardiac output is concerned may exceed 100 per minute, it is important to consider that heart rate is one of the major determinants of myocardial oxygen consumption and that at more rapid heart rates myocardial energy needs can be elevated to levels that adversely affect ischemic myocardium. Therefore, in patients with AMI, the optimal rate is usually somewhat lower, in the range of 80 beats/min.

A second factor to consider in assessing the hemodynamic consequences of a particular arrhythmia is the loss of atrial transport function, i.e., the atrial "kick." [688] Studies in patients without AMI have demonstrated that loss of atrial transport decreases left ventricular output by 15 to 20 per cent.[689] However, in patients with reduced diastolic left ventricular compliance of any cause (including AMI), atrial systole is of greater importance for left ventricular filling. In patients with AMI, atrial systole boosts end-diastolic volume by 15 per cent, end-diastolic pressure by 29 per cent, and stroke volume by 35 per cent (Fig. 39–24).[690]

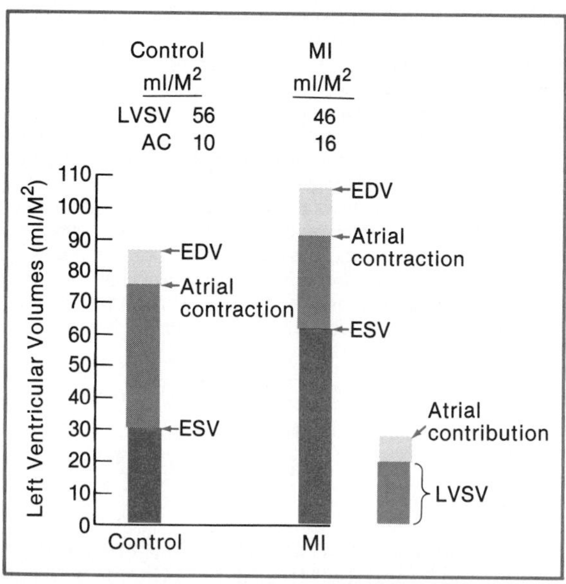

FIGURE 39–24. Average end-diastolic volumes (EDV), end-systolic volumes (ESV), left ventricular stroke volumes (LVSV), and atrial contribution (AC) in a control group of patients and in patients after myocardial infarction (MI). (From Rahimtoola, S. H., et al.: Left atrial transport function in myocardial infarction. Am. J. Med. *59*:686, 1975.)

BRADYARRHYTHMIAS

SINUS BRADYCARDIA

(See also p. 674)

Sinus bradycardia is the most common arrhythmia occurring during the early phases of AMI, and it is particularly frequent in patients with inferior and posterior infarction.[691,692] Observations in mobile coronary care units indicate that 25 to 40 per cent of patients with AMI have electrocardiographic evidence of sinus bradycardia within the first hour after the onset of symptoms; however, 4 hours after infarction commences, the incidence of sinus bradycardia has declined to 15 to 20 per cent.[682] The cause of the vagotonia and resultant bradycardia and hypotension accompanying AMI is not entirely clear. One factor appears to be stimulation of cardiac vagal afferent receptors (which are more common in the inferoposterior than the anterior or lateral portions of the left ventricle) with resulting efferent cholinergic stimulation of the heart. The phenomenon is a manifestation of the Bezold-Jarisch reflex.[693] This reflex is mediated by the vagus nerves and occurs during thrombolytic reperfusion, particularly of the right coronary artery.[514] Often sinus bradycardia is a component of a vasovagal or vasodepressor response, which may be intensified by severe pain as well as by morphine, and may be related to vasovagal syncope (p. 875).

The clinical significance of sinus bradycardia is debated. On the one hand, this arrhythmia is a risk factor during the very early phase of AMI and predisposes the patient to the development of repetitive ventricular arrhythmias and hypotension. On the other hand, it has been suggested on the basis of data obtained in experimental infarction and from some clinical observations that the increased vagal tone that produces sinus bradycardia during the early phase of AMI may actually be protective, perhaps because it reduces myocardial oxygen demands.[692] Thus the acute mortality rate appears to be as low in patients with sinus bradycardia as in patients without this arrhythmia.

MANAGEMENT. This depends upon the timing and severity, and on other clinical manifestations. Isolated sinus bradycardia, unaccompanied by hypotension or ventricular ectopy, should be observed rather than treated initially. In the first 4 to 6 hours following infarction, if the sinus rate is extremely slow (under 40/min), administration of intravenous atropine in aliquots of 0.3 to 0.6 mg every 3 to 10 minutes (with a total dose not exceeding 2 mg) to bring heart rate up to approximately 60/min often abolishes the premature ventricular beats commonly associated with this degree of sinus bradycardia. Atropine often contributes to restoration of arterial pressure and hence coronary perfusion, and should be employed if hypotension accompanying any degree of sinus bradycardia is present. The favorable effects of atropine may be accompanied by regression of ST-segment elevation. Elevation of the lower extremities will also often elevate arterial pressure by redistributing blood from the systemic venous bed to the thorax, thereby augmenting ventricular preload, cardiac output, and arterial pressure.

Sinus bradycardia occurring more than 6 hours after the onset of the AMI is often transitory, is caused by sinus node dysfunction or atrial ischemia rather than vagal hyperactivity, is usually not accompanied by hypotension, and does not usually predispose to ventricular arrhythmias. Treatment is not required unless ventricular performance is compromised or the administration of a beta-adrenoceptor blocker or high doses of antiarrhythmic drugs (which may slow the sinus rate further) is planned. When atropine is ineffective and the patient is symptomatic and/or hypotensive, electrical pacing is indicated (Chap. 25). In patients with depressed ventricular performance, who require the "atrial kick," atrial pacing or atrioventricular sequential pacing is superior to simple ventricular pacing.[694]

CONDUCTION DISTURBANCES: ATRIOVENTRICULAR AND INTRAVENTRICULAR BLOCK

Ischemic injury can produce blocks at any level of the atrioventricular or intraventricular conduction system. Such blocks may occur in the atrioventricular node, producing various grades of AV block; in either main bundle branch, producing right or left bundle branch block; and in the anterior and posterior divisions of the left bundle, producing left anterior or left posterior (fascicular) divisional blocks. Disturbances of conduction can, of course, occur in various combinations. The mechanisms and recognition of intraventricular conduction disturbances are discussed in Chapter 5 and of atrioventricular conduction disturbances in Chapter 24.

FIRST-DEGREE AV BLOCK (see also p. 711). First-degree AV block (Fig. 24–40, p. 711) occurs in 4 to 14 per cent of patients with AMI admitted to coronary care units. His bundle electrocardiographic studies have shown that almost all patients with first-degree AV block have disturbances in conduction *above* the bundle of His, i.e., intranodal. The localization of the site of block is important, since development of complete heart block and ventricular asystole is restricted almost exclusively to those patients with first-degree block in whom the conduction disturbance is *below* the bundle of His[695]; this occurs more commonly in patients with anterior infarction and in those with associated bifascicular block.[696]

First-degree AV block generally does not require specific treatment. However, if digitalis intoxication is suspected as the cause, this drug should be discontinued. Beta blockers and calcium antagonists (other than nifedipine) prolong AV conduction and may be responsible for first-degree AV block as well. However, discontinuation of these drugs in the setting of AMI has the potential of increasing ischemia and ischemic injury. Therefore, in the presence of first-degree block alone, the clinician may consider decreasing the dosage of these drugs but for this reason alone should not discontinue them. Only if higher-degree block or hemodynamic impairment occurs should these agents be stopped. If the block is a manifestation of excessive vagotonia and is associated with sinus bradycardia and hypotension, administration of atropine, as already outlined, may be helpful. In all circumstances, careful surveillance is important in view of the possibility of progression to higher degrees of block.[697]

SECOND-DEGREE AV BLOCK (see also p. 712). **Mobitz Type I, or Wenckebach.** Mobitz type I block (Fig. 24–43, p. 712) occurs in 4 to 10 per cent of patients with AMI admitted to coronary care units and accounts for about 90 per cent of all patients with AMI and second-degree AV block. This type of block (1) generally occurs within the AV node, (2) is usually associated with narrow QRS complexes, (3) is presumably secondary to ischemic injury, (4) occurs more commonly in patients with inferior than anterior myocardial infarction, (5) is usually transient and does not persist for more than 72 hours after infarction, (6) may be intermittent, and (7) rarely progresses to complete AV block. First-degree and type I second-degree AV block do not appear to affect survival, are most commonly associated with occlusion of the right coronary artery, and are caused by ischemia of the AV node.

Specific therapy also is not required in patients with second-degree AV block of the Mobitz type I variety when the ventricular rate is adequate and ventricular irritability, heart failure, and bundle branch block are absent. However, if these complications develop or if the heart rate falls below approximately 50 beats/min, immediate treatment with a temporary pacemaker is indicated.

Mobitz Type II. This is a rare conduction defect (Fig. 24–44, p. 712) following AMI, occurring in only 10 per cent of all cases of second-degree block[681]; thus, the overall incidence of Mobitz type II block after infarction is less than 1 per cent. In contrast to Mobitz type I block, type II second-degree block (1) usually originates from a lesion in the conduction system below the bundle of His, (2) is associated with a wide QRS complex, (3) often but not invariably reflects trifascicular block with impaired conduction distal to the bundle of His, (4) often progresses suddenly to complete AV block, and (5) is almost always associated with anterior rather than inferior infarction.

Because of its potential for progression to complete heart block, Mobitz type II second-degree AV block should be treated with a temporary demand pacemaker with the rate set at approximately 60 beats/min.

COMPLETE (THIRD-DEGREE) AV BLOCK (see also p. 714). The atrioventricular conduction system has a dual blood supply, the AV branch of the right coronary artery and the septal perforating branch from the left anterior descending coronary artery.[698] Therefore, complete AV block can occur in patients with either anterior or inferior infarction. Complete AV block develops in 5 to 8 per cent of patients with AMI. As with other forms of AV block, the prognosis depends on the anatomical location of the block in the conduction system and the size of the infarction.

In general, complete heart block in patients with inferior infarction results from an intranodal or prenodal lesion[699] and develops gradually, often progressing from first-degree or type I second-degree block. The escape rhythm is usually stable without asystole and often junctional, with a rate exceeding 40/min and a narrow QRS complex in 70 per cent of cases and a slower rate and wide QRS in the others. This form of complete AV block is often transient and resolves in a week.[696] The mortality is approximately 15 per cent unless right ventricular infarction is present, in which case the mortality associated with complete AV block may be more than doubled.[700]

In patients with anterior infarction, third-degree AV block often occurs suddenly, 12 to 24 hours after the onset of infarction, although it is usually preceded by intraventricular block and often a Mobitz type II pattern (not first-degree or Mobitz type I) AV block. Such patients have unstable escape rhythms with wide QRS complexes and rates less than 40 beats/min; ventricular asystole may occur quite suddenly. The mortality in this group of patients is extremely high, approximately 70 to 80 per cent.[701]

Prognosis. The prognosis for patients with AV block complicating AMI depends on the extent and secondarily on the anatomical site of the myocardial injury.[698] Thus, patients with inferior infarction often have concomitant ischemia or infarction of the AV node secondary to hypoperfusion of the AV node artery. However, the His-Purkinje system usually escapes injury in such individuals. Patients with inferior MI who develop AV block usually have lesions in both the right and left anterior descending arteries.[702] Likewise, patients with inferior MI and AV block have larger infarcts and more depressed right ventricular and left ventricular function than do patients with inferior infarct and no AV block. As already noted, junctional escape rhythms with narrow QRS complexes occur commonly in this setting. Hemodynamic derangements are often mild in these patients, and mortality is only slightly increased. In patients with anterior infarction, AV block usually develops as a result of extensive septal necrosis that involves the bundle branches. The high mortality in this group of patients with slow idioventricular rhythm and wide QRS complexes is the consequence of extensive myocardial necrosis resulting in severe left ventricular failure and often shock.

While data suggest that *complete* AV block is not an *independent* risk factor for mortality,[705] whether temporary transvenous pacing per se improves survival of patients with AMI remains controversial. Some investigators contend that ventricular pacing is useless when employed to correct complete AV block in patients with *anterior* infarction in view of the poor prognosis in this group regardless of therapy. We agree with others,[698,706] however, that ventricular or atrioventricular sequential pacing is indicated in essentially *all* patients with AMI with complete AV block. Pacing is likely to protect against transient hypotension with its attendant risks of extending infarction and precipitating malignant ventricular arrhythmias. Also, pacing protects against asystole, a particular hazard in patients with anterior infarction and infranodal block. Improved survival with pacing probably occurs in only a small fraction of patients with complete AV block and anterior wall infarcts, since the extensive destruction of the myocardium that almost invariably accompanies this condition results in a very high mortality rate, even in paced patients.

Given these considerations, an extremely large series of patients would be required to demonstrate the small reduction of mortality that might be achieved by pacing. The absence of data supporting such an effect, however, by no means excludes the possibility that it may be present. While it is generally agreed that pacing is indicated in patients with *inferior* wall infarction and complete AV block, it is of particular importance if the ventricular rate is very slow (<45 beats/min), if ventricular irritability or hypotension is present, or if pump failure develops; atropine is only rarely of value in these patients. Only when complete heart block develops in less than 6 hours after the onset of symptoms is atropine likely to abolish the AV block or cause acceleration of the escape rhythm.[707] In such cases the AV block is more likely to be transient and related to increases in vagal tone rather than the more persistent block seen later in the course of MI, which generally requires cardiac pacing.

INTRAVENTRICULAR BLOCK. Intraventricular conduction disturbances, i.e., block within one or more of the three subdivisions (fascicles) of the His-Purkinje system (the anterior and posterior divisions of the left bundle and the right bundle, p. 131), occur in 10 to 20 per cent of patients with AMI. The right bundle branch and the left posterior division have a dual blood supply from the left anterior descending and right coronary arteries, whereas the left anterior division is supplied by septal perforators originating from the left anterior descending coronary artery. Not all conduction blocks observed in patients with AMI can be considered to be complications of infarcts, since almost half are already present at the time the first ECG is recorded, and they may represent antecedent disease of the conduction system.

Isolated Left Anterior Divisional Block (Fig. 5–18, p. 130). This occurs in 3 to 5 per cent of patients with AMI,[708,709] and in an additional 5 per cent of patients with associated right bundle branch block and AMI.[708] Mortality is increased in these patients, although not as much as in patients with other forms of conduction block.

Left Posterior Divisional Block. This occurs in only 1 to 2 per cent of patients with AMI admitted to coronary care units. The posterior fascicle is larger than the anterior fascicle, and, in general, a larger infarct is required to block it. As a consequence, mortality is markedly increased.[708] Complete AV block is not a frequent complication of *either* form of isolated divisional block.

Right Bundle Branch Block. This defect alone occurs in approximately 2 per cent of patients with AMI and frequently leads to AV block because it is often a new lesion, associated with anteroseptal infarction. The mortality is high even if complete AV block does not occur.[681,708–711]

Bifascicular Block. The combination of right bundle branch block with either left anterior or posterior divisional block or the combination of left anterior and posterior divisional blocks (i.e., left bundle branch block) is known as bidivisional or bifascicular block (p. 132). If new block occurs in two of the three divisions of the conduction system, the risk of developing complete AV block is quite high.[681,708] Mortality is also high because of the occurrence of severe pump failure secondary to the extensive myocardial necrosis required to produce such an extensive intraventricular block.[712] Left bundle branch block occurs in approximately 5 per cent of patients with AMI. Although the latter defect progresses to complete AV block only half as frequently as does right bundle branch block, it is associated with as high a mortality as right bundle branch block and the other two forms of bifascicular block,[681,708,710,711] and with a high late mortality. Patients with intraventricular conduction defects, particularly right bundle branch block, account for the majority of patients who develop ventricular fibrillation late in their hospital stay. However, the high mortality in these patients occurs even in the absence of AV block and appears to be related to cardiac failure and massive infarction rather than to the conduction disturbance. Preexisting bundle branch block or divisional block is less often associated with the development of complete heart block in patients with AMI than are conduction defects acquired during the course of the infarct.[710] Bidivisional block in the presence of prolongation of the P-R interval (first-degree AV block) may indicate disease of the third subdivision rather than disease of the AV node. In such cases, termed trifascicular block, nearly 40 per cent will progress to complete heart block, a risk that is considerably greater than the risk of complete heart block without first-degree AV block.[706]

Complete bundle branch block (either left or right), the combination of right bundle branch block and left anterior divisional (fascicular) block, and any of the various forms of trifascicular block are all more often associated with anterior than inferoposterior infarction. All these forms are more frequent with large infarcts and in older patients and have a higher incidence of other accompanying arrhythmias than is seen in patients without bundle branch block.[711]

Use of Pacemakers in Acute Myocardial Infarction

(See also p. 728)

TEMPORARY PACING. Just as is the case for complete AV block, transvenous ventricular pacing has not resulted in statistically demonstrable improvement in prognosis among patients with AMI who develop intraventricular conduction defects. However, temporary pacing is advisable in certain of these patients because of the high risk of developing complete AV block. This includes patients with *new* bilateral (bifascicular) bundle branch block, i.e., right bundle branch block with left anterior or posterior divisional block and alternating right and left bundle branch block; first-degree AV block adds to this risk. Isolated new block in only one of the three fascicles even with P-R prolongation and preexisting bifascicular block and normal P-R interval poses somewhat less risk; these patients should be monitored closely, with insertion of a temporary pacemaker deferred unless higher-degree AV block occurs.

The risk of developing complete heart block following AMI can be predicted on the basis of results of an analysis of several large series of well-characterized patients with AMI.[712] The presence (new or preexisting) of any of the following conduction disturbances was considered a risk factor: first-degree AV block, Mobitz type I second-degree AV block, Mobitz type II second-degree AV block, left anterior hemiblock, left posterior hemiblock, right bundle branch block, and left bundle branch block. Each risk factor was assigned a score of 1, and the risk score was calculated as the sum of these electrocardiographic risk factors. The incidence of *complete heart block* occurred as follows: risk score *0*, 1.2 to 6.8 per cent incidence; risk score *1*, 7.8 to 10.4 per cent incidence; risk score *2*, 25.0 to 30.1 per cent incidence; and risk score *3*, 36 or greater per cent incidence.[712]

We believe that failure to demonstrate improved prognosis statistically does not belie the potential value of pacemaker therapy; it probably reflects the overriding impact on mortality of the extensive infarction responsible for the development of the conduction abnormality and the large number of patients required to permit statistical documentation of reduction of mortality.

Temporary pacing in AMI has been successfully employed for the last 2 decades. In assessing the need for temporary pacing (Table 39–10), the clinician must keep in mind that

TABLE 39-10 SUGGESTED USE OF TEMPORARY PACING WITH AMI

	STRENGTH OF INDICATION
Rate Disturbances	
Sinus bradycardia without hypotension, VEA, angina, left ventricular failure, or syncope	−
Sinus bradycardia with any of the above despite atropine	+
Accelerated idioventricular rhythm	−
Idioventricular rhythm with bradycardia, and hypotension or rate <45	+
Recurrent sick sinus syndrome, prolonged sinus pauses	+
Ventricular tachycardia (especially overdrive pacing for torsades de pointes)	+
Conduction Disturbances	
First-degree AV block	−
Second-degree AV block	
Mobitz I without bradycardia or hypotension	−
Mobitz I with bradycardia and hypotension	+
Mobitz II	++
Complete (third-degree) AV block	++
Isolated new or preexisting LAH, LPH, *or* RBBB	−
New LBBB	+
New bifascicular block*	++
Preexisting bifascicular block	−†
Asystole	++

Indications are graded as −, temporary pacing not indicated; +, temporary pacing should be considered, particularly if other therapeutic maneuvers have failed or if emergency pacer insertion would be difficult or logistically impossible at some other time (e.g., skilled personnel not always available); ++, temporary pacing should be instituted.

VEA = ventricular ectopic activity, AV = atrioventricular, LAH = left anterior hemiblock, LPH = left posterior hemiblock, RBBB = right bundle branch block, LBBB = left bundle branch block.

*Bifascicular block includes alternating right and left bundle branch block, right bundle branch block with left axis deviation, right bundle branch block with right axis deviation, and left bundle branch block with P-R interval prolongation.

†If duration of block is uncertain or if preexisting block occurs with new first-degree AV block, stronger consideration should be given.

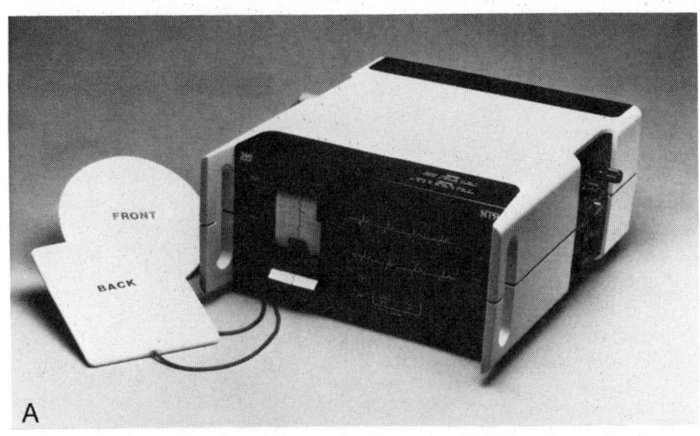

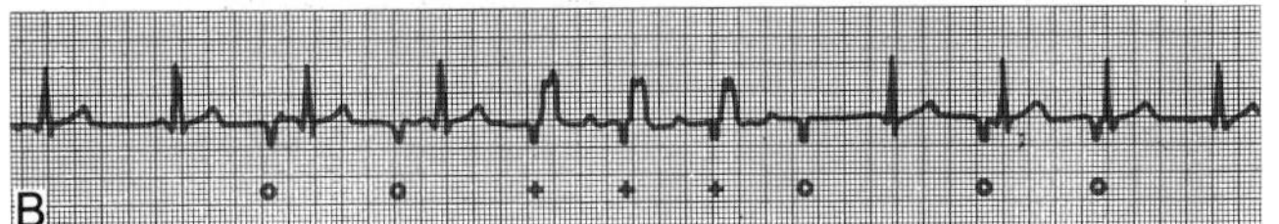

FIGURE 39–25. *A*, Noninvasive temporary pacing device shown with patient electrodes. The electrodes are self-adhering and applied to the left precordium (front) and posteriorly (back). The pacemaker includes an oscilloscopic monitor and strip recorder. Sensitivity, output, and rate adjustments can be made from the controls on the side of the device. *B*, Electrocardiographic strip during pacing with capture (+); also shown is the pacing artifact (0) when output of the pacer is lowered so as not to capture. The pacer rate is approximately 80 beats/min; the patient's intrinsic rate is approximately 60 beats/min. (Courtesy of P. Zoll, M.D.)

between 10 and 20 per cent of patients develop pacemaker-related complications.[713] A pericardial friction rub is heard in approximately 5 per cent of patients but does not necessarily indicate cardiac perforation, nor is such a finding an indication for withdrawal of the pacemaker electrode. Arrhythmias requiring cardioversion, right ventricular perforation, and local infectious complications occur in 1 to 3 per cent of cases.[713] Pacemaker malfunction also occurs rather frequently and is, in part, related to the experience of the clinical team in managing the device and its insertion.

Although external temporary cardiac pacing was introduced in 1952,[714] its widespread clinical use has not occurred until relatively recently, due to technical refinements making the technique safe, quickly applicable, and relatively well tolerated. Noninvasive external temporary cardiac pacing is now possible routinely in conscious patients and is acceptable to many but not all patients because of the discomfort[715] (Fig. 39–25). Used in a standby mode, it is virtually free of complications and contraindications and provides an important alternative to transvenous endocardial pacing. However, until its effectiveness has been more clearly documented, its routine use should be reserved for patients with moderate (or less) risk of complete heart block. Furthermore, once continuous pacing is required, external pacing is generally not well tolerated for more than minutes to hours. In such situations, it should be replaced by a temporary transvenous pacemaker.

PERMANENT PACING. The question of permanent pacing in survivors of AMI associated with conduction defects is still controversial[710,716,717] (Table 39–11). Patients with inferior infarction with *transient* type II second-degree block or complete AV block without an associated intraventricular conduction defect do not appear to require permanent pacing. Some contend that prophylactic pacing makes little difference in the long-term survival of patients with AMI and bundle branch block complicated by transient high-degree block.[718] On the other hand, in a retrospective multicenter study, survivors of AMI and bundle branch block who experienced transient high-degree (Mobitz type II second-degree, or third-degree) block had a high incidence of recurrent high-degree AV block and sudden death, and this incidence was reduced by insertion of a permanent demand pacemaker.[706,710] Thus, these findings suggest a role for prophylactic permanent pac-

TABLE 39-11 SUGGESTED USE OF PERMANENT PACING FOLLOWING AMI

	STRENGTH OF INDICATION
Transient AV conduction disturbances in the absence of intraventricular conduction defects	−
Transient advanced* AV block and associated bundle branch block	+
Persistent first degree AV block with new bundle branch block	+
Persistent advanced* AV block	++

Indications are graded as −, permanent pacing not indicated; +, permanent pacing frequently used but opinion is divided (certain patients in this category warrant further testing, such as Holter monitoring or measurement of H-V conduction time before decision can be made); ++, permanent pacing indicated (insertion of pacemaker should take place before hospital discharge).

* Advanced heart block is defined as Mobitz II second-degree AV block or third-degree (complete) AV block.

ing in patients with AMI and bundle branch block with transient high-degree atrioventricular block.

The question of the advisability of permanent pacemaker insertion is complicated by the fact that not all sudden deaths in this population are due to recurrent high-degree block. A high incidence of late in-hospital ventricular fibrillation occurs in coronary care unit survivors with anteroseptal myocardial infarction complicated by either right or left bundle branch block.[719] If the propensity for this arrhythmia continued, ventricular fibrillation rather than asystole due to failure of atrioventricular conduction and of the infranodal pacemaker could be responsible for late sudden death.

Long-term pacing is often helpful when complete heart block persists throughout the hospital phase in a patient with acute myocardial infarction, or when sinus node function is impaired markedly, or when Mobitz II second- or third-degree block occurs intermittently. When block is associated with newly acquired bundle branch block or other criteria of impairment of conduction system function, prophylactic long-term pacing may be justified as well. Thus, despite the difficulty of proving that long-term pacing improves survival after MI because of the high mortality associated with extensive infarction frequently responsible for high degrees of heart block, prophylactic long-term pacing is prudent.

ASYSTOLE. This arrhythmia has been reported to occur in 1 to 14 per cent of patients with AMI admitted to coronary care units.[681] This wide variation in incidence reflects differences in the definition of this event. The lower incidence rates include only patients who develop asystole either as a primary event or following abnormalities of atrioventricular or intraventricular conduction, whereas the higher rates include patients who develop asystole as a terminal complication. In either event, the mortality is very high, ranging upward from 90 per cent.[681]

The presence of apparent ventricular asystole on monitor displays of continuously recorded electrocardiograms may be misleading, since the mechanism may in fact be fine ventricular fibrillation. Because of the predominance of ventricular fibrillation as the cause of cardiac arrest in this setting, initial therapy should include electrical countershock, even if definitive electrocardiographic documentation of this arrhythmia is not available. In the rare instance in which asystole can be documented to be the responsible electrophysiological disturbance, immediate transthoracic pacing (or stimulation with a transvenous pacemaker if one is already in place) is indicated. In this situation temporary noninvasive pacing with an external stimulating device may be life-saving.[715]

SUPRAVENTRICULAR TACHYARRHYTHMIAS

SINUS TACHYCARDIA (see also p. 673). Almost one-third of patients with an AMI will develop sinus tachycardia at some time during the first few days after the infarction,[681] an arrhythmia that may be associated with transient hypertension or hypotension and augmented sympathetic activity. The most common causes of sinus tachycardia are anxiety, persistent pain, and left ventricular failure. Other causes include fever, pericarditis, hypovolemia, atrial infarction, pulmonary embolism, and the administration of cardioaccelerator drugs such as atropine, epinephrine, or dopamine. Sinus tachycardia is particularly common in patients with anterior infarction. It is an undesirable rhythm in patients with AMI, since it results in an augmentation of myocardial oxygen consumption, as well as a reduction in the time available for coronary perfusion. Persistent sinus tachycardia may signify persistent heart failure and under these circumstances is a poor prognostic sign associated with an excess mortality. An underlying cause should be sought and appropriate treatment instituted, e.g., analgesics for pain, diuretics for heart failure, oxygen, beta blockers and nitroglycerin for ischemia, and aspirin for fever or pericarditis.

Administration of beta-adrenoceptor blocking agents, in the dosage and manner described on page 645, may be helpful in the treatment of sinus tachycardia, particularly when this arrhythmia is a manifestation of a hyperdynamic circulation, which is seen particularly in young patients with an initial MI without extensive cardiac damage. However, beta blockade is contraindicated in patients in whom the sinus tachycardia is a manifestation of hypovolemia or pump failure, the latter reflected by a systolic arterial pressure below 100 mm Hg, rales involving more than one-third of the lung fields, a pulmonary capillary wedge pressure exceeding 20 to 25 mm Hg, or a cardiac index below approximately 2.3 liters/min/m^2.

ATRIAL PREMATURE CONTRACTIONS (see also p. 377). Atrial premature contractions are relatively common after MI, occurring in up to half of all patients.[681,720,721] Atrial premature contractions, and the atrial tachyarrhythmias (paroxysmal supraventricular tachycardia, atrial flutter, and atrial fibrillation) that they often herald, may be caused by atrial distention secondary to increases in left ventricular diastolic pressure, by pericarditis with its associated atrial epicarditis, or, less commonly, by ischemic injury to the atria[722] and sinus node. Atrial premature beats per se are not associated with an increase in mortality,[721] and cardiac output is unaffected. Occasionally an atrial premature beat may initiate ventricular tachycardia or even ventricular fibrillation in the presence of AMI.

Premature atrial contractions require no specific therapy and may indicate atrial dilatation, excessive autonomic stimulation, or the presence of overt or occult heart failure. If they are related to heart failure, they often respond to treatment of this condition.

PAROXYSMAL SUPRAVENTRICULAR TACHYCARDIA (see also pp. 487 and 1684). This arrhythmia occurs in 2 to 11 per cent of patients with AMI.[721,723] It tends to be both transient and recurrent.[720] Its deleterious effects result from the elevation of myocardial oxygen consumption and the impairment of ventricular performance consequent to the rapid ventricular rate; it is associated with an increase in mortality.

Aggressive management is indicated for paroxysmal supraventricular tachycardia because of the rapid rate. Augmentation of vagal tone by manual carotid sinus stimulation may restore sinus rhythm. Intravenous verapamil is preferable to the use of alpha-adrenoceptor agonists to increase arterial pressure and activate carotid sinus baroreceptors. Although the latter is an acceptable form of therapy for paroxysmal supraventricular tachycardia under other circumstances, it can be hazardous in patients with AMI. Although digitalis glycosides may be useful in augmenting vagal tone, thereby terminating the arrhythmia, their effect is often delayed. Most rapidly acting is intravenous adenosine, which has recently been released for the treatment of supraventricular tachycardia. This agent should be *avoided* in MI patients with a low blood pressure because it is prone to cause hypotension. Accordingly, low-energy DC countershock or rapid atrial stimulation via a transvenous intraatrial electrode should be utilized if hemodynamic decompensation occurs or if the rhythm is refractory to conventional measures. *Paroxysmal atrial tachycardia with AV block* may be a manifestation of digitalis intoxication and should be treated by withholding this drug and instituting potassium therapy, when it is accompanied by hypokalemia.

ATRIAL FLUTTER AND FIBRILLATION (see also pp. 679 and 682). Atrial flutter is the least common major atrial arrhythmia associated with AMI, occurring in only 1 to 3 per cent of all patients.[721] As in patients who develop this arrhythmia in the absence of infarction, atrial flutter is usually associated with 2:1 atrioventricular block. Since the atrial rate ranges from 250 to 350 beats/min, the ventricular rate is usually 125 to 175 beats/min. Atrial flutter is usually transient and is a consequence of augmented sympathetic stimulation of the atria, often occurring in patients with left ventricular failure or pulmonary emboli. Atrial flutter often intensifies hemodynamic deterioration.[681,682,720]

Atrial fibrillation is far more common than flutter, occurring in 10 to 15 per cent of patients with AMI.[682,720,723] As with atrial premature contractions and atrial flutter, fibrillation is usually transient and tends to occur in patients with left ventricular failure but is also observed in patients with pericarditis and ischemic injury to the atria; it occurs more frequently following anterior than inferior infarction and appears to be a consequence of left atrial ischemia in the majority of cases.[724] The increased ventricular rate and the loss of the atrial contribution to left ventricular filling—i.e., the atrial kick—result in a significant reduction in cardiac output. Both atrial flutter and fibrillation are more common during the first 24 hours after infarction than later and are associated with increased mortality, particularly in patients with anterior wall infarction. However, because they are more common in patients with clinical and hemodynamic manifestations of extensive infarction and a poor prognosis, their *independent* contributions to increased mortality appear to be minor.[721,725] Unfortunately, their management is complicated by frequent recurrence, particularly when they result from left atrial dilatation secondary to left ventricular failure.

Management. Atrial flutter and fibrillation in patients with AMI are treated in a manner similar to that in other settings (pp. 681 and 683). However, because of the possibility that a rapid ventricular rate can increase infarct size and because of the important role played by atrial contraction in the support of cardiac output in patients with AMI (Fig. 39–24), treatment must be prompt, especially when the ventricular rate exceeds 100/min. *Digitalis glycosides* are the principal agents used to slow the ventricular response. Digitalis may be supplemented by small intravenous doses of a beta blocker, which also prolongs the AV nodal refractory period: 1 to 4 mg of propranolol in divided doses is often quite effective in reducing the ventricular rate and is well tolerated even in patients with mild heart failure and a rapid ventricular rate. Reduction of the rate of ventricular response to atrial fibrillation may be achieved also with verapamil administered intravenously via bolus injections of 60 to 120 μg/kg, followed by a continuous infusion of 2.5 to 5.0 μg/kg/min, although caution must be exercised to avoid systemic arterial hypotension. On the other hand, when hemodynamic decompensation is prominent, electrical cardioversion is indicated with anterior and laterally placed paddles,[726] beginning with 25 watt-seconds for atrial flutter and 50 watt-seconds for atrial fibrillation, with gradual increase if the initial shock is not successful.

An additional important option for the treatment of atrial flutter is the use of rapid atrial stimulation via a transvenous intraatrial electrode (p. 682); in contrast to DC cardioversion, this technique can be employed in the presence of possible digitalis intoxication, is less prone than DC countershock to elicit bradycardia after conversion to sinus rhythm, provides control of ventricular rate via atrial or ventricular pacing should this be necessary, and can be reapplied with less difficulty than cardioversion, should the patient experience recurrent atrial flutter. Following restoration of sinus rhythm, attention should be directed to the management of the underlying cause, usually heart failure, and to the prevention of recurrences, with antiarrhythmic agents such as quinidine. Patients with recurrent episodes should be treated with oral anticoagulants.

JUNCTIONAL RHYTHMS (see also p. 685). Sustained junctional rhythms fall into three categories:

1. *AV junctional rhythm* at a rate of 35 to 60 beats/min in which the AV junctional tissue simply assumes the role of the dominant pacemaker when the sinus node is depressed.
2. *Accelerated junctional rhythm* in which increased rhythmicity of the junctional tissue usurps the role of pacemaker, usually at a rate of 70 to 130 beats/min.

These two arrhythmias are often transient, occur during the first 48 hours of the infarction, usually develop and terminate gradually, and are characterized by QRS complexes that resemble those of normally conducted beats. Retrograde P waves may be evident, or atrioventricular dissociation may occur, with the junctional rate slightly in excess of the underlying sinus rate. Disagreement exists concerning the prognostic implications of these arrhythmias; some observers attach a poor prognosis to these arrhythmias, whereas others believe that they are benign.[720,727] However, in patients with relatively slow junctional rhythm, the process is generally a benign protective escape rhythm and is commonly seen among patients with a slow sinus rate in the presence of inferior myocardial infarction.

3. *Paroxysmal junctional tachycardia* usually produces rates between 160 and 220 beats/min.[720] This arrhythmia is uncommon in AMI, occurring in only 1 to 2 per cent of patients. In contrast to accelerated junctional rhythms, episodes of paroxysmal junctional tachycardia commence and terminate abruptly, thereby resembling other forms of paroxysmal supraventricular tachycardia, and they often occur in the presence of left ventricular failure, ischemia of the conduction system, or digitalis excess. When intraventricular conduction defects are present, it may be difficult to distinguish paroxysmal atrial or junctional tachycardia from ventricular tachycardia. The hemodynamic and prognostic significance of paroxysmal junctional tachycardia is similar to that for paroxysmal atrial tachycardia except that the atrial kick is lost with the junctional rhythm. As indicated above, the loss of atrial transport function may be tolerated poorly. When a junctional rhythm is present and there is hemodynamic impairment, transvenous sequential atrioventricular pacing may be required to facilitate ventricular performance and maintain adequate peripheral perfusion.

VENTRICULAR ARRHYTHMIAS

VENTRICULAR PREMATURE BEATS (VPBs) (see also p. 701). Although VPBs are very frequent, indeed almost universal[728] in the presence of AMI, the value of the so-called warning arrhythmias in the prediction of ventricular fibrillation is not clear. It was believed that warning arrhythmias—defined as frequent VPBs (more than five per minute), VPB's with multiform configuration, early coupling (the "R-on-T" phenomenon), and repetitive patterns in the form of couplets or salvos—presage ventricular fibrillation. However, it is now clear that they are present in as many patients who develop fibrillation as those who do not.[234] Several reports have shown that primary ventricular fibrillation (see below) occurs without antecedent warning arrhythmias in 40 to 83 per cent of cases.[728,729] On the other hand, frequent and complex VPBs are commonly observed in patients with AMI who never develop ventricular fibrillation.[728a,729]

Prognosis. The significance of early coupling ("R-on-T" phenomenon) has been reassessed in experimental[730] and clinical[729] studies. These have shown that ventricular tachyarrhythmias in patients with AMI are often initiated by a VPB that does *not* fall on an antecedent T wave. In fact, a majority of ventricular tachycardias in patients with AMI appear to be initiated by a *late*-coupled VPB.[731] In two clinical reports on electrocardiographic antecedents of primary ventricular fibrillation, 45 per cent[728] and 41 per cent[729] of episodes of ventricular fibrillation, respectively, were initiated by a late-coupled VPB. However, in one study[732] frequent VPBs showing the R-on-T phenomenon did appear to herald the development of ventricular fibrillation but not of ventricular tachycardia. Thus, the prognostic value, if any, of various forms of VPBs in AMI remains unclear.

Management. Historically, a large number of randomized trials have compared the routine (including prehospital[733]) administration of several potent antiarrhythmic drugs—lidocaine, quinidine, procainamide, and disopyramide, as well as beta-adrenoceptor blocking agents—against placebo.[734] All of these agents reduced the frequency of ventricular premature contractions, and in the case of lidocaine, routine administration lowered the incidence of ventricular fibrillation in some studies,[733,735,736] but not in all.[737] None of the agents administered in this fashion, however, conclusively reduced mortality.[738-740]

Frequent ventricular premature contractions occurring very soon after the onset of MI, particularly during the first hour, may depend primarily on reentry rather than on increased automaticity.[741] At this time, lidocaine, which impairs conduction in ventricular myocardium and diminishes automaticity, may be somewhat less effective than it is later.[738] When, at the very inception of an infarction, ventricular premature contractions are encountered in the presence of sinus tachycardia, augmented sympathoadrenal stimulation is often a contributing factor, and may be improved by beta-adrenoceptor blockade. In fact, early administration of an intravenous beta blocker is effective in reducing the incidence of ventricular fibrillation in evolving MI.[639,641] The effectiveness of beta-adrenoceptor blocking drugs under these circumstances may, in fact, play a role in the reduction in sudden deaths reported in patients who have recovered from AMI and are at high risk of recurrence.[645,647] The dosages and modes of administration as well as contraindications to beta blockade are discussed on pp. 645–646.

Lidocaine (see also p. 639). In the past, lidocaine was administered routinely to patients with AMI and "warning arrhythmias" including frequent ventricular premature contractions (>6/min), multiform premature contractions, extrasystoles occurring in pairs or salvos, and early premature contractions (R-on-T). On the basis of results of a recent trial[739] and pooled data from over 9000 patients,[740] this strategy can no longer be recommended. Furthermore, the complications of lidocaine prophylaxis might actually outweigh any small potential benefit, so that universal prophylaxis may actually be detrimental (Fig. 39–26). Lidocaine should be reserved for patients in whom sustained and/or symptomatic ventricular arrhythmias have occurred, for patients who cannot be managed with electrocardiographic monitoring, and possibly also for patients given thrombolytic agents because of the high incidence of "reperfusion" arrhythmias.

The pharmacology and pharmacokinetics of lidocaine are discussed on page 777. With regimens depending on continuous infusion alone, therapeutic blood levels (1.5 to 5 μg/ml) are reached only after several hours because of the short half-life of the drug. Therefore, a loading dose of 100 mg or 1.5 mg/kg should be given intravenously as a bolus injection at the time of admission or during the patient's transportation to the hospital, followed in 5 to 10 minutes by an injection of 0.5 mg/kg. An intravenous infusion should be started concomitantly; a dose of 50 μg/kg/min in patients without heart failure, hypotension, or primary hepatic dysfunction and of 20 μg/kg/min in patients with any of these problems is advised.[742] Intramuscular injections into the deltoid or gluteal muscles with conventional syringes and needles do not achieve therapeutic concentrations as promptly as do intravenous injections.

The maintenance dose of lidocaine should be adjusted within the range of 1 to 4 mg/min to reduce sharply or abolish premature ventricular contractions. It should be recognized that the metabolism of lidocaine is slowed not only in patients with heart failure or hypotension but also in those with diminution of hepatic blood flow due to effects of pharmacological agents such as propranolol.[743] The rate of infusion should be lower in patients taking cimetidine and in patients with renal failure. Therefore, careful titration is needed to avoid toxicity, manifested primarily by central nervous system hyperactivity, as well as by depression of intraventricular and atrioventricular conduction and cardiac contractility. Saturation of an extravascular pool normally occurs after a continuous infusion of approximately 3 hours, at which time blood levels will increase despite maintenance of a constant infusion rate.[744] At this time, it may be desirable to reduce the rate of administration by about 25 per cent.

Procainamide (see also p. 777). When ventricular premature contractions compromise hemodynamics and persist despite administration of lidocaine, or when lidocaine is contraindi-

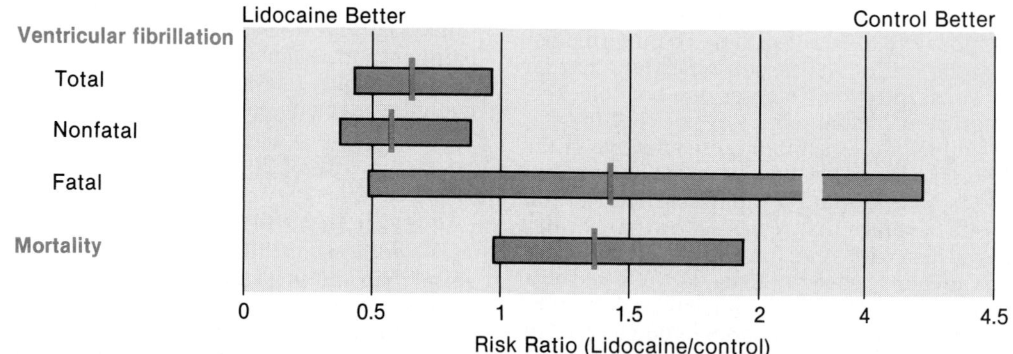

FIGURE 39–26. Pooled results of 14 randomized controlled trials of lidocaine in patients with suspected acute myocardial infarction suggest that the drug increases mortality despite reducing the risk of ventricular fibrillation. Patients received the drug intravenously (nine trials) or by intramuscular injection (five trials) and were followed for roughly the length of treatment (24 to 48 hours of IV administration, a few hours for IM). The narrow vertical bars represent the risk ratio derived from the pooled data and the broad horizontal bars show the 95% confidence limits for these ratios. (Adapted from Antman, E. M., and Braunwald, E.: Acute MI: Management in the 1990s. Hosp. Pract. July 15, 1990, p. 73.)

cated for other reasons (e.g., allergy), administration of procainamide intravenously in bolus doses of approximately 1 to 2 mg/kg intravenously over intervals of 5 minutes to a cumulative dose of approximately 1000 mg, followed by maintenance therapy with an intravenous infusion (20 to 80 μg/kg/min), may be effective. In patients with AMI, suppression of premature ventricular beats occurs at lower plasma concentrations of procainamide than are required in patients with chronic heart disease. This difference appears to reflect an electrophysiological difference, with the myocardium being more sensitive to the drug, rather than a change in procainamide pharmacokinetics, which is apparently normal in patients with AMI.[745]

Other Drugs. Other drugs such as tocainide[746] and propafenone[747] appear to be as effective as lidocaine for suppressing premature ventricular beats. Ventricular premature contractions that are unresponsive to lidocaine, procainamide, or tocainide in approximately the first 6 hours following AMI, particularly in the presence of sinus tachycardia, may be responsive to beta-adrenoceptor blocking agents.

Although phenytoin (Dilantin) (p. 641) (50 to 100 mg intravenously at 5 to 10 minute intervals to a total of 1000 mg) may diminish ventricular arrhythmia, it does not confer protection against ventricular fibrillation either in the first few hours[748] or later in the course of AMI.

The prognostic significance of VPBs in the postmyocardial infarction period continues to be controversial. Although there is little correlation between ventricular arrhythmias occurring in the early hours or days of AMI and those observed in the late postinfarction period,[749] frequent VPBs or ventricular tachycardia after hospital discharge are an independent risk factor for sudden death (p. 771).[750,751]

Because frequent and repetitive ventricular premature contractions are an independent risk factor for sudden cardiac death following AMI,[750,751] and because previous trials of antiarrhythmic agents to suppress ventricular ectopy in such patients have been flawed or inconclusive, a large placebo-controlled, double-blinded, multicenter study was initiated in 1987. This trial, known as the Cardiac Arrhythmia Suppression Trial (CAST), used the drugs flecainide, encainide, and moricizine to suppress ventricular arrhythmias in MI patients who were asymptomatic or mildly symptomatic. With over 1400 patients randomized and an average follow-up of 10 months, the flecanide and encainide arms of the trial were terminated prematurely because of a marked and unexpected increase (3.6 fold) in sudden cardiac death or arrest, and an increase in total mortality (2.5 fold) in the *treatment* groups[752] (Fig. 39–27). The important implications of this study have been much discussed.[753–755] They suggest that chronic prophylactic antiarrhythmic treatment of asymptomatic ventricular ectopy is *not* indicated after AMI, and specifically that type IC agents have powerful proarrhythmic effects that may entail risk with such drugs, particularly in patients who have recovered from AMI.

ACCELERATED IDIOVENTRICULAR RHYTHM (Fig. 24–35, p. 707). Commonly defined as a ventricular rhythm with a rate of 60 to 110 (or 125) beats/min,[756] and frequently called "slow ventricular tachycardia," this arrhythmia is seen in 8 to 20 per cent of patients with AMI, usually in the first 2 days, and seems to be equally common in anterior and inferior infarctions. About half of all episodes of accelerated idioventricular rhythm are manifested as an escape rhythm occurring during slowing of the sinus rhythm or gradual speeding of the ventricular pacemaker; the other half of accelerated idioventricular rhythms are initiated by a premature beat. Most episodes are of short duration, and the arrhythmia may terminate abruptly, slow gradually before termination, or be overdriven by acceleration of the basic cardiac rhythm. Variation of the rate is common. Accelerated idioventricular rhythms in patients with AMI probably result from enhanced automaticity of Purkinje fibers. In contrast to rapid ventricular tachycardia, accelerated idioventricular rhythms are thought not to affect prognosis.[234,756] However, accelerated idioventricular

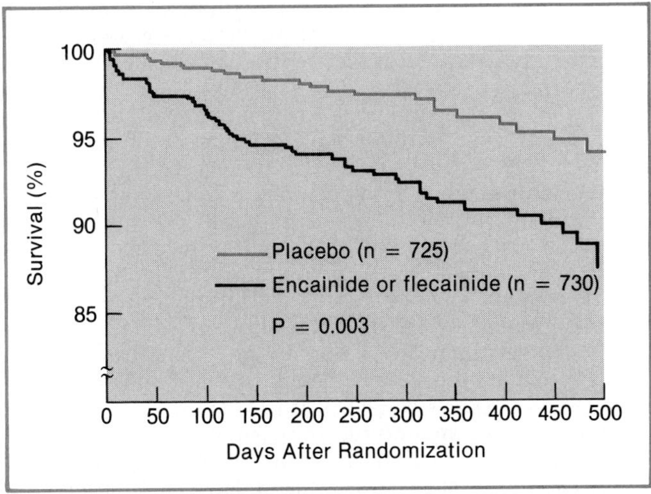

FIGURE 39–27. Survival among 1455 patients randomly assigned to receive encainide or flecainide, or matching placebo, from the Cardiac Arrhythmia Suppression Trial (CAST). The calculations were based on all causes of death. The nominal *p* value was based on a traditional two-sided log-rank test adjusted for multiple groups. A similarly significant difference in survival between groups was seen when only cardiac deaths were considered. (Reprinted by permission from the Cardiac Arrhythmias Suppression Trial [CAST] Investigators: Preliminary report: Effect of encainide and flecainide on mortality in a randomized trial of arrhythmia suppression after myocardial infarction. N. Engl. J. Med. *321*:406, 1989.)

rhythms are frequently associated with episodes of rapid ventricular tachycardia, and in many patients increased automaticity is manifested at times as accelerated idioventricular rhythms and at other times as ventricular tachycardia.

The need for treatment of this arrhythmia is controversial. Since these rhythms may deteriorate into ventricular tachycardia and since they may compromise cardiac function because of impairment of the physiological sequential relationship between atrial and ventricular contraction, it may be prudent to treat them by accelerating the sinus rate with atropine or atrial pacing or by suppressing the ventricular pacemaker with the administration of lidocaine intravenously. However, there is no definitive evidence that this arrhythmia, when left untreated, increases the incidence of either ventricular fibrillation or death.[757]

VENTRICULAR TACHYCARDIA (see also p. 658). This arrhythmia is generally defined as three or more consecutive ventricular ectopic beats occurring at a frequency exceeding 120 beats/min. It appears with a circadian variability similar to that seen with other phenomena associated with AMI, namely an increased incidence during the awake hours (Fig. 39–14, p. 1214).[758] The reported incidence of ventricular tachycardia in AMI is in the range of 10 to 40 per cent.[234,681] When this arrhythmia occurs within the first 24 hours, it is often precipitated by a late VPB and is generally transient and benign. Ventricular tachycardia occurring late in the course of AMI is more common in patients with transmural infarction and left ventricular dysfunction, is sustained, usually induces marked hemodynamic deterioration, and is associated with a relatively high hospital mortality rate—40 to 50 per cent.[681,759] However, the relative contribution to the high mortality rate of this arrhythmia per se, compared with that of the underlying impairment of left ventricular performance due to extensive infarction, is not clear.[759a] In addition, the long-term mortality in patients who exhibit ventricular tachycardia in the late hospital phase of AMI is greatly increased.[760]

Hypokalemia increases the risk of all ventricular tachycardia.[761] Low serum potassium should be identified quickly after a patient's admission for AMI and should be treated promptly. During the course of the patient's hospitalization, care should be taken to insure that the serum potassium level remains consistently above 4.0 mEq/liter. Care should be taken to identify and treat hypomagnesemia as well. Rapid abolition of ventricular tachycardia in patients with AMI is mandatory because of its deleterious effect on pump function and because it frequently deteriorates into ventricular fibrillation. When the ventricular rate is rapid (>150/min) and/or there is a decline in arterial pressure, a single attempt at "thump-version," i.e., striking a sharp blow to the precordium, is indicated (p. 775). If this maneuver is unsuccessful, it should be followed immediately by synchronized DC countershock, beginning with relatively low energies, i.e., 10 watt-seconds. When the ventricular rate is very rapid and synchronization is not possible, a defibrillatory impulse of 100 to 200 watt-seconds should be delivered. When the ventricular rate is slower than approximately 150/min and the arrhythmia is well tolerated hemodynamically, a brief (15 to 20 min) trial of treatment with lidocaine or procainamide, using the loading doses described on pages 636 and 639, is in order. If these measures are unsuccessful, an infusion of bretylium tosylate (1 to 2 mg/min) may be tried. After reversion to sinus rhythm, every effort should be made to correct underlying abnormalities such as hypoxia, hypotension, acid-base or electrolyte disturbances, and digitalis excess. Recurrent or refractory ventricular tachycardia may respond to aneurysm resection, encircling endocardial ventriculotomy, or endocardial resection with or without coronary artery bypass grafting (p. 1236); these surgical procedures are generally reserved for use until after the acute phase.[762–764]

VENTRICULAR FIBRILLATION (see also p. 709). This arrhythmia occurs in 4 to 18 per cent of patients with AMI treated in coronary care units.[728,729] It occurs with equal incidence in patients with anterior and with inferior Q-wave infarctions[234] and is rare in patients with non-Q-wave infarction. This arrhythmia may occur in three settings in hospitalized patients with AMI. (Its occurrence as a mechanism of sudden death is discussed in Chapter 26.) *Primary* ventricular fibrillation, responsible for more than 80 per cent of all instances of this arrhythmia, occurs suddenly and unexpectedly in patients with no or few signs or symptoms of left ventricular failure. Approximately 60 per cent of episodes occur within 4 hours and 80 per cent within 12 hours of the onset of symptoms. *Secondary* ventricular fibrillation, on the other hand, is the final phase of a progressive downhill course with left ventricular failure and cardiogenic shock.[681] So-called *late* ventricular fibrillation usually occurs 1 to 6 weeks following AMI. Patients with intraventricular conduction defects and anterior wall infarction, patients with persistent sinus tachycardia, atrial flutter, or fibrillation early in the clinical course, and those with right ventricular infarction who require ventricular pacing[765] all are at higher risk for suffering late *in-hospital* ventricular fibrillation than patients without these features. A recent large study has confirmed that the increase in mortality associated with late ventricular fibrillation (Fig. 39–28) is fully explained by the presence of heart failure in this group.[766]

Coronary care unit survivors with anteroseptal infarction complicated by right or left bundle branch block are particularly vulnerable to this late complication.[767] Those patients discharged alive with an anterior MI complicated by ventricular fibrillation face a much worse prognosis than those with inferior MI and ventricular fibrillation. In a case-controlled study, cumulative mortality at 5-year follow-up for the anterior MI group (54 per cent) was twice that for the inferior MI group (26 per cent).[768]

The effect of *primary* ventricular fibrillation on prognosis continues to be debated.[765,769] The MILIS study showed that it does not have an adverse effect,[769] while the first GISSI trial suggested that excess mortality due to primary ventricular fibrillation occurred only during the hospital phase but not thereafter.[770] On the other hand, *secondary* ventricular fibrillation occurring in association with marked left ventricular failure or hypotension clearly entails a dire prognosis, with only 20 to 25 per cent of patients surviving hospitalization.[757] The prognosis is intermediate in so-called late in-hospital ventricular fibrillation.[234] In the latter two forms it is the impairment of cardiac function consequent to the loss of contracting myocardium rather than the arrhythmia per se that is responsible for the poor prognosis.

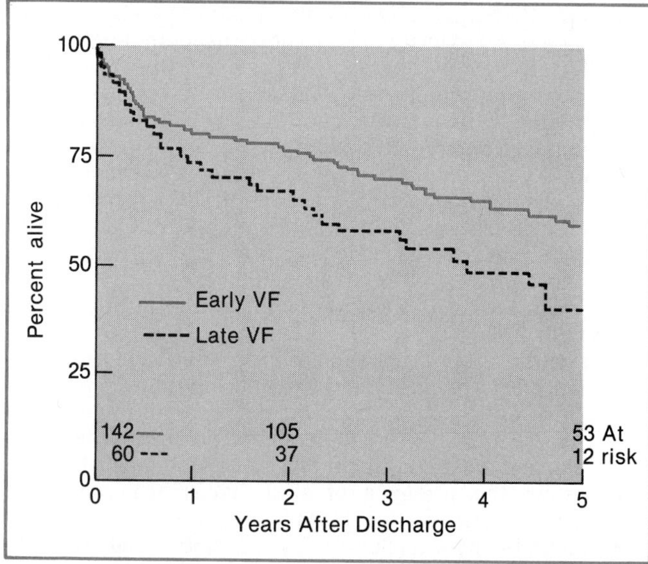

FIGURE 39–28. Kaplan-Meier survival curves from study of 422 consecutive patients discharged alive after acute myocardial infarction complicated by ventricular fibrillation (VF). (From Jeusen G.V.H., et al.: Prognosis of late versus early ventricular fibrillation in acute myocardial infarction. Am. J. Cardiol. *66*:10, 1990.)

Procainamide, lidocaine,[733,735] and the beta-adrenoceptor blockers propranolol[639] and metoprolol[771] administered prophylactically have all been reported to reduce the incidence of primary ventricular fibrillation in hospitalized patients. However, they may not reduce overall mortality substantially because treatment of this arrhythmia is so successful in an efficient coronary care unit.

Management. The treatment of ventricular fibrillation is *electrical countershock*, implemented as rapidly as possible. The likelihood of successful restoration of an effective cardiac rhythm declines rapidly with time after the onset of uncorrected ventricular fibrillation. Irreversible brain damage may occur within 1 to 2 minutes, particularly in elderly patients. Despite the superficial appeal of "thump-version," which may sometimes terminate ventricular tachycardia (as opposed to fibrillation), no time should be lost before treating patients with ventricular fibrillation by means of electrical countershock.

Prompt electrical countershock generally interrupts fibrillation and restores an effective cardiac rhythm in patients under direct medical observation in the coronary care unit. When ventricular fibrillation occurs outside of an intensive care unit, resuscitative efforts are much less likely to be successful, primarily because the time interval between the onset of the episode and institution of definitive therapy tends to be prolonged. Since closed-chest cardiopulmonary resuscitation with external cardiac compression provides only a marginal cardiac output even under optimal circumstances, countershock should be implemented as soon as possible after the detection of ventricular fibrillation rather than deferred under the mistaken impression that adequate circulatory and respiratory support can be maintained in the interim. Failure of electrical countershock to restore an effective cardiac rhythm is due almost always to rapidly recurrent ventricular tachycardia or ventricular fibrillation, to electromechanical dissociation, or, very rarely, to electrical asystole.

Ventricular fibrillation often recurs rapidly and repeatedly when the metabolic milieu of the heart has been compromised by severe or prolonged hypoxemia, acidosis, electrolyte abnormalities, or digitalis intoxication. Under these conditions, continued cardiopulmonary resuscitation, prompt implementation of pharmacological and ventilatory maneuvers designed to correct these abnormalities, treatment with antiarrhythmic agents such as lidocaine, and rapidly repeated attempts with electrical countershock may be effective. Even though repeated shocks with excessive energy may damage the myocardium[772] and elicit arrhythmias,[773] speed is essential and prompt efforts with high-intensity shocks (generally 300 to 400 watt-seconds initially) are justified. When ventricular fibrillation persists without documented interruption by electrical countershock, the intracardiac administration of epinephrine (up to 10 ml of a 1:10,000 concentration) or calcium gluconate (up to 15 ml of 10 per cent calcium gluconate) may facilitate success in a subsequent attempt. Conversion of fine to coarse ventricular fibrillation by either or both of these drugs may augur well for subsequent successful defibrillation.

Successful interruption of ventricular fibrillation or prevention of refractory recurrent episodes may be facilitated by administration of *bretylium tosylate*, 5 mg/kg intravenously, repeated 20 minutes later if necessary (p. 648).[774] When synchronous cardiac electrical activity is restored by countershock, but contraction is ineffective—i.e., during electromechanical dissociation, the usual underlying cause is very extensive myocardial ischemia or necrosis or rupture of the ventricular free wall or septum.[775,776] If rupture has not occurred, intracardiac administration of calcium gluconate or epinephrine may facilitate restoration of an effective heartbeat. Another antifibrillatory agent is amiodarone (p. 646). It has a slow onset of action; therefore, its principal role may prove to be in the *prevention* rather than treatment of ventricular fibrillation.

Hemodynamic Disturbances in Acute Myocardial Infarction

More than one and a half decades ago Swan, Forrester, and their associates measured the cardiac output and wedge pressure simultaneously in a large series of patients with AMI and identified four major hemodynamic subsets of patients (Table 39-12): (1) patients with normal perfusion and without pulmonary congestion (normal cardiac output and normal wedge pressure); (2) patients with normal perfusion and pulmonary congestion (normal cardiac output and elevated wedge pressure); (3) patients with decreased perfusion but without pulmonary congestion (reduced cardiac output and normal wedge pressure); and (4) patients with decreased perfusion and pulmonary congestion (reduced cardiac output and elevated wedge pressure).[777] Although this classification has proved to be quite useful, patients frequently pass from one category to another with therapy and, sometimes, even apparently spontaneously.

HEMODYNAMIC SUBSETS. These are usually reflected in the patient's clinical status. Hypoperfusion usually becomes evident clinically when the cardiac index falls below approximately 2.2 liters/min/sq meter, whereas pulmonary congestion is noted when the wedge pressure exceeds approximately 20 mm Hg. However, approximately 25 per cent of patients with cardiac indices less than 2.2 liters/min/sq meter and 15 per cent of patients with elevated pulmonary capillary wedge pressures are not recognized clinically. Discrepancies in hemodynamic and clinical classification of patients with AMI arise for a variety of reasons. Patients may exhibit "phase lags" as clinical pulmonary congestion develops or resolves, symptoms secondary to chronic obstructive pulmonary disease may be confused with those resulting from pulmonary congestion, or longstanding left ventricular dysfunction may mask signs of hypoperfusion secondary to compensatory vasoconstriction.[777]

The hemodynamic subsets shown in Table 39-12 allow for rational approaches to therapy as indicated in Table 39-13. The goals of hemodynamic therapy are to maintain ventricular performance, support blood pressure, and protect jeopardized myocardium. Since these goals occasionally may be at cross purposes, careful recognition of the hemodynamic profile, as assessed clinically or as available from hemodynamic monitoring, is required before optimal therapeutic interventions can be chosen.

INVASIVE HEMODYNAMIC MONITORING (see also p. 617 and Table 39-4 p. 1226). Hemodynamic assessment becomes possible once the patient reaches the hospital. An estimation of the presence or absence of gross abnormalities in cardiac index and left ventricular filling pressure can be made on the basis of clinical examination in approximately 80 per cent of patients. However, as noted above, severe depression of cardiac index and/or elevation of left ventricular filling pressure may be unsuspected in as many as 15 per cent of patients when estimates are based exclusively on clinical criteria.[440]

In patients with *clinically uncomplicated AMI*, invasive hemodynamic monitoring is not necessary, since the status of the circulation can be assessed by careful clinical evaluation. This ordinarily consists of monitoring of heart rate and rhythm, measurement of systemic arterial pressure by cuff, obtaining chest roentgenograms to detect heart failure, careful and repeated auscultation of the lung fields for pulmonary congestion, measurement of urine flow, examination of the skin and mucous membranes for evidence of the adequacy of perfusion, and arterial sampling for pO_2, pCO_2, and pH when hypoxemia or metabolic acidosis is suspected.

Invasive monitoring ordinarily consists of inserting an arterial line for the continuous measurement of arterial pressure and a balloon flotation catheter for measurement of pulmonary artery, pulmonary artery occlusive (equivalent to pulmonary wedge), and right atrial pressures, and cardiac output by thermodilution. In patients with hypotension, a Foley

TABLE 39-12 HEMODYNAMIC SUBSETS IN ACUTE MYOCARDIAL INFARCTION

CLINICAL SUBSET	CARDIAC INDEX (liter/min/sq meter)	PULMONARY CAPILLARY WEDGE PRESSURE (mm Hg)	MORTALITY (%)
I. No pulmonary congestion or peripheral hypoperfusion	**2.7 ± 0.5**	**12 ± 7**	**2.2**
II. Isolated pulmonary congestion	**2.3 ± 0.4**	**23 ± 5**	**10.1**
III. Isolated peripheral hypoperfusion	**1.9 ± 0.4**	**12 ± 5**	**22.4**
IV. Both pulmonary congestion and hypoperfusion	**1.6 ± 0.6**	**27 ± 8**	**55.5**

From Forrester, J. S., et al.: Medical therapy of acute myocardial infarction by application of hemodynamic subsets. N. Engl. J. Med. *295*:1404, 1976. Reprinted by permission of the New England Journal of Medicine.

al.: Patients with cardiogenic shock had lost an average of 51 per cent of the left ventricular myocardium (range: 35 to 68 per cent), whereas in a group of patients with AMI who died suddenly from arrhythmias and who had never been in cardiogenic shock, necrosis averaged 23 per cent (range: 14 to 31 per cent) of the left ventricle.[781]

Patients who die as a consequence of cardiogenic shock usually develop this complication while in the hospital. These individuals often have "piecemeal" necrosis, progressive myocardial necrosis from marginal extension of their infarct into an ischemic zone bordering on the infarction. This is generally associated with persistent elevation of CK-MB. Early deterioration in left ventricular function secondary to apparent extension of infarction may, in some cases, result from *expansion* of the necrotic zone of myocardium without actual *extension* of the necrotic process (p. 1219). Shearing forces that develop during ventricular systole can disrupt necrotic myocardial muscle bundles, with resultant expansion and thinning of the akinetic zone of myocardium, which in turn results in deterioration of overall left ventricular function.

At autopsy, patients with cardiogenic shock consistently demonstrate marginal extension of recent areas of infarction (Fig. 39–18) (p. 1228).[780,781] Additionally, focal areas of necrosis are frequently found in regions of the left and right ventricles that are not adjacent to the major area of recent infarction.[780] Such extensions and focal lesions are probably in part the result of the shock state itself, since they can also be found in the hearts of patients dying of noncardiogenic shock. Infarction of the ischemic periinfarction zone can be precipitated by a number of factors that adversely affect the supply of oxygen or the metabolic demand in this zone of myocardium. These adverse factors include a reduction of coronary perfusion pressure and an augmentation of myocardial oxygen demand resulting from the local release of catecholamines from ischemic adrenergic nerve endings in the heart as well as from circulating endogenous or infused catecholamines. Patients with rupture of the ventricular septum or of a papillary muscle can also exhibit cardiogenic shock. These patients often have smaller infarcts than do those with cardiogenic shock secondary to ventricular failure without a mechanical lesion. The prognosis is better in such patients, since the smaller infarct allows their left ventricle to support the circulation once the mechanical defect has been corrected surgically.

PATHOPHYSIOLOGY. The shock state in patients with AMI appears to be the result of a vicious circle, demonstrated in Figure 39–11, p. 1210. According to this formulation, coronary obstruction leads to myocardial ischemia, which impairs myocardial contractility and ventricular performance. This, in turn, reduces arterial pressure and therefore coronary perfusion pressure, leading to further ischemia and extension of necrosis until the left ventricle has insufficient contracting myocardium to sustain life. The progressive nature of the myocardial insult in this syndrome is reflected in the stuttering and progressive evolution of elevations in the plasma enzyme–time activity curves of markers specific for myocardial injury. Consideration of this vicious circle also points to the hazard of hypovolemic hypotension in patients with AMI but without cardiogenic shock; hypotension reduces coronary perfusion and thereby may enhance necrosis.

At autopsy, more than two-thirds of patients with cardiogenic shock demonstrate stenosis of 75 per cent or more of the luminal diameter of all three major coronary vessels, usually including the left anterior descending coronary artery.[782] Almost all patients with cardiogenic shock are found to have thrombotic occlusion of the artery supplying the major region of recent infarction.[780,781]

For many years the incidence of cardiogenic shock following AMI was about 15 per cent. Recent series have suggested that its incidence has fallen to about 7 per cent.[783] While this is in part related to newer interventional techniques, such as intraaortic balloon pumps and coronary angioplasty,[784] it is probable that medical therapy with thrombolysis and early treatment of ongoing ischemia are also responsible for this improvement.[783,785] Although the onset of shock is generally early in the course of AMI, when shock does develop later, it usually is due to infarct extension.[783]

MANAGEMENT OF LEFT VENTRICULAR FAILURE

Invasive hemodynamic monitoring is essential to guide therapy of patients with severe left ventricular failure.

AVOIDANCE OF HYPOXEMIA. The treatment of left ventricular failure with AMI requires meticulous attention to ventilation, since hypoxemia can impair the function of ischemic tissue at the margin of the infarct and thereby contribute to establishing or perpetuating the vicious circle (Fig. 39–11, p. 1210) The combination of pulmonary vascular congestion (or when it is severe, pulmonary edema), reduced pulmonary compliance, and the respiratory depression that may be associated with excessive doses of analgesics conspires to impair ventilatory function and arterial oxygenation. When in patients with left ventricular failure secondary to AMI arterial oxygen tension cannot be maintained above 60 mm Hg despite inhalation of 100 per cent oxygen delivered at 8 liters/min by mask and the adequate use of bronchodilators, endotracheal intubation, assisted ventilation, and positive pressure should be considered. The improvement of arterial oxygenation and hence myocardial oxygen supply may help to restore ventricular performance. Positive end-expiratory pressure may diminish systemic venous return and reduce effective left ventricular filling pressure. Once a patient is intubated and mechanically ventilated, withdrawal of the support during the recovery phase must be undertaken extremely carefully. Since myocardial ischemia frequently occurs during the return to unsupported spontaneous breathing,[786] the weaning process should be accompanied by careful observation for signs of ischemia and is potentially facilitated by a period of intermittent mandatory ventilation before extubation. Continuous ST-segment monitoring has been recommended for these patients.[786]

When wheezing complicates pulmonary congestion, bronchodilators that act primarily on $beta_2$-adrenoceptors, such as isoetharine or metaproterenol, given as aerosols, or terbutaline, which can be administered subcutaneously or orally, are more desirable than conventional bronchodilators, such as isoproterenol or epinephrine, whose primary effects are on $beta_1$-receptors.

Although positive inotropic agents may be useful, they do *not* represent the *initial* therapy of choice in patients with AMI. Instead, heart failure in this setting is managed most effectively first by reduction of blood volume and ventricular preload, and then, if possible, by lowering afterload. Arrhythmias may contribute to hemodynamic compromise as discussed on page 1240 and should be treated promptly in patients with left ventricular failure.

The use of rotating tourniquets, routine in past years for advanced degrees of pulmonary congestion, is probably ineffective and not recommended.[787]

DIURETICS (see also p. 472). Mild heart failure in patients with AMI frequently responds well to diuretics such as furosemide, administered intravenously in doses of 10 to 40 mg, repeated at 3 to 4 hour intervals if necessary. The resultant reduction of pulmonary capillary pressure reduces dyspnea, and the lowering of left ventricular wall tension that accompanies the reduction of left ventricular diastolic volume diminishes myocardial oxygen requirements and may lead to improvement of contractility and augmentation of the ejection fraction, stroke volume, and cardiac output. The reduction of elevated left ventricular filling pressure may also enhance myocardial oxygen delivery by diminishing the impedance to coronary perfusion attributable to elevated ventricular wall tension. It may also improve arterial oxygenation by reducing pulmonary vascular congestion.

The intravenous administration of furosemide reduces pulmonary vascular congestion and pulmonary venous pressure within 15 minutes, before renal excretion of sodium and water has occurred; presumably this action results from a direct dilating effect of this drug on the systemic arterial bed. It is important not to "overshoot the mark" by reducing left ventricular filling pressure much below 18 mm Hg, the lower range associated with optimal left ventricular performance in AMI, since this may reduce cardiac output further and cause arterial hypotension. Excessive diuresis may also result in hypokalemia, with its attendant risk of digitalis intoxication.

VASODILATORS (see also p. 491). Myocardial oxygen requirements depend on left ventricular wall stress, which in turn is proportional to the product of peak developed left ventricular pressure, volume, and wall thickness. Vasodilator therapy is not currently recommended in patients with uncomplicated AMI (although the results of ongoing trials may alter this) but is useful in patients whose MI is complicated by: (1) heart failure unresponsive to treatment with diuretics, (2) hypertension, (3) mitral regurgitation, or (4) ventricular septal defect. In these patients, treatment with vasodilator agents increases stroke volume and may reduce myocardial oxygen requirements and thereby lessen ischemia. Hemodynamic monitoring of systemic arterial and, in many cases, pulmonary capillary wedge (or at least pulmonary artery) pressure and cardiac output in patients treated with these agents is important. Improvement of cardiac performance and energetics requires three simultaneous effects: (1) reduction of left ventricular afterload, (2) avoidance of excessive systemic arterial hypotension in order to maintain effective coronary perfusion pressure, and (3) avoidance of excessive reduction of ventricular filling pressure with consequent diminution of cardiac output. In general, pulmonary capillary wedge pressure should be maintained at approximately 20 mm Hg and arterial diastolic blood pressure above 60 mm Hg in patients who were normotensive before developing the AMI.

Appropriate doses of vasodilators generally enhance stroke volume and cardiac output, and reduce left ventricular filling pressure and volume and calculated systemic vascular resistance, without causing serious reflex tachycardia. While available data are not conclusive and do not apply to all subsets of patients with AMI, at least one vasodilator, nitroglycerin, when given early in the course of AMI, has been reported also to protect ischemic myocardium and limit infarct size[651] (p. 1237). *Excessive* doses of vasodilators may decrease cardiac output by reducing preload and left ventricular filling pressure below optimal levels or may decrease coronary perfusion by excessive depression of systemic arterial pressure. Compromise of coronary perfusion, in turn, may impair ventricular performance further, extend infarction, and give rise to lethal arrhythmias.

Vasodilator therapy is particularly useful when AMI is complicated by mitral regurgitation or rupture of the ventricular septum. In such patients, vasodilators alone or in combination with intraaortic balloon counterpulsation can sometimes serve as a "holding maneuver" and provide hemodynamic stabilization to permit definitive catheterization and angiographic studies to be carried out and to prepare the patients for early surgical intervention. Because of the precarious state of patients with complicated infarction and the need for meticulous adjustment of dosage, therapy is best initiated with agents that can be administered intravenously and that have a short duration of action, such as nitroprusside,[788,789] nitroglycerin,[790,791] or isosorbide dinitrate.[792] After initial stabilization, medications that may be useful are long-acting nitrates given by mouth, sublingually, or by ointment,[793] and angiotensin-converting enzyme inhibitors[794] such as captopril, or enalapril, which is now available for intravenous use.

Nitroprusside. There has been more experience with the intravenous infusion of sodium nitroprusside in patients with AMI than with other vasodilators. It is generally given initially in doses of 0.5 μg/kg/min,[795] which may be gradually and progressively increased up to 50 μg/kg/min. While it increases stroke volume and cardiac output in patients with AMI and left ventricular failure, nitroprusside diminishes arteriolar resistance and impedance to left ventricular ejection, pulmonary capillary wedge pressure, myocardial oxygen requirements, and sometimes the frequency of ventricular premature contractions. Nitroprusside may augment cardiac output even in patients with cardiogenic shock, if arterial diastolic and coronary perfusion pressures are maintained by concomitant intraaortic balloon counterpulsation.

Nitroglycerin. This drug has been shown in animal experiments to be less likely than nitroprusside to produce a "coronary steal," i.e., to divert blood flow from the ischemic to the nonischemic zone.[790] Therefore, used intravenously, it (or isosorbide dinitrate, which has a similar action[792]) may be a particularly useful vasodilator in patients with AMI.[650-652] Ten to 15 μg/min is infused and the dose is increased by 10 μg/min every 5 minutes until (1) the desired effect (improvement of hemodynamics or relief of ischemic chest pain) is achieved or (2) a decline in systolic arterial pressure to 90 mm Hg, or by more than 15 mm Hg, has occurred. Although both nitroglycerin and nitroprusside lower systemic arterial pressure, systemic vascular resistance, and the heart rate–systolic blood pressure product, the reduction of left ventricular filling pressure is more prominent with nitroglycerin because of its relatively greater effect than nitroprusside on venous capacitance vessels. Nevertheless, in patients with severe left ventricular failure, cardiac output often increases despite the reduction in left ventricular filling pressure produced by nitroglycerin.

Oral Vasodilators. The use of oral vasodilators in the treatment of chronic congestive heart failure is discussed on page 491. In patients who have persistent heart failure, long-term treatment with a converting enzyme inhibitor should be carried out. Studies are under way to determine the efficacy of these agents in patients with left ventricular dysfunction without heart failure. It is hoped that this reduced ventricular load will decrease the remodeling of the left ventricle that occurs commonly in the period after MI and thereby defer the development of heart failure and death therefrom[167] (Fig. 39–12, p. 1211).

DIGITALIS (see also p. 486). Although digitalis increases the contractility and the oxygen consumption of normal hearts, when heart failure is present the diminution of heart size and wall tension frequently results in a net reduction of myocardial oxygen requirements.[796] In animal experiments it fails to improve ventricular performance immediately following experimental coronary occlusion, but salutary effects are elicited when it is administered several days later.[797] The absence of early beneficial effects may be due to the inability of ischemic tissue to respond to digitalis, the already maximal stimulation of contractility of the normal heart by circulating and neuronally released catecholamines, or the dissipation of the force of contraction of normal myocardium into dyskinetic areas.

Although the issue is still controversial, arrhythmias may be increased by digitalis glycosides when they are given to patients in the first few hours after the onset of MI, particularly in the presence of hypokalemia. Also, undesirable peripheral systemic and coronary vasoconstriction may result from the rapid intravenous administration of rapidly acting glycosides such as ouabain.[797]

Administration of digitalis to patients hospitalized with AMI should generally be reserved for the management of supraventricular tachyarrhythmias such as atrial flutter and fibrillation and of heart failure that persists despite treatment with diuretics and vasodilators. There is no indication for its use as an inotropic agent in patients without clinical evidence of left ventricular dysfunction (Killip Class I), and it is too weak an inotropic agent to be relied upon as the principal cardiac stimulant in patients with overt pulmonary edema or cardiogenic shock (Class III or IV). It may, however, be useful as a supplement to vasodilator agents and in the treatment of persistent or recurrent left ventricular failure.[798] Cardiac glycosides appear to become progressively more effective in the treatment of heart failure as the interval from the acute events lengthens; i.e., they are more effective in the treatment of chronic than of acute heart failure secondary to ischemic heart disease. However, the possibility that continued administration of digitalis might contribute to late mortality in the two years following AMI has been raised[799] and debated.[800,801] While it is clear that mortality is greater in patients treated with digoxin after AMI, it is not clear that this increase in mortality is due to digoxin itself or to confounding variables that correlate with use of digoxin.[801] At this time, digoxin would appear to be indicated only if there is overt heart failure and/or supraventricular tachyarrhythmias.

BETA-ADRENOCEPTOR AGONISTS. When left ventricular failure is severe, as manifested by marked reduction of cardiac index (<2 liters/min/sq meter), and pulmonary capillary wedge pressure is at optimal (18 to 24 mm Hg) or excessive (>24 mm Hg) levels despite therapy with diuretics, beta-adrenoceptor agonists are indicated. Although isoproterenol is a potent cardiac stimulant and improves ventricular performance, it should be avoided in the MI patient. It also causes tachycardia and augments myocardial oxygen consumption and lactate production[802]; in addition, it reduces coronary perfusion pressure by causing systemic vasodilation and in animal experiments increases the extent of experimentally induced infarction.[803] Norepinephrine also increases myocardial oxygen consumption because of its peripheral vasoconstrictor as well as positive inotropic actions.

Dopamine (p. 501) and *dobutamine* (p. 502), which is relatively cardioselective and stimulates $beta_1$ receptors, exert predominantly positive inotropic effects and may be particularly useful in patients with AMI and reduced cardiac output, increased left ventricular filling pressure, pulmonary vascular congestion, and hypotension.[804] Fortunately, the potentially deleterious alpha-adrenergic vasoconstrictor effects exerted by *dopamine* occur only at higher doses than those required to increase contractility. Its vasodilating actions on renal and splanchnic vessels and its positive inotropic effects generally improve hemodynamics and renal function.[805] In patients with AMI and severe left ventricular failure, this drug should be administered at a dose of 3 μg/kg/min, while monitoring pulmonary capillary wedge and systemic arterial pressures as well as cardiac output. The dose may be increased stepwise to 20 μg/kg/min, in order to reduce pulmonary capillary wedge pressure to approximately 20 mm Hg and elevate cardiac index to exceed 2 liters/min/sq meter. However, it must be recognized that doses exceeding 5 μg/kg/min activate peripheral alpha receptors and cause vasoconstriction. While concern has been raised that the positive inotropic effect of even low-dose dopamine could extend infarct size, experimental evidence suggests that the enhancement in contractility by dopamine does not increase infarct size or lead to late deterioration of cardiac function even when the drug is administered to acutely reperfused, severely ischemic myocardium.[806]

Dobutamine has a positive inotropic action comparable to that of dopamine but a slightly less positive chronotropic effect,[807] and less vasoconstrictor activity at higher doses. In patients with AMI dobutamine improves left ventricular performance without augmenting enzymatically estimated infarct size.[808] It may be administered in a starting dose of 2.5 μg/kg/min and increased stepwise to a maximum of 30 μg/kg/min. Both dopamine and dobutamine must be given carefully and with constant monitoring of the ECG, systemic arterial pressure, and pulmonary artery or pulmonary artery occlusive pressure and, if possible, with frequent measurements of cardiac output. The dose must be reduced if the heart rate exceeds 100 to 110 beats/min, if supraventricular or ventricular tachyarrhythmias are precipitated, or if ST-segment changes increase.

AMRINONE (p. 503). This is a noncatecholamine, nonglycoside, inotropic, and vasodilating agent that is approved for clinical use parenterally.[809] Experience with it in the setting of AMI is relatively limited, but it appears to be an ideal agent for selected patients with heart failure persisting despite treatment with diuretics, who are not hypotensive and who are likely to benefit from both an enhancement in contractility and afterload reduction. In patients with left ventricular failure following AMI amrinone increases cardiac output while reducing pulmonary wedge pressure and systemic vascular resistance.[810,811] Heart rate increases only at relatively high doses.[811] In MI patients studied, no exacerbation of angina or increased incidence of arrhythmias has been reported.[810] The initial intravenous dosage of amrinone is 0.75 mg/kg infused slowly over several minutes. This is then followed by a continued maintenance infusion started at 5 to 10 μg/kg/min and titrated to the patient's hemodynamic response. The total daily dose should not be greater than 10 mg/kg.[812]

TREATMENT OF CARDIOGENIC SHOCK

(See also p. 579)

When a massive AMI produces profound global impairment of left ventricular function, cardiogenic shock supervenes. This condition is characterized by marked and persistent (>30 min) hypotension with systolic arterial pressure less than 80 mm Hg and a marked reduction of cardiac index (generally <1.8 liters/mm/sq meter) in the face of elevated left ventricular filling pressure (pulmonary capillary wedge pressure >18 mm Hg). Spurious estimates of left ventricular filling pressure based on measurements of the pulmonary artery wedge pressure can occur in the presence of marked mitral regurgitation, in which the tall *v* wave in the left atrial (and pulmonary artery wedge) pressure tracing elevates the mean pressure above left ventricular end-diastolic pressure. Accordingly, mitral regurgitation and other mechanical lesions such as ventricular septal defect, ventricular aneurysm, and pseudoaneurysm must be excluded before the diagnosis of cardiogenic shock due to global impairment of left ventricular function can be established. These potentially catastrophic mechanical complications should be suspected in any patient with AMI in whom circulatory collapse occurs. Immediate hemodynamic and angiographic evaluations are necessary in patients with cardiogenic shock. It is important to exclude these complications because primary therapy of such lesions usually requires immediate operative treatment with intervening support of the circulation by intraaortic balloon counterpulsation.

When the aforementioned mechanical complications are not present, cardiogenic shock is due to global impairment of left ventricular function. While dopamine or dobutamine usually improves hemodynamics in these patients, unfortunately neither appears to improve hospital survival significantly. Similarly, vasodilators have been utilized in an effort to elevate cardiac output and to reduce left ventricular filling pressure. However, by lowering the already markedly reduced coronary perfusion pressure, myocardial perfusion can be compromised further, accelerating the vicious circle illustrated in Figure 39–11 (p. 1210). Vasodilators may nonetheless be employed in conjunction with intraaortic balloon counterpulsation and inotropic agents in an effort to increase cardiac output while sustaining or elevating coronary perfusion pressure.

The systemic vascular resistance is usually elevated in patients with cardiogenic shock, but occasionally resistance is normal, and in a few cases vasodilation actually predominates. When systemic vascular resistance is *not* elevated in patients with cardiogenic shock, norepinephrine (in doses ranging from 2 to 10 μg/min), which has both alpha- and beta-adrenoceptor agonist properties, may be employed to increase diastolic arterial pressure, maintain coronary perfusion, and improve contractility, but, again, there is no definitive evidence that ultimate outcome is affected by this drug.[813] Norepinephrine should be used only when other means, including balloon counterpulsation, fail to maintain arterial diastolic pressure above 50 to 60 mm Hg in a previously normotensive patient. The use of alpha-adrenoceptor agents such as phenylephrine or methoxamine is contraindicated in most patients with cardiogenic shock (unless systemic vascular resistance is inordinately low).

REPERFUSION. Reversal of cardiogenic shock by acute reperfusion has been reported, usually with thrombolytic therapy, emergency PTCA, or a combination of these measures.[599,600,814,815] In a relatively large series of patients, the mortality of cardiogenic shock appears to have been reduced by early angioplasty.[814] Although data from a controlled trial are not available, such therapy appears warranted when suitable coronary anatomy is identified.[784] In several reported cases, cardiogenic shock due to total occlusion of the left main coronary artery was reversed by intravenous thrombolysis with streptokinase.[816,817]

INTRAAORTIC BALLOON COUNTERPULSATION (see also p. 537). Cardiogenic shock due to mechanical defects following AMI (pp. 1256 to 1259) or to severe left ventricular dysfunction may be managed by means of the appropriate use of intraaortic balloon counterpulsation (IABP) when other medical measures fail.[818–821] In present practice, the balloon is inserted percutaneously[822] or, rarely, via an arterial cutdown in the femoral artery and advanced into the thoracic aorta via the femoral artery. Phased pulsations, electrocardiographically synchronized, allow for inflation at the time of closure of the aortic valve and deflation just before the onset of systole. The augmented coronary perfusion pressure during diastole enhances coronary blood flow because coronary vascular resistance is minimal during this portion of the cardiac cycle (Fig. 13–32, p. 375). Since the balloon is deflated throughout systole, the left ventricle ejects against a lower impedance. Hemodynamic changes generally include a 10 to 20 per cent increase in cardiac output, a reduction in systolic and increase in diastolic arterial pressure with little change in mean pressure, a diminution of heart rate, and an increase in urine output.[818,819] The reduction in left ventricular afterload reduces myocardial oxygen consumption, and, as a consequence, anaerobic metabolism and myocardial ischemia are diminished.[819] Favorable effects are sometimes reflected in prompt resolution of electrocardiographic signs of ischemia.

Indications. Intraaortic balloon counterpulsation is utilized in the treatment of AMI in three groups of patients: (1) those whose conditions are hemodynamically unstable and in whom support of the circulation is required for the performance of cardiac catheterization and angiography carried out to assess lesions that are potentially correctable surgically; (2) those with cardiogenic shock that is unresponsive to medical management; and (3) rarely, those with persistent ischemic pain that is unresponsive to treatment with inhalation of 100 per cent oxygen, beta-adrenoceptor blockade, nitrates, and calcium channel blocking agents during the postinfarction state. Unfortunately, among patients with cardiogenic shock, improvement is often only temporary, and "balloon dependence" is common.[818,820] Patients with cardiogenic shock treated with this modality can be successfully weaned from the supporting system only occasionally. Counterpulsation alone does not improve overall mortality, either in patients with or those without a surgically remediable mechanical lesion.[820,821] However, it may be life-saving in allowing the patient to tolerate catheterization and coronary arteriography and to undergo coronary angioplasty or to be brought to the operating room for definitive treatment. Surgical treatment in cardiogenic shock (aside from correcting mechanical abnormalities) may involve bypassing severely obstructed nonoccluded vessels. Occlusion of one major vessel may cause left ventricular dysfunction and hypotension, which can then lead to hypoperfusion and ischemia of myocardium subserved by the other diseased vessels. Left ventricular function may be improved by relief of this ischemia with revascularization. It is possible that left ventricular bypass, a technique that reduces left ventricular oxygen demands more drastically, may ultimately prove to be more effective in improving survival in patients with cardiogenic shock than intraaortic balloon counterpulsation[823]; however, it is still experimental. Emergency percutaneous cardiopulmonary bypass has been utilized in a small series of patients before catheterization.[824] While relatively successful in pilot studies, this complex strategy cannot be widely recommended until tested further.

Noninvasive approaches to circulatory assistance have been developed, such as external devices that apply pressure to the lower extremities during diastole, thereby promoting increased runoff during systole. However, this form of therapy likewise does not alter outcome decisively; its hemodynamic effects are, in fact, less than those of intraaortic counterpulsation.[825]

Complications. These occur infrequently but include damage to or perforation of the aortic wall, ischemia distal to the site of insertion of the balloon in the femoral artery, thrombocytopenia, hemolysis, renal emboli, and mechanical failure such as rupture of the balloon.[677,826] Those at highest risk include patients with peripheral vascular disease, the elderly, and women, particularly if they are small. These factors should be taken into consideration before an attempt to institute intraaortic balloon counterpulsation. Because of the potential for vascular bleeding complications there has been reluctance to use intraaortic pumps in patients who have undergone thrombolytic therapy. However, because of the poor outcome among patients with shock following thrombolysis (usually ineffective thrombolysis), and because balloon counterpulsation can be utilized relatively safely in this group,[827] this modality should be considered in carefully selected patients.

HYPOTENSION SECONDARY TO RIGHT VENTRICULAR INFARCTION

A characteristic hemodynamic pattern (Table 39–14) has been observed in patients with right ventricular infarc-

TABLE 39–14 FEATURES OF RIGHT VENTRICULAR INFARCTION

1. **Inferior-posterior myocardial infarction**
2. **Clinical findings may include:**
   A. Normal or depressed right ventricular function
   B. Shock
   C. Tricuspid regurgitation
   D. Ruptured ventricular septum
3. **Hemodynamic measurements**
   A. Abnormally elevated right atrial pressure
   B. Normal right ventricular and pulmonary artery systolic pressures
   C. Increased ratio of right ventricular to left ventricular filling pressure
   D. Depressed right ventricular function curve
4. **Scintigraphy**
   A. Uptake in right ventricular free wall
   B. Increased right ventricular dimensions and decreased wall motion
5. **Echocardiography**
   A. Increased right ventricular dimension
   B. Absence of pericardial effusion
6. **Cardiac enzymes**
   A. Increased magnitude of enzyme values to left ventricular dysfunction
7. **Cardiac catheterization**
   A. Involvement of right (usually) or left (rarely) circumflex coronary arteries
   B. Right ventricular akinesis
8. **Differential diagnosis**
   A. Hypotension with acute myocardial infarction
   B. Pericardial tamponade
   C. Constrictive pericarditis
   D. Pulmonary embolus

Modified from Rackley, C. E., Russell, R. O., Jr., Mantle, J. A., Rogers, W. J., Papapietro, S. E., and Schwartz, K. M.: Right ventricular infarction and function. Am. Heart J. *101*:215, 1981.

tion,[26,828] which frequently accompanies inferior left ventricular infarction,[704] or rarely occurs in isolated form.[829,830] Right-heart filling pressures (central venous, right atrial, and right ventricular end-diastolic pressures) are elevated while left ventricular filling pressure is normal or only slightly raised[779]; right ventricular systolic and pulse pressures are decreased, and cardiac output is often markedly depressed. Rarely, this disproportionate elevation of right-sided filling pressure causes right-to-left shunting through a patent foramen ovale.[831] This possibility should be considered in patients with right ventricular infarction who have unexplained systemic hypoxemia. The finding of an elevation in atrial natriuretic factor in this condition has led to the suggestion that abnormally high levels of this peptide might be, in part, responsible for the hypotension seen with right ventricular infarction.[832]

DIAGNOSIS. Many patients with the combination of normal left ventricular filling pressure and depressed cardiac index in fact have right ventricular infarcts (with accompanying inferior left ventricular infarcts). The hemodynamic picture may superficially resemble that seen in patients with pericardial disease (Chap. 45).[779] In it are seen elevated right ventricular filling pressure; steep, right atrial y descent; and an early diastolic dip and plateau (square root sign) in the right ventricular pressure tracing. Moreover, Kussmaul's sign (page 1484) and pulsus paradoxus (page 1474) may be present in patients with right ventricular infarction. In fact, Kussmaul's sign in the setting of inferior wall AMI is highly predictive of right ventricular involvement. The ECG may provide the first clue that right ventricular involvement is present in the patient with inferior wall MI (Fig. 39–16, p. 1221). Most patients with right ventricular infarction have ST-segment elevation in lead V_4R (right precordial lead in V_4 position).[340,833] Transient elevation of the ST segment in any of the right precordial leads may occur with right ventricular MI and the presence of ST-segment elevation of 0.1 mV or more in any one or combination of leads V_4R, V_5R, or V_6R in patients with the clinical picture of acute MI is highly sensitive and specific for the diagnosis of right ventricular MI.[339,340]

Echocardiography. This technique is helpful in the differential diagnosis[834] because in right ventricular infarction—in contrast to pericardial tamponade—no significant quantities of pericardial fluid are seen. On two-dimensional echocardiography, abnormal wall motion of the right ventricle as well as right ventricular dilatation and depression of the right ventricular ejection fraction can be noted.[834,835] Gated equilibrium radionuclide angiography also is useful for recognizing right ventricular MI.[26,836] Serial scintigraphic studies have shown that some degree of recovery of an initially depressed right ventricular ejection fraction is the rule with right ventricular myocardial infarction,[26,837,838] whereas this is not necessarily true for left ventricular ejection fraction.

Hemodynamics. Loss of atrial transport in patients with right ventricular infarction can result in marked reductions in stroke volume and arterial blood pressure.[837] As already noted, disproportionate elevation of the right-sided filling pressure compared with the left side is the hemodynamic hallmark of right ventricular infarction. Therefore, ventricular pacing, when required, may fail to increase cardiac output, and atrioventricular sequential pacing may be required.[694,839] In general, the hemodynamic importance of right ventricular infarction in patients with inferior infarction is reflected in the observations of Marmor et al. They noted that although infarct sizes (reflected in CK release curves) were similar in patients with anterior and inferior infarcts, the former had severe depression of the left ventricular ejection fraction and the latter had more severe depression of the right ventricular ejection fraction.[840]

TREATMENT. In patients with hypotension due to right ventricular MI, hemodynamics may be improved by a combination of expanding plasma volume to augment right ventricular preload and cardiac output and, when left ventricular failure is present, arterial vasodilators. The initial therapy for hypotension in patients with right ventricular infarction should almost always be volume expansion. However, if hypotension has not been corrected after one or more liters of fluid has been administered briskly, consideration should be given to hemodynamic monitoring with a pulmonary artery catheter, because further volume infusion may be of little use and may produce pulmonary congestion.[443] Vasodilators reduce the impedance to left ventricular outflow and in turn left ventricular diastolic, left atrial, and pulmonary (arterial) pressures, thereby lowering the impedance to right ventricular outflow and enhancing right ventricular output. A remarkably high survival rate of 60 per cent, albeit in a small series of patients with right ventricular infarction and serious and prolonged hypotension, emphasizes the importance of recognition and vigorous medical therapy of this cause of serious hypotension in MI.[841]

Right ventricular infarction is common among patients with inferior left ventricular infarction. Therefore, otherwise unexplained systemic arterial hypotension or diminished cardiac output, or marked hypotension in response to small doses of nitroglycerin,[432] in patients with inferior infarction should lead to the prompt consideration of this diagnosis. In view of the importance of atrial transport, patients requiring pacing should have atrial or atrioventricular sequential pacing.[694,839] Replacement of the tricuspid valve has been carried out in the treatment of severe tricuspid regurgitation secondary to right ventricular infarction.[842]

MECHANICAL CAUSES OF HEART FAILURE AND SHOCK FOLLOWING ACUTE MYOCARDIAL INFARCTION

MYOCARDIAL RUPTURE

The most dramatic complications of AMI are those that involve tearing or rupture of acutely infarcted tissue. The clinical characteristics of these lesions vary considerably and depend on the site of rupture, which may involve the papillary muscles, the interventricular septum, or the free wall of either ventricle. The overall incidence of these complications is hard to assess because clinical and autopsy series differ considerably.[843,844] However, as a group they are probably responsible for about 15 per cent of all deaths from AMI.[843,845,845a] A large autopsy study suggests that the incidence of myocardial rupture has increased since the late 1960's, with a current rate of 31 per cent among necropsied cases.[844] The prior use of corticosteroids or nonsteroidal antiinflammatory agents has been implicated as predisposing to rupture as a result of impaired healing. Controversy remains about the actual relationship between the use of such agents and the frequency of rupture, with several series suggesting a correlation of rupture with their use[846,847] and others not.[843,845] Conversely, the *early* use of thrombolytic therapy appears to reduce the incidence of cardiac rupture,[848,849] an effect that is responsible in part for improved survival with effective thrombolysis. A recent detailed analysis[849] of many trials has, however, raised the possibility that *late* thrombolytic therapy may actually increase the risk of cardiac rupture despite improving overall survival. The comparative clinical profile of these complications, as gathered from different studies, is shown in Table 39–15.

Rupture of the Free Wall

Rupture of the free wall of the infarcted ventricle (Fig. 39–30) occurs in up to 10 per cent of patients dying in the hospital of AMI. Thinness of the apical wall, marked intensity of necrosis at the terminal end of the blood supply, poor collateral flow, the shearing effect of muscular contraction against an inert and stiffened necrotic area, and aging of the myocardium with laceration of the myocardial microstructure have all been proposed as the local factors that lead to rupture.[850–852]

The following are some features that characterize this serious complication of AMI. Rupture of the free wall:

1. Occurs more frequently in the elderly and possibly more frequently in women than in men with infarction[845];

TABLE 39-15 CLINICAL PROFILE OF MECHANICAL COMPLICATIONS OF MYOCARDIAL INFARCTION

VARIABLE	VENTRICULAR SEPTAL DEFECT	FREE WALL RUPTURE	PAPILLARY MUSCLE RUPTURE
Age (mean, years)	63	69	65
Days post-MI	3-5	3-6	3-5
Anterior MI	66%	50%	25%
New murmur	90%	25%	50%
Palpable thrill	Yes	No	Rare
Previous MI	25%	25%	30%
Echocardiographic findings			
2D	Visualize defect	May have pericardial effusion	Flail or prolapsing leaflet
Doppler	Detect shunt	—	Regurgitant jet in LA
PA catheterization	Oxygen step-up in RV	Equalization of diastolic pressure	Prominent V wave in PCW tracing
Incidence	2-4%	Up to 10%	1%
Mortality			
Medical	90%	90%	90%
Surgical	50%	Case reports	40-90%

MI = myocardial infarction, VSD = ventricular septal defect, 2D = two-dimensional, LA = left atrium, PA = pulmonary artery, RV = right ventricle, PCW = pulmonary capillary wedge.
Modified from Labovitz, A. J., et al.: Mechanical complications of acute myocardial infarction. Cardiovasc. Rev. Rep. 5:948, 1984.

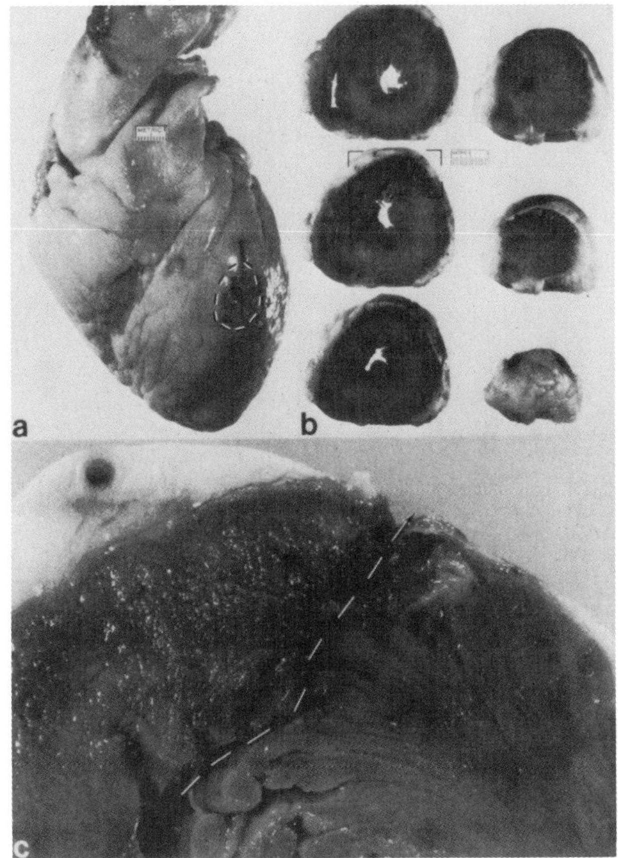

FIGURE 39-30. Heart of a 76-year-old woman who developed chest pain 14 hours before death. Her electrocardiogram showed changes of an anterior wall acute myocardial infarction. At necropsy, 300 ml of clotted blood was present in the pericardial sac. *A*, View of the anterior aspect of the heart showing the increased subepicardial adipose tissue and the rupture site (dotted circle). *B*, View of transverse cuts of the cardiac ventricles showing the acute myocardial infarct on the anterior left ventricular wall and the rupture site. *C*, Close-up view of the slice in brackets in *B* showing the acute myocardial infarct and the rupture site (arrow). (From Mann, J. M., and Roberts, W. C.: Rupture of the left ventricular free wall during acute myocardial infarction: Analysis of 138 necropsy patients and comparison with 50 necropsy patients with acute myocardial infarction without rupture. Am. J. Cardiol. *62*:847, 1988.)

2. May be more common in hypertensive than normotensive patients[845,850];
3. Occurs approximately seven times more frequently in the left than the right ventricle and seldom occurs in the atria;
4. Usually involves the anterior or lateral walls[853] of the ventricle in the area of the terminal distribution of the left anterior descending coronary artery;
5. Is usually associated with a relatively large transmural infarction involving at least 20 per cent of the left ventricle[843];
6. Occurs between 1 day and 3 weeks, but most commonly 1 to 4 days, following infarction;
7. Is usually preceded by infarct expansion, i.e., thinning and a disproportionate dilatation within the softened necrotic zone[173];
8. Most commonly results from a distinct tear in the myocardial wall or a dissecting hematoma that perforates a necrotic area of myocardium (Fig. 39-31);
9. Usually occurs near the junction of the infarct and the normal muscle;
10. Occurs less frequently in the center of the infarct, but when rupture occurs here, it is usually during the second rather than the first week following the infarct;
11. Rarely occurs in a hypertrophied ventricle or in an area of extensive collateral vessels[851];
12. Most often occurs in patients without previous infarction.[843,853]

Rupture of the free wall of the left ventricle usually leads to hemopericardium and death from cardiac tamponade. Occasionally, rupture of the free wall of the ventricle occurs as the first clinical manifestation in patients with undetected or silent myocardial infarction, and then it may be considered a form of "sudden cardiac death" (Chap. 26).

The course of rupture varies from catastrophic, with an acute tear leading to immediate death, to slow and incomplete, leading to late rupture or formation of a false aneurysm.[854] In either case, survival depends on the recognition of this complication, hemodynamic stabilization of the patient —usually with inotropic agents and/or intraaortic balloon pump—and most importantly on immediate surgical repair.[855,856] Survival has occasionally been reported even in the most dire of circumstances, i.e., when the diagnosis is correctly made within moments of rupture, and through a well-coordinated operating room effort, the patients were placed on cardiopulmonary bypass within 1 hour and the defects then successfully repaired.[856,857]

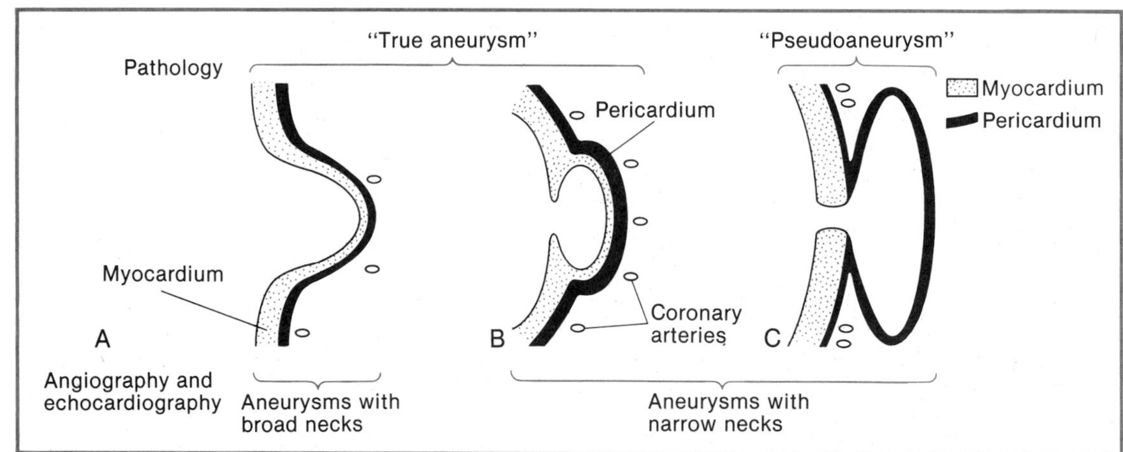

FIGURE 39–31. Pathological difference between true and pseudo-aneurysms. As can be seen in *B*, a narrow neck may occur with true aneurysms. A narrow neck may be a marker of higher risk for rupture, but it does not necessarily indicate that a pseudoaneurysm is present. (From Davies, M. J.: Ischemic ventricular aneurysm: True or false? Br. Heart J. *60*:95, 1990.)

Incomplete rupture of the heart may occur when organizing thrombus and hematoma, together with pericardium, seal a rupture of the left ventricle and thus prevent the development of hemopericardium (Fig. 39–31). With time, this area of organized thrombus and pericardium can become a small left ventricular diverticulum, or a large pseudoaneurysm that maintains communication with the cavity of the left ventricle.[858] In contrast to true aneurysms, which always contain some myocardial elements in their walls, the walls of false aneurysms are composed of organized hematoma and pericardium and lack any elements of the original myocardial wall. False aneurysms can become quite large, even equaling the true ventricular cavity in size, and they communicate with the left ventricular cavity through a narrow neck. Frequently, false aneurysms contain significant quantities of old and recent thrombus, superficial portions of which can cause arterial emboli. False aneurysms can drain off a portion of each ventricular stroke volume exactly as do true aneurysms. The diagnosis of pseudoaneurysm can usually be made by two-dimensional echocardiography (Fig. 4–88, p. 97) and contrast angiography, although at times differentiation between true and false aneurysms may be difficult by any imaging technique.[858a]

DIAGNOSIS. The recognition of rupture usually is first suggested by the development of sudden profound right heart failure associated with shock, often rapidly leading to electromechanical dissociation. Immediate pericardiocentesis will confirm the diagnosis and relieve the pericardial tamponade, at least momentarily. If the patient's condition is relatively stable, echocardiography may help in establishing the diagnosis of tamponade. Under the most favorable conditions, cardiac catheterization can be carried out, not necessarily to confirm the diagnosis of rupture but to delineate the coronary anatomy. This is helpful so that, in addition to ventricular repair, coronary artery bypass surgery can be performed in patients in whom high-grade lesions are seen. In situations in which hemodynamics are critically compromised, establishment of the diagnosis should be followed immediately by surgery for resection of the necrotic and ruptured myocardium with primary reconstruction. When rupture is subacute and a pseudoaneurysm is suspected or present, prompt elective surgery is indicated because rupture of the pseudoaneurysm occurs relatively frequently.[858,859]

Rupture of the Interventricular Septum

Although rupture of the interventricular septum appears to be less common than rupture of the free wall at autopsy,[850,860] our clinical experience is often otherwise,[843] perhaps because death usually is not immediate, and patients frequently can reach a referral center at which this complication is treated. The perforation usually is single (Fig. 39–32) and ranges in length from one to several centimeters. It may be a direct through-and-through hole or may be more irregular and serpiginous.[861,862] The size of the defect determines the magni-

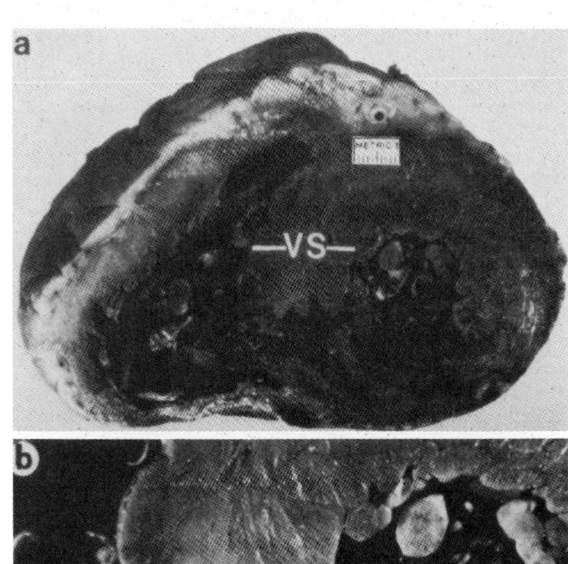

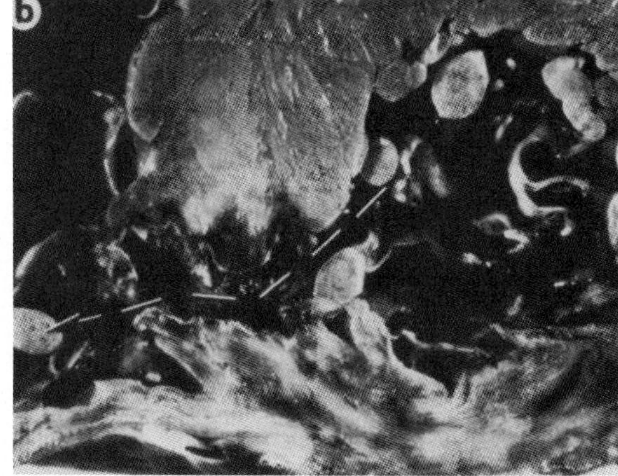

FIGURE 39–32. Heart of a 76-year-old woman who died 2 days after the onset of AMI. Her electrocardiogram had revealed an inferoposterior infarct and her course was complicated by complete heart block. *A*, View of the most basal transverse cut of the cardiac ventricles showing the posterior acute myocardial infarct and the posterior ventricular septal defect. VS = ventricular septum. *B*, Close-up view of the rupture site (arrow). (From Mann, J. M., and Roberts, W. C.: Acquired ventricular septal defect during acute myocardial infarction: Analysis of 38 unoperated necropsy patients and comparison with 50 unoperated necropsy patients without rupture. Am. J. Cardiol. 62:8, 1988.)

tude of the left-to-right shunt and the extent of hemodynamic deterioration, which in turn affects the likelihood of survival. The development of shock and the likelihood of survival appear to depend critically on impairment of right ventricular function.[860,863,864] As in rupture of the free wall of the ventricle, transmural infarction underlies rupture of the ventricular septum. Rupture of the septum with an anterior infarction tends to be apical in location, whereas inferior infarctions are associated with perforation of the basal septum and with a worse prognosis.[663,864] Virtually all patients have multivessel coronary artery disease, with the majority exhibiting lesions in all of the major vessels.[860]

The development of ruptured interventricular septum is usually heralded by the appearance of a new harsh, loud holosystolic murmur that is heard best at the lower left and usually right sternal borders. A thrill may occur with the murmur. Biventricular failure generally ensues within hours to days. Confirmation of the diagnosis usually requires insertion of a pulmonary artery balloon catheter to document the left-to-right shunt. The defect can also be recognized by two-dimensional echocardiography with color flow Doppler imaging.[865,866,866a]

Catheter placement of an umbrella-shaped device within the ruptured septum has been reported to stabilize the conditions of critically ill patients with acute septal rupture following AMI.[867]

Rupture of a Papillary Muscle

Partial or total rupture of a papillary muscle is a rare but often fatal complication of transmural MI[868] (Fig. 39–33). Inferior wall infarction can lead to rupture of the posteromedial papillary muscle, which occurs more commonly than rupture of the anterolateral muscle, a consequence of anterolateral MI.[869,870] Rupture of a right ventricular papillary muscle is rare but can cause massive tricuspid regurgitation and right ventricular failure. Complete transection of a left ventricular papillary muscle is incompatible with life because the sudden massive mitral regurgitation that develops cannot be tolerated. Rupture of a portion of a papillary muscle, usually the tip or head of the muscle, resulting in severe, although not necessarily overwhelming, mitral regurgitation is much more frequent. Unlike rupture of the ventricular septum, which occurs with large infarcts, papillary muscle rupture occurs with a relatively small infarction in approximately one-half of the cases seen.[868] The extent of coronary artery disease in these patients sometimes is modest as well.[869]

In a small number of patients, rupture of more than one cardiac structure is noted clinically[871] or at postmortem examination; all possible combinations of rupture of the free left ventricular wall, the interventricular septum, and papillary muscles have been described.[861]

As with patients who have a ruptured ventricular septal defect, those with papillary muscle rupture manifest a new holosystolic murmur followed by the development of increasingly severe heart failure. In both situations the murmur may become softer or disappear as arterial pressure falls. Mitral regurgitation due to partial or complete rupture of a papillary muscle may be promptly recognized echocardiographically.[872] Color flow Doppler imaging is particularly helpful in distinguishing acute mitral regurgitation from a ventricular septal defect in the setting of AMI.[873] Therefore, an echocardiogram should be obtained immediately on any patient in whom the diagnosis is suspected, because hemodynamic deterioration can ensue rapidly. Echocardiography also often permits differentiation of papillary muscle rupture from other, generally less severe forms of mitral regurgitation that occur with AMI.[874]

Hemodynamic Findings and Management in Ventricular Septal Rupture and Mitral Regurgitation

It may be difficult, on clinical grounds, to distinguish between acute mitral regurgitation and rupture of the ventricular septum in patients with AMI who suddenly develop a loud systolic murmur.[875] This differentiation can be made most readily by color flow Doppler echocardiography. In addition, a right-heart catheterization with a balloon-tipped catheter can readily distinguish between these two complications. As already noted, patients with ventricular septal rupture demonstrate a "step-up" in oxygen saturation in blood samples from the right ventricle and pulmonary artery compared with those from the right atrium. Patients with acute mitral regurgitation lack this step-up; they may demonstrate tall *v* waves in both

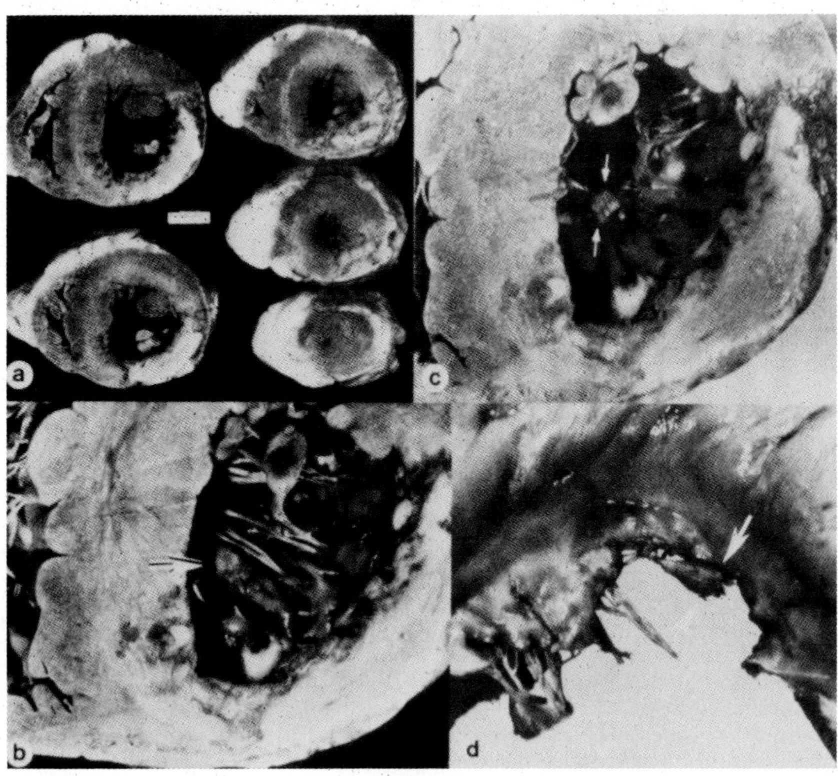

FIGURE 39–33. **This 76-year-old woman had a large posterior wall acute myocardial infarction with incomplete rupture of the posteromedial papillary muscle. *A*, Ventricular transverse slices from base (top left) to apex (bottom left) demonstrating the extent of the infarction. *B* and *C*, Close-up of the basal portion of the left ventricle showing a portion of the ruptured posteromedial papillary muscle (arrows). *D*, Opened mitral valve showing the ruptured papillary muscle head (arrows) and the tangled chordae tendineae. (From Barbour, D. J., and Roberts, W. C.: Rupture of a left ventricular papillary muscle during acute myocardial infarction: Analysis of 22 necropsy patients. Reprinted with permission of the American College of Cardiology. J. Am. Coll. Cardiol. *8*:558, 1986.)**

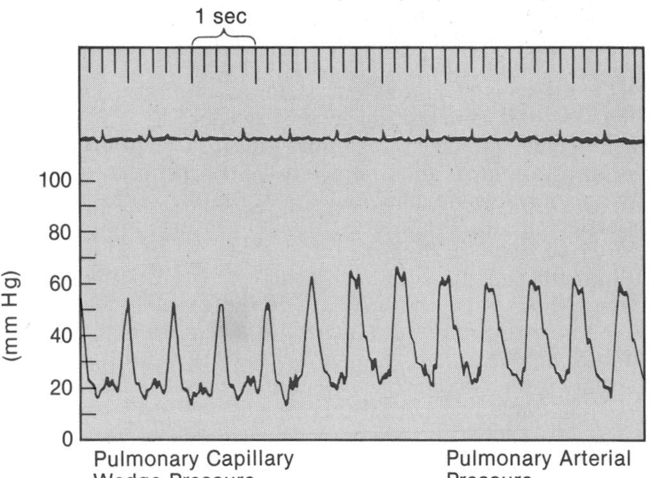

FIGURE 39-34. Acute mitral regurgitation secondary to ruptured chord from infarcted papillary muscle in a 45-year-old man. Tracing shows mitral regurgitation, tall *v* waves in pulmonary capillary wedge and pulmonary artery tracings. (Courtesy of Ira S. Ockene, M.D.)

the pulmonary capillary and the pulmonary arterial pressure tracings (Fig. 39-34). However, patients with septal rupture may also develop large *v* waves and thus the presence of this finding is not necessarily useful in an individual patient. Cardiac output is usually significantly decreased in both conditions.

Invasive monitoring, which is essential in these patients, also allows for the critically important assessment of right ventricular function. Right and left ventricular filling pressures (right atrial pressure and pulmonary capillary wedge pressure) dictate fluid administration and the use of diuretics, while measurements of cardiac output and mean arterial pressure are obtained for calculation of systemic vascular resistance as a guide for vasodilator therapy. This therapy, generally using nitroprusside, should be instituted as early as possible once hemodynamic monitoring is available. This may be critically important for stabilizing the patient's condition in preparation for further diagnostic studies and surgical repair. If vasodilator therapy is not tolerated or if it fails to achieve hemodynamic stability, intraaortic balloon counterpulsation should be rapidly instituted.

Surgical Treatment of Hemodynamic Impairment

Operative intervention is most successful in patients with AMI and circulatory collapse when a surgically correctable mechanical lesion can be identified and repaired, such as ventricular septal defect.[876] In such patients the circulation should at first be supported by intraaortic balloon pulsation and a positive inotropic agent such as dopamine or dobutamine in combination with a vasodilator, unless the patient is hypotensive. Operation should not be delayed in patients with a correctable lesion who require pharmacological and/or mechanical (counterpulsation) support (Fig. 39-35).[876-879] Such patients frequently develop a serious complication—infection, adult respiratory distress syndrome, extension of the infarct, or renal failure—if operation is delayed. Surgical survival is predicted by early operation, short duration of shock, and mild degrees of right and left ventricular impairment.[876,878,879] When the hemodynamic status of a patient with one of these mechanical lesions complicating an AMI remains stable *after* the patient has been weaned from pharmacological and/or mechanical support, occasionally it may be desirable to postpone operation for 2 to 4 weeks to allow some healing of the infarct to occur. Surgical repair may involve either repair of a ventricular septal defect, correction of mitral regurgitation, or insertion of a prosthetic mitral valve, usually accompanied by coronary revascularization.

LEFT VENTRICULAR ANEURYSM

A ventricular aneurysm, which is a circumscribed, noncontractile outpouching of the left ventricle, develops in 8 to 15 per cent of patients who survive a myocardial infarction.[880,881] The wall of the aneurysm is thin in comparison with the rest of the left ventricle (Figs. 39-31 and 39-36), and it is usually composed of fibrous tissue as well as necrotic muscle, occasionally mixed with viable myocardium.[882] Aneurysm formation presumably occurs when intraventricular tension stretches the noncontracting infarcted heart muscle, thus producing infarct expansion,[173] a relatively weak, thin layer of necrotic muscle, and fibrous tissue that bulges with each cardiac contraction. With the passage of time, the wall of the aneurysm becomes more densely fibrotic, but it continues to bulge with systole, thus "stealing" some of the left ventricular stroke volume during each systole.

When an aneurysm is present after anterior MI, there is generally a total occlusion of a poorly collateralized left anterior descending coronary artery.[883] An aneurysm is rarely seen with multivessel disease when there are either extensive collaterals or a nonoccluded left anterior descending artery.[883,884] Aneurysms usually range from 1 to 8 cm in diameter.[880] They occur approximately four times more often at the apex and in the anterior wall than in the inferoposterior wall.[880] The overlying pericardium is usually densely adherent to the wall of the aneurysm, which may even become partially calcified after several years. Rarely, a true left ventricular aneurysm ruptures soon after its development. In iso-

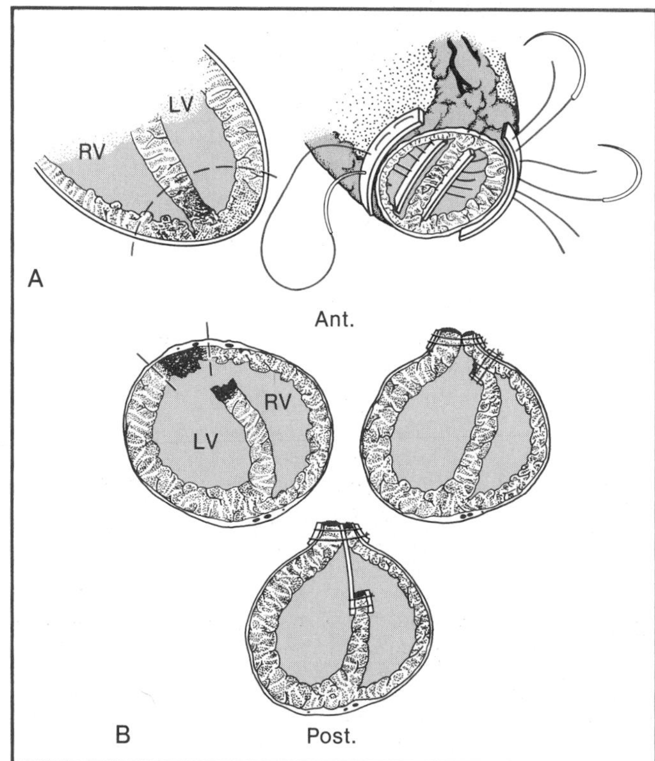

FIGURE 39-35. *A*, Closure of apical ventricular septal rupture. The infarcted apex is resected, and the remaining viable myocardium of the septum and the left and right ventricular free walls are buttressed together using Teflon felt inside and outside the ventricle. *B*, Closure of a ventricular septal rupture with an extensive anterior infarct. The septum is reconstructed with a heavy Dacron patch that is sewn to the base of remaining septum using Teflon bolsters on both sides. The free edge of the patch is then brought out and the left and right ventricular free walls are attached to it. Ant. = anterior; LV = left ventricle; Post = posterior; RV = right ventricle. (Reproduced with permission from Kopf, G. S., Meshkov, A., Laks, H., Hammond, G. L., and Geha, A. S.: Changing patterns in the surgical management of ventricular septal rupture after myocardial infarction. Am. J. Surg. *143*:465, 1982.)

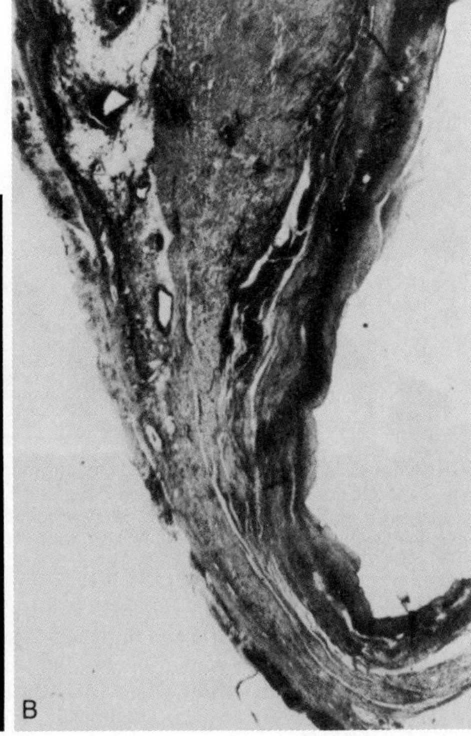

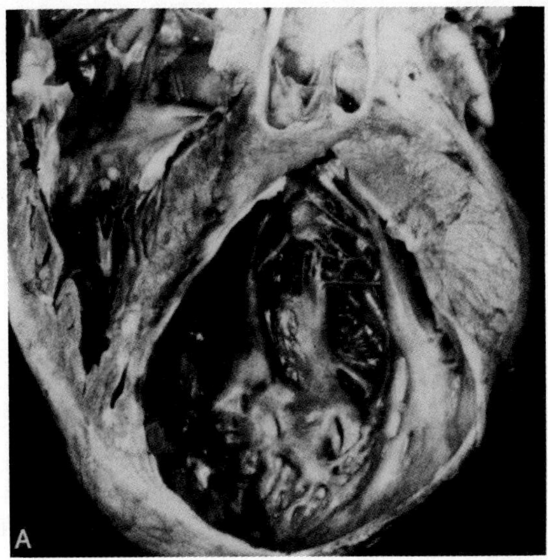

FIGURE 39-36. Example of true left ventricular aneurysm. ***A,*** **Aneurysm complicating an anterior infarction. The ventricular portion of the heart, cut in frontal section and viewed from in front, shows the left ventricle to the left of the right ventricle. The aneurysm is thin-walled and has a fibroelastic lining.** ***B,*** **Photomicrograph of aneurysm. Epicardium is to the left. This low-power view shows virtual molding of the aneurysm at the edge of an infarct. The aneurysm displays endocardial fibrosis and some mural thrombosis. Elastic tissue stain, ×5. (From Edwards, B. S., and Edwards, J. E.: Pathology of acute myocardial infarction.** ***In*** **Francis, G. S., and Alpert, J. S. [eds.]: Modern Coronary Care. Boston, Little, Brown and Co., 1990, p. 64.)**

lated cases this may be due to a degree of early myocardial rupture interrupted by subepicardial aneurysm formation, susceptible to later complete rupture. Late rupture, when the true aneurysm has become stabilized by the formation of dense fibrous tissue in its wall, almost never occurs.[858]

Mortality in patients with a left ventricular aneurysm is up to six times higher than in patients without aneurysms, even when compared to that in patients with comparable left ventricular ejection fraction.[885] Death in these patients is often sudden and presumably related to the high incidence of ventricular tachyarrhythmias that occur with aneurysms.

The presence of persistent ST-segment elevation in an electrocardiographic area of infarction, classically thought to suggest aneurysm formation, actually indicates a large infarct but does not necessarily imply an aneurysm.[886] The diagnosis of aneurysm is best made noninvasively by an echocardiographic study (Fig. 4-85, p. 95), by radionuclide ventriculography, or at the time of cardiac catheterization by left ventriculography. With the loss of shortening from the area of the aneurysm, the remainder of the ventricle is required to compensate. With relatively large aneurysms, complete compensation is impossible. The stroke volume falls, or if maintained, it is at the expense of an increase in end-diastolic volume, which in turn leads to increased wall tension and myocardial oxygen demand. Heart failure may ensue, and angina may appear or worsen.

TREATMENT. Aggressive management of AMI, including coronary thrombolysis, may diminish the incidence of ventricular aneurysms. Surgical aneurysmectomy generally is successful only if there is relative preservation of contractile performance in the nonaneurysmal portion of the left ventricle.[887] In such circumstances, when the operation is performed for worsening heart failure or angina, operative mortality is relatively low and clinical improvement can be expected.[887] Aneurysmectomy and special procedures carried out to control ventricular tachyarrhythmias occurring with left ventricular aneurysms are described on page 658.

OTHER COMPLICATIONS OF ACUTE MYOCARDIAL INFARCTION

LEFT VENTRICULAR THROMBUS AND ARTERIAL EMBOLISM

Mural thrombi (Fig. 39-37) are common in patients succumbing to AMI.[888] In one report, 44 per cent of 924 patients dying of AMI were found to have mural thrombi attached to the endocardium overlying the infarct[889]; thrombi are more common in patients with large than small infarcts and are more frequent in nonsurvivors than in survivors. They are almost universally located in the left ventricle, particularly at its apex. With extensive transmural infarction of the septum, however, mural thrombi may overlie infarcted myocardium in both ventricles. As noted earlier, mural thrombus is rather common in a ventricular aneurysm or pseudoaneurysm. Clinical series suggest that the incidence of left ventricular thrombi identified echocardiographically is 20 to 40 per cent, with the vast majority occurring in anterior MI[378,890-893] (Fig. 4-91, p. 98).[378,890-893] Computed tomography may be even more sensitive than echocardiography for the identification of intracardiac thrombi[348] (Fig. 11-37, p. 330). Mural thrombi have been found to be more frequent in patients treated with beta-adrenoceptor blockade after AMI.[894]

Although a mural thrombus adheres to the endocardium overlying the infarcted myocardium, superficial portions of it can become detached and produce systemic arterial emboli. Approximately half of patients with mural thrombi at autopsy also have evidence of systemic emboli.[881] Serial echocardiographic studies suggest that the incidence of emboli from documented mural thrombi in AMI is about 5 per cent,[895] but it is highly variable (0 to 25 per cent) even when a mural thrombus has been identified.[890-893] Occasionally, embolism from a mural thrombus is the presenting symptom with the underlying myocardial infarction either silent or overlooked. Prospec-

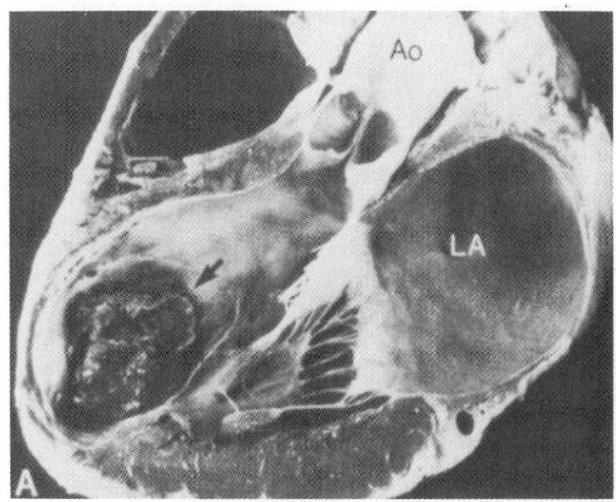

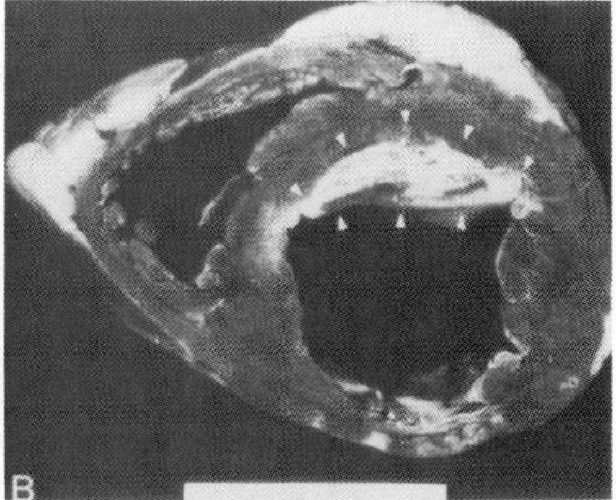

FIGURE 39-37. Postinfarction left ventricular mural thrombus. *A*, Recent thrombus (arrow) with central ulceration. Systemic embolization occurred in this patient. *B*, Old organized thrombus (arrowheads) adjacent to area of infarction. (From Edwards, W. D.: Pathology of myocardial infarction and reperfusion. *In* Gersh, B. J., and Rahimtoola, S. H. [eds.]: Acute Myocardial Infarction. New York, Elsevier, 1991, p. 29.)

tive studies have suggested that patients who develop a mural thrombus early (within 48 to 72 hours of infarction) have an extremely poor early prognosis.[878,892] In one series, over 90 per cent of the patients developing a thrombus within 48 hours died, all of causes related to the large infarction (shock, reinfarction, rupture, and ventricular tachyarrhythmia), while none had clinical evidence of emboli from the left ventricular thrombus.[378] Only 1 of the 24 patients with thrombus had a clinically apparent embolic episode. (None of the patients were receiving anticoagulation therapy.)

MANAGEMENT. It is not entirely clear whether heparinization or a combination of thrombolytic therapy with heparin prevents emboli from left ventricular thrombi,[890,895-897] although both heparin and thrombolytic therapy reduce the incidence or extent of mural thrombi.[898,899] Recommendations for anticoagulation vary considerably,[890,900-903] and thrombolysis has precipitated fatal embolization.[893] Nevertheless, prudent anticoagulation for 3 to 6 months with warfarin is advocated for many patients with demonstrable mural thrombi.[904,905] It is not our practice to recommend routine anticoagulation, even if a left ventricular thrombus is present, *unless*: (1) an embolic event has already occurred or (2) the thrombus appears highly mobile and/or markedly protuberant and shaggy on the echocardiogram.[891,893,906]

Antiplatelet therapy, while probably not capable of affecting thrombus size in most patients, may prevent further platelet deposition on existing thrombi.[907] Because it is generally so benign, antiplatelet therapy is therefore recommended for most patients with left ventricular thrombi in whom systemic anticoagulation is not undertaken. Independent of therapy, early spontaneous regression of a thrombus occurs in 20 per cent or more of patients,[378,891] while systemic thrombolytic therapy causes echocardiographic regression or disappearance of the thrombus in most patients so treated.[908]

VENOUS THROMBOSIS AND EMBOLISM

Almost all pulmonary emboli originate from thrombi in the veins of the lower extremities (Chap. 48); much less commonly, they originate from mural thrombi overlying an area of infarction in the right ventricle. Bed rest and heart failure predispose to venous thrombosis and subsequent pulmonary embolism, and both of these factors occur commonly in patients with AMI, particularly those with large infarcts. Several decades ago, at a time when patients with AMI were subjected to prolonged periods of bed rest, significant pulmonary embolism was found in more than 20 per cent of patients with MI at autopsy,[909] and massive pulmonary embolism accounted for 10 per cent of deaths from AMI.[889] In recent years, with early mobilization and the widespread use of low-dose anticoagulant prophylaxis, pulmonary embolism has become an uncommon cause of death in this condition.

POSTINFARCTION ISCHEMIA AND INFARCT EXTENSION

POSTINFARCTION ANGINA. *Angina* developing within the first 10 days following AMI is disconcerting to patients and physicians alike. In many patients, it responds to rest, nitroglycerin, beta-adrenoceptor blockade, and calcium channel antagonists,[904] just as does classic angina. In a minority of patients, postinfarction angina may be refractory to treatment and occurs at rest or is provoked by minimal activity, meals, or emotional upset. This represents a form of unstable angina (p. 1334). When accompanied by ST-T–wave changes in the same area where Q waves have appeared, it may be due to coronary spasm,[911] to occlusion of an initially patent vessel, or to reocclusion of a recanalized one.

Regardless of whether postinfarction angina is persistent or limited, its presence is important, for both short- and long-term mortality is higher among such patients.[331,912,913] For this reason we concur with the recommendation of others[914] that most patients who develop spontaneous angina early after AMI should undergo cardiac catheterization and coronary arteriography to assess their suitability for a revascularization procedure.

Exercise stress testing, particularly when used with stress-thallium scintigraphy, may be helpful in discerning whether chest pain following an AMI is due to ischemia. However, such tests should usually be avoided if symptoms have been persistent, accompanied by ECG changes, or have occurred at rest or with minimal activity. Positron-emission tomography has proved useful for recognizing hypoperfused but viable myocardium following AMI,[915] and its sensitivity is improved further when dual isotope imaging (with thallium and indium antimyosin) is utilized.[916] Early dipyridamole-thallium imaging performed within 4 days of AMI may be able to predict further in-hospital ischemia.[917]

INFARCT EXTENSION

Extension of the infarct occurs in approximately 7 to 10 per cent of patients with AMI during the first 10 days[912,918] and in closer to 20 per cent in patients who have undergone thrombolytic therapy.[919] In the latter group it is due to reocclusion. One study employing echocardiograms every 48 hours or less found extension in over 50 per cent of a selected group of patients with anterior MI.[920] While this incidence may be high, it is probable that many episodes of extension are unrecognized. It is frequently difficult to distinguish postinfarction angina from infarct extension. The latter is usually associated with more severe and prolonged discomfort, and *persistent* electrocardiographic changes (ST-T changes or QRS changes or both) may occur. It is generally defined as reelevation or reappearance of CK-MB in the serum after the initial peak. Neither chest pain nor the ECG provides accurate markers for recognizing infarct extension, as both occur in only about half of patients with extension. The majority of patients with cardiogenic shock have developed infarct extension.[781] In a prospective study of patients, it was found that mortality in those experiencing extension is more than double that noted in patients in whom extension did not occur.[921] Marmor reported that infarct extension occurred most frequently in obese females and was most common in patients with nontransmural infarction.[922] It is apparently more common in patients with diabetes mellitus, a previous MI, and in those with an early peaking CK-MB curve (<15 hours),[918] but it is not predictable from the angiographic appearance of the coronary artery early after infarction—at least when thrombolytic therapy has been given.[919] Presumably, the higher mortality associated with infarct extension is related to the larger mass of myocardium whose function becomes compromised.

PERICARDIAL EFFUSION AND PERICARDITIS

(See also p. 1495–1496)

PERICARDIAL EFFUSION. This is common after AMI. Effusions are generally detected echocardiographically, and their incidence varies with technique, criteria, and laboratory expertise. They occur in approximately 17 to 25 per cent of patients after MI.[923-925] Effusions are more common with anterior MI and with larger infarcts and when congestive failure is present.[923,925] This finding cannot be viewed as a complication because it does not necessarily lead to clinical problems. (When tamponade occurs, it is usually due to ventricular rupture or hemorrhagic pericarditis.)

The reabsorption rate of a postinfarction pericardial effusion is slow, with resolution often taking several months. The presence of an effusion does not indicate that pericarditis is present; although they may occur together, the majority of effusions occur without other evidence of pericarditis.[926]

PERICARDITIS. When secondary to transmural AMI, pericarditis may produce pain as early as the first day and as late as 6 weeks after MI. The pain of pericarditis may be confused with that resulting from persistent ischemia or extension of the infarct or both. Transmural myocardial infarction, by definition, extends to the epicardial surface and is responsible for causing local pericardial inflammation. Although transitory pericardial friction rubs are relatively common among patients with transmural infarction within the first 48 hours, the pain or electrocardiographic changes occur much less often. In one recent study of 423 consecutive patients with AMI, 31 (7.3 per cent) developed a pericardial friction rub, but only one patient had electrocardiographic changes diagnostic of acute pericarditis[267] (p. 1470). Pericarditis is more common in males, among patients with Q-wave infarction, and in those with congestive heart failure.[267,927] Fibrinous or serofibrinous pericarditis may be seen in up to 15 per cent of patients with AMI at autopsy, while clinical studies also suggest the presence of active pericarditis in 10 to 20 per cent of patients,[927,928] whereas pericardial effusion without evidence of pericarditis is far more common.[923] The discomfort of pericarditis usually becomes worse during a deep inspiration, but it may be somewhat relieved when the patient sits up and leans forward (Chap. 45).

Pericarditis generally occurs between the second and fourth days after the infarction. In some patients with diffuse pericarditis, an accompanying pericardial effusion may be large, but tamponade is rare, and as noted earlier no effusion is present in the majority of patients. Occasionally, hemorrhagic effusion with cardiac tamponade develops after myocardial infarction in patients who have been treated with anticoagulants.[929] Late pericardial constriction due to anticoagulant-induced hemopericardium has been reported.[930] While anticoagulation clearly increases the risk for hemorrhagic pericarditis early after MI, this complication has not been reported with sufficient frequency during heparinization or following thrombolytic therapy to warrant *absolute* prohibition of such agents when a rub is present. In cases in which continuation or initiation of anticoagulant therapy is *strongly* indicated (such as during cardiac catheterization or following coronary angioplasty), particularly careful attention is warranted to the clotting parameters and the duration of anticoagulation, and in observation for clinical signs of possible tamponade.

DRESSLER SYNDROME. Also known as the *postmyocardial infarction syndrome,*[269,270] this usually occurs 2 to 10 weeks after infarction. Its incidence is difficult to define because it often blends imperceptibly with the more common early postmyocardial infarction pericarditis. This incidence has decreased dramatically since the use of chronic anticoagulation has fallen out of favor and since antiinflammatory agents are used more vigorously. However, it has probably not disappeared completely as some have contended.[931,932] At autopsy, patients with this syndrome usually demonstrate localized fibrinous pericarditis[928] containing polymorphonuclear leukocytes.[269] The syndrome is treated with aspirin 650 mg, as often as every 4 hours. Other nonsteroidal antiinflammatory agents are best avoided in the AMI patient because of their potential to impair infarct healing,[933] to cause ventricular rupture,[934] and to increase coronary vascular resistance.[935] In occasional patients full-dose steroids are necessary to control what may be very severe symptoms.

Convalescence, Discharge, and Postmyocardial Infarction Care

(See also Chap. 42)

For the patient with an uncomplicated AMI, washing and personal care should be assisted by an attendant during the first 2 to 4 days. If the convalescence continues uneventfully, limited ambulation within the room can be begun on the third or fourth day. Once early ambulatory activities are begun, advancement in the activity should depend on the patient's condition. Activity can then increase progressively, and a shower may be allowed some time after the sixth day. In an era characterized by encouragement of earlier physical activity after AMI, investigators regularly have failed to identify any complication of early ambulation. One recent small study demonstrated that early "vigorous mobilization" (monitored brisk 10 to 15 minute walks from day 4 onward) produced no changes in ventricular volumes, heart rate, or cardiac output in a group of low-risk AMI patients compared with controls managed in a more conventional manner.[936] While concern has been raised from studies in animals[937,938] that such early activity might unfavorably influence ventricular remodeling, perhaps by causing infarct extension, there is no evidence to suggest that this concern is valid, and early mobilization does appear warranted in most stable AMI patients.

Prolonged hospitalization and enforced bed rest for any illness may lead to complications (particularly in elderly patients) such as constipation, decubitus ulcers, excessive resorption of bone with formation of renal calculi, atelectasis, thrombophlebitis, pulmonary emboli, urinary retention, mild anemia due to repetitive blood sampling for diagnostic tests, impaired oral intake of fluids, bleeding from the gastrointestinal tract due to stress ulcers, and deconditioning of cardiovascular reflex responses to postural changes. Because of the precarious status of the heart recovering from AMI, avoidance of such complications is of primary importance. For example, constipation may lead to straining, transitory reduction of venous return and diminution of cardiac output, impaired coronary perfusion, and ventricular arrhythmias, occasionally culminating in ventricular fibrillation. Early use of a bedside commode, stool softeners, and a bed-chair regimen appears to be useful in avoiding many of the difficulties encountered previously among patients confined to bed for several weeks.

TIMING OF HOSPITAL DISCHARGE

The time of discharge from the hospital is variable. It may be as early as 6 or 7 days after admission for patients who experience no complications, who can be followed readily at home, and for whom the family setting is conducive to convalescence.[939] Most complications that would preclude early discharge occur within the first day or so of admission; therefore, patients suitable for early discharge can be identified early during the hospitalization.[940] Ordinarily, discharge of patients without complications is deferred until approximately 7 to 8 days following infarction, at a time when the patient has become fully ambulatory. For patients who have experienced a complication, discharge is deferred until their condition has been stable for several days and it is clear that they are responding appropriately to necessary medications such as antiarrhythmic agents, vasodilators, or positive inotropic agents, or that they have undergone the appropriate work-up for recurrent ischemia.

TRIALS INVOLVING EARLY DISCHARGE. Several controlled trials and many uncontrolled trials of early discharge after AMI have been conducted.[940,940a] None have shown any increase in risk with early discharge, and some have actually shown significantly worse mortality and morbidity in the group discharged later,[941] although this may have been due to confounding variables. When considered together, the studies of early discharge are quite encouraging. Results involving 892 patients in 8 different trials of discharge between 7 and 14 days after admission for AMI suggest that there is no unfavorable effect on mortality and morbidity.[940] A multivariant statistical technique to determine risk of discharge for individual patients has been proposed.[942] Using 19 clinical variables, this technique was developed with the following assumptions: discharge would take place when the risk of a serious complication occurring in the 2 weeks following discharge was below 5 per cent, and when the risk of death in the first 30 days after admission for AMI was also less than 5 per cent. Tested retrospectively in over 1000 patients and prospectively in almost 200 patients, this statistical system confirmed that about 50 per cent of patients could be discharged safely after 5 days, and that up to a 20 per cent saving in hospitalization days could be obtained.[942] More recently, very early discharge (after *3 days*) has been reported without apparent clinical complications.[943] Furthermore, early discharge appeared to promote an earlier return to work and some degree of savings in hospital and professional costs. While conclusions from this study are intriguing, they are limited to a carefully selected group of patients, almost all of whom underwent cardiac catheterization with reperfusion by either thrombolytic therapy or coronary angioplasty. Whether the same savings would occur with the same degree of safety in patients not undergoing catheterization and reperfusion remains to be seen.[944]

While early discharge certainly is feasible for the majority of patients with uncomplicated MI, an attempt should be made before hospital discharge to identify patients at considerable risk of reinfarction or cardiac death. This usually involves noninvasive testing, which may lead to cardiac catheterization and coronary arteriography and, if indicated, to coronary revascularization. Much can be said for accomplishing such procedures, if necessary, before hospital discharge. Furthermore, since we do not yet know with certainty that vigorous exercise does not adversely affect scar formation or ventricular remodeling, an early increase in physical activity should be minimized by strict instructions to the patient and family concerning the gradual resumption of activity after discharge. In fact, patients with poor left ventricular function following relatively large anterior MI have been shown to have infarct expansion and greater shape distortion of the left ventricle after a late exercise program (beginning 15 weeks after AMI).[945] Thus, in patients with extensive degrees of ventricular dysfunction, exercise should be undertaken with caution and monitoring.

COUNSELING. Before discharge from the hospital, all patients should receive detailed instruction concerning physical activity. Initially, this activity should consist of ambulation at home but avoidance of isometric exercise such as lifting; several rest periods should be taken daily. In addition, the patient should be given fresh nitroglycerin tablets and instructed in their use and should receive careful instructions about the use of any other medication prescribed. As convalescence progresses, graded resumption of activity should be encouraged. Many approaches have been utilized, ranging from formal rigid guidelines to general advice advocating moderation and avoidance of any activity that evokes symptoms. *Sexual counseling* is often overlooked during recovery from MI[946] and should also be included as part of the educational process. Such counseling should begin early after AMI and should include the recommendation that sexual activity be resumed after successful completion of either early submaximal or later symptom-limited exercise stress testing.[947]

There is some evidence that behavior alteration is possible after recovery from MI and that this may improve prognosis.[948,949] A cardiac rehabilitation program with supervised physical exercise and an educational component has been recommended for most MI patients following discharge.[950,951] While the overall clinical benefit of such programs continues to be debated,[952,953] there is little question that most people derive considerable knowledge and psychological security from such interventions. The physical and psychological aspects of rehabilitation of patients convalescing from AMI are discussed in Chapter 42.

SECONDARY PREVENTION OF MYOCARDIAL INFARCTION

The concept of secondary prevention of reinfarction and death after recovery from an AMI has been investigated actively during the past $2\frac{1}{2}$ decades. Problems in proving the efficacy of various interventions have been related both to the ineffectiveness of certain strategies and to the difficulty in proving a benefit as mortality and morbidity have improved following AMI. Nevertheless, patients who survive the initial course of AMI are at increased risk due to coronary artery disease and its complications; therefore, it is imperative that efforts be made to reduce this risk.[954] While secondary prevention drug trials generally have tested one form of therapy against placebo in an attempt to demonstrate a benefit of that therapy, the physician must remember that disciplined clinical care of the individual patient is far more important than rote use of an agent found beneficial in the latest drug trial.[955]

In reviewing the results of any secondary prevention trial, the clinician must consider several issues before deciding on its relevance to a particular patient: (1) Was the intervention begun immediately (once AMI was identified) or was it applied later, and what is the relationship of its expected effectiveness to this timing? (2) Were patients in the trial similar to the patient for whom the intervention is contemplated, or would the specific patient under consideration have been excluded from the trial, thus rendering the trial's conclusion less meaningful for that particular patient? (3) Is there some reason to anticipate that the intervention being considered might be unusually risky in certain patients for whom it may be used (e.g., beta-adrenoceptor blockers in a patient with a history of obstructive lung disease)? (4) Once the intervention is started, how long should it be continued, or is this information unavailable because studies have not been ongoing for a sufficient time? (5) What is the underlying risk that the individual patient faces? As detailed on pages 1267 to 1270, patients with low risk can be separated from those with higher risk. In interventional strategies, the level of risk should be taken into consideration when any therapy, particularly if it is to be long term, is contemplated.

It is likely that secondary prevention efforts are, in fact, responsible in part for the remarkable decline in mortality and morbidity[12] in patients with coronary artery disease, although the magnitude of the impact is not clear.

RISK FACTOR REDUCTION. Efforts to improve survival and the quality of life after MI that relate to modification of known risk factors are considered in Chapter 37. Of the risk factors considered, cessation of smoking and control of hypertension are probably most important. It has been shown that within 2 years of quitting smoking, the risk of a nonfatal MI in these former smokers falls to a level compatible with that in never-smokers.[956] Being hospitalized for an AMI is a powerful motivation for patients to cease cigarette smoking, and this is an ideal time to encourage that clearly beneficial change. It is also an ideal time to begin to treat hypertension, to counsel patients to achieve optimal body weight, and to consider various strategies to improve the patient's lipid profile. Unfortunately, unless prior values of total cholesterol and HDL cholesterol are known, or unless measurements are obtained within the first 24 to 48 hours,[312-314] reliable values necessary to guide therapy will not be available until approximately 2 to 3 months after the MI. However, that is not too late to evaluate the lipid profile and to begin appropriate therapeutic measures as outlined in Chapter 37. Following a step I AHA diet (p. 1224) during the initial hospitalization and until the lipids have been evaluated is appropriate. As discussed in Chapter 42, cardiac rehabilitation efforts that include exercise programs and the teaching of stress reduction techniques are also likely to have an impact on secondary prevention.[952,953] However, despite the general desirability of these measures, for many patients with AMI, particularly the elderly, it is unlikely that much change in the underlying coronary atherosclerosis will take place with their institution.

Beta-Adrenoceptor Blockers

These drugs have been the most intensively investigated agents for secondary prevention following AMI. Numerous studies have now shown that beta blocker administration improves survival after AMI, and as a result, prescribing patterns for these agents have changed dramatically.[957] The first post-MI beta blocker trial was reported by Snow in 1965,[958] arousing a great deal of interest. Of the many beta blocking agents tested since then, propranolol,[642,959] metoprolol,[482,960] timolol,[961] and oxprenolol[962] have been tried in the greatest number of patients. Large trials with timolol, propranolol, and metoprolol have demonstrated that these drugs improve survival in a wide spectrum of postinfarction patients and also reduce the incidence of sudden death and reinfarction. Results with oxprenolol, a beta blocker with intrinsic sympathomimetic activity (ISA), are far less encouraging, with at least one trial of this agent appearing to show a slight adverse effect on mortality.[647] Structure in the various trials has varied considerably, making comparisons exceedingly difficult.[647] While increasingly rigorous trial design and analysis have allowed for more definitive conclusions, controversy continues regarding optimal selection of patients, variety of beta blocker, initial route (intravenous followed by oral vs. oral vs. intravenous), and timing of administration.[16]

Although differences in trials have made it statistically unsound to pool data from studies, one useful strategy, known as meta-analysis, has been to compare by graphs estimates of the mortality benefit (or lack of benefit) and the trial's 95 per cent confidence limits.[16,647,963] This form of analysis has been applied to beta blocker trials to demonstrate both the mode of benefit and the effect of ancillary properties of the beta blocker. It appears that improved mortality is related primarily to the prevention of sudden death and that, while there is no difference between cardioselective and noncardioselective beta blockers, agents with ISA are markedly less beneficial than those without ISA.[647]

ADVERSE EFFECTS. While adverse effects have required withdrawal of the beta blocker in approximately 10 per cent of patients, most of these effects can be ameliorated by varying the choice of beta blocker, reducing the dosage, or discontinuing the medication if necessary. There has been natural concern that, because of the beta blockers' negative inotropic effect, heart failure would complicate the administration of these agents to patients after AMI. Although a slight excess of clinical heart failure has been reported in some trials,[647] this difference appears to be at most trivial. Most studies have excluded patients with heart failure at entry, but even those including patients with mild failure do not show any increase in either death or subsequent heart failure.[647] Subgroup analysis of patients from the Norwegian timolol study showed a more marked ability to prevent sudden death in patients with cardiac enlargement than in patients with normal heart size.[964] In the BHAT trial propranolol decreased the incidence of sudden death by 13 per cent in patients without heart failure and by 47 per cent in patients who had prior failure.[965] Early administration of beta blockers may reduce the incidence of heart failure by improving ischemia and by preventing reinfarction. At least one of the large trials suggests that this concept may be accurate. In the Göteborg metoprolol trial, a similar percentage of patients developed heart failure after AMI (27 per cent in the metoprolol group and 30 per cent in the control group), but significantly less diuretic was required among metoprolol-treated patients than among controls.[966] The results of the Beta-Blocker Pooling Project, in which data were examined from 9 separate studies involving more than 10,000 patients, suggest a highly significant reduction in overall mortality among treated patients *with* pump or mechanical failure compared with patients on placebo with such failure.[967] The relative benefit of beta blockers following thrombolytic therapy has been well studied in only one trial.[3] Early intravenous metoprolol reduced the incidence of recurrent ischemia and early reinfarction but did not affect 1-year survival or alter left ventricular function.

The mechanism by which beta blockers improve survival is not completely clear. It is likely that many factors are important, including control of hypertension and ischemia, an antiarrhythmic effect, perhaps an antiplatelet effect, an improvement in scar size, and possibly vascularity of the myocardium.[647] Blockade of the direct toxic effect of adrenergic stimulation on the myocardium may also be important. Since neither cardioselectivity or membrane-stabilizing activity appears to be requisite, the mechanism of beneficial effect appears to be due to a "class effect," i.e., it is secondary to beta blockade itself. The reduction in mortality is seen in all age groups and for all types of infarction.

RECOMMENDATIONS. On the basis of currently available evidence, patients without a contraindication to beta blockade (asthma, moderate or severe congestive heart failure, bradyarrhythmias) should have prophylactic treatment with beta blockers initiated after AMI. The dosage should be sufficient to blunt the heart rate response through stress or exercise. Since, in different trials, therapy has been initiated over a wide range of starting times (from hours to weeks) it is impossible to know which time is best from the available data. However, since the safety of early administration of beta blockers has been well documented,[958,960] it is reasonable to suggest that beta blocker administration should begin as early as possible, certainly before hospital discharge, as long as contraindications are not present. Since much of the impact in preventing mortality occurs in the first few weeks, not only is an excess degree of caution unwarranted, but delay may lead to failure to prevent a proportion of early deaths.[647] It is unclear how long patients should be treated. While it is reasonable to conclude that treatment need not extend beyond the period when mortality curves no longer diverge, this rationale is problematic: Will discontinuation of therapy lead to increasing mortality in some patients? Do mortality curves actually continue to diverge? Will continuing the drug lead to some degree of continued protection?

There are, in fact, conflicting data regarding the benefit of continuing therapy beyond 2 years. Late follow-up of a large metoprolol trial showed no significant difference in mortality at 5 years of treatment, even though a significant difference had existed at 2 years.[968] However, 6-year follow-up of the Norwegian timolol study showed lower cardiac mortality in the treated group, even 2 to 3 years after the study drug had been withdrawn.[961] Finally, in another trial, patients withdrawn from metoprolol demonstrated increased mortality following drug withdrawal.[969] Taken together, these studies suggest that therapy should be continued for at least 2 years.[16,970] At that time, if the beta blocker is well tolerated and if there is no reason to discontinue therapy, such therapy probably should be continued in most patients.

The 1 to 2 per cent overall reduction in mortality in postinfarction patients that would come from long-term use of beta blockers and secondary prevention may seem small, but it is comparable to the reduction in mortality achieved by long-term antihypertensive therapy, and would result in the saving of approximately 6000 lives per year in the United States.[647] While it should not be considered "ethically imperative" to treat all postinfarction patients, the fact that over 35,000 patients have been randomized into placebo-controlled beta blocker trials does make it important that the clinician be aware of the results of these trials, and at least consider beta blocker therapy in all patients, including the elderly, who survive MI.[647,971] The cost-effectiveness of such therapy in medium- or high-risk persons compares very favorably with many other accepted interventions such as coronary bypass surgery, angioplasty, and lipid-lowering therapy.[972] Beta blockers should not be given to patients who have clear contraindications, and *probably* need not be given to patients with an *extremely* good prognosis (first AMI, good ventricular function, no angina, negative stress test, and no complex ventricular ectopy) in whom a mortality rate of approximately 1 per cent per year can be anticipated.[973] Among such patients, long-term beta blockers do not appear to offer a benefit.[974]

Anticoagulants

(see also p. 1780)

There are at least three theoretical reasons for anticipating that anticoagulants might be beneficial in the management of AMI: (1) Since the coronary occlusion responsible for the AMI is often due to a thrombus (p. 1206), anticoagulants might be expected to halt or slow progression and to prevent the development of new thrombi elsewhere in the coronary arterial tree. (2) Anticoagulants might be expected to diminish the formation of mural thrombi and resultant systemic embolization. (3) Anticoagulants might be expected to reduce the incidence of venous thrombosis and pulmonary embolization.

After several decades of evaluation, the weight of evidence now suggests that anticoagulants appear to have a favorable effect on late mortality and reinfarction among patients hospitalized with AMI[975-978] (Fig. 39–38). While salutary effects on the underlying coronary disease and its progression have not been clearly demonstrated with conventional anticoagulant drugs, it is possible that they decrease the incidence of cerebral emboli resulting from mural thrombi (p. 1821).[969] In addition, the administration of heparin in doses sufficient to influence activation of factor X without affecting conventional laboratory tests of the coagulation system has in the past substantially diminished the incidence of deep vein thrombosis,[980] thereby reducing the incidence of pulmonary emboli. Whether anticoagulant therapy produces this benefit today, with earlier ambulation and discharge of patients, has not been retested. Nevertheless, it appears advisable to administer minidose heparin (5000 units subcutaneously) every 8 to 12 hours in the absence of specific contraindications.[981] The drug should be continued until 2 to 3 days before hospital discharge, although it is recognized that in patients with uncomplicated AMI there is no clear evidence that it reduces mortality. In any event, patients treated with thrombolytic agents require heparin therapy.

In patients at high risk of embolism (e.g., those with ventricular aneurysm, marked obesity, cardiogenic shock, low output state, present or past thrombophlebitis, arterial or pulmonary embolism), in the absence of contraindications, anticoagulant treatment does exert a favorable effect on survival, and full-dose anticoagulation with heparin is indicated (e.g., intravenous administration of 10,000 units, followed by continuous infusion of 1000 units per hour) to maintain the clotting time and partial thromboplastin time at 1.5 to 2.0 times normal. After 5 to 7 days of therapy, warfarin or continued administration of subcutaneous, adjusted doses of heparin may be employed if conditions exist that suggest that venous thrombosis and embolism are likely to recur. These include continued or worsening heart failure, persistent thrombophlebitis, and the need for prolonged bed rest.

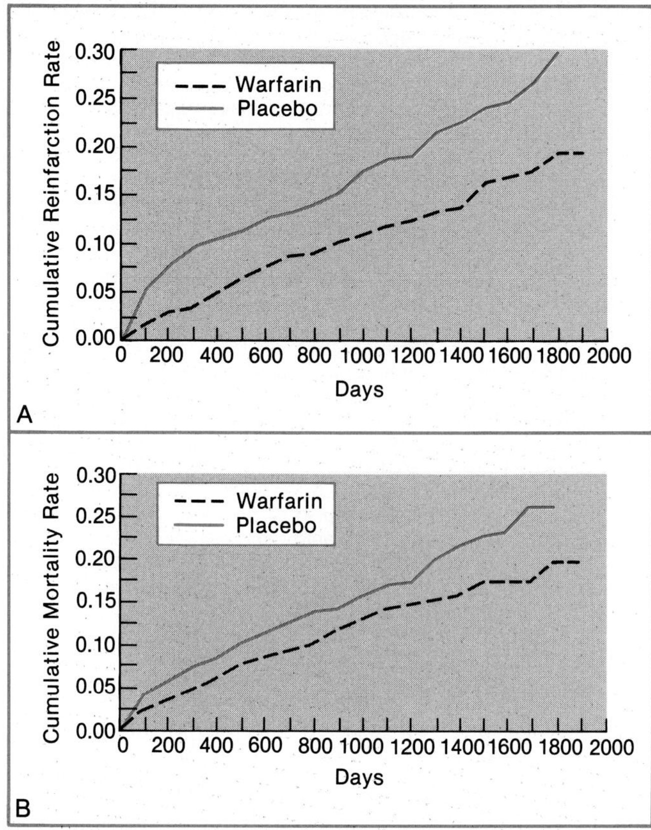

FIGURE 39–38. Cumulative rates of reinfarction (*A*) and death from all causes (*B*) according to original treatment assignment from randomized study of warfarin in 1214 patients with AMI. Treatment began a mean of 27 days after infarction. (Reprinted by permission from Smith, P., et al.: The effect of warfarin on mortality and reinfarction after myocardial infarction. N. Engl. J. Med. *323*:147, 1990.)

As anticoagulation does clearly reduce the occurrence of thromboembolic complications, it is reasonable to use chronic anticoagulants in patients in the posthospital phase with specific indications, including thrombophlebitis, a history of pulmonary or systemic embolism, evidence of a mural thrombus in the left ventricle on two-dimensional echocardiography (Fig. 4–91, p. 98), and severe heart failure.[982] As both warfarin and aspirin have now been shown to be of long-term benefit but have not been compared directly, the choice of one over the other must be based on individual physician preferences and patient characteristics.

Antiplatelet Agents

(See also p. 1340)

Secondary prevention trials with antiplatelet agents are based on the theory that platelets play a role in MI and sudden death. Thrombi may be composed of platelet aggregates at the site of an atherosclerotic coronary artery narrowing, and aggregates may obstruct the coronary microcirculation, inducing coronary vasospasm through the release of the vasoconstrictor thromboxane A_2. Platelets may also play a role in atherogenesis (p. 1337). In two different careful reviews of the major secondary prevention aspirin trials performed over the last 15 years, opposite conclusions were reached about the efficacy of aspirin after AMI.[983,984] Although seven of the eight trials reviewed showed a lower mean mortality with aspirin, the difference was statistically significant in only one (Table 58–3, p. 1785). However, pooling of the data suggests that aspirin prophylaxis could result in at least a 10 to 15 per cent reduction in total deaths and a 20 to 30 per cent reduction in reinfarction.[983,995] Accordingly, in the absence of contraindications to aspirin administration, particularly the history of peptic ulcer disease or gastrointestinal bleeding, we recommend 80 to 325 mg aspirin daily, which can be administered as an enteric-coated tablet. This dosage should minimize the risk of accompanying gastrointestinal side effects; the cost is low and inconvenience trivial. Despite the use of sulfinpyrazone in earlier trials,[986] there is no reason to anticipate that its antiplatelet effect is superior to aspirin's,[985] and it may, in fact, be less effective. Therefore, use of sulfinpyrazone in place of aspirin is not recommended. The addition of dipyridamole to aspirin for possible potentiation of antiplatelet effect has not convincingly improved on the effect of aspirin alone[987]; therefore, coadministration of dipyridamole also is not recommended.[985]

Other Measures

The effectiveness of secondary prevention with other agents, including calcium antagonists, nitrates, antiarrhythmics, lipid-lowering drugs, prostacyclin analogs, and thromboxane synthetase inhibitors, requires further investigation.

CALCIUM ANTAGONISTS. Studies of verapamil[670] and nifedipine[662,998] have failed to show any clear benefit with the *early* administration of these agents. In fact, three studies[663-665] have actually shown a higher early mortality when nifedipine was given early to patients with threatened or acute MI. Therefore, nifedipine cannot be recommended for secondary prevention following AMI, and, in fact, should probably be avoided in most patients.[989] Although diltiazem also showed no benefit in one large trial,[666] a subgroup analysis suggests that it may actually be harmful in patients with preexisting left ventricular dysfunction, while a parallel study showed potential benefit (reduction in reinfarction) in patients with non-Q wave infarction (Fig. 38-39).[990] This finding has led some to recommend diltiazem for patients with non-Q-wave MI.[991] Finally, verapamil also has produced mixed results, with one recent study showing a favorable long-term effect in patients free of heart failure.[667]

NITRATES. These agents are widely prescribed prophylactically to patients following AMI, usually for prevention of recurrent ischemia. However, controlled trials to test the long-term efficacy of this strategy have not been carried out; therefore, such an approach cannot be recommended on a routine basis. In one retrospective study, patients treated with long-acting nitrates had a significantly lower mortality (10 versus 26 per cent) than those not receiving this therapy.[992] This observational study cannot be used as justification for applying such therapy to all patients unless a specific indication such as continuing angina is present.

ANTIARRHYTHMICS. While it has been recognized for decades that antiarrhythmic therapy can control atrial and ventricular arrhythmias effectively in many patients, careful reviews of clinical trials have failed to suggest that routine use of these agents would be of any benefit.[993,994] Such agents have never been shown conclusively to reduce long-term mortality following AMI,[995] and certain agents (e.g., flecainide and encainide) appear to increase mortality,[752] as discussed on p. 643) (Fig. 39-27). Accordingly, the routine use of antiarrhythmic agents cannot be recommended. Whether subgroups with complex arrhythmias, particularly if they are symptomatic, should be treated remains unanswered by such studies, yet treatment of such patients with antiarrhythmic agents does seem reasonable in the absence of contraindications or newer data to the contrary.

Recently early treatment of AMI patients with intravenous magnesium (in patients with normal baseline magnesium levels) has been shown to reduce 1-year mortality, partly on the basis of a nearly 50 per cent reduction in arrhythmias.[996] This intriguing finding awaits confirmation before such therapy can be widely recommended.

RISK FACTOR MODIFICATION. This strategy applied universally after AMI has not been shown convincingly to affect long-term mortality and morbidity and is the subject of several large ongoing controlled studies. However, three trials are worthy of note. In the first, late follow-up (at a mean of 15 years) from the Coronary Drug Project, begun in 1966, has revealed lower mortality among patients treated with niacin to induce favorable effects on serum lipids.[997] Remarkably, this benefit was seen nearly 9 years after termination of the study, when patients were no longer taking niacin. The second, a recent trial from Sweden, demonstrated that clofibrate and nicotinic acid administered together reduced overt recurrent *ischemic* heart disease by 28 per cent at 5 years.[998] Third, it is known that type A behavior (an excessive sense of time urgency and easily aroused hostility, p. 1152) can be improved by training techniques, and it has been reported, although not yet confirmed, that the use of such techniques following AMI may reduce significantly the risk of recurrent AMI and sudden death.[999] It is clearly prudent to follow strategies known to improve long-term cardiac risks such as encouraging smoking cessation, control of diabetes and hypertension if present, and treatment of elevated serum cholesterol or other prognostically unfavorable lipid profiles.[1000]

RISK STRATIFICATION FOLLOWING MYOCARDIAL INFARCTION

Both short-term and long-term survival after AMI depend on a number of factors,[1001,1002] (Table 39-16) the most important of which is the state of left ventricular function. Additional importance is ascribed to the severity and extent of the obstructive lesions in the coronary vascular bed perfusing residual viable myocardium.[1003,1004] In other words, survival relates to the quantity of myocardium that has become necrotic and the quantity at risk of becoming necrotic. At one extreme, the prognosis is best for the patient with normal intrinsic coronary vessels whose completed infarction constitutes a small fraction (less than 5 per cent) of the left ventricle as a consequence of a coronary embolus and who has no jeopardized myocardium. At the other extreme is the patient with a massive infarct who is in cardiogenic shock and whose residual viable myocardium is perfused by markedly obstructed vessels; obviously, progression of atherosclerosis or lowering of perfusion pressure in these vessels will impair the function and viability of the residual myocardium on which left ventricular function depends. The situation may not be hopeless even in such a patient, however, since revascularization may reduce the threat to the jeopardized myocardium.

CLINICAL FACTORS. Soon after coronary care units were instituted, it became apparent that left ventricular function is an important early determinant of survival. Thus, Killip divided patients into four groups on the basis of the clinical severity of left ventricular failure as assessed by physical examination at the time of admission to the coronary care unit. As noted in Table 39-12, hospital mortality from AMI depends directly on the severity of left ventricular dysfunction present at the time of admission.[1005] Similarly, Peel[1006] and Norris[1007] and their collaborators developed clinical prognos-

TABLE 39-16 ADVERSE RISK FACTORS AFTER ACUTE MYOCARDIAL INFARCTION

1. Congestive heart failure (clinical, hemodynamic, or radiographic)
2. Left ventricular ejection fraction less than 0.04
3. Large infarct size (estimated by enzymes, technetium-99m radionuclide scan, electrocardiographic QRS mapping, or echocardiographic techniques)
4. New bundle branch block (any type, including fascicular blocks)
5. Mobitz II second-degree or third-degree heart block
6. Anterior infarction
7. Reinfarction or infarct extension
8. Ventricular fibrillation or ventricular tachycardia
9. Ventricular premature beats (especially if frequent or complex)
10. Supraventricular arrhythmias (other than sinus bradycardia)
11. Abnormal signal-averaged electrocardiogram
12. Inducible sustained monomorphic ventricular tachycardia during electrophysiologic study
13. Postinfarction angina
14. Inability to perform exercise testing
15. Angina pectoris, ST-segment elevation or depression, abnormal blood pressure response, or ventricular ectopy induced by exercise testing
16. Diabetes mellitus
17. Hypertension or loss of preexisting hypertension
18. Age greater than 70 years
19. Female gender

Adapted from Hessen, S. E., and Brest, A. N.: Risk profiling the patient after acute myocardial infarction. *In* Pepine, C. J. (ed.): Acute myocardial infarction. Philadelphia, F. A. Davis, 1989, p. 284.

tic indices for patients with AMI. Although they used historical, electrocardiographic, and radiological data to predict hospital mortality, evidence of left ventricular failure heavily weigh these indices in the direction of poor prognosis.

Certain demographic and historical factors are associated with a poor prognosis after infarction, including female sex,[1008,1008a] age greater than 70 years,[1009,1010] a history of diabetes mellitus,[1011] hypertension, prior angina pectoris, and previous MI.[1012–1014] *Diabetes mellitus*, in particular, appears to confer a three- to fourfold increase in risk[1015,1016]; whether this is due to accelerated atherosclerosis or some other characteristic induced by the diabetic state (such as a larger infarct size[1017]) is unclear.[1018] Surviving diabetic patients also experience a more complicated postmyocardial infarction course than nondiabetic ones, including a greater incidence of postinfarction angina, infarct extension, and heart failure.[1011] Isolated elevation of systolic blood pressure and combined systolic and diastolic hypertension are also unfavorable prognostic factors.[1019] Interestingly, however, patients whose blood pressure falls after AMI seem to have a worse prognosis than those whose blood pressure increases or remains unchanged.[1019] There is also greater mortality after anterior wall MI than after inferior MI, even when corrected for infarct size.[1020,1021] As has already been discussed, infarct extension (p. 1262) influences prognosis adversely. Poor prognosis comes from the loss of viable myocardium with the resulting larger area of infarction creating a greater compromise in overall ventricular function. Postinfarction angina generally connotes a less favorable prognosis because it indicates the presence of jeopardized myocardium[1022]; however, if it is due to coronary artery spasm rather than critical organic obstruction, prognosis may be relatively good.[1023] In the current era of aggressive revascularization, early postinfarction angina often leads to early interventions that tend to improve outcome, diminishing the long-term impact and significance of angina early after AMI. Silent postinfarction ischemia detected by ambulatory monitoring is associated with the same unfavorable prognosis as symptomatic ischemia after AMI.[1024]

Although the incidence of unrecognized MI is less than that of clinically apparent MI,[258] the long-term prognosis from unrecognized infarction appears to be similar to, and as serious as, that following recognized infarction.[1025] Although the risk of angina recurring after an unrecognized MI is less than after a clinically apparent MI, the incidence of late stroke and heart failure may be even greater among patients with unrecognized MI.[1025]

Increasingly sophisticated statistical techniques have been applied to risk assessment following AMI. Madsen et al. have developed a discriminate function analysis score based on the presence or absence of four factors: heart failure, ventricular tachycardia, AV block, and previous infarction or extension of infarction.[1026] The accuracy of this score has been tested in several different populations and is useful for predicting both the risk of reinfarction and that of death following AMI.[1026] This group has also shown that reliable long-term prediction of outcome is possible using data from the first 24 hours of hospitalization,[1027] without a substantial increase in accuracy when further data from the rest of the hospitalization are added.[1028] Finally, they have applied these data to the development of a decision scheme for the selection of patients for coronary angiography after AMI,[1029] suggesting that the procedure be avoided in patients with a low 1-year mortality and recommending it for patients at higher risk.

As the widespread use of thrombolytic therapy is relatively recent, less is known about specific short- and long-term prognostic characteristics in patients having received such therapy. However, in studies carried out thus far, important risk factors appear to be no different in this group of patients from those in patients not undergoing thrombolysis.[1030,1031] The TIMI group has identified a series of clinical factors that can be detected at the time of presentation and used to help select patients at particularly high risk of death in the first 6 weeks following AMI[1031] (Table 39–6, p. 1232).

HEMODYNAMICS AND VENTRICULAR FUNCTION. Physiological evidence of compromised left ventricular function also correlates with hospital mortality in AMI, as already discussed. Thus, patients with hemodynamic (elevated pulmonary capillary wedge pressure and/or depressed cardiac index) or ventriculographic (depressed ejection fraction and elevated end-systolic volume by radionuclide angiography) evidence of left ventricular failure have a worse prognosis than patients without these findings.[1032,1033] Acute pulmonary edema with AMI, even if due to diastolic dysfunction and associated with a normal ejection fraction, can be used to identify a high-risk group.[1034]

Left ventricular ejection fraction may be the most easily assessed measurement of left ventricular function, and this measurement is extremely useful for risk stratification (Fig. 39–40). Further prognostic information can be obtained by the accurate assessment of end-systolic volume, which is an index superior even to ejection fraction for prediction of survival following AMI.[157] In patients with a low left ventricular ejection fraction, the measurement of exercise capacity is useful for further identifying those individuals at particularly high risk.[1035] Likewise, since a low ejection fraction per se is predictively highly variable, it is useful to know that patients with a *good* exercise capacity in this group fare far better than those who cannot perform more than modest exercise.[1036]

The presence or absence of concomitant right ventricular dysfunction with AMI (usually with inferior MI) does *not* appear to influence long-term outcome.[1037] The *chest roentgenogram* is of prognostic value because patients with cardiomegaly after infarction do not fare as well as individuals without this feature.

Because impaired ventricular function generally is a manifestation of the cumulative extent of myocardial damage sustained, one important determinant of prognosis is *infarct size*. This may be determined from an analysis of CK (or CK-MB) samples obtained at frequent intervals[273] or less accurately from the peak enzyme level. Thus, patients with markedly elevated plasma enzyme levels (CK > 2000 IU) often manifest left ventricular failure with concomitant poor prognosis. Furthermore, prognosis for as long as 4 years after an initial infarction is related to infarct size estimated from plasma CK time-activity curves at the time of the acute episode.[308] However, some patients with low peak CK levels may represent a higher-risk group with an increased incidence of late cardiac events, presumably due to jeopardized but noninfarcted myocardium.[1038] A large defect or multiple defects on a thallium-201 perfusion scintigram obtained early in the course of AMI, also presumably related to infarct size, is associated with a high incidence of mortality or subsequent cardiac events.[1032,1033] Similarly, patients with large infarcts on technetium-99m scintigrams have an adverse prognosis.[1039]

Experimental evidence suggests that an intervention aimed at improving ventricular function and ventricular remodeling after AMI (p. 1210), such as vasodilator therapy with captopril, may lessen ventricular dilatation and improve survival in the chronic phase of infarction.[167] A clinical trial is now under way to assess the possible benefit of this strategy in patients. Thus, in the future, ways may be found to improve upon the altered prognosis associated with large infarcts and compromised ventricular function.

Q-WAVE VERSUS NON-Q-WAVE INFARCTION (Table 39–17). Myocardial infarction occurring without the development of new Q waves has been called subendocardial, nontransmural, and non-Q-wave infarction. However, the correlation between the electrocardiographic findings of transmural or subendocardial myocardial infarction and the pathological counterparts is not good.[326] Indeed, many patients with pathological transmural infarctions have no Q waves or loss of R waves and vice versa. Consequently, it has been suggested that the description of MI based on electrocardiographic findings be confined to what is actually observed on the electrocardiogram—that is, "Q-wave" and "non-Q-wave" infarctions.

TABLE 39-17 DIFFERENCES IN PATIENTS WITH Q-WAVE AND NON-Q-WAVE MYOCARDIAL INFARCTION (MI)

CHARACTERISTIC	Q-WAVE MI	NON-Q-WAVE MI
Prevalence	60–70% of infarcts	30–40% of infarcts
Prior infarction	Rare	Frequent
Occluded infarct-related artery	75–80%	10–20%
Coronary collaterals	Less prominent	More prominent
ST-segment elevation	80%	40%
Peak creatine kinase	Higher	Lower
Ejection fraction	Lower	Higher
Wall motion	More dysfunction	Less dysfunction
Postinfarction ischemia	Less common	More common
Early infarction	~8%	~40%
In-hospital mortality	7–15%	5–10%
3-year mortality	10–30%	10–30%
Effect of medications		
Thrombolytic agents	Beneficial	Not established
β-Adrenergic blockers	Beneficial	Not established
Calcium channel blockers	Possibly detrimental	Possibly beneficial (diltiazem)

Adapted from Lavie, C. L., et al.: Acute myocardial infarction: Initial manifestations, management, prognosis. Mayo Clin. Proc. *65*:531, 1990.

The early (hospital) mortality in patients with Q-wave infarcts is approximately 1½ to 2 times that in patients with non-Q-wave infarcts,[451,1040,1041] unless early recurrent infarction or infarct extension occurs, in which case mortality is similar to that for both groups.[451] Patients with non-Q-wave infarction tend to have smaller infarcts initially and only infrequently have total occlusions of the infarct-related vessel when compared with patients with Q-wave infarction.[1041] Consistent with this finding are a lower incidence of heart failure early after infarction (as a consequence of a lesser degree of ventricular function impairment), and more frequent angina (related to the presence of preserved myocardium with marginal blood supply).[1040-1042] However, uncomplicated non-Q-wave infarctions are not benign conditions.[329,1040-1044] Thus, 60 per cent of these patients have critical obstruction in two or three of the major coronary arteries, and frequently go on to develop an acute Q-wave infarction within 12 months of the non-Q-wave infarct.[1040,1041] In one series almost half of the patients with non-Q-wave infarction developed unstable angina during a follow-up period averaging 11 months.[1045] In others, the incidence of infarct extension or early recurrent infarction was high.[1040,1041] In-hospital extension of a non-Q-wave infarction appears to increase long-term risk, with a doubling of 1-year mortality in one study.[1046]

Thus, it is clear that patients with non-Q-wave infarctions have a natural history different from that in patients with Q-wave infarction. The former may be considered a relatively unstable condition associated with a lower initial mortality rate but a higher risk of later infarction. The differing early and late risk patterns cancel each other out, to a certain extent, when overall long-term mortality is considered, because at late follow-up (1 to 3 years), both Q-wave and non-Q-wave MI patients have similar morbidities and mortalities.[1040,1044,1047,1048] The recognition of differences between the early natural histories of these two forms of infarction suggests the need for a more aggressive diagnostic approach including a careful noninvasive search for ischemia and often coronary arteriography perhaps followed by early coronary angioplasty[1049] or surgical treatment even in selected asymptomatic patients who have sustained an acute non-Q-wave infarction.[1044,1050]

Despite the logic inherent in this approach, there is no firm evidence that this strategy influences the course favorably, although it has been shown that the calcium antagonist diltiazem may be effective in preventing early recurrent MI and angina following non-Q-wave infarction. A multicenter study of this intervention in over 500 randomized patients showed a 50 per cent reduction in the cumulative incidence of such events after infarction (Fig. 39-39).[990] Patients with non-Q-wave infarction at greatest risk, who would appear likely to benefit most from the aforementioned interventions, include those with persistent ST-T-segment depression during hospitalization[1051] and those with spontaneous ischemia[1052] or ischemia provoked by stress testing.[1044,1053,1053a]

Patients with evidence of recurrent ischemia after infarction (regardless of location or ECG configuration) should receive medical therapy (bedrest, oxygen, nitrates, beta blockers, and calcium antagonists as tolerated) and should have coronary arteriography and be considered for revascularization (Chap. 40). However, it is particularly important to carefully follow symptomatic patients with non-Q-wave infarction because of the frequent presence of jeopardized but viable myocardium in such patients. Symptoms of recurrent angina or findings on noninvasive testing compatible with exercise-induced ischemia should be pursued vigorously and treated appropriately.[1050]

ELECTROCARDIOGRAM. Patients whose ECG demonstrates persistent advanced heart block (e.g., Mobitz type II, second-degree, or third-degree atrioventricular block) or new intraventricular conduction abnormalities (bifascicular or trifascicular) in the course of an AMI have a worse prognosis than do patients without these abnormalities. The influence of high degrees of heart block is particularly important in patients with right ventricular infarction, for such patients have a markedly increased mortality.[700] Other electrocardiographic findings that augur poorly for the postinfarction patient are repetitive ventricular ectopic activity (Table 39-9) (couplets, runs), persistent horizontal or downsloping ST-segment depression and Q waves in multiple leads, atrial arrhythmias (especially atrial fibrillation), voltage criteria for left ventricular hypertrophy, and an abnormal signal-averaged electrocardiogram (on a specially filtered and processed QRS complex).[1054-1057]

ST-segment depressions in leads other than those with acute Q waves are also a poor prognostic sign; for example, patients with acute inferior wall infarcts who demonstrate ST-segment depressions in precordial leads have a worse prognosis than do patients without this finding. There is con-

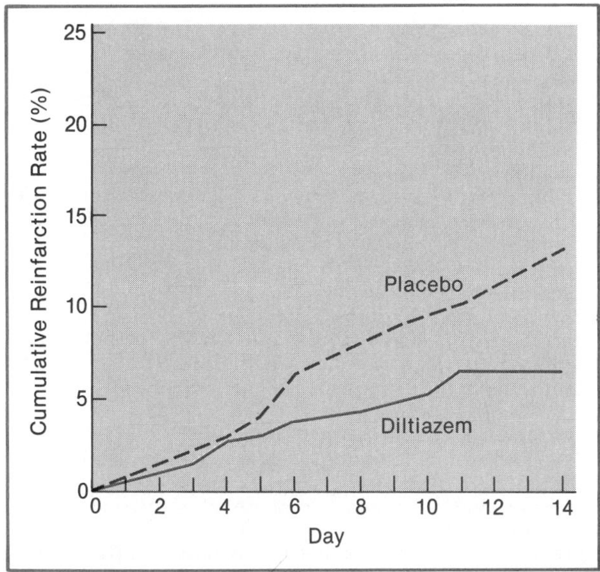

FIGURE 39-39. Life-table cumulative reinfarction rate, according to treatment group, from randomized study of 576 patients with non-Q-wave myocardial infarction. (Reprinted by permission from Gibson, R. S., et al.: Diltiazem and reinfarction in patients with non-Q-wave myocardial infarction. N. Engl. J. Med. *315*:423, 1986.)

troversy concerning whether these ST-segment depressions reflect reciprocal electrical changes, associated disease of the left anterior descending coronary artery, or, most likely, a larger inferior infarct.[332,333,335] Similarly, patients who develop angina during the first 10 days following infarction, with new electrocardiographic changes distant from the acute infarct, i.e., angina "at a distance," have a distinctly worse prognosis than do patients having postinfarct angina with ischemia in the infarct zone.[331]

LATE POSTINFARCT ASSESSMENT OF PROGNOSIS

Following recovery from AMI—i.e., by 10 days to 6 weeks after the event—long-term prognosis can be evaluated by ambulatory electrocardiographic monitoring and exercise testing,[1058,1059] with a recent survey suggesting that the vast majority employ at least the latter in most postinfarction patients.[1060] The development of ST-segment abnormalities, typical angina or exercise limitation by dyspnea at low levels of exercise (heart rate <120 beats/min or exercise duration <6 minutes on the Bruce protocol [p. 163]), and major (>2 mm) ST-segment depression and a stress-induced fall in blood pressure at any level of exercise all signify a poor prognosis.[1061-1063] A predischarge submaximal exercise test is useful for early risk stratification and can detect ischemia and arrhythmias among patients in whom these clinical features were not necessarily apparent during their hospital stay.[1059,1061,1064] A maximal stress test performed 4 to 6 weeks later may identify a greater number of patients with residual myocardial ischemia,[1066,1067] although this is controversial.[1063] Radionuclide angiography,[1067,1068] echocardiography,[1069] and thallium scintigraphy,[1066,1067] as well as coronary arteriography and left ventriculography, can provide additional important prognostic information.[1059] The high-risk variables which can be identified with noninvasive testing are shown in Table 39–18. Invasive tests are ordinarily carried out only if the patient is symptomatic or if the noninvasive tests suggest a poor prognosis and if the results of these examinations would alter the management (Chap. 40).[1029] A progressive increase in 1-year mortality is seen as ejection fraction, as measured by radionuclide angiography during hospitalization, falls below

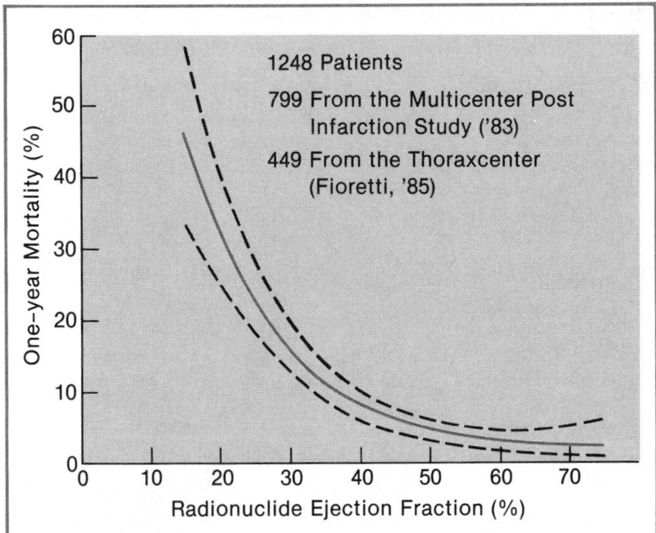

FIGURE 39–40. One-year mortality as a function of radionuclide ejection fraction (per cent) measured at hospital discharge after acute myocardial infarction. The solid line between the *dashed lines* indicates the corresponding 95 per cent confidence interval. The calculations are based on pooled data from the Multicenter Postinfarction Study and the Thoraxcenter. (From Serray, P. W., et al.: Preservation of global and regional left ventricular function after early thrombolysis in acute myocardial infarction. Reprinted with permission of the American College of Cardiology. J. Am. Coll. Cardiol. *7*:729, 1986.)

0.40 (Fig. 39–40).[1070] Evidence indicates that electrical instability, as reflected in frequent, multiple, or complex ventricular extrasystoles, and left ventricular dysfunction, as reflected in a depressed left ventricular ejection fraction (<40 per cent) 10 days after the occurrence of an AMI, are independent risk factors[1071]; the presence of either risk factor was associated with an increased 15-month mortality.[1072]

Despite the clear prognostic importance of severe ventricular ectopy when detected during in-patient bedside or ambulatory monitoring, studies utilizing invasive programmed ventricular stimulation have provided conflicting evidence that ventricular arrhythmias provoked by this technique have any prognostic significance.[1073,1074] Patients who develop sustained ventricular tachycardia or fibrillation spontaneously in the early recovery period are at increased risk of sudden cardiac death following hospital discharge. Control of ventricular arrhythmias in such patients, by medical and (if necessary) surgical therapy, may improve long-term mortality but has not been shown definitely to do this.[1075] When considered together, the combination of clinical factors, radionuclide ejection fraction, and the results of ambulatory monitoring can provide an accurate assessment of prognosis—not surprisingly, the more risk factors present, the greater mortality at any time following AMI (Fig. 39–41).[15,1059,1070]

Use of readily available clinical variables[1076] and exercise electrocardiography is probably sufficient for risk stratification in most patients following AMI. The additional techniques of echocardiography, with or without dipyridamole[1076a] radionuclide angiography, thallium-201 scintigraphy (if necessary with dipyridamole[1077]), and ambulatory electrocardiography should probably be reserved for (1) patients who cannot undergo exercise electrocardiography, (2) those in whom it is not diagnostic, e.g. patients with left bundle branch block, and (3) those who are already thought to be at relatively high risk and in whom a search for specific risks (e.g. ventricular arrhythmia, myocardial dysfunction, or left ventricular thrombus) is appropriate and might lead to specific forms of therapy.[1059,1066,1078]

RECOMMENDATIONS. While there are many different strategies for the overall assessment of prognosis following

TABLE 39–18 HIGH-RISK EXERCISE TEST AND IMAGING VARIABLES AFTER ACUTE MYOCARDIAL INFARCTION

Exercise ECG Stress Testing
Failure to reach target heart rate (120–130 beats per minute)
Failure to achieve >3 METS
Failure to increase systolic blood pressure by ≥10 mm Hg
Exercise-induced ST-segment depression (>1.0 mm)
Inducible angina
Exercise Thallium-201 Scintigraphy
Multiple perfusion defects in more than one vascular region (for example, left anterior descending and circumflex zones)
Presence of thallium-201 redistribution
Increased lung thallium-201 uptake
Exercise-induced LV cavity dilation
Exercise Radionuclide Angiography
Decrease of >5% in LV ejection fraction from rest to exercise
Absolute exercise LV ejection fraction <50%
Exercise-induced increase in end-systolic volume
Rest Radionuclide Imaging
Resting LV ejection fraction <45%
Extensive resting thallium-201 or technetium-99m isonitrile persistent defects
Large areas of technetium pyrophosphate or indium-111 antimyosin antibody uptake
Large nitrogen-13 ammonia defect with no fluorine-18 2-deoxyglucose uptake

LV = left ventricular.
Adapted from Beller, G. A.: Radionuclide imaging in acute myocardial infarction. *In* Gersh, B. J., and Rahimtoola, S. H.: Acute myocardial infarction. New York, Elsevier, 1991, p. 192. By permission of the publisher.

results from left ventricular dysfunction, reflecting damaged myocardium as well as provokable ischemia, reflecting myocardium at risk.[1079] The strategy outlined is directed at identifying patients at more than low risk who can expect some benefit from anticipated interventions. Unfortunately, in patients at greatest risk—those with very severe left ventricular dysfunction—most currently available medical and surgical therapies are of little long-term benefit.

The general approach outlined in Figure 39–43 has been recommended by a combined American Heart Association and American College of Cardiology Task Force[1080] to help select patients for invasive investigations. Three different strategies can be employed depending upon physician preferences for an early symptom-limited stress test (Strategy I), combined early submaximal stress testing and later symptom-limited testing (Strategy II), or early discharge without stress testing followed by a relatively early (3-week) symptom-limited exercise test with or without thallium evaluation (Strategy III). Our own approach is as follows: In the first 5 days of hospitalization invasive or noninvasive testing generally is not performed in patients with uncomplicated AMI. However, if ischemia recurs after the first 24 hours, at any time before discharge, and if the patient is a suitable candidate for revascularization, consideration is given to proceeding with early cardiac catheterization and coronary arteriography to define the coronary anatomy and assess left ventricular function. Following AMI, symptoms secondary to left ventricular dysfunction are treated medically unless accompanied by evidence of reversible ischemia (angina, electrocardiographic changes, and/or reversible thallium-201 defects on imaging following an exercise stress test).

Before hospital discharge, patients without evidence of overt pump failure or ischemia and whose overall medical condition permits (e.g., excluding the very elderly or those with serious associated systemic diseases) undergo noninvasive testing. For most patients this means limited exercise stress (treadmill or bicycle) electrocardiography combined with thallium imaging for those with marked resting ECG abnormalities, or radionuclide ventriculography for those in whom an assessment of left ventricular function has not been obtained already (by echocardiography, for example).

Patients at high risk of recurrent MI or death should have cardiac catheterization and coronary arteriography. This includes patients with angina induced at a low level of exercise, particularly if associated with marked ECG changes (ST depressions >0.2 mV or serious electrical instability). Others in this category are those with a large reversible defect on thallium-201 imaging and those with an exercise-induced fall in left ventricular ejection fraction (more than 5 to 10 per cent)

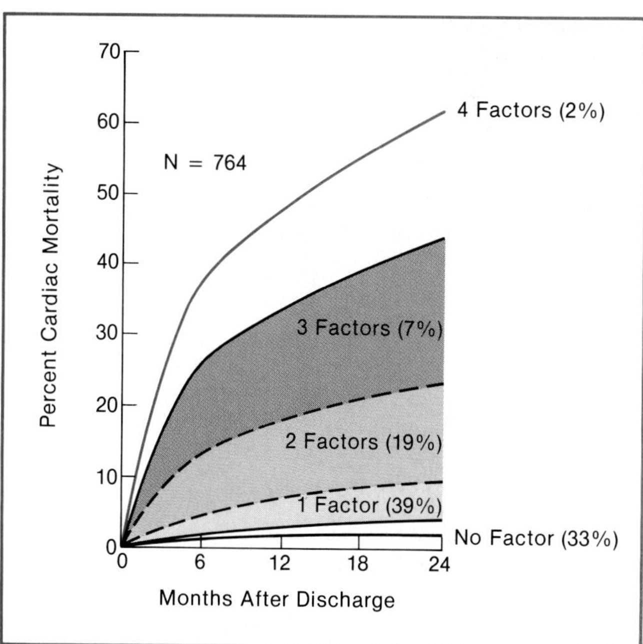

FIGURE 39–41. Mortality curves and zones of risk, according to number of risk factors. Individual risk factors included New York Heart Association functional classes II through IV (not class I) before admission, pulmonary rales, occurrence of 10 or more ventricular ectopic depolarizations per hour, and a radionuclide ejection fraction below 0.40. The variation of risk within each zone reflects the spectrum of relative risk for individual factors as well as the range of multiplicative risks for combinations of two and three factors. The numbers in the parentheses denote the percentage of the population with the specified number of factors. (Reprinted by permission from The Multicenter Post-infarction Research Group: Risk stratification and survival after myocardial infarction. N. Engl. J. Med. *309*:331, 1983.)

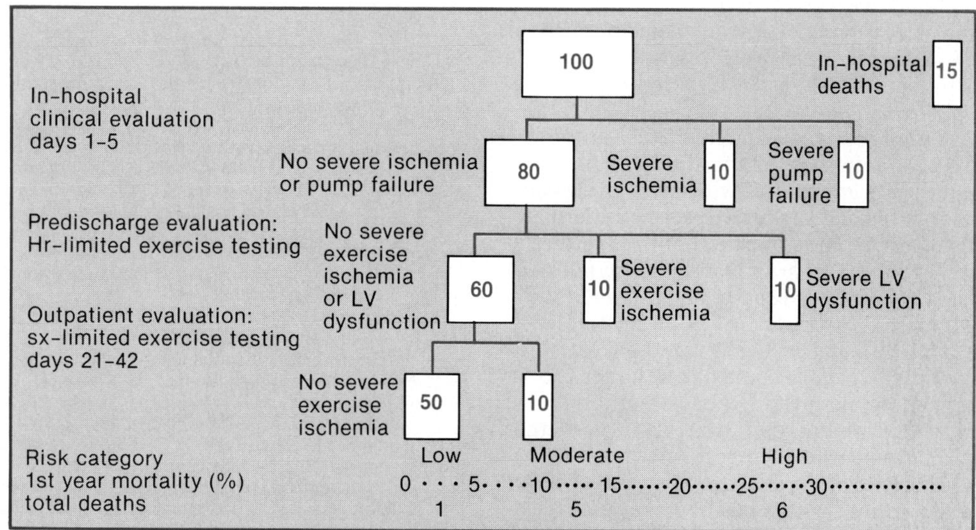

FIGURE 39–42. Prognostic stratification after acute myocardial infarction. The size of each patient subset (numbers in boxes) in the algorithm is approximate and will vary according to the patient population. Stratification of patients into the three main risk categories (low, moderate, and high) is based on the extent of myocardial ischemia (MI) and left ventricular (LV) dysfunction. A variety of clinical observations and tests may be used to detect these abnormalities at various times after acute myocardial infarction. Hr = heart rate, LV = left ventricle, SX = symptom. (Reprinted by permission from DeBusk, R. F., et al.: Identification and treatment of low-risk patients after acute myocardial infarction and coronary-artery bypass graft surgery. N. Engl. J. Med. *314*:161, 1986.)

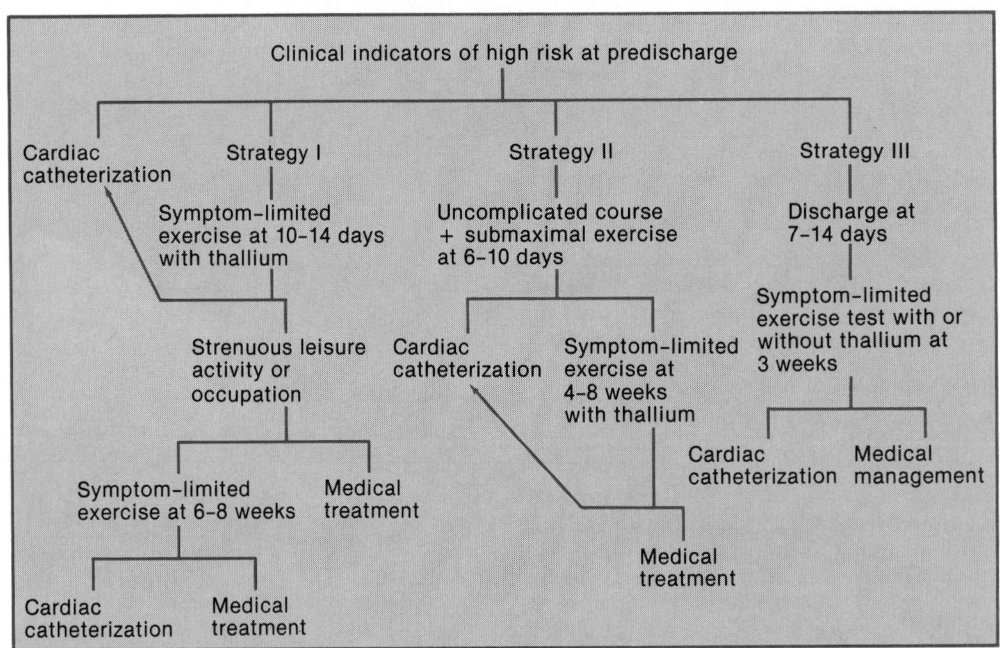

FIGURE 39-43. Strategies for predischarge or early postdischarge exercise evaluation. (From: A report of the American College of Cardiology/American Heart Association Task Force on Assessment, Diagnostic and Therapeutic Cardiovascular Procedures [Subcommittee to Develop Guidelines for the Early Management of Patients with Myocardial Infarction]: Guidelines for the early management of patients with acute myocardial infarction. Reprinted with permission of the American College of Cardiology. J. Am. Coll. Cardiol. *16*:249, 1990.)

on radionuclide ventriculography. If exercise testing is negative or only mildly positive, the patient may be discharged.

The predischarge exercise test is useful not only for the detection of ischemia, arrhythmias, or symptoms of left ventricular dysfunction, but it also serves the patient and physician as a useful guide in developing activity recommendations and limitations for the early post-MI period. Patients with ventricular ectopy during hospitalization and those with severe left ventricular dysfunction should generally undergo ambulatory electrocardiographic monitoring before discharge as well. If symptomatic ventricular arrhythmias are detected, we recommend treatment with antiarrhythmic agents, recognizing that the value of this approach has not been established definitively. If high-grade ventricular ectopy occurs without symptoms, invasive electrophysiology evaluation may be indicated (p. 1351).

Four to six weeks after hospital discharge, further noninvasive testing, including maximal (symptom-limited) exercise stress testing, is appropriate for patients who are suitable candidates for revascularization (and have not already undergone such therapy). This would include those patients not already selected for invasive work-up by prior testing, those not suffering from associated debilitating diseases and those not very elderly—in other words, all patients for whom the results of noninvasive testing might lead to a change in the treatment program and for whom that change could affect the prognosis favorably. Catheterization and arteriography should be performed in patients whose noninvasive work-up suggests the presence of remaining jeopardized myocardium following AMI.[1081,1082a] Proceeding with an invasive work-up is therefore a consideration in any patient with a positive exercise stress test in the post-MI period. However, angiography is most strongly indicated in patients who have an exercise-induced fall in blood pressure, signs or symptoms of ischemia at a low workload, more than 0.2 mV of ST-segment depression on exercise electrocardiography, large (or multiple) reversible defects on thallium-201 imaging (or lung accumulation of thallium), or a marked fall in left ventricular ejection fraction with exercise radionuclide ventriculography.

REFERENCES

1. American Heart Association: 1990 Heart Facts. Dallas, American Heart Association National Center, p. 1.
2. National Center for Health Statistics. Utilization of short stay hospitals, United States, 1987. Vital Health Stat. *31*:197, 1987.
3. The TIMI Study Group: Comparison of invasive and conservative strategies after treatment with intravenous tissue plasminogen activator in acute myocardial infarction. Results of the Thrombolysis in Myocardial Infarction (TIMI) Phase II Trial. N. Engl. J. Med. *320*:618, 1989.
4. Califf, R. M., Topol, E. J., George, B. S., et al.: One-year outcome after therapy with tissue plasminogen activator: Report from the Thrombolysis and Angioplasty in Myocardial Infarction trial. Am. Heart J. *119*:777, 1990.
5. Weinstein, M. C., and Stason, W. B.: Cost-effectiveness of interventions to prevent or treat coronary heart disease. Annu. Rev. Public Health *6*:41, 1985.
6. Wittels, E. H., Hay, J. W., and Gotto, A. M.: Medical costs of coronary artery disease in the United States. Am. J. Cardiol. *65*:432, 1990.
7. Sawitz, E., Showstack, J. A., Chow, J., et al.: The use of in-hospital physician services for acute myocardial infarction. Changes in volume and complexity over time. JAMA *259*:2419, 1988.
8. Pell, S., and Fayerweather, W. E.: Trends in the incidence of myocardial infarction and in associated mortality and morbidity in a large employed population, 1957–1983. N. Eng. J. Med. *312*:1005, 1985.
9. Pryor, D. B., Harrell, F. E. Jr., Lee, et al.: An improving prognosis over time in medically treated patients with coronary artery disease. Am. J. Cardiol. *52*:444, 1983.
10. Elveback, L. R., and Connolly, D. C.: Coronary heart disease in residents of Rochester, Minnesota. V. Prognosis of patients with coronary heart disease based on initial manifestation. Mayo Clin. Proc. *60*:305, 1985.
11. Gomez-Martin, O., Folsom, A. R., Kottke, T. E., et al.: Improvement in long-term survival among patients hospitalized with acute myocardial infarction, 1970 to 1980. N. Engl. J. Med. *316*:1353, 1987.
12. Goldman, L., and Cook, E. F.: The decline in ischemic heart disease mortality rates. An analysis of the comparative effects of medical interventions and changes in lifestyle. Ann. Intern. Med. *101*:825, 1984.
13. Beaglehole, R.: Medical management and the decline in mortality from coronary heart disease. Br. Med. J. *292*:33, 1986.
14. Kuller, L. H., Traven, N. D., Rutan, G. H., et al.: Marked decline of coronary heart disease mortality in 35 44-year-old white men in Allegheny County, Pennsylvania. Circulation *80*:261, 1989.
15. Ong, L., Green, S., Reiser, P., and Morrison, J.: Early prediction of mortality in patients with acute myocardial infarction: A prospective study of clinical and radionuclide risk factors. Am. J. Cardiol. *57*:33, 1986.
16. Yusuf, S., Wittes, J., and Friedman, L.: Overview of results of randomized clinical trials in heart disease. 1. Treatments following myocardial infarction. JAMA *260*:2088, 1988.

17. Rude, R. E., Muller, J. E., and Braunwald, E.: Efforts to limit the size of myocardial infarcts. Ann. Intern. Med. *95*:736, 1981.
18. Lange, L. G., and Sobel, B. E.: Pharmacological salvage of myocardium. Annu. Rev. Pharmacol. Toxicol. *22*:115, 1982.
19. Sobel, B.: Coronary thrombolysis and the new biology. J. Am. Coll. Cardiol. *14*:850, 1989.
20. Califf, R. M., and Ohman, E. M.: Thrombolytic therapy: Overview of clinical trials. Coronary Artery Disease *1*:23, 1990.

PATHOLOGY

21. Braunwald, E.: The aggressive treatment of acute myocardial infarction. Circulation *71*:1087, 1985.
21a. Freifeld, A. G., Schuster, E. H., and Bulkley, B. H.: Nontransmural versus transmural myocardial infarction. Am. J. Med. *75*:423, 1983.
22. DeWood, M. A., Stifter, W. F., Simpson, C. S., et al.: Coronary arteriographic findings soon after non-Q wave myocardial infarction. N. Engl. J. Med. *315*:417, 1986.
23. Miller, R. D., Burchell, H. B., and Edwards, J. E.: Myocardial infarction with and without acute coronary occlusion: A pathologic study. Arch. Intern. Med. *88*:597, 1951.
24. Ambrose, J. A., Tannenbaum, M. A., Alexopoulos, D., et al.: Angiographic progression of coronary artery disease and the development of myocardial infarction. J. Am. Coll. Cardiol. *12*:56, 1988.
25. Haupt, H. M., Hutchins, G. M., and Moore, G. W.: Right ventricular infarction: Role of the moderator band artery in determining infarct size. Circulation *67*:1268, 1983.
26. Shah, P. K., Maddahi, J., Berman, D. S., et al.: Scintigraphically detected predominant right ventricular dysfunction in acute myocardial infarction: Clinical and hemodynamic correlates and implications for therapy and prognosis. J. Am. Coll. Cardiol. *6*:1264, 1985.
27. Forman, M. B., Wilson, B. H., Sheller, J. R., et al.: Right ventricular hypertrophy is an important determinant of right ventricular infarction complicating acute inferior left ventricular infarction. J. Am. Coll. Cardiol. *10*:1180, 1987.
28. Kopelman, H. A., Forman, M. B., Wilson, B. H., et al.: Right ventricular myocardial infarction in patients with chronic lung disease: possible role of right ventricular hypertrophy. J. Am. Coll. Cardiol. *5*:1302, 1985.
29. Lowe, T. E., and Wartman, W. B.: Myocardial infarction. Br. Heart J. *6*:115, 1944.
30. Bloor, C. M.: Cardiac Pathology. Philadelphia, J. B. Lippincott Co., 1978, p. 176.
31. Mallory, G. K., White, P. D., and Salcedo-Salger, J.: The speed of healing of myocardial infarction: A study of the pathological anatomy in seventy-two cases. Am. Heart J. *18*:647, 1939.
32. Buja, L. M., and Willerson, J. T.: Clinicopathologic correlates of acute ischemic heart disease syndromes. Am. J. Cardiol. *47*:343, 1981.
33. Schlesinger, M. J., and Reiner, L.: Focal myocytolysis of the heart. Am. J. Pathol. *31*:443, 1955.
34. Bouchardy, B., and Majno, G.: Histopathology of early myocardial infarcts. Am. J. Physiol. *74*:301, 1974.
35. Kloner, R. A., Ganote, C. E., Whalen, D. A., Jr., and Jennings, R. B.: Effect of a transient period of ischemia on myocardial cells: Fine structure during the first few minutes of reflow. Am. J. Pathol. *74*:399, 1974.
36. Willerson, J. T., Hillis, L. D., and Buja, L. M.: Ischemic Heart Disease. New York, Raven Press, 1982, 374 pp.
37. Kloner, R. A., Rude, R. E., Carlson, N., et al.: Ultrastructural evidence of microvascular damage and myocardial cell injury after coronary artery occlusion: Which comes first? Circulation *62*:945, 1980.
38. Kloner, R. A., DeBoer, L. W. V., Carlson, N., and Braunwald, E.: The effect of verapamil on myocardial ultrastructure during and following release of coronary artery occlusion. Exp. Mol. Pathol. *36*:277, 1982.
39. Caulfield, J., and Klionsky, B.: Myocardial ischemia and early infarction. An electron microscopic study. Am. J. Pathol. *35*:489, 1959.
40. Jennings, R. B., and Ganote, C. E.: Structural change in myocardium during acute ischemia. Circ. Res. *35*(Suppl. 3):156, 1974.
41. Kloner, R. A., Fishbein, M. C., Hare, C. M., and Maroko, P. R.: Early ischemic ultrastructural and histochemical alterations in the myocardium of the rat following coronary artery occlusion. Exp. Mol. Pathol. *30*:129, 1979.
42. Baroldi, G.: Different types of myocardial necrosis in coronary heart disease: A pathophysiologic review of their functional significance. Am. Heart J. *89*:742, 1975.
43. Hutchins, G. M., and Bulkley, B. H.: Correlation of myocardial contraction band necrosis and vascular patency: A study of coronary artery bypass graft anastomoses at branch points. Lab. Invest. *36*:642, 1977.
44. Kloner, R. A., Ellis, S. G., Lange, R., and Braunwald, E.: Studies of experimental coronary artery reperfusion: effects on infarct size, myocardial function, biochemistry, ultrastructure and microvascular damage. Circulation *68*(Suppl I):8, 1983.
45. Matsuda, M., Fujiwara, J., Onodera, T., et al.: Quantitative analysis of infarct size, contraction band necrosis, and coagulation necrosis in human autopsied hearts with acute myocardial infarction after treatment with selective intracoronary thrombolysis. Circulation *76*:981, 1987.
46. Herrick, J. B.: Clinical features of sudden obstruction of the coronary arteries. JAMA *59*:2015, 1912.
47. Blumgart, H. L., Schlesinger, M. J., and Davis, D.: Studies on the relation of the clinical manifestations of angina pectoris, coronary thrombosis, and myocardial infarction to the pathologic findings with particular reference to the significance of the collateral circulation. Am. Heart J. *19*:1, 1940.
48. Friedberg, C. K., and Horn, H.: Acute myocardial infarction not due to coronary artery occlusion. JAMA *112*:1675, 1939.
49. Roberts, W. C., Potkin, B. N., Solus, D. E., and Reddy, S. G.: Mode of death, frequency of healed and acute myocardial infarction, number of major epicardial coronary arteries severely narrowed by atherosclerotic plaque, and heart weight in fatal atherosclerotic coronary artery disease: analysis of 889 patients studied at necropsy. J. Am. Coll. Cardiol. *15*:196, 1990.
50. Betriu, A., Castaner, A., Sanz, G. A., et al.: Angiographic finding 1 month after myocardial infarction: A prospective study of 259 survivors. Circulation *65*:1099, 1982.
51. Ellis, S., Alderman E., Cain, K., et al.: Prediction of risk of anterior myocardial infarction by lesion severity and measurement method of stenoses in the left anterior descending coronary distribution: a CASS registry study. J. Am. Coll. Cardiol. *11*:908, 1988.
52. Ellis, S., Alderman E. L., Cain, K., et al.: Morphology of left anterior descending coronary territory lesions as a predictor of anterior myocardial infarction: A CASS registry study. J. Am. Coll. Cardiol. *13*:1481, 1989.
53. Little, W. C., Constantinescu, M., Applegate, R. J., et al.: Can coronary angiography predict the site of a subsequent myocardial infarction in patients with mild-to-moderate coronary artery disease? Circulation *78*:1157, 1988.
54. Rackley, C. E., Russell, R. O., Jr., Mantle, J. A., et al.: Right ventricular infarction and function. Am. Heart J. *101*:215, 1981.
55. deFeyter, P. J., van den Brand, M., Serruys, P. W., and Wijns, W.: Early angiography after myocardial infarction: What have we learned? Am. Heart J. *109*:194, 1985.
56. DeWood, M. A., Spores, J., and Notske, R., Mouser, L. T., Burroughs, R., Golden, M. S., and Lang, H. T.: Prevalence of total coronary occlusion during the early hours of transmural myocardial infarction. N. Engl. J. Med. *303*:897, 1980.
57. Ganz, W., Buchbinder, N., Marcus, H., et al.: Intracoronary thrombolysis in evolving myocardial infarction. Am. Heart J. *101*:4, 1981.
58. Ong, L., Reiser, P., Coromilas, J., et al.: Left ventricular function and rapid release of creatine kinase MB in acute myocardial infarction: Evidence for spontaneous reperfusion. N. Engl. J. Med. *309*:1, 1983.
59. DeWood, M. A., Notske, R. N., Simpson, C. S., et al.: Prevalence and significance of spontaneous thrombolysis in transmural myocardial infarction. Eur. Heart J. *6*:33, 1985.
59a. Pichard, A. D., Ziff, C., Rentrop, P., et al.: Angiographic study of infarct-related coronary artery in the chronic stage of acute myocardial infarction. Am. Heart J. *106*:687, 1983.
60. Willerson, J. T., Campbell, W. B., Winniford, M. D., et al.: Conversion from chronic to acute coronary artery disease: Speculation regarding mechanisms. Am. J. Cardiol. *54*:1349, 1984.
61. Alpert, J. S.: Coronary vasomotion, coronary thrombosis, myocardial infarction and the camel's back. J. Am. Coll. Cardiol. *5*:617, 1985.
62. Muller, J. E., Tofler, G. H., and Stone, P. H.: Circadian variation and triggers of onset of acute cardiovascular disease. Circulation *79*:733, 1989.
63. Kragel, A. H., Reddy, S. G., Wittes, J. T., and Roberts, W. C.: Morphometric analysis of the composition of atherosclerotic plaques in the four major epicardial coronary arteries in acute myocardial infarction and in sudden coronary death. Circulation *80*:1747, 1989.
64. Roberts, W. C.: Qualitative and quantitative comparison of amounts of narrowing by atherosclerotic plaques in the major epicardial coronary arteries at necropsy in sudden coronary death, transmural acute myocardial infarction, transmural healed myocardial infarction and unstable angina pectoris. Am. J. Cardiol. *64*:324, 1989.
65. Levin, D. C., and Fallon, J. T.: Significance of the angiographic morphology of localized coronary stenoses: Histopathologic correlations. Circulation *66*:316, 1982.
66. Ridolfi, R. L., and Hutchins, G. M.: Relationship between coronary artery lesions and myocardial infarcts: Ulceration of atheroslcerotic plaques precipitating coronary thrombosis. Am. Heart J. *93*:468, 1977.
67. Falk, E.: Plaque rupture with severe pre-existing stenosis precipitating thrombosis: Characteristics of coronary atherosclerotic plaque underlying fatal occlusion thrombi. Br. Heart J. *50*:127, 1983.
68. Davies, M. J., and Thomas, A. C.: Plaque fissuring—the cause of acute myocardial infarction, sudden ischemic death, and crescendo angina. Br. Heart J. *53*:363, 1985.
69. Falk, E.: Morphologic features of unstable atherothrombotic plaques underlying acute coronary syndrome. Am. J. Cardiol. *63*:114E, 1989.
70. Wilson, R. F., Holida, M. D., and White, C. W.: Quantitative angiographic morphology of coronary stenoses leading to myocardial infarction or unstable angina. Circulation *73*:286, 1986.
71. Mandelkorn, J. B., Wolf, N. M., Singh, S., et al.: Intracoronary thrombus in nontransmural myocardial infarction and in unstable angina pectoris. Am. J. Cardiol. *52*:1, 1983.
72. Davies, M. J., and Thomas, A.: Thrombosis and acute coronary-artery lesions in sudden cardiac ischemic death. N. Engl. J. Med. *310*:1137, 1984.
73. Fox, K. A. A., Bergmann, S. R., Mathias, C. J., et al.: Scintigraphic detection of coronary artery thrombi in patients with acute myocardial infarction. J. Am. Coll. Cardiol. *4*:975, 1984.
74. Trip, M. D., Cats, V. M., Van Capelle, F. J. L., and Vreenken, J.: Platelet hyperactivity and prognosis in survivors of myocardial infarction. N. Engl. J. Med. *322*:1549, 1990.

195. Vetter, N. J., Adams, W., Strange, R. C., and Oliver, M. F.: Initial metabolic and hormonal response to acute myocardial infarction. Lancet *1*:284, 1974.
196. Bertel, O., Buhler, F. R., Baitsch, G., et al.: Plasma adrenaline and noradrenaline in patients with acute myocardial infarction. Relationship to ventricular arrhythmias in varying severity. Chest *82*:64, 1982.
197. Taylor, S. H., Majid, P. A., Saxton, C., and Sharma, B.: Insulin secretion in heart failure. Am. Heart J. *83*:281, 1972.
198. Ceremuzynski, L.: Hormonal and metabolic reactions evoked by acute myocardial infarction. Circ. Res. *48*:767, 1981.
199. Bellodi, G., Manicardi, V., Malavasi, V., et al.: Hyperglycemia and prognosis of acute myocardial infarction in patients without diabetes mellitus. Am. J. Cardiol. *64*:885, 1989.
200. Jefferson, L. S., Rannels, D. E., Munger, B. L., and Morgan, H. E.: Insulin in the regulation of protein turnover in heart and skeletal muscle. Fed. Proc. *33*:1098, 1974.
201. Opie, L. H.: Metabolism of free fatty acids, glucose, and catecholamines in acute myocardial infarction: Relation to myocardial ischemia and infarct size. Am. J. Cardiol. *36*:938, 1975.
201a. Rouleau, J. L., Dagerais, G-R., Packer, M., et al.: Selective activation of neurohormonal systems in post-infarction left ventricular dysfunction. J. Am. Coll. Cardiol. *17*:21A, 1991.
202. Karlsberg, R. P., Cryer, P. E. and Roberts, R.: Serial plasma catecholamine response early in the course of clinical acute myocardial infarction: relationship to infarct extent and mortality. Am. Heart J. *102*:24, 1981.
203. Wiersinga, W. M., Lie, K. I., and Touber, J. L.: Thyroid hormones in acute myocardial infarction. Clin. Endocrinol. *14*:367, 1981.
204. Kahana, L., Keidar, S., Sheinfeld, M., and Palant, A.: Endogenous cortisol and thyroid hormone levels in patients with acute myocardial infarction. Clin. Endocrinol. *19*:131, 1983.
205. Steele, P., Rainwater, J., and Vogel, R.: Abnormal platelet survival time in men with myocardial infarction and normal coronary arteriogram. Am. J. Cardiol. *41*:60, 1978.
206. Dorn, G. W., II, Liel, N., Trask, J. L., et al.: Increased platelet thromboxane A_2/prostaglandin H_2 receptors in patients with acute myocardial infarction. Circulation *81*:212, 1990.
207. Laursen, B., and Gormsen, J.: Spontaneous fibrinolysis demonstrated by immunological technique. Thromb. Diath. Haemorrh. *17*:42, 1967.
208. Handin, R. I., McDonough, M., and Lesch, M.: Elevation of platelet factor 4 in acute myocardial infarction: Measurement by radioimmunoassay. J. Lab. Clin. Med. *91*:340, 1978.
209. Smitherman, T. C., Milam, M., Woo, J., et al.: Elevated beta thromboglobulin in peripheral venous blood of patients with acute myocardial ischemia: Direct evidence for enhanced platelet reactivity in vivo. Am. J. Cardiol. *48*:395, 1981.
210. Eisenberg, P., Sherman, L. A., Schechtman, K., et al.: Fibrinopeptide A: a marker for acute coronary thrombosis. Circulation *71*:912, 1985.
211. Rapold, H. J., Kuemmerli, H., Weiss, M., et al.: Monitoring of fibrin generation during thrombolytic therapy of acute myocardial infarction with recombinant tissue-type plasminogen activator. Circulation *79*:980, 1989.
212. Eisenberg, P. R., Sherman, L., Rich, M., et al.: Importance of continued activation of thrombin reflected by fibrinopeptide A to the efficacy of thrombolysis. J. Am. Coll. Cardiol. *7*:1255, 1986.
213. Eisenberg, P. R., Miletich, J. E., Sobel, B. E., and Jaffe, A. S.: Differential effects of activation of prothrombin by streptokinase compared with urokinase and tissue-type plasminogen activator (t-PA). Thromb. Res. *50*:707, 1988.
214. Cowan, D. H.: Acquired disorders of platelet function. *In* Colman, R. W., Hirsch, J., Marker, V. J., and Salzman, E. W. (eds.): Hemostasis and Thrombosis: Basic Principles and Clinical Practice. Philadelphia, J. B. Lippincott Co., 1982, pp. 516–524.
215. Marcus, A. J., Safier, L. B., Ullman, H. L., et al.: Inhibition of platelet function in thrombosis. Circulation *72*:698, 1985.
216. Fantone, J. C., and Ward, P. A.: Role of oxygen-derived free radicals and metabolites in leukocyte-dependent inflammatory reactions. Am. J. Physiol. *107*:397, 1982.
217. Engler, R. L., Dahlgren, M. D., Morris, D. D., et al.: Role of leukocytes in response to acute myocardial ischemia and reflow in dogs. Am. J. Physiol. *251*:H314, 1986.
217a. Acute Myocardial Infarction. *In* Fowler, N. O.: Diagnosis of Heart Disease. New York, Springer-Verlag, 1991, pp. 207–238.
218. Hershberg, P. I., Wells, R. E., and McGandy, R. B.: Hematocrit and prognosis in patients with acute myocardial infarction. JAMA *219*:855, 1972.
219. Kok, F. J., Hofman, A., Witteman, J.C.M., et al.: Decreased selenium levels in acute myocardial infarction. JAMA *261*:1161, 1989.
220. Kok, F. J., Schrijver, J., Hofman, A., et al.: Low vitamin B6 status in patients with acute myocardial infarction. Am. J. Cardiol. *63*:513, 1989.
221. Tomoda, H.: Atrial natriuretic peptide in acute myocardial infarction. Am. J. Cardiol. *62*:1122, 1988.
222. Robalino, B. D., Petrella, R. W., Jubran, F. Y., et al.: Atrial natriuretic factor in patients with right ventricular infarction. J. Am. Coll. Cardiol. *15*:546, 1990.

CLINICAL FEATURES

223. Phipps, C.: Contributory causes of coronary thrombosis. JAMA *106*:761, 1936.
224. Tofler, G. H., Stone, P. H., Maclure, M., et al.: Analysis of possible triggers of acute myocardial infarction (The MILIS Study). Am. J. Cardiol. *66*:22, 1990.
225. Smith, C., Sauls, H. C., and Ballew, J.: Coronary occlusion: A clinical study of 100 patients. Ann. Intern. Med. *17*:681, 1942.
226. French, A. J., and Dock, W.: Fatal coronary arteriosclerosis in young soldiers. JAMA *124*:1233, 1944.
227. Fitzhugh, G., and Hamilton, B. E.: Coronary occlusion and fatal angina pectoris: Study of the immediate causes and their prevention. JAMA *100*:475, 1933.
228. Matsuda, M., Matsuda, Y., Ogawa, H., et al.: Angina pectoris before and during acute myocardial infarction: Relation to degree of physical activity. Am. J. Cardiol. *55*:1255, 1985.
229. Knapp, R. B., Topkins, M. J., and Artusio, J. F., Jr.: The cerebrovascular accident and coronary occlusion in anesthesia. JAMA *182*:332, 1962.
230. Levine, H. D.: Acute myocardial infarction following wasp sting. Report of two cases and critical survey of the literature. Am. Heart J. *91*:365, 1976.
231. Maseri, A., L'Abbate, A., Baroldi, G., et al.: Coronary vasospasm as a possible cause of myocardial infarction. A conclusion derived from the study of "preinfarction" angina. N. Engl. J. Med. *299*:1271, 1978.
232. Jenkins, C. D.: Recent evidence supporting psychologic and social risk factors for coronary disease. N. Engl. J. Med. *294*:987, 1976.
233. Rahe, R. H., Romo, M., Bennett, L., and Siltanen, P.: Recent life changes, myocardial infarction, and abrupt coronary death. Arch. Intern. Med. *133*:221, 1974.
234. Norris, N. M.: Myocardial Infarction. New York, Churchill Livingstone, 1982, 322 pp.
235. Muller, J. E., Stone, P. H., Turi, Z. G., et al.: Circadian variation in the frequency of onset of acute myocardial infarction. N. Engl. J. Med. *313*:1315, 1985.
236. Mitler, M. M., and Kripke, D. F.: Circadian variation in myocardial infarction. N. Engl. J. Med. *314*:1187, 1986.
237. Goldberg, R. J., Brady, P., Muller, J. E., et al.: Time of onset of symptoms of acute myocardial infarction. Am. J. Cardiol. *66*:140, 1990.
238. Myocardial infarction community registers: Results of a WHO international collaborative study coordinated by the regional office for Europe. In: Public Health In Europe, No. 5. Copenhagen: Regional Office for Europe (World Health Organization), 1976, pp. 1–230.
239. Muller, J. E., Stone, P. H., Turi, Z. G., et al.: Circadian variation in the frequency of sudden cardiac death. Circulation *75*:131, 1987.
240. Tsementzis, S. A., Gill, J. S., Hitchcock, E. R., et al.: Diurnal variation of and activity during the onset of stroke. Neurology *17*:901, 1985.
241. Quyyumi, A. A., Mockus, L., Wright, C., and Fox, K. M.: Morphology of ambulatory ST segment changes in patients with varying severity of coronary artery disease: investigation of the frequency of nocturnal ischemia and coronary spasm. Br. Heart J. *53*:186, 1985.
242. Rocco, M. B., Barry, J., Campbell, S., et al.: Circadian variation of transient myocardial ischemia in patients with coronary artery disease. Circulation *75*:395, 1987.
243. Willich, S. N., Linderer, T., Wegscheider, K., et al.: Increasing morning incidence of myocardial infarction in the ISAM study: absence with prior β-adrenergic blockade. Circulation *80*:853, 1989.
244. Ridker, P. M., Manson, J. E., Buring, J. E., et al.: Circadian variation of acute myocardial infarction and the effect of low-dose aspirin in a randomized trial of physicians. Circulation *82*:897, 1990.
245. Hjalmarson, A., Gilpin, E. A., Nicod, P., et al.: Differing circadian patterns of symptom onset in subgroups of patients with acute myocardial infarction. Circulation *80*:267, 1989.
246. Alonzo, A. M., Simon, A. B., and Feinleib, M.: Prodromata of myocardial infarction and sudden death. Circulation *52*:1056, 1975.
247. Muller, D. W. M., Topol, E. J., Califf, R. M., et al.: Relationship between antecedent angina pectoris and short-term prognosis after thrombolytic therapy for acute myocardial infarction. Am. Heart J. *119*:224, 1990.
248. Harper, R. W., Kennedy, G., DeSanctis, R. W., and Hutter, A. M., Jr.: The incidence and pattern of angina prior to acute myocardial infarction: a study of 577 cases. Am. Heart J. *97*:178, 1979.
249. Rogers, D. E.: Some observations on having a coronary. The Pharos of Alpha Omega Alpha *49*:12, 1986.
250. Baker, P.: Suspected myocardial infarction: Early diagnostic value of analgesic requirements. Br. Med. J. *290*:27, 1985.
251. Malliani, A., and Lombardi, F.: Consideration of the fundamental mechanisms eliciting cardiac pain. Am. Heart J. *103*:575, 1982.
252. Malliani, A.: The elusive link between transient myocardial ischemia and pain. Circulation *73*:201, 1986.
253. Ganz, W., Geft, I., Shah, P. K., et al.: Intravenous streptokinase in evolving acute myocardial infarction. Am. J. Cardiol. *53*:1209, 1984.
254. Ingram, D. A., Fulton, R. A., Portal, R. W., and Aber, C. P.: Vomiting as a diagnostic aid in acute ischemic cardiac pain. Br. Med. J. *281*:636, 1980.
255. Sleight, P.: Cardiac vomiting. Br. Heart J. *46*:5, 1981.
256. Uretsky, B. F., Farquhar, D. S., Borezin, A., and Hood, W. B.: Symptomatic myocardial infarction without chest pain: Prevalence and clinical course. Am. J. Cardiol. *40*:498, 1977.
257. Appels, A., Hoppener, P., and Mulder, P.: A questionnaire to assess premonitory symptoms of myocardial infarction. Int. J. Cardiol. *17*:15, 1987.
258. Margolis, J. R., Kannel, W. B., Feinleib, M., et al.: Clinical features of unrecognized myocardial infarction: Silent and symptomatic. Eighteen year follow-up: The Framingham Study. Am. J. Cardiol. *32*:1, 1973.

259. Yano, K., and MacLean, C. J.: The incidence and prognosis of unrecognized myocardial infarction in the Honolulu, Hawaii, Heart Program. Arch. Intern Med. *149*:1528, 1989.
260. Bean, W. B.: Masquerade of myocardial infarction. Lancet *1*:1044, 1977.
261. Chadda, K. D., Lichstein, E., Gupta, P. K., and Choy, R.: Bradycardia-hypotension syndrome in acute myocardial infarction. Reappraisal of the overdrive effects of atropine. Am. J. Med. *59*:158, 1975.
262. Webb, S. W., Adgey, A. A., and Pantridge, J. F.: Autonomic disturbance at onset of acute myocardial infarction. Br. Med. J. *818*:89, 1982.
263. The International Study Group: In-hospital mortality and clinical course of 20,891 patients with suspected acute myocardial infarction randomised between alteplase and streptokinase with or without heparin. Lancet *2*:71, 1990.
264. Gadsboll, N., Hoilund-Carlsen, P. F., Nielsen, G. G., et al.: Symptoms and signs of heart failure in patients with myocardial infarction: Reproducibility and relationship to chest x-ray, radionuclide ventriculography and right heart catheterization. Eur. Heart J. *10*:1017, 1989.
265. Riley, C. P., Russell, R. O., Jr., and Rackley, C. E.: Left ventricular gallop sound and acute myocardial infarction. Am. Heart J. *86*:598, 1973.
266. Case Records of the Massachusetts General Hospital (Case 49-1986). N. Engl. J. Med. *315*:1533, 1986.
267. Krainin, F. M., Flessas, A. P., and Spodick, D. H.: Infarction-associated pericarditis. Rarity of diagnostic electrocardiogram. N. Engl. J. Med. *311*:1211, 1984.
268. Galve, E., Garcia-Del-Castillo, H., Evangelista, A., et al.: Pericardial effusion in the course of myocardial infarction: Incidence, natural history, and clinical relevance. Circulation *73*:294, 1986.
269. Dressler, W.: The post-myocardial infarction syndrome: A report of 44 cases. Arch Intern. Med. *103*:28, 1959.
270. Lichstein, E., Arsura, E., Hollander, G., Greengart, A., and Sanders, M.: Current incidence of postmyocardial infarction (Dressler's) syndrome. Am. J. Cardiol. *50*:1269, 1982.
271. Thompson, P. L., and Robinson, J. S.: Stroke after acute myocardial infarction: Relation to infarct size. Br. Med. J. *2*:457, 1978.
272. Sobel, B. E., and Shell, W. E.: Serum enzyme determinations in the diagnosis and assessment of myocardial infarction. Circulation *45*:471, 1972.
273. Lee, T. H., and Goldman, L.: Serum enzyme assays in the diagnosis of acute myocardial infarction. Ann. Intern. Med. *105*:221, 1986.
274. Shell, W. E., Kjekshus, J. K., and Sobel, B. E.: Quantitative assessment of the extent of myocardial infarction in the conscious dog by means of analysis of serial changes in serum creatine phosphokinase activity. J. Clin. Invest. *50*:2614, 1971.
275. Vasudevan, G., Mercer, D. W., and Varat, M. A.: Lactic dehydrogenase isoenzyme determination in the diagnosis of acute myocardial infarction. Circulation *57*:1055, 1978.
276. Weidner, N.: Laboratory diagnosis of acute myocardial infarct. Usefulness of determination of lactate dehydrogenase (LDH)-1 level and the ratio of LDH-1 to total LDH. Arch. Pathol. Lab. Med. *106*:375, 1982.
277. Fisher, M. L., Kelemen, M. H., Collins, D., et al.: Routine serum enzyme tests in the diagnosis of acute myocardial infarction. Arch. Intern. Med. *143*:1541, 1983.
278. Reis, G. J., Kaufman, H. W., Horowitz, G. L., and Pasternak, R. C.: Usefulness of lactate dehydrogenase and lactate dehydrogenase isoenzymes for diagnosis of acute myocardial infarction. Am. J. Cardiol. *61*:754, 1988.
279. Herlitz, J.: Time lapse from estimated onset of acute myocardial infarction to peak serum enzyme activity. Clin. Cardiol. *7*:433, 1984.
280. Ong, L., Reiser, P., Coromilas, J., et al.: Left ventricular function and rapid release of creatine kinase MB in acute myocardial infarction: Evidence for spontaneous reperfusion. N. Engl. J. Med. *309*:1, 1983.
281. Blanke, H., von Hardenberg, D., Cohen, M., et al.: Patterns of creatine kinase release during acute myocardial infarction after nonsurgical reperfusion: Comparison with conventional treatment and correlation with infarct size. J. Am. Coll. Cardiol. *3*:675, 1984.
282. Horie, M., Yasue, H., Omote, S., et al.: A new approach for the enzymatic estimation of infarct size: Serum peak creatine kinase and time to peak creatine kinase activity. Am. J. Cardiol. *57*:76, 1986.
283. Roberts, R., and Sobel, B. E.: Isoenzymes of creatine phosphokinase and diagnosis of myocardial infarction. Ann. Intern. Med. *79*:741, 1973.
284. Godfrey, N. F., Halter, D. G., Minna, D. A., et al.: Thoracic outlet syndrome mimicking angina pectoris with elevated creatine phosphokinase values. Chest *83*:461, 1983.
285. Tsung, S. H.: Several conditions causing elevation of serum CK-BB. Am. J. Clin. Pathol. *75*:711, 1981.
286. Apple, F. S., Rogers, M. A., Sherman, W. M., and Ivy, J. L.: Comparison of serum creatine kinase and creatine kinase MB activities post marathon race versus post myocardial infarction. Clin. Chim. Acta *138*:111, 1984.
287. Jaffe, A. S., Garfinkel, B. T., Ritter, C. S., and Sobel, B. E.: Plasma MB creatine kinase after vigorous exercise in professional athletes. Am. J. Cardiol. *53*:856, 1984.
288. Ingwall, J. S., Kramer, M. F., Fifer, M. A., et al.: The creatine kinase system in normal and diseased human myocardium. N. Engl. J. Med. *313*:1050, 1985.
289. Morelli, R. L., Carlson, D. J., Emilson, B., et al.: Serum creatine kinase MM isoenzyme sub-bands after acute myocardial infarction in man. Circulation *67*:1283, 1983.
290. Roberts, R.: Reperfusion and the plasma isoforms of creatine kinase isoenzymes: a clinical perspective. J. Am. Coll. Cardiol. *9*:464, 1987.
291. Puleo, P. R., Guadagno, P. A., Roberts, R., et al.: Early diagnosis of acute myocardial infarction based on assay for subforms of creatine-kinase-MB. Circulation *82*:759, 1990.
292. Puleo, P. R., Perryman, B., Bresser, M. A., et al.: Creatinine kinase isoform analysis in the detection and assessment of thrombolysis in man. Circulation *75*:1162, 1987.
293. Abendschein, D., Seacord, L. M., Nohara, R., et al.: Prompt detection of myocardial injury by assay of creatine kinase isoforms in initial plasma samples. Clin. Cardiol. *11*:661, 1988.
294. Nohara, R., Myears, D. W., Sobel, B. E., and Abendschein, D. R.: Optimal criteria for rapid detection of myocardial reperfusion by creatinine kinase MM isoforms in the presence of residual high-grade stenosis. J. Am. Coll. Cardiol. *14*:1067, 1989.
295. Roberts, R., Gowda, K. S., Ludbrook, P. A., and Sobel, B. E.: Specificity of elevated serum MB creatine phosphokinase activity in the diagnosis of acute myocardial infarction. Am. J. Cardiol. *36*:433, 1975.
296. Cooperating investigators from the MILIS study group: Electrocardiographic, enzymatic and scintigraphic criteria of acute myocardial infarction as determined from study of 726 patients (MILIS study). Am. J. Cardiol. *55*:1463, 1985.
297. Roberts, R., Sobel, B. E., and Parker, C. W.: Radioimmunoassay for creatine kinase isoenzymes. Science *194*:855, 1976.
298. Clyne, C. A., Medeiros, L. J., and Marton, K.: The prognostic significance of immunoradiometric CK-MB assay (IRMA) diagnosis of myocardial infarction in patients with low total CK and elevated MB isoenzymes. Am. Heart J. *118*:901, 1989.
299. McGrath, R. B., and Revtyak, G.: Secondary myocardial injuries. Crit. Care Med. *12*:1024, 1984.
300. Roberts, R., Sobel, B. E., and Ludbrook, P. A.: Determination of the origin of elevated plasma CPK after cardiac catheterization. Cathet. Cardiovasc. Diagn. *2*:239, 1976.
301. Klein, M. S., Coleman, R. E., Weldon, C. S., et al.: Concordance of electrocardiographic and scintigraphic criteria of myocardial injury after cardiac surgery. J. Thorac. Cardiovasc. Surg. *71*:934, 1976.
302. Smith, J. L., Ambos, D., Gold, H. K., et al.: Enzymatic estimation of myocardial infarct size when early creatinine kinase values are not available. Am. J. Cardiol. *51*:1294, 1983.
303. Hong, R. A., Licht, J. D., Wei, J. Y., et al.: Elevated CK-MB with normal total creatine kinase in suspected myocardial infarction: Associated clinical findings and early prognosis. Am. Heart J. *111*:1041, 1986.
304. Heyndrickx, G. R., Amano, J., Kenna, T., et al.: Creatine kinase release not associated with myocardial necrosis after short periods of coronary artery occlusion in conscious baboons. J. Am. Coll. Cardiol. *6*:1299, 1985.
305. Yusuf, S., Collins, R., Lin, L., et al.: Significance of elevated MB isoenzyme with normal creatine kinase in acute myocardial infarction. Am. J. Cardiol. *59*:245, 1987.
306. Grande, P., Hansen, B. F., Christiansen, C., and Naestoft, J.: Estimation of acute myocardial infarct size in man by serum CK-MB measurements. Circulation *65*:756, 1982.
307. Hori, M., Inoue, M., Fukui, S., et al.: Correlation of ejection fraction and infarct size estimated from the total CK released in patients with acute myocardial infarction. Br. Heart J. *41*:433, 1979.
308. Geltman, E. M., Ehsani, A. A., Campbell, M. K., et al.: The influence of location and extent of myocardial infarction on long-term ventricular dysrhythmia and mortality. Circulation *60*:805, 1979.
309. Tamaki, S., Murakami, T., Kadota, K., et al.: Effects of coronary artery reperfusion on relation between creatine kinase-MB release and infarct size estimated by myocardial emission tomography with thallium-201 in man. J. Am. Coll. Cardiol. *2*:1031, 1983.
310. Goldberger, E., Alesio, J., and Woll, F.: The significance of hyperglycemia in myocardial infarction. N.Y. State Med. J. *45*:391, 1945.
311. Tan, M. H., Wilmshurst, E. G., Gleason, R. E., and Soeldner, J. S.: Effect of posture on serum lipids. N. Engl. J. Med. *289*:416, 1973.
312. Gore, J. M., Goldberg, R. J., Matsumoto, A. S., et al.: Validity of serum total cholesterol level obtained within 24 hours of acute myocardial infarction. Am. J. Cardiol. *54*:722, 1984.
313. Ryder, R.E.J., Hayes, T. M., Mulligan, I. P., et al.: How soon after myocardial infarction should plasma lipid values be assessed? Br. Med. J. *289*:1651, 1984.
314. Ronnemaa, T., Viikari, J., Irjala, K., and Peltola, O.: Marked decrease in serum HDL cholesterol level during acute myocardial infarction. Acta Med. Scand. *207*:161, 1980.
315. Isakov, A., Shapira, I., Burke, M., and Almog, C.: Serum myoglobin levels in patients with ischemic myocardial insult. Arch. Intern. Med. *148*:1762, 1988.
316. Kagen, L., Scheidt, S., and Butt, A.: Serum myoglobin in myocardial infarction: The "staccato phenomenon." Is acute myocardial infarction in man an intermittent event? Am. J. Med. *62*:86, 1977.
317. Ellis, A. K., Little, T., Masud, A.R.Z., et al.: Early noninvasive detection of successful reperfusion in patients with acute myocardial infarction. Circulation *78*:1352, 1988.
318. Eastham, R. D., and Morgan, E. H.: Plasma-fibrinogen levels in coronary-artery disease. Lancet *2*:1196, 1963.
319. Savage, R. M., Wagner, G. S., Ideker, R. E., et al.: Correlation of postmortem anatomic findings with electrocardiographic changes in patients with myocardial infarction. Circulation *55*:279, 1977.
320. Cooksey, J. D., Dunn, M., and Massie, E.: Clinical Vectorcardiography and Electrocardiography. 2nd ed. Chicago, Year Book Medical Publishers, 1977, p. 361.
321. Seyal, M. S., and Swiryn, S.: True posterior myocardial infarction. Arch. Intern. Med. *143*:983, 1983.
322. Jaarsma, W., Visser, C. A., Van Eenige, J., and Roos, J. P.: Left ventricular

wall motion with and without Q-wave disappearance after acute myocardial infarction. Am. J. Cardiol. 59:516, 1987.
323. Coll, S., Betriu, A., De Flores, T., et al.: Significance of Q-wave regression after transmural acute myocardial infarction. Am. J. Cardiol. 61:739, 1988.
324. Haiat, R., Worthington, F. X., Castellanos, A., and Lemberg, L.: Unusual normalization of the electrocardiogram on the 6th day of myocardial infarction. J. Electrocardiol. 4:363, 1971.
325. Goldberger, A. L.: Myocardial Infarction. St. Louis, C. V. Mosby, 1984, pp. 29–146.
326. Phibbs, B.: "Transmural" versus "subendocardial" myocardial infarction: An electrocardiographic myth. J. Am. Coll. Cardiol. 1:561, 1983.
327. Levine, H. D.: Subendocardial infarction in retrospect: Pathologic, cardiographic, and ancillary features. Circulation 72:790, 1985.
328. Spodick, D. H.: Q-wave infarction versus S-T infarction: Nonspecificity of electrocardiographic criteria for differentiating transmural and nontransmural lesions. Am. J. Cardiol. 51:913, 1983.
329. Zema, M. J.: Q wave, S-T segment, and T wave myocardial infarction. Am. J. Med. 78:391, 1985.
330. Goldberg, R. J., Gore, J. M., Alpert, J. S., and Dalen, J. E.: Non-Q wave myocardial infarction: Recent changes in occurrence and prognosis—a community-wide perspective. Am. Heart J. 113:273, 1987.
331. Schuster, E. H., and Bulkley, B. H.: Early postinfarction angina. Ischemia at a distance and ischemia in the infarct zone. N. Engl. J. Med. 305:1101, 1981.
332. Ferguson, D. W., Pandian, N., Kioschos, J. M., et al.: Angiographic evidence that reciprocal ST-segment depression during acute myocardial infarction does not indicate remote ischemia: Analysis of 23 patients. Am. J. Cardiol. 53:55, 1984.
333. Mukharji, J., Murray, S., Lewis, S. E., et al.: Is anterior ST depression with acute transmural inferior infarction due to posterior infarction? J. Am. Coll. Cardiol. 4:28, 1984.
334. Mirvis, D. M.: Physiologic bases for anterior ST segment depression in patients with acute inferior wall myocardial infarction. Am. Heart J. 116:1308, 1988.
335. Little, W. C., Rogers, E. W., and Sodums, M. T.: Mechanism of anterior ST segment depression during acute inferior myocardial infarction. Ann. Intern. Med. 100:26, 1984.
336. Lew, A. S., Weiss, A. T., Shah, P. K., et al.: Precordial ST segment depression during acute inferior myocardial infarction: Early thallium-201 scintigraphic evidence of adjacent posterolateral or inferoseptal involvement. J. Am. Coll. Cardiol. 5:203, 1985.
337. Chou, T., Van Der Bel-Kahn, J., Allen, J., et al.: Electrocardiographic diagnosis of right ventricular infarction. Am. J. Med. 70:1175, 1981.
338. Lopez-Sendon, J., Coma-Canella, I., Alcasena, S., et al.: Electrocardiographic findings in acute right ventricular infarction: Sensitivity and specificity of electrocardiographic alterations in right precordial leads V4R, V3R, V1, V2, and V3. J. Am. Coll. Cardiol. 6:1273, 1985.
339. Braat, S. H., Brugada, P., DeZwaan, C., et al.: Value of electrocardiogram in diagnosing right ventricular involvement in patients with an acute inferior wall myocardial infarction. Br. Heart J. 49:368, 1983.
340. Robalino, B. D., Whitlow, P. L., Underwood, D. A., and Salcedo, E. E.: Electrocardiographic manifestations of right ventricular infarction. Am. Heart J. 118:138, 1989.
341. Geft, I. L., Shah, P. K., Rodriguez, L., et al.: ST elevations in leads V1 to V5 may be caused by right coronary artery occlusion and acute right ventricular infarction. Am. J. Cardiol. 53:991, 1984.
342. Lew, A. S., Maddahi, J., Shah, P. K., et al.: Factors that determine the direction and magnitude of precordial ST-segment deviations during inferior wall acute myocardial infarction. Am. J. Cardiol. 55:883, 1985.
343. Lieu, C. K., Greenspan, G., and Piccirillo, R. T.: Atrial infarction of the heart. Circulation 23:331, 1961.
344. Silvertssen, E., Hoel, B., Bay, G., and Jorgensen, L.: Electrocardiographic atrial complex and acute atrial myocardial infarction. Am. J. Cardiol. 31:450, 1973.
345. Timmis, A. D., Fowler, M. D., Burwood, R. J., et al.: Pulmonary oedema without critical increase in left atrial pressure in acute myocardial infarction. Br. Med. J. 283:636, 1981.
346. Field, B. J., Russell, R. O., Jr., Moraski, R. E., et al.: Left ventricular size and function and heart size in the year following myocardial infarction. Circulation 50:331, 1974.
347. Brattler, A., Karliner, J. S., Higgins, C. B., et al.: The initial chest x-ray in acute myocardial infarction. Prediction of early and late mortality and survival. Circulation 61:1004, 1980.
348. Foster, C. J., Sekiya, T., Love, H. G., et al.: Identification of intracardiac thrombus: comparison of computed tomography and cross-sectional echocardiography. Br. J. Radiol. 60:327, 1987.
349. Rumberger, J. A., and Lipton, M. J.: Ultrafast cardiac CT scanning. Cardiol. Clin. 7:713, 1989.
350. Gibson, R. S., Taylor, G. J. Watson, D. D., et al.: Predicting the extent and location of coronary artery disease during the early postinfarction period by quantitative thallium-201 scintigraphy. Am. J. Cardiol. 47:1010, 1981.
351. Khaw, B. A., Gold, H. K., Yasuda, T., et al.: Scintigraphic quantification of myocardial necrosis in patients after intravenous injection of myosin-specific antibody. Circulation 74:501, 1986.
352. Hashimoto, T., Kambara, H., Fudo, T., et al.: Non-Q wave versus Q wave myocardial infarction: regional myocardial metabolism and blood flow assessed by positron emission tomography. J. Am. Coll. Cardiol. 12:88, 1988.
353. Johnson, L. L., Seldin, D. W., Becker, L. C., et al.: Antimyosin imaging in acute transmural myocardial infarction: Results of a multicenter clinical trial. J. Am. Coll. Cardiol. 13:27, 1989.
354. Becker, L.: Technetium-99m isonitrile tomography in patients with acute myocardial infarction: measurement of myocardial salvage by thrombolysis. J. Am. Coll. Cardiol. 15:315, 1990.
355. Gibbons, R. J., Verani, M. S., Behrenbeck, T., et al.: Feasibility of tomographic 99mTc-hexakis-2-methoxy-2-methylopropyl, isonitrile imaging for the assessment of myocardial area at risk and the effect of treatment in acute myocardial infarction. Circulation 80:1277, 1989.
355a. Christian, T. F., Clements, I. P., and Gibbons, R. J.: Noninvasive identification of myocardium at risk in patients with acute myocardial infarction and nondiagnostic electrocardiograms with technetium-99m-Sestamibi. Circulation 83:1615, 1991.
356. Santoro, G. M., Bisi, G., Sciagra, R., et al.: Single photon emission computed tomography with technetium-99m hexakis 2-methoxyisobutyl isonitrile in acute myocardial infarction before and after thrombolytic treatment: Assessment of salvaged myocardium and prediction of late functional recovery. J. Am. Coll. Cardiol. 15:301, 1990.
357. Johnston, D. L., Thompson, R. C., Liu, P., et al.: Magnetic resonance imaging during acute myocardial infarction. Am. J. Cardiol. 57:1059, 1986.
358. Johns, J. A., Leavitt, M. B., Newell, J. B., et al.: Quantitation of acute myocardial infarct size by nuclear magnetic resonance imaging. J. Am. Coll. Cardiol. 15:143, 1990.
359. Johnston, D. L., Mulvagh, S. L., Cashion, R. W., et al.: Nuclear magnetic resonance imaging of acute myocardial infarction within 24 hours of chest pain onset. Am. J. Cardiol. 64:172, 1989.
360. Ratner, A. V., Okada, R. D., Newell, J. B., and Pohost, G. M.: The relationship between proton nuclear magnetic resonance relaxation parameters and myocardial perfusion with acute coronary arterial occlusion and reperfusion. Circulation 71:823, 1985.
361. Reeves, R. C., Evanochko, W. T., and Pohost, G. M.: Potential approaches to evaluating the cardiovascular system using NMR. Prog. Cardiovasc. Dis. 29:53, 1986.
362. Wisenberg, G., Finnie, K. J., Jablonsky, G., et al.: Nuclear magnetic resonance and radionuclide angiographic assessment of acute myocardial infarction in a randomized trial of intravenous streptokinase. Am. J. Cardiol. 62:1011, 1988.
363. Kloner, R. A., and Parisi, A. F.: Acute myocardial diagnostic and prognostic applications of two-dimensional echocardiography. Circulation 75:521, 1987.
364. Lindvall, K., Erhardt, L., and Sjögren, A.: Serial M-mode echocardiographic mapping in myocardial infarction: A quantitative evaluation of left ventricular wall motion abnormalities. Clin. Cardiol. 6:220, 1983.
365. Corya, B. C., Rasmussen, S., Knoebel, S. B., and Feigenbaum, H.: Echocardiography in acute myocardial infarction. Am. J. Cardiol. 36:1, 1975.
366. Feigenbaum, H., Corya, B. C., Dillon, J. C., et al.: Role of echocardiography in patients with coronary artery disease. Am. J. Cardiol. 37:775, 1976.
367. Peels, C. H., Visser, C. A., Funke Kupper, A. J., et al.: Usefulness of two-dimensional echocardiography for immediate detection of myocardial ischemia in the emergency room. Am. J. Cardiol. 65:687, 1990.
368. Mann, D. L., Gillam, L. D., and Weyman, A. E.: Cross-sectional echocardiographic assessment of regional left ventricular performance and myocardial perfusion. Prog. Cardiovasc. Dis. 23:1, 1986.
369. Oh, J. K., Miller, F. A., Shub, C., Reeder, G. S., and Tajik, A. J.: Evaluation of acute chest pain syndromes by two-dimensional echocardiography. Its potential application in the selection of patients for acute reperfusion therapy. May Clin. Proc. 62:59, 1987.
370. Berning, J., and Steensgaard-Hansen, F.: Early estimation of risk by echocardiographic determination of wall motion index in an unselected population with acute myocardial infarction. Am. J. Cardiol. 65:567, 1990.
371. Sabia, P., Afrookteh, A., Touchstone, D. A., et al.: Superiority of regional dyssynergy in the emergency room diagnosis of acute myocardial infarction: A prospective study utilizing two-dimensional echocardiography. Circulation (in press).
372. Parisi, A. F., Nieminen, M., O'Boyle, J. E., et al.: Enhanced detection of the evolution of tissue changes after acute myocardial infarction using color-coded two-dimensional echocardiography. Circulation 66:764, 1982.
373. Otto, C. M., Stratton, J. R., Maynard, C., et al.: Echocardiographic evaluation of segmental wall motion early and late after thrombolytic therapy in acute myocardial infarction: The Western Washington Tissue Plasminogen Activator Emergency Room Trial. Am. J. Cardiol. 65:132, 1990.
374. Weiss, J. L., Bulkley, B. H., Hutchins, G. M., and Mason, S. J.: Two-dimensional echocardiographic recognition of myocardial injury in man: Comparison with postmortem studies. Circulation 63:401, 1981.
375. Barrett, J. J., Charuzi, Y., and Corday, E.: Ventricular aneurysm: Cross sectional echocardiographic approach. Am. J. Cardiol. 46:1133, 1980.
376. Catherwood, E., Mintz, G. S., Kotler, M. N., et al.: Two-dimensional echocardiographic recognition of left ventricular pseudoaneurysm. Circulation 62:294, 1980.
377. Donaldson, R. M., and Ballester, M.: Echocardiographic visualization of the anatomic causes of mitral regurgitation resulting from myocardial infarction. Postgrad. Med. J. 58:257, 1982.
378. Spirito, P., Bellotti, P., Chiarella, F., et al.: Prognostic significance and natural history of left ventricular thrombi in patients with acute ante-

rior myocardial infarction: A two-dimensional echocardiographic study. Circulation *72*:774, 1985.

379. Nishimura, R. A., Miller, F. A., Callahan, M. J., et al.: Doppler echocardiography: theory, instrumentation, technique, and application. Mayo Clin. Proc. *60*:321, 1985.
380. Smyllie, J. H., Sutherland, G. R., Geuskens, R., et al.: Doppler color flow mapping in the diagnosis of ventricular septal rupture and acute mitral regurgitation after myocardial infarction. J. Am. Coll. Cardiol. *15*:1449, 1990.
381. Harrison, M. R., MacPhail, B., Gurley, J. C., et al.: Usefulness of color Doppler flow imaging to distinguish ventricular septal defect from acute mitral regurgitation complicating acute myocardial infarction. Am. J. Cardiol. *64*:697, 1989.
382. Chandrantna, P. A., Nanna, M., McKay, C., et al.: Determination of cardiac output by transcutaneous continuous-wave ultrasonic Doppler computer. Am. J. Cardiol. *53*:234, 1984.
383. Maroko, P. R., Libby, P., Covell, J. W., et al.: Precordial ST-T segment elevation mapping: an atraumatic method for assessing alterations in the extent of myocardial ischemic injury. Am. J. Cardiol. *29*:227, 1972.
384. Lekven, J., Chatterjee, K., Tyberg, J. V., and Parmley, W. W.: Influence of left ventricular dimensions on endocardial and epicardial QRS amplitude and ST segment elevations during acute myocardial ischemia. Circulation *61*:679, 1980.
385. Ideker, R. E., Wagner, G. S., Ruth, W. K., et al.: Evaluation of a QRS scoring system for estimating myocardial infarct size. II. Correlation with quantitative anatomic findings for anterior infarcts. Am. J. Cardiol. *49*:1604, 1982.
386. Roark, S. F., Ideker, R. E., Wagner, G. S., et al.: Evaluation of a QRS scoring system for estimating myocardial infarct size. III. Correlation with quantitative anatomic findings for inferior infarcts. Am. J. Cardiol. *51*:382, 1983.
387. Cowan, M. J., Bruce, R. A., and Reichenbach, D. D.: Validation of a computerized QRS criterion for estimating myocardial infarction size and correlation with quantitative morphologic measurements. Am. J. Cardiol. *57*:60, 1986.
388. Roberts, R.: Enzymatic estimation of infarct size. Thrombolysis induced its demise: will it now rekindle its renaissance? Circulation *81*:707, 1990.
389. Morrison, J., Coromilas, J., Munsey, D., et al.: Correlation of radionuclide estimates of myocardial infarction size and release of creatine kinase-MB in man. Circulation *62*:277, 1980.
390. Hackel, D. B., Reimer, K. A., Ideker, R. E., et al.: Comparison of enzymatic and anatomic estimates of myocardial infarct size in man. Circulation *70*:824, 1984.
391. Armstrong, W. F., West, S. R., Dillon, J. C., and Feigenbaum, H.: Assessment of location and size of myocardial infarction with contrast-enhanced echocardiography. II. Application of digital imaging techniques. J. Am. Coll. Cardiol. *4*:141, 1984.
392. Force, T., Kemper, A., Perkins, L., et al.: Overestimation of infarct size by quantitative two-dimensional echocardiography: The role of tethering and of analytic procedures. Circulation *63*:1360, 1986.
393. Corbett, J. R., Lewis, S. E., Wolfe, C. L., et al.: Measurement of myocardial infarct size by technetium pyrophosphate single-photon tomography. Am. J. Cardiol. *54*:1231, 1984.
394. Volpini, M., Giubbini, R., Gei, P., et al.: Diagnosis of acute myocardial infarction by indium-111 antimyosin antibodies and correlation with the traditional techniques for the evaluation of extent and localization. Am. J. Cardiol. *63*:7, 1989.
395. Grande, P., Hindman, N. B., Saunamaki, K., et al.: A comprehensive estimation of acute myocardial infarct size using enzymatic, electrocardiographic and mechanical methods. Am. J. Cardiol. *59*:1239, 1987.

MANAGEMENT

395a. Wenger, N. K., Hellerstein, H. K., Blackburn, H., and Castranova, S. J.: Physician practice in the management of patients with uncomplicated myocardial infarction: Changes in the past decade. Circulation *65*:421, 1982.
396. Ericcson, C-G., Lindvall, B., Olsson, G., et al.: Trends in coronary care. A retrospective study of patients with myocardial infarction treated in coronary care units. Acta Med. Scand. *227*:507, 1988.
397. Gore, J. M., Goldberg, R. J., and Alpert, J. S.: The increased use of diagnostic procedures in patients with acute myocardial infarction. A community-wide perspective. Arch. Intern. Med. *147*:1729, 1987.
398. Antman, E. M., and Rutherford, J. D.: Coronary Care Medicine. Boston, Martinus Nijhoff, 1986, p. 20.
398a. Gibler, W. B., Kereiakes, D. J., Dean, E. N., et al.: Prehospital diagnosis and treatment of acute myocardial infarction: A North-South perspective. Am. Heart J. *121*:1, 1991.
399. Herlitz, J., Hartford, M., Blohm, M., et al.: Effect of a median campaign on delay times and ambulance use in suspended acute myocardial infarction. Am. J. Cardiol. *64*:90, 1989.
400. Maynard, C., Althouse, R., Olsufka, M., et al.: Early versus late hospital arrival for acute myocardial infarction in the Western Washington Thrombolytic Therapy Trials. Am. J. Cardiol. *63*:1296, 1989.
401. British Heart Foundation Working Group: Role of the general practitioner in managing patients with myocardial infarction: impact of thrombolytic treatment. Br. Med. J. *299*:555, 1989.
402. Pantridge, J. R., and Geddes, J. S.: Diseases of the cardiovascular system. Management of acute myocardial infarction. Br. Med. J. *2*:168, 1976.
403. Dean, N. C., Haug, P. J., and Hawker, P. J.: Effect of mobile paramedic units on outcome in patients with myocardial infarction. Ann. Emerg. Med. *17*:1034, 1988.
404. Dillon, J. C., Vasu, C. M., Berman, D. S., et al.: Thirteenth Bethesda Conference—Task Force III: Diagnostic Procedures. Am. J. Cardiol. *50*:377, 1982.
405. Cobb, L. A., Baum, R. S., Alvarez, H., III, and Schaffer, W. A.: Resuscitation from out-of-hospital ventricular fibrillation: 4 years' follow-up. Circulation *51*(Suppl. III):223, 1975.
406. Lewis, R. P., Lanese, R. R., Stang, J. M., et al.: Reduction of mortality from prehospital myocardial infarction by prudent patient activation of mobile coronary care system. Am. Heart J. *103*:123, 1982.
407. Crampton, R. S., Aldrich, F. R., Gascho, J. A., et al.: Reduction of prehospital, ambulance and community coronary death rates by the community-wide emergency cardiac care system. Am. J. Med. *58*:151, 1975.
408. Capone, R. J., Visco, J., Curwen, E., and VanEvery, S.: The effect of early prehospital transtelephonic coronary intervention on morbidity and mortality: experience with 284 postmyocardial infarction patients in a pilot program. Am. Heart J. *107*:1153, 1984.
409. Pressley, J. C., Wilson, B. H., Severance, H. W., et al.: Basic emergency medical care of patients with acute myocardial infarction: Initial prehospital characteristics and in-hospital complications. J. Am. Coll. Cardiol. *4*:487, 1984.
410. Gotsman, M. S.: Prehospital thrombolysis in acute myocardial infarction: is it feasible, practical and safe? Intensive Care World *5*:9, 1988.
411. Califf, R. M., and Harrelson-Woodlief, S. L.: At home thrombolysis. J. Am. Coll. Cardiol. *15*:937, 1990.
412. Weiss, A. T., Fine, D. G., Applebaum, D., et al.: Prehospital coronary thrombolysis. A new strategy in acute myocardial infarction. Chest *92*:124, 1987.
413. The Thrombolysis Early in Acute Heart Attack Trial Study Group: Very early thrombolytic therapy in suspected acute myocardial infarction. Am. J. Cardiol. *65*:401, 1990.
414. Roth, A., Barbash, G. I., Hod, H., et al.: Should thrombolytic therapy be administered in the mobile intensive care unit in patients with evolving myocardial infarction? A pilot study. J. Am. Coll. Cardiol. *15*:932, 1990.
415. Castaigne, A. D., Herve, C., Duval-Moulin, A-M., et al.: Prehospital use of APSAC: results of a placebo-controlled study. Am. J. Cardiol. *64*:30A, 1989.
416. Weaver, W. D., Eisenberg, M. S., Martin, J. S., et al.: Myocardial Infarction Triage and Intervention Project—Phase I: patient characteristics and feasibility of prehospital initiation of thrombolytic therapy. J. Am. Coll. Cardiol. *15*:925, 1990.
417. Lee, T. H., and Goldman, L.: The coronary care unit turns 25: Historical trends and future directions. Ann. Intern. Med. *108*:887, 1988.
418. Morris, A. L., Nernberg, V., Roos, N. P., et al.: Acute myocardial infarction: Survey of urban and rural hospital mortality. Am. Heart J. *105*:44, 1983.
419. Hill, J. D., Hampton, J. R., and Mitchell, J.R.A.: A randomized trial of home-versus-hospital management for patients with suspected myocardial infarction. Lancet *1*:837, 1978.
420. Fesmire, F. M., Percy, R. F., Wears, R. L., and MacMath, T. L.: Risk stratification according to the initial electrocardiogram in patients with suspected acute myocardial infarction. Arch. Intern. Med. *149*:1294, 1989.
421. Brush, J. E., Brand, D. A., Acampora, D., et al.: Use of the initial electrocardiogram to predict in-hospital complications of acute myocardial infarction. N. Engl. J. Med. *312*:1137, 1985.
422. Lee, T. L., Cook, E. F., Weisberg, M., et al.: Acute chest pain in the emergency ward: identification and evaluation of low risk patients. Arch. Intern. Med. *145*:65, 1985.
423. Goldman, L., Weinberg, M., Weisberg, M., et al.: A computer-derived protocol to aid in the diagnosis of emergency room patients with acute chest pain. N. Engl. J. Med. *307*:588, 1982.
424. Pozen, M. W., D'Agostino, R. B., Mitchell, J. B., et al.: The usefulness of a predictive instrument to reduce inappropriate admissions to the coronary care unit. Ann. Intern. Med. *92*:238, 1980.
425. Fineberg, H., Scadden, D., and Goldman, L.: Management of patients with a low probability of acute myocardial infarction: Cost-effectiveness of alternatives to coronary care unit admission. N. Engl. J. Med. *310*:1301, 1984.
426. McGregor, M.: The coronary care unit. A lack of consensus. Am. J. Med. *78*:378, 1985.
427. Lee, T. H., Rouan, G. W., Weisberg, M. D., et al.: Sensitivity of routine clinical criteria for diagnosing myocardial infarction within 24 hours of hospitalization. Ann. Intern. Med. *106*:181, 1987.
428. Weingarten, S., Ermann, B., Bolus, R., et al.: Early "step-down" transfer of low-risk patients with chest pain. A controlled interventional trial. Ann. Intern. Med. *113*:283, 1990.
429. Herlitz, J., Hjalmarson, A., and Waagstein, F.: Treatment of pain in acute myocardial infarction. Br. Heart J. *61*:9, 1989.
430. Mikolich, J. R., Nicoloff, N. B., Robinson, P. H., and Logue, H. B.: Relief of refractory angina with continuous intravenous infusion of nitroglycerin. Chest *77*:375, 1980.
431. Come, P. C., and Pitt, B.: Nitroglycerin-induced severe hypotension and bradycardia in patients with acute myocardial infarction. Circulation *54*:624, 1976.
432. Ferguson, J. J., Diver, D. J., Boldt, M., and Pasternak, R. C.: Significance of

nitroglycerin-induced hypotension with acute myocardial infarction. Am. J. Cardiol. *64*:311, 1989.

433. Zelis, R., Mansour, E. J., Capone, R. J., and Mason, D. T.: The cardiovascular effects of morphine: The peripheral capacitance and resistance vessels in human subjects. J. Clin. Invest. *54*:1247, 1974.

434. Fillmore, S. J., Shapiro, M., and Killip, T.: Arterial oxygen tension in acute myocardial infarction. Serial analysis of clinical state and blood gas changes. Am. Heart J. *79*:620, 1970.

435. Madias, J. E., and Hood, W. B., Jr.: Reduction of precordial ST-segment elevation in patients with anterior myocardial infarction by oxygen breathing. Circulation *53*(Suppl. I):198, 1976.

436. Richterova, A., Herlitz, J., Holmberg, S., et al.: Goteborg metoprolol trial: effects on chest pain. J. Cardiol. *53*:32D, 1984.

436a. Yusuf, S., Held, P., and Furberg, C.: Update of effects of calcium antagonists in myocardial infarction or angina in light of the second Danish verapamil infarction trial (DAVIT-II) and other recent studies. Am. J. Cardiol. *67*:1295, 1991.

437. Kirschenbaum, J. M., Koner, R. A., Antman, E., and Braunwald, E.: Use of an ultrashort acting β blocker in patients with acute myocardial ischemia. Circulation *72*:873, 1985.

438. Levine, S. A., and Lown, B.: "Armchair" treatment of acute coronary thrombosis. JAMA *148*:1365, 1952.

439. Swan, H.J.C., Ganz, W., Forrester, J. S., et al.: Catheterization of the heart in man with use of a flow-directed balloon-tipped catheter. N. Engl. J. Med. *283*:447, 1970.

440. Rackley, C. E., Satler, L. F., Pearle, D. L., et al.: Use of hemodynamic measurements for management of acute myocardial infarction. *In* Rackley, C. E. (ed.): Advances in Critical Care Cardiology. Philadelphia, F. A. Davis Co., 1986, pp. 3–16.

441. Weisel, R. D., Berger, R. L., and Hechtman, H. B.: Measurement of cardiac output by thermodilution. N. Engl. J. Med. *292*:682, 1975.

442. McMichan, J. C., Baele, P. L., and Wignes, M. W.: Insertion of pulmonary artery catheters—a comparison of fiberoptic and nonfiberoptic catheters. Crit. Care Med. *12*:517, 1984.

443. Gewirtz, H., Gold, H. K., Fallon, J. T., et al.: Role of right ventricular infarction in cardiogenic shock associated with inferior myocardial infarction. Br. Heart J. *42*:719, 1979.

444. Shell, W. E., DeWood, M. A., Peter, T., et al.: Comparison of clinical signs and hemodynamic state in the early hours of transmural myocardial infarction. Am. Heart J. *104*:521, 1982.

445. Goldenheim, P. D., and Kazemi, H.: Cardiopulmonary monitoring of critically ill patients. N. Engl. J. Med. *311*:776, 1984.

446. Eisenberg, P. R., Jaffe, A. S., and Schuster, D. P.: Clinical evaluation compared to pulmonary artery catheterization in the hemodynamic assessment of critically ill patients. Crit. Care Med. *12*:549, 1984.

447. Robin, E. D.: The cult of the Swan-Ganz catheter. Ann. Intern. Med. *103*:445, 1985.

448. Robin, E. D.: Death by pulmonary artery flow–directed catheter (editorial). Time for a moratorium? Chest *92*:727, 1987.

449. Gore, J. M., Goldberg, R. J., Spodick, D. H., et al.: A community-wide assessment of the use of pulmonary artery catheters in patients with acute myocardial infarction. Chest *92*:721, 1987.

450. Graboys, T. B.: In-hospital sudden death after coronary care unit discharge: A high risk profile. Arch. Intern. Med. *135*:512, 1975.

451. Marmor, A., Geltman, E. M., Schechtman, K., et al.: Recurrent myocardial infarction: Clinical predictors and prognostic implications. Circulation *66*:415, 1982.

452. Lie, K. I., Liem, K. L., Schuilenburg, R. M., et al.: Early identification of patients developing late in-hospital ventricular fibrillation after discharge from the Coronary Care Unit. Am. J. Cardiol. *41*:674, 1978.

453. Starling, M. R., Crawford, M. H., Kennedy, G. T., and O'Rourke, R. A.: Treadmill exercise tests predischarge and 6-week postmyocardial infarction to detect abnormalities of known prognostic value. Ann. Intern. Med. *94*:721, 1981.

454. Sellier, P., Plat, F., Corona, P., et al.: Prognostic significance of angina pectoris recurring soon after myocardial infarction. Eur. Heart J. *9*:447, 1988.

455. Severance, H. W., Jr., Morris, K. G., and Wagner, G. S.: Criteria for early discharge after acute myocardial infarction. Validation in a community hospital. Arch. Intern. Med. *142*:39, 1982.

456. Resnekov, L.: The intermediate care unit—a stage in continued coronary care. Br. Heart J. *39*:357, 1977.

457. Weinberg, S. L.: Intermediate coronary care—observations on the validity of the concept. Chest *73*:154, 1978.

458. van der Laarse, A., van Leeuwen, F. T., Krul, R., et al.: The size of infarction as judged enzymatically in 1974 patients with acute myocardial infarction. Relation with symptomatology, infarct localization and type of infarction. Int. J. Cardiol. *19*:191, 1988.

459. Page, D. L., Caulfield, J. B., Kastor, J. A., et al.: Myocardial changes associated with cardiogenic shock. N. Engl. J. Med. *285*:133, 1971.

460. Gutovitz, A. L., Sobel, B. E., and Roberts, R.: Progressive nature of myocardial injury in selected patients with cardiogenic shock. Am. J. Cardiol. *41*:469, 1978.

461. Rogers, W. J., McDaniel, H. G., Smith, L. R., et al.: Correlation of angiographic estimates of myocardial infarct size and accumulated release of creatine kinase MB isoenzyme in man. Circulation *56*:199, 1977.

462. Holman, B. L., Chisholm, R. J., and Braunwald, E.: The prognostic implications of acute myocardial infarct scintigraphy with 99m Tc-pyrophosphate. Circulation *57*:320, 1978.

463. Geltman, E. M., Ehsani, A. A., Campbell, M. K., et al.: The influence of location and extent of myocardial infarction on long-term ventricular dysrhythmia and mortality. Circulation *60*:805, 1979.

464. Sobel, B. E., and Shell, W. E.: Jeopardized, blighted and necrotic myocardium. Circulation *47*:215, 1973.

465. Braunwald, E., and Maroko, P. R.: The reduction of infarct size—an idea whose time (for testing) has come. Circulation *50*:206, 1974.

466. Yusuf, S., Collins, R., Peto, R., et al.: Intravenous and intracoronary fibrinolytic therapy in acute myocardial infarction: Overview of results on mortality, reinfarction and side effects from 33 randomized control trials. Eur. Heart J. *6*:556, 1985.

467. Kubler, W., and Doorey, A.: Reduction of infarct size. An attractive concept: useful—or possible—in human? Br. Heart J. *53*:5, 1985.

468. Christlieb, I. Y., Clark, R. E., and Sobel, B. E.: Three-hour preservation of the hypothermic globally ischemic heart with nifedipine. Surgery *90*:947, 1981.

469. Weisfeldt, M. L.: Reperfusion and reperfusion injury. Clin. Res. *35*:13, 1987.

470. Engler, R., and Gilpin, E.: Can superoxide dismutase alter myocardial infarct size? Circulation *79*:1177, 1989.

470a. Murohara, Y., Yui, Y., Hattori, R., and Kawai, C.: Effects of superoxide dismutase on reperfusion arrhythmias and left ventricular function in patients undergoing thrombolysis for anterior wall acute myocardial infarction. Am. J. Cardiol. *67*:765, 1991.

471. Corr, P. B., Snyder, D. W., Lee, B. I., et al.: Pathophysiological concentrations of lysophosphatides and the slow response. Am. J. Physiol. *12*:187, 1982.

472. Schaper, W., and Pasyk, S.: Influence of collateral flow on the ischemic tolerance of the heart following acute and subacute coronary occlusion. Circulation *53*(Suppl. I):57, 1976.

473. Braunwald, E.: Coronary artery spasm as a cause of myocardial ischemia. J. Lab. Clin. Med. *97*:299, 1981.

474. Maseri, A., L'Abbate, A., Baroldi, G., et al.: Coronary vasospasm as a possible cause of myocardial infarction. N. Engl. J. Med. *299*:1271, 1978.

475. Koiwaya, Y., Torii, S., Takeshita, A., et al.: Postinfarction angina caused by coronary arterial spasm. Circulation *65*:275, 1982.

476. Williams, D. O., Amsterdam, E. A., Miller, R. R., and Mason, D. T.: Functional significance of coronary collateral vessels in patients with acute myocardial infarction: Relation to pump performance, cardiogenic shock and survival. Am. J. Cardiol. *37*:345, 1976.

477. Baker, J. T., Bramlet, D. A., Lester, R. M., et al.: Myocardial infarction extension: Incidence and relationship to survival. Circulation *65*:918, 1982.

478. Hutter, A. M., Jr., DeSanctis, R. W., Flynn, T., and Yeatman, L. A.: Nontransmural myocardial infarction. A comparison of hospital and late clinical course of patients with that of matched patients with transmural anterior and transmural inferior myocardial infarction. Am. J. Cardiol. *48*:595, 1981.

479. Kao, W., Khaja, F., Goldstein, S., and Gheorghiade, M.: Cardiac event rate after non-Q-wave acute myocardial infarction and the significance of its anterior location. Am. J. Cardiol. *64*:1236, 1989.

480. Shell, W. E., and Sobel, B. E.: Protection of jeopardized ischemic myocardium by reduction of ventricular afterload. N. Engl. J. Med. *291*:481, 1974.

481. Derrida, J. P., Sal, R., and Chiche, P.: Nitroglycerin infusion in acute myocardial infarction. N. Engl. J. Med. *297*:336, 1977.

482. Hjalmarson, A., Herlitz, J., Malek, I., et al.: Effect on mortality of metoprolol in acute myocardial infarction. Lancet *2*:823, 1981.

483. Yusuf, S., Ramsdale, E., Peto, R., et al.: Early intravenous atentolol treatment in suspected acute myocardial infarction. Preliminary report of a randomized trial. Lancet *2*:73, 1980.

484. Braunwald, E., Muller, J. E., Kloner, R. A., and Maroko, P. R.: Role of beta-adrenergic blockade in the therapy of patients with myocardial infarction. Am. J. Med. *74*:113, 1983.

485. Chatterjee, K., and Parmley, W. W.: Vasodilator therapy for acute myocardial infarction and chronic congestive heart failure. J. Am. Coll. Cardiol. *1*:133, 1983.

486. Lavie, C. J., Gersh, B. J., and Chesebro, J. H.: Reperfusion in acute myocardial infarction. Mayo Clin. Proc. *65*:549, 1990.

487. Ginks, W. R., Sybers, H. D., Maroko, P. R., et al.: Coronary artery reperfusion: II. Reduction of myocardial infarct size at 1 week after the coronary occlusion. J. Clin. Invest. *51*:2717, 1972.

488. Smith, G. T., Soeter, J. R., Haston, H. H., and McNamara, J. J.: Coronary reperfusion in primates: Serial electrocardiographic and histologic assessment. J. Clin. Invest. *54*:1420, 1974.

489. Deloche, A., Fabiani, J. N., Camilleri, J. P., et al.: The effect of coronary artery reperfusion on the extent of myocardial infarction. Am. Heart J. *93*:358, 1977.

490. Bergmann, S. R., Lerch, R. A., Fox, K.A.A., et al.: The temporal dependence of beneficial effects of coronary thrombolysis characterized by positron tomography. Am. J. Med. *73*:573, 1982.

491. Reimer, K. A., and Jennings, R. B.: The wavefront phenomenon of myocardial ischemic cell death. II. Transmural progression of necrosis within the framework of ischemic bed size (myocardium at risk) and collateral flow. Lab. Invest. *40*:633, 1979.

492. Cheauvechai, C., Effler, D. B., Loop, F. D., et al.: Emergency myocardial revascularization. Am. J. Cardiol. *32*:901, 1973.

493. Chazov, E. I., Mateeva, L. S., Mazaev, A. V., et al.: Intracoronary administration of fibrinolysin in acute myocardial infarction. Ter. Arkh. *48*:8, 1976.

494. Rentrop, P., DeVivie, E. R., Karsch, K. R., and Kreuzer, H.: Acute coronary occlusion with impending infarction as an angiographic complication relieved by a guide-wire recanalization. Clin. Cardiol. *1*:101, 1978.

495. Califf, R. M., Topol, E., and Gersh, B. J.: From myocardial salvage to patient salvage in acute myocardial infarction: The role of reperfusion therapy. J. Am. Coll. Cardiol. *14*:1382, 1989.
496. Kloner, R. A., Ellis, S. G., Lange, R., and Braunwald, E.: Studies of experimental coronary artery reperfusion: Effects on infarct size, myocardial function, biochemistry, ultrastructure and microvascular damage. Circulation *68*(Suppl I):8, 1983.
497. Schwartz, F., Schuler, G., Katus, H., et al.: Intracoronary thrombolysis in acute myocardial infarction: duration of ischemia as a major determinant of late results after recanalization. Am. J. Cardiol. *50*:933, 1982.
498. Sheehan, F. H., Mathey, D. G., Schofer, J., et al.: Factors that determine recovery of left ventricular function after thrombolysis in patients with acute myocardial infarction. Circulation *71*:1121, 1985.
499. Sheehan, F. H., Braunwald, E., Canner, P., et al.: The effect of intravenous thrombolytic therapy on left ventricular function: A report on tissue-type plasminogen activator and streptokinase from the thrombolysis in myocardial infarction (TIMI Phase I) trial. Circulation *75*:817, 1987.
500. Kurnik, P. B., Courtois, M. R., and Ludbrook, P. B.: Diastolic stiffening induced by acute myocardial infarction is reduced by early reperfusion. J. Am. Coll. Cardiol. *12*:1029, 1988.
501. Gruppo Italiano Per Lo Studio Della Streptochinasi Nell'infarcto Miocardico (GISSI): Effectiveness of intravenous thrombolytic treatment in acute myocardial infarction. Lancet *1*:397, 1986.
502. ISIS 2 Collaborative Group: Randomized trial of intravenous streptokinase, oral aspirin, both, or neither among 17,187 cases of suspected acute myocardial infarction: ISIS 2. Lancet *2*:349, 1988.
503. Saito, Y., Yasuno, M., Ishida, M., et al.: Importance of coronary collaterals for restoration of left ventricular function after intracoronary thrombolysis. Am. J. Cardiol. *55*:1259, 1985.
504. Nayler, W. G., and Elz, J. S.: Reperfusion injury: Laboratory artifact or clinical dilemma? Circulation *74*:215, 1986.
504a. Forman, M. B., Virmani, R., and Puett, D. W.: Mechanisms and therapy of myocardial reperfusion injury. Circulation *81*(Suppl. *IV*):IV–69, 1990.
505. Braunwald, E., and Kloner, R. A.: Myocardial reperfusion: A double-edged sword? J. Clin. Invest. *76*:1713, 1985.
506. Kloner, R. A., Ganote, C. E., and Jennings, R. B.: The "no-reflow" phenomenon after temporary coronary occlusion in the dog. J. Clin. Invest. *54*:1496, 1974.
507. Laffel, G. L., and Braunwald, E.: Thrombolytic therapy. A new strategy for treatment of acute myocardial infarction. N. Engl. J. Med. *311*:710, 1984.
508. Waller, B. F., Rothbaum, D. A., Pinkerton, C. A., et al.: Status of the myocardium and infarct-related coronary artery in 19 necropsy patients with acute recanalization using pharmacologic (streptokinase, r-tissue plasminogen activator), mechanical (percutaneous transluminal coronary angioplasty) or combined types of reperfusion therapy. J. Am. Coll. Cardiol. *9*:785, 1987.
509. Gertz, S. D., Kalan, J. M., Kragel, A. H., et al.: Cardiac morphologic findings in patients with acute myocardial infarction treated with recombinant tissue plasminogen activator. Am. J. Cardiol. *65*:953, 1990.
510. Mattfeldt, T., Schwarz, F., Schuler, G., et al.: Necropsy evaluation in seven patients with evolving acute myocardial infarction treated with thrombolytic therapy. Am. J. Cardiol. *54*:530, 1984.
510a. Carrea, F. P., and Lesnefsky, E. J., Repine, J. E., et al.: Reduction of canine myocardial infarct size by a diffusible reactive oxygen metabolite scavenger. Circ. Res. *68*:1652, 1991.
511. Werns, S. W., Shea, M. J., and Lucchesi, B. R.: Free radicals and myocardial injury: Pharmacologic implications. Circulation *74*:1, 1986.
512. TIMI Study Group: Comparison on invasive and conservative strategies following tissue plasminogen activator in acute myocardial infarction: Results of the Thrombolysis in Myocardial Infarction (TIMI-II) trial. N. Engl. J. Med. *320*:618, 1989.
513. Roberts, R., Rogers, W. J., Mueller, H. S., et al.: Immediate versus deferred *β* blockade following thrombolytic therapy in patients with acute myocardial infarction: Results of the Thrombokysis in Myocardial Infarction (TIMI) II-B Study. Circulation *83*:422, 1991.
514. Wei, J. Y., Markis, J. E., Malagold, M., and Braunwald, E.: Cardiovascular reflexes stimulated by reperfusion of ischemic myocardium in acute myocardial infarction. Circulation *67*:796, 1983.
515. Cercek, B., and Horvat, M.: Arrhythmias with brief, high-dose intravenous streptokinase infusion in acute myocardial infarction. Eur. Heart J. *6*:109, 1985.
516. Goldberg, S., Greenspan, A. J., Urban, P. L., et al.: Reperfusion arrhythmia: a marker of restoration of antegrade flow during intracoronary thrombolysis for acute myocardial infarction. Am. Heart J. *105*:26, 1983.
517. Califf, R. M., O'Neil, W., Stack, R. S., et al.: Failure of simple clinical measurements to predict perfusion status after intravenous thrombolysis. Ann. Intern. Med. *658*:108, 1988.
518. Wilber, D., Walton, J., O'Neill, W., et al.: Effects of reperfusion on complete heart block complicating anterior myocardial infarction. J. Am. Coll. Cardiol. *4*:1315, 1984.
519. Selzer, A.: Does thrombolytic therapy reduce infarct size? J. Am. Coll. Cardiol. *13*:1431, 1989.
519a. Deshmukh, P., Winters, S. L., and Gomes, J. A.: Frequency and significance of occult late potentials on the signal-averaged electrocardiogram in sustained ventricular tachycardia after healing of acute myocardial infarction. Am. J. Cardiol. *67*:806, 1991.
520. Braunwald, E.: Editorial Comment. Coronary artery patency in patients with myocardial infarction. J. Am. Coll. Cardiol. *16*:1550, 1990.
521. Fortin, D. F., and Califf, R. M.: Long-term survival from acute myocardial infarction: salutary effect of an open coronary vessel. Am. J. Med. *88*:1–9N, 1990.
521a. Bonaduce, D., Petretta, M., Villari, B., et al.: Effects of late administration of tissue-type plasminogen activator on left ventricular remodeling and function after myocardial infarction. J. Am. Coll. Cardiol. *16*:1561, 1990.
522. Grines, C. L., O'Neill, W. W., Anselmo, E. G., et al.: Comparison of left ventricular function and contractile reserve after successful recanalization by thrombolysis versus rescue percutaneous transluminal coronary angioplasty for acute myocardial infarction. Am. J. Cardiol. *62*:352, 1988.
523. Schroder, R., Neuhaus, K., Linderer, T., et al.: Impact of late coronary artery reperfusion on left ventricular function one month after acute myocardial infarction (results from the ISAM study). Am. J. Cardiol. *64*:878, 1989.
524. Agress, C. M., Jacobs, H. I., Clark, W. G., et al.: Intravenous trypsin in experimental acute myocardial infarction (abst). J. Pharmacol. Exp. Ther. *110*:1, 1952.
525. Fletcher, A. P., Alkjaersig, N., Smyriotis, F. E., and Sherry, S.: The treatment of patients suffering from early myocardial infarction with massive and prolonged streptokinase therapy. Trans. Assoc. Am. Phys. *71*:287, 1958.
526. Rentrop, P., Blanke, H., Marsch, K. R., et al.: Acute myocardial infarction: intracoronary application of nitroglycerin and streptokinase in combination with transluminal recanalization. Clin. Cardiol. *2*:354, 1979.
527. Khaja, F., Walton, J. A., Brymer, J. F., et al.: Intracoronary fibrinolytic therapy in acute myocardial infarction, report of a prospective randomized trial. N. Engl. J. Med. *308*:1305, 1983.
528. Tiefenbrunn, A. J., and Sobel, B. E.: The impact of coronary thrombolysis on myocardial infarction. Fibrinolysis *3*:1, 1989.
529. European Cooperative Study Group for Streptokinase Treatment in Acute Myocardial Infarction: Streptokinase in acute myocardial infarction. N. Engl. J. Med. *301*:797, 1979.
530. Fry, E.T.A., and Sobel, B. E.: Coronary thrombosis. *In* Zipes, D. P., and Rowlands, D. J. (eds.): Progress in Cardiology. Vol. II. Philadelphia, Lea & Febiger, 1990, pp. 199–239.
531. Anderson, J. L.: Reperfusion, patency, and reocclusion with anistreplase (APSAC) in acute myocardial infarction. Am. J. Cardiol. *64*:12A, 1989.
532. Sherry, S.: Unresolved clinical pharmacologic questions in thrombolytic therapy for acute myocardial infarction. J. Am. Coll. Cardiol. *12*:519, 1988.
533. Anderson, J. L., Rothbard, R. L., Hackworthy, R. A., et al.: Multicenter reperfusion trial of intravenous anisoylated plasminogen activator complex (APSAC) in acute myocardial infarction: controlled comparison with intracoronary streptokinase. J. Am. Coll. Cardiol. *11*:1153, 1988.
533a. Becker, R. C., Corrao, J. M., Harrington, R., et al.: Recombinant tissue-type plasminogen activator: Current concepts and guidelines for clinical use in acute myocardial infarction. Part 1. Am. Heart J. *121*:220, 1991.
533b. Becker, R. C., and Harrington, R.: Recombinant tissue-type plasminogen activator: Current concepts and guidelines for clinical use in acute myocardial infarction. Part II. Am. Heart J. *121*:627, 1991.
534. Topol, E. J., and Califf, R. M.: Tisue plasminogen activator: Why the backlash? J. Am. Coll. Cardiol. *13*:1477, 1989.
535. The TIMI Study Group: The thrombolysis in myocardial infarction (TIMI) trial. Phase I Findings. N. Engl. J. Med. *312*:932, 1985.
536. Verstraete, M., Bory, M., Collen, D., et al.: Randomised trial of intravenous recombinant tissue-type plasminogen activator versus intravenous streptokinase in acute myocardial infarction. Lancet *I*:842, 1985.
537. Chesebro, J. H., Knatterud, G., Roberts, R., et al.: Thrombolysis in myocardial infarction (TIMI) trial, phase I: a comparison between intravenous tissue plasminogen activator and intravenous streptokinase. Circulation *76*:142, 1987.
538. White, H. D., Rivers, J. T., Maslowski, A. H., et al.: Effect of intravenous streptokinase as compared with that of tissue plasminogen activator on left ventricular function after first myocardial infarction. N. Engl. J. Med. *320*:817, 1989.
539. Magnani, B., for the PAIMS Investigators: Plasminogen Activator Italian Multicenter Study (PAIMS): Comparison of intravenous recombinant single-chain human tissue-type plasminogen activator (rt-PA) with intravenous streptokinase in acute myocardial infarction. J. Am. Coll. Cardiol. *13*:19, 1989.
540. Collen, D.: Coronary thrombolysis: Streptokinase or recombinant tissue–type plasminogen activator? Ann. Intern. Med. *112*:529, 1990.
540a. Data presented at American College of Cardiology Annual Scientific Sessions, Atlanta, 1991.
541. Baim, D. S., Braunwald, E., Feit, F., et al.: The thrombolysis in myocardial infarction (TIMI) trial phase II: Additional information and perspectives. J. Am. Coll. Cardiol. *15*:1188, 1990.
542. Braunwald, E.: Thrombolytic reperfusion of acute myocardial infarction: resolved and unresolved issues. J. Am. Coll. Cardiol. *12*:85A, 1988.
543. Mauri, F., Gasparini, M., Barbonaglia, L., et al.: Prognostic significance of the extent of myocardial injury in acute myocardial infarction treated by streptokinase (the GISSI Trial). Am. J. Cardiol. *63*:1291, 1989.
544. Meinertz, T., Kasper, W., Schumacher, M., et al.: The German multicenter trial of anisoylated plasminogen activator complex versus heparin for acute myocardial infarction. Am. J. Cardiol. *62*:347, 1988.
545. Gruppo Italiano Per Lo Studio Della Streptochinasi Nell'Infarto Miocar-

650. Derrida, J. P., Sal, R., and Chiche, P.: Favorable effects of prolonged nitroglycerin infusion in patients with acute myocardial infarction. Am. Heart J. *96*:833, 1978.
651. Jugdutt, B. I., and Warnica, J. W.: Intravenous nitroglycerin therapy to limit myocardial infarct size, expansion, and complications. Effect of timing, dosage, and infarct location. Circulation *78*:906, 1988.
652. Bussman, W. D., Passek, D., Seidel, W., and Kaltenbach, M.: Reduction of CK and CK-MB indexes of infarct size by intravenous nitroglycerin. Circulation *63*:615, 1981.
653. Flaherty, J. T., Becker, L. C., Bulkley, B. H., et al.: A randomized prospective trial of intravenous nitroglycerin in patients with acute myocardial infarction. Circulation *68*:576, 1983.
654. Osuna, P. B., Moreno, M. G., Jimenez, A. A., et al.: Isosorbide dinitrate sublingual therapy for inferior myocardial infarction: Randomized trial to assess infarct size limitation. Am. J. Cardiol. *55*:330, 1985.
655. Shah, R., Bodenheimer, M. M., Banka, V. S., and Helfant, R. H.: Nitroglycerin and ventricular performance: Differential effect in the presence of reversible and irreversible asynergy. Chest *70*:473, 1976.
656. Shook, T. L., Kirschenbaum, J. M., Hundley, R. F., et al.: Ethanol intoxication complicating intravenous nitroglycerin therapy. Ann. Intern. Med. *101*:498, 1984.
657. Kaplan, K. J., Taber, M., Teagarden, J. R., et al.: Association of methemoglobinemia and intravenous nitroglycerin administration. Am. J. Cardiol. *55*:181, 1985.
658. Jugdutt, B. I., and Warnica, J. W.: Tolerance with low dose intravenous nitroglycerin therapy in acute myocardial infarction. Am. J. Cardiol. *64*:581, 1989.
659. Levy, W. E., Katz, R. J., Ruffalo, R. L., et al.: Potentiation of the hemodynamic effects of acutely administered nitroglycerin by methionine. Circulation *78*:640, 1988.
660. Abrams, J.: Nitrates. Med. Clin. North Am. *72*:1, 1988.
661. Skolnick, A. E., and Frishman, W. H.: Calcium channel blockers in myocardial infarction. Arch. Intern. Med. *149*:1669, 1989.
662. Sirnes, P. A., Overskeid, K., Pederson, T. R., et al.: Evolution of infarct size during the early use of nifedipine in patients with acute myocardial infarction: The Norwegian Nifedipine Multicenter Trial. Circulation *70*:738, 1984.
663. Muller, J. E., Morrison, J., Stone, P. H., et al.: Nifedipine therapy for patients with threatened and acute myocardial infarction: A randomized, double-blind, placebo-controlled comparison. Circulation *69*:740, 1984.
664. Erbel, R., Pop, T., Meinertz, T., et al.: Combination of calcium channel blocker and thrombolytic therapy in acute myocardial infarction. Am. Heart J. *115*:529, 1988.
665. Report of the Holland Interuniversity Nifedipine/Metoprolol Trial (HINT) Research Group: Early treatment of unstable angina in the coronary care unit: a randomised, double-blind, placebo-controlled comparison of recurrent ischaemia and thrombolytic therapy in patients treated with nifedipine or metoprolol or both. Br. Heart J. *56*:400, 1986.
666. The Multicenter Diltiazem Postinfarction Trial Research Group: The effect of diltiazem on mortality and reinfarction after myocardial infarction. N. Engl. J. Med. *319*:385, 1988.
667. The Danish Study Group on Verapamil in Myocardial Infarction: Effect of verapamil on mortality and major events after acute myocardial infarction (the Danish Verapamil Infarction Trial II—DAVIT II). Am. J. Cardiol. *66*:779, 1990.
668. Renard, M., Sterling, I., Van Camp G., et al.: Comparison of the effect of intravenous diltiazem and a placebo on hemodynamics and blood gases in the acute phase of myocardial infarction. Ann. Cardiol. Angiol. *36*:509, 1987.
669. Kloner, R. A., and Braunwald, E.: Effects of calcium antagonists on infarcting myocardium. Am. J. Cardiol. *59*:84B, 1987.
670. Held, P. H., Yusuf, S., and Furberg, C. D.: Calcium channel blockers in acute myocardial infarction and unstable angina: an overview. Br. Med. J. *299*:1187, 1989.
671. Mantle, J. A., Rogers, W. J., McDaniel, H. G., et al.: Metabolic support of mechanical performance in myocardial infarction in man—a randomized clinical trial of glucose-insulin-potassium. Am. J. Cardiol. *43*:395, 1979.
672. Rogers, W. J., Segall, P. H., McDaniel, H. G., et al.: Prospective randomized trial of glucose-insulin-potassium in acute myocardial infarction. Am. J. Cardiol. *43*:801, 1979.
673. Heng, M. K., Norris, R. M., Singh, B. N., and Barratt-Boyes, C.: Effects of glucose and glucose-insulin-potassium on haemodynamics and enzyme release after acute myocardial infarction. Br. Heart J. *39*:748, 1977.
674. Powell, W. J., Jr., Daggett, W. M., Magro, A. E., et al.: Effects of intra-aortic balloon counterpulsation on cardiac performance, oxygen consumption, and coronary blood flow in dogs. Circ. Res. *26*:753, 1970.
675. Leinbach, R. C., Gold, H. K., Harper, R. W., et al.: Early intraaortic balloon pumping for anterior myocardial infarction without shock. Circulation *58*:204, 1978.
676. Flaherty, J. T., Becker, L. C., Weiss, J. L., et al.: Results of a randomized prospective trial of intraaortic balloon counterpulsation and intravenous nitroglycerin in patients with acute myocardial infarction. J. Am. Coll. Cardiol. *6*:434, 1985.
677. Alderman, J. D., Gabliani, G. I., McCabe, C. H., et al.: Incidence and management of limp ischemia with percutaneous wire-guided intraaortic balloon catheters. J. Am. Coll. Cardiol. *9*:524, 1987.
678. Werns, S. W., Shea, M. J., Driscoll, E. M., et al.: The independent effects of oxygen radical scavengers on canine infarct size reduction by superoxide dismutase but not catalase. Circ. Res. *56*:895, 1985.
679. Myers, M. L., Bolli, R., Lekich, R. F., et al.: Enhancement of recovery of myocardial function by oxygen free-radical scavengers after reversible regional ischemia. Circulation *72*:915, 1985.
680. Shechter, M., Hod, H., Marks, N., et al.: Beneficial effects of magnesium sulfate in acute myocardial infarction. Am. J. Cardiol. *66*:271, 1990.

ARRHYTHMIAS

681. Meltzer, L. E., and Cohen, H. E.: The incidence of arrhythmias associated with acute myocardial infarction. *In* Meltzer, L. E., and Dunning, A. J. (eds.): Textbook of Coronary Care. Philadelphia, Charles Press, 1972.
682. Pantridge, J. F., and Adgey, A.A.J.: Pre-hospital coronary care. The mobile coronary care unit. Am. J. Cardiol. *24*:666, 1969.
683. Hinkel, L. E., Jr., Carver, S. T., and Stevens, M.: The frequency of asymptomatic disturbances of cardiac rhythm and conduction in middle-aged men. Am. J. Cardiol. *24*:629, 1969.
684. Bloor, C. M., Ehsani, A., White, F. C., and Sobel, B. E.: Ventricular fibrillation threshold in acute myocardial infarction and its relation to myocardial infarct size. Cardiovasc. Res. *9*:468, 1975.
685. Roque, F., Amuchastegui, L. M., Lopez Morillos, M. A., et al.: Beneficial effects of timolol on infarct size and late ventricular tachycardia in patients with myocardial infarction. Circulation *76*:610, 1987.
686. Corr, P. B., and Gillis, R. A.: Autonomic neural influences on the dysrhythmias resulting from myocardial infarction. Circ. Res. *43*:1, 1978.
687. Barber, M. J., Mueller, T. M., Davies, B. G., et al.: Interruption of sympathetic and vagal-mediated afferent responses by transmural myocardial infarction. Circulation *72*:623, 1985.
688. Lassers, B. E., Anderton, J. L., George, M., et al.: Hemodynamic effects of artificial pacing in complete heart block complicating acute myocardial infarction. Circulation *38*:308, 1968.
689. Ruskin, J., McHale, P. A., Harley, A., and Greenfield, J. C., Jr.: Pressure-flow studies in man; effects of atrial systole on left ventricular function. J. Clin. Invest. *49*:472, 1970.
690. Rahimtoola, S. H., Ehsani, A., Sinno, M. Z., et al.: Left atrial transport function in myocardial infarction: Importance of its booster function. Am. J. Med. *59*:686, 1975.
691. Adgey, A.A.J., Alley, J. D., Geddes, J. S., et al.: Acute phase of myocardial infarction. Lancet *2*:501, 1971.
692. Graner, L. E., Gershen, B. J., Orlando, M. M., and Epstein, S. E.: Bradycardia and its complications in the pre-hospital phase of acute myocardial infarction. Am. J. Cardiol *32*:607, 1973.
693. Mark, A. L.: The Bezold-Jarisch reflex revisited: Clinical implications of inhibitory reflexes originating in the heart. J. Am. Coll. Cardiol. *1*:90, 1983.
694. Topol, E. J., Goldschlager, N., Ports, T. A., et al.: Hemodynamic benefit of atrial pacing in right ventricular myocardial infarction. Ann. Intern. Med. *96*:594, 1982.
695. Damato, A. N., and Lau, S. H.: Clinical value of the electrogram of the conduction system. Prog. Cardiovasc. Dis. *13*:119, 1970.
696. Rotman, M., Wagner, G. S., and Wallace, A.G.P.: Bradyarrhythmias in acute myocardial infarction. Circulation *45*:703, 1972.
697. Norris, R. M., and Mercer, C. J.: Significance of idioventricular rhythms in acute myocardial infarction. Prog. Cardiovasc. Dis. *16*:455, 1974.
698. Fisch, G. R., Zipes, D. P., and Fisch, C.: Bundle branch block and sudden death. Prog. Cardiovasc. Dis. *23*:187, 1980.
699. Bilbao, F. J., Zabalza, I. E., Vilanova, J. R., and Froupe, J.: Atrioventricular block in posterior acute myocardial infarction. A clinicopathologic correlation. Circulation *75*:733, 1987.
700. Mavric, Z., Zaputovic, L., Matana, A., et al.: Prognostic significance of complete atrioventricular block in patients with acute inferior myocardial infarction with and without right ventricular involvement. Am. Heart J. *119*:823, 1990.
701. Kostuk, W. J., and Beanlands, D. S.: Complete heart block associated with acute myocardial infarction. Am. J. Cardiol. *26*:380, 1970.
702. Bassan, R., Maia, I. G., Bozza, A., Amino, J.G.C., and Santos, M.: Atrioventricular block in acute inferior wall myocardial infarction: Harbinger of associated obstruction of the left anterior descending coronary artery. J. Am. Coll. Cardiol. *8*:773, 1986.
703. Sagiura, T., Iwasaka, T., Takahashi, N., et al.: Factors associated with late onset of advanced atrioventricular block in acute Q wave inferior infarction. Am. Heart J. *119*:1008, 1990.
704. Berger, P. B., and Ryan, T. J.: Inferior myocardial infarction. High-risk subgroups. Circulation *81*:401, 1990.
705. Nicod, P., Gilpin, E., Dittrich, H., et al.: Long-term outcome in patients with inferior myocardial infarction and complete atrioventricular block. J. Am. Coll. Cardiol. *12*:589, 1988.
706. Hindman, M. C., Wagner, G. S., JaRo, M., et al.: The clinical significance of bundle branch block complicating acute myocardial infarction. 2. Indications for temporary and permanent pacemaker insertion. Circulation *58*:689, 1978.
707. Feigl, D., Ashkenazy, J., and Kishon, Y.: Early and late atrioventricular block in acute inferior myocardial infarction. J. Am. Coll. Cardiol. *4*:35, 1984.
708. Mullins, C. B., and Atkins, J. M.: Prognoses and management of ventricular conduction blocks in acute myocardial infarction. Mod. Concepts Cardiovasc. Dis. *45*:129, 1976.
709. Scheinman, M. M., and Gonzalez, R. P.: Fascicular block and acute myocardial infarction. JAMA *244*:2646, 1980.

710. Hindman, M. C., Wagner, G. S., JaRo, M., et al.: The clinical significance of bundle branch block complicating acute myocardial infarction. I. Clinical characteristics, hospital mortality and one-year follow-up. Circulation *58*:679, 1978.
711. Dubois, C., Pierard, L. A., Smeets, J.-P., et al.: Short- and long-term prognostic importance of complete bundle-branch complicating acute myocardial infarction. Clin. Cardiol. *11*:292, 1988.
712. Lamas, G. A., Muller, J. E., Turi, Z. G., et al.: A simplified method to predict occurrence of complete heart block during acute myocardial infarction. Am. J. Cardiol. *57*:1213, 1986.
713. Hynes, J. K., Holmes, D. R., Jr., and Harrison, C. E.: Five-year experience with temporary pacemaker therapy in the coronary care unit. Mayo Clin. Proc. *58*:122, 1983.
714. Zoll, P.: Resuscitation of the heart in ventricular standstill by external electrical stimulation. N. Engl. J. Med. *247*:768, 1952.
715. Zoll, P. M., Zoll, R. H., Falk, R. H., et al.: External noninvasive temporary cardiac pacing: Clinical trials. Circulation *71*:937, 1985.
716. Frye, R. L., Collins, J. J., DeSanctis, R. W., et al.: Guidelines for permanent cardiac pacemaker implantation. J. Am. Coll. Cardiol. *4*:434, 1984.
717. ACC/AHA Task Force on Assessment of Diagnostic and Therapeutic Cardiovascular Procedures (Subcommittee on Pacemaker Implantation): Guidelines for permanent cardiac pacemaker implantation. J. Am. Coll. Cardiol. 4:434, 1984.
718. Ginks, W. R., Sutton, R., Oh, W., and Leatham, A.: Long-term prognosis after acute inferior infarction with atrioventricular block. Br. Heart J. *39*:186, 1977.
719. Wilson, C., and Adgey, A.A.J.: Survival of patients with late ventricular fibrillation after acute myocardial infarction. Lancet *2*:214, 1974.
720. DeSanctis, R. W., Block, P., and Hutter, A. M.: Tachyarrhythmias in myocardial infarction. Circulation 45:681, 1972.
721. Berisso, M. Z., Carratino, L., Ferroni, A., et al.: Frequency, characteristics and significance of supraventricular tachyarrhythmias detected by 24-hour electrocardiographic recording in the late hospital phase of acute myocardial infarction. Am. J. Cardiol. *65*:1064, 1990.
722. Gordon, S., Finck, D. R., Perera, R. D., Levine, J., and Barnes, S. J.: Atrial infarction complicating an acute inferior myocardial infarction. Arch. Intern. Med. *144*:193, 1984.
723. James, T. N.: Myocardial infarction and atrial arrhythmias. Circulation *24*:761, 1961.
724. Hod, H., Lew, A. S., Keltai, M., et al.: Early atrial fibrillation during evolving myocardial infarction: A consequence of impaired left atrial perfusion. Circulation 75:146, 1987.
725. Goldberg, R. J., Seeley, D., Becker, R. C., et al.: Impact of atrial fibrillation on the in-hospital and long-term survival of patients with acute myocardial infarction: a community-wide perspective. Am. Heart J. *119*:996, 1990.
726. Kerber, R. E., Jensen, S. R., Grayzel, J., et al.: Elective cardioversion: Influence of paddle-electrode location and size on success rates and energy requirements. N. Engl. J. Med. *305*:658, 1981.
727. Konecke, L. L., and Knoebel, S. B.: Nonparoxysmal junctional tachycardia complicating acute myocardial infarction. Circulation *45*:367, 1972.
728. Weinberg, B., and Zipes, D.: Strategies to manage the post-MI patient with ventricular arrhythmias. Clin. Cardiol. *12*(Suppl. III):86, 1989.
728a. Lee, K. J., Wellens, H.J.J., Dorsnar, E., and Durrer, D.: Observations on patients with primary ventricular fibrillation complicating acute myocardial infarction. Circulation *52*:755, 1975.
729. El-Sherif, N., Myerburg, R. J., Scherlag, B. J., et al.: Electrocardiographic antecedents of primary ventricular fibrillation. Value of the R-on-T phenomenon in myocardial infarction. Br. Heart J. *38*:415, 1976.
730. El-Sherif, N., Scherlag, B. J., and Lazzara, R.: Electrode catheter recordings during malignant ventricular arrhythmias following experimental acute myocardial ischemia. Evidence for reentry due to conduction delay and block in ischemic myocardium. Circulation *51*:1003, 1975.
731. DeSoyza, N., Meacham, D., Murphy, M. L., et al.: Evaluation of warning arrhythmias before paroxysmal ventricular tachycardia during acute myocardial infarction in man. Circulation *60*:814, 1979.
732. Campbell, R.W.F., Murray, A., and Julian, D. G.: Relation of ventricular arrhythmias to ventricular fibrillation. Br. Heart J. *43*:109, 1980.
733. Koster, R. W., and Dunning, J.: Intramuscular lidocaine for prevention of lethal arrhythmias in the prehospitalization phase of acute myocardial infarction. N. Engl. J. Med. *313*:1105, 1985.
734. Josephson, M. E.: Treatment of ventricular arrhythmias after myocardial infarction. Circulation *74*:653, 1986.
735. Lie, K. I., Wellens, H. J., and Van Capelli, F. J.: Lidocaine in the prevention of primary ventricular fibrillation. A double-blind randomized study of 212 consecutive patients. N. Engl. J. Med. *291*:1324, 1974.
736. DeSilva, R. E., Hennekens, C. H., Lown, B., and Casscells, S. W.: Lidocaine prophylaxis in acute myocardial infarction: An evaluation of methodology. Lancet *1*:855, 1981.
737. Dunn, H. M., McComb, J. M., Kinney, C. D., et al.: Prophylactic lidocaine in the early phase of suspected myocardial infarction. Am. Heart J. *110*:353, 1985.
738. May, G. S., Furberg, C. D., Eberlein, K. A., and Geraci, B. J.: Secondary prevention after myocardial infarction. A review of short-term acute phase trials. Prog. Cardiovasc. Dis. *25*:335, 1983.
739. Wyse, D. G., Kellen, J., and Rademaker, A. W.: Prophylactic versus selective lidocaine for early ventricular arrhythmias of myocardial infarction. J. Am. Coll. Cardiol. *12*:507, 1988.
740. Hine, L. K., Laird, N., Hewitt, P., and Chalmers, T. C.: Meta-analytic evidence against prophylactic use of lidocaine in acute myocardial infarction. Arch. Intern. Med. *149*:2694, 1989.
741. Mehra, R., Zeiler, R. H., Gough, W. B., and El-Sherif, N.: Reentrant ventricular arrhythmias in the later myocardial infarction period. 9. Electrophysiologic-anatomic correlation of reentrant circuits. Circulation *67*:11, 1983.
742. Lopez, L. M., Mehta, J. L., Robinson, J. D., and Roberts, R. J.: Optimal lidocaine dosing in patients with myocardial infarction. Therap. Drug Monitoring *4*:271, 1982.
743. Feely, J., Wade, D., McAllister, C. B., et al.: Effect of hypotension on liver blood flow and lidocaine disposition. N. Engl. J. Med. *307*:866, 1982.
744. LeLorier, J., Grenon, D., Latour, Y., et al.: Pharmacokinetics of lidocaine after prolonged intravenous infusions in uncomplicated myocardial infarction. Ann. Intern. Med. *87*:700, 1977.
745. Kessler, K. M., Kayden, D. S., Estes, D. M., et al.: Procainamide pharmacokinetics in patients with acute myocardial infarction or congestive heart failure. J. Am. Coll. Cardiol. *7*:1131, 1986.
746. Keefe, D. L., Williams, S., Torres, V., et al.: Prophylactic tocainide or lidocaine in acute myocardial infarction. Am. J. Cardiol. *57*:527, 1986.
747. Rehnqvist, N., Ericsson, G. G., Ericsson, S., et al.: Comparative investigation of the antiarrhythmic effect of propafenone and lidocaine in patients with ventricular arrhythmias during acute myocardial infarction. Acta Med. Scand. *216*:525, 1984.
748. Lown, B., and Wolf, M.: Approaches to sudden death from coronary heart disease. Circulation *44*:130, 1971.
749. Wenger, T. L., Bigger, J. T., Jr., and Merrill, G. S.: Ventricular arrhythmias in the late hospital phase of acute myocardial infarction. Circulation *52*:110, 1975.
750. Moss, A. J., De Camilla, J. J., Davis, H. P., and Bayer, L.: Clinical significance of ventricular ectopic beats in the early post-hospital phase of myocardial infarction. Am. J. Cardiol. *39*:635, 1977.
751. Mukharji, J., and MILIS Study Group: Risk factors for sudden death after acute myocardial infarction. Am. J. Cardiol. *54*:31, 1984.
752. The Cardiac Arrhythmia Suppression Trial (CAST) Investigators: Preliminary report: effect on encainide and flecainide on mortality in a randomized trial of arrhythmia suppression after myocardial infarction. N. Engl. J. Med. *321*:405, 1989.
753. Ruskin, J. N.: The cardiac arrhythmia suppression trial (CAST). N. Engl. J. Med. *321*:386, 1989.
754. Pratt, C. M., and Moye, L. A.: The cardiac arrhythmia suppression trial: background, interim results and implications. Am. J. Cardiol. *65*:20B, 1990.
755. Task Force of the Working Group on Arrhythmias of the European Society of Cardiology: CAST and beyond: implications of the cardiac arrhythmia suppression trial. Circulation *81*:1123, 1990.
756. Sclarovsky, S., Strasberg, B., Martonovich, G., and Agmon, J.: Ventricular rhythms with intermediate rates in acute myocardial infarction. Chest *74*:180, 1978.
757. Bigger, J. T., Jr., Dresdale, R. J., Heissenbuttel, R. H., et al.: Ventricular arrhythmias in ischemic heart disease: Mechanism, prevalence, significance, and management. Prog. Cardiovasc. Dis. *19*:255, 1977.
758. Lucente, M., Rebuzzi, A. G., Lanza, G. A., et al.: Circadian variation of ventricular tachycardia in acute myocardial infarction. Am. J. Cardiol. *62*:670, 1988.
759. Kleiman, R. B., Miller, J. M., Buxton, A. E., et al.: Prognosis following sustained ventricular tachycardia occurring early after myocardial infarction. Am. J. Cardiol. *62*:528, 1988.
759a. El-Sherif, N., Gough, W. B., and Restivo, M.: Reentrant ventricular arrhythmias in the late myocardial infarction period: Mechanism by which a short-long-short cardiac sequence facilitates the induction of reentry. Circulation *83*:268, 1991.
760. Bigger, J. T., Jr., Weld, F. M., and Rolnitzky, L. M.: Prevalence, characteristics and significance of ventricular tachycardia (three or more complexes) detected with ambulatory electrocardiographic recording in the late hospital phase of acute myocardial infarction. Am. J. Cardiol. *48*:815, 1981.
761. Nordehaug, J. E., Johannessen, K. A., and von der Lippe, G.: Serum potassium concentration as a risk factor of ventricular arrhythmias early in acute myocardial infarction. Circulation *71*:645, 1985.
762. Wald, R. W., Waxman, M. B., Corey, P. N., et al.: Management of intractable ventricular tachyarrhythmias after myocardial infarction. Am. J. Cardiol. *44*:329, 1979.
763. Guiraudon, G., Fontaine, G., Frank, R., et al.: Encircling endocardial ventriculotomy: A new surgical treatment for life-threatening tachycardias resistant to medical treatment following myocardial infarction. Ann. Thorac. Surg. *26*:438, 1978.
764. Bourke, J. P., Hilton, C. J., McComb, J. M., et al.: Surgery for control of recurrent life-threatening ventricular tachyarrhythmias within 2 months of myocardial infarction. J Am. Coll. Cardiol. *16*:42, 1990.
765. Schwartz, P. J., Zaza, A., Grazi, S., et al.: Effect of ventricular fibrillation complicating acute myocardial infarction on long-term prognosis: importance of the site of infarction. Am. J. Cardiol. *56*:384, 1985.
766. Jensen, G.V.H., Torp-Pedersen, C., Kober, L., et al: Prognosis of late versus early ventricular fibrillation in acute myocardial infarction. Am. J. Cardiol. *66*:10, 1990.
767. Lie, K. I., Liem, K. L., Schuilenburg, R. M., et al.: Early identification of patients developing late in-hospital ventricular fibrillation after discharge from the coronary care unit. Am. J. Cardiol. *41*:674, 1978.
768. Sclarovsky, S., Zafrir, N., Strasberg, B., et al.: Ventricular fibrillation complicating temporary ventricular pacing in acute myocardial in-

farction: significance of right ventricular infarction. Am. J. Cardiol. *48*:1160, 1981.

769. Toffler, G. H., Stone, P. H., Muller, J. E., et al.: Prognosis after myocardial infarction complicated by ventricular fibrillation. Circulation *74*(Suppl. II):304, 1986.
770. Volpi, A., Cavalli, A., Franzosi, M. G., et al.: One-year prognosis of primary ventricular fibrillation complicating acute myocardial infarction. Am. J. Cardiol. *63*:1174, 1989.
771. Ryden, L., Ariniego, R., Arnman, K., et al.: A double-blind trial of metoprolol in acute myocardial infarction. Effects on ventricular tachyarrhythmias. N. Engl. J. Med. *308*:614, 1983.
772. Ehsani, A., Ewy, G. A., and Sobel, B. E.: Effects of electrical countershock on serum creatine phosphokinase (CPK) isoenzyme activity. Am. J. Cardiol. *37*:12, 1976.
773. Abboud, F. M., Pansegrau, D. G., and Mark, A. L.: Autonomic responses to ventricular defibrillation. *In* Proceedings, Cardiac Defibrillation Conference, Purdue University, West Lafayette, Ind., 1975.
774. Heissenbuttel, R. H., and Bigger, J. T., Jr.: Bretylium tosylate, a newly available antiarrhythmic drug for ventricular arrhythmias. Ann. Intern. Med. *91*:229, 1979.
775. Bellotto, F., Forman, R., and Buja, G.: Electromechanical dissociation in the acute myocardial infarction. A review of the literature shows the need for a codified definition. J. Electrophys. *2*:517, 1988.
776. Charlap, S., Kahlam, S., Lichstein, E., and Frishman, W.: Electromechanical dissociation: diagnosis, pathophysiology, and management. Am. Heart J. *118*:355, 1989.

HEMODYNAMIC DISTURBANCES

777. Forrester, J. S., Diamond, G., Chatterjee, K., and Swan, H.J.C.: Medical therapy of acute myocardial infarction by application of hemodynamic subsets. N. Engl. J. Med. *295*:1356, 1976.
777a. Noble, R. J.: Myocardial infarction with hypotension. Chest *99*:1012, 1991.
778. Dwyer, E. M., Greenberg, H. M., Steinberg, G., and the Multicenter Postinfarction Research Group: Clinical characteristics and natural history of survivors of pulmonary congestion during acute myocardial infarction. Am. J. Cardiol. *63*:1423, 1989.
779. Coma-Canella, I., Lopez-Sendon, J., and Gamallo, C.: Low output syndrome in right ventricular infarction. Am. Heart J. *98*:613, 1979.
780. Page, D. L., Caulfield, J. B., Kastor, J. A., et al.: Myocardial changes associated with cardiogenic shock. N. Engl. J. Med. *285*:133, 1971.
781. Alonso, D. R., Scheidt, S., Post, M., and Killip, T.: Pathophysiology of cardiogenic shock; quantification of myocardial necrosis, clinical, pathologic and electrocardiographic correlation. Circulation *48*:588, 1973.
782. Wackers, F. J., Lie, K. I., Becker, A. E., et al.: Coronary artery disease in patients dying from cardiogenic shock or congestive heart failure in the setting of acute myocardial infarction. Br. Heart J. *38*:906, 1976.
783. Hands, M. E., Rutherford, J. D., Muller, J. E., et al.: The in-hospital development of cardiogenic shock after myocardial infarction: Incidence, predictors of occurrence, outcome and prognostic factors. J. Am. Coll. Cardiol. *14*:40, 1989.
784. Gunnar, R. M.: Cardiogenic shock complicating acute myocardial infarction. Circulation *78*:1508, 1988.
785. Killip, T.: Cardiogenic shock complicating myocardial infarction. J. Am. Coll. Cardiol. *14*:47, 1989.
786. Rasanen, J., Nikki, O. P., and Heikkila, J.: Acute myocardial infarction complicated by respiratory failure. The effects of mechanical ventilation. Chest *85*:21, 1984.
787. Roth, A., Hochenberg, M., Keren, G., et al.: Are rotating tourniquets useful for left ventricular preload reduction in patients with acute myocardial infarction and heart failure? Ann. Emer. Med. *16*:764, 1987.
788. Cohn, J. N., Franciosa, J. A., Francis, G. S., et al.: Effect of short-term infusion on sodium nitroprusside in mortality rate in acute myocardial infarction complicated by left ventricular failure. Results of a Veterans Administration Cooperative Study. N. Engl. J. Med. *306*:1129, 1982.
789. Passamani, E. R.: Nitroprusside in myocardial infarction. N. Engl. J. Med. *306*:1168, 1982.
790. Chiariello, M., Gold, H. K., Leinbach, R. C., et al.: Comparison between the effects of nitroprusside and nitroglycerin on ischemic injury during acute myocardial infarction. Circulation *54*:766, 1976.
791. Flaherty, J. T.: Intravenous nitroglycerin. Johns Hopkins Med. J. *151*:36, 1982.
792. Rabinowitz, B., Tamari, I., Elazar, E., and Neufeld, H. N.: Intravenous isosorbide dinitrate in patients with refractory pump failure and acute myocardial infarction. Circulation *65*:771, 1982.
793. Franciosa, J. A., Mikulic, E., Cohn, J. N., et al.: Hemodynamic effects of orally administered isosorbide dinitrate in patients with congestive heart failure. Circulation *50*:1020, 1974.
794. Cohn, J. N.: Editorial—Progress in vasodilator therapy for heart failure. N. Engl. J. Med. *302*:1414, 1980.
795. Franciosa, J. A., Guiha, N. H., Limas, C. J., et al.: Improved left ventricular function during nitroprusside infusion in acute myocardial infarction. Lancet *1*:650, 1972.
796. Covell, J. W., Braunwald, E., Ross, J., Jr., and Sonnenblick, E. H.: Studies on digitalis. XVI. Effects on myocardial oxygen consumption. J. Clin. Invest. *45*:1535, 1966.
797. Ross, J., Jr., Waldhausen, J. S., and Braunwald, E.: Studies on digitalis. I. Direct effects on peripheral vascular resistance. J. Clin. Invest. *39*:930, 1960.
798. Marchionni, N., Pini, R., Vannucci, A., et al.: Hemodynamic effects of digoxin in acute myocardial infarction in man: A randomized controlled trial. Am. Heart J. *109*:63, 1985.
799. Moss, A. J., Davis, H. T., Conrad, D. L., et al.: Digitalis-associated cardiac mortality after myocardial infarction. Circulation *64*:1150, 1981.
800. Muller, J. E., Turi, Z. G., Stone, P. H., et al.: Digoxin therapy and mortality after myocardial infarction. Experience in the MILIS study. N. Engl. J. Med. *314*:265, 1986.
801. Bigger, J. T., Jr., Fleiss, J. L., Rolnitzky, L. M., et al.: Effects of digitalis treatment on survival after acute myocardial infarction. Am. J. Cardiol. *55*:623, 1985.
802. Mueller, H., Ayres, S. M., Giannelli, S., Jr., et al.: Effect of isoproterenol, L-norepinephrine, and intra-aortic counterpulsation on hemodynamics and myocardial metabolism in shock following acute myocardial infarction. Circulation *45*:335, 1972.
803. Shell, W. E., and Sobel B. E.: Deleterious effects of increased heart rate on infarct size in the conscious dog. Am. J. Cardiol. *31*:474, 1973.
804. Ichard, C., Ricome, J. L., Rimailho, A., et al.: Combined hemodynamic effects of dopamine and dobutamine in cardiogenic shock. Circulation *67*:620, 1983.
805. Holzer, J., Karliner, J. S., O'Rourke, R. A., et al.: Effectiveness of dopamine in patients with cardiogenic shock. Am. J. Cardiol. *32*:79, 1973.
806. Arnold, J.M.O., Braunwald, E., Sandor, T., and Kloner, R. A.: Inotropic stimulation of reperfused myocardium with dopamine: Effects on infarct size and myocardial function. J. Am. Coll. Cardiol. *6*:1026, 1985.
807. Tuttle, R. R., and Mills, J.: Development of a new catecholamine to selectively increase cardiac contractility. Circ. Res. *36*:185, 1975.
808. Maekawa, K., Liang, C-S., and Hood, W. B., Jr.: Comparison of dobutamine and dopamine in acute myocardial infarction. Effects of systemic hemodynamics, plasma catecholamines, blood flows and infarct size. Circulation *67*:750, 1983.
809. Mancini, D., LeJemtel, T., and Sonnenblick, E.: Intravenous use of amrinone for the treatment of the failing heart. Am. J. Cardiol. *56*:8B, 1985.
810. Taylor, S. H., Verma, S. P., Hussain, M., et al.: Intravenous amrinone in left ventricular failure complicated by acute myocardial infarction. Am. J. Cardiol. *56*:29B, 1985.
811. Verma, S. P., Silke, B., and Taylor, S. H.: Hemodynamic dose-response effects of amrinone in left ventricular failure complicating myocardial infarction. Br. J. Clin. Pharmacol. *19*:540P, 1985.
812. Colucci, W. S., Wright, R. F., and Braunwald, E.: New positive inotropic agents in the treatment of congestive heart failure. N. Engl. J. Med. *314*:349, 1986.
813. Mueller, H., Ayres, S. M., Gregory, J. J., et al.: Hemodynamics, coronary blood flow, and myocardial metabolism in coronary shock: Response to L-norepinephrine and isoproterenol. J. Clin. Invest. *49*:1885, 1970.
814. Lee, L., Bates, E. R., Pitt, B., et al.: Percutaneous transluminal coronary angioplasty improves survival in acute myocardial infarction complicated by cardiogenic shock. Circulation *78*:1345, 1988.
815. Sotolongo, R. P., Smith, M. L., and Margolis, W. S.: Coronary angioplasty in emergency treatment of myocardial infarction. Texas Heart Inst. J. *17*:31, 1990.
816. Lew, A., Weiss, A. T., Shah, P. K., et al.: Extensive myocardial salvage and reversal of cardiogenic shock after reperfusion of the left main coronary artery by intravenous streptokinase. Am. J. Cardiol. *54*:450, 1984.
817. Alosilla, C. E., Bell, W. W., Ferree, J., and De La Torre, A.: Thrombolytic therapy during acute myocardial infarction due to sudden occlusion of the left main coronary artery. J. Am. Coll. Cardiol. *5*:1253, 1985.
818. Corral, C. H., and Vaughn, C. C.: Intraaortic balloon counterpulsation: An eleven-year review and analysis of determinants of survival. Texas Heart Inst. J. *13*:39, 1986.
819. Mueller, H., Ayres, S. M., Conklin, E. F., et al.: The effects of intra-aortic counterpulsation on cardiac performance and metabolism in shock associated with acute myocardial infarction. J. Clin. Invest. *50*:1885, 1971.
820. Johnson, S. A., Scanlon, P. J., Loeb, H. S., et al.: Treatment of cardiogenic shock in myocardial infarction by intraaortic balloon counterpulsation and surgery. Am. J. Med. *62*:687, 1977.
821. O'Rourke, M. F., Norris, R. M., Campbell, T. J., et al.: Randomized controlled trial of intraaortic balloon counterpulsation in early myocardial infarction with acute heart failure. Am. J. Cardiol. *47*:815, 1981.
822. Goldberg, M. J., Rubenfire, M., Kantrowitz, A., et al.: Intraaortic balloon pump insertion: A randomized study comparing percutaneous and surgical techniques. J. Am. Coll. Cardiol. *9*:515, 1987.
823. Pae, W. E., Jr., and Pierce, W. S.: Temporary left ventricular assistance in acute myocardial infarction and cardiogenic shock. Rationale and criteria for utilization. Chest *79*:692, 1981.
824. Shawl, F. A., Domanski, M. J., Hernandez, T. J., and Punja, S.: Emergency percutaneous cardiopulmonary bypass support in cardiogenic shock from acute myocardial infarction. Am. J. Cardiol. *64*:967, 1989.
825. Gowda, S. K., Gillespie, T. A., Byrne, J. D., et al.: Effects of external counterpulsation on enzymatically estimated infarct size and ventricular arrhythmia. Br. Heart J. *40*:308, 1978.
826. Isner, J. M., Cohen, S. J., Viruari, R., et al.: Complications of the intra-aortic balloon counterpulsation device: Clinical and morphologic observations in 45 necropsy patients. Am. J. Cardiol *45*:250, 1980.
827. Goodwin, M., Hartmann, J., McKeever, L., et al.: Safety of intraaortic balloon counterpulsation in patients with acute myocardial infarction receiving streptokinase intravenously. Am. J. Cardiol. *64*:937, 1989.
828. Dell-Italia, L. J., Lembo, N. J., Starling, M. R., et al.: Hemodynamically important right ventricular infarction. Follow-up evaluation of right

ventricular systolic function at rest and during exercise with radionuclide ventriculography and respiratory gas exchange. Circulation 75:996, 1987.

829. Roberts, N., Harrision, D. G., Reimer, K. A., et al.: Right ventricular infarction with shock but without significant left ventricular infarction: A new clinical syndrome. Am. Heart J. 110:1047, 1985.

830. Forman, M. B., Goodin, J., Phelan, B., et al.: Electrocardiographic changes associated with isolated right ventricular infarction. J. Am. Coll. Cardiol. 4:640, 1984.

831. Bansal, R. C., Marsa, R. J., Holland, D., et al.: Severe hypoxemia due to shunting through a patent foramen ovale: A correctable complication of right ventricular infarction. J. Am. Coll. Cardiol. 5:188, 1985.

832. Robalino, B. D., Petrella, R. W., Jubran, F. Y., et al.: Atrial natriuretic factor in patients with right ventricular infarction. J. Am. Coll. Cardiol. 15:546, 1990.

833. Braat, S. H., Brugada, P., DeZwaan, C., et al.: Right and left ventricular ejection fraction in acute inferior wall infarction with or without ST segment elevation in lead V4R. J. Am. Coll. Cardiol. 4:940, 1984.

834. Lopez-Sendon, J., Garcia-Fernandez, M. A., Coma-Canella, I., et al.: Segmental right ventricular function after acute myocardial infarction: Two-dimensional echocardiographic study in 63 patients. Am. J. Cardiol. 51:390, 1983.

835. Arditti, A., Lewin, R. F., Hellman, C., et al.: Right ventricular dysfunction in acute inferoposterior myocardial infarction. An echocardiographic isotopic study. Chest 87:307, 1985.

836. Starling, M. R., Dell'italia, L. J., Chaudhuri, T. K., et al.: First transit and equilibrium radionuclide angiography in patients with inferior transmural myocardial infarction: Criteria for the diagnosis of associated hemodynamically significant right ventricular infarction. J. Am. Coll. Cardiol. 4:923, 1984.

837. Dell'italia, L. J., Starling, M. R., Crawford, M. H., et al.: Right ventricular infarction: Identification by hemodynamic measurements before and after volume loading and correlation with noninvasive techniques. J. Am. Coll. Cardiol. 4:931, 1984.

838. Yasuda, T., Okada, R. D., Leinbach, R. C., et al.: Serial evaluation of right ventricular dysfunction associated with acute inferior myocardial infarction. Am. Heart J. 119:816, 1990.

839. Matangi, M. F.: Temporary physiologic pacing in inferior wall acute myocardial infarction with right ventricular damage. Am. J. Cardiol. 59:1207, 1987.

840. Marmor, A., Geltman, E. M., Biello, D. R., et al.: Functional response to the right ventricle to myocardial infarction: Dependence on the site of left ventricular infarction. Circulation 64:1005, 1981.

841. Lorell, B., Leinbach, R. C., Pohost, G. M., et al.: Right ventricular infarction. Clinical diagnosis and differentiation from cardiac tamponade and pericardial constriction. Am. J. Cardiol. 43:465, 1979.

842. Korr, K. S., Lewvinson, H., Bough, E. W., et al.: Tricuspid valve replacement for cardiogenic shock after acute right ventricular infarction. JAMA 244:1958, 1980.

843. Pohjola-Sintonen, S., Muller, J. E., Stone, P. H., et al.: Ventricular septal and free wall rupture complicating acute myocardial infarction: Experience in the Multicenter Investigation of Limitation of Infarct Size. Am. Heart J. 117:809, 1989.

844. Reddy, S. G., and Roberts, W. C.: Frequency of rupture of the left ventricular free wall or ventricular septum among necropsy cases of fatal acute myocardial infarction since introduction of coronary care units. Am. J. Cardiol. 63:906, 1989.

845. Shapira, I., Isakov, A., Burke, M., and Almong, C. H.: Cardiac rupture in patients with acute myocardial infarction. Chest 92:219, 1987.

845a. Pappas, P. J., Cernaianu, A. C., Baldino, W. A., et al.: Ventricular free-wall rupture after myocardial infarction. Chest 99:892, 1991.

846. Silverman, H. S., and Pfeifer, M. P.: Relation between use of anti-inflammatory agents and left ventricular free wall rupture during acute myocardial infarction. Am. J. Cardiol. 59:363, 1987.

847. Bulkley, B. H., and Roberts, W. C.: Steroid therapy during acute myocardial infarction: A cause of delayed healing and of ventricular aneurism. Am. J. Med. 56:244, 1974.

848. Gertz, S. D., Kragel, A. H., Kalan, J. M., et al.: Comparison of coronary and myocardial morphologic findings in patients with and without thrombolytic therapy during fatal first acute myocardial infarction. Am. J. Cardiol. 66:904, 1990.

849. Honan, M. B., Harrell, F. E., Reimer, K. A., et al.: Cardiac rupture, mortality and the timing of thrombolytic therapy: a meta-analysis. J. Am. Coll. Cardiol. 16:359, 1990.

850. Edmondson, H. A., and Hoxie, H. J.: Hypertension and cardiac rupture: Clinical and pathological study of 72 cases, in 13 of which rupture of the interventricular septum occurred. Am. Heart J. 24:719, 1942.

851. London, R. E., and London, S. B.: Rupture of the heart. A critical analysis of 47 consecutive autopsy cases. Circulation 31:202, 1965.

852. Kassis, E., Vogelsang, M., and Lyngoborg, K.: Cardiac rupture complicating myocardial infarction. A study concerning early diagnosis and possible management. Dan. Med. Bull. 48:164, 1981.

853. Mann, J. M., and Roberts, W. C.: Rupture of the left ventricular free wall during acute myocardial infarction: Analysis of 138 necropsy patients and comparison with 50 necropsy patients with acute myocardial infarction without rupture. Am. J. Cardiol. 62:847, 1988.

854. Balakumaran, K., Verbaan, C. J., Essed, C. E., et al.: Ventricular free wall rupture: sudden, subacute, slow, sealed and stabilized varieties. Eur. Heart J. 5:282, 1984.

855. Coma-Canella, I., Lopez-Sendon, J., Gonzalez, L. N., and Ferrufino, O.: Subacute left ventricular free wall rupture following acute myocardial infarction: Bedside hemodynamics, differential diagnosis, and treatment. Am. Heart J. 106:278, 1983.

856. Pifarre, R., Sullivan, H. J., Grieco, J., et al.: Management of left ventricular rupture complicating myocardial infarction. J. Thorac. Cardiovasc. Surg. 86:441, 1983.

857. McMullan, M. H., Kilgore, T. L., Dear, H. D., and Hindman, S. H.: Sudden blowout rupture of the myocardium after infarction: Urgent management. J. Thorac. Cardiovasc. Surg. 89:259, 1985.

858. Vlodaver, Z., Coe, J. L., and Edwards, J. E.: True and false left ventricular aneurysms. Circulation 51:567, 1975.

858a. Lascault, G., Reeves, F., and Drobinski, G.: Evidence of the inaccuracy of standard echocardiographic and angiographic criteria used for the recognition of true and "false" left ventricular inferior aneurysms. Br. Heart J. 60:125, 1988.

859. Shabbo, F. P., Dymond, D. S., Rees, G. M., and Hill, I. M.: Surgical treatment of false aneurysm of the left ventricle after myocardial infarction. Thorax 38:25, 1983.

860. Radford, M. J., Johnson, R. A., Daggett, W. M., et al.: Ventricular septal rupture: A review of clinical and physiologic features and an analysis of survival. Circulation 64:545, 1981.

861. Edwards, B. S., Edwards, W. D., and Edwards, J. E.: Ventricular septal rupture complicating acute myocardial infarction: Identification of simple and complex types in 53 autopsied hearts. Am. J. Cardiol. 54:1201, 1984.

862. Mann, J. M., and Roberts, W. C.: Acquired ventricular septal defect during acute myocardial infarction: analysis of 38 unoperated necropsy patients and comparison with 50 unoperated necropsy patients without rupture. Am. J. Cardiol. 62:8, 1988.

863. Moore, C. A., Nygaard, T. W., Kaiser, D. L., et al.: Postinfarction ventricular septal rupture: the importance of location of infarction and right ventricular function in determining survival. Circulation 74:45, 1986.

864. Cummings, R. G., Reimer, K. A., Califf, R., et al.: Quantitative analysis of right and left ventricular infarction in the presence of postinfarction ventricular septal defect. Circulation 77:33, 1988.

865. Bansal, R. C., Eng, A. K., and Shakudo, M.: Role of two-dimensional echocardiography, pulsed, continuous wave and color flow Doppler techniques in the assessment of ventricular septal rupture after myocardial infarction. Am. J. Cardiol. 65:852, 1990.

866. Helmcke, F., Mahan, E. F., Nanda, N. C., et al.: Two-dimensional echocardiography and Doppler color flow mapping in the diagnosis and prognosis of ventricular septal rupture. Circulation 81:1775, 1990.

866a. Fortin, D. F., Sheikh, K. H., and Kisslo, J.: The utility of echocardiography in the diagnostic strategy of postinfarction ventricular septal rupture: A comparison of two-dimensional echocardiography versus Doppler color flow imaging. Am. Heart J. 121:25, 1991.

867. Lock, J. E., Block, P. C., McKay, R. G., et al.: Transcatheterization closure of ventricular septal defects. Circulation 78:361, 1988.

868. Nishimura, R. A., Schaff, H. V., Shub, C., et al.: Papillary muscle rupture complicating acute myocardial infarction: Analysis of 17 patients. Am. J. Cardiol. 51:373, 1983.

869. Barbour, D. J., and Roberts, W. C.: Rupture of a left ventricular papillary muscle during acute myocardial infarction: Analysis of 22 necropsy patients. J. Am. Coll. Cardiol. 8:588, 1986.

870. Coma-Canella, I., Gamallo, C., Onsurbe, P. M., and Jadraque, L. M.: Anatomic findings in acute papillary muscle necrosis. Am. Heart J. 118:1188, 1989.

871. Lader, E., Colvin, S., and Tunick, P.: Myocardial infarction complicated by rupture of both ventricular septum and right ventricular papillary muscle. Am. J. Cardiol. 52:424, 1983.

872. Come, P. C., Riley, M. F., Weintraub, R., et al.: Echocardiographic detection of complete and partial papillary muscle rupture during acute myocardial infarction. Am. J. Cardiol. 56:787, 1985.

873. Harrison, M. R., MacPhail, B., Gurley, J. C., et al.: Usefulness of color Doppler flow imaging to distinguish ventricular septal defect from acute mitral regurgitation complicating myocardial infarction. Am. J. Cardiol. 64:697, 1989.

874. Ballester, M., Tasca, R., Marin, L., et al.: Different mechanisms of mitral regurgitation in acute and chronic forms of coronary heart disease. Eur. Heart J. 4:557, 1983.

875. Meister, S. G., and Helfant, R. H.: Rapid bedside differentiation of ruptured interventricular septum from acute mitral insufficiency. N. Engl. J. Med. 287:1024, 1972.

876. Jones, M. T., Schofield, P. M., Dark, J. F., et al.: Surgical repair of acquired ventricular septal defects: Determinants of early and late outcome. J. Thorac. Cardiovasc. Surg. 93:680, 1987.

877. Miller, D. C., and Stinson, E. B.: Surgical management of acute mechanical defects secondary to myocardial infarction. Am. J. Surg. 141:677, 1981.

878. Held, A. C., Cole, P. L., Lipton, B., et al.: Rupture of the interventricular septum complicating acute myocardial infarction: a multicenter analysis of clinical findings and outcome. Am. Heart J. 116:1330, 1988.

879. Norell, M. S., Gershlick, A. H., Pillai, R., et al.: Ventricular septal rupture complicating myocardial infarction: Is earlier surgery justified? Eur. Heart J. 8:1281, 1987.

880. Abrams, D. L., Edelist, A., Luria, M. H., and Miller, A. J.: Ventricular aneurysm: A reappraisal based on a study of 65 consecutive autopsied cases. Circulation 27:164, 1963.

881. Faxon, D. P., Ryan, T. J., Davis, K. B., et al.: Prognostic significance of angiographically documented left ventricular aneurysm from the Coronary Artery Surgery Study (CASS). Am. J. Cardiol. 50:157, 1982.

882. Schlichter, J., Hellerstein, H. K., and Katz, L. N.: Aneurysm of the heart: A correlative study of 102 proved cases. Medicine 33:43, 1954.

883. Forman, M. D., Collins, H. W., Kipelman, H. A., et al.: Determinants of left ventricular aneurysm formation after anterior myocardial infarction: A clinical and angiographic study. J. Am. Coll. Cardiol. *8*:1256, 1986.
884. Hirai, T., Fujita, M., Nakajima, H., et al.: Importance of collateral circulation for prevention of left ventricular aneurysm formation in acute myocardial infarction. Circulation *79*:791, 1989.
885. Meizlish, J. L., Berger, H. J., Plankey, M., et al.: Functional left ventricular aneurysm formation after acute anterior transmural myocardial infarction: Incidence, natural history, and prognostic implications. N. Engl. J. Med. *311*:1001, 1984.
886. Lindsay, J., Jr., Dewey, R. C., Talesnick, B. S., and Nolan, N. G.: Relation of ST-segment elevation after healing of acute myocardial infarction to the presence of left ventricular aneurysm. Am. J. Cardiol. *54*:84, 1984.
887. Brawley, R. K., Magovern, G. J., Jr., Gott, V. L., et al.: Left ventricular aneurysmectomy. Factors influencing postoperative results. J. Thorac. Cardiovasc. Surg. *85*:712, 1983.
888. Visser, C. A., Kan, G., Lie, K. I., and Durrer, D.: Incidence and one-year follow-up of left ventricular thrombus following acute myocardial infarction: An echocardiographic study of 96 patients. J. Am. Coll. Cardiol. *1*:648, 1983.
889. Hellerstein, H. K., and Martin, J. W.: Incidence of thromboembolic lesions accompanying myocardial infarction. Am. Heart J. *33*:443, 1947.
890. Nihoyannopoulos, P., Smith, G. C., Maseri, A., and Foale, R. A.: The natural history of left ventricular thrombus in myocardial infarction: a rationale in support of masterly inactivity. J. Am. Coll. Cardiol. *14*:903, 1989.
891. Jugdutt, B. I., and Sivaram, C. A.: Prospective two-dimensional echocardiographic evaluation of left ventricular thrombus and embolism after acute myocardial infarction. J. Am. Coll. Cardiol. *13*:554, 1989.
892. Funke Kupper, A. J., Verheugt, F.W.A., Peels, C. H., et al.: Left ventricular thrombus incidence and behavior studied by serial two-dimensional echocardiography in acute anterior myocardial infarction: left ventricular wall motion, systemic wall motion, systemic embolism and oral anticoagulation. J. Am. Coll. Cardiol. *13*:1514, 1989.
893. Keren, A., Goldberg, S., Gottlieb, S., et al.: Natural history of left ventricular thrombi: their appearance and resolution in the posthospitalization period of acute myocardial infarction. J. Am. Coll. Cardiol. *15*:790, 1990.
894. Johannessen, K. A., Nordehaug, J. E., and von der Lippe, G.: Increased occurrence of left ventricular thrombi during early treatment with timolol in patients with acute myocardial infarction. Circulation *75*:151, 1987.
895. Gueret, P., Dubourg, O., Ferrier, A., et al.: Effects of full-dose heparin anticoagulation on the development of left ventricular thrombosis in acute transmural myocardial infarction. J. Am. Coll. Cardiol. *8*:419, 1986.
896. Sharma, B., Carvalho, A., Wyeth, R., and Franciosa, J. A.: Left ventricular thrombi diagnosed by echocardiography in patients with acute myocardial infarction treated with intracoronary streptokinase followed by intravenous heparin. Am. J. Cardiol. *56*:422, 1985.
897. Nordrehaug, J. E., Johannessen, K. A., and von der Lippe, G.: Usefulness of high-dose anticoagulants in preventing left ventricular thrombus in acute myocardial infarction. Am. J. Cardiol. *55*:1941, 1985.
898. Turpie, A.G.G., Robinson, J. G., Doyle, D. J., et al.: Comparison of high-dose with low-dose subcutaneous heparin to prevent left ventricular mural thrombosis in patients with acute transmural anterior myocardial infarction. N. Engl. J. Med. *320*:352, 1989.
899. Motro, M., Keren, G., Hod, H., et al.: Incidence of left ventricular thrombi formation after thrombolytic therapy with recombinant tissue plasminogen activator, heparin, and aspirin in patients with acute myocardial infarction. Am. J. Cardiol. *(in press)*.
900. Halperin, J. L., and Fuster, V.: Left ventricular thrombus and stroke after myocardial infarction: toward prevention or perplexity? J. Am. Coll. Cardiol. *14*:912, 1989.
901. Weintraub, W. S., and Ba'albaki, H. A.: Decision analysis concerning the application of echocardiography to the diagnosis and treatment of mural thrombi after anterior wall acute myocardial infarction. Am. J. Cardiol. *64*:708, 1989.
902. Stein, B., Fuster, V., Halperin, J. L., and Chesebro, J. H.: Antithrombotic therapy in cardiac disease. An emerging approach based on pathogenesis and risk. Circulation *80*:1501, 1989.
903. Kouvaras, G., Chronopoulos, G., Soufras, G., et al.: The effects of long-term antithrombotic treatment on left ventricular thrombi in patients after an acute myocardial infarction. Am. Heart J. *119*:73, 1990.
904. Kouvaras, G., Chronopoulos, G., Soufras, G., et al.: The effect of long-term antithrombotic treatment on left ventricular thrombi in patients after an acute myocardial infarction. Am. Heart J. *119*:73, 1990.
905. Halperin, J. L., and Fuster, V.: Left ventricular thrombi and cerebral embolism. N. Engl. J. Med. *320*:392, 1989.
906. Visser, C. A., Kan, G., Meltzer, R. S., et al.: Embolic potential of left ventricular thrombus after myocardial infarction: A two-dimensional echocardiographic study of 119 patients. J. Am. Coll. Cardiol. *5*:1276, 1985.
907. Stratton, J. R., and Ritchie, J. L.: The effects of antithrombotic drugs in patients with left ventricular thrombi: Assessment with indium-111 platelet imaging and two-dimensional echocardiography. Circulation *69*:561, 1984.
908. Kremer, P., Fiebig, R., Tilsner, V., et al.: Lysis of left ventricular thrombi with urokinase. Circulation *72*:112, 1985.
909. Eppinger, E. C., and Kennedy, J. A.: The cause of death in coronary thrombosis, with special reference to pulmonary embolism. Am. J. Med. Sci. *195*:104, 1938.
910. Stone, P., and Muller, J. E.: Nifedipine therapy for recurrent ischemic pain following myocardial infarction. Clin. Cardiol. *5*:223, 1982.
911. Koiwaya, Y., Torii, S., Takeshita, A., et al.: Postinfarction angina caused by coronary arterial spasm. Circulation *65*:275, 1982.
912. Bosch, X., Theroux, P., Waters, D. D., et al.: Early postinfarction ischemia: Clinical, angiographic, and prognostic significance. Circulation *75*:988, 1987.
913. Benhorin, J., Andrews, M. L., Carleen, E. D., et al.: Occurrence, characteristics, and prognostic significance of early postacute myocardial infarction angina pectoris. Am. J. Cardiol. *62*:679, 1988.
914. Epstein, S. E., Palmeri, S. T., and Patterson, R. E.: Evaluation of patients after acute myocardial infarction. Indications for cardiac catheterization and surgical intervention. N. Engl. J. Med. *307*:1467, 1982.
915. Brunken, R., Tillisch, J., Schwaiger, M., et al.: Regional perfusion, glucose metabolism, and wall motion in patients with chronic electrocardiographic Q wave infarctions: Evidence for persistence of viable tissue in some infarct regions by positron emission tomography. Circulation *73*:951, 1986.
916. Johnson, L. L., Seldin, D. W., Keller, A. M., et al.: Dual isotope thallium and indium antimyosin SPECT imaging to identify acute infarct patients at further ischemic risk. Circulation *81*:37, 1990.
917. Brown, K. A., O'Meara, J., Chambers, C. E., and Plante, D. A.: Ability of dipyridamole-thallium-201 imaging one to four days after acute myocardial infarction to predict in-hospital and late recurrent myocardial ischemic events. Am. J. Cardiol. *65*:160, 1990.
918. Muller, J. E., Rude, R. E., Braunwald, E., et al.: Myocardial recurrence, outcome, and risk factors in the Multicenter Investigation of Infarct Size. Ann. Intern. Med. *108*:1, 1988.
919. Ellis, S. G., Topol, E. J., George, B. S., et al.: Recurrent ischemia without warning. Analysis of risk factors for in-hospital ischemic events, following successful thrombolysis with intravenous tissue plasminogen activator. Circulation *80*:1159, 1989.
920. Isaacsohn, J. L., Earle, M. G., Kemper, A. J., and Parisi, A. F.: Postmyocardial infarction pain and infarct extension in the coronary care unit: Role of two-dimensional echocardiography. J. Am. Coll. Cardiol. *11*:246, 1988.
921. Baker, J. T., Bramlet, D. A., Lester, R. M., et al.: Myocardial infarct extension: Incidence and relationship to survival. Circulation *65*:918, 1982.
922. Marmor, A., Sobel, B. E., and Roberts, E.: Factors presaging early recurrent myocardial infarction ("extension"). Am. J. Cardiol. *48*:603, 1981.
923. Pierard, L. A., Albert, A., Henrard, L., et al.: Incidence and significance of pericardial effusion in acute myocardial infarction as determined by two-dimensional echocardiography. J. Am. Coll. Cardiol. *8*:517, 1986.
924. Charlap, S., Greenberg, S., Greengart, A., et al.: Pericardial effusion early in acute myocardial infarction. Clin. Cardiol. *12*:252, 1989.
925. Sugiura, T., Iwasaka, T., Takayama, Y., et al.: Factors associated with pericardial effusion in acute Q wave myocardial infarction. Circulation *81*:477, 1990.
926. Somolinos, M., Violán, S., Sanz, R., and Marrero, P.: Early pericarditis after acute myocardial infarction: A clinical echocardiographic study. Crit. Care Med. *15*:648, 1987.
927. Tofler, G. H., Muller, J. E., Stone, P. H., et al.: Pericarditis in acute myocardial infarction: Characterization and clinical significance. Am. Heart J. *117*:86, 1989.
928. Lichstein, E., Liu, H.-M., and Gupta, P.: Pericarditis complicating acute myocardial infarction: incidence of complications and significance of electrocardiogram on admission. Am. Heart J. *87*:246, 1974.
929. Blau, N., Shen, B. A., Pittman, D. E., and Joyner, C. E.: Massive hemopericardium in a patient with post-myocardial infarction syndrome. Chest *71*:549, 1977.
930. Karim, A. H., and Salomon, J.: Constrictive pericarditis after myocardial infarction. Sequelae of anticoagulant-induced hemopericardium. Am. J. Med. *79*:389, 1985.
931. Lichstein, E., Arsura, E., Hollander, G., et al.: Current incidence of postmyocardial infarction (Dressler's) syndrome. Am. J. Cardiol. *50*:1269, 1982.
932. Northcote, R. J., Hutchinson, S. J., and McGuinness, J. B.: Evidence for the continued existence of the postmyocardial infarction (Dressler's) syndrome. Am. J. Cardiol. *53*:1201, 1984.
933. Brown, E. J., Jr., Kloner, R. A., Schoen, F. J., et al.: Scar thinning due to ibuprofen administration following experimental myocardial infarction. Am. J. Cardiol. *51*:877, 1983.
934. Silverman, H. S., and Pfeifer, M. P.: Relation between use of anti-inflammatory agents and left ventricular free wall rupture during acute myocardial infarction. Am. J. Cardiol. *59*:363, 1987.
935. Friedman, P. L., Brown, E. J., Jr., Gunther, S., et al.: Coronary vasoconstrictor effect of indomethacin in patients with coronary artery disease. N. Engl. J. Med. *305*:1171, 1981.

CONVALESCENCE, DISCHARGE, AND POST-MI CARE

936. Rowe, M. H., Jelinek, M. V., Liddell, N., and Hugens, M.: Effect of rapid mobilization on ejection fractions and ventricular volumes after acute myocardial infarction. Am. J. Cardiol. *63*:1037, 1989.
937. Kloner, R. A., and Kloner, J. A.: The effect of early exercise on myocardial infarct scar formation. Am. Heart J. *106*:1009, 1983.
938. Hammerman, H., Kloner, R. A., Alker, K. U., et al.: Effects of transient increased afterload during experimentally induced acute myocardial infarction in dogs. Am. J. Cardiol. *55*:566, 1985.
939. Madsen, E. B.: Time of discharge for patients with acute myocardial infarction. Cardiovasc. Rev. Rep. *4*:1301, 1983.

940. Pryor, D. B., Hindman, M. C., Wagner, G. S., et al.: Early discharge after acute myocardial infarction. Ann. Intern. Med. *99*:528, 1983.

940a. Mark, D., Sigmon, K., Topol, E. J., et al.: Identification of acute myocardial infarction patients suitable for early hospital discharge after aggressive interventional therapy. Circulation *83*:1186, 1991.

941. Abraham, A. S., Sever, Y., Weinstein, M., et al.: Value of early ambulation in patients with and without complications after acute myocardial infarction. N. Engl. J. Med. *292*:719, 1975.

942. Madsen, E. B., Hougaard, P., Gilpin, E., and Pedersen, S.: The length of hospitalization after acute myocardial infarction determined by risk calculation. Circulation *68*:9, 1983.

943. Topol, E. J., Burek, K., O'Neill, W. W., et al.: A randomized controlled trial of hospital discharge three days after myocardial infarction in the era of reperfusion. N. Engl. J. Med. *318*:1083, 1988.

944. Bates, E. R., and Topol, E. J.: Early hospital discharge in the myocardial reperfusion era. Clin. Cardiol. *12*(Suppl. III):65, 1989.

945. Jugdutt, B. I., Michorowski, B. L., and Kappagoda, C. T.: Exercise training after anterior Q wave myocardial infarction: Importance of regional left ventricular function and topography. J. Am. Coll. Cardiol. *12*:362, 1988.

946. Papadopoulos, C.: A survey of sexual activity after myocardial infarction. Cardiovasc. Med. *3*:821, 1978.

947. Tardif, G. S.: Sexual activity after a myocardial infarction. Arch. Phys. Med. Rehabil. *70*:763, 1989.

948. Friedman, M., Thoresen, C. E., Gill, J. J., et al.: Feasibility of altering type A behavior pattern after myocardial infarction. Recurrent coronary prevention project study: Methods, baseline results and preliminary findings. Circulation *66*:83, 1982.

949. Powell, L. H., and Thoresen, C. A.: Effects of type A behavioral counseling and severity of prior acute myocardial infarction on survival. Am. J. Cardiol. *62*:1159, 1988.

950. Health and Public Policy Committee, American College of Physicians: Cardiac Rehabilitation Services. Ann. Intern. Med. *109*:671, 1988.

951. Squires, R. W., Gau, G. T., Miller, T. D., et al.: Cardiovascular rehabilitation: Status, 1990. Mayo Clin. Proc. *65*:731, 1990.

952. Greenland, P., and Chu, J. S.: Efficacy of cardiac rehabilitation services, with emphasis on patients after myocardial infarction. Ann. Intern. Med. *109*:650, 1988.

953. O'Connor, G. T., Buring, J. E., Yusuf, S., et al.: An overview of randomized trials of rehabilitation with exercise after myocardial infarction. Circulation *80*:234, 1989.

954. Moss, A. J., and Benhorin, J.: Prognosis and management after a first myocardial infarction. N. Engl. J. Med. *322*:743, 1990.

955. Taylor, S. H.: Secondary prevention after myocardial infarction: Facts and fallacies. J. Cardiovasc. Pharmacol. *6*:5914, 1984.

956. Rosenberg, L., Kaufman, D. W., Helmrich, S. P., and Shapiro, S.: The risk of myocardial infarction after quitting smoking in men under 55 years of age. N. Engl. J. Med. *313*:1511, 1985.

957. Myers, M. G.: Changing patterns in drug therapy for ischemic heart disease. Can. Med. Assoc. J. *312*:644, 1984.

958. Snow, P.J.D.: Effect of propranolol in myocardial infarction. Lancet *2*:735, 1965.

959. Beta Blocker Heart Attack Study Group: The Beta-Blocker Heart Attack Trial. JAMA *246*:2073, 1981.

960. Herlitz, J., Elmfeldt, D., Holmberg, S., et al.: Goteborg metoprolol trial: Mortality and causes of death. Am. J. Cardiol. *53*:9D, 1984.

961. Pedersen, T. R., and the Norwegian Multicenter Study Group: Six-year follow-up of the Norwegian multicenter study on timolol after acute myocardial infarction. N. Engl. J. Med. *313*:1055, 1985.

962. Taylor, S. H., Silke, B., Ebbutt, A., et al.: A long-term prevention study with oxprenolol in coronary heart disease. N. Engl. J. Med. *307*:1293, 1982.

963. May, G. S.: A review of acute-phase beta-blocker trials in patients with myocardial infarction. Circulation *67*(Suppl. I):21, 1983.

964. Gundersen, T.: Secondary prevention after myocardial infarction: subgroup analysis of patients at risk in the Norwegian timolol multicenter study. Clin. Cardiol. *8*:253, 1985.

965. Chadda, K., Goldstein, S., Byington, R., and Curb, J. D.: Effect of propranolol after acute myocardial infarction in patients with congestive heart failure. Circulation *73*:503, 1986.

966. Herlitz, J., Hjalmarson, A., Holmberg, S., et al.: Development of congestive heart failure after treatment with metoprolol in acute myocardial infarction. Br. Heart J. *51*:539, 1984.

967. Beta-Blocker Pooling Project Research Group: The Beta-Blocker Pooling Project (BBPP): subgroup findings from randomized trials in post-infarction patients. Eur. Heart J. *9*:8, 1988.

968. Herlitz, J., Hjalmarson, A., Swedberg, K., et al.: Effects on mortality during five years after early intervention with metoprolol in suspected acute myocardial infarction. Acta Med. Scand. *223*:227, 1988.

969. Olsson, G., Oden, A., Johansson, L., et al.: Prognosis after withdrawal of chronic postinfarction metoprolol treatment: A 2–7 year follow-up. Eur. Heart J. *9*:365, 1988.

970. Goldstein, S.: Review of beta blocker myocardial infarction trials. Clin. Cardiol. *12*(Suppl. III):54, 1989.

971. Gundersen, T., Abrahamsen, A. M., Kjekshus, J., and Ronnevik, P. K.: Timolol-related reduction in mortality and reinfarction in patients ages 65–77 years surviving acute myocardial infarction. Circulation *66*:1179, 1982.

972. Goldman, L., Sia, S.T.B., Cook, E. F., et al.: Costs and effectiveness of routine therapy with long-term beta-adrenergic antagonists after acute myocardial infarction. N. Engl. J. Med. *319*:152, 1988.

973. Ahumada, G. G.: Identification of patients who do not require beta antagonists after myocardial infarction. Am. J. Med. *76*:900, 1984.

974. Lopressor Intervention Trial Research Group: The Lopressor Intervention Trial: multicentre study of metoprolol in survivors of acute myocardial infarction. Eur. Heart J. *8*:1056, 1987.

975. Modan, B., Shani, M., Schor, S., and Modan, M.: Reduction of hospital mortality from acute myocardial infarction by anticoagulant therapy. N. Engl. J. Med. *292*:1359, 1975.

976. Horwitz, R. I., and Feinstein, A. R.: The application of therapeutic trial principles to improve the design of epidemiologic research: A case-control study suggesting that anticoagulants reduce mortality in patients with myocardial infarction. J. Chron. Dis. *34*:575, 1981.

977. Turpie, A.G.G.: Anticoagulant therapy after acute myocardial infarction. Am. J. Cardiol. *65*:20C, 1990.

978. Smith, P., Arnesen, H., and Holme, I.: The effect of warfarin on mortality and reinfarction after myocardial infarction. N. Engl. J. Med. *323*:147, 1990.

979. Anticoagulants in acute myocardial infarction: Results of a cooperative clinical trial. JAMA *225*:724, 1973.

980. Wray, R., Maurer, B., and Shillingford, J.: Prophylactic anticoagulant therapy in the prevention of calf-vein thrombosis after myocardial infarction. N. Engl. J. Med. *288*:815, 1973.

981. Pitt, A., Anderson, S. T., Habersberger, P. G., and Rosengarten, D. S.: Low dose heparin in the prevention of deep thromboses in patients with acute myocardial infarction. Am. Heart J. *99*:574, 1980.

982. Goldberg, R. J., Gore, J. J., Dalen, J. E., and Alpert, J. S.: Long-term anticoagulant therapy after acute myocardial infarction. Am. Heart J. *109*:616, 1985.

983. Elwood, P. C.: Aspirin in the prevention of myocardial infarction: Current status. Drugs *28*:1, 1984.

984. Friedewald, W. T., Furberg, C. D., and May, G. S.: Aspirin and myocardial infarction. Cardiovasc. Rev. Rep. *5*:1285, 1984.

985. Antiplatelet Trialists' Collaboration: Secondary prevention of vascular disease by prolonged antiplatelet treatment. Br. Med. J. *296*:320, 1988.

986. Anturane Reinfarction Trial Research Group: Sulfinpyrazone in the prevention of sudden death after myocardial infarction. N. Engl. J. Med. *302*:250, 1980.

987. Klimt, C. R., Knatterud, G. L., Stamler, J., and Meier, P.: Persantine-aspirin reinfarction study. Part II. Secondary coronary prevention with persantine and aspirin. J. Am. Coll. Cardiol. *7*:251, 1986.

988. Israeli Sprint Study Group: Secondary Prevention Reinfarction Israel Nifedipine Trial (SPRINT). A randomized intervention trial of nifedipine in patients with acute myocardial infarction. Eur. Heart J. *9*:354, 1988.

989. Roberts, R.: Review of calcium antagonists trials in acute myocardial infarction. Clin. Cardiol. *12*(Suppl. III):41, 1989.

990. Gibson, R. S., Boden, W. E., Theroux, P., et al.: Diltiazem and reinfarction in patients with non-Q wave infarction. N. Engl. J. Med. *315*:423, 1986.

991. Gibson, R. S.: Management of acute non-Q-wave myocardial infarction: Role of prophylactic pharmacotherapy and indications for predischarge coronary arteriography. Clin. Cardiol. *12*(Suppl. III):26, 1989.

992. Rapport, E.: Influence of long-acting nitrate therapy on the risk of reinfarction, sudden death, and total mortality in survivors of acute myocardial infarction. Am. Heart J. *110*:276, 1985.

993. May, G. S., Furberg, C. D., Eberlein, K. A., and Geraci, B. J.: Secondary prevention after myocardial infarction: A review of short-term acute phase trials. Prog. Cardiovasc. Dis. *25*:335, 1983.

994. May, G. S., Eberlein, K. A., Furberg, C. D., et al.: Secondary prevention after myocardial infarction: A review of long-term trials. Prog. Cardiovasc. Dis. *25*:331, 1982.

995. Gottleib, S. H., Achuff, S. C., Mellits, E. D., et al.: Prophylactic antiarrhythmic therapy of high-risk survivors of myocardial infarction: Lower mortality at 1 month but not at 1 year. Circulation *75*:792, 1987.

996. Rasmussen, H. S., Gronbaek, M., Cintin, C., et al.: One-year death rate in 270 patients with suspected acute myocardial infarction, initially treated with intravenous magnesium or placebo. Clin. Cardiol. *11*:377, 1988.

997. Canner, P. L., Berge, K. G., Weuger, N. K., et al.: Fifteen-year mortality in Coronary Drug Project patients: Long-term benefits with niacin. J. Am. Coll. Cardiol. *8*:1245, 1986.

998. Carlson, L. A., and Rosenhaumer, G.: Reduction of mortality in the Stockholm ischaemic heart disease secondary prevention study by combined treatment with clofibrate and nicotinic acid. Acta Med. Scand. *223*:405, 1988.

999. Freidman, M., Thoresen, C. E., Gill, J. J., et al.: Alteration of type A behavior and its effect on cardiac recurrences in post myocardial infarction patients: Summary results of the recurrent coronary prevention project. Am. Heart J. *112*:653, 1986.

1000. Rossouw, J. E., Lewis, B., and Rifkind, B. M.: The value of lowering cholesterol after myocardial infarction. N. Engl. J. Med. *323*:1112, 1990.

1001. Madsen, E. B., Hougaard, P., and Gilpin, E.: Dynamic evaluation of prognosis from time-dependent variables in acute myocardial infarction. Am. J. Cardiol. *51*:1579, 1983.

1002. DeBusk, R. F., for the Health and Public Policy Committee of the Clinical Efficacy Assessment Subcommittee, American College of Physicians: Evaluation of patients after recent acute myocardial infarction. Ann. Intern. Med. *110*:485, 1989.

1003. Taylor, G. J., Humphries, J. O., Mellits, E. D., et al.: Predictors of clinical course, coronary anatomy and left ventricular function after recovery from acute myocardial infarction. Circulation *62*:960, 1980.

1004. Norris, R. M., Barnaby, P. F., Brandt, P.W.T., et al.: Prognosis after recov-

40

Chronic Ischemic Heart Disease

by JOHN D. RUTHERFORD, M.B., Ch.B., and EUGENE BRAUNWALD, M.D.

Chronic ischemic heart disease is usually due to obstruction of the coronary arteries, which in turn most commonly results from atherosclerosis; the pathogenesis of atherosclerosis is described in Chapter 36 and factors that predispose to this condition in Chapter 37. The importance of ischemic heart disease in contemporary society is attested to by the almost epidemic number of persons afflicted—especially when this number is compared with the anecdotal reports of its occurrence in the medical literature before this century. Ischemic heart disease causes more deaths, disability, and economic loss in industrialized nations than any other group of diseases.

In this century a dramatic increase in coronary heart disease mortality has occurred, with a peak being reached in the late 1960's in most industrialized countries. Since then a continuing downward trend in coronary heart disease mortality has been noted in North America, Belgium, Finland, Israel, Japan, Australia, and New Zealand. In contrast, in most Eastern European countries and in the U.S.S.R. and Sweden, death rates from coronary heart disease are still increasing.[1] In the United States, coronary artery disease (CAD) is the leading cause of death, and in 1989 there were an estimated 27.7 million physician visits for this diagnosis.[2] In 1987, the total economic impact of coronary heart disease amounted to an estimated \$43 billion.[2] Despite major declines in mortality, coronary heart disease still causes over half a million deaths annually. It is estimated that 3.1 per cent of Americans (about 7 million) have clinically active coronary heart disease.

Community-based studies carried out in Rochester, Minnesota showed that the incidence of CAD increased until 1959, fell to the level recorded in 1954 over the next 5 years, and thereafter slowly declined until 1969.[3,4] These observations applied to angina pectoris, myocardial infarction, and sudden unexpected death, with the greatest decline being noted in the incidence of sudden death. This fall in the incidence of CAD was followed a decade later by lowering of the overall annual mortality rate and probably was a contributing factor. The 5-year survival of patients with angina pectoris improved from 75 per cent in the years 1950 to 1970 to 87 per cent during 1970 to 1975. The Allegheny County Coronary Heart Disease Mortality Study, ongoing since 1970, showed a decline in coronary heart disease mortality from 91 to 40 deaths per 100,000 per year in the years 1970 to 1972 to 1985 to 1986, respectively.[5] Two-thirds of this decline was related to a decline in sudden deaths, and it was concluded that primary prevention had contributed substantially to this decline.[5] Mortality rate among diabetics did not decline during the 17 years of the study, and the proportion of diabetics with CAD deaths actually increased.

It remains to be seen whether the decline in CAD mortality (in the countries in which it has been observed) is due to a reduction in incidence, a change in case fatality rates, or both of these factors. Whereas changing incidence might suggest that preventive programs are having an impact, changing case fatality rates suggest improvements in medical and surgical management of patients known to have CAD.

The widespread decline in mortality secondary to CAD noted in different countries with different health systems and in all age groups appears to be real rather than the result of changes in methods of classifying patients. Studies in Rochester already mentioned[3] suggest that both the incidence and the case fatality rates may be falling. The fact that the population rates of CAD can change substantially over the course of several years provides a strong argument that efforts to prevent and/or treat the disease have the potential for success.[5,6]

There is no uniform presenting syndrome for chronic ischemic heart disease. Although chest discomfort is usually the predominant symptom in chronic (stable) or unstable angina and acute myocardial infarction, syndromes of ischemic heart disease also occur in which ischemic chest discomfort is absent or not prominent. These include asymptomatic (silent) myocardial ischemia, cardiac arrhythmias, and congestive heart failure. There are also nonatherosclerotic causes of obstructive coronary artery disease.[6a] Myocardial ischemia may also occur in the absence of CAD (as in aortic valve disease, hypertrophic cardiomyopathy, and syphilitic aortitis), and CAD may occur with these other forms of heart disease. Finally, the various syndromes characteristic of ischemic heart disease may complicate noncardiac disease, e.g., coronary atherosclerosis occurs commonly in patients with chronic renal failure requiring dialysis (p. 1863).

Chronic Stable Angina Pectoris

CLINICAL MANIFESTATIONS

CHARACTERISTICS OF ANGINA (see also p. 4). Angina pectoris is a discomfort in the chest or adjacent areas, which is caused by myocardial ischemia and is associated with a disturbance of myocardial function but without myocardial necrosis.[7] Heberden's initial description of the chest discomfort as conveying a sense of "strangling and anxiety" is still remarkably pertinent, although adjectives frequently used to describe this distress include "vise-like," "constricting," "suffocating," "crushing," "heavy," and "squeezing." In other patients, the quality of the sensation is more vague and may be described as a mild pressure-like discomfort or an uncomfortable numb sensation. The site of the discomfort is usually retrosternal, but radiation is common and usually occurs down the ulnar surface of the left arm; commonly the right arm and the outer surfaces of both arms are also involved[8,8a] (Fig. 1–1, p. 6). Sampson and Cheitlin have documented the large number of regions that can be sites of radiation, with neck, jaw, and throat pain observed most commonly.[9] The location of pain does not reliably identify the specific coronary artery involved.[10] Discomfort above the mandible or below the epigastrium due to angina is rare. Anginal "equivalents" (i.e., symptoms of myocardial ischemia other than angina) such as breathlessness, faintness, fatigue, and eructations have also been reported. A history of abnormal exertional dyspnea may be an early indicator of CAD even when angina is absent or there is no electrocardiographic evidence of ischemic heart disease.[11] Pain seldom occurs only in the left pectoral area, and a discomfort lasting all day is unlikely to be cardiac ischemia unless it is caused by myocardial infarction or an uncorrected arrhythmia. It is characteristic that patients with angina usually prefer to rest, sit, or stop walking during attacks.[7]

MECHANISM. The mechanism responsible for angina pectoris is complex and not fully understood. For example, the specific substance that actually stimulates sympathetic afferents and begins the series of interactions that culminate in chest discomfort has not been identified. Some evidence favors agents that are released from cells as a result of transient ischemia, such as adenosine,[12] bradykinin, histamine, or serotonin.[13] Acidosis or elevated potassium concentration in the involved tissues may trigger release of these substances to which the sensory end-plates of the intracardiac sympathetic nerves appear to be particularly sensitive. The end-plates are the receptors of a network of unmyelinated nerves that lie between cardiac muscle fibers and that are also found around coronary vessels, travel to a cardiac plexus, and then ascend to the sympathetic ganglia (C7–T4). Impulses are transmitted to corresponding spinal ganglia, then via the spinal cord to the thalamus, and finally to the cerebral cortex.

The discomfort of myocardial ischemia is perceived in various regions of the chest because it is "referred" to the corresponding peripheral dermatomes that supply afferent nerves to the same segment of the spinal cord as the heart. A plausible explanation is that a common pool of secondary neurons can be stimulated by somatic and visceral afferent impulses. If visceral stimuli are excessive, the nearby intermediate neurons that are receptors for somatic impulses may be excited, and the discomfort will then be perceived as being cutaneous in origin. Thus, pain impulses can be referred to the medial aspects of the arm via common connections to the brachial plexus and can be referred to the neck via connections with the cervical roots.

It is not clear why some patients with clear-cut evidence of ischemic heart disease experience no chest discomfort; diabetics appear to have a higher frequency of "silent" ischemia, perhaps because of autonomic denervation.[14] In some patients chest pain disappears after a myocardial infarction, even though other evidence of transient ischemia, such as ST-segment depression, may persist. It is postulated that in these patients the nerve endings may have been damaged as a result of the infarction. Patients with reproducible evidence of myocardial ischemia may or may not experience chest pain with each episode. Ambulatory electrocardiography has revealed that the majority of patients with angina also experience numerous episodes of silent ischemia, i.e., ST-segment and T-wave changes identical to those occurring during typical angina but unaccompanied by chest discomfort. These episodes are accompanied by reductions of myocardial perfusion, as measured by uptake of radioactive rubidium.[15] The frequency of episodes of silent ischemia is reduced by treatment with nitrates, beta blockers, and calcium antagonists, supporting the contention that they represent instances of myocardial ischemia (p. 1347). It has been suggested that patients with silent myocardial ischemia may have an altered central modulation of pain perception. This hypothesis is supported by the observations that, compared with patients who develop angina during myocardial ischemia, those who have silent ischemia have a higher dental pain threshold and, once the pain threshold is reached, feel it less intensely.[16] Other studies have suggested that the higher the endorphin level induced after exercise the less likely angina is to occur.[17]

FEATURES OF ANGINAL DISCOMFORT. The fact that the discomfort of angina is not uniform and that other entities can mimic it often makes the differential diagnosis of chest pain difficult[7,8] (see Table 1–1, p. 3). Constant[18] has suggested that physicians should ask specific questions to differentiate "nonanginal chest pain" from angina. He notes that some of the characteristics of *nonanginal* discomfort are episodes lasting less than 5 seconds or greater than 20 to 30 minutes; discomfort that is aggravated or precipitated by one deep breath; discomfort precipitated by a single movement of the trunk or arm; discomfort relieved within a few seconds of lying horizontally; discomfort relieved within a few seconds of one or two swallows of food or water; discomfort localized to a very small area, e.g., an area the size of the tip of a finger; pain associated with tenderness of the chest wall (unless the anginal pain is referred to a site of previous chest wall trauma). Differentiating the discomfort resulting from noncardiac disorders from angina pectoris is usually possible when the quality of the pain and its duration, precipitating factors, and associated symptoms are taken into consideration[9] (Table 1–3, p. 5). Thus, the typical anginal episode usually begins gradually and reaches maximum intensity over a period of minutes before dissipating—usually as a result of cessation of the activity that precipitated it. Noncoronary causes should be considered in patients with sharp, stabbing, or burning chest pain that comes and goes in a matter of seconds or with a dull, continuous ache in the chest that lasts for more than 30 minutes. Similarly, changes in posture do not usually affect immediately the discomfort of myocardial ischemia, and this maneuver helps to distinguish angina from pericardial disease or hiatus hernia.

Angina Due to Increased Oxygen Demand. In typical angina, the pain is related to an increase in myocardial oxygen demand, most commonly brought about by physical activity; the *rate* at which a task is carried out is also important. Hurrying is particularly likely to precipitate angina, as are efforts involving motion of the hands over the head. Emotion or eating, particularly when combined with physical activity, commonly causes angina, as do a variety of other factors, including the excessive metabolic demands imposed by chills and fever, thyrotoxicosis, tachycardia from any cause, severe anemia, and hypoglycemia. In all of these conditions, underlying fixed coronary artery obstruction is usually present, and the other factors (e.g., exercise, fever) increase the activity of the heart, stimulate myocardial oxygen needs in the presence of a fixed and limited oxygen supply, and thus precipitate ischemia and chest discomfort.

Angina Due to Transient Decreased Oxygen Supply. There is increasing evidence, however, that angina may also be caused by transient reductions of oxygen supply as a consequence of coronary vasoconstriction.[19,20] As pointed out on page 1164, the coronary arterial bed is well innervated, and a variety of stimuli alter coronary tone. There is a reciprocal relationship between the severity of dynamic and organic obstruction required to cause myocardial ischemia. Thus, in the occasional patient with no organic lesions, severe dynamic obstruction alone can cause myocardial ischemia and resultant angina. On the other hand, in patients with severe fixed obstruction to coronary flow, only a minor increase in dynamic obstruction is necessary for blood flow to fall below a critical level and cause myocardial ischemia (Fig. 38–21, p. 1175). Nonocclusive intracoronary thrombi are another cause of myocardial ischemia, although usually of angina at rest (unstable angina) rather than chronic stable angina.

FIXED COMPARED WITH VARIABLE-THRESHOLD ANGINA. The variability of the threshold for angina differs among patients. In patients with fixed-threshold angina precipitated by increased oxygen demands, with few if any dynamic (vasoconstrictive) components, the level of physical activity required to precipitate angina is relatively constant. Characteristically, these patients can predict with some precision the amount of physical activity that causes angina, e.g., walking up exactly two and a half flights of stairs. When these patients are tested on a treadmill or bicycle, the pressure-rate product that elicits angina and/or electrocardiographic evidence of ischemia is constant or almost so.

Patients with variable-threshold angina,[20a] the majority of whom have atherosclerotic coronary arterial narrowing, but in whom dynamic obstruction caused by vasoconstriction plays an important role in causing myocardial ischemia, typically have "good days," when they are capable of substantial physical activity, and "bad days," when even minimal activity can cause clinical and/or electrocardiographic evidence of myocardial ischemia or when angina occurs at rest. Often, even in the course of a single day, they may be capable of substantial physical activity at one time, while at another time minimal activity will result in angina. Patients with variable-threshold angina often complain of angina precipitated by cold temperatures, emotion, and meals and occasionally of angina occurring at rest or nocturnally. It is presumed that coronary vasoconstriction contributes to the development of angina under these circumstances. In many patients with stable angina, cold does not lower the ischemic threshold; however, others give a history that angina is more readily provoked by the cold and in them the ischemic threshold is lowered by cold.[21] Both beta blockers and calcium antagonists prolong the time to exercise-induced ischemia both at normal and cold temperatures.[21] The anginal threshold tends to be lower in the morning than in the afternoon, correlating with the angiographic finding of smaller coronary arterial lumina at that time of day. However, even in patients with angina at rest and nocturnal angina, an increase in myocardial oxygen demand may play a role.[22]

The term *mixed angina* has been suggested by Maseri to describe the many patients who fall between these two extremes of fixed threshold and variable threshold angina[23] (Fig. 38–21, p. 1175).

Changes in the blood pressure–heart rate product (the double product) provide an approximation of alterations of myocardial oxygen requirements (p. 1163). In patients with effort-induced, fixed-threshold angina, the specific threshold at which ischemia develops (as reflected in angina and/or ST-segment depression) is a function of the myocardial oxygen requirements. As the activity of the left ventricle (and therefore its oxygen consumption) increases, a point is reached at which perfusion distal to a critical coronary arterial obstruction cannot supply sufficient oxygen to the myocardium perfused by the obstructed artery; ischemia and angina ensue.

Observations in patients experiencing angina under circumstances other than exercise help to explain the pathophysiological bases of angina. For example, as already indicated, some patients with ischemic heart disease characteristically experience angina on exposure to cold weather or during or after meals. A cold environment has been shown to increase peripheral resistance at rest and during exercise.[24] The rise in arterial pressure, by augmenting myocardial oxygen requirements, lowers the threshold for the development of angina. An alternative, or additional, explanation is the development of cold-induced coronary vasoconstriction. The reduction in exercise capacity during or after meals has been explained by a more rapid rise in heart rate and blood pressure after meals as compared with before meals,[25] but the postprandial increase in myocardial oxygen needs may not be sufficient to explain the development of ischemia, and a dynamic component, i.e., coronary vasoconstriction, may also be involved.[26] Similarly, during angina induced by emotion, heart rate and blood pressure (and therefore myocardial oxygen needs) rise but usually not to the level required to produce angina during exercise. Therefore, a dynamic component probably plays a role here as well.[27]

Relief of anginal discomfort is usually afforded by rest and by sublingual use of nitroglycerin; indeed, the response to this drug is often a useful diagnostic tool.[28] A delay of more than 5 to 10 minutes before relief is obtained suggests that the pain is not ischemic in origin. As described by Levine, carotid sinus pressure can also often bring about rapid alleviation of discomfort.[29] Some patients experience loss of angina when they continue to exercise, a phenomenon described as "walk-through" angina.[30]

In atypical angina the precipitating factors may be similar to those of typical angina, but the quality of the discomfort is different (sharp and stabbing, for example); or, if the quality of the discomfort is angina-like, the precipitating causes are unusual, such as varying body positions; or the discomfort may be typical in quality and occur only at rest but may not be accompanied by characteristic ST-segment changes. Nonanginal chest pain has neither the quality of typical angina nor its usual precipitating causes.

GRADING OF ANGINA PECTORIS. A system of grading effort angina proposed by the Canadian Cardiovascular Society in 1972 has gained widespread acceptance.[31] This grading system is the New York Heart Association (NYHA) functional classification, modified to allow independent observers to categorize patients in more precise terms. The Specific Activity Scale described by Goldman et al.[32] is also useful in estimating symptomatic severity. These systems are described in Table 1–6 (p. 11). An anginal "score" describing the frequency, associated electrocardiographic or ST-segment changes, and whether or not the angina is stable or progressive or nocturnal can add significant, independent prognostic information over and above the patient's age, gender, and knowledge of left ventricular function and coronary anatomy.[33]

CLINICAL-PATHOLOGICAL CORRELATIONS. The incidence of CAD in subsets of patients with typical angina, atypical angina, and nonanginal chest pain has been estimated by Diamond and Forrester to be about 90 per cent, 50 per cent, and 16 per cent, respectively, while the incidence of CAD in asymptomatic middle-aged adults is estimated to be 3 to 4 per cent.[34] While the clinical manifestations of ischemia tend to be more severe in patients with multivessel than single-vessel disease,[35] in any individual patient the extent of the underlying disease cannot be predicted from the severity, nature, duration, or quality of the discomfort. Perhaps the best examples of this lack of clinical-pathological correlation are two subgroups of patients who have been well characterized: those with advanced obstructive CAD and so-called silent ischemia (p. 1347) and some with Prinzmetal's angina who may have episodes of excruciating angina yet have minimal or no coronary atherosclerosis (p. 1342).

For comparable degrees of obstructive CAD, as defined arteriographically, asymptomatic or minimally symptomatic patients have a better prognosis than do those with severe angina.[36] When infarction (without angina) is the first manifestation of ischemic heart disease, it is often associated with single-vessel disease; when infarction has been preceded by angina, two- or three-vessel disease is usually present. Gender also appears to influence the clinical expression of CAD. Among women, angina pectoris is by far the most frequent clinical expression, as compared with men, in whom fatal and nonfatal myocardial infarction are more common.[37]

DIFFERENTIAL DIAGNOSIS OF CHEST PAIN

(Table 1–1, p. 3 and Fig. 40–1)

The differentiation of various disorders from CAD is challenging because, as has already been noted, the severity of the chest pain and the seriousness of the underlying disorder are not necessarily related. Compounding the difficulty in differential diagnosis is the common myth that pain in the left arm or left side of the chest is an ominous sign signifying the presence of CAD. However, a host of disorders can cause these types of discomfort.

ESOPHAGEAL DISORDERS. These may produce symptoms that can mimic myocardial ischemia.[38,39] Abnormal regurgitation of acid from the stomach to the esophagus—esophageal reflux—is relatively common. This can cause inflammation of the esophageal mucosa and is often associated with retrosternal burning—"heartburn"—indigestion, and/or gaseous eructations. Esophageal spasm also may cause constant retrosternal discomfort of uniform intensity or severe spasmodic pain during or after swallowing. These symptoms are intermittent and often accompanied by

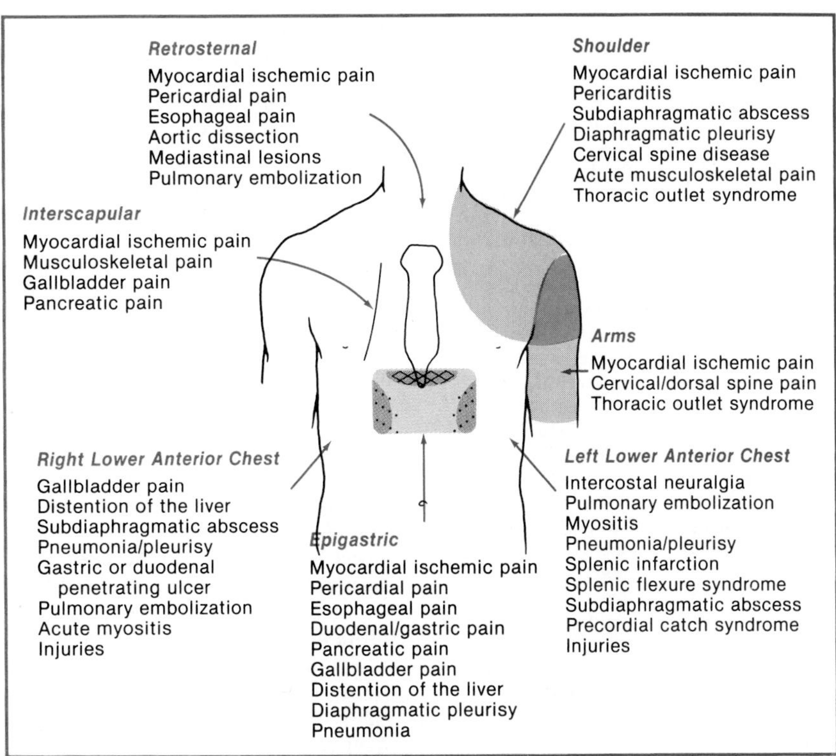

FIGURE 40–1. **Differential diagnosis of chest pain according to location where pain starts. Serious intrathoracic or subdiaphragmatic diseases are usually associated with pains that begin in the left anterior chest, left shoulder or upper arm, the interscapular region, or the epigastrium. The scheme is not all-inclusive, e.g., intercostal neuralgia occurs in locations other than the left, lower anterior chest area. (From Miller, A. J.: Diagnosis of Chest Pain. New York, Raven Press, 1988, p. 175.)**

difficulty in swallowing, although the pain may occur spontaneously at times. While esophageal disorders may produce substernal "burning," features more suggestive of esophageal than anginal pain include a background of continuous aching, discomfort that is not associated with exercise, and a pain disturbing sleep and occurring in association with other esophageal symptoms. Like angina, discomfort caused by esophageal spasm is often relieved by nitroglycerin (although not usually in less than 3 minutes). Unlike angina, esophageal pain is often also relieved by milk, antacids, foods, or occasionally warm liquids[18] (Table 40–1).

Acid regurgitation, or acid-induced esophageal spasm, as a cause of chest pain may be investigated by alternate infusions of dilute acid and normal saline via a nasogastric catheter with the tip at the level of the midesophagus (Bernstein test). In patients with subjective and objective evidence of gastroesophageal acid reflux, acid infusion readily produces pain within 2 to 4 minutes; however, pain may continue for more than 20 minutes in patients after the acid infusion is stopped despite the fact that the esophageal pH returns to normal much earlier.[40] Acid reflux into the esophagus can also be recognized by recording pH from an electrode at the tip of a catheter inserted into the distal esophagus.[41]

TABLE 40-1 SIMILARITIES AND DIFFERENCES BETWEEN ESOPHAGEAL AND CARDIAC PAIN

	SIMILARITIES OF CARDIAC AND ESOPHAGEAL PAIN	DISTINGUISHING FEATURES OF ESOPHAGEAL PAIN
Location	Mid or lower retrosternal. May be a severe epigastric pain with radiation up to neck.	High epigastric, behind xiphoid process or in low retrosternal area.
Nature	Heaviness, squeezing, tightness or burning. Can be associated with weakness, diaphoresis, and anxiety.	Often burning or perceived as spasm. Heartburn is frequent association. Can be associated with increased salivation. Dysphagia occurs.
Radiation	Upward toward throat. May radiate to left neck, shoulder, or arm.	Tends to ascend but not radiate to left side. Radiation to both shoulders and/or arms is less frequent. When pain begins in lower retrosternal area it often radiates down to epigastrium.
Precipitants	After eating. Angina is more likely with physical activity after eating.	After eating; certain foods—alcohol, coffee, spices. Less likely to be brought on by exertion. Can be precipitated by change in posture, e.g., by lying down.
Duration	Can last a short duration (2 to 10 min).	May last hours; may wax and wane.
Relieving factors	May be relieved or eased by nitroglycerin, standing, and relaxing.	

Modified from Miller, A. J.: Diagnosis of Chest Pain. New York, Raven Press, 1988, pp. 74–76.

Gastric reflux is often associated with hiatus hernia, which can be diagnosed radiographically. In patients with hiatus hernia, postprandial distress is most marked in the recumbent position, a feature that helps to differentiate it from angina pectoris. The differentiation between esophageal pain and angina is complicated by the observation that infusion of acid into the esophagus of patients with CAD can increase the rate-pressure product, can cause angina as well as electrocardiographic evidence of ischemia, and can cause pain indistinguishable from angina in patients with absence of or infrequent reflux symptoms.[42] Also, esophageal stimulation with acid will lower the threshold for exertional angina pectoris, especially in patients who have concurrent, regular esophageal symptoms.[43]

In patients with retrosternal chest pain of unclear cause, esophageal motility disorders are not uncommon[44,45] and should be specifically excluded or confirmed, if possible. In addition to chest pain, the majority of such patients have dysphagia. While barium studies may reveal motility problems, esophageal manometry may reveal diffuse esophageal spasm, increased pressure at the lower esophageal sphincter, and other disorders. Provocative pharmacological agents such as ergonovine[45] and methacholine[44] may provoke esophageal pain and manometric signs of spasm (in patients with normal coronary arteries). Surgical or medical therapy of esophageal reflux will improve symptoms in patients with normal coronary arteries whose experience of chest pain coincides with documented episodes of reflux (using esophageal pH monitoring).[41] While esophageal disease is frequent in patients with retrosternal chest pain of unclear cause, CAD occurs concomitantly in approximately 10 per cent of such patients. Thus, the diagnosis of CAD cannot be dismissed in such patients.[39]

BILIARY COLIC. This symptom is sometimes confused with angina pectoris. It is usually caused by a rapid rise in biliary pressure due to obstruction of the cystic or bile duct. The pain is steady, usually lasts 2 to 4 hours, and subsides spontaneously without any symptoms between attacks.[46] It is usually most intense in the right upper abdomen but may also be felt in the epigastrium, left abdomen, or precordium. This discomfort is often referred to the scapula, may radiate around the costal margin to the back, or rarely may be felt in the shoulder, suggesting diaphragmatic irritation. Although nausea and vomiting are common, the relationship of the pain to meals is variable. While a history of dyspepsia, flatulence, fatty food intolerance, and indigestion may be associated with cholelithiasis, these symptoms are also commonly experienced by the general population. Ultrasound is quite accurate in diagnosing gallstones and allows determination of gallbladder size, thickness, and whether or not the bile ducts are dilated.[46] Failure to opacify the gallbladder on oral cholecystography may indicate nonfunction due to disease.

Distention of the splenic flexure of the colon can also mimic anginal pain, but, unlike angina, relief of symptoms often follows a bowel movement.

COSTOSTERNAL SYNDROME. In 1921, Tietze first described a syndrome of local pain and tenderness, usually limited to the anterior chest wall, associated with swelling of the costal cartilages. This condition causes pain that can resemble angina pectoris. The full-blown Tietze syndrome, i.e., pain associated with tender swelling of the costochondral junctions, is uncommon, whereas costochondritis causing tenderness of the costochondral junctions (without swelling) is relatively common.[47] Pain on palpation of these joints is a useful clinical sign. Local pressure should be applied routinely to the anterior chest wall during the examination of the patient being evaluated for angina pectoris. Treatment of costochondritis usually consists of reassurance and antiinflammatory agents.

CERVICAL RADICULITIS. This may occur as a constant ache, sometimes resulting in a sensory deficit. The pain may be related to motion of the neck, just as motion of the shoulder triggers attacks of pain due to bursitis. A hyperalgesic area of skin, noted by running the finger down the back and exerting pressure, may lead to the suspicion of thoracic root pain.[18] Occasionally, pain mimicking angina can be due to compression of the brachial plexus via cervical ribs. Physical examination may also detect pain brought about by movement of an arthritic shoulder, a calcified shoulder tendon, and the like. The musculoskeletal disorders that can mimic angina include subacromial bursitis and costochondritis.

OTHER CAUSES OF ANGINA-LIKE PAIN. *Acute myocardial infarction* (Chap. 39) is usually associated with prolonged (> 30 minutes), severe pain that apart from duration and intensity may be similar to angina pectoris. It is associated with characteristic electrocardiographic and enzyme findings.

Severe pulmonary hypertension may be associated with exertional chest pain with the characteristics of angina pectoris (p. 806). Other associated symptoms include dyspnea on exertion, dizziness, and exertional syncope. Associated findings on physical examination, such as a parasternal lift, palpable and loud pulmonary component of the second sound, and right ventricular hypertrophy on the electrocardiogram usually are readily recognized.

Pulmonary embolism (Chap. 48) causes chest pain that is usually associated with dyspnea.[48] Associated pleuritic pain suggests pulmonary infarction, and a history of exacerbation of the pain with inspiration with findings of a pleural friction rub usually readily distinguish this from angina pectoris.

The pain of *acute pericarditis* (p. 1469) at times may be difficult to distinguish from angina pectoris. However, pericarditis tends to occur in younger patients than does angina, and the diagnosis depends on chest pain, a pericardial friction rub, and electrocardiographic changes. The chest pain usually is sudden in onset, severe and persistent, and is intensified by coughing, swallowing, and inspiration. Relief may be obtained by sitting up and leaning forward: palpation of the trapezius ridge often causes discomfort. A pericardial friction rub can be detected in most patients if listened for carefully, at different times, with the patient in different positions. Early widespread ST-segment elevation may be present.

In many of the disorders just mentioned, angina pectoris can usually be excluded by a careful history and physical examination. It must be emphasized, however, that chronic ischemic heart disease can and frequently does coexist with any of these other disorders and that noncardiac disease can trigger a true anginal attack in a patient with coronary artery disease.

PHYSICAL EXAMINATION

GENERAL EXAMINATION. In the patient with chronic ischemic heart disease and angina pectoris, the general examination may be entirely normal or may reveal the presence of risk factors for the development of coronary atherosclerosis. Inspection of the eyes, especially in men,[49] may reveal a *corneal arcus*, and examination of the skin may reveal xanthomas (Figs. 2–3, p. 17 and 37–10, p. 1138, and 37–11, p. 1139). In men, the size of the corneal arcus appears to correlate positively with age and levels of cholesterol and low-density lipoproteins.[50] The corneal arcus is not known to regress in humans and is unaffected by a reduction in the level of lipids.[51] *Xanthelasma*, in which lipid deposits are intracellular, appears to be promoted by increased levels of triglycerides and a relative deficiency of high-density lipoproteins. In the Lipid Research Clinic's study,[51] the incidence of both xanthelasma and corneal arcus increased with age and was highest in patients with Type II hyperlipoproteinemia and usually low in those with the Type IV phenotype (Ch. 37). In young persons, the presence of both xanthelasma and corneal arcus is closely correlated and identifies persons with plasma lipoprotein abnormalities. Adjusted-odds ratios for the presence of ischemic heart disease in individuals with xanthelasma and corneal arcus generally are increased.

There appears to be some correlation between CAD and *diagonal earlobe crease*, except in native American Indians, Orientals, and children with Beckwith-Wiedemann syndrome (exomphalos, macroglossia, giantism).[52] It has been observed that there is often a unilateral diagonal earlobe crease in younger persons with CAD that becomes bilateral with advancing age.[53] Some believe that it develops along with CAD,[53] and pathological studies have linked diagonal earlobe creases and cardiovascular mortality.[54] Since the incidence of both diagonal earlobe creases and CAD increases with age,[55] it is not a very helpful clinical finding in persons over the age of 50 years.

The *blood pressure* may be chronically elevated or may rise acutely (along with the heart rate) during an anginal attack. Changes in blood pressure may precede (and precipitate) or follow (and be caused by) the anginal episode. Other features of the general physical examination that are important to seek are abnormalities of the arterial pulses and of the venous system. Major abnormalities of the carotid artery pulse, or bruits, associated with cerebral symptoms usually will lead to carotid ultrasonography and perhaps arteriography. Abnormality to palpation of the peripheral arterial pulses (femoral and popliteal) or the presence of bruits is not as accurate as are actual measurements of limb perfusion.[56] However, the positive correlation of CAD with carotid and peripheral arterial disease makes physical examination of these vessels, including palpation of the dorsalis pedis and posterior tibial pulses, an important part of the examination. Retinal arteriolar changes (p. 15) are common in patients with diabetes mellitus or hypertension and CAD. An abnormal light reflex is quite common, while abnormal vessel tortuosity and decreased caliber are less sensitive but more specific signs.

Evaluation of the patient's venous system, particularly in the legs, may have an important bearing on the type of grafting procedure employed in subsequent coronary artery surgery.

CARDIAC EXAMINATION. This may supply useful clues to both the diagnosis of ischemic heart disease and the functional state of the myocardium. First, the presence of murmurs of hypertrophic cardiomyopathy or aortic valve disease suggests that the ischemic chest pain may be due to conditions other than (or in addition to) CAD (Chaps. 2 and 3). Second, certain findings such as a third or loud fourth heart sound suggest ischemia as the basis for chest pain if other obvious cardiac diseases are absent. These sounds are common in patients with angina at rest, and their frequency is increased during handgrip exercise,[57] even if the latter does not precipitate angina pectoris. These sounds and pulsations are related to the functional state of the left ventricle, particularly its pressure and compliance during diastole (p. 370). In patients with moderate to severe left ventricular dysfunction, a sustained apical cardiac impulse is common. A palpable presystolic impulse may be more indicative of moderate than severe left ventricular dysfunction.[58] While a fourth heart sound may be recorded phonocardiographically in many apparently normal subjects over the age of 45, we agree with Tavel[59] that a clear, loud fourth heart sound accompanied by a palpable presystolic wave is an abnormal finding. It is not specific for ischemic heart disease but may be elicited in other conditions associated with left ventricular hypertrophy such as aortic stenosis, hypertrophic cardiomyopathy, and hypertension, in which left ventricular compliance is reduced (p. 50).

Paradoxical splitting of the second heart sound (p. 47) may occur transiently during an anginal attack and appears to be related to asynergy and prolongation of left ventricular contraction resulting in delayed closure of the aortic valve.

When patients with CAD lie in the left lateral recumbent position, dyskinetic bulges at the apex may be palpated or recorded by means of apexcardiography; these bulges correspond to dyskinetic areas and often complement the auscultatory findings of diastolic filling sounds. A transient apical systolic murmur is quite common in CAD and has been attributed to reversible papillary muscle dysfunction secondary to transient myocardial ischemia; when persistent, such murmurs may be due to fibrosis, often a manifestation of subendocardial infarction. These murmurs are more prevalent in patients with extensive coronary artery disease, especially those with prior myocardial infarction and left ventricular dysfunction. The systolic murmur may assume a variety of configurations (early, late, or holosystolic) and may be accentuated by exertion or during angina. A midsystolic click, often followed by a late systolic murmur characteristic of mitral regurgitation produced by mitral valve prolapse (Fig. 34–23, p. 1034), also occurs in patients with CAD. A diastolic murmur or a continuous murmur is an uncommon finding and has been attributed to turbulent flow across a proximal coronary artery stenosis.[60]

LABORATORY TESTS IN CHRONIC STABLE ANGINA

ELECTROCARDIOGRAM

(See also Chap. 5)

The resting electrocardiogram is normal in approximately one-third of patients with chronic stable angina pectoris. Patients with normal tracings at rest may have severe angina, but they usually have not previously suffered extensive infarction. When the electrocardiogram is abnormal, the most common findings are nonspecific ST-T changes with or without evidence of prior transmural infarction; however, a variety of conduction disturbances, most frequently left bundle branch block and left anterior fascicular block, have also been reported. When left bundle branch block is found in patients with chronic ischemic heart disease, it is often associated with marked impairment in left ventricular function,[61] presumably reflecting multivessel CAD and myocardial damage. The finding of incomplete right bundle branch block does not appear to be associated with an increased risk of death from CAD.[62] A variety of arrhythmias, especially ventricular premature beats, may be present, but they are not specific for identifying CAD. Abnormal Q waves are relatively specific but insensitive indicators of myocardial necrosis.

Interval electrocardiograms may reveal the development of Q-wave infarctions that are unrecognized clinically either by patients or their physicians. Such electrocardiographic abnormalities have as serious a prognosis as clinically recognized infarctions.[63] The increasing use of ambulatory electrocardiographic monitoring has shown that many patients with symptomatic myocardial ischemia also have episodes of silent ischemia that would otherwise go unrecognized during normal daily activities (p. 1347).

Exercise Electrocardiography

(See Chap. 6)

For appropriate application of noninvasive tests, it is important to consider Bayes' theorem (pp. 169 and 1697), which states that while the reliability of any test is defined by its sensitivity and specificity,* its predictability depends on the prevalence of the disease in the population under study (Table 54–2, p. 1697).

DIAGNOSIS OF CORONARY ARTERY DISEASE. Exercise electrocardiography is of limited value in predicting the *presence or absence* of CAD after other easily obtainable clinical data have been taken into account, e.g., the presence or absence of typical anginal symptoms, the presence or absence of Q waves, a clinical history of acute myocardial infarction, a history of cigarette smoking, elevated cholesterol level, and age.[64] However, the recording of an electrocardiogram during and after exercise—especially if angina is precipitated—is valuable in assessing the severity and prognosis of CAD.[65-67] Nonetheless, the exercise electrocardiogram may be of diagnostic value in several circumstances:

1. In patients with a chest pain syndrome and a normal resting electrocardiogram, we believe that a standard electrocardiographic exercise test is useful for detection of significant CAD.[67a]

2. Certain symptomatic and electrocardiographic responses during exercise testing suggest the presence of critical obstruction in one or more coronary arteries. The presence of *typical* anginal chest pain alone, in the absence of ST-segment changes, has a high predictive value for the detection of CAD.[67] However, the most useful exercise electrocardiographic variable for the detection of CAD is the ST-segment shift.[68] If typical chest discomfort occurs during the test associated with ≥ 1 mm ST-segment depression (of horizontal or downsloping nature) the predictive value for the detection of CAD is 90 per cent, and if > 2 mm ST-segment depressions coexist with typical chest discomfort, this is virtually diagnostic of significant CAD.[67] In the absence of typical angina pectoris, downsloping or horizontal ST-segment depressions ≥ 1 mm have a predictive value of 70 per cent, and ST depressions of ≥ 2 mm have a predictive value of 90 per cent for the detection of one or more significant coronary arterial narrowings.

3. An exercise test associated with a hypotensive response, i.e., a drop in systolic blood pressure during exercise below the preexercise value (in the absence of known major ventricular dysfunction), has an 80 per cent predictive value for the detection of significant CAD.[69]

4. Exercise-induced bundle branch block is relatively rare, is usually found in patients with significant CAD,[70-72] and is associated with a high incidence of critical obstruction of the proximal left anterior descending coronary artery.

5. The persistence of ST-segment changes at lower heart rates during the recovery period than the rate at which they develop represents additional evidence supporting the presence of significant CAD.[73]

6. Exercise test predictors of multivessel coronary artery disease include exercise-induced hypotension,[74,75] ST-segment changes ≥ 2 mm, a low work capacity or duration of exercise (which reflects the functional state of the left ventricle),[76] and persistent ST-segment depressions, especially beyond 5 minutes, in the recovery phase. Indeed, early onset of ST-segment depression, its long persistence following exercise, and, most importantly, its shape (downsloping or horizontal) are all strongly associated with multivessel CAD[77] (Fig. 40–2).

7. Failure to achieve a normal heart rate response to exer-

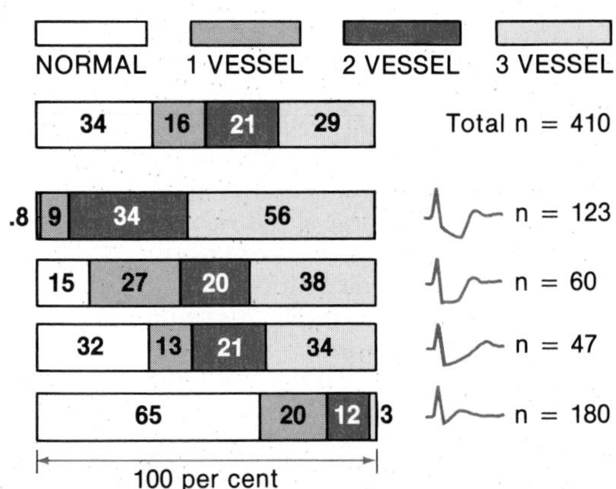

FIGURE 40–2. Relation between the type of ST-segment response in an exercise test and the extent of coronary artery disease. All numbers represent percentages. The total study population is represented at the top. Downsloping ST segments are highly specific for coronary disease, with only one false-positive response (0.8 per cent) encountered; most patients with this response (90 per cent) have double- and triple-vessel involvement. Neither the horizontal nor the slowly upsloping ST segments aid in identifying severe disease. A small percentage (15 per cent) of patients with entirely normal treadmill tests have double- and triple-vessel disease. (From Goldschlager, N., et al.: Treadmill stress tests as indicators of presence and severity of coronary artery disease. Ann. Intern. Med. *85*:277, 1976.)

*For definitions of these terms, see Table 6–2, p. 168.

cise (chronotropic incompetence) is also frequently observed in patients with multivessel or extensive CAD.[78,79] A low maximal heart rate associated with ST-segment depression increases the likelihood of the presence of CAD.[78]

8. Ventricular ectopic activity may be provoked during exercise testing, and if it is "high grade" (e.g., ventricular tachycardia, multiform ventricular ectopy) the likelihood that the patient has abnormal ventricular function or severe CAD is increased.[80]

ASSESSMENT OF PROGNOSIS. Several points should be considered in utilizing the electrocardiographic stress test to evaluate prognosis in patients *known* to have CAD.

1. One of the most important prognosticators derived from exercise electrocardiography is exercise duration or capacity. In symptom-limited exercise tests, *even in the presence of > 2 mm ST-segment depression*, patients who continue to exercise into stage 4 of a standard Bruce protocol have an excellent prognosis.[65,80a] In an 8-year follow-up of medically treated patients with angiographically confirmed CAD and a positive exercise test, the duration of exercise correlated significantly with survival—patients reaching stage 4 of a Bruce protocol had a survival rate of 93 per cent, compared with those terminating their exercise in stage 1 who had a survival rate of only 45 per cent.[66] This direct relationship between exercise duration and long-term survival held regardless whether the exercise test was terminated because of dyspnea, fatigue, or angina.[80b] Coronary artery revascularization appears to improve survival in comparison to medical treatment alone in patients with a positive exercise test and short exercise duration.[80c]

2. Exercise-induced hypotension not only correlates with left main CAD or multivessel disease[69,74,75] but also, in patients with evidence of ischemia during exercise testing who have a remote history of myocardial infarction, it indicates a threefold increased risk for subsequent death or myocardial infarction.[69]

3. Early onset of angina with ST-segment depression is associated with a greater likelihood of myocardial infarction or coronary death.[81] In patients with known left ventricular dysfunction and multivessel coronary artery disease, the possibility of subsequent acute myocardial infarction or sudden death may be greater in patients who exhibit silent myocardial ischemia during exercise testing than in those who develop angina.[82] Therefore, in patients who exhibit substantial myocardial ischemia at levels of activity that they would normally exceed in daily living but *who do not have symptoms of angina, i.e., patients who have a defective anginal warning system*, an aggressive attitude should be adopted toward investigation and possible revascularization for prognostic reasons.

INFLUENCE OF ANTIANGINAL THERAPY. Antianginal pharmacological therapy reduces the sensitivity of exercise testing as a screening tool for left main coronary disease or three-vessel disease.[83] Beta blockade will increase the exercise duration and suppress, diminish, or delay the appearance of ST-segment depression and thus obscure the diagnostic interpretation of exercise testing.[84] In patients receiving antianginal medications, a positive exercise test will have the usual implications for management. However, a negative exercise test in patients receiving antianginal drugs does not exclude significant and possibly life-threatening myocardial ischemia. Therefore, if the purpose of the exercise test is to *diagnose* ischemia, it should be performed, if possible, in the absence of antianginal medications. The advisability of withdrawing medications in an individual patient before exercise testing is a matter of judgment. Unless the patient has severe angina, sublingual nitroglycerin for 1 or 2 days is likely to be sufficient to control symptoms if other therapy is withdrawn. For long-acting nitrates, calcium antagonists, and short-acting beta blockers, stopping the medications the day before testing usually will suffice. Two or three days are required for patients receiving long-acting beta blockers. However, if the purpose of the exercise test is to identify safe levels of daily activity, the test should be carried out while the patient is taking medications.

INCONCLUSIVE TESTS. In view of the relatively low sensitivity (approximately 75 per cent) of exercise stress electrocardiography in the diagnosis of CAD, a negative result does not exclude this diagnosis. However, it makes three-vessel or left main disease much less likely. Conversely, an adequate maximum exercise test—one achieving more than 85 per cent of predicted maximal heart rate—is unlikely to occur in patients with three-vessel or left main CAD.

A major limitation of the sensitivity of the exercise electrocardiogram is that it cannot be interpreted in many patients. This includes patients who are incapable of reaching the level of exercise required for near-maximal effort (85 per cent or more of maximal predicted heart rate), particularly those receiving beta-adrenoceptor blockers or those who develop fatigue, leg cramps, or dyspnea, and patients with abnormalities in the baseline electrocardiogram, including those taking digitalis. In patients with vascular, orthopedic, or neurological conditions who cannot perform leg exercise, the usual alternative tests considered include dipyridamole (or adenosine)-thallium imaging[85-87,87a] (p. 277), Holter monitoring to detect changes in ST segments (p. 1347), or, if appropriate, diagnostic coronary angiography.

RADIONUCLIDE IMAGING

STRESS THALLIUM-201 MYOCARDIAL PERFUSION IMAGING (see also p. 227). In this technique, the radionuclide is injected at peak exercise and the image is obtained several minutes later when the patient is at rest; it demonstrates the regional perfusion pattern that existed during the stress of exercise. Defects represent either areas of stress-induced impairment of blood flow or infarction. If a delayed image is obtained 2 to 3 hours later and the initial defect persists, it is probably due to an infarction. On the other hand, if it exhibits delayed uptake (i.e., redistribution), it probably represents an area of ischemic, transiently hypoperfused but viable myocardium. An electrocardiogram is ordinarily obtained at rest and during the various stages of exercise. Thus, stress thallium scintigraphy provides more information than exercise stress electrocardiography.[87b]

Since a stress thallium scan cannot ordinarily be performed in a physician's office and it is a relatively expensive test (three to four times the cost of a regular exercise electrocardiogram) requiring injection of a radionuclide, certain issues should be considered:

1. A regular exercise electrocardiogram should almost always be obtained first in patients with chest pain and a *normal resting electrocardiogram* for screening and detection of CAD. Stress thallium-201 scintigraphy should not be used as a screening test in populations in whom the prevalence of coronary disease is low or moderate since the sensitivity of exercise thallium imaging is approximately 70 to 85 per cent and the specificity is only 50 to 60 per cent.[88]

2. Thallium scanning is, in essence, either positive or negative and has little quantitative value in determining the number of vessels with significant coronary disease. However, in patients with an abnormal baseline electrocardiogram (e.g., left bundle branch block or right bundle branch block), a history of infarction, or a history of revascularization (by percutaneous transluminal coronary angioplasty or coronary bypass grafting) when the test is being used to assess whether significant stress-induced myocardial ischemia exists, thallium perfusion imaging may be the test of choice. In patients with single-vessel CAD, exercise thallium-201 perfusion imaging appears more sensitive in detecting CAD than an electrocardiographic exercise test[89] and will give information about the location and extent of the perfusion deficit. However, in most patients with single-vessel CAD (except those with a very proximal left anterior descending coronary artery stenosis) the prognosis is good.

3. Thallium scan results do not establish or exclude the

diagnosis of CAD with certainty. However, in patients with chest pain and normal findings during exercise thallium testing, the prognosis is excellent[90,91] even if angiography has demonstrated underlying CAD.[92]

4. If multiple thallium-201 redistribution defects are observed with exercise, especially if associated with abnormal lung uptake (reflecting a sudden rise in left ventricular diastolic pressure), multivessel or left main CAD causing significant ischemia is usually present.[93,93a] The finding of a larger left ventricle on the immediate post-stress image than on the delayed image, i.e., transient ischemic dilatation of the ventricle, is a highly specific marker of multivessel disease and left ventricular dysfunction.[94]

5. Single photon emission computed tomography (SPECT) offers an advantage over conventional planar thallium-201 imaging by providing a three-dimensional view of the myocardium and enhancement of lesion contrast.[95]

6. If a patient cannot perform a routine exercise test, dipyridamole-(or adenosine-[96]) induced maximal coronary vasodilation, when used in conjunction with thallium myocardial imaging (p. 277), offers sensitivity and specificity for the detection of CAD comparable to that of exercise thallium imaging and is relatively safe.[96a] Imaging 45 minutes after administration of oral dipyridamole is effective in unmasking regions of underperfused but viable myocardium.[97] A single high oral dose of dipyridamole (300 mg) followed by quantitative SPECT resulted in a sensitivity of approximately 92 per cent and specificity of 80 per cent in the diagnosis of CAD.[87]

Because thallium scintigraphy has certain disadvantages (unavailable in a physician's office, relatively costly, difficult to interpret), we generally proceed with exercise electrocardiography in the assessment of known or suspected chronic stable angina in patients with a normal resting electrocardiogram. In patients with major electrocardiographic conduction abnormalities at rest (left or right bundle branch block) and in patients with a history of infarction or revascularization in whom the significance of ST-segment changes may be difficult to assess and in whom we are primarily concerned with the consequences of CAD on regional perfusion during exercise, we would often proceed directly to stress thallium-201 myocardial perfusion imaging. In this situation, information concerning the location of ischemia, the extent of ischemia (presence or absence of multiple defects), irreversible ventricular damage (fixed defects), and ventricular dysfunction is useful clinically. In patients who cannot exercise we utilize dipyridamole-induced coronary vasodilation in conjunction with thallium myocardial imaging[85,86] or Holter monitoring of ST segments,[98] depending on the clinical circumstance.

EXERCISE RADIONUCLIDE ANGIOGRAPHY. Since two-dimensional (2-D) echocardiography at rest or during exercise (p. 96) may provide excellent information about ventricular function, radionuclide angiography has a somewhat diminished role in the assessment of patients with CAD than heretofore. It is unusual to use this test for the detection of CAD, but it can provide important information about the influence of known CAD on ventricular function at rest or the functional reserve of the ventricle. Normally, exercise should be associated with an increase in left ventricular ejection fraction of 5 per cent or more. The combination of failure of this normal rise in ejection fraction with exercise and development of new regional wall motion abnormalities is highly specific for CAD.[99]

It is important to realize that the failure of left ventricular ejection fraction to increase during exercise *unaccompanied* by regional wall motion abnormalities is a nonspecific finding that can occur in patients with conditions other than ischemic heart disease, including cardiomyopathy, valvular heart disease, and hypertension, and in some normal individuals receiving beta-adrenoceptor blocker. In patients unable to perform standard exercise testing, dipyridamole radionuclide ventriculography[100] may provide an alternative to ST-segment Holter monitoring, dipyridamole-thallium imaging, or coronary angiography in the detection of CAD.

Clinical Application of Noninvasive Tests

(See also p. 168)

In asymptomatic persons or in those with nonanginal chest pain who are being screened or examined for CAD, i.e., patients in whom the pretest likelihood of coronary disease is low (less than 15 per cent), a normal exercise electrocardiogram excludes, for practical purposes, ischemic heart disease. However, if in such a patient there is an abnormal exercise electrocardiographic test, several alternatives exist. If the patient demonstrates excellent exercise capacity (i.e., to stage IV of a Bruce protocol or the equivalent) then, since the likelihood of left main coronary disease or multivessel CAD is slight and the prognosis is excellent, the patient may be observed without further testing. If, on the other hand, the patient has an early abnormal exercise electrocardiogram, exercise-induced hypotension, or very poor work capacity, coronary angiography is generally indicated to determine whether or not left main CAD or severe multivessel disease with left ventricular dysfunction exists. If the patient falls into an intermediate category (a moderately positive exercise test) then a thallium scan may provide further information. If both the exercise electrocardiogram and thallium perfusion scan are abnormal, the likelihood of significant CAD exceeds 80 per cent. If there is a discrepancy in the results of the two tests, one may either proceed to coronary arteriography or follow up the patient medically, depending on the clinical circumstances.

In patients with atypical angina, if two noninvasive tests are abnormal, the likelihood of CAD exceeds 95 per cent; if both tests are normal, this likelihood falls below 5 per cent. When test results are discordant, they should be evaluated in the light of the level of exercise achieved as well as the degree of positivity (e.g., the presence of accompanying symptoms, the depth of the ST-segment response, the heart rate at which it occurred, and the persistence of the ST-segment response on the stress electrocardiogram; the size and number of perfusion defects on the stress perfusion scintigram; and the magnitude of the exercise-induced change in ejection fraction and regional wall-motion disorder on the exercise radionuclide angiogram). Thus, for example, a patient with a normal exercise electrocardiogram who develops multiple large perfusion defects on a thallium-201 scintigram (accompanied by chest pain at a heart rate of 130 beats/min) has a much greater likelihood of having ischemic heart disease than one who has a normal exercise electrocardiogram and develops a single small perfusion defect without chest pain at a heart rate of 185 beats/min.

In patients with typical angina (i.e., those with a high pretest likelihood of disease), noninvasive testing is most valuable for estimating the extent and severity of CAD and thereby the prognosis. The development of exertional hypotension, marked or prolonged ST-segment depression at low work levels and/or heart rate, striking decreases in ejection fraction and wall motion abnormalities, and large or multiple defects or lung uptake on the exercise thallium scintigram all point to severe multivessel disease in patients at high risk of subsequent coronary events, including sudden death.[101]

OTHER LABORATORY TESTS IN PATIENTS WITH KNOWN CORONARY ARTERY DISEASE

ECHOCARDIOGRAPHY (see also p. 95). Two-dimensional echocardiography allows visualization of large portions of the left ventricle, and serial recordings may detect wall-motion abnormalities due to transient myocardial ischemia. Echocardiography performed immediately after exercise (p. 96) is useful in the detection of wall-motion abnormalities and may enhance the diagnostic yield of a treadmill exercise test by providing information regarding functional reserve of the ventricles in addition to the usual information about exercise capacity, ST-segment changes, and the like.[102] Exercise echocardiography is moderately sensitive (75 to 90 per cent) and highly specific in detecting CAD in patients with normal ventricular wall motion at rest.[103] The test is also highly reproducible.[104] Adequate images can be obtained in more than 85 per cent of patients, and post-peak exercise imaging does not result in failure to detect significant CAD, because ventricular wall-motion abnormalities do not usually normalize immediately.[105] The development of wall-motion abnormalities detected by exercise echocardiography is closely related to the severity of coronary artery stenoses, measured by quantitative angiography.[106]

For patients who cannot exercise on a treadmill or bicycle, transesophageal atrial pacing combined with 2-D echocardiography[107] or dipyridamole–2-D echocardiographic testing may be utilized.[108,109] The development of wall-motion abnormalities and/or angina following the administration of intravenous dipyridamole predicts subsequent cardiac events.[108] During follow-up, cumulative survival rates free of cardiac events over 3 years were 92 per cent for patients with a normal dipyridamole–echocardiography test, 68 per cent for patients who had a positive test with a high dose of dipyridamole, and 50 per cent for patients with a positive test with a low dose of dipyridamole.[108]

It is unclear where exercise echocardiography will eventually fit into the overall scheme of available tests to evaluate CAD. Because, compared with radionuclide ventriculography, it is inexpensive, can be performed in a physician's office, and does not require injection of isotope, it is likely to be used widely. Two-dimensional echocardiography has also been used for defining obstructive lesions of the left main coronary artery[110] (Fig. 4–87, p. 96).

BIOCHEMICAL TESTS. Serum levels of cardiac enzymes (p. 1218) are normal in angina pectoris and serve to differentiate these patients from those with acute myocardial infarction. One of the striking features of chronic ischemic heart disease in relatively young persons is the frequency with which certain metabolic abnormalities are detected. Since hypercholesterolemia and carbohydrate intolerance are recognized as risk factors for the development of ischemic heart disease, the incidence of these abnormalities, particularly in patients under the age of 50 years, is impressive (Chap. 37). Over 90 per cent of patients under the age of 50 with angiographically proven ischemic heart disease have carbohydrate intolerance of either Type II or IV hyperlipoproteinemia.[111,112]

CHEST ROENTGENOGRAM. This is usually within normal limits in patients with chronic ischemic heart disease. However, coronary artery calcification detected fluoroscopically may be more diagnostic of CAD than was once thought, especially in young people. More than 90 per cent of patients with coronary artery calcification were found to have critical coronary artery obstruction; however, coronary calcification on fluoroscopy is not a very sensitive test, since it is found in only 40 per cent of patients with angiographically documented CAD.[113] When fluoroscopic evidence of coronary calcification is present in combination with a positive exercise test, the probability of finding CAD on coronary angiography is very high. Ultrafast computed tomography is more sensitive than fluoroscopy in detecting and quantifying coronary artery calcium.[114]

CATHETERIZATION, ANGIOGRAPHY, AND CORONARY ARTERIOGRAPHY

Although the clinical examination and noninvasive techniques described above are extremely valuable in establishing the diagnosis of ischemic heart disease and, in many instances, the prognosis as well, the definitive diagnosis of CAD and a precise assessment of its anatomical severity and its effects on cardiac performance require cardiac catheterization (Chap. 7), coronary arteriography (Chap. 9), and left ventricular angiography. Among patients with chronic stable angina pectoris referred to cardiologists, coronary arteriography usually reveals relatively equal distribution (approximately 25 per cent each) of critical (> 70 per cent luminal diameter) narrowing of one, two, and three of the major coronary arteries. Five to 10 per cent of patients have obstruction of the left main coronary artery (these patients have a higher complication rate[115]), and in approximately 15 per cent no critical obstruction is detectable (Chap. 9). Total occlusion of at least one major coronary artery is more common in patients with chronic angina who have a history of prior infarction than in those without such a history.

Coronary artery ectasia, i.e., patulous, aneurysmal dilatation involving most of the length of a major epicardial coronary artery, is present in approximately 2 per cent of patients with obstructive CAD. This angiographic lesion does not appear to affect symptoms, survival, or the incidence of myocardial infarction.[116] Coronary ectasia should be distinguished from discrete *coronary artery aneurysms*, which are almost *never* found in arteries without severe stenoses, are most common in the left anterior descending coronary artery, and are usually associated with extensive CAD.[117] These discrete atherosclerotic coronary artery aneurysms do not appear to rupture, and their resection is not warranted.

The functional significance of *collateral vessels* (p. 1164) is unclear. They may protect against myocardial infarction when total occlusion occurs, provided they are of adequate size.[118] Thus, patients with a total occlusion of a major epicardial artery may have well-developed collateral vessels and normal ventricular function, i.e., no evidence of myocardial infarction. Thus, well-developed coronary collaterals may protect against resting ischemia even in the presence of total occlusion, but they may fail to meet the increased needs of exercise and therefore may not abolish exertion-induced angina. Patients with abundant collateral vessels appear to suffer smaller myocardial infarctions.[119,120]

Myocardial bridging of coronary arteries (Fig. 9–25, p. 253) is observed in angiographically normal coronary arteries and normally does not constitute a hazard for the patient. Occasionally, compression of a portion of a coronary artery by a myocardial bridge can be associated with clinical manifestations of myocardial ischemia during strenuous physical activity and may even initiate malignant ventricular arrhythmias.[121,121a]

Ventricular relaxation (p. 438), as reflected in the early diastolic ventricular filling rate, may be impaired at rest. Diastolic filling becomes even more abnormal (slowed) during exercise, when ischemia intensifies.

The frequency of abnormal left ventricular dynamics at rest, i.e., elevations of left ventricular end-diastolic pressure and reduced cardiac output, increases with the number of vessels exhibiting critical narrowing and with the number of prior infarctions,[122] but there is a great deal of overlap among individual patients so that the severity of coronary arterial disease cannot be predicted from these two measurements. The left ventricular end-diastolic pressure may be elevated because of reduced ventricular compliance, left ventricular systolic failure, or a combination of these two processes[123]; both impaired systolic and diastolic function may occur as a consequence of acute, reversible ischemia and chronic scar formation. The elevation of left ventricular diastolic pressure has its clinical correlate in the presence of diastolic (third and fourth) heart sounds. In many patients with normal hemodynamics in the basal state, abnormalities of left ventricular function can be elicited by dynamic or isometric exercise. Elevations of left ventricular end-diastolic pressure usually occur before the patient complains of chest discomfort and before there is electrocardiographic ST-segment depression.

Pacing-induced and post-pacing angina and/or ST-segment depression can also be observed in the catheterization laboratory. This form of stress testing is especially useful for combined hemodynamic-metabolic-ventriculographic studies[124] because quantitative left ventricular angiography and myocardial lactate metabolism can be obtained during or immediately after pacing, uncomplicated by an elevation of systemic arterial lactate levels, as occurs in dynamic exercise. When atrial pacing to induce ischemia is carried out in patients with chronic angina secondary to obstructive CAD, elevations in ventricular end-diastolic pressure occur frequently and usually in association with the development of angina and at a reproducible heart rate–blood pressure product.[124] Impaired ventricular relaxation and increased regional diastolic myocardial stiffness have also been demonstrated during pacing-induced ischemia[125] and represent one component of the altered diastolic properties of the ischemic ventricle (p. 1179).

LEFT VENTRICULAR FUNCTION. Left ventricular dysfunction can be detected with greatest accuracy by means of biplane contrast ventriculography. Global abnormalities of left ventricular function are expressed in elevations of left ventricular end-diastolic and end-systolic volumes and depression of the ejection fraction (p. 424). However, abnormalities of *regional* wall motion (hypokinesia, akinesia, or dyskinesia; Fig. 9–55, p. 272) are more sensitive, specific, and characteristic of CAD, since the latter is usually regional in distribution. Also, hyperkinetic contraction of nonischemic myocardium may compensate for hypokinetic or akinetic ischemic or necrotic myocardium, thereby maintaining normal or almost-normal *global* left ventricular function, despite marked depression of function in one region of the ventricle.[126]

Left ventricular function (global or regional) may be normal at rest in patients with chronic CAD without previous myocardial infarction but become abnormal during or after stress (exercise, pacing). While in most instances resting abnormalities of left ventricular function signify irreversible damage, i.e., prior infarction or acute ischemia, chronic hypoperfusion sufficient to maintain the viability but not the contractility of the myocardium can result in persistent ventricular dysfunction, a condition termed "myocardial hibernation"[127,128,128a] (p. 1176). This form of reversible left ventricular dysfunction may or may not be accompanied by angina pectoris or electrocardiographic changes of ischemia. The reversibility of this form of left ventricular dysfunction is reflected in long-term improvement after revascularization (by surgery or percutaneous transluminal coronary angioplasty) or transiently after an inotropic stimulus (postextrasystolic) potentiation[129] or the infusion of a sympathomimetic amine.[130]

Histopathological studies of myocardial biopsy specimens obtained at the time of coronary artery bypass operations have demonstrated that those segments that exhibit reversible asynergy at angiography are made up predominantly of histologically normal myocardium, while the segments that do not exhibit response to inotropic stimuli exhibit marked muscle loss and replacement by fibrous tissue.[131] The more responsive areas are usually better perfused, either by the native coronary artery or by collateral vessels, and are associated with a lower frequency of electrocardiographic Q waves.[132] The most severe aspect of left ventricular asynergy is the well-demarcated aneurysm, which not only exhibits contractile failure but also is unable to resist expansion during ventricular systole; in other words, it exhibits dyskinesis (paradoxical pulsation).

In addition to demonstrating areas of asynergy, left ventriculography may also show mitral valve prolapse, which occurs in 20 to 25 per cent of patients with obstructive CAD[133] and probably results from impaired contractility of the ventricular myocardium and papillary muscles.

Coronary Blood Flow and Myocardial Metabolism. Abnormal myocardial metabolism has also been documented by means of cardiac catheterization in patients with chronic stable angina. With a catheter in place in the coronary sinus, arterial and coronary venous lactate measurements are obtained at rest and after suitable stresses, such as the infusion of isoproterenol[134] or pacing.[135] Since lactate is a byproduct of anaerobic glycolysis, its production by the heart and subsequent appearance in coronary sinus blood is a reliable sign of myocardial ischemia (p. 1182). When combined with coronary arteriography, this technique may be helpful in localizing significant coronary obstructive lesions and myocardial ischemia.[136]

Coronary flow reserve (maximum flow divided by resting flow, p. 1173) has been measured in patients at cardiac catheterization with coronary sinus thermodilution, Doppler-tipped catheters, and digital subtraction angiography.[137] This invasive measurement is relatively imprecise. Another approach to obtain this variable is by means of quantitative coronary arteriography, which incorporates per cent narrowing with other measurements, including lumen area and vessel length derived by automated border recognition and densitometry. These dimensions can be integrated into a single number, stenosis flow reserve, which if it is below 2.0 to 2.5 is usually associated with clinical manifestations of ischemia, most commonly exertional angina.[137] If this technique is coupled with positron-emission tomography (p. 302), a complete description of the arterial narrowing and its metabolic consequences may be obtained.

Studies of endothelial function in the human coronary circulation (p. 1168) may reveal evidence of a diffuse abnormality of endothelial function even in the presence of angiographically normal coronary arteries.[138,139] An abnormal response, i.e., vasoconstriction, of coronary endothelium to a variety of vasoactive stimuli such as acetylcholine may precede the angiographic recognition of CAD.[139a]

RIGHT-HEART PRESSURE MEASUREMENTS. The value of right-heart catheterization in patients primarily undergoing routine evaluation for CAD has been questioned. It reveals previously unsuspected abnormalities such as right-sided pressure elevations or pulmonary hypertension in only 20 per cent of patients, and the data from right-sided catheterization alter management infrequently.[140] Therefore, routine right-sided catheterization is usually unnecessary in patients with a normal cardiac examination who are undergoing routine, diagnostic coronary angiography, if an echocardiogram has already been obtained and the clinician believes that CAD represents the patient's major cardiac problem.

MANAGEMENT

The management of chronic stable angina involves four aspects: (1) correction of specific coronary risk factors, discussed in Chapter 37; (2) general and nonpharmacological methods, with particular attention toward adjustment of the patient's life style; (3) various specific medications used to treat angina; and (4) revascularization by percutaneous transluminal angioplasty and coronary bypass surgery.

GENERAL MEASURES

General measures include the treatment of hypertension (Chap. 29), which not only is a risk factor for the development and progression of atherosclerosis but also causes cardiac hypertrophy, augments myocardial oxygen requirements, and thereby intensifies myocardial ischemia in patients with obstructive coronary disease. Attainment of an ideal body weight is particularly important in obese patients in whom weight reduction raises the threshold for and may even abolish angina pectoris.

It is imperative for patients with chronic CAD who are cigarette smokers to discontinue this practice. Among patients with angiographically documented CAD, cigarette smokers have a higher 5-year mortality and relative risk of infarction or sudden death than those who have quit smoking,[141] and smoking cessation lessens the risk of adverse coronary events in both older and younger persons with CAD.[142] Habitual smokers who survive out-of-hospital cardiac arrest have a lower incidence of recurrent arrest at 3 years if they stop smoking than do patients who continue to smoke.[143]

There appears to be a strong association between the risk of myocardial infarction and smoking,[144,145] and this risk appears related more to the number of cigarettes smoked per day than to the duration of smoking. Within a few years of stopping smoking this risk of infarction returns to a level similar to that in men who have never smoked.[146] These observations should

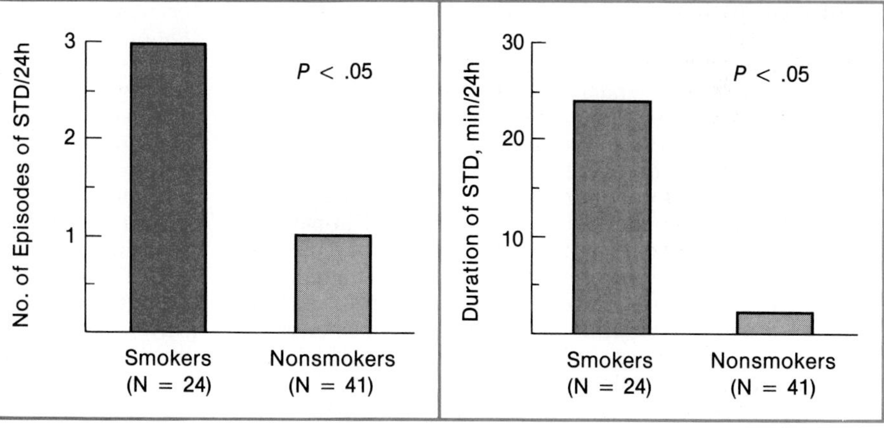

FIGURE 40–3. Influence of smoking on myocardial ischemia. Patients with chronic stable angina and a positive exercise test underwent continuous ambulatory monitoring to quantify the ischemic ST depression during daily life. The frequency of episodes of ischemia was 3 times greater and the duration of ischemia was 12 times longer in smokers than in nonsmokers. The histograms show the median number of episodes (left) and median duration of significant ST-segment depression (STD) (right) during 24 hours in 24 smokers and 41 nonsmokers. (From Barry, J., et al.: Effect of smoking on the activity of ischemic heart disease. JAMA *261*:398, 1989. Copyright 1989, American Medical Association.)

serve as a strong stimulus for discontinuing smoking. They suggest that cigarette smoking may be responsible for ischemic events other than through progression of atherosclerosis. Indeed, while cigarette smoking may increase myocardial oxygen demands and 24-hour energy expenditure (by approximately 10 per cent),[147] it can also cause reductions in coronary blood flow[148] due to an alpha-adrenergically mediated increase in coronary artery tone and increase myocardial ischemia (Fig. 40–3).[149,150]

Cigarette smoking also appears to interfere with the efficacy of antianginal drugs. Improvement in exercise tolerance and a reduction in angina pectoris were noted when cigarette smoking was discontinued while patients were receiving therapy with a beta blocker and nifedipine.[151] Active and passive cigarette smoking,[152] the inhalation of smog and carbon monoxide, and ascent to high altitude all lower the threshold for angina, and their avoidance represents an important aspect of therapy. Symptoms may be aggravated[153] or exercise performance impaired[153,154] in patients with chronic stable angina who encounter some specific environmental situations (traffic tunnels, houses with defective gas furnaces, and closed automobiles during heavy highway traffic).[154] The mechanism of symptom aggravation or exercise impairment is probably decreased oxygen delivery to the myocardium. Every effort must be made to avoid these aggravating stimuli.

In addition, fever, anemia, thyrotoxicosis, infection, tachycardia, hypoxemia (which occurs in acute and chronic pulmonary disease), and certain drugs used to treat noncardiac diseases (such as amphetamines and isoproterenol mists) all increase myocardial oxygen needs and may precipitate or intensify angina; cocaine can cause coronary spasm (p. 1167). These conditions and drugs must be eliminated. Congestive heart failure (by causing cardiac dilatation) and cardiac tachyarrhythmias can increase myocardial oxygen needs. Their treatment, as outlined in Chapters 17 and 24, will frequently diminish the frequency and severity of angina.

COUNSELING AND CHANGES IN LIFE STYLE. Effective communication with both the patient with angina pectoris and the family is essential. The psychosocial issues faced by the patient who develops chronic stable angina for the first time are similar to, although usually less intense than, those experienced by the patient with an acute myocardial infarction. Many patients have an unrealistically gloomy perception of their prognosis; they should be offered a realistic appraisal, together with an understandable explanation of the pertinent clinical features of the disease.

An important aspect of the physician's role is to counsel patients in the kind of work they can do, in their leisure activities, eating habits, vacation plans, and the like. It is desirable, if possible, to consult with the closest member(s) of the family, both to ensure an accurate and full assessment of the patient's activities and to inform the family of what can be expected in the course of the patient's illness.

Certain changes in life style may be helpful, such as modifying strenuous activities if they constantly and repeatedly produce angina. These changes may be minor in many instances. For example, golfing could be modified to include use of a golf cart instead of walking. Many activities, such as shopping or climbing stairs, need not be discontinued; often, it is merely necessary to perform them more slowly or to pause for brief periods of rest. The patient with chronic stable angina should avoid excessive fatigue and exhaustion; one or two regular rest periods during each day are often helpful. While it is desirable to minimize the number of bouts of angina, an occasional episode is not to be feared; indeed, unless patients occasionally reach their anginal threshold, they may not appreciate the extent of their exercise capacity. The vast majority of patients with chronic stable angina should not be treated as invalids. Often the propensity for angina actually declines, perhaps as a result of the development of collaterals or because of training effects, discussed later.

Eliminating or reducing the factors that precipitate anginal episodes is of obvious importance. Patients learn their usual threshold by trial and error. Since many anginal episodes are precipitated by increases in the mechanical activity of the heart (due to increases in myocardial oxygen consumption), the patient should avoid sudden bursts of activity, particularly after long periods of rest. Chronic angina exhibits a circadian rhythm (Fig. 39–14, p. 1214) characterized by a lower anginal threshold shortly after arising.[155] Therefore, morning activities such as showering, shaving, and dressing should be done at a slower pace, and if necessary with use of prophylactic nitroglycerin. The stress of sexual intercourse is ordinarily approximately equal to that of climbing one flight of stairs at a normal pace or of any activity that induces a heart rate of approximately 120 beats/min. With proper precautions, i.e., commencing more than 2 hours postprandially and taking an additional dose of a short-acting beta blocker 1 hour before and nitroglycerin 15 minutes before, the majority of patients with chronic stable angina are able to continue a satisfactory sexual life.

Just as there is a role for exercise in the management of CAD, so is there a role for rest, especially in situations in which angina has become frequent or severe. Marked restriction of activity or even complete bed rest, in addition to drug therapy, may be necessary to control symptoms. In less critical situations, merely reducing the amount of time spent working or increasing the rest periods will have a beneficial effect. For example, a long lunch break including a short nap may be beneficial. It may be helpful for the patient to use a face mask or scarf to cover the mouth or nose in cold weather. A hot, humid environment may also precipitate angina, and air conditioning may be a necessity rather than a luxury for patients with ischemic heart disease. Large meals can have a similar effect if they are followed by exertion. An effort should be made to minimize emotional outbursts, since they too increase myocardial oxygen requirements and sometimes induce coronary vasoconstriction. Occasionally antianxiety drugs or sedation may be useful.

PREVENTION OF MYOCARDIAL (RE)INFARCTION. A variety of measures are used widely in patients with chronic stable angina to prevent acute myocardial infarction and reinfarction (p. 1264). These include discontinuation of smoking, reduction of low-density lipoprotein cholesterol and elevated blood pressure, and the administration of antiplatelet agents and beta blockers. Some of these measures, such as discontinuation of smoking and administration of beta blockers and aspirin,[156] have been shown to improve survival in patients who have experienced infarction and to reduce the incidence of reinfarction. Others have been shown to reduce the incidence of first infarctions in normal persons, or those at high risk, but there is less information on their ability to improve clinical outcome in patients with chronic stable angina. While it would be extremely helpful to obtain such information, it is current policy to advise patients with chronic stable angina to cease smoking (p. 1303), assume an ideal body weight, and control blood pressure.

In men with chronic stable angina but no prior history of myocardial infarction who took aspirin, there was an 87-per cent reduction in the risk of myocardial infarction during 5 years of follow-up.[157] Therefore, in patients with chronic stable angina without contraindications to the drug, the administration of low-dose aspirin (160 mg/day or 325 mg every other day) may be beneficial in reducing the subsequent incidence of myocardial infarction. There is no evidence that long-term use of anticoagulants is indicated in these patients.

Whether beta blockers have any value in preventing infarction and sudden death in patients with chronic stable angina, as they do in patients after myocardial infarction, is not clear. However, since the beneficial effects observed in the post-myocardial infarction population (p. 1254) also possibly occur in the chronic stable angina group, it seems sensible to administer the drugs when angina or hypertension or both are present in these patients and when these drugs are well tolerated. Perhaps the antiarrhythmic and antiischemic effects exhibited by patients with recent myocardial infarction treated with beta blockers also occur in patients with chronic stable angina.

While strong effort should be made to bring total and LDL cholesterol to optimal levels in patients with chronic stable angina, it is not clear that intense dietary and pharmacological measures need be undertaken in the elderly (> 70 years). Men with CAD, thought to be at high risk for subsequent cardiovascular events, underwent intensive lipid-lowering therapy over a $2\frac{1}{2}$-year period and demonstrated a reduced frequency of progression of coronary lesions, reduced incidence of adverse events (death, myocardial infarction, or revascularization), and increased frequency of regression of coronary lesions compared with patients assigned to conventional therapy.[158] This suggests that efforts to lower lipids in patients with a high-risk profile are justified and that this may influence favorably their long-term outcome.

EXERCISE (see also Chapter 42). The *conditioning effect of exercise* on skeletal muscles allows the patient to develop a greater workload at any level of total body oxygen consumption. The conditioning effect of exercise on the heart, by decreasing the heart rate at any level of exercise, allows a higher cardiac output to be achieved at any level of myocardial oxygen consumption. The combination of these two effects of exercise conditioning permits the patient with chronic stable angina to increase physical performance substantially following institution of a continuing exercise program. The reduced pressure-rate product lowers myocardial oxygen requirements during exertion and enables the patient with CAD to perform at higher workloads before reaching the ischemic threshold.[159] Therefore, physical conditioning reduces the amount of oxygen needed by the heart for any given amount of total body work. An example of this effect is seen in the study of Redwood et al. carried out in patients with chronic stable angina. They reported that a 6-week training program improved exercise performance by reducing the responses of heart rate and arterial pressure to bicycle exercise and by prolonging the duration of exercise before angina occurred.[160] Patients with chronic ischemic heart disease may achieve a greater ejection fraction at equivalent workloads after training.

The psychological benefits of exercise are difficult to evaluate. However, exercise conditioning programs may be quite helpful in increasing the self-confidence of patients with chronic CAD (as they do in patients recovering from acute myocardial infarction). The question whether or not exercise accelerates the development of collateral vessels in patients with chronic CAD is unsettled.[161]

For all of the aforementioned reasons, patients are urged to participate in regular exercise programs—usually walking (see below)—in conjunction with their drug therapy. Patients who are involved in exercise programs usually are also more likely to be health conscious, to pay attention to diet and weight, and to discontinue cigarette smoking. Thus, in addition to a conditioning effect on skeletal and cardiac muscle, regular dynamic exercise provides the patient with a feeling of well-being, an important consideration in the management of any chronic disease.

The rationale and specific details for establishing an exercise program in patients with CAD are outlined in Chapter 42. Despite the many favorable effects of regular physical exercise in patients with chronic stable angina enumerated above, it must be acknowledged that there is no hard evidence that such programs improve survival or reduce the need for surgery in these patients.

NITRATES

(See also pp. 497 and 1172)

MECHANISM OF ACTION. Although the clinical effectiveness of amyl nitrite in angina pectoris was first described in 1867 by Brunton, organic nitrates are still the most common medications physicians employ to treat patients with this condition. The action of these agents is to relax vascular smooth muscle. The vasodilator effects of nitrates are evident in both systemic (including coronary) arteries and veins in normal subjects and in patients with ischemic heart disease, but they appear to be predominant in the venous circulation.[162] The decrease in venous tone reduces the return of blood to the heart and reduces preload and ventricular dimensions,[163] which in turn reduces wall tension and afterload. The actions of nitrates to reduce both preload and afterload make them useful in the treatment of heart failure as well as angina pectoris.

Posture is important in evaluating the hemodynamic effects of nitrates. In a patient in the supine position, venous return is normally greater while exercise tolerance and the anginal threshold are lower than in the upright position. The hemodynamic and angina-relieving effects of nitrates are most marked when patients are sitting or standing, i.e., when these drugs can reduce preload, and their hemodynamic effect resembles those of phlebotomy. By reducing the heart's mechanical activity, volume, and oxygen consumption, nitrates increase exercise capacity in patients with ischemic heart disease, i.e., a greater total body workload can be achieved before the anginal threshold is reached.

EFFECTS ON THE CORONARY CIRCULATION. A vasodilating effect of the nitrates on the larger (conductance) coronary arteries can be readily demonstrated, and there is evidence, obtained from quantitative, computer-assisted measurements of coronary arterial diameter, that nitroglycerin causes dilatation of epicardial stenoses. These are often eccentric lesions, and nitroglycerin causes relaxation of smooth muscle in the wall of the coronary artery that is not encompassed by the plaque. Even a small increase in the narrowed arterial lumen can produce a significant reduction in resistance to blood flow across the narrowed lesion (Fig. 40–4).[164]

Studies in experimental animals with coronary obstruction

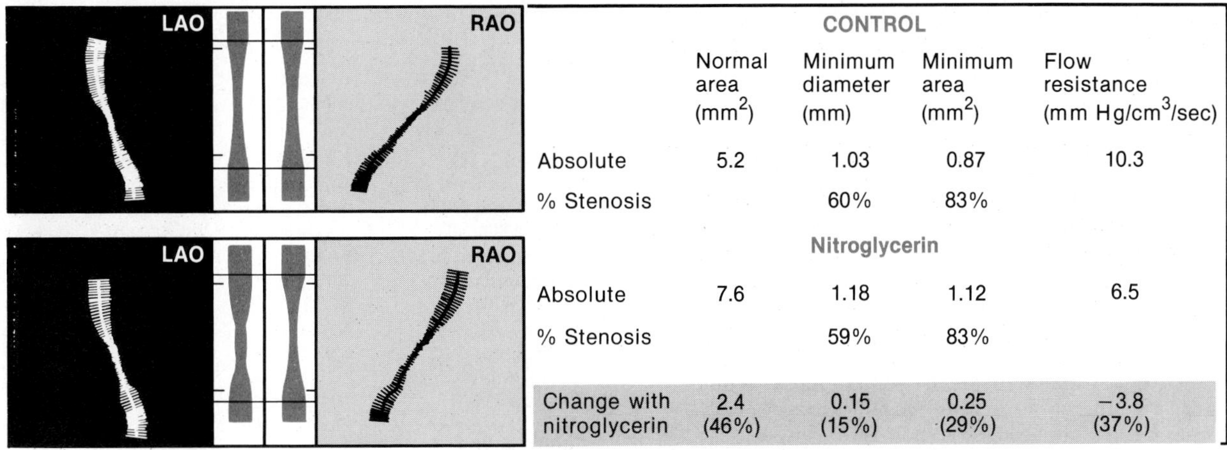

	Normal area (mm^2)	Minimum diameter (mm)	Minimum area (mm^2)	Flow resistance (mm Hg/cm^3/sec)
CONTROL				
Absolute	5.2	1.03	0.87	10.3
% Stenosis		60%	83%	
Nitroglycerin				
Absolute	7.6	1.18	1.12	6.5
% Stenosis		59%	83%	
Change with nitroglycerin	2.4 (46%)	0.15 (15%)	0.25 (29%)	−3.8 (37%)

FIGURE 40–4. A representative computer printout of segmental stenosis images and dimensional data for prenitroglycerin and postnitroglycerin (0.4 mg, sublingual) angiograms of this 60 per cent mid-right coronary artery stenosis. Each value is averaged from 8 estimates. LAO = left anterior oblique; RAO = right anterior oblique. (From Brown, B. G., et al.: The mechanisms of nitroglycerin action: Stenosis vasodilation as a major component of the drug response. Circulation *64:*1089, 1981, by permission of the American Heart Association, Inc.)

have shown that nitroglycerin causes redistribution of blood flow from normally perfused to ischemic areas, particularly in the subendocardium,[165] perhaps mediated in part by an increase in collateral blood flow[166] and in part by a lowering of ventricular diastolic pressure, reducing subendocardial compression. The results of studies of nitroglycerin on coronary blood flow have been conflicting. Some studies in patients have reported increased blood flow after sublingual or intravenous nitroglycerin,[167] but most report no change or reduced flow.[168–170] However, since myocardial oxygen demands fell, the net effect on oxygen balance became favorable. In studies employing intracoronary injection of xenon-133[171] (as well as in retrograde perfusion studies performed during coronary bypass surgery), regional myocardial blood flow in areas perfused by stenotic coronary arteries rose after administration of nitroglycerin when well-developed collaterals supplying those regions were present. Atrial pacing studies indicate that after nitroglycerin the heart can be paced to higher rates before angina occurs. The nitrates have also been shown to improve ventricular wall motion in patients with ischemic heart disease, as demonstrated by contrast ventriculography,[172] echocardiography, and radionuclide ventriculography, at rest and during exercise.[173]

MECHANISM OF ANTIANGINAL ACTION. This action of the nitrates is complex (Fig. 40–5). Nitrates are not considered to exert a direct effect on the contractile state of the heart, although heart rate may rise reflexly as a consequence of the decline in blood pressure. When beta blockers are administered concurrently, the reflex tachycardia accompanying the nitrate-induced hypotension is blunted. Apparently, one action is to reduce the mechanical activity of the heart through the previously noted systemic effects, with subsequent reduction in left ventricular wall tension (which results from the simultaneous nitrate-induced reduction of arterial pressure and ventricular volume) and of myocardial oxygen consumption. Reduced left ventricular diastolic pressure may also decrease the resistance to coronary blood flow. It is probable that the cardiac actions of the nitrates—dilating epicardial stenoses, dilating coronary collateral vessels, and reducing ventricular diastolic pressure and thereby lowering extravascular resistance to endocardial perfusion—all act to increase oxygen delivery to ischemic myocardium. In the final analysis, some combination of a nitrate-induced reduction of myocardial oxygen requirements and increased oxygen delivery to the ischemic area relieves or prevents the development of myocardial ischemia in patients with chronic stable angina.

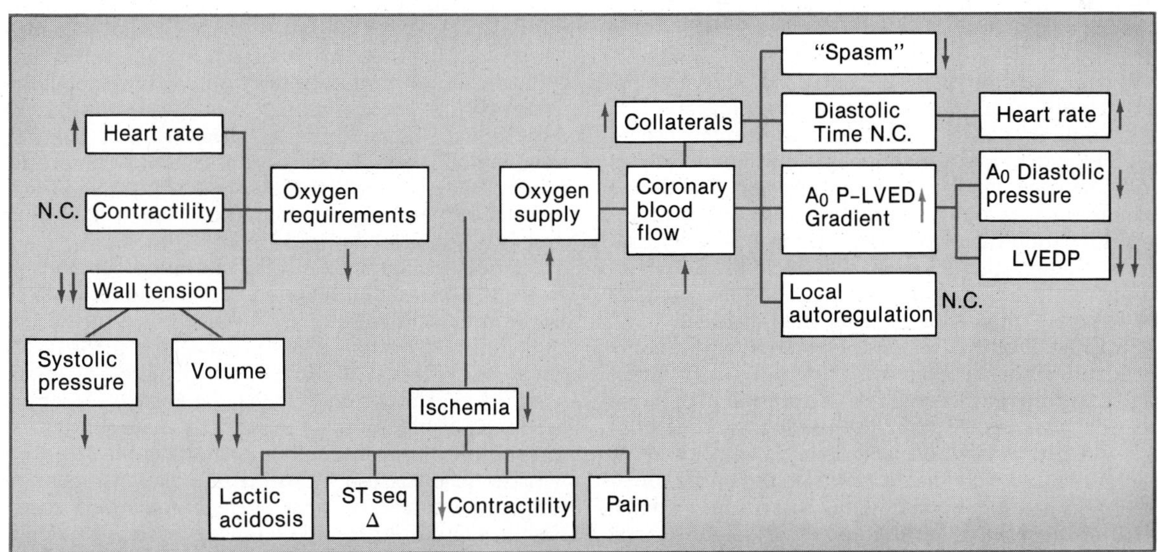

FIGURE 40–5. Factors influencing balance between myocardial oxygen requirements *(left)* and supply *(right)*. Arrows indicate effects of nitrates. In relieving angina pectoris, nitrates exert favorable effects by reducing oxygen requirements and increasing supply. Although a reflex increase in heart rate would tend to reduce the time for coronary flow, dilation of collaterals and enhancement of the pressure gradient for flow to occur as the LVEDP falls tend to increase coronary flow. AoP = aortic pressure; LVEDP = left ventricular end-diastolic pressure; NC = no change. (From Frishman, W. H.: Pharmacology of the nitrates in angina pectoris. Am. J. Cardiol. *56:*81, 1985.)

Assessment of the relative importance of these two actions of nitroglycerin (reducing oxygen demand and increasing oxygen supply) has been complicated by the differing results of studies on the effects of intracoronary nitroglycerin. Any effect of the drug administered by this route must derive from its direct action on the coronary vascular bed, i.e., by improving myocardial oxygen supply; some studies have demonstrated a beneficial effect of intracoronary nitroglycerin,[164] while others have not. It is of interest that smoking-induced coronary vasoconstriction is prevented by nitroglycerin and calcium antagonists.[174] Perhaps the principal action of nitrates differs in different patients; in patients with a strong coronary vasoconstrictive component to their angina their principal action may be to increase oxygen delivery to ischemic myocardium, while in patients with relatively fixed lesions and constant-threshold angina their principal action may be to reduce myocardial oxygen demands.

Cellular Mechanism of Action. Nitrates have the ability to cause vasodilation whether or not endothelium is intact.[175] After entering the vascular smooth muscle cell, nitrates are converted to reactive nitric oxide–free radical (NO) or S-nitrosothiols, which activate intracellular guanylate cyclase to produce cyclic guanosine monophosphate (GMP),[162,175] which in turn triggers smooth muscle relaxation.[176] Sulfhydryl (SH) groups are required for both the formation of NO and the stimulation of guanylate cyclase, and nitroglycerin-induced vasodilation can be enhanced by prior administration of *N*-acetylcysteine, an agent that increases the availability of sulfhydryl groups.[177] This action of *N*-acetylcysteine potentiates the peripheral hemodynamic responses[177] and the coronary vasodilator effect of nitroglycerin[178] and reverses the partial tolerance to the coronary vasodilator effect of nitroglycerin.[179]

Types of Preparations and Routes of Administration

Nitroglycerin administered sublingually remains the drug of choice for treatment of acute anginal episodes. A transient but effective concentration of the drug rapidly appears in the circulation because sublingual administration avoids first-pass hepatic metabolism. The half-life of nitroglycerin itself is brief, and it is rapidly converted to two inactive metabolites, both of which are found in the urine after nitroglycerin administration. The liver possesses large amounts of hepatic glutathione organic nitrate reductase, but there is also evidence that blood vessels (veins and arteries) may metabolize nitrates directly. Thus, within 30 to 60 minutes hepatic breakdown has abolished the hemodynamic and clinical effects. Nitroglycerin is also available in a variety of other forms (Table 40–2).

The usual sublingual dosage is 0.3 to 0.6 mg, and most patients respond within 5 minutes to one or two 0.3-mg tablets. If symptoms are not relieved by a single dose, additional doses of 0.3 mg may be taken at 5-minute intervals, but no more than 1.2 mg should be used within a 15-minute period. The development of tolerance is rarely a problem with intermittent usage (see below). Sublingual nitroglycerin is especially useful when it is taken prophylactically shortly before activities are begun that are likely to cause angina. Used for this purpose, it may prevent angina for up to 30 to 40 minutes.

ADVERSE REACTIONS. These are common and include headache, flushing, and hypotension. The last is only rarely severe but can be potentially dangerous if the chest pain is due to a myocardial infarction rather than angina and arterial pressure has already declined because of pump failure and/or a vagal reaction or hypovolemia. In addition, the partial pressure of oxygen in arterial blood may fall after large doses of nitroglycerin because of a ventilation-perfusion imbalance due to inability of the pulmonary vascular bed to constrict in areas of alveolar hypoxia and thereby redirect perfusion to less hypoxic tissues.[180] *Methemoglobinemia* is a rare complication of very large doses of nitrates (p. 1761). Commonly used doses of nitrates cause small elevations of methemoglobin that probably are not of clinical significance.

TABLE 40-2 DOSAGE AND KINETICS OF NITROGLYCERIN AND LONG-ACTING NITRATES

MEDICATION	USUAL DOSAGE	ONSET OF ACTION	DURATION OF ACTION
Aerosol NTG	0.4 mg	2–5 min	10–30 min
NTG ointment (2%)	½–2 inches	20–60 min	3–8 hr
Sublingual NTG	0.3–0.6 mg	2–5 min	10–30 min
Oral NTG (SR)	2.5–9 mg	30–45 min	2–8 hr*
Transdermal NTG	5–15 mg	30–60 min	8–14 hr
Transmucosal NTG	1–3 mg	2–5 min	3–5 hr*
Oral ISDN	5–30 mg	15–30 min	3–6 hr
Oral ISDN (SR)	40 mg	30–60 min	6–10 hr
Sublingual and chewable ISDN	2.5–10 mg	3–15 min	1–2 hr
Oral ISMN	10–40 mg	30 min	6–8 hr
Oral ISMN (SR)	40–100 mg	30 min	6–10 hr
Sublingual and chewable ET	5–15 mg	3–15 min	2 hr
Oral ET	10 mg	30 min	Variable
Oral PET	10–40 mg	30 min	3–6 hr
Oral PET (SR)	30–80 mg	Slow	6–10 hr

* Duration of action lengthens with increasing dosage.

ET = erythrityl tetranitrate; ISDN = isosorbide dinitrate; ISMN = isosorbide-5-mononitrate (not available in the U.S.); NTG = nitroglycerin; PET = pentaerythrityl tetranitrate; SR = sustained release.

PREPARATIONS. Nitroglycerin tablets tend to lose their potency, especially if exposed to light, and should be kept in dark containers. Other nitrate preparations are available in sublingual, buccal, oral, spray, and ointment form (Table 40–2). Isosorbide dinitrate and other long-acting preparations are available in 2.5- and 5.0-mg sublingual tablets, 10-mg buccal (chewable) form, and 5-, 10-, and 20-mg tablets for oral use, as well as in 40-mg (sustained-release) capsules. An oral nitroglycerin spray that dispenses metered, aerosolized doses of 0.4 mg may be better absorbed than the sublingual form in patients with dry mucosal membranes. It can also be quickly sprayed onto, or under, the tongue with one hand and has a 3-year shelf life. For prophylaxis, the spray should be used 5 to 10 minutes before attack-provoking activities.[181]

Isosorbide Dinitrate. Isosorbide dinitrate is an effective antianginal agent but has low bioavailability after oral administration, because it undergoes rapid hepatic metabolism[182] and there are marked variations in plasma concentrations after oral administration. It has two metabolites (one has a potent vasodilator action) that are cleared less rapidly than the parent drug and are excreted unchanged in the urine.

Isosorbide-5-mononitrate,[183] an active metabolite of the dinitrate (not yet available in the United States), is completely bioavailable, since it does not undergo first-pass hepatic metabolism. Plasma levels of isosorbide-5-mononitrate reach their peak between 30 minutes and 2 hours, and the drug has a plasma half-life of 4 to 6 hours. A single 20-mg tablet still exhibits activity 8 hours after administration.

Partial or complete nitrate tolerance develops with regimens of isosorbide dinitrate when it is administered as 30 mg three or four times daily.[184,185] When this drug is used, a dosage schedule should be adopted that allows a 10- to 12-hour nitrate-free interval.[164,186–188] If the drug is administered on a three-times daily schedule (e.g., at 8 AM, 1 PM, and 6 PM), the antianginal benefit lasts for approximately 6 hours, and the magnitude of the antianginal benefit decreases with each successive dose.[185] Isosorbide dinitrate, like nitroglycerin, dilates both atherosclerotic and normal epicardial coronary segments, including diseased segments in small and medium-size arteries.[189] The drug has been shown to augment the increased exercise response observed with beta-adrenoceptor blockers.[190] While oral nitrates are not especially potent agents, they can reduce the incidence of anginal attacks and the need for sublingual nitroglycerin as well as raise the threshold of activity required for the development of angina.

TOLERANCE. Partial or complete nitrate tolerance develops with transdermal nitroglycerin patches,[191] once-daily applications of sustained-release isosorbide dinitrate ointment,[192] and regimens of isosorbide dinitrate administered 30 mg four times daily,[184] and 20 to 30 mg three times daily (at 8 AM, 1 PM, and 6 PM).[185] Thus, any regimen using frequent doses of long-acting nitrates (three or more times daily), continuous delivery systems (intravenous nitroglycerin or transdermal nitroglycerin patches) or long-acting (sustained-release) preparations *will result in tolerance unless there is a 10- to 12-hour nitrate-free interval.*[162,186–188,192a] Nitroglycerin administered by the buccal route does not result in tolerance and, even after 2 weeks of therapy, there is no diminished efficacy when buccal nitroglycerin is administered three times daily.[193] Even in patients who are already tolerant to long-acting oral nitrate therapy, intermittent doses of sublingual nitroglycerin will be effective.[194] Transdermal nitroglycerin patches will retain their efficacy provided patients have a 12-hour nitrate-free interval every 24 hours.[188]

The most commonly accepted hypothesis for the development of nitrate tolerance is that a depletion of intracellular sulfhydryl cofactors occurs in the metabolic conversion of nitroglycerin to nitric oxide or S-nitrosothiols, a conversion necessary for the activation of guanylate cyclase.[192,195,196] It is also possible that nitrate therapy is associated with increased catecholamine release and activation of the renin-angiotensin system, which might oppose the effect of nitrate-induced vasodilation.[195,196] It has been shown that if the sulfhydryl groups of the nitrate receptors are replenished by compounds such as N-acetylcysteine[177] or made more available by methionine,[197] then nitrate tolerance can be partially reversed[177] or the hemodynamic effects of intravenous nitroglycerin can be potentiated.[197]

Topical Nitroglycerin. Nitroglycerin ointment (15 mg/inch) is efficacious when applied (mostly commonly to the chest) in strips of 0.5 to 2.0 inches. Delay in the onset of action is approximately 30 minutes. Since it is effective for 4 to 6 hours, this form of the drug is particularly useful in patients with severe angina or unstable angina who are confined to bed and chair. Nitroglycerin ointment also may be used prophylactically after retiring by patients with nocturnal angina. Skin permeability increases with increased hydration, and absorption is also enhanced if the paste is covered with plastic whose edges are taped to the skin.

Transdermal Nitroglycerin Patches. A silicone gel or polymer matrix is impregnated with nitroglycerin, and absorption is then maintained for 24 to 48 hours at a rate determined by various methods of preparation, including a semipermeable membrane placed between the drug reservoir and the skin. The release rate of the patches varies from 2.5 to 15 mg/24 hours. Relatively low doses (2.5 mg to 5 mg/24 hours) may not produce sufficient plasma and tissue concentrations to sustain consistent, effective antianginal effects.[198]

A meta-analysis of randomized clinical trials of nitroglycerin patches suggested that in doses of 5 to 10 mg/24 hours exercise duration was improved early after administration, but by 24 hours the effect of nitroglycerin on exercise performance was attenuated by nitrate tolerance.[199] However, a regimen in which transdermal nitroglycerin was applied for 12 hours, and removed for 12 hours, improved exercise performance for 8 to 12 hours after application of the patch. After 1 month of such therapy, responsiveness to transdermal nitroglycerin remained virtually unchanged.[188] Therefore, after application of a transdermal nitroglycerin patch one can expect therapeutic efficacy (improved exercise performance) for 8 to 12 hours, and provided a substantial nitrate-free interval (of 10 to 12 hours) exists every 24-hour period, sustained improvement in exercise performance may be maintained. If a state of tolerance has been induced, a nitrate-free interval will restore responsiveness. If large, intermittent doses of transdermal or oral nitrates are employed (equivalent to 20 mg/24 hours of a transdermal patch), it is possible that rebound angina may occur during the nitrate-free period.[188,192]

WITHDRAWAL OF NITRATES. Because of the possibility of nitrate dependence, nitrate therapy should be withdrawn carefully. In individuals exposed to industrial doses of nitroglycerin, nitrate tolerance, nitrate dependence, and withdrawal symptoms may cause serious problems. During the manufacture of dynamite, substantial levels of nitrates are often present in the atmosphere and can be absorbed from the skin and lungs. After an acute response of headache, hypotension, palpitations, and gastrointestinal disturbance, adaptation occurs. Withdrawal from this environment may result in angina unrelated to exertion or emotion. In fact, spontaneous coronary vasospasm and acute myocardial infarction have been documented during a period of withdrawal.[200] A less dramatic, but far more common, form of nitrate withdrawal is observed in patients whose angina is intensified after discontinuation of large doses of long-acting nitrates.

BETA-ADRENOCEPTOR BLOCKING AGENTS

(See also p. 862)

These drugs constitute a cornerstone of therapy for effort-induced chronic stable angina. In the United States, four beta-adrenoceptor blocking drugs have been approved for the treatment of *angina*: atenolol, metoprolol, nadolol, and propranolol. A number of studies have shown that beta-adrenoceptor blockers, in doses that are generally well tolerated, reduce the frequency of anginal episodes and raise the anginal threshold, both when given alone and when added to other antianginal agents. The salutary action of these drugs, which have a chemical structure resembling that of isoproterenol and other beta-adrenoceptor agonists, depends on their ability to cause competitive inhibition of the effects of neuronally released and circulating catecholamines on beta-adrenoceptors.[201] In this manner, these drugs attenuate the cardiac responses to adrenergic stimulation (chiefly increases in heart rate and contractility). Thus, beta blockers reduce myocardial oxygen demands primarily during activity or excitement when surges of increased sympathetic activity occur. Effects on heart rate and myocardial contractility at rest are less prominent because of the lower adrenergic drive to the heart in the basal state. Beta-adrenoceptor blockers also lower myocardial oxygen needs by reducing arterial pressure, and they are extremely useful antihypertensive agents (p. 862).

Coronary vasoconstriction during the cold pressor test has been shown to be potentiated by beta-adrenergic receptor blockers in patients with coronary artery disease[202] but intracoronary administration of propranolol does not cause coronary vasoconstriction of epicardial vessels at rest or during exercise.[203] In clinical practice the potential adverse influence of unopposed increased alpha-receptor–mediated coronary artery tone associated with beta-blocker therapy is not a problem, except in some patients with variant angina (p. 1344).

Continuous ambulatory electrocardiographic and intraarterial blood pressure monitoring during normal daily activities of patients with chronic stable effort angina suggest that many ischemic events may be precipitated by transient impairment of regional myocardial perfusion rather than increases in myocardial oxygen demand.[20a] Beta blockers significantly reduce episodes of transient myocardial ischemia in these patients.[204]

CHARACTERISTICS OF DIFFERENT BETA BLOCKERS. The differing pharmacological properties of these agents affect their clinical effects (Table 40–3).

Selectivity. Two major subtypes of beta receptors, designated $beta_1$, and $beta_2$,[205] are present in different proportions in different tissues. $Beta_1$ receptors predominate in the heart, and their stimulation leads to an increase in heart rate and A-V conduction and contractility, whereas stimulation of these receptors leads to the release of renin in juxtaglomerular cells and lipolysis in adipocytes. $Beta_2$ stimulation results in bronchodilation, vasodilatation, and glycogenolysis.

The beta blockers have been classified according to their

TABLE 40-3 PHARMACOKINETICS AND PHARMACOLOGY OF SOME BETA-ADRENOCEPTOR BLOCKERS

	DRUG									
	Atenolol	Metoprolol	Nadolol	Pindolol	Propranolol	Timolol	Propranolol HCl	Propranolol LA	Acebutolol	Labetalol
Extent of absorption (%)	≃50	>95	≃30	>90	90	>90	>90	>90	≃70	>90
Extent of bioavailability (% of dose)	≃40	≃50	≃30	≃90	≃30	75	≃30	≃20	≃50	≃25
Beta-blocking plasma concentration	0.2–0.5 μg/ml	50–100 ng/ml	50–100 ng/ml	50–100 ng/ml	50–100 ng/ml	5–10 ng/ml	50–100 ng/ml	20–100 ng/ml	0.2–2.0 μg/ml	0.7–3.0 μg/ml
Protein binding (%)	<5	12	≃30	57	93	≃10	93	93	30–40	≃50
Lipophilicity*	Low	Moderate	Low	Moderate	High	Low	High	High	Low	Low
Elimination half-life (hr)	6 to 9	3 to 4	14 to 25	3 to 4	3.5 to 6.0	3 to 4	3–4	10	3–4‡	≃6
Urinary recovery of unchanged drug (% of dose)	≃40	≃3	70	≃40	<1	≃20	<1	<1	≃40	<1
Total urinary recovery (% of dose)	>95	>95	70	>90	>90	65	>90	>90	>90	>90
Drug accumulation in renal disease	Yes	No	Yes	No	No	No	No	No	Yes§	No
Predominant route of elimination†	RE (mostly unchanged)	HM	RE	RE (≃40% unchanged) and HM	HM	RE (≃20% unchanged) and HM	HM	HM	HM§	HM
Active metabolites	No	No	No	No	Yes	No	Yes	Yes	Yes	No
β_1-blocker potency ratio (propranolol = 1)	1.0	1.0	1.0	6.0	1.0	6.0	1.0	1.0	0.3	0.3
Relative β_1 sensitivity	+	+	0	0	0	0	0	0	Yes	0
Intrinsic sympathetic activity	0	0	0	+	0	0	0	0	+	0
Membrane-stabilizing activity	0	0	0	+	++	0	++	++	+	0
Usual maintenance dose	50–100 mg/qd	50–100 mg/qid	40–80 mg/qd	5–20 mg/tid	60 mg/qid	20 mg/bid	60 mg/qid	80–160 mg/qd	200–600 mg/bid	100–600 mg/bid

*Determined by the distribution ratio between octanol and water.
†RE = renal excretion; HM = hepatic metabolism.
‡Half-life of the active metabolite, diacetolol, is 12 to 15 hours.
§Acebutolol is mainly eliminated by the liver, but its major metabolite, diacetolol, is excreted by the kidney.
Modified from Frishman, W. H., et al.: Antianginal agents, Part 2: β-Blockers. Hosp. Formul. *21*:62, 1986.

relative cardioselectivity, i.e., $beta_1$-blocking properties. *Nonselective* beta-blocking drugs (propranolol, nadolol, oxprenolol, penbutolol, pindolol, sotalol, timolol, carteolol) block both $beta_1$ and $beta_2$ receptors, whereas *cardioselective* beta blockers (atenolol, betaxolol, bevantolol, esmolol, metoprolol) produce selective blockade of $beta_1$ receptors, while having lesser effects on $beta_2$ receptors. Thus, cardioselective beta blockers will reduce myocardial oxygen demands while tending not to block bronchodilation, vasodilatation, or glycogenolysis. As the dosages administered are increased, this cardioselectivity diminishes.[206] Since cardioselectivity is only relative, the use of cardioselective beta blockers in doses sufficient to prevent angina may still cause bronchoconstriction in some susceptible patients. Some drugs with beta-blocking properties also have the ability to cause vasodilatation. These include labetalol (an alpha-adrenergic blocking agent and a $beta_2$ agonist, p. 866), carvedilol (a direct vasodilator with $beta_1$- and $beta_2$-blocking activity), and dilevalol (the R,R isomer of labetalol that causes vasodilation due to $beta_2$-agonist activity and has $beta_1$- and $beta_2$-receptor competitive antagonist properties). Such agents are useful in the treatment of hypertension.

Membrane-Stabilizing Activity. This property refers to the "quinidine-like" effect of certain beta blockers that reduce the rate of rise of the cardiac action potential (p. 358). The clinical relevance of this effect is questionable because it is observed only at concentrations far exceeding therapeutic levels of the beta blockers that exhibit this action at all (propranolol, acebutolol).

Intrinsic Sympathomimetic Activity. Beta blockers with intrinsic sympathomimetic activity (acebutolol, carteolol, celiprolol, dilevalol, oxprenolol, penbutolol, pindolol) are "partial agonists" and produce blockade by shielding beta receptors from more potent beta agonists. Pindolol and acebutolol produce low-grade beta stimulation when sympathetic activity is low (at rest), while under conditions of stress and exercise, when sympathetic activity is high, partial agonists behave more like conventional beta blockers.

Pindolol causes little if any lowering of heart rate, depression of A-V conduction, or depression of contractility at rest but still blocks the effects of exercise on these variables. Its partial agonist activity also induces bronchodilation.[207] In patients with severe symptoms and nocturnal angina, agents with partial agonist activity may not be as effective at reducing heart rate or the frequency, duration, and magnitude of ambulatory ST-segment changes (monitored over 48 hours) or increasing the duration of exercise.[208]

Potency. This is the ability of beta blockers to inhibit the tachycardia produced by isoproterenol. All drugs are considered in reference to propranolol, which is given a value of 1.0 (Table 40–3). Timolol and pindolol are the most potent agents, while acebutolol and labetalol are the least.

Lipid Solubility. The hydrophilicity or lipid solubility of beta blockers is a major determinant of their absorption and metabolism. The lipid-soluble (lipophilic) beta blockers, propranolol, metoprolol, and pindolol (Table 40–3), are readily absorbed from the gastrointestinal tract. They are metabolized predominantly by the liver, have a relatively short half-life, and usually require administration twice or more daily to achieve continuing pharmacological effects. The water-soluble beta blockers (hydrophilic), atenolol, sotalol, and nadolol, are not as readily absorbed from the gastrointestinal tract, are not as extensively metabolized, have relatively long plasma half-lives, and can be administered once daily. Thus, in patients with renal or hepatic dysfunction the lipid-insoluble agents may be preferable.

Lipid-insoluble beta blockers are less likely to cross the blood-brain barrier; central nervous system side effects of beta blockers include depression, sleep disturbances, nightmares, fatigue, and weakness. While beta blockers with increased lipid solubility, such as pindolol and metoprolol, cross the blood-brain barrier more readily, there is no direct, consistent correlation between this property and central nervous system side effects.[209,210] For example, atenolol and metoprolol cause a similar degree of central nervous system effects despite large differences in lipid solubility[210] and, while the lipid-soluble agents propranolol, pindolol, and metoprolol cause more sleep interruptions and restlessness than either placebo or atenolol, other measures of mood and psychomotor and sexual function do not appear to correlate with lipid solubility.[211] Overall, atenolol (low lipid solubility) and metoprolol (moderate lipid solubility) may be useful if central nervous system side effects are a problem with other beta blockers.

Alpha-Adrenoceptor Blocking Activity. The alpha-blocking potency of labetalol is approximately 20 per cent of its beta-blocking potency, and it is also one of the weaker beta blockers compared with propranolol[212] (Table 40–3). Its combined alpha- and beta-blocking effects make it a particularly useful antihypertensive agent (p. 866), especially in patients with hypertension and angina. During exercise testing in normotensive patients with angina, labetalol prolonged exercise duration and blunted the exercise-induced tachycardia and increases in arterial pressure.[213]

Oxidation Phenotype. Metoprolol and propranolol are lipid-soluble beta blockers noted for the variability of their pharmacokinetics, drug metabolism, and pharmacodynamics. It has been found that the oxidative metabolism of metoprolol exhibits the debrisoquin type of genetic polymorphism (p. 630) and that poor hydroxylators, or metabolizers (up to 10 per cent of Caucasians), have significant prolongation of the elimination half-life of the drug as compared with extensive hydroxylators, or metabolizers. Thus, angina might be controlled by a single daily dose of metoprolol in poor metabolizers, whereas extensive metabolizers require the same dose two or three times a day.[214] Therefore, clinicians should be aware that if a patient exhibits an exaggerated clinical response (e.g., extreme bradycardia) following administration of metoprolol, propranolol, or other lipid-soluble beta blockers, it may be the result of prolongation of the elimination half-life due to slow oxidative metabolism of the drug.

First-Pass Effects. The lipid-soluble beta blockers are usually rapidly absorbed from the gastrointestinal tract and metabolized extensively by the liver (first-pass metabolism) before they reach the systemic circulation. Drugs such as propranolol and metoprolol have extensive first-pass metabolism, while timolol and pindolol have moderate first-pass metabolism. If either metoprolol or propranolol is administered intravenously, a much higher concentration reaches the bloodstream, and therefore intravenous dosing has much greater potency than oral dosing.

Effects on Serum Lipids. In general, beta blocker therapy (with agents without intrinsic sympathomimetic activity [ISA]) usually causes no significant changes in total or LDL cholesterol but increases triglycerides and decreases HDL.[215,216] The most commonly studied drug has been propranolol, which can increase plasma triglyceride concentrations by up to 50 per cent and reduce HDL cholesterol by approximately 15 per cent.[215] (Sotalol, a drug without ISA, increases total cholesterol, triglycerides, and LDL cholesterol and also decreases HDL cholesterol.) Two drugs possessing ISA, acebutolol and pindolol, do not significantly change total cholesterol, triglycerides, or LDL cholesterol, but pindolol *increases* serum HDL cholesterol. The clinical importance of these changes in serum lipids after long-term administration of beta blockers for either hypertension or angina is unknown, but obviously physicians should be aware that beta blockers may affect the serum lipid profile of their patients and should take this into account when monitoring long-term therapy.[215,216]

DOSAGE. For optimal results, the dosage of beta blocker should be carefully titrated. In the case of propranolol, it is useful to start with 80 mg of propranolol daily (20 mg four times a day) or comparable doses of other blockers. It should be realized that with such a dosage regimen 24 to 48 hours will be required for the drug to reach levels of 100 ng/ml needed to achieve the physiological effect usually required to achieve an antianginal effect, i.e., to reduce resting heart rate to 50 to 60 beats/min and to cause increase of less than 20 beats/min with modest exercise (e.g., climbing one flight of stairs) and to produce 70 to 80 per cent reduction in the tachycardia induced by strenuous exercise on a treadmill.[217] The usual dosage of propranolol ranges from 80 to 320 mg/day, but some patients require (and tolerate) doses as high as 1000 mg daily.

ADVERSE EFFECTS AND CONTRAINDICATIONS. These drugs are well tolerated by the majority of patients with angina pectoris. Most of the adverse reactions are a consequence of their beta-blocking properties and include cardiac effects (severe sinus bradycardia, sinus arrest, AV block, reduced left ventricular contractility), bronchoconstriction, fatigue, mental depression, nightmares, gastrointestinal upset, sexual dysfunction, intensification of insulin-induced hypoglycemia, cutaneous reactions, and withdrawal syndrome.[218] Lethargy, weakness, and fatigue may be caused by reduced cardiac output or may arise from a direct effect on the central nervous system. Nightmares, depression, and very rarely even psychotic reactions may occur. Bronchoconstriction results from a blockade of $beta_2$ receptors in the tracheobronchial tree (Table 40–4). As a consequence, asthma and chronic obstructive lung disease are contraindications to the use of such agents. As already noted, cardioselectivity of beta blockers such as metoprolol and atenolol is only relative, and the use of such drugs in dosages sufficient to prevent angina may still cause bronchoconstriction in susceptible patients. In general, therefore, a history of asthma or wheezing probably constitutes a contraindication to the use of beta blockers. Other side effects include skin rash, fever, gastrointestinal symptoms (nausea, diarrhea, or constipation), and pharyngitis. In patients who already have impaired left ventricular function, congestive heart failure may be intensified, an effect that can be counteracted by the use of digitalis or diuretics.

Beta blockers should *not* be used in patients with bradyarrhythmias of any kind unless a pacemaker is in place. In patients with partial AV block, they may impair conduction further. Blockade of noncardiac $beta_2$ receptors inhibits

TABLE 40-4 CONTRAINDICATIONS TO USE OF NITRATES, CALCIUM CHANNEL ANTAGONISTS, AND BETA-ADRENOCEPTOR BLOCKING AGENTS

	NITRATES	VERAPAMIL	DILTIAZEM	NIFEDIPINE	BETA BLOCKER
Aortic stenosis (severe)	1	2	2	3	2
Asthma	0	0	0	0	3
A-V conduction defects	0	3	2	0	2
Congestive heart failure	0	3	3	2	3
Coronary spasm	0	0	0	0	1
Hypersensitivity or idiosyncrasy	3	3	3	3	3
Hypotension (BP < 90 mm Hg systolic)	3	3	3	3	3
Peripheral arterial disease and Raynaud's	0	0	0	0	2
Pregnancy	2(C)	2(C)	2(C)	2(C)	2(**)
Sick sinus syndrome	0	2	2	0	2
Sinus bradycardia	0	2	2	0	2
Unstable angina (in absence of beta blocker)	0	1	0	3	0

LEVEL OF CONTRAINDICATION: 3 = contraindication; 2 = relative contraindication; 1 = possible contraindication; 0 = no contraindication.
FDA CATEGORIES:
(B) = FDA Category B. Either animal reproduction studies have not demonstrated a fetal risk but there are no controlled studies in women, or animal reproduction studies have shown an adverse effect that was not confirmed in controlled studies in women in the first trimester.
(C) = FDA Category C. Either studies in animals have revealed adverse effects on the fetus and there are no controlled studies in women, or studies in women and animals are not available. Drugs should be given only if the potential benefit justifies the potential risk to the fetus.
(D) = FDA Category D. There is positive evidence of human fetal risk, but the benefits from use in pregnant women may be acceptable despite the risk. There will be an appropriate statement in the "warnings" section of the label.
(**). FDA Categories for Beta-Adrenergic Blocking Agents: FDA Category B = atenolol, metoprolol; FDA Category C = nadolol, timolol, pindolol, labetalol, and acebutolol; FDA Category D = propranolol.

catecholamine-induced glycogenolysis so that noncardioselective beta blockers can impair the defense to insulin-induced hypoglycemia. Blockage of vascular beta$_2$ receptors also inhibits the vasodilating effects of catecholamines in peripheral blood vessels and leaves the constrictive (alpha-adrenergic) receptors unopposed and thereby enhances vasoconstriction. Noncardioselective beta blockers may precipitate episodes of Raynaud's phenomenon in patients with this condition and may cause uncomfortable coldness of the distal extremities. In patients with peripheral vascular disease, reduced flow to the limbs may occur.[219]

In patients with chronic stable angina, abrupt withdrawal of beta-adrenoceptor blocking agents can result in increased total ischemic activity, as detected by ambulatory monitoring. This may be caused by a return to the previously high levels of myocardial oxygen demand while the underlying atherosclerotic process had progressed.[218] Occasionally this can precipitate unstable angina and rarely even provoke myocardial infarction. Although experimental evidence suggests that there may be increased myocardial sensitivity to catecholamines upon withdrawal of beta-adrenoreceptor blockade,[220] this may have limited biological and clinical importance; in patients without cardiac failure, it has never been proved that up-regulation of myocardial beta$_1$ receptors occurs during long-term beta blocker therapy. If abrupt withdrawal of beta blockers is required, patients should be instructed to reduce exertion, manage anginal episodes with sublingual nitroglycerin, and/or substitute a calcium antagonist.

Drug interactions involving beta blockers also occur. Most of the available information relates to propranolol, but detailed information regarding other beta blockers is available[221] (Table 40–5).

TABLE 40-5 INTERACTIONS OF BETA-ADRENOCEPTOR BLOCKING AGENTS WITH OTHER DRUGS

PHARMACOKINETIC INTERACTIONS

1. Cimetidine:	**Reduces hepatic metabolism of beta blockers; increased plasma levels of beta blockers and serum half-life prolonged. Bradycardia may be excessive.** ***Management:*** **Monitor heart rate and reduce dose of one or both drugs.**
2. Aluminum hydroxide gel:	**Delay or reduction in GI absorption with reduced plasma levels of beta blocker.** ***Management:*** **Take drugs at different times or increase beta blocker dose.**
3. Barbiturates:	**Induction of hepatic enzymes enhances metabolism of beta blockers and reduces plasma levels.** ***Management:*** **Avoid barbiturates or increase beta blocker dosage.**
4. Lidocaine:	**Propranolol therapy reduces hepatic clearance of lidocaine; serum lidocaine levels may increase, and toxicity may ensue.** ***Management:*** **Monitor plasma lidocaine concentration and reduce dosage if appropriate.**

PHARMACODYNAMIC INTERACTIONS

1. **Verapamil: Hypotension, bradycardia, negative inotropic responses and abnormal A-V conduction are all additive with beta blockers. Avoid concurrent use (especially in patients with depressed left ventricular function). Monitor patients carefully if concurrent use unavoidable.**
2. **Epinephrine: Hypertension (and reflex bradycardia) result from unopposed alpha-vasoconstrictive effects of epinephrine.**
3. **Aminophylline: By phosphodiesterase inhibition, aminophylline increases cyclic AMP. Antagonism results from concurrent use with beta blockers.**
4. **Antidiabetic agents: Propranolol may induce hypoglycemia (reduced glycogenolysis), hyperglycemia (inhibition of insulin release); hypertension (release of endogenous epinephrine with hypoglycemia and unopposed alpha-vasoconstrictor effects ensue), absence of tachycardia with hypoglycemia. Avoid beta blockers in diabetics if possible. Cardioselective agents preferable.**
5. **Clonidine: Sudden withdrawal (and norepinephrine release) may result in severe hypertension if unopposed alpha-adrenergic tone exists because of beta-adrenergic blockade.** ***Management:*** **Withdraw beta blockers before clonidine.**
6. **Cyclopropane: Combined effects of cyclopropane and beta blockade may result in depression of LV function.**

OTHER INTERACTIONS

1. **Indomethacin: May reduce antihypertensive effect of beta blockers.**
2. **Ergot alkaloids: With beta blockers may cause excessive vasoconstriction.**
3. **Tricyclic antidepressants: May inhibit the bradycardia and negative inotropic effects of beta blockers.**
4. **Monoamine oxidase inhibitors: Enhance hypotensive effect of beta blockers.**
5. **Tubocurarine, succinylcholine, and pancuronium: Potentiate muscle relaxation when used with beta blockers.**

CALCIUM ANTAGONISTS

(See also p. 867)

The critical role played by calcium ions in the normal contraction of cardiac and vascular smooth muscle is discussed on page 357. Despite their chemical heterogeneity, the major action of these drugs is to interfere with the entry of calcium into myocytes and vascular smooth muscle cells.[222–224,224a] These agents are effective in the treatment of chronic stable angina, either alone or in combination with beta-adrenoceptor blockers and nitrates.[225–227] Calcium antagonists appear to be beneficial in controlling angina and improving exercise tolerance in patients with chronic stable angina due to coronary atherosclerosis as well as in patients with Prinzmetal's variant angina (p. 1344) and those in whom angina results from abnormal, small coronary arteries with limited vasodilator reserve.[228]

Five calcium antagonists—nifedipine, verapamil, diltiazem, nicardipine, and bepridil—are approved in the United States by the FDA for the treatment of angina pectoris (Table 40–6). All of these agents are effective in causing relaxation of vascular smooth muscle in both the systemic arterial and coronary arterial beds. In addition, the antagonism of entry of calcium into myocardium results in a negative inotropic effect. Peripheral vascular dilation is more prominent than the negative inotropic effects of the dihydropyridines—nifedipine and nicardipine—and to a lesser extent of diltiazem; verapamil's effects on the heart and vascular bed are approximately evenly balanced.

A large number of so-called second-generation calcium antagonists have been developed. They are mainly dihydropyridine derivatives and most have longer plasma half-lives and greater vascular selectivity than the prototypical agent, nifedipine (Table 40–7).[223] Several of these agents have potentially useful features. *Amlodipine*, which is less lipid soluble than nifedipine, has slow, smooth onset and ultralong duration of action (plasma half-life = 36 hours). It causes marked coronary and peripheral dilation and may be useful in the treatment of hypertension and angina. *Nicardipine* has a similar half-life to nifedipine (2 to 4 hours), but intravenous administration is easier because it is water soluble without associated light sensitivity. It also appears to have greater vascular selectivity.

Other compounds have interesting possibilities. *Bepridil* is a less specific calcium antagonist that interacts with the dihydropyridine binding site as well as having sodium channel blocking effects. This agent markedly prolongs the atrial refractory period and thus has some potential use in the treatment of atrial arrhythmias as well as angina, although it is also arrhythmogenic and causes Q-T prolongation and torsades de pointes.

TABLE 40-6 PHARMACOKINETICS OF CALCIUM ANTAGONISTS USED COMMONLY FOR ANGINA TREATMENT*

	DILTIAZEM	NICARDIPINE	NIFEDIPINE	NIFEDIPINE GITS	VERAPAMIL
Usual adult dose	IV: 0.075 to 0.15 mg/kg Oral: 30–90 mg tid or qid	IV: 10–15 mg/hr for 30 min then 3–5 mg/hr Oral: 20–30 mg tid	SL: 10–30 mg tid or qid Oral: 10–30 mg tid or qid	Oral: 30–90 mg daily	IV: 0.075 to 0.15 mg/kg Oral: 80–120 mg tid or qid
Per cent absorbed	80–90	~100	90	>90	90
Extent of bioavailability (% of dose)	40–70	30	65–75	45–70	20–35
Onset of action	Oral: <15 min	<20 min	SL: <3 min Oral: <20 min	Approximately 6 hr	IV: ~2 min Oral: 2 hr
Peak effect	Oral: 30 min	1 hr	Oral: 1–2 hr	After 6 hr	IV: 3–5 min Oral: 3–4 hr
Therapeutic serum levels (ng/ml)	50–200	30–50	25–100	25–100	80–300
Protein binding (%)	70–80	>95	95	95	80–90
Elimination half-life (hr)	3.5–6.0	2.0–4.0	2.0–5.0	2.0–5.0	3.0–7.0†
Elimination	60% metabolized by liver; remainder excreted by kidneys		High first-pass hepatic metabolism		85% eliminated by first-pass hepatic metabolism
Urinary recovery of unchanged drug (% of dose)	2–4	<1	1–2	1–2	3–4
Active metabolites	Yes‡	No	No	No	Yes§

*All agents approved by FDA for treatment of angina pectoris.
†4.5–12 hr with multiple dosing.
‡Desacetyl-diltiazem has 25–50% activity of parent compound.
§Norverapamil has 20% activity of parent compound.
GITS = gastrointestinal therapeutic system, IV = intravenous, SL = sublingual.

Perhexiline maleate is a less specific calcium antagonist that does not interact with the dihydropyridine binding site. It may be useful in refractory angina, but infrequently causes unpredictable serious hepatic and neurological toxicity.[228a] However, if plasma levels are maintained in the 150 to 600 ng/ml range, these toxicities are usually avoidable.

Studies in experimental animals, both in primates and nonprimates, have suggested that calcium antagonists might have an antiatherogenic effect, and recent human studies support this.[229,230] In a multicenter, randomized trial utilizing quantitative arteriography, patients showing mild coronary artery disease developed significantly fewer new lesions taking nifedipine than did patients taking placebo.[229] Preexisting lesions did not appear to be affected, however. Another study comparing the effects of nifedipine, propranolol, and isosorbide dinitrate on angiographic progression and regression of coronary arterial narrowing also showed that patients receiving nifedipine developed fewer new lesions than patients taking the other two agents over a 2-year period.[230] Prolonged follow-up in such studies will be required to determine whether these angiographic observations will be accompanied by clinical benefits.

NIFEDIPINE. This dihydropyridine is particularly effective in reducing the contractility of smooth muscle, especially vascular smooth muscle. The dose is 10 mg orally every 8 hours, increased stepwise to 20 mg every 6 hours, guided by the blood pressure response. The dosage of 160 mg daily is considered to be maximal. An extended-release formulation of nifedipine utilizes the gastrointestinal therapeutic system (GITS) of drug delivery (Table 40–6). The formulation is designed to deliver 30, 60, or 90 mg of nifedipine in a single daily dose at a relatively constant rate over a 24-hour period, and patients can be readily switched from nifedipine capsules to the nearest total daily dose of the extended-release preparation,[231] which is useful for the treatment of chronic stable angina, vasospastic angina, and hypertension.

Nifedipine is a more potent vasodilator than either diltiazem or verapamil. Although its in vitro actions on myocardium and specialized cardiac tissue, i.e., the sinoatrial and AV nodes, are similar to those of the other agents, the concentration required to reproduce effects on these tissues is not reached in vivo because of the early appearance of its powerful vasodilating effects. Thus, in clinical practice the potential negative chronotropic, inotropic, and dromotropic (on A-V conduction) effects of nifedipine are seldom a problem.

In patients with chronic stable angina, maximally tolerated doses of nifedipine result in a significant increase in heart rate at rest and at peak exercise and also in a reduced resting systolic blood pressure but have no effect on the blood pressure achieved at peak exercise. Compared with placebo the duration of a symptom-limited treadmill exercise is prolonged following nifedipine administration.[232] The beneficial effects of nifedipine in the treatment of angina result from its capacity to reduce myocardial oxygen needs consequent to afterload reduction, and to increase myocardial oxygen delivery consequent to its dilating action on the coronary vascular bed. In conscious animals, nifedipine has been shown to dilate both large coronary arteries and coronary resistance vessels.[233] Nifedipine decreases left ventricular afterload, while ejection fraction, velocity of circumferential fiber shortening, heart rate, and cardiac index all show slight reflex increases; these increases can be blocked by simultaneous administration of beta-adrenoceptor blockers. In patients with elevated left ventricular end-diastolic pressures and volumes, nifedipine reduces these variables and enhances ejection fraction more than it does in patients with normal baseline left ventricular function.[234]

Adverse Effects. These occur in 15 to 20 per cent of patients; they lead to discontinuation of medication in about 5 per cent (Table 40–8). Most adverse effects are related to the systemic vasodilation and include headache, dizziness, flushing, hypotension, and troublesome leg edema (not related to heart failure). Gastrointestinal side effects, including nausea, epigastric pressure, and vomiting, are noted in approximately 5 per cent of patients. Occasionally, nifedipine aggravates angina, presumably by lowering arterial pressure excessively with subsequent reflex tachycardia, in patients with extremely severe, fixed coronary obstructions. For this reason, combined therapy of nifedipine with a beta blocker is particularly effective in the treatment of chronic stable angina and is superior to nifedipine alone.[226,227] Most of the adverse effects are reduced by use of the extended-release preparations.

A comparison of the side effects of nifedipine with those of other calcium antagonists is shown in Table 40–8. Because of its potent vasodilator effects, nifedipine is *contraindicated* (Table 40–4) in patients who are hypotensive or who have severe aortic valve stenosis and also in patients with unstable angina who are not taking a beta blocker, in whom reflex-mediated increases in heart rate may be harmful. In patients with mild left ventricular dysfunction, sinus bradycardia, sick sinus syndrome, and AV block (particularly if a beta-adrenoceptor blocking agent is concurrently administered and additional drug therapy of angina is indicated), nifedipine is the calcium antagonist of choice.[226] This is because in the clinical dosage range tolerated it has fewer negative effects on myocardial contractility or on the specialized automatic and con-

TABLE 40-7 SECOND-GENERATION CALCIUM ANTAGONISTS AND RELATED COMPOUNDS

AGENTS	POSSIBLE USES	CHARACTERISTICS
DIHYDROPYRIDINES		
Amlodipine	Hypertension, angina	Ultra long acting, plasma half-life = 36 hr. Marked coronary and peripheral dilator properties with minimal changes in inotropy, chronotropy, and cardiac conduction. Slow, smooth onset of action (less lipid soluble than nifedipine).
Felodipine	Hypertension, ? angina, ? CHF	Medium action duration, plasma half-life = 8 hr. Vascular selectivity without negative chronotropic and inotropic effects clinically. Increases serum digoxin levels.
Isradipine	Hypertension, angina, ? CHF	Medium action duration, plasma half-life = 8 hr. Vascular selectivity without negative chronotropic and inotropic effects clinically. No change in serum digoxin levels. Can cause arthralgia.
Nicardipine	Angina, hypertension	Short action duration, plasma half-life = 4–5 hr or less. Water soluble without light sensitivity (IV administration easier). Vascular selectivity, ? greater effect on coronaries, no clinically significant negative inotropic effects.
Nimodipine	Early stroke and subarachnoid hemorrhage	Short action duration, plasma half-life = 5 hr. Possibly more selective for cerebral than peripheral vessels.
Nisoldipine	Hypertension, angina, ? CHF	Medium action duration, plasma half-life = 8–11 hr. Possibly more selective as a vasodilator than nifedipine. Highly specific for slow calcium channel.
Nitrendipine	Hypertension, ? angina, ? CHF	Medium action duration, plasma half-life = 7–8 hr. Vascular selectivity without clinically significant negative inotropic effects and less reflex tachycardia. Pure calcium antagonist with some agonist properties. Increases serum digoxin levels.
OTHER COMPOUNDS		
Bepridil	Angina, ? atrial arrhythmias	Ultra long acting, plasma half-life = 40 hr. Combined sodium-calcium channel blockade. Marked prolongation of atrial refractory period. Arrhythmogenic, causing prolonged Q-T and torsades de pointes.
Perhexiline maleate	Refractory angina	Unclear mechanism of action, but current hypothesis is a drug-induced shift in myocardial metabolism. Hepatic and neurologic toxicity is usually avoidable by maintaining drug levels in 150–600 ng/ml range.
VERAPAMIL-LIKE AGENTS		
Anipamil	Hypertension	Long half-life, ? minimal effect on A-V conduction.

TABLE 40-8 SIDE EFFECTS OF ANTIANGINAL DRUGS*

	HYPOTENSION FLUSHING, HEADACHE	LEFT VENTRICULAR DYSFUNCTION	DECREASED HEART RATE ATRIOVENTRICULAR BLOCK†	GASTROINTESTINAL SYMPTOMS	BRONCHOCONSTRICTION‡
Beta blockers	0	++	+++	+	+++
Nitrates	+++	0	0	0	0
Diltiazem	+	+	+	0	0
Nifedipine	+++	0	0	0	0
Verapamil	+	+	++	++	0

*0 = absent; + = mild; ++ = moderate; +++ = sometimes severe.
†In patients with sick sinus node syndrome or conduction system disease.
‡In patients with obstructive lung disease.
Reprinted by permission from Braunwald, E.: Mechanism of action of calcium channel blocking agents. N. Engl. J. Med. *307*:1618, 1982.

TABLE 40-9 DRUG INTERACTIONS WITH CALCIUM ANTAGONISTS

	VERAPAMIL	NIFEDIPINE	DILTIAZEM
Beta-adrenergic blockers (negative inotropic and chronotropic effects)	2(+)[A]		2(+)
Carbamazepine (inhibition of hepatic metabolism)	3(+)		1(+)
Cimetidine (increased bioavailability of calcium antagonists)	3(+)	3(+)	3(+)
Cyclosporine (increased plasma levels of cyclosporine)	2(+)	1(−)?	2(+)
Digoxin (increased plasma digoxin levels)	3(+)	1(+)	1(+)
Disopyramide (sinus node depression)	1(+)		1(+)
Lithium carbonate (after plasma levels of lithium)	1(−)		2(+)
Neuromuscular blocking agents (verapamil potentiates action)	3(+)		
Phenobarbital (hepatic enzyme inducer)	3(−)		
Phenytoin (causes peak nifedipine levels to rise)		2(+)	
Prazosin (excessive hypotension)	2(+)	3(+)	
Quinidine (*hypotension and bradycardia, decreased serum quinidine)**	2(+)*	2(−)**	
Rifampin and sulfinpyrazone (hepatic enzyme inducers)	3(−)		
Theophylline (after pharmacological effects of theophylline)	1(+)	1(+/−)	1(+)

Modified from Pieho, R. W., et al.: Drug interactions with calcium-entry blockers. Circulation 75 (Suppl. V): 181, 1987, by permission of the American Heart Association, Inc.

(−) = decreased drug effect; (+) = increased drug effect (e.g., verapamil and beta blockers will interact so that the negative inotropic and chronotropic effects of verapamil will be increased significantly); 3 = significant, common interaction; 2 = significant, uncommon interaction; 1 = reported interaction of questioned significance; ? = debated response; A = the intravenous administration of a beta blocker while a patient is taking verapamil orally (or vice versa) may be hazardous.

duction systems than does verapamil or diltiazem. Nonetheless, in patients with left ventricular dysfunction all calcium antagonists—even nifedipine—can precipitate heart failure.[235] In patients already receiving maximal doses of nitrates and beta blocker therapy, the addition of nifedipine (80 to 100 mg/day) has been shown to improve diastolic function of the left ventricle at rest and during exercise.[236] However, in patients with severe left ventricular dysfunction, the addition of nifedipine may precipitate left ventricular failure. Nifedipine *interacts* significantly with prazosin (resulting in excessive hypotension), cimetidine, and phenytoin (resulting in increased bioavailability of nifedipine) and may result in reduced plasma quinidine levels (Table 40–9).

VERAPAMIL (see also p. 648). The usual starting dose of verapamil for oral administration is 40 to 80 mg three times daily. It may later be increased to 80 to 120 mg three or four times daily to a maximum dose of 480 mg/day (Table 40–6). Sustained-release capsules of verapamil are available (60 mg, 90 mg, and 120 mg), and starting doses are 60 to 120 mg twice daily with a usual optimal dose range of 240 to 360 mg/day.

Parenteral verapamil dilates the systemic and coronary resistance vessels without clearly increasing myocardial metabolic demands. In addition, it has been shown to dilate large conductance vessels in both normal and diseased arterial segments, although this effect is not as potent as that of nitroglycerin. Verapamil appears to decrease myocardial oxygen demand without any change in the anginal threshold, i.e., in the rate-pressure product at the onset of angina. Trials comparing verapamil with a beta blocker (usually propranolol) in the treatment of effort-related angina have shown that the drugs are comparable in producing dose-dependent reductions in the frequency of anginal episodes. In a comparison of propranolol (480 mg/day) and verapamil (320 mg/day), the latter was found to be a more effective antianginal agent than the former, although the combination of both drugs resulted in better exercise capacity than did either alone.[237]

Verapamil accelerates left ventricular diastolic filling at rest and during exercise in patients with chronic stable angina (and hypertrophic cardiomyopathy [p. 1313]), whereas beta blockade does not have this effect.[237] Despite the marked negative inotropic effects of verapamil in isolated cardiac muscle preparations, changes in contractility are modest in patients with normal cardiac function. However, in patients with cardiac dysfunction, verapamil, like beta blockade, may reduce cardiac output and elevate left ventricular filling pressure.

In clinical doses, verapamil also inhibits calcium influx into specialized cardiac cells, sometimes causing slowing of heart rate and A-V conduction; it may cause slight P-R prolongation. Although the drug depresses sinus node automaticity, the systemic vasodilator effects of the drug activate reflexes that counteract or minimize this effect. Verapamil is therefore contraindicated in patients with sick sinus syndrome, A-V conduction abnormalities, or congestive heart failure and in patients with suspected digitalis toxicity.

Verapamil interacts significantly with a number of other drugs (Table 40–9). Intravenous verapamil should not be used together with an orally administered beta blocker nor should a beta blocker be administered intravenously in patients receiving oral verapamil, and certainly intravenous verapamil and intravenous beta blockade should not ordinarily be used together. The bioavailability of verapamil is increased by cimetidine and carbamazepine, while verapamil may increase plasma levels of cyclosporine and digoxin and may be associated with excessive hypotension with both quinidine and prazosin. Hepatic enzyme inducers such as phenobarbital may reduce the effects of verapamil.

Adverse effects of verapamil are noted in approximately 10 per cent of patients and relate to systemic dilation (hypotension and facial flushing), gastrointestinal symptoms (constipation and nausea), and central nervous system reactions such as headache and dizziness.

DILTIAZEM. The dosage of diltiazem is 30 to 60 mg four times daily, although higher doses are sometimes needed.[238]

Diltiazem's actions are intermediate between those of nifedipine and verapamil. In clinically useful doses its vasodilator effects are somewhat less profound than nifedipine's, while its cardiac depressant action (on the sinoatrial and AV nodes and myocardium) may be less than those of verapamil. This profile may explain the remarkably low incidence of adverse effects of diltiazem. This drug is a systemic vasodilator, lowering arterial pressure at rest and during exertion and increasing the workload required to produce myocardial ischemia, but there is some evidence that the drug may also increase myocardial oxygen delivery.[239] Although diltiazem causes little vasodilation of epicardial coronary arteries under basal conditions, it may enhance perfusion of the subendocardium distal to a flow-limiting coronary stenosis[240]; it also blocks exercise-induced coronary vasoconstriction.[241,242] In patients with ischemic heart disease, diltiazem reduces afterload and depresses myocardial systolic function, although it improves left ventricular relaxation.[243] Studies in patients during tachycardia-induced angina pectoris suggest that the major benefit of diltiazem is related to reduction of myocardial oxygen demand rather than to enhancing myocardial oxygen delivery.[244] In patients with chronic stable angina receiving maximally tolerated doses of diltiazem there is a significant reduction in heart rate at rest, but there is no effect on peak blood pressure achieved during exercise, and the duration of symptom-limited treadmill exercise is prolonged.[232]

Diltiazem is a highly efficacious antianginal agent with minimal side effects when given to patients with angina pectoris that persists despite nitrate and beta blocker therapy.[245] High doses of diltiazem (mean dose 340 mg) have been shown to be a safe addition to maximally tolerated doses of isosorbide dinitrate and a beta blocker, causing increases in exercise tolerance and resting and exercise left ventricular ejection fraction without increasing side effects.[238] The combination of high doses of diltiazem with beta blockers is more effective in reducing symptoms and improving exercise capacity without increasing adverse effects than is the use of diltiazem alone.[244,246] The combination of diltiazem and nifedipine may be effective in patients who do not respond adequately to either agent alone.[247,248]

Like verapamil, diltiazem should be used with caution in patients with sick sinus syndrome and advanced degrees of AV block and left ventricular dysfunction. Diltiazem has *interactions* with other drugs, including beta-adrenergic blocking agents (with enhanced negative inotropic and chronotropic effects) and cimetidine (which increases the bioavailability of diltiazem), and diltiazem has been associated with increased plasma levels of cyclosporine, carbamazepine, and lithium carbonate. Diltiazem may cause excess sinus node depression if administered with disopyramide (Table 40–9).

SELECTION OF DRUGS FOR THE TREATMENT OF CHRONIC STABLE ANGINA

Verapamil (360 mg/day) and diltiazem (360 mg/day) appear to be equipotent antianginal agents and similar in efficacy to propranolol (320 mg/day). Nifedipine 60 mg/day appears to be equivalent to propranolol 160 to 240 mg/day. Diltiazem and verapamil, which reduce resting heart rate, appear to be more effective as single drugs for angina than is nifedipine, which causes reflex sympathetic stimulation; both diltiazem and verapamil appear to be safe and effective alternatives to beta blockers.[249]

RELATIVE ADVANTAGES OF BETA BLOCKERS AND CALCIUM ANTAGONISTS. There is some controversy whether a calcium antagonist or a beta blocker should be employed first in the treatment of chronic stable angina in patients in whom more than an occasional sublingual nitroglycerin tablet is required. Both classes of agents are effective. Long-term administration of beta-adrenoceptor blockers has been found to prolong life in patients after acute myocardial infarction.[249a] In general, however, agents without intrinsic sympathomimetic activity increase serum triglycerides[216] and decrease HDL cholesterol with uncertain long-term consequences. Long-term administration of calcium antagonists has not been shown definitively to improve long-term survival following acute myocardial infarction, although diltiazem apparently is effective in preventing severe angina and early reinfarction after non-Q-wave infarction,[250] and verapamil reduces reinfarction rates.[251] Nifedipine has been associated with the development of fewer new coronary artery lesions[229,230] in patients with coronary artery disease.

The choice of which agent to initiate therapy is influenced by a number of clinical factors:

1. Whether the patient's anginal threshold is fixed or variable, as discussed on page 1294. When there is a relatively fixed anginal threshold, it is presumed that myocardial ischemia is caused primarily by an increase in myocardial oxygen needs during exercise in the face of a fixed supply, and a beta blocker would usually be considered first (Table 40–10). Conversely, in patients with variable-threshold angina in whom reductions of myocardial blood supply may be caused by alterations in coronary vasomotor tone, a calcium antagonist may be preferable to a beta blocker.
2. If a patient is suspected of having variant angina (p. 1342) then calcium antagonists are clearly preferred, since occasionally beta blockers may aggravate angina under these circumstances.
3. The presence of moderate to severe left ventricular dysfunction in patients with angina limits the therapeutic options (Table 40–11). Obviously, cardiac failure may be controlled with diuretics, digitalis, and angiotensin-converting enzyme inhibitors, and nitrates can be used for angina. However, when cardiac failure is treated and angina persists, other agents may be required. Nifedipine and diltiazem are reasonable choices if the left ventricular ejection fraction is greater than 30 per cent and overt cardiac failure does not exist. Verapamil and beta blockers are more likely to be associated with adverse effects under these circumstances.
4. In patients with a history of asthma or chronic obstructive lung disease and/or with wheezing on clinical examination (in whom beta blockers, even relatively selective agents, are contraindicated), calcium antagonists and nitrates should be selected for the treatment of angina.

TABLE 40-10 EFFECTS OF ANTIANGINAL AGENTS ON INDICES OF MYOCARDIAL OXYGEN SUPPLY AND DEMAND*

		BETA-ADRENOCEPTOR BLOCKERS						
		ISA†		Cardio-Selective		CALCIUM ANTAGONISTS		
INDEX	NITRATES	*No*	*Yes*	*No*	*Yes*	*Nifedipine*	*Verapamil*	*Diltiazem*
Supply								
Coronary resistance								
Vascular tone	↓↓	↑	0	↑	0↑	↓↓↓	↓↓↓	↓↓↓
Intramyocardial diastolic tension	↓↓↓	↑	0	↑	↑	↓↓	0↑	0
Coronary collateral circulation	↑	0	0	0	0	↑	0	↑
Duration of diastole	0(↓)	↑↑↑	0↓	↑↑↑	↑↑↑	0↑(↓↓)	↑↑↑(↓)	↑↑(↓)
Demand								
Intramyocardial systolic tension								
Preload	↓↓↓	↑	0	↑	↑	↓0	↑0↓	0↓
Afterload (peripheral vascular resistance)	↓	↑	↑	↑↑	↑	↓↓	↓	↓
Contractility	0(↑)	↓↓↓	↓	↓↓↓	↓↓↓	↓(↑↑)‡	↓↓(↑)‡	↓(↑)‡
Heart rate	0(↑)	↓↓↓	0↓	↓↓↓	↓↓↓	0(↑↑)	↓↓(↑)	↓↓(↑)

*↑ = increase, ↓ = decrease, 0 = little or no definite effect. Number of arrows represents relative intensity of effect. Symbols in parentheses indicate reflex-mediated effects.

†ISA = intrinsic sympathomimetic activity.

‡Effect of calcium entry blockers on left ventricular *contractility*, as assessed in the intact animal model. The net effect on *left ventricular performance* is variable, being influenced by alterations in afterload, reflex cardiac stimulation, and the underlying state of the myocardium.

From Shub, C., et al.: Selection of optimal drug therapy for the patient with angina pectoris. Mayo Clin. Proc. *60*:539, 1985.

TABLE 40-11 RECOMMENDED DRUG THERAPY (CALCIUM ANTAGONIST VS. BETA BLOCKER) IN PATIENTS WHO HAVE ANGINA IN CONJUNCTION WITH OTHER MEDICAL CONDITIONS*

CLINICAL CONDITION	RECOMMENDED DRUG (ALTERNATIVE DRUG)
Cardiac arrhythmias and conduction abnormalities	
Sinus bradycardia	Nifedipine
Sinus tachycardia (not due to cardiac failure)	Beta blocker
Supraventricular tachycardia	Verapamil or beta blocker
Atrioventricular block	Nifedipine
Rapid atrial fibrillation (with digitalis)	Verapamil or beta blocker
Ventricular arrhythmias	Beta blocker (±group 1 antiarrhythmic agent)
Left ventricular dysfunction	
Congestive heart failure	
Mild (LVEF ≥ 40%)	Nifedipine (verapamil, diltiazem, or beta blockers cautiously)
Moderate to severe (LVEF < 40%)	Nifedipine (cautiously, in combination with other therapy)
Left-sided valvular heart disease†	
Aortic stenosis (mild)‡	Beta blocker
Aortic insufficiency	Nifedipine
Mitral regurgitation	Nifedipine
Mitral stenosis§	Beta blocker
Miscellaneous medical conditions	
Systemic hypertension	Beta blocker (calcium antagonists)
Severe preexisting headaches	Beta blockers (verapamil or diltiazem)
COPD with bronchospasm or asthma	Nifedipine, verapamil, or diltiazem
Hyperthyroidism	Beta blocker
Raynaud's syndrome	Nifedipine
Claudication	Nifedipine, verapamil, or diltiazem (low-dose $beta_1$ blocker or beta-ISA)
Depression	Nifedipine, verapamil, or diltiazem
Neurasthenia or fatigue states	Nifedipine, verapamil, or diltiazem
Insulin-dependent diabetes mellitus	Nifedipine, verapamil, or diltiazem (low-dose $beta_1$ or beta-ISA)

From Shub, C., et al.: Selection of optimal drug therapy for the patient with angina pectoris. Mayo Clin. Proc. *60*:539, 1985.

* Beta-ISA = beta blocker with intrinsic sympathomimetic activity such as pindolol or acebutolol; COPD = chronic obstructive pulmonary disease; LVEF = left ventricular ejection fraction.

† Surgical therapy should be considered for patients with severe valvular heart disease; beta blockers are not routinely used in patients with valvular heart disease and left ventricular failure.

‡ Vasodilators may increase aortic valve gradient, and beta blockers can cause left ventricular failure. Any of these drugs should be used with extreme caution in patients with severe aortic stenosis.

§ If congestive heart failure (associated with normal left ventricular function) occurs in a patient with angina, severe mitral stenosis, and rapid atrial fibrillation, a beta blocker (in combination with digitalis) may be used to decrease the heart rate.

5. In patients with sick sinus syndrome, sinus bradycardia, or significant A-V conduction disturbances, nifedipine or nicardipine is the calcium antagonist of choice, and beta blockers and verapamil are often contraindicated and should be used only with great caution.

6. If patients have significant, symptomatic peripheral arterial disease, calcium antagonists are preferred over beta blockers.

7. In patients with new-onset or rapidly progressive angina or rest angina, i.e., unstable angina, nifedipine should not be used as the initial and only agent, but rather treatment should be initiated with nitrates, diltiazem, verapamil, or beta blockers to avoid the reflex-mediated tachycardia associated with nifedipine alone that may aggravate unstable angina. Nifedipine is, however, helpful when added to a beta blocker under this circumstance.

8. Beta blockers should usually be avoided in patients with significant depressive illness, a history of sexual dysfunction, or a history of sleep disturbance, nightmares, fatigue, or lethargy.

9. Hypertensive patients with angina pectoris do well with either beta blockers or calcium antagonists, since both agents have antihypertensive effects.

10. When treated with a beta blocker, patients with significant ambulatory asymptomatic ischemia appear to have a reduction in the number and duration of ischemic episodes as compared with results of calcium antagonist therapy.[252]

11. Verapamil is an effective alternative to beta-adrenergic blocking drugs for the treatment of chronic stable angina and may offer advantages over beta blockers in patients with fatigue, depression, impotence, memory loss, or bronchospasm.[237] Diltiazem is less likely than verapamil to exacerbate A-V conduction disturbances, is effective compared with nifedipine at reducing the frequency of angina attacks, and seems to be associated with fewer adverse reactions than nifedipine.[253]

COMBINATION THERAPY. A combination of a beta-adrenoceptor blocker, calcium antagonist, and long-acting nitrate may be employed. The hemodynamic spectrum of action of beta blockers, long-acting nitrates, and calcium antagonists is sufficiently different to suggest that combination therapy might be useful, and indeed it is, in patients with severe angina (Tables 40–4 and 40–8).

When adrenergic blockers and calcium antagonists are to be used together in the treatment of angina pectoris, a number of practical issues should be considered:

1. The combination of a beta blocker and calcium antagonist is not consistently better than the use of a beta blocker (or calcium antagonist) alone if the single agent is administered in a maximum tolerated dose.

2. However, if angina persists despite optimal doses of a beta blocker, then the addition of a calcium antagonist is likely to reduce angina and improve exercise performance.[254]

3. The addition of a beta blocker to either verapamil or diltiazem therapy does not appear to enhance antianginal efficacy,[227] although the addition of a beta blocker does seem to enhance the effects of nifedipine.

4. In patients with moderate or severe left ventricular dysfunction, sinus bradycardia, or A-V conduction disturbances, combination therapy with calcium antagonists and beta blockers either should be avoided or initiated with caution.[255,256] In patients with conduction system disease, the preferred combination is nifedipine and a beta blocker. The negative inotropic effects of calcium antagonists are not usually a problem in combined therapy with low doses of beta blockers but can become significant with high doses of beta blockers. Under these circumstances, nifedipine and nicardipine are the agents of choice. However, it should be noted that both nifedipine and diltiazem used alone can cause deterioration of left ventricular function in patients with treated cardiac failure.

5. The combination of nifedipine (or nicardipine) and long-acting nitrates is usually not optimal, since both are potent vasodilators.

Following (or simultaneously with) the general measures described on page 1302, we believe that it is usually advisable to initiate drug therapy of chronic stable angina with sublingual nitroglycerin (and aspirin). If the patient requires more than approximately three or four tablets per week either a beta blocker or calcium antagonist should be added, depending on the profile of the patient, as outlined above. The dosage of the drug selected is then raised progressively as efficacy and side effects are monitored and alternative agents added only if angina persists or side effects become a problem. With the recognition that all longer acting forms of oral or transdermal nitrate therapy provoke tolerance, regimens utilizing these agents are designed to allow a nitrate-free interval of about 10 hours. This is readily achieved with intermittent, transdermal nitrate therapy or careful dosage schedules of long-acting oral nitrates. At times, lower doses of triple-drug therapy (a long-acting nitrate, a beta blocker, and a calcium antagonist) are used early in the treatment plan if the patient can tolerate only low doses of the chosen agents. If symptoms persist despite these approaches and if there are no contraindications, myocardial revascularization is then considered.

In decisions about the management of individual patients with angina, the effects of the antianginal agents on indices of myocardial oxygen supply and demand should be considered.[257] When angina pectoris exists with other conditions that can complicate drug therapy, such as asthma and diabetes mellitus, the choice of therapy should be made especially carefully (Table 40–11).

GUIDELINES FOR MEDICAL TREATMENT OF CHRONIC STABLE ANGINA

Risk factor modification is most important in patients with chronic stable angina under the age of approximately 65 years. This is most easily accomplished by cessation of cigarette smoking and treatment of hypertension and low-density hyperlipoproteinemia. There is increasing evidence that *marked* reduction of elevated serum cholesterol levels will cause the regression of atheroma, but it is not yet clear that lowering a total cholesterol < 240 mg/dl and an LDL cholesterol < 175 mg/dl is of benefit in patients with chronic stable angina. At this time we recommend treatment above these thresholds but recognize that the results of ongoing trials may dictate an alteration of these limits. Perhaps currently available methods of diet and drug therapy may slow the progression of the disease. Similarly, the relationship between maintenance of blood sugar within the normal range in diabetics and preventing vascular disease is far from settled.

In mild chronic stable angina, drug therapy may be limited to sublingual nitroglycerin on an "as necessary" basis if pain episodes are relatively infrequent (once or twice a week). It should also be used prophylactically in situations known to precipitate angina. If nitroglycerin is required on a daily basis, either long-acting nitrate preparations or moderate doses of a beta blocker or a calcium antagonist may be employed. The doses of the drugs will depend on how well they are tolerated and on the clinical response. Resting heart rate should be lowered to 50 to 60 beats/min, and heart rate during ordinary activity should be below 100 beats/min. The clinical response can often be estimated by an improvement in exercise tolerance or the degree of ST-segment depression during a standard treadmill test. If the patient is still symptomatic at high doses of either a beta blocker or a calcium antagonist, then the other agent should be added. The relative advantages and disadvantages of the different agents have been discussed. Whichever is selected, a relatively low dose is given to begin and dosage is increased gradually.

There is no unanimity of opinion concerning when a patient with chronic angina pectoris should undergo cardiac catheterization, coronary arteriography, and left ventriculography. Some physicians take a more aggressive posture with patients under 50 years of age, with the hope of finding a lesion that demands revascularization; others prefer to wait for development of refractoriness to medical therapy, regardless of the patient's age. We believe that the use of noninvasive tests, as outlined on page 1298, can be extremely helpful in identifying patients with chronic stable angina at high risk of coronary events or early death; if there are no contraindications to coronary revascularization in such patients, they should undergo coronary arteriography, as should patients for whom medical therapy fails.

PERCUTANEOUS TRANSLUMINAL CORONARY ANGIOPLASTY

(See also Chap. 41)

With improved equipment and an increasing number of experienced operators, the primary success rate of coronary angioplasty (PTCA) has improved over the last 10 years, and the number of procedures performed has risen rapidly. Thus, PTCA is playing an increasingly important role in the treatment of chronic stable angina.[258,258a]

PATIENT SELECTION. PTCA should, in general, be carried out in patients with symptomatic angina, objective evidence of myocardial ischemia, and anatomical features on coronary arteriography that make them suitable for complete or nearly complete revascularization (Table 40–12). Ideally, such patients should also be suitable surgical candidates; however, selected patients with severe chronic angina who are not appropriate for surgical treatment (e.g., with advanced pulmonary or renal disease, and advanced age with infirmity) may be considered for PTCA. In such patients, PTCA may be undertaken as a palliative procedure and may, on occasion, be useful even in those with multivessel disease in whom all lesions are not suitable for dilatation.

The optimal lesion for PTCA in a patient with chronic stable angina pectoris involves a single, proximal coronary artery (but not at the coronary ostium) that is easily accessible. It is concentric, smooth, noncalcified, short (less than 0.5 cm), subtotal, and occupies a straight portion of the artery that has no side branches and that supplies an area of myocardium "protected" by distal collateral vessels.[258] PTCA of such lesions has a primary success rate of greater than 90 per cent.[259] If at the end of the procedure there is less than 30 per cent residual narrowing or a pressure gradient of less than 15 mm Hg at the site of the coronary lesion, there is a high chance of symptomatic relief.[259,260] However, PTCA is being carried out with increasing frequency in lesions that are eccentric, calcified, less accessible, and totally occluded.[261] Each of these factors reduces the chance of primary success and adds to the risk of the procedure.[261a]

RISKS. The NHLBI PTCA Registry, examining a cohort of 1801 patients treated in 1985 to 1986, compared with a cohort examined from 1977 to 1981, showed that in the latter period patients were older and had an increased incidence of multivessel coronary disease (double- or triple-vessel disease in 51 per cent), and more patients had depressed left ventricular function or a history of prior infarction. Despite these differences in patient population, the risk of PTCA appeared to decrease. The most significant decreases in complication rates were a fall in the incidence of coronary spasm from 5.0 to 1.3 per cent and a decreased requirement for emergency coronary artery bypass grafting from 5.8 to 3.5 per cent. In-hospital mortality rates depended on the extent of coronary disease (0.2 per cent for single-vessel disease, 0.9 per cent for

TABLE 40-12 INDICATIONS FOR CORONARY ANGIOPLASTY

GENERALLY ACCEPTED INDICATIONS
Chronic stable angina unresponsive to medical therapy or unstable angina:
1. With objective evidence of myocardial ischemia
2. With normal or mildly reduced left ventricular function
3. With significant coronary artery stenoses involving one or two coronary arteries
EVOLVING INDICATIONS
1. Chronic stable angina unresponsive to medical therapy with multivessel disease
2. Acute myocardial infarction complicated by continuing unstable angina or cardiogenic shock
3. No angina, or mild angina, taking medical therapy, and with a strongly positive exercise test
4. Angina in patients with a recent coronary artery occlusion (less than 3 months)
5. Angina after coronary bypass surgery
6. Documented variant angina, taking medical therapy, with significant "fixed" coronary stenoses
7. Angina in inoperable/high-risk patients
RELATIVE CONTRAINDICATIONS
1. No angina or mild angina without evidence of myocardial ischemia
2. Significant left main coronary artery stenosis
3. Coronary artery stenoses with <50% diameter narrowing
4. Chronic, total coronary artery occlusions older than 3 months
5. Severe left ventricular dysfunction (ejection fraction <25%)

Adapted from Report of the ISFC/WHO Task Force on Coronary Angioplasty. Circulation *78*:780, 1988, by permission of the American Heart Association, Inc.

double-vessel disease, and 2.2 per cent for triple-vessel disease). The factors that showed an association with increased mortality included age greater than 64 years, female gender, new-onset angina, congestive heart failure, multivessel disease and left main coronary artery disease.[262] Even in patients with refractory angina and severe left ventricular dysfunction, both symptomatic and angiographic improvement can be accomplished in up to 90 per cent of patients, but major events (death, infarction, and emergency bypass surgery) may occur in about 8 per cent of patients.[263] Careful documentation of the risks of elective PTCA performed by experienced operators has shown that almost 90 per cent of procedures will be uneventful.

With steerable catheter systems, which are now used routinely, independent clinical predictors of *acute closure* are female gender, the presence of thrombus near the stenosis, stenosis occurring at a major bend or branch point, other stenoses in the same vessel, and the presence of multivessel disease.[264] At the time of the procedure the presence of an intimal tear or dissection, a post-PTCA stenosis of 35 per cent or more or a transtenotic gradient of 20 mm Hg or more, and the use of prolonged heparin infusion after PTCA were all associated with a higher incidence of acute closure.[264] Of particular importance is the observation that the presence of angiographic intimal dissection after PTCA substantially increases the immediate risk of a major complication.[264] The independent risk factors for in-hospital death following acute closure (<0.2 per cent in experienced centers) included female gender, the presence of multivessel disease, and collateral vessels *arising* from the vessel dilated.[265]

MULTIVESSEL PTCA. The overall clinical success rate of multivessel PTCA (angiographic success, clinical improvement, and absence of a major complication) initially is 83 to 95 per cent,[266–269,269a] with a mortality rate of 0.4 to 2.8 per cent.[266,267,270,270a] There is clinical recurrence or restenosis in approximately 30 per cent of patients during follow-up of 6 months or more,[266,268,270] even when initial technical success (at least a 35-per cent reduction in degree of stenosis and a decrease in the transstenotic gradient to 15 mm Hg or less) is seen in 89 per cent of vessels dilated.[266] The need for urgent revascularization surgery has been reported in 1 to 2.8 per cent,[266,268,270] and a major event (myocardial infarction, death, and need for emergency coronary artery surgery) occurred in 4 to 9 per cent of patients undergoing PTCA in two or more major epicardial vessels.[266,270] The acute occlusion rate of multivessel angioplasty has been reported as 2.9 per cent per patient and 1.7 per cent per vessel and is often linked to a hypotensive event occurring during dilation of the second vessel.[271]

Adverse procedural outcome is more likely in patients with high-grade (80 to 99 per cent) diameter stenoses, excessive tortuosity or a bend > 60 degrees, or in patients with chronic, total occlusion.[270a] Delayed closure (1 to 24 hours after PTCA) is usually related to intimal dissection.[271] Follow-up at 1 year reveals that approximately 80 per cent of patients who have undergone multivessel angioplasty exhibit continued improvement in symptoms[267] and may not experience death, myocardial infarction, or the need for revascularization surgery[267]; 5-year survival is nearly 90 per cent after initially successful PTCA.[269] Incomplete revascularization following multivessel PTCA may be associated with an increased restenosis rate, recurrence of angina, morbid events, and the need for coronary surgery.[272–274] Analyses of the degree of revascularization in patients with multivessel disease suggest that, while patients with one or more severe residual stenoses are more likely to require coronary artery revascularization surgery during follow-up, the risk of myocardial infarction or death is not different from that in patients who have no residual stenoses following successful angioplasty.[275,276]

RESTENOSIS. The risk of restenosis of a lesion is approximately 30 per cent[260,276a] within the first 6 months of the procedure,with angina recurring in the majority of patients with significant restenoses. Restenosis following successful PTCA appears to follow intimal hyperplasia in the dilated portion of the vessel.[277,277a] One factor that seems to increase the frequency of restenosis following PTCA is continued smoking.[266,278] While aspirin and dipyridamole do not appear to reduce the 6-month rate of restenosis after successful PTCA, they appear to reduce the incidence of transmural infarction during, or soon after, the procedure.[279]

Some factors suggestive of high risk for a second restenosis after a repeat PTCA include a lesion longer than 14 mm, the need to have an additional coronary artery dilated at the time of repeat PTCA, and a short interval between the initial and second angioplasty.[280,280a] Restenosis rates after third or fourth angioplasty procedures for recurrent restenosis are higher than those for initial procedures and approximate 50 per cent.[281] Emergency surgery will be required in 3 to 4 per cent[259,262] of patients undergoing elective PTCA (for severe coronary artery dissection, occlusion, or intractable angina) and is usually associated with higher morbidity and mortality[282] than routine coronary artery bypass grafting. An essential requirement for any institution performing PTCA is the immediate availability of surgical revascularization.

Left main coronary artery lesions are usually associated with significant disease elsewhere in the coronary arteries and thus present major potential risks, both at the time of PTCA and later if restenosis occurs. In our view, attempts at PTCA of patients with left main coronary lesions are almost always contraindicated unless some protection is provided by a patent graft to the circumflex or anterior descending coronary arteries.

If left ventricular function is impaired, successful reperfusion by PTCA can improve both systolic[283] and diastolic[284] function, even though the risks of the procedure are increased. Indeed, significant long-term improvement in coronary artery dynamics (equivalent to the results of coronary artery surgery) is seen following successful PTCA.[285] This improvement is reflected in improved myocardial function during exercise[286] and long-term improvements in symptoms.[259,272–274, 287,288]

PREVIOUS BYPASS SURGERY. Patients who have previously undergone coronary artery bypass surgery with recurrent angina can benefit from PTCA of the native coronary circulation and of the venous grafts to improve symptomatic status and avoid the need for reoperation.[289] Better long-term results are achieved with dilatation of distal graft lesions than of those located proximally or in the body of the graft. Angiographic success can approach 90 per cent at the distal site of the graft insertion, 70 per cent in the midportion, and 55 per cent proximally.[290] Cardiac complications occur in approximately 5 to 7 per cent,[289–291,291a] and the complication and recurrence rates of stenoses are significantly higher when PTCA is attempted in saphenous vein grafts failing 3 or more years after implantation than in those failing sooner after coronary artery surgery.[289,291,291a] Even totally occluded coronary arteries can be dilated,[292–294] especially if there is a short segment of occluded artery of known short duration.[293]

Invariably, a number of issues should be considered as the risks and benefits of PTCA are balanced against those of coronary artery surgery in individual patients. There are no absolute rules, but the following questions should be considered:

1. How experienced is the angioplasty team, and is there adequate surgical back-up?
2. How "favorable" is the lesion?
3. What are the potential consequences of abrupt total occlusion of the vessel to be dilated?
4. What are the chances of achieving adequate revascularization?

These factors involve judgment and discussion among cardiologists, surgeons, patients, and their families.

LASER ANGIOPLASTY (see also p. 1374). Successful vaporization of an atherosclerotic plaque (into its elementary components—water vapor, carbon dioxide, and other combustion byproducts) has been reported. Pulsed lasers[295] and excimer systems (which operate in the near-ultraviolet range) have the potential for minimizing adjacent thermal injury, and with the development of hydrophilic wires may become widely applicable with minimal risk of perforation of the vessel wall. Recent clinical reports of percutaneous excimer laser coronary angioplasty[296–298,298a] suggest that atheroma can be safely ablated, and with careful patient selection excimer laser angioplasty may become either a useful sole procedure or an adjunctive procedure to routine balloon coronary angioplasty.[296–298] This form of therapy is in a developmental phase, and issues remain, such as vessel restenosis and the development of flexible optical fibers or fiber bundles that can also achieve an adequate-sized lumen following the irradiation.[295]

CORONARY ATHERECTOMY (see also p. 1374). Directional, transluminal coronary atherectomy excises atherosclerotic plaque, whereas balloon angioplasty commonly disrupts plaque and separates it from the media. Early clinical studies suggest that the immediate angiographic results and incidence of serious complications are comparable to those of conventional balloon angioplasty.[299,300] As with balloon angioplasty, there is, however, a high incidence of early restenosis.[299] It remains to be established whether or not atherectomy provides long-term benefit relative to conventional PTCA.

CORONARY STENTS. These are discussed on page 1373.

CORONARY ARTERY BYPASS SURGERY

OPERATIVE PROCEDURE

When the decision has been reached to proceed with coronary artery bypass grafting (CABG), administration of beta-adrenoceptor blockers, nitrates, and calcium antagonists is continued until operation. Most surgeons perform coronary artery surgery using cardiopulmonary bypass at moderate hypothermia (24° to 32°C) with hemodilution. A motionless heart is achieved by continuous aortic cross-clamping with profound cardiac hypothermia and cardioplegia induced with cold potassium solution. Simultaneous topical and core myocardial hypothermia (such as achieved by direct injection of cold solutions into the coronary arteries) has been recommended to provide uniform myocardial cooling. Rapid diastolic cardiac arrest is the aim, and in the United States the most commonly used agent to achieve this is a highly concentrated solution of potassium chloride. Both crystalloid and blood cardioplegic solutions have been used with success.[301]

VENOUS CONDUITS. The saphenous vein is mainly used for distal branches of the right and circumflex coronary arteries and for sequential grafts to these vessels and diagonal branches[302] (Figs. 40–6 and 40–7). In emergency situations, many surgeons prefer the saphenous vein, which can be harvested and grafted more rapidly than the internal mammary artery. Arm vein grafts are not as effective as either saphenous veins or internal mammary artery grafts.[303,304] Since 8 to 12 per cent of saphenous vein grafts occlude in the early postoperative period, increasing attention has been directed to technical aspects of the procedure: avoidance of excessive distending pressures and atraumatic harvesting are employed to reduce intimal and medial injury of the graft.[302] When sequential vein grafts are used, the first side-to-side anastomosis has a higher patency rate than the more distal ones, and the terminal end-to-side anastomosis (end of saphenous vein to side of coronary artery) has the least favorable outcome. Indeed, the patency rate of such a distal anastomosis is lower than the patency rate of a single graft to the same vessel.[305]

INTERNAL MAMMARY ARTERY BYPASS GRAFTS. In patients under the age of 65 years, the internal mammary artery (also known as the internal thoracic artery) usually is remarkably free of atheroma. When it is grafted to a coronary artery, it appears to be virtually immune to the development of intimal hyperplasia, which is almost universally seen in aortocoronary vein grafts, and atherosclerotic changes in this vessel develop in only a small percentage of patients after coronary artery surgery. The internal mammary artery is delicate, and great care has to be taken to mobilize the vessel

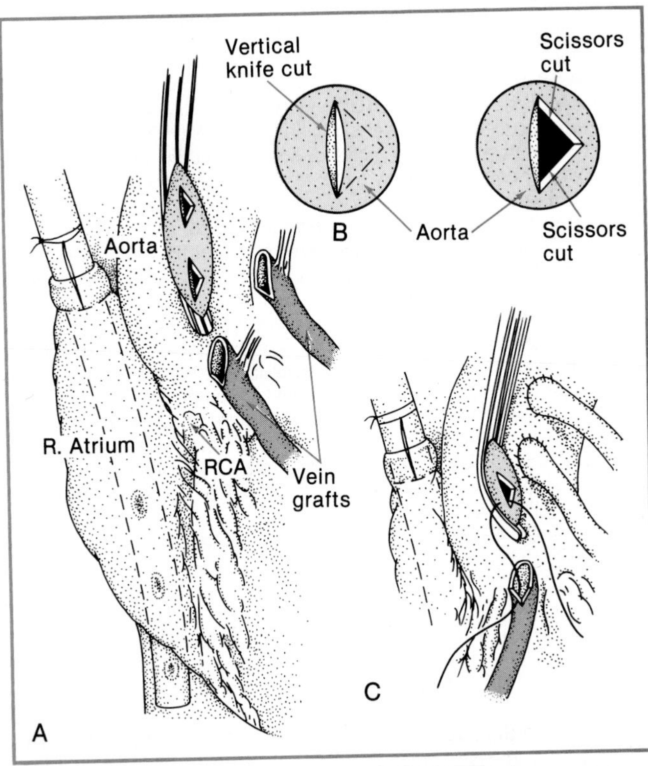

FIGURE 40–6. The aorticovenous anastomosis in a coronary arterial–saphenous vein bypass graft. *A* shows the direction of the anastomotic site for left-sided grafts; *B* shows details of aortic orifices; *C* shows the direction of right coronary artery (RCA) grafts. (From Cohn, L. H.: Surgical techniques of emergency coronary revascularization. *In* Cohn, L. H. [ed.]: The Treatment of Acute Myocardial Ischemia: An Integrated Medical-Surgical Approach. Mt. Kisco, N.Y., Futura Publishing Co., 1979, p. 87.)

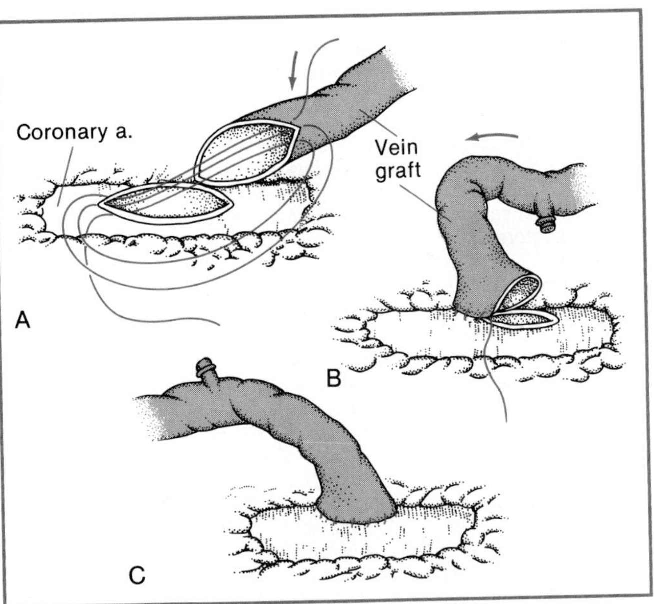

FIGURE 40–7. The venocoronary anastomosis to the proximal portion of the arteriotomy. (From Cohn, L. H.: Surgical techniques of emergency coronary revascularization. *In* Cohn, L. H. [ed.]: The Treatment of Acute Myocardial Ischemia: An integrated Medical-Surgical Approach. Mt. Kisco, N.Y., Futura Publishing Co., 1979, p. 87.)

without traumatizing it (Fig. 40–8).[306] This prolongs the operative time and often involves entry into the pleural space. Therefore, the internal mammary artery is not often used for emergency surgery. Comparative morphologic and angiographic studies of internal mammary arteries and saphenous vein bypass grafts that have been implanted long-term show that accelerated atherosclerosis occurs commonly in saphenous vein grafts but is extremely rare in internal mammary artery grafts. The media of the internal mammary artery may derive nourishment from the lumen rather than from vasa vasorum. Endothelium-dependent relaxation is more pronounced in the internal mammary artery than in vein grafts,[307] which may allow flow-dependent autoregulation to occur. The diameter of the internal mammary artery graft usually is a closer match to that of the recipient coronary artery than the diameter of a saphenous vein.

In contrast to the 40- to 60-per cent patency for vein grafts at 10 to 12 years following coronary surgery, that of internal mammary artery grafts exceeds 90 per cent.[308] However, fibrointimal proliferation may occasionally develop in internal mammary artery grafts and cause internal mammary artery narrowing and may be a factor in late graft closure.[309]

The improved 10-year survival described by Loop et al.[310] in patients who received an internal mammary artery graft to the anterior descending coronary artery alone, or combined with one or more saphenous vein grafts, compared with survival in patients who had only saphenous vein bypass grafts (Fig. 40–9) has been confirmed.[311,312] Indeed, in patients who receive an internal mammary artery graft to the left anterior descending coronary artery, the risk of dying is reduced by approximately 35 per cent compared to that in patients revascularized with vein grafts.[308] Most surgeons now believe that whenever it is technically feasible, internal mammary artery grafting is the preferable treatment (at least for lesions of the anterior descending coronary artery).

Multiple internal mammary artery grafts, which are technically more demanding and usually require more operative time compared with single internal mammary artery grafts (with or without concurrent vein grafts), do not appear to be associated with different operative mortality or morbidity than single internal mammary artery grafts, and intermediate (4-year) survival is similar (Fig. 40–10).[313]

OTHER CONDUITS. Other arterial conduits used for coro-

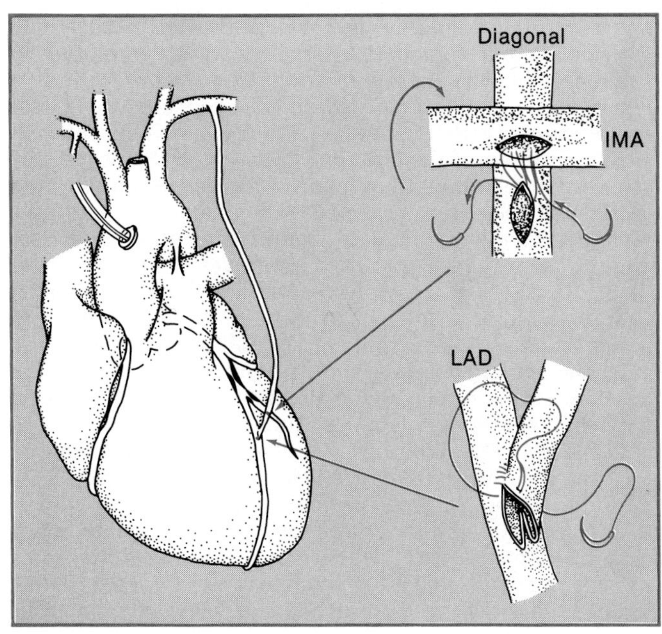

FIGURE 40-8. Internal mammary grafting: In situ left internal mammary artery (IMA) graft to the left anterior descending artery (end-to-side) and diagonal branch (side-to-side) employing the diamond anastomotic technique to the latter. The details show the IMA pedicle rolled up over the diagonal coronary artery to facilitate exposure and use of continuous suture. (From Jones, E. L.: Extended use of the internal mammary coronary artery bypass. J. Cardiac Surg. *1*:13, 1986.)

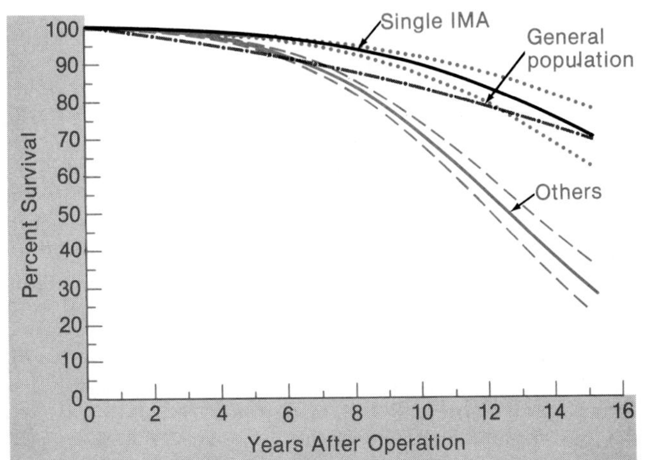

FIGURE 40-9. Survival of patients with extensive three-vessel disease according to whether or not a single internal mammary artery graft (IMA) to the left anterior descending coronary artery was used as a conduit in addition to whatever vein grafts were necessary. "General population" refers to an age, race, and gender-matched general population from government statistics and "Others" refers to patients revascularized without a single internal mammary artery graft applied to the left anterior descending coronary artery. These data strongly suggest that having a single IMA graft applied to the left anterior descending coronary artery is beneficial to survival in patients with extensive three-vessel coronary artery disease. (Modified from Kirklin J. W., et al.: Summary of a consensus concerning death and ischemic events after coronary artery bypass grafting. Circulation *79*[Suppl. I]:81, 1989, by permission of the American Heart Association, Inc.)

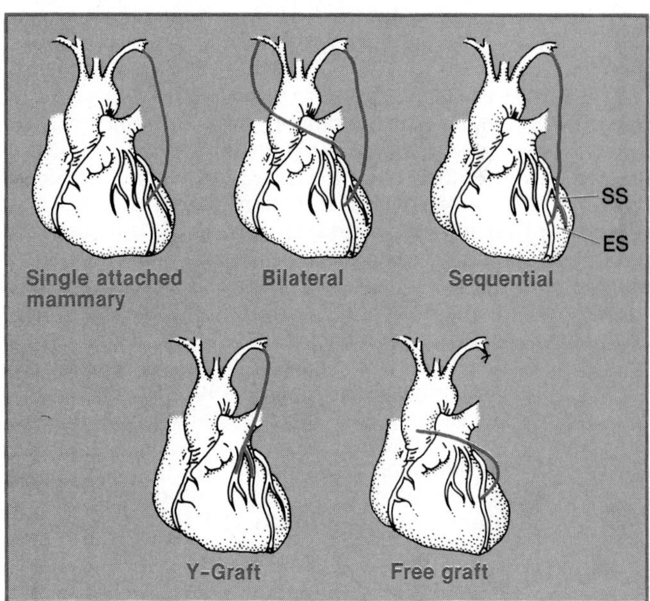

FIGURE 40-10. Different types of internal mammary artery grafts. A single attached internal mammary artery graft (either the right or left) remains attached proximally to the subclavian artery and is connected to the coronary arteries. Bilateral internal mammary artery grafts (right and left) are joined end to side to coronary arteries. Sequential internal mammary artery grafts consist of an attached or free internal mammary artery with one or more side-to-side anastomoses and one end-to-side anastomosis. The internal mammary artery Y graft has two terminal branches of either the attached or free internal mammary artery sutured to two coronary arteries. A free internal mammary graft is placed by transecting the right or left internal mammary artery near its origin in the subclavian artery, and the proximal artery is anastomosed to the aorta with the distal end to the coronary artery. (From Tector, A. J., et al.: Expanding the use of the internal mammary artery to improve patency in coronary artery bypass grafting. J. Thorac. Cardiovasc. Surg. *91*:9, 1986.)

nary artery revascularization include the gastroepiploic artery,[314-316] which appears to be able to provide an adequate coronary artery supply even during exercise.[315] The radial artery is associated with poor patency rates,[314] and technical difficulty preparing the splenic artery for use as a graft has led to its disuse. The use of arm, allogeneic veins, and synthetic conduits have all been associated with relatively poor patency.[314]

MILD OBSTRUCTION. Intraoperative studies have shown that native arteries with less than 50 per cent luminal diameter obstruction often have minimal, if any, pressure gradients across the lesions and little difference in blood flow through the artery distal to the graft when the bypass graft is opened.[317] Patients with higher-grade obstructions usually have greater pressure gradients across the lesions, and flow through artery may increase significantly when the bypass graft is opened.

THE DISTAL VASCULATURE. The state of the distal coronary arterial vasculature is also important. Late patency of grafts is related to coronary arterial runoff, as determined by the diameter of the coronary artery into which the graft is inserted, the size of the distal vascular bed, and, to a lesser degree, the severity of coronary atherosclerosis distal to the site of insertion of the graft.[318,319] The highest graft patency rates are found when the lumina of the vessels distal to the graft insertion are greater than 1.5 mm in diameter, perfuse a large peripheral vascular bed, and are free of atheroma occluding more than 25 per cent of the vessel lumen. Vessel diameters measured at coronary arteriography correlate satisfactorily with those obtained at operation.[319] Whenever there is a question about the ability of a vessel to accept a graft, the surgeon should (consistent with patient safety) attempt the anastomosis because symptomatic improvement depends on the completeness of revascularization.[320]

FLOW RATES. When measured at the time of operation, flow rates through saphenous vein grafts average nearly 70 ml/min. Those in which the flow is less than 45 ml/min—and especially less than 25 ml/min—are frequently associated with graft closure, which is less common at flow rates exceeding 45 ml/min.[321] The possible causes for reduced flow include subcritical obstruction of the coronary artery; a technically poor anastomosis, with narrowing of the lumen due to kinking of the vessel or pinching at the site of the anastomosis; and a small myocardial mass perfused by the graft, which may in turn be due to diseased distal vasculature.

OTHER SURGICAL PROCEDURES FOR ISCHEMIC HEART DISEASE. Replacement of the aortic or mitral valve or both (Chap. 34) and left ventricular aneurysmectomy (p. 1350) may be performed with or without associated bypass grafting in patients with CAD. When valve replacement or aneurysmectomy is carried out as the sole procedure in such patients, it is usually because of the presence of heart failure refractory to medical management. These procedures add to the operative risk of bypass grafting, presumably because of the prolongation and greater technical complexity of the procedure, as well as because they are usually carried out on patients with left ventricular failure who are poor operative risks.

RESULTS OF SURGERY

OPERATIVE MORTALITY. As Kirklin et al. have pointed out, risk factors for death following coronary artery surgery are (1) preoperative factors related to CAD (severe or unstable angina, recent acute myocardial infarction, hemodynamic instability, left ventricular dysfunction, extent of CAD, and presence of left main coronary artery disease); (2) preoperative factors related to aggressiveness of the arteriosclerotic process, as reflected in associated carotid or peripheral vascular disease; (3) preoperative biological factors, (older age at operation, diabetes mellitus and perhaps female gender); (4) intraoperative factors (intraoperative ischemic damage and failure to use internal mammary artery grafts); and (5) environmental or institutional factors, including the specific surgeon and treatment protocols used.[311]

Operative mortality for the treatment of stable and unstable angina pectoris has been declining steadily despite the fact that with the extensive application of PTCD surgeons are operating on greater numbers of sicker, older patients with worse ventricular function and more extensive CAD.[322,323] During the last 10 years excellent operative results have been obtained even in patients with CAD and impaired ventricular function.[324-329] It is noteworthy that in patients of small stature (which probably correlates with small cardiac size and small coronary arteries), operative mortality is significantly increased and relief of angina is not as complete. In some series, operative mortality is 0.2 to 0.3 per cent.[330,331] However, *multi-institutional* results suggest hospital death rates of 6.5 per cent in community hospitals and 2.1 to 3.7 per cent in university hospitals.[311] Incremental risk factors for hospital death include increasing age, recent or previous myocardial infarction, left ventricular dysfunction,[311] left main coronary artery disease (operative mortality 3.8 per cent compared with 2.6 per cent in patients with three-vessel disease),[332,332a] hemodynamic instability or cardiogenic shock, and the use of saphenous vein graft only.[311]

It has become increasingly clear that the use of internal mammary artery grafts (whether or not combined with vein grafts) is associated with reduced hospital and long-term mortality (Fig. 40–9).[311] The major areas of management that have been responsible for the currently low operative mortality of coronary artery surgery involve measures during both the intraoperative and perioperative periods. Improved anesthetic techniques, intraoperative protection of myocardium, conduit selection and preservation, blood conservation, perioperative hemodynamic monitoring, pharmacological left ventricular unloading, intraaortic balloon assistance, and arrhythmia control have all contributed.[301] In patients with active ischemia, cardiogenic shock, or extremely poor left ventricular function, operative mortality may be reduced when the intraaortic balloon is used to support the circulation during the perioperative period.[333]

There is still considerable variability in the results of various surgical groups, and the physician considering the referral of a particular patient for surgical treatment must be aware of the recent results obtained by the surgical group selected.

PERIOPERATIVE COMPLICATIONS (see also Chap. 53). Perioperative morbidity has increased because of larger numbers of higher-risk patients.[323] Greater numbers of patients with associated disease (hypertension, cerebrovascular disease), recent infarction, extensive coronary artery disease, and impaired ventricular function are being operated upon.[333a] Previous bypass surgery has become a more significant predictor of mortality with respect to time,[323] but there has also been a significant increase in patients undergoing emergency operation with associated increased mortality.[323,333a]

Myocardial Infarction. This complication occurs in approximately 2 to 5 per cent of elective coronary revascularizations.[330,331,334,335] In the Coronary Artery Surgery Study (CASS) trial, carried out between 1975 and 1979, the perioperative infarction rate, defined as the appearance of Q waves in the perioperative period, was reported as 6.4 per cent.[334] The incidence of perioperative infarction is usually related to the obstruction of a graft and correlates with the number of bypass grafts. Therefore, meticulous attention to anastomosis of the graft to the coronary artery is vital. Although the loss of any viable myocardium obviously is undesirable, in most patients the perioperative infarcts are small. In patients experiencing a perioperative myocardial infarction, perioperative mortality is higher, and in those with residual depressed left ventricular function (left ventricular ejection fraction <40 per cent) and inadequate revascularization, the long-term prognosis is poorer.[336]

Intellectual Dysfunction. It is common for patients to show impaired cognitive function early following coronary artery bypass surgery. This occurs in the absence of evidence of a perioperative stroke.[337] It is important that the physician reassure the patient and family that this is usually a temporary phenomenon.[338]

Hypertension. This complication can occur in up to one-third of all patients after coronary artery surgery (p. 841). The mechanism is unclear, but it may be related to increased levels of circulating catecholamines and renin. With the use of agents such as calcium antagonists,[339] sodium nitroprusside,[339] or nitrates[340] in the perioperative period, it rarely presents a problem. Esmolol, a short-acting beta-blocking agent (p. 864) appears to be equally effective in reducing systolic and diastolic pressures and also slows heart rate.[341] It is important that hypertension be adequately controlled to prevent myocardial ischemia, cardiac failure, and excessive perioperative bleeding.

Intraventricular Conduction Disturbances. In general, patients with CAD who develop fascicular conduction disturbances have diffuse myocardial disease and an unfavorable prognosis. The subsequent causes of death are ventricular arrhythmias and cardiac failure. However, in one series of patients, the development of new perioperative ventricular conduction disturbances did not worsen the long-term survival rate.[342]

Complications in the Obese. Physicians, nurses, and physiotherapists involved in the perioperative care of obese patients are well aware of the need for aggressive chest physiotherapy and the potential problems with persistent immobilization. While obesity per se does not appear to increase significantly the operative mortality,[343] it is associated with a higher incidence of complications, including sternotomy dehiscence,[344] impaired leg wound healing following saphenous vein excision,[345] postoperative hypertension, and bronchoconstriction.[343]

SYMPTOMATIC RESULTS. Major relief of angina pectoris occurs in most appropriately selected patients after coronary artery surgery.[346–350] Approximately three-quarters of patients will be free from ischemic events (return of angina, occurrence of a myocardial infarction, or sudden death) for 5 years after coronary artery surgery, and nearly half of patients for at least 10 years (Fig. 40–11).[311] However, by 15 years only about 15 per cent of patients can be expected to remain free of an ischemic event.

Return to full employment has been disappointing in many series.[351] Factors that adversely affect the prospects of patients returning to work include increasing age,[352,353] postoperative angina,[352–354] and either unemployment or a period of disability before surgery.[352,353] Approximately half of patients will return to presurgery levels of household activity,[355] and most will experience improved physical and sexual functional status from presurgery levels.[356] However, with time there is a falloff in symptomatic benefit, and there is a suggestion that by 10 years after coronary vein graft surgery the relief of symptoms and improved exercise performance noted at 5 years have decreased to levels seen in medically treated patients.[357]

GRAFT PATENCY RATE AND CHANGES IN NATIVE CIRCULATION. Experimental studies and observations in patients suggest that there are several consecutive phases of disease development in venous aortocoronary artery bypass grafts (Fig. 40–12).

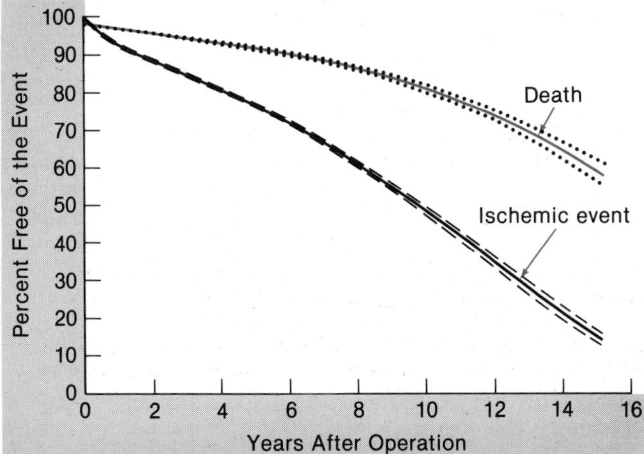

FIGURE 40–11. Freedom from the first ischemic event (angina, myocardial infarction, or sudden death) after coronary artery bypass grafting for ischemic heart disease. Freedom from death (the survivorship) is depicted, as is freedom from the first ischemic event after primary, isolated coronary artery bypass graft surgery for ischemic heart disease using any type of conduit (saphenous vein grafts and internal mammary grafts). In considering freedom from the first ischemic event, patients dying before the development of this event of causes other than sudden death (e.g., accidental death, cancer) have been censored at the time of death. (Modified from Kirklin J. W., et al.: Summary of a consensus concerning death and ischemic events after coronary artery bypass grafting. Circulation *79*[Suppl. I]:81, 1989, by permission of the American Heart Association, Inc.)

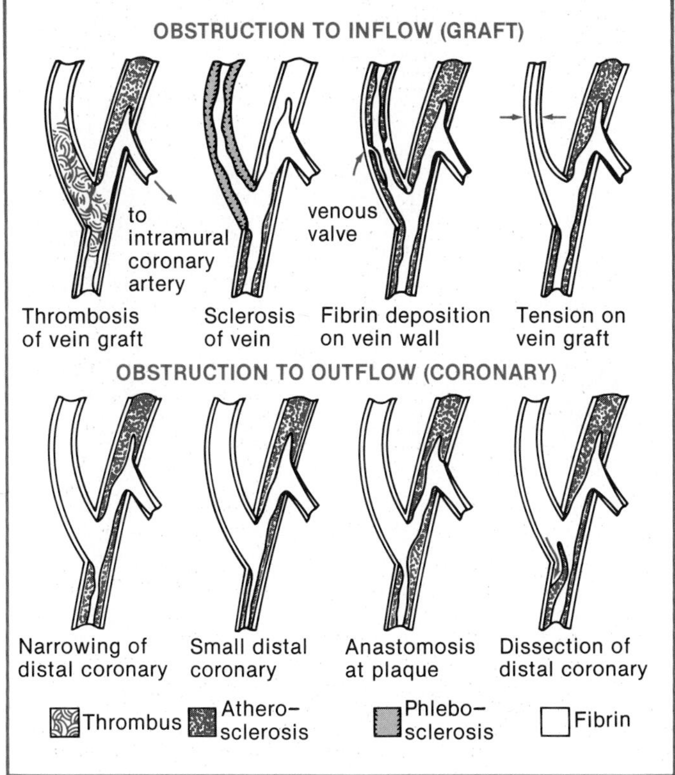

FIGURE 40–12. Anatomical and technical factors that can produce obstruction of a vein graft *(top)* and of arterial outflow *(bottom)*. (From Spray, T. L., and Roberts, W. C.: Morphologic observations in biologic conduits between aorta and coronary artery. *In* Rahimtoola, S. [ed.]: Coronary Bypass Surgery. Philadelphia, F. A. Davis, Co., 1977, p. 11.)

Early Occlusion. Early occlusion (prior to hospital discharge) occurs in 8 to 12 per cent of venous grafts, and by 1 year 12 to 20 per cent of vein grafts have become occluded.[302,305] Technical factors may cause closure at the proximal or distal anastomoses; both kinks due to excessive length and tension due to insufficient length may promote occlusion. Graft flow and distal vessel runoff are also important. Atheroma at the arteriotomy site may predispose to early occlusion. Perioperative platelet inhibitor therapy with both high-[358] and low-dose[359] aspirin and dipyridamole appears to diminish the rate of early occlusion.

Intermediate Phase. In vein grafts that have been implanted in the arterial circulation for 1 month to 1 year, there is substantial endothelial denudation and proliferation and migration of medial cells to the intima. These events are promoted by aggregation of platelets and growth factor secretion.[302] Intimal thickening and hyperplasia appear, but this process is not prevented by platelet inhibitor therapy. Histological studies of grafts that occlude within 1 year show either substantial thrombosis with minimal intima-medial changes or marked intimal hyperplasia and superimposed thrombus.[360] This accelerated process of intimal hyperplasia is an early stage of atherosclerotic plaque formation and is believed to occur because of an interaction between platelets and other circulating cells and chronic, mild endothelial damage. If the proliferation is severe and localized (as may occur at the site of the anastomosis between the grafts and the recipient artery), total occlusion can occur within 1 year.

Atherosclerosis in Venous Bypass Grafts. Beyond the first year, a histological picture occurs that is indistinguishable from that of arterial atherosclerotic disease (Fig. 40–13).[361] Some investigators believed that, as in native arteries, the development of atherosclerosis in vein grafts is a continuum starting from platelet deposition and advancing to smooth muscle cell proliferation and finally to lipid incorporation into the plaque. By 10 years, nearly one-half of venous grafts patent at 5 years have become occluded.[302,361a]

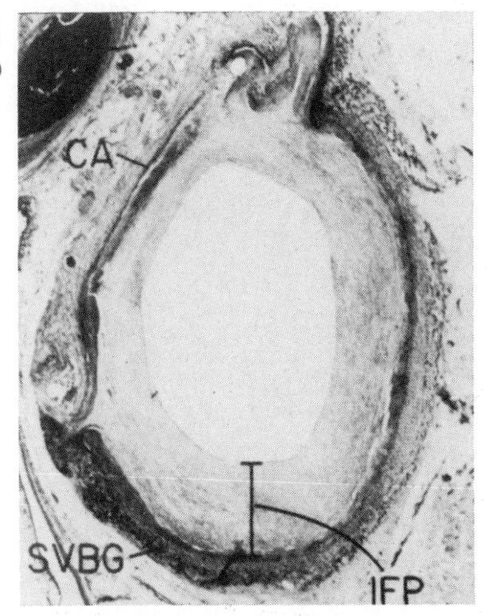

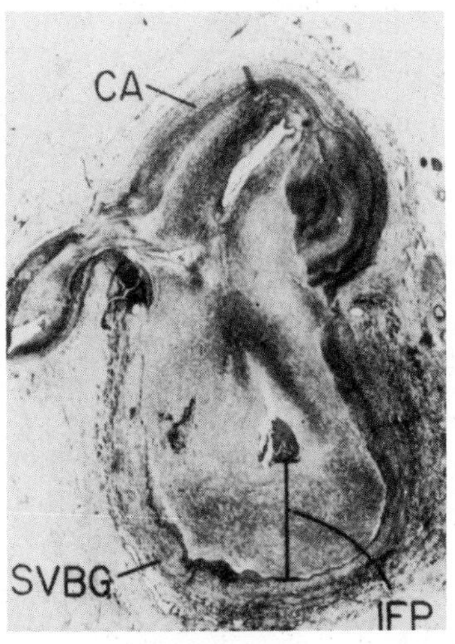

FIGURE 40–13. **Postmortem histological sections through coronary artery (CA) anastomosis sites of saphenous vein bypass grafts (SVBG) show extensive fibrous tissue proliferation in the grafts' intimal layers. In the graft at *left,* the circumferential intimal fibrous plaque (IFP) developed in 5 months. In the graft at *right,* the process resulted in greater than 90 per cent stenosis 8 months after implantation. With time, such fibrous plaques may become infiltrated with lipids and calcium and increasingly resemble atherosclerotic plaques. (From Bulkley, B. H.: Why coronary bypass grafts fail: Early and late pathologic changes. J. Cardiovasc. Med. *5*:1025, 1980.)**

Nongrafted Coronary Arteries. While determination of graft patency usually involves postoperative angiography, radionuclide techniques assessing myocardial perfusion may also indicate graft patency.[362] Serial imaging after coronary surgery may identify patients with a greater or lesser likelihood of graft occlusion. In patients who have no recurrent angina, the absence of new thallium-perfusion defects correlates well with graft patency. In contrast, the development of new perfusion defects in addition to the return of typical or atypical chest pain indicates a high probability of graft occlusion.[362] Contrast-enhanced computer tomography also may be used to assess patency of saphenous vein grafts (Fig. 9–47, p. 267). Disease progression in nongrafted arteries (worsening of a preexisting lesion or appearance of a new diameter narrowing of greater than 49 per cent) can occur at a rate of 18 to 38 per cent over 5 to 10 years.[363–365] The rate of disease progression appears highest in arterial segments already showing evidence of disease.[364]

Late Occlusion. By the end of the first year, the overall occlusion rate per distal anastomosis is between 12 and 20 per cent (and the chance of one or more distal anastomoses being occluded in an individual patient with multiple venous grafts is approximately 45 per cent).[305,358,366] The occlusion rate decreases substantially beyond the first year to an annual rate of 2 per cent.[302] The attrition rate for grafts between 6 and 11 years after operation increases to 4 per cent per year.[305] Thus, the overall occlusion rate per distal anastomosis is 25 to 30 per cent at 5 to 7 years and 40 to 50 per cent at 10 years.

The risk of disease progression (appearance of a new lesion ≥50 per cent diameter stenosis or worsening of a preexisting lesion) is between three and six times higher in grafted native coronary arteries than in ungrafted native arteries,[363] and it is higher in arteries with patent grafts than in arteries with occluded grafts.[363] In the Veterans Administration Cooperative Study, the progression of disease in native grafted arteries was most often to total occlusion.[363] In general, progression usually occurs proximal to the site of graft insertion.[363,364] These data suggest that bypassing an artery with minimal disease, even if initially successful, may ultimately be harmful to the patient, who incurs both the risk of graft closure and the increased risk of accelerated obstruction of the native vessel.

Effects of Therapy on Vein Graft Occlusion and Native Vessel Progression. A meta-analysis of clinical trials suggests that antiplatelet or anticoagulant therapy after coronary artery bypass surgery may prevent graft occlusions.[367]

In a prospective randomized double-blind trial, dipyridamole (started 48 hours before operation) plus aspirin (started 7 hours after operation) was compared with placebo treatment. The daily maintenance therapy was dipyridamole 75 mg and aspirin 325 mg orally three times a day. Within 1 month of operation 3 per cent of vein-graft distal anastomoses were occluded in the treated patients compared to 10 per cent in the placebo group.[358] At angiography performed 1 year after operation, 11 per cent of vein-graft distal anastomoses were occluded in the treated group and 25 per cent in the placebo group.[366] It is possible, however, that dipyridamole is not an essential component of this treatment[368,368a] and that much lower doses of aspirin (40 to 80 mg/day) may be sufficient.

A Veterans Administration Cooperative Study Group has also examined the effect of specific antiplatelet therapy on vein graft[365,369] and internal mammary artery graft patency[370] after coronary artery bypass grafting. In this study, 772 patients were randomized to receive aspirin (325 mg once a day), aspirin (325 mg three times a day), aspirin plus dipyridamole (325 and 75 mg together three times a day), sulfinpyrazone (267 mg three times a day), or placebo.[369] In all aspirin subgroups, one 325-mg aspirin dose was given 12 hours before surgery and maintained thereafter according to the assigned regimen, but in other groups all therapy was started 48 hours before operation. Patients receiving aspirin required more reoperations for postoperative bleeding (6.6 per cent) compared with patients not receiving aspirin (1.7 per cent).[370a] All aspirin-containing therapeutic regimens improved vein graft patency compared with placebo.[369] Early graft patency rates were 94 per cent for aspirin daily, 92 per cent for aspirin three times daily, 92 per cent for aspirin and dipyridamole, and 90 per cent for dipyridamole alone compared with 85 per cent for placebo. At 1 year the graft occlusion rate in all the aspirin groups combined was 16 per cent compared with 23 per cent for the placebo group.[365] At 1 year the patency rate for all internal mammary artery grafts was 93 per cent (versus 90 per cent for all vein grafts to the left anterior descending artery) and aspirin therapy did not alter this.[370]

Effects of Hypercholesterolemia. It has been observed that LDL cholesterol levels are higher and HDL cholesterol levels are lower 11 years after operation in patients with atherosclerotic vein grafts than in patients with normal grafts.[371] Seventy-nine per cent of patients without new atherosclerotic lesions had normal lipid and normal plasma LDL apoprotein levels compared with only 8 per cent of patients whose grafts showed new atherosclerotic lesions. In addition, patients with elevated serum Lp(a) (p. 1129) have an increased risk of developing vein graft stenosis after coronary bypass surgery.[372] Successful lowering of total and LDL cholesterol and raising of HDL cholesterol (using a combination of colestipol and niacin) reduced the appearance of new lesions in coronary vein grafts as well as in the native coronary vessels.[373] Since late closure of venous grafts is invariably associated with atherosclerotic changes and is linked to continued smoking following surgery,[374] it is important for patients and physicians to work hard to maintain ideal body weight, reduce total and LDL cholesterol levels, and permanently cease smoking following coronary artery surgery.

LATE SURVIVAL. The large randomized trials of coronary artery surgery have provided detailed information of late survival (p. 1318). These studies predate the widespread use of the internal thoracic artery for revascularization, the use of PTCA, the use of aspirin, and an increasingly aggressive approach to the treatment of elevated levels of LDL cholesterol. Despite these improvements in medical and surgical management, preoperative left ventricular dysfunction continues to have a profound influence on both operative mortality and long-term survival. The beneficial influence of using the internal mammary artery as a conduit has been seen on early surgical mortality[311,330] and on later mortality.[308,311,312,330] Twelve-year follow-up in the European Coronary Surgery Study Group[375] suggests that the long-term benefits of surgery tend to be greater in patients at higher risk, i.e., patients over 50 years of age, with infarction on the preoperative electrocardiogram, a markedly ischemic response to exercise testing, and peripheral arterial disease. During short-term follow-up, there appears to be no significant difference with respect to relief of symptoms or survival between diabetics and nondiabetics,[376] although studies of patients with peripheral vascular disease show a cumulative 5-year survival of only 43 per cent for diabetics compared with 78 per cent for nondiabetics.[377] The results of coronary artery surgery in patients aged 35 or younger showed excellent actuarial survival rates of 94 per cent at 5 years and 85 per cent at 10 years despite the severity of the underlying disease and the rapidity of the atherosclerotic process in these patients.[378] However, during longer follow-up, atherosclerosis of the venous grafts becomes an increasingly important problem in these patients.[379]

COMPARISON OF MEDICAL AND SURGICAL THERAPY OF CHRONIC STABLE ANGINA PECTORIS

Prognostic Considerations

OBSERVATIONS WITHOUT ANGIOGRAPHIC ASSESSMENT. Prior to the widespread use of aspirin, beta blockers, and efforts to lower cholesterol in patients with CAD, the Framingham Study revealed that the average annual mortality of patients with chronic stable angina was 4 per cent.[380] Remission of angina may occur in up to one-third of patients with angina of recent onset. However, if the condition has been present for several years, remission is unusual. Survivors of myocardial infarction had a 5 per cent annual mortality after the first postinfarction year.[380] Others have reported similar,[381] higher,[382] and lower mortality rates.[383] In a long-term follow-up study of 586 men who had survived an attack of unstable angina or acute infarction and who were treated conservatively, the survival at 5 years was 80 per cent, at 10 years 61 per cent, and at 15 years 43 per cent.[383]

The severity of angina pectoris has some influence on the survival of patients with CAD. In a patient population with normal ventricular function and a similar extent of coronary disease, those with severe angina (perhaps reflecting, albeit indirectly, the severity of ischemia) have a worse prognosis.[384] Data from the Veterans Administration Study have shown that clinical factors such as the severity of symptoms, the presence of ST-segment depression on the resting electrocardiogram, and a history of either myocardial infarction or hypertension all adversely affect outcome in medically treated patients, particularly if two or more factors are present.[385] The European Coronary Study Group showed that an abnormal resting electrocardiogram and peripheral vascular disease also adversely affect survival in medically managed patients with chronic coronary artery disease.[347] Others have reported the adverse influence of hypertension on prognosis in patients with established CAD, and cigarette smoking appears to increase the incidence of sudden death. Cardiomegaly on a routine chest x-ray examination and the presence of a third sound on physical examination have adverse effects on prognosis because they reflect more extensive myocardial damage.[386]

PROGNOSIS BASED ON ANGIOGRAPHIC CRITERIA. In studies using angiographic criteria for prognostic evaluation, the two important variables are left ventricular function and the severity and extent of CAD. In general, the extent of left ventricular dysfunction is a more important determinant of prognosis than the extent and severity of CAD.[387] The follow-up of patients in the CASS Registry has allowed accurate study of survival of medically treated patients with angiographically assessed CAD. Both the number of major coronary arteries with severe obstruction and the degree of depression of left ventricular ejection fraction were independent risk factors, the latter exerting the dominant influence.[388] These two risk factors are synergistic in that the adverse effects on prognosis of impaired ventricular function are more pronounced as the number of stenotic vessels increases (Fig. 40–14).

Studies in *symptomatic* patients have revealed that if only *one* of the three major coronary arteries has more than 50 per cent stenosis, the annual mortality rate will be approximately 2 per cent.[389] The importance to survival of the *quantity of* myocardium that is jeopardized is reflected in the observation that an obstructive lesion proximal to the first septal perforator of the left anterior descending coronary artery was associated with a 5-year survival of 90 per cent, compared with 98 per cent in patients with more distal lesions.[389] The survival rate of patients with isolated right CAD at 5 years appeared to be higher (96 per cent) than in patients with disease of the left anterior descending coronary artery (92 per cent). The overall survival of nonsurgically treated patients with left anterior descending and left circumflex CAD was not significantly different, but both were less than the survival of patients with isolated right CAD.[389] The risk of cardiac events does not appear to be related to the presence or absence of collateral vessels in patients with one-vessel coronary disease[390]; however, even in patients with single-vessel disease, left ventricular ejection fraction was the baseline descriptor most strongly associated with survival.

In symptomatic patients or survivors of infarction, if two of the major arteries exhibit severe stenosis, the 5-year mortality is approximately 9 per cent, and if all three vessels are stenotic it rises to approximately 15 per cent.[330,391] In an observational study of patients with obstructive coronary disease who initially were treated medically, 15-year survival rates were 48, 28, 18, and 9 per cent for patients with single-, double-, triple-, and left main vessel disease, respectively.[392] In addition to the number of vessels involved, the severity of obstruction is also important. Prognosis in patients with 50- to 75 per cent narrowing is better than in those with more than 75 per cent narrowing.[393]

High-grade lesions of the left main coronary artery are particularly life threatening.[394] Mortality among medically treated patients has been reported as 29 per cent at 18 months,[395] 39 per cent at 2 years,[396] and 43 per cent at 5 years.[397] Survival is better for patients having a 50 to 70 per cent stenosis (1- and 3-year survivals of 91 per cent and 66 per cent, respectively) than for patients with a greater than 70 per cent left main coronary artery stenosis (1- and 3-year survivals of 72 and 41 per cent)[394] (Fig. 40–15). Furthermore, a number of characteristics found at catheterization or noninvasive examination are predictors of an adverse prognosis in patients with 70 per cent or greater left main coronary artery stenosis; these include chest pain at rest, ST-T wave changes on the resting electrocardiogram, cardiomegaly on the chest roentgenogram, a history of congestive heart failure, findings of left ventricular dysfunction at catheterization, and elevation of the arterial-mixed venous oxygen difference.[394]

The severity of symptoms is a useful prognostic factor in conjunction with arteriographic findings. In asymptomatic or mildly symptomatic patients with one- or two-vessel disease, the prognosis is excellent, and the annual mortality is approximately 1.5 per cent. In patients with three-vessel disease with good exercise capacity (achievement of 85 per cent predicted heart rate or workload of 100 watts or more), the annual mortality rate also is only 4 per cent, but in those with poor exercise capacity it is much higher.[398] During exercise testing in the CASS randomized study (a group of patients with mild angina or history of infarction and a left ventricular ejection fraction of >35 per cent), the presence of exercise-induced angina identified patients who had a survival advantage over

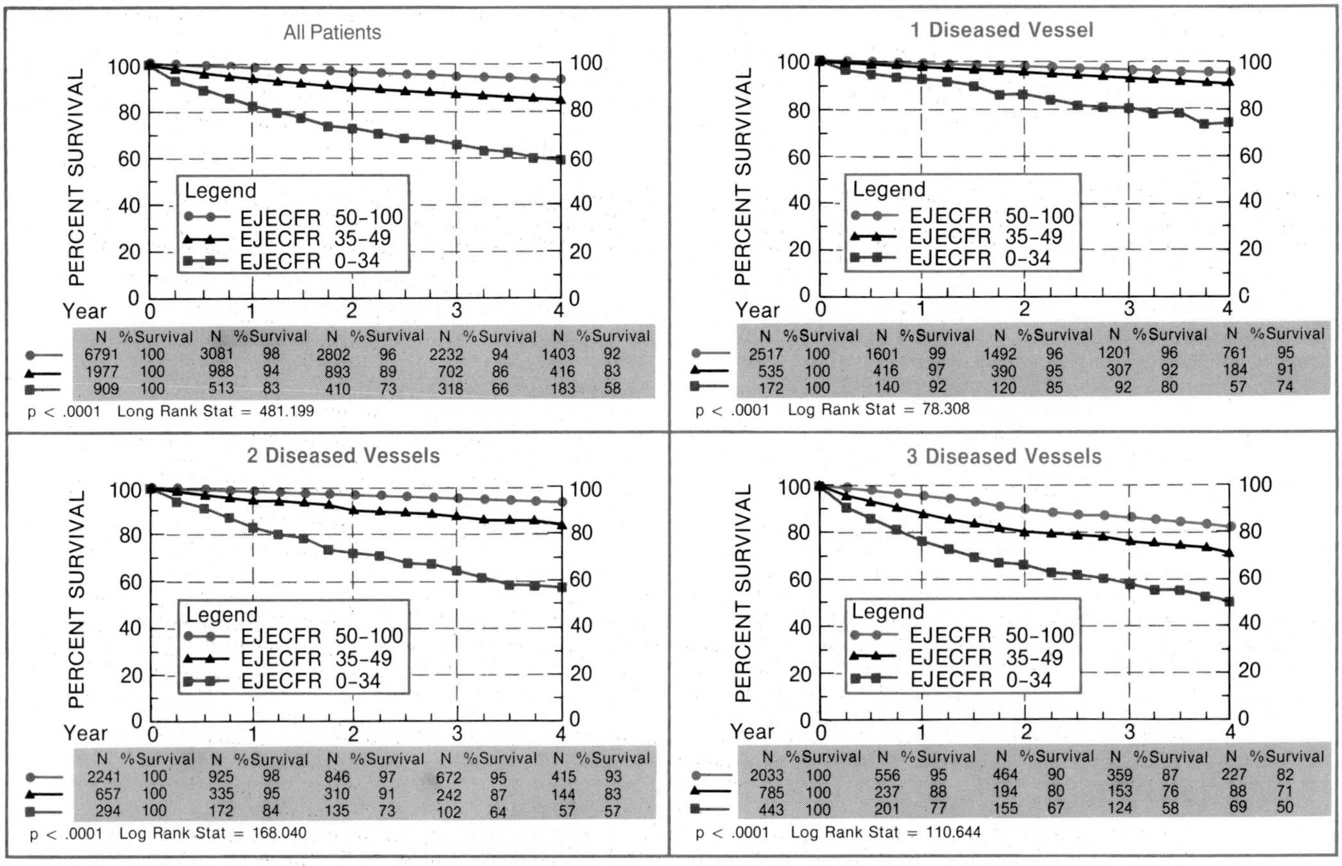

All Patients

EJECFR	Year 0 N	%Survival	Year 1 N	%Survival	Year 2 N	%Survival	Year 3 N	%Survival	Year 4 N	%Survival
50-100	6791	100	3081	98	2802	96	2232	94	1403	92
35-49	1977	100	988	94	893	89	702	86	416	83
0-34	909	100	513	83	410	73	318	66	183	58

p < .0001 Long Rank Stat = 481.199

1 Diseased Vessel

EJECFR	Year 0 N	%Survival	Year 1 N	%Survival	Year 2 N	%Survival	Year 3 N	%Survival	Year 4 N	%Survival
50-100	2517	100	1601	99	1492	96	1201	96	761	95
35-49	535	100	416	97	390	95	307	92	184	91
0-34	172	100	140	92	120	85	92	80	57	74

p < .0001 Log Rank Stat = 78.308

2 Diseased Vessels

EJECFR	Year 0 N	%Survival	Year 1 N	%Survival	Year 2 N	%Survival	Year 3 N	%Survival	Year 4 N	%Survival
50-100	2241	100	925	98	846	97	672	95	415	93
35-49	657	100	335	95	310	91	242	87	144	83
0-34	294	100	172	84	135	73	102	64	57	57

p < .0001 Log Rank Stat = 168.040

3 Diseased Vessels

EJECFR	Year 0 N	%Survival	Year 1 N	%Survival	Year 2 N	%Survival	Year 3 N	%Survival	Year 4 N	%Survival
50-100	2033	100	556	95	464	90	359	87	227	82
35-49	785	100	237	88	194	80	153	76	88	71
0-34	443	100	201	77	155	67	124	58	69	50

p < .0001 Log Rank Stat = 110.644

FIGURE 40–14. Effect of the anatomical extent of obstructive coronary artery disease and left ventricular function on survival in medically treated patients in the CASS Registry. Survival of medically treated patients with no significant obstructive disease was 97 per cent, in contrast to 92 per cent, 84 per cent, and 68 per cent of patients with one-, two-, and three-vessel disease, respectively. In patients with less than 50 per cent left main coronary artery obstruction and measured ejection fraction (EJEC FR), the effect of decreasing ejection fraction on survival is evident, even when the probability of survival is already high, as in patients with one or two obstructed arteries. As the severity of arterial disease increases, the impact of left ventricular dysfunction is even greater upon survival. (From Mock, M. B., et al.: Survival of medically treated patients in the Coronary Artery Surgery [CASS] Registry. Circulation *66*:562, 1982, by permission of the American Heart Association, Inc.)

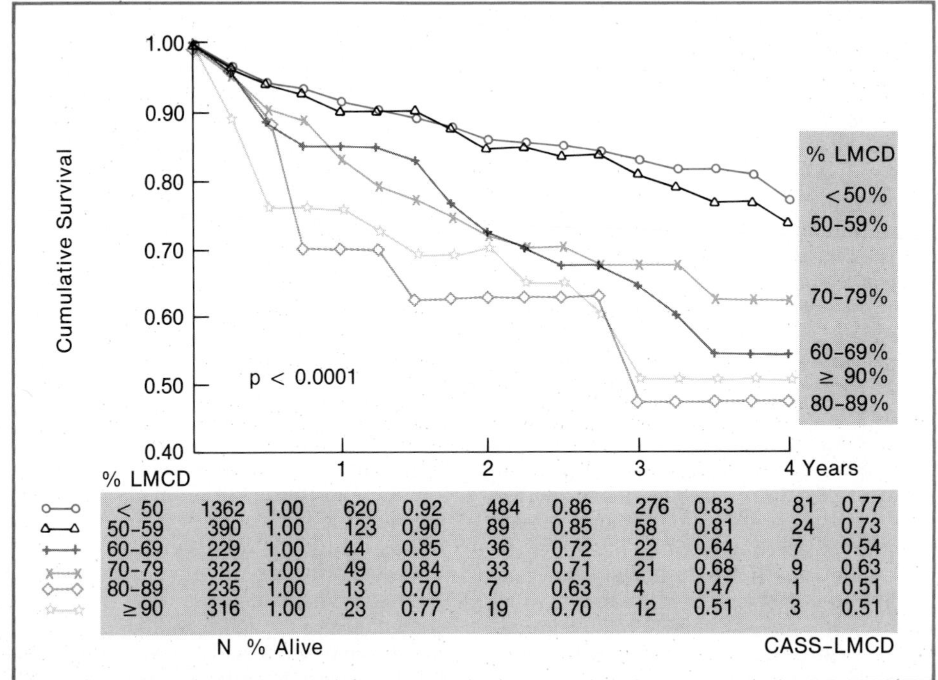

% LMCD	Year 0 N	% Alive	Year 1 N	% Alive	Year 2 N	% Alive	Year 3 N	% Alive	Year 4 N	% Alive
< 50	1362	1.00	620	0.92	484	0.86	276	0.83	81	0.77
50–59	390	1.00	123	0.90	89	0.85	58	0.81	24	0.73
60–69	229	1.00	44	0.85	36	0.72	22	0.64	7	0.54
70–79	322	1.00	49	0.84	33	0.71	21	0.68	9	0.63
80–89	235	1.00	13	0.70	7	0.63	4	0.47	1	0.51
≥90	316	1.00	23	0.77	19	0.70	12	0.51	3	0.51

FIGURE 40–15. Survival curves for medically treated patients with left main coronary artery disease. The cumulative survival rates of nonsurgically treated patients with left main coronary artery disease (LMCD) in the CASS Registry analyzed according to per cent intraluminal narrowing are demonstrated. The survival curves separate when the degree of angiographically assessed stenosis exceeds 60 per cent, so that patients with a lesser degree of narrowing have relatively favorable long-term prognosis. (From Chaitman, B. R., et al.: Effect of coronary bypass surgery on survival patterns in subsets of patients with left main coronary artery disease. Am. J. Cardiol. *48*:765, 1981.)

7 years if assigned to surgical therapy (94 per cent), compared with medical therapy (87 per cent).[399]

The assessment of ventricular function and extent and severity of CAD have been major influences in determining our understanding of the natural history of CAD and have been of help in selecting patients for surgical therapy. Taken together, the available information suggests that the volume of myocardium perfused by critically narrowed vessels and the rate of progression of coronary atherosclerosis are the principal determinants of prognosis in patients with CAD. The likelihood that stable atherosclerotic plaque will develop into an ulcerated plaque leading to coronary thrombosis and development of electrical instability also affects prognosis.

EXERCISE ELECTROCARDIOGRAPHY AND OTHER NONINVASIVE TESTS FOR PROGNOSTIC EVALUATION. The aims of exercise electrocardiographic testing, thallium scintigraphy, and exercise radionuclide ventriculography are to provide data about ventricular function and the quantity of myocardium that becomes ischemic during stress. In this manner, an assessment of the patient's functional status and the quantity of "jeopardized" myocardium can be assessed. In patients in whom left ventricular function and coronary anatomy have also been defined, exercise stress testing can provide important additional prognostic information.

By means of the CASS Registry, 30 clinical and exercise variables were analyzed in 4083 patients with defined ventricular function and coronary anatomy to assess factors of prognostic importance.[400] The *duration* of exercise and the *ST-segment response* emerged as the most important exercise test variables. In a subgroup of 570 patients with three-vessel coronary disease and preserved left ventricular function, the probability of survival at 4 years ranged from 53 per cent for patients able to achieve only stage I of exercise to 100 per cent for patients able to exercise into stage V of the standard or modified Bruce protocol. Patients showing less than 0.1 mV of ST-segment depression who could exercise into stage III of the Bruce protocol or higher had an annual mortality of 1 per cent or less, while those with at least 0.1 mV ST-segment depression who could not complete stage I had an annual mortality of 5 per cent or more (Table 40–13).

STRESS THALLIUM-201 MYOCARDIAL PERFUSION IMAGING (see also p. 1270). Exercise thallium scintigraphy may be helpful in identifying areas of myocardium in which ischemia may be induced and that may benefit from revascularization. Predictors of adverse prognosis following thallium-201 scintigraphy performed during exercise, or after administration of dipyridamole, include a delayed tracer redistribution, multiple large perfusion defects, and abnormal lung uptake.[93] The disadvantages of thallium-201 scintigraphy include the high cost, the long time required for imaging, interpretation difficulties, and poor imaging in obese persons. The patient has to be able to attain a sufficient level of exercise before a normal perfusion pattern can be assumed confidently to indicate no significant underlying coronary artery disease, although dipyridamole can be employed in patients with severe exercise limitations.

EXERCISE RADIONUCLIDE ANGIOGRAPHY (see also p. 1300). A number of studies suggest that the exercise left ventricular ejection fraction is one of the best prognostic predictors of major future cardiac events or of high-risk CAD.[401] In patients with known CAD, if the left ventricular ejection fraction during exercise fails to rise appropriately or if it falls, it suggests that a substantial segment of myocardium has become ischemic, and correlates with multivessel disease, left main coronary artery disease, and a high mortality over the next 2 years.[401] During preoperative evaluation patients who had the most profound exercise-induced left ventricular dysfunction prior to myocardial revascularization had improved survival, compared to those treated medically,[402,403] while those with a normal ejection fraction response to exercise did not.

In patients whose left ventricular function and coronary anatomy have been defined, the demonstration of ischemia or jeopardized myocardium may have a profound bearing on management. In a study of minimally symptomatic patients with preserved resting left ventricular function and three-vessel disease, evidence of impaired exercise capacity combined with the demonstration of inducible myocardial ischemia (as manifested by a decrease in ejection fraction during exercise) identified those at high risk of death during medical therapy.[404] Patients who did not manifest ischemia during exercise by radionuclide angiography or exercise electrocardiography had an excellent prognosis compared with those with impaired exercise capacity, especially if it occurred at a low workload (Fig. 40–16).

Initial Results

RELIEF OF ANGINA PECTORIS. As early as 1972, a committee of the American Heart Association indicated that the most widely accepted indication for surgical revascularization was "significant disability from moderate to severe angina pectoris, unresponsive to optimal medical care."[404a] Two decades later angina pectoris remains the principal indication; however, coronary bypass surgery is now being carried out in increasing numbers of patients with multivessel coro-

TABLE 40-13 RISK STRATIFICATION BY EXERCISE TESTING

STUDY	PATIENTS (N)	RISK CLASSIFICATION: Low	Intermediate	High
McNeer et al. Circulation *57*:64, 1978	1472	<1 mm ST ↓ FS ≥ IV Peak HR ≥ 160 beats/min		≥1 mm ST ↓ FS I or II
Bruce et al. (Seattle Heart Watch) Circulation *60*:638, 1979	2001	<1 mm ST ↓ No LV dysfunction	≥1 mm ST ↓ No LV dysfunction	FS ≤ I Peak SBP <130 mm Hg, Cardiomegaly
Dagenais et al. Circulation *65*:452, 1982	107	≤2 mm ST ↓ FS ≥ IV	≤2 mm ST ↓ FS ≥ III	≥2 mm ST ↓ FS ≤ I
Schneider et al. Am. J. Cardiol. *50*:682, 1982	80			>1 mm ST ↓ FS I or II
Weiner et al. Am. Heart J. *105*:749, 1983	292	≤2 mm ST ↓ No LV dysfunction		LV dysfunction or ≥2 mm ST ↓ beginning in stage I
Weiner et al. (CASS) J. Am. Coll. Cardiol. *3*:772, 1984	4083	<1 mm ST ↓ FS ≥ III	≥1 mm ST ↓ FS ≥ III	≥1 mm ST ↓ FS I ≤ I

N = number; FS = final exercise stage (Bruce protocol); LV = left ventricular; SBP = systolic blood pressure; HR = heart rate; CASS = Coronary Artery Surgery Study.

From Deering, T. F., and Weiner, D. A.: Prognosis of patients with coronary artery disease. J. Cardiopulmon. Rehabil. 5:325, 1985.

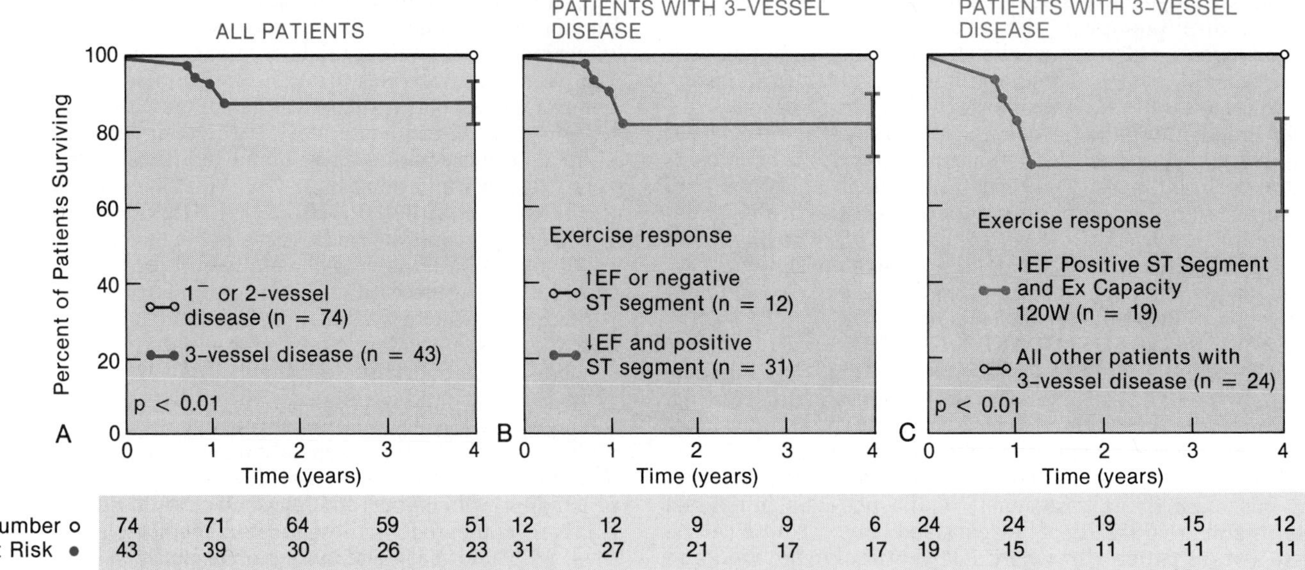

FIGURE 40–16. Influence of anatomical severity of coronary artery disease, reversible ischemia, and exercise capacity on survival in mildly symptomatic patients with coronary artery disease and left ventricular ejection fractions greater than 40 per cent. Survival curves are shown for patients with three-vessel disease as compared with those with one- or two-vessel disease *(A)*; patients with three-vessel disease and an increase in ejection fraction (EF) or a negative ST-segment response to exercise as compared with those with three-vessel disease and both a decreased ejection fraction and a positive ST-segment response with exercise *(B)*; and patients with three-vessel disease and a decrease in ejection fraction during exercise, a positive ST-segment response, and exercise capacity of 120 watts or less as compared with all other patients with three-vessel disease *(C)*. The number of patients with potential follow-up at each time is shown for each group. Evidence of impaired exercise capacity associated with evidence of reversible myocardial ischemia defines a group of patients with three-vessel disease with an adverse prognosis long-term. (Reprinted with permission from Bonow, R. O., et al.: Exercise-induced ischemia in mildly symptomatic patients with coronary artery disease and preserved left ventricular function. N. Engl. J. Med. *311*:1339, 1984.)

nary disease and either mild to moderate symptoms, left ventricular dysfunction, or poor exercise tolerance, because of the apparent improval in survival in these groups. Patients with unstable angina[405] and left ventricular dysfunction as well as survivors of acute myocardial infarction[406] are also undergoing revascularization with increasing frequency.

Relief of angina pectoris occurs in up to 95 per cent of patients with chronic stable angina following coronary artery surgery. More than half of the patients become totally asymptomatic, at least initially. Most of the others exhibit substantial symptomatic relief.[346] The major randomized trials have all demonstrated greater relief of angina, better exercise performance, and a lower requirement for antianginal medications for surgically as opposed to medically treated patients 5 years postoperatively.[347–349] There is a reoperation rate of 6 to 8 per cent per year for recurrence of symptoms.[407] After 5 years, about three-quarters of patients can be predicted to be free from an ischemic event (return of angina, occurrence of myocardial infarction, or sudden death), about half remain free for approximately 10 years, and about 15 per cent for 15 or more years.[311] Compared with medical therapy, the overall advantages of angina relief, increased physical activity, and reduced use of antianginal medications are less apparent 10 years after coronary surgery[408]; symptomatic improvement is best maintained in those patients with the most complete revascularization.

For patients with persistent angina despite adequate medical therapy and for those who cannot tolerate the usual antianginal medications and who are not ideal candidates for PTCA, coronary artery surgery provides excellent symptomatic relief.[408a] With increasing use of internal mammary artery grafts, long-term relief of angina and freedom from subsequent cardiac events will improve, compared with previous patient populations who have received coronary artery vein grafts alone.

Long-Term Survival

Analyses from the Duke Database suggest changing survival benefits of coronary revascularization over time. In the present era, refinements in surgical care have improved survival after revascularization for patients with one-, two-, and three-vessel disease.[409] One important factor is the use of the internal mammary artery (IMA) graft to the left anterior descending coronary artery, in addition to other vein grafts as needed (Fig. 40–9, p. 1319).[311] Early[311,312] and later mortality[311,312,330] are both improved by the use of internal mammary grafting. By 10 years, the survival in typical patients with extensive three-vessel disease in whom the IMA graft is used to revascularize the left anterior descending artery is 89 per cent compared to 71 per cent when other conduits are used.[311] By 15 years, a further divergence in the survival curves is apparent. The lessons learned from the historical randomized trials of coronary artery surgery will be amended with time because of the known attenuation of survival advantage of surgical therapy (using only venous conduits) after 5 or 7 years in the subgroups of patients for whom it was shown initially to be beneficial (Fig. 40–17) and the slower attrition rate of internal mammary artery grafts over very long-term follow-up. Bilateral internal mammary artery grafts, sequential internal mammary artery anastomoses, and free internal mammary artery grafts have all been used since the large randomized trials were carried out[306,308] (Fig. 40–9). These latter studies also predated the widespread use of percutaneous transluminal coronary angioplasty and platelet inhibiting agents.

LEFT MAIN CORONARY ARTERY STENOSIS. There is general agreement that surgical treatment improves survival in patients with left main coronary artery obstruction[410,411] (Fig. 40–15). As already pointed out, the presence of left main coronary artery stenosis does not define a homogeneous population.[394] Coronary bypass surgery appears to confer the most benefit on patients with severe degrees of left main coronary

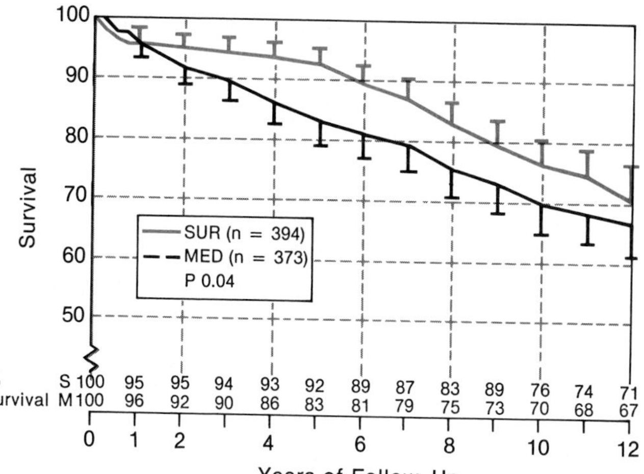

FIGURE 40–17. Cumulative survival curves for patients in the European Coronary Surgery Study. Twelve-year cumulative survival rates and 95 per cent confidence intervals for all patients randomly assigned to either surgical treatment (SUR,S), or medical therapy (MED,M). N denotes number of patients, and % survival denotes percentage surviving. The cumulative survival rate among patients who had early surgical treatment was significantly higher than those who had only medical treatment throughout the observation period. The significant difference in survival noted at 5 years between the two treatment groups (92 per cent medical treatment vs. 83 per cent surgical treatment) gradually decreased but remained significant at 10 years. After 5 years, the patients originally assigned to surgical treatment fared worse, and the benefit of early surgical treatment gradually decreased. The net result of these changes in the two treatment groups is a considerably smaller difference in survival rates at 10 and 12 years as compared with 5 years. (Reprinted with permission from Varnauskas E., and the ECSSG: Twelve-year follow-up of survival in the randomized European Coronary Surgery Study. N. Engl. J. Med. *319*:332, 1988.)

artery disease and/or those patients with impaired left ventricular function. However, it is still beneficial in all patients with left main coronary stenoses greater than 50 per cent and for patients with normal left ventricular function.[411]

There is continuing debate whether there is a "left main equivalent," which has a natural history similar to that of left main coronary disease. The condition in question may consist of disease in the proximal portions of both the left anterior descending and left circumflex coronary arteries. We believe that the ominous nature of significant left main coronary disease exists because a single event (rupture of a single plaque) can cause infarction of a large quantity of myocardium. While combined disease of the proximal left anterior descending and circumflex coronary arteries does identify a subgroup of high-risk patients, the prognosis is not as poor as for those with left main coronary artery disease.[412] Nevertheless, patients with combined stenoses of 70 per cent or more in the left anterior descending coronary artery, before the first septal perforator, and in the proximal circumflex coronary artery before the first obtuse marginal branch who have impaired ventricular function appear to have improved longevity and less angina following revascularization surgery than if they are treated medically.[413] Not unexpectedly, the CASS Registry demonstrated that 96 per cent of patients with ≥50 per cent left main coronary artery stenoses were symptomatic and that the advantages of revascularization were equivalent in both symptomatic and asymptomatic patients with disease affecting this vessel.[397]

ONE-, TWO-, OR THREE-VESSEL CORONARY ARTERY DISEASE WITH OR WITHOUT IMPAIRED VENTRICULAR FUNCTION. Current clinical practice has been shaped by three major randomized trials in which patients were enrolled between 1972 and 1979, and follow-up has continued since then. In considering these studies today it is important to recognize that major improvements have taken place in both medical and surgical treatment, as well as in the postsurgical medical treatment of patients with coronary artery disease in the 13 to 20 years since patients were entered into these trials. Nonetheless, some of the lessons they have taught us endure.

THE VETERANS ADMINISTRATION COOPERATIVE STUDY. This study prospectively examined the effects of coronary artery surgery as opposed to medical treatment in 686 adult males, randomly allocated to surgical or medical management in 1972 to 1974.[385,414–417] The patients were males who had stable angina pectoris of at least 6 months' duration, electrocardiographic evidence of either prior infarction or ischemia at rest or during exercise, significant coronary disease of at least one major coronary artery with a graftable distal segment, and a left ventricular ejection fraction greater than 25 to 30 per cent.

By 7 years after randomization, survival rates were 70 per cent with medical treatment and 77 per cent with surgical treatment ($p = 0.043$), but by 11 years the rates were 57 and 58 per cent, respectively, presumably because of later occlusion of the venous grafts.[417] Retrospective analyses have revealed that coronary artery surgery appears to confer an advantage in survival over medical therapy in patients at high clinical risk (having two or more of the following: NYHA Class III or IV, a history of hypertension, previous myocardial infarction, and ST-segment depression on the resting electrocardiogram). It also appeared to confer an advantage in a high angiographic risk group (impaired left ventricular function and three-vessel coronary artery disease).

The Veterans Administration Study investigators have summarized their long-term survival results as follows: coronary artery surgery did *not* significantly improve *overall* survival in patients without left main disease, while a significant survival benefit was seen with surgery at 5 to 7 years in subgroups of patients with multiple clinical and angiographic risk factors. This benefit diminished gradually when follow-up was extended to 11 years. The majority of patients who did not belong to high-risk subgroups derived no survival benefit from surgical treatment at any time.[416]

THE EUROPEAN CORONARY SURGERY STUDY GROUP. Men under the age of 65 with mild or moderately severe chronic stable angina (57 per cent were in Class I or II Canadian Cardiovascular Society and 42 per cent were in Class III), significant stenoses of at least two major coronary arteries, and good left ventricular function (ejection fraction greater than 50 per cent) were randomized to medical or surgical treatment between 1973 and 1976.[347,418] At 8 years of follow-up the policy of early surgery improved survival significantly compared with medical treatment in the total population (89 vs. 80 per cent), in the subgroup with three-vessel disease (92 vs. 77 per cent), and in the patients with two-vessel disease in which one of the diseased vessels was the proximal segment of the left anterior descending coronary artery (90 vs. 79 per cent) (Fig. 40–18).

There was no significant difference in survival between medical and surgical treatment in patients with one-vessel disease and in those with two-vessel disease without stenosis of the proximal left anterior descending coronary artery (Fig. 40–19). At 12 years of follow-up, it was apparent that the improvement in survival in patients treated surgically had become attenuated after 5 years and the percentage of patients surviving decreased more rapidly in the surgically treated patients (Fig. 40–17).[375] Nevertheless, the diminishing difference between the survival curves still favored surgical over medical treatment after 12 years (71 per cent vs. 67 per cent, respectively). The presence of proximal left anterior descending coronary artery stenosis as a component of two- or three-vessel disease was the outstanding predictor of poor prognosis with medical therapy and improved outcome with surgery.[375]

CORONARY ARTERY SURGERY STUDY (CASS). Patients age 65 or younger with mild angina or with a myocardial infarction more than 3 weeks previously were randomized to medical or surgical therapy between 1975 and 1979 if they had significant, operable coronary artery disease.[324,325,334] After 10 years, cumulative survival for CASS patients as a whole showed no significant difference in medical versus surgical 10-year survival (79 per cent vs. 82 per cent, respectively).[419] A significant advantage favoring initial surgical assignment was observed in patients with ejection fractions between 35 per cent and 50 per cent (medical, 61 per cent vs. surgical, 79 per cent; $p = 0.01$) (Fig. 40–20).[419] The CASS Registry observational studies have shown that in patients with mild[420] or severe[384,421] angina, surgery improves survival in patients with three-vessel disease regardless whether ventricular function is normal or depressed. However, in patients with more extensive disease and the worst ventricular function,[421] survival may be improved to an even greater extent by surgery. Other studies have also suggested that patients who demonstrate the most severe ischemia-induced ventricular dysfunction during exercise are most likely to benefit subsequently with respect to survival, relief of pain, and improvement in exercise capacity.[402,403,422]

TREATMENT OF PATIENTS WITH SEVERELY DEPRESSED LEFT VENTRICULAR FUNCTION. Studies have compared medical and surgical therapy in CAD patients with severely depressed left ventricular function.[326,327,329] In a

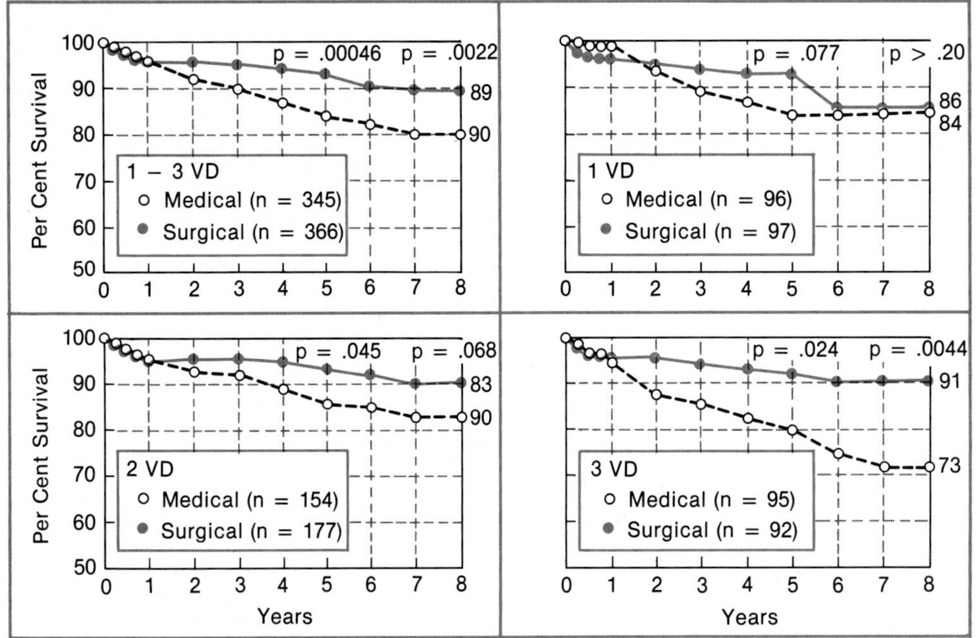

FIGURE 40–18. Cumulative survival curves for patients in the European Coronary Surgery Study. To compare the European prospective randomized coronary surgery study with other studies, a cohort of 711 patients was identified as having greater than 75 per cent obstruction in one, two, or three vessels. A significant improvement in survival with surgery was found in the total cohort and in the subgroup with three-vessel disease; however, there was no significant difference in survival between the two treatments in patients with one-vessel disease and those with two-vessel disease without proximal left anterior descending stenosis. (From Varnauskas, E., and the European Coronary Surgery Study Group: Survival, myocardial infarction, and employment status in a prospective, randomized study of coronary bypass surgery. Circulation *72*[Suppl. V]:90, 1985, by permission of the American Heart Association, Inc.)

FIGURE 40–19. Cumulative survival for the subgroup of patients with double-vessel disease (2 VD group) in the European Coronary Study Group when disease is defined as 75 per cent or greater narrowing and is subdivided by the presence or absence of disease in the proximal segment of the left anterior descending coronary artery (LAD). This retrospective analysis suggests that surgery may confer an advantage over medical therapy in patients with two-vessel disease in whom both narrowings are greater than 75 per cent of luminal diameter, and one of them is the proximal segment of the left anterior descending coronary artery. (From Varnauskas, E., and European Coronary Surgery Study Group: Survival, myocardial infarction, and employment status in a prospective, randomized study of coronary bypass surgery. Circulation *72*[Suppl. V]:90, 1985, by permission of the American Heart Association, Inc.)

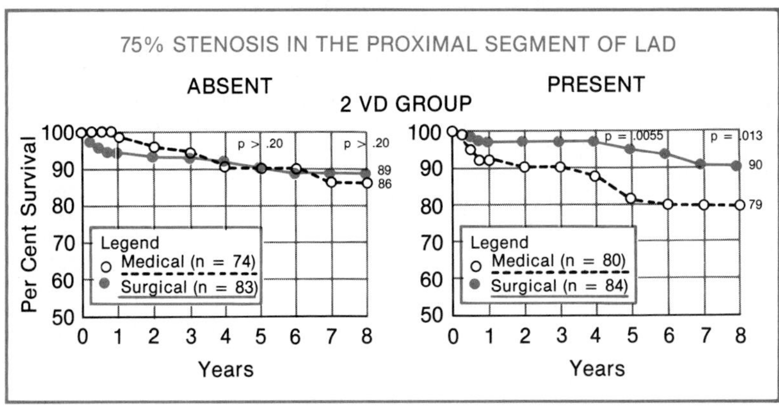

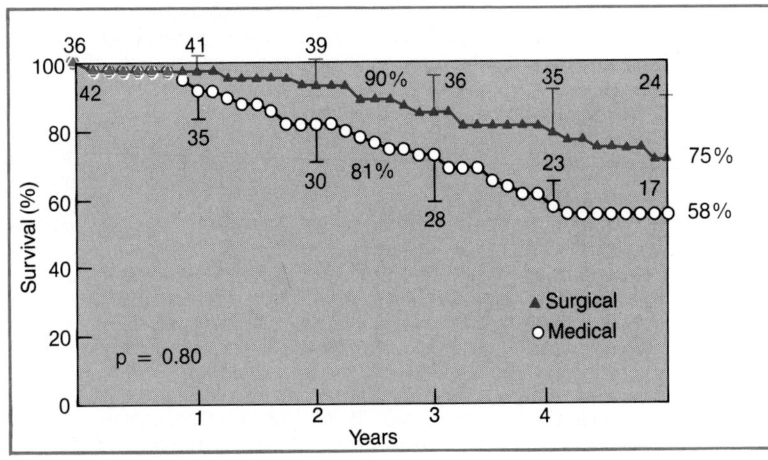

FIGURE 40–20. Survival of patients with three-vessel coronary disease and left ventricular dysfunction. Ten-year follow-up of survival in the Coronary Artery Surgery Study (CASS) in the subset of patients with an ejection fraction of less than 50 per cent and three-vessel coronary disease. Patients with left ventricular dysfunction exhibit long-term benefit from an initial strategy of surgical treatment, and this is particularly evident in patients with three-vessel coronary disease who show a survival benefit after 10 years with initial surgical treatment (75 per cent) vs. medical treatment (58 per cent). (From Alderman E. L., et al.: Ten-year follow-up of survival and myocardial infarction in the randomized Coronary Artery Surgery Study. Circulation *82*:1629, 1990, by permission of the American Heart Association, Inc.)

CASS Registry study[423] surgical treatment was shown to prolong survival, particularly in patients with ejection fractions below 0.26 (Fig. 40–21). In another study examining the late results of surgical and medical therapy for patients with coronary artery disease and resting ejection fractions of less than 36 per cent, 7-year survival and freedom from nonfatal infarction were greater in the surgically than in the medically treated patients. Surgical treatment also was associated with improved survival in the patients with an ejection fraction of 25 per cent or less.[326] These studies, together with observations made by the Duke group (Fig. 40–22) suggest that if operative mortality is lower than approximately 7 per cent, surgery is likely to offer an advantage over medical therapy in terms of survival and relief of anginal symptoms in patients with ischemic myocardium and severely depressed left ventricular function.

Despite the advantage of surgical as opposed to medical therapy in patients with left ventricular dysfunction,[424] the relationship between poor surgical outcome and preoperative clinical evidence of congestive heart failure is well recog-

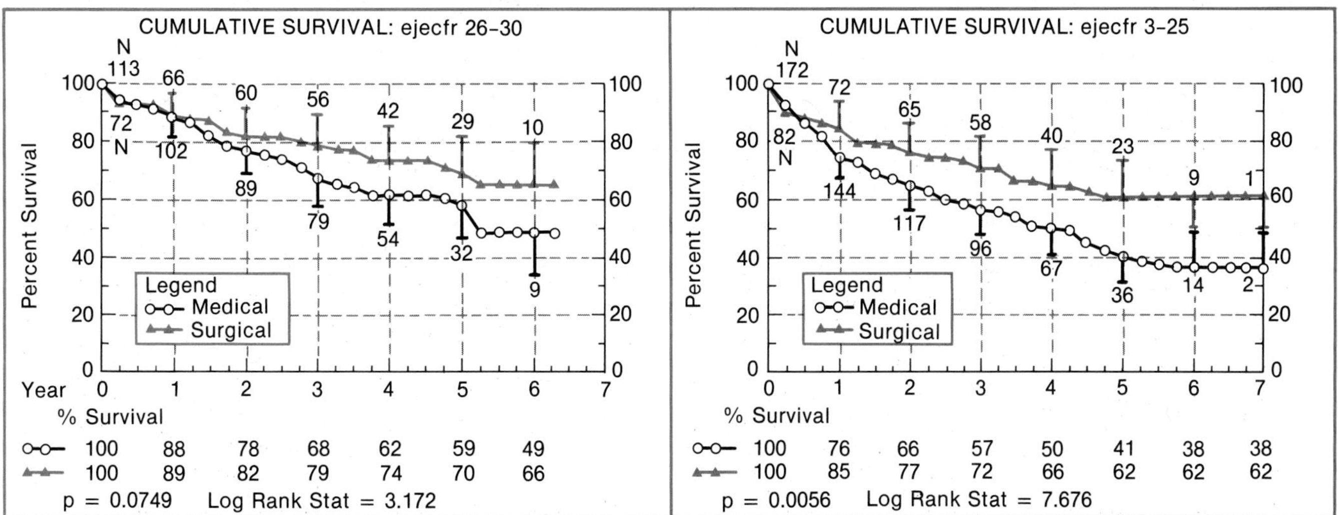

FIGURE 40–21. Life table cumulative survival curves for patients with severe left ventricular dysfunction. A CASS Registry study identified 420 medically treated and 231 surgically treated patients (coronary graft plus myocardial surgery in 30 per cent) who had severe left ventricular dysfunction manifested by an ejection fraction below 0.36 and markedly abnormal wall motion. Life table cumulative survivals for patients with an ejection fraction (ejecfr) of 0.26 to 0.30 *(left panel),* and for patients with ejection fractions of 0.03 to 0.25 *(right panel)* are shown. The survival curves are adjusted for all other significant prognostic variables. The P values associated with each analysis are shown in the bottom left corner of the figures. Surgical benefit was most apparent for patients with ejection fractions below 0.26 who had a 43-per cent 5-year survival with medical treatment vs. a 63-per cent 5-year survival with surgery. Surgically treated patients experienced substantial symptomatic benefit compared with medically treated patients if their presenting symptoms were predominantly angina; however, there was no relief of symptoms caused primarily by heart failure. The operative mortality in this high-risk subset was 6.9 per cent. (From Alderman, E. L., et al.: Results of coronary artery surgery in patients with poor left ventricular function [CASS]. Circulation *68:*785, 1983, by permission of the American Heart Association, Inc.)

nized. Clinical descriptors, such as a history of heart failure (particularly if such a history predominates over a history of angina pectoris), pulmonary rales, previous need of a diuretic or digitalis, and a cardiothoracic ratio of 0.50 or more, are all associated with a significantly higher operative risk. In the CASS and the CASS Registry,[332] there was increasing operative mortality with increasing left ventricular dysfunction. Patients with normal or near-normal left ventricular function had an operative mortality rate of 2 per cent and a 5-year survival of 92 per cent. Patients with moderate impairment had an operative mortality of 4.2 per cent and a 5-year survival of 80 per cent, and in those with poor ventricular function the operative mortality was 6.2 per cent and 5-year survival 65 per cent. Thus, while left ventricular dysfunction indicates higher surgical risk than normal ventricular function, such patients also have more to gain from surgery.

ASSESSMENT OF CONTRACTILE RESERVE. In patients with impaired left ventricular function it may be useful to estimate ejection fraction and left ventricular wall motion in the basal state as well as after inotropic stimulation or afterload reduction to show enhancement of otherwise depressed wall motion.[128–130] The term *contractile reserve* is used to describe the ability of ventricular wall segments that contract abnormally in the basal state to exhibit augmented contractility, often with an increase in overall ejection fraction in response to a suitable stimulus. Zones of the myocardium responding to inotropic stimulation or to a decrease in afterload may improve functionally after revascularization[129] (Fig. 40–23). Methods for assessing the contractile reserve of potentially viable myocardium include use of postextrasystolic potentiation during left ventricular angiography[129]; the response of left ventricular ejection fraction to an inotropic stimulus such as an epinephrine infusion[130]; evidence of delayed uptake of thallium-201 after exercise testing in a dysfunctional region of myocardium, which suggests that it is viable[424a]; and, finally, positron emission tomography, which shows glucose utilization by the myocardium (p. 1182). Regions of myocardium with abnormal motion and preserved glucose uptake are likely to be viable, in contrast to regions with diminished uptake that are likely to be irreversibly damaged.[425] Nesto et al. have reported that survival following revascularization is better among patients whose ejection fraction rose by more than 10 per cent when stimulated by either epinephrine or postextrasystolic potentiation than in those in whom this failed to occur.[130] The demonstration of augmentation of contractility acutely, and similar improvement after revascularization, is related to the finding that many hypokinetic (and even akinetic) areas of ventricular wall are composed either of ischemic, although viable, muscle or of a mixture of the latter and fibrous scar. The viable muscle is capable of responding to the inotropic stimulation, and its contraction may also respond to improved perfusion after operation.[131] In contrast, necrotic tissue obviously cannot be stimulated to contract by any pharmacological or hemodynamic intervention or by improved perfusion.

In patients with poor left ventricular function and poor contractile reserve (less than 10 per cent increase in ejection fraction with inotropic stimulation), perioperative mortality is high and long-term survival is poorer than in patients with equally depressed left ventricular function but with normal contractile reserve.[129–131] There are now a number of studies demonstrating that revascularization surgery will increase the ejection fraction at rest[426,427] and after exercise.[428] Regional wall-motion abnormalities have also shown improvement after revascularization surgery.[427,429,430] Percutaneous transluminal coronary angioplasty has also been shown to improve ischemic left ventricular dysfunction.[431,432]

MYOCARDIAL STUNNING AND HIBERNATION. Two related pathophysiological conditions termed myocardial stunning (prolonged but temporary postischemic ventricular dysfunction without myocardial necrosis) and myocardial hibernation (persistent left ventricular dysfunction when myocardial perfusion is chronically reduced but is still sufficient to maintain the viability of tissue) have been defined (pp. 1176 to 1178). In myocardial stunning there may be abnormalities of systolic and/or diastolic ventricular function. The stunned myocardium is viable and exhibits contractile reserve. There are a number of clinical situations in which myocardial stunning occurs, including delayed recovery of ventricular dysfunction after successful thrombolytic therapy administered

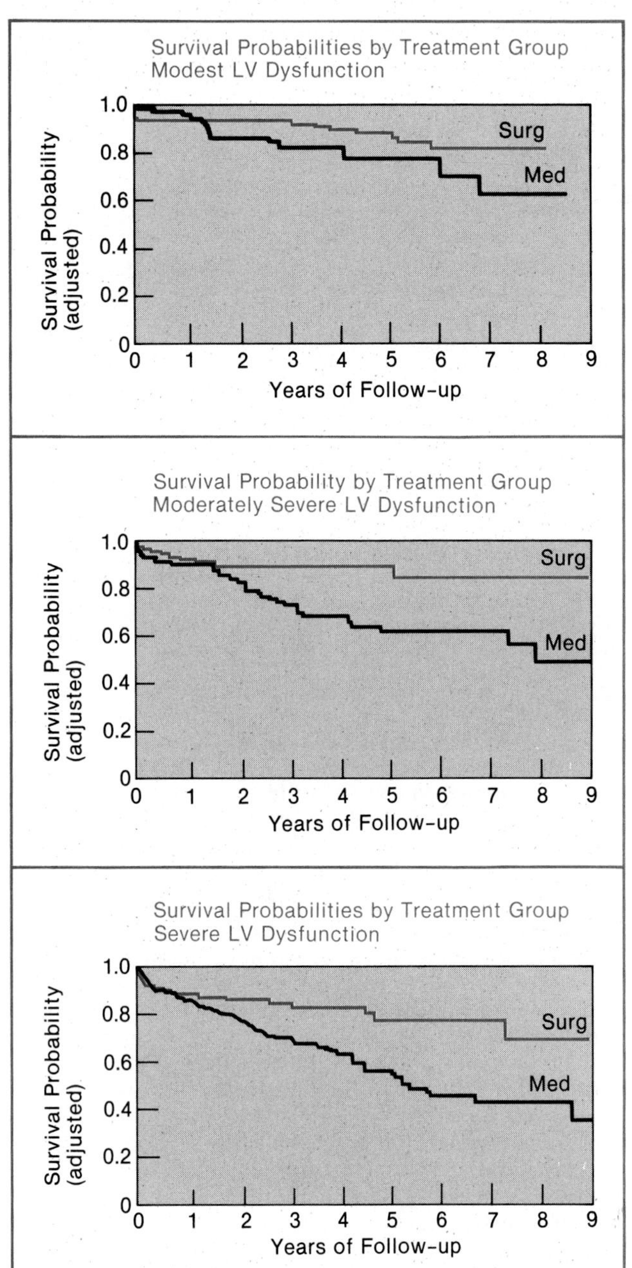

FIGURE 40–22. Survival of medically vs. surgically treated patients with left ventricular dysfunction. Patients undergoing first cardiac catheterization at Duke University Medical Center between 1976 and 1983 for any symptom of coronary artery disease with a 75 per cent or greater stenosis of at least one major coronary segment and a left ventricular ejection fraction of 40 per cent or less were reviewed. The survival curves were constructed from standard life table calculations after adjustment for differences in baseline prognostic factors, when appropriate, with the Cox proportional hazards model. Adjusted Kaplan-Meier survival estimates (survival probability) and time (years of follow-up) of the study population are divided according to baseline left ventricular ejection fraction. Med = medically treated; Surg = surgically treated. The upper panel shows upper tertile of ejection fraction (median ejection fraction 38 per cent). The middle panel shows mid tertile of ejection fraction (median ejection fraction 32 per cent). The lower panel shows lower tertile of ejection fraction (median ejection fraction 24 per cent). Surgical survival benefit was apparent in each third of the study group; however it appeared greater in those patients with moderate to severe left ventricular dysfunction than in those with only modest left ventricular dysfunction. (From Bounous E. P., et al.: Surgical survival benefits for coronary disease patients with left ventricular dysfunction. Circulation *78*[Suppl. I]:151, 1988, by permission of the American Heart Association, Inc.)

during evolving acute myocardial infarction,[126] alterations in diastolic properties of the ventricle following percutaneous transluminal coronary angioplasty,[433] and following relief of ischemia caused by coronary vasospasm[434] or exercise.[435] In addition, delayed recovery of ventricular dysfunction following successful coronary artery bypass graft surgery may be explained by the disappearance of myocardial stunning.[436]

Hibernating myocardium results from months or years of ischemia, and ventricular dysfunction persists until blood flow is restored.[436a,436b] Hibernating myocardium can be associated with abnormal systolic and/or diastolic ventricular function; the dysfunction is reversible and the myocardium exhibits contractile reserve. In these patients the predominant clinical feature of myocardial ischemia may be elevation of left ventricular diastolic pressure and dyspnea secondary to ventricular systolic and/or diastolic dysfunction. Symptoms resulting from chronic left ventricular dysfunction may be inappropriately ascribed to myocardial necrosis and scarring when they may, in fact, be reversed when the chronic ischemia is relieved by coronary revascularization.[436c]

Surgical Results in Patients With Left-Ventricular Dysfunction. Surgical revascularization appears to confer the greatest advantage in those patients with the most severe anginal symptoms, the most severe left ventricular dysfunction (Fig. 40–22), and the most extensive coronary artery disease.[437] While the risk of operation is higher in patients with depressed left ventricular function, it has been found that patients with moderately impaired[324] and even severely impaired left ventricular function[326,423] may have improved long-term survival as compared with similar patients with CAD treated medically.[329,437,438] Indeed, patients with the worst ventricular function may show the most striking symptomatic and functional response to revascularization[423] and a greater survival advantage.[437] Since the prognosis with medical therapy is so poor in these patients, they have the most to gain from surgical treatment. Furthermore, in patients with a history of heart failure and three-vessel CAD, coronary artery surgery may reduce the incidence of sudden death, compared with those receiving medical therapy.[439]

It is helpful to evaluate heart failure secondary to CAD to determine whether the patient's myocardium exhibits contractile reserve. If it does, and the anatomy is appropriate, we recommend surgical treatment, recognizing that higher than usual risks are involved. When the myocardium fails to exhibit contractile reserve and when the patient has a history (and/or electrocardiographic findings) of extensive or multiple infarctions (and/or electrocardiographic findings) and no or little angina, it probably offers little benefit and is associated with substantial risk.

CONCLUSIONS. In considering which groups of patients are likely to achieve greater survival benefit from coronary artery surgery rather than medical therapy, the large randomized trials and CASS Registry studies all contribute important information. Clearly, coronary artery surgery is a procedure that prolongs survival in patients with significant left main coronary artery disease and those patients with multivessel disease associated with clinical or catheterization evidence of impaired ventricular function. In patients with moderately severe, stable angina pectoris and normal left ventricular function, the European study suggests that if several factors such as age greater than 50 years, an abnormal electrocardiogram at rest, ST-segment depression greater than 1.5 mm during exercise, and peripheral arterial disease are present (Table 40–14), coronary angiography should be performed. In such patients with three-vessel disease or coronary artery stenoses of greater than 75 per cent reduction in luminal diameter in the proximal left anterior descending coronary artery and one other major vessel, surgery appears superior to medical therapy.

Surgery also appears to have an advantage over medical therapy in patients with no or mild symptoms and three-vessel disease and impaired ventricular function. Other clinical risk factors in patients with three-vessel disease and either

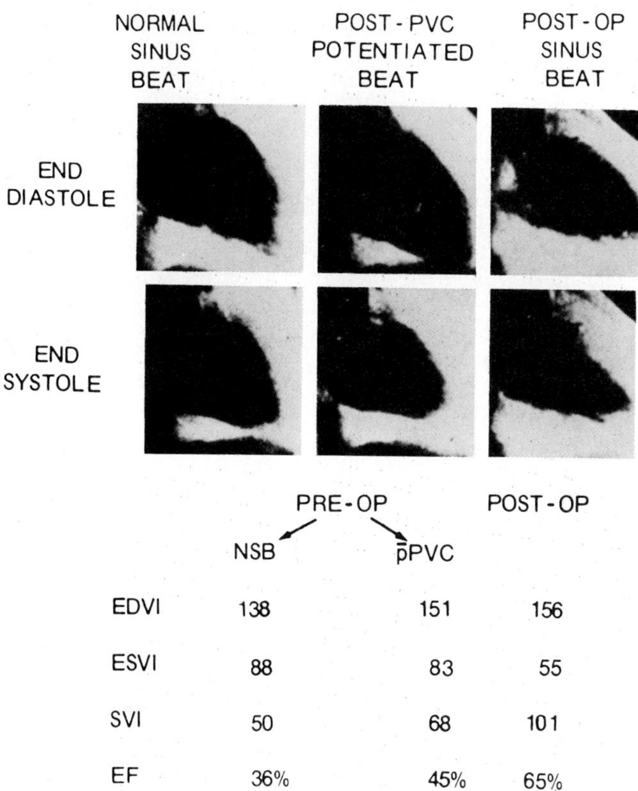

FIGURE 40–23. Examples of the ventriculographic analysis performed to evaluate the effects of an inotropic stimulus, including some of the calculations made. p̄PVC = premature ventricular contraction; PRE-OP = preoperative; POST-OP = postoperative; NSB = normal sinus beat; p̄PVC = after premature ventricular contraction; EDVI = end-diastolic volume index (ml/m²); ESVI = end-systolic volume index (ml/m²); SVI = stroke volume index (ml/m²); EF = ejection fraction. (From Popio, K. A., et al.: Post extrasystolic potentiation as a predictor of potential myocardial viability. Am. J. Cardiol. *39:*944, 1977.)

normal or impaired ventricular function that might lead to surgical rather than medical therapy include severe angina pectoris (Class III or IV NYHA), a history of myocardial infarction or hypertension, and resting ST-segment depression on the electrocardiogram. There is no evidence that surgical therapy confers any survival advantage over medical therapy in patients with two-vessel disease (which does not include severe proximal involvement of the left anterior descending coronary artery) and single-vessel disease. Patients in this latter category are being treated with increasing frequency by PTCA. As yet there is no evidence to suggest that the benefits of successful dilatation outweigh the risks of the procedure or whether any survival advantage is conferred upon such patients by PTCA. Patients with a left anterior descending stenosis of more than 50 per cent that is rough and long may have a greater risk of future myocardial infarction and therefore may be candidates for surgical revascularization.[440] There is some evidence that among patients with one- or two-vessel CAD and impaired left ventricular function, those who either have no change in their ejection fraction with exercise or a peak exercise ejection fraction less than 30 per cent have poor long-term survival.[441] If this subset of patients has angina and evidence of ischemia at a low or moderate level of exercise then they too *may* benefit from surgical revascularization.

The randomized trials of coronary bypass surgery have also suggested that both medical and surgical treatments have improved over time. In patients with angiographically confirmed three-vessel CAD treated medically, the annual mortality in the late 1960's was 11.4 per cent. Fifteen years later in the CASS it was only 2.1 per cent. (It is not clear how similar these two patient groups were.) For patients who have less than severe angina or who are free of angina after a recent infarction, if ventricular function is normal, surgical therapy does not appear to confer any benefits over medical therapy in terms of long-term survival for those with one-, two-, or three-vessel coronary disease. Surgical therapy may confer some survival advantage to patients with three-vessel and with two-vessel disease involving the proximal left anterior descending coronary artery if moderate angina pectoris exists, if the left ventricular ejection fraction decreases during exercise,[422] or if there is a positive symptom-limited exercise test in stage I or II of a standard Bruce protocol (or its equivalent) associated with 1.5 mm or greater ST-segment electrocardiographic depression (Table 40–15).

For patients with CAD whose dominant symptom is angina pectoris and who have severely depressed left ventricular function (ejection fraction ≤35 per cent), surgery appears to offer survival advantages if they can also be demonstrated to have critically narrowed vessels which perfuse viable myocardium. In patients whose dominant symptoms are heart failure without angina and diffuse poor contraction of the left ventricle without contractile reserve, revascularization is unlikely to be beneficial.

In patients with chronic stable angina who do not satisfy the indications for operation shown in Table 40–15, there is no evidence that survival is improved. Bypass grafting is usually associated with some small risk (<1 per cent mortality, 5 per cent incidence of perioperative infarction), and progressive attrition of venous grafts occurs, particularly after 5 years.[305] Therefore it is suggested that in patients with normal ventricular function and mild to moderate symptoms with medical therapy, bypass surgery be postponed until the symptoms warrant consideration of this intervention.

OCCURRENCE OF MYOCARDIAL INFARCTION. The major randomized trials of patients with mild to moderate angina and absence of major left ventricular dysfunction suggested that the likelihood of occurrence of myocardial infarction after 5 to 10 years of follow-up was similar in medically and surgically treated patients.[418,419,442,443] In the CASS, in which the perioperative myocardial infarction rate was 6.4 per cent, surgery did not appear to prevent the occurrence of subsequent infarction. In the same study, the reported annual risk of nonfatal myocardial infarction (Q-wave) was 2.2 per cent per year with medical treatment compared with 2.8 per cent per year with surgical treatment.[443] In an attempt to ascertain whether the risk of subsequent myocardial infarction might be prevented by surgical revascularization in patients at higher risk for ischemic events (i.e., those with severe angina and three-vessel coronary artery disease), a CASS Registry study was performed.[444] During a 6-year follow-up period, 21 per cent of the medical patients and 13 per cent of the surgical patients had a new myocardial infarction, and the fatality rate of first new myocardial infarctions was 45 per cent for the medically treated patients and 16 per cent for the surgi-

TABLE 40-14 FIVE-YEAR SURVIVAL IN MEDICALLY MANAGED PATIENTS WITH TWO- OR THREE-VESSEL CORONARY ARTERY DISEASE

	RISK FACTORS			5-YEAR SURVIVAL (%)	
PROXIMAL LAD STENOSIS	ST Depression >1.5 mm With Exercise	Peripheral Vascular Disease	Abnormal Resting ECG	2-Vessel Disease	3-Vessel Disease
−	−	−	−	98	96
+	−	−	−	94	92
+	+	−	−	88	83
+	+	+	−	69	60
+	+	+	+	−	40

LAD = Left anterior descending coronary artery.

From Rutherford, J. D.: Coronary artery surgery, 1984. N. Z. Med. J. *97:*813, 1984. Adapted from European Surgery Study Group: Long-term results of prospective, randomized study of coronary artery bypass surgery in stable angina pectoris. Lancet 2:1173, 1982.

TABLE 40-15 INDICATIONS FOR CORONARY REVASCULARIZATION IN PATIENTS WITH CHRONIC STABLE ANGINA

1. Angina pectoris that is severe, disabling, or interfering with life style on maximally tolerated medical therapy.
2. Results of noninvasive stress testing indicate extensive inducible ischemia, poor functional capacity, associated with critical (>70%) obstruction in one or more vessels.
3. Left main coronary artery stenosis (>60%).
4. Critical obstruction (>70%) in three major coronary arteries with:
   a. Resting left ventricular dysfunction, or
   b. Normal resting left ventricular function + evidence of inducible ischemia or a poor exercise tolerance.
5. Critical obstruction of proximal left anterior descending artery with significant obstruction of one other major vessel + moderate angina pectoris and/or inducible ischemia.

cally treated patients ($p < 0.0001$). After adjustment for left ventricular dysfunction and the extent of CAD, 86 per cent of surgical and 73 per cent of medical patients were free of new myocardial infarction at 6 years ($p < 0.0001$). The advantage of surgical treatment was particularly evident in patients with stenoses of the left anterior descending coronary artery of 70 per cent or greater and moderate or severe impairment of left ventricular function, as well as those patients with two proximal coronary artery narrowings. This observational study suggests that coronary artery revascularization reduces the incidence of subsequent myocardial infarction in patients at high risk for subsequent ischemic events (those with severe angina, three-vessel CAD, or left anterior descending coronary artery stenoses). The risk of death following subsequent myocardial infarction also appears to be lower in the patients who underwent revascularization.[444a]

PATIENT SELECTION FOR CORONARY ARTERY SURGERY

To undergo coronary artery bypass grafting, patients with chronic stable angina must usually meet certain clinical criteria.[444b] A plan for work-up and management of patients with mild to moderate angina is shown in Figure 40–24.

The most widely accepted indication for coronary artery bypass surgery in patients with chronic stable angina is significant disability from symptoms despite optimal medical care.[408a] Although this disability usually results from the CAD itself, it may be related to the side effects of the medication required to control the discomfort of myocardial ischemia, or patients may find taking large amounts of medication intolerable. Lastly, if the level of angina pectoris on a medical regimen clearly interferes with a patient's work, recreational activity, or life expectations, a recommendation for coronary artery surgery may be entirely appropriate.

Optimal medical care, as described earlier (p. 1302), involves achievement of satisfactory body weight, control of medical conditions such as thyrotoxicosis or anemia that might intensify myocardial ischemia, maintenance of normal blood pressure, assessment and control of arrhythmias (particularly in patients with impaired ventricular function), and treatment of metabolic abnormalities such as carbohydrate intolerance and hyperlipidemia. Abstinence from smoking is encouraged, and a range of medications including beta blockers, short- and long-acting nitrates, and calcium antagonists is used to control symptoms.

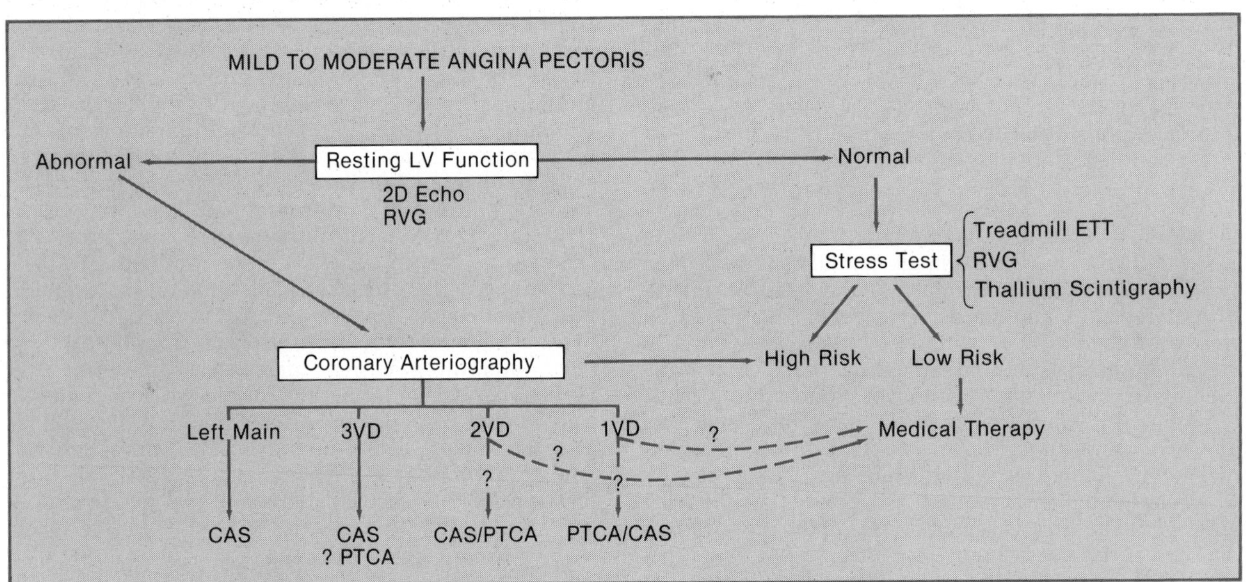

FIGURE 40–24. Management of patients with mild to moderate angina pectoris. Since coronary artery disease prognosis is worse in patients with left ventricular (LV) dysfunction, it is important to assess resting LV function (most readily accomplished noninvasively by either two-dimensional echocardiography [2D-echo] or radionuclide ventriculography [RVG].) If LV function is abnormal at rest, coronary angiography should be performed; if normal, some form of stress testing should be performed, e.g., treadmill exercise testing, radionuclide ventriculography at rest and during exercise, and thallium scintigraphy (with exercise or dipyridamole).

If there is evidence of significant exercise-induced ischemia or LV dysfunction, coronary arteriography should be performed. If stress is accomplished that is equivalent to or greater than completion of stage III of a Bruce protocol treadmill test without evidence of significant exercise-induced ischemia or LV dysfunction, a trial of medical therapy is reasonable. If this approach is used, the results of coronary arteriography will lead to logical management choices. For all patients with significant (> 60 per cent) left main coronary artery disease and for most with significant (> 70 per cent) three-vessel coronary artery disease (3VD), coronary artery surgery (CAS) is advised. With significant two- (2VD) and one-vessel disease (1VD), the options of CAS, percutaneous transluminal angioplasty (PTCA), or medical therapy will be considered.

In patients with critical obstruction of the proximal left anterior descending artery with significant obstruction of one other major vessel and moderate angina pectoris and/or inducible ischemia, either CAS or PTCA is usually advised. In patients with significant one-vessel coronary artery disease, the decision for CAS, PTCA, or medical therapy is made individually. Either PTCA or CAS is favored in those with results of noninvasive testing indicating extensive inducible ischemia, poor functional capacity, and a critical (> 70 per cent) obstruction present. (Adapted from Corne, R. A.: Risk stratification in stable angina pectoris [editorial]. Am. J. Cardiol. *59*:695, 1987.)

In the early 1970's most patients selected for operation were in functional Classes III and IV, but now patients with three-vessel disease and left ventricular dysfunction at rest or inducible by exercise, regardless of the severity or even the presence of symptoms, are appropriately undergoing coronary artery surgery.

WOMEN AS SURGICAL CANDIDATES. Symptomatic relief following revascularization surgery in women is not as good initially or as well sustained as it is in men.[323] In the CASS, 15 institutions carried out isolated coronary artery bypass grafting on 6258 men and 1153 women from 1975 to 1980. The operative mortality in men was 1.9 per cent, while the operative mortality for women undergoing coronary artery bypass grafting at the same institutions, during the same period, was 4.5 per cent. When matched for age, severity of angina, and the extent of coronary atherosclerosis, women appear to have twice the operative mortality of men.[445] Elderly women have a particularly high operative mortality.[323] After 2 years of follow-up, women were shown to have lower overall graft patency rates, and at 5 to 10 years postoperatively they had a higher incidence of recurrent angina than did men.[445] Women's smaller physical size and the smaller diameter of grafted coronary arteries may be responsible for this poorer response[446]; operative mortality increases in both men and women as physical size decreases.

CORONARY ARTERY BYPASS GRAFTING IN THE ELDERLY. During the past decade the hospital mortality of coronary artery surgery in the elderly (65 years or older) has declined to between 2.7 and 7.7 per cent.[447–450] In general, mortality is greater in patients over 75 years,[448,451] and women in this age group may be at even higher risk of hospital death than men. Variables predictive of perioperative mortality are the same as in younger patients and include rest angina,[451] the presence of 70 per cent or more severe stenosis of the left main coronary artery, severe left ventricular dysfunction,[447,448,451] and the presence of one or more associated medical diseases.[448,452] Compared with younger patients, the elderly spend more time in the hospital[449] and are more prone to complications,[449] which include cerebrovascular accidents, sternal dehiscence, and respiratory failure.[451] These complications, in turn, are associated with a higher perioperative mortality.[448,450,452a] However, angina is relieved or diminished in approximately 80 to 90 per cent of patients[451] more than 65 years of age, and the 5-year survival is generally excellent.[447,451] Thus, advanced age per se is not a contraindication to surgery.

REOPERATION. Six to 10 per cent of coronary artery surgery procedures are now reoperations.[407,453] Operative mortality rates for repeat coronary artery surgery are two to three times those of the initial procedure and range from 2 to 10 per cent[407,453–455,455a] for second operations and up to 15 per cent for third or more reoperations.[456] The reasons for reoperation include recurrence of angina due to primary graft failure (in approximately half of patients[407,455]), progression of disease with or without graft failure in 20 to 30 per cent,[407,455] and incomplete initial revascularization in the remainder.[407,455] At the time of reoperation, patients generally have more extensive CAD,[407,456] and the revascularization achieved at a second operation is less optimal,[455,456] which is reflected in an onset of recurrent angina at an earlier time than after initial cardiac revascularization surgery (Fig. 40–25).[407,455,456] The perioperative myocardial infarction rate in reoperations is approximately 10 per cent.[455] However, late survival is excellent, with 85 to 95 per cent of patients being alive at 5 years,[407,455,457] 89 per cent of patients being alive at 7 years[457] and 70 to 80 per cent at 10 years. Since long-term patency of internal mammary artery grafts is better than of vein grafts, if it is technically feasible this is the preferred conduit for both initial and repeat coronary artery surgery revascularization.

PATIENTS WITH ASSOCIATED CAROTID, ABDOMINAL AORTIC, AND PERIPHERAL VASCULAR DISEASE. The incidence of carotid arterial disease in patients undergoing coronary artery surgery varies from 2 to 12 per cent. Postoperative strokes occur in 2 to 3 per cent of all patients following coronary revascularization, but in patients with known carotid disease it may occur in up to 20 per cent.[458] Conversely, myocardial infarction is responsible for a substantial number of late deaths following carotid endarterectomy. The risk factors for the development of stroke after coronary bypass grafting are increasing age, preexisting cerebrovascular disease, severe atheroma of the ascending aorta, prolonged cardiopulmonary bypass, and severe perioperative hypotension.[459]

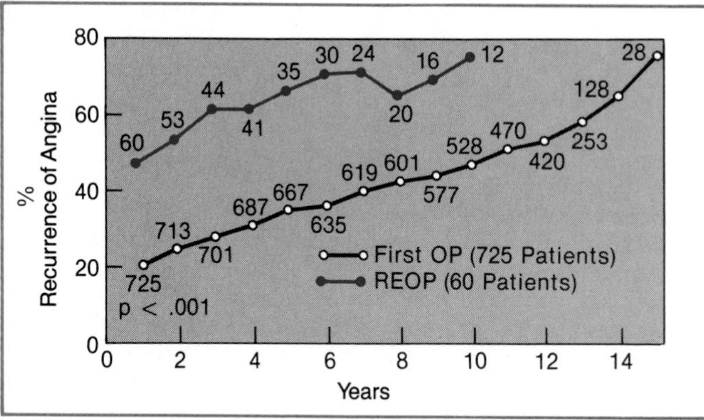

FIGURE 40–25. Recurrence of angina after initial operation and reoperation for coronary artery disease. Of 743 consecutive patients undergoing an initial coronary artery bypass procedure between 1970 and 1973, 64 patients required reoperation for angina recurrence and were followed up for 15 years or less (mean 6.2 years). Plot of annual recurrence of angina (%) and time (years) after initial operation (FIRST OP) and reoperation (REOP). The absolute numbers of patients at risk each year are indicated. There was less relief of angina in the first year after reoperation than after initial operation, but thereafter the annual increases in recurrence of angina were similar. Thus, less relief of angina after reoperation is predominantly attributable to early return of angina in the first postoperative year, rather than an accelerated return of angina in subsequent years, suggesting diffuse atherosclerosis is the cause of continuing angina rather than further progression of coronary artery lesions or occurrence of graft failure. (From Cameron A., et al.: Reoperation for coronary artery disease: 10 years of clinical follow-up. Circulation *78*[Suppl. I]:158, 1988, by permission of the American Heart Association, Inc.)

When patients with asymptomatic carotid bruits have coronary artery bypass surgery the risk for stroke appears to be unaltered by prophylactic carotid endarterectomy.[460] Noninvasive diagnostic testing is recommended for patients with neurological symptoms and anterior-circulation transient ischemic attacks or previous minor strokes if coronary artery surgery is contemplated. For those patients who previously had minor strokes, selective carotid angiography can be performed directly, because they have a higher likelihood of a surgically approachable carotid lesion.[460] It is clear that the presence of carotid bruits increases the risk of stroke after coronary bypass surgery (2.9 per cent), but this risk is small and comparable to the reported risk of stroke from carotid endarterectomy.[461–463]

Simultaneous carotid-coronary operations should be considered in patients with symptomatic carotid disease with bilateral carotid arterial obstructions and concurrent unstable angina, left main coronary artery obstruction, or diffuse multivessel coronary artery disease. Combined coronary and carotid arterial[464] and coronary arterial and abdominal aortic[465] procedures can be performed with mortality and morbidity similar to that of isolated surgery on the carotid artery and abdominal aorta. Most patients with asymptomatic cervical bruits or mild to moderate carotid artery obstruction can undergo coronary artery surgery alone with a low incidence of perioperative stroke.[466] In patients with unstable angina and a prior stroke the perioperative risk of neurological injury may be increased, and decisions need to be made on a case-by-case basis. Asymptomatic, unilateral, internal carotid artery stenosis or occlusion does not appear to increase the stroke risk during coronary artery surgery.[467]

Coronary artery disease is commonly associated with peripheral vascular disease and is the leading cause of mortality and morbidity in the perioperative period of patients undergoing peripheral vascular surgery.[468] Commonly these patients have major exercise limitations because of peripheral vascular insufficiency, and they may have significant CAD. However, their angina is masked by the limitation in their physical activities. Routine exercise testing may be impossible. In patients admitted for nonemergency surgery on the abdominal aorta or vessels of the lower extremities, preoperative thallium imaging after administration of dipyridamole may identify ischemic myocardium. With this technique, one-half of patients with thallium redistribution had cardiac events, whereas there were no such events in patients whose thallium scan was either normal or showed only persistent defects.[469] These findings suggest that patients with redistribution following dipyridamole-thallium imaging should be considered for preoperative coronary angiography and possible myocardial revascularization to avoid perioperative myocardial infarction or ischemia and possibly to improve survival. Ambulatory electrocardiographic monitoring of patients undergoing peripheral vascular surgery has shown that the finding of preoperative ischemia (ST-segment deviations) is the most significant correlate of postoperative cardiac events and assessing cardiac risk in patients undergoing elective peripheral vascular surgery. The absence of ischemia during such monitoring indicates that the patient has a very low risk for cardiac events perioperatively.[98]

HEART FAILURE AND MYOCARDIAL INFARCTION. In the absence of severe angina, patients with overt heart failure secondary to myocardial infarctions are not good candidates for coronary revascularization. However, in patients in whom left ventricular failure is due to chronically ischemic but not irreversibly damaged tissue, regardless of the presence or absence of pain, surgical revascularization can improve left ventricular function. The most striking improvement in clinical manifestations of heart failure and survival in these patients is seen in those with the most severe ventricular dysfunction. Patients with overt heart failure should be studied carefully to exclude a mechanical lesion such as mitral regurgitation or a ventricular aneurysm, which is usually amenable to surgical treatment.

Elsewhere are discussed indications for coronary revascularization in patients with CAD and unstable angina (p. 1340, cardiogenic shock secondary to acute myocardial infarction (p. 1255), and intractable ventricular arrhythmias (p. 656).

Unstable Angina

Unstable angina (previously also known as preinfarction angina, crescendo angina, [acute] coronary insufficiency, and intermediate coronary syndrome) is important clinically because of its frightening and disabling nature and the distinct possibility that it heralds acute myocardial infarction.[469a] Pathological studies of patients with this syndrome who do not develop an acute fatal myocardial infarction are rare, but those that are available usually reveal multivessel disease but a low incidence of recent occlusive thrombi. These findings suggest that coronary vasospasm, transient platelet aggregation, and/or nonocclusive thrombi play a role in the development of the acute ischemic episodes occurring in the presence of severe obstructive organic disease.[470] Thus, ischemic heart disease may really represent a spectrum of severities, with acute transmural infarction at one end of the spectrum, ranging successively through acute subendocardial infarction, unstable angina, chronic stable angina, with occasional silent ischemia at the other end of the spectrum.

DEFINITION. In addition to the absence of clear-cut electrocardiographic and cardiac enzyme changes diagnostic of a myocardial infarction, the currently used definition of unstable angina pectoris depends on the presence of one or more of the following three historical features, accompanied by electrocardiographic changes: (1) crescendo angina (more severe, prolonged, or frequent) superimposed on a preexisting pattern of relatively stable, exertion-related angina pectoris; (2) angina pectoris at rest as well as with minimal exertion; or (3) angina pectoris of new onset (usually within 1 month), which is brought on by minimal exertion. The ischemic episodes of unstable angina pectoris can be related to obvious precipitating factors, such as anemia, infection, thyrotoxicosis, or cardiac arrhythmias and the condition is then called secondary unstable angina (Table 40–16). Prinzmetal's ("variant") angina is a different entity and is discussed on page 1342. The syndrome of unstable angina describes a heterogeneous population of patients. They may be patients with single- or multivessel coronary artery disease, they may or may not have a history of prior myocardial infarction, they may have unstable angina while receiving no medical therapy, or they may be suffering severe, transient episodes of ischemia despite a combination of medications including full doses of nitrates, calcium antagonists, beta blockers, and intravenous heparin.

To categorize the heterogeneous population of patients who get unstable angina, a classification has been suggested that focuses on three important issues: (1) the severity of the clinical manifestations, (2) the clinical circumstances in which the unstable angina occurs, and (3) whether or not the sympto-

TABLE 40-16 CLASSIFICATION OF UNSTABLE ANGINA

	SEVERITY
Class I	**New-onset, severe, or accelerated angina.** Patients with angina of less than 2 months' duration, severe or occurring three or more times per day, or angina that is distinctly more frequent and precipitated by distinctly less exertion. No rest pain in the last 2 months.
Class II	**Angina at rest. Subacute.** Patients with one or more episodes of angina at rest during the preceding month but not within the preceding 48 hr.
Class III	**Angina at rest. Acute.** Patients with one or more episodes at rest within the preceding 48 hr.
	CLINICAL CIRCUMSTANCES
Class A	**Secondary unstable angina.** A clearly identified condition extrinsic to the coronary vascular bed that has intensified myocardial ischemia, e.g., anemia, infection, fever, hypotension, tachyarrhythmia, thyrotoxicosis, hypoxemia secondary to respiratory failure.
Class B	**Primary unstable angina.**
Class C	**Postinfarction unstable angina (within 2 weeks of documented myocardial infarction).**
	INTENSITY OF TREATMENT
1.	**Absence of treatment or minimal treatment.**
2.	**Occurring in presence of standard therapy for chronic stable angina (conventional doses of oral beta blockers, nitrates, and calcium antagonists).**
3.	**Occurring despite maximally tolerated doses of all three categories of oral therapy, including intravenous nitroglycerin.**

Modified from Braunwald, E.: Unstable angina: A classification. Circulation *80*:410, 1989, by permission of the American Heart Association, Inc.

matic ischemic episodes are accompanied by transient electrocardiographic changes[471] (Table 40–16). This classification notes whether or not rest pain is present, whether the episodes have occurred within the preceding 48 hours, and whether the unstable angina is provoked by conditions such as anemia, fever, infection, and tachyarrhythmias. It is also proposed that the amount of therapy administered be taken into account. Thus, a patient who experiences recurrent angina at rest, with transient ST-segment depression, several days after an acute myocardial infarction despite maximally tolerated doses of standard therapy (including intravenous nitroglycerin) would be Class III, C, 3. (Class III involves angina at rest, acute; C: postinfarction unstable angina; 3: occurring despite maximally tolerated doses of all three categories of oral therapy, including intravenous nitroglycerin.) While this is a clinical classification, it can be related to underlying disease. For example, Class III patients (with recent rest angina) are more likely to have intracoronary thrombus, and anticoagulants or perhaps thrombolytic therapy may be of greater value in such patients but of less value in patients in Classes I and II.

CLINICAL AND LABORATORY FINDINGS

SYMPTOMS. The chest discomfort in this syndrome is similar in quality to that of classic effort-induced angina, although it is often more intense, is usually described as pain, may persist for as long as 30 minutes, and occasionally awakens the patient from sleep. Longer episodes of ischemic pain are usually associated with acute myocardial infarction. The usual therapeutic regimen of bed rest and nitroglycerin administration often provides only temporary or incomplete relief. Several clues should alert the physician to a changing anginal pattern and the development of unstable angina; these include an abrupt and persistent reduction in the threshold of physical activity that provokes angina; an increase in the frequency, severity, and duration of angina; radiation of the discomfort to an additional or new site; and onset of new associated features such as diaphoresis, nausea, or palpitation.

The proportion of patients with unstable angina who have angina of new onset, a crescendo pattern superimposed on stable angina, or rest angina varies among different series and depends on how the observers defined the syndrome. Patients in whom unstable angina is superimposed on longstanding, stable angina often have multivessel disease, while patients with new onset of severe angina may have a strong dynamic (vasoconstrictive) component superimposed on fixed obstructive disease involving only a single coronary artery.

PHYSICAL EXAMINATION. This may reveal transient diastolic (third and fourth) heart sounds and a dyskinetic apical impulse suggesting left ventricular dysfunction, or a transient systolic murmur of mitral regurgitation during or immediately after an ischemic episode. These findings are nonspecific, since they may also be present in patients with chronic angina pectoris or acute myocardial infarction.

ELECTROCARDIOGRAM

Twelve-Lead Electrocardiogram. Transient deviations of the ST segment (depression or elevation) and/or T-wave inversions occur commonly but not universally in unstable angina. Usually these changes clear completely or partially with the relief of pain. Persistence of these electrocardiographic changes for more than 6 to 12 hours may suggest that a non-Q-wave infarction has occurred.

If patients have a typical history of chronic stable angina pectoris or established CAD (previous myocardial infarction, abnormal coronary arteriograms, or a history of a positive noninvasive stress test) before the development of symptoms of unstable angina, the diagnosis of unstable angina may be made with reliability if typical symptoms exist, even in the absence of electrocardiographic changes. It is in the subgroup of patients without evidence of previous CAD and no electrocardiographic change associated with pain that the diagnosis may be inaccurate. Also, in these patients no underlying CAD may be found at coronary arteriography.

Ischemic chest pain is not a reliable or sensitive marker of transient acute myocardial ischemia. Episodes of primary reduction in coronary blood flow may be associated with variable and minor electrocardiographic changes that precede symptoms of pain or discomfort.[472] In continuously monitored patients who demonstrated large falls in coronary sinus oxygen saturation, reflecting changes in myocardial blood flow, when the ischemic episodes were associated with chest pain (10 of 37) the pain always occurred 50 to 120 seconds after the onset of the ST-T changes.[472] Evaluation of the admission 12-lead electrocardiogram allows some risk stratification of patients admitted to the hospital with unstable angina. Patients with electrocardiographic ST-segment deviations (either depressions or elevations) are more likely to have a subsequent unfavorable hospital outcome (myocardial infarction, death, or the need for revascularization) than patients with no ST-segment deviations.[473]

Holter Monitoring. When continuous electrocardiographic monitoring is performed, many patients with unstable angina have a high incidence of ischemic electrocardiographic changes without accompanying symptoms, i.e., silent ischemia.[15,474–477] Recent studies suggest that more than 85 to 90 per cent of these ischemic episodes detected by Holter monitoring techniques are not associated with angina.[473,478] Furthermore, the presence of a significant degree of ischemia, detected by Holter monitoring, serves as a predictor of unfavorable outcome during hospital admission[473,479] and during follow-up (Fig. 40–26).[478,480] Holter monitoring appears to be more sensitive than ST-segment changes seen on the admission 12-lead electrocardiogram in predicting unfavorable outcome.[473] Ischemic electrocardiographic changes occurring without symptoms also correlate with transient reductions in myocardial perfusion and abnormalities of ventricular func-

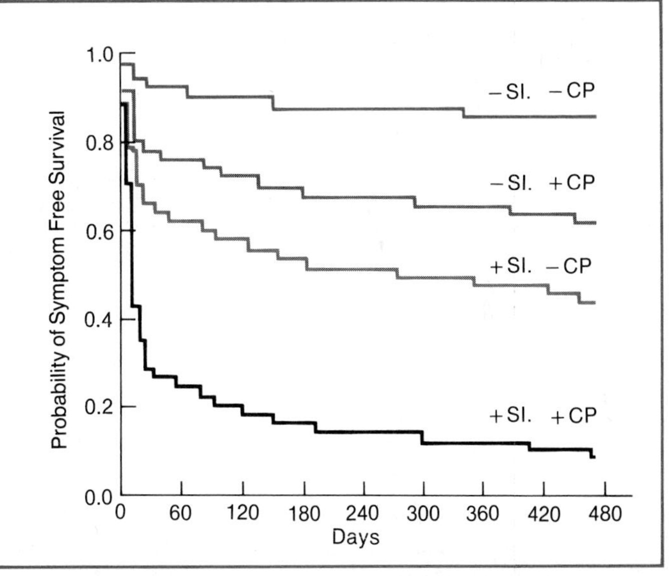

FIGURE 40–26. Symptom-free survival following unstable angina. Seventy patients with the clinical diagnosis of unstable angina treated with combination, triple-drug medical therapy were monitored electrocardiographically for silent ischemia for a 48-hour period, and the occurrence of chest pain during this period was documented. During follow-up, the influence of silent ischemia (SI) and recurrent chest pain (CP) on adverse outcome was assessed by Cox's hazard function analysis demonstrating the risk for death, myocardial infarction, or revascularization for recurrent symptoms. There was a five-fold relative risk for adverse outcomes associated with the presence of silent ischemia during the first 48 hours after the onset of unstable angina and a three-fold relative risk associated with the occurrence of chest pain during the initial 2 days of treatment for unstable angina. If both variables were present, the relative risk for experiencing an adverse outcome was increased by a factor of 15. (From Gottlieb S. O., et al.: Silent ischemia predicts infarction and death during 2 year follow-up of unstable angina. Reprinted with permission from the American College of Cardiology. J. Am. Coll. Cardiol. *10:*756, 1987.)

tion.[15,475,476] Episodes of silent ischemia may persist and still be a sign of adverse prognosis in patients with unstable angina who are treated with conventional antianginal agents and whose symptoms are controlled.[478] Therefore, in patients with unstable angina, predischarge Holter monitoring may be helpful in detecting continuing ischemia and stratifying patients into groups who need early angiography and revascularization and groups who can continue on a conservative medical therapy regimen.[480] In the majority of patients adverse clinical outcomes are most likely within the first 2 to 4 months after hospitalization.[479,480]

STANDARD LABORATORY TESTS. Findings on chest roentgenogram, serum cholesterol level, and carbohydrate tolerance are similar to those observed in patients with chronic stable angina (p. 1298). Unlike acute myocardial infarction, nonspecific indicators of gross tissue necrosis, such as leukocytosis and fever, are usually absent. Cardiac enzymes are not abnormally elevated; when cardiac-specific enzymes are elevated, by definition the diagnosis is acute myocardial infarction and not unstable angina.

CARDIAC CATHETERIZATION AND CORONARY ARTERIOGRAPHY

Coronary arteriographic findings in patients with unstable angina vary according to the population being studied.[480a] In a population of male patients included in a randomized Veterans Administration study on unstable angina, 18 per cent had one-vessel coronary disease, 35 per cent had two-vessel coronary disease, and 46 per cent had three-vessel coronary disease. Similarly, in a population of patients from the CASS registry who received surgical therapy for unstable angina, 50 per cent had three-vessel coronary disease and 14 per cent had significant left main coronary artery stenoses.[481] However, in patients with new-onset unstable angina, and no previous history of myocardial infarction or chronic stable angina, there is a higher incidence of single-vessel disease (43 per cent versus 27 per cent) and a lower incidence of three-vessel disease (23 per cent versus 35 per cent) compared to patients with chronic stable angina.[482] The left anterior descending coronary artery is the most commonly affected vessel in patients with unstable (as well as chronic stable) angina. The collateral circulation appears less well developed in patients with unstable angina than in those with chronic stable angina, an arteriographic impression that is supported by findings at operation in which retrograde flow, measured directly by cannulation of the opened artery, was less in patients with unstable angina than in those with chronic stable angina.[483] The incidence of normal coronary arteriograms among patients with unstable angina varies among different series and averages 10 to 15 per cent. No obvious explanation other than coronary spasm, the spontaneous lysis of a coronary thrombus, or the presence of a lesion overlooked on coronary arteriography exists for this finding.

CORONARY MORPHOLOGY. Autopsy studies of patients with CAD suggest that the subset of patients with unstable angina can have the most severe and extensive CAD.[484] Such studies also have shown that about 70 per cent of specimens of diseased arterial segments with significant narrowings (greater than or equal to 50 per cent diameter loss) have an eccentric, residual arterial lumen that is partially circumscribed by an arc of at least 60 degrees of normal arterial wall.[485,486] The presence of this pliable, muscular elastic arc of normal wall provides a mechanism whereby variations in intraluminal pressure and/or vasomotor tone may alter lumen caliber and thus flow resistance. In patients with unstable angina, postmortem angiograms, histological examinations, and coronary arteriograms display eccentric stenoses with scalloped or overhanging edges more frequently than in patients with chronic stable angina (Fig. 9–64, p. 264).[487] In contrast, lesions with concentric, symmetrical narrowing, or asymmetrical narrowing with smooth borders and a broad neck are more common in patients with stable angina. In patients with known coronary artery anatomy and stable angina pectoris who were restudied after an episode of acute unstable angina, it appeared in most instances that acute progression had occurred from a previously insignificant lesion. Also, the eccentric lesion (type II lesion, that is, eccentrically placed convex stenosis with a narrow neck due to one or more overhanging edges or irregular, scalloped borders, or both [p. 263]) is the most common morphological feature of disease progression. This finding may represent either a disrupted atherosclerotic plaque or a partially lysed thrombus, or the combination.[487]

Plaque fissuring has been implicated in acute coronary syndromes, including acute myocardial infarction (p. 1205) and unstable angina.[488] The type of plaque most likely to undergo fissuring is one with an eccentrically situated pool of extracellular lipid (cholesterol) contained within the intima (Fig. 39–9, p. 1206). This pool is separated from the blood in the lumen of the artery by a cap of fibrous tissue covered by endothelium.[488] The cap seems most likely to tear at the lateral margin of the plaque where it is attached to more normal intima. Blood enters the lipid cavity from the lumen, and because of the thrombogenicity of the subendothelial tissues that are exposed a thrombus develops within the plaque itself. This thrombus can expand the volume of the plaque, but subsequently the tear may reseal, restabilize, and heal. Plaque fissures heal by smooth muscle proliferation that can contribute to an increase in the severity of chronic obstruction.[489] Some episodes of plaque fissuring are followed by the development of thrombus within the coronary arterial lumen. Pathological as well as coronary arteriographic studies have suggested the presence of subtotally occlusive coronary arterial thrombi in patients with unstable angina.[490–493]

Coronary angioscopy has revealed complex plaques or thrombi not detected by coronary angiography in such patients.[494] In patients presenting early after the onset of rest angina, coronary arteriography has shown a 40 per cent inci-

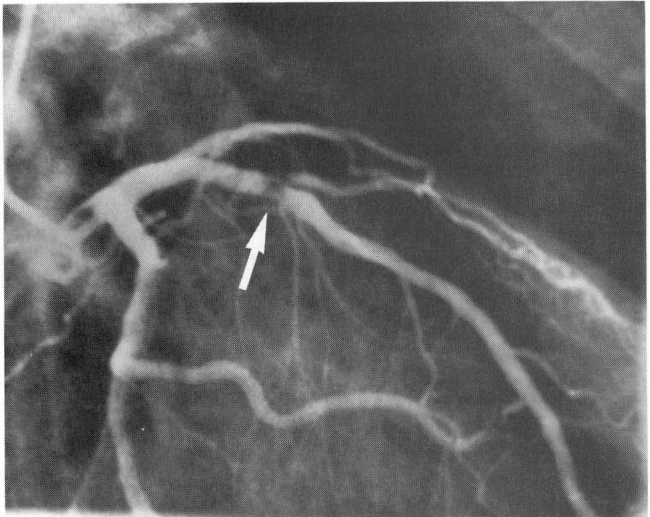

FIGURE 40–27. Coronary artery thrombus in a patient with unstable angina. A 60-year-old man was admitted to the hospital with a history of crescendo angina and prolonged rest pain. He had electrocardiographic T-wave inversions in leads V_2-V_5, I, aV_L and no abnormalities of serial cardiac enzymes. After 72 hours of hospital treatment with aspirin, heparin, and beta blocker therapy he had a further episode of rest pain associated with 5- to 8-mm anterior ST-segment elevations. Coronary angiography was performed, and the left coronary artery (right anterior oblique caudal projection) is shown. In the left anterior descending coronary artery, at the level of the second diagonal branch, an irregular hazy filling defect is present (arrow). It is surrounded by angiographic contrast medium and extends into the diagonal branch itself. After 4 further days of heparin and antianginal therapy, a repeat coronary angiogram was obtained, and the size of the intracoronary filling defect had decreased, confirming that it was a coronary thrombus.

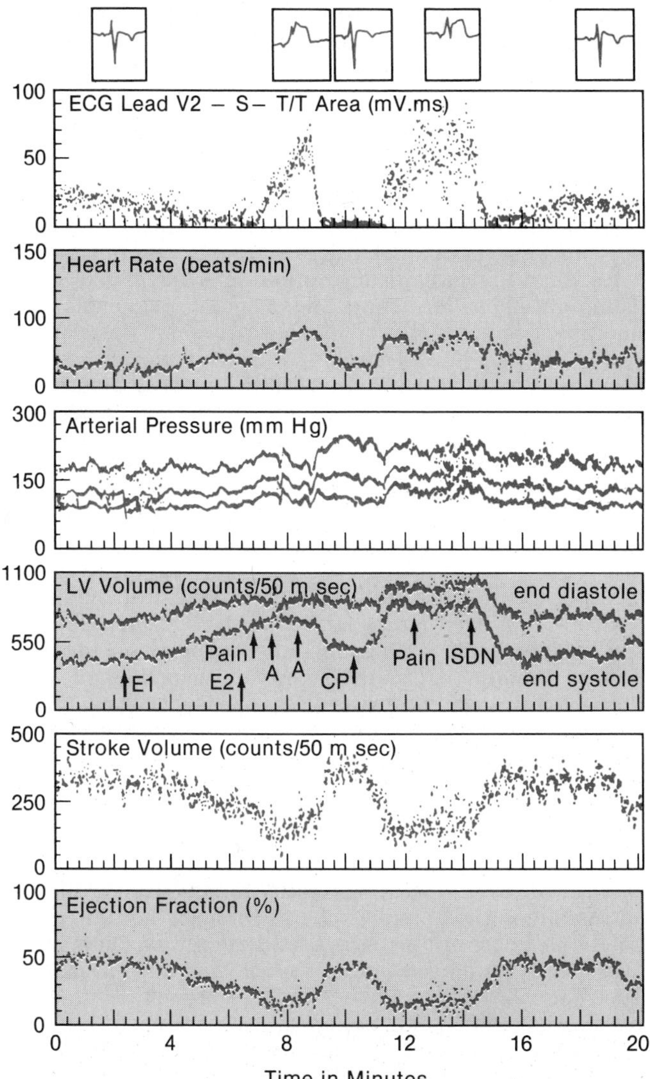

FIGURE 40-28. Changes in ventricular volume and function associated with myocardial ischemia. During spontaneous and ergometrine-induced ST-segment elevation, changes (from *top* to *bottom*) in ECG, heart rate, arterial pressure, left ventricular volume, stroke volume, and ejection fraction are parametrically displayed. E1 = ergometrine 0.025 mg IV; E2 = ergometrine 0.05 mg IV; A = amyl nitrite; CP = cold pressor test; ISDN = isosorbide dinitrate 2.5 mg IV. The small dose of ergometrine led to abrupt, severe left ventricular dilatation with reduction in stroke volume and ejection fraction. ST-segment elevation and pain were late events. Amyl nitrite administration led to resolution of all manifestations of the attack with left ventricular volume returning almost to the basal level. Cold pressor stimulation caused prompt recurrence of ST-segment elevation with extreme left ventricular dilatation and pain, and the episode was completely abolished by isosorbide dinitrate. (From Davies G. J., et al.: Sequence and magnitude of ventricular volume changes in painful and painless myocardial ischemia. Circulation *78*:310, 1988, by permission of the American Heart Association, Inc.)

dence of coronary thrombi (Fig. 40-27).[493] Cardiac events (death, myocardial infarction, and the need for urgent revascularization) were more frequent in patients with coronary thrombus (73 per cent), complex coronary morphology (55 per cent), or multivessel disease (58 per cent) than in patients without these angiographic features (17 per cent, 31 per cent, and 7 per cent, respectively). Similarly, intracoronary thrombi were present in 75 per cent of patients requiring urgent coronary arteriography for persistent angina later during admission.[493] Therefore, coronary thrombus is commonly present in patients with rest angina and appears to be an angiographic predictor of subsequent adverse cardiac events. It is not difficult to conceive that alterations in coronary artery tone at the site of irregular plaques may initiate and/or be exacerbated by local formation of subtotally occlusive thrombi with resulting intensification of angina. In patients with well-formed coronary collaterals, total thrombotic occlusion of a coronary artery may lead to unstable angina without myocardial infarction.

Findings on left ventriculography are similar to those in patients with chronic stable angina and generally show good wall motion between episodes of acute ischemia, except of course in patients who have had prior myocardial infarction. During episodes of acute ischemia, localized areas of asynergy are present, and stroke volume and ejection fraction decline, while left ventricular end-systolic and end-diastolic volumes rise, as does left ventricular filling pressure; nitroglycerin restores both global and regional left ventricular function (Fig. 40-28).

PATHOPHYSIOLOGY

Most patients with unstable angina have severe obstructive CAD; episodes of myocardial ischemia can be precipitated by either an increase in myocardial oxygen demand and/or a reduction in supply.[473] Episodes of spontaneous (rest) angina can be preceded by arterial hypertension and/or tachycardia, which lead to increases in myocardial oxygen requirements. In patients with fixed atherosclerotic obstructive lesions, a primary reduction of myocardial oxygen supply (due to either coronary vasoconstriction, i.e., a further reduction in lumen diameter consequent to transient vasoconstrictor influences, or perhaps to platelet thrombi) may also be responsible for many cases of angina at rest and not merely those associated with Prinzmetal's angina (in which there is abnormal severe spasm of a proximal coronary artery [p. 1342]).

In many patients with unstable angina who are continuously monitored, an interesting sequence of events has been demonstrated (Fig. 40-28). First, there is a reduction of coronary sinus oxygen saturation (which, in the presence of constant myocardial oxygen needs, signifies a reduction of coronary blood flow). This is followed by the characteristic electrocardiographic changes discussed above, and only then does chest discomfort appear. Secondary to the latter, blood pressure and/or heart rate may rise.[472] Thus, in many patients with rest angina, ischemia appears to be precipitated by a reduction in oxygen supply rather than an increase in oxygen demand. It is also possible that in some instances an increase in myocardial oxygen demand and a reduction in supply occur simultaneously. Thus, in some patients with Prinzmetal's angina, coronary vasoconstriction has been observed to occur during exercise.[495] This is an example of simultaneous augmentation of myocardial oxygen needs with concurrent reduced availability. A similar mechanism may be operative in some patients with unstable angina.

Mechanisms contributing to the reduction of oxygen supply, and therefore to the precipitation of ischemic episodes in patients with unstable angina who have severe underlying obstructive CAD, include progression of atherosclerosis, platelet aggregation, thrombosis, and coronary vasoconstriction.

PROGRESSION OF ATHEROSCLEROSIS. Evidence exists that the development of unstable angina may be associated with more marked recent progression in the extent and severity of CAD than that seen in patients with chronic stable angina. Such progression appears to occur as commonly in areas that are minimally diseased as in segments that are initially severely narrowed.[496]

PLATELET AGGREGATION. There is substantial evidence to support the role of platelet aggregation in the precipitation of ischemic episodes in patients with unstable angina. Animal models have shown that spontaneous decreases in coronary blood flow through coronary artery stenoses may be due to episodic platelet aggregation (which may transiently occlude a partially constricted coronary artery) and that these cyclic reductions in coronary blood flow can be prevented by aspirin.[497] This suggests that platelet aggregation rather than fibrin deposition may cause the observed cyclic reductions of coronary flow. Platelets and the coronary vascular endothelium interact in a complex manner; platelets produce the proaggregatory and vasoconstrictive thromboxane A_2 (p. 1173), while the normal endothelium produces antiaggregatory prostacyclin (prostaglandin I_2), tissue plasminogen activator (t-PA), and endothelial-derived relaxing factor (p. 263). It is likely that other factors such as change in sympathetic vascular tone and the activation of platelet receptors (alpha$_2$-adrenergic and serotonergic) may promote platelet aggregation. It has been speculated that the abrupt conversion from chronic stable to unstable angina may result from the more intense myocardial ischemia initiated by platelet aggregation[498] and coronary vasoconstriction resulting from the local accumulation of thromboxane A_2 and serotonin, and also from reductions in the local concentrations of endothelially derived vasodilators and inhibitors of platelet aggregation.[499]

In patients with unstable angina who have had pain within 24 hours, the finding of elevated metabolites of thromboxane A_2 in plasma and urine suggests that local thromboxane release may be associated with the episodes of unstable angina.[498] The reductions in coronary blood flow in canine preparations with marked obstruction appear to be abolished by platelet inhibitors, including aspirin, sulfinpyrazone, prostacyclin, ibuprofen, and indomethacin but not by heparin, nitroglycerin, or papaverine.[500] Again this suggests that they are mediated by platelet aggregation rather than by vasospasm or fibrin deposition. Furthermore, four separate clinical trials have now shown that aspirin can protect against death and nonfatal acute myocardial infarction in patients with unstable angina.[501-504] Finally, in patients with unstable angina who suffer sudden death, aggregates of platelet emboli have been found in small intramyocardial vessels. These occur in segments of myocardium immediately downstream from a major epicardial coronary artery containing an atheromatous plaque that has undergone fissuring and on which mural thrombus had developed.[490]

THROMBOSIS. In addition to platelet aggregation, the presence of an active thrombotic process in patients with unstable angina is suggested by increased serum concentrations of fibrin-related antigen, and D-dimer (the principal breakdown fragment of fibrin) in patients with unstable angina, changes that do not occur in patients with chronic stable angina.[505] Several clinical studies have shown that when coronary angiography is performed in patients with unstable angina, intracoronary filling defects having the appearance of thrombi are commonly found[492,493,506]; coronary angioscopy has confirmed this interpretation.[494] Furthermore, when thrombolytic therapy is given to patients with unstable angina and recent pain, a reduction in the severity of coronary stenosis, dissolution of intracoronary filling defects, and opening of an occluded artery have all been observed.[506,507] The associations of persistent rest pain, intracoronary thrombus, and adverse outcome have also been noted.[493,506] Finally, postmortem observations in many patients with unstable angina have suggested an ongoing thrombotic process in a major coronary artery during the period of unstable angina. This process culminates in total vascular occlusion, which causes infarction and/or sudden death.[491]

CORONARY SPASM OR ALTERATIONS IN VASOMOTOR TONE. Quantitative angiography in patients with unstable angina has shown vasomotor hyperreactivity localized to regions of preexisting coronary atheroma.[508] Also, clinical studies have reported large-vessel coronary spasm as a cause of ST-segment elevation in such patients.[509] Postmortem studies have shown that in the majority of significantly diseased coronary arteries a portion of the circumference is circumscribed by normal arterial walls.[485,486] Because of this and because unstable angina pectoris is a dynamic, multifactorial process, it is likely that a normal pliable muscular elastic arc of vessel wall provides a mechanism whereby normal (vasoconstriction) or abnormally intense (vasospasm) increases in vasomotor tone may affect lumen caliber and thus flow resistance.[509a] Alterations in coronary artery tone at the site of plaques may initiate and/or be exacerbated by local formation of platelet thrombi with resulting ischemia. Endothelial injury may be responsible for abnormal responses in coronary vasomotor tone to a variety of stimuli.[509] Even in patients with minimal disease of the coronary arteries, there may be an abnormal response to endothelium-dependent stimuli,[510] and dilatation of large coronary arteries in response to increases in coronary blood flow (flow-dependent coronary artery dilatation) may be impaired in atherosclerotic vessels,[511-514] probably reflecting endothelial dysfunction.

It is likely that progression of atherosclerosis, platelet aggregation, thrombus formation, and changes in vasomotor tone may operate either alone or together at different times in individual patients. The syndrome of unstable angina is a complex, dynamic one that may be interrupted by a variety of measures aimed at modifying these processes. Furthermore, unstable angina is often a precursor of myocardial infarction, and both conditions may occur suddenly and may share a common pathological link.

NONINVASIVE TESTS

Most patients who are hospitalized with unstable angina will, after initial therapy of bed rest, oxygen, analgesics, aspirin or heparin, nitrates, beta-adrenoceptor blocking drugs, and/or calcium antagonists, become asymptomatic quite quickly, and their electrocardiographic signs of continuing ischemia will disappear. During this period, serial electrocardiographic and enzyme evaluations will confirm that no infarction has taken place, thereby differentiating them from patients with acute myocardial infarction. Noninvasive tests may help determine whether or not angiography should be performed urgently.

EXERCISE TESTING. Exercise testing after stabilization of symptoms and before discharge from the hospital can be safely performed in patients admitted with unstable angina who have become asymptomatic.[515] When large numbers of such patients are studied, those with a normal resting electrocardiogram and an exercise stress test negative for ischemia have a 5-year survival greater than 95 per cent.[516] While such patients with chest pain but no changes on resting electrocardiograms or evidence of ischemia during exercise testing, are at very low risk for coronary events, the presence of chest pain at a low rate-pressure product associated with ST-segment changes during exercise testing identifies patients at high risk for subsequent morbid and fatal events.[515,516]

TWO-DIMENSIONAL ECHOCARDIOGRAPHY. This examination may reveal transient abnormalities of ventricular wall motion. Persistent abnormalities of wall motion are associated with an adverse prognosis.[517]

THALLIUM SCINTIGRAPHY. Abnormal thallium images indicating resting hypoperfusion of viable myocardium have been demonstrated to occur more commonly in patients with rapidly worsening exertional angina than in patients with chronic stable angina.[518,518a] In patients with rest angina, the combination of thallium defects and washout abnormalities has a sensitivity of 67 per cent for detecting coronary stenoses and a specificity of 59 per cent.[519] Detection of a reversible thallium defect by intravenous dipyridamole thallium scintigraphy can serve as a predictor of adverse cardiac events.[520] Exercise thallium testing performed when unstable angina had stabilized demonstrated that thallium defect size was a useful predictor of the extent of coronary artery disease[521] and of patients at higher risk for subsequent fatal and morbid events.[521a]

MANAGEMENT

INDICATIONS FOR CATHETERIZATION AND ANGIOGRAPHY. As is the case in patients with chronic stable angina, several questions need to be resolved: How will these tests aid in further management? In which patients should they be performed? What are the risks involved? Are any special precautions necessary? Although there is no unanimity of opinion regarding the answers, we believe that in most instances coronary arteriography is very helpful in the management of patients with unstable angina. For patients in whom medical therapy fails, i.e., who have continued episodes of ischemia at rest or with minimal exertion despite medical therapy described below, coronary arteriography should be carried out as soon as possible after the hemodynamic condition has been stabilized, unless there are obvious contraindications to possible angioplasty or coronary bypass surgery. On the other hand, in patients who respond to medical therapy, we recommend stress electrocardiography (and possibly a thallium scan). If these tests are strongly positive for myocardial ischemia, catheterization and coronary arteriography should be carried out.

Catheterization and arteriography are helpful in that they identify several subgroups of patients with unstable angina pectoris and can thus be used to dictate therapy: (1) Patients with left main coronary artery disease—the most life-threatening form of the disease—in whom urgent surgery is indicated. (2) Patients with multivessel obstructive disease without a clear "culprit" lesion and who are not suitable for angioplasty. Unless there are contraindications, we recommend that operation be planned on a semiurgent basis (within 10 days) after the patient's hemodynamic condition has stabilized. (3) Patients with left ventricular dysfunction and multivessel disease who should be revascularized to improve long-term survival. (4) A small number of patients (about 10 per cent of all patients with unstable angina) with no demonstrable CAD, in whom the prognosis appears to be excellent with medical management and in whom no further surgical consideration is necessary. In some of these patients, coronary spasm is responsible for the angina, and this can be established by provocative testing at the time of coronary arteriography (p. 1336); intensification of therapy with nitrates and calcium antagonists would then be indicated. (5) Patients with single-vessel or double-vessel disease with a discrete narrow proximal lesion (i.e., "culprit" lesion) amenable to percutaneous transluminal angioplasty (p. 1316). (6) Patients with diffuse distal CAD unsuitable for angioplasty or bypass grafting.

Which patients are unsuitable for cardiac catheterization and coronary arteriography? Obviously, patients who are suffering from another serious life-threatening illness with a poor prognosis do not require study. Advanced age per se is not considered a contraindication. The risks of coronary arteriography may be somewhat greater in patients with unstable angina than in those with chronic stable angina, but the addition of intraaortic balloon counterpulsation has reduced mortality to near zero. Maximal medical therapy, as described later, should be maintained up to and continued through the time of cardiac catheterization and arteriography.

Opinion is divided whether or not these procedures are necessary in patients in whom unstable angina has come under control and in whom severe ischemia cannot be provoked by a low level stress test. This question is currently being addressed in a large randomized clinical trial (TIMI III).

APPROACH TO MANAGEMENT. Unstable angina pectoris is a serious, potentially dangerous condition, and its management must be approached with this in mind. The patient should be admitted to the hospital and immediately placed at bed rest. Removal from an emotionally taxing situation, the presence of a quiet atmosphere, physical and emotional rest, the physician's reassurance, mild sedation, and antianxiety drugs are all helpful and will diminish or relieve episodes of rest pain in perhaps half of all patients. A vigorous effort must be undertaken immediately to diagnose and treat conditions that may be responsible for transient increases in myocardial oxygen demands, such as infection, fever, thyrotoxicosis, anemia, arrhythmias, exacerbation of preexisting heart failure, concurrent illnesses (particularly of the pulmonary tract, leading to coughing and hypoxemia, and acute gastrointestinal disturbances, causing vomiting, retching, or severe diarrhea), tachyarrhythmias (that increase myocardial oxygen demand), and severe bradyarrhythmias that reduce myocardial perfusion. Control of these aggravating factors will be helpful in 10 to 15 per cent of patients. Placing the bed into the reverse Trendelenburg position (feet down) is a simple measure that may be helpful, as may the inhalation of 100 per cent oxygen during periods of pain.

The electrocardiogram should be monitored continuously; diagnostic tests to rule out a myocardial infarction should include serial CK-MB enzymes. Invasive monitoring is usually not necessary unless a serious hemodynamic disturbance is suspected. Frequent radionuclide angiograms, thallium perfusion scans, and two-dimensional echocardiograms, although useful in elucidating the mechanism and consequences of unstable angina, are not especially helpful in immediate management and may actually be harmful in that they disturb the patient's rest.

NITRATES. These are a mainstay of therapy. In addition to frequently relieving and preventing recurrence of pain, they have been shown to improve global and regional left ventricular function. Nitrates may be given sublingually, orally, topically, or intravenously, and they may be of the short- or long-acting variety. Intravenous nitroglycerin offers the advantage of more consistent control of ischemic episodes during the first 24 hours of treatment. An additional advantage of intravenous nitroglycerin in patients already receiving standard therapy of oral or topical nitrates and beta-blocking drugs is that it will reduce the number of anginal episodes, reduce the need for sublingual nitroglycerin and for analgesics. A dosage schedule designed to reduce mean arterial pressure by 10 per cent is a safe and effective way of treating unstable angina unresponsive to standard medical therapy.[522]

Nitroglycerin is relatively stable when stored in glass containers; however, plastic bags should be avoided because the drug is absorbed by the plastic. Polyvinylchloride tubing also has a great affinity for nitroglycerin.[523] Therefore, the quantity of nitroglycerin delivered to the patient may be much less than that ordered. Several companies offer a non-polyvinylchloride infusion set with preparations of intravenous nitroglycerin. Also, commercial preparations of intravenous nitroglycerin contain alcohol in quantities of 0.01 to 0.14 ml/mg of nitroglycerin, so that when large doses of the agent are administered the quantity of alcohol delivered may be substantial. Acute gout has been described in patients receiving intravenous nitroglycerin, and it has been postulated that the alcohol content of the preparation may have altered serum uric acid levels.[524] It has been demonstrated that platelets taken from patients treated with intravenous nitroglycerin exhibit attenuated aggregation responses ex vivo, and this effect depends on the adequacy of reduced intracellular thiol stores.[525] The combined administration of intravenous nitroglycerin and the sulfhydryl (SH) donor N-acetylcysteine (NAC) may augment the clinical efficacy of nitroglycerin but increase the risk of development of hypotension.[526] Pharmacological tolerance to continuous intravenous nitroglycerin therapy develops within 24 hours.[179,527]

BETA-ADRENOCEPTOR BLOCKERS. The role of beta-adrenoceptor blockade in the treatment of unstable angina pectoris is being reexamined because many episodes of myocardial ischemia in these patients are *not* preceded by increases in heart rate or blood pressure, which are the major determinants of myocardial oxygen consumption. However, immediately after the onset of ischemia, increases in heart rate and blood pressure commonly occur and may perpetuate the ischemia.[528]

Several randomized trials have placed the role of beta blockers in the treatment of unstable angina pectoris into better perspective. In unstable angina patients who have not previously been receiving beta blocker therapy, the addition of a beta blocker[529,530] or the combination of a beta blocker and nitrates[531] appears to reduce symptoms of recurrent ischemia[529–531] and the occurrence of myocardial infarction.[529,530] In patients already receiving nitrates and calcium antagonists, the addition of beta blockers reduces the frequency and duration of both symptomatic and silent ischemic episodes.[532] Propranolol and diltiazem may provide equivalent relief of symptoms, and the incidence of death, infarction, and the need for coronary artery surgery appears equal in patients treated with these.[533] In patients already taking a beta blocker with continuous episodes of angina at rest, the addition of nifedipine appears to provide additional symptomatic benefit.[529-531]

In conclusion, in patients not already receiving beta blockers who present with unstable angina, either a beta blocker alone,[529,530] a combination of a beta blocker and nitrates,[531] or a beta blocker with nifedipine would appear to be the preferred treatment regimen. Propranolol and diltiazem appear equivalent in providing symptomatic relief without any difference in adverse events.[533] When rapid beta blockade is desired to reduce angina by lowering heart rate and/or blood pressure, intravenous esmolol (p. 864) is efficacious and safe, even in patients with compromised left ventricular function.[534,535] Resolution of drug effect occurs within 20 to 30 minutes of discontinuing esmolol.

In patients who are already taking a beta blocker at the time unstable angina develops, the drug should be continued unless contraindications are present. The dosage of beta blockers should be adjusted so that the resting heart rate is reduced to between 50 and 60 beats/min. This usually requires 240 to 320 mg of propranolol per day (or the equivalent for other beta blockers). Beta blockade may improve pulmonary congestion if the elevated pulmonary venous pressure is due to an ischemia-induced reduction of left ventricular compliance or left ventricular systolic failure. Rarely, heart failure may be precipitated by beta blockade in patients with previous infarction. In this situation the drug should be discontinued or the dose reduced and treatment with diuretics instituted.

CALCIUM ANTAGONISTS. A systematic overview of all randomized trials of calcium antagonists in unstable angina suggests that they do not prevent the development of acute myocardial infarction or reduce mortality.[536] A large, randomized, double-blind, placebo-controlled comparison of recurrent ischemia in patients with unstable angina treated with nifedipine or metoprolol, or both, was terminated prematurely because it appeared that nifedipine therapy alone might have been associated with more nonfatal myocardial infarctions within the first 48 hours of treatment than therapy with metoprolol alone or a combination of nifedipine and metoprolol.[529,530] Studies of patients with unstable angina have suggested that the addition of nifedipine to beta blocker therapy[531] or to a combination of nitrates and beta blockers[537] is useful in relieving angina[531] and reducing the subsequent short-term risk of death, myocardial infarction, or the need for urgent coronary artery surgery.[537] We believe that unless contraindicated a calcium antagonist should be added to nitrates and a beta blocker in patients with continuing ischemia.

ANTICOAGULANTS AND ANTIPLATELET DRUGS. The potential importance of platelet activation and thrombus formation in the pathogenesis and the clinical outcome of unstable angina[488,492,493,506] has led to management strategies that include heparin[503,538] and aspirin.[501-504] Theroux et al.[503] have shown in a double-blind, placebo-controlled trial in patients with unstable angina that heparin alone (1000 units per hour), aspirin alone (325 mg twice daily), and their combination are effective in reducing subsequent in-hospital cardiac events. In patients receiving placebo therapy, myocardial infarction occurred in 12 per cent, compared with 0.8 per cent in patients receiving heparin, in 3 per cent of patients receiving aspirin, and in 1.6 per cent of patients receiving a combination of aspirin and heparin. Recurrent angina also occurred less frequently in the heparin-treated group. Thus, both heparin and aspirin appeared to reduce the incidence of myocardial infarction in patients presenting with unstable angina, but neither agent, taken as the sole therapy, appeared better than the other. The limited sample size precluded the evaluation of the effect of treatment on mortality. Long-term administration of aspirin to patients with unstable angina reduces the incidence of nonfatal myocardial infarction and death.[501,502]

THROMBOLYTIC THERAPY. There is no agreement whether thrombolytic therapy plays a role in the clinical management of unstable angina. However, this question is currently being addressed by a large randomized trial (TIMI III).

INTRAAORTIC BALLOON COUNTERPULSATION (see also p. 580). This mode of therapy is considered when others have failed, and it is usually effective in stabilizing the patient's condition, both symptomatically and hemodynamically.[539] Intraaortic balloon counterpulsation is usually initiated either before or during coronary arteriography with a view to continuing it through revascularization.[540] This technique is useful primarily because it allows the safe performance of coronary arteriography and ensures that the patient goes to coronary artery surgery or PTCA under optimal conditions. Local complications related to intraaortic balloon placement are more common in the elderly, women, and diabetics.[541]

REVASCULARIZATION. PTCA. In patients with unstable angina, successful PTCA results in immediate abolition of ischemic episodes as well as improvement in both regional and global ischemic left ventricular dysfunction.[542] Patients with less than 50 per cent residual stenoses 6 months after PTCA often show sustained improvement in their functional status and myocardial perfusion 4 to 6 years later.[543] In large series of patients with unstable angina in whom PTCA is attempted, single-vessel CAD is present in 60 to 80 per cent.[544-546] The initial success rate of dilation of significant stenoses is 83 to 93 per cent.[544-549] Procedure-related myocardial infarction occurs in approximately 8 per cent of patients,[544-548] and in-hospital mortality is usually less than 1 per cent.[544,548] If PTCA is performed early after the *onset* of unstable angina, the complication rate is higher and the success rate is lower.[549a] Patients with unstable angina appear to be at higher risk of developing a myocardial infarction at the time of PTCA than do patients with chronic stable angina.[546,547] The risk factors for a procedure-related complication include severe degrees of stenosis,[548] the presence of thrombus and either ST-segment elevations, or persistent T-wave inversions on the electrocardiogram.[548]

The incidence of restenosis following PTCA appears to be similar in patients with unstable angina to those with chronic stable angina (approximately 30 per cent).[548-550] The risk factors for restenosis in patients with unstable angina appear to be multifactorial and include poor perfusion beyond the "culprit" lesion,[549] multiple irregularities in the vessel being dilated,[549] the presence of intraluminal thrombus,[549] involvement of the left anterior descending coronary artery,[548,549] and the presence of collateral vessels.[548] Urgent coronary artery surgery may be required in up to 10 per cent of patients.[548] Despite these problems, 18-month and 5-year survival are greater than 95 per cent[551] and approximately three-fourths of patients remain free of angina following successful angioplasty.[544,551] There is a myocardial infarction rate of 6 to 14 per cent during long-term follow-up,[546,551] which does not differ substantially from that following PTCA for chronic stable angina.[546]

Surgical Therapy. In patients with uncontrolled unstable angina (who have not suffered recent myocardial infarction) the operative mortality for coronary artery surgery is 3.7 per cent (approximately twice that observed in patients with chronic stable angina pectoris), the incidence of perioperative myocardial infarction is 10 per cent, and postoperative low cardiac output (patients requiring inotropic or intraaortic balloon support) is seen in 16 per cent of patients.[405] In patients observed for 7 to 10 years, either minimal angina or no angina is found in 80 per cent of patients, and survival at 5 years is approximately 90 per cent and at 10 years approximately 80 per cent.[405] It is estimated that the annualized rate of late nonfatal myocardial infarction is 3 to 4 per cent per year. In the Veterans Administration Cooperative Study that com-

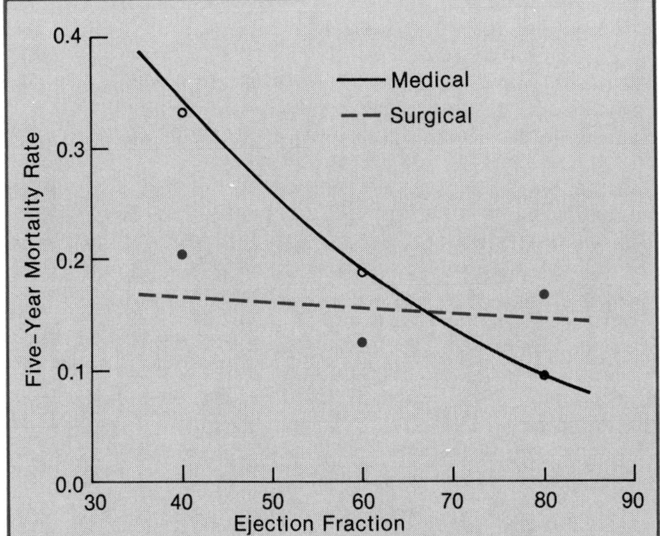

FIGURE 40–29. Mortality following medical and surgical treatment of unstable angina using ejection fraction as a continuous variable. Curves computed by logistic regression analysis based on 5-year mortality of 468 patients with unstable angina randomized to medical (open circles) and surgical (closed circles) therapy. The mean observed per cent mortality is illustrated for ejection fraction intervals 0.30–0.49, 0.50–0.69, and > 0.70. The worse the ejection fraction, the poorer the survival in medically treated patients; thus, surgery should be recommended for patients with unstable angina and reduced ejection fraction for three-vessel coronary artery disease suitable for surgical revascularization because it offers improved 5-year survival. (From Parisi A. F., et al.: Medical compared with surgical management of unstable angina: 5-year mortality and morbidity in the Veterans Administration Study. Circulation *80*:1176, 1989, by permission of the American Heart Association, Inc.)

pared medical and surgical treatment for unstable angina pectoris,[552] no difference in 2-year mortality was seen in patients randomized to medical versus surgical therapy, although as is the case in patients with chronic stable angina, in patients with low ejection fractions surgical therapy conferred a survival advantage.[552] In patients with a left ventricular ejection fraction less than 50 per cent, the cumulative 3-year mortality for surgical patients was 6.1 per cent vs. 17.6 per cent for medical patients ($p = 0.039$), representing a 65-per cent reduction in mortality with surgery.[553] Furthermore, at 5-year follow-up, patients with abnormal left ventricular function and three-vessel coronary disease had a survival of 75 per cent if treated medically and 89 per cent if treated surgically (Fig. 40–29).[554] The cumulative 5-year rate of repeat hospitalizations for cardiac reasons was lower in patients treated with surgery and the quality of their life appeared to be better.[554a] Interestingly, survival of patients whose ejection fractions were greater than 69 per cent was better with medical treatment.[553]

Thus, surgery appears to be the treatment of choice for patients with unstable angina pectoris, abnormal left ventricular function, and extensive CAD.[554] Risk factors for increased operative mortality in patients undergoing coronary artery bypass grafting for unstable angina include clinical and angiographic markers of left ventricular dysfunction[481,555] and the need for an intraaortic balloon for preoperative control of angina.[555] In patients who have postinfarction unstable angina, the independent predictors of perioperative mortality include the presence of an anterior transmural myocardial infarction and the need for preoperative intraaortic balloon pumping for either continuing angina or congestive heart failure.[539] In patients who have undergone coronary bypass grafting and later develop unstable angina, the risk of subsequent death and myocardial infarction is greater because they are less suitable candidates for further revascularization.[556]

The role of coronary arteriography and reperfusion and the timing of such therapy remain controversial. The choice of reperfusion technique depends on the findings in an individual patient, the local expertise, and experience. If a patient has received intensive medical therapy for a 48-hour period and there is persistent evidence of continuing ischemia, it is our policy to proceed with catheterization and coronary arteriography. Intraaortic balloon counterpulsation is often instituted either before or during cardiac catheterization if the patient exhibits any hemodynamic instability. If the patient has single-vessel disease and well-maintained left ventricular function, then PTCA is performed, if technically feasible. On the other hand, in patients in whom there is evidence of left main coronary disease, ventricular dysfunction, or multivessel disease and the anatomy is suitable for bypass grafting, operation is performed immediately.

Patients who respond to intensive medical therapy are gradually ambulated. If angina on mild effort recurs despite maximal medical therapy, coronary arteriography is performed, and PTCA or bypass grafting is carried out as in patients who did not respond to medical therapy initially. Patients who improve on medical management without recurrence of pain undergo exercise stress testing, often with ^{201}thallium, before hospital discharge. In many patients, the results of these tests will be positive and angiography is performed.[518] If the provocative tests are not indicative of high risk the patient may be discharged from the hospital.

PROGNOSIS

Unstable angina and acute myocardial infarction are closely related pathogenetically and clinically. While the majority of patients with acute myocardial infarction reported a prodrome of more intense or longer periods of angina, i.e., unstable angina shortly before infarction, the opposite is not the case, i.e., only a minority of patients with unstable angina pectoris develop early infarction. While patients with unstable angina may present difficult management problems, it is generally recognized that most *do not* in fact develop myocardial infarction over the short term. Documentation of all cardiac admissions to coronary and intensive care units in Hamilton, Ontario, over the 1-year period 1979–1980 revealed that in 811 patients admitted with unstable angina, hospital mortality was 1.5 per cent (compared with 17 per cent for acute myocardial infarction), 1-year mortality was 9.2 per cent (compared to 27 per cent for acute myocardial infarction), and only 16 per cent of the patients who died with unstable angina did so during the initial hospitalization. Repeat hospital admission occurred in 28 per cent of patients with unstable an-angina.[557] Patients with unstable angina who appear to have a worse prognosis and to be at high risk for adverse events while in the hospital include those of advanged age[518,557] with continuing rest pain and intracoronary thrombi,[493] and those with complex coronary morphology or multivessel disease.[493] Significant ischemia detected by Holter monitoring during hospitalization confers an immediate unfavorable outcome,[473,478,479] which extends to a follow-up of 2 years.[480]

Adverse events (death, myocardial infarction, or recurrent unstable angina) are most likely to occur in the first 2 to 4 months after discharge from the hospital.[479,480] Predischarge exercise testing shows that those patients whose exercise is limited by pain or who exhibit ST-segment depression or can achieve only a low rate-pressure product are likely to have a worse prognosis during 1 year of follow-up.[518] As already noted, revascularization is ordinarily the treatment of choice for patients presenting with unstable angina who are subsequently found to have abnormal ventricular function and extensive CAD[554]; 5-year survival is 75 per cent in such patients treated medically and 89 per cent if treated surgically.[554]

Variant Angina Pectoris (Prinzmetal's Angina)

In 1959, Prinzmetal et al. described an unusual syndrome of cardiac pain that occurs almost exclusively at rest, usually is *not* precipitated by physical exertion or emotional stress, and is associated with electrocardiographic ST-segment elevations.[558] This syndrome, now known as *Prinzmetal's*, or *variant, angina*, may be associated with acute myocardial infarction, severe cardiac arrhythmias, including ventricular tachycardia, and fibrillation, as well as sudden death.

MECHANISM

Variant angina pectoris has been demonstrated convincingly to be due to coronary artery spasm. The latter is a transient, abrupt, *marked* reduction in the diameter of an epicardial (or large septal) coronary artery resulting in myocardial ischemia in the absence of any preceding increases in myocardial oxygen demand (reflected in elevations of heart rate or blood pressure). This reduction in diameter can usually be reversed by nitroglycerin and can occur in either normal or diseased coronary arteries. The striking reduction in luminal diameter is usually focal and involves one or occasionally more than one site. The focal, severe vasospasm of Prinzmetal's angina should not be confused with vasoconstriction of both the large and small coronary resistance vessels, a normal response to stimuli such as cold exposure. The latter response is much less intense and occurs diffusely throughout the coronary vascular bed. In patients with Prinzmetal's angina, basal coronary artery tone may be increased. While responses to ergonovine and nitrates are greater in spastic segments of the coronary arteries, there is also hypersensitivity to vasoconstrictor stimuli throughout the entire coronary artery tree.[559] Sites of spasm in Prinzmetal's angina are often adjacent to atheromatous plaques. It has been suggested that in these patients the basic abnormality, i.e., coronary artery spasm, may be hypercontractility of the arterial wall associated with the atherosclerotic process itself.[560] Other mechanisms suggested include endothelial injury (which reverses the dilator response to a variety of stimuli, e.g., acetylcholine [p. 1169]), and hypercontractility of vascular smooth muscle due to vasoconstrictor mitogens, leukotrienes, serotonin,[560a] and higher local concentrations of blood-borne vasoconstrictors in areas of neovascularized atherosclerotic plaques.

During episodes of severe ischemia in patients with variant angina, coronary spasm associated with myocardial ischemia may induce stasis and result in fibrinogen-fibrin conversion in the coronary vessels with elevated levels of plasma fibrinopeptide A, an index of fibrin formation.[561] Furthermore, there appears to be a significant circadian variation in plasma levels of fibrinopeptide A, with the peak levels occurring from midnight to early morning in parallel with the frequency of the ischemic attacks in patients with variant angina.[562] Heparin suppressed the circadian variation and elevation of the plasma fibrinopeptide A levels but did *not* suppress the variant anginal attacks themselves. Therefore, increased plasma fibrinopeptide A levels, and thus, increased thrombin activity, appear to be the *result* rather than the *cause* of variant anginal attacks.[562] In support of the possibility that vasoactive substances may have a role in the pathogenesis of coronary spasm is the observation that an excessive number of mast cells have been noted in the adventitia of a vasospastic artery of a young patient succumbing to coronary artery spasm[563] and the occurrence of coronary artery spasm in carcinoid heart disease.[564]

Several studies suggest that magnesium ions play a role in the pathogenesis of attacks of variant angina. In patients with variant angina, magnesium sulfate has been shown to terminate cold-pressor–induced anginal attacks and prevent induction of further attacks.[565] Magnesium has also been shown to suppress variant anginal attacks induced by hyperventilation[566] and exercise.[567] Finally, in an anorexic patient with intractable variant angina unresponsive to calcium antagonists and nitrates, intravenous magnesium sulfate prevented coronary spasm from being induced by ergonovine; subsequently, oral magnesium oxide stabilized the patient.[568]

Cocaine, which blocks the presynaptic uptake of the neurotransmitters norepinephrine and dopamine, not only causes alpha-adrenergically mediated coronary constriction when administered intranasally (near the dose used for topical anesthesia),[569] but there also appears to be a high incidence of spontaneous, silent myocardial ischemia in cocaine addicts (detected by Holter monitoring) during the early stages of withdrawal.[570] Obviously, clinicians must consider the possibility that coronary vasoconstriction may be mediated by therapeutic or illicit cocaine usage in patients with suspected coronary artery spasm.

CLINICAL MANIFESTATIONS

The history differs from that of typical angina; the principal finding is angina *at rest*. However, in contrast to the situation in many patients with unstable angina and the rest pain, the latter usually has not progressed from an earlier period in which pain occurred with decreasing levels of effort. Although exercise capacity is usually well preserved, some patients experience typical pain and ST-segment elevations not only at rest but during or after exertion as well. The anginal discomfort may be extremely severe, is generally referred to as "pain," and is accompanied by syncope, the latter presumably caused by arrhythmias. Attacks of variant angina tend to be clustered between midnight and 8 AM.[562] Patients studied with 48-hour Holter electrocardiograms, even those without clinically apparent angina pectoris, show more frequent abnormalities in the morning than in the afternoon.[571]

Clinical features do not reliably differentiate patients with Prinzmetal's angina with normal or mildly abnormal coronary arteriograms from those with fixed severe coronary obstruction. A large percentage of the latter are heavy smokers. This supports the observations that cigarette smoking may influence vasomotor tone.[572] These patients often have a combination of fixed-threshold exertion-induced angina with ST-segment depression and variant angina (rest angina with ST-segment elevation). Rarely, variant angina develops following coronary artery bypass grafting,[573] and coronary artery spasm has also been observed intraoperatively after the application of coronary vein grafts. In a few patients, variant angina appears to be a manifestation of a generalized vasospastic disorder associated with attacks of migraine and Raynaud's phenomenon and has been reported in association with aspirin-induced asthma.[574] Patients with Prinzmetal's angina tend to be younger than patients with chronic stable angina or unstable angina, and the male preponderance in the latter group is not evident.[575] In some patients there appears to be a distinct relationship between emotional distress and episodes of coronary vasospasm. Alcohol withdrawal may precipitate variant angina,[576] and alcohol administration may prevent coronary spasm.[577] Variant angina has been reported to be provoked by therapy with 5-fluorouracil[579,580] and by cyclophosphamide (p. 1759).[578]

Although patients with Prinzmetal's angina are often heavy cigarette smokers, on physical examination they do not usually exhibit the risk factors for coronary atherosclerosis. Cardiac examination is usually normal in the absence of ischemia (unless the patient has suffered a previous myocardial infarction) but often reveals signs of dyskinesis and impaired left ventricular function during episodes of myocardial ischemia.

ELECTROCARDIOGRAM. The key to the diagnosis of variant angina lies in the development of ST-segment elevations with pain (Fig. 40–30). In some patients, episodes of ST-segment depression follow episodes of ST-segment elevation and are associated with T-wave changes. The phenomenon of

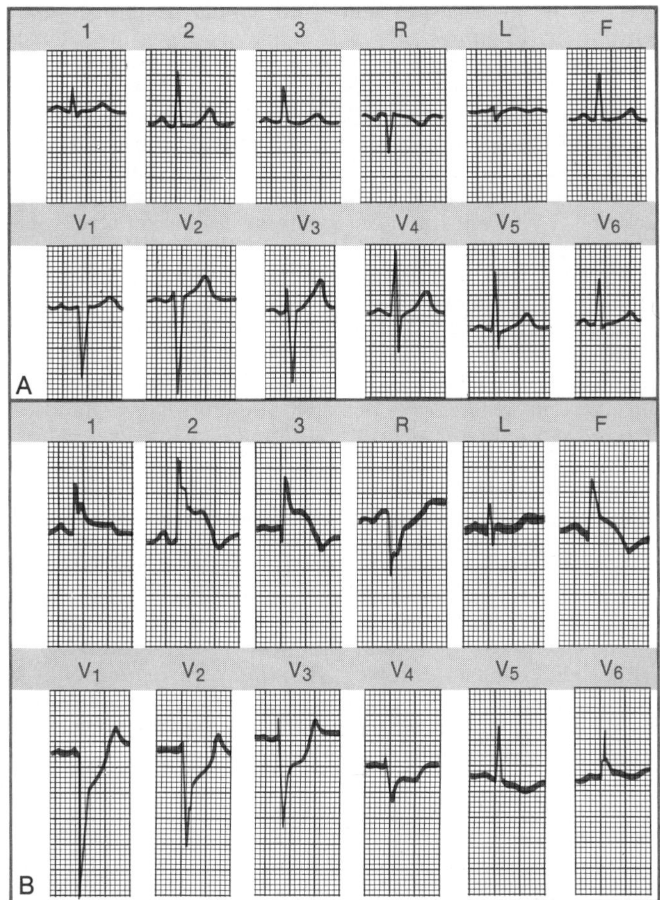

FIGURE 40-30. **ECG *(A)* prior to an episode of Prinzmetal's angina and *(B)* during an episode of Prinzmetal's angina. ST segments are now markedly elevated in the inferior leads, with reciprocal depression in the anterior leads. After nitroglycerin was given, the electrocardiogram returned to baseline. (From Berman, N. D., et al.: Prinzmetal's angina with coronary artery spasm. Angiographic, pharmacologic, metabolic and radionuclide perfusion studies. Am. J. Med. *60*:727, 1976.)**

ST-segment and T-wave alternans[581] may be ominous (it is the result of ischemic conduction delay) and may be associated with potentially lethal ventricular arrhythmias.[582] The presence of R-wave "growth" may also be associated with the occurrence of ventricular arrhythmias.[583] Many patients exhibit multiple episodes of asymptomatic ST-segment deviation (silent ischemia). The ST-segment deviations may be present in any leads; however, the concurrent presence of ST-segment elevations in both the inferior and anterior leads (reflecting extensive ischemia) is associated with an increased risk of sudden death.[584]

Transient conduction disturbances may occur during episodes of ischemia.[585,586] The development of ventricular ectopic activity associated with episodes of spontaneous variant angina is always a serious clinical problem. Ventricular ectopic activity is more likely to be associated with ST-segment elevations,[587] is more frequent during longer episodes of ischemia, and is often associated with ST-segment and T-wave alternans.[583] Myocardial cell damage, as reflected by the release of small quantities of CK-MB, may occur in the absence of persistent electrocardiographic changes in patients with prolonged attacks of Prinzmetal's angina, and transient Q waves have been observed.[588]

Exercise testing in patients with variant angina is of limited value since the response is so variable. Approximately equal numbers of patients show ST-segment elevation, ST-segment depression, or no change in ST segments during exercise, reflecting the variability of the underlying fixed CAD in some patients, the absence of significant lesions in others, and the provocation of spasm by exercise in a few.

In contrast to the finding in patients with chronic stable (effort-induced) angina, episodes of Prinzmetal's angina often occur at rest or during mild exertion and are not usually preceded by increases in heart rate, arterial pressure, or myocardial contractility—all of which increase cardiac work or oxygen consumption. Spasm of a proximal coronary artery with resultant transmural ischemia, first postulated as the cause of variant angina, has been convincingly documented arteriographically (Fig. 9-62, p. 262). Exercise-induced ST-segment elevation can be associated with partial or total obstruction of large epicardial arteries in a manner similar to episodes observed during spontaneous or ergonovine-induced angina.[589,590] This suggests that coronary spasm may have a common mechanism despite being initiated by different stimuli. Echocardiographic studies performed during episodes of spontaneous variant angina have demonstrated abnormalities in ventricular function that precede the onset of symptoms of angina and electrocardiographic changes.[591]

The coronary anatomy in patients with Prinzmetal's angina has been defined both at autopsy and during coronary arteriography. Severe proximal coronary atherosclerosis of at least one major vessel occurs in approximately two-thirds of patients, and in them spasm usually occurs within 1 cm of the organic obstruction. The remainder have normal coronary arteries in the absence of ischemia. Spasm may occur at one or more sites in one artery or in multiple arteries simultaneously[592] and it is most common in the right coronary artery. Patients with variant angina with normal coronary arteriograms are more likely to have purely nonexertional angina and ST-segment elevations involving inferior leads. In contrast, patients with variant angina who have organic obstructive lesions with superimposed coronary artery spasm often have associated effort-induced angina and ischemia in anterolateral leads. Patients with no or mild fixed coronary obstruction tend to experience a more benign course than do patients with associated severe obstructive lesions.

THE ERGONOVINE TEST. A number of provocative tests for coronary spasm have been developed. Of these, the ergonovine test is the most sensitive and useful. Ergonovine maleate, an ergot alkaloid that stimulates both alpha-adrenergic and serotonergic receptors and therefore exerts a direct constrictive effect on vascular smooth muscle,[593] has been used to induce coronary artery spasm in patients with Prinzmetal's angina. Coronary arteries that constrict spontaneously appear to be abnormally sensitive to this agent. When administered intravenously in doses ranging from 0.05 to 0.40 mg, ergonovine provides a sensitive and specific test for provoking coronary artery spasm.[594] There is some correlation between the dose of ergonovine required to induce a positive test and the frequency of spontaneous attacks.[595] In low doses and in carefully controlled clinical situations, ergonovine is a relatively safe drug, but prolonged coronary artery spasm precipitated by ergonovine may cause myocardial infarction. Because of this hazard, it is recommended that ergonovine be administered only to patients in whom coronary arteriography has demonstrated normal or nearly normal coronary arteries and in gradually increasing doses, beginning with a very low dose.

The ergonovine test should be carried out only in a setting where appropriate resuscitative equipment, drugs, and personnel are readily available, usually in the cardiac catheterization laboratory, so that the angiographic diagnosis of spasm can be made and intracoronary nitroglycerin can be administered to abolish the spasm. Some investigators have also found that the ergonovine test can be carried out safely in the coronary care unit, with a positive test being reflected in the development of chest pain and ST-segment elevation; however, the safety of the test in this setting has not been firmly established. The normal response of the coronary arterial bed to larger doses (0.40 mg) of ergonovine is a diffuse reduction in arterial caliber by approximately 30 per cent.

In patients whose atypical chest pain is being evaluated (in

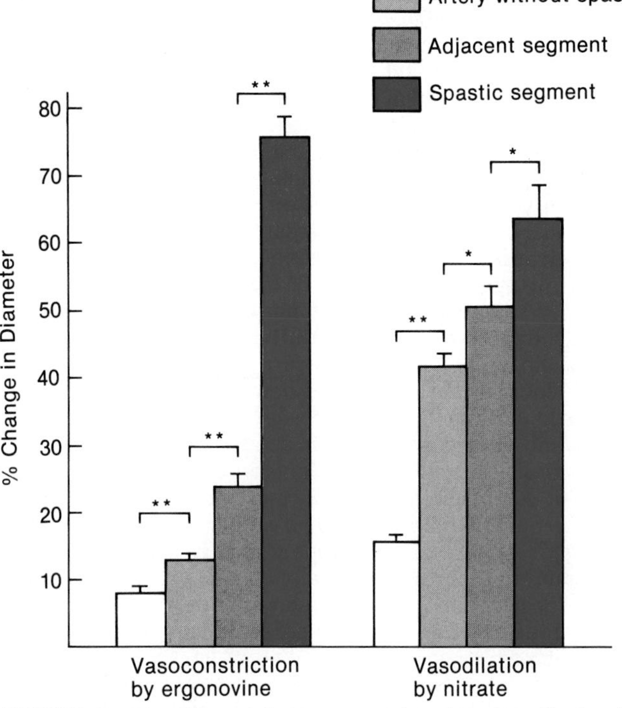

FIGURE 40–31. Changes in coronary artery tone in patients with coronary spasm in response to ergonovine and nitrates. A retrospective analysis was performed involving 159 patients who had undergone diagnostic coronary angiography with the ergonovine provocative test and who had normal coronary arteries or fixed lesions with < 40 per cent diameter reduction after nitrate administration. Per cent vasoconstriction after ergonovine (left panel) and vasodilation after nitrates (right panel) were compared among the spastic segments, adjacent segments, and segments of the coronary arteries without spasm in the vasospastic angina group, and the combined segments in the non-angina group. * $P < 0.05$; ** $P < 0.01$. Thus, in patients with vasospastic angina, coronary artery responses to both ergonovine and nitrate were greater in the spastic segments than in other segments. (From Hoshio, A., et al.: Significance of coronary artery tone in patients with vasospastic angina. Reprinted with permission of the American College of Cardiology. J. Am. Coll. Cardiol. *14*:604, 1989.)

the absence of a strongly positive exercise test and of evidence of organic coronary artery obstruction) who do *not* have Prinzmetal's angina, sequential intravenous bolus infusions of ergonovine maleate result in progressive nonspecific reductions in coronary dimensions. These vasoconstrictor responses appear to be accentuated in women and in patients with intimal coronary arteriographic irregularities suggesting the existence of minor atherosclerotic disease.[596] This dose-dependent phenomenon differs from the abnormal response in Prinzmetal's angina, which is characterized by severe focal spasm, usually at much lower doses of the agent (Fig. 40–31). The sensitivity of the ergonovine test is high in patients with active disease (who have at least one attack daily) and lower in patients with sporadic episodes of variant angina.[597]

HYPERVENTILATION. This stimulus has also been demonstrated to provoke some episodes of variant angina,[561,566,568,593,597,598] electrocardiographic ST-segment elevations,[561,568,597,598] angiographic evidence of coronary artery spasm,[593] and ventricular arrhythmias.[593,597,598] In patients with active disease who have at least one daily attack of variant angina, the sensitivity of hyperventilation was 95 per cent compared with 100 per cent for ergonovine. However, in patients with sporadic attacks of angina, hyperventilation has a lower sensitivity than ergonovine and, therefore, a limited diagnostic value.[597]

ACETYLCHOLINE. Intracoronary injections of acetylcholine have been shown to induce severe coronary spasm in patients with variant angina. (This should not be confused with the mild diffuse constriction that acetylcholine induces in patients with abnormal coronary endothelium.) Because this method allows induction of spasm separately in the left and right coronary arteries, it is useful in patients with known multivessel disease or spasm. In such patients, the use of intracoronary acetylcholine has been shown to be sensitive, reliable,[599] and safe.[600] Indeed, the sensitivity (90 per cent) and the specificity (99 per cent) of acetylcholine for induction of coronary spasm[599] is comparable to ergonovine testing.

Methacholine, a parasympathomimetic drug, and *dopamine*,[601] a catecholamine, can also induce coronary artery spasm. Like ergonovine, these agents are capable of producing marked coronary artery spasm both in patients with variant angina who have severe underlying arteriosclerotic coronary artery narrowing and in those without such fixed stenoses. Exercise, the cold pressor test, and induced alkalosis can all cause coronary spasm in patients with variant angina, but none of these tests is as sensitive as ergonovine. Catheter-induced coronary ostial spasm is nonspecific and not helpful in the diagnosis of Prinzmetal's angina.

MYOCARDIAL PERFUSION STUDIES. Localization of the myocardial perfusion defect to an area perfused by a coronary artery in which spasm can be demonstrated by arteriography has been reported using intravenous thallium-201,[602] and a reduction in coronary sinus flow during episodes of spasm has also been noted. These studies support the relationship between coronary spasm and the resultant myocardial perfusion and ischemia.

MANAGEMENT

There are several important differences between the optimal management of Prinzmetal's angina and chronic stable angina.

1. Patients with both forms of angina usually respond well to nitrates; sublingual or intravenous nitroglycerin often abolishes attacks of variant angina promptly, and long-acting nitrates are useful in preventing attacks.[603] However, the mechanism of action of the drugs may differ in the two types of angina. As already discussed (p. 1305), in chronic (effort-induced) stable angina, one important action of the nitrates appears to involve reducing myocardial oxygen needs. In Prinzmetal's angina, the nitrates abolish or prevent myocardial ischemia by exerting a direct vasodilating effect on the spastic coronary arteries.

2. In patients with chronic stable angina pectoris, beta-adrenoceptor blockade is usually beneficial, but the response in patients with Prinzmetal's angina is variable. Some, particularly those with associated fixed lesions, exhibit a reduction in the frequency of exertion-induced angina caused primarily by augmentation of myocardial oxygen requirements. In others, however, propranolol or any nonselective beta-adrenoceptor blocker may actually be detrimental, since blockade of the $beta_2$ receptors, which subserve coronary dilation, allows unopposed alpha-receptor–mediated coronary artery vasoconstriction to occur; the duration of episodes of vasotonic angina can be prolonged by propranolol.

3. In contrast to beta blockers, the calcium antagonists have been found to be extremely effective in preventing the coronary artery spasm of variant angina.[575,604] These drugs, along with long- and short-acting nitrates, are the mainstay of therapy in Prinzmetal's angina. Similar efficacy rates have been noted for nifedipine, diltiazem, and verapamil. Rarely, a patient will respond to only one of these three agents, and even less commonly simultaneous administration of two or even three antagonists is required.[605] A multicenter trial with nifedipine has shown dramatic reductions in the frequency of episodes and in the need for nitroglycerin. Because calcium antagonists act through a different mechanism than do nitrates, the vasodilatory actions of these classes of drugs may be additive. There have been reports suggesting a rebound of symptoms when nifedipine, verapamil, and diltiazem[606] are

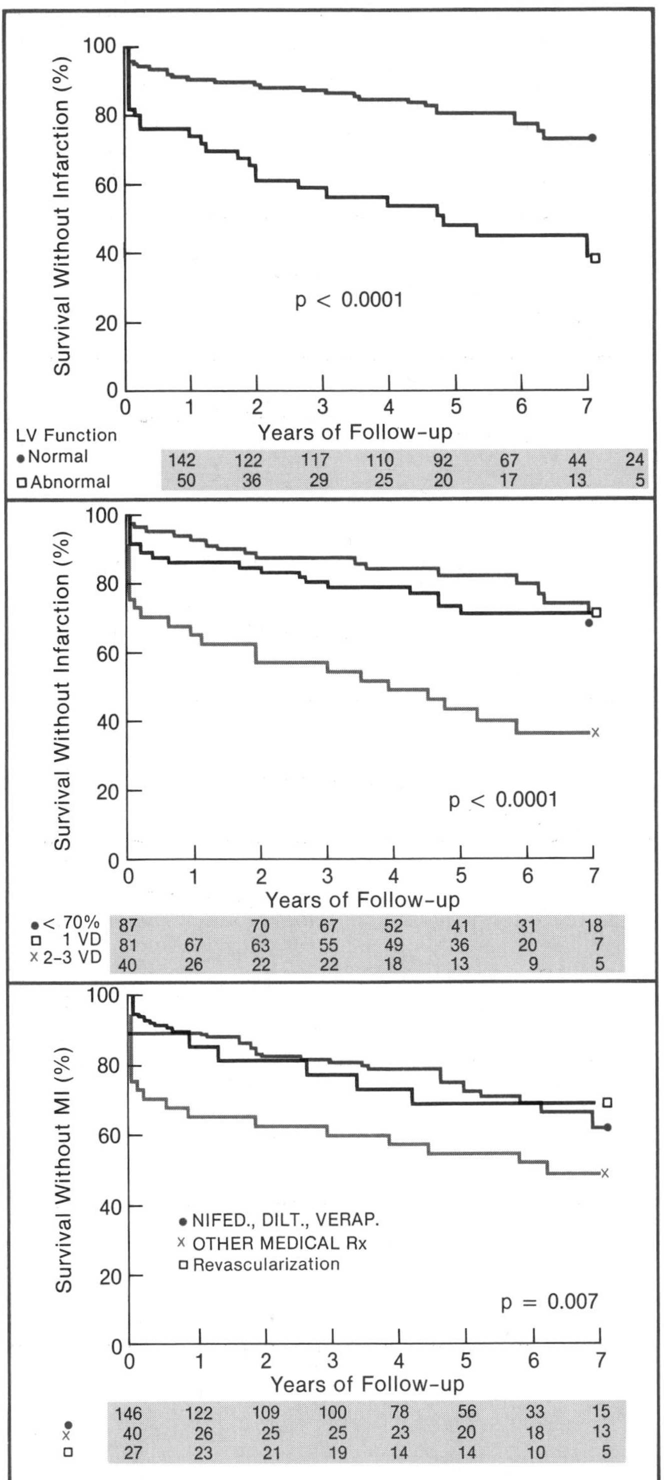

FIGURE 40–32. Event-free 7-year survival of patients with variant angina; 217 consecutive patients with variant angina were observed for 7 years. Top panel: Survival without myocardial infarction is compared in patients with normal (closed circle) and abnormal (open squares) left ventricular function. The number of patients completing each year without an endpoint event are listed. Middle panel: Survival without infarction in patients with no stenoses of 70 per cent or greater (closed circles), those with one-vessel disease (open squares), and those with multivessel involvement (X 2-3 VD). Bottom panel: Influence of treatment on survival without infarction. Patients initially treated with nifedipine, diltiazem, or verapamil (closed circles) had a better outcome than patients receiving other medical treatment (X). Too few patients underwent bypass surgery or coronary angioplasty (open square, revascularization) to assess the value of these interventions. Thus, impaired ventricular function, the presence of multivessel coronary artery disease, and medical therapy not including calcium antagonists were all adverse factors for long-term survival in patients with variant angina. (From Walling, A., et al.: Long-term prognosis of patients with variant angina. Circulation *76*:990, 1987, by permission of the American Heart Association, Inc.)

discontinued. Calcium antagonists ordinarily should be used in maximally tolerated doses.

The *natural history* of Prinzmetal's angina is characterized by cyclic periods of frequent spasm that alternate with asymptomatic periods. After 6 to 12 months of therapy, gradual tapering of the calcium antagonist with careful observation may be considered. Complete remission of variant angina, documented by both Holter recordings and ergonovine testing, has been demonstrated typically in patients who have had a shorter duration of symptoms and who have either shown normal or nonsignificantly diseased coronary arteries.[607]

4. *Prazosin*, a selective alpha-adrenoceptor blocker (p. 864), has also been found to be of value in patients with Prinzmetal's angina.[608] Aspirin, helpful in unstable angina (p. 1340), may actually increase the severity of ischemic episodes in patients with Prinzmetal's angina, because aspirin in high dosage inhibits biosynthesis of the naturally occurring coronary vasodilator prostaglandin I_2.[609] Provocation of asthma and variant angina by aspirin in the same patient has been reported.[574]

5. PTCA may be helpful in patients with variant angina[610] who have discrete proximal noncalcified obstructive lesions in a single major coronary artery. Calcium antagonists should be continued for at least 6 months following successful angioplasty. In patients with isolated coronary artery spasm without accompanying obstructive disease, PTCA and coronary artery bypass surgery are *not* indicated. In patients with Prinzmetal's angina who require coronary artery bypass surgery because of significant organic narrowings of the coronary arteries, the addition of verapamil to the priming solution for bypass appears to be effective in preventing perioperative coronary vasospasm.[611] Furthermore, internal mammary artery bypass grafts do not appear to show the hyperreactivity of the coronary arteries of patients with variant angina.[612]

PROGNOSIS

Many patients with Prinzmetal's angina go through an acute, active phase, with frequent episodes of angina and cardiac events during the first 6 months after their presentation. Over this period, nonfatal myocardial infarction occurs in up to 20 per cent of patients and death in up to 10 per cent.[613,614] Patients with variant angina who develop serious arrhythmias, ventricular tachycardia, ventricular fibrillation, high-degree atrioventricular block, or asystole during spontaneous episodes of pain have higher maximal ST-segment elevations and are at a higher risk for sudden death.[615] Patients with severe obstructive coronary artery lesions are at greater risk for persistent anginal symptoms, acute myocardial infarction, and death.[613,614] In most patients who survive an infarction or the initial 3- to 6-month period, the condition stabilizes and there is a tendency for symptoms and cardiac events to diminish with time. In patients who experience such remissions, cautious tapering or discontinuation of calcium antagonists may be attempted. For reasons that are not clear, some patients, after a relatively quiescent period of months or even years, experience a recrudescence of vasospastic activity with frequent and severe episodes of ischemia. Fortunately these patients respond to re-treatment with calcium antagonists.

Long-term survival at 5 years is excellent (89 to 97 per cent).[616,617] The extent and severity of CAD[614,616,617] and the activity of the disease[616,617] have an adverse influence on long-term survival free of myocardial infarction (Fig. 40–32). Calcium antagonist therapy improves long-term survival.[617] Overall patients without significant obstructive CAD have an excellent prognosis.[618]

Chest Pain With Normal Coronary Arteriogram

The syndrome of angina or angina-like chest pain with a normal coronary arteriogram is an important clinical entity to be differentiated from classic ischemic heart disease caused by coronary atherosclerosis.[619] In this condition, sometimes referred to as *syndrome X*, the prognosis is usually excellent[620-621a]—contrasted with that in patients with coronary atherosclerosis—and its recognition is of clinical importance. Patients with chest pain who have normal coronary arteriograms may constitute as many as 10 to 20 per cent of those undergoing coronary arteriography because of the strong suspicion of angina. The cause of the syndrome is unknown. True myocardial ischemia, reflected in the production of lactate by the myocardium during exercise or pacing, is present in some of these patients.[622]

INADEQUATE VASODILATOR RESERVE (see also p. 1173). Several studies suggest that many patients with chest pain with angiographically normal coronary arteries and no evidence of large vessel spasm, even after an ergonovine challenge, demonstrate an abnormally reduced capacity to decrease coronary resistance and increase coronary flow in response to atrial pacing.[623] This abnormality appears to affect the smaller resistance vessels that are not visible angiographically, while the large proximal conductance vessels appear to be normal. This abnormal vasodilator reserve may be associated with exercise-induced regional wall-motion abnormalities and abnormalities of resting diastolic function.[624] Such patients, with low coronary flow reserve, may exhibit abnormalities of myocardial perfusion detectable noninvasively with positron emission tomography.[625] Some patients have an abnormally reduced dilator response of distal coronary arteries to the physiological dilator stimulus of exercise and also a reduced dilator capacity of the resistance vessels following administration of dipyridamole.[626] This same patient population also has an impairment of vasodilator reserve in forearm vessels[627] and airway hyperresponsiveness,[627a] suggesting that not only is their coronary circulation affected but also their peripheral arterial circulation.

In patients with hypertension and secondary left ventricular hypertrophy with angina pectoris and a normal coronary arteriogram, a reduced coronary blood flow response to dipyridamole has been observed. Similarly, patients with dilated cardiomyopathy and angiographically normal coronary arteries also exhibit impaired vasodilator responses to both rapid atrial pacing and pharmacological stimuli with an increased sensitivity to the vasoconstrictor effects of ergonovine.[628] Other patients with angina and normal coronary arteries are found on extensive investigation to have a cardiomyopathy—either hypertrophic[629] or dilated—and in these cases reduced perfusion, especially of the subendocardium, may be responsible for myocardial ischemia and angina. This finding correlates well with the autopsy observation of thickening of the walls of the coronary arterioles in hypertrophy obstructive cardiomyopathy.[630]

OTHER CAUSES. Patients with psychogenic chest pain, neurocirculatory asthenia, and DaCosta syndrome may also manifest chest pain and have normal coronary arteries.

CLINICAL FEATURES. The syndrome of angina or angina-like chest pain with normal large coronary arteries occurs more frequently in women, while obstructive CAD is found more commonly in men. Fewer than half of the patients with chest pain and normal coronary arteriograms have typical angina pectoris; the majority have a variety of forms of atypical chest pain.

In some patients with minimal or no coronary disease, an exaggerated preoccupation with personal health is associated with continued chest pain,[631] and panic disorder may account for a proportion of such patients.[632] Bass and Wade found that two-thirds of patients with chest pain and normal coronary arteries have predominantly psychiatric disorders.[633] Others have reported that the incidence of CAD is extremely low in patients with atypical chest pain who are anxious and/or depressed.[634] At the time of cardiac catheterization, it has been observed that patients with syndrome X seem unusually sensitive to intracardiac instrumentation, with typical chest pain being consistently produced by direct right atrial stimulation and saline infusion.[635]

PHYSICAL AND LABORATORY FINDINGS. Abnormal physical findings indicative of ischemia, such as precordial bulges, gallop sounds, and murmurs of mitral regurgitation, are uncommon. The resting electrocardiogram may be normal, but nonspecific ST-T abnormalities are often observed. Commonly, perusal of serial electrocardiograms during multiple episodes of chest pain reveals no significant change from baseline. A minority, approximately 20 per cent of patients with chest pain and normal coronary arteriograms, have positive exercise tests. However, many patients with this chest pain syndrome fail to complete the exercise test, discontinuing because of fatigue or mild chest discomfort. Left ventricular function is usually normal at rest and after pacing,[622] unlike the situation in obstructive CAD in which function often becomes impaired during stress. However, a small percentage of patients with chest pain and normal coronary arteries exhibit lactate production and ST-segment depression during exercise (signifying ischemia). Some patients show abnormal myocardial perfusion reserve,[625] but there is no consistent pattern of abnormal myocardial blood flow, although coronary vasodilator reserve may be impaired.[623,624]

In patients with persistent chest pain syndrome and normal coronary arteries, esophageal abnormalities should be considered (p. 1295). Such patients may show either motility disorders of the esophagus or abnormal reflux. In patients whose experience of chest pain coincides with documented reflux, either surgical or medical therapy may give gratifying relief of symptoms.[636]

Important prognostic information on patients with either normal or near-normal coronary arteriograms has been obtained from the CASS Registry.[621] In patients with an ejection fraction of at least 50 per cent, the 7-year survival rate was 96 per cent for patients with a normal arteriogram and 92 per cent for those whose arteriographic study revealed mild disease (less than 50 per cent luminal stenosis). In such patients, an ischemic response to exercise was not associated with increased mortality although a history of smoking or hypertension was. Over follow-up periods of 4 to 6 years,[637,638] symptoms of angina, exercise test evidence of ischemia, and 24-hour ST-segment monitoring of ischemia can all persist relatively unchanged,[637] adversely affecting life style but with a seemingly benign prognosis. In some patients who have either constant or rate-dependent left bundle branch block during exercise there is significant deterioration of left ventricular function over a several-year follow-up, suggesting that they may comprise a subgroup of patients with a cardiomyopathy.[638] Inhibition of adenosine receptors by aminophylline appears to exert a beneficial effect on exercise-induced chest pain and ischemia-like electrocardiographic changes in patients with syndrome X.[639]

In *summary*, there are a number of possible explanations in patients having chest pain and normal coronary arteriograms. Sometimes review of angiography will reveal that significant CAD actually does exist (i.e., incorrect interpretation of angiograms with a false-negative result). When there is no evidence of coronary artery narrowing, even after ergonovine, other causes of pain may be defined (e.g., esophageal disease, mitral valve prolapse syndrome), although often other causes cannot be found even after exhaustive tests. However, a group of patients exists who have normal coronary arteries, symptoms of angina, evidence of ischemia, and abnormal coronary flow reserve with exercise.

MANAGEMENT. This should focus on the explanation of the relatively benign nature of the condition to the patient, psychological counseling, and analgesics to provide pain relief. Calcium antagonists appear to be effective in reducing the frequency and severity of angina and improving exercise tolerance in most patients with chest pain resulting from abnormal vasodilator reserve.[640] Aminophylline administration may be useful in some patients.[639] However, some patients continue to remain disabled with long-term chest discomfort. This can lead to multiple medical consultations and be responsible for a great deal of anxiety. Behavioral therapy may teach the patient with pain how to function more effectively, although unfortunately chronic symptoms may persist.

Ischemic Heart Disease in Which Discomfort Is Not The Dominant Symptom

SILENT MYOCARDIAL ISCHEMIA

There appear to be two forms of silent myocardial ischemia. The first and less common form, designated type I silent ischemia, occurs in patients with severe CAD who do not experience angina at any time; indeed, some of these patients do not even experience pain in the course of myocardial infarction. Epidemiological studies of sudden death (p. 756), clinical and postmortem studies of patients with silent myocardial infarction, and studies of patients with chronic angina pectoris suggest that many individuals with extensive coronary artery obstruction do not have angina pectoris in any of its recognized forms (stable, unstable, or variant).[641] These individuals, representative of type I silent ischemia, may be considered to have a defective anginal "warning system." Both the patient and physician may be unaware of the presence of ischemic heart disease until a fatal event ensues or an old infarction is detected on routine electrocardiogram. The second and much more frequent form, designated type II silent ischemia, occurs in patients with the usual forms of chronic stable angina, unstable angina, or Prinzmetal's angina. When carefully monitored, patients with type II are shown to have some episodes of ischemia that are associated with chest discomfort and other episodes that are not—i.e., episodes of silent ischemia. The term "total ischemic burden" refers to all episodes of myocardial ischemia, both symptomatic and asymptomatic.[642,642a]

During long-term follow-up in the Framingham Study, one-quarter of patients who developed myocardial infarction had unrecognized infarctions, detected only by pathological Q waves on routine 2-yearly electrocardiogram, and of these approximately half were truly silent.[63] In other patients, a myocardial infarction is the first clinical manifestation of ischemic heart disease, although postmortem or angiographic studies indicate that severe coronary atherosclerosis must have existed prior to the infarction yet the patient had never complained of angina. Such patients with silent ischemia may be identified prior to such an event because of cardiac arrhythmias or abnormal electrocardiograms (occasionally at rest, more commonly during exercise) or by means of coronary arteriography performed as a result of a positive exercise test.

AMBULATORY ELECTROCARDIOGRAPHY. The extensive use of ambulatory electrocardiographic monitoring has led to a greater appreciation of the frequency of "silent" ischemia.[642a] It has become apparent that anginal pain is a poor indicator of, and underestimator of, the frequency of significant cardiac ischemia.[642] Episodic hemodynamic changes indicative of myocardial ischemia (increasing left ventricular end-diastolic pressure and decreasing left ventricular ejection fraction with exercise) occur in patients with CAD, irrespective of the occurrence of angina pectoris.[643] Ambulatory studies in patients with chronic stable angina have also emphasized that, while increases in myocardial oxygen demand lead to ischemia, in many episodes of ischemia, both symptomatic and silent, heart rate is *not* accelerated and arterial pressure does *not* rise, suggesting that reductions in myocardial supply make an important contribution to the initiation of ischemia in such patients.[644] With the use of frequency-modulated ambulatory electrocardiographic recordings, it has been found that transient ST-segment depression of 0.1 mV or greater that lasts for more than 30 seconds is a very rare finding in normal subjects.[645] However, in patients known to have CAD there is a strong correlation between such transient ST-segment depression and independent measurements of regional myocardial perfusion and ischemia using rubidium-82 uptake measured by positron-emission tomography.[15] Perfusion defects occurred in the same myocardial segment during painful and silent episodes of ST-segment depression. These responses were significantly different from those observed in normal subjects studied similarly (Fig. 40–33).

Analyses of ambulatory electrocardiograms in patients with angina (exertion induced, and occurring at rest) suggest that the majority of ischemic episodes occurring during normal daily activities are asymptomatic (Fig. 40–34) (type II silent ischemia). Episodes of ST-segment depression, both symptomatic and silent, exhibit a circadian rhythm and are more common in the morning.[646] Nocturnal ST-segment changes are almost invariably an indicator of two- or three-vessel CAD or left main stem stenosis.[647]

MECHANISM OF SILENT ISCHEMIA. It is unclear why some episodes of myocardial ischemia are silent while others are symptomatic. It has been suggested that patients who have no episodes of symptomatic ischemia have a higher pain threshold.[16] Some, although not all, studies suggest that silent episodes may reflect less severe ischemia with less evidence of left ventricular dysfunction.[476] Among patients who experience both symptomatic and asymptomatic ischemia, the ST-segment changes recorded by ambulatory electrocardiographic monitoring are similar, although there is a tendency for symptomatic episodes to be accompanied by longer periods of ST-segment deviation and more marked ST depressions[647]; however, there is considerable overlap between symptomatic and asymptomatic episodes. In keeping with the increased incidence of silent myocardial infarction in patients with diabetes mellitus, there is a greater incidence of asymptomatic ischemia in patients with CAD and type II diabetes mellitus than in nondiabetic patients.[648]

Smokers with CAD may have profound asymptomatic disturbances of regional myocardial perfusion and ST-segment depressions during smoking.[649] Mental stress can also induce silent myocardial ischemia in patients with CAD.[650] Pharmacological agents that reduce or abolish episodes of symptomatic ischemia, i.e., nitrates, beta blockers[651] and calcium antagonists,[642] also reduce or abolish episodes of silent ischemia. It is not clear whether abolition of silent ischemia should be the endpoint of therapy and whether this will influence prognosis favorably, but patients with continuing ischemia despite treatment have a high risk of cardiac death.[652] Monitoring of patients with unstable angina pectoris also identifies a subset of patients with a worse long-term prognosis.[478–480] Elderly men frequently have asymptomatic silent ischemia, and if during these episodes they have ST-segment depressions greater than 0.1 mV, they have a higher relative risk of fatal or nonfatal myocardial infarction. When they also have a history

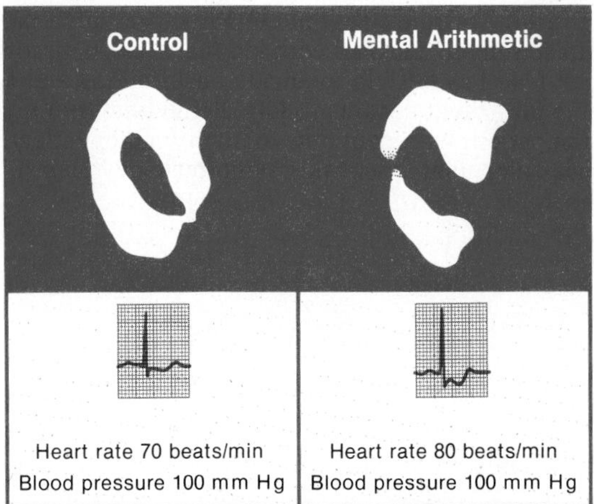

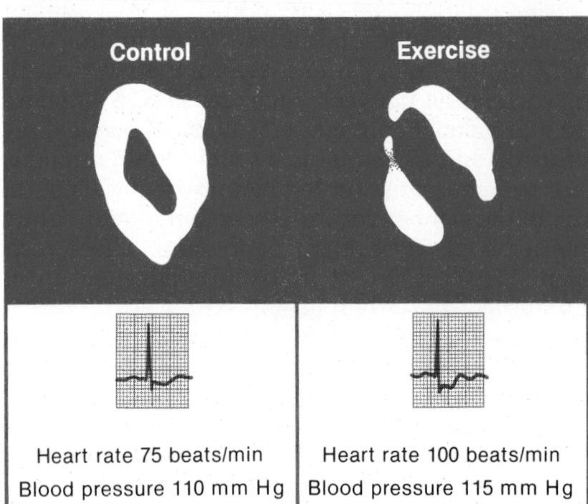

FIGURE 40–33. Tomographic slices of the myocardium recorded using positron-emission tomography in a patient with chronic stable angina, a positive exercise test, and proven coronary artery disease. The information from the heart is obtained from the short-lived tracer rubidium-82, which provides a measure of the distribution and changes in regional myocardial perfusion. The first image (control, *top left*) shows uniform perfusion to the posterior wall, free wall, anterior wall, and septum of the left ventricle. Regional myocardial perfusion during mental arithmetic *(top right)* shows a regional decrease in myocardial perfusion to the left ventricular free wall accompanied by ST-segment depression but not associated with chest pain. The second control image *(bottom left)* shows a return of myocardial perfusion to normal. During exercise *(bottom right)* there is recurrence of ischemia in the same area of the myocardium in which a perfusion abnormality occurred during the stress of mental arithmetic. With exercise, there were both ST-segment depression and symptoms of angina pectoris. Thus in this patient the ischemia provoked by mental arithmetic (asymptomatic) and exercise (symptomatic) showed similar ST-segment depression and myocardial perfusion abnormalities. (From Deanfield, J. E., et al.: Silent myocardial ischemia due to mental stress. Lancet *2:*1001, 1984.)

of CAD, the risk is even greater.[653] In patients with stable CAD and positive exercise tests for myocardial ischemia, the presence of ischemia on ambulatory monitoring is a significant additional predictor of adverse outcome (Fig. 40–35).[654] Asymptomatic patients with positive thallium exercise tests have been treated in an uncontrolled manner with PTCA as the primary therapy for silent ischemia; whether this approach has any merit will be unknown until the results of controlled clinical trials become available.[655]

DETECTION. As of this writing, the detection of patients with CAD without angina (type I silent ischemia) is largely fortuitous. It is likely that screening of populations on a mass basis for silent ischemia would be extraordinarily costly. In Norway, an effort to detect such patients was carried out using a combination of screening techniques (questionnaires, resting and exercise electrocardiograms) in over 2000 asymptomatic and presumably healthy men aged 40 to 50 years.[656] Overall, less than 4 per cent of this population had silent myocardial ischemia, with more than 75 per cent luminal stenosis of one or more coronary arteries. This figure is close to the 4 to 5 per cent of the population estimated by others to be the size of this subgroup.[641] Exercise testing appears to identify the majority of patients likely to have significant ischemia during their daily activities[657,657a] and remains the most important screening test for significant CAD (p. 167).

However, many patients with type I asymptomatic ischemia have been identified because of an asymptomatic positive exercise electrocardiogram obtained following myocardial infarction[658] or asymptomatic ST-segment deviation on an ambulatory (Holter) electrocardiogram.[659] In these patients with a defective anginal warning system it would appear to be useful to obtain coronary arteriograms. Consideration should be given to eliminating silent ischemia by antiischemic pharmacotherapy (nitrates, beta blockers, and Ca^{++} antagonists).[659a] If frequent episodes persist despite optimal drug therapy, critically obstructive lesions may be treated by revascularization (PTCA or surgery) so that severe asymptomatic ischemia is not induced repeatedly during normal life. Whether or not such an approach will improve survival has yet to be determined.

HEART FAILURE

Manifestations of congestive heart failure are common in patients with CAD, but it may be the dominant feature in some patients, especially those who have sustained prior myocardial infarctions and in whom the ischemic focus may have become replaced by fibrous scar, with disappearance or reduction of the angina. The three most common causes of congestive heart failure are (1) left ventricular aneurysm, (2) mitral regurgitation due to papillary muscle dysfunction, and (3) an inadequate quantity of normally contracting myocardium. The last may be secondary to extensive myocardial infarction, a large quantity of viable but "hibernating" myocardium, multiple scars and patchy fibrous replacement of myocardium, or a combination of these.

LEFT VENTRICULAR ANEURYSM

This is usually defined as a segment of the ventricular wall that exhibits paradoxical (dyskinetic) systolic expansion. It involves almost exclusively the left ventricle, most commonly

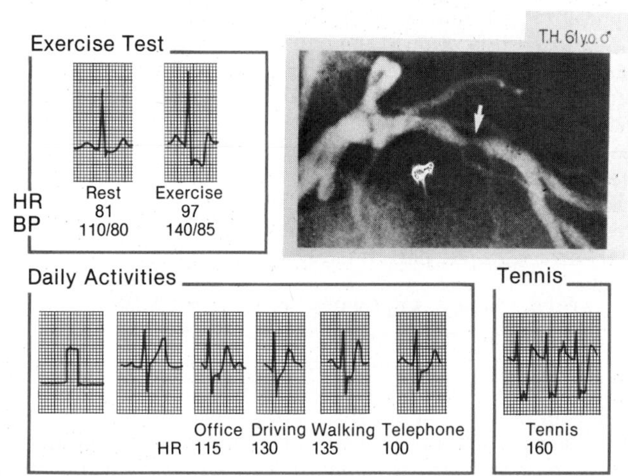

FIGURE 40–34. The ambulatory ECGs and coronary angiograms of a severe left anterior descending stenosis in a patient with fatigue (but not angina) during a tennis match. In stage II of a treadmill exercise test (Bruce protocol), 4 mm of ST-segment depression were seen in lead V_5. Ambulatory Holter monitoring of lead V_5 demonstrates ischemic ST-segment depressions during a number of ordinary activities, e.g., walking, telephoning. During a game of tennis, marked ST-segment depression was recorded when the patient was asymptomatic. (From Nabel, E. G., et al.: Characteristics and significance of ischemia detected by ambulatory electrocardiographic monitoring. Circulation *75*[Suppl. II]:74, 1987, by permission of the American Heart Association, Inc.)

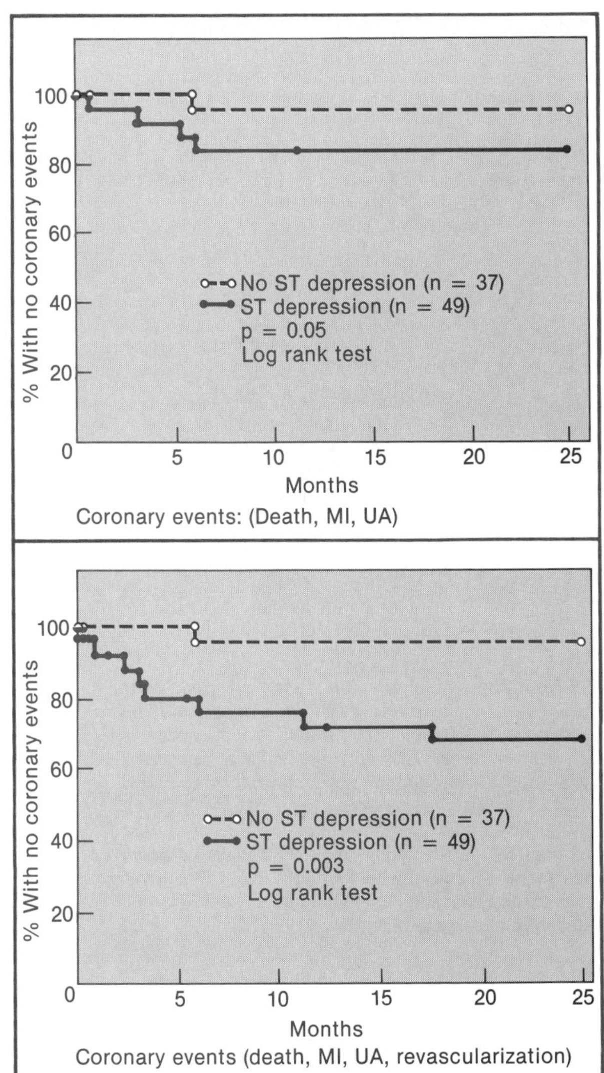

FIGURE 40-35. Prognostic importance of silent ischemia in patients with stable coronary artery disease. Ambulatory monitoring of the ECG was performed in 86 patients with stable coronary artery disease and positive exercise tests for myocardial ischemia. Monitoring was performed after withdrawal of antianginal medications. Prospective follow-up was obtained during routine medical care as prescribed by physicians who were unaware of the monitor results. Kaplan-Meier curves comparing the probability of not experiencing (top panel) an acute ischemic event (death, myocardial infarction, unstable angina), and (bottom panel) progressive ischemic events (acute events or revascularization for worsening symptoms) during follow-up for the 37 patients without ST-segment depression (open circles) and the 49 patients with ST-segment depression (closed circles) as detected by ambulatory monitoring. The presence of ischemia detected by ambulatory monitoring in patients with stable symptoms was common and identified a high-risk group for the development of subsequent unfavorable outcomes while receiving routine medical treatments. (From Rocco, M. B., et al.: Prognostic importance of myocardial ischemia detected by ambulatory monitoring in patients with stable coronary artery disease. Circulation *78*:877, 1988, by permission of the American Heart Association, Inc.)

the anterior or apical segments. In vitro length-tension studies of tissue taken from human ventricular aneurysms have demonstrated that chronic fibrous aneurysms interfere with ventricular performance principally through loss of contractile tissue and that the extent of expansion and "lost work" by the normal left ventricle is minor. These might be considered to be anatomical aneurysms (Fig. 40-36). In contrast, aneurysms made up largely of a mixture of scar tissue and viable myocardium or of thin scar tissue produce a mechanical disadvantage by a combination of paradoxical expansion and loss of effective contraction; these might be considered to be functional aneurysms. *False aneurysms* (pseudoaneurysms), which represent localized myocardial rupture, in which the hemorrhage is limited by pericardial adhesions (Fig. 39-31, p. 1258), have a mouth that is considerably smaller than the maximal diameter.

The frequency of ventricular aneurysm after myocardial infarction depends on the incidence of transmural myocardial infarction and congestive heart failure in the population studied. Left ventricular aneurysm can also result from myocardial infarction secondary to blunt chest trauma.[660] Anterior aneurysms are often associated with total occlusion of the left anterior descending coronary artery, and a poor collateral blood supply,[661] but are unusual in the presence of multivessel disease with a good collateral circulation or a patent anterior descending coronary artery.[662]

Over 80 per cent of left ventricular aneurysms are located anterolaterally near the apex, with approximately 5 to 10 per cent located posteriorly. Most anterior aneurysms are true aneurysms, whereas nearly half of the posterior aneurysms are false aneurysms. Three-quarters of patients with aneurysms have multivessel CAD.[663] Almost half of patients with moderate or large aneurysms have symptoms of heart failure, with or without associated angina. One-third have severe angina alone, and approximately 15 per cent have symptomatic ventricular arrhythmias. Mural thrombi are found in almost half of patients with chronic left ventricular aneurysms. Systemic embolic events in patients with thrombi in left ventricular aneurysms occur infrequently and tend to occur within the initial 4 to 6 months after infarction. Thrombi within the left ventricle can be detected by angiography and two-dimensional echocardiography (Figs. 4-91, p. 98 and 39-37, p. 1262). Available data are insufficient to suggest that long-term anticoagulant treatment is routinely indicated to prevent systemic embolization beyond the first 6 months after infarction.[664] Some patients with ventricular aneurysms have intractable life-threatening ventricular arrhythmias requiring operation (p. 656).[665]

DETECTION. Diagnostic clues to the presence of aneurysm include persistent ST-segment elevations on the electrocardiogram and a characteristic contour (bulge) of the silhouette of the left ventricle on a chest roentgenogram. These findings, when clear-cut, are relatively specific, but they have limited sensitivity. Radionuclide ventriculography and two-dimensional echocardiography can demonstrate ventricular aneurysm more readily. Color-flow echocardiographic imaging is useful in establishing the diagnosis of left ventricular pseudoaneurysm, since flow "in and out" of the aneurysm as well as abnormal flow within the aneurysm can be detected, and subsequent pulsed Doppler imaging can reveal a "to-and-fro" pattern with characteristic respiratory variation of the peak systolic velocity.[666] Computed tomography and magnetic resonance imaging are reliable noninvasive techniques for the identification of left ventricular aneurysms (Fig. 11-5, p. 314) and screening for resectability.[667] However, biplane left ventriculography remains the most precise method available for outlining a left ventricular aneurysm, assessing septal motion, and determining the quantity of functioning residual myocardium.

The motion of the interventricular septum, as assessed by echocardiography, is also of importance in evaluating the function of residual myocardium. Patients with akinesis of the interventricular septum tend to have less favorable outcomes following operation than patients who exhibit septal motion. On the other hand, patients who exhibit the most paradoxical systolic movement of the aneurysm tend to do better after operation than those showing akinesis.[668]

LEFT VENTRICULAR ANEURYSMECTOMY. Indications for this procedure include congestive heart failure, refractory ventricular tachycardia, recurrent thromboembolism, and refractory angina.[669] A large left ventricular aneurysm in a patient with symptoms of heart failure, particularly if angina pectoris is also present, is an indication for operation. The operative mortality rate for left ventricular

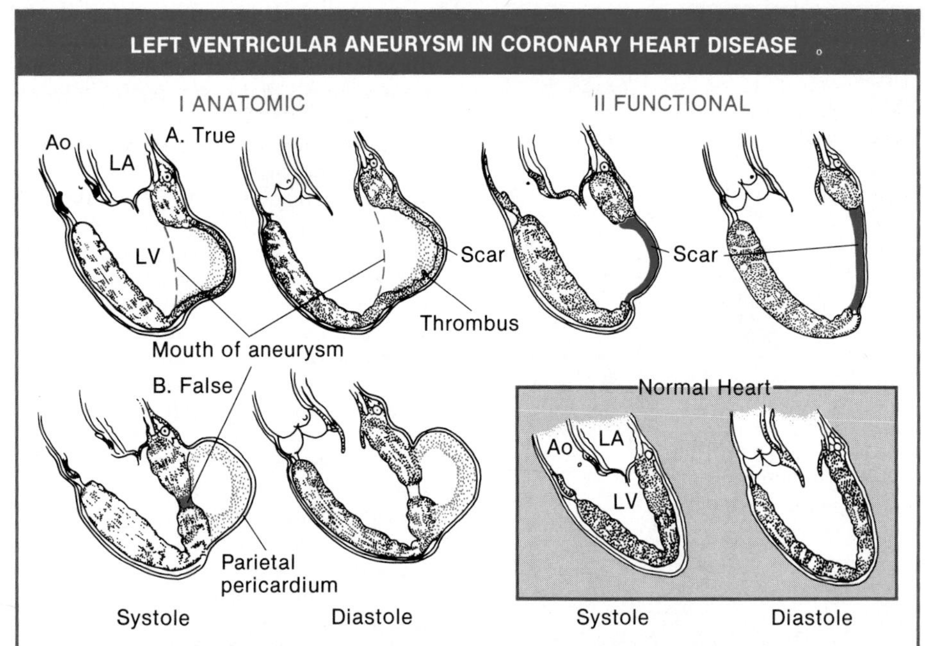

FIGURE 40–36. Hearts in systole and diastole with true and false anatomical and functional left ventricular aneurysms and healed myocardial infarction. A normal heart in systole and diastole is shown for comparison. The true anatomical left ventricular aneurysm protrudes during both systole and diastole, has a mouth that is as wide as or wider than the maximal diameter, has a wall that was formerly the wall of the left ventricle, and is composed of fibrous tissue with or without residual myocardial fibers. A true aneurysm may or may not contain thrombus and almost never ruptures once the wall is healed. The false anatomical left ventricular aneurysm protrudes during both systole and diastole, has a mouth that is considerably smaller than the maximal diameter of the aneurysm and represents a myocardial rupture site, has a wall made up of parietal pericardium, virtually always contains thrombus, and often ruptures. The functional left ventricular aneurysm protrudes during ventricular systole but not during diastole and consists of fibrous tissue with or without myocardial fibers. (From Cabin, H. S., and Roberts, W. C.: Left ventricular aneurysm, intraaneurysmal thrombus and systemic embolus in coronary heart disease. Chest *77*:586, 1980.)

aneurysmectomy is approximately 10 per cent (ranging from 2 to 19 per cent).[669,670] Risk factors for early death include poor left ventricular function,[663,670] resection of an akinetic rather than a dyskinetic aneurysm,[669] recent myocardial infarction,[671] the presence of mitral regurgitation,[672] and intractable ventricular arrhythmias.[670,671] Operation carries a particularly high risk in patients with symptoms of severe heart failure, a low-output state, a requirement for more than 80 mg of furosemide daily, and akinesis of the interventricular septum. Akinesia or dyskinesia of the posterior basal segment of the left ventricle and significant right coronary artery stenoses are additional risk factors.[663] Coronary revascularization is frequently carried out along with aneurysmectomy, especially in patients in whom angina accompanies heart failure.[663,669]

Risk factors for poor late survival following surgery include incomplete revascularization, impaired systolic function of the basal segments of the ventricle and of the septum not involved by the aneurysm, presence of a huge aneurysm with only an inadequate quantity of residual viable myocardium, and the presence of dominant symptoms of cardiac failure rather than angina pectoris (Fig. 40–37).[663] Improvement in left ventricular function has been reported in survivors 1[671] to 3[672] years following resection of left ventricular aneurysms complicated by cardiac failure. A concomitant improvement in exercise performance also occurs, particularly in patients who undergo complete revascularization.[671] After 5 years, 70 to 80 per cent of survivors are in NYHA Class I or II, with a 10-year actuarial survival of 69 per cent in patients undergoing left ventricular aneurysmectomy and revascularization, compared with 57 per cent in those undergoing left ventricular aneurysmectomy alone.[673] Right ventricular dysfunction is relatively common in patients with left ventricular aneurysm and may not be improved by surgery.

True ventricular aneurysms do not rupture, and operative excision is carried out to improve the clinical manifestations (most often heart failure but sometimes also angina, embolization, and life-threatening tachyarrhythmias). Pseudoaneurysms, on the other hand, do rupture frequently, and they should therefore be resected on an urgent basis as soon as the diagnosis is established.

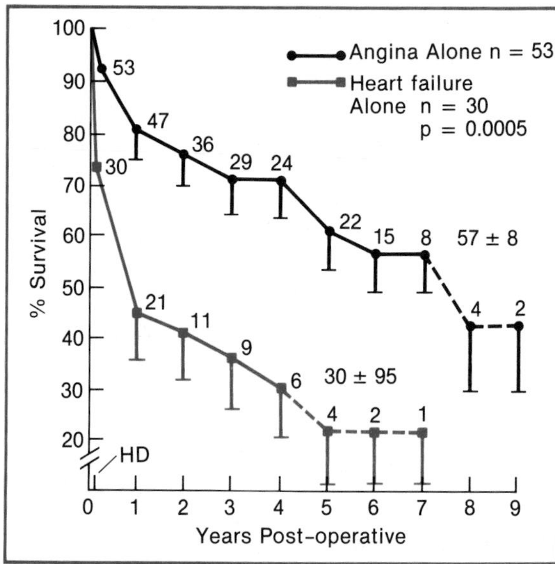

FIGURE 40–37. Survival curves for surgically treated patients with left ventricular aneurysm. Those patients complaining of angina rather than heart failure before operation have a more favorable long-term survival. The numbers of patients at risk are noted. (From Barratt-Boyes, B. G., et al.: The results of surgical treatment of left ventricular aneurysms: An assessment of risk factors affecting early and late mortality. J. Thorac. Cardiovasc. Surg. *87*:87, 1984.)

MITRAL REGURGITATION

Rupture of a papillary muscle, or of the head of a papillary muscle, usually causes severe acute mitral regurgitation in the course of an acute myocardial infarction (Fig. 39–33, p. 1259). Chronic mitral regurgitation in patients with ischemic heart disease is caused, most commonly, by papillary muscle dysfunction due to ischemia or fibrosis (Fig. 34–10, p. 1019) and/or by dilatation of the mitral annulus; many of the latter patients have ventricular aneurysms. Most patients with chronic CAD and mitral regurgitation have suffered a prior myocardial infarction, but the frequency of this syndrome (as with aneurysm) varies depending on the population studied. Clinical features that help to identify mitral regurgitation due to papillary muscle dysfunction as the cause of acute pulmonary edema or of milder symptoms of left-sided failure include a typical loud systolic heart murmur and demonstration of a flail mitral valve leaflet on echocardiography. The latter is the preferred diagnostic technique, since the timing and duration of the murmur are variable. Instead of being only mid to late systolic, as was originally thought, murmurs may be holosystolic or early systolic. Doppler echocardiography is helpful in assessing the severity of the regurgitation (p. 83).

The left atrium is usually not greatly enlarged unless severe mitral regurgitation has been present for more than 6 months. The electrocardiogram is nonspecific, and most patients have angiographic evidence of multivessel CAD. In patients with moderate to severe ischemic mitral regurgitation, variables influencing long-term survival include age, comorbid disorders (renal failure or pulmonary dysfunction), ventricular dysfunction, the need for intensive care management, and the extent of CAD.[674] In patients with posterior papillary muscle dysfunction resulting from acute myocardial infarction, reperfusion therapy with thrombolysis or PTCA may be attempted initially since urgent surgery often has a very high hospital mortality. In patients with rupture of a papillary muscle or, more frequently, one or more heads of a papillary muscle, immediate valve surgery is required provided the various descriptors of prognosis suggest a reasonable chance of satisfactory outcome.[675] Medical therapy is preferred in patients with generalized, severe ventricular dysfunction.

ISCHEMIC CARDIOMYOPATHY

Burch and colleagues used the term *ischemic cardiomyopathy* to describe the condition in which CAD results in severe myocardial dysfunction, with clinical manifestations often indistinguishable from those of primary dilated cardiomyopathy (p. 1398).[676] The fact that manifestations of cardiac dysfunction such as dyspnea or heart failure rather than anginal pain may be the predominant feature of ischemic myocardium is now well known. Observations have confirmed that in ambulatory patients with CAD the occurrence or frequency of angina pectoris is an inaccurate indicator of significant cardiac ischemia[474,645,651] and of ventricular dysfunction occurring during exertion.[643] Thus, symptoms of heart failure (caused by ischemic myocardial dysfunction, diffuse fibrosis, and multiple infarctions, alone or in combination) rather than a single discrete ventricular aneurysm may dominate the clinical picture. In some patients with chronic CAD, angina may be the principal clinical manifestation at one time but later diminishes or even disappears as heart failure becomes more prominent. Other patients have no history of angina or myocardial infarction (type I silent ischemia, p. 1347) and it is in this subgroup that ischemic cardiomyopathy may be confused with dilated cardiomyopathy.

The electrocardiogram may also be misleading. Myocardium with apparent electrocardiographic evidence of infarction, namely, pathological Q waves and diminished R wave height, can be successfully reperfused with improvement in myocardial function. Further evidence that electrocardiographic Q waves may overlie ischemic, rather than necrotic, myocardium is provided by the observation that Q waves may be induced by exercise and subsequently disappear with rest.[677]

Long-term reduction of myocardial perfusion may cause persistent left ventricular dysfunction without tissue necrosis as long as myocardial flow is sufficient to maintain the myocardium viable but inadequate to sustain normal or even subnormal contractile function ("hibernating myocardium," pp. 1176 and 1329).[128] Thus, hibernating myocardium, which can be the basis of or play a role in the development of ischemic cardiomyopathy, can result from chronic ischemia and persist until blood flow is restored. The concept of myocardial hibernation is a useful one because symptoms resulting from chronic left ventricular dysfunction may be incorrectly thought to result from necrotic and scarred myocardium rather than from a reversible ischemic process. For this reason, attempts have been made to decide whether cardiac dysfunction is irreversible (due to necrosis) or potentially reversible (due to ischemia). If myocardial contractility can be improved by an inotropic stimulus such as postextrasystolic potentiation or the infusion of a sympathomimetic amine, it is said to exhibit contractile reserve (p. 1329). Hibernating myocardium may be present in patients with known or suspected CAD with a degree of cardiac dysfunction or heart failure not readily accounted for by other possible causes, e.g., cardiomyopathy of other etiology, longstanding hypertension, and prior myocardial infarctions.

In patients with heart failure in whom myocardial hibernation is suspected, cardiac catheterization and coronary arteriography should be carried out to assess hemodynamic parameters, ventricular function, and coronary anatomy. If myocardium exhibiting a contractile defect is supplied by stenotic coronary arteries or collateral vessels, it is helpful to determine whether it exhibits contractile reserve. If ventricular function improves with inotropic stimulation it is possible that revascularization carried out by surgery[128,130,429] or coronary angioplasty[263] may result in improved ventricular function and survival.[324,326,327,427]

The outlook for patients with ischemic cardiomyopathy treated medically is quite poor, and revascularization or cardiac transplantation may be considered.[679] Associated ventricular arrhythmias occurring in patients with ischemic cardiomyopathy usually are an ominous sign. Patients with diffuse disease have the worst outlook, with a slightly better clinical course being observed in patients with isolated wall-motion disorders.

CARDIAC ARRHYTHMIAS

Many patients with CAD and serious cardiac arrhythmias have other manifestations of active myocardial ischemia, such as acute myocardial infarction. Various degrees of ventricular ectopic activity are the most common arrhythmias. The frequency and severity of ventricular arrhythmias induced during exercise tests and ambulatory monitoring correlate, in general, with the degree of arteriographically documented CAD. Patients with severe left ventricular dysfunction associated with multivessel disease have more high-grade ectopic activity than do those with normal ventricular function and single-vessel disease. In some patients with CAD, cardiac arrhythmias are the predominant manifestation of their disease. That there is a substantial subgroup of patients with CAD and occult arrhythmias is suggested by the frequency with which sudden death is the first manifestation of ischemic heart disease (Ch. 26).

When arrhythmias are the predominant clinical manifestation, they are also the main focus of therapeutic interventions. This ordinarily involves pharmacological therapy, but in cases of drug failure, the implementation of an automatic cardiovascular defibrillator surgical therapy may be useful. Surgical revascularization in survivors of cardiac arrest can reduce the subsequent inducibility of ventricular arrhythmias in approximately one-half of patients, but advanced age and poor ventricular function are adverse prognostic indicators.[680]

Nonatheromatous CAD may also result from congenital abnormalities in the origin or distribution of the coronary arteries (p. 254). The most important of these are anomalous origin of a coronary artery (usually the left) from the pulmonary artery, origin of both coronary arteries from either the right or left sinus of Valsalva, and coronary arteriovenous fistula. Anomalous origin of either the left main coronary artery or right coronary artery from the aorta with subsequent coursing between the aorta and pulmonary trunk is a rare and sometimes fatal coronary arterial anomaly.[681]

Dissection of a coronary artery is often a postmortem finding. Two-thirds of the described cases have occurred in women, and one-half of these were associated with the postpartum state.[682] In patients who survive spontaneous coronary artery dissection, there is a 20-per cent mortality over the next 3 years. In general, coronary revascularization is recommended, particularly in patients who have ongoing ischemia.

A number of inherited connective tissue disorders are associated with myocardial ischemia.[6a] These include the Marfan syndrome (aortic dissection; p. 1641), Hurler syndrome (coronary obstruction; p. 1646), homocystinuria (coronary artery thrombosis; p. 1644), Ehlers-Danlos syndrome (coronary arterial dissection; p. 1643), and pseudo xanthoma elasticum (accelerated CAD; p. 1644). Kawasaki disease, the mucocutaneous lymph node syndrome, may cause coronary artery aneurysms and ischemic heart disease in children (p. 997). On rare occasions Takayasu disease (p. 1544) is associated with angina, myocardial infarction, and cardiac failure resulting from hypertension, aortic regurgitation, or annuloaortic ectasia in patients under the age of 40 years.[683] The average age of onset of symptoms is 24 years, and event-free survival at 10 years after diagnosis is approximately 60 per cent.[683]

Perhaps the most common cause of nonatheromatous CAD resulting in myocardial ischemia is the syndrome of angina-like pain despite normal coronary arteriograms, i.e., so-called syndrome X, which is discussed earlier in this chapter (p. 1346). Myocardial ischemia *not* caused by coronary atherosclerosis can also result from embolism, as in infective endocarditis (Chap. 35); implanted prosthetic heart valves (Ch. 34); primary tumors of the heart (Ch. 45); calcific emboli from calcified aortic valves; and emboli from mural thrombi. Luetic aortitis may also produce myocardial ischemia by causing obstruction of coronary ostia (p. 1548). Occasionally, a mass of amorphous, calcified material accumulates at the sinotubular ridge, i.e., the junction of the sinus and tubular portions of the ascending aorta, most commonly near the right aortic sinus. Complications can include coronary ostial stenosis or embolism to an epicardial coronary artery resulting from the lesion overhanging the ostium or invading the wall of the aorta at the site of the coronary artery takeoff.[684] Important CAD associated with systemic lupus erythematosus has been reported, but is rare.

Cardiac transplant–associated coronary arteriosclerosis (p. 528) is frequently observed in cardiac transplant survivors. It is a rapidly evolving, concentric, diffuse arteriosclerosis involving epicardial and intramural coronary vessels and appears to have an inconstant association with coronary risk factors. Suggested etiologic factors include opportunistic infection (cytomegalovirus infection), immunosuppressive therapy, and elevated lipid levels. Acute myocardial infarction can result and is usually not accompanied by chest pain or typical electrocardiographic changes. However infarction in these patients is associated with a high mortality rate, and, at anatomical examination, diffuse disease of the coronary arteries and multiple foci of nontransmural cardiac infarction.[685] It is likely that the initiating mechanism is in some way immunologically mediated, and intense research is continuing in this area.

An interesting nonatherosclerotic ischemic syndrome has been described in workers in the nitrate industry who apparently experience nitrate withdrawal symptoms on weekends, presumed to be secondary to coronary spasm when there is no counterstimulation to the vasoconstriction that they undergo as an adaptation to the vasodilating actions of the high concentrations of nitrates to which they are exposed.[686]

Acknowledgment

Dr. Peter Cohn was an author of this chapter in the first three editions of this book. He has had a lasting influence on its organization and contents. The authors gratefully acknowledge the secretarial help of Lisa McHale.

REFERENCES

INTRODUCTION

1. Marmot, M. G.: Interpretation of trends in coronary heart disease mortality. Acta Med. Scand. (Suppl.) *701*:58, 1985.
2. National Heart, Lung, and Blood Institute: Morbidity from coronary heart disease in the United States. NHLBI Data Fact Sheet, June, 1990.
3. Connolly, D. C., Oxman, A. J., Nobrega, F. T., et al: Coronary heart disease in residents of Rochester, Minnesota, 1950–1975. I. Background in study design. Mayo Clinic Proc. *56*:661, 1981.
4. Elveback, L. R., Connolly, D. C., and Kurland, L. T.: Coronary heart disease in residents of Rochester, Minnesota, 1950–1975. II. Mortality, incidence, and survival. Mayo Clin. Proc. *56*:665, 1981.
5. Kuller, L. H., Traven, N. D., Rutan, G. H., et al.: Marked decline of coronary heart disease mortality in 35–44-year old white men in Allegheny County, Pennsylvania. Circulation *80*:261, 1989.
6. WHO Expert Committee: Prevention of coronary heart disease. Tech. Rep. Ser. WHO No. 678, 1982.
6a. Virmani, R, and Forman, M. B.: Nonatherosclerotic ischemic heart disease. 1st ed. New York, Raven Press, 1989.

CHRONIC STABLE ANGINA PECTORIS

7. Matthews, M. B., and Julian, D. G.: Angina pectoris: Definition and description. *In* Julian, D. G. (ed.): Angina Pectoris. 2nd ed. New York, Churchill Livingstone, 1985, p. 2.
8. Christie, L. G., Jr., and Conti, C. R.: Systematic approach to evaluation of angina-like chest pain: Pathophysiology and clinical testing with emphasis on objective documentation of myocardial ischemia. Am. Heart J. *102*:897, 1981.
8a. Angina pectoris. *In* Fowler, N.O.: Diagnosis of Heart Disease. New York, Springer-Verlag, 1991, pp. 187–206.
9. Sampson, J. J., and Cheitlin, M. D.: Pathophysiology and differential diagnosis of cardiac pain. Prog. Cardiovasc. Dis. *13*:507, 1971.
10. Lichstein, E., Breitbart, S., Shani, J., et al.: Relationship between location of chest pain and site of coronary artery occlusion. Am. Heart J. *115*:564, 1988.
11. Cook, D. G., and Shaper, A. G.: Breathlessness, angina pectoris and coronary artery disease. Am. J. Cardiol. *63*:921, 1989.
12. Crea, F., Pupita, G., Galassi, A. R., et al: Role of adenosine in pathogenesis of anginal pain. Circulation *81*:164, 1990.
13. Del Banco, P. L., Bel Bene, E., and Sicuteri, F.: Heart pain. *In* Bonica, J. J. (ed.): Advances in Neurology. Vol. 4. New York, Raven Press, 1974, p. 375.
14. Umachandran, V., Ranjadaylan, K., Ambepityia, G., et al.: The perception of angina in diabetes: Relation to somatic pain threshold and autonomic function. Am. Heart J. *121*:1649, 1991.
15. Deanfield, J., Shea, M., Ribeiro, P., et al: Transient ST-segment depression as a marker of myocardial ischemia during daily life. Am. J. Cardiol. *54*:1195,1984.
16. Falcone, C., Sconocchia, R., Guasti, L., et al: Dental pain threshold and angina pectoris in patients with coronary artery disease. J. Am. Coll. Cardiol. *12*:348, 1988.
17. Sheps, D. S., Adams, K. F., Hindliter, A., et al.: Endorphins are related to pain perception in coronary artery disease. Am. J. Cardiol. *59*:523, 1987.
18. Constant, J.: The clinical diagnosis of nonanginal chest pain: The differentiation of angina from nonanginal chest pain by history. Clin. Cardiol. *6*:11, 1983.
19. Hillis, L. D., and Braunwald, E.: Coronary artery spasm. N. Engl. J. Med. *299*:695, 1978.
20. Ganz, P., Abben, R. P., and Barry, W. H.: Dynamic variations in resistance of coronary arterial narrowings in angina pectoris at rest. Am. J. Cardiol. *59*:66, 1987.
20a. Maseri, A.: Medical therapy of chronic stable angina pectoris. Circulation *82*:2258, 1990.
21. Juneau, M., Johnstone, M., Dempsey, E., and Waters, D. D.: Exercise-induced myocardial ischemia in a cold environment. Effect of antianginal medications. Circulation *79*:1015, 1989.
22. Quyyumi, A. A., Mockus, L. J., Wright, C. A., and Fox, K. M.: Mechanisms of nocturnal angina pectoris: Importance of increased myocardial oxygen demand in patients with severe coronary artery disease. Lancet *1*:1207, 1984.
23. Maseri, A.: Mixed angina pectoris. Am. J. Cardiol. *56*:30E, 1985.

24. Epstein, S. E., Stampfer, M., Beiser, G. D., et al: Effect of a reduction in environmental temperature on the circulatory response to exercise in man. Implications concerning angina pectoris. N. Engl. J. Med. *280*:7, 1969.
25. Goldstein, R. E., Redwood, D. R., Beiser, G. D., and Epstein, S. E.: Alterations in the circulatory response to exercise following a meal and their relationship in postprandial angina pectoris. Circulation *44*:90, 1971.
26. Figueras, J., Singh, B. N., Ganz, W., and Swan, H.J.C.: Hemodynamic and electrocardiographic accompaniments of resting postprandial angina. Br. Heart J. *42*:402, 1979.
27. Schiffer, F., Hartley, L. H., Schulman, C. L., and Abelmann, W. H.: Evidence for emotionally induced coronary arterial spasm in patients with angina pectoris. Br. Heart J. *44*:62, 1980.
28. Horowitz, L. D., Herman, M. V., and Gorlin, R.: Clinical response to nitroglycerin as a diagnostic test for coronary artery disease. Am. J. Cardiol. *29*:149, 1972.
29. Levine, S. A.: Carotid sinus massage: A new diagnostic test for angina pectoris. JAMA *182*:1332, 1962.
30. Joy, M., Cairns, A. W., and Sprigings, D.: Observations on the warm up phenomenon in angina pectoris. Br. Heart J. *58*:116, 1987.
31. Campeau, L.: Grading of angina pectoris. Circulation *54*:522, 1976.
32. Goldman, L., Hashimoto, B., and Cook, E. F.: Comparative reproducibility and validity of systems for assessing cardiovascular functional class: Advantages of a new specific activity scale. Circulation *64*:1227, 1981.
33. Califf, R. M., Mark, D. B., Harrell, F. E., et al.: Importance of clinical measures of ischemia in the prognosis of patients with documented coronary artery disease. J. Am. Coll. Cardiol. *11*:20, 1988.
34. Diamond, G. A., and Forrester, J. S.: Analysis of probability as an aid in the clinical diagnosis of coronary artery disease. N. Engl. J. Med. *300*:1350, 1979.
35. Welch, C. C., Proudfit, W. L., and Sheldon, W. C.: Coronary arteriographic findings in 1000 women under age 50. Am. J. Cardiol. *35*:211, 1975.
36. Cohn, P. F., Harris, P., Barry, W. H. et al.: Prognostic importance of anginal symptoms in angiographically defined coronary artery disease. Am. J. Cardiol. *47*:233, 1981.
37. Reunanen, A., Suhonen, O., Aromaa, A., et al.: Incidence of different manifestations of coronary heart disease in middle-aged Finnish men and women. Acta Med. Scand. *218*:19, 1985.
38. Davies, H. A., Jones, D. B., Rhodes, J., and Newcombe, R. G.: Anginal-like esophageal pain: Differentiation from cardiac pain by history. J. Clin. Gastroenterol. *7*:477, 1985.
39. Conte, M. R., Orzan, F., Magnacca, M., et al.: Atypical chest pain: Coronary or esophageal disease? Int. J. Cardiol. *13*:135, 1986.
40. Winnan, G. R., Meyer, C. T., and McCallum, R. W.: Interpretation of the Bernstein Test: A reappraisal of criteria. Ann. Intern. Med. *96*:320, 1982.
41. DeMeester, T. R., O'Sullivan, G. C., Bermudez, G., et al.: Esophageal function in patients with angina-type chest pain and normal coronary angiograms. Ann. Surg. *196*:488, 1982.
42. Mellow, M. H., Simpson, A. G., Watt, L., et al.: Esophageal acid perfusion in coronary artery disease. Gastroenterology *85*:306, 1983.
43. Davies, H. A., Rush, E. M., Lewis, M. J., et al.: Oesophageal stimulation lowers exertional angina threshold. Lancet *1*:1011, 1985.
44. Lee, M. G., Sullivan, S. N., Watson, W. C., and Melendez, L. J.: Chest pain—esophageal, cardiac, or both? Am. J. Gastroenterol. *80*:320, 1985.
45. Eastwood, G. L., Weiner, B. H., Dickerson, W. J., et al.: Use of ergonovine to identify esophageal spasm in patients with chest pain. Ann. Intern. Med. *94*:768, 1981.
46. Hargrove, M. D.: Gallbladder disease and chest pain. CV Dis & Chest Pain *2*:3, 1987.
47. Epstein, S. E., Gerber, L. H., and Borer, J. S.: Chest wall syndrome. A common cause of unexpected cardiac pain. JAMA *241*:2793, 1979.
48. Bettmann, M. A., and Salzman, E. W.: Current concepts in the diagnosis of pulmonary embolism. Mod. Concepts Cardiovasc. Dis. *53*:1, 1984.
49. Pe'er J., Vidaurri, J., Halfon, S. T., et al.: Association between corneal arcus and some of the risk factors for coronary artery disease. Br. J. Ophthalmol. *67*:795, 1983.
50. Winder, A. F.: Relationship between corneal arcus and hyperlipidaemia is clarified by studies in familial hypercholesterolaemia. Br. J. Ophthalmol. *67*:789, 1983.
51. Segal, P., Insull, W., Chambless, L. E., et al.: The association of dyslipoproteinemia with corneal arcus and xanthelasma. The Lipid Research Clinic's Program Prevalence Study. Circulation *73*:108, 1986.
52. Elliot, W. J.: Ear lobe crease and coronary artery disease. 1,000 patients and review of the literature. Am. J. Med. *75*:1024, 1983.
53. Kaukola, S.: The diagonal ear-lobe crease, heredity and coronary heart disease. Acta Med. Scand. (Suppl.)*668*:60, 1982.
54. Kirkham, N., Murrells, T., Melcher, D. H., and Morrison, E. A.: Diagonal earlobe creases and fatal cardiovascular disease: A necropsy study. Br. Heart J. *61*:361, 1989.
55. Brady, P. M., Zive, M. A., Goldberg, R. J., et al.: A new wrinkle to the earlobe crease. Arch. Intern. Med. *147*:65, 1987.
56. Criqui, M. H., Coughlin, S. S., and Fronek, A.: Noninvasively diagnosed peripheral arterial disease as a predictor of mortality: Results from a prospective study. Circulation *72*:768, 1985.
57. Cohn, P. F., Thompson, S., Strauss, W., et al.: Diastolic heart sounds during static (handgrip) exercise in patients with chest pain. Circulation *47*:1217, 1973.
58. Ranganathan, N., Juma, Z., and Sivaciyan, V.: The apical impulse in coronary heart disease. Clin. Cardiol. *8*:20, 1985.
59. Tavel, M. E.: the fourth heart sound—a premature requiem? Circulation *49*:4, 1974.
60. Sangster, J. F., and Oakley, C. M.: Diastolic murmur of coronary artery stenosis. Br. Heart J. *35*:840, 1973.
61. Hamby, R. I., Weissman, R. H., Prakash, M. N., and Hoffman, I.: Left bundle branch block: A predictor of poor left ventricular function in coronary artery disease. Am. Heart J. *106*:471, 1983.
62. Liao, Y., Emidy, L. A., Dyer, A., et al.: Characteristics and prognosis of incomplete right bundle branch block: An epidemiologic study. J. Am. Coll. Cardiol. *7*:492, 1986.
63. Kannel, W. B., and Abbott, R. D.: Incidence and prognosis of unrecognized myocardial infarction. N. Engl. J. Med. *311*:1144, 1984.
64. Goldman, L., Cook, E. F., Mitchell, N., et al.: Incremental value of the exercise test for diagnosing the presence or absence of coronary artery disease. Circulation *66*:945, 1982.
65. Dagenais, G. R., Rouleau, J. R., Christen, A., and Fabia, J.: Survival of patients with a strongly positive exercise electrocardiogram. Circulation *65*:452, 1982.
66. Bogaty, P., Dagenais, G. R., Cantin, B., et al.: Prognosis in patients with a strongly positive exercise electrocardiogram. Am. J. Cardiol. *64*:1284, 1989.
67. Weiner, D. A., McCabe, C., Hueter, D. C., et al.: The predictive value of anginal chest pain as an indicator of coronary disease during exercise testing. Am. Heart J. *96*:458, 1978.
67a. Wilson, R. F., Marcus, M. L., Christensen, B. V., et al.: Accuracy of exercise electrocardiography in detecting physiologically significant coronary arterial lesions. Circulation *83*:412, 1991.
68. Detrano, R., Gianrossi, R., Mulvihill, D., et al.: Exercise-induced ST segment depression in the diagnosis of multivessel coronary disease: A meta analysis. J. Am. Coll. Cardiol. *14*:1501, 1989.
69. Dubach, P., Froelicher, V. F., Klein, J., et al.: Exercise-induced hypotension in a male population. Criteria, causes and prognosis. Circulation *78*:1380, 1988.
70. Boran, K. G., Oliveros, R. A., Boucher, C. A., et al.: Ischemia-associated intraventricular conduction disturbances during exercise testing as a predictor of proximal left anterior descending coronary artery disease. Am. J. Cardiol. *51*:1098, 1983.
71. Vasey, C., O'Donnell, J., Morris, S., and McHenry, P.: Exercise-induced left bundle branch block and its relation to coronary artery disease. Am. J. Cardiol. *56*:892, 1985.
72. Williams, M. A., Esterbrooks, D. I., Nair, C. K., et al.: Clinical significance of exercise-induced bundle branch block. Am. J. Cardiol. *61*:346, 1988.
73. Okin, P. M., Ameisen, O., and Kligfield, P.: Recovery-phase patterns of ST segment depression in the heart rate domain. Identification of coronary artery disease by the rate-recovery loop. Circulation *80*:533, 1989.
74. Stone, P. H., LaFolette, E. L., and Cohn, K.: Patterns of exercise treadmill test performance in patients with left main coronary artery disease: Detection dependent on left coronary dominance or coexistent dominant right coronary disease. Am. Heart J. *104*:13, 1982.
75. Nygaard, T. W., Gibson, R. S., Ryan, J. M., et al.: Prevalence of high-risk thallium-201 scintigraphic findings in left main coronary artery stenosis: Comparison of patients with multiple-and single-vessel coronary artery disease. Am. J. Cardiol. *53*:462, 1984.
76. Bartel, A. L., Behar, V. S., Peter, R. H., et al.: Graded exercise stress tests in angiographically documented coronary artery disease. Circulation *49*:348, 1974.
77. Goldschlager, N., Selzer, A., and Cohn, K.: Treadmill stress tests as indicators of presence and severity of coronary artery disease. Ann. Intern. Med. *85*:282, 1976.
78. Hlatky, M. A., Pryor, D. B., Harrell, F. E., Jr., et al.: Factors affecting sensitivity and specificity of exercise electrocardiography. Am. J. Med. *77*:64, 1984.
79. Weins, R. D., Lafia, P., Marder, C. M., et al.: Chronotropic incompetence in clinical exercise testing. Am. J. Cardiol. *54*:74, 1984.
80. McHenry, P. L., Morris, S. N., Kavalier, M., and Jordan, J. W.: Comparative study of exercise-induced ventricular arrhythmias in normal subjects and patients with documented coronary artery disease. Am. J. Cardiol. *37*:609, 1976.
80a. Podrid, P. J., Graboys, T. B., and Lown, B.: Prognosis of medically treated patients with coronary-artery disease with profound ST-segment depression during exercise testing. N. Engl. J. Med. *305*:1111, 1981.
80b. Dagenais, G. R., Rouleau, J. R., Hochart, P., et al.: Survival with painless strongly positive exercise electrocardiogram. Am. J. Cardiol. *62*:892, 1988.
80c. Weiner, D. A., Ryan, T. J., McCabe, C. H., et al.: The role of exercise testing in identifying patients with improved survival after coronary artery bypass surgery. J. Am. Coll. Cardiol. *8*:741, 1986.
81. Cole, J. R., and Ellestad, M. H.: Significance of chest pain during treadmill exercise: Correlation with coronary events. Am. J. Cardiol. *41*:227, 1978.
82. Weiner, D. A., Ryan, T. J., McCabe, C., et al.: Risk of developing an acute myocardial infarction or sudden coronary death in patients with exercise-induced silent myocardial ischemia. A report from the coronary artery surgery study (CASS) registry. Am. J. Cardiol. *62*:1155, 1988.
83. Mukharji, J., Kremers, M., Lipscomb, K., and Blomqvist, C. G.: Early positive exercise test and extensive coronary disease: Effect of antianginal therapy. Am. J. Cardiol. *55*:267, 1985.
84. Ho, S. W. -C., McComish, M. J., and Taylor, R. R.: Effect of beta-adrenergic blockade on the results of exercise testing related to the extent of coronary artery disease. Am. J. Cardiol. *55*:258, 1985.
85. Severi, S., and Michelassi, C.: Prognostic impact of stress testing in coronary artery disease. Circulation *83*:(Suppl. III):82, 1991.
86. Younis, L. T., Byers, S., Shaw, L., et al.: Prognostic importance of silent

myocardial ischemia detected by intravenous dipyridamole thallium myocardial imaging in asymptomatic patients with coronary artery disease. J. Am. Coll. Cardiol. *14*:1635, 1989.

87. Borges-Neto, S., Mahmarian, J. J., Jain, A., et al.: Quantitative thallium-201 single photon emission computed tomography after oral dipyridamole for assessing the presence, anatomic location and severity of coronary artery disease. J. Am. Coll. Cardiol. *11*:962, 1988.

87a. Coyne, E. P., Belvedere, D. A., Vande Streek, P. R., et al.: Thallium-201 scintigraphy after intravenous infusion of adenosine compared with exercise thallium testing in the diagnosis of coronary artery disease. J. Am. Coll. Cardiol. *17*:1289, 1991.

87b. Brown, K. A.: Prognostic value of thallium-201 myocardial perfusion imaging: A diagnostic tool comes of age. Circulation *83*:363, 1991.

88. Gould, K. L.: How accurate is thallium exercise testing for the diagnosis of coronary disease. J. Am. Coll. Cardiol. *14*:1487, 1989.

89. Port, S. C., Oshima, M., Ray, G., et al.: Assessment of single-vessel coronary artery disease: Results of exercise electrocardiography, thallium-201 myocardial perfusion imaging and radionuclide angiography. J. Am. Coll. Cardiol. *6*:75, 1985.

90. Wackers, F. J. T., Russo, D. J., Russo, D., and Clements, J. P.: Prognostic significance of normal quantitative planar thallium-201 stress scintigraphy in patients with chest pain. J. Am. Coll. Cardiol. *6*:27, 1985.

91. Koss, J. H., Kobren, S. M., Grunwald, A. M., and Bodenheimer, M. M.: Role of exercise thallium-201 myocardial perfusion scintigraphy in predicting prognosis in suspected coronary artery disease. Am. J. Cardiol. *59*:531, 1987.

92. Pamelia, F. X., Gibson, R. S., Watson, D. D., et al.: Prognosis with chest pain and normal thallium-201 exercise scintigrams. Am. J. Cardiol. *55*:920, 1985.

93. Gill, J. B., Ruddy, T. D., Newell, J. B., et al.: Prognostic importance of thallium uptake by the lungs during exercise in coronary artery disease. N. Engl. J. Med. *317*:1485, 1987.

93a. Pollock, S. G., Abbott, R. D., Boucher, C. A., et al.: A model to predict multivessel coronary artery disease from the exercise thallium-201 stress test. Am. J. Med. *90*:345, 1991.

94. Weiss, A. T., Berman, D. S., Lew, A. S., et al.: Transient ischemic dilation of the left ventricle on stress thallium-201 scintigraphy: A marker of severe and extensive coronary artery disease. J. Am. Coll. Cardiol. *9*:752, 1987.

95. Kiat, H., Berman, D. S., and Maddahi, J.: Comparison of planar and tomographic exercise thallium-201 imaging methods for the evaluation of coronary artery disease. J. Am. Coll. Cardiol. *13*:613, 1989.

96. Coyne, E. P., Belvedere, D. A., Vande Streek, P. R., et al.: Thallium-201 scintigraphy after intravenous infusion of adenosine compared with exercise thallium testing in the diagnosis of coronary artery disease. J. Am. Coll. Cardiol. *17*:1289, 1991.

96a. Ranhosky, A., Kempthorne-Rawson, J., and the Intravenous Dipyridamole Thallium Imaging Study Group: The safety of intravenous dipyridamole thallium myocardial perfusion imaging. Circulation *81*:1205, 1990.

97. Kaul, S., Kiess, M., Liu, P., et al.: Comparison of exercise electrocardiography and quantitative thallium imaging for one-vessel coronary artery disease. Am. J. Cardiol. *56*:257, 1985.

98. Raby, K. E., Goldman, L., Creager, M. A., et al.: Correlation between preoperative ischemia and major cardiac events after peripheral vascular surgery. N. Engl. J. Med. *321*:1296, 1989.

99. Gibbons, R. J., Fyke, F. E., Clements, I. P., et al.: Noninvasive identification of severe coronary disease using exercise radionuclide angiography. J. Am. Coll. Cardiol. *11*:28, 1988.

100. Cates, C. U., Kronenberg, M. W., Collins, H. W., and Sandler, M. P.: Dipyridamole radionuclide ventriculography: A test with high specificity for severe coronary artery disease. J. Am. Coll. Cardiol. *13*:841, 1989.

101. Kaul, S., Lilly, D. R., Gascho, J. A., et al.: Prognostic utility of the exercise thallium-201 test in ambulatory patients with chest pain: Comparison with cardiac catheterization. Circulation *77*:745, 1988.

102. Armstrong, W. F., O'Donnell, W. F., Dillon, J. C., et al.: Complementary value of two-dimensional exercise echocardiography to routine treadmill exercise testing. Ann. Intern. Med. *105*:829, 1986.

103. Ryan, T., Vasey, C. G., Presti, C. F., et al.: Exercise echocardiography: Detection of coronary artery disease in patients with normal left ventricular wall motion at rest. J. Am. Coll. Cardiol. *11*:993, 1988.

104. Oberman, A., Fan, P.-H., Nanda, N. C., et al.: Reproducibility of two-dimensional echocardiography. J. Am. Coll. Cardiol. *14*:923, 1989.

105. Armstrong, W. F.: Exercise echocardiography: Ready, willing and able. J. Am. Coll. Card. *11*:1359, 1988.

106. Sheikh, K. H., Bengtson, J. R., Helmy, S., et al.: Relation of quantitative coronary lesion measurements to the development of exercise-induced ischemia assessed by exercise echocardiography. J. Am. Coll. Cardiol. *15*:1043, 1990.

107. Lim, T.-J., Nanto, S., Masuyama, T., et al.: Visualization of subendocardial myocardial ischemia with myocardial contrast echocardiography in humans. Circulation *79*:233, 1989.

108. Picano, E., and Lattanzi, F.: Dipyridamole echocardiography. Circulation *83*(Suppl. III):19, 1991.

109. Picano, E., Lattanzi, F., and L'Abbate, A.: Present application, practical aspects, and future issues on dipyridamole echocardiography Circulation *83*(Suppl. III)111, 1991.

110. Ryan, T., Armstrong, W. F., and Feigenbaum, H.: Prospective evaluation of the left main coronary artery using digital two-dimensional echocardiography. J. Am. Coll. Cardiol. *7*:807, 1986.

111. Neinle, R. A., Levy, R. I., Frederickson, D. S., and Gorlin, R.: Lipid and carbohydrate abnormalities in patients with angiographically documented coronary artery disease. Am. J. Cardiol. *24*:178, 1969.

112. Falsetti, H. L., Schnatz, J. D., Greene, D. G., and Bunelli, I. L.: Lipid and carbohydrate studies in coronary artery disease. Circulation *37*:184, 1968.

113. Margolis, J. R., Chan, J. T. T., Kong, Y., et al: The diagnostic and prognostic significance of coronary artery calcification. A report of 800 cases. Radiology *127*:609, 1980.

114. Agatston, A. S., Janowitz, W. R., Hildner, F., et al.: Quantification of coronary artery calcium using ultrafast computed tomography. J. Am. Coll. Cardiol. *15*:827, 1990.

115. Gordon, P. R., Abrams, C., Gash, A. K., and Carabello, B. A.: Pericatheterization risk factors in left main coronary artery stenosis. Am. J. Cardiol. *59*:1080, 1987.

116. Hartnell, G. G., Parnell, B. M., and Pridie, R. B.: Coronary artery ectasia: Its prevalence and clinical significance in 4993 patients. Br. Heart J. *54*:392, 1985.

117. Tunick, P. A., Slater, J., Kronzon, I., et al.: Discrete atherosclerotic coronary artery aneurysms: A study of 20 patients. J. Am. Coll. Cardiol. *15*:279, 1990.

118. Agarwal, J. B., and Helfant, R. H.: Functional importance of coronary collateral circulation. Int. J. Cardiol. *4*:94, 1983.

119. Newman, P. E.: The coronary collateral circulation: Determinants and functional significance in ischemic heart disease. Am. Heart J. *102*:431, 1981.

120. Gregg, D. E., and Patterson, R. E.: Functional importance of the coronary collaterals. N. Engl. J. Med. *303*:1404, 1980.

121. Kracoff, O. H., Ovsyshcher, I., and Gueron, M.: Malignant course of a benign anomaly: Myocardial bridging. Chest *92*:1113, 1987.

121a. Bestetti, R. B., Costa, R. S., Kazava, D. K., and Oliveira, J. S. M.: Can isolated myocardial bridging of the left anterior descending coronary artery be associated with sudden death during exercise? Acta Cardiologica *XLVI*:27, 1991.

122. Moraski, R. E., Russell, R. O., Jr., Smith, M., and Rackley, C. E.: Left ventricular function in patients with and without myocardial infarction and one, two or three vessel coronary artery disease. Am. J. Cardiol. *35*:1, 1975.

123. Mann, T., Brodie, B. R., Grossman, W., and McLaurin, L. P.: Effect of angina on the left ventricular diastolic pressure-volume relationship. Circulation *35*:761, 1977.

124. Helfant, R. H., Forrester, J. S., Hampton, J. R., et al.: Coronary heart disease. Differential hemodynamic, metabolic, and electrocardiographic effects in subjects with and without angina pectoris during atrial pacing. Circulation *42*:601, 1970.

125. Bourdillon, P. D., Lorell, B. H., Mirsky, I., et al.: Increased regional myocardial stiffness of the left ventricle during pacing-induced angina in man. Circulation *67*:316, 1983.

126. Stack, R. S., Phillips, H. R., Grierson, D. S., et al.: Functional improvement of jeopardized myocardium following intracoronary streptokinase infusion in acute myocardial infarction. J. Clin. Invest. *72*:84, 1983.

127. Rahimtoola, S. H.: A perspective on the three large multicenter randomized clinical trials of coronary bypass surgery for chronic stable angina. Circulation *72*(Suppl. V):123, 1985.

128. Braunwald, E., and Rutherford, J. D.: Reversible ischemic left ventricular dysfunction: Evidence for the "hibernating myocardium." J. Am. Coll. Cardiol. *8*:1467, 1986.

128a. Marban, E.: Myocardial stunning and hibernation. The physiology behind the colloquialisms. Circulation *83*:681, 1991.

129. Popio, K. A., Gorlin, R., Bechtel, D., and Levine, J. A.: Postextrasystolic potentiation as a predictor of potential myocardial viability: Preoperative analyses compared with studies after coronary bypass surgery. Am. J. Cardiol. *39*:944, 1977.

130. Nesto, R. W., Cohn, L. H., Collins, J. J., Jr, et al.: Inotropic contractile reserve: A useful predictor of increased 5-year survival and improved postoperative left ventricular function in patients with coronary artery disease and reduced ejection fraction. Am. J. Cardiol. *50*:39, 1982.

131. Bodenheimer, M. M., Banka, V. S., Hermann, G. A., et al.: Reversible asynergy: Histopathologic and electrographic correlations in patients with coronary artery disease. Circulation *53*:792, 1976.

132. Banka, V. S., Bodenheimer, M. M., and Helfant, R. H.: Determinants of reversible asynergy: The native coronary circulation. Circulation *52*:810, 1975.

133. Verani, M. S., Carroll, R. J., and Falsetti, H. L.: Mitral valve prolapse in coronary artery disease. Am. J. Cardiol. *37*:1, 1976.

134. Herman, M. V., Elliott, W. C., and Gorlin, R.: An electrocardiographic, anatomic, and metabolic study of zonal myocardial ischemia in coronary heart disease. Circulation *35*:834, 1967.

135. Gertz, E. W., Wisneski, J. A., Neese, R., et al.: Myocardial lactate metabolism: Evidence of lactate release during net chemical extraction in man. Circulation *63*:1273, 1981.

136. Cannon, P. J., Weiss, M. B., and Sciacca, R. R.: Myocardial blood flow in coronary artery disease: Studies at rest and during stress with inert gas washout techniques. Prog. Cardiovasc. Dis. *20*:95, 1977.

137. Gould, K. L.: Identifying and measuring severity of coronary artery stenosis. Circulation *78*:237, 1988.

138. Harrison, D. G.: From isolated vessels to the catheterization laboratory. Studies of endothelial function in the coronary circulation of humans. Circulation *80*:703, 1989.

139. Werns, S. W., Walton, J. A., Hsia, H. H., et al.: Evidence of endothelial

dysfunction in angiographically normal coronary arteries of patients with coronary artery disease. Circulation *79*:287, 1989.

139a. Zeiher, A. M., Drexler, H., Wollschläger, H., et al.: Modulation of coronary vasomotor tone in humans. Progressive endothelial dysfunction with different early stages of coronary atherosclerosis. Circulation *83*:391, 1991.

140. Hill, J. A., Miranda, A. A., Keim, S. G., et al.: Value of right-sided cardiac catheterization in patients undergoing left-sided catheterization for evaluation of coronary artery disease. R_2 Management of Chronic Stable Angina Am. J. Cardiol. *65*:590, 1990.

Management of Chronic Stable Angina

141. Kronmal, R. A., Oberman, A., Frye, R. L., and Killip, T., III: Effect of cigarette smoking on survival of patients with angiographically documented coronary artery disease. Report from CASS Registry. JAMA *255*:1023, 1986.

142. Hermanson, B., Omenn, G. S., Kronmal, R. A., et al.: Beneficial six-year outcome of smoking cessation in older men and women with coronary artery disease. Results from the CASS Registry. N. Engl. J. Med. *319*:1365, 1988.

143. Hallstom, A. P., Cobb, L. A., and Ray, R.: Smoking as a risk factor for recurrence of sudden cardiac arrest. N. Engl. J. Med. *314*:271, 1986.

144. Rogot, E., and Murray, J. L.: Smoking and causes of death among U.S. veterans: 16 years of observation. Public Health Rep. *95*:213, 1980.

145. Kannel, W. B., Castelli, W. P., and McNamara, P. M.: Cigarette smoking and risk of CHD: Epidemiologic clues to pathogenesis: The Framingham Study. N.C.I. Mongr. *28*:9, 1968.

146. Kaufman, D. W., Helmich, S. P., and Shapiro, S.: The risk of myocardial infarction after quitting smoking in men under 55 years of age. N. Engl. J. Med. *313*:1511, 1985.

147. Hofstetter, A., Schutz, Y., Jequier, E., and Wahren, J.: Increased 24-hour energy expenditure in cigarette smokers. N. Engl. J. Med. *314*:79, 1986.

148. Nicod, P., Rehr, R., Winniford, M. D., et al.: Acute systemic and coronary hemodynamic and serologic responses to cigarette smoking in long-term smokers with atherosclerotic coronary artery disease. J. Am. Coll. Cardiol. *4*:964, 1984.

149. Winniford, M. D., Wheelan, K. R., Kremers, M. S., et al.: Smoking-induced coronary vasoconstriction in patients with atherosclerotic coronary artery disease: Evidence for adrenergically mediated alterations in coronary artery tone. Circulation *73*:662, 1986.

150. Winniford, M. D., Jansen, D. E., Reynolds, G. A., et al.: Cigarette smoking-induced coronary vasoconstriction in atherosclerotic coronary artery disease and prevention by calcium antagonists and nitroglycerin. Am. J. Cardiol. *59*:203, 1987.

151. Deanfield, J., Wright, C., Kirkler, S., et al.: Cigarette smoking and the treatment of angina with propranolol, atenolol, and nifedipine. N. Engl. J. Med. *310*:951, 1984.

152. Aronow, W. S.: Effect of passive smoking on angina pectoris. N. Engl. J. Med. *299*:21, 1978.

153. Adams, K. F., Koch, G., Chatterjee, B., et al.: Acute elevation of blood carboxyhemoglobin to 6% impairs exercise performance and aggravates symptoms in patients with ischemic heart disease. J. Am. Coll. Cardiol. *12*:900, 1988.

154. Alldred, E. N., Bleecker, E. R., Chaitman, B. R., et al.: Short-term effects of carbon monoxide exposure on the exercise performance of subjects with coronary artery disease. N. Engl. J. Med. *321*:1426, 1989.

155. Rocco, M. B., Barry J., Campbell, S., et al.: Circadian variation of transient myocardial ischemia in patients with coronary artery disease. Circulation *75*:395, 1987.

156. Hennekens, C. H., Buring, J. E., Sandercock, P., et al.: Aspirin and other antiplatelet agents in the secondary and primary prevention of cardiovascular disease. Circulation *80*:749, 1989.

157. Ridker, P. M., Manson, J. E., Gaziano, J. M., et al.: Low-dose aspirin therapy for chronic stable angina. A randomized clinical trial. Ann. Intern. Med. *114*:835, 1991.

158. Brown, G., Albers, J. J., Fisher, L. D., et al.: Regression of coronary artery disease as a result of intensive lipid-lowering therapy in men with high levels of apolipoprotein B. N. Engl. J. Med. *323*:1289, 1990.

159. Ferguson, R. J., Taylor, A. W., Cote, P., et al.: Skeletal muscle and cardiac changes with training in patients with angina pectoris. Am. J. Physiol. *243*:H830, 1982.

160. Redwood, D. R., Rosing, D. R., and Epstein, S. E.: Circulatory and symptomatic effects of physical training in patients with coronary artery disease and angina pectoris. N. Engl. J. Med. *286*:959, 1972.

161. Ehsani, A. A., Biello, D. R., Schultz, J., et al.: Improvement of left ventricular contractile function by exercise training in patients with coronary artery disease. Circulation *74*:350, 1986.

162. Parker, J. O.: Nitrate therapy in stable angina pectoris. N. Engl. J. Med. *316*:1635, 1987.

163. Williams, J. F., Jr., Glick, G., and Braunwald, E.: Studies on cardiac dimensions in intact unanesthetized man. V. Effects of nitroglycerin. Circulation *32*:76, 1965.

164. Brown, B. G., Bolson, E., Petersen, R. B., et al.: The mechanisms of nitroglycerin action: Stenosis vasodilation as a major component of the drug response. Circulation *64*:1089, 1981.

165. Bache, R. J., Ball, R. M., Cobb, F. R., et al.: Effects of nitroglycerin on transmural myocardial blood flow in the unanesthetized dog. J. Clin. Invest. *55*:1219, 1975.

166. Cohen, M. V., Downey, J. M., Sonnenblick, E. H., and Kirk, E. S.: The effects of nitroglycerin on coronary collaterals and myocardial contractility. J. Clin. Invest. *52*:2836, 1973.

167. Cowan, C., Duran, P.V.M., Corsini, G., et al.: The effects of nitroglycerin on myocardial blood flow in man. Measured by coincidence counting and bolus injections of 84-rubidium. Am. J. Cardiol. *24*:154, 1969.

168. Parker, J. O., West, R. O., and DiGiorgi, S.: The effect of nitroglycerin on coronary blood flow and the hemodynamic response to exercise in coronary artery disease. Am. J. Cardiol. *27*:59, 1971.

169. Ganz, W., and Marcus, H. S.: Failure of intracoronary nitroglycerin to alleviate pacing-induced angina. Circulation *46*:880, 1972.

170. Bernstein, L., Friesinger, G. C., Lichtlen, P. R., and Ross, R. S.: The effect of nitroglycerin on the systemic circulation in man and dog. Circulation *33*:107, 1966.

171. Cohn, P. F., Maddox, D. E., Holman, B. L., et al.: Effect of sublingually administered nitroglycerin on regional myocardial blood flow in patients with coronary artery disease. Am. J. Cardiol. *39*:672, 1977.

172. Dove, J. T., Shah, P. M., and Schreiner, B. F.: Effects of nitroglycerin on left ventricular wall motion in coronary artery disease. Circulation *49*:682, 1974.

173. Borer, J. S., Bacharach, S. L., Green, M. V., et al.: Effect of nitroglycerin on exercise-induced abnormalities of left ventricular regional function and ejection fraction in coronary artery disease. Assessment by radionuclide cineangiography in symptomatic and asymptomatic patients. Circulation *57*:314, 1978.

174. Winniford, M. D., Jansen, D. E., Reynolds, G. A., et al.: Cigarette smoking-induced coronary vasoconstriction in atherosclerotic coronary artery disease and prevention by calcium antagonists and nitroglycerin. Am. J. Cardiol. *59*:203, 1987.

175. Murad, F.: Cyclic guanosine monophosphate as a mediator of vasodilation. J. Clin. Invest. *78*:1, 1986.

176. Ignarro, L. J., Lippton, H., Edwards, J. C., et al.: Mechanism of vascular smooth muscle relaxation by organic nitrates, nitrites, nitroprusside, and nitric oxide: Evidence for the involvement of S-nitrosothiols as active intermediates. J. Pharmacol. Exp. Ther. *218*:739, 1981.

177. Horowitz, J. D., Antman, E. M., Lorell, B. H., et al.: Potentiation of the cardiovascular effects of nitroglycerin by *N*-acetylcysteine. Circulation *68*:1247, 1983.

178. Winniford, M. D., Kennedy, P. L., Wells, P. J., and Hillis, L. D.: Potentiation of nitroglycerin-induced coronary dilatation by *N*-acetylcysteine. Circulation *73*:138, 1986.

179. May, D. C., Popma, J. J., Black, W. H., et al.: In vivo induction and reversal of nitroglycerin tolerance in human coronary arteries. N. Engl. J. Med. *317*:805, 1987.

180. Hales, C. A., and Westphal. D.: Hypoxemia following the administration of sublingual nitroglycerin. Am. J. Med. *65*:911, 1978.

181. Parker, J. O., Vankoughnett, K. A., and Farrell, B.: Nitroglycerin lingual spray: Clinical efficacy and dose response relation. Am. J. Cardiol. *57*:1, 1986.

182. Needleman, P., Lang, S., and Johnson, E. M., Jr.: Organic nitrates: Relationship between biotransformation and rational angina pectoris therapy. J. Pharmacol. Exp. Ther. *181*:489, 1972.

183. Belder, M. A., Schneeweiss, A., and Camm, A. J.: Evaluation of the efficacy and duration of action of isosorbide mononitrate in angina pectoris. Am. J. Cardiol. *65*:6J, 1990.

184. Thadani, U., Fung, H. L., Darke, A. C., and Parker, J. O.: Oral isosorbide dinitrate in angina pectoris: Comparison of duration of action and dose-response relation during acute and sustained therapy. Am. J. Cardiol. *49*:411, 1982.

185. Bassan, M. M.: The daylong pattern of the antianginal effect of long-term three times daily administered isosorbide dinitrate. J. Am. Coll. Cardiol. *16*:936, 1990.

186. Abrams, J.: Interval therapy to avoid nitrate tolerance: Paradise regained? Am. J. Cardiol. *64*:931, 1989.

187. Schaer, D. F., Buff, l. A., and Katz, R. J.: Sustained antianginal efficacy of transdermal nitroglycerin patches using an overnight 10-hour nitrate-free interval. Am. J. Cardiol. *61*:46, 1988.

188. Demots, H., and Glasser, S. P.: Intermittent transdermal nitroglycerin therapy in the treatment of chronic stable angina. J. Am. Coll. Cardiol. *13*:786, 1989.

189. Badger, R. S., Brown, B. G., Gallery, C. A., et al.: Coronary artery dilation and hemodynamic responses after isosorbide dinitrate therapy in patients with coronary artery disease. Am. J. Cardiol. *56*:390, 1985.

190. Bassan, M. M., and Weiler-Ravell, D.: The additive antianginal action of oral isosorbide dinitrate in patients receiving propranolol. Magnitude and duration of effect. Chest *83*:233, 1983.

191. Colditz, G. A., Halvorsen, K. T., and Goldhaber, S. Z.: Randomized clinical trials of transdermal nitroglycerin systems for the treatment of angina: A meta-analysis. Am. Heart J. *116*:174, 1988.

192. Parker, J. O.: Intermittent transdermal nitroglycerin therapy in the treatment of chronic stable angina. J. Am. Coll. Cardiol. *13*:794, 1989.

192a. Elkayam, U.: Tolerance to organic nitrates: evidence, mechanisms, clinical relevance, and strategies for prevention. Ann. Intern. Med. *114*:667, 1991.

193. Parker, J. O., Vankoughnett, K. A., and Farrell, B.: Comparison of buccal nitroglycerin and oral isosorbide dinitrate for nitrate tolerance in stable angina pectoris. Am. J. Cardiol. *56*:724, 1985.

194. Lee, G., Mason, D. T., and DeMaria, A. N.: Effects of long-term oral administration of isosorbide dinitrate on the antianginal response to nitroglycerin. Am. J. Cardiol. *41*:82, 1978.

195. Marcus, F. I.: The rapid onset of nitrate tolerance. J. Am. Coll. Cardiol. *16*:941, 1990.
196. Packer, M.: What causes tolerance to nitroglycerin? The 100 year old mystery continues. J. Am. Coll. Cardiol. *16*:932, 1990.
197. Levy, W. S., Katz, R. J., and Wasserman, A. G.: Methionine restores the venodilative response to nitroglycerin after the development of tolerance. J. Am. Coll. Cardiol. *17*:474, 1991.
198. Armstrong, P. W., Armstrong, J. A., and Marks, G. S.: Blood levels after sublingual nitroglycerin. Circulation *59*:585, 1979.
199. Parker, J. O., Vankoughnett, K. A., and Fung, F.-L.: Transdermal isosorbide dinitrate in patients receiving propranolol. Magnitude and duration of effect. Chest *83*:233, 1983.
200. Przybojewski, J. Z., and Heyns, M. H.: Acute coronary vasospasm secondary to industrial nitroglycerin withdrawal. S. Afr. Med. J. *63*:158, 1983.
201. Watanabe, A. G.: Recent advances in knowledge about beta-adrenergic receptors: Application to clinical cardiology. J. Am. Coll. Cardiol. *1*:82, 1983.
202. Kern, M. J., Ganz, P., Horowitz, J. D., et al.: Potentiation of coronary vasoconstriction by beta adrenergic blockade in patients with coronary artery disease. Circulation *67*:1178, 1983.
203. Gaglione, A., Hess, O. M., Corin, W. J., et al.: Is there coronary vasoconstriction after intracoronary beta-adrenergic blockade in patients with coronary artery disease. J. Am. Coll. Cardiol. *10*:299, 1987.
204. Chierchia, S., Muiesan, L., Davies, A., et al.: Role of the sympathetic nervous system in the pathogenesis of chronic stable angina. Implications for the mechanism of action of β-blockers. Circulation *82*(Suppl. 11):71, 1990.
205. Lands, A. M., Arnold, A., McAuliff, J. P., et al.: Differentiation of receptor systems activated by sympathomimetic amines. Nature *214*:597, 1967.
206. Conolly, M. E., Kersting, F., and Dollery, C. T.: The clinical pharmacology of beta-adrenoreceptor blocking drugs. Prog. Cardiovasc. Dis. *19*:203, 1976.
207. Kostis, J. B., Frishman, W., Hosler, M. H., et al.: Treatment of angina pectoris with pindolol: The significance of intrinsic sympathomimetic activity of beta blockers. Am. Heart J. *104*:496, 1982.
208. Quyyumi, A. A., Wright, C., Mockus, L., and Fox, K. M.: Effect of partial agonist activity in beta blockers in severe angina pectoris: A double-blind comparison of pindolol and atenolol. Br. Med. J. *289*:951, 1984.
209. Drayer, D. E.: Lipophilicity, hydrophilicity and the central nervous system side effects of beta-blockers. Pharmacotherapy *7*:87, 1987.
210. Gengo, F. M., Huntoon, L., and McHugh, W. B.: Lipid-soluble and water-soluble β-blockers. Comparison of the central nervous system depressant effect. Arch. Intern. Med. *147*:39, 1987.
211. Kostis, J. B., and Rosen, R. C.: Central nervous system effects of the β-adrenergic-blocking drugs: The role of ancillary properties. Circulation *75*:204, 1987.
212. Frishman, W., and Halprin, S.: Clinical pharmacology of the new beta-adrenergic blocking drugs. VII. New horizons in beta-adrenoceptor blocking therapy—labetalol. Am. Heart J. *98*:660, 1979.
213. Prida, X.E., Hill, J. A., and Feldman, R. L.: Systemic and coronary hemodynamic effects of combined alpha- and beta-adrenergic blockade (Labetolol) in normotensive patients with stable angina pectoris and positive exercise test responses. Am. J. Cardiol. *59*:1084, 1987.
214. Lennard, M. S.: The polymorphic oxidation of beta-adrenoceptor antagonists. Pharmacol. Ther. *41*:461, 1989.
215. Lehtonen, A.: Effect of beta blockers on blood lipid profile. Am. Heart J. *109*:1192, 1985.
216. Northcote, R. J., Todd, I. C., and Ballantyne, D.: Beta blockers and lipoproteins: A review of current knowledge. Scott Med. J. *31*:220, 1986.
217. Rutherford, J. D., Singh, B. N., Ambler, P. K., and Norris, R. M.: Plasma propranolol concentration in patients with angina and acute myocardial infarction. Clin. Exp. Pharmacol. Physiol. *3*:297, 1976.
218. Miller, R. R., Olson, H. G., Amsterdam, E. A., and Mason, D. T.: Propranolol withdrawal rebound phenomenon. Exacerbation of coronary events after abrupt cessation of antianginal therapy. N. Engl. J. Med. *293*:416, 1975.
219. Hiatt, W. R., Stoll, S., and Nies, A. S.: Effect of beta-adrenergic blockers on the peripheral circulation in patients with peripheral vascular disease. Circulation *72*:1226, 1985.
220. Cooper, G., Kent, R. L., McGonigle, P., and Watanabe, A.: Beta adrenergic receptor blockade of feline myocardium. Cardiac mechanics, energetics, and beta adrenoceptor regulation. J. Clin. Invest. *77*:441, 1986.
221. Cardiology Drug Facts, 1989. 1st ed. St. Louis. C.V. Mosby.
222. Opie, L. H.: Calcium channel antagonists. A Review. Part 1. Fundamental properties: Mechanisms, classification, sites of action. Cardiovasc, Drugs Ther. *I*:411, 1987.
223. Opie, L. H.: Calcium channel antagonists. Part V. Second generation agents. Cardiovasc. Drugs Ther. *2*:191, 1988.
224. Wood, A. J. J.: Calcium antagonists. Pharmacologic differences and similarities. Circulation *80*(Suppl. IV):184, 1989.
224a. Hurwitz, L., Partridge, L. D., and Leach, J. K. (eds.): Calcium Channels: Their Properties, Functions, Regulation, and Clinical Relevance. Boca Raton, FL, CRC Press, 1991.
225. Stone, P. H., Turi, Z., Muller, J. E., et al.: Experience with nifedipine in 845 patients with refractory angina pectoris. J. Am. Coll. Cardiol. *1*:596, 1983.
226. Strauss, W. E., and Parisi, S. F.: Combined use of calcium-channel and beta-adrenergic blockers for the treatment of chronic stable angina. Ann. Intern. Med. *109*:570, 1988.
227. Packer, M.: Combined beta-adrenergic and calcium-entry blockade in angina pectoris. N. Engl. J. Med. *320*:709, 1989.
228. Cannon, R. O., Watson, R. M., Rosing, D. R., and Epstein, S. E.: Efficacy of calcium channel blocker therapy for angina pectoris resulting from small-vessel coronary artery disease and abnormal vasodilator reserve. Am. J. Cardiol. *56*:242, 1985.
228a. Cole, P. L., Beamer, A. D., McGowan, N., et al.: Efficacy and safety of perhexiline maleate in refractory angina. A double-blind placebo-controlled clinical trial of a novel antianginal agent. Circulation *81*:1260, 1990.
229. Lichtlen, P. R., Hugenholtz, P. G., Raffenbleul, W. et al.: Retardation of angiographic progression of coronary artery disease by nifedipine. Results of the International Nifedipine Trial on Antiatherosclerotic Therapy (INTACT). Lancet *335*:1109, 1990.
230. Loadi, A., Polese, A., Montorsi, P., et al.: Comparison of nifedipine, propranolol and isosorbide dinitrate on angiographic progression and regression of coronary arterial narrowings in angina pectoris. Am. J. Cardiol. *64*:433, 1989.
231. Extended-release nifedipine: Effective 24-hour treatment for hypertension and angina. Hosp. Formul. (Suppl. A) *25*:2, 1990.
232. Wallace, W. A., Wellington, K. L., Murphy, G. W., and Liang, C.-S.: Comparison of antianginal efficacies and exercise hemodynamic effects of Nifedipine and Diltiazem in stable angina pectoris. Am. J. Cardiol. *63*:414, 1989.
233. Vatner, S. F., and Hintze, T. H.: Effects of a calcium-channel antagonist on large and small coronary arteries in conscious dogs. Circulation *66*:579, 1982.
234. Ludbrook, P. A., Tiefenbrunn, A. J., Reed, F. R., and Sobel, B. E.: Acute hemodynamic responses to sublingual nifedipine: Dependence on left ventricular function. Circulation *65*:489, 1982.
235. Elkayam, U., Amin, J., Mehra, A., et al.: A prospective, randomized, double-blind, crossover study to compare the efficacy and safety of chronic nifedipine therapy with that of isosorbide dinitrate and their combination in the treatment of chronic congestive heart failure. Circulation *82*:1954, 1990.
236. White, H. D., Polak, J. F., Wynne, J., et al.: Addition of nifedipine to maximal nitrate and beta-adrenoreceptor blocker therapy in coronary artery disease. Am. J. Cardiol. *55*:1303, 1985.
237. Leon, M. B., Rosing, D. R., Bonow, R. O., et al.: Clinical efficacy of verapamil alone and combined with propranolol in treating patients with chronic stable angina pectoris. Am. J. Cardiol. *48*:131, 1981.
238. Boden, W. E., Bough, E. W., Reichman, M. J., et al.: Beneficial effects of high-dose diltiazem in patients with persistent effort angina on beta blockers and nitrates: A randomized, double-blind, placebo-controlled cross-over study. Circulation *71*:1197, 1985.
239. Wagniart, P., Feguson, R. J., Chaitman, B. R., et al.: Increased exercise tolerance and reduced electrocardiographic ischemia with diltiazem in patients with stable angina pectoris. Circulation *66*:23, 1982.
240. Bache, R. J.: Effects of calcium entry blockade on myocardial blood flow. Circulation *80*(Suppl. IV):40, 1989.
241. Nonogi, H., Hess, O. M., Ritter, M., et al.: Prevention of coronary vasoconstriction during dynamic exercise in patients with coronary artery disease. J. Am. Coll. Cardiol. *12*:892, 1988.
242. Rossen, J. D., Simonetti, I., Marcus, M. L., et al.: The effect of diltiazem on coronary flow reserve in humans. Circulation *80*:1240, 1989.
243. Murakami, T., Hess, O. M., and Krayenbuehl, H. P.: Left ventricular function before and after diltiazem in patients with coronary artery disease. J. Am. Coll. Cardiol. *5*:723, 1985.
244. DeServi, S., Ferrario, M., Ghio, S., et al.: Effects of diltiazem on regional coronary hemodynamics during atrial pacing in patients with stable exertional angina: Implications for mechanism of action. Circulation *73*:1248, 1986.
245. O'Hara, M. J., Khurmi, N. S., Bowles, M. J., and Raftery, E. B.: Diltiazem and propranolol combination for the treatment of chronic stable angina pectoris. Clin. Cardiol. *10*:115, 1987.
246. Strauss, W. E., and Parisi, A. F.: Superiority of combined diltiazem and propranolol therapy for angina pectoris. Circulation *71*:951, 1985.
247. Frishman, W., Charlap, S., Kimmel, B., et al.: Diltiazem, nifedipine, and their combination in patients with stable angina pectoris: effects on angina, exercise tolerance, and the ambulatory electrocardiographic ST segment. Circulation *77*:774, 1988.
248. Toyosaki, N., Toyo-Oka, T., Natsume, T., et al.: Combination therapy with diltiazem and nifedipine in patients with effort angina pectoris. Circulation *77*:1370, 1988.
249. Van Dijk, R. B., Lie, K. I., and Crijns, H.J.G.M.: Diltiazem in comparison with metoprolol in stable angina pectoris. Eur. Heart J. *9*:1194, 1988.
249a. Hampton, J. R.: Secondary prevention of acute myocardial infarction with beta-blocking agents and calcium antagonists. Am. J. Cardiol. *66*;3c, 1990.
250. Gibson, R. S., Boden, W. E., Theroux, P., et al.: Diltiazem and reinfarction in patients with non-Q-wave myocardial infarction. Results of a double-blind, randomized, multicenter trial. N. Engl. J. Med. *315*:423, 1986.
251. The Danish Study Group on Verapamil in Myocardial Infarction: Effect of Verapamil on mortality and major events after acute infarction (The Danish Verapamil Infarction Trial II-DAVIT II). Am. J. Cardiol. *66*:779, 1990.
252. Stone, P. H., Gibson, R. S., Glasser, S. P., et al. (The ASIS Study Group): Comparison of propranolol, diltiazem, and nifedipine in the treatment of ambulatory ischemia in patients with stable angina. Differential effects on ambulatory ischemia, exercise performance, and anginal symptoms. Circulation *82*:1962, 1990.
253. Klinke, W. P., Kvill, L., Dempsey, E. E., and Grace, M.: A randomized double-blind comparison of diltiazem and nifedipine in stable angina. J. Am. Coll. Cardiol. *12*:1562, 1988.

254. Nesto, R. W., White, H. D., Wynne, J., et al.: Comparison of nifedipine and isosorbide dinitrate when added to maximum propranolol therapy in stable angina pectoris. Am. J. Cardiol. *60*:256, 1987.
255. Packer, M., Meller, J., Medina, N., et al.: Hemodynamic consequences of combined beta-adrenergic and slow calcium channel blockade in man. Circulation *65*:660, 1982.
256. Kieval, J., Kirsten, E. B., Kessler, K. M., et al.: The effects of intravenous verapamil on hemodynamic status of patients with coronary artery disease receiving propranolol. Circulation *65*:653, 1982.
257. Shub, C.: Stable angina pectoris. 3. Medical treatment. Mayo Clin. Proc. *65*:256, 1990.
258. Ellis, S. G., Cowley, M. J., DiSciascio, G., et al.: Determinants of 2-year outcome after coronary angioplasty in patients with multivessel disease on the basis of comprehensive preprocedural evaluation: Implications for patient selection. Circulation *83*:1905, 1991.
258a. Wong, J. B., Sonnenberg, F. A., Salem, D. N., and Pauker, S. G. P.: Myocardial revascularization for chronic stable angina. Ann. Intern. Med. *113*:852, 1990.
259. Cowley, M. J., Vetrovec, G. W., DiSciascio, G., et al.: Coronary angioplasty of multiple vessels: Short-term outcome and long-term results. Circulation *72*:1314, 1985.
260. Leimgruber, P. P., Roubin, G. S., Hollman, J., et al.: Restenosis after successful coronary angioplasty in patients with single-vessel disease. Circulation *73*:710, 1986.
261. Melchior, J. P., Meier, B., Urban, P., et al.: Percutaneous transluminal coronary angioplasty for chronic total coronary arterial occlusion. Am. J. Cardiol. *59*:535, 1987.
261a. Savage, M. P., Goldberg, S., Hirshfeld, J. W., et al.: Clinical and angiographic determinants of primary coronary angioplasty success. J. Am. Coll. Cardiol. *17*:22, 1991.
262. Holmes, D. R., Holubkov R., Vlietstra R. E., and the Coinvestigators of the NHLBI Transluminal Coronary Angioplasty Registry: Comparison of the complications during percutaneous transluminal coronary angioplasty from 1977 to 1981 and from 1985 to 1986. J. Am. Coll. Cardiol. *12*:1149, 1988.
263. Kohli, R. S., DiSciascio, G., Cowley, M. J., et al.: Coronary angioplasty in patients with severe left ventricular dysfunction. J. Am. Coll. Cardiol. *16*:807, 1990.
264. Ellis, S. G., Roubin, G. S., King, S. B., et al.: Angiographic and clinical predictors of acute closure after native vessel coronary angioplasty. Circulation *77*:372, 1988.
265. Ellis, S. G., Roubin, G. S., King, S. B., et al.: In-hospital cardiac mortality after acute closure after coronary angioplasty: Analysis of risk factors from 8,207 procedures. J. Am. Coll. Cardiol. *11*:211, 1988.
266. Stammen, F., Piessens, J., Vrolix, M., et al.: Immediate and short-term results of a 1988–1989 coronary angioplasty registry. Am. J. Cardiol. *67*:253, 1991.
267. Deligonul, U., Vandormael, M. G., Kern, M. J., et al.: Coronary angioplasty: A therapeutic option for symptomatic patients with tow and three vessel coronary disease. J. Am. Coll. Cardiol. *11*:1173, 1988.
268. DiSciascio, G., Cowley, M. J., Vetrovec, G. W., et al.: Triple vessel coronary angioplasty: Acute outcome and long-term results. J. Am. Coll. Cardiol. *12*:42, 1988.
269. Vandormael, M., Deligonul, U., Taussig, S., and Kern, M. J.: Predictors of long-term cardiac survival in patients with multivessel coronary artery disease undergoing percutaneous transluminal coronary angioplasty. Am. J. Cardiol. *67*:1, 1991.
269a. Thompson, R. C., Holmes, D. R., Gersh, B. J., et al.: Percutaneous transluminal coronary angioplasty in the elderly: Early and long-term results. J. Am. Coll. Cardiol. *17*:1245, 1991.
270. O'Keefe, J. H., Rutherford, B. D., McConohay, D. R., et al.: Multivessel coronary angioplasty from 1980 to 1989: Procedural results and long-term outcome. J. Am. Coll. Cardiol. *16*:1097, 1990.
270a. Ellis, S. G., Vandormael, M. G., Cowley, M. J., et al.: Coronary morphologic and clinical determinants of procedural outcome with angioplasty for multivessel coronary disease. Implications for patient selection. Circulation *82*:1193, 1990.
271. Gaul, G., Hollman, J., Simpfendorfer, C., and Franco, I.: Acute occlusion in multiple lesion coronary angioplasty: Frequency and management. J. Am. Coll. Cardiol. *123*:283, 1989.
272. Mabin, T. A., Holmes, D. R., Jr., Smith, H. E., et al.: Follow-up clinical results in patients undergoing percutaneous transluminal coronary angioplasty. Circulation *71*:754, 1985.
273. Vandormael, M. G., Chaitman, B. R., Ischinger, T., et al.: Immediate and short-term benefit of multilesion coronary angioplasty: Influence of degree of revascularization. J. Am. Coll. Cardiol. *6*:983, 1985.
274. Reeder, G. S., Vlietstra, R. E., Mock, M. B., et al.: Comparison of angioplasty and bypass surgery in multivessel coronary artery disease. Int. J. Cardiol. *10*:213, 1986.
275. Reeder, G. S., Holmes, D. R., Detre, K., et al.: Degree of revascularization in patients with multivessel coronary disease: A report from the NHLBI Percutaneous Transluminal Coronary Angioplasty Registry. Circulation *77*:638, 1988.
276. Bell, M. R., Bailer, K. R., Reeder, G. S., et al.: Percutaneous transluminal angioplasty in patients with multivessel coronary disease: How important is complete revascularization for cardiac event-free survival? J. Am. Coll. Cardiol. *16*:553, 1990.
276a. Topol, E. J., and Faxon, D. P.: Symposium on restenosis: From basic studies to clinical trials. J. Am. Coll. Cardiol. *17*:Suppl B, 1991, 199 pp.
277. Popma, J. J., and Topol, E. J.: Factors influencing restenosis after coronary angioplasty. Am. J. Med. *88*:16N, 1990.
277a. Nobuyoshi, M., Kimura, T., Ohishi, H., et al.: Restenosis after percutaneous transluminal coronary angioplasty: Pathologic observations in 20 patients. J. Am. Coll. Cardiol. *17*:433, 1991.
278. Galan, K. M., Deligonul, U., Kern, M. J., et al.: Increased frequency of restenosis in patients continuing to smoke cigarettes after percutaneous transluminal coronary angioplasty. Am. J. Cardiol. *61*:260, 1988.
279. Schwartz, L., Bourassa, M. G., Lesperance, J., et al.: Aspirin and dipyridamole in the prevention of restenosis after transluminal coronary angioplasty. N. Engl. J. Med. *318*:1714, 1988.
280. Black, A.J.R., Anderson, H. V., Roubin, G. S., et al.: Repeat coronary angioplasty: Correlates of a second restenosis. J. Am. Coll. Cardiol. *11*:714, 1988.
280a. Hollman, J.: What does pathology teach us about recurrent stenosis after coronary angioplasty? J. Am. Coll. Cardiol. *17*:440, 1991.
281. Teirstein, P. S., Hoover, C. A., Ligon, R. W., et al.: Repeat coronary angioplasty: Efficacy of a third angioplasty for a second restenosis. J. Am. Coll. Cardiol. *13*:291, 1989.
282. Talley, J. D., Weintraub, W. S., Roubin, G. S., et al.: Failed elective percutaneous transluminal coronary angioplasty requiring coronary artery bypass surgery. Circulation *82*:1203, 1990.
283. Bentivoglio, L. G., Van Raden, M. J., Kelsey, S. F., and Detre, K. M.: Percutaneous transluminal coronary angioplasty (PTCA) in patients with relative contraindications: Results of the National Heart, Lung, and Blood Institute PTCA Registry. Am. J. Cardiol. *53*(Suppl. 1):82C, 1984.
284. Bonow, R. O., Kent, K. M., Rosing, D. R., et al.: Improved left ventricular diastolic filling in patients with coronary artery disease after percutaneous transluminal coronary angioplasty. Circulation *66*:1159, 1982.
285. Bates, E. R., Aueron, F. M., Legrand, V., et al.: Comparative long-term effects of coronary artery bypass graft surgery and percutaneous transluminal coronary angioplasty on regional coronary flow reserve. Circulation *72*:833, 1985.
286. Kent, K. M., Bonow, R. O., Rosing, D. R., et al.: Improved myocardial function during exercise after successful percutaneous transluminal coronary angioplasty. N. Engl. J. Med. *306*:441, 1982.
287. Gruentzig, A. R., King, S. B., Schlumpf, M., and Siegenthaler, W.: Long-term follow-up after percutaneous transluminal coronary angioplasty. The early Zurich experience. N. Engl. J. Med. *316*:1127, 1987.
288. Berger, E., Williams, D. O., Reinert, S., and Most, A. S.: Sustained efficacy of percutaneous transluminal coronary angioplasty. Am. Heart J. *111*:233, 1986.
289. Webb, J. G., Myler, R. K., Shaw, R. E., et al.: Coronary angioplasty after coronary bypass surgery: Initial results and late outcome in 422 patients. J. Am. Coll. Cardiol. *16*:812, 1990.
290. Cooper, I., Ineson, N., Demirtas, E., et al.: Role of angioplasty in patients with previous coronary artery bypass surgery. Cathet. Cardiovasc. Diagn. *16*:81, 1989.
291. Platko, W. P., Hollman, J., Whitlow, P. L., and Franco, I.: Percutaneous transluminal angioplasty of saphenous graft stenosis: Long-term followup. J. Am. Coll. Cardiol. *14*:1645, 1989.
291a. Plokker, H. W. T., Meester, B. H., and Serruys, P. W.: The Dutch experience in percutaneous transluminal angioplasty of narrowed saphenous veins used for aortocoronary arterial bypass. Am. J. Cardiol. *67*:361, 1991.
292. Serruys, P. W., Umans, V., Heyndrickx, G. R., et al.: Elective PTCA of totally occluded coronary arteries not associated with acute myocardial infarction; short-term and long-term results. Eur. Heart J. *6*:2, 1985.
293. Kereiakes, D. J., Selmon, M. R., McAuley, B. J., et al.: Angioplasty in total coronary artery occlusion: Experience in 76 consecutive patients. J. Am. Coll. Cardiol. *6*:526, 1985.
294. DiSciascio, G., Vetrovec, G. W., Cowley, M. J., and Wolfgang, T. C.: Early and late outcome of percutaneous transluminal coronary angioplasty for subacute and chronic total coronary occlusion. Am. Heart J. *111*:833, 1986.
295. Isner, J. M., Rosenfield, K., and Losordo, D. W.: Excimer laser atherectomy. The greening of Sisyphus. Circulation *81*:2018, 1990.
296. Karsch, K. R., Haase, K. K., Voelker, W., et al.: Percutaneous coronary excimer laser angioplasty in patients with stable and unstable angina pectoris. Circulation *81*:1849, 1990.
297. Veith, F. J., Bakal, C. W., Cynamon, J., et al.: Early experience with the smart laser in treatment of atherosclerotic occlusion. Am. Heart J. *121*:1531, 1991.
298. Sanborn, T. A., Bittl, J. A., Hershman, R. A., and Siegel, R. M.: Percutaneous coronary excimer laser-assisted angioplasty: Initial multicenter experience in 141 patients. J. Am. Coll. Cardiol. (Suppl. B) *17*:169B, 1991.
298a. Sanborn, T. A., Torre, S. R., Sharma, S. K., et al.: Percutaneous coronary excimer laser-assisted balloon angioplasty: Initial clinical and quantitative angiographic results in 50 patients. J. Am. Coll. Cardiol. *17*:94, 1991.
299. Hillis, L. D.: Efficacy and safety of coronary balloon angioplasty and directional atherectomy. Circulation *82*:305, 1990.
300. Safian, R. D., Gelbfish, J. S., Erny, R. E., et al.: Coronary atherectomy. Clinical, angiographic, and histological findings and observations regarding potential mechanisms. Circulation *82*:69, 1990.

CORONARY ARTERY BYPASS SURGERY

301. Kaiser, G. C.: CABG 1984: technical aspects of bypass surgery. Circulation *72*(Suppl. V):46, 1985.
302. Grondin, C. M., Campeau, L., Thornton, J. C., et al.: Coronary artery bypass grafting with saphenous vein. Circulation *79*(Suppl. I):24, 1989.
303. Preito, I., Basil, E. F., and Abdulnou, R. E.: Upper extremity vein graft for aortocoronary bypass. Ann. Thorac. Surg. *37*:218, 1984.

304. Stoney, W. S., Alford, W. C., Burrus, G. R., et al.: The fate of arm vein grafts used for coronary artery bypass grafts. J. Thorac. Cardiovasc. Surg. *88*:522, 1984.
305. Campeau, L., Enjalbert, M., Lesperance, J., et al.: Atherosclerosis and late closure of aortocoronary saphenous vein grafts: Sequential angiographic studies at 2 weeks, 1 year, 5 to 7 years, and 10 to 12 years after surgery. Circulation *68*(Suppl. II):1, 1983.
306. Green, G. E.: Use of internal thoracic artery for coronary artery grafting. Circulation *79*(Suppl. I):30, 1989.
307. Luscher, T. F., Diederich, D., Siebenmann, R., et al.: Difference between endothelium-dependent relaxation in arterial and in venous coronary bypass grafts. N. Engl. J. Med. *319*:462, 1988.
308. Loop, F. D., Lytle, B. W., and Cosgrove, D. M.: New arteries for old. Circulation *79*(Suppl. I):40, 1989.
309. Shelton, M. E., Forman, M. B., Virmani, R., et al.: A comparison of morphologic and angiographic findings in long-term internal mammary artery and saphenous vein bypass grafts. J. Am. Coll. Cardiol. *11*:297, 1988.
310. Loop, F. D., Lytle, B. W., Cosgrove, D. M., et al.: Influence of the internal mammary artery graft on 10-year survival and other cardiac events. N. Engl. J. Med. *314*:1, 1986.
311. Kirklin, J. W., Naftel, D. C., Blackstone, E. H., and Pohost, G. M.: Summary of a consensus concerning death and ischemic events after coronary artery bypass grafting. Circulation *79*(Suppl. I):81, 1989.
312. Cameron, A., Davis, K. B., Green, G. E., et al.: Clinical implications of internal mammary bypass grafts: The Coronary Artery Surgery Study experience. Circulation *77*:815, 1988.
313. Morris, J. J., Smith, R., Glower, D. D., et al.: Clinical evaluation of single versus multiple mammary artery bypass. Circulation *82*(Suppl. IV):214, 1990.
314. Foster, E. D., and Kranc, M. A.: Alternative conduits for aortocoronary bypass grafting. Circulation *79*(Suppl. I):34, 1989.
315. Kusukawa, J., Hirota, Y., Kawamura, K., et al.: Efficacy of coronary artery bypass surgery with gastroepiploic artery. Assessment with thallium-201 myocardial scintigraphy. Circulation *79*(Suppl. I):135, 1989.
316. Mills, N. L., and Everson, C. T.: Right gastroepiploic artery: A third arterial conduit for coronary artery bypass. Ann. Thorac. Surg. *47*:706, 1989.
317. Smith, S. C., Jr., Gorlin, R., Herman, M. V., et al.: Myocardial blood flow in man. Effect of coronary collateral circulation and coronary artery bypass surgery. J. Clin. Invest. *51*:2556, 1972.
318. Lesperance, J., Bourassa, M. G., Biron, P., et al.: Aorta to coronary artery saphenous vein grafts. Preoperative angiographic criteria for successful surgery. Am. J. Cardiol. *30*:459, 1972.
319. Rosch, J., Dotter, C. T., Antonovic, R., et al.: Angiographic appraisal of distal vessel suitability for aortocoronary bypass graft surgery. Circulation *48*:202, 1973.
320. Cukingnan, R. A., Carey, J. S., Wittig, J. H., and Brown, B. G.: Influence of complete coronary revascularization on relief of angina. J. Thorac. Cardiovasc. Surg. *79*:188, 1980.
321. Grondin, C. M., Lapage, G., Castoguay, Y. R., et al.: Aortocoronary bypass graft. Initial blood flow through the graft, and early postoperative patency. Circulation *44*:815, 1971.
322. Califf, R. M., Harrell, F. E., Lee, K. L., et al.: The evolution of medical and surgical therapy for coronary artery disease. A 15-year perspective. JAMA *261*:2077, 1989.
323. Christakis, G. T., Ivanov, J., Weisel, R. D., et al.: The changing pattern of coronary artery bypass surgery. Circulation *80*(Suppl. I):151, 1989.
324. Passamani, E., Davis, K. B., Gillespie, M. J., Killip, T., and the CASS principal investigators and their associates: A randomized trial of coronary artery bypass surgery. Survival of patients with a low ejection fraction. N. Engl. J. Med. *312*:1665, 1985.
325. Killip, T., Passamani, E., Davis, K., and the CASS Principal Investigators and their Associates: Coronary artery surgery study (CASS): A randomized trial of coronary bypass surgery. Eight-year follow-up and survival in patients with reduced ejection fraction. Circulation *72*(Suppl. V):102, 1985.
326. Pigott, J. D., Kouchoukos, N. T., Oberman, A., and Cutter, G. R.: Late results of surgical and medical therapy for patients with coronary artery disease and depressed left ventricular function. J. Am. Coll. Cardiol. *5*:1036, 1985.
327. Vigilante, G. J., Weintraub, W. S., Klein, L. W., et al.: Improved survival with coronary bypass surgery in patients with three-vessel coronary disease and abnormal left ventricular function. Matched case-control study in patient with potentially operable disease. Am. J. Med. *82*:697, 1987.
328. Mock, M. B., Fisher, L. D., Holmes, D. R., et al.: Comparison of effects of medical and surgical therapy on survival in severe angina pectoris and two-vessel coronary artery disease with and without left ventricular dysfunction. A coronary artery surgery study registry study. Am. J. Cardiol. *61*:1198, 1988.
329. Bounous, E. P., Mark, D. B., Pollock, B. G., et al.: Surgical survival benefits for coronary disease patients with left ventricular dysfunction. Circulation *78*(Suppl. I):151, 1988.
330. Proudfit, W. L., Kramer, J. R., Goormastic, M., and Loop, F. D.: Survival of patients with mild angina or myocardial infarction without angina; A comparison of medical and surgical treatment. Br. Heart J. *59*:641, 1988.
331. Daily, P. O.: Early and 5-year results for coronary artery bypass grafting. A benchmark for percutaneous transluminal coronary angioplasty. J. Thorac. Cardiovasc. Surg. *96*:67, 1989.
332. Myers, W. O., Davis, K., Foster, E. D., Maynard, C., and Kaiser, G. C.: Surgical survival in the Coronary Artery Surgery Study (CASS) Registry. Ann. Thorac. Surg. *40*:245, 1985.
332a. Gomberg, J., Klein, L. W., Seelaus, P., et al.: Surgical revascularization of left main coronary artery stenosis: Determinants of perioperative and long-term outcome in the 1980s. Am. Heart J. *116*:440, 1988.
333. Bolooki, H.: Emergency cardiac procedures in patients in cardiogenic shock due to complications of coronary artery disease. Circulation *79*(Suppl. I):137, 1989.
333a. Naunheim, K. S., Fiore, A. C., Wadley, J. J., et al.: The changing profile of the patient undergoing coronary artery bypass surgery. J. Am. Coll. Cardiol. *11*:494, 1988.
334. CASS Principal Investigators and their Associates: Coronary Artery Surgery Study (CASS): A randomized trial of coronary artery bypass surgery. Survival data. Circulation *68*:939, 1983.
335. Chaitman, B. R., Alderman, E. L., Sheffield, L. T., et al.: Use of survival analysis to determine the clinical significance of new Q waves after coronary bypass surgery. Circulation *67*:302, 1983.
336. Force, T., Hibberd, P., Weeks, G., et al.: Perioperative myocardial infarction after coronary artery bypass. Clinical significance and approach to risk stratification. Circulation *82*:903, 1990.
337. Shaw, P. J., Bates, D., Cartlidge, N.E.F., et al.: Early intellectual dysfunction following coronary bypass surgery. Q. J. Med. *58*:59, 1986.
338. Raymond, M., Conklin, C., Schaeffer, J., et al.: Coping with transient intellectual dysfunction after coronary bypass surgery. Heart Lung *13*:531, 1984.
339. Mullen, J. C., Miller, D. R., Weisel, R. D., et al.: Postoperative hypertension: A comparison of diltiazem, nifedipine, and nitroprusside. J. Thorac. Cardiovasc. Surg. *96*:122, 1988.
340. Durkin, M. A., Thys, D., Morris, R. B., et al.: Control of perioperative hypertension during coronary artery surgery. A randomized double-blind study comparing isosorbide dinitrare and nitroglycerin. Eur. Heart J. *9*:A-181, 1988.
341. Gray, R. J., Bateman, T. M., Czer, L.S.C., et al.: Use of esmolol in hypertension after cardiac surgery. Am. J. Cardiol. *56*:49F, 1985.
342. Tuzcu, E. M., Emre, A., Goormastic, M., et al.: Incidence and prognostic significance of intraventricular conduction abnormalities after coronary bypass surgery. J. Am. Coll. Cardiol. *16*:607, 1990.
343. Koshal, A., Hendry, P., Roman, S. V., and Keon, W. J.: Should obese patients not undergo coronary artery surgery? Can. J. Surg. *28*:331, 1985.
344. McDonald, W. S., Brame, M., Sharp, C., and Eggerstedt, J.: Risk factors for median sternotomy dehiscence in cardiac surgery. South. Med. J. *82*:1361, 1989.
345. Utley, J. R., Thomason, M. E., Wallace, D. J., et al.: Preoperative correlates of impaired wound healing after saphenous vein excision. J. Thorac. Cardiovasc. Surg. *98*:147, 1989.
346. Rutherford, J. D., Whitlock, R. M. L., McDonald, B. W., et al.: Multivariate analysis of the long-term results of coronary artery bypass grafting performed during 1976 and 1977. Am. J. Cardiol. *57*:1264, 1986.
347. European Coronary Surgery Study Group: Long-term results of prospective randomized study of coronary artery bypass surgery in stable angina pectoris. Lancet *2*:1173, 1982.
348. CASS Principal Investigators and their Associates: Coronary Artery Surgery Study (CASS): A randomized trial of coronary artery bypass surgery. Quality of life in patients randomly assigned to treatment groups. Circulation *68*:951, 1983.
349. Hultgren, H. M., Peduzzi, P., Detre, K., Takaro, T., and the study participants: The 5-year effect of bypass surgery on relief of angina and exercise performance. Circulation *72*(Suppl. V):79, 1985.
350. Johnson, W. D., Kayser, K. L., and Pedraza, P. M.: Angina pectoris and coronary bypass surgery: Patterns of prevalence and recurrence in 3105 consecutive patients followed up to 11 years. Am. Heart J. *108*:1190, 1984.
351. Wenger, N. K.: Rehabilitation of the coronary patient: status 1986. Prog. Cardiovasc. Dis. *29*:181, 1986.
352. Hymowitz, Z., Freiman, I., Borman, J., et al.: Work status before and after coronary artery bypass surgery. Publ. Health (Lond.) *99*:367, 1985.
353. Misra, K. K., Kazanchi, B. N., Davies, G. J., et al.: Determinants of work capability and employment after coronary artery surgery. Eur. Heart J. *6*:176, 1985.
354. Sergeant, P., Lesaffire, E., Flameng, W., and Suy, R.: How predictable is the postoperative work resumption after aortocoronary bypass surgery? Acta Cardiologica *41*:41, 1986.
355. Hall, R.: Coronary artery bypass long-term follow-up on 22,284 consecutive patients. Circulation *68*(Suppl. II):20, 1983.
356. Stanton, B., Jenkins, C. D., Savageau, J. A., and Thurer, R. L.: Functional benefits following coronary artery bypass graft surgery. Ann. Thorac. Surg. *37*:286, 1984.
357. Peduzzi, P., Hultgren, H., Thomsen, J., and Detre, K.: Ten-year effect of medical and surgical therapy on quality of life: Veterans Administration Cooperative Study of Coronary Artery Surgery. Am. J. Cardiol. *59*:1017, 1987.
358. Chesebro, J. H., Clements, I. P., Fuster, V., et al.: A platelet-inhibitor drug trial in coronary-artery bypass operations. Benefit of perioperative dipyridamole and aspirin therapy on early postoperative vein-graft patency. N. Engl. J. Med. *307*:73, 1982.
359. Sanz, G., Pajaron, A., Alegria, E., et al.: Prevention of early aortocoronary bypass occlusion by low-dose aspirin and dipyridamole. Circulation *82*:765, 1990.
360. Vlodaver, Z., and Edwards, J. E.: Pathologic changes in aortic-coronary arterial saphenous vein grafts. Circulation *44*:719, 1971.
361. Lie, J. T., Lawrie, G. M., and Morris, G. C.: Aortocoronary bypass saphenous vein graft atherosclerosis. Am. J. Cardiol. *40*:906, 1977.
361a. Fitzgibbon, G. M., Leach, A. J., Kafka, H. P., and Keon, W. J.: Coronary

bypass graft fate: Long-term angiographic study. J. Am. Coll. Cardiol. *17*:1075, 1991.

362. Rasmussen, S. L., Nielsen, S. L., Amtorp, O., et al.: 201-Thallium imaging as an indicator of graft patency after coronary artery bypass surgery. Eur. Heart J. *5*:494, 1984.
363. Kroncke, G. M., Kosolcharoen, P., Clayman, J. A., et al.: Five-year changes in coronary arteries of medical and surgical patients of the Veterans Administration randomized study of bypass surgery. Circulation *78*(Suppl. I):144, 1988.
364. Hwang, M. H., Meadows, W. R., Palac, R. T., et al.: Progression of native coronary artery disease at 10 years: Insights from a randomized study of medical versus surgical therapy for angina. J. Am. Coll. Cardiol. *16*:1066, 1990.
365. Goldman, S., Copeland, J., Moritz, T., et al.: Saphenous vein graft patency 1 year after coronary artery bypass surgery and effects of antiplatelet therapy: Results of a Veterans Administration Cooperative Study. Circulation *80*:1190, 1989.
366. Chesbro, J. H., Fuster, V., Elveback, L. R., et al.: Effect of dipyridamole and aspirin on late vein-graft patency after coronary bypass operations. N. Engl. J. Med. *310*:209, 1984.
367. Henderson, W. G., Goldman, S., Copeland, J. G., et al.: Antiplatelet or anticoagulant therapy after coronary artery bypass surgery. A meta-analysis of clinical trials. Ann. Intern. Med. *111*:743, 1989.
368. Fitzgerald, G. A.: Dipyridamole. N. Engl. J. Med. *316*:1247, 1987.
368a. Gavaghan, T. P., Gebski, V., and Baron, D. W.: Immediate postoperative aspirin improves vein graft patency early and late after coronary artery bypass graft surgery. A placebo-controlled, randomized study. Circulation *83*:1526, 1991.
369. Goldman, S., Copeland, J., Moritz, T., et al.: Improvement in early saphenous vein graft patency after coronary artery bypass surgery with antiplatelet therapy: Results of a Veterans Administration Cooperative Study. Circulation *77*:1324, 1988.
370. Goldman, S., Copeland, J., Moritz, T., et al.: Internal mammary and saphenous vein graft patency. Circulation *82*(Suppl. IV):237, 1990.
370a. Sethi, G. K., Copeland, J. G., Goldman, S., et al.: Implications of preoperative administration of aspirin in patients undergoing coronary artery bypass grafting. J. Am. Coll. Cardiol. *15*:15, 1990.
371. Campeau, L., Enjalbert, M., Lesperance, J., et al.: The relation of risk factors to the development of atherosclerosis in saphenous-vein bypass grafts and the progression of disease in the native circulation. A study 10 years after aortocoronary bypass surgery. N. Engl. J. Med. *311*:1329, 1984.
372. Hoff, H. F., Beck, G. J., Skibinski, C. I., et al.: Serum LP(A) level as a predictor of vein graft stenosis after coronary artery bypass surgery in patients. Circulation *77*:1238, 1988.
373. Blankenhorn, D. H., Nessim, S. A., Johnson, R. L., et al.: Beneficial effects of combined colestipol-niacin therapy on coronary atherosclerosis and coronary vein bypass grafts. JAMA *257*:3233, 1987.
374. Solymoss, B. C., Nadeau, P., Millette, D., and Campeau, L.: Late thrombosis of saphenous vein bypass grafts related to risk factors. Circulation *78*(I):140–143, 1988.
375. Varnauskas, E., and The European Coronary Surgery Study Group: Twelve-year follow-up of survival in the randomized European Coronary Surgery Study. N. Engl. J. Med. *319*:332, 1988.
376. Devineni, R., and McKenzie, F. N.: Surgery for coronary artery disease in patients with diabetes mellitus. Can. J. Surg. *28*:367, 1985.
377. Hertzer, N. R., Young, J. R., Beven, E. G., et al.: Late results of coronary bypass in patients with peripheral vascular disease. II. Five-year survival according to sex, hypertension, and diabetes. Cleve. Clin. J. Med. *54*:15, 1987.
378. Lytle, B. W., Kramer, J. R., Golding, L. R., et al.: Young adults with coronary atherosclerosis: 10-year results of surgical myocardial revascularization. J. Am. Coll. Cardiol. *4*:445, 1984.
379. Fitzgibbon, G. M., Hamilton, M. G., Leach, A. J., et al.: Coronary artery disease and coronary bypass grafting in young men: Experience with 138 subjects 39 years of age and younger. J. Am. Coll. Cardiol. *9*:977, 1987.
380. Kannel, W. B., and Feinlieb, M.: Natural history of angina pectoris in the Framingham study: Progress and survival. Am. J. Cardiol. *29*:154, 1972.
381. Frank, C. W., Weinblatt, W., and Shapiro, S.: Angina pectoris in men: Prognostic significance of related medical factors. Circulation *47*:509, 1973.
382. Vedin, A., Wilhelmsson, C., Elmfeldt, D., et al.: Death and non-fatal reinfarctions during two years' follow-up after myocardial infarction. Acta Med. Scand. *198*:353, 1975.
383. Graham, i., Mulcahy, R., Hickey, N., et al.: Natural history of coronary heart disease: A study of 586 men surviving an initial acute attack. Am. Heart J. *105*:249, 1983.
384. Kaiser, G. C., Davis, K. B., Fisher, L. D., et al.: Survival following coronary artery bypass grafting in patients with severe angina pectoris (CASS). J. Thorac. Cardiovasc. Surg. *89*:513, 1985.
385. Detre, K., Peduzzi, P., Murphy, M., et al.: Effect of bypass surgery on survival in patients with low- and high-risk groups delineated by the use of simple clinical variables. Circulation *63*:1329, 1981.
386. Harlan, W. R., Oberman, A., Grimm, R., and Rosati, R. A.: Chronic congestive heart failure in coronary artery disease: Clinical criteria. Ann. Intern. Med. *86*:133, 1977.
387. Sanz, G., Castaner, A., Betriu, A., et al.: Determinants of prognosis in survivors of myocardial infarction. A prospective clinical angiographic study. N. Engl. J. Med. *306*:1065, 1982.
388. Mock, M. B., Ringqvist, I., Fisher, L. D., et al.: Survival of medically treated patients in the Coronary Artery Surgery Study (CASS) Registry. Circulation *66*:562, 1982.
389. Califf, R. M., Tomabechi, Y., Lee, K. L., et al.: Outcome in one-vessel coronary artery disease. Circulation *67*:283, 1983.
390. Nestico, P. F., Hakki, A. -H., Meissner, M. D., et al.: Effect of collateral vessels on prognosis in patients with one-vessel coronary artery disease. J. Am. Coll. Cardiol. *6*:1257, 1985.
391. Humphries, J. O., Kuller, L., Ross, R. S., et al.: Natural history of ischemic heart disease in relation to angiographic findings. Circulation *49*:489, 1974.
392. Proudfit, W. J., Bruschke, A. V. G., MacMillan, J. P., et al.: Fifteen-year survival study of patients with obstructive coronary artery disease. Circulation *68*:986, 1983.
393. Harris, P. J., Behar, V. S., Conley, M. J., et al.: The prognostic significance of 50 per cent coronary stenosis in medically treated patients with coronary artery disease. Circulation *62*:240, 1980.
394. Conley, M. J., Ely, R. L., Kisslo, J., et al.: The prognostic spectrum of left main stenosis. Circulation *57*:947, 1978.
395. Conti, C. R., Selby, J. H., and Christie, L. G.: Left main coronary artery stenosis: Clinical spectrum, pathophysiology and management. Progr. Cardiovasc. Dis. *22*:73, 1979.
396. Talano, J., Scanlon, P., Meadows, W., et al.: Influence of surgery on survival in 145 patients with left main coronary artery disease. Circulation *51, 52*(Suppl. I):105, 1975.
397. Taylor, H. A., Deumite, N. J., Chaitman, B. R., et al.: Asymptomatic left main coronary artery disease in the coronary artery surgery study (CASS) registry. Circulation *79*:1171, 1989.
398. Kent, K. M., Rosing, D. R., Ewels, C. J., et al.: Prognosis of asymptomatic or mildly symptomatic patients with coronary artery disease. Am. J. Cardiol. *49*:1823, 1982.
399. Ryan, T. J., Weiner, D. A., McCabe, C. H., et al.: Exercise testing in the Coronary Artery Surgery Study randomized population. Circulation *72*(Suppl. V):31, 1985.
400. Weiner, D. A., Ryan, T. J., McCabe, C. H., et al.: Prognostic importance of a clinical profile and exercise test in medically treated patients with coronary artery disease. J. Am. Coll. Cardiol. *3*:772, 1984.
401. Lee, K. L., Pryor, D. B., Pieper, K. S., et al.: Prognostic value of radionuclide angiography in medically treated patients with coronary artery disease. A comparison with clinical and catheterization variables. Circulation *82*:1705, 1990.
402. Jones, R. H., Floyd, R. D., Austin, E. H., and Sabiston, D. C.: The role of radionuclide angiography in the preoperative prediction of pain relief and prolonged survival following coronary artery bypass grafting. Ann. Surg. *197*:743, 1983.
403. Kronenberg, M. W., Pederson, R. W., Harston, W. E., et al.: Left ventricular performance after coronary artery bypass surgery. Ann. Intern. Med. *99*:305, 1983.
404. Bonow, R. O., Kent, K. M., Rosing, D. R., et al.: Exercise-induced ischemia in mildly symptomatic patients with coronary artery disease and preserved left ventricular function. N. Engl. J. Med. *311*:1339, 1984.
404a. Report of Inter-Society Commission for Heart Disease Resources: Optimal resources for coronary artery surgery. Circulation *46*:A–325, 1972.
405. Kaiser, G. C., Schaff, H. V., and Killip, T.: Myocardial revascularization for unstable angina pectoris. Circulation *79*(Suppl. I):60, 1989.
406. Kouchoukos, N. T., Murphy, S., Philpott, T., et al.: Coronary artery bypass grafting for postinfarction angina pectoris. Circulation *79*(Suppl. I):68, 1989.
407. Cameron, A., Kemp, H. G., and Green, G. E.: Reoperation of coronary artery disease. 10 years of clinical follow-up. Circulation *78*(Suppl. I):158, 1988.
408. Rogers, W. J., Coggin, J., Gersh, B. J., et al.: Ten-year follow-up quality of life in patients randomized to receive medical therapy or coronary artery bypass graft surgery. The coronary artery surgery study (CASS). Circulation *82*:1647, 1990.
408a. American College of Cardiology/American Heart Association Task Force on Assessment of Diagnostic and Therapeutic Cardiovascular Procedures (Subcommittee on Coronary Artery Bypass Graft Surgery): Guidelines and indications for coronary artery bypass graft surgery. J. Am. Coll. Cardiol. *17*:543, 1991.
409. Pryor D. B., Harrell, F. E., Rankin, S. J., et al.: The changing survival benefits of coronary revascularization over time. Circulation *76*(Suppl. V):13, 1987.
410. Takaro, T., Pifarre, R., and Fish, R.: Left main coronary artery disease. Progr. Cardiovasc. Dis. *28*:229, 1985.
411. Chaitman, B. P., Fisher, L. D., and Bourassa, M. G.: Effect of coronary bypass surgery on survival patterns in subsets of patients with left main coronary artery disease. Report of the Collaborative Study in Coronary Artery Surgery (CASS). Am. J. Cardiol. *48*:765, 1981.
412. Califf, R. M., Conley, M. J., Behar, V. S., et al.: "Left main equivalent" coronary artery disease: Its clinical presentation and prognostic significance with nonsurgical therapy. Am. J. Cardiol. *53*:1489, 1984.
413. Chaitman, B. R., Davis, K. B., Kaiser, G. C., et al.: The role of coronary bypass surgery for "left main equivalent" coronary disease: The Coronary Artery Surgery Study Registry. Circulation *74*(Suppl. III):17, 1986.
414. Detre, K. M., Takaro, T., Hultgren, H., Peduzzi, P., and the Study Participants: Long-term mortality and morbidity results of the Veterans Administration randomized trial of coronary artery bypass surgery. Circulation *72*(Suppl. V):84, 1985.
415. Peduzzi, P., Detre, K., Murphy, M. L.: Ten-year incidence of myocardial infarction and prognosis after infarction: Department of Veterans Af-

fairs Cooperative study of coronary artery bypass surgery. Circulation 83:747, 1991.

416. Detre, K., Peduzzi, P., Scott, S. M., and Davies, B.: Long-term survival results in medically and surgically randomized patients. Progr. Cardiovasc. Dis. 28:235, 1985.

417. The Veterans Administration Coronary Artery Bypass Surgery Cooperative Study Group: Eleven-year survival in the Veterans Administration randomized trial of coronary bypass surgery for stable angina. N. Engl. J. Med. 311:1333, 1984.

418. Varnauskas, E., and the European Coronary Surgery Study Group: Survival, myocardial infarction, and employment status in a prospective randomized study of coronary bypass surgery. Circulation 72(Suppl. V):90, 1985.

419. Alderman, E. L., Bourassa, M. G., Cohen, L. S., et al.: Ten-year follow-up of survival and myocardial infarction in the randomized coronary artery surgery study. Circulation 82:1629, 1990.

420. Myers, W. O., Martshfield, W. I., Gersh, B. J., et al.: Medical versus early surgical therapy in patients with triple-vessel disease and mild angina pectoris: A CASS registry study of survival. Ann. Thorac. Surg. 44:471, 1987.

421. Myers, W. O., Schaff, H. V., Gersh, B. J., et al.: Improved survival of surgically treated patients with triple vessel coronary artery disease and severe angina pectoris. J. Thorac. Cardiovasc. Surg. 97:487, 1989.

422. Iskandrian, A. S., Hakki, A.-H., Goel, I. P., et al.: The use of rest and exercise radionuclide ventriculography in risk stratification in patients with suspected coronary artery disease. Am. Heart J. 110:864, 1985.

423. Alderman, E. L., Fisher, L. D., Litwin, P., et al.: Results of coronary artery surgery in patients with poor left ventricular function (CASS). Circulation 68:785, 1983.

424. Nwasokwa, O. N., Koss, J. H., Friedman, G. H., et al.: Bypass surgery for chronic stable angina: Predictors of survival benefit and strategy for patient selection. Ann. Intern. Med. 114:1035, 1991.

424a. Bonow, R. O., Dilsizian, V., Cucolo, A., and Bacharach, S. L.: Identification of viable myocardium in patients with chronic coronary artery disease and left ventricular dysfunction: Comparison of thallium scintigraphy with reinjection and PET imaging with 18F-fluorodeoxyglucose. Circulation 83:26, 1991.

425. Tillisch, J., Brunken, R., Marshall, R., et al.: Reversibility of cardiac wall-motion abnormalities predicted by positron tomography. N. Engl. J. Med. 314:884, 1986.

426. Shanes, J. G., Kondos, G. T., Levitsky, S., et al.: Coronary artery obstruction: A potentially reversible cause of dilated cardiomyopathy. Am. Heart J. 110:173, 1985.

427. Shearn, D. L., and Brent, B. N.: Coronary artery bypass surgery in patients with left ventricular dysfunction. Am. J. Med. 80:405, 1986.

428. Lim, Y. L., Kalff, V., Kelly, M. J., et al.: Radionuclide angiographic assessment of global and segmental left ventricular function at rest and during exercise after coronary artery bypass graft surgery. Circulation 66:972, 1982.

429. Kolibash, A. J., Goodenow, J. S., Bush, C. A., et al.: Improvement of myocardial perfusion and left ventricular function after coronary artery bypass grafting patients with unstable angina. Circulation 59:66, 1979.

430. Topol, E. J., Weiss, J. L., Guzman, P. A., et al.: Immediate improvement of dysfunctional myocardial segments after coronary revascularization: Detection by intraoperative transesophageal echocardiography. J. Am. Coll. Cardiol. 4:1123, 1984.

431. Cohen, M., Charney, R., Hershman, R., et al.: Reversal of chronic ischemic myocardial dysfunction after transluminal coronary angioplasty. J. Am. Coll. Cardiol. 12:1193, 1988.

432. Carlson, E. B., Cowley, M. J., Wolfgang, T. C., and Vetrovec, G. W.: Acute changes in global and regional rest left ventricular function after successful coronary angioplasty: Comparative results in stable and unstable angina. J. Am. Coll. Cardiol. 13:1262, 1989.

433. Wijns, W., Serruys, P. W., Slager, C. J., et al.: Effect of coronary occlusion during percutaneous transluminal angioplasty in humans on left ventricular chamber stiffness and regional diastolic pressure-radius relations. J. Am. Coll. Cardiol. 7:455, 1986.

434. Mathias, P., Kerin, N. Z., Blevins, R. D., et al.: Coronary vasospasm as a cause of stunned myocardium. Am. Heart J. 113:383, 1987.

435. Robertson, W. S., Feigenbaum, H., Armstrong, W. F., et al.: Exercise echocardiography: A clinically practical addition in the evaluation of coronary artery disease. J. Am. Coll. Cardiol. 6:1085, 1983.

436. Ballantyne, C. M., Verani, M. S., Short, H. D., et al.: Delayed recovery of severely "stunned" myocardium with the support of a left ventricular assist device after coronary artery bypass graft surgery. J. Am. Coll. Cardiol. 10:710, 1987.

436a. Ross, J., Jr.: Myocardial perfusion-contraction matching: Implications for coronary heart disease and hibernation. Circulation 83:1076, 1991.

436b. Lewis, S. J., Sawada, S. G., Ryan, T., et al.: Segmental wall motion abnormalities in the absence of clinically documented myocardial infarction: Clinical significance and evidence of hibernating myocardium. Am. Heart. J. 121:1088, 1991.

436c. Bonow, R. O., Dilsizian, V., Cuocolo, A., and Bacharach, S. L.: Identification of viable myocardium in patients with chronic coronary artery disease and left ventricular dysfunction: Comparison of thallium scintigraphy with reinjection and PET imaging with ^{18}F-fluorodeoxyglucose. Circulation 83:26, 1991.

437. Gersh, B. J., Califf, R. M., Loop, F. D., et al.: Coronary bypass surgery in chronic stable angina. Circulation 79(Suppl. I):46, 1989.

438. Balu, V., Szmedra, L., Dean, D., and Bhayana, J.: Long-term survival of patients with low ejection fraction. Tex. Heart Inst. J. 15:44, 1988.

439. Holmes, D. R., Davis, K. B., Mock, M. B., et al.: The effect of medical and surgical treatment on subsequent sudden cardiac death in patients with coronary artery disease: A report from the Coronary Artery Surgery Study. Circulation 73:1254, 1986.

440. Ellis, S., Alderman, E. L., Cain, K., et al.: Morphology of left anterior descending coronary artery lesions as a predictor of anterior myocardial infarction. A CASS Registry Study. J. Am. Coll. Cardiol. 13:1481, 1989.

441. Mazzotta, G., Bonow, R. O., Pace, L., et al.: Relation between exertional ischemia and prognosis in mildly symptomatic patients with single or double vessel coronary artery disease and left ventricular dysfunction at rest. J. Am. Coll. Cardiol. 13:567, 1989.

442. Murphy, M. L., Meadows, W. R., Thomsen, J., et al.: The effect of coronary artery bypass surgery on the incidence of myocardial infarction and hospitalization. Progr. Cardiovasc. Dis. 28:309, 1986.

443. CASS principal investigators and their associates: Myocardial infarction and mortality in the Coronary Artery Surgery Study (CASS) randomized trial. N. Engl. J. Med. 310:750, 1984.

444. Myers, W. O., Schaff, H. V., Fisher, L. D., et al.: Time to first new myocardial infarction in patients with severe angina and three-vessel disease comparing medical and early surgical therapy: A CASS registry study of survival. J. Thorac. Cardiovasc. Surg. 95:382, 1988.

444a. Peduzzi, P., Detre, K., Murphy, M. L., et al.: Ten-year incidence of myocardial infarction and prognosis after infarction. Department of Veterans Affairs Cooperative Study of Coronary Artery Bypass Surgery. Circulation 83:747, 1991.

444b. Kirklin, J. W., Akins, C. W., Blackstone, E. H., et al.: ACC/AHA guidelines and indications for coronary artery bypass graft surgery. A report of the American College of Cardiology/American Heart Association Task Force on assessment of diagnostic and therapeutic cardiovascular procedures. Circulation 83:1125, 1991.

445. Loop, F. D., Golding, L. R., Macmillan, J. P., et al.: Coronary artery surgery in women compared with men: analyses or risks and long-term results. J. Am. Coll. Cardiol. 1:383, 1983.

446. Fisher, L. D., Kennedy, J. W., Davis, K. B., et al.: Association of sex, physical size, and operative mortality after coronary artery bypass in the Coronary Artery Surgery Study (CASS). J. Thorac. Cardiovasc. Surg. 84:334, 1982.

447. Gersh, B. J., Kronmal, R. A., Schaff, H. V., et al.: Comparison of coronary artery bypass surgery and medical therapy in patients 65 years of age or older. N. Engl. J. Med. 313:217, 1985.

448. Montague, N. T., Kouchoukos, N. T., Wilson, T.A.S., et al.: Morbidity and mortality of coronary bypass grafting in patients 70 years of age and older. Ann. Thorac. Surg. 39:552, 1985.

449. Roberts, A. J., Woodhall, D. D., Conti, C. R., et al.: Mortality, morbidity, and cost-accounting related to coronary artery bypass graft surgery in the elderly. Ann. Thorac. Surg. 39:426, 1985.

450. Rose, D. M., Gelbfish, J., Jacobowitz, I. J., et al.: Analysis of morbidity and mortality in patients 70 years of age and over undergoing isolated coronary artery bypass surgery. Am. Heart J. 110:361, 1985.

451. Ennabli, K., and Pelletier, L. C.: Morbidity and mortality of coronary artery surgery after the age of 70 years. Ann. Thorac. Surg. 42:197, 1986.

452. Rich, M. W., Keller, A. J., Schechtman, K. B., et al.: Increased complications and prolonged hospital stay in elderly cardiac surgical patients with low serum albumin. Am. J. Cardiol. 63:714, 1989.

452a. Hammermeister, K. E., Burchfiel, C., Johnson, R., and Grover, F. L.: Identification of patients at greatest risk for developing major complications at cardiac surgery. Circulation 82(Suppl. IV):380, 1990.

453. Foster, E. D., Fisher, L. D., Kaiser, G. C., et al.: Comparison of operative mortality and morbidity results for initial and repeat coronary artery bypass grafting: The Coronary Artery Surgery Study (CASS) Registry experience. Ann. Thorac. Surg. 38:563, 1984.

454. Lamas, G. A., Mudge, G. H., Collins, J. J., et al.: Clinical response to coronary reoperations. J. Am. Coll. Cardiol. 8:274, 1986.

455. Osaka, S., Barratt Boyes, B. G., Brandt, P. W., et al.: Early and late results of re-operation for coronary artery disease: A 13-year experience. Aust. N. Z. J. Surg. 58:537, 1988.

455a. Verheul, H. A., Moulijn, A. C., Hondema, S., et al.: Late results of 200 repeat coronary artery bypass operations. Am. J. Cardiol. 67:24, 1991.

456. Brenowitz, J. B., Johnson, D., Kayser, K. L., et al.: Coronary artery bypass grafting for the third time or more. Results of 150 consecutive cases. Circulation 78(Suppl. I):166, 1988.

457. Schaff, H. V., Orzulak, T. A., Gersh, B. J., et al.: The morbidity and mortality of reoperation for coronary artery disease and analysis of late results with use of actuarial estimate of event-free interval. J. Thorac. Cardiovasc. Surg. 85:508, 1983.

458. Brener, B. J., Brief, D. K., Alpert, J., et al.: A four-year experience with preoperative noninvasive carotid evaluation of 2,026 patients undergoing cardiac surgery. J. Vasc. Surg. 1:326, 1984.

459. Gardner, T. J., Horneffer, P. J., Manolio, T. A., et al.: Stroke following coronary artery bypass grafting: A ten-year study. Ann. Thorac. Surg. 40:574, 1985.

460. Feussner, J. R., and Matchar, D. B.: When and how to study the carotid arteries. Ann. Intern. Med. 109:805, 1988.

461. Reed, G. L., Singer, D. E., Picard, E. H., DeSanctis, R.: Stroke following coronary-artery bypass surgery. A case-control estimate of the risk from carotid bruits. N. Engl. J. Med. 319:1246, 1988.

462. Beebe, H. G., Clagett, G. P., DeWeese, J. A., et al.: Assessing risk associated with carotid endarterectomy. Circulation 79:472, 1989.

463. Grotta, J. C.: Current medical and surgical therapy for cerebrovascular disease. N. Engl. J. Med. 317:1505, 1987.

464. Babu, S. C., Shah, P. M., Singh, B. M., et al.: Coexisting carotid stenosis in patients undergoing cardiac surgery: Indications and guidelines for simultaneous operations. Am. J. Surg. *150*:207, 1985.
465. David, T. E.: Combined cardiac and abdominal aortic surgery. Circulation *72*(Suppl. II):18, 1985.
466. Jones, E. L., Craver, J. M., Michalik, R. A., et al.: Combined carotid and coronary operations: When are they necessary? J. Thorac. Cardiovasc. Surg. *87*:7, 1984.
467. Furlan, A. J., and Craciun, A. R.: Risk of stroke during coronary artery bypass graft surgery in patients with internal carotid artery disease documented by angiography. Stroke *16*:797, 1985.
468. Debakey, M. E., and Lawrie, G. M.: Combined coronary artery and peripheral vascular disease: Recognition and treatment. J. Vasc. Surg. *1*:605, 1984.
469. Boucher, C. A., Brewster, D. C., Darling, R. C., et al.: Determination of cardiac risk by dipyridamole-thallium imaging before peripheral vascular surgery. N. Engl. J. Med. *312*:389, 1985.

UNSTABLE ANGINA

469a. Bleifeld, W., Hamm, C. W., and Braunwald, E. (eds.): Unstable Angina. New York, Springer-Verlag, 1990, 270 pp.
470. Collins, P., and Fox, K. M.: Pathophysiology of angina. Lancet *1*:94, 1990.
471. Braunwald, E.: Unstable angina. A classification. Circulation *80*:410, 1989.
472. Chierchia, S., Brunelli, C., Simonetti, I., et al.: Sequence of events in angina at rest: Primary reduction in coronary blood flow. Circulation *61*:759, 1980.
473. Langer, A., Freeman, M. R., and Armstrong, P. W.: ST segment shift in unstable angina: Pathophysiology and association with coronary anatomy and hospital outcome. J. Am. Coll. Cardiol. *13*:1495, 1989.
474. Deanfield, J. E., Maseri, A., Selwyn, A. P., et al.: Myocardial ischaemia during daily life in patients with stable angina: Its relation to symptoms and heart rate changes. Lancet *2*:753, 1983.
475. Cohn, P. F., Brown, A. J., Jr., Wynne, J., et al.: Global and regional left ventricular ejection fraction abnormalities during exercise in patients with silent myocardial ischemia. J. Am. Coll. Cardiol. *1*:931, 1983.
476. Chierchia, S., Lazzari, M., Freedman, B., et al.: Impairment of myocardial perfusion and function during painless myocardial ischemia. J. Am. Coll. Cardiol. *1*:924, 1983.
477. Campbell, S., Barry, J., Rocco, M. B., et al.: Features of the exercise test that reflect the activity of ischemic heart disease out of hospital. Circulation *74*:72, 1986.
478. Nademanee, K., Intrachot, V., Josephson, M. A., et al.: Prognostic significance of silent myocardial ischemia in patients with unstable angina. J. Am. Coll. Cardiol. *10*:1, 1987.
479. Gottlieb, S. O., Weisfeldt, M. L., Ouyang, P., et al.: Silent ischemia as a marker for early unfavorable outcomes in patients with unstable angina. N. Engl. J. Med. *314*:1214, 1986.
480. Gottlieb, S. O., Weisfeldt, M. L., Ouyang, P., et al.: Silent ischemia predicts infarction and death during 2 years follow-up of unstable angina. J. Am. Coll. Cardiol. *10*:756, 1987.
480a. Bugiardini, R., Pozzati, A., Borghi, A., et al.: Angiographic morphology in unstable angina and its relation to transient myocardial ischemia and hospital outcome. Am. J. Cardiol. *67*:460, 1991.
481. McCormick, J. R., Schick, E. C., Jr., McCabe, C. H., et al.: Determinants of operative mortality and long-term survival in patients with unstable angina. The CASS experience. J. Thorac. Cardiovasc. Surg. *89*:683, 1985.
482. Roberts, K. B., Califf, R. M., Harrell, F. E., Jr., et al.: The prognosis for patients with new-onset angina who have undergone cardiac catheterization. Circulation *68*:970, 1983.
483. Parker, F. B., Jr., Neville, J. F., Jr., Hanson, E. C., and Webb, W. R.: Retrograde and antegrade pressures and flows in preinfarction syndrome. Circulation *50*(Suppl. II):122, 1974.
484. Roberts, W. C.: Qualitative and quantitative comparison of amounts of narrowing by atherosclerotic plaques in the major epicardial coronary arteries at necropsy in sudden coronary death, transmural acute myocardial infarction, transmural healed myocardial infarction and unstable angina pectoris. Am. J. Cardiol. *64*:324, 1989.
485. Freudenberg, H., and Lichtlen, P. R.: The normal segment in coronary stenosis—a postmortem study. Z. Kardiol. *70*:863, 1981.
486. Saner, G. E., Gobel, F. L., Salomonowitz, E., et al.: The disease-free wall in coronary atherosclerosis: Its relation to degree of obstruction. J. Am. Coll. Cardiol. *6*:1096, 1985.
487. Fuster, V., Stein, B., Ambrose, J. A., et al.: Atherosclerotic plaque rupture and thrombosis. Evolving concepts. Circulation *82*(Suppl. II):47, 1990.
488. Davies, M. J., and Thomas, A. C.: Plaque fissuring—The cause of acute myocardial infarction, sudden ischaemic death, and crescendo angina. Br. Heart J. *53*:363, 1985.
489. Moise, A., Theroux, P., Taeymans, Y., et al.: Unstable angina and progression of coronary atherosclerosis. N. Engl. J. Med. *309*:685, 1983.
490. Davies, M. J., Thomas, A. C., Knapman, P. A., and Hangartner, J. R.: Intramyocardial platelet aggregation in patients with unstable angina suffering sudden ischemic cardiac death. Circulation *73*:418, 1986.
491. Falk, E.: Unstable angina with fatal outcome: Dynamic coronary thrombosis leading to infarction and/or sudden death. Circulation *71*:699, 1985.
492. Ambrose, J. A., Hjemdahl-Monsen, C., Borrico, S., et al.: Quantitative and qualitative effects of intracoronary streptokinase in unstable angina and non-Q infarction. J. Am. Coll. Cardiol. *9*:1156, 1987.
493. Freeman, M. R., Williams, A. E., Chisholm, R. J., and Armstrong, P. W.: intracoronary thrombus and complex morphology in unstable angina. Relation to timing of angiography and in-hospital cardiac events. Circulation *80*:17, 1989.
494. Sherman, C. T., Litvack, F., Grundfest, W., et al.: Coronary angioscopy in patients with unstable angina pectoris. N. Engl. J. Med. *315*:913, 1986.
495. Speechia, G., De Servi, S., Falcon, C., et al.: Coronary arterial spasm as a cause of exercise-induced ST-segment elevation in patients with variant angina. Circulation *59*:948, 1979.
496. Haft, J. I., Haik, B. J., Goldstein, J. E., and Brodyn, N. E.: Development of significant coronary artery lesions in areas of minimal disease. A common mechanism for coronary disease progression. Chest *94*:731, 1988.
497. Folts, J. D., Crowell, E. B., and Rowe, G. G.: Platelet aggregation in partially obstructed vessels and its elimination with aspirin. Circulation *54*:365, 1976.
498. Grande, P., Grauholt, A.-M., and Madsen, J. K.: Unstable angina pectoris. Platelet behaviour and prognosis in progressive angina and intermediate coronary syndrome. Circulation *81*:(Suppl. I):16, 1990.
499. Willerson, J. T., Golino, P., Eidt, J., et al.: Specific platelet mediators and unstable coronary artery lesions. Experimental evidence and potential clinical implications. Circulation *80*:198, 1989.
500. Folts, J. D., Gallagher, K., and Rowe, G. G.: Blood flow reductions in stenosed canine coronary arteries: Vasospasm or platelet aggregation. Circulation *65*:248, 1982.
501. Lewis, H. D., Davis, J. W., Archibald, D. G., et al.: Protective effects of aspirin against acute myocardial infarction and death in men with unstable angina. N. Engl. J. Med. *309*:396, 1983.
502. Cairns, J. A., Gent, M., Singer, J., et al.: Aspirin, sulfinpyrazone, or both in unstable angina. Results of a Canadian multicenter trial. N. Engl. J. Med. *313*:1369, 1985.
503. Theroux, P., Ouimet, H., McCans, J., et al.: Aspirin, heparin, or both to treat unstable angina. N. Engl. J. Med. *319*:1105, 1988.
504. The RISC Group: Risk of myocardial infarction and death during treatment with low-dose aspirin and intravenous heparin in men with unstable coronary artery disease. Lancet *336*:827, 1990.
505. Kruskal, J. B., Commerford, P. J., Franks, J. J., et al.: Fibrin and fibrinogen related antigens in patients with stable and unstable coronary artery disease. N. Engl. J. Med. *317*:1361, 1987.
506. Zalewski, A., Shi, Y., Nardone, D., et al.: Evidence for reduced fibrinolytic activity in unstable angina at rest: Clinical, biochemical, and angiographic correlates. Circulation *83*:1685, 1991.
507. Gold, H. K., Johns, J. A., Leinbach, R. C., et al.: A randomized, blinded, placebo-controlled trial of recombinant human tissue-type plasminogen activator in patients with unstable angina pectoris. Circulation *75*:1192, 1987.
508. Brown, B. G., Bolson, E. L., and Dodge, H. T.: Dynamic mechanisms in human coronary stenosis. Circulation *70*:917, 1984.
509. Chesebro, J. H., Fuster, V., and Webster, M.W.I.: Endothelial injury and coronary vasomotion (editorial). J. Am. Coll. Cardiol. *14*:1191, 1989.
509a. Kaski, J. C., Tousoulis, D., Heider, A. W., et al.: Reactivity of eccentric and concentric coronary stenoses in patients with chronic stable angina. J. Am. Coll. Cardiol. *17*:627, 1991.
510. Zeiher, A. M., Drexler, H., Wollschlaeger, H., et al.: Coronary vasomotion in response to sympathetic stimulation in humans: Importance of the functional integrity of the endothelium. J. Am. Coll. Cardiol. *14*:1181, 1989.
511. Drexler, H., Zeiher, A. M., Wollschlager, H., et al.: Flow-dependent coronary artery dilatation in humans. Circulation *80*:466, 1989.
512. Cox, D. A., Vita, J. A., Treasure, C. B., et al.: Atherosclerosis impairs flow-mediated dilation of coronary arteries in humans. Circulation *80*:458, 1989.
513. Hodgson, J.M.B, and Marshall, J. J.: Direct vasoconstriction and endothelium-dependent vasocilation. Mechanisms of acetylcholine effects on coronary flow and arterial diameter in patients with nonstenotic coronary arteries. Circulation *79*:1043, 1989.
514. Vita, J. A., Treasure, C. B., Ganz, P., et al.: Control of shear stress in the epicardial coronary arteries of humans: Impairment by atherosclerosis. J. Am. Coll. Cardiol. *14*:1193, 1989.
515. Swahn, E., Areskog, M., Berglund, U., et al.: Predictive importance of clinical findings and a predischarge exercise test in patients with suspected unstable coronary artery disease. Am. J. Cardiol. *59*:208, 1987.
516. Severi, S., Orsini, E., Marraccini, P., et al.: The basal electrocardiogram and the exercise stress test in assessing prognosis in patients with unstable angina. Eur. Heart J. *4*:441, 1988.
517. Nixon, J. V., Brown, C. N., and Smitherman, T. C.: Identification of transient and persistent segmental wall motion abnormalities in patients with unstable angina by two-dimensional echocardiography. Circulation *65*:1497, 1982.
518. Brown, K. A., Okada, R. D., Boucher, C. A., et al.: Serial thallium-201 imaging at rest in patients with unstable and stable angina pectoris: Relationship of myocardial perfusion at rest to presenting clinical syndrome. Am. Heart J. *106*:70, 1983.
518a. Zhu, Y. Y., Chung, W. S., Botvinick, E. H., et al.: Dipyridamole perfusion scintigraphy: the experience with its application in one hundred seventy patients with known or suspected unstable angina. Am. Heart J. *121*:33, 1991.
519. Freeman, M. R., Williams, A. E., Chisholm, R. J., et al.: Role of resting thallium 201 perfusion in predicting coronary anatomy, left ventricular wall motion, and hospital outcome in unstable angina pectoris. Am. Heart J. *117*:306, 1989.
520. Younis, L. T., Byers, S., Shaw, L., et al.: Prognostic value of intravenous

dipyridamole thallium scintigraphy after an acute myocardial ischemic event. Am. J. Cardiol. *64*:161, 1989.

521. Freeman, M. R., Chisholm, R. J., and Armstrong, P. W.: Usefulness of exercise electrocardiography and thallium scintigraphy in unstable angina pectoris in predicting the extent and severity of coronary artery disease erratum published in Am. J. Cardiol. *63*:392, 1989. Am. J. Cardiol. *62*:1164, 1988.

521a. Brown, K. A.: Prognostic value of thallium-201 myocardial perfusion imaging in patients with unstable angina who respond to medical treatment. J. Am. Coll. Cardiol. *17*:1053, 1991.

522. Lin, S.-G., and Flaherty, J. T.: Crossover from intravenous to transdermal nitroglycerin therapy in unstable angina pectoris. Am. J. Cardiol. *56*:742, 1985.

523. Baaske, D. M., Amann, A. H., Wagenknecht, D. M., et al.: Nitroglycerin compatibility with intravenous fluid filters, containers, and administration sets. Am. J. Hosp. Pharm. *37*:201, 1980.

524. Necoechea, A.J.C., Camacho, J. P., Gil, D., et al.: Acute gouty arthritis and intravenous nitroglycerin. Arch. Intern. Med. *148*:2505, 1988.

525. Stamler, J., Cunningham, M., Loscalzo, J.: Reduced thiols and the effect of intravenous nitroglycerin on platelet aggregation. Am. J. Cardiol. *62*:377, 1988.

526. Horowitz, J. D., Henry, C. A., Syrjanen, M. L., et al.: Combined use of nitroglycerin and N-acetylcysteine in the management of unstable angina pectoris. Circulation *77*:787, 1988.

527. Jugdutt, B. I., and Warnica, J. W.: Tolerance with low dose intravenous nitroglycerin therapy in acute myocardial infarction. Am. J. Cardiol. *64*:581, 1989.

528. Figueras, J., Singh, B. N., Ganz, W., et al.: Mechanism of rest and nocturnal angina: Observations during continuous hemodynamic and electrocardiographic monitoring. Circulation *59*:955, 1979.

529. Hint Research Group: Early treatment of unstable angina in the coronary care unit: A randomized, double blind, placebo controlled comparison of recurrent ischaemia in patients treated with nifedipine or metoprolol or both. Br. Heart J. *56*:400, 1986.

530. Tijssen, J. G., and Lubsen, J.: Early treatment of unstable angina with nifedipine and metoprolol—the HINT trial. J. Cardiovasc. Pharmacol. *12*(Suppl. 71):1988.

531. Muller, J. E., Turi, Z. G., Pearle, D. L., et al.: Nifedipine and conventional therapy for unstable angina pectoris: A randomized, double-blind comparison. Circulation *69*:728, 1984.

532. Gottlieb, S. O., Weisfeldt, M. L., Ouyang, P., et al.: Effect of the addition of propranolol therapy with nifedipine for unstable angina pectoris: A randomized, double-blind, placebo-controlled trial. Circulation *73*:331, 1986.

533. Theroux, P., Taeymans, Y., Morissette, D., et al.: A randomized study comparing propranolol and diltiazem in the treatment of unstable angina. J. Am. Coll. Cardiol. *5*:717, 1985.

534. Wallis, D. E., Pope, C., Littman, W. J., and Scanlon, P. J.: Safety and efficacy of esmolol for unstable angina pectoris. Am. J. Cardiol. *62*:1033, 1988.

535. Kirshenbaum, J. M., Kloner, R. F., McGowan, N., and Antman, E. M.: Use of an ultrashort-acting beta-receptor blocker (esmolol) in patients with acute myocardial ischemia and relative contraindications to beta-blockade therapy. J. Am. Coll. Cardiol. *12*:773, 1988.

536. Held, P. H., Yusuf, S., and Furberg, C. D.: Calcium channel blockers in acute myocardial infarction and unstable angina: An overview. Br. Med. J. *2*:1187, 1989.

537. Gerstenblith, G., Ouyang, P., Achuff, S. C., et al.: Nifedipine in unstable angina: A double-blind, randomized trial. N. Engl. J. Med. *306*:885, 1982.

538. Telford, A. M., and Wilson, C.: Trial of heparin versus atenolol in prevention of myocardial infarction in intermediate coronary syndrome. Lancet *1*:1225, 1981.

539. Gardner, T. J., Stuart, R. S., Greene, P. S., and Baumgartner, W. A.: The risk of coronary bypass surgery for patients with postinfarction angina. Circulation *79*(Suppl. I):79, 1989.

540. Szatmary, L. J., Marco, J., Fajadet, J., and Caster, L.: The combined use of diastolic counterpulsation and coronary dilation in unstable angina due to multivessel disease under unstable hemodynamic conditions. Int. J. Cardiol. *19*:59, 1988.

541. Kantrowitz, A., Wasfie, T., Freed, P. S., et al.: Intraaortic balloon pumping 1967 through 1982: Analysis of complications in 733 patients. Am. J. Cardiol. *57*:976, 1986.

542. de Feyter, P. J., Suryapranata, H., Serruys, P. W., et al.: Effects of successful percutaneous transluminal coronary angioplasty on global and regional left ventricular function in unstable angina pectoris. Am. J. Cardiol. *60*:993, 1987.

543. Danchin, N., Haouzi, A., Amor, M., et al.: Sustained improvement in myocardial perfusion four to six years after PTCA in patients with a satisfactory angiographic result, six months after the procedure. Eur. Heart J. *9*:454, 1988.

544. Leeman, D. E., McCabe, C. H., Faxon, D. P., et al.: Use of percutaneous transluminal coronary angioplasty and bypass surgery despite improved medical therapy for unstable angina pectoris. Am. J. Cardiol. *61*:38G, 1988.

545. Timmis, A. D., Griffin, B., Crick, J. C., and Sowton, E.: Early percutaneous transluminal coronary angioplasty in the management of unstable angina. Int. J. Cardiol. *14*:25, 1987.

546. Kamp, O., Beatt, K. J., De Feyter, P. J., et al.: Short-, medium-, and long-term follow-up after percutaneous transluminal coronary angioplasty for stable and unstable angina pectoris. Am. Heart J. *117*:991, 1989.

547. Perry, R. A., Seth, A., Hunt, A., and Shiu, M. F.: Coronary angioplasty in unstable angina and stable angina: A comparison of success and complications. Br. Heart J. *60*:367, 1988.

548. De Feyter, P. J., Suryapranata, H., Serruys, P. W., et al.: Coronary angioplasty for unstable angina: immediate and late results in 200 consecutive patients with identification of risk factors for unfavorable early and late outcome. J. Am. Coll. Cardiol. *12*:324, 1988.

549. Halon, D. A., Merdler, A., Shefer, A., et al.: Identifying patients at high risk for restenosis after percutaneous transluminal coronary angioplasty for unstable angina pectoris. Am. J. Cardiol. *64*:289, 1989.

549a. Myler, R. K., Shaw, R. E., Stertzer, S. H., et al.: Unstable angina and coronary angioplasty. Circulation *82*(Suppl. II):88, 1990.

550. Steffenino, G., Meier, B., Finci, L., and Ruitshauer, W.: Followup results of treatment of unstable angina by coronary angioplasty. Br. Heart J. *57*:416, 1987.

551. Talley, J. D., Hurst, J. W., King, S., et al.: Clinical outcome 5 years after attempted percutaneous transluminal coronary angioplasty in 427 patients. Circulation *77*:820, 1988.

552. Luchi, R. J., Scott, S. M., Deupree, R. H., and the principal investigators and their associates of Veterans Administration Cooperative Study No. 28: Comparison of medical and surgical treatment for unstable angina pectoris. N. Engl. J. Med. *316*:977, 1987.

553. Scott, S. M., Luchi, R. J., Deupree, R. H., and the Veterans Administration Unstable Angina Cooperative Study Group: Veterans Administration Cooperative Study for treatment of patients with unstable angina. Results in patients with abnormal left ventricular function. Circulation *78*(Suppl. I):113, 1988.

554. Parisi, A. F., Khuri, S., Deupree, R. H., et al.: Medical compared with surgical management of unstable angina. 5-Year mortality and morbidity in the Veterans Administration Study. Circulation *80*:1176, 1989.

554a. Booth, D. C., Deupree, R. H., Hultgren, H. N., et al.: Quality of life after bypass surgery for unstable angina. 5-year follow-up results of a Veterans Affairs Cooperative Study. Circulation *83*:87, 1991.

555. Naunheim, K. S., Fiore, A. C., Arango, D. C., et al.: Coronary artery bypass grafting for unstable angina pectoris: Risk analysis. Ann. Thorac. Surg. *47*:569, 1989.

556. Waters, D., Walling, A., Roy, D., et al.: Previous coronary artery bypass grafting as an adverse prognostic factor in unstable angina pectoris. Am. J. Cardiol. *58*:465, 1986.

557. Cairns, J. A., Singer, J., Gent, M., et al.: One year mortality outcomes of all coronary and intensive care unit patients with acute myocardial infarction, unstable angina or other chest pain in Hamilton, Ontario, a city of 375,000 people. Can. J. Cardiol. *5*:239, 1989.

VARIANT ANGINA PECTORIS (PRINZMETAL'S ANGINA)

558. Prinzmetal, M., Kennamer, R., Merliss, R., et al.: A variant form of angina pectoris. Am. J. Med. *27*:375, 1959.

559. Hoshio, A., Kotare, H., and Mashiba, H.: Significance of coronary artery tone in patients with vasospastic angina. J. Am. Coll. Cardiol. *14*:604, 1989.

560. Ganz, P., and Alexander, R. W.: New insights into the cellular mechanisms of vasospasm. Am. J. Cardiol. *56*:11E, 1985.

560a. McFadden, E. P., Clarke, J. G., Davies, G. J., et al.: Effect of intracoronary serotonin on coronary vessels in patients with stable angina and patients with variant angina. N. Engl. J. Med. *324*:648, 1991.

561. Irie, T., Imaizumi, T., Matuguchi, T., et al.: Increased fibrinopeptide A during anginal attacks in patients with variant angina. J. Am. Coll. Cardiol. *14*:589, 1989.

562. Ogawa, H., Yasue, H., Oshima, S., et al.: Circadian variation of plasma fibrinopeptide A level in patients with variant angina. Circulation *80*:1617, 1989.

563. Forman, M. B., Oates, J. A., Robertson, D., et al.: Increased adventitial mast cells in a patient with coronary spasm. N. Engl. J. Med. *313*:1138, 1985.

564. Topol, E. J., and Fortuin, N. J.: Coronary artery spasm and cardiac arrest in carcinoid heart disease. Am. J. Med. *77*:950, 1984.

565. Cohen, L., and Kitzes, R.: Prompt termination and/or prevention of cold-pressor-stimulus-induced vasoconstriction of different vascular beds by magnesium sulfate in patients with Prinzmetal's angina. Magnesium *5*:144, 1986.

566. Miyagi, H., Yasue, H., Okumura, K., et al.: Effect of magnesium on anginal attack induced by hyperventilation in patients with variant angina. Circulation *79*:597, 1989.

567. Kugiyama, K., Yasue, H., Okumura, K., et al.: Suppression of exercise-induced angina by magnesium sulfate in patients with variant angina. J. Am. Coll. Cardiol. *12*:1177, 1988.

568. Tanabe, K., Noda, K., Masaka, A., et al.: Variant angina due to deficiency of intracellular magnesium by anorexia nervosa. Kokyu To Junkan *37*:467, 1989.

569. Lange, R. A., Cigarroa, R. G., Yancy, C. W., et al.: Cocaine-induced coronary-artery vasoconstriction. N. Engl. J. Med. *321*:1557, 1989.

570. Nademanee, K., Gorelick, D. A., Josephson, M. A., et al.: Myocardial ischemia during cocaine withdrawal. Ann. Intern. Med. *111*:876, 1989.

571. Waters, D. D., Muller, D., Bouchard, A., et al.: Circadian variation in variant angina. Am. J. Cardiol. *54*:61, 1984.

572. Winniford, M. D., Jansen, D. E., Reynolds, G. A., et al.: Cigarette smoking-induced coronary vasoconstriction in atherosclerotic coronary artery disease and prevention by calcium antagonists and nitroglycerin. Am. J. Cardiol. *59*:203, 1987.

573. Waters, D. D., Theroux, P., Crittin, J., et al.: Previously undiagnosed variant angina as a cause of chest pain after coronary artery bypass surgery. Circulation *61*:1159, 1980.

574. Habbab, M. A., Szwed, S. A., and Haft, J. I.: Is coronary arterial spasm part of the aspirin-induced asthma syndrome? Chest *90*:141, 1986.
575. Antman, E., Muller, J., Goldberg, S., et al.: Nifedipine therapy for coronary-artery spasm. Experience in 127 patients. N. Engl. J. Med. *302*:12, 1980.
576. Pijls, N. J., and van der Werf, T.: Prinzmetal's angina associated with alcohol withdrawal. Cardiology *75*:226, 1988.
577. Matsuguchi, T., Araki, H., Nakamura, N., et al.: Prevention of vasospastic angina by alcohol ingestion: Report of 2 cases. Angiology *39*:394, 1988.
578. Stefenelli, T., Zielinski, C. C., Mayr, H., and Scoheithauer, W.: Prinzmetal's angina during cyclophosphamide therapy. Eur. Heart J. *9*:1155, 1988.
579. Kleiman, N. S., Lehane, D. E., Geyer, C.E.J., et al.: Prinzmetal's angina during 5-flurouracil chemotherapy. Am. J. Med. *82*:566, 1987.
580. Mancuso, L., Bondi, F., Marchi, S., et al.: Cardiac toxicity of 5-fluorouracil. Report of a case of spontaneous angina. Tumori *72*:121, 1986.
581. Chockalingham, V., Jaganathan, V., Chandrasekar, P. V., et al.: A case of ST-segment and T-wave alternans. Arch. Intern. Med. *143*:1792, 1983.
582. Salerno, J. A., Previtali, M., Panciroli, C., et al.: Ventricular arrhythmias during acute myocardial ischaemia in man. The role and significance of R-ST-T alternans and the prevention of ischaemic sudden death by medical treatment. Eur. Heart J. *7* (Suppl. A):63, 1986.
583. Bayes de Luna, A., Carreras, F., Cladellas, M., et al.: Holter ECG study of the electrocardiographic phenomena in Prinzmetal angina attacks with emphasis on the study of ventricular arrhythmias. J. Electrocardiol. *18*:267, 1985.
584. Yasue, H., Takizawa, A., Nagao, M., et al.: Long-term prognosis for patients with variant angina and influential factors. Circulation *78*:1, 1988.
585. Ortega, C. J., Garcia, N. F., Malillos, M., and Sanchez, F. A.: Transient left posterior hemiblock during Prinzmetal's angina culminating in acute myocardial infarction. Chest *84*:638, 1983.
586. Ortega, C. J., and Paylos, J.: Transient right bundle branch block and left anterior hemiblock during Prinzmetal's angina. J. Electrocardiol. *16*:419, 1983.
587. Gabliani, G. I., Winniford, M. D., Fulton, K. L., et al.: Ventricular ectopic activity with spontaneous variant angina: Frequency and relation to transient ST-segment deviation. Am. Heart J. *110*:40, 1985.
588. Meller, J., Conde, C. A., Donoso, E., and Dack, S.: Transient Q waves in Prinzmetal's angina. Am. J. Cardiol. *35*:691, 1975.
589. Matsuda, Y., Ozaki, M., Ogawa, H., et al.: Coronary arteriography and left ventriculography during spontaneous and exercise-induced ST-segment elevation in patients with variant angina. Am. Heart J. *106*:509, 1983.
590. Crea, F., Davies, G., Romeo, F., et al.: Myocardial ischemia during ergonovine testing: Different susceptibility to coronary vasoconstriction in patients with exertional and variant angina. Circulation *69*:690, 1984.
591. Distante, A., Rovai, D., Picano, E., et al.: Transient changes in left ventricular mechanics during attacks of Prinzmetal's angina: An M-mode echocardiographic study. Am. Heart J. *107*:465, 1984.
592. Bell, M. R., Lapeyre, A. C., and Bove, A. A.: Angiographic demonstration of spontaneous diffuse three vessel coronary artery spasm. J. Am. Coll. Cardiol. *14*:523, 1989.
593. Yokoyama, M., Akita, H., Hirata, K-I., et al.: Supersensitivity of isolated coronary artery to Ergonovine in a patient with variant angina. Am. J. Med. *89*:507, 1990.
594. Winniford, M. D., Johnson, S. M., Mauritson, D. R., and Hillis, L. D.: Ergonovine provocation to assess efficacy of long-term therapy with calcium antagonists in Prinzmetal's variant angina. Am. J. Cardiol. *51*:684, 1983.
595. Waters, D. D., Szlachcic, J., Theroux, P., et al.: Ergonovine testing to detect spontaneous remissions of variant angina during long-term treatment with calcium antagonists drugs. Am. J. Cardiol. *47*:179, 1981.
596. Kimball, B. P., LiPreti, V., and Aldridge, H. E.: Quantitative arteriographic responses to ergonovine provocation in subjects with atypical chest pain. Am. J. Cardiol. *64*:778, 1989.
597. Previtali, M., Ardissino, D., Barberis, P., et al.: Hyperventilation and ergonovine tests in Prinzmetal's variant angina pectoris in men. Am. J. Cardiol. *63*:17, 1989.
598. Mortensen, S. A., Vilhelmsen, R., and Sande, E.: Nonpharmacological provocation of coronary vasospasm. Experience with prolonged hyperventilation in the coronary care unit. Eur. Heart J. *4*:391, 1983.
599. Okumura, K., Yasue, H., Matsuyama, K., et al.: Sensitivity and specificity of intracoronary injection of acetylcholine for the induction of coronary artery spasm. J. Am. Coll. Cardiol. *12*:883, 1988.
600. Okumura, K., Yasue, H., Horio, Y., et al.: Multivessel coronary spasm in patients with variant angina: A study with intracoronary injection of acetylcholine. Circulation *77*:535, 1988.
601. Crea, F., Chierchia, S., Kaski, J. C., et al.: Provocation of coronary spasm by dopamine in patients with active variant angina pectoris. Circulation *74*:262, 1986.
602. Maseri, A., Parodi, O., Severi, S., and Pesola, A.: Transient transmural reduction of myocardial blood flow, demonstrated by thallium-201 scintigraphy, as a cause of variant angina. Circulation *54*:280, 1976.
603. Ginsburg, R., Lamb, I. H., Schroeder, J. S., et al.: Randomized double-blind comparison of nifedipine and isosorbide dinitrate therapy in variant angina pectoris due to coronary artery spasm. Am. Heart J. *103*:44, 1982.
604. Beller, G.: Calcium antagonists in the treatment of Prinzmetal's angina and unstable angina pectoris. Circulation *80*(Suppl. IV):78, 1989.
605. Prida, Z. E., Gelman, J. S., Feldman, R. L., et al.: Comparison of diltiazem and nifedipine alone and in combination in patients with coronary artery spasm. J. Am. Coll. Cardiol. *9*:412, 1987.
606. Pesola, A., Lauro, A., Gallo, R., et al.: Efficacy of diltiazem in variant angina. Results of a double-blind crossover study in CCU by Holter monitoring. The possible occurrence of a withdrawal syndrome. G. Ital. Cardiol. *17*:329, 1987.
607. Previtali, M., Panciroli, C., Ardissino, D., et al.: Spontaneous remission of variant angina documented by Holter monitoring and ergonovine testing in patients treated with calcium antagonists. Am. J. Cardiol. *59*:235, 1987.
608. Tzivoni, D., Keren, A., Benhorin, J., et al.: Prazosin therapy for refractory variant angina. Am. Heart J. *105*:262, 1983.
609. Miwa, K., Kambara, H., and Kawai, C.: Effect of aspirin in large doses on attacks of variant angina. Am. Heart J. *105*:351, 1983.
610. Corcos, T., David, P. R., Bourassa, M. G., et al.: Percutaneous transluminal coronary angioplasty for the treatment of variant angina. J. Am. Coll. Cardiol. *5*:1046, 1985.
611. Katsumoto, K., and Niibori, T.: Prevention of coronary spasms during aorto-coronary (A-C) bypass surgery for variant angina and effort angina with ST elevation. J. Cardiovasc. Surg. *29*:343, 1988.
612. Kitamura, S., Morita, R., Kawachi, K., et al.: Different responses of coronary artery and internal mammary artery bypass grafts to ergonovine and nitroglycerin in variant angina. Ann. Thorac. Surg. *47*:756, 1989.
613. Waters, D. D., Miller, D., Szlachcic, J., et al.: Factors influencing the long-term prognosis of treated patients with variant angina. Circulation *68*:258, 1983.
614. Mark, D. B., Califf, R. M., Morris, K. G., et al.: Clinical characteristics and long-term survival of patients with variant angina. Circulation *69*:880, 1984.
615. Miller, D. D., Waters, D. D., Szlachcic, J., and Theroux, P.: Clinical characteristics associated with sudden death in patients with variant angina. Circulation *66*:588, 1982.
616. Walling, A., Waters, D. D., Miller, D. D., et al.: Long-term prognosis of patients with variant angina. Circulation *76*:990, 1987.
617. Yasue, H., Takizawa, D., Nagao, M., et al.: Long-term prognosis for patients with variant angina and influential factors. Circulation *78*:1, 1988.
618. Shimokawa, H., Nagasawa, K., Irie, T., et al.: Clinical characteristics and long-term prognosis of patients with variant angina. A comparative study between western and Japanese populations. Int. J. Cardiol. *18*:331, 1988.

CHEST PAIN WITH NORMAL CORONARY ARTERIOGRAM

619. Hutchison, S. J., Poole-Wilson, P. A., and Henderson, A. H.: Angina with normal coronary arteries: A review. Q. J. Med. *72*:677, 1988.
620. Papanicolaou, M. N., Califf, R. M., Hlatky, M. A., et al.: Prognostic implications of angiographically normal and insignificantly narrowed coronary arteries. Am. J. Cardiol. *58*:1181, 1986.
621. Kemp, H. G., Kronmal, R. A., Vlietstra, R. E., et al.: Seven-year survival of patients with normal or near normal coronary arteriograms: A CASS Registry study. J. Am. Coll. Cardiol. *7*:479, 1986.
621a. Maseri, A., Crea, F., Kaski, C., and Crake, T.: Mechanisms of angina pectoris in syndrome X. J. Am. Coll. Cardiol. *17*:499, 1991.
622. Camici, P., Marraccini, P., Lorenzoni, R., et al.: Coronary hemodynamics and myocardial metabolism in patients with syndrome X: Response to pacing stress. J. Am. Coll. Cardiol. *17*:1461, 1991.
623. Cannon, R. O., III, Schenke, W. H., Quyyumi, A., et al.: Comparison of exercise testing with studies of coronary flow reserve in patients with microvascular angina. Circulation *83*(Suppl. III):77, 1991.
624. Cannon, R. O., Bonow, R. O., Bacharach, S. L., et al.: Left ventricular dysfunction in patients with angina pectoris, normal epicardial coronary arteries, and abnormal vasodilator reserve. Circulation *71*:218, 1985.
625. Geltman, E. M., Henes, C. G., Senneff, M. J., et al.: Increased myocardial perfusion at rest and diminished perfusion reserve in patients with angina and angiographically normal coronary arteries. J. Am. Coll. Cardiol. *16*:586, 1990.
626. Bortone, A. S., Hess, O. M., Eberli, F. R., et al.: Abnormal coronary vasomotion during exercise in patients with normal coronary arteries and reduced coronary flow reserve. Circulation *79*:516, 1989.
627. Sax, F. L., Cannon, R. O., Hanson, C., and Epstein, S. E.: Impaired forearm vasodilator reserve in patients with microvascular angina. N. Engl. J. Med. *317*:1366, 1987.
627a. Cannon, R. O. III, Peden, D. B., Berkebile, C., et al.: Airway hyperresponsiveness in patients with microvascular angina: Evidence for a diffuse disorder of smooth muscle responsiveness. Circulation *82*:2011, 1990.
628. Cannon, R. O., Cunnion, R. E., Parrillo, J. E., et al.: Dynamic limitation of coronary vasodilator reserve in patients with dilated cardiomyopathy and chest pain. J. Am. Coll. Cardiol. *10*:1190, 1987.
629. Pasternac, A., Noble, J., Streulens, Y., et al.: Pathophysiology of chest pain in patients with cardiomyopathies and normal coronary arteries. Circulation *65*:778, 1982.
630. Spray, T. L., Maron, B. J., Morrow, A. G., et al.: Clinical pathologic conference. A discussion on hypertrophic cardiomyopathy. Am. Heart J. *95*:511, 1978.
631. Wielgosz, A. T., Fletcher, R. H., McCants, C. B., et al.: Unimproved chest pain in patients with minimal or no coronary disease: A behavioral phenomenon. Am. Heart J. *108*:67, 1984.
632. Beitman, B. D., Mukerji, V., Lamberti, J. W., et al.: Panic disorder in

patients with chest pain and angiographically normal coronary arteries. Am. J. Cardiol. *63*:1399, 1989.
633. Bass, C., and Wade, C.: Chest pain with normal coronary arteries. A comparative study of psychiatric and social morbidity. Psychol. Med. *14*:51, 1984.
634. Channer, K. S., James, M. A., Papouchado, M., and Rees, J. R.: Anxiety and depression in patients with chest pain referred for exercise testing. Lancet *2*:820, 1985.
635. Shapiro, L. M., Crake, T., and Poole-Wilson, P. A.: Is altered cardiac sensation responsible for chest pain in patients with normal coronary arteries? Clinical observation during cardiac catheterisation. Br. Med. J. *296*:170, 1988.
636. DeMeester, T. R., O'Sullivan, G. C., Bermudez, G., et al.: Esophageal function in patients with angina-type chest pain and normal coronary angiograms. Ann. Surg. *196*:488, 1982.
637. Pupita, G., Kaski, J. C., Galassi, A. R., et al.: Long-term variability of angina pectoris and electrocardiographic signs of ischemia in syndrome X. Am. J. Cardiol. *64*:139, 1989.
638. Opherk, D., Schuler, G., Wetterauer, K., et al.: Four-year follow-up study in patients with angina pectoris and normal coronary arteriograms ("syndrome X"). Circulation *80*:1610, 1989.
639. Emdin, M., Picano, E., Lattanzi, F., and L'Abbate, A.: Improved exercise capacity with acute aminophylline administration in patients with syndrome X. J. Am. Coll. Cardiol. *14*:1450, 1989.
640. Cannon, R. O., Watson, R. M., Rosing, D. R., and Epstein, S. E.: Efficacy of calcium channel blocker therapy for angina pectoris resulting from small-vessel coronary artery disease and abnormal vasodilator reserve. Am. J. Cardiol. *56*:242, 1985.

ISCHEMIC HEART DISEASE IN WHICH DISCOMFORT IS NOT THE DOMINANT SYMPTOM

641. Parmley, W. W.: Prevalence and clinical significance of silent myocardial ischemia. Circulation *80*(Suppl. IV):68, 1989.
642. Mulcahy, D., Keegan, J., Crean, P., et al.: Silent ischemia in chronic stable angina: A study of its frequency and characteristics in 150 patients. Br. Heart J. *60*:417, 1988.
642a. Kellermann, J. J., and Braunwald, E. (eds.): Silent Myocardial Ischemia: A Critical Appraisal. Basel, Karger, 1990, 358 pp.
643. Hirzel, H. O., Leutwyler, R., and Kralyenbuehl, H. P.: Silent myocardial ischemia: Hemodynamic changes during dynamic exercise in patients with proven coronary artery disease despite absence of angina pectoris. J. Am. Coll. Cardiol. *6*:275, 1985.
644. Chierchia, S., Smith, G., Morgan, M., et al.: Role of heart rate in pathophysiology of chronic stable angina. Lancet *2*:1353, 1984.
645. Deanfield, J. E., Ribiero, P., Oakley, K., et al.: Analysis of ST-segment changes in normal subjects: Implications for ambulatory monitoring in angina pectoris. Am. J. Cardiol. *54*:1321, 1984.
646. Rocco, M. B., Barry, J., Campbell, S., et al.: Circadian variation of transient myocardial ischemia in patients with coronary artery disease. Circulation *75*:395, 1987.
647. Quyyumi, A. A., Mockus, L., Wright, C., and Fox, K. M.: Morphology of ambulatory ST-segment changes in patients with varying severity of coronary artery disease. Investigation of the frequency of nocturnal ischaemia and coronary spasm. Br. Heart J. *53*:186, 1985.
648. Langer, A., Freeman, M. R., Josse, R. G., et al.: Detection of silent myocardial ischemia in diabetes mellitus. Am. J. Cardiol. *67*:1073, 1991.
649. Deanfield, J. E., Shea, M. J., Wilson, R. A., et al.: Direct effects of smoking on the heart: Silent ischemic disturbances of coronary flow. Am. J. Cardiol. *57*:1005, 1986.
650. Rozanski, A., Bairy, C. N., Krantz, D. S., et al.: Mental stress and the induction of silent myocardial ischemia in patients with coronary artery disease. N. Engl. J. Med. *318*:1005, 1988.
651. Deedwania, P. C., and Carbajal, E. V.: Prevalence and patterns of silent myocardial ischemia during daily life in stable angina patients receiving conventional antianginal drug therapy. Am. J. Cardiol. *65*:1090, 1990.
652. Yeung, A. C., Barry, J., Orav, J., et al.: Effects of asymptomatic ischemia on long-term prognosis in chronic stable coronary disease. Circulation *83*:1598, 1991.
653. Hedblad, B., Juul-Moller, S., Svensson, K., et al.: Increased mortality in men with ST segment depression during 24 h ambulatory long-term ECG recording. Eur. Heart J. *10*:149, 1989.
654. Rocco, M. B., Nabel, E. G., Campbell, S., et al.: Prognostic importance of myocardial ischemia detected by ambulatory monitoring in patients with stable coronary artery disease. Circulation *78*:877, 1988.
655. Bergin, P., Myler, R. K., Shaw, R. E., et al.: Transluminal coronary angioplasty in the treatment of silent ischemia. Cathet. Cardiovasc. Diagn. *15*:223, 1988.
656. Erikssen, J., Enge, I., Forfang, K., and Storstein, O.: False-positive diagnostic tests and coronary angiographic findings in 105 presumably healthy males. Circulation *54*:371, 1976.
657. Mulcahy, D., Keegan, J., Sparrow, J., et al.: Ischemia in the ambulatory setting—the total ischemic burden: Relation to' exercise testing and investigative and therapeutic implications. J. Am. Coll. Cardiol. *14*:1166, 1989.
657a. Miranda, C. P., Lehmann, K. G., Lachterman, B., et al.: Comparison of silent and symptomatic ischemia during exercise testing in men. Ann. Intern. Med. *114*:649, 1991.
658. Weiner, D. A.: The diagnostic and prognostic significance of an asymptomatic positive exercise test. Circulation *75*(Suppl. II):20, 1987.
659. Yeung, A. C., Barry, J., and Selwyn, A. P.: Silent ischemia after myocardial infarction. Prognosis, mechanism and intervention. Circulation *82*(Suppl. II):143, 1990.
659a. Hill, J. A., Gonzalez, J. I., Kolb, R., and Pepine, C. J.: Effects of atenolol alone, nifedipine alone and their combination on ambulant myocardial ischemia. Am. J. Cardiol. *67*:671, 1991.
660. Grieco, J. G., Montoya, A., Sullivan, H. J., et al.: Ventricular aneurysm due to blunt chest injury. Ann. Thorac. Surg. *47*:322, 1989.
661. Hirai, T., Fujita, M., Nakajima, H., et al.: Importance of collateral circulation for prevention of left ventricular aneurysm formation in acute myocardial infarction. Circulation *79*:791, 1989.
662. Forman, M. B., Collins, H. W., Kopelman, H. A., et al.: Determinants of left ventricular aneurysm formation after anterior myocardial infarction: A clinical and angiographic study. J. Am. Coll. Cardiol. *8*:1256, 1986.
663. Barratt-Boyes, B. G., White, H. D., Agnew, T. M., et al.: The results of surgical treatment of left ventricular aneurysms: An assessment of the risk factors affecting early and late mortality. J. Thorac. Cardiovasc. Surg. *87*:87, 1984.
664. Meltzer, R. S., Visser, C. A., and Fuster, V.: Intracardiac thrombi and systemic embolization. Ann. Intern. Med. *104*:689, 1986.
665. Stephenson, L. W., Hargrove, W. C., Ratcliffe, M. B., et al.: Surgery for left ventricular aneurysm. Early survival with and without endocardial resection. Circulation *79*(Suppl. X):1, 1989.
666. Sutherland, G. R., Smyllie, J. H., and Roelandt, J. R.: Advantages of colour flow imaging in the diagnosis of left ventricular pseudoaneurysm. Br. Heart J. *61*:59, 1989.
667. Marcus, M. L., Stanford, W., Hajduczok, Z. D., and Weiss, R. M.: Ultrafast computed tomography in the diagnosis of cardiac disease. Am. J. Cardiol. *64*:54E, 1989.
668. Mangschau, A.: Akinetic versus dyskinetic left ventricular aneurysms diagnosed by gated scintigraphy: Difference in surgical outcome. Ann. Thorac. Surg. *47*:746, 1989.
669. Couper, G. S., Bunton, R. W., Birjiniuk, V., et al.: Relative risks of left ventricular aneurysmectomy in patients with akinetic scars versus true dyskinetic aneurysms. Circulation *82*(Suppl. IV):248, 1990.
670. Cosgrove, D. M., Lytle, B. W., Taylor, P. C., et al.: Ventricular aneurysm resection. Circulation *79*(Suppl. I):97, 1989.
671. Mangschau, A., Forfang, K., Rootwelt, K., and Frysaker, T.: Improvement in cardiac performance and exercise tolerance after left ventricular aneurysm surgery: A prospective study. Thorac. Cardiovasc. Surg. *36*:320, 1988.
672. Louagie, Y., Alouini, T., Lesperance, J., and Pelletier, L. C.: Left ventricular aneurysm complicated by congestive heart failure: An analysis of long-term results and risk factors of surgical treatment. J. Cardiovasc. Surg. *30*:648, 1989.
673. Olearchyk, A. S., Lemole, G. M., and Spagna, P. M.: Left ventricular aneurysm. Ten years' experience in surgical treatment of 244 cases. Improved clinical status, hemodynamics, and long-term longevity. J. Thorac. Cardiovasc. Surg. *88*:544, 1984.
674. Rankin, J. S., Hickey, M. S., Smith L. R., et al.: Ischemic mitral regurgitation. Circulation *79*(Suppl. I):116, 1989.
675. Replogle, R. L., and Campbell, C. D.: Surgery for mitral regurgitation associated with ischemic heart disease. Circulation *79*(Suppl. I):122, 1989.
676. Burch, G. E., Giles, T. D., and Colcolough, H. L.: Ischemic cardiomyopathy. Am. Heart J. *79*:291, 1970.
677. Bateman, T. M., Czer, L.S.C., Gray, R. J., et al.: Transient pathologic Q waves during acute ischemic events: An electrocardiographic correlate of stunned but viable myocardium. Am. Heart J. *106*:1421, 1983.
678. Shanes, J. G., Kondos, G. T., Levitsky, S., et al.: Coronary artery obstruction: A potentially reversible cause of dilated cardiomyopathy. Am. Heart J. *110*:173, 1985.
679. Kron, I. L., Flanagan, T. L., Blackbourne, L. H., et al.: Coronary revascularization rather than cardiac transplantation for chronic ischemic cardiomyopathy. Ann. Surg. *210*:348, 1989.
680. Kelly, P., Ruskin, J. N., Vlahakes, G. J., et al.: Surgical coronary revascularization in survivors of prehospital cardiac arrest: Its effect on inducible ventricular arrhythmias and long-term survival. J. Am. Coll. Cardiol. *15*:267, 1990.
681. Kragel, A. H., and Roberts, W. C.: Anomalous origin of either the right or left main coronary artery from the aorta with subsequent coursing between aorta and pulmonary trunk: Analysis of 32 necropsy cases. Am. J. Cardiol. *62*:771, 1988.
682. DeMaio, S. J., Kinsella, S. H., and Silverman, M. E.: Clinical course and long-term prognosis of spontaneous coronary artery dissection. Am. J. Cardiol. *64*:471, 1989.
683. Subramanyan, R., Joy, J., and Balakrishnan, K. G.: Natural history of aortoarteritis (Takayasu's disease). Circulation *80*:429, 1989.
684. Tveter, K. J., and Edwards, J. E.: Calcified aortic sinotubular ridge: A source of coronary ostial stenosis or embolism. J. Am. Coll. Cardiol. *12*:1510, 1988.
685. Gao, S. Z., Schroeder, J. S., Hunt, S. A., et al.: Acute myocardial infarction in cardiac transplant recipients. Am. J. Cardiol. *64*:1093, 1989.
686. Lange, R. L., Reid, M. S., Tresch, D. D., et al.: Nonatheromatous ischemic heart disease following withdrawal from chronic industrial nitroglycerin exposure. Circulation *46*:666, 1972.

Interventional Catheterization Techniques: Percutaneous Transluminal Balloon Angioplasty, Valvuloplasty, and Related Procedures

by DONALD S. BAIM, M.D.

From 1950 through the 1970's essentially all cardiac catheterizations were performed to evaluate individual disease states, to guide medical therapy, or to provide a road map for cardiac surgical repair (see Chaps. 7 and 9). In the 1980's, however, cardiac catheterization began to play an increasingly important role in *treating* as well as *diagnosing* cardiovascular lesions. In the 1990's this new application of catheterization-based treatment has become known as "interventional" cardiology, which may involve delivery of mechanical, thermal, microsurgical, or light energy to cardiovascular lesions by means of specialized percutaneously inserted catheters. The end result may be to open stenotic blood vessels or cardiac valves, or to close undesired channels for blood flow, in an effort to achieve a physiological correction of the underlying cardiac pathology comparable to that obtained by traditional surgical techniques. If such a correction is possible (as it now is in one-half of the patients requiring coronary revascularization), it may be obtained frequently at a fraction of the expense, disability, and discomfort of surgery. The explosive growth of this area has already had a major impact on health care delivery and is likely to increase as these interventional techniques continue to mature. The delivery through catheters of electric currents to the heart and specialized conduction tissue for therapeutic purposes is another application of interventional catheterization and is described on pages 651 and 776.

Treatment of Vascular Stenosis

The development of vascular angiography made it possible to visualize atherosclerotic and fibromuscular stenoses in various arterial beds. In the course of such angiographic procedures, Dotter et al. noted that it was frequently possible to pass first a guidewire and then a catheter or rigid dilator through an area of stenosis in the iliac-femoral system, thereby enlarging the lumen and improving antegrade blood flow (Fig. 41–1).[1–3] While the so-called *Dotter technique* was used to some extent in Europe between 1964 and 1974,[4] its application was limited by the trauma to the artery which resulted from exertion of axial force on the stenosis, and the local complications which were related to the percutaneous introduction of the large-caliber rigid dilators. In 1974 Gruentzig and Kumpe modified the technique by substituting a balloon-tipped catheter for the rigid dilator.[5] This nonelastomeric balloon catheter could be introduced and passed across the stenosis in its smaller collapsed state and then inflated to a predetermined size with liquid contrast material in order to achieve the desired enlargement in luminal caliber (Fig. 41–2). Balloon angioplasty (the so-called *Gruentzig technique*) was applied first to peripheral[5] and then to renal arterial stenoses.[6] In 1977, after cadaver and intraoperative studies during bypass surgery, percutaneous balloon angioplasty was extended to stenoses of the epicardial coronary arteries.[7] Balloon angioplasty—albeit with many technical refinements—still constitutes the core of interventional cardiology and has provided major encouragement for the subsequent development of a variety of other interventional techniques for application in the heart and extracardiac vasculature.

PERCUTANEOUS TRANSLUMINAL CORONARY ANGIOPLASTY (PTCA)

EARLY EXPERIENCE. Between 1977 and 1980 coronary angioplasty used the original Gruentzig catheter,[7] a two-lumen device in which one

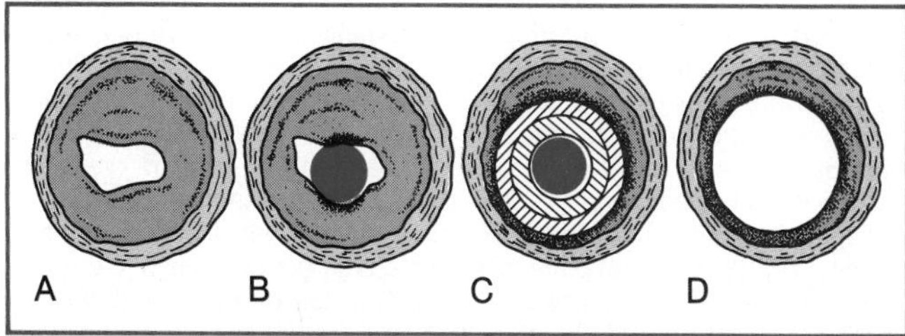

FIGURE 41–1. The Dotter technique. Cross sections of a stenotic arterial lumen are shown at baseline *(A)*, during the passage of the initial catheter *(B)*, during the passage of the coaxial dilators *(C)*, and after the procedure *(D)*. Note the improvement in luminal diameter without enlargement of the outer vessel caliber, suggesting compaction of the atheroma as the mechanism of dilatation. (From Dotter, C. T., Rosch, J., and Judkins, M. P.: Transluminal dilatation of atherosclerotic stenosis. Surg. Gynecol. Obstet. *127*:794, 1968.)

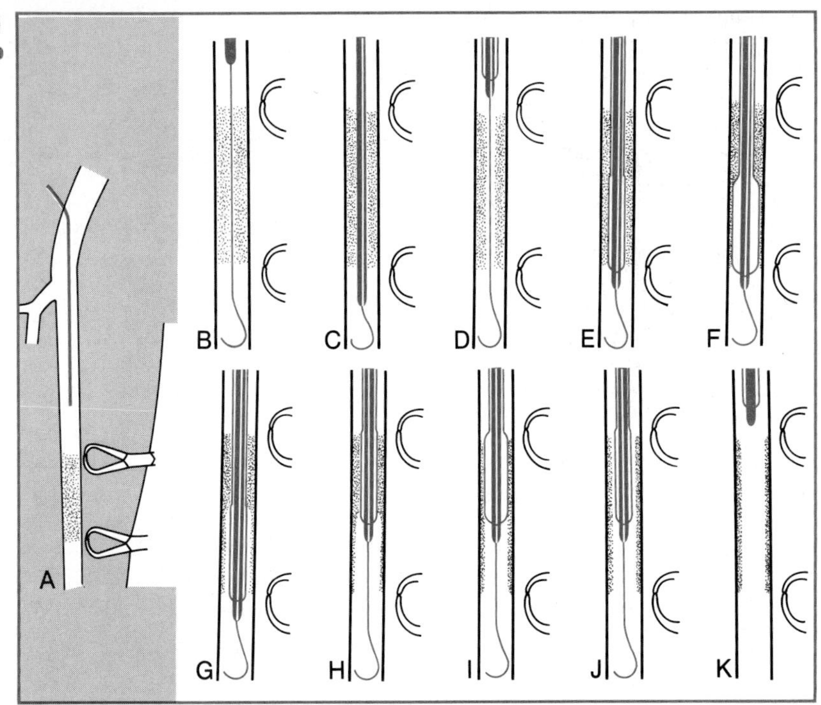

FIGURE 41–2. The Gruentzig technique. This series of diagrams depicts the application of balloon angioplasty to the treatment of a totally occluded peripheral artery *(A)*. After diagnostic angiography a guidewire *(B)* and an angiographic catheter *(C)* are passed through the area of total occlusion. This creates a lumen for passage of the deflated dilatation catheter *(D, E)*. The dilatation balloon is then inflated at several points throughout the stenotic lumen (*F* to *I*), resulting in improvement in vessel patency *(J, K)*. Again note the absence of enlargement in the outer diameter, suggesting compaction of atherosclerotic material as the mechanism for luminal enhancement. (From Gruentzig, A., and Kumpe, D. A.: Technique of percutaneous transluminal angioplasty with the Gruentzig balloon catheter. Am. J. Radiol. *132*:547, 1979.)

lumen was used to inflate and deflate the polyvinylchloride (PVC) balloon, while the second lumen was used to monitor pressure or inject radiographic contrast material through a port near the catheter tip. A short segment of flexible guidewire was attached to the tip of the dilatation catheter. Although this guidewire reduced the chance of intimal dissection and subintimal passage, it could not be reshaped or manipulated once introduced into the patient, sharply limiting the ability to advance the dilatation catheter beyond all but the most proximal coronary stenoses. Moreover, the large diameter of these early balloon catheters in their deflated state (0.060 inch, or 1.5 mm) made it difficult to cross severe or inelastic stenoses, since the diameter of the deflated balloon was frequently larger than that of the stenotic lumen (i.e., 0.6 mm for an 80 per cent stenosis of a typical 3-mm diameter coronary artery). To deal with this problem, the dilatation catheter had to be advanced through a large (No. 8 or 9 French, 2.7 or 3.0 mm outer diameter), stiff "guiding catheter" positioned in the coronary ostium. The third limitation of the original Gruentzig catheter was its comparatively low balloon rupture pressure (6 atm, or 90 psi), which made it difficult to dilate rigid lesions adequately. In an effort to mitigate these problems, early angioplasty operators attempted to select patients considered to have "soft" rather than rigid lesions (as reflected by recent onset of anginal symptoms and absence of calcification of the lesion on fluoroscopy), and particularly those patients whose lesions were located in the proximal coronary segments.

To define better the results, complications, and long-term efficacy of this new technique, the National Heart, Lung, and Blood Institute (NHLBI) established a PTCA Registry in 1979.[8] Candidates for PTCA were selected to have severe enough angina to warrant consideration of bypass surgery, objective evidence of myocardial ischemia, and coronary anatomy (proximal, subtotal, discrete, concentric, noncalcified stenosis of a single coronary artery) thought to be approachable with the limited equipment then available. Although such patients were believed to represent fewer than 5 to 10 per cent of the symptomatic coronary artery disease population, more than 3,000 patients underwent PTCA before the Registry was closed in late 1981. Despite the careful selection of ideal candidates, the primary success rate of PTCA in the original Registry was less than 60 per cent, with failure to cross the stenosis with the dilatation system in 29 per cent and failure to dilate the stenosis in 12 per cent of patients attempted. Two other important problems were identified: (1) approximately 6 per cent of patients required emergency bypass to correct acute, severe myocardial ischemia which resulted from abrupt reclosure of the dilated artery, and (2) between 20 and 30 per cent of patients with an initially successful procedure experienced return of angina owing to angiographically evident renarrowing ("restenosis") of the dilated segment within 6 months after the procedure.

TECHNICAL ADVANCES. Shortly after the original NHLBI Registry was closed, a variety of technical improvements in PTCA equipment,[9,10] coupled with the availability of more experienced operators, facilitated major improvements in the overall success of PTCA.[10a] The original dilatation catheter was redesigned so that the guidewire now extended the entire length of the dilatation catheter, allowing the wire to be advanced, withdrawn, reshaped, or steered during the procedure (Fig. 41–3).[11] Although these specialized guidewires are only 0.010 to 0.018 inch (0.3 to 0.5 mm) in diameter, sophisticated engineering has allowed the fabrication of devices with soft atraumatic tips, excellent torque control, and superb radiographic visibility. Current guidewires can be manipulated across stenoses located virtually anywhere in the coronary tree, and then serve as a "railroad track" over which advancement of the dilatation catheter can be performed. Special "exchange-length" guidewires (300 cm long) can be left positioned in the distal coronary artery as one balloon catheter is withdrawn and a second is inserted, or as contrast injection is

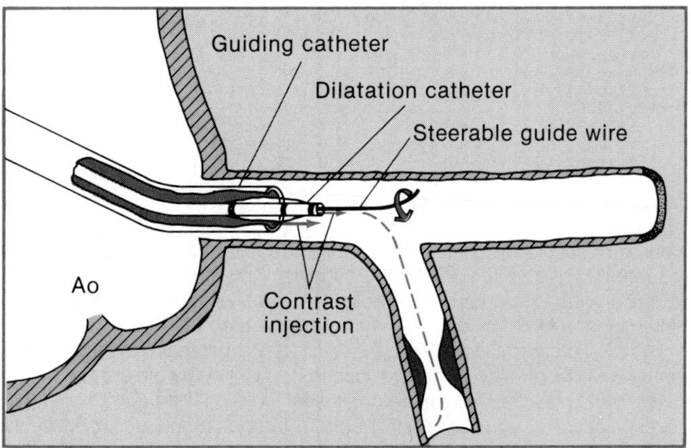

FIGURE 41–3. Movable guidewire dilatation system. The dilatation catheter is shown here at the end of a large (No. 8 or 9 French, 2.7- or 3.0-mm) guiding catheter, which is positioned at the ostium of the involved vessel. The soft, yet steerable guidewire is then advanced through the central lumen of the dilatation catheter and directed through and beyond the target lesion. The position of this guidewire relative to coronary branches and lesions can be revealed by contrast injection through the guiding catheter or through the central lumen of the dilatation catheter. Once the guidewire has been successfully positioned, it serves as a "track" over which the dilatation catheter itself can be advanced. (From Baim, D. S.: Coronary angioplasty. *In* Grossman, W., and Baim, D. S. [eds.]: Cardiac Catheterization, Angiography and Intervention. 4th ed. Philadelphia, Lea and Febiger, 1991.)

PLATE 9

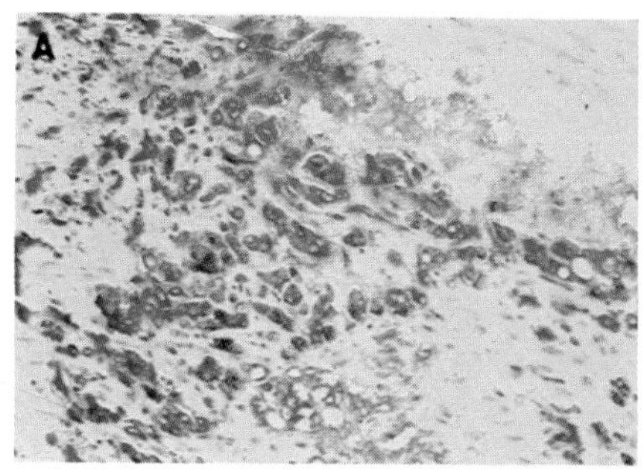

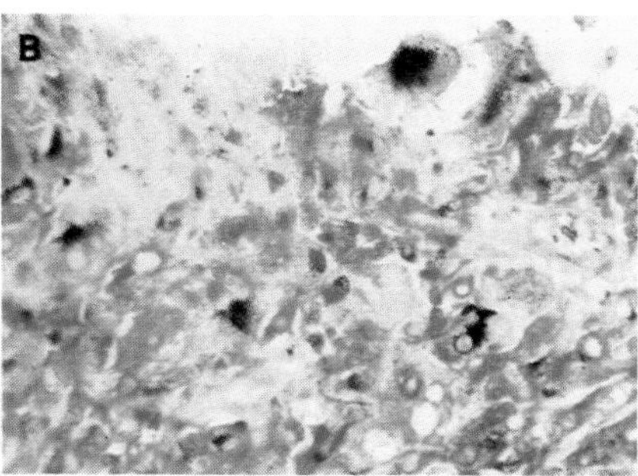

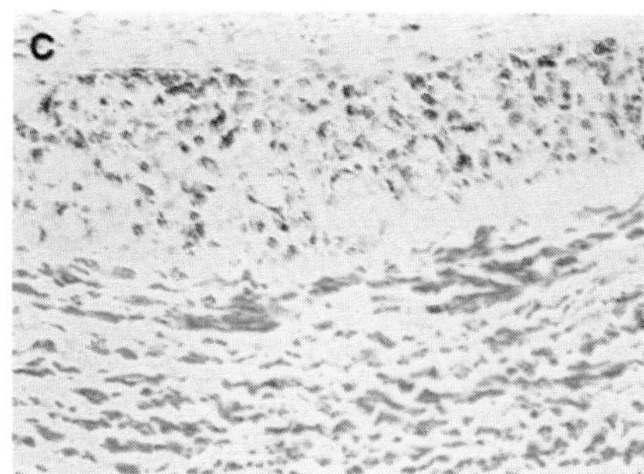

FIGURE 36–12 (See page 1115)

Double-immunostained preparations demonstrating the distribution of PDGF-B chain in methacarn-fixed, deparaffinized sections of advanced lesions of atherosclerosis from a high-level hypercholesterolemic nonhuman primate fed a hypercholesterolemic diet for one year. The sections were stained with a monoclonal antibody specific for PDGF-B-chain protein, and with cell-type-specific monoclonal antibodies for macrophages *(A, B)* or smooth muscle *(C)*, with IGSS and avidin-biotin immunoalkaline-phosphatase procedures.

A) PDGF-B chain (black, granular reaction product) is localized to HAM56-positive macrophages (red reaction product).

B) Positive cells at higher magnification.

C) PDGF-B chain (black, granular reaction product) and HHF35-positive smooth muscle cells (red reaction product) are identified in nonoverlapping cell populations. All sections were counterstained with methyl green. *A* and *C* original magnifications, X250; *B* original magnification, X400. (From Ross, R., Masuda, J., Raines, E.W., et al.: Localization of PDGF-B protein in macrophages in all phases of atherogenesis. Science 248:1009, 1990. © Copyright 1990 by the American Association for the Advancement of Science.

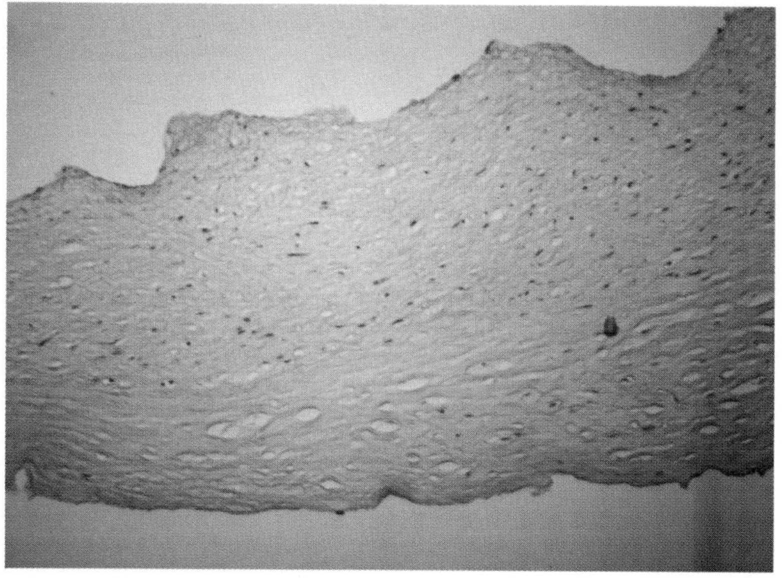

FIGURE 41–14 (See page 1372)

Histology of restenosis. This sample was obtained by directional coronary atherectomy from a patient who developed recurrent symptoms and angiographic restenosis 4 months after laser balloon angioplasty. There is a homogeneous population of smooth muscle cells showing a proliferative rather than contractile phenotype, wihch have grown within the initial treated lumen to renarrow the flow channel. Similar histological findings are apparent in postmortem specimens and atherectomy specimens in patients with restenosis after diverse coronary interventions. (From Safian, R. D., et al.: Coronary atherectomy: Clinical, angiographic and histologic findings and observations regarding mechanism. Circulation *82*:69, 1990, by permission of the American Heart Association, Inc.)

PLATE 10

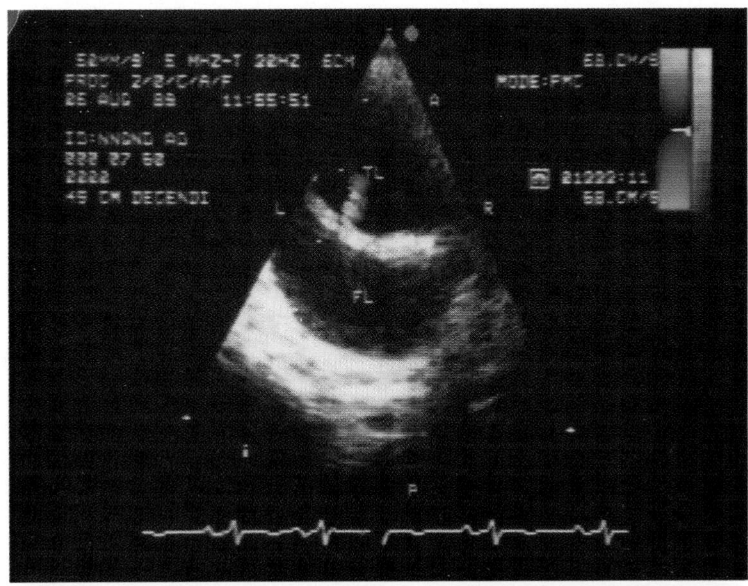

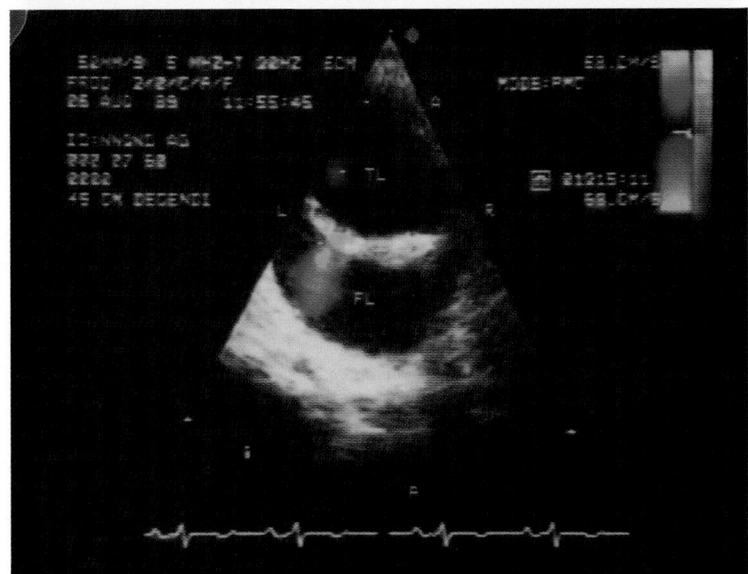

FIGURE 47–11 (See page 1538)

Transesophageal echocardiographic image of an aortic dissection, demonstrating a large false lumen posteriorly in the ascending aorta. Communication between the true lumen (TL) and false lumen (FL) is present. Bidirectional flow is demonstrated by transesophageal color Doppler echocardiography in these images of the descending aorta. The red jet indicates flow into true lumen from the false lumen; the blue jet indicates flow into the false lumen.

performed through the guiding catheter to assess adequacy of dilatation. Improvements in the design of dilatation catheters[10] have led to the development of devices with deflated diameters as small as 0.025 inch (0.60 mm), inflated diameters between 2.0 and 4.0 mm, and the ability to tolerate inflation pressures as high as 20 atm (300 psi). These devices can be used to cross and dilate even the most rigid stenoses. Specialized "balloon-on-a-wire" catheters are available with deflated profiles as small as 0.020 inch (0.5 mm) to allow dilatation of the most severe or most distal lesions.

The impact of these improvements in angioplasty catheters and guidewires was evident in PTCA Registry II,[12] which collected information on patients treated during 1985 and 1986 at 14 centers that had participated in the original Registry. Analysis demonstrated an improved success rate of 85 per cent, with concomitant reduction in the incidence of emergency bypass surgery to 3.5 per cent.[13] While the procedural mortality for patients with single-vessel disease had decreased compared to the original Registry (from 0.9 to 0.2 per cent), overall procedural mortality remained approximately 1 per cent because Registry II included more patients with multivessel disease (mortality 1.7 per cent). One-year follow-up of 838 patients with single-vessel disease showed a low incidence of death (1.6 per cent) and myocardial infarction (1.9 per cent), although repeat angioplasty (18.1 per cent) and bypass surgery (6.2 per cent) were required to treat restenosis or disease progression.[14] With the exception of a slight further increase in success (to 90 per cent) and reduction in emergency bypass surgery (to 2 per cent) as the result of further refinements in equipment and technique since 1986, the results of Registry II can be taken to reflect those obtainable by conventional balloon angioplasty at the time of this writing.

CURRENT TECHNIQUE

Patients undergoing coronary angioplasty are usually admitted to the hospital the day before or the morning of the procedure. Prior catheterization and exercise test data are reviewed, and a dilatation strategy is developed detailing the specific lesions, the sequence, and the equipment to be used for dilatation. The procedure—including the likelihood of successful dilatation, abrupt reclosure with emergency surgery, and late restenosis—is discussed with the patient and the family. Consent forms for both PTCA and possible emergency coronary artery bypass surgery are signed. Patients are proscribed from oral intake after midnight and asked to bathe with an antiseptic scrub. Aspirin (325 mg/day), dipyridamole (200 mg/day), and a calcium antagonist are added to existing medical therapy.

At the time of PTCA appropriate vascular access (by way of either brachial artery cutdown or femoral artery puncture) is obtained (Fig. 7–1, p. 182), and a guiding catheter is positioned at the ostium of the involved coronary artery. A venous catheter for monitoring right heart pressure and/or temporary ventricular pacing is usually placed, and full systemic anticoagulation is achieved using 10,000 units of intravenous heparin. Baseline angiography is performed to clarify any uncertainties (e.g., location of side branches relative to the target stenosis) and to document continued suitability of the lesion for dilatation. The guidewire is then passed across the target lesion and positioned in the distal segment of the involved vessel. A dilatation catheter comparable in size to the adjacent normal artery is advanced into the lesion and adequately pressurized to expand the balloon to its full diameter. Adequate dilatation is confirmed by repeat angiography and/or measurement of the translesional pressure gradient, after which the dilated segment is observed over 5 to 10 minutes to document the stability of the result. Additional lesions may then be dilated according to the predetermined dilatation strategy. The effect of heparin is allowed to wear off before removal of the vascular sheaths, although intravenous heparin infusion may be resumed for 24 to 48 hours if significant intimal dissection is present at the dilatation site. After 8 to 24 hours of bed rest, the patient is ambulated and discharged.

Discharge medications typically include aspirin 325 mg/day and short-term (6 weeks) therapy with a calcium channel blocker.[15] The patient is scheduled for an exercise tolerance test during the following month but may typically return to work within 1 week of a successful and uncomplicated coronary angioplasty. A follow-up exercise tolerance test should be performed at 6 months (or sooner if anginal symptoms recur) to detect restenosis of the dilated segment(s). Annual exercise testing and continued attention to risk factor reduction are generally indicated in these coronary patients at high risk of additional coronary arterial lesions.

INDICATIONS

(See also pp. 1316–1317)

The indication for PTCA is myocardial ischemia (Table 41–1) owing to coronary stenosis(es) deemed suitable for this procedure.[16,17] With the advantage of improved guidewires, dilatation catheters, and guiding catheters, a high success rate is achieved despite the inclusion of patients with progressively more challenging anatomical and clinical disease.

ANATOMICAL INDICATIONS. Whereas PTCA was originally limited to proximal stenoses, more distal, eccentric, and calcified lesions are now approached on a routine basis.[9] Angioplasty of such lesions, however, is generally associated with less favorable results in terms of a lower success rate and/or a higher complication rate[18] than expected with an "ideal" lesion. This pattern is reflected in the ad hoc lesion grading system (Table 41–2) proposed by the AHA/ACC Task Force,[16] but also validated in a retrospective sample of multivessel angioplasty patients.[19] Lesions involving *coronary bifurcations*—previously avoided because of the 14 per cent incidence of "snowplow" occlusion of the side branch (Fig. 41–4)[20]—can now be dilated using the "kissing-balloon"[21] or double-wire (Fig. 41–5)[22] technique to preserve both the main and the side-branch lumina. *Totally occluded coronary arteries* are also approachable by PTCA, to revascularize areas of viable myocardium supplied by inadequate collateral flow (Fig. 41–6) or to provide collateral flow to other stenotic ves-

TABLE 41–1 INDICATIONS FOR AND CONTRAINDICATIONS TO PTCA

CLINICAL INDICATIONS FOR PTCA

Significant stenosis of one or more major epicardial arteries, which subtend at least a moderate-sized area of viable myocardium, in a patient who has:

1. **Recurrent ischemic episodes after myocardial infarction or major ventricular arrhythmia,**
2. **Angina that has not responded adequately to medical therapy,**
3. **Clear evidence of myocardial ischemia on resting, ambulatory, or exercise electrocardiography, or**
4. **Objective evidence of myocardial ischemia that increases the overall risk of required noncardiac surgery.**

ABSOLUTE OR RELATIVE CONTRAINDICATIONS TO PTCA

High-risk anatomy (including significant left main artery disease) in which vessel closure would likely result in hemodynamic collapse,

Severe, diffuse, and/or extensive coronary artery disease better treated surgically,

Target lesion morphology (type C) associated with an anticipated success <60%, unless PTCA is the only reasonable treatment option,

No coronary stenosis >50% diameter reduction,

No objective or compelling clinical evidence of myocardial ischemia, or

Absence of on-site surgical back-up, qualified PTCA operators, or adequate radiographic imaging equipment.

TABLE 41-2 ANTICIPATED SUCCESS IN VARIOUS LESIONS ACCORDING TO MORPHOLOGICAL TYPES

TYPE A LESION (HIGH [>85%] SUCCESS WITH LOW RISK)	
Discrete (<10 mm long)	Little or no calcification
Concentric	Less than total occlusion
Readily accessible	Not ostial
Nonangulated segment	No major branch involvement
Smooth contour	Absence of thrombus
TYPE B LESION (MODERATE [60-85%] SUCCESS WITH MODERATE RISK)	
Tubular (10-20 mm long)	Moderate calcification
Eccentric	Total occlusion <3 months
Moderate tortuosity	Ostial location
Moderate (45°-90°) angle	Treatable bifurcation lesion
Irregular contour	Some thrombus present
TYPE C LESION (LOW [<60%] SUCCESS WITH HIGH RISK)	
Diffuse (>20 mm long)	Total occlusion >3 months
Excessive tortuosity or angulation	Bifurcation with nonprotectable side branch
Degenerated vein graft	

(After Ryan, T. J., et al.[16])

sels undergoing dilatation (Fig. 41-7).[23] Although the primary success rate in dilatation of chronic total occlusions remains lower than that for other stenotic lesions (75 per cent for occlusions less than 3 months old and below 50 per cent for older occlusions), dilatation of total occlusions now accounts for 10 to 20 per cent of PTCA volume in large centers.[24]

An increasing number of patients with multivessel coronary artery disease are undergoing PTCA as an alternative to bypass surgery (Fig. 41-7). These patients account for more than half of those entered into the 1985-86 Registry, although fewer than two-thirds of patients identified as having multivessel *disease* actually underwent multivessel *dilatation*.[12] Preliminary data suggest that many patients with multivessel coronary artery disease may derive substantial clinical benefit from successful PTCA, but multivessel disease clearly imposes several additional difficulties to those of single-vessel disease. These include: (1) longer duration of the procedure and greater usage of radiographic contrast material, (2) more diffuse myocardial ischemia if abrupt reclosure should occur, (3) a greater chance that not all significant coronary lesions will be successfully dilated (incomplete revascularization), and (4) a greater chance that recurrent angina will develop owing to restenosis of a dilated segment or progression of disease in one or more undilated segments.[14] These difficulties affect both the selection of patients for and the performance of

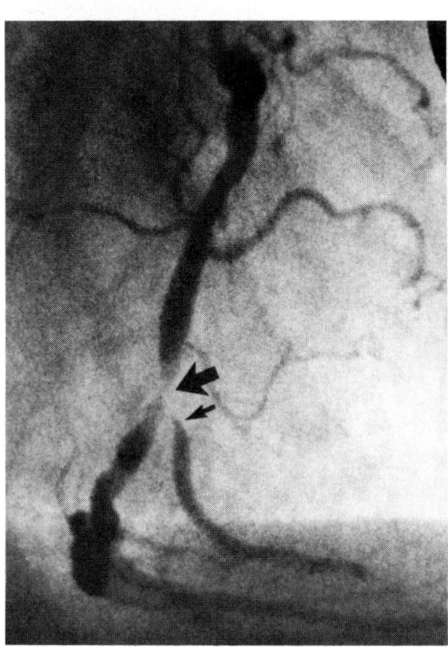

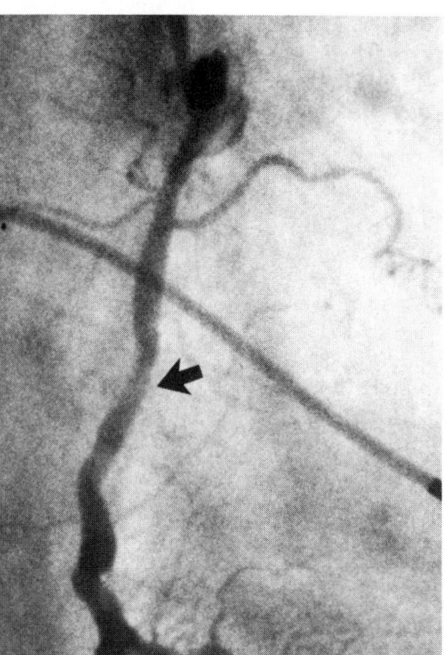

FIGURE 41-4. The "snowplow" effect. The left panel shows severe stenosis of the midportion of the right coronary artery (large arrow), from which a proximally diseased right ventricular branch (small arrow) originates. After PTCA (right panel), dilatation of the right coronary lesion has been achieved at the expense of occlusion of the right ventricular side branch. (From Baim, D. S.: Percutaneous transluminal angioplasty. *In* Petersdorf, R. G., et al. [eds.]: Harrison's Principles of Internal Medicine, Update VI. New York, McGraw-Hill Book Co., 1985.)

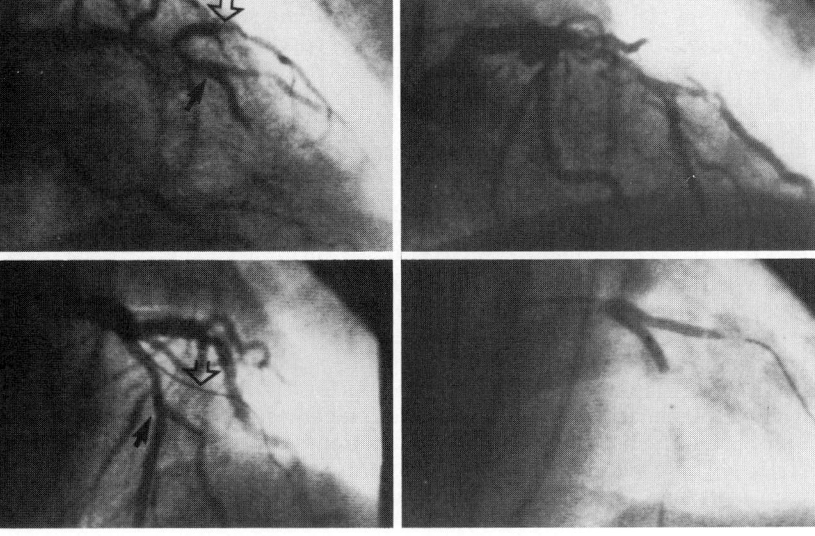

FIGURE 41-5. "Double-wire" and "kissing-balloon" techniques. To avoid occlusion of an involved branch, two guidewires are placed: one into the distal left anterior descending, and one into the involved diagonal. Repeated alternate balloon inflation in the two vessels resulted in alternating occlusion. With resort to a kissing-balloon approach, two balloons were inflated simultaneously to achieve patency of both vessels. (From Baim, D. S.: Coronary angioplasty. *In* Grossman, W., and Baim, D. S. [eds.]: Cardiac Catheterization, Angiography, and Intervention. 4th ed. Philadelphia, Lea and Febiger, 1991.)

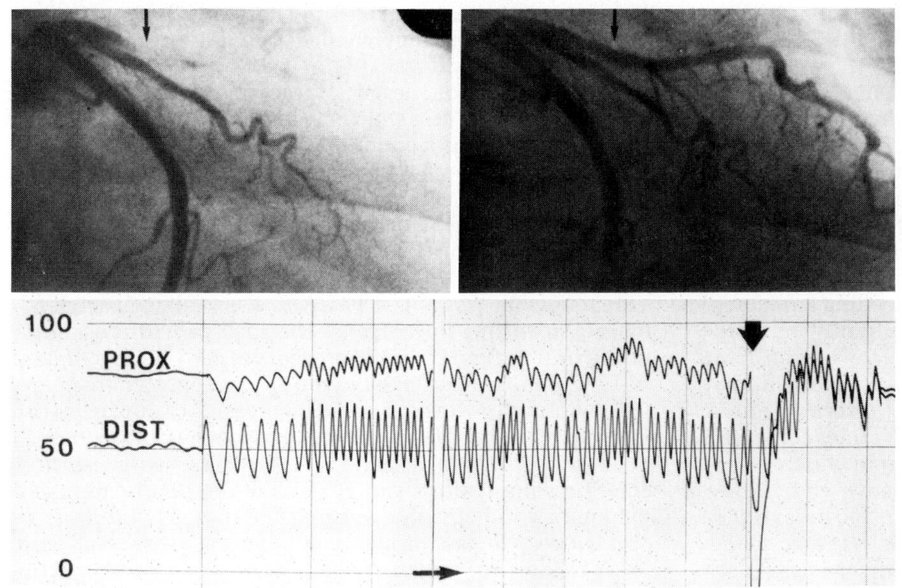

FIGURE 41–6. Angioplasty of a totally occluded coronary artery. Baseline angiography *(upper left)* shows total occlusion of the proximal left anterior descending. Prominent collateral filling of the distal vessel was evident during right coronary injection (not shown). Despite the presence of total occlusion of the involved vessel, this lesion was successfully crossed and dilated, with the result shown in the *upper right*. The *bottom panel* shows measurement of the "proximal" aortic and "distal" intracoronary pressure during inflation and after deflation (bold arrow) of the dilatation catheter. Note the presence of a high distal occluded coronary artery pressure (50 mm Hg), consistent with good collateral function, and the resolution of the pressure difference between the proximal and distal sampling sites after balloon deflation (residual transstenotic gradient 5 mm Hg). (From Dervan, J. P., Baim, D. S., Cherniles, J., and Grossman, W.: Transluminal angioplasty of occluded coronary arteries: Use of a movable guidewire system. Circulation *68:*776, 1983, by permission of the American Heart Association, Inc.)

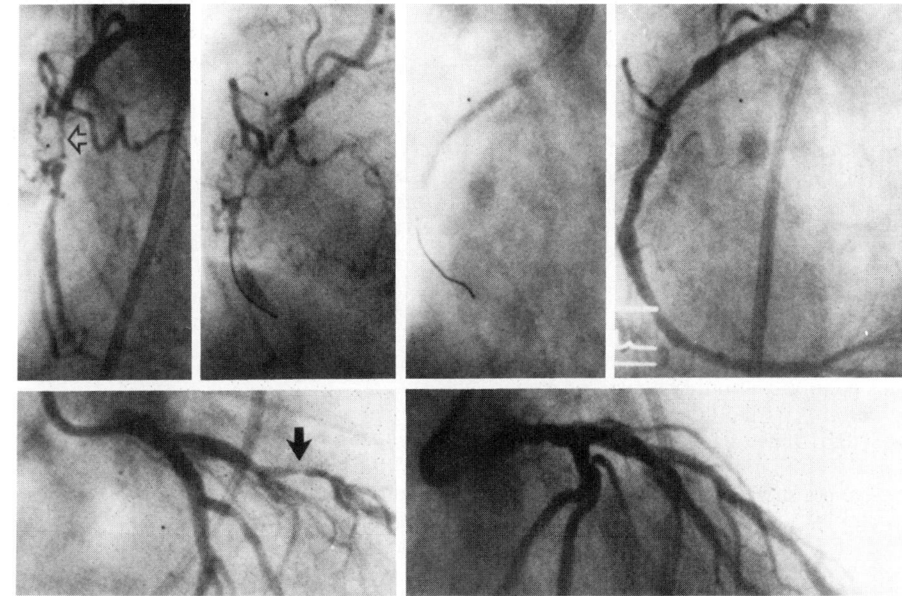

FIGURE 41–7. "Boot strap" two-vessel dilatation. *Upper panel* shows functionally occluded mid-right coronary artery, with filling of the distal vessel by way of bridging (right-to-right) and left-to-right collaterals. Successful dilatation of this lesion *(upper right)* restored antegrade flow in the right coronary artery and allowed reversal of the left-to-right collaterals to support the left anterior descending territory during dilatation of that vessel (bold arrow). (From Baim, D. S.: Coronary angioplasty. *In* Grossman, W. [ed.]: Cardiac Catheterization, Angiography, and Intervention. 4th ed. Philadelphia, Lea and Febiger, 1991.)

the actual PTCA procedure. The operator must decide which lesions are responsible for the patient's symptoms (the "culprit" lesions[25]) and therefore must be dilated, which lesions are mild enough to be left alone, what the sequence of dilatations should be, and whether a suboptimal result in one lesion necessitates deferral of other dilatations to a separate sitting (a "staged" multivessel PTCA procedure). These issues must be addressed on a case-by-case basis, but the general goal of PTCA in a patient with multivessel disease is to dilate all lesions which narrow the diameter of major coronary segments by more than 70 per cent. Milder lesions can be dilated easily, but such dilatation is not usually required to control symptoms and still entails some risk of abrupt reclosure or accelerated restenosis.[26] If natural progression of these mild lesions leads to recurrent ischemic symptoms, they can be addressed in a subsequent procedure. Given these uncertainties about PTCA in multivessel disease, an adequately controlled comparison of PTCA with bypass surgery—as in the Bypass Angioplasty Revascularization Intervention (BARI) Trial currently being conducted—will be required to establish the optimal application of PTCA in this important patient population.

CLINICAL INDICATIONS. At the same time PTCA has been applied to progressively more difficult *anatomical* situations, it has also been applied to a broader spectrum of *clinical* disease states. Whereas PTCA was initially used largely in patients with chronic, stable angina, it is now used increasingly in patients with more unstable patterns, i.e., new onset, rest, or preinfarction angina (p. 1340).[27] Between one-half and three-quarters of such patients are anatomically suitable for PTCA, particularly if revascularization can be limited to dilatation of one or more severe "culprit" lesions responsible for the unstable clinical picture[28] without attempting revascularization of other milder lesions, small branches, or chronic total occlusions. In many instances PTCA can be performed in patients with unstable angina as an extension of the initial diagnostic catheterization procedure.[29] A tendency toward an increased incidence of ischemic complications initially reported for PTCA in the unstable angina population can be reduced by several days of intravenous heparin infusion prior to attempted dilatation.[30]

Acute Myocardial Infarction (see also p. 1316). The majority of patients with acute myocardial infarction have anatomical features that make them suitable for PTCA, either after or instead of thrombolytic therapy. While current thrombolytic regimens are capable of restoring patency to more than 75 per cent of infarct-related arteries within 90 minutes of initiation of therapy, patients typically are left with at least moderate stenosis of the infarct vessel, which makes them prone to reocclusion, reinfarction, or subsequent angina. Angioplasty can generally be performed safely in acute myocardial infarction, and it was initially thought that routine catheterization and angioplasty of such patients following thrombolytic therapy might reduce the incidence of subsequent adverse events. Several studies (including the Thrombolysis in Myocardial Infarction or TIMI IIA trial), however, have shown that routine *immediate* catheterization and angioplasty increase the risk of procedure-related complications (bleeding and emergency bypass surgery) without improving mortality, reinfarction, or left ventricular function.[31] Similarly, the overall TIMI II study has shown that even routine *delayed* (18 to 48 hours) catheterization and angioplasty fail to affect favorably either in-hospital or 1-year mortality or reinfarction rates compared to a *conservative* strategy (watchful waiting) in which catheterization and PTCA are reserved for patients who exhibit recurrent spontaneous or exercise-induced myocardial ischemia.[32] Although it has not yet been compared to the conservative TIMI strategy in a controlled trial, *primary* angioplasty (e.g., angioplasty without prior thrombolytic therapy) appears able to safely restore patency of the infarct artery.[33] It may be of particular value in patients with contraindications to thrombolytic therapy, who present within 4 to 6 hours of symptom onset to an institution with skilled angioplasty operators and in-house surgical standby.

Post Bypass. A rapidly growing indication for PTCA is seen in patients with *recurrent angina following bypass surgery*, who may undergo dilation of a lesion in a saphenous vein[34,35,35a] or internal mammary[36] graft or of a lesion in a previously grafted or ungrafted native coronary artery.[34] Saphenous vein graft lesions occurring within 1 year of surgery are typically due to local intimal hyperplasia and dilate quite nicely, albeit with a relatively high (50 per cent) restenosis rate. Atherosclerotic graft lesions occurring several years after surgery are more friable, and are prone to disruption with distal embolization during attempted angioplasty. Recently occluded grafts pose special problems with distal thromboembolization and long-term patency, so that PTCA of such vessels generally should be avoided.[37]

Patients with other factors increasing the risk of bypass surgery (advanced age[38] or other medical problems) may be offered PTCA of unprotected left main lesions or diffuse three-vessel coronary disease that would otherwise be rejected for angioplasty in favor of bypass surgery.[39] When it is necessary to perform angioplasty on patients at high risk because of poor left ventricular function, the procedure may be performed with the temporary assistance of intraaortic balloon counterpulsation[40] or percutaneous cardiopulmonary support.[41]

At the other end of the spectrum, some patients with *milder anginal symptoms* (Canadian Heart Class I or II) may be subjected to catheterization followed by dilatation of one or more severe underlying lesions, rather than continuing with medical antianginal therapy. Although such patients constitute less than 20 per cent of those currently subjected to PTCA,[42] it should be pointed out that there is no evidence that PTCA is superior to medical therapy for this patient group in terms of longevity, freedom from subsequent myocardial infarction, or reduced long-term health costs.

ECONOMIC AND REGULATORY IMPLICATIONS

The rapidly growing role of PTCA is reflected in current statistics. An estimated 250,000 PTCA procedures are being performed annually, compared with approximately the same number of coronary artery bypass operations. From another perspective, the current utilization of PTCA is reflected in the revascularization outcome of patients undergoing first-time diagnostic catheterizations for coronary artery disease. Approximately 60 per cent of such patients are referred for revascularization, which consists of nearly equal numbers of PTCA and surgical bypass procedures.[42,43] Because PTCA can be performed for approximately one-half to one-third the in-hospital cost of bypass surgery, with a shorter length of stay and convalescent period, it is being increasingly favored by third-party payers. Most cost studies, however, do not factor in the hidden expenses of standby bypass surgery or the late expenses associated with treatment of restenosis, so that the magnitude of this cost savings may be somewhat less than expected.[44] Finally, both the success rate of PTCA and the resultant cost savings depend heavily on the experience and track record of the individual operator.

Standards for training in PTCA as a specialized part of fellowship are being developed[45] and include 150 procedures during training and 50 to 100 procedures per year to maintain the PTCA skills of individuals who have already entered practice. It is clear, however, that not all invasive cardiologists can or should perform PTCA, particularly complex procedures in which lack of ongoing experience is associated with less satisfactory results.[46] Moreover, because of the requirements for high-quality radiographic imaging and in-house cardiac surgical back-up to deal promptly with abrupt vessel reclosure, PTCA is likely to continue to be restricted to a fraction of the hospitals which currently perform diagnostic cardiac catheterization.

COMPLICATIONS

Like any cardiac catheterization procedure, PTCA is associated with risks relating to arrhythmia, arterial embolization, contrast agent toxicity, or vascular injury at the catheter entry site.[47,47a] One relatively unique complication, however, relates to the process by which angioplasty enlarges the stenotic coronary lumen. While angioplasty was initially thought to rely on compression of the atherosclerotic plaque[1,2,5] (Figs. 41–1 and 41–2), experimental studies disclose neither significant compression nor embolization of plaque elements.[48] Instead, the majority of improvement in vessel lumina appears to result from "cracking" and outward displacement of the plaque, associated with local plastic stretching of the media and adventitia (Fig. 41–8).[49,50] The use of a nonelastomeric balloon with an inflated diameter comparable to the diameter of the normal lumen adjacent to the stenotic segment is usually sufficient to achieve adequate dilatation. Use of a larger balloon increases the likelihood of excessive vessel trauma or

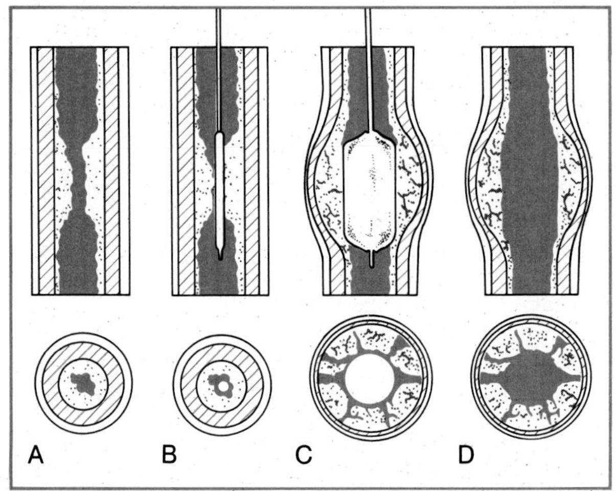

FIGURE 41–8. **Current concept of the mechanism of balloon dilatation. Serial panels show the baseline stenosis *(A)*, passage of the deflated balloon catheter *(B)*, balloon inflation *(C)*, and the postdilatation appearance *(D)*, as drawn in longitudinal and transverse cross-sectional views. Balloon inflation *(panel C)* is associated with fracture and outward displacement of the atherosclerotic plaque, as well as plastic stretching of the media and adventitia. The result *(panel D)* is enlargement of the lumen owing to expansion of the entire vessel wall, rather than compaction of atherosclerotic material. (From Castaneda-Zuniga, W. R., et al.: The mechanism of balloon angioplasty. Radiology *135*:565, 1980.)**

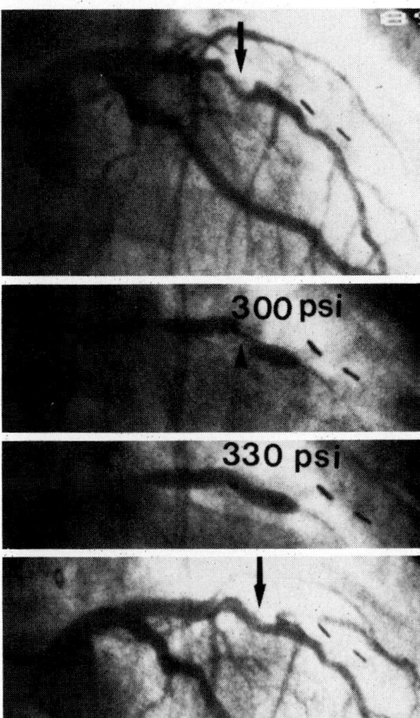

FIGURE 41-9. Angioplasty of a rigid lesion using a high-pressure balloon. This calcified stenosis in the midportion of the left anterior descending artery resisted dilatation at 300 psi (20 atm), but ultimately dilated at 330 psi with an acceptable result. Such rigid lesions are uncommon (<5 per cent) among angioplasty attempts. (From Baim, D. S.: Coronary angioplasty. *In* Grossman, W., and Baim D. S. [eds.]: Cardiac Catheterization, Angiography, and Intervention. 4th ed. Philadelphia, Lea and Febiger, 1991.)

vessel rupture precipitated by overdilatation.[51,52] Particularly rigid lesions may require inflation of the balloon to high pressure (10 to 20 atm, 150 to 300 psi) to achieve this result (Fig. 41-9), while eccentric lesions may require use of a slightly oversized balloon catheter, repeated inflations, or prolonged (1 minute) inflations to overcome the intrinsic elasticity of the normal arterial wall opposite the atherosclerotic plaque.[53] Although usually associated with transient left ventricular dysfunction,[54] these repeated transient coronary occlusions are usually well tolerated hemodynamically and do not cause serious arrhythmias. If limiting angina develops during balloon inflation in those patients who do not have good collateral flow to the dilated vessels, use of an autoperfusion balloon or distal Fluosol infusion through the inflated balloon[55] may help control temporary ischemia.

In the process of achieving adequate dilatation, neither too little nor too much "controlled injury" should be inflicted on the vessel wall. It is therefore important to monitor the adequacy of dilatation closely during the procedure, either by repeated angiographic examination of the dilated segment or by ongoing estimation of the residual translesional gradient,[56] i.e., the difference between mean aortic pressure and the mean coronary pressure distal to the dilated segment measured through the central lumen of the deflated balloon catheter (Fig. 41-6). Residual stenosis of less than 50 per cent and residual translesional gradients below 15 mm Hg are indicative of a successful procedure, although better results (30 per cent stenosis, or a 2-mm lumen in a 3-mm vessel) are commonly achieved.

Even when the dilatation has been successful, the vascular injury associated with PTCA is often evident in the radiographic appearance of intimal dissection at the dilatation site (Fig. 41-10). Patients with dissection may have some chest discomfort due to local vessel trauma, but limited dissection does not usually interfere with antegrade flow and goes on to heal by reendothelialization within 6 weeks of the dilatation procedure.

ABRUPT RECLOSURE. In approximately 4 per cent of patients—particularly those undergoing dilatation of long (more than 2 cm), eccentric, or curved stenotic segments—local injury produces more extensive dissection.[57] This may (in conjunction with local vasospasm or thrombus formation) progress to abrupt vessel closure within 30 minutes of dilatation.[18,58] Half the vessels which manifest abrupt reclosure can be reopened by redilatation[59] (Fig. 41-11), but the other half (or approximately 2.5 per cent of the total PTCA attempts) currently require emergency surgery if vessel closure recurs and is associated with clinical and electrocardiographic evidence of myocardial ischemia.[60] Management of this complication necessitates prompt availability of an experienced cardiac surgical team and highlights the need for close cooperation between interventional cardiologists and their surgical colleagues. Although most patients requiring emergency surgery recover uneventfully,[61] up to half still sustain some degree of a myocardial infarction despite prompt revascularization, contributing heavily to the 0.4 per cent mortality associated with elective PTCA. Management of abrupt reclosure has been improved recently with the advent of special perfusion or "shunt" catheters[62] (Fig. 41-12), which can be placed across the occluded segment to permit perfusion of the distal bed while surgical control of the situation is being achieved. Better understanding of the dilatation process may allow more predictable responses and lower the incidence of significant dissection, while newer adjunctive techniques, e.g., the use of even more prolonged balloon inflations, thermal welding of the dissection plane, or placement of an intraluminal vascular stent (Fig. 41-12), may allow more consistent reversal of the reclosure phenomenon (see below). These advances may reduce further the incidence of emergency coronary bypass grafting and might even obviate the need for in-house surgical standby during PTCA procedures.

RESTENOSIS. Enhanced understanding of the biology of angioplasty will be required to prevent restenosis of the dilated segment. After successful PTCA there should be no clinical, electrocardiographic, or thallium perfusion evidence of myocardial ischemia,[63,64] but in approximately 20 per cent of patients, evidence of myocardial ischemia reappears within 6 months of the dilatation, coupled with angiographic evidence of restenosis of the dilated segment (Fig. 41-13). An additional 5 to 10 per cent of patients may remain free of recurrent symptoms but demonstrate partial angiographic renarrowing of the dilated segment. Some clinical parameters—severe baseline stenosis, incomplete dilatation, unstable angina with a brief duration of symptoms, male gender, stenosis of the left anterior descending coronary artery, ostial stenosis, uncontrolled vasospasm at the dilatation site,[65,66] a soft lesion which dilates without visible dissection, or early asymptomatic perfusion defects after PTCA[67]—are associated with a higher incidence of late restenosis.

Animal studies suggest that post-PTCA restenosis results from platelet adhesion to the area of endothelial damage at the

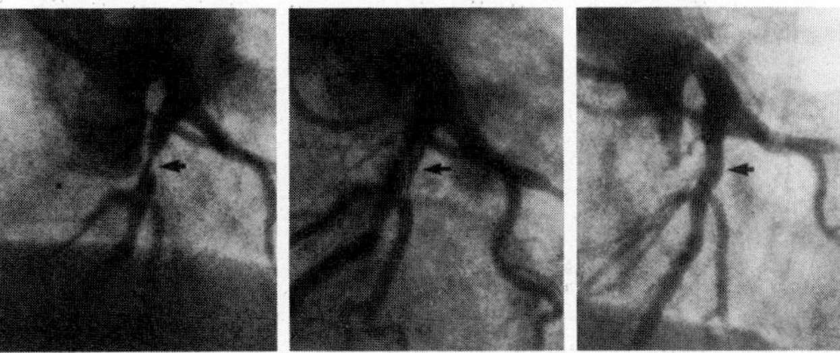

FIGURE 41-10. Intimal dissection during successful dilatation. Examination of the mid-left anterior descending artery (arrow) before *(left panel)* and immediately after (center panel) successful dilatation shows both enlargement of luminal caliber and the presence of two linear filling defects within the vessel lumen. This localized dissection did not impede antegrade flow and healed to leave an essentially normal vessel at 3-month restudy (right panel). (From Baim, D. S.: Percutaneous transluminal angioplasty. *In* Petersdorf, R. G., et al. [eds.]: Harrison's Principles of Internal Medicine, Update VI. New York, McGraw-Hill Book Co., 1985.)

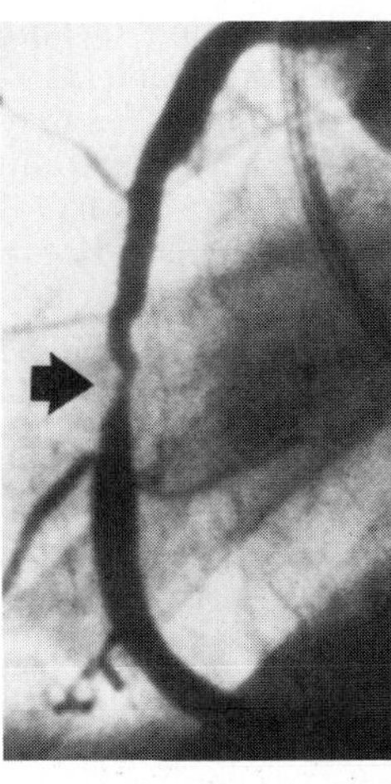

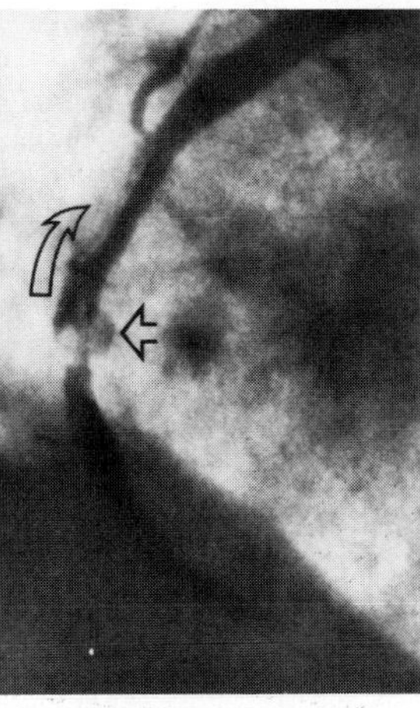

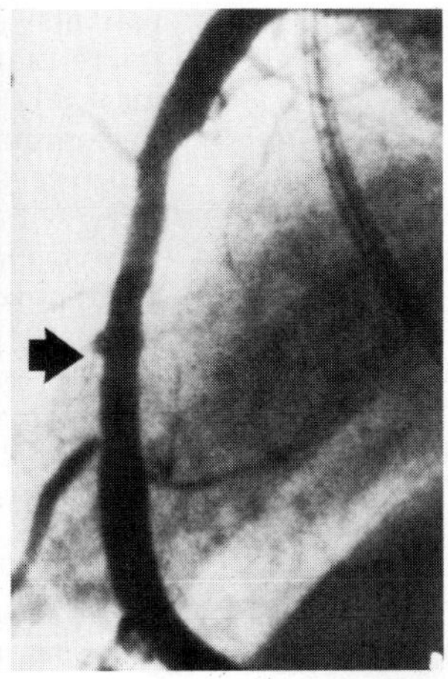

FIGURE 41-11. Dissection leading to abrupt closure. Baseline angiography (left panel) shows an eccentric lesion in the midportion of the right coronary artery. After dilatation with a 3.0-mm balloon (center panel) there is extensive dissection and imminent abrupt closure manifest as delayed propagation of distal contrast. Prolonged (10 minutes) inflation of a slightly larger 3.5-mm balloon catheter reestablished stable patency. (From Baim, D. S.: Coronary angioplasty. *In* Grossman, W., and Baim, D. S. [eds.]: Cardiac Catheterization, Angiography, and Intervention. 4th ed. Philadelphia, Lea and Febiger, 1991.)

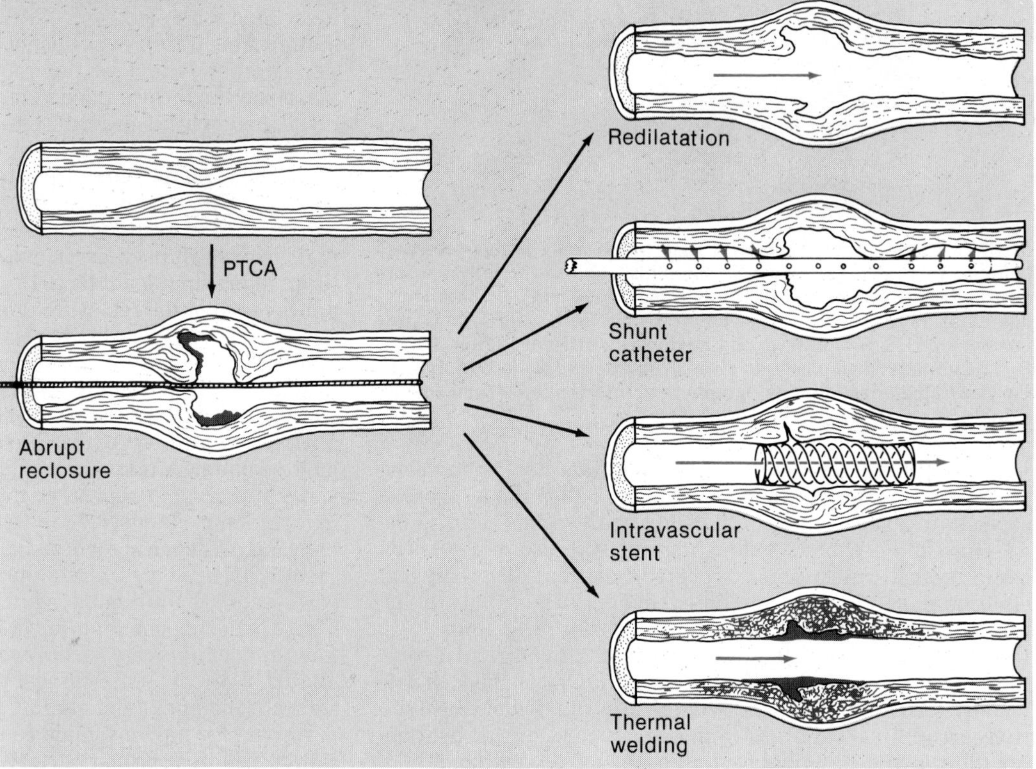

FIGURE 41-12. Current alternatives for the management of abrupt reclosure. Abrupt reclosure owing to local dissection and accompanying thrombosis or spasm occurs in approximately 5 per cent of vessels treated with PTCA (left panel). Although such vessels were previously allowed to remain completely occluded during preparations for emergency bypass surgery (see color plate 9), four alternative management strategies have now been developed: *Redilatation* using multiple, prolonged inflations of the balloon catheter is successful in remolding the dissected vessel into a stable patent configuration in approximately one-half of the cases of abrupt reclosure. In the remaining cases a *shunt catheter* can be positioned within the occluded segment, over an exchange-length guidewire. Arterial blood can enter this catheter through side holes located proximal to the point of occlusion and exit through side holes located distally, to maintain perfusion of the distal vessel as the patient is transported to the operating room. The catheter is then removed after the local delivery of cardioplegic solution and before placement of the aortic cross clamp. Two investigational approaches to abrupt reclosure include placement of an *intravascular stent* which can be delivered into the affected segment over a dilatation catheter and expanded to the caliber of the adjacent normal vessel by balloon inflation. This prevents the dissection flaps from acutely compromising lumen caliber and permits long-term patency and reendothialization in the presence of anticoagulant drugs. *Thermal welding* uses a laser-heated balloon catheter to coagulate and seal the local dissection and maintain vessel patency without placement of a prosthetic material.

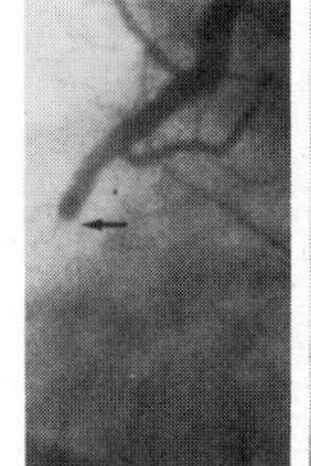

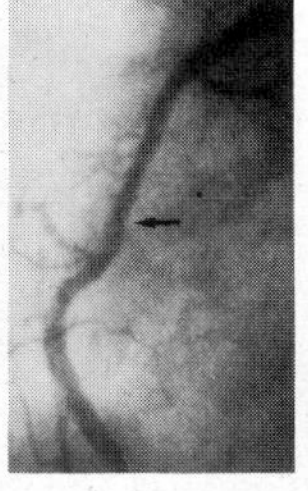

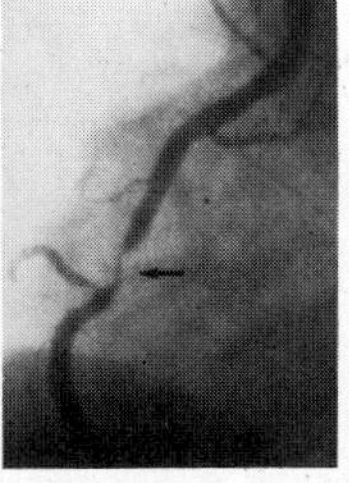

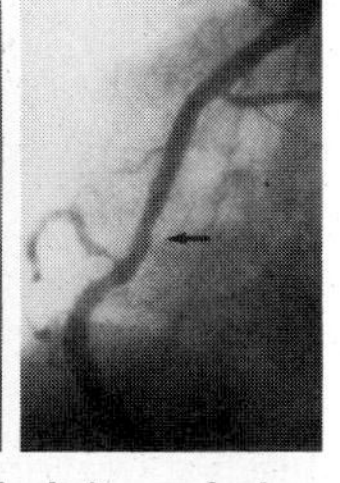

FIGURE 41-13. Restenosis of a dilated segment. The left panels show the appearance of a totally occluded mid-right coronary artery before and immediately after successful dilatation. Despite the absence of residual stenosis, this patient experienced recurrent symptoms 6 weeks after the procedure. Repeat catheterization (right panels) showed severe recurrence of the original lesion, which was successfully redilated. Restenosis developed again 6 weeks later (not shown), but this patient has now remained entirely asymptomatic for more than 4 years after a successful third dilatation. (From Baim, D. S.: Coronary angioplasty. In Grossman, W., and Baim, D. S. [eds.]: Cardiac Catheterization, Angiography, and Intervention. 4th ed. Philadelphia, Lea & Febiger, 1991.)

dilatation site, with subsequent release of potent smooth muscle vasoconstrictors and mitogens, such as platelet-derived growth factor (PDGF).[62] According to this hypothesis, restenosis represents a human correlate of the arterial injury technique used to create atherosclerotic plaques in experimental animals.[68a,68b] In support of this, postmortem and atherectomy[69] studies show that areas of restenosis tend to have a different, more proliferative histological appearance compared with the underlying primary plaque (color plate 9). This proliferative process (rather than simple recoil of the dilated vessel wall) is also favored by the angiographic finding of sta-

FIGURE 41-14. See color plate 9.

bility of the luminal diameter within the first month after PTCA, followed by subsequent progressive narrowing.[70,71]

On the other hand, adjunctive therapy with currently available antiplatelet agents (aspirin and dipyridamole) has failed to decrease the incidence of restenosis in PTCA patients, despite a favorable effect in some animal models. Clinical trials with other antiplatelet agents (prostacyclin analogs,[73] omega-3 fatty acids)[74] have similarly failed to show any consistent effect on restenosis. Other more potent antiplatelet agents[75-77] are currently being developed and may be at least partially effective if the platelet-triggered hypothesis is correct. A second avenue includes a search for pharmacological blockers of PDGF or techniques to leave behind a smoother and less platelet-attractive surface (thermal "smoothing" or mechanical plaque resection) in an effort to decrease the restenosis rate. Thus far, any favorable effects of new devices on restenosis appear to be the result of a larger initial lumen rather than reduction in intimal hyperplasia.[78] In the meantime, patients who have undergone successful PTCA should have their clinical symptoms and exercise test performance monitored closely over the 6 months following the procedure.

If clinical evidence of restenosis develops, repeat catheterization, including repeat PTCA, is the best management (Fig. 41–13). Repeat PTCA is almost always successful and is preferable to relying on intensified medical therapy alone, since the restenotic lesion may progress rapidly and produce escalating symptoms. Restenosis may develop in 30 to 40 per cent of patients after repeat PTCA, necessitating a third (or even a fourth) dilatation before long-term patency is secured.[79,80] If symptoms and signs of restenosis do not develop within 6 months of the dilatation procedure, they are unlikely to do so in future years, although anginal symptoms may develop because of progression of disease at other sites and require additional dilatation procedures.[64] Routine follow-up angiography is not clinically justified after PTCA, except in special situations (high-risk patients, commercial pilots). With the use of repeat PTCA for management of restenosis and progressive disease at other sites, fewer than 10 per cent of patients undergoing initially successful dilatation will require bypass surgery during the next several years.[8]

NEWER TECHNIQUES FOR TREATING VASCULAR STENOSIS

While essentially all experience in the treatment of coronary stenoses has involved the use of balloon dilatation, a number of other methods are under investigation.[81,81a] Given the advanced state and evident success of balloon dilatation, these methods must strive for the following goals: (1) to improve the crossing rate for difficult (e.g., totally occluded) lesions; (2) to dilate elastic, rigid, or diffusely diseased segments predictably; (3) to minimize or correct local injury responsible for abrupt vessel reclosure; and (4) to remove plaque and/or leave behind a smoother luminal surface in an effort to reduce the incidence of late restenosis.[82]

CORONARY STENTING. The concept of placing an intraluminal prosthesis to scaffold the treated vessel (stent) and maintain patency was advanced by Dotter more than 20 years ago[83] but has only recently become a therapeutic reality in the management of coronary artery disease.[83a] All current stents are made from polished metal wires or tubes and fall into two broad classes: (1) self-expanding stents (e.g., the Medinvent Wallstent), and (2) balloon-expandable stents (e.g., the Palmaz-Schatz or Gianturco-Roubin stent).[84,85] Regardless of design, use of all these devices presents difficulties in successful placement, prevention of thrombosis on the stent surface, and avoidance of excessive late intimal hyperplasia that can restrict the flow.[85a,85b]

Coronary stents remain investigational but have been implanted in more than 2,000 patients worldwide at the time of this writing. With suitable refinement of the delivery system, stent implantation can be accomplished in more than 97 per cent of patients with relatively focal (<15 mm length) lesions. Because of the relative absence of elastic recoil, stent placement results in the creation of a large and smooth lumen whose diameter approximates or even slightly exceeds that of the adjacent reference segment, regardless of the underlying lesion morphology (eccentricity, ulceration, or friable plaque in an aged saphenous vein bypass graft)[86-89] (Fig. 41–15). Both mild intimal flaps and the more severe dissections responsible for post-PTCA abrupt vessel closure can be controlled by stent placement. Given the inherent thrombogenicity of current metallic stents, aggressive anticoagulation with heparin, aspirin, dipyridamole, and low molecular weight dextran (dextran 40) is generally required to prevent immediate thrombosis.[84] This is followed by continued heparin infusion until effective anticoagulation with oral warfarin is established, and given concurrently with aspirin and dipyridamole. Interruption of this regimen within the first 2 weeks after stent placement (i.e., to manage bleeding from the gastrointestinal system or the vascular puncture site) carries an incidence of subacute stent thrombosis as great as 15 per cent. On the other hand, removal of the vascular sheath on uninterrupted anticoagulation engenders a 5 to 10 per cent incidence of vascular complications requiring surgical correction under local anesthesia. Warfarin therapy may be discontinued in approximately 8 weeks, at which time the stent is fully endothelialized. Antibiotic prophylaxis for dental procedures is also imperative until the stent is fully endothelialized.

The fibrocellular layer that forms over the stent at the blood interface is typically 0.2 to 0.5 mm thick at 8 weeks, with some subsequent thinning as it matures further. By 6 months, this local intimal hyperplasia has caused the typical stented coronary lumen to lose 1 mm in luminal diameter, which is equivalent to a 30 per cent diameter stenosis in a 3-mm vessel. While the restenosis rate (defined as the fraction of patients with a stenosis > 60 per cent) may be as low as 15 to 20 per cent for stented vessels, it is important to emphasize that this appears to be because the larger stented lumen can tolerate more late loss due to intimal hyperplasia rather than because a stented vessel develops less local hyperplasia.[78]

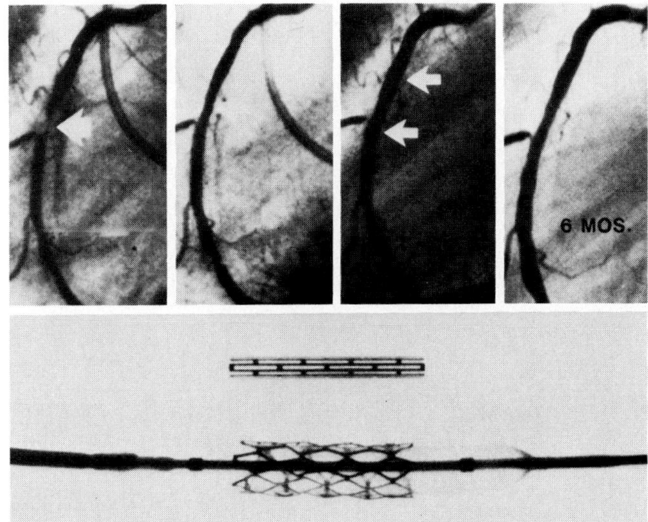

FIGURE 41–15. **Placement of an intracoronary stent. This patient had an eccentric restenosis of the midportion of the right coronary artery *(left panel)*. After predilation with a 3.0-mm balloon *(left center)*, moderate (35 per cent) stenosis remained because of elastic recoil of the vessel wall. Placement of a single Palmaz-Schatz balloon-expandable stent *(right center)* allowed further enlargement of the vessel lumen. While there was some loss of luminal caliber due to intimal hyperplasia within the stent at 6-month routine follow-up angiography *(right panel)*, the degree of stenosis was 32 per cent and the exercise test showed no evidence of ischemia. The stent itself is shown *(bottom panel)* in both its original and expanded configurations. (From Levine, M. J., et al.: Clinical and angiographic results of balloon-expandable intracoronary stents in right coronary artery stenoses. J. Am. Coll. Cardiol. *16*:332, 1990.)**

ATHERECTOMY. While both conventional balloon angioplasty and coronary stenting work by outward displacement of plaque, several catheter designs have been developed to actually remove plaque mass. The first of these designs was the side-cutting directional atherectomy catheter designed by Simpson et al.[90,90a] It consists of a cylindrical metal chamber in which a 10 mm long window has been cut. On the outside of the chamber opposite the window, a small (1.8 mm) balloon is affixed. Low-pressure balloon inflation serves to press the window against the diseased vessel wall. Any plaque that prolapses into the cylinder is then cut free by a cup-shaped cutter and trapped in the tip of the catheter, allowing it to be removed from the body.

After trials of this concept in diseased peripheral arteries,[91] a coronary design entered clinical testing in 1988.[69] By mid 1990, more than 1,200 patients had been treated, with favorable rates of acute success (88 per cent) and emergency surgery (3 per cent). Perforation has been reported in 0.5 to 0.7 per cent of atherectomy-treated vessels, particularly when atherectomy is used in an effort to retrieve an extensive dissection that has developed following conventional PTCA. Treated vessels have a smoother surface and less residual stenosis than do vessels treated with conventional angioplasty,[92] and the technique appears to be particularly useful in larger (>3 mm diameter) noncalcified vessels with ostial, eccentric, or ulcerated lesions less than 20 mm in length (Fig. 41–16). Weighing shows a mean removed plaque sample weight of approximately 20 mg, suggesting that only part of the luminal improvement results from tissue removal per se.[69] The remainder of the improvement appears to result from "facilitated angioplasty" in which mechanical dilatation takes place within the bases of the initial atherectomy cuts. The restenosis rate for directional coronary atherectomy is currently 20 to 30 per cent, but has not yet been compared to that of conventional angioplasty in a randomized trial. The Simpson atherectomy system was approved by the Food and Drug Administration for general use in the coronary circulation in mid 1990.

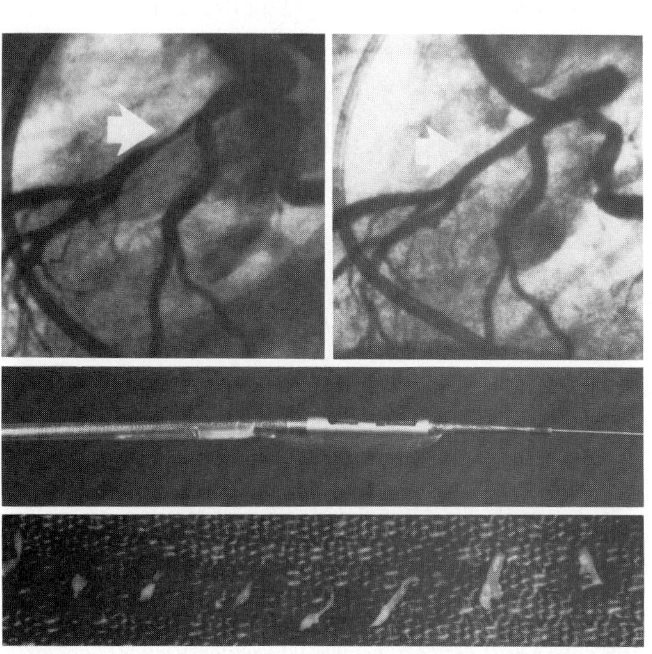

FIGURE 41–16. Directional coronary atherectomy. This patient had an eccentric restenosis lesion *(upper left)* of the left anterior descending artery following conventional angioplasty. This lesion was treated by directional coronary atherectomy using a No. 6 French device *(middle)*, with removal of the specimens shown *(bottom)*, producing a smooth lumen without residual stenosis. There was slight stenosis evident at routine 6-month angiography *(upper right)* (presumably the result of local intimal hyperplasia), but no evidence of regional ischemia. (From Safian, R. D., et al.: Coronary atherectomy: Clinical, angiographic and histologic findings and observations regarding mechanism. Circulation *82*:69, 1990.)

There has been less experience to date with two other atherectomy systems. The *end-cutting design* developed by Stack et al.[93] uses blades mounted on the tip of a rotating catheter to cut free fragments of plaque, which are then suctioned out of the body through the central lumen of the catheter. In the absence of mechanical advantage (i.e., a balloon catheter), this device typically cannot provide a larger lumen than the physical diameter of the cutter (2 mm), so that postatherectomy balloon angioplasty may be required to adequately treat larger vessels. The *Rotablator* developed by Auth et al. utilizes fine diamond chips mounted on the leading surface of a metal burr, which is rotated rapidly (100,000 rpm) as it is advanced down the diseased vessel over a guidewire.[94,95,95a] Plaque ground free from the lesion is pulverized into fragments averaging 25 μm in diameter. These fragments are generally well tolerated by the distal coronary circulation, although they may cause transient ischemia if generated in excessive size or number by aggressive cutting. Except in vessels of smaller diameter, subsequent PTCA is commonly required to achieve adequate lumen, and restenosis rates appear to be 30 to 40 per cent. Both devices seem to be particularly useful in smaller, diffusely diseased vessels.

LASER ANGIOPLASTY. Lasers emitting any of several wavelengths from the infrared to the ultraviolet bands can be used to deliver energy to the stenotic vessel by means of fiberoptic catheters. The fundamental goal of laser angioplasty is the direct ablation of plaque material.[96] This usually produces associated prothrombotic thermal charring and surrounding acoustic ("blast") injury of the adjacent vessel wall when the comparatively long wavelength lasers used in our medical applications ($CO_2 = 10.6\ \mu$, Nd:YAG $= 1.06\ \mu$, argon $= 0.5\ \mu$), are employed, but there is some evidence that the shorter wavelength excimer laser (less than 0.3 μ) achieves ablation of plaques with less surrounding thermal and acoustic injury.[96,97] Similar effects may be obtained by rapid-pulsing, high-energy lasers of longer wavelengths. Clinical trials with the excimer laser in the coronary circulation have utilized multifiber catheters that are advanced over a guidewire.[98,99] Because of the limited diameter of the catheter, these devices are most effective in smaller-diameter vessels or as pretreatment devices before conventional balloon dilatation. There is experimental evidence that the luminal surface present after excimer laser treatment is less thrombogenic than that seen after thermal injury as might be produced by a continuous-wave laser of longer wavelength.[100] Although the use of an over-the-wire system prevents use as a device to cross total occlusions, perforation appears to be much less frequent than was the case with earlier bare-fiber laser approaches. To date, a modified delivery system, plaque staining, or the use of fluorescence-guided ablation[101] has not overcome *that* limitation of laser ablation.

Another use of laser energy is as a thermal source to intentionally heat the diseased vessel segment. The so-called hot-tip design utilized a metal cap placed over the end of the laser fiber, which was heated to several hundred degrees during laser activation. Clinical trials, however, suggest that much of the ability of this device to cross chronic total occlusions in the peripheral circulation was the result of its mechanical properties rather than tip heating.[102] On the other hand, the "laser balloon" catheter developed by Spears et al.[103] uses a diffusing fiber wrapped around the central core of a balloon catheter to deliver Nd:YAG laser energy to the vessel wall during balloon inflation. It appears to be at least partially effective in overcoming vessel elasticity and providing a smooth luminal surface despite preexisting dissections or flaps (Fig. 41–17), but has thus far been associated with a restenosis rate of 35 to 50 per cent. If the restenosis limitation can be overcome, other thermal sources might be employed in a similar fashion.[104]

OTHER APPROACHES TO TOTAL OCCLUSIONS. Difficulty in crossing a chronically occluded segment constitutes one of the main remaining limitations of conventional angioplasty[24] and has thus been a driving force for device development. Modifications of mechanical force[105,106] appear to offer

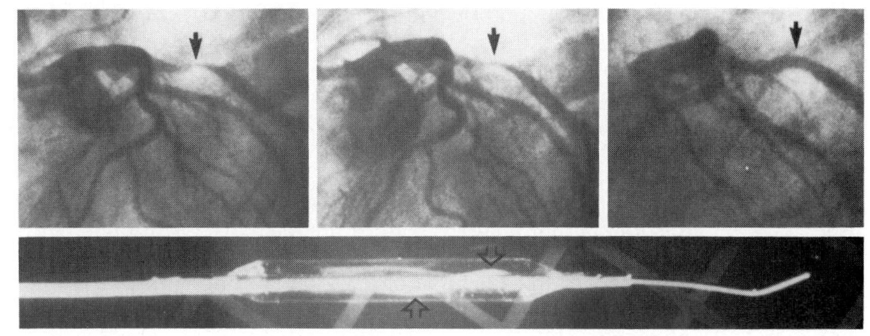

FIGURE 41-17. **Laser balloon angioplasty. An eccentric lesion in the circumflex *(left)* responded elastically to conventional angioplasty using a 3.0-mm balloon *(center)*. Following treatment with an identical-size laser balloon with 20 sec of Nd:YAG delivery during balloon inflation, adequate to heat the vessel wall to 80 to 90°C, wide luminal patency was obtained *(right)*. The design of the Spears laser balloon is shown *(bottom)* with a diffusing fiber wrapped helically around the balloon central shaft.**

some increase in crossing rate without a significant increase in vessel perforation. Because an ablative laser system usable in this situation is lacking, other alternatives utilizing ultrasonic energy are currently being explored.[107,108]

ANGIOPLASTY OF OTHER (NONCORONARY) ARTERIES

Most interventional techniques have been developed and tested in peripheral vessels (femoral or iliac arteries).[1,5,90,106,109] The number of peripheral angioplasty procedures, however, remains much smaller than the number of coronary angioplasties because of a lack of established referral pattern among the involved (medical, surgical, radiological) specialties, general lack of knowledge about interventional alternatives to vascular surgery, and lack of enthusiasm for angiography in patients with ischemic syndromes milder than rest pain.[110,111] In general, the results of peripheral angioplasty are similar to those described for PTCA. Primary success rates for peripheral arterial balloon dilatation exceed 95 per cent for the iliac and 87 per cent for the femoral arteries, with a 5-year restenosis rate which varies from 10 per cent for iliac vessels up to 40 per cent for smaller popliteal vessels.[112-114] Peripheral lesions, however, are more likely to be long (up to 10 cm) or totally occluded, in comparison to coronary arterial lesions. These technical challenges, coupled with better end-organ tolerance of ischemia and the absence of cardiac tamponade as a complication of vessel perforation or rupture, have fostered more aggressive trials of mechanical, thermal, or laser techniques in the peripheral circulation.

As in coronary angioplasty, peripheral angioplasty of technically suitable lesions may offer significant clinical and economic benefits over surgical repair, particularly since patients with peripheral vascular disease frequently have other cardiac or pulmonary disease that increases the risk of general anesthesia. Because peripheral angiography is viewed as a preparation for vascular surgery, however, only a small fraction of patients with mildly or moderately symptomatic peripheral vascular disease are currently offered the option of peripheral angioplasty.[110]

Dilatation of atherosclerotic or fibromuscular stenoses in the *renal arteries* followed peripheral angioplasty as an application of balloon angioplasty (Fig. 41-18).[6] Renal artery angioplasty continues to be applied with excellent short- and long-term success as an alternative to vascular surgery in patients with renovascular hypertension (p. 835) or renal insufficiency as the result of anatomically suitable stenoses in the main artery or its principal branch.[115,116] Overall, patients with hypertension due to fibromuscular renal arterial disease have an excellent chance of cure (70 per cent), improvement (20 per cent), and lower risk of restenosis (10 to 20 per cent), compared to patients with atherosclerotic renal arterial disease in whom the chances of cure (25 per cent), improvement (40 per cent), and restenosis (40 to 70 per cent) are less favorable. Still, the incidence of major complications from renal angioplasty is low, and these results compare quite favorably with those of renovascular surgery.

In their original paper,[1] Dotter and Judkins predicted that interventional techniques would ultimately be applied to a variety of other vascular territories, including the *brachiocephalic and cerebral circulation*. Although the underlying disease processes (atherosclerosis and fibromuscular disease) are similar to those treated by balloon angioplasty in other vascular beds, carotid lesions are more likely to exhibit ulceration and adherent thrombus. At the same time, the brain is less tolerant of microembolic debris than any other end organ, Balloon angioplasty, however, continues to be used in inoper-

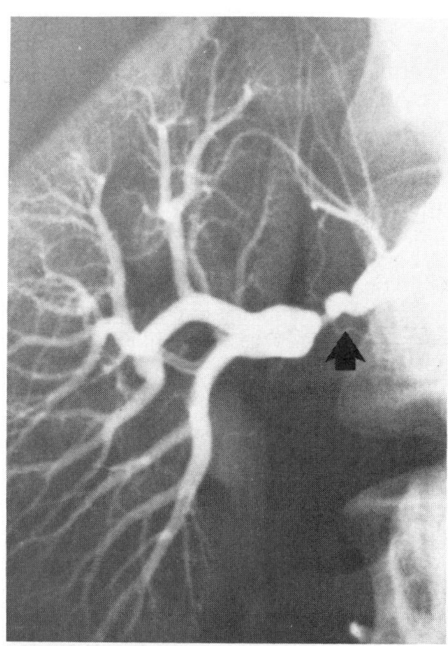

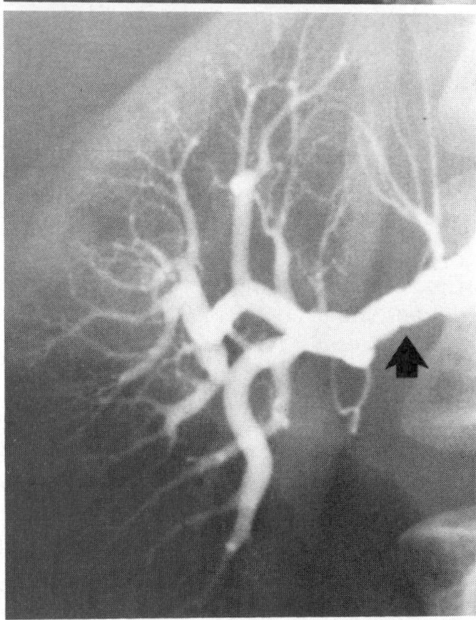

FIGURE 41-18. **Renal artery angioplasty. *Top,* Severe stenosis of the right renal artery (arrow) due to fibromuscular disease in a patient with refractory hypertension. *Bottom,* Luminal caliber improved after successful dilatation. (Courtesy of Ducksoo Kim, M.D.)**

able lesions of the posterior circulation and in small numbers of patients with stenosis of the extracranial carotid artery.[117,118] Still, use of these applications is likely to increase rapidly over the next decade, since surgical correction of cerebrovascular disease is performed in approximately 100,000 patients per year in the United States and continues to be associated with significant morbidity.

Balloon dilatation of other stenotic vessels has also been used. This includes dilatation of stenoses in pulmonary arteries or veins and vascular shunts.[119-121] A conventional catheter is generally used to cross the target stenosis and place an exchange-length guidewire. The conventional catheter is then removed, and replaced by a balloon dilatation catheter of appropriate diameter. Because of the elasticity of most congenital stenoses, balloon diameters of 10 to 12 mm (slightly larger than the adjacent normal segment) may be required to produce significant dilatation. Balloon dilatation has also been used to maintain patency of the *ductus arteriosus* in children with cyanotic congenital heart disease and to treat *coarctation of the aorta.* The site of coarctation is crossed with a guidewire, which permits advancement of a diagnostic catheter for performance of baseline angiography and calculation of the aortic diameter adjacent to the area of narrowing. A balloon catheter with a diameter 1 or 2 mm less than that of the normal segment is then advanced over the guidewire, positioned within the stenotic segment, and inflated with dilute contrast material. Successful procedures are marked by at least a 30 per cent increase in the diameter of the treated segment and at least a 50 per cent reduction in the associated pressure gradient. Because primary dilatation of coarctation is associated with a significant incidence of late aneurysm formation,[122] it may be appropriate to reserve balloon dilatation for recurrent stenoses which develop after primary surgical repair (p. 921).[123,124]

Treatment of Valvular Stenosis

PULMONARY BALLOON VALVULOPLASTY

Pulmonary valvular stenosis (p. 931), a relatively common congenital cardiac lesion, was traditionally corrected by surgical "valvuloplasty," i.e., incision of fused commissures under direct vision. Beginning in 1982 pediatric cardiologists began using balloon dilatation catheters with inflated diameters 1 to 2 mm larger than the annulus size (20 to 25 mm) to produce similar commissural splitting by way of a closed transluminal approach.[126] This procedure has been quite successful, with a reduction of the pulmonic valve gradient to approximately one-third of its baseline value. Given the high success rate and low incidence of complication, balloon valvuloplasty has essentially replaced open surgical repair for valvular pulmonic stenosis (p. 933). Application of balloon valvuloplasty for the treatment of *congenital* aortic stenosis has also been reported (p. 1043), with a 70 per cent reduction in valve gradient and no significant increase in aortic regurgitation.[127]

MITRAL BALLOON VALVULOPLASTY

In contrast to *congenital* pulmonic or aortic stenosis, it was believed that adult *acquired* rheumatic and/or calcific stenosis of the mitral or aortic valves would *not* be amenable to balloon valvuloplasty because of (1) the more rigid structure of such lesions, (2) the potential for systemic embolization of valve debris, and (3) the potential for creating severe regurgitation. In 1985, however, balloon valvuloplasty was first applied to young adult patients with acquired (rheumatic) mitral stenosis, using a transseptal approach,[128] and the technique has become widely adapted as an alternative to surgical repair or replacement of stenotic mitral valves.[126]

TECHNIQUE. After puncture of the intraatrial septum with a needle and long sheath (Fig. 7–5, p. 184), a small balloon flotation catheter is advanced from the left atrium to the left ventricle. While it was once common to then advance this catheter across the aortic valve into the descending aorta (Fig. 41–19), a position near the apex of the left ventricle is easier to obtain and adequate for most mitral valvuloplasty procedures. An exchange-length (260 cm) guidewire is then positioned through this catheter to allow removal of the balloon flotation catheter and advancement of a small (8 mm) dilatation catheter for enlargement of the opening made in the intraatrial septum. This step is required to facilitate passage of the larger (23- to 25-mm diameter) valvuloplasty balloon through the intraatrial septum and across the stenotic mitral valve. Inflation of this larger balloon results in separation of the fused commissures analogous to the earlier surgical technique of closed or open mitral commissurotomy. Subsequent variations of the technique have included the use of two smaller (12 to 18 mm) balloon catheters, which can be advanced individually across the atrial septum and then inflated simultaneously within the mitral orifice[126] or use of a single compliant dumbbell-shaped balloon.[129]

After these encouraging results in young adults with rheumatic mitral stenosis, similar procedures were attempted in adult patients with more rigid calcific lesions (p. 1017). Using this technique, it has been possible to achieve physiologically

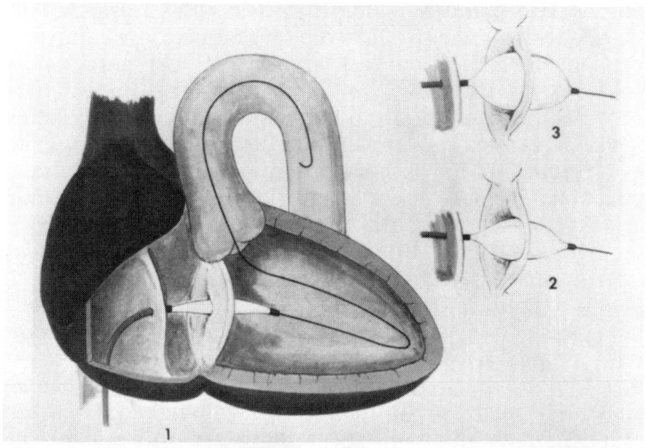

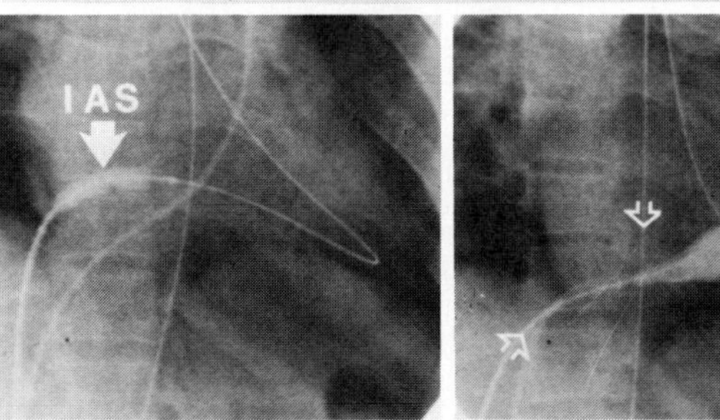

FIGURE 41–19. Mitral balloon valvuloplasty. The *top panel* shows the transseptal approach to mitral valvuloplasty, while the *bottom panel* shows radiographic frames obtained during an actual procedure. After dilatation of the intraatrial septum (IAS) by an 8-mm balloon catheter, a 25-mm dilatation catheter is advanced into the mitral valve orifice (MVO) and inflated. Note the appearance of a "waist" corresponding to the impression of the stenotic mitral orifice on the partially inflated dilatation catheter. This waist resolved with full inflation of the balloon, associated with an increase in mitral valve area from 0.9 to 1.6 cm². The path of the guidewire from right atrium to left atrium, to left ventricle, to descending aorta is shown by the open arrows.

adequate enlargement of the mitral orifice area (from 0.9 to 2.0 cm^2). Overall procedural mortality is 1 to 2 per cent, with cardiac perforation by the transseptal needle, guidewire, or dilatation catheter in approximately 1 per cent of patients. A significant increase in the degree of mitral regurgitation is uncommon, as are systemic emboli in patients preselected by transesophageal echocardiography for absence of left atrial thrombus and pretreated with oral warfarin for 2 to 3 months before attenuated valvuloplasty. Approximately 20 per cent of patients show evidence of a small ($<2:1$) left-to-right shunt at the atrial level, owing to dilatation of the atrial septal puncture during passage of the valvuloplasty balloon. Approximately half of these shunts resolve spontaneously by the time of follow-up catheterization.[130] This minor complication should become even less common as improved technology permits the production of valvuloplasty balloons with smaller collapsed profiles. Similarly, balloon catheters capable of more rapid inflation and deflation will be of value in minimizing the period of systemic arterial hypotension which invariably results from transient occlusion of left ventricular inflow during balloon inflation.

RESULTS. Early (6- to 12-month) follow-up studies have demonstrated preservation of the improved mitral orifice and similar physiological improvements (fall in filling pressures and pulmonary vascular resistance) to those seen after surgical correction of mitral stenosis.[128,131] Both the early and late (1 year) hemodynamic result can be predicted by an "echocardiographic score" in which four unfavorable features (poor leaflet mobility, valvular thickening, subvalvular thickening, and valvular calcification) are each assigned a value of 1 to 4. Patients with a cumulative score below 8 have a greater than 90 per cent chance of a good initial result (valve area > 1.5 cm^2) and a low chance (4 per cent) of significant restenosis at 1 year. In contrast, patients with a cumulative score of 8 to 16 have only a 50 per cent chance of a good initial result and a 70 per cent chance of restenosis at 1 year.[126] This pattern may relate to a greater contribution of separation of commissural fusion in patients with pliable leaflets versus a more limited benefit obtained by leaflet cracking and transient stretching of the mitral valve annulus in patients with more rigid valvular and subvalvular structures.

AORTIC BALLOON VALVULOPLASTY

(See also p. 1043)

With evident success of balloon valvuloplasty in the treatment of acquired mitral stenosis and of congenital aortic stenosis in children (p. 925), attention has now been turned to dilatation of calcific aortic stenosis in the adult. This disorder is the principal indication for most of the approximately 20,000 aortic valve replacements performed each year in the United States. Narrowing of the valve orifice is due to a combination of an underlying congenital structural abnormality (e.g., a bicuspid aortic valve), commissural fusion, and stiffening of the leaflets by extensive calcium deposition. Postmortem and intraoperative balloon dilatations have demonstrated separation of fused commissures, increased leaflet pliability due to microfractures and macrofractures through the calcium deposits, and transient stretching of the aortic annulus.[133] These findings suggested that percutaneous aortic valvuloplasty might be possible in advanced aortic stenosis. By 1990 this procedure had been performed in more than 1,000 patients, using principally the retrograde approach (Fig. 41–20).[126]

TECHNIQUE. A conventional catheter is advanced retrogradely across the stenotic valve and into the left ventricle. Through this catheter an exchange-length guidewire is then positioned in the left ventricular apex and used to advance a series of balloon dilatation catheters (12, 15, 18, 20, and, occasionally, 23 mm in diameter) across the stenotic valve. Each balloon is inflated several times using dilute liquid radiographic contrast material. Maintenance of the balloon within

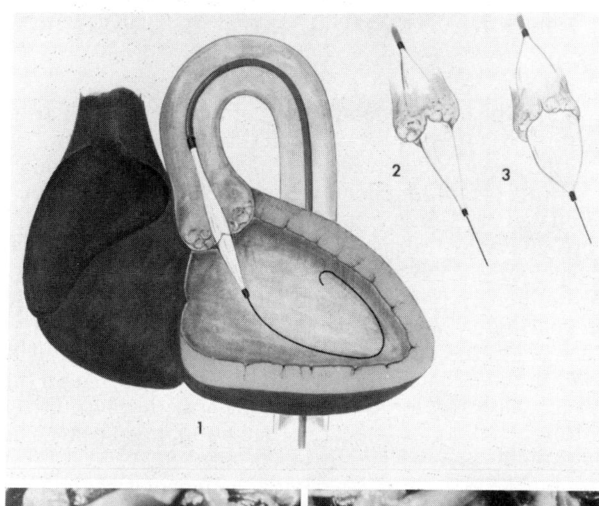

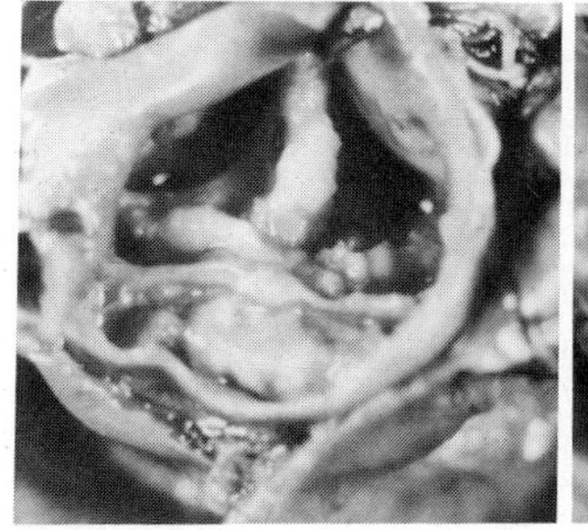

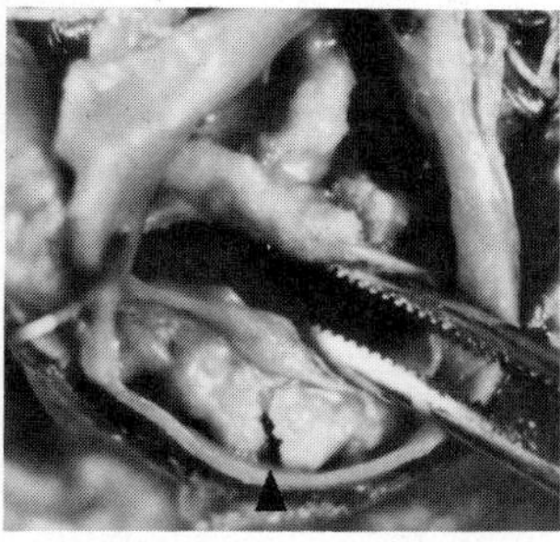

FIGURE 41–20. **Aortic balloon valvuloplasty. The *top panel* shows the retrograde approach to aortic valvuloplasty, while the *bottom panels* show the gross appearance of a stenotic aortic valve before (*left*) and after (*right*) postmortem balloon valvuloplasty. Note the fracture through the large calcified nodule (arrow) and the overall improvement in leaflet compliance.**

the aortic orifice during inflation is difficult because of a tendency for the balloon to be ejected by the force of left ventricular contraction but is facilitated by the use of catheters with longer (i.e., 6-cm rather than 3-cm) balloon segments. In patients with peripheral vascular disease, aortic balloon valvuloplasty can be performed using an antegrade (transseptal) approach, similar to that used for mitral valvuloplasty.

RESULTS. The magnitude of orifice improvement during aortic valvuloplasty (from 0.6 to 0.9 cm^2, peak gradient from 60 to 30 mm Hg) appears to be less than that seen with mitral valvuloplasty, but is usually adequate to produce marked improvement in clinical status, filling pressures, and left ventricular performance in patients with severe resting symptoms caused by critical aortic stenosis.[133a,134] Procedural mortality is 5 per cent[134a]; other problems include systemic emboli (1.5 per cent), worsened aortic regurgitation (1 per cent), and vascular injury at the access site (5 to 10 per cent). Balloon inflation seems to cause less hemodynamic compromise than is seen during mitral dilatation because some left ventricular ejection can occur between the inflated balloon and the aortic commissures.

While aortic balloon valvuloplasty is likely to play an increasing role in the treatment of patients whose poor left ventricular function, advanced age, or other medical problems place them at high risk for surgical aortic valve replacement,[135,136,136a] improvement in the orifice area is less than that usually obtained with a valve replacement, and an unacceptably high fraction of patients show evidence of poor long-term (24-month) results[136b] by death (30 to 40 per cent), repeat valvuloplasty (20 per cent), or valve replacement (15 to 20 per cent). Since the predominant effect is by leaflet cracking and annulus stretching, changes in technique (e.g., the use of larger-diameter balloons) have increased the incidence of complications without providing better immediate or long-term results. Valve replacement is thus still preferred in patients with severe aortic stenosis who are candidates for surgery.

Some of the earliest applications of interventional cardiology were in patients with congenital heart disease.[121] In 1966 Rashkind described passage of a balloon catheter through a preexisting patent foramen ovale, followed by withdrawal of the inflated balloon to create a functional atrial septal defect in patients with transposition of the great arteries (p. 941), tricuspid atresia, pulmonic atresia, mitral atresia, total anomalous pulmonary venous return, or a single ventricle.[137] Sixteen years later Park and coworkers modified this technique by use of a catheter with a surgical blade, which can be deployed in the left atrium after transseptal puncture and then used to incise the atrial septum during withdrawal.[138] The resulting atrial septal defect can then be enlarged using a balloon catheter as described by Rashkind.

In addition to the creation or enlargement of vascular channels, pediatric cardiologists have also developed devices for closing aberrant vascular channels. Rashkind developed a "double-disc" prosthesis which can be passed across an unwanted atrial septal defect, ventricular septal defect, or patent ductus arteriosus[139-141] (Fig. 41-21). The first disc is deployed on the far side of the defect and then held in place by three spring struts, as the remaining disc and struts are pulled back across the defect and deployed on its near side. The result is sealing of the defect between two layers of prosthetic material.

Methods have also been developed for preoperative closure of unwanted systemic-pulmonary collateral vessels in patients undergoing correction of tetralogy of Fallot, using preformed steel coils or detachable balloons embolized into the unwanted vessel through a catheter delivery system[121,142,143] (Fig. 41-22). These approaches—similar to those used by vascular radiologists to treat arteriovenous malformations or actively bleeding vessels in other beds—lead to occlusion of the target vessel by local thrombosis.

SUMMARY

After the first tentative exploration of mechanical dilatation in the peripheral arterial circulation, the past 15 years have seen the explosive growth of interventional techniques for the treatment of a number of common cardiovascular diseases. Of these techniques, balloon dilatation is the most highly developed. It provides a safe and effective alternative to bypass surgery in up to one-half of patients requiring revascularization of coronary, renal, or peripheral arterial lesions. Extension of this technique to valvular stenosis is of clear value in selected patients and has already made some inroads into current surgical practice. Newer interventional techniques, such as the use of stents, mechanical atherectomy, and thermal or ablative laser devices, have demonstrated early feasibility and will almost certainly enhance one or more existing applications or create entirely new applications for interventional cardiology.

At a time of rising health care costs and an aging population, these interventional techniques frequently offer the chance of equivalent symptomatic improvement with less discomfort, disability, and expense than conventional surgery. As with all new techniques, however, careful validation of their utility in comparison with existing medical and surgical techniques will be necessary to insure their optimal use in patient care.

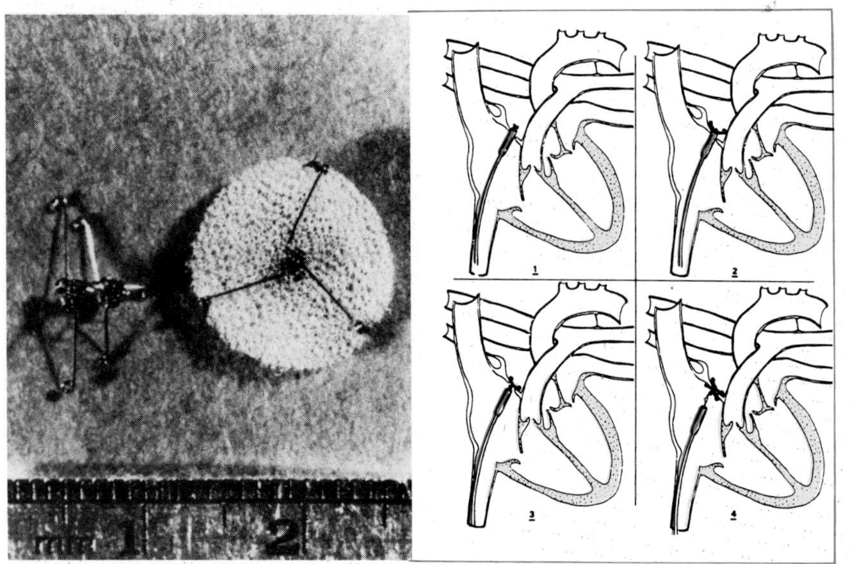

FIGURE 41-21. Closure of an atrial septal defect with the Rashkind double-disc occluder. The Rashkind occluder consists of cloth discs mounted on two pairs of back-to-back spring arms *(left)*. The entire device is collapsed for loading into a delivery catheter, which is in turn positioned across the defect. Following extrusion and expansion of the distal arms, the delivery catheter is partially withdrawn so that the proximal arms can be deployed on the near side of the septum.

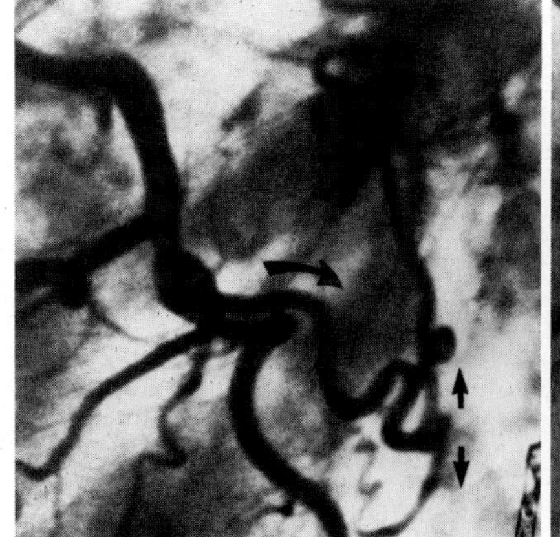

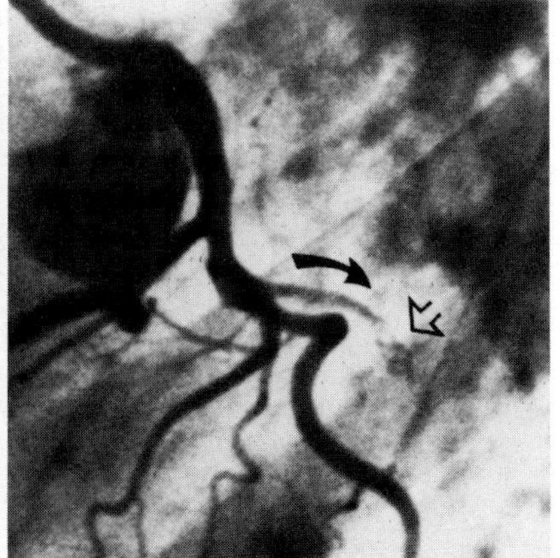

FIGURE 41-22. Coil embolization of a coronary-artery-to-pulmonary-artery fistula. This patient had ischemic chest pain presumed to be due to a persistent fistula from a left atrial branch of the circumflex to the left lower pulmonary artery *(curved arrow, left)*, many years following surgical correction of tetralogy. Following placement of a single Gianturco occlusion coil *(open arrow, right)* and selective injection of thrombin, flow through the fistula ceased within 10 minutes.

REFERENCES

TREATMENT OF VASCULAR STENOSIS

1. Dotter, C. T., and Judkins, M. P.: Transluminal treatment of arteriosclerotic objection: Description of a new technique and a preliminary report of its application. Circulation *30*:654, 1964.
2. Dotter, C. T., Rosch, J., and Judkins, M. P.: Transluminal dilatation of atherosclerotic stenosis. Surg. Gynecol. Obstet. 127:794, 1968.
3. Dotter, C. T.: Transluminal angioplasty: A long view. Radiology *135*:561, 1980.
4. Zeitler, E., Schoop, W., and Zahnow, W.: The treatment of occlusive arterial disease by transluminal catheter angioplasty. Radiology *99*:19, 1971.
5. Gruentzig, A., and Kumpe, D. A.: Technique of percutaneous transluminal angioplasty with the Gruentzig balloon catheter. Am. J. Radiol. *132*:547, 1979.
6. Gruentzig, A., Kuhlmann, U., Vetter, W., et al.: Treatment of renovascular hypertension with percutaneous transluminal dilatation of a renal-artery stenosis. Lancet 1:801, 1978.

PERCUTANEOUS TRANSLUMINAL CORONARY ANGIOPLASTY

7. Gruentzig, A. R., Senning, A., and Siegenthaler, W. E.: Non-operative dilatation of coronary artery stenosis—percutaneous transluminal coronary angioplasty. N. Engl. J. Med. *301*:61, 1979.
8. Kent, K. M., Mullin, S. M., and Passamani, E. R. (eds.): Proceedings of the National Heart, Lung, and Blood Institute workshop on the outcome of percutaneous transluminal angioplasty (June 7–8, 1983). Am. J. Cardiol. *53*:1C, 1984.
9. Baim, D. S.: Coronary angioplasty. *In* Grossman, W., and Baim, D. S. (eds.): Cardiac Catheterization, Angiography, and Intervention, 4th ed. Philadelphia, Lea & Febiger, 1991.
10. Avedissian, M. G., Killeavy, E. S., Garcia, J. M., and Dear, W. E.: Percutaneous transluminal coronary angioplasty: A review of current balloon dilatation systems. Cathet. Cardiovasc. Diagn. *18*:263, 1989.

10a. Stammen, F., Piessens, J., Vrolix, M., et al.: Immediate and short-term results of a 1988–1989 coronary angioplasty registry. Am. J. Cardiol. *67*:253, 1991.

11. Simpson, J. B., Baim, D. S., Robert, E. W., and Harrison, D. C.: A new catheter system for coronary angioplasty. Am. J. Cardiol. *49*:1216, 1982.
12. Detre, K., Holubkov, R., Kelsey, S., et al.: Percutaneous transluminal coronary angioplasty in 1985–1986 and 1977–1981: The NHLBI Registry. N. Engl. J. Med. *318*:265, 1988.
13. Holmes, D. R., Holubkov, R., Vlietstra, R. E., et al.: Comparison of complications during percutaneous transluminal coronary angioplasty from 1977 to 1981 and from 1985 to 1986: The NHLBI PTCA Registry. J. Am. Coll. Cardiol. *12*:1149, 1988.
14. Detre, K., Holubkov, R., Kelsey, S., et al.: One year follow-up results of the 1985–1986 National Heart, Lung, and Blood Institute's Percutaneous Transluminal Coronary Angioplasty Registry. Circulation *80*:421, 1989.
15. Popma, J. J., and Dehmer, G. J.: Care of the patient after coronary angioplasty. Ann. Intern. Med. *110*:547, 1989.
16. Ryan, T. J., Faxon, D. P., Gunnar, R. M., et al.: Guidelines for percutaneous transluminal coronary angioplasty—A report of the ACC/AHA Task Force on assessment of diagnostic and therapeutic cardiovascular procedures. J. Am. Coll. Cardiol. *12*:529, 1988.
17. Bourassa, M. G., Alderman, E. L., Bertrand, M., et al.: Report of the joint ISFC/WHO task force on coronary angioplasty. Circulation *78*:780, 1988.
18. Ellis, S. G., Roubin, G. S., King S. B., et al.: Angiographic and clinical predictors of acute closure after native vessel coronary angioplasty. Circulation *77*:372, 1988.
19. Ellis, S. G., Vandormael, M. G., Cowley, M. J., et al.: Coronary morphologic and clinical determinants of procedural outcome with angioplasty for multivessel coronary artery disease. Circulation *82*:1193, 1990.
20. Meier, B., Gruentzig, A. R., King, S. B., et al.: Risk of side branch occlusion during coronary angioplasty. Am. J. Cardiol. *53*:10, 1984.
21. Meier, B.: Kissing balloon coronary angioplasty. Am. J. Cardiol. *54*:918, 1984.
22. Weinstein, J. S., Baim, D. S., Sipperly, M. E., et al.: Salvage of branch vessels during bifurcation lesion angioplasty—acute and long-term follow-up. Cathet. Cardiovasc. Diagn. *22*:1, 1991.
23. Dervan, J. P., Baim, D. S., Cherniles, J., and Grossman, W.: Transluminal angioplasty of occluded coronary arteries: Use of a movable guide wire system. Circulation *68*:776, 1983.
24. Stone, G. W., Rutherford, B. D., McConahay, D. R., et al.: Procedural outcome of angioplasty for total coronary occlusion: An analysis of 971 lesions in 905 patients. J. Am. Coll. Cardiol. *15*:849, 1990.
25. Wohlgelernter, D., Cleman, M., Highman, H. A., and Zaret, B. L.: Percutaneous transluminal coronary angioplasty of the "culprit lesion" for the management of unstable angina pectoris in patients with multivessel coronary artery disease. Am J. Cardiol. *58*:460, 1986.
26. Ischinger, T., Gruentzig, A. R., Hollman, J., King, S., et al.: Should coronary arteries with less than 60% diameter stenosis be treated by angioplasty? Circulation *68*:148, 1983.
27. de Feyter, P. J.: Coronary angioplasty for unstable angina. Am. Heart J. *118*:860, 1989.
28. Leeman, D., McCabe, C. H., Faxon, D. P., et al.: Use of percutaneous transluminal coronary angioplasty and bypass surgery despite improved medical therapy for unstable angina pectoris. Am. J. Cardiol. *61*:38G, 1988.
29. Feldman, R. L., Macdonald, R. G., Hill, J. A., et al.: Coronary angioplasty at the time of initial cardiac catheterization. Cathet. Cardiovasc. Diagn. *12*:219, 1986.
30. Laskey, M. A., Deutsch, E., Barnathan, E., and Laskey, W. K.: Influence of heparin therapy on percutaneous transluminal coronary angioplasty outcome in unstable angina pectoris. Am. J. Cardiol. *651*:425, 1990.
31. Rogers, W. J., Baim, D. S., Gore, J. M., et al.: Comparison of immediate invasive, delayed invasive and conservative strategies following tissue plasminogen activator—results of the Thrombolysis in Myocardial Infarction (TIMI) Phase IIA trial. Circulation *81*:1457, 1990.
32. The TIMI Study Group: Comparison of invasive and conservative strategies after treatment with intravenous tissue plasminogen activator: Results of the thrombolysis in myocardial infarction (TIMI) phase II trial. N. Engl. J. Med. *320*:618, 1989.
33. O'Keefe, J. H., Rutherford, B. D., McConahay, D. R., et al.: Early results and long-term outcome of direct coronary angioplasty for acute myocardial infarction in 500 consecutive patients. Am. J. Cardiol. *64*:1221, 1989.
34. Pinkerton, C. A., Slack, J. D., Orr, C. M., et al.: Percutaneous transluminal angioplasty in patients with prior myocardial revascularization surgery. Am. J. Cardiol. *61*:15G, 1988.
35. Cote, G., Myler, R. K., Stertzer, S. H., et al.: Percutaneous transluminal angioplasty of stenotic coronary artery bypass grafts: 5 years' experience. J. Am. Coll. Cardiol. *9*:8, 1987.

35a. Plokker, H.W.T., Meester, B. H., and Serruys, P. W.: The Dutch experience in percutaneous transluminal angioplasty of narrowed saphenous veins used for aortocoronary arterial bypass. *(In press.)*

36. Shimshak, T. M., Giorgi, L. V., Johnson, W. L., et al.: Application of percutaneous transluminal angioplasty to the internal mammary artery graft. J. Am. Coll. Cardiol. *12*:1205, 1988.
37. de Feyter, P. J., Serruys, P., van den Brand, M., et al.: Percutaneous transluminal angioplasty of totally occluded venous bypass graft: A challenge that should be resisted. Am. J. Cardiol. *64*:88, 1989.
38. Holt, G. W., Sugrue, D. D., Bresnahan, J. F., et al.: Results of percutaneous transluminal coronary angioplasty for unstable angina in patients 70 years of age and older. Am. J. Cardiol. *61*:994, 1988.
39. O'Keefe, J. H., Hartzler, G. O., Rutherford, B. D., et al.: Left main coronary angioplasty—early and late results of 127 acute and elective procedures. Am. J. Cardiol. *54*:144, 1989.
40. Kahn, J. E., Rutherford, B. D., McConahay, D. R., et al.: Supported "high-risk" coronary angioplasty using intraaortic balloon counterpulsation. J. Am. Coll. Cardiol. *15*:1151, 1990.
41. Vogel, R. A., Shawl, F., Tommaso, C., et al.: Initial report of the National Registry of Elective Cardiopulmonary Bypass Supported Coronary Angioplasty. J. Am. Coll. Cardiol. *15*:23, 1990.
42. Baim, D. S., and Ignatius, E. J.: Use of percutaneous transluminal coronary angioplasty: Results of a current survey. Am. J. Cardiol. *61*:3G, 1988.
43. Weintraub, W. S., Jones, E. L., King, S. B., et al.: Changing use of coronary angioplasty and coronary bypass surgery in the treatment of chronic coronary artery disease. Am. J. Cardiol. *65*:183, 1990.
44. Black, A. J. R., Roubin, G. S., Sutor, C., et al.: Comparative costs of percutaneous transluminal coronary angioplasty in multivessel coronary artery disease. Am. J. Cardiol. *62*:809, 1988.
45. Ryan, T. J., Klocke, F. J., Reynolds, W. A., et al.: Clinical competence in percutaneous transluminal coronary angioplasty—a statement for physicians from the ACP/ACC/AHA Task Force on Clinical Privileges in Cardiology. Circulation *81*:2041, 1990.
46. Hamad, N., Pichard, A. D., Lyle, H. R. P., Lindsay, J.: Results of percutaneous transluminal coronary angioplasty by multiple, relatively low frequency operators: 1986–1987 experience. Am. J. Cardiol. *61*:1229, 1988.
47. Wyman, R. M., Safian, R. D., Portway, V., et al.: Current complications of diagnostic and therapeutic cardiac catheterization. J. Am. Coll. Cardiol. *12*:1400, 1988.

47a. Plante, S., Laarman, G., de Feyter, P. J., et al.: Acute complications of percutaneous transluminal coronary angioplasty for total occlusion. Am. Heart J. *121*:417, 1991.

48. Sanborn, T. A., Faxon, D. P., Waugh, D., et al.: Transluminal angioplasty in experimental atherosclerosis: Analysis for embolization using an in vivo perfusion system. Circulation *66*:917, 1982.
49. Sanborn, T. A., Faxon, D. P., Haudenschild, C., et al.: The mechanism of transluminal angioplasty: Evidence for formation of aneurysms in experimental atherosclerosis. Circulation *68*:1136, 1983.
50. Castaneda-Zuniga, W. R., Formanek, A., Tadavarthy, M., et al.: The mechanism of balloon angioplasty. Radiology *135*:565, 1980.
51. Roubin, G. S., Douglas, J. S., King, S. B., et al.: Influence of balloon size on initial success, acute complications, and restenosis after percutaneous transluminal coronary angioplasty. A prospective randomized study. Circulation *78*:557, 1988.
52. Saffitz, J. E., Rose, T. E., Oaks, J. B., and Roberts, W. C.: Coronary artery rupture during coronary angioplasty. Am. J. Cardiol. *51*:902, 1983.
53. Kaltenbach, M., Beyer, J., Walter, S., et al.: Prolonged application of pressure in transluminal angioplasty. Cathet. Cardiovasc. Diagn. *10*:213, 1984.
54. Wijns, W., Serruys, P. W., Slager, C. J., et al.: Effect of coronary occlusion during percutaneous transluminal angioplasty in humans on left ventricular chamber stiffness and regional diastolic pressure-radius relations. J. Am. Coll. Cardiol. *7*:455, 1986.

55. Kent, K. M., Cleman, M. W., Cowley, M. J., et al.: Reduction of myocardial ischemia during percutaneous transluminal coronary angioplasty with oxygenated Fluosol. Am. J. Cardiol. *66*:279, 1990.
56. Anderson, H. V., Roubin, G. S., Leimgruber, P. P., et al.: Measurement of transstenotic pressure gradient during percutaneous transluminal coronary angioplasty. Circulation *73*:1223, 1986.
57. Black, A. J. R., Namay, D. L., Niederman, A. L., et al.: Tear or dissection after coronary angioplasty—morphologic correlates of an ischemic complication. Circulation *79*:1035, 1989.
58. Fischell, T. A., Derby, G., Tse, T. M., and Stadius, M. L.: Coronary artery vasoconstriction after percutaneous transluminal coronary angioplasty: A quantitative arteriographic analysis. Circulation *78*:1323, 1988.
59. Sinclair, I. N., McCabe, C. H., Sipperly, M. E., and Baim, D. S.: Predictors, therapeutic options and long-term outcome of abrupt reclosure. Am. J. Cardiol. *61*:61G, 1988.
60. Detre, K. M., Holmes, D. R., Holubkov, R., et al.: Incidence and consequences of periprocedural occlusion: The 1985–86 National Heart, Lung, and Blood Institute's Percutaneous Transluminal Coronary Angioplasty Registry. Circulation *82*:739, 1990.
61. Talley, J. D., Weintraub, W. S., Roubin, G. S., et al.: Failed elective percutaneous transluminal coronary angioplasty requiring coronary artery bypass surgery: In-hospital and late clinical outcome at 5 years. Circulation *82*:1203, 1990.
62. Sundrum, P., Harvey, J. R., Johnson, R. G., et al.: Benefit of the perfusion catheter for emergency coronary artery grafting after failed percutaneous transluminal coronary angioplasty. Am. J. Cardiol. *63*:282, 1989.
63. Wilson, R. F., Johnson, M. R., Marcus, M. L., et al.: The effect of coronary angioplasty on coronary flow reserve. Circulation *77*:873, 1988.
64. Gruentzig, A. R., King, S. B., III, Schlumpf, M., and Siegenthaler, W.: Long-term follow-up after percutaneous transluminal coronary angioplasty. N. Engl. J. Med. *316*:1127, 1987.
65. Bertrand, M. E., LaBlanche, J. M., Thieuleux, F. A., et al.: Comparative results of percutaneous transluminal coronary angioplasty in patients with dynamic versus fixed coronary stenosis. J. Am. Coll. Cardiol. *8*:504, 1986.
66. Ellis, S. G., Roubin, G. S., King, S. B., et al.: Importance of stenosis morphology in the estimation of restenosis risk after elective percutaneous transluminal angioplasty. Am. J. Cardiol. *63*:30, 1989.
67. Hardoff, R., Shefer, A., Gips, S., et al.: Predicting late restenosis after coronary angioplasty by very early (12–14 h) thallium-201 scintigraphy: Implications with regard to mechanisms of late coronary restenosis. J. Am. Coll. Cardiol. *15*:1486, 1990.
68. Liu, M. W., Roubin, G. S., and King, S. B.: Restenosis after coronary angioplasty: Potential biologic determinants and the role of intimal hyperplasia. Circulation *79*:1374, 1989.
68a. Veda, M., Becker, A. E., Tsukada, T., et al.: Fibrocellular tissue response after percutaneous transluminal coronary angioplasty. An immunocyto-chemical analysis of the cellular composition. Circulation *83*:1327, 1991.
68b. Forrester, J. S., Fishbein, M., Helfant, R., and Fagin, J.: A paradigm for restenosis based on cell biology: clues for the development of new preventive therapies. J. Am. Coll. Cardiol. *17*:758, 1991.
69. Safian, R. D., Gelbfish, J. S., Erny, R. E., et al.: Coronary atherectomy: Clinical, angiographic and histologic findings and observations regarding mechanism. Circulation *82*:69, 1990.
70. Nobuyoshi, M., Kimura, T., Nosaka, H., et al.: Restenosis after successful percutaneous transluminal coronary angioplasty: Serial angiographic follow-up of 220 patients. J. Am. Coll. Cardiol. *12*:616, 1988.
71. Beatt, K. J., Serruys, P. W., and Hugenholtz, P. G.: Restenosis after coronary angioplasty: New standards for clinical studies. J. Am. Coll. Cardiol. *15*:491, 1990.
72. Schwartz, L., Bourassa, M. G., Lesperance, J., et al.: Aspirin and dipyridamole in the prevention of restenosis after percutaneous transluminal coronary angioplasty. N. Engl. J. Med. *318*:1714, 1988.
73. Knudtson, M. L., Flintoft, V. F., Roth, D. L., et al.: Effect of short-term prostacyclin administration on restenosis after percutaneous transluminal coronary angioplasty. J. Am. Coll. Cardiol. *15*:691, 1990.
74. Reis, G. J., Boucher, T. M., Sipperley, M. E., et al.: Randomised trial of fish oil for prevention of restenosis after coronary angioplasty. Lancet *2*:1777, 1989.
75. Coller, B. S., Folts, J. D., Smith S. R., et al.: Abolition of in vivo platelet thrombus formation in primates with monoclonal antibodies to the platelet GPIIb/IIIa receptor: Correlation with bleeding time, platelet aggregation, and blockage of GPIIb/IIIa receptors. Circulation *80*:1766, 1989.
76. Jang, I. K., Gold, H. K., Ziskind, A. A., et al.: Prevention of platelet-rich arterial thrombosis by selective thrombin inhibition (argatroban). Circulation *81*:219, 1990.
77. Heras, M., Chesboro, J. H., Webster, M. W. I., et al.: Hirudin, heparin and placebo during deep arterial injury in the pig. Circulation *82*:1476, 1990.
78. Kuntz, R. E., Schmidt, D. A., Levine, M. J., et al.: Importance of post-procedure luminal diameter on restenosis following new coronary intervention. Circulation *82*: III-314, 1990.
79. Black, A. J. R., Anderson, H. V., Roubin, G. S., et al.: Repeat coronary angioplasty: Correlates of a second restenosis. J. Am. Coll. Cardiol. *11*:714, 1988.
80. Teirstein, P. S., Hoover, C. A., Ligon, R. W., et al.: Repeat coronary angioplasty: Efficacy of a third angioplasty for a second restenosis. J. Am. Coll. Cardiol. *13*:291, 1989.
81. Waller, B. F.: "Crackers, breakers, stretchers, drillers, scrapers, shavers, burners, welders and melters"—the future treatment of atherosclerotic coronary artery disease. A clinical-morphologic assessment. J. Am. Coll. Cardiol. *13*:969, 1989.
81a. Topol, E. J.: Promises and pitfalls of new devices for coronary artery disease. Circulation *83*:689, 1991.
82. Baim, D. S., Detre, K., and Kent, K.: Problems in the development of new devices for coronary intervention—Possible role for a multicenter registry. J. Am. Coll. Cardiol. *14*:1389, 1989.
83. Dotter, C. T.: Transluminally placed coil-spring endarterial tube grafts: Long-term patency in canine popliteal artery. Invest Radiol. *4*:329, 1969.
83a. Goy, J-J., Sigwart, U., Vogt, P., et al.: Long-term follow-up of the first 56 patients treated with intracoronary self-expanding stents (the Lausanne Experience) Am. J. Cardiol. *67*:569, 1991.
84. Schatz, R. A.: A view of vascular stents. Circulation *79*:445, 1989.
85. Ellis, S. G., and Topol, E. J.: Intracoronary stents: Will they fulfill their promise as an adjunct to angioplasty? J. Am. Coll. Cardiol. *13*:1425, 1989.
85a. Schatz, R. A., Baim, D. S., Leon, M., et al: Clinical experience with the Palmaz-Schatz coronary stent—initial results of a multicenter study. Circulation *83*: 148, 1991.
85b. Serruys, P. W., Strauss, B. H., Beatt, K. J., et al.: Angiographic follow-up after placement of a self-expanding coronary-artery stent. N. Engl. J. Med. *324*: 13, 1991.
86. Levine, M. J., Leonard, B. M., Nash, I. D., et al.: Clinical and angiographic results of balloon-expandable intra-coronary stents in right coronary artery stenoses. J. Am. Coll. Cardiol. *16*:332, 1990.
87. Roubin, G. S., King, S. B., Douglas, J. S., et al.: Intracoronary stenting during percutaneous transluminal coronary angioplasty. Circulation *81*:IV92, 1990.
88. Sigwart, U., Puel, J., Mirkovitch, V., et al.: Intravascular stents to prevent occlusion and restenosis after transluminal angioplasty. N. Engl. J. Med. *316*:701, 1987.
89. Urban, P., Sigwart, U., Gold, S., et al.: Intravascular stenting for stenosis of aortocoronary venous bypass grafts. J. Am. Coll. Cardiol. *13*:1085, 1989.
90. Hinohara, T., Selmon, M. R., Robertson, G. C., et al.: Directional atherectomy—new approaches for treatment of obstructive coronary and peripheral vascular disease. Circulation *81*:IV79, 1990.
90a. Hinohara, T., Rowe, M., Robertson, G. C., et al.: Effect of lesion characteristics on outcome of directional coronary atherectomy. J. Am. Coll. Cardiol. *17*:1112, 1991.
91. von Polnitz, A., Nerlich, A., Berger, H., and Hofling, B.: Percutaneous peripheral atherectomy: Angiographic and clinical follow-up of 60 patients. J. Am. Coll. Cardiol. *15*:682, 1990.
92. Rowe, M. H., Hinohara, T., White, N. W., et al.: Comparison of dissection rates and angiographic results following directional coronary atherectomy and coronary angioplasty. Am. J. Cardiol. *66*:49, 1990.
93. Stack, R. S., Quigley, P. J., Sketch, M. J., et al.: Extraction atherectomy. *In* Topol, E. J. (ed.): Textbook of Interventional Cardiology. Philadelphia, W. B. Saunders Company, 1990.
94. Zacca, N. M., Raizner, A. E., Noon, G. P., et al.: Treatment of symptomatic peripheral atherosclerotic disease with a rotational atherectomy device. Am. J. Cardiol. *63*:77, 1989.
95. Fourrier, J. L., Bertrand, M. E., Auth, D. C., et al.: Percutaneous coronary rotational atherectomy in humans. Preliminary report. J. Am. Coll. Cardiol. *14*:1278, 1989.
95a. Buchbinder, M., Warth, D., O'Neill, W., et al.: Multicenter registry of percutaneous coronary rotational ablation using the rotablator. J. Am. Coll. Cardiol. *17*:31A(abstr), 1991.
96. Litvak, F., Grundfest, W. S., Segalowitz, J., et al.: Interventional cardiovascular therapy by laser and thermal angioplasty. Circulation *81*:IV109, 1990.
97. Isner, J. M., Donaldson, R. F., Deckelbaum, L. J., et al.: The excimer laser: Gross, light microscopic and ultrastructural analysis of potential advantages for use in laser therapy of cardiovascular disease. J. Am. Coll. Cardiol. *6*:1102, 1985.
98. Karsch, K. R., Haase, K. K., Voelker, W., et al.: Percutaneous excimer coronary angioplasty in patients with stable and unstable angina pectoris. Circulation *81*:1849, 1990.
99. Litvak, F., Grundfest, W. S., and Goldenberg, T.: Percutaneous excimer laser coronary angioplasty of aortocoronary saphenous vein grafts. J. Am. Coll. Cardiol. *14*:803, 1989.
100. Sanborn, T. A., Alexopoulos, D., Marmur, J. D., et al.: Coronary excimer laser angioplasty: Reduced complications and indium-111 platelet accumulation compared with thermal laser angioplasty. J. Am. Coll. Cardiol. *16*:502, 1990.
101. Leon, M. B., Almagor, Y., Bartorelli, A. L., et al.: Fluorescence-guided laser-assisted balloon angioplasty in patients with femoropopliteal occlusions. Circulation *81*:143, 1990.
102. Tobis, J., Smolin, M., Mallery, J., et al.: Laser-assisted thermal angioplasty in human peripheral artery occlusions: Mechanism of recanalization. J. Am. Coll. Cardiol. *13*:1547, 1989.
103. Spears, J. R., Reyes, V. P., Wynne, J., et al.: Percutaneous coronary laser balloon angioplasty: Initial results of a multicenter experience. J. Am. Coll. Cardiol. *16*:293, 1990.
104. Lee, B. J., Becker, G. J., Waller, B. F., et al.: Thermal compression and molding of atherosclerotic vascular tissue with use of radiofrequency

energy: Implications for radiofrequency balloon angioplasty. J. Am. Coll. Cardiol. *13*:1167, 1989.
105. Meier, B.: Chronic total occlusion angioplasty. Cathet. Cardiovasc. Diagn. *17*:212, 1989.
106. Vallbracht, C., Lierman, D., Prignitz, I., et al.: Results of low speed rotational angioplasty for chronic peripheral occlusions. Am. J. Cardiol. *62*:935, 1988.
107. Rosenschein, U., Bernstein, J. J., DiSegni, E., et al.: Experimental ultrasonic angioplasty: Disruption of atherosclerotic plaques and thrombi in vitro and arterial recanalization in vivo. J. Am. Coll. Cardiol. *15*:711, 1990.
108. Siegel, R. J., Fishbein, M. C., Forester, J., et al.: In vivo ultrasound arterial recanalization of atherosclerotic total occlusions. J. Am. Coll. Cardiol. *15*:345, 1990.
109. Palmaz, J. C., Garcia, O. J., Schatz, R. A., et al.: Placement of balloon-expandable intraluminal stents in iliac arteries: First 171 procedures. Radiology *174*:969, 1990.
110. Doubilet, P., and Abrams, H. L.: The cost of underutilization—percutaneous transluminal angioplasty for peripheral vascular disease. N. Engl. J. Med. *310*:95, 1984.
111. Zairns, C. K.: The vascular wars of 1988: The enemy is met. JAMA *261*:416, 1989.
112. Gallins, A., Mahler, F., Probst, P., and Nachbur, B.: Percutaneous transluminal angioplasty of the lower limbs: A 5-year follow-up. Circulation *70*:619, 1984.
113. Hewes, R. C., White, R. I., Murray, R. R., et al.: Long-term results of superficial femoral artery angioplasty. A. J. R. *146*:1025, 1986.
114. Rooke, T. W., Stanson, A. W., Johnson, C. M., et al.: Percutaneous transluminal angioplasty in the lower extremities: A 5-year experience. Mayo Clin. Proc. *62*:85, 1987.
115. Sos, T. A., Pickering, T. G., Saddekni, S., et al.: The current role of renal angioplasty in the treatment of renovascular hypertension. Urol. Clin. North Am. *11*:503, 1984.
116. Martin, L. G., Price, R. B., Casarella, W. J., et al.: Percutaneous angioplasty in clinical management of renovascular hypertension: Initial and long-term results. Radiology *155*:629, 1985.
117. Motarjeme, A., Keifer, J. W., and Zuska, A. J.: Percutaneous transluminal angioplasty of the vertebral arteries. Radiology *139*:715, 1981.
118. Tsai, F. Y., Matovich, V., Hieshima, G., et al.: Percutaneous transluminal angioplasty of the carotid artery. Am. J. Neurol. Radiol. *7*:349, 1986.
119. Rothman, A., Perry, S. B., Keane, J. F., and Lock, J. E.: Early results and follow-up of balloon angioplasty for branch pulmonary artery stenoses. J. Am. Coll. Cardiol. *15*:1109, 1990.
120. Marx, G. R., Allen, H. D., Ovitt, T. W., and Hanson, W.: Balloon dilation angioplasty of Blalock-Taussig shunts. Am. J. Cardiol. *62*:824, 1988.
121. Mullins, C. E.: Pediatric and congenital therapeutic cardiac catheterization. Circulation *79*:1153, 1989.
122. Tynan, M., Finley, J.P., Fontes, V., et al.: Balloon angioplasty for the treatment of native coarctation: Results of the valvuloplasty and angioplasty for congenital anomalies registry. Am. J. Cardiol. *65*:790, 1990.
123. Cooper, S. G., Sullivan, I. D., and Wren, C.: Treatment of recoarctation: Balloon dilation angioplasty. J. Am. Coll. Cardiol. *14*:413, 1989.
124. Rao, P. S.: Which aortic coarctations should we dilate? Am. Heart J. *117*:987, 1989.

TREATMENT OF VALVULAR STENOSIS

125. Stanger, P., Cassidy, S. C., Girod, D. A., et al.: Balloon pulmonary valvuloplasty: Results of the valvuloplasty and angioplasty of congenital anomalies registry. Am. J. Cardiol. *65*:775, 1990.
126. Block, P. C., and Palacios, I. F.: Aortic and mitral balloon valvuloplasty: The United States experience. *In* Topol, E. J. (ed.): Textbook of Interventional Cardiology. Philadelphia, W. B. Saunders Company, 1990.
127. Rochini, A. P., Beekman, R. H., Shachar, G. B., et al.: Balloon aortic valvuloplasty: Results of the valvuloplasty and angioplasty congenital anomalies registry. Am. J. Cardiol. *65*:784, 1990.
128. Lock, J. E., Khalilullah, M., Shrivastava, S., et al.: Percutaneous catheter commissurotomy in rheumatic mitral stenosis. N. Engl. J. Med. *313*:1515, 1985.
128a. Kirklin, J. W.: Percutaneous balloon versus surgical closed commissurotomy for mitral stenosis. *(In press.)*
128b. Tuzcu, E. M., Block, P. C., and Palacios, I. F.: Comparison of early versus late experience with percutaneous mitral balloon valvuloplasty. J. Am. Coll. Cardiol. *17*:1121, 1991.
129. Nobuyoshi, M., Hamasaki, N., Kimura, T., et al.: Indications, complications, and short-term clinical outcome of percutaneous transvenous mitral commissurotomy. Circulation *80*:782, 1989.
130. Casale, P., Block, P. C., O'Shea, J. P., and Palacios, I. F.: Atrial septal defect after percutaneous mitral balloon valvuloplasty: Immediate results and follow-up. J. Am. Coll. Cardiol. *15*:1300, 1990.
131. Hermann, H. C., Kleaveland, J. P., Hill, J. A., et al.: The M-Heart Percutaneous Balloon Mitral Valvuloplasty Registry: Initial results and early follow-up. J. Am. Coll. Cardiol. *15*:1221, 1990.
132. Palacios, I. F., Block, P. C., Wilkins, G. T., and Weyman, A. E.: Follow-up of patients undergoing percutaneous mitral balloon valvotomy: Analysis of factors determining restenosis. Circulation *79*:573, 1989.
133. Letac, B., Gerber, L. I., and Koning, R.: Insights on the mechanism of balloon valvuloplasty in aortic stenosis. Am. J. Cardiol. *62*:1241, 1988.
133a. McKay, R. G.: The Mansfield Scientific Aortic Valvuloplasty Registry. Overview of acute hemodynamic results and procedural complications. J. Am. Coll. Cardiol. *17*:485, 1991.
134. Safian, R. D., Berman, A. D., Diver, D. J., et al.: Balloon aortic valvuloplasty in 170 consecutive patients. N. Engl. J. Med. *319*:125, 1988.
134a. Homes, D. R., Jr., Nishimura, R. A., and Reeder, G. S.: In-hospital mortality after balloon aortic valvuloplasty: Frequency and associated factors. J. Am. Coll. Cardiol. *17*:189, 1991.
135. Berland, J., Squavin, T., Lefebvre, E., et al.: Percutaneous balloon valvuloplasty in patients with severe aortic stenosis and low ejection fraction. Circulation *79*:1189, 1989.
136. Levine, M. J., Berman, A. D., Safian, R. D., et al.: Palliation of valvular aortic stenosis by balloon valvuloplasty as preparation for noncardiac surgery. Am. J. Cardiol. *62*:1309, 1988.
136a. Nishimura, R. A., Holmes, D. R., Jr., Michela, M. A., et al.: Follow-up of patients with low output, low gradient hemodynamics after percutaneous balloon aortic valvuloplasty: The Mansfield Scientific Aortic Valvuloplasty Registry. J. Am. Coll. Cardiol. *17*:828, 1991.
136b. Bashore, T. M., Davidson, C. J., and the Mansfield Scientific Aortic Valvuloplasty Registry Investigators: Follow-up recatheterization after balloon aortic valvuloplasty. J. Am. Coll. Cardiol. *17*:1188, 1991.
137. Rashkind, W. J.: Transcatheter treatment of congenital heart disease. Circulation *67*:711, 1983.
138. Park, S. C., Neches, W. H., Mullins, C. E., et al.: Blade atrial septostomy: Collaborative study. Circulation *66*:258, 1982.
139. Lock, J. E., Cockerham, J. T., Keane, J. F., et al.: Transcatheter umbrella closure of congenital heart defects. Circulation *75*:593, 1987.
140. Lock, J. E., Block, P. C., McKay, R. G., et al.: Transcatheter closure of ventricular septal defects. Circulation *78*:361, 1988.
141. Dyck, J. D., Benson, L. N., Smallhorn, J. F., et al.: Catheter occlusion of the persistently patent ductus arteriosus. Am. J. Cardiol. *62*:1089, 1988.
142. Gewillig, M., van der Hauwaert, L., and Daenen, W.: Transcatheter occlusion of high-flow Blalock-Taussig shunts with a detachable balloon. Am. J. Cardiol. *65*:1518, 1990.
143. Miranda, A. A., Hill, J. A., Mickle, J. P., and Quisling, R. G.: Balloon occlusion of an internal mammary artery to anterior interventricular vein fistula. Am. J. Cardiol. *65*:257, 1990.

42

Rehabilitation of Patients With Coronary Artery Disease

by CHARLES DENNIS, M.D.

Cardiac rehabilitation has traditionally focused on physical reconditioning and risk factor modification for patients recovering from myocardial infarction and coronary artery bypass surgery. Advances in the treatment of coronary artery disease and new data supporting the efficacy of secondary prevention measures have broadened the indications for cardiac rehabilitation services and increased the number of patients who may benefit from these services. Currently only 10 per cent of patients who might benefit from cardiac rehabilitation participate in formal programs.[1] A wider application of these services could potentially reduce the morbidity and mortality of coronary heart disease.

Cardiac rehabilitation has short- and long-term goals. The short-term goals include physical reconditioning sufficient for resumption of customary activities, education of patients and family about the disease process, and psychological support during the early recovery phase of the illness. The long-term goals include identifying and treating risk factors that influence the progression of disease, teaching and reinforcing the health behaviors that improve prognosis, optimizing physical conditioning, and facilitating a return to occupational and avocational activities. Cardiac rehabilitation must be both comprehensive and individualized. The most important factors to be considered in development of a program of rehabilitation are disease severity, medical and surgical therapy, risk factors, physical condition, vocational status, and emotional state.

EXERCISE IN CARDIAC REHABILITATION

PHYSICAL RECONDITIONING

FACTORS INFLUENCING PHYSICAL CAPACITY. Peak exercise capacity is defined as the maximum ability of the cardiovascular system to deliver oxygen to exercising skeletal muscle and of the exercising muscle to extract oxygen from the blood. The most accurate measure of exercise capacity is the maximal oxygen uptake ($\dot{V}O_{2\,max}$), representing the liters of oxygen transported from the lungs per minute and used by skeletal muscle at peak effort. Because measurement of $\dot{V}O_{2\,max}$ is cumbersome, multiples of resting oxygen consumption (METS) are used clinically. One MET equals 3.5 ml oxygen uptake per kilogram body weight per minute and represents the approximate metabolic cost to stand quietly. Exercise tests are calibrated to approximate MET requirements at each stage. The MET capacity on treadmill testing usually overestimates the $\dot{V}O_{2\,max}$ for cardiac patients.[2]

The degree of physical incapacity following a cardiac event is related to several factors: physical capacity prior to the event; treatments such as bed rest and medications; intravascular volume depletion; left ventricular dysfunction; residual myocardial ischemia; age; other noncardiac medical problems; and symptoms experienced by the patient during physical activity. Distinguishing the influence of each factor can be difficult, but recognizing their potential effects on physical capacity is paramount to minimizing iatrogenic effects and developing a conditioning program.

IATROGENIC AND PHYSIOLOGICAL FACTORS. While early mobilization is more common than in the past, bed rest remains the initial standard of care for most cardiac patients. Bed rest causes decrements in $\dot{V}O_{2\,max}$ of 9 to 30 per cent for several reasons.[3–5] Bed rest causes intravascular volume depletion. Absence of orthostatic stress of upright posture decreases venous capacitance vessel tone and blunts the normal postural vasomotor reflexes. These changes lead to diminished venous return, postural hypotension, and tachycardia.[6] Skeletal muscle mass decreases 10 to 15 per cent with a week of bed rest.[7] Pulmonary abnormalities resulting from bed rest include diminished lung volume and vital capacity and an increased respiratory exchange ratio.[8] Anaerobic metabolism occurs at lower levels of work in individuals placed at bed rest for a week or more. Vigorous exercise training in the supine position during bed rest fails to prevent the deterioration in upright exercise capacity. However, as little as 3 hours of daily upright posture significantly diminishes the deconditioning effects of bed rest.[4,5]

Chronotropic incompetence, the inability to achieve the age-predicted heart rate response to exercise, is common in patients with coronary artery disease.[9] The etiology is not clearly defined but appears to be related to loss of normal vagal reflexes during exercise.[10] Peak heart rate can decrease as much as 25 per cent in the first few weeks after myocardial infarction. Because the heart rate response to exercise is quantitatively the most important mechanism for increasing cardiac output, chronotropic incompetence significantly lowers $\dot{V}O_{2\,max}$. Chronotropic incompetence improves spontaneously over the first 3 to 8 weeks following myocardial infarction, leading to increases in $\dot{V}O_{2\,max}$ even in the absence of formal exercise training.[11]

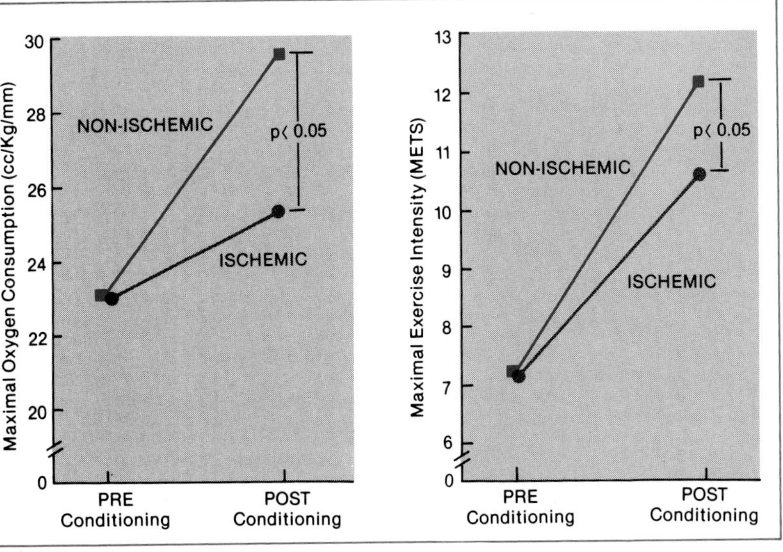

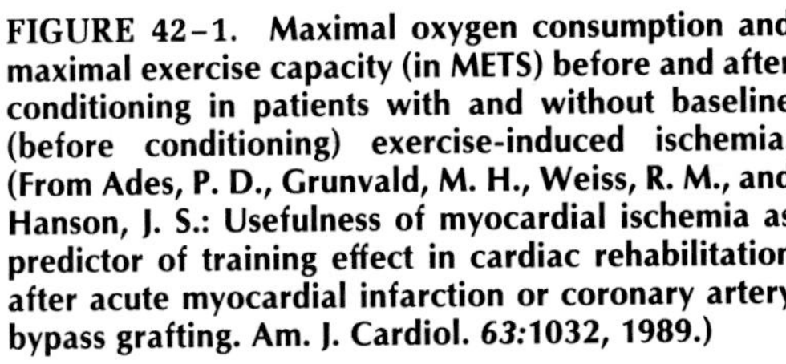

FIGURE 42–1. Maximal oxygen consumption and maximal exercise capacity (in METS) before and after conditioning in patients with and without baseline (before conditioning) exercise-induced ischemia. (From Ades, P. D., Grunvald, M. H., Weiss, R. M., and Hanson, J. S.: Usefulness of myocardial ischemia as predictor of training effect in cardiac rehabilitation after acute myocardial infarction or coronary artery bypass grafting. Am. J. Cardiol. *63:*1032, 1989.)

LEFT VENTRICULAR DYSFUNCTION. Left ventricular dysfunction would be expected to impair physical capacity. However, most measures of ventricular performance at rest and during exercise, including left ventricular end-diastolic dimension, velocity of circumferential fiber shortening, systolic time intervals, and ejection fraction,[12] correlate poorly with exercise performance. In patients with left ventricular dysfunction, the two factors most predictive of low exercise capacity are chronotropic incompetence and early onset of anaerobic metabolism during exercise.[13] Central and peripheral mechanisms may preserve exercise capacity even when left ventricular dysfunction is severe. These include a preserved chronotropic response to exercise, increasing stroke volume, ventricular dilation, decreasing peripheral vascular resistance, increased levels of circulating catecholamines, and the ability to tolerate markedly elevated pulmonary artery wedge pressures.[14] Some of these mechanisms may be stimulated by exercise training, whereas others remain unchanged. Because the common clinical measures of resting left ventricular function do not predict exercise capacity, exercise testing is necessary to assess the functional limitation.

MYOCARDIAL ISCHEMIA. If large areas of myocardium become ischemic with exercise, patients may be limited by angina, dyspnea, and/or fatigue. Dyspnea and fatigue in the absence of angina may reflect left ventricular dysfunction at rest or exercise-induced ischemic left ventricular dysfunction, leading to elevated pulmonary vascular pressures and/or inadequate cardiac output.[15] Angina may also limit exercise performance in the absence of exercise-induced left ventricular dysfunction. Because the severity of anginal discomfort and the perception of the discomfort vary among patients, the same severity of myocardial ischemia may limit some patients and be tolerated by others. Amelioration of symptomatic and asymptomatic ischemia by medication may improve exercise capacity even in the absence of formal exercise training[16] (Fig. 42–1).

OTHER FACTORS. Concomitant illnesses, such as chronic obstructive pulmonary disease and peripheral vascular disease, can limit the exercise capacity before the effects of ischemia or left ventricular dysfunction are manifested. The common cardiovascular drugs, including nitrates, beta blockers, and calcium antagonists, increase the exercise capacity by increasing coronary blood flow, decreasing myocardial oxygen demand, or improving hemodynamics during exercise.[17,18]

EFFECTS OF EXERCISE TRAINING

SKELETAL MUSCLE. The primary physiological effects of exercise training are on skeletal muscle performance. Improved skeletal muscle performance is directly related to increases in capillary density, oxidative enzyme content, and increased numbers of mitochondria. These changes increase skeletal muscle perfusion and the efficiency of oxygen extraction.[19]

MYOCARDIAL PERFORMANCE. There is no convincing evidence that low- or moderate-intensity exercise training substantially improves myocardial performance. However, exercise training does cause modest improvements in thallium perfusion.[20,21] Diminished exercise-induced ST-segment abnormalities,[22] increased ejection fraction and stroke volume, and increased ischemic threshold have also been demonstrated with exercise training.[23] Whether these improvements reflect primary effects on myocardial performance or secondary effects due to changes in hemodynamics or skeletal muscle efficiency is debatable. Postulated mechanisms of primary cardiac effects include improved coronary blood flow, development of collateral circulation, and improved oxygen extraction and utilization by myocardium[20–23] (Fig. 42–2).

OTHER EFFECTS. Exercise training lowers heart rate and blood pressure at rest and at submaximal exercise, increases

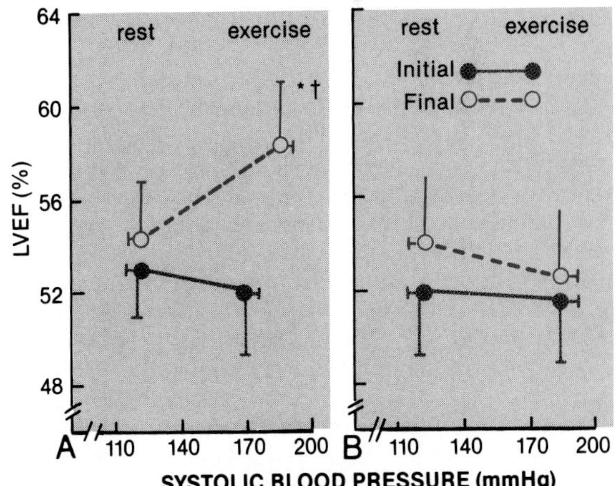

FIGURE 42–2. Effect of training on left ventricular ejection fraction (LVEF). *A,* In the training group, LVEF at rest was not significantly changed after training. During maximal exercise, LVEF increased significantly (*$p < .01$) above the resting level after (○) but not before (●) training. During maximal exercise, LVEF was significantly higher (†$p < .001$) after training despite the attainment of higher systolic blood pressure ($p < .001$). *B,* In the nonexercising patients, LVEF did not change with exercise initially (●) or 12 months later (○). Systolic blood pressure values were also similar. Data are mean ± SE for 25 trained *(A)* and 14 untrained patients *(B)*. (From Ehsani, A. A., Biello, D. R., Schultz, J., et al.: Improvement of left ventricular contractile function by exercise training in patients with coronary artery disease. Circulation *74:*350, 1986, by permission of the American Heart Association, Inc.)

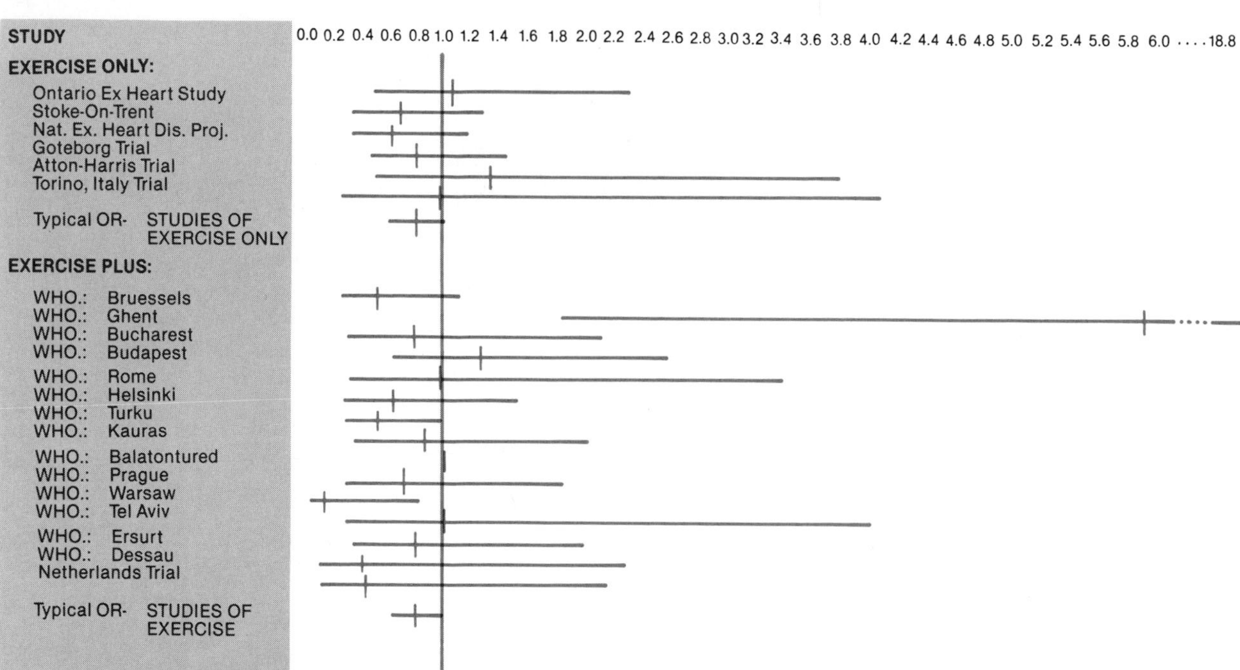

FIGURE 42-3. Chart of effects of pooling from randomized trials of cardiac rehabilitation on the estimate of mortality 3 years after randomization. Short vertical lines indicate the point estimates; horizontal lines depict the 95 per cent confidence intervals. (From O'Connor, G. T., Buring, J. E., Yusuf, S., et al.: An overview of randomized trials of rehabilitation with exercise after myocardial infarction. Circulation *80*:234, 1989, by permission of the American Heart Association, Inc.)

peak MET capacity, and increases both endurance and strength. The lower the initial MET capacity, the greater the benefit in most patients.[19,24,25] Patients with a combination of myocardial ischemia and resting left ventricular dysfunction are less likely to benefit from short-term exercise training.[26] Treatment with beta blockers does not prevent a training effect in patients with coronary heart disease,[27] although some studies indicate that the training effect may be blunted.[28] Other benefits of exercise include weight reduction, improved glucose tolerance in diabetic patients, improved HDL cholesterol levels, and psychological benefits, including a greater confidence to resume customary activities more quickly.[29]

MORBIDITY AND MORTALITY. Exercise training has not been shown definitively to reduce morbidity or mortality in patients with coronary heart disease. Only 1 of 22 individual randomized trials of cardiac rehabilitation with exercise training demonstrated a statistically significant reduction in cardiovascular mortality.[30] However, all other studies were limited by inadequate sample size, short follow-up, or crossovers after randomization. Two recent analyses using data pooled from several studies showed that overall mortality and cardiovascular mortality, defined as fatal reinfarction or sudden death, were reduced by 20 to 25 per cent in patients randomized to exercise training (Fig. 42-3). Nonfatal reinfarction rates were similar in exercise and control groups.[31,32] The magnitude of benefit is similar to that seen in the randomized trials of prophylactic beta blockade after myocardial infarction,[33] suggesting that exercise training may be equally beneficial.

SELECTION OF PATIENTS FOR EXERCISE TESTING AND TRAINING

(See also Chap. 6)

PATIENTS ELIGIBLE FOR EXERCISE TRAINING. Exercise training is usually recommended for patients recovering from myocardial infarction or coronary artery bypass graft surgery. Other patients may also benefit, including those with chronic stable angina or compensated congestive heart failure and those recovering from coronary angioplasty, valve surgery, or cardiac transplantation.[19,25,34] Exercise prescription should be based on the results of electrocardiographically monitored exercise tests. Therefore, patients ineligible for exercise testing because of severe angina, uncompensated congestive heart failure, or uncontrolled arrhythmias are not candidates for exercise training. Other limiting noncardiac illnesses such as chronic obstructive pulmonary disease, peripheral vascular disease, stroke, and orthopedic disease do not necessarily obviate exercise testing and training, because specialized techniques such as arm crank ergometry can be used.[35,36]

EXERCISE TESTING. Exercise testing to a symptom or sign limit should be performed as soon after a cardiac event as the patient's condition permits. In uncomplicated cases, testing can be performed 14 to 21 days after myocardial infarction, 14 to 28 days after cardiac surgery, and 3 to 10 days after coronary angioplasty.[37] The advisability of early testing and training after myocardial infarction has been questioned because of experimental and clinical evidence showing abnormal myocardial scar formation, especially in large anterior myocardial infarctions.[38] The clinical relevance of these findings is uncertain and should probably not preclude the current clinical approach.[39] Exercise testing is performed somewhat later after cardiac surgery to minimize the detrimental effects of wound healing and pulmonary dysfunction on exercise performance.

Submaximal exercise testing is commonly used prior to or soon after hospital discharge because of the perceived safety of such testing compared to maximal testing. Maximal testing is then performed at 6 to 8 weeks following hospital discharge. However, there is no evidence that submaximal testing is safer than symptom-limited testing in properly selected patients,[40] and there are disadvantages to submaximal testing. Patients may be inappropriately limited in their customary activities and in exercise training if submaximal testing is used to evaluate physical capacity.[41-43] Return to work may be significantly delayed.[43]

Because exercise capacity is reduced in patients recovering from a cardiac event, a modified treadmill protocol should be used. The Bruce protocol increases by 2 or 3 METS at each stage and quickly surpasses the average capacity of patients recovering from a cardiac event. The modified Naughton protocol starts at a lower MET workload and increases at increments of 1 MET. This gradual progression is better tolerated and provides a more accurate assessment of MET capacity. The usual symptomatic endpoints are dyspnea and fatigue, whereas moderate angina, dizziness, and claudication occur less commonly. Signs that are important endpoints include high-grade ventricular arrhythmias, such as triplets; a fall in systolic blood pressure of 20 mm Hg compared to the previous stage; marked ischemia; and blank facies, suggesting decreased cerebral perfusion.

While the exercise test is the basis of the exercise prescription, certain test results contraindicate exercise training. Severe exercise-induced ischemia, arrhythmias, or left ventricular dysfunction must be corrected before patients are allowed to exercise. Exercise testing should be repeated after treatment to confirm that the abnormalities have resolved. Less severe abnormalities that occur at high heart rates and workloads are not necessarily contraindications to exercise therapy, especially if patients are receiving maximal medical therapy and no other treatment options are available. In those instances, the exercise prescription is modified as discussed below, and more intensive surveillance is used during exercise training.

EXERCISE PRESCRIPTION

INDIVIDUALIZED PRESCRIPTION. The exercise prescription is individualized, based upon the results of the symptom-limited exercise test. The components of the prescription are summarized by the acronym FIT—frequency, intensity, and time. The minimum frequency needed to improve cardiovascular fitness is three times weekly. The intensity is most easily prescribed as a target heart rate. The time or duration of exercise is usually 30 to 60 minutes for each session, but is individually determined.[29,44]

The intensity is based on the peak heart rate achieved during exercise testing. The conditioning effect is a balance between the intensity and duration of exercise. A low intensity is prescribed initially to allow the patient to complete 1 hour sessions without excessive fatigue. A target heart rate of 65 per cent of the peak predicted heart rate is a common starting point. In some instances, especially after cardiac surgery, the resting pulse is high and 65 per cent of the peak heart rate places the target rate near the resting pulse. In those cases, a slightly higher initial target of 75 per cent may be used. Alternatively, 40 to 50 per cent of the difference between the peak and the resting heart rate may be calculated and added to the resting pulse to determine the target. For convenience, the target is given as a 10-sec count. Patients should be taught to measure their pulse during exercise.

COMPONENTS OF EXERCISE SESSIONS. Exercise sessions, whether performed individually or in a group, should last 1 hour. Each session includes a warm-up period, a period of aerobic and muscular conditioning, and a cool-down period. A 10-minute warm-up includes stretching and light calisthenics to prevent musculoskeletal injury and gradually increase the heart rate. A 40-minute conditioning period is best spent in aerobic exercise such as walking, jogging, and bicycling during the first several weeks of the training program. Swimming is excellent aerobic exercise but creates problems with surveillance, pulse monitoring, and response in the event of a cardiovascular emergency. The exercise session is concluded with a 10-minute cool-down using stretching exercises similar to those in the warm-up period. This is especially important in coronary patients, in whom ventricular arrhythmias are commonly precipitated by abrupt cessation of moderate- or high-intensity exercise.[45]

Aerobic conditioning rather than strength training is emphasized in the first several weeks of exercise training. Arm training, especially isometric exercise, is usually proscribed in the early training period because it causes a disproportionate increase in blood pressure compared to heart rate[46] and may compromise sternal wound healing in the first 4 to 6 weeks after cardiac surgery. Standard exercise programs emphasizing dynamic leg training by walking, jogging, and bicycling also increase arm strength and endurance even without specific arm training.[47] If arm and shoulder strength training is important, patients can begin using light hand weights during walk-jog exercises early in the exercise program.

Circuit training, which refers to a series of weight-lifting exercises using moderate weight loads and frequent repetition, emphasizes muscular conditioning in both upper and lower extremities and may be advantageous to some patients later in their training program.[48] This is especially true of those patients who perform a significant amount of upper extremity work in their occupation. The major disadvantage of circuit training is the need for more elaborate equipment.

ADVANCING THE PRESCRIPTION. The Borg scale of Rate of Perceived Exertion (RPE)[49] is a useful tool for advancing the exercise prescription during training. As shown in Table 42–1, the RPE scale gives a numerical value to a perceived level of exertion. Patients should exercise at an RPE of 13 to 15. As patients become more fit, the RPE will fall and the intensity of exercise may then be increased. The target is usually increased by 5 to 10 per cent of the peak heart rate. Ultimately, patients should be able to exercise at 85 per cent of their peak heart rate for the entire session; most patients reach this intensity within 8 to 12 sessions.

Follow-up treadmill testing should be performed 4 to 8 weeks after the beginning of exercise training. Many patients will achieve significantly higher heart rates on subsequent testing. Higher achieved heart rates are related to improvements in chronotropic incompetence in some patients and the ability to achieve a maximal cardiovascular effort in others previously limited by severe skeletal muscle deconditioning.[11] The follow-up treadmill test can be used to advance the exercise prescription for most patients and to allow some to graduate to lower levels of surveillance during exercise.

PATIENTS WITH MYOCARDIAL ISCHEMIA. Patients with exercise-induced myocardial ischemia should receive optimal therapy to eliminate or ameliorate the problem. Some patients will still show evidence of ischemia. Assuming that ischemia does not occur at extremely low workloads, these patients may still exercise safely as long as their target heart rate remains well below that at which ischemia occurs.[50] Limiting the maximal target heart rate to 10 beats per minute below that at which ischemic abnormalities occur is useful clinically. Increased surveillance during exercise, as with continuous ECG monitoring, is also recommended in the initial stages of exercise training.

TABLE 42–1 BORG SCALE OF RATE OF PERCEIVED EXERTION (RPE)[49]

LEVEL OF EXERTION	VALUE
Very, very light	6 7 8
Very light	9 10
Light	11 12
Somewhat hard	13 14
Hard	15 16
Very hard	17 18
Very, very hard	19 20

Data from Borg, G., and Linderholm, H.: Exercise performance and perceived exertion in patients with coronary insufficiency, arterial hypertension and vasoregulatory asthenia. Acta Med. Scand. *187*:17, 1970.

PATIENTS WITH HEART FAILURE. Patients with heart failure are at higher risk for complications related to exercise but also tend to have the most significant improvements from exercise training. Supervised exercise training has been shown to be safe in patients with heart failure.[25,26,50] The exercise prescription must often be modified for heart failure patients because of limited endurance. Shorter periods of aerobic training, lower target heart rates, and intermittent rest periods can all be used to limit the degree of fatigue felt by these patients. The ultimate target heart rate should also be kept 10 beats per minute below that at which significant symptoms of dyspnea and fatigue occur on exercise testing.

PATIENTS WITH ARRHYTHMIAS. Patients with arrhythmias present a significant challenge to the clinician because of controversies regarding therapy and the uncertainty of the safety of exercise. No definitive data are available regarding the safety of exercise in patients with arrhythmias. The usual clinical approach to cardiac rehabilitation in patients with severe exercise-induced arrhythmias is to exclude them from exercise training until suppression of the arrhythmia is achieved. Higher levels of surveillance are recommended during exercise, using continuous ECG monitoring. Longitudinal studies have shown that arrhythmia frequency and grade are unchanged by exercise training.[51] Stable patterns of arrhythmia during ECG-monitored exercise training are often used as evidence to allow patients to begin supervised, unmonitored exercise. However, the safety of this approach has not been documented.

RISKS OF EXERCISE TRAINING

Exercise training is not without risks. The greatest risk of exercise lies in patients with untreated or unrecognized left ventricular dysfunction, myocardial ischemia, or ventricular arrhythmias. In patients with these abnormalities who have received optimal therapy, the greatest risk lies in exercising at or above the level at which the abnormalities can be elicited by exercise testing.[52] For this reason, the maximum target heart rate used in exercise training must be lower than the heart rate at which abnormalities become evident on testing.

PATIENT SELECTION AND SURVEILLANCE. Safe exercise training is best assured by proper selection of patients and adequate surveillance during exercise. Patients at high risk for cardiovascular complications during exercise have one or more of the characteristics listed in Table 42–2.[34,52,53] In such patients the abnormality should be ameliorated or corrected before starting the exercise program. If the abnormality cannot be corrected, the risks and benefits of exercise training should be carefully considered. If an exercise program is recommended, the highest level of surveillance during exercise is required. There are some patients in whom the risks of exercise outweigh the benefits despite optimal medical therapy. Such patients should be informed of the risks and counseled not to exercise.

The highest level of surveillance is supervised group exercise with continuous electrocardiographic monitoring. Approximately 15 to 25 per cent of patients eligible for exercise training have one or more of the characteristics in Table 42–2 and require continuous electrocardiographic monitoring.[34,53] The next level of surveillance is unmonitored group exercise training supervised by health professionals with Advanced Cardiac Life Support certification. Patients without high-risk characteristics and those who improve during electrocardiographic monitored training can participate in supervised, unmonitored group training.[53] Very low-risk patients can safely exercise independently after learning the principles of pulse monitoring and symptom recognition. In general, low-risk patients have an exercise capacity of 8 METS or more without symptoms or signs of left ventricular dysfunction, myocardial ischemia, or ventricular arrhythmias. These criteria may be used to graduate patients from supervised programs.[54]

All patients should be taught to monitor their pulse and recognize symptoms during exercise. The concepts of the target heart rate and RPE are conveyed and reinforced during group exercise sessions. These principles and concepts will guide patients in independent, safe, and effective exercise after completion of a formal exercise program. Patients who are unable or unwilling to follow the exercise prescription should receive higher levels of surveillance.

SAFETY OF SUPERVISED PROGRAMS. Despite the potential for cardiovascular complications during exercise training, supervised exercise programs have an extremely good safety record. In a survey of 167 programs, the incidence of fatal events per million patient hours of exercise was 1.3, of myocardial infarction 3.4, and of resuscitated cardiac arrests 8.9. There were no significant differences in these rates for small compared to large programs or continuously electrocardiographically monitored compared to intermittently monitored programs.[55] The event rates in this study were significantly lower than in a survey performed a decade earlier.[56] The reasons for improvement are speculative. Improved risk stratification, improved revascularization and medical therapy, more rigorous standards for cardiac rehabilitation programs, and increased awareness of the necessity for monitoring high-risk patients may all have contributed to the improved safety record.

TABLE 42–2 INDICATIONS FOR CONTINUOUS ECG MONITORING DURING EXERCISE TRAINING

CLINICAL INDICATION	OBJECTIVE SIGNS
Severe left ventricular dysfunction	Ejection fraction <30%
Complex ventricular arrhythmia (at rest or exercise induced)	Lown grade 4 or 5
Hypotensive response to exercise	Systolic drop of 20 mm Hg or more at increasing load
Complicated myocardial infarction	Cardiogenic shock Congestive heart failure
Severe exercise-induced ischemia	ST-segment depression ≥ 2 mV Angina at a workload ≤ 5 METS
Low functional capacity	Peak workload ≤ 5 METS
Prior cardiac arrest	
Inability to self-monitor heart rate	

SECONDARY PREVENTION

(See also Chap. 37)

Increasing evidence supports the widespread application of specific measures to prevent recurrence of cardiac disease after a first cardiac event. In the short term, abstinence from cigarette smoking is extremely effective in reducing morbidity and mortality. In the long term, reduction in serum lipid abnormalities appears to slow the progression of coronary atherosclerosis and may improve the outcome. While controversial, treatment of certain behavioral manifestations, such as Type A behavior, may exert a positive influence on prognosis. There is no definitive evidence that the treatment of hypertension and diabetes positively influences prognosis *after* a cardiac event, although the standard of care is to treat these conditions vigorously.

CIGARETTE SMOKING

(See also p. 1302)

RISKS. Cigarette smoking is an established risk factor for the development of angina and myocardial infarction[57] and increases the risk for recurrence of infarction and death.[58] In survivors of myocardial infarction who continue to smoke, the rate of recurrence of infarction and cardiac death is twice that in patients who quit smoking. The risk of a second cardiac event declines rapidly after cessation of smoking. Within 3 years of ceasing smoking, the risk of reinfarction is approximately the same in ex-smokers and in survivors who never smoked.[57-59]

PATHOPHYSIOLOGY. The pathophysiology underlying the increased risk for death and reinfarction is uncertain. Platelet aggregation, thrombosis, coronary spasm, and diminished coronary and collateral flow reserve have all been implicated. Coronary flow reserve is significantly lower in smokers than nonsmokers, with heavier smokers having greater reductions than lighter smokers.[60] Fibrinogen levels are significantly higher in smokers than in nonsmokers and increase the primary risk of myocardial infarction.[61] Although the degree of coronary atherosclerosis is not strongly correlated with smoking habits, the risk for myocardial infarction in smokers is strongly correlated with the extent of coronary artery disease and plasma cholesterol levels.[59]

ETIOLOGY OF TOBACCO DEPENDENCE. Smoking is a complex behavior with physiological, psychological, and sociological roots. There are several theories regarding the etiology of tobacco dependence, although no single theory is adequate to explain all aspects of smoking behavior. Physiological dependence on nicotine causes acute craving for cigarettes with abrupt cessation of smoking. Smoking is a habit that minimizes negative emotions such as distress, anger, and fear. It may also be used as a coping mechanism to transfer such negative emotions into socially acceptable behavior. Finally, a smoking habit may have deep sociological origins, such as modeling behavior after parents and peers.[62]

SMOKING CESSATION PROGRAMS. Demographic and psychological factors identify patients more likely to continue smoking after a cardiac event. Lower occupational and educational levels, smoking a greater number of cigarettes, increasing age, and higher rates of alcohol consumption are demographic factors associated with continued smoking. Psychological factors such as a less negative attitude regarding smoking, higher anxiety levels, and a low sense of personal control over life events predict smokers who are less likely to quit smoking after a cardiac event.[62,63]

Smoking cessation is facilitated by treating both the physiological and psychological aspects of the habit. The association between cardiac disease and smoking is well known to the lay public. Myocardial infarction or coronary surgery is a sufficient impetus for 20 to 60 per cent of patients to stop smoking. Patients who receive strong advice from health professionals to stop smoking are more likely to quit and remain abstinent than those who do not receive advice.[64] This is particularly true of individuals who believe that they are at personal risk if they continue smoking. Unfortunately, the high acute cessation rates are also associated with high recidivism rates in the absence of interventions to maintain abstinence.

Hospital confinement for myocardial infarction or coronary surgery usually provides sufficient time for the psychological manifestations of nicotine withdrawal such as irritability, emotionality, inability to concentrate, nausea, and headache to resolve. In patients who continue to crave cigarettes, nicotine dependence is strong, and more gradual nicotine withdrawal may be necessary.[59]

Nicotine withdrawal can be managed by tapering cigarette smoking, gradually changing to lower-nicotine cigarettes, and substituting chewing of nicotine gum. A 2-mg dose of nicotine gum gives average serum nicotine levels of 12 ng/ml compared to 35 to 54 ng/ml from cigarette smoke. This level is usually sufficient to blunt the craving for nicotine, although in heavier smokers higher doses of oral nicotine appear to be more effective.[65] Nicotine gum is prescribed as needed, up to 30 doses per day. The average patient uses 10 doses daily, and the frequency of dosing declines over a 1- to 3-month period. If the patient is still dependent on the gum after 6 months, it is likely being used as a cigarette substitute rather than an aid to abstinence. Aversive techniques, such as smoke holding or rapid puffing, may also be effective in nicotine-dependent patients.

The most effective programs for smoking abstinence address both the physiological and psychological dependence on cigarettes. The prescription of nicotine gum alone does not significantly increase the long-term abstinence rate.[66] Smoking is usually linked to other behaviors, such as eating or talking on the telephone. It is also more common in particular situations, such as stressful activities or social situations.

Teaching patients to recognize the high-risk behaviors or situations in which the desire to smoke is likely is the first step in maintaining abstinence. Using techniques of self-control or substitution of healthful behaviors for smoking assists the patients in abstaining from smoking.[67] Enlisting the social support of family, friends, and coworkers reinforces the nonsmoking behavior. Long-term abstinence rates of up to 70 per cent have been achieved with formal programs.[67,68]

Serum Lipids

(See also p. 1116)

PRIMARY AND SECONDARY PREVENTION. Data from laboratory, epidemiological, and clinical studies have established the role of serum lipids in the genesis of coronary atherosclerosis. There is compelling evidence that reducing serum cholesterol reduces the risk of a primary cardiac event. The Coronary Primary Prevention Trial demonstrated that lowering serum cholesterol with cholestyramine decreased the risk of cardiovascular death and nonfatal myocardial infarction in men with serum cholesterol in the 90th percentile who had no evidence of coronary disease.[69,70] Similar results were obtained in patients treated with gemfibrozil.[71]

The data are less clear regarding the effects of cholesterol reduction on the risk for second cardiac events. Nicotinic acid treatment after myocardial infarction was associated with lower cardiovascular mortality and nonfatal reinfarction rates in the Coronary Drug Project.[72] No other data are yet available definitively linking treatment of increased serum cholesterol with reduction in cardiovascular risk.

PROGRESSION OF ATHEROSCLEROSIS. Progression of atherosclerosis has been linked with higher rates of cardiovascular complications after a first cardiac event.[73] Slowing the progression or causing regression of atherosclerosis would potentially result in a reduction in cardiovascular complications.

Several trials have used quantitative coronary angiography to evaluate the effects of diet and drug therapy on coronary atherosclerosis. The Leiden Intervention Trial evaluated the effect of a vegetarian diet and found that 46 per cent of participants showed no progression of coronary atherosclerosis.[74] The Cholesterol Lowering Atherosclerosis Study was a randomized, placebo-controlled study of the effect of diet plus niacin and colestipol versus diet plus placebo on coronary atherosclerosis in patients who had previously undergone coronary artery bypass surgery. Progression of disease was significantly reduced in native vessels and bypass grafts in the treatment compared to the placebo group. Regression of atherosclerosis was observed in 16.2 per cent of the treatment group as compared to 3.6 per cent of the placebo group. Clinical outcomes were better in the drug group, although the sample size was insufficient to demonstrate an improvement in mortality.[75]

Similar though less conclusive findings were seen in a randomized trial of diet plus cholestyramine versus diet plus placebo in patients with Type II hyperlipidemia and overt coronary disease.[76] These trials suggest that diet and drug therapy can slow the progression of coronary atherosclerosis but do not necessarily reduce morbidity and mortality.

NATIONAL CHOLESTEROL EDUCATION PROGRAM. An expert panel developed recommendations for the evaluation and treatment of hypercholesterolemia that have been publicized as the National Cholesterol Education Program. Low-, moderate-, and high-risk categories of serum cholesterol were established, and treatment within each category was recommended.[77] High-risk patients were those with elevated LDL-cholesterol levels and two or more cardiac risk factors or clinically manifested coronary artery disease. Most patients eligible for cardiac rehabilitation who also have elevated cholesterol levels would be in the high-risk group.

In patients with coronary artery disease, the panel recommends that total cholesterol greater than 200 mg/dl be evaluated with a lipoprotein analysis. Patients with LDL-cholesterol levels greater than 130 mg/dl are recommended for dietary treatment. Patients with LDL-cholesterol greater than 160 mg/dl are recommended for drug therapy in addition to dietary treatment. In both instances, the goal is to reduce LDL-cholesterol below 130 mg/dl. The first-choice drugs are those known to lower LDL-cholesterol that have also lowered the risk of a primary cardiac event.[77] Cholestyramine, colestipol, nicotinic acid, and gemfibrozil all meet these criteria.

The recommendations of the panel have been criticized in some areas. Specific therapy for low HDL-cholesterol levels was not recommended, despite the known increased coronary risk associated with this finding. Data from one primary prevention trial found that increasing the HDL level with gemfibrozil lowered coronary risk independent of any lowering of LDL levels.[71]

No specific recommendations were made regarding modifications of the recommendations in older patients. The benefits of cholesterol treatment in the elderly have been questioned.[78] While drug treatment is recommended at lower LDL-cholesterol levels in patients who manifest coronary disease, some have suggested that the recommendations are too conservative in this subgroup.[79] The panel clearly advises that the guidelines be applied according to the clinical judgments of practicing physicians.[77]

DIETARY TREATMENT. The approach to the dietary treatment of hypercholesterolemia is to lower the intake of total fat, saturated fat, and cholesterol and to achieve ideal weight. A two-step dietary approach is recommended, with the first step restricting total fat to 30 per cent and saturated fat to 10 per cent of caloric intake and cholesterol to 300 mg daily. If the first step is not sufficient to reach desired goals, the second step restricts saturated fat to 7 per cent and cholesterol to 200 mg. A 4- to 12-week period of dietary modification is recommended with at least one reevaluation of serum lipids.[77] The dietary evaluation and treatment plan is best developed by a dietitian with the patient and spouse. Food purchasing and preparation should be emphasized in addition to selection of low-fat and low-cholesterol foods. Information should be provided on selection of foods in restaurants. The cardiac rehabilitation team reinforces the cholesterol management guidelines during rehabilitation sessions.

DRUG TREATMENT. If dietary intervention and exercise are insufficient to meet the goals of treatment of hypercholesterolemia, specific drug therapy should be initiated. The effect of other cardiovascular drugs that may increase serum lipids, such as beta blockers and thiazide diuretics, should be considered. Selection of specific lipid-lowering agents is discussed on page 1142.

EFFECTS OF CARDIAC REHABILITATION. The effect of exercise on serum cholesterol is not clear. Conflicting reports are probably related to the failure of studies to control for effects of changes in body weight, diet, and intensity of exercise.[80] In general, low- to moderate-intensity exercise has little influence on total cholesterol. However, most reports are consistent in demonstrating that all intensities and durations of exercise increase HDL-cholesterol levels.[81] Weight loss resulting from calorie and fat restriction in conjunction with exercise usually results in decreased LDL levels.[80,81]

Other influences are less clear. While moderate alcohol consumption has been associated with a decreased prevalence of coronary heart disease,[83] the reason is unclear. The effects of fish oils are similarly unclear. High concentrations of omega-3 fatty acids either reduce hepatic synthesis of VLDL or increase catabolism. Through this effect, LDL levels may be reduced, especially in hypercholesterolemic states in which VLDL levels are elevated.[84]

PSYCHOLOGICAL FACTORS

COMMON PSYCHIATRIC PROBLEMS. Most professionals providing cardiac rehabilitation believe that exercise training and related services produce significant psychological benefits. In particular, anxiety and depression are improved, and patients have a greater sense of well-being. However, there are few well-performed studies demonstrating psychological benefits of cardiac rehabilitation in the absence of specific interventions, such as stress management or group therapy.[85] In patients with disabling psychiatric symptoms, specific treatment with medications or psychotherapy is indicated. The most common of these symptoms are delirium in the acute setting[86] and anxiety or depression during early recovery.[87] Two areas in which specific interventions might be helpful as an adjunct to cardiac rehabilitation are self-efficacy and Type A behavior.

SELF-EFFICACY. Acute cardiac illnesses have many psychosocial sequelae, including medical restrictions on even the most routine of activities such as driving, climbing stairs, and lifting. These restrictions are reinforced by family, friends, and coworkers, who perceive a poor prognosis and are concerned that physical and emotional stress can further damage the heart. If the patient has a poor understanding of his illness, fear of recurrent cardiac problems leads to a sense of loss of control and a lack of confidence to resume customary activities. This lack of confidence can be a significant impediment to the resumption of a full and active life style.

"Self-efficacy" is a psychological term used to describe how an individual's judgment regarding his capacity for performance of a task or action is an important determinant of whether he will attempt the task or action.[88] Self-efficacy reflects confidence and is highly predictive of action. Self-efficacy for specific tasks can be rated on confidence scales of 0 to 100 per cent. For example, self-efficacy scales that predict whether a coronary patient will be successful with a regular exercise program have been validated for physical activity.[89] The most common areas of low self-efficacy for coronary patients are physical exertion, emotional stress, and sexual activity.[88]

Self-efficacy can be increased in coronary patients by four methods: persuasion, information, vicarious experience, and enactive techniques. Using exercise as an example, physicians can persuade patients that they are capable of exercising. Patients can be informed about what sensations to expect with exercise, so they do not misread normal physiological responses such as tachycardia as grave symptoms. Vicarious experiences can be shared by other patients who have successfully undertaken an exercise program. The most powerful method for increasing exercise self-efficacy is the performance of a supervised exercise test.[88,89]

Self-efficacy is a useful measure for predicting potential success for other important behavioral changes, such as smoking cessation,[67] dietary modification, and exercise training.[89,90] In circumstances of low self-efficacy, informative, persuasive, vicarious, and enactive techniques to raise self-efficacy are helpful for increasing the success rate for behavioral change. Spousal perceptions are equally important. Self-efficacy scales that rate a spouse's perception of the patient's potential for success with a particular task are also highly predictive of success or failure. Support and encouragement by the spouse in behavior change are extremely important for success. Spousal self-efficacy can be raised by means of techniques similar to those used for patients.[88,91]

TYPE A BEHAVIOR. While Type A behavior, i.e., behavior characterized by excesses of competitiveness, pace, and aggressiveness, has been recognized as a risk factor for the development of coronary artery disease,[92] its effect on the prognosis of coronary disease is unknown. Conflicting results are reported in several studies, although there are limitations in each. The major limitations are the populations studied, the instruments used to classify behavior, the duration of follow-up, and the endpoints studied.[93,94] One of the most important concepts that has emerged from the Type A controversy is recognition that the construct probably reflects a collection of behaviors, not all of which are related to either the development or the prognosis of coronary disease. Of the three primary characteristics of Type A behavior—competitive achievement striving, time urgency, and hostility—only the last appears to be independently related to coronary disease outcomes.[95]

Despite the controversy regarding the effect of Type A behavior on prognosis, there is evidence from one intervention trial that modifying Type A behavior reduces risk of recurrent cardiac events in patients recovering from myocardial infarction. The Recurrent Coronary Prevention Project randomized a group of 862 men who had experienced a myocardial infarction to either a control group receiving cardiological counseling or an intervention group receiving cardiological counseling and Type A behavioral counseling. Type A behavior patterns were significantly reduced in the intervention group as compared to the control group. The rate of recurrent cardiac events over 3 years was 13 per cent in control patients and 7.2 per cent in intervention patients. This significant reduction in event rate was primarily related to a reduction in nonfatal myocardial infarctions in the intervention group.[96] The risk reduction is on the same order of magnitude as the benefit of prophylactic beta blockade after myocardial infarction.[33] The results from this single study are encouraging and warrant further investigation of treatment of Type A behavior.

VOCATIONAL REHABILITATION

The cost of cardiovascular disability is high. The direct cost of care for patients with heart disease is estimated at $85 billion annually in the United States.[97,98] Indirect costs, due to goods and services not provided because of cardiovascular illness, are several times greater. Indirect costs can be significantly reduced by increasing the numbers of patients who return to work and shortening the interval between a cardiac event and return to work.

FACTORS RELATED TO EMPLOYMENT. Employment after a cardiac event is related to demographic, medical, and psychosocial factors. Patients unemployed at the time of a cardiac event, those over 60 years of age, and those with blue-collar jobs are significantly less likely to work after the event. Unemployment for 3 months or more before a cardiac event is common in patients with more severe cardiac disease but also may be related to psychological or social causes for unemployment. Retirement and disability benefits are more easily obtained after age 60, encouraging patients to leave the work force. Blue collar workers, especially those who are unskilled, are easily replaced in the work force and consequently lose their jobs more commonly after a cardiac event.[99] After a cardiac event, the medical condition of the patient and the advice provided by the physician regarding return to work are the most important factors influencing the rate of reemployment in previously employed patients.

In the absence of demographic and psychosocial impediments, physicians play a pivotal role in the return-to-work decision.[100] The physician must first ensure that the risk of a cardiovascular complication is low and will not be increased by returning to work and then must determine if the patient has the physical capacity to perform his occupational work. Finally the physician must provide explicit advice regarding the timing of return to work and any work restrictions that the patient and employer must follow.

FACILITATING REEMPLOYMENT. In the majority of patients recovering from cardiac surgery or myocardial infarction, a careful clinical evaluation and a symptom-limited treadmill test are sufficient to guide the physician in the return-to-work decision. Accurate methods to stratify the risk of recurrent coronary events rely on clinical information obtained during hospitalization and specialized testing performed during or shortly after hospitalization. More than half of patients surviving myocardial infarction have no symptoms or signs of congestive heart failure or myocardial ischemia. Their risk of cardiac death, myocardial infarction, or unstable angina in the year following the primary event is less than 10 per cent. A symptom-limited exercise capacity on treadmill testing of 7 METS or more without ischemia lowers the risk to less than 3 per cent.[101]

The treadmill test also establishes peak physical capacity, which can be related to the patient's occupational work. Individuals can sustain 6 to 8 hours of continuous effort at 40 per cent of their peak MET capacity. Continuous work tolerance declines at higher levels, averaging 4 hours at 60 per cent of peak capacity and 2 hours above 60 per cent of peak capacity.[102] Table 42–3 lists the MET requirements for selected occupational and recreational activities.[103] The average job has an energy requirement well under 5 METS, meaning that a peak capacity of 7 to 10 METS is sufficient for most individuals to perform their occupational work.[102] Only 16 per cent of Americans perform jobs requiring manual labor, and that percentage declines rapidly with age.[104] Most manual labor jobs require only intermittent high-energy expenditure, which significantly prolongs work tolerance.

Intensive physical reconditioning is not necessary for the average patient to return to work. In patients with very low functional capacity and those with higher physical requirements of their job, an exercise training program can hasten their return to work. Unless the patient's job requires lifting and carrying of moderate to heavy loads, the standard aerobic training described previously is sufficient to expedite return to work. In specialized circumstances, exercise programs that include upper extremity isometric training can be provided. Work simulation and specialized training programs may be helpful in unusual circumstances. In the particular circumstance of jobs affecting public safety, such as pilots, police, and fire fighters, more stringent requirements regarding return to work are legislated.[105]

The average interval between uncomplicated myocardial infarction and return to work is 70 to 90 days; it averages 80 to

TABLE 42–3 ESTIMATES OF ENERGY REQUIREMENTS OF AVOCATIONAL AND OCCUPATIONAL TASKS[103]

CATEGORY	SELF-CARE OR HOME	OCCUPATIONAL	RECREATIONAL	PHYSICAL CONDITIONING
Very light < 3 METS < 10 ml/kg/min < 4 kcal	Washing, shaving, dressing, desk work, writing; washing dishes; driving auto	Sitting (clerical, assembly), standing (store clerk, bartender); driving truck, operating crane	Shuffleboard, horseshoes, bait casting, billiards, archery, golf (cart)	Walking (2 mph), stationary bicycle (very low resistance), very light calisthenics
Light 3–5 METS 11–18 ml/kg/min 4–6 kcal	Cleaning windows, raking leaves, weeding, power lawn mowing, waxing floors (slowly), painting, carrying objects (15–30 lb)	Stocking shelves (light objects), light welding, light carpentry, machine assembly, auto repair, paper hanging	Dancing (social and square), golf (walking), sailing, horseback riding, volleyball (6 man), tennis (doubles)	Walking (3–4 mph), level bicycling (6–8 mph), light calisthenics
Moderate 5–7 METS 18–25 ml/kg/min 6–8 kcal	Easy digging in garden, level lawn mowing, climbing stairs (slowly), carrying objects (30–60 lb)	Carpentry (exterior home building), shoveling dirt, using pneumatic tools	Badminton (competitive), tennis (singles), snow skiing (downhill), light backpacking, basketball, skating (ice and roller), horseback riding (gallop)	Walking (4.5–5 mph), bicycling (9–10 mph), swimming (breast stroke)
Heavy 7–9 METS 25–32 ml/kg/min 8–10 kcal	Sawing wood, heavy shoveling, climbing stairs (moderate speed), carrying objects (60–90 lb)	Tending furnace, digging ditches, pick and shovel	Canoeing, mountain climbing, fencing, paddleball, touch football	Jog (5 mph), swim (crawl stroke), rowing machine, heavy calisthenics, bicycling (12 mph)
Very heavy > 9 METS > 32 ml/kg/min > 10 kcal	Carrying loads upstairs, carrying objects (> 90 lb), climbing stairs (quickly), shoveling heavy snow, shoveling 10 min (16 lb)	Lumberjack, heavy laborer	Handball, squash, ski touring over hills, vigorous basketball	Running (≥ 6 mph), bicycle (≥ 13 mph or up steep hills), rope jumping

From Haskell, W. L.: Design and implementation of cardiac conditioning programs. *In* Wenger, N. K., and Hellerstein, H. F. (eds.): Rehabilitation of the Coronary Patient. New York, John Wiley & Sons, pp. 214–215.

100 days after uncomplicated coronary surgery.[100,102,106] These intervals can be substantially shortened with a coordinated approach using risk stratification, treadmill testing, and explicit physician advice regarding the timing of return to work. In employed patients without high-risk clinical characteristics or severe treadmill ischemia, the time from myocardial infarction was shortened from 75 to 51 days in a randomized trial of an early-return-to-work intervention. Recurrent cardiac events averaged 3.5 per cent in the 6 months after infarction and were no higher in patients returning to work earlier than in those returning to work later. Although this study did not include a special intervention for patients performing manual labor, the intervention was as successful in the 11 per cent of the population performing manual labor as it was in the sedentary workers. Higher-risk patients with evidence of congestive heart failure or myocardial ischemia accounted for 23 per cent of all employed patients under the age of 60 and were specifically excluded from the study. Return-to-work decisions in such patients must be individualized.

BENEFITS OF REEMPLOYMENT. The benefits of early return to work are primarily financial; however, the psychological benefits, while more difficult to identify, must not be overlooked. In the trial discussed previously, patients randomized to the return-to-work intervention earned $2100 more than patients randomized to usual care in the 6 months following myocardial infarction. While not specifically examined, financial benefits to employers probably accrued, including increased productivity and reduced costs of temporary employees and disability insurance payments.[107] Interventions that increase the numbers of patients returning to work and shorten the interval between the illness and reemployment will have the greatest impact on reducing the economic burden of cardiovascular disability.

ORGANIZATION OF CARDIAC REHABILITATION SERVICES

For most patients, cardiac rehabilitation begins in the hospital following a cardiac event and continues for several months thereafter. Cardiac rehabilitation has traditionally been provided in phases with activity guidelines based upon the time since the cardiac event. While phased rehabilitation provides a framework, individual patients will progress more slowly or quickly depending upon their age, condition prior to their cardiac event, the severity of illness, and motivation. The rehabilitation program should be individualized to facilitate a rate of recovery commensurate with the patient's status.[108]

INPATIENT REHABILITATION

Hospitalization has been significantly shortened for patients recovering from myocardial infarction and cardiac surgery. Inpatient rehabilitation must make patients self-sufficient in the activities of daily living in a short period of time. Patients must be able to recognize important cardiac symptoms, obtain medical care appropriately, and take prescribed medications. The behavioral changes required for secondary prevention may be introduced in the hospital but are mainly deferred until patients are at home.

EARLY MOBILIZATION. Early mobilization reduces the detrimental effects of bed rest, as discussed previously,[3-7] and maximizes the rate at which customary activities can be resumed. In the coronary care unit, assisted range-of-motion exercises can be initiated in the first 24 to 48 hours for most patients. Patients whose condition is stable should be encouraged to sit in a chair for increasing periods each day to minimize intravascular volume depletion, skeletal muscle deconditioning, and orthopedic impairment. Self-care activities such as shaving, oral hygiene, and sponge bathing can be undertaken in the intensive care unit. These activities have a low MET requirement (Table 42–3) and encourage patients to resume more activities quickly.[103] There is no specific time frame in which these activities should take place, other than as soon as tolerated by patients within the context of their medical and surgical care.

GRADUATED PHYSICAL ACTIVITY. A graduated program of physical and self-care activities can begin upon transfer from the intensive care unit. Upright posture should be encouraged as much as tolerated. Patients should walk with assistance at least twice daily. While some inpatient programs suggest walking specific distances each day,[108] ambulation can be based upon the patient's tolerance. In that way, patients are neither pushed beyond their tolerance nor held back in their recovery. The target heart rate and RPE scale can be used to individualize the intensity and time of activity. For each session, standing heart rate and blood pressure are obtained, followed by 5 minutes of range-of-motion and flexibility exercises. Patients are then assisted with walking at a rate that keeps the pulse within the range of resting pulse plus 20 beats/min and the RPE less than 14. Most patients will tolerate a minimum of 5 minutes of walking the first day. As long as the pulse and RPE remain within these limits, walking time can be increased until patients are walking for 30 minutes twice daily. At that point, the walking sessions should include stair climbing to ensure that patients can perform that task at home. Patients able to walk unassisted for 30 minutes and climb stairs have sufficient strength and endurance for most activities of daily living.

EDUCATION AND COUNSELING. During the periods of assisted ambulation, the nurse or physical therapist teaches patients how to count their pulse and recognize important symptoms. Before hospital discharge, patients are taught how to obtain emergency medical care; learn the names, dosages, effects, and side-effects of their medications; and have specific questions answered regarding their cardiac status. Basic information regarding the risk factors for coronary disease should be presented, with emphasis on those that affect the patient.

At the time of hospital discharge, patients should receive very specific advice about resumption of activities at home. To exercise safely at home, the patient should be able to count the pulse accurately and understand the use of the RPE scale. Even common sense knowledge should not be presumed by the health professionals caring for the patient. The spouse should receive the advice with the patient because the retention of information by hospitalized patients is limited, and most disagreements between patient and spouse in the early recovery period are related to perceptions of medical advice given.[109,110] A simple approach to providing guidelines for physical activities is to treat them as forms of exercise. Patients can use the rule of resting pulse plus 20 beats/min for most household activities. The patient will learn quickly the heart rate response to each activity and be confident in undertaking such activities at home. Patients should be told what restrictions are placed on common activities, such as climbing stairs, lifting, driving, socializing with visitors, shopping, and walking outdoors. Individual patients may have more specific questions.

Activities that involve more mental than physical stress, such as driving, socializing, and shopping, concern patients and family at the time of hospital discharge. In studies of patients recovering from myocardial infarction who underwent psychological stress testing using standard techniques, the mean resting heart rate rose less than 10 beats/min and the mean systolic blood pressure rose less than 15 mm/Hg with the most stressful intervention. In every case the hemodynamic response to psychological stress was substantially lower than to treadmill exercise testing. In a subset of patients with exercise-induced ST-segment depression, none developed ischemic responses to psychological stress testing.[111] These data suggest that the psychological stress of usual social activities is unlikely to precipitate significant cardiovascular abnormalities in the early recovery period.

EARLY POSTDISCHARGE REHABILITATION AND EXERCISE TRAINING

ACTIVITIES BEFORE EXERCISE TESTING. The interval between hospital discharge and formal cardiac rehabilitation should be as brief as possible. During this period, patients can continue their walking program as it was prescribed in the hospital. They should walk a minimum of 30 minutes twice daily at a target heart rate within the range of resting pulse plus 20 beats/min at an RPE of less than 14. Patients able to tolerate that duration of walking should be encouraged to add a third session or increase the two sessions to 45 minutes each. Secondary prevention efforts can begin, since patients are motivated and have time to begin to make behavioral changes. Initial visits with a dietitian can be scheduled if weight loss or cholesterol reduction is necessary. A smoking abstinence program can begin during this period. Patients should be provided with resources to teach them about coronary disease and risk factor management.

RECOMMENDATIONS FOLLOWING EXERCISE TESTING. A postdischarge exercise test is a good focal point for the subsequent rehabilitation effort. The formal exercise prescription can then be given. Goals for weight loss, serum cholesterol reduction, smoking cessation, and return to work can be established. In the absence of significant abnormalities on the treadmill test, patients may begin most customary activities such as driving, sexual activity, and light lifting. Although lifting is often proscribed for 6 to 8 weeks after myocardial infarction and cardiac surgery, studies suggest that lifting and carrying of moderate loads are not dangerous after uncomplicated myocardial infarction and cardiac surgery. In patients recovering from myocardial infarction, static lifting of 25 to 50 lb and combined static lifting and dynamic treadmill walking were associated with similar or lower double products compared to dynamic treadmill walking alone. In these studies, there was no evidence of myocardial ischemia induced by static lifting alone.[112,113] In another study, static lifting to a double product that elicited ischemia on dynamic treadmill walking was not associated with myocardial ischemia. The conclusion of that study was that the increased diastolic blood pressure response of static lifting increased coronary blood flow and prevented myocardial ischemia.[114]

SEXUAL ACTIVITY. The most common sexual problems of coronary patients are reduction or absence of libido, avoidance of sexual activity even if libido has recovered, impotence, and premature or delayed ejaculation in men. The causes of sexual dysfunction include preexisting conditions, fear of precipitating a cardiac event, depression, and medications, especially beta blockers and diuretics. In addition, the sexual partner may believe that sexual activity could precipitate a cardiac event and therefore may avoid sexual activity. Because patients are reluctant to discuss sexual dysfunction, the physician should address issues of sexuality and consider the effects of medications on sexual drive.[115]

The hemodynamic response to sexual intercourse has been evaluated in patients recovering from myocardial infarction. The maximal heart rate during sexual intercourse averages 120 beats/min, which approximates maximal heart rates attained in the performance of other customary activities.[116] The hemodynamic response to sexual activity is far greater with an unfamiliar than a familiar partner, in unfamiliar settings, and after excessive eating and alcohol consumption.[115] The exercise test can be used to gauge the potential cardiac stress of sexual activity. Patients without significant treadmill abnormalities can be advised to resume sexual activity gradually. Masturbation and mutual caressing can be initiated first, followed by progression to sexual intercourse. Cardiac work associated with sexual intercourse can be minimized by adopting relaxed positions such as side-to-side rather than top-and-bottom postures, which increase the isometric work.[115–117] Patients should be told to report symptoms such as angina, prolonged dyspnea, excessive fatigue, or tachycardia lasting more than 10 minutes after intercourse. In sedentary individuals, such symptoms may be the only manifestation of exercise-induced or left ventricular dysfunction.

OUTPATIENT REHABILITATION PROGRAMS

Formal cardiac rehabilitation programs typically have both a medical director and a program director. The medical director is a physician, whereas the program director may be trained in a variety of disciplines. The rehabilitation team is multidisciplinary and includes nurses, physical therapists, exercise physiologists, dietitians, vocational counselors, and psychologists. When smaller programs cannot support the broad range of services, a referral network that includes all of the disciplines is necessary. Adequate facilities for outpatient exercise training are needed. If high-risk patients are included, continuous electrocardiographic monitoring must be available. Equipment and training for cardiopulmonary resuscitation are mandatory.

EXERCISE TRAINING. Exercise training guidelines were presented earlier. The type of exercise program the patient enters depends upon medical condition, physical capacity, risk, and ability to self-monitor exercise. Most patients can benefit from group exercise programs. The standard group training program provides three sessions weekly for 8 to 12 weeks. Some patients require more prolonged training, while others may progress to independent exercise more quickly. In such groups, proper techniques of exercise training can be reinforced, and patients can learn how to perform safe and effective exercise independently. The group setting is also an opportunity for patients to receive reliable information from health professionals regarding coronary disease and risk factor modification. While difficult to quantitate, there is an obvious benefit of the social support provided by interactions with other patients in various stages of recovery from coronary illness.[118] Group exercise sessions are often the focal point for the development of educational programs and support groups.

RISK FACTOR MODIFICATION. A comprehensive program of cardiac rehabilitation should combine exercise training with risk factor modification. Smoking abstinence programs and dietary counseling are the two most important additional services a program should provide. Continued reinforcement of the principles of risk factor modification improves compliance with behavioral programs.[85,110]

Current evidence suggests that cardiac rehabilitation programs offering exercise training and facilitation of smoking abstinence and cholesterol lowering can improve the morbidity and mortality in coronary artery disease. Cardiac rehabilitation programs can also facilitate functional recovery. Early risk stratification, including treadmill testing, can identify patients requiring further treatment and hasten the resumption of customary activities of low-risk patients. Education and counseling can improve psychosocial outcomes. Significant economic benefits can be realized when vocational rehabilitation is included in a cardiac rehabilitation program. As the principles of cardiac rehabilitation become more broadly applied, larger numbers of patients with coronary disease will benefit medically, socially, and psychologically.

REFERENCES

EXERCISE IN CARDIAC REHABILITATION

1. Leon, A. S., Certo, C., Comoss, P., et al.: Scientific evidence of the value of cardiac rehabilitation with emphasis on patients following myocardial infarction: I. Exercise conditioning component. J. Cardiopulm. Rehabil. *10*:79, 1990.
2. Roberts, J. M., Sullivan, M., Froelicher, V. F., et al.: Predicting oxygen uptake from treadmill testing in normal subjects and coronary artery disease patients. Am. Heart J. *108*:1454, 1984.
3. Saltin, B., Blomquist, G., Mitchell, J. H., et al.: Response to exercise after bedrest and after training. Circulation *38*:1, 1968.
4. Convertino, V., Hung, J., Goldwater, D., et al.: Cardiovascular responses to exercise in middle-aged men after 10 days of bedrest. Circulation *65*:134, 1982.

5. Convertino, V. A., Goldwater, D. J., and Sandler, H.: Bedrest-induced peak VO_2 reduction associated with age, gender, and aerobic capacity. Aviat. Space Environ. Med. *57*:17, 1986.
6. Fareeduddin, K., and Abelmann, W. H.: Impaired orthostatic tolerance after bedrest in patients with acute myocardial infarction. N. Engl. J. Med. *280*:345, 1969.
7. Dudley, G. A., Gollnick, P. D., Convertino, V. A., et al.: Changes of muscle function and size with bedrest. Physiologist *32*:S65, 1989.
8. Landin, R. J., Linnemeier, T. S., Rothbaum, D. A., et al.: Exercise testing and training in the elderly. *In* Wenger, N. K., and Brest, A. N. (eds.): Exercise and the Heart. 2nd ed. Philadelphia, F. A. Davis Co., 1985, p. 206.
9. Wiens, R. D., Lafia, P., Marder, C. M., et al.: Chronotropic incompetence in clinical exercise testing. Am. J. Cardiol. *54*:74, 1984.
10. Thoren, P. N.: Activation of left ventricular receptors with nonmedullated vagal afferent fibers during occlusion of a coronary artery in the cat. Am. J. Cardiol. *37*:146, 1976.
11. Haskell, W. L., and DeBusk, R.: Cardiovascular responses to repeated treadmill exercise testing soon after myocardial infarction. Circulation *60*:1247, 1979.
12. Franciosa, J. A.: Lack of correlation between exercise capacity and indexes of resting left ventricular performance in heart failure. Am. J. Cardiol. *47*:33, 1981.
13. Higginbotham, M. B., Morris, K. G., and Conn, E. H.: Determinants of variable exercise performance among patients with severe left ventricular dysfunction. Am. J. Cardiol. *51*:52, 1983.
14. Litchfield, R. L., Kerber, R. E., Benge, W., et al.: Normal exercise capacity in patients with severe left ventricular dysfunction: Compensatory mechanisms. Circulation *129*:134, 1982.
15. Ben-Ari, E., Fisman, E. Z., Pines, A., et al.: Painful versus silent myocardial ischemia during leg and arm exercise testing in stable angina pectoris. Am. J. Cardiol. *64*:300, 1989.
16. Ades, P. A., Grunvald, M. H., Weiss, R. M., et al.: Usefulness of myocardial ischemia as predictor of training effect in cardiac rehabilitation after acute myocardial infarction or coronary artery bypass grafting. Am. J. Cardiol. *63*:1032, 1989.
17. Wenger, N. K.: Cardiovascular drugs: Effects on exercise testing and exercise training of the coronary patient. Cardiovasc. Clin. *15*:133, 1985.
18. Ho, S. W. C., McComish, M. H., and Taylor, R. R.: Effect of beta-adrenergic blockade on the results of exercise testing related to the extent of coronary artery disease. Am. J. Cardiol. *55*:258, 1985.
19. Franklin, B. A., Wrisley, D., Johnson, S., et al.: Chronic adaptations to physical conditioning in cardiac patients. Clin. Sports Med. *3*:471, 1984.
20. Froelicher, V. F., Jensen, D., Atwood, E., et al.: Cardiac rehabilitation: Evidence for improvement in myocardial perfusion and function. Arch. Phys. Med. Rehabil. *61*:517, 1980.
21. Hung, J., Gordon, E. P., Houston, N., et al.: Changes in rest and exercise myocardial perfusion and left ventricular function 3 to 26 weeks after clinically uncomplicated acute myocardial infarction: Effects of exercise training. Am. J. Cardiol. *54*:943, 1984.
22. Rogers, M. A., Yamamoto, C., Hagberg, J. M., et al.: The effect of 7 years of intense exercise training on patients with coronary artery disease. J. Am. Coll. Cardiol. *10*:321, 1987.
23. Ehsani, A. A., Biello, D. R., Schultz, R., et al.: Improvement in left ventricular contractile function in patients with coronary artery disease. Circulation. *74*:350, 1986.
24. Laslett, L., Paumer, L., and Amsterdam, E. A.: Exercise training in coronary artery disease. Cardiol. Clin. *5*:211, 1987.
25. Dubach, P., and Froelicher, V. F.: Cardiac rehabilitation for heart failure patients. Cardiology *76*:368, 1989.
26. Squires, R. W., Lavie, C. J., Brandt, T. R., et al.: Cardiac rehabilitation in patients with severe ischemic left ventricular dysfunction. Mayo Clin. Proc. *62*:997, 1987.
27. Laslett, L. J., Paumer, L., Scott-Baier, P., et al.: Efficacy of exercise training in patients with coronary artery disease who are taking propranolol. Circulation *68*:1029, 1983.
28. Ciske, P. E., Dressendorfer, R. H., Gordon, S., et al.: Attenuation of exercise training effects in patients taking beta blockers during early cardiac rehabilitation. Am. Heart J. *112*:1016, 1986.
29. Health and Public Policy Committee, American College of Physicians: Cardiac rehabilitation services. Ann. Intern. Med. *109*:671, 1988.
30. Kallio, V., Hamalainen, H., Hakkila, J., et al.: Reduction in sudden deaths by a multifactorial intervention programme after acute myocardial infarction. Lancet *2*:1091, 1979.
31. Oldridge, N. B., Guyatt, G. H., Fischer, M. E., et al.: Cardiac rehabilitation after myocardial infarction. Combined experience of randomized clinical trials. JAMA *260*:945, 1988.
32. O'Connor, G. T., Buring, J. E., Yusuf, S., et al.: An overview of randomized trials of rehabilitation with exercise after myocardial infarction. Circulation *80*:234, 1989.
33. Yusuf, S., Peto, R., Lewis, J., et al.: Beta blockade during and after myocardial infarction: An overview of randomized trials. Prog. Cardiovasc. Dis. *27*:335, 1985.
34. Position paper on cardiac rehabilitation. Recommendations of the American College of Cardiology. J. Am. Coll. Cardiol. *7*:451, 1986.
35. Acker, J., and Martin, D.: Angina and ST-segment depression during treadmill and arm ergometer testing in patients with coronary artery disease. Phys. Ther. *68*:195, 1988.
36. Levandoski, S. G., Sheldahl, L. M., Silke, N. A., et al.: Cardiorespiratory responses of coronary artery disease patients to arm and leg cycle ergometry. J. Cardiopulm. Rehabil. *10*:39, 1990.
37. Detrano, R., and Froelicher, V. F.: Exercise testing: Uses and limitations considering recent studies. Prog. Cardiovasc. Dis. *31*:173, 1988.
38. Jugdutt, B. S., Michorowski, B. L., and Kappagoda, C. T.: Exercise training after anterior Q wave myocardial infarction: Importance of regional left ventricular function or topography. J. Am. Coll. Cardiol. *12*:362, 1988.
39. Iskandrian, A. S.: Exercise training after anterior Q wave myocardial infarction: Harmful or beneficial? J. Am. Coll. Cardiol. *12*:373, 1988.
40. Hamm, L. F., Stull, G. A., and Crow, R. S.: Exercise testing early after myocardial infarction: Historic perspective and current uses. Prog. Cardiovasc. Dis. *28*:463, 1986.
41. Sullivan, I. D., Davies, D. W., and Sowton, E.: Submaximal exercise testing early after myocardial infarction: Difficulty of predicting coronary anatomy and left ventricular performance. Br. Heart J. *53*:180, 1985.
42. Weiner, D. A.: Predischarge exercise testing after myocardial infarction: Prognostic and therapeutic features. Cardiovasc. Clin. *15*:95, 1985.
43. DeBusk, R. F., and Dennis, C. A.: "Submaximal" predischarge exercise testing after acute myocardial infarction: Who needs it? Am. J. Cardiol. *55*:499, 1985.
44. Coplan, N. L., Gleim, G. W., and Nicholas, J. A.: Principles of exercise prescription for patients with coronary artery disease. Am. Heart J. *112*:145, 1986.
45. Fagan, E. T., Wayne, V. S., and McConachy, D. L.: Serious ventricular arrhythmias in a cardiac rehabilitation programme. Med. J. Aust. *141*:421, 1984.
46. Hanson, P., and Nagle, F.: Isometric exercise: Cardiovascular responses in normal and cardiac populations. Cardiol. Clin. *5*:157, 1987.
47. Ben-Ari, E., Kellermann, J. J., Rothbaum, D. A., et al.: Effects of prolonged intensive versus moderate leg training on the untrained arm exercise response in angina pectoris. Am. J. Cardiol. *59*:231, 1987.
48. Kelemen, M. H., Stewart, K. J., Gillilan, R. E., et al.: Circuit weight training in cardiac patients. J. Am. Coll. Cardiol. *7*:38, 1986.
49. Borg, G., and Linderholm, H.: Exercise performance and perceived exertion in patients with coronary insufficiency, arterial hypertension and vasoregulatory asthenia. Acta Med. Scand. *187*:17, 1970.
50. Arvan, S.: Exercise performance of the high risk acute myocardial infarction patient after cardiac rehabilitation. Am. J. Cardiol. *62*:197, 1988.
51. Laslett, L., Baier, P. S., and Paumer, L.: Ventricular ectopy frequency and complexity are not altered by exercise training in coronary disease patients. Cardiology *70*:284, 1983.
52. Van Camp, S. P., and Peterson, R. A.: Identification of the high risk cardiac rehabilitation patient. J. Cardiopulm. Rehabil. *9*:103, 1989.
53. Greenland, P., and Chu, J. S.: Efficacy of cardiac rehabilitation services. With emphasis on patients after myocardial infarction. Ann. Intern. Med. *109*:650, 1988.
54. DeBusk, R. F., Haskell, W. L., Miller, N. H., et al.: Medically directed at-home rehabilitation soon after clinically uncomplicated acute myocardial infarction: A new model for patient care. Am. J. Cardiol. *55*:251, 1985.
55. Van Camp, S. P., and Peterson, R. A.: Cardiovascular complications of outpatient cardiac rehabilitation programs. JAMA *256*:1160, 1986.
56. Haskell, W. L.: Cardiovascular complications during exercise training of cardiac patients. Circulation *57*:920, 1978.

SECONDARY PREVENTION

57. Rosenberg, L., Kaufman, D. W., Helmrich, S. P., et al.: The risk of myocardial infarction after quitting smoking in men under 55 years of age. N. Engl. J. Med. *313*:1511, 1985.
58. Ronnevik, P. K., Gundersen, T., and Abrahamsen, A. M.: Effect of smoking habits and timolol treatment on mortality and reinfarction in patients surviving acute myocardial infarction. Br. Heart J. *54*:134, 1985.
59. Sachs, D. P. L.: Cigarette smoking: Health effects and cessation strategies. Clin. Geriatr. Med. *2*:337, 1986.
60. Klein, L. W., Pichard, A. D., Holt, J., et al.: Effects of tobacco smoking on the coronary circulation. J Am. Coll. Cardiol. *1*:421, 1983.
61. Wilhelmsen, L., Svardsudd, K., Korsan-Bengfsen, K., et al.: Fibrinogen as a risk factor for stroke and myocardial infarction. N. Engl. J. Med. *311*:501, 1984.
62. Ockene, J. K., Hosmer, D., Rippe, J., et al.: Factors affecting cigarette smoking status in patients with ischemic heart disease. J. Chron. Dis. *38*:985, 1985.
63. Wilcox, N. S., Prochaska, J. O., Velicer, W. F., et al.: Subject characteristics as predictors of self-change in smoking. Addict. Behav. *10*:407, 1985.
64. Nett, L. M.: The physician's role in smoking cessation: A present and future agenda. Chest *97*:28S, 1990.
65. McNabb, M. E., Ebert, R. V., and McCusker, K.: Plasma nicotine levels produced by chewing nicotine gum. JAMA *248*:865, 1982.
66. Hjalmarson, A. I.: Effect of nicotine chewing gum in smoking cessation: A randomized, placebo-control double-blind study. JAMA *252*:2835, 1984.
67. Taylor, C. B., Houston-Miller, N., Haskell, W. L., et al.: Smoking cessation after acute myocardial infarction: The effects of exercise training. Addict. Behav. *13*:331, 1988.
68. Garvey, A. J., Heinold, J. W., and Rosner, B.: Self-help approaches to smoking cessation: A report from the normative aging study. Addict. Behav. *14*:23, 1989.
69. Lipid Research Clinics Program: The lipid research clinics coronary primary prevention trial results: I. Reduction in incidence of coronary heart disease. JAMA *251*:351, 1984.
70. Lipid Research Clinics Program: The lipid research clinics coronary pri-

mary prevention trial results: II. The relationship of reduction in incidence of coronary heart disease to cholesterol lowering. JAMA *251*:365, 1984.
71. Frick, M. H., Elo, O., Haapa, K., et al.: Primary-prevention trial with gemfibrozil in middle-aged men with dyslipidemia. Safety of treatment, changes in risk factors and incidence of coronary heart disease. N. Engl. J. Med. *317*:1237, 1987.
72. Canner, P. L., Berge, K. G., Wenger, N. K., et al.: Fifteen year mortality in Coronary Drug Project patients: Long-term benefit with niacin. J. Am. Coll. Cardiol. *8*:1245, 1986.
73. Moise, A., Bourassa, M. G., Theroux, P., et al.: Prognostic significance of progression of coronary artery disease. Am. J. Cardiol. *55*:941, 1985.
74. Artzenius, A. C., Krombout, D., Barth, J. D., et al.: Diet, lipoproteins and progression of coronary atherosclerosis: The Leiden intervention trial. N. Engl. J. Med. *312*:805, 1985.
75. Blankenhorn, D. H., Nessim, S. A., Johnson, R. L., et al.: Beneficial effects of combined colestipol-niacin therapy on coronary atherosclerosis and coronary venous bypass grafts. JAMA *257*:3233, 1987.
76. Brensike, J. F., Levy, R. I., Kelsey, S. F., et al.: Effects of therapy with cholestyramine on progression of coronary atherosclerosis: Results of the NHLBI type II coronary intervention study. Circulation *69*:313, 1984.
77. The expert panel: Report of the National Cholesterol Education Program expert panel on detection, evaluation and treatment of high blood cholesterol in adults. Arch. Intern. Med. *184*:36, 1988.
78. Garber, A. M.: Where to draw the line against cholesterol. Ann. Intern. Med. *111*:625, 1989.
79. Roberts, W. C.: Lipid-lowering after an atherosclerotic event. Am. J. Cardiol. *65*:16F, 1990.
80. Tran, Z. V., and Weltman, A.: Differential effects of exercise on serum lipid and lipoprotein levels seen with changes in body weight. JAMA *254*:919, 1985.
81. Krauss, R. M.: Exercise, lipoproteins, and coronary artery disease. Circulation *79*:1143, 1989.
82. Dyer, A. R., Stamler, J., Paul, O., et al.: Alcohol consumption and seventeen year mortality in the Chicago Western Electric Company Study. Prev. Med. *9*:78, 1980.
83. Haskell, W. L., Camargo, C., Williams, P. T., et al.: The effect of cessation and resumption of moderate alcohol intake on serum high-density-lipoprotein subfractions: A controlled study. N. Engl. J. Med *310*:805, 1984.
84. Phillipson, B. E., Rothrock, D. W., Connor, W. E., et al.: Reduction of plasma lipids, lipoproteins and apoproteins by dietary fish oils in patients with hypertriglyceridemia. N. Engl. J. Med. *312*:1210, 1985.
85. Godin, G.: The effectiveness of interventions in modifying behavioral risk factors of individuals with coronary heart disease. J. Cardiopulm. Rehabil. *9*:223, 1989.
86. Stern, T. A.: Psychiatric management of acute myocardial infarction in the coronary care unit. Am. J. Cardiol. *60*:59J, 1987.
87. Tesar, G. E., and Hackett, T. P.: Psychiatric management of the hospitalized cardiac patient. *In* Krantz, D. S., and Blumenthal, J. A. (eds.). Behavioral Assessment and Management of Cardiovascular Disorders. Sarasota, Fla., Professional Resource Exchange, Inc., 1987.
88. Bandura, A.: Self-efficacy mechanism in human agency. Am. Psychol. *37*:122, 1982.
89. Ewart, G. K., Taylor, B., Reese, L. B., et al.: Effects of early postmyocardial infarction exercise testing on self-perception and subsequent physical activity. Am. J. Cardiol. *51*:1076, 1983.
90. Ewart, C. K., Stewart, K. J., Gillilan, R. E., et al.: Self-efficacy mediates strength gains during circuit weight training in men with coronary artery disease. Med. Sci. Sports Exerc. *18*:531, 1986.
91. Taylor, C. B., Bandura, A., Ewart, C. K., et al.: Exercise testing to enhance wives' confidence in their husbands' cardiac capability soon after clinically uncomplicated acute myocardial infarction. Am. J. Cardiol. *55*:635, 1985.
92. The Review Panel on Coronary-Prone Behavior and Coronary Heart Disease: Coronary-prone behavior and coronary heart disease: A critical review. Circulation *63*:1199, 1981.
93. Mathews, K. A., and Haynes, S. G.: Type A behavior pattern and coronary disease risk: Update and critical evaluation. Am. J. Epidemiol. *123*:923, 1986.
94. Ragland, D. R., and Brand, R. J.: Type A behavior and mortality from coronary heart disease. N. Engl. J. Med. *318*:65, 1988.
95. Williams, R. B.: Refining the Type A hypothesis: Emergence of the hostility complex. Am. J. Cardiol. *60*:27J, 1987.
96. Friedman, M., Thoresen, C. E., Gill, J. J., et al.: Alteration of Type A behavior and its effect on cardiac recurrences in postmyocardial infarction patients: Summary results of the recurrent coronary prevention project. Am. Heart J. *112*:653, 1986.
97. American Heart Association: 1989 Heart Facts. Dallas, American Heart Association, 1988.
98. Wittels, E. H., Hay, J. W., and Gotto, A. M.: Medical costs of coronary artery disease in the United States. Am. J. Cardiol. *65*:432, 1990.
99. Guillette, W., Judge, R. D., Koehn, E., et al.: Committee report on economic, administrative and legal factors influencing the insurability and employability of patients with ischemic heart disease: 20th Bethesda conference. J. Am. Coll. Cardiol. *14*:1010, 1989.
100. Dennis, C., Houston-Miller, N., Schwartz, R. G., et al.: Early return to work after uncomplicated myocardial infarction: Results of a randomized trial. JAMA *260*:214, 1988.
101. Pryor, D. B., Bruce, R. A., Chaitman, B. R., et al.: Task force I: Determination of prognosis in patients with ischemic heart disease: 20th Bethesda conference. J. Am. Coll. Cardiol. *14*:1016, 1989.
102. Haskell, W. L., Brachfeld, N., Bruce, R. A., et al.: Task force II: Determination of occupational working capacity in patients with ischemic heart disease: 20th Bethesda conference. J. Am. Coll. Cardiol. *14*:1025, 1989.
103. Haskell, W. L.: Design and implementation of cardiac conditioning programs. *In* Wenger, N. K., and Hellerstein, H. K. (eds.): Rehabilitation of the Coronary Patient. New York. John Wiley & Sons, 1978, pp. 214–215.
104. Bureau of Labor Statistics. Handbook of Labor Statistics. Washington, D.C. U.S. Department of Labor, 1988.
105. DeBusk, R. F.: Determination of cardiac impairment and disability: 20th Bethesda conference. J. Am. Coll. Cardiol. *14*:1043, 1989.
106. Smith, G. R., and O'Rourke, D. F.: Return to work after a first myocardial infarction: A test of multiple hypotheses. JAMA *259*:1673, 1988.
107. Picard, M. H., Dennis, C., Schwartz, R. G., et al.: Cost-benefit of early return to work after uncomplicated myocardial infarction. Am. J. Cardiol. *63*:1308, 1989.

ORGANIZATION OF REHABILITATION SERVICES

108. Wenger, N. K., and Brest, A. N., (eds). Exercise and the Heart. 2nd ed. Philadelphia, F. A. Davis Co., 1985.
109. Beckie, T.: A supportive-educative telephone program: Impact on knowledge and anxiety after coronary artery bypass graft surgery. Heart Lung *18*:46, 1989.
110. Wiggins, N. C.: Education and support for the newly diagnosed cardiac family: A vital link in rehabilitation. J. Adv. Nurs. *14*:63, 1989.
111. De Busk, R. F., Taylor, C. B., and Agras, W. C.: Comparison of treadmill exercise testing and psychologic stress testing soon after myocardial infarction. Am. J. Cardiol. *43*:907, 1979.
112. DeBusk, R. F., Valdez, R., Houston, N., and Haskell, W.: Cardiovascular responses to dynamic and static effort soon after myocardial infarction: Application to occupational work assessment. Circulation *58*:368, 1978.
113. Wilke, N. A., Sheldahl, S. G., Levandoski, S. G., et al.: Weight carrying versus handgrip exercise testing in men with coronary artery disease. Am. J. Cardiol. *64*:736, 1989.
114. Bertagnoli, K., Hanson, P., and Ward, A.: Attenuation of exercise-induced ST depression during combined isometric and dynamic exercise in coronary artery disease. Am. J. Cardiol. *65*:314, 1990.
115. Cooper, A. J.: Myocardial infarction and advice on sexual activity. Practitioner *229*:575, 1985.
116. Tardif, G. S.: Sexual activity after a myocardial infarction. Arch. Phys. Med. Rehabil. *70*:763, 1989.
117. Papadopoulos, C., Shelley, S. I., Piccolo, M., et al.: Sexual activity after coronary bypass surgery. Chest *90*:681, 1986.
118. Fontana, A. F., Kerns, R. D., Rosenberg, R. L., et al.: Support, stress, and recovery from coronary heart disease: A longitudinal causal model. Health Psychol. *8*:175, 1989.

43

The Cardiomyopathies and Myocarditides: Toxic, Chemical, and Physical Damage to the Heart

by JOSHUA WYNNE, M.D., and EUGENE BRAUNWALD, M.D.

The cardiomyopathies constitute a group of diseases, often of unknown etiology, in which the dominant feature is involvement of the heart muscle itself.[1] They are unique in that they are not the result of ischemic,[2]* hypertensive, congenital, valvular, or pericardial diseases (Table 43–1). While the diagnosis of cardiomyopathy requires the exclusion of these etiological factors, the features of cardiomyopathy are often sufficiently distinctive—both clinically and hemodynamically—to allow a positive diagnosis to be made.[1] With increasing awareness of this condition by clinicians, along with improvements in diagnostic techniques, cardiomyopathy is being recognized as a significant cause of morbidity and mortality.[1,3] Whether the result of improved recognition or of other factors, the incidence of cardiomyopathy appears to be increasing.[3,4]

A variety of schemes have been proposed for classifying the cardiomyopathies.[1,5,6] Perhaps the most widely recognized classification scheme is that promulgated by the World Health Organization.[5] In this scheme, the term *cardiomyopathy* is restricted to diseases solely involving the heart muscle that are of unknown cause; other diseases that affect the myocardium but are of known cause or are part of a generalized systemic disorder are termed *specific heart muscle diseases.*[5,6] While conceptually sound, this classification system may be overly rigid for the clinician, because the *clinical* features of a given cardiomyopathy are often identical to those of one of the specific heart muscle diseases.[1] We prefer to use the term *secondary cardiomyopathy* to identify those patients with a specific heart muscle disease that clinically closely simulates an idiopathic or "primary" cardiomyopathy. Three basic categories of functional impairment have been described (Table 43–2 and Fig. 43–1): (1) *dilated* (formerly called congestive), characterized by ventricular dilatation, contractile dysfunction, and often symptoms of congestive heart failure; (2) *hypertrophic,* recognized by inappropriate left ventricular hypertrophy, often with asymmetrical involvement of the septum, usually with preserved or enhanced contractile function; and (3) *restrictive,* marked by impaired diastolic filling, in some cases with endocardial scarring of the ventricle. The distinctions between these three functional categories are not absolute, and there is often overlap; in particular, patients with hypertrophic cardiomyopathy also have increased wall stiffness (as a consequence of the myocardial hypertrophy) and thus present some of the features of a restrictive cardiomyopathy.

ENDOMYOCARDIAL BIOPSY

Evaluation of the pediatric or adult patient suspected of suffering from a cardiomyopathy has been facilitated by the use of endomyocardial biopsy (p. 1489).[7–9] Using a flexible bioptome, the clinician easily and safely may obtain tissue samples from the right (and occasionally left) ventricle via a transvenous (or transarterial) approach (Fig. 43–2). The availability of disposable transfemoral bioptomes has further facilitated endomyocardial biopsy.[7] Two-dimensional echocardiography may help guide the placement of the bioptome and reduce radiation exposure.[10] Endomyocardial biopsy results in a small tissue sample (average size 1–4 mm), and multiple

* The term *ischemic cardiomyopathy* refers to the condition in which ischemic heart disease causes diffuse fibrosis or multiple infarctions and leads to heart failure with left ventricular dilatation; it may or may not be associated with angina pectoris (p. 1351).

TABLE 43-1 IMPORTANT CAUSES OF CARDIOMYOPATHY AND MYOCARDITIS

1. **Inflammatory**
   a. Infective
      Viral
      Rickettsial
      Bacterial
      Mycobacterial
      Spirochetal
      Fungal
      Parasitic
   b. Noninfective
      Collagen diseases
      Granulomatous
      Kawasaki
2. **Metabolic**
   a. Nutritional
      Thiamine
      Kwashiorkor
      Pellagra
      Scurvy
      Hypervitaminosis D
      Obesity
      Selenium deficiency
      Carnitine deficiency
   b. Endocrine
      Acromegaly
      Thyrotoxicosis
      Myxedema
      Uremia
      Cushing's disease
      Pheochromocytoma
      Diabetes mellitus
   c. Altered metabolism
      Gout
      Oxalosis
      Porphyria
   d. Electrolyte imbalance
3. **Toxic**
   a. Cobalt
   b. Alcohol
   c. Bleomycin
   d. Adriamycin
   e. Phenothiazines and antidepressants
   f. Antimony compounds
   g. Carbon monoxide
   h. Lead
   i. Emetine and dehydroemetine
   j. Chloroquine
   k. Lithium
   l. Cyclophosphamide
   m. Hydrocarbons
   n. Catecholamines
   o. Phosphorus
   p. Mercury
   q. Insect stings
   r. Snake bites
   s. Paracetamol
   t. Reserpine
   u. Corticosteroids
   v. Cocaine
   w. Methylsergide
4. **Infiltrative**
   a. Amyloidosis
   b. Hemochromatosis
   c. Neoplastic
   d. Glycogen storage disorders
   e. Sarcoidosis
   f. Mucopolysaccharidosis
   g. Fabry disease
   h. Whipple disease
   i. Gaucher disease
   j. Sphingolipidoses
5. **Fibroplastic**
   a. Endomyocardial fibrosis
   b. Endocardial fibroelastosis
   c. Löffler's fibroplastic endocarditis
   d. Carcinoid
6. **Hematological**
   a. Sickle cell anemia
   b. Polycythemia vera
   c. Thrombotic thrombocytopenic purpura
   d. Leukemia
7. **Hypersensitivity**
   a. Methyldopa
   b. Penicillin
   c. Sulfonamides
   d. Tetracycline
   e. Phenindione
   f. Phenylbutazone
   g. Antituberculous drugs
   h. Giant cell myocarditis
   i. Cardiac transplant rejection
8. **Genetic**
   a. Hypertrophic cardiomyopathy
      With gradient
      Without gradient
   b. Neuromuscular
      Duchenne muscular dystrophy
      Facioscapulohumeral muscular dystrophy
      Limb-girdle dystrophy of Erb
      Myotonia dystrophica
      Friedreich's ataxia
      Kearns-Sayre syndrome
      Nemaline cardiomyopathy
      Multicore cardiomyopathy
9. **Miscellaneous acquired**
   a. Postpartum cardiomyopathy
   b. Obesity
10. **Idiopathic**
   a. Idiopathic dilated cardiomyopathy
   b. Idiopathic restrictive cardiomyopathy
   c. Idiopathic hypertrophic cardiomyopathy
   d. Idiopathic right ventricular cardiomyopathy
11. **Physical agents**
   a. Heat stroke
   b. Hypothermia
   c. Radiation
   d. Tachycardia

samples are often required, because pronounced topographic variations may be found within the myocardium.[11] It remains controversial as to which patients should be subjected to biopsy, but there is general agreement that biopsy may be of benefit in certain specific situations (Table 43-3).[7,11] Although on occasion endomyocardial biopsy may identify a specific etiological agent in an individual patient with cardiac disease of uncertain cause (Tables 43-4 and 43-5), the clinical utility of routine biopsy in cardiomyopathy remains uncertain, particularly since no definitive pattern has been found in dilated cardiomyopathy (Table 43-6 and Fig. 43-2).[7,11] Although interpretation of biopsy specimens had been plagued by a high degree of interobserver variability, the recent adoption of a near-universally accepted set of histological definitions, the *Dallas criteria*, appears to have substantially improved agreement.[7,11,12] It is hoped that newer histochemical and molecular biological techniques may expand further the diagnostic utility of endomyocardial biopsy.[7]

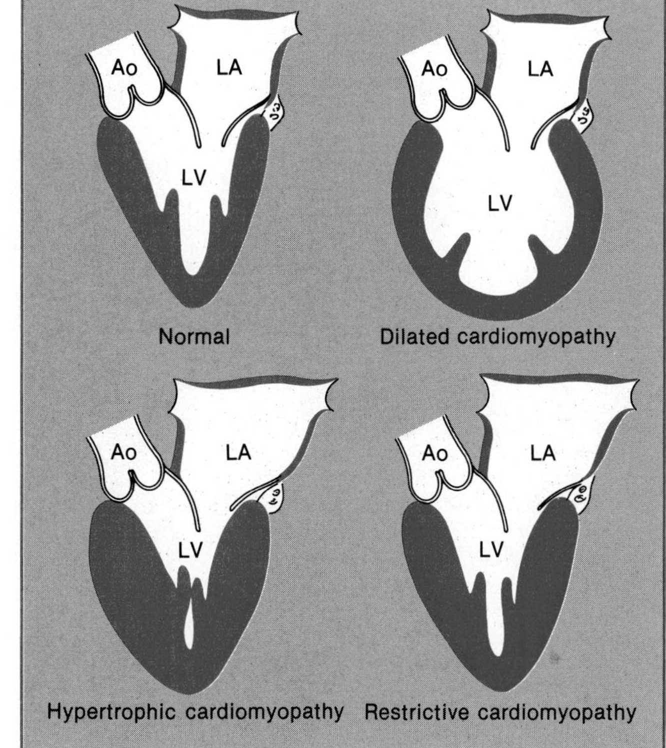

FIGURE 43-1. Diagram comparing three morphologic types of cardiomyopathies of unknown cause. Ao = Aorta, LA = left atrium, LV = left ventricle. (From Waller, B. F.: Pathology of the cardiomyopathies. J. Am. Soc. Echocardiog. *1*:4, 1988.)

TABLE 43-2 FUNCTIONAL CLASSIFICATION OF THE CARDIOMYOPATHIES

	DILATED	RESTRICTIVE	HYPERTROPHIC
Symptoms	Congestive heart failure, particularly left-sided Fatigue and weakness Systemic or pulmonary emboli	Dyspnea, fatigue Right-sided congestive heart failure Signs and symptoms of systemic disease: amyloidosis, iron storage disease, etc.	Dyspnea, angina pectoris Fatigue, syncope, palpitations
Physical Examination	Moderate to severe cardiomegaly; S_3 and S_4 Atrioventricular valve regurgitation, especially mitral	Mild to moderate cardiomegaly: S_3 or S_4 Atrioventricular valve regurgitation; inspiratory increase in venous pressure (Kussmaul's sign)	Mild cardiomegaly Apical systolic thrill and heave; brisk carotid upstroke S_4 common Systolic murmur that increases with Valsalva maneuver
Chest Roentgenogram	Moderate to marked cardiac enlargement, especially left ventricular Pulmonary venous hypertension	Mild cardiac enlargement Pulmonary venous hypertension	Mild to moderate cardiac enlargement Left atrial enlargement
Electrocardiogram	Sinus tachycardia Atrial and ventricular arrhythmias ST-segment and T-wave abnormalities Intraventricular conduction defects	Low voltage Intraventricular conduction defects AV conduction defects	Left ventricular hypertrophy ST-segment and T-wave abnormalities Abnormal Q waves Atrial and ventricular arrhythmias
Echocardiogram	Left ventricular dilatation and dysfunction Abnormal diastolic mitral valve motion secondary to abnormal compliance and filling pressures	Increased left ventricular wall thickness and mass Small or normal-sized left ventricular cavity Normal systolic function Pericardial effusion	Asymmetrical septal hypertrophy (ASH) Narrow left ventricular outflow tract Systolic anterior motion (SAM) of the mitral valve Small or normal-sized left ventricle
Radionuclide Studies	Left ventricular dilatation and dysfunction (RVG)	Infiltration of myocardium (^{201}Tl) Small or normal-sized left ventricle (RVG) Normal systolic function (RVG)	Small or normal-sized left ventricle (RVG) Vigorous systolic function (RVG) Asymmetrical septal hypertrophy (RVG or ^{201}Tl)
Cardiac Catheterization	Left ventricular enlargement and dysfunction Mitral and/or tricuspid regurgitation Elevated left- and often right-sided filling pressures Diminished cardiac output	Diminished left ventricular compliance "Square root sign" in ventricular pressure recordings Preserved systolic function Elevated left- and right-sided filling pressures	Dimished left ventricular compliance Mitral regurgitation Vigorous systolic function Dynamic left ventricular outflow gradient

RVG = Radionuclide ventriculogram; ^{201}Tl = thallium-201

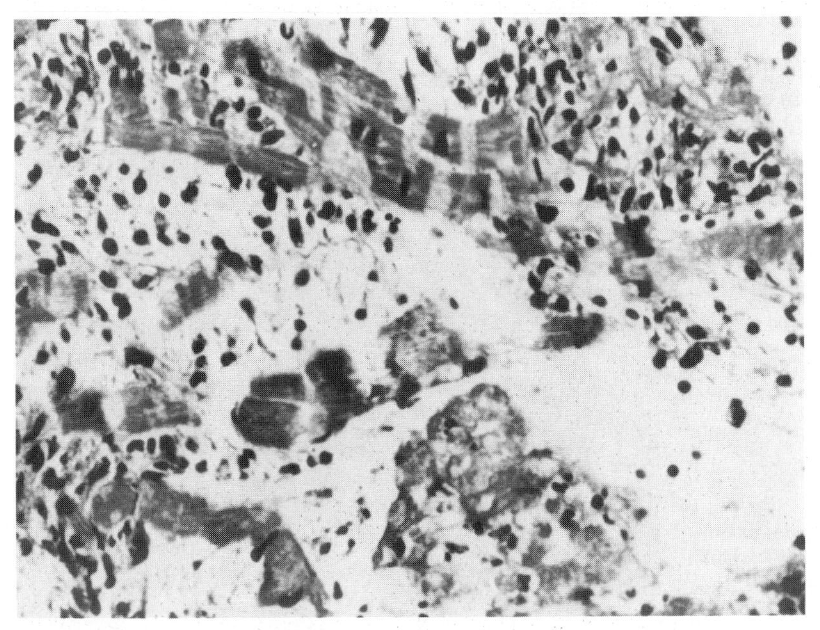

FIGURE 43-2. Endomyocardial biopsy in myocarditis (hematoxylin and eosin, original magnification ×100). Diffuse mononuclear cellular infiltrate with loss and necrosis of myocytes is present. (From Salvi, A., Di Lenarda, A., Dreas, L., et al.: Immunosuppressive treatment in myocarditis. Int. J. Cardiol. *22*:329, 1989.)

TABLE 43-3 CLINICAL INDICATIONS FOR ENDOMYOCARDIAL BIOPSY

Definite
- Monitoring of cardiac allograft rejection
- Monitoring of anthracycline cardiotoxicity

Possible
- Detection and monitoring of myocarditis
- Diagnosis of secondary cardiomyopathies
- Differentiation between restrictive and constrictive heart disease

Uncertain
- Unexplained, life-threatening ventricular tachyarrhythmias
- AIDS
- Formulation of prognosis in idiopathic dilated cardiomyopathy

From Mason, J. W., and O'Connell, J. B.: Clinical merit of endomyocardial biopsy. Circulation *79*:971, 1989, reprinted by permission of the American Heart Association, Inc.

TABLE 43-4 SPECIFIC DIAGNOSES THAT CAN BE CONFIRMED BY MYOCARDIAL BIOPSY

Cardiac allograft rejection	Fabry disease of the heart	Henoch-Schönlein purpura
Myocarditis	Carcinoid disease	Rheumatic carditis
Giant cell myocarditis	Irradiation injury	Chagasic cardiomyopathy
Doxorubicin cardiotoxicity	Glycogen storage disease	Chloroquine cardiomyopathy
Cardiac amyloidosis	Cardiac tumors of cardiac origin	Lyme carditis
Cardiac sarcoidosis	Cardiac tumors of noncardiac origin	Carnitine deficiency cardiomyopathy
Cardiac hemochromatosis	Kearns-Sayre syndrome	Right ventricular lipomatosis
Endocardial fibrosis	Cytomegalovirus infection	Hypereosinophilic syndrome
Endocardial fibroelastosis	Toxoplasmosis	

From Mason, J. W., and O'Connell, J. B.: Clinical merit of endomyocardial biopsy. Circulation *79*:971, 1989, reprinted by permission of the American Heart Association, Inc.

TABLE 43-5 ENDOMYOCARDIAL BIOPSY DIAGNOSES FOR WHICH THERE IS A PROVEN THERAPY

Cardiac rejection*	Endocardial fibrosis*	Certain malignancies involving the heart
Cardiac sarcoidosis*	Incipient anthracycline cardiotoxicity*	Carnitine deficiency cardiomyopathy
Giant cell myocarditis*	Cardiac hemochromatosis	Lyme carditis
Hypereosinophilic syndrome involving the heart*	Certain infections involving the heart	

*Diagnoses that usually cannot reliably be made without cardiac biopsy.

From Mason, J. W., and O'Connell, J. B.: Clinical merit of endomyocardial biopsy. Circulation *79*:971, 1989, reprinted by permission of the American Heart Association, Inc.

TABLE 43-6 ENDOMYOCARDIAL BIOPSY CHARACTERISTICS

DILATED CARDIOMYOPATHY
- Light microscopy
  - Increase in myofiber size
  - Attenuation of cells
  - Hyperchromatic, irregular shaped nuclei
  - Interstitial, focal, perivascular fibrosis
- Electron microscopy
  - Hypertrophic changes
    - Increased number of sarcomeres and mitochondria
    - Large, lobulated nuclei
    - Z-band abnormalities
    - Irregular invaginations of sarcolemma
    - Widened, convoluted, intercalated discs
  - Degenerative changes
    - Myofilament loss
    - Aggregation of glycogen and mitochondria
    - Pleomorphic mitochondria
    - Myelin figures, lipid vacuoles

HYPERTROPHIC CARDIOMYOPATHY
- Light microscopy
  - Endocardial thickening and fibrosis
  - Marked myocardial hypertrophy
  - Large, bizarre nuclei
  - Myofiber disorganization
  - Interstitial fibrosis
- Electron microscopy
  - Myofibrillar disarray
  - Increased side-to-side junctions
  - Increased cell branching
  - Increased glycogen

MYOCARDITIS
- Light and electron microscopy
  - Inflammatory infiltrate, usually lymphocytic
  - Necrosis or degeneration of adjacent myocytes
  - Uninvolved, normal myocardium
  - Absence of severe chronic myocardial changes

From Leatherbury, L., Chandra, R. S., Chapiro, S. R., and Perry, L. W.: Value of endomyocardial biopsy in infants, children, and adolescents with dilated or hypertrophic cardiomyopathy and myocarditis. Reprinted from the American College of Cardiology. J. Am. Coll. Cardiol. *12*:1547, 1988.

IDIOPATHIC DILATED CARDIOMYOPATHY

Dilated cardiomyopathy (DCM) is a syndrome characterized by cardiac enlargement and impaired systolic function of one or both ventricles. While formerly it was called congestive cardiomyopathy, the term *dilated cardiomyopathy* is now preferred, since the earliest abnormality usually is ventricular enlargement and systolic contractile dysfunction, with congestive heart failure often (but not invariably) developing later. In an occasional patient, the predominant finding is that of contractile dysfunction with only a mildly dilated left ventricle.[13]

Although the cause is not definable in many cases, more than 75 specific diseases of heart muscle can produce the clinical manifestations of DCM.[1] It is likely that this condition represents a final common pathway that is the end result of myocardial damage produced by a variety of toxic, metabolic, or infectious agents. Alcohol, for example, may lead to severe cardiac dysfunction and may produce clinical, hemodynamic, and pathological findings identical to those present in idiopathic dilated cardiomyopathy (see p. 1402). The course of idiopathic dilated cardiomyopathy is usually one of progressive deterioration, with three-fourths of patients dying within 5 years after the onset of symptoms, although a minority improve, with a reduction in cardiac size and longer survival (Fig. 43-3).[13] A variety of clinical predictors of patients at enhanced risk of death in DCM have been identified (Table 43-7).[1,14-24] However, the predictive reliability of any single feature is not high. Because of considerable variability, it may be difficult to predict with any accuracy the clinical course and outcome in any individual patient.[25] Surprisingly, there is not a good correlation between the extent of impairment of ventricular function and symptoms or mortality,[26] although once advanced biventricular failure has developed, the prognosis is poor.[27] Specific endomyocardial biopsy morphological findings may offer some predictive information regarding prognosis.[25] Children with DCM appear to have a prognosis similar to that of comparable adults; it is controversial whether age at presentation in childhood has any prognostic significance.[28,29]

PATHOLOGY

POSTMORTEM EXAMINATION. This reveals enlargement and dilatation of all four chambers; the ventricles are more dilated than the atria[30] (Fig. 43-4). While the thickness of the ventricular wall is increased in some cases, the degree of hypertrophy is often inadequate for the severe dilatation present.[31] The development of left ventricular hypertrophy appears to have a protective or beneficial role in dilated cardiomyopathy, because it may serve to reduce systolic wall stress and protect against further cavity dilatation.[1,32] Scars, usually small, occasionally are found in the left or right ventricle.[30] The cardiac valves are intrinsically normal, and intracavitary thrombi, particularly in the ventricular apex, are common.[31] The coronary arteries are usually normal. The right ventricle is preferentially involved in some cases of dilated cardiomyopathy, sometimes on a familial basis.

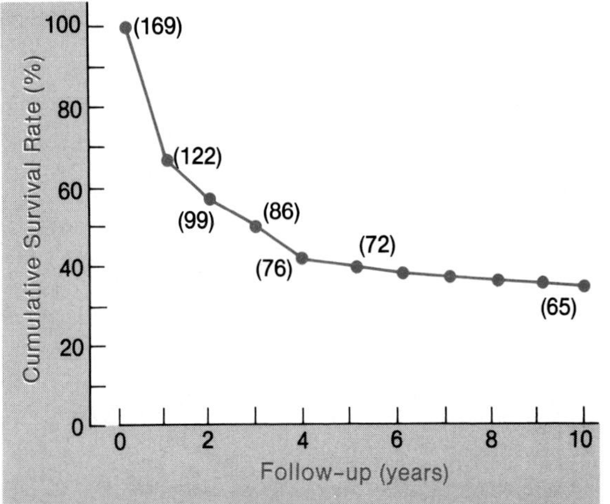

FIGURE 43-3. Ten-year survival curve of 169 patients with dilated cardiomyopathy. Numbers in parentheses are patients alive at the beginning of interval. (From Diaz, R. A., Obasohan, A., and Oakley, C. M.: Prediction of outcome in dilated cardiomyopathy. Br. Heart J. *58*:393, 1987.)

TABLE 43-7 FACTORS ASSOCIATED WITH REDUCED SURVIVAL IN DILATED CARDIOMYOPATHY

S_3
Left ventricular conduction delay
Elevation of filling pressures
Absence of left ventricular thickening
Age > 55 years
Cardiac enlargement
Depressed cardiac output
Depressed ejection fraction
Depressed serum sodium levels
Elevated serum norepinephrine levels
Functional class
Ventricular arrhythmias
Large thallium defects
Myocardial biopsy findings
Ventricular shape (more spherical)

HISTOLOGICAL EXAMINATION. Microscopic study reveals extensive areas of interstitial and perivascular fibrosis, particularly involving the left ventricular subendocardium. Small areas of necrosis and cellular infiltrate are seen on occasion, but these typically are not prominent features.[30,31,33] Some myocardial cells are hypertrophied, while others are atrophied (Fig. 43-5).[31] Cardiac biopsy specimens obtained during life by a transvenous or transthoracic approach demonstrate a variety of similar abnormalities, including interstitial fibrosis, cellular infiltrates, cellular hypertrophy, and myocardial cell degeneration.[34,34a,34b] No viruses or other etiological agents have been identified with any regularity in tissue from patients with DCM. Particularly disappointing has been the failure to identify any immunological, histochemical, morphological, ultrastructural, or microbiological markers that might be used to establish the diagnosis of idiopathic dilated cardiomyopathy or to clarify its cause.

ETIOLOGY

It is likely that DCM represents a common expression of myocardial damage that has been produced by a variety of as yet unestablished myocardial insults. While the cause or causes remain unclear,[35] at least four conditions, if not etiologically linked, appear to lower the threshold for the development of cardiomyopathy, and it is possible that in some cases a combination of factors results in severe myocardial damage. Chronic excessive ingestion of alcohol (p. 1402), pregnancy (Chap. 59), systemic hypertension (Chap. 28), and a variety of infections (pp. 1425 to 1434) may each be associated with myocardial dysfunction and congestive failure and are important causes of secondary DCM. Cigarette smoking has also been found to be associated with DCM,[36] independent of its important role as a risk factor in the development of ischemic heart disease.

The precise etiology of contractile dysfunction at the cellular level in patients with DCM remains unclear. While abnormalities in calcium handling by cardiomyopathic tissue is a common finding,[36a] the cause is unestablished.[37] There is a

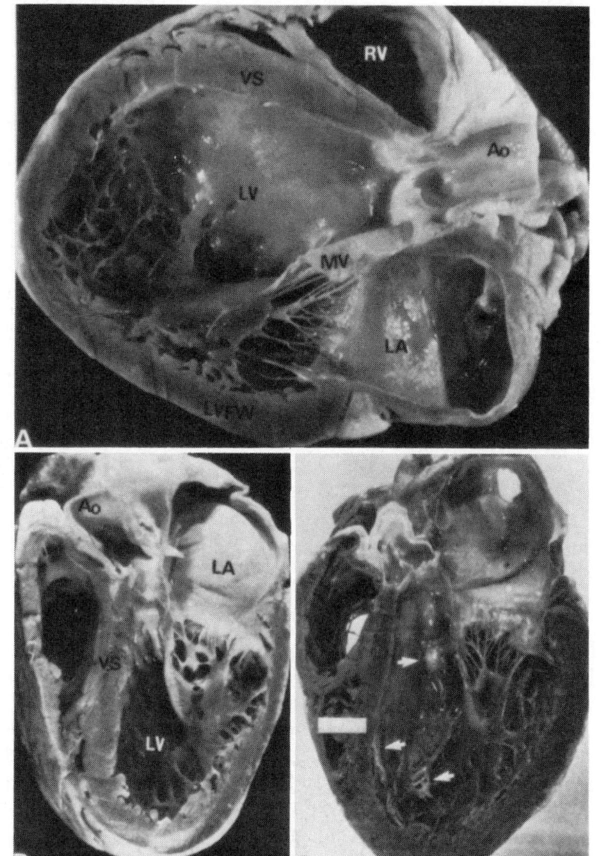

FIGURE 43–4. *A–C*, Three different hearts from patients with dilated cardiomyopathy cut in tomographic planes simulating two-dimensional echocardiographic parasternal long-axis views. In each case, left ventricle (LV) is markedly dilated, but chamber walls vary in thickness. *C*, Whitish endocardial plaques (arrows) ("milk spots") probably represent organized thrombus. Ao = Aorta, LA = left atrium, LVFW = left ventricular free wall, MV = mitral valve, RV = right ventricle, VS = ventricular septum. (From Waller, B. F.: Pathology of the cardiomyopathies. J. Am. Soc. Echocardiog. *1*:4, 1988.)

reduction in density of membrane-associated beta-adrenoceptors[38,39] that may be a consequence of the development of anti-beta-adrenoreceptor autoantibodies.[40,41] An alteration in the signal transmission pathway by which the receptors stimulate the contractile apparatus appears likely to occur.[42,43] It seems that there is enhanced inhibition of this system in DCM patients, perhaps accounting for their depressed contractile function.[44]

Regardless of possible cellular causes of contractile dysfunction in DCM, there has been wide speculation that an episode of subclinical viral myocarditis initiates an autoimmune reaction that culminates in the development of full-blown DCM.[45–47] While this hypothesis is inviting, it remains largely unsupported; it has been estimated that only 15 per cent of patients with myocarditis progress to DCM.[48] Little evidence exists to suggest prior viral infections in most patients with unequivocal cardiomyopathy.[49] However, there are patients who exhibit the clinical features of DCM in whom endomyocardial biopsy reveals evidence of an inflammatory myocarditis. The reported frequency of finding evidence of an inflammatory infiltrate in DCM varies widely and undoubtedly depends largely on criteria used for diagnosis; using rigorous criteria, only about 5 to 10 per cent of patients with DCM have biopsy evidence of myocarditis.[46,49–51] Other evidence favoring the concept that DCM is a postviral disorder includes the presence of high antibody viral titers,[48] viral-specific RNA sequences,[52] and apparent viral particles[48] in patients with "idiopathic" dilated cardiomyopathy. Dilated cardiomyopathy has been reported as *peripartum cardiomyopathy* when it occurs in this period. This condition is discussed on p. 1798.

Although the findings have not been completely reproducible, abnormalities of both humoral and cellular immunity have been found in patients with DCM, and there is a suggestion of an association with specific HLA antigens.[53] Circulating antimyocardial antibodies[54–57] and abnormalities of various T cells, including cytotoxic T cells, suppressor T lymphocytes, and natural killer cells,[1] have been found in some,[58–62] but not all,[63] studies. It has been suggested that these putative immunological abnormalities may be the consequence of prior viral myocarditis. Viral components may be incorporated into the cardiac sarcolemma, only to serve as an antigenic source that directs the immune response to attack the myocardium.[48]

A variety of other possible causes has been proposed, although none is accepted as *the* cause of DCM (Table 43–8). Thus, endocrine abnormalities as well as the effects of chemicals or toxins, notably doxorubicin, have been suggested as possible etiological factors.[64] It has been suggested that microvascular hyperreactivity (spasm) may lead to myocellular necrosis and scarring, with resultant heart failure, although this remains speculative.[1] From a clinical standpoint, the more important causes of secondary DCM include alcohol, cocaine, human immunodeficiency virus, metabolic abnormalities,

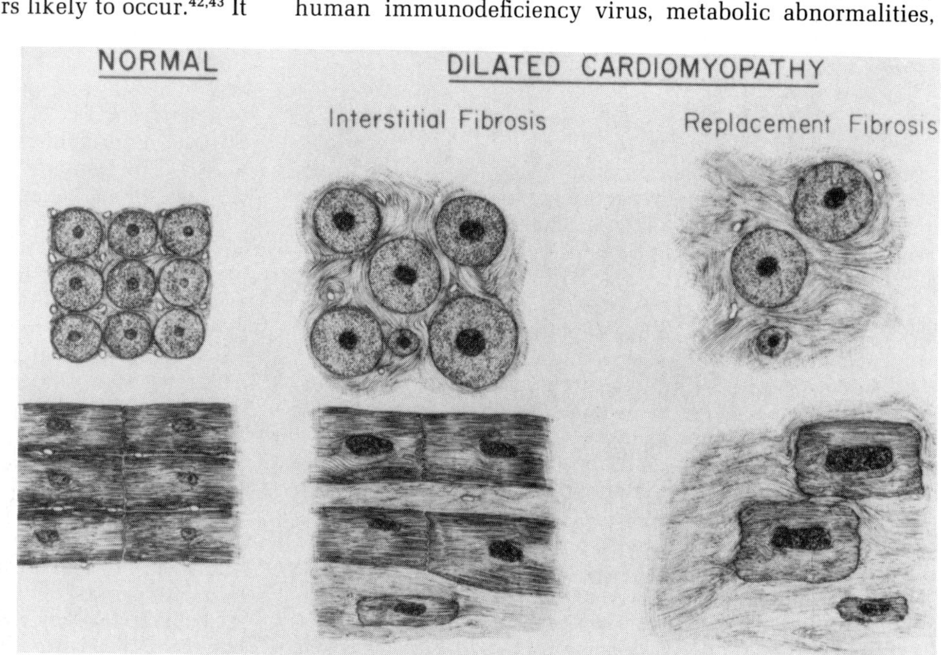

FIGURE 43–5. Diagram showing the various findings commonly observed in sections of left ventricular wall in patients with idiopathic dilated cardiomyopathy. Some myocardial cells are larger than normal, others are smaller than normal and others have been replaced by fibrous tissue, which also is increased in the interstitium between the myocardial cells. (From Roberts, W. C., Siegel, R. J., and McManus, B. M.: Idiopathic dilated cardiomyopathy: Analysis of 152 necropsy patients. Am. J. Cardiol. *60*:1340, 1987.)

TABLE 43-8 POSSIBLE CAUSES OR PRECIPITATING FACTORS IN DILATED CARDIOMYOPATHY

Hereditary
X-linked
Nutritional and related deficiencies
Thiamine deficiency
Selenium deficiency
Carnitine deficiency
Hypophosphatemia
Hypocalcemia
Toxins and drugs
Ethanol
Anthrocyclines
5-Fluorouracil
Vasoactive agents and microvascular spasm
Decreased coronary flow reserve
Tachyarrhythmia
Calcium overload
Hypocalcemia
Oxygen free radical damage
Pregnancy
Infection
Viral myocarditis
HIV virus
Subacute and chronic myocarditis
Immune/autoimmune mechanisms
Degeneration of cardiac ganglia
Alterations in cardiac cytoskeleton

Adapted from Abelmann, W. H., and Lorell, B. H.: The challenge of cardiomyopathy. Reprinted by permission of the American College of Cardiology. J. Am. Coll. Cardiol. *13*:1219, 1989.

and the cardiotoxicity of a variety of anticancer drugs (especially Adriamycin and 5-fluorouracil).

In contrast to hypertrophic cardiomyopathy, in which it is common, familial transmission is rare in DCM. Occasional instances of autosomal dominant as well as X-linked inheritance in DCM have been reported[65-70]; one intriguing familial metabolic deficiency is that of carnitine, with improvement occurring in the myopathy with carnitine repletion.[71]

An increase of the α subunits of the inhibitory guanine nucleotide-binding protein ($G_{i\alpha}$) has been reported to occur in the membranes of myocytes from failing hearts[72] (Fig. 13–11, p. 360). This abnormality has been shown to be more profound in myocardial membranes from hearts with dilated than in those with ischemic cardiomyopathy.[73] This increase in $G_{i\alpha}$ is associated with a striking reduction of basal adenylate cyclase activity and of the positive inotropic effects of isoproterenol and of the phosphodiesterase inhibitor milrinone (p. 505). These findings suggest that the increase of $G_{i\alpha}$ might contribute to the reduced effects of endogenous catecholamines in DCM.

CLINICAL MANIFESTATIONS

HISTORY. Symptoms usually develop gradually in patients with DCM. Some patients may be asymptomatic yet have left ventricular dilatation for months or even years.[74,75] An unrecognized illness may result in left ventricular dilatation, which is clinically recognized only years later when symptoms develop or when routine chest roentgenography demonstrates cardiomegaly. Other patients, after recovery from what appears to be a systemic viral infection, develop symptoms of heart failure for the first time. In still others, severe heart failure develops acutely during an episode of myocarditis; while some recovery occurs, chronic manifestations of diminished cardiac reserve persist and heart failure reappears months or years later. Although patients of any age may be affected, the disease is most common in middle age and is more frequent in men than in women.

The most striking symptoms are those of left ventricular failure. Fatigue and weakness due to diminished cardiac output are common. Exercise intolerance is common and relates, at least in part, to reduced skeletal muscle perfusion as well as histological and biochemical alterations in the exercising muscle groups.[76-78] Right heart failure is a late and ominous sign and is associated with a particularly poor prognosis (p. 445). Chest pain occurs in one-fourth to one-half of patients and may suggest concomitant ischemic heart disease.[79] There is a reduction in the vasodilator reserve of the coronary microvasculature in DCM, suggesting that subendocardial ischemia may play a role in the genesis of chest pain despite angiographically normal coronary arteries.[80] Chest pain secondary to pulmonary embolism and abdominal pain secondary to congestive hepatomegaly are frequent in the late stages of the illness.

PHYSICAL EXAMINATION. This usually reveals variable degrees of cardiac enlargement and findings of congestive heart failure. The systolic blood pressure is usually normal or low, and the pulse pressure is narrow, reflecting a diminished stroke volume. Pulsus alternans (p. 24) is common when severe left ventricular failure is present. The jugular veins are frequently distended. Prominent *a* and *v* waves are visible—the latter a late manifestation of the presence of tricuspid valvular regurgitation. The liver may be engorged and pulsatile. Peripheral edema and ascites may be present. Wheezing resulting from bronchospasm may be found, apparently as a consequence of bronchial hyperresponsiveness and dilatation of the bronchial vessels.[81]

The precordium usually reveals left and, occasionally, right ventricular impulses, but the heaves are not sustained, as they are in patients with considerable ventricular hypertrophy. The apical impulse is usually displaced laterally, reflecting left ventricular dilatation. A presystolic *a* wave may be palpable. The second heart sound is usually normally split, although paradoxical splitting (p. 47) may be detected in the presence of left bundle branch block, an electrocardiographic finding that is not unusual in dilated cardiomyopathy. If pulmonary hypertension is present the pulmonary component of the second heart sound may be accentuated, and the splitting may be narrow. Presystolic gallop sounds (S_4) often precede the development of overt congestive heart failure. Ventricular gallops (S_3) are the rule once cardiac decompensation occurs, and a summation gallop is often heard when there is tachycardia. Systolic murmurs are common and are usually due to mitral or, less commonly, tricuspid valvular regurgitation.[74] Mitral regurgitation results from enlargement and abnormal motion of the mitral annulus; ventricular dilatation with resultant distortion of the geometry of the subvalvar apparatus ("papillary muscle dysfunction") plays a lesser role.[82-84] Gallop sounds and regurgitant murmurs can often be elicited or intensified by isometric handgrip exercise with its attendant enhancement of systemic vascular resistance and impedance to left ventricular outflow (p. 62). Systemic emboli resulting from dislodgment of intracardiac thrombi from the left atrium and ventricle and pulmonary emboli that originate in the venous system of the legs are common late complications. Specific abnormalities of blood flow in the left ventricle can be detected by Doppler ultrasonography in patients with echocardiographically demonstrable thrombi.[85]

NONINVASIVE EXAMINATION. To identify potentially reversible secondary causes of dilated cardiomyopathy, several basic screening biochemical tests are often indicated, including determination of serum phosphorus (hypophosphatemia), serum calcium (hypocalcemia), serum creatinine and urea nitrogen (uremia), and serum iron (hemochromatosis).[86] The *chest roentgenogram* usually reveals left ventricular enlargement, although generalized cardiomegaly is often seen. Left ventricular failure may result in signs of pulmonary venous hypertension (i.e., pulmonary vascular redistribution) as well as interstitial and even alveolar edema.[86] Pleural effusions may be present, and the azygos vein and superior vena cava may be dilated when right heart failure supervenes. The *electrocardiogram* often shows sinus tachycardia when heart failure is present. The entire spectrum of atrial and ventricular tachyarrhythmias and atrioventricular conduction disturbances may be seen. Poor R-wave progression and intraventricular conduction abnormalities, especially left bundle branch block, are common.[87] Anterior Q waves may be present when there is extensive left ventricular fibrosis, even without a discrete myocardial scar.[87] ST-segment and T-wave abnormalities are common, as are P-wave changes, especially left atrial abnormality.[87] Ambulatory Holter monitoring often demonstrates ventricular arrhythmias, with about half of monitored patients with DCM exhibiting nonsustained ventricular tachycardia.[88] There is no consensus that complex or frequent ventricular arrhythmias predict sudden (presumably arrhythmic) death, although they do appear to predict total mortality.[89-91] Perhaps ventricular arrhythmias as detected on Holter monitoring are a marker for the extent of myocardial damage in DCM and therefore are *associated* with sudden death without necessarily being its *cause*.[89] In rare cases, particularly in children, recurrent and/or incessant supraventricular or ventricular tachyarrhythmias may actually be the *cause* (rather than the result) of ventricular dysfunction.[92-94] In those cases, restoration of sinus rhythm or slowing of the heart rate may be therapeutic.

Two-dimensional and Doppler *echocardiography* are useful in assessing the degree of impairment of left ventricular function and for excluding concomitant valvular or pericardial disease (Chap. 4).[86] In addition to examining all four cardiac valves for evidence of structural or functional abnormalities, echocardiography allows evaluation of the size of the ventricular cavity and thickness of the ventricular walls and estimation of ventricular function. A pericardial effusion may sometimes be demonstrated. Doppler studies are useful in delineating the severity of mitral (and tricuspid) regurgitation.[74,86,95] *Thallium-201 imaging* at rest may be helpful in distinguishing left ventricular enlargement caused by DCM from that caused by coronary artery disease,[96] although there is not complete agreement on this point.[74,86] However, newer experimental isotopes and positron scanning show great promise for the future[97,98] (Chap. 11). Scanning with gallium or antimyosin antibody may help to identify patients more likely to have myocarditis on biopsy.[99-101]

Radionuclide ventriculography, like echocardiography, reveals increased end-diastolic and end-systolic left ventricular volumes, reduced ejection fractions in both ventricles, and wall-motion abnormalities.[74] In many cases, however, it is not necessary to carry out serial *batteries* of noninvasive tests in order to follow patients with DCM and evaluate their response to treatment.

CARDIAC CATHETERIZATION AND ANGIOCARDIOGRAPHY. The left ventricular end-diastolic, left atrial, and pulmonary artery wedge pressures are usually elevated. Modest degrees of pulmonary arterial hypertension are common.[74] Advanced cases may demonstrate right ventricular dilatation and failure as well, with resultant elevation of the right ventricular end-diastolic, right atrial, and central venous pressures.

Left ventriculography demonstrates enlargement of this chamber, typically with diffuse reduction in wall motion. Segmental wall motion abnormalities during systole and diastole are not uncommon and may simulate the angiographic findings in ischemic heart disease.[102] However, prominent localized wall disorders are more characteristic of ischemic heart disease, while diffuse, global dysfunction is more typical of DCM. The ejection fraction is reduced and the end-systolic volume is increased as a result of the impairment of left ventricular contractility. Sometimes left ventricular thrombi may be visualized within the left ventricle as intracavitary filling defects. Mild mitral regurgitation is often present. On occasion, it may be difficult to distinguish left ventricular dilatation secondary to severe mitral regurgitation from DCM with secondary mitral regurgitation.

Coronary arteriography usually reveals normal vessels, although coronary dilatory capacity may be impaired.[79,80] This examination may be of particular value in patients with abnormal Q waves on the electrocardiogram or regional left ventricular wall motion abnormalities on noninvasive testing. Coronary arteriography helps to distinguish between myocardial infarction as a result of obstructive coronary artery disease and extensive localized myocardial fibrosis secondary to severe DCM in the absence of coronary artery obstruction.

MANAGEMENT

Since the cause of idiopathic dilated cardiomyopathy is unknown, specific therapy is not possible. Treatment, therefore, is for heart failure, as discussed in Chapter 17. Physical, dietary, and pharmacological interventions may help to control symptoms; only cardiac transplantation (Chap. 18) and specific vasodilator therapy (enalapril and hydralazine plus nitrates) have been shown to prolong life.[1,103-105] Because of the possible link between DCM, microvascular circulatory abnormalities, and abnormal myocardial calcium handling, the use of calcium antagonists is of interest. Diltiazem in particular appears to be safe and preliminary results regarding clinical utility are encouraging, although myocardial depression is an important potential side effect of the calcium antagonists as a group.[1,106] Diuretics may improve symptoms of pulmonary congestion and sometimes can lower ventricular filling pressures without compromising cardiac output.[107]

Certain treatment considerations specific to DCM are worthy of discussion. Because of recent evidence that activation of the sympathetic nervous system may have deleterious cardiac effects (rather than being an important compensatory mechanism as traditionally thought), beta-adrenoceptor blockade (usually with metoprolol) has been suggested as a means to prolong survival.[108] Results to date have been generally favorable, and improvement in symptoms (sometimes dramatic) and survival have been suggested.[108-111] Beta-adrenoceptor blockade has been surprisingly well tolerated, with infrequent aggravation of heart failure (which, on occasion, may be profound). The mechanism of beneficial action of beta blockers may relate to five factors: (1) negative chronotropic effect with reduced myocardial oxygen demand, (2) reduced myocardial damage due to catecholamines, (3) improved diastolic relaxation, (4) inhibition of sympathetically mediated vasoconstriction, and (5) increase in myocardial beta-adrenoceptor density.[112] Assessment of the true clinical efficacy of beta-adrenergic blockage and its impact on mortality in DCM must await the results of an ongoing multicenter trial.[113]

While there is no evidence that antiarrhythmic agents prolong life or prevent sudden death in DCM, it is appropriate to use them in the treatment of symptomatic arrhythmias.[26] Because of the adverse effects of most available agents, many of which depress myocardial contractility and have a proarrhythmic effect (Chap. 23), treatment should be individualized, with both efficacy and toxicity carefully monitored.[114] Unfortunately, electrophysiological testing is of limited utility in DCM, since it is positive in a minority of patients at risk. The lack of inducibility of ventricular tachyarrhythmias does not identify a low-risk group, and pharmacological suppression of provoked arrhythmias does not necessarily predict freedom from recurrences.[115-117] The recording of late potentials by the signal-averaged electrocardiogram has not proved to be especially helpful either.[118] Implantation of the internal defibrillator (p. 750) should be considered in appropriate candidates with symptomatic ventricular tachyarrhythmias. Even in the absence of controlled clinical trials demonstrating their efficacy,[119] anticoagulants are recommended in patients with DCM and heart failure.[120] Anticoagulants should be so used even without direct clinical or echocardiographic evidence of thrombus formation if there are no specific contraindications to these agents.[1,121] In those patients with chronic heart failure secondary to DCM and lymphocytic infiltrate on myocardial biopsy, treatment with corticosteroids and immunosuppressive agents has been advocated. Prednisone therapy does not appear to have a clinically important effect on symptoms, exercise performance, or ejection fraction (in more than just the short term) and is associated with significant complications in half the patients so treated.[122,123] Routine clinical use of immunosuppressive therapy thus cannot be recommended at present, although it is being tested in a prospective randomized clinical trial at the time of this writing.

Surgical repair, mitral annuloplasty, or replacement of regurgitant valves has been attempted in some patients in whom progressive atrioventricular valvular regurgitation (almost always mitral) appeared to result in progressive cardiac enlargement and failure. The results of operation are usually less than satisfactory because of the degree of preexisting cardiac dysfunction and damage. In appropriate patients, cardiac transplantation may be an alternative (Ch. 18), with a 5-year survival rate of about 80 per cent compared with less than 5 per cent in nontransplanted patients.[124]

ALCOHOLIC CARDIOMYOPATHY

Chronic excessive consumption of alcohol may be associated with congestive heart failure, hypertension, arrhythmias, and sudden death; it is the major cause of secondary, nonischemic dilated cardiomyopathy in the Western world.[125,126] It is estimated that two-thirds of the adult population use alcohol to some extent, and more than 10 per cent are heavy users. Therefore, it is not surprising that alcoholic cardiomyopathy is a major problem.[126] Whereas the course in many cases of idiopathic dilated cardiomyopathy relentlessly goes downhill, ceasing consumption of alcohol early in the course of alcoholic cardiomyopathy may halt the progression or even reverse left ventricular contractile dysfunction.[1,127,128]

The consumption of alcohol may result in myocardial damage by three basic mechanisms: (1) a presumed direct toxic effect of alcohol or of its metabolites; (2) nutritional effects, most commonly in association with thiamine deficiency which leads to beriberi heart disease (p. 461); and (3) rarely, toxic effects due to additives in the alcoholic beverage (cobalt)[129,130] (p. 1403). There had been speculation that alcohol caused myocardial damage only through dietary deficiencies, but it is now clear that alcoholic cardiomyopathy occurs in the absence of nutritional deficiencies.[131]

Typical Oriental beriberi may coexist with alcoholic cardiomyopathy, although it is no longer seen with any frequency.[126,130] The distinguishing features of each include peripheral vasodilatation and high output heart failure, often right-sided, in the former and reduced contractility with typically left-sided low output failure in the latter.[1]

Alcohol results in acute as well as chronic depression of myocardial contractility and may produce demonstrable cardiac dysfunction even when ingested by normal individuals in quantities consumed in social drinking[132,133]; compensatory mechanisms such as vasodilatation or sympathetic stimulation are invoked and they may mask the direct myocardial depression produced by alcohol.[130,133,134]

The mechanism of the cardiac depression produced by alcohol remains unclear, and a direct causal relationship between alcohol and the development of cardiomyopathy, while highly likely, has not been proved. In acute studies, alcohol and its metabolite acetaldehyde have been shown to interfere with a number of membrane and cellular functions that involve the transport and binding of calcium, mitochondrial respiration, myocardial lipid metabolism, myocardial protein synthesis, and myofibrillar ATPase.[130,131,135-137] Studies in isolated ferret papillary muscles have shown that ethanol in concentrations similar to those occurring in intoxicated humans depresses myocardial contractility by interfering with excitation-contraction coupling through inhibition of the interaction between calcium and the myofilaments.[138] The accumulation of metabolites of ethanol in the myocardium may interfere with normal myocardial lipid metabolism and may play a role in the pathogenesis of alcohol-induced myocardial damage.[139] The roles that other associated electrolyte imbalances (hypokalemia, hypophosphatemia, hypomagnesemia) may play in alcohol-mediated damage have not been clarified.[131] The major unanswered question is precisely how these metabolic effects result in persistent myocardial injury.

PATHOLOGY. The gross and microscopic pathological findings are nonspecific and similar to those observed in idiopathic dilated cardiomyopathy, although certain ultrastructural details suggest alcoholic cardiomyopathy.[140] Edema of the vascular wall and perivascular fibrosis of the intramyocardial coronary arteries has been observed, and it has been suggested that the myocardial damage in alcoholic cardiomyopathy may be the result of ischemia produced by disease of the small intramural coronary arteries.

Clinical Manifestations

Alcoholic cardiomyopathy most commonly occurs in men 30 to 55 years of age who have been heavy consumers of whiskey, wine, or beer, usually for more than 10 years.[126,140a] While alcoholic cardiomyopathy may be observed in the homeless, malnourished, "skid row" alcoholic man who is a candidate for and often suffers from alcoholic cirrhosis, many patients are well-nourished individuals of middle and even upper socioeconomic status without liver disease or peripheral neuropathy. Therefore, unless a high index of suspicion is maintained, it may be easy to miss a history of alcohol abuse. Persistent questioning of the patient and particularly the relatives of patients with unexplained cardiomegaly or cardiomyopathy is often required to elicit a history of alcoholism.

It is frequently possible to demonstrate mild depression of cardiac function in chronic alcoholics even before cardiac dysfunction becomes clinically manifested.[141] Abnormalities of both systolic function (reduced ejection fraction) and diastolic function (increased myocardial wall stiffness) have been demonstrated in alcoholic patients without cardiac symptoms by a variety of invasive and noninvasive techniques.[141-142a] The typical findings are those of left ventricular dilatation, with reduced ejection fraction.[131] While overt alcoholic liver disease and cardiac involvement often do not occur together, even cirrhotic patients without signs or symptoms of heart disease have inducible evidence of asymptomatic myocardial disease.[141,142]

The development of symptoms may be insidious, although some patients have acute and florid left-sided congestive heart failure. A paroxysm of atrial fibrillation is a relatively frequent initial presenting finding.[130] More advanced cases involve findings of biventricular failure, with left ventricular dysfunction usually dominating. Dyspnea, orthopnea, and paroxysmal nocturnal dyspnea are frequently observed. Palpitations and syncope due to tachyarrhythmias, usually supraventricular, are occasionally present. Angina pectoris does not occur unless there is concomitant coronary artery disease or aortic stenosis.

PHYSICAL EXAMINATION. This usually reveals a narrow pulse pressure, often with an elevated diastolic pressure secondary to excessive peripheral vasoconstriction. There is cardiomegaly, and protodiastolic (S_3) and presystolic (S_4) gallop sounds are common. An apical systolic murmur of mitral regurgitation due to papillary muscle dysfunction is often found. The severity of right heart failure varies, but jugular venous distention and peripheral edema are common. A concomitant skeletal muscle myopathy is a frequent finding.[131,135]

LABORATORY EXAMINATION. The *chest roentgenogram* in the advanced case demonstrates considerable cardiac enlargement (Fig. 43-6), pulmonary congestion, and pulmonary venous hypertension (p. 217). Pleural effusions are often seen. *Electrocardiographic abnormalities* are common and are frequently the only indication of alcoholic heart disease during the preclinical phase. Alcoholic patients without other evidence of heart disease often are seen after developing palpitations, chest discomfort, or syncope typically following a binge of alcohol consumption on a weekend, particularly during the year-end holiday season. This is dubbed the "holiday heart syndrome." The most common arrhythmia observed is atrial fibrillation, followed by atrial flutter and frequent ventricular premature contractions.[143] Alcohol consumption may even predispose to atrial fibrillation or flutter in nonalcoholics.[131,143] Hypokalemia may play a role in the genesis of some of these arrhythmias. Supraventricular arrhythmias are also frequently observed in patients with overt alcoholic cardiomyopathy. Sudden, unexpected death is not uncommon in young adult alcoholics, and it is likely that ventricular fibrillation is responsible.[144]

Atrioventricular conduction disturbances (most commonly first degree heart block), bundle branch block, left ventricular hypertrophy, and repolarization abnormalities are common electrocardiographic findings.[126,130,145] Prolongation of the Q-T

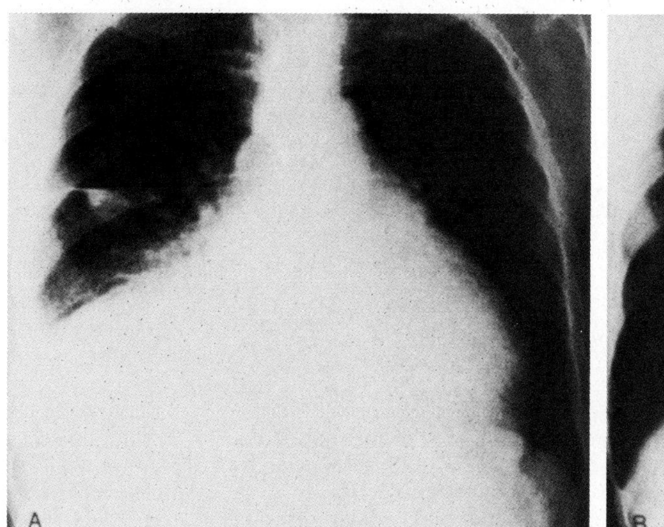
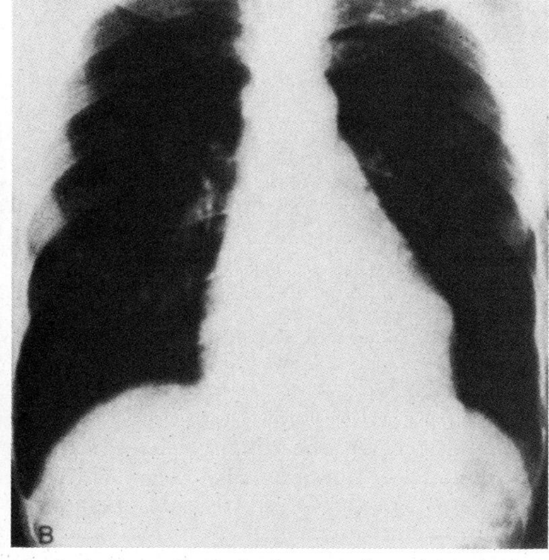

FIGURE 43-6. Chest radiographs of a 36-year-old man with alcoholic cardiomyopathy. *A*, Before abstention, there was marked cardiomegaly and a right pleural effusion. *B*, After 6 weeks of abstention the radiograph was virtually normal. (From Stevenson, L. W., and Perloff, J. K.: The dilated cardiomyopathies: Clinical aspects. Cardiol. Clin. *6*:194, 1988.)

interval is noted frequently. ST-segment and T-wave changes are often restored to normal within several days after cessation of alcohol consumption.

The hemodynamic findings observed at cardiac catheterization and the assessment of left ventricular function by noninvasive methods (echocardiography and isotope angiography) resemble those found in idiopathic dilated cardiomyopathy.

The *natural history* of alcoholic cardiomyopathy depends on the drinking habits of the patient. Total abstinence in the early stages of the disease may lead to resolution of the manifestation of congestive heart failure and a return of heart size toward normal,[127,130] although patients with severe heart failure may show no improvement in function or prognosis. Continued alcohol consumption leads to further myocardial damage and fibrosis, with the development of refractory congestive heart failure. Death may also be due to arrhythmia, heart block, and systemic or pulmonary embolism.

MANAGEMENT. The key to the long-term treatment of alcoholic cardiomyopathy is *immediate and total abstinence*, as early in the course of the disease as possible.[146] This may be quite effective (Table 43-6). The prognosis in patients who continue to drink, particularly if they have been symptomatic for a long period, is poor.[130] In the overall population of patients with alcoholic cardiomyopathy, between 40 and 50 per cent succumb within a 3- to 6-year period.[130,145] Prolonged bed rest is also thought to result in functional improvement, although its major benefit may simply be the decreased alcohol consumption.[130]

The management of acute episodes of congestive heart failure is similar to that of idiopathic dilated cardiomyopathy. For patients with severe congestive heart failure, it is prudent to administer thiamine on the chance that beriberi may be contributing to the heart failure. Whether to use chronic anticoagulation (as is usually recommended for idiopathic dilated cardiomyopathy) is controversial[129,143]; we usually do not prescribe coumadin for risk of bleeding due to noncompliance, trauma, and overanticoagulation due to hepatic dysfunction. Animal studies have suggested that ribose and verapamil may improve the myocardial depression found in alcoholic cardiomyopathy,[147,148] but their efficacy in humans is not established.

COBALT CARDIOMYOPATHY

A previously unrecognized syndrome of fulminating congestive heart failure appeared in the mid-1960's, first in Canada, and subsequently in the United States and Europe.[130] The disease was found in people who drank a particular brand of beer to which cobalt sulfate had been added as a foam stabilizer. After cobalt had been removed from the process, no more cases of the disease were reported.

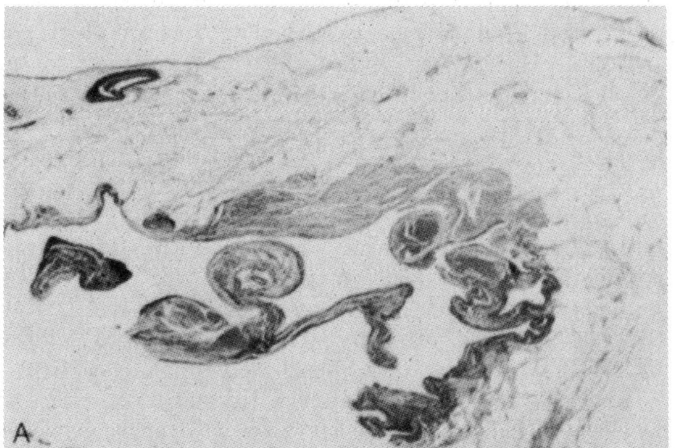
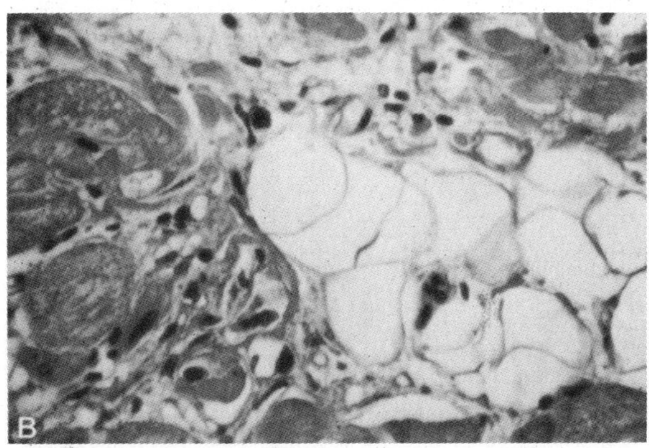

FIGURE 43-7. *A*, Section through the anterior free wall of the right ventricle in a patient with right ventricular cardiomyopathy and sudden death, showing massive lipomatous infiltration (azan, ×5). *B*, Closeup of residual myocardium, showing histological evidence of myocardial degeneration and lipomatous infiltration (hematoxylin-eosin, ×300). (Reproduced by permission from Thiene, G., Nava, A., Corrado, D., et al.: Right ventricular cardiomyopathy and sudden death in young people. N. Engl. J. Med. *318*:129, 1988.)

RIGHT VENTRICULAR CARDIOMYOPATHY (ARRHYTHMOGENIC RIGHT VENTRICULAR DYSPLASIA)

Right ventricular cardiomyopathy is marked by partial or total replacement of right ventricular muscle by adipose or fibrous tissue (Fig. 43–7) and may be associated with ventricular tachyarrhythmias of right ventricular origin (left bundle branch configuration of the QRS)[149–151] (p. 706). The cause of the myocardial changes is unclear—both congenital and acquired factors have been suggested,[150] although probably it is distinct from Uhl's disease, which is marked by extreme thinning of the ventricular wall. Typical clinical features include male predominance, normal physical examination, symptoms of palpitations and syncope, and a risk of sudden death.[149–152] Noninvasive and invasive evaluation demonstrates a dilated, poorly contractile right ventricle, usually with a normal left ventricle.[149–155] Antiarrhythmic therapy appears to control the ventricular arrhythmias, but the influence of therapy on the risk of sudden death is unknown.[149,151,152,156] Electrode catheter ablation (p. 654) has also been successful in patients with drug-resistant ventricular tachycardia.[157]

Hypertrophic Cardiomyopathy

Although first described over one hundred years ago, the unique features of hypertrophic cardiomyopathy (HCM) were not studied systematically until the late 1950's.[158–163] Characteristic findings are inappropriate myocardial hypertrophy, often predominantly involving the interventricular septum of a nondilated left ventricle, with hyperdynamic ventricular function.[161] A distinctive clinical feature was soon recognized in some patients with HCM: a dynamic pressure gradient in the subaortic area that divided the left ventricle into a high-pressure apical region and a lower-pressure subaortic region. Hence the terms *idiopathic hypertrophic subaortic stenosis (IHSS)* and muscular subaortic stenosis were suggested, although subsequent findings have indicated that most patients (probably about three-quarters) do not, in fact, ever have obstruction to left ventricular outflow. Since hypertrophy often occurs in the absence of a pressure gradient, the characteristic feature of HCM is myocardial hypertrophy that is out of proportion to the hemodynamic load. Importantly, valvular aortic stenosis or systemic hypertension usually is absent.

The physiological characteristics of HCM differ substantially from those of dilated cardiomyopathy (Table 43–9). The most characteristic pathophysiological abnormality in HCM is *diastolic* dysfunction[158] (see also p. 402 and p. 446). Thus, HCM is characterized by abnormal stiffness of the left ventricle during diastole, with resultant impaired ventricular filling. This abnormality in diastolic relaxation results in elevation of the left ventricular end-diastolic pressure with resulting pulmonary congestion and dyspnea, the most common symptom in HCM, despite typically hyperdynamic left ventricular function. The disease appears to be genetically transmitted in somewhat more than half the patients as a single gene autosomal dominant trait[162] with variable expression and penetrance.[163,164] In the remainder of patients, the disease appears to occur spontaneously.[165] Evidence of the disease is found in about one-fourth of the first-degree relatives of a patient with HCM; in many of the relatives the disease is milder than in the propositus, the degree of hypertrophy is less and it is more localized, and outflow gradients are usually lacking.[164,166] Symptoms are often absent or minimal, and the disease is detected only by echocardiography. The overall prevalence of HCM is low, and has been estimated to average between 0.02 and 0.2 per cent of the population.[4,167]

TABLE 43–9 DIFFERENCES IN SYSTOLIC AND DIASTOLIC FUNCTION IN DILATED (CONGESTIVE) AND HYPERTROPHIC CARDIOMYOPATHY

	DILATED CARDIOMYOPATHY	HYPERTROPHIC CARDIOMYOPATHY
Left ventricular volume		
End-diastolic	Increased	Normal
End-systolic	Markedly increased	Decreased
Left ventricular mass	Increased	Markedly increased
Mass/volume ratio	Decreased	Increased
Systolic function		
Ejection fraction	Decreased	Normal or increased
Myocardial shortening	Decreased	Increased
Wall stress	Increased	Decreased
Diastolic function		
Chamber stiffness	Decreased	Increased
Myocardial stiffness	Increased	Increased

From Chatterjee, K.: Pathophysiology of cardiomyopathy. *In* Giles, T. D., and Sander, G. E. (eds.): Cardiomyopathy. Middleton, MA, PSG Publishing Co., 1988, p. 65.

PATHOLOGY

MACROSCOPIC EXAMINATION. This typically discloses a marked increase in myocardial mass, and the ventricular cavities are small (Figs. 43–1 and 43–8).[161] The left ventricle is usually more involved with the hypertrophic process than is the right.[168] The atria are dilated and often hypertrophied,[169] reflecting the high resistance to filling of the ventricles caused by diastolic dysfunction and the effects of atrioventricular valve regurgitation. The pattern and extent of left ventricular hypertrophy in HCM vary greatly from patient to patient, and a characteristic feature is heterogenicity in the amount of hypertrophy evident in different regions of the left ventricle.[161] A typical feature found in more than half of the patients with HCM is disproportionate involvement of the interventricular septum and anterolateral wall compared with the posterior segment of the free wall of the left ventricle.[161,170] When hypertrophy is largely localized to the septum, the process has been called asymmetric septal hypertrophy (ASH). Other patterns of hypertrophy are not uncommon, including concentric left ventricular hypertrophy, with symmetrical thickening of the left ventricle, involving the septum and free wall equally. This variant may occasionally be seen in patients with the genetically transmitted as well as the sporadic forms of hypertrophic cardiomyopathy.[161] In some patients with HCM there is substantial hypertrophy in unusual locations, such as the posterior portion of the septum, the posterobasal free wall, and the midventricular level.[170–172] Asymmetric left ventricular hypertrophy is not limited to HCM; 5 to 10 per cent of adult patients with other acquired or congenital defects (especially associated with right ventricular pressure overload) may present with nonuniform, especially septal, hypertrophy.[161]

Apical HCM. A variant with predominant involvement of the apex is common in Japan and is estimated to represent a quarter of Japanese HCM patients.[173] In other parts of the world, apical HCM is uncommon.[174] Typical features include a characteristic spade-like configuration of the left ventricle during angiographic study,[175] giant negative T waves in the precordial electrocardiographic leads, the absence of an intraventricular pressure gradient, mild symptoms, and a generally benign course.[173,176]

Two variants of HCM are seen particularly in elderly women. The first, termed hypertensive hypertrophic cardiomyopathy of the elderly, is characterized by severe concentric left ventricular hypertrophy and small left ventricular cavity size, and is associated with hypertension.[177–180] The second

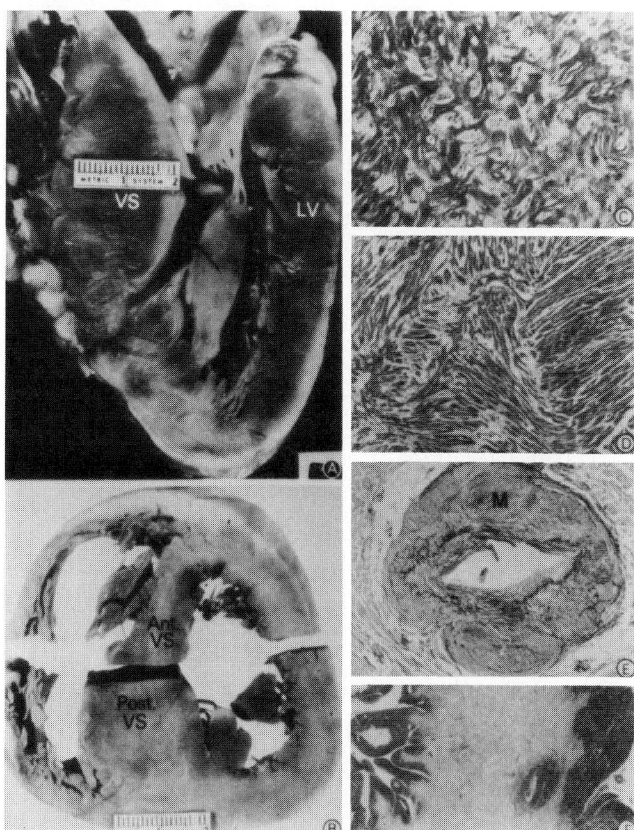

FIGURE 43-8. Morphological components of the underlying disease process in hypertrophic cardiomyopathy. *A*, Gross heart specimen sectioned in a cross-sectional plane similar to that of the echocardiographic (parasternal) long axis. The pattern of left ventricular hypertrophy is asymmetric, with wall thickening confined primarily to the anterior ventricular septum (VS), which bulges into the left ventricular outflow tract. LV denotes left ventricular free wall. (Reproduced from Maron and Roberts with the permission of the publisher.) *B*, Heart specimen with a different pattern of hypertrophy; here marked left ventricular wall thickening is localized to the posterior portion of the ventricular septum (Post. VS), whereas the anterior septum (Ant. VS) is only minimally thickened. (Reproduced from Maron with the permission of the publisher.)

***C* and *D*, Histology characteristic of the left ventricle in hypertrophic cardiomyopathy. In *C*, the septal myocardium shows a markedly disordered architecture with adjacent hypertrophied cardiac muscle cells arranged at perpendicular and oblique angles to each other. In *D*, bundles of hypertrophied cells show a disorganized, interwoven arrangement; *E*, Intramural coronary artery with an apparently narrowed lumen and thickened wall due primarily to medial (M) hypertrophy; *F*, Extensive scarring of ventricular septum that is transmural in distribution. (Reproduced by permission from Maron, B. J., Bonow, R. O., Cannon, R. O., et al.: Hypertrophic cardiomyopathy: Interrelations of clinical manifestations, pathophysiology, and therapy. N. Engl. J. Med. *316*:780, 1987.)**

presentation also is marked by an especially small left ventricular cavity but with relatively mild hypertrophy; other findings include marked anterior displacement of the mitral valve, extensive submitral (annular) calcification, a left ventricular outflow gradient, and the late appearance of severe and progressive symptoms.[181] In contrast to young patients with HCM, the elderly patient is more likely to show a localized septal bulge just below the aortic valve and is less likely to have marked abnormalities in the orientation and curvature of the septum.[182]

A variety of disparate conditions may present similar gross morphological features of HCM, including hyperparathyroidism, infants of diabetic mothers, neurofibromatosis, generalized lipodystrophy, lentiginosis, pheochromocytoma, Friedreich's ataxia, and Noonan syndrome.[161,183-186] Rarely, the findings may be simulated by amyloid or tumor involvement of the septum.[187]

HISTOLOGY. Microscopic findings in HCM are distinctive, with myocardial hypertrophy and gross disorganization of the muscle bundles resulting in a characteristic whorled pattern; abnormalities are found in the cell-to-cell arrangement (disarray), and disorganization of the myofibrillar architecture within a given cell[163,188] (Fig. 43-8). Fibrosis is usually prominent[189] and may be extensive enough to produce grossly visible scars.[161] Foci of disorganized cells are often interspersed between areas of hypertrophied but otherwise normal-appearing muscle cells. While abnormally arranged cardiac muscle cells initially were considered specific for HCM, it is now recognized that they may be found in a variety of acquired and congenital heart conditions.[161] What is unique about the disarray in HCM is its ubiquity and frequency. Almost all HCM patients have some degree of disarray and most have involvement of 5 per cent or more of the myocardium; in contrast, disarray in non-HCM patients (when it occurs) usually involves only about 1 per cent of the myocardium (Fig. 43-9).[161]

Abnormal intramural coronary arteries, with a reduction in the size of the lumen and thickening of the vessel wall, are common in HCM,[190] occurring in over 80 per cent of patients (Fig. 43-8).[161,191] This abnormality occurs most frequently in the ventricular septum; it also has been observed in infants who died of this condition and could represent a congenital component of the condition. The prominence of abnormal intramural coronary arteries in areas of extensive myocardial fibrosis is consistent with the hypothesis that these abnormalities may be responsible for the development of myocardial ischemia.[191]

ETIOLOGY

The cause of the myocardial hypertrophy in HCM remains unknown. There are suggestive data linking abnormal myocardial calcium kinetics and specific features of HCM, particularly the abnormalities of diastolic function.[158,192,193] Abnormal calcium fluxes with a resultant increase in intracellular calcium concentration appear to occur as a consequence of an increase in the number of calcium channels.[194] This in turn produces (in an as yet undefined process) hypertrophy and cellular disarray.[192]

Other suggested etiologies of HCM include (1) abnormal sympathetic stimulation because of heightened responsiveness of the heart to or excessive production of circulating

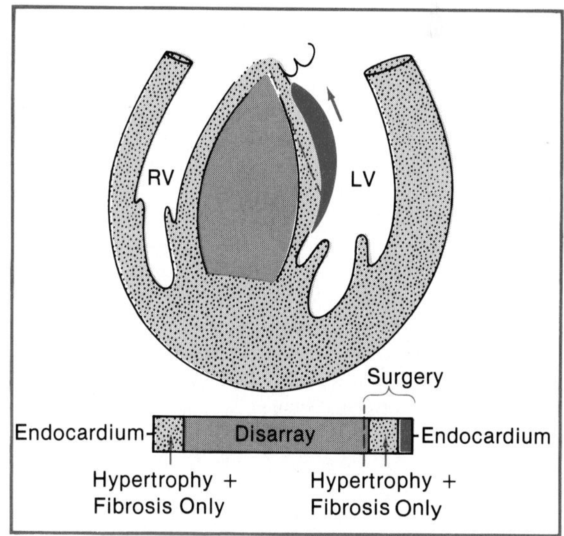

FIGURE 43-9. Diagrammatic representation showing usual location of myocyte disarray in interventricular septum in hypertrophic cardiomyopathy. This explains why disarray is usually deep or absent in septectomy specimen, and why endomyocardial biopsy (3-mm maximum dimension) is also unlikely to sample zone of disarray. RV = right ventricle, LV = left ventricle. (From Tazelaar, H. D., and Billingham, M. E.: The surgical pathology of hypertrophic cardiomyopathy. Arch. Pathol. Lab. Med. *111*:257, 1987.)

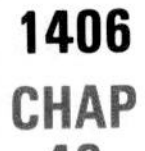

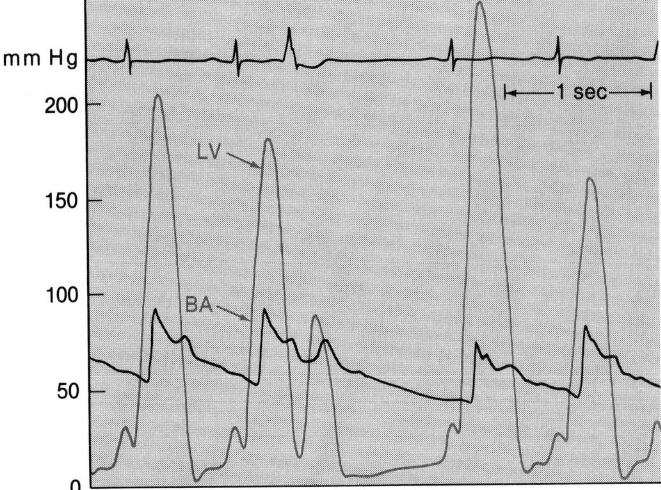

FIGURE 43–10. Simultaneous pressures recorded in the left ventricle (LV) and brachial artery (BA) in a patient with HCM. During the post-premature contraction beat, the pulse pressure in the brachial artery is less than in the control beats. (From Braunwald, E., et al.: Idiopathic hypertrophic subaortic stenosis. Circulation *30*(Suppl. IV):78, 1964, by permission of the American Heart Association, Inc.)

catecholamines[195–197] or reduced neuronal uptake of cardiac norepinephrine[198]; (2) abnormally thickened intramural coronary arteries that do not dilate normally and lead to myocardial ischemia, with resultant fibrosis and abnormal compensatory hypertrophy[197]; (3) subendocardial ischemia, possibly related to abnormalities of the microcirculation, that depletes the energy stores essential for the sequestration of calcium during diastole, resulting in persistent interaction of the contractile elements during diastole and attendant increased diastolic stiffness[199]; and (4) structural abnormalities, including a catenoid configuration of the septum, that lead to myocardial cell hypertrophy and disarray.[197,200]

Mutation of the Myosin Heavy-Chain Gene. Seidman and her collaborators have reported the existence of a gene located on 14 q 1, (i.e., the long arm of the 14th chromosome in the band closest to the centromere) and termed it *FHC-1* (for familial hypertrophic cardiomyopathy); it was believed to be responsible for HCM in two families. Subsequently they found this to be the gene encoding for myosin heavy chain (MHC). Sequencing of this gene in one family with HCM revealed that the abnormality was caused by a gene duplication in which the α and β MHC genes were fused and present in an extra copy. In the second family, there was a point mutation in the β MHC sequence that alters the myosin's arginine to glutamine. Both of these mutations affect the polypeptides crucial to the structure of myofibrils and might be responsible for the myocyte and myofibrillar disarray characteristic of familial HCM.[201–204] Thus, it would appear that the structural organization of the α and β cardiac MHC genes may predispose them to genetic events that produce these two (and perhaps other) mutations, which are ultimately responsible for familial HCM. Seidman et al. have also reported that familial HCM is a genetically heterogeneous disease,[205] i.e., it can be caused by genetic defects in at least two loci. However, the genetic heterogeneity does *not* appear to explain the clinical variability. Further, they have suggested that mutations of the cardiac MHC genes occurring in the myocardial precursor cells of an individual might be responsible for sporadic cases of HCM that would cause a similar phenotype without being responsible for transmission through the germ line (and therefore would not cause familial HCM) (see also pp. 1636 and 1637).

While a genetic test might be developed that could permit early detection of the disease, the demonstrated genetic heterogeneity will require identification of the other gene(s) responsible and ultimately a battery of genetic tests.

PATHOPHYSIOLOGY

SYSTOLE. Since the initial descriptions of hypertrophic cardiomyopathy, the feature that has attracted the greatest attention is the dynamic pressure gradient (Fig. 43–10). While this pressure gradient was initially thought to be due to a muscular sphincter action in the subaortic region or was an artifact, it appears to be related to further narrowing of an already small outflow tract (narrowed by the prominent septal hypertrophy and possibly abnormal location of the mitral valve) by systolic anterior motion (SAM) of the mitral valve against the septum.[206,207]

There continues to be considerable controversy about the cause and significance of the outflow gradient.[161,208,209] Central to the disagreement is whether there is true obstruction to left ventricular ejection or whether the pressure gradient is simply the consequence of vigorous ventricular emptying.[210,211] Most favor the view that a true mechanical impediment to left ventricular ejection occurs when outflow gradients are present and is the result of distal portions of the mitral valve apparatus moving anteriorly across the outflow tract and contacting the ventricular septum in mid-systole.[161,210,212–217] It is likely that the mitral valve is displaced anteriorly because of Venturi effects or as a result of the increased ejection velocities produced by the abnormal left ventricular outflow tract orientation and geometry (Fig. 43–11).[211,216]

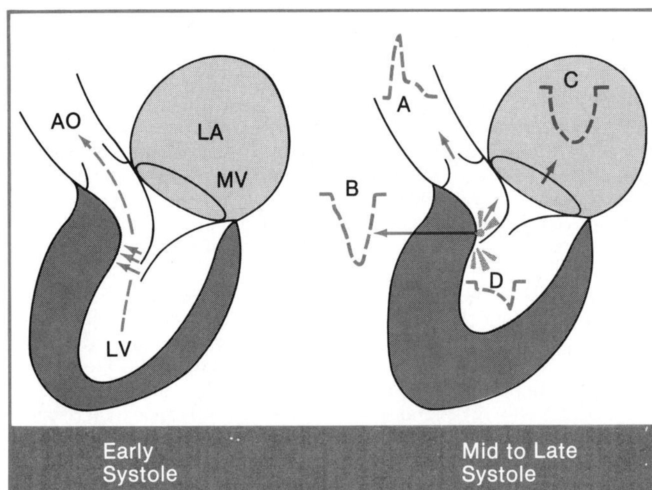

FIGURE 43–11. Left panel illustrates proposed mechanism of mitral leaflet systolic anterior motion (SAM) in early systole in hypertrophic cardiomyopathy (HCM). Ventricular septal hypertrophy causes narrowed outflow tract, as result of which ejection velocity is rapid and path of ejection (dashed line) is closer to mitral leaflets (MV) than is normal. This results in Venturi forces (three short oblique arrows in outflow tract) drawing anterior and/or posterior mitral leaflets toward septum. Subsequent mitral leaflet septal contact results in obstruction to left ventricular (LV) outflow and concomitant mitral regurgitation as seen on right panel. By midsystole, SAM septal contact is well established, causing marked narrowing of LV outflow tract with obstruction to outflow. LA = left atrium.

Proximal to level of SAM-septal contact, converging lines indicate acceleration of jet just proximal to obstruction and narrowing of jet width that occurs. Distal to obstruction, arrow and diverging lines indicate high velocity flow that emanates from site of SAM-septal contact, directed posterolaterally at considerable angle from normal path of aortic outflow. In late systole, although forward flow continues into outflow tract and aorta (AO), the volume of flow is much less than in early nonobstructed systole. Typical Doppler flow velocities that can be recorded are shown.

In right panel, *A*, Integrated Doppler flow signal in ascending aorta; *B*, High outflow tract velocity recorded by continuous wave (CW) Doppler at site of SAM-septal contact; *C*, Presence of mitral regurgitation recorded by CW Doppler; *D*, Late systolic velocity peak that can be recorded in apical region of LV. (From Wigle, E. D.: Hypertrophic cardiomyopathy: A 1987 viewpoint. Circulation *75*:312, 1987, by permission of the American Heart Association, Inc.)

TABLE 43-10 PROPOSED CAUSES OF ISCHEMIA IN HCM DESPITE NORMAL EPICARDIAL CORONARY ARTERIES

Increased muscle mass
Inadequate capillary density
Elevated diastolic filling pressures
Abnormal intramural coronary arteries
Impaired vasodilatory reserve
Systolic compression of arteries
Enhanced myocardial oxygen demand (increased wall stress)

DIASTOLE. Most patients with HCM demonstrate abnormalities of diastolic function whether or not a gradient is present and whether or not they are symptomatic.[210,218] These abnormalities of diastolic filling are largely independent of the extent and distribution of myocardial hypertrophy; patients with mild and apparently localized hypertrophy may demonstrate prominent diastolic dysfunction, suggesting that the myopathic process occurs in ventricular regions that are not macroscopically hypertrophied.[219] Diastolic dysfunction in turn leads to increased filling pressure despite a normal or small left ventricular cavity size and appears to result from abnormalities of left ventricular relaxation and distensibility.[161,210,220] Early diastolic filling is impaired when relaxation is prolonged,[221] perhaps related to abnormal calcium kinetics, subendocardial ischemia, or the abnormal loading conditions found in HCM.[161,222,223] Late diastolic filling is altered when left ventricular distensibility is impaired; as a consequence, filling pressures rise. HCM may cause abnormal distensibility because of fibrosis[191] or cellular disorganization.[161]

MYOCARDIAL ISCHEMIA. Myocardial ischemia is common and multifactorial in HCM (Table 43-10 and Fig. 43-12).[161,210,224-228] Major causes include impaired vasodilator reserve (perhaps related to the thickened and narrowed small intramural coronary arteries found in HCM, see also p. 1405)[190]; increased oxygen demand, especially in patients with outflow gradients; and elevated filling pressures with resultant subendocardial ischemia.[210,224]

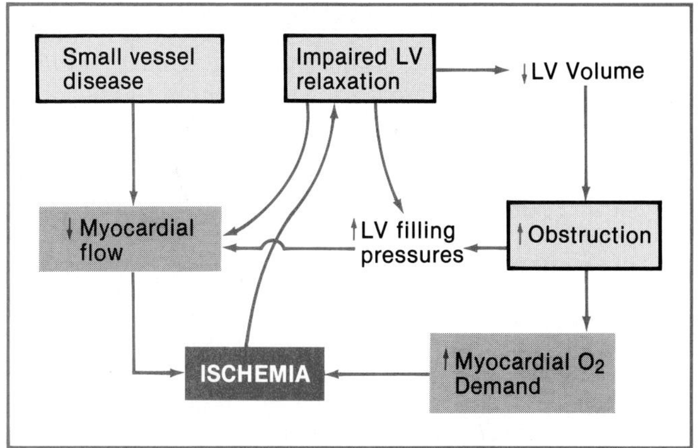

FIGURE 43-12. Determinants of ischemia in hypertrophic cardiomyopathy. (From Maron, B. J., and Epstein, S. E.: Hypertrophic cardiomyopathy: Pathophysiology and therapy. *In* Braunwald, E. (ed.): Heart Disease: A Textbook of Cardiovascular Medicine. 3rd ed. Philadelphia, W. B. Saunders Company, Update No. 7, pp. 157-168, 1989.)

CLINICAL MANIFESTATIONS

SYMPTOMS. The majority of patients with HCM are asymptomatic or only mildly symptomatic[229] and often are identified during screening of relatives of a patient with HCM. Unfortunately, the first clinical manifestation of the disease in such individuals may be sudden death. The disease is identified most often in adults in their 30's and 40's; it occurs more often than commonly suspected in elderly patients.[229,229a] The condition has been observed at necropsy in stillborns and both clinically and pathologically in octogenarians. The importance of recognizing this disorder in children at the earliest possible time is highlighted by the higher mortality rate in younger patients; death is often sudden and unexpected.[230] Because syncope and sudden death have been associated with competitive sports and severe exertion in patients with HCM, it is important to diagnose this condition so that these activities may be proscribed. A particularly high index of suspicion of this condition must be maintained to make the clinical diagnosis in the elderly, since their symptoms may easily be confused with those of coronary artery or aortic valve disease. The disease is slightly more common in men,[229] although women may be more likely to be severely disabled and may initially present at a younger age than men.[231]

The clinical picture varies considerably, ranging from the asymptomatic relative of a patient with recognized HCM who has a slightly abnormal echocardiogram but no other manifestation of the illness to the patient with incapacitating symptoms.[230] There is a general relationship between the extent of hypertrophy and the severity of symptoms, but the relationship is not absolute, and some patients have severe symptoms with only mild and apparently localized hypertrophy, and vice versa.[232-234] There is a complex interaction between left ventricular hypertrophy, left ventricular pressure gradient, diastolic dysfunction, and myocardial ischemia that accounts for the great variability in symptoms from patient to patient (Fig. 43-13).

The most common symptom is *dyspnea*, occurring in up to 90 per cent of symptomatic patients, which is largely a consequence of the elevated left ventricular diastolic (and therefore left atrial and pulmonary venous) pressure, which results largely from impaired ventricular filling owing to diastolic dysfunction.[229,230] Angina pectoris (found in about three-fourths of symptomatic patients), fatigue, and presyncope and syncope are also common. Palpitations, paroxysmal nocturnal dyspnea, overt congestive heart failure, and dizziness are found less frequently, although severe congestive heart failure culminating in death may be seen. Exertion tends to exacerbate many of the symptoms.[235] A variety of mechanisms may contribute to the production of angina pectoris. It is at least in part the result of an imbalance between oxygen supply and demand as a consequence of the greatly increased myocardial mass. Transmural infarction may occur in the absence of narrowing in the extramural coronary arteries.[210] Narrowing of the small coronary arteries may contribute to myocardial ischemia,[191,224] particularly during exertion, and perhaps

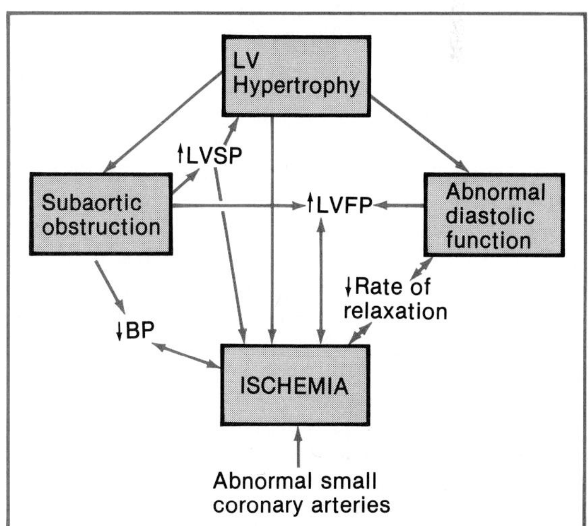

FIGURE 43-13. Pathophysiological and hemodynamic interrelations between left ventricular (LV) hypertrophy, subaortic obstruction, diastolic dysfunction, and myocardial ischemia in hypertrophic cardiomyopathy. The symptoms in any given patient reflect the complex interactions among these pathophysiological mechanisms. LVSP = left ventricular systolic pressure, LVFP = left ventricular filling pressure, BP = blood pressure. (Reproduced by permission from Maron, B. J., Bonow, R. O., Cannon, R. O., et al.: Hypertrophic cardiomyopathy: Interrelations of clinical manifestations, pathophysiology, and therapy. N. Engl. J. Med. *316*:780, 1987.)

20 per cent of older patients with hypertrophic cardiomyopathy may have concurrent atheromatous obstructive coronary artery disease. Impaired diastolic relaxation may produce subendocardial ischemia as a result of prolonged maintenance of wall tension with a concomitant slower-than-normal decrease in the impedance to coronary blood flow. Syncope may result from inadequate cardiac output with exertion or from cardiac arrhythmias. It occurs most commonly in young patients with small left ventricular chamber size and evidence of ventricular tachycardia on Holter monitoring.[236] Near-syncopal ("graying out") spells that occur in the erect posture and that can be relieved by immediately lying down are common. However, in contrast to valvular aortic stenosis, syncope or near-syncope may not be an ominous finding in adult patients with HCM; some patients have a history of such episodes dating back many years without deterioration. In children and adolescents, however, presyncope and syncope identify patients at increased risk of sudden death (see Natural History below).

PHYSICAL EXAMINATION. This may be normal in asymptomatic patients without gradients, particularly those with the apical variant of HCM, save for a left ventricular lift and a loud fourth heart sound, but there are usually prominent findings in patients with a left ventricular outflow tract pressure gradient. The apical precordial impulse is often displaced laterally and is usually abnormally forceful and enlarged. Because of decreased left ventricular compliance, a prominent presystolic apical impulse which results from forceful atrial systole is often present.[230] This may result in a double apical impulse as a result of the prominent *a* wave. A more characteristic but less frequently recognized abnormality is a triple apical beat, the third impulse being a late systolic bulge that occurs when the heart is nearly empty and is performing near-isometric contraction. These findings may be readily recorded by apexcardiography (Fig. 2–17, p. 27).

A systolic thrill may be present (Table 2–1, p. 26), is most frequently palpable at the apex or along the lower left sternal border, and bears only a rough relationship to the severity of the pressure gradient.[231] The jugular venous pulse may demonstrate a prominent *a* wave, reflecting diminished right ventricular compliance secondary to the massive hypertrophy of the ventricular septum. The carotid pulse typically rises briskly and then declines in midsystole as the gradient develops, followed by a secondary rise. This may be well appreciated on physical examination and can be demonstrated more clearly by means of indirect pulse tracings (Fig. 2–14, p. 24).

The first heart sound is normal and is often preceded by a fourth heart sound that corresponds to the apical presystolic impulse.[231] The second heart sound is usually normally split. In some patients, however, it is narrowly split and in others, particularly those with severe outflow gradients, paradoxical splitting may be noted.[231] A third heart sound is common but does not have the same ominous significance as in patients with valvular aortic stenosis. Systolic ejection sounds relating to rapid acceleration of blood flow may be found on occasion. The auscultatory hallmark of HCM associated with an outflow gradient is a systolic murmur that is typically harsh and crescendo-decrescendo in configuration (Fig. 2–17, p. 27); it usually commences well after the first heart sound and is best heard between the apex and the left sternal border. It often radiates well to the lower sternal border, the axillae, and base of the heart but not into the neck vessels. In patients with large gradients, the murmur usually reflects both outflow tract turbulence and concomitant mitral regurgitation, while in patients without gradients, turbulence in the outflow tract is the only cause. Accordingly, the murmur is often more holosystolic and blowing at the apex and in the axillae (probably due to mitral regurgitation) and midsystolic and harsher along the lower sternal border (due to flow across the outflow tract).[231]

The murmur is labile in intensity and duration, and a variety of maneuvers may be utilized to augment or suppress it (Table 2–8, p. 38, and Fig. 2–27, p. 40).[237] A diastolic rumbling murmur, reflecting increased transmitral flow, may occur in patients with marked mitral regurgitation. The murmur of aortic regurgitation is observed only occasionally in patients with HCM, although mild aortic regurgitation can be demonstrated by Doppler echocardiography in one-third of patients.[238] It may develop after operation to correct the outflow gradient[239] or following infective endocarditis.

It is important to emphasize the features of physical examination that permit differentiation of HCM from fixed orifice obstruction, most commonly due to valvular aortic stenosis (Tables 2–1, p. 26 and 34–11, p. 1039). The character of the carotid pulse and features of the murmur are most useful in this regard. Because there is obstruction to left ventricular emptying from the beginning of systole with fixed valvular stenosis, the carotid upstroke is slowed and of low amplitude (pulsus parvus et tardus). With HCM, initial ejection of blood from the left ventricle is actually enhanced, and therefore the arterial upstroke is brisk. The murmur of HCM, as opposed to that of aortic stenosis, can be reliably identified by its increase with the Valsalva maneuver and during squatting-to-standing action, and its decrease during standing-to-squatting action, passive leg elevation, and handgrip[231] (Table 43–11). Other features that may be helpful but are of considerably less significance are the location of the murmur (it radiates along the carotid arteries in valvular aortic stenosis but not in HCM), and the location of the systolic thrill (most prominent in the second right intercostal space in valvular aortic stenosis and in the fourth interspace along the left sternal border in HCM).

ELECTROCARDIOGRAM. This is usually abnormal in HCM and invariably so in symptomatic patients with left ventricular outflow gradients. Entirely normal electrocardiograms are seen in only about 15 per cent of patients and usually are found in the presence of only localized left ventricular hypertrophy. The most common abnormalities are ST-segment and T-wave abnormalities, followed by evidence of left ventricular hypertrophy, with QRS complexes that are tallest in the midprecordial leads.[240,241] There may be progressive electrocardiographic evidence of hypertrophy over time. Giant negative T-waves in the midprecordial leads of Japanese patients are characteristic of HCM involving the apex,[242] but such a pattern in the West may be found with HCM involving segments other than the apex.[242] Prominent, abnormal Q waves are relatively common, occurring in 20 to 50 per cent of patients. The Q-wave abnormalities often involve the inferior

TABLE 43–11 EFFECTS OF INTERVENTIONS ON OUTFLOW GRADIENT AND SYSTOLIC MURMUR IN HCM

	CONTRACTILITY	PRELOAD	AFTERLOAD
Increase in Gradient and Murmur			
Valsalva maneuver (during strain)	—	↓	↓
Standing	—	↓	—
Postextrasystole	↑	↑	—
Isoproterenol	↑	↓	↓
Digitalis	↑	↓	—
Amyl nitrite	— then ↑	↓ then ↑	↓
Nitroglycerin	—	↓	↓
Exercise	↑	↑	↑
Tachycardia	↑	↓	—
Hypovolemia	↑	↓	↓
Decrease in Gradient and Murmur			
Mueller maneuver	—	↑	↑
Valsalva overshoot	—	↑	↑
Squatting	—	↑	↑
Alpha-adrenocepter stimulation (phenylephrine)	—	—	↑
Beta-adrenocepter blockade	↓	↑	—
General anesthesia	↓	—	—
Isometric handgrip	—	—	↑

↑ = increase; ↓ = decrease; — = no major change.

(II, III, aV_1) and/or lateral (V_4-V_6) leads. They appear to be due to depolarization of myopathic cells in the septum that have abnormal electrophysiological properties.[243] A variety of other electrocardiographic abnormalities may occur, including abnormal electrical axis (usually left-axis deviation) and P-wave abnormalities (usually left atrial enlargement). Accessory atrioventricular pathways have been found in HCM, although they are uncommon.[244,245] Clinically significant abnormalities of AV conduction are uncommon but may cause syncope.[246]

Although a hemodynamic mechanism may play a role in the death of patients with HCM (particularly the young), many deaths, particularly those that are known to have been sudden, are probably due to an arrhythmia.[161,247,248] Because of the systolic and diastolic abnormalities in this disorder, rhythm disturbances are less well tolerated.

Ventricular arrhythmias are common in patients with HCM, occurring in over three-fourths of patients undergoing continuous ambulatory electrocardiographic monitoring.[230,249] Ventricular tachycardia is found in about one-fourth of the patients studied, and in some it is a harbinger of subsequent sudden death.[161,229,230] A similar spectrum of arrhythmias may be detected in those asymptomatic relatives of patients with HCM who themselves have the disease (often undiagnosed). Ventricular tachycardia occurs with greater frequency in patients with more pronounced hypertrophy.[250] Treadmill testing may expose arrhythmias that are not present at rest, although continuous ambulatory monitoring is superior in detecting repetitive ventricular tachyarrhythmias. Supraventricular tachycardia may be found in one-fourth to one-half of patients.[249]

Atrial fibrillation occurs in 5 to 15 per cent of patients, and the resultant loss of the atrial contribution to the filling of a hypertrophied, stiff ventricle may result in clinical deterioration. Treatment is often effective in controlling symptoms and restoring sinus rhythm; if this is done, long-term survival usually is not jeopardized.[251-253] The signal-averaged electrocardiogram may prove to be helpful in identifying patients at increased risk of sustained or lethal ventricular arrhythmia, although additional studies are necessary.[254]

Electrophysiological Testing. The role of electrophysiological studies in identifying HCM patients at increased risk of sudden death is evolving.[247,255-258a] These studies identify a variety of abnormalities in HCM patients (Table 43-12), but most important is their ability to induce ventricular tachycardia in two-thirds of patients with syncope or aborted sudden death, compared with 10 per cent in other HCM patients.[256]

CHEST ROENTGENOGRAM. The findings on radiographic examination are variable; heart size, principally the left ventricle, may range from normal to markedly enlarged, but there is little correlation between heart size and the severity of the outflow tract gradient. Left atrial enlargement is frequently observed, especially when significant mitral regurgitation is present. Aortic root enlargement and valvular calcification are not seen unless associated diseases are present, although calcification of the mitral annulus is common in HCM.

ECHOCARDIOGRAPHY. Because echocardiography combines the attributes of high resolution and no known risk, it has been widely utilized in the evaluation of hypertrophic cardiomyopathy (Figs. 4-95, 4-96, and 4-97, p. 100). The two-dimensional study is now standard; M-mode echocardiography may be used as an adjunctive modality.[161] It is useful in the study of patients with suspected HCM and also in the screening of relatives of patients in whom this condition has been documented. The echocardiogram is of value in identifying and quantifying morphological (i.e., distribution of septal hypertrophy) as well as functional features (e.g., hypercontractile left ventricle).

The cardinal echocardiographic feature of HCM is left ventricular hypertrophy. Although the characteristic feature is hypertrophy of the septum and anterolateral free wall, the echocardiogram is useful in identifying involvement of other left ventricular locations, including portions of the free wall and the apex.[161] There is considerable variability in the degree and pattern of hypertrophy; in most patients, there is variation in the extent of hypertrophy from left ventricular region to region.[161] Maximal hypertrophy of the septum often occurs midway between the base and apex of the left ventricle. The finding of a thickened septum that is at least 1.3 to 1.5 times the thickness of the posterior wall when measured in diastole just prior to atrial systole has been the time-honored criterion for the diagnosis of asymmetrical septal hypertrophy (ASH). The septum not only is relatively thicker than the posterior wall but is typically at least 15 mm in thickness (normal $\leq$ 11 mm).

TABLE 43-12 ELECTROPHYSIOLOGICAL ABNORMALITIES IN HCM PATIENTS

Abnormal study	**81%**
Sinoatrial dysfunction	**66%**
Sustained ventricular tachycardia	**43%**
His-Purkinje dysfunction	**30%**
Accessory pathway	**5%**

Adapted from Fananapazir, L., Tracy, C. M., Leon, M. B., et al.: Electrophysiologic abnormalities in patients with hypertrophic cardiomyopathy: A consecutive analysis in 155 patients. Circulation *80*:1259, 1989, reprinted by permission of the American Heart Association, Inc.

An unusual echocardiographic pattern consisting of a ground-glass appearance has been noted in portions of the hypertrophied myocardium in HCM. Even when abnormalities are not apparent on visual inspection, quantitative texture analysis often identifies them in HCM patients.[259] It has been speculated that this pattern may be related to the abnormal cellular architecture and myocardial fibrosis that has been noted in pathological studies.[259]

A second echocardiographic feature often found in hypertrophic cardiomyopathy in addition to left ventricular hypertrophy is narrowing of the left ventricular outflow tract, which is formed by the interventricular septum anteriorly and the anterior leaflet of the mitral valve posteriorly. The mitral valve apparatus is positioned abnormally close to the septum, possibly the result of the posterior bulging of the septum.[260] When HCM is associated with a pressure gradient, there is abnormal systolic anterior motion (SAM) of the anterior leaflet, and occasionally the posterior leaflet of the mitral valve (Fig. 43-11; also see Fig. 4-95*A*, p. 100).[260,261] Although the role of SAM in *producing* the gradient is controversial, there is a close relationship between the degree of SAM and the size of the outflow gradient. Prolonged interventricular septal contact of the mitral apparatus is limited to HCM with resting pressure gradients, and there is a close temporal relationship between the onset of the pressure gradient and the onset of septal apposition of the mitral apparatus.

Three explanations have been offered for SAM: (1) the mitral valve is *pulled* against the septum by contraction of the papillary muscles, because of the abnormal location and orientation of these muscles resulting from septal hypertrophy[262]; (2) the mitral valve is *pushed* against the septum (perhaps by the left ventricular posterior wall) because of its abnormal position in the outflow tract; and (3) the mitral valve is drawn toward the septum because of the lower pressure that occurs as blood is ejected at a high velocity through a narrowed outflow tract (Venturi effect).[261] SAM of the mitral valve and dynamic left ventricular gradients is not pathognomonic of HCM but may be found in a variety of other conditions, including hypercontractile states, left ventricular hypertrophy, transposition of the great arteries, and infiltration of the septum. Even mild degrees of left ventricular hypertrophy may be associated with SAM and outflow gradients, particularly under conditions of enhanced sympathetic tone.[263,264] In many cases in conditions other than HCM, SAM is due to buckling of the chordae tendineae rather than to movement of the anterior mitral valve leaflet as occurs in HCM (although the chordae tendineae and papillary muscles may contribute to SAM in HCM).

Several other echocardiographic findings may be present: (1) a small left ventricular cavity; (2) reduced septal motion and thickening during systole, particularly of the upper septum (presumably because of the disarray of the myofibrillar architecture and abnormal contractile function); (3) normal or increased motion of the posterior wall; (4) a reduced rate of closure of the mitral valve in mid-diastole secondary to a decrease in left ventricular compliance or abnormal transmitral flow during diastole; (5) mitral valve prolapse; and (6) partial systolic closure or, more commonly, coarse systolic fluttering of the aortic valve related to turbulent blood flow in the outflow tract. The echocardiographic findings that accompany a left ventricular outflow tract gradient (SAM and aortic valve partial closure) may be quite labile, and provocative measures such as the Valsalva maneuver, pharmacologically induced vasodilatation with amyl nitrite, stimulation of contractility with isoproterenol, or an induced premature ventricular contraction may be required to precipitate the findings.

Abnormalities of diastolic function may be demonstrated by echocardiography in many patients with HCM, independent of the presence or absence of a systolic pressure gradient. The isovolumetric relaxation time, measured from aortic valve closure to mitral valve opening, is frequently prolonged and the peak velocity of left ventricular filling is reduced.[265] Because the septum is typically hypokinetic, the rate of left ventricular filling is determined primarily by the rate of free wall thinning. While there is a general relationship between the extent of hypertrophy and the severity of abnormalities of diastolic function, even nonhypertrophied regions of the HCM ventricle appear to contribute to the impairment of diastolic function seen in HCM.[266]

Doppler ultrasound has confirmed the virtual ubiquity of mitral regurgitation when an outflow gradient is present[267] and has accurately measured the magnitude of the outflow tract gradient.[268] Doppler color flow imaging reveals mitral regurgitation, most prominent in late systole, with the appearance of turbulent flow in the left ventricular outflow tract; in one study, the velocity of the latter was correlated with the degree of SAM, supporting the concept of left ventricular outflow tract obstruction.[269]

RADIONUCLIDE SCANNING. These techniques are gaining popularity in the evaluation of HCM. Thallium-201 myocardial imaging, particularly when tomographic imaging is performed, permits direct determination of the relative thicknesses of the septum and free wall and may be of particular value when technical constraints limit the reliability of echocardiographic evaluation in a given patient with presumed HCM. The utility of rest and exercise thallium-201 scintigraphy in identifying patients with HCM whose angina pectoris is due to obstructive epicardial coronary artery disease is controversial; at least in some patients, thallium-201 defects suggestive of regional myocardial ischemia are found despite angiographically normal coronary arteries.[225,270] Fixed defects, probably indicative of myocardial scarring, occur primarily in patients with impaired systolic function.[161,225] Gated radionuclide ventriculography with blood pool labeling permits the evaluation of not only the size but also the motion of the septum and left ventricle. Disproportionate thickening of the upper septum is a distinctive scintigraphic feature that may be seen in the steep left anterior oblique view. As with the echocardiogram, abnormal diastolic filling of the ventricle has been observed in patients with HCM (both with and without gradients) by computer analysis of the blood pool scan.[271]

HEMODYNAMICS

Cardiac catheterization discloses diminished diastolic left ventricular compliance and in some patients a systolic pressure gradient, when present, within the body of the left ventricle, which is separated from a subaortic chamber by the thickened septum and the anterior leaflet of the mitral valve that abuts the septum[211] (Fig. 43–10). The pressure gradient may be quite labile and may vary between 0 and 175 mm Hg. The pressure tracing may, on occasion, demonstrate a pattern of pulsus alternans.[272] The arterial pressure tracing may demonstrate a "spike and dome" configuration similar to the carotid pulse recording.[211] As a consequence of diminished left ventricular compliance, the mean and particularly the *a* wave in the left atrial pressure pulse and the left ventricular end-diastolic pressures are usually elevated. Artifactual outflow gradients may occur if the left ventricular catheter becomes entrapped in the trabeculae of a markedly hypertrophied left ventricle.[207] Proper technique and choice of catheters with side holes should clarify the mechanism of such gradients. Cardiac output may be depressed in patients with longstanding severe gradients. In the majority of patients it is normal; occasionally it is elevated.

Hemodynamic abnormalities in HCM are not limited to the left heart. Approximately one-fourth of patients demonstrate pulmonary hypertension, which is usually mild but in some cases may be moderate to severe. This may be due to elevated mean left atrial pressures. A pressure gradient in the right ventricular outflow tract occurs in approximately 15 per cent of patients who have obstruction to left ventricular outflow[231] and appears to result from muscular contraction of the infundibulum. Right atrial and right ventricular end-diastolic pressures may be slightly elevated.

LABILITY OF GRADIENT. A feature characteristic of HCM is the variability and lability of the left ventricular outflow gradient. A given patient may demonstrate a large outflow gradient on one occasion but have none at another time. In some patients without a resting gradient, it may be temporarily provoked. Three basic mechanisms are involved in the production of dynamic gradients, all of which act by reducing ventricular volume and presumably accentuate the apposition of the anterior mitral leaflet against the septum: (1) increased contractility, (2) decreased preload, and (3) decreased afterload. In a minority of patients with HCM, the gradient is midventricular[273] and may be intensified by increased contractility, which exerts a direct muscular sphincteric action. The stimuli that provoke or intensify left ventricular outflow tract gradients in HCM generally improve myocardial performance in normal subjects and in patients with most other forms of heart disease. Conversely, reductions in contractility or increases in preload or afterload, which increase left ventricular dimensions, reduce or abolish the left ventricular outflow gradient.

Alterations in the magnitude of the gradient are reflected by changes in the findings on physical examination (Table 43–11), noninvasive tests, and left heart catheterization. *It is this dynamic characteristic of HCM that distinguishes it from the discrete forms of obstruction to ventricular outflow.* An increase in the gradient usually results in a louder murmur, a longer ejection period with a more characteristic spike and dome configuration in the carotid pulse, and more flagrant echocardiographic evidence of SAM of the anterior mitral leaflet. In some patients, the intensity of the murmur may *not* track with the gradient, perhaps because in many cases the murmur reflects mitral regurgitation (at least in part).[274]

A number of bedside procedures may be useful in the evaluation of suspected hypertrophic cardiomyopathy.[237] Perhaps the most helpful is sudden standing from a squatting position. Squatting results in an increase in venous return and an increase in aortic pressure, which increases ventricular volume, diminishing the gradient and decreasing the intensity of the murmur. Sudden standing has the opposite effects and results in accentuation of the gradient and the murmur. The Valsalva maneuver is another useful bedside technique for eliciting or exacerbating the gradient. Following a transient increase in arterial pressure that usually lasts for four or five cardiac cycles after the onset of the strain coincident with an increase in heart rate, the arterial systolic and pulse pressures and ventricular volume decline, and the gradient (and murmur) increase. Following release of the strain, there is a compensatory overshoot of arterial pressure and venous return and cardiac slowing, all of which increase ventricular volume and reduce the magnitude of the gradient and the murmur. In occasional patients, there may be paradoxical attenuation of the systolic murmur despite an increase in the pressure gradient, presumably related to a critical reduction in stroke volume. Inhalation of amyl nitrite also intensifies the murmur and the abnormality of the arterial pulse. The murmur of

HCM is attenuated by passive leg elevation, handgrip, and sudden squatting from a standing position.[237]

One of the most potent stimuli for enhancing the gradient is *postextrasystolic potentiation* (p. 380), which may occur following a spontaneous premature contraction or be induced by mechanical stimulation with a catheter. The resultant increase in contractility in the beat following the extrasystole is so marked that it outweighs the otherwise salutary effect of increased ventricular filling caused by the compensatory pause and produces an increase in the gradient and often of the murmur as well. A characteristic change often occurs in the directly recorded arterial pressure tracing, which, in addition to displaying a more marked spike and dome configuration, exhibits a pulse pressure that fails to increase as expected or actually decreases (Fig. 43–10). This is one of the more reliable signs of dynamic obstruction of the left ventricular outflow tract. In some patients, the postextrasystolic murmur is attenuated despite an increase in the outflow gradient, apparently because in this setting the murmur (a hybrid of outflow tract turbulence and mitral regurgitation) is mirroring to a greater degree changes in the degree of mitral regurgitation rather than changes in the outflow tract gradient.[274]

Digitalis glycosides and the beta-adrenoceptor agonist isoproterenol augment the gradient, because they increase myocardial contractility, whereas nitroglycerin and amyl nitrite exaggerate the gradient by decreasing arterial pressure and ventricular volume.[275] Hypovolemia (as a result of hemorrhage or overly aggressive diuresis) may also provoke overt obstruction to left ventricular outflow. The intensity of the murmur and the left ventricular outflow gradient may be decreased by beta-adrenoceptor blockade, although the effect of the latter is often not dramatic and is of most hemodynamic benefit in protecting against the *increase* in the gradient that may be provoked by exercise. In most patients the severity of mitral regurgitation and the intensity of the apical blowing regurgitant murmur vary with the degree of obstruction of left ventricular outflow.

ANGIOCARDIOGRAPHY. Left ventriculography shows a hypertrophied ventricle; when an outflow gradient is present, the anterior leaflet of the mitral valve moves anteriorly during systole and encroaches upon the outflow tract. Associated with this motion of the leaflet is mitral regurgitation, which appears to be a constant finding in patients with gradients. The left ventricular cavity is often small, and systolic ejection is typically vigorous, resulting in virtual obliteration of the cavity at end systole, although the apparent hypercontractile state may relate more to reduced afterload (end-systolic wall stress) than to enhanced inotropy.[276] The papillary muscles are often prominent and may fill the left ventricular cavity in late systole. In patients with apical involvement, the extensive hypertrophy may convey a spade-like configuration to the left ventricular angiogram.[174]

It is often helpful to supplement angiographic evaluation of the left ventricle with simultaneous right ventriculography in a cranially angulated LAO projection in order to obtain optimal visualization of the size, shape, and configuration of the interventricular septum.[277] The left septal surface either is flat or bulges into the left ventricular cavity at its mid or lower portion, in contrast to the normal findings of the septum curving toward the right ventricle.

In patients over 45 years of age, obstructive coronary artery disease is rather common, although the symptoms of ischemic pain are indistinguishable from those of patients with normal coronary angiograms and HCM.[278] The left anterior descending and septal perforator coronary arteries may demonstrate phasic narrowing during systole (myocardial bridging) in the absence of fixed obstructive lesions.[279]

NATURAL HISTORY

The clinical course in HCM is varied; in many patients symptoms are absent or mild, remain stable, and in some instances improve (Fig. 43–14) over a period of 5 to 10 years. The annual attrition is about 3 per cent a year in adults, and 6 per

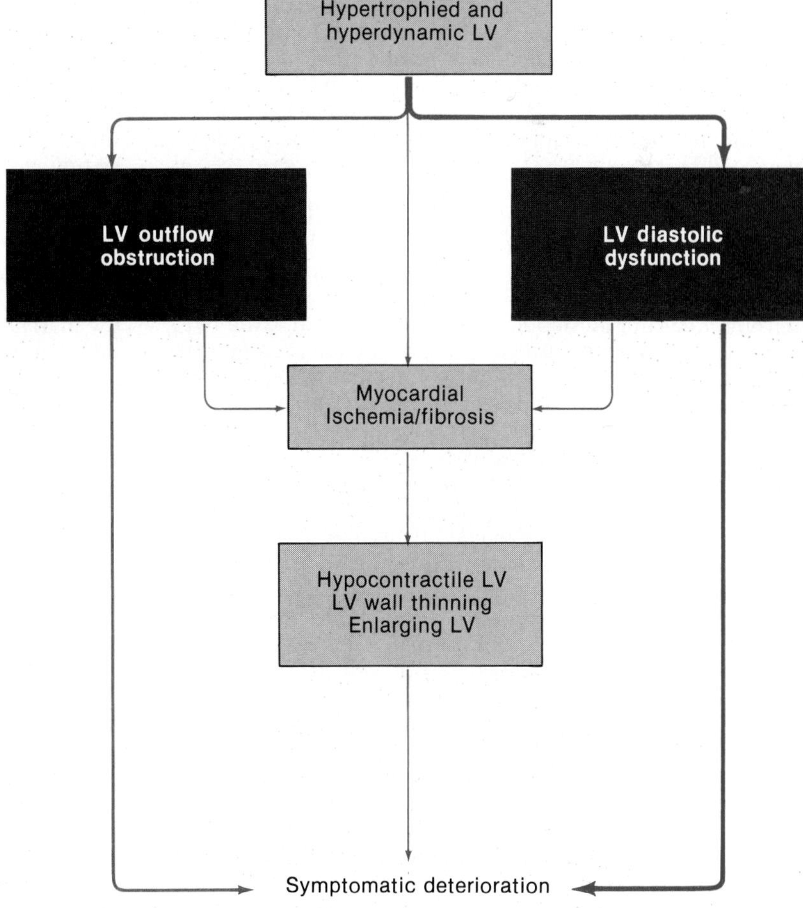

FIGURE 43–14. Possible evolution of disease state in hypertrophic cardiomyopathy. Patients with hypertrophic cardiomyopathy initially have a hypertrophied and hyperdynamic left ventricle. Approximately 20 per cent of patients exhibit left ventricular outflow gradient that can lead to progressive symptomatic deterioration. Patients with gradients, as well as many other patients without them, may have left ventricular diastolic dysfunction that can also lead to progressive symptomatic deterioration. Patients can also proceed through a course characterized by progressive myocardial fibrosis. This may lead to an enlarging and hypocontractile left ventricle and associated symptomatic deterioration. (From Maron, B. J., and Epstein, S. E.: Hypertrophic cardiomyopathy: Pathophysiology and therapy. *In:* Braunwald, E. (ed.): Heart Disease: A Textbook of Cardiovascular Medicine. 3rd ed. Philadelphia, W. B. Saunders Company, Update No. 7, pp. 157–168, 1989.)

cent a year in children[280]; clinical deterioration (aside from sudden death) is usually slow.[161,247,280] Although symptoms are unrelated to the severity or even the presence of a gradient,[210,281] the percentage of severely symptomatic patients does increase with age.[231,280] The onset of atrial fibrillation usually leads to an increase in symptoms, and prompt cardioversion (often pharmacological) is usually indicated.[251] Pregnancy is generally well tolerated, although maternal death has been reported.[282]

Progression of HCM to left ventricular dilatation and dysfunction[283] without a gradient, i.e., dilated cardiomyopathy, occurs in upward of 10 per cent of patients.[210] It appears to result, at least in part, from wall thinning and scar formation as a consequence of myocardial ischemia caused by small vessel coronary artery disease.[284] The extent of left ventricular hypertrophy usually remains stable over time, although a minority of patients may develop increasing degrees of hypertrophy.[285] In some children, the pattern of HCM may develop despite a previous normal echocardiogram; this does not appear to occur in adults.[286] Its occurrence does emphasize that a single normal echocardiogram does *not* exclude HCM in a child or adolescent; cellular disarray and the attendant risk of sudden death may be present even in the absence of left ventricular hypertrophy.[234,287] A marker for the later appearance of clinical HCM may be an initially abnormal electrocardiogram demonstrating increased QRS voltage.[288] Substantial changes in the magnitude of the gradient occur in a small proportion of patients. Both the appearance (or intensification) of a gradient are usually accompanied by an increase in symptoms.[289]

Sudden Death. Death is most often sudden in HCM and may occur in previously asymptomatic patients, in individuals who were unaware they had the disease, or in patients with an otherwise stable course.[231,280] Those features that most reliably identify high-risk patients include young age (<30 years) at diagnosis and family history of HCM with sudden death.[280] The presence or severity of an outflow tract gradient,[290] the degree of functional limitation, and symptoms in general do not correlate with the risk of death.[161] A history of syncope is ominous in children,[247,280,291-293] although not so much in adults. In adults, the single most useful marker of increased risk is nonsustained ventricular tachycardia (NSVT) on 48-hour electrocardiographic monitoring, although most patients (perhaps 75 per cent) with NSVT do *not* die suddenly.[161,210,247,280] In children, the mechanism of death may be different, since preexisting ventricular arrhythmias are much less common.[294] Perhaps in some patients, especially the young, the precipitating event is hemodynamic rather than primarily arrhythmic in origin.[247] Sudden death often occurs during exercise, and strenuous exertion should probably be proscribed in all patients with HCM whether or not symptoms are prominent. Unsuspected HCM is the most common abnormality found at autopsy in young competitive athletes who die suddenly.[295] The development of atrial fibrillation also may be a poor prognostic sign. The degree of left ventricular hypertrophy does not appear to correlate well with prognosis, since patients with massive hypertrophy are often no more than minimally symptomatic and appear to have no more malignant courses than do patients with moderate hypertrophy.[232,247] Sudden death is unlikely, however, in asymptomatic or mildly symptomatic patients with mild hypertrophy.[296]

It is presumed, but not established, that sudden death is due to a ventricular arrhythmia, although atrial arrhythmias may play a role in sensitizing the heart so that ventricular arrhythmias appear subsequently.

MANAGEMENT

Management of patients with HCM is directed toward alleviation of symptoms, prevention of complications, and reduction in the risk of death (Fig. 43-15). Whether asymptomatic patients should be treated is unestablished, because no adequate controlled studies are available.[210] However, reversible thallium perfusion defects develop during exercise in half of the asymptomatic patients with HCM,[225] and most of these defects can be improved by the use of verapamil.[297] *Digitalis glycosides* should generally be avoided unless atrial fibrillation or systolic dysfunction develops.[161] *Diuretics* were previously thought to be contraindicated for fear of precipitating or worsening the outflow gradient. More recent experience indicates that cautious use of diuretics often helps reduce symptoms of pulmonary congestion, particularly when combined with beta-adrenergic blockers or calcium antagonists.[161,298] *Beta-adrenergic agonists* may improve diastolic filling but should not be used because they may produce ischemia[299] and usually worsen the outflow gradient.

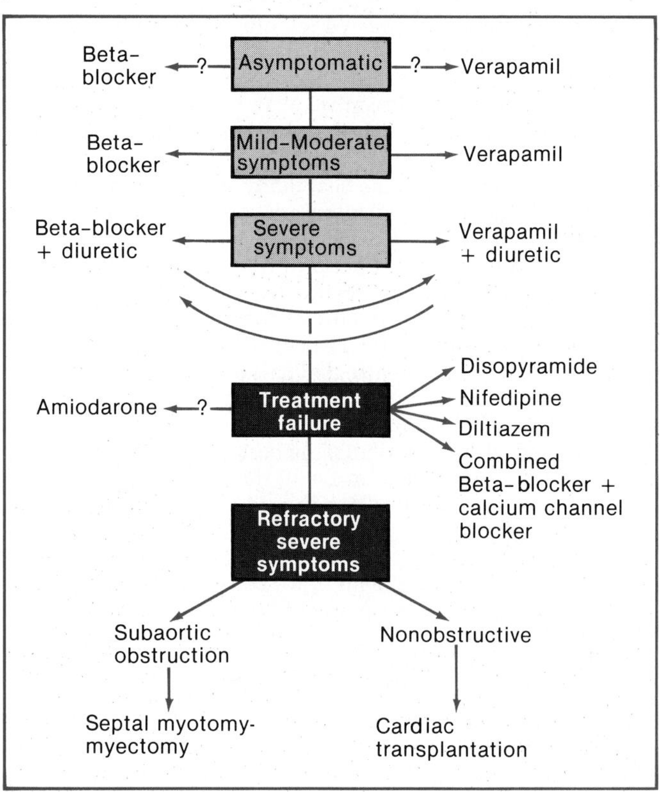

FIGURE 43-15. Therapeutic strategies for patients with hypertrophic cardiomyopathy. Question marks indicate treatment recommendations that are largely unresolved. (From Maron, B. J., and Epstein, S. E.: Hypertrophic cardiomyopathy: Pathophysiology and therapy. *In* Braunwald, E. (ed.): Heart Disease: A Textbook of Cardiovascular Medicine. 3rd ed. Philadelphia, W. B. Saunders Company, Update No. 7, pp. 157-168, 1989.)

BETA-ADRENOCEPTOR BLOCKERS. These drugs are the mainstay of medical therapy. With their use, angina, dyspnea, and presyncope may all be improved.[161] Beta blockade may prevent the increase in outflow obstruction that accompanies exercise, although resting gradients are largely unchanged.[298] It decreases the determinants of myocardial oxygen consumption and thus angina pectoris, and perhaps exerts an antiarrhythmic action. Angina pectoris generally responds more favorably to treatment with a beta blocker than does dyspnea.[5] It has also been suggested that beta blockade may prevent sudden death, but its efficacy for this purpose has not been established.[280] Beta blockade also blunts the chronotropic response, thus limiting the demand for increased myocardial oxygen delivery. Beta-adrenoceptor blockade previously was thought to have a beneficial effect on diastolic ventricular filling, but it now appears that any benefit is simply the consequence of a slower heart rate.[161,298] The overall clinical response to beta blockade is variable, however, since only about one-third to two-thirds of patients experience symptomatic improvement[161]; a double-blinded, properly controlled test of this therapy has not been reported. It is reasonable to try large doses of propranolol (greater than 320 mg per day) in patients without contraindications who have not experienced adequate symptomatic improvement with conventional doses. Some patients so treated experience symptomatic improvement and improved exercise capacity.[161]

CALCIUM ANTAGONISTS. These are an increasingly popular alternative to beta-adrenoceptor blockade in the management of HCM[300]; most of the experience has been with verapamil, with more limited use of nifedipine and diltiazem. There is no clear consensus whether therapy should be initiated first with a beta-adrenergic or a calcium antagonist. Exercise performance in particular may be improved when patients are changed from a beta-adrenoceptor blocker to verapamil. Both the hypercontractile systolic function and the abnormalities of diastolic filling may be related to abnormal calcium kinetics, and drugs that block the inward transport of calcium across the myocardial cell membrane may be able to rectify both abnormalities.

Verapamil has been the most widely utilized calcium-channel blocking agent in this condition.[301] Its use was suggested, at least in part, by the observation that it produces a protective and beneficial effect in the hereditary cardiomyopathy of the Syrian hamster, a condition marked by intracellular calcium overload, in which propranolol is ineffective.[197] Although the vasodilator effects of verapamil should not be helpful in HCM, it appears that by depressing myocardial contractility, verapamil can decrease the left ventricular outflow gradient when given intravenously or orally. Perhaps more important from a symptomatic point of view, verapamil improves diastolic filling in HCM,[302,303] at least in part by reducing asynchronous regional diastolic performance.[304] Verapamil appears to improve diastolic filling by improved relaxation rather than by changes in left ventricular diastolic stiffness; at any given diastolic volume, filling pressure is reduced. While variable clinical responses have been reported with verapamil, about two-thirds or more of patients show increased exercise capacity and an improved symptomatic status.[301,305,306] Sustained symptomatic improvement has been noted with the long-term administration of verapamil in ambulatory patients,[303] although important adverse effects, including sudden death, have been observed in a small fraction of patients so treated. Complications with verapamil include suppression of sinus node automaticity and inhibition of atrioventricular conduction, vasodilatation, and negative inotropic effects. These side effects may culminate in hypotension, pulmonary edema, and death; there is a suggestion that antiarrhythmic agents, especially quinidine, may exacerbate the deleterious hemodynamic effects of verapamil. Because of these adverse effects, it has been suggested that verapamil should not be used, or be used only with extreme caution, in patients with high left ventricular filling pressure or symptoms of paroxysmal nocturnal dyspnea or orthopnea. Unfortunately, these are usually the patients who are in greatest need of therapy. In addition, patients with abnormalities of electrical impulse generation or conduction should not receive verapamil unless a pacemaker is in place. We favor initiation of therapy with doses of 240 to 360 mg/day, increasing as needed to higher doses (480 mg/day).

Nifedipine has also been used in HCM, and it may have advantages over verapamil, since it causes less depression of atrioventricular conduction, although it is a more potent vasodilator. Reports of its effect on diastolic function have shown inconsistent results.[161,298,307,308] Nifedipine may also alleviate the chest pain in these patients. Combined administration of nifedipine and propranolol may be of benefit in some patients, particularly those with outflow gradients. However, it should be recognized that the potent vasodilator effects of nifedipine may lead to systemic hypotension and an increase in the outflow gradient,[308] and in high doses it may depress left ventricular function.[309]

Diltiazem has also shown beneficial effects in HCM, producing improved diastolic function.[310] Although the data are not conclusive, there are suggestive findings that calcium-channel blocker therapy may promote regression of left ventricular hypertrophy with a reduction in muscle mass.[311]

OTHER NONSURGICAL MEASURES. *Disopyramide*, an antiarrhythmic drug that alters calcium kinetics, has produced symptomatic improvement and abolition of the pressure gradient in patients with HCM, presumably as a consequence of depression of left ventricular systolic performance.[312-315] Long-term experience with disopyramide is limited, particularly in asymptomatic patients and those without outflow gradients.[161,298]

Beta-adrenoceptor blockers, calcium antagonists, and the conventional antiarrhythmic agents do not appear to suppress serious ventricular arrhythmias or reduce the frequency of supraventricular arrhythmias.[280] However, *amiodarone* is effective in the treatment of both supraventricular and ventricular tachyarrhythmias in HCM without significantly affecting left ventricular function.[316] Although there is some belief that amiodarone improves prognosis in HCM,[317,318] only limited and inconclusive data are available. We do not favor empiric use of amiodarone (or other antiarrhythmic agents for that matter) and share the concern[210] about possible proarrhythmic effects[318a,b] and potential toxicity.[298] In high-risk patients or those surviving a cardiac arrest, insertion of an implantable cardioverter-defibrillator should be considered.[319]

Strenuous exercise should be avoided because of the risk of sudden death; it is the major cause of a fatal outcome in HCM cardiomyopathy. Even though there are many individuals with subclinical HCM who exercise vigorously, the risk of sudden death is sufficiently real that competitive sports are proscribed in patients with marked hypertrophy or other factors believed to be associated with increased risk; e.g., marked left ventricular hypertrophy or a history of sudden death in relatives with HCM, evidence of a marked outflow gradient (>40 mm Hg at rest), and important supraventricular or ventricular arrhythmias.[320] Atrial fibrillation should usually be pharmacologically or electrically converted because of the hemodynamic consequences of loss of the atrial contribution to ventricular filling in this disorder. Infective endocarditis may occur in about 5 per cent of patients, and antibiotic prophylaxis is indicated.[231] The infection usually occurs on the aortic valve or mitral apparatus, on the endocardium, or at the site of the contact lesion on the septum; thus, chronic endocardial trauma may provide a nidus for subsequent infection. Anticoagulants should be given to patients with chronic atrial fibrillation when no contraindication exists.

SURGICAL TREATMENT. A variety of surgical procedures aimed at reducing the outflow gradient have been developed and are most commonly utilized in the markedly symptomatic patient who has not responded well to medical management.[321,321a,321b] The most popular operation for HCM consists of excising a portion of the hypertrophied septum (Figs. 43-16 and 43-17). A transaortic approach with septal myotomy-myectomy is the most widely utilized procedure, although left transventricular as well as combined transaortic and left ventricular approaches have also been employed successfully.[321] Operative management is facilitated by intraoperative echocardiography,[322] and operative mortality is now ≤5 per cent.[321,323] Operation often relieves the obstruction (Fig. 43-18) as well as the mitral regurgitation.[324] The reduction in left ventricular systolic pressure produced by the operation leads to reduced myocardial oxygen demands, especially during stress.[325] Patients over the age of 65 as well as under the age of 10 years have undergone successful operations with benefits and risks comparable to those in the usual patient.[326] Surgery results in long-term improvement in symptoms and exercise capacity in about 70 per cent of patients.[161,327] Furthermore, septal myotomy-myectomy does not produce important impairment of global left ventricular function at rest or during exercise. Myotomy-myectomy may be combined with other necessary operative procedures (particularly coronary artery bypass grafting and mitral valve replacement), although the risk is increased somewhat.[328] Although mitral valve replacement is performed in fewer centers, the long-term results also have been favorable (Fig. 43-18), with symptomatic benefit and an improvement in

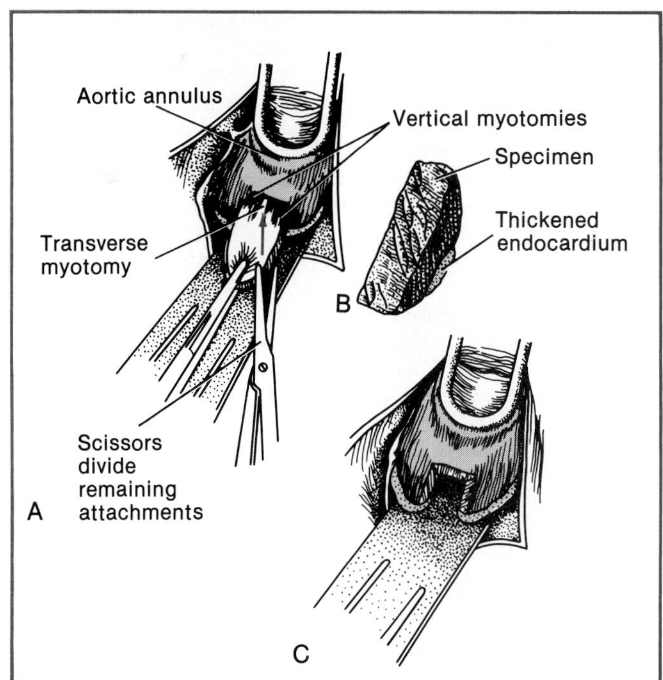

FIGURE 43-16. Illustration of standard ventricular septal myotomy-myectomy operation performed through an aortotomy. *A*, Two vertical and parallel incisions are made in the most basal portion of ventricular septum about 1 cm apart. A third incision is made transversely, connecting the initial two parallel myotomies. Attachments of the muscle bar to the septum are divided. *B*, This segment of muscle is isolated and excised. *C*, At completion of the myotomy-myectomy operation, a rectangular channel is created, about 1 cm wide, 1 cm deep, and 4 cm long, extending from a point 5 to 10 mm below the aortic annulus to a point just distal to the systolic contact between the distal portion of mitral valve leaflets and ventricular septum. In some patients, additional tissue may be resected from the margins of the channel to achieve greater enlargement of the left ventricular outflow tract. (From McIntosh, C. L., and Maron, B. J.: Current operative treatment of obstructive hypertrophic cardiomyopathy. Circulation *78*:487, 1988, reprinted by permission of the American Heart Association, Inc.)

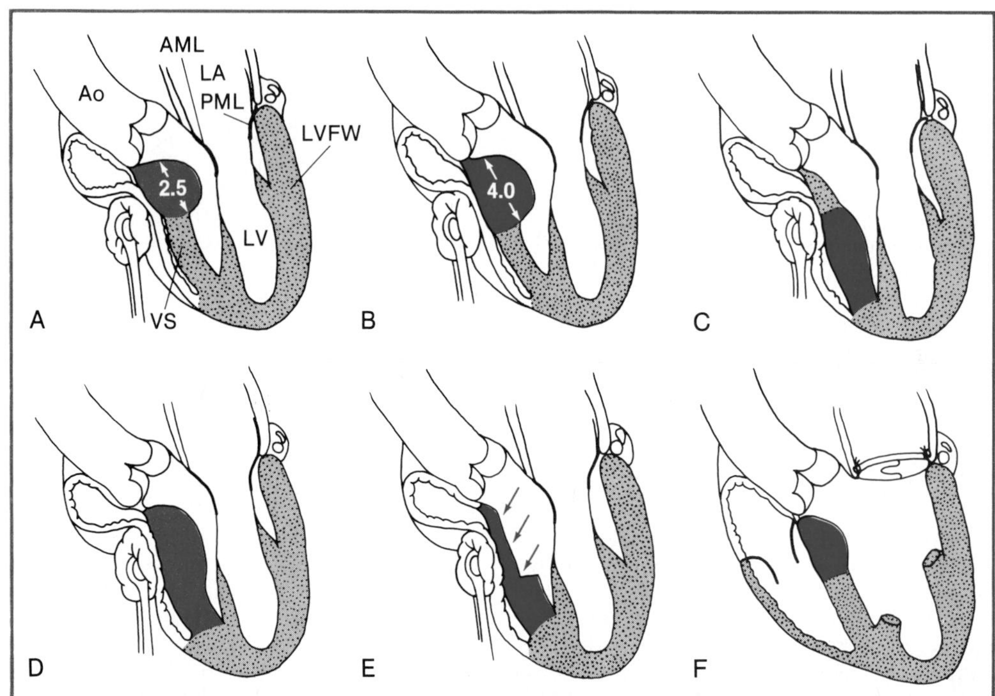

FIGURE 43-17. Illustration of the morphological spectrum of hypertrophic cardiomyopathy and importance of the distribution of ventricular septal (VS) thickening to the myotomy-myectomy operation (shown in diastole). *A*–*D*. Different distributions of ventricular septal hypertrophy in the longitudinal cross-sectional plane; thickened areas of septum are denoted in red. *A*, Septal hypertrophy is quite localized to the most proximal 2 cm of the anterior basal septum. *B*, Hypertrophy involves the upper and midseptal areas, extending over the proximal 4 cm of anterior septum. *C*, Basal portion of the anterior ventricular septum is relatively thin, whereas substantially increased septal thickness is evident at the point of systolic contact between mitral valve and septum as well as in the more distal portion of the septum. *D*, Hypertrophy is more diffuse and involves the entire septum homogeneously. *E*, Completed myotomy-myectomy channel (arrows) created in the same left ventricle that is depicted in *D*, extending from near the aortic annulus to just beyond the mitral valve tips. *F*, Low-profile disc prosthesis implanted in the mitral position after the native mitral valve has been removed from a patient with relatively thin ventricular septum. AML = anterior mitral leaflet, Ao = aorta, LA = left atrium, LV = left ventricle, LVFW = left ventricular free wall, PML = posterior mitral leaflet. (From McIntosh, C. L., and Maron, B. J.: Current operative treatment of obstructive hypertrophic cardiomyopathy. Circulation *78*:487, 1988, reprinted by permission of the American Heart Association, Inc.)

hemodynamics.[329–332] The rationale for this operation is that it abolishes obstruction by preventing systolic anterior movement (SAM) of the mitral valve (p. 100). It appears to be of particular value in patients with less than severe (18 mm) thickness of the upper septum or other atypical septal morphology, in those with previous myotomy-myectomy with persistent severe symptoms and obstruction, as well as in patients with independent intrinsic mitral valve disease.[331] In appropriate candidates not responding to maximal standard medical and surgical therapy, cardiac transplantation may be an option.[333]

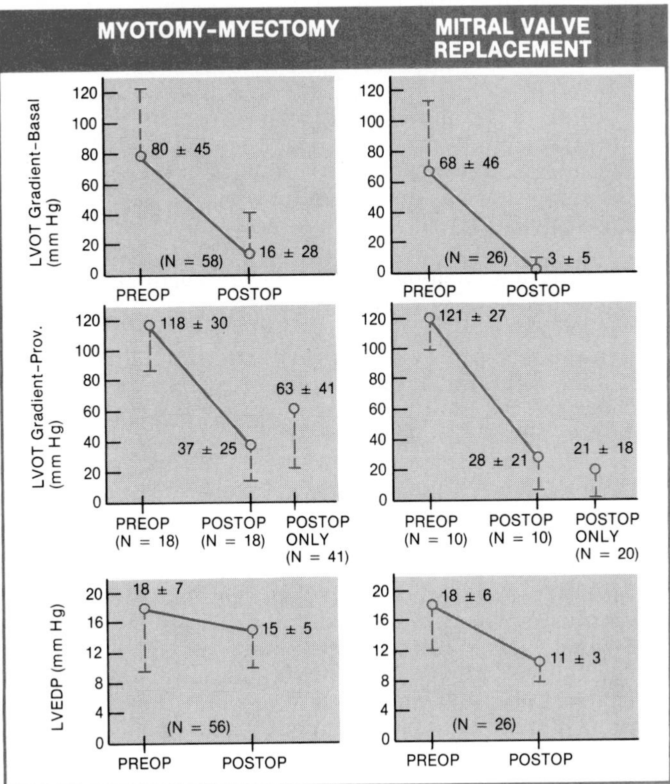

FIGURE 43–18. Plots of hemodynamic alterations associated with ventricular septal myotomy-myectomy (*left*) and mitral valve replacement (*right*) in patients with hypertrophic cardiomyopathy operated on at the National Institutes of Health from 1982 to 1988. Data are from 84 patients (among a total of 156 undergoing operation) who had both preoperative studies and a second cardiac catheterization 6 to 12 months after operation. Data are mean ± SD. LVEDP = left ventricular end-diastolic pressure, LVOT = left ventricular outflow tract, PROV = provocable (with infusion of isoproterenol). PREOP = preoperative patients, POSTOP = postoperative patients, POSTOP ONLY, patients in whom the subaortic gradients recorded under basal conditions preoperatively were 100 mm Hg or more so that measurements of provocable gradients in the catheterization laboratory were not considered to be clinically justified. Therefore, in these patients, provocable gradients were only measured postoperatively at a time when the basal gradient was either absent or small. (From McIntosh, C. L., and Maron, B. J.: Current operative treatment of obstructive hypertrophic cardiomyopathy. Circulation *78*:487, 1988, reprinted by permission of the American Heart Association, Inc.)

Restrictive and Infiltrative Cardiomyopathies

Of the three major functional categories of the cardiomyopathies (dilated, hypertrophic, and restrictive), the restrictive are the least common in Western countries, although secondary forms of restrictive cardiomyopathy such as endomyocardial disease (see p. 1421) are common in specific geographic regions.[334] The hallmark of the restrictive cardiomyopathies is abnormal diastolic function; the ventricular walls are excessively rigid and impede ventricular filling. Contractile function, on the other hand, is often relatively unimpaired. Thus, restrictive cardiomyopathy bears some functional resemblance to constrictive pericarditis, which is also characterized by normal or near-normal systolic function but abnormal ventricular filling.[334–336] Differentiation of the two conditions is mandatory because of the potential for successful surgical treatment of the latter.[337,338]

A variety of specific pathological processes may result in restrictive cardiomyopathy, although the cause often remains unknown. Myocardial fibrosis, infiltration, or endomyocardial scarring is usually responsible for the abnormal diastolic behavior. Myocardial involvement with amyloid is a common cause of secondary restrictive cardiomyopathy in the Western world, although it can be caused by a variety of other conditions (Table 43–13).[334,339]

Some patients may manifest the features of a restrictive cardiomyopathy and yet exhibit the pathological findings of left ventricular hypertrophy and fibrosis; certainly ventricular hypertrophy, especially hypertrophic cardiomyopathy can cause diminished ventricular compliance but not restrictive cardiomyopathy per se. Findings include biatrial dilatation, often with thrombi in the atrial appendages, and normal left ventricular cavity size.[340] Rare patients may present with findings of restrictive physiology but without fibrosis, infiltration, or other pathological findings demonstrable in the heart. It has been suggested that a defect in myocardial relaxation is present in these patients.[334] Unlike dilated and especially hypertrophic cardiomyopathy, restrictive cardiomyopathy is only rarely familially linked.[341,342]

HEMODYNAMICS. The clinical and hemodynamic features of restrictive heart disease simulate those of chronic constrictive pericarditis; endomyocardial biopsy, CT scanning (Fig. 11–9, p. 317), and especially MR imaging (Fig. 11–31, p. 328) may be particularly useful in differentiating the two diseases by demonstrating myocardial scarring or infiltration (biopsy) or thickening of the pericardium (CT and MR imaging).[334–337,340,343–345] With the use of these modalities,

TABLE 43–13 CLASSIFICATION OF THE RESTRICTIVE CARDIOMYOPATHIES

MYOCARDIAL
- A. Noninfiltrative
  - Idiopathic
  - Scleroderma
- B. Infiltrative
  - Amyloid
  - Sarcoid
  - Gaucher disease
  - Hurler disease
- C. Storage diseases
  - Hemochromatosis
  - Fabry disease
  - Glycogen storage diseases

ENDOMYOCARDIAL
- Endomyocardial fibrosis
- Hypereosinophilic syndrome
- Carcinoid
- Metastatic malignancies
- Radiation
- Anthracycline toxicity

exploratory thoracotomy should be required rarely if at all.[337] The characteristic hemodynamic feature in both conditions is a deep and rapid early decline in ventricular pressure at the onset of diastole, with a rapid rise to a plateau in early diastole.[343] This dip and plateau has been termed the "square root" sign (Fig. 45–14, p. 1483) and is manifested in the atrial pressure tracing as a prominent *y* descent followed by a rapid rise and plateau. The x descent may also be rapid, and the combination results in the characteristic M or W waveform in the atrial pressure tracing. The *a* wave is prominent and often is of the same amplitude as the *v* wave.[343] Both systemic and pulmonary venous pressures are elevated, although patients with restrictive heart disease typically have left ventricular filling pressures that exceed right ventricular filling pressure by more than 5 mm Hg, and this difference is accentuated by exercise.[337] In this respect they differ from patients with constrictive pericarditis, in whom diastolic pressures are similar in both ventricles, usually differing by not more than 5 mm Hg. The pulmonary artery systolic pressure is often greater than 45 mm Hg in patients with restrictive cardiomyopathy but is lower in constrictive pericarditis.[334,337] Furthermore, the plateau of the right ventricular diastolic pressure is usually at least one-third of the peak right ventricular systolic pressure in patients with constrictive pericarditis, while it is frequently less in restrictive cardiomyopathy.[334]

CLINICAL MANIFESTATIONS. Exercise intolerance is frequent because of the inability of patients with restrictive cardiomyopathy to increase their cardiac output by tachycardia without further compromising ventricular filling.[337] Weakness and dyspnea are often prominent. Exertional chest pain may be prominent in a small fraction of patients but is usually absent. Particularly in advanced cases, an elevated central venous pressure, with peripheral edema, enlarged liver, ascites, and anasarca may be present.[337] *Physical examination* may reveal jugular venous distention, and an S_3, S_4, or both. An inspiratory increase in venous pressure (Kussmaul sign, p. 1482) may be seen. However, in contrast to constrictive pericarditis, the apex impulse is usually palpable.[334]

Various ancillary laboratory findings in addition to endomyocardial biopsy, CT scanning, and MR imaging may be useful in distinguishing between constrictive and restrictive disease. While pericardial calcification is neither absolutely sensitive nor specific for constrictive pericarditis (p. 1485), its presence in a patient in whom the differential diagnosis rests between restrictive cardiomyopathy and constrictive pericarditis lends strong support to the latter diagnosis.[337] The echocardiogram may demonstrate thickening of the left ventricular wall and an increase of left ventricular mass in patients with infiltrative disease causing restrictive cardiomyopathy.[334] The pattern of filling of the left ventricle differs in the two conditions, as can be demonstrated by digitized echocardiograms,[346] transthoracic[347,348] and transesophageal Doppler[349] ultrasound, and radionuclide ventriculography (Fig. 43–19).[350,351] In patients with constrictive pericarditis, respiratory variations in left ventricular isovolumic relaxation time and peak mitral valve velocity in early diastole are prominent; however, this finding is not present in patients with restrictive cardiomyopathy (or in normal subjects).[348]

The prognosis in restrictive cardiomyopathy is one of relentless symptomatic progression; only 10 per cent of patients are alive at 10 years.[340] No specific therapy (other than symptomatic) is available,[340] although there is speculation that calcium antagonists may be of some value.[334]

AMYLOIDOSIS

ETIOLOGY AND TYPES. Amyloidosis is a disease complex that results from deposition of unique twisted β-pleated sheet fibrils formed from various proteins by several different pathogenic mechanisms.[334,352] Amyloid may be found in almost any organ, but clinically evident disease does not appear unless there is extensive infiltration. Several classifications systems have been used to characterize the different clinical presentations of amyloidosis. The condition with the traditional designation of *primary amyloidosis* is now known to be caused by the production of an amyloid protein composed of portions of immunoglobulin light chain (designated AL) by a monoclonal population of plasma cells, often as a consequence of multiple myeloma. *Secondary amyloidosis* is due to the production of a nonimmunoglobulin protein, termed AA.[352] Six different forms of *familial amyloidosis* are recognized; they result from the production of a prealbumin protein, and generally present in one of three clinical presentations: progressive neuropathy, cardiomyopathy, or nephropathy.[352] *Senile systemic amyloidosis* also is due to the production of a prealbumin protein and is becoming increasingly common as the average age of the population increases. Scattered deposits of amyloid localized to the aorta or atria

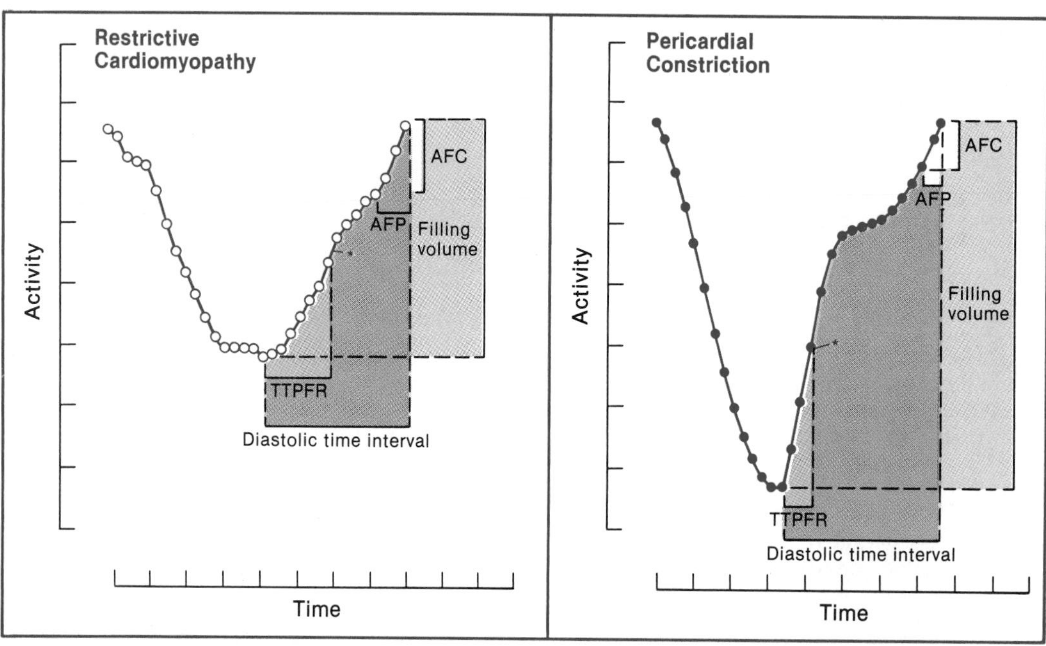

FIGURE 43–19. Time-activity curves showing ventricular emptying and filling for a patient with restrictive cardiomyopathy (*left*), and a patient with pericardial constriction (*right*). Note the slow initial filling in restrictive cardiomyopathy and the rapid initial filling in constriction. * = Peak filling rate, AFC = atrial filling contribution, AFP = atrial filling period, TTPFR = time to peak filling rate. (From Aroney, C. N., Ruddy, T. D., Dighero, H., et al.: Differentiation of restrictive cardiomyopathy from pericardial constriction: Assessment of diastolic function by radionuclide angiography. Reprinted by permission from the American College of Cardiology. J. Am. Coll. Cardiol. *13*:1007, 1989.)

are virtually ubiquitous in individuals over the age of 80; one-fourth have diffuse cardiac involvement.[353] Small deposits of amyloid may often be found in the pulmonary vessels or the vessels of other organs as well.

CARDIAC AMYLOIDOSIS

Involvement of the heart is a common finding and is the most frequent cause of death in amyloidosis associated with an immunocyte dyscrasia.[353] Clinically apparent heart disease is present in one-third to one-half of patients, although the heart is virtually always involved when studied pathologically.[352,353] In secondary amyloidosis, on the other hand, clinically significant cardiac involvement is uncommon (10 per cent or less); the myocardial deposits are typically small and perivascular and usually do not result in significant myocardial dysfunction.[353] Familial amyloidosis is only occasionally associated with overt cardiac involvement and then usually only late in the course of the disease. The clinical course is usually dominated by neurological or renal dysfunction.[353] Cardiac involvement in senile amyloidosis varies from small atrial deposits that do not result in functional impairment to extensive ventricular involvement with resultant cardiac failure.[353]

Cardiac amyloidosis occurs more commonly in men than in women, and it is rare before the age of 30 years.[352,354] Even in the familial form, the onset of clinical cardiac disease usually does not occur before the age of 35 years and generally occurs much later in life.[354]

PATHOLOGY. The pathological findings often include mild atrial enlargement, usually without significant ventricular dilatation (Fig. 43–20). The walls of both ventricles are typically firm, rubbery, noncompliant, and thickened.[334,353,354] Amyloid is present between the myocardial fibers,[353] (Fig. 43–21) with extensive deposition in the papillary muscles occurring commonly. Serial sections of the sinoatrial and atrioventricular nodes and the bundle branches may disclose amyloid deposits, particularly in the familial forms, although fibrosis of these structures is perhaps more common.[354] In addition, endocardial involvement of the atria and ventricles is frequent (Fig. 43–20). Amyloidosis often results in focal thickening of or deposits on the cardiac valves, but these abnormalities do not appear to interfere with valvular function, other than to produce murmurs. The intramural coronary arteries and veins frequently contain amyloid deposits in the media and adventitia, occasionally compromising the lumina of the vessels.[353,354]

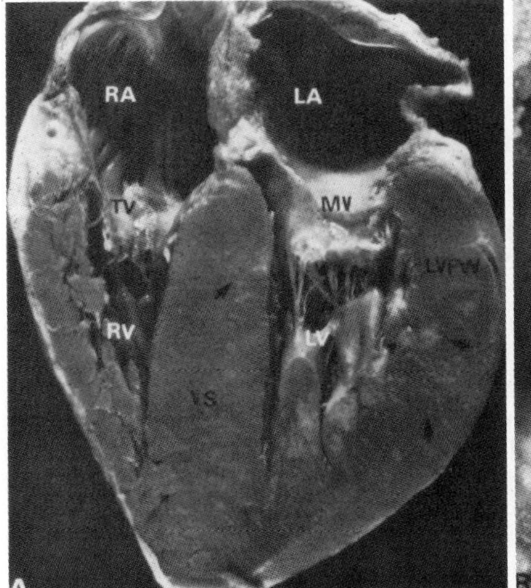

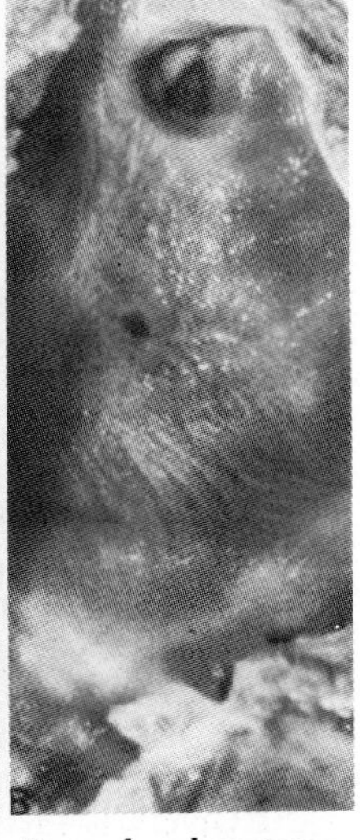

FIGURE 43–20. Amyloid heart disease. ***A,*** **Four-chamber tomographic view of heart showing asymmetrically thickened ventricular septum (VS) compared with left ventricular free wall (LVFW) and grossly visible myocardial and valvular amyloid deposits (arrows).** ***B,*** **Close-up of left atrium showing characteristic "gritty" endocardium of cardiac amyloidosis. LA = left atrium, LV = left ventricle, MV = mitral valve, RA = right atrium, RV = right ventricle, TV = tricuspid valve. (From Waller, B. F.: Pathology of the cardiomyopathies. J. Am. Soc. Echocardiog.** ***1*****:4, 1988.)**

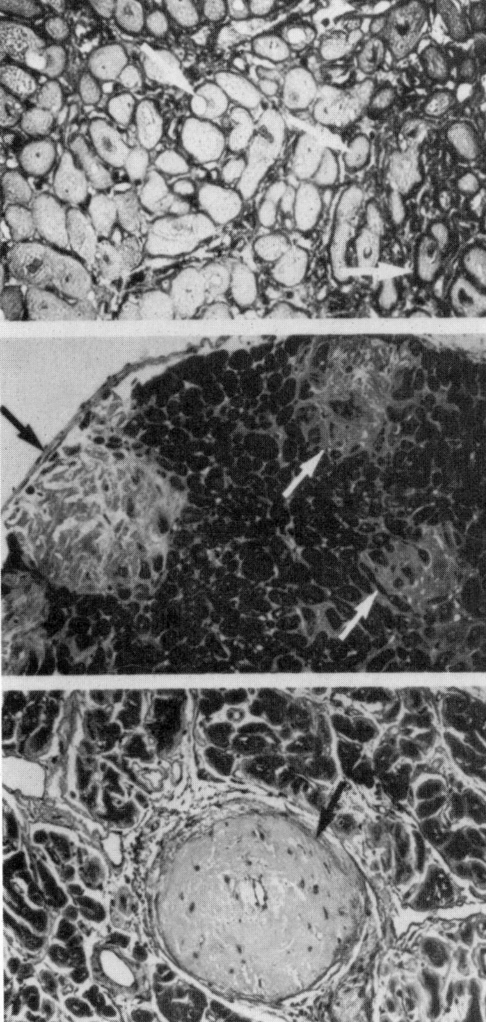

FIGURE 43–21. Patterns of cardiac amyloid deposition. ***Top,*** **pericellular (arrows);** ***middle,*** **nodular (arrows); and** ***bottom,*** **vascular (arrow). (Top, sulfated alcian blue, ×270; middle and bottom, hematoxylin-eosin, ×135.) (From Pellikka, P. A., Holmes, D. R., Edwards, W. D., et al.: Endomyocardial biopsy in 30 patients with primary amyloidosis and suspected cardiac involvement. Arch. Intern. Med.** ***148*****:662, 1988.)**

CLINICAL MANIFESTATIONS. Involvement of the cardiovascular system by amyloidosis occurs in four general forms.

1. The most common presentation of cardiac amyloidosis is that of *restrictive cardiomyopathy.*[353] Right-sided findings dominate the clinical presentation; peripheral edema is a prominent finding while paroxysmal nocturnal dyspnea and orthopnea are absent. Amyloid infiltration of the myocardium results in increased stiffness of the myocardium, producing the characteristic diastolic dip and plateau (square root sign) in the ventricular pressure pulse that may simulate constrictive pericarditis. In contrast to the accelerated early left ventricular diastolic filling found in constrictive pericarditis, cardiac amyloidosis is marked by an impaired rate of early diastolic filling, because of the stiffness of the ventricle.

2. A second common presentation is congestive heart failure due to *systolic dysfunction,* which occurs in many patients. Hemodynamic evidence of restriction of ventricular filling may not be prominent in these patients. The course of this form of the disease is often one of relentless progression, usually poorly responsive to treatment. Angina pectoris occurs on occasion and may be due to amyloid involvement of the coronary arteries or to concomitant atherosclerotic disease.[353,354]

3. *Orthostatic hypotension* is the third mode of presentation, occurring in about 10 per cent of cases. Although most likely

due to amyloid infiltration of the autonomic nervous system or of blood vessels (p. 1647), amyloid deposition in the heart and adrenals may contribute to this manifestation. Hypovolemia as a result of the nephrotic syndrome secondary to renal amyloidosis may aggravate the postural hypotension.[353]

4. An *abnormality of cardiac impulse formation and conduction* is the fourth and least common mode of presentation and may result in arrhythmias and conduction disturbances.[353] Sudden death, presumably arrhythmic in origin, is relatively common.[353,354]

Physical examination often reveals findings of congestive heart failure, especially right-sided; a systolic murmur due to atrioventricular valvular regurgitation may be present.[353] Particularly in patients with the restrictive cardiomyopathic presentation, jugular venous distention, a protodiastolic gallop, hepatomegaly, peripheral edema, and a narrow pulse pressure are found.[334] A fourth heart sound is uncommon, presumably due to amyloid infiltration of the atrium. Patients typically are normotensive or hypotensive; even previously hypertensive individuals usually have a fall in blood pressure as the disease progresses.[353]

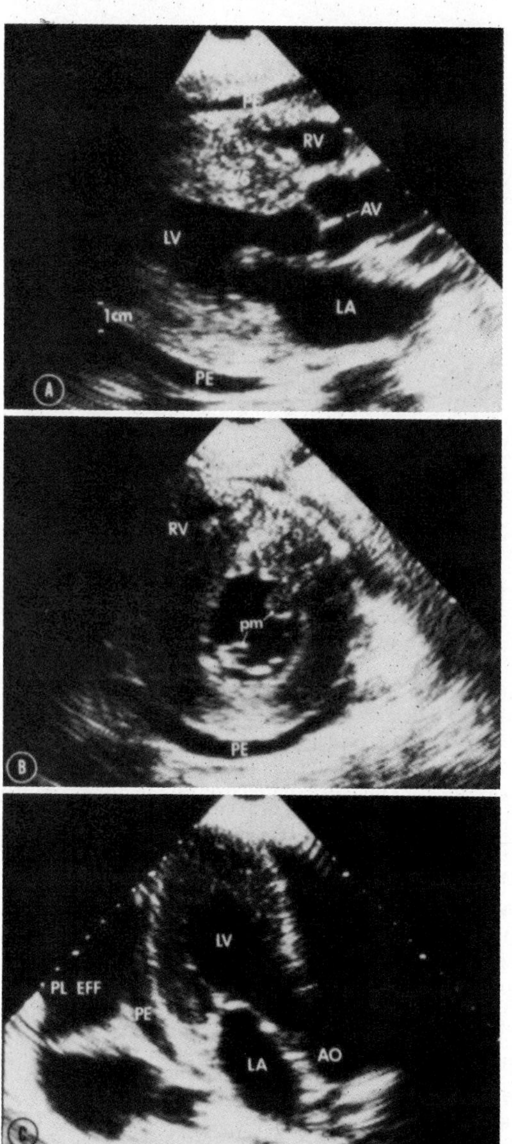

FIGURE 43–22. Parasternal long (A) and short axis (B) and apical long-axis (C) views show typical echocardiographic features of advanced cardiac amyloidosis. Note normal left ventricular cavity size and markedly thickened ventricular walls (ventricular septum = 22 mm, posterior wall = 18 mm, and right ventricular free wall = 15 mm) and the characteristic granular sparkling appearance. Small pericardial effusion (PE) and left pleural effusion (PL EFF) are also present. AO = Aorta, AV = aortic valve, LA = left atrium, LV = left ventricle, pm = papillary muscles, RV = right ventricle, VS = ventricular septum. (From Klein, A. L., Oh, J. K., Miller, F. A., et al.: Two-dimensional and Doppler echocardiographic assessment of infiltrative cardiomyopathy. J. Am. Soc. Echocardiog. *1*:48, 1988.)

The *chest roentgenogram* usually shows cardiomegaly in patients with systolic dysfunction, although heart size may be normal in patients with the restrictive form. Pulmonary congestion may be prominent in patients with congestive heart failure. Pleural effusions are common.[334,353] The *electrocardiogram* is often abnormal; however, the most characteristic feature is diffusely diminished voltage,[353] occurring in approximately half the patients. Myocardial infarction is often simulated because of small or absent R waves in right precordial leads or, less frequently, by Q waves in the inferior leads. Left-axis deviation is seen in more than half the patients.[353] Arrhythmias, particularly atrial fibrillation, are common, although they rarely are the presenting feature of cardiac amyloidosis.[353] Complex ventricular arrhythmias are found frequently in patients with cardiac amyloidosis, and in some may be a harbinger of sudden death.[353,355] Various forms of AV conduction defects are often seen.[353] Abnormalities of AV conduction appear to be particularly common in familial amyloidosis with polyneuropathy.[356] Sinus node involvement is common, and the clinical and electrocardiographic features of the sick sinus syndrome may be present (p. 677).

Echocardiography (Figs. 43–22 and 4–98, p. 101) in advanced cases most commonly reveals increased thickness of the walls of the ventricles, small ventricular chambers, dilated atria, thickening of the interatrial septum, and impaired left ventricular function.[334,353,357,358] Early preclinical unsuspected cardiac involvement may be detectable only by echocardiography or Doppler ultrasound (see below).[334,359] Although the cardiac valves may be thickened, they usually move normally. A pericardial effusion is common but rarely results in tamponade. The appearance of the thickened cardiac walls is often distinctive on two-dimensional echocardiography, demonstrating a granular sparkling texture, presumably due to the amyloid deposit.[353,360] The echocardiographic appearance probably results from the presence of nodules containing amyloid and collagen,[361] and digital image analysis techniques are able to identify a unique tissue signature in cardiac amyloidosis.[259,362] In some cases the pattern of increased wall thickness is nonuniform and may resemble HCM with ASH.[187,353,363] Echocardiographic demonstration of thick left ventricular walls with concomitant low voltage on the electrocardiogram appears to distinguish cardiac amyloidosis from pericardial disease or left ventricular hypertrophy, and this distinctive voltage/mass ratio is characteristic of myocardial infiltration by the amyloid fibrils[334,358,364] (except in the familial forms). Doppler ultrasound[359,365] and radionuclide ventriculography[366] routinely demonstrate abnormalities of diastolic function.[367,367a]

Scintigraphy with technetium-99m-pyrophosphate (p. 315) is often strongly positive with prominent cardiac involvement, although in a minority of cases it is inexplicably falsely negative.[353,368] Positive scans tend to correlate with extensive cardiac involvement; scans are usually negative when the echocardiogram does not demonstrate abnormalities, as well as in the secondary forms of amyloidosis.[353]

Computed tomography may suggest the presence of myocardial amyloid when diffuse ventricular thickening is associated with a radiographic myocardial density lower than that seen when myocardial hypertrophy exists alone; the clinical utility of this modality is uncertain as of this writing.[353]

DIAGNOSIS. Whereas 2 or 3 decades ago the clinical diagnosis of systemic amyloidosis was made correctly antemortem only 25 per cent of the time, with more recent clinical awareness of the disease and the utilization of *biopsy techniques* the diagnosis is now made antemortem in the majority of cases. An abdominal fat aspirate has been the single most useful diagnostic procedure, combining the attributes of ease of performance, sensitivity, and safety.[352,353] Biopsy of rectum, gingiva, bone marrow, liver, kidney, and various other tissues has

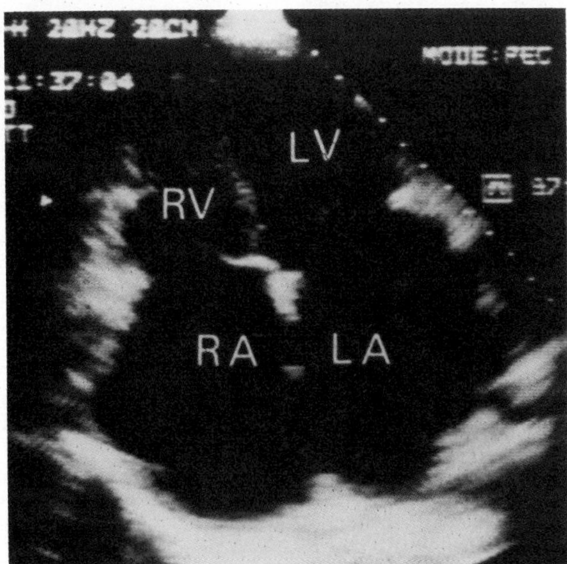

FIGURE 43–23. **Two-dimensional echocardiogram (four-chamber apical view) in a 15-year-old boy with idiopathic restrictive cardiomyopathy reveals small right (RV) and left (LV) ventricular cavities with markedly dilated right (RA) and left (LA) atria. (From Child, J. S., and Perloff, J. K.: The restrictive cardiomyopathies. Cardiol. Clin. 6:294, 1988.)**

also been employed. Endomyocardial biopsy of the right or left ventricles may be helpful in establishing the diagnosis of cardiac amyloidosis if the abdominal fat aspirate is negative.[334,353]

MANAGEMENT. The treatment of cardiac amyloidosis is generally unsatisfactory and ineffective,[352] although it is speculated that alkylating agents may have some role.[353,355] Digitalis glycosides should be used with caution because patients with cardiac amyloidosis appear to be particularly sensitive to digitalis preparations, and the use of ordinary doses may lead to serious arrhythmias; this may relate to selective binding of digoxin to amyloid fibrils in the myocardium.[353] Similarly, nifedipine binds to amyloid fibrils[369]; its use and that of the other calcium antagonists may lead to exacerbation of congestive heart failure symptoms due to an enhanced negative inotropic effect.[352,370] Insertion of a permanent pacemaker may be beneficial in patients with symptomatic conducting system disease.[353] Careful use of low doses of diuretics and vasodilators may afford some symptomatic benefit,[353] but there is a real risk of hypotension with use of these agents.

INHERITED INFILTRATIVE DISORDERS CAUSING CARDIOMYOPATHY

The intramyocardial accumulation or infiltration of an abnormal metabolic product may result in abnormal systolic contractile performance. However, it may also impair the filling of the ventricles, thereby adding a restrictive component. A variety of infiltrative diseases, often inherited, may result in this hemodynamic picture, including the glycogenoses (p. 1645), the mucopolysaccharidoses (p. 1637), Fabry disease, and Gaucher disease.

FABRY DISEASE

Fabry disease (angiokeratoma corporis diffusum universale) is an X-linked disorder of glycosphingolipid metabolism due to a deficiency of the enzyme ceramide trihexosidase.[371] It is characterized by an intracellular accumulation of a neutral glycolipid, with prominent involvement of the skin and kidneys as well as the myocardium. *Histological examination* often reveals widespread involvement of the myocardium, vascular endothelium, conducting tissues, and valves—particularly the mitral valve.[372] The major clinical manifestations of the disease result from the accumulation of the glycolipid substrate in endothelial cells, with eventual occlusion of small arterioles.[373] The accumulation of the glycolipid occurs in the lysosomes of the cardiac tissues and is responsible for the multiple cardiovascular manifestations of Fabry disease.[374] Symptomatic cardiovascular involvement occurs eventually in most affected males, while female carriers are usually asymptomatic or only minimally symptomatic, but on occasion may have severe cardiac involvement.[371] Systemic hypertension, renovascular hypertension, mitral valve prolapse, and congestive heart failure are common clinical manifestations. Altered vasomotor activity is found in Fabry disease, resulting in a Reynaud-like picture. Electrocardiographic abnormalities include left ventricular hypertrophy, P-wave abnormalities, conduction defects, and arrhythmias.[374–376] The echocardiogram usually reveals increased left ventricular wall thickness, presumably the result of glycolipid deposition, which may simulate hypertrophic cardiomyopathy and mitral valve prolapse.[374,375] Differentiation from other restrictive or hypertrophic processes (such as cardiac amyloidosis) may not be possible on echocardiographic grounds but may be possible with nuclear magnetic resonance imaging.[374] Endomyocardial biopsy may be of considerable value in making a definitive diagnosis,[374,377] and a low alpha-galactosidase activity in leukocytes is also helpful diagnostically.

Whether renal transplantation prevents progressive cardiac involvement in Fabry disease is not clear.[378]

GAUCHER DISEASE

Gaucher disease is an uncommon, inherited disorder of glycosyl ceramide metabolism. It is secondary to a deficiency of the enzyme beta-glucosidase and results in accumulation of cerebrosides in the spleen, liver, bone marrow, lymph nodes, brain, and myocardium. Diffuse interstitial infiltration of the left ventricle by cells laden with cerebroside occurs in Gaucher disease, associated with reduced left ventricular compliance and cardiac output. Clinical evidence of cardiac involvement is uncommon, but when present it is characterized by left ventricular dysfunction, hemorrhagic pericardial effusion, increase in left ventricular wall mass, and calcification of the left-sided valves.[379–382]

HEMOCHROMATOSIS AND HEMOSIDEROSIS (See also p. 1646.)

Hemochromatosis is characterized by excessive deposition of iron in a variety of parenchymal tissues (heart, liver, gonads, and pancreas). It may occur (1) as a familial or idiopathic disorder, (2) in association with a defect in hemoglobin synthesis resulting in ineffective erythropoiesis, (3) in chronic liver disease, and (4) with excessive oral intake of iron over many years. While patients who have iron deposits in the myocardium almost always have deposits in other organs (e.g., liver, spleen, pancreas, bone marrow), the severity of myocardial involvement varies widely and only roughly parallels that in other organs.[383] Cardiac involvement leads to a mixed dilated/restrictive cardiomyopathic presentation, with both systolic and diastolic dysfunction.[384]

Pathological Findings

(Fig. 57–7 p. 1748.) These consist of a dilated heart with thickened ventricular walls. Myocardial iron deposits are found within the sarcoplasmic reticulum,[385] and are most common in the subepicardial region, followed by the subendocardial region, and are least common in the midmyocardial wall.[386] They are more extensive in ventricular than in atrial myocardium. Involvement of the cardiac conducting system is common.[385] Myocardial degeneration and fibrosis may also occur.

The severity of myocardial dysfunction is proportional to the quantity of iron present in the myocardium.[386] Extensive deposits of cardiac iron (particularly those grossly visible at postmortem examination) are invariably associated with cardiac dysfunction—usually chronic congestive heart failure, which is often the cause of death. Extensive cardiac deposits usually occur in patients who receive more than 100 blood transfusions (unless there is associated iron loss due to bleeding).

Clinical Manifestations

These vary widely, depending on the extent of myocardial involvement. Some patients remain asymptomatic despite echocardiographic evidence of myocardial involvement, which is expressed as normal or increased left ventricular wall thickness, chamber enlargement and contractile dysfunction.[384,386,387] In such cases, a variety of noninvasive techniques, including exercise radionuclide ventriculography, may demonstrate early subclinical myocardial involvement in which treatment is most effective.[384,387,388] Symptomatic cardiac involvement is usually associated with electrocardiographic abnormalities, including ST-segment and T-wave changes, as well as supraventricular arrhythmias; these electrocardiographic changes correlate with the degree of iron deposits in the heart.[384] Atrioventricular conduction disturbances and ventricular arrhythmias are uncommon.

Cardiac involvement usually is evident from the clinical and echocardiographic features; endomyocardial biopsy may be useful to confirm (but not exclude) the diagnosis.[384,386] The diagnosis is aided by finding elevated plasma iron levels (180 to 300 μg/dl; normal = 50 to 150), a normal or low total iron-binding capacity (200 to 300 μg/dl; normal = 250 to 370), and markedly elevated values for saturation of transferrin (80 to 100 per cent; normal = 22 to 46 per cent), serum ferritin (900 to 6000 ng/ml; normal = 3 to 180), urinary iron (9 to 23 mg/24 hr; normal = 0 to 2), and liver iron (600 to 1800 μg/100 mg dry wt; normal = 30 to 140).[389] Repeated phlebotomies or the use of the chelating agent desferrioxamine may be clinically beneficial.[384,390] (For further discussion of the treatment of iron storage disease see p. 1748.).

SARCOIDOSIS

Sarcoidosis is a granulomatous disorder of unknown etiology, characterized by multisystem involvement. Infiltration of the lungs, reticuloendothelial system, and skin usually dominates the clinical picture, but virtually any tissue may be affected. The most important manifestation results from pulmonary involvement. This often leads to diffuse fibrosis that may result in fatal right heart failure. Primary cardiac involvement is not often recognized clinically, although it may be demonstrated at autopsy in 20 to 30 per cent of cases of sarcoid, most of which demonstrate generalized sarcoidosis.[391-394] Clinical manifestations of sarcoid heart disease are present in less than 5 per cent of patients, although myocardial involvement may result in heart block, congestive heart failure, ventricular arrhythmias, and sudden death, particularly in youngsters.[391] Myocardial sarcoidosis may have restrictive as well as congestive features, since cardiac infiltration by sarcoid granulomas results not only in increased stiffness of the ventricular wall but diminished systolic contractile function as well. Myocardial sarcoidosis typically affects young or middle-aged adults of either sex; there is usually evidence of generalized sarcoidosis.[393,395]

Pathology

The typical pathological feature of sarcoidosis is the presence of noncaseating granulomas, which occur in many organs. They infiltrate the myocardium and may eventually become fibrotic scars.[395] The granulomas may involve any region of the heart, although the left ventricular free wall and the interventricular septum are the most common sites, and extensive granulomas and scar tissue in the cephalad portion of the interventricular septum is a constant finding in patients with abnormalities of the conduction system.[395,396] Cardiac effects may range from a few scattered lesions to extensive involvement.[397] Because of the variable cardiac involvement, myocardial biopsy may be positive in only about half of the patients, and therefore a negative biopsy by no means excludes the diagnosis.[398,399] Transmural involvement is common, and large portions of the ventricular wall may be replaced by sarcoid tissue, which may lead to aneurysm formation.[395] While involvement of small coronary artery branches may be found in sarcoidosis, the pathophysiological importance of this observation remains unclear.

CLINICAL MANIFESTATIONS. Sudden death is the most feared and unfortunately one of the more common manifestations of cardiac sarcoidosis.[394-396] Conduction disturbances and congestive heart failure are common manifestations of symptomatic involvement in nonfatal cases, but many patients are apparently asymptomatic despite extensive cardiac involvement.[392-394] Syncope is common and may reflect paroxysmal arrhythmias or conduction disturbances.[334] Atrial and ventricular arrhythmias, especially ventricular tachycardia, are observed frequently.[334] While cor pulmonale as a consequence of pulmonary sarcoidosis accounts for some of the symptoms of heart failure, many symptoms are caused by direct myocardial involvement by granulomas and scar tissue, and the patients show the clinical features of restrictive or dilated cardiomyopathy.[334] Symptoms of myocardial sarcoid may be present for variable lengths of time; however, the disease may progress rapidly to death, and in some patients the interval from the onset of the cardiac symptoms to death is measured in months.[394] Survival may be considerably longer, however.[393,400]

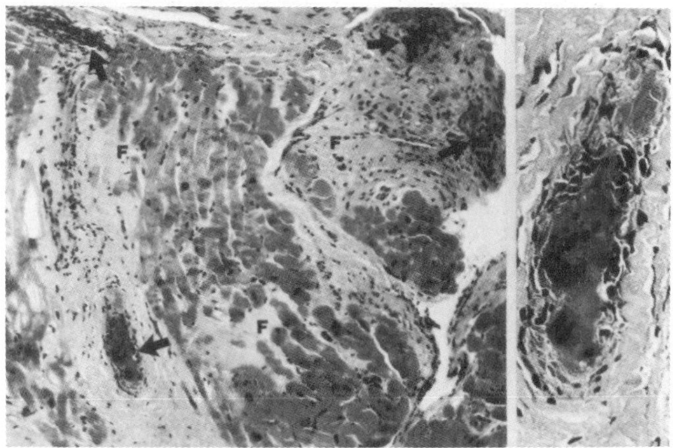

FIGURE 43-24. Under low magnification (left panel) this endomyocardial biopsy sample from a patient with sarcoid shows several foci of intense inflammation (arrows), as well as a marked interstitial infiltrate of mononuclear cells. There is abundant interstitial fibrosis (F). On high power magnification (right panel), a giant cell is clearly discernible in one granuloma. Hematoxylin-phloxine-saffron stain. (Left panel, original magnification ×125; right panel, original magnification ×325.) (From Ratner, S. J., Fenoglio, J. J., and Ursell, P. C.: Utility of endomyocardial biopsy in the diagnosis of cardiac sarcoidosis. Chest *90*:528, 1986.)

Cardiac dysfunction is often severe and progressive. Occasionally, patients with extensive involvement develop overt left ventricular aneurysms.[396,400] Pericardial effusions are rare in patients with sarcoidosis.[401,402]

The *physical examination* may reveal findings of extracardiac sarcoid or may be totally normal. A systolic murmur reflecting mitral regurgitation is common. This appears to be more the result of left ventricular dilatation or infiltration than of direct sarcoid involvement of the papillary muscles.

The *electrocardiogram* is frequently abnormal in patients with known sarcoid and most commonly demonstrates T-wave abnormalities.[393] Sarcoidosis appears to have an affinity for involvement of the AV junction and bundle of His, and

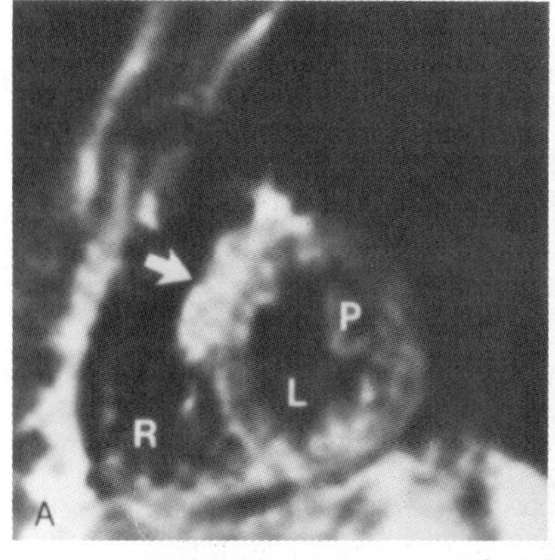

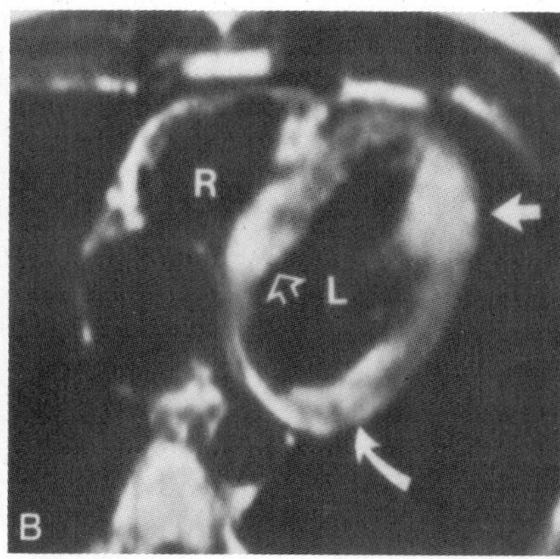

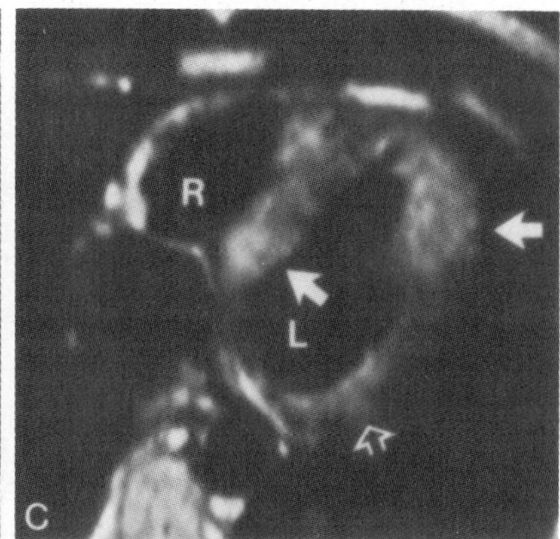

FIGURE 43-25. *A,* Gated cardiac MR image in an oblique sagittal plane from a patient with cardiac sarcoid shows a discrete, high-intensity mass (arrow) arising from basal portion of septum. R = right ventricle, L = left ventricle, P = posterolateral papillary muscle. *B,* Gated cardiac MR image in transverse plane shows discrete high-intensity masses in myocardium of basal portion of septum (open arrow), anterolateral wall (straight closed arrow), and posterolateral wall (curved arrow). *C,* With additional imaging, the normal myocardium has a relative decrease in signal intensity whereas masses (solid arrows) have a higher intensity. Third lesion in posterolateral left ventricle wall (open arrow) is seen better. (From Riedy, K., Fisher, M. R., Belic, N., and Koenigsberg, D. I.: MR imaging of myocardial sarcoidosis. Am. J. Roentgenol. *151*:915, 1988.)

thus varying degrees of intraventricular or AV block are common.[393] With extensive myocardial involvement, pathological Q waves may appear and simulate myocardial infarction.[393] Characteristic features of *echocardiography* include left ventricular dilatation and dysfunction, often with regional wall motion abnormalities suggestive of ischemic heart disease.[393,400]

DIAGNOSIS. In many cases the diagnosis may be suspected in patients with bilateral hilar lymphadenopathy on chest roentgenogram in whom there is clinical or electrocardiographic evidence of myocardial disease. Endomyocardial biopsy may be useful in establishing the diagnosis (Fig. 43–24).[403] Myocardial imaging with thallium-201 may also be helpful in demonstrating segmental perfusion defects that may be due to sarcoid infiltration of the myocardium; there also is speculation that they may reflect a derangement in the microcirculation.[392] Imaging may also indicate the presence of right ventricular hypertrophy in patients with right ventricular overload due to pulmonary fibrosis and pulmonary hypertension. Uptake of technetium pyrophosphate and gallium in myocardial sarcoidosis may aid in the diagnosis, as may nuclear magnetic imaging (Fig. 43–25).[402]

MANAGEMENT. The treatment of myocardial sarcoidosis is difficult. Arrhythmias are often refractory to antiarrhythmic drugs. Permanent pacing may be helpful. While the matter is not settled, it appears that corticosteroids may be of some benefit in treating the conduction disturbances, arrhythmias, and myocardial dysfunction of sarcoidosis.[334,404] Since the risk of sudden death appears to be greatest in patients with extensive myocardial involvement, it may be reasonable to attempt to halt the progression of the disease with steroids before irreversible fibrosis occurs. Formation of a ventricular aneurysm may be a possible side effect of steroid use.[334,396] Insertion of an implantable cardioverter-defibrillator may be considered in appropriate patients at high risk of sudden death.[396]

ENDOMYOCARDIAL DISEASE

Endomyocardial disease (EMD) is a common form of restrictive cardiomyopathy in equatorial Africa and is encountered with less frequency in South America, Asia, and nontropical countries, including the United States.[334,405–408] It is marked by intense endocardial fibrotic thickening of the apex and subvalvular regions of one or both ventricles that results in obstruction to inflow of blood into the respective ventricle, thus producing restrictive physiology. Two variants of the disease have been described, one occurring principally in tropical countries (termed endomyocardial fibrosis, EMF), and the other in temperate countries (Löffler endocarditis parietalis fibroplastica).

Although long considered separate entities, if only because Löffler endocarditis is marked by intense tissue and often peripheral eosinophilia, there is now general agreement that EMF and Löffler endocarditis are different manifestations of the same disease, since the pathological findings in advanced cases are identical.[405–409] Despite the pathological similarities, there are differences in clinical presentation. In addition to the geographic differences, the temperate form of the disease (Löffler endocarditis) acts as a more aggressive and rapidly progressive disorder, affecting principally males, and is associated with hypereosinophilia, thromboembolic phenomena, and generalized arteritis.[410] EMF, conversely, shows no sex predilection, occurs in younger patients, and usually is not associated with an intense eosinophilia.[411]

It has also been postulated that Löffler endocarditis and EMF are different phases in a progressive disease that results from the toxic effect of eosinophils on the heart.[405,412–414] Under this formulation, an initial hypereosinophilia of whatever cause results in damage to the myocardium that produces the first phase of EMD: a necrotic phase, marked by an intense myocarditis, rich in eosinophils, and with an associated arteritis (i.e., Löffler endocarditis). This initial phase occurs within the first few months of illness. It appears to be followed by a thrombotic stage, occurring about a year after initial presentation, during which the myocarditis has receded, nonspecific thickening of the myocardium is beginning, and there is a variable degree of superimposed thrombus formation. The last stage is one of fibrosis, presenting all of the features of EMF.[405,409] The three stages—necrotic, thrombotic, and fibrotic—have been defined on the basis of postmortem material, and it is not suggested that each patient with advanced disease (manifested by EMF) has necessarily passed through the earlier phases.

The possible role of *eosinophils* in the production of the cardiac abnormalities has intrigued investigators for years.[410,412–414] Eosinophils may damage tissues by direct invasion or the release of toxic substances.[409,415] The presence of degranulated peripheral eosinophils in patients with Löffler endocarditis suggests that the protein constituents of the eosinophil's granule may be cardiotoxic,[412,416] producing first the necrotic phase of EMD, followed by the thrombotic and fibrotic phases after the disappearance of the initial eosinophilia.[405,415]

Since the clinical manifestations of EMD demonstrate geographical and clinical differences, Löffler endocarditis and EMF will be discussed separately, even though they could be part of the same disease continuum.

LÖFFLER ENDOCARDITIS

Hypereosinophilic Syndrome

Marked eosinophilia of any cause may be associated with endomyocardial disease. The typical patient who presents with Löffler endocarditis is a man in his fourth decade who lives in a temperate climate and has the hypereosinophilic syndrome (i.e., persistent eosinophilia with $\geq$ 1500 eosinophils/mm^3 for at least 6 months or until death, with evidence of organ involvement).[334,410,412,417] Cardiac involvement in the hypereosinophilic syndrome is the rule, occurring in more than three-fourths of patients.[410,417] Hypereosinophilia and cardiac involvement is also seen in the Churg-Strauss syndrome, which is differentiated by asthma, nasal polyposis, and a necrotizing vasculitis. The cause of the eosinophilia in most patients with Löffler endocarditis is unknown, although in some it may be the result of leukemia, or it may be reactive (that is, secondary to various parasitic, allergic, granulomatous, hypersensitivity, or neoplastic disorders[410,417]). The relationship of the eosinophilia to possible parasitic infestation is unclear.[417]

PATHOLOGY. In the hypereosinophilic syndrome, a variety of organs are usually involved besides the heart, including the lungs, bone marrow, and brain.[334] Cardiac involvement is often biventricular, with mural endocardial thickening of the inflow portions and apex of the ventricles. Histological findings include variable degrees of (1) an acute inflammatory eosinophilic myocarditis involving the myo- and endocardium; (2) thrombosis, fibrinoid change, and inflammatory reaction involving small intramural coronary vessels; (3) mural thrombosis, often containing eosinophils; and (4) fibrotic thickening of up to several millimeters.[412]

CLINICAL MANIFESTATIONS. The principal clinical features include weight loss, fever, cough, skin rash, and congestive heart failure. Although early cardiac involvement may be asymptomatic, overt cardiac dysfunction occurs in more than half the patients and may be right- and/or left-sided.[412] Cardiomegaly, often without overt symptoms of congestive heart failure, may be present, and the murmur of mitral regurgitation is common.[417] Systemic embolism is frequent and may lead to neurological and renal dysfunction. Death is usually due to congestive heart failure, often with associated renal, hepatic, or respiratory dysfunction.

LABORATORY EXAMINATION. The *chest roentgenogram* may reveal cardiomegaly and pulmonary congestion or, less commonly, pulmonary infiltrates. The *electrocardiogram* most commonly shows nonspecific ST-segment and T-wave abnormalities.[417] Arrhythmias, especially atrial fibrillation, and conduction defects, particularly right bundle branch block, may also be present.[412]

The *echocardiogram* commonly demonstrates localized thickening of the posterobasal left ventricular wall, with absent or markedly limited motion of the posterior leaflet of the mitral valve.[334,412] There may be obliteration of the apex by thrombus. Enlargement of the atria may be seen,[418] along with Doppler ultrasound evidence of AV valve regurgitation. The endocardium may be unusually echo-reflective as a consequence of fibrosis.[405]

The *hemodynamic consequences* of the dense endocardial scarring seen in Löffler endocarditis are those of a restrictive cardiomyopathy, as already described (p. 1415), with abnormal diastolic filling due to increased stiffness of the ventricles and a reduction in the size of the ventricular cavity by organized thrombus. Systolic performance usually is largely preserved. Atrioventricular valvular regurgitation may occur because of involvement of the supporting apparatus of the mitral or tricuspid valves.[412] *Cardiac catheterization* reveals markedly elevated ventricular filling pressures, and there may be evidence of tricuspid or mitral regurgitation. A characteristic feature on angiocardiography is largely preserved systolic function with obliteration of the apex of the ventricles. The diagnosis is often confirmed by percutaneous endomyocardial biopsy.[412]

TREATMENT. Medical therapy during the course of early Löffler endocarditis, and surgical therapy during the later phases of fibrosis, may have a positive effect on symptoms and survival. Corticosteroids appear to have a beneficial effect on acute myocarditis,[412] and together with cytotoxic drugs (hydroxyurea in particular), may improve survival substantially.[296,412,417,418] Routine cardiac therapy with digitalis, diuretics, afterload reduction, and anticoagulation as indicated are adjuncts in the management of these patients. Surgical therapy appears to offer significant palliation of symptoms once the fibrotic stage has been reached.[296,417,419]

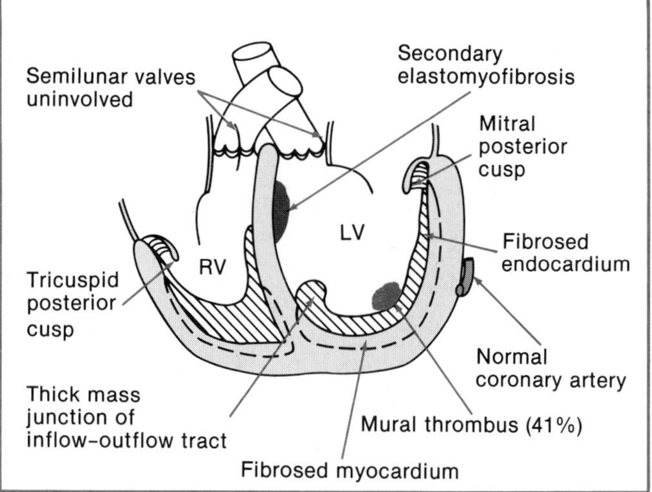

FIGURE 43–26. Cardiac lesions of endomyocardial fibrosis. (From Davies, J. N. P.: Endomyocardial fibrosis. *In* Giles, T. D., and Sander, G. E.: Cardiomyopathy. Littleton, MA, PSG Publishing Co., 1988, p. 188.)

ENDOMYOCARDIAL FIBROSIS

Endomyocardial fibrosis (EMF) occurs most commonly in tropical and subtropical Africa, particularly Uganda and Nigeria. It is typified by fibrous endocardial lesions of the inflow portion of the right or left ventricle or both and often involves the atrioventricular valves, resulting in regurgitation (Fig. 43–26).[406] It is a relatively frequent cause of heart failure and death in equatorial Africa, accounting for 10 to 20 per cent of deaths due to heart disease.[334,405]

While most prominent in Africa, it is also found in tropical and subtropical regions in the rest of the world, including India, Brazil, Colombia, and Sri Lanka.[406] EMF is most common in specific ethnic groups, notably the Rwanda tribe in Uganda, and in people of low socioeconomic status.[406,420] The disease is equally frequent in both sexes, and, although most common in children and young adults, its reported age range is from 4 to 70 years of age.[334,406,411] It is most common in blacks, but cases have been reported occasionally in whites in temperate climates, rarely in the absence of prior residence in tropical areas.[405]

PATHOLOGY

A pericardial effusion, which may be quite large, may be present.[406] The heart is normal in size or slightly enlarged, but massive cardiomegaly does not occur. The right atrium is often dilated, and in patients with severe right ventricular involvement there may be massive enlargement of this chamber. Indentation of the right border of the heart above the apex as a result of apical scarring may occur.[406]

Combined right and left ventricular disease occurs in about half the cases, with pure left ventricular involvement occurring in 40 per cent and pure right ventricular involvement in the remaining 10 per cent of patients who are examined post mortem.[334] When affected, the right ventricle exhibits extensive, dense, fibrous thickening of the inflow tract and apex, with involvement of the papillary muscles and chordae tendineae. Involvement of the right ventricle may lead to obliteration of the apex, with a mass of thrombus and fibrous tissue filling the cavity.[406] The tricuspid valve is often pulled down and distorted by the fibrous process involving the supporting structures.[421] Right atrial thrombi occur commonly. Left ventricular involvement is similar, with fibrosis extending from the apex up the inflow portion of the left ventricle to the posterior mitral valve leaflet. The anterior leaflet of the mitral valve and the outflow portion of the left ventricle are usually spared.[421] Thrombi often overlie the endocardial lesions, and widely distributed endocardial calcific deposits may occur.[422] The coronary arteries are uninvolved, as is the remainder of the body.[334]

Microscopically, the involved endocardium demonstrates a thick layer of collagen tissue on top of a layer of loosely arranged connective tissue.[406] Septa composed of fibrous and granulation tissue extend for variable distances into the myocardium.[334] Interstitial edema is often present, but there is no cellular infiltration. Small patches of fibroelastosis may occur in both ventricular outflow tracts beneath the semilunar valves but are thought to be a secondary phenomenon due to local trauma rather than a result of the basic pathological process.[406]

CLINICAL MANIFESTATIONS

As already noted, EMF may involve both ventricles or either ventricle selectively; left-sided involvement results in symptoms of pulmonary congestion, while predominant right-sided disease may present features of a restrictive cardiomyopathy and therefore simulate constrictive pericarditis. There is often regurgitation of one or both atrioventricular valves. The onset of the disease is usually insidious, but it is sometimes ushered in by an acute febrile illness. Rarely, the disease appears to stabilize, and survival for up to 12 years has been observed, but it is usually relentlessly progressive. Death is due to progressive myocardial failure, often associated with pulmonary congestion, infection, or infarction. The most important immediate cause of death is sudden, unexpected cardiovascular collapse, presumably arrhythmic in origin.[334] Survival appears to be unrelated to site of predominant involvement (right or left ventricle), although those patients presenting in advanced right-sided failure have a worse prognosis than do other patients.[411]

RIGHT VENTRICULAR EMF. Pure or predominant right ventricular involvement is characterized by fibrous obliteration of the right ventricular apex that diminishes the capacity of this chamber. The fibrosis often extends to the supporting apparatus of the tricuspid valve, resulting in tricuspid regurgitation. Therefore, clinical manifestations in patients with right-sided involvement include an elevated jugular venous pressure, a prominent *v* wave, and a rapid *y* descent. A protodiastolic gallop sound may be heard along the lower sternal border,[406] reflecting right ventricular dysfunction. The liver is usually large and pulsatile, and ascites, splenomegaly, and peripheral edema are common. Pulmonary congestion is not present in the absence of left-sided involvement, and the pulmonary artery and pulmonary capillary wedge pressures are normal. A pericardial effusion, which is sometimes quite large, may be present. The right atrium is often enlarged, sometimes massively so.

Laboratory Findings. The *electrocardiogram* is usually abnormal, with diminished QRS voltage (probably resulting from the presence of a pericardial effusion), ST-segment and T-wave abnormalities, and findings of right atrial enlargement, especially a qR pattern in lead V_1.[423] Atrial fibrillation is common.[406] The *chest roentgenogram* demonstrates cardiac enlargement, usually with gross prominence of the right atrium and a pericardial effusion.[406] Calcification in the region of the right ventricular apex may be found.[424] *Echocardiography* may demonstrate right ventricular thickening, obliteration of the apex, dilated atrium, strong echoes emanating from the endocardial surface, and abnormal septal motion in patients with tricuspid regurgitation.[405,406,425] At *angiography* the right ventricular apex is characteristically not visualized because of obliteration by the fibrous endocardium, but tricuspid regurgitation, right atrial enlargement, and filling defects in the right atrium due to intraatrial thrombi are sometimes seen.[334,405] Early angiographic changes that may be present before advanced disease develops include a change in the endocardial appearance, small apical filling defects, and mild tricuspid regurgitation.[406]

LEFT VENTRICULAR EMF. With predominant *left-sided* involvement, the endomyocardial fibrosis invades the apex of the ventricle and usually the chordae tendineae or the posterior mitral valve leaflet as well, leading to mitral regurgitation.[405] The murmur may be confined to late systole, as is characteristic of the papillary muscle dysfunction type of murmur, or it may be pansystolic. Findings of pulmonary hypertension may be prominent. A protodiastolic gallop is commonly heard.[405]

Laboratory Findings. The *electrocardiogram* usually shows T-wave abnormalities and diminished QRS voltage in the presence of a pericardial effusion, although left ventricular hypertrophy may be present.[334] There may be findings of left atrial abnormality.[406] As with right-sided involvement, atrial fibrillation often is present. *Echocardiographic* features include thickening and reduced motion of the posterobasal wall and posterior mitral leaflet, increased echo-reflectivity of the endocardium, preserved systolic wall motion in the presence of apical obliteration, dilated atrium, and Doppler ultrasound evidence of mitral regurgitation (Fig. 43–27).[405,406,425] *Cardiac catheterization* often reveals pulmonary hypertension, with elevated left ventricular filling pressures and a reduced cardiac index.[426] The left ventriculogram usually shows mitral regurgitation, and a filling defect due to an intracavitary thrombus within the ventricle may be seen on occasion[334] (Fig. 43–28). Coronary arteriography does not reveal obstructive disease.

BIVENTRICULAR EMF. This form of endomyocardial fibrosis occurs more frequently than either isolated right- or left-sided disease.[427] If there is more than minimal right ventricular involvement, severe pulmonary hypertension does not occur, and the right-sided findings dominate the clinical presentation. The typical patient with biventricular involvement may have the features of right ventricular endomyocardial fibrosis, as already described, with only a mitral regurgitant murmur to suggest left ventricular involvement. Systemic embolization may occur in up to 15 per cent of patients; infective endocarditis is even less frequent and is found in less than 2 per cent.

DIAGNOSIS

This is based on the presence in an individual of the typical clinical and laboratory features, particularly angiography, from the appropriate geographical area. Eosinophilia is usually not a prominent feature and when present may reflect associated parasitic infestation. *Endomyocardial biopsy* may occasionally be helpful in establishing the diagnosis.[405] However, this risks dislodging a mural thrombus, with resultant embolization, and left-sided biopsy is *not* recommended. In addition, because the disease is often focal, the biopsy may miss the pathological process, particularly if a right ventricular biopsy is performed in a patient with isolated left-sided disease.

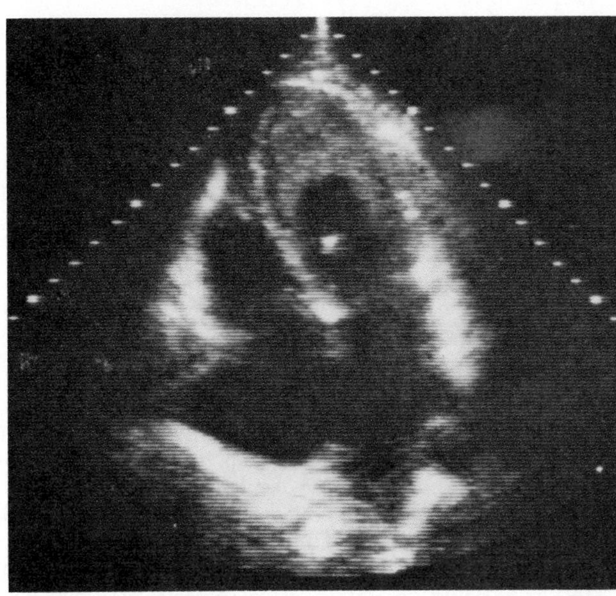

FIGURE 43–27. Apical four-chamber echocardiogram in endomyocardial fibrosis with typical left ventricular apical obliteration. Contrast injection (agitated saline solution) showed right ventricular apical obliteration also. Doppler examination showed moderate mitral regurgitation, severe tricuspid regurgitation, and pulmonary hypertension. (From Acquatella, H., and Schiller, N. B.: Echocardiographic recognition of Chagas' disease and endomyocardial fibrosis. J. Am. Soc. Echocardiog. *1*:60, 1988.)

MANAGEMENT

The medical treatment of EMF is often difficult and not particularly effective. In patients with advanced disease, the outlook is poor, with a 35 to 50 per cent 2-year mortality.[411,427] Substantially better survival may be seen in less symptomatic patients who have milder forms of the disease.[427,428] Digitalis glycosides may be helpful in controlling the ventricular rate in patients with atrial fibrillation, but the response of congestive symptoms is disappointing. Diuretics are not particularly helpful in the treatment of ascites. Once endomyocardial disease has reached the fibrotic stage, surgery offers the possibility of symptomatic improvement and is the treatment of choice.[334] Operative excision of the fibrotic endocardium and replacement of the mitral and/or tricuspid valves have led to substantial symptomatic improvement, especially with predominant left-sided involvement.[421,423,426,428] Mitral valve repair, rather than replacement, can be accomplished in some patients.[421] Postoperative catheterization has also provided objective evidence of hemodynamic improvement with a reduction in ventricular filling pressures, an increase in cardiac output, and normalization of the angiographic appearance.[421,426] Operative mortality has been high, running between 15 and 25 per cent in the larger series.[421,423,426,428]

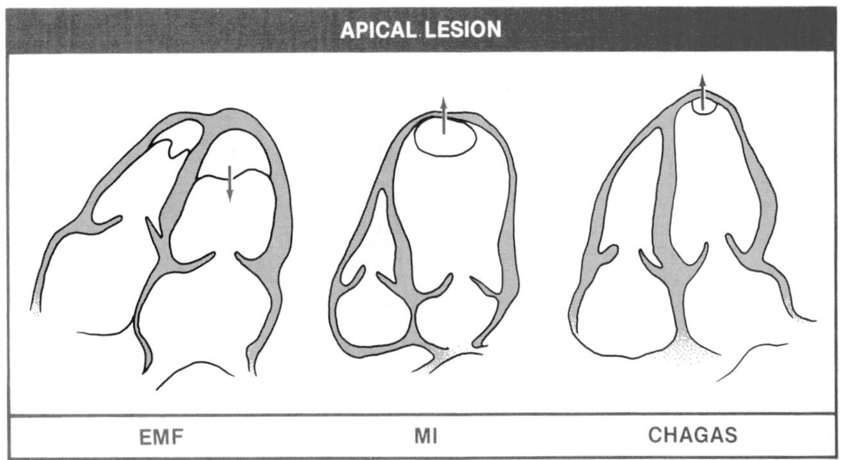

FIGURE 43–28. Differences in the apical lesion between endomyocardial fibrosis (EMF), myocardial infarction (MI), and Chagas' heart disease. Both apices can be affected in EMF, but typically LV function is preserved or hypercontractile, and LV obliteration moves inward. In apical MI, dyskinetic apex frequently is combined with septal or anterior wall motion abnormalities, depending on extent of disease of left anterior descending coronary artery. "Neck" of dyskinetic area tends to be large. In chronic Chagas' disease, although apical aneurysm can be as large as in ischemic heart disease, some patients may have typical "small" neck aneurysm. When apical dyskinesis without aneurysm is found, its appearance cannot be used to differentiate between ischemic or Chagas' disease. Chagas' disease with isolated apical aneurysm typically spares all but most apical portion of septum. In Chagas' disease, RV apical dyskinesis or aneurysm may also be present. (From Acquatella, H., and Schiller, N. B.: Echocardiographic recognition of Chagas' disease and endomyocardial fibrosis. J. Am. Soc. Echocardiog. *1*:60, 1988.)

ENDOCARDIAL FIBROELASTOSIS

(See p. 994)

CARCINOID HEART DISEASE

ETIOLOGY AND PATHOLOGY. The carcinoid syndrome is caused by a metastasizing carcinoid tumor and is characterized by cutaneous flushing, diarrhea, bronchoconstriction, and endocardial plaques composed of a unique type of fibrous tissue. The vasomotor, bronchoconstrictor, and cardiac manifestations are undoubtedly related to circulating humoral substances secreted by the tumor,[429] although the precise substance(s) responsible remains to be elucidated. Virtually all patients develop diarrhea and flushing, while cardiac abnormalities occur in over two-thirds; clinically apparent and severe right-sided disease is seen in a quarter.[430,431]

Sixty to 90 per cent of tumors arise in the appendix, while the rest originate in the ileum, stomach, duodenum, other areas of the gastrointestinal tract, and bronchus.[429] Carcinoid tumors of the ileum are the most likely to metastasize, with involvement of the regional lymph nodes and liver. Also, it is usual that only carcinoid tumors that invade the liver result in carcinoid heart disease.[432] The cardiac lesions may be related to large circulating quantities of serotonin (5-hydroxytryptamine), bradykinin, or other substances secreted by the tumor,[430] which are usually inactivated by the liver, lungs, and brain. Hepatic metastases apparently allow large quantities of tumor products to reach the heart without being inactivated by the liver. Left-sided cardiac involvement occurs in about one-third of patients with fatal cardiac carcinoid; when it occurs, it typically is of little hemodynamic significance, in contrast to right-sided involvement.[429] Many of the left-sided findings are minor; it has been suggested that they are similar to those seen in age-matched normal subjects and do not necessarily indicate carcinoid disease.[430] The preferential right-sided involvement presumably is related to inactivation of the offending humoral substance(s) by the lungs. In rare cases, significant left-sided valvular disease develops, perhaps related to passage of blood directly from the right to the left side of the heart through a patent foramen ovale.[433]

The characteristic *pathological* findings are fibrous plaques that involve the "downstream" aspect of the tricuspid and pulmonic valves, the endocardium of the cardiac chambers, and the intima of the venae cavae, pulmonary artery, and coronary sinus.[429] The fibrous tissue in the plaques results in distortion of the valves, leading to pulmonic stenosis and tricuspid regurgitation, sometimes with some degree of stenosis.[429] Histologically, the plaques consist of deposits of fibrous tissue located superficially on the endocardium with little or no extension into the underlying layers. Ultrastructural and immunohistochemical studies have demonstrated that the plaques are composed of smooth muscle cells embedded in a stroma rich in acid mucopolysacharides and collagen.[434]

CLINICAL MANIFESTATIONS. *Physical examination* usually reveals a systolic murmur along the left sternal border, produced by tricuspid regurgitation; in some cases, there may be concomitant pulmonic stenosis. A murmur of pulmonary regurgitation may be found as well.[429,435]

The *chest roentgenogram* may reveal enlargement of the heart; the pulmonary artery trunk is typically of normal size, without evidence of poststenotic dilatation as occurs in congenital pulmonic stenosis. No specific *electrocardiographic pattern* is diagnostic of carcinoid heart disease,[430] although low voltage is often present. Evidence of right atrial enlargement may be seen on occasion, but electrocardiographic evidence of right ventricular hypertrophy is usually lacking. Nonspecific ST-segment and T-wave abnormalities and intraventricular conduction block may be seen.[430] *Echocardiography* may reveal evidence of tricuspid and/or pulmonary valve thickening, along with right atrial and right ventricular dilatation (Fig. 43-29).[430-431]

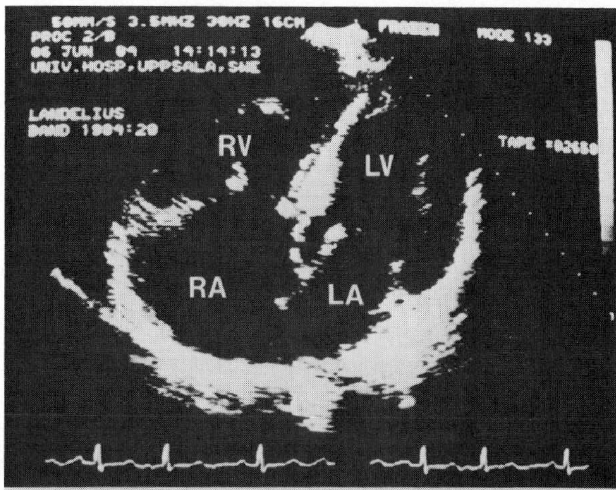

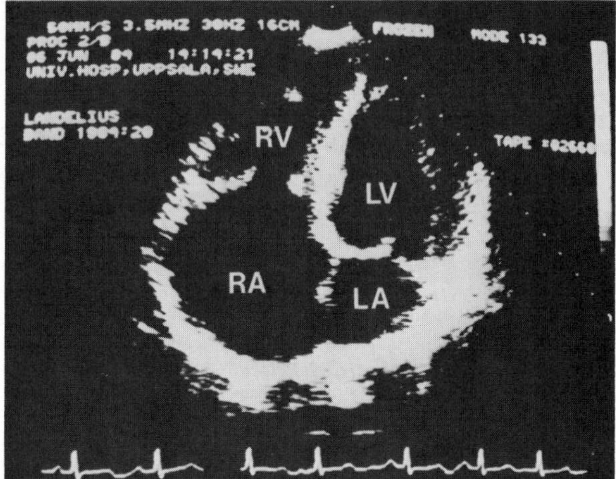

FIGURE 43-29. Echocardiographic apical four-chamber view of a patient with carcinoid heart disease. *Top,* Diastolic frame. *Bottom,* Systolic frame. Note prominent enlargement of right heart cavities and pronounced immobility of tricuspid valve leaflets as compared with the mitral leaflets. LA = left atrium, LV = left ventricle, RA = right atrium, RV = right ventricle. (From Lundin, L., Norheim, I., Landelius, J., et al.: Carcinoid heart disease: Relationship of circulating vasoactive substances to ultrasound detectable cardiac abnormalities. Circulation *77*:264, 1988, reprinted by permission of the American Heart Association, Inc.)

The *hemodynamic findings* most commonly encountered are those of tricuspid regurgitation (p. 1055) and occasionally pulmonic stenosis. Some patients with the carcinoid syndrome appear to be in a hyperkinetic state, which may lead to high-output heart failure.

MANAGEMENT. In patients with mild congestive heart failure this consists of digitalis and diuretics. Some of the vasomotor symptoms may be controlled with alpha-adrenoceptor blockers and serotonin antagonists. Surgical replacement of the tricuspid valve and pulmonic valvotomy or valvectomy may be beneficial in severely symptomatic patients with serious valvular dysfunction.[436]

OBESITY AND HEART DISEASE

(See p. 1150)

DIABETIC CARDIOMYOPATHY

(See p. 1139)

When the heart is involved in an inflammatory process, often caused by an infectious agent, myocarditis is said to be present. The inflammation may involve the myocytes, interstitium, vascular elements, and/or pericardium; involvement of the latter structure is discussed in Chapter 45.

Myocarditis has been described during and following a wide variety of viral, rickettsial, bacterial, protozoal, and metazoal diseases; indeed, virtually any infectious agent may produce cardiac inflammation[437,438] (Table 43–14). Infectious agents cause myocardial damage by three basic mechanisms: (1) invasion of the myocardium[439]; (2) production of a myocardial toxin, e.g., diphtheria,[440] and (3) immunologically mediated myocardial damage.[439] The principal mechanism of heart involvement in viral myocarditis is believed to be a cell-mediated immunological reaction to new cell surface changes or a new antigen related to the virus, and not merely resulting from cell damage caused by viral replication.[441,442] Additional evidence for an immune-mediated mechanism is the demonstration of a marked increase in major histocompatibility complex antigen expression in the biopsy specimens from patients with myocarditis.[443] Antibodies against intracellular components may also play a role.[444] Although often mistakenly limited to inflammation due to an infective agent, myocarditis may also be caused by allergic reactions and pharmacological agents, as well as occurring during the course of some systemic diseases such as vasculitis.[440]

Myocarditis may be an acute or a chronic process and may occur during the peripartum period (p. 1798). In North America, viruses are presumed to be the most common agents producing myocarditis, while in South America, Chagas' disease (produced by *Trypanosoma cruzi*) is far more common.[437] The identification of the specific etiological agent responsible for infectious myocarditis usually rests on the associated extracardiac findings, since the cardiovascular signs and symptoms are often nonspecific. The histological findings vary, depending on the stage of the disease, the mechanism of myocardial damage, and the specific etiological agent. Myocardial involvement may be focal or diffuse, but the myocardial lesions are generally randomly distributed in the heart, and thus the clinical consequences depend to a large extent on the size and number of the lesions.[437] However, a single small lesion may have profound consequences if it is located within the cardiac conducting system. The histological findings are usually nonspecific (except for some parasitic and granulomatous forms of myocarditis), and with certain exceptions (Table 43–4), myocardial biopsy seldom elucidates the specific etiological agent.[445]

TABLE 43–14 PRINCIPAL INFECTIOUS ETIOLOGICAL AGENTS ASSOCIATED WITH MYOCARDITIS

BACTERIAL INFECTIONS	
Streptococcal	Brucellosis
Staphylococcal	Diphtheria
Pneumococcal	Salmonellosis
Meningococcal	Tuberculosis
Hemophilus	Tularemia
Gonococcal	
SPIROCHETAL INFECTIONS	
Leptospirosis	Relapsing fever
Lyme disease	Syphilis
FUNGAL INFECTIONS	
Aspergillosis	Coccidioidomycosis
Actinomycosis	Cryptococcosis
Blastomycosis	Histoplasmosis
Candidiasis	
PARASITIC INFECTIONS	
Cysticercosis	Trichinosis
Schistosomiasis	Trypanosomiasis
Toxoplasmosis	Visceral larva migrans
RICKETTSIAL INFECTIONS	
Rocky Mountain spotted fever	Scrub typhus
Q fever	Typhus
VIRAL INFECTIONS	
Adenovirus	Mycoplasma pneumoniae
Arbovirus	Poliomyelitis
Coxsackievirus	Psittacosis
Cytomegalovirus	Respiratory syncytial virus
Echovirus	Rabies
Encephalomyocarditis virus	Rubella
Hepatitis	Rubeola
Human immunodeficiency virus	Vaccina
Infectious mononucleosis	Varicella
Influenza	Variola
Mumps	Yellow fever

Adapted from Marboe, C. C., and Fenoglio, J. J.: Pathology and natural history of human myocarditis. Pathol. Immunopathol. Res. 7:226, 1988.

INFECTIOUS MYOCARDITIS

CLINICAL MANIFESTATIONS. The clinical expression of myocarditis ranges from the asymptomatic state secondary to focal inflammation to fulminant fatal congestive heart failure due to diffuse myocarditis.[437,438] An initial episode of viral myocarditis, perhaps unrecognized and forgotten, may be the initial event that eventually culminates in an "idiopathic" dilated cardiomyopathy.[439] In experimental animals, the structural and functional myocardial alterations that follow viral myocarditis may persist well beyond the stage of viral replication and myocardial inflammatory response,[439] and the late changes resemble those of dilated cardiomyopathy.[440]

The outcome after viral myocarditis is quite variable,[437] perhaps related to differing genetic susceptibility of individual patients.[446] In most patients, the event is entirely self-limited and often unrecognized.[440,447] More overt myocarditis may result in acute congestive heart failure.[439] In others, unrecognized myocarditis may be the cause of arrhythmias in what appears to be a structurally normal heart.[448] Some patients with chest pain and angiographically normal coronary arteries may have had subclinical myocarditis at some point in the past. Most intriguing is the possibility that viral myocarditis may culminate in dilated cardiomyopathy, presumably as a consequence of viral-mediated immunological cardiac damage.[56,296,437,441–444,446]

While transient electrocardiographic abnormalities suggesting myocardial involvement are noted in many patients with infectious diseases, most patients do not have other clinical manifestations of myocarditis.[447] It is postulated that these electrocardiographic changes reflect subclinical myocardial involvement. That unrecognized myocardial involvement occurs with systemic infections is supported by histological evidence of myocarditis during routine postmortem examinations of subjects believed to be free of prior cardiac disease.[448–450] Some degree of myocardial involvement, often subepicardial in location, also frequently occurs in patients with acute pericarditis.[451]

Since myocardial involvement is subclinical in most acute infectious diseases, the majority of patients have no specific complaints referable to the cardiovascular system[447]; the presence of myocarditis is often inferred from the ST-segment and T-wave changes on the electrocardiogram.[439] From a clinical viewpoint, myocardial involvement is associated with nonspecific symptoms, including fatigue, dyspnea, palpitations, and precordial discomfort.[440] Chest pain usually reflects associated pericarditis, but precordial discomfort suggestive of myocardial ischemia is occasionally observed. In some cases, the clinical presentation (with chest pain, electrocardiographic abnormalities, increased muscle enzyme levels, and regional wall motion abnormalities) may simulate an acute myocardial infarction;[452] in others, transient coronary vasospasm has been invoked.[453]

Physical Examination. Tachycardia is usual and may be out of proportion to the temperature elevation.[439] The first heart sound is often muffled, and a protodiastolic gallop may be present. A transient apical systolic murmur may appear,[440] but diastolic murmurs are rare. Clinical evidence of congestive heart failure occurs only in the more severe cases.[439,440] The heart is usually normal in size in the clinically silent cases, but it may be dilated in patients with congestive heart failure. Pulmonary and systemic emboli may occur.

Laboratory Findings. *Electrocardiographic* abnormalities are usually transient and occur far more frequently than does clinical myocardial involvement.[439] The most common changes are abnormalities of the ST segment and T wave, but atrial and in particular ventricular arrhythmias, atrioventricular (AV) and intraventricular conduction defects, and, rarely, Q waves may be seen.[439] Complete AV block is usually transient and resolves without sequelae, but it is occasionally a cause of sudden death in patients with myocarditis.[440] On *radiological examination,* heart size may range from normal to markedly enlarged, and pulmonary congestion may be present in patients with fulminant disease.[440] *Echocardiography* demonstrates some degree of left ventricular dysfunction (surprisingly often regional in nature) in many patients with clinical myocarditis, although wall motion may be normal. Often findings may include increased wall thickness, left ventricular thrombi, and abnormal diastolic filling despite normal systolic function.[454,455] *Radionuclide scanning* after the administration of gallium-67, indium-111 anti-myosin antibody, or technetium-99m pyrophosphate may identify inflammatory and necrotic changes characteristic of myocarditis, as may nuclear magnetic resonance imaging.[101,456–460]

DIAGNOSIS. This is often predicated on the identification of the associated systemic illness and its characteristic features.[447] The diagnosis of viral myocarditis is supported by the identification of the virus in stool, throat washings, blood, myocardium, or pericardial fluid, or by a distinct (usually fourfold) increase in virus neutralizing antibody, complement-fixation, or hemagglutination inhibition titers, but cultures usually are negative and serological tests nondiagnostic.[411] Even in fatal cases, isolation of virus from the myocardium at necropsy is unusual.[437,438] cDNA clones representing various regions of the Coxsackie B virus–specific RNA sequences have been used to detect and quantify virus-specific sequences in tissue.[52] *Endomyocardial biopsy* frequently is used to confirm the diagnosis of myocarditis. A borderline or negative biopsy does not exclude the diagnosis,[461,462] and, if clinically indicated, a repeat biopsy may be appropriate and diagnostic.[463]

PATHOLOGY. Patients with or dying of myocarditis demonstrate a wide spectrum of gross and histological changes, reflecting the range of disease seen clinically. Grossly, the hearts in acute cases are flabby, with focal hemorrhages; in chronic cases, the heart is enlarged and hypertrophied.[440] The histological hallmark of myocarditis is an inflammatory myocardial infiltrate, with associated evidence of myocyte damage.[12,438,440] The inflammatory infiltrate may be composed of a variety of cell types, including polymorphonuclear cells, lymphocytes, macrophages, plasma cells, eosinophils, and/or giant cells.[440] In bacterial myocarditis, polymorphonuclear cells predominate; in viral infections, lymphocytes predominate; and in hypersensitivity myocarditis, eosinophils are seen in abundance.[440] Routine histological examination of the heart rarely provides a specific diagnosis, although in some instances electron microscopic and immunofluorescent techniques may allow elucidation of a specific etiology.

MANAGEMENT. Therapy is often supportive and is usually directed at the more prominent systemic manifestations of the disease. The demonstration of a particular predilection for involvement of the AV conducting system in some forms of myocarditis[439] suggests that patients with suspected myocarditis should be observed closely for any evidence of conduction abnormality. Since exercise intensifies the damage from myocarditis in experimental animals, adequate rest is important.[464–466] Congestive heart failure responds to routine management, including digitalization and diuresis, although patients with myocarditis appear to be particularly sensitive to digitalis, and toxicity should be watched for. Significant arrhythmias should be treated with antiarrhythmic agents, although beta-adrenoceptor blockers are probably best avoided in view of their negative inotropic action.[467] The use of corticosteroids is controversial.[467a] Although corticosteroids were previously thought to be proscribed in acute viral myocarditis (because increased tissue necrosis and viral replication have been demonstrated following their use in experimental myocarditis), their use in a small number of patients has not been associated with similar dire short-term consequences.[440] Nonsteroidal antiinflammatory agents—indomethacin, salicylates, and ibuprofen,[468,469] along with cyclosporine[470–472a]—are contraindicated during the acute phase of viral myocarditis (the first 2 weeks), because they increase myocardial damage. On the other hand, nonsteroidal antiinflammatory agents appear to be safe in the late phase of myocarditis.[469,473] In experimental models of myocarditis, the converting enzyme inhibitor captopril has beneficial effects in the acute phase of myocarditis; human data are not yet available.[474,474a] Bed rest (or at least restricted activity) is advisable, because exercise in experimental animals with myocarditis is deleterious.[440]

It is hoped that effective antiviral agents,[475,476] immunosuppressive agents, or antilymphocyte monoclonal antibodies for treating viral myocarditis will be available soon for clinical use.[477,478] It may also be possible, in the future, to treat patients with myocarditis with agents that stimulate production of interferon, since this substance affords protection against the effects of viral myocarditis, at least in experimental animals.[479–481] Antibiotics may also be employed with benefit in infections caused by atypical pneumonia and psittacosis.

VIRAL MYOCARDITIS

There are approximately two dozen viruses that may be associated with clinical evidence of myocarditis[440] (Table 43–14). The myocarditis characteristically develops after a lag period of several weeks following the initial systemic infection, suggesting involvement of an immunological mechanism. In animals, a variety of factors appears to enhance susceptibility to myocardial damage, including radiation, malnutrition, steroids, exercise, and previous myocardial injury. Viral myocarditis may be particularly virulent in infants and in pregnant women.[439]

COXSACKIE VIRUS. Both Coxsackie A and B viruses may produce myocarditis, although infection with Coxsackie B is more common, and this agent is the most frequent cause of viral myocarditis.[439] The myocardium appears to be particularly susceptible to the effects of this virus because of the apparent affinity of myocardial membrane receptors for the viral particles.[439] Necropsy often demonstrates a pericardial effusion, pericarditis, cardiac enlargement, and a predominantly mononuclear inflammatory infiltrate, with necrosis of the atrial and ventricular myocardium. In some cases, focal myocardial necrosis simulating myocardial infarction is seen, despite normal coronary arteries.[452]

Although most infections are probably benign, self-limited, and subclinical,[439] Coxsackie myocarditis appears to be particularly virulent in the neonate.[482] In most infections in adults, the other clinical manifestations of viral involvement, such as pleurodynia, myalgia, upper respiratory tract symptoms, and arthralgias, predominate. Severe cases in the adult are characterized by myopericardial involvement with pleuritic or pericarditic chest pain, palpitations, and fever. Many patients with overt myocardial involvement develop congestive heart failure with cardiomegaly and pulmonary edema.

The *electrocardiogram* is virtually always abnormal, with ST-segment and T-wave changes and arrhythmias, often ventricular in origin; AV conduction disturbances are common.[482] Blood levels of myocardial enzymes (serum glutamic oxaloacetic transaminase, creatine kinase) may be normal or elevated, reflecting the absence or presence of variable degrees of myocardial necrosis. *Echocardiography* may reveal diffuse and regional left ventricular wall motion abnormalities[454] that usually improve or disappear over time.

Most patients recover completely within weeks, although the electrocardiogram and ventricular function may require months to return to normal.[483] Rarely, Coxsackie myocarditis is fatal in adults.[484] Some patients become symptomatic following resolution of the infection, and they may present years later with dilated cardiomyopathy.[485,486] Occasionally, patients appear to recover completely only to develop symptoms subsequently.[487]

Treatment is symptomatic, and despite occasional postmortem evidence of intracardiac thrombi, anticoagulation should probably be avoided because of the risk of a hemorrhagic pericardial effusion. Bed rest is indicated during the acute course of myocarditis, but there is no convincing evidence that a period of prolonged rest after apparent resolution of the acute process is useful. Heart failure and cardiac arrhythmias are treated in the usual fashion.

CYTOMEGALOVIRUS. Unrecognized infection with cytomegalovirus (CMV) is extremely common in childhood,[488] and the majority of the adult population have antibodies to CMV. Primary infection after the age of 35 years is uncommon, and generalized infection usually occurs only in immunosuppressed patients with neoplastic disease, after transplantation and with HIV infection.[489,490] The cardiovascular manifestations in adults are generally limited to asymptomatic and transient electrocardiographic changes.[488] Symptomatic cardiac involvement is rare, although a hemorrhagic pericardial effusion or myocarditis with left ventricular dysfunction and attendant congestive heart failure may occur.[488-492] The diagnosis of CMV myocarditis may be suggested by the presence of viral inclusions in myocardial biopsy specimens and confirmed by the detection of viral DNA in the myocardium.[493] While fatalities are unusual, when they do occur histological examination of the heart may reveal focal lymphocytic infiltration and fibrosis.[494]

DENGUE. Although previous dengue epidemics often were associated with symptomatic cardiac involvement, more recent outbreaks have been associated with fewer apparent cardiac complications.[495] Nonspecific electrocardiographic repolarization abnormalities are common but typically benign and transient.[495,496] Transient ventricular arrhythmias may be seen on occasion. Frank myocarditis and clinically significant cardiac involvement appear to be more common in some of the related hemorrhagic fevers, especially those due to arenaviruses.[497]

HEPATITIS. Clinical cardiac involvement in hepatitis is rare; an occasional patient may develop fulminant myocarditis with congestive heart failure, hypotension, and death.[498,499] The characteristic *pathological changes* in the myocardium associated with viral hepatitis are minute foci of necrosis of isolated muscle bundles, often surrounded by lymphocytes, and a diffuse serous inflammation.[498] The ventricles may be dilated, with petechial hemorrhages. Hemorrhage into the myocardium may be a conspicuous finding.[498] Myocardial damage may be produced indirectly through an immune-mediated mechanism or directly by viral invasion of the heart.[498]

Symptomatic myocarditis is generally observed in the first to third week of illness. Patients may have dyspnea, palpitations, and anginal chest pain; fatalities have been reported.[498,500] *Electrocardiographic changes,* including bradycardia, ventricular premature beats, and ST-segment and T-wave changes, may be seen during the course of hepatitis.[498] These abnormalities are usually transient and asymptomatic, although congestive heart failure, cardiomegaly, and sudden death have been reported.[498,499]

Human Immunodeficiency Virus (HIV)

Heart involvement (Table 43–15) in the acquired immunodeficiency syndrome (AIDS) may consist of metastatic involvement from Kaposi's sarcoma (Fig. 43–30), a wide variety of infective and nonspecific forms of myocarditis (Fig. 43–31), pericarditis with or without an effusion, endocarditis, and dilated cardiomyopathy (Fig. 43–32). Cardiac involvement occurs in about one-quarter to one-half of patients (on the basis of echocardiographic, endomyocardial biopsy, and autopsy findings); however, it leads to clinically apparent heart disease in only approximately 10 per cent.[501-513] When there are clinical manifestations, congestive heart failure is the most common finding and is due to left ventricular dilatation and dysfunction, simulating a dilated cardiomyopathy.[505-509] Because of the frequency of opportunistic pulmonary infections, dyspnea may be attributed incorrectly to lung disease rather than congestive heart failure; echocardiography may be useful in identifying left ventricular dysfunction as the cause of the dyspnea.[504,509] Other common clinical and echocardiographic findings that result in symptoms in a minority of patients include pericardial effusion (usually but not invariably without cardiac tamponade), ventricular arrhythmias,

TABLE 43–15 CARDIAC LESIONS IN AIDS

MYOCARDITIS
- Opportunistic infections
  - *Pneumocystis carinii*
  - *Mycobacterium* tuberculosis
  - *Mycobacterium avium-intracellulare*
  - *Cryptococcus neoformans*
  - *Aspergillus fumigatus*
  - *Candida albicans*
  - *Histoplasma capsulatum*
  - *Coccidioides immitis*
  - *Toxoplasma gondii*
  - Herpes simplex
- Viral agents
  - Cytomegalovirus
  - Human immunodeficiency virus (HIV)
- Lymphocytic myocarditis
- Noninflammatory myocardial necrosis
  - Microvascular spasm?

ENDOCARDITIS
- Marantic endocarditis (nonbacterial thrombotic endocarditis)
- Healed bacterial endocarditis
- Aspergillus endocarditis

PERICARDITIS
- Infectious
  - Tuberculous
  - Herpes simplex
- Noninfectious
- Pericardial effusion

CARDIOMEGALY
- Right ventricular hypertrophy or dilation
- Biventricular dilation (dilated cardiomyopathy)

VASCULAR LESIONS
- Arteriopathy
- Myocardial infarction

MALIGNANCY
- Kaposi's sarcoma
- Malignant lymphoma

TOXIC LESIONS
- Drug-induced
  - Drugs used in combating opportunistic infections
  - Anti-HIV drugs

From Acierno, L. J.: Cardiac complications in acquired immunodeficiency syndrome (AIDS): A review. Reprinted by permission of the American College of Cardiology. J. Am. Coll. Cardiol. *13*:1144, 1989.

repolarization changes on the electrocardiogram, marantic endocarditis, and right ventricular dilatation and hypertrophy.[502,504,505,507,508,514]

Pathological cardiac findings in AIDS patients are common, with myocarditis the most frequent.[501,507,508,510,511] While opportunistic infections caused by a wide variety of viral, fungal, parasitic, and bacterial pathogens account for some cases of myocarditis, most are unexplained but are suspected to be related to the human immunodeficiency virus (HIV) itself.[508] Isolation of HIV from the myocardium has added further credence to this speculation.[515] It has been speculated that the HIV-related myocarditis may result in the dilated cardiomyopathy found in some patients.[516] Other important postmortem findings include pericardial effusions, right and/or left ventricular dilatation, and nonbacterial thrombotic endocarditis.[507,508,517]

Treatment of AIDS-associated heart disease may afford some degree of symptomatic improvement. Relief of cardiac tamponade, therapy for infective myocarditis, and treatment of congestive heart failure have resulted in at least short-term palliation.[509,518]

INFECTIOUS MONONUCLEOSIS. Evident cardiac involvement in infectious mononucleosis is extremely rare, although nonspecific ST-segment and T-wave abnormalities may be seen.[519] In rare cases, pericarditis and myocarditis (even simulating a myocardial infarction)[520] may be present.[519,521]

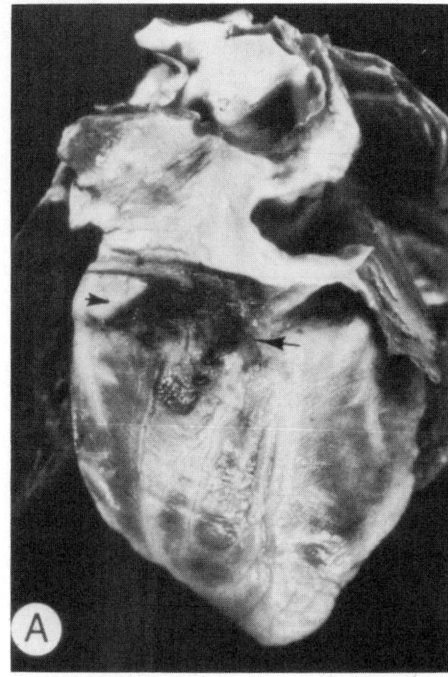

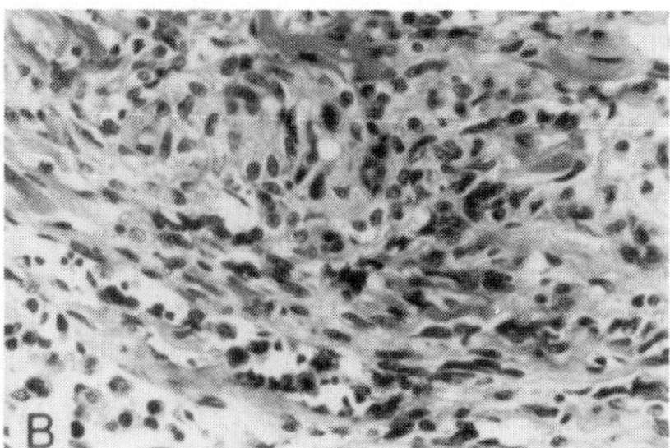

←

FIGURE 43-30. Kaposi's sarcoma involving the heart in AIDS. *A*, Gross photography of tumor invading the epicardium and superficial myocardium (arrows). *B*, Kaposi's sarcoma of the epicardium. Slit-like vascular clefts (characteristic of Kaposi's sarcoma) were abundant. (Hematoxylin and eosin; original magnification ×250.) (From Lewis, W.: AIDS: Cardiac findings from 115 autopsies. Prog. Cardiovasc. Dis. *32*:207, 1989.)

→

FIGURE 43-31. Example of lymphocytic myocarditis showing myocyte necrosis in AIDS patient (×400, reduced by 5 per cent). (From Baroldi, G., Corallo, S., Moroni, M., et al.: Focal lymphocytic myocarditis in acquired immunodeficiency syndrome (AIDS): A correlative morphologic and clinical study in 26 consecutive fatal cases. Reprinted by permission from the American College of Cardiology. J. Am. Coll. Cardiol. *12*:463, 1988.).

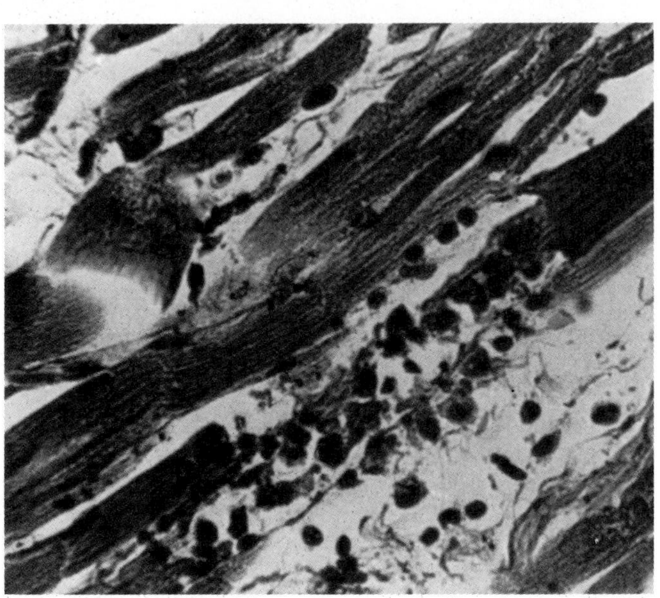

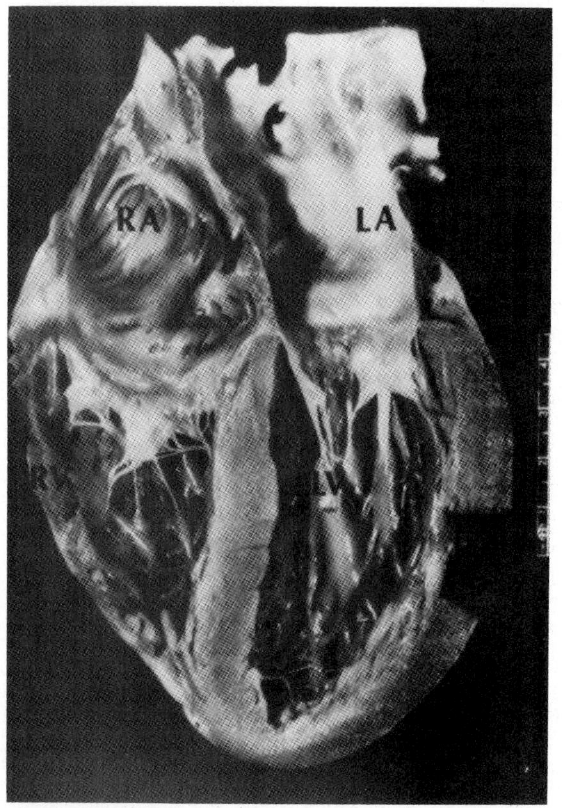

←

FIGURE 43-32. Marked dilatation of all four chambers of the heart in a patient with AIDS. LA = left atrium, RA = right atrium. (Reproduced by permission from Cohen, I. S., Anderson, D. W., Virmani, R., et al.: Congestive cardiomyopathy in association with the acquired immunodeficiency syndrome. N. Engl. J. Med. *315*:628, 1986.)

INFLUENZA. Although clinically apparent myocarditis is rare in influenza, the presence of preexisting cardiovascular disease greatly increases the risk of morbidity and mortality.[522,523] Postmortem findings in fatal cases include biventricular dilatation,[476] with evidence of a mononuclear infiltrate,[524] especially in perivascular areas.

Cardiac involvement typically occurs within 1 to 2 weeks of the onset of the illness and may be severe, sometimes contributing to mortality.[476] The *clinical manifestations* include dyspnea, palpitations, anginal chest pain, arrhythmia, and heart failure: there may be concomitant involvement of the pericardium.[476,525] Sinus tachycardia or, less commonly, sinus bradycardia may be seen. The *electrocardiogram* may show transient ST-segment and T-wave abnormalities, conduction defects, and even complete AV block[526]; death may be associated with massive hemorrhagic pulmonary edema due to viral or bacterial involvement of the lungs.[527]

LASSA FEVER. Lassa fever, a major cause of death in West Africa that is caused by an arenavirus, often is associated with electrocardiographic abnormalities[528] that may represent subclinical myocardial involvement. More than half the patients demonstrate nonspecific repolarization changes and low voltage.[528] Pericardial involvement may occur.[529] *Pathological findings* include myocardial congestion, edema, and a mononuclear cellular infiltrate.[530] In most cases, however, the putative cardiac involvement does not appear to play a major clinical role.[528]

MUMPS. Myocardial involvement during the course of mumps is rarely recognized.[531,532] The hearts of only a few patients with mumps have come to postmortem examination and they have been found to be both dilated and hypertrophied. Histologically, there is diffuse interstitial fibrosis, with infiltration of mononuclear cells and areas of focal necrosis.[531]

Cardiac involvement is usually unrecognized clinically, and the diagnosis of myocarditis is based on nonspecific electrocardiographic changes.[531] Transient ST-segment and T-wave abnormalities are most common, but extrasystoles and AV conduction block may occur.[531-533] Myocarditis generally occurs in the first week of illness and is transient, in most cases resolving within several weeks. A few patients develop precordial chest pain, dyspnea, palpitations, and fatigue; cardiomegaly and congestive heart failure occur on occasion.[531-534] Tachycardia, a transient apical systolic murmur, and protodiastolic gallop may be present.[531-533]

POLIOMYELITIS. Myocarditis is a frequent finding in fatal cases of poliomyelitis, particularly during epidemics,[537] occurring in half or more of all patients dying with this disease; death may be sudden.[538] While myocardial involvement is usually focal and minimal in extent, some patients with bulbar disease succumb early in the course of the illness, often with cardiovascular collapse.[537,539] These patients all have viral infection of the medulla and severe systemic vasoconstriction that leads to pulmonary edema. Myocarditis appears to contribute to the heart failure.[537] The *electrocardiogram* is frequently abnormal, with ST-segment and T-wave abnormalities, prolongation of the P-R and Q-T intervals,[540] premature contractions, tachycardia, and atrial fibrillation. *Treatment* is symptomatic, with aggressive support of pulmonary function; tracheostomy and prolonged mechanical ventilatory support may be required. Fortunately, this disease has been largely eliminated by immunization.

RESPIRATORY SYNCYTIAL VIRUS. Although respiratory syncytial virus is an important cause of respiratory disease, particularly in children, it rarely results in cardiac involvement.[542] Congestive heart failure and complete heart block have been seen on occasion.[543,544]

RUBELLA AND RUBEOLA. Congenital cardiovascular lesions may develop in the offspring when *rubella* is contracted by the mother during the first trimester of pregnancy, with persistent ductus arteriosus and pulmonary artery maldevelopment as prominent anomalies. Rare cases of myocarditis occur, with attendant conduction defects and heart failure.[545]

In *rubeola,* transient electrocardiographic abnormalities, including prolongation of the P-R interval, ST-segment and T-wave changes, AV conduction abnormalities, and ventricular tachycardia, have been reported.[546,547] Congestive heart failure occurs on rare occasions, and its appearance is a poor prognostic sign, often indicating a fatal outcome.[548] Histological examination of the heart in fatal cases has revealed evidence of myocarditis characterized predominantly by a perivascular lymphocytic infiltrate.[547]

VARICELLA. Clinical myocarditis is a rare finding in varicella, although unsuspected myocarditis is common in fatal varicella.[549] Occasionally a patient may develop overt evidence of myocarditis with congestive heart failure.[549-552] Histological findings include rare but characteristic intranuclear inclusion bodies within the myocardial cells, along with interstitial edema, cellular infiltrates, and myonecrosis. The electrocardiogram may show conduction abnormalities; sudden death occurs rarely.

VARIOLA AND VACCINIA. Cardiac involvement following smallpox is rare, although several cases of myocarditis associated with acute cardiac failure and death have been reported.[553] Myocarditis with pericardial effusion and congestive heart failure has also been observed as a complication of smallpox vaccination[554]; an immunological mechanism has been suggested and dramatic responses to steroids have been reported. The histological changes include a mixed mononuclear infiltrate, with interstitial edema and occasional degenerating or necrotic muscle bundles.[555]

RICKETTSIAL MYOCARDITIS

The rickettsial diseases frequently are associated with evidence of myocardial involvement, but usually it is subclinical. Transient ST-segment and T-wave alterations in particular are observed commonly. The circulatory collapse that may accompany these diseases is largely a manifestation of abnormalities of the peripheral vascular bed, but a myocardial component may also be present. The basic histopathological process is vasculitis, with a periarterial interstitial infiltrate.

Q FEVER. Endocarditis is the most common cardiac manifestation of infection with *R. burnettii* (Q fever). Myocarditis is not a prominent feature,[556] although dyspnea and chest pain, perhaps reflecting associated pericarditis, occur frequently. The electrocardiogram may demonstrate transient ST-segment and T-wave changes as well as paroxysmal ventricular arrhythmias. Abnormalities of the immune system have been implicated in the pathogenesis of the disease.[557,558]

ROCKY MOUNTAIN SPOTTED FEVER. Clinical evidence of myocarditis is more common than often appreciated in Rocky Mountain spotted fever (caused by *R. rickettsii*), and the heart is often involved in the multisystem damage that occurs as the result of a widespread vasculitis.[559-561] Unsuspected left ventricular dysfunction is common, and echocardiographic evidence of dysfunction may persist in some patients.[559]

SCRUB TYPHUS. Myocarditis is common during the course of scrub typhus (tsutsugamushi disease, caused by *R. tsutsugamushi*).[562] The histological findings are those of a focal panvasculitis involving the small blood vessels. Myocardial necrosis is unusual, but hemorrhage into the heart and subepicardial petechiae may occur. Clinical evidence of myocardial involvement typically is not severe and is usually not associated with residual cardiac damage.[562,563] The electrocardiogram may show nonspecific ST-segment and T-wave abnormalities, as well as first degree AV block. A protodiastolic gallop and apical systolic murmur suggestive of mitral regurgitation are occasionally found.[562]

BACTERIAL MYOCARDITIS

BRUCELLOSIS. Cardiac involvement in the course of brucellosis is uncommon, usually consisting of endocarditis.[564-566] Myocardial involvement, when it occurs, is manifested by T-wave changes and prolongation of AV conduction.[566,567] An occasional patient develops fulminant myocarditis, with a lymphocytic and polymorphonuclear infiltrate.[566,567]

CLOSTRIDIA. Cardiac involvement is common in patients with clostridial infections with multiple organ involvement.[568] The myocardial damage results from the toxin elaborated by the bacteria, but the precise actions of the toxin remain to be elucidated.[569] The *pathological findings* are distinctive, with gas bubbles usually present in the myocardium. Areas of degenerated muscle fibers are apparent, but an inflammatory infiltrate is usually absent.[568] *C. perfringens* may cause myocardial abscess formation with myocardial perforation and resultant purulent pericarditis.[570]

DIPHTHERIA. Myocardial involvement is one of the most serious complications of diphtheria and occurs in up to 20 per cent of cases.[571] Indeed, myocardial involvement is the most common cause of death in this infection, and half of the fatal cases demonstrate cardiac involvement.[571] Cardiac damage is due to the liberation by the diphtheria bacillus of a toxin that inhibits protein synthesis by interfering with the transfer of amino acids from soluble RNA to polypeptide chains under construction.

Pathological findings include a flabby and dilated heart with a myocardium that has a "streaky" appearance. Microscopic examination reveals characteristic fatty infiltration of the myocytes,[571] often with an interstitial inflammatory infiltrate, myocytolysis, and hyaline necrosis of muscle fibers. With time, fibrosis and hypertrophy of the remaining myocardial cells develop. The conduction system is often involved.

Typically, *clinical* signs of cardiac dysfunction appear at the end of the first week of the illness. Cardiomegaly and severe congestive heart failure are often present. A protodiastolic gallop and pulmonary congestion may be prominent features. Elevation of the serum transaminase levels may be seen; a high level is associated with a poor prognosis. Sudden circulatory failure and death may occur. Many patients develop ST-segment and T-wave abnormalities, but atrial and ventricular arrhythmias and conduction defects may also occur.[571] Persistently abnormal electrocardiograms are common following diphtheritic myocarditis, as are cardiomegaly and symptoms of reduced cardiac reserve. Some patients recover fully.

Because of the serious effects of the toxin on the myocardium, antitoxin should be administered as rapidly as possible.[571] Antibiotic therapy is of less urgency. General supportive measures are indicated. Overt congestive heart failure may be resistant to therapy with cardiac glycosides. The development of complete AV block is a serious complication, but it may be amenable to treatment with a transvenous pacemaker. Corticosteroids do not appear to have any place in the treatment of the cardiac abnormalities[572]; treatment with carnitine seems to reduce the incidence of heart failure and the need for pacemaker, and to lower mortality.[573]

INFECTIVE ENDOCARDITIS. Myocardial infection is frequently observed as a consequence of infective endocarditis (Chap. 35).

LEGIONNAIRES' DISEASE. Although pneumonia, rhabdomyolysis, renal failure, and hepatic as well as central nervous system involvement are common with *Legionella pneumophila,* overt cardiac involvement is not. Occasional electrocardiographic changes may be noted, consisting primarily of ST-segment and T-wave abnormalities; ventricular arrhythmias may be seen.[574] Rarely, pericardial effusion or myocarditis with evidence of myocardial necrosis and congestive heart failure may be seen.[575]

MENINGOCOCCUS. Myocardial involvement is common during the course of fatal meningococcal infections but is less commonly recognized in the usual case.[576,577] *Pathological findings* include hemorrhagic myocardial lesions, occasionally associated with intracellular organisms.[577] An interstitial myocarditis composed of lymphocytes, plasma cells, and polymorphonuclear leukocytes is often observed, occasionally with myonecrosis.[577]

Meningococcal myocarditis may result in congestive heart failure, which may be fatal, as well as in pericardial effusion with tamponade.[576,578,579] Death may also occur suddenly and be associated with involvement of the AV node.[577] It is advisable to monitor the heart rhythm of patients with meningococcemia. In milder cases, transient electrocardiographic abnormalities, principally ST-segment and T-wave changes, are often seen and may resolve completely with time.[579]

MYCOPLASMA PNEUMONIAE. Electrocardiographic abnormalities are not uncommon during the course of atypical pneumonia; when carditis occurs, it may be serious, and, rarely, fatal.[535] Nonspecific ST-segment and T-wave abnormalities are the most common manifestation of cardiac involvement. The electrocardiographic findings usually resolve within 1 to 2 weeks. A cell-mediated myocarditis has been postulated as the cause of the changes.[535] Pericarditis may be a prominent finding, and congestive heart failure is occasionally seen.[535,536] A protodiastolic gallop and pericardial friction rub may be noted in occasional cases. No specific treatment for the cardiovascular involvement is usually indicated. Complete recovery is the rule in most patients, although occasional patients may have persistent sequelae, including arrhythmias.[536]

PSITTACOSIS. Myocarditis complicating psittacosis is a relatively common occurrence and is characterized by congestive heart failure and acute pericarditis.[541] *Pathological changes* include fibrinous pericarditis as well as endocarditis and myocarditis. Fever, chest pain, electrocardiographic changes, cardiomegaly, systemic emboli, tachycardia, and hypotension may occur. While most patients recover completely, fatalities have been reported in a small fraction.[541] The systemic infection may be treated effectively with tetracycline, but the effect of the antibiotic on the myocardium is unknown.

SALMONELLA. Symptomatic myocardial involvement during salmonella infections is rare,[580,581] although electrocardiographic abnormalities are often seen, suggesting subclinical myocarditis. *Postmortem findings* in salmonella myocarditis may reveal a shaggy, fibrinous pericarditis and, in some cases, evidence of endocarditis.[582] Myocardial petechiae and hemorrhagic necrosis may occur, with evidence of biventricular dilatation. A polymorphonuclear leukocytic infiltrate with evidence of coronary arteritis may be found. The arteritis may lead to thrombosis, infarction, and death. Other cardiovascular complications include infected mural thrombi, occasionally resulting in pulmonary and systemic emboli, and mycotic aneurysms.[582] Myocardial abscesses often develop and may rupture, producing fatal cardiac tamponade. Myocarditis with congestive heart failure occurs most commonly in children who are severely ill with salmonellosis, and it is associated with a high mortality.[583] When myocarditis occurs, it often develops rapidly, with evidence of biventricular failure, tachycardia, a protodiastolic gallop, an apical systolic murmur of mitral regurgitation, and peripheral edema.

Electrocardiographic abnormalities include ST-segment and T-wave changes, prolonged P-R or Q-T intervals, and low QRS voltage.[580,582,584]

STREPTOCOCCUS. The most commonly detected cardiac finding following beta-hemolytic streptococcal infection is acute rheumatic fever, which is discussed in detail in Chapter 56.

Involvement of the heart by the streptococcus may produce a myocarditis that is distinct from acute rheumatic carditis. It is characterized by an interstitial infiltrate composed of mononuclear cells with occasional polymorphonuclear leukocytes[585]; the infiltrate may be focal or diffuse and may be localized to the subendocardial or perivascular region. There may be small areas of myocardial necrosis.[585] *Electrocardiographic abnormalities,* including prolongation of the P-R and Q-T intervals, occur frequently.[586] While these abnormalities are rarely associated with other clinical manifestations of myocardial involvement, sudden death, conduction disturbances, and arrhythmias may occur.[585,586]

TUBERCULOSIS. Tuberculous involvement of the myocardium (not as a complication of tuberculous pericarditis) is extremely rare, particularly since the introduction of drugs effective against tuberculosis.[587,588] Most cases of myocardial tuberculosis are clinically silent and are diagnosed only at autopsy.[587] Tuberculous involvement of the myocardium may lead to arrhythmias, including atrial fibrillation and ventricular tachycardia, complete AV block, congestive heart failure, left ventricular aneurysms, and sudden death.[587,588]

WHIPPLE DISEASE

Intestinal lipodystrophy, or Whipple disease, may be associated with myocardial involvement, and PAS-positive macrophages may be found in the myocardium, pericardium, and heart valves of patients with this disorder.[589,590] Coronary artery lesions, with smooth muscle necrosis, panarteritis, and medial scarring, are not rare.[591] Unusually, patients may develop pulmonary hypertension.[592] Electron microscopy has demonstrated rod-shaped structures in the myocardium similar to those found in the small intestine, and it has been suggested that they are the causative agent of the myocardial abnormalities. There may be an associated inflammatory infiltrate and foci of fibrosis.[589] The valvular fibrosis may be severe enough to result in aortic regurgitation and mitral stenosis.[591] While asymptomatic, nonspecific electrocardiographic changes are most common; systolic murmurs, pericarditis, and even overt congestive heart failure may occur.[590] Antibiotic therapy appears to be effective in treating the basic disease; however, relapses can occur, often more than 2 years after initial diagnosis.[593,594]

SPIROCHETAL INFECTIONS

LEPTOSPIROSIS (WEIL DISEASE). Cardiac involvement is common in fatal leptospirosis,[595] and almost half of all patients demonstrate transient ST-segment and T-wave abnormalities.[596] The *pathological findings* include petechiae or larger foci of hemorrhage, often located in the epicardium.[597] An interstitial myocardial infiltration, often subendocardial in location, may occur, with involvement of the papillary muscles. Involvement of the AV conduction system, aortitis, and coronary arteritis may be prominent features. The most common manifestations of cardiac involvement are ST-segment and T-wave changes; atrial and ventricular arrhythmias, sinus bradycardia, and conduction defects may occur.[596,598,599] Cardiomegaly, pulmonary congestion, a protodiastolic gallop, pericarditis, and symptoms of congestive heart failure occur rarely.[596]

LYME CARDITIS. Lyme disease is caused by a tickborne spirochete *(Borrelia burgdorferi).*[600] The disease is found principally in areas of tick distribution including most of the United States, Europe, and the Far East.[601] It usually begins during the summer months with a characteristic skin rash (erythema chronicum migrans), followed in weeks to months by neurological, joint, or cardiac involvement; some clinical manifestations may persist for years.[603]

About 10 per cent of patients with Lyme disease develop evidence of transient cardiac involvement, the most common manifestation being variable degrees of AV block.[602,603] The location of the block appears to be at the level of the atrioventricular node.[600] Syncope due to complete heart block is frequent with cardiac involvement, since often there is an asso-

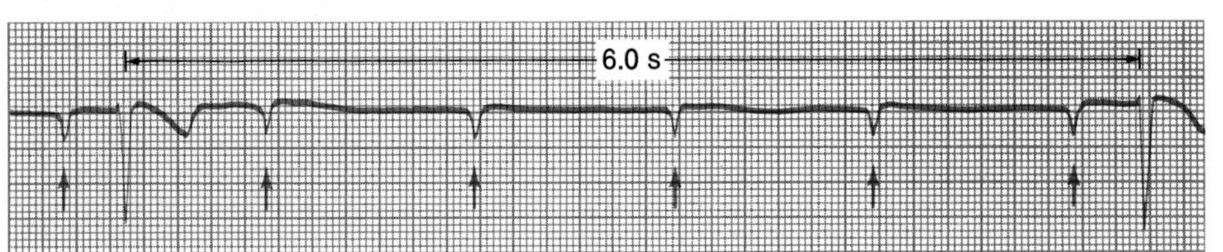

FIGURE 43–33. Complete atrioventricular block with 6-second ventricular asystole in patient with Lyme carditis. P waves, indicated by arrows, are regular at a rate of 50 per minute. (From McAlister, H. F., Klementowicz, P. T., Andrews, C., et al.: Lyme carditis: An important cause of reversible heart block. Ann. Intern. Med. *110*:339, 1989.)

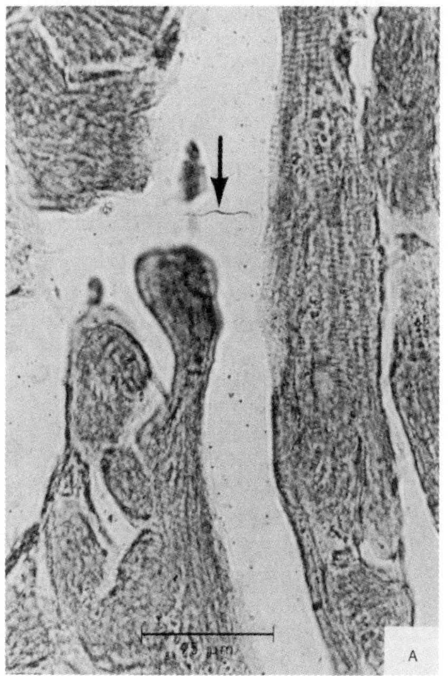

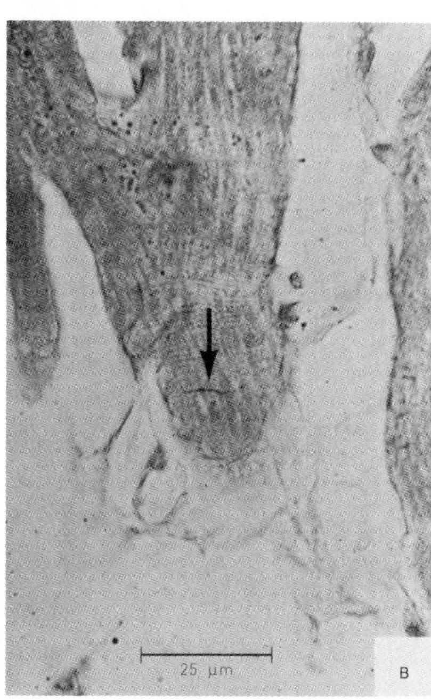

FIGURE 43–34. Human myocardium infected with *B. burgdorferi* (modified Steiner's silver stain). A spirochetal organism is shown in the endomysial space (arrow, Panel A) and apparently within the myocardial cell (arrow, Panel B). (Reprinted with permission from Stanek, G., Klein, J., Bittner, R., and Glogar, D.: Isolation of *Borrelia burgdorferi* from the myocardium of a patient with longstanding cardiomyopathy. N. Engl. J. Med. *322*:249, 1990.)

ciated depression of ventricular escape rhythms (Fig. 43–33).[600,604] Ventricular tachycardia occurs uncommonly. Diffuse ST-segment and T-wave abnormalities and transient, usually asymptomatic left ventricular dysfunction may be found in some patients, although cardiomegaly or symptoms of congestive heart failure are rare. A positive[600,601] gallium or indium antimyosin antibody scan may point to suspected cardiac involvement in this disease.[605,606] The demonstration of spirochetes in myocardial biopsies of some patients with Lyme carditis (Fig. 43–34) suggests that the cardiac manifestations are due to a direct toxic effect, although there is speculation that immune-mediated mechanisms may be involved as well.[600,607]

The value of specific therapy in Lyme carditis remains uncertain; however, it is thought that treating the early manifestations of the disease may prevent development of late complications. Patients with second degree or complete heart block should be hospitalized and should undergo continuous electrocardiographic monitoring. Temporary transvenous pacing may be required for up to a week or longer in patients with high-grade block.[600] Although the efficacy of antibiotics in carditis is unestablished, they are utilized routinely (intravenous penicillin G, 20 million units per day, or oral tetracycline, 250 mg four times a day).[600] Whether antiinflammatory agents (salicylates, corticosteroids) can ameliorate heart block is also not clear.[604]

RELAPSING FEVER. Many infections are currently observed in Ethiopia. During pandemics, mortality may be particularly high, reaching 70 per cent, although sporadic cases are often more benign.[608] Cardiac involvement is a common complication and is often implicated as a cause of death. AV conduction defects occur frequently and may be responsible for sudden death, although tachyarrhythmias have also been implicated.[608] Numerous petechiae are observed with a diffuse histiocytic interstitial infiltrate, particularly around small arterioles in the left ventricle.

SYPHILIS. Aortitis is the most common manifestation of luetic involvement of the cardiovascular system. Aortic regurgitation and coronary ostial narrowing are associated findings. Syphilitic involvement of the myocardium itself in the form of gumma formation is rare and is usually unsuspected clinically. Involvement of the interventricular septum may result in damage to the conducting system and AV block.[609] Gummae may also impinge on the heart valves and interfere with their function.[610]

FUNGAL INFECTIONS OF THE HEART

Cardiac fungal infections occur most frequently in patients with malignant disease and/or those receiving chemotherapy, steroids, radiation, or immunosuppressive therapy. Cardiac surgery, intravenous drug abuse, and infection with HIV are also predisposing factors for fungal cardiac involvement.[611]

ACTINOMYCOSIS. Myocarditis is a rare complication of actinomycotic infection, occurring in less than 2 per cent of patients.[612] However, cardiac involvement is quite serious when it does occur. Involvement of the heart most commonly is the result of direct extension of disease within the thorax.[612,613] Initially the pericardium is invaded, with eventual obliteration of the pericardial space. The myocardium may be involved by extension of the pericardial process. Myocardial seeding is less common.[612] The myocardial lesion is a suppurative, necrotizing abscess containing the organism, surrounded by granulation tissue. Both right- and left-sided failure are common manifestations. A pericardial rub may be heard, sometimes associated with clinical evidence of a pericardial effusion or constriction.[612,613]

ASPERGILLOSIS. Myocardial involvement is not uncommon in generalized aspergillosis, and when it occurs it is usually fatal.[614] It is being encountered increasingly in the immunocompromised patient.[615] On pathological examination, myocardial necrosis and infarction caused by thrombosis of vessels that contain fungal mycelia are commonly seen, along with myocardial abscesses and pericardial involvement.[614] The electrocardiogram may be normal in the face of significant myocardial damage but T-wave changes may be present. The *diagnosis* of aspergillus infection is often difficult. Identification of aspergillus through open lung biopsy, aspiration lung biopsy, transtracheal aspiration, or bronchial brush technique may be successful. Treatment with antifungal agents often is unsuccessful.[614]

BLASTOMYCOSIS. Involvement of the heart by the fungus is quite uncommon, even in the immunocompromised heart. When involvement occurs, it is most often by direct extension from the pericardium.

CANDIDIASIS. Disseminated monilial infections are common opportunistic infections, particularly in the compromised host.[616] Endocarditis is the most frequent manifestation of cardiac involvement (p. 1494), occurring most commonly in cardiac surgical patients or drug addicts, although multiple abscesses of the myocardium may occur as associated or independent findings.[617] Complete heart block may be caused by microabscesses of the conduction system.[616]

COCCIDIOIDOMYCOSIS. Involvement of the heart is rare in patients with generalized coccidioidomycosis.[618] The hearts may be grossly normal, although epicardial lesions with resultant pericarditis are common, and progression to constrictive pericarditis may occur (p. 1494). A nonspecific, focal interstitial, and perivascular cellular infiltrate with associated muscle fiber degeneration and interstitial edema is commonly found, although granulomas containing fungi are also seen sometimes.

CRYPTOCOCCOSIS. Cryptococcal infection of the myocardium occurs most commonly in immunocompromised patients with disseminated malignancy or HIV infection.[619] *Pathological examination* may show cardiac dilatation, with epithelial granulomas, giant cells, and an inflammatory infiltrate.[619] When congestive heart failure occurs, pulmonary congestion and muffled heart sounds may be found on physical examination, and cardiomegaly on the chest roentgenogram.[619] The *electrocardiogram* may show first-degree AV block and T-wave inversions; ventricular arrhythmias have been observed.

HISTOPLASMOSIS. Cardiac involvement in histoplasmosis is rare and usually is related to mediastinal fibrosis, the most serious complication of histoplasmosis.[620,621] Pericarditis with effusion may occur[620] (p. 1489) and superior vena caval obstruction has been observed.[621] Myocardial involvement occurs less frequently, although atrial arrhythmias and T-wave abnormalities have been reported.

PROTOZOAL MYOCARDITIS

Trypanosomiasis (Chagas' Disease)

Chagas' disease is caused by the protozoan *Trypanosoma cruzi*. The major cardiovascular manifestation is an extensive myocarditis that typically becomes evident years after the initial infection. The disease is prevalent in Central and South America, particularly in Brazil, Argentina, and Chile, where it is a major public health problem. Perhaps 20 million people in South America may be infected with the parasite.[622] In rare cases, the disease may be found in nonendemic areas as a consequence of transfusion with contaminated blood products.[623]

The natural history of Chagas' disease is characterized by three phases: acute, latent, and chronic. During the *acute phase*, the disease is transmitted to humans (usually below the age of 20 years)[624,625] through the bite of a reduviid bug (subfamily Triatominae), which harbors the parasite in its gastrointestinal tract. This insect acquires the disease from feeding on infected animals, including the armadillo, raccoon, opossum, and skunk as well as domestic dogs and cats. The reduviid bug, popularly known in Argentina as "vinchuca," meaning "to let oneself drop," lives in the walls and roofs of houses and, during nocturnal feedings, drops from the ceiling onto the sleeping person below. The bug then often bites the person around the eyes, and infection of the human host occurs when the trypanosomes in the animal's feces gain entry through abraded skin or through the conjunctivae. Occasionally, this results in unilateral periorbital edema and swelling of the eyelid, termed *Romaña's sign*,[626] while entry through the skin may result in a lesion called a *chagoma*. Transmission may occur through blood transfusions as well as congenitally.

ACUTE TRYPANOSOMIASIS. Following inoculation, the protozoa multiply and then migrate widely throughout the body. In about 1 per cent of cases an acute illness occurs.[625]

Pathological examination during the acute phase often reveals parasites in the cardiac fibers with a marked cellular infiltrate, particularly around cardiac cells that have ruptured and released the parasites.[627] Involvement may extend into the endocardium, resulting in thrombus formation, and into the epicardium, resulting in pericardial effusion. The pathogenesis of the myocardial lesions of acute Chagas' disease appears to relate in large part to immune lysis by antibody and cell-mediated immunity directed against antigens released from *T. cruzi*–infected cells, which become adsorbed onto the surface of infected and noninfected host cells. In experimental acute Chagas' disease there are generalized alterations of the adenylate cyclase complex, but the significance of this observation is not clear.[628]

Clinical Manifestations. These include fever, muscle pains, sweating, hepatosplenomegaly, myocarditis with congestive heart failure, and, occasionally, meningoencephalitis. Most patients recover, and their symptoms resolve over several months. Young children most commonly develop clinical acute disease and generally are more seriously ill than adults.

CHRONIC TRYPANOSOMIASIS. The disease then enters a *latent phase* without clinical symptoms; however, there is evidence of early and progressive subclinical cardiomyopathy. Electrocardiographic changes often appear at this stage and are a marker for the eventual clinical heart disease and increased mortality to become evident later.[624] At an average of 20 years after the initial (and usually unrecognized) infestations, approximately 30 per cent of infected individuals develop findings of *chronic Chagas' disease*, the manifestations of which cover a wide spectrum from asymptomatic but seropositive patients through those with electrocardiographic abnormalities to those with advanced disease characterized by cardiomegaly, congestive heart failure, arrhythmias, thromboembolic phenomena, atypical chest pain, right bundle branch block, and sudden death.[629–632] In the advanced stage, cardiac dilatation typically involves all the cardiac chambers, although right-sided enlargement may predominate. Even those individuals whose only clinical evidence of the disease is seropositivity often have subclinical cardiac involvement that may be demonstrated by endomyocardial biopsy.[633]

The central paradox in the pathogenesis of this disorder is the negative correlation between the severity of disease and the level of parasitemia. It is not unusual to be unable to detect parasites in patients dying of Chagas' disease.[634] An autoimmune mechanism has been proposed,[634,635] although this has by no means been established.[636] It appears (at least in an animal model) that self-reactive cytotoxic T lymphocytes develop following the initial infection, and these lymphocytes are able to lyse normal host cells, perhaps related to cross-reacting antigens of *T. cruzi* and striated muscle.[1,637,638] A variety of antibodies against myocyte sarcoplasmic reticulum, laminin, and other constituents have also been implicated in the pathogenesis of Chagas' myocarditis. It is thought that the acute phase results in the release from parasite-modified host cells of self components that are immunogenic.[639] Another hypothesis suggests that cardiac parasympathetic denervation leads to eventual chronic Chagas' disease.[640,641]

Pathology. Nerves and autonomic ganglia are frequently abnormal, and megaesophagus and megacolon may occur; less commonly, there is dilatation of the stomach, duodenum, ureter, and bronchi. Different strains of *T. cruzi* may account for the geographic differences in the expression of Chagas' disease; in Brazil, megaesophagus and megacolon are common, but these conditions are unusual in Venezuela.[634] Lesions of the cardiac nerves are routinely found in patients with chronic Chagas' disease, with evidence of cardiac parasympathetic denervation.[642] Pathological cardiac findings include cardiac enlargement with dilatation and hypertrophy of all cardiac chambers. The left ventricular apex is often thin and bulging, resembling an aneurysm[643] (Fig. 43–35). Thrombus formation is frequent and may fill much of the apex; the right atrium also frequently contains thrombus. It has been suggested that this characteristic apical aneurysm may be the result of intravascular platelet aggregation leading to focal myocardial necrosis.[644]

The microscopic findings are principally those of extensive fibrosis, particularly of the left ventricle.[624] A chronic cellular infiltrate composed of lymphocytes, plasma cells, and macrophages is often present. Preferential involvement of the right bundle branch and the anterior fascicle of the left bundle branch by inflammatory and fibrotic changes explains the frequent occurrence of right bundle branch and left anterior fascicular block.[624] The basement membranes of capillaries,

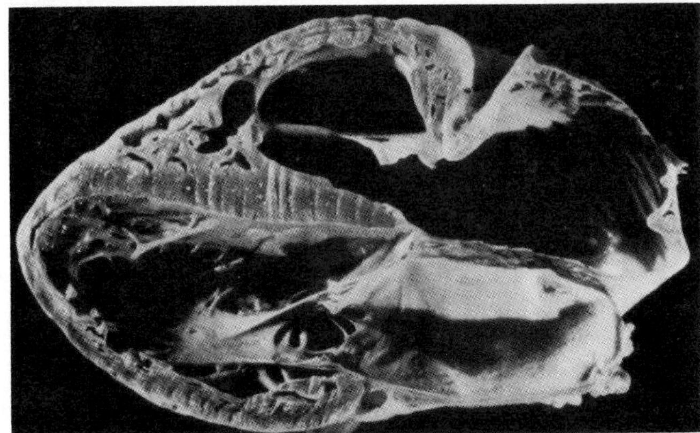

FIGURE 43–35. Long-axis autopsy section of heart from patient who had congestive heart failure caused by chronic Chagas' heart disease. Left ventricular apical and posteroapical thinning and fibrosis with relative septal sparing are evident. Coronary arteries were normal. (From Acquatella, H., Schiller, N. B., Puigbo, J. J., et al.: Circulation *62*:790, 1980, reprinted with permission of the American Heart Association, Inc.)

vascular smooth muscle cells, and myocytes are thickened.[645] Parasites may be identified in one-fourth of patients; the frequency with which they are found depends upon the diligence of the search for them.

Clinical Manifestations. Chronic progressive heart failure, often predominantly right-sided, is the rule in advanced cases. Thus, while pulmonary congestion is occasionally noted, the usual findings generally include fatigue due to diminished cardiac output, peripheral edema, ascites, and hepatic congestion. Tricuspid regurgitation is often present, particularly in patients with severe right-sided heart failure, although mitral regurgitation is frequently present as well. The second heart sound is widely split, often with an accentuated pulmonic component, reflecting the combined effects of right bundle branch block and pulmonary hypertension. Autonomic dysfunction is common,[646] with marked abnormalities in the expected reflex changes in heart rate produced by various maneuvers.[647,648]

The *chest roentgenogram* often demonstrates severe cardiomegaly, with or without pulmonary venous hypertension. *Electrocardiographic abnormalities* are the rule[631] particularly in patients who are seroreactive to *T. cruzi* antigen, with right bundle branch block and left anterior hemiblock being the most common changes in patients with chronic Chagas' disease.[43,646,649] ST-segment and T-wave abnormalities are common, while Q waves involving the inferior leads, P-wave abnormalities, and AV block are occasionally seen. Early in the disease, the electrocardiogram may be normal or nearly so. Administration of the antiarrhythmic agent ajmaline may precipitate the appearance of electrocardiographic abnormalities and thus identify patients with as yet clinically silent cardiac involvement. Furthermore, electrophysiological testing of asymptomatic patients, even those with normal electrocardiograms, may demonstrate abnormalities of the conducting system in the majority.

Ventricular arrhythmias are a prominent feature of chronic Chagas' disease.[630] Frequent ventricular premature depolarizations, often with multiple morphologies, are seen frequently, and bouts of ventricular tachycardia may occur.[649] Ventricular arrhythmias are particularly common during and following exercise, occurring in the majority of patients subjected to stress electrocardiographic testing (including some without any clinical evidence of cardiac involvement). Ventricular tachycardia induced by electrophysiological testing is most common in patients with evidence of conduction abnormalities on the electrocardiogram, low ejection fraction and apical left ventricular aneurysm.[639] Syncope and sudden death due to ventricular fibrillation are a constant threat and may develop even before cardiomegaly or heart failure. Sinus bradycardia may also be seen, even in patients with severe heart failure when a tachycardia would be expected, presumably related to cardiac autonomic dysfunction. Atrial arrhythmias, including atrial fibrillation, may also occur. Thromboembolic phenomena are a frequent complication,[643] occurring in more than 50 per cent of the patients.

The *echocardiographic findings* in advanced cases are those of a dilated cardiomyopathy (Fig. 43–28) with dilatation, increased end-diastolic and end-systolic volumes, and reduced ejection fraction, often with enlargement of the left atrium and right ventricle. Diastolic filling of the left ventricle is frequently abnormal, even in those without other clinical or echocardiographic evidence of cardiac involvement.[650,651] In the majority of advanced cases, the echocardiographic appearance is distinctive, with left ventricular posterior wall hypokinesis and relatively preserved interventricular septal motion; an apical aneurysm is often seen on two-dimensional echocardiography. Ten to 15 per cent of asymptomatic patients demonstrate apical dyskinesis.[622]

Radionuclide ventriculography may, like echocardiography, demonstrate right or left ventricular wall motion abnormalities in the absence of an overall depression of global ventricular function.[652]

Left ventricular cineangiography in advanced cases shows a dilated, hypokinetic left ventricle with a large apical aneurysm containing intracavitary thrombus, often with evidence of mitral regurgitation. *Coronary angiography* is usually normal, although abnormalities of the coronary microcirculation have been suggested as the cause of the clinical manifestations of Chagas' disease.[653]

The *complement-fixation* test (Machado-Guerreiro test) is useful in diagnosis; it has high sensitivity and specificity for the identification of chronic Chagas' disease. Also used in diagnosis are the indirect immunofluorescent antibody, the enzyme-linked immunosorbent assay (ELISA), and the hemagglutination tests.[654] Another test that is occasionally useful is the detection of parasites in the blood of patients with chronic Chagas' disease (which occurs in 30 to 40 per cent of cases) by means of *xenodiagnosis*.[625] The patient is bitten by reduviid bugs bred in the laboratory; the subsequent identification of parasites in the intestine of the insect is proof of infection in the human host.

TREATMENT. The management of Chagas' disease remains difficult; although slowly progressive at first, once cardiac decompensation develops there is usually a rapid and inexorable progression to death, which is usually due to arrhythmia, congestive failure, and systemic thromboembolism.[649,655] Major efforts are aimed at interrupting transmission of the parasite to humans; such vector control methods have been generally successful.[622,623,646,656] They may prevent not only the initial infection but also superinfection that may play a role in determining the severity of the resulting cardiomyopathy.[622] Amiodarone appears to be particularly effective in controlling the ubiquitous ventricular arrhythmias seen in Chagas' disease, although whether this translates into improved survival remains unestablished.[625] Anticoagulation may be of some benefit in preventing recurrent thromboembolic episodes. While antiparasitic agents such as nifurtimox and benzimidazole are effective in reducing parasitemia, there is no evidence that they are efficacious in curing the disease.[654] A promising avenue of approach appears to be immunoprophylaxis, although a clinically useful vaccine is not yet available.[626] Insertion of an implantable cardioverter-defibrillator[657] and heart transplantation have been performed in a few patients but are not practical options for the vast majority of patients.

AFRICAN TRYPANOSOMIASIS. African sleeping sickness, due to *Trypanosoma gambiense* or *T. rhodesiense,* may be associated with myocardial abnormalities, although they are usually of less functional significance than in so-called American trypanosomiasis (Chagas' disease).[658] *T. rhodesiense,* in particular, may lead to cardiac failure,[658] although the central nervous system findings (excessive somnolence) usually dominate the clinical picture.

Pathological examination often reveals pericardial fluid.[658] The heart is not as greatly dilated and hypertrophied as it is in Chagas' disease and may appear grossly to be normal. There is often epicardial thickening with a cellular exudate composed of lymphocytes, plasma cells, and histiocytes. The myocardium typically displays a diffuse interstitial infiltrate, often with zones of patchy fibrosis and interstitial edema.[659]

Nonspecific *electrocardiographic* changes, commonly ST-segment and T-wave abnormalities and prolongation of the Q-T interval, are observed in at least half the patients.[658] Unlike Chagas' disease, arrhythmias and conduction disturbances are usually not prominent features and the arterial pressure is usually normal. Some of the patients have asymptomatic cardiomegaly,[658] although both pulmonary congestion and peripheral edema have been reported.

TOXOPLASMOSIS. *Toxoplasma* infections are caused by an obligate intracellular parasite *(T. gondii);* both congenital and acquired forms may occur.[660] Symptomatic acquired toxoplasmic infections involving the heart are uncommon. They occur most commonly in immunosuppressed patients with malignant diseases, and occasionally in patients with acquired immune deficiency syndrome and following cardiac or bone marrow transplantation.[661,662] An inflammatory infiltrate, often with eosinophils and variable degrees of edema and degeneration of the muscle bundles, and pericardial effusion are often present.[663–665]

Most adult cases are asymptomatic, but *Toxoplasma* infections may produce a severe, fatal disease with multisystem involvement.[661] Toxoplasmic myocarditis, often with pericarditis, may occur as an isolated disease process or as part of a multisystem disseminated disease.[665,666] Manifestations may include arrhythmia (atrial and ventricular), AV block, pericarditis, and heart failure.[660] Large pericardial effusions may be seen on occasion.[663] Diagnosis may be aided by endomyocardial biopsy.[662]

Treatment is with a combination of pyrimethamine and triple sulfonamides, but the response to therapy is variable.[661,662] Corticosteroids may be helpful in treating arrhythmias or conduction defects.

MALARIA. While myocardial changes may be demonstrated during the course of malaria, particularly with *Plasmodium falciparum,* clinical findings to indicate cardiac involvement are rare.[667] The heart generally demonstrates few gross abnormalities. The principal findings are histological. The capillaries are often filled and even distended with an accumulation of parasites, sometimes totally occluding the lumen of the vessels. Thrombosis of the capillaries and ischemic myocardial changes may be seen.[667] Focal myocardial damage may be present, along with an interstitial infiltrate composed of lymphocytes, plasma cells, and macrophages.[667] In rare cases, cardiac failure may contribute to or even cause death.[667] Slight ST-segment and T-wave changes on the electrocardiogram may be the only clinical indications of myocardial involvement.

METAZOAL MYOCARDIAL DISEASE

ECHINOCOCCUS (HYDATID CYST). *Echinococcus* is endemic in many sheep-raising areas of the world, particularly Argentina, Uruguay, New Zealand, Greece, North Africa, and Iceland, but cardiac involvement in hydatid disease is uncommon, occurring in less than 2 per cent of cases.[668,669] The usual host of *Echinococcus granulosus* is the dog, but human beings may serve as intermediate hosts (rather than the sheep, the usual intermediate host) if they accidentally ingest ova from contaminated dog feces.

When cardiac involvement is present, the cysts usually are intramyocardial in the interventricular septum or left ventricular free wall; involvement of the right ventricle or atrium may occur.[668] Involvement of the tricuspid valve may be seen on occasion,[668] and pericardial involvement with compression of the heart is not uncommon.[668] In most cases, a single cardiac cyst is present.[668,669]

A myocardial cyst may degenerate and calcify, develop daughter cysts, or rupture. Rupture of the cyst is the most dreaded complication; rupture into the pericardium may result in acute pericarditis, which may progress to chronic constrictive pericarditis. Rupture into the cardiac chambers may result in systemic or pulmonary emboli.[669] Rapidly progressive pulmonary hypertension may occur with rupture of right-sided cysts, with subsequent embolization of hundreds of scolices into the pulmonary circulation.[668] The liberation of hydatid fluid into the circulation may produce profound, fatal circulatory collapse due to an anaphylactic reaction to the protein constituents of the fluid.[686]

Symptoms depend on the location, size and integrity of the cyst; patients may be asymptomatic or in profound circulatory collapse.[668,669] The *electrocardiogram* may reflect the location of the cyst; T-wave changes and loss of QRS voltage may occur with left ventricular involvement, while AV conduction defects or right bundle branch block may be seen with involvement of the interventricular septum. Chest pain is usually due to rupture of the cyst into the pericardial space with resultant pericarditis. Large cystic masses may sometimes produce right-sided obstruction.[668,669]

Diagnosis. Recognition of an echinococcal cyst of the heart is a relatively simple matter if there is evidence of cysts in other organs, particularly the liver and lung. However, a cardiac cyst may be an isolated, solitary finding. The *chest roentgenogram* frequently shows an abnormal cardiac silhouette or a calcified lobular mass adjacent to the left ventricle. Although computed tomography and nuclear magnetic resonance imaging may aid in the detection and localization of heart cysts, two-dimensional echocardiography is thought to be the best choice.[668,670] *Eosinophilia,* present in some patients, is a useful adjunctive finding. The *Casoni skin test* is not very helpful because both false-positive and false-negative results occur. Serological tests, including hemagglutination and complement-fixation, are more useful.[671]

Management. Until recently, treatment for hydatid disease was limited to surgical excision. Experience suggests that the benzimidazole derivative mebendazole may be somewhat useful in the medical management of this disease.[669] Because of the significant risk of rupture of the cyst and its attendant serious and sometimes fatal consequences, surgical excision is generally recommended, even for asymptomatic patients. The surgical results have been generally favorable.

VISCERAL LARVA MIGRANS. People are occasional accidental hosts of the roundworm infestations of dogs due to *Toxocara canis* but cardiac involvement is rare. Most cases occur in children 1 to 3 years of age.[672] Myocarditis may occur in association with invasion of the myocardium by larvae.[672] The myocardial lesions include granulomas or extensive inflammatory infiltrates (often with eosinophils) with foci of muscle necrosis.[672] Congestive failure and death may occur, although asymptomatic cardiac involvement may be seen as well.[672]

SCHISTOSOMIASIS AND RELATED DISEASES. Direct cardiac involvement in schistosomiasis, heterophyiasis, and cysticercosis is distinctly unusual. The principal cardiovascular manifestation of schistosomiasis is right heart overload as a consequence of embolization of the ova to the pulmonary vasculature, with attendant pulmonary hypertension.

TRICHINOSIS. Infestation with *Trichinella spiralis* is a common human finding. Mild myocarditis is frequent and may be responsible for the majority of fatilities.[673] Less frequently, death is due to pulmonary embolism secondary to venous thrombosis as well as encephalitis.[673]

Although the parasite frequently invades the heart, it does not usually encyst there, and it is rare to find larvae or larval fragments in the myocardium.[673] Nonetheless, *pathological findings* at autopsy may be impressive. The heart may be dilated and flabby and a pericardial effusion may be present. A prominent focal infiltrate composed of lymphocytes and eosinophils, with interstitial edema, hyperemia, and scattered hemorrhages, is commonly found.[673] Areas of muscle degeneration and necrosis are present. The lesions may be due to toxic effects of the products produced in the course of the host reaction.

Clinical Manifestations. Myocarditis usually is mild and goes unnoticed, but in occasional cases it is manifested by congestive heart failure and chest pain, usually appearing around the third week of the disease, when the general constitutional symptoms are abating.[673] Physical examination may be normal, or there may be gross cardiomegaly with severe congestive heart failure. Sudden death may occur, usually in the fourth to eighth week of the illness.

Electrocardiographic abnormalities may be detected in one-fourth of patients with trichinosis and parallel the time course of clinical cardiac involvement, initially appearing in the second or third week and usually resolving by the seventh week of the illness.[674] The most common electrocardiographic abnormalities are repolarization abnormalities and conduction defects.[674] The electrocardiographic changes usually resolve completely.

The definitive *diagnosis* is based on the demonstration of larval forms in tissue biopsy samples, usually of the gastrocnemius muscle.[674] Eosinophilia, when present, is a supportive finding. The skin test is usually but not invariably positive. Treatment is with corticosteroids; dramatic improvement in cardiac function has been reported following their use.[673,674]

TOXIC, CHEMICAL, IMMUNE, AND PHYSICAL DAMAGE TO THE HEART

A wide variety of substances other than infectious agents may act on the heart and damage the myocardium. In some cases, the damage is acute, transient, and associated with evidence of an inflammatory infiltrate with myocyte necrosis (such as with arsenicals and lithium); in other cases, a hypersensitivity reaction occurs, without evidence of necrosis (as with sulfonamides).[675] Other agents that damage the myocardium may lead to chronic changes with resulting histological evidence of fibrosis and a clinical picture of a dilated cardiomyopathy. Furthermore, many offending stimuli may be associated with both acute and chronic phases (e.g., alcohol, Adriamycin). The response often is related to the dose and rate of exposure.

Numerous chemicals and drugs (both industrial and therapeutic) may lead to cardiac damage and dysfunction. Several physical agents (e.g., radiation and excessive heat) may also result in myocardial damage. Furthermore, myocardial involvement may be evident in a variety of systemic diseases, which are described in Part V of this book.

COCAINE (see also p. 1207). The illicit use of this drug is often associated with chest pain, diaphoresis, and palpitations.[676] In a minority of cases, there is evidence of myocardial ischemia or infarction as a consequence of heightened myocardial oxygen demand (increased blood pressure and heart rate), coronary vasoconstriction, accelerated atherosclerosis, or thrombotic occlusion of the coronary artery.[676–679] Associated clinical findings include ventricular arrhythmias, sudden death in some persons, and reversible ventricular myocardial depression (Fig. 43–36).[680–685] Myocarditis, contraction band necrosis, and thickening of the intramural coronary arteries have been found on histological study.[686–689] A variety of mechanisms have been invoked to explain the cardiovascular effects of cocaine, including vasoconstrictor, hypersensitivity, sympathomimetic, and direct actions (Fig. 43–37).[682] Treatment is empirical; beta-adrenergic blockers, combined alpha- and beta-adrenergic blockers, and calcium antagonists have been advocated but without any definite demonstration of their efficacy.[676]

INTERFERON ALPHA. Interferon alpha is a leukocyte-derived protein used therapeutically to treat malignancies and perhaps HIV infections. Cardiotoxicity, usually consisting of hypotension, tachycardia, and transient arrhythmias, occurs in a minority of patients (perhaps up to 10 per cent).[689,690] Several patients have developed congestive heart failure and the clinical picture of a dilated cardiomyopathy during interferon alpha

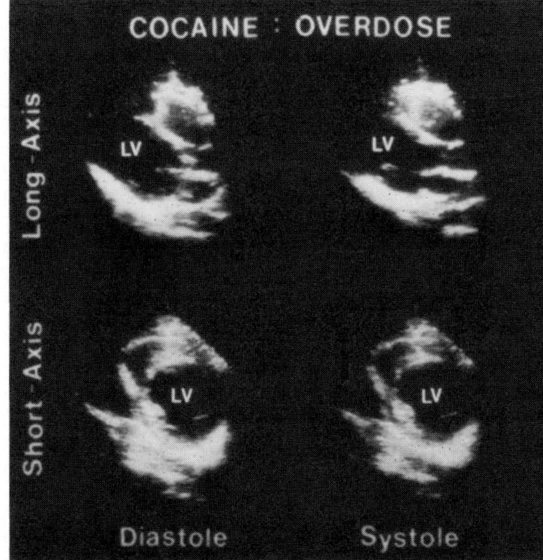

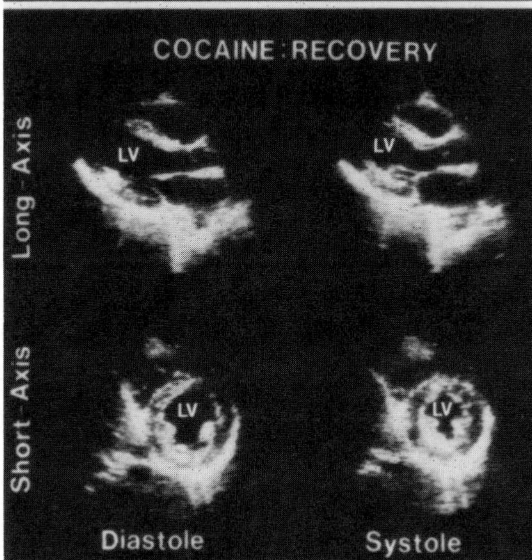

FIGURE 43-36. Two-dimensional echocardiograms recorded in long-axis and short-axis views during systole and diastole in a patient with cocaine cardiotoxicity. *Top,* Echocardiogram recorded shortly after overdose of cocaine shows dilated, globally hypocontractile left ventricle (LV). *Bottom,* Echocardiogram recorded during recovery period shows nondilated left ventricle with markedly improved left ventricular ejection performance. (From Chokshi, S. K., Moore, R., Pandian, N. G., and Isner, J. M.: Reversible cardiomyopathy associated with cocaine intoxication. Ann. Intern. Med. *111*:1039, 1989.)

therapy; in at least some patients, cardiomyopathy resolves rapidly with discontinuation of interferon.[690,691]

TRICYCLIC ANTIDEPRESSANTS. Although sudden death, disturbances in rhythm, and abnormalities of AV conduction may be seen with the tricyclic antidepressants, particularly when taken as an overdose, important depression of left ventricular function is usually not seen, even in patients with preexisting heart disease.[692] It is not clear whether there is a synergistic depression of ventricular function when a tricyclic antidepressant is given with another drug (such as an antiarrhythmic) that also has negative inotropic effects.[693] Postural hypotension may be exacerbated, however, and heart block precipitated in patients with preexisting conduction system disease.[694]

INTERLEUKIN-2 (see also p. 1760). The lymphokine interleukin-2, an antineoplastic agent, has significant cardiovascular toxicity, the most prominent of which is a diffuse capillary leak syndrome with hypotension and oliguria.[695] In about 5 per cent of patients, additional cardiotoxicity is seen,[696] consisting of myocardial ischemia,[695] infarction,[696,697] injury,[698,699] arrhythmias, and eosinophilic myocarditis.[696,700]

PHENOTHIAZINES. The phenothiazines may be associated with a variety of cardiac disturbances, including electrocardiographic changes, atrial and ventricular arrhythmias, and sudden death.[701] Postural hypotension may also be seen.[693] The cardiac effects are largely dose-dependent. Electrocardiographic abnormalities may be seen with as little as 200 mg of thioridazine per day and consist of lengthening of the Q-T interval and T-wave changes. Prolongation of the Q-T interval may set the stage for the emergence of ventricular arrhythmias, particularly torsades de pointes (p. 707).[701] Higher doses may lead to frank T-wave inversion and increase in the amplitude of the U wave. Changes in the P wave, QRS complex, and ST segment are usually absent. The electrocardiographic abnormalities and arrhythmias resolve with discontinuation of the drug, usually within 48 hours.

Pathological changes in the hearts of patients who have received psychotropic drugs and who have died suddenly include the deposition of acid mucopolysaccharide between muscle bundles in periarteriolar regions as well as the conduction system, with myofibrillar degeneration, and endothelial proliferation in the smaller blood vessels, although a direct causal relatonship between drug administration and cardiomyopathic changes is only inferential.[693] A variety of explanations have been invoked for apparent cardiac damage, including direct toxic effects of the phenothiazines on the myocardium, stimulation of higher autonomic centers, and changes in circulating or myocardial levels of catecholamines.

EMETINE. Cardiovascular changes are common with the use of emetine, a drug often employed in the treatment of amebiasis and schistosomiasis, presumably because of its prolonged duration of action and consequent potential for accumulation with resultant toxicity.[693] Myocardial lesions may be observed in some but not all patients at autopsy, and similar cardiac damage is noted in experimental animals given emetine.[702] The myocardial lesions consist of myofibrillar degeneration and necrosis,[702] with an interstitial infiltrate of mononuclear cells and histiocytes.

The *electrocardiogram,* which may be abnormal in 50 per cent of treated patients, most commonly shows reduced T-wave amplitude or inversion. Prolongation of the Q-T interval and ST-segment shifts may also be seen, although abnormalities of the P wave, P-R segment, and QRS complex are infrequent. The electrocardiographic changes usually resolve within weeks or months after cessation of treatment. Sinus tachycardia and hypotension may also be seen, although clinical evidence of myocardial toxicity is usually lacking. Only rare fatalities have been reported. *Dehydroemetine* results in electrocardiographic abnormalities similar to those of emetine, but they are less prominent and of shorter duration.

Emetine and dehydroemetine therapy should be discontinued upon appearance of clinical evidence of cardiac toxicity, but treatment may be continued cautiously if electrocardiographic changes are the only manifestation.

METHYSERGIDE. The widespread fibrotic reactions seen with this drug can also involve the heart. Up to 1 per cent of patients treated long-term may develop typically left-sided valvular lesions resulting in stenosis and regurgitation.[693] Fibrotic endocardial and pericardial lesions are also seen on occasion, producing a hemodynamic picture of restrictive and constrictive disease.[703]

CHLOROQUINE. This drug has been widely used in the prophylaxis and treatment of a variety of parasitic and other diseases and has potent

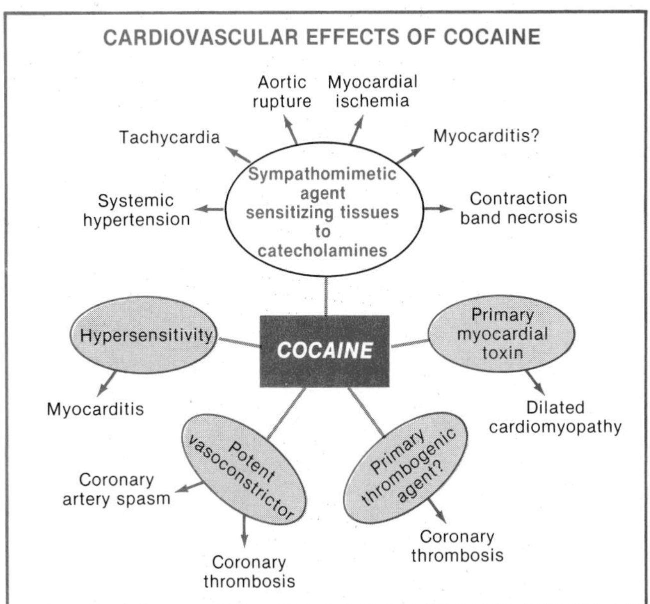

FIGURE 43-37. Diagram showing the effects of cocaine on the heart. (From Waller, B. F.: Cocaine and the heart. Indiana Med. *81*:956, 1988.)

toxic cardiac effects, which appear to be related to its ability to inhibit cellular respiration by blocking the Krebs cycle.[704] It is a myocardial depressant in large doses,[705] although routine doses are not usually associated with clinical evidence of cardiac dysfunction.[704] Electrocardiographic changes may be seen and are similar to those seen with emetine, although they are less pronounced and of shorter duration. In toxic doses, chloroquine may result in depressed cardiac output, bradycardia, arrhythmias, heart block, and death.[704] Characteristic changes are found on endomyocardial biopsy.[704,706]

ANTIMONY COMPOUNDS. Various antimony compounds, such as stibophen and tartar emetic, have been widely used in the treatment of schistosomiasis; less toxic agents are now becoming available. The antimony compounds are associated with electrocardiographic changes in almost all patients.[707] Typical *electrocardiographic changes* include prolongation of the Q-T interval with flattening or inversion of T waves.[707] ST-segment shifts and P-wave changes may be seen, although the QRS complex usually demonstrates no abnormality. The majority of patients do not demonstrate cardiac findings, although chest pain, bradycardia, hypotension, ventricular arrhythmias (including paroxysmal ventricular tachycardia), and sudden death may occur.[707,708]

LITHIUM. Lithium carbonate, used in the treatment of manic-depressive disorders, is associated with T-wave changes in one-fourth or more of patients who receive the drug.[709] Clinical evidence of myocardial involvement is usually lacking, although intoxication with lithium may be associated with ventricular arrhythmias, symptomatic sinus node abnormalities, atrioventricular conduction disturbances, congestive heart failure, and in rare cases, death.[709] In fatal lithium toxicity, the heart is said to be dilated, with evidence of myofibrillar degeneration associated with a lymphocytic interstitial infiltrate and fibrosis, although there is no definite proof that these changes are due to lithium.[709]

HYDROCARBONS. Ingestion of hydrocarbons may result in fragmentation and vacuolization of the muscle fibers with loss of cross-striations.[710] Electrocardiographic changes, arrhythmias, and cardiomegaly may occur. Involvement of the central nervous, renal, hepatic, and pulmonary systems may dominate the clinical presentation and obscure the myocardial damage, which may well contribute to the mortality of hydrocarbon ingestion.[710]

The *fluorinated hydrocarbons,* commonly used as aerosol propellants, appear to be cardiac toxins, contrary to their reputation of being inert. In animal preparations, at least, the aerosol propellants cause ventricular tachyarrhythmias, depress myocardial contractility, and lower systemic vascular resistance and arterial pressure.[711] These cardiovascular effects may be involved in the sudden deaths seen in individuals who abuse aerosols for their psychotropic effect.[711]

CATECHOLAMINES. A severe reversible dilated cardiomyopathy has been observed in conjunction with pheochromocytoma, and the myocardial damage has been attributed to high levels of circulating catecholamines[64,712] (p. 1839). Similar changes have been demonstrated in experimental animals treated with prolonged infusions of L-norepinephrine. Catecholamines also may produce acute myocarditis, with focal myocardial necrosis, inflammation, epicardial hemorrhages, tachycardia, and arrhythmias,[713] as well as indications of a hypertrophic cardiomyopathy.[712] Similar findings have been described with excessive use of beta-adrenergic agonist inhalants and methylxanthines in the treatment of decompensated pulmonary disease.[714]

A variety of mechanisms have been suggested. A direct toxic effect may be involved, or the damage may be secondary to relative tissue hypoxia because of heightened metabolic demands.[715] Alternatively, the damage may result from changes in autonomic tone, enhanced lipid mobility, calcium overload, damaging effects of catecholamine oxidation products, or increased sarcolemmal permeability.[715-718] Aspirin and dipyridamole appear to offer some protection against experimental myocardial necrosis by catecholamines, suggesting that platelet aggregation plays a major role.

LEAD. The prominent features in lead poisoning generally center on the gastrointestinal and central nervous systems. However, myocardial involvement may contribute to or be the principal cause of death in some cases.[719] Electrocardiographic changes, atrioventricular conduction defects, and overt congestive heart failure may occur.[719] The electrocardiographic and myocardial changes appear to be reversible with chelation therapy.[719]

CARBON MONOXIDE. Both acute and chronic carbon monoxide toxicity can occur. While central nervous system findings usually dominate the clinical presentation, significant and occasionally fatal cardiac abnormalities may be present.[720] Because carbon monoxide has a higher affinity for hemoglobin than does oxygen, reduced amounts of oxygen are delivered to the tissues. Thus, the cardiac toxicity may be partially caused by myocardial hypoxia, but a direct toxic effect of the gas on myocardial mitochondria may play an even more important role.[721,722] The *histological features* include focal areas of necrosis, most marked in the subendocardium. Focal perivascular infiltrates and punctate hemorrhages are also seen.[722]

Cardiac involvement may appear promptly after exposure or it may be delayed for up to several days. Palpitations, sinus tachycardia, and various arrhythmias, including ventricular extrasystoles and atrial fibrillation, are common.[723] Bradycardia and AV block may occur in more severe cases.[723] In patients with ischemic heart disease, angina pectoris and myocardial infarction may be precipitated. Electrocardiographic ST-segment and T-wave abnormalities are quite common. Transient right and/or left ventricular wall motion abnormalities may be present.[722] Administration of 100 per cent oxygen, bed rest, and surveillance for serious rhythm or conduction abnormalities will usually permit rapid recovery.

HYPOCALCEMIA (see also pp. 150 and 1841). In rare patients with chronic hypocalcemia (often due to hypoparathyroidism), congestive heart failure may occur and resolve only when the serum calcium level is raised.[724,725] Rapid transfusion of citrated blood can produce hypocalcemia and reversible myocardial depression,[726] as can ambulatory peritoneal dialysis in patients with chronic renal failure.[727]

HYPOPHOSPHATEMIA. A form of reversible left ventricular dysfunction may be seen with severe hypophosphatemia. Restoration of the serum phosphate level to normal results in hemodynamic recovery,[728] although the modest reduction in levels usually seen is associated with normal function.[729]

HYPOMAGNESEMIA. Focal cardiac necrosis is found in experimental magnesium deficiency and may account for the supraventricular and ventricular arrhythmias and electrocardiographic changes that are seen clinically. The ventricular arrhythmias are particularly likely to occur when hypomagnesemia complicates digitalis toxicity.[730,731]

TAURINE DEFICIENCY. A deficiency of taurine, an amino acid found in high concentration in cardiac and retinal tissue, produces a dilated cardiomyopathy in cats that is reversible with oral taurine supplementation.[732] Whether a similar condition exists in humans is unestablished; this has been the subject of speculation.[733]

CARNITINE DEFICIENCY. Carnitine, an essential cofactor for the oxidation of fatty acids, produces a hypertrophic or dilated cardiomyopathy in children when deficient.[71,734-736] Carnitine supplementation can lead to symptomatic and functional improvement[735-738]; determination of carnitine levels therefore is important in children with unexplained cardiomyopathy.[737] Myocardial carnitine levels are reduced in the hearts of patients with dilated cardiomyopathy, but the significance of this observation is unknown at present.[71]

SELENIUM DEFICIENCY. Dietary deficiency of the trace element selenium appears to be one of the principal factors responsible for a form of dilated cardiomyopathy endemic to certain rural areas in China that are deficient in selenium, although others have questioned the etiological role played by selenium.[739] Termed *Keshan disease,* it affects mainly children and young women and apparently is prevented by the prophylactic administration of sodium selenite tablets.[739] A similar cardiomyopathy, occasionally fatal, may be found in Occidentals subjected to prolonged parenteral hyperalimentation.[740]

SCORPION STING. The venom of the scorpion is mainly neurotoxic, but cardiac findings may be prominent and even fatal, particularly in children.[741-744] Hearts are normal on gross examination with prominent microscopic changes usually but not invariably present, particularly in the subendocardial regions and papillary muscles.[745] Degeneration and necrosis of muscle fibers are noted, with interstitial edema and a mononuclear infiltrate. The histological features of scorpion sting suggest high levels of circulating catecholamines and are similar to those seen with experimental catecholamine infusion and in pheochromocytoma.[742] The parasympathetic system appears to be stimulated as well.[742]

The *electrocardiogram* often initially shows tall peaked T waves that progress to inversions and ST-segment shifts. Q waves may appear, and the Q-T interval is usually prolonged.[746] Atrial, junctional, and ventricular arrhythmias may occur. Tachycardia, hypertension, anxiety, diaphoresis, and pulmonary edema—findings resembling those of a massive catecholamine effect—are striking in many patients.[745,746] A smaller number of patients are seen in shock with peripheral vascular collapse. Most deaths are due to pulmonary edema, presumably the result of left ventricular dysfunction.[746a] Occasionally, sudden and unexpected deaths occur in a smaller percentage of patients, presumably as a consequence of arrhythmias. Adrenergic blocking agents and the use of specific antivenom appear to be useful in the management of the cardiovascular manifestation of scorpion stings.[744,747]

WASP AND SPIDER STINGS. Stings by the vespine wasps may lead to hypotension, circulatory collapse, and cyanosis, manifestations of anaphylaxis.[748] Occasional patients may have chest pain and clinical findings compatible with acute myocardial infarction.[748] The mechanism of myocardial damage is unclear; perhaps it merely reflects necrosis from profound hypotension, although a direct toxic effect on the myocardium or an indirect effect on the coronary arteries may be involved.[748]

SNAKE BITE. Cardiac complications are usually not prominent features of snake bites, and the clinical picture is usually dominated by the neurological, hematological, and vascular damage produced by the snakebite toxin.[749,750] Myocardial involvement is seen on occasion and may rarely contribute to morbidity and mortality. T-wave abnormalities are the most common manifestation of myocardial involvement, although ST-segment depression, QRS prolongation, and AV conduction defects may also be seen.[751] The electrocardiographic changes are usually transient, but when persistent they are attributed to direct myocardial damage due to the toxin. Death may occur from circulatory collapse, myocardial depression, or myocardial infarction due to hypotension and coronary artery thrombosis. Coronary artery vasospasm may also be involved.[752-754]

ARSENIC. Arsenicals are currently utilized in pesticides. Myocardial involvement may be seen in both acute and chronic poisoning; the heart may be dilated, with accumulation of pericardial fluid.[755] Multiple local and confluent areas of subepicardial and subendocardial hemorrhage are characteristic findings.[755] The myocardium is usually abnormal, with evidence of a perivascular mononuclear infiltrate.[756]

Clinically unrecognized, toxic, interstitial myocarditis is reflected in T-wave inversions and ST-segment depressions, along with prolongation of the Q-T interval.[755,756] The electrocardiographic changes usually revert to normal within 2 to 4 weeks. The electrocardiographic abnormalities appear to resolve more rapidly when BAL (British antilewisite, dimercaprol) is utilized in therapy.[755,756]

CYCLOPHOSPHAMIDE (see also p. 1759). High doses of cyclophosphamide have been associated with electrocardiographic changes, congestive heart failure, and death from hemorrhagic myocarditis.[757] In the majority of patients treated a reversible decrease of QRS voltage and systolic function is seen, often asymptomatic, although more than 20 per cent may succumb owing to myopericarditis.[758] The myocardial damage appears to result from direct endothelial damage and resultant fibrin microthrombi in the capillaries.

AZIDE. Sodium azide, a chemical preservative that interferes with oxidative phosphorylation, may produce fatal acute cardiotoxicity when accidentally ingested.[759] Pathological findings include marked interstitial edema and myofibrillar degeneration. Clinical features include arrhythmias, myocardial ischemia, left ventricular dysfunction, and hypotension.[759]

PARACETAMOL. Paracetamol, a phenacetin metabolite, may result in massive liver necrosis.[760] On occasion it also results in fatty degeneration and focal necrosis of the myocardium after an overdose.[760]

5-FLUOROURACIL. This antineoplastic agent has been associated with cardiotoxicity manifested by chest pain, electrocardiographic changes, and arrhythmia.[761-764] Swelling of myocardial fibers without an inflammatory infiltrate has been found at necropsy.[763]

DAUNORUBICIN AND ADRIAMYCIN (see p. 1756).

HYPERSENSITIVITY

Hypersensitivity to a variety of agents may result in allergic reactions that involve the myocardium. In addition to anaphylaxis and serum sickness, allergies to a variety of drugs (most commonly the sulfonamides, the penicillins, and methyldopa) or other sensitizers may lead to an allergic myocarditis, characterized by eosinophilia, and a perivascular infiltration of the myocardium by eosinophils, multinucleated giant cells, and leukocytes[765] (Table 43–16). Hypersensitivity myocarditis is rarely recognized clinically and is often first discovered at postmortem examination, although it is occasionally diagnosed on endomyocardial biopsy.[765] Since some of the clinical courses of patients are marked by sudden death (presumably arrhythmic in origin), it is likely that undiagnosed hypersensitivity myocarditis may have significant clinical effects[766,767] (Table 43–17). Because of the significant deleterious effects, a high index of suspicion for this condition should be maintained; in one unusual case, penicillin residue in pet food led to hypersensitivity myocarditis in a young child.[766] Therapy includes discontinuation of the offending agent, and corticosteroids and/or immunosuppression therapy in severe cases.[765]

TABLE 43–16 PRINCIPAL DRUGS CAPABLE OF CAUSING HYPERSENSITIVITY MYOCARDITIS

Antibiotics	**Antiinflammatory**
Amphotericin B	Indomethacin
Ampicillin	Oxyphenbutazone
Chloramphenicol	Phenylbutazone
Penicillin	**Diuretics**
Tetracycline	Acetazolamide
Streptomycin	Chlorthalidone
Sulfonamides	Hydrochlorothiazide
Sulfadiazine	Spironolactone
Sulfisoxazole	**Others**
Anticonvulsants	Amitriptyline
Phenindione	Methyldopa
Phenytoin	Sulfonylureas
Carbamazepine	Tetanus toxoid
Antituberculous	
Isoniazid	
Paraaminosalicylic acid	

From Kounis, N. G., Zavras, G. M., Soufras, G. D., and Kitrou, M. P.: Hypersensitivity myocarditis. Ann. Allergy *62*:71, 1989.

TABLE 43–17 CLINICAL FEATURES OF HYPERSENSITIVITY MYOCARDITIS

Cardiac symptoms
Chest discomfort
Dyspnea
Palpitations
Cardiac signs
Irregular pulse
Elevated jugular venous pressure
Gallop rhythm
Electrocardiographic signs
Sinus tachycardia
ST segment elevation
ST segment depression
T-wave inversion
Right bundle branch block
Left bundle branch block
Atrioventricular block
Ventricular tachycardia
Laboratory findings
Increased cardiac enzymes (especially CK-MB)
Cardiomegaly in the chest roentgenogram
Dilated cardiac chambers in echocardiogram
Eosinophils, atypical lymphocytes, and giant cells in biopsy

From Kounis, N. G., Zavras, G. M., Soufras, G. D., and Kitrou, M. P.: Hypersensitivity myocarditis. Ann. Allergy *62*:71, 1989.

METHYLDOPA. Although hepatitis is the most frequently encountered serious adverse reaction to methyldopa, sudden and unexpected death has been reported in a number of patients found at necropsy to have had an unsuspected myocarditis.[765] The *histological findings* have the characteristics of an allergic myocarditis, showing an interstitial inflammatory infiltrate with abundant eosinophils, a vasculitis, and focal myocardial necrosis. Electrocardiographic changes include sinus bradycardia, sinus pauses, and first- and second-degree AV block.[768]

PENICILLIN. Allergic reactions to penicillin are fairly common, but myocardial involvement is rare.[766] *Histological findings* consist of a perivascular and interstitial infiltrate composed of eosinophils and mononuclear cells.[766] Both myocardial infarction and pericarditis may occur and account for some of the electrocardiographic changes.[766,767] Transient electrocardiographic changes may be the only manifestation of cardiac involvement, with sinus tachycardia, ST-segment elevation, and T-wave inversion.[766]

SULFONAMIDES. Sulfonamides may result in myocardial damage owing to a hypersensitivity vasculitis as well as a myocarditis.[767] In fatal cases eosinophilic myocarditis, sometimes with granulomas, usually can be demonstrated. While usually clinically silent, severe and even fatal congestive heart failure may occur.[765] Electrocardiographic changes are usually absent, but nonspecific ST-segment and T-wave abnormalities may be seen.

TETRACYCLINE. Allergic reactions to antibiotics of the tetracycline class include fever, tachycardia, and first degree AV block. Postmortem findings include cardiac dilatation, fibrinoid muscle cell degeneration, and a diffuse interstitial and perivascular infiltrate.[769]

PHENINDIONE. Marked congestive heart failure with cardiomegaly and pulmonary edema has been reported following the use of phenindione. The electrocardiogram may show sinus tachycardia, low QRS voltage, and T-wave inversion.[769]

ANTITUBERCULOUS DRUGS. Most reactions to antituberculous drugs consist of a fever, rash, or both, but serious and fatal cardiac reactions may occur on rare occasions. *Paraaminosalicylic acid* may lead to the development of interstitial edema, acute inflammatory infiltrate, refractory congestive heart failure, hypotension, and ventricular irritability.[770]

Streptomycin has been implicated as an unusual cause of myocarditis. Pathological findings may include cardiac dilatation, myocarditis with necrosis, hemorrhage, and a fibrinous pericardial effusion.[770] Clinically, it may be associated with chest pain, dyspnea, fever, and rash, followed by collapse and death.

GIANT CELL MYOCARDITIS

Giant cell myocarditis is a rare disease of unknown etiology characterized by the presence of multinucleated giant cells in the myocardium. (It is included here because of the possibility that it may be of immune or autoimmune etiology.) Variously called acute isolated myocarditis and granulomatous myocarditis, this condition is typically a rapidly fatal disease, often of young to middle-aged adults.[771,772,772a] *Pathological findings* are usually impressive. The ventricles are dilated, and mural thrombi may be present.[773] A serpiginous area of myocardial necrosis may be seen involving the right as well as the left ventricle.[772] Multinucleated giant cells are found, particularly at the margins of the areas of myocardial necrosis; the giant cells appear to be of macrophage, rather than myocyte origin.[774] An extensive inflammatory infiltrate is present within the necrotic areas, composed of eosinophils, histiocytes, and other cells.[772]

Although giant cell myocarditis appears to be associated with thymoma, systemic lupus erythematosus, and thyrotoxicosis, the cause of the disease remains obscure.[772,774] In many ways the clinical features suggest a viral myocarditis except for the rapid and virulent course. However, despite careful investigation there has been no serological or bacteriological evidence of an infectious etiology.[772] Sarcoid, syphilis, and tuberculosis have all been proposed as possible causes, although these usually present distinctive histological features. It has also been suggested that the cause is an autoimmune reaction,[772] although little evidence aside from the histological findings supports this view.

Both sexes are equally affected; the onset is typically rapid, with dyspnea, chest pain, orthopnea, and hypotension.[772,775] Fever is usually present, with electrocardiographic evidence of widespread myocardial involvement. Sinus tachycardia, left bundle branch block, atrial and ventricular arrhythmias, complete heart block, and findings suggesting acute myocardial necrosis may be seen.[775] Overt congestive heart failure and sudden death may occur.[772] Therapy (other than cardiac transplantation) is invariably unsuccessful, although corticosteroids and immunosuppressive agents have been used.[772a] It has been suggested that cyclosporine might be more effective.[772]

PHYSICAL AGENTS

HEAT STROKE. This condition results from failure of the thermoregulatory center following exposure to high ambient temperature and is manifested principally by hyperpyrexia and central nervous system dysfunction. However, cardiovascular abnormalities (usually electrocardiographic) appear to be common; pulmonary edema and right ventricular dysfunction may occur,[776] along with hypotension and circulatory collapse. *Pathological changes* include dilatation of the right side of the heart, particularly the right atrium. Hemorrhages of the subendocardium and the subepicardium are frequently seen at necropsy and often involve the interventricular septum and posterior wall of the left ventricle.[776] Histological findings include degeneration and necrosis of muscle fibers as well as interstitial edema.[776] Possible factors responsible for myocardial damage include direct thermal injury, myocardial hypoxia secondary to circulatory collapse, decreased coronary blood flow, and metabolic abnormalities resulting from widespread injury to other organs.

Sinus tachycardia is invariably present, while atrial and ventricular arrhythmias are usually absent. Transient prolongation of the Q-T interval may be seen, along with ST-segment and T-wave abnormalities. It may take up to several months for these repolarization abnormalities to resolve. Serum enzyme levels may be elevated and may reflect myocardial damage, at least in part.[776]

HYPOTHERMIA. Low temperature may also result in myocardial damage. Cardiac dilatation may occur with epicardial petechiae and subendocardial hemorrhages. Microinfarcts are present in the ventricular myocardium, and fatty changes are common. The lesions are not due to the low temperature per se but appear to be the result of the circulatory collapse, hemoconcentration, capillary sludging, and depressed cellular metabolism that accompany hypothermia. Clinical manifestations of hypothermia include sinus bradycardia, conduction disturbances, atrial (and occasionally ventricular) fibrillation, and a characteristic deflection of the terminal portion of the QRS pattern (Osborne wave).[777,778]

RADIATION. The employment of ionizing radiation during radiotherapy or, less commonly, after radiation accidents, may result in a variety of acute and chronic cardiac complications including pericarditis with effusion, tamponade, and constriction; coronary artery fibrosis and myocardial infarction; valvular abnormalities; myocardial fibrosis; and conduction disturbances.[779-782] While the heart is thought to be one of the organs most resistant to the effects of radiation, damage to the pericardium (p. 1754), myocardium, and endocardium occurs.[783] Although radiation probably results in some degree of tissue damage in all patients, clinically significant cardiac involvement occurs in the minority of patients. Radiation-induced cardiac damage is related to the dose of radiation, the mass of heart irradiated, and the dose schedule of the radiation.

The late cardiac damage that may follow irradiation appears to result from a long-lasting injury of the capillary endothelial cells, which leads to cell death, capillary rupture, and microthrombi.[780] Because of this damage to the microvasculature, ischemia results and is followed by myocardial fibrosis. In addition to microvascular damage, the major epicardial coronary arteries may become narrowed, especially at the ostia.[780,781,784,785]

Only an occasional patient manifests acute cardiac abnormality clinically with radiation therapy; typically this consists of acute pericarditis.[786] A mild, transient, asymptomatic depression of left ventricular function may be seen early after radiation therapy.[779] The more common clinical expressions of radiation heart disease occur months or years after the exposure.[786] The pericardium is the most common site of clinical involvement, with findings of chronic pericardial effusion or pericardial constriction. Myocardial damage occurs less frequently and is characterized by myocardial fibrosis with or without endocardial fibrosis or fibroelastosis. Left and/or right ventricular dysfunction at rest or with exercise appears to be a common, albeit usually asymptomatic, finding 5 to 20 years after radiation therapy, especially in those in whom the now-outmoded technique of a single anteroposterior port was used.[787]

REFERENCES

1. Abelmann, W. H., and Lorell, B. H.: The challenge of cardiomyopathy. J. Am. Coll. Cardiol. *13*:1219, 1989.
2. Cardiomyopathy. *In* Fowler, N. O.: Diagnosis of Heart Disease. New York, Springer-Verlag, 1991, pp. 239–255.
3. Gillum, R. F.: The epidemiology of cardiomyopathy in the United States. *In* Zipes, D. P., and Rowlands, D. J. (eds.): Progress in Cardiology. Philadelphia, Lea and Febiger, 1989, p. 11.
4. Codd, M. B., Sugrue, D. D., Gersh, B. J., and Melton, L. J., III: Epidemiology of idiopathic dilated and hypertrophic cardiomyopathy. Circulation *80*:564, 1989.
5. WHO Technical Report Series: Cardiomyopathies. Report of a WHO expert committee. Technical Report Series *697*:7, 1984.
6. Goodwin, J. F.: Classification of nonhypertrophic cardiomyopathies. *In* Zipes, D. P., and Rowlands, D. J. (eds.): Progress in Cardiology. Philadelphia, Lea and Febiger, 1989, p. 3.
7. Mason, J. W., and O'Connell, J. B.: Clinical merit of endomyocardial biopsy. Circulation *79*:971, 1989.
8. Yoshizato, T., Edwards, W. D., Alboliras, E. T., et al.: Safety and utility of endomyocardial biopsy in infants, children and adolescents: A review of 66 procedures in 53 patients. J. Am. Coll. Cardiol. *15*:436, 1990.
9. Schmeltz, A. A., Apitz, J., Hort, W., and Maisch, B.: Endomyocardial biopsy in infants and children: Experience in 60 patients. Pediatr. Cardiol. *11*:15, 1990.
10. Miller, L. W., Labovitz, A. J., McBride, L. A., et al.: Echocardiography-guided endomyocardial biopsy: A 5-year experience. Circulation *78*:99, 1988.
11. Lie, J. T.: Myocarditis and endomyocardial biopsy in unexplained heart failure: A diagnosis in search of a disease (editorial). Ann. Intern. Med. *109*:525, 1988.
12. Aretz, H. T., Billingham, M. E., Edwards, W. D., et al.: Myocarditis: A histopathologic definition and classification. Am. J. Cardiovasc. Pathol. *1*:3, 1987.

DILATED CARDIOMYOPATHY

13. Keren, A., Gottlieb, S., Tzivoni, D., et al.: Mildly dilated congestive cardiomyopathy. Use of prospective diagnostic criteria and description of the clinical course without heart transplantation. Circulation *81*:506, 1990.
14. Stevenson, L. W.: Dilated Cardiomyopathy: Principles and Prognosis. *In* Zipes, D. P., and Rowlands, D. J. (eds.): Progress in Cardiology. Philadelphia, Lea and Febiger, 1989, p. 51.
15. Diaz, R. A., Obasohan, A., and Oakley, C. M.: Prediction of outcome in dilated cardiomyopathy. Br. Heart J. *58*:393, 1987.
16. Stevenson, L. W., Fowler, M. B., Schroeder, J. S., et al.: Poor survival of

patients with idiopathic cardiomyopathy considered too well for transplantation. Am. J. Med. *83*:871, 1987.
17. Romeo, F., Pelliccia, F., Cianfrocca, C., et al.: Determinants of end-stage idiopathic dilated cardiomyopathy: A multivariate analysis of 104 patients. Clin. Cardiol. *12*:387, 1989.
18. Romeo, F., Pelliccia, F., Cianfrocca, C., et al.: Predictors of sudden death in idiopathic dilated cardiomyopathy. Am. J. Cardiol. *63*:138, 1989.
19. Juilliere, Y., Danchin, N., Briancon, S., et al.: Dilated cardiomyopathy: Long-term follow-up and predictors of survival. Int. J. Cardiol. *21*:269, 1988.
20. Douglas, P. S., Morrow, R., Ioli, A., and Reichek, N.: Left ventricular shape, afterload and survival in idiopathic dilated cardiomyopathy. J. Am. Coll. Cardiol. *13*:311, 1989.
21. Tanganelli, P., Di Lenarda, A., Bianciardi, G., et al.: Correlation between histomorphometric findings on endomyocardial biopsy and clinical findings in idiopathic dilated cardiomyopathy. Am. J. Cardiol. *64*:504, 1989.
22. Tamai, J., Nagata, S., Nishimura, T., et al.: Hemodynamic and prognostic value of thallium-201 myocardial imaging in patients with dilated cardiomyopathy. Int. J. Cardiol. *24*:219, 1989.
23. Keogh, A. M., Baron, D. W., and Hickie, J. B.: Prognostic guides in patients with idiopathic or ischemic dilated cardiomyopathy assessed for cardiac transplantation. Am. J. Cardiol. *65*:903, 1990.
24. Chetty, S., and Mitha, A. S.: Arrhythmias in idiopathic dilated cardiomyopathy. A preliminary study. S. Afr. Med. J. *77*:190, 1990.
25. Figulla, H. R., Rahlf, G., Nieger, M., et al.: Spontaneous hemodynamic improvement or stabilization and associated biopsy findings in patients with congestive cardiomyopathy. Circulation *71*:1095, 1985.
26. Natural history of dilated cardiomyopathy (editorial). Lancet *1*:248, 1986.
27. Oakley, C.: Importance of right ventricular function in congestive heart failure. Am. J. Cardiol. *62*:14A, 1988.
28. Griffin, M. L., Hernandez, A., Martin, T. C., et al.: Dilated cardiomyopathy in infants and children. J. Am. Coll. Cardiol. *11*:139, 1988.
29. Chen, S-C., Nouri, S., Balfour, I., et al.: Clinical profile of congestive cardiomyopathy in children. J. Am. Coll. Cardiol. *15*:189, 1990.
30. Roberts, W. C., Siegel, R. J., and McManus, B. M.: Idiopathic dilated cardiomyopathy: Analysis of 152 necropsy patients. Am. J. Cardiol. *60*:1340, 1987.
31. Ferrans, V. J.: Pathologic anatomy of the dilated cardiomyopathies. Am. J. Cardiol. *64*:9C, 1989.
32. Kuroda, T., Shiina, A., Suzuki, O., et al.: Prediction of prognosis of patients with idiopathic dilated cardiomyopathy: A comparison of echocardiography with cardiac catheterization. Jpn. J. Med. *28*:180, 1989.
33. Klein, L. W., and Horowitz, L. N.: Familial right ventricular dilated cardiomyopathy associated with supraventricular arrhythmias. Am. J. Coll. Cardiol. *62*:482, 1988.
34. Tazelaar, H. D., and Billingham, M. E.: Leukocytic infiltrates in idiopathic dilated cardiomyopathy. A source of confusion with active myocarditis. Am. J. Surg. Pathol. *10*:405, 1986.
34a. Edwards, W. D.: Cardiomyopathies. Hum. Pathol. *18*:625, 1987.
34b. Schaper, J., Froede, R., Hein, S., et al.: Impairment of the myocardial ultrastructure and changes of the cytoskeleton in dilated cardiomyopathy. Circulation *83*:504, 1991.
35. Bender, J. R.: Idiopathic dilated cardiomyopathy: An immunologic, genetic, or infectious disease, or all of the above? Circulation *83*:704, 1991.
36. Hartz, A. J., Anderson, A. J., Brooks, H. L., et al.: The association of smoking with cardiomyopathy. N. Engl. J. Med. *311*:1201, 1984.
36a. Wikman-Coffelt, J., Stefenelli, T., Wu, S. T., et al.: $[Ca^{2+}]_i$ Transients in the cardiomyopathic hamster heart. Circ. Res. *68*:45, 1991.
37. Movsesian, M. A., Bristow, M. R., and Krall, J.: Ca^{2+} uptake by cardiac sarcoplasmic reticulum from patients with idiopathic dilated cardiomyopathy. Circ. Res. *65*:1141, 1989.
38. Brodde, O. E., Zerkowski, H. R., Doetsch, N., et al.: Myocardial beta-adrenoceptor changes in heart failure: Concomitant reduction in beta 1- and beta 2-adrenoceptor function related to the degree of heart failure in patients with mitral valve disease. J. Am. Coll. Cardiol. *14*:323, 1989.
39. Vago, T., Bevilacqua, M., Norbiato, G., et al.: Identification of alpha 1-adrenergic receptors on sarcolemma from normal subjects and patients with idiopathic dilated cardiomyopathy: Characteristics and linkage to GTP-binding protein. Circ. Res. *64*:474, 1989.
40. Limas, C. J., Goldenberg, I. F., and Limas, C.: Autoantibodies against beta-adrenoceptors in human idiopathic dilated cardiomyopathy. Circ. Res. *64*:97, 1989.
41. Limas, C. J., Goldenberg, I. F., and Limas, C.: Effect of cardiac transplantation on anti-beta-receptor antibodies in idiopathic dilated cardiomyopathy. Am. J. Cardiol. *63*:1134, 1989.
42. Bohm, M., Gierschik, P., Jakobs, K. H., et al.: Localization of a "postreceptor" defect in human dilated cardiomyopathy. Am. J. Cardiol. *64*:812, 1989.
43. Limas, C. J., Goldenberg, I. F., and Limas, C.: Influence of anti-beta-receptor antibodies on cardiac adenylate cyclase in patients with idiopathic dilated cardiomyopathy. Am. Heart J. *119*:1322, 1990.
44. Maisel, A. S., Michel, M. C., Isel, P. A., et al.: Pertussis toxin treatment of whole blood: A novel approach to assess G protein function in congestive heart failure. Circulation *81*:1198, 1990.
45. Muir, P., Nicholson, F., Tilzey, A. J., et al.: Chronic relapsing pericarditis and dilated cardiomyopathy: Serological evidence of persistent enterovirus infection. Lancet 1:804, 1989.
46. O'Connell, J. B., and Mason, J. W.: Immunosuppressive therapy in experimental and clinical myocarditis. Pathol. Immunopathol. Res. *7*:292, 1988.
47. Shabetai, R.: Myocarditis and dilated cardiomyopathy: Twins or distant relatives? Cardiology *76*:332, 1989.
48. O'Connell, J. B.: Immunosuppression for dilated cardiomyopathy (editorial). N. Engl. J. Med. *321*:1119, 1989.
49. Fallon, J. T.: Myocarditis and dilated cardiomyopathy: Different stages of the same disease? Cardiovasc. Clin. *18*:155, 1988.
50. Maisch, N., Bauer, E., Hufnagel, G., et al.: The use of endomyocardial biopsy in heart failure. Eur. Heart J. *9*:59, 1988.
51. Popma, J. J., Cigarroa, R. G., Buja, L. M., and Hillis, L. D.: Diagnostic and prognostic utility of right-sided catheterization and endomyocardial biopsy in idiopathic dilated cardiomyopathy. Am. J. Cardiol. *63*:955, 1989.
52. Bowles, N. E., Rose, M. L., Taylor, P., et al.: End-state dilated cardiomyopathy. Persistence of enterovirus RNA in myocardium at cardiac transplantation and lack of immune response. Circulation *80*:1128, 1989.
53. Limas, C. J., and Limas, C.: HLA antigens in idiopathic dilated cardiomyopathy. Br. Heart J. *62*:379, 1989.
54. Limas, C. J., Limas, C., Kubo, S. H., and Olivari, M. T.: Anti-beta-receptor antibodies in human dilated cardiomyopathy and correlation with HLA-DR antigens. Am. J. Cardiol. *65*:483, 1990.
55. Obrador, D., Ballester, M., Carrio, I., et al.: High prevalence of myocardial monoclonal antimyosin antibody uptake in patients with chronic idiopathic dilated cardiomyopathy. J. Am. Coll. Cardiol. *13*:1289, 1989.
56. Schulze, K., Becker, B. F., and Schultheiss, H. P.: Antibodies to the ADP/ATP carrier, an autoantigen in myocarditis and dilated cardiomyopathy, penetrate into myocardial cells and disturb energy metabolism in vivo. Circ. Res. *64*:179, 1989.
57. Caforio, A.L.P., Bonifacio, E., Stewart, J. T., et al.: Novel organ-specific circulating cardiac autoantibodies in dilated cardiomyopathy. J. Am. Coll. Cardiol. *15*:1527, 1990.
58. Sanderson, J. E., Koech, D., Iha, D., and Ojiambo, H. P.: T-lymphocyte subsets in idiopathic dilated cardiomyopathy. Am. J. Cardiol. *55*:755, 1985.
59. Franceschini, R., Messina, V., Petillo, A., et al.: Humoral immunity and lymphocyte subpopulations in patients with dilated cardiomyopathy. Int. J. Cardiol. *8*:113, 1985.
60. Anderson, J. L., Carlquist, J. F., and Higashikubo, R.: Quantitation of lymphocyte subsets by immunofluorescence flow cytometry in idiopathic dilated cardiomyopathy. Am. J. Cardiol. *55*:1550, 1985.
61. Lowry, P. J., Thompson, R. A., and Littler, W. A.: Cellular immunity in congestive cardiomyopathy. The normal cellular immune response. Br. Heart J. *53*:394, 1985.
62. Tatsunori, I., Katsutoshi, Y., Ono, S., et al.: Dilated cardiomyopathy associated with natural killer cell deficiency. Am. Heart J. *115*:1326, 1988.
63. Lowry, P. J., Gammage, M. D., Gentle, T. A., et al.: Suppressor T lymphocyte function in patients with idiopathic congestive cardiomyopathy. Br. Heart J. *57*:458, 1987.
64. Imperato-McGinley, J., Gautier, T., Ehlers, K., et al.: Reversibility of catecholamine-induced dilated cardiomyopathy in a child with a pheochromocytoma. N. Engl. J. Med. *316*:793, 1987.
65. Graber, H. L., Unverferth, D. V., Baker, P. B., et al.: Evolution of a hereditary cardiac conduction and muscle disorder: A study involving a family with six generations affected. Circulation *74*:21, 1986.
66. Berko, B. A., and Swift, M.: X-linked dilated cardiomyopathy. N. Engl. J. Med. *316*:1186, 1987.
67. Valentine, H. A., Hunt, S. A., Fowler, M. B., et al.: Frequency of familial nature of dilated cardiomyopathy and usefulness of cardiac transplantation in this subset. Am. J. Cardiol. *63*:959, 1989.
68. Urie, P. M., and Billingham, M. E.: Ultrastructural features of familial cardiomyopathy. Am. J. Cardiol. *62*:325, 1988.
69. Schmidt, M. A., Michels, V. V., Edwards, W. D., and Miller, F. A.: Familial dilated cardiomyopathy. Am. J. Med. Genet. *31*:135, 1988.
70. Fragola, P. V., Autore, C., Picelli, A., et al.: Familial idiopathic dilated cardiomyopathy. Am. Heart J. *115*:912, 1988.
71. Regitz, V., Shug, A. L., and Fleck, E.: Defective myocardial carnitine metabolism in congestive heart failure secondary to dilated cardiomyopathy and to coronary, hypertensive and valvular heart disease. Am. J. Cardiol. *65*:755, 1990.
72. Feldman, A. M., Cates, A. E., Veazey, W. B., et al.: Increase of the 40,000-mol wt pertussis toxin substrate (G Protein) in the failing human heart. J. Clin. Invest. *82*:189, 1988.
73. Böhm, M., Gierschik, P., Jakobs, K-H, et al.: Increase in $G_{1\alpha}$ in human hearts with dilated but not ischemic cardiomyopathy. Circulation *82*:1249, 1990.
74. Rahko, P. S., and Orie, J. E.: The clinical presentation and laboratory evaluation of congestive and ischemic cardiomyopathies. Cardiovasc. Clin. *19*:75, 1988.
75. Stewart, R.A.H., McKenna, W. J., and Oakley, C. M.: Good prognosis for dilated cardiomyopathy without severe heart failure or arrhythmia. Q. J. Med. New Series *74*:309, 1990.
76. Roubin, G. S., Anderson, S. D., Shen, W. F., et al: Hemodynamic and metabolic basis of impaired exercise tolerance in patients with severe left ventricular dysfunction. J. Am. Coll. Cardiol. *15*:986, 1990.
77. Sullivan, M. J., Green, H. J., and Cobb, F. R.: Skeletal muscle biochemistry and histology in ambulatory patients with long-term heart failure. Circulation *81*:518, 1990.
78. Caforio, A. L. P., Rossi, B., Risaliti, R., et al.: Type 1 fiber abnormalities in skeletal muscle of patients with hypertrophic and dilated cardiomyopathy: Evidence of subclinical myogenic myopathy. J. Am. Coll. Cardiol. *14*:1464, 1989.
79. Cannon, R. O., Cunnion, R. E., Parrillo, J. E., et al.: Dynamic limitation of

coronary vasodilator reserve in patients with dilated cardiomyopathy and chest pain. J. Am. Coll. Cardiol. *10*:1190, 1987.

80. Treasure, C. B., Vita, J. A., Cox, D. A., et al.: Endothelium-dependent dilation of the coronary microvasculature is impaired in dilated cardiomyopathy. Circulation *81*:722, 1990.
81. Cabanes, L. R., Weber, S. N., Matran, R., et al.: Bronchial hyperresponsiveness to methacholine in patients with impaired left ventricular function. N. Engl. J. Med. *320*:1317, 1989.
82. Dickerman, S. A., and Rubler, S.: Mitral and tricuspid valve regurgitation in dilated cardiomyopathy. Am. J. Cardiol. *63*:629, 1989.
83. Feldman, M. D., and Beller, G. A.: Is secondary mitral regurgitation in congestive heart failure a marker of clinical importance? J. Am. Coll. Cardiol. *15*:181, 1990.
84. Keren, G., Sonnenblick, E. H., and LeJemtel, T. H.:Mitral anulus motion: Relation to pulmonary venous and transmitral flow in normal subjects and in patients with dilated cardiomyopathy. Circulation *78*:621, 1988.
85. Maze, S. S., Kotler, M. N., and Parry, W. R.: Flow characteristics in the dilated left ventricle with thrombus: Qualitative and quantitative Doppler analysis. J. Am. Coll. Cardiol. *13*:873, 1989.
86. Uretsky, B. F.: Diagnostic considerations in the adult patient with cardiomyopathy or congestive heart failure. Cardiovasc. Clin. *19*:35, 1988.
87. Wilensky, R. L., Yudelman, P., Cohen, A. I., et al.: Serial electrocardiographic changes in idiopathic dilated cardiomyopathy confirmed at necropsy. Am. J. Cardiol. *62*:276, 1988.
88. Milechman, G., and Scheinman, M. M.: Ventricular dysrhythmias and sudden death in dilated cardiomyopathy. *In* Zipes, D. P., and Rowlands, D. J. (eds.): Progress in Cardiology. Philadelphia, Lea and Febiger, 1989, p. 85.
89. Anderson, D. P., Freedman, R. A., and Mason, J. W.: Sudden death in idiopathic dilated cardiomyopathy (editorial). Ann. Intern. Med. *107*:104, 1987.
90. Liem, L. B., and Swerdlow, C. D.: Value of electropharmacologic testing in idiopathic dilated cardiomyopathy and sustained ventricular tachyarrhythmias. Am. J. Cardiol. *62*:611, 1988.
91. Hofmann, T., Meinertz, T., Kasper, W., et al.: Mode of death in idiopathic dilated cardiomyopathy: A multivariate analysis of prognostic determinants. Am. Heart J. *116*:1455, 1988.
92. Rakovec, P., Lajovic, J., and Dolenc, M.: Reversible congestive cardiomyopathy due to chronic ventricular tachycardia. PACE *12*:542, 1989.
93. Sarembock, I. J., Horak, A. R., and Commerford, P. J.: Tachycardia-induced reversible left ventricular dysfunction: A report of 2 cases. S. Afr. Med. J. *73*:484, 1988.
94. Peters, K. G., and Kienzle, M. G.: Severe cardiomyopathy due to chronic rapidly conducted atrial fibrillation: Complete recovery after restoration of sinus rhythm. Am. J. Med. *85*:242, 1988.
95. Vanoverschelde, J., Raphael, D. A., Robert, A. R., and Cosyns, J. R.: Left ventricular filling in dilated cardiomyopathy: Relation to functional class and hemodynamics. J. Am. Coll. Cardiol. *15*:1288, 1990.
96. Iskandrian, A. S., Hakki, A. H., and Kane, S.: Resting thallium-201 myocardial perfusion patterns in patients with severe left ventricular dysfunction: Differences between patients with primary cardiomyopathy, chronic coronary artery disease, or acute myocardial infarction. Am. Heart J. *11*:760, 1986.
97. Eisenberg, J. D., Sobel, B. E., and Geltman, E. M.: Differentiation of ischemic from nonischemic cardiomyopathy with positron emission tomography. Am. J. Cardiol. *59*:1410, 1987.
98. Mody, F. V., Brunken, R. C., Stevenson, L. W., et al.: Differentiating cardiomyopathy of coronary artery disease from nonischemic dilated cardiomyopathy utilizing positron emission tomography J. Am. Coll. Cardiol. *17*:373, 1991.
99. Bouhour, J. B., Helias, J., de Lajartre, A. Y., et al.: Detection of myocarditis during the first year after discovery of a dilated cardiomyopathy by endomyocardial biopsy and gallium-67 myocardial scintigraphy: Prospective multicentre French study of 91 patients. Eur. Heart J. *9*:520, 1988.
100. O'Connell, J. B., and Mason, J. W.: Diagnosing and treating active myocarditis. West. J. Med. *150*:431, 1989.
101. Yasuda, T., Palacios, I. F., Dec, G. W., et al.: Indium-111 monoclonal antimyosin imaging in the diagnosis of acute myocarditis. Circulation *76*:306, 1987.
102. Sunnerhagen, K. S., Bhargava, V., and Shabetai, R.: Regional left ventricular wall motion abnormalities in idiopathic dilated cardiomyopathy. Am. J. Cardiol. *65*:364, 1990.
103. Cohn, J. N., Archibald, D. G., Ziesche, S., et al.: Effect of vasodilator therapy on mortality in chronic congestive heart failure. Results of Veterans Administration Cooperative Study. N. Engl. J. Med. *314*:1547, 1986.
104. Massin, E. K.: Current treatment of dilated cardiomyopathy. Texas Heart Inst. J. *18*:41, 1991.
105. CONSENSUS Trial Study Group: Effects of enalapril on mortality in severe congestive heart failure. N. Engl. J. Med. *316*:1429, 1987.
106. Figulla, H. R., Rechenberg, J. V., Wiegand, V., et al.: Beneficial effects of long-term diltiazem treatment in dilated cardiomyopathy. J. Am. Coll. Cardiol. *13*:653, 1989.
107. Stevenson, L. W., and Tillisch, J. H.: Maintenance of cardiac output with normal filling pressures in patients with dilated heart failure. Circulation *74*:1303, 1986.
108. Waagstein, F., Caidahl, K., Wallentin, I., et al.: Long-term beta-blockade in dilated cardiomyopathy. Effects of short- and long-term metoprolol treatment followed by withdrawal and readministration of metoprolol. Circulation *80*:551, 1989.
109. Heilbrunn, S. M., Shah, P., Bristow, M. R., et al.: Increased beta-receptor density and improved hemodynamic response to catecholamine stimulation during long-term metoprolol therapy in heart failure from dilated cardiomyopathy. Circulation *79*:483, 1989.
110. Gilbert, E. M., Anderson, J. L., Deitchman, D., et al.: Long-term beta-blocker vasodilator therapy improves cardiac function in idiopathic dilated cardiomyopathy: A double-blind, randomized study of bucindolol versus placebo. Am. J. Med. *88*:223, 1990.
111. Leung, W. H., Lau, C. P., Wong, C. K., et al.: Improvement in exercise performance and hemodynamics by labetalol in patients with idiopathic dilated cardiomyopathy. Am. Heart J. *119*:884, 1990.
112. Fowler, M. B., and Bristow, M. R.: Rationale for beta-adrenergic blocking drugs in cardiomyopathy. Am. J. Cardiol. *55*:120D, 1985.
113. Lee, H. R., O'Connell, J. B., and Mason, J. W.: Immunosuppression and beta-blockade in heart failure. Cardiol. Clin. *7*:171, 1989.
114. Parmley, W. W., and Chatterjee, K.: Congestive heart failure and arrhythmias: An overview. Am. J. Cardiol. *57*:34B, 1986.
115. Kulick, D. L., Bhandari, A. K., Hong, R., et al.: Effect of acute hemodynamic decompensation on electrical inducibility of ventricular arrhythmias in patients with dilated cardiomyopathy and complex nonsustained ventricular arrhythmias. Am. Heart J. *119*:878, 1990.
116. Milner, P. G., Dimarco, J. P., and Lerman, B. B.: Electrophysiological evaluation of sustained ventricular tachyarrhythmias in idiopathic dilated cardiomyopathy. PACE *11*:562, 1988.
117. Constantin, L., Martins, J. B., Kienzle, M. G., et al.: Induced sustained ventricular tachycardia in nonischemic dilated cardiomyopathy: Dependence on clinical presentation and response to antiarrhythmic agents. PACE *12*:776, 1989.
118. Fauchier, J. P., Cosnay, P., Moquet, B., et al.: Late ventricular potentials and spontaneous and induced ventricular arrhythmias in dilated or hypertrophic cardiomyopathies. A prospective study about 83 patients. PACE *11*:1974, 1988.
119. Falk, R. H.: A plea for a clinical trial of anticoagulation in dilated cardiomyopathy. Am. J. Cardiol. *65*:914, 1990.
120. Goodwin, J. F.: Clinical decisions in the management of the cardiomyopathies. Pract. Therapeut. *38*:988, 1989.
121. Kyrle, P. A., Korninger, C., Gossinger, H., et al.: Prevention of arterial and pulmonary embolism by oral anticoagulants in patients with dilated cardiomyopathy. Thromb. Haemost. *54*:521, 1985.
122. Parrillo, J. E., Cunnion, R. E., Epstein, S. E., et al.: A prospective, randomized, controlled trial of prednisone for dilated cardiomyopathy. N. Engl. J. Med. *321*:1061, 1989.
123. Latham, R. D., Mulrow, J. P., Virmani, R., et al.: Recently diagnosed idiopathic dilated cardiomyopathy: Incidence of myocarditis and efficacy of prednisone therapy. Am. Heart J. *117*:876, 1989.
124. Heck, C. F., Shumway, S. J., and Kaye, M. P.: The Registry of the International Society for Heart Transplantation: Sixth official report—1989. J. Heart Transplant. *8*:271, 1989.
125. Walsh, T. K., and Vacek, J. L.: Ethanol and heart disease. An underestimated contributing factor. Postgrad. Med. *79*:60, 1986.
126. Regan, T. J.: Alcoholic cardiomyopathy. *In* Zipes, D. P., and Rowlands, D. J. (eds.): Progress in Cardiology. Philadelphia, Lea and Febiger, 1989, p. 129.
127. Pavan, D., Nicolosi, G. L., Lestuzzi, C., et al.: Normalization of variables of left ventricular function in patients with alcoholic cardiomyopathy after cessation of excessive alcohol intake: An echocardiographic study. Eur. Heart J. *8*:535, 1987.
128. Auffermann, W., Wu, S., Parmley, W. W., et al.: Reversibility of chronic alcohol cardiac depression: 31P magnetic resonance spectroscopy in hamsters. Magn. Reson. Med. *9*:343, 1989.
129. Davidson, M. D.: Cardiovascular effects of alcohol. West. J. Med. *151*:430, 1989.
130. McCall, D.: Alcohol and the cardiovascular system. Curr. Probl. Cardiol. *12*:351, 1987.
131. Urbano-Marquez, A., Estruch, R., Navarro-Lopez, F., et al.: The effects of alcoholism on skeletal and cardiac muscle. N. Engl. J. Med. *320*:409, 1989.
132. Lang, R. M., Borow, K. M., Neumann, A., and Feldman, T.: Adverse cardiac effects of acute alcohol ingestion in young adults. Ann. Intern. Med. *102*:742, 1985.
133. Kelbaek, H., Heslet, L., Skagen, K., et al.: Cardiac function after alcohol ingestion in patients with ischemic heart disease and cardiomyopathy: A controlled study. Alcohol Alcohol. *23*:17, 1988.
134. Kelbaek, H.: Acute effects of alcohol and food intake on cardiac performance. Prog. Cardiovasc. Dis. *23*:347, 1990.
135. Diamond, I.: Alcoholic myopathy and cardiomyopathy (editorial). N. Engl. J. Med. *72*:458, 1989.
136. Feldman, A. M., Levine, M. A., Cates, A. E., et al.: Multiple effects of ethanol on cardiac adenylate cyclase. J. Cardiovasc. Pharmacol. *13*:774, 1989.
137. Preedy, V. R., and Peters, T. J.: Synthesis of subcellular protein fractions in the rat heart in vivo in response to chronic ethanol feeding. Cardiovasc. Res. *23*:730, 1989.
138. Guarnieri, T., and Lakatta, E. G.: Mechanism of myocardial contractile depression by clinical concentrations of ethanol. J. Clin. Invest. *85*:1462, 1990.
139. Laposata, E. A., and Lange, L. G.: Presence of nonoxidative ethanol metabolism in human organs commonly damaged by ethanol abuse. Science *231*:497, 1986.
140. Tsiplenkova, V. G., Vikhert, A. M., and Cherpachenko, N. M.: Ultrastructural and histochemical observations in human and experimental alcoholic cardiomyopathy. J. Am. Coll. Cardiol. *8*:22A, 1986.

140a. Cerqueira, M. D., Harp, G. D., Ritchie, J. L., et al.: Rarity of preclinical alcoholic cardiomyopathy in chronic alcoholics over 40 years of age. Am. J. Cardiol. *67*:183, 1991.
141. Dancy, M., Leech, G., Bland, J. M., et al.: Preclinical left ventricular abnormalities in alcoholics are independent of nutritional status, cirrhosis, and cigarette smoking. Lancet *I*:1122, 1985.
142. Ahmed, S. S., Howard, M., ten Hove, W., et al.: Cardiac function in alcoholics with cirrhosis: Absence of overt cardiomyopathy—myth or fact? J. Am. Coll. Cardiol. *3*:696, 1984.
142a. Kupari, M., Koskinen, P., and Suokas, A.: Left ventricular size, mass and function in relation to the duration and quantity of heavy drinking in alcoholics. Am. J. Cardiol. *67*:274, 1991.
143. Regan, T. J.: Alcohol and the cardiovascular system (editorial). West. J. Med. *151*:454, 1989.
144. Vikert, A. M., Tsiplenkova, V. G., and Cherpachenko, N. M.: Alcoholic cardiomyopathy and sudden cardiac death. J. Am. Coll. Cardiol. *8*:3A, 1986.
145. Kinney, E. L., Wright, R. J., and Caldwell, J. W.: Risk factors in alcoholic cardiomyopathy. Angiology *40*:270, 1989.
146. Milgaard, H., Kristensen, B. O., and Baandrup, U.: Importance of abstention from alcohol in alcoholic heart disease. Int. J. Cardiol. *26*:373, 1990.
147. Clay, M. A., Stewart-Richardson, P., Tassett, D. M., and Williams, J. F.: Chronic alcoholic cardiomyopathy. Protection of the isolated ischaemic working heart by ribose. Biochem. Int. *17*:791, 1988.
148. Wu, S., White, R., Wikman-Coiffelt, J., et al.: The preventive effect of verapamil on ethanol-induced cardiac depression: Phosphorus-31 nuclear magnetic resonance and high-pressure liquid chromatographic studies of hamsters. Circulation *75*:1058, 1987.
149. Blomstrom-Lundqvist, C., Sabel, K-G., and Olsson, S. B.: A long term follow up of 15 patients with arrhythmogenic right ventricular dysplasia. Br. Heart J. *58*:477, 1987.
150. Thiene, G, Nava, A., Corrado, D., et al.: Right ventricular cardiomyopathy and sudden death in young people. N. Engl. J. Med. *318*:129, 1988.
151. Mohan, J. C., Chutani, S. K., Sethi, K. K., et al.: Dominant right ventricular dilated cardiomyopathy: Clinical, echocardiographic and haemodynamic profile. Indian Heart J. *41*:177, 1989.
152. Brandt, J., Hofvendahl, S., Ljungdahl, L., et al.: Non-invasive recognition of arrhythmogenic right ventricular dysplasia. Acta Med. Scand. *223*:281, 1988.
153. Chiddo, A., Locuratolo, N., Gaglione, A., et al.: Right ventricular dysplasia: Angiographic study. Eur. Heart J. *10*:42, 1989.
154. Hirooka, Y., Urable, Y., Imaizumi, T., et al.: The usefulness of equilibrium radionuclide ventriculography in the diagnosis of arrhythmogenic right ventricular dysplasia and a report of cases of a familial occurrence. Jpn. Circ. J. *52*:511, 1988.
155. Scognamiglio, R., Fasoli, G., Nava, A., et al.: Contribution of cross-sectional echocardiography to the diagnosis of right ventricular dysplasia at the asymptomatic stage. Eur. Heart J. *10*:538, 1989.
156. Lemery, R., Brugada, P., Janssen, J., et al.: Nonischemic sustained ventricular tachycardia: Clinical outcome in 12 patients with arrhythmogenic right ventricular dysplasia. J. Am. Coll. Cardiol. *14*:96, 1989.
157. Fontaine, G., Frank, R., Rougier, I., et al.: Electrode catheter ablation of resistant ventricular tachycardia in arrhythmogenic right ventricular dysplasia. Heart Vessels *5*:172, 1990.

HYPERTROPHIC CARDIOMYOPATHY

158. Braunwald, E.: Hypertrophic cardiomyopathy—continued progress. N. Engl. J. Med. *320*:800, 1989.
159. Hypertrophic cardiomyopathy. *In* Fowler, N. O.: Diagnosis of heart disease. New York, Springer-Verlag, 1991, pp. 256–267.
160. Morrow, A. G., and Braunwald, E.: Functional aortic stenosis: A malformation characterized by resistance to left ventricular outflow without anatomic obstruction. Circulation *20*:181, 1959.
161. Maron, B. J., Bonow, R. O., Cannon, R. O., et al.: Hypertrophic cardiomyopathy: Interrelations of clinical manifestations, pathophysiology, and therapy. N. Engl. J. Med. *316*:780, and 844, 1987.
162. Jarcho, J. A., McKenna, W., Pare, J.A.P., et al.: Mapping a gene for familial hypertrophic cardiomyopathy to chromosome 14q1. N. Engl. J. Med. *321*:1372, 1989.
163. Maron, B. J., and Mulvihill, J. J.: The genetics of hypertrophic cardiomyopathy. Ann. Intern. Med. *105*:610, 1986.
164. Greaves, S. C., Roche, A.H.G., Neutze, J. M., et al.: Inheritance of hypertrophic cardiomyopathy: A cross sectional and M mode echocardiographic study of 50 families. Br. Heart J. *58*:259, 1987.
165. Autore, C., Fragola, P. V., Picelli, A., et al.: Equivocal and borderline myocardial hypertrophy in relatives of patients with hypertrophic cardiomyopathy: Possible implications in genetics of the disease. Cardiology *75*:348, 1988.
166. Maron, B. J., Nichols, P. F., Pickle, L. W., et al.: Patterns of inheritance in hypertrophic cardiomyopathy: Assessment by M-mode and two-dimensional echocardiography. Am. J. Cardiol. *53*:1087, 1984.
167. Hada, Y., Sakamoto, T., Amano, K., et al.: Prevalence of hypertrophic cardiomyopathy in a population of adult Japanese workers as detected by echocardiographic screening. Am. J. Cardiol. *59*:183, 1987.
168. McKenna, W. J., Kleinebenne, A., Nihoyannopoulos, P., and Foale, R.: Echocardiographic measurement of right ventricular wall thickness in hypertrophic cardiomyopathy: Relation to clinical and prognostic features. J. Am. Coll. Cardiol. *11*:351, 1988.
169. Motamed, H. E., and Roberts, W. C.: Frequency and significance of mitral anular calcium in hypertrophic cardiomyopathy: Analysis of 200 necropsy patients. Am. J. Cardiol. *60*:877, 1987.
170. Maron, B. J.: Asymmetry in hypertrophic cardiomyopathy: The septal to free wall thickness ratio revisited. Am. J. Cardiol. *55*:835, 1985.
171. Wakasugi, S., Shibata, N., Kobayashi, T., et al.: Thallium-201 imaging in a patient with mid-ventricular hypertrophic obstructive cardiomyopathy. J. Nucl. Med. *29*:1738, 1988.
172. Zoghbi, W. A., Haichin, R. N., and Quinones, M. A.: Mid-cavity obstruction in apical hypertrophy: Doppler evidence of diastolic intraventricular gradient with higher apical pressure. Am. Heart J. *116*:1469, 1988.
173. Maron, B. J.: Apical hypertrophic cardiomyopathy: The continuing saga. J. Am. Coll. Cardiol. *15*:91, 1990.
174. Louie, E. K., and Maron, B. J.: Apical hypertrophic cardiomyopathy: Clinical and two-dimensional echocardiographic assessment. Ann. Intern. Med. *106*:663, 1987.
175. Gosselin, G., Pasternac, A., Lesperance, J., et al.: Apical hypertrophic cardiomyopathy: Clinical and angiographic characteristics of the first Canadian series. Can. J. Cardiol. *4*:258, 1988.
176. Webb, J. G., Sasson, Z., Rakowski, H., et al.: Apical hypertrophic cardiomyopathy: Clinical follow-up and diagnostic correlates. J. Am. Coll. Cardiol. *15*:83, 1990.
177. Topol, E. J., Traill, T. A., and Fortuin, N. J.: Hypertensive hypertrophic cardiomyopathy of the elderly. N. Engl. J. Med. *312*:277, 1985.
178. Shapiro, L. M.: Hypetrophic cardiomyopathy in the elderly. Br. Heart J. *63*:265, 1990.
179. Karam, R., Lever, H., and Healy, B. P.: Hypertensive hypertrophic cardiomyopathy or hypertrophic cardiomyopathy with hypertension? A study of 78 patients. J. Am. Coll. Cardiol. *13*:580, 1989.
180. Pearson, A. C., Gudipati, C. V., and Labovitz, A. J.: Systolic and diastolic flow abnormalities in elderly patients with hypertensive hypertrophic cardiomyopathy. J. Am. Coll. Cardiol. *12*:989, 1988.
181. Lewis, J. F., and Maron, B. J.: Elderly patients with hypertrophic cardiomyopathy: A subset with distinctive left ventricular morphology and progressive clinical course late in life. J. Am. Coll. Cardiol. *13*:36, 1989.
182. Lever, H. M., Karam, R. F., Currie, P. J., and Healy, B. P.: Hypertrophic cardiomyopathy in the elderly: Distinctions from the young based on cardiac shape. Circulation *79*:580, 1989.
183. Rheuban, K. S., Blizzard, R. M., Parker, M. A., et al.: Hypertrophic cardiomyopathy in total lipodystrophy. J. Pediatr. *109*:301, 1986.
184. Fitzpatrick, A. P., and Emanuel, R. W.: Familial neurofibromatosis and hypertrophic cardiomyopathy. Br. Heart J. *60*:247, 1988.
185. Davies, M. J.: Hypertrophic cardiomyopathy: One disease or several? Br. Heart J. *63*:263, 1990.
186. Symons, C., Fortune, F., Greenbaum, R. A., and Dandona, P.: Cardiac hypertrophy, hypertrophic cardiomyopathy, and hyperparathyroidism—an association. Br. Heart J. *54*:539, 1985.
187. Eriksson, P., Backman, C., Eriksson, A., et al.: Differentiation of cardiac amyloidosis and hypertrophic cardiomyopathy: A comparison of familial amyloidosis with polyneuropathy and hypertrophic cardiomyopathy by electrocardiography and echocardiography. Acta Med. Scand. *221*:39, 1987.
188. Davies, M. J.: The current status of myocardial disarray in hypertrophic cardiomyopathy (editorial). Br. Heart J. *51*:361, 1984.
189. Factor, S. M., Butany, J., Sole, M. J., et al.: Pathologic fibrosis and matrix connective tissue in the subaortic myocardium of patients with hypertrophic cardiomyopathy. J. Am. Coll. Cardiol. *17*:1343, 1991.
190. Tanaka, M., Fujiwara, H., Onodera, T., et al.: Quantitative analysis of narrowings of intramyocardial small arteries in normal hearts, hypertensive hearts, and hearts with hypertrophic cardiomyopathy. Circulation *75*:1130, 1987.
191. Maron, B. J., Wolfson, J. K., Epstein, S. E., and Roberts, W. C.: Intramural ("small vessel") coronary artery disease in hypertrophic cardiomyopathy. J. Am. Coll. Cardiol. *8*:545, 1986.
192. Pearce, P. C., Hawkey, C., Symons, C., and Olsen, E. G.: Role of calcium in the induction of cardiac hypertrophy and myofibrillar disarray. Experimental studies of a possible cause of hypertrophic cardiomyopathy. Br. Heart J. *54*:420, 1985.
193. Gwathmey, J. K., Copelas, L., MacKinnon, R., et al.: Abnormal intracellular calcium handling in myocardium from patients with end-stage heart failure. Circ. Res. *60*:70, 1987.
194. Wagner, J. A., Sax, F. L., Weisman, H. F., et al.: Calcium-antagonist receptors in the atrial tissue of patients with hypertrophic cardiomyopathy. N. Engl. J. Med. *320*:755, 1989.
195. Koga, Y., Itaya, M., and Toshima, H.: Increased cardiovascular response to epinephrine in hypertrophic cardiomyopathy. Jpn. Heart J. *26*:727, 1985.
196. Olsen, E. G.: An endocrine experimental model for myofibrillar disarray as found in hypertrophic cardiomyopathy. J. Mol. Cell. Cardiol. *17*:35, 1985.
197. Lawson, J.W.R.: Hypertrophic cardiomyopathy: Current views on etiology, pathophysiology, and management. Am. J. Med. Sci. *294*:191, 1987.
198. Brush, J. E., Jr., Eisenhofer, G., Garty, M., et al.: Cardiac norepinephrine kinetics in hypertrophic cardiomyopathy. Circulation *79*:836, 1989.
199. Ogata, Y., Hiyamuta, K., Terasawa, M., et al.: Relationship of exercise- or pacing-induced ST segment depression and myocardial lactate metabolism in patients with hypertrophic cardiomyopathy. Jpn. Heart J. *27*:145, 1986.
200. Hirzel, H. O., Tuchschmid, C. R., Schneider, J., et al.: Relationship between myosin isoenzyme composition, hemodynamics, and myocardial structure in various forms of human cardiac hypertrophy. Circ. Res. *57*:729, 1985.

201. Jarcho, J. A., McKenna, W., Pare, J.A.P., et al.: Mapping a gene for familial hypertrophic cardiomyopathy to chromosome 14q1. N. Engl. J. Med. *321*:1372, 1989.
202. Tanigawa, G., Jarcho, J. A., Kass, S., et al.: A molecular basis for familial hypertrophic cardiomyopathy: An α/β cardiac myosin heavy chain hybrid gene. Cell *62*:991, 1990.
203. Geisterfer-Lowrance, A.A.T., Kass, S., Tanigawa, G., et al.: A molecular basis for familial hypertrophic cardiomyopathy: A β cardiac myosin heavy chain gene missense mutation. Cell *62*:999, 1990.
204. Solomon, S. D., Geisterfer-Lowrance, A.A.T., Vosberg, H-P., et al.: A locus for familial hypertrophic cardiomyopathy is closely linked to the cardiac myosin heavy chain genes, CRI-L436, and CRI-L329 on chromosome 14 at q11-q12. Am. J. Hum. Genet. *47*:389, 1990.
205. Solomon, S. D., Jarcho, J. A., McKenna, W., et al.: Familial hypertrophic cardiomyopathy is a genetically heterogeneous disease. J. Clin. Invest. *86*:993, 1990.
206. Wigle, E. D.: Hypertrophic cardiomyopathy: A 1987 viewpoint. Circulation *75*:311, 1987.
207. Come, P. C., Riley, M. F., Carl, L. V., and Lorell, B.: Doppler evidence that true left ventricular-to-aortic pressure gradients exist in hypertrophic cardiomyopathy. Am. Heart J. *116*:1253, 1988.
208. Criley, J. M., and Siegel, R. J.: Has "obstruction" hindered our understanding of hypertrophic cardiomyopathy? Circulation *72*:1148, 1985.
209. Pasipoularides, A.: Clinical assessment of ventricular ejection dynamics with and without outflow obstruction. J. Am. Coll. Cardiol. *15*:859, 1990.
210. Maron, B. J., and Epstein, S. E.: Hypertrophic cardiomyopathy: Pathophysiology and therapy. *In* Braunwald, E. (ed.): Heart Disease: A Textbook of Cardiovascular Medicine. 3rd ed. Philadelphia, W. B. Saunders Company. Update No. 7, pp. 157–168, 1989.
211. Murgo, J. P.: The hemodynamic evaluation in hypertrophic cardiomyopathy: Systolic and diastolic dysfunction. Cardiovasc. Clin. *19*:193, 1988.
212. Maron, B. J., and Epstein, S. E.: Clinical significance and therapeutic implications of the left ventricular outflow tract pressure gradient in hypertrophic cardiomyopathy. Am. J. Cardiol. *58*:1093, 1986.
213. Bonow, R. O.: Left ventricular ejection dynamics and outflow obstruction in hypertrophic cardiomyopathy. J. Am. Coll. Cardiol. *13*:1280, 1989.
214. Sasson, Z., Henderson, M., Wilansky, S., et al.: Causal relation between the pressure gradient and left ventricular ejection time in hypertrophic cardiomyopathy. J. Am. Coll. Cardiol. *13*:1275, 1989.
215. Bryg, R. J., Pearson, A. C., Williams, G. A., and Labovitz, A. J.: Left ventricular systolic and diastolic flow abnormalities determined by Doppler echocardiography in obstructive hypertrophic cardiomyopathy. Am. J. Cardiol. *59*:925, 1987.
216. Hoit, B. D., Penonen, E., Dalton, N., and Sahn, D. J.: Doppler color flow mapping studies of jet formation and spatial orientation in obstructive hypertrophic cardiomyopathy. Am. Heart J. *117*:1119, 1989.
217. Stewart, W. J., Schiavone, W. A., Salcedo, E. E., et al.: Intraoperative Doppler echocardiography in hypertrophic cardiomyopathy: Correlation with the obstructive gradient. J. Am. Coll. Cardiol. *10*:327, 1987.
218. Maron, B. J., Spirito, P., Green, K. J., et al.: Noninvasive assessment of left ventricular diastolic function by pulsed Doppler echocardiography in patients with hypertrophic cardiomyopathy. J. Am. Coll. Cardiol. *10*:733, 1987.
219. Spirito, P., and Maron, B. J.: Relation between extent of left ventricular hypertrophy and diastolic filling abnormalities in hypertrophic cardiomyopathy. J. Am. Coll. Cardiol. *15*:808, 1990.
220. Wigle, E. D.: Impaired left ventricular relaxation in hypertrophic cardiomyopathy: Relation to extent of hypertrophy. J. Am. Coll. Cardiol. *15*:814, 1990.
221. Alvares, R. F., Shaver, J. A., Gamble, W. H., and Goodwin, J. F.: Isovolumic relaxation period in hypertrophic cardiomyopathy. J. Am. Coll. Cardiol. *3*:71, 1984.
222. Betocchi S., Bonow, R. O., Bacharach, S. L., et al.: Isovolumic relaxation period in hypertrophic cardiomyopathy: Assessment by radionuclide angiography. J. Am. Coll. Cardiol. *7*:74, 1986.
223. Brutsaert, D. L., Rademakers, F. E., and Sys, S. U.: Triple control of relaxation: Implications in cardiac disease. Circulation *69*:190, 1984.
224. Cannon, R. O., Schenke, W. H., Maron, B. J., et al.: Differences in coronary flow and myocardial metabolism at rest and during pacing between patients with obstructive and patients with nonobstructive hypertrophic cardiomyopathy. J. Am. Coll. Cardiol. *10*:53, 1987.
225. O'Gara, P. T., Bonow, R. O., Maron, B. J., et al.: Myocardial perfusion abnormalities in patients with hypertrophic cardiomyopathy: Assessment with thallium-201 emission computed tomography. Circulation *76*:1214, 1987.
226. Ikeda, H., Shimamatsu, M., Yoshiga, O., et al.: Impaired myocardial perfusion in patients with hypertrophic cardiomyopathy: Assessment with digital subtraction coronary arteriography. Heart Vessels *4*:170, 1988.
227. Fine, D. G., Clements, I. P., and Callahan, M. J.: Myocardial stunning in hypertrophic cardiomyopathy: Recovery predicted by single photon emission computed tomographic thallium-201 scintigraphy. J. Am. Coll. Cardiol. *13*:1415, 1989.
228. Grover-McKay, M., Schwaiger, M., Krivokapich, J., et al.: Regional myocardial blood flow and metabolism at rest in mildly symptomatic patients with hypertrophic cardiomyopathy. J. Am. Coll. Cardiol. *13*:317, 1989.
229. Spirito, P., Chiarella, F., Carratino, L., et al.: Clinical course and prognosis of hypertrophic cardiomyopathy in an outpatient population. N. Engl. J. Med. *320*:749, 1989.
229a. Shaver, J. A., Salerni, R., Curtiss, E. I., and Follansbee, W. P.: Clinical presentation and noninvasive evaluation of the patient with hypertrophic cardiomyopathy. Cardiovasc. Clin. *19*:149, 1988.
230. Brigden, W.: Hypertrophic cardiomyopathy. Br. Heart J. *58*:299, 1987.
231. Frank, S., and Braunwald, E.: Idiopathic hypertrophic subaortic stenosis. Clinical analysis of 126 patients with emphasis on the natural history. Circulation *37*:759, 1968.
232. Louie, E. K., and Maron, B. J.: Hypertrophic cardiomyopathy with extreme increase in left ventricular wall thickness: Functional and morphologic features and clinical significance. J. Am. Coll. Cardiol. *8*:57, 1986.
233. Spirito, P., Maron, B. J., Bonow, R. O., and Epstein, S. E.: Severe functional limitation in patients with hypertrophic cardiomyopathy and only mild localized left ventricular hypertrophy. J. Am. Coll. Cardiol. *8*:537, 1986.
234. McKenna, W. J., Steward, J. T., Nihoyannopoulos, P., et al.: Hypertrophic cardiomyopathy without hypertrophy: Two families with myocardial disarray in the absence of increased myocardial mass. Br. Heart J. *63*:281, 1990.
235. Frenneaux, M. P., Porter, A., Caforio, A. L., et al.: Determinants of exercise capacity on hypertrophic cardiomyopathy. J. Am. Coll. Cardiol. *13*:1521, 1989.
236. Nienaber, C. A., Hiller, S., Spielmann, R. P., et al.: Syncope in hypertrophic cardiomyopathy: Multivariate analysis of prognostic determinants. J. Am. Coll. Cardiol. *15*:948, 1990.
237. Lembo, N. J., Dell-Italia, L. J., Crawford, M. H., and O'Rourke, R. A.: Bedside diagnosis of systolic murmurs. N. Engl. J. Med. *318*:1572, 1988.
238. Shiota, T., Sakamoto, T., Takenaka, K., et al.: Aortic regurgitation associated with hypertrophic cardiomyopathy: A colour Doppler echocardiographic study. Br. Heart J. *62*:171, 1989.
239. Sasson, Z., Prieur, T., Skrobik, Y., et al.: Aortic regurgitation: A common complication after surgery for hypertrophic obstructive cardiomyopathy. J. Am. Coll. Cardiol. *13*:63, 1989.
240. Maron, B. J., Wolfson, J. K., Ciro, E., and Spirito, P.: Relation of electrocardiographic abnormalities and patterns of left ventricular hypertrophy identified by two-dimensional echocardiography in patients with hypertrophic cardiomyopathy. Am. J. Cardiol. *51*:189, 1983.
241. Dollar, A. L., and Roberts, W. C.: Usefulness of total 12 lead QRS voltage compared with other criteria for determining left ventricular hypertrophy in hypertrophic cardiomyopathy: Analysis of 57 patients studied at necropsy. Am. J. Med. *87*:377, 1989.
242. Alfonso, F., Annopoulos, P. N., Stewart, J., et al.: Clinical significance of giant negative T waves in hypertrophic cardiomyopathy. J. Am. Coll. Cardiol. *15*:965, 1990.
243. Cosio, F. G., Moro, C., Alonso, M., et al.: The Q waves of hypertrophic cardiomyopathy: An electrophysiologic study. N. Engl. J. Med. *302*:96, 1980.
244. Henderson, M. A., Ruddy, T. D., Makowski, H., and Wigle, E. D.: Left ventricular hypertrophy by ECG in hypertrophic cardiomyopathy. J. Am. Coll. Cardiol. *1*:693, 1983.
245. McKenna, W. J., Borggrefe, M., England, D., et al.: The natural history of left ventricular hypertrophy in hypertrophic cardiomyopathy: An electrocardiographic study. Circulation *66*:1233, 1982.
246. Khair, G. Z., and Bamrah, V. S.: Syncope in hypertrophic cardiomyopathy. I. Association with atrioventricular block. Am. Heart J. *110*:1081, 1985.
247. McKenna, W. J., and Camm, A. J.: Sudden death in hypertrophic cardiomyopathy: Assessment of patients at high risk. Circulation *80*:1489, 1989.
248. Nicod, P., Polikar, R., and Peterson, K. L.: Hypertrophic cardiomyopathy and sudden death. N. Engl. J. Med. *318*:1255, 1988.
249. Lazzeroni, E., Domenicucci, S., Finardi, A., et al.: Severity of arrhythmias and extent of hypertrophy in hypertrophic cardiomyopathy. Am. Heart J. *118*:734, 1989.
250. Spirito, P., Watson, R. M., and Maron, B. J.: Relation between extent of left ventricular hypertrophy and occurrence of ventricular tachycardia in hypertrophic cardiomyopathy. Am. J. Cardiol. *60*:1137, 1987.
251. Robinson, K., Frenneaux, M. P., Stockins, B., et al.: Atrial fibrillation in hypertrophic cardiomyopathy: A longitudinal study. J. Am. Coll. Cardiol. *15*:1279, 1990.
252. Greenspan, A. M.: Hypertrophic cardiomyopathy and atrial fibrillation: A change of perspective. J. Am. Coll. Cardiol. *15*:1286, 1990.
253. Pelliccia, F., Cianfrocca, C., Cristofani, R., et al.: Electrocardiographic findings in patients with hypertrophic cardiomyopathy. J. Electrocardiol. *23*:213, 1990.
254. Cripps, T. R., Counihan, P. J., Frenneaux, M. P., et al.: Signal-averaged electrocardiography in hypertrophic cardiomyopathy. J. Am. Coll. Cardiol. *15*:956, 1990.
255. Bahl, V. K., Kaul, U., Dev, V., and Bhatia, M. L.: Electrophysiologic evaluation of patients with hypertrophic cardiomyopathy. Int. J. Cardiol. *25*:87, 1989.
256. Fananapazir, L., Tracy, C. M., Leon, M. B., et al.: Electrophysiologic abnormalities in patients with hypertrophic cardiomyopathy: A consecutive analysis in 155 patients. Circulation *80*:1259, 1989.
257. Kuck, K. H., Kunze, K. P., Schluter, M., et al.: Programmed electrical stimulation in hypertrophic cardiomyopathy. Eur. Heart J. *9*:177, 1988.
258. Watson, R. M., Schwartz, J. L., Maron, B. J., et al.: Inducible polymorphic ventricular tachycardia and ventricular fibrillation in a subgroup of patients with hypertrophic cardiomyopathy at high risk for sudden death. J. Am. Coll. Cardiol. *10*:761, 1987.
258a. Fananapazir, L., and Epstein, S. E.: Hemodynamic and electrophysiologic evaluation of patients with hypertrophic cardiomyopathy surviving cardiac arrest. Am. J. Cardiol. *67*:280, 1991.
259. Lattanzi, F., Spirito, P., Picano, E., et al.: Quantitative assessment of ultra-

sonic myocardial reflectivity in hypertrophic cardiomyopathy. J. Am. Coll. Cardiol. 17:1085, 1991.
260. Madeira, H. C.: The mitral valve in hypertrophic cardiomyopathy—an echocardiographic approach. Postgrad. Med. J. 62:563, 1986.
261. Moro, E., tenCate, F. J., Leonard, J. J., et al.: Genesis of systolic anterior motion of the mitral valve in hypertrophic cardiomyopathy: An anatomical or dynamic event? Eur. Heart J. 8:1312, 1987.
262. Cape, E. G., Simon, D., Jimoh, A., et al.: Chordal geometry determines the shape and extent of systolic anterior mitral motion: In vitro studies. J. Am. Coll. Cardiol. 13:1438, 1989.
263. Miller, W., Walsh, R., and McCall, D.: Eosinophilic heart disease presenting with features suggesting hypertrophic obstructive cardiomopathy. Cathet. Cardiovasc. Diag. 13:185, 1987.
264. Maron, B. J., Epstein, S. E., Bonow, R. O., et al.: Obstructive hypertrophic cardiomyopathy associated with minimal left ventricular hypertrophy. Am. J. Cardiol. 53:377, 1984.
265. Gidding, S. S., Snider, R., Rocchini, A. P., et al.: Left ventricular diastolic filling in children with hypertrophic cardiomyopathy: Assessment with pulsed Doppler echocardiography. J. Am. Coll. Cardiol. 8:310, 1986.
266. Spirito, P., Maron, B. J., Chiarella, F., et al.: Diastolic abnormalities in patients with hypertrophic cardiomyopathy: Relation to magnitude of left ventricular hypertrophy. Circulation 72:310, 1985.
267. Gardin, J. M., Dabestani, A., Glasgow, G. A., et al.: Echocardiographic and Doppler flow observations in obstructed and nonobstructed hypertrophic cardiomyopathy. Am. J. Cardiol. 56:614, 1985.
268. Sasson, Z., Yock, P., Hatle, L. K., et al.: Doppler echocardiographic determination of the pressure gradient in hypertrophic cardiomyopathy. J. Am. Coll. Cardiol. 11:752, 1988.
269. Nishimura, R. A., Tajik, A. J., Reeder, G. S., and Seward, J. B.: Evaluation of hypertrophic cardiomyopathy by Doppler color flow imaging: Initial observations. Mayo Clin. Proc. 61:631, 1986.
270. von Dohlen, T. W., Prisant, L. M., and Frank, M. J.: Significance of positive or negative thallium-201 scintigraphy in hypertrophic cardiomyopathy. Am. J. Cardiol. 64:498, 1989.
271. Chikamori, T., Dickie, S., Poloniecki, J. D., et al.: Prognostic significance of radionuclide-assessed diastolic function in hypertrophic cardiomyopathy. Am. J. Cardiol. 65:478, 1990.
272. Cannon, R. O., Schenke, W. H., Bonow, R. O., et al.: Left ventricular pulsus alternans in patients with hypertrophic cardiomyopathy and severe obstruction to left ventricular outflow. Circulation 73:276, 1986.
273. Blazer, D., Kotler, M. N., Parry, W. R., et al.: Noninvasive evaluation of mid-left ventricular obstruction by two-dimensional and Doppler echocardiography and color flow Doppler echocardiography. Am. Heart J. 114:1162, 1987.
274. Kramer, D. S., French, W. J., and Criley, J. M.: The postextrasystolic murmur response to gradient in hypertrophic cardiomyopathy. Ann. Intern. Med. 104:772, 1986.
275. Sheikh, K. H., Pearce, F. B., and Kisslo, J.: Use of Doppler echocardiography and amyl nitrite inhalation to characterize left ventricular outflow obstruction in hypertrophic cardiomyopathy. Chest 97:389, 1990.
276. Pouleur, H., Rousseau, M. F., van Eyll, C., et al.: Force-velocity-length relations in hypertrophic cardiomyopathy: Evidence of normal or depressed myocardial contractility. Am. J. Cardiol. 52:813, 1983.
277. Kishimoto, C., Kadota, K., Sakurai, T., et al.: Improved evaluation of hypertrophic cardiomyopathy by biventriculography with axial projection. Am. Heart J. 110:77, 1985.
278. Cokkinos, D. V., Krajcer, Z., and Leachman, R. D.: Coronary artery disease in hypertrophic cardiomyopathy. Am. J. Cardiol. 55:1437, 1985.
279. Kimball, B. P., LiPreti, V., Bui, S., and Wigle, E. D.: Comparison of proximal left anterior descending and circumflex coronary artery dimensions in aortic valve stenosis and hypertrophic cardiomyopathy. Am. J. Cardiol. 65:767, 1990.
280. McKenna, W. J.: The natural history of hypertrophic cardiomyopathy. Cardiovasc. Clin. 19:135, 1988.
281. Aron, L. A., Hertzeanu, H. L., Fisman, E. Z., et al.: Prognosis of nonobstructive hypertrophic cardiomyopathy. Am. J. Cardiol. 67:215, 1991.
282. Shah, D. M., and Sunderji, S. G.: Hypertrophic cardiomyopathy and pregnancy: Report of a maternal mortality and review of literature. Obstet. Gynecol. Surv. 40:444, 1985.
283. Fighali, S., Krajcer, Z., Edelman, S., and Leachman, R. D.: Progression of hypertrophic cardiomyopathy into a hypokinetic left ventricle: Higher incidence in patients with midventricular obstruction. J. Am. Coll. Cardiol. 9:288, 1987.
284. Spirito, P., Maron, B. J., Bonow, R. O., and Epstein, S. E.: Occurrence and significance of progressive left ventricular wall thinning and relative cavity dilatation in patients with hypertrophic cardiomyopathy. Am. J. Cardiol. 60:123, 1987.
285. Domenicucci, S., Lazzeroni, E., Roelandt, J., et al.: Progression of hypertrophic cardiomyopathy. A cross sectional echocardiographic study. Br. Heart J. 53:405, 1985.
286. Maron, B. J., Spirito, P., Wesley, Y., and Arce, J.: Development and progression of left ventricular hypertrophy in children with hypertrophic cardiomyopathy. N. Engl. J. Med. 315:610, 1986.
287. Maron, B. J., Kragel, A. H., and Roberts, W. C.: Sudden death in hypertrophic cardiomyopathy with normal left ventricular mass. Br. Heart J. 63:308, 1990.
288. Panza, J. A., and Maron, B. J.: Relation of electrocardiographic abnormalities to evolving left ventricular hypertrophy in hypertrophic cardiomyopathy during childhood. Am. J. Cardiol. 63:1258, 1989.
289. Ciro, E., Maron, B. J., Bonow, R. O., et al.: Relation between marked changes in left ventricular outflow tract gradient and disease progression in hypertrophic cardiomyopathy. Am. J. Cardiol. 53:1103, 1984.
290. Romeo, F., Pelliccia, F., Cristofani, R., et al.: Hypertrophic cardiomyopathy: Is a left ventricular outflow tract gradient a major prognostic determinant? Eur. Heart J. 11:233, 1990.
291. Romeo, F., Cianfrocca, C., Pelliccia, F., et al.: Long-term prognosis in children with hypertrophic cardiomyopathy: An analysis of 37 patients aged ≤ 14 years at diagnosis. Clin. Cardiol. 13:101, 1990.
292. Nienaber, C. A., Hiller, S., Spielmann, R. P., et al.: Syncope in hypertrophic cardiomyopathy: Multivariate analysis of prognostic determinants. J. Am. Coll. Cardiol. 15:948, 1990.
293. Brandenburg, R. O.: Syncope and sudden death in hypertrophic cardiomyopathy. J. Am. Coll. Cardiol. 15:962, 1990.
294. McKenna, W. J., Franklin, R. C., Nihoyannopoulos, P., et al.: Arrhythmia and prognosis in infants, children and adolescents with hypertrophic cardiomyopathy. J. Am. Coll. Cardiol. 11:147, 1988.
295. Maron, B. J., Epstein, S. E., and Roberts, W. C.: Causes of sudden death in competitive athletes. J. Am. Coll. Cardiol. 7:204, 1986.
296. Spirito, P., and Maron, B. J.: Relation between extent of left ventricular hypertrophy and occurrence of sudden cardiac death in hypertrophic cardiomyopathy. J. Am. Coll. Cardiol. 15:1521, 1990.
297. Udelson, J. E., Bonow, R. O., O'Gara, P. T., et al.: Verapamil prevents silent myocardial perfusion abnormalities during exercise in asymptomatic patients with hypertrophic cardiomyopathy. Circulation 79:1052, 1989.
298. Bonow, R. O., Maron, B. J., Leon, M. B., et al.: Medical and surgical therapy of hypertrophic cardiomyopathy. Cardiovasc. Clin. 19:221, 1988.
299. Udelson, J. E., Cannon, R. O., Bacharach, S. L., et al.: Beta-adrenergic stimulation with isoproterenol enhances left ventricular diastolic performance in hypertrophic cardiomyopathy despite potentiation of myocardial ischemia. Comparison to rapid atrial pacing. Circulation 79:371, 1989.
300. Chatterjee, K.: Calcium antagonist agents in hypertrophic cardiomyopathy. Am. J. Cardiol. 59:146B, 1987.
301. Hopf, R., and Kaltenbach, M.: Ten-year results and survival of patients with hypertrophic cardiomyopathy treated with calcium antagonists. Z. Kardiol. 76:137, 1987.
302. Bonow, R. O., Dilsizian, V., Rosing, D. R., et al.: Verapamil-induced improvement in left ventricular diastolic filling and increased exercise tolerance in patients with hypertrophic cardiomyopathy: Short- and long-term effects. Circulation 72:853, 1985.
303. Shaffer, E. M., Rocchini, A. P., Spicer, R. L., et al.: Effects of verapamil on left ventricular diastolic filling in children with hypertrophic cardiomyopathy. Am. J. Cardiol. 61:413, 1988.
304. Bonow, R. O., Vitale, D. F., Maron, B. J., et al.: Regional left ventricular asynchrony and impaired global left ventricular filling in hypertrophic cardiomyopathy: Effect of verapamil. J. Am. Coll. Cardiol. 9:1108, 1987.
305. Bonow, R. O.: Effects of calcium-channel blocking agents on left ventricular diastolic function in hypertrophic cardiomyopathy and in coronary artery disease. Am. J. Cardiol. 55:172B, 1985.
306. Kaltenbach, M., and Hopf, R.: Treatment of hypertrophic cardiomyopathy: Relation to pathological mechanisms. J. Mol. Cell. Cardiol. 2:59, 1985.
307. Yamakado, T., Okano, H., Higashiyama, S., et al.: Effects of nifedipine on left ventricular diastolic function in patients with asymptomatic or minimally symptomatic hypertrophic cardiomyopathy. Circulation 81:593, 1990.
308. Richardson, P. J.: Calcium antagonists in cardiomyopathy. Br. J. Clin. Pract. 42:4, 1988.
309. Betocchi, S., Bonow, R. O., Cannon, R. O. III, et al.: Relation between serum nifedipine concentration and hemodynamic effects in nonobstructive hypertrophic cardiomyopathy. Am. J. Cardiol. 61:830, 1988.
310. Iwase, M., Sobotata, I., Takagi, S., et al.: Effects of diltiazem on left ventricular diastolic behavior in patients with hypertrophic cardiomyopathy: Evaluation with exercise pulsed Doppler echocardiography. J. Am. Coll. Cardiol. 9:1099, 1987.
311. Rosing, D. R., Idanpaan-Heikkila, U., Maron, B. J., et al.: Use of calcium-channel blocking drugs in hypertrophic cardiomyopathy. Am. J. Cardiol. 55:185B, 1985.
312. Sherrid, M., Delia, E., and Dwyer, E.: Oral disopyramide therapy for obstructive hypertrophic cardiomyopathy. Am. J. Cardiol. 62:1085, 1988.
313. Cokkinos, D. V., Salpeas, D., Ioannou, N. E., and Christoulas, S.: Combination of disopyramide and propranolol in hypertrophic cardiomyopathy. Can. J. Cardiol. 5:33, 1989.
314. Pollick, C., Kimball, B., Henderson, M., and Wigle, E. D.: Disopyramide in hypertrophic cardiomyopathy. I. Hemodynamic assessment after intravenous administration. Am. J. Cardiol. 62:1248, 1988.
315. Duncan, W. J., Tyrrell, M. J., and Bharadwaj, B. B.: Disopyramide as a negative inotrope in obstructive cardiomyopathy in children. Can. J. Cardiol. 7:81, 1991.
316. Sugrue, D. D., Dickie, S., Myers, M. J., et al.: Effects of amiodarone on left ventricular ejection and filling in hypertrophic cardiomyopathy as assessed by radionuclide angiography. Am. J. Cardiol. 54:1054, 1984.
317. McKenna, W. J., Oakley, C. M., Krikler, D. M., and Goodwin J. F.: Improved survival with amiodarone in patients with hypertrophic cardiomyopathy and ventricular tachycardia. Br. Heart J. 53:412, 1985.
318. Counihan, P. J., and McKenna, W. J.: Low-dose amiodarone for the treatment of arrhythmias in hypertrophic cardiomyopathy. J. Clin. Pharmacol. 29:436, 1989.
318a. Fananapazir, L., Leon, M. B., Bonow, R. O., et al.: Sudden death during empiric amiodarone therapy in symptomatic hypertrophic cardiomyopathy. Am. J. Cardiol. 67:169, 1991.

318b. Fananapazir, L., and Epstein, S. E.: Value of electrophysiologic studies in hypertrophic cardiomyopathy treated with amiodarone. Am. J. Cardiol. *67*:175, 1991.
319. Cecchi F., Maron, B. J., and Epstein, S. E.: Long-term outcome of patients with hypertrophic cardiomyopathy successfully resuscitated after cardiac arrest. J. Am. Coll. Cardiol. *13*:1283, 1989.
320. Maron, B. J., Gaffney, F. A., Jeresaty, R. M., et al.: Task force III: Hypertrophic cardiomyopathy, other myopericardial diseases and mitral valve prolapse. J. Am. Coll. Cardiol. *6*:1215, 1985.
321. McIntosh, C. L., and Maron, B. J.: Current operative treatment of obstructive hypertrophic cardiomyopathy. Circulation *78*:487, 1988.
321a. Seiler, C., Hess, O. M., Schoenbeck, M., et al.: Long-term follow-up of medical versus surgical therapy for hypertrophic cardiomyopathy: A retrospective study. J. Am. Coll. Cardiol. *17*:634, 1991.
321b. Chahine, R. A.: Surgical versus medical therapy of hypertrophic cardiomyopathy: Is the perspective changing? J. Am. Coll. Cardiol. *17*:643, 1991.
322. Surgical treatment of hypertrophic obstructive cardiomyopathy. Lancet *1*:358, 1989.
323. Mohr, R., Schaff, H. V., Danielson, G. K., et al.: The outcome of surgical treatment of hypertrophic obstructive cardiomyopathy: Experience over 15 years. J. Thorac. Cardiovasc. Surg. *97*:666, 1989.
324. Cooper, M. M., Tucker, E., McIntosh, C. L., et al.: Effect of left ventricular septal myectomy on concurrent mitral regurgitation. Ann. Thorac. Surg. *48*:251, 1989.
325. Cannon, R. O., McIntosh, C. L., Schenke, W. H., et al.: Effect of surgical reduction of left ventricular outflow obstruction on hemodynamics, coronary flow, and myocardial metabolism in hypertrophic cardiomyopathy. Circulation *79*:766, 1989.
326. Mohr, R., Schaff, H. V., Puga, F. J., and Danielson, G. K.: Results of operation for hypertrophic obstructive cardiomyopathy in children and adults less than 40 years of age. Circulation *80*:191, 1989.
327. Williams, W. G., Wigle, E. D., Rakowski, H., et al.: Results of surgery for hypertrophic obstructive cardiomyopathy. Circulation *76*:V104, 1987.
328. Siegman, I. L., Maron, B. J., Permut, L. C., et al.: Results of operation for coexistent obstructive hypertrophic cardiomyopathy and coronary artery disease. J. Am. Coll. Cardiol. *13*:1527, 1989.
329. Leachman, R. D., Krajcer, Z., Azic, T., and Cooley, D. A.: Mitral valve replacement in hypertrophic cardiomyopathy: Ten-year follow-up in 54 patients. Am. J. Cardiol. *60*:1416, 1987.
330. Walker, W. S., Reid, K. G., Cameron, E.W.J., et al.: Comparison of ventricular septal surgery and mitral valve replacement for hypertrophic obstructive cardiomyopathy. Ann. Thorac. Surg. *48*:528, 1989.
331. Krajcer, Z., Leachman, R. D., Cooley, D. A., et al.: Mitral valve replacement and septal myomectomy in hypertrophic cardiomyopathy: Ten-year follow-up in 80 patients. Circulation *78*:35, 1988.
332. McIntosh, C. L., Greenberg, G. J., Maron, B. J., et al.: Clinical and hemodynamic results after mitral valve replacement in patients with obstructive hypertrophic cardiomyopathy. Ann. Thorac. Surg. *47*:236, 1989.
333. Warren, S. E., Cohn, L. H., Schoen, F. J., et al.: Advanced diastolic heart failure in familial hypertrophic cardiomyopathy managed with cardiac transplantation. J. Appl. Cardiol. *3*:415, 1988.

RESTRICTIVE AND INFILTRATIVE CARDIOMYOPATHY

334. Child, J. S., and Perloff, J. K.: The restrictive cardiomyopathies. Cardiol. Clin. *6*:289, 1988.
335. Schoenfeld, M. H., Supple, E. W., Dec, G. W., et al.: Restrictive cardiomyopathy versus constrictive pericarditis: Role of endomyocardial biopsy in avoiding unnecessary thoracotomy. Circulation *75*:1012, 1987.
336. Hirota, Y. Shimizu, G., Kita, Y., et al.: Spectrum of restrictive cardiomyopathy: Report of the national survey in Japan. Am. Heart J. *120*:188, 1990.
337. Restrictive cardiomyopathy or constrictive pericarditis? (editorial) Lancet 15:372, 1987.
338. Wilmshurst, P. T., and Katritsis, D.: Restrictive cardiomyopathy (editorial). Br. Heart J. *63*:323, 1990.
339. Webb-Peploe, M. M.: Obliterative and restrictive cardiomyopathies. Eur. Heart J. 9:159, 1988.
340. Hosenpud, J. D.: Restrictive cardiomyopathy. *In* Zipes, D. P., and Rowlands, D. J. (eds.): Progress in Cardiology. Philadelphia, Lea and Febiger, 1989, p. 91.
341. Aroney, C., Bett, N., and Radford, D.: Familial restrictive cardiomyopathy. Aust. N.Z. J. Med. *18*:877, 1988.
342. Fitzpatrick, A. P., Shapiro, L. M., Rickards, A. F., and Poole-Wilson, P. A.: Familial restrictive cardiomyopathy with atrioventricular block and skeletal myopathy. Br. Heart J. *63*:114, 1990.
343. Shabetai, R.: Pathophysiology and differential diagnosis of restrictive cardiomyopathy. Cardiovasc. Clin. *19*:123, 1988.
344. Sechtem, U., Tscholakoff, D., and Higgins, C. B.: MRI of the abnormal pericardium. Am. J. Roentgenol. *147*:245, 1986.
345. Sechtem, U., Higgins, C. B., Sommerhoff, B. A., et al.: Magnetic resonance imaging of restrictive cardiomyopathy. Am. J. Cardiol. *59*:480, 1987.
346. Morgan, J. M., Raposo, L., Clague, J. C., et al.: Restrictive cardiomyopathy and constrictive pericarditis: Non-invasive distinction by digitised M mode echocardiography. Br. Heart J. *61*:29, 1989.
347. Appleton, C. P., Hatle, L. K., and Popp, R. L.: Demonstration of restrictive ventricular physiology by Doppler echocardiography. J. Am. Coll. Cardiol. *11*:757, 1988.
348. Hatle, L. K., Appleton, C. P., and Popp, R. L.: Differentiation of constrictive pericarditis and restrictive cardiomyopathy by Doppler echocardiography. Circulation *79*:357, 1989.
349. Schiavone, W. A., Calafiore, P. A., and Salcedo, E. E.: Transesophageal Doppler echocardiographic demonstration of pulmonary venous flow velocity in restrictive cardiomyopathy and constrictive pericarditis. Am. J. Cardiol. *63*:1286, 1989.
350. Gerson, M. C., Colthar, M. S., and Fowler, N. O.: Differentiation of constrictive pericarditis and restrictive cardiomyopathy by radionuclide ventriculography. Am. Heart J. *118*:114, 1989.
351. Aroney, C. N., Ruddy, T. D., Dighero, H., et al.: Differentiation of restrictive cardiomyopathy from pericardial constriction: Assessment of diastolic function by radionuclide angiograhy. J. Am. Coll. Cardiol. *13*:1007, 1989.
352. Gertz, M. A., and Kyle, R. A.: Primary systemic amyloidosis—a diagnostic primer. Mayo Clin. Proc. *64*:1505, 1989.
353. Falk, R. H.: Cardiac amyloidosis. *In* Zipes, D. P., and Rowlands, D. J. (eds.): Progress in Cardiology. Philadelphia, Lea and Febiger, 1989, p. 143.
354. Smith, T. J., Kyle, R. A., and Lie, J. T.: Clinical significance of histopathologic patterns of cardiac amyloidosis. Mayo Clin. Proc. *59*:547, 1984.
355. Olson, L. J., Gertz, M. A., Edwards, W. D., et al.: Senile cardiac amyloidosis with myocardial dysfunction: Diagnosis by endomyocardial biopsy and immunohistochemistry. N. Engl. J. Med. *317*:738, 1987.
356. de Freitas, A. F.: The heart in Portuguese amyloidosis. Postgrad. Med. J. *62*:601, 1986.
357. Klein, A. L., Oh, J. K., Miller, F. A., et al.: Two-dimensional and Doppler echocardiographic assessment of infiltrative cardiomyopathy. J. Am. Soc. Echocardiogr. *1*:48, 1988.
358. Falk, R. H., Plehn, J. F., Deering, T., et al.: Sensitivity and specificity of the echocardiographic features of cardiac amyloidosis. Am. J. Cardiol. *59*:418, 1987.
359. Kinoshita, O., Hongo, M., Yamada, H., et al.: Impaired left ventricular diastolic filling in patients with familial amyloid polyneuropathy: A pulsed Doppler echocardiographic study. Br. Heart J. *61*:198, 1989.
360. Hongo, M., and Ikeda, S. I.: Echocardiographic assessment of the evolution of amyloid heart disease: A study with familial amyloid polyneuropathy. Circulation *73*:249, 1986.
361. Eriksson, P., Eriksson, A., Backman, C., et al.: Highly refractile myocardial echoes in familial amyloidosis with polyneuropathy. Acta Med. Scand. *217*:27, 1985.
362. Pinamonti, B., Picano, E., Ferdeghini, E. M., et al.: Quantitative texture analysis in two-dimensional echocardiography: Application to the diagnosis of myocardial amyloidosis. J. Am. Coll. Cardiol. *14*:666, 1989.
363. Presti, C. F., Waler, B. F., and Armstrong, W. F.: Cardiac amyloidosis mimicking the echocardiographic appearance of obstructive hypertrophic myopathy. Chest *93*:881, 1988.
364. Cueto-Garcia, L., Reeder, G. S., Kyle, R. H., et al.: Echocardiographic findings in systemic amyloidosis: Spectrum of cardiac involvement and relation to survival. J. Am. Coll. Cardiol. *6*:737, 1985.
365. Klein, A. L., Hatle, L. K., Burstow, D. J., et al.: Doppler characterization of left ventricular diastolic function in cardiac amyloidosis. J. Am. Coll. Cardiol. *13*:1017, 1989.
366. Hongo, M., Fujii, T., Hirayama, J., et al.: Radionuclide angiographic assessment of left ventricular diastolic filling in amyloid heart disease: A study of patients with familial amyloid polyneuropathy. J. Am. Coll. Cardiol. *13*:48, 1989.
367. Plehn, J. F., and Friedman, B. J.: Diastolic dysfunction in amyloid heart disease: Restrictive cardiomyopathy or not? J. Am. Coll. Cardiol. *13*:54, 1989.
367a. Klein, A. L., Hatle, L. K., Talierco, C. P., et al.: Prognostic significance of Doppler measures of diastolic function in cardiac amyloidosis: A Doppler echocardliography study. Circulation *83*:808, 1991.
368. Hongo, M., Hirayama, J., Fujii, T., et al.: Early identification of amyloid heart disease by technetium-99m-pyrophosphate scintigraphy: A study with familial amyloid polyneuropathy. Am. Heart J. *113*:654, 1987.
369. Gertz, M. A., Skinner, M., Connors, L. H., et al.: Selective binding of nifedipine to amyloid fibrils. Am. J. Cardiol. *55*:1646, 1985.
370. Gertz, M. A., Falk, R. H., Skinner, M., et al.: Worsening of congestive heart failure in amyloid heart disease treated by calcium channel-blocking agents. Am. J. Cardiol. *55*:1645, 1985.
371. Hozumi, I., Nishizawa, M., Ariga, T., and Miyatake, T.: Biochemical and clinical analysis of accumulated glycolipids in symptomatic heterozygotes of angiokeratoma *corporis diffusum* (Fabry's disease) in comparison with hemizygotes. J. Lipid Res. *31*:335, 1990.
372. Sakurabab, H., Yanagawa, Y., Igarashi, T., et al.: Cardiovascular manifestations in Fabry's disease. Clin. Genetics *29*:276, 1986.
373. Goldman, M. E., Cantor, R., Schwartz, M. F., et al.: Echocardiographic abnormalities and disease severity in Fabry's disease. J. Am. Coll. Cardiol. *7*:1157, 1986.
374. Matsui, S., Murakami, E., Takekoshi, N., et al.: Myocardial tissue characterization by magnetic resonance imaging in Fabry's disease. Am. Heart J. *117*:472, 1989.
375. Tanaka, H., Adachi, K., Yamashita, Y., et al.: Four cases of Fabry's disease mimicking hypertrophic cardiomyopathy. J. Cardiol. *18*:705, 1988.
376. Yokoyama, A., Yamazoe, M., and Shibata, A.: A case of heterozygous Fabry's disease with a short PR interval and giant negative T waves. Br. Heart J. *57*:296, 1987.
377. Iwase, M., Yamauchi, K., Maeda, M., et al.: Echocardiographic findings in a case of Fabry's disease with aortic regurgitation and complete AV block, and in his family members. J. Cardiol. *18*:589, 1988.
378. Kramer, W., Thormann, J., Mueller, K., and Frenzel, H.: Progressive cardiac involvement by Fabry's disease despite successful renal allotransplantation. Int. J. Cardiol. *7*:72, 1985.
379. Casta, A., Hayden, K., and Wolf, W. J.: Calcification of the ascending aorta

and aortic and mitral valves in Gaucher's disease. Am. J. Cardiol. *54*:1390, 1984.
380. Platzker, Y., Pisman, E. Z., Pines, A., and Kellermann, J.: Unusual echocardiographic pattern in Gaucher's disease. Cardiology *72*:144, 1985.
381. Wilson, E. R., Barton, N. W., and Barranger, J. H.: Vascular involvement in type 3 neuronopathic Gaucher's disease. Arch. Pathol. Lab. Med. *109*:82, 1985.
382. Laks, Y., and Passwell, J.: The varied clinical and laboratory manifestations of type II Gaucher's disease. Acta Paediatr. Scand. *76*:378, 1987.
383. Barosi, G., Arbustini, E., Gavazzi, A., et al.: Myocardial iron grading by endomyocardial biopsy. A clinico-pathologic study on iron overloaded patients. Eur. J. Haematol. *42*:382, 1989.
384. Rahko, P. S., Salerni, R., and Uretsky, B. F.: Successful reversal by chelation therapy of congestive cardiomyopathy due to iron overload. J. Am. Coll. Cardiol. *8*:436, 1986.
385. Olson, L. J., Edwards, W. D., McCall, J. T., et al.: Cardiac iron deposition in idiopathic hemochromatosis: Histologic and analytic assessment of 14 hearts from autopsy. J. Am. Coll. Cardiol. *10*:1239, 1987.
386. Olson, L. J., Edwards, W. D., Holmes, D. R., Jr., et al.: Endomyocardial biopsy in hemochromatosis: Clinicopathologic correlates in six cases. J. Am. Coll. Cardiol. *13*:116, 1989.
387. Dabestani, A., Child, J. S., Henze, E., et al.: Primary hemochromatosis: Anatomic and physiologic characteristics of the cardiac ventricles and their response to phlebotomy. Am. J. Cardiol. *54*:153, 1984.
388. Furth, P. A., Futterweit, W., and Gorlin, R.: Refractory biventricular heart failure in secondary hemochromatosis. Am. J. Med. Sci. *290*:209, 1985.
389. Powell, L. W., and Isselbacher, K. J.: Hemochromatosis. *In* Wilson, J. D., et al. (eds.): Harrison's Principles of Internal Medicine. New York, McGraw-Hill, 1990, p. 1825.
390. Strohmeyer, G., Niederau, C., and Stremmel, W.: Survival and causes of death in hemochromatosis. Observations in 163 patients. Ann. N.Y. Acad. Sci. *526*:245, 1988
391. Lewin, R. F., Mor, R., Spitzer, S., et al.: Echocardiographic evaluation of patients with systemic sarcoidosis. Am. Heart J. *110*:116, 1985.
392. Tellier, P., Paycha, F., Antony, I., et al.: Reversibility by dipyridamole of thallium-201 myocardial scan defects in patients with sarcoidosis. Am. J. Med. 85:189, 1988.
393. Burstow, D. J., Tajik, A. J., Bailey, K. R., et al.: Two-dimensional echocardiographic findings in systemic sarcoidosis. Am. J. Cardiol. *63*:478, 1989.
394. Stewart, R. E., Graham, D. M., Godfrey, G. W., et al.: Rapidly progressive heart failure resulting from cardiac sarcoidosis. Am. Heart J. *115*:1324, 1988.
395. Temple-Camp, C. R.: Sarcoid myocarditis: A report of three cases. N.Z. Med. J. *102*:501, 1989.
396. Bajaj, A. K., Kopelman, H. A., and Echt, D. S.: Cardiac sarcoidosis with sudden death: Treatment with the automatic implantable cardioverter defibrillator. Am. Heart J. *116*:557, 1988.
397. Freiman, D. G.: The pathology of sarcoidosis. Semin. Roentgenol. *20*:327, 1985.
398. Fleming, H. H.: Sarcoid heart disease (editorial). Br. Med. J. *292*:1095, 1986.
399. Lemery, R., McGoon, M. D., and Edwards, W. D.: Cardiac sarcoidosis: A potentially treatable form of myocarditis. Mayo Clin. Proc. *60*:549, 1985.
400. Valantine, H., McKenna, W. J., Nihoyannopoulos, P., et al.: Sarcoidosis: A pattern of clinical and morphological presentation. Br. Heart J. *57*:256, 1987.
401. Diderholm, E., Eklund, A., Orinius, E., and Widstrom, O.: Exudative pericarditis in sarcoidosis. A case report and echocardiographic study. Sarcoidosis *6*:60, 1989.
402. Riedy, K., Fisher, M. R., Belic, N., and Koenigsberg, D. I.: MR imaging of myocardial sarcoidosis. Am. J. Roentgen. *151*:915, 1988.
403. Ratner, S. J., Fenoglio, J. J., Jr., and Ursell, P. C.: Utility of endomyocardial biopsy in the diagnosis of cardiac sarcoidosis. Chest *90*:528, 1986.
404. Ishikawa, T., Kondoh, H., Nakagawa, S., et al.: Steroid therapy in cardiac sarcoidosis: Increased left ventricular contractility concomitant with electrocardiographic improvement after prednisolone. Chest *85*:445, 1984.
405. Moodie, D. S., Baum, J. E., Gill, C. C., and Ratliff, N. B.: Endomyocardial fibrosis: Diagnosis and surgical treatment of two cases occurring in the United States. Cleveland Clin. Q. *53*:159, 1986.
406. Valiathan, M. S., Balakrishnan, K. G., and Kartha, C. C.: A profile of endomyocardial fibrosis. Indian J. Pediatr. *54*:229, 1987.
407. Valiathan, S. M., and Kartha, C. C.: Endomyocardial fibrosis—the possible connexion with myocardial levels of magnesium and cerium. Int. J. Cardiol. *28*:1, 1990.
408. Valiathan, M. S., Kartha, C. C., Eapen, J. T., et al.: A geochemical basis for endomyocardial fibrosis. Cardiovasc. Res. *23*:647, 1989.
409. Frustaci, A., Abdulla, A. K., Possati, G., and Manzoli, U.: Persisting hypereosinophilia and myocardial activity in the fibrotic stage of endomyocardial disease. Chest *96*:674, 1989.
410. Spry, C. J. F.: The pathogenesis of endomyocardial fibrosis: The role of the eosinophil. Springer Semin. Immunopathol. *11*:471, 1989.
411. Gupta, P. N., Valiathan, M. S., Balakrishnan, K. G., et al.: Clinical course of endomyocardial fibrosis. Br. Heart. J. *62*:450, 1989.
412. Olsen, E.G.J., and Spry, C.J.F.: Relation between eosinophilia and endomyocardial disease. Prog. Cardiovasc. Dis. *27*:241, 1985.
413. Shah, A. M., Brutsaert, D. L., Meulemans, A. L., et al.: Eosinophils from hypereosinophilic patients damage endocardium of isolated feline heart muscle preparations. Circulation *81*:1081, 1990.
414. Sasano, H., Virmani, R., Patterson, R. H., et al.: Eosinophilic products lead to myocardial damage. Hum. Pathol. *20*:850, 1989.
415. Tai, P. C., Ackerman, S. J., Spry, C. J., et al.: Deposits of eosinophil granule proteins in cardiac tissues of patients with eosinophilic endomyocardial disease. Lancet *21*:643, 1987.
416. Spry, C. J., Weetman, A. P., Olsson, I., et al.: The pathogenesis of eosinophilic endomyocardial disease in patients with carcinomas of the lung. Heart Vessels *1*:162, 1985.
417. Arnold, M., McGuire, L., and Lee, J. C.: Loeffler's fibroplastic endocarditis. Pathology *20*:79, 1988.
418. Hendren, W. G., Jones, E. L., and Smith, M. D.: Aortic and mitral valve replacement in idiopathic hypereosinophilic syndrome. Ann. Thorac. Surg. *46*:570, 1988.
419. Blake, D. P., Palmer, I. E., and Olinger, G. N.: Mitral valve replacement in idiopathic hypereosinophilic syndrome. J. Thorac. Cardiovasc. Surg. *89*:630, 1985.
420. Olsen, E.G.J.: Pathology of nonhypertrophic cardiomyopathies. *In* Zipes, D. P., and Rowlands, D. J. (eds.): Progress in Cardiology. Philadelphia, Lea and Febiger, 1989, p. 23.
421. Metras, D., Coulibaly, A. Q., and Quattara, K.: Recent trends in the surgical treatment of endomyocardial fibrosis. J. Cardiovasc. Surg. *28*:607, 1987.
422. Lengyel, M., Arvay, A., and Palik, I.: Massive endocardial calcification associated with endomyocardial fibrosis. Am. J. Cardiol. *56*:815, 1985.
423. Martinez, E. E., Venturi, M., Buffolo, E., et al.: Operative results in endomyocardial fibrosis. Am. J. Cardiol. *63*:627, 1989.
424. Siegel, R. J., and Fishbein, M. C.: Detection of endocardial calcium in endomyocardial fibrosis by computed tomography. Am. J. Cardiol. *60*:420, 1987.
425. Pawzy, M. E., Ziady, G., Halim, M., et al.: Endomyocardial fibrosis: Report of eight cases. J. Am. Coll. Cardiol. *5*:983, 1985.
426. Valiathan, M. S., Balakrishnan, K. G., Sankarkumar, R., and Kartha, C. C.: Surgical treatment of endomyocardial fibrosis. Ann. Thorac. Surg. *43*:68, 1987.
427. Barretto, A. C., da Luz, P. L., de Oliveira, S. A., et al.: Determinants of survival in endomyocardial fibrosis. Circulation *80*(Suppl. I): 177, 1989.
428. Mady, C., Pereira Barretto, A. C., de Oliveira, S. A., et al.: Effectiveness of operative and nonoperative therapy in endomyocardial fibrosis. Am. J. Cardiol. *15*:1281, 1989.
429. Ross, E. M., and Roberts, W. C.: The carcinoid syndrome: Comparison of 21 necropsy subjects with carcinoid heart disease to 15 necropsy subjects without carcinoid heart disease. Am. J. Med. *79*:339, 1985.
430. Lundin, L., Norheim, I., Landelius, J., et al.: Carcinoid heart disease: Relationship of circulating vasoactive substances to ultrasound-detectable cardiac abnormalities. Circulation *77*:264, 1988.
431. Lundin, L., Landelius, J., Andren, B., and Oberg, K.: Transesophageal echocardiography improves the value of cardiac ultrasound in patients with carcinoid heart disease. Br. Heart J. *64*:190, 1990.
432. Artaza, A., Beiner, J. H., Gonzalez, M., et al.: Carcinoid heart disease: Report of a case secondary to a pure carcinoid tumor of the ovary. Eur. Heart J. *6*:800, 1985.
433. Millward, M. J., Blake, M. P., Byrne, M. J., et al.: Left heart involvement with cardiac shunt complicating carcinoid heart disease. Aust. N.Z. J. Med. *19*:716, 1989.
434. Lundin, L., Funa, K., Hansson, H. E., et al.: Histochemical and immunohistochemical morphology of carcinoid heart disease. Pathol. Res. Pract. *187*:73, 1991.
435. Tornebrandt, K., Eskilsson, J., and Nobin, H.: Heart involvement in metastatic carcinoid disease. Clin. Cardiol. *9*:13, 1986.
436. Lundin, L., Hansson, H. E., Landelius, J., and Oberg, K.: Surgical treatment of carcinoid heart disease. J. Thorac. Cardiovasc. Surg, *100*:552, 1990.

MYOCARDITIS

437. Weinstein, C., and Fenoglio, J. J.: Myocarditis. Hum. Pathol. *18*:613, 1987.
438. Peters, N. S., and Poole-Wilson, P. A.: Myocarditis—continuing clinical and pathologic confusion. Am. Heart J. *121*:942, 1991.
439. Reyes, M. P., and Lerner, A. M.: Coxsackievirus myocarditis—with special reference to acute and chronic effects. Prog. Cardiovasc. Dis. *27*:373, 1985.
440. Marboe, C. C., and Fenoglio, J. J.: Pathology and natural history of human myocarditis. Pathol. Immunopathol. Res. *7*:226, 1988.
441. Gauntt, C. J., Godeny, E. K., and Lutton, C. W.: Host factors regulating viral clearance. Pathol. Immunopathol. Res. *7*:251, 1988.
442. Leslie, K. O., Schwarz, J., Simpson, K., and Huber, S. A.: Progressive interstitial collagen deposition in *Coxsackievirus* B3–induced murine myocarditis. Am. J. Pathol. *136*:683, 1990.
443. Herskowitz, A, Ahmed-Ansari, A., Neuman, D. A., et al.: Induction of major histocompatibility complex antigens within the myocardium of patients with active myocarditis: A nonhistologic marker of myocarditis. J. Am. Coll. Cardiol. *15*:624, 1990.
444. Wenger, N. K.: Myocarditis. *In* Zipes, D. P., and Rowlands, D. J. (eds.): Progress in Cardiology. Philadelphia, Lea and Febiger, 1989, p. 43.
445. Olsen, E. G. J.: Interpretation of endomyocardial biopsies: Infectious agents. Am. J. Cardiovasc. Pathol. *2*:329, 1989.
446. Herskowitz, A., Wolfgram, L. J., Rose, N. R., and Beisel, K. W.: Coxsackievirus B_3 murine myocarditis: A pathologic spectrum of myocarditis in genetically defined inbred strains. J. Am. Coll. Cardiol. *9*:1311, 1987.
447. Abelmann, W. H.: Myocarditis and dilated cardiomyopathy (editorial). West. J. Med. *150*: 458, 1989.
448. Hosenpud, J. D., McAnulty, J. H., and Niles, N. R.: Unexpected myocardial disease in patients with life threatening arrhythmias. Br. Heart J. *56*:55, 1986.

449. Claydon, S. M.: Myocarditis as an incidental finding in young men dying from unnatural causes. Med. Sci. Law *29*:55, 1989.
450. Phillips, M., Robinowitz, M., Higgins, J. R., et al.: Sudden cardiac death in Air Force recruits. A 20-year review. JAMA *21*:2696, 1986.
451. Karjalainen, J., and Heikkila, J.: "Acute pericarditis": Myocardial enzyme release as evidence for myocarditis. Am. Heart J. *111*:546, 1986.
452. Miklozek, C. L., Crumpacker, C. S., Royal, H. D., et al.: Myocarditis presenting as acute myocardial infarction. Am. Heart J. *115*:768, 1988.
453. Ferguson, D. W., Farwell, A. P., Bradley, W. A., and Rollings, R. C.: Coronary artery vasospasm complicating acute myocarditis: A rare association. West J. Med. 148:664, 1988.
454. Pinamonti, B., Alberti, E., Cigalotto, A., et al.: Echocardiographic findings in myocarditis. Am. J. Cardiol. *62*:285, 1988.
455. Arvan, S., and Manalo, E.: Sudden increase in left ventricular mass secondary to acute myocarditis. Am. Heart J. *116*:200, 1988.
456. Khaw, B. A., and Haber, E.: Imaging necrotic myocardium: Detection with 99mTc-pyrophosphate and radiolabeled antimyosin. Cardiol. Clin. *7*:577, 1989.
457. Rezkalla, S., Kloner, R. A., Khaw, B. A., et al.: Detection of experimental myocarditis by monoclonal antimyosin antibody Fab fragment. Am. Heart J. *117*:391, 1989.
458. Matsumori, A., Ohkusa, T., Matoba, Y., et al.: Myocardial uptake of antimyosin monoclonal antibody in a murine model of viral myocarditis. Circulation *79*:400, 1989.
459. Wakafugi, S., Kajiya, S., Hayakawa, M., et al.: Ga-67 myocardial scintigraphy in patients with acute myocarditis. Jpn. Circ. J. *51*:1373, 1987.
460. Chandraratna, P. A., Bradley, W. G., Kortman, K. E., and Minagoe, S.: Detection of acute myocarditis using nuclear magnetic resonance imaging. Am. J. Med. *83*:1144, 1987.
461. Chow, L. H., Radio, S. J., Sears, T. D., and McManus, B. M.: Insensitivity of right ventricular endomyocardial biopsy in the diagnosis of myocarditis. J. Am. Coll. Cardiol. *14*:915, 1989.
462. Hauck, A. J., Kearney, D. L., and Edwards, W. D.: Evaluation of postmortem endomyocardial biopsy specimens from 38 patients with lymphocytic myocarditis: Implications for role of sampling error. Mayo Clin. Proc. *64*:1235, 1989.
463. Dec, G. W., Fallon, J. T., Southern, J. F., and Palacios, I.: "Borderline" myocarditis: An indication for repeat endomyocardial biopsy. J. Am. Coll. Cardiol. *15*:283, 1990.
464. Ilback, N. G., Fohlman, J., and Friman, G.: Exercise in coxsackie B3 myocarditis: Effects on heart lymphocyte subpopulations and the inflammatory reaction. Am. Heart J. *117*:1298, 1989.
465. Lerner, A. M.: A new continuing fatigue syndrome following mild viral illness: A proscription to exercise. Chest *94*:901, 1988.
466. Kiel, R. J., Smith, F. E., Chason, J., et al.: Coxsackievirus B3 myocarditis in C3H/HeJ mice: Description of an inbred model and the effect of exercise on virulence. Eur. J. Epidemiol. *5*:348, 1989.
467. Rezkalla, S., Kloner, R. A., Khatib, G., et al.: Effect of metoprolol in acute coxsackievirus B3 murine myocarditis. J. Am. Coll. Cardiol. *12*:412, 1988.
467a. Chan, K. Y., Iwahara, M., Benson, L. N., et al.: Immunosuppressive therapy in the management of acute myocarditis in children: A clinical trial. J. Am. Coll. Cardiol. *17*:458, 1991.
468. Rezkalla, S., Khatib, G., and Khatib, R.: Coxsackievirus B3 murine myocarditis: Deleterious effects of nonsteroidal anti-inflammatory agents. J. Lab. Clin. Med. *107*:393, 1986.
469. Rezkalla, S. H., and Kloner, R. A.: Management strategies in viral myocarditis. Am. Heart J. *117*:706, 1989.
470. O'Connell, J. B., Reap, E. A., and Robinson, J. A.: The effects of cyclosporine on acute murine Coxsackie B3 myocarditis. Circulation *73*:353, 1986.
471. Monrad, E. S., Matsumori, A., Murphy, J. C., et al.: Therapy with cyclosporine in experimental murine myocarditis with encephalomyocarditis virus. Circulation *73*:1058, 1986.
472. Kishimoto, C., and Abelmann, W. H.: Absence of effects of cyclosporine on myocardial lymphocyte subsets in Coxsackievirus B3 myocarditis in the aviremic stage. Circ. Res. *65*:934, 1989.
472a. Kishimoto, C., Thorp, K. A., and Abelmann, W. H.: Immunosuppression with high doses of cyclophosphamide reduces the severity of myocarditis but increases the mortality in murine coxsackievirus B3 myocarditis. Circulation *82*:982, 1990.
473. Rezkalla, S., Khatib, R., Khatib, G., et al.: Effect of indomethacin in the late phase of coxsackievirus myocarditis in a murine model. J. Lab. Clin. Med. *112*:118, 1988.
474. Rezkalla, S., Kloner, R. A., Khatib, G., and Khatib, R.: Beneficial effects of captopril in acute coxsackievirus B3 murine myocarditis. Circulation *81*:1039, 1990.
474a. Rezkalla, S., Kloner, R. A., Khatib G., and Khatib, R.: Effect of delayed captopril therapy on left ventricular mass and myonecrosis during acute coxsackievirus murine myocarditis. Am. Heart J. *120*:1377, 1990.
475. Ray, C. G., Icenogle, T. B., Minnich, L. L., et al.: The use of intravenous ribavirin to treat influenza virus–associated acute myocarditis. J. Infect. Dis. *159*:829, 1989.
476. Chan, K. Y., Iwahara, M., Benson, L. N., et al.: Immunosuppressive therapy in the management of acute myocarditis in children: A clinical trial. J. Am. Coll. Cardiol. *17*:458, 1991.
477. Gilbert, E. M., O'Connell, J. B., Hammond, M. E., et al.: Treatment of myocarditis with OKT3 monoclonal antibody (letter). Lancet *1*:759, 1988.
478. Kishimoto, C., and Abelmann, W. H.: Monoclonal antibody therapy for prevention of acute coxsackievirus B3 myocarditis in mice. Circulation *79*:1300, 1989.
479. Kishimoto, C., Crumpacker, C. S., and Abelmann, W. H.: Prevention of murine coxsackie B3 viral myocarditis and associated lymphoid organ atrophy with recombinant human leucocyte interferon alpha A/D. Cardiovasc. Res. *22*:732, 1988.
480. Matsumori, A., Tomioka, N., and Kawai, C.: Protective effect of recombinant alpha interferon on coxsackievirus B3 myocarditis in mice. Am. Heart J. *115*:1229, 1988.
481. Matsumori, A., Crumpacker, C. S., and Abelmann, W. H.: Prevention of viral myocarditis with recombinant human leukocyte interferon alpha A.D. in a murine model. J. Am. Coll. Cardiol. *9*:1320, 1987.
482. Wolfgram, L. J., and Rose, N. R.: Coxsackievirus infection as a trigger of cardiac autoimmunity. Immunol. Res. *8*:61, 1989.
483. Rozkovec, A., Cambridge, G., King, M., and Hallidie-Smith, K. A.: Natural history of left ventricular function in neonatal Coxsackie myocarditis. Pediatr. Cardiol. *6*:151, 1985.
484. Read, R. B., Ede, R. J., Morgan-Capner, P., et al.: Myocarditis and fulminant hepatic failure from coxsackievirus B infection. Postgrad. Med. J. *61*:749, 1985.
485. Remes, J., Helin, M., Vaino, P., and Rautio, P.: Clinical outcome and left ventricular function 23 years after acute coxsackie virus myopericarditis. Eur. Heart J. *11*:182, 1990.
486. Levi, G., Scalvini, S., Volterrani, M., et al.: Coxsackie virus heart disease: 15 years after. Eur. Heart J. *9*:1303, 1988.
487. O'Connell, J. B., and Robinson J. A.: Coxsackie viral myocarditis. Postgrad. Med. J. *61*:1127, 1985.
488. Biton, A., and Herman, J.: Perimyocarditis. Report on an unusual cause. Postgrad. Med. *85*:77, 1989.
489. Gonwa, T. A., Capehart, J. E., Pilcher, J. W., and Alivizatos, P. A.: Cytomegalovirus myocarditis as a cause of cardiac dysfunction in heart transplant recipient. Transplantation *47*:197, 1989.
490. Shabtai, M., Luft, B., Waltzer, W. C., et al.: Massive cytomegalovirus pneumonia and myocarditis in a renal transplant recipient: Successful treatment with DHPG. Transplant Proc. *20*:562, 1988.
491. Markin, R. S., Hollins, S., Wood, R. P., and Shaw, B. W., Jr.: Main autopsy finding in liver transplant patients. Mod. Pathol. *2*:339, 1989.
492. Schindler, J. M., and Neftel, K. A.: Simultaneous primary infection with HIV and CMV leading to severe pancytopenia, hepatitis, nephritis, perimyocarditis, myositis, and alopecia totalis. Klin. Wochenschr. *68*:237, 1990.
493. Powell, K.F.H., Bellamy, A. R., Catton, M. G., et al.: Cytomegalovirus myocarditis in a heart transplant recipient: Sensitive monitoring of viral DNA by the polymerase chain reaction. J. Heart Transplant *8*:465, 1989.
494. Giampalmo, A., Ardoino, S., Borghesi, M. R., et al.: Anatomo-pathologic findings in 25 autopsy cases of AIDS. Pathologica *81*:1, 1989.
495. George, R.: Dengue haemorrhagic fever in Malaysia: A review. Southeast Asian J. Trop. Med. Pub. Hlth. *18*:278, 1987.
496. Songco, R. S., Hayes, C. G., Leus, C. D., and Manaloto, C.O.R.: Dengue fever/dengue haemorrhagic fever in Filipino children: Clinical experience during the 1983–1984 epidemic. Southeast Asian J. Trop. Med. Pub. Hlth. *18*:284, 1987.
497. Milei, J., and Bolomo, N. J.: Myocardial damage in viral hemorrhagic fevers. Am. Heart. J. *104*:1385, 1982.
498. Ursell, P. C., Habib, A., Sharma, P., et al.: Hepatitis B virus and myocarditis. Hum. Pathol. *15*:481, 1984.
499. Singh, D. S., Gupta, P. R., Gupta, S. S., et al.: Cardiac changes in acute viral hepatitis in Varanasi (India): Case reports. J. Trop. Med. Hyg. *92*:243, 1989.
500. Mahapatra, R. K., and Ellis, G. H.: Myocarditis and hepatitis B virus. Angiology *36*:116, 1985.
501. Blanchard, D. G., Hagenhoff, C., Chow, L. C., et al.: Reversibility of cardiac abnormalities in human immunodeficiency virus (HIV)-infected individuals: A serial echocardiographic study. J. Am. Coll. Cardiol. *17*:1270, 1991.
502. Levy, W. S., Simon, G. L., Rios, J. C., and Ross, A. M.: Prevalence of cardiac abnormalities in human immunodeficiency virus infection. Am. J. Cardiol. *63*:86, 1989.
503. Raffanti, S. P., Chiaramida, A. J., Sen, P., et al.: Assessment of cardiac function in patients with the acquired immunodeficiency syndrome. Chest *93*:592, 1988.
504. Himelman, R. B., Chung, W. S., Chernoff, D. N., et al.: Cardiac manifestations of human immunodeficiency virus infection: A two-dimensional echocardiographic study. J. Am. Coll. Cardiol. *13*:1030, 1989.
505. Corallo, S., Mutinelli, M. R., Moroni, M., et al.: Echocardiography detects myocardial damage in AIDS: Prospective study in 102 patients. Eur. Heart J. *9*:887, 1988.
506. Monsuez, J-J., Kinney, E. L., Vittecoq, D., et al.: Comparison among acquired immune deficiency syndrome patients with and without clinical evidence of cardiac disease. Am. J. Cardiol. *62*:1311, 1988.
507. Lewis, W.: AIDS: Cardiac findings from 115 autopsies. Prog. Cardiovasc. Dis. *32*:207, 1989.
508. Anderson, D. W., Virmani, R., Reilly, J. M., et al.: Prevalent myocarditis in necropsy in the acquired immunodeficiency syndrome. J. Am. Coll. Cardiol. *11*:792, 1988.
509. Reilly, J. M., Cunnion, R. E., Anderson, D. W., et al.: Frequency of myocarditis, left ventricular dysfunction and ventricular tachycardia in the acquired immune deficiency syndrome. Am. J. Cardiol. *62*:789, 1988.
510. Baroldi, G., Corallo, S., Moroni, M., et al.: Focal lymphocytic myocarditis in acquired immunodeficiency syndrome (AIDS): A correlative morphologic and clinical study in 26 consecutive fatal cases. J. Am. Coll. Cardiol. *12*:463, 1988.
511. Acierno, L. J.: Cardiac complications in acquired immunodeficiency syndrome (AIDS): A review. J. Am. Coll. Cardiol. *13*:1144, 1989.

512. Grody, W. W., Cheng, L., and Lewis, W.: Infection of the heart by the human immunodeficiency virus. Am. J. Cardiol. *66*:203, 1990.
513. Anderson, D. W., and Virmani, R.: Emerging patterns of heart disease in human immunodeficiency virus infection. Hum. Pathol. *21*:253, 1990.
514. Stewart, J. M., Kaul, A., Gromisch, D. S., et al.: Symptomatic cardiac dysfunction in children with human immunodeficiency virus infection. Am. Heart. J. *117*:140, 1989.
515. Calabrese, L. H., Proffitt, M. R., Yen-Lieberman, B., et al.: Congestive cardiomyopathy and illness related to the acquired immunodeficiency syndrome (AIDS) associated with isolation of retrovirus from myocardium. Ann. Intern. Med. *107*:691, 1987.
516. Coplan, N. L., and Bruno, M. S.: Acquired immunodeficiency syndrome and heart disease: The present and the future. Am. Heart J. *117*:1175, 1989.
517. Bharati, S., Joshi, V. V., Connor, E. M., et al.: Conduction system in children with acquired immunodeficiency syndrome. Chest *96*:406, 1989.
518. Kinney, E. L., Monsuez, J-J., Kitzis, M., and Vittecoq, D.: Treatment of AIDS-associated heart disease. Angiology *40*:970, 1989.
519. Frishman, W., Kraus, M. E., Zabkar, J., et al.: Infectious mononucleosis and fatal myocarditis. Chest *72*:535, 1977.
520. Tyson, A. A., Jr., Hackshaw, B. T., and Kutcher, M. A.: Acute Epstein-Barr virus myocarditis simulating myocardial infarction with cardiogenic shock. South. Med. J. *82*:1184, 1989.
521. Hudgins, J. M.: Infectious mononucleosis complicated by myocarditis and pericarditis. JAMA *235*:2626, 1976.
522. Cate, T. R.: Clinical manifestations and consequences of influenza. Am. J. Med. *82*:15, 1987.
523. Sprenger, M. J., Van Naelten, M. A., Mulder, P. G., and Masurel, N.: Influenza mortality and excess deaths in the elderly, 1967–1982. Epidemiol. Infect. *103*:633, 1989.
524. Engblom, E., Ekfors, T. O., Meurman, O. H., et al.: Fatal influenza A myocarditis with isolation of virus from the myocardium. Acta Med. Scand. *213*:75, 1983.
525. Proby, C. M., Hackett, D., Gupta, S., and Cox, T. M.: Acute myopericarditis in influenza A infection. Q. J. Med. *60*:887, 1986.
526. Drescher, J., Zink, P., Verhagen, W., et al.: Recent influenza virus A infections in forensic cases of sudden unexplained death. Arch. Virol. *92*:63, 1987.
527. Ruben, F. L., and Cate, T. R.: Influenza pneumonia. Semin. Respir. Infect. *2*:122, 1987.
528. Cummins, D., Bennett, D., Fisher-Hoch, S. P., et al.: Electrocardiographic abnormalities in patients with Lassa fever. J. Trop. Med. Hyg. *92*:350, 1989.
529. McCormick, J. B., King, I. J., Webb, P. A., et al.: Lassa fever: A case-control study of the clinical diagnosis and course. J. Infect. Dis. *155*:445, 1987.
530. Walker, D. H., McCormick, J. B., Johnson, K. M., et al.: Pathologic and virologic study of fatal Lassa fever in man. J. Infect. Dis. *107*:349, 1982.
531. Ozkutlu, S., Soylemezoglu, O., Calikoglu, A. S., et al.: Fatal mumps myocarditis. Jpn. Heart J. *30*:109, 1989.
532. Ward, S. C., Wiselka, M. J., and Nicholson, K. G.: Still's disease and myocarditis associated with recent mumps infection. Postgrad. Med. J. *64*:693, 1988.
533. Chaudary, S., and Jaski, B. E.: Fulminant mumps myocarditis. Ann. Intern. Med. *110*:569, 1989.
534. Baandrup, U., and Mortensen, S. A.: Fatal mumps myocarditis. Acta Med. Scand. *216*:331, 1984.
535. Chen, S. C., Tsai, C. C., and Nouri, S.: Carditis associated with mycoplasma pneumoniae infection. Am. J. Dis. Child. *140*:471, 1986.
536. Murray, B. J.: Nonrespiratory complications of *M. pneumoniae* infection. Am. Fam. Physician *37*:127, 1988.
537. Hildes, J. A., Schaberg, A., and Alcock, A.U.W.: Cardiovascular collapse in acute poliomyelitis. Circulation *12*:986, 1955.
538. Dunne, J. W., Harper, C. G., and Hilton, J. M.: Sudden infant death syndrome caused by poliomyelitis. Arch. Neurol. *41*:775, 1984.
539. Teloth, H. A.: Myocarditis in poliomyelitis. Arch. Pathol. *55*:408, 1953.
540. Weinstein, L., and Shelokov, A.: Cardiovascular manifestations of acute poliomyelitis. N. Engl. J. Med. *244*:281, 1951.
541. Page, S. R., Stewart, J. T., and Bernstein, J. J.: A progressive pericardial effusion caused by psittacosis. Br. Heart J. *60*:87, 1988.
542. Pahl, E., and Gidding, S. S.: Echocardiographic assessment of cardiac function during respiratory syncytial virus infection. Pediatrics *81*:830, 1988.
543. Menahem, S., and Uren, E. C.: Respiratory syncytial virus and heart block —cause and effect? Aust. N.Z. J. Med. *15*:55, 1985.
544. Martin, J. T., Kugler, J. D., Gumbiner, G. H., et al.: Refractory congestive heart failure after ribavirin in infants with heart disease and respiratory syncytial virus. Nebr. Med. J. *75*:23, 1990.
545. Thanopoulos, B. D., Rokas, S., Frimas, C. A., et al.: Cardiac involvement in postnatal rubella. Acta Paediatr. Scand. *78*:141, 1989.
546. Goldfield, M., Bayer, N. H., and Weinstein, L.: Electrocardiographic changes during the course of measles. J. Pediatr. *46*:30, 1955.
547. Degen, J. A.: Visceral pathology in measles: A clinicopathologic study of 100 cases. Am. J. Med. Sci. *194*:104, 1937.
548. Weinstein, L.: Cardiovascular manifestations in some of the common infectious diseases. Mod. Concepts Cardiovasc. Dis. *23*:229, 1954.
549. Lorber, A., Zonis, Z., Maisuls, E., et al.: The scale of myocardial involvement in varicella myocarditis. Int. J. Cardiol. *20*:257, 1988.
550. Woolf, P. K., Chung, T. S., Stewart, J., et al.: Life-threatening dysrhythmias in varicella myocarditis. Clin. Pediatr. *26*:480, 1987.
551. Ettedgui, J. A., Ladusans, E., and Bamford, M.: Complete heart block as a complication of varicella. Int. J. Cardiol. *14*:362, 1987.
552. Wagner, D. C., and Murphy, T. V.: Varicella myocarditis. Pediatr. Infect. Dis. J. *9*:360, 1990.
553. Anderson, T., Foulis, M. A., Grist, N. R., and Landsman, J. B.: Clinical and laboratory observations in a smallpox outbreak. Lancet *1*:1248, 1951.
554. Matthews, A. W., and Griffiths, I. D.: Post-vaccinal pericarditis and myocarditis. Br. Heart J. *36*:1043, 1974.
555. Finley-Jones, L. R.: Fatal myocarditis after vaccinations for smallpox. N. Engl. J. Med. *270*:41, 1964.
556. Schmeer, N., Krauss, H., Werth, D., and Schiefer, H. G.: Serodiagnosis of Q fever by enzyme-linked immunosorbent assay (ELISA). Zentralbl. Bakteriol. Mikrobiol. Hyg. *267*:57, 1987.
557. Maisch, B.: Rickettsial perimyocarditis — a follow-up study. Heart Vessels *2*:55, 1986.
558. Koster, F. T., Williams, J. C., and Goodwin, J. S.: Cellular immunity in Q fever: Specific lymphocyte unresponsiveness in Q fever endocarditis. J. Infect. Dis. *152*:1283, 1985.
559. Marin-Garcia, J., and Barrett, F. F.: Myocardial function in Rocky Mountain spotted fever: Echocardiographic assessment. Am. J. Cardiol. *51*:341, 1983.
560. Marin-Garcia, J., and Mirvis, D. M.: Myocardial disease in Rocky Mountain spotted fever: Clinical, functional, and pathologic findings. Pediatr. Cardiol. *5*:149, 1984.
561. Marin-Garcia, J.: Left ventricular dysfunction in Rocky Mountain spotted fever. Clin. Cardiol. *6*:501, 1983.
562. Ganjoo, R. K., Sharma, S, N. and Roy, A. K.: Typhus myocarditis (letter). J. Assoc. Physicians India *37*:357, 1989.
563. Brown, G. W., Shirai, A., Jegathesan, M., et al.: Febrile illness in Malaysia —an analysis of 1,629 hospitalized patients. Am. J. Trop. Med. Hyg. *33*:311, 1984.
564. Valliattu, J., Shuhaiber, H., Kiwan, Y., et al.: Brucella endocarditis. Report of one case and review of the literature. J. Cardiovasc. Surg. *30*:782, 1989.
565. Lubani, M., Sharda, D., and Helin, I.: Cardiac manifestations in brucellosis. Arch. Dis. Child. *61*:569, 1986.
566. Gur, H., Gefel, D., and Tur-Kaspa, R.: Transient electrocardiographic changes during two episodes of relapsing brucellosis. Postgrad. Med. J. *60*:544, 1984.
567. Jubber, A. S., Gunawardana, D. R., and Lulu, A. R.: Acute pulmonary edema in Brucella myocarditis and interstitial pneumonitis. Chest *97*:1008, 1990.
568. Roberts, W. C., and Beard, G. W.: Gas gangrene of the heart in clostridial septicemia. Am. Heart J. *74*:482, 1967.
569. Stevens, D. L., Troyer, B. E., Merrick, D. T., et al.: Lethal effects and cardiovascular effects of purified alpha- and theta-toxins from *Clostridium perfringens*. J. Infect. Dis. *157*:272, 1988.
570. Guneratre, P.: Gas gangrene (abscess) of heart. N. Y. State J. Med. *75*:1766, 1975.
571. Havaldar, P. V., Patil, V. D., Siddibhavi, B. M., et al.: Fulminant diphtheritic myocarditis. Indian Heart J. *41*:265, 1989.
572. Thisyakorn, U., Wongvanich, J., and Kumpens, V.: Failure of corticosteroid therapy to prevent diphtheritic myocarditis or neuritis. Pediatr. Infect. Dis. *3*:126, 1984.
573. Ramos, H. C., Elias, P. R., Barrucand, L., et al.: The protective effect of carnitine in human diphtheric myocarditis. Pediatr. Res. *18*:815, 1984.
574. Castellani Pastoris, M., Nigro, G., and Middulla, M.: Arrhythmia or myocarditis: A novel clinical form of *Legionella pneumophila* infection in children without pneumonia. Eur. J. Pediatr. *144*:157, 1985.
575. Friedland, L., Syndman, D. R., Weingarden, A. S., et al.: Ocular and pericardial involvement in Legionnaires' disease. Am. J. Med. *77*:1105, 1984.
576. Brasier, A. R., Macklis, J. D., Vaughan, D., et al.: Myopericarditis as an initial presentation of meningococcemia. Unusual manifestation of infection with serotype W135. Am. J. Med. *82*:641, 1987.
577. Sandler, M. A., Pincus, P. S., Weltman, M. D., et al.: Meningococcaemia complicated by myocarditis. A report of 2 cases. S. Afr. Med. J. *75*:391, 1989.
578. Ejlertsen T., Vesterlund, T., and Schmidt, E. B.: Myopericarditis with cardiac tamponade caused by Neisseria meningitides serogroup W135. Eur. J. Clin. Microbiol. Infect. Dis. *7*:403, 1988.
579. Monsalve, F., Rucabado, L., Salvador, A., et al.: Myocardial depression in septic shock caused by meningococcal infection. Crit. Care Med. *12*:1021, 1984.
580. Kovoor, P., Mathew, M., Abraham, T., and Taneja, P. K.: Enteric fever complicated by myocarditis, hepatitis and shock. J. Assoc. Physicians India *36*:353, 1988.
581. Delapenha, R. A., Greaves, W. L., Mani, V., and Frederick, W. R.: Typhoid fever with unusual clinical features (letter). South. Med. J. *81*:417, 1988.
582. Siwach, S. B., and Nand, N.: Cardiovascular complications of enteric fever. Angiology *34*:436, 1983.
583. Le-Van-Diem, A. K.: Typhoid fever with myocarditis. Am. J. Trop. Med. Hyg. *23*:218, 1974.
584. Dhar, K. L., Adlakha, A., and Phillips, P. J.: Recurrent seizures and syncope, ventricular arrhythmias with reversible prolonged Q-Tc interval in typhoid myocarditis. J. Indian Med. Assoc. *85*:336, 1987.
585. Karjalainen, J.: Streptococcal tonsillitis and acute nonrheumatic myopericarditis. Chest *95*:359, 1989.
586. Caraco, J., Arnon, R., and Raz, I.: Atrioventricular block complicating acute streptococcal tonsillitis. Br. Heart J. *59*:389, 1988.
587. Rose, A. G.: Cardiac tuberculosis. A study of 19 patients. Arch. Pathol. Lab. Med. *111*:422, 1987.
588. Picard, R., Vinceneux, Ph., Lim, D. Q., et al.: Heart failure due to myocardial tuberculosis. Report of three cases. Sem. Hôp. Paris *64*:1991, 1988.

589. Southern, J. F., Moscicki, R. A., Magro, C., et al.: Lymphedema, lymphocytic myocarditis, and sarcoid-like granulomatosis. Manifestations of Whipple's disease. JAMA *261*:1467, 1989.
590. Sossai, P., DeBoni, M., and Cielo, R.: The heart and Whipple's disease (letter). Int. J. Cardiol. *23*:275, 1989.
591. James, T. N., and Bulkley, B. H.: Abnormalities of the coronary arteries in Whipple's disease. Am. Heart J. *105*:481, 1983.
592. Morrison, D. A., Gay, R. G., Feldshon, D., and Sampliner, R. E.: Severe pulmonary hypertension in a patient with Whipple's disease. Am. J. Med. *79*:263, 1985.
593. Keinath, R. D., Merrell, D. E., Vlietstra, R., and Dobbins, W. O., III: Antibiotic treatment and relapse in Whipple's disease. Long-term follow-up of 88 patients. Gastroenterology *88*:1867, 1985.
594. Feldman, M.: Whipple's disease. Am. J. Med. Sci. *291*:56, 1986.
595. de Brito, T., Morais, C. F., Yasuda, P. H., et al.: Cardiovascular involvement in human and experimental leptospirosis: Pathologic findings and immunohistochemical detection of leptospiral antigen. Ann. Trop. Med. Parasitol. *81*:207, 1987.
596. Lee, M. G., Char, G., Dianzumba, S., and Prussia, P.: Cardiac involvement in severe leptospirosis. West Indian Med. J. *35*:295, 1986.
597. De Biase, L., De Curtis, G., Paparoni, S., et al.: Fatal leptospiral myocarditis. G. Ital. Cardiol. *17*:992, 1987.
598. Ram, P., and Chandra, M. S.: Unusual electrocardiographic abnormality in leptospirosis: Case reports. Angiology *36*:477, 1985.
599. Winearls, C. G., Chan, L., Coghlan, J. D., et al.: Acute renal failure due to leptospirosis: Clinical features and outcome in six cases. Q. J. Med. *53*:487, 1984.
600. McAlister, H. F., Klementowicz, P. T., Andrews, C., et al.: Lyme carditis: An important cause of reversible heart block. Ann. Intern. Med. *110*:339, 1989.
601. Stanek, G., Klein, J., Bittner, R., and Glogar, D.: Isolation of *Borrelia burgdorferi* from the myocardium of a patient with longstanding cardiomyopathy. N. Engl. J. Med. *322*:249, 1990.
602. van der Linde, M. R., Crijns, H.J.G.M., and Lie, K. I.: Transient complete AV block in Lyme disease: Electrophysiologic observations. Chest *96*:219, 1989.
603. van der Linde M. R., Crijns, H.J.G.M., de Koning, J., et al.: Range of atrioventricular conduction disturbances in Lyme borreliosis: A report of four cases and review of other published reports. Br. Heart J. *63*:162, 1990.
604. Vlay, S. C., Dervan, J. P., Elias, J., et al.: Ventricular tachycardia associated with Lyme carditis. Am. Heart J. *121*:1558, 1991.
605. Rienzo, R. J., Morel, D. E., Prager, D., et al.: Gallium-avid Lyme myocarditis. Clin. Nuc. Med. *12*:475, 1987.
606. Kimball, S. A., Janson, P. A., and LaRaia, P. J.: Complete heart block as the sole presentation of Lyme disease. Arch. Intern. Med. *149*:1897, 1989.
607. DeKoning, J., Hoogkamp-Korstanje, J.A.A., van der Linde, M. R., and Crijns, H.J.G.M.: Demonstration of spirochetes in cardiac biopsies of patients with Lyme disease. J. Infect. Dis. *160*:150, 1989.
608. Wengrower, D., Knobler, H., Gillis, S., Chajek-Shaul, T.: Myocarditis in tick-borne relapsing fever. J. Infect. Dis. *149*:1033, 1984.
609. Doscia, J. L., Fisco, J. M., and Brace, W. T.: Complete heart block due to a solitary gumma. Am. J. Cardiol. *13*:553, 1964.
610. Spain, D. M., and Johannsen M. W.: Three cases of localized gummatous myocarditis. Am. Heart J. *241*:689, 1942.
611. Atkinson, J. B., Robinowitz, M., McAllister, H. H., et al.: Cardiac infections in the immunocompromised host. Cardiol. Clin. *2*:671, 1984.
612. Nahass, R. G., Scholz, P., Mackenzie, J. W., and Gocke, D. J.: Chronic constrictive pericarditis. A case report and review of the literature. Arch. Intern. Med. *149*:1202, 1989.
613. Slutzker, A. D., and Claypool, W. D.,: Pericardial actinomycosis with cardiac tamponade from a contiguous thoracic lesion. Thorax *44*:442, 1989.
614. Schwartz, D. A.: Aspergillus pancarditis following bone marrow transplantation for chronic myelogenous leukemia. Chest *95*:1338, 1989.
615. Andersson, B. S., Luna, M. A., and McCredie, K. B.: Systemic aspergillosis as cause of myocardial infarction. Cancer *58*:2146, 1986.
616. Hall J. C., and Giltman, L. I.: Candida myocarditis in a patient with chronic active hepatitis and macronodular cirrhosis. J. Tenn. Med. Assoc. *79*:473, 1986.
617. Atkinson, J. B., Connor, D. H., Robinowitz, M., et al.: Cardiac fungal infections: Review of autopsy findings in 60 patients. Hum. Pathol. *15*:935, 1984.
618. Vartivarian, S. E., Coudron, P. E., and Markowitz, S. M.: Disseminated coccidioidomycosis. Unusual manifestations in a cardiac transplantation patient. Am. J. Med. *83*:949, 1987.
619. Lafont, A., Wolff, M., Marche, C., et al.: Overwhelming myocarditis due to *Cryptococcus neoformans* in an AIDS patient (letter). Lancet 14:1145, 1987.
620. Loyd, J. E., Tillman, B. F., Atkinson, J. B., and Des Prez, R. M.: Mediastinal fibrosis complicating histoplasmosis. Medicine *67*:295, 1988.
621. Garrett, H. E., Jr., and Roper, C. L.: Surgical intervention in histoplasmosis. Ann. Thorac. Surg. *42*:711, 1986.
622. Acquatella, H., Catalioti, F., Gomez-Mancebo, J. R., et al.: Long-term control of Chagas disease in Venezuela: Effects on serologic findings, electrocardiographic abnormalities, and clinical outcome. Circulation *76*:556, 1987.
623. Grant, I. H., Gold, J.W.M., Wittner, M., et al.: Transfusion-associated acute Chagas' disease acquired in the United States. Ann. Intern. Med. *111*:849, 1989.
624. Maguire, J. H., Hoff, R., Sherlock, I., et al.: Cardiac morbidity and mortality due to Chagas' disease: Prospective electrocardiographic study of a Brazilian community. Circulation *75*:1140, 1987.
625. Morris, S. A., Tanowitz, H. B., Wittner, M., and Bilezikian, J. P.: Pathophysiological insights into the cardiomyopathy of Chagas' disease. Circulation *82*:1900, 1990.
626. Hudson, L., and Britten, V.: Immune response to South American trypanosomiasis and its relationship to Chagas' disease. Br. Med. Bull. *41*:175, 1985.
627. Palacios-Pru, E., Carrasco, H., Scorza, C., and Espinoza, R.: Ultrastructural characteristics of different stages of human chagasic myocarditis. Am. J. Trop. Med. Hyg. *41*:29, 1989.
628. Morris, S. A., Tanowitz, H., Factor, S. M., et al.: Myocardial adenylate cyclase activity in acute murine Chagas' disease. Circ. Res. *62*:800, 1988.
629. Bestetti, R. B., Ramos, C. P., Godoy, R. A., and Oliveira, J. S.: Chronic Chagas' heart disease in the elderly: A clinicopathologic study. Cardiology *74*:344, 1987.
630. Carrasco, H. A., Guerrero, L., Prada, H., et al.: Ventricular arrhythmias and left ventricular myocardial function in chronic chagasic patients. Int. J. Cardiol. *28*:35, 1990.
631. Casado, J., Davila, D. F., Donis, J. H., et al.: Electrocardiographic abnormalities and left ventricular systolic function in Chagas' heart disease. Int. J. Cardiol. *27*:55, 1990.
632. Rossi, M. A.: Microvascular changes as a cause of chronic cardiomyopathy in Chagas' disease. Am. Heart J. *1220*:233, 1990.
633. Carrasco, H. A., Palacios-Pru, E., Dagert deScorza, C., et al.: Clinical, histochemical, and ultrastructural correlation in septal endoymocardial biopsies from chronic chagasic patients: Detection of early myocardial damage. Am. Heart J. *113*:716, 1987.
634. Oliveira, J. S. M., and Marin-Neto, J. A.: Parasympathetic impairment in Chagas' heart disease: Cause or consequence (editorial)? Int. J. Cardiol. *21*:153, 1988.
635. Levin, M. J., Mesri, E., Benarous, R., et al.: Identification of major *Trypanosoma cruzi* antigenic determinants in chronic Chagas' heart disease. Am. J. Trop. Med. Hyg. *41*:530, 1989.
636. Higuchi, M. deL., Lopes, E. A., Saldanha, L. B., et al.: Immunopathologic studies in myocardial biopsies of patients with Chagas' disease and idiopathic cardiomyopathy. Rev. Inst. Med. Trop. Sao Paulo *28*:87, 1986.
637. Acosta, A. M., and Santos-Buch, C. A.: Autoimmune myocarditis induced by *Trypanosoma cruzi*. Circulation *71*:1255, 1985.
638. Morato, M. J., Brener, Z., Cancado, J. R., et al.: Cellular immune responses of chagasic patients to antigens derived from different *Trypanosoma cruzi* strains and clones. Am. J. Trop. Med. Hyg. *35*:505, 1986.
639. Sadigursky, M., von Kreuter, B. F., Ling, P. Y., and Santos-Buch, C. A.: Association of elevated anti-sarcolemma, anti-idiotype antibody levels with the clinical and pathologic expression of chronic Chagas myocarditis. Circulation *80*:1269, 1989.
640. Fuenmayor, A. J., Rodriguez, L., Torres, A., et al.: Valsalva maneuver: A test of the functional state of cardiac innervation in chagasic myocarditis. Int. J. Cardiol. *18*:351, 1988.
641. Davila, D. F., Donis, J. H., Navas, M., et al.: Response of heart rate to atropine and left ventricular function in Chagas' heart disease. Int. J. Cardiol. *21*:143, 1988.
642. Oliveira, J.S.M.: A natural human model of intrinsic heart nervous system denervation: Chagas' cardiopathy. Am. Heart J. *110*:1092, 1985.
643. Acquatella, H., and Schiller, N. B.: Echocardiographic recognition of Chagas' disease and endomyocardial fibrosis. J. Am. Soc. Echo. *1*:60, 1988.
644. Abelmann, W. H.: The dilated cardiomyopathies: Experimental aspects. Cardiol. Clin. *6*:219, 1988.
645. Ferrans, V. J., Milei, J., Tomita, Y., and Storino, R. A.: Basement membrane thickening in cardiac myocytes and capillaries in chronic Chagas' disease. Am. J. Cardiol. *61*:1137, 1988.
646. Maguire, J. H., Hoff, R., Sleigh, A. C., et al.: An outbreak of Chagas' disease in southwestern Bahia, Brazil. Am. J. Trop. Med. Hyg. *35*:931, 1986.
647. Marin-Neto, J. A., Maciel, B. C., Gallo, L., Jr., et al.: Effect of parasympathetic impairment on the haemodynamic response to handgrip in Chagas's heart disease. Br. Heart J. *55*:204, 1986.
648. Junqueira, L. F., Jr., Gallo, L., Jr., Manco, J. C., et al.: Subtle cardiac autonomic impairment in Chagas' disease detected by baroreflex sensitivity testing. Braz. J. Med. Biol. Res. *18*:171, 1985.
649. de Paola, A.A.V., Horowitz, L. N., Miyamoto, M. H., et al.: Angiographic and electrophysiologic substrates of ventricular tachycardia in chronic chagasic myocarditis. Am. J. Cardiol. *65*:360, 1990.
650. Combellas, I., Puigbo, J. J., Acquatella, H., et al.: Echocardiographic features of impaired left ventricular diastolic function in Chagas's heart disease. Br. Heart J. *53*:298, 1985.
651. Caeiro, T., Amuchastegui, L. M., Moreyra, E., and Gibson, D. G.: Abnormal left ventricular diastolic function in chronic Chagas' disease: An echocardiographic study. Int. J. Cardiol. *9*:417, 1985.
652. Marin-Neto, J. A., Marzullo, P., Sousa, A. C., et al.: Radionuclide angiographic evidence for early predominant right ventricular involvement in patients with Chagas' disease. Can. J. Cardiol. *4*:231, 1988.
653. Factor, S. M., Cho, S., Wittner, M., and Tanowitz, H.: Abnormalities of the coronary microcirculation in acute murine Chagas' disease. Am. J. Trop. Med. Hyg. *34*:246, 1985.
654. Kirchhoff, L. V.: Is *Trypanosoma cruzi* a new threat to our blood supply? Ann. Intern. Med. *111*:773, 1989.
655. Espinosa, R., Carrasco, H. A., Belandria, F., et al.: Life expectancy analysis in patients with Chagas' disease: Prognosis after one decade (1973–1983). Int. J. Cardiol. *8*:45, 1985.
656. Schofield, C. J.: Control of Chagas' disease vectors. Br. Med. Bull. *41*:187, 1985.
657. de Paola, A. A., Horowitz, L. N., Miyamoto, M. H., et al.: Automatic im-

plantable defibrillator with VVI pacemaker in a patient with chronic Chagas myocarditis and total atrioventricular block. Am. Heart J. *118*:415, 1989.
658. Tsala Mbala, P., Blackett, K., Mbonifor, C. L., et al.: Functional and immunologic involvement in human African trypanosomiasis caused by *Trypanosoma gambiense*. Bull. Soc. Pathol. Exot. Filiales *81*:490, 1988.
659. Holmes, P. H.: Pathophysiology of parasitic infections. Parasitology *94*:S29, 1987.
660. McCabe, R. E., Brooks, R. G., Dorfman, R. F., and Remington, J. S.: Clinical spectrum in 107 cases of toxoplasmic lymphadenopathy. Rev. Infect. Dis. *9*:754, 1987.
661. Jehn, U., Fink, M., Gundlach, P., et al.: Lethal cardiac and cerebral toxoplasmosis in a patient with acute myeloid leukemia after successful allogenic bone marrow transplantation. Transplantation *38*:430, 1984.
662. Luft, B. J., Billingham, M., and Remington, J. S.: Endomyocardial biopsy in the diagnosis of toxoplasmic myocarditis. Tranplant. Proc. *18*:1871, 1986.
663. Adair, O. V., Randive, N., and Krasnow, N.: Isolated toxoplasma myocarditis in acquired immune deficiency syndrome. Am. Heart J. *118*:856, 1989.
664. Tschirhart, D., and Klatt, E. C.: Disseminated toxoplasmosis in the acquired immunodeficiency syndrome. Arch. Pathol. Lab. Med. *112*:1237, 1988.
665. Tolat, D., and Kim, H. S.: Toxoplasmosis of the brain and heart: Autopsy report of a patient with AIDS. Tex. Med. *85*:40, 1989.
666. Permanyer-Miralda, G., Sagrista-Sauleda, J., and Soler-Soler, J.: Primary acute pericardial disease: A prospective series of 231 consecutive patients. Am. J. Cardiol. *56*:623, 1985.
667. Sharma, S. N., Mohapatra, A. K., and Machave, Y. V.: Chronic falciparum cardiomyopathy (letter). J. Assoc. Physicians India *35*:251, 1987.
668. Oliver, J. M., Sotillo, J. F., Dominguez, F. J., et al.: Two-dimensional echocardiographic features of echinococcosis of the heart and great blood vessels: Clinical and surgical implications. Circulation *78*:327, 1988.
669. Russo, G., Tamburino, C., Cuscuna, S., et al.: Cardiac hydatid cyst with clinical features resembling subaortic stenosis. Am. Heart J. *117*:1385, 1989.
670. Desnos, M., Brochet, E., Cristofini, P., et al.: Polyvisceral echinococcosis with cardiac involvement imaged by two-dimensional echocardiography, computed tomography and nuclear magnetic resonance imaging. Am. J. Cardiol. *59*:383, 1987.
671. Barnard, P. M., MacGregor, L. A., and Weich, H. F. H.: Premere Eichinococcus-sist van die hart 'n Gevalbespreking. S. Afr. Med. J. *76*:275, 1989.
672. Dao, A. H., and Virmani, R.: Visceral larva migrans involving the myocardium: Report of two cases and review of literature. Pediatr. Pathol. *6*:449, 1986.
673. Ursell, P. C., Habib, A., Babchick, O., et al.: Myocarditis caused by *Trichinella spiralis* (letter). Arch. Pathol. Lab. Med. *108*:4, 1984.
674. Lopez-Lozano, J. J., Garcia Merino, J. A., and Liano, H.: Bilateral facial paralysis secondary to trichinosis. Acta Neurol. Scand. *78*:194, 1988.
675. Starling, R. C., and Unverferth, D. V.: Value of endomyocardial biopsy: Indications and applications. *In* Zipes, D. P., and Rowlands, D. J. (eds.): Progress in Cardiology. Philadelphia, Lea and Febiger, 1989, p. 33.

TOXIC, CHEMICAL, IMMUNE AND PHYSICAL DAMAGE

676. Brody, S. L., Slovis, C. M., and Wrenn, K. D.: Cocaine-related medical problems: Consecutive series of 233 patients. Am. J. Med. *88*:325, 1990.
677. Lange, R. A. Cigarroa, R. G., Yancy, C. W., et al.: Cocaine-induced coronary-artery vasoconstriction. N. Engl. J. Med. *321*:1557, 1989.
678. Isner, J. M., and Chokshi, S. K.: Cocaine and vasospasm. N. Engl. J. Med. *321*:1604, 1989.
679. Dressler, F. A., Malekzadeh, S., and Roberts, W. C.: Quantitative analysis of amounts of coronary arterial narrowing in cocaine addicts. Am. J. Cardiol. *65*:303, 1990.
680. Przywara, D. A., and Dambach, G.: Direct actions of cocaine on cardiac cellular electrical activity. Circ. Res. *65*:185, 1989.
681. Chokshi, S. K., Moore, R., Pandian, N. G., and Isner, J. M.: Reversible cardiomyopathy associated with cocaine intoxication. Ann. Intern. Med. *111*:1039, 1989.
682. Waller, B. F.: Cocaine and the heart. Indiana Med. *81*:956, 1988.
683. Fraker, T. D., Jr., Temesy-Armos, P. N., Brewster, P. S., and Wilkerson, R. D.: Mechanism of cocaine-induced myocardial depression in dogs. Circulation *81*:1012, 1990.
684. Abel, F. L., Wilson, S. P., Zhao, R. R., and Fennell, W. H.: Cocaine depresses the canine myocardium. Circ. Shock *28*:309, 1989.
685. Inoue, H., and Zipes, D. P.: Cocaine-induced supersensitivity and arrhythmogenesis. J. Am. Coll. Cardiol. *11*:867, 1988.
686. Majid, P. A., Patel, B., Kim, H-S., et al.: An angiographic and histologic study of cocaine-induced chest pain. Am. J. Cardiol. *65*:812, 1990.
687. Peng, S-K., French, W. J., and Pelikan, P. C. D.: Direct cocaine cardiotoxicity demonstrated by endomyocardial biopsy. Arch. Pathol. Lab. Med. *113*:842, 1989.
688. Isner, J. M., and Chokshi, S. K.: Cardiovascular complications of cocaine. Curr. Prob. Cardiol. *16*:538, 1991.
689. Karch, S. B., and Billingham, M. E.: The pathology and etiology of cocaine-induced heart disease. Arch. Pathol. Lab. Med. *112*:225, 1988.
690. Deyton, L. R., Walker, R. E., Kovacs, J. A., et al.: Reversible cardiac dysfunction associated with interferon alpha therapy in AIDS patients with Kaposi's sarcoma. N. Engl. J. Med. *321*:1246, 1989.
691. Cohen, M. C., Huberman, M. S., and Nesto, R. W.: Recombinant alpha$_2$ interferon-related cardiomyopathy. Am. J. Med. *85*:549, 1988.
692. Levin, R., Burtt, D. M., Levin, W. A., and Ginsberg, M. B.: Ventricular fibrillation in a tetraplegic patient who had a therapeutic level of a tricyclic antidepressant. Paraplegia *23*:354, 1985.
693. Horowitz, J. D.: Drugs that induce heart problems. Which agents? What effects? J. Cardiovasc. Med. *8*:308, 1983.
694. Orme, M. L.: Antidepressants and heart disease (editorial). Br. Med. J. *289*:1, 1984.
695. Margolin, K., Raynor, A., Hawkins, M., et al.: Interleukin-2 and lymphokine-activated killer cell therapy and solid tumors: Analysis and toxicity and management guidelines. J. Clin. Oncol. *7*:486, 1989.
696. Schuchter, L. M., Hendricks, C. B., Holland, K. H., et al.: Eosinophilic myocarditis associated with high-dose interleukin-2 therapy. Am. J. Med. *88*:439, 1990.
697. Nora, R., Abrams, J., and Silverman, H.: Myocardial infarction in patients receiving high-dose recombinant interleukin-2. N. Engl. J. Med. *316*:275, 1987.
698. Osanto, S., Cluitmans, F. H., Franks, H. A., and Cleton, F. J.: Myocardial injury after interleukin-2 therapy. Lancet *2*:48, 1988.
699. Gaynor, E., Vitek, L., Sticklin, L., et al.: The hemodynamic effects of treatment with interleukin-2 and lymphokine-activated killer cells. Ann. Intern. Med. *109*:953, 1988.
700. Samlowski, W. E., Ward, J. H., Craven, C. M., and Freedman, R. A.: Severe myocarditis following high-dose interleukin-2 administration. Arch. Pathol. Lab. Med. *113*:838, 1989.
701. Raehl, C. L., Patel, A. K., and LeRoy, M.: Drug-induced torsade de pointes. Clin. Pharm. *4*:675, 1985.
702. Khan, M. Y., Haider, B., and Thind, I. S.: Emetine-induced cardiomyopathy in rabbits. J. Submicrosc. Cytol. *15*:495, 1983.
703. Harbin, A. D., Gerson, M. C., and O'Connell, J. B.: Simulation of acute myopericarditis by constrictive pericardial disease with endomyocardial fibrosis due to methylsergide therapy. J. Am. Coll. Cardiol. *4*:196, 1984.
704. Ratliff, N. B., Estes, M. L., Myles, J. L., et al.: Diagnosis of chloroquine cardiomyopathy by endomyocardial biopsy. N. Engl. J. Med. *316*:191, 1987.
705. McAllister, H. A., Jr., Ferrans, V. J., Hall, R. J., et al.: Chloroquine-induced cardiomyopathy. Arch. Pathol. Lab. Med. *111*:953, 1987.
706. Estes, M. L., Ewing-Wilson, D., Chou, S. M., et al.: Chloroquine neuromyotoxicity. Clinical and pathologic perspective. Am. J. Med. *82*:477, 1987.
707. Chulay, J. D., Spencer, H. C., and Mugambi, M.: Electrocardiographic changes during treatment of leishmaniasis with pentavalent antimony (sodium stibogluconate). Am. J. Trop. Med. Hyg. *34*:702, 1985.
708. Winship, K. A.: Toxicity of antimony and its compounds. Adverse Drug React. Acute Poisoning Rev. *6*:67, 1987.
709. Brady, H. R., and Horgan, J. H.: Lithium and the heart: Unanswered questions. Chest *93*:166, 1988.
710. James, F. W., Kaplan, S., and Benzig, G., 3rd: Cardiac complications following hydrocarbon ingestion. Am. J. Dis. Child. *121*:431, 1971.
711. Cunningham, S. R., Dalzell, G. W. N., McGirr, P., and Khan, M. M.: Myocardial infarction and primary ventricular fibrillation after glue sniffing. Br. Med. J. *294*:739, 1987.
712. Scott, I., Parkes, R., and Cameron, D. P.: Phaeochromocytoma and cardiomyopathy. Med. J. Austr. *148*:94, 1988.
713. Ferry, D. R., Henry, R. L., and Kern, M. J.: Epinephrine-induced myocardial infarction in a patient with angiographically normal coronary arteries. Am. Heart J. *111*:1193, 1986.
714. Nino, A. F., Berman, M. M., Gluck, E. H., et al.: Drug-induced left ventricular failure in patients with pulmonary disease: Endomyocardial biopsy demonstration of catecholamine myocarditis. Chest *92*:732, 1987.
715. Rona, G.: Catecholamine cardiotoxicity. J. Mol. Cell. Cardiol. *17*:291, 1985.
716. Panagia, V., Pierce, G. N., Dhalla, K. S., et al.: Adaptive changes in subcellular calcium transport during catecholamine-induced cardiomyopathy. J. Mol. Cell. Cardiol. *17*:411, 1985.
717. Downing, S. E., and Lee, J. C.: Contribution of alpha-adrenoceptor activation to the pathogenesis of norepinephrine cardiomyopathy. Circ. Res. *52*:471, 1983.
718. Opie, L. H., Walpoth, B., and Barsacchi, R.: Calcium and catecholamines: Relevance to cardiomyopathies and significance in therapeutic strategies. J. Mol. Cell. Cardiol. *17*:21, 1985.
719. Kopp, S. J., Barron, J. T., and Tow, J. P.: Cardiovascular actions of lead and relationship to hypertension: A review. Environ. Hlth. Perspec. *78*:91, 1988.
720. Kurppa, K., Hietanen, E., Klockars, M., et al.: Chemical exposures at work and cardiovascular morbidity. Atherosclerosis, ischemic heart disease, hypertension, cardiomyopathy and arrhythmias. Scand. J. Work Environ. Hlth. *10*:381, 1984.
721. Penney, D. G.: A review: Hemodynamic response to carbon monoxide. Environ. Hlth. Perspec. *77*:121, 1988.
722. McMeekin, J. D., and Finegan, B. A.: Reversible myocardial dysfunction following carbon monoxide poisoning. Can. J. Cardiol. *3*:118, 1987.
723. Marius-Nunez, A. L.: Myocardial infarction with normal coronary arteries after acute exposure to carbon monoxide. Chest *97*:491, 1990.
724. Levine, S. N., and Rheams, C. N.: Hypocalcemic heart failure. Am. J. Med. *78*:1033, 1985.
725. Rimailho, A., Bouchard, P., Schaison, G., et al.: Improvement of hypocalcemic cardiomyopathy by correction of serum calcium level. Am. Heart J. *109*:611, 1985.
726. Bashour, T. T., Ryan, C., Kabbani, S. S., and Crew, J.: Hypocalcemic acute

resulted in an increase in the detection of primary cardiac tumors,[131] in many cases prior to the onset of clinical signs or symptoms.

Two-dimensional echocardiography may facilitate the differentiation between left atrial thrombus and myxoma, because the former typically produces a layered appearance and is generally situated in the posterior portion of the atrium, whereas the latter is often mottled in appearance and rarely occurs in the posterior portion of the atrium. In some atrial myxomas, areas of echolucency may be seen within the tumor mass, corresponding to areas of hemorrhage within the tumor. Since these areas of echolucency are not found in thrombotic or infective lesions, this finding may be of value in the differential diagnosis of an intraatrial mass. Continuous-mode Doppler ultrasonography may be useful for evaluating the hemodynamic consequences of valvular obstruction or incompetence caused by cardiac tumors.[140]

Transesophageal Echocardiography. (see Fig. 4–106, p. 105 and 44–5). This approach provides an unimpeded view of both atria[140a] and the atrial septum. Growing experience with the use of this approach to visualize atrial tumors has suggested that it may be superior to transthoracic echocardiography in certain patients.[22,23] Potential advantages of transesophageal echocardiography include improved resolution of the tumor and its attachment (Fig. 44–5), the ability to detect some masses not visualized by transthoracic echocardiography, and improved visualization of right atrial tumors.[22] Although transesophageal echocardiography does not appear warranted on a routine basis, it should be considered when the transthoracic study is suboptimal or confusing.

RADIONUCLIDE IMAGING. Gated blood pool scanning has been used to identify atrial, ventricular, and intramural tumors.[15] Radionuclide ventriculography generally has a lower rate of resolution than does echocardiography or contrast injection angiography and therefore may be less sensitive for the detection of small filling defects. However, radionuclide ventriculography may provide clear visualization of filling defects in some cases when other methods are nondiagnostic, particularly in the case of ventricular or intramural tumors. In some cases, gated blood pool scanning may provide more detailed information regarding myocardial geometry and tumor size and location than that obtained by echocardiography. Mobile left atrial tumors may be seen to prolapse into the left ventricle during diastole. Thus, gated blood pool scanning may, in some cases, provide information complementary to that obtained by echocardiography. In some cases in which the cardiac tumor was not evident by routine static or dynamic radionuclide imaging, it has been possible to delineate the tumor and its movement during a cardiac cycle by use of a computer-generated composite functional image.[15]

COMPUTED TOMOGRAPHY. CT of the heart has been used to demonstrate cardiac tumors[17] (Fig. 11–11, p. 319). Although more experience will be necessary to establish its role, certain advantages are apparent. These include a high degree of tissue discrimination, which may allow definition of the degree of intramural tumor extension; evaluation of the extracardiac structures; and the ability to construct images in any plane. Resolution appears to be improved substantially by gating the computed tomographic acquisition to the cardiac cycle.[17] At present CT appears to be most useful in the evaluation of suspected tumors of the heart to determine the degree of myocardial invasion and the involvement of pericardial and extracardiac structures.

MAGNETIC RESONANCE IMAGING. MRI may be of considerable value in the detection and delineation of cardiac tumors and in some cases may depict the size, shape, and surface characteristics of the tumor more clearly than two-dimensional echocardiography.[18–21] The larger field of view with MRI (Fig. 44–6) provides better definition of tumor prolapse, secondary valve obstruction, and cardiac chamber size than does two-dimensional echocardiography.

OTHER NONINVASIVE METHODS. Cardiac tumors cannot be diagnosed by phonocardiography, apexcardiography, or jugular venous or carotid pulse analysis. However, when valvular or myocardial disease is suspected on clinical grounds, certain atypical findings may raise the question of cardiac tumor. The intensity of the systolic or diastolic murmur caused by a left atrial myxoma is often exquisitely sensitive to positional change, a finding atypical of valvular heart disease. S_1 may be delayed as a consequence of an elevated left atrial pressure, as in mitral stenosis. It is often intense and widely split, and an early systolic sound may occur, representing tumor movement toward the atrium during systole. In addition, a tumor "plop" may be present about 100 msec after S_2, which appears to result from the sudden tension of the tumor stalk as it prolapses into the left ventricle during diastole or from the tumor striking the myocardium. The tumor plop *precedes* the end of the rapid filling wave of the apexcardiogram and can thereby be differentiated from an S_3; as noted, it usually occurs later than an opening snap. Systolic time intervals are usually consistent with a reduced stroke volume. Apexcardiography often shows a deep notch on the upstroke which occurs at the time of extrusion of the tumor through the mitral valve in early systole.

Right atrial tumors may also result in a widely split S_1 and an early systolic sound. The S_2 may be paradoxically split as a result of early pulmonic valve closure. A tumor plop and systolic and diastolic murmurs which are increased by inspiration may also occur with right atrial tumors. The jugular venous pulse tracing may reflect obstruction of the tricuspid orifice, demonstrating an accentuated *a* wave, attenuation of the *x* descent, or an early, broad *v* wave.

ANGIOGRAPHY

Cardiac catheterization and selective angiocardiography are not necessary in all cases of cardiac tumors, since, as already discussed, in many cases adequate preoperative information may be obtained by echocardiography, CT, or MRI. However, several circumstances exist in which the risk and expense of cardiac catheterization are outweighed by the supplemental information it may provide. These situations include cases in which (1) noninvasive evaluation has not been adequate in defining fully tumor location or attachment; (2) all four cardiac chambers have not been adequately visualized noninvasively; (3) a malignant cardiac tumor is considered likely; or (4) other cardiac lesions may coexist with a cardiac tumor and possibly dictate a different surgical approach. For instance, when a malignant cardiac tumor is suspected, cardiac angiography may provide valuable information regarding the degree of myocardial, vascular, and/or pericardial invasion. Likewise, in certain cases, such as the presence of pulmonary hypertension or the coexistence of significant valvular or coronary artery lesions, cardiac catheterization and angiography may provide information that significantly affects the surgical approach.[141]

The major angiographic findings in patients with cardiac tumors include (1) compression or displacement of cardiac chambers or large vessels, (2) deformity of cardiac chambers, (3) intracavitary filling defects, (4) marked variations in myocardial thickness, (5) pericardial effusion, and (6) local alterations in wall motion.[151,152] Displacement of the cardiac chambers or the great vessels without deformation of the internal contour may be observed in both benign and malignant tumors, whereas deformation of a cardiac chamber usually indicates an infiltrating malignant lesion.[152] The most frequent angiographic findings are intracavitary filling defects, which may be either fixed or mobile. Fixed defects may be lobulated or appear as a coarse nodularity of the myocardium often difficult to distinguish from a mural thrombus. Such defects may reflect endocardial tumors with broad attachments or intramural tumors with intracavitary extension. Mobile intracavitary defects are usually pedunculated tumors, typically myxomas, although the stalk may be difficult to visualize. Such tumors may prolapse into the AV valve orifice during diastole or, in the case of ventricular tumors, into the left ventricular outflow tract during systole. An atrial ball thrombus may mimic a pedunculated tumor, but is more likely to be associated with clot in the atrial appendage.

A localized increase in myocardial wall thickness, especially when accompanied by a pericardial effusion, suggests an infiltrating malignant tumor. It is often difficult to differentiate myocardial thickening from pericardial effusion, but this may be aided by observation of the thickness of the right atrial wall. Since the right atrial wall is seldom infiltrated by tumor, the finding of right atrial thickening to greater than 5 mm suggests a pericardial effusion.[133] In myocardial infiltration, localized areas of disordered wall motion may also be noted by cineangiography. Coronary arteriography may in some cases allow visualization of the vascular supply of the tumor, thus demarcating the extent of tumor invasion, the source of its blood supply, and its relation to the coronary arteries.[142,143] However, the vascular pattern of cardiac tumors has not proved to be a useful sign of malignancy.[133]

False-negative angiographic studies generally occur when the diagnosis is not suspected prior to catheterization. False positive studies are most often the result of thrombus, but may also be produced by many entities, such as streaming of non-opaque venous blood, a hematoma in the atrial septum, an aneurysm of the muscular or membranous ventricular septum, Bernheim syndrome, congenital septal dysplasia, and hydatid cysts of the interventricular septum.[133]

The major risk of angiography is peripheral embolization due to dislodgement of a fragment of tumor or of an associated thrombus.[133,144] Therefore, the thorough evaluation of all cardiac chambers by *noninvasive* methods prior to catheterization is recommended in patients suspected of having cardiac tumors so that contrast material can be injected into the chamber proximal (upstream) to the location of the tumor. The transseptal approach to the left atrium (p. 184) is particularly hazardous because of the frequent occurrence of left atrial myxomas in the region of the fossa ovalis.

Growing experience with digital subtraction angiography (p. 1567) indicates that it can provide important diagnostic information in patients with atrial or ventricular tumors having intracavitary projections. The ability to image intracavitary structures during injection of contrast material from a remote site eliminates the risk of catheter-induced tumor embolization and may play an important role in the diagnosis and characterization of a cardiac tumor, particularly in patients in whom the other noninvasive techniques are not technically satisfactory.

TREATMENT AND PROGNOSIS

BENIGN TUMORS

Operative excision is the treatment of choice for most benign cardiac tumors and in many cases results in a complete cure.[11,12,145-147] Although many tumors are histologically benign, all cardiac tumors are potentially lethal as a result of intracavitary or valvular obstruction, peripheral embolization, and disturbances of rhythm or conduction. Unfortunately, it is not unusual for patients to die or experience a major complication while awaiting operation, and therefore it is mandatory to carry out the operation promptly after the diagnosis has been established.[148]

Although some epicardial tumors may be removed without the aid of extracorporeal circulation, most intramural and intracavitary tumors must be excised under direct vision, with use of the heart-lung machine. Closed approaches, although occasionally used in the past, are not now recommended because of increased risk of dislodging tumor fragments. In addition, excision cannot be as complete, and adequate inspection of the other cardiac chambers for additional tumors is not possible.

The dislodgment of tumor fragments constitutes a major risk of operation and may result in peripheral emboli or the dispersion of micrometastases, which may seed peripherally. To reduce this risk, manipulation of the heart prior to cardiopulmonary bypass should be minimized. Some surgeons recommend that venous cannulation for cardiopulmonary bypass be performed via the femoral or azygos vein rather than through the right atrium to avoid dislodging an unsuspected right atrial tumor. In addition, the tumor should be removed en bloc when possible, and the chamber then irrigated well with saline.

ATRIAL MYXOMAS. Numerous reports document complete cure of left and right atrial myxomas with follow-up periods of 10 to 15 years.[11,12,146-152] In about 1 to 5 per cent of cases a recurrence or second cardiac myxoma has been reported following resection of the initial myxoma.[67,153] Possible causes of the second tumor include incomplete excision of the original tumor with regrowth, growth from a second "pretumorous" focus, i.e., metasynchronous, or intracardiac implantation from the original tumor. Because of the first two possibilities, some surgeons have advocated excision of the entire region of the fossa ovalis and repair of the resultant atrial septal defect to remove presumably high concentrations of "pretumor" cells thought to be located in that region.[150] In one case, the large size of a myxoma, together with its location on the posterior left atrial wall, necessitated complete removal of the heart, followed by autotransplantation, i.e., reimplantation of the patient's excised heart.[153] Laser photocoagulation of a 1 cm area around the stalk attachment site has also been suggested as a way of eradicating pretumorous cells without the necessity of creating an atrial septal defect.[154] Other surgeons have reported equally successful long-term recurrence-free periods with simple excision of the tumor and a small rim at the base.[80] It now appears that in approximately 7 per cent of patients with (1) a familial history of cardiac myxoma, (2) features of the complex of lentigines and other abnormalities described on p. 1454, or (3) synchronous tumor appearance (i.e., multiple tumors at the time of presentation), the incidence of a second tumor occurring at some time in the future is in the range of 12 to 22 per cent, as compared to approximately 1 per cent for patients with sporadic atrial myxoma.[67] It is believed that tumor recurrence in these cases is from a second pretumorous focus of cells. In these high-risk patients, a careful search for multiple tumors preoperatively and more extensive resection of the underlying endocardium, atrial septum, or both is recommended. Careful echocardiographic follow-up for detection of metasynchronous tumors is recommended[67] in all patients following resection of a myxoma. Regardless of the extent of tumor resection performed, such patients should receive periodic long-term follow-up by cross-sectional echocardiography.

OTHER BENIGN TUMORS. Although the majority of operations for cardiac tumors have been performed for atrial myxomas owing to their high frequency, successful excision has also been reported for ventricular myxomas, as well as most other types of benign cardiac tumor, including rhabdomyoma, hamartoma, fibroma, lipoma, hemangioma, and papillary fibroelastoma.[107,155-160] The major surgical considerations in excision of ventricular tumors include preservation of adequate ventricular myocardium, maintenance of proper atrioventricular valve function, and preservation of as much of the conduction system as possible. Often, however, papillary muscles, chordae tendineae, or the AV conduction system must be sacrificed during the resection of a tumor, thereby necessitating replacement of the atrioventricular valve, implantation of a pacemaker, or both. In one case, extensive involvement of the heart by a fibrous histiocytoma that replaced 60 per cent of the left ventricle was treated successfully by cardiac transplantation.[161]

MALIGNANT TUMORS

Operation is not an effective treatment for the great majority of primary malignant tumors of the heart because of the large mass of cardiac tissue involved or the presence of metastases. The major role for surgery in such cases is to establish a diagnosis in order to exclude the possibility of a curable benign tumor. Nevertheless, in some cases palliation of hemodynamics and/or constitutional symptoms and extension of life may be achieved by aggressive therapy. Survivals of from 1 to 3 years have been reported following partial resection, chemotherapy, radiation therapy, or various combinations of these modalities.[126,162–167] In some instances, localized recurrences have been eliminated by multiple operations. Some success in palliation of symptoms has been reported following the combination of chemotherapy and radiation therapy[165] and radiation therapy alone.[168] Lymphosarcoma of the heart frequently responds to chemotherapy, radiation therapy, or both.[169,170] Unfortunately, many other reports indicate a failure to alter the course of cardiac sarcomas despite various combinations of surgery, chemotherapy, and radiation therapy.

REFERENCES

HISTORICAL PERSPECTIVE

1. Straus, R., and Merliss, R.: Primary tumors of the heart. Arch. Pathol. *39*:74, 1945.
2. Fine, G.: Neoplasms of the pericardium and heart. *In* Gould, S. E. (ed): Pathology of the Heart and Blood Vessels. Springfield, Ill., Charles C Thomas, 1968, p. 851.
3. Heath, D.: Pathology of cardiac tumors. Am. J. Cardiol. *21*:315, 1968.
4. Lammers, R. J., and Bloor, C. M.: Pathology of cardiac tumors. *In* Kapoor, A. S. (ed.): Cancer of the Heart. New York, Springer-Verlag, 1986, p. 1.
5. Urba, W. J., and Longo, D. L.: Primary solid tumors of the heart. *In* Kapoor, A. S. (ed.): Cancer of the Heart. New York, Springer-Verlag, 1986, p. 62.
6. Smith, C.: Tumors of the heart. Arch. Pathol. Lab. Med. *110*:1, 1986.
7. Mahaim, I.: Les Tumeurs et les Polypes de Coeur: Étude Anatomo-Cliniqué. Paris, Masson, 1945.
8. Barnes, A. R., Beaver, D. C., and Snell, A. M.: Primary sarcoma of the heart: Report of a case with E. C. G. and pathological studies. Am. Heart J. *9*:480, 1934.
9. Goldberg, H. P., Glenn, F., Dotter, C. T., and Steinberg, I.: Myxoma of the left atrium. Diagnosis made during life with operative and postmortem findings. Circulation *6*:762, 1952.
10. Crafoord, C. L.: Case report. *In* Lam, C. R. (eds.): Proceedings. International Symposium on Cardiovascular Surgery. Philadelphia, W. B. Saunders Company, 1955, p. 202.
11. Reece, I. J., Cooley, D. A., Frazier, O. H., et al.: Cardiac tumors. Clinical spectrum and prognosis of lesions other than classical benign myxoma in 20 patients. J. Thorac. Cardiovasc. Surg. *88*:439, 1984.
12. Guiloff, A. K., Flege, J. B., Callard, G. M., et al.: Surgery of left atrial myxomas. Report of eleven cases and review of literature. J. Cardiovasc. Surg. *27*:194, 1986.
13. Effert, S., and Domanig, E.: The diagnosis of intra-atrial tumor and thrombi by the ultrasonic echo method. Ger. Med. Mon. *4*:1, 1959.
14. Fyke, F. E., Seqard, J. B., Edwards, W. D., et al.: Primary cardiac tumors: Experience with 30 consecutive patients since the introduction of two-dimensional echocardiography. J. Am. Coll. Cardiol. *5*:1465, 1985.
15. Bough, E., Bodem, W., Gandsman, E., et al.: Radionuclide diagnosis of left atrial myxoma with computer-generated functional images. Am. J. Cardiol. *52*:1365, 1986.
16. Tamari, I., Goldberg, H. L., Moses, J. W., et al.: Left atrial myxoma: Diagnosis by digital substraction intravenous angiography. Cathet. Cardiovasc. Diagn. *12*:26, 1986.
17. Jack, C. M., Cleland, J., and Geddes, J. S.: Left atrial rhabdomyosarcoma and the use of digital gated computed tomography in its diagnosis. Br. Heart J. *55*:305, 1986.
18. Freedberg, R. S., Kronzon, I., Rumancik, W. M., and Liebeskind, D.: The contribution of magnetic resonance imaging to the evaluation of intracardiac tumors diagnosed by echocardiography. Circulation *77*:96, 1988.
19. Brown, J. J., Barakos, J. A., and Higgins, C. B.: Magnetic resonance imaging of cardiac and paracardiac masses. J. Thorac. Imaging *4*:58, 1989.
20. Rienmuller, R., Lloret, J. L., Tiling, R., et al.: MR imaging of pediatric cardiac tumors previously diagnosed by echocardiography. J. Comput. Assist. Tomogr. *13*:621, 1989.
21. Lund, J. T., Ehman, R. L., Julsrud, P. R., et al.: Cardiac masses: assessment by MR imaging. Am. J. Roentgenol. *152*:469, 1989.
22. Obeid, A. I., Marvasti, M., Parker, F., and Rosenberg, J.: Comparison of transthoracic and transesophageal echocardiography in diagnosis of left atrial myxoma. Am. J. Cardiol. *63*:1006, 1989.
23. Dittmann, H., Voelker, W., Karsch, K. R., and Seipel, L.: Bilateral atrial myxomas detected by transesophageal two-dimensional echocardiography. Am. Heart J. *118*:172, 1989.

CLINICAL PRESENTATION

24. Goodwin, J. F.: Symposium on cardiac tumors. The spectrum of cardiac tumors. Am. J. Cardiol. *21*:307, 1968.
25. MacGregor, G. A., and Cullen, R. A.: The syndrome of fever, anaemia and high sedimentation rate with an atrial myxoma. Br. Med. J. *5*:158, 1959.
26. Huston, K. A., Combs, J. J., Lie, J. T., and Guiliani, E. R.: Left atrial myxoma simulating peripheral vasculitis. Mayo Clin. Proc. *53*:752, 1978.
27. Levinson, J. P., and Kincaid, O. W.: Myxoma of the right atrium associated with polycythemia. N. Engl. J. Med. *264*:1187, 1961.
28. Vuopio, P., and Nikkila, E. A.: Hemolytic anemia and thrombocytopenia in a case of left atrial myxoma associated with mitral stenosis. Am. J. Cardiol. *17*:585, 1966.
29. Jourdan, M., Bataille, R., Sequin, J., et al.: Constitutive production of interleukin-6 and immunologic features in cardiac myxomas. Arthritis Rheum. *33*:398, 1990.
30. Curry H. L. F., Mathews, J. A., and Robinson, J.: Right atrial myxoma mimicking a rheumatic disorder. Br. Med. J. *1*:542, 1967.
31. Savige, J. A., Yeung, S. P., Davies, D. J., et al.: Anti-neutrophil cytoplasmic antibodies associated with atrial myxoma. Am. J. Med. *85*:755, 1988.
32. Graham, S. L., and Sellers, A. L.: Atrial myxoma with multiple myeloma. Arch. Intern. Med. *139*:116, 1979.
33. Wens, R., Goffin, Y., Pepys, M. B., et al.: Left atrial myxoma associated with systemic AA amyloidosis. Arch. Intern. Med. *149*:453, 1989.
34. Leonhardt, E. T. G., and Kullenberg, K. P. G.: Bilateral atrial myxomas with multiple arterial aneurysms—A syndrome mimicking polyarteritis nodosa. Am. J. Med. *62*:792, 1977.
35. Byrd, W. E., Matthews, O. P., and Hunt, R. E.: Left atrial myxoma presenting as a systemic vasculitis. Arthritis Rheum. *23*:240, 1980.
36. Feldman, A. R., and Keeling, J. H.: Cutaneous manifestation of atrial myxoma. J. Am. Acad. Dermatol. *21*:1080, 1989.
37. Quinn, T. J., Condini, M. A., and Harris, A. A.: Infected cardiac myxoma. Am. J. Cardiol. *53*:381, 1984.
38. Transden, T. M., Prichard, J. G., and Storz, S. O.: *Streptococcus viridans* bacteremia associated with atrial myxoma. Am. Heart J. *110*:180, 1985.
39. Silverman, J., Olwin, J. S., and Graettinger, J. S.: Cardiac myxomas with systemic mobilization. Circulation *26*:99, 1962.
40. Koikkalainen, K., Kostiainen, S., and Luosto, R.: Left atrial myxoma revealed by femoral embolectomy. Scand. J. Thorac. Cardiovasc. Surg. *11*:33, 1977.
41. Yufe, R., Karpati, G., and Carpenter, S.: Cardiac myxoma: A diagnostic challenge for the neurologist. Neurology *26*:1060, 1976.
42. Schweiger, M. J., Hafer, J. G., Jr., Brown, R., and Gianelly, R. E.: Spontaneous cure of infected left atrial myxoma following embolization. Am. Heart J. *99*:630, 1980.
43. Gonzalez, A., Altieri, P. I., Marquez, E., et al.: Massive pulmonary embolism associated with right ventricular myxoma. Am. J. Med. *69*:795, 1980.
44. Heath, D., and Mackinnon, J.: Pulmonary hypertension due to myxoma of the right atrium. With special reference to the behavior of emboli of myxoma in the lung. Am. Heart J. *68*:227, 1964.
45. Semb, B. K., Wexels, J. C., Vatne, K., and Bjornstad, P. G.: Angiographic and echocardiographic observations in surgical patients with atrial myxoma. Cardiovasc. Intervent. Radiol. *8*:119, 1985.
46. Rath, S., Har-Zahav, Y., Battler, A., et al.: Coronary arterial embolus from left atrial myxoma. Am. J. Cardiol. *54*:1392, 1984.
47. Branch, C. L., Jr., Laster, D. W., and Kelley, D. L., Jr.: Left atrial myxoma with cerebral emboli. Neurosurgery *16*:675, 1985.
48. Verkkala, K., Kupari, M., Maamies, T., et al.: Primary cardiac tumors—operative treatment of 20 patients. Thorac. Cardiovasc. Surg. *37*:361, 1989.
49. Weerasena, N. A., Groome, D., Pollock, J. G., and Pollock, J. C.: Atrial myxoma as the cause of acute lower limb ischemia in a teenager. Scott. Med. J. *34*:440, 1989.
50. Reed, R. J., Utz, M. P., and Terezakis, N.: Embolic and metastatic cardiac myxoma. Am. J. Dermatopathol. *11*:157, 1989.
51. Michael, A. S., Mikhael, M. A., and Christ, M.: Myxoma of the heart presenting with recurrent episodes of hemorrhagic cerebral infarction: MR findings. J. Comput. Assist. Tomogr. *13*:123, 1989.
52. Knepper, L. E., Biller, J., Adams, H. P., Jr., and Bruno, A.: Neurologic manifestations of atrial myxoma. A 12-year experience and review. Stroke *19*:1435, 1988.
53. Panidis, I. P., Kotler, M. N., Mintz, G. S., and Ross, J.: Clinical and echocardiographic features of right atrial masses. Am. Heart J. *107*:745, 1984.
54. Harvey, W. P.: Clinical aspects of cardiac tumors. Am. J. Cardiol. *21*:328, 1968.
55. James, T. N., and Galakhov, I.: De subitaneis mortibus XXVI. Fatal electrical instability of the heart associated with benign congenital polycystic tumor of the atrioventricular node. Circulation *56*:667, 1977.
56. Nishida, K., Kamijima, G., and Nagayama, T.: Mesothelioma of the atrioventricular node. Br. Heart J. *53*:468, 1985.
57. Strauss, W. E., Asinger, R. W., and Hodges, M.: Mesothelioma of the AV node: Potential utility of pacing. PACE *11*:1296, 1988.
58. Lantz, D. A., Dougherty, T. H., and Lucca, M. J.: Primary angiosarcoma of the heart causing cardiac rupture. Am. Heart J. *118*:186, 1989.
59. Greenwood, W. F.: Profile of atrial myxoma. Am. J. Cardiol. *21*:367, 1968.
59a. Mitral Stenosis and Left Atrial Myxoma. *In* Fowler, N. O.: Diagnosis of Heart Disease. New York, Springer-Verlag, 1991, pp. 146–159.
60. Gershlick, A. H., Leech, G., Mills, P. G., and Leatham, A.: The loud first heart sound in left atrial myxoma. Br. Heart J. *52*:403, 1984.
61. Bass, N. M., and Sharratt, G. J. P.: Left atrial myxoma diagnosed by echocardiography with observations on tumor movement. Br. Heart J. *35*:1332, 1973.
62. Waxler, E. B., Kawai, N., and Kasparian, H.: Right atrial myxoma: Echocardiographic, phonocardiographic and hemodynamic signs. Am. Heart J. *82*:251, 1972.
63. Talley, R. C., Baldwin, B. J., Symbas, P. N., and Nutter, D. O.: Right atrial myxoma. Unusual presentation with cyanosis and clubbing. Am. J. Med. *48*:256, 1970.
64. Keren, A., Chenzbruna, A., Schuger, L., et al.: The etiology of tumor plop in a patient with huge right atrial myxoma. Chest *95*:1147, 1989.
65. Hada, Y., Wolfe, C., Murry, C. F., and Craige, E.: Right ventricular myxoma. Case report and review of phonocardiographic and auscultatory manifestations. Am. Heart J. *100*:871, 1980.

66. Bulkley, B. H., and Hutchins, G. M.: Atrial myxomas: A fifty year review. Am. Heart J. *97*:639, 1979.
67. McCarthy, P. M., Piehler, J. M., Schaff, H. V., et al.: The significance of multiple, recurrent, and "complex" cardiac myxomas. Thorac. Cardiovasc. Surg. *91*:389, 1986.
68. Carney, J. A.: Differences between nonfamilial and familial cardiac myxoma. Am. J. Surg. Pathol. 9:53, 1985.
69. Davison, E. T., Mumford, D., Zaman, Q., and Horowitz, A.: Left atrial myxoma in the elderly. Report of four patients over the age of 70 and review of the literature. J. Am. Geriatr. Soc. *34*:229, 1986.
70. Gosse, P., Herpin, D., Roudant, R., et al.: Myxoma of the mitral valve diagnosed by echocardiography. Am. Heart J. *111*:803, 1986.
71. Bennett, W. S., Skelton, T. N., and Lehan, P. H.: The complex of myxomas, pigmentation and endocrine overactivity. Am. J. Cardiol. *65*:399, 1990.
72. Carney, J. A., Gordon, J., Carpenter, P. C., et al.: The complex of myxomas, spotty pigmentation, and endocrine overactivity. Medicine *64*:270, 1985.
73. Rhodes, A. R., Silverman, R. A., Harrist, T. J., and Perez-Atayde, A. R.: Mucocutaneous lentigines, cardiomucocutaneous myxomas, and multiple blue nevi: The "LAMB" syndrome. Am. Acad. Dermatol. *10*:72, 1984.
74. Peterson, L. L., and Serrill, W. S.: Lentiginosis associated with a left atrial myxoma. Am. Acad. Dermatol. *10*:337, 1984.
75. Vidaillet, H. J., Jr., Seward, J. B., Fyke, E., and Tajik, A. J.: NAME syndrome (nevi, atrial myxoma, myxoid neurofibroma, ephelides): A new and unrecognized subset of patients with cardiac myxoma. Minn. Med. *67*:695, 1984.
76. Carney, J. A., Hruska, L. S., Beauchamp, G. D., and Gordon, H.: Dominant inheritance of the complex of myxomas, spotty pigmentation and endocrine overactivity. Mayo Clin. Proc. *61*:165, 1986.
77. Michels, V. V.: A new inherited syndrome with cardiac, cutaneous, and endocrine involvement. Mayo Clin. Proc. *61*:224, 1986.
78. Vidaillet, H. J., Jr., Seward, J. B., Fyke, F. E. et al.: "Syndrome myoxma": a subset of patients with cardiac myxoma associated with pigmented skin lesions and peripheral and endocrine neoplasms. Br. Heart J. *57*:247, 1987.
79. McCarthy, P. M., Schaff, H. V., Winkler, H. Z., et al.: Deoxyribonucleic acid ploidy pattern of cardiac myxomas. Another predictor of biologically unusual myxomas. J. Thorac. Cardiovasc. Surg. *98*:1083, 1989.
80. Sayler, W. R., Page, D. L., and Hutchins, G. M.: The development of cardiac myxomas and papillary endocardial lesions from mural thrombus. Am. Heart J. *89*:4, 1975.
80a. Seidman, J. D., Berman, J. J., Hitchcock, C. L., et al.: DNA analysis of cardiac myxomas: Flow cytometry and image analysis. Hum. Pathol. *22*:494, 1991.
81. Tanimura, A., Tanaka, S., Kitazono, M., and Kosuga, K.: The surface lining of cells of cardiac myxoma. Light, electron microscopic and immunohistochemical observation. Acta Pathol. Jpn. *35*:667, 1986.
82. Boxer, M. E.: Cardiac myxoma: An immunoperoxidase study of histogenesis. Histopathology *8*:861, 1984.
83. Landon, G., Ordonez, N. G., and Guarda, L. A.: Cardiac myxomas. An immunohistochemical study using endothelial, histiocytic, and smooth-muscle cell markers. Arch. Pathol. Lab. Med. *110*:116, 1986.
84. McComb, R. D.: Heterogeneous expression of factor VIII/von Willebrand factor by cardiac myxoma cells. Am. J. Surg. Pathol. *8*:539, 1984.
85. Tanimura, A., Kitazono, M., Nagayama, K., et al.: Cardiac myxoma: Morphologic, histochemical, and tissue culture studies. Hum. Pathol. *19*:316, 1988.
86. Govoni, E., Severi, B., Cenacchi, G., et al.: Ultrastructural and immunohistochemical contribution to the histogenesis of human cardiac myxoma. Ultrastruct. Pathol. *12*:221, 1988.
87. Takagi, M.: Ultrastructural and immunohistochemical characteristics of cardiac myxoma. Acta Pathol. Jpn. *34*:1099, 1984.
88. Hannah, H., Eisemann, G., Hiszcyniskyj, R., Wimsky, M., and Cohen, R.: Invasive atrial myxoma. Documentation of malignant potential of cardiac myxoma. Am. Heart J. *104*:881, 1982
89. Chen, K. T.: Carcinosarcoma of the heart. Am. Surg. Oncol. *27*:48, 1984.
90. Seo, I. S., Warner, T. F. C. S., Colyer, R. A., and Winkler, F. R.: Metastasizing atrial myxoma. Am. J. Surg. Pathol. *4*:391, 1980.
91. Budzilovich, G., Aleksic, S., Greco, A., et al.: Malignant cardiac myxoma with cerebral metastases. Surg. Neurol. *11*:461, 1979.
91a. Kotani, K., Matsuzawa, Y., Funahashi, T., et al.: Left atrial myxoma metastasizing to the aorta, with intraluminal growth causing renovascular hypertension. Cardiology *78*:72, 1991.
92. Ferrans, V. J., and Roberts, W. C.: Structural features of cardiac myxomas. Hum. Pathol. *4*:111, 1973.
93. Feldman, P. S., Horvath, E., and Kovacs, K.: An ultrastructural study of seven cardiac myxomas. Cancer *40*:2216, 1977.
94. Zhang, P. F., Jones, J. W., and Anderson, W. R.: Cardiac myxomas correlative study by light, transmission, and scanning electron microscopy. Am. J. Cardiovasc. Pathol. *2*:295, 1989.
95. Wold, L. E., and Lie, J. T.: Scanning electron microscopy of intracardiac myxoma. Mayo Clin. Proc. *56*:198, 1981.
96. Topol, E. J., Bierm, R. O., and Reitz, B. A.: Cardiac papillary fibroelastoma and stroke. Am. J. Med. *80*:129, 1986.
97. Pomerance, A.: Papillary "tumours" of the heart valves. J. Pathol. Bacteriol. *81*:135, 1961.
98. Lichtenstein, H. L., Lee, J. C. K., and Stewart, S.: Papillary tumor of the heart: Incidental finding at surgery. Hum. Pathol. *10*:473, 1979.
99. Fenoglio, J. J., McAllister, H. A., and Ferrans, V. J.: Cardiac rhabdomyoma: A clinicopathologic and electron microscopic study. Am. J. Cardiol. *38*:241, 1976.
100. Bruni, C., Prioleau, P. G., Ivey, H. H., and Nolan, S. P.: New fine structural features of cardiac rhabdomyoma: A case report. Cancer *46*:2068, 1980.
101. Takatoh, H., Iwamoto, H., Ikezu, M., et al.: Cardiac rhabdomyoma. A case report with reference to atrial natriuretic peptide. Acta Pathol. Jpn. *38*:95, 1988.
102. Shrivastava, S., Jacks, J. J., White, R. S., and Edwards, J. E.: Diffuse rhabdomyomatosis of the heart. Arch. Pathol. Lab. Med. *101*:78, 1977.
103. Bass, J. L., Breningstall, G. N., and Swaiman, K. F.: Echocardiographic incidence of cardiac rhabdomyoma in tuberous sclerosis. Am. J. Cardiol. *55*:137, 1985.
104. Gibbs, J. L.: The heart and tuberous sclerosis. An echocardiographic and electrocardiographic study. Br. Heart J. *54*:596, 1985.
105. Howanitz, E. P., Teske, D. W., Qualman, S. J., et al.: Pedunculated left ventricular rhabdomyoma. Ann. Thorac. Surg. *41*:443, 1986.
106. Van der Hauwaert, L. G.: Cardiac tumours in infancy and childhood. Br. Heart J. *33*:125, 1971.
107. Feldman, P. S., and Meyer, M. W.: Fibroelastic hamartoma (fibroma) of the heart. Cancer *38*:314, 1976.
108. Jones, K. L., Wolf, P. L., Jensen, P., et al.: The Gorlin syndrome: A genetically determined disorder associated with cardiac tumor. Am. Heart J. *111*:1013, 1986.
109. Takahashi, K., Imamura, Y., Ochi, T., et al.: Echocardiographic demonstration of an asymptomatic patient with left ventricular fibroma. Am. J. Cardiol. *53*:981, 1984.
110. deRuiz, M., Potter, J. L., Stavinoha, J., et al.: Real-time ultrasound diagnosis of cardiac fibroma in a neonate. J. Ultrasound Med. *4*:367, 1985.
111. Prior, J. T.: Lipomatous hypertrophy of cardiac interatrial septum. Arch. Pathol. *78*:11, 1964.
112. Hutter, A. M., Jr., and Page, D. L.: Atrial arrhythmias and lipomatous hypertrophy of the cardiac interatrial septum. Am. Heart J. *82*:16, 1971.
113. Simons, M., Cabin, H. S., and Jaffer, C. C.: Lipomatous hypertrophy of the atrial septum: Diagnosis by combined echocardiography and computerized tomography. Am. J. Cardiol. *54*:465, 1984.
114. Chao, J. C., Reyes, C. V., and Hwang, M. H.: Cardiac hemangioma. South Med. J. *83*:44, 1990.
115. Cox, J. N., Friedli, B., Mechmeche, M., et al.: Teratoma of the heart. Virchows Arch. (A) *402*:163, 1983.
116. Duray, P. H., Mark, E. J., Barwick, K. W., et al.: Congenital polycystic tumor of the atrioventricular node. Arch. Pathol. Lab. Med. *109*:30, 1985.
117. Linder, J., Shelburne, J. D., Sorge, J. P., et al.: Congenital endodermal heterotopia of the atrioventricular node: Evidence for the endodermal origin of so-called mesotheliomas of the atrioventricular node. Hum. Pathol. *15*:1093, 1984.
118. David, T. E., Lenkei, S. C., Marquez-Julio, A., et al.: Pheochromocytoma of the heart. Ann. Thorac. Surg. *41*:98, 1986.
119. Hodgson, S. F., Sheps, S. G., Subramanian, R., et al.: Catecholamine-secreting paraganglioma of the interatrial septum. Am. J. Med. *77*:157, 1984.
120. Shemin, R. J., Marsh, J. D., and Schoen, F. J.: Benign intracardiac thyroid mass causing right ventricular outflow tract obstruction. Am. J. Cardiol. *56*:828, 1985.
121. Whorton, C. M.: Primary malignant tumor of the heart. Cancer *2*:245, 1949.
121a. Burke, A. P., and Virmani, R.: Osteosarcomas of the heart. Am. J. Surg. Pathol. *15*:289, 1991.
122. Goldberg, H. P., and Steinberg, I.: Primary tumors of the heart. Circulation *11*:963, 1955.
123. Glancy, L., Morales, J. B., and Roberts, W. C.: Angiosarcoma of the heart. Am. J. Cardiol. *21*:413, 1968.
124. Janigan, D. T., Husain, A., and Robinson, N. A.: Cardiac angiosarcomas. A review and a case report. Cancer *57*:852, 1986.
125. Keohane, M. E., Lazzam, C., Halperin, J. L., et al.: Angiosarcoma of the left atrium mimicking myxoma. Case report. Hum. Pathol. *20*:599, 1989.
126. Yang, H.-Y., Wasielewski, J. F., Lee, E., and Paik, Y. K.: Angiosarcoma of the heart: Ultrastructural study. Cancer *47*:72, 1981.
127. Hui, K. S., Green, L. K., and Schmidt, W. A.: Primary cardiac rhabdomyosarcoma: Definition of a rare entity. Am. J. Cardiovasc. Pathol. *2*:19, 1988.
128. Proctor, M. S., Tracy, G. P., and Von Koch, L.: Primary cardiac B-cell lymphoma. Am. Heart J. *118*:179, 1989.
129. Bleisch, N., and Kraus, F.: Polypoid sarcoma of the pulmonary trunk. Cancer *46*:314, 1980.

DIAGNOSTIC TECHNIQUES

130. Oldershaw, P. J., Sutton, M. St. J., and Gibson, R. V.: Long asymptomatic period of atrial myxomas. Thorax *35*:70, 1980.
131. Roberts, W. C.: The echocardiographic diseases. Am. J. Cardiol. *64*:1084, 1989.
132. Steiner, R. E.: Radiologic aspects of cardiac tumors. Am. J. Cardiol. *21*:344, 1968.
133. Abrams, H. L., Adams, D. F., and Grant, H. A.: The radiology of tumors of the heart. Radiol. Clin. North Am. *9*:299, 1971.
134. Sabot, G., Fauvel, J. M., and Bounhoure, J. P.: Echocardiographic diagnosis of mobile left ventricular tumour. Br. Heart J. *42*:113, 1979.
135. Nanda, N. C., Barold, S. S., Gramiak, R., et al.: Echocardiographic features of right ventricular outflow tumor prolapsing into the pulmonary artery. Am. J. Cardiol. *40*:272, 1977.

136. Green, S. E., Joynt, L. E., Fitzgerald, P. J., et al.: In vivo ultrasonic tissue characterization of human intracardiac masses. Am. J. Cardiol. *51*:231, 1983.

137. Duncan, W. J., Rowe, R. D., Freedom, R. M., et al.: Space-occupying lesions of the myocardium: Role of two-dimensional echocardiography in detection of cardiac tumors in children. Am. Heart J. *104*:780, 1982.

137a. Wrisley, D., Rosenberg, J., Giambartolomei, A., et al.: Left ventricular myxoma discovered incidentally by echocardiography. Am. Heart J. *121*:1554, 1991.

138. Charuzi, Y., Bolger, A., Beeder, C., and Lew, A. S.: A new echocardiographic classification of left atrial myxoma. Am. J. Cardiol. *55*:614, 1985.

139. Dennis, M. A., Appareti, K., Manco-Johnson, M. L., et al.: The echocardiographic diagnosis of multiple fetal cardiac tumors. Ultrasound Med. *4*:327, 1985.

140. Panidis, I. P., Mimtz, G. S., and McAllister, M.: Hemodynamic consequences of the left atrial myxomas as assessed by Doppler ultrasound. Am. Heart J. *111*:927, 1986.

140a. Lyons, S. V., McCord, J., and Smith, S.: Asymptomatic giant right atrial myxoma: Role of transeophageal echocardiography in management. Am. Heart J. *121*:1555, 1991.

141. Fueredi, G. A., Knechtges, T. E., and Czarnecki, D. J.: Coronary angiography in atrial myxoma: Findings in nine cases. Am. J. Roentgenol. *152*:737, 1989.

142. Singh, R. N., Burkholder, J. A., and Magovern, G. J.: Coronary arteriography as an aid in left atrial myxoma diagnosis. Cardiovasc. Intervent. Radiol. *7*:40, 1984.

143. Weyne, A. E., Heyndrickx, G. R., Cuvelier, C. C., et al.: Cardiac imaging techniques in the diagnosis of angiosarcoma of the heart: report of two cases. Postgrad. Med. J. *61*:271, 1985.

144. Pendyck, F., Pierce, E. C., Baron, M. G., and Lukban, S. B.: Embolization of left atrial myxoma after transseptal cardiac catheterization. Am. J. Cardiol. *30*;569, 1972.

TREATMENT AND PROGNOSIS

145. Becker, R. C., Loeffler, J. S., Leopold, K. A., and Underwood, D. A.: Primary tumors of the heart: A review with emphasis on diagnosis and potential treatment modalities. Semin. Surg. Oncol. *1*:161, 1985.

146. Murphy, M. C., Sweeney, M. S., Putnam, J. B., Jr., et al.: Surgical treatment of cardiac tumors: a 25-year experience. Ann. Thorac. Surg. *49*:612, 1990.

147. Dapper, F., Gorlach, G., Hoffmann, C., et al: Primary cardiac tumors—clinical experiences and late results in 48 patients. Thorac. Cardiovasc. Surg. *36*:80, 1988.

148. Semb, B. K.: Surgical considerations in the treatment of cardiac myxoma. J. Thorac. Cardiovasc. Surg. *87*:251, 1984.

149. Marvasti, M. A., Obeid, A. I., Potts, J. L., and Parker, F. B.: Approach in the management of atrial myxoma with long-term follow-up. Ann. Thorac. Surg. *38*:53, 1984.

150. Waller, D. A., Ettles, D. F., Saunders, N. R., and Williams, G.: Recurrent cardiac myxoma: The surgical implications of two distinct groups of patients. Thorac. Cardiovasc Surg. *37*:226, 1989.

151. Bortolotti, U., Maraglino, G., Rubino, M., et al.: Surgical excision of intracardiac myxomas: A 20-year follow-up. Ann. Thorac. Surg. *49*:449, 1990.

152. Larsson, S., Lepore, V., and Kennergren, C.: Atrial myxomas: Results of 25 years' experience and review of the literature. Surgery *105*:695, 1989.

153. Scheld, H. H., Nestle, H. W., Kling, D., et al.: Resection of a heart tumor using autotransplantation. Thorac. Cardiovasc. Surg. *36*:40, 1988.

154. Mesnildrey, P., Bloch, G., Cachera, J. P., and Piwnica, A.: Atrial myxoma: A new surgical approach using neodymium: yttrium-aluminum-garnet laser photocoagulation. J. Thorac. Cardiovasc. Surg. *98*:313, 1989.

155. Parks, F. R., Adams, F., and Longmire, W. P.: Successful excision of a left ventricular hamartoma. Circulation *26*:1316, 1962.

156. Etches, P. C., Gribbin, B., and Gunning, A. J.: Echocardiographic diagnosis and successful removal of cardiac fibroma in 4-year old child. Br. Heart J. *43*:360, 1980.

157. Goldman, S., Lortscher, R., and Pappas, G.: Surgical treatment for rhabdomyoma of the right atrium causing arrhythmias. J. Thorac. Cardiovasc. Surg. *89*:802, 1985.

158. Corno, A., deSimone, G., Catena, G., and Marcelletti, C.: Cardiac rhabdomyoma: Surgical treatment in the neonate. Thorac. Cardiovasc. Surg. *87*:1984.

159. Foster, E. D., Spooner, E. W., Farina, M. A., et al.: Cardiac rhabdomyoma in the neonate: Surgical treatment. Ann. Thorac. Surg. *37*:249, 1984.

160. Orringer, M. B., Sisson, J. C., Glazer, G., et al.: Surgical treatment of cardiac pheochromocytomas. J. Thorac. Cardiovasc. Surg. *89*:753, 1985.

161. Key, T. C., Resnik, R., Dittrich, H. C., and Reisner, L. S.: Successful pregnancy after cardiac transplantation. Am. J. Obstet. Gynecol. *160*:367, 1989.

162. Marvasti, M. A., Bove, E. L., Obeid, A. I., et al.: Primary osteosarcoma of left atrium: Complete surgical excision. Ann. Thorac. Surg. *40*;402, 1985.

163. Sharma, S., Tendolkar, A., and Parulkar, G. B.: Angiosarcoma of the heart. Am. Heart J. *109*:601, 1985.

164. Vergnon, J. M., Vincent, M., Perinetti, M., et al.: Chemotherapy of metastatic primary cardiac sarcomas. Am. Heart J. *110*;682, 1985.

165. Hollingworth, J. H., and Sturgill, B. C.: Treatment of primary angiosarcoma of the heart. Am. Heart J. *78*:254, 1969.

166. Potter, R., Baumgart, P., Greve, H., Schnepper, E.: Primary angiosarcoma of the heart. Thorac. Cardiovasc. Surg. *37*:374, 1989.

167. Dichek, D. A., Holmvang, G., Fallon, J. T., et al.: Angiosarcoma of the heart: Three year survival and follow-up by nuclear magnetic resonance imaging. Am. Heart J. *115*:1323, 1988.

168. Allaire, F. J., Grimm, C. A., Taylor, L. M., and Pfaff, J. P.: Primary hemangioendothelioma of the heart. Rocky Mt. Med. J. *61*:34, 1964.

169. Terry, L. N., and Kilgerman, M. M.: Pericardial and myocardial involvement by lymphomas and leukemias. The role of radiotherapy. Cancer *25*:1003, 1970.

170. Garfein, O. B.: Lymphosarcoma of the right atrium: Angiographic and hemodynamic documentation of response to chemotherapy. Arch. Intern. Med. *135*:325, 1975.

45

Pericardial Disease

by BEVERLY H. LORELL, M.D., and EUGENE BRAUNWALD, M.D.

ANATOMY

The pericardium forms a strong flask-shaped sac with short tubelike extensions that enclose the origins of the aorta and its junction with the aortic arch, the pulmonary artery where it branches, the proximal pulmonary veins, and venae cavae. Fibrous tissue of the pericardium actually blends with adventitia of the great arteries to form very strong attachments. In addition, the pericardium has firm ligamentous attachments anteriorly to the sternum and xiphoid process, posteriorly to the vertebral column, and inferiorly to the diaphragm.[1,1a]

The human pericardium receives its arterial blood supply from small branches of the aorta and internal mammary and musculophrenic arteries. The pericardium is innervated by the vagus, left recurrent laryngeal nerve, and esophageal plexus and also has rich sympathetic innervation from the stellate and first dorsal ganglia and the cardiac, aortic, and diaphragmatic plexuses. The phrenic nerves course over the pericardium en route to the diaphragm. The afferent nerves responsible for pain perception appear to be transmitted via the phrenic nerve entering the spinal cord at C4–C5.[1] Peripheral sensory fibers that enter the dorsal root ganglia at C8–T2 supply both the brachial plexus and the pericardium, which provides a possible morphological explanation for referred pericardial pain.[2]

THE TWO LAYERS OF THE PERICARDIUM. The pericardium is composed of a fibrous outer layer and an inner serous membrane composed of a single layer of mesothelial cells. The inner serous layer is intimately attached to the surface of the heart and epicardial fat to form the visceral pericardium, and this inner serous membrane reflects back on itself to line the outer fibrous layer to form the parietal pericardium.

The pericardium has two major serosal tunnels: the transverse sinus, which lies posterior to the great arteries and anterior to the atria and superior vena cava, and the oblique sinus, which lies posterior to the left atrium so that the posterior left atrial wall is actually separated from the pericardial space. The serous visceral pericardium is attached to the parietal pericardium by delicate connective tissue with elastin fibers. The parietal pericardium is composed of collagen fibers interlaced with extensive elastic fibers, which are wavy during childhood and become progressively straighter with age, suggesting that young pericardia are more compliant than those of the elderly.

ELECTRON MICROSCOPY. This reveals that exuberant microvilli and long, single cilia project from the serous mesothelium composing the visceral pericardium and the inner lining of the parietal pericardium (Fig. 45–1),[3] which increase markedly the surface area available for fluid transport. Both microvilli and cilia provide a specialized surface to permit movement of the pericardial membranes over each other during each cardiac cycle and to permit the pericardium to accommodate changes in cardiac shape during contraction. In addition, numerous small fenestrations or pores less than 50 μ in diameter provide direct communication between the pericardial and pleural cavities in mammals.[4]

PERICARDIAL FLUID. The human pericardium normally contains up to 50 ml of clear fluid. The visceral pericardium is believed to be the source of normal pericardial fluid and of excessive fluid in disease states. Normal pericardial fluid appears to be an ultrafiltrate of plasma, since electrolytes are present in pericardial fluid in concentrations compatible with such an ultrafiltrate; protein concentrations are about one-third those of the plasma, and albumin is present in a higher ratio in pericardial fluid, reflecting its lower molecular weight. Current data suggest that drainage of the pericardial space occurs both by the thoracic duct via the parietal pericardium and by the right lymphatic duct via the right pleural space.

Pericardial fluid also contains phospholipids that serve as a lubricant to reduce friction between the surfaces of the parietal pericardium and the visceral pericardium.[5] The pericardium appears to produce prostaglandins in response to physiological stimuli that may modulate efferent cardiac sympathetic stimulation and alter cardiac electrophysiological properties.[6] The clinical implications of this potential regulatory effect of the pericardium on electrical conduction of the heart are not yet known.

FUNCTIONS OF THE PERICARDIUM

The pericardium's ligamentous attachments help to fix the heart anatomically and prevent excessive motion with changes in body position. The pericardium also reduces friction between the heart and surrounding organs and provides a barrier against the extension of infection and malignancy from contiguous organs to the heart itself. The role of the pericardium in the regulation of the circulation is controversial, since congenital absence of the pericardium is not associated with overt disturbances of cardiac function. However, observations in both dogs and humans indicate that the pericardium may play a role in (1) the distribution of hydrostatic forces on the heart, (2) the prevention of acute cardiac dilatation, and (3) diastolic coupling of the two ventricles (p. 1468).

The normal pericardium is relatively stiff, and the relationship between pressure within the pericardium and total intrapericardial volume, which is the sum of the volume of the heart itself and the reserve volume of the surrounding pericardial sac, appears as a steep curve when plotted on a graph.[1]

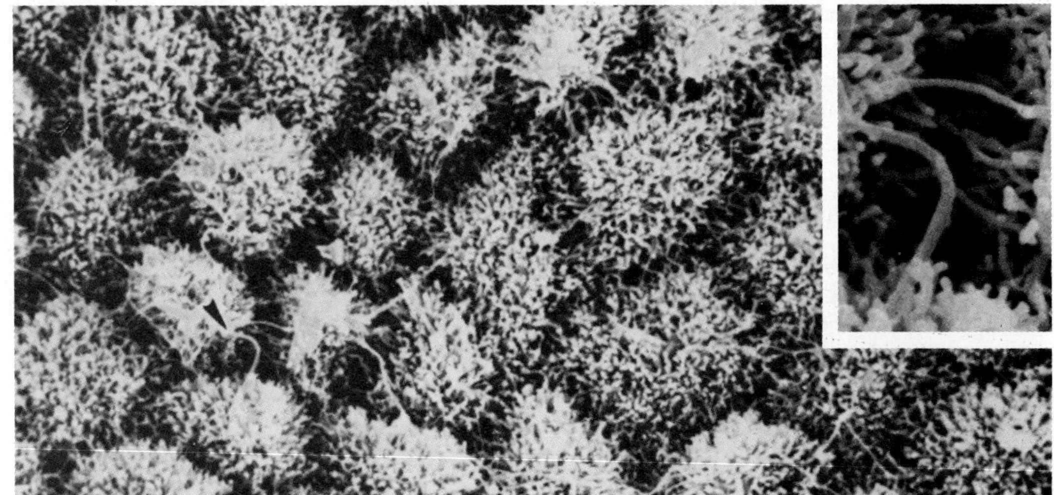

FIGURE 45-1. Scanning electron micrograph of human parietal pericardium. The mesothelial cells are covered with microvilli, and long individual cilia (arrow) are also present. Insert shows cilia at higher magnification. (From Ishihara, T., et al.: Histologic and ultrastructural features of normal human parietal pericardium. Am. J. Cardiol *46*:744, 1980.)

Once the pericardium is filled, intrapericardial pressure rises sharply as volume is increased (Fig. 45-2). Thus, the stiffness of the pericardium increases when load is increased, and then it becomes almost inextensible. Although much of our knowledge regarding the physiological role of the pericardium has been derived from experimental studies in dogs, it is important to recognize that the human pericardium is about three times as thick and much less distensible than canine pericardium.[7] Usually, the pericardial sac is filled with a thin film of fluid distributed throughout the pericardial space in such a way that the pericardial reserve volume is not exceeded. This permits respiratory and postural changes in cardiac volume and total intrapericardial volume to occur without significant changes in intrapericardial pressure. When measured with a fluid-filled or micromanometer-tipped catheter, pericardial pressure is nearly equal to intrapleural pressure and varies from -5 to $+5$ cm H_2O during the respiratory cycle.[8]

INTRAPERICARDIAL PRESSURE. Normal intrapericardial pressure is zero or negative. This has major implications for our understanding of the influence of pericardial pressure on the transmural distending pressure of the cardiac chambers and the operation of the Frank-Starling mechanism in the beat-to-beat regulation of stroke volume.[9] The transmural distending pressure of either ventricle is the difference between intracardiac and intrapericardial pressures and is independent of gravity. When intrapericardial pressure is assumed to be negative, normally a substantial transmural distending pressure would be expected to exist across both ventricles. For example, when left ventricular end-diastolic pressure is +8 mm Hg and intrapericardial pressure is -2 mm Hg relative to atmosphere, the actual left ventricular distending pressure would be $8-(-2)=10$ mm Hg, and when right ventricular end-diastolic pressure is 4 mm Hg and intrapericardial pressure is -2 mm Hg relative to atmosphere, the actual right ventricular distending pressure would be $4-(-2)=6$ mm Hg.

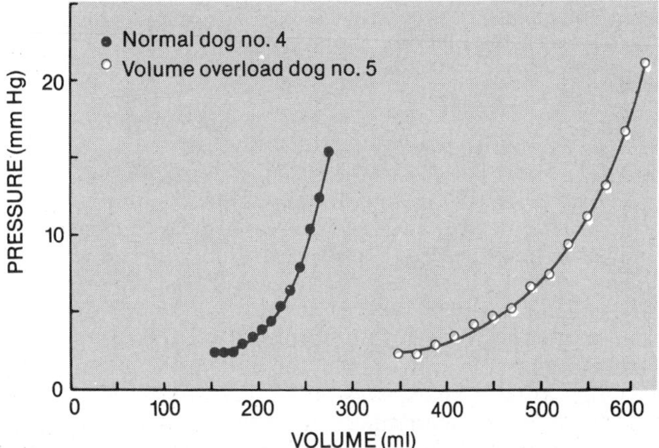

FIGURE 45-2. Pericardial pressure-volume curves from a normal dog *(left)* and from a dog with chronic volume overload *(right)*. Note that the normal pressure-volume curve *(right)* is initially flat but becomes extremely steep as total volume within the pericardium increases. In response to chronic cardiac dilatation, the pericardium enlarges in size and mass such that the pericardium can accomodate a large volume at low pressure *(right curve)*. (From Freeman, G. L., and LeWinter, M. M.: Pericardial adaptations during chronic dilation in dogs. Circ. Res. *54*:294, 1984.)

Studies using micromanometer pressure measurements support the view that pericardial pressure is usually very low and thus exerts only a small influence on the average transmural distending pressure of the heart as long as pericardial reserve volume is not exceeded by volume loading.[8] Under normal conditions, it is clear that the pericardium does influence the pattern of venous return and ventricular filling that occurs in every cardiac cycle. Ventricular ejection is accompanied by abrupt descent of the atrioventricular junction (the "base" of the heart) and a reduction in right atrial pressure, manifest by the x descent* in the right atrial pressure pulse as well as by a decline in intrapericardial pressure. These changes result in a surge of venous return during systole, particularly when ventricular and pericardial pressures are increased. This acceleration of venous return during systolic ejection is diminished by opening of the pericardium.

When the volume of the heart or other contents of the pericardial sac increase and exceed the elastic limits of the pericardium during diastole, the heart is shifted to the steep portion of the curve relating intrapericardial pressure and volume, resulting in marked increases in intrapericardial and intracardiac pressures. However, the difference between the two pressures, i.e., the transmural pressure, usually declines. In the extreme case of cardiac tamponade, in which both intrapericardial and intracardiac pressures are markedly increased, the transmural pressure distending the ventricles may fall precipitously toward zero, resulting in decreased ventricular diastolic volumes and preload. These findings, taken together, support the classic view that the pericardium is a distensible "loosely fitting" sac that modestly affects stroke volume by changes in intrapericardial pressure and

*It is recognized that the descent in venous pressure after the *a* wave is usually termed the x descent and, after the *c* wave, the x' descent. In this chapter, the major systolic venous pressure descent after the *a* and *c* waves will be termed the x descent.

transmural pressure and exerts a substantial influence only at higher ventricular and pericardial pressures.

CHALLENGES TO THE "CLASSIC VIEW." This classic view has been seriously challenged by Smiseth and coworkers,[10] who contend that the use of either fluid-filled or micromanometer catheters underestimates pericardial pressure and its influence on transmural distending pressures in normal hearts. They have shown in dogs that the measurement of the *surface contact pressure* of the pericardium against the heart using a flat balloon is more accurate than a fluid-filled catheter in estimating the actual pericardial pressure (the fall in left ventricular pressure observed immediately after opening the pericardium in the absence of any change in chamber volume). Observations from dogs and from humans indicate that when the amount of fluid in the pericardial sac is small, pericardial pressure measured in this way is much higher than intrathoracic pressure or pericardial pressure measured with a fluid-filled or micromanometer catheter, whereas pericardial pressures measured by either a balloon or fluid-filled catheter are similar when a substantial volume of pericardial fluid (40 to 50 ml) is present.[11,12] Thus the controversy regarding the concept of pericardial surface contact pressure does not detract from the accuracy or the clinical utility of measuring intrapericardial pressure with a catheter in patients with large pericardial effusions and cardiac tamponade.

However, these arguments profoundly challenge classic views regarding the normal physiology of the heart and the accurate measurement of the transmural pressure of each ventricle. These studies have emphasized that intrapericardial surface contact pressure is not zero or negative and, to the contrary, is virtually equal to right atrial pressure.[10,11] A further assumption is that differences in pericardial surface contact pressure do not exist over different chambers of the heart. This analysis indicates that left ventricular transmural pressure in normal hearts should be estimated by subtracting right atrial pressure rather than intrathoracic pressure. It also carries the remarkable implication that the transmural distending pressure of the normal right ventricle is extremely small, and negligible or zero at end-diastole.

Experiments by Santamore et al.[13] and Slinker et al.[14] have modified this concept and indicate that closed flat-balloon catheters probably exaggerate the constraining pressure exerted by the normal pericardium on the surface of the heart. Experiments examining right ventricular and left ventricular pressure-volume relationships in arrested canine hearts showed that although right ventricular transmural pressure is always less than left ventricular transmural pressure over the physiological range, measurable right ventricular transmural pressure is always present in the absence of the pericardium even at low volumes, and right heart transmural pressure increases with increments in ventricular volume. In the canine heart the contribution of the pericardium to right ventricular diastolic pressure is substantial (greater than 50 per cent) only at right ventricular filling pressures greater than 10 mm Hg. In addition, experiments indicate that the pressure exerted by the pericardium on the surface of the heart is not uniform over different regions of the heart.[15]

Taken together, these experiments suggest that right atrial pressure cannot be used to estimate precisely the pericardial constraint or to calculate transmural pressures of either ventricle in the normal heart. Furthermore, pericardial catheter measurements tend to underestimate while pericardial balloons tend to overestimate pericardial pressure, which appears to be within the range of 0.2 to 3 mm Hg under normal physiological conditions. Finally, these experiments confirm that the pericardium modifies the filling and intracavitary pressures of both ventricles, particularly when cardiac distention occurs.

LIMITATION OF CARDIAC DISTENTION. The relatively nondistensible pericardium may help to limit acute distention of the heart. This was appreciated as early as 1898 by Bernard, who used a pump to increase pressure in excised hearts with and without the pericardium and noted that hearts unsupported by the pericardium ruptured at lower pressures than did hearts with intact pericardia.[16] Subsequent studies in dogs demonstrated that the pericardium restrains right and left ventricular filling, so that ventricular volume is greater at any given ventricular pressure with the pericardium removed than with the pericardium intact. Thus, acute changes in intracardiac and total intrapericardial volume result in an upward shift of both the left and right ventricular pressure-volume relationships, which is in part mediated by the restraining effect of the pericardium and an increase in intrapericardial pressure.[14,17,18] As ventricular volumes increase, the proportional contribution of the pericardium to end-diastolic pressure of the thin-walled right ventricle increases relative to that of the left ventricle.[14] Thus, as the heart is distended, the pericardium makes a greater contribution to right ventricular end-diastolic pressure than to left ventricular end-diastolic pressure.

The hemodynamic effects of acute volume loading and vasodilators are in part mediated by pericardial constraint. Shirato et al.[19] demonstrated that acute volume loading with dextran in dogs with intact pericardia resulted in an upward shift in the left ventricular pressure–segment length relation, i.e., left ventricular pressure was higher at any given segment length while the reduction of venous return and cardiac volume by means of nitroprusside administration shifted the curves downward toward control levels (Fig. 45–3). This occurred because nitroprusside and other vasodilators that decrease right heart filling reduce the total volume occupied by the heart within the pericardial space and thus reduce the restraining of the left ventricle by the pericardium; in turn, this causes a downward shift of the left ventricular pressure-volume relation so that a given left ventricular volume is associated with lower left ventricular diastolic pressure. After pericardiectomy, volume loading results in a rightward shift in the pressure-segment length relation and, after nitroprusside, a leftward shift along a single curve.[19] When the effect of the pericardium is eliminated by plotting left ventricular transmural pressure versus segment length, the points during all interventions fall along a single curve. Smiseth et al.[20] have extended these findings and have shown that the opposite effects of angiotensin (upward shift) and nitroprusside (downward shift) of the left ventricle pressure-volume relation depend on changes in intrapericardial pressure mediated by shifts in blood volume from the heart to systemic vascular beds.

A restraining effect of the pericardium has been observed early in the course of chronic volume overloading induced by formation of arteriovenous shunts in dogs prior to enlargement of the pericardium by stretch or hypertrophy. However,

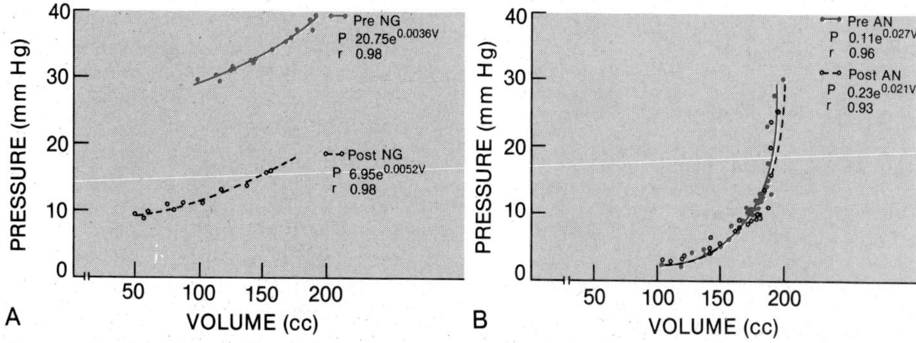

FIGURE 45–3. Left ventricular pressure-volume curves in man (*A*) before and after nitroglycerin (NG) and (*B*) before and after amyl nitrite (AN). Nitroglycerin, which causes venodilation and reduces total intrapericardial volume, shifts the curve downward and leftward. In contrast, the curves before and after amyl nitrite, which causes arterial dilation, can be superimposed. (From Ludbrook, P. A., et al.: Influence of right ventricular hemodynamics on left ventricular diastolic pressure-volume relations in man. Circulation *59*:21, 1979, by permission of the American Heart Association, Inc.)

this restraining effect was not apparent in dogs studied late during the course of chronic volume overload.[21] This occurs because chronic left ventricular enlargement and hypertrophy are accompanied by an increase in the compliance of the pericardial chamber and an increase in total pericardial volume due to the addition of new pericardial tissue.[22] In addition to its effects on ventricular filling, pericardial pressure also appears to influence indices of isovolumic relaxation of the left ventricle. Frais et al.[23] showed that alterations in the asymptote and time constant of left ventricular pressure decay (tau) in dogs subjected to volume loading vary with changes in intrapericardial pressure.

These observations suggest that shifts in the left and right ventricular diastolic pressure-volume relations following volume loading or vasodilator administration are largely due to changes in intrapericardial pressure. However, the pericardium does not affect *intrinsic* myocardial compliance; neither does it account for changes in the left ventricular diastolic pressure-volume relationship observed during ischemia.[24]

VENTRICULAR INTERDEPENDENCE. The pericardium also contributes to diastolic coupling between the two ventricles. The distention of one ventricle alters the distensibility of the other, even in the absence of the pericardium.[25] This effect appears to be mediated in part by shared encircling muscle bands and by the interventricular septum, which tends to bulge into the left ventricle, causing a change in the shape of the left ventricle when the right ventricle is distended.[26] In the absence of the pericardium, large increases in right ventricular volume and pressure are required to cause an appreciable increase in left ventricular filling pressure.[27] In contrast, the presence of an intact pericardium markedly accentuates the coupling between ventricular diastolic pressures.[28] When right ventricular volume and pressure are increased with the normal pericardium intact, right and left ventricular filling pressures are closely correlated, and left ventricular volume is smaller than in the absence of the pericardium. In the absence of the pericardium, cardiac distensibility is primarily related to properties of the myocardium. This effect of the pericardium on the interaction between the two ventricles is accentuated in experimental constrictive pericarditis when the distensibility of the pericardium is decreased.[29] This effect of the pericardium on diastolic ventricular interaction is present at normal filling pressures and becomes of increasing importance at high right ventricular filling pressures. During volume loading in normal conscious dogs, it has been shown that pericardial pressure exerts a disproportionately greater effect on the thin-walled right ventricle, which suggests that the pericardium couples diastolic function of the two ventricles via its influence on right ventricular filling and geometry.[8,14]

Although normal pericardium does not appear to contribute importantly to the interaction of the ventricles during systole at normal filling pressures,[30] it does influence global and regional systolic function during conditions of acute distention of the heart.[31,32] Kanazawa et al.[31] showed that removal of the pericardium in dogs caused insignificant changes in stroke volume, whereas removal of the pericardium during volume loading caused a substantial increase in stroke volume associated with an increase in end-diastolic segment length and systolic excursion. Although pericardial pressure was not measured, it is likely that this increase in stroke volume was due to the Frank-Starling mechanism via an increase of the transmural distending pressure of the ventricle following removal of the pericardium. Furthermore, during volume overload, the pericardium caused an upward shift in the left ventricular end-systolic pressure-volume relationship in the absence of a change in inotropic state. Pericardial constraint also appears to modify regional systolic function during acute right ventricular pressure overload and distention. Goto et al.[32] found that acute right ventricular loading in dogs results in nonuniform decreases in regional left ventricular shortening, an effect that is enhanced by the presence of the pericardium.

The pericardium also appears to limit maximal body oxygen consumption by limiting stroke volume and cardiac output during maximal exercise in conscious dogs.[33] These observations suggest that the normal pericardium exerts a restraining effect and modifies ventricular interaction during systole at high ventricular filling pressures.

In *summary*, there is experimental evidence from canine studies that the pericardium limits acute distention of the heart, mediates changes in the relationship between ventricular pressure and volume, and enhances the effect that distention of one ventricle has on the diastolic pressure-volume relations of the contralateral ventricle.

FUNCTIONS OF THE PERICARDIUM IN HUMANS. There is substantial evidence that the restraining effects of the pericardium are clinically relevant. For example, in humans after pericardiotomy, there is a downward shift of the left ventricular pressure-volume curve that is increasingly prominent as left ventricular volume increases.[34] Similarly, routine pericardial closure after open-heart surgery has been shown to result in an increase in right heart filling pressure associated with a reduction in left ventricular diastolic cavity dimension and cardiac output, whereas opening of the pericardium causes the opposite effects.[35] In addition, angiotensin, nitroprusside, and nitroglycerin infusions, which alter intracardiac volume, cause acute shifts in the left ventricular diastolic pressure-volume relation in humans,[36] an effect that has been shown in animal studies to depend on the presence of the constraint of the pericardium.[20] Ludbrook demonstrated in humans that the downward shift in the left ventricular pressure-volume curve that occurs during nitroglycerin administration is not observed with amyl nitrite, which alters aortic pressure but has little acute effect on intrapericardial volumes (Fig. 45–3).[36,37] After pericardiotomy and loss of the restraining effect of the pericardium, the human left ventricular pressure-volume curve is not altered by nitroprusside administration.[38] These observations indicate that the beneficial effects of interventions such as nitroprusside infusion, in which an augmentation of stroke volume may be observed at a lower ventricular filling pressure, are in part due to an alteration of apparent cardiac distensibility mediated by reducing the restraining effect of the pericardium.[39]

The pericardium may also provide a significant restraining effect on acute cardiac dilatation during acute volume loading in humans.[40] Extrapolating the findings of dog experiments may underestimate the restraining effect of the human pericardium during acute volume loading, since normal human pericardium is thicker and shows much greater viscous responses than canine pericardium.[7] In patients, volume overload due to acute mitral regurgitation is sometimes associated with striking elevation and equilibration of diastolic pressures in all four cardiac chambers similar to that observed in constrictive pericardial disease (p. 1486), but these findings do not appear to be present in patients with chronic volume overload.[41] Similarly, acute right ventricular infarction is sometimes associated with elevation and equilibration of diastolic right and left ventricular pressures[42] that have been shown experimentally to be related to the elevation of intrapericardial pressure.[43]

The role of the pericardium in the pathogenesis of chronic heart failure in patients is controversial and not yet well understood. Although compensatory enlargement and increased capacitance of the pericardium is likely to occur in humans with chronic cardiac enlargement, it is feasible that acute increases in venous return in patients with heart failure could increase the effects of the pericardium on ventricular diastolic and systolic function. Consistent with this hypothesis, Janicki studied the effects of the augmentation of venous return by exercise in 61 patients with chronic heart failure and deduced that pericardial constraint became evident when stroke volume abruptly became invariant and a similar increment in right and left heart filling pressures occurred during progressive exercise.[44] In this study, pericardial constraint became evident during exercise in half of the patients. Thus, it appears that the pericardium can be an important determinant of the limits of systolic pump function and result in the coupling of right and left ventricular diastolic pressures in patients with heart failure.

Acute Pericarditis

Acute pericarditis is a syndrome due to inflammation of the pericardium characterized by chest pain, a pericardial friction rub, and serial electrocardiographic abnormalities. The incidence of pericardial inflammation detected in several autopsy series ranges from 2 to 6 per cent, whereas pericarditis is diagnosed clinically in only about 1 of 1000 hospital admissions. This suggests that pericarditis is frequently inapparent clinically, although it may occur in the presence of a vast number of medical and surgical disorders (Table 45–1). The most common causes of the syndrome of acute pericarditis include idiopathic or viral pericarditis, uremia, bacterial infection, acute myocardial infarction, pericardiotomy associated with cardiac surgery, tuberculosis, neoplasm, and trauma. All types of pericarditis are more common in men than in women, and in adults compared with young children. The relative frequency of causes of pericarditis depend on the clinical setting. Presumed viral or idiopathic pericarditis is common in an outpatient setting, while pericarditis related to trauma, neoplasm, and uremia, is seen more frequently in tertiary hospitals.

The *pathological changes* of acute pericarditis are those of acute inflammation, including the presence of polymorphonuclear leukocytes, increased pericardial vascularity, and deposition of fibrin. Inflammation may also involve the superficial myocardium, and fibrinous adhesions may form between the pericardium and epicardium and between the pericardium and adjacent sternum and pleura. The visceral pericardium may also react to acute injury by exudation of fluid. The pathological and clinical features of specific causes of pericarditis are discussed later in this chapter. This section will focus on clinical features common to acute pericarditis of many causes.

TABLE 45–1 CAUSES OF PERICARDITIS

1. **IDIOPATHIC (nonspecific)**
2. **VIRAL INFECTIONS: Coxsackie A virus, Coxsackie B virus, echovirus, adenovirus, mumps virus, infectious mononucleosis, varicella, hepatitis B, AIDS (acquired immunodeficiency syndrome)**
3. **TUBERCULOSIS**
4. **ACUTE BACTERIAL INFECTION: pneumococcus, staphylococcus, streptococcus, gram-negative septicemia, *Neisseria meningitidis, Neisseria gonorrhoeae*, tularemia, *Legionella pneumophila***
5. **FUNGAL INFECTIONS: histoplasmosis, coccidioidomycosis, *Candida*, blastomycosis**
6. **OTHER INFECTIONS: toxoplasmosis, amebiasis, mycoplasma, *Nocardia*, actinomycosis, echinococcosis, Lyme disease**
7. **ACUTE MYOCARDIAL INFARCTION**
8. **UREMIA: untreated uremia; in association with hemodialysis**
9. **NEOPLASTIC DISEASE: lung cancer, breast cancer, leukemia, Hodgkin's disease, lymphoma**
10. **RADIATION**
11. **AUTOIMMUNE DISORDERS: acute rheumatic fever, systemic lupus erythematosus, rheumatoid arthritis, scleroderma, mixed connective tissue disease, Wegener granulomatosis, polyarteritis nodosa**
12. **OTHER INFLAMMATORY DISORDERS: sarcoidosis, amyloidosis, inflammatory bowel disease, Whipple disease, temporal arteritis, Behçet disease**
13. **DRUGS: hydralazine, procainamide, diphenylhydantoin, isoniazid, phenylbutazone, dantrolene, doxorubicin, methysergide, penicillin (with hypereosinophilia)**
14. **TRAUMA: including chest trauma; hemopericardium following thoracic surgery; pacemaker insertion; cardiac diagnostic procedures; esophageal rupture; pancreatic-pericardial fistula**
15. **DELAYED POSTMYOCARDIAL-PERICARDIAL INJURY SYNDROMES:**
    a. **Postmyocardial infarction (Dressler) syndrome**
    b. **Postpericardiotomy syndrome**
16. **DISSECTING AORTIC ANEURYSM**
17. **MYXEDEMA**
18. **CHYLOPERICARDIUM**

TABLE 45–2 PERICARDIAL VERSUS ISCHEMIC PAIN

	ISCHEMIA	PERICARDITIS
Location	**Retrosternal; left shoulder, arm**	**Precordium; left trapezius ridge**
Quality	**Pressure, burning, buildup**	**Sharp, pleuritic; or dull, oppressive**
Thoracic motion	**No effect**	**Increased by breathing, rotating thorax**
Duration	**Angina; 1 or 2 to 15 min Unstable angina: ½ hr to hrs**	**Hours or days**
Effort	**Stable angina: usually Unstable angina or infarction: usually not**	**No relation**
Posture	**No effect; may sit, belch, use Valsalva or knee-chest position for relief**	**Leaning forward for relief; aggravated by recumbency**

From Fowler N. O.: Acute pericarditis. In Fowler, N. O. (ed.): The Pericardium in Health and Disease. Mt. Kisco, NY, Futura Publishing Co., 1985, p. 158.

HISTORY. *Chest pain* is frequently the chief complaint of patients with acute pericarditis; its quality and location are variable. Pain is often localized to retrosternal and left precordial regions and frequently radiates to the trapezius ridge and neck (Table 45–2). Occasionally it may be localized to the epigastrium, mimicking an "acute abdomen," or have a dull or oppressive quality, with radiation to the left arm similar to the ischemic pain of myocardial infarction. The pain is often aggravated by lying supine, coughing, deep inspiration, and swallowing and is eased by sitting up and leaning forward. Sometimes it is noted with each heartbeat. The pain associated with pericarditis may arise from inflammation of both the pericardium and the adjacent pleura, accounting for the pleuritic nature of the discomfort. Pericardial pain may also be provoked by stretch of the pericardial sac due to the presence of intrapericardial fluid.

Acute pericarditis may also cause *dyspnea*. This symptom is related in part to the need to breathe shallowly to avoid pericardiopleuritic chest pain. Dyspnea may be aggravated by the presence of fever or by the development of a large pericardial effusion that compresses adjacent bronchi and pulmonary parenchyma. Additional symptoms such as cough, sputum production, or weight loss may be due to an underlying systemic disease such as tuberculosis or uremia.

PHYSICAL EXAMINATION. The *pericardial friction rub* (p. 60) is the pathognomonic physical finding of acute pericarditis. It is a scratching, grating, high-pitched sound, described by Laennec's associate Victor Collin as "the squeak of leather of a new saddle under the rider." Although the sound is believed to arise from friction between the roughened pericardial and epicardial surfaces, a loud pericardial rub may also be heard in the presence of scant or large pericardial effusions.[45] The pericardial friction rub is classically described as having three components that are related to cardiac motion during atrial systole (presystole), ventricular systole, and rapid ventricular filling in early diastole. Spodick's prospective analysis of the pericardial friction rub revealed that the presystolic component is present in about 70 per cent of cases, while a ventricular systolic component is the loudest and most easily heard component, present in almost all cases.[46] The rapid diastolic filling component is detected less frequently and may be slurred into that of atrial contraction, resulting in a biphasic "to-and-fro" rub. In this series, a true three-component rub was detected about half the time and at

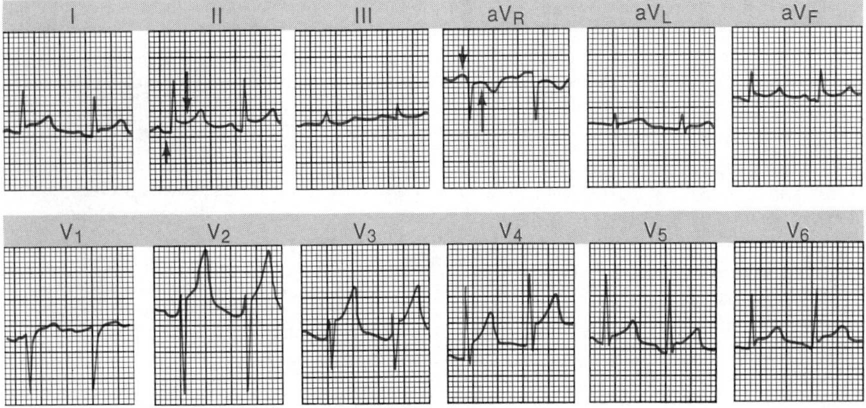

FIGURE 45-4. Stage I electrocardiographic changes from a patient with acute pericarditis. Diffuse ST-segment elevation, which is concave upward, is present in all leads except aV_R and V_1. (A short P-R interval unrelated to acute pericarditis is also present.) Depression of the PR segment, an electrocardiographic abnormality that is common in patients with acute pericarditis, is not evident because of the short P-R interval.

the lower left sternal border. The single-component rub is the least common but is likely to be the auscultatory finding in patients with atrial fibrillation.

An important feature of the pericardial friction rub is that it is often evanescent and may change in quality from one examination to the next. Detection of the rub is aided by listening with the stethoscope diaphragm applied firmly to the chest at the lower left sternal border during inspiration and full expiration with the patient sitting up and leaning forward. Occasionally, rubs may be detected with the patient lying supine with arms extended above the head during inspiration or suspended respiration. The single-component pericardial friction rub may be mistaken for a systolic murmur or tricuspid or mitral regurgitation. A pericardial rub may also be confused with the crunch of air in the mediastinum or the artifact of skin scratching against the stethoscope. Pericardial friction rubs may be differentiated from murmurs by (1) the use of exercise to permit detection of a classic three-component rub, (2) the failure of a rub to radiate widely or to vary in timing and duration with inspiration or a change in posture in a manner characteristic of regurgitant murmurs, and (3) by the confirmatory finding of typical electrocardiographic and echocardiographic changes of pericarditis.

ELECTROCARDIOGRAM (see also p. 158). Serial electrocardiograms are extremely helpful in confirming the diagnosis of acute pericarditis. Electrocardiographic changes can occur a few hours or days after the onset of pericardial pain, and the electrocardiographic diagnosis of acute pericarditis is made by detecting the serial appearance of four stages of abnormalities of the ST segments and T waves (Fig. 45-4).[47,48] The etiology of these changes is believed to be related to an actual current of injury caused by superficial myocardial inflammation or epicardial injury. There are four stages in the evolution of acute pericarditis (Table 45-3). Stage I electrocardiographic changes accompany the onset of chest pain and are virtually diagnostic of acute pericarditis. These comprise ST-segment elevation, which, unlike the pattern of ST-segment elevation in acute myocardial infarction, is concave upward and usually present in all leads except aVr and V1. The T waves are usually upright in the leads with ST-segment elevation. The ST-segment axis in the frontal plane also differs in these two conditions and is reported to range from 30 to 60 degrees in acute pericarditis, unlike acute anterior myocardial infarction in which the ST-segment axis varies from 100 to 120 degrees.[49] Stage II occurs several days later and represents the return of ST segments to baseline, accompanied by T-wave flattening. This change in the ST segments usually occurs prior to the appearance of T-wave inversion. In contrast, T waves in acute myocardial infarction often become inverted before the ST segments return to baseline. Stage III is characterized by inversion of the T waves so that the T-wave vector becomes directed opposite to the ST-segment vector. T-wave inversion is generally present in most leads and is not associated with the loss of R-wave voltage or the appearance of Q waves. These features help to differentiate this stage of nonspecific T-wave inversion from changes associated with the evoiution of transmural or subendocardial myocardial infarction. Stage IV represents the reversion of T-wave changes to normal, which may occur up to weeks or months later. T-wave inversion may occasionally persist indefinitely in patients with chronic pericardial inflammation due to tuberculosis, uremia, or neoplastic pericardial disease.

Electrocardiographic abnormalities appear in about 90 per cent of cases of acute pericarditis,[47,50] and the finding of typical Stage I changes or a classic evolution of all four stages can be diagnostic even when other clinical features of pericarditis are misleading. All four stages are detected in about 50 per cent of patients with acute pericarditis. In addition, depression of the PR segment occurs in about 80 per cent of patients with acute pericarditis.[47] Depression of the PR segment occurs during the early stages of ST-segment elevation or T-wave inversion, is usually present in both limb and precordial leads, and may reflect abnormal atrial repolarization due to atrial inflammation.

TABLE 45-3 FOUR-STAGE ("TYPICAL") ECG EVOLUTION OF ACUTE PERICARDITIS

SEQUENCE	LEADS OF "EPICARDIAL" DERIVATION (I, II, aV_L, aV_F, V_{3-6})			LEADS REFLECTING "ENDOCARDIAL" POTENTIAL aV_R, OFTEN V_1, SOMETIMES V_2		
Stage	J-ST*	T Waves	PR Segment	ST Segment	T Waves	PR Segment
I	Elevated	Upright	Depressed or isoelectric	Depressed	Inverted	Elevated or isoelectric
II early	Isoelectric	Upright	Isoelectric or depressed	Isoelectric	Inverted	Isoelectric or elevated
II late	Isoelectric	Low to flat to inverted	Isoelectric or depressed	Isoelectric	Shallow to flat to upright	Isoelectric or elevated
III	Isoelectric	Inverted	Isoelectric	Isoelectric	Upright	Isoelectric
IV	Isoelectric	Upright	Isoelectric	Isoelectric	Inverted	Isoelectric

* J-ST = junction of S (or T) wave with the end of the QRS complex.
Modified from Spodick, D. H.: Electrocardiographic changes in acute pericarditis. Am. J. Cardiol. *33*:470, 1974.

Variations of the patterns already described are present in slightly less than 50 per cent of patients with pericarditis and include (1) isolated PR-segment depression, (2) the absence of one or more stages of the ST-segment and T-wave changes, (3) evolution of Stage I (ST-segment elevation) directly to Stage IV (reversion of T waves to normal), (4) persistence of T-wave inversion, (5) appearance of ST-segment changes in only a few leads, (6) the appearance of marked T-wave inversion before the ST segments returned to baseline, and (7) the absence of any serial electrocardiographic changes whatsoever.[51] Regional ST-segment deviation may be confused with electrocardiographic changes of regional myocardial ischemia. ST-segment elevation in the right precordial leads has been described in acute pericarditis.[52] The frequency of acute right precordial ST-segment elevation in acute pericarditis has not been systematically studied, and this finding could cause confusion with acute right ventricular infarction.

In addition to the features already described that help to distinguish the ST-segment changes of pericarditis from those of acute myocardial infarction, the changes of Stage I must also be differentiated from the electrocardiographic variant of normal early repolarization (p. 117).[53] This pattern is usually seen in young males, in whom the clinical syndrome of pain and dyspnea suggesting acute pericarditis is absent; PR-segment depression is occasionally present but is uncommon, and most importantly, the electrocardiogram does not evolve through a pattern of the return of ST segments to baseline followed by T-wave inversion. An ST-segment/T wave ratio greater than 0.25 in lead V_6 also appears to discriminate patients with acute pericarditis from those with the normal variant of early repolarization.[54]

Sinus tachycardia is common and may be present in the absence of other contributing factors, such as fever or hemodynamic compromise.[55] Other atrial arrhythmias are infrequent in uncomplicated acute pericarditis and suggest the presence of underlying heart disease.[56] Atrioventricular block, bundle branch block, and ventricular tachycardia are not features of acute pericarditis, and these findings suggest the presence of extensive myocardial inflammation, fibrosis, or acute ischemia.

THE CHEST ROENTGENOGRAM. This is of little diagnostic value in uncomplicated acute pericarditis. If acute pericarditis is complicated by the appearance of a large pericardial effusion, the chest roentgenogram may show both enlargement and changes in configuration of the cardiac silhouette. The chest roentgenogram may provide clues to the underlying etiology of the pericarditis, as in the case of pericarditis secondary to tuberculosis, or malignant disease. Pleural effusions occur in about one-fourth of patients with pericarditis and are usually left-sided in contrast to patients with heart failure in whom right pleural effusions predominate.[50,57] The echocardiogram is at present the most sensitive and accurate tool in the detection and quantification of pericardial fluid and is discussed on pages 102 and 103.

RADIONUCLIDE SCANS. Technetium 99m pyrophosphate scans[58] and gallium radionuclide scans have also been reported to be useful in detecting acute pericarditis,[59] but their sensitivity and specificity have not been clearly established.

BLOOD TESTS. Acute pericarditis is often associated with nonspecific indicators of inflammation, including leukocytosis and elevation of the sedimentation rate. Cardiac isoenzymes are usually normal, but modest elevation of the MB fraction of creatine phosphokinase may occur in the presence of epicardial inflammation accompanying acute pericarditis.[60] For this reason, cardiac isoenzymes cannot always be used to differentiate between acute pericarditis and acute myocardial infarction, particularly non Q-wave infarction.

Based on the history, including recent travel, physical examination, and clinical setting, some patients may require more extensive diagnostic tests to clarify the possibility of an underlying systemic disease. Because of the serious consequences of missing the diagnosis of tuberculous pericarditis, screening for tuberculosis with a tuberculin skin test and a control skin test to exclude anergy is reasonable for patients with acute pericarditis in geographic areas and in patient populations with a low pretest risk of having a positive tuberculin skin test.

Other diagnostic tests that may be indicated in individual patients are based on the clinical presentation: (1) blood cultures to exclude associated possible infective endocarditis and bacteremia; (2) acute and convalescent cultures of blood, urine, throat, and feces, if available from the hospital laboratory, to evaluate a suspected viral etiology; (3) HIV test to evaluate the possibility of acquired immunodeficiency syndrome and unusual pathogens in patients with a compatible clinical syndrome; (4) fungal serological tests to evaluate a suspected fungal etiology in patients from endemic areas or in immunocompromised patients; (5) ASO titer in children with suspected rheumatic fever; (6) cold agglutinins to exclude a mycoplasma etiology; (7) heterophile antibody test to exclude mononucleosis; (8) immunofluorescent antibody titers for toxoplasmosis; (9) TSH, T4, and T3 to exclude hypothyroidism; (10) BUN and creatinine to exclude uremic etiology; and (11) antinuclear antibody titer (ANA) and rheumatoid factor, to exclude systemic lupus erythematosus and rheumatoid arthritis.

AORTIC DISSECTION. In middle-aged and elderly patients, close attention should be paid to the history, chest roentgenogram, and echocardiogram for evidence of prior aortic dissection, since subacute inflammatory pericarditis following the slow penetration of blood into the pericardial space can be the initial presentation of aortic dissection.[61]

PERICARDIOCENTESIS AND PERICARDIAL BIOPSY. The issue of the additional diagnostic yields of pericardiocentesis or pericardial biopsy has been addressed by a prospective study of 231 patients with acute pericarditis of inapparent cause.[62] Noninvasive clinical and laboratory studies as described above were done in all patients, while diagnostic pericardiocentesis was done if clinical illnesss and an effusion lasted more than 1 week, and diagnostic biopsy was done if clinical illness lasted more than 3 weeks. This strategy yielded a diagnosis in 14 per cent of patients, which in the majority warranted specific therapy (bacterial pericarditis, tuberculosis, toxoplasmosis, unsuspected malignant disease). The diagnostic yield was substantial when pericardiocentesis or pericardiectomy with biopsy was done to relieve cardiac tamponade (39 and 54 per cent, respectively), and only 5 per cent when these procedures were done only for diagnostic reasons. This experience suggests that there is a higher likelihood of establishing an etiologic diagnosis in patients who develop cardiac tamponade than in those with uncomplicated acute pericarditis, and therapeutic pericardiocentesis or pericardiectomy should always be accompanied by a rigorous examination of fluid or tissue for occult malignant disease or infection. In the immunocompetent patient with uncomplicated acute pericarditis who does not have cardiac tamponade, diagnostic pericardiocentesis or biopsy has a very low yield and is not justified. Pericardiocentesis should be performed for diagnostic reasons in the absence of cardiac tamponade only in patients in whom there is an urgent need to confirm a diagnosis of suspected purulent pericarditis.

MANAGEMENT. The first step in the management of acute pericarditis consists of establishing whether the pericarditis is related to an underlying problem that requires specific therapy. Nonspecific therapy of an initial episode of pericarditis should include bed rest until pain and fever have disappeared, since activity may cause worsening of symptoms. Initial observation in the hospital is warranted for almost all patients with acute pericarditis to exclude an associated myocardial infarction or a pyogenic process and to watch for the development of tamponade, which occurs in about 15 per cent of patients with acute pericarditis.[62]

The pain of pericarditis usually responds to nonsteroidal antiinflammatory agents such as aspirin (650 mg orally every 3 to 4 hours) or indomethacin (25 to 50 mg orally 4 times daily). When pain is severe and does not respond to this therapy within 48 hours, corticosteroids may be employed. If prednisone is used, large doses, such as 60 to 80 mg daily in divided doses, should be given. After 5 to 7 days, if the patient has been free of symptoms for several days, antiinflammatory agents should be tapered. Owing to the adverse consequence of long-term steroid therapy, it is desirable to avoid their use for pain control whenever possible. When long-term steroid administration is needed to control pain and other evidence of inflammation, alternate-day therapy should be attempted. Patients in whom steroids cannot be discontinued may tolerate tapering of steroids and weaning to nonsteroidal antiinflammatory agents.

Antibiotics should be used only to treat documented purulent pericarditis. Oral anticoagulants should not be administered during the acute phase of pericarditis of any cause. If anticoagulants must be continued owing to the presence of a mechanical prosthetic heart valve, we recommend use of intravenous heparin, the action of which can be promptly reversed with protamine, and both physical examination and echocardiography should be performed at regular intervals to watch closely for the development of a pericardial effusion under pressure.

NATURAL HISTORY. Viral pericarditis, idiopathic pericarditis, post-myocardial infarction pericarditis, or the post-pericardiotomy syndrome are usually self-limited; clinical and laboratory signs of inflammation abate after 2 to 6 weeks. Sagrista-Sauleda et al.[63] have observed, by physical examination and noninvasive recordings, that about 9 per cent of patients with acute idiopathic pericarditis and pericardial effusion develop signs of mild cardiac constriction within the first 30 days after onset of the illness when signs of acute pericarditis and the effusion have already abated. These findings spontaneously disappear within 3 months and indicate that the development of transient constrictive physiology may occur during the resolution of acute pericardial inflammation.

The most troublesome complication is the development of recurrent episodes of pericardial inflammation at intervals of weeks or months after the initial episode. In two series of patients with acute pericarditis, between 20 and 28 per cent of patients experienced recurrent episodes of pericarditis with severe chest pain.[50,63] The majority of patients can be managed by reinstitution of high-dose nonsteroidal antiinflammatory agents and very gradual tapering over several months to discontinuation or alternate-dose therapy. In rare patients, disabling chest pain associated with fever may recur over a period of years and require steroid administration for pain relief.[64] Pericardiectomy has been proposed for the relief of refractory relapsing pericarditis,[65] but pericardiectomy is not always followed by relief of pain.[64,66]

Pericarditis can also be complicated by the development of disabling or life-threatening hemodynamic complications due to cardiac compression. These include (1) the development of pericardial effusion under pressure, resulting in cardiac tamponade; (2) the development of fibrosis and/or calcification of the pericardium, resulting in chronic constrictive physiology; and (3) a combination of both effusive and constrictive pericardial disease.

Pericardial Effusion

Pericardial effusion may develop as a response to injury of the parietal pericardium with all causes of acute pericarditis. It may be clinically silent, but if the accumulation of fluid causes intrapericardial pressure to increase, resulting in cardiac compression, the symptoms of cardiac tamponade develop. The development of increased intrapericardial pressure secondary to pericardial effusion depends on several factors: (1) the absolute volume of the effusion, (2) the rate of fluid accumulation, and (3) the physical characteristics of the pericardium itself. The pericardial space in humans normally contains between 15 and 50 ml of fluid. If additional fluid accumulates slowly, the pericardium stretches; the pericardial sac can accommodate up to 2 liters without elevation of intrapericardial pressure. However, the normal unstretched pericardial sac can accommodate the rapid addition of only 80 to 200 ml of fluid and still remain on the flat portion of the curve relating intrapericaridial pressure and volume (Fig. 45–2). If additional fluid is rapidly added to a volume exceeding about 150 to 200 ml, a marked rise of intrapericardial pressure occurs. Intrapericardial pressure may also increase markedly after the accumulation of a smaller amount of fluid if the pericardium is excessively stiff because of fibrosis or tumor infiltration.

PERICARDIAL EFFUSION WITHOUT CARDIAC COMPRESSION

HISTORY. Patients who develop pericardial effusion without elevation of intrapericardial pressure may have no symptoms whatsoever. Occasionally these patients complain of a constant oppressive dull ache or pressure in the chest. Large pericardial effusions may cause symptoms by mechanical compression of adjacent structures, including dysphagia from esophageal compression, cough due to bronchial/tracheal compression, dyspnea from lung compression with subsequent atelectasis, hiccups due to phrenic nerve compression, or hoarseness due to recurrent laryngeal nerve compression. Nausea and a sense of abdominal fullness may be present from pressure on adjacent abdominal viscera.

PHYSICAL EXAMINATION. A small pericardial effusion in the absence of an increase in intrapericardial pressure may result in no specific physical findings, whereas a large effusion may produce several characteristic physical findings. First, the heart sounds may be muffled owing to the interposition of fluid between the chest wall and the cardiac chambers. Compression of the base of the left lung by pericardial fluid produces Ewart's sign, i.e., a patch of dullness on auscultation beneath the angle of the left scapula. Rales may be heard over the lung fields secondary to compression of lung parenchyma. Abnormalities of the arterial pulse, systemic blood pressure, and jugular venous pulse do not occur when a large pericardial effusion is present without significant elevation of the intrapericardial pressure.

CHEST ROENTGENOGRAM. Enlargement of the cardiac silhouette usually does not occur until at least 250 ml of fluid have accumulated in the pericardial space. Therefore, a normal or unchanged chest roentgenogram does not exclude the presence of a hemodynamically important pericardial effusion. This examination may suggest the presence of a percardial effusion if there is a rapid increase in the size of the cardiac silhouette in the presence of clear lung fields. In some cases the heart may assume a globular or water-bottle shape, blurring the contours along the left cardiac border and obscuring the hilar vessels. Loculated effusions may have a cyst-like appearance (Fig. 45–5).

The parietal pericardial and epicardial fat layers are normally separated by 1 to 2 mm. The presence of effusion may result in more marked separation of the pericardial fat lines,

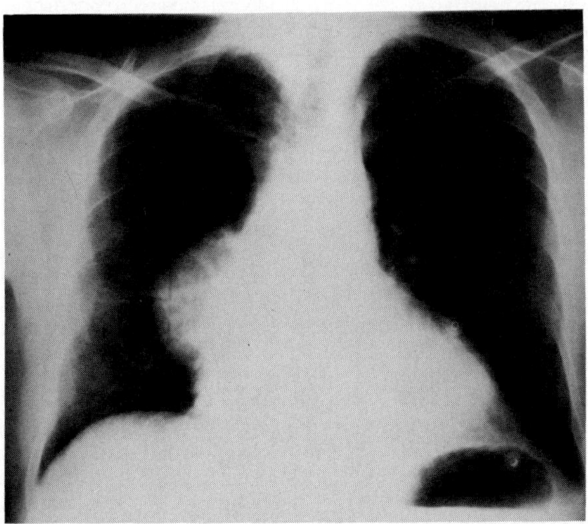

FIGURE 45–5. Posteroanterior chest roentgenogram from a patient with recurrent pericarditis and a loculated pericardial effusion that was subsequently drained surgically. In this patient, the loculated pericardial effusion simulated the roentgenographic appearance of a pericardial cyst.

apparent on high-quality frontal or lateral chest films in about 25 per cent of patients with pericardial effusions.[67] Fluoroscopy may reveal the absence of or weak pulsations and the absence of any changes in the size and shape of the cardiac silhouette during inspiration. These findings are especially useful in the cardiac catheterization laboratory when perforation of the heart is suspected. Computed tomography (p. 317) has also been used to image pericardial effusions, and magnetic resonance imaging (p. 327) can identify effusions, characterize an effusion as hemorrhagic, differentiate fluid from epicardial fat, and delineate other pathology including pericardial thickening and intrapericardial masses[68] (Fig. 11–31, p. 328).

ELECTROCARDIOGRAM. The electrocardiogram may reveal the nonspecific findings of a reduction in QRS voltage and flattening of the T waves as fluid accumulates within the pericardial space.[69] Electrical alternans suggests the presence of massive pericardial effusion and cardiac tamponade.

ECHOCARDIOGRAPHY (see also p. 102). This is the most accurate, rapid, and widely used technique for evaluating pericardial effusion, in following the accumulation or resolution of fluid over time, and in assessing the functional status of the cardiac valves and myocardium. Recognition of pericardial fluid depends on the acoustical differences among the pericardium, cardiac muscle, and pericardial fluid. Accumulation of pericardial fluid results in the appearance of an echo-free space between the posterior left ventricular wall and posterior parietal pericardium and between the anterior wall of the right ventricle and adjacent echoes of the parietal pericardium and chest wall. Posterior and anterior epicardial fat can simulate this echocardiographic appearance of pericardial effusion. M-mode echocardiography appears to be sufficiently sensitive to detect as little as 20 ml of pericardial fluid.[70]

The incidence of small pericardial effusions detected by echocardiography in asymptomatic subjects ranges between 8 and 15 per cent.[71,72] In normal pregnant women, a substantial subset (43 per cent) has been found to have asymptomatic pericardial effusions that resolve within the first weeks after delivery.[72]

Although the quantification of pericardial effusions by echocardiography is not precise, several guidelines of assessment are helpful. Very small effusions are likely to be imaged only posteriorly, with separation of the pericardial and epicardial echoes only in systole. Small-to-moderate-sized effusions are likely to be imaged only posteriorly, with the presence of an echo-free space throughout the cardiac cycle. Pericardial effusions of approximately 300 ml can usually be imaged both anteriorly and posteriorly. Moderate to large effusions may be associated with excessive swinging motion of the heart and the false-positive appearance of mitral valve prolapse and anterior septal motion. Usually, the echo-free space representing a pericardial effusion disappears behind the left atrium owing to the absence of fluid in the oblique pericardial sinus. However, in massive effusions, fluid may also collect in the oblique sinus, resulting in an echo-free space behind the left atrium as well as the left ventricle.

M-mode echocardiography is usually adequate to diagnose pericardial effusion, but occasionally the diagnosis may be confused with a left pleural effusion, giant left atrium, pulmonary infiltrate, or retrograde hiatal hernia. Two-dimensional echocardiography is particularly useful in identifying a loculated pericardial effusion.[73] Blood in the pericardial space can often be differentiated from an effusion of lower acoustical density, and two-dimensional echocardiography is useful in identifying rapidly the presence of hemopericardium with or without thrombus formation secondary to cardiac invasive procedures.[74]

MANAGEMENT. The clinical signficance of any pericardial effusion depends on (1) the presence or absence of hemodynamic embarrassment due to increased intrapericardial pressure and (2) the presence and nature of the underlying systemic disease. The use of echocardiography to establish the diagnosis of pericardial effusion is warranted in suspected cases of acute pericarditis, since the presence of effusion is suggestive, although not diagnostic, of pericardial inflammation. Pericardiocentesis (p. 1490) is not indicated unless there is evidence of cardiac compression due to cardiac tamponade or unless analysis of pericardial fluid is necessary to establish a diagnosis such as acute bacterial pericarditis.

CHRONIC PERICARDIAL EFFUSION

Chronic pericardial effusions persisting for more than 6 months may occur in any form of pericardial disease. Often they are surprisingly well tolerated, with no symptoms of cardiac compression, and are discovered when a routine chest roentgenogram discloses an unexpectedly large cardiac silhouette. Chronic pericardial effusions are particularly likely to be found in patients with previous idiopathic or viral pericarditis, uremic pericaditis, and pericarditis secondary to myxedema or neoplasm. Chronic pericardial effusions can also occur in association with ascites and pleural effusions in the setting of chronic salt and water retention of many causes, including chronic heart failure, nephrotic syndrome, and hepatic cirrhosis.[75] Massive idiopathic chronic pericardial effusion is reported to be the initial presentation in about 3 per cent of patients with primary pericardial disease, with predominance in women.[76] The management of chronic pericardial effusion depends in part on the etiology, and occult hypothyroidism should always be excluded. Stable and apparently idiopathic effusions in asymptomatic patients usually require no specific treatment except for avoidance of anticoagulants.

PERICARDIAL EFFUSION WITH CARDIAC COMPRESSION: CARDIAC TAMPONADE

An increase in intrapericardial pressure secondary to fluid accumulation within the pericardial space results in cardiac tamponade, which is characterized by (1) elevation of intracardiac pressures, (2) progressive limitation of ventricular diastolic filling, and (3) reduction of stroke volume and cardiac output.

PATHOPHYSIOLOGY

When intrapericardial pressure is measured using a conventional fluid-filled catheter, usually it is quite close to intrapleural pressure and several millimeters of mercury lower than right and left ventricular diastolic pressures. As already noted (p. 1466), recent studies using special catheters with closed flat balloons indicate that the *constraint* pressure exerted by the normal pericardium is very close to right atrial pressure.[13] However, this controversy regarding the accurate measurement of normal pericardial pressure does not limit the use of fluid-filled catheters in patients with cardiac tamponade, because intrapericardial pressure can be accurately measured by either technique once about 50 ml of free fluid is present in the pericardial space. When the addition of fluid into the pericardial space causes intrapericardial pressure to rise to the level of the right atrial and right ventricular diastolic pressures, the transmural pressure distending these chambers declines to close to zero and cardiac tamponade occurs. The rise of right atrial and intrapericardial pressures is less marked in the presence of hypovolemia, and therefore cardiac tamponade may be masked when hypovolemia is present. Further accumulation of intrapericardial fluid causes both intrapericardial and right ventricular diastolic pressures to rise together to the level of left ventricular diastolic pressure, and all three pressures subsequently rise together in association with a fall in systemic arterial pressure. If left ventricular diastolic pressure is markedly elevated owing to preexisting left ventricular disease, cardiac tamponade occurs when right atrial and right ventricular diastolic and pericardial pressures equalize but at a lower level than the left ventricular diastolic pressure.[77]

CONSEQUENCES OF CARDIAC TAMPONADE. Equalization of intrapericardial and ventricular filling pressures results in markedly diminished transmural distending pressures and diastolic volumes of both ventricles and a fall in stroke volume.[78,79] The reduction in stroke volume is initially compensated for by reflex increases in adrenergic tone; both tachycardia and increases in ejection fraction initially help to maintain forward cardiac output.[78] The importance of the adrenergic support of the heart is reflected in the finding that when beta-adrenergic blockade is carried out in cardiac tamponade, ejection fraction and stroke volume decline.[80] Systemic vascular resistance increases so that, at first, systemic arterial pressure is maintained at the expense of cardiac output. Acute increases in pericardial volume and pressure also reflexly induce a marked decrease in urinary sodium excretion,[81] associated with the inhibition of release of atrial natriuretic factor.[82] With severe cardiac tamponade, as cardiac output declines, compensatory mechanisms are no longer sufficient to maintain systemic arterial pressure, and perfusion of vital organs becomes impaired; reduced coronary perfusion causes selective hypoperfusion of the subendocardium.[83] The superimposition of myocardial ischemia during cardiac tamponade could further compromise left ventricular stroke volume. In extreme cardiac tamponade, transmural diastolic ventricular pressures may actually be less than zero, suggesting that ventricular filling occurs by diastolic suction.[84] Sinus bradycardia, mediated by the cardiac depressor branches of the vagus nerve and by the nonvagal mechanism of sinoatrial node ischemia, may also occur during severe cardiac tamponade.[85] Profound bradycardia often occurs during severe hypotension and precedes the development of electrical-mechanical dissociation and death.

Cardiac tamponade also alters the dynamics of systemic venous return and cardiac filling. Normally, one surge of systemic venous return occurs during ventricular ejection coincident with the systolic x descent of the venous pressure pulse, and a second surge occurs during right atrial emptying with the opening of the tricuspid valve in diastole, corresponding to the *y* descent. In cardiac tamponade, the heart is compressed throughout the cardiac cycle. During ejection, intracardiac volume decreases, resulting in a transient fall in both intrapericardial and right atrial pressures, manifest as the x descent, which is accompanied by a surge of systemic venous return into the right atrium. However, in early diastole the total volume within the pericardial space remains elevated despite opening of the tricuspid valve; intrapericardial pressure remains elevated and equal to or exceeds early diastolic right atrial pressure so that transmural distending pressure is close to zero or negative. As a result, the usual surge of systemic venous return during early diastole is abolished, right atrial emptying is impeded, and the right atrium is compressed or partially collapsed during diastole. These events are graphically reflected in the right atrial or systemic venous waveform in cardiac tamponade, in that the systolic x descent is prominent while the early diastolic y descent is usually completely absent or attenuated.

REGIONAL TAMPONADE. The individual chambers of the heart resist external compressive force differently, and the magnitude of hemodynamic deterioration during cardiac tamponade critically depends on the specific region of the heart that is compressed during diastole. Fowler and Gable[86] studied regional cardiac tamponade in dogs and showed that isolated tamponade of the right or left ventricle has little hemodynamic effect and that a substantial fall in cardiac output and aortic pressure occurs only when the atria (and intrapericardial veins) are also compressed. A subsequent study of regional tamponade in dogs has shown that right atrial and right ventricular compression causes greater depression of cardiac output and aortic pressure than does left heart compression.[87] In patients with cardiac tamponade, compression of the right heart chambers is likely to be more important than left atrial compression, since pericardial fluid is often not present behind the left atrium during cardiac tamponade, and echocardiographic studies of patients with cardiac tamponade indicate that the presence of left atrial and left ventricular diastolic collapse is variable.[88] For the normal thin-walled right atrium and right ventricle, the critical buckling pressure consists of a negative transmural pressure of only 0.05 to 0.1 mm Hg.[12] This critical difference between pericardial and right atrial or right ventricular diastolic pressure can occur when pericardial pressure is lower than that of the thick-walled left ventricle, whereas right ventricular collapse may be absent in the presence of severe right ventricular hypertrophy.[89]

RIGHT ATRIAL AND VENTRICULAR COLLAPSE. During the development of tamponade, collapse of the right atrium and right ventricle initially occurs only in early diastole in association with delayed diastolic filling of the right ventricle and a modest fall in cardiac output without hypotension or overt hemodynamic deterioration (Fig. 45–6)[89,90] Pandiastolic right atrial and ventricular buckling occurs when pericardial pressure equals or exceeds right atrial and ventricular pressures throughout diastole so that the ventricles may fill only during atrial systole. This stage is accompanied by a severe reduction in ventricular volumes, a failure of compensatory mechanisms, and hypotension.[89,90] In this setting, pulsus alternans may occur because of beat-to-beat variation in right ventricular output and left ventricular filling.[90] During hypovolemia with low right heart pressures, right ventricular collapse occurs at low intrapericardial pressures while volume expansion delays the development of right ventricular diastolic collapse and hemodynamic deterioration until a higher intrapericardial pressure is achieved.[90,91] Singh et al.[92] have obtained simultaneous hemodynamics and two-dimensional echocardiographic measurements in patients undergoing pericardiocentesis and have shown that hemodynamic improvement first occurs at the point of disappearance of right ventricular diastolic collapse, which is followed by the subsequent disappearance of right atrial collapse and further improvement in cardiac output during continued pericardiocentesis.

PULSUS PARADOXUS. Inspiration and the transmission of negative intrathoracic pressure to the pericardial space further alter the dynamics of right and left ventricular filling and are responsible for pulsus paradoxus, the inspiratory fall of aortic systolic pressure greater than 10 mm Hg (Fig. 45–7). The finding of weakening of the arterial pulse during inspiration was described by Kussmaul in 1873 as the apparent *paradox* of the disappearance of the pulse during inspiration despite persistence of the heartbeat. It should be emphasized that pulsus paradoxus is in fact an exaggeration of the normal inspiratory decline of left ventricular stroke volume by about 7 per cent and of systemic arterial pressure by 3 per cent.[93] Inspiration is normally accompanied by an increase in diastolic dimensions of the right ventricle, a small decrease in left ventricular di-

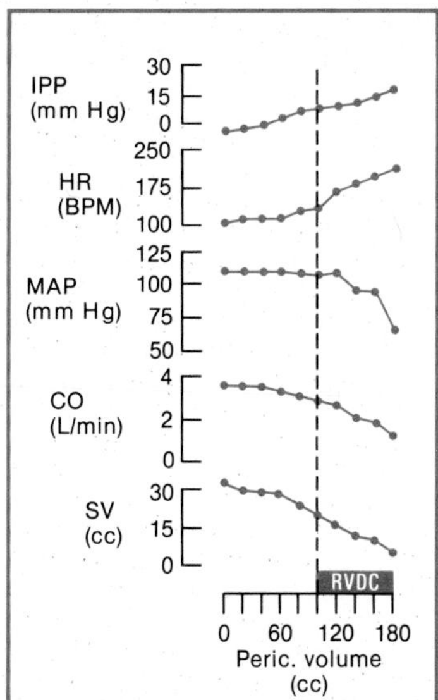

FIGURE 45–6. Hemodynamic measurements from a dog with experimental cardiac tamponade in which two-dimensional echocardiograms showed right ventricular diastolic collapse (RVDC). Mean intrapericardial pressure (IPP) continuously rose as pericardial volume increased, accompanied by a progressive decline of stroke volume (SV). At the time RVDC was first detected, mean arterial pressure (MAP) was well preserved, cardiac output (CO) had only modestly declined, and a compensatory increase in heart rate (HR) was present. Mean arterial pressure fell rapidly late in the course of cardiac tamponade in the decompensated phase. (From Leimgruber, P. P., et al.: The hemodynamic derangement associated with right ventricular diastolic collapse in cardiac tamponade: An experimental echocardiographic study. Circulation 68:612, 1983, by permission of the American Heart Association, Inc.)

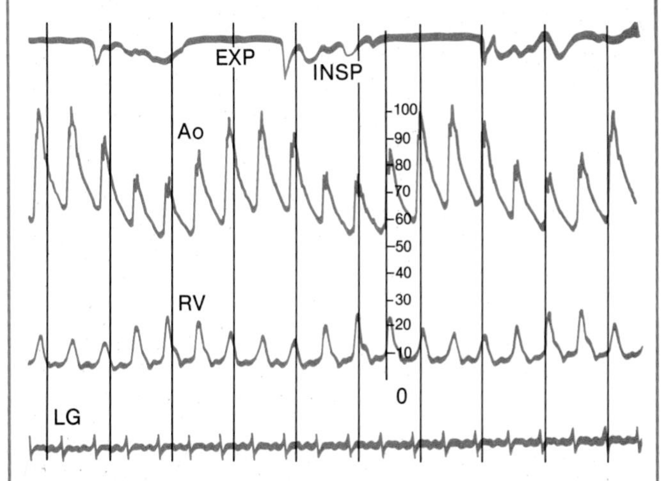

FIGURE 45-7. Recording of aortic (Ao) and right ventricular (RV) pressures in a patient with cardiac tamponade complicated by hypovolemia. Pulsus paradoxus is evident as a marked inspiratory decline in aortic systolic and pulse pressures during inspiration (INSP). RV pressure variation is out of phase with aortic pressure. Note that the RV waveform does not show a dip-and-plateau configuration. (From Shabetai, R., et al.: The hemodynamics of cardiac tamponade and constrictive pericarditis. Am. J. Cardiol. *26*:480, 1970.)

mension, and increased velocity of flow from the venae cavae into the right atrium.[94,95] Pulsus paradoxus in cardiac tamponade appears to result from an exaggeration of these normal findings.

Measurement of intracardiac pressures and flow during experimental tamponade[96] and in humans during cardiac tamponade[93,97] have demonstrated that inspiration causes a decrease in intrapericardial and right atrial pressures. This results in augmentation of flow from the venae cavae into the right atrium and right ventricle and augmentation of pulmonary artery flow and pulmonary artery systolic pressure. The increase in venous return flow during inspiration results in a marked and exaggerated increase in right ventricular dimensions accompanied by a reduction in left ventricular dimensions and flattening and displacement of the septum toward the left ventricle.[98] On the left side of the heart, left atrial and left ventricular diastolic pressures fall, accompanied by a fall in aortic flow and systolic arterial pressure. Thus, *pulsus paradoxus in cardiac tamponade is critically dependent on the inspiratory augmentation of systemic venous return and right ventricular filling.*

Shabetai et al. demonstrated that when experimental cardiac tamponade was induced in dogs, pulsus paradoxus did not develop when either the right heart was bypassed or right ventricular volume was strictly controlled.[96] These experiments also demonstrated that traction on the heart by the diaphragm was not an essential mechanism. These observations indicate that pulsus paradoxus in cardiac tamponade depends on the inspiratory expansion of right-heart filling at the expense of left-heart filling (Fig. 45-8).

The importance of respiratory preload variation is supported by recent observations in patients with cardiac tamponade that showed that left ventricular transmural diastolic pressure falls to or below zero during inspiration.[12] An additional factor that may contribute to the inspiratory fall of left ventricular stroke volume and systolic arterial pressure is a transient reduction in the gradient between the pulmonary venous circulation and the left heart during inspiration causing inspiratory pooling of blood in the lungs (Fig. 45-9).[99] Also the underfilled left ventricle may be operating on the steep ascending limb of the Starling curve so that any inspiratory reduction of left ventricular filling results in marked depression of left ventricular stroke volume and systolic pressure.[100] Pulsus paradoxus is occasionally observed in constrictive pericarditis and restrictive heart disease, and the latter mechanisms may account for its presence in these disorders.

Pulsus paradoxus has also been observed in severe lung disease and massive pulmonary embolism.[101,102] Under these circumstances, pulsus paradoxus is probably related to the transmission of excessively negative intrathoracic pressure during inspiration to the aorta, inspiratory pooling of right ventricular stroke volume in the lungs, and exaggerated right-heart filling with an associated decrease in left-heart filling during inspiration. Pulsus paradoxus may be absent in cardiac tamponade when left ventricular hypertrophy or heart failure causes a marked elevation of left ventricular diastolic pressure so that the two ventricles are unequally compressed. This may occur in atrial septal defect when the increase in systemic venous return during inspiration is shared between the two sides of the heart, and in aortic regurgitation when there is a major component of left ventricular filling that is independent of respiratory variation.[77,103] Pulsus paradoxus may also be absent in the presence of pulmonary hypertension and right ventricular hypertrophy that impedes the inspiratory increase in right ventricular filling; in this unusual clinical situation, the depression of left ventricular diastolic filling and cardiac outcome may depend on regional compression of the left ventricle.[104]

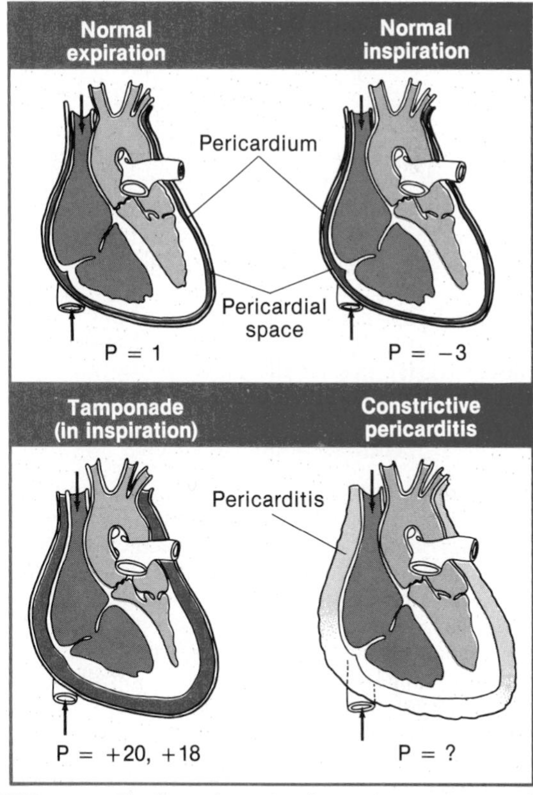

FIGURE 45-8. The hemodynamic effects of respiration. In the normal heart *(upper panel),* inspiration results in a fall in intrathoracic and intrapericardial pressure from +1 to −3 mm Hg, which causes an increase in venous return (heavy black arrows) and a slight increase in right ventricular size at the expense of a slight decrease in left ventricular size due to displacement of the interventricular septum from right to left. During cardiac tamponade *(lower left panel),* inspiration causes a fall in the elevated intrapericardial pressure from +20 to +18 mm Hg. Although both the right and left heart volumes are diminished owing to compression by the pericardial effusion, the inspiratory fall in intrapericardial pressure results in an increase in venous return (heavy black arrow), an increase in right heart volume due to septal bulging, and a further decrease in left heart volume. In constrictive pericarditis *(lower right panel),* the inspiratory fall in intrathoracic pressure is not transmitted to the heart, since the pericardial space is obliterated. For this reason, there is minimal or no increase in venous return (light black arrows) during inspiration. (From Shabetai, R.: The Pericardium. New York, Grune & Stratton, 1981, p. 244.)

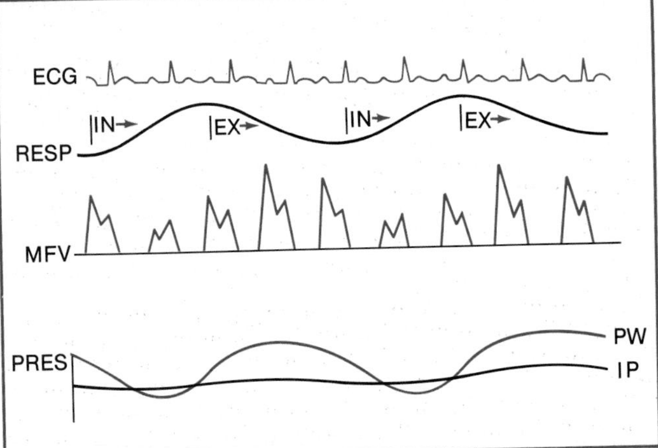

FIGURE 45–9. Relation between mitral flow velocity (MFV) and pericardial and pulmonary wedge pressures. The first beat after the onset of inspiration is associated with a reduced pressure gradient between the pulmonary venous circulation and intrapericardial (and left ventricular diastolic) pressures, which results in an abrupt reduction in mitral flow velocity, as shown, and an increase in tricuspid flow velocity. Opposite changes occur with the onset of expiration. ECG = electrocardiogram, RESP = respiratory phase determined by a nasal thermistor, IN = inspiration, EX = expiration, PRES = pressure, PW = pulmonary capillary wedge, IP = intrapericardial. (From Appleton, C. P., et al.: Cardiac tamponade and pericardial effusion: Respiratory variation in transvalvular flow velocities studied by Doppler echocardiography. J. Am. Coll. Cardiol. *11*:1020, 1988.)

ETIOLOGY

Cardiac tamponade may occur with almost any cause of pericarditis and may exist in either an acute or a chronic form. The distributions of the causes of acute cardiac tamponade in a city hospital between 1963 and 1980[105] and at our institution between 1984 and 1988 are noted in Table 45–4. In these contemporary series the most frequent causes of cardiac tamponade were neoplasm, idiopathic or viral pericarditis, and uremia, followed by pericarditis associated with myocardial infarction, invasive cardiac diagnostic procedures, purulent bacterial infection, and tuberculosis.

CLINICAL MANIFESTATIONS

The triad of (1) a decline in systemic aterial pressure; (2) elevation of systemic venous pressure; and (3) a small, quiet heart was described by the thoracic surgeon Claude S. Beck in 1935.[106] These three features are typical of cardiac tamponade from sudden intrapericardial hemorrhage due to penetrating heart wounds from trauma or invasive diagnostic cardiac procedures, aortic dissection, and intrapericardial rupture of an aortic or cardiac aneurysm. This syndrome develops when the pericardium is not enlarged or stretched, so that the addition of less than 200 ml of fluid or blood causes intrapericardial pressure to rise abruptly to above 20 to 30 mm Hg. In cases that are not immediately fatal, both cardiac output and arterial pressure fall, accompanied by tachycardia and tachypnea. The patient may be stuporous or agitated and restless, and the additional important finding of pulsus paradoxus may be difficult to appreciate when profound hypotension is present. Jugular venous pressure is usually markedly elevated. Precordial heart activity is usually not palpable, and heart sounds are distant or inaudible. Cold, clammy extremities and anuria may be present.

Patients in whom cardiac tamponade develops slowly differ from those with cardiac tamponade due to cardiac penetration or rupture. In the setting of more slowly developing cardiac tamponade, patients usually appear acutely ill but not in extremis, and the major complaint is usually dyspnea.[105] Studies of acute cardiac tamponade in dogs have shown that the elevation of intrapericardial pressure results in the accumulation of interstitial fluid without the development of alveolar edema or hypoxemia.[107] Thus the sensation of dyspnea experienced by many patients with cardiac tamponade may be due to lung stiffening from increased interstitial fluid that increases the work of breathing. Chest pain may also be present. In patients with chronic development of tamponade, additional systemic symptoms may include weight loss, anorexia, and profound weakness.

PHYSICAL EXAMINATION. Jugular venous distention was the most common physical finding in a series of 56 medical patients whose cardiac tamponade was diagnosed at the bedside.[105] In addition to absolute elevation of the systemic venous pressure, a characteristic waveform consisting of a prominent systolic x descent and absence of diastolic y descent can often be appreciated at the bedside. Other common physical findings include tachypnea (80 per cent), tachycardia (77 per cent), pulsus paradoxus (77 per cent), pulsus paradoxus with total inspiratory disappearance of the brachial pulse and Korotkoff sounds (23 per cent), pericardial friction rub (29 per cent), hepatomegaly (55 per cent), and diminished heart sounds (34 per cent). It is noteworthy that systolic arterial hypotension, consisting of a systolic pressure less than 100 mm Hg, was present in a minority (36 per cent), and the majority of patients were alert, with warm extremities and preservation of urine output.[105]

Pulsus Paradoxus (see p. 24). The finding of pulsus paradoxus is crucial in making the diagnosis of cardiac tamponade, since most patients with slowly developing cardiac tamponade do not have the classic physical findings of a small, quiet heart and severe hypotension. Pulsus paradoxus can be detected on physical examination as an inspiratory decrease in the amplitude of the palpated pulse in the femoral or carotid arteries. Total paradox, i.e., complete disappearance of the palpated pulse during inspiration, occurs during very severe cardiac tamponade or tamponade combined with hypovolemia. The magnitude of the paradoxical pulse can be accurately quantified by means of an intraarterial catheter but may be estimated by cuff sphygmomanometry. The cuff should be inflated 20 mm Hg above systolic pressure and slowly deflated until the Korotkoff sounds are heard only during expiration. The cuff should then be deflated to the point at which Korotkoff sounds are heard equally well in inspiration and expiration. The difference between these pressures is the estimated magnitude of pulsus paradoxus.

Other disorders with systemic venous distention, pulsus paradoxus, and clear lungs that can be confused with cardiac tamponade include obstructive pulmonary disease, constrictive pericarditis, restrictive cardiomyopathy, and massive pulmonary embolism. Pulsus paradoxus is occasionally noted

TABLE 45–4 COMMON CAUSES OF CARDIAC TAMPONADE

DISORDER	%	%
	1980	1988
Malignant disease	32	58
Idiopathic pericarditis	14	14
Uremia	9	14
Acute cardiac infarction (receiving heparin)	9	
Diagnostic procedures with cardiac perforation	7.5	
Bacterial	7.5	5
Tuberculosis	5	1
Radiation	4	
Myxedema	4	
Dissecting aortic aneurysm	4	
Postpericardiotomy syndrome	2	
Systemic lupus erythematosus	2	2
Cardiomyopathy (receiving anticoagulants)	2	6

Modified from Guberman, B. A., et al.: Cardiac tamponade in medical patients. Circulation 64:633, 1981, by permission of the American Heart Association, Inc., and from Levina, M. J., et al.: Implications of echocardiographically-assisted diagnosis of pericardial tamponade in contemporary medical patients. J. Am. Coll. Cardiol. 17: 59, 1991.

during severe hypovolemia due to hemorrhagic or septic shock, but jugular venous distention is usually absent.[108] Cardiac tamponade may be confused with shock due to right ventricular infarction with jugular venous distention and clear lungs.[42] However, the hemodynamics of right ventricular infarction are more like those of pericardial constriction than of tamponade (p. 1482).

LOW-PRESSURE TAMPONADE. The clinical findings may be further modified in patients with so-called *low-pressure cardiac tamponade* in whom jugular venous distention is absent and the right atrial pressure is low. This syndrome, which occurs in the setting of hypovolemia, represents an early stage in the development of cardiac tamponade in which accumulation of a pericardial effusion causes intrapericardial pressure to rise and equilibrate with low right heart diastolic filling pressures. Pericardiocentesis reduces intrapericardial pressure and causes the separation of right atrial and intrapericardial pressures. Low-pressure cardiac tamponade has been reported in patients with tuberculosis and neoplastic pericarditis complicated by severe dehydration.[109]

TENSION PNEUMOPERICARDIUM. This condition causes hemodynamic changes similar to those of acute hemorrhagic cardiac tamponade.[110] It is being increasingly recognized as a cause of cardiac tamponade with high mortality in infants during mechanical ventilation and in adults as a result of penetrating chest trauma, gastric and esophageal rupture, carcinomatous bronchopericardial fistula, gas production from contiguous infection, and diagnostic procedures such as sternal bone marrow aspiration.[110,111] Characteristic clinical findings include muffled heart sounds, bradycardia, and shifting tympany over the precordium. Unique auscultatory findings can be detected, including a metallic cracking sound, and the bruit de moulin, which was described in the first report of pneumopericardium in 1844 by Bricheteau as "the noise made by floats of a mill wheel as they strike the water,"[112] and which indicates the presence of both air and fluid in the pericardial space.

LABORATORY STUDIES

CHEST ROENTGENOGRAM. There are no roentgenographic features diagnostic of cardiac tamponade. The heart may appear completely normal in size in cardiac tamponade that develops from acute hemopericardium due to cardiac rupture or laceration. On the other hand, if an effusion that accumulates more slowly to more than approximately 250 ml is responsible, the cardiac silhouette may be enlarged with a water bottle configuration (Fig. 8–43, p. 231). This finding suggests the presence of a large pericardial effusion but supplies no information about its hemodynamic significance. In patients with cardiac tamponade due to tension pneumopericardium, the chest roentgenogram usually shows that the heart is surrounded by air delineated by a strip of soft tissue extending up the aorta consisting of the pericardium.

ELECTROCARDIOGRAM. The electrocardiographic abnormalities seen in acute cardiac tamponade include those of acute pericarditis and pericardial effusion *per se* (p. 158). The development of electrical alternans is a more specific indicator of pericardial tamponade and reflects pendular swinging of the heart within the pericardial space.[113] This may not be the only mechanism, since two-dimensional echocardiographic findings suggest that electrical alternans may be related to a beat-to-beat alteration of right and left ventricular filling.[90] Electrical alternans may also occur in constrictive pericarditis, in tension pneumothorax, after myocardial infarction, and with severe cardiac muscle dysfunction. However, the appearance of electrical alternans in a patient with a known pericardial effusion is highly suggestive of cardiac tamponade —a finding that has been confirmed in experimental cardiac tamponade.[114] Electrical alternans of the QRS complex may occur in a 2:1 or 3:1 pattern. Alternans is usually limited to the QRS complex, but alternans of the P wave, QRS complex, and T wave may rarely occur in extreme cardiac tamponade. Both the abnormal heart motion within the pericardial sac and electrical alternans disappear when pericardial fluid is aspirated.

ECHOCARDIOGRAM (see also p. 102 and Fig. 4–102, p. 103). In patients with jugular venous distention and the possibility of cardiac tamponade, echocardiography is extremely useful and should be performed prior to consideration of pericardiocentesis.[115,116] In a rare patient who is in extremis from the extremely rapid development of cardiac tamponade, the physician may have to rely on the history and physical findings to make a judgment about the need for pericardiocentesis. If echocardiography is readily available and the patient with suspected cardiac tamponade is not moribund, obtaining an echocardiogram will increase the likelihood of diagnosing cardiac tamponade correctly and will prevent inappropriate and potentially lethal attempts at pericardiocentesis or pericardiotomy. First, the echocardiogram helps to document the presence and magnitude of pericardial effusion. The absence of echocardiographic evidence of pericardial effusion virtually excludes the diagnosis of cardiac tamponade (with the important exception of the postoperative cardiac surgery patient in whom loculated fluid or thrombus may cause cardiac compression). Second, the echocardiogram can rapidly differentiate cardiac tamponade from other causes of systemic venous hypertension and hypotension, including constrictive pericarditis, cardiac muscle dysfunction, and right ventricular infarction. The appearance of dense echoes in the pericardial space or extrinsic to the pericardium suggests the presence of compression by material other than free fluid. Echocardiograms can often detect both massive extracardiac hematoma and extrinsic compression of the heart by tumor, which can cause cardiac compression with the physiology of cardiac constriction or cardiac tamponade.

Two-dimensional and Doppler echocardiography can provide additional clues that pericardial effusion is associated with cardiac tamponade. The presence of pulsus paradoxus is associated with sudden leftward motion of the septum during inspiration and an exaggerated increase in right ventricular size with a reciprocal decrease in left ventricular size.[99,116–118] This characteristic respiratory variation in ventricular preload can also be detected by the Doppler ultrasound findings of exaggerated tricuspid and pulmonic flow velocities and reduction of peak mitral flow velocity with the onset of inspiration and the opposite changes after the onset of expiration (Fig. 45–9).[119–121] When the inspiratory reduction in left ventricular filling is extreme, the aortic valve may close prematurely or fail to open[122] and mitral valve opening may be delayed until atrial systole. *Diastolic right atrial and right ventricular compression* or collapse occur early during the development of cardiac tamponade[88–92] (Fig. 45–10). Left atrial diastolic collapse can also occur when pericardial fluid is present behind the left atrium.[88] Right ventricular diastolic collapse appears to be more predictive of cardiac tamponade than pulsus paradoxus, particularly during hypovolemia,[123,124] and these echocardiographic signs may be reversed by volume expansion.[125] Right ventricular diastolic collapse may be absent in the presence of right ventricular hypertrophy. Thus, the echocardiographic findings of pericardial effusion, an inspiratory increase in right ventricular dimensions, and right atrial and ventricular diastolic collapse strongly suggest the diagnosis of cardiac tamponade. However, these changes are not 100 per cent sensitive or specific,[88,90,92,123] and experimental studies indicate that a single echocardiogram cannot always predict the presence or severity of cardiac tamponade.[126] Radionuclide and contrast angiography can also detect right ventricular and right atrial collapse and compression of the superior vena cava as it enters the pericardium,[127] but these findings, while suggestive of cardiac tamponade, also lack complete sensitivity and specificity.

Furthermore, hemodynamic observations at our institution in a consecutive series of 50 patients with suspected cardiac tamponade and echocardiographic evidence of right atrial and ventricular diastolic collapse showed that these echocardio-

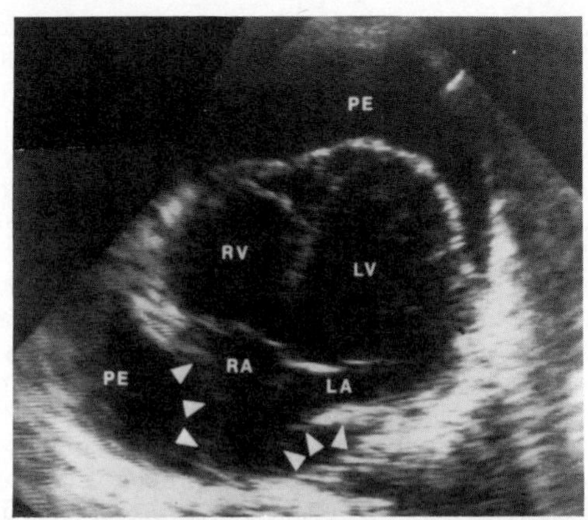

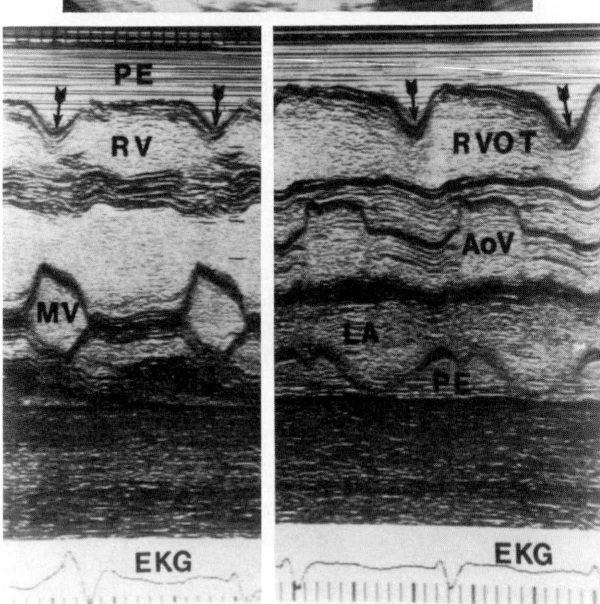

FIGURE 45-10. Two-dimensional *(upper panel)* and M-mode *(lower panels)* echocardiograms from a patient with a malignant pericardial effusion and cardiac tamponade. The two-dimensional image shows a large pericardial effusion (PE) adjacent to the borders of the right ventricle (RV), right atrium (RA), and left ventricle (LV). The effusion is sufficiently large that fluid is also present behind the left atrium (LA). Diastolic compression (white arrows) of both the right and left atria is present. The M-mode images also show striking diastolic compression (dark arrows) of the right ventricle during diastole when the mitral valve (MV) is open and compression of the right ventricular outflow tract (RVOT) in early to mid diastole after aortic valve (AoV) closure.

graphic findings were uniformly associated with elevation of pericardial pressure and the near equilibration of right atrial and right ventricular pressures[128] (Fig. 45-11). However, right heart diastolic collapse was associated with a wide spectrum of hemodynamic derangement, including a subset of patients with minimal elevation of right atrial pressure and the preservation of a normal cardiac output and systemic arterial pressure. Thus, the recognition of patients with cardiac tamponade by echocardiography requires complementary clinical and hemodynamic assessment to distinguish patients with milder degrees of cardiac compression from those with hemodynamic decompensation who require urgent drainage of pericardial fluid. It must be emphasized that cardiac tamponade is a clinical, not an echocardiographic nor a radionuclide, diagnosis that is established definitively by documentation of the elevation and equilibration of intrapericardial and right atrial pressures and the reversal of these findings by evacuation of pericardial fluid.

CARDIAC CATHETERIZATION

Cardiac catheterization is invaluable in establishing the hemodynamic importance of pericardial effusion. Except in extreme emergencies, such as when the patient is moribund, we prefer to catheterize the right heart and pericardial space in conjunction with pericardiocentesis. Cardiac catheterization (1) provides absolute confirmation of the diagnosis of cardiac tamponade; (2) quantitates the hemodynamic compromise; (3) guides pericardiocentesis by documenting that pericardial aspiration is associated with hemodynamic improvement; and (4) permits the detection of coexisting hemodynamic problems, including left ventricular failure, effusive-constrictive pericarditis (p. 1487), and unsuspected pulmonary hypertension in patients with malignant effusions.

Cardiac catheterization typically demonstrates elevation of right atrial pressure with a characteristic preserved systolic *x* descent and absence of or a diminutive diastolic *y* descent. When intrapericardial and right atrial pressures are recorded simultaneously, both are elevated and virtually identical (Fig. 45-12); both pressures fall during inspiration, and intrapericardial pressure may fall slightly below right atrial pressure during systolic ejection at the time of the *x* descent. If intrapericardial pressure is not elevated, and if right atrial and intrapericardial pressures are not virtually identical, the diagnosis of cardiac tamponade must be reconsidered.

Right ventricular mid-diastolic pressure is elevated and equal to right atrial and intrapericardial pressures and lacks the dip-and-plateau configuration characteristic of constrictive percarditis. Since right ventricular and pulmonary artery systolic pressures are equal to the sum of the pressure developed by the right ventricle plus the intrapericardial pressure, right ventricular and pulmonary artery systolic pressures are usually moderately elevated, in the range of 35 to 50 mm Hg. In the case of severe cardiac compression, right ventricular systolic pressure may be reduced and only slightly higher than right ventricular diastolic pressure.

Usually the pulmonary capillary wedge pressure and left ventricular diastolic pressure are elevated and equal to intrapericardial pressure when recorded simultaneously. During expiration, the pulmonary capillary wedge pressure is usually

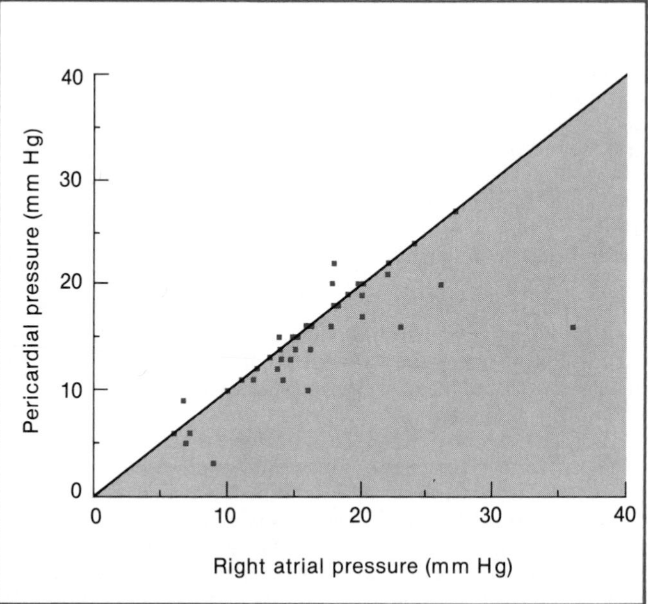

FIGURE 45-11. Relationship between simultaneous measurements of right atrial pressure and intrapericardial pressure in 50 consecutive medical patients with the echocardiographic finding of right atrial diastolic collapse. Although these patients had near-equilibration of right atrial and intrapericardial pressures, the echocardiographic finding of right atrial diastolic collapse was associated with variable degrees of cardiac compression, and 56 per cent of patients had preservation of both a normal cardiac index and systemic arterial pressure. (From Levine, M. J., et al.: Implications of echocardiographically assisted diagnosis of pericardial tamponade in contemporary medical patients: Detection prior to hemodynamic embarrassment. Reprinted by permission of the American College of Cardiology. J. Am. Coll. Cardiol. *17*:59, 1991.)

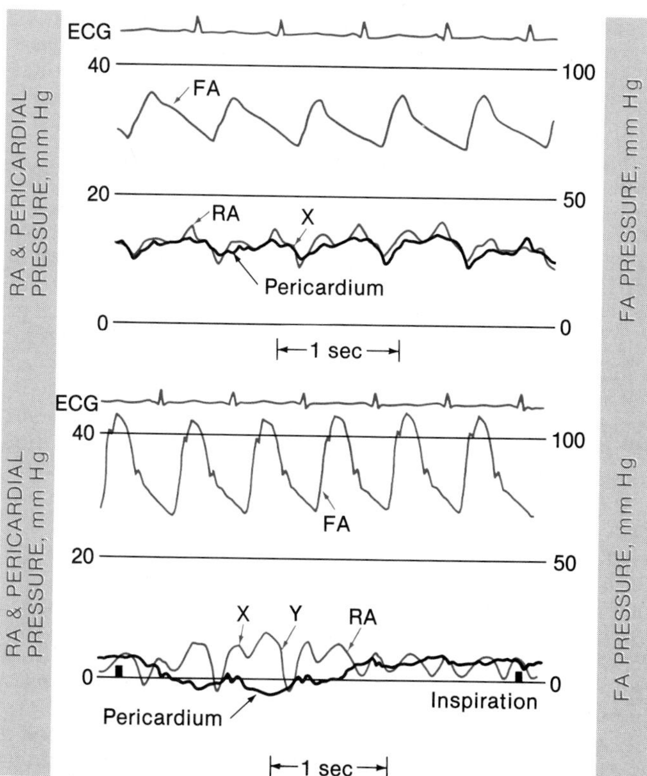

FIGURE 45–12. Simultaneous right atrial (RA) and intrapericardial pressures (scale 0 to 40 mm Hg) and femoral artery pressure (scale 0 to 100 mm Hg) from a patient with decompensated cardiac tamponade. Before pericardiocentesis *(upper panel),* systemic hypotension is present, and there is elevation and equalization of right atrial and intrapericardial pressures. Note that a systolic *x* descent is present, but the diastolic *y* descent is absent, suggesting that right atrial emptying is impeded by compression of the right ventricle in early diastole. After aspiration of about 300 ml of pericardial fluid *(lower panel),* cardiac tamponade is relieved as shown by the restoration of intrapericardial pressure to zero, the restoration of right atrial pressure to a normal level, and the improvement in systemic arterial pressure. The right atrial tracing shows the appearance of a diastolic *y* descent, which indicates the relief of cardiac compression and restoration of normal right atrial emptying in early diastole. Although this degree of fluid aspiration relieved tamponade physiology, an additional 1,500 ml of fluid was subsequently aspirated from the pericardial space. (Modified from Lorell, B. H., and Grossman, W.: Profiles in constrictive pericarditis, restrictive cardiomyopathy, and cardiac tamponade. *In* Grossman, W., and Baim, D. S. (eds.): Cardiac Catheterization, Angiography and Intervention. Philadelphia, Lea and Febiger, 1991, p. 644.)

slightly higher than intrapericardial pressure, resulting in a pressure gradient that promotes left-heart filling. During inspiration, the pulmonary capillary wedge pressure may transiently decrease more than intrapericardial pressure such that the pressure gradient between the pulmonary venous circulation and the left heart is reduced or absent. In patients with severe underlying left ventricular dysfunction or hypertrophy and elevation of the left ventricular diastolic pressure, cardiac tamponade can be present when intrapericardial and right atrial pressures are equal but lower than left ventricular diastolic pressure. Depending on the severity of cardiac compression, left ventricular systolic and aortic pressures may be normal or reduced.

Pulsus paradoxus can be easily documented by intraarterial catheterization and pressure measurement. Simultaneous recording of systemic arterial and right ventricular pressures shows that the inspiratory pressure variation is out of phase (Fig. 45–7). Stroke volume is usually markedly depressed. Cardiac output may be normal, owing to the compensatory effect of tachycardia, or it may be markedly reduced when cardiac tamponade is severe; systemic vascular resistance is usually elevated.

Angiographic studies add no additional information if echocardiographic findings suggestive of cardiac tamponade were obtained prior to cardiac catheterization. In an otherwise normal heart, right and left ventricular end-diastolic volumes are usually reduced with normal or increased ejection fractions.

Aspiration of pericardial fluid results initially in the lowering of the identical intrapericardial, right atrial, right ventricular, and left ventricular diastolic pressures, followed by a fall of intrapericardial pressure below right atrial pressure and reappearance of the *y* descent in the right atrial waveform (Fig. 45–12). Further aspiration causes intrapericardial pressure to fall to a mean level of zero and to fluctuate with changes in intrathoracic pressure. Since the pressure-volume curve of the pericardium is steep, the initial aspiration of 50 to 100 ml of pericardial fluid usually leads to striking reduction in intrapericardial pressure, marked improvement in systemic arterial pressure and cardiac output, and abolition of pulsus paradoxus. The reduction of intrapericardial pressure is often followed by diuresis, related both to the augmentation of cardiac output and the release of atrial natriuretic factor.[81,82,129]

If intrapericardial pressure falls to zero or becomes negative and right atrial pressure remains elevated, *effusive-constrictive pericarditis* (p. 1489) should be strongly considered, especially in patients with underlying neoplasm or prior radiation. Other causes of continued elevation of right atrial pressure after successful pericardiocentesis include the coexistence of cardiac tamponade and preexisting left ventricular dysfunction causing, in turn, pulmonary hypertension and right atrial hypertension, tricuspid valve disease, and restrictive cardiomyopathy. In patients with suspected malignant disease, pulmonary hypertension due to pulmonary microvascular tumor is an important cause of persistent elevation of right atrial pressure and the failure to relieve dyspnea after complete drainage of the pericardial space.[130]

The distinction between cardiac tamponade and the superior vena cava syndrome must always be made in patients with neoplastic disease in whom these lesions may occur singly or together. In patients with obstruction of the superior vena cava, cardiac tamponade may be suspected from the presence of elevated jugular venous pressure and pulsus paradoxus due to respiratory distress. In this condition (without accompanying cardiac tamponade), pressure in the superior vena cava is markedly elevated, with dampened pulsations, and exceeds right atrial and inferior vena cava pressures. Two-dimensional and Doppler echocardiography may not be successful in distinguishing between these conditions because cardiac tamponade as well as other causes of elevated central venous pressure may modify the appearance and respiratory fluctuation of flow in the venae cavae.[121,131] If elevation of jugular venous pressure persists after relief of cardiac tamponade in patients with neoplastic disease, obstruction of the superior vena cava, as reflected in a pressure gradient between the superior vena cava and right atrium, should be sought. Superior vena caval obstruction may be amenable to radiation therapy.

PERICARDIOCENTESIS

Hemodynamic support during preparation of the patient for pericardiocentesis or pericardiotomy should include administration of intravenous fluid, blood, plasma, or saline. The rationale for volume expansion is that it has been shown to delay the appearance of right ventricular diastolic collapse and hemodynamic deterioration.[91] In experimental cardiac tamponade, administration of norepinephrine and isoproterenol[132] has produced an increase in cardiac output. The vasodilators hydralazine and nitroprusside have also been employed in experimental cardiac tamponade to promote an increase in cardiac output secondary to the reduction of elevated systemic resistance.[133] The administration of vasodilators in conjunction with volume expansion must be done with extreme caution in patients with cardiac tamponade, since it may be hazardous in patients with borderline or frank hypotension. Positive-pressure ventilation should be avoided whenever possible because it has been shown to depress cardiac output further in patients with cardiac tamponade.[134]

Pericardial fluid under pressure causing tamponade can be evacuated by (1) percutaneous pericardiocentesis using a needle or catheter, (2) pericardiotomy via a subxiphoid incision, or (3) partial or extensive surgical pericardiectomy. Considerable controversy exists regarding the exact indications for pericardiocentesis[112] although the procedure has been performed extensively since its initial demonstration in 1840 by the Viennese physician Franz Schuh. The benefits of pericardiocentesis include the rapid relief of cardiac tamponade and the opportunity to obtain accurate hemodynamic measurements before and after pericardial aspiration. The major risk of percutaneous pericardiocentesis is laceration of the heart, coronary arteries, or lung. Prior to the 1970's, pericardiocentesis was usually performed blindly at the bedside using a sharp needle without hemodynamic or echocardiographic monitoring, and the risk of death or life-threatening complications appeared to be as high as 20 per cent.[135]

TECHNIQUE. The modern approach is exemplified by the Stanford experience in 123 patients.[136] In the majority of patients, pericardiocentesis was performed by a cardiologist in the cardiac catheterization laboratory using a subxiphoid approach under fluoroscopic guidance with hemodynamic and electrocardiographic monitoring. In this experience, five deaths occurred in association with pericardiocentesis; nonfatal hemopericardium developed in an additional five patients. Pericardiocentesis in this study was successful in obtaining pericardial fluid in 106 of 123 patients. Importantly, the probability of success in safely obtaining fluid was directly related to the size of the pericardial effusion, since fluid was obtained in 93 per cent of patients with large effusions located both anteriorly and posteriorly on echocardiogram but in only 58 per cent with a small posterior pericardial effusion. In 23 patients a specific etiological diagnosis was possible from analysis of the pericardial fluid. Cardiac tamponade was successfully relieved by pericardiocentesis in 61 per cent, while the remainder required subsequent surgical drainage owing either to failure to relieve tamponade or to recurrence after pericardiocentesis. Surgery was most frequently required in patients with acute traumatic hemopericardium (p. 1503). An unsuspected physiological cause of increased systemic venous pressure other than simple cardiac tamponade was documented in 40 per cent of the patients studied, including effusive-constrictive pericarditis in 17 per cent, congestive heart failure in 16 per cent, and coexisting neoplastic superior vena caval obstruction in 5 per cent. Similar experiences regarding the efficacy and safety of pericardiocentesis have been reported by ourselves[128] and others.[137,138]

Two-dimensional echocardiography is useful in guiding pericardiocentesis. Callahan et al.[139] have reported their experience in 132 consecutive pericardiocenteses guided by two-dimensional echocardiography. Pericardiocentesis was successful in obtaining pericardial fluid in 95 per cent of the procedures. There were no deaths, one pneumothorax, and three minor complications. Partial or complete surgical pericardiectomy was subsequently required in 25 per cent of patients for recurrent effusion, chronic relapsing pericarditis, or effusive-constrictive disease. Two-dimensional echocardiographic guidance is particularly helpful in percutaneous pericardiocentesis in patients with loculated pericardial effusion after cardiac surgery.[140]

RISKS AND COMPLICATIONS. Thus, pericardiocentesis is now safer than it was a decade ago, and when the procedure is performed by an experienced operator, the risk of developing a life-threatening complication is only about 0 to 5 per cent.[128,136–141] The procedure is most likely to be successful and uncomplicated when performed in patients with clear-cut echocardiographic evidence of a large effusion with an anterior clear space of 10 mm or more. Cardiac tamponade associated with malignant pericardial effusion or prior radiation therapy can often be managed with pericardiocentesis alone or with a combination of pericardiocentesis, radiation therapy, and local or systemic chemotherapy.[128,136] This therapeutic approach may be preferable in patients with advanced malignant disease when it is desirable to avoid major surgery that is not definitive.

These recent experiences with pericardiocentesis indicate that the procedure should usually be performed in conjunction with hemodynamic measurements, including right heart and intrapericardial pressures, to (1) document the presence of the physiological changes of cardiac tamponade prior to attempted pericardiocentesis and (2) exclude other important coexisting causes of elevated jugular venous pressure, such as effusive-constrictive disease, superior vena caval obstruction, and left ventricular failure. There is rarely justification for performing blind needle pericardiocentesis at the bedside in the absence of optimal hemodynamic monitoring or of a prior echocardiogram documenting the presence of a large anterior and posterior effusion.

Pericardiocentesis is likely to be either complicated or unsuccessful in improving hemodynamics in patients with (1) acute traumatic hemopericardium in which blood enters the pericardial space as rapidly as it can be aspirated, (2) a small pericardial effusion judged to be less than 200 ml in size, (3) absence of an anterior effusion based on echocardiogram, (4) a loculated effusion, or (5) clot and fibrin as well as fluid filling the mediastinal or pericardial space postoperatively. Acute hemopericardium secondary to laceration, puncture of the heart, or leaking left ventricular or aortic aneurysm is likely to recur rapidly after pericardiocentesis. This procedure should be used only as an emergency temporizing measure prior to surgical pericardial exploration in which repair of the heart or aorta may be necessary.[142] Surgical drainage is also usually preferred in patients with tamponade caused by purulent pericarditis to permit extensive drainage and in patients with suspected or known tuberculous pericarditis to permit bacteriological and histological examination of pericardial biopsy specimens. A very rare complication that may occur after the relief of cardiac tamponade is the development of sudden ventricular dilatation[143] and acute pulmonary edema.[144] The mechanism is probably a sudden increase in pulmonary venous blood flow following the relief of pericardial compression in the presence of underlying ventricular dysfunction.

PROCEDURE OF COMBINED CATHETERIZATION AND PERICARDIOCENTESIS

We prefer the following method of combined catheterization and pericardiocentesis, which allows documentation of increased intrapericardial pressure and assessment of hemodynamic improvement after pericardiocentesis.[145] In contrast to traditional bedside sharp-needle pericardiocentesis, this method utilizes a soft catheter for pericardial aspiration and eliminates the prolonged presence of a sharp needle in the pericardial sac, thereby minimizing the risk of cardiac laceration. If possible, pericardiocentesis should be performed in a cardiac procedure laboratory where radiographic and hemodynamic monitoring facilities are optimal and by cardiologists experienced with hemodynamic measurements and the procedure itself. Before the procedure, the patient's blood should be typed and crossmatched and the cardiac surgery team alerted.

Pericardiocentesis is performed after the recording of baseline hemodynamic variables and cardiac output. Since the equilibration of right and left ventricular diastolic pressures is an important feature of cardiac tamponade, it is often desirable to catheterize both sides of the heart and to record right atrial and right ventricular pressures simultaneously with left ventricular pressure. Care should be taken to use equisensitive transducers and to avoid an underdamped catheter-transducer system. Before pericardiocentesis, the transducer system that will be used to record intrapericardial pressure should be leveled with the other transducers, calibrated, and connected to a short length of fluid-filled tubing and a stopcock.

PATIENT POSITION AND ROUTE. Pericardiocentesis is carried out with the patient's thorax and head tilted up, which enhances the pooling of the effusion anteriorly and inferiorly. Although multiple sites have been advocated for pericardiocentesis, we strongly prefer the subxiphoid route, since it is extrapleural and avoids the coronary, pericardial, and internal mammary arteries. The skin is shaved, cleansed, and prepared in aseptic fashion, and the skin and subcutaneous tissue are anesthetized with 1 per

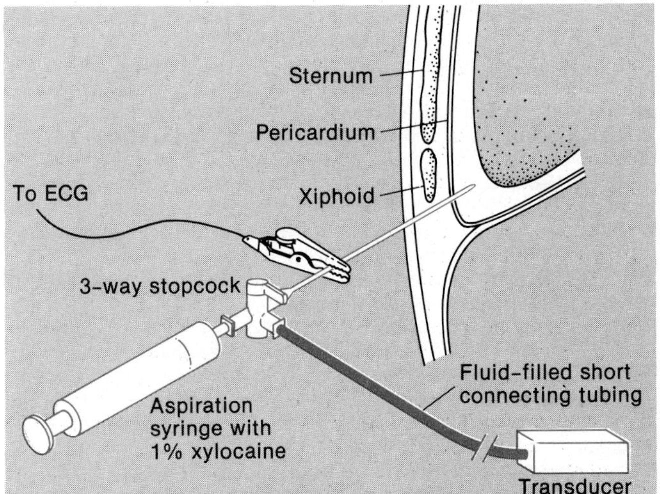

FIGURE 45-13. Pericardiocentesis using the subxiphoid approach, which avoids the major epicardial vessels. A hollow needle, which is attached via a stopcock to an aspiration syringe and to a short length of connecting tubing to a transducer, is used to enter the pericardial space. When fluid is initially aspirated, the pressure waveform at the needle tip should be briefly examined to confirm that the needle tip is in the pericardial space. A floppy-tipped guidewire is then passed through the hollow needle, the needle is exchanged for a soft flexible catheter with end and side holes to facilitate safe and thorough drainage of the pericardial sac. (Modified from Lorell, B. H., and Grossman, W.: Profiles in constrictive pericarditis, restrictive cardiomyopathy, and cardiac tamponade. *In* Grossman, W., and Baim, D. S. (eds.): Cardiac Catheterization, Angiography and Intervention. Philadelphia, Lea and Febiger, 1991, p. 643.)

cent lidocaine. The skin is pierced with a No. 11 blade, 0.5 cm below and to the left of the xiphoid process, and the subcutaneous tissues are spread with a small curved clamp.

A long, 8-inch, thin-walled No. 18-gauge pointed needle (pericardiocentesis kit, Mansfield Scientific, Inc., Mansfield, MA) is attached via a stopcock to a hand-held syringe containing 1 per cent lidocaine. One port of the stopcock is connected to the short length of fluid-filled tubing and the transducer that will be used to measure pericardial pressure (Fig. 45-13). The thin-walled needle commonly used for lumbar puncture is not adequate because its long sharp bevel poses some hazard. The metal hub of the needle may be attached by a sterile connector to the V lead of an electrocardiographic machine, and the electrocardiogram should be continuously recorded. *It is essential that the electrocardiogrpahic apparatus have equipotential grounding with no chance of a current wave that could induce ventricular fibrillation.* If this condition cannot be assured, it is safer to omit electrocardiographic monitoring from the needle.

The needle is directed posteriorly until the tip passes posterior to the bony cage. The hub of the needle is then pressed toward the diaphragm, and the needle is advanced with a 15-degree posterior tilt, either directly toward the patient's head or toward the right or left shoulder. As the needle is smoothly and slowly advanced, the operator periodically attempts to aspirate fluid and then injects a small amount of lidocaine to clear the needle and to provide anesthesia of the deep tissues. The needle is advanced until the pericardial membrane is felt to "give" and pericardial fluid is aspirated or until ST-segment elevation and ventricular premature beats appear on the electrocardiogram, indicating that the needle has reached the epicardium. In the latter case, the needle is promptly and smoothly withdrawn while the operator attempts to aspirate pericardial fluid until the needle lies within the fluid-filled pericardial space and the ECG changes disappear. If fluid cannot be freely aspirated, the needle is slowly withdrawn out of the body, avoiding lateral motion; the needle is flushed and the procedure repeated.

If hemorrhagic fluid is freely aspirated and it is not clear whether the needle is in the ventricle, atrium, or pericardial space, a few milliliters of contrast medium may be injected under fluoroscopic observation. If the contrast medium instantly swirls and disappears, the needle is within a cardiac chember; in contrast, the appearance of sluggish layering of contrast medium inferiorly indicates that the needle is correctly positioned. When fluid can be freely aspirated, the stopcock is turned into its transducer and needle tip, and phasic right atrial pressures are simultaneously displayed. If the needle tip is in the pericardial space, pericardial and right atrial pressures should be equal with identical waveforms. A soft floppy-tip 0.038-inch guidewire is then passed through the hollow needle so that its tip lies within the pericardial space, as confirmed by fluoroscopy. A soft tapered large-bore lumen No. 6 French or 7 French catheter with multiple sideholes and an end hole is advanced over the guidewire, the guidewire is removed, and a few millimeters of fluid are aspirated. The catheter is then promptly connected to the prepared transducer, and intrapericardial pressure is recorded simultaneously with right atrial and systemic arterial pressure to document the presence of cardiac tamponade.

THE PERICARDIAL FLUID. Fluid samples are then aspirated from the catheter and sent for analysis of protein, amylase, glucose, and cholesterol content; hematocrit and white blood cell count; and bacteriological culture for aerobic and anaerobic bacteria, tuberculosis, and fungi. In most cases, a generous sample of fluid should also be sent in a heparinized container for cytological examination. Right atrial, systemic arterial, and intrapericardial pressures should then be recorded periodically as aliquots of fluid are removed—not only until intrapericardial pressure falls to zero but until no further fluid can be aspirated; intrapericardial pressure may return to normal levels after removal of only 50 to 100 ml of fluid in the presence of an effusion of 1 to 2 liters. In our experience, extremely thorough drainage can be accomplished by connecting the intrapericardial catheter via sterile noncollapsible tubing to a stoppered sterile glass bottle with a vacuum. This should be done only when a soft catheter is in the pericardial space, since vacuum suction would be hazardous with sharp needle drainage. When no further fluid can be aspirated or drained, cardiac output and systemic arterial pressure as well as right atrial, right ventricular, and left ventricular (or pulmonary capillary wedge) pressures should be recorded, the last three simultaneously. The jugular veins should also be examined.

Successful relief of cardiac tamponade is documented by (1) the fall of intrapericardial pressure to levels of −3 and +3 mm Hg, (2) the fall of elevated right atrial pressure and separation between right- and left-heart filling pressures, (3) augmentation of cardiac output, and (4) disappearance of pulsus paradoxus. The presence of continued elevation and equilibration of right and left ventriclar diastolic pressures with the appearance of a prominent *y* descent in the right atrial pressure tracing strongly suggests the presence of constricting pericardium due to effusive-constrictive pericarditis (p. 1489). Jugular venous distention despite a fall in right atrial pressure should raise the question of coexisting superior vena caval obstruction, particularly in patients with known or suspected malignant disease.

Some cardiologists advocate the routine injection of a small volume of CO_2 or air into the pericardial space to outline the pericardium at the end of the procedure. This procedure has not been shown to be of aid in identifying unsuspected tumor masses,[136] and we do not advocate it. When the pericardial space is nearly obliterated, there is also the risk of injecting gas into a pleural cavity or cardiac chamber or the production of air tamponade.

It is often desirable to leave the intrapericardial catheter in place for several hours to permit repeated aspiration of fluid if cardiac tamponade recurs or to allow instillation of a nonabsorbable corticosteroid or antineoplastic agent in special cases. The catheter may be sutured securely to the skin and attached via a three-way stopcock to a closed drainage system. If the fluid is hemorrhagic or rich in fibrin, the catheter must be cleared frequently with a few millimeters or fluid. Dilute heparin may be instilled into the catheter to prevent clotting. The catheter should usually be removed after 24 to 48 hours because of the risk of introducing infection and producing iatrogenic purulent pericarditis. However, in some patients, continuous catheter drainage for several days has been reported to be necessary and effective in relieving cardiac tamponade.[139,146,147] Percutaneous pericardial drainage in infants and children can be done without complications using a modification of this approach in which a catheter is inserted over a curved guidewire into the pericardial space under fluoroscopic control.[147]

Following pericardiocentesis, the majority of patients should be observed for about 24 hours in an intensive care setting for recurrence of cardiac tamponade. It is frequently helpful to obtain an echocardiogram soon after pericardiocentesis to establish the appearance of the heart and pericardium following aspiration.

PERICARDIECTOMY AND PERICARDIOTOMY

Surgical evacuation of pericardial fluid under pressure can be accomplished for patients who do not require extensive pericardial excision with the subxiphoid limited pericardiotomy. Subxiphoid pericardiotomy can usually be performed under local anesthesia.[142,148] In patients who are not in extremis, the procedure is usually done without initial palliative pericardiocentesis so that the pericardial sac is distended. After a small longitudinal incision is made below the xiphoid process through the linea alba, the diaphragm and pericardium are dissected away from the sternum, and the diaphragm is retracted inferiorly to permit direct exposure of the anterior pericardium. The tense parietal pericardium is visualized, a small incision is made in the pericardium, a small segment of pericardium is resected for drainage, and a tube is inserted into the pericardial space for extrathoracic drainage by gravity into a sterile container.

The use of the term *subxiphoid pericardial window*[142] to describe this operation should probably be avoided, since it creates confusion with a limited pericardiectomy, which is often referred to as a pleuropericardial window or pericardial window. A limited pericardiectomy[149] via a left hemithorax drains the pericardial cavity into the left hemithorax, and all accessible pericardial tissue is not excised. In a complete pericardiectomy the pericardium is resected from the right phrenic nerve to the left pulmonary veins (sparing the left phrenic nerve) and from the great vessels to the mid-diaphragm, while a partial pericardiectomy is limited by the great vessels.[150]

The relative efficacy of these surgical approaches has been reviewed in two recent large series.[149,150] The overall 30-day surgical mortality ranged from 12.5 to 15.5 per cent, and was higher in patients with malignant than benign effusions. The subxiphoid pericardiotomy has some advantages over extensive formal pericardiectomy in that it is simpler and shorter, permits both drainage of pericardial fluid and examination of a small pericardial biopsy specimen, and can usually be performed safely using local anesthesia in critically ill patients.[148] However, in comparison with a significantly higher risk of reoperation for recurrent tamponade or constrictive disease within a few months after surgery.[149] This suggests that the less invasive subxiphoid pericrdiotomy should be chosen as a palliative procedure in patients who are critically ill with limited expected survival. The left thoracotomy partial pericardiectomy appears to offer none of the advantages of the subxiphoid pericardiotomy and is associated with higher operative mortaity.[150] Complete pericardiectomy is usually recomended for the surgical treatment of patients with effusive-constrictive pericardial disease or loculated effusion who are in good general condition and who are expected to survive more than a few months.

PERICARDIOSCOPY. With use of a flexible fiberoptic bronchoscope or endoscope, this procedure has been reported as an adjunct to subxiphoid pericardiotomy following the drainage of the effusion in the operating room.[151,152] Pericardioscopy permits visualization of the parietal pericardium and epicardium on the anterior, posterior, and inferior surfaces of the heart and allows selective biopsies beyond the small region of pericardium that is usually accessible with a subxiphoid incision.

PERICARDIAL BIOPSY. Endrys et al.[153] described a technique for percutaneous pericardial biopsy using an endomyocardial bioptome inserted via a curved sheath after percutaneous pericardiocentesis and distention of the pericardial space with air. These techniques offer new approaches for obtaining diagnostic information in patients with suspected malignant or infectious pericardial disease, but the efficacy and safety of these approaches in comparison with surgical exploration and pericardial biopsy are not yet established.

Constrictive Pericarditis

Constrictive pericarditis is present when a fibrotic, thickened, and adherent pericardium restricts diastolic filling of the heart. It usually begins with an initial episode of acute pericarditis, which may not be detectable clinically, characterized by fibrin deposition, often with a pericardial effusion. This then slowly progresses to a subacute stage of organization and resorption of the effusion, followed by a chronic stage consisting of fibrous scarring and thickening of the pericardium with obliteration of the pericardial space. In the majority of cases, the visceral and parietal layers become completely fused, but in a few cases, the constricting process is produced primarily by the visceral pericardium (epicardium). In the chronic stage of constrictive pericarditis, calcium deposition may contribute to thickening and stiffening of the pericardium. Constrictive pericarditis is usually a symmetrical scarring process that produces uniform restriction of the filling of all heart chambers. Rare cases of strictly localized pericardial thickening have been reported, including constricting bands in the atrioventricular groove surrounding the semilunar valve rings, or in the aortic groove, right ventricular outflow tract, and venae cavae.[154,155]

PATHOPHYSIOLOGY

In classic constrictive pericarditis, the heavily fibrosed or calcified pericardium restricts diastolic filling of all chambers of the heart and determines the diastolic volume of the heart. The symmetrical constricting effect of the pericardium results in elevation and equilibrium of diastolic pressures in all four cardiac chambers (as well as of pulmonary capillary wedge pressures). In early diastole when intracardiac volume is less than that defined by the stiff pericardium, diastolic filling is unimpeded, and early diastolic filling occurs abnormally rapidly because venous pressure is elevated. Rapid early diastolic filling is abruptly halted when the intracardiac volume reaches the limit set by the noncompliant pericardium.

Instantaneous plots of ventricular volume versus time in patients with constrictive pericarditis have shown that virtually all filling of the ventricle occurs very early in diastole. This abnormal pattern of diastolic filling is reflected in the characteristic dip-and-plateau waveforms in both right and left ventricles (Fig. 45–14). The early diastolic dip corresponds to the period of excessively rapid diastolic filling, while the plateau phase corresponds to the period of mid and late diastole when there is little additional ventricular volume expansion. Since the atria are equilibrated with the ventricles in early diastole, the jugular venous waveform and right and left atrial waveforms show a prominent and deep diastolic *y* descent. The systolic x descent is usually also present, and the venous waveform may therefore exhibit a characteristic M or W configuration.

A bimodal pattern of systemic venous return occurs in constrictive pericarditis with an acceleration of systemic venous blood flow from the venae cavae into the right atrium during both ventricular systolic ejection and early diastole. The greatest acceleration of venous blood flow occurs during early diastole simultaneous with the *y* descent. This contrasts with the normal filling pattern, in which a bimodal pattern of systemic venous return also is present, but the major surge of venous return occurs during systole. The pattern of systemic venous return in constrictive pericarditis also contrasts with that in cardiac tamponade. Cardiac compression is present throughout diastole in cardiac tamponade, so that the diastolic surge of venous return is blunted, and the venous pressure tracing shows absence of or blunted diastolic *y* descent and a preserved x descent.

KUSSMAUL'S SIGN. Another striking abnormality of constrictive pericarditis is the failure of intrathoracic pressure changes during respiration to be transmitted to the pericardial space and intracardiac chambers. As a consequence, during inspiration, systemic venous and right arterial pressures do not fall and venous flow into the right atrium does not increase, in contrast to the situation in normal subjects and patients with cardiac tamponade (Fig. 45–8). In some patients, systemic venous pressure may actually increase with inspiration, i.e., *Kussmaul's sign*.[156] This finding may occur in other disorders such as chronic right ventricular failure and restrictive cardiomyopathy, in which right atrial and systemic venous pressures also are markedly elevated. However, Kussmaul's sign does *not* occur in acute cardiac tamponade, in which the inspiratory fall in intrathoracic pressure is transmitted to the fluid-filled pericardial space.[157] Pulsus paradoxus (p. 1474) is also less common in constrictive pericarditis than in cardiac tamponade, in which the mechanism is thought to be largely the exaggerated increase in right ventricular filling during inspririation at the expense of left ventricular filling. The presence of an inspiratory fall in arterial pressure greater than 10 mm Hg suggests the presence of a tense

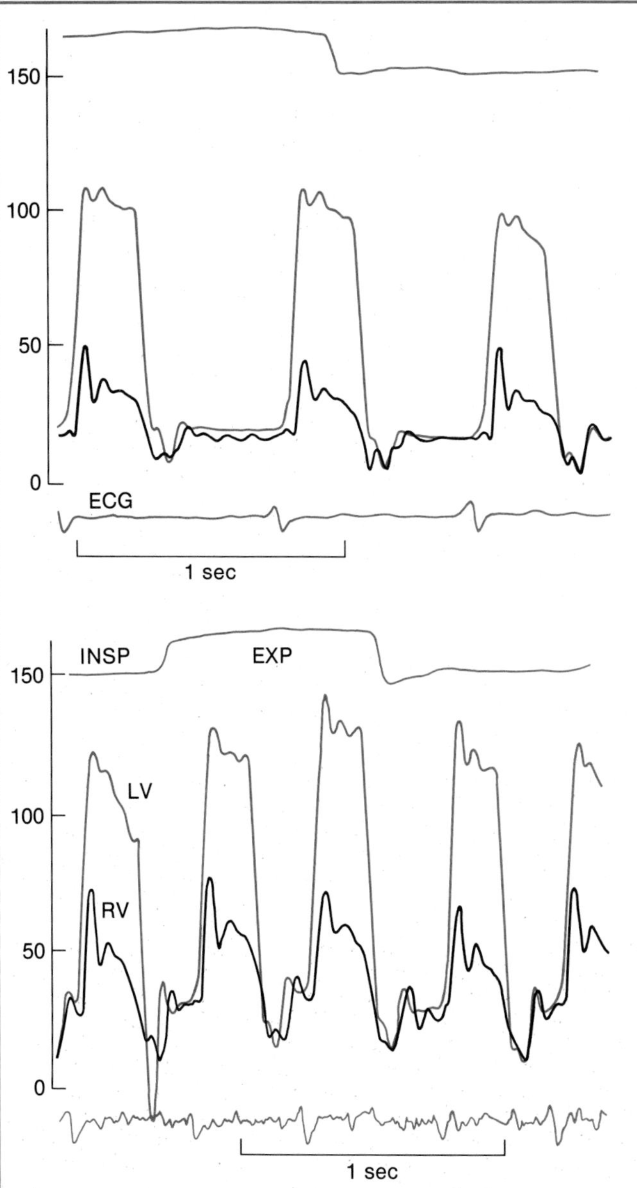

FIGURE 45-14. Left (LV) and right ventricular (RV) pressure recordings from a patient with constrictive pericarditis illustrating that the presence of tachycardia partially obscures evaluation of the diastolic waveforms. The long diastole following a premature beat allows recognition of equilibration of ventricular diastolic pressures before the a wave, as well as detection of a dip-and-plateau configuration of the waveforms. (From Lorell, B. H., and Grossman, W.: Profiles in constrictive pericarditis, restrictive cardiomyopathy, and cardiac tamponade. *In* Grossman, W. (ed.): Cardiac Catheterization and Angiography. Philadelphia, Lea and Febiger, 1986, p. 430.)

pericardial effusion or coexisting pulmonary disease with an exaggerated inspiratory fall in intrathoracic pressure.

Restriction of diastolic filling ultimately results in compensatory renal retention of sodium and water that contributes further to the increase in systemic venous pressure and initially serves to maintain diastolic filling of the ventricles despite pericardial compression. The inhibition of the release of atrial natriuretic factor may contribute to renal fluid retention.[158] In some cases, the pericardial scar is so dense that diastolic ventricular volumes are reduced, which may cause stroke volume and then cardiac output to fall despite compensatory tachycardia. The presence of reduced cardiac output, tachycardia, and elevated right and left heart filling pressures may simulate myocardial failure, and classic ventricular performance curves may show reduced left ventricular stroke volume relative to elevated left ventricular filling pressure. However, systolic contraction of the ventricles and the intrinsic contractile state of the myocardium are usually normal or nearly so.[159] In severe cases of constrictive pericarditis, myocardial systolic function may also be depressed, owing to myocardial atrophy, fibrosis, or compression of superficial coronary arteries in the fibrotic pericardium resulting in myocardial ischemia.[160-162] Although the presence of coexisting cardiomyopathy is usually a factor predictive of a poor outcome after pericardiectomy (p. 1503), a striking improvement of left ventricular ejection fraction may occasionally occur after stripping of a fibrotic and thick pericardium.[163]

SUBACUTE NONCALCIFIC PERICARDITIS. Pathophysiological and hemodynamic findings in patients with subacute noncalcific pericarditis may differ from those in patients with chronic constrictive pericarditis in whom the pericardium resembles a rigid shell. Hancock has suggested that the presence of a thick fluid-fibrin layer in the process of organization leads to relatively elastic compression of the heart, which may be compared to "wrapping the heart tightly with rubber bands." [164] The pathophysiological disturbance caused by this nonrigid fibroelastic form of constrictive pericarditis is similar to that in cardiac tamponade, since fibroelastic constriction compresses the heart continuously throughout the cardiac cycle, and respiratory changes in intrathoracic pressure usually are transmitted to the cardiac chambers.[164] Thus, patterns of ventricular filling and waveforms in the subacute form of fibroelastic compression tend to resemble those of cardiac tamponade rather than of constrictive pericarditis and include a systemic venous waveform with a predominant *x* descent or equal *x* and *y* descents, an inconspicuous early diastolic dip in the ventricular waveform, an inspiratory fall in systemic venous and right atrial pressures, and the presence of pulsus paradoxus (Table 45-5).

ETIOLOGY

Tuberculosis was formerly the leading cause of constrictive pericarditis in Western nations as reported in the classic series

TABLE 45-5 CLINICAL AND HEMODYNAMIC FEATURES OF COMPRESSIVE PERICARDIAL DISEASE

	CARDIAC TAMPONADE	SUBACUTE "ELASTIC" CONSTRICTION	CHRONIC "RIGID" CONSTRICTION
Duration of symptoms	Hours to days	Weeks to months	Months to years
Chest pain, friction rub	Usual	Recent past	Remote
Pulsus paradoxus	Prominent	Usually prominent	Slight or absent
Kussmaul's sign	Absent	Usually absent	Often present
Early diastolic knock	Absent	Usually absent	Often present
Heart size on chest roentgenogram	Usually enlarged	Usually enlarged	Usually normal, sometimes enlarged
Pericardial calcification	Absent	Rare	Often present
Abnormal P waves or atrial fibrillation	Absent	Absent	Often present
Venous (right atrial) waveform	X or Xy	Xy or XY	XY or xY
Pericardial effusion	Always present	Often present	Absent

X and Y = prominent x and y descents, respectively, x and y = inconspicuous x and y descents.
Modified from Hancock, E. W.: On the elastic and rigid forms of constrictive pericarditis. Am. Heart J. *100*:917, 1980.

of Paul[165] and Andrews[166] and their coworkers. In disadvantaged nations, this is still true,[167] whereas with the advent of antituberculosis therapy this disease now accounts for 15 per cent or less of cases in developed nations.[168,169] The largest number of cases of constrictive pericarditis today are of unknown etiology (42 per cent) and attributed to earlier clinically inapparent viral pericarditis.[169] In the past decade, constrictive pericarditis after cardiac surgery has emerged as an important cause (p. 1688). In a series of consecutive patients with constrictive pericarditis seen at Stanford from 1970 to 1985, postsurgical pericarditis accounted for 11 per cent of all cases but constituted 29 per cent of cases between 1980 and 1985.[169] In this series, constrictive pericarditis following mediastinal radiation therapy accounted for 30 per cent of cases, with an average latency period of 11 years after radiotherapy. Other nontubercular causes include chronic renal failure treated with hemodialysis (p. 1868); connective tissue disorders, including rheumatoid arthritis and systemic lupus erythematosus (p. 1501); and neoplastic pericardial infiltration or encasement of the heart due mostly commonly to lung cancer, breast cancer, Hodgkin's disease, and lymphoma. Constrictive pericarditis can develop after incomplete drainage of purulent pericarditis (p. 1494) and as a complication of fungal infections (p. 1494) and parasitic infections (p. 1495). It may occasionally follow pericarditis associated with acute myocardial infarction and the postpericardiotomy syndrome, (p. 1503), and in association with pulmonary asbestosis.[170]

CONSTRICTIVE PERICARDITIS IN CHILDREN (see also p. 1493). Constrictive pericarditis is far less common in children than in adults and may rarely occur following a viral syndrome in a child mistakenly thought to have hepatitis or a protein-losing enteropathy. When constrictive pericarditis occurs in young children, tuberculosis should be strongly considered, since it was a proved or highly likely cause in 56 per cent of 84 children with constrictive pericarditis reported in the literature.[171] Nontraumatic hemopericardium has been reported in children and young adults with congenital bleeding disorders complicated by a second process such as endocarditis or viral syndrome, and constrictive pericarditis has occurred following pericardial bleeding due to congenital afibrinogenemia.[172] The newly described familial syndrome of pericarditis, arthritis, and camptodactyly (flexion contractures) is a rare cause of constrictive pericarditis in children and young adults.[173] A rare congenital cause of constrictive pericarditis is *mulibrey nanism*, an autosomal recessive disorder characterized by dwarfism, constrictive pericarditis, abnormal fundi, and fibrous dysplasia of the long bones.[174,175]

CLINICAL FEATURES

In patients in whom systemic venous and right atrial pressures are modestly elevated (10 to 15 mm Hg), left ventricular filling pressure is also usually only modestly elevated. In this setting, symptoms secondary to systemic venous congestion such as edema, abdominal swelling, and discomfort due to ascites and passive hepatic congestion may predominate. Vague abdominal symptoms such as postprandial fullness, dyspepsia, flatulence, and anorexia may also be present. When both right and left heart filling pressures are elevated to the level of 15 to 30 mm Hg, symptoms of pulmonary venous congestion, such as exertional dyspnea, cough, and orthopnea, are present. Pleural effusions and elevation of the diaphragm due to ascites may also contribute to dyspnea. Severe fatigue, weight loss, and muscle wasting suggest the presence of fixed or reduced cardiac output.

PHYSICAL EXAMINATION. The single most important finding is elevation of jugular venous pressure. If the neck is examined casually, or if the patient is examined supine so that jugular venous pressure is measured above the angle of the jaw, this important clue to the presence of constrictive pericarditis may be missed. A prominent feature of the elevated jugular venous pressure is the rapidly collapsing negative wave of the diastolic *y* descent. In patients in sinus rhythm, both x and y descents can be distinguished; the x descent is synchronous with while the diastolic y descent is out of phase with the carotid pulse. These features may be difficult to detect in patients with tachycardia, tachypnea, or arrhythmia. It may also be difficult to distinguish between right heart failure due to tricuspid regurgitation and chronic constrictive pericarditis by neck vein examination at the bedside. The finding of Kussmaul's sign (an inspiratory increase in systemic venous pressure) is difficult to appreciate at the bedside and may be confused with exaggerated amplitude of the venous waves during inspiration.

The arterial pulse may be normal or show diminished pulse pressure. Severe pulsus paradoxus is uncommon in rigid constrictive pericarditis and rarely exceeds 10 mm Hg unless pericardial fluid under pressure is also present. Systolic retraction of the apical impulse occurs in the majority of patients and usually consists of an unobtrusive diffuse precordial movement. The most impressive abnormality during auscultation is the diastolic pericardial knock, an early diastolic sound that is often heard along the left sternal border in rigid constrictive pericarditis, infrequently heard in subacute constrictive pericarditis of the fibroelastic variety, and not heard in pure cardiac tamponade.[157] The pericardial knock usually occurs 0.09 to 0.12 second after A_2 and corresponds in timing to the sudden cessation of ventricular filling and the premature diastolic plateau of the diastolic ventricular volume curve[176] (Fig. 45–15). The pericardial knock tends to occur earlier and to have a higher acoustic frequency than the typical S_3 gallop sound, and therefore it may be confused with the opening snap of mitral stenosis. Widening of the split between the aortic and pulmonic components of the second heart sound may occur in constrictive pericarditis. This is attributed to (1) a fixed right ventricular stroke volume during inspiration due to pericardial compression and (2) premature aortic valve closure due to a transitory inspiratory decrease in left ventricular stroke volume.

Hepatomegaly is usually present, and prominant hepatic pulsations that conform to the jugular venous pulse can be

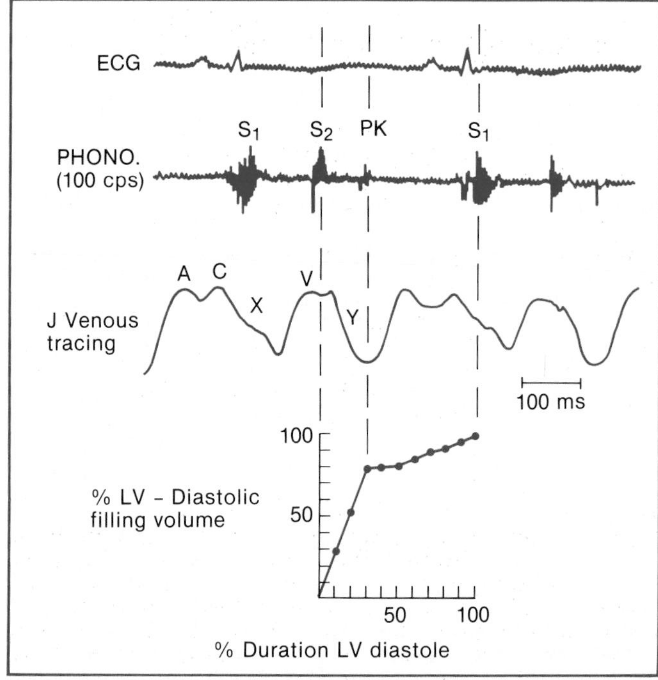

FIGURE 45–15. Electrocardiogram (ECG), phonocardiogram (PHONO), jugular venous pulse tracing, and left ventricular (LV) diastolic filling curve in a patient with constrictive pericarditis and pericardial knock (PN). The pericardial knock (PK) occurs simultaneously with the nadir of the diastolic *y* descent and sudden plateau of the LV filling curve. (From Tyberg, T. I., et al.: Genesis of pericardial knock in constrictive pericarditis. Am. J. Cardiol. *46*:570, 1980.)

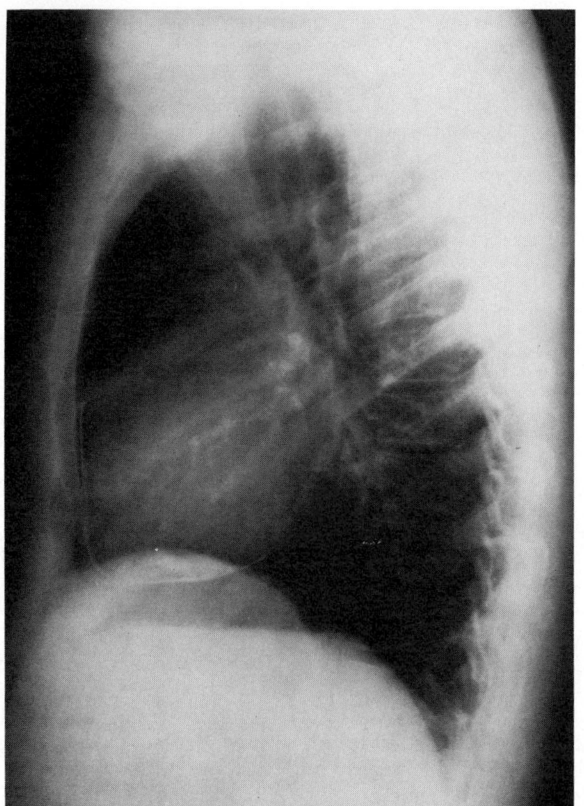

FIGURE 45-16. Lateral chest roentgenogram showing calcification of the pericardium in a patient with chronic constrictive pericarditis of idiopathic (postviral) etiology. The eggshell rim of pericardial calcification is often best appreciated in the lateral projection.

TABLE 45-6 RADIOLOGICAL FEATURES OF CONSTRICTIVE PERICARDITIS

Normal heart size	33%
Enlarged heart	67%
Calcified pericardium	43%
Pleural effusion	83%
Pulmonary venous congestion	86%
Left atrial enlargement	85%

Modified from Pulvaneswary, M., et al.: Constrictive pericarditis. Clinical, hemodynamic, and radiologic correlation. Australas. Radiol. *26*:53, 1982.

detected in 70 per cent of patients[177] (Fig. 2-7, p. 19). Other evidence of hepatic dysfunction secondary to passive liver congestion and diminished cardiac output may include ascites, icterus, spider angiomas, and palmar erythema. In young patients with competent venous valves, edema of the extremities may be noticeably absent in the presence of marked abdominal distention. Older patients with longstanding constrictive pericarditis may have enormous ascites and massive edema of the scrotum, thighs, and calves.[177a] In contrast, the upper torso and arms may show evidence of marked muscle wasting and cachexia.

CHEST ROENTGENOGRAM (see also p. 230). The cardiac silhouette may be small, normal, or enlarged. Cardiac enlargement may be apparent because of coexisting pericardial effusion, the contribution of an enormously thickened pericardium, or preexisting cardiac chamber enlargement or hypertrophy. The right superior mediastinum may be prominent as a result of engorgement of the superior vena cava, and left atrial enlargement is common.[178] Extensive calcification of the pericardium is present in approximately half the patients and raises the possibility of a tubercular etiology. The location of calcification is helpful in distinguishing between pericardial and myocardial aneurysm calcium, since pericardial calcification is predominantly located over the right heart chambers and in the atrioventricular grooves, whereas isolated calcification of the left ventricular apex or posterior wall suggests left ventricular aneurysm.[179] However, this finding is not specific for constrictive pericarditis in that *a calcified pericardium is not necessarily a constricted one.* The lateral chest film is particularly useful for the detection of pericardial calcium in the atrioventricular groove or along the anterior and diaphragmatic surfaces of the right ventricle (Fig. 45-16). Fluoroscopy may be helpful in distinguishing pericardial calcification from calcium within the wall of a myocardial aneurysm or thrombus or within the mitral or aortic valves, mitral annulus, or coronary arteries. Pleural effusions are present in about 60 per cent of patients, and unexplained persistent pleural effusion can be the presenting manifestation.[180] Since left atrial pressure is commonly elevated to 15 to 30 mm Hg, there may be evidence of redistribution of blood flow, while Kerley's B lines or infiltrates suggestive of frank pulmonary edema are rare (Table 45-6).

ELECTROCARDIOGRAM. Electrocardiographic findings include low QRS voltage, generalized T-wave inversion or flattening, and left atrial abnormalities suggestive of P mitrale (Fig. 45-17). Atrial fibrillation occurs in less than half the patients with constrictive pericarditis and is thought to be related to longstanding elevation of atrial pressures and atrial enlargement. In a postmortem study of constrictive pericarditis, Levine noted that atrioventricular block, intraventricular conduction defects, and pseudoinfarction patterns with deep wide Q waves seemed to be related to an extension of calcification into the myocardium and around the coronary arteries, compromising coronary blood flow.[161] An unusual pattern that simulates right ventricular hypertrophy with right-axis deviation may be present in about 5 per cent of patients and due to dense pericardial scar overlying the right ventricle in association with compensatory dilation and hyperkinesis of the outflow tract.[181,182]

ECHOCARDIOGRAM. One distinct M-mode echocardiographic pattern of pericardial thickening in constrictive pericarditis consists of two parallel lines representing the visceral and parietal pericardia separated by a clear space of at least 1 mm; another consists of multiple dense echoes.[183] Extreme respiratory variation in the depth of the pulmonic valve *a* wave[184] and premature pulmonic valve opening secondary to a high right ventricular early diastolic pressure may be present,[185] but these changes are also seen in other disorders with high right ventricular early diastolic pressure, such as tricuspid and pulmonic regurgitation. Other M-mode echocardiographic abnormalities include abrupt posterior motion of the interventricular septum in early diastole, coinciding with the pericardial knock, abrupt posterior motion during atrial systole,[185] and reduced amplitude of left ventricular posterior wall motion.[186] Engle et al.[187] reviewed M-mode echocardiograms from 40 patients with proven constrictive pericarditis and 40 normal subjects. They observed that normal left ventricular size, left atrial enlargement, flattened diastolic ventricular wall motion, and abnormal septal motion were

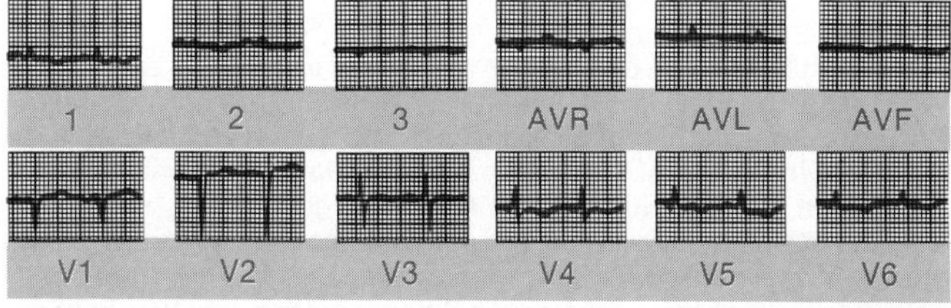

FIGURE 45-17. Electrocardiogram from a patient with surgically proven constrictive pericarditis and normal coronary arteries who had symptoms of chronic fatigue, dyspnea, and chest pain. The electrocardiogram is notable for the presence of a wide, notched P wave and diffuse T-wave inversion. These changes were initially mistakenly thought to be related to coronary insufficiency.

found in most patients, but no single feature was diagnostic of constrictive pericarditis. Computer-assisted digitization of M-mode echocardiograms may be useful in distinguishing the abnormal rapid early diastolic filling of constrictive pericarditis from the more delayed filling pattern of restrictive cardiomyopathy.[188]

Two-dimensional echocardiography in constrictive pericarditis shows an immobile and dense appearance of the pericardium, abrupt displacement of the interventricular septum during early diastolic filling ("septal bounce"), prominent early diastolic filling, and an abnormal contour of the junction of the left ventricle and left atrial posterior wall.[189] Dilatation of the hepatic veins and inferior vena cava,[190] intense and spontaneous contrast in the inferior vena cava,[191] and distention of the inferior vena cava with blunted respiratory fluctuations in diameter ("plethora")[192] have also been described in patients with constrictive pericarditis. Himelman et al.[192] reviewed the diagnostic value of pericardial adhesions, septal bounce, and vena cava plethora and noted that false-positive findings occurred in patients with pacemakers or bundle branch block after pericardiotomy, and with other causes of right heart failure. Studies in an experimental dog model and in patients have confirmed that two-dimensional echocardiography can demonstrate abnormal early diastolic filling but greatly overestimates pericardial thickness.[193]

Doppler echocardiography of the engorged hepatic vein has been reported to show a *W*-wave pattern that corresponds to the characteristic pattern of right atrial filling and consists of rapid forward flow during early diastole, abrupt deceleration and subsequent reverse flow before the *a* wave, and a second wave of rapid forward flow during early systolic ejection with reverse flow in late systole[194] (Fig. 45–18).

CT AND MR IMAGING (see also Fig. 11–9, p. 317). CT has also emerged as a valuable tool in the evaluation of suspected constrictive pericarditis. The technique is especially useful in identifying pericardial thickening and in identifying other

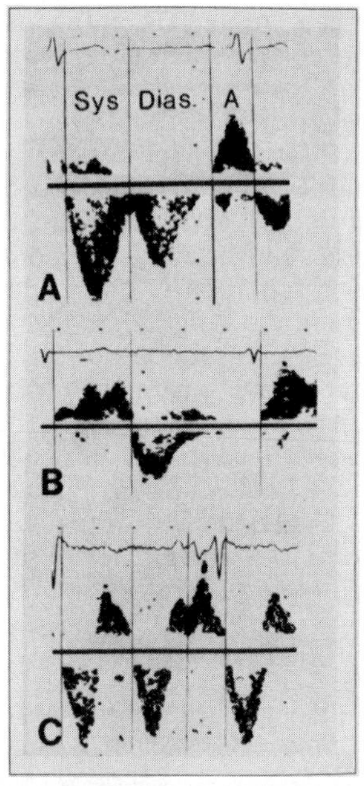

FIGURE 45–18. Pulsed Doppler recordings of central venous flow velocities in the hepatic vein. In *panel A*, a recording of a normal subject shows a normal pattern of biphasic flow with downward deflection of the signal indicative of a normal pattern of biphasic forward flow in systole and diastole with transient reversal of flow during atrial contraction. In *panel B*, a recording of a patient with severe tricuspid regurgitation shows holosystolic reverse flow. In *panel C*, a recording of a patient with constrictive pericarditis shows rapid forward flow in early systole and subsequent reverse flow in late systole, and an abbreviated signal of rapid forward flow in early diastole with abrupt deceleration and subsequent reverse flow that begins in mid-diastole before the *a* wave. (From von Bibra, H., et al.: Diagnosis of constrictive pericarditis by pulsed Doppler echocardiography of the hepatic vein. Am. J. Cardiol. *63*:483, 1989.)

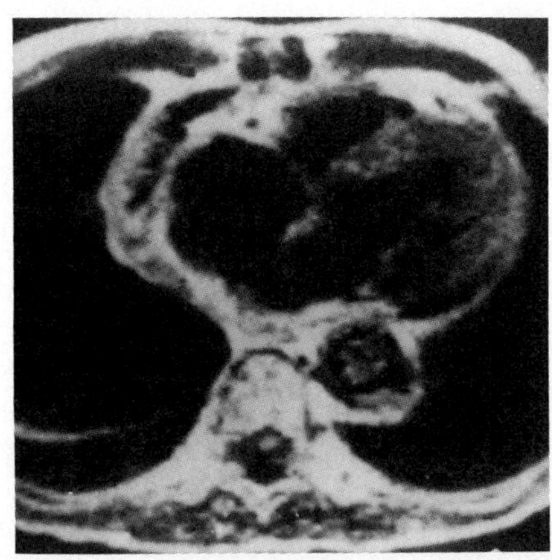

FIGURE 45–19. Magnetic resonance image from a patient with constrictive uremic pericarditis shows irregular thickening of the visceral and parietal pericardial layers, which are separated by low-intensity fluid, overlying the enlarged right atrium. Pericardial fluid is also present behind the left ventricle, which is hypertrophied. (From Soulen, R. L., et al.: Magnetic resonance imaging of constrictive pericardial disease. Am. J. Cardiol. *55*:480, 1985.)

findings compatible with constrictive pericarditis, including dilation of the venae cavae and deformation of the right ventricle.[195,196] Nonvisualization of the left ventricular posterolateral wall by computed tomography suggests coexisting myocardial fibrosis or atrophy and may predict a poor outcome following pericardiectomy.[197]

Experience with MR imaging in patients with constrictive pericarditis suggests that it can detect pericardial thickening, dilation of the venae cavae and hepatic veins, and narrowing of the right ventricle[196,198] (Fig. 45–19). All of these findings are suggestive of constrictive pericarditis.

The use of noninvasive imaging techniques to assist in discrimination between constrictive pericarditis and restrictive cardiomyopathy is discussed later in this chapter (p. 1488).

OTHER LABORATORY FINDINGS. Other abnormal laboratory findings may be present as a result of chronic elevation of right atrial pressure causing passive congestion of the liver, kidneys, and gastrointestinal tract. These include depressed serum albumin, elevated serum globulin, elevated conjugated and unconjugated serum bilirubin, and abnormal hepatocellular function tests. In patients with hepatomegaly and ascites, liver biopsy may show histological features similar to the Budd-Chiari syndrome, including hepatic venule thrombi and ductular proliferation.[199] Chylous ascites may occur because of impedance of lymphatic drainage due to central venous hypertension.[200] Protein-losing enteropathy may be evident from the presence of albumin in the stool and lymphangiectasis on small-bowel biopsy.[201] Elevated systemic venous pressure may also produce variable degrees of albuminuria as well as pronounced protein loss consistent with the nephrotic syndrome.[202] Nonspecific evidence of the presence of chronic disease such as normocytic and normochromic anemia may be found.

DIFFERENTIAL DIAGNOSIS. Constrictive pericarditis should be suspected in patients with jugular venous distention, unexplained pleural effusion, hepatomegaly, systemic edema, or ascites. It must be distinguished from superior vena caval obstruction, nephrotic syndrome, hepatic and intraabdominal disease due to malignancy, and other cardiac causes of right atrial hypertension, including restrictive cardiomyopathy, tricuspid stenosis, tricuspid regurgitation, hypertrophic cardiomyopathy, and right atrial myxoma. It may be extremely difficult to distinguish patients with constrictive pericarditis from those with restrictive physiology due to amyloidosis, sarcoidosis, radiation injury, hemochromatosis, and the hypereosinophilic syndrome, which may involve pericardium as well as the myocardium.[203–205] Both constrictive pericarditis and restrictive cardiomyopathy may show the electrocardiographic changes of atrial fibrillation, left atrial abnormalities, and diffuse low QRS voltage with T-wave flattening. The presence of atrioventricular block and conduction disturbances simulating myocardial infarction favors the diagnosis of restrictive cardiomyopathy. Echocardiography in some patients with restrictive cardiomyopathy may show abnormal thickening of the ventricular myocardium or a peculiar "sparkling" appearance when amyloidosis is present.[206] The simultaneous use of electrocardiography and echocardiography to demonstrate a reduction of the voltage/mass ratio has been described in patients with amyloid restrictive cardiomyopathy in whom diffuse low QRS voltage is associated with increased thickness of the left ventricular wall due to amyloid deposition.[207]

In the presence of findings suggestive of constrictive pericarditis, right- and left-heart catheterization should be performed to document the presence of constrictive physiology and to exclude other causes of right atrial hypertension. Diuresis should be avoided prior to catheterization, since hypovolemia may obscure the characteristic hemodynamic findings. Cardiac catheterization and angiography, often with endomyocardial biopsy, are usually helpful in discriminating between constrictive pericarditis and restrictive cardiomyopathy in many patients, but in a minority exploratory thoracotomy may be required.

CARDIAC CATHETERIZATION AND ANGIOGRAPHY

Cardiac catheterization is useful in the assessment of patients suspected of having constrictive pericarditis to (1) document the presence of elevation and equilibration of diastolic filling pressures, (2) assess the effect of constrictive pericarditis on stroke volume and cardiac output, (3) evaluate myocardial systolic function, (4) assist in the difficult discrimination between constrictive pericarditis and restrictive cardiomyopathy, and (5) exclude compression of the coronary arteries or regional outflow tract compression by the fibrotic pericardium.

Catheterization of both the right and left ventricles should be performed to permit simultaneous recording of right and left heart filling pressures. Typical findings include the elevation and virtual identity (within 5 mm Hg) of right atrial, right ventricular diastolic, left atrial (pulmonary capillary wedge), and left ventricular diastolic pressures before the *a* wave. Right atrial pressure is characterized by a preserved systolic x descent, a prominent early diastolic *y* descent, and *a* and *v*

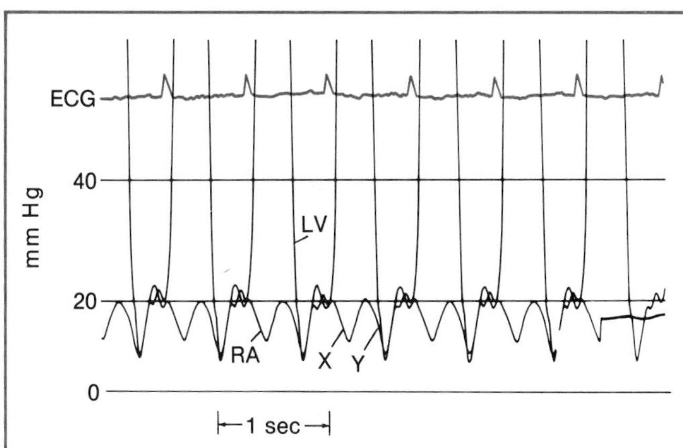

FIGURE 45–20. Simultaneous left ventricular (LV) and right atrial (RA) pressure recordings from a patient with constrictive pericarditis showing that both pressures are elevated and virtually equal throughout diastole. The prominent diastolic *y* descent in the right atrial waveform indicates that right atrial emptying is rapid and unimpeded in early diastole. In contrast, the *y* descent is absent or attenuated in cardiac tamponade because cardiac compression limits right ventricular filling throughout diastole. (From Lorell, B. H., and Grossman, W.: Profiles in constrictive pericarditis, restrictive cardiomyopathy, and cardiac tamponade. *In* Grossman, W., and Baim, D. S. (ed.): Cardiac Catheterization and Angiography. Philadelphia, Lea and Febiger, 1986, p. 440.)

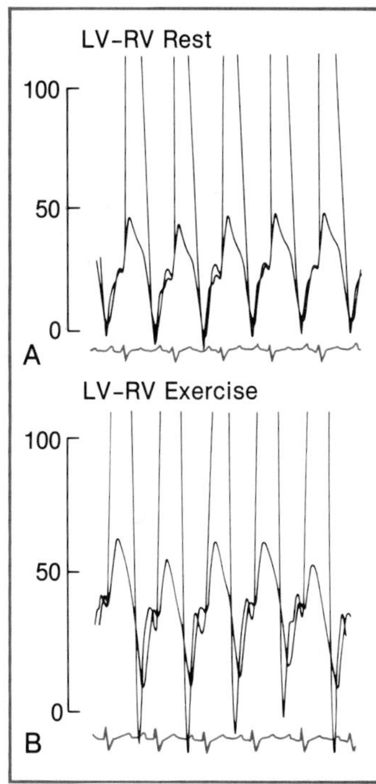

FIGURE 45–21. Representative left (LV) and right ventricular (RV) pressure tracings obtained at rest (*A*) and during exercise (*B*) from a patient with constrictive pericarditis. The diastolic equalization of pressures that is present at rest persists during exercise when the diastolic pressure of both ventricles is substantially higher. (From Robbins, M. A., et al.: Resting and exercise hemodynamics in constrictive pericarditis and a case of cardiac amyloidosis mimicking constriction. Cathet. Cardiovasc. Diagn. 9:463, 1983.)

waves that are small and equal in height and result in the typical M or W configurations (Fig. 45–20). Both the right and left ventricular diastolic pressures show an early diastolic dip followed by a plateau. This sign may be obscured by the presence of tachycardia, although the equilibration of diastolic pressures persists during exercise (Fig. 45–21), and by the damping effect of connecting tubes or bubbles within the catheters and transducers. Right ventricular and pulmonary artery systolic pressures are usually modestly elevated, in the range of 35 to 40 mm Hg, and rarely exceed 60 mm Hg. When hemodynamics in the baseline state are unremarkable, the rapid infusion of about 1000 ml of warmed saline over 6 to 8 minutes may unmask these findings in the rare patient with occult constrictive pericarditis.[208]

Careful recordings during respiration show that mean right atrial pressure fails to decrease normally or actually rises during inspiration. Since inspiration is associated with transient pooling of blood within the pulmonary bed and reduction in right ventricular afterload, inspiration causes a fall in pulmonary artery and right ventricular systolic pressures, pulmonary capillary wedge pressure, and left ventricular diastolic pressure. Because constrictive pericarditis is not associated with marked inspiratory swings in right ventricular filling, pulsus paradoxus is usually absent or less prominent than that observed in cardiac tamponade. Both cardiac output and stroke volume are low-normal or depressed. When they are depressed, compensatory tachycardia and elevation of systemic vascular resistance may be found.

The left ventricular angiogram usually demonstrates that left ventricular end-systolic and end-diastolic volumes are normal or decreased. In the absence of myocardial fibrosis or inflammation, both isovolumic and ejection phase indices of systolic function are normal.[159,209] Venous angiography may demonstrate dilatation of the superior vena cava and straightening of the right heart border; pericardial thickening may be detectable. These findings contrast with those of cardiac tamponade in which diastolic compression of the superior vena cava and right atrium is present. Coronary angiography may demonstrate that the coronary arteries are within the cardiac silhouette rather than on the surface of the heart, and rarely, diastolic pinching or external compression of the coronary arteries may be detected.[210] In rare patients, careful hemodynamic measurements may demonstrate the presence of regional pericardial constriction causing pulmonary outflow tract obstruction, which can be confirmed by right ventricular angiography.[154,155,211]

HEMODYNAMIC DIFFERENTIATION AMONG CONSTRICTIVE PERICARDITIS, CARDIAC TAMPONADE, AND RESTRICTIVE CARDIOMYOPATHY

Although both constrictive pericarditis and tamponade are characterized by elevation and equilibrium of right and left ventricular diastolic pressures, several hemodynamic features differ. In contrast to patients with constrictive pericarditis, patients with cardiac tamponade demonstrate (1) marked pulsus paradoxus, (2) a fall in right atrial pressure during inspiration, (3) elevation of intrapericardial pressure, (4) a right atrial pressure tracing with a predominant x descent and absence of or an attenuated y descent, and (5) lack of a prominent dip-and-plateau pattern in the right and left ventricular pressure pulses.

The findings of cardiac catheterization help to differentiate some but not all patients with constrictive pericarditis from those with restrictive cardiomyopathy (Table 45–7) due to amyloidosis, radiation injury, hemochromatosis, or other causes. In both conditions, right and left ventricular diastolic pressures are elevated, stroke volume and cardiac output are depressed, left ventricular end-diastolic volume is normal or decreased, and diastolic filling is impaired. A diagnosis of restrictive cardiomyopathy is more likely when marked right ventricular systolic hypertension is present (pressure > 60 mm Hg), and left ventricular diastolic pressure exceeds right ventricular diastolic pressure at rest or during exercise by more than 5 mm Hg.[212] However, in some patients with restrictive cardiomyopathy, hemodynamics at rest and during exercise may be indistinguishable from constrictive pericarditis, with equilibration of right and left ventricular diastolic pressures and a predominant dip-and-plateau pattern in the ventricular waveforms.[145,213–215]

TABLE 45–7 CONSTRICTIVE PERICARDITIS VERSUS RESTRICTIVE CARDIOMYOPATHY

	CONSTRICTIVE PERICARDITIS	RESTRICTIVE CARDIOMYOPATHY
S_3 gallop	Absent	May be present
Pericardial knock	May be present	Absent
Palpable systolic apical impulse	Absent	May be present
Pericardial calcification	Present 50%	Absent
Pulsus paradoxus	May be present	May be present
Equal RV and LV diastolic pressures	Usually present	LV > RV
Rate of LV filling	80% in first half of diastole	40% in first half of diastole
PEP/LVET	Av. 0.31	Av. 0.48 (congestive failure)
CAT scan, echo, MRI	Thickened pericardium	Normal pericardium

Modified from Fowler, N. O.: Constrictive pericarditis. *In* Fowler, N. O. (ed.): The Pericardium in Health and Disease. Mt. Kisco, NY, Futura Publishing Co., 1985, p. 319.

Angiographically, straightening of the right heart border may be present in both conditions, and thickening of the heart border may be detected as a result of either pericardial or myocardial thickening.[216] The finding of a depressed left ventricular ejection fraction in the presence of a small heart has been suggested as a discriminating feature of restrictive cardiomyopathy.[216] However, the left ventricular ejection fraction may be normal in some patients with restrictive cardiomyopathy and, conversely, is occasionally reduced in patients with constrictive pericarditis.[213,214]

Frame-by-frame analysis of left ventricular filling using left ventricular angiograms has been suggested as a method for distinguishing between constrictive pericarditis and restrictive cardiomyopathy.[217] In constrictive pericarditis, early dia-

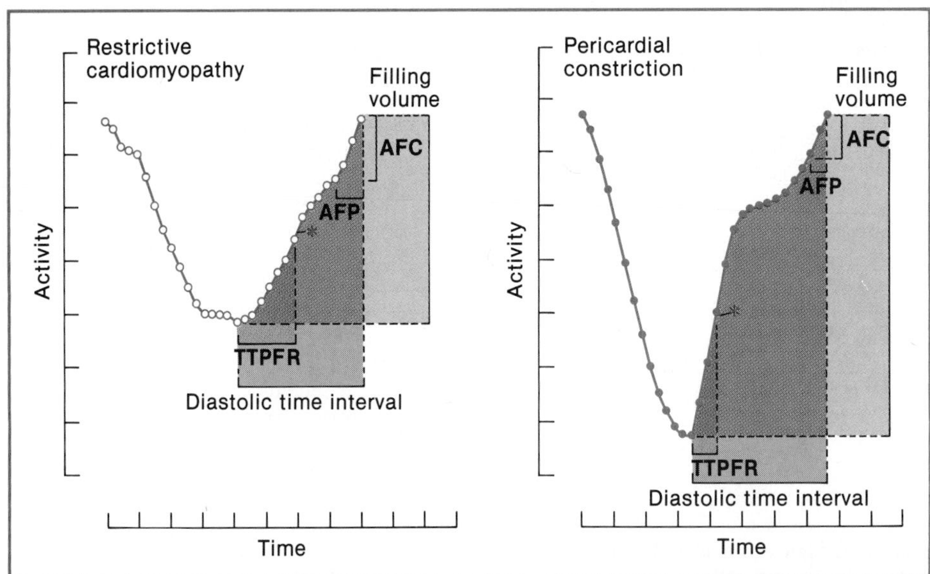

FIGURE 45–22. Time-activity curves obtained using first-pass radionuclide angiography in a patient with restrictive cardiomyopathy *(left panel)* and a patient with constrictive pericarditis *(right panel)*. The curve for the patient with constrictive pericarditis is characterized by an increased peak filling rate and an increased extent of ventricular filling, which occurs in early diastole, in contrast with the curve for the patient with restrictive cardiomyopathy that shows a "sluggish" pattern of diastolic filling with slower peak filling rate, a longer time to peak filling rate, and an enhanced atrial contribution to total left ventricular filling volume. * = peak filling rate; AFC = atrial filling contribution; TTPFR = time to peak filling rate. (From Aroney, C. N., et al.: Differentiation of restrictive cardiomyopathy from pericardial constriction: Assessment of diastolic function by radionuclide angiography. J. Am. Coll. Cardiol.*13*:1007, 1989.)

stolic filling tends to be excessively rapid in contrast to restrictive cardiomyopathy, in which early diastolic filling is slower than normal with greater dependence on the atrial contribution to filling. The discrimination between these patterns of left ventricular filling in constrictive pericarditis versus restrictive cardiomyopathy has also been accomplished using noninvasive methods, including the assessment of diastolic filling by radionuclide angiography[218] (Fig. 45–22), digitized M-mode echocardiography,[219] and Doppler echocardiography.[220,221] The use of transthoracic Doppler echocardiography for the analysis of respiratory changes in transvalvular flow velocities[221] and the use of transesophageal Doppler echocardiography to analyze patterns of pulmonary venous flow velocity during respiration[222] have been proposed to distinguish between these conditions. However, the predictive value of these approaches has not yet been established prospectively. Nor has the value of the assessment of filling patterns been clarified in the troublesome patient with suspected restrictive cardiomyopathy who has a dip-and-plateau ventricular waveform that simulates constrictive physiology and itself suggests a pattern of rapid and abruptly attenuated diastolic filling.

ENDOMYOCARDIAL BIOPSY. This technique is very useful in documenting the presence of specific causes of restrictive physiology such as amyloidosis or myocarditis in patients in whom constrictive pericarditis and restrictive cardiomyopathy cannot be differentiated at cardiac catheterization.[213,223] However, normal biopsy findings do not exclude the presence of restrictive cardiomyopathy.[214] Furthermore, pericardial involvement may coexist with several causes of restrictive physiology, including amyloid heart disease, radiation-induced myopathy, and hypereosinophilic syndrome.[169,203-205,224,225] In a minority of patients, exploratory thoracotomy with careful examination of both pericardial and myocardial biopsy specimens is warranted. These examinations will differentiate constrictive pericarditis, a condition that is usually treatable surgically, from restrictive cardiomyopathy, in which treatment is usually expectant.

MANAGEMENT OF CONSTRICTIVE PERICARDITIS

Chronic constrictive pericarditis is a progressive disease without spontaneous reversal of either pericardial thickening or abnormal symptoms and hemodynamics. A minority of patients may survive for many years with modest jugular venous distention and peripheral edema that is controlled by the judicious use of diet and diuretics. The majority of patients who are symptomatic and come to medical attention, however, become progressively more disabled by weakness, ascites, and peripheral edema and subsequently suffer the complications of severe cardiac cachexia. Treatment for constrictive pericarditis is complete resection of the pericardium (p. 1482), which achieves excision of the pericardium from the anterior and inferior surfaces of the right ventricle and the diaphragmatic and anterolateral surfaces of the left ventricle extending to the great vessels and to or across the atrioventricular grooves. Attention must also be paid to the presence of right atrial thrombosis in association with constrictive pericarditis, which should be managed with thrombectomy at the time of pericardiectomy.[226] Changes in technique have included the use of median sternotomy rather than left thoracotomy, cardiopulmonary bypass to permit greater mobilization of the heart,[227] and performance of pericardiectomy earlier in the course of the disease prior to the appearance of cardiac cachexia and dense pericardial calcification. Ultrasonic debridement using an ultrasonic surgical aspiration device has been reported to be a useful adjunct to the complete surgical removal of densely calcified and adherent pericardium.[228]

RESULTS OF PERICARDIECTOMY. In 1980, Culliford et al. reported an operative mortality of 15 per cent with a range of 6 to 25 per cent in over 300 reported cases of pericardiectomy.[229] In over 700 cases reported in 11 series since 1981, the average operative mortality was 11 per cent and ranged from 7 to 19 per cent.[149,230-235] A low-output syndrome occurs in 14 to 28 per cent of patients in the immediate postoperative period, and risk factors predictive of in-hospital mortality and low-output syndrome include the degree of preoperative disability (functional Class III or IV) and severity of constriction as indicated by marked elevation of right ventricular end-diastolic pressure.[230,233] Among patients who survive the operation, symptomatic improvement can be expected in about 90 per cent and complete relief of symptoms in about 50 per cent of patients.[230,231,233-236] Careful actuarial analysis of long-term survival has been available in large series from the Mayo Clinic[230] and Stanford,[233] which have reported a 5-year survival of 84 and 74 per cent, respectively. Long-term survival and symptomatic relief do not appear to be influenced by age, choice of median sternotomy or left thoracotomy, or transient low-output syndrome postoperatively. However, overall outcome is unfavorably influenced by the presence of severe preoperative functional disability (NYHA Class III or IV, diuretic use), renal insufficiency in the preoperative state, the presence of extensive nonresectable calcifications, incomplete pericardial resection, and the presence of radiation pericarditis, which is commonly complicated by myocardial fibrosis and restrictive myocardial disease. These considerations indicate that pericardiectomy should be performed early in the course of constrictive pericarditis in symptomatic patients, since the development of severe clinical disability is associated with a poor surgical outcome.

Pericardiectomy should probably not be routinely attempted in very elderly patients with severe liver dysfunction, cachexia, densely calcified pericardium, and massive cardiac enlargement indicative of underlying myocardial damage or in patients with limited life expectancy. Patients with known or suspected tubercular pericarditis should be treated with multidrug antituberculosis therapy for 2 to 4 weeks before operation; if the diagnosis is confirmed, these drugs should be continued for 6 to 12 months after pericardiectomy.

Striking hemodynamic and symptomatic improvement is apparent in some patients immediately after operation. In others, symptomatic improvement and resolution of elevated jugular venous pressure and abnormal filling patterns may be delayed for weeks to months.[237] This delayed or inadequate response to pericardiectomy has been attributed to incomplete pericardial resection, myocardial damage by the inflammatory process,[230,233] and the development of recurrent cardiac compression by mediastinal inflammation and fibrosis.[238,239] The role of unrecognized constriction by an epicardial peel (visceral pericardium) as a cause for a poor response to pericardiectomy was described by Harrington in 1944[240] and subsequently confirmed.[241] The importance of visceral constriction has also been underscored by the Stanford experience in which 59 per cent of cases had involvement of the visceral pericardium (epicardium) and required visceral decortication.[233] When there is little change in size of the heart or fall in intracardiac pressures after removal of the parietal pericardial layer, consideration should be given to epicardial dissection.

EFFUSIVE-CONSTRICTIVE PERICARDITIS

Effusive-constrictive pericarditis is the condition of a tense pericardial effusion in the presence of visceral pricardial constriction.[242,243] *The hallmark of this condition is continued elevation of right atrial pressure after the aspiration of pericardial fluid and restoration of intrapericardial pressure to zero.* This entity may represent a stage in the development of classic constrictive pericarditis. The most common causes of effusive-constrictive pericarditis are the same as for chronic constrictive pericarditis (p. 1483) and include idiopathic or presumed viral pericarditis, tuberculosis, neoplastic infiltration of the pericardium, and mediastinal irradiation.[243] Symptoms are nonspecific and include atypical chest pain and a heavy underprivileged or immunosuppressed. It is noteworthy that tuberculous pericarditis may develop during chemotherapy for pulmonary tuberculosis.[290] In a minority of patients with pericarditis, a definitive diagnosis of a tuberculous origin may be made by culture or histological demonstration of tuberculosis outside the pericardium (sputum, gastric wash, pleural fluid, liver or bone marrow biopsy). A definitive diagnosis can be made by isolation of the bacillus from the pericardial fluid or pericardial biopsy. It is difficult to establish a definitive bacteriological diagnosis because of the low yield of the bacillus when pericardial fluid is examined by acid-fast stain on microscopy; the failure of the bacillus to grow on appropriate media or in guinea pigs, even in patients with known tuberculous pericardial effusion; and the need to observe bacterial cultures for at least 8 weeks. The probability of obtaining a definitive diagnosis is greatest if both pericardial fluid and a pericardial biopsy specimen are examined early in the effusive stage.[286,291] However, it must be emphasized that a normal pericardial biopsy result does not exclude tuberculous pericarditis, since in some patients examination of the entire pericardium removed at pericardiectomy or autopsy is required to demonstrate clear-cut evidence of tuberculosis.[286,292] Furthermore, the finding of granulomas and caseous material without viable bacilli is also not diagnostic of tuberculous pericarditis, since these findings can be present in chronic pericardial disease due to rheumatoid arthritis and sarcoidosis. The measurement of a high level of adenosine deaminase activity (>45 units/liter) in pleural or pericardial fluid, although not diagnostic, is supportive of a diagnosis of tuberculous pericarditis.[286,293,294]

It may be necessary to make a presumptive clinical diagnosis of tuberculous pericarditis in severely ill patients with a large hemorrhagic pericardial effusion, a positive tuberculin skin test, and systemic symptoms such as weight loss and anorexia, even when examinations of the pericardial fluid and biopsy do not reveal tuberculosis. In such patients, clinical improvement may occur after initiation of antituberculosis chemotherapy. It should be emphasized that the tuberculin skin test alone is not a reliable indicator of tuberculous pericarditis, since it may be negative in as many as 30 per cent of patients with documented tuberculosis due to anergy, and is positive in about 30 to 40 per cent of patients with acute idiopathic pericarditis and benign natural history.[62,168] Making a presumptive clinical diagnosis of tuberculous pericarditis requires careful judgment, since, on the one hand, treatment should not be withheld from seriously ill patients, while, on the other, it is not prudent to commit patients with nontuberculous effusions to a prolonged course of multiple-drug antituberculosis therapy. The systematic approach suggested by Permanyer-Miralda et al. (p. 1471) appears to have a high likelihood of identifying patients with tuberculous pericarditis with a very low risk of either missing active tuberculosis or inappropriately applying blind antituberculous therapy.[62] This strategy remains to be validated in other populations.

MANAGEMENT. In the era before antituberculosis chemotherapy, tuberculous pericarditis was rapidly fatal, with an early mortality rate greater than 80 per cent; the remaining patients had a protracted course of months to years with frequently fatal outcome due to miliary tuberculosis or constrictive pericarditis. Since the introduction of early chemotherapy, mortality from acute tuberculous pericarditis has fallen to less than 50 per cent, but the effectiveness of antituberculosis chemotherapy in preventing the development of constrictive pericarditis is controversial.[276,282–285] In a recent series of 294 consecutive patients with acute pericarditis, 13 patients were shown to have tuberculous pericarditis and 7 (54 per cent) developed constrictive pericarditis requiring pericardiectomy.[286]

Treatment of tuberculous pericarditis includes hospitalization with bedrest and particular attention to findings of physical examination, electrocardiography, and echocardiography that suggest the development of an enlarging pericardial effusion and tamponade or constrictive pericarditis. Initial chemotherapy should usually consist of a three-drug regimen, such as oral isoniazid, oral ethambutol, and intramuscular streptomycin. The use of corticosteroids has been advocated to reduce pericardial inflammation and enhance resorption of pericardial effusion.

In a controlled trial in South Africa, 143 patients with tuberculous pericarditis and clinical signs of constrictive physiology were randomized to receive antitubercular drug therapy with prednisolone or placebo added during the first 11 weeks of treatment.[295] In this trial, clinical improvement occurred more rapidly, and there was a lower mortality at 24 months (4 versus 11 per cent) and a lower requirement for pericardiectomy (21 versus 30 per cent) in the prednisolone versus placebo-treated cohort. The use of steroids earlier in the course of tuberculous pericarditis before the development of constrictive physiology has not been studied in a clinical trial. We believe that corticosteroids should be reserved for critically ill patients with recurrent large effusion who do not respond to antituberculosis drugs alone.

In patients with documented cardiac tamponade or with a large pericardial effusion seen on the echocardiogram, the effusion should be drained initially by percutaneous pericardiocentesis with continued catheter drainage. Pericardiectomy should be performed after 4 to 6 weeks of antituberculosis drug therapy if patients develop large recurrent effusions or cardiac compression due to effusive-constrictive disease or early constrictive pericarditis.[271,276,277,283,295] Pericardiectomy should be performed early in the course in patients with clinical and hemodynamic evidence of chronic cardiac compression with anticipation of a good outcome. In a South African study of 113 patients with severe constrictive tuberculous pericarditis, 97 per cent were discharged from the hospital; in the majority, hepatomegaly and edema promptly resolved, whereas resolution of venous congestion required 2 to 3 months in some patients.[287] Mortality is higher among patients who undergo pericardiectomy at the late stage of calcific pericardial constriction.[276,287]

BACTERIAL (PURULENT) PERICARDITIS

Although the clinical spectrum of bacterial purulent pericarditis has changed over the past four decades, mortality remains high. Since the introduction of antibiotics in the 1940's, the incidence of bacterial pericarditis detected at autopsy has decreased.[295,296] Before 1943, purulent pericarditis occurred primarily as a complication of pneumococcal pneumonia or empyema and uncontrolled pleuropulmonary disease due to staphylococci or streptococci. During the antibiotic era, there has been a decline in the incidence of pneumococcal and streptococcal pericarditis, although these organisms continue to cause purulent pericarditis.[297] Acute self-limited pericarditis has also been observed in young adults with acute streptococcal tonsillitis in the absence of rheumatic fever.[298] The incidence of hospital-acquired penicillin-resistant staphylococcal pericarditis in post-thoracotomy patients has increased, and there is a widened spectrum of organisms responsible for bacterial pericarditis, including non-group A streptococcus[299] the gram-negative bacilli (*Proteus, Escherichia coli, Pseudomonas, Klebsiella*),[296] *Brucella melitensis*,[300] *Salmonella* species,[301,302] *Neisseria gonorrhoeae*,[303] *Hemophilus influenzae*,[304] *Francisella tularensis*,[305] anaerobic organisms,[306,307] and other unusual pathogens.[308–310] It is now established that *Neisseria meningitidis*, particularly from serogroup C and W, can cause either a primary infection of the pericardium in the absence of meningitis, or secondary pericarditis complicating meningitis and sepsis.[311–313] *Legionella pneumophila*, the causative organism in legionnaire's disease, has been reported as a cause of purulent pericarditis associated with pneumonia and as a primary infection.[314,315] Important predisposing factors for the development of purulent pericarditis include a preexisting pericardial effusion as in uremic pericarditis, as well as immunosuppression due to burns, immunotherapy, lymphoma, leukemia, or AIDS.

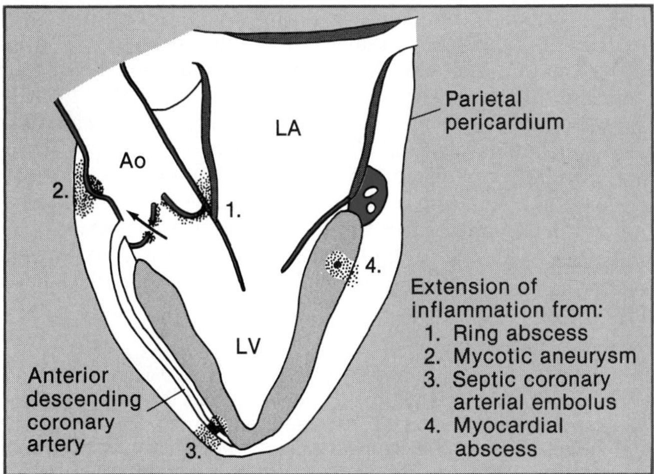

FIGURE 45-23. The pathogenesis of pericarditis in infective endocarditis. Ao = aorta; LV = left ventricle; LA = left atrium. (From Roberts, W. C., and Spray, T. L.: Pericardial heart disease: A study of its causes, consequences, and morphologic features. *In* Spodick, D. H. (ed.): Pericardial Diseases. Philadelphia, F. A. Davis Co., 1976, p. 31.)

The routes of pericardial infection have also changed. Direct pulmonary extension of bacterial pneumonia or empyema now accounts for only about 20 per cent of cases of purulent pericarditis.[307] Today, purulent pericarditis tends to occur in adults via (1) contiguous spread from an early postoperative infection after thoracic surgery or trauma, (2) infection related to infective endocarditis, (3) extension from a subdiaphragmatic suppurative source, and (4) hematogenous spread during bacteremia. In patients with endocarditis, bacterial pericarditis is a life-threatening complication that is detected ante mortem in about 1 of 25 patients with endocarditis,[316] in about 1 of 8 patients with endocarditis studied at autopsy, and in a higher percentage of those with staphylococcal endocarditis.[296] In such patients, bacterial pericarditis may develop (1) by extension from a valve ring abscess, (2) by rupture of an aneurysm, (3) by extension from a myocardial abscess, or (4) from a septic coronary embolus[317,318] (Fig. 45-23). An infected myocardial infarction or aortic aneurysm may also be a source for the development of purulent bacterial pericarditis.[319] Extension of a subdiaphragmatic abscess into the pericardial space is a rare source of purulent pericarditis.[320]

BACTERIAL PERICARDITIS IN CHILDREN. In children, the most common organisms include *Staphylococcus aureus* followed by *Hemophilus influenzae* and *Neisseria meningitis.*[321,322] *Hemophilus influenzae* pericarditis has been increasingly recognized in young children and is usually characterized by a mild prodromal illness followed by the rapid development of cardiac compression and death due to pericardial effusion.[323] Pediatric illnesses associated with the development of bacterial pericarditis include pharyngitis, pneumonia, meningitis, otitis media, impetigo, endocarditis, and bacterial arthritis.[321] The development of bacterial pericarditis in infants and children carries a high mortality—approaching 70 per cent, depending on the organism, and the risk of extremely rapid early development of constrictive pericarditis.[321,324] The high mortality in children appears to be reduced by early diagnosis and combined treatment with parenteral antibiotics and open surgical pericardial drainage, if effusion recurs after initial pericardiocentesis.[321,324] Following this contemporary approach of parenteral antibiotics and early drainage of purulent fluid, a series of purulent pericarditis in children reported a mortality of 18 per cent.[322]

PATHOLOGY. Bacterial pericarditis is usually frankly suppurative by the time it is detected clinically. The inflammation may result in organization and dense adhesions with a loculated pericardial effusion followed by obliteration of the pericardial space, thickening, and eventual calcification of the pericardium. In some patients, the inflammation may involve the adjacent sternum, pleura, and diaphragm with formation of dense adhesions between the parietal pericardium and contiguous structures. The evolution of this inflammatory process has been studied in an animal model of pericarditis caused by the injection of heat-killed staphylococci into the pericardial space.[325]

CLINICAL FEATURES. Bacterial pericarditis is usually an acute fulminant illness of only a few days' duration. In one series,[307] the mean duration of symptoms prior to hospitalization was only 3 days. High fevers, shaking chills, night sweats, and dyspnea are common. In most patients the symptom of typical pericardial chest pain is absent. Tachycardia is present in nearly all patients, but a pericardial friction rub is present in less than half. In many cases the pericarditis remains unsuspected because of the dominant presence of symptoms and signs related to an underlying known infection, such as pneumonia or mediastinitis following complicated thoracic surgery or trauma. The appearance of new jugular venous distention and pulsus paradoxus may be the first evidence of pericardial involvement, and these ominous signs reflect the development of cardiac tamponade due to the acute accumulation of suppurative fluid under pressure. In one series, cardiac tamponade developed acutely in 38 per cent of patients with previously unsuspected purulent pericarditis and contributed to death in the majority.[307]

Laboratory Findings. These usually include a leukocytosis with a marked leftward shift. The chest roentgenogram usually shows enlargement of the cardiac shadow and, less commonly, widening of the mediastinum. In the majority of cases the roentgenogram shows evidence of underlying pneumonia, empyema, or mediastinitis. Electrocardiographic changes typically include ST-segment and T-wave changes characteristic of pericarditis in the majority of patients.[307] The appearance of electrical alternans suggests the possibility of cardiac tamponade. In patients with suspected infective endocarditis, the appearance of a prolonged P-R interval, atrioventricular dissociation, or bundle branch block is strong evidence of extension of infection from the valve ring into the adjacent myocardium. The latter is an important predisposing factor for the development of pericarditis, especially in patients with staphylococcal endocarditis.[307]

Pericardial Fluid. This usually shows polymorphonuclear leukocytosis and sometimes frank pus. Pericardial glucose levels are usually depressed, and the protein content is increased; lactate dehydrogenase values may also be markedly elevated.

Purulent bacterial pericarditis should be suspected in a debilitated patient with unexplained high spiking fevers, dyspnea, markedly elevated white blood cell count, and an increase in the size of the cardiac silhouette on chest roentgenogram. The key to the diagnosis, which unfortunately is frequently not made before death, is a high index of suspicion. An echocardiogram should be promptly obtained to look for evidence of a new pericardial effusion and/or loculation of fluid with adhesions.

Natural History. Despite the lower incidence of purulent bacterial pericarditis in the antibiotic era, overall survival continues to be extremely poor, averaging about 30 per cent in modern series.[307,326] The poor prognosis stems in large part from failure of clinical diagnosis before death. In patients treated only with antibiotics without pericardial drainage, the rapid unsuspected development of a large pericardial effusion may result in sudden cardiovascular collapse and death due to cardiac tamponade. The high mortality from purulent pericarditis can be reduced substantially through the institution of both appropriate parenteral antibiotic therapy and early complete surgical drainage.[307,322,326] Early surgical drainage of the pericardium may help to prevent the complication of constrictive pericarditis. Successful treatment of bacterial endocarditis with long-term simple catheter drainage of the pericardial space has been reported, but experience with this approach is limited.[327]

Meningococcal Pericarditis. The pericardium may become infected early during meningococcal sepsis (in the presence or absence of meningitis), causing purulent pericarditis with cardiac tamponade, as described earlier. In these cases the pericardial fluid is frankly purulent, and viable organisms can usually be isolated. In addition, sterile pericarditis may occur late in the convalescent period in association with arthritis, pleuritis, and ophthalmitis. This syndrome appears to have an immunological etiology, does not require further antibiotic therapy if the primary infection has been adequately treated, and responds to antiinflammatory agents. Febrile, self-limited polyserositis with pericarditis has also been reported after effective treatment of sepsis due to *Staphylococcus aureus*,[328] and in young adults with acute streptococcal tonsillitis in the absense of rheumatic fever.[298]

MANAGEMENT. Suspicion of the presence of purulent pericardial fluid is an indication to explore the pericardial space. This may be done by percutaneous pericardiocentesis only if there is echocardiographic evidence of a large anterior and posterior pericardial effusion that may be safely tapped or, preferably, by a generous subxiphoid pericardiotomy with thorough pericardial drainage. Both pericardial fluid and pericardial tissue should be immediately studied by means of Gram-stained, acid-fast, and fungal smears by an experienced examiner. The fluid should then be cultured for aerobic and anaerobic bacteria with appropriate antibiotic sensitivity testing and for fungi and tuberculosis. Pericardial fluid should also be examined; the number of white blood cells, the differential count, hematocrit, and glucose and protein content should be determined. Cultures of blood, sputum, and recent surgical wounds should also be obtained.

Results of Gram-staining of the pericardial fluid should be used in the selection of antibiotic therapy. If the effusion is purulent but no organisms can be easily identified and tuberculosis is not considered likely, therapy should be initiated with both a semisynthetic antistaphylococcal antibiotic and an aminoglycoside. Depending on the results of the cultures of the pericardial fluid and blood, antibiotic therapy may then be modifed. High concentrations of antibiotics can be achieved in pericardial fluid, so that instillation of antibiotics into the pericardial space is not warranted.[329] However, systemic antibiotics alone are inadequate treatment, and prompt and thorough surgical drainage of the pericardium is essential in almost all patients with bacterial pericarditis.[307,323] Percutaneous aspiration of a large effusion may be extremely helpful in making an initial bacteriological diagnosis and initiating therapy, and percutaneous aspiration followed by catheter drainage is sometimes effective in preventing recurrent effusion.[327,330] However, purulent pericardial effusions are likely to recur, and more extensive surgical drainage may be needed in some patients after antibiotic therapy has been initiated. Open drainage, through creation of a subxiphoid pericardiotomy, is usually adequate when the diagnosis is made early and when the pericardial fluid is thin and the pericardium minimally thickened. This procedure is also the preferred route of drainage in severely disabled patients, since it can be performed under local anesthesia and avoids the pleural cavities. In a patient with a thick purulent effusion and dense adhesions with loculation, extensive pericardiectomy is needed to achieve adequate drainage and to prevent development of constrictive pericarditis,[296,307,324,331] which can occur very early after presentation.[332]

FUNGAL PERICARDITIS

ETIOLOGY AND PATHOPHYSIOLOGY. Histoplasmosis is the most common cause of fungal pericarditis. This diagnosis should be considered in young and otherwise healthy patients suspected of having acute viral or tuberculous pericarditis who live in the Ohio or Mississippi River Valley or the Western Appalachians, where the fungus is endemic.[333] In these areas, histoplasmosis is acquired by inhalation of spores during small rural outbreaks from bird or bat droppings and during major urban outbreaks related to excavation and building demolition. Coccidioidomycosis pericarditis occurs in patients who have inhaled chlamydospores from soil or dust in areas of the American Southwest, particularly the San Joaquin Valley, and Argentina, where it is endemic.[334] Other fungal infections responsible for pericarditis incude aspergillosis, blastomycosis, and those caused by *Candida albicans* and *Candida tropicalis*.[335-338] Groups at increased risk for the development of fungal pericarditis consequent to disseminated infection include drug addicts, patients who are immunosuppressed or who have received potent broad-spectrum antibiotics, and patients recovering from complicated open-heart surgery.

Histoplasmosis pericarditis most commonly develops as a noninfectious inflammatory response to infection confined to adjacent mediastinal lymph nodes and rarely by direct or hematogenous infection in patients with disseminated infection.[333,339] The isolation of organisms from pericardial fluid is unusual, and its predilection for young immunocompetent males suggests that self-limited histoplasmois pericarditis usually represents a sterile immune reaction. Pericarditis due to fungi other than histoplasmosis may occur as a complication of open-heart surgery in adults and children as a result of spread from contiguous infected lymph nodes or pulmonary lesions or hematogenous dissemination in immunosuppressed patients with fungal sepsis.

PATHOLOGY. Pericardial fluid may accumulate extremely rapidly and to massive quantities in patients with histoplasmosis. The fluid can be serous or hemorrhagic with increased protein content and polymorphonuclear leukocytosis. In cases of fungal pericarditis due to agents other than *Histoplasma*, exudative pericardial effusions may accumulate more slowly, so that an effusion may be present for months. Histoplasmosis and other fungal pericardial effusions occasionally become organized, with pericardial thickening, the appearance of granulomas and multinucleated giant cells, and the development of a constricting, calcified pericardium.[333,339]

Histoplasmosis in patients with disseminated infection may rarely cause infection of the myocardium and endocardium as well as of the pericardium.[339] Similarly, aspergillosis, candidiasis, and coccidioidomycosis may cause pericarditis in the context of pulmonary infection, endocarditis, and myocardial abscess.[336,337] Therefore, cardiac decompensation in patients with fungal pericarditis may be due either to the presence of cardiac compression from a pericardial effusion or a constricting pericardium or to an underlying myocardial infection.

CLINICAL FEATURES. The clinical course of histoplasmosis pericarditis is now better understood from two large urban outbreaks in which 6.3 per cent of 712 patients with clinically recognized histoplasmosis had acute pericarditis.[333] Almost all of the patients had a preceding respiratory illness, and pericardial pain and typical electrocardiographic changes at presentation. The chest roentgenogram was always abnormal, an enlarged cardiac silhouette was present in 95 per cent, and pleural effusions and intrathoracic adenopathy were present in two-thirds of the patients. Notably, the "classic" manifestations of histoplasmosis—acute self-limited disseminated infection or severe cavity pulmonary infection—were absent. However, more than 40 per cent of patients had hemodynamic compromise or frank cardiac tamponade consistent with other reports.[333,339] Histoplasmosis pericarditis can rarely occur in the less common setting of severe prolonged disseminated infection evident by fever, anemia, leukopenia, and the syndrome of pneumonitis progressing to pulmonary cavitation, massive hepatomegaly, meningitis, myocarditis, or endocarditis. Severe disseminated infections are especially likely to occur in young infants, elderly males, and immunosuppressed patients.

Coccidioidomycosis Pericarditis. This condition does not occur in the brief self-limited influenza-like form of the infection but is instead a complication of the progressive disseminated form of coccidiodomycosis.[334] Blacks, Filipinos, and Chicanos appear to be especially vulnerable to the development of disseminated coccidioidomycosis. These patients are usually chronically ill and debilitated, with fever, weight loss, and the complications of pulmonary cavitations with lymphadenopathy, osteomyelitis, and meningitis. In immunocompromised patients, the insidious appearance of symptoms of fungal pericarditis and underlying myocardial infection may initially be overlooked because attention is focused on symptoms related to underlying lymphoma, leukemia, or known valvular endocarditis. Physical findings suggestive of cardiac compression (jugular venous distention, hypotension, pulsus paradoxus) may be the first clues to the diagnosis of fungal pericarditis.

DIAGNOSIS.

Histoplasmosis Pericarditis. In young and otherwise healthy adults with evidence of pericarditis, a presumptive clinical diagnosis of histoplasmosis pericarditis can be made on the basis of (1) residence or travel in an endemic area, (2) an elevated complement fixation titer of at least 1:32, and (3) a positive immunodiffusion test.[333] Most patients do not show a progressive rise in titer, since pericarditis usually occurs after initial mild or asymptomatic pneumonitis such that titers are high when first measured. Histoplasmin skin tests are not helpful, and their use may falsely elevate antibody titers.[333] *Histoplasma* may be isolated from specimens from invasive biopsies of mediastinal nodes, but cultures or methenamine silver stains rarely identify the organism in extrapulmonary sites such as the liver, bone marrow, and pericardium in patients with benign, self-limited form of pericarditis. Histoplasmosis pericarditis that occurs in the setting of severe disseminated infection must be differentiated from sarcoidosis, tuberculosis, Hodgkin's disease, and brucellosis. Histological tissue examination and culture are important in disseminated progressive histoplasmosis, and in this setting the organism may be isolated from extrapericardial sites such as the bone marrow, exudate from ulcers, or sputum by inoculation on Sabouraud's medium or by guinea pig inoculation with subsequent subculture of the spleen.

Coccidioidomycosis Pericarditis. A presumptive diagnosis of coccidioidomycosis pericarditis is made in a patient with pericarditis who has (1) a history of dust exposure in an endemic area in the American Southwest, California Central Valley, or South America, (2) a characteristic clinical picture of disseminated coccidioidomycosis involving the lungs and other organs, (3) the appearance of a positive serum precipitin test early in the infection followed by a rising positive complement-fixation antibody titer, and (4) microscopic evidence of the characteristic spherule in biopsy material. A definitive diagnosis is made by culture identification of the organism on Sabouraud's medium. Coccidioidin skin tests are often negative in the presence of progressive disseminated disease.

Other Fungal Pericarditis. If pericarditis due to other fungal organisms is suspected, appropriate complement-fixing antibody titers should be measured. Serology and precipitin tests for *candida* are not sensitive or specific, and the diagnosis of candida pericarditis depends on growth of the fungus from several sites other than superficially contaminated catheters in association with immunosuppression or complicated cardiac surgery.[337] Depending on the clinical setting, it may be important to obtain pericardial fluid and a pericardial biopsy specimen. It must be emphasized that the microscopic finding of granulomas alone is nonspecific and may occur in tuberculosis, fungal and parasitic infections, and sarcoid involvement of the pericardium. Therefore, histological documentation of the characteristic appearance of the fungus and subsequent culture identification are important.

MANAGEMENT. *Histoplasmosis pericarditis* is generally a benign illness that resolves within 2 weeks and does not require treatment with amphotericin.[333] Nonsteroidal antiinflammatory drugs or steroids appear to shorten the duration of chest pain, fever, pericardial friction rub, and effusion.[333] Patients should always be hospitalized, since histoplasmosis may cause the rapid development of massive effusions with acute cardiac tamponade that require emergency pericardiocentesis or pericardiectomy.[333,339] Although pericardial calcification and pericardial constriction have been reported in histoplasmosis pericarditis, these complications are uncommon. Intravenous amphotericin B is required only for patients with histoplasmosis pericarditis and severe systemic disease.

In *nonhistoplasmosis fungal pericarditis* the diagnosis is rarely made before death. Spontaneous remissions do not occur; infection progresses until the patient dies either of the underlying disease or of fungal pericardial and myocardial involvement. Survival from nonhistoplasmosis fungal pericarditis has been reported in occasional patients treated with parenteral antifungal therapy and surgical drainage by pericardiectomy.[337,340] Drug therapy for pericarditis associated with disseminated coccidioidomycosis, aspergillosis, and blastomycosis consists of prolonged intravenous therapy with amphotericin B. The South American form of blastomycosis may require the addition of a sulfonamide. Candida pericarditis associated with fungal sepsis and disseminated infection is treated with amphotericin B, in addition to pericardiectomy.[337] In many cases of nonhistoplasmosis fungal pericarditis, chronic pericardial fungal infection progresses to severe pericardial constriction or, less commonly, cardiac tamponade. Therefore, depending on the patient's underlying medical condition, pericardiectomy is usually indicated. Intrapericardial instillation of antifungal agents has not proved helpful in these diseases. The serious toxicity associated with prolonged amphotericin B administration underscores the importance of making a definitive diagnosis after histological examination or culture.

Pericarditis complicated by the development of cardiac tamponade and chronic constrictive pericarditis may also be caused by *Actinomyces israelii* and *Nocardia asteroides*, which are intermediate forms between fungi and bacteria.[341-343] These organisms may cause indolent infections and invasion of the pericardium from thoracic, abdominal, or cervicofascial abscesses.

OTHER INFECTIOUS PERICARDITIS

The parasite *Toxoplasma gondii*, which is usually acquired by accidental cyst ingestion in endemic areas, is a cause of myocarditis, acute pericarditis, and chronic pericardial effusion.[344] The prevalence of *Toxoplasma* as a cause of acute pericarditis of unknown origin may be underestimated.[62] Other parasitic causes include amebiasis,[345-347] schistosomiasis,[348] and echinococcosis.[349-351] The diagnosis of amebic pericarditis is facilitated by the demonstration of multiple cystic lesions in the region of the pericardium by chest roentgenography and two-dimensional echocardiography.[346,347] Uncommon causes of parasitic pericarditis include dracunculosis,[352] cysticercosis, and filariasis.[353] These unusual infections rarely cause acute cardiac tamponade but may cause chronic constrictive pericarditis. The spirochetes *Borrelia burgdorferi* and *Babesia microti* are newly recognized as a cause of fatal myopericarditis in association with Lyme disease.[354-356] The psittacosis agent, *Chlamydia psittaci,* an obligate intracellular parasite-like bacterium that causes a febrile pneumonitis via bird-to-human transmission, is also a rare cause of effusive pericarditis.[357]

PERICARDITIS FOLLOWING ACUTE MYOCARDIAL INFARCTION

(See also p. 1263)

Pericarditis is a common occurrence during the first few days after acute myocardial infarction. The incidence of early postmyocardial infarction pericarditis varies from 6 to 25 per cent, although a much higher incidence is detected at autopsy.[358-360] In a prospective study of 703 patients with acute myocardial infarction, pericarditis, defined by the detection of a pericardial friction rub, occurred in 25 per cent of patients with transmural infarction and in 9 per cent of patients with subendocardial (non-Q wave) infarction.[361] Almost all patients with acute transmural myocardial infarction are found to have evidence of a localized fibrinous pericarditis overlying the infarction at autopsy, whereas fibrinous pericarditis is detected in about 10 per cent of patients with subendocardial infarction (non-Q wave infarction) at autopsy.[362] Pericarditis is more prevalent in anterior than in inferior infarction[361] and also occurs following lateral and predominant right ventricular infarction. Other forms of pericardial involvement after myocardial infarction include acute pericardial hemorrhage secondary to cardiac rupture and the late occurrence of Dressler syndrome (p. 1263).

CLINICAL FEATURES. Pericarditis is recognized clinically by the appearance of a pericardial friction rub within 12 hours to 10 days after acute myocardial infarction. In most patients with postinfarction pericarditis, a pericardial friction rub appears on the first, second, or third day after infarction.[359-361] In about 70 per cent of patients, the presence of a pericardial rub is accompanied by pleuritic or positional chest pain.[361] There is usually a slight temperature elevation, but pneumonitis is uncommon. Appearance of a new friction rub more than 10 days after acute infarction probably represents the onset of Dressler syndrome[359] or pericarditis complicating a second infarction. Since pericardial friction rubs are notoriously evanescent, serial auscultatory evaluation of patients in various positions in a quiet room is important for detection. Pericardial rubs with a single systolic component heard near the apex may be confused with a new murmur of mitral regurgitation due to papillary muscle dysfunction or rupture. Postinfarction pericarditis does not directly cause hemodynamic deterioration unless pericardial effusion under pressure develops, causing cardiac tamponade.

In a series of patients with early postinfarction pericarditis,[359] and in a series of patients with acute infarction and pericardial effusion,[363] the use of heparin did not appear to be associated with increased risk. However, hemorrhagic cardiac tamponade related to the use of anticoagulants has been reported as a rare complication in patients with postinfarction pericarditis.[364,365] Constrictive pericarditis has been reported as a sequel of hemopericardium after infarction.[366,367] Acute thrombolytic therapy of acute infarction with streptokinase or tissue plasminogen activator followed by intravenous heparin has not yet been reported to promote the development of hemopericardium after infarction.

The typical diagnostic electrocardiographic changes of acute pericarditis are extremely rare in early postinfarction pericarditis,[360] and the electrocardiogram cannot be used to confirm the diagnosis in this setting. The finding of a small pericardial effusion in a post-myocardial infarction patient in the absence of hemodynamic compromise is also not pathognomonic of acute postinfarction pericarditis. Galve et al. found that a small pericardial effusion could be detected in 28 per cent of patients early after acute infarction in comparison with 8 per cent of asymptomatic patients with unstable angina and 5 per cent of normal subjects.[363] The presence of pericardial effusion correlates highly with the presence of extensive infarction and congestive failure, but not with clinical pericarditis reflected in the appearance of a pericardial rub or pain. Patients who develop pericarditis after infarction experience a more complicated hospital course and more extensive myocardial damage compared to patients without pericarditis, as evidenced by higher myocardial MB-CK enzyme levels and lower ejection fraction.[361] The development of congestive heart failure and a high Killip class are more common in patients with postinfarction pericarditis.[358,359,361] The development of atrial tachyarrhythmias is also more common in patients with pericarditis following infarction.[361,368,369] The appearance of acute postinfarction pericarditis *per se* does not appear to affect adversely the in-hospital mortality after acute infarction.[358–361] However, pericarditis does appear to be associated with an increase in 12-month mortality, which is probably accounted for by its association with larger infarct size and lower ejection fraction.[361]

Postinfarction pericarditis without cardiac compression must be differentiated from acute stress ulcer, acute pulmonary embolism, and, most importantly, from recurrent myocardial ischemia. Myocardial ischemic pain can usually be differentiated from the pain of postinfarction pericarditis by (1) obvious amelioration of the pain by nitroglycerin and (2) the appearance of new regional ST-segment and T-wave changes with reciprocal changes.

Cardiac Tamponade. The development of cardiac tamponade in patients with myocardial infarction may be related to pericardial hemorrhage secondary to pericarditis or to myocardial rupture within the first 3 days after infarction. Both situations may be associated with cardiovascular collapse, the appearance of dense echoes in the pericardial space or two-dimensional echocardiogram, and an abrupt increase in heart size on the chest roentgenogram. Pericardiocentesis may successfully relieve postinfarction hemorrhagic cardiac tamponade in occasional patients.[370] Massive cardiac hemorrhage secondary to cardiac rupture is usually followed by the rapid development of electromechanical dissociation and death, although survivors have been reported after subacute rupture managed with pericardiocentesis and surgical repair.[371,372] The development of a chronic myocardial rupture (pseudoaneurysm) with effusive-constrictive pericarditis is a rare complication of extensive silent infarction with postinfarction pericarditis.[373]

Acute cardiac tamponade secondary to postinfarction pericarditis must also be differentiated from cardiogenic shock without intrapericardial hemorrhage due to an acute ventricular septal defect or mitral regurgitation. In the setting of an inferior myocardial infarction, the appearance of hypotension, pulsus paradoxus, and jugular venous distention may be related to massive right ventricular infarction rather than to cardiac tamponade. Echocardiographic findings of right ventricular enlargement without a significant pericardial effusion and catheterization findings suggestive of constrictive physiology (right atrial waveform with steep *y* descent) rather than cardiac tamponade (right atrial waveform with attenuated *y* descent) help to differentiate these entities and prevent possibly disastrous attempts at pericardiocentesis.

MANAGEMENT. Postinfarction pericarditis may produce mild symptoms that require no specific therapy or severe chest pain that persists for several days. If the pain is severe, high-dose aspirin will relieve pain within 48 hours in most patients. A short course of prednisone may be required in patients whose pain does not improve after a 48-hour trial of nonsteroidal antiinflammatory agents.[374]

There is experimental evidence that indomethacin, ibuprofen, and multiple large doses of corticosteroids interfere with the conversion of the myocardial infarct into a scar, so that thinning of the myocardial wall occurs.[375] Myocardial rupture has been observed in a patient during ibuprofen use for postinfarction percarditis,[376] and there is evidence of a higher incidence of pericardial rupture in postmyocardial infarction patients who receive nonsteroidal antiinflammatory drugs. Therefore, these drugs should be employed with great caution in patients with acute myocardial infarction. Fortunately, aspirin does not appear to cause any of these adverse effects, and postinfarction pericarditis usually responds well to aspirin. Accordingly, we favor use of this drug.

UREMIC PERICARDITIS

(See also p. 1868)

ETIOLOGY. Pericarditis is a frequent and serious complication of chronic renal failure. Before the advent of dialysis, uremic pericarditis was detected in about half of the patients with untreated chronic renal failure and was usually a harbinger of death. Uremic pericarditis is now detected clinically in up to 20 per cent of uremic patients who require chronic dialysis.[377,378] Uremic pericarditis tends to be a complication that occurs either prior to initiation of dialysis or during the first few months of therapy.

The etiology of uremic pericarditis is unknown. Viral causes have been proposed,[379] but there is no consistent evidence to suggest a viral etiology in the majority of cases of uremic pericarditis. The occasional observation of a seasonal clustering of episodes of pericarditis in uremic patients is consistent with a viral etiology. Specific etiological factors, including purulent bacterial infections, are common in patients with uremic pericarditis, and it is unwise to assume that pericarditis in a patient with several renal disease is simply related to uremia. Toxic catabolic nitrogen metabolites and secondary hyperparathyroidism have been suggested mechanisms responsible for uremic pericarditis. This suggestion is supported by the observations that uremic pericarditis is rare in patients with acute mild renal failure and that uremic pericarditis often improves with initiation of dialysis in previously untreated patients. However, there is no clear correlation between the development of pericarditis and the levels of catabolic metabolites in uremic patients. It has also been proposed that pericarditis in dialysis patients may reflect an immunological response. Some support for this hypothesis comes from Maisch and Kochsiek's observations that 64 per cent of 25 patients with chronic uremia and pericarditis had complement-fixing antimyolemmal antibodies with cytolytic properties for cardiac tissue, whereas antimyocardial antibodies were rarely detected in patients with acute renal failure due to surgery or trauma.[380] It is possible that etiological factors in nondialyzed patients differ from those in patients undergoing regular dialysis. In the latter group, systemic and regional heparinization during dialysis itself may exacerbate uremic pericarditis by promoting the tendency of vascular pericardial granulation tissue to bleed into the pericardial space.

Acute uremic pericarditis is characterized by the appearance of shaggy, hemorrhagic, fibrinous exudate on both parietal and visceral pericardial surfaces with little acute inflammatory cellular reaction. In some patients, the friable pericardial surface may bleed, giving rise to hemorrhagic pericardial effusion. Subacute or chronic constrictive pericarditis may develop, coincident with organization of the effusion and formation of thick adhesions within the pericardial space.[381]

CLINICAL FEATURES. The development of pericarditis in patients undergoing dialysis is of clinical importance, since it may (1) cause disability or life-threatening cardiac tamponade in patients who are otherwise well compensated when undergoing dialysis, (2) compromise the status of patients who are candidates for renal transplantation, and (3) cause hemodynamic complications during routine dialysis. Patients with uremic pericarditis usually come to attention because of the development of chest pain. A pericardial friction rub is present on initial presentation in nearly 90 per cent of patients. Fever, leukocytosis, and tachycardia are frequent but nonspecific findings. Dyspnea and cardiac enlargement on the chest roentgenogram are common, but these findings can be related to underlying myocardial dysfunction and volume overload. Uremic pericarditis with a large pericardial effusion may first come to clinical attention when an otherwise asymptomatic patient becomes hypotensive and confused upon fluid removal during ultrafiltration. This occurs because volume depletion may cause an abrupt fall in systemic blood pressure when ventricular filling is already compromised by the presence of a large, tense pericardial effusion. Uremic pericarditis can also present as acute or subacute tamponade with the findings of jugular venous distention, hypotension, and pulsus paradoxus. In a study of 1058 patients undergoing dialysis over a 14-year period, acute cardiac tamponade developed in 17 per cent of 161 episodes of uremic pericarditis.[378]

Echocardiography. The presence of a small pericardial effusion is common in uremic patients, and in the absence of typical pericardial pain and friction rubs it is not diagnostic of pericarditis. Asymptomatic pericardial effusions of small to moderate size occur in 36 to 62 per cent of uremic patients who require dialysis and appear to be related to volume overload and clinical congestive heart failure.[382,383] On the other hand, the presence of a large anterior and posterior pericardial effusion in patients with uremic pericarditis that persists after about 10 days of intensive dialysis is associated with a high likelihood of requiring intervention to relieve tamponade.[377,378,382,384] The presence of a large pericardial effusion in association with echocardiographic findings of right atrial and right ventricular collapse is highly suggestive of cardiac tamponade in a patient with uremic pericarditis. Prior to consideration of pericardiostomy or pericardiectomy, it is important to document that these clinical findings are indeed related to the hemodynamics of cardiac tamponade (elevation and equilibration of pericardial, right and left heart filling pressures) rather than to underlying congestive cardiomyopathy, ischemic heart disease, or excessively vigorous ultrafiltration. It must be remembered that pulsus paradoxus may be absent in uremic patients with cardiac tamponade and coexisting left ventricular failure and elevated left ventricular filling pressures.

MANAGEMENT. Uremic patients who develop symptomatic pericarditis prior to the initiation of dialysis almost always respond to the initiation of vigorous dialysis.[377,382] In patients with acute uremic pericarditis with a large pericardial effusion, a period of 10 days to 3 weeks is usually required for resolution of the effusion after initiation of intensive dialysis.[377,385] In contrast, less than half of patients with asymptomatic pericardial effusions show resolution of effusion after initiation of dialysis.[382] No treatment is required for small, asymptomatic pericardial effusions that can be followed simply by serial echocardiography.[383]

Treatment of symptomatic uremic pericarditis that develops in patients more than 3 months after the initiation of chronic dialysis is controversial, and mutliple approaches have been advocated. About two-thirds of the patients who develop effusive uremic pericarditis following the initiation of dialysis will respond to a program of intensification of dialysis and regional heparinization. The remainder are likely to require operative drainage of the pericardium.[377,386,387] Factors that predict that the strategy of intensive dialysis is likely to fail include the presence of large anterior and posterior effusions, high fever, leukocytosis with left shift, and clinical evidence of the development of cardiac tamponade, such as hypotension and jugular venous distention.[378,385,388] Nonsteroidal antiinflammatory drugs have been widely advocated as therapy for patients with uremic pericarditis. A randomized, double-blind comparison of indomethacin versus placebo in symptomatic patients with uremic pericarditis showed that indomethacin reduced the duration of fever, but it had no significant effect on the duration of chest pain, pericardial rub, pericardial effusion, or need for relief of tamponade, which occurred in 20 per cent of patients.[389] The complications of long-term steroid administration limit its usefulness in the treatment of recurrent uremic pericarditis.

Pericardiocentesis with an indwelling catheter followed by instillation of a nonresorbable steroid into the epicardial space has also been advocated,[390] but this procedure has been complicated by the development of purulent pericarditis.[391] A single pericardiocentesis followed by a one-time instillation of triamcinolone appears to be effective and may eliminate the need for prolonged catheter drainage.[392] There are reports of repetitive pericardiocenteses with low morbidity and mortality in uremic patients,[393] but other series have reported substantial mortality as a consequence of pericardiocentesis.[377] The presence of a friable visceral pericardium may increase the risk of traumatic intrapericardial hemorrhage in uremic pericarditis, and the status of many patients is also compromised by the presence of left ventricular dysfunction. These considerations warrant special caution during the performance of pericardiocentesis in uremic patients, and this procedure probably should be carried out only by experienced personnel in an optimal environment.

Surgical Treatment. The surgical treatment of uremic patients with pericardial effusions with a subxiphoid pericardiostomy or limited pericardiectomy (window) performed through a left thoracotomy is effective in relieving cardiac tamponade. These approaches do not appear to be associated with an appreciable risk of developing recurrent effusions or constriction.[394,395] The intrapericardial instillation of steroids during surgical drainage has also been advocated,[385] although there is no evidence that this offers any advantage over thorough drainage alone.

Early surgical intervention in uremic patients with a large pericardial effusion has been advocated as a prophylactic measure to prevent the development of cardiac tamponade and to allow the procedures to be carried out at a time when the patient's condition is clinically stable. We feel that this approach is excessively aggressive, since many symptomatic uremic patients with pericardial effusions respond well to intensification of dialysis.

We advocate that patients with hemodynamic instability and with hemodynamic evidence of cardiac tamponade and echocardiographic evidence of a large anterior and posterior effusion may be treated by percutaneous catheter pericardiocentesis with continued catheter drainage of the pericardial sac for 24 to 48 hours. Subxiphoid pericardiotomy or limited pericardiectomy is reserved for patients with hemodynamic instability associated with recurrent pericardial effusions following pericardiocentesis or with loculated pericardial effusions.

NEOPLASTIC PERICARDITIS

(See also p. 1760)

PATHOLOGY. At autopsy, the pericardium is involved in 5 to 15 per cent of patients with malignant neoplasm.[396,397] Lung cancer, breast cancer, leukemia, Hodgkin's disease, and non-Hodgkin's lymphoma account for about 80 per cent of reported cases of malignant pericarditis.[396–402] Other malignant diseases reported to lead to pericardial involvement include gastrointestinal cancer, ovarian cancer, cervical cancer, sarcoma, thymoma, and melanoma[403–406] (Table 45–8). In children the most common etiologic factors are non-Hodgkin's lymphoma, neuroblastoma, sarcomas, and Wilms' tumor,[402] whereas pericardial teratomas are a rare cause of hydrops fetalis in utero and in neonates.[407–409] Primary malignant neoplasms of the pericardium are rare and are predominantly due to mesothelioma, including that arising after asbestos and fiberglass exposure,[410–412] and, less frequently, to benign localized fibrous mesothelioma, malignant fibrosarcoma, angiosarcoma, and benign and malignant teratomas.[413–416] Rare primary neoplasms of the pericardium occasionally have been reported in association with congenital developmental disorders such as tuberous sclerosis.[417] Catecholamine-secreting pheochromocytoma is a rare primary neoplasm of the pericardium.[418]

TABLE 45–8 CAUSES OF TUMORS METASTATIC TO THE PERICARDIUM

PRIMARY MALIGNANT NEOPLASM	FREQUENCY (%)
Lung carcinoma	40
Breast carcinoma	22
Gastrointestinal carcinoma	3
Other carcinomas	6
Leukemia and lymphoma	15
Melanoma	3
Sarcoma	4
Other (including malignant mesothelioma, germ cell tumors)	7

Relative frequency of neoplasms metastatic to the pericardium in 1315 patients.

Data from Goodie, R. B.: Secondary tumors of the heart and pericardium. Br. Heart J. *17*:183, 1955; and Scott, R. W., and Garvin, C. F.: Tumors of the heart and pericardium. Am. Heart J. *17*:431, 1939.

Pericardial metastases may involve the heart in several ways: (1) extension and attachment to the pericardium of a malignant mediastinal mass, (2) nodular tumor deposits from hematogenous or lymphatic spread, (3) diffuse pericardial thickening and infiltration with tumor, and (4) local infiltration of the pericardium.[398] In the majority of cases, the epicardium and myocardium are *not* involved.

Neoplastic pericarditis may cause several syndromes of cardiac compression. Neoplastic involvement of the pericardium may result in serosanguineous or hemorrhagic effusions, which may develop extremely rapidly, causing acute or subacute cardiac tamponade. Pericardial involvement by tumors such as sarcomas, mesotheliomas, and melanomas can also erode the cardiac chamber or intrapericardial blood vessels, causing acute pericardial distention and abrupt fatal cardiac tamponade. A rare cause of hemorrhagic effusion and cardiac tamponade is intrapericardial extramedullary hematopoiesis associated with preleukemic conditions and with Philadelphia chromosome–positive chronic myeloid leukemia.[419,420] Cardiac compression may also occur as a consequence of the development of both thickened pericardium and pericardial effusion under pressure (effusive-constrictive pericarditis), or it may be caused by thickening of the pericardium produced by tumor encasement of the heart, causing the physiology of constrictive pericarditis.

Not all pericardial effusions associated with mediastinal cancer are malignant. Asymptomatic pericardial effusions are common in patients with mediastinal lymphoma and Hodgkin's disease.[421] These evanescent effusions are frequently detected during staging procedures and presumably develop as a result of impaired lymphatic drainage. Fracp et al. have observed that small, clinically unsuspected pericardial effusions detectable by echocardiography are common in women with metastatic breast cancer.[422] In a prospective study of 38 women with metastatic breast cancer in whom echocardiography was done on a routine basis, 53 per cent were found to have small pericardial effusions that did not progress to cause hemodynamic embarrassment in any patient. It is uncertain whether small pericardial effusions in asymptomatic women with metastatic breast cancer are due to indolent malignant pericardial involvement or impaired lymphatic drainage.

CLINICAL FEATURES. Neoplastic pericarditis is often totally asymptomatic and detected only as an incidental finding at autopsy. However, it is the most common specific cause of acute pericarditis in developed countries. In a prospective series of patients with acute pericarditis of unknown cause, a diagnostic protocol revealed an unsuspected malignant etiology in 5 per cent of patients.[61] In patients with undiagnosed cancer, leukemia, or primary pericardial tumors, cardiac tamponade can be the initial manifestation.[398,412,423] In patients with known malignancy, symptoms resulting from pericardial involvement may be incorrectly attributed to the underlying neoplasm, so that malignant pericarditis is not suspected until symptoms and signs of severe cardiac compression appear.

In patients with malignant pericarditis, dyspnea is by far the most common symptom.[398,401,424] Other frequent symptoms and physical findings include chest pain, cough, orthopnea, and hepatomegaly. Distant heart sounds and a pericardial friction rub are rarely detected, which is in part probably due to a low index of suspicion.[398,424] In the majority of patients the diagnosis is made only when there is evidence of cardiac compression of frank cardiac tamponade, manifest as jugular venous distention, pulsus paradoxus, and hypotension. These findings occur more frequently with neoplastic pericarditis than in patients with an underlying neoplasm and idiopathic or radiation-induced pericarditis.[398]

The chest roentgenogram is abnormal in more than 90 per cent of patients with malignant pericarditis and may show pleural effusion, cardiac enlargement, mediastinal widening, a hilar mass, or, less commonly, an irregular nodular contour of the cardiac silhouette.[398,401] The electrocardiogram is usually abnormal but nonspecific, showing tachycardia, ST- and T-wave changes, low QRS voltage, and occasionally atrial fibrillation. In occasional patients, persistent tachycardia or electrocardiographic changes are the initial findings that lead to the diagnosis.[424] Electrocardiographic findings that are rarely seen in pericarditis, such as atrioventricular conduction disturbances, suggest malignant invasion of the myocardium and conduction system.

DIAGNOSIS. Patients with cancer and pericarditis benefit from a systematic evaluation, and these patients should not be summarily assumed to have a preterminal condition. The diagnosis of malignant pericarditis depends on both documentation of pericardial inflammation and substantiation that pericarditis is due to neoplasm. It is often not appreciated that in approximately half the patients with symptomatic pericarditis and neoplastic disease there is a nonmalignant cause; most commonly the condition is due to prior radiation or to idiopathic causes.[136,398] Many patients with advanced neoplastic disease are immunosuppressed as a consequence of their malignant disease and/or therapy and are therefore also at risk for tuberculous and fungal pericarditis. In a series of 140 patients with acute leukemia, pericarditis was diagnosed clinically or at autopsy in eight patients; it was caused by malignant disease in only one patient and by bacterial, fungal, or tuberculous pericarditis in the other patients.[425] Acute pericarditis has also been rarely reported as a complication of intravenous administration of the chemotherapeutic agents Adriamycin and daunorubicin.

In patients with the acquired immunodeficiency syndrome, the differential diagnosis is complex and includes involvement of the pericardium with Kaposi's sarcoma[426] as well as opportunistic infections with fungus or atypical acid-fast bacilli. Neoplastic pericarditis with cardiac compression must be differentiated from other causes of jugular venous distention, hepatomegaly, and peripheral edema in cancer patients. The most important of these are (1) underlying left ventricular dysfunction secondary to prior cardiac disease or adriamycin cardiac toxicity, (2) superior vena caval obstruction, (3) malignant hepatic involvement with portal hypertension, and (4) microvascular tumor spread in the lungs with secondary pulmonary hypertension.

Echocardiography often provides critical information about the presence and size of a pericardial effusion and the thickness and motion of the pericardium and may suggest the presence of abnormal diastolic filling of the heart due to cardiac compression. Two-dimensional echocardiography may be helpful in the detection of irregular undulating masses that protrude into the pericardial space and define the presence of pericardial space-occupying lesions.[427] Computed tomography and magnetic resonance imaging can also detect the presence of pericardial effusions and, in some instances, may give added information regarding the presence and location of space-occupying masses within the pericardium and adjacent mediastinum and lungs.[410,414,428,429]

We recommend that pericardiocentesis using the catheter drainage technique (p. 1480) should be performed in conjunction with cardiac catheterization in cancer patients with suspected cardiac tamponade in whom a large pericardial effusion is documented by echocardiography. Two additional diagnoses should always be systematically evaluated during cardiac catheterization in these patients. (1) Superior vena caval obstruction may coexist with malignant cardiac tamponade and contribute to the development of facial edema and jugular venous distention and should be systematically excluded at cardiac catheterization in cancer patients. (2) Cyanosis, hypoxemia, and elevation of the pulmonary vascular resistance are not features of cardiac tamponade, and pulmonary microvascular tumor (lymphangitic tumor) should be strongly suspected in a patient with these findings, hypoxemia, or persistent dyspnea following pericardiocentesis. Support for this diagnosis can be obtained at the same setting as pericardiocentesis and right-heart catheterization by obtaining a sample of blood from the pulmonary capillary wedge position for cytological analysis using the right-heart catheter.[430]

The appearance of the pericardial fluid does not differentiate among neoplastic, radiation, or idiopathic causes. Since treatment strategies differ, it is necessary to carry out a meticulous cytological examination of pericardial fluid in an attempt to differentiate malignant pericarditis from radiation-induced or idiopathic pericarditis. Cytological examination of pericardial fluid is diagnostic of a malignant neoplasm in about 85 per cent of the cases of malignant pericarditis.[136,398,431,432] False-negative cytological diagnoses are uncommon in carcinomatous pericarditis but occur more commonly with involvement by lymphoma or mesothelioma.[431,432] The measurement of carcinoembryonic antigen (CEA) may add to the diagnostic yield of the examination of pericardial fluid in patients with suspected neoplastic pericarditis; open pericardial biopsy may be required if the results of cytological examination of pericardial fluid are normal. If a sufficiently large biopsy specimen is obtained, open pericardial biopsy should provide a histological diagnosis in up to 90 per cent of cases. However, false-negative diagnoses may occur if only a small tissue sample is obtained, and in critically ill patients open pericardial biopsy is not without risk.

In patients with echocardiographic evidence of a thickened pericardium and the physical findings of cardiac compression (jugular venous distention, edema, ascites, and hepatomegaly), cardiac catheterization is useful for documenting the presence of constrictive physiology before a decision is made to proceed with aggressive surgical intervention, i.e., extensive pericardiectomy.

NATURAL HISTORY. If cardiac tamponade can be avoided or successfully treated, the mere presence of neoplastic pericarditis does not imply that death is imminent. Since lung cancer and breast cancer are by far the most common causes of malignant pericarditis with cardiac tamponade, both the management strategy and subsequent natural history usually depend on the type of underlying malignant disease. The natural history of neoplastic pericarditis in patients treated for cardiac tamponade was studied using a Kaplan-Meier analysis in two series.[150,398] In both series, the mean survival was 4 months with 25 per cent surviving 1 year. We studied the outcome of a consecutive series of 29 patients with malignant pericardial effusion and tamponade managed with pericardiocentesis in whom the 1-year survival rate was 17 per cent compared with 91 per cent for 21 patients with nonmalignant effusion.[128] These series indicate that a subset of about 25 per cent of patients with cardiac tamponade due to malignant pericarditis who are managed surgically or with pericardiocentesis will enjoy 1 year survival or better. Furthermore, the outcome in patients with malignant pericarditis due to breast cancer is strikingly better than that in patients with lung cancer or other metastatic carcinomas. Following surgical treatment of cardiac tamponade in lung cancer patients, Piehler et al. reported that the mean survival was only 3.5 months in contrast with breast cancer patients in whom mean survival was 9 months with survivorship extending to more than 5 years.[150] In one series of breast cancer patients with malignant pericarditis managed with pericardiectomy or pericardiotomy, the overall median survival was 17 months.[422] A similar prolonged survival in patients with malignant effusion due to breast cancer has been reported by others.[398,432,434–436]

MANAGEMENT. Decisions about the management of neoplastic pericardial effusion depend on the underlying condition of the patient, the presence or absence of clinical manifestations related to cardiac compression, and the prognosis and treatment options available for the specific histology and stage of the underlying malignant disease. At one end of the spectrum are debilitated patients with end-stage malignant disease for whom there is no promising treatment option for the underlying malignant disease and for whom the prognosis is bleak. In this setting, diagnostic procedures should be as brief and painless as possible, and intervention should be directed toward alleviation of symptoms with a goal of improving the quality of the remaining days or weeks of life. In these patients, pericardiocentesis with catheter drainage is indicated for immediate relief of severe dyspnea, chest pain, or orthopnea. At centers experienced in catheter pericardiocentesis, neoplastic cardiac tamponade can be safely relieved with pericardiocentesis in 90 to 100 per cent of cases with a low (< 2 per cent) risk of major complications.[105,128,397,436,437] At centers with a high complication rate with pericardiocentesis or if cardiac tamponade recurs, palliation can be achieved with an equally high success rate and low morbidity by a subxiphoid pericardiotomy under local anesthesia.[150,397] The more invasive and debilitating partial pericardiectomy (window) done via a left thoracotomy has also been advocated, but this procedure appears to have no advantage as a palliative procedure over a subxiphoid pericardiotomy and should rarely be done in patients with end-stage malignancy.[150]

When the general prognosis of the patient is better, several more aggressive treatment options are available, the goals of which are (1) relief of cardiac tamponade, (2) prevention of recurrence of the malignant effusion, and (3) treatment or prevention of constrictive pericardial disease.

In patients with asymptomatic pericardial effusion who have a treatment option of effective chemotherapy or hormonal therapy directed against the underlying malignant disease, treatment with systemic agents alone can be attempted while progression of the effusion is observed by means of echocardiography. In patients with cardiac tamponade and large effusions secondary to neoplastic pericarditis, pericardiocentesis with thorough catheter drainage in combination with systemic chemotherapy can be attempted. Based on small series of patients, the instillation of multiple chemotherapeutic agents, radioisotopes, and lymphokine-activated killer cells into the pericardial space following pericardiocentesis or surgical drainage has been advocated, with the aim being sclerosis of the pericardial membranes and obliteration of the pericardial space.[424,437–441] However, in comparison with complete catheter or surgical pericardial drainage, there is *no* convincing evidence to date from either a large collective experience or prospective trial to indicate that instillation of drugs into the pericardial space alters the outcome. Side effects of instillation of intrapericardial agents include chest pain, nausea, high fever, and atrial arrhythmias.

External-beam radiation therapy is an important option for patients with radiosensitive tumors who have not yet received extensive mediastinal or cardiac radiation as a treatment modality. Approximately half the patients with malignant pericarditis due to a variety of primary tumors respond to this form of treatment.[436,442] In one series, malignant pericardial effusion improved significantly in 11 of 16 patients with breast cancer, while 6 of 7 patients with malignant pericarditis secondary to leukemia or lymphoma improved with cardiac radiation.

In cancer patients whose overall condition is good and who develop recurrent symptomatic effusions after pericardiocentesis, a limited subxiphoid pericardiotomy should probably not be chosen when the goal is definitive therapy. The procedure has a much higher likelihood of being followed by recurrent tamponade, constriction, or reoperation than does extensive pericardiectomy, and tamponade almost always recurs in less than a year after operation.[150] Since one of four patients with malignant effusive pericarditis is likely to survive at least 1 year, extensive surgical pericardiectomy should be strongly considered in cancer patients with recurrent effusions or pericardial constriction who have (1) potential response to systemic cancer therapy or (2) one or more years of expected survival.

RADIATION PERICARDITIS

ETIOLOGY. Radiation injury to the heart and pericardium is an important complication of radiation therapy used in breast carcinoma, Hodgkin's disease, and non-Hodgkin's lymphoma. Factors that influence the development of radiation-induced heart disease include (1) the radiation dose;

(2) the duration and fractionation of therapy; (3) the volume of the heart included in the radiation field; (4) the use of a ^{60}Co source, with inhomogeneous dose distribution, in comparison with a linear accelerator source; and (5) anterior weighting of the radiation dose.[443,444] When at least 60 per cent of the cardiac silhouette is included within the treatment beam, as occurs in mantle field therapy of patients with Hodgkin's disease, the risk of radiation-induced pericarditis is about 5 to 7 per cent when a dose less than 4000 rads is delivered over 4 weeks and rises sharply in incidence above this dose.[443–446] When the whole pericardium is included in the field, the incidence of pericarditis is about 20 per cent, while the use of a subcarinal block that shields the heart decreases the risk to about 2.5 per cent.[447] This observation has been confirmed in a contemporary series of 590 patients who received mantle irradiation as initial treatment for Hodgkin's disease at the Joint Center for Radiation Therapy; 2.2 per cent of patients developed postirradiation pericarditis.[445]

In patients with Hodgkin's disease who receive radiation therapy using a ^{60}Co source or anterior weighting of the beam, which results in a higher dose to the pericardium, the incidence of pericarditis rises to about 20 per cent.[448] It approaches 50 per cent when a fluid challenge is used to unmask occult constrictive pericarditis.[449] In breast cancer radiation therapy in which the volume of the heart included in the field is usually less than 30 per cent, the incidence of radiation-induced pericarditis is less than 5 per cent, with a tolerance for up to 6000 rads given over 6 weeks.[443]

Pericardial injury may occur during the course of treatment or, more commonly, months later. In one series, 92 per cent of cases in patients presenting with pericardial effusions occurred within 12 months after completion of the course of radiation therapy.[450] However, it is now recognized that radiation pericarditis manifesting as chronic pericardial effusion or constrictive pericarditis may become apparent many years after radiation therapy.[443,446,448–451] In a series of patients with postirradiation constrictive pericarditis referred for pericardiectomy at Stanford, recent cases appeared to have a longer latent period between radiotherapy and presentation with constrictive pericarditis (4.7 years for cases during 1970 to 1980, versus 11 years for cases in 1980 to 1985).[169] The risk and latency period for the later development of constrictive pericarditis in children undergoing mediastinal irradiation is not known. In a study of 17 children observed for 72 months after radiation therapy for Hodgkin's disease, 47 per cent had prominent pericardial thickening on echocardiograms without overt evidence of cardiac constriction.[452]

PATHOLOGY. Radiation pericarditis is associated with fibrin deposition and pericardial fibrosis (Fig. 45–24). The acute inflammatory stage may be accompanied by a pericardial effusion that can be serous, serosanguineous, or hemorrhagic with a high protein and lymphocyte content.[443] The inflammation and initial effusion may resolve spontaneously. Alternatively, the effusion may organize and progress to a stage of dense fibrinous adhesions with gradual obliteration of the pericardial space, thickening of the pericardium, and proliferation of small blood vessels within the pericardium associated with a chronic pericardial effusion or a constricting pericardium. The visceral pericardium may also become fibrotic and thickened, and radiation pericarditis is a common cause of effusive-constrictive pericardial disease. Radiation injury represents an important cause of constrictive pericarditis in children, in whom progression from pericarditis to constriction is otherwise rare.[453]

It is important to recognize that radiation may occasionally injure the heart itself, causing interstitial myocardial fibrosis, valvular thickening, endothelial proliferation, and fibrotic thickening of small intramyocardial arteries. Radiation may also cause premature atherosclerosis of the epicardial coronary arteries.[443,454]

The most important consequence of radiation-induced myocardial fibrosis is the development of restrictive cardiomyopathy, which may coexist with constrictive pericarditis

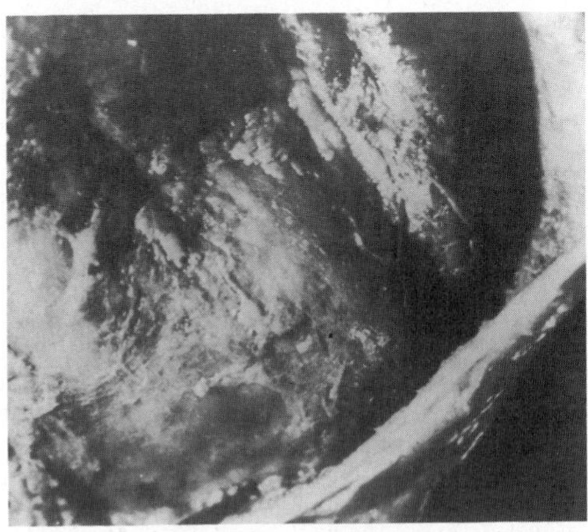

FIGURE 45–24. **Anterior surface of the heart from a patient treated with radiation to the mediastinum 29 years before for a malignant thymoma. There is marked thickening of the parietal pericardium which is reflected away from the heart (right), and a thick fibrinous exudate is present on the epicardial surface of the heart. (From Stewart, J. R., and Fajardo, L. F.: Radiation-induced heart disease. Prog. Cardiovasc. Dis. *27*:173, 1984.)**

and contribute to inadequate relief of symptoms of pulmonary and venous congestion and poor survival after pericardiectomy.

CLINICAL FEATURES. The *acute* form of pericarditis is seldom evident clinically. It usually occurs in the context of irradiation of bulky mediastinal tumor adjacent to the pericardium, which suggests that acute pericarditis is largely related to inflammatory necrosis of the adjacent tumor. Patients may have a syndrome of acute pericarditis consisting of fever, pericardial pain, anorexia, malaise, a pericardial friction rub, and electrocardiographic abnormalities. Acute pericarditis that occurs during radiation therapy usually abates rapidly, does not preclude completion of planned treatment, and correlates poorly with the risk of late pericardial damage.

In the *delayed* form of pericardial injury, the onset of symptoms is usually within 12 months but varies from 4 months to more than 20 years. It may present as the syndrome of acute idiopathic pericarditis or as an asymptomatic pericardial effusion with a coexisting pleural effusion on the chest roentgenogram. In about half of the patients, there is some degree of cardiac compression associated with dyspnea, jugular venous distention, and pulsus paradoxus due to delayed chronic pericardial effusion. The importance of this mode of presentation is underscored by the fact that radiation-induced pericardial effusion now accounts for 10 per cent of patients who undergo surgical drainage of the pericardium.[149,150] In the Stanford experience,[443] about 20 per cent of patients with delayed pericardial injury progress to development of chronic pericarditis that requires pericardiectomy. These patients may present years after radiation therapy with the insidious onset of fatigue, dyspnea, systemic edema, and jugular venous distention due to the development of constrictive pericarditis.[453,454] The clinical recognition and consequences of this delayed form of pericardial injury have become increasingly important as patients with breast cancer and Hodgkin's disease have prolonged survival and cures.

DIAGNOSIS. Radiation-induced pericarditis with pericardial effusion is most often confused with pericarditis due to the underlying malignant disease. However, patients with malignant pericardial effusion are more likely to have massive effusions and cardiac tamponade, and cytological examination of pericardial fluid can identify a malignant origin in about 85 per cent of cases.[398] When symptoms referable to the pericardium occur years after apparently successful treatment of Hodgkin's disease or lymphoma, the pericarditis is much more likely to be related to radiation injury than to recurrent mediastinal malignant disease. Similarly, the development of pericarditis with effusion in women with treated breast cancer with no evidence of metastatic disease is likely to be related to prior radiation, radiation-induced hypothyroidism, or idiopathic (viral) inflammation.[422] Occasionally, histological examination of the pericardium or pericardial fluid may be required to differentiate between radiation-induced pericarditis and recurrent metastatic disease in the pericardium.

MANAGEMENT. Patients in whom an asymptomatic pericardial effusion develops after radiation therapy may be followed up by physical examination and serial echocardiography without the institution of specific therapy. Percutaneous pericardiocentesis by skilled operators should be limited to the treatment of cardiac tamponade or to drainage of a large pericardial effusion when cytological examination is required for management. Radiation-induced thyroid dysfunction occurs in about 25 per cent of patients who undergo mantle irradiation,[445] and hypothyroidism should always be excluded as a cause of effusive pericarditis following radiation therapy. Systemic corticosteroids should be reserved for patients with severe intractable pain or life-threatening effusive disease because of the well-documented risk of unmasking latent radiation-induced lung or heart injury when steroids are withdrawn.[455]

Surgical Treatment. Pericardiectomy is required for that small number of symptomatic patients with large recurrent pericardial effusion or severe effusive-constrictive or constrictive pericarditis. The surgical experience at the Mayo Clinic has shown that late constriction developed in 75 per cent of patients with radiation-induced pericarditis who underwent drainage with a limited left thoracic partial pericardiectomy (window).[150] These data are supported by others[149,233] and suggest that extensive pericardiectomy should be performed in patients with severe effusive or effusive-constrictive radiation-induced pericarditis whose prognosis is otherwise favorable. Operative mortality for pericardiectomy in patients after radiation therapy is 21 per cent, compared with a rate of about 8 per cent in patients with idiopathic constrictive pericarditis.[169] Actuarial analysis has shown that the 5-year survival rate of patients after pericardiectomy for postirradiation pericarditis is 51 per cent, which is inferior to the 83 per cent 5-year survival rate of other patients who underwent pericardiectomy.[233] Factors that contribute to a poor outcome include failure to resect constricting visceral pericardium (epicardium), and underlying myocardial injury and fibrosis causing advanced restrictive cardiomyopathy.[233,456,457] Prospective studies are needed to elucidate the potential role of endomyocardial biopsy for the assessment of myocardial injury and fibrosis to aid in discriminating patients with radiation-induced constrictive pericarditis with a high probability of experiencing a good outcome following pericardiectomy from those with a low probability.

PERICARDITIS RELATED TO HYPERSENSITIVITY OR AUTOIMMUNITY

ACUTE RHEUMATIC FEVER (see also p. 1721)

During the 19th century, acute rheumatic fever was believed to be the most common cause of pericarditis, and it was recognized that rheumatic pericarditis could occur independently of overt rheumatic endocarditis.[458] The condition is now uncommon, but occasionally the development of a pericardial friction rub or effusion is the initial clue to the presence of rheumatic carditis.

PATHOPHYSIOLOGY. Rheumatic pericarditis is characterized by fibrin deposition that can be accompanied by a fibrinous, serofibrinous, or purulent exudate.[458,459] The pericardial reaction usually resolves spontaneously. The deposition of IgG, IgM, and complement on the pericardial surface during active pericarditis has been reported,[459] but it is still unclear whether pericarditis occurs as an immune-mediated mechanism or simply as nonspecific inflammation associated with underlying myocarditis. The development of chronic calcification and constrictive pericarditis, although reported, is very rare.[460]

CLINICAL FEATURES. Rheumatic pericarditis usually occurs at the onset of the initial episode of acute rheumatic fever and may be asymptomatic or associated with typical pericardial pain and other symptoms of acute rheumatic fever, including fever, malaise, and arthralgias (p. 1727). When present, pericarditis usually indicates extensive pancarditis. The diagnosis of rheumatic pericarditis is based on the presence of pericardial chest pain, a pericardial friction rub, or echocardiographic evidence of pericardial effusion in association with the usual serological and clinical criteria for acute rheumatic fever (p. 1728). In children, the onset of pericarditis, which is otherwise rare in this age group, should prompt a rigorous search for evidence of acute rheumatic fever.[460,461] The combination of pericarditis, fever, arthralgias, and rash in a child or young adult may be mistaken for a viral exanthem, Lyme disease, infectious endocarditis, juvenile rheumatoid arthritis, systemic lupus erythematosus, Henoch-Schönlein purpura, Crohn's disease, or sickle cell crisis.

MANAGEMENT. The treatment of rheumatic pericarditis is that of acute rheumatic fever and includes bed rest and penicillin as well as digoxin, if myocardial failure is present. Chest pain associated with rheumatic pericarditis should be treated with aspirin, as described on page 1471. Rarely, corticosteroids are required. Small or moderate-sized pericardial effusions usually resolve spontaneously, and pericardiocentesis should not be performed solely for diagnostic reasons in a patient with documented acute rheumatic fever.

PERICARDITIS ASSOCIATED WITH SYSTEMIC LUPUS ERYTHEMATOSUS (see also p. 1734)

Pericarditis usually occurs during flare-ups of disease activity in patients with systemic lupus erythematosus (SLE) and is the most common cardiovascular manifestation of the disease.[462] Pericarditis is detected clinically in about 20 to 40 per cent of these patients during the course of their disease.[462] Echocardiographic abnormalities can be detected in a higher percentage of these patients, but the clinical significance of this is unclear.[463] The incidence of pericarditis in autopsied patients averages about 62 per cent and ranges from 43 to 100 per cent, whereas the incidence of myocarditis in autopsy series is about 40 per cent.[464,465] The inflammatory process may cause fibrinous or effusive pericarditis with the rare occurrence of pathognomonic hematoxylin bodies in the visceral pericardium. Pericardial fluid may be serous or grossly hemorrhagic with a high protein content, low glucose content, and white cell count below 10,000/mm^3 (composed primarily of polymorphonuclear leukocytes). Low pericardial fluid complement levels relative to normal serum values have been reported, but caution must be used in interpreting this finding, since total hemolytic complement levels appear to be normally low in pericardial fluid.[462,466] Cardiospecific antimyosin, antisarcolemmal, and antipericardial antibodies associated with elevated creatine phosphokinase levels have been detected in the serum of a patient with SLE and severe chronic pericarditis prior to steroid treatment and pericardiectomy.[467]

CARDIAC TAMPONADE. This occurs in less than 10 per cent of patients with SLE and clinically recognized pericarditis, while the development of constrictive pericarditis has been reported but is rare.[462,468,469,470] Occasionally, cardiac tamponade is the presenting manifestation of SLE.[470,471] Pericarditis due to SLE may be accompanied by other cardiac lesions, including verrucous endocarditis, inflammation and necrosis involving the conduction system, and coronary artery vasculitis.[462,464]

CLINICAL FEATURES. Pericarditis should be suspected when patients with SLE develop pleuritic chest pain, a pericardial rub, or an enlarging cardiac silhouette on the chest roentgenogram. *Electrocardiographic abnormalities* are those characteristic of acute pericarditis. Since pericarditis usually occurs during periods of active disease, there is typically evidence of increased disease activity on blood tests for complement fixation levels, antinuclear antibodies, lupus erythematosus cell preparations, and sedimentation rate. The *chest roentgenogram* may show enlargement of the cardiac silhouette, pleural effusions, and parenchymal infiltrates. The *echocardiogram* may show evidence of a new pericardial effusion, suggesting the presence of pericardial inflammation. Since many patients with SLE are treated with immunosuppressive drugs, corticosteroids, and cytotoxic agents, a careful physical examination, blood cultures, and tuberculin skin test should be obtained to search for evidence of purulent, fungal, or tuberculous pericarditis. Except when purulent pericarditis is strongly suspected, it is not necessary to confirm the clinical diagnosis of SLE pericarditis by performing pericardiocentesis.

MANAGEMENT. In the majority of patients, pericarditis subsides when the systemic disease becomes inactive following treatment with corticosteroids or immunotherapy. The unusual complication of cardiac tamponade can ordinarily be treated with pericardiocentesis and usually does not require surgical intervention (i.e., pericardiotomy or pericardiectomy). However, since the development of acute cardiac tamponade is unpredictable, symptomatic patients with SLE pericarditis should be hospitalized and under close observation.

RHEUMATOID ARTHRITIS (see also p. 1732)

Although pericarditis is detected at autopsy in up to 50 per cent of patients with rheumatoid arthritis, the clinical incidence of symptomatic pericarditis is less than 10 per cent.[472,473] Based on echocardiographic criteria for the presence of a pericardial effusion, possible effusive pericarditis has been detected in 50 per cent of patients with chronic nodular rheumatoid arthritis, in 15 per cent of patients with typical non-nodular rheumatoid arthritis, and in no patients with typical non-nodular rheumatoid arthritis, and in no patients of comparable age with osteoarthritis.[474] Pericarditis tends to appear in patients with other evidence of severe rheumatoid arthritis, including extensive joint deformity, subcutaneous rheumatoid nodules, pneumonitis, and positive serum rheumatoid factor. On rare occasions, rheumatoid pancarditis with pericarditis can occur in patients with otherwise quiescent well-controlled rheumatoid arthritis.[475] Rheumatoid pericarditis in adults can cause cardiac tamponade and has been recognized as a cause of effusive-constrictive pericarditis and constrictive pericarditis.[243,472,473,476,477] Pericarditis, and the complication of cardiac tamponade, may occur with or without evidence of active joint involvement in children with juvenile rheumatoid arthritis[478-480] and in adults with juvenile rheumatoid arthritis (adult Still's disease).[481-483]

PATHOLOGY. Typical pathological changes in the pericardium are those of nonspecific fibrous thickening of the visceral and parietal pericardium with adhesions. Rarely, small, necrotic granulomatous nodules are detected on the epicardial surface that are histologically identical to the subcutaneous, rheumatoid nodule. Pericardial effusions, whose characteristics are similar to those of pleural effusions associated with rheumatoid arthritis pericarditis, are usually serous or hemorrhagic, with greater than 5 gm/dl of protein, glucose levels less than 45 mg/dl, high cholesterol levels, and white blood cell counts ranging from 20,000 to 90,000/mm^3.[472,473] Soluble immune complexes, positive latex fixation titers, and low complement levels in the pericardial fluid as well as immune complex and complement deposits in pericardial vessels with plasma cell infiltration have also been described.[484] Acute pericarditis may progress to cause diffusely constricting fibrotic pericarditis and can coexist with other cardiac lesions, including granulomatous aortic and mitral valve deformity causing chronic aortic or mitral insufficiency.

CLINICAL FEATURES. Rheumatoid arthritis is often associated with fever, precordial chest pain, and dyspnea in association with a pericardial friction rub. Pericarditis commonly coexists with exacerbation of joint inflammation and pleuritis, manifest on the chest roentgenogram as a unilateral or bilateral pleural effusion in about 65 per cent of cases. Children with juvenile rheumatoid arthritis and pericarditis commonly show transient pulmonary infiltrates.[478,479] The *ECG* usually shows nonspecific ST-segment and T-wave changes. The presence of atrioventricular block in patients with rheumatoid pericarditis probably reflects rheumatoid myocardial involvement. On *echocardiography* a pericardial effusion is present in approximately half of patients with nodular rheumatoid arthritis,[472,474,485] but its presence does not always correlate with the presence of symptomatic pericarditis. In some patients, two-dimensional echocardiography can demonstrate the presence of dense fibrinous strands in the pericardial space.[486]

CARDIAC TAMPONADE AND CONSTRICTION. Although rheumatoid pericarditis is usually self-limited and benign, cardiac tamponade may develop abruptly in 3 to 25 per cent of patients[472]; it has been reported as a complication of sudden steroid withdrawal[487] and in association with intravenous anticoagulant therapy.[488] An uncommon but major complication is the rapid onset of subacute effusive-constrictive pericarditis.[472,484] The development of chronic constrictive pericarditis is a well-recognized complication that is more prevalent in men than in women.[243,472,477,489,490]

MANAGEMENT. Patients with symptomatic pericarditis may be treated with aspirin or other nonsteroidal antiinflammatory agents, as described on page 1471.

Pericardiocentesis is indicated for relief of a large anterior-posterior effusion causing cardiac tamponade. Although intrapericardial steroid instillation has been advocated,[491] there is no clear evidence that steroids alter the natural history of effusions or prevent the development of the constrictive pericarditis. There is now an extensive experience in the *surgical management* of rheumatoid pericarditis, and patients with connective tissue disorders (predominantly rheumatoid arthritis) now constitute between 4 and 20 per cent of patients undergoing pericardiectomy.[169,231,232] In patients with documented effusive-constrictive or constrictive pericarditis, pericardiectomy can provide gratifying hemodynamic and symptomatic improvement.[169,232,472,489,490]

PROGRESSIVE SYSTEMIC SCLEROSIS

(see also p. 1736)

Pericardial involvement is found at autopsy in about 50 percent of patients with progressive systemic sclerosis (scleroderma), while pericarditis is detected clinically in about 10 per cent.[492-494] While the pathogenesis of scleroderma pericarditis is unknown, it has been suggested that increased collagen formation by fibroblasts, in combination with tissue hypoxia, may result in aberrant collagen metabolism. Histological changes include nonspecific fibrotic pericardial thickening with adhesions and perivascular inflammatory cells. Pericardial effusions can be detected by means of echocardiography in about 40 per cent of patients with scleroderma, but in the majority of patients a small pericardial effusion is not associated with symptoms.

When present, the pericardial effusion is straw colored and characterized by a protein content greater than 5 gm/dl, low cell count, and—in contrast with the characteristics of pericardial effusions in SLE and rheumatoid arthritis—the absence of autoantibodies, low complement levels, and immune complexes. Pericardial involvement is often associated with sclerodermatous infiltration of the heart, causing restrictive cardiomyopathy, arrhythmias, and conduction abnormalities.[493]

Scleroderma pericardial disease may present as an acute syndrome resembling viral myocarditis, with fever, chest pain, and pericardial friction rub, and nonspecific electrocardiographic ST- and T-wave changes. In other cases, patients develop a chronic pericardial effusion or pericardial constriction with symptoms of right and left atrial hypertension, cardiomegaly, and pleural effusions on the chest roentgenogram, and low QRS voltage on the electrocardiogram.

MANAGEMENT. There is no definitive treatment for scleroderma pericarditis. Patients with the syndrome of acute pericarditis may be treated with aspirin, as described on pages 1471 and 1496. Rarely, pericardial effusions with cardiac tamponade may develop, necessitating pericardiocentesis.[495] Patients with constrictive pericarditis may require pericardiectomy. Severe recurrent constrictive pericarditis has also been reported as a complication of idiopathic retroperitoneal and mediastinal fibrosis, which are regional expressions of a systemic sclerosing disease.[496] It is especially important to perform cardiac catheterization in patients with scleroderma and suspected cardiac tamponade or constrictive pericarditis, since dyspnea and systemic venous hypertension may be related to sclerodermatous cardiac involvement or to pulmonary hypertension secondary to pulmonary fibrosis. The development of symptomatic pericarditis in patients with scleroderma is ominous, since the 5-year survival rate is about 25 per cent when isolated pericardial or other cardiac involvement is present and about 75 per cent in patients without heart, lung, or kidney involvement.[497]

PERICARDITIS IN OTHER CONNECTIVE TISSUE DISORDERS

Acute pericarditis with pericardial effusions occurs in about 30 per cent of patients with mixed connective tissue and may coexist with other cardiac abnormalities, including myocarditis, conduction systemic degeneration, and intimal hyperplasia of the coronary arteries.[498,499] Cardiac involvement, including pericarditis, is less common in these patients than in patients with systemic sclerosis (scleroderma) or rheumatoid arthritis.

Pericarditis may rarely develop in other connective tissue disorders, including Sjögren's syndrome, dermatomyositis,[500] ankylosing spondylitis,[501] Wegener's granulomatosis,[502] Reiter's syndrome,[503] severe serum sickness,[504] and Felty's syndrome.[505] Pericarditis associated with polyarteritis nodosa may occur in patients who are hepatitis B antigen-positive. It also occurs in disorders of possible autoimmune etiology, including temporal arteritis,[506,507] inflammatory bowel disease,[508,509] Kawasaki's disease,[510] familial Mediterranean fever,[511] Whipple's disease,[512] celiac disease,[513] eosinophilic fasciitis,[514] Behçet's disease, and myasthenia gravis.[515] Amyloidosis is well known as a cause of infiltrative restrictive myopathy, the hemodynamics of which may mimic constrictive pericarditis (p. 1416), but it may also involve the pericardium.[224,225]

Cardiac involvement is present at autopsy in about 25 per cent of patients with sarcoidosis and can involve the pericardium in the absence of significant myocardial infiltration.[516] Sarcoidosis can be a rare cause of cardiac tamponade and constrictive pericarditis;[517,518] in the latter case, the findings of pericardial thickening with noncaseating granulomas may cause confusion with tuberculous or fungal pericarditis (Fig. 45–25).

DRUG- AND TOXIN-RELATED PERICARDITIS

Pericarditis occurs in about 25 per cent of patients with procainamide-related and 2 per cent of those with hydralazine-related development of the SLE syndrome.[519] In these patients, pericarditis may occasionally be complicated by the development of cardiac tamponade or the rapid development of pericardial constriction.[520] Other drugs that may produce pericarditis in association with the drug-induced syndrome of SLE include reserpine, methyldopa, isoniazid, and diphenylhydantoin.[519,521]

Other drugs appear to produce pericarditis through separate mechanisms. Pericarditis has been reported as a complication of a hypersensitivity reaction with peripheral eosinophilia after administration of penicillin[522] and cromolyn sodium.[523] The mechanisms of drug-induced pericarditis following administration of 6-amino-9-D-psicofuranosylpurine,[524] minoxidil,[525] dantrolene sodium,[526] and practolol[527] are not understood. Pericarditis has also been observed in association with polymer fume fever, a syndrome of pleuritis and noncardiogenic pulmonary edema that occurs following inhalation of fumes from the burning of polytetrafluoroethylene (Teflon).[528] Methysergide is well recognized as a cause of constrictive pericarditis as part of a generalized process of mediastinal fibrosis.[529] The

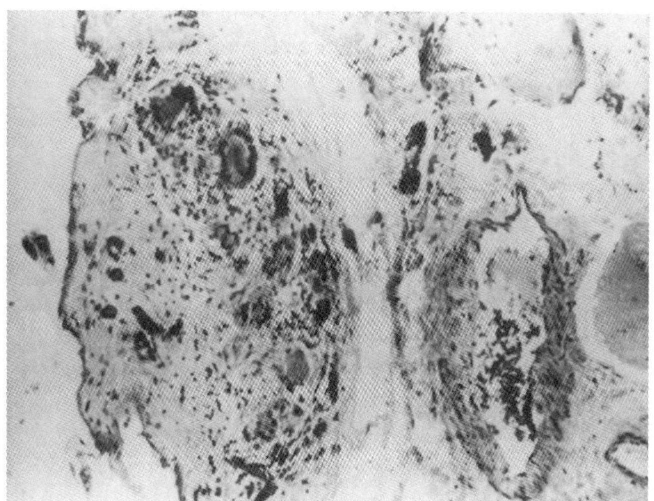

FIGURE 45–25. Photomicrograph of a pericardial biopsy specimen from a patient with cardiac tamponade secondary to cardiac sarcoidosis showing a noncaseating granuloma with several giant cells (250×). (From Verkleeren, J. L., et al.: Cardiac tamponade secondary to sarcoidosis. Am. Heart J. *106*:601, 1983.)

anthracycline neoplastic agents doxorubicin and daunorubicin may cause acute pericarditis as well as myocardial inflammation,[530] and pericarditis has also been reported in association with the use of cytosine arabinoside.[531] Pericarditis has similarly been noted as a foreign body reaction to the presence of silicone[532] and talc[533] within the pericardial space, in association with cardiac iron deposition and pericardial fibrosis in thalassemia,[534] and as a toxic response to scorpionfish sting.[535]

Acute drug-related pericarditis usually resolves when the offending drug is discontinued, and improvement may be accelerated by administration of corticosteroids. The rare development of chronic constrictive pericarditis may be treated by pericardiectomy.

Postmyocardial Infarction (Dressler) Syndrome

(See also p. 1495)

Dressler syndrome is an acute illness with fever, pericarditis, and pleuritis, possibly of autoimmune origin, that occurs weeks to months after an acute myocardial infarction.[536] A similar syndrome of fever and pericarditis has been reported in six patients following pulmonary embolism with infarction.[537] Today, a distinction is usually made between acute postinfarction pericarditis, which occurs during the first week after infarction (p. 1263), and Dressler syndrome, which usually appears 2 to 3 weeks after infarction, with a range of 1 week to several months. Dressler estimated that this syndrome occurred in up to 4 per cent of patients after acute myocardial infarction[538]; however, a more recent series from the same hospital indicates that the incidence of the Dressler syndrome has markedly decreased.[539]

The etiology of Dressler syndrome is unknown. The association of symptoms and the appearance of antimyocardial antibodies has led to the hypothesis that an autoimmune mechanism, with or without a latent viral infection, is the etiologic factor,[539] while some workers have concluded that the development of antimyocardial antibodies is not specific for the presence of Dressler syndrome.[539,540] Leakage of blood into the pericardial space is another proposed mechanism, and the current lower incidence of the syndrome may reflect less use of oral anticoagulants in the postinfarction period.[539] It is likely that there are common factors in the pathogenesis of Dressler syndrome and the postpericardiotomy syndrome, both of which have the following features: (1) an initial insult of endothelial cell injury and entry of blood into the pericardial space; (2) a delayed response after the initial insult, consisting of fever and inflammation of the pericardial surfaces; (3) development of antiheart antibodies; (4) a dramatic response to antiinflammatory agents; and (5) a tendency for recurrence.

PATHOLOGY. The histology of the pericardium usually reveals a nonspecific inflammation with fibrin deposition. In contrast to the acute pericarditis following myocardial infarction in which pericardial inflammation is often patchy, overlying the regions of infarction, the pericarditis in Dressler syndrome is usually diffuse.

CLINICAL FEATURES. Patients characteristically have severe malaise, fever, chest pain, and pleurisy.[538,541] The chest pain may be severe enough initially to cause both patient and physician to consider that it is caused by a second myocardial infarction or postinfarction angina.[542] Dressler syndrome is occasionally the initial presentation of a previously undiagnosed infarction.[543] *Physical examination* often discloses a pericardial friction rub and sometimes a pleural friction rub as well. The chest roentgenogram commonly reveals an enlarged cardiac silhouette secondary to pericardial effusion associated with pleural effusions[538] and, occasionally, transient pulmonary infiltrates. The *echocardiographic* evidence of pericardial effusion in the absence of other symptoms is not diagnostic of Dressler syndrome, since asymptomatic small pericardial effusions occur in about one of four patients after myocardial infarction.[363] *Electrocardiographic* abnormalities usually consist of serial ST-segment and T-wave changes strongly suggestive of acute pericarditis, but the electrocardiogram may not be helpful in patients with persistent repolarization abnormalities following infarction. Blood tests usually reveal the nonspecific findings of an increased erythrocyte sedimentation rate and peripheral leukocytosis. Tests for antimyocardial antibodies are not widely available or established as a means of confirming the diagnosis. Gallium scanning has been reported to be ineffective in identifying patients with pericarditis due to Dressler syndrome.[544]

Dressler syndrome can usually be discriminated from recurrent myocardial infarction by (1) the characteristics of the chest pain and its failure to improve with nitroglycerin; (2) the absence of new Q waves on the ECG; and (3) the absence of a marked rise in the CK-MB band. Small increases in cardiac enzyme levels may occur in pericarditis when the underlying epicardium is involved. Dressler syndrome must also be distinguished from hemorrhagic pericarditis secondary to chronic systemic anticoagulation.

MANAGEMENT. A single episode of Dressler syndrome is usually self-limited, but the syndrome does tend to recur. The onset of severe pericarditis usually warrants hospital admission and observation for the development of cardiac tamponade.[545] Oral anticoagulants should be discontinued because of the risk of pericardial hemorrhage. As in other patients with acute pericarditis, patients with severe symptoms with fever and chest pain usually benefit from bed rest and treatment with aspirin or a nonsteroidal antiinflammatory agent. Recurrent episodes of Dressler syndrome may respond only to corticosteroids and occasionally require complete pericardiectomy for relief of intractable pericardial pain or prevention of recurrence. Cardiac tamponade in the absence of anticoagulant therapy can usually be managed with pericardiocentesis.[545] Constrictive pericarditis is a well-recognized complication of Dressler syndrome that may be relieved by pericardiectomy.[546,547]

Postpericardiotomy Syndrome

ETIOLOGY. The postpericardiotomy syndrome is identified by the appearance of fever, pericarditis, and pleuritis more than 1 week after a cardiac operation in which the pericardium has been opened and manipulated. This syndrome was first recognized in patients after mitral commissurotomy for rheumatic heart disease, and it was initially believed to represent reactivation of rheumatic fever.[548] Subsequently, it was realized that the syndrome could occur following cardiac operations in patients without rheumatic heart disease and that the common denominator appeared to be wide incision and manipulation of the pericardium.[549] An identical clinical syndrome has been reported following cardiac perforation by a catheter or transvenous pacemaker, blunt chest trauma, percutaneous diagnostic left ventricular puncture, and epicardial pacemaker implantation.[550] The incidence of postpericardiotomy syndrome following cardiac surgery ranges from 10 to 40 per cent in various series and is higher in children than in adults.[551-553] The observation of a 31 per cent incidence of postpericardiotomy syndrome in patients undergoing cardiac surgery for the Wolff-Parkinson-White syndrome clearly indicates that pericardial damage prior to surgery is not a contributing factor.[553] Furthermore, pericardial drainage techniques do not appear to affect the frequency of development of the syndrome after cardiac surgery.[554]

Analogous to the Dressler syndrome, the etiology of postpericardiotomy syndrome is hypothesized to be an autoimmune reaction directed against the epicardium, possibly in concert with a new or reactivated viral infection. Studies by Engle and colleagues have demonstrated that antiheart antibodies appear in the serum of some patients who undergo pericardiotomy and that there is a positive correlation between the level of the titers and the incidence of the syndrome.[552] Approximately 70 per cent of patients with the postpericardiotomy syndrome and high antiheart antibody titers also develop a fourfold or higher rise in titer against one or more viral antigens, while in patients without the postpericardiotomy syndrome, a rise in viral titers occurs in only 8 per cent of those with normal antiheart antibody titers and in only 19 per cent of those with low levels of antiheart antibody titers; these findings suggest that viral infection may be a triggering or permissive factor. The postpericardiotomy syndrome is rare in children under 2 years of age who undergo cardiac surgery, a finding that may be related to the short exposure time to viruses or to protective maternal antibodies transmitted via the placenta. The development of pleuritis and pleural effusions is believed to reflect involvement of the pleura adjacent to the inflamed pericardium; involvement of serous membranes distant from the heart is uncommon.

PATHOLOGY. There are no pathognomonic histological features of postpericardiotomy syndrome. The presence of blood in the pericardial space adjacent to an injured epicardium may result in later development of pericardial adhesions, thickening of the pericardial membranes, and occasionally fibrinous obliteration of the pericardial space, causing pericardial constriction. Pericardial effusions in patients with postpericardiotomy syndrome may be straw colored, serosanguineous, or frankly hemorrhagic, with a protein content greater than 4.5 gm/dl and a white blood cell count between 3,000 and 8,000/mm^3 (composed of both lymphocytes and granulocytes).[555]

CLINICAL FEATURES. Patients typically develop an acute illness characterized by fever, malaise, and chest pain that usually begins during the second or third postoperative week (Fig. 45–26). In some cases, the fever may reflect a continuation of the more common problem of fever in the first week after operation. The chest pain is typical of acute pericarditis (p. 1469) and usually has a pleuritic quality. Nonspecific signs of inflammation, including an elevated sedimentation rate and polymorphonuclear leukocytosis, may also be present. Noncardiac pulmonary edema may also occur.[555a]

Physical examination often reveals a pericardial friction rub. It should be noted that the friction rub present in almost all patients during the first few days after cardiac surgery disappears in most patients who do not develop postpericardiotomy syndrome by the end of the first postoperative week. The *chest roentgenogram* demonstrates left-sided or bilateral pleural effusions in about two-thirds of patients, pulmonary infiltrates in about one-tenth, and transient enlargement of the cardiac silhouette in half.[553] The *ECG* shows nonspecific ST-segment and T-wave changes and episodic atrial tachyarrhythmias. *Echocardiography* is useful in monitoring the appearance and size of a pericardial effusion and in detecting evidence of cardiac compression such as right atrial collapse.

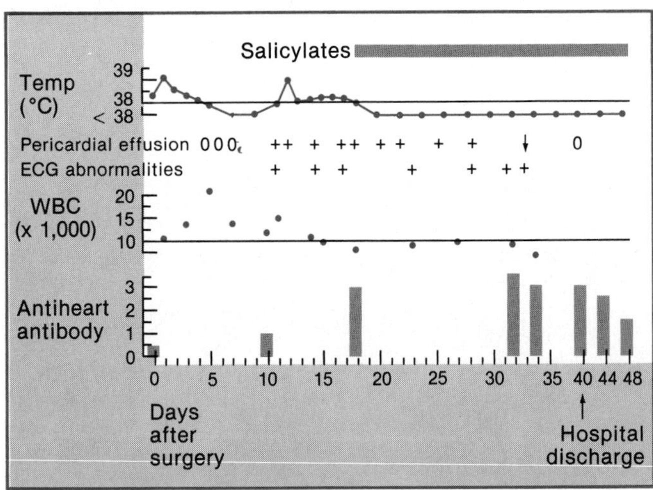

FIGURE 45–26. Representative clinical course of a child with the postpericardiotomy syndrome after cardiac surgery. Note that a febrile illness associated with effusive pericarditis, electrocardiographic changes, and leukocytosis began about 10 days after surgery. The administration of salicylates was followed by prompt relief of fever and pericarditis. The antiheart antibody titer, which was initially high, subsequently declined. (From Engle, M. A., et al.: The postpericardiotomy syndrome. 25 years' experience. J. Cardiovasc. Med. *4*:321, 1984.)

However, it should be noted that pericardial effusions are extremely common after cardiac surgery, occurring in 56 to 84 per cent of patients within the first 10 days.[556] Thus, the diagnosis of postpericardiotomy syndrome is made on clinical grounds based on recognition of the distinctive features of the syndrome in the postoperative patient. Other causes of postoperative fever, including infection, as well as the viral-induced postperfusion syndrome of atypical lymphocytosis, fever, and hepatosplenomegaly, must be excluded.[557]

MANAGEMENT. The postpericardiotomy syndrome is a self-limited but often prolonged and disabling illness. Fever and severe chest pain are usually relieved by aspirin or nonsteroidal antiinflammatory drugs. Corticosteroids should be reserved for patients in whom fever and chest pain are not relieved within 48 hours by other antiinflammatory agents. Recurrences tend to appear during the first 6 months after surgery.

Cardiac tamponade is an important and well-recognized complication of the postpericardiotomy syndrome.[555,558,559] In one large series of adult patients who survived cardiac surgery, almost 1 per cent developed cardiac tamponade an average of 49 days after surgery, in association with fever, a pericardial friction rub, and pericardial chest pain typical of the postpericardiotomy syndrome.[555] In contrast to the important role of anticoagulation in early postoperative bleeding after cardiac surgery, the use of anticoagulants did not appear to be a prerequisite for the development of cardiac tamponade in association with the postpericardiotomy syndrome. Cardiac tamponade can be managed conservatively by pericardiocentesis followed by the administration of antiinflammatory agents.[555] Patients with recurrent tamponade require surgical drainage and pericardiectomy. Percutaneous pericardiocentesis should not be attempted in patients with echocardiographic evidence of only a small posterior effusion, a loculated effusion, or an effusion with dense echoes suggesting the presence of both thrombus and free fluid. Constrictive pericarditis is a rare complication that may occur months to years after the postpericardiotomy syndrome.

POSTOPERATIVE HEMOPERICARDIUM. Acute cardiac tamponade and pericardial constriction in the absence of typical features of the postpericardiotomy syndrome also occur secondary to hemopericardium following cardiac surgery and perforation of the heart during cardiac catheterization, pacemaker insertion, pericardiocentesis, and coronary artery angioplasty.[560-563] Acute pericarditis without frank cardiac perforation has been reported in 0.5 per cent of 981 patients who underwent angioplasty, and this complication may be secondary to occult epicardial-pericardial hematoma formation.[564] Other invasive procedures that have been reported to cause hemopericardium and cardiac tamponade include percutaneous aortic and mitral valvuloplasty,[565] sternal bone marrow aspiration,[566] esophagoscopy,[567] and mediastinoscopy.[568] Endoscopic sclerotherapy for esophageal varices is a new cause of both acute hemopericardium and the later development of pericarditis associated with chest pain and the development of cardiac tamponade.[569,570]

In some patients, cardiac tamponade following invasive cardiac procedures and cardiac surgery has been successfully managed with pericardiocentesis alone.[555,571] However, the development of early and late postoperative tamponade is commonly due to the combination of free fluid and organizing thrombus, which usually requires open surgical drainage of the pericardial space. Postoperative cardiac tamponade and thrombus formation can cause localized compression of the heart and have been reported to cause right ventricular outflow obstruction.[572,573]

CONSTRICTIVE PERICARDITIS. This condition is being increasingly recognized as a complication of cardiac surgery and may occur in patients in whom the pericardium is left open but in situ.[574–577] The time from cardiac surgery to definitive diagnosis usually is about 1 year but ranges from less than 1 month to more than 15 years.[575–577] In one review of 5207 adults who underwent cardiac surgery, 0.2 per cent (11 patients) developed constrictive pericarditis, documented by cardiac catheterization, an average of 82 days after operation.[574] An incidence of 0.2 to 0.3 per cent has also been observed in other series.[575]

Etiology. Povidone-iodine irrigation of the heart is postulated to be a triggering factor in some patients. This factor has been absent in most reports, and it is likely that intrapericardial hemorrhage and serosal injury are major contributing factors.[574] In the series of 45 patients reported by Killian et al., transient postpericardiotomy syndrome may have been a contributing factor in about 60 per cent of the patients.[576] There is now strong evidence that postoperative constrictive pericarditis can involve bypass grafts and can contribute to premature graft closure as well as damage to grafts during pericardiectomy.[577–579] The development of constrictive pericarditis, possibly related to both occult hemopericardium and the development of a foreign body reaction to the epicardial patch electrodes, has been observed several months after the placement of automatic implantable cardioverter-defibrillators (AICD).[580] Acute pericarditis as manifested as localized, progressive fibrosis adjacent to the patch electrodes has been found in virtually all patients who have undergone autopsy after AICD placement.[581]

Important clinical features in patients with postsurgical constrictive pericarditis include dyspnea, chest pain, jugular venous distention, pedal edema, and increased roentgenographic heart size, while echocardiographic evidence of pericardial thickening with a posterior pericardial effusion is present in the majority. Magnetic resonance imaging and computed tomography are useful in showing pericardial thickening in some patients.

MANAGEMENT. In patients in whom this syndrome is suspected, the diagnosis of constrictive pericarditis should be confirmed at cardiac catheterization before the pericardium is explored (p. 1478). The majority of these patients (about 85 per cent) improve after undergoing extensive pericardiectomy and are found to have hemorrhage-induced fibrosis of the pericardium, usually associated with a posterior organized hematoma.[575,576] The operative mortality for pericardiectomy in these patients is high, ranging from 5 to 14 per cent.[575]

OTHER FORMS OF PERICARDIAL DISEASE

Myxedema Pericardial Disease

(See also page 1834)

Myxedema is frequently associated with myopathy; pericardial effusion also occurs in up to one-third of patients.[582,583] Since myxedematous patients frequently have ascites, pleural effusions, and uveal edema, it has been suggested that pericardial effusion may be related to a combination of sodium and water retention, slow lymphatic drainage, and increased capillary permeability with protein extravasation.[584] The pericardial fluid is usually clear or straw-colored, with elevated protein and cholesterol concentrations and few leukocytes or red blood cells. Pericardial fluid usually accumulates very slowly and may achieve enormous volumes—as much as 5 to 6 liters. Occasionally, the pericardial effusion may resemble a viscous jelly rather than a clear fluid. Myxedematous pericardial effusions usually do not cause symptoms. Often attention is called to the heart by the finding of unsuspected marked cardiomegaly on a chest roentgenogram, and a large pericardial effusion is occasionally the presenting feature of hypothyroidism.[585]

Since infants and elderly patients with hypothyroidism may be asymptomatic, this etiologic factor should always be excluded in these patients with pericardial effusion of unknown cause. Hypothyroidism should also be considered as the cause of pericardial effusion in patients following mediastinal radiation therapy, in whom 25 per cent develop radiation-induced thyroid dysfunction.[445] The *ECG* often shows nonspecific abnormalities, including low QRS voltage and flattened or inverted T waves, due to either myxedematous heart disease or pericardial effusion. In myxedematous patients with cardiac compression from a pericardial effusion, the expected compensatory tachycardia may be absent.

Myxedematous pericardial effusions tend to regress slowly and ultimately disappear over a period of months after patients have been treated with thyroid replacement and have returned to the euthyroid state.[582,585] Cardiac tamponade has been reported, but it is a rare complication.[585–587]

Cholesterol Pericarditis

Cholesterol pericarditis results from pericardial injury associated with deposition of cholesterol crystals and a mononuclear cell inflammatory reaction consisting of foam cells, macrophages, and giant cells. The presence of cholesterol crystals in the pericardial space is believed to provoke a chronic inflammatory response that results in effusion and may ultimately lead to the development of constrictive pericarditis. A pericardial effusion that contains microscopic cholesterol crystals typically has a glittering "gold" appearance. The similarities in the lipid and cholesterol contents of pericardial fluid and serum in some patients with cholesterol pericarditis suggest that simple transudation may explain the high cholesterol content in the pericardial space.

MANAGEMENT. The management of patients with cholesterol pericarditis includes detection and treatment of any underlying predisposing condition associated with the development of cholesterol pericarditis, such as tuberculous, rheumatoid, or myxedematous pericarditis or hypercholesterolemia. However, in the majority of cases, cholesterol pericarditis occurs in the absence of a clear underlying disease.[588] Cholesterol pericardial effusions are usually large, but since they develop slowly, cardiac tamponade is an unusual complication.[589] Pericardiectomy is indicated in the unlikely event of cardiac tamponade as well as in the treatment of massive cholesterol pericardial effusion, which may cause dyspnea and chest pain.[590] The development of constrictive pericarditis requiring pericardiectomy has been reported but is extremely rare.[591]

Chylopericardium

Idiopathic chylopericardium is rare, and chylopericardium is usually associated with mechanical obstruction of the thoracic duct or its drainage into the left subclavian vein resulting from (1) surgical or traumatic rupture of the thoracic duct or (2) lymphatic blockage by neoplasms, tuberculosis, or congenital lymphangiomatosis.[592,593] Thoracic duct obstruction with failure of adequate collateral drainage then results in reflux of chyle through lymphatics draining the pericardium. Most patients with chylopericardium are asymptomatic and come to clinical attention when a large, slowly accumulating pericardial effusion is detected on chest roentgenogram or echocardiogram. The presence of a connection between a damaged thoracic duct and the pericardial space can be established by lymphangiography and radionuclide lymphangiography with technetium-99m antimony sulfur colloid, as well as by the recovery of ingested Sudan III, a lipophilic dye, from pericardial aspirate.[592,593] Computed tomography may demonstrate density compatible with fat in the pericardial space.[594] The pericardial fluid is usually milky white with a high cholesterol and triglyceride content, protein content greater than 3.5 gm/dl, and microscopic fat droplets demonstrated with a Sudan III stain.[593] Lymphopericardium, which is due to pericardial angiomas as part of generalized lymphangiectasis, is characterized by clear pericardial fluid.

Cardiac tamponade and constrictive pericarditis are rare complications.[593,594] Chylopericardium has been reported as a rare cause of cardiac tamponade after cardiac surgery.[595,596] The management of symptomatic chylopericardium consists of efforts to reduce the likelihood of recurrence. These include ingestion of a diet rich in medium-chain triglycerides or, if this is unsuccessful, in ligation of the thoracic duct and parietal pericardiectomy to evacuate chylous fluid and prevent reaccumulation.[593,596]

Traumatic Pericarditis

(See also p. 1518)

In addition to penetrating or nonpenetrating cardiac trauma (Chap. 46), other important causes of traumatic pericarditis include rupture of the esophagus into the pericardial space, which may occur from esophageal erosion secondary to esophageal carcinoma or sudden rupture of the esophageal contents into the pericardial space in Boerhaave's syndrome, or as a complication of esophagogastrectomy. Traumatic pericarditis due to esophageal rupture is usually followed by intense erosive pericardial inflammation and infection. Esophageal rupture or perforation may also be followed by the development of an esophagopericardial fistula.[597] These disorders usually require immediate surgical intervention and are associated with a high mortality, although medical management with spontaneous fistula closure has been reported.[597] Pericarditis may also occur secondary to pancreatitis associated with a pericardial effusion with high amylase content and, rarely, the development of cardiac tamponade or a pancreatic-pericardial fistula.[598,599] The incidence of occult pericardial effusion in patients with acute alcoholic pancreatitis is significantly higher (47 per cent) than in control subjects (11 per cent).[598] The development of fistulas to the pericardium in response to ulcer formation, malignant disease, or surgery may occur from other sites, including the stomach,[600] biliary tract,[601] colon,[602] and bronchi.[603]

Pericardial trauma may also give rise to unusual traumatic syndromes, including cardiovascular collapse following herniation of the heart through a rent in the pericardium caused by trauma, or prior pericardiotomy mimicking congenital partial absence of the pericardium with cardiac subluxation,[604,605] and intrapericardial diaphragmatic hernia.[606] Diagnosis of cardiac herniation can be made by computed tomography and magnetic resonance imaging.[605,607] Life-threatening cardiac herniation may also occur following radical left pneumonectomy with partial pericardial resection.[608]

Pericardial Cysts

Pericardial cysts are rare developmental anomalies and are typically located at the right costophrenic angle.[609] Unusual locations include the left costophrenic angle, hilum, and superior mediastinum at the level of the aortic arch. They are usually unilocular and filled with clear liquid, giving rise to the term *springwater cysts.*

Pericardial cysts usually do not cause symptoms or unusual physical findings. Rarely, chest pain may occur owing to torsion of the cyst. These lesions typically come to medical attention as an unsuspected finding of a round, sharply defined mass along the right cardiac border on a chest roentgenogram. The size of the cyst in asymptomatic patients may vary over time.[610,611] In most cases, a cyst can be differentiated from solid tumor or aneurysm by two-dimensional echocardiography or CT (Fig. 45–27).[611] When a suspected pericardial cyst is in an unusual location, angiography may occasionally be needed to discriminate a cyst from an aneurysm or pseudoaneurysm. Pericardial cysts located at the right costophrenic angle can be accurately diagnosed and treated by percutaneous aspiration under fluoroscopic guidance.[612] Because long-term follow-up studies have shown that most asymptomatic patients do not develop symptoms, most patients should be managed conservatively, without surgical exploration.[613]

Other benign developmental abnormalities of the pericardium include benign intrapericardial teratomas and intrapericardial bronchial cysts, which can be identified by computed tomography.[614]

Congenital Absence and Defects of the Pericardium

Congenital absence of the pericardium was first described anatomically by Realdus Columbus in 1559, but its antemortem detection did not occur until 1959.[615] In patients with pericardial agenesis, the anomaly usually involves a partial defect of the left-sided pericardium, which is potentially lethal, in 70 per cent; total absence in 9 per cent; partial absence of the right-sided pericardium, and absence of the inferior pericardium, in 17 per cent.[616] There is a 3 : 1 male/female predominance among patients with pericardial defects, and about 30 per cent have other congenital anomalies, including atrial septal defect, bicuspid aortic valve, bronchogenic cysts, or pulmonic sequestration. A familial occurrence of congential absence of the pericardium has been reported.[617]

Total absence of the pericardium is not usually associated with symptoms. Occasionally the patient may complain of chest discomfort and palpitations. The etiology of these symptoms is unknown, but they may be related to torsion of the great vessels due to excess mobility of the heart. Most asymptomatic patients come to attention because of an unexplained heart murmur or abnormal chest roentgenogram. The extremely rare complication of acute chest pain due to strangulation of the heart between the diaphragm and the pulmonary ligament has been reported.[618]

TOTAL ABSENCE. Patients with total absence of the left pericardium often have widened splitting of the second heart sound, a hyperdynamic precordial impulse, leftward displacement of the apical impulse, and a systolic murmur at the upper left sternal border that may be related to turbulent blood flow in an unusually mobile heart. ECG abnormalities include right-axis deviation due to levoposition of the heart, incomplete right bundle branch block, clockwise displacement of the QRS transition zone of the precordial leads, and tall and peaked P waves in the right precordial leads.[619]

The standard posteroanterior view of the chest roentgenogram reveals marked leftward displacement of the cardiac silhouette, prominence of the main pulmonary artery, and interposition of radiolucent lung tissue between the aorta and main pulmonary artery or between the left hemidiaphragm and inferior cardiac border. This anomaly must be differentiated from other conditions that cause prominence of the left hilum or pulmonary artery on the standard chest film, including pulmonic valve stenosis, atrial septal defect, idiopathic dilatation of the pulmonary artery, and hilar adenopathy.

M-mode *echocardiographic findings* simulate those seen in right ventricular volume overload, including dilatation of the right ventricle and paradoxical anterior motion of the septum in systole, which is an artifact related to exaggerated cardiac rotation. Two-dimensional echocardiography can demonstrate localized bulging of the left ventricular contour and the drop-off of pericardial echoes.[620] Radionuclide perfusion imaging can be used to confirm the diagnosis by demonstration of a wedge of lung tissue between the heart and left hemidiaphragm;[621] computed tomography and magnetic resonance imaging can also be used to detect absence of the left pericardium by demonstrating visibility of the right pericardium and absence of the left pericardium, absence of the preaortic recess, and the abnormal presence of a wedge of lung between the aorta and pulmonary artery.[622,623]

Findings at cardiac catheterization are usually normal. Diagnostic left pneumothorax has been used in the past to outline the pericardium, but this procedure is hazardous and is now rarely needed to make the diagnosis of complete absence of the left pericardium if radiological and noninvasive imaging findings are compatible with the diagnosis. Cardiac catheterization with angiography is indicated only if there is a strong suspicion of associated congenital anomalies requiring surgical correction. Usually no specific therapy is required for management of complete absence of the left-sided pericardium.

PARTIAL ABSENCE. Partial left-sided pericardial defects may be complicated by herniation of the left atrial appendage, atrium, or left ventricle through the defect, associated with chest pain, syncope, and sudden death from cardiac strangulation.[624–627] The chest roentgenogram usually shows the nonspecific finding of prominence of the second arch of the left heart border, which must be distinguished from pulmonary artery dilation or aneurysm of the left atrial appendage.[628] Two-dimensional echocardi-

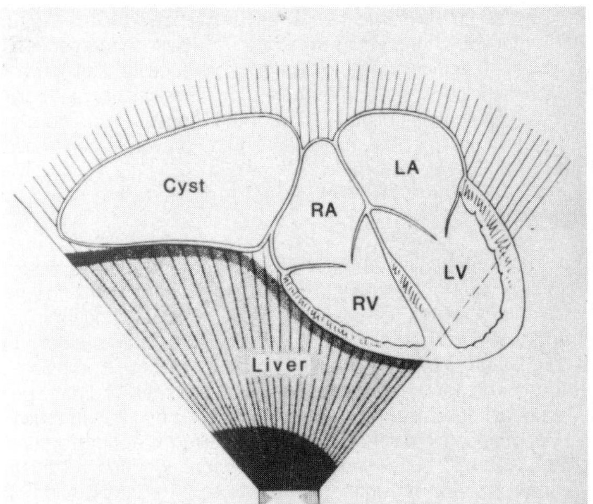

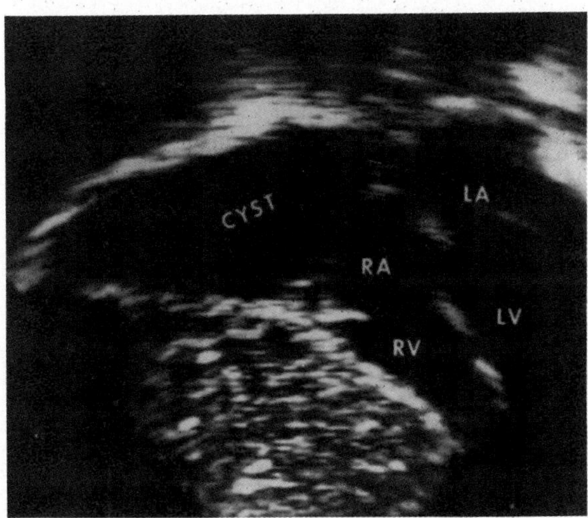

FIGURE 45–27. Two-dimensional subcostal echocardiographic appearance of a well-demarcated benign pericardial cyst adjacent to the right atrial (RA) wall. (From Hynes, J. K., et al.: Two-dimensional echocardiographic diagnosis of pericardial cyst. Mayo Clin. Proc. *58*:60, 1983.)

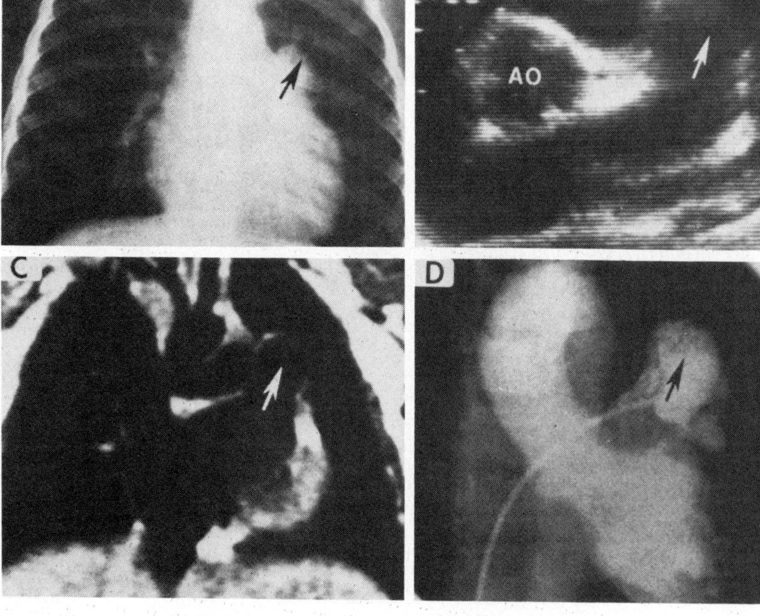

FIGURE 45–28. Noninvasive diagnostic features of partial absence of the left pericardium. The chest roentgenogram (*A*) shows knoblike prominence of the left atrial appendage (arrow). The short-axis cross-sectional 2-D echocardiogram (*B*) shows an enlarged left atrial appendage (arrow) extending beyond the pulmonary artery. The frontal plane magnetic resonance image (*C*) shows enlargement and lateral protuberance of the left atrial appendage (arrow). A contrast cineangiogram (*D*) with the catheter positioned across a patent foramen ovale in the left atrial appendage shows a characteristic wedge of lung between the aorta and pulmonary artery and confirms the herniation of the left atrial appendage (arrow). (From Altman, C. A., et al.: Noninvasive diagnostic features of partial absence of the pericardiaum. Am. J. Cardiol. *63*:1536, 1989.)

ography and magnetic resonance imaging are helpful in demonstrating dilation of the left atrial appendage that extends beyond the pulmonary artery (Fig. 45–28).[628,629] Pulmonary artery angiography with follow-through of contrast opacification to the left heart is the standard method of definitively demonstrating herniation of the left atrium or left atrial appendage beyond the left heart border.[628,629] Partial herniation of the heart and diastolic collapse and compression of the coronary arteries through the defect is a complication of this anomaly that uncommonly may contribute to the development of chest pain and coronary artery strictures.[630,631]

The even rarer anomaly of partial right-sided pericardial defect may be associated with inspiratory right-sided chest pain secondary to herniation of the right atrium and right ventricle through the defect or herniation of lung into the pericardial cavity. The chest roentgenogram may show an unusual protuberance of the right heart border, and technetium-99m cardiac blood pool imaging may demonstrate that the abnormal contour of the right heart border fills simultaneously with the right atrium.[632] Right atrial angiography in the left anterior oblique projection is helpful in documenting herniation of the right atrium and right ventricle through the pericardial defect. Surgical treatment of partial left- or right-sided pericardial defects is usually indicated to relieve symptoms and prevent cardiac strangulation. The defect may be approached by excision of the atrial appendage, pericardioplasty, or pericardiectomy.[633]

REFERENCES

ANATOMY AND FUNCTIONS

1. Pericardial Diseases. *In* Fowler, N. O.: Diagnosis of Heart Disease. New York, Springer-Verlag, 1991, pp. 292–313.
1a. Holt, J. P.: The normal pericardium. Am. J. Cardiol. *26*;455, 1970.
2. Alles, A., and Dom, R. M.: Peripheral sensory nerve fibers that dichotomize to supply the brachium and the pericardium in the rat. Brain Res. *342*:382, 1985.
3. Ishihara, T., Ferrans, V. J., Jones, M., et al.: Histologic and ultrastructural features of normal human parietal pericardium. Am. J. Cardiol. *46*:744, 1980.
4. Fukuo, Y., Nakatani, T., Shinohara, H., and Matsuda, T.: Pericardium of rodents: Pores connect the pericardial and pleural cavities. Anat. Res. *220*:132, 1988.
5. Hills, B. A., and Butler, B. D.: Phospholipids identified on the pericardium and their ability to impart boundary lubrication. Ann. Biomed. Eng. *13*:573, 1985.
6. Miyazaki, T., Pride, H. P., and Zipes, D. P.: Prostaglandins in the pericardial fluid modulate neural regulation of cardiac electrophysiological properties. Circ. Res. *66*:163, 1990.
7. Lee, M. D., Fung, Y. C., Shabetai, R., and LeWinter, M. M.: Biaxial mechanical properties of human pericardium and canine comparisons. Am. J. Physiol. *253*:H75, 1987.
8. Tyson, G. S., Jr., Maier, G. W., Olsen, C. O., et al.: Pericardial influences on ventricular filling in the conscious dog. Circ. Res. *54*:173, 1984.
9. Shabetai, R.: Pericardial and cardiac pressure. Circulation *77*:1, 1988.
10. Smiseth, O. A., Frais, M. A., Kingma, I., et al.: Assessment of pericardial constraint in dogs. Circulation *71*:158, 1985.
11. Smiseth, O. A., Frais, M. A., Kingma, I., et al.: Assessment of pericardial constraint: The relation between right ventricular filling pressure and pericardial pressure measured after pericardiocentesis. J. Am. Coll. Cardiol. *7*:307, 1986.
12. Boltwood, C. M., Jr.: Ventricular performance related to transmural filling pressure in clinical tamponade. Circulation *73*:428, 1987.
13. Santamore, W. P., Constantinesco, M., and Little, W. C.: Direct assessment of right ventricular transmural pressure. Circulation *75*:744, 1987.
14. Slinker, B. K., Ditchey, R. V., Bell, S. P., and LeWinter, M. M.: Right heart pressure does not equal pericardial pressure in the potassium chloride arrested canine heart in situ. Circulation *7G*:357, 1987.
15. Hoit, B. D., Lew, W. Y., and LeWinter, M.: Regional variation in pericardial contact pressure in the canine ventricle. Am. J. Physiol. *255*:H1370, 1988.
16. Bernard, H. L.: The functions of the pericardium. J. Physiol. *22*:43, 1898.
17. Junemann, M., Smiseth, O. A., Refsum, H., et al.: Quantification of effect of pericardium on LV diastolic PV relation in dogs. Am. J. Physiol. *252*:H963, 1987.
18. Gilbert, J. C., and Glantz, S. A.: Determinants of ventricular filling and of the diastolic pressure-volume relation. Circ. Res. *64*:827, 1989.
19. Shirato, K., Shabetai, R., Bhargave, V., et al.: Alteration of the left ventricular diastolic pressure-segment length relation produced by the pericardium. Circulation *57*:1191, 1978.
20. Smiseth, O. A., Manyari, D. E., Lima, J. A., et al.: Modulation of vascular capacitance by angiotensin and nitroprusside: A mechanism of changes in pericardial pressure. Circulation *76*:875, 1987.
21. LeWinter, M. M., and Pavelec, R.: Influence of the pericardium on left ventricular end-diastolic pressure-segment relations during early and later stages of experimental chronic volume overload in dogs. Circ. Res. *50*:501, 1982.
22. Freeman, G. L., and LeWinter, M. M.: Pericardial adaptations during chronic cardiac dilation in dogs. Circ. Res. *54*:294, 1984.
23. Frais, M. A., Bergman, D. W., Kingma, I., et al.: The dependence of the time constant of left ventricular isovolumic relaxation (tau) on pericardial pressure. Circulation *81*:1071, 1990.
24. Serizawa, T., Carabello, B. A., and Grossman, W.: Effect of pacing induced ischemia on left ventricular diastolic pressure-volume relations in dog with coronary stenosis. Circ. Res. *46*:430, 1980.
25. Taylor, R. R., Covell, J. W., Sonnenblick, E. H., and Ross, J., Jr.: Dependence of ventricular distensibility on filling of the opposite ventricle. Am. J. Physiol. *213*:711, 1967.
26. Brinker, J. A., Weiss, J. L., Lappe, D. L., et al.: Leftward septal displacement during right ventricular loading in man. Circulation *61*:626, 1980.
27. Lorell, B. H., Palacios, I., Daggett, W. M., et al.: Right ventricular distention and left ventricular compliance. Am. J. Physiol. *240*:H87, 1981.
28. Hoit, B. D., Dalton, N., Bhargava, V., and Shabetai, R.: Pericardial influences on right and left ventricular filling dynamics. Circulation Res. *68*:197, 1991.
29. Santamore, W. P., Bartlett, R., Van Buren, S. J., et al.: Ventricular coupling in constrictive pericarditis. Circulation *74*:597, 1986.
30. Mangano, D. T.: The effect of the pericardium on ventricular systolic function in man. Circulation *61*:352, 1980.
31. Kanazawa, M., Shirato, K., Ishikawa, K., et al.: The effect of pericardium on the end-systolic pressure-segment length relationship in canine left ventricle in acute volume overload. Circulation *68*:1290, 1983.
32. Goto, Y., Slinker, B. K., and LeWinter, M. M.: Nonhomogeneous left ventricular regional shortening during acute right ventricular pressure overload. Circ. Res. *65*:43, 1989.
33. Stray-Gendersen, J., Musch, T. I., Haidet, G. C., et al.: The effect of pericardiectomy on maximal oxygen consumption and maximal cardiac output in untrained dogs. Circ. Res. *58*:523, 1986.
34. Ringertz, H. G., Misbach, G. A., and Tyberg, J. V.: Effect of the normal pericardium on the left ventricular diastolic pressure-volume relationship. Acta Radiol. *22*:529, 1981.

35. Jarvinen, A., Peltola, K., Rasanen, J., and Heikkila, J.: Immediate hemodynamic effects of pericardial closure after open-heart surgery. Scand. J. Thorac. Cardiovasc. Surg. *21*:131, 1987.
36. Ludbrook, P. A., Byrne, J. D., Kurnik, P. B., and McKnight, R. C.: Influence of reduction of preload and afterload by nitroglycerin on left ventricular diastolic pressure-volume relations and relaxation in man. Circulation *56*:937, 1977.
37. Ludbrook, P. A., Byrne, J. D., and McKnight, R. C.: Influence of right ventricular hemodynamics on left ventricular diastolic pressure-volume relations in man. Circulation *59*:21, 1979.
38. Wong, C. Y., and Spotnitz, H. M.: Effect of nitroprusside on end-diastolic pressure-diameter relations of the human left ventricle after pericardiotomy. J. Thorac. Cardiovasc. Surg. *82*:350, 1981.
39. Ross, J., Jr.: Acute displacement of the diastolic pressure-volume curve of the left ventricle: Role of the pericardium and the right ventricle. Circulation *59*:32, 1979.
40. Lee, M. J., and Boughner, D. R.: Mechanical properties of human pericardium. Circ. Res. *57*:475, 1985.
41. Bartle, S. H., and Hermann, H. J.: Acute mitral regurgitation in man. Hemodynamic evidence and observations indicating an early role for the pericardium. Circulation *36*:839, 1967.
42. Lorell, B. H., Leinbach, R. C., Pohost, G. M., et al.: Right ventricular infarction. Am. J. Cardiol *43*:465, 1979.
43. Goldstein, J. A., Vlahakes, G. H., Verrier, E. D., et al.: The role of right ventricular systolic dysfunction and elevated intrapericardial pressure in the genesis of low output in experimental right ventricular infarction. Circulation *65*:513, 1982.
44. Janicki, J. S.: Influence of the pericardium and ventricular interdependence on left ventricular diastolic and systolic function in patients with heart failure. Circulation 81(Suppl. II):15, 1990.

ACUTE PERICARDITIS

45. Markiewicz, W., Brik, A., Brook, G., et al.: Pericardial rub in pericardial effusion: Lack of correlation with amount of fluid. Chest *77*:643, 1980.
46. Spodick, D. H.: Pericardial rub: Prospective, multiple observer investigation of pericardial friction rub in 100 patients. Am. J. Cardiol. *35*:357, 1975.
47. Spodick, D. H.: Diagnostic electrocardiographic sequences in acute pericarditis: Significance of PR segment and PR vector changes. Circulation *48*:575, 1973.
48. Surawicz, B., and Lasseter, K. C.: Electrocardiogram in pericarditis. Am. J. Cardiol. *26*:471, 1970.
49. Kouvaras, G., Soufras, G., Chronopoulos, G., et al.: The ST segment as a differential diagnostic feature between acute pericarditis and acute inferior myocardial infarction. Angiology *41*:207, 1990.
50. Toriya Martinez, R. N., and Gonzalez Hermosillo, J. A.: Acute nonspecific pericarditis. Arch. Inst. Cardiol. Mex. *57*:307, 1987.
51. Bruce, M. A., and Spodick, D. H.: Atypical electrocardiogram in acute pericarditis: Characteristics and prevalence. J. Electrocardiol. *13*:61, 1980.
52. Carson, W.: Maximal spatial ST vector of ST segment elevation in the right praecordial leads on electrocardiogram due to acute pericarditis. Eur. Heart J. *9*:665, 1988.
53. Wanner, W. R., Schaal, S. F., Bashore, T. M., et al.: Repolarization variant vs. acute pericarditis. A prospective electrocardiographic and echocardiographic evaluation. Chest *83*:180, 1983.
54. Ginzton, L. E., and Laks, M. M.: The differential diagnosis of acute pericarditis. Circulation *65*:1004, 1982.
55. Dressler, N.: Sinus tachycardia complicating and outlasting pericarditis. Am. Heart J. *72*:422, 1966.
56. Spodick, D. H.: Frequency of arrhythmias in acute pericarditis determined by Holter monitoring. Am. J. Cardiol. *53*:842, 1984.
57. Weiss, J. M., and Spodick, D. H.: Association of left pleural effusion with pericardial disease. N. Engl. J. Med. *308*:696, 1983.
58. Olson, H. G., Lyons, K. P., Aronow, W. S., et al.: Technetium-99m stannous pyrophosphate myocardial scintigrams in pericardial disease. Am. Heart. J. *99*:459, 1980.
59. Martin, P., Devriendt, J., Goffin, Y., and Verhas, M.: Gallium 67 scintigraphy in fibrinous pericarditis associated with bacterial endocarditis. Eur. J. Nucl. Med. *7*:192, 1982.
60. Karjalainen, J., and Heikkila, J.: Acute pericarditis: Myocardial enzyme release as evidence for myocarditis. Am. Heart J. *111*:546, 1986.
61. Saner, H. E., Gobel, F. L., Nicoloff, D. M., and Edwairds, J. E: Aortic dissection presenting as pericarditis. Chest. *91*:71, 1987.
62. Permanyer-Miralda, G., Sagrista-Sauleda, J., and Soler-Soler, J.: Primary acute pericardial disease: A prospective series of 231 consecutive patients. Am. J. Cardiol. *56*:623, 1985.
63. Sagrista-Sauleda, J., Permanyer-Miralda, G., Candell-Riera, J., et al.: Transient cardiac constriction: An unrecognized pattern of evolution in effusive acute idiopathic pericarditis. Am. J. Cardiol. *59*:961, 1987.
64. Fowler, N. O., and Harbin, A. D.: Recurrent pericarditis: Follow-up of 31 patients. J. Am. Coll. Cardiol. *7*:300, 1986.
65. Hatcher, C. R., Logue, R. B., Logan, W. D., et al.: Pericardiectomy for recurrent pericarditis. J. Thorac, Cardiovasc. Surg. *62*:371, 1971.
66. Permanyer-Miralda, G., Sagrista-Sauleda, J., Shabetai, R., et al.: Acute pericardial disease: An approach to etiologic diagnosis and treatment. *In* Soler-Soler, J., Permanyer-Miralda, G., and Sagrista-Sauleda, J. (eds.): Pericardial Disease: New Insights and Old Dilemmas. Dordrecht, The Netherlands, Kluwer Academic Publishers, 1990, pp. 193–214.

PERICARDIAL EFFUSION

67. Carsky, E. W., Mauceri, R. A., and Azimi, F.: The epicardial fat pad sign: Analysis of frontal and lateral chest radiographs in patients with pericardial effusion. Radiology *137*:303, 1980.
68. Miller, S. W.: Imaging pericardial disease. Radiol. Clin. North. Am. *27*:1113, 1989.
69. Unverferth, D. V., Williams, T. E., and Fulkerson, P.K.: Electrocardiographic voltage in pericardial effusion. Chest *75*:157, 1979.
70. Horowitz, M. S., Schultz, C. S., and Stinson, E. B.: Sensitivity and specificity of echocardiographic diagnosis of pericardial effusion. Circulation *50*:239, 1974.
71. Berger, M., Bobak, K., Jelveh, M., and Goldberg, E.: Pericardial effusion diagnosed by echocardiography. Clinical and electrocardiographic findings. Chest *74*:174, 1978.
72. Enein, M., Zina, A. A., Kassem, M., and el-Tabbakh, G.: Echocardiography of the pericardium in pregnancy. Obstet. Gynecol. *69*:851, 1987.
73. Friedman, M. J., Sahn, D. J., and Haber, K.: Two-dimensional echocardiography and B-mode ultrasonography for the diagnosis of loculated pericardial effusion. Circulation *60*:1644, 1979.
74. Iliceto, S., Amtonelli, G., Sorino, M., et al.: Two-dimensional echocardiographic recognition of complications of cardiac invasive procedures Am. J. Cardiol. *53*:846, 1984.
75. Shah, A., and Variyam, E.: Pericardial effusion and left ventricular dysfunction associated with ascites secondary to hepatic cirrhosis. Arch. Intern. Med. *148*:585, 1988.
76. Soler-Soler, J.: Massive chronic idiopathic pericardial effusion. *In* Soler-Soler, J., Permanyer-Miralda, G., and Sagrista-Sauleda, J. (eds.): Pericardial Disease: New Insights and Old Dilemmas. Dordrecht, The Netherlands, Kluwer Academic Publishers, 1990, pp. 153–165.
77. Reddy, P. S., Curtiss, E. I., O'Toole, J. D., and Shaver, J. A.: Cardiac tamponade: Hemodynamic observations in man. Circulation *58*:265, 1978.
78. Spodick, D. H.: The normal and diseased pericardium: Current concepts of pericardial physiology, diagnosis, and treatment. J. Am. Coll. Cardiol. *1*:240, 1983.
79. Manyari, D. E., Kostuk, W. J., and Purves, P.: Effect of pericardiocentesis on right and left ventricular function and volumes in pericardial effusion. Am. J. Cardiol. *52*:159, 1983.
80. Pegram, B. L., Kardon, M. B., and Bishop, V. S.: Changes in left ventricular internal diameter with increasing pericardial pressure. Cardiovasc. Res. *9*:707, 1975.
81. Osborn, J. L., and Lawton, M. T.: Neurogenic antinatriuresis during development of acute cardiac tamponade. Am. J. Physiol. *250*:H195, 1986.
82. Mancini, G. B. J., McGillem, M. J., Bates, E. R., et al.: Hormonal responses to cardiac tamponade: Inhibition of release of atrial natriuretic factor despite elevation of atrial pressures. Circulation *76*:884, 1987.
83. Wechsler, A. S., Auerbach, B. J., Graham, T. C., and Sabiston, D. C.: Distribution of intramyocardial blood flow during pericardial tamponade: Correlation with microscopic anatomy and intrinsic myocardial contractility. J. Thorac. Cardiovasc. Surg. *68*:847, 1974.
84. Brecher, G. A.: Critical review of recent work on ventricular diastolic suction. Circ. Res. *6*:554, 1958.
85. Kostreva, D. R., Castaner, A., Pedersen, D. H., and Kampine, J. P.: Nonvagally mediated bradycardia during cardiac tamponade or severe hemorrhage. Cardiology *68*:65, 1981.
86. Fowler, N. O., and Gabel, M.: The hemodynamic effects of cardiac tamponade: Mainly the result of atrial, not ventricular, compression. Circulation *71*:154, 1985.
87. Fowler, N. O., Gabel, M., and Buncher, C. R.: Cardiac tamponade: A comparison of right versus left heart compression. J. Am. Coll. Cardiol. *12*:187, 1988.
88. Kronton, I., Cohen, M. L., and Winer, H. E.: Diastolic atrial compression: A sensitive echocardiographic sign of cardiac tamponade. J. Am. Coll. Cardiol. *2*:770, 1983.
89. Leimgruber, P. P., Klopfenstein, H. S., Wann, L. S., and Brooks, H. L.: The hemodynamic derangement associated with right ventricular diastolic collapse in cardiac tamponade: An experimental echocardiographic study. Circulation *68*:612, 1983.
90. Gaffney, F. A., Keller, A. M., Peshock, R. M., et al.: Pathophysiologic mechanisms of cardiac tamponade and pulsus alternans shown by echocardiography. Am. J. Cardiol *53*:1162, 1984.
91. Klopfenstein, H. S., Cogswell, T. L., Bernath, G. A., et al.: Alternations in intravascular volume affect the relation between right ventricular diastolic collapse and the hemodynamic severity of cardiac tamponade. J. Am Coll. Cardiol. *6*:1057, 1985.
92. Singh, S., Wann, L. S., Schuchard, G. H., et al.: Right ventricular and right atrial collapse in patients with cardiac tamponade—a combined echocardiographic and hemodynamic study. Circulation *70*:966, 1984.
93. Ruskin, J., Bache, R. J., Rembert, J. C., and Greenfield, J. C., Jr.: Pressure-flow studies in man: Effect of respiration on left ventricular stroke volume. Circulation *48*:79, 1973.
94. Goldblatt, A., Harrison, D. C., Glick, G., and Braunwald, E.: Studies on cardiac dimensions in intact, unanesthetized man. II. Effects of respiration. Circ. Res. *13*:448, 1963.
95. Wexler, L., Bergel, D. H., Gabe, I. T., et al.: Velocity of blood flow in normal human venae cavae. Circ. Res. *23*:349, 1968.
96. Shabetai, R., Fowler, N. O., Fenton, J. C., and Masangkay, M.: Pulsus paradoxus. J. Clin. Invest. *44*:1882, 1965.
97. Shabetai, R., Fowler, N. O., and Gueron, M.: The effects of respiration on aortic pressure and flow. Am. Heart J. *65*:525, 1963.

98. Settle, H. P., Adolph, R. J., Fowler, N. O., et al.: Echocardiographic study of cardiac tamponade. Circulation *56*:951, 1977.
99. Gonzales, M. S., Basnight, M. A., Appleton, C. P., et al.: Experimental pericardial effusion: relation of abnormal respiratory variation in mitral flow velocity to hemodynamics and diastolic right heart collapse. J. Am. Coll. Cardiol. *17*:239, 1991.
100. Friedman, H. S., Sakurai, H., and Lajam, F.: Pulsus paradosus: A manifestation of marked reduction of left ventricular end-diastolic volume in cardiac tamponade. J. Thorac. Cardiovasc. Surg. *79*:74, 1980.
101. Cohen, S. I., Kupersmith, J., Aroesty, J., and Rowe, J. W.: Pulsus paradoxus and Kussmaul's sign in acute pulmonary embolism. Am. J. Cardiol. *32*:271, 1973.
102. Settle, H. P., Jr., Engel, P. J., Fowler, N. O., et al.: Echocardiographic study of the paradoxical arterial pulse in chronic obstructive lung disease. Circulation *62*:1297, 1980.
103. Winer, H. E., and Kronzon, I.: Absence of paradoxical pulse in patients with cardiac tamponade and atrial septal defects. Am. J. Cardiol. *44*:378, 1979.
104. Frey, M. J., Berko, B., Palevsky, H., et al.: Recognition of cardiac tamponade in the presence of severe pulmonary hypertension. Ann. Intern. Med. *111*:615, 1989.
105. Guberman, B. A., Fowler, N. O., Engel, P. J., et al.: Cardiac tamponade in medical patients. Circulation *64*:633, 1981.
106. Beck, C. S.: Two cardiac compression triads. J.A.M.A. *104*:714, 1935.
107. Sznajder, J. I., Evander, E., Pollak, E. R., et al.: Pericardial effusion causes interstitial pulmonary edema in dogs. Circulation *76*:843, 1987.
108. Cohn, J. N., Pinkerson, A. L., and Tristani, F. E.: Mechanism of pulsus paradoxus in clinical shock. J. Clin Invest. *46*:1774, 1967.
109. Labib, S. B., Udelson, J. E., and Pandian, N. G.: Echocardiography in low pressure cardiac tamponade. Am. J. Cardiol. *63*:1156, 1989.
110. Johnston,S. L., and Oliver, R. M.: Cardiac tamponade due to pneumopericardium. Thorax *43*:482, 1988.
111. Katzir, D., Klinovsky, E., Kent, V., et al.: Spontaneous pneumopericardium: Case report and review of the literature. Cardiology *76*:305, 1989.
112. Bricheteau: Observat d'hydropneumopercarde accompane d'un fluctuation perceptible a l'orielle. Arch. Gen. Med. *4*:334, 1844.
113. Usher, B. W., and Popp, R. L.: Electrical alternans: Mechanism in pericardial effusion. Am. Heart. J. *83*:459, 1972.
114. Friedman, H. S., Lajam, F., Calderon, J., et al.: Electrocardiographic features of experimental cardiac tamponade in closed-chest dogs. Eur. J.Cardiol. *6*:311, 1977.
115. Mazurek, B., Jehle, D., and Martin, M.: Emergency department echocardiography in the diagnosis and therapy of cardiac tamponade. J. Emerg. Med. *9*:27, 1991.
116. Chuttani, K., Pandian, N. G., Mohanty, P. K. et al.: Left ventricular diastolic collapse: An echocardiographic sign of regional cardiac tamponade. Circulation *83*:1999, 1991.
117. Kronzon, I., Cohen, M. J., and Winer, H. E.: Contribution of echocardiography to the understanding of the pathophysiology of cardiac tamponade. J. Am. Coll. Cardiol. *1*:1180, 1983.
118. D'Cruz, I. A., Cohen, H. C., Prabhus, R., and Glick, G.: Diagnosis of cardiac tamponade by echocardiography (changes in mitral valve motion and ventricular dimensions with special reference to paradoxical pulse). Circulation *52*:460, 1975.
119. Appleton, C. P., Hatle, L. K., and Popp, R. L.: Cardiac tamponade and pericardial effusion: Respiratory variation in transvalvular flow velocities studied by Doppler echocardiography. J. Am. Coll. Cardiol. *11*:1020, 1988.
120. Leeman, D. E., Levine, M. J., and Come, P. C.: Doppler echocardiography in cardiac tamponade: Exaggerated respiratory variation in transvalvular blood flow velocity integrals. J. Am. Coll. Cardiol. *11*:572, 1988.
121. Burstow, D. J., Jae, K. O., Baileys, K. R., et al.: Cardiac tamponade: Characteristic Doppler observations. Mayo Clin. Proc. *64*:312, 1989.
122. Shindler, D. M., Reddy, K., Shindler, O. I., and Kostis, J. B.: Failure of the aortic valve to open during inspiration in cardiac tamponade. Chest *82*:797, 1982.
123. Singh, S., Wann, L. S., Klopfenstein, H. S., et al.: Usefulness of right ventricular diastolic collapse in diagnosing cardiac tamponade and comparison to pulsus paradoxus. Am. J. Cardiol. *57*:652, 1986.
124. Cogswell, T. L., Bernath, G. A., Wann, L. S., et al.: Effects of intravascular volume on the value of pulsus paradoxus and right ventricular diastolic collapse in predicting cardiac tamponade. Circulation *72*:1076, 1985.
125. Tunick, P. A., Nachamie, M., and Kronzon, I.: Reversal of echocardiographic signs of pericardial tamponade by transfusion. Am. Heart J. *119*:199, 1990.
126. Martins, J. B., and Kerber, R. E.: Can cardiac tamponade be diagnosed by echocardiography? Circulation *60*:737, 1979.
127. Miller, S. W., Feldman, L., Palacios, I., et al.: Compression of the superior vena cava and right atrium in cardiac tamponade. Am. J. Cardiol. *50*:1287, 1982.
128. Levine, M. J., Lorell, B. H., Diver, D. J., and Come, P. C.: Implications of echocardiographically assisted diagnosis of pericardial tamponade in contemporary medical patients: Detection prior to hemodynamic embarrassment. J. Am. Coll. Cardiol. *17*:59, 1991.
129. Northridge, D. B., McMurray, J., Ray, S., et al.: Release of atrial natriuretic factor after pericardiocentesis for malignant pericardial effusion. Br. Med. J. *299*:603, 1989.
130. Safian, R. D., Come, S. E., Kadin, M., and Lorell, B. H.: Antemortem diagnosis of pulmonary microvascular tumor. Cathet. Cardiovasc. Diagn. *17*:112, 1989.
131. Himelman, R. B., Kircher, B., Rockey, D. C., and Schiller, N. B.: Inferior vena cava plethora with blunted respiratory response: A sensitive echocardiographic sign of cardiac tamponade. J. Am. Coll. Cardiol. *12*:1470, 1988.
132. Fowler, N. O., and Holmes, J. C.: Hemodynamic effect of isoproterenol and norepinephrine in acute cardiac tamponade. J. Clin. Invest. *48*:502, 1969.
133. Kerber, R. E., Jascho, J. A., Litchfield, R., et al.: Hemodynamic effects of volume expansion and nitroprusside compared with the pericardiocentesis in patients with cardiac tamponade. N. Engl. J. Med. *306*:929, 1982.
134. Moller, C. T., Schoonbee, C. G., and Rosendorff, C.: Hemodynamics of cardiac tamponade during various modes of ventilation. Br. J. Anaesth. *51*:409, 1979.
135. Kilpatrick, Z. M., and Chapman, C. B.: On pericardiocentesis. Am. J. Cardiol. *16*:722, 1965.
136. Krikorian, J. G., and Hancock, E. W.: Pericardiocentesis. Am. J. Med. *65*:808, 1978.
137. Kaiser, E., and Loewenneck, H.: Pericardial puncture. The most favorable anatomical approach. Munch. Med. Wochenschr. *123*:1697, 1981.
138. Heilerh, B., Anderes, U., and Follath, F.: Diagnosis and therapy of cardiac tamponade. An analysis of 50 patients. Schweiz. Med. Wochenschr. *111*:735, 1981.
139. Callahan, J. A., Seward, J. B., Nishimura, R. A., et al.: Two-dimensional echocardiographically guided pericardiocentesis: Experience in 117 consecutive patients. Am. J. Cardiol. *55*:476, 1985.
140. Pandian, N. G., Brockway, B., Simonetti, J. et al.: Pericardiocentesis under two-dimensional echocardiographic guidance in loculated pericardial effusion. Ann. Thorac. Surg. *45*:99, 1988.
141. Morgan, C. D., Marshall, S. A., and Ross, J. R.: Catheter drainage of the pericardium: Its safety and efficacy. Can. J. Surg. *32*:331, 1989.
142. Aron, D. C., Richardson, J. D., Webb, G., et al.: Subxiphoid pericardial window in patients with suspected traumatic pericardial tamponade. Ann. Thorac. Surg. *23*:545, 1977.
143. Armstrong, N. F., Feigenbaum, H., and Dillon, J. C.: Acute right ventricular dilation and echocardiographic volume overload following pericardiocentesis for relief of cardiac tamponade. Am. Heart J. *107*:1266, 1984.
144. Glasser, F., Fein, A. M., Feinsilver, S. H., et al.: Non-cardiogenic pulmonary edema after pericardial drainage for cardiac tamponade. Chest *94*:869, 1988.
145. Lorell, B. H., and Grossman, W: Profiles in constrictive pericarditis, restrictive cardiomyopathy, and cardiac tamponade. *In* Grossman, W., and Baim, D. S. (eds.): Cardiac Catheterization, Angiography, and Intervention. 4th ed. Philadelphia, Lea and Febiger, 1991, pp. 633–653.
146. Erdman, S., Levinsky, L., Derivi, E., and Levy, M. J.: Closed pericardial drainage for relief of cardiac tamponade. Thorac. Cardiovasc. Surg. *34*:66, 1986.
147. Lock, J. E., Bass, J. L., Kulif, F. J., and Fuhrman, B. P.: Chronic percutaneous pericardial drainage with modified pigtail catheters in children. Am. J. Cardiol. *53*:1179, 1984.
148. Sinzobahamvya, N.: Results of subxiphoid pericardiostomy in pericardial effusion. Acta Chir. Belg. *88*:175, 1988.
149. Palatianos, G. M., Thurer, R. J., and Kaiser, G. A.: Comparison of effectiveness and safety of operations on the pericardium. Chest *88*:30, 1985.
150. Piehler, J. M., Pluth, J. R., Schaff, H. V., et al: Surgical management of effusive pericardial disease. J. Thorac. Cardiovasc. Surg. *90*:506, 1986.
151. Little, A. G., and Ferguson, M. K.: Pericardioscopy as adjunct to pericardial window. Chest *89*:53, 1986.
152. Millaire, A., Wurtz, A., Brullard, B., et al.: Value of pericardioscopy in pericardial effusion. Arch. Mal. Coeur *81*:1071, 1988.
153. Endrys, J., Simo, M., Shafie, M. Z., et al: New nonsurgical technique for multiple pericardial biopsies. Cathet. Cardiovasc. Diagn. *15*:92, 1988.

CONSTRICTIVE PERICARDITIS

154. Nishimura, R. A., Kazmier, F. J., Smith, H. C., and Danielson, G. K.: Right ventricular outflow obstruction caused by constrictive pericardial disease. Am. J. Cardiol. *55*:1447, 1985.
155. Nigri, A., Mangieri, E., Martuscelli, E., et al.: Pulmonary trunk stenosis due to constriction by a pulmonary band. Am. Heart J. *114*:448, 1987.
156. Meyer, T. E., Sareli, P., Marcus, R. H., et al.: Mechanism underlying Kussmaul's sign in chronic constrictive pericarditis. Am. J. Cardiol. *64*:1069, 1989.
157. Hancock, E. W.: Constrictive pericarditis: Modern view of diagnosis and management. J. Cardiovasc. Med. *41*:367, 1980.
158. Wolozin, M. W., Ortola, F. V., Spodick, D. H., and Seifter, J. L.: Release of atrial natriuretic factor after pericardiectomy for chronic constrictive pericarditis. Am. J. Cardiol. *62*:1323, 1988.
159. Gaasch, W. H., Peterson, K. L., and Shabetai, R.: Left ventricular function in chronic constrictive pericarditis. Am. J. Cardiol. *34*:107, 1974.
160. Dines, D. E., Edwards, J. E., and Burchell, H. B.: Myocardial atrophy in constrictive pancarditis. Proc. Staff Meet. Mayo Clin. *33*:93, 1958.
161. Levine, H. D.: Myocardial fibrosis in constrictive pericarditis. Electrocardiographic and pathologic observations. Circulation *48*:1268, 1973.
162. Gregory, M. A., Whitton, I. D., and Cameron, E. W.: Myocardial ischemia in constrictive pericarditis: A morphometric and electron microscopic study. Br. J. Exp. Pathol. *65*:365, 1984.
163. Nichols, D. A., and Peter, R. H.: Constrictive pericarditis as a late complication of meningococcal pericarditis. Am. J. Cardiol. *55*:1442, 1985.

164. Hancock, E. W.: On the elastic and rigid forms of constrictive pericarditis. Am. Heart J. *100*:917, 1980.
165. Paul, O., Castleman, B., and White, P. D.: Chronic constrictive pericarditis: A study of 53 cases. Am. J. Med. Sci. *216*:361, 1948.
166. Andrews, G.W.S., Pickering, G. W., and Sellors, T. H.: The aetiology of constrictive pericarditis with special reference to tuberculous pericarditis, together with a note on polyserositis. Q. J. Med. *17*:291, 1948.
167. Bashi, V. V., Ravikumar, J. S., Jairaj, P. S., et al.: Early and late results of pericardiectomy in 118 cases of constrictive pericarditis. Thorax *43*:637, 1988.
168. Blake, S., Bonar, S., O'Neill, H., et al: Aetiology of chronic constrictive pericarditis. Br. Heart J. *50*:273, 1983.
169. Cameron, J., Oesterle, S. N., Baldwin, J. C., and Hancock, E. W.: The etiologic spectrum of constrictive pericarditis. Am. Heart J. *113*:354, 1987.
170. Fischbein, L., Namade, M., Sachs, R. N., et al: Chronic constrictive pericarditis associated with asbestosis. Chest *94*:646, 1988.
171. Van der Horst, R. L.: Pericardial calcification in childhood. Cardiovasc. Radiol. *1*:265, 1978.
172. Bonische, C. H., and Jaffe, J. P.: Spontaneous severe constrictive pericarditis in congenital afibrinogenemia: Mechanism, evaluation and successful surgical management. Am. Heart J. *101*:503, 1981.
173. Laxer, R. M., Cameron, B. J., Chaisson, D., et al.: The camptodactyly-arthropathy-pericarditis syndrome: Case report and literature review. Arthritis Rheum. *29*:439, 1986.
174. Voorhees, M. L., Husson, G. S., and Blackman, M. S.: Growth failure with pericardial constriction. The syndrome of mulibrey nanism. Am. J. Dis. Child. *130*:1146, 1976.
175. Cotton, J. B., Rebelle, C., Bosnio, A., et al.: Familial intrauterine nanism with constrictive pericarditis: The Mulibrey syndrome. Pediatric *43*:197, 1988.
176. Tyberg, T. I., Goodyer, A. V. N., and Langou, R. A.: Genesis of pericardial knock in constrictive pericarditis. Am. J. Cardiol. *46*:570, 1980.
177. Manga, P., Vythilingum, S., and Mitha, A. S.: Pulsatile hepatomegaly in constrictive pericarditis. Br. Heart J. *52*:465, 1984.
177a. Anand, I. S., Ferrari, R., Kalra, G. S., et al.: Pathogenesis of edema in constrictive pericarditis. Circulation *83*:1880, 1991.
178. Plus, G. E., Brower, A. J., and Clagett, O. T.: Chronic constrictive pericarditis: Roentgenologic findings in 35 surgically proved cases. Proc. Staff Meet. Mayo Clinic. *32*:555, 1957.
179. MacGregor, J. H., Chen, J. T., Chiles, C. et al: The radiographic distinction between pericardial and myocardial calcifications. Am. J. Roentgenol. *148*:675, 1987.
180. Tomaselli, G., Gamsu, G., and Stolberg, M. S.: Constrictive pericarditis presenting as pleural effusion of unknown origin. Arch. Intern. Med. *149*:201, 1989.
181. Chesler, E., Mitha, A. S., and Matisonn, R. E.: The ECG of constrictive pericarditis—Pattern resembling right ventricular hypertrophy. Am. Heart J. *91*:420, 1979.
182. Fukuda, K., Nakamura, Y., Ogawa, S., et al.: Constrictive pericarditis with electrocardiographic evidence of right ventricular hypertrophy. Chest *96*:691, 1989.
183. Schnittger, I, Bowden, R. E., Abrams, J., and Popp, R. L.: Echocardiography: Pericardial thickening and constrictive pericarditis. Am. J. Cardiol. *42*:388, 1978.
184. Doi, Y. L., Sugiura, T., and Spodick, D. H.: Motion of pulmonic valve and constrictive pericarditis. Chest *80*:513, 1981.
185. Tei, C., Child, J. S., Tanaka, H., and Shah, P. M.: Atrial systolic notch on the interventricular septal echogram: An echocardiographic sign of constrictive pericarditis. J. Am. Coll. Cardiol. *1*:907, 1983.
186. Trappe, H. J., Herrmann, G., Daniel, W. G., et al.: Reduced diastolic left ventricular posterior wall motion in patients with constrictive pericarditis: Incidence, hemodynamic and clinical correlations. Int. J. Cardiol. *20*:53, 1988.
187. Engle, P. J., Fowler, N. O., Tei, C. W., et al.: M-mode echocardiography in constrictive pericarditis. J. Am. Coll. Cardiol. *6*:471, 1985.
188. Janos, G. G., Arjunan, K., Meyer, R. A., et al.: Differentiation of constrictive pericarditis and restrictive cardiomyopathy using digitized echocardiography. J. Am. Coll. Cardiol. *1*:541, 1983.
189. D'Cruz, I. A., Dick, A., Gross, C. M., et al.: Abnormal left ventricular–left atrial posterior wall contour: A new two-dimensional echocardiographic sign in constrictive pericarditis. Am. Heart J. *118*:128, 1989.
190. Lewis, B. S.: Real time two-dimensional echocardiography in constrictive pericarditis. Am. J. Cardiol. *49*:1789, 1982.
191. Hjemdahl-Monson, C. E., Daniels, J., Kaufman, D., et al.: Spontaneous contrast in the inferior vena cava in a patient with constrictive pericarditis. J. Am. Coll. Cardiol. *4*:165, 1984.
192. Himelman, R. B., Lee, E., and Schiller, N. B.: Septal bounce, vena cava plethora, and pericardial adhesion: Informative two-dimensional echocardiographic signs in the diagnosis of pericardial constriction. J. Am. Soc. Echocadiogr. *1*:333, 1988.
193. Pandian, N. G., Skorton, D. J., Kieso, R. A., and Kerber, R. E.: Diagnosis of constrictive pericarditis by two-dimensional echocardiography: Studies in a new experimental model and in patients. J. Am. Coll. Cardiol. *4*:1164, 1984.
194. Von Bibra, H., Schober, K., Jenni, R., et al.: Diagnosis of constrictive pericarditis by pulsed Doppler echocardiography of the hepatic vein. Am. J. Cardiol. *63*:483, 1989.
195. Sutton, F. J., Whitney, N. O., and Applefeld, M.M.: The role of echocardiography and computed tomography in the evaluation of constrictive pericarditis. Am. Heart J. *109*:350, 1985.
196. Nishimura, R. A., Connolly, D. C., Parkin, T. W., and Stanson, A. W.: Constrictive pericarditis: Assessment of current diagnostic procedures. Mayo Clin. Proc. *60*:397, 1985.
197. Reinmuller, R., Doppman, J. L., Lossner, J. et al.: Constrictive pericardial disease: Prognostic significance of a nonvisualized left ventricular wall. Radiology *156*:753, 1985.
198. Soulen, R. L., Stark, D. D., and Higgins, C. B.: Magnetic resonance imaging of constrictive pericardial disease. Am. J. Cardiol. *55*:480, 1985.
199. Solano, F. X., Young, E., Talamo, T. S., and Dekker, A: Constrictive pericarditis mimicking Budd-Chiari syndrome. Am. J. Med. *80*:113, 1986.
200. Savage, M. P., Munoz, S. J., Herman, W. M., and Kusiak, V. M.: Chylous ascites caused by constrictive pericarditis. Am. J. Gastroenterol. *82*:1088, 1987.
201. Wilkinson, P., Pinto, B., and Senior, J. R.: Reversible protein-losing enteropathy with intestinal lymphangiectasia, secondary to chronic constrictive pericarditis. N. Engl. J. Med. *273*:1178, 1965.
202. Pastor, B. H., and Cahn, M.: Reversible nephrotic syndrome resulting from constrictive pericarditis. N. Engl. J. Med. *262*:872, 1960.
203. Wasserman, A. J., Richardson, D. W., Baird, C. L., and Wyso, E. M.: Cardiac hemochromatosis simulating constrictive pericarditis. Am. J. Med. *32*:316, 1962.
204. Arrillo, J. E., Borer, J. S., Henry, W. L., et al.: The cardiovascular manifestations of the hypereosinophilic syndrome. Am. J. Med. *67*:572, 1979.
205. Lui, C. Y., and Makoui, C.: Severe constrictive pericarditis as an unsuspected cause of death in a patient with idiopathic hypereosinophilic syndrome and restrictive cardiomyopathy. Clin. Cardiol. *11*:502, 1988.
206. Siguera-Filho, A. G., Cunha, C. L. P., Tajik, A. J., et al.: M-mode and two-dimensional echocardiographic features in cardiac amyloidosis. Circulation *63*:188, 1981.
207. Carroll, J. D., Gaasch, W. H., and McAdam, K.P.W.J.: Amyloid cardiomyopathy: Characterization by a distinctive voltage/mass ratio. Am. J. Cardiol. *49*:9, 1982.
208. Bush, C. A., Stang, J. M., Wooley, C. G., and Kilman, J.: Occult constrictive pericardial disease. Diagnosis by rapid volume expansion and correction by pericardiectomy. Circulation *56*:924, 1977.
209. Lewis, B. S., and Gotsman, M. S.: Left ventricular function in systole and diastole in constrictive pericarditis. Am. Heart J. *86*:23, 1973.
210. Goldberg, E., Stein, J., Berger, M., and Berdoff, R. L.: Diastolic segmental coronary artery obliteration in constrictive pericarditis. Cathet. Cardiovasc. Diagn. *7*:197, 1981.
211. Vallance, P.J.T., Gray, H. H., and Oldershaw, P. J.: Diagnostic features of localised pericardial constriction. Int. J. Cardiol. *20*:416, 1988.
212. Meaney, E., Shabetai, R., and Bhargava, V.: Cardiac amyloidosis, constrictive pericarditis and restrictive cardiomyopathy. Am. J. Cardiol. *38*:547, 1976.
213. Swanton, R. H., Brooksby, I.A.B., Davies, M. J., et al.: Systolic and diastolic ventricular function in cardiac amyloidosis. Studies in six cases diagnosed with endomyocardial biopsy. Am. J. Cardiol. *39*:658, 1977.
214. Benotti, J. R., Grossman, W., and Cohn, P. F.: Clinical profile of restrictive cardiomyopathy. Circulation *61*:1206, 1980.
215. Robbins, M. A., Pizzarello, R. A., Stechel, R. P., et al.: Resting and exercise hemodynamics in constrictive pericarditis and a case of cardiac amyloidosis mimicking constriction. Cathet. Cardiovasc. Diagn. *9*:463, 1983.
216. Chew, C., Ziady, G., Raphael, M. J., and Oakley, C. M.: The functional defect in amyloid heart disease. Am. J. Cardiol. *36*:438, 1975.
217. Tyberg, T. I., Goodyer, A.V.N., Hurst, V. W., et al.: Left ventricular filling in differentiating restrictive amyloid cardiomyopathy and constrictive pericarditis. Am. J. Cardiol. *47*:791, 1981.
218. Aroney, C. M., Ruddy, T. D., Dighero, H., et al.: Differentiation of restrictive cardiomyopathy from pericardial constriction. J. Am. Coll. Cardiol. *13*:1007, 1989.
219. Morgan, J. M., Raposo, L., Chow, W. H., and Oldershaw, P. J.: Restrictive cardiomyopathy and constrictive pericarditis: Non-invasive distinction by digitised M mode echocardiography. Br. Heart J. *61*:29, 1989.
220. Klein, A. L., Oh, J. K., Miller, F. A., et al.: Two-dimensional and Doppler echocardiographic assessment of infiltrative cardiomyopathy. J. Am. Soc. Echocardiogr. *1*:48, 1988.
221. Hatle, L. K., Appleton, C. P., and Popp, R. L.: Differentiation of constrictive pericarditis and restrictive cardiomyopathy by Doppler echocardiography. Circulation *79*:357, 1989.
222. Schiavone, W. A., Calafiore, P. A., and Salcedo, E. E.: Transesophageal Doppler echocardiographic demonstration of pulmonary venous flow velocity in restrictive cardiomyopathy and constrictive pericarditis. Am. J. Cardiol. *63*:1286, 1989.
223. Schoenfeld, M. H., Supple, E. W., Dec, G. W., et al.: Restrictive cardiomyopathy versus constrictive pericarditis: Role of endomyocardial biopsy in avoiding unnecessary thoracotomy. Circulation *75*:1012, 1987.
224. Broadarick, S., Paine, R., Higa, E., and Carmichael, K. A.: Pericardial tamponade—A new complication of amyloid heart disease. Am. J. Med. *73*:133, 1982.
225. Kern, M. J., Lorell, B. H., and Grossman, W.: Cardiac amyloidosis masquerading as constrictive pericarditis. Cathet. Cardiovasc. Diagn. *8*:629, 1982.
226. Katagiri, M., Tanabe, Y., Takahashi, M., and Kasuya, S.: Right atrial thrombosis: Association with constrictive pericarditis. Ann. Thorac. Surg. *49*:145, 1990.
227. Copeland, J. G., Stinson, E. B., Griepp, R. B., and Shumway, N. E.: Surgical treatment of chronic constrictive pericarditis using cardiopulmonary bypass. J. Thorac. Cardiovasc. Surg. *69*:236, 1975.
228. Johnson, R. G., Thurer, R. L., Lorell, B. H., and Weintraub R. M.: Ultrasonic

debridement of calcified pericardium in constrictive pericarditis. Ann. Thorac. Surg. *48*:855, 1989.
229. Culliford, A. T., Lipton, M., and Spencer, F. C.: Operation for chronic constrictive pericarditis: Do the surgical approach and degree of pericardial resection influence the outcome significantly? Ann. Thorac. Surg. *29*:146, 1980.
230. McCaughlin, B. C., Schaff, H. V., Piehler, J. M., et al.: Early and late results of pericardiectomy for constrictive pericarditis. J. Thorac. Cardiovasc. Surg. *89*:340, 1985.
231. Robertson, J. M., and Mulder, D. G.: Pericardiectomy: A changing scene. Am. J. Surg. *148*:86, 1984.
232. Aagaard, M. T., and Haraldsted, V. Y.: Chronic constrictive pericarditis treated with total pericardiectomy. Thorac. Cardiovasc. Surg. *32*:311, 1984.
233. Siefert, F. C., Miller, C. D., Oesterle, S. N., et al.: Surgical treatment of constrictive pericarditis: Analysis of outcome and diagnostic error. Circulation 72 (Suppl. 2):264, 1985.
234. Astrudillo, R., and Ivert, T.; Late results after pericardiectomy for constrictive pericarditis via left thoracotomy. Scand. J. Thorac. Cardiovasc. Surg. *23*:115, 1989.
235. Bashi, I., Ravikumar, J. S., Jairaj, P. S., et al.: Early and late results of pericardiectomy in 118 cases of constrictive pericarditis. Thorax *43*:637, 1988.
236. Potwar, S. A., Arsiwala, S S., Bhosle, K. N., and Mehta, V. I.: Surgical treatment of chronic constrictive pericarditis. Indian Heart J. *41*:30, 1989.
237. Viola, A R.: The influence of pericardiectomy on the hemodynamics of chronic constrictive pericarditis. Circulation *48*:1038, 1973.
238. Pick, R. A., Joswig, B. C., and Bloor, C. M.: Recurrent cardiac constriction after pericardiectomy. Arch. Intern. Med. *144*:2061, 1984.
239. Kashani, I. A., Higgins, C. B., and Utley, J. R.: Inflammatory constriction following complete pericardiectomy in tuberculous constrictive pericarditis. Clin. Pediatr. *22*:219, 1983.
240. Harrington, S. W.: Chronic constrictive pericarditis. Partial pericardiectomy and epicardiolysis in 24 cases. Ann. Surg. *120*:468, 1944.
241. Walsh, T. J., Baughman, K. L., Gardner, T. J., and Bulkley, B. H.: Constrictive epicarditis as a cause of delayed or absent response to pericardiectomy. J. Thorac. Cardiovasc. Surg. *83*:126, 1982.
242. Spodick, D. H., and Kumar, S.: Subacute constrictive pericarditis with cardiac tamponade. Dis. Chest *54*:62. 1968.
243. Hancock, E. W.: Subacute effusive constrictive pericarditis. Circulation *43*:183, 1971.
244. Martin, R. P., Bowden, R., Filly, K., and Popp, R. L.: Intrapericardial abnormalities in patients with pericardial effusion. Circulation *61*:568, 1980.

SPECIFIC FORMS OF PERICARDITIS

Viral Pericarditis

245. Brodie, H. R., and Marchessault, V.: Acute benign pericarditis caused by Coxsackie virus group B. N. Engl. J. Med. *262*:1278, 1960.
246. Celers, J., Celers, P., and Bertocchi, A.: Non-polio enterovirus in France from 1974 to 1985. Pathol. Biol. *36*:1221, 1988.
247. Kleinfeld, M., Milles, S., and Lidsky, M.: Mumps pericarditis: Review of the literature and report of a case. Am. Heart J. *55*:153, 1958.
248. Cheng, T. C.: Severe chest pain due to infectious mononucleosis. Postgrad. Med. *73*:149, 1983.
249. Williams, A. J., Freemont, A. J., and Barnett, D. B.: Pericarditis and arthritis complicating chicken pox. Br. J. Clin. Pract. *37*:226, 1983.
250. Adler, R., Takahashi, M., and Wright, H. T., Jr.: Acute pericarditis associated with hepatitis B infection. Pediatrics *61*:716, 1978.
251. Fink, C., Schaad, V. B., and Socker, F. P.: Pericarditis as a complication of rubella. Schweiz. Med. Wochenschr. *117*:28, 1987.
252. Beaman, M. H., and Hung, J.: Pericarditis associated with tick-borne Q fever. Aust. N. Z. J. Med. *19*:254, 1989.
253. Tellez, A, Romero, J. M., and Leon, P.: Pericarditis caused by Q fever. Rev. Clin. Esp. *181*:340, 1987.
254. Linz, D. H., Tolle, S. W., and Elliot, D. L.: Mycoplasma pneumoniae. Experience at a referral center. West. J. Med. *140*:895, 1984.
255. Balaguer, A, Boronat, M., and Carrascosa, A.: Successful treatment of pericarditis associated with *Mycoplasma pneumoniae* infection. Pediatr. Infect. Dis. J. *9*:141, 1990.
256. Malu, K., Longo-Mbenza, B., Lurhuma, Z., and Odio, W.:Pericarditis and the acquired immune deficiency syndrome. Arch. Mal. Coeur. *81*:207, 1988.
257. Acierno, L. J.: Cardiac complications in acquired immune deficiency syndrome (AIDS): A review. J. Am. Coll. Cardiol. *13*:1144, 1990.
258. Fink, L., Reichek, N., and St. John Sutton, M. G.: Cardiac abnormalities in acquired immune deficiency syndrome. Am. J. Cardiol. *54*:1161, 1984.
259. Biton, A., and Herman, J.: Perimyocarditis. Report on an unusual cause. Postgrad. Med. *85*:77, 1989.
260. Kassab, A., Demoulin, J. C., Vanlancker, M. A., et al.: Cytomegalovirus hemopericarditis. Acta Cardiol. *42*:69, 1987.
261. Einsele, H., Ehninger, G., Vallbracht, A., et al.: Isolated pericardial relapse following allogeneic bone marrow transplantation for acute myelogenous leukemia. Bone Marrow Transplant.*4*:323, 1989.
262. Cammarosano, C., and Lewis, W.: Cardiac lesions in acquired immune deficiency syndrome (AIDS). J. Am. Coll. Cardiol. *5*:703, 1985.
263. Scott, P. J., Conway, S. P., and DaCosta, P.: Cardiac tamponade complicating cytomegalovirus pericarditis in a patient with AIDS. J. Infect. *20*:92, 1990.
264. Cohen, I. S., Anderson, D. W., Virmani, R. et al.: Congestive cardiomyopathy in association with the acquired immunodeficiency syndrome. N. Engl. J. Med. *315*:628, 1986.
265. Toma, E., Poisson, M., Claessens, M. R., et al.: Herpes simplex type 2 pericarditis and bilateral facial palsy in a patient with AIDS. J. Infect. Dis. *160*:553, 1989.
266. Cooper, D.K.C., and Sturridge, M. F.: Constrictive pericarditis following Coxsackie virus infection. Thorax *31*:472, 1976.
267. Frisk, G., Torfason, E. G., and Diderholm, H.: Reverse immunoassays of IgM and IgG antibodies to Coxsackie B viruses in patients with acute myopericarditis. J. Med. Virol. *14*:191, 1984.
268. Riecansky, I., Schreinerova, Z., Egnerova, A., et al: Incidence of coxsackie virus infection in patients with dilated cardiomyopathy. Cor. Vasa *31*:325, 1989.
269. Muir, P., Nicholson, F., Tilzey, A. J., et al.: Chronic relapsing pericarditis and dilated cardiomyopathy: Serologic evidence of persistent enterovirus infection. Lancet *15*:804, 1989.
270. Yoneda, S., Ohte, N., Samoto, T., et al.: Two cases of viral myocarditis and one case of viral pericarditis. Jpn. Circ. J. *46*:1222, 1982.

Tuberculous Pericarditis

271. Larneu, A. J., Tyers, G. F., Williams, E. H., and Derrick, J. R.: Recent experience with tuberculous pericarditis. Ann. Thorac. Surg. *29*:464, 1980.
272. Pogliani, E. M., Cortellaro, M., Foa, P., et al.: Cyclosporin A in the treatment of severe aplastic anemia: Description of a case complicated by the development of tuberculous pericarditis during treatment. Am. J. Hematol. *30*:257, 1989.
273. Dalli, E., Quesada, A., Juan, G., et al: Tuberculous pericarditis as the first manifestation of acquired immune deficiency syndrome. Am. Heart J. *114*:905, 1987.
274. Kinney, E. L., Monsuez, J. J., Kitzis, M. and Vittecog, D.: Treatment of AIDS-related heart disease. Angiology *40*:970, 1989.
275. D'Cruz, I. A., Sengupta, E. E., Abrahams, C., et al.: Cardiac involvement, including tuberculous pericardial effusion, complicating acquired immune deficiency syndrome, Am. Heart J. *5*:1100, 1986.
276. Desai, H. N.: Tuberculous pericarditis: A review of 100 cases. S. Afr. Med. J. *55*:877, 1979.
277. Strang, J.I.G: Tuberculous pericarditis in Transkei. Clin. Cardiol. *5*:667, 1984.
278. Gooi, H. C. and Smith, J. M.: Tuberculous pericarditis in Birmingham. Thorax *33*:94, 1978.
279. Peel, A.A.F.: Tuberculous pericarditis. Br. Heart J. *10*:195, 1948.
280. Auerbach, O.: Pleural, peritoneal, and pericardial tuberculosis. Am. Rev. Tuberc. *61*:845, 1950.
281. Maisch, B., Maisch, S., and Kocksiek, K.: Immune reactions in tuberculous and chronic constrictive pericarditis. Am. J. Cardiol. *50*:1007, 1982.
282. Schrire, V.: Experience with pericarditis of Groote Schuur Hospital, Cape Town; An analysis of one hundred and sixty cases over a six-year period. S. Afr. Med. J. *33*:810, 1959.
283. Hageman, J. H., D'Esopo, N. D., and Glenn, W.W.L.: Tuberculosis of the pericardium: A long-term analysis of forty-four cases. N. Engl. J. Med. *270*:327, 1964.
284. Long, E., Younes, M., Patton, N., and Hershfield, E.: Tuberculous pericarditis: Long-term outcome in patients who received medical therapy alone. Am. Heart J. *117*:1133, 1989.
285. Quale, J. M., Lipschik, G. Y., and Heurich, A. E.: Management of tuberculous pericarditis. Ann. Thorac. Surg. *43*:653, 1987.
286. Sagrista-Sauleda, J., Permanyer-Miralda, G., and Soler-Soler, J.: Tuberculous pericarditis: Ten year experience with a prospective protocol for diagnosis and treatment. J. Am. Coll. Cardiol. *11*:724, 1988.
287. Fennell, W.M.P.: Surgical treatment of constrictive tuberculous pericarditis. S. Afr. Med. J. *62*:353, 1982.
288. Agrawal, S., Radhakrishnan, S., and Sinha, N.: Echocardiographic demonstration of resolving intrapericardial mass in tuberculous pericardial effusion. Int. J. Cardiol. *26*:240, 1990.
289. Lin, D. S., and Tipton, R. E.: Ga-67 cardiac uptake. Clin. Nucl. Med. *8*:603, 1983.
290. Hirasing, R. A., and Van Bel, F.: Tuberculous pericarditis developing during chemotherapy. Eur. J. Resp. Dis. *63*:73, 1982.
291. Barr, J. F.: The use of pericardial biopsy in establishing etiologic diagnosis in acute pericarditis. Arch. Intern. Med. *96*:693, 1955.
292. Cheitlin, M. D., Serfos, L. J., Sbar, S. S., and Glosser, S. P.: Tuberculous pericarditis: Is limited pericardial biopsy sufficient for diagnosis? Am. Rev. Resp. Dis. *98*:287, 1968.
293. Ocana, I., Martinez Vasquez, J. M., Sugura, R. M., et al.: Adenosine deaminase in pleural fluids: A test for the diagnosis of tuberculous pleural effusion. Chest *84*:51, 1983.
294. Martinez Vasquez, J. M., Ribera, E., Ocana, I., et al.: Adenosine deaminase activity in tuberculous pericarditis. Thorax *41*:888, 1986.

Bacterial (Purulent) Pericarditis

295. Strang, J. I., Kakaza, H. H., Gibson, D. G., et al.: Controlled trial of prednisolone as adjuvant in the treatment of tuberculous constrictive pericarditis in Transkei. Lancet *2*:1418, 1987.
296. Klacsmann, P. B., Bulkley, B. H., and Hutchins, G. M: The changed spectrum of purulent pericarditis. An 86 year autopsy experience in 200 patients. Am. J. Med. *63*:666, 1977.

297. Berk, S. L., Rice, P. A., Reynolds, C. A., and Finland, M.: Pneumococcal pericarditis: A persisting problem in contemporary diagnosis. Am. J. Med. *70*:247, 1981.
298. Karjalainen, J.: Streptococcal tonsillitis and acute nonrheumatic myopericarditis. Chest *95*:359, 1989.
299. Marsa, R. J., Blomquist, I. K., Bansal, R. C., et al.: Acute pericarditis due to group C Streptococcus: Report of a medically treated case. Am. J. Med. *86*:474, 1989.
300. Rivera, J. M., Garcia-Bragado, F., Gomez, F. A., et al.: Brucellar pericarditis. Infection *16*:254, 1988.
301. Haggman, D. L., Rehm, S. J., Moodie, D. S., and MacKenzie, A. H.: Nontyphoidal Salmonella pericarditis: A case report and review of the literature. Pediatr. Infect. Dis. *5*:259, 1986.
302. Sanchez-Guerrero, J., and Alarcon-Segovia, D.: Salmonella pericarditis with tamponade in systemic lupus erythematosus. Br. J. Rheumatol. *29*:69, 1990.
303. Vietzke, W. M.: Gonococcal arthritis with pericarditis. Arch. Intern. Med. *117*:270, 1966.
304. Iggo, R., and Higgins, R.: Bilateral empyema and purulent pericarditis due to Haemophilus influenzae capsular type b. Thorax *43*:582, 1988.
305. Evans, M. E., Gregory, D. W., Schaffner, W., and McGee, Z. A.: Tularemia: A 30-year experience with 88 cases. Medicine *64*:251, 1985.
306. Finley, R. W., and Marr, J. J.: Anaerobic bacterial abscess following myocardial infarction. Am. J. Med. *78*:513, 1985.
307. Rubin, R. H., and Moellering, R. C., Jr.,: Clinical, microbiologic, and therapeutic aspects of purulent pericarditis. Am. J. Med. *59*:68, 1975.
308. Holoshitz, J., Schneider, M., Yaretsky, A., et al.: Listeria monocytogenes pericarditis in a chronically hemodialyzed patient. Am. J. Med. Sci. *288*:34, 1984.
309. Kahn, M. Y.: Subacute constrictive pericarditis from Serratia marcescens. Hum. Pathol. *14*:1089, 1983.
310. Lieber, I. H., Rensimer, E. R., and Ericsson, C. D.: Campylobacter pericarditis in hypothyroidism. Am. Heart J. *102*:462, 1981.
311. Blaser, M. J., Reingold, A. L., Alsever, R. N., and Hightower, A.: Primary meningococcal pericarditis: A disease of adults associated with serogroup C Neisseria meningitidis. Rev. Infect. Dis. *6*:625, 1984.
312. Ejlertsen, T., Vesterlund, T., and Schmidt, E. B.: Myopericarditis with cardiac tamponade caused by Neisseria meningitidis serogroup W135. Eur. J. Clin. Microbiol. Infect. Dis. *7*:403, 1988.
313. Brasier, A. R., Macklis, J. D., Vaughan, D., et al.: Myopericarditis as an initial presentation of meningococcemia. Unusual manifestation of infection with serotype W135. Am. J. Med. *82*:641, 1987.
314. Luck, P. C., Helbig, J. H., Wunderlich, E., et al.: Isolation of Legionella Pneumophila serogroup 3 from pericardial fluid in a case of pericarditis. Infection *17*:388, 1989.
315. Svendsen, J. H., Jonsson, V., and Niebuhr, V.: Combined pericarditis and pneumonia caused by Legionella infection. Br. Heart J. *58*:663, 1987.
316. Pititalot, J. P., Allal, J., Thomas, P., et al.: Cardiac complications of infectious endocarditis. Ann. Med. Interne *136*:539, 1985.
317. Weinstein, L.: Life-threatening complications of infective endocarditis and their management. Arch. Intern. Med. *146*:953, 1986.
318. Suzuki, S., Tajimi, T., Takeshita, A., et al.: Isolated right heart purulent pericarditis forming a large mediastinal mass. Chest *93*:667, 1988.
319. Olson, L. J., Edwards, W. D., Olney, B. A., et al.: Hemorrhagic cardiac tamponade: A clinicopathologic correlation. Mayo Clin. Proc. *59*:785, 1984.
320. Horton, J. M., and Tucker, W. S., Jr.: Pericarditis with effusion and tamponade complicating left subdiaphragmatic abscess. West. J. Med. *149*:213, 1988.
321. Hier-Madsen, K., Suanamaki, K. I., Wulff, J., et al.: Purulent pericarditis in children. Review and case report. Scand. J. Thorac. Cardiovasc. Surg. *19*:185, 1985.
322. Sinzobahamvya, N., and Ikeogu, M. O.: Purulent pericarditis. Arch. Dis. Child. *62*:696, 1987.
323. Fyfe, D. A., Hagler, D. J., Puga, F. J., and Driscoll, D. J.: Clinical and therapeutic aspects of Hemophilus influenzae pericarditis in pediatric patients. Mayo Clin. Proc. *59*:415, 1984.
324. Chun, P. K., and Rocchini, A. P.: Occult constrictive pericarditis in infancy. Chest *78*:648, 1980.
325. Leak, L. V., Ferrans, V. J., Cohen, S. R., et al.: Animal model of acute pericarditis and its progression to pericardial fibrosis and adhesions: Ultrastructural studies. Am. J. Anat. *180*:373, 1987.
326. Gould, K., Barnett, J. A., and Sanford, J. P.: Purulent pericarditis in the antibiotic era. Arch. Intern. Med. *134*:923, 1974.
327. Bouwels, L., Jansen, E., Janssen, J., et al.: Successful long-term catheter drainage in an immunocompromised patient with purulent pericarditis. Am. J. Med. *83*:581, 1987.
328. Miller, G. C., and Witham, A. C.: Delayed febrile pleuropericarditis after sepsis. Ann. Intern. Med. *79*:194, 1973.
329. Tan, J. S., Holmes, J. C., Fowler, N. O., et al.: Antibiotic levels in pericardial fluid. J. Clin. Invest. *53*:7, 1974.
330. Biancaniello, T. M., Anagnostipoulos, C. E., Bernstein, H. E., and Proctor, C.: Purulent meningococcal pericarditis: Chronic percutaneous drainage with a modified catheter aided by echocardiography. Clin. Cardiol. *8*:542, 1985.
331. Morgan, R. J., Stephenson, L. W., Woolf, P. K., et al.: Surgical treatment of purulent pericarditis in children. J. Thorac. Cardiovasc. Surg. *85*:527, 1983.
332. Laaban, J. P., d'Orbcastel, O. R., Prudent, J., et al.: Primary pneumococcal pericarditis complicated by acute constriction. Intensive Care Med. *10*:155, 1984.

Fungal Pericarditis

333. Wheat, L. J., Stein, L., Corya, B. C., et al.: Pericarditis as a manifestation of histoplasmosis during two large urban outbreaks. Medicine *62*:110, 1983.
334. Chapman, M. G., and Kaplan, L.: Cardiac involvement in coccidioidomycosis. Am. J. Med. *23*:87, 1957.
335. Ross, E. M., Macher, A. M., and Roberts, W. C.: Aspergillus fumigatus thrombi causing total occlusion of both coronary arterial ostia, all four major coronary arteries and coronary sinus and associated with purulent pericarditis. Am. J. Cardiol. *56*:499, 1985.
336. Schwartz, D. A.: Aspergillus pancarditis following bone marrow transplantation for chronic myelogenous leukemia. Chest *95*:1338, 1989.
337. Kraus, W. E., Valenstein, P. N., and Corey, G. R.: Purulent pericarditis caused by Candida: Report of three cases and identification of high-risk populations as an aid to early diagnosis. Rev. Infect. Dis. *10*:34, 1988.
338. Glower, D. D., Douglas, J. M., Jr., Gaynor, J. W., et al.: Candida mediastinitis after a cardiac operation. Ann. Thor. Surg. *49*:157, 1990.
339. Prager, R. L., Burney, D. P., Waterhouse, G., and Bender, H. W., Jr.: Pulmonary, mediastinal, and cardiac presentations of histoplasmosis. Ann. Thorac. Surg. *30*:385, 1980.
340. Kaufman, L. D., Seifert, F. C., Eilbott, D. J. et al.: Candida pericarditis and tamponade in a patient with systemic lupus erythematosus. Arch. Intern. Med. *148*:715, 1988.
341. Holtz, H. A., Lavery, D. P., and Kapila, R.: Actinomycetales infection in the acquired immunodeficiency syndrome. Ann. Intern. Med. *102*:203, 1985.
342. Ramsdale, D. R., Gautam, P. C., Perera, B., and Charles, R. G.: Cardiac tamponade due to actinomycosis. Thorax *39*:473, 1984.
343. Nahass, R. G., Scholz, P., MacKenzie, J. W., and Gocke, D. J.: Chronic constrictive pericarditis. A case report and review of the literature. Arch. Intern. Med. *149*:1202, 1989.
344. Sagrista-Sauleda, J., Permanyer-Miralda, G., Juste-Sanchez, C., et al.: Huge chronic pericardial effusion caused by Toxoplasma gondii. Circulation *66*:895, 1982.
345. Baid, C. S., Varma, A. R., and Lakhotia, M.: A case of subacute effusive constrictive pericarditis with a probable amoebic etiology. Br. Heart J. *58*:296, 1987.
346. Blackett, K.: Amoebic pericarditis. Int. J. Cardiol. *21*:183, 1988.
347. Strang, J. I.: Two-dimensional echocardiography in the diagnosis of amoebic pericarditis. S. Afr. Med. J. *71*:328, 1987.
348. van der Horst, R.: Schistosomiasis of the pericardium. J. R. Soc. Trop. Med. Hyg. *73*:243, 1979.
349. Chens, W.: Hydatid cysts in the pericardium—a new case and review of the literature. J. Thorac. Cardiovasc. Surg. *30*:56, 1982.
350. Hafid, F., Maiza, E., Hammoudi, D., et al: Hydatid cyst of the pericardium and diaphragm. Pediatrie *44*:331, 1989.
351. De Martini, M., Nador, F., Binda, A., et al.: Myocardial hydatid cyst ruptured into the pericardium: Cross-sectional echocardiographic study and surgical treatment. Eur. Heart J. *9*:819, 1988.
352. Kinare, S. G., Parulkar, G. B., and Sen, P. K.: Constrictive pericarditis resulting from dracunculosis. Br. Med. J. *1*:845, 1962.
353. Charon, A., and Sinha, K.: Constrictive pericarditis following filiariasis. Indian Heart J. *25*:213, 1973.
354. Marcus, L. C., Steere, A. C., Duray, P. H., et al.: Fatal pancarditis in a patient with coexistent Lyme disease and babesiosis. Intern. Med. *103*:374, 1985.
355. Lorcerie, B., Boutron, M. C., Portier, H., et al.: Pericardial manifestations of Lyme disease. Ann. Med. Interne *138*:601, 1987.
356. Veyssier, P., Davous, N., Kaloustian, E, et al.: Cardiac involvement in Lyme disease. Rev. Med. Interne *8*:357, 1987.
357. Page, S. R., Stewart, J. T., and Bernstein, J. J.: A progressive pericardial effusion caused by psittacosis. Br. Heart J. *60*:87, 1988.

Pericarditis Following Acute Myocardial Infarction

358. Dubois, C., Smeets, J. P., Demoulin, J. C., et al.: Frequency and clinical significance of pericardial friction rubs in the acute phase of myocardial infarction. Eur. Heart. J. *6*:766, 1985.
359. Lichstein, E., Arsura, E., Hollander, G., et al.: Current incidence of postmyocardial infarction (Dressler's) syndrome. Am. J. Cardiol. *50*:1269, 1982.
360. Krainin, F. M., Flessas, A. P., and Spodick, D. H.: Infarction-associated pericarditis. N. Engl. J. Med. *311*:1211, 1984.
361. Tofler, G. H., Muller, J. A., Stone, P. H., et al.: Pericarditis in acute myocardial infarction: Characterization and clinical significance. Am. Heart J. *117*:86, 1989.
362. Levine, H. D.: Subendocardial infarction in retrospect: Pathologic, cardiographic, and ancillary features. Circulation *72*:790, 1985.
363. Galve, E., Garcia-del-Castillo, H., Evangelista, A., et al.: Pericardial effusion in the course of myocardial infarction: Incidence, natural history, and clinical relevance. Circulation *73*:294, 1986.
364. Aarseth, S, and Lange, H. F.: The influence of anticoagulant therapy on the occurrence of cardiac rupture and hemopericardium following heart infarction: I. A study of 89 cases of hemopericardium. Am. Heart J. *56*:250, 1958.
365. Lange, H. F., and Aarseth, S: The influence of anticoagulant therapy on the occurrence of cardiac rupture and hemopericardium following heart infarction. II. A controlled study of a selected treated group based on 1,044 autopsies. Am. Heart J. *56*:257, 1958.

366. Karim, A. M., and Solomon, J.: Constrictive pericarditis after myocardial infarction. Am. J. Med. *79*:389, 1985.
367. Low, R. I., Arthur, A., Kelly, P. B., and Takeda, P. A: Clotted hemopericardium post myocardial infarction presenting as effusive constrictive pericarditis. Am. Heart J. *109*:905, 1985.
368. Liberthson, R. R., Salisbury, K. W., and Hutter, A. M., Jr.: Atrial tachyarrhythmias in acute myocardial infarction. Am. J. Med. *60*:956, 1976.
369. Liem, K. L., Durrer, D, and Lie, K. L.: Pericarditis in acute myocardial infarction. Lancet *2*:1004, 1975.
370. Limaye, S. B., and Stubberfield, J.: Cardiac tamponade following infarction: Management with pericardiocentesis and surgery. Aust. N. Z. J. Med. *15*:446, 1985.
371. Coma-Canella, I., Lopez-Sendon, J., Gonzalez-Garcia, A, and Jadraque, L. M.: Hemodynamic effect of dextran, dobutamine, and pericardiocentesis in cardiac tamponade secondary to subacute heart rupture. Am. Heart J. *114*:78, 1987.
372. Stryjer, D., Friedensohn, A., and Hendler, A.: Myocardial rupture in acute myocardial infarction: Urgent management. Br. Heart J. *59*:73, 1988.
373. Sehgal, E., Sherman, W., Isom, O.W., et al.: Left ventricular pseudoaneurysm causing superior vena caval obstruction and effusive-constrictive pericarditis. J. Nucl. Med. *28*:918, 1987.
374. Berman, J., Haffajee, C. I., and Alpert, J. S.: Therapy of symptomatic pericarditis after myocardial infarction: Retrospective and prospective studies of aspirin, indomethacin, prednisone, and spontaneous resolution. Am. Heart J. *101*:750, 1981.
375. Hammerman, H., Kloner, R. A., Schoen, F. J., et al.: Indomethacin-induced scar thinning following experimental myocardial infarction. Circulation *67*:1290, 1983.
376. Boden, W. E., and Sadaniantz, A.: Ventricular septal rupture during ibuprofen therapy for pericarditis after acute myocardial infarction. Am. J. Cardiol. *55*:1631, 1985.

Uremic Pericarditis

377. Suki, W. N.: Pericarditis. Kidney Int. (Suppl.) *24*:510, 1988.
378. Rutsky, E. A., and Rostand, S. G.: Treatment of uremic pericarditis and pericardial effusion. Am. J. Kidney Dis. *10*:2, 1987.
379. Joffe, P., and Johannesen, A. C.: Uraemic pericarditis, an epidemic disease? Dan. Med. Bull. *34*:117, 1987.
380. Maisch, B., and Kochsiek, K.: Humoral immune reactions in uremic pericarditis. Am. J. Nephrol. *3*:264, 1983.
381. Lindsay, J., Jr., Crawley, I. S., and Callaway, G. M.: Chronic constrictive pericarditis following uremic hemopericardium. Am. Heart J. *79*:390, 1970.
382. Frommer, J. P., Young, J. B., and Ayus, J. C.: Asymptomatic pericardial effusion in uremic patients: Effect of long-term dialysis. Nephron *39*:296, 1985.
383. Yoshida, K., Shiina, A., Asano, Y. and Hosoda, S.: Uremic pericardial effusion: Detection and evaluation of uremic pericardial effusion by echocardiography. Clin. Nephrol. *13*:260, 1980.
384. Leehey, D. J., Daugirdas, J. T., Popli, S., et al.: Predicting need for surgical drainage of pericardial effusion in patients with end-stage renal disease. Int. J. Artif. Organs *12*:618, 1989.
385. Morlans, M.: Pericardial involvement in end stage renal disease. *In* Soler-Soler, J., Permanyer-Miralda, G., and Sagrista-Sauleda, J.: Pericardial Disease: New Insights and Old Dilemmas. Dordrecht, The Netherlands, Kluwer Academic Publishers, 1990, p. 123–139.
386. Masson, J. F., Maes, M. L., and Zilberman, C.: Pericarditis in chronic renal insufficiency treated by periodic hemodialysis. Rev. Med. Intern. *2*:447, 1981.
387. Kwasnik, E. M., Koster, J. K., Lazarus, J.M., et al.: Conservative management of uremic pericardial effusions. J. Thorac. Cardiovasc. Surg. *76*:629, 1978.
388. Rotler, M. N., and Swartz, C.: Predicting success of intensive dialysis in the treatment of uremic pericarditis. Am. J. Med. *76*:38, 1984.
389. Spector, D, Alfred, H., Seidlecki, M., and Briefel, G.: A controlled study of the effect of indomethacin in uremic pericarditis. Kidney Int. *24*:663, 1983.
390. Buselmeir, T. J., Davin, T. D., and Simmons, R. L.: Treatment of intractable uremic pericardial effusion: Avoidance of pericardiectomy with local steroid instillation. JAMA *240*:1358, 1978.
391. Feinroth, M. V., Goldstein, E J., Josephson, A., and Friedman, E. A.: Infection complicating intrapericardial steroid instillation in uremic pericarditis. Clin. Nephrol. *15*:331, 1981.
392. Quigg, R. J., Idelson, B. A., Yoburn, D. C., et al.: Local steroids in dialysis-associated pericardial effusion. Arch. Intern. Med. *145*:2249, 1985.
393. Beaudry, C., Nakamoto, S., and Koloff, W. J.: Uremic pericarditis and cardiac tamponade in chronic renal failure. Ann. Intern. Med. *64*:990, 1966.
394. Frame, J. R., Lucas, S. K., Pederson, J. A., and Elkins, R. C.: Surgical treatment of pericarditis in the dialysis patient. Am. J. Surg. *146*:300, 1983.
395. Prager, R. L., Wilson, C. H., and Bender, H. W., Jr.: The subxiphoid approach to pericardial disease. Ann. Thorac. Surg. *34*:6, 1982.

Neoplastic Pericarditis

396. Mukai, K., Shinkai, T., Tominaga, K., and Shimosato, Y.: The incidence of secondary tumors of the heart and pericardium: A ten-year study. Jpn. J. Clin. Oncol. *18*:195, 1988.
397. Press, O. W., and Livingston, R.: Management of malignant pericardial effusion and tamponade. JAMA. *257*:1088, 1987.
398. Posner, M. R., Cohen, G. I., and Skarin, A. T.: Pericardial disease in patients with cancer. Am. J. Med. *71*:407, 1981.
399. Roberts, W. C., Bodey, G. P., and Wertlake, P. T.: The heart in acute leukemia: A study of 420 autopsy cases. Am. J. Cardiol. *21*:388, 1968.
400. Roberts, W. C., Glancy, D. L., and DeVita, V. T.:Heart in malignant lymphoma (Hodgkin's disease, lymphosarcoma, reticulum cell sarcoma and mycosis fungoides): A study of 196 autopsy cases. Am. J. Cardiol. *22*:85, 1968.
401. Thurber, D. L., Edwards, J. E., and Achor, R. W.: Secondary malignant tumors of the pericardium. Circulation *26*:228, 1962.
402. Chan, H. S., Sonley, M. J., Moes, C. A., et al.: Primary and secondary tumors of childhood involving the heart, pericardium, and great vessels. Cancer *56*:825, 1985.
403. Wilding, G., Green, H. L., Longo, D. L., and Urba, W. J.: Tumors of the heart and pericardium. Cancer Treat. Rev. *15*:165, 1988.
404. Rudoff, J., Percy, R., Benrubi, G., and Ostrowski, M. L.: Recurrent squamous cell carcinoma of the cervix presenting as cardiac tamponade: Case report and subject review. Gynecol. Oncol. *34*:226, 1989.
405. Malviya, V. K., Casselberry, J. M., Parekh, N., and Deppe, G.: Pericardial metastases in squamous cell cancer of the cervix. J. Reprod. Med. *35*:49, 1990.
406. Venegas, R. J., and Sun, N. C.: Cardiac tamponade as a presentation of malignant thymoma. Acta Cytol. *32*:257, 1988.
407. Skyggebjerg, K. D.: Hydrops fetalis caused by intrapericardial teratoma. Acta Obstet. Gynecol. Scand. *67*:653, 1988.
408. Webber, H. S., Kleinman, C. S., Hellenbrand, W. E., et al.: Development of a benign intrapericardial tumor between 20 and 40 weeks of gestation. Pediatr. Cardiol. *9*:153, 1988.
409. Brabham, K. R., and Roberts, W. C.: Cardiac-compressing intrapericardial teratoma at birth. Am. J. Cardiol. *63*:386, 1989.
410. Gossinger, H. D., Siostrzonek, P., Zangeneh, M., et al.: Magnetic resonance imaging finding in a patient with pericardial mesothelioma. Am. Heart J. *115*:1321, 1988.
411. Lund, O., Hansen, O. K., Ardest, S., and Baandrup, V.: Primary malignant pericardial mesothelioma mimicking left atrial myxoma. Scand. J. Thorac. Cardiovasc. Surg. *21*:273, 1987.
412. Pasqual, M. A., Povar, J., Munoz, J. R., et al.: Pericardial mesothelioma. Rev. Esp. Cardiol. *42*:559, 1989.
413. el-Naggar, A. K., Ro, J. Y., Ayala, A. G., et al.: Localized fibrous tumor of the serosal cavities. Immunohistochemical, electron microscopic, and flow-cytometric DNA study. Am. J. Clin. Pathol. *92*:561, 1989.
414. Kim, E. E., Wallace, S., Abello, R., et al.: Malignant cardiac fibrous histiosarcomas and angiosarcomas: MR features. J. Comput. Assist. Tomogr. *13*:627, 1989.
415. Montalescot, G., Chapelon, C., Drobinski, G., et al.: Diagnosis of primary cardiac sarcoma. Report of 4 cases and review of the literature. Int. J. Cardiol. *20*:209, 1988.
416. Meissner, A., Kirch, W., Regensburger, D., et al.: Intrapericardial teratoma in an adult. Am. J. Med. *84*:1089, 1988.
417. Naramoto, A, Itoh, N., Nakano, M., and Shigematsu, H.: An autopsy case of tuberous sclerosis associated wth primary pericardial mesothelioma. Acta Pathol. Jpn. *39*:400, 1989.
418. Shimoyama, Y., Kawada, K., and Imamura, H.: A functioning intrapericardial paraganglioma (pheochromocytoma). Br. Heart J. *57*:380, 1987.
419. Haedersdal, C., Hasselbalch, H., Devantier, A., and Saunamaki, K.: Pericardial haematopoiesis with tamponade in myelofibrosis. Scand. J. Haematol. *34*:270, 1985.
420. Shih, L. Y., Lin, F. C., and Kuo, T. T.: Cutaneous and pericardial extramedullary hematopoiesis with cardiac tamponade in chronic myeloid leukemia. Am. J. Clin. Pathol. *89*:693, 1988.
421. Markiewicz, W., Gladstein, E., London, E. J., and Popp, R. L.: Echocardiographic detection of pericardial effusion and pericardial thickening in malignant lymphoma. Radiology *123*:161, 1977.
422. Fracp, M. B., Ingle, J. N., Giuliani, E. R., et al.: Pericardial effusion in women with breast cancer. Cancer *60*:263, 1987.
423. Lopez, J. M., Delgado, J. L., Tovar, E., and Gonzalez, A. G.: Massive pericardial effusion produced by extracardiac malignant neoplasms. Arch. Intern. Med. *143*:1815, 1983.
424. Theologides, A.: Neoplastic cardiac tamponade. Semin. Oncol. *5*:181, 1978.
425. Nowicka, J., Haus, O., Dzik, T., et al.: Pericarditis in the course of acute leukemia. Folia Haematol. *114*:220, 1987.
426. Steigman, C. K., Anderson, D. W., Macher, A. M., et al.: Fatal cardiac tamponade in acquired immunodeficiency syndrome with epicardial Kaposi's sarcoma. Am. Heart. J. *116*:1105, 1988.
427. Engberding, R., Schulze-Waltrup, N., Grosse-Heitmeyer, W., and Stoll, V.: Transthoracic and transesophageal 2-D echocardiography in the diagnosis of peri- and paracardiac tumors. Dtsch. Med. Wochenschr. *112*:49, 1987.
428. Pizzarello, R. A., Goldberg, S. M., Goldman, M. A., et al.: Tumor of the heart diagnosed by magnetic resonance imaging. J. Am. Coll. Cardiol. *5*:989, 1985.
429. Brown, J. J., Barakos, J. A., and Higgins, C. B.: Magnetic resonance imaging of cardiac and paracardiac masses. J. Thorac. Imaging *4*:58, 1989.
430. Safian, R. D., Come, S. E., Kadin, M., and Lorell, B. H.: Use of pulmonary capillary wedge aspirates for the antemortem diagnosis of pulmonary microvascular tumor. Cathet. Cardiovasc. Diagn. *17*:112, 1989.
431. King, D. T., and Nieberg, R. K.: The use of cytology to evaluate pericardial effusions. Ann. Clin. Lab. Sci. *9*:18, 1979.

432. Yazdi, H. M., Hajdu, S. I., and Melamed, M. R.: Cytopathology of pericardial effusions. Acta Cytol. J. *24*:401, 1980.
433. Tatsuda, M., Yamamura, H., Yamamoto, R., et al.: Carcinoembryonic antigens in the pericardial fluid of patients with malignant pericarditis. Oncology *41*:328, 1984.
434. Yancik, R., Reis, L. G., and Yates, J. W.: Breast cancer in aging women. A population-based study of contrasts in stage, surgery, and survival. Cancer *63*:976, 1989.
435. Carter, C. L., Allen, C., and Henson, D. E.: Relation of tumor size, lymph node status, and survival in 24,740 breast cancer cases. Cancer *63*:181, 1989.
436. Sundareswaren, R., Marshall, A. J., Pickard, J. G., and Tyrrell, C. J.: Pericardiocentesis and systemic cytotoxic therapy in the management of cardiac tamponade secondary to disseminated breast carcinoma. Br. Heart J. *60*:162, 1988.
437. Shepherd, F. A., Morgan, C., Evans, W. K., et al.: Medical management of malignant pericardial effusion by tetracycline sclerosis. Am. J. Cardiol. *60*:1161, 1987.
438. Hawkins, J. W., and Vacek, J. L.: What constitutes definitive therapy of malignant pericardial effusion? "Medical" versus surgical treatment. Am. Heart. J. *118*:428, 1989.
439. Florentino, M. V., Daniele, O., Morandi, P., et al.: Intrapericardial instillation of platin in malignant pericardial effusion. Cancer *62*:1904, 1988.
440. Figoli, F., Zanette, M. L., Tirelli, V., et al.: Pharmacokinetics of VM26 given intraperitoneally or intravenously in patients with malignant pericardial effusion. Cancer Chemother. Pharmacol. *20*:239, 1987.
441. Ueno, Y., Kohgo, Y., Sasagawa, Y., et al.: A case of pericarditis carcinomatosa showing good response following local transfer of lymphokine-activated killer cells. Gan To Kagaku Ryoho *14*:2579, 1987.
442. Cham, W. C., Freiman, A. H., and Carstens, P. H. B.: Radiation therapy of cardiac and pericardial metastases. Ther. Radiol. *114*:701, 1975.
443. Stewart, J. R., and Fajardo, L. F.: Radiation-induced heart disease: An update. Prog. Cardiovasc. Dis. *27*:173, 1984.

Radiation Pericarditis

444. Cosset, J. M., Henry-Amar, M., Girinski, T., et al.: Late toxicity of radiotherapy in Hodgkin's disease. The role of fraction size. Acta Oncol *27*:123, 1988.
445. Tarbell, N. J., Thompson, L., and Mauch, P.: Thoracic irradiation in Hodgkin's disease: Disease control and long-term complications. Int. J. Radiat. Oncol. Biol. Phys. *18*:275, 1990.
446. Mill, S. B., Baglan, R. J., Kurichety, P., et al.: Symptomatic radiation-induced pericarditis in Hodgkin's disease. Int. J. Radiat. Oncol. Biol. Phys. *10*:2061, 1984.
447. Carmel, R. J., and Kaplan, H. S.: Mantle irradiation in Hodgkin's disease. Cancer *37*:2813, 1976.
448. Coltart, R. S., Roberts, J. T., Thom, C. H., and Petch, M. C.: Severe constrictive pericarditis after single 16 MeV anterior mantle irradiation for Hodgkin's disease. Lancet *1*:488, 1985.
449. Applefeld, M. M., Slawson, R. G., Spicer, K. M., and Singleton, R. T.: Long-term cardiovascular evaluation of patients with Hodgkin's disease treated by thoracic mantle radiation therapy. Cancer Treat. Rep. *66*:1003, 1982.
450. Martin, R. G., Ruckdeschel, J. C., Chang, P., et al.: Radiation-related pericarditis. Am. J. Cardiol *35*:216, 1975.
451. Applefeld, M. M., Slawson, R. G., Hall-Craigs, M., et al.: Delayed pericardial disease after radiotherapy. Am. J. Cardiol. *47*:210, 1981.
452. Green, D. M., Gingell, R. L., Pearce, J., et al.: The effect of mediastinal irradiation on cardiac function of patients treated during childhood and adolescence for Hodgkin's disease. J. Clin. Oncol. *5*:239, 1987.
453. Greenwood, R. D., Rosenthal, A., Cassedy, R., et al.: Constrictive pericarditis in childhood due to mediastinal irradiation. Circulation *50*:1033, 1974.
454. Brosius, F. C., Waller, B. F., and Roberts, W. C.: Radiation heart disease. Am. J. Med. *70*:519, 1981.
455. Castellino, R. A., Gladstein, E., and Turbow, M. M.: Latent radiation injury of lungs or heart activated by steroid withdrawal. Ann. Intern. Med. *80*:593, 1974.
456. Morton, D. L., Kagan, A. R., Roberts, W. C., et al.: Pericardiectomy for radiation-induced pericarditis with effusion. Ann. Thorac. Surg. *8*:195, 1969.
457. Ni, Y., von Segesser, L. K., and Turina, M.: Futility of pericardiectomy for postirradiation constrictive pericarditis? Ann. Thorac. Surg. *49*:445, 1990.

PERICARDITIS RELATED TO HYPERSENSITIVITY OR AUTOIMMUNITY

458. Osler, W.: The Principles and Practice of Medicine. New York, D. Appleton and Company, 1892, p. 273.
459. Persellin, S. T., Ramirez, G., and Moatamed, F.: Immunopathology of rheumatic pericarditis. Arthritis Rheum. *25*:1054, 1982.
460. Przybojewski, J. Z.: Rheumatic constrictive pericarditis. A case report and review of the literature. S. Afr. Med. J. *59*:682, 1981.
461. Rathore, M. H., and Barton, L. L.: Acute rheumatic pericarditis. Pediatr. Infect. Dis. J. *8*:183, 1989.
462. Ansari, A., Larson, P. H., and Bates, H. D.: Cardiovascular manifestations of systemic lupus erythematosus: Current perspective. Prog. Cardiovasc. Dis. *27*:421, 1985.
463. Chang, R. W.: Cardiac manifestation of systemic lupus erythematosus. Clin. Rheum. Dis. *8*:197, 1982.
464. Doherty, N. E., and Siegel, R. J.: Cardiovascular manifestations of systemic lupus erythematosus. Am. Heart. J. *110*:1257, 1985.
465. Bulkley, B. H., and Roberts, W. C.: The heart in systemic lupus erythematosus and the changes induced in it by corticosteroid therapy. Am. J.Med. *58*:243, 1975.
466. Kinney, E., Wynn, J., Hinton, D. M., et al.: Pericardial-fluid complement. Normal values. Am. J. Clin. Pathol. *72*:972, 1979.
467. Wolf, R. E., King, J. W., and Brown, T. A.: Antimyosin antibodies and constrictive pericarditis in lupus erythematosus. J. Rheumatol. *15*:1284, 1988.
468. Jacobsen, E. J., and Reza, M. J.: Constrictive pericarditis in systemic lupus erythematosus. Demonstration of immunoglobulins in the pericardium. Arthritis Rheum. *21*:972, 1978.
469. Starkey, R. H., and Hahn, B. H.: Rapid development of constrictive pericarditis in a patient with systemic lupus erythematosus. Chest *63*:448, 1973.
470. Ehrenfeld, M., Asman, A., Shpilberg, O., and Samra, Y.: Cardiac tamponade as the presenting manifestation of systemic lupus erythematosus. Am. J. Med. *86*:626, 1989.
471. Porcel, J. M., Selva, A., Tornos, M. P., et al.: Resolution of cardiac tamponade in systemic lupus erythematosus with indomethacin. Chest *96*:1193, 1989.
472. Thadani, U., Iveson, J. M., and Wright, V.: Cardiac tamponade, constrictive pericarditis and pericardial resection in rheumatoid arthritis. Medicine *54*:261, 1975.
473. Escalante, A., Kaufman, R. L., Quismorio, F. P., Jr., et al.: Cardiac compression in rheumatoid arthritis. Semin. Arthritis Rheum. 20:148, 1990.
474. Kirk, J., and Cosh, J.: The pericarditis of rheumatoid arthritis. Q. J. Med. *38*:397, 1969.
475. Sigel, L. H., and Friedman, H. D.: Rheumatoid pancarditis in a patient with well controlled rheumatoid arthritis. J. Rheumatol. *16*:368, 1989.
476. Stables, R. H., Campbell, S., and Ormerod, O.J.M.: Haemopericardium in rheumatoid arthritis. Int. J. Cardiol. *23*:268, 1989.
477. Breut, C., Drouelle, S., Lognone, S., et al.: Complications of rheumatoid pericarditis: Constriction and tamponade. Presse Med. *18*:1151, 1989.
478. Alukal, M. K., Costello, P. B., and Green, F. A.: Cardiac tamponade in systemic juvenile rheumatoid arthritis requiring emergency pericardiectomy. J. Rheumatol. *11*:222, 1984.
479. Newman, B., Park, S. C., and Oh, K. S.: Coexistent transient pulmonary edema and pericardial effusion. Pediatr. Radiol. *18*:455, 1988.
480. Bagga, A., Kabra, S. K., Shankar, V., and Kalra, V.: Cardiac tamponade in juvenile rheumatoid arthritis. Indian Pediatr. *25*:875, 1988.
481. Esdaile, J. M., Tannenbaum, H., and Hawkins, D.: Adult Still's disease. Am. J. Med. *68*:825, 1980.
482. Jamieson, T. W.: Adult Still's disease complicated by cardiac tamponade. JAMA *249*:2065, 1983.
483. Shimomoto, H., Imaizumi, K., Mizoguchi, K., and Ikeda, T.: A case of adult Still's disease with severe pulmonary complications. Nippon Kyobu Shikkan Gakkai Zasshi *27*:1092, 1989.
484. Butman, S., Espinoza, L. R., Carpio, J. D., and Osterland, C. K.: Rheumatoid pericarditis. Rapid deterioration with evidence of local vasculitis. JAMA *238*:2394, 1977.
485. Parkash, R., Atassi, A., Poske, R., and Rosen, K. M.: Prevalence of pericardial effusion and mitral valve involvement in patients with rheumatoid arthritis without cardiac symptoms. N. Engl. J. Med. *289*:597, 1973.
486. Lam, D., and Rapaport, E.: Two-dimensional echocardiographic demonstration of intrapericardial fibrinous strands in rheumatoid pericarditis. Am. Heart J. *114*:442, 1987.
487. Mathew, P. K.: Pericardial tamponade secondary to sudden steroid withdrawal in chronic rheumatoid arthritis. Chest *75*:532, 1977.
488. Cotton, D. W., Cooper, C., Searle, M., et al.: Fatal cardiac tamponade complicating anticoagulant therapy in rheumatoid arthritis. Clin. Exp. Rheumatol. *5*:367, 1987.
489. Thould, A. K.: Constrictive pericarditis in rheumatoid arthritis. Ann. Rheum. Dis. *45*:89, 1986.
490. Keith, T. A.: Chronic constrictive pericarditis in association with rheumatoid disease. Circulation *25*:477, 1962.
491. Nakano, T., Konishi, T., Yamamuro, M., et al.: Cardiac tamponade in rheumatoid arthritis. Successful treatment with intrapericardial steroid administration. Jpn. Heart J. *28*:287, 1987.
492. Nassar, W. K., Miskin, M. E., and Rosenbaum, D.: Pericardial and myocardial disease in progressive systemic sclerosis. Am. J. Cardiol. *22*:538, 1968.
493. Janosik, D. L., Osborn, T. G., Moore, T. L., et al.: Heart disease in systemic sclerosis. Semin. Arthritis Rheum. *19*:191, 1989.
494. Smith, J. W., Clements, P. J., Levisman, J., et al.: Echocardiographic features of progressive systemic sclerosis. Am. J. Med. *66*:28, 1979.
495. Uhl, G. S., and Kippes, G. M.: Pericardial tamponade in systemic sclerosis (scleroderma). Br. Heart J. *42*:345, 1979.
496. Hanley, P. C.: Constrictive pericarditis associated with combined retroperitoneal and mediastinal fibrosis. Mayo Clin. Proc. *59*:300, 1984.
497. Medsger, T. A., Jr., Masi, A. T., and Rodnan, G. P.: Survival with systemic sclerosis (scleroderma). A life-table analysis of clinical and demographic factors in 309 patients. Ann. Intern. Med. *75*:369, 1971.
498. Alpert, M. A., Goldberg, S. H., Singsen, B. H., et al.: Cardiovascular complications of mixed connective tissue disease in adults. Circulation *69*:1182, 1983.
499. Purice, S., Luca, R., Vintila, M., et al.: Cardiac involvement in progressive

systemic sclerosis and polymyositis: A comparative study in 116 patients. Med. Interne 27:209, 1989.
500. Tamir, R., Pick, A. J., and Theodor, E.: Constrictive pericarditis complicating dermatomyositis. Ann. Rheum. Dis. 47:961, 1988.
501. Shah, A., and Askari, A. D.: Pericardial changes and left ventricular function in ankylosing spondylitis. Am. Heart J. 113:1529, 1987.
502. Maryhew, N. L., Bache, R. J., and Messner, R. P.: Wegener's granulomatosis with acute pericardial tamponade. Arthritis Rheum. 31:300, 1988.
503. Csonka, G. W., and Oates, J. K.: Pericarditis and electrocardiographic changes in Reiter's syndrome. Br. Med. J. 1:866, 1957.
504. Goldman, M. J., and Lau, F. Y. K.: Acute pericarditis associated with serum sickness. N. Engl. J. Med. 250:278, 1954.
505. Shapiro, L., and Buckingham, R. B.: Septic rheumatoid pericarditis complicating Felty's syndrome. Arthritis Rheum. 24:1435, 1981.
506. Clementz, G. L., Gold, F., Khaiser, N., et al.: Giant cell arteritis associated with pericarditis and pancreatic insufficiency in a patient with psoriatic arthritis. J. Rheumatol. 16:128, 1989.
507. Sonnenblick, M., Nesher, G., and Rosin, A.: Nonclassical organ involvement in temporal arteritis. Semin. Arthritis Rheum. 19:183, 1989.
508. Granot, E., Rottem, M., and Rein, A. J.: Carditis complicating inflammatory bowel disease in children. Case report and review of the literature. Eur. J. Pediatr. 148:203, 1988.
509. Birnbaum, Y., and Shpirer, Z.: Cardiac involvement in inflammatory bowel disease. Harefuah 1:235, 1989.
510. Cullen, S., Duff, D. F., Denham, B., and Ward, O. C.: Cardiovascular manifestations in Kawasaki disease. Ir. J. Med. Sci. 158:253, 1989.
511. Erol, C., Sonel, A., Candan, I., et al.: Pericardial involvement in familial Mediterranean fever. Postgrad. Med. J. 64:453, 1988.
512. Crake, T., Sandie, G. I., Crisp, A. J., and Record, C. O.: Constrictive pericarditis and intestinal hemorrhage due to Whipple's disease. Postgrad. Med. J. 59:194, 1983.
513. Dawes, P. T., and Atherton, S. T.: Coeliac disease presenting as recurrent pericarditis. Lancet 1:1021, 1981.
514. Naschitz, J. E., Yeshurun, D., Miselevich, I., and Boss, J. H.: Colitis and pericarditis in a patient with eosinophilic fasciitis. A contribution to the multisystem nature of eosinophilic fasciitis. J. Rheumatol. 16:688, 1989.
515. Wanner, W. R., Williams, T. E., Fulkerson, P. K., et al.: Postoperative pericarditis following thymectomy for myasthenia gravis. A prospective study. Chest 83:647, 1983.
516. Silverman, K. J., Hutchins, G. M., and Bulkley, B. H.: Cardiac sarcoid: A clinicopathologic study of 84 unselected patients with systemic sarcoidosis. Circulation 58:1204, 1978.
517. Garrett, J., O'Neill, H., and Blake, S.: Constrictive pericarditis associated with sarcoidosis. Am. Heart J. 107:394, 1984.
518. Diderholm, E., Eklund, A., Orinius, E., and Widstrom, O.: Exudative pericarditis in sarcoidosis. Sarcoidosis 6:60, 1989.
519. Alarcon-Segovia, D.: Drug-induced lupus syndromes. Mayo Clin. Proc. 44:664, 1969.
520. Browning, C. A., Bishop, R. L., Heilpern, R. J., et al.: Accelerated constrictive pericarditis in procainamide-induced systemic lupus erythematosus. Am. J. Cardiol. 53:376, 1984.
521. Harrington, T. M., and Davis, D. E.: Systemic lupus-like syndrome induced by methyldopa therapy. Chest 79:696, 1981.
522. Schoenwetter, A. H, and Silber, E. N.: Penicillin hypersensitivity, acute pericarditis and eosinophilia. J.A.M.A. 191:136, 1965.
523. Slater, E. E.: Cardiac tamponade and peripheral eosinophilia in a patient receiving cromolyn sodium. Chest 73:878, 1978.
524. Yates, R. C., and Olson, K. B.: Drug-induced pericarditis. Report of three cases due to 6-amino-9-D-psicofuranosylpurine. N. Engl. J. Med. 265:274, 1961.
525. Krehlik, J. M., Hindson, D. A., Crowley, J. J., Jr., and Knight, L. L.: Minoxidil-associated pericarditis and fatal cardiac tamponade. West. J. Med. 143:527, 1985.
526. Miller, D. H., and Haas, L. F.: Pneumonitis, pleural effusion and pericarditis following treatment with dantrolene. J. Neurol. Neurosurg. Psychiatry 47:553, 1984.
527. Lipworth, B. J., and Oakley, D. G.: Surgical treatment of constrictive pericarditis due to practolol. A case report. J. Cardiovasc. Surg. 29:408, 1988.
528. Haugtomt, H., and Haerem, J.: Pulmonary edema and pericarditis after inhalation of teflon fumes. Tidsskr. Nor. Laegeforen 109:584, 1989.
529. Harbin, A. D., Gerson, M. C., and O'Connell, J. B.: Simulation of acute myopericarditis by constrictive pericardial disease with endomyocardial fibrosis to methysergide therapy. J. Am. Coll. Cardiol. 4:196, 1984.
530. Bristow, M. R., Thompson, P. D., Martin, R. P., et al.: Early anthracycline toxicity. Am. J. Med. 65:823, 1978.
531. Cazin, B., Gorin, N. C., Laporte, J. P., et al.: Cardiac complications after bone marrow transplantation. Cancer 57:2061, 1986.
532. Ratliff, N. B., McMahon, J. T., Shirey, E. K., and Groves, L. K.: Silicone pericarditis. Cleve. Clin. Q. 51:185, 1984.
533. Fraker, T. D., Jr., Walsh, T. E., Morgan, R. J., and Kim, K.: Constrictive pericarditis after the Beck operation. Am. J. Cardiol. 54:931, 1984.
534. Sonakul, D., Thakerngpol, K., and Pocaree, P.: Cardiac pathology in 76 thalassemic patients. Birth Defects 23:177, 1988.
535. Abdun Nur, D., Marcus, C. S., and Russell, F. E.: Pericarditis associated with scorpionfish (Scorpaena buttata) sting. Toxicon 19:579, 1981.
536. Dressler, W.: A postmyocardial infarction syndrome. Preliminary report of a complication resembling idiopathic recurrent benign pericarditis. JAMA 160:1379, 1956.
537. Jerjes-Sanchez, C., Ibarra-Perez, C., Ramirez-Rivera, A., et al.: Dressler-like syndrome after pulmonary embolism and infarction. Chest 92:115, 1987.
538. Dressler, W.: The post-myocardial infarction syndrome. A report of forty-four cases. Arch. Intern. Med. 103:28, 1959.
539. Van der Geld, H.: Anti-heart antibodies in the post-pericardiotomy and the post-myocardial infarction syndrome. Lancet 2:617, 1964.
540. Liem, K. L., ten Veen, J. H., Lie, K. I., et al.: Incidence and significance of heart muscle antibodies in patients with acute myocardial infarction and unstable angina. Acta Med. Scand. 206:473, 1971.
541. Weiser, N. J., Kantor, M., and Russell, H. K.: Post-myocardial infarction syndrome. Circulation 20:371, 1959.
542. Holloway, J. D.: Post-infarction pericarditis. Chronic symptoms in a middle-aged man. Postgrad. Med. 15:57, 1989.
543. Streifer, J., Pitlik, S., Dux, S., et al.: Dressler's syndrome after right ventricular infarction. Postgrad. Med. J. 60:298, 1984.
544. Hutchison, S. J., McKillop, J. H., and Hutton, I.: Failure of gallium-67 citrate imaging to diagnose post-myocardial infarction (Dressler's) syndrome. Eur. J. Nucl. Med. 13:52, 1987.
545. Hertzeanu, H., Almog, C., and Algom, M.: Cardiac tamponade in Dressler's syndrome. Cardiology 70:31, 1983.
546. Goldhaber, S. Z., Lorell, B. H., and Green, L. H.: Constrictive pericarditis. A case requiring pericardiectomy following Dressler's postmyocardial infarction syndrome. J. Thorac. Cardiovasc. Surg. 81:793, 1981.
547. Kanawaty, D. S., Burggraf, G. W., and Abdollah, H.: Constrictive pericarditis and anemia post myocardial infarction. Can. J. Cardiol. 5:147, 1989.
548. Soloff, L. A., Zatuchni, J., Janton, D. H., et al.: Reactivation of rheumatic fever following mitral commissurotomy. Circulation 8:481, 1953.
549. Engle, M. A., and Ito, T.: The postpericardiotomy syndrome. Am. J. Cardiol. 7:73, 1961.
550. Peters, R. W., Scheinman, M. M., Raskin, S., and Thomas, A. N.: Unusual complications of epicardial pacemakers. Am. J. Cardiol. 45:1088, 1980.
551. Livelli, F. D., Jr., Johnson, R. A., McEnany, M. T., et al.: Unexplained in-hospital fever following cardiac surgery: Natural history, relationship to postpericardiotomy syndrome and a prospective study of therapy with indomethacin versus placebo. Circulation 57:968, 1978.
552. Engle, M. A., Gay, W. A., Jr., Zabriskie, J. B., and Senterfit, L. B.: The postpericardiotomy syndrome: 25 years' experience. J. Cardiovasc. Med. 4:321, 1984.
553. Kaminsky, M. E., Rodan, B. A., Osborne, D. R., et al.: Postpericardiotomy syndrome. Am. J. Radiol. 138:503, 1982.
554. DeSaulniers, D., Gervais, N., and Rouleau, J.: Does pericardial drainage decrease the frequency of the postpericardiotomy syndrome? Can. J. Surg. 24:265, 1981.
555. Ofori-Krakye, S. K., Tyberg, T. I., Geha, A. S., et al.: Late cardiac tamponade after open heart surgery: Incidence, role of anticoagulants in its pathogenesis and its relationship to the postpericardiotomy syndrome. Circulation 63:1323, 1981.
555a. Kassanoff, A. H., and Martirossian, M. G.: Postpericardiotomy and post-myocardial infarction syndrome presenting as noncardiac pulmonary edema. Chest 99:1410, 1991.
556. Weitzman, L. B., Tinkler, W. P., Kronzon, I., et al.: The incidence and natural history of pericardial effusion after cardiac surgery—an echocardiographic study. Circulation 69:506, 1984.
557. Wheeler, E. O., Turner, J. D., and Scannell, J. G.: Fever, splenomegaly, and atypical lymphocytes. A syndrome observed after cardiac surgery utilizing a pump oxygenator. N. Engl. J. Med. 266:454, 1962.
558. Berger, R. L., Loveless, G., and Warner, O.: Delayed and latent postcardiotomy tamponade: Recognition and nonoperative treatment. Ann. Thorac. Surg. 12:22, 1971.
559. King, T. E., Jr., Stelzner, T. J., and Sahn, S. A.: Cardiac tamponade complicating the postpericardiotomy syndrome. Chest 83:500, 1983.
560. Gehl, L., Iskandrian, A. S., Goel, I., et al.: Cardiac perforation with tamponade during cardiac catheterization. Cathet. Cardiovasc. Diagn. 8:293, 1982.
561. B-Lundqvist, C., Olsson, S. B., and Varnauskas, E.: Transseptal left heart catheterization: A review of 278 studies. Clin. Cardiol. 9:21, 1986.
562. Foster, C. J.: Constrictive pericarditis complicating an endocardial pacemaker. Br. Heart J. 47:497, 1982.
563. Goldbaum, T. S., Jacob, A. S., Smith, D. F., et al.: Cardiac tamponade following percutaneous transluminal coronary angioplasty. Cathet. Cardiovasc. Diagn. 11:413, 1985.
564. Slack, J. D., Pinkerton, C. A., and Nassar, W. K.: Acute pericarditis after percutaneous transluminal coronary angioplasty. Am. J. Cardiol. 55:843, 1985.
565. Koller, H.: Pericardial tamponade as a lethal complication following dilation of aortic valve stenosis. Wien Med. Wochenschr. 137:255, 1987.
566. Bichel, J.: Serious complications of sternal puncture. Ugeskr. Laeger 151:442, 1989.
567. Mellon, J. K., Galvin, J. F., Bowe, P. C., et al.: Oesophago-pericardial fistula and cardiac tamponade after oesophagoscopy. Eur. J. Cardiothorac. Surg. 2:282, 1988.
568. Puhakka, H. J.: Complications of mediastinoscopy. J. Laryngol. Otol. 103:312, 1989.
569. Knauer, C. M., and Fogel, M. R.: Pericarditis: Complication of esophageal sclerotherapy. A report of three cases. Gastroenterology 93:287, 1987.
570. Brown, D. L., and Luchi, R. J.: Cardiac tamponade and constrictive pericarditis complicating endoscopic sclerotherapy. Arch. Intern. Med. 147:2169, 1987.
571. Lindenau, K. F., Warnke, H., and Bergmann, U.: Cardiac tamponade following open heart surgery. Zentralbl. Chir. 104:1345, 1979.
572. Marx, P., Jaffe, C., Laks, H., and Wolfson, S.: Delayed post-cardiac-surgery

tamponade producing localized right atrial compression. Cathet Cardiovasc. Diagn. *7*:275, 1981.

573. Huwer, H., Vokmer, I., and Dyckmans, J.: Late pericardial tamponade after aortic and mitral valve replacement. Thorac. Cardiovasc. Surg. *36*:54, 1988.
574. Ng, A. S. H., Dorosti, K., and Sheldon, W. C.: Constrictive pericarditis following cardiac surgery—Cleveland Clinic experience: Report of 12 cases and review. Cleve. Clin. Q. *50*:39, 1984.
575. Cimino, J. J., and Kogan, A. D.: Constrictive pericarditis after cardiac surgery: Report of three cases and review of the literature. Am. Heart J. *118*:1292, 1989.
576. Killian, D. M., Furiasse, J. G., Scanlon, P. J., et al.: Constrictive pericarditis after cardiac surgery. Am. Heart J. *118*:563, 1989.
577. Ribiero, P., Sapsford, R., Evans, T., et al.: Constrictive pericarditis as a complication of coronary artery bypass surgery. Br. Heart J. *51*:205, 1984.
578. Kabbani, S. S., Bashour, T., Ellertson, D. G., et al.: Constrictive pericarditis following myocardial revascularization: A possible cause of graft occlusion. Am. Heart J. *110*:493, 1985.
579. Bewtra, C., and Schultz, R. D.: Constrictive calcific pericarditis following coronary arterial bypass surgery. Hum. Pathol. *16*:522, 1985.
580. Almassi, G. H., Chapman, R. D., Troup, P. J., et al.: Constrictive pericarditis associated with patch electrodes of the automatic implantable cardioverter-defibrillator. Chest *92*:369, 1987.
581. Singer, I., Hutchins, G. M., Mirowski, M., et al.: Pathologic findings related to the lead system and repeated defibrillations in patients with the automatic implantable cardioverter-defibrillator. J. Am. Coll. Cardiol. *10*:382, 1987.
582. Kerber, R. E., and Sherman, B.: Echocardiographic evaluation of pericardial effusion in myxedema. Incidence and biochemical and clinical correlations. Circulation *52*:823, 1975.
583. Hardisty, C. A., Naik, D. R., and Munro, D. S.: Pericardial effusion in hypothyroidism. Clin. Endocrinol. *13*:349, 1980.
584. Parving, H., Hansen, J. M., Nielsen, S. V., et al.: Mechanisms of edema formation in myxedema-increased protein extravasation and relatively slow lymphatic drainage. N. Engl. J. Med. *301*:460, 1981.
585. Zimmerman, J., Yahalom, J., and Bar-On, H.: Clinical spectrum of pericardial effusion as the presenting feature of hypothyroidism. Am. Heart J. *106*:770, 1983.
586. Das, S., Lieberman, A. N., and Schussler, G. C.: Prolonged persistence of a large pericardial effusion and hemodynamic evidence of cardiac tamponade during treatment of myxedema. Clin. Cardiol. *5*:459, 1982.
587. Manolis, A. S., Varriale, P., and Ostrowski, R. M.: Hypothyroid cardiac tamponade. Arch. Intern. Med. *147*:1167, 1987.
588. Rosenbau, D. L., and Yu, P. N.: Idiopathic cholesterol pericarditis with effusion. Am. Heart J. *70*:515, 1965.
589. Van Buren, P. C., and Roberts, W. C.: Cholesterol pericarditis and cardiac tamponade with congenital hypothyroidism in adulthood. Am. Heart J. *119*:697, 1990.
590. Ridenhouse, C. E., and Kiphart, R. J.: Idiopathic cholesterol pericarditis treatment with pericardiectomy. Ann. Thorac. Surg. *4*:360, 1967.
591. Stanley, R. J., Subramanian, R., and Lie, J. T.: Cholesterol pericarditis terminating as constrictive calcific pericarditis. Follow-up study of patient with 40-year history of disease. Am. J. Cardiol. *46*:511, 1980.
592. Bhatti, M. A., Ferrante, J. W., Gielchinsky, I., and Norman, J. C.: Pleuropulmonary and skeletal lymphagiomatosis with chylothorax and chylopericardium. Ann. Thorac. Surg. *40*:398, 1985.
593. Rose, D. M., Colvin, S. B., Danilowicz, D., and Isom, O. W.: Cardiac tamponade secondary to chylopericardium following cardiac surgery: Case report and review of the literature. Ann. Thorac. Surg. *34*:333, 1982.
594. Morishita, Y., Taira, A., Furoi, A., et al.: Constrictive pericarditis secondary to primary chylopericardium. Am. Heart J. *109*:373, 1985.
595. Pereira, W. M., Kalil, R. A., Prates, P. R., and Nesralla, I. A.: Cardiac tamponade due to chylopericardium after cardiac surgery. Ann. Thorac. Surg. *46*:572, 1988.
596. Bar-El, Y., Smolinksy, A., and Yellin, A.: Chylopericardium as a complication of mitral valve replacement. Thorax *44*:74, 1989.
597. Naggar, C. Z., Daly, P. A., Burke, M. J., and Swartz, M. R.: Successful medical management of esophagopericardial fistula. Heart Lung *16*:47, 1987.
598. Variyam, E. P., and Shah, A.: Pericardial effusion and left ventricular function in patients with acute alcoholic pancreatitis. Arch. Intern. Med. *147*:923, 1987.
599. Jones, B., Haponik, E. F., and Katz, R.: Fibrinous pericarditis: An uncommon complication of acute pancreatitis. South. Med. J. *80*:377, 1987.
600. Letoquart, J. P., Fasquel, J. L., L'Huillier, J. P., et al.: Gastropericardial fistula. Review of the literature apropos of an original case. J. Chir. *127*:6, 1990.
601. Song, Z. L.: Cholangiothoracic fistulae. Chung Hua Wai Ko Tsa Chih *27*:269, 1989.
602. Isolauri, J., and Markkula, H.: Recurrent ulceration and colopericardial fistula as late complications of colon interposition. Ann. Thorac. Surg. *44*:84, 1987.
603. Ali, I., and Beg, M. H.: Traumatic bronchopericardial fistula presenting as cardiac tamponade. J. Thorac. Cardiovasc. Surg. *95*:740, 1988.
604. Aho, A. J., Vanttinen, E. A., and Nelimarkka, O. I.: Rupture of the pericardium with luxation of the heart after blunt trauma. J. Trauma *27*:560, 1987.
605. Rothschild, P. A., Tarver, R. D., Boyko, O. B., and Conces, D. J., Jr.: MR diagnosis of herniation of the left ventricle through a pericardial window. Comput. Radiol. *11*:15, 1987.
606. Callejas, M. A., Mestres, C. A., Catalan, M., and Sanchez-Lloret, J.: Traumatic intrapericardial diaphragmatic rupture. Thorac. Cardiovasc. Surg. *32*:376, 1984.
607. Kirsch, J. D., and Escarous, A.: CT diagnosis of traumatic pericardium rupture. J. Comput. Assist. Tomogr. *13*:523, 1989.
608. Cassorla, L., and Katz, J. A.: Management of cardiac herniation after intrapericardial pneumonectomy. Anesthesiology *60*:362, 1984.
609. Feigin, D. S., Fenoglio, J. J., McAllister, H. A., and Madewell, J. E.: Pericardial cysts: A radiologic-pathologic correlation and review. Radiology *125*:15, 1977.
610. Kruger, S. R., Michaud, J., and Cannom, D. S.: Spontaneous resolution of a pericardial cyst. Am. Heart J. *109*:1390, 1985.
611. Hynes, J. K., Tajik, A. J., Osborn, M. J., et al.: Two-dimensional echocardiographic diagnosis of pericardial cyst. Mayo Clin. Proc. *58*:60, 1983.
612. Klatte, E. C., and Yune, H. Y.: Diagnosis and treatment of pericardial cysts. Radiology *104*:541, 1972.
613. Unverferth, D. V., and Wooley, C. F.: The differential diagnosis of paracardiac lesions: Pericardial cysts. Cathet. Cardiovasc. Diagn. *5*:31, 1979.
614. Moncada, R., Baglia, K., Moguillansky, S. J., et al.: CT diagnosis of congenital intrapericardial masses. J. Comput. Assist. Tomogr. *9*:56, 1985.
615. Ellis, K., Leeds, N. E., and Himmelstein, A.: Congenital deficiencies in partial pericardium: Review of two new cases including successful diagnosis by plain roentgenography. Am. J. Roentgenol. *82*:125, 1959.
616. Letanche, G., Gayet, C., Souguet, P. J., et al.: Agenesis of the pericardium: Clinical, echocardiographic and MRI aspects. Rev. Pneumol. Clin. *44*:105, 1988.
617. Taysi, K., Hartmann, A. F., Shackelford, G. D., and Sundarum, V.: Congenital absence of the pericardium in a family. Am. J. Med. Genet. *21*:77, 1985.
618. Gehlmann, H. R., and van Ingen, G. J.: Symptomatic congenital complete absence of the left pericardium. Case report and review of the literature. Eur. Heart J. *10*:670, 1989.
619. Inoue, H., Fujii, J., Mashima, S., and Marao, S.: Pseudo right atrial overloading pattern in complete defect of the left pericardium. J. Electrocardiol. *14*:413, 1981.
620. Candan, I., Erol, C., and Sonel, A.: Cross sectional echocardiographic appearance in presumed congenital absence of the left pericardium. Br. Heart. J. *55*:405, 1986.
621. D'Altoria, R. A., and Caro, J. Y.: Congenital absence of the left pericardium detected by imaging of the lung: Case report. J. Nucl. Med. *18*:267, 1977.
622. Gutierrez, F. R., Shackelford, G. D., McKnight, R. C., et al.: Diagnosis of congenital absence of left pericardium by MR imaging. J. Comput. Assist. Tomogr. 9:551, 1985.
623. Millaire, A., Goullard, L., Tison, E., et al.: Unilateral agenesis of the pericardium. Arch. Mal. Coeur. *83*:275, 1990.
624. Saito, R., and Hotta, F.: Congenital pericardial defect associated with cardiac incarceration: Case report. Am. Heart J. *100*:866, 1980.
625. Chapman, J. E., Rubin, J. W., Gross, C. M., and Janssen, M. E.: Congenital absence of pericardium: An unusual cause of atypical angina. Ann. Thorac. Surg. *45*:191, 1988.
626. Jones, J. W., and McManus, B. M.: Fatal cardiac strangulation by congenital partial pericardial defect. Am. Heart. J. *107*:183, 1984.
627. Auch-Schweik, W., Bonzel, T., Krause, T., et al.: Differential diagnosis of chest pain and diagnostic findings in pericardial defects combined with coronary artery disease. Clin. Cardiol. *11*:650, 1988.
628. Altman, C. A., Ettedgui, J. A., Wozney, P., and Beerman, L. B.: Noninvasive diagnostic features of partial absence of the pericardium. Am. J. Cardiol. *63*:1536, 1989.
629. Ruys, F., Paulus, W., Stevens, C., and Brutsaert, D.: Expansion of the left atrial appendage is a distinctive cross-sectional echocardiographic feature of congenital defect of the pericardium. Eur. Heart J. *4*:738, 1983.
630. Wolff, F., Fritz, A., Dumeny, P., and Eisenmann, B.: Diastolic coronary prolapse in partial left pericardial agenesis. Arch. Mal. Coeur. *80*:206, 1987.
631. Amiri, A., Weber, C., Schlosser, V., and Meinertz, T. H.: Coronary artery disease in a patient with a congenital pericardial defect. Thorac. Cardiovasc. Surg. *37*:379, 1989.
632. Minocha, G. K., Falicov, R. E., and Nijensohn, E.: Partial right-sided congenital pericardial defect with herniation of the right atrium and right ventricle. Chest *76*:484, 1979.
633. Bernal, J. M., Lepiedra, J. O., Gonzalez, I., et al.: Angiocardiographic demonstration of a partial defect of the pericardium with herniation of the left atrium and ventricle. J. Cardiovasc. Surg. *27*:344, 1986.

Traumatic Heart Disease

by PETER F. COHN, M.D., and EUGENE BRAUNWALD, M.D.

Unfortunately, traumatic heart disease is still regarded as an uncommon and even esoteric form of heart disease of interest primarily to emergency physicians or those in the military service. That this is not the case is attested to by the statistics—violent injury accounts for the majority of deaths in persons under 40 years of age,[1] and among these victims cardiac trauma is one of the leading causes of death.[2,3] For example, chest injuries are directly responsible for more than 25 per cent of the 50,000 to 60,000 deaths that result annually from automobile accidents and contribute significantly to another 25 per cent of these deaths.[4] The increasing frequency of physical violence has also resulted in a corresponding increase in the incidence of traumatic heart disease, especially in *young adult males*. These are the most frequent victims, since they are more likely to have automobile and motorcycle accidents, to incur injuries while performing heavy labor, and to be involved in or victims of acts of physical violence.

There is, regrettably, no evidence that the frequency of these mishaps is declining. At Boston City Hospital, for example, the annual incidence of penetrating wounds of the heart rose from 2.8 cases during the period from 1956 through 1964 to 8.0 cases from 1965 through 1976.[5] In Houston,[6] a 30-year analysis of 4459 patients with cardiovascular injuries (86 per cent of whom were males) showed a steady rise between 1958 (averaging 27 patients/yr) and 1988 (213 patients/yr) (Table 46–1). In addition, the incidence of medically related cardiac trauma is also rising, such as increased use of intravascular and intracardiac catheters leading to penetrating injuries of the heart and great vessels, and resuscitative cardiac massage causing a variety of nonpenetrating injuries of these organs.

The two principal, immediate consequences of cardiac injury are *exsanguinating hemorrhage* and *cardiac tamponade*. Effective treatment has resulted in an increasing number of immediate survivors, and later sequelae—including myocardial infarction, ventricular aneurysm and pseudoaneurysm, ventricular septal defect, valvular damage, recurrent pericarditis, and constrictive pericarditis—are becoming far more common. Serious cardiac trauma is frequently overlooked in patients with nonpenetrating injury, particularly when other structures such as the thoracic cage and lungs are obviously damaged. Such oversight can be tragic, because the lethal consequences of cardiac injury may suddenly emerge after the superficial injuries have been attended to. Clearly, a much higher index of suspicion of this possibility is necessary if the increasing magnitude of this problem is to be halted and reversed.

NONPENETRATING CARDIAC INJURY

Nonpenetrating injuries result from the effects of external physical forces, but it is important to recognize that these forces need not necessarily be applied directly to the chest, since injuries to the heart and great vessels may also occur with trauma to other parts of the body. Parmley et al. have summarized the mechanisms of nonpenetrating injuries to the heart as follows: (1) direct force against the chest; (2) bidirectional force against the thorax; (3) indirect forces resulting in a marked increase in intravascular pressure, as from sudden compression in the abdomen and lower extremities; (4) decelerative forces; (5) blast forces; (6) concussive forces; and (7) combinations of these.[6]

The most common cause of nonpenetrating injury in civilian life is probably that directly related to *vehicular impact*,[7] either by direct compression, usually with the steering wheel squeezing the heart between the sternum and the spine, or by indirect compression. Causes of nonpenetrating injuries other than automobile and motorcycle accidents include direct blows to the chest by any kind of blunt object or missile, such as a clenched fist and various kinds of sporting equipment, as well as by the kicks of animals, falls, and cardiac resuscitative procedures. Fractures of the bony structures of the chest wall are *not* necessary accompaniments of cardiac injury in any of these situations. This point is of critical importance, since *the absence of such obvious injuries following trauma should by no*

TABLE 46–1 ETIOLOGY OF CARDIOVASCULAR INJURIES PER 5-YEAR TIME INTERVAL

Etiology	1958–63	1964–69	1970–73	1974–78	1979–83	1984–88	Total
Gunshot wound	42	236	436	501	625	456	2296
Stab/laceration	64	110	161	229	362	463	1389
Blunt trauma	1	17	58	90	62	76	304
Shotgun wound	1	15	45	55	61	37	214
Iatrogenic	1	1	0	0	4	25	31
Other/unknown	54	20	111	25	3	12	225
Total	163	399	811	900	1117	1069	4459

From Mattox, K. L., et al.: Five thousand seven hundred sixty cardiovascular injuries in 4459 patients: Epidemiologic evolution 1958 to 1987. Ann. Surg. *209*:698, 1989.

TABLE 46-2 TYPES OF CARDIAC INJURY FROM BLUNT TRAUMA

A. MYOCARDIUM
1. Contusion
2. Laceration
3. Rupture
4. Septal perforation
5. Aneurysm, pseudoaneurysm
6. Hemopericardium, tamponade
7. Thrombosis, systemic embolism

B. PERICARDIUM
1. Pericarditis
2. Postpericardiotomy syndrome
3. Constrictive pericarditis
4. Pericardial laceration
5. Hemorrhage
6. Cardiac herniation

C. ENDOCARDIAL STRUCTURES
1. Rupture of papillary muscle
2. Rupture of chordae tendineae
3. Rupture of atrioventricular and semilunar valves

D. CORONARY ARTERY
1. Thrombosis
2. Laceration
3. Fistula

From Jackson, D. H., and Murphy, G. W.: Nonpenetrating cardiac trauma. Mod. Conc. Cardiovasc. Dis. 45:123, 1976, by permission of the American Heart Association, Inc.

means exclude the possibility of nonpenetrating injury to the heart. The clinical manifestations may not be apparent for days or even weeks after the accident.

Pathological findings following nonpenetrating cardiac injury usually include some degree of *pericarditis,* which may be associated with the late development of *pericardial constriction.* Changes in the heart itself range from minute ecchymotic areas in the subepicardium or subendocardium to transmural contusions with edematous, fragmented, or necrotic muscle fibers, surrounded at first by red blood cells and invaded soon thereafter by polymorphonuclear leukocytes. The external appearance of the heart may be misleading in the case of nonpenetrating injury, since large areas of intramural contusion, including involvement of the interventricular septum, may not be apparent.[4,8] In patients who survive the injury, healing is by scar formation resembling that following acute myocardial infarction, and post-traumatic aneurysms resembling postinfarction aneurysms may develop.[9] The types of cardiac injury resulting from blunt (nonpenetrating) trauma are listed in Table 46-2, the most severe forms being rupture of the aortic or mitral valve and rupture of the interventricular septum or even of the free wall of a cardiac chamber. While these injuries are frequently fatal, fortunately they constitute only a small fraction of all nonpenetrating injuries (Table 46-3).

PERICARDIUM

Injury to the pericardium in blunt trauma may range from contusion to laceration or rupture. Whether the pericardium tears or not, some degree of traumatic pericarditis is found at autopsy or operation in most patients sustaining severe blunt trauma of the chest, especially of the precordial area. Parmley et al. reported pericardial laceration or rupture in 249 of 546 autopsy cases of nonpenetrating trauma to the heart,[6] but it should be noted that this rarely occurs as an isolated lesion (Table 46-3) and is usually associated with cardiac contusion and even more serious cardiac injury. On the basis of a series of experiments in a canine model, in which 14 of 18 dogs receiving sublethal blunt chest trauma developed pericardial rents, DeMuth et al. suggested that a higher frequency of pericardial tears than is generally appreciated occurs in survivors of chest trauma.[10] Herniation of the heart or a portion of it through the defect may result from such injuries.[11] Clinically, a rent in the pericardium can occur as a consequence of blunt trauma, and delayed herniation of the heart through the rent may then compromise circulatory function acutely.

CLINICAL FEATURES AND DIAGNOSIS. Clinically, traumatic pericarditis is manifested by the development of a typical pericardial friction rub and ST-T–wave changes on the electrocardiogram characteristic of pericarditis (p. 1470). During and immediately following the acute episode, the major problem is not the pericarditis itself but its most common complications, i.e., hemopericardium and resultant tamponade, discussed on p. 1473. Commonly, the patient is restless, with hypotension, oliguria or anuria, distant heart sounds, and pulsus paradoxus. There is usually diffuse low voltage on the electrocardiogram. Pericardial fluid on the echocardiogram (p. 1473) is a key finding.[12]

TREATMENT AND PROGNOSIS. As a rule, uncomplicated pericarditis secondary to cardiac trauma simply resolves. Tamponade, however, requires emergency operative treatment, as discussed below. Recurrent pericardial effusions sometimes associated with chest pain and fever, i.e., the so-called postcardiotomy syndrome, occur in a small number of patients. The cause of this syndrome is not clear (p. 1473). Although patients with recurrent effusion usually respond to aspirin or nonsteroidal antiinflammatory agents, occasionally glucocorticosteroids are necessary. *Constrictive pericarditis* (p. 1482) occurs as a rare complication of traumatic pericarditis, with or without recurrent effusions.

MYOCARDIUM

CONTUSION. Myocardial contusion usually produces no significant symptoms and often goes unrecognized. At times, manifestations of the injury are masked by injury to the chest wall or other organs.[13–16] This is important because as many as 75 per cent of patients with myocardial contusion can have

TABLE 46-3 NONPENETRATING CARDIAC TRAUMA

TYPE AND/OR SITE OF INJURY	NUMBER OF CASES	CASES COMBINED WITH AORTIC RUPTURE	TOTAL
Rupture	273	80	353
Right ventricle	56	10	66
Left ventricle	46	13	59
Right atrium	35	6	51
Left atrium	24	2	26
IV septum	25(20*)	7(4*)	30(24*)
IA septum	18(10*)	5(3*)	25(13*)
Multiple chamber ruptures	69	37	106 128
Contusion/laceration	105	24	
Pericardial laceration	18	18	36
Hemopericardium	13	12	25
Valvular laceration/rupture	1(2†)	0(4†)	1(6†)
Aortic valve	1(1†)	0(2†)	1(3†)
Pulmonic valve	0(4†)	0	0(4†)
Tricuspid valve	0(8†)	0	0(8†)
Mitral valve	0(8†)	0(1†)	0(9†)
Mitral and tricuspid valves	0(1†)	0(1†)	0(2†)
Coronary artery laceration/ rupture	0(7†)	1(2†)	1(9†)
Papillary muscle laceration/ rupture	1(23†)	0	1(23†)
TOTAL	411	135	546

Numbers in parentheses indicate more significant associated cardiac injuries (tabulated in another column).
* Associated with other sites of cardiac rupture.
† Combined with cardiac rupture or other cardiac injury.
From Parmley, L. F., et al.: Nonpenetrating traumatic injury of the heart. Circulation 18:371, 1958, by permission of the American Heart Association, Inc.

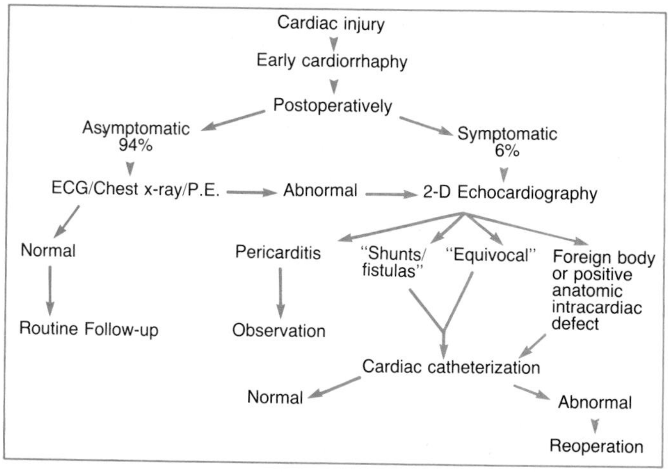

Cardiac injury
Early cardiorrhaphy
Postoperatively
Asymptomatic 94%
Symptomatic 6%
ECG/Chest x-ray/P.E. → Abnormal → 2-D Echocardiography
Normal → Routine Follow-up
Pericarditis → Observation
"Shunts/fistulas"
"Equivocal"
Foreign body or positive anatomic intracardiac defect
Cardiac catheterization
Normal
Abnormal → Reoperation

FIGURE 46–1. A recommended decision schema for post-traumatic cardiac evaluation. Following cardiac injury repair is generally carried out by simple cardiorrhaphy. This algorithm shows a suggested approach to detect residual damage following emergency cardiorrhaphy. (From Mattox, K. L., et al.: Cardiac evaluation following heart injury. J. Trauma *25*:758, © by Williams and Wilkins, 1985.)

signs of external chest injury.[17] Thus there is a higher frequency of diagnosis of cardiac contusion associated with increasing awareness of the lesion.

Clinical Features and Diagnosis. The most common symptom of myocardial contusion is precordial pain resembling that of myocardial infarction, but the pain from other sites of chest trauma can confuse the clinical picture.[15,17] As with myocardial infarction, nitroglycerin and related drugs have little effect in relieving the pain. The *electrocardiogram* probably represents one of the most helpful tools for recognizing contusion of the left ventricle. Either nonspecific ST-T abnormalities or the classic findings of pericarditis are the most common changes noted. Initially, electrocardiographic signs of deeper injury to the myocardium, i.e., pathological Q waves, may be dwarfed by pericardial inflammation; only as the latter subsides does injury to the myocardium become more evident. However, because the possibility of cardiac trauma is often not considered in trauma victims, an electrocardiogram is often not recorded immediately on patients with chest injuries and the diagnosis may be missed. Just as in acute myocardial infarction, serial findings, i.e., the evolution of Q waves and the subsidence of the ST-segment and T-wave abnormalities, are of critical importance. The sensitivity and specificity of electrocardiographic findings are less than 100 per cent, however; hence the need for additional tests.

A recommended decision schema for evaluating cardiac injury immediately after early cardiorrhaphy is depicted in Figure 46–1.

SERUM ENZYMES. *Since enzyme levels* may be elevated by trauma to noncardiac as well as to cardiac tissue, they too are of limited diagnostic value. With the widespread availability of reliable measurements of the MB band of creatine kinase (CK), the presence or absence of cardiac necrosis can be better documented in patients with blunt trauma.[18] Indeed, with the electrocardiogram and CK-MB as screening tests, the detection of myocardial contusion has increased from 7 to 17 per cent in patients with blunt chest trauma entering the Henry Ford Hospital.[19] Similarly, at the Mayo Clinic 58 of 291 such patients (20 per cent) had elevations of CK-MB.[20] However, false-positive elevations of the CK-MB isoenzyme can also be seen if the total CK is greater than 20,000 units; this can occur after massive injury to skeletal muscle.

RADIONUCLIDE IMAGING (see Chap. 10). Myocardial perfusion is reduced in areas of myocardial contusion.[18] Chiu et al. have used technetium-labeled pyrophosphate to demonstrate images of positive uptake that were then correlated with postmortem angiograms showing extravasation of contrast material.[21] Images usually became negative 1 week after the trauma. Contused myocardium concentrates ^{99m}Tc-pyrophosphate in amounts comparable to those observed in ischemic injury. Scanning following injection of radioactive thallium to detect areas of reduced perfusion and of labeled pyrophosphate to locate areas of recent necrosis may be expected to identify patients with myocardial damage following blunt trauma, to localize this damage, and to indicate the extent of the damage. Radionuclide ventriculography often shows a reduced ventricular ejection fraction in such patients.[22] These tests show changes similar to those observed in patients with acute myocardial infarction (Chap. 39). Sutherland et al.[22] used radionuclide ventriculography to define focal defects in ventricular wall motion. They subgrouped the 43 patients whom they studied into those with right ventricular abnormalities (18), left ventricular abnormalities (4), biventricular abnormalities (6), and neither kind (15). They described the state of right ventricular pump function using modified ventricular function curves and found it to be surprisingly well preserved (Fig. 46–2). Schamp et al. also found a high (83 per cent) frequency of right ventricular abnormalities in the 40 patients they studied.[23]

ECHOCARDIOGRAPHY. In addition to identifying pericardial effusion, *two-dimensional echocardiography* is also useful in evaluating cardiac injuries, including myocardial contusion. Such findings as abnormal wall motion and chamber enlargement can be detected with this technique.[24] Echocardiography is useful when the patient with suspected cardiac injury first undergoes testing, as well as after emergency thoracotomy and cardiac repair in an effort to detect residual cardiac damage. When confirmed with pulsed-Doppler echocardiography, intracardiac shunts and regurgitant lesions can be demonstrated.

ARRHYTHMIAS. A wide variety of arrhythmias is common with areas of extensive contusion,[25] and ventricular tachycardia that degenerates into ventricular fibrillation represents a frequent cause of death in these patients. The precise mechanism responsible for these arrhythmias has not been defined, but in the dog, increasing frequencies of ventricular premature beats were observed with increasing grades of trauma.[13] In addition, both atrioventricular and intraventricular conduction defects, as well as sinus node dysfunction, are seen.[26,27] In contrast to acute myocardial infarction, cardiac contusion rarely leads to severe *heart failure* unless massive damage to a valve or rupture of the interventricular septum has

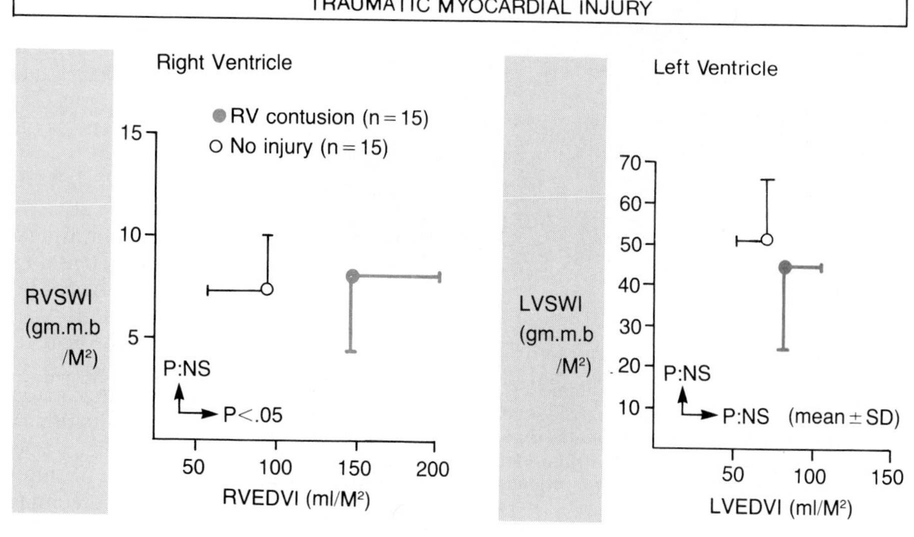

FIGURE 46–2. Left and right ventricular (LV and RV) myocardial function curves in 43 patients who sustained acute myocardial contusion complicating blunt chest injury. Patients with RV contusion (●) maintained an RV stroke work index (RVSWI) similar to that of patients without RV contusion (○) by virtue of a larger RV end-diastolic volume index (RVEDVI) (preload). Hence, RV performance was well-maintained albeit at a greater preload and the two groups of patients appeared to have identical LV function. NS = not significant; SD = standard deviation. (From Sutherland, G. R., et al.: Hemodynamic adaptation to acute myocardial contusion complicating blunt chest injury. Am. J. Cardiol. *57*:291, 1986.)

occurred.[28] However, some impairment of right and/or left ventricular function, as reflected in depressed ejection fractions and ventricular function (myocardial performance) curves, may be found.[22,29] In the animal model, alcohol ingestion potentiates the effect of blunt trauma on the myocardium.[30] This gives added strength to the warning not to mix drinking and driving.

Treatment and Prognosis. In this era of progressively earlier ambulation of patients with acute myocardial infarction, a similar approach appears to be reasonable after several days of close observation for myocardial contusion. Several groups have concluded that in trauma patients in stable condition, contusion neither increases the complication rate nor necessitates intensive care unit monitoring.[31,32] Hossack et al. have even questioned the need for routine imaging studies.[33] From the point of view of physical activity, we recommend treating these patients in a manner similar to that for those with acute myocardial infarction with comparable extent of myocardial damage (Chap. 39). However, *treatment with anticoagulants and obviously with thrombolytics is contraindicated,* since intramyocardial or intrapericardial hemorrhage may be precipitated or exacerbated. Atrial fibrillation, when present, usually reverts to sinus rhythm spontaneously. If it does not, digitalis glycosides may be used to slow the ventricular rate and may also cause reversion to sinus rhythm. Chest pain is best treated with analgesics; nonsteroidal anti-inflammatory agents are not advised because they might interfere with myocardial healing (p. 1215).

As already noted, the prognosis from complete or partial recovery is generally excellent, but these patients require careful follow-up, since late complications, ranging from ventricular arrhythmias to cardiac rupture, may occur. Coronary occlusion[34–36] aorto–right atrial fistula,[37] and ventricular aneurysms (Fig. 46–3)[9] are occasional sequelae, and there is no agreement about whether or not surgical resection of the last-named is required. It is our policy to use the presence of heart failure as an indication for operation of aneurysms analogous to that in patients with postinfarct aneurysms (p. 1260). Pseudoaneurysms, however, require immediate repair (p. 227).

Although many analogies can be drawn between the cardiac necrosis caused by trauma and that caused by ischemic heart disease, a number of critically important differences must be emphasized. Patients with acute myocardial infarction secondary to coronary artery disease generally have diffuse, obstructive, gradually progressive coronary atherosclerosis, are frequently middle-aged or elderly, and may have underlying heart disease such as that secondary to prolonged hypertension or diabetes mellitus; patients with traumatic myocardial contusion generally have normal coronary vessels and only a discrete area of myocardial damage; most often, they are young and without underlying cardiovascular illness. Hence, the long-term prognosis in surviving patients with myocardial necrosis secondary to trauma tends to be far better than in patients with myocardial infarction secondary to atherosclerotic coronary artery disease.

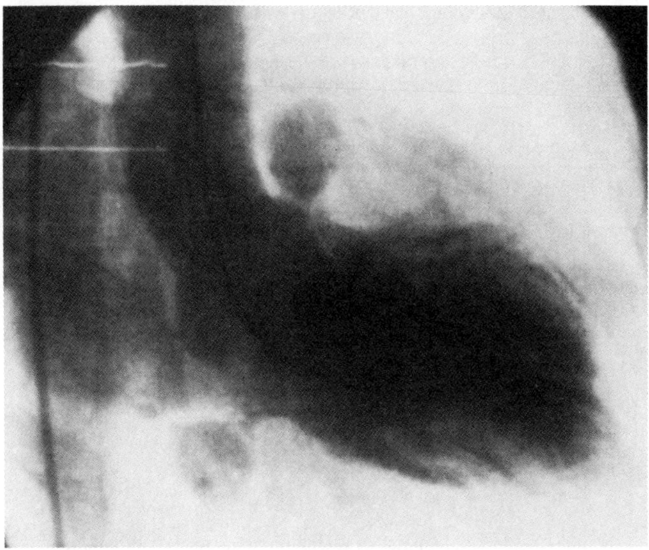

FIGURE 46–3. Right anterior oblique left ventriculogram. Submitral aneurysms appear as saccular narrow-necked structures at superior and inferior portions of mitral annulus during diastole. Top of inferior aneurysm is compressed by left atrium. (From Matthews, R. V., et al.: Chest trauma and subvalvular left ventricular aneurysms. Chest *95*:474, 1989.)

CARDIAC RUPTURE. There appear to be two mechanisms of cardiac rupture: (1) acute laceration due to compression of the heart by direct force,[38] and (2) contusion and hemorrhage that proceed to necrosis, softening, and rupture several days following the trauma. Rupture of a cardiac chamber usually, but not always, results in immediate death. It is this minority of patients that survive the initial trauma that must be assessed and treated immediately in the emergency room setting.

Clinical Features and Diagnosis. In the patient who survives the first few minutes of cardiac rupture, the clinical picture of cardiac tamponade described above is common. Although ventricular rupture is far more common than is atrial rupture,[3] the latter occurs particularly following automobile accidents. Rupture of the interventricular septum should be suspected in patients who develop severe congestive heart failure immediately or within several days of the trauma, together with a new holosystolic murmur along the left sternal border; however, trauma to the mitral valve apparatus, which may be manifested with a similar picture clinically, must be excluded. On the basis of a series of 546 autopsy cases of nonpenetrating injury to the heart, the incidence of rupture of the ventricular septum has been estimated by Parmley et al. to be almost 10 per cent, with a similar number of patients experiencing rupture of the atrial septum (Table 46–3).[6] These lesions may occur without other serious cardiac injuries, but occasionally other abnormalities are present, including valve cusp perforations and a variety of intracardiac shunts.[39] Although the predilection for perforation of the ventricular septum is highest at the apex, any portion of the muscular septum may be involved, and multiple perforations are not uncommon. The diagnosis of ventricular septal defect and of damage to the mitral valve apparatus can be confirmed by means of catheterization, demonstration of an oxygen step-up in the right ventricle, left ventricular angiography,[40] as well as by color-flow Doppler echocardiography[24] (p. 1523).

Treatment and Prognosis. Patients with external rupture of the heart obviously require emergency surgery if they are to have any chance of survival. Although operation should not be postponed, pericardiocentesis and expansion of the intravascular volume can be carried out while the most rapid preparations possible for operation are undertaken. Successful surgical treatment of external cardiac rupture has been reported in a small number of cases.[41] In contrast, patients with rupture of the interventricular septum do not always require emergency operation. Indeed, many defects are small, with minimal left-to-right shunts, and may even heal spontaneously. If heart failure develops subsequently, as occurs in many patients, surgical correction should be carried out promptly and is often successful.

COMPLICATIONS OF CARDIAC RESUSCITATION

Closed-chest (external) cardiac massage (p. 776) is generally thought to be safe and simple—so much so that it is included as part of the cardiopulmonary resuscitation technique taught to lay persons. What is not sufficiently appreciated is that the procedure itself can result in serious complications, which may go unrecognized because many of the patients succumb to the cardiac arrest itself.[42] Even at postmortem examination, the complications may be improperly attributed to the underlying cardiac disease.

Rupture of the left ventricle is a more common complication of cardiac massage than is rupture of the right ventricle.

However, rupture of either chamber may occur and may be life-threatening if the patient survives the arrhythmia that necessitated massage in the first place. Since in most instances external resuscitation is performed for patients with myocardial infarction, it may not always be clear whether the left ventricular rupture preceded the massage or occurred as a consequence of it.

Rupture of right ventricular papillary muscles with acute tricuspid regurgitation has also been reported as a complication of closed-chest cardiac massage,[43] as has rupture of the atria and aorta and dissecting hematoma of a coronary artery.[44] A variety of noncardiovascular traumatic lesions, such as fracture of the sternum, hemothorax, pneumothorax, and laceration of abdominal organs may occur. Because of the efficacy of cardiopulmonary resuscitation and its increasing use by paramedical personnel and laymen, an increasing number of such complications may be anticipated in the future. This increased incidence will be stemmed only by educational programs for all individuals likely to employ this technique.

PENETRATING CARDIAC INJURY

Penetrating cardiac injuries occurring in civilian life are due to a variety of objects, such as bullets, knives, ice picks, and the like. The demographics of penetrating cardiac trauma in Jefferson County, Alabama were reviewed by Naughton, et al.[45] As with blunt trauma, male victims predominated and gunshot wounds were the major mechanism of injury. Penetrating injuries may also be due to the inward displacement of ribs or sternal fragments accompanying chest injuries. The chamber most commonly involved in this type of injury is the right ventricle because of its anterior position, followed, in descending order of frequency, by the left ventricle, the right atrium, and the left atrium.[46] However, penetrating wounds of the precordium are not the only types of wounds that may result in cardiac injury. Occasionally, wounds of other areas of the chest, as well as of the neck and upper abdomen, are associated with penetration of the heart. In addition, intravenous or intracardiac catheters may fracture and become impaled within the walls of a great vessel or cardiac chamber (Chap. 7). Migration of an indwelling venous catheter into the pulmonary artery, which may ultimately lead to perforation of this vessel, is another complication that has increased in frequency with its widespread use in intensive care units. Formerly, thoracotomy was necessary to remove these catheter fragments, but catheters with snares and other devices are now available for this purpose.[47,48]

Perforation of the right ventricle with a transvenous pacing electrode is not uncommon, but tamponade is rare. During cardiac catheterization, perforation of the thin-walled right atrium or outflow tract of the right ventricle has been reported. Such patients usually require only careful observation, but when tamponade occurs, immediate drainage is mandatory.[49] Coronary angioplasty[50] and endomyocardial biopsy[51,52] can also result in tamponade. Dissection of the aorta or arch vessels has been reported as a complication of retrograde arterial catheterization and occasionally is also severe enough to require operative intervention.

Penetrating wounds of the heart often result in laceration of the pericardium, sometimes occurring alone but usually associated with laceration of the myocardium itself. One or more chambers but also the cardiac valves and their accessory structures, as well as the interventricular and interatrial septa, may be perforated. Cardiac tamponade resulting from pneumopericardium has been reported.[53] When laceration of the pericardium occurs as an isolated lesion, acute compromise of cardiac function resulting from herniation of the heart may be the presenting manifestation. Occasionally, low-velocity missiles may penetrate the cardiac chambers but may be retained within the myocardium.

The most common penetrating injuries resulting from physical violence are stab and gunshot wounds.[45,54] The former do not necessarily cause extensive cellular destruction adjacent to the wound; they resemble surgical incisions, and transmural wounds in the thick-walled left ventricle may actually seal quickly without disastrous consequences. In contrast, bullet wounds are associated with bleeding that is not usually self-limited and extensive cellular destruction in and adjacent to the path of the bullet. When a coronary artery is lacerated or perforated, myocardial infarction may ensue.

CLINICAL FEATURES AND DIAGNOSIS. The clinical picture of a penetrating wound of the heart depends on several factors, including the object responsible for the injury (e.g., bullet, knife, ice pick), the size of the wound, and the precise location of the structures injured. Pericardial laceration occurring by itself is uncommon and of relatively little significance unless infection supervenes. Rather, the injuries to underlying cardiac structures usually determine the clinical presentation, course, and choice of treatment. However, the nature of the pericardial wound is important, i.e., whether or not the wound is open and allows free drainage of intrapericardial blood. If the pericardium remains open and extravasated blood can pass freely into the pleural cavities or mediastinum, cardiac tamponade will not develop, at least initially, and the presenting signs and symptoms will be those of hemorrhage and hemothorax. On the other hand, if the pericardium does *not* permit free drainage because its opening has been obliterated by a blood clot, adjacent lung tissue, or other structures, or because a flap develops in the pericardial rent, immediate exsanguination may be averted, but tamponade may occur minutes or hours later. In some instances, blood accumulates both intra- and extrapericardially.

Whether the hemorrhage is intra- or extrapericardial, its severity can often be surmised from the clinical picture. Traumatic penetrating lesions of the heart are usually associated with injuries to the lungs and other organs, which may predominate at first; a high index of suspicion of cardiac penetration is necessary when patients are evaluated following thoracic or upper abdominal trauma. Although extensive injuries to the pericardium and underlying heart are usually immediately fatal or result in shock, delayed clinical manifestations of cardiac injury as a result of hemorrhage, infection, retained foreign bodies, or arrhythmias may become apparent after the other bodily injuries have been attended to. Failure to give serious consideration to the possibility that *cardiac* damage has occurred in a patient with obvious noncardiac trauma may lead to an unanticipated catastrophe.

Although echocardiography is extremely valuable in the recognition of pericardial effusion[12,24,27,55] (p. 102), foreign bodies in the heart,[56] and intracardiac shunts,[12,24,57,58] it is not always readily available in an emergency setting. When agitation, cool and clammy skin, neck vein distention, pulsus paradoxus, and other classic findings of tamponade (considered earlier) are present, the diagnosis can be relatively simple; in patients without such typical findings, the clinical picture may be attributed to blood loss, especially since volume expansion can improve the hemodynamic state, at least temporarily. Whether or not pericardiocentesis should be performed as a diagnostic test is controversial. If nonclotting blood is obtained, the diagnosis of hemopericardium is confirmed, and the accompanying decompression may constitute effective, albeit temporary, initial treatment. If the pericardiocentesis is negative, however, cardiac tamponade cannot be ruled out. Since, as discussed below, the primary management in any event is thoracotomy, it seems pointless to waste valuable time with pericardial aspiration unless there is doubt regarding the diagnosis.

TREATMENT. The definitive treatment of cardiac wounds *accompanied by severe hemorrhage* is immediate thoracotomy and cardiorrhaphy.[59] Although multiple pericardiocenteses are no longer considered a substitute for thoracotomy in the treatment of cardiac wounds associated with cardiac tamponade, there may still be a role for pericardial aspiration *while the patient is being prepared for operation.* Algorithms for management of patients with penetrating

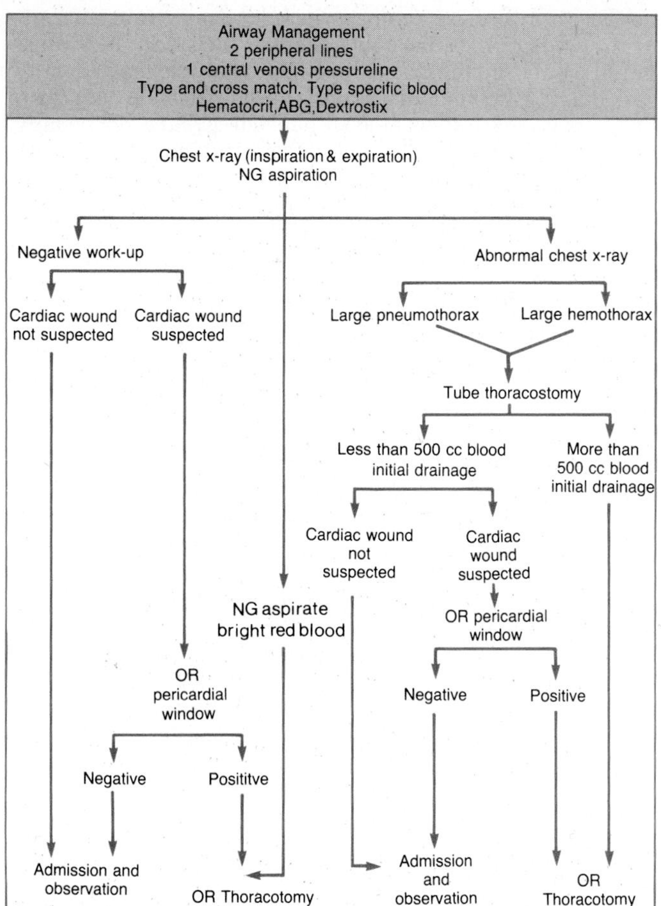

FIGURE 46-4. Algorithm for management of penetrating chest wound with stable vital signs on admission. ABG = arterial blood gases; NG = nasogastric. (From Karrel, R., et al.: Emergency diagnosis, resuscitation, and treatment of acute penetrating cardiac trauma. Ann. Emerg. Med. *11*:504, 1982.)

chest wounds—with either stable or unstable vital signs—have been proposed (Figs. 46-4 and 46-5). The availability in many hospitals of surgical teams and equipment for cardiopulmonary bypass has permitted the safe and effective repair of many penetrating injuries of the heart. Marshall and associates[54] described a 10½-year experience with 47 patients admitted after penetrating cardiac trauma (stab wounds and gunshot wounds); 46 underwent immediate surgery and 10 died. The one patient who refused surgery also died, resulting in a total mortality of 11/47, or 23 per cent. Mortality was 26 per cent in patients with shunts and 15 per cent in those with tamponade.

Occasionally, thoracotomy may be performed in moribund patients for whom general anesthesia is unnecessary. However, adequate ventilation must be maintained. Administration of antibiotics and tetanus prophylaxis should also be instituted as routine measures. Operative treatment includes repair of the pericardium, myocardium, aorta, and valves as well as of any lacerations of the coronary arteries. At operation, the heart and great vessels should be thoroughly examined for the presence of multiple wounds. When the bullet has penetrated the anterior wall of the heart, the posterior wall should always be inspected for an exit wound before the chest is closed. Many victims of penetrating cardiac injury, young and otherwise in good health, can withstand relatively long periods of hypoperfusion without irreversible brain, renal, or cardiac damage. Therefore, one should err on the side of aggressive attempts at resuscitation in patients who arrive moribund in the operating room. Retained foreign bodies in the heart are less of a problem in civilian than in military injuries, because shootings in civilian life usually occur at short range and thus result in through-and-through wounds.

There is disagreement concerning whether or not retained foreign bodies should be removed. Certainly, if the projectile is accessible, it should be removed; echocardiography (Fig. 46-6) can be helpful in locating foreign bodies.[56,60] If deemed not dangerous, they can probably be left in place, although there is some risk of later infection, pain, aneurysm formation, or migration of the foreign body.[60,61] In addition, dealing with a patient who is preoccupied with the knowledge that he has a foreign body retained in or close to the heart may present some difficulty; indeed, anxiety can become excessive, impairing the patient's function more than the physical damage and, occasionally, becoming an indication for reoperation and extraction of the object. The serious consequences of a foreign body embolus from the left ventricle also encourage a more aggressive surgical policy toward foreign bodies lodged in that chamber than in the right ventricle. Foreign bodies embedded at strategic points in great vessels may erode the vessel and cause potentially severe hemorrhage or may embolize[60] and should, if possible, be removed.

Late complications of penetrating wounds of the heart are quite common and include post-traumatic pericarditis and infection as well as arrhythmias, ventricular septal defect, and ventricular aneurysm.

PROGNOSIS. The outlook following a penetrating wound depends, first and foremost, on the extent of the injury. Gunshot wounds of the heart are more usually fatal than are stab wounds, while among the latter, knife wounds are more serious than are ice pick wounds. Salvage rates are lower in patients with extrapericardial hemorrhage compared with tamponade and also with penetrating wounds involving thin-walled structures such as the atria or the pulmonary artery, since they rarely seal off spontaneously, whereas injury

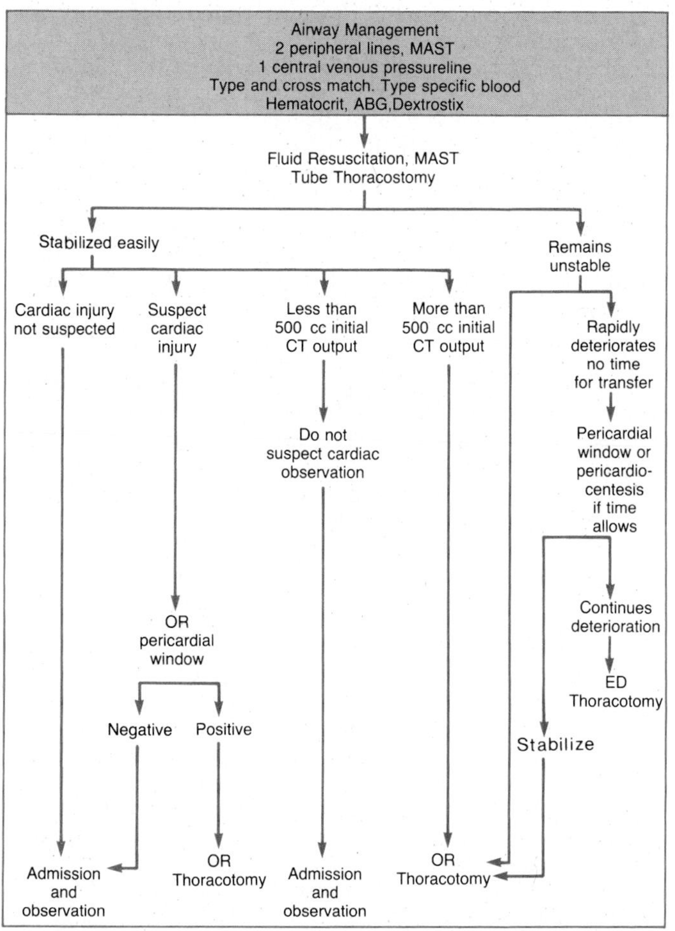

FIGURE 46-5. Algorithm for penetrating chest wound with unstable vital signs on admission. MAST = military anti-shock trousers. (From Karrel, R., et al.: Emergency diagnosis, resuscitation, and treatment of acute penetrating cardiac trauma. Ann. Emerg. Med. *11*:504, 1982.)

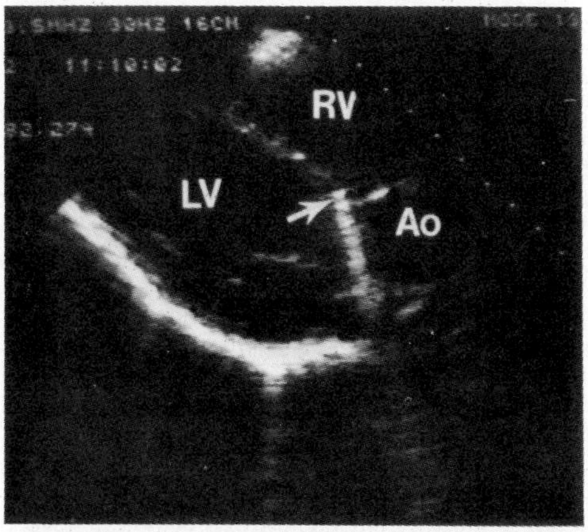

FIGURE 46-6. Two-dimensional echocardiographic image in the left parasternal long-axis view. A bullet fragment (arrow) is located high in the interventricular septum and has the typical appearance of such missiles with dense trailing reverberations. Ao = aortic root; LV = left ventricle; RV = right ventricle. (From Hassett, A., et al.: Utility of echocardiography in the management of patients with penetrating missile wounds of the heart. Reprinted with permission of the American College of Cardiology. J. Am. Coll. Cardiol. *7*:1151, 1986.)

to the ventricles is associated with distinctly higher survival. The state of consciousness and the extent of damage, if any, to the central nervous system at the time the patient is brought to the hospital also affect prognosis. It is clear that delay in performing the initial thoracotomy also adversely influences the chances for survival.

Rupture of the interventricular septum (Fig. 46-7) is often a late complication of penetrating injury as it is with blunt injury. Asfaw et al. described 12 patients with stab wounds who presented with cardiac tamponade and who had epicardial and pericardial wounds that were repaired at thoracotomy.[62] Days to years later, septal defects were diagnosed, but only four patients were symptomatic enough to warrant subsequent reoperation for closure of the defect. Residual injuries requiring reoperation can often be detected with color-flow Doppler echocardiography.[24]

Patients with preexisting valvular heart disease may be at higher risk than those with normal valves for the development of valvular injury following blunt trauma. Parmley et al. cited a 9 per cent incidence of valvular injury in their report of 546 cases of nonpenetrating chest trauma (Table 46-3).[6] Damage to the aortic valve is by far the most common of these lesions (Fig. 46-8). (Parmley's series appears to be an exception in this regard.) This is followed, in order, by damage to the mitral and tricuspid valves, presumably owing to the higher pressures generated by blunt trauma to the aorta. Indeed, sustained damage of the aortic valve should be suspected in any patient without a history of heart disease who presents with a heart murmur after severe blunt trauma to the chest. Damage to cardiac valves may also occur as a consequence of penetrating wounds of the heart, but, in contrast to the damage caused by nonpenetrating injury, these are rarely solitary lesions.[63,64] Blunt chest trauma has also been reported to cause bioprosthetic valve dysfunction.[65,66]

CLINICAL FEATURES AND DIAGNOSIS. New, loud, musical murmurs are characteristic of injury to the valves and their supporting structures. The combination of a high-pitched diastolic blowing murmur with a widened pulse pressure following blunt trauma to the chest suggests rupture of the *aortic valve*. The murmur and the hemodynamic consequences of the rupture may not appear for several days following the trauma. Aortic regurgitation may also occur transiently owing to perivalvular edema or hemorrhage.

Rupture of the *mitral valve* or of a papillary muscle appears to occur as a consequence of sudden obstruction of left ventricular outflow due to blunt injury in early diastole. It is usually associated with the development of precordial pain and a loud, harsh holosystolic murmur that radiates to the apex. Fulminant pulmonary edema quickly develops; compensation in those patients with lesser degrees of regurgitation due to torn leaflets or chordae tendineae may remain for longer periods of time, although they may eventually show signs of decompensation.

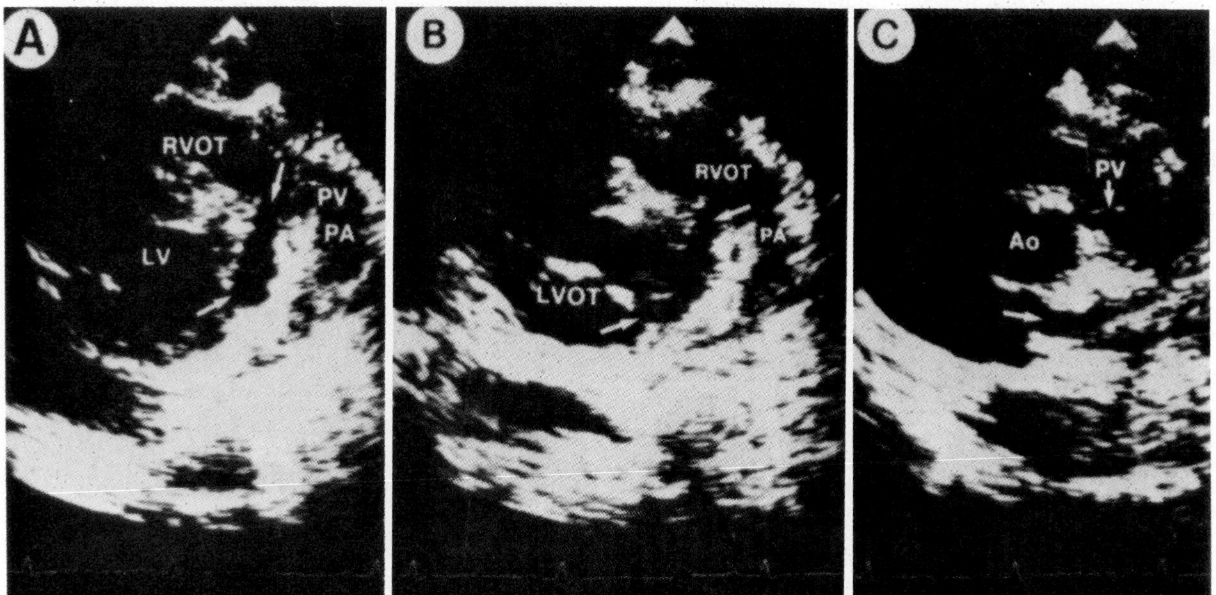

FIGURE 46-7. Two-dimensional echocardiogram from the parasternal short-axis position in a patient with a ventricular septal defect caused by knife stabbing. *A,* A defect is seen in the interventricular septum (arrows) between the left ventricle (LV) and the right ventricular outflow tract (RVOT) just proximal to the pulmonary valve (PV). *B,* At a slightly higher level the defect originates in the left ventricular outflow tract (LVOT) and exits in the distal right ventricular outflow tract. *C,* At an even higher level, but just below the aorta (Ao) and left atrium, a portion of the defect is seen (arrow). PA = pulmonary artery. (From Goldfarb, M. S., et al.: Two-dimensional Doppler echocardiographic diagnosis of a traumatic intracardiac shunt. Am. J. Cardiol. *57*:494, 1986.)

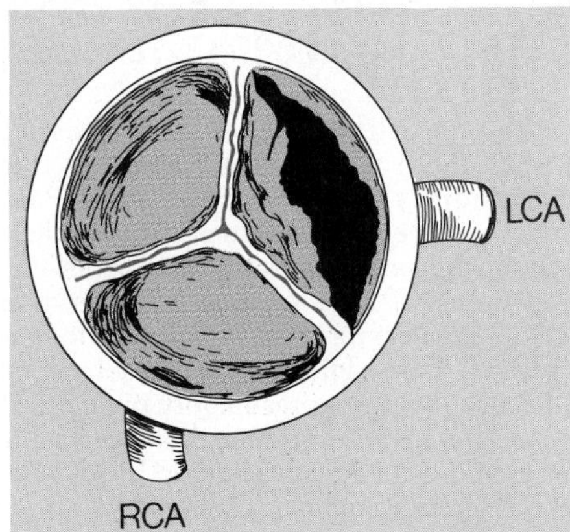

FIGURE 46-8. Diagram showing avulsion of the left coronary cusp of the aortic valve due to blunt chest trauma. (From Devineni, R., and McKenzie, F. N.: Avulsion of a normal aortic valve cusp due to blunt chest injury. J. Trauma *24*:910, © by Williams and Wilkins, 1984.)

Rupture of the *tricuspid valve* is not as rare as previously thought[67,68] and is more benign than mitral valve rupture, with symptoms ranging from fatigue to ascites and edema. Physical findings can be striking, with prominent systolic venous pulsations, hepatic pulsations, and a typical holosystolic murmur with inspiratory accentuation.

TREATMENT AND PROGNOSIS. The prognosis depends largely on the severity of the regurgitation. Since the lesion usually develops suddenly, the ventricle does not have the opportunity to adapt to this burden, as it does in most forms of chronic valvular regurgitation. Obviously, the baseline condition of the ventricle prior to the trauma, the presence of other injuries occurring simultaneously, and the severity of the regurgitation affect the heart's ability to tolerate the insult. When effective surgical treatment is not possible, survival without the need for operation is not uncommon in patients with mild or moderate regurgitation. With severe left ventricular failure due to a ruptured mitral valve or papillary muscle, however, early surgery is mandatory.

The diagnosis of acute left ventricular failure may be difficult immediately after serious trauma, because fractured ribs and pulmonary contusions may be blamed for the shortness of breath and dyspnea. When left ventricular failure develops slowly or the lesion is not hemodynamically significant, as with lesser degrees of injury, medical therapy may suffice. Hemorrhage into a papillary muscle may cause late necrosis and delayed rupture, and these patients must be observed carefully.

Post-traumatic *tricuspid* regurgitation appears to have a more benign course, and many patients survive for long periods with supportive treatment. However, when failure does occur, valve replacement is the procedure of choice.

INJURIES TO THE CORONARY ARTERIES AND GREAT VESSELS

CORONARY ARTERIES

Transmural myocardial infarctions have been reported following blunt trauma, (including trauma to the head)[69] but angiographic confirmation of coronary obstruction is uncommon, and, when found, its relationship to preexisting coronary atherosclerosis may be difficult to determine. When infarction occurs, it may not be clear whether it results directly from myocardial contusion, from trauma to a coronary artery, or from some combination of these two processes. In many cases of myocardial infarction, preexisting coronary artery disease has been present, and it is reasonable to postulate that the injury dislodges a plaque, which then obstructs the vessel completely. However, it is also possible that a normal coronary artery becomes occluded, by either a traumatically induced intimal tear or hemorrhage.[70] Indeed, coronary arteriography has provided strong evidence that myocardial infarction follows blunt chest trauma in previously asymptomatic persons with normal vessels except for complete obstruction of the vessel supplying the infarcted area (Fig. 46-9).[36] The complications of myocardial infarction—arrhythmias, pump failure, and late development of aneurysms—are similar when the lesion has an atherosclerotic basis, and treatment is similar as well. However, it may be anticipated that *following survival from the initial episode, the long-term prognosis will be more favorable in patients with traumatic damage of a coronary artery,* because the remaining vessels are usually normal. There are exceptions, however.[71]

ANEURYSM. Left ventricular *aneurysm and pseudoaneurysm* following injury to the coronary arteries can lead to ventricular rupture, cardiac failure, embolism, or arrhythmia. Operative intervention is indicated in the presence of a pseudoaneurysm, in which the myocardium has actually ruptured but in which a thrombus, fibrous tissue, and/or pericardium prevent exsanguination, since external rupture—an event that is usually fatal—is likely to occur ultimately if the condition is left untreated. Pseudoaneurysm can often be differentiated from true aneurysm by contrast or radionuclide angiography (p. 1349).

FISTULA. Formation of an *arteriovenous fistula* is an unusual complication of traumatic damage of a coronary artery.[72] Injury to the right coronary artery is more commonly followed by an arteriovenous fistula than is injury to the left. The venous side of the fistula may be the coronary sinus, the great cardiac vein (Fig. 46-10), the right atrium, or the right ventricle; in the last instance, the fistula should be termed an "arteriocameral fistula." The murmur in traumatic coronary arteriovenous or arteriocameral fistula is usually loud, widely radiating, and continuous; the electrocardiogram frequently shows transmural myocardial infarction, and the roentgenogram exhibits cardiomegaly with increased pulmonary vascularity. In patients who do not undergo surgical repair, symptoms of congestive heart failure and chest pain are frequent unless the shunt is minimal.

Espada et al. reported nine patients with *coronary artery lacerations* among a series of 76 penetrating wounds of the heart, including seven patients with stab wounds and two with gunshot wounds.[73] The left anterior descending coronary artery is the vessel most commonly involved, and at operation, the treatment of choice is suture-ligation of the cut vessel with coronary artery bypass grafting if the lacerated vessel is large and the lesion is a proximal one. Angiography is not advised in the emergency setting, as it is with nonpenetrating trauma. However, postoperative angiography is useful in localizing the presence of possible residual injuries such as a coronary arteriocameral fistula.

INJURIES TO THE GREAT VESSELS (See also p. 1551)

Rupture of the aorta is one of the most common traumatic lesions involving the heart or great vessels. In one of every six automobile accident victims dying from blunt chest trauma the aorta is ruptured.[74] To a lesser extent, aortic rupture also occurs with falls from heights and other types of crushing injuries.[75] Rupture occurs in the isthmus in 90 per cent of

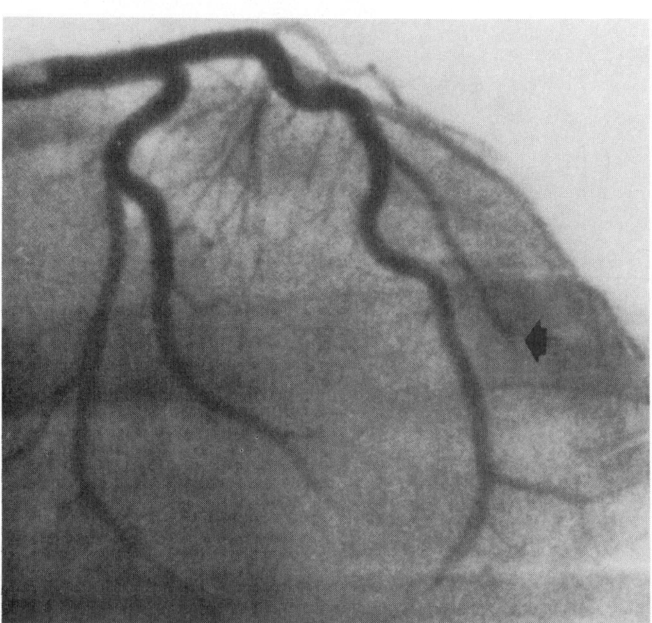

FIGURE 46-9. Coronary angiography of the left coronary artery (RAO projection) 3 days after an auto accident shows a nonocclusive thrombus in the left main artery and distal occlusion of the left anterior descending coronary artery (arrow) and of a diagonal branch. (From Unterberg, C., et al.: Traumatic thrombosis of the left main coronary artery and myocardial infarction caused by blunt chest trauma. Clin. Cardiol. *12*:672, 1989. Copyrighted and reprinted with permission of Clinical Cardiology Publishing Co., Inc., and/or the Foundation for Advances in Medicine and Science.)

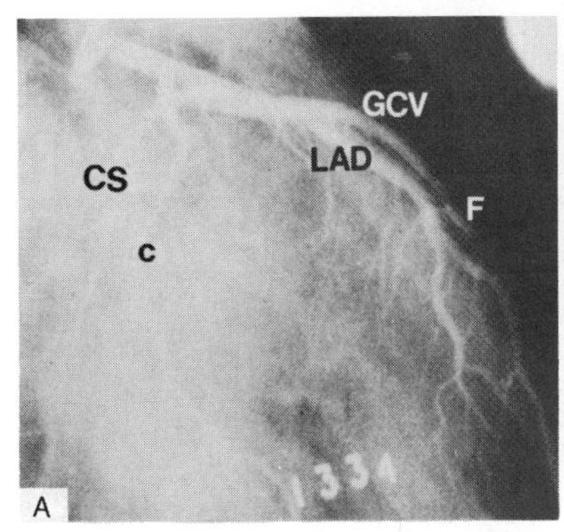

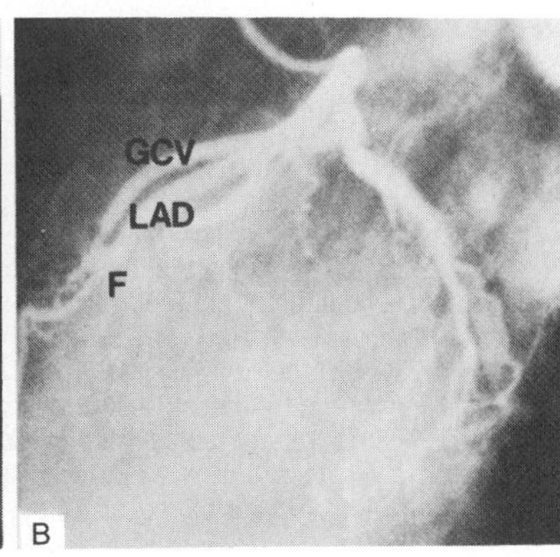

FIGURE 46-10. Left coronary arteriograms *(A)* in the right anterior oblique projection and *(B)* in the left anterior oblique projection in a patient six weeks after a penetrating chest injury. The fistula (F) can be seen arising from the second diagonal branch of the left anterior descending coronary artery (LAD) with early opacification of the great cardiac vein (GCV) and coronary sinus (CS). C = circumflex branch. (From Martin, R., et al.: Late pericardial tamponade and coronary arteriovenous fistula after trauma. Br. Heart J. *55*:216, 1986.)

cases. Multiple tears may be present in some patients, and in others the edges of the torn aorta may be separated by several centimeters, producing a mediastinal hematoma or pseudoaneurysm.

It has been estimated that 10 to 20 per cent of patients with ruptured aortas live long enough to be treated successfully under ideal circumstances, which include a high level of awareness of the possibility of aortic rupture in victims of automobile accidents as well as a well-coordinated team approach.[76] As with cardiac injury, rupture of the aorta may be overshadowed by injuries to other organs, and the diagnosis may be overlooked.[77] Common clinical and radiological findings are listed in Table 46-4. Patients with aortic rupture often complain of pain in the back in addition to the chest, as do patients with aortic dissection (p. 1535). If the expanding mediastinal hematoma or false aneurysm narrows the aortic lumen, or if the torn intima and media cause partial aortic obstruction, ischemia of the spinal cord and kidneys may ensue. A systolic murmur may be heard in the midscapular region, and widening of the superior mediastinum is visible on the chest roentgenogram (Fig. 47-23, p. 1550) along with other findings.[78,79]

A diagnostic triad that occurs in well over half the cases of ruptured aorta consists of (1) increased arterial pressure and pulse amplitude in the upper extremities, (2) decreased pressure and pulse amplitude in the lower extremities, and (3) radiological evidence of widening of the superior mediastinum.[80] Chronic rupture of the aorta may be manifested by hoarseness, dysphagia, and cough. The diagnosis can be confirmed by aortography, which should be performed as soon as the nature of the injury is suspected. CT scanning is *not* a useful screening procedure;[80] aortography is very useful for diagnosing and localizing the injury. The entire thoracic aorta and its branches should be visualized so as not to overlook a rupture occurring at an unusual site or multiple sites of rupture (Fig. 46-11).[82]

PENETRATING TRAUMA TO THE GREAT VESSELS. This is usually the result of bullet or stab wounds and occurs most commonly in conjunction with cardiac wounds. Cardiac tamponade is a frequent complication of injury to the intrapericardial segment of one of the great vessels, but when it is extrapericardial, massive hemothorax is usually the presenting finding. The superior vena cava, trachea, or esophagus or some combination of these structures may be compressed if a large mediastinal hematoma forms as a result of bleeding. Injury to the innominate or carotid arteries may compress these vessels, with resultant neurological signs. An arteriovenous fistula may develop with symptoms of congestive heart failure accompanied by a systolic or, more commonly, a continuous murmur.[83] These fistulous connections may also involve the systemic and pulmonary vessel.[84] Blunt trauma has also been reported to cause transection of the inferior vena cava.[85]

Penetrating injury to the great vessels should be suspected in any patient in whom a projectile traverses the mediastinum and is suggested by radiological evidence of a widened mediastinum. Aortography should be performed immediately, provided that emergency thoracotomy for shock or tamponade can be deferred briefly. Immediate operation, sometimes using a heparinized shunt between the ascending and descending aorta, should be carried out as soon as the diagnosis of thoracic aortic disruption has been established.[86] Pickard et al. described their experi-

TABLE 46-4 CLINICAL AND RADIOLOGICAL FINDINGS IN PATIENTS WITH AORTIC INJURY

A. CLINICAL FINDINGS	PERCENTAGE OF PATIENTS
Bone fractures (other than ribs)	75
External evidence of thoracic injury	66
Upper extremity hypertension	30-45
Systolic murmur	20-45
Dyspnea	10
Paralysis	10
Back pain	7
Dysphagia	4
B. RADIOLOGICAL FINDINGS	**PERCENTAGE OF PATIENTS**
Abnormal aortic outline	100
Mediastinal widening	50-100
NG tube displaced to right	100
Displaced SVC	85
Left apical cap	65-93
Opacification of AP clear space	60
First or second rib fractures	50
Depressed left bronchus	35-80
Pneumothorax/pneumomediastinum	35-50
Hemothorax	20-65
Displaced right paraspinous line	15-55
Pulmonary contusion	15-50
Displaced left paraspinous line	15-25
Deviation of trachea to right	10-55

SVC = superior vena cava; NG = nasogastric; AP = anteroposterior.
Adapted from Barcia, T. C., and Livoni, J. P.: Indications for angiography in blunt thoracic trauma. Radiology *147*:15, 1983.

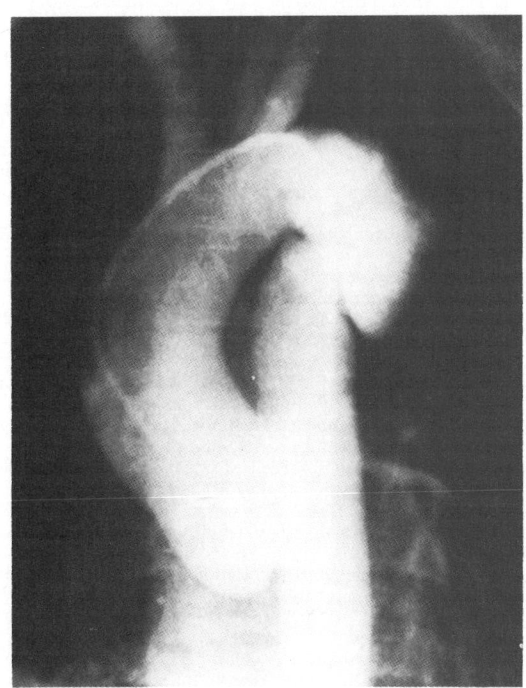

FIGURE 46-11. In a 27-year-old male, acute false and irregular aneurysm of the thoracic aorta just distal to the left subclavian artery. (Reproduced with permission from Andresen, J., and Axelsen, F.: Traumatic rupture of the thoracic aorta. Scand. J. Thorac. Cardiovasc. Surg. *14*:281, 1980.)

ence with 22 patients with transection of the descending thoracic aorta secondary to blunt trauma who reached the hospital alive; five patients died shortly after admission, three died in the operating room, three died within 30 days of operation, and one died more than 1 year after the injury.[87] Ten patients were long-term survivors. A Dacron tube graft was utilized to bridge the defect in the majority of patients.

In order to avoid the problem inherent in heparinization, i.e., bleeding from what are often multiple sites of trauma, tears of the descending thoracic aorta may often be repaired without cardiopulmonary bypass by simple aortic cross-clamping, as long as the cross-clamp time is restricted to less than 30 minutes.[88,89] An experienced surgeon can interpose a graft into the aorta with a total occlusion time ranging from 13 to 21 minutes, and ischemic injury to the spinal cord or kidneys should not occur. This technique may be aided by the intravenous administration of nitroprusside, which can maintain proximal aortic systolic pressure below 140 mm Hg.

Antiadrenergic agents such as guanethidine, reserpine, and propranolol, which have been utilized in the treatment of spontaneous dissection of the aorta (p. 1540), may also have a role in treatment of patients with aortic rupture if, for logistical reasons, operation must be deferred.

REFERENCES

1. Committee on Trauma and Committee on Shock: Accidental death and disability: The neglected diseases of modern society. Washington, D.C., National Academy of Sciences, 1965, p. 5.
2. Cheitlin, M. D.: Cardiovascular trauma. Circulation *65*:1529, 1982, and Circulation *66*:244, 1982.
3. Mayfield, W., and Hurley, E. J.: Blunt cardiac trauma. Am. J. Surg. *148*:162, 1984.
4. Sherman, M. M., Saini, V. K., Yarnoz, M. D., Ramp, J., Williams, L. F., and Berger, R. L.: Management of penetrating heart wounds. Am. J. Surg. *135*:553, 1978.
5. Mattox, K. L., Feliciano, D. V., Burch, J., et al.: Five thousand seven hundred sixty cardiovascular injuries in 4459 patients: Epidemiologic evolution 1958 to 1987. Ann. Surg. *209*:698, 1989.

NONPENETRATING CARDIAC INJURY

6. Parmley, L. F., Manion, W. C., and Mattingly, T. W.: Nonpenetrating traumatic injury of the heart. Circulation *18*:371, 1958.
7. Glock, Y., Massabuau, P., and Puel, P.: Cardiac damage in non-penetrating chest injuries. J. Cardiovasc. Surg. *30*:27, 1989.
8. Rothstein, R. J.: Myocardial contusion. J.A.M.A. *250*:2189, 1983.
9. Matthews, R. V., French, W. J., and Criley, J. M.: Chest trauma and subvalvular left ventricular aneurysms. Chest *95*:474, 1989.
10. DeMuth, W. E., Lerner, E. H., and Liedtke, A. J.: Nonpenetrating injury of the heart: An experimental model. J. Trauma *13*:639, 1973.
11. Clifford, R. P., and Gill, K. S.: Traumatic rupture of the pericardium with dislocation of the heart. Injury *16*:123, 1984.
12. Miller, F. A., Jr., Seward, J. B., Gersh, B. J., et al.: Two-dimensional echocardiographic findings in cardiac trauma. Am. J. Cardiol. *50*:1022, 1982.
13. Lau, V.-K., Viano, D. C., and Doty, D. B.: Experimental cardiac trauma—Ballistics of a captive bolt pistol. J. Trauma *21*:39, 1982.
14. Pandian, N. G., Skorton, D. J., Doty, D. B., and Kerber, R. E.: Immediate diagnosis of acute myocardial contusion by two-dimensional echocardiography: Studies in a canine model of blunt chest trauma. J. Am. Coll. Cardiol. *2*:488, 1983.
15. Tenzer, M. L.: The spectrum of myocardial contusion: A review. J. Trauma *25*:620, 1985.
16. Frazee, R. C., Mucha, P., Jr., Farnell, M. B., and Miller, F. A., Jr.: Objective evaluation of blunt cardiac trauma. J. Trauma *26*:510, 1986.
17. Snow, N., Richardson, J. D., and Flint, L. M., Jr.: Myocardial contusion: Implications for patients with multiple traumatic injuries. Surgery *92*:744, 1982.
18. Kumar, S. A., Puri, V. K., Mittal, V. K., and Cortez, J.: Myocardial contusion following nonfatal blunt chest trauma. J. Trauma *23*:327, 1983.
19. Torres-Mirabal, P., Gruenberg, J. C., Brown, R. S., and Obeid, F. N.: Spectrum of myocardial contusion. Am Surg. *48*:383, 1982.
20. Frazee, R. C., Mucha, P., Jr., Farnell, M. B., and Miller, F. A., Jr.: Objective evaluation of blunt cardiac trauma. J. Trauma *26*:510, 1986.
21. Chiu, C. L., Roelofs, J. D., Go, R. T., et al.: Coronary angiographic and scintigraphic findings in experimental cardiac contusion. Radiology *116*:679, 1975.
22. Sutherland, G. R., Cheung, H. W., Holliday, R. L., et al.: Hemodynamic adaptation to acute myocardial contusion complicating blunt chest injury. Am. J. Cardiol. *57*:291, 1986.
23. Schamp, D. J., Plotnick, G. D., Croteau, D., et al.: Clinical significance of radionuclide angiographically-determined abnormalities following acute blunt chest trauma. Am. Heart J. *116*:500, 1988.
24. Mattox, K. L., Limacher, M. C., Feliciano, D. V., et al.: Cardiac evaluation following heart injury. J. Trauma *25*:758, 1985.
25. Fox, K. M., Rowland, E., Krikler, D. M., et al.: Electrophysiological manifestations on nonpenetrating cardiac trauma. Br. Heart J. *43*:458, 1980.
26. Cooperman, Y., Low, S., and Laniado, S.: Traumatic heart block. PACE *12*:25, 1989.
27. Bognolo, D. A., Rabow, F. I., Vijayanagar, R. R., and Eckstein, P. F.: Traumatic sinus node dysfunction. Ann. Emerg. Med. *11*:319, 1982.
28. Évora, P. R. B., Ribeiro, P. J. F., Brasil, J. C. F., et al.: Late surgical repair of ventricular septal defect due to nonpenetrating chest trauma: Review and report of two contrasting cases. J. Trauma *25*:1007, 1985.
29. Torres-Mirabal, P., Gruenberg, J. C., Talbert, J. G., and Brown, R. S.: Ventricular function in myocardial contusion: A preliminary study. Crit. Care Med. *10*:19, 1982.
30. Desiderio, M. A.: The potentiation of the response to blunt cardiac trauma by ethanol in dogs. J. Trauma *26*:467, 1986.
31. Dubrow, T. J., Mihalka, J., Eisenhauer, D. M., et al.: Myocardial contusion in the stable patient: What level of care is appropriate? Surgery *106*:267, 1989.
32. Soliman, M. H., and Waxman, K.: Value of a conventional approach to the diagnosis of traumatic cardiac contusion after chest injury. Crit. Care Med. *15*:218, 1987.
33. Hossack, K. F., Moreno, C. A., Vanway, C. W., and Burdick, D. C.: Frequency of cardiac contusion in nonpenetrating chest injury. Am. J. Cardiol. *61*:391, 1988.
34. Watt, A. H., and Stephens, M. R.: Myocardial infarction after blunt chest trauma incurred during rugby football that later required cardiac transplantation. Br. Heart J. *55*:408, 1986.
35. Espinosa, R., Badui, E., Castaño, R., and Madrid, R.: Acute posterior wall myocardial infarction secondary to football chest trauma. Chest *88*:928, 1985.
36. Unterberg, C. Buchwald, A., and Viegand, V.: Traumatic thrombosis of the left main coronary artery and myocardial infarction caused by blunt chest trauma. Clin. Cardiol. *12*:672, 1989.
37. Chang, H., Chu, S-H., and Lee, Y-T.: Traumatic aorto-right atrial fistula after blunt chest injury. Ann. Thorac. Surg. *45*:778, 1989.
38. Getz, B. S., Davies, E., Steinberg, S. M., et al.: Blunt cardiac trauma resulting in right atrial rupture. J.A.M.A. *255*:761, 1986.
39. Hines, G. L., Doyle, E., and Acinapura, A. J.: Post-traumatic ventricular septal defect, mitral insufficiency, and multiple coronary cameral fistulas. J. Trauma *17*:234, 1977.
40. Pickard, L. R., Mattox, K. L., and Beall, A. C., Jr.: Ventricular septal defect from blunt chest injury. J. Trauma *20*:329, 1980.
41. Leavitt, B. J., Meyer, J. A., Morton, J. R., et al.: Survival following nonpenetrating traumatic rupture of cardiac chambers. Ann. Thorac. Surg. *44*:532, 1987.
42. Eisenberg, M. S., Horwood, B. T., Cummins, R. O., et al.: Cardiac arrest and resuscitation: A tale of 29 cities. Ann. Emerg. Med. *19*:179, 1990.
43. Gerry, J. L., Bulkley, B. H., and Hutchins, G. M.: Rupture of the papillary muscle of the tricuspid valve. A complication of cardiopulmonary resuscitation and a rare cause of tricuspid insufficiency. Am. J. Cardiol. *40*:825, 1977.
44. Baker, P. B., Keyhani-Rofagha, S., Graham, R. L., and Sharma, H. M.: Dissecting hematoma (aneurysm) of coronary arteries. Am. J. Med. *80*:317, 1986.

PENETRATING CARDIAC INJURY

45. Naughton, M. J., Brissie, R. M., Bessey, P. Q., et al.: Demography of penetrating cardiac trauma. Ann Surg. *209*:676, 1989.
46. Fallahnejad, M., Kutty, A. C. K., and Wallace, H. W.: Secondary lesions of penetrating cardiac injuries. Ann. Surg. *191*:228, 1980.
47. Auge, J. M., Oriol, A., Serra, C., and Crexells, C.: The use of pigtail catheters for retrieval of foreign bodies from the cardiovascular system. Cathet. Cardiovasc. Diagn. *10*:625, 1984.
48. McIvor, M. E., Kaufman, S. L., Satre, R., et al.: Search and retrieval of a radiolucent foreign object. Cath. Cardiovasc. Diagn. *16*:19, 1989.
49. Gehl, L., Iskandriann, A. N., Goel, I., et al.: Cardiac perforation with tamponade during cardiac catheterization. Cathet. Cardiovasc. Diagn. *8*:293, 1982.
50. Goldbaum, T. S., Jacob, A. S., Smith, D. F., et al.: Cardiac tamponade following percutaneous transluminal coronary angioplasty: Four case reports. Cathet. Cardiovasc. Diagn. *11*:413, 1985.
51. Przybojewski, J. Z.: Endomyocardial biopsy: a review of the literature. Cathet. Cardiovasc. Diagn. *11*:287, 1985.
52. Anastasious-Nana, M. I., O'Connell, J. B., Nanas, J. N., et al.: Relative efficiency and risk of endomyocardial biopsy: Comparisons in heart transplant and nontransplant patients. Cath. Cardiovasc. Diagn. *16*:7, 1989.
53. Cummings, R. G., Wesly, R. L. R., Adams, D. H., and Lowe, J. E.: Pneumopericardium resulting in cardiac tamponade. Ann. Thoracic Surg. *37*:511, 1984.
54. Marshall, W. G., Jr., Bell, J. L., and Kouchoukos, N. T.: Penetrating cardiac trauma. J. Trauma *24*:147, 1984.
55. Whye, D., Barish, R., Almquist, T., et al.: Echocardiographic diagnosis of acute pericardial effusion in penetrating chest trauma. Am. J. Emerg. Med. *6*:21, 1988.
56. Hassett, A. Moran, J., Sabiston, D. C., and Kisslo, J.: Utility of echocardiography in the management of patients with penetrating missile wounds of the heart. J. Am. Coll. Cardiol. *7*:1151, 1986.
57. Miller, J. T., Richards, K. L., Miller, J. F., and Crawford, M. H.: Doppler echocardiographic determination of the cause of a systolic murmur following penetrating chest trauma. Am. Heart J. *111*:988, 1986.
58. Goldfarb, M. S., Walpole, H. T., Jr., Landolt, C. C., et al.: Two-dimensional Doppler echocardiographic diagnosis of a traumatic intracardiac shunt. Am. J. Cardiol. *57*:494, 1986.

59. Martin, L. F., Mavroudis, C., Dyess, D. L., et al.: The first 70 years' experience managing cardiac disruption due to penetrating and blunt injuries at the University of Louisville. Am. Surg. *52*:14, 1986.
60. Bergin, P. J.: Aortic thrombosis and peripheral embolization after thoracic gunshot wound diagnosed by transesophageal echocardiography. Am. Heart J. *119*:688, 1990.
61. Alsofrom, D. J., Marcus, N. H., Seigel, R. S., et al.: Shotgun pellet embolization from the chest to the middle cerebral arteries. J. Trauma *22*:155, 1982.
62. Asfaw, I., Thoms, N. W., and Arfulu, A.: Interventricular septal defects from penetrating injuries of the heart. A report of 12 cases and review of the literature. J. Thorac. Cardiovasc. Surg. *69*:450, 1975.
63. Rustad, D. G., Hopeman, A. R., Murr, P. C., and VanWay, C. W., III: Aorta-cardiac fistula with aortic valve injury from penetrating trauma. J. Trauma *26*:266, 1986.
64. Werne, C., Sagraves, S. G., and Costa, C.: Mitral and tricuspid valve rupture from blunt trauma sustained during a motor vehicle collision. J. Trauma *29*:15, 1989.
65. Reinfeld, H. B., Agatston, A. S., Robinson, M. J., and Hildner, F. J.: Bioprosthetic mitral valve dysfunction following blunt chest trauma. Am. Heart J. *111*:800, 1986.
66. Rumisek, J. D., Robonowitz, M., Virmani, R., et al.: Bioprosthetic heart valve rupture associated with trauma. J. Trauma *26*:276, 1986.
67. Eskilsson, J.: Tricuspid insufficiency caused by nonpenetrating chest trauma: Report of two cases diagnosed by Doppler cardiography. Acta Med. Scand. *218*:347, 1985.
68. Gayet, C., Pierre, B., Delahaye, J-P., et al.: Traumatic tricuspid insufficiency: An underdiagnosed disease. Chest *92*:429, 1987.
69. Bashour, T. T., Morelli, R. L., Cunningham, T., and Budge, W. R.: Acute coronary thrombosis following head trauma in a young man. Am. Heart J. *119*:676, 1990.
70. Sabbah, H. N., Mohyi, J., and Stein, P. D.: Coronary arteriography in dogs following blunt cardiac trauma: A longitudinal assessment. Cath. Cardiovasc. Diagn. *15*:155, 1988.
71. Watt, A. H., and Stephens, M. R.: Myocardial infarction after blunt chest trauma incurred during rugby football that later required cardiac transplantation. Br. Heart J. *55*:408, 1986.
72. Martin, R., Mitchell, A., and Dhalla, N.: Late pericardial tamponade and coronary arteriovenous fistula after trauma. Br. Heart J. *55*:216, 1986
73. Espada, R., Whisennard, H. H., Mattox, K. L., and Beall, A. C., Jr.: Surgical management of penetrating injuries to the coronary arteries. Surgery *78*:755, 1975.
74. Greendyke, R. M.: Traumatic rupture of the aorta. Special reference to automobile accidents. J.A.M.A. *195*:527, 1966.
75. Shaikh, K. A., Schwab, C. W., and Camishion, R. C.: Aortic rupture in blunt trauma. Am. Surg. *52*:47, 1986.
76. Ayella, R. J., Hankins, J. R., Turney, S. Z., and Cowley, R. A.: Ruptured thoracic aorta due to blunt trauma. J. Trauma *17*:199, 1977.
77. Barcia, T. C., and Livoni, J. P.: Indications for angiography in blunt thoracic trauma. Radiology *147*:15, 1983.
78. Gundry, S. R., Burney, R. E., Mackenzie, J. R., et al.: Assessment of mediastinal widening associated with traumatic rupture of the aorta. J. Trauma *23*:293, 1983.
79. Heystraten, F. M., Rosenbusch, G., Kingma, L. M., et al.: Chest radiography in acute traumatic rupture of the thoracic aorta. Acta Radiolog. *29*:411, 1988.
80. Symbas, P. N., Tyras, D. H., Ware, R. E., and Hatcher, C. R., Jr.: Rupture of the aorta. A diagnostic triad. Ann. Thorac. Surg. *15*:405, 1973.
81. Miller, F. B., Richardson, J. D., Thomas, H. A., et al.: Role of CT in diagnosis of major arterial injury after blunt thoracic trauma. Surgery *106*:596, 1989.
82. Kirsh, M. M., Orringer, M. B., Behrendt, D. M., et al.: Management of unusual traumatic ruptures of the aorta. Surg. Gynecol. Obstet. *146*:365, 1978.
83. Machiedo, G. W., Jain, K. M., Swan, K. G., et al.: Traumatic aorto-caval fistula. J. Trauma *23*:243, 1983.
84. Arom, K. V., and Lyons, G. W.: Traumatic pulmonary arteriovenous fistula. J. Thorac. Cardiovasc. Surg. *70*:918, 1975.
85. Peitzman, A. B., Udekwu, A. O., Pevec, W., and Albrink, M.: Tansection of the inferior vena cava from blunt thoracic trauma: Case reports. J. Trauma *29*:534, 1989.
86. Akins, C. W., Buckley, M. J., Daggett, W., et al.: Acute traumatic disruption of the thoracic aorta: A ten-year experience. Ann. Thorac. Surg. *31*:305, 1981.
87. Pickard, L. R., Mattox, K. L., Espada, R., et al.: Transection of the descending thoracic aorta secondary to blunt trauma. J. Trauma *17*:749, 1977.
88. Vasko, J. S., Raess, D. H., Williams, T. E., Jr., et al.: Nonpenetrating trauma to the thoracic aorta. Surgery *82*:400, 1977.
89. Turney, S. Z., Attar, S., Ayella, R., et al.: Traumatic rupture of the aorta. A five-year experience. J. Thorac. Cardiovasc. Surg. *72*:727, 1976.

47

Diseases of the Aorta

by KIM A. EAGLE, M.D., and ROMAN W. DE SANCTIS, M.D.

THE NORMAL AORTA

FUNCTION. Appropriately called "the greatest artery" by the ancients, the aorta is admirably suited for its task. This thin but large and remarkably tough vessel must absorb the impact of 2.5 to 3 billion heartbeats in an average lifetime while carrying roughly 200,000,000 liters of blood to the body.

Arteries can be categorized as either "conductance" or "resistance" vessels. Conductance vessels are the conduits for blood, and the aorta is the ultimate conductance vessel. It is composed of three layers: a thin, inner tunica intima; a thick middle layer, the tunica media; and a rather thin outer layer, the tunica adventitia. The strength of the aorta lies in the tunica media, which is composed of laminated but intertwining sheets of elastic tissue arranged in a spiral manner that affords maximum tensile strength. As thin as it is, the wall of the aorta can withstand the experimental pressure of thousands of millimeters of mercury without bursting. In contrast to peripheral arteries, the aortic media contains very little smooth muscle, although there is a network of some smooth muscle and collagen between the elastic layers. This tremendous accretion of elastic tissue in the aorta gives it not only great tensile strength but also elasticity, which serves a vital circulatory role. The aortic intima is a thin, delicate layer lined by endothelium and easily traumatized. The adventitia contains mainly collagen but also houses the important vasa vasorum and lymphatics, which nourish the aortic wall.

As systole develops, part of the force generated by the contracting ventricle is converted into potential energy stored in the wall of the aorta as it is distended by the blood ejected into it. In diastole, this potential energy in the stretched aortic wall is transformed into kinetic energy as the resilient aorta decompresses, and the force that is created acts against the column of blood contained within the lumen. With a competent aortic valve proximally, the blood is propelled distally into the arterial bed. Thus, the aorta plays a major role in circulating the blood after it is delivered into the aorta by the heart. The pulse wave itself with its milking effect is transmitted along the aorta to the periphery at a speed of about 5 meters per second. This is much faster than the velocity of the intraluminal blood, which travels only 40 to 50 cm per second.

The systolic pressure developed within the aorta is a function of the volume of blood ejected into the aorta, the compliance or distensibility of the aorta, and the resistance to blood flow. Resistance is determined primarily by the tone in the peripheral muscular arteries and arterioles and to a slight extent by the inertia of the column of blood in the aorta when systole commences. The aorta and its branches tend to stiffen with age, accounting for the increase in systolic blood pressure with advancing age.

In addition to its conductance and pumping functions, the aorta plays a role in the control of systemic vascular resistance and heart rate. Pressure-responsive receptors analogous to those in the carotid sinus lie in the ascending aorta and the aortic arch and send afferent signals to the vasomotor center in the brain stem by way of the vagus nerves. Raising the aortic pressure causes reflex bradycardia and reduction of systemic vascular resistance, whereas lowering the pressure increases the heart rate and systemic resistance.

ANATOMICAL CONSIDERATIONS. The *ascending aorta* in a normal adult is about 3 cm wide at its origin from the base of the heart and extends 5 to 6 cm cephalad to join the aortic arch. Normally, the ascending aorta lies just to the right of the midline. Its proximal portion is within the pericardial cavity. Nearby structures include the pulmonary trunk in front and the left atrium, right pulmonary artery, and right main stem bronchus behind.

The *arch of the aorta* gives rise to all the brachiocephalic vessels. It courses slightly leftward in front of the trachea and then proceeds dorsally and inferiorly above the left main stern bronchus to the left of the trachea and esophagus. The arch assumes almost a directly anteroposterior orientation in the superior mediastinum. Other closely related structures are the left phrenic and vagus nerves to the left of the arch; inferiorly lie the bifurcation of the pulmonary trunk and most of the left lung. The left recurrent laryngeal nerve also loops underneath it distally.

The *descending thoracic aorta* is the continuation of the aorta beyond the arch. It lies in the posterior mediastinum to the left of the vertebral column, gradually courses in front of the vertebral column as it descends, occupying a position behind the esophagus, and passes through the diaphragm, usually at the level of the 12th thoracic vertebra.

A small but important segment called the *aortic isthmus* is the point at which the arch and descending thoracic aorta join. This is where coarctations of the aorta are usually located, and it is also the point at which the mobile portion of the aorta—the ascending aorta and arch—becomes relatively fixed to the thorax by the pleural reflections, intercostal arteries, and left subclavian artery. The aorta is especially vulnerable to trauma at this point.

The *abdominal aorta* forms the continuation of the thoracic aorta, giving off the important splanchnic vessels and ending in the aortic bifurcation at the level of the 4th lumbar vertebra.

EXAMINATION OF THE AORTA

Unless the aorta is abnormally enlarged, the only location at which it can be palpated is in the abdomen. The ease with which it can be felt depends largely on the body habitus and on the pulse pressure; it is readily felt in thin individuals. It is quite sensitive to pressure. Auscultation usually is unrevealing in aortic diseases, except for occasional bruits at sites of narrowing of the aorta or its tributary branches. Diseases of the proximal ascending aorta sometimes involve the aortic valve, with resultant aortic insufficiency.

Chest roentgenography and fluoroscopy are valuable and simple procedures for assessing the aorta. Normally, the ascending aorta is not visible on the direct anteroposterior chest roentgenogram. The aortic arch is seen as the aortic "knob" or "knuckle" in the superior mediastinum just to the left of the vertebral column (Fig. 8–6, p. 205). The edge of the descending thoracic aorta can often be recognized to the left of the spine.

On the lateral chest roentgenogram, the proximal ascending aorta can be seen as an indistinct shadow in the middle mediastinum arising from the base of the heart. The ascending

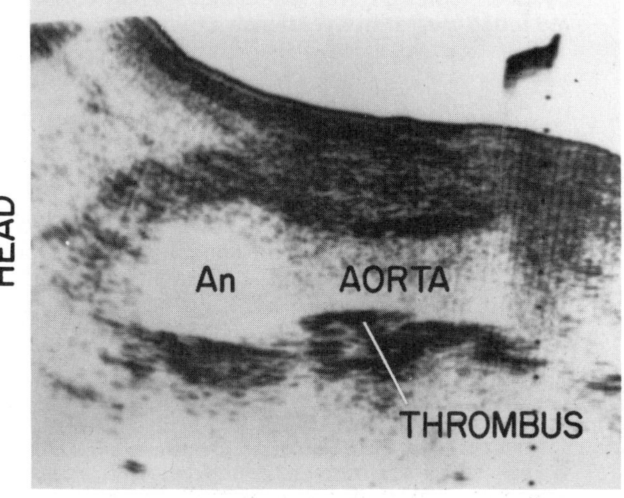

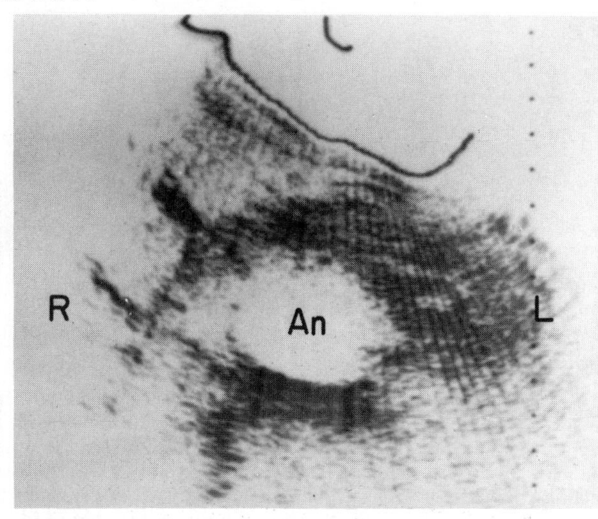

FIGURE 47-1. Cross-sectional echocardiograms of an abdominal aortic aneurysm in a 62-year-old man. *Left,* Lateral view showing a 5-cm aneurysm (An), with dilatation of the aorta distal to the aneurysm. The widened aorta is visualized down to the aortic bifurcation. Note the thrombus in the wall of the aneurysm. The dense echoes between the aneurysm and skin are made up of subcutaneous fat, muscle, and mesenteric contents. *Right,* Echocardiogram with the ultrasound beam oriented in the anteroposterior direction showing the aneurysm clearly. R and L indicate the patient's right and left sides. The distance between each of the dots aligned vertically on the right in both scans represents 1 cm. (Courtesy of Rob Kirkpatrick, M.D., Department of Radiology, Massachusetts General Hospital, Boston.)

aorta and arch are best demonstrated in a left anterior oblique projection—a view that should always be included when disease of the thoracic aorta is suspected (Fig. 8-15, p. 214).

Calcification in the aortic knob is often present, particularly in older people and patients with hypertension. It has little significance. Arteriosclerosis often results in extensive aortic calcification. The location of aortic calcification is useful in the differential diagnosis of aortic disease. Syphilis causes calcification predominantly of the ascending aorta, whereas arteriosclerotic calcification is ordinarily densest in the arch and the descending thoracic and abdominal aorta. Aneurysms of the abdominal aorta can often be seen radiographically if they are calcified. A lateral film of the abdomen is the most useful view for demonstrating them.

Normally, the aorta tends to elongate and widen slightly with age, a process which is accelerated by hypertension. Aneurysms, of course, appear as localized dilatations of the aorta. It is sometimes difficult to distinguish aneurysms from other mediastinal masses. In such cases fluoroscopy or real-time ultrasound may be very helpful by showing the presence or absence of pulsations in the mass.

Angiographic study of the aorta is of critical importance in the evaluation of aortic diseases. Aneurysms, aortic dissections, and occlusive disease of the aorta and its arterial branches can usually be readily demonstrated by a contrast study. With technical improvements in digital subtraction angiography, performed by venous injection of contrast material, adequate aortic definition should be possible while obviating catheterization of the aorta. However, this technique is limited by poor spatial resolution, artifacts caused by patient movement, and difficulty in defining anatomical detail because of overlapping blood vessels.[1]

Ultrasonography is a very important tool in the diagnosis of aortic disease (p. 106). The presence or absence of an abdominal aortic aneurysm can be definitively established by this simple noninvasive technique. In particular, two-dimensional echocardiography is extremely accurate in both diagnosing and sizing abdominal aortic aneurysms (Fig. 47-1) and can also provide valuable information about the location and size of aortic root aneurysms. Transesophageal echocardiography, particularly when combined with Doppler color flow imaging, now allows the highly accurate ultrasound assessment of both proximal and distal aortic dissection.[2,3]

Computed tomographic scanning of the body (CT scan), enhanced by intravenous injection of contrast material, is an excellent technique for noninvasive visualization of the aorta (Fig. 47-2, and Fig. 11-16, p. 320). CT scans are particularly useful for the diagnosis and sizing of thoracic and abdominal aortic aneurysms and for the diagnosis of aortic dissection and traumatic aneurysms of the aorta.[4-7] The CT scan is even more accurate than ultrasonography in determining the size of abdominal aortic aneurysms.[8] Magnetic resonance imaging (MRI) is another excellent noninvasive technique for evaluating aortic disease (Fig. 11-46, p. 336). It has advantages over CT scanning in that imaging can be performed in multiple planes (i.e., coronal and sagittal planes) and contrast agents are

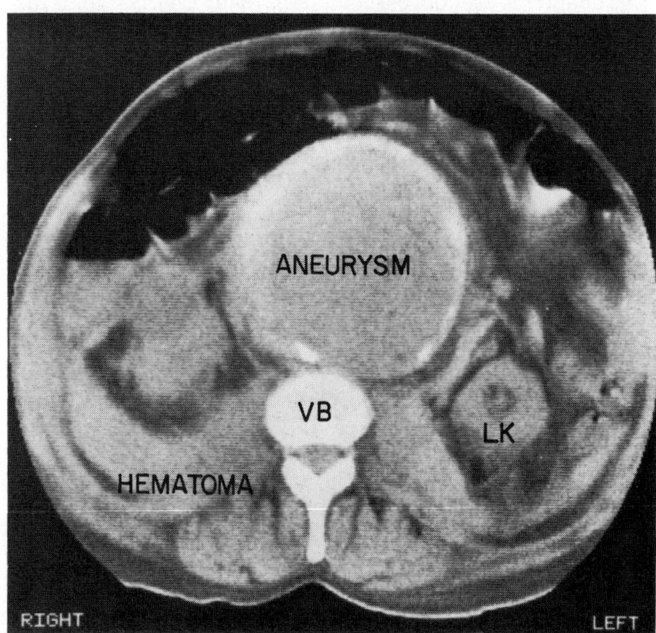

FIGURE 47-2. Abdominal CT scan showing a large, leaking abdominal aortic aneurysm. The aneurysm measures approximately 11 cm in diameter and abuts the vertebral body (VB) posteriorly. The light areas in the periphery of the aneurysm are calcific deposits in the aortic wall. The lower pole of the left kidney is identified (LK); behind the right kidney is a retroperitoneal hematoma. (Courtesy of Jack Wittenberg, M.D., Department of Radiology, Massachusetts General Hospital, Boston.)

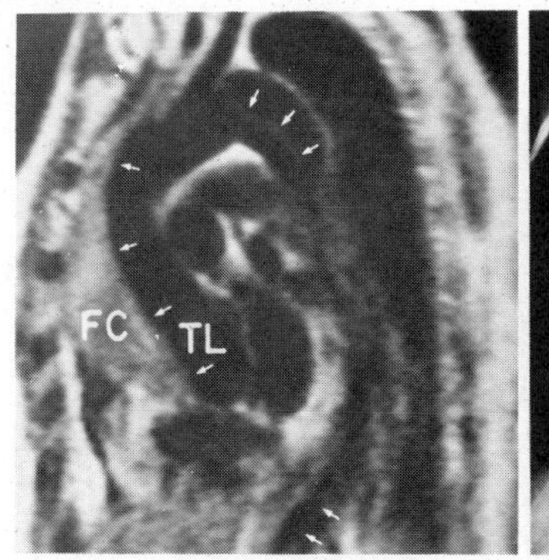

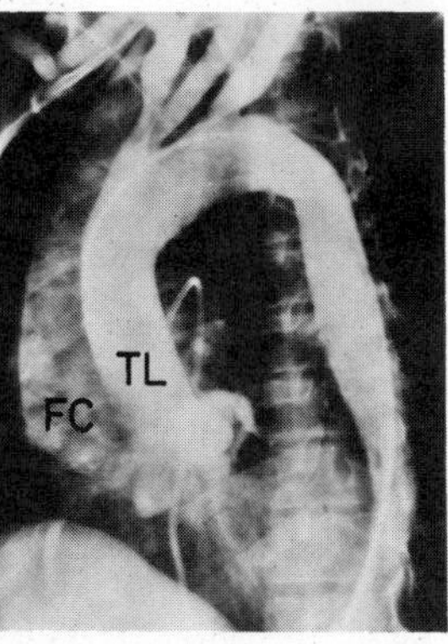

FIGURE 47–3. Nuclear magnetic resonance image in long axis (left), with corresponding aortogram (right) in a 55-year-old woman with a Type A dissection. The arrows indicate the partition between the false channel (FC) of the dissection and the true lumen (TL) of the aorta. The dissection extends into the descending thoracic aorta. The false channel shows up densely in the NMR scan because of stagnant blood blow within it. (Courtesy of Robert E. Dinsmore, M.D., Massachusetts General Hospital, Boston. NMR scan from Dinsmore, R. E., et al.: A. J. R. *146:*1286, 1986.)

unnecessary. Many studies confirm its accuracy in locating and sizing aortic aneurysms and dissections (Fig. 47–3).[9–16]

PATHOGENESIS OF DISEASES OF THE AORTA

Diseases of the aorta are either congenital or acquired.[16a] Congenital defects in turn are either gross anatomical abnormalities, such as coarctation, right aortic arch, anomalous arterial branches, double aortic arches, and so on, or histological disorders, such as degenerative abnormalities in the aortic wall that predispose to later problems (e.g., cystic medial degeneration in the Marfan syndrome and other inherited connective tissue disorders).

The only congenital gross anatomical disease considered in this chapter is pseudocoarctation (p. 1549). *Coarctation* is discussed on pages 920, 967, and 1550. All other conditions discussed either are acquired or result from congenital histological changes in the aortic wall.

Acquired diseases of the aorta are primarily the result of degenerative changes in the aortic wall. Prominent among the factors that lead to this degeneration are aging, arteriosclerosis, hypertension, and specific infectious, inflammatory, or autoimmune diseases that involve the aorta focally or diffusely. Some of these processes may affect the aortic root, with resultant aortic insufficiency, or the major arterial branches arising from the aorta. The importance of the velocity at which blood is ejected from the left ventricle (dV/dt) as a major shearing stress on the aortic wall has also been emphasized as promoting aortic dissection.

Some patients with aortic aneurysms have been shown to have decreased ratios of type III collagen as compared with type I collagen.[16b] In these instances it is not unusual to find a family history of aneurysm, particularly in women, with up to 18 per cent of first-degree relatives affected.[16c,16d] Several investigators have proposed that polymorphic variants in collagen type III genes are responsible for these observations, much as has been seen in Ehlers-Danlos Type IV syndrome.[16e]

Arteriosclerosis is especially important in the pathogenesis of aortic aneurysms. Hypertension may be particularly important in causing diseases of the aorta. Experimental work suggests that hypertension leads to structural aortic changes that may accelerate medial degeneration in certain patients; may decrease the blood flow in the vasa vasorum, with resultant ischemia of the aortic wall; and may initiate a response that stiffens the aorta and serves to perpetuate the hypertensive state. Although some degree of aortic medial degeneration is common with aging, the extent and severity of these changes are much greater in hypertensive individuals.[17–19]

ARTERIOSCLEROTIC AORTIC ANEURYSMS

ABDOMINAL AORTIC ANEURYSMS

Approximately three-fourths of all arteriosclerotic aortic aneurysms are confined to the abdominal aorta. Normally, in the adult, the aorta measures 2 cm in diameter at the level of the celiac axis and 1.8 cm just below the renal arteries; it then tapers slightly to the iliac vessels. Most abdominal aneurysms arise in the area between the renal arteries and the aortic bifurcation. Clinically significant aneurysms measure 4 cm or more in diameter.

ETIOLOGY AND PATHOGENESIS. Abdominal aortic aneurysms arise in areas of dense atherosclerosis. The atherosclerotic process erodes the aortic wall, destroying the medial elastic elements.[20] This causes weakening of the aortic wall and eventually leads to fusiform or, rarely, saccular dilation of the abdominal aorta. As the aorta widens, tension in the wall of the aorta rises in accordance with Laplace's law, which states that tension is proportional to the product of pressure and radius. Further widening results in greater tension, which in turn leads to acceleration in the rate of enlargement of the aneurysm. A vicious circle is thus established and produces dilatation that is often rapidly progressive. Hypertension may also contribute to the pathogenesis of these aneurysms. Epidemiological studies suggest that there is a familial occurrence of abdominal aortic aneurysms.[21]

Most abdominal aortic aneurysms arise just below the renal arteries and extend to, and often involve, the aortic bifurcation. Only 2 to 5 per cent of abdominal aortic aneurysms are suprarenal, and these usually result from the distal extension of a thoracic aneurysm into the abdomen. As aneurysms expand they may compress contiguous structures. Laminated thrombi frequently form in areas of stagnant flow within the aneurysm. Thrombotic and arteriosclerotic debris may embolize distally (p. 1551) and compromise the circulation of tributary arteries. Finally, the aneurysm may rupture. Of those aneurysms which do rupture, 80 per cent rupture retroperitoneally, and most of the remainder rupture into the periotoneal cavity, causing rapid circulatory collapse.[22] Rarely, an aneurysm may rupture into the inferior vena cava, iliac vein, or renal vein.[23,24]

CLINICAL MANIFESTATIONS. The majority of abdominal aneurysms are asymptomatic and are discovered on routine physical examination or on a routine abdominal roentgenogram.[25] Aneurysms may cause a sense of fullness in the epigastrium. If pain is present, it is usually located in the hypogastrium and lower back. The pain is usually steady, with a gnawing quality, and may last for hours or days at a time. In contrast to musculoskeletal back pain, it is not affected by movement, although patients may be more comfortable in certain positions, such as with the legs drawn up. Some astute patients may suspect an aneurysm by recognizing an abnormal pulsation of the aorta, as when lying down reading a book perched on the abdomen. Expansion and impending rupture are heralded by the development of pain, often of sudden onset, which is characteristically constant, severe, and located in the back or lower abdomen, sometimes with radiation into the groin, buttocks, or legs. Actual rupture is associated with the abrupt onset of back pain with abdominal pain and tenderness. Most patients have a palpable, pulsatile abdominal mass and many are hypotensive.[26]

Many aneurysms can be detected on physical examination, although even large aneurysms may be difficult or impossible to detect in obese individuals. When palpable, a pulsatile mass extending variably from between the xiphoid process to the umbilicus may be appreciated. Owing to difficulty in distinguishing the abdominal aorta from surrounding structures by palpation, the size of an aneurysm tends to be overestimated on physical examination. Moreover, it may sometimes be difficult to differentiate a tortuous, ectatic aorta from true aneurysmal dilatation. Aneurysms are often sensitive to palpation and may be quite tender if they are rapidly expanding or about to rupture. Aneurysms should always be palpated cautiously, particularly if they are tender.

Associated occlusive arterial disease is sometimes present in the femoral pulses and distal pulses in the legs or feet. Bruits arising from associated narrowed arteries may be heard over the aneurysm. Rarely, an aneurysm may expand in such a way as to occlude the inferior vena cava or one of the iliac veins, resulting in venous congestion and edema in one or both legs. Occasionally an arteriovenous fistula may be formed by spontaneous rupture into the inferior vena cava, iliac vein, or renal vein and a syndrome of hemodynamic collapse and acute high-output cardiac failure results.[24,27]

Patients who suffer rupture of an abdominal aortic aneurysm are critically ill.[28] Hemorrhagic shock may ensue rapidly and is manifested by hypotension, vasoconstriction, mottled skin, diaphoresis, mental obtundation, oliguria, and terminally by arrhythmias and cardiac arrest.[26] Retroperitoneal hemorrhage may be signaled by hematomas in the flanks and groin. Rupture into the abdominal cavity may result in abdominal distention, whereas rupture into the duodenum presents as massive gastrointestinal hemorrhage.

DIAGNOSIS AND SIZING OF ANEURYSMS. Currently, aneurysms may be detected and their size estimated by seven methods: (1) physical examination, (2) routine roentgenography, (3) abdominal ultrasound, (4) abdominal aortic angiography, (5) digital subtraction angiography, (6) CT scan, and (7) MRI.

Brewster and colleagues have carefully compared results on physical examination, routine roentgenography, two-dimensional echocardiography, and aortic angiography for sizing abdominal aortic aneurysms.[29] *Physical examination* is clearly the least accurate. *Lateral x-ray examination* of the lumbar spine is inexpensive and reliably detects the outline of the aneurysm if its wall is calcified (Fig. 47–4). However, this is not the case in at least one-fourth of all patients with aneurysms, so that these cannot be visualized radiographically.[30] *Cross-sectional ultrasound* is very accurate and is easily and atraumatically performed (Fig. 47–1). Refinements in ultrasonic techniques have permitted precise definition of the aortic adventitial border. Thus, abdominal ultrasound is currently the simplest and best way to detect and size an abdominal aortic aneurysm.

Abdominal aortic angiography is less accurate in predicting size because the full width of an aneurysm may be masked by the presence of nonopacified mural thrombus. Moreover, angiography carries with it a small but definite risk of complications, including hematoma, localized dissection, infection, embolization, and renal failure. Nevertheless, when angiography is performed by experienced hands, morbidity from the procedure is minimal, and valuable information is often gleaned from it. Thus, in a survey of 190 patients, angiography of the aorta and distal circulation resulted in only minor complications in 2 per cent; averted an incorrect diagnosis in 11 per cent; revealed extension of the aneurysm above the renal arteries in 5 per cent; showed renal artery stenosis in 22 per cent and atypical renal arterial anatomy in 17 per cent; delineated significant occlusive vascular disease in 48 per cent; and demonstrated associated aneurysms of the iliac, hypogastric, femoral, and popliteal vessels in 50 per cent.[31] Thus, aortography—if performed by experienced angiographers—is currently recommended for patients in whom there is any question of a correct diagnosis, for hypertensive patients with possible renal arterial disease, when the extent of the aneurysm is unclear, and for patients with suspected associated occlusive or aneurysmal diseases. In fact, at our institution, it is done routinely in most patients under consideration for surgery in order to facilitate perioperative management.

Experience with *digital subtraction angiography* (p. 1567) is still being accumulated, and it is hoped that this technique will eventually yield information as detailed as that provided by aortography, while eliminating the need for intraarterial injection. *CT scanning* has proved to be as useful and accurate as ultrasound in the diagnosis and measurement of abdominal aortic aneurysms (Fig. 47–2). Additional advantages over ultrasound are that it provides better definition of the intraluminal characteristics of the aneurysm and relationships to surrounding structures such as renal arteries, retroperitoneum, and spine.[4] It also provides potentially useful information about other abdominal organs.[4] However, it does involve the use of radiation and is more costly and time-consuming than ultrasound. Studies of MRI (p. 332) (Fig. 47–3) demonstrate close correlation between this technique and both CT scanning and ultrasound with regard to estimating the size of aneurysms and their relationship to the renal and iliac arteries. Its major limitations have included prolonged imaging time and a greater cost. However, the newer generation magnets may require much less imaging time than older models. For these reasons, ultrasound remains the procedure of choice for the screening of patients with suspected aneurysms.

NATURAL HISTORY. There is a crucial relationship between the size of aneurysms and their natural history, which is why it is so important to determine their width. Half of all aneurysms greater than 6 cm in diameter rupture within 1 year, compared with 15 to 20 per cent of aneurysms less than 6

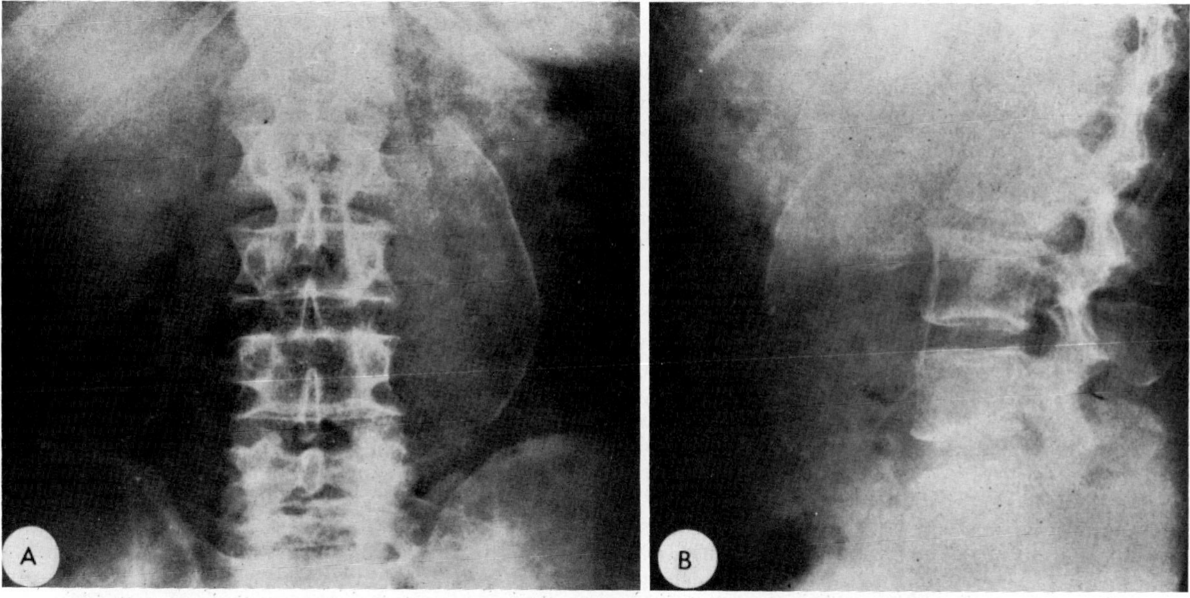

FIGURE 47–4. Anteroposterior *(A)* and lateral *(B)* views of the lumbar spinal column and the abdomen, disclosing a soft tissue mass with curvilinear calcification. (From Estes, J. E., Jr.: Abdominal aortic aneurysm: A study of one hundred and two cases. Circulation *2*:261, 1950, by permission of the American Heart Association, Inc.)

cm.[32] In a review of 24,000 consecutive autopsies, Darling et al. found that in aneurysms 10 cm or larger the incidence of rupture was 60 per cent; for those 7 to 10 cm the incidence was 45 per cent; and for those measuring 4 to 7 cm the rate was 25 per cent.[33] Two recent reports suggest an "average" aneurysm expansion rate of 0.4 to 0.5 cm in diameter per year,[34,35] while another population-based study suggested an average expansion rate of 0.21 cm in diameter per year.[36] Despite this seeming discrepancy, all three studies confirm that the rate of aneurysm expansion increases as aneurysms become larger and the risk of rupture becomes prohibitive (more than 25 per cent) when aneurysm diameter exceeds 4 to 5 cm.

SURGICAL MANAGEMENT. At present, elective surgery is advised for all abdominal aortic aneurysms 6 cm in diameter or wider, assuming that surgical risks are not prohibitive because of other medical problems. The management of asymptomatic aneurysms less than 6 cm in diameter remains controversial. Pasch and coworkers have argued that elective resection of such lesions would result in the saving of lives and is economically viable because it obviates the tremendously costly care associated with aneurysm rupture.[37] Cooley has argued that improvements in surgical management of acute rupture now allow salvage of nearly 80 per cent of patients,[38] but the experience of others would appear to favor elective resection of aneurysms larger than 4 cm in otherwise good surgical candidates.[32,33] In poor-risk patients with aneurysms of 4 to 6 cm, close follow-up is advised, with immediate surgery if the aneurysm expands or shows signs of impending rupture, such as the sudden onset of pain.

Surgery consists of resection of the aneurysm and insertion of a synthetic prosthesis, usually of Dacron. Sometimes a simple tube graft is all that is necessary, although frequently the operation must be carried distally into one or both iliac arteries in order to excise the aneurysm completely. With large aneurysms, much of the wall of the aneurysm may be left in situ ("intrasaccular approach of Creech"). This reduces the need for extensive dissection, thereby decreasing aortic cross-clamping time, and has significantly ameliorated the problem of postoperative sexual dysfunction.

Expanding or ruptured abdominal aortic aneurysms are true surgical emergencies. In the case of rupture, patients can sometimes be stabilized by using a compression G-suit, a garment that may diminish the rate of bleeding by exerting counterforce externally against the abdomen. However, operation must be undertaken as soon as possible.

Perioperative Management. Advances in perioperative management have improved survival rates in patients undergoing surgical resection of abdominal aortic aneurysms. Many of these patients have significant heart disease, and monitoring of arterial blood pressure, cardiac output, cardiac filling pressures, and urine output may help enormously in their operative management. These measurements provide a valuable guide to volume replacement. So-called "declamping shock" has been virtually eliminated by volume replacement guided by monitored pressures. This term is applied to a syndrome characterized by marked hypotension upon release of the aortic cross clamp at the completion of surgery; the cause is believed to be pooling of blood in the dilated distal vascular bed and release of vasodepressor substances that have accumulated during surgery distal to the aortic clamp. The use of vasodilators such as nitroprusside or intravenous nitroglycerin may also improve and protect cardiac function by attenuating the changes in left ventricular afterload caused by clamping and unclamping the aorta.[39] Administration of mannitol and potent loop diurectics such as intravenous furosemide has reduced the frequency of postoperative renal failure.[40] The occurrence of renal failure postoperatively in patients with ruptured abdominal aortic aneurysms has correlated with very poor survival rates. Autotransfusion has led to less frequent occurrence of hepatitis and fewer transfusion reactions,[41] and antibiotic coverage has reduced the frequency of infections. Hypothermia has been better controlled, and better understanding of the clotting system has improved management of hemostasis.

Many patients with abdominal aortic aneurysms are heavy smokers and have serious chronic obstructive lung disease. Such patients have benefited greatly from improvements in postoperative respiratory care. Preoperative preparation of pulmonary patients is also important, and smokers should abstain from tobacco use for at least 1 month before surgery.

If there is evidence of carotid artery disease in patients facing elective aneurysm resection, preoperative evaluation and surgery for critical carotid stenoses, if indicated, have resulted in fewer strokes. In patients with severe coronary artery disease, it may be important to evaluate the extent of coronary narrowing before aneurysm resection. Since half the perioperative deaths in this setting are due to myocardial infarction,[42] Hertzer and others have recommended routine coronary angiography and selective coronary bypass surgery before aneurysm resection in patients with severe correctable coronary disease.[43] Studies by Boucher et al.[44] and Eagle et al.[45] have suggested that dipyridamole-thallium cardiac scanning (p. 1712) is an effective noninvasive means of identifying patients at highest risk for perioperative ischemic events. In recent reports, these investigators have shown that further preoperative testing is unnecessary in patients without overt clinical evidence of left ventricular dysfunction, coronary artery disease, or diabetes.[46] However, in patients with one or more of these clinical markers, dipyridamole-thallium testing is quite useful in separating patients into low- and high-risk categories.[46] In particular, patients with thallium redistribution in multiple segments of myocardium are at highest risk.[47] It is in this subgroup that coronary angiography and selective bypass surgery or coronary artery angioplasty, is likely to be most helpful.[48] Others have evaluated exercise stress testing[49] (Chap. 6), gated blood pool scanning,[50] and Holter monitoring for silent ischemia[51] to identify patients at high risk. Further experience with these methods and their comparison with each other is necessary before the best and most cost-effective ways of assessing cardiac risk can be determined.

In cases of associated severe renal artery stenosis causing renin-dependent hypertension or jeopardizing renal function, simultaneous renal artery reconstruction is often performed.[52]

OPERATIVE RISK. The risk of operation obviously depends on the general status of the patient and on whether the aneurysm has ruptured. Prompt recognition and immediate operation for patients with rupture have markedly improved survival. In low-risk patients, the mortality from the elective resection of abdominal aortic aneurysms should be 2 to 5 per cent. With expanding aneurysms, mortality is 5 to 15 per cent, and with rupture, mortality has reached a plateau at approximately 50 per cent, the major determinant of survival being the speed with which surgery is accomplished.[40,52–54]

Age and preexisting cardiac, pulmonary, cerebrovascular, and/or renal diseases all add to the surgical risk. Congestive heart failure, diabetes, and evidence of coronary artery disease are particularly important, whereas advanced age per se should not be a deterrent to surgery in an otherwise healthy patient.[45,55]

An alternative to aneurysmectomy for patients at very high risk has been reported by Karmody et al.[56] This group has combined thrombosis of the aortic aneurysm with right axillary to bilateral femoral artery bypass conduits. Thrombosis of the aneurysm usually followed the interruption of flow below the aortic bifurcation achieved by ligation of the iliac outflow vessels. If the aneurysm did not thrombose within 72 hours, the iliac outflow vessels responsible for continued patency were identified by angiography and were occluded by intraarterial injection of bucrylate. Although the perioperative and late mortality in these patients was high (17 deaths among 42 patients), the deaths were related mostly to associated diseases and not to the operative procedure itself.

The statistics showing better survival with elective resection of aneurysms are impressive. From several reports, the 5-year survival rate is only 5 to 10 per cent in patients with unexcised aneurysms larger than 6 cm compared with over 50 per cent for those who undergo resection and 80 per cent for the age-matched "normal" population. *Late* survival is unaffected by whether the aneurysm was electively resected, acute, or ruptured.[54] With aneurysms smaller than 6 cm, the 5-year unoperated survival rate is about 50 per cent, as opposed to 60 to 70 per cent for those who undergo resection.[57]

COMPLICATIONS. The rate of late complications of aneurysmectomy is approximately 10 per cent.[58,59] These complications include stenosis or occlusion of the prosthetic graft, false aneurysm formation, enteric fistula formation, infection, and rupture. Patients with graft occlusion usually have evidence of prior distal vascular disease that impedes aortic runoff. *Occlusions* occur mainly at the sites of anastomosis, and patients usually develop ischemic symptoms distal to the graft site. These stenoses may be amenable to correction by balloon catheter angioplasty.[60] *False aneurysms* may be caused by infection but others arise spontaneously and present as expanding masses in the groin, abdomen, or lower back. *Enteric fistulas* are caused by rupture of the graft into the duodenum, resulting in gastrointestinal hemorrhage, and are associated with a high mortality. This complication can occur anywhere from 1 day to several years after operation, and the diagnosis must be suspected in any patient who has undergone abdominal aneurysmectomy and who presents with melena, hematemesis, hematochezia, or abdominal pain.[24,61,62] Recognition is obtained by gastrointestinal series, endoscopy, colonoscopy, or angiography. *Infections* most commonly are seen as a painful or tender groin mass, with or without a draining sinus. Recommended therapy involves administration of antibiotics, removal of the infected prosthetic material, and reestablishment of the circulation by an alternate route, usually axillofemoral bypass.

Attention has been called to the occasional occurrence of *colonic ischemia* following aneurysm surgery, caused by the intraoperative sacrifice of the inferior mesenteric artery in patients with concomitantly diseased superior or mesenteric and hypogastric arteries, resulting in inadequate perfusion of the colon.[63] This complication is best avoided by paying careful attention to collateral blood flow to the colon, maintaining adequate blood pressure during surgery, and handling the distal colon carefully at the time of operation. If necessary, reimplantation of the inferior mesenteric artery can be performed if collateral circulation is inadequate. Doppler ultrasound measurement of inferior mesenteric arterial flow or direct measurement of the inferior mesenteric arterial stump pressure may be useful in identifying patients likely to benefit from such reimplantation.[63]

THORACIC AORTIC ANEURYSMS

About one-fourth of all arteriosclerotic aneurysms involve the thoracic aorta. Dilatation may occur anywhere along the thoracic aorta—that is, the ascending segment, the arch, or the descending portion; the latter two sites are the more common ones. This contrasts with luetic aneurysms, which are located predominantly in the ascending aorta. Sometimes the entire aorta is ectatic, with localized aneurysms at many sites in both the thoracic and the abdominal aorta. Aneurysms of the descending thoracic aorta not infrequently extend into the abdominal aorta, creating a thoracoabdominal aneurysm.

PATHOGENESIS. The pathogenesis of arteriosclerotic aneurysms is identical to that of aneurysms in the abdominal aorta. The arteriosclerotic process leads to weakening of the aortic wall, medial degeneration, and localized dilatation. Hypertension often coexists and contributes to both undermining the strength of the aortic wall and expansion of the aneurysm. In the thorax, localized saccular aneurysms are somewhat more common than circumferential or fusiform aneurysms. The natural history of thoracic aneurysms differs somewhat from that of abdominal aortic aneurysms in that spontaneous rupture without warning is less common, because evidence of a growing thoracic aneurysm is usually afforded by symptoms caused by compression of the surrounding structures.[64]

CLINICAL MANIFESTATIONS. Thoracic aneurysms are frequently associated with widespread atherosclerosis, particularly of the renal, cerebral, and coronary arteries. In fact, the consequences of arterial obliterative disease in these other areas may dominate the clinical picture.

Symptoms and signs of thoracic aneurysms are related to their size and location and are caused primarily by their impingement upon adjacent structures. Thus, tracheal deviation, wheezing, cough, dyspnea, stridor, hemoptysis, recurrent pneumonitis, and intrapulmonary hemorrhage are the direct result of compression of the tracheobronchial tree and contiguous lung, especially the left main stem bronchus, by aneurysms of the descending thoracic aorta. Occasionally, an asymptomatic arch aneurysm will be visible or palpable rising above the suprasternal notch. Hoarseness may follow compression of the recurrent laryngeal nerve. Arch aneurysms sometimes produce a tracheal tug. Dysphagia arises from pressure against the nearby esophagus. The superior vena caval syndrome can develop as a consequence of obstruction of venous return from the superior vena cava or innominate veins.

Pain is due to compression and erosion of adjacent musculoskeletal structures. It is usually steady and boring—occasionally pulsating—and may be extremely severe. Erosion of the sternum and right thoracic cage may result from large aneurysms of the ascending aorta, while erosion of the vertebral column and posterior left ribs may result from descending thoracic aortic aneurysms. Visible and pulsatile masses are evident when aneurysms reach and begin to erode through the chest wall. Rupture of an aneurysm is heralded by the dramatic onset of excruciating pain, usually in the area where some pain had existed previously.

DIAGNOSIS. Most thoracic aortic aneurysms are readily visible on chest roentgenograms, with fluoroscopy helping to differentiate an aneurysm from other types of mediastinal masses, such as neoplasms. However, some aneurysms are small, especially saccular aneurysms, and may rupture without having been visible on chest roentgenogram (Fig. 47–5).

Aortic angiography is clearly the definitive procedure for outlining an aneurysm to make a diagnosis and to reveal the anatomical features of the aneurysm (Fig. 47–6). It should be performed in all patients under consideration for surgical repair. Although digital subtraction angiography continues to undergo evaluation as an alternative to conventional angiography, its inability to define the anatomy of small arteries (such as coronary arteries) and susceptibility to motion artifact limit its general application at this time.[1] CT scanning (Fig. 11–15, p. 320) enhanced by the use of a contrast medium can be used to identify and size aneurysms of both the ascending and the descending thoracic aorta.[4] Alternatively, significant aneurysms of either the ascending or the descending thoracic aorta can be defined by cross-sectional ultrasonography, but in the thoracic aorta, unlike the abdominal aorta, this technique is not as accurate as the CT scan, especially in the descending thoracic aorta. Transesophageal echocardiography has emerged as a better ultrasonographic method for imaging the thoracic aorta. Studies suggest that it is comparable to CT scanning in defining thoracic aneurysms (Fig. 4–13, p. 69). MRI is also an excellent technique that does not require administration of contrast agents. It is very reliable in defining the infarct and size of thoracic aneurysms.[9,11]

NATURAL HISTORY. Data for natural history of arteriosclerotic thoracic aortic aneurysms are somewhat scanty, but, as with abdominal aneurysms, ultimate survival is related to the size of the aneurysms. Thoracic aneurysms greater than 7 cm in diameter are more prone to rupture than are smaller ones.[64] Aneurysms that indicate expansion by producing

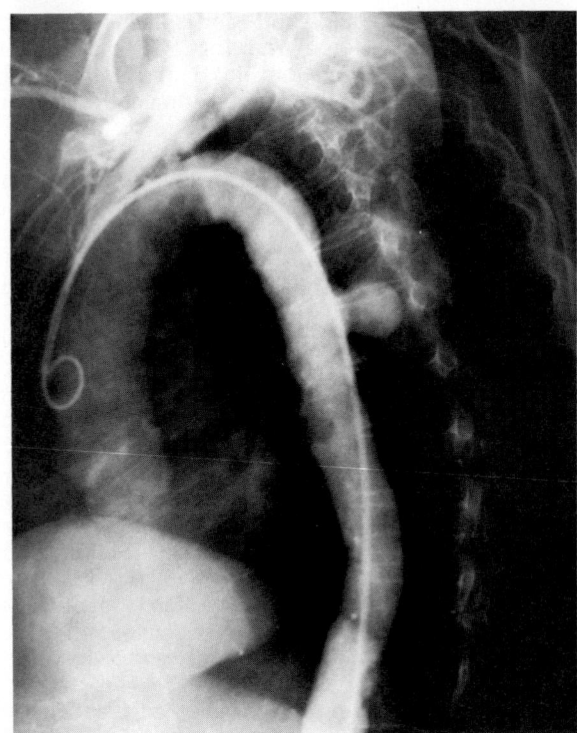

FIGURE 47–5. A localized saccular aneurysm in the descending thoracic aorta is clearly shown in the aortic angiogram of this 62-year-old man. The aneurysm had leaked, and a faint halo caused by the hematoma can be seen surrounding the aneurysm. The routine chest film appeared normal in this patient. (Courtesy of Christos Athanasoulis, M.D., and Arthur Waltman, M.D., Section of Vascular Radiology, Massachusetts General Hospital, Boston.)

symptoms of compression of surrounding structures are obviously diagnosed and treated earlier than aneurysms at "silent" sites. As noted, thoracic aneurysms are frequently associated with severe generalized arteriosclerosis, and many patients die of complications of arteriosclerosis before an aneurysm can rupture. When aneurysms do pursue a natural course, it has been found that symptomatic aneurysms are more prone to rupture than are asymptomatic ones. In the classic natural history study by Joyce et al., patients with symptomatic thoracic aneurysms had a 27 per cent 5-year survival compared with 58 per cent in asymptomatic patients. One-third of the deaths were attributed to rupture, while more than half were caused by complications of arteriosclerosis unrelated to the aneurysm.[65]

MANAGEMENT. Historically, surgical therapy once consisted of the introduction of long lengths of thrombogenic wire into an aneurysm, with the resultant thrombus buttressing the wall of the aneurysm. Direct wrapping of the aneurysm has also been tried. Currently, surgical excision is the procedure of choice whenever possible and is advised for aneurysms measuring 7 cm or more in diameter in the ascending and descending thoracic aorta. Clearly, even smaller aneurysms should be resected if they are producing symptoms. The aggressiveness with which surgical repair is undertaken depends greatly upon the general condition of the patient. The surgical procedure must be tailored to the specific aneurysm. Saccular aneurysms can sometimes be excised directly without resection of the aorta. Fusiform aneurysms in the ascending and descending thoracic aorta are best resected and replaced with a prosthetic tubular sleeve of appropriate size. Total cardiopulmonary bypass is necessary for the removal of ascending aortic aneurysms, and partial bypass to support the circulation distal to the aneurysm is often advisable in resection of descending thoracic aortic aneurysms. A temporary shunt (Gott shunt) may be used from the proximal aorta to the aorta beyond the aneurysm to divert blood around the site of the aneurysm while it is being repaired,[66] although the use of such adjuncts is less important than are the nature and extent of the aneurysm in determining the incidence of postoperative complications.[67]

The use of a composite graft consisting of a Dacron tube with a prosthetic aortic valve sewn into one end represents a major advance in therapy of proximal aortic aneurysms extending to the aortic annulus and associated with aortic regurgitation. The valve and graft are sewn into the annulus, and the coronary arteries are reimplanted into the Dacron aortic graft or onto separate Dacron tubes.[68,69] (Fig. 47–16).

Fusiform aneurysms of the arch have been successfully excised surgically; however, the risks of operation in this area are high. Arch aneurysmectomy requires excision of the aneurysm and in some instances reimplantation of all the brachiocephalic vessels. Each of these important arteries is selectively perfused by local cannulation while they are being reimplanted. Alternatively, resection of the aneurysm using profound hypothermia and circulatory arrest, a technique that is now favored by many surgical groups, has been used successfully.[70,71] In some centers both selective cerebral perfusion and hypothermic cardiopulmonary bypass are utilized.[72]

Surgical results have improved considerably in recent years, with a nearly 90 per cent survival rate for the elective resection of ascending and descending thoracic aortic aneurysms being reported in most major centers.[68,69,73,74] Moreno-Cabral reported a 94 per cent early and an 80 per cent late survival rate[75] in 214 patients with arteriosclerotic aneurysms of the ascending aorta. In a report on 82 patients with thoraco-

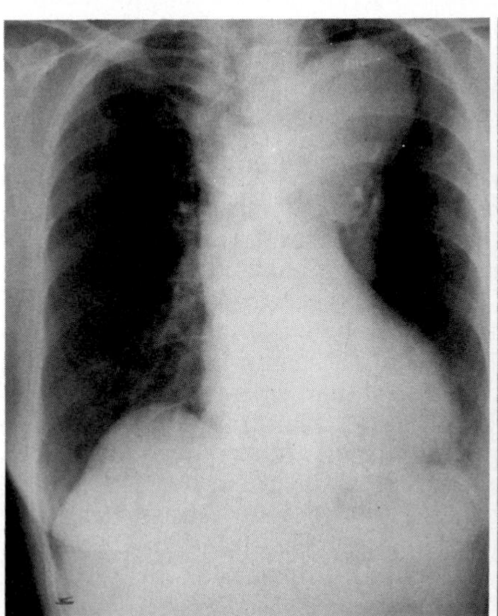

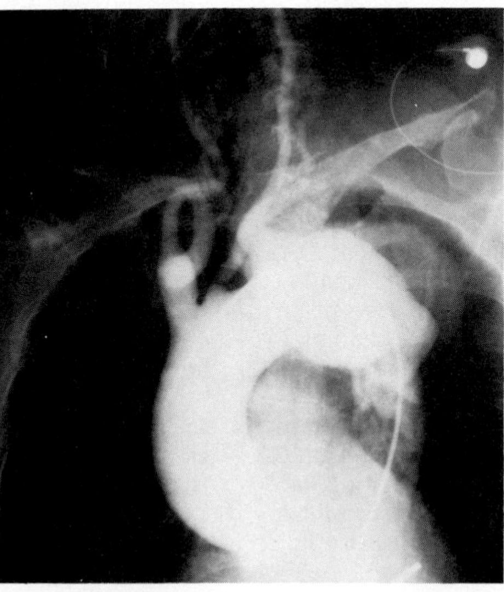

FIGURE 47–6. *Left,* Posteroanterior chest roentgenogram in a 66-year-old woman with an arteriosclerotic aneurysm of the descending thoracic aorta. *Right,* Aortographic appearance in the left oblique anterior projection. The aneurysm arises just at the site of origin of the left subclavian artery. Thrombus is evident in the outer wall of the aneurysm on the angiogram. (Courtesy of Christos Athanasoulis, M.D., and Arthur Waltman, M.D., Section of Vascular Radiology, Massachusetts General Hospital, Boston.)

abdominal aneurysms, the survival rate was 94 per cent.[76] More recently, in a large series of patients with aneurysm and/or dissection involving the ascending aorta or arch, Crawford reported a 91 per cent 30-day and 66 per cent 5-year survival.[74]

Major complications of the operation are technical, especially hemorrhage from tearing of the diseased aorta. A catastrophic complication of resection of descending thoracic aortic aneurysms is paraplegia from inadvertent interruption of the arterial blood supply to the spinal cord. This problem has been reduced by maintaining distal aortic perfusion during surgery[77]; by reducing the period of aortic cross clamping; by removal of minimal segments of aorta with the attendant intercostal arteries, especially in the areas of T7 through T9; by prompt treatment of hypertension in the proximal aorta, which elevates cerebrospinal fluid pressure, thus reducing collateral blood flow to the spinal cord; and possibly by perfusion cooling of the spinal cord during surgery. Recent studies report that the spinal cord is injured in at least 5 per cent of patients despite these and other precautions.[68,73,78,79]

Complications of associated arteriosclerosis, such as myocardial infarction, cerebrovascular infarcts, and renal failure, often manifest themselves under the massive physiological stress of surgery. The most frequent causes of early postoperative deaths are myocardial infarction, congestive heart failure, stroke, renal failure, hemorrhage, respiratory failure, and sepsis. Advanced age, emergency operation, prolonged aortic cross-clamp time, extent of aneurysm, diabetes, previous aortic operation, aneurysm symptoms, and intraoperative hypotension are the most important factors determining early perioperative morbidity and mortality.[75] Late postoperative deaths are usually associated with cardiac complications, aneurysm rupture respiratory failure, or stroke.[74,75] Aneurysm rupture may be due to aneurysm formation at the graft margins or formation of aneurysms at other aortic sites.[73]

Many patients with arteriosclerotic aneurysms are heavy smokers, and pulmonary complications are frequent. The left lung may be severely traumatized by compression during resection of large aneurysms of the descending thoracic aorta, a complication that may seriously jeopardize the patient's survival, particularly if there is underlying pulmonary disease.

Widespread aneurysmal dilatation of the aorta often precludes operation, although there are reports of successful surgical replacement of essentially the entire diseased thoracic and abdominal aorta. Associated diseases—especially pulmonary—preclude any operation in still others. Although it seems logical to reduce blood pressure vigorously in patients with aneurysms and to reduce the velocity of ventricular ejection, the long-term impact of such therapy on retarding the expansion of aneurysms and improving survival is unknown.

AORTIC DISSECTION

Acute aortic dissection is a relatively common catastrophic illness and occurs at the rate of at least 2000 new cases per year in the United States.[80-82] Over the past two decades, great strides have been made in the diagnosis and the medical and surgical treatment of this highly lethal disease.[74,83,83a] It has been cogently pointed out that the term *dissecting hematoma* describes this entity more accurately than does the commonly used term dissecting aneurysm. More recently, the simpler term *aortic dissection* has gained favor.

Aortic dissection is caused by the sudden development of a tear in the aortic intima, opening the way for a column of blood driven by the force of the arterial pressure to enter the aortic wall, destroying the media and stripping the intima from the adventitia for variable distances along the length of the aorta.[84] It is uncertain whether the primary event in aortic dissection is rupture of the intima, with secondary dissection into the media, or hemorrhage within a diseased media followed by disruption of the subjacent intima and subsequent propagation of the dissection through the intimal tear (Fig. 47–7). However, occasional cases of extensive aortic dissection can occur without any identifiable intimal tear.[85]

The manifestations of aortic dissection in any given patient are determined by its path as it progresses through the aorta. Thus, the circulation of any major artery arising from the aorta may be compromised; disruption of the support of the aortic valve by extension into the aortic root may cause aortic incompetence; and finally the dissecting column may rupture through the adventitia anywhere along the aorta, although the two most common sites of rupture are the pericardial space and the left pleural cavity.

CLASSIFICATION. Most classification schemes for aortic dissection are based upon the fact that over 95 per cent of all dissections arise in one of two locations: (1) the ascending aorta within several centimeters of the aortic valve and (2) the descending thoracic aorta, usually just beyond the origin of the left subclavian artery at the site of the ligamentum arteriosum.[81] The widely used classification of DeBakey et al. recognizes three groups (Fig. 47–8). Types I and II both begin in the ascending aorta: Type I extends beyond the ascending aorta and arch, whereas Type II is confined to the ascending aorta.

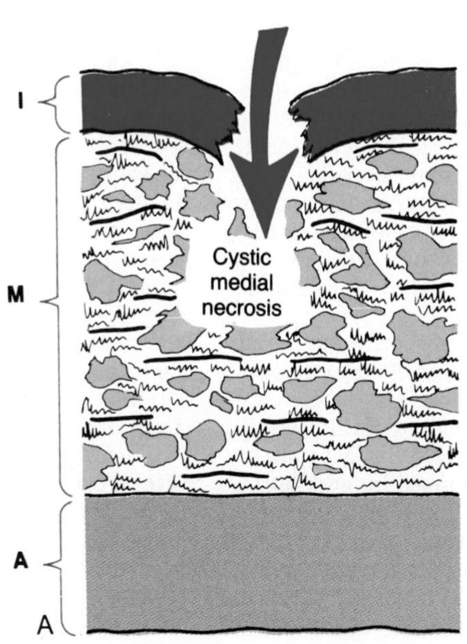

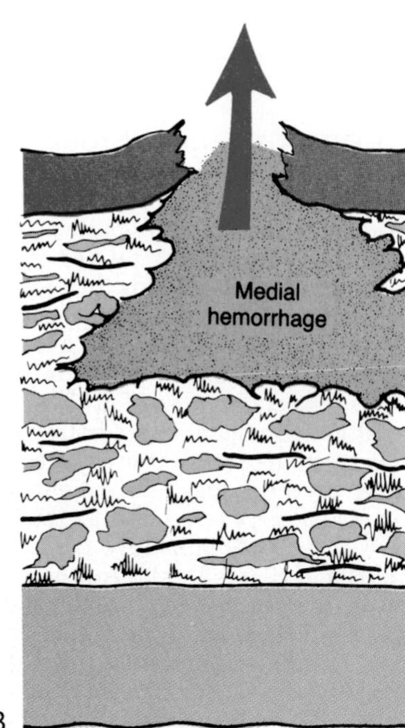

FIGURE 47–7. Proposed mechanisms of initiation of aortic dissection. In both cases, cystic medial necrosis is present. In *A*, an intimal tear is the initial event, allowing aortic blood to enter the media. In *B*, the primary event is hemorrhage into the media, with secondary rupture of the overlying intima. I = intima; M = media; A = adventitia.

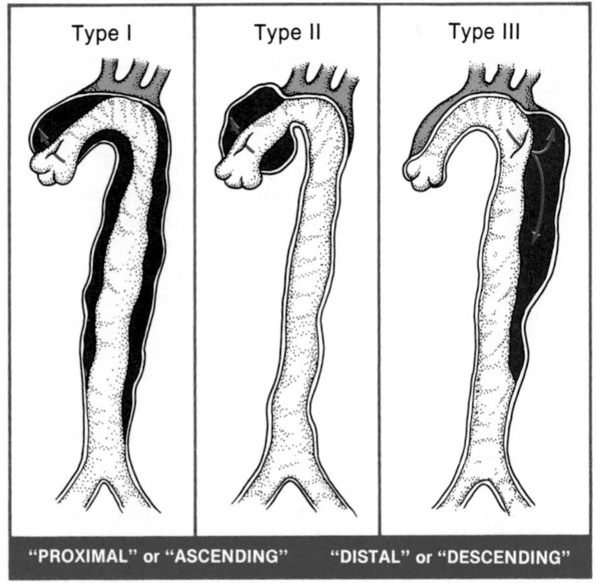

FIGURE 47-8. The DeBakey classification of aortic dissections.

Type III originates in the descending thoracic aorta and usually propagates distally for a variable distance. It uncommonly extends retrograde into the arch and ascending aorta. In Type IIIa dissection, the process is limited to the thoracic aorta, while a IIIb designation connotes extension of the dissection below the diaphragm.[86]

Another classification, based upon approach to therapy and proposed by Daily et al., delineates two types, A and B.[87] Type A includes all proximal dissections and those distal dissections that extend retrograde to involve the arch and ascending aorta; Type B refers to all other distal dissections without proximal extension.

Since the behavior and managment of Types I and II dissections are similar, many investigators, including ourselves, have adopted a simple two-category classification into "proximal" (DeBakey Types I and II) and "distal" (DeBakey Type III) dissections.[88] "Ascending" and "descending" have also been used synonymously with "proximal" and "distal." Proximal dissections occur more frequently than distal dissections in a ratio of almost two to one in autopsy series.[89] However, because proximal dissections are more rapidly lethal, many clinical series report larger numbers of patients with distal than proximal dissection.[88,90]

Other occasional sites of origin include the aortic arch and the abdominal aorta. Furthermore, individual arteries may be the locus of isolated dissection, especially the coronary and carotid arteries.[91-93]

ETIOLOGY AND PATHOGENESIS. Degeneration of the aortic media is believed to be the prerequisite for the development of aortic dissection.[81-84,94] Usually, this consists of deterioration of the collagen and elastic tissue, often with cystic changes. This process, termed cystic medial necrosis or degeneration, most often is the result of chronic stress against the aortic wall, such as might occur with longstanding hypertension. Indeed, hypertension is an important contributing factor to aortic dissection and is found in well over half of all cases, especially those of distal dissection.

Although medial degeneration is part of the normal aging process in the aorta, these changes are qualitatively and quantitatively much greater in patients with aortic dissection. Cystic medial degeneration is an intrinsic feature of the hereditary defects of connective tissue, especially the Marfan (p. 1641) and Ehlers-Danlos (p. 1643) syndromes. Indeed, aortic dissection—especially proximal dissection—is a frequent and serious complication of the Marfan syndrome. However, cystic medial degeneration and aortic dissection may occur in the absence of an associated phenotypic syndrome.[95] Certain congenital cardiovascular abnormalities, especially coarctation of the aorta and bicuspid aortic valves, predispose to aortic dissection. A combination of bicuspid aortic valve, cystic medial degeneration, and aortic root dissection in the absence of the Marfan syndrome has been described.[96] Recent reports of aortic dissection in patients with Noonan syndrome and Turner syndrome have also appeared.[97,98] Also, a family in which nine members developed aortic dilatation or dissection over two generations has recently been described.[99] Cystic medial degeneration appears to be a common theme in all these patients.

An unexplained relationship exists between pregnancy and aortic dissection (p. 1801). About half of all aortic dissections in women under the age of 40 occur during pregnancy, usually in the last trimester.[100,101] Isolated coronary artery dissection also usually occurs during pregnancy.

In older patients, dissections occasionally originate by way of perforation through an intimal atheromatous plaque. Trauma almost never causes a classic aortic dissection, although a localized tear in the region of the aortic isthmus is not uncommon following massive chest trauma. Rarely, dissection of the aorta is a complication of other forms of vasculitis, including granulmatous arteritis (p. 1547).

Although strenuous physical exertion and emotional stress have been linked to aortic dissection, such a relationship is not usual. In a series of 124 cases of aortic dissection that we reviewed, we found such a history in only 14 per cent.[88]

The role played by chemicals toxic to connective tissue in the etiology of dissecting aneurysm in human beings is unknown. It is well known that the seeds of *Lathyrus odoratus* (sweet pea), which contain aminopropionitrile, cause cystic medial degeneration and aortic dissection in rats.[102] We have encountered a proximal dissection in a young man with no obvious predisposing factors other than prolonged industrial exposure to dimethyl hydrazine, a connective tissue toxin.[88]

CLINICAL MANIFESTATIONS

Aortic dissection afflicts men more frequently than women in a ratio of approximately two to one and has a peak incidence in the sixth and seventh decades, with a range from childhood well into the 90's.[103] Patients with proximal dissection are on the average somewhat younger. By far the most common presenting symptom of aortic dissection is *severe pain*, which is found in over 90 per cent of cases.[104] In fact, those patients without pain usually have suffered some disturbance of consciousness as a result of the dissection that renders them unable to perceive pain. Nonetheless, painless dissection can and does occur rarely.[105]

Cataclysmic in onset, the pain of aortic dissection is often as severe at its inception as it ever becomes. This feature contrasts with that of myocardial infarction, where the pain usually has a crescendo-like onset. The pain of dissection may be all but unbearable, forcing the patient to writhe in agony or to pace restlessly in an attempt to gain some measure of relief. Several features of the pain may arouse suspicion of aortic dissection. The quality of the pain as described by the patient is often morbidly appropriate to the actual event. Adjectives such as "tearing," "ripping," and "stabbing" are frequently used. Another important characteristic of the pain of aortic dissection is its tendency to migrate from its point of origin to other sites, following the path of the dissecting hematoma as it extends through the aorta. This feature was noted in 70 per cent of our cases.[88] Vasovagal manifestations, such as a drenching sweat, apprehension, nausea, vomiting, and faintness, are common at the outset.

The location of pain may be of some help in suggesting the site of origin.[88] Pain felt maximally in the anterior thorax is more frequent with proximal dissection, whereas pain that is most severe in the interscapular area is much more common with a distal site of origin. Although pain may be felt simultaneously in the anterior and posterior chest with both proximal and distal dissection, the *absence* of posterior interscapular pain strongly militates against a distal dissection, since over 90 per cent of patients with distal dissection report some back pain. Pain in the neck, throat, jaw, or teeth often occurs in dissections involving the ascending aorta or arch.

Less common modes of presentation include congestive heart failure with or without associated chest pain, cerebrovascular accidents, syncope, paraplegia, and pulse loss with or without ischemic pain. Heart failure usually results from severe aortic regurgitation secondary to the dissection. The occurrence of syncope in aortic dissection may bear special significance. Syncope without focal neurological signs occurred in 6 of 124 patients in our series. In each case, there was evidence for rupture of the dissection into the pericardial cavity with cardiac tamponade.[88]

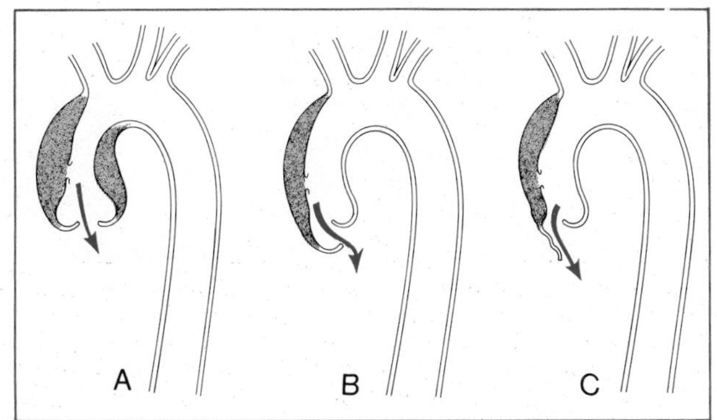

FIGURE 47-9. **Mechanisms of aortic regurgitation in proximal dissecting aortic aneurysm. *A,* A circumferential tear pulls the annulus apart, preventing the leaflets from coapting. *B,* With asymmetrical dissection, pressure from the hematoma depresses one leaflet below the line of closure of the other. C, The annular support is disrupted, resulting in a flail aortic leaflet and aortic regurgitation.**

Diagnosis

PHYSICAL FINDINGS. The diagnosis of aortic dissection can often be made with reasonable assurance from the *physical examination* alone. Patients with aortic dissection may appear to be in shock; however, the blood pressure when measured is frequently elevated. More than half the patients with distal dissection are hypertensive on initial presentation. Hypotension usually results from cardiac tamponade, intrapleural or intraperitoneal rupture, or dissection of the brachiocephalic vessels resulting in "pseudohypotension," i.e., the inability to measure the blood pressure accurately because of occlusion of the brachial arteries.

Those physical findings most typically associated with aortic dissection, namely, pulse deficits, aortic insufficiency, and neurological manifestations, are more characteristic of proximal than distal dissection. Pulse abnormalities, which include the absence, diminution, or reduplication of pulses, occur in approximately one-half of patients with proximal dissection and most commonly involve the brachiocephalic vessels. Pulse deficits are much less common in patients with distal dissection and tend to involve the left subclavian and femoral arteries, although the femoral vessels are equally affected by the distal propagation of a proximal dissection. Pulses may be lost either by direct compression of the lumen of an artery through extension of the dissection into it or by blockade due to a flap of intima overlying the vessel orifice. Rarely, intimointimal intussusception may occur.[106] Whatever the cause, pulse deficits in aortic dissection may be transitory, owing to decompression of the hematoma by distal reentry into the true lumen or by movement of the intimal flap away from the occluded orifice.

Aortic regurgitation is an important feature of proximal dissection and occurs in over 50 per cent in most series.[107] It was present in two-thirds of our patients with proximal dissection.[88] When aortic regurgitation is present in patients with distal dissection, it most commonly antedates the dissection and results from preexisting dilatation of the aortic root due to severe hypertension or annuloaortic ectasia. The murmur of aortic regurgitation in aortic dissection often has a musical quality and may be heard better along the right than the left sternal border. It may wax and wane, the intensity varying directly with the height of the arterial blood pressure. Depending upon the severity of the regurgitation, other peripheral signs of aortic incompetence may be present, such as collapsing pulses and a wide pulse pressure. There are three mechanisms of aortic regurgitation in proximal dissection (Fig. 47-9). First, the dissection may dilate the aortic root, widening the annulus so that aortic leaflets are unable to coapt in diastole; second, in an asymmetrical dissection, pressure from the dissecting hematoma may depress one leaflet below the line of closure of the others; and third, the annular support of the leaflets or the leaflets themselves may be torn so as to render the valve incompetent.

As noted, patients with proximal dissection sometimes have heart failure, which is almost always due to the sudden onset of severe aortic insufficiency. In rare cases, the congestive failure may be so severe as to mask the murmur and other usual signs of aortic regurgitation. In a few such patients whom we have encountered, the presence of disproportionately bounding pulses in the face of severe heart failure, coupled with a history highly suggestive of aortic dissection, served as a clue to the correct diagnosis.

Neurological deficits associated with aortic dissection include cerebrovascular accidents, ischemic peripheral neuropathy, ischemic paraparesis, and disturbances of consciousness. Each of these is more common with proximal dissection, but deficits in the lower extremities are equally frequent in proximal and distal dissection.

Other occasionally encountered clinical manifestations of aortic dissection include pulsation of one of the sternoclavicular joints, Horner syndrome due to compression of the superior cervical sympathetic ganglion, vocal cord paralysis and hoarseness from pressure against the left recurrent laryngeal nerve, superior mediastinal syndrome from superior vena caval compression,[108] pulsating neck masses, tracheal or bronchial compression with bronchospasm,[81] hemorrhage into the tracheobronchial tree with hemoptysis,[109] hematemesis due to perforation into the esophagus,[110] heart block from retrograde burrowing of a dissection into the interatrial septum and thence down to the AV node,[111] and a continuous murmur due to rupture into the right atrium or ventricle.[112] Pleural effusions result from rupture of the dissection into one of the pleural spaces—usually the left—or simply from an exudative inflammatory reaction around the involved aorta. Additional complications may result from occlusion of important arteries by the dissection. Mesenteric infarction, renal infarction with severe renovascular hypertension, and myocardial infarction (seen in 1 to 2 per cent of patients with proximal dissection) are among the more serious occlusive events. Occasionally, high fever results, presumably from the release of pyrogenic substances from the hematoma or from associated effusions.

A variety of conditions may mimic aortic dissection. These include myocardial infarction, acute aortic regurgitation without dissection, thoracic nondissecting aneurysm, musculoskeletal pain, mediastinal tumors, pericarditis, and coronary insufficiency.[113] Confusion usually arises in these conditions when chest pain suggesting aortic dissection is coincidentally associated with other clinical manifestations of that entity, such as aortic regurgitation, deficient pulses, neurological abnormalities, or an abnormally widened aortic contour.[113]

Routine laboratory studies are not very helpful in making the diagnosis of aortic dissection. Anemia may develop from significant hemorrhage or sequestration of blood in the false channel. A mild to moderate polymorphonuclear leukocytosis (10,000 to 14,000/mm^3) is common. Lactic acid dehydro-

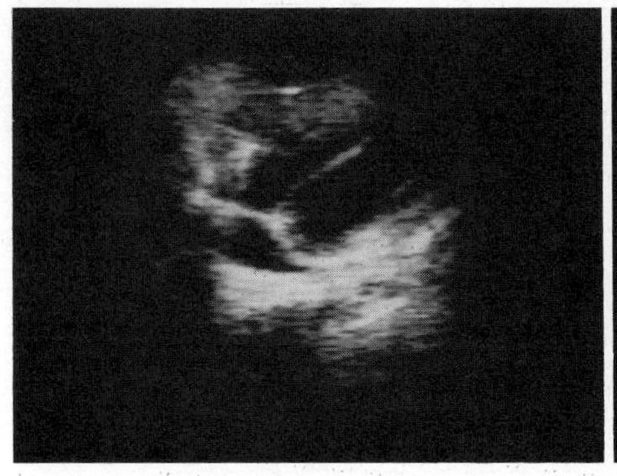

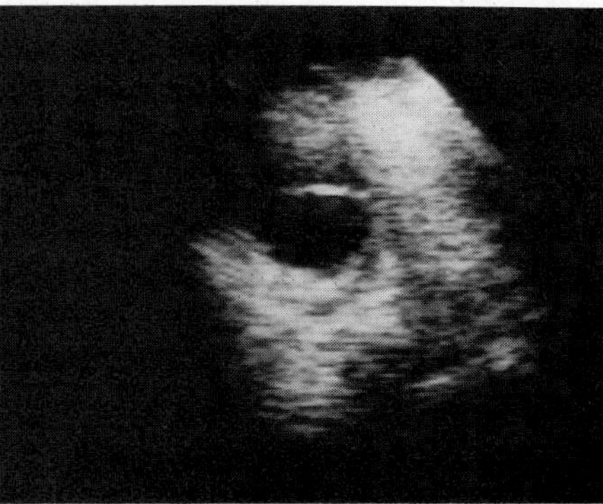

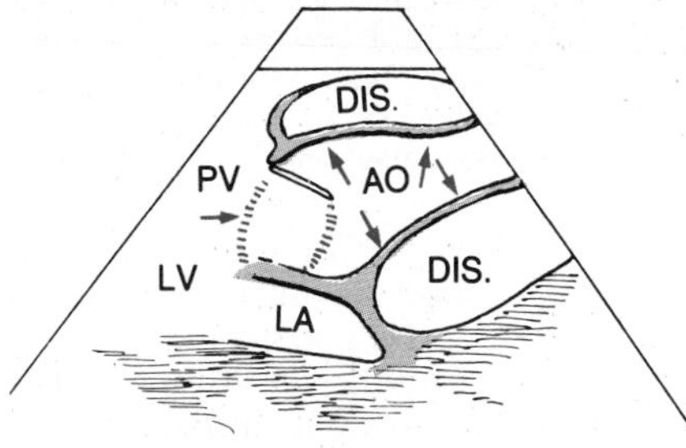

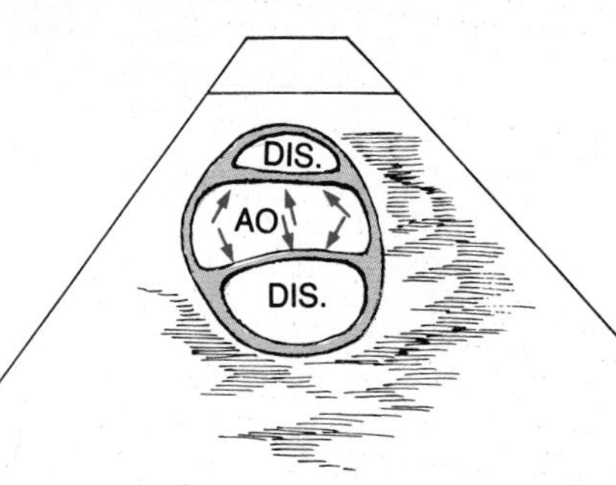

FIGURE 47-10. Cross-sectional echogram of the proximal aorta in a 63-year-old woman with dissection of the proximal aorta occurring 12 years after implantation of a Starr-Edwards aortic valve prosthesis. A, Parasternal long-axis recording. B, Short-axis recording. The actual recordings are shown above, and diagrammatic representations of the findings are pictured below. The echodense prosthetic valve (PV) is easily seen on the long-axis recording. Surrounding the aorta (AO) is the false channel of the dissection (DIS). (From Weyman, A. E.: Cross-sectional Echocardiography. Philadelphia, Lea and Febiger, 1982.)

genase (LDH) and bilirubin levels are sometimes elevated because of hemolysis of blood trapped within the false lumen. Serum glutamic oxaloacetic transaminase (SGOT) and creatine phosphokinase (CK or CK-MB) values are usually normal. Disseminated intravascular coagulation has been reported rarely.[114] The electrocardiogram frequently shows left ventricular hypertrophy from preexistent hypertension and usually the absence of acute ischemic changes. The absence of electrocardiographic changes of myocardial ischemia or infarction in a patient with severe chest pain is a helpful point in the differential diagnosis from myocardial infarction.

IMAGING TECHNIQUES: ULTRASOUND, CT, AND MRI. Diagnostic ultrasound (M-mode), in combination with cross-sectional (2-D) echocardiography, is helpful in the detection of a proximal dissection by revealing a widened aortic root, with delineation of the dissecting hematoma[115-117] (Figs. 4-109 and 47-10). The delineation of descending aortic dissection is now possible using transesophageal ultrasound (Fig. 47-11). One large multicenter study reported a sensitivity and specificity of 99 and 98 per cent respectively with transesophageal echocardiography in the diagnosis of aortic dissection.[118,118a] The addition of Doppler color flow imaging can identify sites of communication between true and false lumen and define flow characteristics in both lumina. CT scanning with contrast injection (Fig. 11-15, p. 320) is quite accurate in defining both ascending and descending dissections, provided that there is identification of a false lumen to distinguish the dissection from a fusiform aneurysm.[116,119] MRI is another noninvasive technique that may be useful in defining aortic dissection. Identification of an intimal flap is possible in most cases, as is characterization of the extent of the dissection and involvement of major branch vessels.[9-12,122] Unlike CT scanning, it does not require administration of potentially toxic contrast material. Its major limitations are necessity for prolonged imaging time, cost, and inability to use metallic objects such as medication pumps, pacemakers, and others in and around the magnet. Although ultrasounds, CT, and MRI clearly offer the advantage of noninvasive diagnosis,[120,121] angiography is generally required to define the full extent of the dissection, to outline the relationship of the dissection to the major aortic branches, to evaluate aortic valve competency, and to identify the site of the intimal tear. However, these noninvasive techniques—especially the CT scan or MRI—are quite useful in the long-term follow-up of treated patients with aortic dissection to detect evidence of localized aneurysm formation. Chest roentgenography or two-dimensional echocardiography and aortic angiography provide the most substantive laboratory tests for initial suspicion and definitive diagnosis, respectively. Chest roentgenography almost always

Figure 47-11. See color plate 10

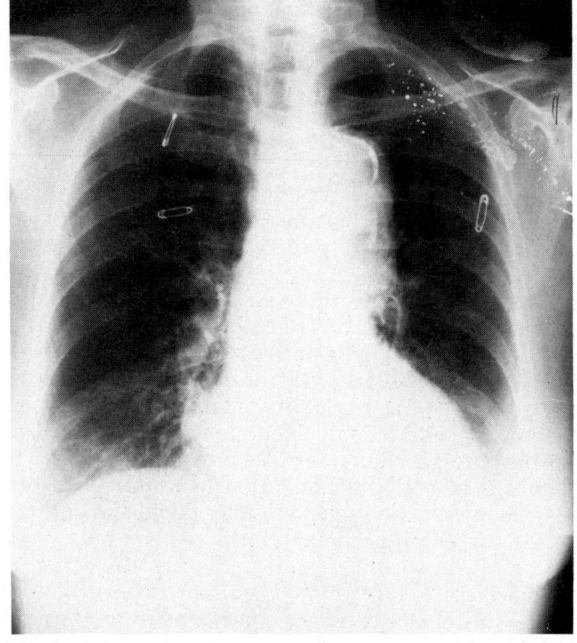

FIGURE 47-12. "Calcium sign" in distal dissection in an 80-year-old woman with longstanding hypertension. Note the marked separation of the calcification in the aortic knob and descending thoracic aorta from the outer wall of the aorta. This distance is normally no greater than 0.5 cm.

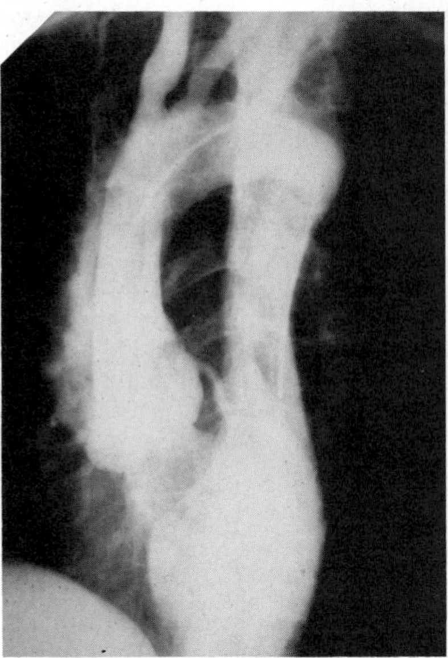
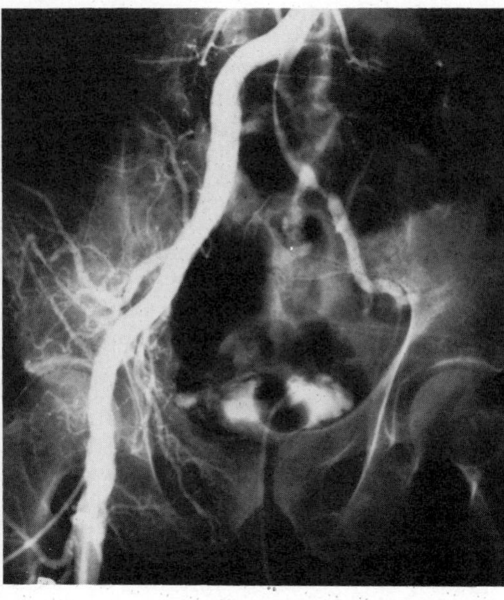

FIGURE 47–13. *Left,* Thoracic aortogram in the left anterior oblique projection showing a dissection beginning in the ascending aorta and spiraling through the aortic arch into the descending aorta. The false lumen can be faintly visualized. *Right,* Angiogram of the distal aorta showing virtual obstruction of the left iliac artery by the dissection. (Courtesy of Christos Athanasoulis, M.D., and Arthur Waltman, M.D., Section of Vascular Radiology. Massachusetts General Hospital, Boston.)

reveals an abnormally widened aortic contour. A localized bulge may overlay the site of origin, and the aortic silhouette may be widened wherever the dissection extends. If the aortic knob is calcified, separation of the intimal calcification from the adventitial border exceeding 1 cm (the "calcium sign") is virtually pathognomonic of aortic dissection (Fig. 47–12). Tracheal deviation or a left pleural effusion may be seen. Comparison with previous films is most helpful. On the other hand, it is possible for extensive aortic dissection to occur without radiographic abnormalities. For suspected proximal dissection, two-dimensional echocardiography can be rapidly performed and frequently will show the dissection.

AORTIC ANGIOGRAPHY. The single most important study in the diagnosis of aortic dissection is *aortic angiography.* Although originally performed by injection of contrast material into the pulmonary artery, with aortic opacification following the pulmonary venous phase, retrograde angiography is now the method of choice. The hazards of this approach have proved minimal, provided the catheter is carefully inserted and contrast material is not injected into the false channel. Aortic angiography has three objectives: (1) to establish a definite diagnosis, (2) to identify the site of origin of the dissection, and (3) to delineate the extent of the dissection and the distal circulation to vital organs (Figs. 47–13 and 47–14).

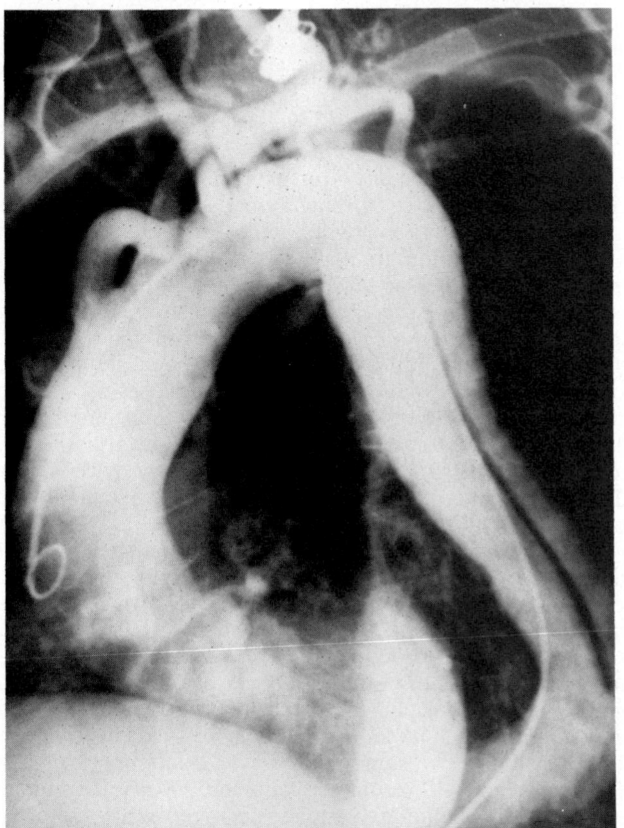

FIGURE 47–14. Left oblique anterior view of the aorta outlined angiographically showing a distal aortic dissection in a 63-year-old man. The true and false channels are clearly seen. The false channel is heavily opacified.

One additional feature to be assessed by angiography is the degree to which the false channel is opacified. There is evidence that the prognosis in medically treated patients is better in those with a nonopacified false channel, presumably an indication of thrombus formation in the channel that may serve to buttress the wall of the dissected aorta.[123] Although highly accurate, angiography is not without occasional pitfalls in the detection of aortic dissection.[113] Angiography may fail to show a dissection if there is faint opacification of the false lumen, unusual tearing of the intima, a small and localized dissection, or equal simultaneous opacification of both channels.[124] Nevertheless, when properly obtained and interpreted, angiograms provide a definite diagnosis in almost every case, and the procedure is well tolerated by even critically ill patients.

MANAGEMENT

Therapy for aortic dissection is directed at halting the progression of the dissecting hematoma, since fatal complications arise not from the intimal tear itself but rather from the subsequent course taken by the dissection.[125] Without treatment, aortic dissection is highly fatal. In a collective review of long-term survival in untreated aortic dissection, more than one-fourth of all patients were dead within 24 hours, more than one-half died within the first week, more than three-fourths died within 1 month, and more than 90 per cent died within 1 year.[126]

The first surgical approach to aortic dissection was the so-called fenestration procedure in which the dissected aorta was incised and a distal communication was created between the true and false channels, thereby decompressing the false lumen.[127,128] Definitive surgical therapy was pioneered by DeBakey and colleagues in the early 1950's.[129] Its principles are to excise the intimal tear, obliterate the false channel by oversewing aortic edges, reconstitute the aorta with or without interposition of a synthetic graft, and, in the case of proximal dissection, restore aortic valve competence by resuspension of the displaced aortic leaflets or by prosthetic aortic valve replacement.

Aggressive medical treatment of aortic dissection was first advocated by Wheat, Palmer, and collaborators.[130] They established two goals for pharmacological therapy: (1) reduction of the systolic blood pressure, and (2) diminution of the velocity of left venticular ejection (dV/dt), which is thought to be a major stress acting upon the aortic wall that contributes to the genesis and propagation of aortic dissection. Originally introduced for patients too ill to withstand surgery, medical therapy now forms the basis for the initial treatment of virtually all patients with aortic dissection before definitive diagnosis by angiography and serves as primary long-term therapy in additional subsets of patients.

EARLY EMERGENCY TREATMENT. All patients in whom there is a strong suspicion of aortic dissection should be admitted immediately to an intensive care unit, where blood pressure, cardiac rhythm, central venous pressure, urine output, and, when necessary, pulmonary wedge pressure and cardiac output can be monitored. Initial therapeutic goals are the elimination of pain and the reduction of systolic blood pressure to 100 to 120 mm Hg (mean of 60 to 75 mm Hg) or to the lowest level commensurate with adequate vital organ (cardiac, renal, and cerebral) perfusion. Simultaneously, arterial dV/dt, which reflects the velocity of left ventricular ejection, should be reduced by beta-adrenergic blockade regardless of whether systolic hypertension or pain is present.

For acute reduction of arterial pressure, the potent vasodilator sodium nitroprusside is very effective, mixed as 50 to 100 mg in 500 ml of 5 per cent dextrose in water and infused initially at 25 to 50 μg/min, with dosages varying according to blood pressure response. Side effects include nausea, restlessness, somnolence, hypotension, and cyanide or thiocyanate toxicity, which can develop after more than 48 hours of continuous use. Sodium nitroprusside alone can cause an increase in dV/dt, which can potentially contribute to propagation of the dissection.[131] Thus, adequate simultaneous beta-adrenergic blockade is essential when this drug is used.[132]

If sodium nitroprusside is ineffective or poorly tolerated, the ganglionic blocking agent trimethaphan (Arfonad), mixed as 500 mg to 2.0 gm in 500 ml of 5 per cent glucose and water, can be used. The initial infusion rate is 1 mg/min, with the dose titrated against the blood pressure response, which is enhanced by the orthostatic maneuver of elevating the head of the bed. Limitations in the use of this powerful agent include severe hypotension, tachyphylaxis, somnolence, and sympathoplegia with urinary retention, constipation, ileus, and pupillary dilation. In contrast to sodium nitroprusside, trimethaphan depresses dV/dt, which should provide a relative advantage in the treatment of aortic dissection. However, its unpleasant side effects and rapid tachyphylaxis have relegated this drug to a position of second choice in acute therapy in most centers.

To reduce dV/dt acutely, propranolol or a comparable intravenous beta blocker should be used in incremental doses of 1 mg intravenously every 5 minutes until there is evidence of satisfactory beta blockade, usually indicated by a pulse rate of 60 to 80 beats/min in the acute setting. A test dose of 0.5 mg intravenously is advised. The maximum initial total dose should not exceed 0.15 mg/kg. Additional propranolol should be given intravenously every 4 to 6 hours in order to maintain adequate beta blockade, as reflected in heart rate, usually in dosages somewhat lower than the initial amount, i.e., 2 to 6 mg. In chronic stable dissection, propranolol (or an alternative beta blocker) can be started orally, using 20 to 40 mg every 6 hours. Propranolol is contraindicated in the presence of bradycardia, asthma, or heart failure. Since propranolol was the first generally available beta-adrenoceptor blocking drug, it is the one that has been used most widely in aortic dissection. However, there is good reason to believe that other beta blockers are equally effective if used in equivalent doses. In particular, those which are cardioselective, such as atenolol and metoprolol, may be preferable in patients with chronic obstructive lung disease or a history of bronchial asthma. Labetalol, a recently released alpha- and beta-adrenergic receptor blocker (p. 1308), has great promise for the treatment of aortic dissection.[133] It combines selective alpha blockade and nonselective beta blockade, which lowers both blood pressure and dV/dt.

Labetalol is given intravenously in a first dose of 5 to 20 mg; further doses of 20 to 40 mg can be administered every 10 to 15 minutes until blood pressure returns to usual levels or a total dose of 300 mg has been given.

Refractory hypertension can follow occlusion of one or both renal arteries, with resultant release of large amounts of renin. In this situation, the intravenous ACE inhibitor, enalapril, may be quite effective in doses of 1 to 2 mg every 4 to 6 hours.

The initial experience with calcium-channel antagonists in the treatment of aortic dissection is encouraging. Use of these agents in managing hypertensive crisis has been favorable (p. 870).[134] Sublingual nifedipine has been used successfully to treat refractory hypertension associated with aortic dissection.[135] The combined vasodilator and negative inotropic effects of these drugs are ideally suited for this disease. Once the patient's condition is stabilized, angiography should be performed for a definitive diagnosis. Angiography should be performed as soon as possible after admission, unless a life-threatening complication such as aortic rupture, free aortic regurgitation, cardiac tamponade, or compromise of a vital organ has supervened. If any of these potentially lethal problems arises, surgery must be undertaken immediately, with angiography performed if possible while the operating room is being readied.

DEFINITIVE SUBSEQUENT THERAPY. Despite minor variations from center to center, a reasonable consensus as to the definitive therapy of aortic dissection has evolved over the past two decades. Although either medical or surgical therapy can be associated with an extremely successful outcome, it can be generally stated that *surgical results are superior to medical results in acute proximal dissection*, and, conversely, *medical therapy offers a relative advantage over surgery in most cases of uncomplicated acute distal dissection.*[136–138] These differences are based largely upon the disparate natural history of proximal and distal disease. Even minute progression of a proximal dissection poses potentially devastating consequences such as pulse loss, aortic regurgitation, neurological compromise, or cardiac tamponade. Thus, immediate surgical repair promises a better outcome. In contrast, patients with distal dissection are for the most part older and have a relatively increased incidence of advanced atherosclerotic or cardiopulmonary disease, thus rendering their surgical risks considerably higher. Medical therapy has proved to be quite effective in this group. Agreement on these principles is not unanimous, with some investigators advocating surgical treatment of all acute dissections, both proximal and distal.[138] However, a recent study involving patients from both Duke and Stanford has shown that medical therapy provides equivalent outcome to surgical treatment of uncomplicated distal dissection.[139]

A hospital survival of approximately 80 to 90 per cent has been reported for patients with acute proximal dissection treated surgically and 80 per cent for those with acute distal dissection treated medically.[139,140] Hospital survival for patients with chronic dissection (defined as presentation 2 weeks or more after the onset of dissection) treated either surgically—usually because of aortic insufficiency or an enlarging aneurysm—or medically exceeds 90 per cent.[136–138,140,141] The somewhat poorer results for surgically treated patients with acute dissection are mostly attributable to complications that have already occurred as a result of the dissection before definitive therapy,[137] although the fragility of the aortic wall in acute dissection often presents a serious problem to surgeons, adding to the risks of operation. The

TABLE 47–1 INDICATIONS FOR DEFINITIVE SURGICAL AND MEDICAL THERAPY IN AORTIC DISSECTION

Surgical
1. Treatment of choice for acute proximal dissection
2. Treatment for acute distal dissection complicated by the following:
   a. Progression with vital organ compromise
   b. Rupture or impending rupture (e.g., saccular aneurysm formation)
   c. Aortic regurgitation (rare)
   d. Retrograde extension into the ascending aorta
   e. Dissection in Marfan syndrome

Medical
1. Treatment of choice for uncomplicated distal dissection
2. Treatment for stable, isolated arch dissection
3. Treatment of choice for stable chronic dissection (uncomplicated dissection presenting 2 weeks or later after onset)

better survival in patients with chronic dissection derives from this same principle, i.e., they have already selected themselves out as a group destined to do well because they have survived the initial high mortality that occurs within the first 2 weeks of onset of the dissection.[136,137] The results of long-term follow-up will be discussed below.

The generally advocated *indications for definitive surgical therapy* are summarized in Table 47–1. Note that occasional patients with proximal dissection who refuse surgery or for whom surgery is contraindicated by age or prior debilitating illness can be treated successfully by medical therapy. Moreover, both early and late medical therapy are usually required in *all* patients, inlcuding those treated surgically, to provide stabilization initially and to protect against later redissection.

SURGICAL THERAPY. Although the precise timing of surgery in patients without life-threatening complications is somewhat controversial, prompt repair is generally recommended to prevent even minimal progression of the dissection that might lead to further complications.[137a] Surgical risk for all patients is obviously increased by age; associated diseases, especially pulmonary emphysema; aneurysm leakage; cardiac tamponade; shock; or vital organ compromise as a result of such conditions as myocardial infarction, cerebrovascular accident, and particularly renal failure.[138]

As noted, the usual objectives of definitive surgical therapy are excision of the intimal tear and obliteration of entry into the false lumen by suturing together the edges of the dissected aorta proximally and distally. Aortic continuity is then reestablished either by joining the edges of the aorta directly or by interposing a prosthetic sleeve graft between the two ends of the aorta (Fig. 47–15). Determining the routes of perfusion of vital organs distal to the surgical site by preoperative angiography may be of importance. For example, one or both renal arteries occasionally are found to be fed from the false lumen, in which case the false channel at the distal end of the surgically transected aorta might be left unclosed.

There is growing consensus favoring more aggressive surgical repair of dissections involving the proximal aorta, regardless of the site of intimal tear, to prevent extension and rupture into the pericardial cavity. This applies even if the dissection originates in the distal aorta and extends proximally.[138,140]

When aortic regurgitation complicates aortic dissection, simple decompression of the false channel may be all that is necessary to resuspend the leaflets and restore valvular competence. However, most surgeons have become increasingly aggressive about replacing the aortic valve if it appears that even moderate aortic regurgitation will be present after the leaflets are decompressed. This avoids the high risk of having to replace the aortic valve in a second operation through a diseased aorta at some later date.

For repair of a proximal dissection, total cardiopulmonary bypass is necessary. On occasion, because of extensive dissection of the aorta, it may be difficult to find a safe site for placement of a perfusion cannula. In rare cases, we have had to abandon plans for surgical repair of a proximal dissection for this reason. In the repair of dissections of the descending thoracic aorta, support of the distal circulation may be necessary and can be achieved either by partial left heart bypass or by using a conduit that carries blood from the proximal to the distal aorta, circumventing the site of the dissection.

The actual operative procedure itself, in aortic dissection, is technically demanding. The wall of the diseased aorta is often

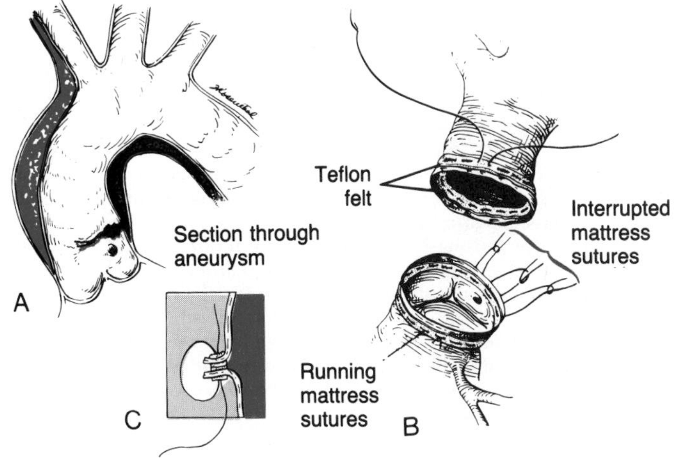

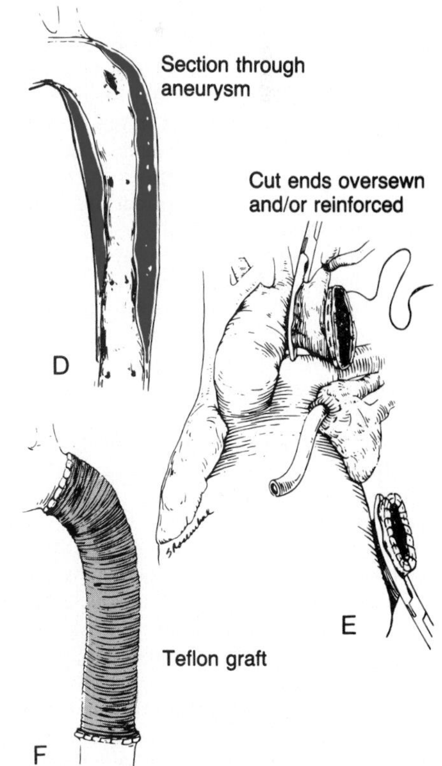

FIGURE 47–15. Several steps in the surgical repair of a proximal (*A, B,* and *C*) and a distal (*D, E,* and *F*) aortic dissection. *A* and *D* show the dissections and the intimal tears. *B,* The aorta has been transected, and the ends of the aorta have been oversewn to obliterate the false lumen and have been buttressed with Teflon felt to prevent the sutures from tearing through the fragile tissue. *C,* The aortic ends are brought together in such a way that the Teflon is again used to reinforce the suture line between the two ends of the aorta or between the aorta and a sleeve graft, if such a graft is necessary for reconstitution of the aorta. *E* shows resection of a distal dissection, with a Teflon graft interposed in *F.* (*D, E,* and *F* reprinted by permission from Austen, W. G., and DeSanctis, R.: Surgical treatment of dissecting aneurysm of the thoracic aorta. N. Engl. J. Med. *272*:1314, 1965.)

friable, and the repair must be performed with meticulous care. The use of Teflon felt to buttress the wall and prevent sutures from tearing through the fragile aorta has represented a significant technical advance (Fig. 47–15*B*). An alternate surgical approach consists of the wrapping of an unstable arch dissection with Dacron.[142] Bleeding, infection, and pulmonary or renal insufficiency consititute the most common early complications of surgical therapy. Spinal cord ischemia with resultant paraplegia due to inadvertent interruption of blood supply from the anterior spinal or intercostal arteries is a rare but dreaded consequence. Late complications include progressive aortic regurgitation if the aortic valve has not been replaced, localized aneurysm formation, and redissection at the original site of repair or at an independent secondary site.[143]

Several innovative techniques for the surgical treatment of aortic dissection have been reported. One utilizes an intraluminal sutureless prosthesis.[144,145] Another, applied especially to distal but also to proximal dissection, consists of bypassing the dissected aorta with a Dacron sleeve, ligating the aorta at the site of proximal extension of the dissection, and creating reversal of flow in the distal aorta to perfuse the major arterial branches arising from the dissected segment.[146] Tanabe and coworkers have inserted strips of Ivalon sponge in the false channel, with the intention of stimulating the organization of blood and the formation of thrombus, thus strengthening the wall of the dissected aorta.[147] Finally, Carpentier and colleagues have reported the use of a gelatin-resorcin-formaldehyde glue to stick the dissected layers of proximal aortic dissections together, thus avoiding the necessity of prosthetic graft replacement.[148] These techniques have been used in only small numbers of patients, and long-term follow-up is lacking.

In proximal dissection, when the aorta is fragile and badly torn, replacement of the aorta and the aortic valve using a composite graft into which the coronary arteries are reimplanted has been a valuable technique (Fig. 47–16).[66]

MEDICAL THERAPY. Indications for *definitive* medical therapy are summarized in Table 47–1. Clearly, operation must be performed if there is medical failure, such as rupture or impending rupture, progression of the dissection with vital organ compromise, aortic regurgitation, or inability to control pain or blood pressure with drugs. Although we prefer medical therapy for low-risk patients with stable distal dissection, some centers advise surgery in this group as well.[136,143] Controlled studies of medical versus surgical treatment of comparable patients with distal dissection are lacking. Because of the extreme difficulty of surgery involving aortic arch dissections, medical therapy is usually advocated in those rare dissections that originate in the arch, with operative intervention reserved for serious complications that might occur on medical treatment.

Medical therapy is recommended for patients with chronic dissection, defined as a stable aortic dissection that has occurred 2 or more weeks prior to presentation, unless late complications of the dissection, such as aortic insufficiency or localized aneurysm formation, necessitate surgery.

Complications of medical therapy include severe hypotension related to the drugs, with possible precipitation of acute tubular necrosis, cerebrovascular accident, or myocardial infarction.[137]

Late follow-up of patients leaving the hospital with treated aortic dissection shows an actuarial survival rate not much worse than that of individuals of comparable age without dissection; there are no significant differences in these patients between those with proximal vs. distal dissection, acute vs. chronic dissection, or medical vs. surgical treatment.[137] Thus, initially successful surgical or medical therapy is usually sustained on long-term follow-up. Late complications include redissection, aortic regurgitation, and localized aneurysm formation.

Long-term medical therapy to control hypertension and reduce dV/dt is indicated for all patients who have sustained an

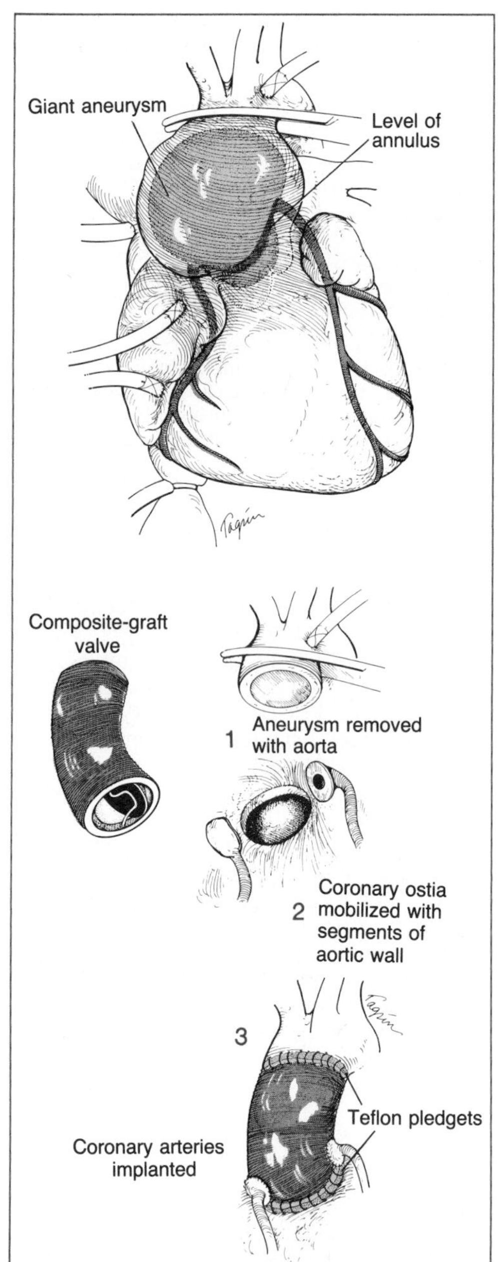

FIGURE 47–16. Technique for the composite graft replacement of an aneurysm of the ascending aorta. *Top,* The aneurysm is shown, involving the sinuses of Valsalva. The patient is on total cardiopulmonary bypass. *Bottom,* The composite graft is shown, with a low profile, tilting-disc prosthesis attached to its inferior end. (1) The aneurysm is resected with the aortic valve; (2) The coronary ostia have been excised, and mobilized with a button or aortic wall; (3) The composite graft has been secured into place using Teflon felt reinforcement for the suture line, and the coronary arteries have been reimplanted as the graft. In the method of Bentall, the composite graft is sewn inside the incised aneurysm, which is left in situ. The coronary ostia are then anastomosed directly to the graft.

aortic dissection, regardless of whether they have received definitive surgical or medical therapy. Systolic blood pressure should be controlled at or below a level of 130 to 140 mm Hg, or even lower if tolerated. Preferred agents are those with a negative inotropic as well as hypotensive effect, such as beta blockers and calcium-channel antagonists, together with a diuretic if necessary to control blood pressure. Hydralazine and minoxidil increase cardiac output and arterial dV/dt and should be used only in the presence of adequate beta blockade. Angiotensin-converting enzyme inhibitors and other drugs such as clonidine and guanabenz are powerful antihypertensive agents and should be useful, especially in combination with beta blockers.

Follow-up of patients who have sustained an aortic dissection should include careful and repeated physical examinations, periodic chest roentgenograms, and CT or MRI scans if localized aneurysm formation is suspected.

ANNULOAORTIC ECTASIA

In a number of patients with pure aortic regurgitation the cause is idiopathic dilatation of the proximal aorta and the aortic annulus. The term *annuloaortic ectasia* was first used by Ellis et al. in 1961 to describe this clinicopathological condition.[149] The entity has been subsequently recognized with increasing frequency and makes up about 5 to 10 per cent of the population of patients who currently undergo aortic valve replacement for pure aortic regurgitation.

ETIOLOGY AND PATHOGENESIS. The common pathological feature shared by patients with annuloaortic ectasia is that of severe degenerative changes (usually cystic medial necrosis) in the wall of the afflicted aorta. Some degree of cystic medial necrosis with annuloaortic ectasia is found in virtually all cases of Marfan syndrome.[150] In fact, it can be severe and is a frequent cause of death from fatal aortic rupture or dissection in this syndrome (p. 1641). There is some evidence to suggest that abnormalities in collagen cross linkage may play a role in this phenomenon,[151] while others have identified abnormalities in elastin.[152] In most reported series of patients with annuloaortic ectasia, however, patients with classic Marfan syndrome have been excluded. Careful examination of patients with annuloaortic ectasia usually reveals that about one-fourth to one-half have other stigmata of Marfan syndrome, indicating that many patients represent a forme fruste of that connective tissue disorder. In a clinicogenetic study of 18 patients with severe aortic regurgitation and dilatation of the ascending aorta but without other evidence of the Marfan syndrome except on pathological examination of the aorta, Emanuel et al. reported that 37.3 per cent of 126 first-degree relatives had one or more stigmata of Marfan syndrome.[153] Thus, it appears that many of these patients have primarily the aortic abnormalities of Marfan syndrome without the other manifestations of the disease. In summary, then, patients with annuloaortic ectasia appear to fall into three groups: (1) those with classic Marfan syndrome, (2) those with a forme fruste of Marfan syndrome, and (3) those with cystic medial necrosis and no obvious underlying cause.

As the media degenerates, the aorta widens. The aortic root is involved, and the annulus dilates, drawing the aortic leaflets apart and leading to aortic regurgitation. The weakened aorta may dissect and this may aggravate the aortic regurgitation.

CLINICAL MANIFESTATIONS. Men predominate over women in virtually all series by a ratio of anywhere between 2 and 8 to 1. Patients without obvious Marfan syndrome usually are encountered in the fourth, fifth, and sixth decades with progressively more severe aortic regurgitation. Patients with the classic Marfan syndrome or its forme fruste are generally younger. Some patients with annuloaortic ectasia experience sudden onset and rapid progression of symptoms, which sometimes but not always are due to severe aortic regurgitation secondary to aortic dissection. In the study of Lemon and White, recent aortic root dissection was found in 11 of 25 patients with annuloaortic ectasia who came to surgery.[154] All 11 of these patients had experienced chest pain before operation, although chest pain was also present in several patients without aortic dissection.

The physical examination may reveal abnormal pulsation of the dilated aorta over the 2nd and 3rd right intercostal spaces, especially if the examination is done with the patient sitting and in full expiration. We have seen three patients with annuloaortic ectasia who had pulsation of the right sternoclavicular joint.

There is nothing unique about the signs of aortic regurgitation in patients with annuloaortic ectasia as opposed to those with regurgitation from other causes, except for the greater intensity of the diastolic murmur to the right of the sternum in the former group and to the left in patients with a primary valvular abnormality. Lemon and White did find that the two features—acute or subacute development of symptoms and the presence of chest pain—were more frequent in the group of patients with annuloaortic ectasia than in those with pure valvular aortic regurgitation, presumably on a rheumatic basis.[154] Features of Marfan syndrome should be sought and may be obvious, subtle, or absent.

The chest film usually shows a grossly dilated aortic root and ascending aorta with left ventricular enlargement proportionate to the severity of aortic regurgitation. Calcification in the aortic valve and dilated aorta is usually absent. Echocardiography, CT scan, or MRI demonstrate an abnormally widened aortic root. The huge aorta and aortic regurgitation are easily demonstrated angiographically. Lemon and White identified three types of angiographic aortic enlargement: (1) "pear-shaped" enlargement (56 per cent) (Fig. 47–17), (2) diffuse symmetrical dilatation (27 per cent), and (3) dilatation limited to the sinuses of Valsalva (6 per cent). In our own unpublished experience, aneurysmal dilatation of the sinuses of Valsalva is typically seen in those with Marfan syndrome. The mean maximal aortic diameter in Lemon and White's patients was 7.6 ± 2.7 cm and ranged from 4.8 to 15 cm. This is two to five times the normal aortic diameter. Because dissections are characteristically small, circumscribed, and confined to the ascending aorta, they may not be easy to identify angiographically.

MANAGEMENT. Surgical correction using total cardiopulmonary bypass is usually undertaken for relief of aortic regurgitation when it is severe and responsible for symptoms of left ventricular failure or when the left ventricle or ascending aorta is increasing in size. However, in addition to replacement of the aortic valve, resection of the aneurysmal aorta with insertion of a prosthetic graft is generally required. Some surgeons advise sewing an artificial aortic valve to one end of a long prosthetic sleeve and suturing this in place from the aortic annulus at one end to the ascending aorta where it narrows beyond the aneurysm at the other. This reconstruction necessitates reimplantation of the coronary arteries (Fig. 47–16). In fact, with aneurysmal sinuses of Valsalva, the coronary ostia may be carried cephalad by the enlarging sinuses, again necessitating ligation and reimplantation of the coronary arteries or the construction of saphenous vein bypass conduits from the aorta to the ligated coronary arteries. Because of the magnitude of the operation and the frequently friable tissues

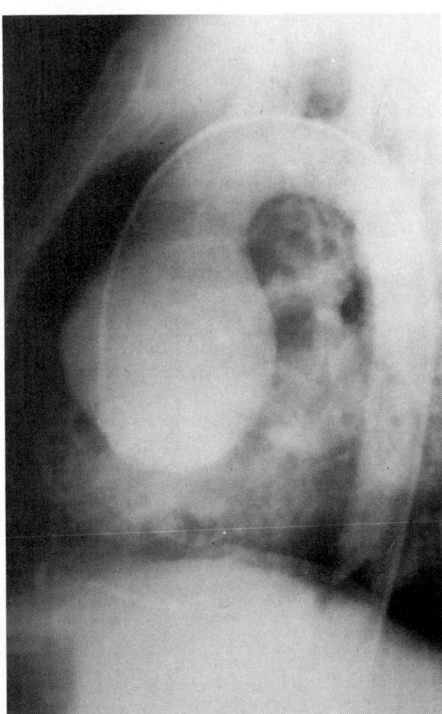

FIGURE 47–17. Lateral aortogram in a man with annuloaortic ectasia. The bulbous, pear-shaped aortic root can be easily seen. The left ventricle is opacified consequent to aortic regurgitation. (Courtesy of Christos Athanasoulis, M.D., and Arthur Waltman, M.D., Section of Vascular Radiology, Massachusetts General Hospital, Boston.)

that make operation difficult, the risks of failure of aortic valve replacement and aneurysm resection are between 10 and 15 per cent in most centers; 5- and 10-year survival rates have been reported at approximately 75 per cent and 55 per cent, respectively.[155,156] Gott et al. reported a 90 per cent 8-year survival in 49 patients operated on for ascending aortic aneurysms associated with Marfan syndrome[157]; they recommend elective repair of the aorta in patients with Marfan syndrome and aortic root diameter greater than 6.0 cm.[157] However, this policy remains controversial.[158] The relative risk of dissection, based on aortic site, appears to be variable. In an echocardiographic study, 3 of 11 patients with annuloaortic ectasia developed dissection during a mean follow-up of 18 months. All three had aortic root diameters exceeding 5.0 cm; however, four other patients with aortic diameters greater than 5.0 cm did not develop dissections.

Although postoperative results in survivors may be excellent, there is a disturbing occurrence of late sudden deaths, mostly from aortic dissection.[159] Late reoperation for adjacent aneurysm formation or dissection is necessary in more than 20 per cent of patients.[156] Death from progressive heart failure and sudden cardiac deaths also occur.

AORTIC ARTERITIS SYNDROMES

Takayasu's Arteritis

This peculiar arteritis was first noted in 1908 by the Japanese ophthalmologist Takayasu, who described a young woman with cataracts and unusual wreathlike arteriovenous anastomoses surrounding the optic papillae. In discussing this case, Takayasu's colleagues called attention to two patients with similar ocular findings who also had absent radial pulses. Subsequently, this disease entity has been described by a variety of terms that reflect some of its many features, such as "aortic arch syndrome," "pulseless disease," "reversed coarctation," "occlusive thromboaortopathy," "young female arteritis," as well as Takayasu's arteritis.[160]

PATHOPHYSIOLOGY AND ETIOLOGY. This disease occurs worldwide, although the majority of cases have been reported from Asia and Africa and most large series consist of Asians, with a heavy predilection for women.[161]

The basic pathological process is that of marked intimal proliferation and fibrosis and fibrous scarring and degeneration of the elastic fibers of the media, with round cell infiltration of variable intensity. However, fibrosis predominates over cellular reaction. The adventitia and intima become markedly thickened and vasa vasorum are destroyed. In its advanced cicatricial stage, the gross appearance of the aorta strikingly resembles the tree-bark–like appearance of luetic aortitis. The proliferative process leads to obliterative luminal changes in the aorta and involved arteries. Localized aneurysm formation, poststenotic dilatation, and calcification in the aortic and arterial walls are late complications. The process most often involves the arch of the aorta and its major branches, usually with changes that are most marked at the points of origin of the arteries from the aorta. It may present as multisegmental aortic disease with areas of normal wall between affected sites, diffuse involvement of the aorta, or disease of individual arteries arising from the aorta. The pulmonary arterial tree may also be affected. In a report from the United States, the most frequently affected arteries were the subclavian (90 per cent), carotid (45 per cent), vertebral (25 per cent), and renal (20 per cent).[162] In another series from the United States, the subclavian arteries, mesenteric arteries, and abdominal aorta were most commonly involved, each in nearly 80 per cent of cases.[163]

Ueno et al. have subdivided the disease into three types, depending upon the sites of involvement[164] (Fig. 47–18). Type I involves primarily the aortic arch and its branches; Type II spares the aortic arch, involving the thoracoabdominal aorta and its branches; Type III combines features of both. Lupi-Herrera and colleagues have suggested a fourth category, Type IV, in which there is pulmonary arterial involvement.[161] In their series of 107 cases, the incidences of the various types were 8, 11, 65, and 45 per cent for Types I, II, III, and IV, respectively.

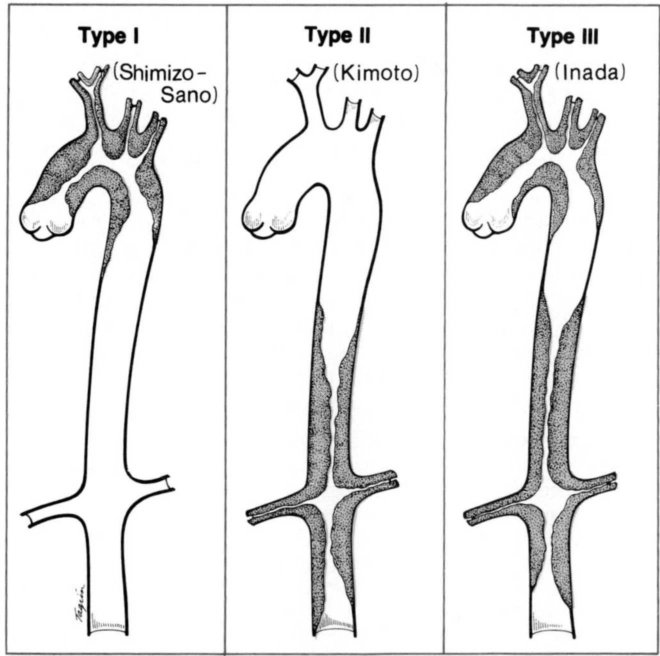

FIGURE 47–18. Types of Takayasu's arteritis. Type I involves primarily the aortic arch and brachiocephalic vessels. Type II affects the thoracoabdominal aorta and particularly the renal arteries. Type III combines features of both Types I and II. Types I and III may be complicated by aortic regurgitation. The eponyms for each type are noted.

A specific etiology for Takayasu's arteritis has not been found.[162] It has been linked to rheumatic fever, streptococcal infections, rheumatoid arthritis, and other collagen vascular diseases. Although giant cells are occasionally found in pathological specimens of vessels involved by the disease, the entity seems clearly distinct from giant cell arteritis, which affects predominantly patients over the age of 50 and involves mainly medium-sized muscular arteries. Although the aortic scarring of advanced Takayasu's arteritis resembles that of syphilis, nothing else suggests a causal relationship. Some investigators have reported a strikingly higher incidence of tuberculin skin reactivity to both *Mycobacterium tuberculosis* and atypical mycobacteria in patients with Takayasu's arteritis compared with the general population, raising the possibility of a relationship to tuberculosis,[165] but this observation has not been confirmed.[163] Although antiaortic antibodies have been detected in patients with this disease, their etiological role is uncertain. Overall, the bulk of evidence favors an autoimmune etiology. It is likely that the arteritis represents the final common pathological expression of a number of different antigenic stimuli in susceptible patients. An association between Takayasu's arteritis and certain HLA subtypes has been reported,[166,167] although the importance of the association remains unclear.[162,163]

CLINICAL MANIFESTATIONS. The disease affects women more frequently than men, in a ratio of 8 to 1. In as many as three-fourths of cases, onset is in the teenage years, although cases beginning in infancy or late middle age have been reported.[161,168,169] More than half the patients with this disease develop an initial systemic illness characterized by symptoms such as fever, anorexia, malaise, weight loss, night sweats, arthralgias, pleuritic pain, and fatigue. Localized pain and tenderness may be noted over affected arteries. This phase subsides, and these patients—as well as those who do not go through this so-called initial "systemic phase"—after a latent period of variable duration show symptoms and signs referable to the obliterative and inflammatory changes in the vessels. These late manifestations include diminished or absent pulses in 96 per cent, bruits in 94 per cent, hypertension in 74 per cent, and heart failure in 28 per cent.[161] The retinopathy originally described by Takayasu is seen in only about 25 per cent and is usually associated with carotid arterial involvement. The ocular process may lead to retinal detachment and loss of vision.

Patients with Types I and III exhibit those findings which are considered to be most typical of this disease, namely "reversed" coarctation of the aorta with absent or diminished upper body pulses and barely detectable blood pressure in the arms, higher pressures in the lower extremities, bruits overlying diseased arteries, manifestations of ischemia at various affected sites, and syncope. Patients with Type II arteritis may have abdominal angina and claudication of the limbs but also tend to develop hypertension because of renal arterial involvement. In fact, hypertension is an extremely important complication of this disease, and it may be difficult to recognize because of the diminished pulsations in the arms. Hypertension appears to arise through several mechanisms, the two most important of which are hemodynamically significant acquired coarctation of the aorta and renal artery stenosis. Decreased aortic capacitance and reduced baroreceptor reactivity may be contributory.[170,171]

Heart failure, when present, is usually seen in very young patients and appears to be a consequence of systemic hypertension. Rarely, aortic regurgitation can also contribute to congestive failure and is due to severe hypertension or to inflammation with scarring of the aortic valve by the inflammatory process.[172] Myocarditis has recently been described in several patients with congestive heart failure without hypertension or aortic regurgitation.[173] Whether this is a frequent cause of heart failure is unknown. The ostia and proximal segments of the coronary arteries can be affected, resulting in angina or myocardial infarction.[174,174a] Rarely, aneurysms are palpable or arteriovenous fistulas occur.[168] Takayasu's arteritis may be a common cause of atypical coarctation syndromes in adults.[175] The frequent absence of antecedent systemic symptoms and the more equal sex distribution of this form of the disease have been stressed. It is also believed that Takayasu's arteritis may be responsible for some cases of what appear to be primary pulmonary hypertension,[176] and occasionally fever of unknown origin.[177]

Laboratory abnormalities during the systemic phase are frequent.[163,165] The sedimentation rate is elevated, and a low-grade leukocytosis and mild anemia of chronic disease are common. These return toward normal when the systemic phase resolves. IgG or IgM values are elevated in more than half the patients. Immune complexes are infrequently present.[162] Other serological abnormalities are common but not specific. These include elevated levels of C-reactive protein, increased antistreptolysin-O titers, the occasional presence of rheumatoid factor and antinuclear antibodies, and elevated fibrinogen levels.[178]

Chest roentgenograms are usually unrevealing, although a rim of calcification is sometimes seen in the walls of the affected arteries. Arteriography reveals typical findings of an irregular intimal surface, with stenosis of the aorta or its tributary arteries, poststenotic dilatations, saccular aneurysms, and even complete occlusion of vessels (Fig. 47–19). Lande and Rossi have described the affected thoracic aorta as having a typical, narrowed, "rat-tail" angiographic appearance (Fig. 47–20).[179]

DIAGNOSIS. Proposed criteria for the clinical diagnosis of Takayasu's arteritis are shown in Table 47–2.[180] An obligatory criterion is age ≤40 years at diagnosis. The two major criteria reflect involvement of either subclavian artery. There are nine minor criteria. A high probability of the disease exists if, in addition to age ≤40 years, the patient meets two major criteria; one major and two or more minor criteria; or four or more minor criteria.[180]

TREATMENT AND PROGNOSIS. Adrenal corticosteroids are often effective in relieving constitutional symptoms and halting progression in patients with the systemic phase of the disease.[162,163] Fever, malaise, and fatigue are often dramatically relieved by steroids, and the sedimentation rate, which is a sensitive indicator of the activity of the disease, falls toward normal. In patients with continued systemic symptoms and/or documented disease progression, cyclophosphamide can be added. This usually results in clinical improvement and the ability to reduce corticosteroids to every other day dosing.[164] The recommended dose of cyclophosphamide is

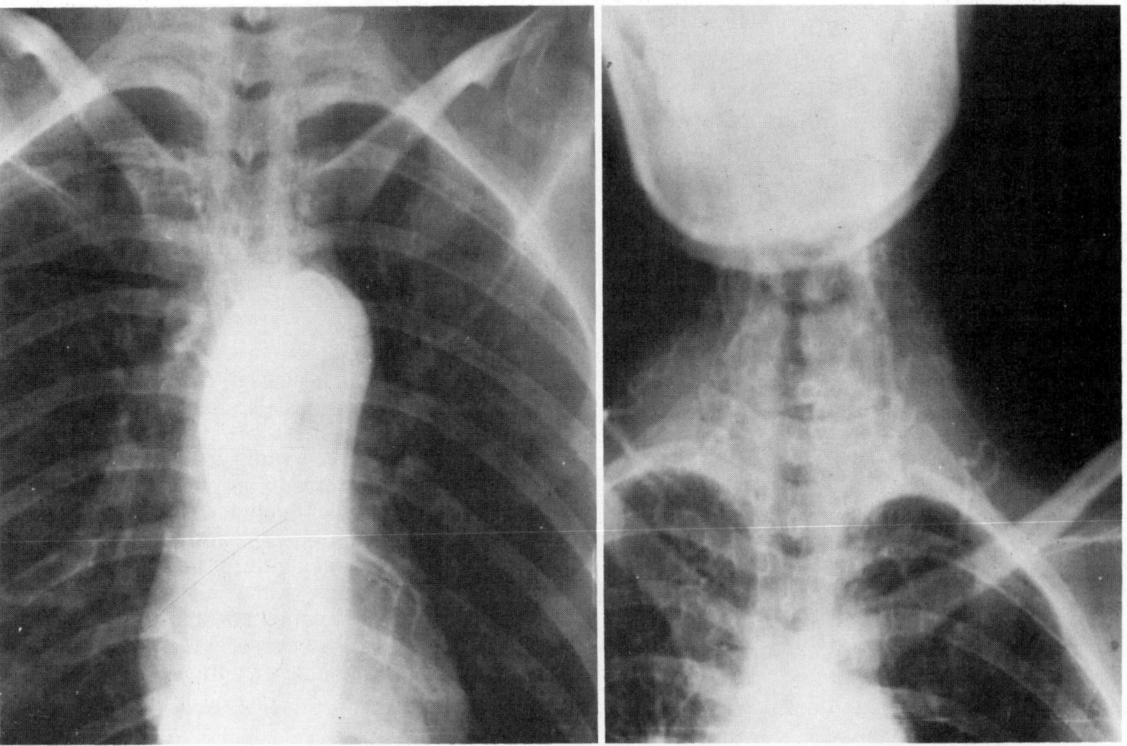

FIGURE 47–19. Thoracic aortogram *(left)* and late films of the head, neck, and upper thorax *(right)* in a 34-year-old Chinese woman with Takayasu's arteritis and no palpable pulses in the upper half of her body. The aortogram shows no direct filling of any of the major arteries arising from the aorta except the coronary arteries. In the delayed film *(right)* collateral channels faintly fill the carotid and vertebral systems.

TABLE 47-2 PROPOSED CRITERIA FOR THE CLINICAL DIAGNOSIS OF TAKAYASU'S DISEASE*

CRITERION	DEFINITION
Obligatory criterion	
Age ≤ 40 yr	Age ≤ 40 yr at diagnosis or at onset of "characteristic signs and symptoms"† of 1 month duration in patient history.
Two major criteria	
1. Left mid subclavian artery lesion	The most severe stenosis or occlusion present in the mid portion from the point 1 cm proximal to the left vertebral artery orifice to that 3 cm distal to the orifice determined by angiography.
2. Right mid subclavian artery lesion	The most severe stenosis or occlusion present in the mid portion from the right vertebral artery orifice to the point 3 cm distal to the orifice determined by angiography.
Nine minor criteria	
1. High ESR	Unexplained persistent high ESR ≥ 20 mm/h (Westergren) at diagnosis or presence of the evidence in patient history.
2. Carotid artery tenderness	Unilateral or bilateral tenderness of common carotid arteries by physician palpation: neck muscle tenderness is unacceptable.
3. Hypertension	Persistent blood pressure ≥ 140/90 mm Hg brachial or ≥ 160/90 mm Hg popliteal at age ≤ 40 yr or presence of the history at age ≤ 40 yr.
4. Aortic regurgitation	By auscultation or Doppler echocardiography or angiography.
or	
Annuloaortic ectasia	By angiography or two-dimensional echocardiography.
5. Pulmonary artery lesion	Lobar or segmental arterial occlusion or equivalent determined by angiography or perfusion scintigraphy; or presence of stenosis, aneurysm, luminal irregularity or any combination in pulmonary trunk or in unilateral or bilateral pulmonary arteries determined by angiography.
6. Left mid common carotid lesion	Presence of the most severe stenosis or occlusion in the mid portion of 5 cm in length from the point 2 cm distal to its orifice determined by angiography.
7. Distal brachiocephalic trunk lesion	Presence of the most severe stenosis or occlusion in the distal third determined by angiography.
8. Descending thoracic aorta lesion	Narrowing, dilation or aneurysm, luminal irregularity, or any combination determined by angiography: tortuosity alone is unacceptable.
9. Abdominal aorta lesion	Narrowing, dilation or aneurysm, luminal irregularity, or any combination and absence of lesion in aortoiliac region consisting of 2 cm of terminal aorta and bilateral common iliac arteries determined by angiography; tortuosity alone is unacceptable.

* The proposed criteria consist of one obligatory criterion, two major criteria, and nine minor criteria. In addition to the obligatory criterion, the presence of two major criteria, or one major and two or more minor criteria, or four or more minor criteria suggests a high probability of the presence of Takayasu's disease.

† "Characteristic signs and symptoms" are explained in the text (Methods). ESR = erythrocyte sedimentation rate.

From Ishikawa, K.: Diagnostic approach and proposed criteria for the clinical diagnosis of Takayasu's arteriopathy J. Am. Coll. Cardiol. *12*:964, 1988.

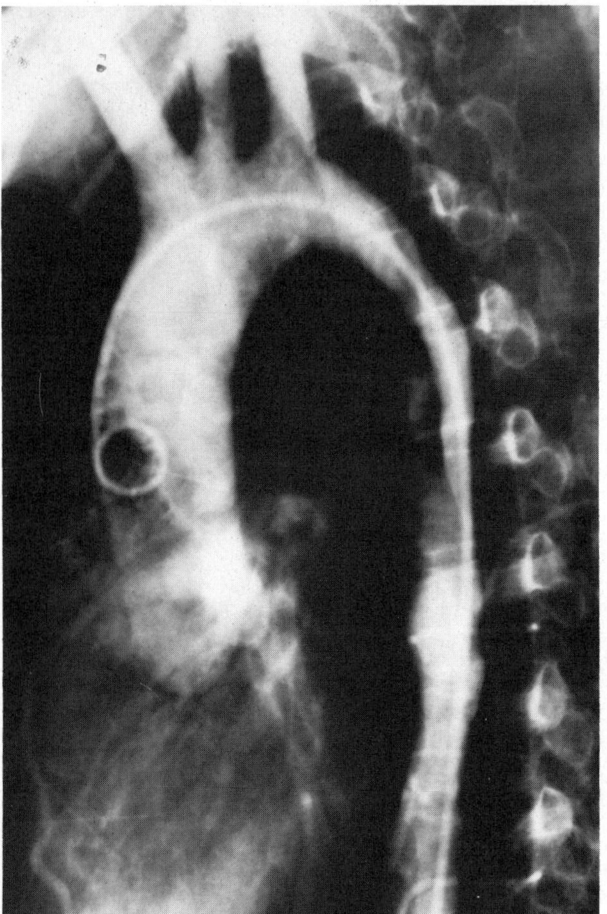

FIGURE 47-20. Aortogram in a 28-year-old Korean man with the clinical features of coarctation of the aorta that proved to be the result of Takayasu's arteritis. Note the typical "rat-tail" angiographic appearance of the descending thoracic aorta.

2 mg/kg/day, adjusted to maintain the peripheral leukocyte count above 3000/mm^3. Anticoagulant drugs, including those of the warfarin family, and drugs that inhibit platelet function, such as aspirin and dipyridamole, are recommended both to treat transient ischemic symptoms and to prevent progression of the disease. Their efficacy is not established. Aggressive treatment of hypertension, when present, is important. In cases related to renovascular disease, the angiotensin-converting enzyme inhibitors may be particularly effective.[181,182] A variety of *surgical treatments* may be needed to deal with late complications of Takayasu's arteritis,[162,163,183,184] including endarterectomy, bypass of obstructed arteries (especially the renal arteries), resection of localized coarctations, excision of saccular aneurysms, and, rarely, aortic valve replacement. Successful use of percutaneous transluminal angioplasty for dilation of stenotic lesions in carotid, subclavian, renal, and mesenteric arteries has also been reported.[163,185]

The course of the disease is unpredictable, but slow progression over a period of months to years is usual. Morbidity and mortality depend upon the presence or absence of severe complications, which include retinopathy, secondary hypertension, aortic regurgitation, and aortic or arterial aneurysms. In several series, uneventful survival over 5 to 7 years was 97 per cent in patients without major complications compared with 59 per cent in patients with complications.[186,187] In a follow-up study, Ishikawa reported 9-year survival of 94 per cent in patients with stable symptoms but 60 to 70 per cent in patients with crescendo symptom patterns.[188] Heart failure and cerebrovascular accidents are common causes of death. However, the combination of corticosteroid therapy, cytotoxic agents, and surgery when needed have led to 5-year survival rates that now may approximate 100 per cent.[162,163]

GIANT CELL ARTERITIS

This disease of unknown cause is predominantly found in elderly people and characteristically involves medium-sized arteries. However, the aorta and its major branches are affected in about 15 per cent of cases.[189] The disease is also referred to as "granulomatous arteritis," "cranial" or "temporal" arteritis, and "arteritis of the aged." It is closely allied to a syndrome characterized by diffuse muscular aching and stiffness called polymyalgia rheumatica.

PATHOPHYSIOLOGY AND ETIOLOGY. The many names given this disease describe its important features. The characteristic pathological lesion that distinguishes it from other arteritis syndromes is granulomatous inflammation of the media of small- to medium-caliber arteries, about the size of the temporal artery, with special predilection for vessels of the head and neck.[190] In addition to granulomas, an inflammatory infiltrate is usually found, composed largely of eosinophils, plasma cells, and other mononuclear cells. Endarteritis is not an important feature, but the mural involvement can lead to obstruction of involved arteries. Rarely, the aortic wall may be weakened by the inflammatory process, leading to localized aneurysm formation, aortic annular dilatation, and aortic regurgitation.[191]

Involvement of the aorta[192] and its major tributaries, when it occurs, usually coexists with the more classic and prevalent syndromes of temporal arteritis and polymyalgia rheumatica, although the aorta may rarely serve as the primary target of this disease.

The etiology of giant cell arteritis is unknown, although the generalized systemic manifestations of the disease and its occasional apparent temporal relationship to prior immunization or a viral illness suggest a possible infectious or autoimmune origin.[193] Klein et al. point out that involvement of the aorta and larger arteries may often arise as corticosteroid therapy for the more classic forms of this disease is being tapered.[189]

CLINICAL MANIFESTATIONS. Giant cell arteritis typically affects patients over the age of 50 and occurs predominantly in women. The disorder is more common in black women and appears to be distinctly uncommon in Hispanics.[194] The classic presentation is a triad of severe headache, marked malaise, and fever. Other common constitutional symptoms include anorexia, weight loss, lassitude, myalgias, and night sweats. Headaches are often intense and almost unbearable. Headache typically occurs over involved arteries, usually the temporal arteries but occasionally the occipital region. The area around the arteries is exquisitely sensitive to pressure, and complaints such as being unable to rest the head comfortably against a pillow, wear a hat, or comb one's hair are common. Claudication in the jaw muscles while chewing occurs in up to two-thirds of patients and is most suggestive of the diagnosis. A serious complication that may occur anywhere in the course of the disease is the onset of blindness from involvement of the ophthalmic artery—blindness that is often irreversible. Visual symptoms ranging from blurring to diplopia and visual loss occur in 25 to 50 per cent of patients. In its milder forms, patients may complain only of generalized muscular aches and pains and unusual fatigue, the syndrome of polymyalgia rheumatica. Blindness in these cases is uncommon. Polymyalgia rheumatica is seen in nearly 40 per cent of patients with giant cell arteritis.[195]

On rare occasions, consequences of involvement of the aorta or its major tributaries may be the first manifestations of the disease, although more typically, when such involvement occurs, it is part of the more generalized syndrome. However, when aortic or major branch disease is present, the symptoms are similar to those of Takayasu's arteritis and are the result of ischemia in the structures supplied by the involved arteries. Specifically, symptoms may include claudication of either upper or lower extremities, paresthesias, Raynaud's phenomenon, abdominal angina, coronary ischemia, transient cerebral ischemic attacks, and aortic arch and great vessel "steal" syndromes. More rarely, aortic aneurysms, aortic regurgitation, and aortic dissection may occur.[196] Interestingly, renal artery involvement is almost never seen, in contrast with Takayasu's arteritis.[189] Rarely, death can occur from aortic rupture or dissection.

On *physical examination*, fever is almost universal and patients appear ill. Involved vessels are thickened and very tender. Indeed, an experienced examiner can make the diagnosis of temporal arteritis with virtual certainty at the bedside simply by palpating an indurated, beaded, tender, temporal artery. Pulses may be lost, and bruits may occur over sites of arterial occlusion. Signs of aortic regurgitation are rarely present.

Laboratory tests may be helpful in making the diagnosis. A very high sedimentation rate is virtually a sine qua non for this disease and is a valuable guide to the activity of the process. A moderate normochromic, normocytic anemia is the rule. Acute phase reactants such as $alpha_2$ globulin are increased, and IgG and C3, and C4 (complement) levels are often elevated.[197]

The *diagnosis* is confirmed by biopsy of an involved artery, usually the temporal artery. In cases of larger vessel and aortic involvement, angiography may serve to differentiate arteritis from arteriosclerosis by the following features, as described by Klein et al.: (1) long, smooth, tapering stenosis alternating with segments of normal or even slightly increased diameter; (2) the absence of irregular ulcerated atheromatous plaques seen in profile; and (3) the more typical anatomical distribution of arteritis to include the subclavian, axillary, and brachial arteries.[189]

MANAGEMENT. High-dose steroid therapy, e.g., 60 to 80 mg of prednisone per day, is recommended in all patients with granulomatous arteritis. The intent of therapy is not only to reverse the disease but also to prevent progression, especially in the ophthalmic arteries, in order to prevent blindness. With constitutional symptoms and the sedimentation rate used as a guide, steroids can usually be reduced gradually to a maintenance dose of 5 to 15 mg/day (or every other day) for 1 to 2 years. The overall course is one of progressive improvement and eventual complete resolution. However, in many patients, the course of the disease may be protracted for months or years. Methotrexate in doses of 7.5 to 12.5 mg per week may be beneficial in patients with steroid-resistant symptoms or can be steroid-sparing in patients needing protracted treatment.[198] Very rarely, surgical resection of an expanding aneurysm or replacement of a regurgitant aortic valve is necessary.[191,196]

OTHER ARTERITIS SYNDROMES

In addition to the aortic inflammation of Takayasu's and giant cell arteritis, isolated aortic regurgitation due to dilatation of the aortic valve ring with associated aortic root involvement may occur during the course of ankylosing spondylitis, psoriatic arthritis, arthritis associated with ulcerative colitis, relapsing polychondritis, and Reiter's syndrome (Chap. 56).[199-201] In addition, aneurysms of the aorta, pulmonary artery, and other major vessels can complicate Behçet's syndrome.[202]

Reported instances of aortitis complicating each of these diseases are rare. For example, it is seen in 1 to 4 per cent of patients with ankylosing spondylitis (p. 1731), and only a small number of well-described cases of Reiter's syndrome with aortic regurgitation have been documented (p. 1732). Nevertheless, the symptoms of aortic regurgitation and resultant heart failure may eventually dominate the clinical picture. In each case of arthritis-associated aortitis, the underlying arthritic disease is particularly fulminant and prolonged, and multiple extraarticular features are usually manifest.

PATHOLOGICAL FEATURES. These appear to be similar in each of the aforementioned diseases. In the early stages of inflammation there is marked dilatation of the aortic valve ring with patchy elastic tissue disruption, an active inflammatory cell infiltrate, and subendothelial fibrosis.[199] These changes are most marked in the aortic root. Later, the proximal ascending aorta appears similar to that in luetic aortitis, with intimal thickening, coarse granular plaque formation, and characteristic obliterative endarteritis of the vasa vasorum. The aortic root dilates but usually without frank aneurysm formation. Early, the aortic valve cusps remain essentially normal and later become thickened and retracted, presumably as a result of the incompetence that arises from root dilatation. Echocardiographic data suggest that patients with subclinical aortitis may be identified by the presence of subaortic fibrous ridging or marked leaflet thickening, even when aortic root dimensions are normal.[203]

The clinical features are those of aortic regurgitation and resemble those of annuloaortic ectasia. However, it is worth noting that the course of this disease is variable. Some patients exhibit a rapid progressive course of cardiac decompensation, whereas others have a more indolent and stable natural history. Thus, the development of aortic regurgitation does not necessarily signify an irreversible downhill course. There is some evidence that the inflammation of the aortic root may be episodic; worsening of aortic regurgitation may also pursue an intermittent course.

Treatment consists of that required for the underlying arthritis or other disease. Aortic valve replacement should be performed when indicated, although special problems may be encountered in these patients. For example, pulmonary function is often impaired in ankylosing spondylitis as a result of rigidity of the thoracic spine and chest wall. In the rare patient with ulcerative colitis who requires aortic valve replacement, a porcine valve is recommended so that anticoagulation will be unnecessary. In contrast to annuloaortic ectasia, replacement of the ascending aorta itself is almost never necessary.

CARDIOVASCULAR SYPHILIS

Once accounting for 5 to 10 per cent of all cardiovascular deaths, syphilitic disease of the heart and aorta has become a rarity in most major medical centers today as a result of aggressive antibiotic treatment of lues in its early stages. Cardiovascular complications occur in approximately 10 per cent of cases of untreated lues. The latent period may extend from 5 to 40 years after the initial spirochetal infection, with a usual time of 10 to 25 years.

PATHOLOGY. The consequences of lues are the direct results of spirochetal infection of the aortic media, thought to occur usually during the secondary phase of the disease, with subsequent inflammation and scarring of the aortic wall. Although the aorta may be invaded anywhere along its course, the most common location is the ascending aorta. It is postulated that this area has a proclivity for syphilitic involvement because it is richer in lymphatics than any other portion of the aorta. The muscular and elastic tissues of the media are destroyed by the spirochetes and the resultant inflammatory process and are replaced by vascular fibrous tissue.

The aortic wall becomes progressively weakened by the inflammatory process, and it may become calcified. Such weakening leads to aneurysmal dilatation. The overlying intima becomes furrowed and wrinkled and is covered with large plaques of a glistening, pearly material. This accounts for the "tree-bark" appearance of the involved aorta characteristic of luetic aortitis.

The infection may extend into the aortic root, resulting in aortic regurgitation due to dilatation of the aortic annulus and separation of the aortic valve commissures. Luetic aortic regurgitation is usually associated with an aortic aneurysm. An obliterative endarteritis may also obstruct the ostia of the coronary arteries. The scarring and injury from lues may progress long after the spirochetal organisms have been eradicated.

There are four categories of syphilitic heart disease[204]: (1) uncomplicated syphilitic aortitis, (2) syphilitic aortic aneurysm, (3) syphilitic aortic valvulitis with aortic regurgitation, and (4) syphilitic coronary ostial stenosis. Based on autopsy studies, about one-third of patients with pathological incidence of cardiovascular lues are asymptomatic; half have a significant aortic aneurysm, and, of these, one-half to one-third have associated aortic regurgitation. Five to 10 per cent will have essentially pure aortic regurgitation, and 26 per cent will have significant luetic coronary ostial stenosis, often in association with aortic regurgitation or an aortic aneurysm.

CLINICAL MANIFESTATIONS. Luetic aneurysms can arise anywhere along the aorta (including the abdomen), but the classical location is in the ascending aorta. They are usually saccular but may be fusiform. In the absence of aortic regurgitation, aneurysms may undergo signifcant enlargement without producing symptoms. Eventually, aneurysms may expand enough to reach, compress, and even erode contiguous structures, particularly the sternum and anterior right thoracic cage in the case of aneurysms of the ascending aorta. A thrusting, pulsating mass may be seen and palpated. Erosion of the bony structures of the chest wall causes pain at the point of involvement. Ascending aortic aneurysms and those involving the arch may produce a tracheal tug, stridor, and dysphagia. Aneurysms elsewhere may cause symptoms from compression of adjacent structures similar to those of any type of aneurysm located in the same area.

Luetic aortic regurgitation tends to occur in older patients with luetic cardiovascular disease, presumably because the disease has been present longer in these individuals. The earliest auscultatory sign of luetic aortic valve involvement is a tambour-like aortic valve closure sound. Because of the dilated aortic root, the murmur of luetic aortic regurgitation may be more prominent along the right sternal border rather than the left. It is often musical in quality and in rare instances of aortic cusp eversion may be particularly loud, with an associated thrill.

Because there is often considerable calcification in the aortic annulus, stiffness of the base of the aortic leaflets, and usually a dilated proximal aorta, a loud systolic ejection murmur, sometimes with a thrill, is often present in luetic aortic valve disease in the absence of any significant aortic stenosis. Also, a loud, slapping ejection sound is sometimes caused by sudden distention of the dilated aorta in early systole.

Luetic aortic regurgitation is associated with an aneurysm of the ascending aorta. Because of concomitant coronary ostial stenosis, angina pectoris may be particularly troublesome. Atrial fibrillation is seen more commonly than in other types of pure aortic regurgitation. Otherwise, the signs and symptoms are typical for those of aortic regurgitation.

DIAGNOSIS. Usually, there is a history of syphilis, and other manifestations of tertiary lues are found in 10 to 30 per cent of patients with cardiovascular syphilis. Fifteen to 30 per cent of patients have negative routine serological tests for syphilis (Wasserman, Hinton, Kahn, Venereal Disease Research Laboratories [VDRL], and Kolmer). On the other hand, serological tests directed against a specific treponema antigen, such as the *Treponema pallidum* immobilization (TPI) test or the fluorescent treponemal antibody absorption (FTA-ABS) test, are almost invariably positive. The chest roentgenogram may afford extremely valuable clues to the diagnosis of luetic aortitis. In sharp contrast to arteriosclerosis, calcification in the ascending aorta proximal to the brachiocephalic vessels is almost always much more extensive than that elsewhere.

Angiography may delineate the aneurysm (Fig. 47–21) and help to quantify the severity of aortic regurgitation. In patients suspected of having coronary ostial stenosis and in any patient with cardiovascular syphilis in whom surgical correction is contemplated, the coronary artery anatomy —and particularly the ostia—should be visualized by angiography if possible.

TREATMENT. All patients with syphilis, including cardiovascular syphilis, who are seen 1 year or more after the initial contact should be given a course of antibiotic therapy aimed at curing the spirochetal infection. Penicillin is still the most effective antibiotic and is given as benzathine penicillin G (Bicillin), 2.4 million units intramuscularly weekly for 3 weeks (total of 7.2 million units). For patients allergic to penicillin, the recommended therapy is doxycycline, 200 mg orally two times daily for 21 days. In penicillin-allergic patients who cannot tolerate doxycycline, the penicillin allergy should be confirmed. In such patients, the alternative regimen is erythromycin, 500 mg orally four times daily for 30 days. Compliance and serological follow-up must be confirmed, especially with the latter regimen.[205] The effectiveness of treatment can be monitored by a decrease in VDRL titer, with the desired result being a fourfold reduction in titer in 12 to 24 months.

Although a course of antibiotics is recommended in any previously untreated patient with cardiovascular syphilis, even those with a negative serology, there is no good evidence that such treatment reverses, or even halts, the progression of aortitis or aortic regurgitation. In cases of cardiovascular syphilis, cerebrospinal fluid examination should also be performed, and, if positive, this too should be followed to assure the adequacy of therapy. Since the efficacy of antibiotics other than penicillin against syphilis is not well studied beyond 1 year, close follow-up of patients treated with these alternative modes is necessary.

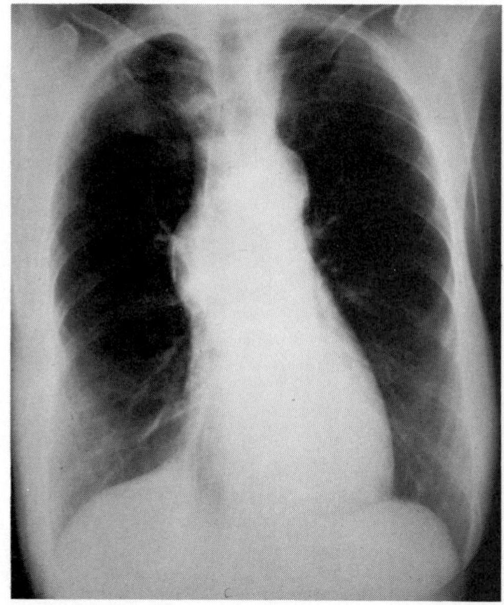
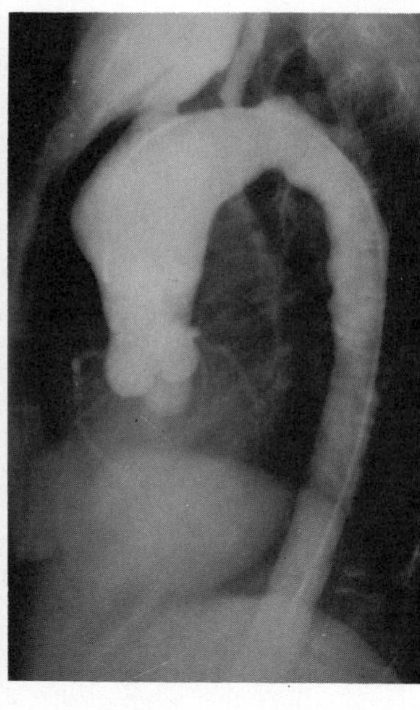

FIGURE 47–21. Films obtained from a 58-year-old woman with luetic aortitis. *Left,* Posteroanterior chest film showing an aneurysm of the ascending aorta with a faint rim of calcification. *Right,* Angiographic appearance of the aneurysm in the lateral view. (Courtesy of Christos Athanasoulis, M.D., and Arthur Waltman, M.D., Section of Vascular Radiology, Massachusetts General Hospital, Boston.)

Indications for excision of the luetic aneurysms are similar to those for other thoracic aortic aneurysms (p. 1533): a diameter of 7 cm or larger or an aneurysm of any size that produces symptoms or is expanding rapidly. Since many luetic aneurysms are saccular, aneurysmorrhaphy is occasionally adequate. However, since ongoing aortitis and scarring are possible, it is probably wiser to replace as much as possible of the diseased aorta with a prosthetic graft. Replacement of the aortic valve is indicated for significant aortic regurgitation, and the results are as good as in aortic regurgitation of other causes. Since the coronary artery disease of syphilis is usually ostial, a localized endarterectomy at the orifices of the coronary arteries may be possible. If an adequate lumen cannot be obtained by endarterectomy, bypass may be necessary.

PSEUDOCOARCTATION

Pseudocoarctation of the aorta is a rare condition resulting from elongation of the aortic arch, with redundancy and kinking of the aorta just distal to the origin of the left subclavian artery at the level of the ligamentum arteriosum.[206,207] Other terms used to describe this entity have included "mild coarctation," "atypical coarctation," or "subclinical coarctation." The etiology is believed to be congenital, with a lack of compression and fusion of certain of the segments of the dorsal aortic root and fourth arch. It is of interest that the incidence and distribution of associated cardiac anomalies parallel those seen in true coarctation. These anomalies include bicuspid aortic valve, sinus of Valsalva aneurysms, ventricular septal defect, corrected transposition, and Turner syndrome.[208,209]

CLINICAL MANIFESTATIONS. The pressure gradient across the deformed area is usually trivial or absent. Thus, the clinical features of true coarctation — upper extremity hypertension, lower extremity hypotension, and the development of collateral arterial circulation — are absent. Physical findings are often those of the associated lesions, although a murmur is sometimes heard over the aortic kink in the interscapular area. With mild degrees of obstruction, blood pressure in the lower extremities may be slightly reduced, and there may be a subtle pulse lag between the radial and femoral arteries.

The entity can usually be recognized on chest roentgenography. The typical appearance is that of a double, rounded density in the left superior mediastinum. Pitfalls in interpreting the x-ray films are common. The upper density, though relatively translucent, represents the uppermost extension of redundant aorta and is often mistaken for tumor or aneurysm. The lower density is the area of the aorta involved by poststenotic dilatation, and it is often misinterpreted as the aortic knob. Calcification may occur in the area of narrowing. Angiography confirms the diagnosis.

SIGNIFICANCE. Problems may arise in pseudocoarctation from the formation of aneurysms either proximal or distal to the kink (Fig. 47–22). Associated aneurysms of the left subclavian artery have been reported.[210] Rarely, thrombus forms at the site of atheromatous degeneration and calcification in the kinked segment.[211] Complete thrombosis can produce a picture mimicking true coarctation, although collateral arterial circulation is notably absent. Thrombus can also propagate directly into tributary vessels or embolize distally. The left subclavian artery is particularly vulnerable because of its proximity to the pseudocoarctation. Infection at the site of aortic narrowing is a rare problem.

TREATMENT. Therapy is necessary only for complications of pseudocoarctation. In the absence of complications, surgical resection is not indicated. If a bruit or pressure gradient is present over an area of pseudocoarctation, antibiotic prophylaxis for endocarditis should be given before dental or surgical procedures.

AORTIC TRAUMA

(See also p. 1524)

Blunt Trauma

Aortic injuries are associated with severe blunt trauma,[212] and they are far from rare. In one autopsy series of fatal automobile accidents, rupture of the aorta was found in one-sixth of all victims.[213]

ETIOLOGY AND PATHOGENESIS. Aortic trauma most commonly results from injuries associated with sudden high-speed deceleration upon impact, such as that resulting from motor vehicle accidents, blast injuries, cave-ins, crush injuries, or severe falls.[213–216] The abrupt deceleration of the body as it crashes to a sudden stop creates enormous shearing forces that act maximally at those points where a highly mobile portion of the aorta joins a fixed segment. Less frequently, pressure or blast injuries may produce rupture of the aorta, believed to be caused by an acute increase in intraaortic pressure generated by the compression of blood contained within the aorta and further increased by the force imparted by cardiac systole.

Although the aorta may be torn anywhere along its length, the most frequent point of rupture (the site in 90 per cent of cases) is in the aortic isthmus at the site of insertion of the ligamentum arteriosum, just distal to the origin of the left subclavian artery. Here, the relatively mobile descending thoracic aorta sweeps dorsally to become fixed to the thoracic cage by the ligamentum arteriosum, the intercostal arteries, and the left subclavian artery. The injury may vary from a minuscule rent in the aortic wall to a complete circumferential transection of all three layers of the aorta. In a series of 296 cases of aortic trauma studied by Parmley et al., a circumferential tear was evident in 80 per cent.[214] If the aorta is partially transected and the patient survives, a localized saccular aneurysm or pseudoaneurysm may subsequently develop at the site of the tear. Pseudoaneurysms may also form between the two ends of a totally transected aorta.

In addition to the aortic isthmus, other areas of injury include the supravalvular portion of the ascending aorta; the innominate artery, which may be avulsed from the aorta; the aortic arch; other portions of the descending thoracic aorta; the abdominal aorta; and combinations of these.[217]

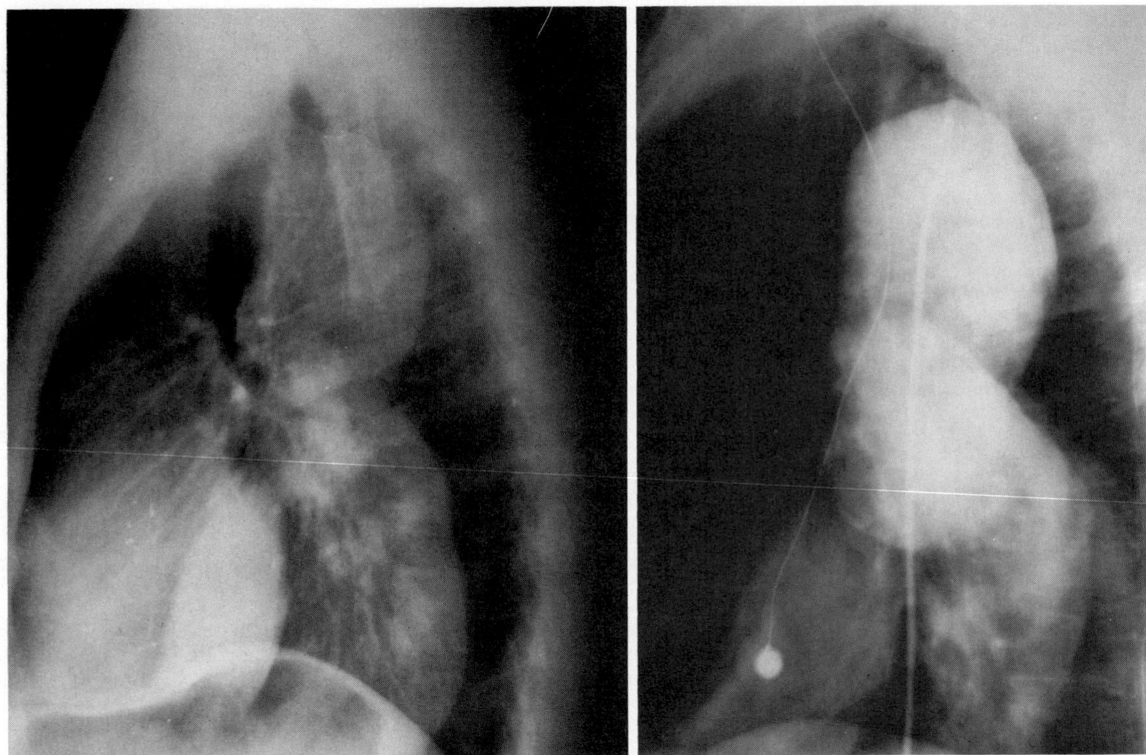

FIGURE 47–22. Pseudocoarctation of the aorta, with aneurysmal dilatation of the aorta proximal and distal to the point of narrowing. *Left,* Lateral chest roentgenogram. *Right,* The aorta is outlined with contrast material.

CLINICAL MANIFESTATIONS. The diagnosis of aortic trauma is often obscured by the presence of other serious injuries, such as central nervous system damage, visceral injury, and multiple skeletal fractures.[218] About two-thirds of patients with aortic rupture have clear-cut evidence of other thoracic trauma, such as chest or cardiac contusions, rib or vertebral fractures, pulmonary contusions, and hemorrhagic pleural effusions. The remaining one-third are surprisingly free of overt evidence of chest wall injury.

Few symptoms are directly attributable to the aortic trauma per se. Pressure from a localized hematoma can cause dyspnea and stridor from tracheal or bronchial compression, dysphagia from esophageal compression, or superior vena caval syndrome from caval compression. Although it is uncommon, the syndrome of so-called "acute coarctation" with upper extremity hypertension, reduced blood pressure in the lower extremities, a systolic murmur over the precordium or in the interscapular area, and a palpable radial-femoral pulse lag is virtually classic for the diagnosis. An interscapular systolic bruit may be heard. Otherwise, the physical examination is relatively unrevealing. Localized aneurysms developing in the aortic isthmus late after trauma may cause hoarseness, cough, and dysphagia from compression of the adjacent recurrent laryngeal nerve, bronchus, and esophagus.

DIAGNOSIS. Because the diagnosis is so frequently overshadowed by the presence of other severe injuries, rupture of the aorta is often overlooked. A *high index of suspicion is crucial, and evidence of aortic trauma should be sought in any patient with severe bodily injuries.* In the absence of classic physical findings—a common situation—the diagnosis is best suspected from the chest roentgenogram, which, if properly obtained and interpreted, is abnormal in over 90 per cent of patients with traumatic aortic rupture. Marsh and Sturm have delineated criteria for rupture of the aorta based upon a 40-degree anteroposterior supine chest film. The numbers on Figure 47–23 correspond to these criteria: (1) mediastinum measuring greater than 8 cm at the level of the aortic knob, (2) shift of the trachea toward the right, (3) blurring of the normally sharp outline of the aorta, (4) obliteration of the medial aspect of the apex of the upper lobe of the left lung, (5) opacification of the clear space between the aorta and pulmonary artery, and (6) depression of the left main stem bronchus below 40 degrees.[219] In a follow-up report, these authors identified indistinct aortic contour, opacification of the clear space between aorta and pulmonary artery, and mediastinal widening (mean diameter = 9.4 cm) as the most sensitive markers for aortic injury.[220] Others have shown that deviation of the trachea (or a nasogastric tube) to the right, depression of the main left bronchus, and widening of the left paraspinal line are also important.[221–223] The concept of increased mediastinal width compared to chest width (m/c ratio) has also been advocated

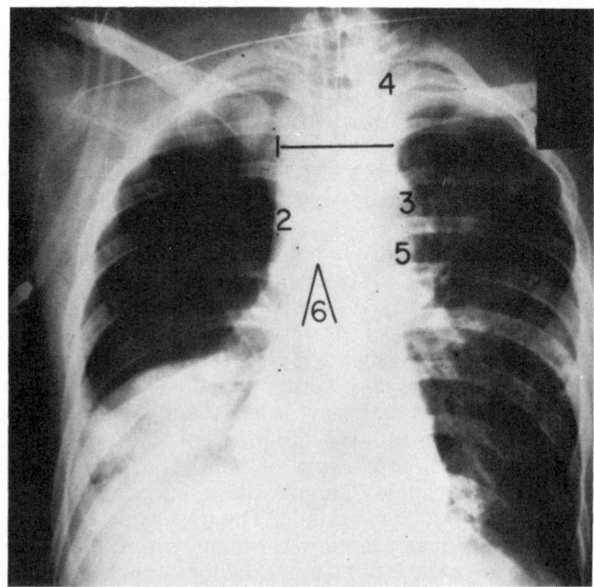

FIGURE 47–23. Aortic trauma. Roentgenographic characteristics of rupture of the proximal descending thoracic aorta in the supine anteroposterior projection (film-to-tube distance = 40 inches). The M/C ratio is 0.32. See text for key to numbers. (From Marsh, D. G., and Sturm, J. T.: Traumatic aortic rupture: Roentgenographic indications for angiography. Ann. Thorac. Surg. *21*:337, 1976.)

as a helpful sign for quantifying the magnitude of mediastinal widening and likelihood of aortic injury.[224] While any m/c ratio greater than 0.20 is considered abnormal, the specificity of the test for identifying patients with aortic injury increases from less than 25 per cent to nearly 90 per cent when the ratio is greater than 0.28. In cases of thoracic trauma, as the ratio increases from 0.25 to 0.28, the threshold for performing angiography should be lower; whenever the m/c ratio exceeds 0.28, additional studies should be carefully considered. It is also important to remember that occasional patients with aortic injury will have no specific signs of mediastinal hemorrhage.[225] CT scanning with contrast injection may confirm the diagnosis and should be performed as expeditiously as possible in a stable patient who has sustained severe chest trauma.[226] Should the diagnosis remain in question or if the patient's condition is unstable, the threshold for performing angiography in suspected cases should be low (Fig. 47–24 and Fig. 46–11, p. 1525). As with chest radiography, CT scanning can occasionally miss severe injuries, including aortic transection.[227]

COURSE AND PROGNOSIS. Approximately 80 per cent of patients with aortic rupture die instantly, although usually from other injuries, such as massive hemorrhage from other sites, trauma to other vital organs, or brain damage. Of those who survive the initial event, death often occurs within the first week from progressive hemorrhage at the site of the aortic tear. However, even with complete transection of the aorta, patients may be remarkably stable. About 2 to 5 per cent of patients with partial tears of the aorta go on to develop a localized aneurysm or pseudoaneurysm over a period of months or years, usually anterior to the aortic isthmus. This may either remain stable or ultimately expand. Such traumatic aneurysms frequently calcify or may become infected.

TREATMENT. The treatment of aortic trauma is operative repair, which should be undertaken as soon as possible once the condition is recognized. Occasionally, other serious injuries make it necessary to delay operation in order to stabilize the patient's condition, but even in the face of other severe trauma, surgery should be performed if there is evidence of progressive hemorrhage from the aorta. Some centers have advocated use of thoracic aortic occlusion with an intraaortic balloon pump to stabilize critically ill patients before definitive surgery.[228] Rupture of the aorta is usually treated by resecting the torn segment of the aorta and interposing a prosthetic graft between the two ends of the aorta. It may be necessary to support the distal circulation with a pump oxygenator or conduit bypass from the left ventricle or proximal aorta to the distal aorta around the rupture in order to reduce ischemic damage to the spinal cord, abdominal viscera, and kidneys.[229,230] Prompt recognition and operation for a ruptured aorta has resulted in survival of nearly 70 per cent of patients with this injury who reach the hospital alive.[218,229,231]

In cases of localized saccular aneurysms developing late after trauma, surgical excision is advised if the patient is an otherwise reasonable operative candidate. Long-term follow-up of patients with such lesions indicates that about half the aneurysms slowly expand and may even rupture. Surgery is curative and can be undertaken at a small risk (1 to 3 per cent).

Penetrating Trauma

Penetrating trauma of the aorta or any of its major arterial trunks is caused by puncture or laceration by missiles or knives, particularly bullet and stab wounds. Massive hemorrhage, often leading to rapidly fatal exsanguination, ensues. The consequences of the trauma depend upon the site and severity of perforation. Thus, perforation of the aorta within the pericardial sac may lead to cardiac tamponade. Perforation of the aorta elsewhere may cause massive hemorrhage, with compression of surrounding structures by the hematoma, such as the vena cava, tracheobronchial tree, and esophagus. Occlusion of a lacerated artery itself or of adjacent vessels may occur, producing focal signs and symptoms such as loss of the right carotid and brachial pulses, with right hemispheric neurological signs in the case of occlusion of the innominate artery. Occasionally, simultaneous penetration of an adjacent artery and vein may cause an arteriovenous fistula, with a resultant continuous murmur, wide pulse pressure, and increased cardiac output.[232,233]

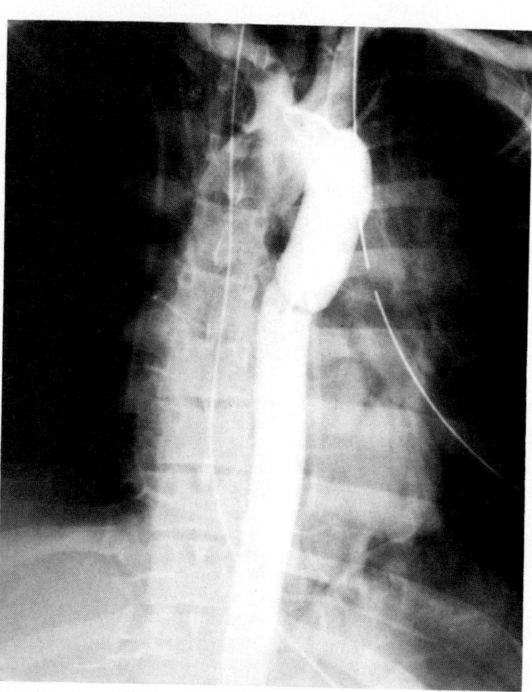

FIGURE 47–24. Thoracic aortogram in a 26-year-old man injured in a motor vehicle accident, showing traumatic transection of the aorta. The site of the tear can be clearly seen. (Courtesy of Robert Dinsmore, M.D., Massachusetts General Hospital, Boston.)

MANAGEMENT. Immediate surgical repair should be undertaken in any patient suspected of having a penetrating wound of the aorta, i.e., one with a missile or stab wound of the chest associated with a wide mediastinum on roentgenogram. If the patient's condition allows it, emergency angiography can usually pinpoint the site of perforation. However, in most patients who survive to reach the hospital, immediate operation for closure of the wound and evacuation of the hematoma is necessary. Similarly, laceration or penetrating wounds of arteries require urgent surgical correction.

AORTIC THROMBOEMBOLIC DISEASE

Aortic Embolism

Between 10 and 25 per cent of peripheral arterial emboli affect the aortic bifurcation, resulting in what are termed "saddle emboli." At least 90 per cent of these emboli originate within the chambers of the left side of the heart; 5 per cent come from the aorta itself, usually from thrombus overlying an arteriosclerotic plaque; and the remainder come from undetermined sites.[234] Rarely, paradoxical systemic embolism from the venous circulation occurs through a patent foramen ovale or atrial septal defect. Conditions that predispose to peripheral embolism are myocardial infarction with mural thrombus, ventricular aneurysm, prosthetic valves, congestive cardiomyopathy, and atrial fibrillation, especially in patients with rheumatic mitral stenosis. So-called "marantic endocarditis" is occasionally encountered in chronically ill patients, especially those with malignant disease, and consists of sterile intracardiac thrombi that may dislodge and travel to distal sites. Other less common conditions that serve to cause arterial emboli are left atrial myxomas and acute and subacute bacterial endocarditis. Emboli in endocarditis are usually small, although large emboli are seen in acute bacterial endocarditis and fungal (*Candida*) endocarditis. This can rarely be seen in disseminated *Aspergillus* infection.[235] An increased tendency to thromboembolism is encountered in women taking contraceptive pills and estrogens; in patients with malignant diseases, particularly carcinoma of the pancreas; and, rarely, in patients with antithrombin III deficiency.[236]

CLINICAL MANIFESTATIONS. Aortic bifurcation embolism is heralded by the sudden onset of excruciating pain in both legs. The pain usually extends distally from the midthigh area but can also involve the buttocks, lumbosacral area, and perineum. Associated with the intense pain are numbness, symmetrical weakness, and paresthesias. Schatz and Stanley have summarized in alliteration this classic presentation as "Pain, Paralysis, Paresthesias, Pulselessness, and Pallor."[237] Additional nonclassic presentations may include sudden onset of bilateral lower extremity weakness, severe hypertension, and acute abdominal pain simulating a perforated viscus.[238]

Examination reveals cold, pale extremities that are cyanotic and often exhibit a mottled, reticulated, reddish-blue appearance. These changes may progress to the blue-black color of gangrene, beginning first in the toes and extending proximally. Pulses are absent below the abdominal aorta. Initially sluggish, capillary filling is ultimately absent. Signs of ischemic neuropathy are present and include diminished or absent deep tendon reflexes, symmetrical weakness, and loss of all modalities of sensation, usually with demarcation at the level of the midthigh. If ischemia persists long enough, there may be myonecrosis with the release of products of muscle breakdown into the bloodstream, causing shock, hypotension, hyperkalemia, myoglobinuria, and acute tubular necrosis. Sepsis may add a serious further dimension to an already desperate problem. If perfusion is not reestablished within hours, death is almost inevitable.

The *differential diagnosis* includes acute aortic thrombosis from arteriosclerotic disease and aortic dissection. With thrombosis, there is usually a history of prior claudication, and an embolic source is lacking. With aortic dissection, a history of severe chest or back pain and an abnormal aortic contour on chest x-ray film usually provide distinguishing features.

The diagnosis is confirmed by angiography. However, most investigators advise prompt surgical intervention without angiography if the diagnosis is strongly suspected, since a delay could lead to irreversible ischemic damage to the limbs.

THERAPY. Most emboli can be removed by using Fogarty balloon-tipped catheters inserted through a transfemoral arterial approach under local anesthesia. In addition to retrieving the embolic material, passage of the Fogarty catheters into the distal arterial bed may result in the removal of any thrombus that may have formed as a result of the stagnant flow beyond the embolus. If the embolus cannot be retrieved with Fogarty catheters, removal by direct transabdominal aortotomy is necessary. Operative mortality ranges from 15 to 30 per cent, with death due to the underlying cardiac disease[238]; limb salvage is estimated at 80 to 90 per cent in most series.[238] Anticoagulation with constant intravenous heparin is instituted upon completion of the operation and is continued until therapeutic levels are achieved with one of the warfarin sodium family of drugs. Depending upon the clinical situation, long-term anticoagulant therapy using warfarin or antiplatelet agents may be required. Reembolization may occur in up to 25 per cent of patients, and some series suggest a reduced incidence if long-term anticoagulants are used. Using the transfemoral approach, surgery can be carried out with a low mortality even in patients whose other disease makes them poor operative risks. Limbs are almost uniformly salvaged if operation is undertaken promptly. All embolic debris should be cultured and examined microscopically. Left atrial myxomas are sometimes first recognized by the pathological examination of embolic specimens.

Aortic Thrombosis

Rarely, primary thrombosis of the distal abdominal aorta may be seen as a result of atheromatous disease or in rare patients with antithrombin III deficiency. In such patients, treatment is generally surgical, although an occasional case of successful balloon catheter dilatation has been reported.[236,239,240] Studies in experimental animals using tissue plasminogen activator (t-PA) for the treatment of aortic thrombotic occlusion suggest that this drug may have a potential role in treating patients with both peripheral emboli and aortic thrombosis.[241]

Atheromatous Emboli

Embolism of atheromatous debris from the disruption of arteriosclerotic plaques in the aorta or its major arterial trunks has been noted with increasing frequency. Usually, such embolism takes the form of showers of microemboli, each between 150 and 600 μm in size, into small arterial branches—an entity that is also termed "cholesterol embolism." However, obstruction of large arteries by embolic arteriosclerotic material may also occur.[242] By far the most common cause of cholesterol embolism is surgery or angiography that involves an atherosclerotic aorta.[243] Atheromatous embolism into the renal and splanchnic vascular beds is common after major abdominal vascular procedures, particularly resection of abdominal aortic aneurysms. Embolism of atheromatous material also occurs as an occasional complication of intraarterial cannulation, cardiac catheterization,[244] and cardiopulmonary bypass. In addition to these iatrogenic causes, however, spontaneously occurring cholesterol embolism is encountered, particularly from the aorta into the femoral-popliteal system. Studies have suggested a causal relationship between cholesterol embolism and anticoagulant therapy, especially long-term anticoagulation with warfarin sodium–type drugs.[245] Presumably, anticoagulation promotes hemorrhage into plaques, leading to their disruption, or prevents the formation of protective thrombus over ulcerated plaques. Finally, atheromatous embolism has followed blunt trauma to the aorta.

CLINICAL MANIFESTATIONS. The consequences of cholesterol embolism depend upon the vascular bed involved as well as the extent to which the small arterial vessels are occluded. Two important complications of cholesterol embolism following abdominal aortic surgery are pancreatitis and renal failure from diffuse microinfarction of the pancreas and kidneys, respectively. Renal failure may be severe and irreversible (p. 1835). Occasionally, cholesterol embolism has been implicated as a cause of severe renovascular hypertension. Gastrointestinal hemorrhage from microinfarction of abdominal viscera is also encountered. Showers of atheromatous emboli may affect the cerebral circulation, producing either focal neurological defects or a diffuse encephalopathic picture. In such cases, shiny cholesterol particles are sometimes visible in the retinal arteries.[246]

Spontaneously occurring cholesterol embolism in the lower extremities is manifested by bilateral pain, livedo reticularis, and purpuric and ecchymotic lesions in the lower legs, feet, and toes. These manifestations may be paroxysmal as emboli intermittently dislodge from their sites of origin. Skin necrosis and ischemic gangrene are common, especially in the toes ("blue toe syndrome").[245,247] With this clinical evidence of severe ischemia, arterial pulses are characteristically well preserved unless there is coincidental peripheral vascular disease.

The clinical picture may mimic that of a vasculitis or septic embolism from neisserial organisms—especially meningococcemia—or bacterial endocarditis. The absence of fever and other signs of systemic illness and the localized distribution of the lesions serve to distinguish cholesterol embolism from these other entities. The diagnosis has been made by muscle biopsy, which may show cholesterol particles in the arterioles.

THERAPY. For the most part, there is no specific treatment for cholesterol microembolism. Careful attention to the prevention of necrosis and infection in the involved extremities is important. Although the amputation of gangrenous digits is occasionally necessary, the ultimate prognosis for recovery is quite good, unless embolism is frequent and recurrent. Pancreatitis often subsides, even though it may be severe. Renal failure may be irreversible.

The use of anticoagulants in the prevention of further embolism is controversial, with some investigators advocating that they be given and others contending that they promote further atheromatous emboli. Overall, it appears that they are not of much value. In instances of recurrent atheromatous embolism, it may be possible to pinpoint the source of the cholesterol particles by angiography and to perform an endarterectomy or to excise the involved segment and replace it with a prosthetic graft. It has been suggested that use of a blood filtering device during aortoiliac reconstruction might reduce or prevent cholesterol embolism in that setting.[248]

AORTIC BACTERIAL INFECTIONS

The term "infected aneurysm" has gradually replaced the original designation of "mycotic aneurysm" used by Osler to define any localized dilation caused by sepsis in the wall of the aorta or any artery and thus to avoid confusion with infections of truly fungal origin. Infection can cause virtually any kind of aneurysmal dilatation, including fusiform, saccular, and false aneurysms. Rupture into the venous system may cause arteriovenous fistulas. Alternatively, infection may arise within preexisting arteriosclerotic aneurysms. Infected aortic aneurysms are rare, with only 1 or 2 cases per year recently being reported from a large general hospital.[249]

PATHOGENESIS. Vascular infection may arise by any of three different mechanisms. First, septic emboli from bacterial endocarditis or diffuse bacteremia may infect normal or diseased tissue. This mechanism of infection has become less frequent owing to the widespread use of effective antibiotics for the control of septicemia. Second, there may be contiguous spread from adjacent abscesses, infected lymph nodes, empyema, and so on. This is the usual cause for rare cases of tuberculous vascular involvement. Third, sepsis may be introduced directly from an external source, such as trauma, intravenous injections, or surgery. The incidence of this type of infection is increasing because of more frequent motor vehicle accidents, the widespread use of intravenous narcotics by drug addicts, and the performance of more intravascular procedures that may produce a portal for infection, such as intraarterial catheterization and intraaortic balloon counterpulsation. With this type of sepsis, the peripheral arteries are obviously more frequently involved than the aorta per se.

Although virtually any organism may infect the arterial tree, certain bacteria seem to have a proclivity for this type of infection. In particular, this is true of the *Salmonella* group, which tends to infect arteriosclerotic aneurysms. *Staphylococcus aureus* was the most common organism identified in a recent series, followed by *Salmonella*.[250]

CLINICAL MANIFESTATIONS. Most patients with infected aortic aneurysms are febrile; the height of the fever depends upon the severity of infection, the organism, and the site of the infection. Extremely high fever and rigors are common. Symptoms may arise from localized expansion of an infected aneurysm, such as dysphagia from esophageal compression and pain in areas contiguous to the infected sac. If palpable, infected aneurysms are almost always tender. A tender and pulsatile mass in a febrile patient should be considered an infected aneurysm until proved otherwise. Jarrett et al. have suggested that infected aortic aneurysms can be differentiated from sterile ones by the presence of fever, relative preponderance in women, tenderness, lack of calcification, and a tendency for early vertebral erosion.[249] With tuberculous involvement, evidence is almost always seen on the chest x-ray. This, coupled with a pulsating mass lesion, should elicit the correct diagnosis.

Sepsis in more peripheral arteries presents most commonly as fever with a palpable, painful, pulsating mass. Symptoms of compression of contiguous structures may also be present, such as arterial regurgitation or a neuropathy. Small abscesses in the distribution of the artery are often seen in staphylococcal infections. The most common sites for infected aneurysms are the following arteries: femoral, abdominal aorta, superior mesenteric, brachial, iliac, and carotid arteries. Together, the femoral arteries and abdominal aorta account for nearly 70 per cent of all mycotic aneurysms.[250]

Leukocytosis, an elevated sedimentation rate, and positive blood cultures are present in most cases. Commonly reported organisms other than *Staphylococcus aureus* and *Salmonella* species are other gram-positive and gram-negative organisms, such as pneumococcus,[251] *Pseudomonas*, and anaerobes. Rarely, fungal infections with *Candida* or *Aspergillus* may occur.[235] Localization of suspected infected aneurysms in a patient with sepsis can be aided by angiography. Valuable information can sometimes be obtained from ultrasound, gallium, and CT scans.[252]

The natural history of infected aneurysms is that of progressive expansion, thinning of the aneurysm wall, and eventual rupture. Jarrett et al. found a more rapid progression in patients with gram-negative infections.[249]

THERAPY. Treatment is always surgical excision combined with appropriate antibiotic or antituberculous chemotherapy. Wide excision of infected tissue is advised.[249,250] Usually a prosthetic tube graft must be inserted if the aorta or a major artery is involved. Early recognition and therapy clearly alter the outcome favorably.

AORTIC TUMORS

One review cites 27 cases of primary aortic tumors recorded in the world's literature.[253] Clearly, secondary tumors can arise from direct extension and invasion from adjacent lung or abdominal neoplasms or from embolic spread. Histological types include fibrosarcoma (most commonly), fibromyxosarcoma, myxosarcoma, fibromyxoma, angiosarcoma, malignant fibrous histiocytoma, leiomyosarcoma, myxoma and endothelioma.[253,254] In the 27 cases of primary aortic tumors, the age of the patients ranged from infancy to 75 years, with a mean of 54 years; male sex predominated by 2:1. Presentation in over half the cases consisted of abdominal or leg pain, proximal hypertension due to the acquired coarctation, decreased femoral pulses, fever, claudication, and occasionally bruits are also seen. Diagnosis is made by the usual noninvasive or angiographic techniques, with key features being the irregular appearance of the lumen and lack of enlargement of the outer diameter of the aorta.

REFERENCES

EXAMINATION OF THE AORTA

1. Grossman, L. B., Buonocore, E. Modic, M. T., and Meaney, T. F.: Digital subtraction angiography of the thoracic aorta. Radiology *150*:323, 1984.
2. Seward, J. B., Khandheria, B. K., Oh, J. K. et al.: Transesophageal echocardiography: Technique, anatomic correlations, implementation, and clinical applications. Mayo Clin. Proc. *63*:649, 1988.
3. Taams, M. A., Gussenhoven, W. J., Schippers, L. A. et al.: The value of transesophageal echocardiography for diagnosis of thoracic aorta pathology. Eur. Heart J. 9:1308, 1988.
4. Brundage, B. H., Rich, S., and Spigos, D.: Computed tomography of the heart and great vessels: Present and future. Ann. Intern. Med. *101*:801, 1984.
5. Singh, H., Fitzgerald, E., and Ruttley, M. S.: Computed tomography: The investigation of choice for aortic dissection? Br. Heart J. *56*:171, 1986.
6. White, R. D., Lipton M. J., Higgins, C. B. et al.: Noninvasive evaluation of suspected thoracic aortic disease by contrast-enhanced computed tomography. Am. J. Cardiol. *57*:282, 1986.
7. Demos, T. C., Posniak, H. V., and Marsan, R. E.: CT of aortic dissection. Semin. Roentgenol. *24*:22, 1989.
8. Gomes, M. N., and Choyke, P. L.: Pre-operative evaluation of abdominal aortic aneurysms: Unltrasound or computed tomography? J. Cardiovasc. Surg. *28*:159, 1987.
9. Dinsmore, R. E., Liberthson, R. R., Wismer, G. L. et al.: Magnetic resonance imaging of thoracic aortic aneurysms: Comparison with other diagnostic techniques. A. J. R. *146*:309, 1986.
10. Valk, P. E., Hale, J. D., Kaufman, L. et al.: MR imaging of the aorta with three dimensional vessel reconstruction: Validation by angiography. Radiology *157*:721, 1985.
11. Glazer, H. S., Gutierrez, F. R., Levitt, R. E. et al.: The thoracic aorta studied by MR imaging. Radiology *157*:149, 1985.
12. Goldman, A. P., Kotler, M. N., Scanlon, M. H. et al.: The complementary role of magnetic resonance imaging, Doppler echocardiography, and computed tomography in the diagnosis of dissecting thoracic aneurysms. Am. Heart J. *111*:970, 1986.
13. Mossard, J. M., Baruthio, J., Germain, P. et al.: Nuclear magnetic reso-

nance in the diagnosis of aortic diseases. Arch. Mal. Coeur. 79:456, 1986.
14. Goldman, A. P., Kotler, M. N., Scanlon, M. H. et al.: Magnetic resonance imaging and two-dimensional echocardiography. Alternative approach to aortography in diagnosis of aortic dissecting aneurysm. Am. J. Med. 80:1225, 1986.
15. Lois, J. F., Gomes, A. S., Brown, K. et al.: Magnetic resonance imaging of the thoracic aorta. Am. J. Cardiol. 60:358, 1987.
16. Gefter, W. B.: Chest applications of magnetic resonance imaging: An update. Radiol. Clin. North Am. 26:573, 1988.
16a. Aortic diseases. In Fowler, N. O.: Diagnosis of Heart Disease. New York, Springer-Verlag, 1991, pp. 375–388.
16b. Powell, J. T., and Greenhalgh, R. M.: Cellular, enzymatic, and genetic factors in the pathogenesis of abdominal aortic aneurysms. J. Vasc. Surg. 1989; 9:297, 1989.
16c. Powell, J. T., and Greenhalgh, R. M.: Multifactorial inheritance of abdominal aortic aneurysm. Eur. J. Vasc. Surg. 1:29, 1987.
16d. Johnston, K. W., and Scobie, T. K.: Multicenter prospective study of monruptured abdominal aortic aneurysms. I. Population and operative management. J. Vasc. Surg. 7:69, 1988.
16e. Tsipouras, P., Byers, P. H., Schwartz, R. C. et al.: Ehlers-Danlos syndrome Type IV: Cosegregation of the phenotype to a COL3AI allele of Type III collagen. Hum. Genet. 74:41, 1986.

PATHOGENESIS OF DISEASES OF THE AORTA

17. Iwatsuki, K., Cardinale, G. J., Spector, S., and Udenfriend, S.: Reduction of blood pressure and vascular collagen in hypertensive rats by β-aminopropionitrile. Proc. Natl. Acad. Sci. USA 74:360, 1977.
18. Schlatmann, T.J.M., and Becker, A. E.: Pathogenesis of dissecting aneurysm of the aorta. Am. J. Cardiol. 39:21, 1977.
19. Heistad, D. D., Marcus, M. L., Law, E. G., Armstrong, M. L., Ehrhardt, J. C., and Abboud, F. M.: Regulation of blood flow to the aortic media in dogs. J. Clin. Invest. 62:133, 1978.
20. Thurmond, A. S., and Semler, H. J.: Abdominal aortic aneurysm: Incidence in a population at risk. J. Cardiovasc. Surg. (Torino) 27:457, 1986.
21. Darling, R. C. III, Brewster, D. C., Darling, R. C. et al.: Are familial abdominal aortic aneurysms different? J. Vasc. Surg. 10:39, 1989.

ARTERIOSCLEROTIC AORTIC ANEURYSMS

22. Darling, R. C.: Ruptured arteriosclerotic abdominal aortic aneurysms. Am. J. Surg. 119:397, 1970.
23. Rantakokko, V., Havia, T., Inberg, M. V., and Vänttinen, E.: Abdominal aortic aneurysms: A clinical and autopsy study of 408 patients. Acta Chir. Scand. 149:151, 1983.
24. Astarita, D., Filippone, D. R., and Cohn, J. D.: Spontaneous major intra-abdominal arteriovenous fistulas: A report of several cases. Angiology 36:656, 1985.
25. Bickerstaff, L. K., Hollier, L. H., Van Peenen, H. J. et al.: Abdominal aortic aneurysms: The changing natural history. J. Vasc. Surg. 1:6, 1984.
26. Crew, J. R., Bashour, T. T., Ellertson, D. et al.: Ruptured abdominal aortic aneurysms: Experience with 70 cases. Clin. Cardiol. 8:433, 1985.
27. Jenkins, A. M., Ruckley, C. V., and Nolan, B.: Ruptured abdominal aortic aneurysm. Br. J. Surg. 73:395, 1986.
28. Martinussen, H. J., Lolk, A., Rohr, N. et al.: Ruptured abdominal aortic aneurysm with fistula into the inferior vena cava. J. Cardiovasc. Surg. (Torino) 27:298, 1986.
29. Brewster, D. C., Darling, R. C., Raines, J. K. et al.: Assessment of abdominal aortic aneurysm size. Circulation 56:164, 1977.
30. Retief, P. J., and Loubser, J. S.: Diagnosis and treatment of abdominal aortic aneurysm. A report of 82 cases. S. Afr. Med. J. 56:67, 1979.
31. Brewster, D. C., Retana, A., Waltman, A. C., and Darling, R. C.: Angiography in the management of aneurysms of the abdominal aorta. Its value and safety. N. Engl. J. Med. 292:822, 1975.
32. Gliedman, M. L., Ayers, W. B., and Vestal, B. L.: Aneurysms of the abdominal aorta and its branches: A study of untreated patients. Ann. Surg. 217:1537, 1982.
33. Darling, R. C., Messina, C. R., Brewster, D. C., and Ottinger, L. W.: Autopsy study of unoperated abdominal aortic aneurysms. The case for early resection. Circulation 56(Suppl. II):161, 1977.
34. Delin, A., Ohlsén, H., and Swedenborg, J.: Growth rate of abdominal aortic aneurysms as measured by computed tomography. Br. J. Surg. 72:530, 1985.
35. Bernstein, E. F., and Chan, E. L.: Abdominal aortic aneurysm in high risk patients. Ann. Surg. 200:255, 1985.
36. Nevitt, M. P., Ballard, D. J., and Hallett, J. W., Jr.: Prognosis of abdominal aortic aneurysms: A population-based study. N. Engl. J. Med. 321:1009, 1989.
37. Pasch, A. R., Ricotta, J. J., May, A. G. et al.: Abdominal aortic aneurysm: The case for elective resection. Circulation 70(Suppl. I):1, 1984.
38. Cooley, D. A., and Carmichael, M. J.: Abdominal aortic aneurysm. Circulation 70(Suppl. I):5, 1984.
39. Shenaq, S. A., Chelly, J. E., Karlberg, et al.: Use of nitroprusside during surgery for thoracoabdominal aortic aneurysm. Circulation 70(Suppl. I):7, 1984.
40. Thompson, J. E., Hollier, L. H., Patman, R. D., and Persson, A. V.: Surgical management of abdominal aortic aneurysms: Factors influencing mortality and morbidity—A 20-year experience. Ann. Surg. 181:654, 1975.
41. Brener, B. J., Raines, J. K., and Darling, R. C.: Intraoperative autotransfusion in abdominal aortic resections. Arch. Surg. 107:78, 1973.
42. Hertzer, N. R.: Fatal myocardial infarction following abdominal aortic aneurysm resection. Three hundred forty-three patients followed 6–11 years postoperatively. Ann. Surg. 192:671, 1980.
43. Hertzer, N. R., Bevin, E. G., Young, J. R. et al.: Coronary artery disease in peripheral vascular patients. Ann. Surg. 199:223, 1984.
44. Boucher, C. A., Brewster, D. C., Darling, R. C. et al.: Determination of cardiac risk by dipyridamole-thallium imaging before peripheral vascular surgery. N. Engl. J. Med. 312:389, 1985.
45. Eagle, K. A., Singer, D. E., Brewster, D. C. et al.: Dipyridamole thallium scans in the preoperative evaluation of patients undergoing vascular surgery. JAMA 257:2185, 1987.
46. Eagle, K. A., Coley, C. M., Newell, J. B. et al.: Combining clinical and thallium data optimizes preoperative assessment of cardiac risk before major vascular surgery. Ann. Intern. Med. 110:859, 1989.
47. Levinson, J. R., Boucher, C. A., Coley, C. M. et al.: Semiquantitative analysis of dipyridamole-^{201}thallium redistribution improves risk stratification before vascular surgery. Am. J. Cardiol. 66:406, 1990.
48. Eagle, K. A., and Boucher, C. A.: Cardiac risk of noncardiac surgery. N. Engl. J. Med. 321:1330, 1989.
49. Leppo, J., Plaja, J., Gionet, M. et al.: The noninvasive evaluation of cardiac risk prior to vascular surgery. Circulation 72(Suppl. III):147A, 1985.
50. Pasternack, P. F., Imparato, A. M., Riles, T. S. et al.: The value of radionuclide angiogram in the prediction of perioperative myocardial infarction in patients undergoing lower extremity revascularization procedures. Circulation 72(Suppl. II):13, 1985.
51. Raby, K. E., Goldman, L., Creager, M. A. et al.: Correlation between preoperative ischemia and major cardiac events after peripheral vascular surgery. N. Engl. J. Med. 321:1296, 1989.
52. Brewster, D. C., Bluth, J., Darling, R. C., and Austen, W. G.: Combined aortic and renal artery reconstruction. Am. J. Surg. 131:457, 1976.
53. Crawford, E. S., Saleh, S. A., Babb, J. W., III et al.: Infrarenal abdominal aortic aneurysm: Factors influencing survival after operation performed over a 25-year period. Ann. Surg. 193:699, 1981.
54. Fielding, J.W.L., Black, J., Ashton, F. et al.: Diagnosis and management of 528 abdominal aortic aneurysms. Br. Med. J. 283:355, 1981.
55. O'Donnell, T. F., Darling, R. C., and Linton, R. R.: Is 80 years too old for aneurysmectomy? Arch. Surg. 111:1250, 1976.
56. Karmody, A. M., Leather, R. P., Goldman, M. et al.: The current position of nonresective treatment for abdominal aortic aneurysm. Surgery 94:591, 1983.
57. Soreide, O., Lillestol, J., Christensen, O. et al.: Abdominal aortic aneurysms: Survival analysis of four hundred thirty-four patients. Surgery 91:188, 1982.
58. Plate, G., Hollier, L. A., O'Brien, P. et al.: Recurrent aneurysms and late vascular complications following repair of abdominal aortic aneurysms. Ann. Surg. 120:590, 1985.
59. Hollier, L. A., Plate, G., O'Brien, P. et al.: Late survival after abdominal aortic aneurysm repair: Influence of coronary artery disease. J. Vasc. Surg. 1:290, 1984.
60. Mitchell, E., Kadir, S., Kaufman, S. L. et al.: Percutaneous transluminal angioplasty of aortic graft stenoses. Radiology 149:439, 1983.
61. O'Donnell, T. F., Scott, G., Shepard, A. et al.: Improvements in the diagnosis and management of aortoenteric fistula. Am. J. Surg. 149:481, 1985.
62. Kierman, P. D., Pairolero, P. C., Hubert, J. P., Jr. et al.: Aortic graft-enteric fistula. Mayo Clin. Proc. 55:731, 1980
63. Ernst, C. B.: Prevention of intestinal ischemia following abdominal aortic reconstruction. Surgery 93:102, 1983.
64. Collins, J. J., Koster, J. K., Cohn, L. H., and Van Devanter, S. H.: Common aortic aneurysms: when to intervene. J. Cardiovasc. Med. 8:245, 1983.
65. Joyce, J. W., Fairbairn, J. F., Kincaid, O. W., and Juergens, J. L.: Aneurysms of the thoracic aorta—A clinical study with special reference to prognosis. Circulation 29:176, 1964.
66. Culliford, A. T., Ayvaliotis, B., Shemin, R. et al.: Aneurysms of the descending aorta. J. Thorac. Cardiovasc. Surg. 85:98, 1983.
67. Livesay, J. J., Cooley, D. A., Ventimiglia, R. A. et al.: Surgical experience in descending thoracic aneurysmectomy with and without adjuncts to avoid ischemia. Ann. Thorac. Surg. 39:37, 1985.
68. Cabrol, C., Pavie, A., Mesnildrey, P. et al.: Long-term results with total replacement of the ascending aorta and reimplantation of the coronary arteries. J. Thorac. Cardiovasc. Surg. 91:17, 1986.
69. Coselli J. S., and Crawford, E. F.: Composite valve-graft replacement of aortic root using separate Dacron tube for coronary artery reattachment. Ann. Thorac. Surg. 47:558, 1989.
70. Antunes, M. J., Colson, P. R., and Kinsley, R. H.: Hypothermia and circulatory arrest for surgical resection of aortic arch aneurysms. J. Thorac. Cardiovasc. Surg. 86:576, 1983.
71. Crawford, E. S., and Snyder, D. M.: Treatment of aneurysms of the aortic arch. J. Thorac. Cardiovasc. Surg. 85:237, 1983.
72. Matsuda, H., Nakano, S., Shirakura, R. et al.: Surgery for aortic arch aneurysm with selective cerebral perfusion and hypothermic cardiopulmonary bypass. Circulation 80(Suppl. I):243, 1989.
73. Pressler, V., and McNamara, J. J.: Aneurysms of the thoracic aorta. J. Thorac. Cardiovasc. Surg. 89:50, 1985.
74. Crawford, E. F., Svensson, L. G., Coselli, J. S. et al.: Surgical treatment of aneurysm and/or dissection of the ascending aorta, transverse aortic arch, and ascending aorta and transverse aortic arch: Factors influencing survival in 717 patients. J. Thorac. Cardiovasc. Surg. 98:659, 1989.
75. Moreno-Cabral, C. E., Miller, C., Mitchell, S. et al.: Degenerative and atherosclerotic aneurysms of the thoracic aorta. J. Thorac. Cardiovasc. Surg. 88:1020, 1984.

76. Crawford, E. S., Snyder, D. M., Cho, G. C., and Roehm, J.O.F., Jr.: Progress in treatment of thoracoabdominal and abdominal aortic aneurysms involving celiac, superior mesenteric, and renal arteries. Ann. Surg. *188*:404, 1978.
77. Verdant, A., Page, A., Cossette, R. et al.: Surgery of the descending thoracic aorta: Spinal cord protection with the Gott shunt. Ann. Thorac. Surg. *46*:147, 1988.
78. Laschinger, J. C., Cunningham, J. N., Nathan, I. N. et al.: Experimental and clinical assessment of the adequacy of partial bypass in maintenance of spinal cord blood flow during operations on the thoracic aorta. Ann. Thorac. Surg. *36*:416, 1983.
79. Crawford, E. S., Mizrahi, E. M., Hess, K. R. et al.: The impact of distal aortic perfusion and somatosensory evoked potential monitoring on prevention of paraplegia after aortic aneurysm operation. J. Thorac. Cardiovasc. Surg. *95*:357, 1988.

AORTIC DISSECTION

80. Wheat, M. W., Jr.: Acute dissecting aneurysms of the aorta: Diagnosis and treatment—1979. Am. Heart J. *99*:373, 1980.
81. Roberts, W. C.: Aortic dissection: Anatomy, consequences, and causes. Am. Heart J. *101*:195, 1981.
82. Doroghazi, R. M., and Slater, E. E. (eds.): Aortic Dissection. New York, McGraw-Hill Book Company, 1983.
83. Cooke, J. P., and Safford, R. E.: Progress in the diagnosis and management of aortic dissection. Mayo Clin. Proc. *61*:147, 1986.
84. Wheat, M. W., Jr.: Pathogenesis of aortic dissection. *In* Doroghazi, R. M., and Slater, E. E. (eds.): Aortic Dissection. New York, McGraw-Hill Book Company, 1983, p. 55.
85. Yamada, T., Tada, S., and Harada, J.: Aortic dissection without intimal rupture: Diagnosis with MR imaging and CT. Radiology *168*:347, 1988.
86. DeBakey, M. E., McCollum, C. H., Crawford, E. S. et al.: Dissection and dissecting aneurysms of the aorta: 20-year follow-up of 527 patients treated surgically. Surgery *92*:1118, 1982.
87. Daily, P. O., Trueblood, H. W., Stinson, E. B. et al.: Management of acute aortic dissection. Ann. Thorac. Surg. *10*:237, 1970.
88. Slater, E. E., and DeSanctis, R. W.: The clinical recognition of dissecting aortic aneurysm. Am. J. Med. *60*:625, 1976.
89. Larson, E. W., and Edwards, W. D.: Risk factors for aortic dissection: A necropsy study of 161 cases. Am. J. Cardiol. *53*:849, 1984.
90. Leonards, J. C., and Hasleton, P. S.: Dissecting aortic aneurysms: A clinicopathological study. Q. J. Med. *48*:55, 1979.
91. Bulkley, B. H., and Roberts, W. C.: Dissecting aneurysm (hematoma) limited to coronary artery. Am. J. Med. *55*:747, 1973.
92. Hochberg, F. H., Bean, C., Fisher, C. M., and Roberson, G. H.: Stroke in a 15-year-old girl secondary to terminal carotid dissection. Neurology *25*:725, 1980.
93. Demaio, S. J., Jr., Kinsella, S. H., and Silverman, M. E.: Clinical course and long-term prognosis of spontaneous coronary artery dissection. Am. J. Cardiol. *64*:471, 1989.
94. Dalen, J. R., Pape, L. A., Cohn, L. H. et al.: Dissection of the aorta: Pathogenesis, diagnosis, and treatment. Prog. Cardiovasc. Dis. *23*:237, 1980.
95. Loeppky, C. B., Alpert, M. A., Hamel, P. C. et al.: Extensive aortic dissection from combined-type cystic medial necrosis in a young man without predisposing factors. Chest *79*:116, 1981.
96. McKusick, V. A., Logue, R. B., and Bahnson, H. T.: Association of aortic valvular disease and cystic medial necrosis of the ascending aorta; report of four instances. Circulation *16*:188, 1957.
97. Shachter, N., Perloff, J. K., and Mulder, D. G.: Aortic dissection in Noonan's syndrome. Am. J. Cardiol. *54*:464, 1984.
98. Price, W. H., and Wilson J.: Dissection of the aorta in Turner's syndrome. J. Med. Genetics *20*:61, 1983.
99. Nicod, P., Bloor, C., Godfrey, M. et al.: Familial aortic dissecting aneurysm. J. Am. Coll. Cardiol. *13*:811, 1989.
100. Pumphrey, C. W., Fay, T., and Weir, I.: Aortic dissection during pregnancy. Br. Heart J. *55*:106, 1986.
101. Williams, G. M., Gott, V. L., Brawley, R. K. et al.: Aortic disease associated with pregnancy. J. Vasc. Surg. *8*:470, 1988.
102. Ponseti, I. V., and Baird, W. A.: Scoliosis and dissecting aneurysm of the aorta in rats fed with *Lathyrus odoratus* seeds. Am. J. Pathol. *28*:1059, 1952.
103. Fikar, C. R., Amrhein, J. A., Harris, J. P., and Lewis, E. R.: Dissecting aortic aneurysm in childhood and adolescence. Clin. Pediatr. *20*:578, 1981.
104. Slater, E. E.: Aortic dissection: Presentation and diagnosis. *In* Doroghazi, R. M., and Slater, E. E. (eds.): Aortic Dissection. New York, McGraw-Hill Book Company, 1983, p. 61.
105. Cohen, S., and Littman, D.: Painless dissecting aneurysm of the aorta. N. Engl. J. Med. *271*:143, 1964.
106. Symbas, P. N., Kelly, T. F., Vlasis, S. E. et al.: Intimo-intimal intussusception and other ususual manifestations of aortic dissection. J. Thorac. Cardiovasc. Surg. *79*:926, 1980.
107. Hirst, A. E., and Gore, I.: The etiology and pathology of aortic regurgitation. *In* Doroghazi, R. M., and Slater, E. E. (eds.): Aortic Dissection. New York, McGraw-Hill Book Company, 1983, p. 13.
108. Riley, D. J., Liv, R. T., and Saxanoff, S.: Aortic dissection: A rare cause of the superior vena cava syndrome. J. Med. Soc. N. J. *78*:187, 1981.
109. McCarthy, C., Dickson, G. H., Besterman, E. M. M. et al.: Aortic dissection with rupture through ductus arteriosus into pulmonary artery. Br. Heart J. *34*:284, 1972.
110. Roth, J. A., and Parekh, M. A.: Dissecting aneurysms perforating the esophagus. N. Engl. J. Med. *299*:776, 1978.
111. Thiene, G., Rossi, L., and Becker, A. E.: The atrioventricular conduction system in dissecting aneurysm of the aorta. Am. Heart J. *98*:447, 1979.
112. Morris, A. L., and Barwinsky, J.: Unusual vascular complications of dissecting thoracic aortic aneurysm. Cardiovasc. Radiol. *1*:95, 1978.
113. Eagle, K. A., Quertermous, T., Kritzer, G. A. et al.: Spectrum of conditions initially suggesting acute aortic dissection but with negative aortograms. Am. J. Cardiol. *57*:322, 1986.
114. ten Cate, J. W., Timmers, H., and Becker, A. E.: Coagulopathy in ruptured or dissecting aortic aneurysms. Am. J. Med. *59*:171, 1975.
115. Granato, J. E., Dee, P., and Gibson, R. S.: Utility of two-dimensional echocardiography in suspected ascending aortic dissection. Am. J. Cardiol. *56*:123, 1985.
116. Perez, J. E.: Noninvasive diagnosis: Computed tomography and ultrasound. *In* Doroghazi, R. M., and Slater, E. E. (eds.): Aortic Dissection. New York, McGraw-Hill Book Company, 1983, p. 133.
117. Iliceto, S., Nanda, N. C., Rizzon, P. et al.: Color Doppler evaluation of aortic dissection. Circulation *75*:748, 1987.
118. Erbel, R., Engberding, R., Daniel, W. et al.: Echocardiography in diagnosis of aortic dissection. Lancet *I*:457, 1989.
118a. Adachi, H., Kyo, S., Takamoto, S., et al.: Early diagnosis and surgical intervention of acute aortic dissection by transesophageal color flow mapping. Circulation *82*(Suppl. IV):IV19, 1990.
119. Thorsen, M. K., San Dretto, M. A., Lawson, T. L. et al.: Dissecting aortic aneurysms: Accuracy of computed tomographic diagnosis. Radiology *148*:773, 1983.
120. Smith, D. C., and Jang, G. C.: Radiological diagnosis and aortic dissection. *In* Doroghazi, R. M., and Slater, E. E. (eds.): Aortic Dissection. New York, McGraw-Hill Book Company, 1983, p. 71.
121. Vasile, N., Mathieu, D., Keita, K. et al.: Computed tomography of thoracic aortic dissection: Accuracy and pitfalls. J. Comput. Assist. Tomogr. *10*:211, 1986.
122. Amparo, E. G., Higgins, C. B., Hricak, L, and Sollitto, R.: Aortic dissection: Magnetic resonance imaging. Radiology *155*:399, 1985.
123. Dinsmore, R. E., Willerson, J. T., and Buckley, M. J.: Dissecting aneurysm of the aorta. Aortographic features affecting prognosis. Diagn. Radiol. *105*:567, 1972.
124. Shuford, W. H., Sybers, R. G., and Weens, H. S.: Problems of the aortographic diagnosis of dissecting aneurysms of the aorta. N. Engl. J. Med. *280*:225, 1969.
125. Collins, J. J., Jr., Koster, J. K., Jr., Cohn, L. H., and VanDevanter S. H.: Common arotic aneurysms: When to intervene. J. Cardiovasc. Med. *8*:245, 1983.
126. Anagnostopoulos, C. E., Prabhakar, M. J. S., and Kittle, C. F.: Aortic dissections and dissecting aneurysms. Am. J. Cardiol. *30*:263, 1972.
127. Gurin, D., Bulmer, J. W., and Derby, R.: Dissecting aneurysms of the aorta. Diagnosis and operative relief of acute arterial obstructions due to this course. N. Y. State J. Med. *35*:1200, 1935.
128. Shaw, R. W.: Acute dissecting aortic aneurysms: Treatment by fenestration of the internal wall of the aneurysm. N. Engl. J. Med. *253*:331, 1955.
129. DeBakey, M. E., Cooley, D. A., and Creech, O., Jr.: Surgical considerations of dissecting aneurysms of the aorta. Ann. Surg. *142*:586, 1955.
130. Wheat, M. W., Jr., Palmer, R. F., Barley, T. D., and Seelman, R. C.: Treatment of dissecting aneurysms of the aorta without surgery. J. Thorac. Cardiovasc. Surg. *50*:364, 1965.
131. Palmer, R. F., and Lasseter, K. C.: Nitroprusside and aortic dissecting aneurysm (letter). N. Engl. J. Med. *294*:1403, 1976.
132. Wheat, M. W.: Intensive drug therapy. *In* Doroghazi, R. M., and Slater, E. E. (eds.): Aortic Dissection. New York, McGraw-Hill Book Company, 1983, p. 165.
133. Grubb, B. P., Sirio, C., and Zelis, R.: Intravenous labetalol in acute aortic dissection. JAMA *258*:78, 1987.
134. Frishman, W. B., Weinberg, P., Peled, H. B. et al.: Calcium entry blockers for the treatment of severe hypertension and hypertensive crisis. Am. J. Med. *77*(Suppl. 2B):35, 1984.
135. White, S. R., and Hall, J. B.: Control of hypertension with nifedipine in the setting of aortic dissection. Chest *88*:781, 1985.
136. Miller, D. C., Stinson, E. B., Oyer, P. E. et al.: The operative treatment of aortic dissections: Experience with 125 patients over a sixteen year period. J. Thorac. Cardiovasc. Surg. *78*:365, 1979.
137. Doroghazi, R. M., Slater, E. E., DeSanctis, R. W. et al.: Long-term survival patients treated with aortic dissection. J. Am. Coll. Cardiol. *3*:1026, 1984.
137a. Svensson, L. G., Crawford, E. S., Hess, K. R., et al.: Dissection of the aorta and dissecting aortic aneurysms: Improving early and long-term surgical results. Circulation *82*(Suppl. IV):IV24, 1990.
138. Miller, D. C., Mitchell, R. C., Oyer, P. E. et al.: Independent determinants of operative mortality for patients with aortic dissections. Circulation *70*(Suppl. I):153, 1984.
139. Glower, D. D., Fann, J. I., Speier, R. H. et al.: Comparison of medical and surgical therapy for uncomplicated descending aortic dissection. Circulation *80*(Suppl. II):24, 1989.
140. Crawford, E. S, Svensson, L. G., Coselli, J. S. et al.: Aortic dissection and dissecting aortic aneurysms. Ann. Surg. *208*:254, 1988.
141. Cachera, J. P., Vouhe, P. R., Loisance, D. Y. et al.: Surgical management of acute dissections involving the ascending aorta. J. Thorac. Cardiovasc. Surg. *82*:576, 1981.
142. Kolff, J., Bates, R. J., Balderman, S. C. et al.: Acute aortic arch dissection: Reevaluation of the indication for medical and surgical therapy. Am. J. Cardiol. *39*:727, 1977.
143. Haverich, A., Miller, D. C., Scott, W. C. et al.: Acute and chronic aortic

dissections—determinants of long-term outcome for operative survivors. Circulation *72*(Suppl. II):22, 1985.
144. Lemole, G. M., Strong, M. D., Spagna, P. M., and Karmilowicz, N. P.: Improved results for dissecting aneurysms: Intraluminal sutureless prosthesis. J. Thorac. Cardiovasc. Surg. *83*:249, 1982.
145. Diehl, J. T., Moon, B., LeClerc, Y. et al.: Acute type A dissection of the aorta: surgical management with the sutureless intraluminal prosthesis. Ann. Thorac. Surg. *43*:502, 1987.
146. Carpentier, A., Deloche, A., Fabiani, J. N. et al.: New surgical approach to aortic dissection: Flow reversal and thromboexclusion. J. Thorac. Cardiovasc. Surg. *81*:659, 1981.
147. Tanabe, T., Hashimoto, M., Sakai, K. et al.: Surgical treatment of aortic dissection: Application of Ivalon sponge to the dissected lumen. Ann. Thorac. Surg. *41*:169, 1986.
148. Fabiani, J. -N., Jebara, V. A., Deloche, A. et al.: Use of surgical glue without replacement in the treatment of type A aortic dissection. Circulation *80*(Suppl. I):264, 1989.

ANNULOAORTIC ECTASIA

149. Ellis, P. R., Cooley, D. A., and DeBakey, M. E.: Clinical consideration and surgical treatment of annulo-aortic ectasia. J. Thorac. Cardiovasc. Surg. *42*:363, 1961.
150. Pyeritz, R. E., and McKusick, V. A.: The Marfan syndrome: Diagnosis and management. N. Engl. J. Med. *300*:772, 1979.
151. Boucek, R. J., Noble, N. L., Gunja-Smith, Z., and Butler, W. T.: The Marfan syndrome: A deficiency of chemically stable collagen cross links. N. Engl. J. Med. *305*:998, 1981.
152. Abraham, P. A., Perejda, A. J., Carnes, W. H., and Uitto, J.: Marfan syndrome: Demonstration of abnormal elastin in the aorta. J. Clin. Invest. *70*:1245, 1982.
153. Emanuel, R., Ng, R.A.L., Marcomichelakis, J. et al.: Formes frustes of Marfan's syndrome presenting with severe aortic regurgitation. Clinicogenetic study of 18 families. Br. Heart J. *39*:190, 1977.
154. Lemon, D. K., and White, C. W.: Annulaortic ectasia: Angiographic, hemodynamic and clinical comparison with aortic valve insufficiency. Am. J. Cardiol. *41*:482, 1978.
155. Miller, D. C., Stinson, E. B., Oyer, P. E. et al.: Concomitant resection of ascending aortic aneurysm and replacement of the aortic valve. J. Thorac. Cardiovasc. Surg. *79*:388, 1980.
156. Svensson, L. G., Crawford, S., Coselli, J. S. et al.: Impact of cardiovascular operation on survival in the Marfan patient. Circulation *80*(Suppl. I):233, 1989.
157. Gott, V. L., Pyeritz, R. E., Magovern, G. J., Jr. et al.: Surgical treatment of aneurysms of the ascending aorta in the Marfan syndrome. Results of composite-graft repair in 50 patients. N. Engl. J. Med. *314*:1070, 1986.
158. Pyeritz, R. E., Gott, V. L., McDonald, G. R. et al.: Surgical repair of the Marfan aorta: Technique, indications, and complications. Johns Hopkins Med. J. *151*:71, 1982.
159. Crawford, E. S.: Marfan's syndrome: Broad spectral surgical treatment of cardiovascular manifestations. Ann. Surg. *198*:487, 1983.

AORTIC ARTERITIS SYNDROMES

160. Takayasu, M.: Case with unusual changes of the central vessels in the retina. Acta Soc. Ophthalmol. Jpn. *12*:554, 1908.
161. Lupi-Herrera, E., Sanchez-Torres, G., Marcushamer, J. et al.: Takayasu's arteritis. Clinical study of 107 cases. Am. Heart J. *93*:94, 1977.
162. Shelhamer, J. H., Volkman, D. J., Parillo, J. E. et al.: Takayasu's arteritis and its therapy. Ann. Intern. Med. *103*:121, 1985.
163. Hall, S., Barr, W., Lie, J. T. et al.: Takayasu arteritis. Medicine *64*:89, 1985.
164. Ueno, A., Awane, G., and Wakahayachi, A.: Successfully operated obliterative brachiocephalic arteritis (Takayasu) associated with the elongated coarctation. Jpn. Heart J. *8*:538, 1967.
165. Kakao, K., Ikeda, M., Kimata, S. et al.: Takayasu's arteritis—Clinical report of 84 cases and immunological studies of 7 cases. Circulation *35*:1141, 1967.
166. Volkman, D. J., Mann, D. L., and Fauci, A. S.: Association between Takayasu's arteritis and a B-cell alloantigen in North Americans. N. Engl. J. Med. *306*:464, 1982.
167. Numano, F., Isohisa, I., Egami, M. et al.: HLA-DR MT and MB antigens in Takayasu disease. Tissue Antigens *21*:208, 1983.
168. Gronemeyer, P. S., and deMello, D. E.: Takayasu's disease with aneurysm of right common iliac artery and iliocaval fistula in a young infant: Case report and review of the literature. Pediatrics *69*:626, 1982.
169. Morooka, S., Saito, Y., Nonaka, Y. et al.: Clinical features of aortitis syndrome in Japanese women older than 40 years. Am. J. Cardiol. *53*:859, 1984.
170. Swinton, N. W., and Cook, G. A.: Systolic hypertension and cardiac mortality of Takayasu's aortoarteritis. Angiology *27*:568, 1976.
171. Takishita, A., Tanaka, S., Orita, G. et al.: Baroflex sensitivity in patients with Takayasu's aortitis. Circulation *55*:803, 1977.
172. Akikusa, B., Kondo, Y., and Muraki, N.: Aortic insufficiency caused by Takayasu's arteritis without usual clinical features. Arch. Pathol. Lab. Med. *105*:650, 1981.
173. Talwar, K. K., Chopra, P., Narula, J. et al.: Myocardial involvement and its response to immunosuppressive therapy in nonspecific aortoarteritis (Takayasu's disease)—a study by endomyocardial biopsy. Int. J. Cardiol. *23*:323, 1988.
174. Cipriano, P. R., Silverman, J. F., Perlroth, M. G. et al.: Coronary arterial narrowing in Takayasu's aortitis. Am. J. Cardiol. *39*:744, 1977.
174a. Hashimoto, Y., Numano, F., Maruyama, Y., et al.: Thallium-201 stress scintigraphy in Takayasu Arteritis. Am. J. Cardiol. *67*:879, 1991.
175. Slater, E. E., and Fallon, J. T.: Upper extremity hypertension in a 28-year-old Korean man. Case Records of the Massachusetts General Hospital. N. Engl. J. Med. *299*:1002, 1978.
176. Lupi, H. E., Sanchez, T. G., Horwitz, S., and Gutierrez, F. E.: Pulmonary artery involvement in Takayasu's arteritis. Chest *67*:69, 1975.
177. Wu, Y.-J.J., Martin, B., Ong, K. et al.: Takayasu's arteritis as a cause of fever of unknown origin. Am. J. Med. *87*:476, 1989.
178. Kanaide H., Takeshita, A., and Nakamura, M.: Etiologic aspects of coagulopathy in Takayasu's aortitis. Am. Heart J. *104*:1039, 1982.
179. Lande, A., and Rossi, P.: The value of total aortography in the diagnosis of Takayasu's arteritis. Radiology *114*:287, 1975.
180. Ishikawa, K.: Diagnostic approach and proposed criteria for the clinical diagnosis of Takayasu's arteriopathy. J. Am. Coll. Cardiol. *12*:964, 1988.
181. Grossman, E., Morag, B., Nussinovitch, N. et al.: Clinical use of captopril in Takayasu's disease. Arch. Intern. Med. *144*:95, 1984.
182. Huddle, K. R., Doodha, M. I., and Mackenzie, M.: Captopril in the treatment of renovascular hypertension secondary to Takayasu's arteritis. S. Afr. Med. J. *69*:58, 1986.
183. Duncan, J. M., and Cooley, D. A.: Surgical consideration in aortitis with special emphasis on Takayasu's arteritis. Texas Heart Inst. J. *10*:233, 1983.
184. Pajari, R., Hekeli, P., and Harjola, P. T.: Treatment of Takayasu's arteritis: An analysis of 29 operated patients. Thorac. Cardiovasc. Surg. *34*:176, 1986.
185. Hodgins, G. W., and Dutton, J. W.: Transluminal dilatation of Takayasu's arteritis. Can. J. Surg. *27*:355, 1984.
186. Ishikawa, K.: Survival and morbidity after diagnosis of occlusive thromboaortopathy (Takayasu's disease). Am. J. Cardiol. *47*:1026, 1981.
187. Subramanyan, R., Joy, J., and Balakrishnan, K. G. Natural history of aortoarteritis (Takayasu's disease). Circulation *80*:429, 1989.
188. Ishikawa, K.: Patterns of symptoms and prognosis in occlusive thromboaortopathy (Takayasu's disease). J. Am. Coll. Cardiol. *8*:1041, 1986.
189. Klein, R. G., Hunder, G. G., Stanson, A. W., and Sheps, S. G.: Larger artery involvement in giant cell (temporal) arteritis. Ann. Intern. Med. *83*:806, 1975.
190. Vincent, F. M., and Vincent, T.: Bilateral carotid siphon involvement in giant cell arteritis. Neurosurgery *18*:773, 1986.
191. Austen, W. G., and Blennerhassett, M. B.: Giant cell aortitis causing an aneurysm of the ascending aorta and aortic regurgitation. N. Engl. J. Med. *272*:80, 1965.
192. Perruquet, J. L., Davis, D. E., and Harrington, T. M.: Aortic arch arteritis in the elderly. An important manifestation of giant cell arteritis. Arch. Intern. Med. *146*:289, 1986.
193. Ghose, M. K., Shensa, S., and Lerner, P. I.: Arteritis of the aged (giant cell arteritis) and fever of unexplained origin. Am. J. Med. *60*:429, 1976.
194. Gonzalez, E. B., Varner, W. T., Lisse, J. R. et al.: Giant-cell arteritis in the southern United States: An 11-year retrospective study from the Texas Gulf Coast. Arch. Intern. Med. *149*:1561, 1989.
195. Chuang, T., Hunder, G. G., Ilstrup, D. M., and Kurland, L. T.: Polymyalgia rheumatica. Ann. Intern. Med. *97*:672, 1982.
196. Salisbury, R. S., and Hazleman, B. L.: Successful treatment of dissecting aortic aneurysm due to giant cell arteritis. Ann Rheum. Dis. *40*:507, 1981.
197. Malmvall, B. E., and Bengtsson, B. A.: Serum levels of immunoglobin and complement in giant cell arteritis. JAMA *236*:1876, 1976.
198. Krall, P. L., Mazanec, D. J., and Wilke, W. S.: Methotrexate for corticosteroid-resistant polymyalgia rheumatica and giant cell arteritis. Cleveland Clin. J. Med. *56*:253, 1989.
199. Paulus, H. E., Pearson, C. M., and Pitts, W.: Aortic insufficiency in five patients with Reiter's syndrome. A detailed clinical and pathologic study. Am. J. Med. *53*:464, 1972.
200. Muna, W. F., Roller, D. H., Craft, J. et al.: Psoriatic arthritis and aortic regurgitation. JAMA *244*:363, 1980.
201. Morgan, S. H., Asherson, R. A., and Hughes, G. V.: Distal aortitis complicating Reiter's syndrome. Br. Heart J. *52*:115, 1984.
202. Park, J. H., Han, M. C., and Bettman, M. A.: Arterial manifestations of Behçet disease. A. J. R. *143*:821, 1984.
203. LaBresh, K. A., Lally, E. V., Sharma, S. C., and Ho, G.: Two-dimensional echocardiographic detection of preclinical aortic root abnormalities in rheumatoid variant diseases. Am. J. Med. *78*:908, 1985.

CARDIOVASCULAR SYPHILIS

204. Heggtveit, H. A.: Syphilitic aortitis. A clinicopathologic autopsy study of 100 cases, 1950 to 1960. Circulation *29*:346, 1964.
205. Center for Disease Control Recommended Treatment Schedules, 1985. The Sexually Transmitted Diseases Advisory Committee. Morbid. Mortal. Weekly Rep. *34*:94s, 1985(Suppl. 4S).
206. Steinberg, I.: Anomalies (pseudocoarctation) of the arch of the aorta—Report of 8 new and review of 8 previously published cases. A. J. R. *88*:73, 1962.
207. Brinsfield, D. E., Shuford, W. M., Plauth, W. H., Jr., and Sybers, R. G.: Congenital anomalies of the aorta. *In* Lindsay, J., Jr., and Hurst, J. W. (eds.): The Aorta. New York, Grune and Stratton, 1979, p. 271.
208. Lajos, T. Z., Meckstroth, C. V., Klassen, K. P., and Sherman, N. J.: Pseudocoarctation of the aorta. A variant or an entity? Chest *58*:571, 1970.

209. Wolf, W. J.: Pseudocoarctation of the aortic arch in a patient with Turner's syndrome. Clin. Cardiol. *9*:A5, 1986.

210. Bahabozorgui, S., Bernstein, R. G., and Frater, R.W.M.: Pseudocoarctation of the aorta associated with aneurysm formation. Chest *60*:616, 1971.

211. Bland, E. F., and Castleman, B.: Vascular collapse in a woman with an unusual calcified ring in the aortic arch. N. Engl. J. Med. *280*:1466, 1969.

AORTIC TRAUMA

212. Shaikh, K. A., Schwab, C. W., Camishion, R. C.: Aortic rupture in blunt trauma. Am. Surg. *52*:47, 1986.

213. Greendyke, R. M.: Traumatic rupture of aorta: Special reference to automobile accidents. JAMA *195*:527, 1966.

214. Parmley, L. F., Mattingly, T. W., Manion, W. C., and Jahnke, E. J.: Nonpenetrating traumatic injury of the aorta. Circulation *17*:1086, 1958.

215. Fleming, A. W., and Green, D. C.: Traumatic aneurysms of the thoracic aorta: Report of 43 patients. Ann. Thorac. Surg. *18*:91, 1974.

216. Shorr, R. M., Crittenden, M., Indeck, M. et al.: Blunt thoracic trauma: Analysis of 515 patients. Ann. Surg. *206*:200, 1987.

217. Faro, R. S., Monson, D. O., Weinberg, M., and Javid, H.: Disruption of aortic arch branches due to nonpenetrating chest trauma. Arch. Surg. *118*:1333, 1983.

218. Sturm, J. T., Billiar, T. R., Dorsey, J. S. et al.: Risk factors for survival following surgical treatment of traumatic aortic rupture. Ann. Thorac. Surg. *39*:418, 1985.

219. March, D. G., and Sturm, J. T.: Traumatic aortic rupture: Roentgenographic indications for angiography. Ann. Thorac. Surg. *21*:337, 1976.

220. Sturm, J. T., Olson, F. R., and Cicero, J. J.: Chest roentgenographic findings in 26 patients with traumatic rupture of the thoracic aorta. Ann. Emerg. Med. *12*:598, 1983.

221. Woodring, J. H., and Dillon, M. L.: Radiographic manifestations of mediastinal hemorrhage from blunt chest trauma. Ann. Thorac. Surg. *37*:171, 1984.

222. Heystraten, F. M., Rosenbusch, G., Kingma, L. M. et al.: Chest radiography in acute traumatic rupture of the thoracic aorta. Acta Radiologica *29*:411, 1988.

223. Mirvis, S. E., Bidwell, J. K., Buddemeyer, E. U. et al.: Value of chest radiography in excluding traumatic aortic rupture. Radiology *163*:487, 1987.

224. Stark, P.: Traumatic rupture of the thoracic aorta: A review. Crit. Rev. Diagn. Imaging *21*:229, 1983.

225. Woodring, J. H., and King, J. G.: The potential effects of radiographic criteria to exclude aortography in patients with blunt chest trauma. J. Thorac. Cardiovasc. Surg. *97*:456, 1989.

226. Brooks, A. P., Olson, L. K., and Shackford, S. R.: Computed tomography in the diagnosis of traumatic rupture of the thoracic aorta. Clin. Radiol. *40*:133, 1989.

227. Miller, F. B., Richardson, J. D., Thomas, H. A. et al.: Role of CT in diagnosis of major arterial injury after blunt thoracic trauma. Surgery *106*:596, 1989.

228. Gupta, B. K., Khaneja, S. C., Flores, L. et al.: The role of intra-aortic balloon occlusion in penetrating abdominal trauma. J. Trauma *29*:861, 1989.

229. Atkins, C. W., Buckley, M. J., Daggett, W. et al.: Acute traumatic disruption of the thoracic aorta: A ten-year experience. Ann. Thorac. Surg. *31*:305, 1981.

230. Marvasti, M. A., Meyer, J. A., Ford, B. E., and Parker, F. B., Jr.: Spinal cord ischemia following operation for traumatic aortic transection. Ann. Thorac. Surg. *42*:425, 1986.

231. Stiles, Q. R., Cohlmia, G. S., Smith, J. H. et al.: Management of injuries of the thoracic and abdominal aorta. Am. J. Surg. *150*:132, 1985.

232. Haskell, R. J., French, W. J., and Harley, D. P.: Traumatic aorto-right ventricular fistula presenting with a diastolic murmur. Am. Heart J. *109*:1110, 1985.

233. Snow, N., and Johnson, P.: Traumatic fistula between the descending thoracic aorta and left main pulmonary artery. J. Trauma *25*:263, 1985.

AORTIC THROMBOEMBOLIC DISEASE

234. Heiskell, C. A., and Conn, J., Jr.: Aortoarterial emboli. Am. J. Surg. *132*:4, 1976.

235. Byard, R. W., Jimenez, C. L., Carpenter, B. F., and Hsu, E.: Aspergillus-related aortic thrombosis. Can. Med. Assoc. J. *136*:155, 1987.

236. Shapiro, M. E., Rodvien, R., Bauer, K. A., and Salzman, E. W.: Acute aortic thrombosis in antithrombin III deficiency. JAMA *245*:1759, 1981.

237. Schatz, I. J., and Stanley, J. C.: Saddle embolus of the aorta. JAMA *235*:1262, 1976.

238. Babu, S. C., Shah, P. M., Sharma, P. et al.: Adequacy of central hemodynamics versus restoration of circulation in the survival of patients with acute aortic thrombosis. Am. J. Surg. *154*:206, 1987.

239. Tegtmeyer, C. J., Wellons, H. A., and Thompson, R. N.: Balloon dilation of the abdominal aorta. JAMA *244*:2636, 1980.

240. Deriu, G. P., and Ballotta, E.: Natural history of ascending thrombosis of the aorta. Am. J. Surg. *145*:652, 1983.

241. Topol, E. J., Ciuffo, A. A., Pearson, T. A. et al.: Thrombolysis with recombinant tissue plasminogen activator in atherosclerotic thrombotic occlusion. J. Am. Coll. Cardiol. *5*:85, 1985.

242. Machleder, H. I., Takiff, H., Lois, J. F., and Holburt, E.: Aortic mural thrombus: An occult source of arterial thromboembolism. J. Vasc. Surg. *4*:473, 1986.

243. Dahlberg, P. J., Frecentese, D. F, and Cogbill, T. H.: Cholesterol embolism: Experience with 22 histologically proven cases. Surgery *105*:737, 1989.

244. Colt, H. G., Begg, R. J., Saporito, J. J. et al.: Cholesterol emboli after cardiac catheterization. Medicine *67*:389, 1988.

245. Hyman, B. T., Landas, S. K., Ashman, R. F. et al.: Warfarin-related purple toes syndrome and cholesterol microembolization. Am. J. Med. *82*:1233, 1987.

ATHEROMATOUS EMBOLI

246. Coppetto, J. R., Lessell, S., Greco, T. P., and Eisenberg, M. S.: Diffuse disseminated atheroembolism. Arch. Ophthalmol. *102*:255, 1984.

247. Fisher, D. F., Clagett, G. P., Brigham, R. A. et al.: Dilemmas in dealing with the blue toe syndrome: Aortic vs. peripheral source. Am. J. Surg. *148*:836, 1984.

248. Robicsek, F.: Prevention of cholesterol embolism (trash foot) during aorto-iliac reconstruction using a blood filtering device. J. Cardiovasc. Surg. (Torino) *27*:63, 1986.

AORTIC BACTERIAL INFECTIONS

249. Jarrett, F., Darling, R. C., Mundth, E. D., and Austen, W. G.: Experience with infected aneurysms of the abdominal aorta. Arch. Surg. *110*:1281, 1975.

250. Brown, S. L., Busuttil, R. W., Baker, J. D. et al.: Bacteriologic and surgical determinants of survival in patients with mycotic aneurysms. J. Vasc. Surg. *1*:541, 1984.

251. Worrell, J. T., Buja, L. M., and Reynolds, R. C.: Pneumococcal aortitis with rupture of the aorta: Report of a case and review of the literature. Am. J. Clin. Pathol. *89*:565, 1988.

252. Vogelzang, R. L., and Sohaey, R.: Infected aortic aneurysms: CT appearance. J. Comput. Assist. Tomog. *12*:109, 1988.

253. Schipper, J., van Oostayen, J. A., den Hollander, J. C., and van Seyen, A. J.: Aortic tumours: Report of a case and review of the literature. Br. J. Radiol. *62*:35, 1989.

AORTIC TUMORS

254. Schmid, E., Port, J. S., Carroll, R. M., and Friedman, N. B.: Primary metastasizing aortic endothelioma. Cancer *54*:1407, 1984.

48

Pulmonary Embolism

by SAMUEL Z. GOLDHABER, M.D., and EUGENE BRAUNWALD, M.D.

Pulmonary embolism (PE) is the third most common cardiovascular disease, after acute ischemic syndromes and stroke. However, venous thromboembolism (VTE) receives less attention than is warranted because PE and deep venous thrombosis (DVT) are managed by physicians in many different specialties (e.g., cardiologists, pulmonologists, hematologists, vascular medicine specialists, vascular surgeons, general internists, and family practitioners). Nevertheless, during the past few years, major advances have been made in optimizing strategies for diagnosis and prevention of this illness, which accounts for approximately 300,000 hospitalizations annually in the United States.[1,2] Unfortunately, PE causes as many as 50,000 deaths per year and, during the past 15 years, the mortality rate has not declined.[3] PE affects men more commonly than women and occurs with increasing frequency in older age groups. However, the death rate is relatively high even among younger patients (Fig. 48–1). Furthermore, recognized cases of VTE constitute only a minority of actual episodes because the diagnosis is elusive and, despite advances in diagnostic imaging, the condition commonly goes undetected until postmortem examination.[4] Therefore, prompt and accurate diagnosis remains the most important step toward managing this illness.[4a] Major controversy and uncertainty persist concerning the proper role of thrombolytic therapy in the overall treatment strategy for PE. Clinical trials are being undertaken to address this important but troublesome issue.

Pathophysiology of Pulmonary Embolism

In 1856, Rudolf Virchow postulated that a triad of factors led to intravascular coagulation: (1) local trauma to the vessel wall, (2) hypercoagulability, and (3) stasis.[5] One useful approach to classifying hypercoagulable states is to consider them as either primary or secondary.[6] Primary hypercoagulable states are usually inherited abnormalities, whereas secondary states are usually acquired clinical conditions associated with an increased risk for PE (Table 48–1).

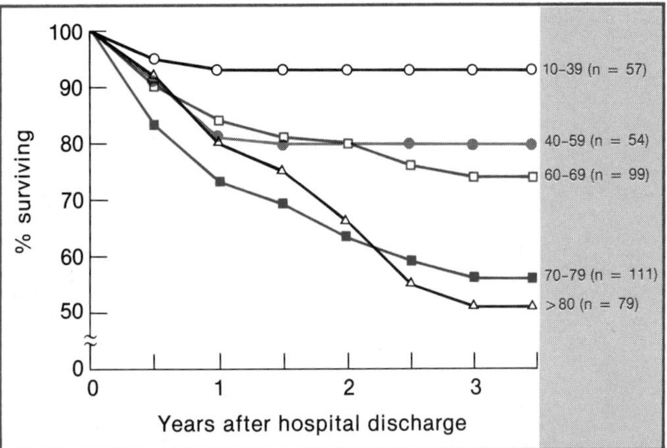

FIGURE 48–1. Age-specific survival rates in 400 patients discharged with the first episode of clinically recognized DVT and/or PE. (From Anderson, F. A., Jr., Wheeler, H. B., Goldberg, R. J., et al.: A population-based perspective of the incidence and case fatality rates of deep vein thrombosis and pulmonary embolism: the Worcester DVT Study. Arch. Intern. Med. *157*:933, 1991.

HYPERCOAGULABLE STATES

(See also Chap. 57)

PRIMARY HYPERCOAGULABLE STATES. Antithrombin III (AT-III) is the major inhibitor of thrombin (which converts circulating fibrinogen to fibrin clot) and other activated clotting factors (Fig. 48–2). The most frequent manifestations of AT-III deficiency are recurrent PE and DVT.[6] Inheritance is autosomal dominant, with partial gene penetration. Congenital deficiencies of protein C (which consumes factors Va and VIIIa and also stimulates fibrinolysis)[7] and protein S (a cofactor for activated protein C) also predispose to recurrent venous thromboembolism at a young age. Defective fibrinolysis, whether due to defective release of tissue plasminogen activator (t-PA)[8] or an excess of t-PA inhibitor,[9] is also associated with venous thrombosis. "Lupus anticoagulant," often encountered in patients without lupus, is usually associated with a prolonged partial thromboplastin time (PTT) but paradoxically increases the risk of venous thromboembolism.[10,11] Lupus anticoagulants are antibodies that interfere with phospholipid-dependent coagulation reactions. Sensitive assays that employ the negatively charged phospholipid cardiolipin as the antigen have identified patients with elevated levels of

TABLE 48-1 HYPERCOAGULABLE STATES

PRIMARY
Antithrombin III deficiency
Protein C deficiency
Protein S deficiency
Lupus anticoagulant
Anticardiolipin antibodies
SECONDARY
Abnormalities of coagulation
Cancer
Pregnancy
Oral contraceptives
Nephrotic syndrome
Abnormalities of platelets
Heparin associated thrombocytopenia
Myeloproliferative disorders
Paroxysmal nocturnal hemoglobinuria
Abnormalities of blood vessels and rheology
Conditions promoting venous stasis (immobilization, postoperative state, obesity, advanced age)
Central venous and long-term in-dwelling catheters
Hyperviscosity (polycythemia, leukemia, sickle cell disease, leukoagglutination)

anticardiolipin antibodies (ACA)—especially IgG and IgM ACA—that are associated with increased frequency of clinical thrombosis and fetal loss.[12,13] Some but not all patients with elevated ACA have demonstrable lupus anticoagulants. The titer of the ACA appears to correlate with the degree of PTT prolongation and with the risk of thrombosis. Investigation of potential primary hypercoagulable states (Table 48-1) has the highest yield in patients younger than 45 years old who have "idiopathic" PE or DVT. Among such patients, approximately 15 per cent may have an identifiable disorder related to defective fibrinolysis or deficiencies in protein C, protein S, or AT-III.[14]

SECONDARY HYPERCOAGULABLE STATES. Some of the most readily recognized risk factors for PE occur in secondary hypercoagulable states (Table 48-1), in which the molecular mechanisms causing thrombosis are not known, as they are in the primary conditions. When investigating the possibility of PE, clinicians may find these clinical settings to be more useful than are symptoms and signs of PE, which are often nonspecific. Among hospitalized patients, the most common setting for PE is after a recent surgical procedure in which vessel trauma is combined with immobilization. Obesity, with its associated venous stasis, may be a long-term risk factor for PE[15] and may also increase the risk of PE among hospitalized patients undergoing surgery.

Neoplastic disease is another well-established risk factor for PE. Patients with known malignancy in whom PE is suspected may have either thrombotic or tumor emboli. Furthermore, PE[16] or DVT[17] (especially bilateral limb DVT) in patients without overt cancer may herald the presence of occult malignancy that will become manifested clinically within the next several years. This suggests that patients with VTE should be screened and followed carefully for cancer when no cause for the PE or DVT is clinically apparent.[18]

PE is also associated with oral contraceptive use and pregnancy,[19] particularly among women confined to bed because of preeclampsia or eclampsia or those who have had a cesarean section.[19] The risk of VTE is actually much greater during the first 6 weeks after delivery than during the pregnancy itself. With respect to maternal mortality, PE is the leading cause (after trauma) and is four times more common than death from hemorrhage or an anesthetic accident and twice as common as death from an ectopic pregnancy or infection.[20]

Indwelling central venous lines can be a nidus for right atrial thrombus that serves as a souce of PE. These catheters are being used with increasing frequency to provide alimentation for chronically ill patients and as venous access for long-term cancer chemotherapy protocols[21,22] (Fig. 48-3). An increasing number of reports have also noted large right atrial thrombi due to acute myocardial infarction, congestive heart failure, atrial fibrillation, or a combination of predisposing factors.[23] In fact, the detection of right atrial thrombus (usually with two-dimensional echocardiography) in most cases should prompt a search for concomitant PE.

DEEP VENOUS THROMBOSIS

RELATIONSHIP OF DVT TO PE. Although the risk of PE among patients with DVT proximal to the calf is high (approxi-

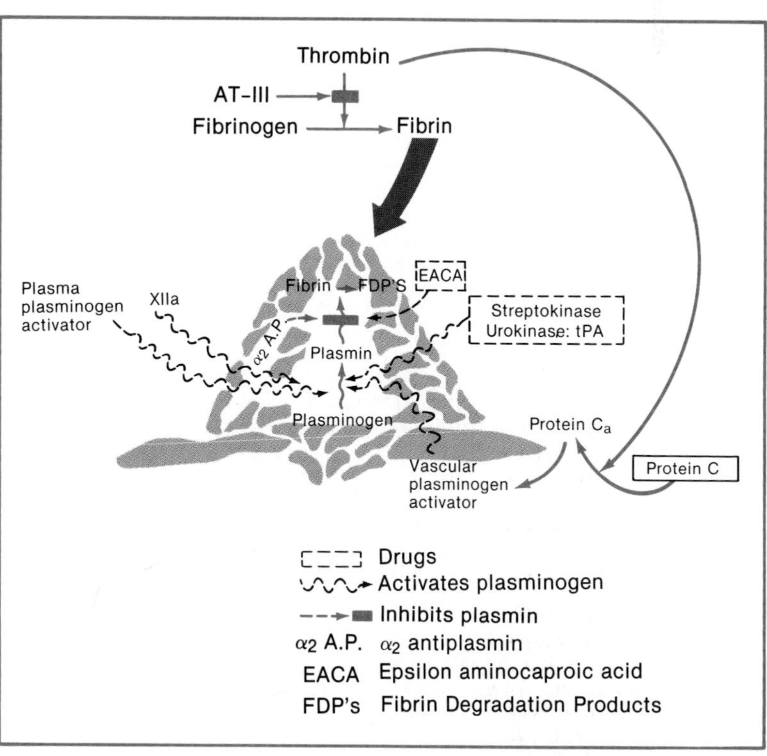

FIGURE 48-2. Schematic view of the fibrinolytic system. Vascular and plasma plasminogen activators as well as pharmacological agents can activate plasmin trapped within the clot. Plasmin dissolves the fibrin clot. Inhibitors of plasmin include alpha²-antiplasmin, also trapped within the clot, and pharmacological agents. (From Stead, R. B.: Regulation of hemostasis. *In* Goldhaber, S. Z. [ed]: Pulmonary Embolism and Deep Venous Thrombosis. Philadelphia, W. B. Saunders Co., 1985, p. 38).

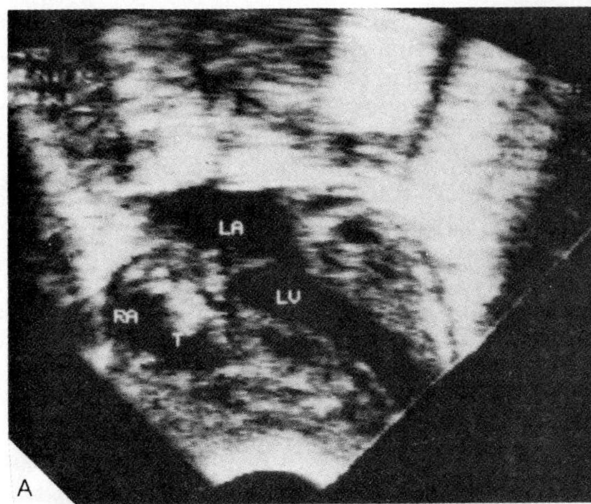

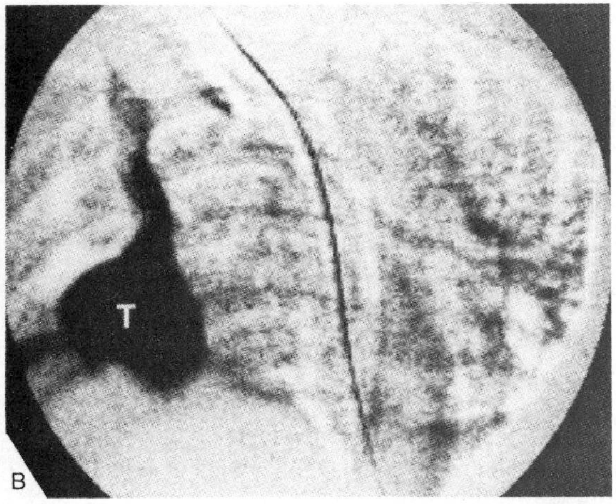

FIGURE 48-3. ***A,*** **Two-dimensional echocardiogram from the subxiphoid position in a 9-month-old boy with *Staphylococcus epidermidis* septicemia and a central hyperalimentation line. A large thrombus (T) can be seen low in the right atrium (RA), just above the tricuspid valve. The mass, acting as a partial ball-valve thrombus, obstructed right ventricular outflow. LA = left atrium; LV = left ventricle. *B,* Digital subtraction angiogram, with contrast material injected through the hyperalimentation catheter. With the catheter tip in the superior aspect of the RA, contrast enters a large cavitary RA thrombus (T), which acts as a cul-de-sac. Thus, contrast cannot be seen in the RA or right ventricle. This thrombus is an ominous nidus for potential pulmonary embolization. (From Fulton, D. R.: Venous thromboembolism in children. *In* Goldhaber, S. Z. [ed.]: Pulmonary Embolism and Deep Venous Thrombosis. Philadelphia, W. B. Saunders Company, 1985, p. 249.)**

mately 50 per cent),[24] this risk is lower (approximately one in three) when DVT remains confined to calf veins.[25] In contrast to leg DVT, superficial thrombophlebitis and upper extremity thrombosis are less often associated with PE.

DIAGNOSIS. DVT often occurs without any symptoms or signs. When present, however, the major symptoms are leg pain, tenderness, and swelling, while the major signs are leg edema, discomfort in the calf upon forced dorsiflexion of the foot (Homans' sign), venous distention of subcutaneous vessels, discoloration, and a palpable cord (i.e., thrombus). Unfortunately, these symptoms and signs are not specific for DVT, so that diagnoses based on clinical findings are often incorrect. Therefore, clinical suspicion of DVT should prompt definitive radiological evaluation.

B-mode Ultrasonography. The introduction of B-mode ultrasonography has revolutionized the diagnosis of DVT. When the ultrasound transducer is placed over the common femoral and popliteal veins, the inability to compress these veins is a highly accurate indication of DVT proximal to the calf.[26] The entire ultrasonographic procedure can be completed on both legs within 15 minutes. At times, thrombus can be demonstrated within the lumen (Fig. 48-4). With more expensive and sophisticated machines, color Doppler imaging can be added to the ultrasound examination, and resolution of calf vein thrombi 1 mm^2 can be achieved.[27] Nevertheless, use of a relatively inexpensive high-resolution real-time scanner equipped with a 5-MHz electronically focused linear-array transducer is adequate for reliable diagnosis of DVT proximal to the calf. Experienced ultrasonographers can often use this machine to image adequately the calf veins as well. B-mode ultrasonography is so reliable, inexpensive, safe, and nontraumatic that it is rapidly supplanting leg phlebography as the "gold standard."

Phlebography. Venography is costly, invasive, and occasionally results in complications such as contrast allergy and contrast-induced phlebitis. Patients with massive leg DVT often have nondiagnostic venograms because the contrast agent simply cannot reach the deep leg veins. Consequently, we reserve phlebography for those situations in which the ultrasound examination is equivocal or, alternatively, when the ultrasound examination is normal despite a high clinical suspicion for DVT.

Impedance Plethysmography (IPG). IPG, which was the most widely used noninvasive test to detect DVT, has been superseded by B-mode ultrasonography. IPG measures changes in electrical resistance caused by obstruction to venous outflow. Two studies have suggested that serial IPG testing repeated three to six times over 10 to 14 days will accurately detect calf vein DVT that extends proximally.[28,29]

TREATMENT. For all cases of DVT proximal to the calf and for symptomatic calf DVT,[30] the usual treatment is initial heparin anticoagulation followed by warfarin therapy. Asymptomatic DVT limited to the calf need not be treated with anticoagulation as long as serial noninvasive monitoring for 2 weeks after diagnosis confirms that the clot has not extended proximally. Anticoagulation reduces the risk of proximal propagation of clot and subsequent PE. Usually, therapy is initiated with a continuous intravenous infusion of heparin, because this appears to be more efficacious than intermittent subcutaneous administration.[31]

The proper role of thrombolytic therapy in the treatment of DVT remains uncertain. Two potential advantages of thrombolysis are the prevention of PE by dissolution in situ of the source of embolization in the pelvic or upper extremity veins or the deep veins of the leg, and the prevention of chronic venous insufficiency. The potential benefits of these preventive measures, neither of which has been proved, must be weighed against the risks of hemorrhage. More than 80 per cent of our DVT patients have a contraindication to thrombolysis. These patients are treated with heparin and warfarin or with an inferior vena caval filter. Among those without contraindications to thrombolysis, we consider the use of thrombolytic therapy followed by a full course of heparin anticoagulation and warfarin. As an adjunctive measure, we prescribe thigh-high compression (30 to 40 mm Hg) stockings to our DVT patients when they ambulate. The stockings help prevent distention of the vein wall and may moderate the syndrome of chronic venous insufficiency that two-thirds of DVT patients treated with standard anticoagulation therapy inevitably experience.[32]

Although chronic anticoagulation (usually for 3 months) is prescribed to avert recurrent VTE, the optimal length of such treatment is unknown. One-fifth of patients with DVT may experience a recurrence despite 3 months of anticoagulation.[33] Therefore, in our practice, we anticoagulate those patients who have no long-term risk factors for 6 months, with (rabbit brain thromboplastin) PT maintained at 15 to 16 sec. For those patients with risk factors such as massive obesity, cancer, and previous DVT, anticoagulants are given for an indefinite period of time.

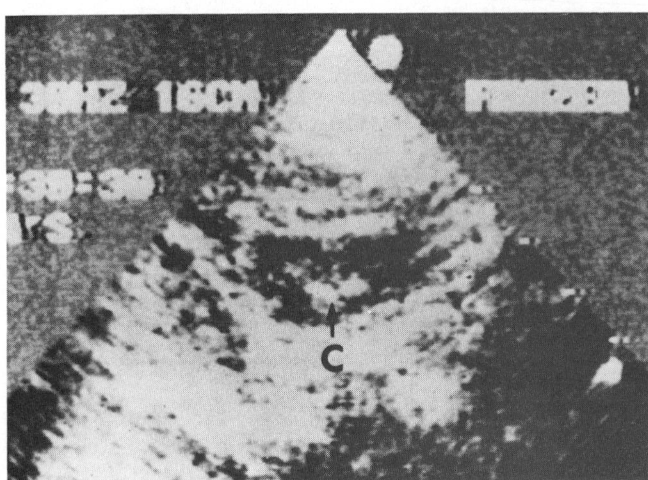

FIGURE 48-4. Left common femoral vein thrombus visualized with high resolution B-mode ultrasonography in a 30-year-old woman. This vein also lacked compressibility. c = clot.

PATHOPHYSIOLOGY

When venous thrombi become dislodged from their site of formation, they flow through the venous system to the pulmonary arterial circulation. If an embolus is extremely large, it may lodge at the bifurcation of the pulmonary artery, forming a "saddle embolus" (Fig. 48–5 *Top*). More commonly, a major pulmonary vessel is occluded (Fig. 48–5 *Bottom*).

The pathophysiological response to acute PE depends on the extent to which pulmonary artery blood flow is obstructed, on preexisting cardiopulmonary disease, and on the release of vasoactive humoral factors from activated platelets that accumulate at the site of new clot (p. 1767). In patients without previous cardiopulmonary disease, right ventricular afterload increases when pulmonary artery obstruction reduces the pulmonary vascular bed by 25 per cent or more. To compensate for this impairment, right ventricular and pulmonary artery pressures rise. As right ventricular afterload increases acutely, this chamber dilates (leading in turn to tricuspid regurgitation) and becomes hypokinetic. These findings can be observed on two-dimensional (Fig. 48–6) and Doppler echocardiography, which can be used to estimate pulmonary artery pressure. As the right ventricle fails, right atrial pressure rises and cardiogenic shock ensues. When cardiac function has been compromised by previous cardiopulmonary illness, relatively smaller emboli obstructing only one or two pulmonary segments can exert a similar hemodynamic effect.

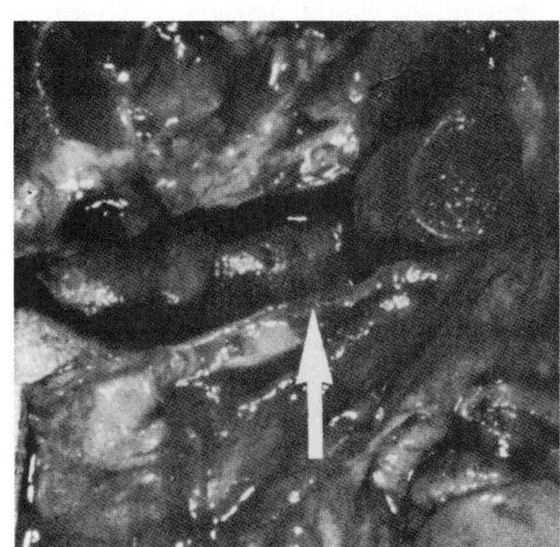

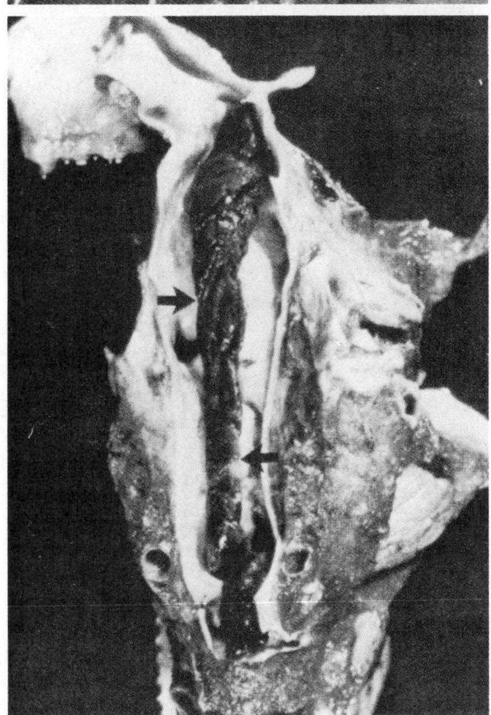

FIGURE 48–5. ***Top,*** **Saddle embolus at the bifurcation of the pulmonary artery.** ***Bottom,*** **Pulmonary embolus in left lower lobe pulmonary artery, with minimal attachment to the wall of the vessel. The embolus was dark red, typical of venous thrombi, and had indentations believed to represent impressions of the venous valves (arrows). (From Godleski, J. J.: Pathology of deep venous thrombosis and pulmonary embolism.** ***In*** **Goldhaber, S. Z. [ed.]: Pulmonary Embolism and Deep Venous Thrombosis. Philadelphia, W. B. Saunders Company, 1985, p. 17.)**

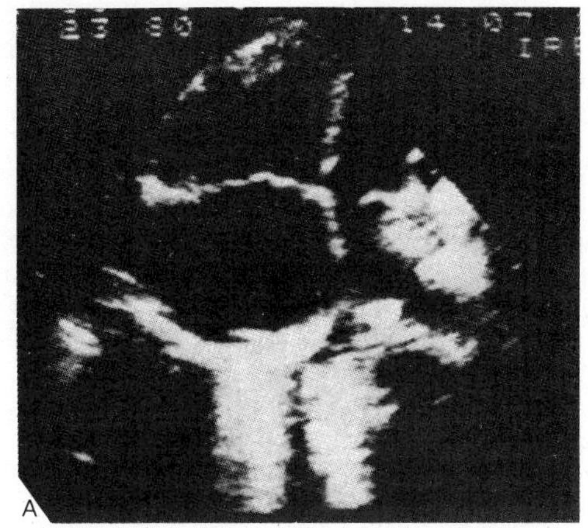

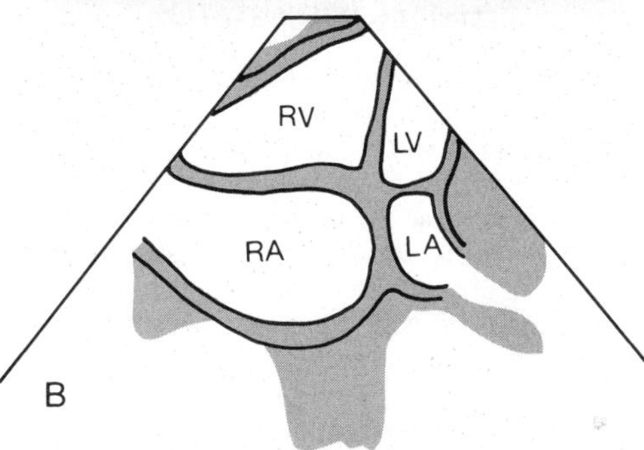

FIGURE 48–6. Apical four-chamber two-dimensional echocardiogram (*A*) and schematic drawing (*B*) from a patient with massive pulmonary embolism. There is marked dilatation of the right atrium (RA) and right ventricle (RV). (The apparent mass in the region of the left atrium (LA) is an imaging defect.) (From Hoagland, P. M.: Massive pulmonary embolism. ***In*** **Goldhaber, S. Z. [ed.]: Pulmonary Embolism and Deep Venous Thrombosis. Philadelphia, W. B. Saunders Company, 1985, p. 187.)**

Although preload, afterload, heart rate, and contractility have traditionally been considered the determinants of left ventricular systolic performance (Chap. 13), acute increases in right ventricular pressure can also affect left ventricular function. In a canine model, acutely induced moderate right ventricular hypertension displaces the interventricular septum toward the left ventricle. Therefore, during pressure overload of the right ventricle, the anatomical juxtaposition of the two ventricles (i.e., ventricular interdependency) results in decreased left ventricular diastolic filling and end-diastolic volume.[34] Increased pericardial restraint during PE may also impair left ventricular function by reducing preload.[35]

Among 14 patients with acute massive PE, echocardiography revealed increased right ventricular end-systolic and end-diastolic areas, reduced right ventricular fractional area contraction, interventricular septal flattening at both end-systole and end-diastole, and markedly decreased left ventricular end-diastolic dimensions. Left ventricular fractional area contraction remained normal. During treatment, the interventricular septum progressively returned to a more normal configuration at both end-systole and end-diastole, and left ventricular diastolic dimension steadily increased. Thus, it appeared that circulatory failure due to massive PE is mediated through a profound decrease in left ventricular preload. Acute dilation of the right ventricle with the concomitant restraining action of the pericardium accounted for the leftward shift of the interventricular septum and reduced left ventricular compliance.[36]

After pulmonary embolization, the release of neurohumoral factors causes pulmonary vasoconstriction and bronchospasm that can affect outcome adversely. Experimental studies suggest that during acute PE the two most important vasoactive humoral factors are serotonin and thromboxane A_2 (TxA_2).[37] Serotonin, a potent neural and smooth muscle agonist, is stored primarily in the dense bodies of platelets and mediates bronchospasm in the small airways, either by direct bronchial smooth muscle constriction or by stimulation of a reflex that induces bronchospasm. Activated platelets also release TxA_2, a potent vasoconstrictor and bronchoconstrictor. Increased dead space and reflex airway constriction from PE result in wasted ventilation. The surfactant concentration can decrease, with attendant alveolar collapse and atelectasis, especially during the first few days after embolization.

Diagnosis of Pulmonary Embolism

CLINICAL PRESENTATION

Clinical suspicion of PE is of paramount importance to guide diagnostic testing. In various autopsy series, rates of overdiagnosis ranged from 32 to 62 per cent, and the rate of underdiagnosis has been reported to be as high as 84 per cent.[38] In the Urokinase-Streptokinase Pulmonary Embolism Trial (UPET), clinical symptoms and signs were tabulated in 327 patients with angiographically documented PE (Table 48–2). Because symptoms and signs often do not help to discriminate between patients with true PE and those with no evidence of PE on the arteriogram,[39] the diagnosis with ventilation-perfusion lung scanning or angiography should be pursued in virtually all cases in which PE is suspected (Fig. 48–7).

DIFFERENTIAL DIAGNOSIS. The wide differential diagnosis justifies the reputation of PE as "The Great Masquerader" (Table 48–3). When established pneumonia (with an infiltrate on chest x-ray), congestive heart failure, or myocardial infarction does not respond to appropriate therapy, it may be prudent to rule out coexisting PE. Recurrent PE can increase pulmonary artery pressure[40] and may be mistaken for primary pulmonary hypertension (p. 806)[41,42] (Table 48–4). Although these two conditions share many similarities, certain other features can be used to differentiate them (Table 48–4).

CLINICAL SYNDROMES OF PE

MASSIVE PE. This can be defined as sufficient obstruction of pulmonary arterial blood flow to cause a substantial increase in right ventricular afterload and consequent elevation of pulmonary arterial systolic pressure. Such patients are at highest risk for sudden death from PE or, over the long term, for chronic pulmonary hypertension due to pulmonary arterial clot that has failed to lyse. The most common features that suggest this diagnosis are syncope, profound dyspnea, cor pulmonale, cardiogenic shock, and cardiac arrest (particularly with electromechanical dissociation). Severe pleuritic chest pain usually indicates that the patient does *not* have massive PE. When syncope occurs, it may at times be caused by associated vagal bradyarrhythmias.[43] Patients also frequently display tachycardia, tachypnea, and cyanosis with distended neck veins; cardiogenic shock (Chap. 21) may be present or incipient. Less common presentations include fever, wheezing, disseminated intravascular coagulation, and paradoxical arterial embolism.[44,45] The differential diagnosis may include septic shock, superior vena caval syndrome, pericardial tamponade (p. 1473), constrictive pericarditis (p. 1486), and right ventricular infarction.

SUBMASSIVE PE. This can be defined as embolism to one or more pulmonary segments *not* accompanied by substantial elevations in right ventricular and pulmonary artery systolic pressures. Although these patients are not likely to succumb to an acute episode, unlysed thrombi in the pulmonary arteries can eventually lead to chronic pulmonary hypertension. The most frequent symptom is pleuritic chest pain.

PULMONARY INFARCTION. With occlusion of small peripheral pulmonary arteries, bronchoconstriction frequently occurs, and collateral blood flow via the bronchial arteries may not be preserved, leading to pulmonary infarction. The clinical diagnosis of pulmonary infarction due to PE cannot be established unless an infiltrate is present on chest X-ray and the usual criteria for PE on lung scan or pulmonary angiography are met. The primary alternative diagnosis based on clinical presentation is pneumonia. Some PE patients with pulmonary infarction present with hemoptysis; virtually all experience intense pleuritic pain but tend to have a unilateral, distal embolism that is less extensive on angiography than in PE patients without pulmonary infarction.[46] Typically, symptoms and signs develop 3 to 7 days after the onset of embolism.

CHRONIC PULMONARY HYPERTENSION. Recurrent PE may cause chronic pulmonary hypertension associated

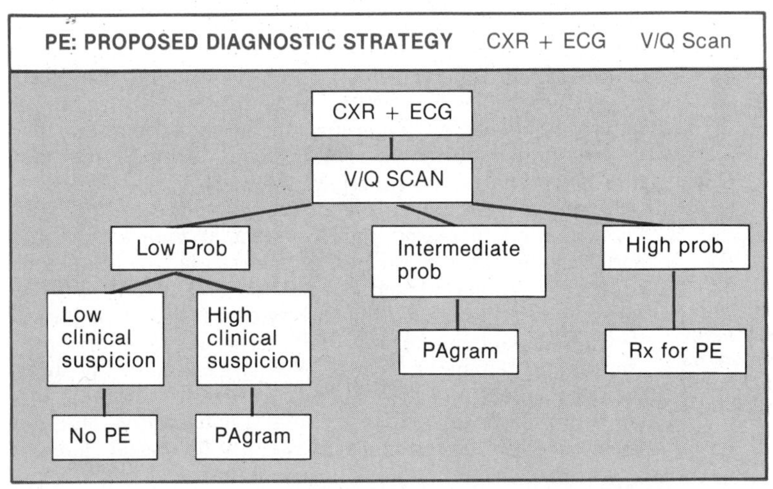

FIGURE 48–7. Diagnostic strategy in suspected pulmonary embolism. CXR = chest x-ray; V/Q = ventilation/perfusion; prob = prob; PAgram = pulmonary arteriogram.

TABLE 48–2 SYMPTOMS AND SIGNS IN 327 PATIENTS WITH PULMONARY EMBOLISM

	PERCENTAGE AFFECTED
SYMPTOMS	
Chest pain	88
Pleuritic chest pain	74
Dyspnea	84
Apprehension	59
Cough	53
Hemoptysis	30
Diaphoresis	36
Syncope	13
SIGNS	
Tachypnea (RR > 16/min)	92
Rales	48
Accentuated 2nd heart sound	53
Tachycardia (HR > 100/min)	44
Fever (Temp > 37.8°C)	43
Phlebitis	32
Cyanosis	19

From Bell, W. R., Simon, T. L., and DeMets, D. L.: The clinical features of submassive and massive pulmonary emboli. Am. J. Med. 52:355, 1977. (Data based on the Urokinase-Streptokinase Pulmonary Embolism Trial.)

TABLE 48–3 DIFFERENTIAL DIAGNOSIS OF PULMONARY EMBOLISM

Myocardial infarction
Pneumonia
Congestive heart failure
Asthma
Chronic obstructive pulmonary disease
Intrathoracic cancer
Rib fracture
Pneumothorax
"Musculoskeletal pain"

with a clinical syndrome of progressive right heart failure and cor pulmonale. This condition tends to develop insidiously when PE either is not diagnosed or is treated inadequately. It is hypothesized that the use of thrombolytic agents to treat PE may reduce the incidence of this complication. On examination, the lung fields may be clear despite the presence of dyspnea, cyanosis, jugular venous distention, *v* waves due to tricuspid regurgitation, hepatic enlargement, ascites, and lower extremity edema. Chronic pulmonary hypertension due to recurrent PE is a feared complication of venous thromboembolism and has a poor prognosis. Nevertheless, it is important to recognize this clinical syndrome so that these patients can be evaluated for potential pulmonary thromboendarterectomy (p. 1574).

NONTHROMBOTIC PE. Sources of nonthrombotic PE[47] include tumor,[48] fat, amniotic fluid,[49] air, and particulate matter such as cotton and catheters.

NONIMAGING MODALITIES

ARTERIAL BLOOD GASES. Hypoxemia, determined by means of arterial blood gas measurement, has traditionally been considered an important screening test for PE. Yet patients suspected of PE who are then found to have normal lung scans or pulmonary angiograms may be as or more hypoxemic than those with documented PE. Conversely, a high arterial PO_2 can cause the physician mistakenly to refrain from pursuing the diagnosis of PE. More recently, it has been suggested that the inaccuracy of hypoxemia can be overcome by analyzing arterial blood gases for the presence of an increased alveolar-arterial oxygen gradient because, in PE, both a ventilation-perfusion mismatch and an increase in true intrapulmonary shunt should increase this gradient.[50] However, others have found that a normal A-a oxygen gradient does not exclude the diagnosis of PE.[51] Therefore, we believe that arterial blood gases, while of value for many aspects of patient care, are so misleading in the investigation of suspected PE that they should not be part of the diagnostic strategy.

ANALYSIS OF PLEURAL FLUID. The results of pleural fluid analysis are so variable[52] that thoracentesis need not be undertaken in patients with suspected PE unless a concomitant infectious process is considered likely. (If thoracentesis has been performed, thrombolytic agents usually should not be administered for 10 days.)

TABLE 48–4 PRIMARY PULMONARY HYPERTENSION (PPH) VS. RECURRENT PE

SIMILARITIES		
Symptoms	Fatigue, dyspnea on exertion—most common Chest pain, syncope, hemoptysis, cyanosis—also common	
Clinical course	Progressive dyspnea, right heart failure	
Hemodynamics	Elevated right heart pressures, normal pulmonary capillary wedge pressure	
DIFFERENCES	**PPH**	**Recurrent PE**
Age	20 to 40 years	>50 years
Female:male ratio	4:1	1:1
Clinical course	Continued downhill	Downhill, with stabilization between episodes
Lung scan	No segmental perfusion defects	Segmental or larger perfusion defects
Pulmonary artery systolic pressure	>60 mm Hg	<60 mm Hg
Pulmonary arteriogram	"Pruning"	Intraluminal filling defects
Confounding problems with arteriogram	Thrombi may occur on or distal to PPH lesions	"Pruning," a common angiographic finding in PPH, can also indicate PE. Arteriogram may not show emboli late in the clinical course
Diagnostic alternatives	Open lung biopsy	Pulmonary angioscopy
Therapy	Isoproterenol Hydralazine Nifedipine Anticoagulation	Anticoagulation IVC interruption Thromboendarterectomy

From Goldhaber, S. Z.: Strategies for diagnosis. *In* Goldhaber, S. Z. (ed.): Pulmonary Embolism and Deep Vein Thrombosis. Philadelphia, W. B. Saunders Company, 1985, p. 89.

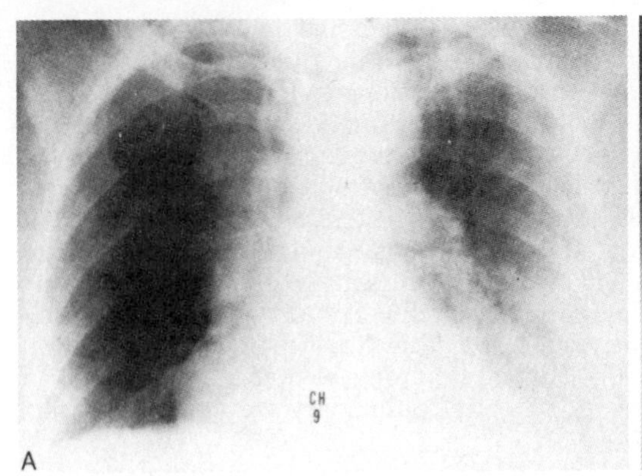

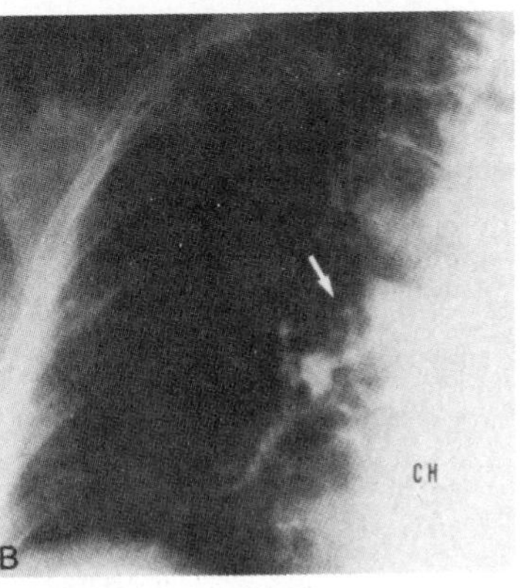

FIGURE 48–8. *A*, Chest x-ray of patient with clinical signs of pulmonary embolism showing marked oligemia (Westermark's sign) in the entire right lobe. *B*, arteriogram from same patient showing massive saddle embolus in the right main pulmonary artery (arrow). (Courtesy of Jack L. Westcott, M.D., The New York Hospital and Cornell University Medical College.)

ELECTROCARDIOGRAM. The electrocardiogram tends to show characteristic abnormalities only in patients with massive PE. Traditional manifestations of acute cor pulmonale such as $S_1Q_3T_3$ (Fig. 5–13, p. 127), right bundle branch block, P pulmonale, or right-axis deviation occurred in 26 per cent of the patients evaluated in the Urokinase Pulmonary Embolism Trial (UPET).[53] Usually, when the electrocardiogram suggests PE, the diagnosis tends to be apparent for other reasons.

BLOOD TESTS. To date, no rapid, inexpensive, and accurate blood test to screen for PE or DVT (analogous to the CK-MB enzyme assays used to diagnose acute myocardial infarction) has been found. The most promising blood test appears to be the D-dimer, which needs further refinement before it becomes a reliable clinical tool. In thrombotic conditions such as PE, endogenous plasmin-mediated proteolysis of cross-linked human fibrin tends to occur, with release of unique products that can be quantified, including D-D and Y-D dimeric fragments. With the use of monoclonal antibodies, immunoassays for human D-dimer have been developed. In a study of 19 patients with angiographically proven PE and 50 patients with completely normal lung scans who were suspected of having PE, elevated levels of D-dimer were present in 89 per cent of patients with PE. However, D-dimer elevation was also present in 56 per cent of patients who did not have PE.[54]

PULMONARY FUNCTION TESTS. PE causes an increase in both the physiological deadspace (V_D) and in the ratio of V_D to tidal volume (V_T). In a study of 16 patients with angiographically diagnosed PE and 29 patients in whom PE was excluded, a $V_D/V_T > 40$ per cent in the presence of a normal spirogram was highly suggestive of PE, whereas a $V_D/V_T < 40$ per cent made the diagnosis of PE very unlikely.[55]

CONVENTIONAL IMAGING MODALITIES

Chest Roentgenography

Occlusion of a lobar or segmental artery will cause a relative local hyperlucency on plain film, with diminished vascular markings (Fig. 48–8). An engorged major hilar artery on a plain film is another important clue to massive PE, especially when serial studies are available. The sudden appearance of a "plump" vessel, particularly the right descending pulmonary artery, may suggest embolic disease. In most cases, hilar signs are right-sided because cardiac and main pulmonary artery shadows make it difficult to visualize left-sided hilar signs. Abrupt tapering or termination of a vessel, termed the "knuckle sign," although rarely noted, can be diagnostic of PE. Nonspecific signs include diminished volume of a lower lobe with displacement of a major fissure or elevation of a hemidiaphragm. Obviously, these findings on chest roentgenography are not diagnostic, but in the proper clinical setting they may increase or even arouse suspicion.[56]

In *pulmonary infarction*, parenchymal consolidation is observed as an increased radiographic density. This finding may be due to actual tissue necrosis or to so-called reversible infarction (i.e., hemorrhage and edema) that clears within 3 to 7 days. However, if infarction leads to necrosis, the average time of resolution is about 3 weeks, usually with permanent residual fibrotic changes. The classic configuration is a homogeneous wedge-shaped density in the peripheral region of the lung with a rounded, convex apex pointing toward the hilum —commonly referred to as "Hampton's hump" (Fig. 48–9).[57] *Absence of an air bronchogram* in a parenchymal consolidation is suggestive of infarction as opposed to a pneumonic process; on the other hand, the *presence* of an air bronchogram is inconclusive because it is sometimes observed in patients with PE.

The chest roentgenogram may also provide an important clue that pulmonary artery hypertension is due to chronic PE when there is right-sided cardiomegaly, mosaic oligemia, or right descending pulmonary artery enlargement.[58] Overall, however, chest roentgenography is an insensitive screening test for PE. Its major diagnostic utility lies in its capacity to suggest diagnoses *other* than PE, such as pneumonia, heart failure, or pneumothorax.

Lung Scanning

Ventilation-perfusion lung scanning is the key diagnostic test in screening for PE.[58a] A normal perfusion scan essentially rules out all but trivial-sized PE and helps direct clinical attention to other diagnostic possibilities. It is usually safe to withhold anticoagulant therapy in patients with suspected PE and normal perfusion scans, regardless of the clinical manifestations; ordinarily, such patients do not need to undergo pulmonary angiography.[59]

For patients with perfusion defects that are segmental or greater in size, normal ventilation on scintigraphy in the same areas as the perfusion defects increases the likelihood of PE. Abnormal scans are usually categorized as having a low, moderate, high, or indeterminate probability for PE. At the Brigham and Women's Hospital, low probability scans are defined as showing multiple subsegmental perfusion defects without a ventilation study, or subsegmental or larger perfusion defects with abnormal ventilation correlating with the perfusion defects (a ventilation-perfusion [$\dot{V}/\dot{Q}$] "match"). Moderate probability scans show multiple subsegmental perfusion defects with normal ventilation, or segmental or larger

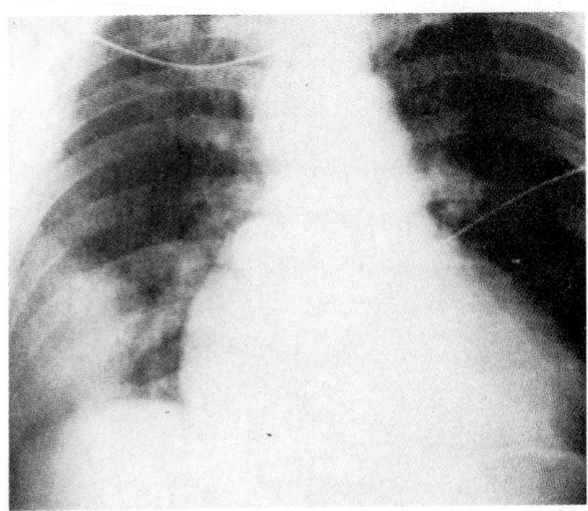

FIGURE 48–9. Posteroanterior chest x-ray of patients with pulmonary embolism showing "Hampton's hump" in right lower lung field, a homogeneous, wedge-shaped density in the peripheral field, convex to the hilum. (Courtesy of Jack L. Westcott, M.D., The New York Hospital and Cornell University Medical College.)

TABLE 48-5 PIOPED: COMPARISON OF SCAN CATEGORY TO ANGIOGRAM FINDINGS

	PULMONARY EMBOLISM			NO	TOTAL
	Present	Absent	Uncertain	ANGIOGRAM	N
Scan Category					
High	102	14	1	7	124
Intermediate	105	217	9	33	364
Low	39	199	12	62	312
Near-normal/normal	5	50	2	74	131
Total	251	480	24	176	931

From the PIOPED Investigators: Value of the ventilation/perfusion scan in acute pulmonary embolism. JAMA *263*:2756, 1990.

perfusion defects without a ventilation study. High probability scans show segmental or larger perfusion defects with normal ventilation ($\dot{V}/\dot{Q}$ "mismatch"). Alternatively, a scan can be high probability with two or more large perfusion defects that are substantially larger than either ventilation or chest x-ray abnormalities. Scans are of indeterminate probability when the chest x-ray either demonstrates COPD or is abnormal in the region(s) of the perfusion defect.

Hull and colleagues at McMaster University in Hamilton, Ontario compared abnormal ventilation-perfusion lung scans with results of pulmonary angiography among patients suspected of having PE.[60] Their findings support the traditional definition of a high-probability lung scan (e.g., 86 per cent accuracy) but they found that 37 of 116 (32 per cent) of their patients with non–high-probability scans also had PE at angiography. More recently, under the auspices of the National Heart, Lung, and Blood Institute, a multicenter study was undertaken to determine the diagnostic usefulness of the ventilation-perfusion lung scan in acute PE.[61,61a] The Prospective Investigation of Pulmonary Embolism Diagnosis (PIOPED) recruited 931 patients, of whom 81 per cent completed mandatory angiography within a day of obtaining an abnormal lung scan. Among the 755 patients who completed angiography, 33 per cent had PE. The most important finding in PIOPED is that of the 251 patients with positive angiograms, only 102 (41 per cent) had high-probability lung scans. Therefore, the sensitivity of high-probability lung scans for PE at angiography is only 41 per cent. Accordingly, if high-probability lung scans are relied upon to establish the diagnosis, PE will not be recognized in more than half (59 per cent) of patients who present with it.

In PIOPED, the positive predictive value of lung scanning for PE at angiography was as follows: 87 per cent for high, 32 per cent for intermediate, 16 per cent for low, and 9 per cent for near-normal scans (Table 48–5). When the "clinical probability" was factored into the interpretation of the lung scan, it was evident that some patients suspected of having PE would not require further work-up before a disposition was made. For example, among patients who had both high-probability lung scans and a clinical suspicion for PE of more than 80 per cent, the likelihood of PE at angiography was 96 per cent. Conversely, among patients who had both a low probability lung scan and a clinical suspicion for PE of less than 20 per cent, the likelihood of PE at angiography was only 4 per cent (Table 48–6). The majority of patients will not fit neatly into either of these categories and, in most circumstances, such as an intermediate- or low-probability scan with high clinical suspicion, the diagnosis of PE should be pursued with angiography (Fig. 48–7). Lung imaging for suspected PE is usually a low-yield strategy, unless the patient has symptoms or signs of DVT or cancer.

Given the limitations of lung scanning, clinicians normally should not defer pulmonary angiography after obtaining a nondiagnostic scan, particularly when the results of the scan differ sharply from the clinical impression obtained by integrating history, symptoms, signs, and findings on the chest roentgenogram and electrocardiogram. Therefore, in estimating the probability of PE, the physician should interpret the lung scan on the basis of clinical assessment of the likelihood of disease.

Pulmonary Angiography

INDICATIONS. When a ventilation-perfusion lung scan is entirely normal, the diagnosis of PE can be excluded reliably. Conversely, when ventilation-perfusion lung scanning indicates a high probability of PE and clinical suspicion is high before scanning, it is not necessary to proceed with pulmonary angiography unless there is some mitigating factor that obscures the diagnosis, such as asthma, intrathoracic cancer, or previous PE. Usually, multiple segmental or lobar perfusion defects in areas of normal ventilation will correspond with angiographically documented PE. (However, if thrombolytic therapy or inferior vena caval interruption is being considered, one may wish to eliminate even the slightest diagnostic uncertainty by obtaining a pulmonary angiogram.) It is also worth emphasizing that perfusion scan findings understate the severity of angiographic and hemodynamic compromise among patients with chronic thromboembolic pulmonary hypertension.[62] For patients with low probability scans, we do not obtain pulmonary angiograms unless clinical suspicion of PE is high.

In general, pulmonary angiography is reserved for patients with nondiagnostic moderate probability or indeterminate lung scans, except when clinical suspicion for PE is high despite low probability scan results. The use of pulmonary angiography is increasing because the limitations of lung scanning and clinical diagnosis are becoming more widely appreciated, especially since results of the McMaster and PIOPED studies were disseminated. However, unless the patient's condition is

TABLE 48-6 PIOPED: PULMONARY EMBOLISM STATUS

	CLINICAL PROBABILITY (%)			
	80–100 No. PE/PTS (%)	20–79 No. PE/PTS (%)	0–19 No. PE/PTS (%)	All Probabilities No. PE/PTS (%)
Scan category				
High	28/29 (96)	70/ 80 (88)	5/ 9 (56)	103/118 (87)
Intermediate	27/41 (66)	66/236 (28)	11/ 68 (16)	104/345 (30)
Low	6/15 (40)	30/191 (16)	4/ 90 (4)	40/296 (14)
Near-normal/normal	0/ 5 (0)	4/ 62 (6)	1/ 61 (2)	5/128 (4)
Total	61/90 (68)	170/569 (30)	21/228 (9)	252/887 (28)

From the PIOPED Investigators: Value of the ventilation/perfusion scan in acute pulmonary embolism. JAMA *263*:2757, 1990.

hemodynamically unstable or unless empirical heparinization is absolutely contraindicated (e.g., active gastrointestinal bleeding), these studies need not be done on an emergency basis.

We do not substitute leg ultrasonography, impedance plethysmography (IPG), or venography for pulmonary angiography unless the patient is pregnant or has an important relative contraindication to angiography such as right atrial thrombus or previous anaphylaxis to contrast agent. In the prospective study by Hull et al.,[60] only 71 per cent of patients with positive pulmonary angiograms had positive venograms; conversely, 33 per cent of patients with normal pulmonary angiograms had positive venograms. Another strategy that we avoid is empirical anticoagulation followed by serial lung scanning to determine whether pulmonary perfusion has improved over time. Such improvement, if observed, could be due to resolving asthma or viral pneumonia as well as PE.

To summarize, except for extenuating circumstances (such as terminal illness, a history of life-threatening anaphylaxis to contrast medium, or pregnancy), we usually recommend pulmonary angiography when lung scans are inconclusive (i.e., moderate or indeterminate probability for PE). We also pursue angiography when our clinical suspicion for the condition is discordant with the result of the lung scan.

PERFORMANCE OF PULMONARY ANGIOGRAPHY

The pulmonary angiogram is the most specific examination available for establishing the clinical diagnosis of PE and serves as a template against which other techniques and approaches are measured.[63] The procedure is generally safe, except in patients who have a contrast allergy, right ventricular end-diastolic pressure more than 20 mm Hg,[64] or amiodarone-induced pulmonary toxicity (p. 646).[65] Newer contrast agents of lower osmolality are less toxic than conventional angiographic dye in patients with pulmonary hypertension.[66] We always employ low osmolar contrast rather than conventional angiographic dye, despite the higher cost of these newer agents. In addition to enhancing patient safety, low osmolar contrast agents virtually abolish the heat sensation and urge to cough. Low osmolar contrast agents may be cost-effective in pulmonary angiography because, unlike conventional contrast agents, the angiographic views almost never have to be repeated because of patient coughing and consequent blurring of the films.

As with any procedure, there is a learning curve for proper and safe performance of pulmonary angiography. Of the 755 patients in PIOPED who completed angiography, the procedure was a contributing cause of death in two (0.3 per cent), both of whom were seriously ill before angiography.[61] At the University of California in San Diego, which has a team of physicians and nurses experienced in managing PE patients with severe chronic pulmonary hypertension, 67 consecutive patients with moderate or severe pulmonary hypertension underwent pulmonary angiography. No major rhythm disturbances or systemic hypotension requiring therapy occurred, and there were no deaths. Thus, pulmonary angiography can be carried out safely despite the presence of severe pulmonary hypertension and right ventricular failure, as long as the procedure is performed by an experienced medical team.[67]

PREPARATION OF THE PATIENT. The rationale for performing this test should be explained to the patient and family. Those with high-probability lung scans should understand that, while there is a 5 to 15 per cent chance that they do not have PE, this determination can be made only with pulmonary angiography. The patient should be told that the procedure may cause discomfort. The injection of conventional contrast medium causes a transient hot, flushed feeling coupled with an almost irresistible urge to cough. Patients should also be informed that pulmonary angiography usually requires between one and four sets of injections in different views (Fig. 48–10).

A history of allergy to contrast medium should be sought. Patients should avoid heavy meals for at least 4 hours before angiography. Heparin can be discontinued for several hours before the procedure. Premedication may include 25 to 50 mg of oral diphenhydramine or 5 to 10 mg of diazepam 30 to 60 minutes before the procedure; when there is a history of adverse reactions to contrast medium, high-dose steroids may be added. If true anaphylaxis to dye has occurred in the past, the decision to proceed with the study must be questioned.

THE ANGIOGRAPHIC PROCEDURE. Our preferred approach is via the right femoral vein. Percutaneous cannulation of the femoral vein permits rapid access to a large vessel and avoids the problems of using small brachial veins, which may be difficult to cannulate with a No. 7 French catheter and which are prone to venospasm. To avoid inadvertent perforation of the right ventricle, a catheter with a pigtail configuration can be used rather than one with a straight end.[68] A pigtail catheter can be manipulated easily into the pulmonary artery in a number of ways: (1) a deflector wire (Cook, Inc., Bloomington, IN) or a curve applied to the stiff end of a 0.038-inch guidewire can be used to bend the catheter in the heart to facilitate its placement into the pulmonary artery (Fig. 48–11); (2) a precurved pigtail catheter such as a Grollman catheter can be used; or (3) a No. 7 French double-lumen Swan-Ganz catheter can be positioned first in the pulmonary artery and can then be replaced by a pigtail catheter over a 0.035 inch-diameter exchange guidewire.

Ordinarily, right atrial, right ventricular, and pulmonary artery pressures are recorded through a pigtail catheter before pulmonary arteriography. Perfusion defects on the lung scan are used to determine which lung to study initially.

Selective angiography should be used rather than main pulmonary artery injection. Once the catheter has been positioned and the patient has been placed in the desired projection, a test dose of 5 to 10 ml is administered. A plain scout film is then obtained to ensure satisfactory exposure and field of view. Before the injection, the patient should be instructed carefully about proper breathing technique and should be reminded to try to suppress the urge to cough. Filming is carried out during maximal inspiration.

Twenty to 25 ml of contrast medium per second is injected for 2 seconds. The exposure rates for this phase are 3 per second for 3 seconds and then 1 per second for the pulmonary venous phase, which occurs 5 to 7 seconds after injection. After the selective pulmonary artery injection, pulmonary artery pressures are rechecked to monitor a possible pulmonary hypertensive response, and systemic arterial pressure should be rechecked to detect potential hypotension. The "large film" method that we use offers high-resolution clarity of vascular detail and versatility in field size. An alternative approach utilizes cineangiography.

INTERPRETING THE ANGIOGRAM. PE cannot be excluded unless the vasculature appears normal on two different oblique views (Fig. 48–10). A definitive diagnosis of PE depends on visualization of a clot. Primary arteriographic signs of emboli are persistent lucent defects without obstruction to flow or a trailing edge of an intraluminal lucency if there is complete obstruction to flow distally. Secondary signs—not diagnostic in themselves but simply indicators of decreased pulmonary perfusion—

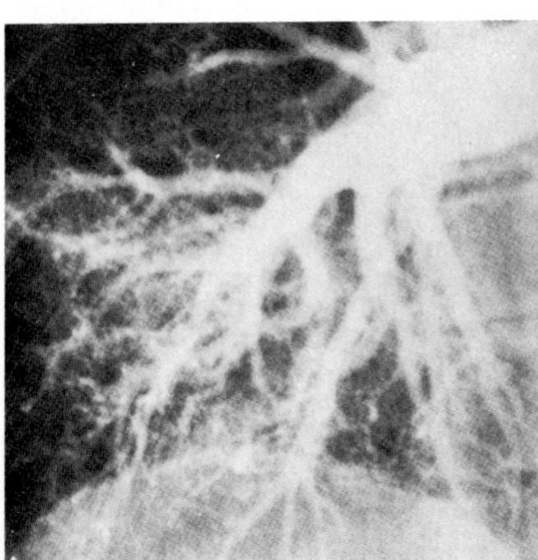

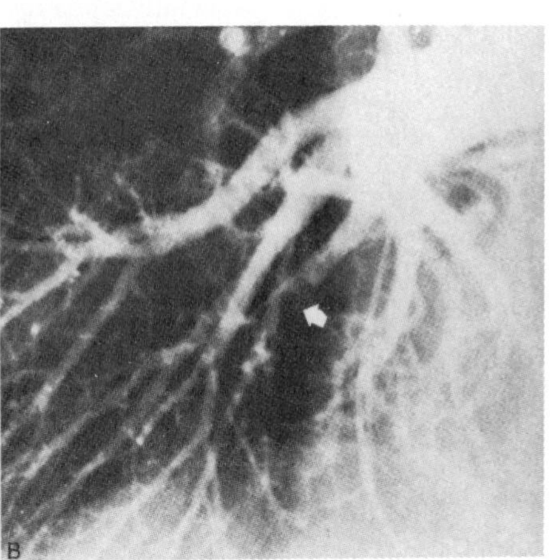

FIGURE 48–10. Selective right pulmonary arteriogram. *A,* Left posterior oblique projection of right lower lobe with normal-appearing pulmonary arteriogram due to overlap of vasculature. *B,* Right posterior oblique projection of the same area exhibiting an intravascular filling defect (arrow) in the artery to the lateral basal segment of the right lower lobe. (Courtesy of Thomas A. Sos, M.D., The New York Hospital and Cornell University Medical Center.)

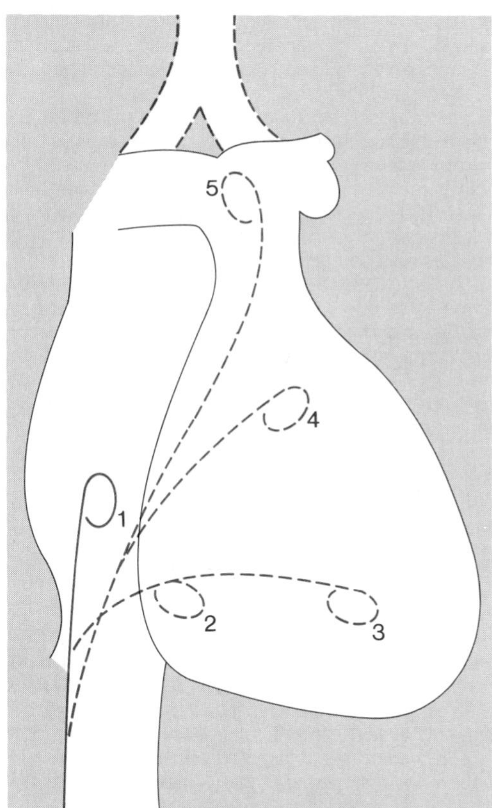

FIGURE 48–11. Technique for pulmonary artery catheterization. The pigtail catheter is advanced into the right atrium (1). A deflector guidewire is inserted into the catheter, the tip of the wire lying immediately proximal to the pigtail loop. The guidewire is deflected using the external handle, so that the catheter is curved toward the tricuspid valve (2). With the deflected guidewire fixed, the catheter is stripped off the wire and into the right ventricle (3). After deflection is released, the catheter will assume a straighter course, pointing toward the right ventricular outflow tract (4). As counterclockwise torque is applied, the catheter is advanced into the main pulmonary artery (5). With further advancement, the catheter will usually enter the left pulmonary artery. To select the right pulmonary artery, the deflector wire can be used to deflect the catheter toward the right, just below the level of the tracheal bifurcation. Pressure measurements are obtained in each right-sided cardiac chamber between each of the maneuvers described here. (From Meyerovitz, M.: How to maximize the safety of coronary and pulmonary angiography in patients receiving thrombolytic therapy. Chest *97*:134S, 1990.)

include areas of avascularity or oligemia, a prolonged arterial phase, tortuosity of peripheral vessels, and delayed visualization of the pulmonary venous circulation. These signs are often associated with PE but can occur in other conditions (e.g., bronchial asthma, severe mitral stenosis with associated pulmonary hypertension, or left ventricular failure) and thus are not specific. A primary sign of embolus is mandatory to prevent false-positive diagnoses. Not all pulmonary artery filling defects or occlusions are due to PE. Other causes include pulmonary Takayasu's arteritis (p. 1544), angiosarcoma, and sarcoidosis.[69]

Angiographic methods for quantitation of the severity of PE have been problematic. The Walsh scoring system,[70] which is most commonly used in the United States, does not take into account impairment of peripheral perfusion. The Miller index,[71] which is commonly used in Europe, can overestimate the extent of pulmonary vascular obstruction among patients with massive PE.

Both methods fail to differentiate adequately between clot size and the degree of vascular occlusion. This limitation can be problematic when a small thrombus causes only a partial filling defect with little effect on blood flow. A newer method for quantitating pulmonary angiograms has been proposed and may be more precise than either the Walsh or Miller indices.[72] However, this newer method appears to be more complex and has not been utilized in any therapeutic trials of PE.

In summary, pulmonary angiography is an underutilized procedure that provides maximal diagnostic accuracy. Because the use of stiff catheters that occasionally cause perforation of the right heart and cardiac tamponade has been abandoned, morbidity at present is predominantly related to toxicity of the contrast agent rather than the catheterization. With proper technique and judicious use of nonionic contrast agents, the mortality rate should not exceed 0.2 to 0.3 per cent.[61,63]

OTHER IMAGING MODALITIES

ECHOCARDIOGRAPHY. The diagnosis of massive PE can sometimes be established by means of two-dimensional echocardiography (Fig. 48–12).[73] The technique of transesophageal two-dimensional echocardiography is particularly well suited for the detection of massive central PE.[74]

Echocardiographic features that suggest acute PE include a dilated, hypokinetic right ventricle, absence of right ventricular hypertrophy, the presence of tricuspid regurgitation with increased flow velocity compatible with mild to moderate elevation of pulmonary arterial systolic pressure, and the absence of important left heart pathological conditions. Features suggestive of chronic pulmonary hypertension that could be caused by chronic PE include a dilated right ventricle that may be hypokinetic, right ventricular hypertrophy, and tricuspid regurgitation with increased flow velocity compatible with moderate to severe elevation of pulmonary arterial systolic pressure.[75]

For patients with dyspnea of unknown cause, it is useful to obtain an echocardiogram. Two-dimensional and Doppler echocardiography can either confirm the presence of left-sided cardiac dysfunction or suggest PE due to the findings of acute pulmonary hypertension.[76]

DIGITAL SUBTRACTION PULMONARY ANGIOGRAPHY (DSA). Although DSA is a useful technique for diagnosing PE in patients suspected of having massive central embolism, it cannot exclude clinically important peripheral PE. Whether DSA remains a research procedure for detecting PE will depend mostly on whether further technological modifications can reduce motion artifacts and improve the images of segmental and subsegmental pulmonary arteries.[77] At present, the only possible niche for DSA performed via a peripheral vein would be in screening patients who present with suspected life-threatening PE.[78]

COMPUTED TOMOGRAPHY (CT). This technique has been used to demonstrate PE[79] and pulmonary infarction.[80] CT scanning should be considered an inadequately validated diagnostic modality that may be appropriate for patients with pulmonary hypertension when the risks associated with conventional angiography are considered prohibitively high. CT scanning is more properly utilized for serial noninvasive evaluation after thrombolysis or surgical embolectomy among patients who have undergone baseline pulmonary angiography.

MAGNETIC RESONANCE IMAGING (MRI). This technique does not image rapidly flowing blood and may therefore be uniquely suited for

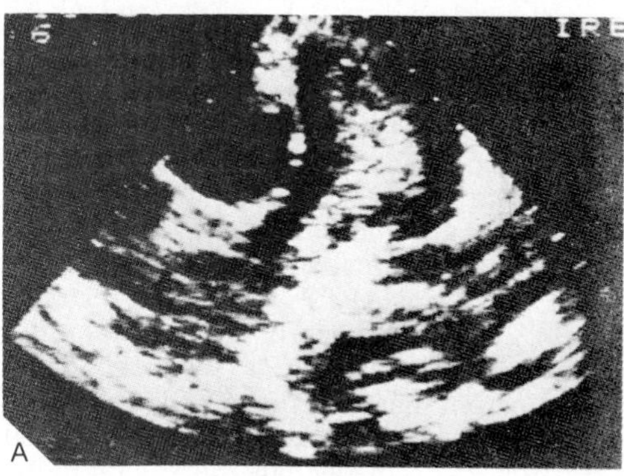

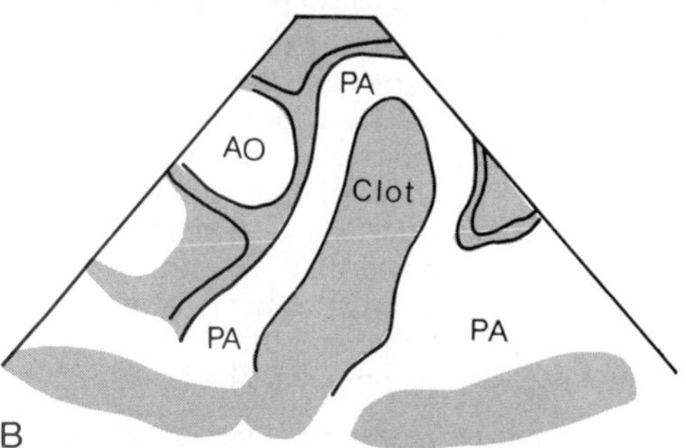

FIGURE 48–12. Two-dimensional echocardiogram in the short-axis parasternal view (*A*) and schematic drawing (*B*) showing a thrombus in the pulmonary artery in a patient with massive pulmonary embolism (seen in Figure 47–4). (From Hoagland, P. M.: Massive pulmonary embolism. *In* Goldhaber, S. Z. [ed.]: Pulmonary Embolism and Deep Venous Thrombosis. Philadelphia, W. B. Saunders Company, 1985, p. 187.)

detecting PE. Initial case reports have been encouraging.[81] The diagnostic niche for MRI may be in differentiating acute from chronic PE.[82]

RADIOISOTOPE IMAGING. The physical half-life of indium-111 (2.8 days) and the biological life of the injected platelet (8 to 10 days) permit imaging of PE and DVT[83] for at least 5 days after injection of the platelet suspension. Therefore, the technique may be useful for surveillance of high-risk patients[84] and for monitoring the therapeutic response once PE and DVT have been detected and treated.[85] However, a prospective study of 65 patients with suspected DVT who underwent indium-111 platelet scintigraphy 2 hours after injection demonstrated a disappointingly low sensitivity of approximately 40 per cent, although the specificity was excellent (greater than 90 per cent) when compared with contrast venography. In this study, the early images were problematic because of slow incorporation of platelets into the thrombi. In addition, limbs with varicose veins and postphlebitic changes presented difficulties in distinguishing platelet uptake into active thrombus.[86]

A promising imaging technique is indium-111–labeled monoclonal antifibrin antibodies for the detection of DVT. A study of 52 patients suspected of having DVT indicated greater than 90 per cent sensitivity in the calf but progressively less accuracy more proximally. The monoclonal antifibrin antibody binds specifically to the amino terminal region of fibrin but does not cross-react with fibrinogen. Diagnosis can be made within 2 hours after injection of the tracer.[87]

Another intriguing isotopic imaging technique utilizes an iodine-125–labeled mutant of tissue plasminogen activator (t-PA) that is fibrinolytically inactive to bind to thrombi. In vitro binding of the mutant t-PA to clots formed from human blood was concentration-dependent, time-dependent, and specific. The rapid clearance of mutant t-PA from the circulation may make it a useful clinical imaging agent. However, to date, in vivo use of this agent has not been reported.[88]

FIBEROPTIC ANGIOSCOPY. After jugular venotomy and insertion of the fiberoptic angioscope into the superior vena cava, the balloon is inflated to displace blood and obtain a clear view. The angioscope is then guided with fluoroscopic assistance into the right heart and main pulmonary artery. Pulmonary artery branches as distal as segmental arteries can be examined. While the technique is complicated to learn, it may be particularly useful in patients with chronic pulmonary hypertension.[89]

Treatment of Pulmonary Embolism

ANTICOAGULATION

Heparin

(See also p. 1761)

Heparin accelerates the action of antithrombin III 1000-fold to prevent further fibrin deposition (Fig. 48–2) and to allow for the body's natural fibrinolytic mechanisms to lyse clot that has already formed. Heparin does *not* dissolve thrombus that already exists. One placebo-controlled randomized trial has been carried out in PE patients.[90] The mortality rate was significantly lower among the treated patients, and the randomized trial was discontinued for ethical reasons. No randomized placebo-controlled trial with heparin has ever been undertaken in DVT.[27]

To achieve an effective antithrombotic state, a certain minimal level of heparin anticoagulation appears necessary. In practice, an effective level of heparin anticoagulation can be inferred from an activated partial thromboplastin time (PTT) that is at least 1½ times greater than the control value.[91]

Unfortunately, physicians tend to administer inadequate doses of heparin to patients with DVT and PE. In a review of physician practices at Vanderbilt University School of Medicine, 60 per cent of patients with venous thromboembolism (VTE) did not have a single PTT greater than 1.5 times control within the first 24 hours of heparin therapy. Not until day 8 of treatment were 90 per cent of the PTTs within the therapeutic range.[92] It is apparent that the usual practice of administering an initial 5000 unit bolus of heparin followed by an initial infusion of 1000 U/hr is inadequate therapy for most patients with VTE. When subtherapeutic PTTs were obtained in this study, physicians responded with modest increases in heparin dosing that were often inadequate to elevate the PTT into the therapeutic range. Conversely, when unacceptably high PTTs were obtained, excessive reductions in heparin dosage caused subtherapeutic PTTs in more than half of the patients.

Patients with DVT and PE have higher heparin requirements than those suspected of VTE who are subsequently proved to have no thrombosis.[93] Among patients with PE, the half-life of heparin is shorter and the clearance of heparin is greater compared with patients who have DVT.[94]

A unique problem is the monitoring of therapy among patients with elevated PTTs at baseline due to the presence of the lupus anticoagulant or anticardiolipin antibodies. Obviously, the usual criterion of a PTT greater than 1½ times control cannot be utilized in this population. To obviate this problem, we measure quantitatively the heparin level by having our chemistry laboratory use an HEPRN pack (Dupont Co., Wilmington, DE) in the automated clinical analyzer used for other chemistry tests. The plasma heparin level is a chromogenic assay based on the inhibition of factor X_a by heparin-activated antithrombin III. The HEPRN pack contains excess factor X_a and, essentially, analyzes the heparin level by means of an anti-factor X_a assay. Blood for this assay should be drawn into a citrated tube, placed on ice, centrifuged within 30 minutes, and analyzed within 4 hours. The therapeutic range for the heparin level is 0.2 to 0.5 U/ml.

For pregnant women with DVT and PE, we treat initially with continuous intravenous heparin and then teach the patient to self-administer full-dose subcutaneous heparin for the remainder of the pregnancy. With subcutaneous injections, peak heparin levels are usually obtained at approximately 3 hours, and the effect may last for 12 hours if the heparin dose is adequate. To monitor the heparin, our target is either a mid-interval PTT of approximately 1.5 times control or a "trough" PTT that is at least several seconds elevated above the upper limit of normal. We have found this approach safe for both the mother and fetus.[95] Although there has been some enthusiasm for administering continuous infusion heparin to pregnant women by utilizing a portable infusion pump,[96] we have abandoned this approach at Brigham and Women's Hospital because of bleeding complications that occurred despite therapeutic PTT levels.[97]

A correlation between hemorrhagic risk and excessively prolonged PTT (e.g., more than 3 times control) seems logical but is not well documented in prospective trials. However, a retrospective analysis of anticoagulated patients at Brigham and Women's Hospital found that bleeding does correlate with the intensity of therapy.[98] Compared with patients whose maximal PTT (or prothrombin time) was less than twice the control value, major bleeding was 3 times as frequent in patients with a maximal PTT (or prothrombin time) that was 2.0 to 2.9 times control and 7.9 times as frequent among patients with a PTT (or prothrombin time) prolonged to 3.0 or more times control. Other independent risk factors for major in-hospital bleeding among anticoagulated patients included the presence of comorbid conditions, age exceeding 60 years, and liver dysfunction that worsened during treatment.

In the majority of studies in which continuous and intermittent infusion of heparin have been compared, the frequency of major hemorrhage was lower with continuous intravenous infusion.[33] However, the patients who were given continuous intravenous heparin infusions tended to receive lower total doses of heparin than those allocated to subcutaneous injections. Theoretically, intermittent intravenous or subcutaneous heparin administration is disadvantageous because it temporarily causes excessive anticoagulation, as reflected by highly elevated peak PTT levels. Therefore, whenever feasible, for patients with suspected acute PE our practice is to administer heparin therapy by continuous intravenous infusion after an initial bolus of heparin.

INITIATION OF HEPARIN THERAPY. Heparin is the cornerstone of treatment for acute PE. Before heparin therapy is begun, the most important first step is to obtain a careful history. In particular, one should consider risk factors such as history of coagulopathy, thrombocytopenia, vitamin K deficiency, older age, underlying diseases, and concomitant drug therapy. The most frequently overlooked portion of the physical examination is a rectal examination for occult blood. The results of the examination should be recorded in the patient's chart. When a stool guaiac examination is equivocal (i.e., "trace"), we proceed with heparin anticoagulation but maintain an even higher state of vigilance than usual for potential bleeding complications.

If results of the history and physical examination are benign, heparin can be started before lung scanning or pulmonary angiography in situations when clinical suspicion of PE is high. However, if a severe bleeding problem is detected, such as active gastrointestinal bleeding, heparin therapy should be withheld and if the diagnosis of PE is confirmed, nonpharmacological treatment with insertion of an inferior vena cava (IVC) filter should be considered. Interestingly, we have modified our practice and no longer automatically place an inferior vena cava filter in patients with nonhemorrhagic brain tumors. Many of these patients can be anticoagulated safely.[99] For patients at high risk of bleeding from heparin, the angiographer should be alerted to the possible need to insert an IVC filter on short notice.

The dosage regimen for achieving optimal heparinization is empirical. For an average-sized adult in whom there is only a modest suspicion of PE, the usual initial dose would be a 5000-unit intravenous bolus followed by a continuous intravenous infusion of 1000 units per hour. In a patient suspected of having massive PE, a more appropriate initial dose is a 10,000-unit bolus followed by an infusion of 1500 units per hour. For maintenance heparin anticoagulation, the PTT should remain 1.5 to 2.5 times the control level and should be checked every 4 hours until the target PTT level is obtained. When the PTT is less than 1.5 times control, the continuous infusion dose should be increased rapidly, by an increment of at least 25 per cent. Conversely, if a PTT level exceeds 3 times the control value, a reduction in the infusion rate of no more than 25 per cent of the dose should be made. Otherwise, if too much of an adjustment is made, a rebound effect to a subtherapeutic level of anticoagulation can be anticipated. In general, heparin infusion rates of 1500 to 2000 units per hour are quite common for achieving adequate anticoagulation, particularly during the first few days of treatment.

COMPLICATIONS. The most important adverse effect of heparin is hemorrhage. Major bleeding during anticoagulation may unmask a previously silent lesion such as bladder or colon cancer. For most cases of moderate bleeding, cessation of heparin therapy will suffice, and the PTT level will usually return to normal within 2 to 3 hours because the half-life of heparin is only 60 to 90 minutes. Resumption of heparin at a lower dose or alternative means of therapy depends on the severity of the bleeding, the risk of recurrent thromboembolism, and the extent to which bleeding may have resulted from excessive anticoagulation (i.e., a PTT greater than 3 times the baseline value). In the event of life-threatening or intracranial hemorrhage, protamine sulfate can be administered when heparin is discontinued. Protamine, a strongly basic protein, will immediately reverse anticoagulant activity by forming a stable complex with the acidic heparin. For life-threatening hemorrhage, the usual dose is approximately 1 mg per 100 units of heparin, administered slowly (e.g., 50 mg over 10 to 30 minutes). Protamine sulfate can cause allergic reactions that vary from mild to life-threatening.[100]

Mild thrombocytopenia that may develop with heparin therapy probably represents a direct, nonimmune-mediated effect of heparin and is not associated with serious clinical consequence. Heparin-associated thrombocytopenia[101] (p. 1782) occurs more frequently with beef lung than with pork gut heparin.[102] The frequency of heparin-associated thrombocytopenia can vary according to the specific lot of heparin that is obtained from the manufacturing plant.[103] When the thrombocytopenia is associated with thrombosis, the condition is immune-mediated and may be life-threatening. Heparin-induced thrombosis can occur even with small doses of prophylactic heparin (e.g., 5000 U subcutaneously every 8 hours).[104] The thrombotic events are often distinctly unusual and may involve the skin[105] or major arteries,[106] such as the femoral or radial arteries.

Patients undergoing prolonged heparin therapy at relatively high doses may develop osteopenia, osteoporosis, and pathological bone fractures.[107,108] In addition, continuous heparin infusion causes aldosterone depression by an unknown mechanism within 4 to 8 days after initiation of therapy.[109] In patients with a normally functioning renin-angiotensin-aldosterone axis, this is probably of no clinical significance, although serum sodium levels may drop slightly. However, it may cause clinically important hyperkalemia in certain patients, such as those with diabetes[110] or renal failure.[111]

Heparin-associated elevations in transaminase levels are being recognized with increasing frequency. The increases occur more often in men, have no relation to whether the heparin is of bovine or porcine origin, and usually do not appear to be associated with clinical toxicity.[112] In our multicentered trial of DVT therapy, it was found that, one week after therapy with heparin alone, patients experienced a mean doubling of serum glutamic oxaloacetic transaminase levels. No similar trend in other measures of liver function (e.g., bilirubin, akaline phosphatase, lactic dehydrogenase) was observed.[101]

Warfarin Sodium

(see p. 1782)

OVERLAP WITH HEPARIN. In the early stage of warfarin administration, the level of protein C falls and this creates a thrombogenic potential. By the overlapping of heparin and warfarin for 4 to 5 days, this theoretically procoagulant effect of warfarin can be counteracted. It is our practice to overlap heparin and warfarin administration for at least 5 days. An Australian study of VTE patients treated everyone initially with heparin and randomly allocated patients to an "early warfarin" or "late warfarin" treatment group. The "early" group initiated warfarin on average after one day of hospitalization. The "late" group began warfarin after 7 days of continuous intravenous heparin. The efficacy and safety of heparin was similar in both groups, and early warfarin treatment shortened overall hospital stay by an average of 4 days.[113] These findings are consistent with the results of a more recent randomized trial at McMaster University. Patients with DVT were treated with either 5 days of heparin (with warfarin begun on the first day) or 10 days of heparin (with warfarin begun on the fifth day). The rate of recurrent DVT and bleeding was the same in both groups.[114] It is our practice to treat with 5 to 7 days of heparin and to initiate warfarin on the first or second hospital day.

DURATION AND INTENSITY OF THERAPY. Chronic anticoagulation is prescribed in PE to avert recurrent venous thromboembolism. In Phase I of UPET, one-fifth of the patients enrolled in the trial suffered recurrent PE during the first 2 weeks of therapy.[115] Recurrence appeared to correlate with lack of adequate intensity of anticoagulation. Although PE patients often receive chronic oral warfarin therapy for 6 months, its optimal duration and intensity are unknown. In patients with a transiently incurred risk for the development of PE, such as an operation, the utility of continuing anticoagulation indefinitely is probably low. However, for patients with a risk factor that is irreversible (i.e., metastatic cancer) or not easily modified (e.g., massive obesity), a stronger case can be made for continuing anticoagulants indefinitely.

The American College of Chest Physicians (ACCP) in conjunction with the National Heart, Lung, and Blood Institute (NHLBI) appointed a special panel to evaluate the indications for anticoagulation in a variety of cardiovascular illnesses. For venous thromboembolism (including DVT and PE) a therapeutic range for oral anticoagulation was determined in which the PT was prolonged 1.3 to 1.5 times the baseline value (using the Simplastin assay).[33] However, this recommendation, which we follow for DVT patients, is based on trials of DVT therapy[116] rather than PE (for which adequate trials are lacking). With regard to duration of therapy, the ACCP-NHLBI group recommended that patients with slowly resolving risk factors (e.g., prolonged immobilization) should be treated for at least 3 months, whereas patients with tumors, AT-III or protein C deficiency, or recurrent venous thromboembolism should be treated indefinitely. The panel implied that no more than 3 months of treatment was necessary for patients with risk factors that are readily reversible, such as estrogen use or transient immobilization.

We usually initiate warfarin therapy with 10 mg daily for 3 days and tend to treat patients with PE more aggressively than those with DVT, in terms of both intensity and duration of anticoagulation, maintaining the PT within the range of 16 to 20 seconds. If risk factors are transient, we treat with warfarin for one year. Otherwise, we advise indefinite anticoagulation.

COMPLICATIONS. The major toxic effect of warfarin is bleeding that tends to be proportional to the intensity of anticoagulation and may be increased by the presence of risk factors such as severe hepatic or renal disease, alcoholism, drug interactions, trauma, malignancy, and known previous bleeding sites in the gastrointestinal tract. A study at Brigham and Women's Hospital demonstrated that the risk of bleeding increases as the PT increases. Of 130 cases of bleeding, 38 per cent were due to remediable lesions, half of which were occult before warfarin administration.[117]

Major life-threatening bleeding requires immediate treatment with enough cryoprecipitate or fresh frozen plasma (FFP, usually 2 units) to normalize the PT and achieve immediate hemostasis.[100] To treat less serious bleeding, vitamin K may be administered parenterally; a dose of 10 mg subcutaneously or intramuscularly will usually reverse the effects of warfarin in 6 to 12 hours. However, this approach will make the patient's condition relatively refractory to warfarin for up to 2 weeks, so that reinstitution of warfarin becomes more difficult.

Minor bleeding with a prolonged PT may merely require interruption of warfarin therapy, without administration of FFP, until the PT has returned to the therapeutic range. If bleeding occurs when the PT is within the therapeutic range, occult malignancy should be suspected and ruled out. Evaluation of patients with minor bleeding and a PT above the therapeutic range is less productive. A study at Boston City Hospital showed that changing from Coumadin to generic warfarin was associated with increased morbidity and increased expense owing to widely fluctuating PT levels.[118] Our practice is to prescribe Coumadin.

Warfarin-induced skin necrosis[119] is a rare but important complication that may be related to a warfarin-induced reduction of protein C. In patients suspected of protein C deficiency, warfarin should be initiated with a lower dose than usual (e.g., 5 mg daily), with full heparin anticoagulation maintained until warfarin's therapeutic effect is achieved.

The "purple toes syndrome" is another rare complication of warfarin that appears to be caused by cholesterol microembolization.[120] In this syndrome, crystals are released from ulcerated atherosclerotic plaques. It appears that warfarin may worsen cholesterol microembolic disease by interfering with the healing of ulcerated atherosclerotic plaques. Therefore, warfarin should be discontinued in patients in whom the purple toes syndrome or other evidence of cholesterol microembolization develops.

During pregnancy, heparin should be used instead of warfarin because warfarin is associated with a 10-fold higher rate of congenital anomalies.[121] The fetus is particularly susceptible to warfarin embryopathy during the sixth through twelfth week of gestation.[122] The main features are saddle nose, nasal hypoplasia, frontal bossing, short stature, stippled epiphyses, optic atrophy, cataracts, mental retardation, and flexion contractures. Intracranial bleeding may also lead to secondary central nervous system deformities. We never prescribe warfarin during any portion of a pregnancy. If pregnancy is diagnosed after the sixth week of gestation, we counsel the parents about the risks of warfarin embryopathy, which occurs in 25 to 30 per cent of fetuses exposed during this vulnerable period of gestation.[122]

Although it was thought that women taking warfarin postpartum could not breast feed, it is now evident that breast feeding can be undertaken safely. The level of warfarin in breast milk is so low (25 ng/ml)[123] that it cannot be detected in the baby's plasma.[123,124]

PROTHROMBIN TIME CONTROL. Most warfarin is administered in the outpatient setting. Until recently, we adjusted the dosage of warfarin on the basis of the plasma PT. When the laboratory telephoned us with PT results, we had to contact patients to either reassure them that their dosing regimen was appropriate or make dosage adjustments. We found that it was quite difficult to explain changes in anticoagulation dosing by telephone. We can now make in-office assessments of warfarin dosing with the Coumatrak (Dupont Co, Wilmington, DE), which provides the PT result in 2 minutes by use of a drop of whole blood obtained from a fingertip puncture.[125] Substantial saving of time has resulted, and patients have left the office with greater peace of mind and with a more accurate understanding of their warfarin dosing regimen. The Coumatrak has also been used at home by anticoagulated patients,[126] much like fingerstick glucose monitors in the management of diabetes mellitus.

THROMBOLYTIC THERAPY

(See also p. 1230 and 1785)

Streptokinase and Urokinase (First-Generation Agents)

Streptokinase (SK) and urokinase (UK) are proteins that indirectly (SK) or directly (UK) activate endogenous plasminogen to form plasmin, which actually lyses clot that has recently formed (Fig. 48–2). In almost all patients, a lytic state will rapidly develop with SK or UK. For SK, the standard regimen to treat PE is 250,000 IU over 30 minutes followed by 100,000 IU per hour for 24 hours. For UK, the standard dose is 4400 IU/kg (i.e., 2000 IU/lb/hr) over 10 minutes followed by 4400 IU/kg/hr (i.e., 2000 IU/lb/hr) for 12 to 24 hours. Although single-bolus therapy with UK has been proposed and appears promising,[127] experience with regimens such as 15,000 IU/kg over 10 minutes has been limited.[128]

Laboratory monitoring is directed toward verifying that the lytic state has been achieved, which is required for drug efficacy. In the presence of a lytic state, there is no need to titrate the dose. The lytic state can be verified by measuring increases in fibrin degradation products, thrombin time, whole blood euglobulin lysis time, PT, or PTT. Among patients with DVT who are treated with SK, an increase in the bleeding time may correlate with thrombolytic efficacy.[129] The most sensitive, widely available test is the thrombin time. Any one of these tests will suffice if the pretreatment value is normal and if a value obtained 4 or more hours after the initiation of fibrinolytic therapy is abnormal. In general, the dosage of the lytic agent can be doubled if a lytic state cannot be documented using standard regimens. Interestingly, the risk of bleeding from SK and UK has not been shown to correlate closely with any specific laboratory abnormality or with the dosage of the lytic agent.[130]

INDICATIONS AND CONTRAINDICATIONS. Whereas heparin acts primarily to prevent thrombus extension, thrombolytic agents promote dissolution of recently formed clots. Only three randomized trials comprising a total of 210 patients have compared SK or UK with heparin for PE treatment.[115,131,132]

In these trials, no reduction in mortality from PE was apparent with SK or UK, even though clots lysed more quickly when these agents were used. In two of the three studies, bleeding complications occurred more often after thrombolysis.[115,132] Increases in pulmonary capillary diffusing capacity and pulmonary capillary blood volume were demonstrated on 2-week and 1-year follow-up in patients treated with SK or UK as compared with heparin-treated patients.[133]

Many patients suspected of having PE receive heparin by continuous infusion while undergoing diagnostic evaluation. After a definitive diagnosis is established, the physician must decide whether to continue heparin anticoagulation or to interrupt heparin treatment for a course of thrombolytic therapy. For patients with venous thromboembolism, the benefit-to-risk ratio of thrombolytic agents is highest in those with massive PE; however, patients with moderate-sized or large emboli may also benefit from this treatment. Heparin should be discontinued several hours before thrombolytic therapy is initiated. Physical handling of the patient and arterial and venous punctures should be minimized because no thrombolytic agent can discriminate between "bad" clot due to PE and "good" clot required for normal hemostasis. Upon discontinuation of SK or UK, heparin should be given by continuous infusion without a loading dose when the thrombin time or

PTT decreases to approximately twice the control value. Contraindications to the use of SK or UK include intracranial or intraspinal disease, recent surgery, or trauma. However, we do not adhere to any upper age limit, and we do not consider the presence of cancer an exclusion criterion.

COMPLICATIONS. Trivial superficial oozing at venipuncture or arterial catheter insertion sites may be considered an index of drug efficacy rather than a complication of thrombolytic therapy. Such bleeding can be controlled with manual compression followed by a pressure dressing. In the UPET, severe bleeding, defined as the need for transfusion of more than 2 units of blood or a decrease in hematocrit of more than 10 points, occurred in 22 of the 82 (27 per cent) UK-treated patients in Phase I. The large amount of blood drawn during the first 24 hours of Phase I (about 200 ml) contributed to the fall in hematocrit; during Phase II,[134] fewer patients (12 per cent) had severe bleeding. In many instances, bleeding occurred at the vascular puncture sites for pulmonary angiography.

Of greatest concern is the risk of intracranial bleeding, which occurs in two to six of every 1000 patients treated with thrombolytic therapy. Retroperitoneal hemorrhage can also be life-threatening because the bleeding is often sustained and brisk, and the source often is difficult to locate. This complication can occur during the femoral catheterization if an artery is inadvertently punctured above the inguinal ligament. Genitourinary and other internal bleeding generally can be well managed; however, if internal bleeding is excessive, therapy should be discontinued. If bleeding is brisk or potentially life-threatening, 10 units of cryoprecipitate should be ordered from the blood bank. Each unit contains 200 to 500 mg of fibrinogen and 80 units of Factor VIII in a volume of 10 to 15 ml. A dose of 10 units will increase the fibrinogen level by about 70 mg/dl and the Factor VIII level by about 30 per cent of normally circulating levels. Cryoprecipitate can be thawed rapidly and should be available within 10 minutes of a request.

In addition, two units of fresh frozen plasma (FFP) should be ordered. FFP, which may take 45 minutes to thaw, is a source of Factors V and VIII as well as alpha $_2$-antiplasmin, fibrinogen, and other active coagulation factors.[100] Minor allergic reactions due to SK or (less often) UK occur occasionally and are manifested by fever and chills. To suppress this reaction, steroids, diphenhydramine (Benadryl), and acetaminophen can be administered prophylactically. If chills occur despite premedication, we have found 50 to 100 mg of intravenous meperidine to be quite effective in suppressing them.

Tissue Plasminogen Activator (t-PA)

(See also p. 1231)

In experimental canine and rabbit models of venous thrombosis, t-PA caused more fibrin-specific thrombolysis and less hemorrhage than did either UK or SK.[135] These experiments have served as the basis for clinical use of t-PA in patients with venous thromboembolism. Its use in acute PE was first reported in a 63-year-old man with massive PE (documented angiographically) who had undergone renal transplantation 5 weeks before t-PA treatment[136]; 30 mg (0.5 mg/kg) of t-PA was infused over 90 minutes through a catheter inserted into the right ventricle. The patient, who had been moribund, recovered dramatically.

In the authors' initial investigation, the short-term efficacy and safety of acutely administered t-PA in acute PE[137,138] were studied. Of 47 patients with angiographically documented PE, 44 had significant clot lysis after 2 to 6 hours of t-PA administered through a peripheral vein. Average pulmonary artery pressures decreased significantly after t-PA therapy, and lung scanning indicated marked improvement in pulmonary perfusion after treatment.[139] In some patients, right ventricular dysfunction and tricuspid regurgitation were documented by Doppler echocardiography before treatment but resolved rapidly after t-PA therapy.[140] In the authors' second PE Trial, the infusion time for t-PA was compressed from 6 to 2 hours. Patients were randomized to a fixed dose of t-PA (100 mg/2 h) or an FDA-approved 24-hour dose of weight-adjusted urokinase. t-PA achieved clot lysis more rapidly (Fig. 48–13*A* and Fig. 48–13*B*) and was safer.[141]

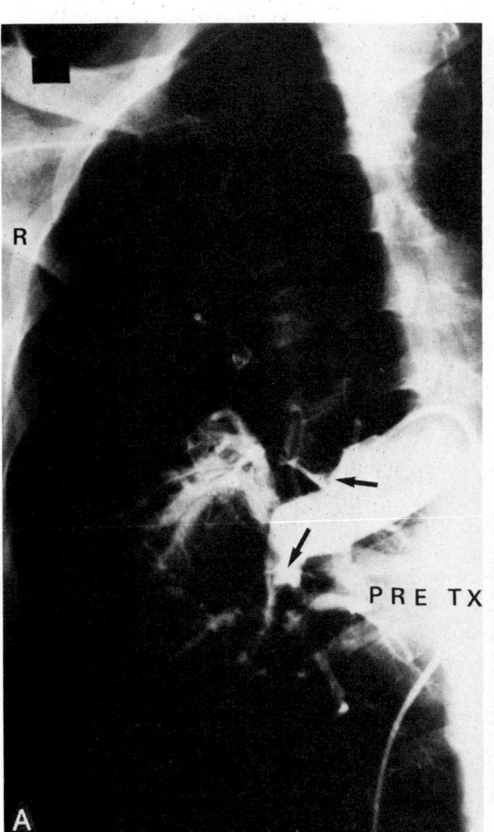

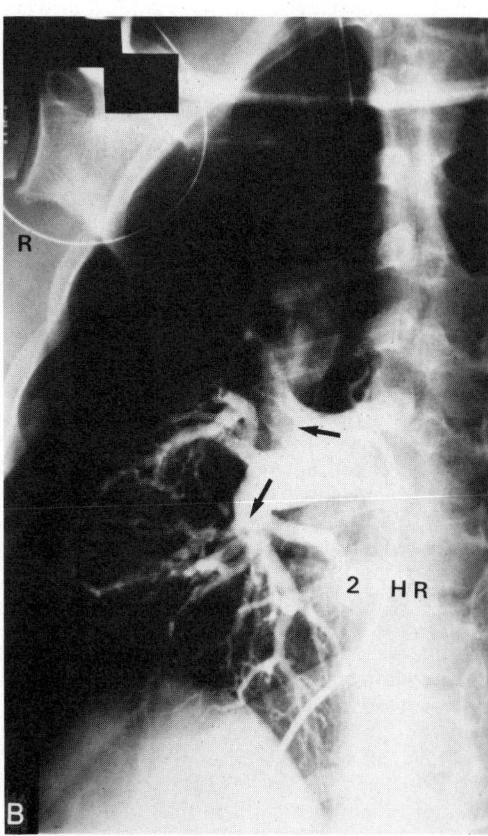

FIGURE 48–13. ***A,*** **Baseline right lung pulmonary angiogram in a 58-year-old man with a 5-day history of dyspnea. Intraluminal clot is visualized in the right upper and lower lobe arteries (arrows) before treatment. The pulmonary artery pressure was 118/40 mm Hg with a mean PA pressure of 65 mm Hg.** ***B,*** **Follow-up pulmonary angiogram demonstrates moderate clot lysis immediately after a 2-hour course of peripheral intravenous t-PA administered in a dose of 100 mg as a continuous infusion. The pulmonary artery pressure is now 53/19 with a mean PA pressure of 34 mm Hg. There has been no change in the systemic arterial pressure. (From Goldhaber, S. Z., Kessler, C. M., Heit, J., et al.: A randomized controlled trial of recombinant tissue plasminogen activator versus urokinase in the treatment of acute pulmonary embolism. Lancet** ***2:*****293, 1988.)**

Recently, Levine et al. published the results of a clinical trial[142] suggesting that weight-adjusted bolus t-PA (0.6 mg/kg ideal body weight with a maximum dose of 50 mg), administered over 2 minutes, can achieve comparable efficacy (assessed by pulmonary reperfusion on pre- and post-treatment perfusion lung scans) to the efficacy we achieved in our prior t-PA vs. urokinase trial[137] and to the pulmonary reperfusion observed in UPET.[115] No major bleeding episodes occurred with bolus t-PA, and there was an approximate one-third decrease from the baseline fibrinogen level at 30 minutes. The theory supporting bolus t-PA as safer than a prolonged infusion is that the bolus is cleared rapidly, thus preventing large amounts of circulating t-PA from interacting with the fibrinogen degradation products (FDPs) of the PE being lysed and therefore limiting the potential of the FDPs to promote fibrinogenolysis.[143–145] Other investigators have studied bolus t-PA in a rabbit jugular vein thrombosis model[146] and in a canine model of PE.[147–149]

Clozel et al.[146] found that the extent of thrombolysis was similar regardless of whether the same dose of t-PA was administered as a bolus or as a continuous 4-hour infusion. Prewitt's group found that the rate of thrombolysis is markedly increased with a 15-minute t-PA infusion compared with a 90-minute infusion, although the total clot lysis was similar in both sets of dogs.[147] However, they found in a subsequent study that a 15-minute t-PA infusion caused more thrombolysis than a 5-minute infusion.[148] This latter study suggests an upper limit to the dose-thrombolytic rate relation with t-PA. In an even more recent study,[149] Prewitt et al. found that a 15-minute infusion of 2 mg/kg of t-PA did not cause significantly more clot lysis than a 15-minute infusion of 1 mg/kg of t-PA. Thus, a bolus of t-PA appears to be a very promising treatment strategy for patients with PE. However, its safety and efficacy have not been tested in a randomized trial against the FDA-approved 100 mg/2 hr regimen of t-PA.

ANTICOAGULATION VS. THROMBOLYTIC THERAPY

Standard therapy for PE has employed heparin anticoagulation followed by warfarin, without thrombolytic therapy. The rationale for anticoagulation therapy is to provide prophylaxis against additional thromboembolic events while natural fibrinolytic mechanisms gradually lyse the previously formed pulmonary artery clot(s). In contrast, the rationale for thrombolytic therapy (followed by anticoagulation) is that thrombolysis actively dissolves clot that has already formed, thereby restoring cardiopulmonary function to normal as quickly as possible.[149a] Thrombolysis relieves the obstruction to pulmonary artery blood flow and thus improves right ventricular function and pulmonary perfusion and reduces pulmonary artery pressures. Lytic therapy may also improve pulmonary function over the long term,[133] may help prevent the development of chronic pulmonary hypertension, and may reduce the source of embolus in the peripheral venous system as well as in the pulmonary artery, thereby preventing recurrent PE.

For patients with major PE who are treated with anticoagulants alone, pulmonary artery clot may fail to resolve in 75 per cent after 1 to 4 weeks[150] and in 50 per cent after 4 months[151] of follow-up. In the UPET, the UK-treated patients initially exhibited significantly greater hemodynamic and anatomical improvement than the heparin-treated patients. However, 7 days after treatment, no difference between the two groups could be demonstrated on lung scans.[115] Unfortunately, no large-scale trial has yet been undertaken to determine whether thrombolytic therapy can reduce the mortality and recurrent PE rate compared with standard heparin treatment.

Although the Food and Drug Administration approved 24-hour SK and 12- to 24-hour UK in 1977 to treat PE, these agents are used only rarely for this condition, probably because of fear of bleeding complications. t-PA (100 mg/2 h) was approved by the FDA in 1990 for use in PE. In 1980, an NIH Consensus Development Conference[152] concluded that thrombolytic therapy was not being utilized often enough for patients with PE who (1) had obstruction of blood flow to a lobe or multiple pulmonary segments or (2) were hemodynamically compromised, regardless of the anatomical size of the PE.[152a] Nevertheless, use of thrombolytic therapy for PE has continued to languish. As of this writing, outside of a research setting, we advocate utilization of thrombolytic therapy according to these NIH guidelines.

ADJUNCTIVE MEDICAL THERAPY

Although the cornerstone of PE treatment involves anticoagulation or thrombolysis, adjunctive measures are also useful. Hypoxia should be treated with supplemental oxygen. In most cases, two to four liters of oxygen via nasal prongs will suffice, but the threshold for intubation and ventilatory support should be low. Right heart failure due to PE should be treated with alpha-range dopamine to alleviate hypotension, dobutamine to increase the cardiac index and stroke index,[153] and possibly amrinone[154] because of its vasodilatory and inotropic properties.

Discomfort due to PE can be intense and can cause chest wall splinting, making the patient susceptible to pneumonia and increased hypoxia owing to poor ventilation. Therefore, pain should be controlled aggressively, with either narcotic analgesia or nonsteroidal antiinflammatory agents. Despite the theoretical concern that nonsteroidal antiinflammatory agents might affect platelet function adversely and predispose to bleeding during anticoagulant or thrombolytic therapy, we use tnese antiinflammatory drugs liberally and find that they are often more effective than narcotics, presumably because the pleuritic pain of PE is due to inflammation. Fever often accompanies PE and not only should be suppressed with acetaminophen but also should lead to a search for accompanying infection, particularly pneumonia.

INFERIOR VENA CAVAL (IVC) INTERRUPTION

INDICATIONS. Most IVC interruption is undertaken with IVC filters, which normally can be inserted percutaneously by an interventional angiographer (Table 48–7). IVC ligation or external clips placed at laparotomy are rarely utilized. However, no randomized clinical trial has compared medical therapy with IVC interruption nor has any study been done to compare the different modes of IVC interruption (i.e., ligation, external clips, filters).[155,156] Certain disadvantages of IVC in-

TABLE 48–7 PERCUTANEOUS INSERTION OF INFERIOR VENAL CAVAL FILTERS

INDICATIONS
1. Anticoagulation contraindicated in patients with known pulmonary emboli:
a. Bleeding, or known risk of bleeding (e.g., gastrointestinal)
b. Patients with complications of anticoagulation (e.g., hemorrhage, heparin-induced thrombocytopenia)
2. Anticoagulation failure despite adequate therapy (e.g., recurrent pulmonary embolism)
3. Prophylactic for high-risk patients:
a. Extensive or progressive deep vein thrombophlebitis
b. Following surgical pulmonary embolectomy
c. Severe pulmonary hypertension; cor pulmonale
CONTRAINDICATIONS (i.e., SURGICAL VENOTOMY PREFERRED)
1. Severe coagulopathy, predisposing to bleeding from the puncture site
2. Anticipated patient noncompliance with post-procedure rest orders (especially with a 24-French filter system)
3. Obstructing thrombus along the available route(s) of insertion

From Goldhaber, S. Z., and Grassi, C. J.: Management of pulmonary embolism. *In* Sabiston, D. C., Jr.: Textbook of Surgery. 14th ed. Philadelphia, W. B. Saunders Company. Update No. 8, pp. 115–127, 1990.

terruption devices should be recognized. First, anticoagulation should be continued whenever possible as adjunctive therapy to help prevent thrombosis at the site of the device and to help prevent limb DVT. Second, if the device becomes occluded with thrombus, large paravertebral venous collateral channels may develop and permit recurrent embolization. Third, it is unknown whether the currently employed interruption devices will cause long-term complications (i.e., perforation or migration). All other implanted devices, whether they be heart valves, pacemakers, or artificial hips, have a lifespan beyond which they require replacement or revision. Therefore, indications for IVC interruption in relatively young patients should be particularly stringent.

LIGATION. There are two possible indications for complete ligation of the inferior vena cava. One is septic embolization, since these emboli are usually small and would pass through all contemporary devices that maintain partial caval patency. In the presence of intravascular sepsis, no foreign material should be placed in the inferior vena cava. However, small emboli should theoretically have little difficulty traversing the collateral circulation around the ligated vessel, and patients with septic pelvic thrombophlebitis can almost always be treated successfully with heparin anticoagulation and antibiotics alone.[157] The second possible use of ligation is the rare case of documented or potential paradoxical embolization[44] because of the devastating neurological effects of even a small paradoxical embolus.

TABLE 48-8 THE "IDEAL" VENA CAVAL FILTER

1. Biocompatible, nonthrombogenic construction
2. High filtering efficiency (large and small emboli)
3. Does not impede flow (e.g., paraxial flow)
4. Rapid percutaneous insertion
   (a) Small caliber
   (b) Release mechanism sample and controlled
   (c) Amenable to repositioning
5. Secure fixation within the vena cava
6. Retrievability

From Goldhaber, S. Z., and Grassi, C. J.: Management of pulmonary embolism. *In* Sabiston, D. C., Jr.: Textbook of Surgery. 14th ed. Philadelphia, W. B. Saunders Company. Update No. 8, pp. 115–127, 1990.

EXTERNAL CLIPS. If a laparotomy is performed, the external clip, such as the Adams-DeWeese device, is preferred to ligation because of its fewer hemodynamic and venous complications and the low frequency of recurrent pulmonary embolization.[158]

TRANSVENOUS DEVICES (Fig. 48–14). Currently, no single type of filter device is ideal (Table 48–8). The Mobin-Uddin filter was used commonly from 1969 to 1977 but is no longer available in the United States. Although the recurrent

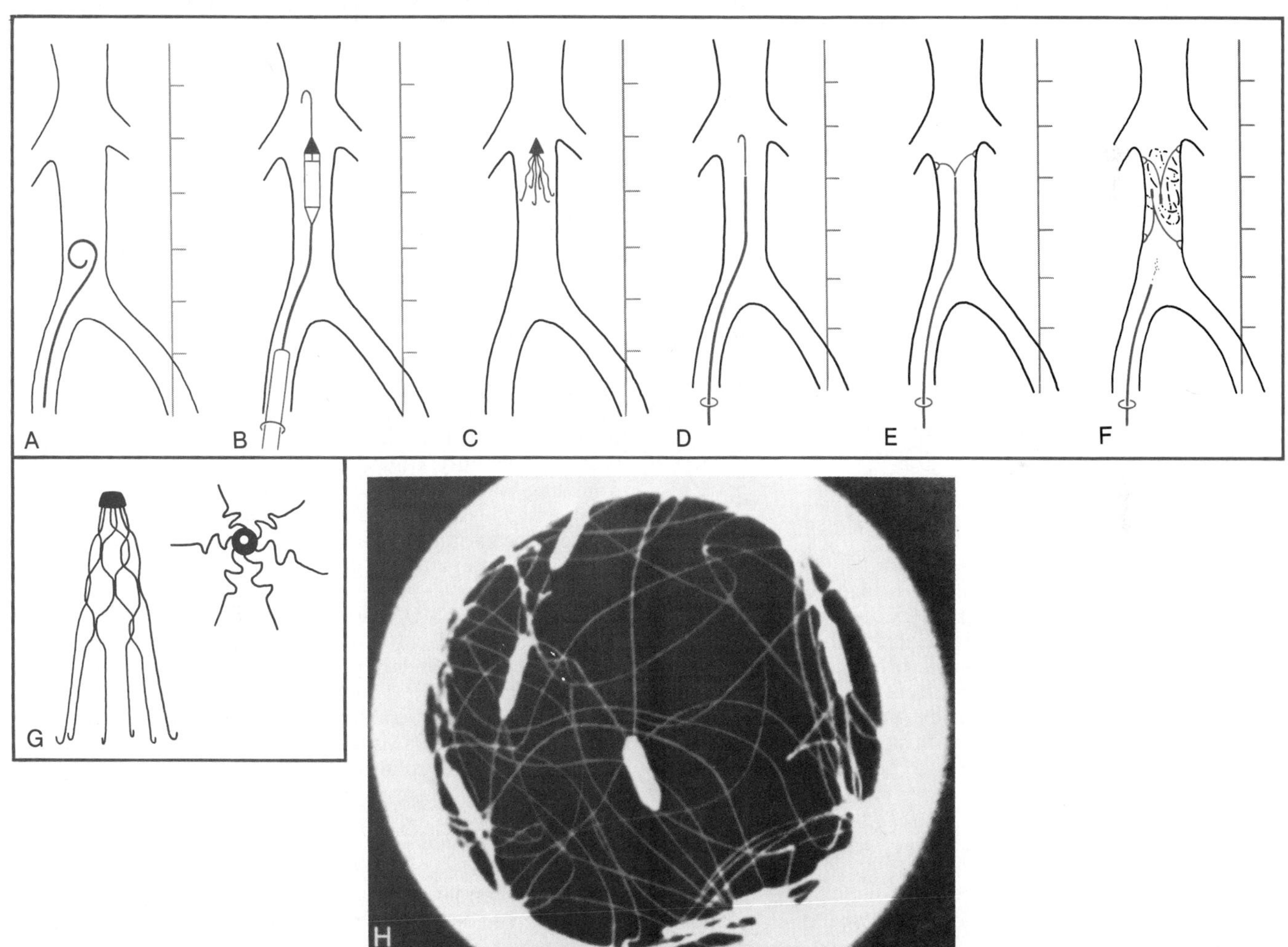

FIGURE 48–14. **Technique for insertion of inferior vena caval filters. *A,* After the vena cavagram is completed with the pigtail catheter, *B,* the filter-introducer system is positioned. *C,* The stainless steel Greenfield filter is released just inferior to the renal veins; alternatively, the following procedure is undertaken if a Bird's Nest filter is preferred to a Greenfield filter. *D,* Following the cavagram, the free-form filter system is inserted over a guidewire, *E,* the Bird's Nest filter is positioned and fixation is started, and, *F,* the mesh is reformed below the renal veins, detached, and the introducer is withdrawn. *G,* Greenfield filter lateral (left hand panel) and axial (right hand panel) views. This device consists of six 0.15 inch stainless steel wires in a conical shape extending from a central hub. These wires form a cone with a maximal apical angle of 35 degrees, and the tips form a circular base with a maximum diameter of 30 mm. At the inferior ends, hooks engage the vena caval wall and prevent filter migration, with the filter apex directed cephalad. *H,* Bird's Nest filter in the axial view demonstrating the mesh-like shape. The filter wire mesh consists of a set of four 25 cm long 0.018 inch stainless steel wires which have preshaped random bends. These are fixed to proximal and distal V-struts, which affix the mesh to the vena caval wall. (From Goldhaber, S. Z., and Grassi, C. J.: Management of pulmonary embolism. *In* Sabiston, D. C., Jr.: Textbook of Surgery. 14th ed. Philadelphia, W.B. Saunders Company. Update No. 8, pp. 115–127, 1990.)**

PE rate was low (0.5 per cent),[159,160] the frequency of IVC occlusion was high, up to 60 per cent. The Adams-DeWeese Teflon vena caval clip is available and is designed to narrow the IVC to four serrated transverse slits, 3 to 5 mm in diameter. However, it is rarely used at this time.

The Greenfield filter (GF) (Medi-Tech, Watertown, MA) (Fig. 48-14*G*), constructed of stainless steel, permits filling of 70 per cent of the filter cone by thrombus with a reduction in its effective cross-sectional area of only 50 per cent.[161,162] With the increased popularity of transfemoral radiological placement and a reported 10 to 24 per cent incidence of clinically symptomatic femoral vein thrombosis,[163,164] the main disadvantage of the GF has been its large 24 French introducer-sheath. Other complications include penetration of the vena caval wall by the filter foot prongs, filter tilting within the vena cava, retroperitoneal hemorrhage, and IVC occlusion in 3 to 5 per cent of cases.[162,164] The frequency of clinically evident recurrent PE averages 2 to 3 per cent.[162,165]

The Gianturco-Roehm Bird's Nest filter (BNF), in clinical trials since 1982 (Cook, Inc., Bloomington, IN), has a small sheath size, 12 French, with an 11 French preloaded filter catheter, thus avoiding the necessity of handling the filter.[166] After the formation of the filter, the wires resemble the shape of a bird's nest (Fig. 48-14*H*). The BNF design has several advantages over the GF. The introducer-sheath is significantly smaller; the freeform mesh of the filtration wire does not suffer from the requirements of centering within the vena caval lumen; and the BNF can accommodate IVCs up to 40 mm in diameter. The reported rate of recurrent PE is 2.7 per cent and the rate of IVC occlusion is 2.9 per cent.[166] At Brigham and Women's Hospital, we now routinely use the BNF instead of the GF.

Utilization of IVC Filters

Patients for whom IVC interruption is recommended are selected carefully (Table 48-7). We advise interruption (almost always with a percutaneously inserted Bird's Nest filter) when a patient with PE cannot tolerate anticoagulation or when adequate anticoagulation does not prevent recurrent PE. However, we usually do not employ these devices prophylactically in patients who have sustained a single large pulmonary embolus that is responding clinically to thrombolysis or anticoagulation.

PULMONARY EMBOLECTOMY

Pulmonary embolectomy can be utilized to treat PE in two different clinical settings: (1) during acute PE in the critically ill patient (i.e., when PE is associated with shock), and (2) to treat disabling dyspnea in patients with chronic pulmonary hypertension due to occult or recurrent PE. In patients with persistent right ventricular failure despite embolectomy, pulmonary artery counterpulsation with a balloon pump may be useful.[167]

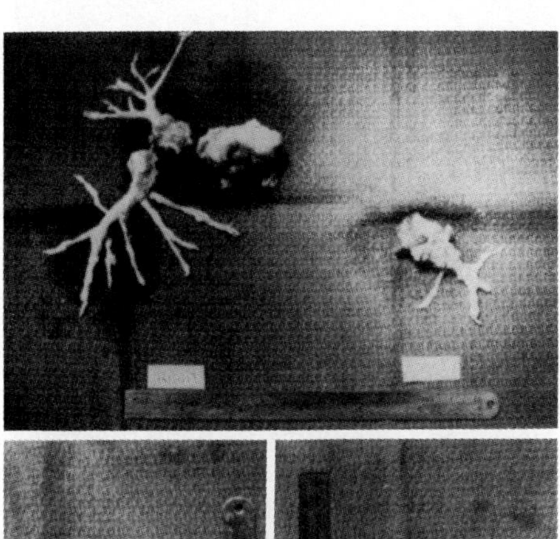

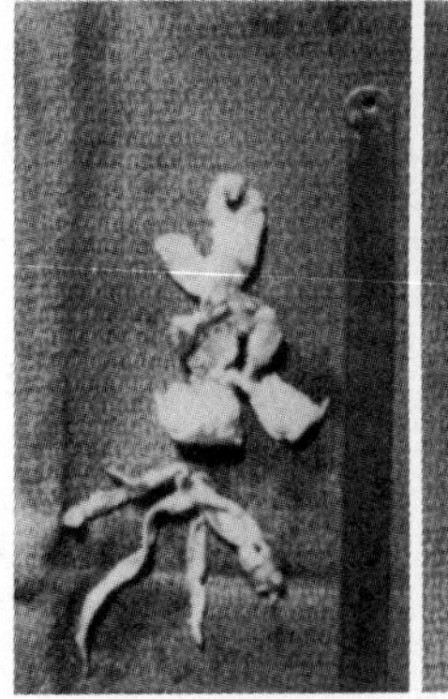

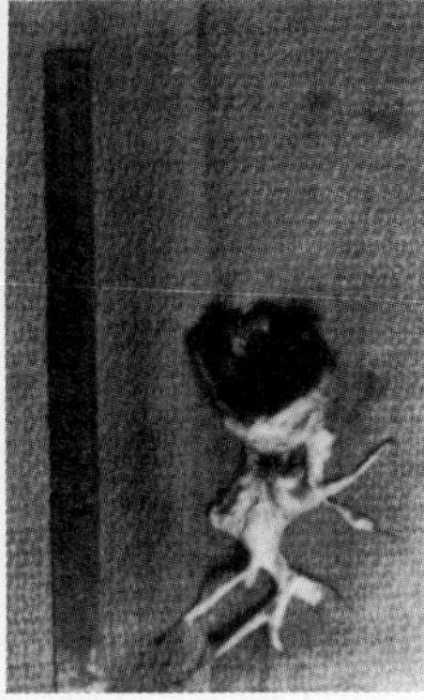

FIGURE 48-15. Large segments of chronic organized clot that were removed from the pulmonary arteries of two patients with excellent results (i.e., they improved from New York Heart Association functional class IV to I). Both patients had had complete obstruction of one pulmonary artery and partial obstruction of the other. (From Utley, J. R.: Pulmonary thromboendarterectomy. *In* Goldhaber, S. Z. (ed.): Pulmonary Embolism and Deep Venous Thrombosis. Philadelphia, W. B. Saunders Company, 1985, p. 278.)

ACUTE PE. Open pulmonary embolectomy[168] is associated with a mortality of approximately 30 per cent and normally should be reserved for patients in extremis in whom thrombolytic therapy is contraindicated or is failing. Embolectomy should also be considered in patients with massive PE due to right atrial or right ventricular thrombus in whom an inferior vena caval filter would be useless, particularly when thrombolytic agents fail to lyse these sources of PE. *Transvenous pulmonary embolectomy* with catheter suction is a promising approach[169,170] that requires further research and development. Another innovative approach involves mechanical fragmentation of PE with a flexible rotating tip catheter.[171] This latter strategy has not been applied clinically as of this writing.

CHRONIC PULMONARY HYPERTENSION (see also p. 790). Recurrent PE can lead to chronic, persistent pulmonary artery clot with attendant pulmonary hypertension, dyspnea, and cor pulmonale.[172] This major complication occurs most often when endogenous fibrinolysis fails and when the diagnosis of recurrent PE is initially overlooked and anticoagulation is withheld for months or even years. Although chronic

TABLE 48-9 AVERAGE HEMODYNAMIC VALUES IN 34 PATIENTS BEFORE AND IMMEDIATELY AFTER THROMBOENDARTERECTOMY AND AT FOLLOW-UP

	PREOPERATIVE	IMMEDIATELY POSTOPERATIVE	FOLLOW-UP*
Mean pulmonary artery pressure (mm Hg)	49	27	24
Mean pulmonary artery systolic press (mm Hg)	80	43	38
Cardiac output (L/min)	3.8	5.9	4.9
Pulmonary vascular resistance (dynes-sec-cm^{-5})	997	230	272

* Follow-up 3 months to 16 years after thromboendarterectomy.

Modified from Moser, K. M., Auger, W. R., and Fedullo, P. F.: Chronic major-vessel thromboembolic pulmonary hypertension. Circulation *81*:1735, 1990, by permission of the American Heart Association.

obstruction of the pulmonary arteries can occur despite prompt anticoagulation, it is probably less frequent when thrombolysis is employed. Chronic pulmonary hypertension due to PE is usually refractory to anticoagulants and thrombolytic agents but can sometimes be managed with pulmonary thromboendarterectomy.[173,174] Surgical success leads to a dramatic reduction in symptoms, with associated improvements noted on lung scanning and pulmonary angiography. Pulmonary thromboendarterectomy produces an early marked reduction of pulmonary hypertension, which is often sustained (Table 48–9). There is an early reduction in the size of the pulmonary artery, right ventricle, right atrium, and inferior vena cava with a normalization of the interventricular septal position. This suggests that some changes in cardiac geometry may be afterload dependent and reversible soon after marked afterload reduction.[175,176] The results of embolectomy tend to be most successful when an embolized thrombus can be removed in large segments that form a cast of the pulmonary vascular tree (Fig. 48–15). In the future, balloon angioplasty may be useful in treating some of these patients.[177]

INDICATIONS FOR PULMONARY EMBOLECTOMY. Despite progress in the technique of pulmonary embolectomy for PE, we regard this operation as a treatment of last resort. For acute massive PE, thrombolytic therapy should be attempted first unless there is an absolute contraindication to its use. For chronic PE, we would not recommend embolectomy unless progressive incapacity due to chronic pulmonary hypertension is well documented. The potential for postoperative rehabilitation must be good, and candidates must be willing to accept the risk of death or of failure to improve that accompanies this "high-stakes" operation.

Prevention of Pulmonary Embolism

RATIONALE

PE is difficult to diagnose, expensive to treat, and occasionally lethal despite therapy. Fortunately, a wide array of effective preventive techniques are available, including pharmacological, mechanical, and combined pharmacological and mechanical measures.[178] Until recently, these measures were widely underutilized. However, with the publication of the 1986 NIH Consensus Development Conference recommendations, the implementation of VTE prophylaxis has become mandatory, from a medicolegal viewpoint, among moderate- and high-risk hospitalized patients.[179] It appears that among postoperative patients, the risk of developing DVT persists after hospital discharge as well.[180] This problem is being addressed by use of prophylactic strategies, such as graduated compression stockings and low-dose warfarin, that are prescribed during the first month after hospital discharge.

PHARMACOLOGICAL AGENTS

LOW-DOSE HEPARIN. The most comprehensive randomized controlled trial of low-dose heparin (5000 units of subcutaneous heparin 2 hours preoperatively and every 8 hours thereafter for 7 days) as postoperative prophylaxis against fatal PE was organized by Kakkar in the International Multicentre Trial (IMT) involving 4121 patients.[181] Eligible patients were over age 40 and were scheduled to undergo elective major surgery. Of the autopsied subjects, 16 controls died of PE versus only two patients in the heparin group. Although more wound hematomas occurred among heparin-treated patients, the number of deaths due to hemorrhage was not increased among those who received heparin. Collins and colleagues have reviewed data from 78 randomized controlled trials with 15,598 patients that have confirmed the IMT result.[182] There was a 40 per cent reduction in nonfatal PE and 64 per cent reduction in fatal PE among heparin-treated patients. The heparin-treated patients also had about one-third as many instances of DVT as control patients, regardless of whether they had undergone general, urological, elective orthopedic, or traumatic orthopedic surgery. There was no significant difference in fatal hemorrhage between the heparin and control groups. Although excessive bleeding was more likely to occur among patients assigned to heparin therapy—especially those who underwent urological procedures—the absolute excess in bleeding was only about 2 per cent.

WARFARIN. In patients at high risk for DVT or PE, low- or moderate-dose warfarin may be appropriate. In a randomized trial at McMaster University, moderate-dose warfarin therapy (target PT of 16 to 18 seconds) reduced the frequency of DVT in patients who had undergone surgery for hip fractures.[185] We use warfarin routinely (in combination with intermittent pneumatic compression) for VTE prophylaxis among patients who undergo total hip replacement, total knee replacement, or osteotomy. Warfarin is initiated the evening before operating in a dose of 5 to 10 mg; 5 mg is given on the night of operation; the dose is then adjusted to achieve a target PT of 15 to 17 seconds. Warfarin is continued after discharge for approximately 1 month.

DEXTRAN. This glucose polymer impairs platelet function by causing decreased platelet aggregability. Dextran 40, with a mean molecular weight of 40,000 (known also as low molecular weight dextran), is approved for prophylaxis against venous thromboembolism. Potential adverse effects include anaphylaxis, volume overload, nephrotoxicity, and (ironically) bleeding. Dextran's efficacy appears comparable to that of low-dose heparin.[183–184] Its particular niche appears to be among patients who require pharmacological VTE prophylaxis but who are unable to receive heparin because of a bleeding problem or previous adverse reaction to heparin, such as heparin-associated thrombocytopenia.

LOW MOLECULAR WEIGHT HEPARIN (LMWH). LMWH, not yet commercially available, has three major potential advantages over unfractionated heparin: (1) a lower frequency of heparin-associated thrombocytopenia, (2) effective prophylaxis with administration only once daily, and (3) a greater efficacy than unfractionated heparin. In a double-blind British study comparing LMWH with unfractionated heparin among 295 patients undergoing elective major abdominal surgery, the rate of DVT as detected on leg scanning with ^{125}I-labeled fibrinogen was 2.5 per cent among those who received LMWH compared with 7.5 per cent among those who received unfractionated heparin ($p < 0.05$).[187] LMWH is also very effective in preventing DVT among patients undergoing elective hip surgery.[188]

ASPIRIN. An overview of antiplatelet trials in the prevention of VTE indicates that antiplatelet therapy is effective in reducing the frequency of DVT by about one-third and in reducing the frequency of PE by about two thirds.[186] However, this finding has not been established in randomized controlled trials of aspirin that focus specifically upon PE as a primary endpoint. Therefore, further data are needed before long-term aspirin prophylaxis can be considered standard therapy for prevention of PE.

MECHANICAL MEASURES

GRADED ELASTIC COMPRESSION STOCKINGS. The most popular type of graded elastic compression is called a TED (thromboembolism-deterrent) stocking. Pressure exerted by the TED stocking is graded: 18 mm Hg at the ankle, 14 mm Hg at midcalf, 8 mm Hg in the popliteal region, 10 mm Hg at the lower thigh, and 8 mm Hg at the upper thigh. Thigh-high TED stockings reduce the frequency of DVT in general surgery patients[189] and appear to be cost-effective as well.[190]

INTERMITTENT PNEUMATIC COMPRESSION (IPC). Intermittent pneumatic compression of the legs (Fig. 48–16) has become an increasingly popular nonpharmacological method for preventing postoperative DVT. IPC devices expel blood from the legs, and the mechanical force may enhance fibrinolytic activity. To test this latter hypothesis, patients undergoing general surgery were randomized either to specially designed intermittent compression devices applied to the *arms* or no prophylaxis. Postoperatively, the frequency of *leg* DVT was assessed with fibrinogen leg scanning. Leg DVT developed in 32 per cent of the control group compared with 14 per cent of the group treated with intermittent arm compression. The reduction of distant thrombosis suggests that an increase in fibrinolytic activity is caused by IPC.[191]

IPC may be even more effective in preventing DVT when graduated compression stockings are used simultaneously.[192] Among patients who have undergone total hip replacement, thigh-high IPC using a sequential compression device has proved efficacy in halving the rate of proximal DVT, from 27 per cent to 14 per cent.[193] IPC has also been proved to be cost-effective in preventing DVT among patients undergoing major orthopedic surgery.[194]

INFERIOR VENA CAVAL (IVC) INTERRUPTION. Interruption of the IVC should be used prophylactically as a preoperative measure only under exceptional circumstances. Patients must be at high risk for PE (e.g., recent prior PE) and must have a contraindication to pharmacological prophylaxis (e.g., active gastrointestinal bleeding, chemotherapy-induced

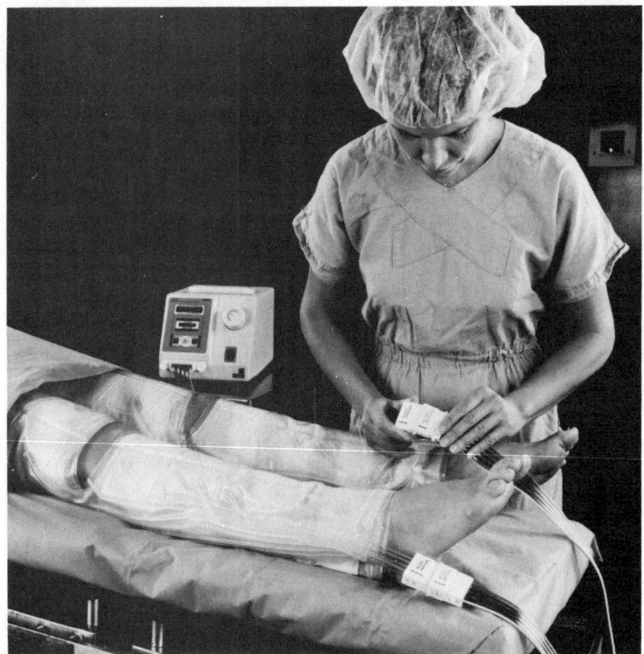

FIGURE 48–16. The Kendall Sequential Compression Device (SCD) expels blood from the legs, and its mechanical force may enhance fibrinolytic activity. The three compartments produce graded sequential compression of the ankles, calves, and thighs, with pressures of 35, 30, and 20 mm Hg, respectively, causing a 240 per cent increase in peak blood flow velocity.

thrombocytopenia, or neurosurgery) and to mechanical prophylaxis (e.g., recent DVT).

COMBINED MODALITIES. No prophylaxis strategy can abolish the risk of DVT. Therefore, combined modalities—especially combined pharmacological and mechanical measures—are useful in VTE prophylaxis, especially among high-risk patients. Among general surgical patients, the combination of heparin plus graduated compression stockings appears particularly effective both in individual trials[195] and in pooled overviews.[196] Among orthopedic surgical patients, the most frequently employed prophylaxis combination is IPC plus low- to moderate-dose warfarin.

RECOMMENDED APPROACH TO PROPHYLAXIS OF PULMONARY EMBOLISM

The NIH Consensus Development Conference on Prevention of Venous Thrombosis and PE has issued recommendations for many specific conditions.[179] Table 48–10 sets forth a general strategy for prevention of PE. However, the intensity of prophylaxis must be assessed separately for each patient on the basis of the patient's level of risk. Therefore, the particular recommendations in Table 48–10 are less important than the idea of providing VTE prophylaxis for every hospitalized patient at high or moderate risk.

SURGICAL PATIENTS

GENERAL SURGERY. Among patients over 40, the average frequency of DVT is 25 per cent based on fibrinogen leg scanning and 19 per cent based on venography in control patients who do not receive prophylaxis. Clinically significant PE occurs in approximately 1.6 per cent of the general surgical population.[179] The NIH Consensus statement recommends prophylaxis in all general surgical patients when any one of the following criteria apply:

- the patient is 40 years of age or older, *or*
- the patient will undergo a surgical procedure of more than 1 hour's duration, *or*
- the patient has cancer, *or*
- the patient has suffered prior PE or DVT

The recommended modality is heparin, 5000 units subcutaneously every 8 to 12 hours, beginning before operation and continuing at least until the patient is ambulatory. Alternative prophylactic modalities include dextran, IPC, and graded compression stockings. Our approach to prophylaxis consists of either graded compression stockings plus low-dose heparin *or* IPC (Table 48–10).

ORTHOPEDIC SURGERY. In hip surgery and knee reconstruction, DVT rates range from 45 to 70 per cent without prophylaxis. Among patients undergoing hip surgery or total knee replacement, the frequency of fatal PE is 1 to 3 per cent.[179,197] Our approach for lower extremity orthopedic surgery is to use both IPC and warfarin.

UROLOGICAL SURGERY. The overall risk of venous thromboembolism in urological surgery is 25 per cent, similar to that in general surgery. Open prostatectomy is associated with a rate of DVT of 40 per cent, whereas for transurethral prostatectomy the rate is 10 per cent.[179] For urological patients, we normally recommend IPC.

GYNECOLOGICAL SURGERY. The guidelines for prophylaxis in benign gynecological surgery are the same as for general surgery. However, patients with gynecological cancer should be considered at high risk for venous thromboembolism and may benefit from the combination of IPC plus warfarin.

NEUROSURGERY. The risk of PE and DVT in neurosurgical patients is similar to that in other surgical high-risk groups. For patients with intracranial or spinal cord lesions, even minor bleeding could have disastrous consequences. Therefore, IPC is recommended.

PREGNANCY. For pregnant women with prior VTE, we assess the level of risk and often attempt to avoid low-dose heparin because of its potential effect of bone demineralization. We recommend that pregnant women at high risk engage in 60 minutes per day of walking, biking, or swimming if feasi-

TABLE 48–10 STRATEGY FOR PE PROPHYLAXIS

CONDITION	STRATEGY
Orthopedic or gynecological cancer surgery	IPC plus low-dose Coumadin
General surgery for patients with prior VTE, cancer, or obesity	IPC *or* graded-compression stockings plus low-dose subcutaneous heparin
General or urological surgery (without prior VTE) or gynecologic surgery for benign condition	Graded-compression stockings plus low-dose subcutaneous heparin *or* IPC
Neurosurgery, eye surgery, or other surgery for patients in whom pharmacological prophylaxis is contraindicated	Graded-compression stockings ± IPC
Pregnancy with prior VTE	Antepartum: graded-compression stockings plus daily exercise program plus serial leg examinations *or* subcutaneous heparin Peripartum: intermittent pneumatic compression plus low-dose subcutaneous heparin Postpartum: Coumadin for 6 weeks
Medical conditions	Graded-compression stockings ± low-dose subcutaneous heparin *or* IPC

IPC = intermittent pneumatic compression; VTE = venous thromboembolism.

ble. We prescribe maternity-style graded compression stockings with high compression levels of 30 to 40 mm Hg. We have these women return for frequent follow-up evaluation during the pregnancy with emphasis on leg examination and ultrasonographic testing. For women who are at very high risk of VTE or who are unable to comply with an exercise program and frequent office visits, we prescribe prophylactic subcutaneous heparin.

MEDICAL PATIENTS

The general medical population has been the least studied group with regard to DVT. These patients are frequently immobilized for prolonged periods; those who have cancer are likely to be hypercoagulable. For patients with nonhemorrhagic stroke, we usually employ IPC; for other medical patients, such as those with chronic congestive heart failure, we usually prescribe graded compression stockings and/or low-dose heparin.

REFERENCES

PATHOPHYSIOLOGY OF PULMONARY EMBOLISM

1. Gillum, R. F.: Pulmonary embolism and thrombophlebitis in the United States, 1970–1985. Am. Heart J. *114*:1262, 1987.
2. Anderson, F. A., Jr., Wheeler, H. B., Goldberg, R. J., et al.: A population-based perspective of the incidence and case-fatality rates of venous thrombosis and pulmonary embolism: The Worcester DVT study. Arch. Intern. Med. *(in press)*.
3. Goldhaber, S. Z.: Pulmonary embolism death rates. Am. Heart J. *115*:1342, 1988.
4. Goldman, L., Sayson, R., Robbins, S., et al.: The value of the autopsy in three medical eras. N. Engl. J. Med. *308*:1000, 1983.

4a. Pulmonary Embolism. *In* Fowler, N. O.: Diagnosis of Heart Disease. New York, Springer-Verlag, 1991, pp. 283–291.

5. Virchow, R.: Gesammelte Abhandlungen zur Wissenschaftlichen Medizin. Frankfurt, Meidinger Sohn, 1856, p. 219.
6. Schafer, A. L.: The hypercoagulable states. Ann. Intern. Med. *102*:814, 1985.
7. Clouse, L. H., and Comp, P. C.: The regulation of hemostasis: The protein C system. N. Engl. J. Med. *314*:1298, 1986.
8. Stead, N. W., Bauer, K. A., Kinney, T. R., et al.: Venous thrombosis in a family with defective release of vascular plasminogen activator and elevated plasma factor VIII/von Willebrand's factor. Am. J. Med. *74*:33, 1983.
9. Pizzo, S. V., Fuchs, H. E., Doman, K. A., et al.: Release of tissue plasminogen activator and its fast-acting inhibitor in defective fibrinolysis. Arch. Intern. Med. *146*:188, 1986.
10. Branch, D. W., Scott, J. R., Kochenour, N. K., and Hershgold, E.: Obstetric complications associated with lupus anticoagulant. N. Engl. J. Med. *313*:1322, 1985.
11. Petri, M., Rheinschmidt, M., Whiting-O'Keefe, Q., et al.: The frequency of lupus anticoagulant in systemic lupus erythematosus. A study of 60 consecutive patients by activated partial thromboplastin time, Russell viper venom time, and anticardiolipin antibody level. Ann. Intern. Med. *106*:524, 1987.
12. Triplett, D. A., Brandt, J. T., Musgrave, K. A., and Orr, C. A.: The relationship between lupus anticoagulants and antibodies to phospholipid. JAMA *259*:550, 1988.
13. Alving, B. M., Barr, C. F., and Tang, D. B.: Correlation between lupus anticoagulants and anticardiolipin antibodies in patients with prolonged activated partial thromboplastin times. Am. J. Med. *88*:112, 1990.
14. Gladson, C. L., Scharrer, I., Hach, V., et al.: The frequency of type I heterozygous protein S and protein C deficiency in 141 unrelated young patients with venous thrombosis. Thromb. Haemost. *59*:18, 1988.
15. Goldhaber, S. Z., Savage, D. D., Garrison, R. J., et al.: Risk factors for pulmonary embolism: The Framingham Study. Am. J. Med. *74*:1023, 1983.
16. Gore, J. M., Appelbaum, J. S., Greene, H. L., et al.: Occult cancer in patients with acute pulmonary embolism. Ann. Intern. Med. *96*:556, 1982.
17. Goldberg, R. J., Seneff, M., Gore, J. M., et al.: Occult malignancy in patients with deep venous thrombosis. Arch. Intern. Med. *147*:251, 1987.
18. Goldhaber, S. Z., Buring, J. E., and Hennekens, C. H.: Cancer and venous thromboembolism. Arch. Intern. Med. *147*:216, 1987.
19. Dixon, J. E.: Pregnancies complicated by previous thromboembolic disease. Br. J. Hosp. Med. *37*:449, 1987.
20. Sachs, B. P., Brown, D.A.J., Driscoll, S. G., et al.: Maternal mortality in Massachusetts: Trends and prevention. N. Engl. J. Med. *316*:667, 1987.
21. Anderson, A. J., Krasnow, S. H., Boyer, M. W., et al.: Hickman catheter clots: A common occurrence despite daily heparin flushing. Cancer Treat. Rep. *71*:651, 1987.
22. Anderson, A. J., Krasnow, S. H., Boyer, M. W., et al.: Thrombosis: The major Hickman catheter complication in patients with solid tumor. Chest *95*:71, 1989.
23. Farfel, Z., Shecter, M., Vered, Z., et al.: Review of echocardiographically diagnosed right heart entrapment of pulmonary emboli-in-transit with emphasis on management. Am. Heart J. *113*:171, 1987.
24. Huisman, M. V., Buller, H. R., ten Cate, J. W., et al.: Unexpected high prevalence of silent pulmonary embolism in patients with deep venous thrombosis. Chest 95:498, 1989.
25. Doyle, D. J., Turpie, A.G.G., Hirsh, J., et al.: Adjusted subcutaneous heparin or continuous intravenous heparin in patients with acute deep vein thrombosis: A randomized trial. Ann. Intern. Med. *107*:441, 1987.
26. Lensing, A.W.A., Prandoni, P., Brandjes, D., et al.: Detection of deep-vein thrombosis by real-time B-mode ultrasonography. N. Engl. J. Med. *320*:342, 1989.
27. Polak, J. F., Cutler, S. S., and O'Leary, D. H.: Deep veins of the calf: Assessment with color Doppler flow imaging. Radiology *171*:481, 1989.
28. Hull, R. D., Hirsh, J., Carter, C. J., et al.: Diagnostic efficacy of impedance plethysmography for clinically suspected deep-vein thrombosis: A randomized trial. Ann. Intern. Med. *102*:21, 1985.
29. Huisman, M. V., Buller, H. R., ten Cate, J. W., and Vreeken, J.: Serial impedance plethysmography for suspected deep venous thrombosis in outpatients. The Amsterdam General Practitioner Study. N. Engl. J. Med. *314*:823, 1986.
30. Lagerstedt, C. I., Olsson, C. -G., Fagher, B. O., et al.: Need for long-term anticoagulant treatment in symptomatic calf-vein thrombosis. Lancet *2*:515, 1985.
31. Hull, R. D., Raskob, G. E., Hirsh, J., et al.: Continuous intravenous heparin compared with intermittent subcutaneous heparin in the initial treatment of proximal-vein thrombosis. N. Engl. J. Med. *315*:1109, 1986.
32. Strandness, D. E., Langlois, Y., Cramer, M., et al.: Long-term sequelae of acute venous thrombosis. JAMA *250*:1289, 1983.
33. Hyers, T. M., Hull, R. D., and Weg, J. G.: Antithrombotic therapy for venous thromboembolic disease. Chest *95*:37S, 1989.
34. Visner, M. S., Arentzen, C. E., O'Connor, M. D., et al.: Alterations in left ventricular three-dimensional dynamic geometry during acute right ventricular hypertension in the conscious dog. Circulation *67*:353, 1983.
35. Belenkie, I., Dani, R., Smith, E. R., and Tyberg, J. V.: Ventricular interaction during experimental acute pulmonary embolism. Circulation *78*:761, 1988.
36. Jardin, F., Dubourg, O., Gueret, P., et al.: Quantitative two-dimensional echocardiography in massive pulmonary embolism: Emphasis on ventricular interdependence and leftward septal displacement. J. Am. Coll. Cardiol. *10*:1201, 1987.
37. Manny, J., and Hechtman, H. B.: Vasoactive humoral factors. *In* Goldhaber, S. Z. (ed.): Pulmonary Embolism and Deep Venous Thrombosis. Philadelphia, W.B. Saunders Company, 1985, p. 283.

DIAGNOSIS OF PULMONARY EMBOLISM

38. Goldhaber, S. Z.: Strategies for diagnosis. *In* Goldhaber, S. Z. (ed.): Pulmonary Embolism and Deep Venous Thrombosis. Philadelphia, W.B. Saunders Company, 1985, p. 79.
39. Stein, P. D., Willis, P. W. III, and DeMets, D. L.: History and physical examination in acute pulmonary embolism in patients without preexisting cardiac or pulmonary disease. Am. J. Cardiol. *47*:218, 1981.
40. Rich, S., Levitsky, S., and Brundage, B. H.: Pulmonary hypertension from chronic pulmonary thromboembolism. Ann. Intern. Med. *108*:425, 1988.
41. Rich, S., Dantzker, D. R., Ayres, S. M., et al.: Primary pulmonary hypertension: A national prospective study. Ann. Intern. Med. *107*:216, 1987.
42. Newman, J. H., and Ross, J. D.: Primary pulmonary hypertension: A look at the future. J. Am. Coll. Cardiol. *14*:551, 1989.
43. Simpson, R. J., Jr., Podolak, R. P., Mangano, C. A., Jr., et al.: Vagal syncope during recurrent pulmonary embolism. J.A.M.A. *249*:390, 1983.
44. Loscalzo, J.: Paradoxical embolism: Clinical presentation, diagnostic strategies, and therapeutic options. Am. Heart J. *112*:141, 1986.
45. Lechat, P., Mas, J. L., Lascault, G., et al.: Prevalence of patent foramen ovale in patients with stroke. N. Engl. J. Med. *318*:1148, 1988.
46. Tsao, M. S., Schraufnagel, D., and Wang, N. -S.: Pathogenesis of pulmonary infarction. Am. J. Med. *72*:599, 1982.
47. Adler, D. S.: Nonthrombotic pulmonary embolism. *In* Goldhaber, S. Z. (ed.): Pulmonary Embolism and Deep Venous Thrombosis. Philadelphia, W.B. Saunders Company, 1985, p. 209.
48. Goldhaber, S. Z., Dricker, E., Buring, J. E., et al.: Clinical suspicion of autopsy-proven thrombotic and tumor pulmonary embolism in cancer patients. Am. Heart J. *114*:1432, 1987.
49. Sperry, K.: Amniotic fluid embolism: To understand an enigma. JAMA *255*:2183, 1986.
50. Cvitanic, O., and Marino, P. L.: Improved use of arterial blood gas analysis in suspected pulmonary embolism. Chest *95*:48, 1989.
51. Overton, D. T., and Bocka, J. J.: The alveolar-arterial oxygen gradient in patients with documented pulmonary embolism. Arch. Intern. Med. *148*:1617, 1988.
52. Bynum, L. J., and Wilson, J. E. III: Characteristics of pleural effusions associated with pulmonary embolism. Arch. Intern. Med. *136*:159, 1976.
53. Stein, P. D., Dalen, J. E., McIntyre, K. M., et al.: The electrocardiogram in acute pulmonary embolism. Prog. Cardiovasc. Dis. *17*:247, 1975.
54. Goldhaber, S. Z., Vaughan, D. E., Tumeh, S. S., and Loscalzo, J.: Utility of cross-linked fibrin degradation products in the diagnosis of pulmonary embolism. Am. Heart J. *116*:505, 1988.

55. Burki, N. K.: The dead space to tidal volume ratio in the diagnosis of pulmonary embolism. Am. Rev. Respir. Dis. *133*:679, 1986.
56. Markisz, J. A.: Radiologic and nuclear medicine diagnosis. *In* Goldhaber, S. Z. (ed.): Pulmonary Embolism and Deep Venous Thrombosis. Philadelphia, W.B. Saunders Company, 1985, p. 41.
57. Hampton, A. O., and Castleman, B.: Correlation of postmortem chest teleroentgenograms with autopsy findings with special reference to pulmonary embolism and infarction. A.J.R. *43*:305, 1940.
58. Woodruff, W. W. III, Hoeck, B. E., Chitwood, W. R., Jr., et al.: Radiographic findings in pulmonary hypertension from unresolved embolism. A.J.R. *144*:681, 1985.
58a. Kelley, M. A., Carson, J. L., Palevsky, H. I., and Schwartz, J. S.: Diagnosing pulmonary embolism: New facts and strategies. Ann. Intern. Med. *114*:300, 1991.
59. Hull, R. D., Raskob, G. E., Coates, G., and Panju, A. A.: Clinical validity of a normal perfusion lung scan in patients with suspected pulmonary embolism. Chest *97*:23, 1990.
60. Hull, R. D., Hirsh, J., Carter, C. J., et al.: Diagnostic value of ventilation-perfusion lung scanning in patients with suspected pulmonary embolism. Chest *88*:819, 1985.
61. The PIOPED Investigators: Value of the ventilation/perfusion scan in acute pulmonary embolism: Results of the prospective investigation of pulmonary embolism diagnosis (PIOPED). JAMA *263*:2753, 1990.
61a. Stein, P. D., Alavi, A., Gottschalk, A., et al.: Usefulness of noninvasive diagnostic tools for diagnosis of acute pulmonary embolism in patients with a normal chest radiograph. Am. J. Cardiol. *67*:1117, 1991.
62. Ryan, K. L., Fedullo, P. F., Davis, G. B., et al.: Perfusion scan findings understate the severity of angiographic and hemodynamic compromise in chronic thromboembolic pulmonary hypertension. Chest *93*:1180, 1988.
63. Kramer, F. L., Teitelbaum, G., and Merli, G. J.: Panvenography and pulmonary angiography in the diagnosis of deep venous thrombosis and pulmonary thromboembolism. Radiol. Clin. North Am. *24*:397, 1986.
64. Perlmutt, L. M., Braun, S. D., Newman, G. E., et al.: Pulmonary arteriography in the high-risk patient. Radiology *162*:187, 1987.
65. Wood, D. L., Osborn, M. J., Rooke, J., and Holmes, D. R.: Amiodarone pulmonary toxicity: Report of two cases associated with rapidly progressive fatal adult respiratory distress syndrome after pulmonary angiography. Mayo Clin. Proc. *60*:901, 1985.
66. Low osmolality contrast agents. Med. Lett. *31*:85, 1989.
67. Nicod, P., Peterson, K., Levine, M., et al.: Pulmonary angiography in severe chronic pulmonary hypertension. Ann. Intern. Med. *107*:565, 1987.
68. Meyerovitz, M.: How to maximize the safety of coronary and pulmonary angiography in patients receiving thrombolytic therapy. Chest *97*:132S, 1990.
69. Cassling, R. J., Lois, J. F., and Gomes, A. S.: Unusual pulmonary angiographic findings in suspected pulmonary embolism. A.J.R. *145*:995, 1985.
70. Walsh, P. N., Greenspan, R. H., Simon, M., et al.: An angiographic severity index for pulmonary embolism. Circulation *47*:II-101, 1973.
71. Miller, G.A.H., Sutton, G. C., Kerr, I.I.H., et al.: Comparison of streptokinase and heparin in treatment of isolated acute massive pulmonary embolism. Br. Med. J. *2*:681, 1971.
72. Simon, M., Sharma, G.V.R.K., and Sasahara, A.A.: An angiographic method for quantitating the severity of pulmonary embolism and the effects of therapy. Int. Angiol. *3*:389, 1984.
73. Kasper, W., Meinertz, T., Henkel, B., et al.: Echocardiographic findings in patients with proved pulmonary embolism. Am Heart J. *112*:1284, 1986.
74. Nixdorff, E., Erbel, R., Drexler, M., and Meyer, J.: Detection of thromboembolus of the right pulmonary artery by transesophageal two-dimensional echocardiography. Am. J. Cardiol. *61*:488, 1988.
75. Come, P. C.: Echocardiographic recognition of pulmonary arterial disease and determination of its cause. Am. J. Med. *84*:384, 1988.
76. Goldhaber, S. Z.: Optimal strategy for diagnosis and treatment of pulmonary embolism due to right atrial thrombus. Mayo Clin. Proc. *63*:1261, 1988.
77. Pond, G. D.: Pulmonary digital subtraction angiography. Radiol. Clin. North Am. *23*:243, 1985.
78. Mussett, D., Rosso, J., Petitprez, P., et al.: Acute pulmonary embolism: Diagnostic value of digital subtraction angiography. Radiology *166*:455, 1988.
79. Chintapalli, K., Thorsen, M. K., Olson, D. L., et al.: Computed tomography of pulmonary thromboembolism and infarction. J. Comput. Assist. Tomogr. *12*:553, 1988.
80. Balakrishnan, J., Meziane, M. A., Siegelman, S. S., and Fishman, E. K.: Pulmonary infarction: CT appearance with pathologic correlation. J. Comput. Assist. Tomogr. *13*:941, 1989.
81. Szucs, R. A., Rehr, R. B., and Tatum, J. L.: Pulmonary artery thrombus detection by magnetic resonance imaging. Chest *95*:232, 1989.
82. Posteraro, R. H., Sostman, H. D., Spritzer, C. E., and Herfkens, R. J.: Cine-gradient–refocused MR imaging of central pulmonary emboli. A.J.R. *152*:465, 1989.
83. Ezekowitz, M. D., Pope, C. F., Sostman, H. D., et al.: Indium-111 platelet scintigraphy for the diagnosis of acute venous thrombosis. Circulation *73*:668, 1986.
84. Clarke-Pearson, D. L., Coleman, R. E., Siegel, R., et al.: Indium-111 platelet imaging for the detection of deep venous thrombosis and pulmonary embolism in patients without symptoms after surgery. Surgery *98*:98, 1985.
85. Ezekowitz, M. D., Pope, C. F., and Smith, E. O.: Indium-111 platelet imaging. *In* Goldhaber, S. Z. (ed.): Pulmonary Embolism and Deep Venous Thrombosis. Philadelphia, W. B. Saunders Company, 1985, p. 261.
86. Farlow, D. C., Ezekowitz, M. D., Rao, S. R., et al.: Early image acquisition after administration of indium-111 platelets in clinically suspected deep venous thrombosis. Am. J. Cardiol. *64*:363, 1989.
87. Jung, M., Kletter, K., Dudczak, R., et al.: Deep vein thrombosis: Scintigraphic diagnosis with in-111-labeled monoclonal antifibrin antibodies. Radiology *173*:469, 1989.
88. Fry, E.T.A., Mack, D. L., Monge, J. C., et al.: Labeling of human clots in vitro with an active-site mutant of t-PA. J. Nucl. Med. *30*:187, 1990.
89. Shure, D., Gregoratos, G., and Moser, K. M.: Fiberoptic angioscopy: Role in the diagnosis of chronic pulmonary arterial obstruction. Ann. Intern. Med. *103*:844, 1985.

TREATMENT OF PULMONARY EMBOLISM

90. Barritt, D. W., and Jordan, S. C.: Anticoagulant drugs in the treatment of pulmonary embolism. A controlled trial. Lancet *1*:1309, 1960.
91. Basu, D., Gallus, A., Hirsh, J., and Cade, J.: A prospective study of the value of monitoring heparin treatment with the activated partial thromboplastin time. N. Engl. J. Med. *287*:324, 1972.
92. Wheeler, A. P., Jaquiss, R.D.B., and Newman, J. H.: Physician practices in the treatment of pulmonary embolism and deep venous thrombosis. Arch. Intern. Med. *148*:1321, 1988.
93. Beaver, B. L., Young, D., and Satiani, B.: Prediction of heparin requirements in acute thromboplastic venous disease. Arch. Surg. *120*:436, 1985.
94. Hirsh, J., van Aken, W. G., Gallus, A. S., et al.: Heparin kinetics in venous thrombosis and pulmonary embolism. Circulation *53*:691, 1976.
95. Ginsberg, J. S., Kowalchuk, G., Hirsh, J., et al.: Heparin therapy during pregnancy. Arch. Intern. Med. *149*:2233, 1989.
96. Brabeck, M. C.: Ambulatory management of thromboembolic disease during pregnancy with continuous infusion heparin. JAMA *257*:1790, 1987.
97. Barss, V. A., Schwartz, P. A., Greene, M. F., et al.: Use of the subcutaneous heparin pump during pregnancy. J. Reprod. Med. *30*:899, 1985.
98. Landefeld, C. S., Cook, E. F., Flatley, M., et al.: Identification and preliminary validation of predictors of major bleeding in hospitalized patients starting anticoagulant therapy. Am. J. Med. *82*:703, 1987.
99. Olin, J. W., Young, J. R., Graor, R. A., et al.: Treatment of deep vein thrombosis and pulmonary emboli in patients with primary and metastatic brain tumors. Arch. Intern. Med. *147*:2177, 1987.
100. Sane, D. C., Califf, R. M., Topol, E. J., et al.: Bleeding during thrombolytic therapy for acute myocardial infarction: Mechanisms and management. Ann. Intern. Med. *111*:1010, 1989.
101. Goldhaber, S. Z., Meyerovitz, M. F., Green, D., et al.: Randomized controlled trial of tissue plasminogen activator in proximal deep venous thrombosis. Am. J. Med. *88*:235, 1990.
102. Rao, A. K., White, G. C., Sherman, L., et al.: Low incidence of thrombocytopenia with porcine mucosal heparin. Arch. Intern. Med. *149*:1285, 1989.
103. Stead, R. B., Schafer, A. I., Rosenberg, R. D., et al.: Heterogeneity of heparin lots associated with thrombocytopenia and thromboembolism. Am. J. Med. *77*:185, 1984.
104. Rankin, J. A.: Heparin-induced thrombosis (white clot syndrome) secondary to prophylactic subcutaneous administration of heparin. Can. J. Surg. *31*:33, 1988.
105. Kelly, R. A., Gelfand, J. A., and Pincus, S. H.: Cutaneous necrosis caused by systemically administered heparin. JAMA *246*:1582, 1981.
106. Cimo, P. L., Moake, J. L., Weinger, R. S., et al.: Heparin-induced thrombocytopenia: Association with a platelet aggregating factor and arterial thromboses. Am. J. Hematol. *6*:125, 1976.
107. Squires, J. W., and Pinch, L. W.: Heparin-induced spinal fractures. JAMA *241*:2417, 1979.
108. de Swien, M., Ward, P. D., Fidler, J., et al.: Prolonged heparin therapy in pregnancy causes bone demineralization. Br. J. Obstet. Gynaecol. *90*:1129, 1983.
109. O'Kelly, R., Magee, F., and McKenna, T. J.: Routine heparin therapy inhibits adrenal aldosterone production. J. Clin. Endocrinol. Metab. *56*:108, 1983.
110. Phelps, K. R., Oh, M. S., and Carroll, H. J.: Heparin-induced hyperkalemia: Report of a case. Nephron *25*:254, 1980.
111. Leekey, D., Gantt, C., and Lim, V.: Heparin-induced hypoaldosteronism —Report of a case. JAMA *246*:2189, 1981.
112. Dukes, G. E., Sanders, S. W., Russo, J., et al.: Transaminase elevations in patients receiving bovine or porcine heparin. Ann. Intern. Med. *100*:646, 1984.
113. Gallus, A., Jackaman, J., Tillett, J., et al.: Safety and efficacy of warfarin started early after submassive venous thrombosis or pulmonary embolism. Lancet *2*:1293, 1986.
114. Hull, R. D., Raskob, G. E., Rosenbloom, D., et al.: Heparin for 5 days as compared with 10 days in the initial treatment of proximal venous thrombosis. N. Engl. J. Med. *322*:1260, 1990.
115. Urokinase Pulmonary Embolism Trial: A National Cooperative Study. Circulation *47* and *48*(Suppl. II):1, 1973.
116. Hull, R., Hirsh, J., Jay, R., et al.: Different intensities of oral anticoagulant therapy in the treatment of proximal-vein thrombosis. N. Engl. J. Med. *307*:1676, 1982.

117. Landefeld, C. S., Rosenblatt, M. W., and Goldman, L.: Bleeding in outpatients treated with warfarin: Relation to the prothrombin time and important remediable lesions. Am. J. Med. *87*:153, 1989.
118. Richton-Hewett, S., Foster, E., and Apstein, C. S.: Medical and economic consequences of a blinded oral anticoagulant brand change at a municipal hospital. Arch. Intern. Med. *148*:806, 1988.
119. Broekmans, A. W., Bertina, R. M., Leoliger, E. A., et al.: Protein C and the development of skin necrosis during anticoagulant therapy. Thromb. Haemost. *49*:251, 1983.
120. Hyman, B. T., Landas, S. K., Ashman, R. F., et al.: Warfarin-related purple toes syndrome and cholesterol microembolization. Am. J. Med. *82*:1233, 1987.
121. Hall, J. G., Pauli, R. M., and Wilson, K. M.: Maternal and fetal sequelae of anticoagulation during pregnancy. Am. J. Med. *68*:122, 1980.
122. Iturbe-Alessio, I., Fonseca, M.D.C., Mutchinik, O., et al.: Risks of anticoagulant therapy in pregnant women with artificial heart valves. N. Engl. J. Med. *315*:1390, 1986.
123. Orme, M.L'E., Lewis, P. J., de Swiet, M., et al.: May mothers given warfarin breast-feed their infants? Br. Med. J. *1*:1564, 1977.
124. McKenna, R., Cole, E. R., and Vasan, U.: Is warfarin sodium contraindicated in the lactating mother? J. Pediatr. *103*:325, 1983.
125. Lucas, F. V., Duncan, A., Jay, R., et al.: A novel whole blood capillary technic for measuring the prothrombin time. Am. J. Clin. Pathol. *88*:442, 1987.
126. Ansell, J., Holden, A., and Knapic, N.: Patient self-management of oral anticoagulation guided by capillary (fingerstick) whole blood prothrombin times. Arch. Intern. Med. *149*:2509, 1989.
127. Dickie, K. J., de Groot, W. J., Cooley, R. N., et al.: Hemodynamic effects of bolus infusion of urokinase in pulmonary thromboembolism. Am. Rev. Respir. Dis. *109*:48, 1974.
128. Petipretz, P., Simmoneau, G., Cerrina, J., et al.: Effects of a single bolus of urokinase in patients with life-threatening pulmonary embolism: A descriptive trial. Circulation *70*:861, 1984.
129. Hirsch, D. R., and Goldhaber, S. Z.: The bleeding time: Its potential utility among patients receiving thrombolytic therapy. Am. Heart J. *119*:158, 1990.
130. Stead, R. B.: Clinical pharmacology. *In* Goldhaber, S. Z. (ed.): Pulmonary Embolism and Deep Venous Thrombosis. Philadelphia, W. B. Saunders Company, 1985, p. 99.
131. Tibbutt, D. A., Davies, J. A., Anderson J. A., et al.: Comparison by controlled clinical trial of streptokinase and heparin in treatment of life-threatening pulmonary embolism. Br. Med. J. *1*:343, 1974.
132. Ly, B., Arnesen, H., Eie, H., and Hol, R.: A controlled clinical trial of streptokinase and heparin in the treatment of major pulmonary embolism. Acta Med. Scand. *203*:465, 1978.
133. Sharma, G.V.R.K., Burleson, V. A., and Sasahara, A. A.: Effect of thrombolytic therapy on pulmonary-capillary blood volume in patients with pulmonary embolism. N. Engl. J. Med. *303*:842, 1980.
134. Urokinase-Streptokinase Embolism Trial: Phase 2 results. A cooperative study. JAMA *229*:1606, 1974.
135. Agnelli, G., Buchanan, M. R., Fernandez, F., et al.: A comparison of the thrombolytic and hemorrhagic effects of tissue-type plasminogen activator and streptokinase in rabbits. Circulation *72*:178, 1985.
136. Bounameaux, H., Vermylen, J., and Collen, D.: Thrombolytic treatment with recombinant tissue-type plasminogen activator in a patient with massive pulmonary embolism. Ann. Intern. Med. *103*:64, 1985.
137. Goldhaber, S. Z., Vaughan, D. E., Markis, J. E., et al.: Acute pulmonary embolism treated with tissue plasminogen activator. Lancet *2*:886, 1986.
138. Goldhaber, S. Z., Meyerovitz, M. F., Markis, J. E., et al.: Thrombolytic therapy of acute pulmonary embolism: Current status and future potential. J. Am. Coll. Cardiol. *10*:96B, 1987.
139. Parker, J. A., Markis, J. E., Palla, A., et al.: Pulmonary perfusion after rt-PA therapy for acute embolism: Early improvement assessed with segmental perfusion scanning. Radiology *166*:441, 1988.
140. Come, P. C., Kim, C., Parker, J. A., et al: Early reversal of right ventricular dysfunction in patients with acute pulmonary embolism after treatment with intravenous tissue plasminogen activator. J. Am. Coll. Cardiol. *10*:971, 1987.
141. Goldhaber, S. Z., Kessler, C. M., Heit, J., et al.: A randomized controlled trial of recombinant tissue plasminogen activator versus urokinase in the treatment of acute pulmonary embolism. Lancet *2*:293, 1988.
142. Levine, M. N., Hirsh, J., Weitz, J., et al.: A randomized trial of a single bolus dosage regimen of recombinant tissue plasminogen activator in patients with acute pulmonary embolism. Chest *98*:1473, 1990.
143. Agnelli, G.: The rationale for bolus t-PA therapy to improve efficacy and safety. Chest *97*:161S, 1990.
144. Agnelli, G., Buchanan, M. R., Fernandez, F., et al: Sustained thrombolysis with DNA-recombinant tissue type plasminogen activator in rabbits. Blood *66*:399, 1985.
145. Agnelli, G., Buchanan, M. R., Fernandez, F., and Hirsh, J.: The thrombolytic and hemorrhagic effects of tissue type plasminogen activator: Influence of dosage regimens in rabbits. Thromb. Res. *40*:769, 1985.
146. Clozel, J-P., Tschopp, T., Luedin, E., and Holvoet, P.: Time course of thrombolysis induced by intravenous bolus or infusion of tissue plasminogen activator in a rabbit jugular vein thrombosis model. Circulation *79*:125, 1989.
147. Shiffman, F., Ducas, J., Hollett, P., et al.: Treatment of canine embolic pulmonary hypertension with recombinant tissue plasminogen activator: Efficacy of dosing regimes. Circulation *78*:214, 1988.
148. Prewitt, R. M., Shiffman, F., Greenberg, D., et al.: Recombinant tissue-type plasminogen activator in canine embolic pulmonary hypertension. Effects of bolus versus short-term administration on dynamics of thrombolysis and on pulmonary vascular pressure-flow characteristics. Circulation *79*:929, 1989.
149. Prewitt, R. M., Hoy, C., Kong, A., et al.: Thrombolytic therapy in canine pulmonary embolism. Comparative effects of urokinase and recombinant tissue plasminogen activator. Am. Rev. Respir. Dis. *141*:290, 1990.
149a. Goldhaber, S. Z.: Recent advances in the diagnosis and lytic therapy of pulmonary embolism. Chest *99*:1735, 1991.
150. Dalen, J. E., Banas, J. S., Brooks, H. L., et al.: Resolution rate of acute pulmonary embolism in man. N. Engl. J. Med. *280*:1194, 1969.
151. Tow, D. E., and Wagner, N. H., Jr.: Recovery of pulmonary artery flow in patients with pulmonary embolism. N. Engl. J. Med. *276*:1053, 1967.
152. Thrombolytic Therapy in Thrombosis: A National Institutes of Health Consensus Development Conference. Ann. Intern. Med. *93*:141, 1980.
152a. Mitchell, J. P., and Trulock, E. P.: Tissue plasminogen activator for pulmonary embolism resulting in shock: Two case reports and discussion of the literature. Am. J. Med. *90*:255, 1991.
153. Jardin, F., Genevray, B., Brun-Ney, D., and Margairaz, A.: Dobutamine: A hemodynamic evaluation in pulmonary embolism shock. Crit. Care Med. *13*:1009, 1985.
154. Spence, T. H., and Newton, W. D.: Pulmonary embolism: Improvement in hemodynamic function with amrinone therapy. South. Med. J. *82*:1267, 1989.
155. Grassi, C. J., and Goldhaber, S. Z.: Interruption of the inferior vena cava for prevention of pulmonary embolism: Transvenous filter devices. Herz *14*:182, 1989.
156. Goldhaber, S. Z., Buring, J. E., Lipnick, R. J., and Hennekens, C. H.: Interruption of the inferior vena cava by clip or filter. Am. J. Med. *76*:512, 1984.
157. Josey, W. E., and Staggers, S. R.: Heparin therapy in septic pelvic thrombophlebitis. A study of 46 cases. Am. J. Obstet. Gynecol. *120*:228, 1974.
158. Askew, A. R., and Gardner, A.M.N.: Long-term follow-up of partial caval occlusion by clip. Am. J. Surg. *140*:441, 1980.
159. Mobin-Uddin, K., Utley, J. R., and Bryant, L. R.: The inferior vena cava umbrella filter. Prog. Cardiovasc. Dis. *17*:391, 1975.
160. McIntyre, A. B., McCready, R. A., Hyde, G. L., and Mattingly, W.: A ten-year follow-up study of the Mobin-Uddin filter for vena cava interruption. Surg. Gynecol. Obstet. *158*:513, 1984.
161. Greenfield, L. J., and Michna, B. A.: Twelve-year clinical experience with the Greenfield vena caval filter. Surgery *104*:706, 1988.
162. Messmer, J. M., and Greenfield, L. J.: Greenfield caval filters: Long-term radiographic follow-up study. Radiology *156*:613, 1985.
163. Kantor, A., Glanz, S, Gordon, D. H., and Sclafani, S.J.A: Percutaneous insertion of the Kimray-Greenfield filter: Incidence of femoral vein thrombosis. A.J.R. *149*:1065, 1987.
164. Pais, S. O., Mirvis, S. E., and De Orchis, D. F.: Percutaneous insertion of the Kimray-Greenfield filter: Technical considerations and problems. Radiology *165*:377, 1987.
165. Geisinger, M. A., Zelch, M. G., and Risius, B.: Recurrent pulmonary emboli after Greenfield filter placement. Radiology *165*:383, 1987.
166. Roehm, J.O.F., Johnsrude, I. S., Barth, M. H., and Gianturco, C.: The Bird's Nest inferior vena cava filter: Progress report. Radiology *168*:745, 1988.
167. Gold, J. P., Shemin, R. J., DiSesa, V. J., et al.: Balloon pump support of the failing right heart. Clin. Cardiol. *8*:599, 1985.
168. Gray, H. H., Morgan, J. M., Paneth, M., and Miller, G.A.H.: Pulmonary embolectomy for acute massive pulmonary embolism: An analysis of 71 cases. Br. Heart J. *60*:196, 1988.
169. Moore, J. H., Jr., Koolpe, H. A., Carabasi, R. A., et al.: Transvenous catheter pulmonary embolectomy. Arch. Surg. *120*:1372, 1985.
170. Feitelberg, S. P., Kahn, S. E., Kotler, M. N., et al.: Transfemoral embolectomy for massive pulmonary embolus and associated myocardial infarction. Am. Heart J. *113*:819, 1987.
171. Stein, P. D., Sabbah, H. N., Basha, M. A., et al.: Mechanical fragmentation of pulmonary thromboemboli in dogs by means of a flexible rotating tip catheter (Kensey catheter). J. Am. Coll. Cardiol. *15*:189A, 1990.
172. Rich, S., Levitsky, S., and Brundage, B. H.: Pulmonary hypertension from chronic pulmonary thromboembolism. Ann. Intern. Med. *108*:425, 1988.
173. Chitwood, W. R., Jr., Lyerly, H. K., and Sabiston, D. C., Jr.,: Surgical management of chronic pulmonary embolism. Ann. Surg. *201*:11, 1985.
174. Moser, K. M., Daily, P. O., Peterson, K., et al.: Thromboendarterectomy for chronic, major-vessel thromboembolic pulmonary hypertension. Immediate and long-term results in 42 patients. Ann. Intern. Med. *107*:560, 1987.
175. Dittrich, H. C., Nicod, P. H., Chow, L. C., et al.: Early changes of right heart geometry after pulmonary thromboendarterectomy. J. Am. Coll. Cardiol. *11*:937, 1988.
176. Moser, K. M., Auger, W. R., Fedullo, P. F.: Chronic major-vessel thromboembolic pulmonary hypertension. Circulation *81*:1735, 1990.
177. Voorburg, J.A.I., Cats, V. M., Buis, B., and Bruschke, A.V.G.: Balloon angioplasty in treatment of pulmonary hypertension caused by pulmonary embolism. Chest *94*:1249. 1988.

PREVENTION OF PULMONARY EMBOLISM

178. Goldhaber, S. Z.: Venous thromboembolism: How to prevent a tragedy. Hospital Practice *23*:164, 1988.

179. NIH Consensus Development Statement. Prevention of venous thrombosis and pulmonary embolism. JAMA *256*:744, 1986.

180. Scurr, J. H., Coleridge-Smith, P. D., and Hasty, J. H.: Deep venous thrombosis: A continuous problem. Br. Med. J. *297*:28, 1988.

181. An International Multicentre Trial: Prevention of fatal postoperative pulmonary embolism by low doses of heparin. Lancet *2*:45, 1975.

182. Collins, R., Scrimgeour, A., Yusuf, S., and Peto, R.: Reduction in fatal pulmonary embolism and venous thrombosis by perioperative administration of subcutaneous heparin: Overview of results of randomized trials in general, orthopedic, and urologic surgery. N. Engl. J. Med. *318*:1162, 1988.

183. Bergqvist, D.: Dextran in the prophylaxis of deep-vein thrombosis. JAMA *258*:324, 1987.

184. Ljungstrom, K. G.: The antithrombotic efficacy of dextran. Acta Chir. Scand. *543*:26, 1988.

185. Powers, P. J., Gent, M., Jay, R. M., et al.: A randomized trial of less intense postoperative warfarin or aspirin therapy in the prevention of venous thromboembolism after surgery for a fractured hip. Arch. Intern. Med. *149*:771, 1989.

186. Anti-platelet Trialists Collaboration: Personal communication.

187. Kakkar, V. V.: Prevention of post-operative venous thromboembolism by a new low molecular weight heparin fraction. Nouv. Rev. Fr. Hematol. *26*:277, 1984.

188. Turpie, A.G.G., Levine, M. N., Hirsh, J., et al.: A randomized controlled trial of low-molecular-weight heparin (enoxaparin) to prevent deep-vein thrombosis in patients undergoing elective hip surgery. N. Engl. J. Med. *315*:925, 1986.

189. Allan, A., Williams, J. T., Bolton, J. P., and Le Quesne, L. P.: The use of graduated compression stockings in the prevention of postoperative deep vein thrombosis. Br. J. Surg. *70*:172, 1983.

190. Oster, G., Tuden, R. L., and Colditz, G. A.: Prevention of venous thromboembolism after general surgery. Cost-effectiveness analysis of alternative approaches to prophylaxis. Am. J. Med. *82*:889, 1987.

191. Knight, M.T.N., and Dawson, R.: Effect of intermittent compression of the arms on deep venous thrombosis in the legs. Lancet. *2*:1265, 1976.

192. Scurr, J. H., Coleridge-Smith, P. D., and Hasty, J. H.: Regimen for improved effectiveness of intermittent pneumatic compression in deep venous thrombosis prophylaxis. Surgery *102*:816, 1987.

193. Hull, R. D., Raskob, G. E., Gent, M., et al.: Effectiveness of intermittent pneumatic leg compression for preventing deep vein thrombosis after total hip replacement. JAMA *263*:2313, 1990.

194. Oster, G., Tuden, R. L., and Colditz, G. A.: A cost-effectiveness analysis of prophylaxis against deep-vein thrombosis in major orthopedic surgery. JAMA *257*:203, 1987.

195. Wille-Jorgensen, P., Thorup, J., Fischer, J. A., et al.: Heparin with and without graded compression stockings in the prevention of thromboembolic complications of major abdominal surgery: A randomized trial. Br. J. Surg. *72*:579, 1985.

PROPHYLAXIS

196. Colditz, G. A., Tuden, R. L., and Oster, G.: Rates of venous thrombosis after general surgery: Combined results of randomized clinical trials. Lancet *2*:143, 1986.

197. Foley, F., Maslack, M. M., Rothman, R. H., et al.: Pulmonary embolism after hip or knee replacement: Postoperative changes on pulmonary scintigrams in asymptomatic patients. Radiology *172*:481, 1989.

Cor Pulmonale

by E. REGIS McFADDEN, Jr., M.D., and EUGENE BRAUNWALD, M.D.

Chronic cor pulmonale is defined as a combination of hypertrophy and dilatation of the right ventricle (RV) secondary to pulmonary hypertension; the latter is caused by disease of the pulmonary parenchyma and/or pulmonary vascular system between the origins of the main pulmonary artery and the entry of the pulmonary veins into the left atrium.[1] *Acute cor pulmonale* is defined as acute right heart strain or overload resulting from the pulmonary hypertension that usually follows massive pulmonary embolism. Cor pulmonale encompasses many disease states with diverse etiologies, pathophysiological mechanisms, and clinical characteristics that have in common only a disturbance of the pulmonary circulation.[2] This chapter focuses on those conditions that produce pulmonary hypertension by acting primarily on the gas-exchanging, neuromuscular, and ventilatory control functions of the respiratory system. Primary pulmonary hypertension and pulmonary thromboembolism, two important causes of cor pulmonale, are discussed in Chaps. 27 and 49, respectively.

ANATOMICAL AND PATHOPHYSIOLOGICAL CORRELATES

RIGHT VENTRICULAR ANATOMY

For the first 3 months of life in infants born at or near sea level, the RV is larger and heavier and has a greater end-diastolic volume than the left.[3,7] With advancing age, the left ventricle (LV) becomes dominant, and in the adult, the right ventricular wall is relatively thin and has a crescentic configuration on cross section. However, in high-altitude dwellers, the situation is different. The degree of RV preponderance, both at birth and for the first 3 months of life, is greater than that seen in low-altitude residents, and the normal regression in size is so delayed that right ventricular enlargement can persist through the first decade.[6] In native adults living above 12,000 feet, 93 per cent of the hearts in a necropsy series showed some degree of right ventricular enlargement.[8] These morphological findings have a close relationship to the hemodynamic characteristics of persons at high altitudes and can be related to the degree of pulmonary arterial hypertension.[9]

Several methods may be used to ascertain the characteristics, presence, and severity of right ventricular hypertrophy; the two traditional methods involve the measurement of ventricular weight and wall thickness. Many investigators believe that wall thickness determinations are not sufficiently precise. Fulton et al. have provided weight criteria that are used widely.[10] In their technique, the RV is dissected free, and the septum is weighed together with the LV. Right ventricular weight can then be described in absolute terms or as a ratio of the LV plus the septum (S) [i.e., (LV + S)/RV]. Using these criteria, a heart is considered normal only if the total ventricular weight is less than 250 gm, the free wall of the RV weighs less than 65 gm in men and 50 gm in women, and the ratio of (LV + S)/RV is between 2.3 : 1 and 3.3 : 1. If left ventricular hypertrophy also is present, the ratio may be within normal limits or even raised. Using this method, Mitchell and colleagues found that the upper limits of normal (as defined by the mean plus 2 standard deviations) in men 40 or more years of age at death were 69 gm for the RV and 203 gm for the LV plus septum. These observers also noted that in their study, right ventricular thickness was a relatively poor index of hypertrophy.[11]

Others have determined muscle fiber size morphometrically and found the distribution of myocardial fiber diameters to be uniform, with a distinct bell-shaped distribution noted for the RV, LV, and septum.[12] In cases of pure RV hypertrophy, the distribution always shifted, so that the mean diameter of the muscle fibers from the RV exceeded that of the septum or normal LV. An example of an enlarged RV in cor pulmonale is shown in Figure 49–1.

RIGHT VENTRICULAR FUNCTION

Because RV hypertrophy occurs most commonly in association with longstanding elevations in pulmonary arterial pressures, an analogy often has been made between the LV in systemic hypertension and the RV in pulmonary hypertension. Because there is no fundamental difference in either the configuration or the pumping action of the two ventricles before birth, the differences that exist in the adult have been attributed to the flow resistances in the respective circula-

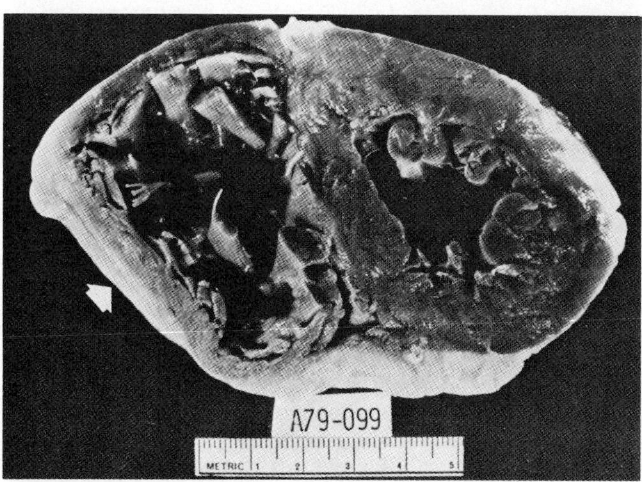

FIGURE 49–1. Cor pulmonale, heart cut in cross section. Notice the rounded contour of the right ventricular cavity (indicated by arrow), which is typical of dilation. The normal right ventricle is a crescent-shaped thin-walled structure. Both hypertrophy and dilatation of the right ventricle are present in this case. (From Taylor, W. E.: Pathology of pulmonary heart disease. *In* Rubin, L. J. [ed.]: Pulmonary Heart Disease. Boston, Martinus Nijhoff, 1984, p. 65.)

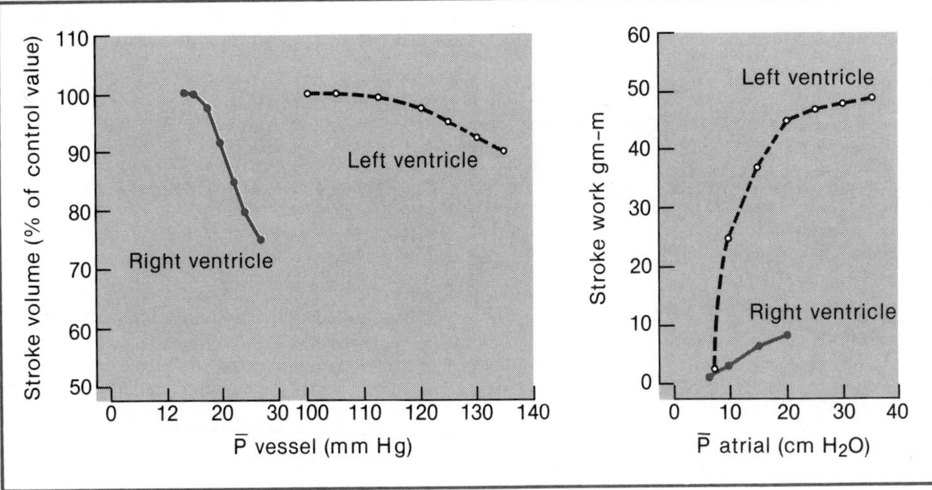

FIGURE 49–2. Effects of increasing preload and afterload on right and left ventricular function. The data in the left panel were obtained by constricting the main pulmonary artery and aorta in dogs. The right panel demonstrates the effect of increasing preloads. RV = right ventricle; LV = left ventricle.

tions.[13] As already noted, the normal adult RV has thin walls and a crescentic shape; its pumping action is akin to that of a bellows working in series with a low-pressure circuit, in contrast to the concentric contraction of the left ventricle.[13–15] Because it is much thinner than the LV, the RV is more compliant,[16] and in comparison with the left, it is better able to handle an increase in volume than in pressure load. The evidence in support of this statement is derived in the main from animal data[17–20] (Fig. 49–2), which contrast the effects of increasing preload and afterload on right and left ventricular function. In the left-hand panel, stroke volume is plotted as a function of various afterloads that were produced by actively constricting the main pulmonary artery and aorta in the dog.[17,18] Small increments in pulmonary artery pressure are associated with sharp decreases in RV stroke volume. In contrast, the LV, which normally works against high initial pressures, continues to maintain stroke volume despite substantial increases in systemic arterial pressure.

The right-hand portion of this figure demonstrates the effects of increasing preload. These ventricular function curves were obtained by volume infusions into the atria of dogs.[20] Note the marked differences in the respective ventricular stroke work that occur as right and left atrial pressures are increased. For a fourfold elevation in filling pressure (i.e., from 5 to 20 cm H_2O), the increase in left ventricular work was about five times that of the right.

In response to chronic pressure loads, significant changes develop in the configuration, mass, and functional characteristics of the RV. The rate at which these occur in humans and the magnitude of the pressures needed to produce them are unknown. Animal studies indicate that alterations in structure and function can be quite rapid after experimental outflow tract obstruction. Spann et al. observed a 71 per cent increase in right ventricular weight in cats 2 days after the pulmonary artery was banded, and within a month, right ventricular weight had risen by 150 per cent of control.[21] Response may not be as rapid in humans but is qualitatively similar.

The lumen of the main pulmonary artery can be reduced acutely by 60 to 80 per cent before aortic pressure declines as a consequence of a fall in cardiac output.[22–24] Because these experiments ignored the effects of neurohumoral compensations that support the systemic circulation, the impression has arisen that the acute right ventricular response is an abrupt, all-or-none event. However, as suggested in Figure 49–2, right ventricular decompensation is really a continuum.[17,20] At right ventricular systolic pressures of 60 to 80 mm Hg, right ventricular dilatation and failure occur with systemic hypotension and hypoperfusion.[25] The rate and/or absolute level of outflow tract obstruction at which these alterations develop can be greatly amplified or attenuated by respectively decreasing or increasing right coronary artery blood flow.[25] The relative roles played by changes in coronary blood flow in acute right heart failure in humans have yet to be determined.

PULMONARY VASCULAR ANATOMY

WALL STRUCTURE. Starting from the pulmonary artery and proceeding distally toward the capillaries, four structural regions can be identified: elastic, muscular, partially muscular, and nonmuscular[29] (Fig. 27–8, p. 800). In keeping with its embryological derivation, the main pulmonary artery and the first five generations are elastic in nature but less so than the aorta and major systemic arteries. These vessels, by definition, have more than five elastic laminae in their media and are more than 2000 μm in diameter in the adult. In the axial pathway, the next three generations are said to be transitional.

Muscular arteries have between 2 and 5 elastic laminae and a continuous muscle coat. These arteries form the majority of vessels in the lung and are found in a diameter range of 150 to 2000 μm in the adult. The medial muscle coat is very thin compared with the arterioles in the systemic circulation. These vessels give way to partially muscular arteries in which the muscle is arranged in a spiral, so that in cross section it appears as a crescent, with the rest of the wall being like a capillary. Nonmuscular arteries are larger than capillaries and range from 30 to 75 μm in diameter in adults. Partially muscular and nonmuscular arteries all lie within the alveolar units in adults. The smallest muscular and partially muscular arteries are thought to represent the resistance arteries.[29]

Although there is great variation in the sizes of arteries that accompany conducting airways such as lobar bronchi, those that follow the respiratory bronchi and alveolar ducts are muscular or partially so.[29] The implications for function of these observations are severalfold. It is known that gas exchange occurs in respiratory bronchi and alveolar ducts through the arteries that accompany these structures.[30] When this information is coupled with the fact that hypoxia acts directly to constrict muscular arteries, it is apparent that this area of the lung has the propensity for active control of pulmonary blood flow. Further, since the spiral of muscle in the partially muscular arteries is directly contiguous with the muscle encircling the larger vessels, retrograde propagation of the hypoxic stimulus can occur in the intracellular pathways of the muscle syncytium,[29] and a wider and more severe response can develop.

INNERVATION. In further contrast to the peripheral circulation, it has proved difficult to demonstrate a nerve supply in the pulmonary circulation. Evidence suggests that although both adrenergic and cholinergic fibers are present, they are sparse in comparison with those innervating systemic vessels of similar size, and their distribution tends to be concentrated in the larger vessels at the hilum.[30,31] Recent data indicate that these nerves contain other neurotransmitters, such as vasoactive intestinal peptide in parasympathetic fibers, substance P, the neurokinins, calcitonin gene-related peptide in sensory fibers, and neuropeptide tyrosine in sympathetic fibers.[32] Some studies in children indicate that the predominant neuropeptide transmitter is tyrosine and that, during growth and development, the relative density of nerve fibers increases only in the arteries of the respiratory unit.[32] In this work, pulmonary hypertension in infants was associated with premature innervation of these arteries.

In *summary,* the structure of the pulmonary circulation is in keeping with its hemodynamics. The thin-walled, sparsely innervated vessels which contain relatively small amounts of smooth muscle (Fig. 27–4, p. 795) do not favor the development of marked vasomotor responses, and, indeed, vasoconstriction alone is not sufficient to overload the RV to the point of producing acute cor pulmonale.[33] Consequently, mechanical obstruction of the pulmonary circulation can be inferred when there is acute cor pulmonale, and structural alterations in the pulmonary vascular bed must be present in the chronic form.

PHYSIOLOGY OF THE PULMONARY CIRCULATION

(See also Chap. 27)

The physiology of the pulmonary circulation is unique from several standpoints. Most of this vascular bed is contained within the parenchyma of the lung, and thus the vessels are subjected to external distending and compressive forces which can act independently of any intrinsic properties of the vessels themselves. In addition, the pulmonary circulation is in series with a pump capable of developing only low pressures, yet it must accommodate the entire cardiac output under all states of physical activity. Consequently, it must adjust to wide variations in blood flow without much change in pressure so as not to overload the RV.

PRESSURE-VOLUME RELATIONS. Historically, it has been thought that the pulmonary circulation is highly distensible and that the vessels dilate to accommodate increases in cardiac output, thus preventing an increase in pulmonary artery pressure in high-flow states.[34,35] Actual measurements of the compliance of the pulmonary vessels have shown that this vascular bed is significantly stiffer than its systemic counterpart,[36,37] and only small increments in blood volume can be accepted by the large pulmonary vessels.[38–41] The major mechanism which accommodates increased blood flow and volume is the recruitment of previously unperfused vessels.[36,42] Morphological evidence suggests that both recruitment and distention occur with an increase in pulmonary blood flow and that the transmural pressures to which the vessel is subjected are what determine which one predominates.[43] In superior portions of the lung where the vessels are collapsed or where alveolar pressure is greater than pulmonary venous pressure, recruitment appears to be the major mechanism. Distention is more important in dependent portions of the lung in which pulmonary venous pressure is greater than alveolar pressure (see below)[30] (Fig. 20–8, p. 555).

PRESSURE-FLOW RELATIONS. Evaluation of the pressure-flow relations of the pulmonary circulation in normal humans at any given lung volume demonstrates a hyperbolic configuration in which large changes in pulmonary blood flow are associated with small elevations in pulmonary artery pressure (Fig. 49–3*A*). The net result is that as flow increases, pulmonary vascular resistance decreases (Fig. 49–3*B*).[33] Consequently, irrespective of whether distention or recruitment occurs, both mechanisms maintain a low-pressure circuit during situations of increased blood flow.

A U-shaped curve describes pulmonary vascular resistance as a function of lung volume (Fig. 49–3*C*).[40] At the extremes of lung volume of full inflation and deflation, vascular resistance is high, and it reaches its nadir at about the resting end-expiratory position (i.e., at functional residual capacity). These findings can be explained by considering the geometry assumed by the alveolar and intrapulmonic but extraalveolar vessels in response to the transmural pressures to which they are exposed.

Because the pulmonary vessels are within the substance of the lung, their dimensions reflect the forces exerted on them by the pulmonary parenchyma. At low lung volumes, the extraalveolar vessels tend to collapse because radial traction no longer supports them. Simultaneously, the alveolar vessels are pulled open by the increased recoil forces generated by the tendency of the alveoli to become smaller. As the lung is inflated to volumes above functional residual capacity, the larger vessels tend to be pulled open, but there is now a progressive increase in the resistance of the small vessels as they are squeezed and lengthened by enlarging alveoli. In addition to this deformation, alterations in alveolar pressure also can influence dynamically the lumina of small vessels. When alveolar pressure is positive, as it is during expiration or with the Valsalva maneuver, vessels are compressed. Alternatively, with negative pressure, as with inspiration or the Mueller maneuver, small vessels are subjected to a proportional distending pressure. It is therefore apparent that alveolar pressure can play a critical role in determining the distribution of pulmonary blood flow and, accordingly, gas exchange.

DETERMINANTS OF PULMONARY GAS EXCHANGE

DISTRIBUTION OF PULMONARY BLOOD FLOW. In the normal human in the upright position, blood flow per unit volume of lung increases progressively from the apex to the base, with flow at the apex being virtually absent[44,45] (Fig. 20–8, p. 555). This distribution is affected by changes of posture and by exercise. When a subject is in the supine position, apical blood flow increases but the basal flow remains virtually unchanged, with the result that the distribution from apex to base becomes almost uniform. In this posture, flow in the posterior or dependent regions exceeds that in the anterior parts. During mild exercise in the upright position, flow to both the upper and the lower zones increases but more so to the upper, so that flow becomes more evenly distributed.

West[44,45] and Permutt and Riley[46] have demonstrated that the pressure-flow relations through the lung can be analogous to those of a "waterfall" or Starling resistor. The basic point of these studies is that the effective pressure drop in the pulmonary vasculature is not always the difference between inflow (pulmonary artery) and outflow (left atrial) pressures but often is between the inflow pressure and the closing pressure of small vessels downstream.

In normal human lungs, pulmonary arterial and venous pressures both increase from superior to dependent regions because of hydrostatic ef-

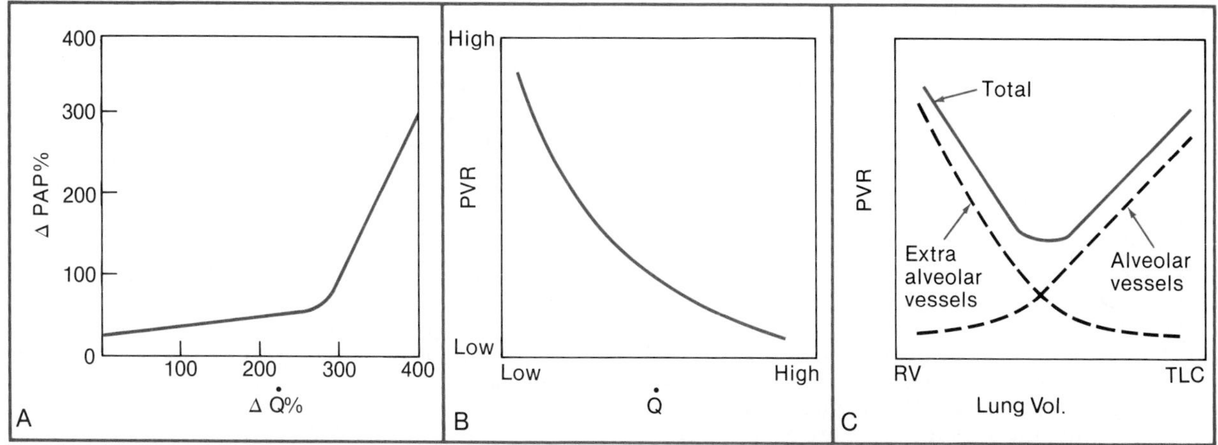

FIGURE 49–3. Some aspects of pulmonary vascular physiology. *A*, Pressure-flow relation. *B*, Resistance-flow relation. *C*, Pulmonary vascular resistance (PVR) as a function of lung volume for the total system and for extraalveolar and alveolar vessels. ΔPAP = percentage of change of mean pulmonary artery pressure from control; ΔQ = percentage of change in cardiac output; 100 = normal cardiac output; RV = residual volume; TLC = total lung capacity.

fects resulting from gravity acting on the blood.[44,45] Alveolar pressures remain essentially constant throughout the lung. Alveolar pressure exceeds venous pressure at a more dependent portion of the lung than does arterial pressure. This results in distribution of blood flow to three major areas.

In the most superior area (zone I), no flow occurs because alveolar pressure exceeds pulmonary arterial pressure. Presumably, this is because thin-walled collapsible vessels are directly exposed to alveolar pressure. In humans, the pulmonary artery pressure is sufficiently high to bring blood to the apex of the lung so that no zone I is present under normal conditions. Flow in the upper segments of the lung may disappear, however, if pulmonary artery pressure falls or if alveolar pressure is elevated, as it is in obstructive airway disease. In the middle zone (zone II), arterial pressure exceeds alveolar pressure, but the latter is greater than venous pressure. Here, flow through the capillaries is proportional to the difference between arterial and alveolar pressure. In the lowest zone, zone III, venous pressure exceeds alveolar pressure, the vessels are held open, and flow is determined in the usual way by the arterial-venous pressure difference. A small zone of reduced flow at the very base of the lung also has been observed and attributed to a possible increase in the interstitial pressure as a consequence of the reduced expansion of the lung parenchyma in the lower zone. This has, therefore, been called zone IV. There is still some uncertainty about the cause of the reduced flow in this area, but the concept of reduction in flow caused by an increased interstitial pressure is almost certainly important in mitral stenosis and may be responsible for the reduction in basilar blood flow observed in that condition.

Distribution of Ventilation

The distribution of ventilation, like that of perfusion, decreases from base to apex in the normal lung, but the rate of change is only about one-third that seen with blood flow.[44] Here, too, gravity plays a role, and changes in posture have an influence. Thus, when normal subjects lie supine, the difference in ventilation between the anatomical upper and lower zones is abolished,[44] and in the inverted lung, the apex ventilates better than the base, so the normal pattern is reversed.

Evaluation of the relative rates of expansion of the upper and lower zones in the upright position reveals different patterns of distribution, depending on the lung volume from which inspiration is initiated.[47] As a consequence of the effect of gravity and the shape of the pressure-volume curve of the lung, when a normal subject takes a breath from functional residual capacity (FRC), ventilation is preferentially distributed to the dependent lung zones. Because blood flow in the resting state also is preferentially distributed to this area, this matching of ventilation to perfusion in different body positions ensures efficient gas exchange under a variety of physiological conditions.

If breathing takes place at lung volumes lower than FRC, the distribution of ventilation is quite different. Because of closure of dependent airways, the most inferior portions of the lung do not ventilate, and all of the inspired gas goes preferentially to the upper zones. The phenomenon of airway closure at low lung volumes has major physiological significance and can produce substantial alterations in ventilation-perfusion relations and arterial hypoxia.[48,49]

Ventilation-Perfusion Ratios

Ventilation-perfusion ($\dot{V}_A/\dot{Q}$) ratios are important because they are the determinants of the gas exchange that occurs in any part of the lung and thereby affect the overall efficiency of the lungs in taking up oxygen and eliminating carbon dioxide.[44] The partial pressure of oxygen in the alveolar gas (and therefore in the end-capillary blood) is set by a balance between the rate of removal by the blood and its rate of replenishment by ventilation. If ventilation is gradually reduced and perfusion maintained to an alveolus, oxygen tension falls and carbon dioxide tension rises. The limit is reached when the unit is not ventilated at all, and the pulmonary venous oxygen and carbon dioxide will be those of mixed venous blood. This is a $\dot{V}_A/\dot{Q}$ relationship of zero and corresponds to the situation in which there is a true anatomical pulmonary arteriovenous shunt (e.g., a pulmonary arteriovenous fistula or a functional one such as produced by atelectasis). By contrast, if perfusion to a normally ventilating alveolus is gradually reduced, the oxygen tension in the venous blood draining this alveolus rises and the partial pressure of carbon dioxide falls. The limit now occurs when the unit is unperfused. This is a $\dot{V}_A/\dot{Q}$ of infinity and is seen in situations in which blood supply is disrupted, such as by pulmonary emboli or other disease in which occlusion of the pulmonary arterial circulation occurs. Between these two extreme examples, a wide range of $\dot{V}_A/\dot{Q}$ abnormalities is possible.

The alveoli hypoventilated in relation to their perfusion (i.e., low $\dot{V}_A/\dot{Q}$ ratio) cause hypoxemia, and their presence has the same effect as mixing venous and arterial blood. This is termed venous admixture or "wasted blood"; it is evaluated clinically by determining the oxygen tension difference between ideal alveolar gas and arterial blood. Normally, venous admixture or "shunt effect" is only about 2 to 3 per cent of the cardiac output, but in severe disease it may rise to 30 per cent or more. The normal alveolar arterial difference of oxygen (A-aDO_2) is 20 mm Hg or less.[50,51]

The alveoli which are hyperventilated in relation to their perfusion (i.e., high $\dot{V}_A/\dot{Q}$ ratio) mainly affect CO_2 elimination. They behave as if part of the inspired gas bypassed the alveoli, so this effect has been called "wasted ventilation" or an increase in "physiological dead space." It is evaluated by comparing mixed expired and arterial CO_2, using the Bohr equation. The physiological dead space normally is less than 30 per cent of the tidal volume.[51,52] In severe lung disease, it can rise to 50 per cent or more. Every pathological condition that directly affects the pulmonary parenchyma or its vascular bed results in mismatched ventilation and blood flow. Consequently, this abnormality is by far the most common cause of arterial hypoxemia in disease states. Both venous admixture and physiological dead space are typically increased in chronic obstructive and infiltrative lung diseases. In pulmonary thromboembolism, an increase in dead space predominates.

In many pulmonary parenchymal diseases, blood supply to poorly ventilated areas tends to be reduced, so that the $\dot{V}_A/\dot{Q}$ ratios are not as low as they would otherwise be. One reason for this is that the local pathological process tends to disturb both ventilation and perfusion by its mechanical effects. Another is local hypoxic vasoconstriction, which shunts blood away from the involved alveoli.[53–55] In the case of thromboembolic phenomena, the regional decreases in CO_2 concentration that occur cause local increases in the resistance of small airways and thus reduce ventilation to the affected region.

Other Causes of Abnormal Arterial Blood Gases

In addition to $\dot{V}_A/\dot{Q}$ inequalities, there are four other causes of arterial hypoxemia: (1) anatomical right-to-left intracardiac or intrapulmonary shunts usually caused by congenital heart disease (Chaps. 31 and 32); (2) reductions in the inspired concentration of oxygen; (3) defects in the diffusion of oxygen from the alveolus to the blood; and (4) alveolar hypoventilation.

Although it was originally thought that measurements of the *diffusing capacity* of the lung for oxygen could demonstrate a specific impairment in the transfer of molecular oxygen across a thickened membrane (i.e., alveolar-capillary block), it is now appreciated that single breath tests of diffusing capacity that use carbon monoxide are profoundly influenced by three variables: (1) the surface area available for diffusion, (2) the volume of blood within the capillaries, and (3) the rate of combination of CO_2 and hemoglobin.[56] Other factors, such as the molecular path for diffusion and the stratified heterogeneity of gas mixtures, also play a role.[57] In addition to the above, steady-state methods also are influenced by regional $\dot{V}_A/\dot{Q}$ relations.[56] Thus these techniques do not measure the thickness of the alveolar-capillary membrane, and in any disease associated with a loss of elastic recoil (loss of surface area through disruption of alveolar walls), marked $\dot{V}_A/\dot{Q}$ heterogeneities or loss of capillary bed will be associated with a reduced "diffusing capacity." Even so, the effect that this has on gas exchange is, at most, small.

ALVEOLAR HYPOVENTILATION. This is a condition in which insufficient gas exchange occurs to meet metabolic demands. It can result from many causes: severe $\dot{V}_A/\dot{Q}$ inequalities; reduced drive from the respiratory center so that the patient "will not breathe"; failure of the patient's respiratory system to act on the information sent from the central nervous system because of severe intrinsic pulmonary disease; or abnormalities of the neuromuscular apparatus of the chest wall or diaphragm.[58] In the latter cases, the patient "cannot breathe." Regardless of cause, the cardinal features of the arterial blood are hypoxemia and hypercapnia, and both must be present to establish the diagnosis. The various diseases associated with alveolar hypoventilation and the mechanisms by which it comes about in each are discussed as examples of chronic cor pulmonale later in this chapter.

EFFECTS OF ALVEOLAR GAS TENSIONS ON THE PULMONARY CIRCULATION

HYPOXIA. The most potent stimulus for the development of pulmonary vasoconstriction is alveolar hypoxia[30,53,54,59]

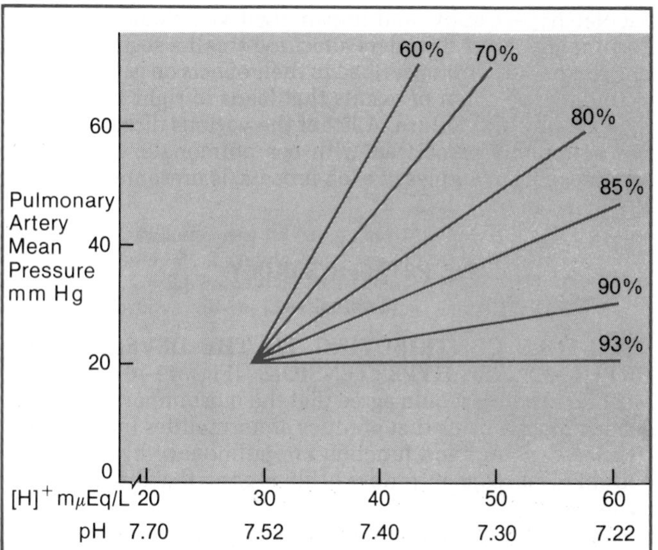

FIGURE 49–4. Relation of arterial oxygen saturation and hydrogen ion concentration to pulmonary artery pressure. (Reproduced from Enson, Y., et al.: The influence of hydrogen ion concentration and hypoxia on the pulmonary circulation. J. Clin. Invest. *43*:1146, 1964, by copyright permission of the American Society for Clinical Investigation.)

(Fig. 27–4, p. 795). Although acute vasoconstriction appears when the alveolar pO_2 is 60 mm Hg or lower, this response is found only in about two-thirds of normal subjects.[60] It is speculated that the subjects who respond to hypoxemia with pulmonary vasoconstriction are those who would be prone to develop chronic cor pulmonale if they developed a disease that interfered with effective alveolar ventilation.[61] The pulmonary constrictor response to hypoxia appears to be locally mediated since it can be elicited both in denervated lungs and isolated perfused lungs.

ACIDOSIS. This also has been shown to produce significant increases in pulmonary vascular resistance as well as to act synergistically with hypoxia.[62] In contrast, an increase in arterial pCO_2 seems to exert no direct effect. Instead, it seems to operate by way of the increase in hydrogen ion concentration that it induces. The interaction of hypoxia and acidemia is clinically important; these two conditions frequently coexist, and their interplay follows a predictable pattern (Fig. 49–4). At minor degrees of oxygen unsaturation, pulmonary artery pressure is relatively insensitive to hydrogen ion concentration, whereas it is extremely sensitive at high levels of unsaturation. On the other hand, when the pH is high, the pressor effect of hypoxia is blunted.

Although the localization of the pulmonary vascular pressor response within the lung is still controversial, most studies indicate that it occurs in partially muscular arteries less than 200 μm in diameter.[29,53,55,63] The mechanism by which hypoxia causes pulmonary arterial smooth muscle to constrict is unclear.

The available information points toward two major alternatives: an indirect effect by which hypoxia might cause endothelial cells to generate various eicosanoids or other cells in the pulmonary parenchyma to release vasoactive substances (e.g., histamine from mast cells), or a direct effect of hypoxia on pulmonary arterial smooth muscle. Other influences may enhance hypoxic pulmonary vasoconstriction. For example, it is possible that extrapulmonic reflexes or the adrenergic neurotransmitter norepinephrine may augment the pressor response.

PULMONARY HYPERTENSION. The precise mechanism by which the resting tone of the pulmonary circulation is controlled is unknown. The smooth muscle and connective tissue elements in the walls of the vessels certainly contribute. The relative roles of other potential controlling factors such as the neuropeptides of the nonadrenergic noncholinergic nervous system, or locally formed or circulating mediators such as the eicosanoids (prostacyclin, thromboxane, leukotrienes), catecholamines (epinephrine, norepinephrine), and autacoids (histamine, bradykinin), and endothelial-derived relaxing and contrasting factors have yet to be explored.[64]

Pulmonary vasoconstriction produces an acute rise in pressure, and it is now known that continuing constriction with pulmonary hypertension of even a few days' duration is associated with structural changes in the vessels.[29] Luminal narrowing is brought about by an increase in the thickness of the medial coat, endothelial swelling, hypertrophy, and the appearance of muscle at more peripheral levels than normal. With continued insult, a reduction in cross-sectional area of the vascular bed develops in association with an increase in RV weight. Although these structural and functional changes occur with all forms of pulmonary hypertension, different time sequences of development or ultrastructural patterns may be seen with different disease processes.

CHRONIC COR PULMONALE

INCIDENCE

Because of its association with chronic lung disease, chronic cor pulmonale is a common type of heart disease.[1,5,7,65] The U.S. Public Health Service estimates that chronic lung disease affects 47 million people in the United States alone and accounts for more than 80,000 deaths every year.[66] Although precise figures on the prevalence of cor pulmonale are lacking, it is possible to appreciate the potential magnitude of the problem by recognizing that chronic bronchitis and emphysema are its most common causes and that these two diseases result in about 30,000 deaths per year.[67] In one study in England, cor pulmonale was responsible for 30 to 40 per cent of all clinical cases of heart failure and of a total of 487 cases of cardiac disease;[68] in the United States 10 to 30 per cent of hospital admissions for congestive heart failure are due to cor pulmonale.[69] Most patients are 45 years of age or older, and men are affected more frequently than women.

The presence of pulmonary hypertension with chronic respiratory disease contributes significantly to mortality. The available data suggest that the severity of pulmonary hypertension correlates more closely with survival than any other variable studied[70–72] (Fig. 49–5). Patients with severe airway obstruction (FEV_1<1 liter) without pulmonary hypertension

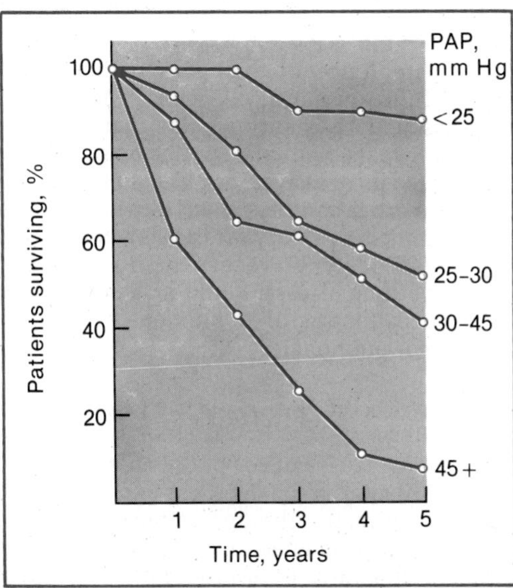

FIGURE 49–5. Correlation between survival (years) and baseline measurement of mean pulmonary arterial pressure (PAP) in patients with chronic bronchitis. (From Bishop, J. M.: Hypoxia and pulmonary hypertension in chronic bronchitis. Prog. Resp. Res. *9*:10, 1975.)

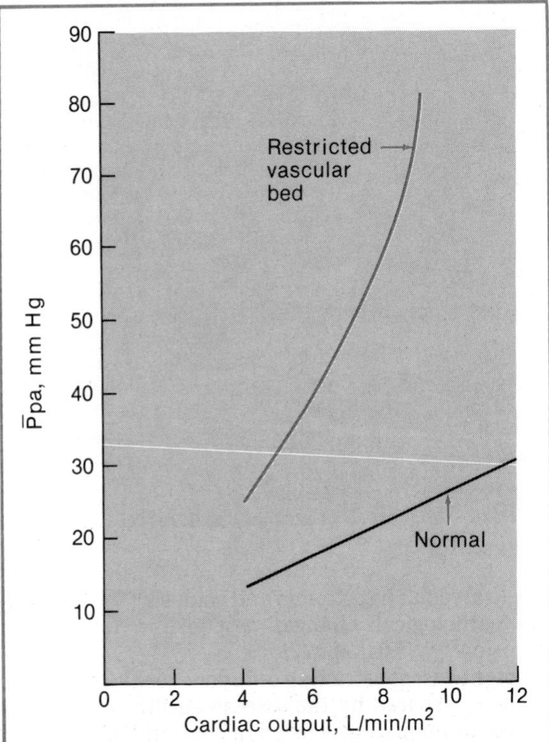

FIGURE 49–8. Pulmonary circulation at sea level, at rest, and during exercise. Restriction of the pulmonary arterial tree causes higher pulmonary arterial pressures at any level of blood flow. (From Fishman, A. P.: Pulmonary hypertension and cor pulmonale. *In* Fishman, A. P.: Pulmonary Diseases and Disorders. 2nd ed. New York, McGraw-Hill Book Co., 1988, p. 999.)

tant role in the development of elevated pulmonary artery pressure and resistance is in congenital heart diseases associated with left-to-right shunts[90] (p. 906): Once established, the anatomical changes in the pulmonary vascular bed may not be completely reversible, even when pulmonary blood flow is restored to normal surgically. Morphological examination of the lungs of patients with congenital cardiac disease and high pulmonary flow shows a gradation of pathological changes that reflects the duration and severity of the condition[90,91] (p. 896).

It is not clear how the above-described pathogenetic mechanisms interrelate in the development of pulmonary hypertension. It is easy to appreciate that the loss of vessels and diffuse constriction of the arterioles with the attendant pathological changes in their walls and lumina can combine to cause a reduction of the pulmonary vascular bed, which in turn causes an increase in pulmonary vascular resistance. These changes need not be manifested at rest as an elevated pulmonary artery pressure. As shown in Figure 49–3, the normal pulmonary vascular bed has the ability to accept large increases in flow without marked increases in pressure, probably through the recruitment of parallel vascular channels. In the case of a restricted vascular bed, this reserve is lost and the patients' physiological response is as though they were starting at the bend of the normal pressure-flow relation (Fig. 49–8). The importance of hypoxia as a determinant of pulmonary artery pressure is demonstrated in Figure 49–9.

Under these circumstances, pressure can rise dramatically with exercise or any other condition that causes pulmonary blood flow to increase. As the secondary changes in the vessels develop with progression of the underlying disease, further raising of pulmonary vascular resistance causes elevation of pulmonary artery pressure, sometimes even at rest. The pressure-flow relation (Fig. 49–3*A*) is shifted upward and to the left, as in a constricted bed, so that small increments in flow produce large increases in pressure over the entire range of cardiac output. It may be inferred that small increases in output are accompanied by large increases in right ventricular work. Increases in viscosity, collateral blood flow, hypoxemia, and acidemia worsen the situation by further increasing pulmonary artery pressure.[70,92,93]

RIGHT VENTRICULAR DYNAMICS. The hemodynamic findings in cor pulmonale depend, to some extent, on the cause and duration of the underlying pathological process. Most patients with relatively mild obstructive lung disease without severe hypoxemia have normal mean right atrial and right ventricular end-diastolic pressures, normal cardiac outputs, normal or slightly elevated pulmonary artery pressures, and slightly elevated pulmonary vascular resistances at rest.[29,70,94–96] Right ventricular ejection fraction, as determined by radionuclide angiography, tends to be normal.[97,98] With exercise, pulmonary artery pressure rises further, right ventricular stroke work increases (Fig. 49–9), and right ventricular ejection fraction falls.[97,98] Relating end-diastolic pressure to stroke work suggests that these patients function on an extension of the normal right ventricular function curve.[99] These findings need not be accompanied by clinical or electrocardiographic evidence of right ventricular hypertrophy,[95] although evidence of right ventricular enlargement may be seen on two-dimensional echocardiography. Acute right ventricular failure can develop in these patients if respiratory failure, hypoxia, and further elevation of pulmonary artery pressure are precipitated by a pulmonary infection.

Progression of the airway obstruction tends to accentuate these findings. As the ventilatory impairment worsens, the hemodynamic alterations, including elevations of the right ventricular end-diastolic and end-systolic volumes, follow.[100,101] At the stage when severe chronic hypoxemia develops, usually in association with chronic hypercapnia, there is moderate pulmonary hypertension at rest, which becomes more severe during exercise in association with abnormal right ventricular filling pressures and function in most patients[70–72,97–102] (Fig. 49–10). Cardiac output tends to be normal or even slightly elevated at rest[103] but increases little with exercise when the patient breathes room air. Oxygen admin-

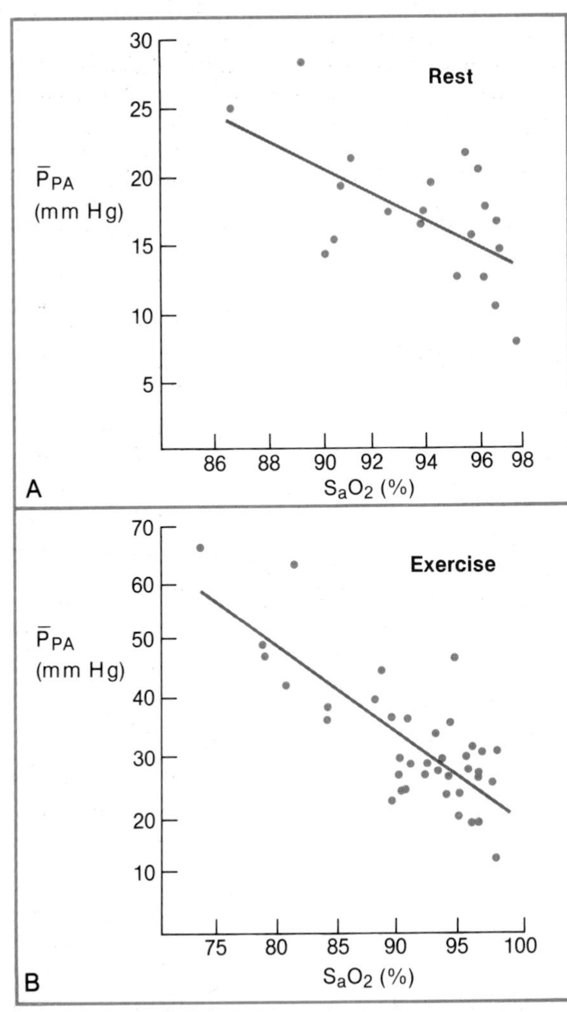

FIGURE 49–9. The correlation between arterial oxygen saturation (SaO_2) and mean pulmonary artery pressures ($\bar{P}_{pa}$) at rest and during exercise in patients with chronic obstructive lung disease. (From Stewart, R. I., et al.: Cardiac output during exercise in patients with COPD. Chest *89*:199, 1986.)

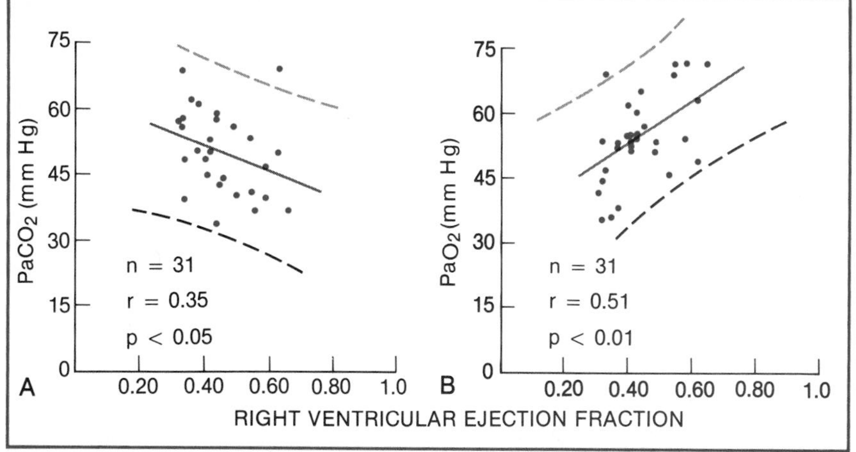

FIGURE 49-10. Relation between arterial carbon dioxide tension (P_{CO_2}) (left panel), arterial oxygen tension (PaO_2) (right panel), and right ventricular ejection fraction in patients with chronic bronchitis and emphysema. These data represent air breathing at rest. (From Flenley, D. C., and Muir, A. L.: Cardiovascular effects of oxygen therapy for pulmonary arterial hypertension. Clin. Chest Med. *4*:297, 1983.)

istration may lower pulmonary artery pressure and raise the right ventricular ejection fraction.[102] Systolic pulmonary artery pressures can reach levels of 80 mm Hg, and these patients are likely to show the clinical and electrocardiographic changes usually ascribed to cor pulmonale. Failure of the RV is associated with an expanded circulating blood volume. In contrast to left ventricular failure, the pulmonary blood volume-total volume ratio remains essentially normal (about 1 to 10) even though red cell mass may be considerably increased.[95] Both circulating plasma volume and lung water increase,[104,105] and each has been shown to decrease as pulmonary artery pressure is lowered with therapy.

LEFT VENTRICULAR DYNAMICS. Abnormally elevated pulmonary venous pressures, with or without overt left ventricular failure, invariably produce alterations in pulmonary mechanics and gas exchange, even in patients with normal lungs. Consequently, left ventricular dysfunction could have deleterious effects in cor pulmonale. Controversy persists about whether the disease affecting the lungs and RV in these patients produces left ventricular disease, or whether the latter results from independent causes.[103] Evidence exists that many patients with cor pulmonale who are over the age of 65 are hypertensive and have reduced left ventricular compliance and/or regional left ventricular wall motion disorders secondary to ischemic heart disease.

The view that disorders of the RV may result in left ventricular disease has gained support from several sources. Animal experiments have shown that (1) right ventricular failure after banding of the pulmonary artery leads to similar morphological and biochemical changes in both cardiac chambers and to reduced contractility of the LV[106-108]; (2) in both isolated hearts and intact animals, alterations in right ventricular compliance or dimensions also change the mechanical properties of the left ventricle, perhaps acting in part through changes in the thickness or position of the interventricular septum (Fig. 49-11)[16,109,110]; and (3) cattle at high altitude with severe pulmonary hypertension have elevated left ventricular end-diastolic pressures.[111] Although these observations are provocative, their relevance to human disease is uncertain.

Autopsy studies have shown that left ventricular hypertrophy frequently occurs in patients with cor pulmonale,[112-114] and left ventricular dysfunction of varying degrees has been observed in vivo.[106,114-116,116a] In all of these investigations, none of the usual causes of left ventricular disease were apparent. Thus, it appears that the structure and function of the left ventricle can become abnormal in association with the pathogenetic mechanisms underlying cor pulmonale. This is probably an uncommon occurrence, and the weight of current evidence indicates that cor pulmonale per se usually does *not* seriously impair left ventricular performance.[70,99,113,117-125]

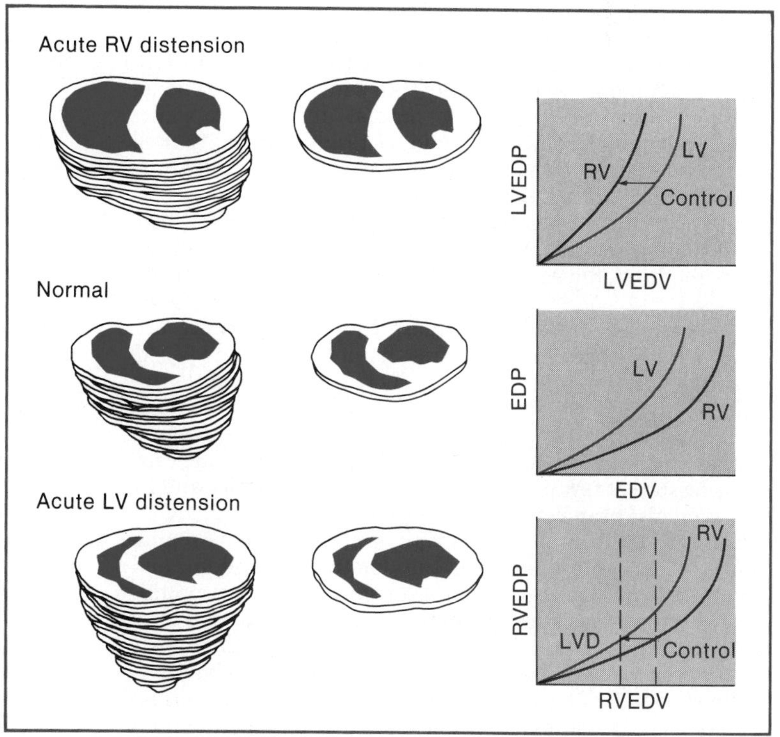

FIGURE 49-11. Alterations in compliance by distention of the contralateral ventricle. Note that acute distention of either ventricle changes not only that ventricle's pressure-volume curve but alters the compliance of the other ventricle as well. The middle graph shows the end-diastolic volume-pressure relations for the right ventricle (RV) and left ventricle (LV). The top graph shows these relations for the LV with a normal RV (right curve) and after the RV has been acutely distended (RVD, left curve). The bottom graph shows the relations for the RV with a normal LV (right curve) and after the LV has been acutely distended (LVD). (From Weber, K. T., et al.: Contractile mechanics and interaction of the right and left ventricles. Am. J. Cardiol. *47*:686, 1981.)

When abnormalities in the latter have been found, they could be explained by a reduction in the apparent distensibility of the left ventricle secondary to right ventricular dilatation (Fig. 49–11),[126,127] by a reduction in right ventricular stroke volume causing diminished left-sided filling, or by independent disease processes such as coronary artery disease aggravated by hypoxemia.[106,125] Given the heterogeneity of the population with cor pulmonale and the variance of its natural history, the controversy will undoubtedly continue. An uncommon syndrome of drug-induced left ventricular failure has been described in patients with chronic lung disease. Some right ventricular endomyocardial biopsies have been compatible with catecholamine myocarditis (p. 1436) in those patients who had been on large doses of adrenergic agonist inhalants and methylxanthines.

CLINICAL MANIFESTATIONS

Chronic Obstructive Pulmonary Disease (COPD)[73,103,123,124]

COPD, by far the most common form of pulmonary parenchymal disease responsible for chronic pulmonary hypertension, consists of chronic bronchitis, emphysema, and in some instances bronchial asthma. Atopic asthma does *not* produce chronic cor pulmonale,[80] and intrinsic, or nonatopic, asthma often is a variant of chronic bronchitis. In this discussion, COPD refers exclusively to chronic bronchitis and/or emphysema.

In most patients with COPD, chronic bronchitis and emphysema coexist, but cor pulmonale is restricted to those with functionally significant airway disease with or without emphysema.[80] This admixture has given rise to a great deal of confusion in terminology in the literature, and until the matter was sorted out by Burrows and colleagues[128] and Mitchell and Filley,[129] the terms bronchitis and emphysema frequently were considered to be synonymous. These workers described fundamental differences in the clinical, physiological, and pathological features of the two conditions and laid the groundwork for a better understanding of these conditions.

CHRONIC BRONCHITIS. It is possible to think of COPD as a continuum, with chronic bronchitis at one extreme and emphysema at the other and the majority of patients having features of both conditions. The distinctions between the two groups are presented in Table 49–3. In the *chronic bronchitis* variety ("blue bloater," "nonfighter"), chronic cough with sputum production, frequently recurring chest infection, secondary erythrocytosis, and repeated bouts of right heart failure are common. Physiologically, the patients have hypoxemia and hypercapnia at rest, normal diffusion capacity, elevated residual volume, functional residual capacity, and airway resistance, with relatively normal values for total lung capacity and pulmonary compliance. Maximum flow rates and forced expiratory volumes are abnormally depressed. The chest roentgenogram shows moderately hyperinflated lungs, increased bronchovascular markings, and sometimes cardiomegaly.

The basic abnormality is widespread but regionally unequal airway obstruction that results in mismatched $\dot{V}_A/\dot{Q}$ relationships. In regions of low $\dot{V}_A/\dot{Q}$ ratios, pulmonary arterial constriction on the basis of hypoxia and/or acidosis occurs. With progression, alveolar hypoventilation develops, the vascular bed becomes constricted, and the pulmonary artery pressure at rest rises. The main pulmonary artery and its two principal branches are enlarged.

EMPHYSEMA. In the emphysematous type ("pink puffer," "fighter"), dyspnea is the dominant symptom, and cough and sputum production are considerably less prominent. Erythrocytosis is uncommon, and right heart failure tends to occur as a terminal event. In keeping with the hyperventilation, the alveolar-arterial gradient for oxygen is abnormally elevated, but arterial oxygen tension usually is normal or only slightly depressed; hypocapnia is common. Standard spirometric indices cannot differentiate this group from those with chronic bronchitis, since the degree of obstruction as measured by this technique may be similar. However, the pink puffer has abnormally low diffusing capacity and greatly increased lung volumes and pulmonary compliance. Roentgenograms of the chest reveal marked pulmonary hyperinflation with flattened diaphragms, oligemia of the peripheral lung fields, and a small heart[130] (Fig. 49–12). With the onset of cor pulmonale, the prominence of the vascular markings increases, but RV enlargement may be difficult to observe.

Although there is some airway disease in this condition, the primary pathological defect is widespread destruction of alveolar septa. As a result, the surface area for gas exchange is lost more or less in proportion to alveolar vessels, and arterial gas tensions can be reasonably well maintained for a period of time by increasing ventilation. The destruction of the parenchyma results in loss of lateral traction of small airways, so that they narrow and collapse. Then the regional distribution of inspired air becomes more impaired, with resultant worsening of the abnormalities in $\dot{V}_A/\dot{Q}$ ratios. These patients ini-

TABLE 49-3 COMPARISON OF THE CLINICAL AND PHYSIOLOGICAL FEATURES OF EMPHYSEMA AND CHRONIC BRONCHITIS

	EMPHYSEMA	CHRONIC BRONCHITIS
Synonyms	Pink puffer Fighter	Blue bloater Nonfighter
Signs and Symptoms		
Cough and sputum	Scant	Marked
Dyspnea at rest	Marked	Usually absent
Recurrent chest infections	Unusual	Frequent
Habitus	Often thin, wasted	Often obese
Cyanosis	No	Yes
Edema	No	Yes
Increased AP diameter of thorax	Marked	Mild
Hyperresonance to percussion	Marked	Mild
Breath sounds	Absent to depressed	Rales and rhonchi
Chest x-ray	Hyperinflation; no cardiomegaly	No hyperinflation; cardiomegaly
Electrocardiogram	RVM uncommon	RVM common
Pulmonary Gas Exchange		
Hematocrit	Normal	Elevated
PaO_2	Slight reduction	Marked reduction
$PaCO_2$	Low or normal	Elevated
Diffusing capacity	Markedly decreased	Normal or slightly reduced
Pulmonary Mechanics		
Expiratory flow rates	Reduced	Reduced
Elastic recoil	Markedly reduced	Normal or slightly reduced
Lung volume	Marked hyperinflation	Mild hyperinflation
Pulmonary Circulation		
Pulmonary hypertension at rest with exercise	None or mild	Marked
Right heart failure	Terminal	Repeated

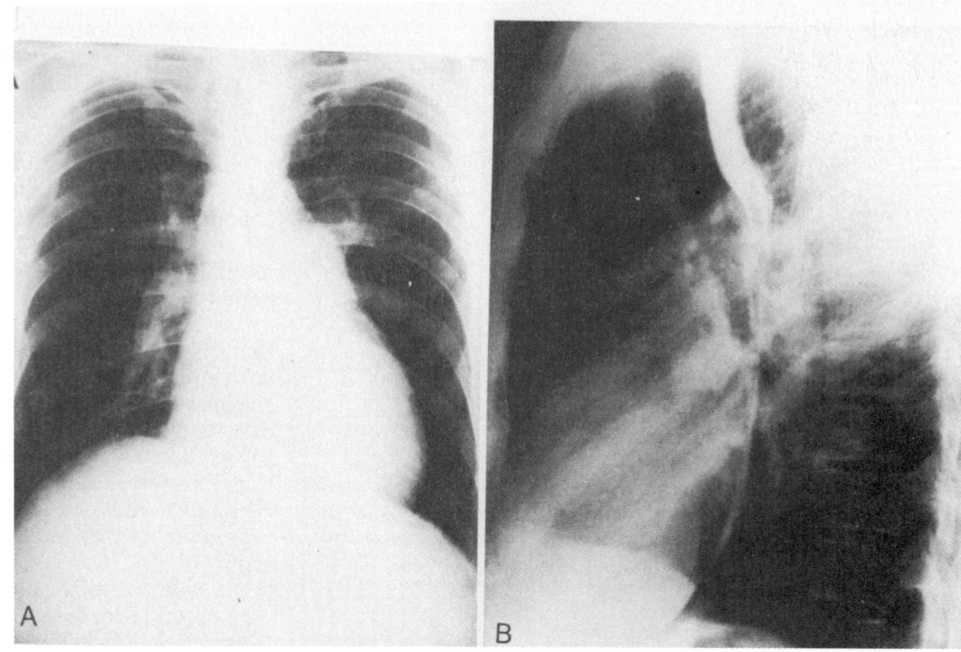

FIGURE 49–12. X-ray changes in cor pulmonale. *A*, Posteroanterior chest x-ray showing cardiomegaly, a definitely enlarged main pulmonary artery, and an enlarged right pulmonary artery. *B*, Lateral chest x-ray shows filling in of the retrosternal space and an enlarged left pulmonary artery. (From Murphy, M. L., Dinh, H., and Nicholson, D.: Chronic cor pulmonale. *In* Bone, R. C. [ed.]: Disease-a-Month, Oct 1989 p. 687.)

tially have a restricted vascular bed, with normal or near-normal pulmonary artery pressures at rest. As their disease process worsens with the development of airway disease and further deterioration of gas exchange, secondary changes in the vasculature occur and resting pulmonary artery hypertension and cor pulmonale develop.

CLINICAL MANIFESTATIONS OF COR PULMONALE WITH HEART FAILURE. These include increasing dyspnea; paroxysmal cough, occasionally with syncope; and fluid retention with edema and sometimes ascites. The distended neck veins exhibit prominent *a* and *v* waves and do not collapse with inspiration. Central cyanosis frequently is present, and hypoxemia, as measured by arterial oxygen saturation, correlates with the pulmonary artery pressure[131] (Fig. 49–8). Pulsus paradoxus (pp. 24 and 1476) may be present. Right ventricular hypertrophy is indicated by a palpable parasternal or subxiphoid heave. On auscultation, a (right-sided) S_3 gallop (heard along the left sternal edge or in the epigastrium and accentuated by inspiration) and a loud pulmonic second sound frequently are present. A holosystolic murmur along the lower left parasternal edge, accentuated by inspiration, usually indicates tricuspid regurgitation; its presence can be confirmed by Doppler echocardiography.[132] These cardiac findings can be evanescent and can develop quickly when acute respiratory failure is superimposed on COPD. Radionuclide techniques have shown that RV ejection fractions are correlated positively with arterial oxygen tension and inversely with arterial pCO_2[133] (Fig. 49–10). Examination of the lungs reveals diffuse inspiratory and expiratory rhonchi and wheezes, and the liver is enlarged and frequently pulsatile. If acute respiratory failure is present in addition, papilledema, confusion, a hyperkinetic circulation, and asterixis also may be present.

It is important to recognize that the hypoxemia of patients with COPD may be profoundly worsened during sleep.[134] This phenomenon may cause a further rise in pulmonary artery pressure and nocturnal cardiac arrhythmias.[135,136] The possible pathogenetic role of these phenomena in the development of cor pulmonale is discussed below.

Treatment

REDUCTION OF AIRWAY OBSTRUCTION. The management of cor pulmonale in COPD is to relieve pulmonary hypertension by improving gas exchange.[136–138] This is accomplished by reducing bronchial smooth muscle constriction, promoting drainage of retained secretions, promptly and vigorously treating respiratory tract infections, and providing supplemental oxygen. The first two goals can be achieved simultaneously with the use of bronchodilators. In addition to relieving smooth muscle spasm, the sympathomimetics also increase mucociliary transport.[139] The net effect of these measures is to reduce airway obstruction and improve the regional distribution of inspired air and, in that manner, $\dot{V}_A/\dot{Q}$ relationships. Methylxanthines may provide benefits above and beyond the usual bronchodilatation, for this class of compounds has been reported to produce favorable hemodynamic effects as well. In one study, the intravenous administration of aminophylline in patients with cor pulmonale was shown to reduce mean pulmonary artery and right and left ventricular end-diastolic pressures significantly without inducing a change in the cardiac index,[140] and in another, right and left ventricular ejection fractions were increased.[141] The use of methylxanthines to improve diaphragmatic function has been in vogue for a number of years. Although this effect does occur, it is quite limited and of questionable clinical significance. Moreover, the effect is nonspecific and also has been observed with beta-adrenergic agonists.

OXYGEN ADMINISTRATION. The administration of supplemental oxygen in a controlled manner represents a major advance in the treatment of cor pulmonale. In acute respiratory failure, supplemental oxygen results in prompt and often dramatic improvement in pulmonary hemodynamics.[70] In fact, long-term oxygen therapy is the only treatment thus far shown to decrease mortality in COPD and to stop the progression of pulmonary hypertension.[142–144] In patients with progressive RV hypertrophy or recurrent heart failure from cor pulmonale associated with severe hypoxemia ($PaO_2 < 50$ mm Hg) and severe pulmonary hypertension, marked improvement has been found when oxygen was administered for 12 to 15 hours per day.[145,146]

Two major controlled studies of different aspects of long-term oxygen therapy in patients with COPD have been carried out. The U.S. (NIH-sponsored) Nocturnal Oxygen Therapy Trial[142] sought to determine if oxygen given for 19 hours a day improved survival over that observed with predominant nocturnal therapy (12 hr/day). The English (MRC) trial, on the other hand, sought to discover whether oxygen administration for 15 to 24 hours of the day had a positive effect on survival as compared with no oxygen.[143] The composite data are contained in Figure 49–13. Survival was poorest in those who did not receive supplemental oxygen and best in those who received it for the longest portion of the day.

According to recent data, survival tends to be greatest in

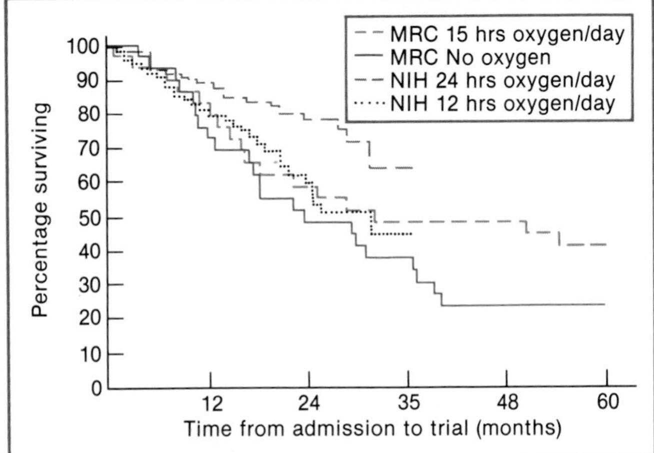

FIGURE 49–13. Survival curves in the MRC (British) and NIH (U.S.) long-term oxygen therapy trials in patients with severe hypoxemia and cor pulmonale. (From Flenley, D. C., and Muir, A. L.: Cardiovascular effects of oxygen therapy for pulmonary arterial hypertension. Clin. Chest Med. *4*:297, 1983.)

younger patients (<60 years of age) with only moderate pulmonary artery hypertension at the time of therapy (mean pulmonary artery pressure <30 mm Hg).[144]

The criterion most commonly used to initiate chronic oxygen therapy is an arterial oxygen tension of 55 mm Hg or less. The inspired oxygen concentration is adjusted to produce a pO_2 of 60 mm Hg or greater. If chronic oxygen therapy is contemplated, it is *mandatory* to demonstrate that the supplemental oxygen will not result in worsening of alveolar hypoventilation with progressive hypercapnia and deterioration of the patient's mental status.

With the widespread availability of pulse oximetry, the place of this technique in the assessment of patients on long-term oxygen therapy is questioned. Although these devices are reasonably accurate under steady-state conditions, they can give false readings during exercise and in the presence of hemodynamic instability, dark skin pigmentation, jaundice, carboxyhemoglobin, and systemic alkalosis.[147] Equally important, pulse oximetry cannot detect acidosis or hypercapnia. Hence arterial blood gases, and not pulse oximetry, should be the means of selecting patients for long-term oxygen therapy. Once the patient's gas exchange is stable on oxygen, oximetry can then be used for monitoring.

VASODILATORS. Another proposed means of reducing pulmonary artery pressure is afterload reduction with vasodilators. This approach assumes that the RV failure seen with COPD results from increased afterload and that a significant feature of the latter is related to active vasoconstriction.[148] A number of drugs have been tried with varying degrees of effectiveness: isoproterenol,[149] phentolamine,[150] diazoxide,[151] prazosin,[152] hydralazine,[153,154] pirbuterol,[155] methyldopa,[156] and the calcium antagonists diltiazem, nifedipine, and nitrendipine.[157–159] During acute testing these have all been reported to improve pulmonary vascular hemodynamics.[160] Hydralazine (Fig. 49–14) and nifedipine appear to be particularly beneficial, and have been found to reduce pulmonary vascular resistance and increase cardiac output in patients with pulmonary hypertension from various causes[153–160] (p. 811). Nifedipine also has been shown to inhibit hypoxic vasoconstriction in patients with acute respiratory failure.[160]

Although there is no question that the aforementioned agents can increase RV stroke volume and reduce pulmonary vascular resistance acutely in patients with severe pulmonary hypertension, unfortunately this hemodynamic benefit does not carry over to the long run. To date, none of these drugs have lead to long-term clinical improvement or to improved survival.[155,157,161,162] In addition, vasodilator therapy can have significant side effects, such as worsening hypoxemia and systemic hypotension.[163] This form of treatment, although theoretically attractive, has not yet lived up to its promise.

OTHER MEASURES. The indications for the use of other therapeutic measures, such as phlebotomy, diuretics, and cardiac glycosides, are considerably less clear. In the case of *phlebotomy*, most older studies have demonstrated an improvement in the subjective complaints related to vascular engorgement, but no evidence of improvement in pulmonary gas exchange, mechanics, or hemodynamics has been found.[164,165] Newer evidence suggests that erythropheresis in patients with secondary polycythemia and cor pulmonale reduces blood viscosity and improves right ventricular function.[166,167] *Diuretics* are commonly used for cor pulmonale with failure, and although there is little question of their effectiveness in reducing fluid retention, there are scant data to demonstrate that they improve pulmonary hemodynamics or gas exchange in the absence of left ventricular decompensation. Excessive use of potent diuretics can aggravate the loss of H^+ and Cl^- induced by chronic hypercapnia and cause a severe metabolic alkalosis. Hence, they should be used sparingly.

The use of *cardiac glycosides* in patients with cor pulmonale is controversial (p. 489). Digitalis apparently is effective in raising cardiac output in patients with cor pulmonale at rest but only at the expense of concomitant increases in pulmonary artery pressures. The consensus is that there is no clear-cut evidence that cardiac glycosides are of substantial benefit *unless left ventricular failure coexists*.[168] Sympathomimetics such as terbutaline may, in addition to their beneficial effects on the tracheobronchial tree, exert a positive inotropic effect.[169]

PROGNOSIS. The outlook for patients with cor pulmonale secondary to COPD is difficult to state with certainty, for it is inextricably linked to the underlying disorder. When cor pulmonale develops in patients with emphysema, life expectancy is quite short, yet patients with bronchitis usually tolerate three to five episodes of failure before ultimately succumbing to the disease. Although long-term survival has been reported after the onset of cor pulmonale with heart failure, the 2- to 3-year survival rates range from 33 to 50 per cent[170–173] but may be improved with continuous oxygen therapy.

In both the NIH and MRC trials cited above, pulmonary vascular resistance and pulmonary artery pressure either declined or remained constant in those patients treated with

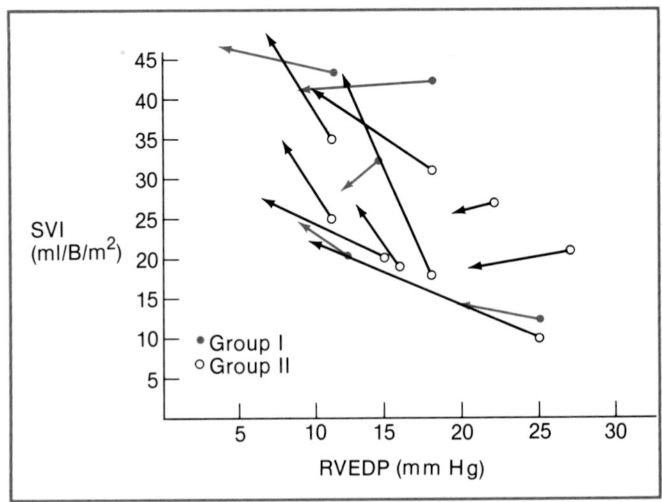

FIGURE 49–14. The relationship between right ventricular end-diastolic pressure (RVEDP) and stroke volume index (SVI) in 14 patients with right ventricular failure treated with oral hydralazine. Circles represent control and arrows represent post-hydralazine measurements. Patients in group I had significant reductions in mean pulmonary arterial pressure, while those in group II did not. (From Rubin, L. J.: Cardiovascular effects of vasodilator therapy for pulmonary arterial hypertension. Clin. Chest Med. *4*:309, 1983.)

TABLE 49-4 CAUSES OF CHRONIC HYPOVENTILATION SYNDROME

(1) Impaired Ventilatory Control
- a. Functional
  - Obesity-hypoventilation syndrome
  - Myxedema
  - Drugs (narcotics, sedatives)
  - Metabolic abnormalities (hypokalemia, hypophosphatemia, hypomagnesemia, metabolic alkalosis)
- b. Structural
  - Brain stem infarction or neoplasm
- c. Idiopathic
  - Primary alveolar hypoventilation

(2) Neuromuscular disorders
- a. Myopathies
  - Muscular dystrophy
- b. Neuropathies
  - Bilateral diaphragm paralysis
  - Poliomyelitis
  - Amyotrophic lateral sclerosis
  - Cervical spinal cord injury
  - Guillain-Barré syndrome
- c. Disorders of neuromuscular junction
  - Myasthenia gravis

(3) Chest-wall Abnormalities
- a. Kyphoscoliosis
- b. Thoracoplasty

(4) Airway Obstruction
- a. Upper airway
  - Tracheal stenosis
  - Obstructive sleep apnea
  - Laryngeal or nasal polyps
  - Tonsillar hypertrophy
- b. Lower airway
  - Chronic obstructive pulmonary disease

(5) Parenchymal Lung Disease
- a. Interstitial lung disease
- b. Surgical resection

From Strumpf, D. A., Millman, R. P., and Hill, N. S.: The management of chronic hypoventilation. Chest *98*:474, 1990.

oxygen, suggesting a stabilization of the disease process. In those not so treated, mean pulmonary pressure and total pulmonary vascular resistance rose, on the average, 3 mm Hg and 100 dynes-sec-cm^{-5} per year, respectively.

Inadequate Ventilatory Drive

(Table 49–4)

The common denominator in this category of disorders causing cor pulmonale is a depressed output from the respiratory center, with resultant generalized alveolar hypoventilation. Cor pulmonale is then the result of pulmonary hypertension caused by chronic hypoxemia and acidemia.

OBESITY-HYPOVENTILATION SYNDROME. The association of extreme obesity with alveolar hypoventilation was originally made by Sir William Osler; Burwell et al. subsequently coined the term "pickwickian syndrome" to describe the combination of obesity, somnolence, plethora, and edema.[174] Despite many investigations, the pathogenesis of the hypoventilation in this syndrome remains obscure.[175] Excessive reduction of chest-wall compliance and muscle weakness secondary to obesity may account in part for this syndrome, but many extremely obese people with these defects do not hypoventilate. These patients may have abnormally low ventilatory responses to hypercapneic and anoxic stimulation, which improve with treatment.[176] Consequently hyposensitivity of the respiratory center with depressed ventilatory drive, whether acquired or preexistent, is probably a background factor.

The primary *treatment* of this disorder consists of weight reduction. The respiratory stimulant progesterone and its congeners have been shown to increase alveolar ventilation so that hypoxemia, hypercapnia, and cor pulmonale all improve substantially.[177,178] This may prove to be a useful adjunct until weight is reduced. If respiratory and cardiac failure are life-threatening, ventilatory assistance may be required.

SLEEP APNEA SYNDROME. After the description of the pickwickian syndrome, variant manifestations such as periodic respirations and hypersomnia were recognized, and it soon became apparent that patients with disturbed respirations during sleep could develop pulmonary hypertension and cor pulmonale.[179,179a] This has been designated the sleep apnea syndrome. Three types of patterns have been recorded (Fig. 49–15): (1) *central apnea,* in which airflow stops in conjunction with cessation of all respiratory muscle effort; (2) *obstructive apnea,* in which upper airway obstruction causes airflow to cease despite continuing or increasing efforts of the inspiratory muscles. The obstruction is believed to result from relaxation or discoordination of the buccal and pharyngeal muscles, from collapse of the walls of the pharynx due to failure of the genioglossus muscle, from greatly enlarged tonsils or adenoids, from backward movement of the tongue during sleep, and from narrowing of the upper airway secondary to marked obesity;[180] and (3) *mixed apnea,* in which airflow and respiratory effort stop early in the episode, followed by a resumption of unsuccessful respiratory effort.[179,180,180a]

The apneic periods, which can occur 40 to 60 times per hour,[180] are associated with phasic hypoxemia and hypercapnia. Alterations in gas exchange may be quite striking, and the pO_2 can fall to 20 to 25 mm Hg with saturations below 50 per cent. Pulmonary and systemic arterial pressures rise with each apneic period, and stroke volume, heart rate, and cardiac output fall.[176] With repetitive episodes, the pulmonary artery pressures progressively increase throughout the night[176] (Fig. 49–16). Hence, pulmonary hypertension is most severe in the morning. During the day, the pressures fall only to rise again with sleep the next night. Eventually hypoxemia, hypercapnia, and pulmonary hypertension become permanent and gradually worsen while the patient is awake.

In association with the fluctuation in gas exchange, patients often have severe bradyarrhythmias and tachyarrhythmias.[181] The former usually occur during periods of apnea, whereas the latter begin with the onset of breathing. The type of arrhythmias found consist of sinus bradycardia, sinus arrest, long asystolic periods (ranging from 2 to 13 seconds), sinoatrial block, premature atrial contractions, atrial fibrillation, ventricular premature beats with bigeminy and trigeminy, multifocal premature beats, and ventricular tachycardia.[181–183] Pulmonary capillary wedge pressures also may increase during periods of apnea.[184] The clinical symptomatology differs, depending on the type, frequency, and intensity of the abnormal, sleep-related respiratory pattern.

The patient rarely reaches the deep stages of sleep because of hypoxic arousal and therefore is chronically sleep-deprived. The other common clinical manifestations are loud

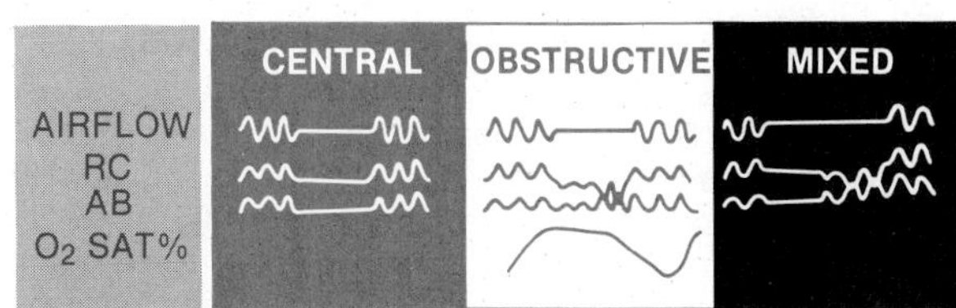

FIGURE 49–15. Schematic representation of the three patterns of apnea that develop during sleep in humans. RC and AB represent ribcage and abdominal displacement, respectively. O_2 sat = oxygen saturation. In each type, airflow at the nose and mouth is absent, indicating apnea. In central apneas, respiratory efforts as measured by the movement of the ribcage and abdomen are absent. During obstructive apneas, the efforts by the chest-wall muscles are present throughout the entire episode. In mixed apneas, both central and obstructive patterns are present. (From Strohl, K. P., et al.: Physiologic basis of therapy for sleep apnea. Am. Rev. Resp. Dis. *134*:791, 1986.)

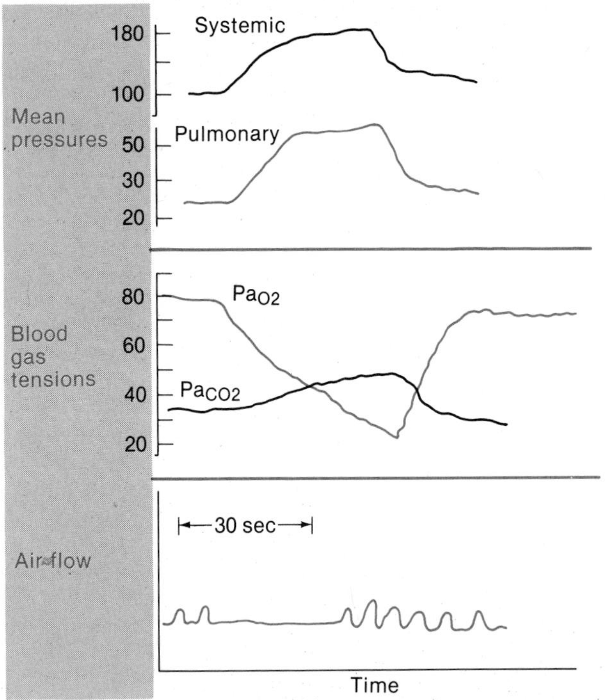

FIGURE 49-16. Schematic representation of hemodynamic and blood gas events during an apneic period. Respiratory pauses are associated with a fall in PaO_2 that usually exceeds the rise in $PaCO_2$. The combined hypoxia and hypercapnia are probably responsible for the rise in pulmonary arterial pressure which occurs with each apnea. Note that baseline pulmonary arterial pressure is slightly higher after the apneic episode. (From Weil, J. V.: Pulmonary hypertension and cor pulmonale in hypoventilating patients. *In* Weir, E. K., and Reeves, J. T. [eds.]: Pulmonary Hypertension. Mount Kisco, N.Y., Futura Publishing Co., 1984, p. 321.)

snoring, abnormal behavior during sleep (somnambulism, tremors, or myoclonus), altered states of consciousness, nocturnal enuresis, morning headache, daytime hypersomnolence, hypnagogic hallucinations, and systemic hypertension (Fig. 49–17). Most patients with sleep apnea are *not obese* and ventilate normally when awake. Patients with obstructive apnea tend to have less severe hypoventilation and fewer hemodynamic abnormalities than do patients with the other varieties. The diagnosis is readily established by performing polysomnography during sleep.

Several well-controlled studies indicate that about 20 per cent of patients with sleep apnea syndrome will have coexistent COPD and that most of these patients will develop pulmonary hypertension.[185,186] Diagnosis of the combined problem can be difficult unless specifically sought, and treatment of both problems is required to control the patient's symptoms.

The cause of sleep apnea is unknown. The weight of current evidence indicates that obstructive apneas occur because of occlusion of the upper airway in the region of the pharynx.[180] Central apneas, on the other hand, may have multiple mechanisms, including sleep-induced alteration in respiratory muscle drive, depressed central ventilatory output, and/or a change in the thresholds for sleep and/or arousal.[180]

Management. Sedatives and antihistamines should be assiduously avoided or withdrawn, and oxygen should be used with caution. Death has followed the use of both narcoleptics and oxygen administered in an uncontrolled manner.[180] Treatment of central apnea consists of respiratory stimulants or nocturnal ventilatory support with respirators.[180] Phrenic nerve or diaphragmatic pacing also has been recommended.[189] In obstructive apnea, tracheostomy and nasal CPAP (continuous positive airway pressure applied to the nose during sleep) are the most commonly used therapeutic modalities.[180] The former bypasses the area of obstruction, whereas the latter is believed to act as a pneumatic splint that prevents upper airway collapse. In an obese patient with obstructive apnea, weight reduction may obviate the need for a permanent tracheal cannula. Removal of enlarged tonsils and/or adenoids or surgical enlargement of the entrance to the airway may be enormously helpful. Nocturnal oxygen therapy may be helpful in some patients by reducing the duration of the apneic periods and decreasing the related arrhythmias but, as already indicated, should be used with care.[187]

PRIMARY ALVEOLAR HYPOVENTILATION. Generalized alveolar hypoventilation in the absence of obesity or intrinsic disease of the lungs, chest wall, or neuromuscular apparatus has been ascribed to a failure of the autonomic control of ventilation. Most cases are acquired and are seen after encephalitis, brain stem surgery, meningitis, and the like, but congenital occurrence has been reported.[188] In this rare condition, the respiratory center does not respond normally to its chemical stimuli, and the patient has a flat or markedly depressed ventilatory–carbon dioxide response curve. An affected patient can improve alveolar ventilation and restore the arterial oxygen and carbon dioxide to normal by voluntary hyperventilation. This syndrome has been called *Ondine's curse*. The pathogenesis and treatment are similar to that outlined for other forms of generalized alveolar hypoventilation. An interesting therapeutic development is long-term pacing of the diaphragm by means of electrical stimulation of the phrenic nerves.[189]

CHRONIC MOUNTAIN SICKNESS. Some acclimatized residents of high altitudes suffer a transient loss of their adaptation after short stays at sea level and, on return to altitude, develop acute pulmonary edema with circulatory and electrocardiographic changes similar to those seen in acute cor pulmonale.[190] Some people who remain at high altitude lose their acclimatization and develop signs and symptoms of generalized alveolar hypoventilation with chronic cor pulmonale. This syndrome is variously called *chronic mountain sickness, soroche*, or *Monge disease*.[191] The mechanism for the hypoventilation is unknown, but it has been postulated that it is due to an adaptation or desensitization of the hypoxic chemoreceptors in the carotid body to chronic hypoxia.[192] The only treatment is removal of the patient to sea level, where pulmonary artery pressure usually falls acutely. With prolonged residence at sea level, polycythemia disappears, and

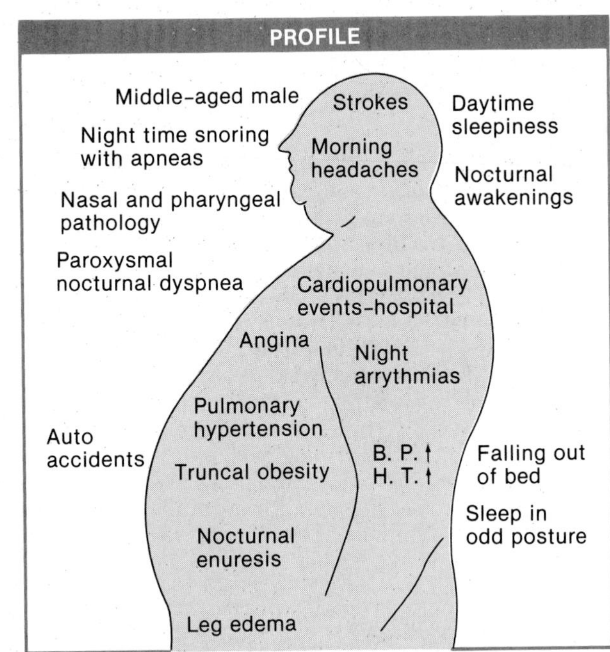

FIGURE 49-17. Clinical profile in patients with hypersomnia-sleep apnea syndromes. BP = blood pressure; HT = hematocrit. (From Burack, B.: The hypersomnia–sleep apnea syndrome: Its recognition in clinical cardiology. Am. Heart J. *107*:543, 1984.)

there is believed to be some involution of the structural changes of the pulmonary vessels.

UPPER AIRWAY OBSTRUCTION. Obstruction of the upper airways may be responsible for an inadequate ventilatory drive, global alveolar hypoventilation, and cor pulmonale. For the most part, this occurs in children,[193] especially black children, who have enlarged tonsils and adenoids; however, cor pulmonale has been reported to follow acute tonsillitis in adults.[194] Other causes include vascular ring (p. 954), macroglossia, micrognathia, laryngotracheomalacia, laryngeal web, Crouzon disease, Hurler syndrome, and severe Pierre Robin syndrome,[195,196] but it also can develop with obstruction of the upper airway during sleep in both children and adults.[197] The mechanism for the hypoventilation is not clear. It has been suggested that an abnormally reactive pulmonary vascular bed, a defect in the central control of respiration, and an interference with normal sleep physiology, as in the sleep apnea syndrome, may play a part, singly or in combination. There is little direct evidence for the first mechanism. However, it is known that ventilatory responsiveness to carbon dioxide is blunted in these patients and that it does not return to normal after therapy.[198]

The clinical features may mimic asthma, but more often the patients display somnolence, respiratory stridor, and recurrent respiratory tract infections. Treatment consists of surgical removal of the obstruction.

PULMONARY VASCULAR DISORDERS (see also Chap. 27). This category consists of diseases such as primary pulmonary hypertension that primarily affect the pulmonary vasculature, with minimal or no parenchymal involvement. These diseases represent the most straightforward pathogenetic sequence in which pulmonary hypertension and RV overloading are consequences of a progressive increase in pulmonary vascular resistance resulting from gradual obliteration of the pulmonary vascular bed. In addition to their pathophysiology, these diseases share in common the symptom of dyspnea and strikingly high pulmonary artery pressures, despite the fact that both vital capacity and pulmonary gas exchange may be only minimally impaired.[199] The latter finding frequently is of considerable diagnostic importance.

Chronic Suppurative Pulmonary Disease Associated with Cor Pulmonale

The two prime examples of chronic suppurative disease associated with chronic cor pulmonale are bronchiectasis and cystic fibrosis.

BRONCHIECTASIS. This chronic inflammatory disease is characterized clinically by cough and the production of copious amounts of purulent sputum and pathologically by cylindrical and saccular dilatation of airways.[200,201] In most patients one can elicit a history of pneumonia developing as a complication of measles, pertussis, or some other contagious disease of childhood. It is thought that bacterial pneumonia and associated atelectasis are responsible for the destruction and dilatation of the bronchial walls. A small percentage of cases are associated with congenital defects such as Kartagener triad and either congenital or acquired defects in immune mechanisms. Cor pulmonale develops in far-advanced cases in which destruction of lung tissue and fibrosis is extensive. The mechanisms for pulmonary hypertension are believed to be capillary loss, hypoxia, and increased bronchial-pulmonary collateral blood flow. Formerly this was a relatively common affliction, but bronchiectasis has decreased considerably in incidence during the past three decades, presumably because of the increasing use of antibiotics.

CYSTIC FIBROSIS. This genetic (autosomal recessive) defect is characterized by the secretion from exocrine glands of thick, tenacious mucus in which the mucopolysaccharide content is relatively insoluble and easily denatured. The lungs are involved to some extent in virtually all patients with the disease, and the thick mucus throughout the tracheobronchial tree partially or completely obstructs air passages, giving rise to focal atelectasis, pneumonia, bronchiectasis, and abscess formation.[202] Cor pulmonale is an important feature in the natural history, and it contributes to 70 per cent of the deaths.[203] Clinical recognition of the cardiac involvement in cystic fibrosis can be difficult in the early stage of the disease. Many investigators use noninvasive radionuclide scanning and/or echocardiography to improve detection.[204] One group has developed an echocardiographic scoring system that provides a method for assessing the progression of the cardiac involvement and for evaluating prognosis.[205] Physiological studies have suggested that hypoxia is the principal stimulus to the production of pulmonary hypertension, and pathological data have supported this.[206-208] In the past, the development of cardiac failure usually presaged death within a few months. In recent years, however, the prognosis has been improving, and a number of patients have survived for considerable periods into their twenties. These patients have been maintained on a vigorous, comprehensive pulmonary care program with postural drainage, antibiotics, and bronchodilators.

Restrictive Lung Diseases

This category encompasses a multitude of diseases which have in common a destruction of functioning pulmonary parenchyma with restriction of the pulmonary vascular bed. The latter results from a physical loss of vessels as well as from intrinsic abnormalities in the lumina and walls of those remaining. Essentially, five types of processes alone or in combination can produce this effect: (1) diffuse interstitial, (2) diffuse alveolar, (3) mixed alveolar-interstitial, (4) chest wall and pleural, and (5) extensive resection of lung tissue with disease in the residual parenchyma. Specific examples of the first three categories are sarcoidosis, radiation fibrosis, connective tissue disorders with primary or secondary lung involvement, fibrosing alveolitis, alveolar proteinosis, pneumoconiosis, and progressive massive fibrosis. The prototypes for the fourth and fifth categories are thoracoplasty for chronic tuberculosis and surgical resections for granulomatous disease or bronchiectasis.

Pulmonary parenchymal disease, especially when complicated by fibrosis of tissue and secondary vascular changes, can lead to severe pulmonary hypertension. As with the other conditions with a restricted vascular bed, the pulmonary hypertension is initially confined to circumstances in which the cardiac output is elevated. As the vascular bed becomes further restricted and the vessels stiffen, pulmonary hypertension persists at rest and intensifies with increased blood flow. As long as hypoxemia remains mild, pulmonary hypertension is modest, but cor pulmonale develops with respiratory failure. Fortunately, the sequence is not inevitable in most patients with these problems. If the pathological process stabilizes, as is often the case, the patient is left with modest pulmonary hypertension at rest, which is usually well tolerated.[59]

PATHOPHYSIOLOGY. In these diseases, the lungs are stiff, with reduced volumes, and minute ventilation is high, with or without an elevated alveolar ventilation. Arterial oxygen tension usually is moderately reduced at rest, but severe hypoxemia may develop with exercise. The diffusing capacity is low and fails to increase normally as cardiac output rises. In contrast to the chronic obstructive syndromes, the correlation between arterial blood gases and pulmonary artery pressure is poor,[209] and there seems to be a parallel deterioration in pulmonary mechanics and hemodynamics.[210] As a general rule, when the vital capacity exceeds 80 per cent of normal, hemodynamics are normal. When vital capacity is between 50 and 80 per cent, vascular resistance is increased and pulmonary artery pressure in the resting state is at the upper limits of normal. When vital capacity is below 50 per cent, pulmonary hypertension usually is present at rest. The role of hypoxic vasoconstriction in these patients has been difficult to clarify. Experimental evidence indicates that the ability of the pulmonary vasculature to respond to alveolar hypoxia is abnormal in diseased regions, so that when hypoxia does occur, blood is shifted toward the affected areas, thus worsening net gas exchange.[18] In any event, the development of severe hypoxemia and carbon dioxide retention heralds the onset of right ventricular failure, which usually is seen late in the course.

CLINICAL FEATURES. In keeping with the pathophysiology, the prominent symptoms of restrictive lung disease are tachypnea at rest and severe dyspnea on exertion. Fine inspiratory rales are found, along with the previously mentioned signs of pulmonary hypertension and right ventricular hypertrophy and/or failure. Early in the course of patients with pulmonary fibrosis, glucocorticoids or immunosuppressive drugs may be helpful if noninfectious inflammatory processes are believed to be present. In the late stages with extensive pulmonary fibrosis, these modalities are unsuccessful; all that can be offered is continuous oxygen therapy, diuretics, and cardiac glycosides. Vasodilator therapy is still experimental but may offer some hope in selected patients.[148] Although many of the diseases in this category progress slowly, once cor pulmonale develops, the prognosis is poor and lung transplantation may be the only hope.

Disorders of the Neuromuscular Apparatus and Chest Wall

These disorders have in common the mechanical failure of the bellows apparatus, through weakness or paralysis of the respiratory muscles or through distortion of the geometry of the thorax. Several factors contribute to the development of cor pulmonale.

FAILURE OF THE NEUROMUSCULAR APPARATUS. Respiratory muscle weakness can result from generalized diseases of muscles such as myopathic infiltrating diseases or muscular dystrophy, but it more commonly follows a neurological disorder, such as a cord lesion at or below the third cervical vertebra, amyotrophic lateral sclerosis, myasthenia gravis, poliomyelitis, or Guillain-Barré syndrome.[199] In all of these diseases, the primary derangement is *generalized alveolar hypoventilation* from mechanical impedance to the movement of the rib cage, diaphragm, or both. The lungs and airways usually are not diseased, although they can become so with retained secretions and multiple aspirations. Although acute respiratory failure is common in these diseases, for cor pulmonale to develop in response to the hypoxic and hypercapneic stimuli the disorder must be chronic; consequently, this complication tends to be seen more often with cord lesions than with the other conditions just noted. Mechanical ventilatory support is the only treatment for the hypoventilation; a cuirass type of respirator is effective in these patients. Along with this, vigorous bronchial toilet facilitates the impaired handling of secretions that frequently coexists.

DIAPHRAGMATIC PARALYSIS. Bilateral diaphragmatic paralysis is an uncommon but insidious and frequently unrecognized cause of cor pulmonale.[211] In the upright position ventilation may be normal or almost so, but with assumption of the supine position gas exchange deteriorates. The diagnosis may be suspected in the patient with supine breathlessness, a disturbed sleep pattern, paradoxical (i.e., inward) motion of the abdomen on inspiration, and a low vital capacity in the erect position. Treatment consists of assisting ventilation when the patient is supine or during sleep. This can easily be accomplished under most circumstances with a rocking bed. When this is inadequate, electrical pacing of the diaphragm may be used.[189] Occasionally, diaphragmatic fatigue can contribute to the respiratory failure of COPD.[212] Bilateral diaphragmatic paralysis can occur after cardiac surgery.[213] The use of ice cardioplegia can damage the phrenic nerves and result in respiratory failure that becomes manifest as soon as the patient is removed from the ventilator postoperatively. This complication usually is transitory, and diaphragmatic function returns.

CHEST-WALL DISORDERS. The common congenital or acquired abnormalities that distort the geometry of the thoracic cage include kyphoscoliosis, pectus excavatum, pectus carinatum, and ankylosing spondylitis; of these, only kyphoscoliosis is associated with cor pulmonale.[214] *Kyphosis* refers to any posterior angulation of the spine, and *scoliosis* consists of a lateral displacement with at least one compensatory curve in the opposite direction. A kyphotic angle exceeding 100 degrees or an angle of scoliosis in excess of 120 degrees may be associated with cor pulmonale.[215] Such marked structural abnormalities of the thorax lead to abnormal positioning and functioning of the respiratory muscles, compression of the lung and pulmonary vasculature, and abnormal gas exchange.[215,216] In addition, it has been suggested that scoliosis interferes with the growth and development of alveoli and pulmonary arteries[217]; dyspnea is the major symptom of these disorders.

Therapy is directed toward avoiding complicating infections; episodes of acute respiratory failure are treated with mechanical ventilation. Surgical improvement of the thoracic deformity often is not associated with a commensurate change in cardiorespiratory function.[218]

NONINVASIVE ASSESSMENT OF COR PULMONALE

Echocardiography

M-mode echocardiography in adults with obstructive airway disease has been disappointing because the pulmonary hyperinflation associated with these conditions frequently precludes adequate visualization of the cardiac valves and chambers. Two-dimensional techniques can overcome this deficiency and permit visualization of right atrial and ventricular cavity dimensions and wall thickness (Fig. 49–18). These parameters are markedly influenced by the state of ventricular function and correlate well with radionuclide parameters of size and function.[219] The right atrium, right ventricle, and pulmonary artery are dilated. The two-dimensional echocardiogram also is useful in excluding left-sided heart disease as a cause of pulmonary hypertension and RV enlargement.

Various echocardiographic techniques available for the noninvasive assessment of pulmonary artery pressure are discussed on p. 80. The most useful of these is the Doppler echocardiographic assessment of the velocity of tricuspid regurgitant blood flow, which, when used in the Bernoulli equation, can be used to determine the right ventricular–right atrial pressure gradient. When this is added to the right atrial pressure, which is assessed clinically, the pulmonary artery systolic pressure can be estimated. This technique is quite useful in the identification of patients with chronic lung disease who have cor pulmonale.[220–224,224a]

Electrocardiographic Findings

(Table 49–5)

In the past, the use of the electrocardiogram to make the diagnosis of cor pulmonale has centered on the electrocardiographic demonstration of right ventricular hypertrophy (p. 126). The classic criteria of a shift of the mean QRS axis to the right (right axis deviation greater than +110 degrees), an R : S ratio in V_1 greater than 1, and an R : S ratio in V_6 of less than 1 were derived from patients with congenital heart disease[225,226] and have proved to be relatively poor criteria of cor pulmonale in patients with chronic obstructive lung disease.[227,228] The reason is that moderate RV hypertrophy is a late manifestation of cor pulmonale and occurs only after prolonged dilatation of the ventricle.[229]

Kilcoyne and associates studied 200 patients with chronic obstructive lung disease and demonstrated that when the arterial oxygen saturation fell below 85 per cent and mean pulmonary pressure rose to 25 mm Hg or greater, one or more of the following changes would develop in the electrocardiogram: (1) a rightward shift of the mean QRS axis of 30 degrees or more from its previous position; (2) inverted, biphasic, or flattened T waves in the right precordial leads; (3) depressed ST segments in leads II, III, and aV_f; and (4) incomplete or complete right bundle branch block.[228]

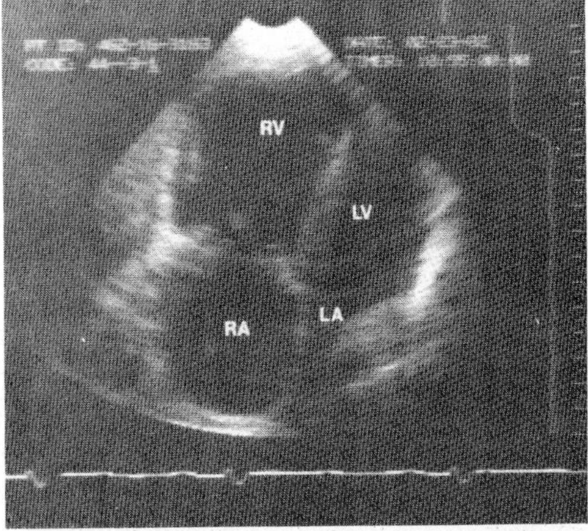

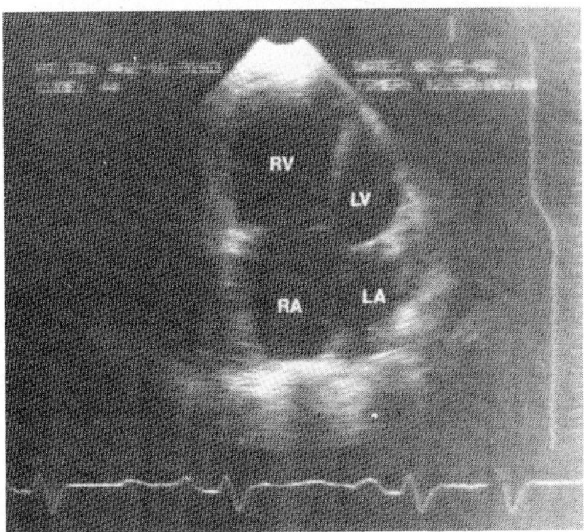

FIGURE 49–18. Echocardiogram from a 47-year-old man with pulmonary hypertension before *(left)* and 48 hours after *(right)* beginning therapy with nifedipine. The right atrium and right ventricle are greatly increased in size before treatment and are reduced in size by therapy. (From Rubin, L. J.: Cardiovascular effects of vasodilator therapy for pulmonary arterial hypertension. Clin. Chest Med. *4*:309, 1983.)

TABLE 49-5 ELECTROCARDIOGRAPHIC CHANGES IN COR PULMONALE

ECG CRITERIA FOR COR PULMONALE WITHOUT OBSTRUCTIVE DISEASE OF THE AIRWAYS*

1. Right-axis deviation with a mean QRS axis to the right of +110°
2. R/S amplitude ratio in $V_1 > 1$
3. R/S amplitude ratio in $V_6 < 1$
4. Clockwise rotation of the electrical axis
5. P-pulmonale pattern
6. S_1Q_3 or $S_1S_2S_3$ pattern
7. Normal voltage QRS

ECG CHANGES IN CHRONIC COR PULMONALE WITH OBSTRUCTIVE DISEASE OF THE AIRWAYS†

1. Isoelectric P waves in lead I or right-axis deviation of the P vector
2. P-pulmonale pattern (an increase in P-wave amplitude in II, III, AV_f)
3. Tendency for right-axis deviation of the QRS
4. R/S amplitude ratio in $V_6 < 1$
5. Low-voltage QRS
6. S_1Q_3 or $S_1S_2S_3$ pattern
7. Incomplete (and rarely complete) right bundle branch block
8. R/S amplitude ratio in $V_1 > 1$
9. Marked clockwise rotation of the electrical axis
10. Occasional large Q wave or QS in the inferior or midprecordial leads, suggesting healed myocardial infarction

*Any one of the first three criteria suffices to raise suspicion of right ventricular hypertrophy. The diagnosis becomes more certain if two or more of these findings are present (2 and 7). The last four criteria commonly occur in cor pulmonale secondary to primary alveolar hypoventilation, interstitial disease of the lung, or pulmonary vascular disease.

†The first seven criteria are suggestive but nonspecific; the last three are more characteristic of cor pulmonale in obstructive disease of the airways.

Reproduced with permission from Holford, F. D.: The electrocardiogram in lung disease. *In* Fishman, A. P. (ed.): Pulmonary Diseases and Disorders. New York, McGraw-Hill Book Co., 1980, p. 140.

With an increase in arterial saturation, these alterations disappeared. The T-wave changes in the right precordial leads and the axis shifts to the right occurred with only modest elevations of pulmonary artery pressure, but if these elevations became more severe, and if recurrences were frequent, then the rightward rotation of the QRS axis and the T-wave changes in the right precordial leads tended to become persistent. If pulmonary function were not improved, true right-axis deviation (a frontal plane axis greater than +90 degrees) and increased R-wave voltage in the right precordial leads developed (Fig. 49–19). Once the latter occurred, the electrocardiogram was less likely to mirror any physiological variability, as reversion of the increased voltage to normal rarely occurred after improvement in arterial blood gases.

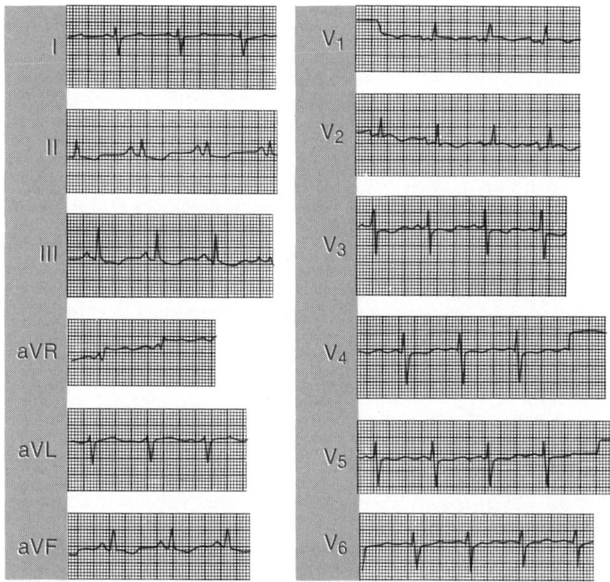

FIGURE 49–19. Electrocardiogram in a patient with emphysema and diffuse lung disease; there is right axis deviation, "P pulmonale," a QR pattern in V_1 and an rS pattern in V_6. (From McGowan, F. X., and Wagner, G. S.: The electrocardiogram in chronic lung disease. *In* Rubin, L. J. [ed.]: Pulmonary Heart Disease. Boston, Martinus Nijhoff, 1984, p. 117.)

Other studies have suggested that clockwise rotation, right-axis deviation, a qR pattern in aV_r, and electrocardiographic evidence of right atrial enlargement (P pulmonale), in that order, also would point to right ventricular hypertrophy in patients with chronic cor pulmonale. Occasionally in chronic obstructive lung disease, the mean QRS axis may be directed posteriorly, superiorly, and to the right, so that there is apparent left-axis deviation in the standard limb leads. This pattern, along with low voltage, most often is associated with emphysema.

The electrocardiogram is far more accurate in detecting RV hypertrophy in patients with primary pulmonary hypertension than it is in detecting such hypertrophy in patients with chronic lung disease. The latter causes flattening of the diaphragms and hyperinflation of the lung, which produces changes in the electrocardiogram resembling right ventricular hypertrophy.[103]

Electrocardiographic features of prognostic importance in severe chronic bronchial obstruction have been outlined by Kok-Jensen.[230] In a study of 288 patients, survival was found to be very poor in patients with a QRS axis of +90 to +180 degrees and an amplitude of the P wave in lead II of 0.20 mV or more; only 37 and 42 per cent, respectively, of the patients with these changes were alive after 4 years.

Arrhythmias. Ambulatory electrocardiograms obtained in 69 stable patients enrolled in the nocturnal oxygen therapy trial described earlier (p. 1591) showed multiple patterns.[231] Ventricular premature beats were found in 83 per cent, ventricular bigeminy in 68 per cent, paired ventricular premature beats in 61 per cent, and nonsustained ventricular tachycardia in 22 per cent of the patients. Sixty-nine per cent had supraventricular tachycardia. Repetitive ventricular arrhythmia occurred in 64 per cent of the patients and tended to be found in those with hypercapnia and edema.

Vectorcardiograms. The vectorcardiogram has been correlated with hemodynamics in patients with COPD, and a linear correlation has been found between terminal rightward QRS forces and mean pulmonary artery pressure during exercise. Because in one such correlation[232] no patient met the electrocardiographic criteria for RV hypertrophy, it was suggested that the vectorcardiogram may be more selective in identifying early hemodynamic abnormalities in the pulmonary circulation.

Radioisotope Imaging

A frequently used radionuclide for RV imaging is thallium-201. The distribution of this isotope is a function of regional myocardial blood flow and myocardial mass, and so only the left ventricle tends to be visualized at rest. Imaging of the right ventricle at rest usually signifies that hypertrophy and dysfunction of the RV are present.[233]

REFERENCES

ANATOMICAL AND PATHOPHYSIOLOGICAL CORRELATES

1. Chronic cor pulmonale: Report of an expert committee. Wld. Hlth. Org. Tech. Rep. Ser. *213*:1, 1961.
2. Chronic Cor Pulmonale. *In* Fowler, N. O.: Diagnosis of Heart Disease. New York, Springer-Verlag, 1991, pp. 268–282.
3. Lewis, T.: Observations upon ventricular hypertrophy with especial reference to preponderance of one or other chamber. Heart 5:367, 1914.
4. Emery, J. L., and Mithal, A.: Weight of cardiac ventricles at and after birth. Br. Heart J. *23*:313, 1961.
5. Keen, E. N.: The post-natal development of the human cardiac ventricles. J. Anat. *89*:484, 1955.
6. Arias-Stella, J., and Recavarren, S.: Right ventricular hypertrophy in native children living at high altitude. Am. J. Pathol. *41*:55, 1962.
7. Mathew, R., Thilenius, O. G., and Arcilla, R. A.: Comparative response of right and left ventricles to volume overload. Am. J. Cardiol. *38*:239, 1976.
8. Recavarren, S., and Arias-Stella, J.: Right ventricular hypertrophy in people born and living at high altitudes. Br. Heart J. *26*:806, 1964.
9. Penaloza, D., Sime, F., Banchero, N., et al.: Pulmonary hypertension in healthy men born and living at high altitudes. Am. J. Cardiol. *11*:150, 1963.
10. Fulton, R. M., Hutchinson, E. C., and Jones, A. M.: Ventricular weight in cardiac hypertrophy. Br. Heart J. *14*:413, 1952.
11. Mitchell, R. S., Stanford, R. E., Silvers, G. W., and Dart, G.: The right ventricle in chronic airway obstruction: A clinicopathologic study. Am. Rev. Respir. Dis. *114*:147, 1976.
12. Ishikawa, S., Fattal, G. A., Popiewicz, J., and Wyatt, J. P.: Functional morphometry of myocardial fibers in cor pulmonale. Am. Rev. Respir. Dis. *105*:358, 1972.
13. Brecher, G. A., and Galletti, P. M.: Functional anatomy of cardiac pumping. *In* Hamilton, A. F., and Dow, P. (eds.): Handbook of Physiology; Circulation. Vol. II. Washington, D.C., American Physiological Society, 1963, p. 759.

14. Visner, M. S., Arentzen, C. E., O'Connor, M. J., et al.: Alterations in left ventricular three-dimensional dynamic geometry and systolic function during acute right ventricular hypertension in the conscious dog. Circulation *67*:353, 1983.
15. Barnard, D., and Alpert, J. S.: Right ventricular function in health and disease. Current Problems in Cardiology *12*:417, 1987.
16. Laks, M. M., Garner, D., and Swan, H. J. C.: Volumes and compliances measured simultaneously in the right and left ventricles of the dog. Circ. Res. *20*:565, 1967.
17. Abel, F. L., and Waldhausen, J. A.: Effects of alterations in pulmonary vascular resistance on right ventricular function. J. Thorac. Cardiovasc. Surg. *54*:886, 1967.
18. Abel, F. L.: Effects of alterations in peripheral resistance on left ventricular function. Proc. Soc. Exp. Biol. Med. *120*:52, 1965.
19. Morrison, D., Goldman, S., Wright, A. L., et al.: The effect of pulmonary hypertension on systolic function of the right ventricle. Chest *84*:250, 1983.
20. Sarnoff, S. J., and Berglund, E.: Ventricular function. I. Starling's law of the heart studied by means of simultaneous right and left ventricular function curves in the dog. Circulation *9*:706, 1954.
21. Spann, J. R., Buccino, R. A., Sonnenblick, E. H., and Braunwald, E. B.: Contractile state of cardiac muscle obtained from cats with experimentally produced ventricular hypertrophy and heart failure. Circ. Res. *21*:341, 1967.
22. Haggart, G. E., and Walker, A. M.: The physiology of pulmonary embolism as disclosed by quantitative occlusion of the pulmonary artery. Arch. Surg. *6*:764, 1923.
23. Gibbons, J. H., Hopkinson, M., and Churchill, E. D.: Changes in the circulation produced by gradual occlusion of the pulmonary artery. J. Clin. Invest. *11*:543, 1932.
24. Fineberg, M. H., and Wiggens, C. J.: Compensation and failure of the right ventricle. Am. Heart J. *11*:255, 1936.
25. Brooks, H., Kirk, E. S., Vokonas, P. S., et al.: Performance of the right ventricle under stress: Relation to right coronary flow. J. Clin. Invest. *50*:2176, 1971.
26. Krahl, V. E.: Anatomy of the mammalian lung. *In* Fenn, O. W., and Rahn, H. (eds.): Handbook of Physiology; Respiration. Vol. I. Washington, D.C., American Physiological Society, 1964, p. 224.
27. Hislop, A., and Reid, L.: Intrapulmonary arterial development during fetal life–branching pattern and structure. J. Anat. *113*:35, 1972.
28. Boyden, E. A., and Tompsett, D. H.: The changing patterns in the developing lungs of infants. Acta Anat. *61*:164, 1965.
29. Meyrick, B., and Reid, L.: Pulmonary hypertension: Anatomic and physiologic correlations. Clin. Chem. Med. *4*:199, 1983.
30. Fishman, A. P.: The normal pulmonary circulation. *In* Fishman, A. P. (ed.): Pulmonary Diseases and Disorders, 2nd ed. New York, McGraw-Hill Book Co., 1991, pp. 975–998.
31. Hebb, C.: Motor innervation of the pulmonary blood vessels of mammals. *In* Fishman, A. P., and Hecht, H. H. (eds.): The Pulmonary Circulation and the Interstitial Space. Chicago, University of Chicago Press, 1969, p. 195.
32. Allen, K. M., Wharton, J., Polak, J. M., and Ghaworth, S. G.: A study of nerves containing peptides in the pulmonary vasculature of healthy infants and children and those with pulmonary hypertension. Br. Heart J. *62*:353, 1989.
33. Fishman, A. P.: Dynamics of the pulmonary circulation. *In* Hamilton, W. F., and Dow, P. (eds.): Handbook of Physiology; Circulation. Vol. II. Washington, D.C., American Physiological Society, 1963, p. 1667.
34. Bard, P.: The pulmonary circulation and respiratory variations in the systemic circulation. *In* Bard, P. (ed.): Medical Physiology. St. Louis, C. V. Mosby, 1961, p. 231.
35. Brofman, B. L., Charms, B. L., Kohn, P. M., et al.: Unilateral pulmonary artery occlusion in man. Control studies. J. Thorac. Surg. *34*:206, 1957.
36. Guyton, A. C.: Circulatory Physiology: Cardiac Output and Its Regulation. Philadelphia, W. B. Saunders Company, 1963.
37. Maseri, A., Caldini, P., Howard, P., et al.: Determinants of pulmonary vascular volume–recruitment versus distensibility. Circ. Res. *31*:218, 1972.
38. Lanari, A., and Agrest, A.: Pressure-volume relationship in the pulmonary vascular bed. Acta Physiol. Lat. Am. *4*:116, 1954.
39. Caro, C. G.: Extensibility of blood vessels in isolated rabbit lung. J. Physiol. (Lond.) *178*:193, 1865.
40. Howell, J. B. L., Permutt, S., Proctor, D. F., and Riley, R. L.: Effect of inflation of the lung on different parts of the pulmonary vascular bed. J. Appl. Physiol. *16*:71, 1961.
41. Engelberg, J., and DuBois, A. B.: Mechanics of pulmonary circulation in isolated rabbit lungs. Am. J. Physiol. *186*:401, 1959.
42. Maseri, A., Caldini, P., Permutt, S., and Zierler, K. L.: Pressure volume relationship in the pulmonary circulation. *In* Widimsky, J., Daum, S., and Herzog, H. (eds.): Progress in Respiration Research. Vol. 5. Basel, S. Karger, 1970, p. 53.
43. Glazier, J. B., Hughes, J. M. B., Maloney, J. E., and West, J. B.: Measurements of capillary dimensions and blood volume in rapidly frozen lungs. J. Appl. Physiol. *26*:65, 1969.
44. West, J. B.: Ventilation/Blood Flow and Gas Exchange. 2nd ed. Philadelphia, F. A. Davis Co., 1970.
45. Zapol, W. M.: Acute respiratory failure in the surgical patient. *In* Fishman, A. P. (ed.): Pulmonary Diseases and Disorders. 2nd ed. New York, McGraw-Hill Book Co., 1991, pp. 2433–2442.
46. Permutt, S., and Riley, R. L.: Hemodynamics of collapsible vessels with tone: The vascular waterfall. J. Appl. Physiol. *18*:924, 1963.
47. Klocke, R. A.: Ventilation, pulmonary blood flow, and gas exchange. *In* Fishman, A. P. (ed.): Pulmonary Diseases and Disorders. 2nd ed. New York, McGraw-Hill Book Co., 1991, pp. 185–198.
48. LeBlanc, P., Ruff, F., and Milic-Emili, J.: Effect of age and body position on airway closure in man. J. Appl. Physiol. *28*:448, 1970.
49. Craig, D. B., Wahba, W. M., Don, H. F., et al.: Closing volume and its relationship to gas exchange in seated and supine position. J. Appl. Physiol. *31*:717, 1971.
50. Lenfant, C.: Measurements of ventilation-perfusion distribution with alveolar-arterial differences. J. Appl. Physiol. *18*:1090, 1963.
51. Raine, J. M., and Bishop, J. M.: A-a difference in O_2 tension and physiologic dead space in normal man. J. Appl. Physiol. *18*:284, 1963.
52. Severinghaus, J. W., and Stupfel, M.: Alveolar dead space as an index of distribution of blood flow in pulmonary capillaries. J. Appl. Physiol. *10*:335, 1957.
53. Grover, R. F.: Chronic hypoxic pulmonary hypertension. *In* Fishman, A. P. (ed.): The Pulmonary Circulation: Normal and Abnormal. Philadelphia, University of Pennsylvania Press, 1990, pp. 283–299.
54. Fishman, A. P.: Hypoxia and its effects on the pulmonary circulation. Circ. Res. *38*:221, 1976.
55. Bergofsky, E. H.: Mechanisms underlying vasomotor regulation of regional pulmonary blood flow in normal and disease states. Am. J. Med. *57*:378, 1974.
56. Bates, D. V., Macklem, P. T., and Christie, R. V.: Respiratory Function in Disease. 2nd ed. Philadelphia, W. B. Saunders Company, 1971, p. 75.
57. Engel, L. A., and Macklem, P. T.: Gas mixing and distribution in the lung. *In* Widdicombe, J. G. (ed.): Respiratory Physiology II. International Review of Physiology. Vol. 14. Baltimore, University Park Press, 1977, p. 37.
58. Sykes, M. K., McNicol, M. W., and Campbell, E. J. M.: Respiratory Failure. Oxford, Blackwell Scientific Publications, 1971, p. 56ff.
59. Habb, P. E., and Durand-Arczynska, W. Y.: Carbon monoxide effects on oxygen transport. *In* Crystal, R. G., et al. (eds.): The Lung: Scientific Foundations. New York, Raven Press, 1991, pp. 1267–1276.
60. Fowler, K. T., and Read, J.: Effect of alveolar hypoxia on zonal distribution of pulmonary blood flow. J. Appl. Physiol. *18*:244, 1963.
61. Lindsay, D. A., and Reed, J.: Pulmonary vascular responsiveness in the prognosis of chronic obstructive lung disease. Am. Rev. Respir. Dis. *105*:242, 1972.
62. Enson, Y., Guintini, C., Lewis, M. L., et al.: The influence of hydrogen ion concentration and hypoxia on the pulmonary circulation. J. Clin. Invest. *43*:1146, 1964.
63. Bergofsky, E. H., Haas, F., and Procelli, R. J.: Determination of the sensitive vascular sites from which hypoxia and hypercapnia elicit rises in pulmonary arterial pressure. Fed. Proc. *27*:1420, 1968.
64. Bergofsky, E. H.: Humoral control of the pulmonary circulation. Ann. Rev. Physiol. *42*:221, 1980.

CHRONIC COR PULMONALE

65. Fishman, A. P.: Pulmonary hypertension and cor pulmonale. *In* Fishman, A. P. (ed.): Pulmonary Diseases and Disorders. 2nd ed. New York, McGraw-Hill Book Co., 1988, pp. 999–1048.
66. U. S. Department of Health and Human Services, National Heart, Lung and Blood Institute, Division of Lung Diseases: Progress report, 1980, p. 121.
67. Respiratory Disease. Task force report on prevention, control and education. Washington, D.C., U.S. Department of Health, Education and Welfare, Public Health Service, National Institute of Health, 1977, p. 83.
68. Stuart-Harris, C. H., Twidle, R. H. S., and Clifton, M. A.: Hospital study of congestive heart failure with special reference to cor pulmonale. Br. Med. J. *2*:201, 1959.
69. Inter-Society Commission for Heart Disease Resources: Primary prevention of pulmonary heart disease. Circulation *41*:A-17, 1970.
70. Burrows, B., Kettel, L. J., Niden, A. H., et al.: Patterns of cardiovascular dysfunction in chronic obstructive lung disease. N. Engl. J. Med. *286*:912, 1972.
71. Bishop, J. M.: Hypoxia and pulmonary hypertension in chronic bronchitis. Prog. Resp. Dis. *9*:10, 1975.
72. Traver, G. A., Cline, M. G., and Burrows, B.: Predictors of mortality in chronic obstructive pulmonary disease. Am. Rev. Respir. Dis. *119*:895, 1979.
73. Fishman, A. P.: Cor pulmonale. Am. Rev. Respir. Dis. *114*:775, 1976.
74. Enson, Y.: Pulmonary heart disease. *In* Baum, G. L. and Wolinsky, E. (eds.): Textbook of Pulmonary Diseases. 4th ed. Boston, Little, Brown, 1989, pp. 1181–1197.
75. Palevesky, H. I., and Fishman, A. P.: Chronic cor pulmonale: Etiology and management. JAMA *263*:2347, 1990.
76. Berbel, L. N., and Miro, R. E.: Pulmonary hypertension in the pathogenesis of cor pulmonale. Cardiovasc. Rev. *4*:359, 1983.
77. Weitzenblum, E., Hirth, C., Duculone, A., et al.: Prognostic value of pulmonary artery pressure in chronic obstructive pulmonary disease. Thorax *36*:752, 1981.
78. Finlay, M., Middleton, H. C., Peake, M. D., and Howard, P.: Cardiac output, pulmonary hypertension, hypoxemia and survival in patients with chronic obstructive airways disease. Eur. J. Respir. Dis. *64*:252, 1983.
79. Wilkinson, M., Langhorne, C. A., Heath, D., et al.: A pathophysiological

study of 10 cases of hypoxia cor pulmonale. Q. J. Med. (New Series) *66*:65, 1988.
80. Thurlbeck, W. M., Henderson, J. A., Fraser, R. G., and Bates, D. V.: Chronic obstructive lung disease. A comparison between clinical, roentgenologic, functional and morphologic criteria in chronic bronchitis, emphysema, asthma and bronchiectasis. Medicine *48*:81, 1970.
81. Edwards, J. E.: Pathology of chronic pulmonary hypertension. Pathol. Annu. *9*:1, 1974.
82. Wagenvoort, C. A., and Wagenvoort, N.: Hypoxic pulmonary vascular lesions in man at high altitude and in patients with chronic respiratory disease. Pathol. Microbiol. *39*:276, 1973.
83. Semmens, M., and Reid, L.: Pulmonary arterial muscularity and right ventricular hypertrophy in chronic bronchitis and emphysema. Br. J. Dis. Chest. *68*:253, 1974.
84. Wagenvoort, C. A., Heath, D., and Edwards, J. E.: The Pathology of the Pulmonary Vasculature. Springfield, Ill., Charles C Thomas, 1964.
85. Roos, A.: Poiseuille's law and its limitation in vascular systems. *In* Grover, R. F. (ed.): Progress in Research in Emphysema and Chronic Bronchitis. Basel, Karger, 1963, p. 32.
86. Wells, R. E., and Merrill, E. W.: Influence of flow properties of blood upon viscosity hematocrit relationships. J. Clin. Invest. *41*:1591, 1962.
87. Rendas, A., Lennar, S., and Reid, L.: Aorto-pulmonary shunts in growing pigs: Functional and structural assessment of the changes in the pulmonary circulation. J. Thorac. Cardiovasc. Surg. *77*:109, 1979.
88. Balchum, O. J., Jung, R. C., Turner, A. F., and Jacobson, G.: Pulmonary artery to vein shunts in obstructive pulmonary disease. Am. J. Med. *43*:178, 1967.
89. Boushy, S. F., North, L. B., and Trice, J. A.: The bronchial arteries in chronic obstructive pulmonary disease. Am. J. Med. *46*:506, 1969.
90. Meyrick, B., and Reid, L.: Ultrastructural findings in lung biopsy material from children with congenital heart defects. Am. J. Pathol. *101*:527, 1980.
91. Rabinovitz, M., Haworth, S., Vanck, Z., et al.: Early pulmonary vascular changes in congenital heart disease studied in biopsy tissue. Hum. Pathol. *11*:499, 1980.
92. Marcus, J. H., McLean, R. L., Duffell, G. M., and Ingram, R. H.: Exercise performance in relation to the pathophysiologic type of chronic obstructive pulmonary disease. Am. J. Med. *49*:14, 1970.
93. Harris, P., Segal, N., and Bishop, J. M.: The relation between pressure and flow in the pulmonary circulation in normal subjects and in patients with chronic bronchitis and mitral stenosis. Cardiovasc. Res. *2*:73, 1968.
94. Seibold, H., Henze, E., Kohler, J., et al.: Right ventricular function in patients with chronic obstructive pulmonary disease. Klin. Wochenschr. *63*:1041, 1985.
95. Kawakami, Y., Kishi, F., Yamamoto, H., and Miyamoto, K.: Relation of oxygen delivery, mixed venous oxygenation and pulmonary hemodynamics to prognosis in chronic obstructive pulmonary disease. N. Engl. J. Med. *308*:1045, 1983.
96. Bergofsky, E. H.: Tissue oxygen delivery and cor pulmonale in chronic obstructive pulmonary disease. N. Engl. J. Med. *308*:1092, 1983.
97. Klinger, J. R., and Hill, N. S.: Right ventricular dysfunction in chronic obstructive pulmonary disease: Evaluation and management. Chest *99*:715, 1991.
98. Olvey, S. K., Redufo, L. A., Stevens, P. M., et al.: First pass radionuclide assessment of right and left ventricular ejection fraction in chronic pulmonary disease. Effect of oxygen upon exercise response. Chest *78*:4, 1980.
99. Khaja, F., and Parker, J. D.: Right and left ventricular performance in chronic obstructive lung disease. Am. Heart J. *82*:319, 1971.
100. Brunet, F., Dhainaut, J. F., Devaux, J. Y., et al.: Right ventricular performance in patients with acute respiratory failure. Intensive Care Med. *14*:474, 1988.
101. Biernacki, W., Flenley, D. C., Muir, A. L., and MacNee, W.: Pulmonary hypertension and right ventricular function in patients with COPD. Chest *94*:1169, 1988.
102. Stewart, R. I., and Lewis, C. M.: Cardiac output during exercise in patients with COPD. Chest *89*:199, 1986.
103. Murphy, M. L., Dinh, H., and Nicholson, D.: Chronic cor pulmonale. Disease-a-Month *35*:653, 1989.
104. Samet, P., Fritts, H. W., Jr., Fishman, A. P., and Cournand, A.: The blood volume in heart disease. Medicine *36*:211, 1957.
105. Turino, G. M., Edelman, N. H., Richards, E. C., and Fishman, A. P.: Extravascular lung water in cor pulmonale. Bull. Physiol. Pathol. Respir. *4*:47, 1968.
106. Meerson, F. Z.: The myocardium in hyperfunction, hypertrophy, and heart failure. Circ. Res. *25*(Suppl. 2):1, 1969.
107. Chidsey, C. A., Kaiser, G. A., Sonnenblick, E. H., et al.: Cardiac norepinephrine stores in experimental heart failure in the dog. J. Clin. Invest. *43*:2386, 1964.
108. Chandler, B. M., Sonnenblick, E. H., Spann, J. F., Jr., and Pool, P. E.: Association of depressed myofibrillar adenosine triphosphatase and reduced contractility in experimental heart failure. Circ. Res. *21*:717, 1967.
109. Kelly, D. T., Spotnitz, H. M., Beiser, G. D., et al.: Effects of chronic right ventricular volume and pressure loading on left ventricular performance. Circulation *44*:403, 1971.
110. Feneley, M. P., Olsen, C. D., Glower, D. D., and Rankin, J. S.: Effect of acutely increased right ventricular afterload on work output from the left ventricle in conscious dogs. Circ. Res. *65*:135, 1989.
111. Hecht, H. H., Kuida, H., and Tsagaris, T. J.: Brisket disease. IV. Impairment of left ventricular function in a form of cor pulmonale. Trans. Assoc. Am. Physicians *75*:263, 1962.
112. Fluck, D. C., Chandrasekar, R. G., and Gardner, F. U.: Left ventricular hypertrophy in chronic bronchitis. Br. Heart J. *28*:92, 1966.
113. Murphy, M. L., Adamson, J., and Hutcheson, F.: Left ventricular hypertrophy in patients with chronic bronchitis and emphysema. Ann. Intern. Med. *81*:307, 1974.
114. Rao, S. B., Cohn, K. E., Eldridge, F. L., and Hancock, E. W.: Left ventricular failure secondary to chronic pulmonary disease. Am. J. Med. *45*:229, 1968.
115. Jezek, V., and Schrijen, F.: Left ventricular function in chronic obstructive pulmonary disease with and without cardiac failure. Clin. Sci. Mol. Med. *45*:267, 1973.
116. Seibold, H., Roth, U., Lippert, R., et al.: Left heart function in chronic obstructive lung disease. Klin. Wochenschr. *64*:433, 1986.
116a. Johnson, G. L., Kanga, J. F., Moffett, C. B., and Noonan, J. A.: Changes in left ventricular diastolic filling patterns by Doppler echocardiography in cystic fibrosis. Chest *99*:646, 1991.
117. Frank, M. J., Weisser, A. B., Moschos, C. B., and Levinson, G. E.: Left ventricular function, metabolism, and blood flow in chronic cor pulmonale. Circulation *48*:798, 1973.
118. Williams, J. F., Childress, R. H., Boyd, D. L., et al.: Left ventricular function in patients with chronic obstructive pulmonary disease. J. Clin. Invest. *47*:1143, 1968.
119. Unger, K., Shaw, D., Karliner, J. S., et al.: Evaluation of left ventricular performance in acutely ill patients with chronic obstructive lung disease. Chest *68*:135, 1975.
120. Steele, P., Ellis, J. H., Jr., Van Dyke, D., et al.: Left ventricular ejection fraction in severe chronic obstructive airways disease. Am. J. Med. *59*:21, 1975.
121. Christianson, L. C., Shah, A., and Fisher, V. J.: Quantitative left ventricular cineangiography in patients with chronic obstructive pulmonary disease. Am. J. Med. *66*:399, 1979.
122. Gabinski, C., Courty, G., Besse, P., and Castaing, R.: Left ventricular function in chronic obstructive lung disease. Bull. Eur. Physiopathol. Resp. *15*:755, 1979.
123. Rubin, L. J.: Clinical evaluation. *In* Rubin, L. J. (ed.): Pulmonary Heart Disease. Boston, Martinus Nijhoff, 1984, p. 107.
124. Murphy, M. L., and Bone, R. C.: Cor Pulmonale in Chronic Bronchitis and Emphysema. Mount Kisco, N.Y., Futura Publishing Co., 1984, 276 pp.
125. Slutsky, A., Hooper, W., Ackerman, W., et al.: Evaluation of left ventricular function in chronic pulmonary disease by exercise gated equilibrium radionuclide angiography. Am. Heart J. *101*:414, 1981.
126. Nino, A. F., Berman, M. M., Gluck, E. H., et al.: Drug-induced left ventricular failure in patients with pulmonary disease: Endomyocardial biopsy demonstration of catecholamine myocarditis: Chest *92*:732, 1987.
127. Lavine, S. J., Tami, L., and Jawad, I.: Pattern of left ventricular diastolic filling associated with right ventricular enlargement. Am. J. Cardiol. *62*:444, 1988.
128. Burrows, B., Fletcher, C. M., Heart, B. E., et al.: Emphysematous and bronchial types of chronic airways obstruction: Clinico-pathological study of patients in London and Chicago. Lancet *1*:830, 1966.
129. Mitchell, R. S., and Filley, G. F.: Chronic obstructive bronchopulmonary disease. I. Clinical features. Am. Rev. Respir. Dis. *89*:360, 1964.
130. Stanford, W., and Galvin, J. R.: The radiology of right heart dysfunction: Chest roentgenogram and computed tomography. J. Thorac. Imag. *4*:7, 1989.
131. Bishop, J. M., and Grass, K. W.: Use of other physiologic variables to predict pulmonary artery pressure in patients with chronic respiratory distress. Multicenter study. Eur. Heart J. *2*:509, 1981.
132. Venditho, M. A., Pisano, D., Simelans, J. P., and Dickerson, C. N.: The incidence of tricuspid valvular regurgitation in patients with severe chronic obstructive pulmonary disease as determined by two-dimensional echocardiography. JAMA *84*:264, 1984.
133. Flenley, D. C., and Muir, A. L.: Cardiovascular effects of oxygen therapy for pulmonary arterial hypertension. Clin. Chem. Med. *4*:297, 1983.
134. Douglas, N. J., Calvertey, P. M. A., Leggett, R. J. E., et al.: Transient hypoxemia during sleep in chronic bronchitis and emphysema. Lancet *1*:1, 1979.
135. Tinlapun, V. G., and Mir, M. A.: Nocturnal hypoxemia and associated electrocardiographic changes in patients with chronic obstructive airway disease. N. Engl. J. Med. *306*:125, 1982.
136. Ingram, R.: Chronic bronchitis, emphysema, and chronic airways obstruction. *In* Wilson, J. E., et al. (eds.): Harrison's Principles of Internal Medicine. 12th ed. New York, McGraw-Hill Book Co., 1991, p. 1074.
137. Rubin, L. J., and Peter, R. H.: Therapy of pulmonary heart disease. *In* Rubin, L. J. (ed.) Pulmonary Heart Disease. Boston, Martinus Nijhoff, 1984, p. 325.
138. Myers, K. E., and Bogden, P. E.: Bronchodilators for patients with chronic heart disease. Postgrad. Med. *86*:324, 1989.
139. McFadden, E. R., Jr.: Inhaled Aerosol Bronchodilators. Baltimore, Williams and Wilkins, 1986, p. 99.
140. Parker, J. O., Kelkar, K., and West, R. S.: Hemodynamic effects of aminophylline in cor pulmonale. Circulation *33*:17, 1966.
141. Matthay, R. A., Berger, H. J., Locke, J., et al.: Effect of aminophylline upon right and left ventricular performance in chronic obstructive pulmonary disease. Noninvasive assessment by radionuclide angiocardiography. Am. J. Med. *65*:903, 1978.
142. Nocturnal Oxygen Therapy Trial Group. Continuous or nocturnal oxygen therapy in hypoxemic chronic obstructive lung disease. A clinical trial. Ann. Intern. Med. *93*:391, 1980.
143. MRC Working Party: Long-term ancillary oxygen therapy in chronic hy-

poxic cor pulmonale complicating chronic bronchitis and emphysema. A clinical trial. Lancet 1:681, 1981.
144. Weitzenblum, E., Sautegeau, A., Ehrhart, M., et al.: Long term oxygen therapy can reverse the progression of pulmonary hypertension in patients with chronic obstructive pulmonary disease. Am. Rev. Respir. Dis. *131*:493, 1985.
145. Hall, J., and Wood, L. D. H.: Oxygen therapy. *In* Crystal, R.G., et al. (eds.): The Lung: Scientific Foundations. New York, Raven Press, 1991, pp. 2143–2154.
146. Morrison, D., Caldwell, J., Lakshminaryan, S., et al.: The acute effects of low flow oxygen and isosorbide dinitrate on left and right ventricular ejection fractions in chronic obstructive pulmonary disease. J. Am. Coll. Cardiol. *2*:652, 1983.
147. Wuertemberger, G., Zielinsky, J., Sliwinsky, P., et al.: Survival in chronic obstructive pulmonary disease after diagnosis of pulmonary hypertension related to long term oxygen therapy. Lung *168*(Suppl.):762, 1990.
148. Rubin, L. J.: Vasodilator therapy (general aspects). *In* Fishman, A. P. (ed.): The Pulmonary Circulation: Normal and Abnormal. Philadelphia, University of Pennsylvania Press, 1990, pp. 479–483.
149. Lupi-Herrera, E., Bialostozky, D., and Sobrino, A.: The role of isoproterenol in pulmonary artery hypertension of unknown etiology. Chest *79*:292, 1981.
150. Ruskin, J., and Hutter, A. M.: Primary pulmonary hypertension treated with oral phentolamine. Ann. Intern. Med. *90*:772, 1979.
151. Klinke, W. P., and Gilbert, J. A. L.: Diazoxide in primary pulmonary hypertension. N. Engl. J. Med. *302*:91, 1980.
152. Vik-Mo, H., Walde, N., Jentoft, H., and Halvorsen, F. J.: Improved haemodynamics but reduced arterial blood oxygenation at rest and during exercise after long-term oral prazosin therapy in chronic cor pulmonale. Eur. Heart J. *6*:1047, 1985.
153. Rubin, L. J., Handel, F., and Peter, R. H.: The effects of oral hydralazine on right ventricular and diastolic pressure in patients with right ventricular failure. Circulation *65*:1369, 1982.
154. Brent, B. N., Berger, J., Matthay, R. A., et al.: Contrasting acute effects of vasodilators (nitroglycerin, nitroprusside and hydralazine) on right ventricular performance in patients with chronic obstructive pulmonary disease and pulmonary hypertension: A combined radionuclide-hemodynamic study. Am. J. Cardiol. *51*:1682, 1983.
155. Biernacki, W., Prince, K., Whyte, K., et al.: The effects of six months of daily treatment with the beta-2 agonist oral pirbuterol on pulmonary hemodynamics in patients with chronic hypoxic cor pulmonale receiving long term oxygen therapy. Am. Rev. Respir. Dis. *139*:492, 1989.
156. Evans, T. W., Waterhouse, J., Finlay, M., et al.: The effects of long-term methyldopa in patients with hypoxic cor pulmonale. Br. J. Dis. Chest *82*:405, 1988.
157. Rubin, L. J., and Moser, K.: Long-term effects of nitrendipine on hemodynamics and oxygen transport in patients with cor pulmonale. Chest *89*:141, 1986.
158. Singh, H., Ebejer, M. J., Higgins, D. A., et al.: Acute haemodynamic effects of nifedipine at rest and during maximum exercise in patients with chronic cor pulmonale. Thorax *40*:910, 1985.
159. Crevey, B. J., Dantzker, D. R., Bower, J. S., et al.: Hemodynamic and gas exchange effects of intravenous diltiazem in patients with pulmonary hypertension. Am. J. Cardiol. *49*:578, 1982.
160. Weir, E. K.: Acute vasodilator testing and pharmacological treatment of primary pulmonary hypertension. *In* Fishman, A. P. (ed.): The Pulmonary Circulation: Normal and Abnormal. Philadelphia, University of Pennsylvania Press, 1990, pp. 485–499.
161. Morley, T. F., Zappasodi, S. J., Belli, A., and Giudice, J. C.: Pulmonary vasodilator therapy for chronic obstructive pulmonary disease and cor pulmonale. Chest *92*:71, 1987.
162. Vestri, R., Philip-Joet, F., Surpas, P., et al.: One year clinical study on niphedipine in the treatment of pulmonary hypertension in chronic obstructive lung disease. Respiration *54*:139, 1988.
163. Packer, M., Greenberg, B., Massiz, B., and Dash, H.: Deleterious effects of hydralazine in patients with pulmonary hypertension. N. Engl. J. Med. *306*:1326, 1982.
164. Dayton, L. M., McCullough, R. E., Scheinhorn, D. J., and Weil, J. V.: Symptomatic and pulmonary response to acute phlebotomy in secondary polycythemia. Chest *68*:785, 1975.
165. Rakita, L., Gillespie, D. G., and Sancetta, S. M.: The acute and chronic effects of phlebotomy on general hemodynamics and pulmonary function of patients with secondary polycythemia associated with pulmonary emphysema. Am. Heart J. *70*:466, 1965.
166. Wallis, P. J. W., Skehan, J. D., Newland, A. C., et al.: Effect of erythropheresis on pulmonary hemodynamics and O_2 transport in patients with secondary polycythemia and cor pulmonale. Clin. Sci. *70*:91, 1986.
167. Erickson, A. D., Golden, W. R., Claunch, B. C., et al.: Acute effects of phlebotomy on right ventricular size and performance in polycythemic patients with chronic obstructive pulmonary disease. Am. J. Cardiol. *52*:163, 1983.
168. Mathur, P. N., Powles, A. C. P., Pugsley, S. O., et al.: Effect of digoxin on right ventricular function in severe chronic airway obstruction. Ann. Intern. Med. *95*:283, 1981.
169. Sunderrajan, E. V., Byron, W. A., McKenzie, W. N., et al.: The effect of terbutaline on cardiac function in patients with stable chronic obstructive lung disease. JAMA *250*:2151, 1983.
170. Gottlieb, L. S., and Balchum, O. J.: Course of chronic obstructive pulmonary disease following first onset of respiratory failure. Chest *63*:5, 1973.
171. Stevens, P. M., Terplan, M., and Knowles, J. H.: Prognosis of cor pulmonale. N. Engl. J. Med. *269*:1289, 1963.
172. Burrows, B., and Earle, R. H.: Course and prognosis of chronic obstructive lung disease. A prospective study of 200 patients. N. Engl. J. Med. *280*:397, 1969.
173. Mitchell, R. S., Webb, N. C., and Filley, G. F.: Chronic obstructive lung disease. III. Factors influencing prognosis. Am. Rev. Respir. Dis. *89*:878, 1964.
174. Burwell, C. S., Robin, E. D., Whaley, R. D., and Bickelman, A. G.: Extreme obesity associated with alveolar hypoventilation—a pickwickian syndrome. Am. J. Med. *21*:811, 1956.
175. Rochester, D. F., and Enson, Y.: Current concepts in the pathogenesis of the obesity-hypoventilation syndrome. Am. J. Med. *57*:402, 1974.
176. Weil, J. V.: Pulmonary hypertension and cor pulmonale in hypoventilating patients. *In* Weir, E. K., and Reeves, J. T. (eds.): Pulmonary Hypertension. Mount Kisco, N.Y., Futura Publishing Co., 1984, p. 321.
177. Lyons, H. A., and Huang, C. T.: Therapeutic use of progesterone in alveolar hypoventilation associated with obesity. Am. J. Med. *44*:881, 1968.
178. Sutton, F. D., Zwillich, C. W., Creagh, C. E., et al.: Progesterone for outpatient treatment of pickwickian syndrome. Ann. Intern. Med. *83*:476, 1975.
179. Cherniack, N. S.: Respiratory dysrhythmias during sleep. N. Engl. J. Med. *305*:325, 1981.
179a. Millman, R. P., and Fishman, A. P.: Sleep apnea syndromes. *In* Fishman, A. P. (ed.): Pulmonary Diseases and Disorders. 2nd ed. New York, McGraw-Hill Book Co., 1991, pp. 1347–1362.
180. Strohl, K. P., Cherniack, N. S., and Gather, B.: Physiologic basis of therapy in sleep apnea. Ann. Rev. Respir. Dis. *134*:791, 1986.
180a. Khoo, M. C. K.: Periodic breathing. *In* Crystal, R. G., et al. (eds.): The Lung: Scientific Foundations. New York, Raven Press, 1991, pp. 1419–1432.
181. Burrek, B.: The hypersomnia-sleep apnea syndrome: Its recognition in clinical cardiology. Am. Heart J. *107*:543, 1984.
182. Guilleminault, C., Cannally, S. J., and Winkler, R. A.: Cardiac arrhythmia and conduction disturbances during sleep in 400 patients with sleep apnea syndrome. Am. J. Cardiol. *52*:490, 1983.
183. Peiser, J., Ovnat, A., Uwyyed, K., et al.: Cardiac arrhythmias during sleep in morbidly obese sleep-apneic patients before and after gastric bypass surgery. Clin. Cardiol. *8*:519, 1985.
184. Buda, A. J., Schroeder, J. S., and Guilleminault, C.: Abnormalities of pulmonary wedge pressures in sleep-induced apnea. Int. J. Cardiol. *1*:67, 1981.
185. Fletcher, E. C., Schaaf, J. W., Miller, J., and Fletcher, J. G.: Long term cardiopulmonary sequelae in patients with sleep apnea and chronic lung disease. Am. Rev. Respir. Dis. *135*:525, 1987.
186. Weitzenblum, E., Krieger, J., Apprill, M., et al.: Daytime pulmonary hypertension in patients with obstructive sleep apnea syndrome. Am. Rev. Respir. Dis. *138*:345, 1988.
187. Martin, R. J., Sanders, M. H., Gray, B. A., and Pennock, B. E.: Acute and long-term ventilatory effects of hyperoxia in the adult sleep apnea syndrome. Am. Rev. Respir. Dis. *125*:175, 1982.
188. Mellins, R. B., Balfour, H. H., Jr., Turino, G. M., and Winters, R. W.: Failure of automatic control of ventilation (Ondine's curse). Medicine *49*:487, 1970.
189. Glenn, W. W. L., Holcomb, W. C., Hogan, J., et al.: Diaphragm pacing by radiofrequency transmission in the treatment of chronic ventilatory insufficiency: Present status. J. Thorac. Cardiovasc. Surg. *66*:505, 1973.
190. Penaloza, D., and Sime, F.: Circulatory dynamics during high altitude pulmonary edema. Am. J. Cardiol. *23*:369, 1969.
191. Penaloza, D., and Sime, F.: Chronic cor pulmonale due to loss of altitude acclimatization (chronic mountain sickness). Am. J. Med. *50*:728, 1971.
192. Severinghaus, J. W., Bainton, C. R., and Carcelen, A.: Respiratory insensitivity to hypoxia in chronically hypoxic man. Respir. Physiol. *1*:308, 1966.
193. Bland, J. W., Edwards, F. K., and Brainsfield, D.: Pulmonary hypertension and congestive heart failure in children with chronic upper airway obstruction. New concepts and etiologic factors. Am. J. Cardiol. *23*:830, 1969.
194. Randall, C. S., Braman, S. S., and Millman, R. P.: Rapid development of cor pulmonale following acute tonsillitis in adults. Chest *95*:462, 1989.
195. Noonan, J. A.: Pulmonary heart disease. Pediatr. Clin. North Am. *18*:1255, 1971.
196. Johnson, G. M., and Todd, D. W.: Cor pulmonale in severe Pierre Robin syndrome. Pediatrics *65*:152, 1980.
197. Glenn, W. W. L., Gee, J. B. L., Cole, D. R., et al.: Combined central alveolar hypoventilation and upper airway obstruction. Treatment by tracheostomy and diaphragm pacing. Am. J. Med. *64*:50, 1978.
198. Ingram, R. H., Jr., and Bishop, J. B.: Ventilatory response to carbon dioxide after removal of chronic upper airway obstruction. Am. Rev. Respir. Dis. *102*:645, 1970.
199. Williams, M. H., Jr., Adler, J. J., and Colp, C.: Pulmonary function studies as an aid in the differential diagnosis of pulmonary hypertension. Am. J. Med. *47*:378, 1969.
200. Glauser, E. M., Cook, C. D., and Harris, C. B. C.: Bronchiectasis. A review of 187 cases in children with follow-up pulmonary function studies in 58. Acta Paediatr. Scand. (Suppl.) *165*:1, 1966.
201. Reid, L.: Reduction in bronchial subdivisions in bronchiectasis. Thorax *5*:233, 1950.
202. Colten, H. R.: Cystic fibrosis. *In* Wilson, J. E., et al. (eds.): Harrison's Principles of Internal Medicine, 12th ed. New York, McGraw-Hill Book Co., 1991, p. 1072.
203. Moss, A. J.: The cardiovascular system in cystic fibrosis. Pediatrics *70*:728, 1982.

204. Moskowitz, W. B., Gewitz, M. H., Heyman, S., et al.: Cardiac involvement in cystic fibrosis: Early noninvasive detection and vasodilator therapy. Ped. Pharmacol. *5*:139, 1985.
205. Lester, L. A., Egge, A. C., Hubbard, V. S., Camerini-Otero, C. S., and Fink, R. J.: Echocardiography in cystic fibrosis: A proposed scoring system. J. Pediatr. *97*:742, 1980.
206. Ryland, D., and Reed, L.: The pulmonary circulation in cystic fibrosis. Thorax *30*:285, 1975.
207. Benesova, D., Voriskova, M., Hrobonova, V., and Vavrova, V.: Cardiovascular complications of cystic fibrosis. Cesk. Pediatr. *38*:458, 1983.
208. Sahilahti, E., and Rapola, J.: Frequent myocardial lesions in Schwachman's syndrome. Eight fatal cases among 16 Finnish patients. Acta Pediatr. Scand. *73*:642, 1984.
209. Emirgil, C., Sobol, B. J., Herbert, W. H., and Trout, K.: The lesser circulation in pulmonary fibrosis secondary to sarcoidosis and its relationship to respiratory function. Chest *60*:371, 1971.
210. Enson, Y., Thomas, H. M., III, Bosken, C. H., et al.: Pulmonary hypertension in interstitial lung disease: Relationship of vascular resistance to abnormal lung structure. Trans. Assoc. Am. Physicians *88*:248, 1975.
211. Newsom Davis, J., Goldman, M., Loh, L., and Casson, M.: Diaphragm function and alveolar hypoventilation. Q. J. Med. *45*:87, 1976.
212. Aubier, M., DeTroyer, A., Sampson, M., et al.: Aminophylline improves diaphragmatic contractility. N. Engl. J. Med. *305*:249, 1981.
213. Chandler, K. W., Rozas, C. J., Kory, R. C., and Goldman, A. L.: Bilateral diaphragmatic paralysis complicating local cardiac hypothermia during open heart surgery. Am. J. Med. *77*:243, 1984.
214. Bergofsky, E. H.: Respiratory failure in disorders of the thoracic cage. Am. Rev. Respir. Dis. *119*:643, 1979.
215. Bergofsky, E. H., Turino, G. M., and Fishman, A. P.: Cardiorespiratory failure in kyphoscoliosis. Medicine *38*:263, 1959.
216. Bijure, J., Grimby, G., Kasalicky, J., Lindh, M., and Nachemson, A.: Respiratory impairment and airway closure in patients with untreated idiopathic scoliosis. Thorax *25*:451, 1970.
217. Davies, G., and Reid, L.: Effect of scoliosis on growth of alveoli and pulmonary arteries and on the right ventricle. Arch. Dis. Child. *46*:623, 1971.
218. Westgate, H. D., and Moe, J. H.: Pulmonary function in kyphoscoliosis before and after correction by the Harrington instrumentation method. J. Bone Joint Surg. *51*:935, 1969.
219. Starling, M. R., Crawford, M. H., Sorensen, S. G., and O'Rourke, R. A.: A new two-dimensional echocardiographic technique for evaluating right ventricular size and performance in patients with obstructive lung disease. Circulation *66*:612, 1982.
220. Ferrazza, A., Marino, B., Giusti, V., et al.: Usefulness of left and right oblique subcostal view of the echo-Doppler investigation of pulmonary arterial blood flow in patients with chronic obstructive pulmonary disease. Chest *98*:286, 1990.
221. Migueres, M., Escamilla, R., Coca, F., et al.: Pulsed Doppler echocardiography in the diagnosis of pulmonary hypertension in COPD. Chest *98*:280, 1990.
222. Himelman, R. B., Abbott, J. A., Lee, E., et al.: Doppler echocardiography and ultrafast cine-computed tomography during dynamic exercise in chronic parenchymal pulmonary disease. Am. J. Cardiol. *64*:528, 1989.
223. Danchin, N., Cornette, A., Henriquez, A., et al.: Two-dimensional echocardiographic assessment of the right ventricle in patients with chronic obstructive lung disease. Chest *92*:229, 1987.
224. Bertoli, L., Mantero, A., Alpago, R., et al.: Value of two-dimensional echocardiography in the identification of pulmonary hypertension in chronic obstructive lung disease. Respiration *55*:193, 1989.
224a. Tramarin, R., Torbicki, A., Marchandise, B., et al.: Doppler echocardiographic evaluation of pulmonary artery pressure in chronic obstructive pulmonary disease. A European multicentre study. Eur. Heart J. *12*:103, 1991.
225. McGowan, F. X., and Wagner, G. S.: The electrocardiogram in chronic lung disease. *In* Rubin, L. J. (ed.): Pulmonary Heart Disease. Boston, Martinus Nijhoff, 1984, p. 117.
226. Goodwin, J. F., and Abdin, Z. N.: The cardiogram of congenital and acquired right ventricular hypertrophy. Br. Heart J. *21*:523, 1959.
227. Phillips, R. W.: The electrocardiogram in cor pulmonale secondary to pulmonary emphysema: A study of 18 cases proved by autopsy. Am. Heart J. *56*:352, 1958.
228. Kilcoyne, M. M., Davis, A. L., and Ferrer, M. I.: A dynamic electrocardiographic concept useful in the diagnosis of cor pulmonale. Circulation *42*:903, 1970.
229. Holford, F. D.: The electrocardiogram in pulmonary disease. *In* Fishman, A. P. (ed.): Pulmonary Diseases and Disorders. 2nd ed. New York, McGraw-Hill Book Company, 1991, pp. 471–478.
230. Kok-Jensen, A.: Simple electrocardiographic features of importance for prognosis in severe chronic bronchial obstruction. Scand. J. Respir. Dis. *56*:273, 1975.
231. Shih, H. T., Webb, C. R., Conway, W. A., et al.: Frequency and significance of cardiac arrhythmias in chronic obstructive lung disease. Chest *94*:44, 1988.
232. Wilson, J. R., Mason, U. G., Bahler, R. C., et al.: Vectorcardiographic detection of early hemodynamic abnormalities in chronic obstructive pulmonary disease. Chest *76*:160, 1979.
233. Shuk, J. W., Walder, J., Oetgen, W., and Thomas, H. M.: Right ventricular visualization by thallium 201 myocardial scintigraphy in chronic obstructive pulmonary disease. South. Med. J. *78*:1435, 1985.

PART IV

BROADER PERSPECTIVES ON HEART DISEASE AND CARDIOLOGIC PRACTICE

50

General Principles of Cardiovascular Cellular and Molecular Biology

by BERNARDO NADAL-GINARD, M.D., Ph.D, and VIJAK MAHDAVI, Ph.D.

As is the case for other organ systems, the development, structure, and function of the cardiovascular system depend on the proper functioning of its constituent cellular elements. Derangement of these cellular functions is at the basis of all cardiovascular disease. Every normal and disordered physiological process at the levels of cell, tissue, and organ is the result of complex biochemical reactions. These biochemical reactions involve proteins that, in turn, are the products of specific genes. Therefore, at some point in the future it should be possible to describe cardiovascular physiological and pathological processes at the cellular, molecular, and genetic levels; this remains an elusive goal for most cardiovascular processes. As a consequence, many diagnostic and therapeutic approaches to cardiovascular disease are still based on empirical observations rather than on an understanding of the precise molecular dysfunction that is at the basis of the disease and the manner in which it is affected by therapeutic agents.

Molecular Biology and the Cardiovascular System

Until recently, the view prevailed that the heart is a relatively static organ biochemically and it therefore did not seem to be either particularly interesting or suitable as a subject for major questions of cellular and molecular biology. As a consequence, the impact of newly developed techniques of recombinant DNA and genetic manipulation on the understanding of the cellular and molecular biology of the heart has lagged behind that of other organs. However, the power of these new techniques and approaches is just beginning to be felt in the field of cardiovascular biology.

MOLECULAR BASIS OF GENE EXPRESSION

All of the genetic information required to produce a human is stored in the nucleus of each cell in the form of deoxyribonucleic acid (DNA). In humans, DNA is packaged in 23 pairs of chromosomes as a double-stranded linear molecule composed of purine (adenosine, *A*, and guanosine, *G*) and pyrimidine (thymidine, *T*, and cytosine, *C*) bases. These bases pair with each other according to Watson and Crick's rules so that an *A*

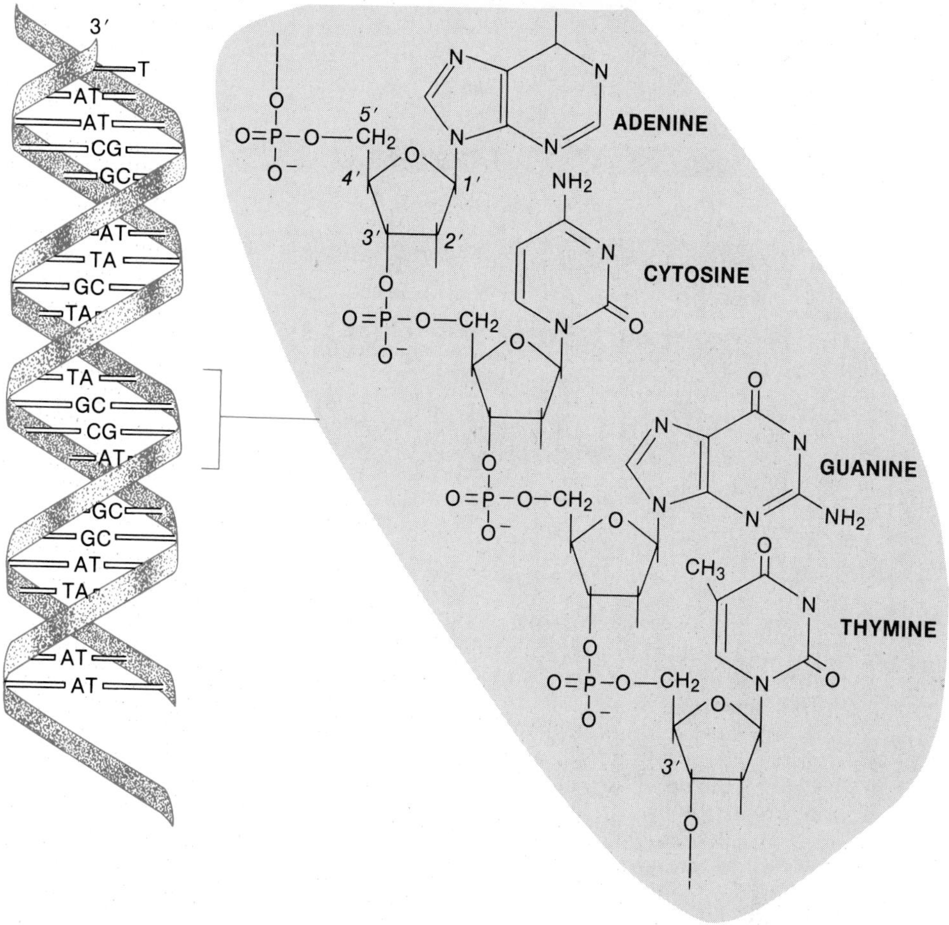

FIGURE 50–1. The structure of DNA. *Left,* a schematic drawing of the DNA double helix, showing the sugar-phosphate backbone as a ribbon, with the bases arranged toward the middle. Note that A always pairs with T and C always pairs with G. *Right,* an expanded view of four nucleotides along one strand, showing the complete chemical structure of the sequence 5′-ACGT-3′. (A nucleotide consists of a sugar, a phosphate group, and an attached base.) Note that the 5′ and 3′ designations, used to indicate the polarity of a DNA strand, refer to the numbering of carbons on the deoxyribose ring. The four nucleotide bases comprising DNA are adenine, cytosine, guanine, and thymine. Adjacent bases in a DNA single-stranded molecule are joined by phosphate group linkages between the 5′ and 3′ carbons of their respective deoxyribose sugar moieties. In DNA, adenine will pair with its complementary nucleotide thymine, and guanine with cytosine, by hydrogen bond formation between their respective purine and pyridamine rings. In this manner, complementary DNA strands pair to form a double helix (*left*). The 5′ to 3′ order of the phosphate linages in the DNA strands of the double helix are reciprocal; i.e., the DNA strands are antiparallel. (From Gelehrter, T. D., and Collins, F. S.: Principles of Medical Genetics. Baltimore, Williams and Wilkins, 1990, p. 10.)

is always paired with a *T* and a *G* with a *C* (Fig. 50–1). As a consequence of this complementary characteristic, knowing the sequence of one strand of DNA allows prediction of the other. In this simple manner, each strand carries the information needed for its faithful duplication and provides the basis for heredity. The rules of base pairing assure that individual cells and whole organisms transmit an identical copy of the DNA sequence stored in the nucleus to their descendants.

The capacity of DNA to store information in a continuous string of *A*s, *T*s, *C*s, and *G*s (the letters of the genetic alphabet) is enormous because the string of DNA is decoded into three letter words called *codons* (Fig. 50–2). Each codon, in turn, specifies either one of the 20 different amino acids that constitute the building blocks of proteins or is used as a punctuation signal to indicate the end of coding information. A *gene* is constituted by the string of bases in the DNA that codes for the amino acid sequence of a protein molecule together with the DNA sequences needed for the regulation of the gene. These regulatory sequences, in general, flank the coding sequences. The gene is the basic functional unit of heredity that is transmitted from one generation to the next.

The simplicity of the system evolved by DNA to store and transmit information is what ensures its accuracy and fidelity. Each second, many millions of cells in the body divide. One of the marvels of DNA is that each time a cell divides, two strands of DNA, each containing approximately one and a half billion bases that have the capacity to code for approximately 100,000 different proteins, are copied faithfully, in a matter of

FIGURE 50–2. The genetic code. The table shows the correspondence (the genetic code) between three-base codons in mRNA and the amino acid inserted into the polypeptide. Amino acids are represented by two types of abbreviations: a three-letter and a single-letter abbreviation. The triplet code of RNA bases that specifies the utilization of amino acids in protein is shown. The triplets are called codons and are "degenerate"; i.e., some amino acids are designated by more than one triplet sequence. All proteins start with a methionine; therefore, its coding sequence, AUG, is also the "start" codon (marked *). Three codons, UAA, UAG and UGA, are "stop" codons and serve to terminate protein translation. The one-letter shorthand notations for the designation of amino acids in primary protein sequences are also shown. Amino acid abbreviations: Ala, alanine; Arg., arginine; Asp, aspartic acid; Cys, cysteine; Gln, glutamine; Glu, glutamic acid; Gly, glysine; His, histidine; Ile, isoleucine; Leu, leucine; Met, methionine; Phe, phenylalanine; Pro, proline; Ser, serine; Thr, threonine; Trp, tryptophan; Tyr, tyrosine; Val, valine. (From Hartl, D. L.: Human Genetics. Hagerstown, MD, Harper and Row, 1983, p. 278.)

THE GENETIC CODE

First nucleotide in codon (5′ end)	Second nucleotide in codon: U			C			A			G		
U	UUU	phe	F	UCU	ser	S	UAU	tyr	Y	UGU	cys	C
	UUC	phe		UCC	ser		UAC	tyr		UGC	cys	
	UUA	leu	L	UCA	ser		UAA	(stop)		UGA	(stop)	
	UUG	leu		UCG	ser		UAG	(stop)		UGG	trp	W
C	CUU	leu	L	CCU	pro	P	CAU	his	H	CGU	arg	R
	CUC	leu		CCC	pro		CAC	his		CGC	arg	
	CUA	leu		CCA	pro		CAA	gln	Q	CGA	arg	
	CUG	leu		CCG	pro		CAG	gln		CGG	arg	
A	AUU	ile	I	ACU	thr	T	AAU	asn	N	AGU	ser	S
	AUC	ile		ACC	thr		AAC	asn		AGC	ser	
	AUA	ile		ACA	thr		AAA	lys	K	AGA	arg	R
	AUG*	met	M	ACG	thr		AAG	lys		AGG	arg	
G	GUU	val	V	GCU	ala	A	GAU	asp	D	GGU	gly	G
	GUC	val		GCC	ala		GAC	asp		GGC	gly	
	GUA	val		GCA	ala		GAA	glu	E	GGA	gly	
	GUG	val		GCG	ala		GAG	glu		GGG	gly	

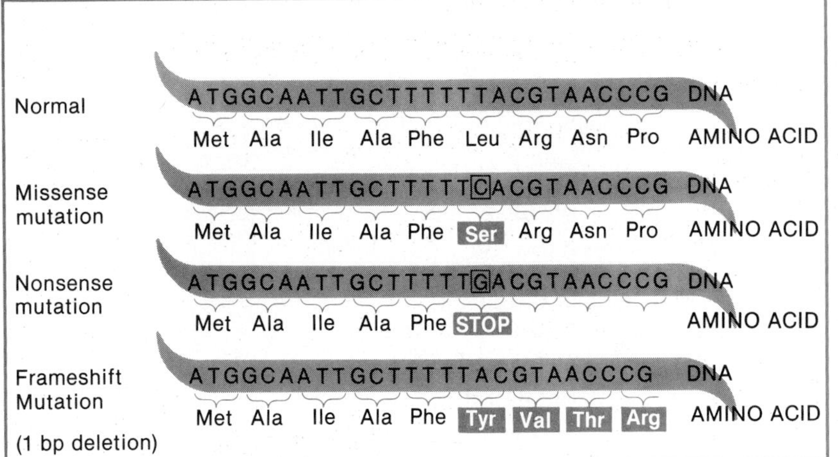

FIGURE 50–3. Examples of mutation; bd = base pair. The "sense" strand DNA sequence of a coding region is shown, together with the encoded amino acid sequence. Three different mutations affecting the second nucleotide of a leucine codon are shown. A missense mutation results in the substitution of an incorrect amino acid, while a nonsense mutation generates a "stop" codon and results in premature termination of protein translation. Addition or deletion of nucleotides can result in a change in the reading frame of the triplet codons (frameshift mutation), and consequently a change in the amino acid sequence of the protein. (From Hartl, D. L.: Human Genetics. Hagerstown, MD, Harper and Row, 1983, p. 22.)

minutes and with (on average) one single mistake. Many of these mistakes are corrected immediately after DNA replication by a "proofreading" system that is an intrinsic part of the DNA replication apparatus.

The errors produced during the replication of DNA that escape the proofreading system are called *mutations.* When mutations occur in somatic cells in most cases they are of little consequence, unless they occur in cells able to amplify the mutation through cell division. Although these mutations are never transmitted to the progeny, they are heritable at the cellular level. (In fact, an increasing number of neoplastic processes are known to originate through this mechanism.) Only when the change in the DNA is present in the reproductive cells does the mutation become transmitted to the progeny. In a genetic sense, therefore, a mutation is a stable and heritable change in the DNA sequence.

Mutations can involve gross rearrangements in the DNA sequence produced by deletions, duplications, and translocations or may involve a single base change in which one base is substituted for another (Fig. 50–3). Many of these point mutations have no detectable physiological and biochemical effects because they do not change the meaning of the codon they affect. This is because of the "degeneracy of the genetic code" in which a given amino acid can be encoded by more than one specific codon; for example, leucine and proline are each encoded by six different codons. Changes in the DNA sequence that do not change the coding content of the gene are called *silent mutations.* When they change the meaning of the codon, they either change the amino acid that is specified (missense mutation) or introduce a stop signal that truncates the coding sequence (nonsense mutation). Many of the human mutations identified so far represent missense mutations that produce an amino acid change in the protein specified by the mutant gene. In some cases, these substitutions have little or no effect on the function of the protein. In other cases, however, the function of the protein is impaired or totally abolished. This latter class of mutations may be responsible for the inherited diseases.

DECODING THE INFORMATION STORED IN DNA

With the exception of the cells of the immune system, all somatic cells contain the same genetic information in their nuclear DNA. In fact, the nucleus of a single somatic cell contains the information necessary to produce a complete organism. However, despite the fact that all cells have the same genotype, multicellular organisms are composed of many different cell types that differ dramatically from one another. These different phenotypes are the result of each cell type making selective use of the common genetic information stored in its nucleus. This selective use of the genome by different cell types at particular stages of development or in different physiological states is the basis of development in general and of cell differentiation in particular. Specific cell types are different from one another because they use specifically different portions of the genome. Genes that are expressed in a single cell type, such as albumin in the hepatocyte, the globin genes in the erythrocyte, and cardiac myosin heavy chain in the myocardium, are cell *type-specific* genes (Fig. 50–4). In addition, all or most cell types share the expression of many genes that are responsible for carrying out the cellular functions necessary for cell survival and proliferation, such as glycolysis, oxidative metabolism, and cell division. This set of common genes is called *housekeeping genes.*

The genetic information that encodes the linear sequence of amino acids in a protein is co-linear with the final protein product; that is, the codons that specify each of the amino acids from the amino to the carboxyl terminus are found in the gene in the same order found in the protein. Surprisingly, with very few exceptions this linear sequence of codons is interrupted by noncoding sequences that disrupt the reading frame of the gene. Consequently, the message specifying a protein encoded by the gene is encrypted in a manner so that it can be read only after the noncoding sequences interspersed between the coding ones have been removed. The sequences containing coding information are called *exons,* because these sequences normally exit the nucleus and accumulate in the cytoplasm. The portions of the gene between the exons are called *introns,* because normally they cannot be transported and remain inside the nucleus (Fig. 50–5). Therefore, in order to decode a gene successfully, the introns need to be removed and the exons joined together to provide an uninterrupted co-linear protein sequence.

TRANSCRIPTION

The selective use by different cells of the genetic information stored in the DNA is made possible because this information is not used directly but is transcribed into a molecule that can be read by the protein synthetic machinery of the cell. By a complex enzymatic process called *transcription,* the double-stranded DNA of each gene expressed in a given cell is copied into a single-stranded ribonucleic acid (RNA) (Fig. 50–6). This molecule of RNA uses the same genetic code as the DNA, but its bases contain the sugar ribose instead of deoxyribose that forms part of DNA. This molecule, which is the intermediate between the gene and the protein, is called *pre-messenger RNA* (pre-mRNA). The pre-mRNA is synthesized in the nucleus of the cell as a faithful copy of the gene and therefore contains both the exons and the introns. After transcription, the introns are removed from each of the transcripts by a process called *pre-mRNA splicing.* After the introns are completely spliced out and further processed in the nucleus, the pre-mRNA has been converted into a mature mRNA that con-

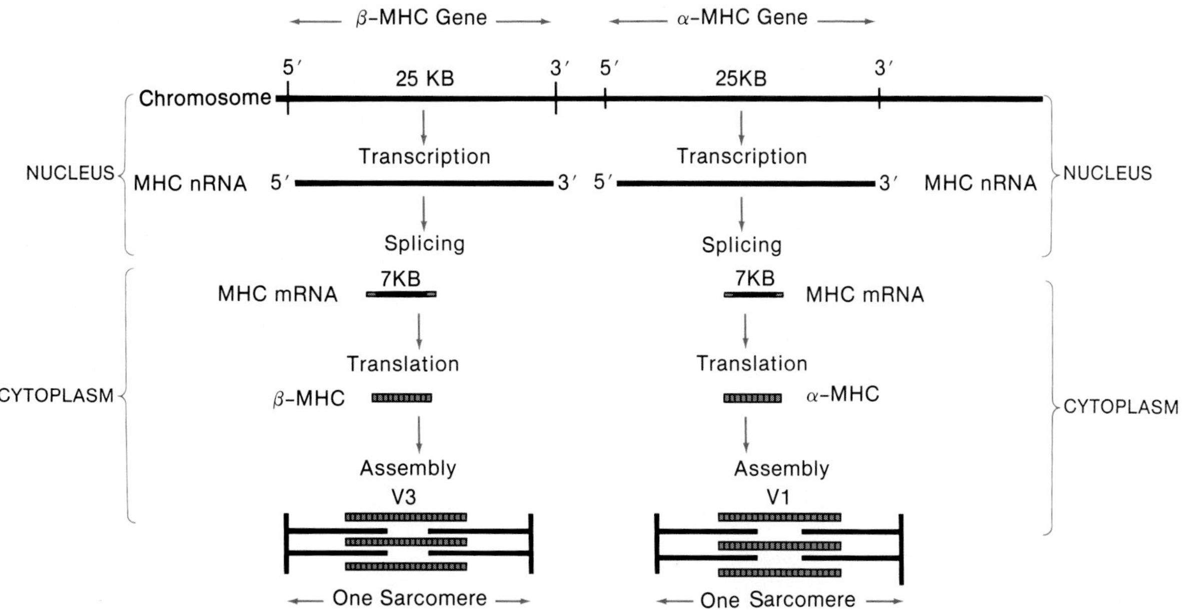

FIGURE 50–4. **Decoding the information stored in the DNA. The steps involved in the regulation of gene expression are illustrated for the cardiac myosin heavy chain (MHC) genes. These genes are organized in tandem on the chromosome, and their expression, at the transcriptional level, is regulated by tissue, developmental, hormonal, physiological, and pathological stimuli. The DNA sequences coding for the α- and β-myosin heavy chains (MHC) are each contained in a 25 kilobase (KB) region of human chromosome 14. A primary RNA transcript (nRNA) is transcribed in the nucleus of cardiocytes. Noncoding sequences are spliced out and the 7 KB mature messenger RNA (mRNA) transported to the cytoplasm. The protein subunit chains are translated from the mRNA on ribosomes and the multimeric myosin proteins are assembled and organized in the sarcomeres. The similarity in DNA sequence of the adjacent MHC genes can lead to mispairing of chromosomes during DNA replication and the generation of deletion mutations. nRNA, nuclear ribonucleic acid or pre-messenger RNA (mRNA); KB, kilobases.**

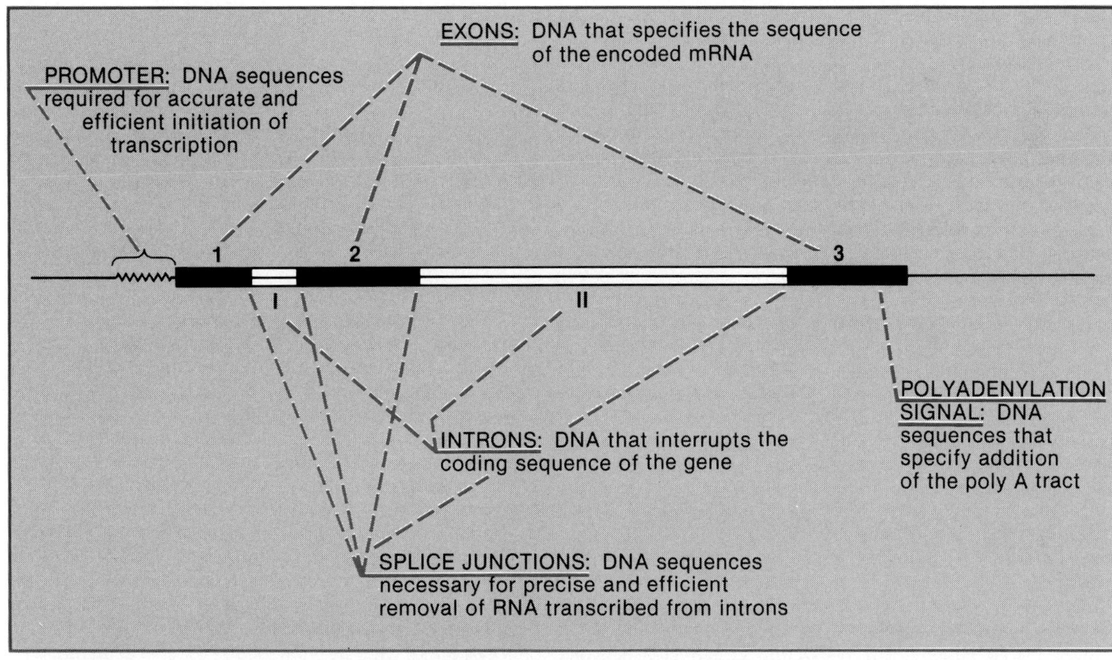

FIGURE 50–5. **Functional elements of the β-globin gene. Expression of β-globin in specific cell lineages is regulated by tissue-specific enhancer sequences, which can be located at a distance from the coding sequences and are not shown. The promoter sequences facilitate binding of RNA polymerase and the initiation of RNA transcription at the mRNA start site. Non-coding intron sequences are present in the primary RNA transcript, but are spliced out of the mature mRNA, which contains only exons. The polyadenylation signal sequence directs the addition of a poly-adenine "tail" to the 3′ end of the mRNA. Mutations that affect β-globin expression have been found in its enhancer, promoter, exon, splice-junction and polyadenylation signal sequences. (From Stamatoyannopoulos, G., Nienhuis, A. W., Leder, P., and Majerus, P. W. (eds): The Molecular Basis of Blood Diseases. Philadelphia, W.B. Saunders Company, 1987, p. 29)**

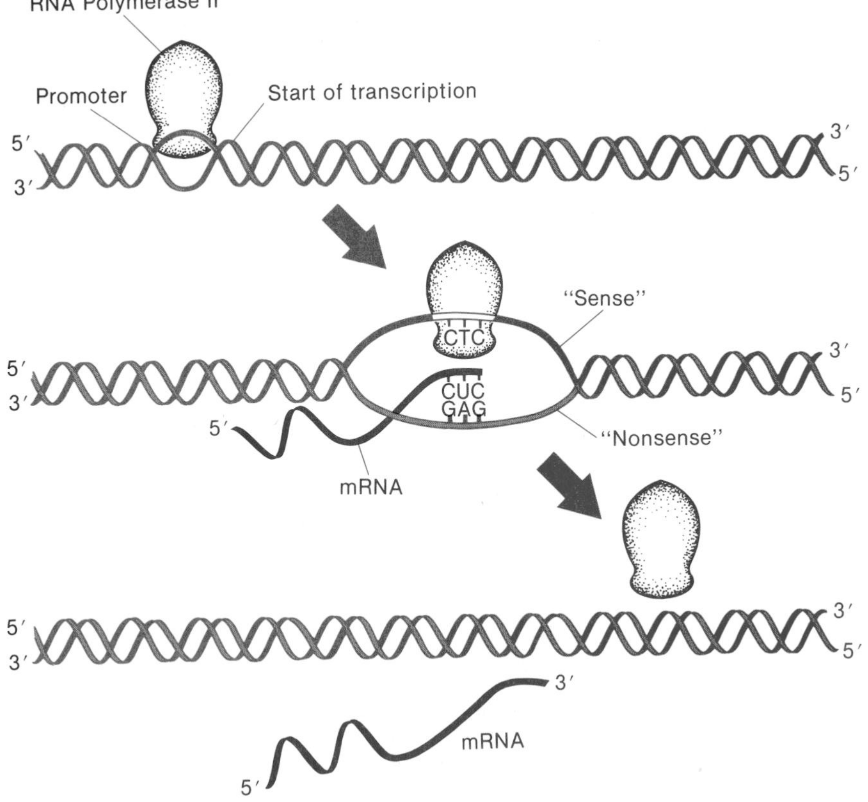

FIGURE 50-6. Schematic drawing of the transcription process. RNA polymerase II recognizes a specific sequence at the 5′ end of a gene (the promoter) and begins to transcribe it into the messenger RNA (mRNA). The mRNA is synthesized in the 5′ to 3′ direction and has the same sequence as the 5′ to 3′ DNA strand, also known as the "sense" strand. The mechanism of RNA formation presumably depends on base pairing of the newly formed RNA with the "nonsense" strand of the DNA, which acts as a template for copying. (From Gelehrter, T. D., and Collins, F. S.: Principles of Medical Genetics. Baltimore, Williams and Wilkins, 1990, p. 14.)

tains a methylated guanosine at its 5′ end (the cap site) and a string of adenosines at the 3′ end, known as the poly(A) tail. This mRNA is then transported to the cytoplasm, where it can be read by the translation machinery and may serve as a template for multiple rounds of translation to generate multiple copies of the protein.

It is now evident that splicing serves an important regulatory function because through this mechanism a single gene can produce several protein isoforms that might have different function or subcellular location. This is so because in some cases exons encoding a particular domain of the protein are present in the gene in several copies, each encoding a different variant of the sequence. These exons can be incorporated into the mature mRNA in different combinations and each will give rise to a different variant of the corresponding protein. The mechanism by which the cell makes selective use of particular exons is called *alternative splicing.* This mode of posttranscriptional gene regulation is particularly prevalent in skeletal and cardiac muscle and plays an important role in the generation of sarcomeric diversity.

The flow of genetic information from the nucleus to the cytoplasm of the cell is ideally suited for two main purposes: selective use and amplification of the genetic information encoded by the DNA. Due to transcription that is specific for the cell, the developmental stage, and the physiological state, the genome common to all cells is used to produce cells with widely different functions. Although most genes are present in the genome in a single copy, their informational content can be amplified several thousandfold by making multiple mRNA copies. Each of these mRNAs is, in turn, further amplified when it undergoes multiple rounds of translation to generate multiple copies of the protein. This amplification mechanism makes it possible for genes such as β-globin and myosin heavy chain to represent a large percentage of the protein content of erythrocytes or cardiac myocytes, respectively, despite the fact that each isoform of these proteins is encoded by a gene present in a single copy per haploid genome. (For further details on these general topics, see references 2 to 4.)

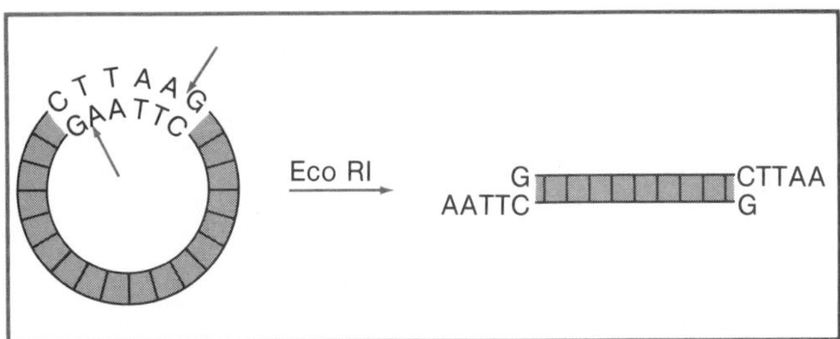

FIGURE 50-7. DNA cloning. The restriction endonuclease EcoR1 will recognize and cut a circular or linear DNA molecule at the palindromic nucleotide sequence 5′-CTTAAg-3′. Since the digestion is asymmetric, the resulting fragments will have overhanging unpaired nucleotides, called "sticky ends," which can pair with a complementary strand and be ligated to form a recombinant DNA molecle. (From Suzuki, D. T., Griffiths, A. J. F., Miller, J. H., and Lewontin, R. C.: An Introduction to Genetic Analysis. 4th ed, New York, W.H. Freeman and Co., 1989, p. 396.)

RECOMBINANT DNA TECHNOLOGY AS A TOOL OF CARDIOVASCULAR BIOLOGY

Although by the early 1970's most of the basic facts about the structure and function of DNA and RNA were known, progress in elucidating the regulatory mechanisms of gene expression was hampered by the inability, with the technology then available, to isolate and purify the DNA and mRNA sequences corresponding to a single gene. It soon became apparent that cloning of particular DNA sequences in bacterial cells would be necessary to produce sufficiently large and homogeneous quantities of DNA to be suitable for the characterization required to understand the regulatory processes. The discovery of restriction endonucleases was crucial in making possible the development of cloning technology. Smith and Wilcox[5] were the first to report a bacterial enzyme able to cut DNA at a specific nucleotide sequence (restriction site). The existence of a large family of these molecules soon became apparent; each molecule recognizes a specific DNA sequence with an extremely high level of specificity and efficiency. Danna and Nathans[6] realized that these specific cuts could be exploited to characterize a DNA molecule by digestion into several fragments with specific restriction enzymes, followed by separation of these fragments according to their electrophoretic mobility. Because individual DNA molecules contain unique sequences, the pattern of digestion provided a set of fragments that was unique for a specific gene. Using this strategy, Danna and Nathans[6] generated the first restriction map of the DNA tumor virus *SV-40* (Fig. 50-7). This accomplishment, together with the discovery of an enzyme that can join separate ends of DNA *(DNA ligase),* opened the way for the cloning of DNA molecules.

GENE CLONING. In 1972 Berg, Boyer, Cohen, and their collaborators[7,8] inserted a fragment of DNA that had been cut with the *E. coli* restriction enzyme Eco RI into a *plasmid vector* that had also been cut with Eco RI. Plasmid vectors are circular DNA molecules that can replicate autonomously in bacterial cells. After ligation of the cohesive ends of the two molecules generated by Eco RI with DNA ligase, a new plasmid

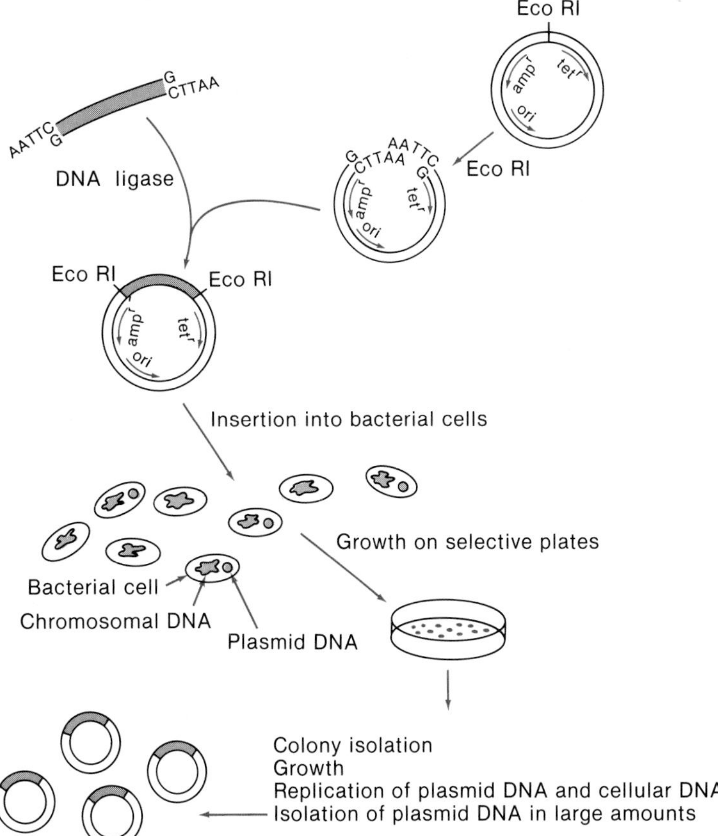

FIGURE 50–8. The process of cloning a DNA fragment into a plasmid cloning vector. A fragment of interest is cut with a restriction endonuclease and ligated into a plasmid vector. The vector contains an origin of replication ("ori") so that it can be grown in bacteria, and an antibiotic resistance gene, so that cells containing the plasmid can be selectively amplified. The recombinant plasmid is mixed with antibiotic-sensitive bacteria that have been treated to permeabilize their cell membranes to facilitate plasmid DNA uptake, a process called bacterial transformation. Bacterial clones carrying the plasmid are antibiotic resistant and grow on selective plates. Individual clones can be grown to abundance in liquid culture, and the recombinant plasmid DNA isolated and purified in quantity. (From Fritsch, E. F., and Maniatis, J.: Methods of Molecular Genetics. *In* Stamatoyannopoulos, G., Nienhuis, A. W., Leder, P., and Majerus, P. W. (eds.): The Molecular Basis of Blood Diseases. Philadelphia, W.B. Saunders Company, 1987, p. 5.)

molecule was produced that contained a piece of foreign DNA. After this recombinant plasmid DNA was reintroduced into bacterial cells (a process called *transformation*), it could be grown and purified in large and homogeneous quantities, taking advantage of the different physical characteristics of plasmid and genomic DNA that allow for their easy separation by physical means. This seemingly simple cloning process, in essence the same that is used today, ushered in the era of recombinant DNA (Fig. 50–8).

USE OF REVERSE TRANSCRIPTASE

A modification of the cloning procedure already outlined was rapidly developed to allow for the cloning of mRNA sequences (Fig. 50–9*A*). This procedure takes advantage of *reverse transcriptase,* the enzyme discovered by Baltimore[9] and Temin[10] and used by RNA viruses to convert the RNA into DNA. By means of this enzyme, the usual flow of genetic information from DNA to RNA that occurs in the cell nucleus can be reversed in the test tube. The single-stranded mRNA molecule that normally is not replicated can be converted into a double-stranded DNA molecule that may be replicated indefinitely. This DNA molecule is a faithful copy of the mRNA and is called *copy DNA (cDNA).* The cDNA produced in this manner, however, cannot be cloned into the plasmid vector, because it is not flanked by restriction enzyme sites. Therefore, compatible cohesive termini on the cDNA and plasmid DNA need to be created in order to ligate the two molecules together. This is accomplished by the thymic enzyme terminal transferase, which is able to incorporate a string of nucleotides at the free end of a DNA molecule. When a string of Gs is added to the ends of the plasmid molecule and a string of Cs is added to the end of the cDNA, because of the base-pairing rules, the two molecules can be annealed together and ligated to form a new recombinant plasmid ready to be amplified when introduced into bacteria (Fig. 50–9*A*).

One of the shortcomings of plasmids as cloning vectors is their low capacity for foreign DNA that allows for the cloning of relatively short sequences. This too has been addressed by the development of new cloning vectors that accommodate quite long DNA sequences. These vectors use bacterial phages or yeast chromosomal sequences as recipients of the foreign DNA sequences. In some cases, vectors are engineered so that the bacteria will produce a protein, or a portion thereof, from the fragment of inserted DNA. To accomplish this, the cDNA sequence is inserted and fused downstream from a bacterial gene that is readily induced by a drug or metabolite (Fig. 50–9*B*). When induced, this gene produces large quantities of the corresponding fusion protein. These *bacterial expression vectors* have the advantage that the gene of interest can be screened using antibodies against the cognate protein or, in some cases, using radiolabeled ligands specific for the protein being cloned. In addition, these vectors are used to produce the corresponding fusion protein in large quantities that can be easily isolated and purified.

GENE ISOLATION

With use of the aforementioned methods, it has become routine practice to isolate genes coding for a large variety of proteins. Once a partial sequence of a protein is known or a specific antibody against it is available, it is possible to produce a synthetic oligonucleotide that contains the codons required to produce the corresponding amino acid sequence (Fig. 50–9*B*). In addition, if the protein is available in small quantities, a synthetic peptide can be produced and used to raise antibodies against this portion of the protein sequence. With these two reagents at hand it is a straightforward task to screen a cDNA or genomic library for the clones that contain the cDNA for this protein using a DNA sequence corresponding to the known amino acid sequence, an antibody against the protein, or a ligand recognized by the protein. This protocol for gene isolation and characterization requires some knowledge of the protein investigated. For this reason, it is called a *direct* method of gene isolation, as compared with the *reverse genetics* method described below that requires no knowledge of the protein sequence or function.

GENE MAPPING

The ready availability of DNA fragments homogeneous in length and sequence allowed the development of efficient techniques of *DNA sequencing.* In 1975 Sanger[11] developed an effective approach to sequencing of single-stranded DNA by elongating nascent DNA chains with DNA polymerase and terminating them at a specific base through incorporating a modified nucleotide that cannot be elongated (a chain terminator). The first complete nucleotide sequence of a natural gene was obtained using this approach. Two years later Maxam and Gilbert[12] developed a different approach to sequencing of double-stranded DNA by specific chemical modification of bases to induce specific cleavages at a particular base. With these two techniques, the sequencing of long genomic and cDNA molecules rapidly became routine. The number of genes sequenced in the following decade runs into the thousands. Further developments and improvements of the Sanger technique[13] have led to the automation of many of the procedures involved in DNA sequencing to the point that sequencing the complete human genome has become a practical goal for the end of the century. However, before this task is accomplished, it will be necessary to produce an accurate and detailed physical map of the human genome.

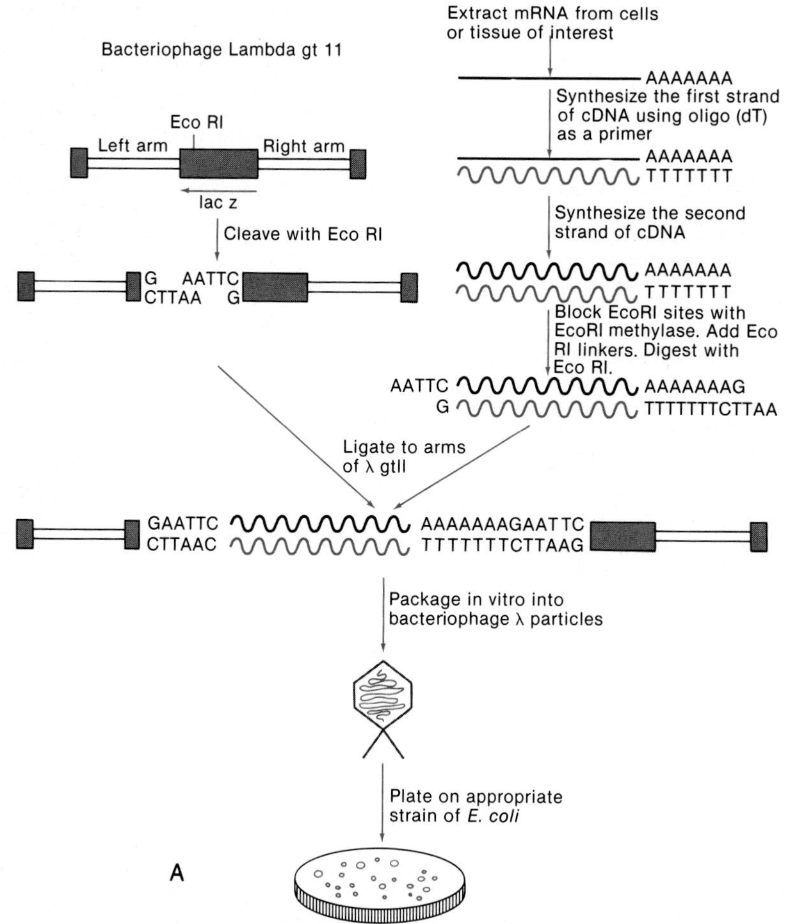

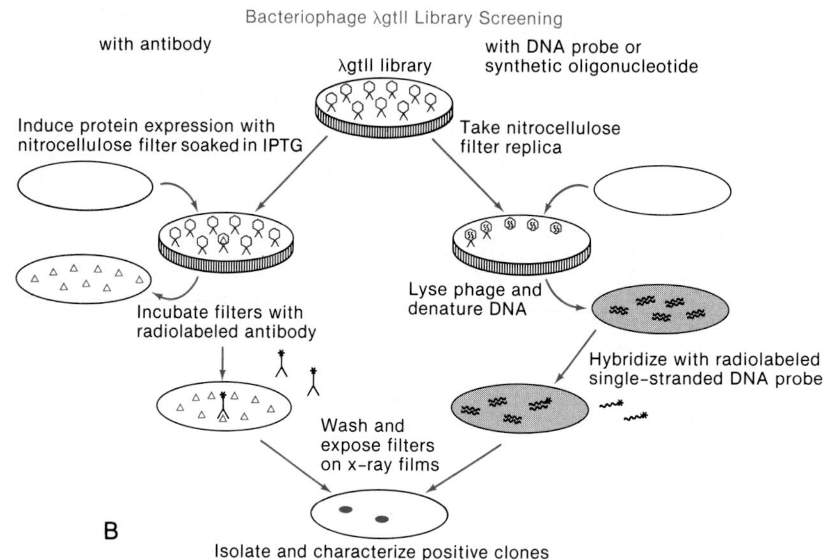

FIGURE 50–9. Cloning in an expression bacteriophage vector. *A.,* The bacteriophage gt11 expression vector contains an Eco R1 cloning site within an inducible gene (lac z or β-galactosidase). A functional coding sequence can be cloned into this site by preparing complementary DNA (cDNA) from messenger RNA using reverse transcriptase. A double-stranded fragment of cDNA can be modified to facilitate cloning by the addition of "linkers" which contain sequences that can be ligated to the "sticky ends" of the vector. Recombinant bacteriophage containing cDNA is mixed in vitro with bacteriophage coat protein, reconstituting infectious virus. *B.,* Recombinant bacteriophage carrying a particular cDNA can be identified by either expression or hybridization screening. Bacteria containing the bacteriophage can be stimulated to make the cDNA-encoded protein by adding an inducer (IPTG) of lac z into which the cDNA has been cloned. The presence of the synthesized protein on nitrocellulose filter replicas of the bacterial plate can be detected by binding of radiolabelled antibodies. Alternatively, recombinant bacteriophage carrying the cDNA sequence can be identified by hybridization to the filter of oligonucleotides or cloned DNA sequences. When a positive signal is detected on the replica filter, the corresponding bacteriophage plaque can be picked from the bacterial plate. The bacteriophage can then be amplified and its DNA characterized by restriction enzyme or DNA sequencing analysis.

RESTRICTION FRAGMENT LENGTH POLYMORPHISMS. The map of the human genome, which is now being constructed, consists of identification of landmarks in human DNA; this process allows the allocation of a given DNA fragment to a specific chromosome and to a particular location within the chromosome. This is accomplished by pinpointing of particular DNA polymorphisms that can differentiate between the two alleles of a given gene. These polymorphisms, called *restriction fragment length polymorphisms* (RFLPs),[14] are a result of the normal variability in the DNA among different individuals that can be recognized by specific restriction endonucleases. On the average, one in every 500 nucleotides has differences between two randomly selected alleles,[15] and approximately 5 per cent of these differences can be detected by restriction enzymes.

A restriction enzyme will cut the DNA at a particular site in one chromosome but not at the same place in the homologous chromosome because of differences in the DNA sequence in the chromosome inherited from each parent. This difference in the restriction enzyme sites is reflected in the size of the DNA fragments generated by the enzyme and visualized on Southern blot testing when hybridized to a DNA probe. The ability of this procedure to distinguish between the paternal and the maternal chromosomes is of great clinical significance. Moreover, it permits the identification of RFLPs that segregate with a particular trait in heterozygous individuals. Therefore, with this technique it is possible to determine whether the pattern of inheritance of a given disorder segregates with a particular chromosome. If this is the case, this particular trait has been mapped to the chromosome. Many different RFLPs for each human chromosome have now been identified; this may facilitate the assignment of any trait that segregates in a large family to a specific chromosome. Because of the abundance of the DNA polymorphisms, when a gene responsible for a disease is cloned, RFLPs may be found within or around the gene that allow distinction between the normal and defective genes in heterozygous individuals.

This process of mapping individual genes in the genome has led to the development of powerful techniques to search for genes whose biochemical function is not known but whose mutation produces a well-defined phenotype. By taking advantage of RFLPs, it is possible, in many cases, to determine which member of a chromosome pair is inherited from the mother and which one has been inherited from the father. Therefore, if a trait is inherited in a mendelian manner in a given family (Chap. 51), when the pattern of inheritance of the disease or trait as well as the origin (paternal or maternal) of each of the chromosomes in the affected and nonaffected members of the family is known, it is possible to map the gene responsible for the trait to a specific chromosome. This may be accomplished even when the function and nature of the gene are unknown. This process is called *gene* or *chromosome mapping.*

Once the chromosome is identified, it is possible to pinpoint the gene in question and isolate its sequence by a process called *chromosome walking.* This approach is known as *reverse genetics* because, in contrast to the direct approach in which the function of the gene and its protein product are already known and used to identify the gene sequences. In this case neither the biochemical function of the gene nor its protein product is known. The normal or abnormal phenotype produced by the gene is the only available clue. The gene is isolated first in order to determine its function. Although this approach is still in its infancy, it holds tremendous promise for the identification of genes responsible for many pathological processes that have obscure and/or complex biochemical nature. Gene mapping has been used to localize the gene responsible for Huntington's chorea,[16] and reverse genetics has been utilized to identify and clone the genes for Duchenne muscular dystrophy[17] and cystic fibrosis.[18]

In the cardiovascular system, reverse genetics using RFLPs has been successfully applied to identify the myosin heavy-chain gene as the locus responsible for certain forms of familial hypertrophic cardiomyopathy in humans[19] (p. 1406), and genetic mapping has been used to identify the locus associated with situs inversus in the iv/iv mouse.[20]

GENE MAPPING BY HYBRIDIZATION

In addition to the RFLP mapping method, a gene can be readily mapped to a chromosome once cDNA and/or genomic sequences of the gene have been cloned, using hybrid chromosome panels or in situ hybridization of the metaphase chromosomes. Hybrid chromosome panels consist of a collection of hybrid cell clones (usually mouse X human hybrid cells). In these combinations, human chromosomes are preferentially and randomly lost from the hybrid cells, and clones that contain only a subset of human chromosomes can be isolated. Panels of these clones are constituted so that it is possible to include and exclude every possible chromosome. DNA from these cells is isolated, digested with a battery of restriction enzymes, separated by gel electrophoresis, and transferred to a membrane support. This is a blotting procedure that can be used for DNA, RNA, or protein. This process, which was first described for analysis of DNA by Southern,[21] is called *Southern blot* when the filter immobilized molecule is DNA, *Northern blot* when it is RNA, and *Western* or *Southwestern blot* when proteins are blotted. The electrophoretically size-separated DNA is then *hybridized* to the radiolabeled cDNA or genomic DNA from the gene to be mapped.

Under the appropriate conditions, the labeled DNA will only hybridize to its cognate sequences blotted to the membrane, despite the fact that it contains DNA from the entire genome. The radiolabeled probe will produce a characteristic pattern of bands that can be visualized when the membrane is exposed to a radiographic film (autoradiograph). In somatic cell hybrid panels, it is possible to distinguish the band produced by hybridization to the mouse genes from the bands produced by the human genes. When the hybridization pattern produced by the human genes is compared with the known chromosome composition of each clone, it is possible to assign the gene sequence to a particular chromosome. An alternative process is to hybridize the radiolabeled cDNA or genomic probe to a mitotic metaphase chromosome spread. The site of hybridization of the probe to the cognate chromosome is visualized by photographic emulsion autoradiography, in which the density of the silver grains indicates not only the chromosomal location of the gene, but also its subchromosomal location.

USE OF CLONED DNA FOR DIAGNOSIS AND TREATMENT OF GENETIC DISORDERS

Substantial progress has been made in identifying genetic loci in humans (Fig. 51–1, p. 1624). In the last edition of McKusick's "Mendelian Inheritance in Man," more than 1500 genes had been mapped to a specific human chromosome.[22] The rate of gene mapping is accelerating rapidly and has now reached more than one gene a day. The valuable contribution of gene mapping to clinical medicine is obvious, although as of this writing it is at the earliest stages of development. However, in the past few years, more than a dozen clinically important genes causative of mendelian-inherited diseases have been mapped, including Huntington's chorea on chromosome 4, adenomatous polyposis of the colon on chromosome 5, cystic fibrosis on chromosome 7, certain forms of familial hypertrophic cardiomyopathy on chromosome 14, retinoblastoma on chromosome 13, neurofibromatosis on chromosome 17, one form of Alzheimer's disease on chromosome 21, and Duchenne muscular dystrophy to the short arm of the X chromosome.

At the time of mapping, there was little information as to the nature of the biochemical defect in some cases. For this reason, there were no reliable diagnostic tests for many of these diseases; moreover, patient testing could not be done during fetal or postnatal life before the appearance of clinical manifestations of the disease. This lack of basic information also made it difficult to design therapeutic approaches to attack the biochemical processes involved or their consequences. However, once the gene had been mapped, it rapidly became possible to use this information for prenatal diagnosis, premorbid diagnosis, and carrier detection for conditions such as cystic fibrosis, muscular dystrophy, and Huntington's chorea, among others.

Despite this progress and the expectations raised by these methods, most of the progress thus far has related to disorders caused by defects in a single gene in which there is a clear mendelian inheritance of the characteristic phenotype.[22] Since many of the significant diseases affecting the cardiovascular system (such as hypertension and atherosclerosis) are *multigenic* and multifactorial, it is not surprising that the impact of the genetic approach in diagnosis and patient management is lagging compared with other areas of medicine, such as immunology, oncology, and metabolism.

MUTATIONS. Two main types of genetic lesions (mutations) are responsible for inherited diseases: gross abnormalities of genes or chromosomes (deletions, insertions, and rearrangements), and a single- or few-base substitution or deletion in critical regions of the gene (point mutations) (Fig. 50–3). The gross abnormalities of genes are the easiest to detect using Southern blot analysis and are simple to explain pathogenetically. The gene does not function because it has been partially or completely deleted or it has been inactivated because an extraneous piece of DNA has been inserted in a crucial area (coding or regulatory). Gross rearrangements can occur in genes that are duplicated in tandem; that is, when there are two quite similar copies of a gene on neighboring regions of the same chromosome. One example of this type of genetic defect involves the α-globin gene cluster, in which rearrangements between the several copies of the α-globin genes can occur by unequal crossover during meiosis, which then gives rise to a mutation that causes α-thalassemia. In the cardiovascular system, affected members of a family with familial hypertrophic cardiomyopathy carry a hybrid myosin heavy-chain (MHC) gene produced by a crossover between the α- and β-MHC genes,[23] which are normally located next to each other on the same chromosome.[24,25]

Point Mutations. Caused by substitution, deletion, or insertion of a single or few nucleotides, point mutations are the most common cause of genetic defect identified so far. Even when they affect only a single nucleotide, these point mutations can have important consequences for the expression of the gene involved. They might completely or partially eliminate the gene product. This can occur because the mutation affects transcription, splicing, or translation of the mRNA. In many cases, however, the effect of the mutation is limited to the substitution of one amino acid for another. The phenotypic consequences of this can be as serious as those of the gross gene rearrangements, or they can be less drastic, depending on the nature of the substitution.

OLIGONUCLEOTIDE PROBES. Point mutations can be identified by restriction enzyme analysis, when the change in nucleotide sequence they produce either creates or abolishes a restriction endonuclease recognition site. At most, 5 to 10 per cent of all point mutations can be detected directly by restriction analysis.[26] For this reason, an alternative method of detection has been devised with synthetic oligonucleotides used as probes to recognize directly the mutated sequence and to distinguish between mutant and normal alleles. These oligonucleotides, specifically tailored for each mutation, will, under optimal conditions, recognize only their identical homologous sequence but will not recognize a sequence that varies at one or more nucleotides. In this manner, the normal gene will be identified only by the normal sequence, while the mutant gene will be recognized only by its mutant counterpart.[27] Although this technique is quite powerful, it has the obvious limitation that it can be used only when the molecular basis of the genetic lesion has already been identified and the proper sequence is known.

In theory, this type of oligonucleotide analysis should allow for the diagnosis of all the known point mutations in a particular gene. In practice, however, its applicability is more limited for several reasons: in many cases of single gene disorders, such as cystic fibrosis[28] and osteogenesis imperfecta,[29] there are many different mutations causing the disease and each family has a different mutation. In other cases, the probes are specific for a single family and cannot be used for anyone else. This is the case for a type of familial hypertrophic cardiomyopathy caused by a single-base substitution in the β-MHC gene.[30]

PRENATAL DIAGNOSIS. Genetic defects, caused by either gross rearrangements or point mutations, can be diagnosed by Southern blot analysis using the methods already described and cloned genes or synthetic oligonucleotides as probes. For this test a significant amount of genomic DNA is needed, which necessitates a long waiting time to grow cells obtained by amniocentesis or chorion villus sampling. These limitations have been eliminated by recently developed methodology. The *polymerase chain reaction* (PCR)[31] allows for the rapid amplification of very small samples of DNA (even a single molecule) by repeated cycles of DNA synthesis using a temperature-resistant DNA polymerase.[32] In this manner, it is possible to amplify a region of a gene starting with the DNA from a single cell or very few cells, followed by hybridization of a diagnostic DNA probe to the amplified DNA. This procedure, which can be completed in a day, has rapidly become the method of choice for the diagnosis of single-gene disorders. The sensitivity and efficiency of the procedure have allowed its application to embryos grown in vitro before implantation in order to identify carriers of known disorders affecting one of the parents. In those cases, a single cell removed from the embryo before transfer to the uterus is sufficient for the procedure. For prenatal diagnosis it is not necessary to know the precise molecular defect that has caused the disease in a given family or individual. It is sufficient to identify the abnormal gene and to be able to follow its pattern of inheritance. As already indicated, in the absence of a cloned gene, the availability of RFLPs located close to the responsible gene is sufficient for this type of analysis.

USE OF CLONED GENES FOR RESEARCH AND THERAPY

Once cDNA clones containing the complete coding sequence for a particular protein have been isolated, they can be used to express the protein product in a variety of cell types. This approach is particularly useful for several purposes: to determine the physiological role of the particular protein, to analyze its structure-function relationships in detail, and to produce large quantities of a natural gene product or its mutants. This is especially useful when these products are synthesized in small amounts by the original source, as is the case for insulin, growth hormone, tissue-type plasminogen activator (t-PA), and erythropoietin, all of which have been produced from cloned DNA and are currently in clinical use.

The advantages of this approach are exemplified by the development of t-PA as a research and therapeutic tool (p. 1231). Although the effect of t-PA as a fibrinolytic agent had been known for several years, its effect on thrombi was tested using t-PA secreted by a tumor cell line in culture.[33] Given the promising results, it became clear that an alternative and more efficient mode of production was required if the role of this substance in acute myocardial infarction was to be assessed. For this reason, the protein secreted by melanoma cell lines was first purified. With use of limited proteolysis followed by peptide sequencing, the sequence of a small portion of the protein was obtained. This sequence was used to synthesize a DNA oligonucleotide containing all possible codon combinations able to code for the t-PA peptide sequence available. This synthetic DNA was used to screen a cDNA library from melanoma cells that contained several hundred thousand different cDNA sequences. Based on the specific hybridization of the synthetic cDNA probes, clones containing the complete sequence coding for t-PA were isolated and remain a source for t-PA production.

Once the cDNA clones have been isolated, it is necessary to produce the corresponding protein. It is possible to carry out the whole process in vitro using cell-free systems that carry out the transcription and translation required to make the protein product. However, this process is quite inefficient and only limited quantities of protein for analytical analyses can be obtained in this manner. To produce large quantities, it is essential to use a host cell capable of using a foreign gene as one of its own. The two most effective expression cell systems use either bacteria or animal cells as the hosts for the cloned gene. In both cases it is important to use strategies that will "trick" the cell into making this foreign gene product in large quantities. In the case of bacteria, the most common strategy is to fuse the cDNA coding for the protein of interest to the coding portion of a gene whose expression can be induced at will to a very high level in response to a drug or metabolite in the medium. In this manner, a fusion protein is obtained that has the amino terminus of the bacterial protein and the carboxyl terminus of the cloned gene; when the host gene is induced, the cloned protein is made in large amounts as a byproduct.

Although recombinant proteins formed by bacteria often have many of the biological functions of the native protein, this is not always the case. Usually, this is because bacterial cells do not produce the postsynthetic modification such as glycosylation or acetylation that is characteristic of the product from animal cells. For this reason, ingredients intended for pharmacological use are commonly produced by expressing the cloned gene in animal cells. To accomplish this, the cloned cDNA to be expressed is ligated to a plasmid vector containing the regulatory sequences (promoter) of an animal gene that is normally expressed at high levels. This DNA is then introduced into the animal cell by a process called *transfection*. In the case of t-PA, it soon became obvious that not enough t-PA could be produced by the transfected cells for clinical trials. To address this problem, Kaufman et al.[35] devised means to produce more t-PA in animal cells by means of the ability of most cells to make multiple copies of the gene coding to dehydrofolate reductase (DHFR) when grown in the presence of the antitumor drug methotrexate.[36] This gene amplification in response to the drug results in the presence of several hundred copies of the DHFR gene in each cell. Kaufman ligated the t-PA cDNA to a cloned DHFR gene in an expression vector. After the gene had been transfected into the host cells, it was amplified by exposing the cells to increasing levels of methotrexate. The augmented DHFR gene sequences produced amplification of the neighboring t-PA cDNA sequences, resulting in a ~100 fold increase in the amount of t-PA secreted into the medium.

The availability of t-PA cDNA sequences has also served to elucidate structure-function relationships in the molecule. By mutation or deletion or both of particular residues or whole domains of the protein, a large number of variant t-PA molecules have been produced. These molecules have different primary structures and/or posttranslational modifications, such as glycosylation, that in many cases change the enzymatic properties or the half-life of the enzyme.

The use of cloned genes for the study of structure-function relationships is a particularly powerful tool for dissection of molecules relevant to the structure and function of the cardiovascular system. Williams et al. used this approach to perform a detailed analysis of the signaling mechanisms involved in the pathway of growth factor signaling using the platelet-derived growth factor (PDGF) receptor as the model system.[37] By this mechanism they elucidated elements in the cellular machinery responsive to receptor stimulation, as well as the structurally and functionally important features of the receptor involved in ligand binding, activation, and interaction with other cellular components.[38] A similar approach has been used by Lefkowitz and colleagues to study the relevant functional elements of the beta-adrenoceptors[39] and Numa et al. for the acetylcholine receptor as well as the sodium and calcium channels,[40] among others.

EXPRESSION OF CLONED GENES IN INTACT ANIMALS. The ability to introduce and target the expression of individual genes to individual cell types and tissues of the living animal or human is one of the most promising developments of molecular biology. Although the value of this technique in analysis of basic mechanisms of gene expression is high, this is overshadowed by its possible practical applications for gene therapy. Brinster and colleagues were the first to demonstrate that it is possible to inject cloned genes into the nucleus of a fertilized egg to produce animals that express the transfected gene (*transgene*) during development and are able to transmit it to their progeny in an inheritable mendelian manner,[41] i.e., the creation of transgenic animals. In most cases the information required to direct the expression of a cloned gene to the proper tissue in which the endogenous gene is expressed is located in the 5′ flanking region of the gene. In this manner, it has been shown that, if a gene containing the 5′ flanking sequences of the atrial natriuretic factor is injected into mouse oocytes, it is exclusively expressed in the cardiac tissues of the resulting mice in a pattern similar to that of the endogenous gene.[42] In these experiments, the transgene responds to physiological stimuli, such as work-overload hypertrophy, in a manner indistinguishable from the natural gene, by reintroduction of its expression in the ventricles of adult animals.[43] A similar result has been obtained with constructs containing the 5′ flanking region of the α-MHC gene. Therefore, with this approach, it is possible to analyze the role of different regulatory sequences in the gene in a natural context, during development and under conditions that are physiologically relevant.

From these experiments it became clear that only selected portions of the gene were required to direct the expression of a foreign gene to the proper cell type. In most, but not all, cases the sequences required and sufficient to direct the proper expression of a gene are located outside the coding regions in the so-called 5′ flanking sequences. These sequences, which contain all of the elements required to direct the proper transcription of the gene, include the promoter sequence and the transcription start site. In some genes many of the important sequences needed for transcription are clustered together in a region of the chromosome and constitute a *tissue-specific enhancer*. These tissue-specific enhancers are the binding sites for transcription factors that are specific for a given cell type or a particular stage of development or both. In some cases these enhancers are not located in the 5′ flanking sequences but rather within the coding region of the gene or at the 3′ flanking region.[44]

These enhancer sequences are able to stimulate (enhance) the expression of any gene even when located at a great distance from the gene. With this type of sequence it has been possible to create hybrid genes and direct their expression to cardiac cells. In this manner the expression of gene products not normally found in the myocardium can be induced. One of the most spectacular outcomes of this approach has resulted from directing the expression of different oncogenes to the myocardium. Unregulated expression of c-myc during development produces cardiac hyperplasia, generating hearts that have an abnormally large number of cells.[45] Even more striking, when the expression of the T antigen oncogene from the simian virus (SV) 40 is directed in mice toward the atria by the atrial natriuretic factor gene promoter and flanking sequences, the resulting mice develop atrial tumors.[46] If the same oncogene is directed toward the atria and ventricle by the α-MHC promoter and flanking sequences, the mice develop atrial and ventricular tumors.[47] The myocardial cells from these hearts are constituted to express the T antigen and have many properties of a tumor cell. However, these properties have been exploited to generate atrial and ventricular myocyte cell lines that cause growth for many passages in tissue culture dishes while retaining many of the differentiated properties of normal cardiac myocytes. The production of these cell strains has been a longstanding goal in the field of cellular and molecular cardiology and should provide a valuable tool to study the biology of these cells.

Gene Therapy

INSERTION OF GENES INTO THE GERM LINE. In addition to its use for the study of gene expression, the potential application of gene transfer technology to correct genetic defects has been obvious for many years and has proved to be successful in experimental animals, when the normal gene was injected into oocytes of mutant animals. In these cases, the gene is present in all cells of the transgenic organism, including the germ cells, and is transmitted to its progeny in a mendelian manner. Obviously, this approach is not feasible in humans because of ethical and practical considerations: the rate of success of this approach is too low, the long-term consequences of harboring the transgene in all cells of the body remain unknown, and tampering with human germ plasm is unacceptable ethically. Therefore, gene therapy in humans is likely to be limited to somatic cells.

INSERTION OF GENES INTO SOMATIC CELLS. Theoretically, a large number of inherited human diseases should be correctable by the introduction of new genes into appropriate cell types. However, since most current models of gene transfer result in the random insertion of the incoming sequence into the genome without correction of the endogenous mutant gene, the ideal candidate diseases are single-gene recessive disorders. A principal requirement for performing somatic gene therapy is the availability of a safe and efficient method of inserting the gene into the appropriate cells. In addition, in the best circumstances the recipient cells should be long lived, so that they produce the permanent correction of the disorder. Therefore, it is not surprising that most of the effort in human gene therapy has been directed toward the introduction of corrective genes into somatic cells. This approach is particularly promising for the correction of hematological disorders because of the relative ease of obtaining stem cells that might be genetically engineered and reintroduced into the body, where they would repopulate the bone marrow and differentiate into different cell types. Combined immunodeficiency caused by adenosine deaminase (ADA) deficiency, beta-thalassemia, and lipid storage diseases such as Gaucher's disease are particularly suitable for this type of therapy. This approach, however, has been hindered by two main problems. First, since the number of target stem cells is quite low, an efficient delivery system is required for this strategy. Second, the transgene needs to be regulated properly during development and in response to different physiological stimuli.

GENE INSERTION USING RETROVIRUSES. In the past few years significant progress has been made in the delivery of genes using a variety of viral vectors. Replication-defective retroviral vectors and cell lines that package the vectors into viral particles have been developed and have proved highly efficient.[48-50] Although thus far the attempts to perform retroviral gene transfer in nonhuman primates have been disappointing, there is evidence that most of the problems hampering progress can be solved.[51] In the meantime, gene transfer has been used to mark autologous tumor-infiltrating lymphocytes (TIL) by means of retrovirus-mediated gene transfer in a series of patients with melanoma. This represents the first report of approved gene transfer in humans and clearly indicates the potential value and relative safety of using retroviral gene markers to study the biology of human cells. As indicated by Rosenberg et al., it should be possible to transduce these TIL cells or other populations of lymphocytes with vectors expressing cytokines or other molecules whose increased concentration would be beneficial.[52]

GENE INSERTION INTO ENDOTHELIAL CELLS. In the cardiovascular system, the endothelial cells appear to be the most promising target for retroviral gene therapy because of their long life and easy accessibility. Nabel et al. demonstrated that endothelial cells genetically modified to express an indicator gene could be used to seed denuded iliofemoral arteries in the in vivo swine model and that they continued to express the indicator gene for at least 4 weeks after implantation.[53] In a similar experiment, Wilson et al. seeded Dacron grafts with endothelial cells genetically engineered to express an indicator gene.[54] The indicator gene was expressed in these carotid artery grafts for at least 5 weeks after implantation. More recently, Dichek et al. seeded endothelial cells that had been modified to produce t-PA onto vascular stents in vitro.[55] The genetically modified endothelial cells continued to express t-PA at significantly higher levels than normal endothelial cells while attached to the stent, and they remained in place when the stent was expanded by balloon dilatation. The number of cells implanted with the stent would not be expected to produce a systemic anticoagulant effect; however, the increased local concentration of t-PA might be sufficient to produce a local thrombolytic effect at the surface of the stents and might make them less subject to thrombosis when implanted in vivo. Although significantly much more data are required to determine the clinical efficacy of this form of gene therapy, it is clear that this approach is potentially useful. Interestingly, catheter-directed delivery of retroviruses to endothelial cells in situ has recently been reported with encouraging results.[56] If this method of delivery proves to be of general applicability, it would simplify greatly this approach to gene therapy and broaden its application.

Recent reports from several laboratories have demonstrated that functional genes can be administered by direct injection into living animals without the use of retroviruses. In some of these cases long-term expression has been obtained in vivo without the need to integrate the foreign gene into the genome of the host cell. The level and duration of expression obtained suggest that these approaches will have scientific and therapeutic applications. Wolff and colleagues demonstrated expression of marker genes following direct injection into skeletal muscle in vivo.[57] Although there was no evidence of integration into the host genome, expression persisted for more than 6 months. Similar results in cardiac muscles using viral promoters to direct the expression of the marker gene were subsequently reported.[58] High levels of expression can be obtained when the marker gene is linked to a myocardial-specific promoter gene sequence as has been demonstrated by several groups, including the authors' own.

HOPES FOR HUMAN GENE THERAPY. Although the studies just mentioned are still in the experimental phase, they provide a glimpse of what is likely to become possible in the near future. It is now clear that many genes coding for physiologically and therapeutically important proteins can be introduced into the cardiovascular system either through the endothelial cells or through direct injection into the myocardium to provide for their local or systemic release in vivo. Proteins that induce angiogenesis, inhibit smooth muscle proliferation, lower plasma levels of cholesterol, affect the thrombogenic properties of the endothelial wall, or produce vasodilation are only a few of the gene products that are candidates for use in gene therapy. Patients with certain forms of cardiomyopathy, such as in muscular dystrophy (p. 1813), may be candidates for direct gene therapy into the myocardium. More tantalizing is the prospect of manipulating the genes responsible for the cell cycle to induce cell division of the differentiated cardiac myocytes at the borders of a ischemic injury to regenerate cardiac muscle. Therefore, "in vivo" gene delivery could allow for creation of customized, discretely localized "cellular factories" in individual patients for the endogenous production of therapeutically efficacious drugs targeted at specific disease processes. Although formidable obstacles such as the regulation of production of gene products obscure the path to routine use of gene therapy in human disease, the first steps down that path recently have been taken successfully.[59]

Molecular Biology of the Cardiac Contractile System

Despite the contributions of molecular biology to the understanding of many processes affecting the cardiovascular system, the cellular and molecular bases of cardiac performance remain poorly understood for the most part. As indicated at the beginning of this chapter, this situation is due, at least in part, to the fact that the myocardium is a less-than-ideal tissue for the application of genetic and molecular approaches.

Given the essential role of the myocardium in the survival of the organism, most of the genetic mutations that significantly affect its development or function or both are likely to be lethal. This feature explains the relatively small number of mutations that affect the myocardium either in humans or animal models described thus far. This contrasts with the large number of mutations affecting blood cells, the endocrine system, and metabolic pathways, among others. The existence of these mutations has provided the means of entry for the molecular dissection of these systems. In addition to the relative unavailability of mutations in the cardiovascular system, the difficulty in obtaining repeated samples of the myocardium from the same animal that are suitable for biochemical and molecular analysis has also slowed progress.

Furthermore, the existence of well-characterized cell lines that can be grown in homogeneous populations and mutated at will are an almost essential requirement for the exploitation of recombinant DNA technology to elucidate regulatory pathways. Given that the cardiac myocyte is a terminally differentiated cell that has lost its ability to replicate in vivo or in vitro shortly after birth,[1] no cell lines with well-defined characteristics of cardiac myocytes have been available until now. The aforementioned combination of characteristics has played an important role in delaying the dissection of the cellular and molecular basis of cardiac performance in physiological and pathological states. Yet it is clear that the application of modern techniques of cellular and molecular biology holds great promise for solving some of the major problems in clinical cardiovascular medicine. In addition, it is becoming increasingly clear that the cardiovascular system in general, and the myocardium in particular, is an excellent model with which to address some broad biological questions that have general significance.

Some recent advances in the understanding of the molecular biology of the cardiac contractile system and its response to physiological and pathological stimuli are presented below. Particular emphasis is placed on the contractile apparatus and on those areas that highlight the extraordinary plasticity of this tissue at the biochemical level and that highlight the insight obtained through new molecular approaches.

THE CARDIAC CONTRACTILE APPARATUS

The sarcomere (Figs. 13–1, p. 353, and 13–4, p. 355) is the basic contractile unit of both the myocardium and skeletal muscle.[60] The contractile properties of the myocardium—in terms of force generated and velocity of contraction—are dependent on the number as well as the biochemical composition of its sarcomeres. The sarcomere, in turn, is made up of seven major proteins and several minor ones organized into thick and thin filaments. The thin filaments, anchored at the Z lines (Fig. 50–10), are formed by a double helix of polymerized sarcomeric actin molecules. In the major groove of this double helix is located a continuous coil of tropomyosin (TM) dimers. Every tropomyosin dimer interacts with seven actins and it is associated with a troponin (Tn) complex (Fig. 13–4, p. 355). Each complex in turn is composed of one molecule of each of the three troponins—T, C, and I. This tropomyosin-troponin complex is responsible for the calcium sensitivity of the contractile apparatus. It regulates the interaction between the heads of the myosin molecule, located in the thick filament, and actin, the main constituent of the thin filament. Although much is known about this interaction, the precise molecular mechanisms responsible for the biochemical-mechanical transduction have not yet been fully elucidated.

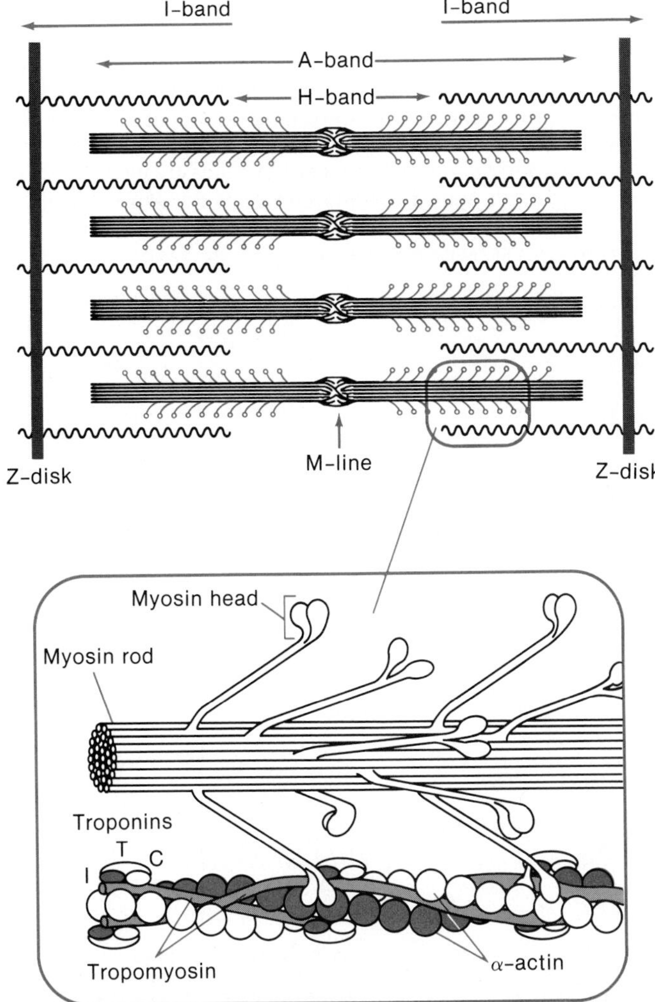

FIGURE 50–10. Structural organization of a sarcomere. Each sarcomere (top panel) is constituted by sets of parallel thick and thin filaments (bottom panel) which partially overlap and are connected to one another.

The thick filament contains the molecular motor of contraction, the myosin heavy chain (MHC). This is a bifunctional molecule that exists in a dimeric form (Fig. 13–5, p. 355). The two functional domains are constituted of the rod portion and the head; the rod is composed of the carboxyl-terminal half of the molecule and is a regular coiled helix responsible for the assembly of myosin into an organized antiparallel thick filament with heads regularly spaced every 14.3 Å at both ends with a bare zone in the middle. The rod carries the load during contraction; its antiparallel organization makes possible the shortening of the sarcomere by pulling together two thin filaments pointing in opposite direction and attached to two neighboring Z lines. During the contraction cycle, the head of MHC—composed of the amino-terminal half of the molecule—interacts directly with the actin molecules in the thin filament and carries the ATPase activity required to produce the physical translocation needed for fiber shortening. The ATPase activity of MHC is modulated by two smaller protein subunits bound to each MHC head—the alkali and essential myosin light chains (MLC). As originally pointed out by Barany, there is a direct correlation between the unloaded maximum velocity of shortening of a muscle fiber (V_{max}) and the actin-activated ATPase activity of its MHC.[61] Although there are some apparent exceptions to this rule, fibers with an MHC with high ATPase activity contract faster than those with a lower enzymatic activity.[62,63] As might be anticipated, there is an inverse correlation between ATPase activity of the MHC in a fiber and the energetic cost to perform a given workload.[62–64] The more rapidly the fiber contracts, the higher the energetic cost of producing the same amount of work. It is clear, therefore, that the *type* of MHC and its ATPase activity present in the sarcomeres are physiologically significant and have a profound effect on the contractile properties of the myocardium.

In addition to the seven major proteins mentioned earlier, the sarcomere contains a number of other proteins, such as α-actinin, C protein, titin, and nebulin,[65,66] that are present in smaller concentrations and are thought to play important roles either in sarcomeric organization or modulation of function. However, with the exception of α-actinin, which is the main constituent of the Z line and serves to anchor the actin filament,[65] the precise function of these minor components of the sarcomere remains to be defined.

The intrinsic properties of the sarcomere are the main determinants of the contractile state. However, a number of other molecules, such as adrenoceptors[67] (p. 363), ion channels[68] (p. 358), Na^+, K^+-ATPase (p. 359), sarcolemmal and sarcoplasmic calcium pumps (p. 361), and sarcoplasmic calcium-release channels,[69–71] are also involved in its modulation. Most of these molecules exert their effect on contractility by directly or indirectly modulating either the availability or the response to calcium by the contractile proteins. Each of the cardiac contractile proteins is a member of a family of *isoforms* that is specific to the cell type and stage of development.

EXPRESSION OF MULTIPLE ISOFORMS

The regulated expression of cell type–specific protein isoforms that are structurally distinct and developmentally regulated is a fundamental characteristic of higher organisms. The molecular mechanisms responsible for the generation of this protein diversity can be broadly categorized into two main systems: those that select a particular gene among the members of a multigene family for expression in a particular cell and those that generate several different isoforms from a single gene. This latter mechanism includes DNA rearrangement and alternative pre-mRNA splicing. Both mechanisms involve the differential use of intragenic sequences that lead to the production of multiple protein isoforms from a single gene. DNA rearrangement appears to be restricted to a quite limited set of genes coding for immunoglobulins and T-cell receptors.[72,73] In contrast, increasing numbers of genes in organisms ranging from insects to humans, including their DNA and RNA viruses, are known to be alternatively spliced.

Alternative pre-mRNA splicing is particularly prevalent in striated muscle, including the myocardium. Among the contractile protein genes, this mode of gene regulation has been documented for alpha- and beta-tropomyosin, troponin T, and the myosin light chains, in addition to a number of other genes.[74,75] Furthermore, the major constituents of the thick (MHCs and MLCs) and thin (actin, tropomyosins, and troponins [C, T, and I]) filaments of mammalian sarcomeres are each encoded by a multigene family of moderate size, ranging from four to eight members.[60,66,76] The expression of each member of these multigene families is regulated at the transcriptional level in a tissue-specific and developmentally regulated manner. The different isoforms of sarcomeric contractile proteins, generated either through the transcription of different genes or from the same gene by alternative pre-mRNA splicing, are able to substitute for one another and when present to combine in the same cell. The restricted combined use of the different members of these multigene families allows for the generation of a moderate number of qualitatively different sarcomere types that exhibit significantly different physiological characteristics, at least in some cases.[66,67,76,77] This potential for the production of different sarcomeres is greatly increased by the generation of multiple protein isoforms by individual MLC and TNT genes. Therefore, in order to understand the mechanisms involved in generating myocardial protein diversity, it is necessary to know the elements responsible for the selective transcription of a given gene in a particular cell type at a particular time in development or physiological state as well as the factors that regulate alternative pre-mRNA splicing in the same cell.

Most of the genes coding for contractile proteins have now been identified; cDNA and genomic sequences have been obtained, mapped to the human genome, and characterized for their potential to generate multiple protein isoforms by alternative splicing. Although some of these genes are closely clustered on the same chromosome, as is the case for the cardiac and skeletal MHCs,[78–80] most other contractile protein gene families are not linked but are scattered on several chromosomes.[81,82] Therefore, although the contractile proteins are assembled in the sarcomere in quite precise stoichiometric quantities, their regulation is of necessity complex, because it involves multiple genes that are located in different regions of the genome that, with few exceptions, do not seem to have common regulatory sequences.

Some of the contractile protein isoforms expressed in the myocardium are shared with skeletal muscle, while others are expressed exclusively in the heart[60,66,67] (Table 50–1). Moreover, for several of these proteins, the atrial and ventricular isoforms are different from one another and both differ from the ones expressed in the conduction system. Although the physiological basis for the selective advantage that has produced this isoform distribution is not apparent from our present understanding of contractility, two main general trends are obvious: (1) the myocardial genes are more likely to be shared with slow than with fast skeletal muscle and (2)

TABLE 50–1 EXPRESSION OF CONTRACTILE PROTEIN GENES IN STRIATED SKELETAL AND CARDIAC MUSCLES OF SMALL MAMMALS

	SKELETAL MUSCLES			VENTRICLE			ATRIUM
	Embryonic/ Neonatal	Adult Fast	Adult Slow	Embryonic	Adult	Pressure Overload Adult	Adult
Myosin heavy chain (MHC)	Embryonic MHC Neonatal MHC	Fast II A MHC Fast II B MHC	Slow I = βMHC	Slow/βMHC	αMHC + ~βMHC	Slow/βMHC + αMHC	α MHC
Myosin light chain (LC)	LC1e LC1f	LC1f LC3f	LC1slow/ cardiac	LC1e	LC1slow/ cardiac	LC1slow/cardiac + LCe	LC1e LC1slow/cardiac
Myosin light chain 2	LC2sk	LC2sk	LC2sk	LC2 cardiac	LC2 cardiac	LC2 cardiac	LC2 cardiac
Tropomyosin	ββ	α/β α/α	α/β	β/α	α/α	α/β	α/α
Troponins T	Fast TnT Slow TnT	Fast TNT	Slow TNT	(Emb)cardiac TNT	(Adult)cardiac TNT		Cardiac TNT
C	c TNC (slow/ cardiac)	skTNC (skeletal)	cTNC	cTNC	cTNC	cTNC	cTNC
I	Fast TNI	Fast TNI	Slow/cardiac TNI	Slow/cardiac TNI	Slow/cardiac TNI		Slow/cardiac
Actin	c α-actin sk α-actin	sk α-actin	sk α-actin	sk α-actin c α-actin	c α-actin	c α-actin sk α-actin	c α-actin
Creatine kinase	BB ck BM ck	MM ck	MM ck	BB ck MM ck	MM ck	MM ck BB ck	

MHC = Myosin heavy chain; each member of this gene family is indicated by a prefix indicating the most common nomenclature used to duplicate the gene. MLC = myosin light chain gene products: LC1e = light chain 1 embryonic, LC1 slow/cardiac = light chain specific for slow and cardiac tissues. LC1f and LC3f are the two products for the myosin light chain 1/3 that is predominantly expressed in fast muscle. LC2sk and LC2 cardiac denote the light chain 2 characteristic of skeletal (sk) and cardiac muscle, respectively. Tropomyosin α and β designate these products of these two genes. α-TM is characteristic of differentiated striated muscle while β is characteristic of the undifferentiated cells. TNC, TNT, TNI indicate troponin C, T, and I, respectively. The prefixes cardiac, skeletal, slow, and embryonic indicate the tissue and or developmental stage in which this gene product is predominantly expressed. cα-Actin and skα-actin indicate the isoform characteristic of adult normal cardiac and skeletal muscle, respectively. Creatine kinase B and M isoform indicate the muscle-specific (M) and nonmuscle (B) isoforms.

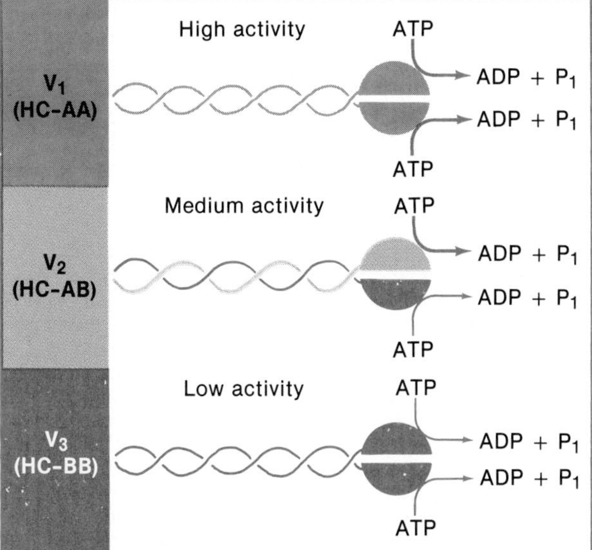

FIGURE 50–11. The three ventricular myosin isoenzymes, designated V1, V2, and V3, originate from combinations of two heavy-chain subunits (HC-A and HC-B), which differ in amino acid sequence. Functionally, these differences are expressed in the level of myosin ATPase activity and contractile performance. Thus, hydrolysis of ATP and release of reaction products are most rapid for V1 and slowest for V3; V2 is intermediate. (From Morkin, E.: Contractile proteins of the heart. Hosp. Pract. *18*:107, 1983.)

embryonic and fetal cardiac isoforms are shared more often with striated muscle than are their adult cardiac counterparts.

ISOFORM SWITCHES IN RESPONSE TO PHYSIOLOGICAL AND PATHOLOGICAL STIMULI

In the ventricles of most mammalian species, including the human, three myosin isoforms have been identified on the basis of their electrophoretic mobility—V1, V2, and V3.[82,83] However, these three myosins are composed of only two distinct types of MHCs, referred to as α and β. V1 and V3 are composed of $\alpha\alpha$ and $\beta\beta$ homodimers, respectively, while V2 is an $\alpha\beta$ heterodimer (Fig. 50–11). These two myosins are produced by two different genes that are closely linked[78,79] and are located on chromosomes 3 and 14 in human and mouse, respectively.[79]

As for all muscle types, the myosin composition of the myocardium is of physiological importance, because the relative distribution of α- and β-MHC is directly correlated with the contractile properties of the heart. The α-MHC, which has high Ca^{++}- and actin-activated ATPase activity,[83,84] is associated with an increased shortening velocity of the cardiac fibers.[84,85] In contrast, the β-MHC, which has lower ATPase activity,[83,84] is associated with slower shortening velocity[84,85] (Fig. 50–12, top). It is therefore interesting that the ratio of these two different cardiac isoforms is developmentally regulated. In the ventricles of all mammalian species studied so far,

CARDIAC MYOSIN HEAVY-CHAIN ISOFORMS

	ATPase activity	Shortening velocity	Efficiency of force production
α-MHC (V_1)	High	Fast	Low
β-MHC (V_3)	Low	Slow	High

ISOFORM SWITCHES

	Thyroid hormone	Exercise	Work overload	Aging
α-MHC (V_1)	↑	↑	↓	↓
β-MHC (V_3)	↓	↓	↑	↑

FIGURE 50–12. Correlation of the ventricular myosin heavy chain phenotype and contractile performance of the myocardium in response to physiological, pathological, and developmental stimuli.

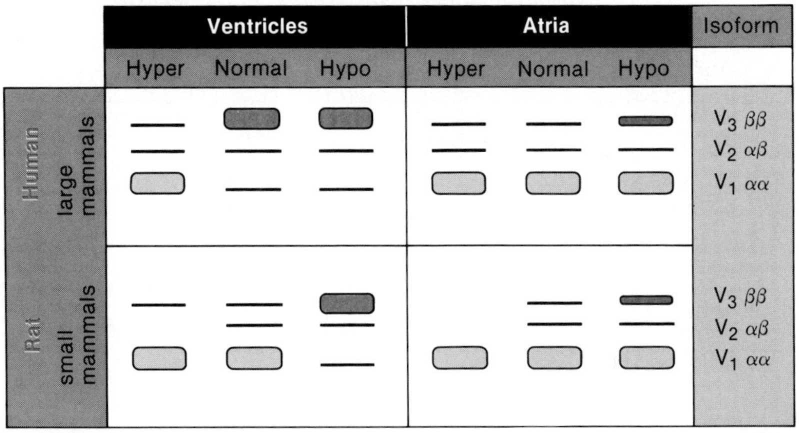

	Ventricles			Atria			Isoform
	Hyper	Normal	Hypo	Hyper	Normal	Hypo	
Human / large mammals							V_3 $\beta\beta$ V_2 $\alpha\beta$ V_1 $\alpha\alpha$
Rat / small mammals							V_3 $\beta\beta$ V_2 $\alpha\beta$ V_1 $\alpha\alpha$

FIGURE 50–13. Effect of thyroid hormone on cardiac myosin expression.

β-MHC is the most abundant isoform in utero until late fetal life.[86] In small mammals such as the rat and mouse, α-MHC increases immediately before birth and becomes the predominant form throughout perinatal and adult life.[86,87] In contrast, in large mammals such as humans, α-MHC is predominant only transiently shortly after birth, with β-MHC then becoming and remaining the most abundant isoform.[86,88] The situation is different in the atria, in which α-MHC is the predominant isoform throughout life in both small and large species[60,87,88] (Fig. 50–13). In all species studied, including humans, the distribution of the cardiac MHC isoforms changes in response to certain pathological and experimental conditions such as work overload,[85,89–92] diabetes,[93] gonadectomy,[94] and, more importantly, changes in thyroid hormone levels (Figs. 50–12 and 50–13).[82,84,87,95,97] These changes are regulated at the level of transcription of the respective genes, because there is a direct correlation between the levels of α- and β-MHC and the corresponding mRNAs[87,97] and between these and the rate of transcription.[98]

REGULATION OF CARDIAC MHC GENES BY THYROID HORMONE

(See also p. 1830)

Thyroid hormone plays a fundamental role in the regulation of the MHC phenotype, both in the myocardium and in skeletal muscle.[97] In mammals at least, all the genes of the striated MHC multigene family are, without exception, responsive to thyroid hormone. Surprisingly, however, whether the hormone induces or represses the expression of a given MHC depends on the gene itself and the muscle in which it is expressed. The same gene can be induced by the hormone in one muscle and repressed in another,[97] indicating that the regulation of this gene family by thyroid hormone is likely to be more complex than described so far for a variety of steroid hormones.[98] In the heart, there is a precise correlation between the levels of circulating thyroid hormone and the relative levels of α- and β-MHC in the ventricles.[87] The expression of α-MHC is dependent on the presence of thyroid hormone (Fig. 50–12, *bottom*). In its absence the α-MHC gene is not transcribed. The converse is true for β-MHC; the expression of this gene is repressed by thyroid hormone and it is induced in hypothyroid states.[87,97] The induction of α-MHC at the time of birth is directly correlated with the surge in the circulating thyroid hormone that occurs at this time.[87] This effect of thyroid hormone on cardiac MHC expression can be directly demonstrated in experimental animals by manipulation of their thyroid state. After surgical or chemical (5-thiouracil) thyroidectomy, the expression of α-MHC is completely suppressed and only β-MHC is expressed in the myocardium. Replacement therapy restores the normal phenotype. On the other hand, hyperthyroid states repress the expression of the β-MHC gene both at the mRNA and protein levels and produce a myocardium constituted exclusively by α-MHC[87,97] (Fig. 50–13). These results are not indirect and are not produced by changes in such factors as metabolic state, or circulating catecholamines. They can be reproduced in isolated tissue slices and cells in culture.[100]

MOLECULAR MECHANISM OF THYROID HORMONE ACTION. This has been elucidated, at least in part, by the demonstration that the c-erb proto-oncogenes (p. 1618) serve as the nuclear receptors for this hormone.[101–104] At least two genes with well-defined tissue-specific expression encode this receptor,[101–103] and each can generate several different isoforms by alternative splicing.[103] The functional properties of some of these alternatively spliced isoforms are quite different, and some have lost their ability to bind T3.[104] It has been proposed recently that some of the isoforms that are impaired in their ability to bind ligand might function as antioncogenes and/or antireceptor molecules[105,106] because of their ability to compete for DNA binding sites. However, due to the absence of ligand binding, they are unable to stimulate transcription.[104–106] It remains to be determined whether this is a general phenomenon. The functional T3 receptors are hormone-dependent transcriptional factors that exercise their effect through binding to a thyroid hormone responsive element (TRE) in the responsive gene.[104,106,107] The TRE for the human and rat β-MHC genes has been determined by a combination of deletion mapping, site-directed mutagenesis, and in vitro and in vivo hormone receptor binding assays.[100,104,108] The two genes have a TRE with identical sequence, and both are able to confer thyroid hormone sensitivity to heterologous genes.[42,46,50] Therefore, the sequence containing the TRE is both required and sufficient to confer T3 responsiveness on a gene.

T3 REPRESSION OF MHC GENES. The mechanism of T3 repression of MHC gene expression is less well understood. Both the human and rat β-MHC genes have sequences with a high degree of homology to the TRE of the α-MHC genes.[100,108] These sequences do not have an effect on the heterologous gene promoters so far tested, and it is not clear whether or not they are specifically recognized by the thyroid hormone receptor. Since these putative TRE sequences in the β-MHC genes are overlapping with the CAAT box sequences,[100] an essential promoter element in these genes, the possibility that T3 exerts its negative regulatory role by sterically hindering the binding of an essential transcription factor is presently being investigated.

The results summarized above demonstrate that thyroid hormone plays an important role in regulating cardiac MHC expression and raise the question of whether this hormone is solely responsible for the regulation of these genes (Fig. 50–14). Several lines of evidence indicate that this is *not* the case. First, it is clear that the α- and β-MHC genes respond to thyroid hormone in a tissue-dependent manner. For example, in the ventricle, the α-MHC gene is exquisitely sensitive to T3 and it is not expressed at all in the hypothyroid state. However, in the atria of the same heart, this gene is practically unresponsive to the hormone. The different behavior in the

GENE SWITCHES IN CARDIAC VENTRICLES

	Fetus & neonates	Normal adult	Work overload	Hypo-thyroid	Hyper-thyroid
Myosin heavy chain	β, α	α	βα	β	α
α-Actin	Skeletal cardiac	Cardiac	Cardiac skeletal	Same as normal adult	
Tropomyosin	α,β	α	α, β		
Na^+, K^+-ATPase	$α_1$, $α_2$	$α_1$	$α_1$, $α_2$		
ANF	+	−	+ +		

FIGURE 50–14. Gene switches in cardiac ventricles.

two tissues is not due to the lack of functional thyroid hormone receptors in the atria, since other genes in this structure are readily responsive to the hormone. A similar phenomenon is apparent for the β-MHC gene. As already indicated, in the ventricle the expression of this gene is repressed by thyroid hormone. Yet in the same animals, its expression continues at almost normal level in the slow fibers of skeletal muscle. Moreover, the TRE of these genes does not explain their tissue specificity because they act as positive regulators of transcription in the presence of receptor and T3, irrespective of the cell type in which they are expressed. In fact, the tissue specificity of these genes is conferred by a combination of positive and negative transcriptional regulatory elements.[108] These other regulatory elements are likely to be responsible for the species-specific differences in the expression of these genes.

WORK-OVERLOAD HYPERTROPHY INDUCES MHC GENE ISOFORM SWITCHES IN THE MYOCARDIUM

The involvement of different regulatory pathways in the expression of the cardiac MHC genes becomes evident when the changes produced by work-overload hypertrophy are analyzed. In small mammals, particularly in rats, in response to a moderate increase in mean aortic pressure (~30 mm Hg) produced by aortic coarctation[109] there is a rapid induction of β-MHC mRNA. This is followed by the appearance of comparable levels of β-MHC protein, in parallel with an increase in left ventricular weight. A similar change is not detectable in larger mammals, including the human, because β-MHC is the predominant isoform expressed in the normal ventricle of such mammals. However, in human atria, which normally express α-MHC, a switch to β-MHC is readily apparent in response to increased pressure.[110] Therefore, the hypertrophied myocardium induces the expression of β-MHC and represses the expression of the α-gene. With respect to the MHC phenotype, it resembles the fetal and hypothyroid states. Yet in these animals the circulating level of thyroid hormone remains normal, and their metabolic state argues against hypothyroidism. Other features argue persuasively that this isoform switch produced in response to work-overload hypertrophy is not regulated through the thyroid hormone pathway.[109]

WORK-OVERLOAD HYPERTROPHY INDUCES MANY FETAL ISOFORMS. The isoform switches produced in response to increased afterload are not limited to MHC. In fact, a general myocardial response to work overload occurs rapidly and affects a number of cellular compartments.[111] This response is characterized by the reexpression of the protein isoforms that are normally expressed in fetal life and normally suppressed in adulthood. This phenomenon has been demonstrated for *all* the gene phenotypes analyzed so far, including other contractile proteins such as skeletal α-actin,[111,112] myosin light chain 1,[113] and tropomyosin[111]; membrane proteins such as Na^+, K^+-ATPase (the cardiac glycoside receptor)[114]; secreted molecules such as atrial natriuretic peptide (ANP)[111]; and those involved in ATP regeneration, such as creatine kinase.[116] With the exception of ANF, all of these examples represent the reexpression of an isoform normally expressed only during fetal and early postnatal life that is later replaced by the corresponding adult isoform. ANF expression in the ventricles is normally suppressed after birth and is not replaced by another isoform. Its expression, however, is rapidly reinduced in response to the hypertrophic stimulus.

From these observations it is clear that myocardial hypertrophy is not only a quantitative phenomenon involving an increase in cardiac mass but, more importantly, it also results in a significant qualitative change in important constituents of the myocardium. In general, these changes produce a muscle that has many of the biochemical characteristics of *fetal* myocardium.

What is the stimulus for this dramatic and concerted change in myocardial gene expression in response to work overload? One possibility is thyroid hormone itself. However, as already indicated, no changes in thyroid hormone levels are detected in these animals. Furthermore, if thyroid hormone were responsible, the normal phenotype could be reestablished in response to thyroid hormone therapy. This is not the case. Thyroid hormone can overcome the effect of pressure overload on MHC gene expression but cannot influence the other phenotypic changes.[109,111] Administration of high doses of T3 in hypertrophic animals produces a rapid de-induction of the β-MHC gene with the concomitant induction of the α-MHC, despite the fact that these animals have a higher degree of hypertrophy than do those with simple hemodynamic overload.[109,111] None of the changes in the expression of other genes are affected by the hormone. These results give further support to the contention that the changes induced by hemodynamic overload are *not* secondary to thyroid hormone changes. However, in the case of the MHC genes, T3 has a dominant effect and can overcome the regulatory mechanisms induced by the hypertrophic stimulus. This behavior highlights the complex interplay that exists between hemodynamic and hormonal stimuli in the expression of myocardial genes.

It is noteworthy that in animals with aortic banding (experimental coarctation), the most commonly used model system, increased afterload, is not the only consequence of the manipulation. Aortic binding might produce an elevation in circulating catecholamine levels and/or activation of the renin-angiotensin system secondary to decreased renal blood flow. Norepinephrine[116,117] and possibly angiotensin II might directly stimulate myocardial cell hypertrophy independently of the hemodynamic effects. The effect of norepinephrine on cardiac cell growth in culture has been shown to be mediated by stimulation of the α_1-adrenoceptor,[116] which couples the hydrolysis of membrane phosphatidylinositol followed by the release of IP_3[118] and activation of protein kinase C (Fig. 13–12, p. 360).[119] Furthermore, phorbol esters, which are direct activators of protein kinase C, can produce hypertrophy and isoform switches when administered to cultured neonatal cardiac cells.[120] However, the fact that the atria and right ventricles of the animals with aortic banding do *not* exhibit the isoform transitions already described strongly suggests that these humoral mechanisms do not play an important role, if they are involved at all, in the processes described here.

MOLECULAR BASIS FOR CERTAIN FORMS OF HYPERTROPHIC CARDIOMYOPATHY

(See p. 1636)

Until recently, not a single mutation for any of the genes coding for contractile proteins had been identified in vertebrates. This contrasts with the large number of mutations with impaired function detected in lower organisms. The lack of phenotypic mutants in vertebrates could be explained by assuming that either most mutations are lethal or that they lack a distinctive phenotype because the mutant isoform is replaced by another from the same multigene family. The latter hypothesis was given credence by the finding of a mouse strain that lacks a functional cardiac α-actin gene. These animals have a normal life span and apparent cardiac performance and express the skeletal α-actin gene in the myocardium at all stages of development and physiological states. This phenotype, together with the changes induced by thyroid hormone and work overload hypertrophy, strongly supports the concept that different isoforms are interchangeable, although they might result in subtle changes in cardiac performance.

For this reason it is surprising that the mutation responsible for certain forms of familial hypertrophic cardiomyopathy maps to the cardiac myosin genes. This disease is a dominant disorder characterized by cardiac hypertrophy, a wide spectrum of clinical symptoms, and a high rate of sudden death (p. 1411). Pathological findings include increased myocardial mass with myocyte and myofibrillar disarray. It has recently been demonstrated that at least two different mutations can produce the disease. In one case there is a novel α/β cardiac MHC hybrid,[23] while in the other a single base pair mutation produces a missense mutation in the β-MHC.[30] From the sequence it appears that both mutant MHCs should be functional, although the mutation maps to an amino acid residue that is conserved in all the MHC sequenced thus far, ranging from unicellular organisms to humans. Although the molecular mechanisms responsible for the production of the anatomical changes in familial hypertrophic cardiomyopathy remain to be elucidated, the dominant character of the phenotype suggests that the assembly of the thick filament is affected by the mutation. Because not all cases of this disease map to the MHC locus, it is likely that mutations in other genes encoding contractile proteins can also produce the same clinical syndrome.

EXPRESSION OF PROTO-ONCOGENES BY WORK OVERLOAD

(See p. 1617)

The cardiac response to normal growth requirements, as well as to work overload, depends on the developmental state of the organ. During fetal and early postnatal life, the demand for an increased cardiac mass is filled mainly by an increase in the number of myocytes (hyperplasia). However, soon after birth, cardiac myocytes lose their ability to divide.[1] Later in life, demand for an increased myocardial mass is met exclusively by an increase in the size of a fixed number of preexisting myocytes. The molecular mechanisms responsible for the loss of replicative ability (terminal differentiation) remain unknown. Genes involved in determining the myogenic lineage and terminal differentiation in skeletal muscle, such as *MyoD*,[121] *myogenin*,[122] and *Mif*[123] that function as tissue-specific transcriptional factors, are *not* involved in the determination and differentiation of the cardiac myocytes, because they are not expressed in these cells. It is likely that a family of genes with functional similarities but with significant sequence divergence from the ones identified in skeletal muscle is responsible for the cardiac phenotype.

What is the mechanism involved in inducing cell growth and isoform switches in response to work overload? The observed reexpression of fetal isoforms in cardiac hypertrophy is reminiscent of the mitogenic response of many differentiated cell types, such as hepatocytes, which often involves the suppression of the adult phenotype and reexpression of the fetal pattern, as is the case in the inhibition of albumin and induction of α-protein expression during liver regeneration.[124] In a general biological context, cardiac hypertrophy could be considered the equivalent of the growth response exhibited by most cell types in response to mitogens. In this particular case the growth response is carried out by terminally differentiated cells (myocytes) that are unable to undergo cell division and have only the hypertrophic response open to them. If this hypothesis were correct, it would be expected that the initial response to the hypertrophic stimuli would mimic early events of cell division induced by growth factors in a large variety of cell types.

One of the early responses of stationary cells to growth stimuli is the induction of a series of *proto-oncogenes*, such as *c-fos* and *c-myc*, among others, that directly or indirectly turn on the cascade of events that leads to cell division. These molecules owe their name to the fact that they are the cellular counterpart of viral oncogenes and their regulation is usually altered in neoplastic cells. Recently, however, it has been demonstrated that these proto-oncogenes are bona fide transcriptional factors that in most cases form part of the normal growth induction machinery of the cell in response to growth stimuli.[125] Furthermore, *c-myc* is able to induce a family of heat shock or stress proteins that are involved in protecting the viability of cells under adverse conditions. This occurs by mechanisms that are not fully elucidated but might affect proper protein folding[126] and/or modulation of gene transcription.[127]

ROLE OF PROTO-ONCOGENES. Not surprisingly, *c-fos* and *c-myc* mRNAs begin to accumulate within 1 hour after the increase in afterload, reach high levels within 3 hours, and return to basal levels in less than 24 hours. Similarly, the mRNA for one of the major stress proteins, HSP 70, is also increased within 30 minutes of increasing aortic pressure.[111] Thus, similar to the mitogenic response of a variety of cell types, induction of the cellular proto-oncogenes and major stress protein genes reflects early changes occurring in the nuclei of myocardial cells in response to acute pressure overload and appears to play an important role in mediating the hypertrophic response. That this factor has a causative role in the hypertrophic response is suggested by the fact that the overexpression of *c-myc* in the myocardium of transgenic animals induces cardiac enlargement and cellular hyperplasia.[128] Several growth factors, including transforming growth factor β (TGFβ) and basic fibroblast growth factor (bFGF), applied to cardiocytes in culture induce a pattern of contractile protein and proto-oncogene expression that is quite similar to that produced by work overload in the intact heart.[127] These results demonstrate that the lack of mitogenic response by cardiac myocytes is not due to a loss of receptors for growth factors. They also give further support to the hypothesis that work overload affects gene expression through mechanisms similar to or shared by the growth factor receptors.

The inability of the cardiocytes to mount a full mitogenic response when challenged by work overload or growth factors remains to be explained, as it does in all other terminally differentiated cells, such as neurons and certain epithelial cells. On the one hand, these cells could have irreversibly lost the expression of some of the genes required to traverse the cell cycle. In that case it should be impossible for them to reenter the cell cycle in response to any stimulus. On the other hand, the terminally differentiated program could induce an inhibitor of the cell cycle. In that case, repression or neutralization of the inhibitor should enable the cells to cycle again. Recently, recessive cellular oncogenes with many of the properties required for this role have been described. One of them, the product of the retinoblastoma (Rb) gene, has been shown to belong to this class. The activity of this gene product is neutralized by certain viral oncogenes: SV40 T antigen[129] and adenovirus EiA.[130] Based on the finding that SV40 T antigen is able to reinduce the ability to cycle to differentiated myotubes,[131] it has been possible to reinduce the cell cycle in terminally differentiated cardiocytes and to create cell lines that express many of the differentiated characteristics. These results suggest the presence of inhibitors in differentiated cardiocytes. Identification of the molecule(s) involved could provide the tool required to induce cardiac muscle regeneration.

WALL STRESS AS A DETERMINANT OF HYPERTROPHY. In various models of cardiac hypertrophy, systolic and diastolic wall stress have been implicated as major determinants of the degree and pattern of hypertrophy during pressure and volume overload.[132] In addition, studies using isolated heart preparations have demonstrated that increased wall tension alone can stimulate protein synthesis[60] directly. Although the precise molecular mechanisms by which wall stress is communicated to the myocyte nucleus remain to be elucidated, the recently discovered stretch-sensitive ion channels[133] provide a likely candidate for the sensor mechanism. These channels could provide a very sensitive measure of wall stress. The ionic changes produced by their opening or closing could trigger a second messenger cascade (perhaps involving IP3) that results in the changes in gene expression already described. The recent demonstration that stretching of isolated cardiocytes in culture induces the changes of contractile gene and proto-oncogene expression[134] described for work overload and growth factors supports this hypothesis.

In physiological terms, the reexpression of the fetal isogenes might be a beneficial adaptation to hemodynamic overload. As a consequence of the changes induced in the thin and thick filaments during cardiac hypertrophy, sarcomeres with significantly different functional properties are produced. For the myocardium, the fetal isoform of MHC has been shown to be energetically more efficient than that of the adult. Moreover, because ANP has potent natriuretic, diuretic, and vasodilatory effects, the marked induction of this molecule in the ventricle in response to increased wall tension might be interpreted as an adaptational response to reduce hemodynamic load imposed on the ventricle.

CONCLUSIONS

It has become apparent that the myocardium is now amenable to cellular and molecular "dissection." It can serve as a good experimental model to address questions that are relevant not only to the cardiovascular system but are also of general biological significance. In addition, it is clear that cardiac hypertrophy is not a simple quantitative increase in ventricular mass but a qualitatively different and heterogeneous process that is influenced strongly by the nature of the hypertrophic stimulus and the developmental stage of the myocardium. Induction of cellular proto-oncogenes that play a role in cell growth in the very early stages of work overload hypertrophy mimics the mitogenic response to growth factors by a variety of cells. The quantitative and qualitative changes in the expression of contractile and regulatory genes that occur later probably represent only a small sample of the changes produced in the myocardium in response to the hypertrophic stimuli. The finding that each fetal gene examined so far is reexpressed in response to pressure overload hypertrophy suggests that reinduction of the fetal program might be a general adaptive process to hemodynamic stress.

Further work is needed, however, to elucidate the precise mechanisms by which the hemodynamic and/or mechanical stimuli are converted into biochemical signals that lead to quantitative as well as qualitative changes in gene expression. A better understanding is also required of the genes involved in converting precursor mesenchymal cells into the cardiogenic pathway, and of the cell-specific transcriptional factors responsible for the expression of cardiac specific genes, as well as of the genes involved in blocking these cells in the terminally differentiated myocytes. This information is essential in order to be able to manipulate the process of cardiac hypertrophy and changes of contractile state to physiological advantage.

REFERENCES

MOLECULAR BIOLOGY AND THE CARDIOVASCULAR SYSTEM

1. Zak, R.: Development and proliferative capacity of cardiac muscle cells. Circ. Res. *35* (Suppl. II):17, 1974.
2. Watson, Hopkins, Roberts, et al.: Molecular Biology of the Gene. 4th Ed. The Benjamin/Cummings Publishing Co., Inc., 1987.
3. Darnell, J., Lodish, H., and Baltimore, D. (eds.): Molecular Cell Biology. New York, Scientific American Books, Inc., 1986.
4. Chien, K. R., and Knowlton, K. V.: Cardiovascular molecular biology. Introduction to the Series. Circulation *80*:219, 1989.
5. Smith, H. O., and Wilcox, K. W.: A restriction enzyme from *Hemophilus influenzae*. Purification and general properties. J. Mol. Biol. *51*:379, 1970.
6. Danna, K., and Nathans, D.: Specific cleavage of simian virus 40 DNA by restriction endonuclease of *Hemophilus influenzae*. Proc. Natl. Acad. Sci. USA *68*:2913, 1971.
7. Cohen, S. N., Chang, A. C., Boyer, M. W., and Melling, R. B.: Construction of biologically functional bacterial plasmids in vitro. Proc. Natl. Acad. Sci. USA *70*:3240, 1973.
8. Jackson, D. A., Symons, R. H., and Berg, P.: Biochemical method for inserting new genetic information into DNA of simian virus 40: Circular SV40 molecules containing lambda phage genes and the galactose operon of *Escherichia coli*. Proc. Natl. Acad. Sci. USA *69*:2904, 1973.
9. Baltimore, D.: Viral RNA-dependent DNA polymerase. Nature *226*:1209, 1970.
10. Temin, H. M., and Mizutani, S.: RNA-dependent DNA polymerase in virions of Rous sarcoma virus. Nature *226*:1211, 1975.
11. Sanger, F., and Coulson, A. R.: A rapid method for determining the sequences in DNA by primed synthesis with DNA polymerase. J. Mol. Biol. *94*:441, 1975.
12. Maxam, A. M., and Gilbert, W.: A new method for sequencing DNA. Proc. Natl. Acad. Sci. USA. *74*:560, 1977.
13. Sanger, F., Nicklen, S., and Coulson, A. R.: DNA sequencing with chain-termination inhibitors. Proc. Natl. Acad. Sci. USA. *74*:5463, 1977.
14. Botstein, D., White, R. L., Skolnick, M., and Davis, R. W.: Construction of a genetic linkage map in man using restriction fragment length polymorphisms. Am J. Hum. Genet. *32*:314, 1980.
15. Mckusick, V. A.: Mapping and sequencing the human genome. N. Engl. J. Med. *320*:910, 1989.
16. Gusella, J. F.: DNA polymorphism and human disease. Annu. Rev. Biochem. *55*:831, 1986.
17. Hoffman, E. P., Brown, R. H., Jr., and Kunkel, L. M.: Dystrophin, the protein product of the Duchenne muscular dystrophy locus. Cell *51*:919–928, 1988.
18. Rommens, J. M., Iannuzzi, M. C., Kerem, Bat-Sheva, et al.: Identification of the cystic fibrosis gene: Chromosome walking and jumping. Science *245*:1059, 1989.
19. Watkins, M. C., Jardro, J. A., Solomon, S. D., et al.: Mapping of the gene for familial hypertrophic cardiomyopathy and analysis of genetic heterogeneity. Eur. Heart J. *11* (Abst. suppl.) 1990.
20. Brueckner, M., D'Eustachio, P., and Horwich, A. L.: Linkage mapping of a mouse gene, iv, that controls left-right asymmetry of the heart and viscera. Proc. Natl. Acad. Sci. USA *86*:5035, 1989.

USE OF CLONED DNA FOR DIAGNOSIS AND TREATMENT OF GENETIC DISORDERS

21. Southern, E.: Detection of specific sequences among DNA fragments separated by gel electrophoresis. J. Mol. Biol. *98*:503, 1975.
22. McKusick, V. A.: Mendelian Inheritance in Man: Catalogs of Autosomal Dominant, Autosomal Recessive, and X-Linked Phenotypes. 9th Ed. Baltimore, Johns Hopkins University Press, 1990.
23. Tanigawa, G., Jarcho, J. A., Kass, S., et al.: A molecular basis for familial hypertrophic cardiomyopathy: An α - β cardiac myosin heavy chain gene. Cell *62*:991, 1990.
24. Mahdavi, V., Chambers, A., and Nadal-Ginard, B.: The ventricular α- and β-MHC genes are linked in the genome and organized according to their developmental expression. Proc. Natl. Acad. Sci. USA. *81*:2626, 1984.
25. Saez, L. J., Gianola, K. M., McNally, E. M., et al.: Human cardiac myosin heavy chain genes and their linkage in the genome. Nucl. Acids Res. *15*:5443, 1989.
26. Antonarakis, S. E.: Diagnosis of genetic disorders at the DNA level. N. Engl. J. Med. *320*:153, 1989.
27. Studenski, A. B., and Wallace, R. B.: Allele-specific hybridization using oligonucleotide probes of very high specific activity: Discrimination of the human β A- and β S-globin genes. DNA *3*:7, 1984.
28. Cutting, G. R., Kasch, L. M., Rosenstein, B. J., et al.: A cluster of cystic fibrosis mutations in the first mucustide-binding fold of the cystic fibrosis conductance regulatory protein. Nature *346*:366, 1990.
29. Sykes, B.: Bone disease cytogenetics. Nature *348*:18, 1990.
30. Geisterfer-Lowrance, A. A. T., Kass, S., Tanigawa, G., et al.: A molecular basis of familial hypertrophic cardiomyopathy. A β cardiac myosin heavy chain missense mutation. Cell *62*:999, 1990.
31. Saiki, R. K., Scharf, S., Faloona, F., et al.: Enzymatic amplification of β-globin genomic sequences and restriction site analysis for diagnosis of sickle cell anemia. Science *230*:1350, 1985.
32. Saiki, R. K., Gelfand, D. H., Staffel, S., et al.: Primer-directed enzymatic amplication of DNA with a thermastable DNA polymerase. Science *239*:487, 1988.
33. Van der Werf, F., Ludbrook, P. A., Bergmann, S. R., et al.: Coronary thrombolysis with tissue-type plasminogen activator in patients with evolving myocardial infarction. N. Engl. J. Med. *310*:609, 1984.
34. Penmica, D., Holmes, W. E., Kohr, W. J., et al.: Cloning and expression of human tissue-type plasminogen activator cDNA in *E. coli*. Nature *301*:214, 1983.
35. Kaufman, R. J., Wasley, L. C., Spilioles, A. J., et al.: Coamplification and coexpression of human-type plasminogen activator and murine dehydrofolate reductase sequences in Chinese hamster ovary cells. Mol. Cell. Biol. *5*:1750, 1985.
36. Alt, K. W., Kellems, R. E., Bertino, J. R., and Schimke, R. T.: Selective multiplication of dehydrofolate reductase genestin methotrexate-resistant variants of cultured murine cells. J. Biol. Chem. *253*:1351, 1978.
37. Yarden, Y., Escobedo, J. A., Kuang, W. J., et al.: Structure of the receptor for platelet-derived growth factor helps define a family of closely related growth factor receptors. Nature *323*:226, 1986.
38. Escobedo, J. A., and Williams, L. T.: A PDGF receptor domain essential for mitogensis but not for many other responses to PDGF. Nature *335*:85, 1988.
39. O'Dowd, B. F., Hnatowich, M., Regan, J. W., et al.: Site directed mutagenesis of the cytoplasmic domains of the human β2-adrenergic receptor. J. Biol. Chem. *263*:1598, 1988.
40. Noda, M., Ikeda, T., Suzuki, M., et al.: Expression of functional sodium channels from cloned cDNA. Nature *322*:826, 1986.
41. Brinster, R. L., Chen, M. Y., Trumbauer, M., et al.: Somatic expression of herpes thymidine kinase in mice following injection of a fusion gene into eggs. Cell *27*:223, 1981.
42. LaPointe, M. C., Wu, J. P., Greenberg, B., and Gardner, D. G.: Upstream sequences confer atrial-specific expression on the human atrial natriuretic factor gene. J. Biol. Chem. *263*:9075, 1988.
43. Seidman, C. E., Wong, D. W., Jarcho, J. A., et al.: *Cis*-Acting sequences that mediate atrial natriuretic factor gene expression. Proc. Natl. Acad. Sci. USA *85*:4104, 1988.
44. Gluzman, Y., and Shenk, T. (eds.): Enhancers and Eukaryotic Gene Expression. Current Communications in Molecular Biology. Cold Spring Harbor Laboratory, 1983.
45. Jackson, T., Allard, M. F., Sreenan, C. M., et al.: The c-myc proto-oncogene regulates cardiac development in transgenic mice. Mol. Cell. Biol. *10*:3709–3716, 1990.
46. Field, L. J.: Atrial natriuretic factor—SV40 T antigen transgenes produce tumors and cardiac arrhythmias in mice. Science *239*:1029, 1988.
47. Steinhelper, M. E., Katz, E., Lanson, N., et al.: Myocardial hyperplasia in transgenic mice. J. Cell Biochem. (abstr.) (Supp. 15C):H14, 1991.

48. Mann, R., Mulligan, R. C., and Baltimore, D.: Construction of a retroviral packaging mutant and its use to produce helper-free defective retrovirus. Cell *33*:153, 1983.
49. Miller, A. D., Jolly, D. J., Friedman, T., and Verma, I. M.: A transmissible retrovirus expressing human hypoxanthine phosphoribosyltransferase (HPRT): Gene transfer into cells obtained from humans deficient in HPRT. Proc. Natl. Acad. Sci. USA *80*:4709, 1983.
50. Dzierzak, E. A., Papayannopoulou, T., and Mulligan, R. C.: Lineage-specific expression of a human β-globin gene in murine marrow transplant recipients reconstituted with retrovirus-transduced stem cells. Nature *331*:35, 1988.
51. Cournoyer, D., and Caskey, C. T.: Gene transfer into humans. A first step. N. Engl. J. Med. *323*:601, 1990.
52. Rosenberg, S. A., Aebersold, P., Cornetta, K., et al.: Gene transfer into humans—immunotherapy of patients with advanced melanoma using tumor-infiltrating lymphocytes modified by retroviral transduction. N. Engl. J. Med. *323*:570, 1990.
53. Nabel, E. G., Plautz, G., Boyce, F. M., et al.: Recombinant gene expression in vivo within endothelial cells of the arterial wall. Science *244*:1342, 1989.
54. Wilson, J. M., Birinyi, L. K., Salomon, R. N., et al.: Implantation of vascular grafts lined with genetically modified endothelial cells. Science *244*:1344, 1989.
55. Dichek, D. A., Neville, R. F., Zwiebel, J. A., et al.: Seeding of intravascular stents with genetically engineered endothelial cells. Circulation *80*:1347, 1989.
56. Nabel, E. G., Plautz, G., and Boice, F. M.: Site-specific gene expression in vivo by direct gene transfer into the arterial wall. Science *249*:1285, 1990.
57. Wolff, J. A., Malone, R. W., Williams, P., et al.: Direct gene transfer into mouse muscle in vivo. Science *247*:1465, 1990.
58. Lin, M., Parmacek, M. S., Marle, G., et al.: Expression of recombinant genes in myocardium in vivo after direct injection of DNA. Circulation *82*:2217, 1990.
59. Swain, J. L.: Gene therapy—A new approach to the treatment of cardiovascular disease. Circulation *80*:1495, 1989.

MOLECULAR BIOLOGY OF THE CARDIAC CONTRACTILE SYSTEM

60. Swynghedauw, B.: Developmental and functional adaptation of contractile proteins in cardiac and skeletal muscles. Physiol. Rev. *66*:710, 1986.
61. Barany, M.: ATPase activity of myosin correlated with speed of muscle shortening. J. Gen. Physiol. *50*(Suppl.):197, 1967.
62. Scheuer, J., and Bhan, A. K.: Cardiac contractile proteins. Adenosine triphosphatase activity and physiological function. Circ. Res. *45*:1, 1979.
63. Schwartz, K., Lecarpentier, Y., Martin et al. Myosin isoenzymic distribution correlates with speed of myocardial contraction. J. Mol. Cell Cardiol. *13*:1071, 1981.
64. Alpert, N. R., and Mulieri, L. A.: Increased myothermal economy of isometric force generation in compensated cardiac hypertrophy induced by pulmonary artery constriction in the rabbit. A characterization of heat liberation in normal and hypertrophied right ventricular papillary muscles. Circ. Res. *50*:491, 1982.
65. Obinata, T., Maruyama, K., Sugita, H., et al.: Dynamic aspects of structural proteins in vertebrate skeletal muscle. Muscle Nerve *4*:456, 1981.
66. Emerson, C., Fischman, D. A., Nadal-Ginard, B., and Siddiqui, M. A. Q. (eds.): Molecular Biology of Muscle Development. UCLA Symposia on Molecular and Cellular Biology. New Series, 29. New York, Alan R. Liss, 1986.
67. Stiles, G. L., and Lefkowitz, R. J.: Cardiac adrenergic receptors. Annu. Rev. Med. *35*:149, 1984.
68. Catterall, W. A.: Molecular properties of voltage-sensitive sodium channels. Annu. Rev. Biochem. *55*:953, 1986.
69. Herrera, V. L., Emanuel, J. R., Ruiz-Opazo, N., et al.: Three differentially expressed Na, K-ATPase α subunit isoforms: Structural and functional implications. J. Cell. Biol. *105*:1855, 1987.
70. MacLennan, D. H., Brandl, C. J., Korczak, B., and Green, N. M.: Amino-acid sequence of a $Ca^{2+} + Mg^{2+}$-dependent ATPase from rabbit muscle sarcoplasmic reticulum, deducted from its complementary DNA sequence. Nature *316*:696, 1985.
71. Brandl, C. J., Green, N. M., Korczak, B., and MacLennan, D. H.: Two Ca^{2+} ATPase genes: Homologies and mechanistic implications of deduced amino acid sequences. Cell *44*:597, 1986.
72. Siu, G., Kronenberg, M., Strauss, E., et al.: The structure, rearrangement, and expression of Dβ gene segments of the murine T-cell antigen receptor. Nature *311*:344, 1984.
73. Honjo, T., and Habu, S.: Origin of immune diversity: Genetic variation and selection. Annu. Rev. Biochem. *54*:803, 1985.
74. Breitbart, R. E., Andreadis, A., and Nadal-Ginard, B.: Alternative splicing: A ubiquitous mechanism for the generation of multiple protein isoforms from single genes. Annu. Rev. Biochem. *56*:467, 1987.
75. Smith, C. W. J., Patton, J. G., and Nadal-Ginard, B.: Alternative splicing in the control of gene expression. Annu. Rev. Genet. *23*:527, 1989.
76. Kedes, L. H., and Stockdale, F. E. (eds.): UCLA Symposia on Molecular and Cellular Biology of Muscle Development. New York, Alan R. Liss, 1988.
77. Pette, D., and Vrbova, G.: Neural control of phenotypic expression in mammalian muscle fibers. Muscle Nerve *8*:676, 1985.
78. Leinwand, L. A., Fournier, R. E., and Nadal-Ginard, B.: TB multigene family for sarcomeric myosin heavy chain in mouse and human DNA: Localization on a single chromosome. Science *221*:766, 1983.
79. Mahdavi, V., Chambers, A. P., and Nadal-Ginard, B.: Cardiac α and β myosin heavy chain genes are organized in tandem. Proc. Natl. Acad. Sci. USA *81*:2626, 1984.
80. Saez, L. J., Gianola, K. M., McNally, E. M., et al.: Human cardiac myosin heavy chain genes and their linkage in the genome. Nucleic Acids Res. *15*:5443, 1987.
81. Czosnek, H., Nudel, U., Shani, M., et al.: The genes coding for the muscle contractile proteins, myosin heavy chain, myosin light chain 2, and skeletal muscle actin are located on three different mouse chromosomes. EMBO J. *1*:1299, 1982.
82. Hoh, J. F., McGrath, P. A., and Hale, P. T.: Electrophoretic analysis of multiple forms of rat cardiac myosin: Effects of hypophysectomy and thyroxine replacement. J. Mol. Cell Cardiol. *10*:1053, 1978.
83. Pope, B., Hoh, J. F., and Weeds, A.: The ATPase activities of rat cardiac myosin isoenzymes. FEBS Lett. *118*:205, 1980.
84. Schwartz, K., Lecarpentier, Y., Martin, J. L., et al.: Myosin isoenzymic distribution correlates with speed of myocardial contraction. J. Mol. Cell Cardiol. *13*:1071, 1981.
85. Lompre, A. M., Schwartz, K., d'Albis, A., et al.: Myosin isoenzyme redistribution in chronic heart overload. Nature *282*:105, 1979.
86. Lompre, A. M., Mercadier, J. J., Wisnewsky, C., et al.: Dev. Biol. *84*:286, 1981.
87. Lompre, A. M., Mahdavi, V., and Nadal-Ginard, B.: Expression of the cardiac ventricular α and β myosin heavy chain genes is developmentally and hormonally regulated. J. Biol. Chem. *259*:6437, 1984.
88. Chizzonite, R. A., and Zak, R.: Regulation of myosin isoenzyme composition in fetal and neonatal rat ventricle by endogenous thyroid hormones. J. Biol. Chem. *259*:12628, 1984.
89. Mercadier, J. J., Lompre, A. M., Wisnewsky, C., et al.: Myosin isoenzyme changes in several models of rat cardiac hypertrophy. Circ. Res. *49*:525, 1981.
90. Gorza, L., Pauletto, P., Pessina, A. C., et al.: Isomyosin distribution in normal and pressure-overloaded rat ventricular myocardium. An immunohistochemical study. Circ. Res. *49*:1003, 1981.
91. Litten, R. Z., 3rd, Martin, B. J., Low, R. B., and Alpert, N. R.: Altered myosin isozyme patterns from pressure-overloaded and thyrotoxic hypertrophied rabbit hearts. Circ. Res. *50*:856, 1982.
92. Scheuer, J., Malhotra, A., Hirsch, C., et al.: Physiologic cardiac hypertrophy corrects contractile protein abnormalities associated with pathologic hypertrophy in rats. J. Clin. Invest. *70*:1300, 1982.
93. Dillmann, W. H.: Diabetes mellitus induces changes in cardiac myosin of the rat. Diabetes *29*:579, 1980.
94. Malhotra, A., Penpargkul, S., Fein, F. S., et al.: The effect of streptozotocin-induced diabetes in rats on cardiac contractile proteins. Circ. Res. *49*:1243, 1981.
95. Everett, A. W., Clark, W. A., Chizzonite, R. A., and Zak, R.: Change in synthesis rates of α and β myosin heavy chains in rabbit heart after treatment with thyroid hormone. J. Biol. Chem. *258*:2421, 1983.
96. Chizzonite, R. A., Everett, A. W., Clark, W. A., et al.: Isolation and characterization of two molecular variants of myosin heavy chain from rabbit ventricle. Change in their content during normal growth and after treatment with thyroid hormone. J. Biol. Chem. *257*:2056, 1982.
97. Izumo, S., Mahdavi, V., and Nadal-Ginard, B.: All members of the MHC multigene family respond to thyroid hormone in a highly tissue-specific manner. Science *231*:597, 1986.
98. Umeda, P. K., Levin, J. E., Shinha, A. M., et al.: *In* Emerson, C., et al. (eds.): Molecular Biology of Muscle Development. New York, Alan R. Liss, 1986, pp. 809–823.
99. Evans, R. M.: The steroid and thyroid hormone receptor superfamily. Science *240*:889, 1988.
100. Mahdavi, V., Koren, G., Michaud, S., et al.: *In* Kedes, L. H., and Stockdale, F. E. (eds.): Cellular and Molecular Biology of Muscle Development. New York, Alan R. Liss, 1989, pp. 369–379.
101. Sap, J., Munoz, A., Damm, K., et al.: The c-erb-A protein is a high-affinity receptor for thyroid hormone. Nature *324*:635, 1986.
102. Weinberger, C., Thompson, C. C., Ong, E. S., et al.: The c-erb-A gene encodes a thyroid hormone receptor. Nature *324*:641, 1986.
103. Thompson, C. C., Weinberger, C., Lebo, R., and Evans, R. M.: Identification of a novel thyroid hormone receptor expressed in the mammalian central nervous system. Science *237*:1610, 1987.
104. Izumo, S., and Mahdavi, V.: Thyroid hormone receptor isoforms generated by alternative splicing differentially activate myosin HC gene transcription. Nature *334*:539, 1988.
105. Damm, K., Thompson, C. C., and Evans, R. M.: Protein encoded by c-erbA functions as a thyroid hormone receptor antagonist. Nature *339*:593, 1989.
106. Koenig, R. J., Lazar, M. A., Hodin, R. A., et al.: Inhbition of thyroid hormone action by a non-hormone binding c-erbA protein generated by alternative mRNA splicing. Nature *337*:659, 1989.
107. Glass, C. K., Franco, R., Weinberger, C., et al.: A c-erb-A binding site in rat growth hormone gene mediates transactivation by thyroid hormone. Nature *329*:738, 1987.
108. Thompson, W. R., Koren, G., Izumo, S., et al.: Molecular recognition of myosin heavy chain switches: A model for study of cardiac gene expression. *In* Clarck, E. B., and Takao, A. (eds.): Developmental Cardiology: Morphogenesis and Function. Mount Kisco, NY, Futura Publishing Co., 1990, pp. 13–25.
109. Izumo, S., Lompre, A. M., Matsuoka, R. et al.: Myosin heavy chain messenger RNA and protein isoform transitions during cardiac hypertrophy. Interaction between hemodynamic and thyroid hormone-induced signals. J. Clin. Invest. *79*:970, 1987.

110. Mercadier, J. J., Bouveret, P., Gorza, L., et al.: Myosin isoenzymes in normal and hypertrophied human ventricular myocardium. Circ. Res. *53*:52, 1983.
111. Izumo, S., Mahdavi, V., and Nadal-Ginard, B.: Proto-oncogene induction and reprogramming of cardiac gene expression produced by pressure overload. Proc. Natl. Acad. Sci. USA *85*:339, 1988.
112. Schwartz, K., Lompre, A. M., Bouveret, P., et al.: Accumulation of skeletal actin mRNA in experimental cardiac hypertrophy. J. Mol. Cell. Cardiol. *17* (Suppl. 3) abstract 22, 1985.
113. Hirzel, H. O., Tuckschmid, C. R., Schneider, J., et al.: Relationship between myosin isoenzyme composition, hemodynamics, and myocardial structure in various forms of human cardiac hypertrophy. Circ. Res. *57*:729, 1985.
114. Cantley, L. C.: Structure and Mechanism of the (Na,K)-ATPase. Curr. Top. Bioenergetics. *11*:201, 1981.
115. Ingwall, J. S., Kramer, M. F., Fifer, M. A., et al.: The creatine kinase system in normal and diseased human myocardium. N. Engl. J. Med. *313*:1050, 1985.
116. Simpson, P.: Norepinephrine-stimulated hypertrophy of cultured rat myocardial cells is an α1-adrenergic response. J. Clin. Invest. *72*:732, 1983.
117. Lacks, M. M., and Morady, F.: Norepinephrine—the myocardial hypertrophy hormone. Am. Heart J. *91*:674, 1976.
118. Berridge, M. J., and Irvine, R. F.: Inositol triphosphate, a novel second messenger in cellular signal transduction. Nature *312*:315, 1984.
119. Nishizuka, Y.: The role of protein kinase C in cell surface signal transduction and tumour promotion. Nature *308*:693, 1984.
120. Simpson, P. C., and Karliner, J. S.: Regulation of cardiac myocyte hypertrophy by a tumor-promoting phorbol ester. Clin. Res. *33*:229A (abstr), 1985.

MOLECULAR BASIS FOR CERTAIN FORMS OF HYPERTROPHIC CARDIOMYOPATHY

121. Lassar, A. B., Paterson, B. M., and Weintraub, H.: Transfection of a DNA locus that mediates the conversion of 10T1/2 fibroblasts to myoblasts. Cell *47*:649, 1986.
122. Wright, W. E., Sassoon, D. A., and Lin, V. K.: Myogenin, a factor regulating myogenesis, has a domain homologous to MyoD. Cell *56*:607, 1989.
123. Braun, T., Buschhausen-Denker, G., Bober, E., et al.: A novel human muscle factor related to but distinct from MyoD1 induces myogenic conversion in 10T1/2 fibroblasts. EMBO J. *8*:701, 1989.
124. Ruoslahti, E., Pihko, H., and Seppala, M.: Alpha-fetoprotein: Immunochemical purification and chemical properties. Expression in normal state and in malignant and nonmalignant liver disease. Transplant Rev. *20*:38, 1974.
125. Johnson, P. F., and McKnight, S. L.: Eukaryotic transcriptional regulatory proteins. Annu. Rev. Biochem. *58*:799, 1989.
126. Rothman, J. E.: Signal-peptide recognition. GTP and methionine bristles (news). Nature *340*:433, 1989.
127. Schneider, M. D., Shih, H. T., and Parker, T. G.: Peptide growth factors and activated oncogenes can selectively induce expression of "fetal" contractile protein genes. J. Mol. Cell. Cardiol. *21*: (Suppl. III) abstract 67.
128. Jackson, T., Allard, M. F., Sreenan, C. M., et al.: The c-myc proto-oncogene regulates cardiac development in transgenic mice. Molec. Cell. Biol. *10*:3709, 1990.
129. DeCaprio, J. A., Ludlow, J. W., Figge, J., et al.: SV40 large tumor antigen forms a specific complex with the product of the retinoblastoma susceptibility gene. Cell *54*:275, 1988.
130. Whyte, P., Buchkovich, K. J., Horowitz, J. M., et al.: Association between an oncogene and an anti-oncogene: the adenovirus E1A proteins bind to the retinoblastoma gene product. Nature *334*:124, 1988.
131. Endo, T., and Nadal-Ginard, B.: *In* Kedes, L. H. and Stockdale, F. E. (eds.): UCLA Symposia on Molecular and Cellular Biology. New Series, vol. 93. New York, Alan R. Liss, 1989, pp. 95–104.
131a. Thompson, R.: Unpublished observation.
132. Grossman, W.: Cardiac hypertrophy: Useful adaptation of pathologic process? Am. J. Med. *69*:576, 1980.
133. Guharay, F., and Sachs, F.: Stretch-activated single ion channel currents in tissue-cultured embryonic chick skeletal muscle. J. Physiol. (Lond.) *352*:685, 1984.
134. Komuro, I., Kurabayashi, M., Takaku, F., and Yazaki, Y.: Expression of cellular oncogenes in the myocardium during the developmental stage and pressure-overloaded hypertrophy of the rat hearts. Circ. Res. *62*:1075, 1988.

51

Genetics and Cardiovascular Disease

by REED E. PYERITZ, M.D., Ph.D.

GENETIC FACTORS IN DISEASE

Genes contribute to both the cause and the pathogenesis of virtually any abnormality of human physiology and behavior including, of course, disorders of the heart and vascular system. This statement carries two messages in addition to the obvious one. First, the pathology associated with even the most "environmental" of causes, such as trauma, malnutrition, and drug abuse, can be defined only in terms of the human body's response to the insult. How the stress of the initial insult is expressed (the *phenotype*) and how the patient suffers and perhaps recovers are, to varying and as yet often poorly defined degrees, dependent on the patient's *genotype*. This idea seems self-evident and verges on the trite, but it is frequently neglected. Some environmental insults, such as massive trauma or poisoning, will be lethal to all, regardless of genotype. Nonetheless, as fields such as *pharmacogenetics* and *ecogenetics* develop, genetic susceptibilities to human disease will be better and more simply defined, and the physician must become increasingly attuned to the importance of the genotype.

Second, the introductory statement stresses that genetic factors play roles in *both* cause and process and that etiology and pathogenesis, while related, are conceptually distinct. For example, the cause of sickle cell anemia is clearly a single mutant gene, whereas whether a patient homozygous for this mutation expresses all, some, or none of the manifestations of the disease is dependent on many other genetic and nongenetic factors. Conversely, the cause of pneumococcal pneumonia is equally evident, but the severity and resolution of the disease depend on the patient's immune competency (which in turn is dependent on genetic and nongenetic factors) as much as on treatment with an antibiotic.

The genotype, therefore, can be detrimental in at least two distinct ways. First, mutant genes can so upset embryology or physiology that a clinical abnormality occurs. Whereas the phenotype of any particular mutation will depend on a host of factors, including which homeostatic systems are available to modulate the action of the defect, the genotype has the principal role in causing the disease. It is this class of mutations that are usually referred to as genetic diseases. Second, a mutation can facilitate the action of an extrinsic cause in producing disease. Inherited susceptibilities are part of the pathogenesis of disease and are what are sought, and often revealed, in taking the patient's family history. Unfortunately, until recently there has been little that the clinician could do to pursue tantalizing facts, such as multiple relatives under age 50 suffering myocardial infarction. The long-touted prospect of detecting a patient's inherited susceptibilities and intervening before irreversible clinical sequelae occur is slowly becoming reality.

DISORDERS DUE TO MICROSCOPIC ALTERATIONS IN CHROMOSOMES

Estimates of the total number of human genes range between 50,000 and 100,000. Two copies (termed *alleles*) of each gene are arrayed along 23 pairs of *chromosomes*. Twenty-two of the chromosomes are called *autosomes* (numbered 1 through 22), while the 23rd pair are the *sex chromosomes*, X and Y. Females have two X chromosomes and males have an X and a Y chromosome. Both autosomal alleles are potentially active in specifying RNA copies of their DNA sequences; whether a gene is active depends on the cell type, developmental stage of the organism, and the regulatory molecules that interact with promoter and enhancer nucleotide sequences that control transcription of the gene. In cells with two X chromosomes (i.e., in all females, in the Klinefelter syndrome in which two X's and one Y occur, and in other rare conditions), only one X is active after early embryogenesis.

Human chromosomes can be examined by culturing cells capable of mitosis; T-lymphocytes obtained from venous blood are the usual source, but fibroblasts, cells from chorionic villi, amniocytes, and leukocyte precursors present in bone marrow are also used clinically. Chromosomes are distinguished from one another by their size, shape (determined by the position of a constriction called the *centromere*, which functions as the attachment of the mitotic apparatus), and characteristic banding pattern as revealed by any of several staining techniques. The chromosomes are photographed, cut out, and arranged in pairs, from 1 through 22 and the sex chromosomes, in a display called the *karyotype.* This display and its interpretation are the end results of a clinical study of a patient's chromosomes. The chromosome constitution of a cell is designated by first specifying the number of chromosomes present (46 being normal in diploid cells), then specifying the sex chromosomes, and finally describing any abnormalities. For example, a normal male is designated 46,XY, and a female with an extra chromosome 21 is designated 46,XX,+21.

Chromosome aberrations, especially too many or too few chromosomes *(aneuploidy),* are extremely common in human embryos; more than one-half of all conceptuses are spontaneously aborted in early pregnancy, and at least one-half of them are aneuploid. Among live-born infants, about 0.5 per cent have a chromosome aberration.

ANEUPLOIDY. Gain or loss of chromosomes generally happens by nondisjunction, or the failure of a homologous pair of chromosomes to separate. Absence of one chromosome is termed *monosomy;* all autosomal monosomies are embryonic lethals, as is presence of only a Y sex chromosome. Presence of three chromosomes is *trisomy,* and presence of an entire extra set of chromosomes (for a total of 69) is *triploidy.* The most common autosomal aneuploidy, trisomy 21 associated with the Down syndrome, and aneuploidy for sex chromosomes are all compatible with survival into adulthood.

CHROMOSOME REARRANGEMENTS. A chromosome can break and rejoin within itself, potentially giving rise to an *inversion* of genetic material. Often no apparent phenotypic effect is seen in people with an inversion, but because inversions may disrupt chromosome pairing during meiosis, their offspring may have more profound aberrations.

DELETIONS AND DUPLICATIONS. Just as their names imply, these aberrations are losses or gains of chromosomal material. Many clinical syndromes have been associated with aberrations of specific chromosome regions.[1,2] The smallest deletion detectable by light microscopy is associated with loss of considerable DNA, on the order of one million base pairs, so more than one gene is potentially disrupted or lost.

A number of conditions, each initially thought to be due to a mutation in a single locus, are associated with small interstitial chromosome deletions (Table 51–1). So rather than pleiotropic manifestations of one mutation, these conditions are likely to be due to the effects of several, and perhaps many, mutations and are therefore called *contiguous gene deletion syndromes.*[3] Such deletions are potentially heritable, and the occurrence of the disorder in a family behaves as a mendelian dominant.

DISORDERS DUE TO CHANGES IN SINGLE NUCLEAR GENES

(See also Chap. 50)

Mutations of genes located on the 22 pairs of autosomes and the two sex chromosomes produce phenotypes inherited according to the two principal tenets of Mendel: alleles segregate and nonalleles assort. The first statement refers to gametes receiving as a result of meiosis only one of the two alleles at a given locus. The second statement describes the results of recombination, the meiotic process of rearranging DNA between the two chromosomes of the pair *(homologous chromosomes);* if two loci are widely spaced along a chromosome, their chances of being separated by recombination are 50–50, and they are said to be *unlinked.*

More than 5000 individual loci have been identified on the basis of the phenotype that mutations in single genes produce. The presumption of single-gene defects is based in most instances on the pattern of inheritance in families; segregation of the phenotype according to mendelian principles is the central piece of evidence. For an increasing number of loci, however, molecular genetic techniques have mapped the phenotype to a single gene, or even revealed the actual alteration in nucleotide sequence.[4,5] The range of known mendelian variation in humans and information about gene mapping and molecular defects are routinely catalogued[6] and available online.[7] Based on current estimates of the size of the human genome, about 5 to 10 per cent of loci have been identified through the effects their mutations have on phenotype.

More than 2000 loci have been mapped to a restricted region of the genome. Many of these loci cause specific mendelian disorders, and the genetic map of these loci represents the "morbid anatomy of the human genome." All of the cardiovascular and hemostatic disorders that have been mapped by early 1991 are shown in Figure 51–1.

Dominance and Recessiveness

These related concepts are characteristics of the phenotype, *not of the gene.* A phenotype is dominant when the patient is *heterozygous* for a mutation, i.e., when one copy of the mutant allele, and one copy of the normal allele, are present; this holds for genes on both autosomes and the X chromosome. A phenotype is recessive when the patient has two mutant alleles at the locus causing the condition. If the mutant alleles are identical, the patient is *homozygous* at that locus, a situation usually present either when the allele is identical by descent through both parents (i.e., the parents had a common ancestor and are *consanguineous)* or when the mutant allele is common in the population (e.g., the most prevalent mutation for cystic fibrosis and the mutation for sickle cell anemia). Biochemical and molecular genetic assessment of mutant alleles has shown that the majority of recessive phenotypes are due to two distinct mutant alleles, a situation termed a *genetic compound,* indicative of the widespread heterogeneity in mutations at each locus. Males have but one X chromosome, and each locus is therefore *hemizygous;* a mutant locus is always expressed in the phenotype of a male. Dominance and recessiveness for X-linked traits refer to expression in heterozygous and homozygous women, respectively.

Whether a disorder is called dominant or recessive depends on how carefully the phenotype is assessed and how it is defined. For example, familial hypercholesterolemia is a relatively common hereditary disorder due to defects in the receptor for low-density lipoprotein (LDL, p. 1128). The vast majority of patients are heterozygous for a mutant allele at the LDLR locus on chromosome 19,[8] and the disease is inherited as a mendelian dominant trait. However, if a man and a woman, each heterozygous for an LDLR mutation, mate, they have a 25 per cent risk of having a child who inherits both of the mutant alleles and will thereby be either homozy-

TABLE 51–1 CONTIGUOUS GENE DELETION SYNDROMES

	LOCUS	CARDIOVASCULAR ABNORMALITIES
Syndromes with Cardiovascular Involvement		
Arteriohepatic dysplasia	**20p11.2**	**Peripheral pulmonic stenosis**
DiGeorge sequence	**22q11**	**Truncus arteriosus, right aortic arch, TOF, PDA**
Miller-Dieker syndrome	**17p13**	**Patent ductus arteriosus ± complex anomalies**
Prader-Willi syndrome	**15q11–q13**	**Cor pulmonale (2° to obesity and central apnea)**
WAGR syndrome	**11p13**	**Hypertension (2° to Wilms tumor)**
Syndromes Without Frequent Cardiovascular Involvement		
Angelman syndrome	**15q11–q13***	
Smith-Magenis syndrome	**17p11.2**	

TOF = tetralogy of Fallot; PDA = patent ductus arteriosus.
WAGR = Wilms tumor, aniridia, genitourinary, and retardation.
* The deletion is indistinguishable from that of the Prader-Willi syndrome; genetic imprinting is thought to account for the phenotypic differences. In Prader-Willi, the deleted chromosome is always the chromosome 15 inherited from father, while in Angelman syndrome, the deletion affects the maternal chromosome 15.

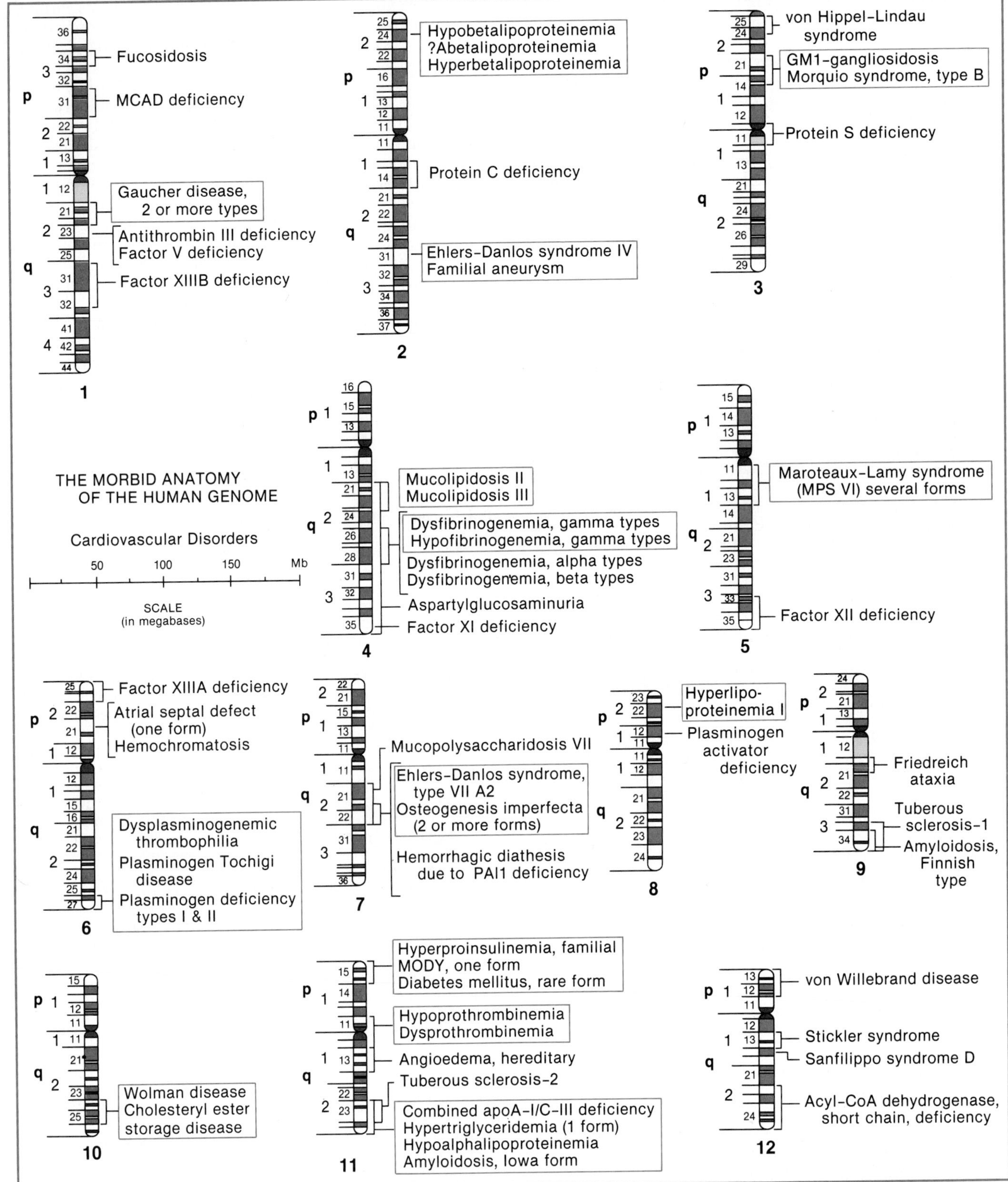

FIGURE 51–1. Chromosomal location of human genes associated with disorders of the cardiovascular system. These 76 genes affect the structure, function, and metabolism of the heart and blood vessels and hemostasis and have been identified by the deleterious effects of mutations. Numerous additional genes that encode structural proteins important to the cardiovascular system have been identified but not yet associated with disease. In the figure, brackets next to the chromosome show the regional localization of the gene causing a particular disorder. Brackets next to two or more disorders indicate that all of the genes causing the disorders map to the same region. Disorders surrounded by boxes are caused by different mutations at the same gene.

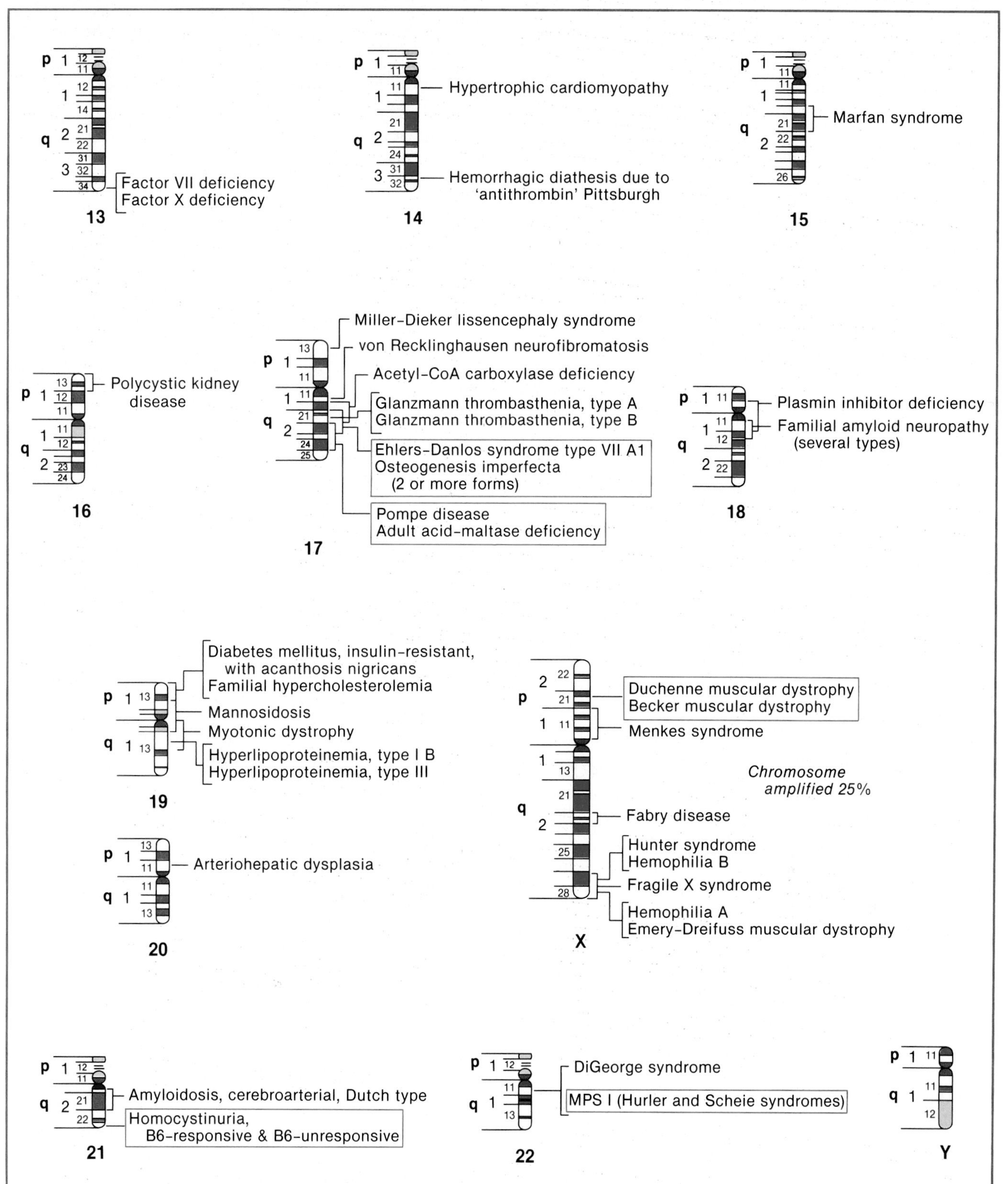

FIGURE 51-1 *Continued*

gous or a genetic compound at the LDLR gene. This child will have a much more severe form of familial hypercholesterolemia (see p. 1145) that is inherited as a mendelian recessive trait. Similarly, homozygosity for the sickle hemoglobin mutation at the β-globin locus on chromosome 11 produces the familiar autosomal recessive disease, sickle cell anemia. However, heterozygosity for the same mutation rarely produces disease but produces sickling of erythrocytes if they are examined under conditions of low oxygen tension; this phenotype is transmitted as a dominant trait.

AUTOSOMAL RECESSIVE INHERITANCE. Nearly all deficiencies of enzymatic activity—the classic inborn errors of metabolism first defined by Archibald Garrod in 1903—cause recessive phenotypes. Most homeostatic systems, which include all metabolic pathways, have sufficient flexibility to function well if one of the enzymatic steps functions at half-normal efficiency, as would occur in heterozygosity for a mutant allele at a structural gene for an enzyme. However, homeostasis cannot cope if two mutant alleles cause a reduction in enzymatic activity to a few percent or less of normal activity. The characteristics of autosomal recessive inheritance, features common to such phenotypes, and a typical pedigree are shown in Figure 51–2.

AUTOSOMAL DOMINANT INHERITANCE. Only a few enzyme deficiencies, but many disorders of development and structure, are inherited as dominant traits. The reasons for this are probably numerous and are certainly poorly understood. One possibility is that developmental homeostasis has a limited repertoire of responses to stress, and when a structural or regulatory macromolecule is reduced to only one-half normal amount, the system cannot cope. Another possibility, illustrated by mutations in procollagen molecules, pertains to gene products that must interact before becoming functional; an aberrant protein combined with a normal one would be a defective multimer, and the effect of being heterozygous for a mutation would be magnified (the concept of *protein suicide*).[9] The characterisitics of autosomal dominant inheritance, features common to many such phenotypes, and a typical pedigree are shown in Figure 51–3.

With the notable exception of Huntington disease, human dominant traits are *incomplete,* in that the heterozygote is less severely affected than the homozygote. Defects of the LDLR are illustrative, in which the heterozygote has classic type IIa hyperlipidemia, while the homozygote has a quantitatively worse form of the same disease.[8] It may well be that homozygosity for most alleles that cause dominant disorders is incompatible with life.

X-LINKED INHERITANCE. The characterisitics of X-linked inheritance, features common to such phenotypes, and a typical pedigree are shown in Figure 51–4. While virtually all diseases due to mutations on the X chromosome are more severe in hemizygous males, women heterozygous for the same mutations often show some manifestations, albeit less severe and of later age of onset. For example, most women carriers of α-galactosidase A deficiency (Fabry's disease) eventually develop cerebrovascular disease or renal failure due to accumulation of sphingolipid.

Mitochondrial Inheritance

Energy generation through oxidative phosphorylation occurs in mitochondria in the cytoplasm of most cell types. Numerous mitochondria, each containing a single chromosome, exist in each cell. Some of the

FIGURE 51–2. *Characteristics of autosomal recessive inheritance*

A single generation affected
Sexes affected equally frequently
Each parent heterozygous (a carrier)
Each offspring of two carriers has a 25% chance of being affected, a 50% chance of being a carrier, and a 25% chance of inheriting neither mutant allele
Two-thirds of clinically normal offspring are carriers
The rarer the phenotype, the greater the likelihood of consanguinity

Characteristics of autosomal recessive phenotypes

Often due to enzyme deficiencies
Often more severe than dominant disorders
Often early age of onset

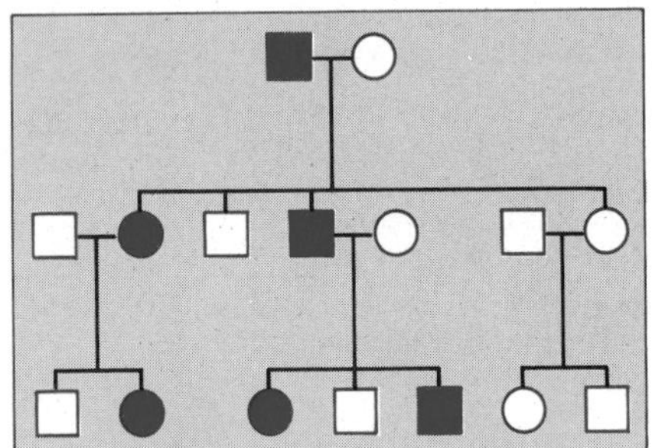

FIGURE 51–3. *Characteristics of autosomal dominant inheritance*

Multiple generations affected
Sexes affected equally frequently
In familial cases, only one parent need be affected
Male-to-male transmission occurs
Offspring of an affected parent have a 50% chance of being affected
Frequency of sporadic cases higher the more severe the condition
Paternal age effect in sporadic cases

Characteristics of autosomal dominant phenotypes

Often associated with malformations
Often pleiotropic
Usually variable
Often less severe than recessive phenotypes
Often age-dependent

FIGURE 51–4. *Characteristics of X-linked inheritance*

No male-to-male transmission
All daughters of affected males are carriers
Sons of a carrier mother have a 50% chance of being affected; daughters have a 50% chance of being carriers
Some mothers of an affected male will not be carriers, but they may have more affected sons if germinal mosaicism is present

Characteristics of X-linked phenotypes

More severe in males
Heterozygous females may be unaffected
Variable, especially in females

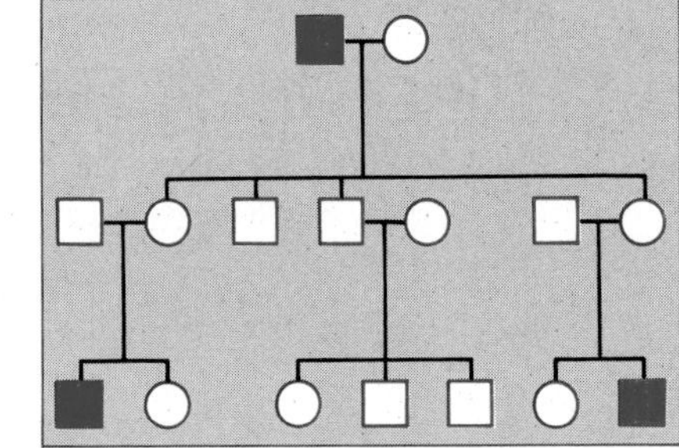

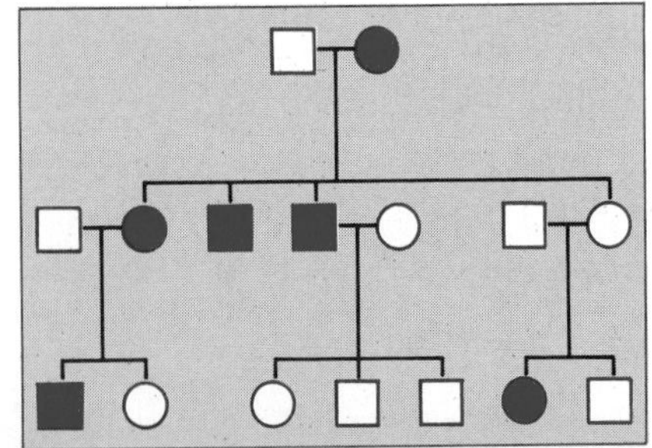

FIGURE 51–5. *Characteristics of disorders due to a mutation of the mitochondrial chromosome*

Sexes equally frequently and severely affected
Transmission only through women; offspring of affected men are unaffected
All offspring of an affected woman may be affected
Variability of expression can be extreme in a family, including apparent nonpenetrance
Phenotypes may be age-dependent

enzymes of oxidative phosphorylation are encoded by genes on the nuclear chromosomes and the proteins transported into the mitochondrion; the rest of the proteins are encoded by genes on the mitochondrial chromosome. Thus, genetic defects of oxidative phosphorylation can be due to mutations of genes on the autosomes or the X chromosome, and the resulting diseases behave as mendelian recessive traits, and to mutations of genes on the mitochondrial chromosome, and the resulting diseases do not behave as mendelian traits.[10,11] The differences are explicable by the events of conception. The spermatocyte contributes virtually no mitochondria to the zygote, and the entire complement of mitochondria that will ever by present in the fetus are derived from the mitochondria already present in the cytoplasm of the oocyte. Thus, phenotypes due to mutations of the mitochondrial chromosome show *maternal inheritance,* the characteristics of which are shown in Figure 51–5.

PRINCIPLES OF CLINICAL GENETICS

PLEIOTROPY. Most mutant alleles have effects on more than one organ system, and a mendelian phenotype frequently displays multiple, often diverse, manifestations.[12] For example, the Marfan syndrome (p. 1641) is defined by abnormalities in the eye, skeleton, skin, heart, and aorta, and until the recent recognition of a defect in extracellular microfibrils,[13] the findings could not be linked either etiologically or pathogenetically.[14]

VARIABILITY. The effect of the same mutant allele on phenotype can be different among people heterozygous (for dominant traits), homozygous (for autosomal recessive traits), or hemizygous (for X-linked traits) for the allele. Variability can be described in terms of the frequency of a particular pleiotropic manifestation among patients with the mutation; the severity of the phenotype; and the age of onset of manifestations. If a person has the mutant allele(s) but shows no phenotypic effect, the trait is called *nonpenetrant.* To an important degree, whether a clinical phenotype is called nonpenetrant or not depends on the sensitivity of the techniques employed for detection. For example, two decades ago, based on bedside examination, cardiovascular abnormalities were thought to affect about half of people with the Marfan syndrome; echocardiography now reveals aortic dilatation in more than 90 per cent. The term *incomplete penetrance* should not be used with reference to individuals but to mean a prevalence of the phenotype in less than 100 per cent of people known to carry the mutation(s). The Holt-Oram syndrome (see p. 1633) is an instructive example. In this autosomal dominant syndrome of reduction anomalies of the upper limb and congenital heart defect, patients in the same family can have only arm anomalies, only a heart defect, or both. Moreover, the severity of the reduction defect varies widely, from a proximally placed thumb to near-total absence of the arm. The cardiac feature is incompletely penetrant because only about 50 per cent of patients have it, but in any individual with the Holt-Oram allele, the heart is either structurally normal or not.

Numerous genetic and environmental factors can affect expression of a gene (Table 51–2), and it is often impossible to determine which of these factors are most important in a specific patient or particular disease. However, the pervasiveness of variable expression emphasizes that phenotypes determined by single genes are to some extent really "multifactorial."

GENETIC HETEROGENEITY. Similar or even identical phenotypes can be due to fundamentally distinct mutations, a phenomenon termed genetic heterogeneity. For example, Marfan syndrome and homocystinuria were long thought to be the same disorder, despite what now appear in retrospect to be obvious differences in inheritance pattern and intelligence.[15] As in the case of these two disorders, the causes may lie in two different genes whose products are functionally distinct. Osteogenesis imperfecta exemplifies a disorder in which mutations in two genes, α1(I) and α2(I) procollagen, can each produce the same phenotype because the two proteins interact to form type I collagen.[16] Genetic heterogeneity is pervasive at the intragenic level of analysis; except for sickle cell anemia, virtually all single-gene disorders are due to a variety of mutations at a given locus.[17–20]

TABLE 51–2 CAUSES OF VARIABILITY OF GENE EXPRESSION

- Genetic background
- Age dependency
- Sex influence
- Sex limitation
- Modifying loci: hypostasis and epistasis
- Gene alteration
  - Somatic mutation
  - Somatic amplification
  - Transpositions and rearrangements
    - Mutations
    - Physiological rearrangements
- Variation in X-inactivation*
- Endogenous complementation*
- Maternal factors
  - Effects of mitochondrial genome
  - Intrauterine environment
- Imprinting
- Exogenous and ecological factors
  - Ecology—temperature, diet
  - Teratogens
  - Medical intervention
  - Chance
  - Chaos

* Pertains to female heterozygotes for X-linked disorders.

NONPATHOLOGICAL VARIATION IN THE CARDIOVASCULAR SYSTEM

CARDIAC STRUCTURE AND PHYSIOLOGY. All aspects of the ontogeny of the cardiovascular system are dictated by the genome. If, as seems most credible, few genes have a large effect and many have small contributions, any specific aspect of "normal" cardiovascular phenotype —size, shape, function—will exhibit multifactorial inheritance. In other words, to the extent that any given phenotype can be quantified, it will show a normal distribution within the population, and near-relatives will be more similar to each other than they will to distant relatives and the rest of the population. The twin method should demonstrate a higher concordance of the trait in monozygotic than dizygotic twins. However, surprisingly few phenotypes have been examined.

Preliminary data on left ventricular dimensions measured echocardiographically showed higher correlations between parent and child than between matched controls, suggesting a genetic contribution[21]; however, as in many such studies, the effect of shared environment was not estimated. In an attempt to minimize environmental contributions, left ventricular sizes of twins who were not exercise trained were compared; the mean intrapair differences in echocardiographic dimensions were less in the monozygotic than in the dizygotic twins and nontwin sibs.[22] The caliber and branch geometry of coronary arteries show familial resemblance, and both parameters are much more similar in monozygotic twins than in other relatives.[23]

Measures of cardiac electrophysiology show familial resemblance. Studies of both nuclear families[24] and twins[25,26] suggest a genetic contribution to resting heart rate, conduction times, and repolarization time. Genetic control of normal cardiovascular function has been especially difficult to study because of the multitude of environmental (training, diet), stochastic (age), and clinical (subtle, unrecognized pathology) issues that confound comparisons of relatives and controls. Thus far, no strong genetic contribution to an individual's response to physical conditioning has emerged.[22]

VASCULAR SYSTEM. All members of certain inbred animal strains show little variation in arterial anatomy, especially branch angles, and considerable variation with other strains of the same species. Except for the study of coronary arterial anatomy already noted,[23] similar studies of humans have not been reported.

One intriguing question of clinical importance is whether certain people are predisposed to arterial spasm and if this susceptibility has a genetic basis. An examination of hereditary pathological and polymorphic variation in factors elaborated by endothelial cells, platelets, and leukocytes to maintain patency of blood vessels, such as prostacyclin, endothelium-derived relaxing factor, and endothelin-1, may prove enlightening.[27,28]

CARDIOVASCULAR DISORDERS ASSOCIATED WITH CHROMOSOME ABERRATIONS

Chromosome aberrations cause primarily structural defects of the cardiovascular system that are evident at birth. The frequency of chromosome aberrations among live-born children with congenital heart defects has been found to range from 5 to 13 per cent.[29,30] Upward of 40 per cent of all fetuses with heart defects detected by ultrasonography at 18 to 20 weeks' gestation have chromosome aberrations; most are spontaneously aborted. Most forms of aneuploidy and most duplications and deletions of more than a chromosome band are associated with defects of the cardiovascular system[32] (Tables 51–1 and 51–3). Exceptions are 47,XXX, 47,XYY, and 47,XXY (Klinefelter syndrome), in which the incidence of congenital heart disease is probably not elevated over the population baseline.

ANEUPLOIDY. How the abnormal phenotypes caused by autosomal aneuploidy develop remains controversial. One view holds that disturbance of the dosage of the genes present on the specific aneuploid chromosome segments is the central issue. The other view is that any aneuploid state disturbs developmental homeostasis in a nonspecific manner. The former theory would predict some distinctiveness of phenotype among the trisomy syndromes that occur in live-born children, whereas the latter would predict shared manifestations. At a coarse level, the clinical pictures are similar, with grave problems of the craniofacies, central nervous system, genitalia, distal limbs, and heart usually present. But when a more refined examination of the phenotypes is obtained, considerable distinctiveness emerges. The three most common autosomal trisomies[8,10,13] can be distinguished readily at the bedside. In all three, membranous ventricular and atrial septal defects are common. However, the detailed accounting of cardiovascular lesions among large numbers of patients with these trisomies reveals important differences that suggest that aneuploidy exerts more than a global effect on development. In this and most other analyses of congenital heart defects, the system of classification based on the presumed pathogenetic mechanisms proves most instructive and is a useful approach to comparing different causative factors (Table 51–4). About one-quarter of the defects in trisomies 13 and 18 are due to cell migration abnormalities, and two-thirds are flow lesions; when combined, these two mechanisms account for considerably more of these classes of defects than in the general population with congenital heart disease. By contrast, in trisomy 21 left-sided flow lesions are much less common, whereas abnormal closure of endocardial cushions is strikingly frequent; indeed, in contrast to endocardial cushion defects without a chromosome 21 anomaly, left-sided flow lesions are rarely seen in Down syndrome patients with endocardial cushion defects.[30,34,35] Furthermore, the high incidence of endocardial cushion defects and low incidence of conotruncal and distal aortic anomalies has suggested a distinct pathogenetic mechanism in trisomy 21, potentially involving cell adhesiveness and the extracellular matrix.[33,36]

TRISOMY 21—DOWN SYNDROME. This most common phenotype due to a human chromosome aberration occurs about once in every 600 births. Most patients have trisomy 21, and the risk of this aberration is exponentially related to maternal age; the risk is lowest for young women and rises steeply after age 35, reaching 4 per cent for women over age 45. A small minority (3 per cent) of Down syndrome results from an extra copy of all or part of the long arm of chromosome 21 translocated to another chromosome. This situation is relatively more common in mothers under age 30. The pheno-

TABLE 51–3 CARDIOVASCULAR MANIFESTATIONS ASSOCIATED WITH CHROMOSOME ABERRATIONS

CHROMOSOME ABERRATION	EPONYM	CARDIOVASCULAR MANIFESTATIONS
Triploidy		
69,XXX (or XXY or XYY)		>50% have CHD: ASD and VSD
Aneuploidy		
+13	Patau	~80% have CHD; 75% of CHD is complex: PDA, VSD, ASD, PS, AS, dextrocardia, CoA
+18	Edwards	~90% have CHD: most CHD is complex: VSD, PDA, ASD, bicuspid PV and AV, CoA
+21	Down	~40% have CHD: ECD, TOF: MVP in ~20%; AR
+8 mosaicism		~25% have CHD, most of little clinical consequence: VSD, PDA, CoA, PS
+9 mosaicism		~70% have CHD, usually complex: VSD, PDA, PLSVC
45,X	Turner	~10% have clinically important CHD: 50% of these have CoA; mild CoA is likely much more common; also AS, ARD, VSD, ASD, dextrocardia
47,XXX		CHD not increased
47,XXY	Klinefelter	CHD possibly slightly increased; ? mild conduction changes; venous thromboembolic disease
47,XYY		CHD not increased; ? mild conduction changes
Deletions		
4p-	Wolf-Hirschhorn	~50% have CHD, usually complex: VSD, ASD, PDA, PS
5p-	Cri du chat	~20% have CHD, usually single: VSD, PDA, ASD, PS
7q-		~20% have CHD, various, often complex
13q-		CHD common, often severe, but depend on region deleted
18p-		CHD uncommon
18q-		~25% have CHD, usually single, of little consequence: VSD, PDA, ASD, PS
ring 18		~20% have CHD: CoA, PA hypoplasia, HLH, PLSVC
Duplications		
4p trisomy		~10% have CHD, usually single: no defect predominates
9 p trisomy		<10% have CHD: VSD, ASD, AS, PS
10p trisomy		~30% have CHD, usually single: no defect predominates
10q24–qter trisomy		~50% have CHD, usually complex: ECD, VSD, TOF
22pter–q11 trisomy or tetrasomy	Cat eye	~50% have CHD, usually complex: TAPVR, VSD, TOF
Other Aberrations		
Marker Xq27.3	Fragile X syndrome	~50% have aortic root dilatation, MVP, or both

CHD = congenital heart defect(s); ASD = atrial septal defect; VSD = ventricular septal defect; PDA = patent ductus arteriosus; PS = valvular pulmonic stenosis; AS = aortic stenosis; CoA = coarctation of aorta; PV = pulmonic valve; AV = aortic valve; ECD = endocardial cushion defect; TOF = tetralogy of Fallot; MVP = mitral valve prolapse; AR = aortic regurgitation; PLSVC = persistence of left superior vena cava; ARD = aortic root dilatation; PA = pulmonary artery; HLH = hypoplastic left heart; TAPVR = totally anomalous pulmonary venous return.

TABLE 51-4 CLASSIFICATION OF CONGENITAL HEART DEFECTS BASED ON PATHOGENETIC MECHANISMS[33]

PATHOGENETIC MECHANISM	EXAMPLES OF DEFECTS
Embryonic blood flow defects	
Left-sided lesions	HLH; bicuspid aortic valve; IAA type A; CoA; PDA
Right-sided lesions	Secundum ASD; PS
Mesenchymal tissue migration defects	TOF; D-TGA
Extracellular matrix defects	ECD
Abnormal cellular death	Ebstein anomaly; muscular VSD
Defects of looping and situs	L-TGA
Abnormalities of targeted growth	TAPVR

HLH = hypoplastic left heart; IAA = interrupted aortic arch; CoA = coarctation of aorta; PDA = patent ductus arteriosus; ASD = atrial septal defect; PS = valvular pulmonic stenosis; TOF = tetralogy of Fallot; TGA = transposition of great arteries; ECD = endocardial cushion defect; VSD = ventricular septal defect; TAPVR = totally anomalous pulmonary venous return.

types of the two forms of Down syndrome do not differ. The phenotype tends to be less severe if the trisomy is mosaic (3 per cent of Down syndrome) as a result of a mitotic nondisjunctional error in the embryo.

The most common causes of morbidity and mortality in Down syndrome patients are congenital heart defects present in 40 to 50 per cent of cases, hematological malignant disease, and duodenal atresia. If the patient either escapes or survives these problems, survival into the fifth decade and beyond is likely, but complicated by progressive dementia of the Alzheimer type. Premature aging may also affect the vasculature, although definitive studies are lacking.

The most characteristic cardiac anomaly in the Down syndrome is a defect of closure of the endocardial cushions. Complicating the clinical problems in such patients and those with simple septal defects is a seeming predisposition to pulmonary hypertension in the face of elevated right-sided flow.[37] About one-third of congenital heart defects are complex, and these patients tend not surprisingly to be the most ill patients. Mitral valve prolapse is found with a frequency exceeding that in age- and sex-matched controls.[38,39] The aortic and pulmonary valve cusps seem predisposed to fenestrations in adulthood.

The medical management of patients with the Down syndrome has undergone evolution to more aggressive measures in recent years. Objections and hesitations on medical, societal, and ethical grounds to operative repair of heart defects in the Down syndrome have been mollified substantially.[40] More follow-up data are becoming available, and early and late postoperative survival in Down syndrome patients appears to be no different from that in other patients with similar defects.[37,40,41]

TRISOMY 18. *Edwards syndrome* is the second most common autosomal trisomy. Most cases are due to meiotic disjunction, and there is a strong relationship to maternal age. Routine prenatal diagnostic testing of women over age 34 could detect at least one-third of all autosomal trisomies, but less than one-half of all women of this advanced age undergo testing. Currently prenatal detection of trisomies followed by termination of pregnancy is having a small but measurable impact on decreasing the incidence of *Down, Edwards, and Patau* syndromes.

Although the severity of the phenotype rarely enables survival beyond a few months, 10 per cent of patients live to 1 year, and a few survive to adulthood, perhaps because of undetected mosaicism for a chromosomally normal cell line. However, central nervous system function is far less than that in the Down syndrome and leads to complex medical management and supportive care for long-term survivors.[42] Cardiovascular defects occur in at least 90 per cent of cases and contribute to death. Complex lesions, usually involving septal defects, dysplastic valves that are rarely hemodynamically important, patent ductus arteriosus, and persistence of the left superior vena cava are common.[43,44] Right ventricular enlargement is common and may indicate not only shunting from left to right, but pulmonary hypertension due to anomalies of the pulmonary vasculature.[43] As in the Down syndrome, transposition of the great arteries is virtually unknown in trisomy 18.[44] Rarely should invasive diagnostic procedures or aggressive supportive measures be undertaken in Edwards syndrome.

TRISOMY 13. *Patau syndrome* occurs in about 0.01 per cent of live births and in progressively higher frequencies in stillbirths and spontaneous abortions. The external phenotype is usually severe, but occasionally not as characteristic as other trisomies; survival beyond a few weeks is rare, and the causes of death involve multiple organ systems, especially the heart. Cardiovascular anomalies are a bit less frequent than in trisomy 18 and have a slightly different spectrum.[32,43] Septal defects are the most common isolated lesions; dextrocardia and bicuspid semilunar valves occur in association with other anomalies.

Patients who survive beyond a month often are mosaic for a chromosomally normal cell line; thus, prognosis is fraught with uncertainty until detailed analysis is completed. Whether invasive cardiological studies are performed or aggressive management undertaken can be determined by the severity of involvement of other organ systems, especially the brain, pending cytogenetic investigation.

TURNER SYNDROME. About one in every 2500 females lacks an X chromosome and has a 45,X karyotype. The frequency of a nonmosaic 45,X karyotype is much higher in spontaneous abortuses than in liveborns, and probably less than 2 per cent of such conceptuses come to term. The clinical phenotype is variable and often mild; the diagnosis is often not suspected until a child's short stature is evaluated or a woman complains of amenorrhea. Many cases are mosaic for cell lines with 46,XX or 46,XY constitutions. A variety of structural aberrations involving the X chromosome can cause partial or complete Turner syndrome.

Among patients with the 45,X karyotype, reported frequencies of congenital cardiovascular defects vary from 20 to 50 per cent, depending on how patients were ascertained. Fifty to 70 per cent of those with cardiovascular defects have clinically important aortic coarctation, usually of the postductal form.[45] As noninvasive imaging studies of asymptomatic patients become routine, the frequency of coarctation may increase. A variety of other cardiac malformations may occur, either singly or combined with coarctation. However, there is strong support for left-sided flow abnormalities as a major pathogenetic mechanism. Bicuspid aortic valve and dilatation of the ascending aorta (with a risk of dissection and histopathology showing elastic fiber disruption) occur even in the absence of coarctation,[46,47] and hypoplastic left heart has been reported.[48] Partial anomalous pulmonary venous drainage without an atrial septal defect is fairly common and should be suspected when right ventricular overload is detected on echocardiography.[49]

Postmortem examination of midtrimester abortuses with 45,X showed a higher incidence of left-sided flow lesions than found at birth, and the authors speculate on an association between the pathogenesis of the cardiovascular anomalies and the uniform presence of lymphatic obstruction at the base of the heart.[45]

Blood pressure elevation is common, even without coarctation or after its repair; a high frequency of renal anomalies is one likely cause, but not the sole explanation, for the prevalence of hypertension.

Women with mosaic karyotypes are less likely to have cardiovascular defects.

CONGENITAL HEART DISEASE

(See Chaps. 31 and 32)

In the past few decades, the reported incidence of structural heart defects in newborns has increased from 5 to 7 per 1000 live births, probably as the result of increased diagnostic sensitivity (especially cross-sectional and Doppler echocardiography and magnetic resonance imaging).[50-54] Supporting this explanation is the lack of change over the same period in the incidence of critical defects at 3.1 to 3.5 per 1000.[50] This enhanced resolving power of noninvasive methods should prove particularly useful in the study of familial structural defects, because apparently unaffected relatives can be evaluated for subclinical evidence of anomalies. Few investigations to date have capitalized on this approach.[55,56]

As is evident from the previous section, gross aberrations of chromosomes produce an extensive and varied array of structural heart disease, an observation as true for spontaneous abortuses as for liveborn children.[57] Unfortunately, the complexity and inscrutability of the human genome severely limit the insight that cytogenetic aberrations provide into etiology and pathogenesis of congenital malformations. This situation is little improved, however, in considering the other two mechanisms by which genes cause congenital heart defects—multifactorial processes and mutations of single genes. The latter group should prove instructive soon, as the protein products of the mutant loci are identified and their normal function and regulation are defined.

MULTIFACTORIAL PROCESSES. The empirical risks of recurrence of congenital heart defects have increased in recent years,[58,59] in keeping with the overall higher incidence noted above. However, this conclusion has been criticized because the studies focused on the offspring of women probands, in whom the recurrence risk appears higher than in men with congenital heart defects.[60] In addition to this unexplained maternal influence, other factors may be at work. For example, improved detection of subtle lesions, more faithful reporting of patients, and the assiduousness of epidemiologists may have shown a systematic variation. It is true that some patients with cardiovascular problems now survive[61,61a] to bear children because of improved medical and surgical care; their offspring might be at increased risk because of the severity of the parents' problems, but some evidence against this idea exists.[62]

As mentioned earlier, the familial aggregation of congenital heart defects has been employed to validate many of the predictions of the threshold liability model of multifactorial inheritance.[56,63-66] In most studies, whether focused on populations or families, defects were classified by their pathology; for example, all ventricular septal defects were considered as one group. There has been bias in reporting families in which one type of defect aggregates, which has led to many reports of "familial atrial septal defect," "familial cardiomyopathy," and so on, without regard to the fact that not all septal defects or cardiomyopathies have the same structure on careful scrutiny, let alone the same cause.

A major advance has been the movement to examine familial aggregation of defects based on presumed pathogenesis.[67-69] The scheme developed by Clark,[33] and since modified and expanded[70] (Table 51–4), has become widely used. Under this approach, some anatomically distinct lesions will be related by common pathogenesis; if it is the pathogenetic mechanism that is under abnormal genetic control, then the occurrence of the distinct defects in the same family would not be troublesome in a genetic model. Alternatively, defects unrelated by pathogenesis would require a different interpretation. This model also focuses on the examination of apparently unaffected relatives and hence increases the chances of detecting subtle manifestations of defective development of cardiovascular structures.

ERRORS IN MESENCHYMAL TISSUE MIGRATION. Included in this category are a wide range of anomalies of the outflow tract, some due to failure of fusion and others due to failure of septation. Relatives of probands with interruption of the aortic arch type B or truncus arteriosus, both uncommon conotruncal malformations, had 2.5 per cent and 6.6 per cent incidences, respectively, of congenital heart defects.[71] Both recurrence rates were higher than expected. The frequency of congenital malformations was much lower in relatives of patients with other forms of interrupted aortic arch. Moreover, relatives of probands with truncus arteriosus and other defects had a recurrence rate of 13 per cent, the majority in the spectrum of conotruncal lesions. Here is an instance in which refined empirical risk data should improve the accuracy of genetic counseling.

Categorizing anatomical defects by presumed pathogenesis emphasizes that all ventricular septal defects are not alike. If there is a strong genetic component to the etiology of tetralogy of Fallot, for example, one might find in close relatives an increased risk not only of tetralogy but of truncus arteriosus and supracristal ventricular septal defects, but not of other forms of septal defects.

FLOW DEFECTS. Left-sided flow lesions comprise a spectrum that includes hypoplastic left heart, congenital aortic stenosis, bicuspid aortic valve, interrupted aortic arch type A, and aortic coarctation. Various components of this spectrum can be present in the same patient.[72] Data from the Baltimore-Washington Infant Study,[73,74] a population-based case-control study of congenital cardiovascular malformations, were used to show that in first-degree relatives of probands with isolated hypoplastic left heart, incidence of bicuspid aortic valve was 12 per cent; most of the cases were asymptomatic and unrecognized before they were detected by echocardiography as part of this investigation.[55] In an exceptional family, four instances of aortic coarctation occurred in four generations.[75]

The association of coarctation of the aorta, bicuspid aortic valve, and dilatation of the ascending aorta, which may occur as part of the *Turner syndrome,*[46] is well known in the general population.[76,77] Several intriguing questions need to be addressed regarding the genetics and pathogenesis of this association. To what extent is the ascending aorta intrinsically abnormal, and hence predisposed to dilate, and to what extent is the dilatation simply a result of abnormal turbulence created by a bicuspid aortic valve? The fact that some patients with this association also have subtle evidence of a systemic connective tissue abnormality, reminiscent of Marfan syndrome, supports the former hypothesis. It will be of interest to extend the study of left-sided flow lesions to include probands with coarctation or congenital aortic stenosis and to evaluate close relatives with techniques capable of detecting the entire range of flow defects.

EXTRACELLULAR MATRIX ABNORMALITIES. Enough is known about the biochemistry and cell biology of cardiac embryology to state with some confidence that the extracellular matrix ("connective tissue") plays an important role. The endocardial cushions have received the most attention as an area where defects in the extracellular matrix might produce malformations.[33] The high frequency of endocardial cushion defects and atrioventricular septal defects in Down syndrome has been noted (p. 1629). Of interest is the finding of increased adhesiveness of fibroblasts from trisomy 21 patients, a phenomenon that could reflect interaction with the extracellular matrix.[78] The distinctiveness of endocardial cushion defects in patients with normal chromosomes and in those with trisomy 21 has been suggested because of differences in associated cardiovascular malformations. However, of six families in which the proband had an endocardial cushion defect, three had recurrence of the same type of defect in a relative, including two with trisomy 21.[69]

SITUS AND LOOPING DEFECTS. This is an area fraught with difficulties of nomenclature, diagnosis, and heterogeneity of both etiology and pathogenesis. In analysis of clinical data, the most informative approach, but clearly arduous because of the large amount of data required, would be to categorize probands and their relatives by the type of situs (solitus, inversus, dextroversion, and levoversion, p. 941), and each of those by the presence or absence of other cardiac and visceral defects. This has not been done on epidemiological cohorts, and in family studies relatives have rarely been subjected to evaluations sufficiently detailed to characterize their phenotypes in detail.[79]

Several mendelian phenotypes point to single genes that have a major effect on determining laterality. In the autosomal recessive *Kartegener syndrome,* a randomization of lateralization of the heart (situs solitus and situs inversus are equally likely in homozygotes)[80] coexists with a defect in ciliary motility, which leads to sinusitis, bronchiectasis, and sperm immotility.[81,82] Not all morphological defects of cilia are associated with aberrations of cardiac situs.[6] Situs inversus with splenic and other cardiac defects, particularly of the position of the great vessels, can be inherited as an autosomal recessive,[83-85] as an autosomal dominant,[86] and as an X-linked recessive.[87,88] Some of the families with these apparently single-gene disorders have concordance of phenotype, but many do not, suggesting that in some cases various types of situs defects, polysplenia, and asplenia are different manifestations of the same mutation.

There is a paucity of data on the recurrence risks of defects in the *cell death* and *abnormal targeted growth* categories. Preliminary data from the Baltimore-Washington Infant Study do not show an increased risk of any cardiovascular defect in the relatives of a proband with a defect in either of these categories.[70]

DISORDERS OF UNCLEAR ETIOLOGY. A number of disorders include an important likelihood of malformation of the cardiovascular system but are of unclear cause (Table 51–5). Familial recurrence is so low as to be *incompatible* with multifactorial inheritance. Several of these disorders deserve comment.

Certain congenital cardiac defects and other malformations occur together more frequently than expected by chance; this *association* of de-

TABLE 51-5 DISORDERS OF UNCERTAIN CAUSE AND INHERITANCE THAT ARE ASSOCIATED WITH A HIGH INCIDENCE OF CARDIOVASCULAR ABNORMALITIES

DISORDER AND PHENOTYPE	MIM NO.*	CARDIOVASCULAR ABNORMALITIES†
Aase syndrome (Congenital anemia, triphalangeal thumbs)	205600	VSD
Bilateral left-sidedness sequence (Polysplenia syndrome)	208530	ASD
Bilateral right-sidedness sequence (Asplenia syndrome; Ivemark syndrome)	208530	Situs inversus, ECD, VSD
CHARGE association (*C*oloboma, *h*eart anomaly, choanal *a*tresia, *r*etardation, *g*enital, and *e*ar anomalies)	214800	TOF, PDA, ECD, VSD
Cornelia de Lange syndrome (Short stature, retardation, synophrys, hypertrichosis, micromelia, genital anomalies)	122470	~20% have CHD: VSD, PDA, ASD, PLSVC, TOF
DiGeorge sequence‡ (Abnormalities of derivatives of 3rd and 4th pharyngeal pouches and 4th branchial arch: hypoplastic thymus with cellular immune deficiency, hyoplastic parathyroids with hypocalcemia)	188400	CHD in ~100%: aortic arch anomalies (especially IAA type B and right-sided aortic arch); PDA, TOF
Goldenhar syndrome (Abnormalities of derivatives of 1st and 2nd branchial arch: hemifacial microsomia, microtia, vertebral anomalies)	141400, 164210, 257700	~50% have CHD: VSD, TOF, PDA, CoA, right-sided aortic arch, PLSVC
Klippel-Feil sequence (Short neck, limited rotation of the head, cervical anomalies)	118100, 148900, 214300	Variable estimates (5–70%) of CHD: VSD, dextrocardia
"Kabuki make-up" syndrome (Dwarfism, peculiar facies, scoliosis, mental retardation)	147920	30% have CHD: ASD, VSD, TOF, CoA, PDA
Pallister-Hall syndrome (Hypothalamic hamartoblastoma, hypopituitarism, imperforate anus, postaxial polydactyly)	146510	ECD
Poland sequence (Unilateral absence of sternocostal pectoralis major, ipsilateral synbrachydactyly)	173800	~10% have dextrocardia or dextroversion
Rubinstein-Taybi syndrome (Short stature, retardation, microcephaly, characteristic facies, broad thumbs)	268600	~20% have CHD: ECD, ASD, TOF, PDA, VSD
VATER association (*V*ertebral defects, *a*nal atresia, *t*racheo-*e*sophageal fistula, *r*adial dysplasia, *r*enal anomaly)	192350	VSD

VSD = ventricular septal defect; ASD = atrial septal defect; TOF = tetralogy of Fallot; PDA = patent ductus arteriosus; ECD = endocardial cushion defect; CHD = congenital heart defect(s); PLSVC = persistence of left superior vena cava; IAA = interrupted aortic arch; CoA = coarctation of aorta; VSD = ventricular septal defect.

* None of these disorders is evidently due to a mutation in a single gene; however, most are listed in Mendelian Inheritance in Man (MIM),[6] and the MIM no. is provided as a ready source to the literature.

† Cardiovascular defects listed in approximate order of decreasing frequency.

‡ Some cases associated with del(22)(q11), raising the possibility of a contiguous gene deletion defect.

fects suggests a common cause, pathogenesis, or both, but the following disorders and those in Table 51–6 remain enigmatic on most of these counts. Designation as a *sequence* implies that some evidence exists for a common developmental problem to account for the features.

CHARGE Association (Table 51–5). Patients with this condition by definition have congenital heart defects.[89,90] The spectrum of cardiovascular malformations suggests not so much a common pathogenetic scheme as a common time of abnormal development. During gestational days 32 to 45, cardiac septation, fusion of the endocardial cushions and membranous ventricular septum, and formation of the outflow tracts and valves occur. An environmental insult or a breakdown in developmental homeostasis during this period could result in the malformation spectrum of this disorder. The defects in other systems could also arise during this embryological window and would be consistent with either environmental or intrinsic factors.

DiGeorge Sequence. This involves developmental anomalies of the

TABLE 51-6 CONGENITAL HEART DEFECTS OCCASIONALLY SHOWING FAMILIAL AGGREGATION CONSISTENT WITH MENDELIAN INHERITANCE

DEFECT	MIM NO.*	DEFECT	MIM NO.
Aneurysm, intracranial berry	105800	Hypoplastic left heart	140500, 241550
Aneurysm, abdominal aortic	100070	Hypoplastic right heart	277200
Angioma	106050, 106070, 206570	Lymphedema, congenital	153000, 153100, 153400, 214900, 247440
ASD, ostium primum	209400		
ASD, ostium secundum	108800, 108900, 178650	Mitral valve prolapse	157700
Bicuspid aortic valve	109730	Patent ductus arteriosus	169100
Cardiomyopathy, dilated	108770, 115200, 115250, 212110	Pulmonary venous return, anomalous	106700
Cardiomyopathy, hypertrophic	192600		
Conotruncal defect	231060	Pulmonic stenosis	126190, 178650, 193520, 265500, 265600, 270460
Dextrocardia	244400, 304750		
Ebstein anomaly	224700	Subaortic stenosis	271950, 271960
Endocardial fibroelastosis	226000, 227280, 305300	Supravalvular aortic stenosis	185500, 194050
Hemangioma	106070, 140800, 140900, 234800	Tetralogy of Fallot	187500
Hemangioma, cavernous	116860, 140850	Ventricle, single	234750

* Data from Mendelian Inheritance in Man.[6]

fourth branchial arch and derivatives of the third and fourth pharyngeal pouches that give rise to the characteristic features. Cardiovascular defects are common, fall into the mesenchymal tissue migration error (conotruncal) spectrum,[33] and frequently cause death in the first month of life. The malformations range from tetralogy of Fallot to ventricular septal defect, truncus arteriosus, patent ductus arteriosus, interrupted aorta, and right aortic arch.[91] Recently several cases have been found to have a small deletion of the proximal long arm of chromosome 22, raising the possibility that this sequence is a contiguous gene deletion syndrome, at least in some instances (Table 51–1).

VATER Association (Table 51–5). This condition has expanded over the years to include *v*ertebral, *v*entricular septal, *a*nal, *t*racheo-*e*sophageal, *r*adial, and *r*enal defects. Omitted from the mnemonic is the single umbilical artery often present.[92,93] Cardiac defects are present in about one-half of patients with more than two components of this association but usually are not life threatening. Although infants with this condition often fail to thrive initially, the long-term prognosis for health and mental function is good, so aggressive management of the multiple malformations is warranted. It is important to separate as soon as possible those patients who have the features of trisomy 18 or 13q- chromosome aberrations, as prognosis in these cases is distinctly unfavorable.

MENDELIAN DISORDERS

Some congenital cardiovascular defects segregate in occasional families as predicted of a mendelian phenotype. There is strong bias favoring reporting such occurrences and an equally strong temptation to conclude that, at least in some cases, the defect is caused by mutation in a single gene. However, rarely and by chance alone, a multifactorial trait will recur in a family in a pattern mimicking mendelian segregation. This potential confusion and the resultant uncertainty in counseling patients and families pertains equally well to disturbances of conduction and rhythm, to various cardiomyopathies, to vascular anomalies, and to hypertension, all discussed subsequently. The true cause of the cardiovascular diseases in such families may not become clarified until each is investigated in detail, perhaps as a result of efforts to map and sequence the entire human genome.

The subject of this section can therefore be parsed into three broad classes of conditions: congenital cardiac defects that occasionally seem to be inherited as mendelian traits (Table 51–6), pleiotropic mendelian syndromes that always or frequently affect the structure of the cardiovascular system (Table 51–7), and mendelian syndromes that occasionally affect the cardiovascular system (Table 51–8).

FAMILIAL ATRIAL SEPTAL DEFECT. Two mendelian forms of atrial septal defect exist as autosomal dominant traits. One has no associated problems and has been described in few pedigrees.[94] Preliminary and unsubstantiated evidence places the gene for this form of secundum atrial septal defect on chromosome 6 linked to the HLA complex.[95]

The second, and more common, condition has atrioventricular conduction delay as the only pleiotropic feature.[96,97] The defect is of the secundum type, and relatives do not seem to be at increased risk of other cardiac malformations. The severity of heart block rarely progresses to third degree. The electrocardiographic abnormality in a patient with apparently sporadic atrial septal defect should prompt a detailed family history and evaluation of close relatives. Attention should be

TABLE 51–7 MENDELIAN DISORDERS WITH CONGENITAL DEFECTS OF CARDIOVASCULAR STRUCTURE AS FREQUENT MANIFESTATIONS

DESCRIPTIVE NAME	EPONYM	MIM NO.*	CARDIOVASCULAR ABNORMALITIES
Adult polycystic kidney disease		173900	MVP, dilated aortic root, intracranial berry aneurysm
Arteriohepatic dysplasia	Alagille syndrome	118450	PPS
Cataract and cardiomyopathy		212350	HCM
Chondroectodermal dysplasia	Ellis–van Creveld syndrome	225500	ASD (ostium primum), common atrium
Deafness, mitral regurgitation, and short stature	Forney syndrome	157800	MR
Familial collagenoma syndrome		115250	DCM
Heart-hand syndrome	Holt-Oram syndrome	142900	ASD (ostium secundum), VSD, MVP, HLH
Keratosis palmoplantaris	Mal de Meleda	248300	DCM, dysrhythmia
Malignant hyperthermia and skeletal defects	King syndrome	145600	malignant hyperthermia → cardiac arrest
	Noonan syndrome	163950	PS, HCM
Pulmonic stenosis and deafness		178651	PS
	Smith-Lemli-Opitz syndrome	270400	PDA, ASD, VSD, TOF, ECD, CoA
Velocardiofacial syndrome	Shprintzen syndrome	192430	TOF, tortuous retinal vasculature

MVP = mitral valve prolapse; PPS = peripheral pulmonic stenosis; HCM = hypertrophic cardiomyopathy; ASD = atrial septal defect; MR = mitral regurgitation; DCM = dilated cardiomyopathy; VSD = ventricular septal defect; HLH = hypoplastic left heart; PS = valvular pulmonic stenosis; PDA = patent ductus arteriosus; TOF = tetralogy of Fallot; ECD = endocardial cushion defect; CoA = coarctation of aorta.

* Data from Mendelian Inheritance in Man.[6]

TABLE 51–8 MENDELIAN DISORDERS WITH CARDIOVASCULAR ABNORMALITIES OCCASIONAL MANIFESTATIONS

SYNDROME	EPONYM	MIM NO.*	CARDIOVASCULAR ABNORMALITIES
Acrocephalosyndactyly type I	Apert syndrome	101200	PS, PPS, VSD, EFE
Acrocephalopolysyndactyly type II	Carpenter syndrome	201000	PDA, VSD, PS, TGV
Hereditary angioedema		106100	Coronary arteritis
Imperforate anus with hand, foot, and ear anomalies	Townes-Brocks syndrome	107480	Sporadic cases have CHD: VSD, ASD
Mandibulofacial dysostosis	Treacher Collins syndrome	154500, 248390	10% have CHD: variable
Neuronal ceroid lipofuscinosis	Batten disease	204200	HCM
Orofacial digital syndrome type II	Mohr syndrome	252100	Variable
Short rib–polydactyly syndrome	Saldino-Noonan syndrome	263530	TGV, ECD, hypoplastic right heart
Thrombocytopenia–absent radius syndrome		274000	TOF

PS = valvular pulmonic stenosis; PPS = peripheral pulmonic stenosis; VSD = ventricular septal defect; EFE = endocardial fibroelastosis; PDA = patent ductus arteriosus; TGV = transposition of great arteries; CHD = congenital heart defect(s); ASD = atrial septal defect; HCM = hypertrophic cardiomyopathy; ECD = endocardial cushion defect; TOF = tetralogy of Fallot.

* Data from Mendelian Inheritance in Man.[6]

directed to the upper limbs, particularly the thumbs, to rule out the Holt-Oram syndrome; radiographic examination of the entire limbs of the proband is helpful on this account.

When patients with atrial septal defect due to aneuploidy (a syndrome with extracardiac features), and one of the autosomal dominant forms are excluded, the recurrence risk of atrial septal defect is about 3 per cent, a value that conforms closely to the multifactorial threshold model.[63,66] Several pleiotropic mendelian conditions have defects of the atrial septum as frequent manifestations.

HOLT-ORAM SYNDROME. This autosomal dominant condition, first elaborated in 1960, shows marked variability within a pedigree.[98] The cardinal manifestations are dysplasia of the upper limbs and atrial septal defect. In heterozygotes for the mutation, arm deformity ranges from undetectable through distally placed thumbs and hypoplastic thenar eminences, triphalangeal thumbs, anomalies of the carpus, and radial aplasia, to phocomelia and hypoplasia of the clavicles and shoulders. Upper extremity deformity is usually bilateral but may be asymmetrical in severity, with the left side the worse.[99] Similarly, the atrial involvement ranges from none to a large secundum defect with early, severe hemodynamic compromise. Other cardiac malformations have been reported, with ventricular septal defects the most frequent. The skeletal and cardiac manifestations are not correlated in individuals, and how a parent is affected is not a reliable predictor of effects on an offspring. Prenatal diagnosis by ultrasound was reported in a fetus with severe limb anomalies;[100] presumably a large septal defect could be detected as well. Other manifestations include dermatoglyphic abnormalities,[98,101] pectus excavatum,[98] hypoplastic peripheral arteries,[99] and cardiac conduction disturbance, the last usually involving the AV node and present in patients with septal defects.[98,99,101] Although the Holt-Oram syndrome bears some resemblance to the VATER association, the clear mendelian nature and lack of more extensive organ system involvement of the former indicate that the two conditions do not represent a pathogenetic spectrum.

The diagnosis of Holt-Oram syndrome is most likely to be missed in a patient with an unknown or unremarkable family history, a secundum septal defect, and minimal or no thumb anomaly. In any "sporadic" case of an atrial septal defect, the patient and the parents should be carefully examined for limb malformations and the family history studied in detail. Detection of a subtle limb defect will alter the recurrence risk in offspring of the proband from the empirical risk of an isolated septal defect of 3 per cent to the 50 per cent of an autosomal dominant trait.

ELLIS–VAN CREVELD SYNDROME (Fig. 51–6). This rare, autosomal recessive chondrodysplasia is found among the old order Amish because of a founder effect and consanguinity. Short stature, metaphyseal dysplasia, dysplastic nails and teeth, and postaxial polydactyly are the pleiotropic manifestations in addition to congenital heart disease.[102] The last is present in more than one-half of homozygotes, and most of the defects affect the atrial septum. The majority are defects of endocardial cushion closure, including ostium primum defects of widely varying size up to a single atrium. This disorder has long been thought to be due to an as yet unknown defect in the extracellular matrix, which would fit with the high frequency of endocardial cushion lesions. However, defects thought due to abnormal embryonic flow (coarctation, hypoplastic left heart, and patent ductus arteriosus) occur in about 20 per cent of cases. Ellis–van Creveld syndrome can be diagnosed prenatally by detection of polydactyly by ultrasonography.

VENTRICULAR SEPTAL DEFECT. This malformation does not seem to be inherited as an isolated mendelian malformation, and no syndromes include it as a common, isolated manifestation. One intriguing pedigree showed maternal transmission of a risk for atrial or ventricular septal defects to at least 11 of 13 offspring; the suggestion was made that phenotype was determined by the mitochondrial chromosome.[103] Subsequent study of the mitochondrial chromosome has not uncovered a candidate gene,[11] and the family has not been studied molecularly. Many other isolated defects have been described in families in patterns suggestive of mendelian inheritance, but only for supravalvular aortic stenosis and mitral valve prolapse is there convincing evidence for the action of a single mutant gene.

SUPRAVALVULAR AORTIC STENOSIS (see also p. 94). This congenital lesion, which may be asymptomatic and detected long after birth because of an ejection murmur, occurs in at least three settings. It can be a sporadic anomaly, a component of Williams syndrome (itself of heterogeneous cause), or an autosomal dominant trait associated with peripheral

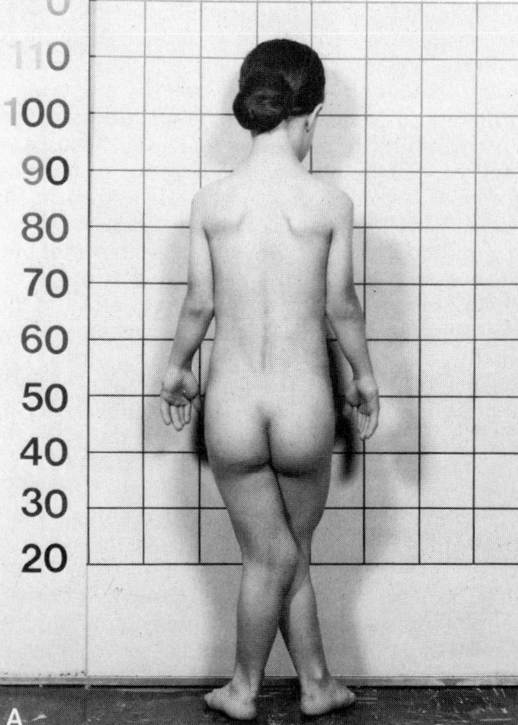

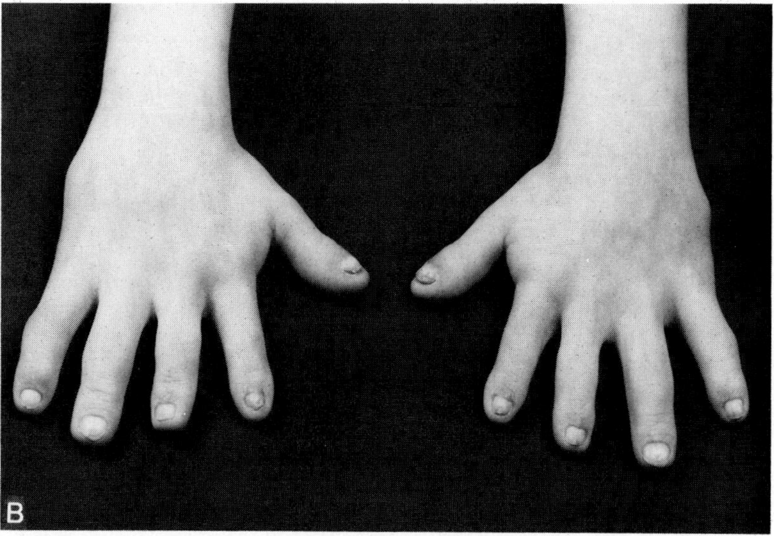

FIGURE 51–6. Ellis–van Creveld syndrome in a young woman. *A*, Note short stature, joint contractures at the elbows, and marked genu valgum. *B*, The fingers are short and the nails dysplastic. Note the protuberances along the ulnar edges of the hands where sixth digits were amputated.

pulmonic stenoses. Cause of the sporadic anomaly is unclear, and counseling about recurrence is difficult. Undetected hypercalcemia during the vulnerable period of gestation or neonatal life has been suggested as one cause.

Williams syndrome is usually sporadic but, in more instances than previously recognized, is a highly variable autosomal dominant condition. The full spectrum includes infantile hypercalcemia, abnormal ("elfin") facies, mental deficiency, short stature, multiple peripheral pulmonic stenoses, and supravalvular aortic stenosis.[104] Occasional cardiovascular manifestations are mitral valve prolapse, bicuspid aortic valve, and hypertension.[105,106] Although patients usually survive the problems of infancy and show catch-up growth, progressive problems of joint contractures, genitourinary and gastrointestinal dysfunction, and psychosocial adjustment define the long-term prognosis.[107] As there are a number of causes of infantile hypercalcemia (including exposure to excessive vitamin D during pregnancy), the clinical entity should be called the Williams phenotype, with the designation "syndrome" reserved for the autosomal dominant variety.

Autosomal dominant supravalvular aortic stenosis is now recognized as an entity distinct from Williams syndrome.[108–110] Mental retardation and abnormal facies should prompt rejection of the diagnosis of this "pure" cardiovascular disorder. Peripheral pulmonary artery stenoses may be present but rarely cause hemodynamic problems. The aortic lesion requires surgery in less than half of patients. Screening of relatives is essential and easily conducted with echocardiography.

MITRAL VALVE PROLAPSE (see also p. 1029). This trait is of heterogeneous cause and pathogenesis; although it has been called the most common abnormality of human heart valves,[111,112] mitral valve prolpase (MVP) is equally clearly not always an "abnormality." Here only the heritable forms of MVP will be discussed. These can be classified into three groups. The first is an autosomal dominant form with minimal extracardiac involvement. The second is an autosomal dominant condition that is clinically variable, and at one end of its spectrum merges with the Marfan syndrome; it could just as well be discussed as a heritable disorder of connective tissue. The third category is composed of the various mendelian syndromes that include mitral valve prolapse as a pleiotropic manifestation.

The first category, which some have called mitral valve prolapse syndrome[113] or familial mitral valve prolapse,[114] includes a condition that is centered on the mitral valve. The development of actual prolapse shows the age- and sex-dependent behavior characteristic of the "idiopathic" form so common in the general population.[114,115] Formal genetic studies confirm *autosomal dominance with variable expression*.[114,115] This category has been partitioned into those patients with billowing of the mitral leaflets and those with excessive systolic mitral annular expansion; because this phenotype breeds relatively true, two distinct autosomal dominant forms may exist.[116] The cause(s) of these entities is unknown.[117] Moreover, when and how the phenotype of this condition can be distinguished from the sporadic cases of MVP and the cases with obvious evidence of a systemic disorder of connective tissue are unclear. The only consistent extracardiac manifestations are excessive arm span in women and relatively low body weight and systolic blood pressure.[118,119]

Many clinical geneticists and cardiologists are referred patients with a suspicion of Marfan syndrome (p. 1641) or Ehlers-Danlos syndrome (p. 1643). Some of these patients do not meet minimal diagnostic criteria for a recognized connective tissue disorder[120] but clearly have extracardiac features consistent with a defect of the extracellular matrix described below. MVP is commonly but not always present; when it is, and evidence of a systemic abnormality of connective tissue is lacking, the patient should be considered as having the condition described in the preceding paragraph, what some call primary mitral valve prolapse.[121] The clinical spectrum of the patients with syndromic MVP includes abnormal striae atrophicae, excessive arm span and leg length, joint hypermobility, pectus excavatum, scoliosis, reduction in thoracic kyphosis ("straight back"), myopia, and mild aortic root dilatation.[122] Aortic dilatation beyond 3 SD above the mean for body surface area, aortic dissection, ectopia lentis, or a family history of any of these three features *removes a* patient from this category. For the remainder of patients, the acronym MASS phenotype, for *m*itral valve, *a*orta, *s*kin, and *s*keletal, describes what certainly is a heterogeneous grouping of patients and families. Aorta is mentioned specifically because of the appropriate concern that progressive dilatation and dissection will occur; in fact, neither has been the case, although prospective evaluation has been brief. Many of the associations between MVP and deformity of the thoracic cage and spontaneous pneumothorax are explained by the MASS phenotype.[123–125]

Finally, as described below, MVP frequently accompanies the Marfan syndrome, several of the Ehlers-Danlos syndromes, and cutis laxa and occurs more often than expected in osteogenesis imperfecta, Larsen syndrome, pseudoxanthoma elasticum, and other mendelian syndromes (see Table 51–11). In addition, occasional families with otherwise unclassified heritable disorders of connective tissue have prominent involvement of the mitral apparatus, with myxomatous deterioration or calcification, or both.[126]

NOONAN SYNDROME. Among the pleiotropic mendelian syndromes that have frequent cardiovascular involvement, the Noonan syndrome is important because of its relatively high prevalence and clinical variability. This autosomal dominant condition has been called the male Turner syndrome in the past because of the short stature, cubitus valgus, neck webbing, congenital lymphedema, and congenital heart defects that coexist in the 45, X Turner syndrome. However, the Noonan syndrome is distinct, not simply because both men and women are affected. Patients with Noonan syndrome often have an unusual deformity of the sternum, mental dullness, hypertelorism, ptosis, and cryptorchidism.[127] The cardiovascular defects, while widely varied, do not include an increased incidence of coarctation of the aorta.[128] Because of the dysmorphism of the facies and the cardiac involvement, Noonan syndrome is often classified, along with Williams, LEOPARD, King, and Watson syndromes, as a cardiofacial syndrome.

The entire phenotype of the Noonan syndrome is highly variable, and affected people can escape clinical problems (or accurate diagnosis), even if they have obvious manifestations.[129] Similarly, a wide range of cardiovascular involvement can occur.[130] *Valvular pulmonic stenosis* was the first defect identified, and Noonan syndrome should always be considered in a patient with this lesion.[131] The valve cusps are thickened and dysplastic, even in the absence of hemodynamic compromise. Obstruction to right-sided flow can also occur in Noonan patients because of pulmonary artery hypoplasia[132] or infundibular subvalvular changes. The latter finding reflects a generalized predisposition to hypertrophic cardiomyopathy, often asymmetrical, that can affect either ventricle.[133,134] Atrial septal defect occurs in about one-third of patients, usually in association with pulmonic stenosis. Ventricular septal defects and patent ductus arteriosus each occur in about 10 per cent. Congenital anomalies of coronary arteries are occasionally and unexpectedly found during evaluation of more obvious defects.[134a] The electrocardiogram often shows left anterior hemiblock and a deep precordial S wave, a pattern not common in pulmonic stenosis of other causes.

Lymphatic dysplasia, especially of the lower limbs, is common but causes clinical difficulties in less than 20 per cent.[127] While evidence of lymphedema often disappears during childhood, chylothorax and a protein-losing enteropathy represent the severe end of the spectrum.[135]

Noonan syndrome shares features with other cardiofacial syndromes, and in sporadic cases (which account for 50 per cent of Noonan syndrome) diagnosis can be difficult. All are *autosomal dominant*, so genetic counseling is somewhat easier. Affected males have reduced reproductive capabilities because of testicular abnormalities. Susceptibility to malignant hyperthermia can be detected by family history, elevated skeletal muscle creatine kinase levels, or muscle biopsy. Despite the relatively high frequency of the Noonan syndrome, estimated up to 1 per 1000, neither its cause nor its pathogenesis is clear. The gene has not been mapped, and interlocus genetic heterogeneity is possible. Intriguing issues that may shed light on these uncertainties are the overlap in phenotype with type I neurofibromatosis[136] (the gene for which is on chromosome 17 and has been cloned) and the frequent coexistence of Noonan syndrome and deficiency of coagulation factor XI.[137]

TERATOGENIC EFFECTS

A teratogen is any agent that adversely affects embryonic or fetal development, such as infectious vectors, radiation, drugs, and other chemicals (Table 51–9). Teratogenic effects on the cardiovascular system are considered in this chapter for several reasons: (1) The phenotypes are often reminiscent of those due to chromosomal aberrations and single-gene mutations. (2) Clinical geneticists and dysmorphologists are involved in diagnosing, managing, and investigating both teratogenic and genetic syndromes. (3) How the organism responds to an encounter with a potential teratogen is largely determined by its genome. The entire field of ecogenetics and part of pharmacogenetics are concerned with these issues.

The abilities to resist disruption of normal human embryogenesis and development involve systems quite distinct from physiologic homeostasis and related only in part with developmental homeostasis. Genetic susceptibilities to teratogens can be illustrated by diverse mechanisms: reduced or inaccurate repair of radiation-induced DNA damage; enhanced receptiveness to viral entry or replication; immune deficiencies that prevent inactivation of infectious vectors or maintenance of immunity; slow inactivation of a compound that exerts a direct deleterious effect; or rapid conversion of an inoffensive drug to a teratogenic metabolite. These types of hereditary variation may be determined by single genes, with susceptibility inherited as a mendelian trait, or by many genes, each of small effect. Either situation can account for the well-known fact that only a fraction of pregnancies exposed to a given agent will be affected adversely. Variation in dose and timing of exposure also confound interpretation of epidemiological and family data. It is not surprising, then, that the actual appearance of the abnormal phenotype is not amenable to traditional pedigree analysis. Rather, examination of the biochemical susceptibilities has proved, and will continue to prove, more enlightening.

TABLE 51–9 CARDIOVASCULAR DEFECTS ASSOCIATED WITH PRENATAL EXPOSURE TO TERATOGENS

TERATOGEN	CARDIOVASCULAR ABNORMALITIES*
Ethanol	~50% have CHD: VSD (~50% close spontaneously), TOF, ASD, ECD, absence of a pulmonary artery
Hydantoin	~10% have CHD: VSD, ASD, PS
Lithium	<3% have Ebstein anomaly
Phenylalanine	~20% have CHD: TOF
Retinoic acid	>50% have CHD: TGA, TOF, VSD, IAA
Rubella	>50% have CHD: PDA with or without ASD, VSD, PPS, IAA
Trimethadione	~50% have CHD: complex combinations most frequent (involving VSD, ASD, PDA, AS, PS), VSD, TOF
Valproic acid	>50% have CHD: left- and right-sided flow lesions: CoA, HLH, ASD, VSD, pulmonary atresia
Vitamin D	supravalvular aortic stenosis is the cardinal manifestation; PPS
Warfarin	~10% have CHD: PDA, PS; rarely, intracranial hemorrhage

CHD = congenital heart defect(s); VSD = ventricular septal defect; TOF = tetralogy of Fallot; ASD = atrial septal defect; ECD = endocardial cushion defect; PS = valvular pulmonic stenosis; TGA = transposition of great arteries; IAA = interrupted aortic arch; PPS = peripheral pulmonic stenosis; PDA = patent ductus arteriosus; AS = aortic stenosis; CoA = coarctation of aorta; HLH = hypoplastic left heart.

* Among patients with the full clinical spectrum associated with each teratogen; cardiovascular defects listed in decreasing order of prevalence.

Some teratogens, such as *warfarin*, have a clear action that explains how the pleiotropic manifestations emerge. The action of other teratogens, such as alcohol, is obscure. Finally, in some teratogenic syndromes, such as that in offspring of women with diabetes mellitus, the actual offensive agent is unclear, and multiple pathogenetic mechanisms seem to pertain.[138,139] Regardless of cause and pathogenetic mechanism, the phenotypes of many teratogens often share manifestations, especially prenatal growth retardation, abnormalities of the craniofacies, and mental retardation. The following syndromes have prominent consequences on the cardiovascular system.

FETAL ALCOHOL SYNDROME. Ethanol is the most common teratogen to which the human embryo and fetus are exposed. The period of greatest vulnerability is during the first trimester, and the risks are clearly related to the amount of alcohol consumed; the risk of the fetal alcohol syndrome occurring in an offspring of a chronic alcoholic woman is 30 to 50 per cent. The features are highly variable and include growth retardation, mild to moderate mental retardation, hyperactivity, short palpebral fissures, a smooth philtrum with a thin upper lip, and small distal phalanges.[140] Congenital heart defects occur in more than one-half of children with the full spectrum of the phenotype; ventricular septal defects are most common and often insignificant, but atrial septal defects, tetralogy of Fallot, and aortic coarctation can occur.

FETAL HYDANTOIN SYNDROME. Virtually all antiseizure medications can affect the fetus. Hydantoin was the first to be identified as a teratogen. The risk to the fetus depends in part on the genotype of the fetus; defects in arene oxidase predisposes to the full syndrome.[141,142] The features include prenatal and postnatal growth retardation, mild mental retardation, a broad face with a short nose, short distal phalanges with small nails, and hip dislocation. Cardiovascular defects, which are an inconstant part of the syndrome, include septal defects, right- and left-sided flow defects, and a single umbilical artery.

RETINOIC ACID EMBRYOPATHY. Isotretinoin was not recognized as a teratogen until after it was licensed for the treatment of acne. The vulnerable period extends from the first week through the fourth month of gestation. The risks of miscarriage and stillbirth are elevated. The phenotype includes anomalies of the craniofacies and gross neuroanatomical disruption. Cardiovascular defects are common and emphasize a variety of conotruncal malformations.[143] Liveborn infants often succumb to the cardiac and brain anomalies. Although the mechanism of action is not certain, vitamin A derivatives such as retinoic acid function as *morphogens* during embryogenesis, serving as signals for cell migration. The fact that the cardiovascular defects are primarily those of rotation and folding suggest disruption of a normal developmental homeostatic system.

WARFARIN EMBRYOPATHY. Coumarin-related vitamin K antagonists are usually prescribed for a variety of cardiovascular problems to women of childbearing age (p. 1805) and can cause a variety of cardiovascular and other organ damage to the fetus. Coumarin interferes with embryogenesis directly when administered during gestational weeks 6 through 9. The most pronounced effects are on cartilage because of inhibition of enzymes of extracellular matrix metabolism. Congenital cardiac defects are perhaps increased in frequency but fit no specific pathogenetic mechanism.[144] The second pattern of coumarin effects involves exposure during the second and third trimester and includes spontaneous abortion, stillbirth, and various central nervous system defects. The last are not due simply to intracranial hemorrhage as was once assumed.[144]

What predisposes to the adverse fetal effects of coumarin remains to be discovered. First, more than 75 per cent of women who take coumarin derivatives throughout pregnancy have normal offspring; reassuring most women while identifying those at risk for adverse effects has obvious advantages. Second, placing all pregnant women on a regimen of heparin is not an acceptable solution, because heparin can cause stillbirth or premature fetal loss in about 20 per cent of exposures, is not as effective as coumarin in some indications for anticoagulation, and is more trouble to administer and regulate.

MATERNAL PKU. The inborn error of metabolism phenylketonuria produces severe mental retardation unless the phenylalanine content of the diet is markedly reduced soon after birth.[145] Deficiency of phenylalanine hydroxylase in the fetus produces no harm because fetal blood levels of phenylalanine are regulated by the heterozygous mother's enzyme. Since neonatal screening for this disease is now routine in all states, virtually all patients receive treatment and grow to adulthood with average intelligence. Many patients discontinue the rigorous dietary therapy during adolescence when the elevated phenylalanine levels have far less deleterious effects. The embryopathy occurs when a woman with homozygous deficiency for phenylalanine hydroxylase becomes pregnant and her fetus is exposed to high levels of the amino acid that overwhelm its ability to metabolize. The result is highly predictable if the mother does not restart dietary restriction of phenylalanine for the entire gestation: moderate to severe mental retardation, prenatal and postnatal growth retardation, microcephaly, and a variety of cardiovascular defects in 15 to 20 per cent.[146] This condition can largely be prevented by effective counseling of female patients with phenylketonuria.

FETAL RUBELLA EFFECTS (see p. 888). About 50 per cent of fetuses become infected with the rubella virus when the mother is infected during the first trimester. Not only does the infected fetus suffer varied and severe interference with development and organogenesis, but it acquires a chronic viral illness that can persist for years. The most common features of the embryopathy are mental deficiency, deafness, cataract, and cardiovascular defects. Patent ductus arteriosus is common as are septal defects. Peripheral pulmonary stenosis and fibromuscular proliferation of medium and small arteries often improve postnatally.

CARDIOMYOPATHIES

(See also Chap. 43)

Each of the three clinical categories of primary cardiomyopathy—hypertrophic, dilated, and restrictive—can be caused by mutations in single genes as judged by mendelian inheritance of a consistent phenotype in multiple families. Many other mendelian disorders also cause cardiomyopathies as a secondary consequence of their basic metabolic disturbance.

HYPERTROPHIC CARDIOMYOPATHY

(See also p. 1404)

In the more than 30 years since the recognition of hypertrophic cardiomyopathy as a clinical entity, many aspects of its natural history, pathology, and management have been substantially clarified.[147] The phenotype is most clearly defined anatomically and histologically and consists of myocardial hypertrophy without secondary cause; cellular and myofiber disarray; myocardial fibrosis; and mediointimal proliferation of small coronary arteries. None of these features is pathognomonic; for example, myofiber disorganization is present in the normal human heart during embryogenesis and in congenital heart defects that place strain on the right-sided circulation.[148]

About half of probands with idiopathic hypertrophic cardiomyopathy of any segment of the left ventricle have affected first-degree relatives, and in those families the phenotype is inherited as an autosomal dominant.[149–151] There is wide variability of expression within a family, in part due to age-dependency of the trait.[151a] Later generations of relatives in adolescence and childhood may not have developed echocardiographic evidence of hypertrophy. Hence, pedigree screening for clinical, counseling, or investigative purposes should not be considered complete until the following criteria are satisfied: two-dimensional echocardiography is used to insure that segmental hypertrophy is detected; a person at risk has a normal echocardiographic study and no evidence of electrocardiographic abnormality or important dysrhythmia after about age 20; and a person of any age has left ventricular hypertrophy without any other explanation, such as hypertension or aortic stenosis.[151b]

In about one-half of families with more than one affected person, the oldest patient appears to be the first affected relative, with neither parent involved.[149,150] Some of these patients may have hypertrophic cardiomyopathy on account of a new mutation rendering them heterozygous; they would have a 50:50 chance of having affected offspring. Others may be phenocopies, that is, have environmental causes of hypertrophy that remain obscure. The possibility of autosomal recessive inheritance has been raised,[147] but convincing pedigrees, in which all parents and offspring of multiple affected sibs have normal echocardiographic findings, have not been found.[149,152]

Given the variability in segmental pattern of hypertrophy within families,[153] the two pedigrees that show *only* apical cardiomyopathy suggest that multiple genetic forms exist.[154] Genetic heterogeneity is also supported by linkage studies that identify potential loci on two different human chromosomes. With cloned DNA probes and restriction fragment site polymorphisms,[5] the phenotype in one large family was linked tightly and with a good statistical power to chromosome band 14q11.[155] Subsequently, the genes for the cardiac α and β myosin heavy chains were linked to the same polymorphism, and are the leading candidates as the site of the basic defect.[155a] However, hypertrophic cardiomyopathy is clearly of heterogeneous genetic cause, as some families show no linkage of the phenotype with 14q11.[155b] In one family, indistinguishable clinically from typical hypertrophic cardiomyopathy, the disease was found only in relatives who had a fragile-site marker on chromosome 16, whereas unaffected relatives lacked the marker.[156] It is possible, but unlikely, that the fragile site itself has something to do with the mutation. More likely the fragile site is close to the gene and therefore serves simply as a pointer, just like the restriction fragment polymorphisms did in the previous example. It is also possible, because the pedigree is relatively small, that the result is fortuitous but incorrect. In appropriate families, availability of tightly linked DNA markers permits prenatal diagnosis and presymptomatic detection superior to echocardiography.

DILATED CARDIOMYOPATHY

(See also p. 1398)

The prevalence of idiopathic dilated cardiomyopathy is about double that of the hypertrophic form.[157] No population-based studies have explored the family history of probands with the dilated, congestive form, and the frequency of hereditary forms is virtually unknown. Although numerous occurrences of familial dilated cardiomyopathy are reported, few investigations have been conducted of an unselected series of probands for clinical and subclinical evidence of cardiac disease.[158] Thus, it is unclear what fraction of patients with idiopathic dilated cardiomyopathy have a mendelian disease, how many have a new mutation for a mendelian disease, and how many have phenocopies of nongenetic causes. Estimates of a positive family history, which could suggest a mendelian condition or a shared environmental cause, range from 7 to 30 per cent.[158–161]

Because of the risk of severe dysrhythmia in dilated cardiomyopathy, early detection of people with the disorder can be life saving. Two-dimensional echocardiography is a sensitive method for detecting affected relatives with subclinical disease. Individuals who have equivocal left ventricular enlargement or dysfunction can have ambulatory electrocardiographic monitoring and, if the diagnosis is still uncertain, can have serial examinations. Certainly every patient with idiopathic dilated cardiomyopathy should have a detailed family history. If any close relative has a history consistent with cardiomyopathy, dysrhythmia, or sudden death at a relatively young age, counseling about the risk of a familial disease and the potential benefits of pedigree screening should be offered.

The majority of instances of familial occurrence fit autosomal dominant inheritance.[161–166] Considerable clinical variability characterizes virtually all pedigrees; variation in severity, clinical phenotype, and age of onset is typical. Several pedigrees suggest autosomal recessive inheritance,[162,167,168] but nonpenetrance and germinal mosaicism are potential explanations for what is really a dominant trait. Recurrence of congestive cardiomyopathy of early onset in an inbred pedigree is more convincing for an autosomal recessive condition.[169] In one pedigree with relatively early onset of symptoms (15 to 21 years of age) in males, much later onset in females, and lack of transmission of cardiomyopathy from father to son (although there was only one opportunity in this family), inheritance is most compatible with X linkage.[170]

The causes of these various hereditary forms of dilated cardiomyopathy are unknown. In some families with autosomal dominant disease, a mild proximal skeletal myopathy of type I fibers coexists with cardiac involvement.[164,171,172] Skeletal muscle changes might serve not only as an early clinical marker of heterozygosity for the mutant gene in some individuals at risk but also indicate that the search for cause should address structural components or metabolites common to both cardiac and skeletal myofibers. Histological examination of myocardium generally shows nonspecific hypertrophy and fibrosis. By electron microscopy, however, mitochondria are distinctly abnormal, a finding not seen in congestive heart failure of other causes.[172,173] Because the inheritance pattern in these cases does not suggest a mutation of the mitochondrial genome, focus could be directed on nuclear genes that encode structural components of the mitochondrion, components of the respiratory chain found in the mitochondrion, or enzymes that regulate and facilitate free fatty acid metabolism in the mitochondrion. As with virtually every common disease, associations with immune response factors have been investigated in dilated cardiomyopathy. Weak associations with HLA-DR loci were found that seemed to predispose to the disease in some cases,[174] but these results remain unconfirmed and unexplained.

In one family, cardiomyopathy developed only in association with pregnancy.[175] Although peripartum cardiomyopathy is a well-recognized, usually sporadic, disorder (see p. 1798), its occurrence in five women in two generations suggests a hereditary predisposition.

RESTRICTIVE CARDIOMYOPATHY

(See also p. 1415)

The pathogenesis of the majority of cases of restrictive cardiomyopathy involves infiltration or replacement of the myocardium or both. The causes are varied and can be nongenetic or genetic; the latter are mostly metabolic diseases with secondary effects on the heart and are summarized in Table 51–10; some are reviewed subsequently. A common form of restrictive cardiomyopathy that has primary genetic forms among many other causes is endocardial fibroelastosis. Other mutations produce restriction through pericardial constriction. Isolated pedigrees of primary myocardial fibrosis without secondary cause and leading to restrictive hemodynamics are not classifiable.[176,177]

ENDOCARDIAL FIBROELASTOSIS (see also p. 944). This abnormality is characterized by thickening of the endocardium, which leads to decreased compliance and impaired diastolic function. Primary forms, discussed here, are unassociated with other cardiac anomalies (Table 51–11). When congenital, endocardial fibroelastosis accounts for somewhat under 10 per cent of childhood deaths from heart disease. In infants there is often an indolent course of failure to thrive, tachypnea, and tachycardia, until a precipitant such as an upper respiratory infection leads to rapid cardiac decompensation. Treatment of children with primary endocardial fibroelastosis is ineffective; cardiac transplantation now offers some hope. Autopsy shows enlargement of the left ventricle and perhaps other chambers, no abnormality of lung vessels, and collapse of the left lower lobe. Histopathological study reveals extensive deposition of extracellular matrix, primarily collagen and elastic fibers, in the endocardium.

X-linked recessive inheritance is the most firmly established of the single-gene causes, and even here there may be heterogeneity. Some pedigrees show mainly small, contracted cardiac chambers, while others have chamber dilatation; both are compatible with the functional pathophysiology described by the term "restrictive." Males are affected earlier and more severely by both forms, with death in infancy not unusual.[178] In other families, the ventricles are dilated, and the condition is distinguished from X-linked dilated cardiomyopathy by the presence of endocardial fibroelastosis and an immune deficiency due to defective granulocyte function in the former.[179] Morphological abnormalities of mitochondria were present on ultrastructural studies of heart and leukocytes. Insufficient longitudinal experience is recorded to know whether females heterozygous for this mutation develop a dilated restrictive cardiomyopathy later in life.

Several pedigrees suggestive of autosomal recessive inheritance of primary endocardial fibroelastosis were reported before the routine availability of laboratory methods to diagnose metabolic derangements, especially defects in fatty acid catabolism.[180-182] Endocardial fibroelastosis can be a prominent finding at autopsy in patients with autosomal dominant dilated cardiomyopathy[183]; whether the endocardial changes are primary, representing yet another mendelian form of this disorder, or secondary is unclear.

CARDIOMYOPATHIES SECONDARY TO OTHER CAUSES

INBORN ERRORS OF METABOLISM. These can affect the left ventricle by various mechanisms and produce diverse anatomical, histological, and functional disturbances. The most common anatomical result is an apparent hypertrophic cardiomyopathy, which is actually *pseudohypertrophic,* because the thickened walls are not due to myocardial cell hypertrophy, but to cellular or interstitial infiltration by metabolites. Abnormalities of both systolic and diastolic function result, outflow obstruction may occur, and in some cases the hemodynamic characteristics resemble a restrictive cardiomyopathy. The offending metabolite may be an incompletely degraded macromolecule such as glycogen (*glycogen storage disorder II* [Pompe's disease] and *glycogen storage disorder III*), proteoglycan and glycosaminoglycan (*mucopolysaccharidoses I, III, IV, VI,* and *VII*), sphingolipid (*Fabry's disease, Tay-Sachs disease, Farber's disease, Refsum's disease,* and *Gaucher's disease*), glycoprotein (*fucosidosis* and *mannosidosis*), and amyloid (*familial amyloidoses I* and *III*) or a small molecule such as iron in *hemochromatosis*. Some of these disorders are discussed later. True myocardial hypertrophy occurs as a part of mendelian syndromes of unclear cause, such as *Noonan syndrome, von Recklinghausen neurofibromatosis,*[184] and *LEOPARD syndrome,*[185,186] and monogenic errors of metabolism, notably those producing *hyperthyroidism* and *pheochromocytoma.* Any of the mendelian disorders that cause hypertension (Table 51–12) may, over time, produce true myocardial hypertrophy.

Dilated cardiomyopathy often results from inborn errors of energy production, especially fatty acid metabolism. Various disorders associated with *carnitine deficiency, mitochondrial* and *peroxisomal dysfunction,* and *muscle dysfunction* can present with symptoms of congestive heart failure or dysrhythmia.

Restrictive cardiomyopathy often occurs with both hemodynamic evidence of impaired diastolic filling and wall thickening; any of the conditions causing pseudohypertrophy of the myocardium can eventually exhibit restrictive pathophysiology. Hemochromatosis and the amyloidoses, both hereditary and acquired forms, are especially likely to present in this manner. Connective tissue replaces myocytes or infiltrates the interstitium in a number of conditions. Fibrosis of the myocardium may cause pseudohypertrophy, but the clinical consequences are more those of restriction. Disorders in this category are those that cause coronary artery disease (*diabetes mellitus,* the *hemoglobinopathies* associated with sickling, *Fabry disease* and the *mucopolysaccharidoses*) and some of the *muscular dystrophies,* in which myocardial fibers are replaced by extracellular matrix. Finally, a number of hereditary conditions are associated with endocardial fibroelastosis (Table 51–11).

CONSTRICTIVE PERICARDITIS (see also Chap. 35). Two rare autosomal recessive disorders include fibrous thickening of the pericardium as a manifestation. In both, signs and symptoms of constrictive pericarditis develop insidiously, and treatment by pericardiotomy is life saving. One condition was first described in Finland and given the name *MULIBREY nanism,* a combination of a mnemonic for *mu*scle, *li*ver, *br*ain, and *ey*e and an archaic word for dwarfism (nanism).[44] Growth failure from an early age is common, and growth does not improve once pericardial constriction is abated. Subsequently, more than a dozen patients, generally with consanguineous parents, have been reported from around the world.[187]

The *arthropathy-camptodactyly syndrome* previously had been reported because of the skeletal and rheumatological manifestations before pericardial effusion and fibrous thickening of the pericardium were recognized as manifestations.[188-190] Its cause is unknown.

TABLE 51-10 MENDELIAN ERRORS OF METABOLISM WITH MANIFESTATIONS IN THE CARDIOVASCULAR SYSTEM

DISORDER	EPONYM OR COMMON NAME	MIM NO.*	PATHOGENESIS	CARDIOVASCULAR INVOLVEMENT	BIOCHEMICAL DEFECT	GENE LOCUS†	ANIMAL MODEL
Aminoacidopathies							
Alkaptonuria	Ochronosis	203500	Deposition of homogentisic acid in connective tissue	AS; atherosclerosis			
Cystinosis, nephropathic type		219800	Lysosomal storage	Hypertension from renal failure, vascular wall thickening	?	?	
Homocystinuria		236200	Unknown	Early CAD; venous thrombosis; pulmonary embolism	Cystathionine-β-synthase	CBS; 21q21-q22.1	
Oxalosis I	Hyperoxaluria	259900	Vascular and tissue accumulation of oxalate	Conduction defect; vascular occlusions; Raynaud phenomenon	Peroxisomal alanine: Glyoxylate aminotransferase	AGT	
Defects in fatty acid metabolism							
Carnitine transport defect	Primary carnitine deficiency	212140	Lipid myopathy; defective energy generation	DCM: ECF	?	?	Syrian hamster
MCAD deficiency		201450	Lipid myopathy; defective energy generation	DCM	Medium-chain acyl-CoA dehydrogenase	ACADM,1p	
LCAD deficiency		201460	Lipid myopathy; defective energy generation	DCM	Long-chain acyl-CoA dehydrogenase	ACADL,7	
Glycogen storage disorders							
GSD I	Pompe	252300	Lysosomal storage	Pseudohypertrophic CM; short P-R interval; ECF	α-1,4-glucosidase	GAA: 17q21-q25	Canine & bovine
GSD II	Adult acid maltase deficiency	232300	Lysosomal storage	Primarily skeletal muscle; respiratory insufficiency; cor pulmonale	α-1,4-glucosidase		
GSD III	Forbes; debrancher deficiency	232400	Intracellular glycogen accumulation fibrosis	Pseudohypertrophic CM	Amylo-1,6-glucosidase		
Phosphorylase kinase deficiency	GSD of the heart		Hypoglycemia	DCM	Phosphorylase kinase		
Glycoproteinoses							
Fucosidosis, severe		230000	Lysosomal storage	Myocardial thickening	α-fucosidase	FUCA1; 1p34	
Fucosidosis, mild		230000	Lysosomal storage	Angiokeratoma	α-fucosidase	FUCA1; 1p34	
Mannosidosis		248500	Lysosomal storage	Myocardial thickening; valvular thickening; conduction disturbance	α-mannosidase	MANB, 19p13.2-12	
Aspartylglycosaminuria		208400	Lysosomal storage	Valvular thickening	Aspartylglycosylamine amino hydrolase	AGA, 4q21-qter	
Mucolipidoses							
ML II	I-cell	252500	Lysosomal storage	Same as MPS IH	Acetylglucosamine-1-phosphotransferase	GNPTA; 4q21-q23	
ML III	Pseudo-Hurler polydystrophy	252500	Lysosomal storage	Valvular thickening and dysfunction, esp. AS, AR	Acetylglucosamine-1-phosphotransferase	GNPTA; 4q21-q23	
Mucopolysaccharidoses							
MPS IH	Hurler	252800	Lysosomal storage	Early CAD; PH and OAD→CP; valvular dysfunction, esp. MR, AR; pseudohypertrophic CM	α-L-iduronidase	IDUA, 22q11-pter	Canine and feline
MPS IS	Scheie	252800	Lysosomal storage	Valvular dysfunction, esp. AS	α-L-iduronidase	IDUA, 22q11-pter	
MPS IH/S	Hurler-Scheie	252800	Lysosomal storage	Same as MPS IH	α-L-iduronidase	IDUA, 22q11-pter	
MPS II	Hunter	209900	Lysosomal storage	Same as MPS IH; less severe in mild MPS II variant	Sulfoiduronate sulfatase	IDS, Xq28	
MPS III A	Sanfilippo A	252900	Lysosomal storage	Valvular thickening and occasional dysfunction	Heparin sulfate sulfatase	?	
MPS III B	Sanfilippo B	252920	Lysosomal storage	Valvular thickening and occasional dysfunction	N-acetyl-α-D-glucosaminidase	?	
MPS III C	Sanfilippo C	252930	Lysosomal storage	Valvular thickening and occasional dysfunction	acetyl-CoA: α-glucosaminidase N-acetyltransferase	?	

TABLE 51-10 MENDELIAN ERRORS OF METABOLISM WITH MANIFESTATIONS IN THE CARDIOVASCULAR SYSTEM *Continued*

DISORDER	EPONYM OR COMMON NAME	MIM NO.*	PATHOGENESIS	CARDIOVASCULAR INVOLVEMENT	BIOCHEMICAL DEFECT	GENE LOCUS†	ANIMAL MODEL
MPS III D	Sanfilippo D		Lysosomal storage	Valvular thickening and occasional dysfunction	N-acetylglucosamine-6-sulfatase	G6S, 12q14	
MPS IV A	Morquio A	253000	Lysosomal storage	Valvular dysfunction, esp. AR	Galactosamine-6-sulfatase		
MPS IV B	Morquio B	253010	Lysosomal storage	Milder than MPS IV A	β-galactosidase		
MPS VI	Maroteaux-Lamy	253200	Lysosomal storage	Same as MPS IH	Arylsulfatase B	5p11-qter	Feline
MPS VII	Sly	253220	Lysosomal storage	Valvular thickening	β-glucuronidase	GUSB;7q	Mouse and canine
Sphingolipidoses							
α-Galactosidase A deficiency	Fabry	301500	Cellular accumulation of trihexosylceramide, esp. endothelium	Early CAD, valvular thickening and dysfunction; pseudohypertrophic CM; short P-R interval; arteriolar occlusion; angiokeratoma	α-galactosidase A	GLA; Xq22	
Ceramidase deficiency	Farber	228000	Histiocytic infiltration	Nodular thickening of valves	Ceramidase	?	
Glucocerebrosidase deficiency	Gaucher, adult form	230800	Cellular accumulation of glucocerebroside	PH→CP; interstitial infiltration of myocytes by Gaucher cells; constrictive pericarditis	β-glucocerebroside	GBA; 1q21	
Miscellaneous disorders							
Acid lipase deficiency	Wolman	278000	↑ Cholesterol; foam cell infiltration	Atherosclerosis	Lysosomal acid lipase	LIPA, 10q	
Acid lipase deficiency	Cholesterol ester storage disease	278000	↑ Cholesterol, foam cell infiltration	Atherosclerosis; PH	Lysosomal acid lipase	LIPA, 10q	
Geleophysic dysplasia		231050	Lysosomal storage	Valvular dysfunction	?		
Hereditary angioedema		106100	Complement and kinin activation	Angioedema	C1 esterase inhibitor	CINH, 11p11.2-q13	
Multiple sulfatase deficiency	Juvenile sulfatidosis	272200	Lysosomal storage		?		

CAD = coronary artery disease; DCM = dilated cardiomyopathy; ECF = endocardial fibroelastosis; CM = cardiomyopathy; AS = aortic stenosis; AR = aortic regurgitation; PH = pulmonary hypertension; OAD = obstructive airway disease; CP = cor pulmonale; MR = mitral regurgitation; GSD = glycogen storage disease.
* Data from Mendelian Inheritance in Man.[6]
† Gene symbol followed by chromosomal locus.

TABLE 51-11 DISORDERS ASSOCIATED WITH RESTRICTIVE CARDIOMYOPATHY

	MIM NO.*
Primary endocardial fibroelastosis	
Familial endocardial fibroelastosis	226000, 305300
Faciocardiorenal syndrome	227280
Secondary endocardial fibroelastosis	
as a relatively common manifestation	
Maternal lupus erythematosus	
Pseudoxanthoma elasticum	177850, 264800
Systemic carnitine deficiency	212140
Trisomy 18	
as a relatively infrequent manifestation	
Cornelia de Lange syndrome	122470
Rubinstein-Taybi syndrome	268600
Secondary infiltrative cardiomyopathy	
Familial amyloidoses I and III	176300
Fabry's disease	301500
Gaucher's disease type I	230800
Glycogen storage disorder II	232300
Glycogen storage disorder III	232400
Hemochromatosis	235200
Mucopolysaccharidosis IH	252800
Mucopolysaccharidosis II	309900

* Data from Mendelian Inheritance in Man.[6]

TABLE 51-12 MENDELIAN CONDITIONS AND MOLECULAR DEFECTS PREDISPOSING TO ATHEROSCLEROSIS

PHENOTYPE	GENE	LOCUS	MIM NO.
Cholesterol ester storage disease	Acid lipase	LIPA; 10q24-q25	278000
Hypoapo A-I; ↓ HDL	Apolipoprotein A-I	APOA1; 11q23-qter	107680
Hyperapo B; ↑ LDL	Apolipoprotein B	APOB; 2p24	107730
Hyperlipoproteinemia Ib; ↓ TG	Apolipoprotein C-II	APOC2; 19q13.1	207750
Hypoapo C-III; low HDL	Apolipoprotein C-III	APOC3; 11q23-qter	107720
Hyperlipoproteinemia III	Apolipoprotein E-II	APOE; 19q13.1	107741
Hyperlipoproteinemia Lp(a)	Apolipoprotein Lp(a)	LPA; 16q26-q27	152200
Hyperlipoproteinemia I; ↑ chylomicrons	Lipoprotein lipase	LPL; 8p22	238600
Hyperlipoproteinemia II; ↑ LDL	LDL receptor	LDLR; 19p13.2-p13.1	143890
Analpha-lipoproteinemia (Tangier disease); ↓ HDL	?	?	205400
Hyperlipidemia V; combined hyperlipidemia	?; probably heterogeneous	?	238400
Hyperlipidemia VI; familial hyperchylomicronemia & hyperprebeta-lipoproteinemia	?; probably heterogeneous	?	238500
Werner syndrome	?	?	277700

PRIMARY DISORDERS OF RHYTHM AND CONDUCTION

Virtually every dysrhythmia and conduction abnormality has been reported to occur in relatives. For example, *familial disturbance of conduction* occurs, without evident cause, at the sinus node,[191-196] atrioventricular node,[197-200] and bundle branches.[201-205] However, understanding the genetics of cardiac electrophysiology has been hampered by several characteristics of this extensive literature: Most families have been small, so that mode of inheritance, or even whether the inheritance is mendelian, is uncertain; many of the families show a mixture of different defects, partly because the disease is progressive[206,207]; and some specific conduction defects are associated with hereditary myocardial diseases, such as hypertrophic cardiomyopathy,[208] atrial cardiomyopathy,[209,210] and familial amyloidosis.[211] As noted earlier, there seems to be genetic control of normal electrical conduction, so it would not be surprising to find mutations in single genes that produced clinically important disturbance.

An important cause of complete heart block, though not mendelian, nonetheless involves genetic factors. The association between rheumatic diseases and heart block was clearly established when the offspring of mothers with acquired disorders of connective tissue, especially lupus erythematosus, were found to have complete heart block.[212-214] Many examples of "autosomal recessive" congenital heart block represent this familial, but nonmendelian, etiology. The risk is not related to severity of the maternal disease but is highest in children of women with antibodies to ribonucleoprotein (anti-Ro[SS-A])[215] and at least one allele for HLA-DR3.[216] Thus, it may be the maternal genotype that determines susceptibility to inflammation of the fetal heart at vulnerable periods, such as gestational weeks 3 to 4 when the atrioventricular node is forming. Genetic susceptibility to inflammation of the atrioventricular node of patients themselves is suggested by the relatively high association of HLA-B27 in adults requiring permanent pacemakers[217,218]; not all of these patients have overt evidence of HLA-B27–associated rheumatic diseases.

Familial dysrhythmia is also not uncommon. Nodal rhythm,[219] ventricular irritability,[220] and tachydysrhythmia associated with accessory atrioventricular pathways[221-223] have been reported in families. Hereditary cardiomyopathies are another cause of familial dysrhythmia, and a notable example is arrhythmogenic right ventricular dysplasia, an autosomal dominant condition with variable expression[224-226] (see also p. 763). In addition to these disorders, several syndromes involving prolongation of the Q-T interval deserve comment.

WARD-ROMANO SYNDROME (see also p. 1640). Familial syncope and sudden death have long been associated with ventricular dysrhythmia, but a distinct syndrome was not recognized until Ward[227] and Romano,[228] working independently nearly three decades ago, reported the characteristic prolonged Q-T interval. Subsequent investigations of numerous families have clearly established that the defect in repolarization is inherited as an *autosomal dominant.* Although a long Q-T_c is consistently present, other abnormalities of conduction also occur, although they may not be evident on the resting electrocardiogram.[229] Ward-Romano syndrome is distinguished from the Jervell and Lange-Nielsen syndrome by inheritance pattern and the absence of hearing deficiency. Early suggestions of linkage of Ward-Romano syndrome to HLA[230] have not been substantiated,[231] and neither the gene locus nor the cause is known. Treatment with beta-adrenergic blockade or an automatic implanted defibrillator is effective. Individuals heterozygous for the mutant gene should be identified through a detailed family history and counseled appropriately.

JERVELL AND LANGE-NIELSEN SYNDROME (see also p. 1640). The association of familial syncope, sudden death, and congenital deafness was codified in 1957,[232] although as with most eponymous syndromes, reports of affected individuals occurred previously. As would be expected for a rare, autosomal recessive condition, the parents of affected children are more likely than average to be consanguineous. Although heterozygotes have normal hearing and no overt primary rhythm disturbance, the Q-T_c intervals may be slightly prolonged.[233] The frequency of a long Q-T_c among deaf children is about 1 per 100, so routine electrocardiographic screening of anyone with congenital deafness is warranted.

Neither the cause nor the pathogenesis is known. Fright and rage clearly precipitate syncope and sudden death, leading to the proposal of autonomic dysfunction as the basic defect. However, allotransplantation of the heart, thereby causing complete denervation, failed to correct the underlying problem in one patient.[234]

DISORDERS OF CONNECTIVE TISSUE

The two broad classes of disorders of connective tissue are those due to mutations in single genes that determine or somehow affect components of the extracellular matrix and those due to extrinsic factors affecting the extracellular matrix, such as rheumatoid arthritis and systemic lupus erythematosus. The former category includes many disorders that affect the cardiovascular system. Susceptibility to so-called acquired disorders of connective tissue is, in part, determined by genes, and this specific aspect will be reviewed. Disorders due to intrinsic factors acting on the extracellular matrix are discussed in Chapter 56.

Mendelian Disorders of the Extracellular Matrix

Close to 200 distinct phenotypes now comprise this category, which was first defined less than four decades ago with fewer than 10 disorders.[235] Several reviews and textbooks describe the phenotypes of many of the conditions, including their frequent cardiovascular matrix (Table 51–13).[16,236-242]

TABLE 51-13 CARDIOVASCULAR MANIFESTATIONS OF HERITABLE DISORDERS OF CONNECTIVE TISSUE

DISORDER		MIM NO.*	CARDIOVASCULAR MANIFESTATIONS
Cutis laxa		219100	PS, PPS, CP
		123700	MVP
Ehlers-Danlos	I	130000	MVP
	II	130010	MVP
	III	130020	MVP
	IV	130050	Arterial rupture, MVP
	VI	225400	MVP
	VIII	130080	MVP
	X	225310	MVP, aortic root dilatation
Osteogenesis imperfecta	I	166200	MVP, mild aortic root dilatation
	II	166210	CP, arterial calcification
	III	259420	MVP
	IV	166220	Aortic root dilatation
Marfan syndrome		154700	MVP, aortic root dilatation, aortic dissection
MASS phenotype		157700	MVP, mild aortic root dilatation
Pseudoxanthoma elasticum		177850	Arteriosclerosis

PS = valvular pulmonic stenosis; PPS = peripheral pulmonic stenosis; CP = cor pulmonale; MVP = mitral valve prolapse
* Data from Mendelian Inheritance in Man.[6]

MARFAN SYNDROME

(See also p. 1627)

This *autosomal dominant* disorder is relatively frequent (~1 per 10,000), occurs in all races and ethnic groups, and is often not diagnosed during life.[243-245] In light of the classic phenotype, failure to diagnose the Marfan syndrome may seem surprising; however, marked clinical variability, age dependency of all of the manifestations, and a high (~30 per cent) rate of new mutation all conspire to make detection of mildly affected, young, sporadic patients challenging.[246] The diagnosis remains based solely on clinical criteria, although progress on defining the biochemical basis[13] and the genetic locus[247] raises the hope of more definitive criteria. Current criteria (Table 51-14) depend on the manifestations in the cardinal organ systems—the eye, the skeleton, the heart, and the aorta—and other systems, and the family history[120] (Fig. 51-7). The presence of manifestations more specific for the Marfan syndrome ("hard criteria"), such as aortic dilatation, aortic dissection in a nonhypertensive young person, ectopia lentis, and dural ectasia, clearly are more important diagnostically than features common in other connective tissue disorders and in the general population, such as scoliosis, joint hypermobility, myopia, and MVP.

The most common cardiovascular features are MVP and dilatation of the sinuses of Valsalva.[243-246,248-250] Associated clinical problems of mitral regurgitation, aortic regurgitation, and aortic dissection account for most of the early mortality that results in an average age of death in the fourth and fifth decades.[251] Children tend to be more severely affected by mitral valve disease,[252-256] while aortic problems are progressive and more likely in adolescence and beyond.

MITRAL VALVE INVOLVEMENT. Mitral valve prolapse is age dependent and more common in women with the Marfan syndrome. The incidence reaches 60 to 80 per cent when patients are studied by two-dimensional echocardiography,[121,257] and generally the valve leaflets have an elongated and redundant appearance. Progression of severity, as judged by appearance or worsening of mitral regurgitation by clinical and echocardiographic criteria, occurs in at least one-quarter of patients,[258] a much higher rate than in MVP found in the general population.[259] The mitral annulus dilates and contributes to the regurgitation, as do stretching and occasional rupture of chordae. About 10 per cent of patients with marked prolapse have calcification of the mitral annulus. Standard treatment for chronic mitral regurgitation is indicated, but coexistent aortic root dilatation usually requires that increasing inotropy be avoided. When mitral regurgitation becomes severe enough to warrant surgical intervention, two considerations must be added to the balance: (1) Repair of the mitral apparatus is often successful in the Marfan syndrome,[260-262] although long-term prospective studies are not yet complete.

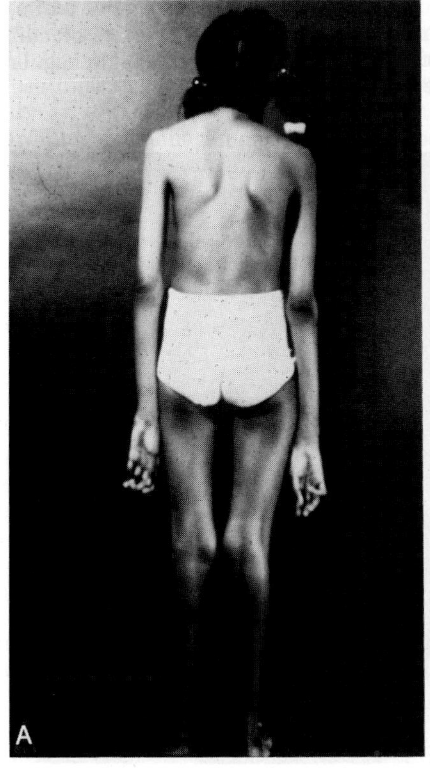

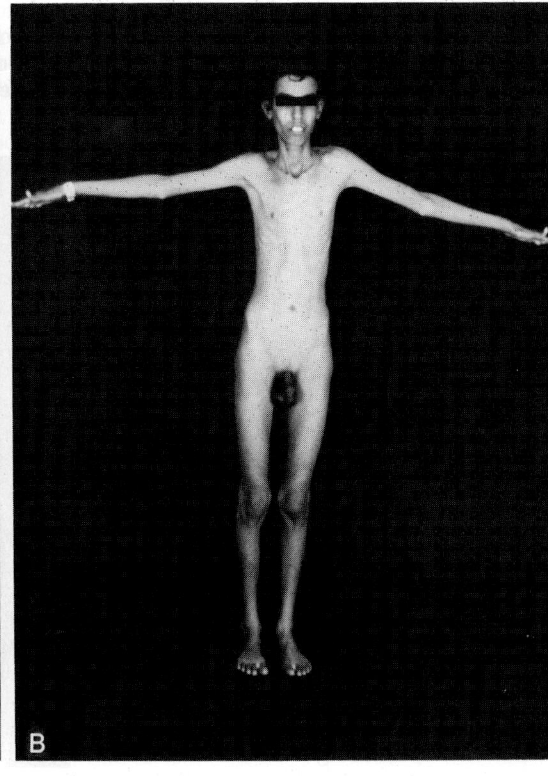

FIGURE 51-7. External phenotype of a boy with Marfan syndrome, showing long extremities and digits, tall stature, and pectus carinatum.

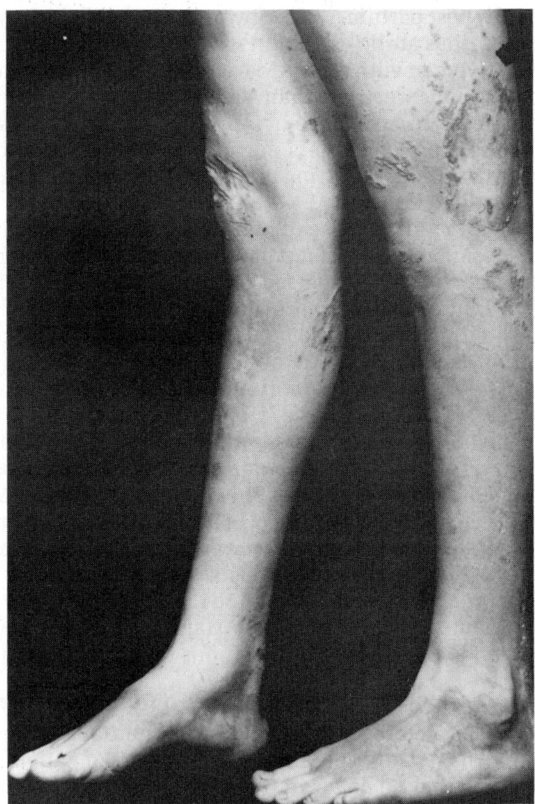

FIGURE 51–9. Legs of a patient with Ehlers-Danlos type IV who died of rupture of the subclavian artery. Note the mild joint hypermobility and the striking dermal abnormalities — elastosis perforans serpiginosa and thin, atrophic scars over areas of recurrent trauma.

PSEUDOXANTHOMA ELASTICUM

This is a clinically variable and genetically heterogeneous disorder of unknown cause. Histopathological examination of affected tissues show fragmentation and calcification of elastic fibers. The skin, the eye, the gastrointestinal system, and the cardiovascular system are the organs most severely affected.[120,236,296] The skin shows highly characteristic raised, yellowish papules (pseudoxanthoma) overlying areas of flexural stress, such as the neck, cubital and popliteal fossae, and groin. Breaks in the elastic lamella, Bruch's membrane of the choroid produce the funduscopic finding of angioid streaks. Gastrointestinal hemorrhage is common and potentially fatal; mucosal arterioles bleed, and because the calcified elastic fibers prevent effective vessel retraction, hemostasis is difficult. Selective arterial embolization was life saving in one instance.[297] The heart is affected in a number of ways. Endocardial fibroelastosis is common, but because primarily the atria are involved, a restrictive cardiomyopathy is uncommon. Mitral valve prolapse may be increased in frequency[298,299] but is rarely a clinical problem. Coronary artery disease with myocardial ischemia and infarction is the major problem and a common cause of early death.[236,300] Elastic and muscular arteries, including the coronaries, develop a type of arteriosclerosis similar to Mönckeberg's; progressive luminal narrowing occurs and can produce complete occlusion. Initially this is most evident at the radial and ulnar arteries, where absence of pulses and a positive Allen test are noted early in the course.[300] Because narrowing progresses slowly, collaterals form, and peripheral ischemia is a late complication. Because the arterial stenoses tend to be diffuse, bypassing them often involves extensive surgery. One patient with marked endocardial fibroelastosis was helped by resection of calcified elastic bands within the left ventricle.[301] Because the basic defect is unknown, no specific treatment is available. Because of a positive association between phenotypic severity and dietary calcium intake, patients can be advised to restrict consumption of dairy products and to avoid calcium supplements.[302] Hypertension and all risk factors for atherosclerosis should be aggressively controlled.

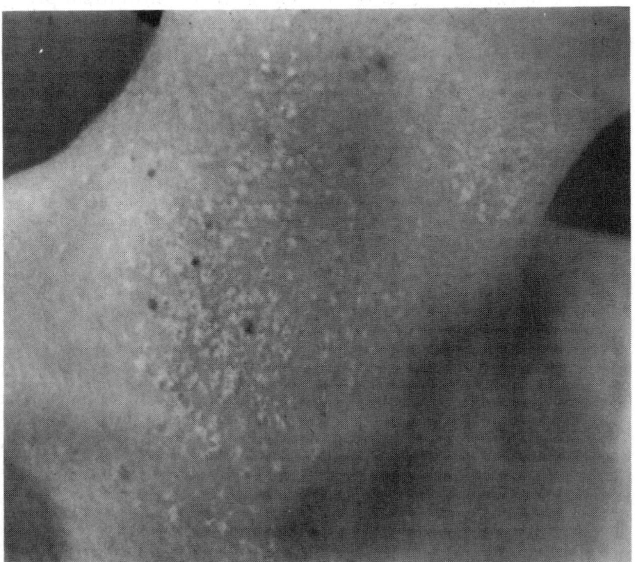

FIGURE 51–10. Skin of a young man with pseudoxanthoma elasticum. The neck is a typical location to notice the raised, yellowish papules from which the name of the condition derives.

GENETIC SUSCEPTIBILITY TO ACQUIRED DISORDERS OF CONNECTIVE TISSUE

Genetic factors are clearly implicated in the susceptibility to many of the rheumatic disorders and to specific complications of specific conditions. The cardiovascular manifestations of these disorders are particularly interesting in this regard (p. 1723). For example, study of HLA-DR antigen frequencies suggests that immune-response factors are involved in the pathogenesis of chronic rheumatic heart disease in blacks.[303]

INBORN ERRORS OF METABOLISM THAT AFFECT THE CARDIOVASCULAR SYSTEM

The hundreds of biochemical defects that affect human metabolism have direct or secondary impact on the cardiovascular system (Table 51–10). Several examples will be reviewed, selected for their relevance to clinical practice or their instructive lessons about pathophysiology.

AMINOACIDOPATHIES

Inborn errors of amino acid metabolism result in the accumulation of precursors and a deficit of end products, either or both of which can be detrimental. In *alkaptonuria*,[304] an intermediate of tyrosine catabolism polymerizes to homogentisic acid, which readily accumulates in the extracellular matrix. Over many years, connective tissue of cartilage, heart valves, and arteries becomes increasingly abnormal. Aortic stenosis and arteriosclerosis are the cardiological sequelae.

Homocystinuria

This condition is caused by a deficiency of cystathionine β-synthase; the pathogenesis of the pleiotropic manifestations is largely unknown.[305] Perhaps the amino acid sulfhydryl groups bind to collagen and other macromolecules and interfere with cross-linking. The clinical features, once confused with the Marfan syndrome, include tall stature, skeletal deformity, ectopia lentis, mental retardation, psychiatric disturbances, and a predilection for venous and arterial thromboses. Those patients with mutations that render the enzyme activity able to be increased by pharmacological doses of pyridoxine are less severely affected; early treatment can prevent most aspects of the phenotype.[306] Patients unresponsive to pyridoxine can be helped by a low-protein diet to reduce intake of methionine.

Myocardial infarction, pulmonary embolism, and stroke are the most common causes of death. The pathogenesis of the vascular complications was once thought to involve abnormal platelet function, but platelet survival in untreated patients is normal.[307] Controversy continues about susceptibility of heterozygotes, who have none of the external phenotype of the disease, to vascular disease.[308-310] Some epidemiological evidence suggests an increased risk of stroke, while challenging individuals with a methionine load appears to identify those who accumulate more homocysteine than normal and who have an increased chance of having atherosclerosis.[311]

DISORDERS OF FATTY ACID METABOLISM

While most organs can metabolize fatty acids when faced with hypoglycemia, only the heart depends on fatty acids as the primary source of energy generation. Thus, it is not surprising that virtually all genetic defects in fatty acid metabolism, including generalized defects in mitochondria and peroxisomes, are associated with myocardial dysfunction. Other substrates—glucose, lactate, and oxaloacetate—also generate energy in myocardial cells by entry into mitochondria and the tricarboxylic acid (Krebs) cycle. Thus, defects in conversion of pyruvate to acetylcoenzyme A and in any point along the tricarboxylic acid cycle and the respiratory chain will have a major impact on myocardial energy generation. Quite likely, some sporadic and familial instances of idiopathic cardiomyopathy may represent undiagnosed or undefined metabolic disorders.

PRIMARY CARNITINE DEFICIENCIES. Carnitine is a required cofactor for entry of long-chain fatty acids into mitochondria and is both synthesized endogenously and available from dietary sources.[312] Deficiency of carnitine effectively blocks metabolism of long-chain fatty acids throughout the body and hepatic metabolism of ketones. Because of their relative dependency on fatty acids, muscle cells, including myocytes, suffer out of proportion to other tissue when carnitine levels are low for any reason. Cytoplasmic inclusions of lipid are characteristic findings in myocytes and hepatocyes.

Several mendelian defects exist leading to actual or relative carnitine deficiency. An autosomal recessive defect in carnitine palmitoyltransferase I leads to a skeletal muscle myopathy with little effect on the heart.[313] So-called systemic carnitine deficiency can be due to a variety of causes: primary deficiency of intake, synthesis, or function, and secondary deficiency, the majority now known to be a result of defects in fatty acid metabolism (especially medium-chain acylcoenzyme A dehydrogenase deficiency).[312,314,315] The latter group of conditions often do not respond to pharmacological doses of carnitine, whereas primary deficiencies often do.[315,316]

Primary carnitine deficiency usually presents in infancy with hypoglycemia, coma, and congestive heart failure due to dilated cardiomyopathy. In the few cases reported, problems largely resolve; they can be prevented from recurring by oral supplementation with l-carnitine[315-317] (p. 1436). Some of the infants with systemic carnitine deficiency have been shown to have a defect in carnitine transport, which leads to excessive urinary loss and which affects muscle but not liver.[315] Thus, muscle cells still may be relatively deficient in carnitine, despite supplementation, and long-term prognosis is uncertain at this time.[315,317]

MITOCHONDRIAL MYOPATHIES (see also Chap. 14). All of the enzymes of fatty acid oxidation are encoded by genes located on nuclear chromosomes, but the components of the electron transport chain are encoded by both nuclear and mitochondrial genes. Several syndromes involving various types of myopathies have been shown to be due to mutations in the mitochondrial chromosome.[11] The *Kearns-Sayre* syndrome includes pigmentary degeneration of the retina, ophthalmoplegia, and cardiomyopathy as its most prominent manifestations; all of the affected tissue have nearly exclusive reliance on oxidative phosphorylation for energy generation. Variations in both the actual mutations and the fraction of abnormal mitochondria in the cells of the different organs (heteroplasmy) account for many of the clinical differences in phenotype, severity, and age of onset among patients with this disorder. Inheritance is maternal for patients with mitochondrial mutations; apparent autosomal recessive and dominant inheritance may indicate that mutations of nuclear genes can impair electron transport similarly to mitochondrial mutations.[6] The disease has been treated with moderate success over the short term with coenzyme Q[318] and with cardiac transplantation in one case.[319]

GLYCOGENOSES

Three of the glycogen storage disorders affect cardiac muscle.

GLYCOGEN STORAGE DISEASE II (see also p. 995). This *autosomal recessive* condition is due to deficiency of the lysosomal enzyme α-1,4-glucosidase and results in the lysosomal accumulation of glycogen in most tissues. Several allelic variants occur.[320,321] The condition with infantile onset is called *Pompe disease*, and cardiac involvement is profound.[322] The infant with Pompe disease appears well initially but soon fails to thrive and develops hypotonia, tachypnea, and tachycardia; the disease progresses during the first year to irreversible congestive heart failure and death from pneumonia or cardiopulmonary failure. Typically, auscultation reveals no murmurs until late in the course when obstruction develops, and hypoglycemia does not appear because the nonlysosomal pathway of glycogen catabolism is intact. The diagnosis is suggested by massive cardiomegaly on examination and chest radiography and by characteristic echocardiographic abnormalities of a short P-R interval and markedly increased QRS voltage.[239] Echocardiography shows tremendously thickened (pseudohypertrophic) ventricles, and Doppler interrogation or catheterization may reveal subaortic and subpulmonic pressure gradients characteristic of obstructive cardiomyopathy.

Reduced diastolic function of a restrictive cardiomyopathy develops eventually, and endocardial fibroelastosis is common.[323,324] With these findings, the diagnosis of Pompe disease is virtually certain, but it can be confirmed by analysis of α-1,4-glucosidase activity in cultured fibroblasts. Prenatal diagnosis is possible by enzymatic assay of amniocytes. Treatment is supportive, but cardiac transplantation could correct the cardiac problem; unfortunately, involvement of other organs, including the lungs, liver, and skeletal muscle might eventually prove just as serious as the cardiomyopathy. Bone marrow transplantation might be a solution if performed early in the course. An animal model of α-1,4-glucosidase deficiency exists in cattle and develops cardiac pathology typical of human Pompe disease.[325]

Cardiomyopathy may develop in the juvenile-onset form of α-1,4-glucosidase deficiency,[326] but it is not invariable because of allelic heterogeneity. In one sibship without cardiac involvement, three brothers had extensive hepatic, skeletal muscle, and arterial smooth muscle accumulation of glycogen, and each died of rupture of a basilar artery aneurysm.[327] The adult-onset form usually presents with insidious onset of respiratory insufficiency, and clinically important cardiac disease is rare.

GLYCOGEN STORAGE DISEASE III (see p. 1638). This autosomal recessive deficiency of amylo-1,6-glucosidase results in infantile- and juvenile-onset syndromes of muscular weakness, wasting, and hepatomegaly. Clinical cardiac disease is not common, although both cytoplasmic (nonlysosomal) and intermyofibril glycogen is routinely present in the heart and causes pseudohypertrophy. The diagnosis has been established by enzymatic assay of an endomyocardial biopsy specimen.[328]

GLYCOGEN STORAGE DISEASE IV. This is caused by deficiency of α-1,4-glucan:α-1,4-glucan 6-glycosyl transferase. It usually causes a fatal disorder of early childhood characterized by hepatic failure; although extensive deposition of polysaccharide occurs in the heart, death intervenes before cardiac symptoms appear. A child who developed exertional dyspnea and exercise intolerance at 7 years was found to have a dilated cardiomyopathy; this enzyme deficiency was diagnosed by endomyocardial biopsy.[329]

CARDIAC PHOSPHORYLASE KINASE DEFICIENCY. A single case of this enzyme deficiency has been reported; deposition of glycogen was confined to the heart, which was massively thickened and enlarged, and had caused the death of the 5-month-old infant.[330]

Glycoproteinoses

As shown in Table 51–10, this group of disorders results in the lysosomal accumulation of a variety of compounds that cannot be catabolized further because of the specific enzyme deficiency. Some have prominent cardiac pathology, generally of pseudohypertrophy and valvular thickening, which present with congestive failure, valvular dysfunction, conduction defects, or dysrhythmia.

HEMATOLOGICAL DISORDERS

(See Chap. 57)

HEMOCHROMATOSIS (See pp. 1419 and 1747). This is an autosomal recessive disorder of unknown cause that results in iron deposition in many tissues, including the myocardium. The manifestations include diabetes mellitus, skin hyperpigmentation, hypogonadism, hepatic failure with cirrhosis, hepatoma, and congestive heart failure; severity is considerably worse, and age of onset earlier, in men because of the autophlebotomy provided by menstruation.[331,332] The gene is located close to the HLA complex on chromosome 6, and presymptomatic diagnosis can be made in a family, even prenatally, by determining HLA antigen haplotypes and performing linkage analysis. Diagnosis in sporadic cases depends on finding increased serum iron, ferritin, and, especially, transferrin saturation in the absence of any obvious cause of excessive iron intake.[333] Fully 10 per cent of the population is heterozygous for the hemochromatosis mutation, suggesting that at an incidence of 2 to 3 per 1000, this disease is underdiagnosed.

Cardiac involvement often appears first as dysrhythmia or congestive heart failure. Dysrhythmia, conduction abnormalities, and low QRS voltage are typical electrocardiographic findings; cardiomegaly is seen on chest radiography, and a dilated cardiomyopathy with reduced systolic function can be documented on echocardiography.[334] Occasional patients have a restrictive pattern on cardiac catheterization.[335]

Treatment by repeated phlebotomy is most effective if begun before organ damage is irreversible. If a patient with congestive heart failure has not yet developed serious compromise in other organs, cardiac transplantation may be contemplated, as may combined heart-liver replacement.

HEMOGLOBINOPATHIES (see p. 1744). *Sickle cell disease* and other hemoglobinopathies associated with sickling can produce ischemia and infarction in multiple organs by occlusion of small vessels; however, the heart is relatively resistant.[336] Nonetheless, the combination of chronic hypoxemia and anemia produces a chronic high-output state that leads to congestive heart failure in many adults. The cardiovascular system can also be compromised by hypertension from renal infarction, pulmonary embolism and infarction (the chest pain of which often causes concern about myocardial ischemia), stroke, and hemosiderosis from chronic transfusions. In addition to a hyperdynamic congestive failure, iron overload is the principal risk to the myocardium in other causes of decreased erythrocyte production *(thalassemias)* and increased erythrocyte consumption *(hemolytic anemias)* requiring repeated transfusions.

MUCOPOLYSACCHARIDOSES AND DISORDERS OF TARGETING LYSOSOMAL ENZYMES

Many of the specific disorders in these two groups share phenotypic manifestations and are caused by various defects in the ability of lysosomes to catabolize proteoglycan and glycosaminoglycan. Short stature, progressive coarsening of facial features, a skeletal dysplasia termed dysostosis multiplex, corneal clouding, and protean effects on the cardiovascular system are common[236,238,337–340,340a] (Fig. 51–11). Only MPS IS

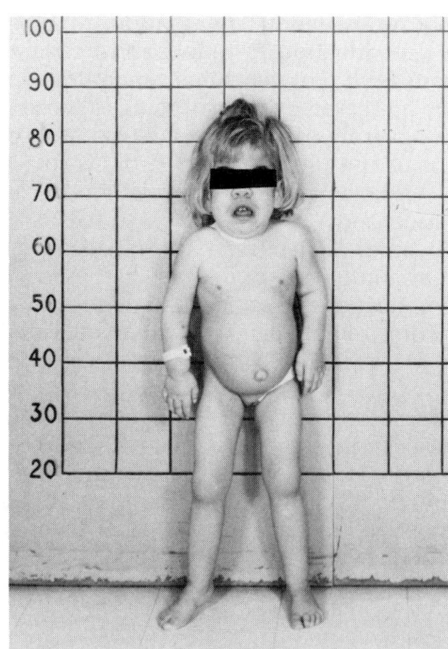

FIGURE 51–11. The Hurler syndrome in a 4-year-old girl. Note short stature and coarse facial features.

(Scheie syndrome), the mild form of MPS II (mild Hunter syndrome), MPS IV (Morquio syndrome), and MPS VI (Maroteaux-Lamy syndrome) have minimal or no mental impairment.

The cardiovascular complications (Table 51–10), which are all progressive and usually insidious, arise from engorgement of cells and tissues with macromolecular storage material.[238,341] First, the ventricular walls become pseudohypertrophic, and systolic function gradually deteriorates. The electrocardiogram shows reduced QRS voltages; rarely is any conduction disturbance present. Second, coronary arteries narrow because of intimal and medial thickening.[342] Myocardial infarction is common in MPS IH and the severe form of MPS II, although the patients are usually too retarded to complain of classic symptoms, and the diagnosis is made post mortem.[343] Third, valve leaflets thicken and cause progressive dysfunction that is oddly specific for individual disorders. For example, aortic stenosis is common in MPS IS, and mitral regurgitation is found frequently in MPS IH and MPS IV. Finally, narrowing of the upper and middle airways causes obstructive apnea, chronic hypoxemia and hypercarbia, pulmonary hypertension, and eventually cor pulmonale.[344,345,345a]

Until recently, treatment of children with those conditions that caused mental retardation has been supportive. Increasing experience with bone marrow transplantation in many of the conditions shows that, in the relatively few survivors of the transplant, somatic accumulation of mucopolysaccharide can be reduced, with clinical improvement in cardiopulmonary function.[337] However, improvement of central nervous system function has been marginal or absent. Nonetheless, bone marrow transplantation may have a role, especially in MPS IV and MPS VI, in which cardiopulmonary compromise can greatly shorten otherwise productive lives. Attempts at cardiovascular surgery, indeed of any procedure requiring general anesthesia, are fraught with risks of difficult intubation, hyperextension of the neck with cervical cord damage (the odontoid process is often hypoplastic), and prolonged efforts to wean from mechanical ventilation.[344]

SPHINGOLIPIDOSES

Fabry Disease

(See also p. 1626)

This X-linked condition deserves comment because the diagnosis is often not made until adulthood when serious end-organ damage has occurred.[346,347] As a result of deficiency of α-galactosidase A, ceramide trihexoside and other glycosphingolipids accumulate in lysosomes of many cells and organs, especially endothelial cells, glomerular and tubular cells of the kidney, and the heart. Microangiopathy causes the characteristic skin lesion, angiokeratoma, and may contribute, along with primary nerve involvement, to acroparesthesias and painful crises. Proteinuria and hypertension precede renal failure, which often has led to death in males and often leads by the fourth decade to the necessity for long-term dialysis or renal transplantation. A successful kidney allograft does not correct the systemic metabolic defect,[348] and the disease usually progresses in other organs.[349]

Structural and functional cardiac involvement is similar qualitatively to that in the mucopolysaccharidoses. Thickening of the myocardium is pseudohypertrophy from deposition of glycosphingolipid in lysosomes; the diagnosis has been made by endocardial biopsy during the evaluation of unexplained ventricular hypertrophy or frank obstructive cardiomyopathy.[350,350a] Chronic hypertension can exaggerate left ventricular dysfunction, as can ischemia and infarction from diffuse luminal narrowing of the coronary arteries. Two-dimensional echocardiography is useful for serial documentation of myocardial function.[351] Although valvular thickening and MVP are common, hemodynamically important mitral regurgitation is not.[351,352] The pulmonary vasculature becomes narrowed and right-sided pressures rise, but cor pulmonale is rarely a problem. The electrocardiogram often shows a shortened P-R interval, increased left ventricular voltages, and dysrhythmia. Medium-sized arteries throughout the body develop luminal narrowing, with cerebrovascular disease the most common cause of death after renal failure.

Heterozygous females generally show some clinical manifestations, especially in the eye, and at much later ages than hemizygous males develop renal, cerebrovascular, and cardiac disease.[346,351–353] Prenatal diagnosis is possible, and a detailed family history and genetic counseling are essential whenever the disease is found. The gene for α-galactosidase A has been cloned, and a variety of mutations identified, illustrating allelic genetic heterogeneity.[350a,354]

Familial Amyloidoses

(See also p. 1451)

A variety of disorders, defined initially by clinical phenotype and due to progressive accumulation of amyloid in organs and tissues, are beginning to be categorized by the underlying biochemical and genetic defects.[6,355] The several conditions termed familial amyloidosis with polyneuropathy, and originally classified as separate autosomal dominant disorders, are now known to be due to different mutations in the same gene encoding transthyretin, a thyroxine- and retinol-binding protein also called prealbumin. Although polyneuropathy dominates the early course during young adulthood, renal failure and restrictive cardiomyopathy supervene later and cause death in most cases. The age of onset, severity, and predilection for kidney and cardiac involvement are determined by the type of mutation, with males affected earlier and more severely.[356–358]

NEUROMUSCULAR DISORDERS

(See Chap. 60)

CARDIAC TUMORS

(See Chap. 44)

The three most common tumors that originate in the heart are myxomas, fibromas, and rhabdomyomas. All occur as part of hereditary syndromes and as sporadic events. The new occurrence of any of these tumors, especially in a child, may represent the first manifestation of a systemic condition, so a detailed general examination and family history are always indicated.[359] For example, 51 to 86 per cent of cardiac rhabdomyomas occur because of tuberous sclerosis.[359a] Tumors due to hereditary disorders tend to be multiple and to recur after resection.

INHERITED DISORDERS OF THE CIRCULATION

Hereditary Hemorrhagic Telangiectasia

This autosomal dominant condition, often called Osler-Rendu-Weber disease, is more common than appreciated. Because of marked intrafamilial- and interfamilial variability, the condition may go undiagnosed in affected patients for years despite mild manifestations.[360] Mucocutaneous telangiectases occur on the tongue, lips, and fingertips most commonly (Fig. 2–4, p. 17). Small and moderate-sized arteriovenous fistulas occur in the nose, leading to recurrent epistaxis, in the gastrointestinal system, where they cause recurrent bleeding and occult anemia, and in the lung, resulting in hypoxemia, hemoptysis, polycythemia, clubbing, paradoxical embolization through the right-to-left shunt, and a hyperdynamic circulation. Less common sites of vascular malformations are the liver[361] and the kidney.[362] Diffuse ectasia of the coronary arteries was noted in one patient.[363]

Patients with this condition, and their close relatives, should be screened for pulmonary arteriovenous malformations through auscultation and a chest x-ray. A low arterial PO_2 should prompt consideration of angiography and therapeutic balloon occlusion of the feeding arteries of any sizable malformation to prevent systemic embolization, especially to the brain.[364] Danazol helps to reduce epistaxis.[365] Neither the biochemical defect nor the gene for hereditary hemorrhagic telangiectasia has been identified, and prenatal diagnosis is not yet possible.

Von Hippel-Lindau Syndrome

The features of this *autosomal dominant* condition involve malformations and abnormal growth of small blood vessels. Retinal angioma, hemangioblastoma of the cerebellum, and hemangioma of the spinal cord occur in association with renal cell carcinoma, pancreatic and epididymal cystadenomas, and pheochromocytoma.[366–369] Secondary hypertension due to renal disease and pheochromocytoma, which is often bilateral, occurs. The basic cause is unclear, but the gene has been mapped to the short arm of chromosome 3, so that prenatal diagnosis by means of linkage analysis is possible.

DISORDERS AFFECTING PRIMARILY ARTERIES

Mendelian disorders are associated with a diverse array of arterial pathology, and some have been described or catalogued earlier in this chapter. This section deals with two categories of disorders caused by a single mutant gene: pleiotropic syndromes better known for affecting organ systems other than the vasculature, and primary abnormalities of arteries.

ADULT POLYCYSTIC KIDNEY DISEASE. In the United States, this relatively common autosomal dominant disease affects a half million people and accounts for about 3 per cent of all long-term hemodialysis. Development of renal cysts is age dependent, and presymptomatic detection of heterozygotes, even by ultrasonography, can be uncertain into adulthood.[369a] About one-half of patients are hypertensive, one-half have hepatic cysts, one-half eventually develop severe renal failure, and an unknown (but probably high) fraction have colonic diverticula. Elevated plasma renin levels contribute to hypertension long before renal failure occurs.[369b] The cardiovascular manifestations include MVP in one-quarter, mild dilatation of the aortic root, occasional thoracic and abdominal aneurysms, and a predisposition to regurgitation of the aortic, mitral, and tricuspid valves.[370–372] The association of diverticula, organ cysts, and cardiovascular lesions reminiscent of, but milder than, the Marfan syndrome suggests an underlying connective tissue disorder.

The most serious vascular problem is typical "berry" aneurysms of the cerebral circulation, which occur in about 10 per cent of heterozygotes but which may remain asymptomatic throughout life. Hypertension predisposes to subarachnoid hemorrhage. How to screen for and treat intracranial aneurysms in patients without neurological symptoms remains controversial, with some advocating angiography and prophylactic surgery,[373] and others concluding that such aggressive management carries more risk than doing nothing.[374] The advent of high-resolution noninvasive screening techniques, such as magnetic resonance imaging, may well have altered the balance, and the analysis is worth repeating.

The gene for most cases of adult polycystic kidney disease has been mapped to a locus, PkD1, on human chromosome 16, but neither the biochemical nor the gene defect is known. In these families, presymptomatic and prenatal diagnoses are possible using DNA probes around the region where the gene is located.[375] In rare families, renal disease is unlinked to chromosome 16 markers,[376] and tends to occur later than in cases due to a mutation of PkD1.[369a]

ARTERIOHEPATIC DYSPLASIA. An autosomal dominant disorder of marked variability, *Alagille syndrome* causes neonatal jaundice and congestive heart failure in the most severely affected infants but may be asymptomatic in heterozygous relatives.[377,378] The cardiovascular findings include peripheral pulmonary artery stenosis in the majority, occasionally associated with septal defects or patent ductus arteriosus. Renal disease may produce hypertension. In some cases, a small deletion of the short arm of chromosome 20 (del[20][p11.2]) has been detected, suggesting the possibility that this complex phenotype is a contiguous gene deletion syndrome.[3]

ARTERIAL ECTASIA AND DISSECTION. Pedigrees abound in which dilatation of the aortic root, aneurysm of the abdominal aorta, aortic dissection without dilatation, or a combination of these problems occurs in an autosomal dominant pattern without evidence of a recognized heritable disorder of connective tissue.[379–381] Because of the variable presentation and natural history of the aortic disease, presymptomatic detection of presumed heterozygotes is uncertain, as is reassurance of relatives at risk who are of childbearing age and would prefer not to pass this condition to offspring. Until recently, no basic defect had been identified. In two families with autosomal dominant transmission of arterial aneurysms and mild increased skin fragility and bruisability, different mutations in the gene encoding type III procollagen have been found.[382,383] Thus, depending on the mutation, deficiency of type III collagen can cause the classic syndrome of Ehlers-Danlos type IV (p. 1643) or a form of the much subtler but just as deadly syndrome, familial arterial rupture. For these families in which the mutations have been defined, reliable presymptomatic and prenatal diagnoses are at hand.

Formal genetic analysis of 91 families ascertained through a proband with abdominal aortic aneurysm suggests an autosomal recessive predisposition exists for late-onset aneurysms.[383a] This study provides a rationale for offering ultrasound screening to sibs of patients with abdominal aortic dilatation.

FAMILIAL ARTERIAL TORTUOSITY. This is a rare, possibly autosomal recessive, condition of unknown cause. Diffuse ectasia of all systemic arteries occurs with, paradoxically, peripheral pulmonic stenoses.[384]

FAMILIAL INTRACRANIAL HEMORRHAGE. In addition to adult polycystic kidney disease, three syndromes predispose to subarachnoid or cerebral hemorrhage. *Berry aneurysms* without pleiotropic manifestations in other organs are a rare, but well documented, autosomal dominant trait.[385,386] A defect in type III collagen has been suggested by linkage analysis, but not by biochemical investigation, in several families.[387]

The *cerebral arterial type of familial amyloidosis* (type VI) is an autosomal dominant condition due to a defect in the proteinase inhibitor cystatin C.[388] This disease is rare outside of Iceland and Holland. The walls of cerebral arteries are thickened by a material resembling amyloid, and the vessels become tortuous and fragile. Recurrent cerebral hemorrhage is common in the fifth and sixth decades.[389]

TABLE 51-15 MENDELIAN DISORDERS ASSOCIATED WITH ABNORMAL BLOOD PRESSURE

DISORDER	MIM NO.*	PATHOGENESIS
Primarily elevated blood pressure		
Adrenal hyperplasia IV	202010	11-β-hydroxylase deficiency → ↑ 11-deoxycorticosterone
Adrenal hyperplasia V	202110	17-α-hydroxylase deficiency → ↑ 11-deoxycorticosterone
Aldosteronism	103900	↑ Aldosterone
Alport syndrome	104200 301050	Renal failure
Amyloidosis, familial visceral (amyloidosis VIII)	105200	Nephropathy
Arterial calcification of infancy	208000	Arteriosclerosis
Arterial fibromuscular dysplasia	135580	Renal artery stenosis → ↑ renin
Arteriohepatic dysplasia	118450	Renal dysplasia; renal arterial stenosis
Bartter syndrome	241200	2° to hyperaldosteronism
Fabry disease	301500	Renal failure; renal arterial stenosis; arteriolar stenosis → ↑ peripheral resistance
Multiple endocrine neoplasia I	131100	Adrenocortical adenoma → ↑ Cushing syndrome
Multiple endocrine neoplasia II	171400	Pheochromocytoma → ↑ catecholamines
Nail-patella syndrome	161200	Nephropathy
Neurofibromatosis type I	162200	Pheochromocytoma → ↑ catecholamines; and renal arterial fibromuscular dysplasia
Paraganglioma	168000	↑ Catecholamines Pheochromocytoma → ↑ catecholamines
Pheochromocytoma, familial	171300	↑ Catecholamines
Polycystic kidney disease, adult	173900 173910	↑ Renin; renal failure
Porphyria, acute intermittent	176000	?, but only during acute attacks
Pseudohypoaldosteronism, type I	264350	Aldosterone receptor deficiency
Pseudohypoaldosteronism, type II	145260	Defective renal secretion of potassium
Pseudoxanthoma elasticum	177850 264800	Arteriosclerosis
Riley-Day syndrome	223900	Dysautonomia
von Hippel-Lindau syndrome	193300	Pheochromocytoma → ↑ catecholamines
Wilms' tumor	194070 194071 194090	?
Primarily low blood pressure†		
Dopamine β-hydroxylase deficiency	223360	↑ Synthesis of epinephrine
Fabry disease	301500	↓ Peripheral vascular tone
Hyperbradykininism	143850	↑ Bradykinin
Pelizaeus-Merzbacher, late-onset	169500	?
Peripheral motor neuropathy and dysautonomia	252320	?
Pheochromocytoma, familial	171300	↑ Catecholamines (epinephrine)
Shy-Drager syndrome	146500	1° Autonomic insufficiency

* Data from Mendelian Inheritance in Man.[6]

† Does not include hypovolemia, obstruction of blood flow, and cardiogeneic causes of hypotension, each of which subsumes numerous hereditary disorders as primary causes.

Familial hemangiomas have been reported infrequently to occur as an autosomal dominant condition.[390] The brain and retina are the principal sites of vascular malformation, although in some pedigrees, cutaneous lesions occur. The intracranial hemangioma can be large and present with varied neurological symptoms, including hemorrhage.

FAMILIAL ARTERIAL OCCLUSIVE DISEASES. *Fibromuscular dysplasia* of the renal and other arteries occurs in *von Recklinghausen neurofibromatosis,* and along with pheochromocytoma can be a cause of hypertension.[391,392] The arterial lesion can occur by itself in families and produce stroke, myocardial infarction, intermittent claudication, and hypertension at young ages ranging down to childhood.[393] Inheritance is most consistent with autosomal dominance.[394,395]

Familial hypoplasia of the carotid arteries,[396] *familial arteriopathy* caused by concentric thickening of systemic and pulmonic arteries,[397] and generalized *arterial calcification of infancy*[398] are all rare, possibly mendelian, syndromes of unknown cause.

FAMILIAL PULMONARY HYPERTENSION (see also p. 804). Primary pulmonary hypertension is occasionally familial.[399-401] Inheritance is most consistent with an autosomal dominant predisposition with sex influence favoring expression in females.[6] The cause is unknown, but molecular defects favoring recurrent microemboli to the pulmonary circulation afford one area to explore.

Pulmonary hypertension can occur in *neurofibromatosis* due to pulmo-

DISORDERS AFFECTING PRIMARILY VEINS

VARICOSE VEINS. Although a familial susceptibility to varicosities of the lower extremity clearly exists, and favors women in a ratio of 2:1, mendelian inheritance has not been confirmed. *Marfan syndrome,* various *Ehlers-Danlos syndromes,* and an autosomal recessive condition featuring distichiasis (a double row of eyelashes)[403] predispose to varicose veins.

ATRETIC VEINS. Some patients with the *Klippel-Trenaunay-Weber syndrome* of cutaneous hemangioma and hemihypertrophy have atresia of the deep venous system.[404] The concomitant superficial varicosities should not be stripped, lest the remaining venous drainage of the lower extremity be removed. This is a confusing syndrome that overlaps with several others; mendelian inheritance is uncertain. Renal arterial aneurysm and hemangioma occurred in one patient.[405]

DISORDERS AFFECTING PRIMARILY LYMPHATICS

Several forms of *hereditary lymphedema* exist, with the best studied inherited as autosomal dominants.[6] An early-onset form bears the eponym *Nonne-Milroy lymphedema* and can cause a protein-losing enteropathy and pleural effusion. *Meige lymphedema* does not appear until about the time of puberty and is most severe in the legs, although one family with late-onset edema had involvement of the arms and face.[406]

GENETIC FACTORS PREDISPOSING TO ATHEROSCLEROSIS

A variety of genetic factors, in addition to the well-studied errors of lipid metabolism clearly predispose to atherosclerosis (Table 51–12; see also Chap. 37). Few genes outside of those involved in lipid metabolism have such an overwhelming impact as to be identifiable from family studies. However, genes that predispose to hypertension and diabetes mellitus, control arterial diameter, reactivity, and branching angles, affect platelet adhesiveness, and regulate endothelial and smooth muscle function can all be considered candidate genes for study in families predisposed to atherosclerosis.

ESSENTIAL HYPERTENSION

The role of genetic factors in essential hypertension is discussed on page 826. Blood pressure is a quantifiable trait that shows continuous variation within the population. Although many genes and environmental factors undoubtedly affect a person's blood pressure, familial transmission of some arbitrarily defined disease "hypertension " follows neither mendelian nor multifactorial inheritance.[407] A variety of cybernetic systems operate to maintain the blood pressure within tolerable limits. When this physiological homeostasis goes awry, or its limits are too lax, pathological and clinical consequences occur.[408]

A number of mendelian conditions, most of which are rare, cause major deviations of blood pressure from an appropriate physiological range (Table 51–15). These disorders are likely to be underdiagnosed.

Acknowledgment

Preparation of this chapter was supported by grant HL35877 from the National Institutes of Health.

REFERENCES

GENETIC FACTORS IN DISEASE

1. deGrouchy, J., and Turleau, C.: Clinical Atlas of Human Chromosomes. 2nd ed. New York, John Wiley & Sons, 1984.
2. Gardner, R. J., and Sutherland, G. R.: Chromosome Abnormalities and Genetic Counseling. New York, Oxford University Press, 1989.
3. Emanuel, B. S.: Molecular cytogenetics: Toward dissection of the contiguous gene syndromes. Am. J. Hum. Genet. *43*:575, 1988.
4. Orkin, S. H.: Molecular genetics and inherited human disease. *In* Scriver, C.R., Beaudet, A. L., Sly, W. S., and Valle, D. (eds.): The Metabolic Basis of Inherited Disease. 6th ed. New York, McGraw-Hill Book Co., 1989, p. 165.
5. White, R. and Lalouel, J. M.: Genetic markers in medicine: DNA sequence variants in the human population reveal genetic basis for metabolic variation. *In* Scriver, C. R., Beaudet, A. L., Sly, W. S., and Valle, D. (eds.): The Metabolic Basis of Inherited Disease. 6th ed. New York, McGraw-Hill Book Co., 1989, p. 277.
6. McKusick, V. A.: Mendelian Inheritance in Man. 9th ed. Baltimore, Johns Hopkins University Press, 1990.
7. McKusick, V. A.: Online Mendelian Inheritance in Man [OMIM™]; contact OMIM User Support, Welch Medical Library, 1830 East Monument Street, Third Floor, Baltimore, MD 21205, Tel: 301-955-7058.
8. Goldstein, J. L., and Brown, M. S.: Familial hypercholesterolemia. *In* Scriver, C. R., Beaudet, A. L., Sly, W. S., and Valle, D. (eds.): The Metabolic Basis of Inherited Disease. 6th ed. New York, McGraw-Hill Book Co., 1989, p. 1215.
9. Prockop, D. J.: Mutations in collagen genes: Consequences for rare and common diseases. J. Clin. Invest. *75*:783, 1985.
10. Clarke, A.: Mitochondrial genome: Defects, disease, and evolution. J. Med. Genet, *27*:451, 1990.
11. Wallace, D. C.: Mitochondrial DNA mutations and neuromuscular disease. Trends Genet. *5*:9, 1989.
12. Costa, T., Scriver, C. R., and Childs, B.: The effect of mendelian disease on human health: A measurement. Am. J. Med. Genet. *21*:231, 1985.
13. Hollister, D. W., Godfrey, M., Sakai, L. Y., et al.: Marfan syndrome: Immunohistologic abnormalities of the elastin-associated microfibrillar fiber system. N. Engl. J. Med. *323*:152, 1990.
14. Pyeritz, R. E.: Pleiotropy revisited: Molecular explanations of a classic concept. Am. J. Med. Genet. *34*:124, 1989.
15. Schimke, R. N., McKusick, V. A., Huang, T., et al.: Homocystinuria. JAMA *193*:87, 1965.
16. Byers, P. H.: Disorders of collagen biosynthesis and structure. *In* Scriver, C. R., Beaudet, A. L., Sly, W. S., and Valle, D. (eds.): The Metabolic Basis of Inherited Disease. 6th ed. New York, McGraw-Hill Book Co., 1989, p. 2805.
17. Antonarakis, S. E., and Kazazian, H. H., Jr.: The molecular basis of hemophilia A in man. Trends Genet. *4*:233, 1988.
18. Kazazian, H. H., Jr., and Boehm, C. D.: Molecular basis and prenatal diagnosis of β-thalassemia. Blood *72*:1107, 1988.
19. Südhof, T. C., Goldstein, J. L., Brown, M. S., et al.: The LDL receptor gene: A mosaic of exons shared with different proteins. Science *228*:815, 1985.
20. Antonarakis, S. E., Waber, P. G., Kittur, A. S., et al.: Hemophilia A: Detection of molecular defects and of carriers by DNA analysis. N. Engl. J. Med. *131*:842, 1985.
21. Diano, R., Bouchard, C., Dumesnil, J., et al.: Parent-child resemblance in left ventricular echocardiographic measurements. Can. J. Appl. Sport. Sci. *5*:4, 1980.
22. Adams, T. D., Yanowitz, F. G., Fisher, A. G., et al.: Heritability of cardiac size: An echocardiographic and electrocardiographic study of monozygotic and dizygotic twins. Circulation *71*:39, 1985.
23. Herrington, D. M., and Pearson, T. A.: Clinical and angiographic similarities in twins with coronary artery disease. Am. J. Cardiol. *59*:366, 1987.
24. Moller, P., and Heiberg, A.: Atrioventricular conduction time—a heritable trait? II. Family studies. Clin. Genet. *18*:454, 1980.
25. Moller, P., Heiberg, A., and Berg, K.: The atrioventricular conduction time—a heritable trait? III. Twin studies. Clin. Genet. *21*:181, 1982.
26. Hawlik, R. J., Garrison, R. J., Fabsitz, R., et al.: Variability of heart rate, P-R, QRS and QT durations in twins. J. Electrocardiol. *13*:45, 1980.
27. Dinerman, J. L., and Mehta, J. L.: Endothelial, platelet and leukocyte interactions in ischemic heart disease: Insights into potential mechanisms and their clinical relevance. J. Am. Coll. Cardiol. *16*:207, 1990.
28. Yang, Z., Richard, V., von Segesser, L., et al.: Threshold concentrations of endothelin-1 potentiate contractions to norepinephrine and serotonin in human arteries: A new mechanism of vasospasm? Circulation *82*:188, 1990.

CARDIOVASCULAR DISORDERS ASSOCIATED WITH CHROMOSOME ABERRATIONS

29. Eriksen, N. L., Buttino, L., and Juberg, R. C.: Congenital pulmonary atresia with intact ventricular septum, tricuspid insufficiency, and patent ductus arteriosus in two sibs. Am. J. Med. Genet. *32*:187, 1989.
30. Ferencz, C., Neill, C. A., Boughman, J. A., et al.: Congenital cardiovascular malformations associated with chromosome abnormalities: An epidemiologic study. J. Pediatr. *114*:79, 1989.
31. Berg, K. A., Clark, E. B., Astemborski, J. A., et al.: Prenatal detection of cardiovascular malformations by echocardiography: An indication for cytogenetic evaluation. Am. J. Obstet. Gynecol. *159*:477, 1988.
32. Schinzel, A. A.: Cardiovascular defects associated with chromosomal aberrations and malformation syndromes. Prog. Med. Genet. *5*:301, 1983.
33. Clark, E. B.: Mechanisms in the pathogenesis of congenital cardiac malformations. *In* Pierpont, M. E. M., and Moller, J. H. (eds): Genetics of Cardiovascular Disease. Boston, Martinus Nijhoff Publishing, 1986, p. 3.
34. Hersh, J. H., Rees, A. H., Bloom, A. S., et al.: Cardiac malformations in trisomy 18 and 13: Specificity or nonspecificity? (abstr.) Proc. Greenwood Genet. Cen. *9*:66, 1990.
35. De Biase, L., Di Ciommo, V., Ballerini, L., et al.: Prevalence of left-sided obstructive lesions in patients with atrioventricular canal without Down syndrome. J. Thorac. Cardiovasc. Surg. *91*:467, 1986.
36. Kurnit, D. M., Aldridge, J. F., Matsuoka, R., et al.: Increased adhesiveness of trisomy 21 cells and atrioventricular canal malformations in Down syndrome: A stochastic model. Am. J. Med. Genet. *20*:385, 1985.
37. Clapp, S., Perry, B. L., Farooki, Z. Q., et al.: Down's syndrome, complete atrioventricular canal, and pulmonary vascular obstructive disease. J. Thorac. Cardiovasc. Surg. *100*:115, 1990.
38. Goldhaber, S. Z., Rubin, I. L., Brown, W., et al.: Valvular heart disease (aortic regurgitation and mitral valve prolapse) among institutionalized adults with Down's syndrome. Am. J. Cardiol. *57*:278, 1986.
39. O'Brien, J. S., Geggel, R., and Feingold, M.: Mitral valve prolapse in Down syndrome (abstr.). Proc. Greenwood Genet. Cen. *9*:96, 1990.
40. Schneider, D. S., Zahka, K. G., Clark, E. B., et al.: Patterns of cardiac care in infants with Down syndrome. Am. J. Dis. Child. *143*:363, 1989.
41. Greenwood, R. D., and Nadas, A. S.: The clinical course of cardiac disease in Down's syndrome. Pediatrics *58*:893, 1976.
42. Van Dyck, D. C., and Allen, M.: Clinical management considerations in long-term survivors with trisomy 18. Pediatrics *58*:893, 1976.
43. Musewe, N. N., Alexander, D. J., Teshima, I., et al.: Echocardiographic evaluation of the spectrum of cardiac anomalies associated with trisomy 13 and trisomy 18. J. Am. Coll. Cardiol. *15*:673, 1990.
44. Van Praagh, S., Truman, T., Firpo, A., et al.: Cardiac malformations in trisomy-18: A study of 41 postmortem cases. J. Am. Coll. Cardiol. *13*:1586, 1989.
45. Lacro, R. V., Lyons Jones, K., and Benirschke, K.: Coarctation of the aorta in Turner syndrome: A pathologic study of fetuses with nuchal cystic hygromas, hydrops fetalis and female genitalia. Pediatrics *81*:445, 1988.
46. Lin, A. E., and Garver, K. L.: Genetic counseling for congenital heart defects. J. Pediatr. *113*:1105, 1988.
47. Allen, D. B., Hendricks, S. A., and Levy, J. M.: Aortic dilation in Turner syndrome. J. Pediatr. *109*:302, 1986.
48. Natowicz, M., and Kelley, R. I.: Association of Turner syndrome with hypoplastic left-heart syndrome. Am. J. Dis. Child. *141*:218, 1987.
49. Moore, J. W., Kirby, W. C., Rogers, W. M., et al.: Partial anomalous pulmonary venous drainage associated with 45,X Turner's syndrome. Pediatrics *86*:273, 1990.

CONGENITAL HEART DISEASE

50. Fixler, D. E., Pastor, P., Chamberlin, M., et al.: Trends in congenital heart disease in Dallas County births: 1971–1984. Circulation *81*:137, 1990.
51. Hagler, D. J., Edwards, W. D., Seward, J. B., et al.: Standardized nomenclature of the ventricular septum and ventricular septal defects, with applications for two-dimensional echocardiography. Mayo Clin. Proc. *60*:741, 1985.
52. Helmcke, F., de Souza, A., Nanda, N. C., et al.: Two-dimensional and color Doppler assessment of ventricular septal defect of congenital origin. Am. J. Cardiol. *63*:1112, 1989.
53. Lowell, D. G., Turner, D. A., Smith, S. M., et al.: The detection of atrial and ventricular septal defects with electrocardiographically synchronized magnetic resonance imaging. Circulation *73*:89, 1986.
54. Simpson, I. A., Sahn, D. J., Valdes-Cruz, L. M., et al.: Color Doppler flow mapping in patients with coarctation of the aorta: New observations and improved evaluation with color flow diameter and proximal acceleration as predictors of severity. Circulation *77*:736, 1988.
55. Brenner, J. I., Berg, K. A., Schneider, D. S., et al.: Cardiac malformations in relatives of infants with hypoplastic left-heart syndrome. Am. J. Dis. Child. *143*:1492, 1989.
56. Pyeritz, R. E., and Murphy, E. A.: The genetics of congenital heart disease: Perspectives and prospects. J. Am. Coll. Cardiol. *13*:1458, 1989.
57. Ursell, P. C., Byrne, J. M., and Strombino, B. A.: Significance of cardiac defects in the developing fetus: A study of spontaneous abortuses. Circulation *72*:1232, 1985.
58. Whittemore, R. Hobbins, J. C., and Engle, M. A.: Pregnancy and its outcome in women with and without surgical treatment of congenital heart disease. *In* Engle, M. A., and Perloff, J. K. (eds.): Congenital Heart Disease After Surgery. New York, Yorke Medical Books, 1983, p. 362.
59. Rose, V. R., Gold, J. M., Lindsay, G., et al.: A possible increase in the incidence of congenital heart defects among the offspring of affected parents. J. Am. Coll. Cardiol. *6*:376, 1985.
60. Nora, J. J., and Nora, A. H.: Update on counseling the family with a first-degree relative with a congenital heart defect. Am. J. Med. Genet. *29*:137, 1988.
61. Boughman, J. A.: Familial risks of congenital heart defects (letter). Am. J. Med. Genet. *29*:233, 1988.
61a. Murphy, J. G., Gersh, B. J., McGoon, M.D., et al.: Long-term outcome after surgical repair of isolated atrial septal defect: Follow-up at 27 to 32 years. N. Engl. J. Med. *323*:1645, 1990.
62. Gold, R.J.M., Rose, V., and Yau, Y.: Severity and recurrence risk of congenital heart defects exemplified by atrial septal defect secundum. Clin. Genet. *32*:148, 1987.
63. Nora, J. J., and Nora, A. H.: Recurrence risks in children having one parent with a congenital heart disease. Circulation *53*:701, 1976.
64. Nora, J. J., and Nora, A. H.: The evolution of specific genetic and environmental counseling in congenital heart disease. Circulation *57*:205, 1978.
65. Nora, J. J., and Nora, A. H.: Genetic epidemiology of congenital heart disease. Prog. Med. Genet. *5*:91, 1983.
66. Sanchez-Cascos, A.: The recurrence risk in congenital heart disease. Eur. J. Cardiol. *7*:197, 1978.
67. Corone, P., Bonaiti, C., Feingold, J., et al.: Familial congenital heart disease: How are the various types related? Am. J. Cardiol. *51*:942, 1983.
68. Boughman, J. A., Berg, K. A., Astemborski, J. A., et al.: Familial risks of congenital heart defect assessed in a population-based epidemiologic study. Am. J. Med. Genet. *26*:839, 1987.
69. Ferencz, C., Boughman, J. A., Neill, C. A., et al.: Congenital cardiovascular malformations: Questions on inheritance. J. Am. Coll. Cardiol. *14*:756, 1989.
70. Maestri, N. E., Beaty, T. H., Liang, K.-Y., et al.: Assessing familial aggregation of congenital cardiovascular malformations in case-control studies. Genet. Epidemiol. *5*:343, 1988.
71. Pierpont, M.E.M., Gobel, J. W., Moller, J. H., et al.: Cardiac malformations in relatives of children with truncus arteriosus or interruption of the aortic arch. Am. J. Cardiol. *61*:423, 1988.
72. Natowicz, M., Chatten, J., Clancy, R., et al.: Genetic disorders and major extracardiac anomalies associated with the hypoplastic left heart syndrome. Pediatrics *82*:698, 1988.
73. Rubin, J. D., Ferencz, C., McCarter, R. J., et al.: Congenital cardiovascular malformations in the Baltimore-Washington area. Md. State Med. J. *34*:1079, 1985.
74. Ferencz, C., Rubin, J. D., McCarter, R. J., et al.: Congenital heart disease: Prevalence at livebirth (The Baltimore-Washington Infant Study). Am. J. Epidemiol. *122*:31, 1985.
75. Beekman, R. H., and Robinow, M.: Coarctation of the aorta inherited as an autosomal dominant trait. Am. J. Cardiol.*56*:818, 1985.
76. McKusick, V. A., Logue, R. B., and Bahnson, H. T.: Association of aortic valvular disease and cystic medial necrosis of the ascending aorta: Report of four instances. Circulation *16*:188, 1957.
77. Lindsay, J., Jr.: Coarctation of the aorta, bicuspid aortic valve and abnormal ascending aortic wall. Am. J. Cardiol. *61*:182, 1988.
78. Wright, T. C., Orkin, R. W., Destrempes, M., et al.: Increased adhesiveness of Down syndrome fetal fibroblasts in vitro. Proc. Natl. Acad. Sci. USA *81*:2426, 1984.
79. Weigel, W. J., Driscoll, D. J., and Michels, V. V.: Occurrence of congenital heart defects in siblings of patients with univentricular heart and tricuspid atresia. Am. J. Cardiol. *64*:768, 1989.
80. Moreno, A., and Murphy, E. A.: Inheritance of Kartagener syndrome. Am. J. Med. Genet. *8*:305, 1981.
81. Afzelius, B. A.: A human syndrome caused by immotile cilia. Science *193*:317, 1976.
82. Afzelius, B. A., and Mossberg, B.: Immotile-cilia syndrome (primary ciliary dyskinesia), including Kartagener syndrome. *In* Scriver, C. R., Beaudet, A. L., Sly, W. S., and Valle D. (eds.): The Metabolic Basis of Inherited Disease. 6th ed. New York, McGraw-Hill Book Co., 1989, p. 2739.
83. Arnold, G. L., Bixler, D., and Girod, D.: Probable autosomal recessive inheritance of polysplenia, situs inversus and cardiac defects in an Amish family. Am. J. Med. Genet. *16*:35, 1983.
84. Czeizel, A.: Familial situs inversus and congenital heart defects. Am. J. Med. Genet. *28*:227, 1987.
85. Zlotogora, J., and Elian, E.: Asplenia and polysplenia syndromes with abnormalities of lateralization in a sibship. J. Med. Genet. *18*:301, 1981.
86. Niikawa, N., Kohsaka, S., Mizumoto, M., et al.: Familial clustering of situs inversus totalis, and asplenia and polysplenia syndrome. Am. J. Med. Genet. *16*:43, 1983.
87. Soltan, H. C., and Li, M. D.: Hereditary dextrocardia associated with congenital heart defects: Report of a pedigree. Clin. Genet. *5*:51, 1974.
88. Mathias, R. S., Lacro, R. V., and Jones, K. L.: X-linked laterality sequence: Situs inversus, complex cardiac defects, splenic defects. Am. J. Med. Genet. *28*:111, 1987.
89. Cyran S. E., Martinez, R., Daniels, S., et al.: Spectrum of congenital heart disease in CHARGE association. J. Pediatr. *110*:576, 1987.
90. Oley, C. A., Baraitser, M., and Grant, D. B.: A reappraisal of the CHARGE associaton. J. Med. Genet. *25*:147, 1988.
91. Freedom, R. M., Rosen, F. S., and Nadas, A. S.: Congenital cardiovascular

disease and anomalies of the third and fourth pharyngeal pouch. Circulation *46*:165, 1972.
92. Temtamy, S. A., and Miller, J. D.: Extending the scope of the VATER associaton: Definition of a VATER syndrome. J. Pediatr. *85*:345, 1974.
93. Weaver, D. D., Mapstone, C. L., Yu, P.: The VATER association: Analysis of 46 patients. Am. J. Dis. Child. *140*:225, 1986.
94. Lynch, H. T., Bachenberg, K., Harris, R. E., et al.: Hereditary atrial septal defect: Update of a large kindred. Am. J. Dis. Child. *132*:600, 1978.
95. Mohl, W., and Mayr, W. R.: Atrial septal defect of the secundum type and HLA. Tissue Antigens *10*:121, 1977.
96. Kahler, R. L., Braunwald, E., Plauth, W. H., Jr., et al.: Familial congenital heart disease. Am. J. Med. *40*:384, 1966.
97. Pease, W. E., Nordenberg, A., and Ladda, R. L.: Genetic counseling in familial atrial septal defect with prolonged atrioventricular conduction. Circulation *53*:759, 1976.
98. Gall, J. C., Stern, A. M., Cohen, M. M., et al.: Holt-Oram syndrome: Clinical and genetic study of a large family. Am. J. Hum. Genet. *18*:187, 1966.
99. Smith, R.R.L., Hutchins, G. M., Sack, G. H., Jr., et al.: Unusual cardiac, renal and pulmonary involvement in Gaucher's disease: Interstitial glucocerebroside accumulation, pulmonary hypertension and fatal bone marrow embolization. Am. J. Med. *65*:352, 1978.
100. Muller, L. M., De Jong, G., and Van Heerden, K.M.M.: The antenatal ultrasonographic detection of the Holt-Oram syndrome. S. Afr. Med. J. *68*:313, 1985.
101. Zhang, K-Z., Sun, Q-B, and Cheng, T. O.: Holt-Oram syndrome in China: A collective review of 18 cases. Am. Heart J. *111*:572, 1986.
102. McKusick, V. A., Egeland, J. A., Eldridge, R., et al.: Dwarfism in the Amish: I. The Ellis-van Creveld syndrome. Bull. Johns Hopkins Hosp. *115*:306, 1964.
103. Sherman, J., Angulo, M., Boxer, R. A., et al.: Possible mitochondrial inheritance of congenital cardiac septal defect (letter). N. Engl. J. Med. *313*:186, 1985.
104. Preus, M.: The Williams syndrome: Objective definition and diagnosis. Clin. Genet. *25*:422, 1984.
105. Maisuls, H., Alday, L. E., and Thuer, O.: Cardiovascular findings in the Williams-Beuren syndrome. Am. Heart J. *114*:897, 1987.
106. Hallidie-Smith, K. A., and Karas, S.: Cardiac anomalies in Williams-Beuren syndrome. Arch. Dis. Child. *63*:809, 1988.
107. Morris, C. A., Demsey, S. A., Leonard, C. O., et al.: Natural history of Williams syndrome: Physical characteristics. J. Pediatr. *113*:318, 1988.
108. Chiarella, F., Bricarelli, F. D., Lupi, G.: Familial supravalvular aortic stenosis: A genetic study. J. Med. Genet. *26*:86, 1989.
109. Ensing, G. J., Schmidt, M. A., Hagler, D. J., et al.: Spectrum of findings in a family with nonsyndromic autosomal dominant supravalvular aortic stenosis: A Doppler echocardiographic study. J. Am. Coll. Cardiol. *13*:413, 1989.
110. Schmidt, M. A., Ensing, G. J., Michels, V. V., et al.: Autosomal dominant supravalvular aortic stenosis: Large three-generation family. Am. J. Med. Genet. *32*:384, 1989.
111. Procacci, P. M., Savran, S. V., Schreiter, S. L., et al.: Prevalence of clinical mitral-valve prolapse in 1169 young women. N. Engl. J. Med. *294*:1086, 1976.
112. Devereux, R. B., Kramer-Fox, R., Shear, M. K., et al.: Diagnosis and classification of severity of mitral valve prolapse: Methodologic, biologic, and prognostic considerations. Am. Heart J. *113*:1265, 1987.
113. Wooley, C. F., and Boudoulas, H.: Mitral valve prolapse: A classification. *In* Boudoulas, H., and Wooley, C. F. (eds.): Mitral Valve Prolapse and the Mitral Valve Prolapse Syndrome. Mt. Kisco, N.Y., Futura Publishing Co., 1988, p. 3.
114. Devereux, R. B., and Kramer-Fox, R.: Inheritance and phenotypic features of mitral valve prolapse. In Boudoulas, H., and Wooley, C. F. (eds.): Mitral Valve Prolapse and the Mitral Valve Prolapse Syndrome. Mt. Kisco, N.Y., Futura Publishing Co., 1988, p. 109.
115. Strahan, N. V., Murphy, E. A., Fortuin, N. J., et al.: Inheritance of the mitral valve prolapse syndrome. Discussion of a three-dimensional penetrance model. Am. J. Med. *74*:967, 1983.
116. Pini, R., Greppi, B., Kramer-Fox, R., et al.: Mitral valve dimensions and motion and familial transmission of mitral valve prolapse with and without mitral leaflet billowing. J. Am. Coll. Cardiol. *12*:1423, 1988.
117. Henney, A. M., Schwartz, R. C., Child, A. H., et al.: Genetic evidence that mutations in the COL1A2, COL3A1 or COL5A2 collagen genes are not responsible for mitral valve prolapse. Br. Heart J. *61*:292, 1989.
118. Hickey, A. J., Narunsky, L., and Wilcken, D.E.L.: Bodily habitus and mitral valve prolapse. Aust. N. Z. J. Med. *15*:326, 1985.
119. Devereux, R. B., Brown, W. T., Lutas, E. M., et al.: Association of mitral valve prolapse with low body weight and low blood pressure. Lancet *2*:792, 1982.
120. Beighton, P., de Paepe, A., Danks, D., et al.: International nosology of heritable disorders of connective tissue, Berlin, 1986. Am. J. Med. Genet. *29*:581, 1988.
121. Roman, M. J., Devereux, R. B., Kramer-Fox, R., et al.: Comparison of cardiovascular and skeletal features of primary mitral valve prolapse and the Marfan syndrome. Am. J. Cardiol. *3*:317, 1989.
122. Glesby, M. J., and Pyeritz, R. E.: Association of mitral valve prolapse and systemic abnormalities of connective tissue: A phenotypic continuum. J.A.M.A. *262*:523, 1989.
123. Hirschfeld, S. S., Rudner, C., Nash, C. L. Jr., et al.: Incidence of mitral valve prolapse in adolescent scoliosis and thoracic kyphoscoliosis. Pediatrics *70*:451, 1982.
124. Chen, W.W.C., Chan, F. L., Wong, P.H.C., et al.: Familial occurrence of mitral valve prolapse: Is this related to the straight back syndrome? Br. Heart J. *50*:97, 1983.
125. Shamberger, R. C., Welch, K. J., and Sanders, S. P.: Mitral valve prolapse associated with pectus excavatum. J. Pediatr. *111*:404, 1987.
126. Rogan, K., Sears-Rogan, P., Vermani, R., et al.: Familial myxomatous valvular disease. Am. J. Cardiol. *63*:1149, 1989.
127. Mendez, H.M.M., and Opitz, J. M.: Noonan syndrome: A review. Am. J. Med. Genet. *21*:493, 1985.
128. Caralis, D. G., Char, F., Graber, J. D., et al.: Delineation of multiple cardiac anomalies associated with the Noonan syndrome in an adult and review of the literature. Johns Hopkins Med. J. *134*:346, 1974.
129. Allanson, J. E., Hall, J. G., Hughes, H. E., et al.: Noonan syndrome: The changing phenotype. Am. J. Med. Genet. *21*:507, 1985.
130. Van Der Hauwaert, L. G., Fryns, J. P., Dumoulin, M., et al.: Cardiovascular malformations in Turner's and Noonan's syndrome. Br. Heart J. *40*:500, 1978.
131. Noonan, J. A., and Ehmke, D. A.: Associated noncardiac malformations in children with congenital heart disease. J. Pediatr. *63*:468, 1963.
132. Pearl, W.: Cardiovascular anomalies in Noonan's syndrome. Chest *71*:677, 1977.
133. Phornphutkul, C., Rosenthal, A., and Nadas, A. S.: Cardiomyopathy in Noonan's syndrome. Br. Heart J. *35*:99, 1973.
134. Battiste, C. E., Feldt, R. H., and Lie, J. T.: Congestive cardiomyopathy in Noonan's syndrome. Mayo Clin. Proc. *52*:661, 1977.
134a. Wong, C.-K., Cheng, C.-H., Lau, C.-P., et al.: Congenital coronary artery anomalies in Noonan's syndrome. Am. Heart J. *119*:396, 1990.
135. Miller, M., and Motulsky, A. G.: Noonan syndrome in an adult family presenting with chronic lymphedema. Am. J. Med. *65*:379, 1978.
136. Quattrin, T., McPherson, E., and Putnam, T.: Vertical transmission of the neurofibromatosis/Noonan syndrome. Am. J. Med. Genet. *26*:645, 1987.
137. Kitchens, C. S., and Alexander, J. A.: Partial deficiency of coagulation factor XI as a newly recognized feature of Noonan syndrome. J. Pediatr. *102*:224, 1983.
138. Khoury, M. J., Becerra, J. E., Cordero, J. F., et al.: Clinical-epidemiologic assessment of patterns of birth defects associated with human teratogens: Application to diabetic embryopathy. Pediatrics *83*:658, 1989.
139. Beckman, D. A., and Brent, R. L.: Mechanisms of teratogenesis. Annu. Rev. Pharmacol. Toxicol. *24*:483, 1984.
140. Jones, K. L.: Fetal alcohol syndrome. Pediatr. Rev. *8*:122, 1986.
141. Finnell, R. H., and Chernoff, G. F.: Genetic background. The elusive component in the fetal hydantoin syndrome. Am. J. Med. Genet. *19*:459, 1984.
142. Strickler, S. M., Dansky, L. V., Miller, M. A., et al.: Genetic predisposition to phenytoin-induced birth defects. Lancet *2*:746, 1985.
143. Lammer, E. J.: Retinoic acid embryopathy. N. Engl. J. Med. *313*:837, 1985.
144. Hall, J. G., Pauli, R. M., and Wilson, K. M.: Maternal and fetal sequelae of anticoagulation during pregnancy. Am. J. Med. *68*:122, 1980.
145. Scriver, C. R., Kaufman, S., and Woo, S.L.C.: The hyperphenylalaninemias. *In* Scriver, C. R., Beaudet, A. L., Sly, W. S., and Valle, D. (eds.): The Metabolic Basis of Inherited Disease, 6th ed. New York, McGraw-Hill Book Co., 1989, p. 495.
146. Lenke, R. R., and Levy, H. L.: Maternal phenylketonuria and hyperphenylalaninemia. N. Engl. J. Med. *303*:1202, 1980.

CARDIOMYOPATHIES

147. Maron, B. J., Bonow, R. O., Cannon, R. O., III, et al.: Hypertrophic cardiomyopathy: Interrelations of clinical manifestations, pathophysiology, and therapy. N. Engl. J. Med. *316*:780;844, 1987.
148. Bulkley, B. H., Weisfeldt, M. L., and Hutchins, G. M.: Asymmetric septal hypertrophy and myocardial fiber disarray: Features of normal, developing, and malformed hearts. Circulation *56*:292, 1977.
149. Maron, B. J., Nichols, P. F., III, Pickle, L. W., et al.: Patterns of inheritance in hypertrophic cardiomyopathy: Assessment by M-mode and two-dimensional echocardiography. Am. J. Cardiol. *53*:1087, 1984.
150. Maron, B. J., and Mulvihill, J. J.: The genetics of hypertrophic cardiomyopathy. Ann. Intern. Med. *105*:610, 1986.
151. ten Cate, F. J., Hugenholtz, P. G., van Dorp, W. G., et al.: Prevalence of diagnostic abnormalities in patients with genetically transmitted asymmetric septal hypertrophy. Am. J. Cardiol. *43*:731, 1979.
151a. Ferraro, M., Scarton, G., and Ambrosini, M.: Cosegregation of hypertrophic cardiomyopathy and a fragile site on chromosome 16 in a large Italian family. J. Med. Genet. *27*:363, 1990.
151b. Epstein, N. D., Lin, H. J., and Fananapazir, L.: Genetic evidence of dissociation (generational skips) of electrical from morphologic forms of hypertrophic cardiomyopathy. Am. J. Cardiol. *66*:627, 1990.
152. Greaves, S. C., Roche, A.H.G., Neutze, J. M., et al.: Inheritance of hypertrophic cardiomyopathy: A cross sectional and M mode echocardiographic study of 50 families. Br. Heart J. *58*:259, 1987.
153. Cirò, E., Nichols, P. F., and Maron, B. J.: Heterogeneous morphologic expression of genetically transmitted hypertrophic cardiomyopathy: Two-dimensional echocardiographic analysis. Circulation *67*:1227, 1983.
154. Penas, M., Fuster, M., Fabregas, R., et al.: Familial apical hypertrophic cardiomyopathy. Am. J. Cardiol. *62*:821, 1988.
155. Jarcho, J. A., McKenna, W., Pare, J.A.P., et al.: Mapping a gene for familial hypertrophic cardiomyopathy to chromosome 14q1. N. Engl. J. Med. *321*:1372, 1989.
155a. Solomon, S. D., Geisterfer-Lowrance, A.A.T., Vosberg, H.-P., et al.: A locus for familial hypertrophic cardiomyopathy is closely linked to the

cardiac myosin heavy chain genes, CRI-L436, and CRI-L329 on chromosome 14 at q11-q12. Am. J. Hum. Genet. *47*:389, 1990.

155b. Solomon, S.D., Jarcho, J. A., McKenna, W., et al.: Familial hypertrophic cardiomyopathy is a genetically heterogeneous disease. J. Clin. Invest. *86*:993, 1990.

156. Ferraro, M., Scarton, G., and Ambrosini, M.: Cosegregation of hypertrophic cardiomyopathy and a fragile site on chromosome 16 in a large Italian family. J. Med. Genet. *27*:363, 1990.

157. Codd, M. B., Sugrue, D. D., Gersh, B. J., et al.: Epidemiology of idiopathic dilated and hypertrophic cardiomyopathy: A population-based study in Olmsted County, Minnesota, 1975–1984. Circulation *80*:564, 1989.

158. Michels, V. V., Moll, P. P., Miller, F. A., et al.: Frequency of familial dilated cardiomyopathy in an unselected series of patients with idiopathic dilated cardiomyopathy (abstr.). Am. J. Hum. Genet. *45*:A55, 1989.

159. Fragola, P. V., Autore, C., Picelli, A., et al.: Familial idiopathic dilated cardiomyopathy. Am. Heart J. *115*:912, 1988.

160. Valantine, H. A., Hunt, S. A., Fowler, M. B., et al.: Frequency of familial nature of dilated cardiomyopathy and usefulness of cardiac transplantation in this subset. Am. J. Cardiol. *63*:959, 1989.

161. Michels, V. V., Driscoll, D. J., and Miller, F. A., Jr.: Familial aggregation of idiopathic dilated cardiomyopathy. Am. J. Cardiol. *55*:1232, 1985.

162. Emanuel, R., Withers, R., and O'Brien, K.: Dominant and recessive modes of inheritance in idiopathic cardiomyopathy. Lancet *2*:1065, 1971.

163. Graber, H. L., Unverferth, D. V., Baker, P. B., et al.: Evolution of a hereditary cardiac conduction and muscle disorder: A study involving a family with six generations affected. Circulation *74*:21, 1986.

164. Gardner, R.J.M., Hanson, J. W., Ionasescu, V. V., et al.: Dominantly inherited dilated cardiomyopathy. Am. J. Med. Genet. *27*:61, 1987.

165. Maclennan, B. A., Tsoi, E. Y., Maguire, C., et al.: Familial idiopathic congestive cardiomyopathy in three generations: A family study with eight affected members. Q. J. Med. *63*:335, 1987.

166. Schmidt, M. A., Michels, V. V., Edwards, W. D., et al.: Familial dilated cardiomyopathy. Am. J. Med. Genet. *31*:135, 1988.

167. Koike, S., Kawa, S., Yabu, K., et al.: Familial dilated cardiomyopathy and human leucocyte antigen: A report of two family cases. Jpn. Heart J. *28*:941, 1987.

168. Przybojewski, J. Z., Vanderwalt, J. J., Vaneeden, P. J., et al.: Familial dilated (congestive) cardiomyopathy. Occurrence in two brothers and an overview of the literature. S. Afr. Med. J. *66*:26, 1984.

169. Goldblatt, J., Melmed, J., and Rose, A. G.: Autosomal recessive inheritance of idiopathic dilated cardiomyopathy in a Madeira Portuguese kindred. Clin. Genet. *31*:249, 1987.

170. Berko, B. A., and Swift, M.: X-linked dilated cardiomyopathy. N. Engl. J. Med. *316*:1186, 1987.

171. Caforio, A.L.P., Rossi, B., and Risaliti, R.: Type 1 fiber abnormalities in skeletal muscle of patients with hypertrophic and dilated cardiomyopathy: Evidence of subclinical myogenic myopathy. J. Am. Coll. Cardiol. *14*:1464, 1989.

172. Hubner, G., and Grantzow, R.: Mitochondrial cardiomyopathy with involvement of skeletal muscles. Virchows Arch *399*:115, 1983.

173. Urie, P. M., and Billingham, M. E.: Ultrastructural features of familial cardiomyopathy. Am. J. Cardiol. *62*:325, 1988.

174. Anderson, J. L., Carlquist, J. F., Lutz, J. R., et al.: HLA A, B and DR typing in idiopathic dilated cardiomyopathy: A search for immune response factors. Am. J. Cardiol. *53*:1326, 1984.

175. Voss, E. G., Reddy, C.V.R., Detrano, R., et al.: Familial dilated cardiomyopathy. Am. J. Cardiol. *54*:456, 1984.

176. Aroney, C., Bett, N., and Radford, D.: Familial restrictive cardiomyopathy. Aust. N. Z. J. Med. *18*:877, 1988.

177. Fitzpatrick, A. P., Shapiro, L. M., Rickards, A. F., et al.: Familial restrictive cardiomyopathy with atrioventricular block and skeletal myopathy. Br. Heart J. *63*:114, 1990.

178. Hodgson, S., Child, A., and Dyson, M.: Endocardial fibroelastosis: Possible X-linked inheritance. J. Med. Genet. *24*:210, 1987.

179. Barth, P. G., Scholte, J. A., Berden, J. A., et al.: An X-linked mitochondrial disease affecting cardiac muscle, skeletal muscle and neutrophil leukocytes. J. Neurol. Sci. *62*:327, 1983.

180. Chen, S.-H, Thompson, M. W., and Rose, V.: Endocardial fibroelastosis: Family studies with special reference to counseling. J. Pediatr. *79*:385, 1971.

181. Hallidie-Smith, K. A., and Olsen, E.G.J.: Endocardial fibro-elastosis, mitral incompetence, and coarctation of abdominal aorta: A report of 3 sibs. Br. Heart J. *30*:850, 1968.

182. Opitz, J. M.: Genetic aspects of endocardial fibroelastosis. Am. J. Med. Genet. *11*:92, 1982.

183. Ross, R. S., Bulkley, B. H., Hutchins, G. M., et al.: Idiopathic familial myocardiopathy in three generations: A clinical and pathologic study. Am. Heart J. *96*:170, 1978.

184. Fitzpatrick, A. P., and Emanuel, R. W.: Familial neurofibromatosis and hypertrophic cardiomyopathy. Br. Heart J. *60*:247, 1988.

185. Sommer, A., Contras, S. B., Craenen, J. M., et al.: A family study of the leopard syndrome. Am. J. Dis. Child. *121*:520, 1971.

186. St. John Sutton, M. G., Tajik, A. J., Giuliani, E. R., et al.: Hypertrophic obstructive cardiomyopathy and lentiginosis: A little known neural ectodermal syndrome. Am. J. Cardiol. *47*:214, 1981.

187. Voorhees, M. L., Hussan, G. S., and Blackman, M. S.: Growth failure with pericardial constriction: The syndrome of mulibrey nanism. Am. J. Dis. Child. *130*:1146, 1976.

188. Martinez-Lavin, M., Buendia, A., Delgado, E., et al.: A familial syndrome of pericarditis, arthritis and camptodactyly. N. Engl. J. Med. *309*:224, 1983.

189. Laxer, R. M., Cameron, B. J., Chaisson, D., et al.: The camptodactyly-arthropathy-pericarditis syndrome: Case report and literature review. Arthritis Rheum. *29*:439, 1986.

190. Bulutlar, G., Yazici, H., Ozdogan, H., et al.: A familial syndrome of pericarditis, arthritis, camptodactyly, and coxa vara. Arthritis Rheum. *29*:436, 1986.

DISORDERS OF RHYTHM AND CONDUCTION

191. Gambetta, M., Weese, J., Ginsburg, M., et al.: Sick sinus syndrome in a patient with familial PR prolongation. Chest *64*:520, 1973.

192. Livesley, B., Catley, P. F., and Oram, S.: Familial sinuatrial disorder. Br. Heart J. *34*:668, 1972.

193. Mackintosh, A. F.: Sinuatrial disease in young people. Br. Heart J. *45*:62, 1981.

194. Nordenberg, A., Varghese, P. J., and Nugent, E. W.: Spectrum of sinus node dysfunction in two siblings. Am. Heart J. *91*:507, 1976.

195. Spellberg, R. D.: Familial sinus node disease. Chest *60*:246, 1971.

196. Caralis, D. G., and Varghese, P. J.: Familial sinoatrial node dysfunction: Increased vagal tone a possible aetiology. Br. Heart J. *38*:951, 1976.

197. Balderston, S. M., Shaffer, E. M., Sondheimer, H. M., et al.: Hereditary atrioventricular conduction defect in a child. Pediatr. Cardiol. *10*:37, 1989.

198. Khorsandian, R. S., Moghadam, A.-N., and Müller, O. F.: Familial congenital A-V dissociation. Am. J. Cardiol. *14*:118, 1964.

199. Wagner, C. W., and Hall, R. J.: Congenital familial atrioventricular dissociation: Report of three siblings. Am. J. Cardiol. *19*:593, 1967.

200. Wolkowicz, J., and Burgess, J. H.: Complete heart block in an Inuit family. Can. J. Cardiol. *4*:352, 1988.

201. Stephan, E.: Hereditary bundle branch system defect: Survey of a family with four affected generations. Am. Heart J. *95*:89, 1978.

202. Steenkamp, W.F.J.: Familial trifascicular block. Am. Heart J. *84*:758, 1972.

203. Mézáros, M., and Czeizel, A.: ECG conduction disturbance in the first-degree relatives of children with ventricular septal defect. Clin. Genet. *19*:298, 1981.

204. Kennel, A. J., Callahan, J. A., Maloney, J. D., et al.: Adult-onset familial infra-Hisian block. Am. Heart J. *102*:447, 1981.

205. Lorber, A., Maisuls, E., and Naschitz, J.: Hereditary right axis deviation: Electrocardiographic pattern of pseudo left posterior hemiblock and incomplete right bundle branch block. Int. J. Cardiol. *20*:399, 1988.

206. Van Der Merwe, P.-L., Weymar, H. W., Torrington, M., et al.: Progressive familial heart block (type I): A follow up study after 10 years. S. Afr. Med. J. *73*:275, 1988.

207. Torrington, M., Weymar, H. W., van der Merwe, P.-L., et al.: Progressive familial heart block: Pt I. Extent of the disease. S. Afr. Med. J. *70*:354, 1986.

208. Kothari, S. S., Agrawal, S. M., and Krishnaswami, S.: Familial complete heart block in hypertrophic cardiomyopathy. Int. J. Cardiol. *20*:294, 1988.

209. Stables, R. H., Bailey, C., and Ormerod, O.J.M.: Idiopathic familial atrial cardiomyopathy with diffuse conduction block. Q. J. Med. *264*:325, 1989.

210. Williams, D. O., Jones, E. L., Nagle, R. E., et al.: Familial atrial cardiomyopathy with heart block. Q. J. Med. *41*:491, 1972.

211. Olofsson, B.-V., Eriksson, P., and Eriksson, A.: The sick sinus syndrome in familial amyloidosis with polyneuropathy. Int. J. Cardiol. *4*:71, 1983.

212. Winkler, R. B., Nora, A. H., and Nora, J. J.: Familial congenital complete heart block and maternal systemic lupus erythematosus. Circulation *56*:1103, 1977.

213. McCue, C. M., Mantakas, M. E., Tingelstad, J. B., et al.: Congenital heart block in newborns of mothers with connective tissue disease. Circulation *56*:82, 1977.

214. Chameides, L., Truex, R. C., Vetter, V., et al.: Association of maternal systemic lupus erythematosus with congenital complete heart block. N. Engl. J. Med. *297*:1204, 1977.

215. Scott, J. S., Maddison, P. J., Taylor, P. V., et al.: Connective-tissue disease, antibodies to ribonucleoprotein, and congenital heart block. N. Engl. J. Med. *309*:209, 1983.

216. Lockshin, M. D., Gibofsky, A., Peebles, C. L., et al.: Neonatal lupus erythematosus with heart block: Family study of a patient with anti-SS-A and SS-B antibodies. Arthritis Rheum. *26*:210, 1983.

217. Bergfeldt, L., and Möller, E.: Complete heart block—another HLA B27 associated disease manifestation. Tissue Antigens *21*:385, 1983.

218. Bergfeldt, L., Vallin, H., and Edhag, O.: Complete heart block in HLA B27 associated disease. Electrophysiological and clinical characteristics. Br. Heart J. *51*:184, 1984.

219. Bacos, J. M., Eagan, J. T., and Orgain, E. S.: Congenital familial nodal rhythm. Circulation *22*:887, 1960.

220. Gault, J. H., Cantwell, J., Lev, M., et al: Fatal familial cardiac arrhythmias. Am. J. Cardiol. *29*:548, 1972.

221. Gulotta, S. J., das Gupta, R., Padmanabhan, V. T., et al.: Familial occurrence of sinus bradycardia, short PR interval, intraventricular conduction defects, recurrent supraventricular tachycardia, and cardiomegaly. Am. Heart J. *93*:19, 1977.

222. Chia, B. L., Yew, F. C., Chay, S. O., et al.: Familial Wolff-Parkinson-White syndrome. J. Electrocardiol. *15*:195, 1982.

223. Vidaillet, H. J., Pressley, J. C., Henke, E., et al.: Familial occurrence of accessory atrioventricular pathways: Preexcitation syndrome. N. Engl. J. Med. *317*:65, 1987.

224. Ibsen, H.H.W., Baandrup, U., and Simonsen, E. E.: Familial right ventricular dilated cardiomyopathy. Br. Heart J. *54*:156, 1985.

225. Laurent, M., Descases, C., Biron, Y., et al.: Familial form of arrhythmogenic right ventricular dysplasia. Am. Heart J. *113*:827, 1987.
226. Ruder, M. A., Winston, S. A., Davis, J. C., et al.: Arrhythmogenic right ventricular dysplasia in a family. Am. J. Cardiol. *56*:799, 1985.
227. Ward, O. C.: A new familial cardiac syndrome in children. J. Ir. Med. Assoc. *54*:103, 1964.
228. Romano, C.: Congenital cardiac arrhythmia. Lancet *1*:658, 1965.
229. Greenspon, A. J., Kidwell, G. A., Barrasse, L. D., et al.: Hereditary long QT syndrome associated with cardiac conduction system disease. PACE *12*:479, 1989.
230. Itoh, S., Munemura, S., and Satoh, H.: A study of the inheritance pattern of Romano-Ward syndrome. Clin. Pediatr. *21*:20, 1982.
231. Weitkamp, L. R., Moss, A. J., Schwartz, P. J., et al.: Analysis of HLA haplotypes in long QT syndrome: withdrawal of the preliminary assignment of LQT to the HLA linkage group (abstr.). Cytogenet. Cell Genet. *51*:1106, 1989.
232. Jervell, A., and Lange-Nielsen, F.: Congenital deaf-mutism, functional heart disease with prolongation of Q-T interval and sudden death. Am. Heart J. *54*:59, 1957.
233. Fraser, G. R., Froggatt, P., and Murphy, T.: Genetical aspects of the cardioauditory syndrome of Jervell and Lange-Nielsen (congenital deafness and electrocardiographic abnormalities). Ann. Hum. Genet. *28*:133, 1964.
234. Till, J. A., Shinebourne, E. A., Pepper, J., et al.: Complete denervation of the heart in a child with congenital long QT and deafness. Am. J. Cardiol. *62*:1319, 1988.

DISORDERS OF CONNECTIVE TISSUE

235. McKusick, V. A.: Heritable Disorders of Connective Tissue. St. Louis, C. V. Mosby Co., 1956.
236. McKusick, V. A.: Heritable Disorders of Connective Tissue, 4th ed. St. Louis, C. V. Mosby Co., 1972
237. Bowen, J., Boudoulas, H., and Wooley, C. F.: Cardiovascular disease of connective tissue origin. Am. J. Med. *82*:481, 1987.
238. Pyeritz, R. E.: Cardiovascular manifestation of heritable disorders of connective tissue. Prog. Med. Genet. *5*:191, 1983.
239. Pyeritz, R. E.: Storage disorders. *In* Pierpont, M. E., and Moller, J. H. (eds.): The Genetics of Cardiovascular Disease. Boston, Martinus Nijhoff Publishing, 1987, p. 215.
240. Pyeritz, R. E.: Heritable disorders of connective tissue. *In* Pierpont, M. E., Moller, J. H. (eds.): The Genetics of Cardiovascular Disease. Boston, Martinus Nijhoff Publishing, 1987, p. 265.
241. Royce, P. M., and Steinmann, B.: Extracellular Matrix and Inheritable Disorders of Connective Tissue. New York, Wiley-Liss *(in press)*.
242. Beighton, P. (ed.): Heritable Disorders of Connective Tissue. 5th ed. St. Louis, C. V. Mosby *(in press)*.
243. McKusick, V. A.: The cardiovascular aspects of Marfan's syndrome: A heritable disorder of connective tissue. Circulation *11*:321, 1955.
244. Pyeritz, R. E., and McKusick, V. A.: The Marfan syndrome—diagnosis and management. N. Engl. J. Med. *300*:772, 1979.
245. Roberts, W. C., and Honig, H. S.: The spectrum of cardiovascular disease in the Marfan syndrome: A clinicomorphologic study of 18 necropsy patients and comparison to 151 previously reported necropsy patients. Am. Heart J. *104*:115, 1982.
246. Pyeritz, R. E.: The Marfan syndrome. *In* Royce, P. M., and Steinmann, B. (eds.) Extracellular Matrix and Inheritable Disorders of Connective Tissue. New York, A. R. Liss *(in press)*.
247. Kainulainen K., Pulkkinen, L., Savolainen, A., et al.: The gene defect causing Marfan syndrome is located in chromosome 15. N. Engl. J. Med. *323*:935, 1990.
247a. Dietz, H. C., Pyeritz, R. E., Hall, B. D., et al.: The Marfan syndrome locus: Confirmation of assignment to chromosome 15 and identification of tightly linked markers at 15q15-q21.3. Genomics *9*:355, 1991.
248. Pyeritz, R. E.: Conference report: First international symposium on the Marfan syndrome. Am. J. Med. Genet. *32*:233, 1989.
249. Marsalese, D. L., Moodie, D. S., Vacante, M., et al.: Marfan's syndrome: Natural history and long-term follow-up of cardiovascular involvement. J. Am. Coll. Cardiol. *14*:422, 1989.
250. Child, J. S., Perloff, J. K., and Kaplan, S.: The heart of the matter: Cardiovascular involvement in Marfan's syndrome. J. Am. Coll. Cardiol. *14*:429, 1989.
251. Murdoch, J. L., Walker, B. A., Halpern, B. L., et al.: Life expectancy and causes of death in the Marfan syndrome. N. Engl. J. Med. *286*:804, 1972.
252. Phornphutkul, C., Rosenthal, A., and Nadas, A. S.: Cardiac manifestations of Marfan syndrome in infancy and childhood. Circulation *47*:581, 1973.
253. Sisk, H. E., Zahka, K. G., and Pyeritz, R. E.: The Marfan syndrome in early childhood: Analysis of 15 patients diagnosed less than 4 years of age. Am. J. Cardiol. *52*:353, 1983.
254. Gross, D. M., Robinson, L. K., Smith, L. T., et al.: Severe perinatal Marfan syndrome. Pediatrics *84*:83, 1989.
255. Geva, T., Hegesh, J., and Frand, M.: The clinical course and echocardiographic features of Marfan's syndrome in childhood. Am. J. Dis. Child. *141*:1179, 1987.
256. Morse, R. P., Rockenmacher, S., Pyeritz, R. E., et al.: Diagnosis and management of Marfan syndrome in infants. Pediatrics *86*:888, 1990.
257. Pyeritz, R. E.: Heritable disorders of connective tissue. *In* Boudoulas, H., and Wooley, C. F. (eds.): Mitral Valve Prolapse and the Mitral Valve Prolapse Syndrome. Mt. Kisco, N. Y., Futura Publishing Co., 1988, p. 129.
258. Pyeritz, R. E., and Wappel, M. A.: Mitral valve dysfunction in the Marfan syndrome. Am. J. Med. *74*:797, 1983.
259. Kolibash, A. J., Jr.: Natural history of mitral valve prolapse. *In* Boudoulas, H., and Wooley, C. F. (eds.): Mitral Valve Prolapse and the Mitral Valve Prolapse Syndrome. Mt. Kisco, N. Y., Futura Publishing Co., 1988, p. 257.
260. Crawford, E. S., and Coselli, J. S.: Marfan's syndrome: Combined composite valve graft replacement of the aortic root and transaortic mitral valve replacement. Ann. Thorac. Surg. *45*:296, 1988.
261. Cohn, L. H. DiSesa, V. J., Couper, G. S., et al.: Mitral valve repair for myxomatous degeneration and prolapse of the mitral valve. J. Thorac. Cardiovasc. Surg. *98*:987, 1989.
262. Gott, V. L., Pyeritz, R. E., Cameron, D., et al.: Ascending aortic aneurysm in the Marfan syndrome: Results of composite graft repair in 100 patients. Ann. Thorac. Surg. *(in press)*.
263. Gott, V. L., Pyeritz, R. E., Magovern, G. J., Jr., et al.: Surgical treatment of aneurysms of the ascending aorta in the Marfan syndrome. Results of composite-graft repair in 50 patients. N. Engl. J. Med. *314*:1070, 1986.
264. Lima, S. D., Lima, J.A.C., Pyeritz, R. E., et al.: Relationship of mitral valve prolapse to left ventricular size in Marfan's syndrome. Am. J. Cardiol. *55*:739, 1985.
265. Lafferty, K., McLean, L., Salisbury, J., et al.: Ruptured abdominal aortic aneurysm in Marfan's syndrome. Postgrad. Med. J. *63*:685, 1987.
266. Pruzinsky, M. S., Katz, N. M., and Green, C. E., et al.: Isolated descending thoracic aortic aneurysm in Marfan's syndrome. Am. J. Cardiol. *51*:1159, 1988.
267. van Ooijen, B.: Marfan's syndrome and isolated aneurysm of the abdominal aorta. Br. Heart J. *59*:81, 1988.
268. Henry, W. L., Gardin, J. M., and Ware, J. H.: Echocardiographic measurements in normal subjects from infancy to old age. Circulation *62*:1054, 1980.
269. Crawford, E. S.: Marfan's syndrome: Broad spectral surgical treatment cardiovascular manifestations. Ann. Surg. *198*:487, 1983.
270. Svensson, L. G., Crawford, E. S., Coselli, J. S., et al.: Impact of cardiovascular operation on survival in the Marfan patient. Circulation *80*:233, 1988.
271. Arn, P. H., Scherer, L. R., Haller, J. A., Jr., et al.: Outcome of pectus excavatum in patients with Marfan syndrome and in the general population. J. Pediatr. *115*:954, 1989.
272. Pyeritz, R. E., Gott, V. L., McDonald, G. R., et al.: Surgical repair of the Marfan aorta: Technique, indications, and complications. Johns Hopkins Med. J. *151*:71, 1982.
273. deSanctis, R., Doroghazi, R. M., Austen, W. G., et al.: Aortic dissection. N. Engl. J. Med. *317*:1060, 1987.
274. Schaefer, S., Peshock, R. M., Malloy, C. R., et al.: Nuclear magnetic resonance imaging in Marfan's syndrome. J. Am. Coll. Cardiol. *9*:70, 1987.
275. Soulen, R. L., Fishman, E., Pyeritz, R. E., et al.: Evaluation of the Marfan syndrome: MR imaging versus CT. Radiology *165*:697, 1987.
276. Crawford, E. S., Crawford, J. L., Stowe, C. L., et al.: Total aortic replacement for chronic aortic dissection occurring in patients with and without Marfan's syndrome. Ann. Surg. *199*:358, 1984.
277. Pyeritz, R. E.: Effectiveness of beta-adrenergic blockade in the Marfan syndrome: Experience over 10 years (abstr.). Am. J. Med. Genet. *32*:245, 1989.
278. Zahka, K. G., Hensley, C., and Glesby, M., et al.: The impact of medical therapy on the cardiovascular prognosis of the Marfan syndrome in early childhood (abstr). J. Am. Coll. Cardiol. *13*:119, 1989.
279. Yin, F.C.P., Brin K. P., Ting, C.-T, et al.: Arterial hemodynamics in the Marfan syndrome. Circulation *79*:854, 1989.
280. Pyeritz, R. E.: Maternal and fetal complications of pregnancy in the Marfan syndrome. Am. J. Med. *71*:784, 1981.
281. Rosenblum, N., Grossman, A., and Gabbe, S.: Failure of serial echocardiographic studies to predict dissection in a pregnant woman with Marfan's syndrome. Am. J. Obstet. Gynecol. *146*:490, 1983.
282. Smith, V. C., Eckenbrecht, P.D., Hankins, G.D.V., et al.: Marfan's syndrome, pregnancy, and the cardiac surgeon. Milit. Med. *154*:404, 1989.
283. Mor-Yosef, S., Younis, J., Granat, J., et al.: Marfan's syndrome in pregnancy. Obstet. Gynecol. Surv. *43*:382, 1988.
284. Ferguson, J. E., II, Ueland, K., Stinson, E. G., et al.: Marfan's syndrome: Acute aortic dissection during labor, resulting in fetal distress and cesarean section, followed by successful surgical repair. Am. J. Obstet. Gynecol. *147*:759, 1983.
285. Cola, L. M., and Lavin, J. P., Jr.: Pregnancy complicated by the Marfan syndrome with aortic arch dissection, subsequent arch replacement and triple coronary artery bypass grafts. J. Reprod. Med. *30*:685, 1985.
286. Bailey, M. K., Hwu-Yun, R., Baker, J. D., III, et al.: Marfan syndrome in the parturient. J. S.C. Med. Assoc. *8*:327, 1989.
287. Sakai, L. Y., Keene, D. R., Engvall, E.: Fibrillin, a new 350-kD glycoprotein, is a component of extracellular microfibrils. J. Cell. Biol. *103*:2499, 1986.
288. Perejda. A. J., Abraham, P. A., Carnes, W. H., et al.: Marfan's syndrome: Structural, biochemical and mechanical studies of the aortic media. J. Lab. Clin. Med. *106*:376, 1985.
289. Becker, A. E.: Medionecrosis aortae. Pathol. Microbiol. *43*:124, 1975.
289a. McGookey, D. J., Pyeritz, R. E., and Byers, P. H.: Marfan syndrome: altered synthesis, secretion or extracellular incorporation of fibrillin. Am. J. Hum. Genet. *47*:A67, 1991.
289b. Magenis, E., and Sakai, L. Y.: The gene for fibrillin maps by *in situ* hybridization to 15q. Genomics *(in press)*.
290. Leier, C. V., Call, T. D., Fulkerson, P. K., et al.: The spectrum of cardiac defects in the Ehlers-Danlos syndrome, types I and III. Ann. Intern. Med. *92*:171, 1980.

291. Jaffe, A. S., Geltman, E. M., Rodey, G. E., et al.: Mitral valve prolapse: A consistent manifestation of type IV Ehlers-Danlos syndrome. Circulation 64:121, 1981.
292. Pyeritz, R. E., Stolle, C. A., Parfrey, N. A., et al.: Ehlers-Danlos syndrome IV due to a novel defect in type III procollagen. Am. J. Med. Genet. 19:607, 1984.
293. Nicholls, A. C., De Paepe, A., Narcisi, P., et al.: Linkage of a polymorphic marker for the type III collagen gene (COL3A1) to atypical autosomal dominant Ehlers-Danlos syndrome type IV in a large Belgian pedigree. Hum. Genet. 78:276, 1988.
294. Fox, R., Pope, F. M., Narcisi, P., et al.: Spontaneous carotid cavernous fistula in Ehlers-Danlos syndrome. J. Neurol. Neurosurg. Psychiat. 51:984, 1988.
295. Rudd, N. L., Nimrod, C., Holbrook, K. A., et al.: Pregnancy complications in type IV Ehlers-Danlos syndrome. Lancet 1:50, 1983.
296. Viljoen, D. L., Pope, F. M., and Beighton, P.: Heterogeneity of pseudoxanthoma elasticum: Delineation of a new form? Clin. Genet. 32:100, 1987.
297. Cunningham, J. R., Lippman, S. M., Renie, W. A., et al.: Pseudoxanthoma elasticum: Treatment of gastrointestinal hemorrhage by arterial embolization and observations of autosomal dominant inheritance. Johns Hopkins Med. J. 147:168, 1980.
298. Lebwohl, M. G., Distefano, D., Prioleau, P. G., et al.: Pseudoxanthoma elasticum and mitral valve prolapse. N. Engl. J. Med. 307:228, 1982.
299. Pyeritz, R. E., Weiss, J. L., Renie, W. A., et al.: Pseudoxanthoma elasticum and mitral-valve prolapse. N. Engl. J. Med. 307:1451, 1982.
300. Goodman, R. M., Smith, E. W., Paton, D., et al.: Pseudoxanthoma elasticum: A clinical and histopathological study. Medicine 42:297, 1963.
301. Challenor, V. F., Conway, N., and Monro, J. L.: The surgical treatment of restrictive cardiomyopathy in pseudoxanthoma elasticum. Br. Heart J. 59:266, 1988.
302. Renie, W. A., Pyeritz, R. E., Combs, J., et al.: Pseudoxanthoma elasticum: High calcium intake in early life correlates with severity. Am. J. Med. Genet. 19:235, 1984.
303. Maharaj, B., Hammond, M. G., Appadoo, B., et al.: HLA-A, B, DR, and DQ antigens in black patients with severe chronic rheumatic heart disease. Circulation 76:259, 1987.

INBORN ERRORS OF METABOLISM THAT AFFECT THE CARDIOVASCULAR SYSTEM

304. La Du, B. N.: Alcaptonuria. *In* Scriver, C. R., Beaudet, A. L., Sly, W. S., and Valle, D. (eds.): The Metabolic Basis of Inherited Disease. 6th ed. New York, McGraw-Hill Book Co., 1989, p. 775.
305. Mudd, S. H., Levy, H. L., and Skovby, F.: Disorders of transsulfuration. *In* Scriver, C. R., Beaudet, A. L., Sly, W. S., and Valle, D. (eds.): The Metabolic Basis of Inherited Disease. 6th ed. New York, McGraw-Hill Book Co., 1989, p. 693.
306. Mudd, S. H., Skovby, F., Levy, H. L., et al.: The natural history of homocystinuria due to cystathionine beta-synthase deficiency. Am. J. Hum. Genet. 37:1, 1985.
307. Hill-Zobel, R. L., Pyeritz, R. E., Scheffel, U., et al.: Kinetics and biodistribution of ^{111}In-labeled platelets in homocystinuria. N. Engl. J. Med. 307:781, 1982.
308. Mudd, S. H.: Vascular disease and homocysteine metabolism (editorial). N. Engl. J. Med. 313:751, 1985.
309. Murphy-Chutorian, D. R., Wexman, M. P., Grieco, A. J., et al.: Methionine intolerance: A possible risk factor for coronary artery disease. J. Am. Coll. Cardiol. 6:725, 1985.
310. Kang, S. S., Wong, P.W.K., Cook, H. Y., et al.: Protein-bound homocyst(e)ine: A possible risk factor for coronary artery disease. J. Clin. Invest. 77:1482, 1986.
311. Wilcken, D. E., and Wilcken, B.: The pathogenesis of coronary artery disease: A possible role for methionine metabolism. J. Clin. Invest. 57:1079, 1976.
312. Roe, C. R., and Coates, P. M.: Acyl-CoA dehydrogenase deficiencies. *In* Scriver, C. R., Beaudet, A. L., Sly, W. S., and Valle, D. (eds.): The Metabolic Basis of Inherited Disease. 6th ed. New York, McGraw-Hill Book Co., 1989, p. 889.
313. Harper, P. S.: The muscular dystrophies. *In* Scriver, C. R., Beaudet, A. L., Sly, W. S., and Valle, D. (eds.): The Metabolic Basis of Inherited Disease. 6th ed. New York, McGraw-Hill Book Co., 1989, p. 2869.
314. Rebouche, C. J., and Engel, A. G.: Carnitine metabolism and deficiency syndromes. Mayo Clin. Proc. 58:533, 1983.
315. Treem, W. R., Stanley, C. A., Finegold, D. N., et al.: Primary carnitine deficiency due to a failure of carnitine transport in kidney, muscle, and fibroblasts. N. Engl. J. Med. 319:1331, 1988.
316. Waber, L. J., Valle, D., Neill, C., et al.: Carnitine deficiency presenting as familial cardiomyopathy: A treatable defect in carnitine transport. J. Pediatr. 101:700, 1982.
317. Tripp, M. E., Katcher, M. L., Peters, H. A., et al.: Systemic carnitine deficiency presenting as familial endocardial fibroelastosis. N. Engl. J. Med. 305:385, 1981.
318. Ogasahara, S., Engel, A. G., Frens, D., et al.: Muscle coenzyme Q deficiency in familial mitochondrial encephalomyopathy. Proc. Natl. Acad. Sci. USA 86:2379, 1989.
319. Channer, K. S., Channer, J. L., Campbell, M. J., et al.: Cardiomyopathy in the Kearns-Sayre syndrome. Br. Heart J. 59:486, 1988.
320. Hers, H.-G., Van Hoof, F., and de Barsy, T.: Glycogen storage diseases. *In* Scriver, C. R., Beaudet, A. L., Sly, W. S., and Valle, D. (eds.): The Metabolic Basis of Inherited Disease. 6th ed. New York, McGraw-Hill Book Co., 1989, p. 425.
321. Bashan, N., Potashnik, R., Barash, V., et al.: Glycogen storage disease type II in Israel. Isr. J. Med. Sci. 24:224, 1988.
322. Ehlers, K. H., Hagstrom, J.W.C., Lukas, D. S., et al.: Glycogen-storage disease of the myocardium with obstruction to left ventricular outflow. Circulation 25:96, 1962.
323. Bharati, S., Serratto, M., Du Brow, I., et al.: The conduction system in Pompe's disease. Pediatr. Cardiol. 2:25, 1982.
324. Bonnici, F., Shapiro, R., Joffe, H. S., et al.: Angiocardiographic and enzyme studies in a patient with type II glycogenosis. S. Afr. Med. J. 58:860, 1980.
325. Robinson, W. F., Howell, J. M., and Dorling, P. R.: Cardiomyopathy in generalised glycogenosis type II in cattle. Cardiovasc. Res. 17:238, 1982.
326. Suzuki, Y., Tsuji, A., Omura, K., et al.: Km mutant of acid alpha-glucosidase in a case of cardiomyopathy without signs of skeletal muscle involvement. Clin. Genet. 33:376, 1988.
327. Makos, M. M., McComb, R. D., Hart, M. N., et al.: Alpha-glucosidase deficiency and basilar artery aneurysm: Report of a sibship. Ann. Neurol. 22:629, 1987.
328. Olson, L. J., Reeder, G. S., Noller, K. L., et al.: Cardiac involvement in glycogen storage disease III. Morphologic and biochemical characterization with endomyocardial biopsy. Am. J. Cardiol. 53:980, 1984.
329. Servidei, S., Metlay, L. A., Chodosh, J., et al.: Fatal infantile cardiopathy caused by phosphorylase b kinase deficiency. J. Pediatr. 113:82, 1988.
330. Eishi, Y., Takemura, T., Sone, R., et al.: Glycogen storage disease confined to the heart with deficient activity of cardiac phosphorylase kinase: a new type of glycogen storage disease. Hum. Pathol. 16:193, 1987.
331. Bothwell, T. H., Charlton, R. W., and Motulsky, A. G.: Hemochromatosis. *In* Scriver, C. R., Beaudet, A. L., Sly, W. S., and Valle, D. (eds.): The Metabolic Basis of Inherited Disease. 6th ed. New York, McGraw-Hill Book Co., 1989, p. 1433.
332. Valberg, L. S., and Ghent, C. N.: Diagnosis and managment of hereditary hemochromatosis. Annu. Rev. Med. 36:27, 1985.
333. Edwards, C. Q.: Early detection of hereditary hemochromatosis. Ann. Intern. Med. 101:707, 1984.
334. Olson, L. J., Baldus, W. P., and Tajik, A. J.: Echocardiographic features of idiopathic hemochromatosis. Am. J. Cardiol. 60:885, 1987.
335. Cutler, D. J., Isner, J. M., Bracey, A. W., et al.: Hemochromatosis heart disease: An unemphasized cause of potentially reversible restrictive cardiomyopathy. Am. J. Med. 69:923, 1980.
336. Weatherall, D. J., Clegg, F. B., Higgs, D. R., et al.: The hemoglobinopathies. *In* Scriver, C. R., Beaudet, A. L., Sly, W. S., and Valle, D. (eds.): The Metabolic Basis of Inherited Disease. 6th ed. New York, McGraw-Hill Book Co., 1989, p. 2281.
337. Neufeld, E. F., and Muenzer, J.: The mucopolysaccharidoses. *In* Scriver, C. R., Beaudet, A. L., Sly, W. S., and Valle, D. (eds.). The Metabolic Basis of Inherited Disease. 6th ed. New York, McGraw-Hill Book Co., 1989, p. 1565.
338. Nolan, C. M., and Sly, W. S.: I-cell disease and pseudo-Hurler polydystrophy: Disorders of lysosomal enzyme phosphorylation and localization. *In* Scriver, C. R., Beaudet, A. L., Sly, W. S., and Valle, D. (eds.): The Metabolic Basis of Inherited Disease. 6th ed. New York, McGraw-Hill Book Co., 1989, p. 1589.
339. Johnson, G. L., Vine, D. L. Cottrill, C. M., et al.: Echocardiographic mitral valve deformity in the mucopolysaccharidoses. Pediatrics 67:401, 1981.
340. Gross, D. M., Williams, J. C., Caprioli, C., et al.: Echocardiographic abnormalities in the mucopolysaccharide storage diseases. Am. J. Cardiol. 61:170, 1988.
340a. John, R. M., Hunter, D., and Swanton, R. H.: Echocardiographic abnormalities in type IV mucopolysaccharidosis. Arch. Dis. Childhood 65:746, 1990.
341. Nelson, J., Shields, M. D., and Mulholland, H. C.: Cardiovascular studies in the mucopolysaccharidoses. J. Med. Genet. 27:94, 1990.
342. Brosius, F. C., III, and Roberts, W. C.: Coronary artery disease in the Hurler syndrome: Qualitative and quantitative analysis of the extent of coronary narrowing at necropsy in six children. Am. J. Cardiol. 47:649, 1981.
343. Renteria, V. G., Ferrans, V. J., and Roberts, W. C.: The heart in the Hurler syndrome: Gross, histologic and ultrastructural observations in five necropsy cases. Am. J. Cardiol. 38:487, 1976.
344. Semenza, G. L., and Pyeritz, R. E.: Respiratory complications of the mucopolysaccharide storage disorders. Medicine 67:209, 1988.
345. Young, I. D., and Harper, P.S.: Long-term complications in Hunter's syndrome. Clin. Genet. 16:125, 1979.
345a. Lenarsky, C., Kohn, D. B., Weinberg, K. I., et al.: Bone marrow transplantation for genetic diseases. Hematol./Oncol. Clin. North Am. 4:589, 1990.
346. Desnick, R. J., and Bishop, D. F.: Fabry disease: α-Galactosidase deficiency; Schindler disease: α-N-acetylgalactosaminidase deficiency. *In* Scriver, C. R., Beaudet, A. L., Sly, W. S., and Valle, D. (eds.): The Metabolic Basis of Inherited Disease. 6th ed. New York, McGraw-Hill Book Co., 1989, p. 1797.
347. Morgan, S. H., and Crawfurd, M. d'A.: Anderson-Fabry disease. A commonly missed diagnosis. Br. Med. J. 297:872, 1988.
348. Spence, M. W., MacKinnon, K. E., Burgess, J. K., et al.: Failure to correct the metabolic defect by renal allotransplantation in Fabry's disease. Ann. Intern. Med. 84:13, 1976.
349. Kramer, W., Thormann, J., Mueller, K., et al.: Progressive cardiac involvement by Fabry's disease despite successful renal allotransplantation. Int. J. Cardiol. 7:72, 1985.
350. Colucci, W. S., Lorell, B. H., Schoen, F. J., et al.: Hypertrophic obstructive cardiomyopathy due to Fabry's disease. N. Engl. J. Med. 307:926, 1982.

350a. von Scheidt, W., Eng., C. M., Fitzmaurice, T. F., et al.: An atypical variant of Fabry's disease with manifestations confined to the myocardium. N. Engl. J. Med. *324*:395, 1991.
351. Goldman, M. E., Cantor, R., Schwartz, M. F., et al.: Echocardiographic abnormalities and disease severity in Fabry's disease. J. Am. Coll. Cardiol. *7*:1157, 1986.
352. Sakuraba, H., Yanagawa, Y., Igarashi, T., et al.: Cardiovascular manifestations in Fabry's disease: A high incidence of mitral valve prolapse in hemizygotes and heterozygotes. Clin. Genet. *29*:276, 1986.
353. Mutoh, T., Senda, Y., Sugimura, K., et al.: Severe orthostatic hypotension in a female carrier of Fabry's disease. Arch. Neurol. *34*:468, 1988.
354. Bernstein, H. S., Bishop, D. F., Astrin, K. H., et al.: Fabry disease: Six gene rearrangements and an exonic point mutation in the alpha-galactosidase gene. J. Clin. Invest. *83*:1390, 1989.
355. Benson, M. D., and Wallace, M. R.: Amyloidosis. *In* Scriver, C. R., Beaudet, A. L., Sly, W. S., and Valle, D. (eds.): The Metabolic Basis of Inherited Disease. 6th ed. New York, McGraw-Hill Book Co., 1989, p. 2439.
356. Benson, M. D., Wallace, M. R., Tejada, E., et al.: Hereditary amyloidosis: Description of a new American kindred with late onset cardiomyopathy: Appalachian amyloid. Arthritis Rheum. *30*:195, 1987.
357. Backman, C., and Olofsson, B. O.: Echocardiographic features in familial amyloidosis with polyneuropathy. Acta Med. Scand. *214*:273, 1983.
358. Eriksson, A., Eriksson, P., Olofsson, B.-O., et al.: The cardiac atrioventricular conduction system in familial amyloidosis with polyneuropathy: A clinico-pathologic study of six cases from Northern Sweden. Acta Pathol. Microbiol. Immunol. Scand. *91*:343, 1983.
359. Vidaillet, H. J., Jr.: Cardiac tumors associated with hereditary syndromes. Am. J. Cardiol. *61*:1355, 1988.
359a. Harding, C. O., and Pagon, R. A.: Incidence of tuberous sclerosis in patients with cardiac rhabdomyoma. Am. J. Med. Genet. *37*:443, 1990.

INHERITED DISORDERS OF THE CIRCULATION

360. Peery, W. H.: Clinical spectrum of hereditary hemorrhagic telangiectasia (Osler-Weber-Rendu disease). Am. J. Med. *82*:989, 1987.
361. Nikolopoulos, N., Xynos, E., and Vassilakis, J. S.: Familial occurrence of hyperdynamic circulation status due to intrahepatic fistulae in hereditary hemorrhagic telangiectasia. Hepatogastroenterology *35*:167, 1988.
362. Cooke, D.A.P.: Renal arteriovenous malformation demonstrated angiographically in hereditary haemorrhagic telangiectasia (Rendu-Osler-Weber disease). J. R. Soc. Med. *79*:744, 1986.
363. Kurnik, P. B., and Heymann, W. R.: Coronary artery ectasia associated with hereditary hemorrhagic telangiectasia. Arch. Intern. Med. *149*:2357, 1989.
364. Terry, P. B., White, J. I., Jr., Barth, K. H., et al.: Pulmonary arteriovenous malformations: Physiologic observations and results of therapeutic balloon embolization. N. Engl. J. Med. *308*:1197, 1983.
365. Haq, A. U., Glass, J., Netchvolodoff, C. V., et al.: Hereditary hemorrhagic telangiectasia and danazol. Ann. Intern. Med. *109*:171, 1988.
366. Green. J. S., Bowmer, M. I., and Johnson, G. J.: Von Hippel-Lindau disease in a Newfoundland kindred. Can. Med. Assoc. J. *134*:133, 1986.
367. Griffiths, D.F.R., Williams, G. T., and Williams, E. D.: Duodenal carcinoid tumours, phaeochromocytoma and neurofibromatosis: Islet cell tumour, phaeochromocytoma and the von Hippel-Lindau complex: Two distinctive neuroendocrine syndromes. Q. J. Med. *245*:769, 1987.
368. Jennings, A. M., Smith, C., Cole, D. R., et al.: Von Hippel-Lindau disease in a large British family: Clinicopathological features and recommendations for screening and follow-up. Q. J. Med. *66*:233, 1988.
369. Lamiell, J. M., Salazar, F. G., and Hsia, Y. E.: Von Hippel-Lindau disease affecting 43 members of a single kindred. Medicine *68*:1, 1989.
369a. Parfrey, P. S., Bear, J. C., Morgan, J., et al.: The diagnosis and prognosis of autosomal dominant polycystic kidney disease. N. Engl. J. Med. *323*:1085, 1990.
369b. Chapman, A. B., Johnson, A., Gabow, P. A., et al.: The renin-angiotensin-aldosterone system and autosomal dominant polycystic kidney disease. N. Engl. J. Med. *323*:1091, 1990.
370. Leier, C. V., Baker, P. B., Kilman, J. W., et al: Cardiovascular abnormalities associated with adult polycystic kidney disease. Ann. Intern. Med. *100*:683, 1984.
371. Hossack, K. F., Leddy, C. L., Johnson, A. M., et al: Echocardiographic findings in autosomal dominant polycystic kidney disease. N. Engl. J. Med. *319*:907, 1988.
372. Chapman, J. R., and Hilson, A.J.W.: Polycystic kidneys and abdominal aortic aneurysms. Lancet *1*:646, 1980.
373. Wakabayashi, T., Fujita, S., Ohbora, Y., et al.: Polycystic kidney disease and inctracranial aneurysms: Early angiographic diagnosis and early operation for the unruptured aneurysm. J. Neurosurg. *58*:488, 1983.
374. Levey, A. S., Pauker, S. G., and Kassirer, J. P.: Occult intracranial aneurysms in polycystic kidney disease: When is cerebral arteriography indicated? N. Engl. J. Med. *308*:986, 1983.
375. Germino, G. G., Barton, N. J., Lamb, J., et al.: Identification of a locus which shows no genetic recombination with the autosomal dominant polycystic kidney disease gene on chromosome 16. Am. J. Hum. Genet. *46*:925, 1990.
376. Elles, R. G., Read, A. P., Hodgkinson, K. A., et al.: Recombination or heterogeneity: Is there a second locus for adult polycystic kidney disease? J. Med. Genet. *27*:413, 1990.
377. Shulman, S. A., Hyams, J. S., Gunta, R., et al.: Arteriohepatic dysplasia (Alagille syndrome): Extreme variability among affected family members. Am. J. Med. Genet. *19*:325, 1984.
378. Mueller, R. F.: The Alagille syndrome (arteriohepatic dysplasia). J. Med. Genet. *24*:621, 1987.
379. Nicod, P., Bloor, C., Godfrey, M., et al.: Familial aortic dissecting aneurysms. J. Am. Coll. Cardiol. *13*:811, 1989.
380. Toyama, M., Amano, A., and Kameda, T.: Familial aortic dissection: A report of rare family cluster. Br. Heart J. *61*:204, 1989.
381. Bixler, D., and Antley, R. M.: Familial aortic dissection with iris anomalies—a new connective tissue disease syndrome? Birth Defects *12*(5):229, 1976.
382. Kontusaari, S. Tromp, G., Kuivaniemi, H., et al.: Inheritance of RNA splicing mutation ($G^{+1\ IVS20}$) in the type III procollagen gene (COL3AI) in a family having aortic aneurysms and easy bruisability: Phenotypic overlap between familial arterial aneurysms and Ehlers-Danlos syndrome type IV. Am. J. Hum. Genet. *47*:112, 1990.
383. Kontusaari, S., Tromp, G., Kuivaniemi, H., et al.: A mutation in the gene for type III procollagen (COL3AI) in a family with aortic aneurysms. J. Clin. Invest. *86*:1465, 1990.
383a. Majumder, P. P., St. Jean, P. L., Ferrell, R. E., et al.: On the inheritance of abdominal aortic aneurysm. Am. J. Hum. Genet. *48*:164, 1991.
384. Welch, J. P., Aterman, K., and Day, E.: Familial aggregation of a 'new' connective disorder, a nosologic problem. Birth Defects *7*(8):204, 1971.
385. Fox, J. L., and Ko, J. P.: Familial intracranial aneurysms: Six cases among 13 siblings. J. Neurosurg. *52*:501, 1980.
386. Halal, F., Mohr, G., Toussi, T., et al.: Intracranial aneurysms: A report of a large pedigree. Am. J. Med. Genet. *15*:89, 1983.
387. De Paepa, A., Van Landeghem, W., De Keyser, F., et al.: Collagen type III deficiency associated with multiple intracranial aneurysms (abstr.) Clin. Genet. *33*:462, 1988.
388. Abrahamson, M.: Human cysteine proteinase inhibitors: Isolation, physiological importance, inhibitory mechanism, gene structure and relation to hereditary cerebral hemorrhage. Scand. J. Clin. Lab. Invest. *48*:21, 1988.
389. Wattendorff, A. R., Bots, G.T.A.M., Went, L. N., et al.: Familial cerebral amyloid angiopathy presenting as recurrent cerebral haemorrhage. J. Neurol. Sci. *55*:121, 1982.
390. Pasyk, K. A., Argenta, L. C., and Erickson, R. P.: Familial vascular malformations: Report of 25 members of one family. Clin. Genet. *26*:221, 1984.
391. Stanley, J. C.: Arterial fibrodysplasia. Arch. Surg. *110*:561, 1975.
392. Kousseff, B. G., and Gilbert-Barness, E. F.: Vascular neurofibromatosis and infantile gangrene. Am. J. Med. Genet. *34*:221, 1989.
393. Petit, H., Bouchez, B., Destee, A., et al.: Familial form of fibromuscular dysplasia of the internal carotid artery. J. Neuroradiol. *10*:15, 1983.
394. Gladstein, K., Rushton, A. R., and Kidd, K. K.: Penetrance estimates and recurrence risks for fibromuscular dysplasia. Clin. Genet. *17*:115, 1980.
395. Rushton, A. R.: The genetics of fibromuscular dysplasia. Arch. Intern. Med. *140*:233, 1980.
396. Austin, J. G., and Stears, J. C.: Familial hypoplasia of both internal carotid arteries. Arch. Neurol. *24*:1, 1971.
397. McDonald, A. H., Gerlis, L. M., and Somerville, J.: Familial arteriopathy with associated pulmonary and systemic arterial stenoses. Br. Heart J. *31*:375, 1969.
398. Van Dyck, M., Proesmans, W., VanHollebeke, E., et al.: Idiopathic infantile arterial calcification with cardiac, renal and central nervous system involvement. Eur. J. Pediatr. *148*:374, 1989.
399. Melmon, K. L., and Braunwald, E.: Familial pulmonary hypertension. N. Engl. J. Med. *269*:770, 1963.
400. Kingdon, H. S., Cohen, L. S., Roberts, W. C., et al.: Familial occurrence of primary pulmonary hypertension. Arch. Intern. Med. *118*:422, 1966.
401. Loyd, J. E., Primm, R. K., and Newman, J. H.: Familial primary pulmonary hypertension: Clinical patterns. Am. Rev. Respir. Dis. *129*:194, 1984.
402. Porterfield, J. K., Pyeritz, R. E., and Traill, T. A.: Pulmonary hypertension and interstitial fibrosis in von Recklinghausen neurofibromatosis. Am. J. Med. Genet. *25*:531, 1986.
403. Goldstein, S., Qazi, Q. H., Fitzgerald, J., et al.: Distichiasis, congenital heart defects and mixed peripheral vascular anomalies. Am. J. Med. Genet. *20*:283, 1985.
404. Lindenauer, S. M.: The Klippel-Trenaunay-Weber syndrome: Varicosity, hypertrophy and hemangioma with no arteriovenous fistula. Ann. Surg. *162*:303, 1965.
405. Campistol, J. M., Agusti, C., Torras, A., et al.: Renal hemangioma and renal artery aneurysm in the Klippel-Trenaunay syndrome. J. Urol. *140*:134, 1988.
406. Herbert, F. A., and Bowen, P. A.: Hereditary late-onset lymphedema with pleural effusion and laryngeal edema. Arch. Intern. Med. *143*:913, 1983.
407. Childs, B.: Causes of essential hypertension. Prog. Med. Genet. *5*:1, 1983.
408. Murphy, E. A., and Pyeritz, R. D.: Homeostasis: VII. A conspectus. Am. J. Med. Genet. *24*:735, 1986.

52

Aging and the Heart

by MYRON L. WEISFELDT, M.D., EDWARD G. LAKATTA, M.D., and GARY GERSTENBLITH, M.D.

CONCEPTS AND THEORIES OF CHANGES WITH AGE

Students of cardiovascular medicine often are presented with two distinct issues concerning the burden imposed on the cardiovascular system by advanced age. The first is that represented by the aged, infirm patient with severe heart failure. At times no clear cause can be defined, and even when one is, the diagnostic and therapeutic management often is more challenging than is the case with the younger patient with the same disease. The issue presented by these patients, therefore, is that the cardiovascular limitations associated with aging itself are significant and often severe. There also is the observation represented by the elderly marathon runner, swimmer, or master athlete whose physical abilities are equal or superior to those of people 30 years younger. The findings in such people suggest that if there is any limitation of cardiovascular reserve imposed by the aging process per se, it is minor. There is some evidence that age-associated musculoskeletal, pulmonary, or psychological factors are more important than cardiovascular consideration in these patients.

AGING, DISEASE, AND LIFE STYLE. Attempts to solve the dilemma posed by the seemingly varied effects of age in the two subject subsets noted above are handicapped by the additional effects of both an increasing prevalence of disease and the altered life style associated with aging. The most prevalent disease, coronary atherosclerosis, is present in up to 60 per cent of elderly people in Western society,[1,2] has a profound effect on measurements of cardiovascular function during stress, but is difficult to diagnose in the absence of overt symptoms or electrocardiographic abnormalities. The most important life style variable is physical activity status. Exercise conditioning and deconditioning studies have indicated that even short periods of changes in physical activity can have a profound influence on cardiovascular function.[3] Toxins from food and chemical exposure (including cumulative effects of cigarette smoking and radiation, as well as malnutrition) are other life style variables whose effects may merge into those of disease. There is considerable evidence, therefore, that changes in the prevalence of disease and altered life style accompanying aging may have accounted for some of the previously described alterations attributed to aging alone.

In summary, changes in cardiovascular function accompanying aging in an unselected population may be due to changes in disease patterns and life style variables as well as those resulting simply from aging. Of the three, aging appears to be the least potent and, therefore, the most difficult to define. Although age-induced changes in cardiac structure, function, and neurohumoral responses do modify cardiovascular function, they are most important clinically when they are superimposed on significant disease or other cardiovascular stresses. The effects of aging alone on cardiovascular function should be examined in the subjects who are free of cardiovascular disease and who have a relatively homogeneous level of physical conditioning. It is relatively easy to exclude people who have symptomatic disease, but identification of atherosclerosis is more difficult in many people because of its high prevalence and because it often is asymptomatic.

INTERPRETATION OF STUDIES OF AGING. The best information concerning aging comes from longitudinal, or repeated, studies of healthy people who have active life styles. Because longitudinal studies require a prolonged time to perform, most aging studies in humans have used cross-sectional methodology. In any aging study it is important to note that data expressed as a ratio (e.g., cardiac index or myosin adenosine triphosphatase activity per milligram protein) may change with age because of changes in the denominator (for the examples given, body mass and total protein content) rather than because of a change in the parameter itself. The interpretation of cross-sectional studies also is limited by the possibility that the older volunteers may represent a subset of the general population selected for longevity and/or high motivational factors.

CARDIOVASCULAR CHANGES IN AGING

After neonatal development, the number of myocardial cells in the heart does not increase.[4] Detailed studies of biochemical and anatomical changes accompanying aging have been performed. It is important, though, to assess the physiological importance of these findings. Although one step in a complex biochemical pathway may be altered with age, the alteration may have no physiological significance if that step does not limit the rate of the overall reaction. Clearly, important general conclusions about cardiovascular aging are as follows:

1. There is moderate hypertrophy of left ventricular myocardium, probably in response to increased arterial vascular stiffness and dropout of myocytes.[5-7]
2. When myocardial hypertrophy occurs, it is out of proportion to capillary and vascular growth.[8]
3. The ability of myocardium to generate tension is well maintained as a result of prolonged duration of contraction and greater stiffness, despite a modest decrease in the velocity of shortening of cardiac muscle.

4. There is a selective decrease in beta-adrenoceptor–mediated inotropic, chronotropic, and vasodilating cardiovascular responses with aging.[9,10]
5. Increased pericardial and myocardial stiffness and delayed relaxation during aging may limit left early ventricular filling during stress,[10a] although end-diastolic volume is not compromised in healthy individuals.

GENERAL THEORIES OF AGING: CARDIOVASCULAR APPLICATION

As organized and discussed by Hayflick,[11] current broadly accepted theories of aging can be grouped by level of integration into genome, physiological, and organ theories. Most work to date on the cardiovascular system has been at the latter two levels.

GENOME THEORIES. The most popular current genome theory proposes that genes are programmed for aging and/or death of the organism.[12–14] Each species as well as cells in culture has what appears to be unmodifiable general boundaries for the duration of survival. Because cardiac function with age does not limit survival in the absence of disease or toxin exposure, little testing of this hypothesis is feasible in the cardiovascular system. Programmed dysfunction or cell destruction may account for neurohormonal regulatory dysfunction, but these notions are remote from the fundamental tenets of the hypothesis. Two other related genomic theories of aging are somatic mutation (related or not to environmental irradiation) and the error theories. Owing to either programmed DNA variability or toxic agents, there is an accumulation of cell components with errors in protein structure and/or sequence. The error theories may not be relevant, however, since searches for such errors have not been successful. In the heart certain aspects of function are so well maintained that it is difficult to use such a general theory to explain the relatively selective cardiovascular age changes.

PHYSIOLOGICAL THEORIES. Physiological theories of aging clearly appear more attractive as explanations for cardiovascular changes.[15–17] One, the cross-linkage theory of aging, points to the importance of time-related changes in the extracellular protein matrix, particularly of collagen and ground substance. Such changes are certainly at the basis of age-associated increases in stiffness of pericardial, valvular, and perhaps myocardial and vascular tissues. Secondary responses probably include myocardial hypertrophy and vascular smooth muscle changes. Neurohormonal changes would be more difficult to explain. Alternatively, physiological theories related to injury by free radicals and/or accumulation of waste product could explain the selectivity of aging changes in terms of selective sensitivity of specific enzymes to free radical injury or specific detrimental effects of waste product buildup, tissue by tissue.

ORGAN THEORIES. Organ theories are attractive in their simplicity and ease of understanding and demonstration. There are two major theories: immunological and neuroendocrine.[17,18] The immunological theory offers an explanation for survival duration characteristics of species in terms of programmed immunological dysfunction leading to autoimmune cellular injury but offers little to explain specific selective changes in the cardiovascular system. The neuroendocrine theory, perhaps in combination with the cross-linkage theory, would provide explanations for many of the observed changes in the characteristics of cardiac function with aging. In the neuroendocrine theory, changes in hypothalamic function, possibly genetically-induced, lead to changes in nerves and mediators. Major alterations in physiological function and the response to stress reflect the long-term and progressive summation effects of changes in individual neurohormonal mediators.

CARDIAC MUSCLE FUNCTION IN AGING

EXCITATION-CONTRACTION COUPLING

Our current understanding of how aging affects the myocardial contraction at the tissue-cellular levels is derived from studies in animal models. In cardiac muscles of senescent animals, contraction and relaxation times are prolonged. Figure 52–1B shows twitch recordings from adult rats (7 months) and aged rats (24 months).[18–28] Prolonged duration of contraction and relaxation can be attributed to alterations in mechanisms that govern excitation-contraction coupling in the heart (p. 357). Excitation of cardiac muscle results in a transient rise in cytosolic [Ca^{++}]. This activates myofilaments which stiffen, shorten, and produce force. The rate of decline in force or muscle lengthening reflects, in part, the rate and time course of decline in [Ca^{++}].

CALCIUM TRANSIENT. The time course of the Ca^{++}–myofilament interaction is a major determinant of duration of contraction and the time course of relaxation. This is determined in part by the extent and rate of myofilament shortening during the contraction, which is itself, in part, determined by the amount of Ca^{++} bound to troponin before the onset of contraction. The extent and rate of myofilament shortening are determined in part by the rate of myofilament hydrolysis of adenosine triphosphate (ATP) and crossbridge cycling rate and in part by the time course of the myoplasmic [Ca^{++}] transient, the duration of which is determined by sarcolemmal depolarization and by the rates of sarcoplasmic reticulum Ca^{++} release and pumping. The myoplasmic [Ca^{++}] transient that follows sarcolemmal depolarization in cardiac muscle has been monitored by injecting the chemiluminescent protein aequorin into multiple cells of that tissue and measuring the light transient that precedes contraction.[28] The duration of the myoplasmic [Ca^{++}] transient, measured as the time course of aequorin luminescence, is prolonged in isometric muscle isolated from aged versus younger adult rats (Fig. 52–1*C*). The myoplasmic free [Ca^{++}] transient results primarily from the sarcoplasmic reticulum Ca^{++} release and is the net result of the amount of Ca^{++} released and the extent of Ca^{++} binding to cell proteins. The rate at which the sarcoplasmic reticulum pumps Ca^{++} is diminished in hearts of senescent versus younger animals (Fig. 52–1*D*),[21,29] and this appears to be a major contributor to the prolonged transient and the prolonged time course of cardiac muscle relaxation. The reduction in sarcoplasmic reticulum Ca^{++} transport rate may be related to a decrease in the density of pump sites, as mRNA coding for the sarcoplasmic reticulum pump protein (Ca^{++} ATPase) is reduced by about 50 per cent in senescent versus younger adult hearts.[30]

The transmembrane action potential of working cardiac muscle from both right and left ventricles of senescent rats is markedly prolonged compared with young controls (Fig. 52–1*A*).[20,24] The magnitude of action potential prolongation in right ventricular isometric muscle from senescent rats is as great as that in left ventricular muscle and as great as that in muscle from experimentally hypertrophied rat hearts.[31] The overshoot and level of depolarization at all relative repolarization times are also greater in older than in younger Wistar rat cardiac muscles.[20] The mechanism for the prolonged action potential appears to be caused by a reduction in outward currents, as the magnitude of the Ca^{++} current (under conditions in which Na^{+} current is blocked) is not markedly changed with age.[32] The larger action potential in intact senescent muscle may serve to reduce Ca^{++} efflux by means of Na/Ca exchange, which is voltage-sensitive and occurs during the action potential of each heartbeat.[33] This would "conserve" cytosolic calcium content and would allow more Ca^{++} to be pumped by the sarcoplasmic reticulum. Alternatively, the changes in the action potential could be the result of age-related differences in the cytosolic [Ca^{++}] transient (i.e., the prolonged [Ca^{++}] transient may cause a prolonged action potential).[34]

DURATION OF CONTRACTION, RELAXATION, AND MUSCLE STIFFNESS. The prolonged time course of the myoplasmic free Ca^{++} transient also may affect other aspects of the cardiac contraction that depend on Ca^{++}–myofilament interactions (i.e., the time to peak force [Fig. 52–1*B*] and the ability of myofilaments to shorten and stiffen at differing times after excitation). The time to peak stiffness and half-relaxation time of peak stiffness are prolonged in senescent versus younger adult cardiac muscle,[23,25,26,35] probably reflecting the prolonged [Ca^{++}] transient and slowed Ca^{++} uptake by the sarcoplasmic reticulum. Muscle stiffness is measured as the ratio of the change in force in response to a length change. Stiffness measured in response to small sinusoidal changes in muscle length made during the contraction has been referred to as "active dynamic" stiffness. The active dynamic stiffness is a linear function of the force and increases as force increases with time during a contraction. The slope coefficient (a) of the active stiffness–force relation, but not its intercept, increases in senescence. Enhanced dynamic stiffness in senescent muscle is present only during contractile activation by Ca^{++}.[23,25] A

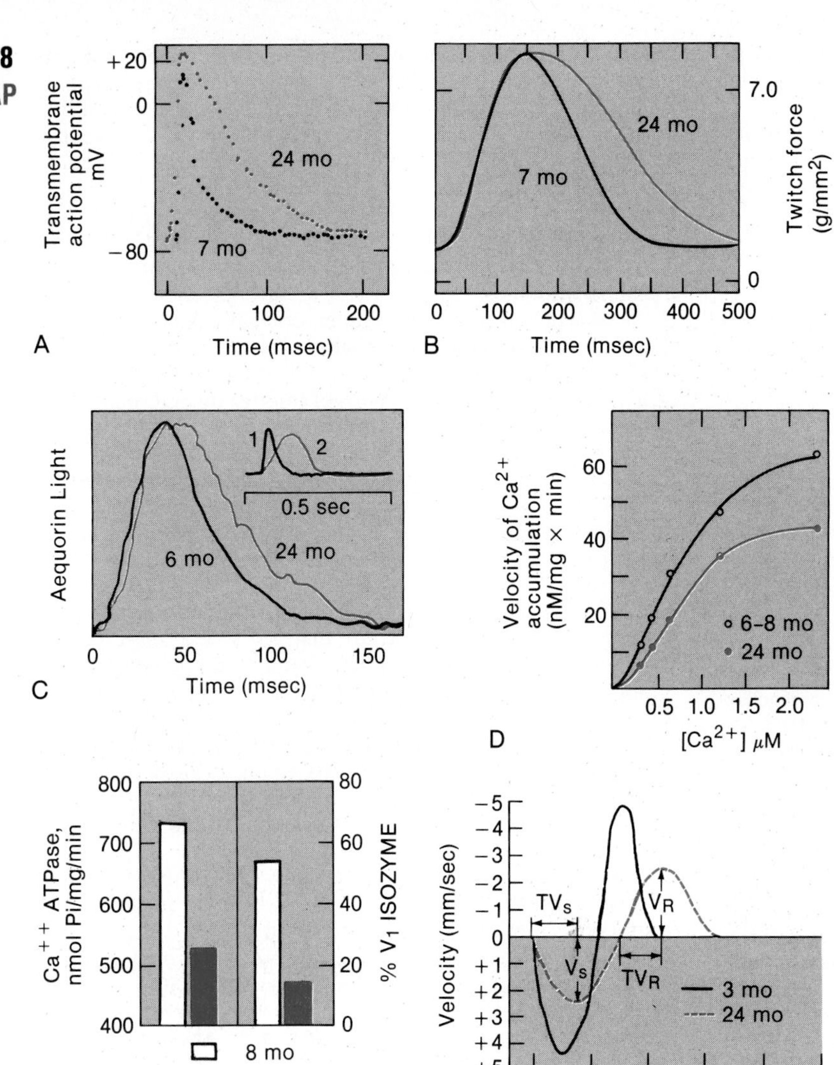

FIGURE 52–1. **Representative data depicting differences in various aspects of excitation-contraction coupling mechanisms in young adult (6 to 9 months) and senescent (24 to 26 months) rat hearts. *A,* Transmembrane action potential,[20] *B,* isometric contraction,[20] *C,* myoplasmic [Ca^{++}] transient,[31] *D,* sarcoplasmic reticulum Ca^{++} uptake rate,[21] *E,* Ca^{++}-stimulated ATPase activity, and myosin isozyme composition (50 per cent) of the heterodimer (V_2) are included in the total percentage of V_1,[23] and *F,* shortening velocity during highly loaded isotonic contractions.[24]**

possible explanation for the increase in the slope stiffness during contraction is as follows: at times during contraction when force is still increasing and myoplasmic [Ca^{++}] is decreasing, myoplasmic [Ca^{++}] remains higher in senescent than in younger muscles. This may result in a relative increase in Ca^{++}–myofilament interaction in senescent versus younger muscles during this phase of contraction, but not at earlier times. The steady-state myofilament response to Ca^{++} is not altered with age, and neither the maximum force nor the shape of the force-pCa relation differs with age.[19]

FORCE GENERATION. The amplitude of the twitch (Fig. 52–1*B*) and aequorin luminescence (Fig. 52–1*C*) do not decline in senescent muscles as long as the [Ca^{++}] in the superfusate is in the physiological range and the rate of stimulation is low. In addition, peak twitch force at relatively low rates of stimulation (6 to 48 min/liter) does not differ with age across a broad range of resting lengths.[18,20,21,24,26–28,31,36–38] Postextrasystolic twitch potentiation during continual paired stimulation also is preserved in senescent muscles.[39] The relatively low rates of stimulation required for studies in papillary muscles do not permit assessment of the extent of Ca^{++} release at rates approaching those in the rat in vivo (e.g., 300 per minute). In addition, the stability of isolated bulk muscle preparations requires that the temperature be maintained typically at 30°C or less. The maintenance of peak twitch force at low stimulation frequencies and temperature in senescent muscle may, in part, result from the prolonged myoplasmic [Ca^{++}] transient (Fig. 52–1*C*). In rat muscles bathed in physiological [Ca^{++}], in the absence of drugs the amplitude of Ca^{++} release and twitch force declines as the stimulation frequency is increased. The magnitude of this decline is not different in senescent and young adult muscles.[28] However, in bathing medium containing higher [Ca^{++}], whereas muscles from younger adult rats are able to produce the same Ca^{++} release and twitch force at low and higher rates of stimulation, at the higher stimulation rate, senescent muscles cannot.[28] In addition, in physiologic bathing Ca^{++} solution, when the coupling interval of paired stimulation is decreased below 200 msec, senescent, but not adult, muscles fail to generate a twitch response to the second stimulus.[26] These deficits of the senescent muscle may be related, in part, to the diminished Ca^{++} pumping rate by sarcoplasmic reticulum in senescent muscle (Fig. 52–1*D*).

CONTRACTILE PROTEINS

(See also p. 406)

A decrease in the rate of ATP hydrolysis has been observed in various contractile protein preparations isolated from the myocardium of aged as compared with younger animals.[19,22,36,40–43] The rate and extent of this decline vary with the particular preparation studied. The Ca^{++}-activated myosin ATPase activity has been found to decline progressively with age from maturation through senescence.[22,36,43a,43b] Myosin ATPase activity is modulated by the myosin heavy chain isoform type.[44] The percentage of the alpha heavy chain myosin (i.e., that which has the most rapid ATP hydrolytic rate [i.e., V_1 isomyosin]) declines progressively with age in rats from maturation through senescence, whereas the proportion of the beta myosin heavy chain with a slower ATP hydrolytic rate (V_3 isoform) progressively increases with age.[22,36] By 24 months of age V_1 constitutes less than 20 per cent of the total myosin content (Fig. 52–1*E*). This shift in myosin isoform (V_1 to V_3) is regulated at the transcriptional level, in part at least, as mRNA levels coding for the alpha and beta heavy chains markedly decrease and increase, respectively, with adult aging.[43a,43b,45]

The myosin isozyme shift to a greater percentage of V_3 with aging is accompanied by a reduction in the velocity of isotonic shortening (Fig. 52–1*F*).[24,40,46] In the isometric contraction, the time to peak tension and duration of the contraction are directly related to the percentage of V_3 or inversely related to the percentage of V_1.[22] The increase in the stiffness during the twitch in senescent versus younger adult rat cardiac muscle[23,25,35] might be related to differences in isozymes.

MORPHOLOGICAL PROPERTIES

The senescent Wistar rat heart exhibits moderate cardiac hypertrophy compared with hearts from young and middle-age animals.[6,35] This occurs in the absence of systemic hypertension.[47] In hearts of male Fischer 344 rats, collagen accumulates in relation to ventricular protein after 3 months of age and continues in that mode with increased age of the animal, leveling off at about 12 per cent at 22 to 26 months, a twofold increase over that at 1 month.[48] With advancing age papillary muscles of the left heart become fibrosed to a greater extent than in the right heart of Fischer rats.[48] In Wistar rats the average left ventricular collagen content doubles between adulthood and senescence.[37] Still, the volume fraction of collagen is less than 5 to 10 per cent of the cardiac mass. Collagen accumulates in intrinsic collagenous structures, including perimysial weaves, coiled perimysial fibers, and struts, where the preexisting fibers are thicker and more extensive. Regions of fibrosis also are increased in size and volume in older animals.[48] In the Sprague-Dawley strain an age-associated increase in the extent of myocardial fibrosis, involving 60 per cent of the rats at the time of spontaneous death, has been observed.[49] This fibrosis appears rather diffuse, with hypertrophied bundles intermingled among the fibrous tissue. The fibrosis is dispersed rather widely within the myocardium, but some concentration is noted in the subendocardial and subepicardial regions.

The majority of the increase in cardiac mass with aging in the Wistar rat can be explained by myocardial cell enlargement. In individual myocytes isolated from Wistar rats of 2, 6 to 9, and 24 to 25 months of age, the average myocyte length measured under high-power light microscopy increased from 133 μm at 2 months to 146 μm at 6 to 9 months to 162 μm at 24 to 25 months of age. The average slack sarcomere length does not vary with age. The average cell volume, measured by means of Coulter counter techniques, approximately doubles between 2 and 24 months.[50] In male Sprague-Dawley rats in the interval between 3 and 10 to 12 months the mean myocyte cell volume per nucleus increases 53 and 26 per cent in the left and the right ventricle, respectively. The total number of myocyte nuclei remains constant in either ventricle. By 19 to 20 months a further (39 per cent) cellular hypertrophy of the left ventricle of the heart occurs found in association with an 18 per cent loss in cell number. Cell loss was accompanied by discrete areas of interstitial and replacement fibrosis in the subendocardium.[7] In contrast to the left ventricle, in the right ventricle no focal myocardial damage was observed, and the measured 35 per cent additional enlargement of myocytes occurred without a change in cell number. These cellular changes in this strain over the age range occurred without an increase in the ratio of heart weight to body weight. Thus the aging left ventricle is composed of a smaller number of hypertrophied cells. As this strain, like the Wistar strain discussed above, is not hypertensive, the stimulus for cell loss and hypertrophy of remaining cells with aging is not known.

PASSIVE MUSCLE PROPERTIES

Classic studies of muscle mechanics denote as "passive"[51] those tissue properties that do not directly depend on excitation. These properties are important because they influence the rate, time course, and extent of shortening and force development. The manner in which the myofilaments are coupled to passive components of the tissue also is a determinant of the viscoelastic properties of muscle.[52,53] Even with detailed information on the amount of collagen, its physical characteristics, and the characteristics of the network weave, direct cause-effect relations between structural and functional alterations are difficult to substantiate.[18]

Estimation of the elastic or viscoelastic modulus is a more meaningful method of assessing passive muscle properties than measurement of resting force at L_{max} or examination of the passive length-tension curve.[54,55] No alteration in passive viscoelastic stiffness parameters can be demonstrated.[23,25,35] In intact ventricles of various species the effect of advanced age on the modulates of viscoelastic stiffness is inconclusive, with no change,[56] an increase,[57,58] and a decrease[59] having been observed.

SIMILARITIES BETWEEN AGING AND EXPERIMENTAL CARDIAC OVERLOAD IN YOUNGER ANIMALS

Many of the changes that occur with senescence in the normotensive rat also occur in the myocardium of younger animals in which experimental hypertension has caused cardiac hypertrophy (cf. ref. 60 for review). The strikingly similar pattern of alteration in excitation-contraction coupling mechanisms in the young hypertensive heart and those occurring in senescence are summarized in Table 52–1. The myocardial hypertrophy in pressure overload is a manifestation of an enhanced net protein synthesis owing to enlargement of a relatively constant number of cardiac myocytes, and reflects global activation of cardiac genes at the translational and posttranslational levels.[61] Because similar changes in cellular ribonucleic acid (RNA) concentration and the rate of protein synthesis have been observed with aging and chronic myocardial overload, it has been suggested that the latter (which usually is accompanied by myocardial hypertrophy) represents "accelerated aging."[62]

There is evidence that the signal that transduces the stress of an enhanced pressure load is mechanical (i.e., stretch or tension).[63–69] In this regard, stimulation of protein synthesis for both systolic and diastolic tension is described by a single linear function.[69] The tension effect may be mediated in part by enhanced coronary flow[70] or hormonal stimulation.[65,66,68,71] There is evidence for an interaction of stretch- and hormone receptor–mediated intracellular signal transduction (e.g., cyclic adenosine monophosphate [cAMP] or phosphatidylinositol turnover[66,72]) or ion flux (e.g., Na^{+}[63]), possibly related to stretch-induced activation of ionic channels.[73] Reorganization of intracellular matrix proteins, desmin and tubulin, also may mediate the stretch response.[74] Additionally, stretch of extracellular matrix and ventricular and cardiac endothelium may lead to the production of growth factors which can initiate protein synthesis.

It is tempting to speculate that because the *pattern* of changes in cell mechanisms occurs in both experimental pressure overload and aging, it may reflect a "logic" within the genome that regulates the expression of multiple genes for cellular adaptation to occur. This particular adaptive constellation allows for an energy-efficient and prolonged contraction. In the hypertensive heart it can be inferred that these adaptations occur in response to an increased afterload; however, with aging, whether the pattern that occurs is adaptive or degenerative is uncertain because the stimuli for these changes remain to be identified. If these changes were to occur in human myocardium with aging, they could easily be attributed to the stiffer arterial system and increases in arterial pressure and impedance. There is no data, however, to indicate that arterial stiffening or vascular impedance occurs with aging in rats, and the changes depicted in Table 52–1 have been described in two strains of rats that do not become hypertensive with aging.[7,47] Although peripheral resistance increases with age in rats, it appears to plateau at 10 to 12 months (cf. ref. 18 for review) and cannot be directly related to the changes in Figure 52–1, which are progressive with advancing age.

The increased left ventricular mass that occurs in the Wistar strain with

TABLE 52–1 ALTERATIONS OF CARDIAC MUSCLE FUNCTION IN AGING AND HYPERTENSION

FUNCTIONAL MEASURE	EXPERIMENTAL LV PRESSURE LOADING	NORMOTENSIVE
Contraction duration	↑	↑
Contraction velocity	↓	↓
Myosin isozyme composition	↓ V_1, ↑ V_3	↓ V_1, ↑ V_3
Sarcoplasmic reticulum Ca^{++} pumping rate	↓	↓
Cytosolic Ca^{++} transient duration	↑ (Ferret)	↑
Myofilament Ca^{++} sensitivity	↔	↔
Action potential repolarization time	↑	↑
β-Adrenergic inotropic response	↓	↓
Cardiac glycoside response	↓	↓

The phenotypic pattern of adult aging bears a striking resemblance to that of experimental pressure loading in young animals and suggests that the molecular mechanisms may be similar in both cases.[60]

aging is largely due to an increase in left ventricular cavity size with the wall thickness appearing to remain normal.[5] Still, as is the case in the young hypertensive rodent, cardiac myocytes become enlarged in the senescent heart, and it may be argued that mechanical hormonal stimulation for cardiac hypertrophic response is present within the aging heart. It may be hypothesized that the dropout of myocardial cells with aging leads to augmented stretch on the remaining cells, and that this is the stimulus for cellular hypertrophy and the adaptive mechanisms that accompany this hypertrophy, as identified for the hypertensive heart, lead to a prolonged efficient contraction. On the other hand, prolonged contraction with aging persists in transplanted, mechanically unloaded atrophied hearts and also in right ventricular muscle in which no cell dropout has been observed.[7]

CHANGES IN THE THYROID STATE. Alterations of thyroid status can produce alterations in the variables depicted in Figure 52–2 (see also Chap. 61). In this regard the changes observed in the aging heart mimic to some extent those observed in the hypothyroid state.[44,75–77] Whether a relative hypothyroid state accompanies aging is uncertain. An age-associated decline in plasma thyroxine levels occurs in at least two rat strains,[22,78] but the magnitude of the decline is small. Still, it has been reported that administration of sufficient thyroxine to restore plasma levels in older rats to those levels that occur in younger rats can abolish the age-associated decline in myosin ATPase activity[78]; however, reversal of the isozyme pattern did not occur with small doses of thyroxine.[78] High doses of thyroxine for a short period of time can increase the myosin V_1 content of senescent hearts but cannot fully restore this to the level observed in the younger heart.[22] Thus failure of cells to respond to thyroxine (e.g., deficits in nuclear receptors or DNA binding sites) may occur with aging and, in part, underlie the pattern of change depicted in Table 52–1.

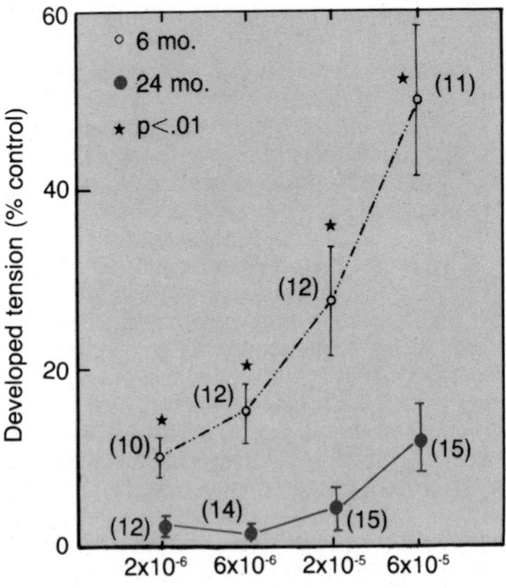

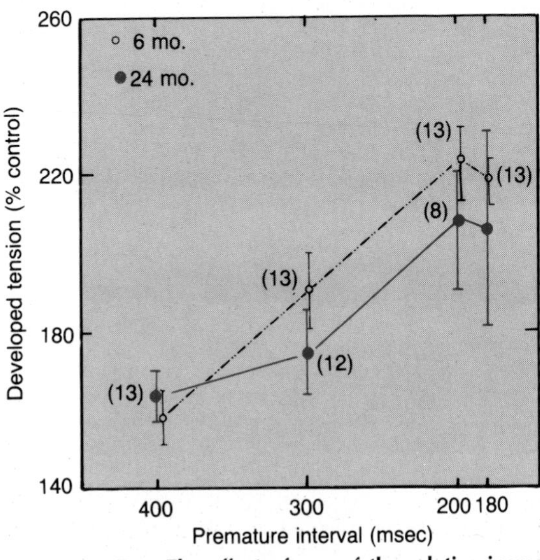

FIGURE 52–2. *Top,* The effect of age of the relative increase on twitch tension in response to incremental concentrations of ouabain in isolated left ventricular trabeculae from 6- to 24-month-old rats. Before drug, twitch tension did not vary with age. *Bottom,* Same muscles show no decrease in inotropic response to post extrasystolic potentiation. (From Gerstenblith, G., et al.: Diminished inotropic responsiveness to ouabain in aged rat myocardium. Circ. Res. *44*:577, 1979, by permission of the American Heart Association, Inc.)

GLUCOSE INTOLERANCE. This has been observed to occur in aged rats[79] and could possibly relate to some of the alterations noted in Table 52–1 because, in rats made diabetic, marked shifts occur in the myosin isoform pattern (increases in V_3 isoform) and in actomyosin and ATPase activity.[80–82] Additionally, the sarcoplasmic reticulum Ca^{++} ATPase activity and Ca^{++} uptake of isolated sarcoplasmic reticulum are depressed in diabetic hearts,[83–85] and the contraction time is prolonged.[86]

PHYSICAL CONDITIONING EFFECTS ON SENESCENT CARDIAC MUSCLE

A reduction of physical activity occurs with age even in rats in captivity.[87,88] Many of the cardiac mechanisms depicted in Figure 52–1 can be modulated by physical conditioning, and physical conditioning of older animals has been shown to modify some of the changes in Table 52–1 but not others.[89]

Chronic exercise in senescent rats abolishes prolonged contraction and reduces the active dynamic stiffness without altering myocardial mass.[24] This chronic (5 months' duration), mild wheel exercise protocol, which was insufficient to alter the body or heart weight in adult (6 to 9 months) and senescent (24 to 26 months) rats at sacrifice, did not alter twitch amplitude in isolated left ventricular trabecular measured across a range of [Ca^{++}] at either age. In the younger animals, this exercise protocol was ineffective in altering the duration of contraction or dynamic stiffness measured during contraction in muscles. In senescent muscles, however, it eliminated the age-associated increase in these parameters to the levels observed in the younger adult muscle. The reduction in both the slope stiffness coefficient and duration of contraction is consistent with an effect of exercise to reduce the duration of the myoplasmic Ca^{++} transient. Indeed, recent studies suggest that the duration of the Ca^{++} transient in senescent cardiac muscle is reduced after chronic exercise.[90] The reduced rate of sarcoplasmic reticulum Ca^{++} sequestration in the senescent heart also can be reversed by chronic physical conditioning.[91]

BIOCHEMICAL CHANGES. A greater relative effect of chronic exercise on some other aspects of cardiac biochemistry in senescent as compared with young adult rat myocardium also has been observed. Although chronic exercise usually does not augment cytochrome *c* oxidase activity in cardiac muscle of younger animals as it does in skeletal muscle,[92] a modest augmentation of cytochrome *c* oxidase has been observed in hearts of senescent animals.[92] This was accompanied by exercise-induced increases in the rates of glutamate-malate, palmitoylcarnitine, and succinate oxidation.[92] Thus, exercise can partially reverse the decline in the oxidation.[92]

Marked age-related declines in cardiac aldolase and superoxide dismutase activities in mice between 9 and 27 months are prevented by chronic exercise begun at 6 months of age and continued into old age.[94] The progressive decline in myocardial Ca^{++}-activated actomyosin ATPase activity that begins during maturation (after 1 month in the rat) and progresses with advancing adult age can be retarded by a chronic (3 months) period of exercise. This relatively small, beneficial effect of exercise, however, was observed only through 12 to 15 months.[94] In older animals that began exercise at 17 to 22 months and were sacrificed at 20 to 25 months, a decline in this ATPase occurred.[95] The altered myosin isoform profile in the senescent heart is not affected by chronic physical conditioning.[96] The insulin resistance of the aging rat also is ameliorated by chronic exercise,[79] as is the response of senescent cardiac muscle to reoxygenation after hypoxia.[97]

RESPONSE OF THE OLDER HEART TO CHRONIC HEMODYNAMIC OVERLOAD

Whereas the relative adaptive response of the senescent versus younger heart to moderate exercise is enhanced, the response to mechanical stresses that evoke substantial myocardial hypertrophy (e.g., pressure or volume overload) appears, in some instances, to be reduced. The extent of hypertrophy after aortic banding,[98] volume overload,[99] or the creation of renal hypertension[36] in senescent rats appears to be reduced. (In the latter study the significance is unclear, because of four groups tested, one younger age group also showed a reduction in the extent of hypertrophy. Additionally, a subsequent study in the same pressure-loading model of the same rat strain observed that the hypertrophic response of senescent heart was not decreased.[100]) The extent to which myosin isoform ATPase activity, action potential, and contraction duration become altered appears to be correlated with the extent of hypertrophy, regardless of age.[36] The hypertrophic response to chronic AV block, causing a 50 per cent reduction in heart rate and 50 per cent hypertrophy, decreases with age and is accompanied by a reduced contractile adaptation.[101] Furthermore, the contractile response to stressful conditions (high pacing rate and high bathing calcium concentration) is reduced in senescent hearts that had responded to mild aortic banding[102] with an appropriate degree of hypertrophy.

Thus it appears that the adaptive reserve capacity with respect to an increase in cardiac mass may become diminished with advancing age. This may indicate that some cardiac adaptations (e.g., an increase in myocyte size or heart size) become utilized with aging such that the reserve capacity of the aged heart to respond to these stressful situations is diminished. This could be in part related to cell death and fibrosis when cell size becomes limiting, owing to ischemia or inadequacy of cell ionic or energy homeostasis for other reasons. A relative reduction in the extent of cardiac hypertrophy in response to a given increment of arterial pressure also could indicate age-associated reduction in the efficiency of global activation of protein synthesis.

DIMINISHED MYOCARDIAL RESPONSE TO BETA-ADRENOCEPTOR STIMULATION

Although the effect of beta-adrenergic agonists to abbreviate the duration of contraction duration is not age-related in isolated cardiac cells, muscle, or perfused rat myocardium, their effect to enhance contractile force is diminished.[27,38,103] Age-related changes that are, in part, distal to the receptor-cyclase system are required to explain the diminished myocardial contractile response to isoproterenol. Neither the number of myocardial beta receptors nor their affinity for antagonists or for isoproterenol appears to be altered with age, and neither basal levels of cAMP nor the increased level achieved during the peak contractile response were age-related. Furthermore, the age-related deficit in enhancement of contractility observed with isoproterenol persisted when dibutyryl cAMP was used as the agonist. Dibutyryl cAMP bypasses the receptor-cyclase system. Neither basal nor stimulated levels of protein kinase activity in the same myocardial preparations in which the contractile responses were studied varied with age. Thus, an explanation for the depressed inotropic response is that one or more steps distal to protein kinase activation differ with age. The possibilities include differences in the extent of phosphorylation of various proteins or differences in ion flux or binding that results from a given level of phosphorylation, or age differences in phosphoprotein phosphatase activity, an enzyme that dephosphorylates proteins and organelles. An age-associated deficit in the ability of norepinephrine to augment troponin I phosphorylation has recently been observed.[104] This was attributed, however, to an apparent net decrease in cAMP production. A 20 per cent increase in phosphoprotein phosphatase activity in the senescent heart has been measured.[38] Enhanced adenosine in coronary effluent isolated from older versus younger rats has been observed and has been related to a reduction in the response to beta-adrenergic stimulation in these hearts.[105] An alternative explanation (i.e., that the Ca^{++}-myofilament interaction that leads to force production is altered with age) can be excluded, since in both intact and skinned preparations[19] the effect of Ca^{++} on force production, from threshold to maximum, is not altered with age.

DIMINISHED RESPONSE TO DIGITALIS GLYCOSIDES

The contractile response to ouabain is diminished in the senescent as compared with the adult myocardium (Fig. 52–2, *top*).[41] The response to paired stimulation (which causes a much greater increase in contractility than ouabain) in the same muscles is not age-related (Fig. 52–2, *bottom*). Thus, the depressed response to ouabain of senescent muscle cannot readily be attributed to a nonspecific failure of the excitation-contraction process, to an inability of the myofilaments to generate additional force, or to a failure in energy necessary for a sustained inotropic response. The mechanism for the effect of age may be at the Na^+, K^+-ATPase receptor (p. 480, i.e., an age-related difference in receptor density, ouabain binding, resultant enzyme inhibition) or in the extent of enhanced Ca^{++} loading caused by this inhibition. The relative ouabain inhibition of Na^+, K^+-ATPase in crude membrane preparations is not dependent on age over the adult range.[41] In the intact senescent (11 to 13 years) beagle, as compared with the adult (1 to 3 years) dog, a decrement in the contractile response to acetylstrophanthidin with no difference in glycoside Na^+, K^+-ATPase inhibition also has been demonstrated.[106]

SUMMARY OF ANIMAL STUDIES

Most information regarding age of the myocardium comes from studies in the rat model. Isometric force production, at least at low frequencies of stimulation, is preserved. There is no clear-cut indication that passive stiffness is increased. Whereas the affinity of the myofibrils for Ca^{++} is preserved in senescent muscle, the inotropic responses to cardiac glycosides and beta-adrenergic stimulation are reduced. The latter may underlie, in part, the alterations in cardiodynamics (i.e., greater utilization of the Frank-Starling mechanism) during vigorous exercise in older men. In senescence, contraction is prolonged in part because the Ca^{++} released into the myoplasm during systole is removed more slowly than in the younger heart. A major cause of this appears to be a reduced rate of Ca^{++} sequestration by the sarcoplasmic reticulum. Although the duration of action potential also is longer in senescent than in younger cardiac muscle, its role in the prolonged contraction is less clear. The action potential changes could reflect age-related changes in the sarcolemmal ionic conductances or be the result of the prolonged myoplasmic Ca^{++} transient. In the older rat heart, myosin isozymes shift to slower forms and ATPase activity declines. These changes appear to underlie the observed decline in shortening velocity in senescent muscle contracting in the isotonic mode. The interrelated alterations in excitation-contraction mechanisms and myofibrillar biochemistry that occur in senescence are adaptive. The same constellation of changes is observed in the myocardium of young rats in which myocardial hypertrophy is induced by chronic hypertension or aortic banding. Some of these changes (e.g., the prolonged contraction duration and decline in sarcoplasmic reticulum pumping ability) can be reversed by chronic exercise in senescent animals.

CARDIAC FUNCTION IN NORMAL AGING HUMANS

The effect of age on cardiac function in humans can be addressed only in the context of the population studied and the variable used to define and measure cardiac function. One of the most consistent findings in studies of the influence of aging is the large variation in the older population for nearly every cardiovascular variable. There are many older people whose measured performance is equal to, or in some instances superior to, their middle-aged counterparts as well as some who are considerably below the mean for their age group. This variation must be related to differences in factors other than age which influence cardiovascular performance. The most important of these are the presence of cardiovascular disease, primarily hypertension and coronary atherosclerosis, and physical conditioning status. Therefore, the results of studies in humans must be related to the certainty of freedom from the effects of superimposed disease and the physical conditioning status of the subjects. This is particularly true when quantitating the "effect of age" on measured left ventricular performance.

ASSESSMENT OF PERFORMANCE

Another equally important consideration is the measured variable. Although maximum oxygen consumption is considered to be the best index of cardiovascular performance, there are several potential difficulties in determining the age effect on this important parameter. The first is that to be certain that any person's oxygen consumption during exercise is the maximum, it is necessary to demonstrate no significant increase in oxygen consumption despite an increase in workload. This often is not found in studies of older age groups, and suggests that musculoskeletal or some other noncardiovascular parameters are limiting exercise before the true maximum oxygen consumption can be achieved. Even if a plateau is reached, it is possible that age differences in muscle mass or in the ability of the muscles to extract and use oxygen may be the limiting factor rather than cardiovascular function per se. This is suggested by recent evidence that age differences in maximum oxygen consumption are minimized or abolished when the values are adjusted for lean body mass.[107]

Studies of "normal" aging have been handicapped until recently by a natural reluctance to use invasive methodology in people who are thought to be free of cardiovascular disease. This resulted in two major limitations in some earlier work. The first is that it was difficult to exclude patients with occult coronary disease. This is an important consideration because the prevalence of autopsy-documented disease is much higher than the prevalence of clinically obvious disease.[2,108,109] Many people thought to be free of coronary disease on screening using routine history, physical examination, and resting electrocardiogram undoubtedly were not. Because there is an age-related increase in the incidence of inapparent disease, many older study participants with latent coronary disease were included in study protocols. A second limitation resulting from the hesitancy to use invasive methodology was an inability to measure central circulatory function (i.e., stroke volume or its determinants, end-diastolic and end-systolic volumes) in relatively large numbers of volunteers. The recent introduction of nuclear cardiology techniques, specifically the use of thallium scintigraphy to diagnose the presence of coronary disease, and gated blood pool scans to measure

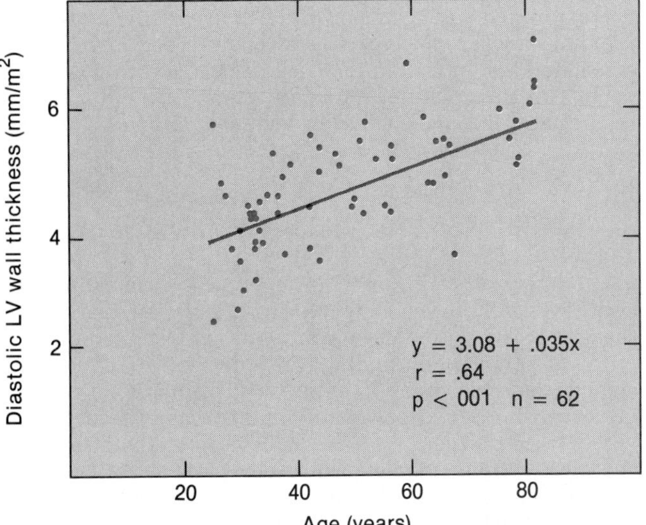

FIGURE 52–3. Linear regression plot of the relationship between age and diastolic left ventricular wall thickness (mm/M²) in male participants of the Baltimore Longitudinal Aging Population. Increased age is associated with mild left ventricular hypertrophy.[116] (From Gerstenblith, G., Frederiksen, J., Yin, V.C.P., et al.: Echocardiographic assessment of a normal adult aging population. Circulation *56*:273, 1977, reprinted by permission of the American Heart Association, Inc.)

cardiac volumes during exercise, provided significant additional information concerning the effect of normal aging on cardiac function during rest and exercise stress.

HEMODYNAMICS AT REST: NO CHANGE IN STROKE VOLUME OR EJECTION FRACTION. Although invasive studies have indicated that aging is associated with a decline in cardiac output at rest,[110–112] these results may have been due to the selection of subjects not free of disease or to the methodology used. Cardiac output may increase more in younger people because of an age difference in the stress response to the invasive procedure itself. Several studies using noninvasive techniques have shown no age-related decrement in cardiac output, heart rate, stroke volume, or ejection fraction at rest.[113–116]

One of the more significant age-associated changes in resting cardiovascular parameters is an increase in systolic arterial pressure (Fig. 28–3, p. 820). This is probably secondary to age-associated changes in arterial stiffening, since the rise in blood pressure varies directly with vascular stiffness in different populations.[117] The increased systolic pressure is probably responsible, in part, for the mild left ventricular hypertrophy associated with aging (Fig. 52–3)[116,118]; it also is seen in laboratory animals, as discussed earlier. This hypertrophy tends to normalize wall stress and may preserve indices of left ventricular function, including resting ejection fraction and the velocity of circumferential fiber shortening.[116] Apart from the increase in systolic pressure, the most striking and consistent change in resting indices is a slowed, delayed, and more heterogeneous pattern of early diastolic filling.[119–121] This is probably due to prolonged cardiac muscle relaxation, and is a consistent characteristic of aging which has been found in many species and experimental preparations, as discussed above. Increased mitral valve stiffness also may play a role. The functional importance of this alteration under normal conditions is not great, since end-diastolic volume is either not age-related or slightly increased with age at rest[113,116,122] and during exercise.[113] However, it probably renders older persons more susceptible to hemodynamic compromise in the presence of a tachycardiac arrhythmic stress[123] or in the presence of superimposed ischemic or hypertensive disease, both of which independently impair diastolic filling.

HEMODYNAMICS DURING EXERCISE: LOWER HEART RATE AND GREATER END-SYSTOLIC AND END-DIASTOLIC VOLUMES. In contrast to the subtle age effect on resting hemodynamic indices, there are more dramatic changes during exercise stress. Most investigators have reported a decline in maximum oxygen uptake and heart rate with aging,[124] even in athletes.[125] Several have reported a decline in exercise cardiac output with increasing age because of a decrease in both heart rate and stroke volume.[111,112] In one study in persons carefully screened to eliminate ischemic heart disease, no age effect was found on cardiac output at comparable and peak workloads because an increase in stroke volume compensated for the decline in heart rate in the older people.[113] In this study end-systolic and end-diastolic volumes also were measured, and the increase in stroke volume was achieved by greater use of the Frank-Starling mechanism (i.e., an increase in end-diastolic volume). Additionally, in younger people there was greater systolic emptying with a decrease in end-systolic volume, as compared with the resting values (Fig. 52–4). Ejection fraction increased more from rest to exercise in younger than in older people. In most older people who were free of disease ejection fraction did increase with exercise, but by only a small amount.

These age-associated changes in the mechanisms used to augment cardiac output with exercise can be interpreted in the light of data showing an age-associated decrease in the inotropic,[27,38] chronotropic,[126] and arterial vasodilating effects of catecholamine stimulation.[127,128] During exercise, heart rate increases less in older people, probably, in part, because of a decreased cardiovascular response to catecholamines (Fig. 52–4). End-systolic volume (Fig. 52–4) also decreases less, owing to a diminished inotropic and vasodilating re-

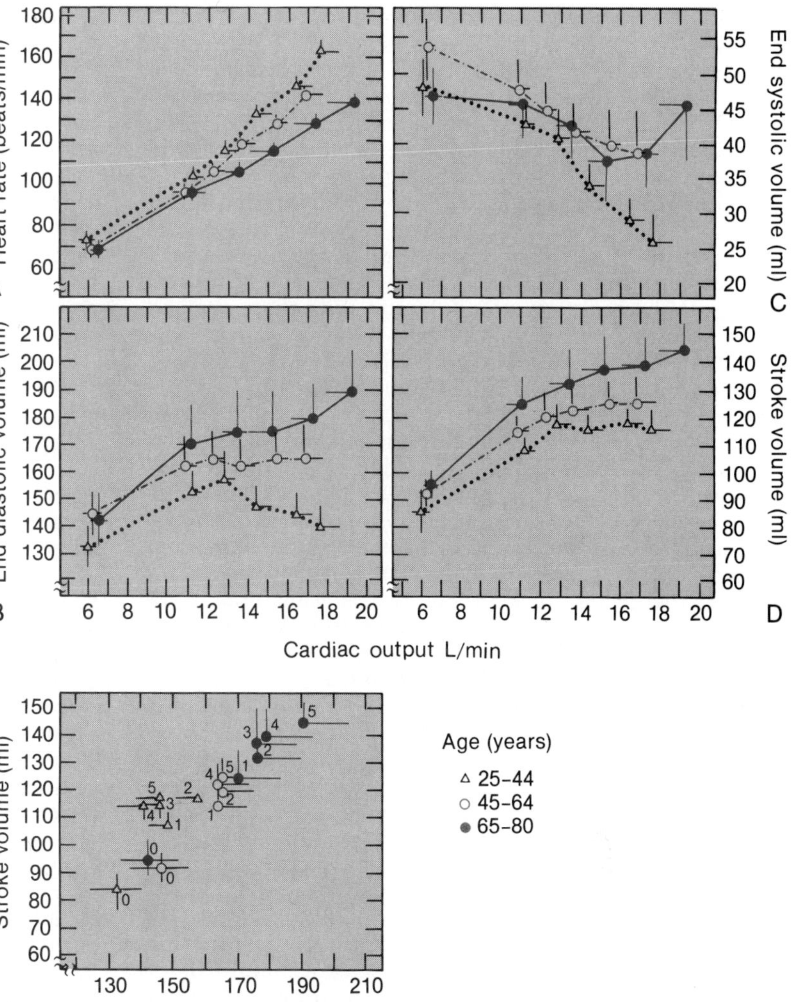

FIGURE 52-4. The relationship between cardiac output (plotted in L/min along the abscissa in Panels A to D) and heart rate (Panel A), end-diastolic volume (Panel B), end-systolic volume (Panel C), and stroke volume (Panel D) and the stroke volume–end-diastolic volume relationship (Panel E) at rest and during graded upright bicycle exercise measured by means of gated blood pool scans. The subjects are divided into three age groups, 25 to 44 years old (n = 22), 45 to 64 years old (n = 23), and 65 to 79 years old (n = 16). The number of subjects able to complete the exercise periods decreased with increasing workload; at a workload of 125 watts, n = 16 in group 1, n = 15 in group 2, and n = 11 in group 3. When the data were analyzed including only those who were able to achieve the 125 watt workload, a similar pattern was observed in all parameters and the significance of the age effect was unchanged. (From Rodeheffer, R. J., Gerstenblith, G., Becker, L. C., et al.: Exercise cardiac output is maintained with advancing age in healthy human subjects: Cardiac dilatation and increased stroke volume compensate for a diminished heart rate. Circulation *69:*203, 1984, reprinted by permission of the American Heart Association, Inc.)

sponse to catecholamines.[113] Finally, the benefit of the Frank-Starling mechanism is unaltered with age and used effectively during exercise to maintain output through a higher stroke volume at a greater end-diastolic volume (Fig. 52–4*B* and *D*).[113] The decrease in catecholamine-mediated effects during exercise is probably not caused by decreased elaboration of catecholamines, since plasma levels are higher, not lower, in humans during exercise.[129]

AGING, DISEASE, AND CARDIAC FUNCTION

ISCHEMIC HEART DISEASE

DIAGNOSIS. The prevalence and severity of coronary atherosclerosis increase so dramatically with age that more than one-half of all deaths in people aged 65 years or older are due to coronary disease and about three-fourths of all deaths from ischemic heart disease occur in the elderly.[130] The diagnosis of ischemic heart disease may be more difficult in the older person, since the prevalence of diagnosed disease[109] is only one-third to one-half the prevalence of autopsy-documented significant atherosclerosis.[108] The lack of classic symptomatology may be related to an age-associated decline in physical activity to the point at which ischemic symptoms are not present. In addition, dyspnea, rather than pain, may be the most prominent feature of the clinical picture in angina as well as infarction (p. 1293),[131] possibly because of the age-related changes in myocardial and pericardial compliance and diastolic relaxation discussed above. The physical examination is of limited usefulness in the diagnosis of ischemic heart disease. It should be remembered, however, that the transient features associated with acute ischemia (i.e., an S_4 gallop, reversed splitting of the second sound, and a systolic murmur owing to mitral regurgitation) often are present in older people, even in the absence of ischemia.[132–134]

Stress testing (Chap. 6) also is useful in the diagnosis of an older patient with suspected coronary disease but with certain caveats. The presence of resting ST-segment abnormalities or the use of digitalis, both of which are more common in the elderly, may invalidate the interpretation of the stress electrocardiogram, and in this setting stress testing using thallium scintigraphy is helpful. Thallium imaging also is helpful when the stress test is unexpectedly negative in an older person whose history suggests the presence of ischemia, since the predictive accuracy of a negative test is low in a population with a high prevalence of disease. Finally, many elderly patients may not be capable of exercising to 85 to 90 per cent of their predicted maximal heart rate. In this setting a thallium scan after dipyridamole administration may provide similar diagnostic information.[135]

MANAGEMENT OF CHRONIC ISCHEMIC HEART DISEASE (see also Chap. 40). The approaches to treatment of angina in older and younger patients are similar. After diagnosis, reversible factors should be identified and treated. Of these, anemia, hyperthyroidism, hypertension, congestive heart failure, and supraventricular arrhythmias may all be more common in the elderly. It also should be remembered that atherosclerosis is a progressive disease, and that although it has been stated that risk factor reduction is less important in the older patient, more recent evidence suggests that both successful treatment of hypertension[136,137] and smoking cessation[138] decrease cardiovascular mortality in the elderly. The use of specific anti-ischemic agents is discussed below. If medical therapy fails to adequately control symptoms, percutaneous transluminal coronary angioplasty (PTCA) should be considered. Although some reports indicate that in-hospital mortality associated with PTCA is higher in older than in younger patients,[139] low mortality (0.8 per cent) also has been reported, which does not differ from that in younger patients.[140] If the coronary anatomy is not suitable for PTCA in patients in whom medical therapy has failed, surgery should be performed. Although coronary bypass is associated with increased perioperative mortality[141] and morbidity and longer duration of hospitalization, as well as increased costs in the older patient,[142] the risks of complications are decreasing[143] and long-term pain relief and survival are good.[143,144] In most patients these results compare favorably with those attained with medical therapy (Fig. 52–5).[145]

MANAGEMENT OF ACUTE MYOCARDIAL INFARCTION (see also Chap. 39). The treatment of acute infarction should be undertaken with the realization that the risk of mortality, congestive heart failure, pulmonary edema, and ventricular rupture is higher in the elderly.[146–148] It is unclear whether the increased incidence of these complications is due to intrinsic age-related changes in the response to the ischemic insult itself, poorer reserve in the remaining noninfarcted regions, perhaps owing to diminished catecholamine responsiveness, the higher prevalence of hypertension, prior myocardial damage, and/or large infarctions. In addition, important topographical changes develop hours to days after an infarction which importantly affect overall mortality and morbidity. Animal and clinical studies have defined regional dilatation and wall thinning at the site of the infarction,[149] and compensatory hypertrophy may occur in the region remote from the infarction. Age-related differences in these architectural changes accompanying an infarction could result from preexisting changes in left ventricular wall thickness,[116,118] peripheral impedance,[127] collagen content,[37] capability of undergoing compensatory hypertrophy, and/or the inflammatory and healing response to the infarct itself.

The demonstration that coronary thrombus is present in a large proportion of patients with early transmural infarction[150] has prompted a number of placebo-controlled randomized studies evaluating the ability of thrombolytic therapy to improve survival.[151–155] These studies also show a several fold, age-related increase in mortality in patients assigned to placebo therapy. Although the magnitude of the benefit confirmed by thrombolytic therapy has been reported to be low in patients over 75 years of age,[151] other studies indicate large survival differences for those over age 65.[152–154] The prevalence of contraindications to thrombolytic treatment increases with age, particularly hypertension, history of stroke, and gastrointestinal bleeding.

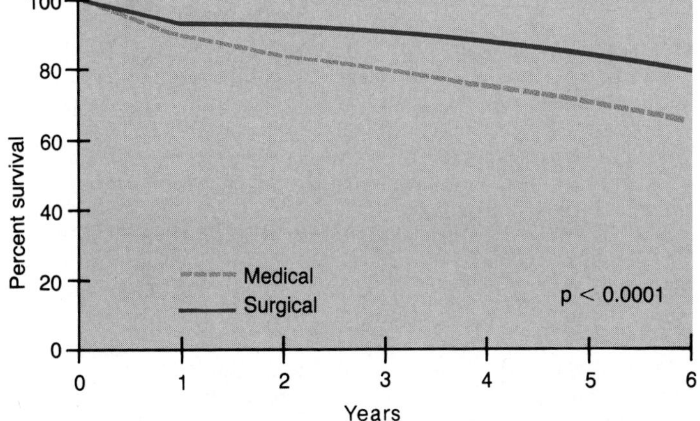

FIGURE 52–5. Cumulative 6-year survival in surgical and medical groups in 1491 patients 65 years or older from the CASS registry. Survival is adjusted for left ventricular wall motion, congestive heart failure, number of diseased vessels, number of associated medical diseases, and age at angiography. (Reprinted with permission from Gersh, B. J., Kronmal, R. A., Schaff, H. V., et al.: Comparison of coronary artery bypass surgery and medical therapy in patients 65 years of age or older. N. Engl. J. Med. *313*:217, 1985.)

Additional considerations regarding treatment of acute myocardial infarction include the higher likelihood of central nervous system side effects from lidocaine[156] and an increased risk of heparin-induced bleeding in older women.[157] The elderly benefit as much as younger patients do from the secondary prevention effects of beta blockade.[158] In a Netherlands multicenter double-blind randomized trial involving more than 800 patients over the age of 60 years, oral anticoagulation was associated with a significantly lower incidence of recurrent myocardial infarction and death.[159] Successful aggressive management of complications, including septal rupture,[160] also has been reported.

ARRHYTHMIAS

(See also Chap. 24)

In part because of the increasing prevalence of hypertension and coronary disease, arrhythmias occur more frequently and more often are associated with hemodynamic compromise in the older age groups. In one study the incidences of supraventricular and ventricular ectopic activity (>100 beats/24 hours of ambulatory monitoring) were 26 per cent and 17 per cent, respectively, in 98 healthy subjects 60 to 85 years of age.[161] Ventricular couplets occurred in 11 per cent but ventricular tachycardia in only 4 per cent of the population. The incidence of asymptomatic ventricular tachycardia on routine treadmill testing in elderly people without other evidence of organic heart disease has been reported to be 4 per cent.[162] These arrhythmias were not associated with symptoms or subsequent sudden death. It should be recognized, however, that arrhythmias may be more ominous in the presence of disease. Even in the absence of disease, slowed and delayed early diastolic relaxation and filling owing to age alone[119,120] may result in greater compromised cardiac output in the older person with a tachyarrhythmia. Any compromise of cardiac output and blood pressure may, in turn, be associated with more critical decreases in cerebral flow in the older patient because of impaired cardiovascular reflex responses to hypotension,[122] an increased likelihood of preexisting cerebrovascular disease, and increased vascular stiffness.

The diagnosis of an arrhythmia in an older patient differs only in that the index of suspicion should perhaps be higher for any complaints relating to transient cerebral ischemia, angina, heart failure, or mental status changes. Long-term ambulatory monitoring often is useful. The urgency of therapy depends on the associated hemodynamic changes, and emergency treatment is the same in all age groups. The routine work-up should include a search for reversible precipitating factors. Some of these, including electrolyte imbalance, digitalis excess, hyperthyroidism, anemia, pulmonary embolism, and congestive heart failure, are more common in the older population. Specific therapy for the arrhythmia is guided by the severity of associated symptoms, the presence and type of underlying heart disease, and the recognition of the age-associated changes in the pharmacokinetics of the antiarrhythmic drugs, as discussed below.

BRADYARRHYTHMIAS. Sinus bradycardia often is present in older people in both the presence and absence of cardiac disease. It may be related to age-associated histological changes in the sinus node, a hypersensitive carotid sinus reflex, or medications, including digitalis, calcium- or beta-blocking drugs, and some other antihypertensives. Evaluation should be undertaken if the patient is symptomatic, and in this instance it is important to determine whether the transient symptoms are in fact caused by the bradyarrhythmia, since other causes for neurological symptoms often are present in this age group. Long-term ambulatory monitoring is most useful in this regard. If the patient is symptomatic, immediate therapy depends on the degree of hemodynamic compromise. Emergency temporary measures, including the administration of atropine and isoproterenol and the insertion of a temporary pacemaker, can be used. If no reversible factors are present, the only effective long-term therapy is permanent pacing. Pacemakers which allow for proper sequencing of atrial and ventricular events may be particularly useful in the elderly because of an increased reliance on late diastolic filling and hence atrial systole.

VALVULAR HEART DISEASE

(See also Chap. 34)

The diagnosis of valvular heart disease in the elderly often is obscured by age-related but benign systolic murmurs,[134] changes in S_2, and increased stiffness of the central arteries. This stiffness may prevent the appearance of the slow anacrotic shoulder and small pulse pressure which would otherwise be seen in significant *aortic stenosis*. The other findings, however, particularly in the presence of a late-peaking systolic murmur, electrocardiographic evidence of left ventricular hypertrophy, and echocardiographic demonstration of valve narrowing and calcification, all retain their significance. Doppler examination may be particularly useful in assessing the severity of obstruction.[163] The usual causes are calcification of a congenitally bicuspid valve and, in those over 75 years of age, degenerative calcification.[164] Aortic valve replacement should be recommended for the usual indications (i.e., syncope, angina, and failure) and is associated with low mortality and excellent results in terms of quality of life.[165,166] Balloon aortic valvuloplasty (p. 1376) provides only palliative relief in patients with aortic stenosis,[167] and should be considered only in those with definite contraindications to surgery.

The diagnosis of *aortic regurgitation* is not more difficult in the older age groups, but the timing of aortic valve replacement may be because of the often benign course of the disease. Surgery usually is recommended only for those patients who continue to be symptomatic on medical therapy.

Mitral stenosis usually is due to rheumatic disease, whereas regurgitation can be due to rheumatic disease as well as calcification of the mitral annulus, mitral valve prolapse (at times with superimposed endocarditis), and ischemic papillary muscle dysfunction. Survival is considerably shortened in the presence of atrial fibrillation and failure,[168] and the results of mitral valve surgery are satisfactory.[169,170] Balloon mitral valvuloplasty in elderly patients with heavily calcified valves is associated with slightly higher morbidity and mortality than in younger patients with pliable valves and no subvalvular stenosis.

HYPERTENSION

(See also Chap. 28)

The importance of the diagnosis and effective treatment of hypertension in the elderly cannot be overemphasized. It is the major remediable risk factor for cardiovascular morbidity and mortality, and successful therapy decreases the incidence of death and cerebrovascular events.[137,171–176,176a,176b] The prevalence of hypertension, defined by a blood pressure of 160/95 or greater, is 30 per cent in elderly men, and an additional 10 to 15 per cent of the total elderly population have isolated systolic hypertension, defined by a systolic pressure exceeding 160 mm Hg and a diastolic of less than 90 mm Hg. Convincing evidence of the effectiveness of therapy for even mild diastolic hypertension in the elderly is provided by the results of the Hypertension Detection and Follow-up Program Trial[136] (a 17.2 per cent reduction in mortality and 45 per cent reduction in cerebrovascular events), the Australian National Blood Pressure Study[172] (a 30 per cent reduction in trial end points), and the European Working Party on High Blood Pressure in the Elderly Trial.[137] In the latter study there were a 38 per cent reduction in cardiac mortality and a 27 per cent reduction in total cardiovascular mortality using an intention-to-treat analysis.

There are no data concerning the effectiveness of therapy for isolated systolic hypertension. However, in view of the fact that systolic blood pressure is the best discriminator of risk in people over age 45[176] and that systolic blood pressure can be controlled effectively with minimal side effects,[177] the Joint National Committee on Detection, Evaluation, and Treatment of High Blood Pressure has recommended that therapy be instituted in the elderly with isolated systolic hypertension.[178]

Thiazides have been used as the step one antihypertensive agent in all of the major trials that have documented a decline in cardiovascular morbidity and mortality. There are several concerns, however, regarding an increase in other cardiovascular risk factors and possibly mortality in patients with baseline electrocardiographic abnormalities.[179] Although beta blockers are effective antihypertensive agents in some populations, elderly patients respond less often than do young hypertensives.[180] Calcium channel antagonists[181] and angiotensin-converting enzyme inhibitors[182] may be especially well suited for use in the older population. They have the potential for effectively controlling blood pressure as either single agents or in combination and also to reduce left ventricular hypertrophy.

The importance of left ventricular hypertrophy as a risk factor for the development of coronary artery disease was reported by Levy et al.[183] in data from the Framingham study. These investigators reported a severalfold increase in the development of coronary disease in elderly hypertensives conferred by the presence of advanced left ventricular hypertrophy. The increase was independent of the risk afforded by pressure elevation alone. A study reported by Schulman et al.[184] compared the ability of the calcium channel blocker verapamil and the beta blocker atenolol to induce regression of left ventricular mass in older hyptertensives and the effect of regression on left ventricular function and diastolic filling parameters. This study showed that the calcium antagonist was better able to induce regression than the beta blocker. In addition, regression was associated with an increase in peak diastolic filling rate and did not handicap either cardiac output or ejection fraction at rest or during mild upright bicycle exercise.

An interesting small group of elderly patients with hypertensive hypertrophic cardiomyopathy also has been described.[185] Females made up more than three-fourths of the reported group, and symptoms consisted primarily of dyspnea and chest pain. The diagnosis is made by echocardiography, which shows exaggerated contractile function, small systolic and diastolic cavity dimensions, and prolonged and reduced early diastolic filling. The importance of the recognition of this patient subset is that therapy with vasodilators was associated with clinical deterioration, whereas patients treated with beta blockers or calcium antagonists were markedly improved.

USE OF CARDIOVASCULAR DRUGS IN THE ELDERLY

As a consequence of the increased prevalence of cardiovascular (and other) diseases in the elderly, the percentage of total expenditures for drugs in this age group is severalfold higher than in the total population.[186] In considering the effects of age on the pharmacokinetics and pharmacodynamics of cardiovascular agents,[187–189] it is important to note the heterogeneity of response in the older population. There are no strict age-related rules, therefore, which apply to the entire geriatric population, and it is clear that the commitment of the physician to assess carefully the therapeutic results and side effects of medical therapy must be greater in older than in younger age groups.

Although age-related changes in gastric pH and absorptive surface have been described, these have relatively unimportant effects for most cardiovascular drugs. The distribution of cardiovascular agents, however, is affected by age-associated decreases in serum albumin[189] and lean body mass[190] and increases in $alpha_1$-acid glycoproteins[191] and body fat.[190] A decrease in albumin results in increased free drug for those agents which are highly protein-bound, which will, in turn, increase plasma concentrations for those agents whose metabolism is independent of the available free drug (e.g., lidocaine and propranolol). An increase in $alpha_1$-acid glycoprotein results in a decrease in the free fractions of acidic drugs such as phenytoin.[191] A change in body mass results in an increased distribution volume for fat-soluble drugs and a decreased distribution volume for water-soluble agents.

The effect of age on metabolism and excretion relates to its effect on renal and hepatic function. The influence of age on renal function has been

100. Buttrick, P., Malhorta, A., Factor, S., et al.: The effect of aging and hypertension on myosin biochemistry and gene expression in the rat heart. Am. J. Physiol. *(in press)*.

101. Walford, G. D., Spurgeon, H. A., and Lakatta, E. G.: Diminished cardiac hypertrophy and muscle performance in older compared to younger adult rats with chronic atrioventricular block. Circ. Res. *63*:502, 1988.

102. Boluyt, M. O., Opiteck, J. A., Esser, K. A., and White, T. P.: Cardiac adaptations to aortic constriction in adult and aged rats. Am. J. Physiol. *257*:H643, 1989.

103. Sakai, M., Danziger, R. S., Spurgeon, H. A., and Lakatta, E. G.: Decreased contractile response to norepinephrine with aging. Circulation *76*(Suppl. IV):153, 1987.

104. Sakai, M., Danziger, R. S., Staddon, J. M., et al.: Decrease with senescence in the norepinephrine-induced phosphorylation of myofilament proteins in isolated rat cardiac myocytes. J. Mol. Cell. Cardiol. *21*:1327, 1989.

105. Dobson, J. G., Jr., Fenton, R. A., and Romano, F. D.: Increased myocardial adenosine production and reduction of beta-adrenergic contractile response in aged hearts. Circ. Res. *66*:1381, 1990.

106. Guarnieri, T., Spurgeon, H. A., Froehlick, J. P., et al.: Diminished inotropic response but unaltered toxicity to acetylstrophanthidin in the senescent beagle. Circulation *60*:1548, 1979.

CARDIAC FUNCTION IN NORMAL AGING HUMANS

107. Fleg, J. L., and Lakatta, E. G.: Loss of muscle mass is a major determinant of the age-related decline in maximal aerobic capacity [abstr.]. Circulation *72*(Suppl. III):464, 1985.

108. Tejada, C., Strong, J. P., Montenegro, M. R., et al.: Distribution of coronary and aortic atherosclerosis by geographic location, race and sex. Lab. Invest. *18*:509, 1968.

109. Kennedy, R. O., Andrews, G. R., and Caird, F. I.: Ischemic heart disease in the elderly. Br. Heart J. *39*:1121, 1977.

110. Brandfonbrener, M., Landowne, M., and Shock, N. W.: Changes in cardiac output with age. Circulation *12*:557, 1955.

111. Strandell, T.: Circulatory studies on healthy old men. Acta Med. Scand. *175*:1, 1964.

112. Conway, J., Wheeler, R., and Sannerstedt, R.: Sympathetic nervous activity during exercise in relation to age. Cardiovasc. Res. *5*:577, 1971.

113. Rodeheffer, R. J., Gerstenblith, G., Becker, L. C., et al.: Exercise cardiac output is maintained with advancing age in healthy human subjects: Cardiac dilatation and increased stroke volume compensate for a diminished heart rate. Circulation *69*:203, 1984.

114. Port, S., Cobb, F. R., Colema, E., and Jones, R. H.: Effect of age on the response of the left ventricular ejection fraction to exercise. N. Engl. J. Med. *303*:1133, 1980.

115. Proper, R., and Wall, F.: Left ventricular stroke volume measurements not affected by chronologic aging. Am. Heart J. *83*:843, 1972.

116. Gerstenblith G., Frederiksen, J., Yin, F.C.P., et al.: Echocardiographic assessment of a normal adult aging population. Circulation *56*:273, 1977.

117. Avolio, A. P., Fa-Quan, D., Wei-Qiang, L., et al.: Effects of aging on arterial distensibility in populations with high and low prevalence of hypertension: Comparison between urban and rural communities in China. Circulation *71*:202, 1985.

118. Sjogren, A. L.: Left ventricular wall thickness determined by ultrasound in 100 subjects without heart disease. Chest *60*:341, 1971.

119. Gerstenblith, G., Fleg, J. L., Becker, L. C., et al.: Maximum left ventricular filling rate in healthy individuals measured by gated blood pool scans: Effect of age. Circulation *68*(Suppl. III):101, 183.

120. Miyatake, K., Okamoto, M., Kinoshita, N., et al.: Augmentation of atrial contribution to left ventricular inflow with aging as assessed by intracardiac Doppler flowmetry. Am. J. Cardiol. *53*:586, 1984.

121. Bonow, R. O., Vitale, D. F., Bacharach, S. L., et al.: Effects of aging on asynchronous left ventricular regional function and global ventricular filling in normal human subjects. J. Am. Coll. Cardiol. *11*:50, 1988.

122. Nixon, J. V., Hallmark, H., Page, K., et al.: Ventricular performance in human hearts aged 61 to 73 yeas. Am. J. Cardiol. *56*:932, 1985.

123. Lima, J.A.C., Weiss, J. L., Guzman, P. A., et al.: Incomplete filling and incoordinate contraction as mechanisms of hypotension during ventricular tachycardia in man. Circulation *68*:928, 1983.

124. Dehn, M. M., and Bruce, R. A.: Longitudinal variations in maximal oxygen intake with age and activity. J. Appl. Physiol. *33*:805, 1971.

125. Hagberg, J. M., Allen, W. K., Seals, D. R., et al.: A hemodynamic comparison of young and older endurance athletes during exercise. J. Appl. Physiol. *58*:2041, 1985.

126. Yin, F.C.P., Raizes, G. S., Guarnieri, T., et al.: Age associated decrease in ventricular response to hemodynamic stress during beta-adrenergic blockade. Br. Heart J. *40*:1349, 1978.

127. Yin, F.C.P., Weisfeldt, M. L., and Milnor, W. R.: The role of aortic input impedance in the decreased cardiovascular response to exercise with aging in the dog. J. Clin. Invest. *68*:28, 1981.

128. Fleisch, J. H., and Hooker, C. S.: The relationship between age and relaxation of vascular smooth muscle in the rabbit and rat. Circ. Res. *38*:243, 1976.

129. Fleg, J. L., Tzankoff, S. P., and Lakatta, E. G.: Age-related augmentation of plasma catecholamines during dynamic exercise in healthy males. J. Appl. Physiol. *59*:1033, 1985.

AGING, DISEASE, AND CARDIAC FUNCTION

130. World Health Organization: World Health Statistics Annual. Geneva, 1979.

131. MacDonald, J. B.: Presentation of acute myocardial infarction in the elderly—a review. Age/Ageing *14*:196, 1984.

132. Spodick, D. H., and Quarry, V. M.: Prevalence of the fourth heart sound by phonocardiography in the absence of heart disease. Am. Heart J. *87*:11, 1974.

133. Slodki, S. J., Hussain, A. T., and Luisada, A. A.: The Q-T interval. III. A study of the second heart sound in old age. J. Am. Geriatr. Soc. *17*:673, 1969.

134. Burch, G. E., and DePlaquale, N. P.: Geriatric cardiology. Am. Heart J. *78*:700, 1969.

135. Lam, J.Y.T., Chaitman, B. R., Glaenzer, M., et al.: Safety and diagnostic accuracy of dipyridamole-thallium imaging in the elderly. J. Am. Coll. Cardiol. *11*:585, 1988.

136. Hypertension Detection and Follow-up Program Cooperative Group: Five-year findings of the Hypertension Detection and Follow-up Program. Mortality by race, sex, and age. J.A.M.A. *242*:2572, 1979.

137. European Working Party on High Blood Pressure in the Elderly: Mortality and morbidity results from the European Working Party on High Blood Pressure in the Elderly Trial. Lancet *1*:1349, 1985.

138. Jajich, C. L., Ostfeld, A. M., and Freeman, D. H.: Smoking and coronary heart disease mortality in the elderly. J.A.M.A. *252*:2831, 1984.

139. Mock, M. B., Holmes, D. R., Vlietstra, R. E., et al.: Percutaneous transluminal coronary angioplasty (PTCA) in the elderly patient: Experience in the National, Heart, Lung and Blood Institute PTCA Registry. Am. J. Cardiol. *53*:89C, 1984.

140. Raizner, A. E., Hust, R. G., Lewis, J. M., et al.: Transluminal coronary angioplasty in the elderly. Am. J. Cardiol. *57*:29, 1986.

141. Gersh, B. J., Kronmal, R. A., Schaff, H. V., et al.: Long-term (5-year) results of coronary bypass surgery in patients 65 years old and older: A report from the Coronary Artery Surgery Study. Circulation *68*(Suppl. II):190, 1983.

142. Roberts, A. J., Woodhall, D. D., Conti, C. R., et al.: Mortality, morbidity, and cost-accounting related to coronary artery bypass graft surgery in the elderly. Ann. Thorac. Surg. *39*:426, 1985.

143. Elayda, M. A., Hall, R. J., Gray, A. G., et al.: Coronary revascularization in the elderly patient. J. Am. Coll. Cardiol. 3:1398, 1984.

144. Kunis, R., Greenberg, H., Yeoh, C. B., et al.: Coronary revascularization for recurrent pulmonary edema in elderly patients with ischemic heart disease and preserved ventricular function. N. Engl. J. Med. *313*:1207, 1985.

145. Gersh, B. J., Kronmal, R. A., Schaff, H. V., et al.: Comparison of coronary artery bypass surgery and medical therapy in patients 65 years of age or older. N. Engl. J. Med. *313*:217, 1985.

146. Letting, C. A., and Silverman, M. E.: Acute myocardial infarction in hospitalized patients over age 70. Am. Heart J. *100*:331, 1980.

147. Williams, B. O., Begg, T. B., Semple, T., and McGuinness, J. B.: The elderly in a coronary care unit. Br. Med. J. *2*:451, 1976.

148. Zerman, F. D., and Rodstein, M.: Cardiac rupture complicating myocardial infarction in the aged. Arch. Intern. Med. *105*:431, 1960.

149. Schuster, E. H., and Bulkley, B. H.: Expansion of transmural myocardial infarction: A pathophysiologic factor in cardiac rupture. Circulation *60*:1532, 1979.

150. DeWood, M. A., Spores, J., Notske, R., et al.: Prevalence of total coronary occlusion during the early hours of transmural myocardial infarction. N. Engl. J. Med. *303*:897, 1980.

151. Gruppo Italiano per lo studio della streptochinasi nell'infarto miocardico (GISSI): Effectiveness of intravenous thrombolytic therapy in acute myocardial infarction. Lancet *1*:397, 1986.

152. Wilcox, R. G., Olsson, C. G., Skene, A. M., et al.: Trial of tissue plasminogen activator for mortality reduction in acute myocardial infarction. Lancet *2*:525, 1988.

153. AIMS Trial Study Group: Effect of intravenous APSAC on mortality after acute myocardial infarction: Preliminary report of a placebo-controlled clinical trial. Lancet *1*:545, 1988.

154. ISIS-2 (Second International Study of Infarct Survival Collaborative Group): Randomized trial of intravenous streptokinase, oral aspirin, both, or neither among 17 187 cases of suspected acute myocardial infarction: Lancet *2*:349, 1988.

155. Guerci, A. D., Gerstenblith, G., Brinker, J. A., et al.: A randomized trial of intravenous tissue plasminogen activator for acute myocardial infarction with subsequent randomization to elective coronary angioplasty. N. Engl. J. Med. *317*:1613, 1987.

156. Lie, K. I., Wellens, H. J., van Capelle, F. J., et al.: Lidocaine in the prevention of primary ventricular fibrillation. N. Engl. J. Med. *291*:1324, 1974.

157. Jick, H., Sloan, D., and Borda, I. T.: Efficacy and toxicity of heparin in relation to age and sex. N. Engl. J. Med. *279*:284, 1968.

158. The Norwegian Multicenter Study Group: Timolol-induced reduction in mortality and reinfarction in patients surviving acute myocardial infarction. N. Engl. J. Med. *304*:801, 1981.

159. Sixty Plus Reinfarction Study Research Group: A double-blind trial to assess long-term oral anticoagulant therapy in elderly patients after myocardial infarction. Lancet *2*:990, 1980.

160. Weintraub, R. M., Thurer, R. L., Wei, J., and Aroesty, J. M.: Repair of postinfarction ventricular septal defect in the elderly. J. Thorac. Cardiovasc. Surg. *85*:191, 1983.

161. Fleg, J. L., and Kennedy, H. L.: Cardiac arrhythmias in a healthy elderly

population: Detection by 24 hour ambulatory electrocardiography. Chest *81*:302, 1982.

162. Fleg, J. L., and Lakatta, E. G.: Prevalence and prognosis of exercise-induced nonsustained ventricular tachycardia in apparently healthy volunteers [abstr.]. Am. J. Cardiol. *54*:762, 184.
163. Berger, M., Berdoff, R. L., Gallerstein, P. E., and Goldberg, E.: Evaluation of aortic stenosis by continuous wave Doppler ultrasound. J. Am. Coll. Cardiol. *3*:150, 1984.
164. Pomerance, A.: Cardiac pathology in the elderly. *In* Noble, R. J., and Rothbaum, D. A. (eds.): Geriatric Cardiology, Cardiovascular Clinics. Philadelphia, F. A. Davis, 1981, p. 9.
165. Hochberg, M. S., Morrow, A. G., Michaelis, L. L., et al.: Aortic valve replacement in the elderly. Encouraging postoperative clinical and hemodynamic results. Arch. Surg. *112*:1475, 1977.
166. Kaplan, O., Yakirevich, V, and Vidne, B. A.: Aortic valve replacement in septuagenarians. Texas Heart Inst. J. *12*:295, 1985.
167. Litvack, F., Jakubowski, A. T., Buchbinder, N. A., and Eigler, N.: Lack of sustained clinical improvement in an elderly population after percutaneous aortic valvuloplasty. Am. J. Cardiol. *62*:270, 1988.
168. Caird, F. I.: Valvular heart disease. *In* Caird, F. I., Dall, J.L.C., and Kennedy, R. D. (eds.): Cardiology in Old Age. New York, Plenum Press, 1976, pp. 231–247.
169. Hochberg, M. S., Derkae, W. M., Conkle, D. M., et al.: Mitral valve replacement in elderly patients. Encouraging postoperative clinical and hemodynamic results. J. Cardiovasc. Thorac. Surg. *77*:422, 1979.
170. Jamieson, W.R.E., Dooner, J., Munro, A. I., et al.: Cardiac valve replacement in the elderly. A review of 320 consecutive cases. Circulation *64*(Suppl. II):177, 1981.
171. Curb, J. D., Borhani, N. O., Schnaper, H., et al.: Detection and treatment of hypertension in older individuals. Am. J. Epidemiol. *121*:371, 1985.
172. Management Committee of the Australian Therapeutic Trial in Mild Hypertension: Treatment of mild hypertension in the elderly. Med. J. Aust. *2*:398, 1981.
173. Kannel, W. B.: Blood pressure and risk of coronary heart disease: The Framingham Study. Dis. Chest *56*:43, 1969.
174. Kannel, W. B., Dawber, T. R., and McGee, N. L.: Perspectives on systolic hypertension. The Framingham Study. Circulation *61*:1179, 1980.
175. Pooling Project Research Group: Relationship of blood pressure, serum cholesterol, smoking, relative weight, and ECG abnormalities to incidence of major coronary events. Final report of the Pooling Project. J. Chron. Dis. *31*:201, 1978.
176. Kannel, W. B.: Blood pressure and development of cardiovascular disease in the aged. *In* Caird, F. I., Randall, J.L.C., and Kennedy, R. D. (eds.): Cardiology in Old Age. New York, Plenum Press, 1976.
176a. Amery, A., and de Schaepdryver, A.: The European working party on high blood pressure in the elderly. Am. J. Med. *90*(Suppl. 3A):15, 1991.
176b. Freis, E. D., for the Veterans Administration Cooperative Study Group on Antihypertensive Agents: Effects of age on treatment results. Am. J. Med. *90*(Suppl. 3A):20S, 1991.
177. Hulley, S. B., Furberg, C. D., Gurland, B., et al.: Systolic Hypertension in the Elderly Program (SHEP): Antihypertensive efficacy of chlorthalidone. Am. J. Cardiol. *56*:913, 1985.
178. Joint National Committee on Detection, Evaluation, and Treatment of High Blood Pressure: The 1984 Report of the Joint National Committee on Detection, Evaluation and Treatment of High Blood Pressure. Arch. Intern. Med. *144*:1045, 1984.
179. Multiple Risk Factor Intervention Trial Research Group: Baseline resting electrocardiographic abnormalities, antihypertensive treatment and mortality in the Multiple Risk Factor Intervention Trial. Am. J. Cardiol. *55*:1, 1985.
180. Buhler, F. R.: Age and cardiovascular response adaptation. Determinants of an antihypertensive treatment concept primarily based on beta-blockers and calcium entry blockers. Hypertension *5*:94, 1983.
181. Massie, B. M., Hirsch, A. T., Inouye, E. K., and Tubau, J. F.: Calcium channel blockers as antihypertensive agents. Am. J. Med. *77*:(Suppl. 4A):135, 1984.
182. Dunn, F. G., Oigman, W., Ventura, H. O., et al.: Enalapril improves systemic and renal hemodynamics and allows regression of left ventricular mass in essential hypertension. Am. J. Cardiol. *53*:105, 1985.
183. Levy, D., Garrison, R. J., Savage, D. D., et al.: Left ventricular mass and incidence of coronary heart disease in an elderly cohort. Ann. Intern. Med. *110*:101, 1989.
184. Schulman, S. P., Weiss, J. L., Becker, L. C., et al.: The effects of antihypertensive therapy on left ventricular mass in elderly hypertensive patients. N. Engl. J. Med. *322*:1350, 1990.
185. Topol, E. J., Traill, T. A., and Fortuin, N. J.: Hypertensive hypertrophic cardiomyopathy of the elderly. N. Engl. J. Med. *312*:277, 1985.

USE OF CARDIOVASCULAR DRUGS IN THE ELDERLY

186. Vestal, R. E., and Dawson, G. W.: Pharmacology and aging. *In* Finch, C. E., and Schneider, E. L. (eds.): Handbook of the Biology of Aging. 2nd ed. New York, Van Nostrand, 1985, p. 744.
187. Greenblatt, D. J., Sellers, E. M., and Shader, R. I.: Drug disposition in old age. N. Engl. J. Med. *306*:1081, 1982.
188. Sjoqvist, F., and Alvan, G.: Aging and drug disposition-metabolism. J. Chron. Dis. *36*:31, 1983.
189. Dybkaer, R., Lauritzen, M., and Krakauer, R.: Relative reference values for clinical chemical and haematological quantities in "healthy" elderly people. Acta Med. Scand. *209*:1, 1981.
190. Bruce, A., Andersson, M., Arvidsson, B., and Isaksson, B.: Body composition. Prediction of normal body potassium, body water and body fat in adults on the basis of body height, body weight and age. Scand. J. Clin. Lab. Invest. *40*:461, 1980.
191. Verbeeck, R. K., Cardinal, J. A., and Wallace, S. M.: Effect of age and sex on the plasma binding of acidic and basic drugs. Eur. J. Clin. Pharmacol. *27*:91, 1984.
192. Rowe, J. W., Andres, R., Tobin, J. D., et al.: Age-adjusted standards for creatinine clearance. Ann. Intern. Med. *84*:567, 1976.
193. Kerremans, A.L.M., and Gribnau, F.W.J.: Changes in pharmacokinetics and in effect of furosemide in the elderly. Clin. Exp. Hyper. [A] *A5*:271, 1983.
194. Vestal, R. E., Wood, A.J.J., and Shand, D. G.: Reduced beta-adrenoceptor sensitivity in the elderly. Clin. Pharmacol. Ther. *26*:181, 1979.

53

Medical Management of the Patient Undergoing Cardiac Surgery

by ELLIOTT M. ANTMAN, M.D.

Advances in cardiac surgery have made the operative repair of a variety of cardiac lesions a viable therapeutic option for an increasing number of patients with cardiovascular disease. The care of the patient undergoing cardiac surgery requires the collaboration of surgeons, cardiologists, anesthesiologists, radiologists, and various other professionals. This chapter summarizes the information required by the cardiologist, whose responsibilities include both preoperative evaluation and postoperative care, especially of the medical complications that may develop. The indications for operation are discussed in the chapters on the individual forms of heart disease.

PREOPERATIVE EVALUATION

PATIENT'S KNOWLEDGE BASE. A sensitive and thoughtful review of the indications for the operation and an explanation of the postoperative procedures will have a calming effect that may translate into a reduced need for antihypertensive and anxiolytic agents perioperatively.[1] The preoperative interview also should be used to assess the patient's potential ability to comply with postoperative medical issues such as anticoagulation and follow-up procedures for permanent pacemakers and implanted defibrillators (see Chap. 25).

TABLE 53–1 IMPORTANT ASPECTS OF PHYSICAL EXAMINATION IN PATIENTS SCHEDULED FOR CARDIAC SURGERY

PORTION OF PHYSICAL EXAMINATION	ABNORMAL FINDING	COMMENT
Head, eyes, ears, nose, throat	Dental caries, ENT infection	Risk of endocarditis in valvular surgery
Chest	Prior radical mastectomy	Previous mastectomy (especially left) may compromise thoracic blood supply[2] and therefore contraindicate use of internal mammary artery as conduit because of lack of patency or possible inadequate sternal wound healing.
Cardiovascular	Murmur of aortic regurgitation	Aortic regurgitation may worsen during cardiopulmonary bypass because of a jet from aortic cannulation; left ventricular distention may ensue. Intraaortic balloon pump contraindicated.
Abdomen	Abdominal aorta	Presence of abdominal aortic aneurysm or significant atherosclerosis may contraindicate use of intraaortic balloon pump.
Extremities	1. Peripheral arterial insufficiency 2. Venous varicosities in lower extremities	1. May prevent use of intraaortic balloon pump. 2. Insufficient venous conduits may be available in lower extremities, necessitating use of arm veins. If this is the case, intravenous lines should not be inserted in the arm veins that will be harvested. For reoperation cases cardiac catheterization should include imaging of the left internal mammary artery; a lesser saphenous venogram also is advisable.
	3. Tinea pedis	3. Increased risk of lower-extremity cellulitis
Neurological	1. Carotid bruits 2. Preoperative neurological deficit(s)	1. Cerebrovascular accident may occur perioperatively. 2. Neurological status may deteriorate postoperatively because of compromised cerebral perfusion.

TABLE 53-2 PREOPERATIVE LABORATORY EVALUATIONS FOR PATIENTS UNDERGOING CARDIAC SURGERY

PREOPERATIVE LABORATORY TEST	ABNORMAL FINDING	COMMENT
Complete blood count	1. Anemia, especially HCt < 35%	1. Anticipate that hemodilution will occur on cardiopulmonary bypass and blood loss will occur intraoperatively. Preoperative RBC transfusions may be needed. In addition, patients with unstable angina, congestive heart failure, aortic stenosis, and left main coronary artery disease should be advised against autologous donation of blood in the preoperative period.
	2. WBC > 10,000	2. Search for possible infection.
Coagulation screen	1. Prolonged bleeding time 2. Elevated PT and/or PTT 3. Thrombocytopenia	All of these laboratory abnormalities suggest that the patient is at risk for bleeding postoperatively and may have excessive chest tube drainage. Corrective measures (e.g., vitamin K, fresh frozen plasma, platelet transfusions) should be considered preoperatively, and surgery may need to be postponed. Hematological consultation may be required if an inherited defect in coagulation (e.g., von Willebrand's factor deficiency) is suspected.
Chemistry profile	1. Elevated BUN/creatinine	1. Abnormal renal function that may worsen in perioperative period (caused by nonpulsatile flow on cardiopulmonary bypass and potential low flow postoperatively); this may necessitate temporary or even permanent hemodialysis.
	2. Potassium <4.0 mEq/liter	2. Hypokalemia will place the patient at risk of arrhythmias perioperatively and should be corrected before induction of anesthesia.
	3. Abnormal liver function tests	3. Patient may clear anesthetic agents as well as other cardioactive drugs more slowly. Low albumin level may indicate a state of relative malnutrition that may need to be corrected with nutritional support perioperatively.
Stool hematest	Positive for occult blood	Because heparinization will take place while on cardiopulmonary bypass apparatus, the patient may be at risk for gastrointestinal (GI) bleeding perioperatively. The source of GI heme loss should be investigated preoperatively, if clinical circumstances permit. The potential for bleeding in the future may influence the choice of prosthetic valve inserted.
Pulmonary function	Reduced VC or prolonged FEV_1	Anticipate longer than usual process of weaning from ventilator postoperatively if FEV_1 < 65% VC or FEV_1 < 1.5–2.0 liters. Obtain baseline arterial blood gas analysis on room air to help guide respiratory management postoperatively.
Thyroid function	These tests are not ordered routinely but should be drawn in cases of suspected hypothyroidism or hyperthyroidism, known thyroid dysfunction on replacement therapy, and in patients with atrial fibrillation who have not undergone evaluation of thyroid function.	1. Hypothyroid patients require prolonged period of ventilatory support postoperatively because of slower clearance of anesthetic agents. 2. Hyperthyroid patients have a hypermetabolic state that places them at increased risk of myocardial ischemia, vasomotor instability, and poorly controlled ventricular rate in atrial fibrillation.
Cardiac catheterization	1. Elevated left ventricular end-diastolic pressure and pulmonary capillary wedge pressure	1. These may remain elevated in the early postoperative period and indicate a need for careful attention to maintenance of adequate preload postoperatively.
	2. Elevated right atrial pressure	2. This may reflect tricuspid regurgitation or right ventricular dysfunction from prior infarction. Such patients require vigorous volume expansion postoperatively to maintain an adequate cardiac output.
	3. Elevated pulmonary artery pressure (and pulmonary vascular resistance)	3. Fixed pulmonary vascular resistance should be suspected when the pulmonary artery diastolic pressure exceeds the mean pulmonary capillary wedge pressure. Vigorous oxygenation and pharmacological support with a pulmonary vasodilator (isoproterenol, prostaglandin E_1) are important in such cases. Patients with a pulmonary artery diastolic pressure equal to the pulmonary capillary wedge pressure usually have a more rapid resolution of pulmonary hypertension postoperatively.
	4. Left ventricular mural thrombus	4. Increased risk of stroke perioperatively.

Hct, hematocrit; RBC, red blood cell; PT, prothrombin time; PTT, partial thromboplastin time; BUN, blood urea nitrogen; VC, vital capacity; FEV_1, volume of air expired at 1 second.

Serious language barriers and lack of a family support system, especially in the elderly patient, can turn a technical surgical success into a postoperative medical failure. Enlistment of support from social workers and nurse practitioners may be essential for minimizing such an unfortunate outcome.

GENERAL MEDICAL CONDITION. Except for life-threatening conditions (e.g., proximal aortic dissection, cardiogenic shock caused by ruptured papillary muscle in acute myocardial infarction, penetrating wound of the heart), it behooves the consulting cardiologist to assess the overall medical condition of the patient and advise the surgical team if postponement of the operation seems warranted. When performing the clinical examination (Table 53–1)[2] and reviewing laboratory data (Table 53–2), particular attention should be paid to the patient's potential for developing one or more of the following complications: (1) bleeding while heparinized on cardiopulmonary bypass; (2) deterioration of renal function; (3) development of arrhythmias because of electrolyte imbalance; (4) sepsis because of incompletely treated pulmonary, urinary tract, or dental infections, or dermatologic infections over the sternum or saphenous vein harvest site; (5) the need for prolonged ventilatory support postoperatively because of underlying pulmonary disease and preoperative malnutrition (cardiac cachexia); and (6) development or exacerbation of a neurological deficit because of carotid artery disease or prior stroke.[3] In cases where perioperative intraaortic balloon pump support may be needed, the status of the ileofemoral circulation should be assessed bilaterally. Preoperative cessation of cigarette smoking should be emphasized. If a delay in elective surgery while preoperative infections, electrolyte disorders, or nutritional deficits are rectified is necessary, the cardiology consultant to the patient and the surgical team are responsible for making this determination.

The *protein-calorie malnutrition* associated with cardiac cachexia has been shown to compromise cardiac function, and is associated with a greater risk of respiratory failure, sepsis, and prolonged hospitalization.[4] If the clinical situation allows, patients diagnosed as having cardiac cachexia should receive 1 to 2 weeks of preoperative nutritional support before undergoing elective cardiac surgery. The general principles of nutritional support in cardiac surgical patients are outlined in Table 53–3.

TABLE 53–3 PRINCIPLES OF NUTRITIONAL SUPPORT IN CARDIAC SURGICAL PATIENTS

I. Recognize nutritionally deficient patient: current weight less than 10% of ideal body weight or a history of loss of >10% of ideal body weight; inadequate daily caloric intake (<1000 calories) for ≥1 week, serum albumin ≤2.5

II. Calculate daily caloric requirements
- A. Determine basal energy expenditure (BEE) in kcal/24 hr from the following Harris-Benedict formulae[5] (where W is ideal body weight in kg, H is height in cm, and A is age in years):

  $BEE_{men} = 66 + (13.7 \times W) + (5 \times H) - (6.8 \times A)$

  $BEE_{women} = 65.5 + (9.6 \times W) + (1.8 \times H) - (4.7 \times A)$
- B. Adjust for level of activity
  1. Add [0.25 × BEE] for hospitalization and postoperative state.
  2. Do not apply activity "factor" for patients who are at a reduced level of physical activity: on ventilator; comatose
- C. Adjust for stress (e.g., fever)
  1. Add [0.13 × BEE] for each 1° C rise in temperature above normal (use [0.07 × BEE]/1° F).
  2. Septic patients may need as much as 0.25–0.45 × BEE added to their daily caloric intake.
- D. Add additional calories if weight gain is desired (e.g., to treat cardiac cachexia): 1000 kcal/day will result in a weight gain of 2 lb/wk. A diet containing 150 kcal: 1 gm of nitrogen should be used (assuming renal or hepatic failure is absent). (Total calories ÷ 150 = # grams of nitrogen; multiply by 6.25 to determine number of grams of protein).

III. Determine route for nutritional support
- A. *Functioning gastrointestinal tract*
  1. Adequate oral intake: provide calculated calories in a diet that is 15–20% protein, 50–60% carbohydrate, and the remainder as fat.
  2. Inadequate oral intake: use enteral feeding to deliver daily caloric requirement (e.g., Osmolite = 1 cal/cc; Ensure Plus = 1.5 cal/cc). If renal or hepatic failure is present, use modified enteral feeding (e.g., Travesorb Renal or Travesorb Hepatic).
- B. *Nonfunctioning gastrointestinal tract or intolerance of enteral feedings*
  1. Normal renal function and can tolerate at least 2500 ml/day: peripheral parenteral nutrition
  2. Renal dysfunction and in need of fluid restriction: insert sterile central line for parenteral nutrition and prescribe central parenteral nutrition or total parenteral nutrition in consultation with nutritional support service. Prescription may need to be modified daily.

TABLE 53–4 PREOPERATIVE RISK FACTORS FOR ADVERSE OUTCOMES IN PATIENTS UNDERGOING CARDIAC SURGERY

I. Increased morbidity and mortality after CABG[6]
- A. Advanced age[6–8]
- B. Female gender*[9]
- C. Left ventricular dysfunction
- D. Symptomatic congestive heart failure
- E. Critical left main stenosis
- F. Urgent or emergency surgery

II. Increased risk of mediastinal infection[11]**
- A. Obesity
- B. Diabetes mellitus (especially if bilateral internal mammary artery grafting is performed)
- C. Malnutrition (see Table 53–3)
- D. Advanced age
- E. Severe pulmonary disease that is likely to lead to prolonged postoperative ventilatory support
- F. Hospitalization for more than 5 days preoperatively

CABG, coronary artery bypass grafting.

* A recent study casts doubt on the significance of female gender as an *independent* risk factor for coronary artery bypass surgery.[10] Women may be referred for surgery later in the course of their disease and undergo operation when they are older and have more advanced disease than do men. Thus differences in functional status and age may account for prior reports of the adverse impact of female gender.

** Highly correlated with increased length of stay and greater hospital costs related to surgery.

The risk factors for morbidity and mortality after coronary revascularization surgery and postoperative mediastinal infection are outlined in Table 53–4. Several centers have noted a higher mortality risk profile of patients referred for cardiac surgery over the past few years, including older persons with complex medical issues (e.g., diabetes mellitus, renal dysfunction) and a history of cardiac surgery.[12,13]

HEMODYNAMIC COMPENSATION. An especially important aspect of the preoperative evaluation of the cardiac surgical patient involves estimating the extent of underlying ventricular dysfunction, using preoperative echocardiography, radionuclide ventriculography, and contrast ventriculography. Careful consideration should be given to the possibility, sometimes occult, of right ventricular dysfunction (Table 53–2).[14] The latter should be suspected in patients with preoperative elevation of pulmonary artery systolic pressure (>60 mm Hg), a history of inferoposterior left ventricular infarction (and possibly associated right ventricular infarction), and longstanding tricuspid regurgitation. Patients with right ventricular dysfunction should be placed on maintenance digitalis and receive supplemental oxygen preoperatively to attempt to lower pulmonary vascular resistance and improve right ventricular systolic performance. Intravenous nitrate infusions in the perioperative period also have been shown to reduce pulmonary hypertension and ameliorate right ventricular failure.[15] Patients with mitral regurgitation and severe heart failure should undergo preoperative afterload reduction with such agents as oral angiotensin converting enzyme (ACE) inhibitors and intravenous sodium nitroprusside to a systolic pressure of about 90 to 100 mm Hg.

RISK OF MYOCARDIAL ISCHEMIA. Many patients with active unstable angina pectoris or critical coronary artery disease (e.g., significant left main coronary artery stenosis or severe three-vessel coronary artery disease), especially if it is associated with left ventricular dysfunction and/or mitral regurgitation, are in a tenuous hemodynamic balance as they proceed to the operating room. Delays while awaiting surgery and the time between the induction of anesthesia and the institution of cardiopulmonary bypass are high-risk periods during which a vicious spiral of myocardial ischemia and low-output syndrome can rapidly develop. Such patients should be protected by an intraaortic balloon pump inserted preoperatively and an infusion of nitroglycerin intraoperatively.[16]

ANESTHESIA FOR CARDIAC SURGERY. The details of the practice of cardiac anesthesia are beyond the scope of this chapter and are available in other sources.[17] As regards the preoperative evaluation, an important consideration relates to the form of anesthesia that may be used in cardiac surgical procedures today. Intravenous morphine in a dose of 1 to 3 mg/kg has been used in association with the inhaled anesthetic nitrous oxide. Although morphine has the advantage of being free of any significant myocardial depression, it does cause vasodilatation (by means of histamine release) and reduces preload and afterload.[18] High-dose synthetic narcotics, such as fentanyl and sufentanil, that do not cause vasodilatation have replaced morphine in many centers. The newer, inhaled anesthetics—enflurane and isoflurane—that have replaced nitrous oxide, still have the potential to cause vasodilatation. Patients with critical aortic stenosis, critical mitral stenosis, and large right-to-left shunts may experience a dramatic reduction in cardiac output as ventricular stroke volume falls with a reduction in preload. Preoperative volume expansion and even administration of vasopressor agents may be necessary to avoid this problem.

STATUS OF CARDIAC RHYTHM. Although supraventricular arrhythmias after cardiac surgery are seldom life-threatening, they frequently jeopardize hemodynamic stability and provoke disturbing symptoms. It is a common preoperative practice in many institutions to administer digitalis prophylactically to patients undergoing cardiac surgery, not only for inotropic support, but also for "control" of the ventricular rate if atrial fibrillation should occur postoperatively.[19,20] The support for this practice is less than compelling. Although the prophylactic use of digoxin has been reported to be "beneficial" by some,[20-22] this is by no means a consistent observation.[19,23] There is little reason to believe that digoxin prevents the development of atrial fibrillation, and indeed, clinical trials do not clearly substantiate either a lower incidence of atrial fibrillation[19] or a slower ventricular rate in atrial fibrillation in digoxin-treated patients.[20] *Furthermore, hypoxia, hypokalemia, and elevated catecholamine levels are common postoperatively, and these may predispose the patient to digoxin toxicity.*[24] Because many patients undergoing cardiac surgery are over age 60, there is likely to be a slower than normal clearance of digoxin, which contributes to the risk of digitalis intoxication.

Attention also has focused on the prophylactic use of beta-adrenoceptor blocking agents.[25] This stems from a number of considerations: (1) there is evidence that a rebound phenomenon after withdrawal of such agents at the time of surgery may contribute to the appearance of arrhythmias in the postoperative period[26]; (2) there is a heightened level of sympathetic nervous system tone in the postoperative period, and this may provoke supraventricular arrhythmias[27]; (3) the therapeutic index for digitalis glycosides is narrow. Clinical trials with several beta blockers have shown a statistically significant reduction not only in the frequency of supraventricular arrhythmias, but also in the severity (duration, speed of ventricular response) of the arrhythmia when it does occur.[23,25-28] In the absence of an ejection fraction less than 30 per cent, severe bronchospastic lung disease, or bradyarrhythmias, we advocate the use of prophylactic beta blockers in patients undergoing coronary artery bypass grafting.[28a]

Insufficient data are available to provide definitive recommendations for prophylaxis against atrial fibrillation in patients undergoing valve surgery. We individualize our recommendations for prophylaxis in such cases, and usually do not start beta blockers in patients who have not been on them chronically preoperatively. Young patients (<40 years) undergoing isolated repair of an atrial septal defect or patent ductus arteriosus need not receive prophylactic beta blockers preoperatively, since they are likely to tolerate a postoperative supraventricular arrhythmia during the time it takes to initiate measures to slow the ventricular rate or terminate the arrhythmia. Suggested doses of beta-adrenoceptor blockers for prophylaxis against atrial fibrillation are as follows: propranolol, 10 to 40 mg every 6 hours; metoprolol, 50 mg every 6 to 12 hours. For patients with depressed left ventricular function who cannot tolerate the negative inotropic effects of beta blockers, digoxin (0.25 to 0.375 mg/day) remains a suitable choice for a prophylactic agent.

Although oral verapamil (40 to 120 mg every 8 hours) also may be considered for prophylaxis against supraventricular arrhythmias, its use for that purpose is less well studied.[29] More commonly, intravenous verapamil is used for the acute postoperative management of supraventricular arrhythmias that may occur despite prophylaxis with other drugs.[30]

With the exception of amiodarone, antiarrhythmic drugs that have been prescribed for hemodynamically compromising ventricular tachyarrhythmias should be continued up to the time of operation because of the risk of "break through" of a potentially lethal ventricular arrhythmia in the preoperative period. Few data support the *initiation* of membrane-active agents such as quinidine and procainamide for prophylaxis against supraventricular arrhythmias; there may even be the potential for harm when such agents are used in the patient with ischemic heart disease.[31] Antiarrhythmic agents that have previously been prescribed for troublesome supraventricular arrhythmias or life-threatening ventricular arrhythmias should be continued up to the time of operation. A possible exception to this is amiodarone, since that agent has been associated with increased difficulty weaning from cardiopulmonary bypass, low cardiac output postoperatively, and a higher risk of hypoxia and bleeding postoperatively.[32,33] The necessity of continuing amiodarone preoperatively should be carefully reviewed. Patients with a documented history of resuscitation from sudden cardiac death should continue to receive amiodarone. In cases where amiodarone was prescribed for a less overtly life-threatening arrhythmia (e.g., atrial fibrillation), we prefer to discontinue the drug if surgery is being performed on an elective basis. Unfortunately adipose tissue stores of amiodarone are extensive with long-term (>1 month) treatment,[34] and electrophysiological effects have been reported for up to 1 year after discontinuation of the medication. No guidelines have been established for a minimum period of withdrawal of amiodarone preoperatively to reduce the perioperative risks noted above, but we advocate at least a 3-month period off the drug before subjecting the patient to elective cardiopulmonary bypass.

BRADYARRHYTHMIAS AND ATRIOVENTRICULAR AND INTRAVENTRICULAR BLOCK. Patients with high-grade (third-degree or type II second-degree) atrioventricular block and hemodynamic compromise (systolic pressure <90 mm Hg) are at high risk for general anesthesia unless a temporary transvenous pacemaker wire is inserted preoperatively.

The specifications (model, mode, and settings) of a permanent pacemaker system and, if possible, a statement as to the pacemaker dependency of the patient should be noted in the medical record. The possibility of postoperative malfunction of the permanent pacing system should be anticipated because of the effects of anesthesia, electrocautery, and surgical manipulation of the leads (e.g., during caval cannulation).[35,36] It is our practice to have the appropriate pacemaker programming equipment available postoperatively, since many problems (e.g., reversion to the VOO mode [p. 746] because of electromagnetic interference from the electrocautery apparatus) can be quickly resolved by interrogation of the generator and reprogramming in the recovery area.

In patients with left bundle branch block preoperatively who are about to undergo aortic or mitral valve replacement, there is an increased risk of permanent complete heart block postoperatively. The surgical team should be alerted to the need for placement of permanent epicardial leads intraoperatively, or plans should be made for implantation of a permanent transvenous pacing system in the early postoperative period if complete heart block develops. In addition to the

TABLE 53–6 ABNORMALITIES OF RESPIRATORY FUNCTION AFTER CARDIAC SURGERY

EFFECTS OF ANESTHESIA, THORACIC SURGERY, AND CARDIOPULMONARY BYPASS ON PULMONARY FUNCTION	POTENTIAL CAUSES
Alveolar dysfunction (e.g., widened alveolar-arterial oxygen gradient because of right-to-left intrapulmonary shunting)	a. Scattered regions of atelectasis with preserved perfusion[50] b. Pulmonary edema (e.g., cardiogenic, noncardiogenic "post pump" alveolar capillary leak)[51] c. Infection d. Inhibition of hypoxic pulmonary vasoconstriction by anesthetic agents[52] e. Exacerbation of ventilation/perfusion mismatch by vasodilating agents used postoperatively (e.g., nitroprusside)
Decreased central respiratory drive	a. General anesthetics b. Narcotic analgesics c. Cerebral insult in perioperative period
Decreased respiratory muscle function	a. Thoracic pain (incision, chest tubes) b. Persistent effects of muscle relaxants c. Age d. Obesity e. Depressed cardiac function f. Primary diaphragmatic dysfunction (e.g., phrenic nerve injury)
Exacerbation of underlying chronic pulmonary disease	a. Increase in airway resistance b. Increased secretions and worsening bronchitis c. Pneumonia

While intubated, the patient should be breathing in the intermittent mandatory ventilation (IMV) mode, and arterial blood gases should be checked every hour for the first 6 hours to ensure adequate oxygenation. Positive end-expiratory pressure (PEEP) often is used to minimize the number of collapsed alveolar segments. PEEP should be used cautiously in patients with obstructive pulmonary disease (risk of pneumothorax from air trapping and barotrauma), and it is contraindicated in patients who have undergone operative procedures in which elevation of the right atrial pressure would be undesirable (e.g., interatrial transposition of venous return, Fontan procedure, superior vena caval–right atrial anastomosis [p. 939]). Initiation of PEEP may not be tolerated in patients with relative hypovolemia and inadequate preload (p. 378).

Guidelines for Weaning. Suggested guidelines for identifying the patient who is ready to be weaned from the ventilator are shown in Table 53–7. The IMV setting is progressively reduced to about 2 to 4 breaths per minute, and then the patient may be given a brief trial of T-tube ventilation (with or without continuous positive airway pressure) before extubation occurs. In certain situations extubation should not take place even if the patient "qualifies" on the basis of pulmonary criteria. These situations include hemodynamic instability, malignant ventricular arrhythmias, and postoperative bleeding that may require reoperation.

SPECIAL PROBLEMS

An increased alveolar-arterial (A-a) gradient postoperatively is a serious problem that demands a thorough evaluation. The ventilator settings should be checked, and a chest radiograph obtained to ascertain the position of the tip of the endotracheal tube (e.g., exclude intubation of the right mainstem bronchus) and to rule out pneumothorax, lobar atelectasis or pneumonia, or a large pleural effusion. Hemodynamic monitoring by means of a pulmonary artery catheter can cause pulmonary hemorrhage because of overinflation of the balloon, and bronchoscopy may need to be performed to diagnose and manage the problem (e.g., occlusion of the bronchus draining the bleeding segment of lung).

PULMONARY EDEMA (see also Chap. 20). The most common cause of pulmonary edema postoperatively is elevated pulmonary venous pressure arising from left ventricular dysfunction and/or a valvular lesion (e.g., mitral regurgitation). Such patients require aggressive diuresis and vasodilator and inotropic support. Mechanical ventilation with PEEP is used until the patient's ventricular function improves.

In a minority of patients pulmonary edema is due to the adult respiratory distress syndrome (ARDS). In its most extreme form, this disorder is associated with a generalized whole-body *postpump syndrome*, characterized by increased capillary permeability, interstitial edema, fever, leukocytosis, renal dysfunction, and hemodynamic collapse. Although the inciting cause of ARDS in some patients may be sepsis, transfusion reactions, or anaphylaxis, in most cases it is the adverse consequences of exposure of the blood to foreign surfaces during prolonged cardiopulmonary bypass. Included among these are platelet clumping and embolization, protein denaturation, liberation of free fat by lipoproteins, and activation of the coagulation cascade, fibrinolytic system, complement system (by way of C3a and C5a), and the kallikrein-bradykinin system. Generation of the anaphylatoxins C3a and C5a mediates leukocyte chemotaxis, aggregation, and enzyme release.[51,54] Pulmonary sequestration of activated leukocytes and platelets occurs with attendant damage to the pulmonary endothelium.[55] There is a direct relation between the duration of cardiopulmonary bypass and the development of the derangements of pulmonary and vascular integrity noted above.[56] Management of ARDS includes mechanical ventilation with PEEP (often for extended periods), minimization of the pulmonary capillary wedge pressure without compromising cardiac output, and nutritional support as needed (Table 53–3).

UNDERLYING CHRONIC LUNG DISEASE. General surgical preparation of patients with obstructive lung disease, including antibiotics, bronchodilators, and cessation of cigarette smoking, has been reported to prevent or diminish respiratory failure from postoperative atelectasis and pneumonia.[57] Inhaled bronchodilators should be continued postoperatively

TABLE 53–7 CRITERIA FOR SUCCESSFUL WEANING FROM VENTILATORY SUPPORT*

Tests of mechanical capability
A. Vital capacity $>10-15$ cc/kg body weight
B. Forced expiratory volume in 1 sec >10 cc/kg body weight
C. Peak inspiratory pressure >-20 to -30 cm H_2O
D. Resting minute ventilation <10 liters/min (can be doubled with maximal voluntary ventilation)
E. Spontaneous respiratory rate under 25 on intermittent mandatory ventilation (IMV) of 6 while resting comfortably, and no apparent increase in work of breathing
Tests of oxygenation capability
A. Alveolar-arterial gradient on 100% O_2 $<300-500$ torr
B. Arterial $Po_2 > 80$ torr in the absence of intracardiac right-to-left shunting when the FIO_2 is ≤ 0.5
C. Arterial $Pco_2 < 45$ and pH >7.37
D. Shunt fraction (Q_s/Q_t) $<10-20\%$
E. Dead space/tidal Volume (V_d/V_t) $<0.55-0.60$

* Modified from Snow, J. C.: Respiration and respiratory care. *In* Snow, J. C. (ed.): Manual of Anesthesia. Boston, Little, Brown, 1977, pp. 317–331; and Kirklin, J. K., Daggett, W. M., and Lappas, D. G.: Postoperative care following cardiac surgery. *In* Johnson, R. A., Haber, E., and Austen, W. G.: The Practice of Cardiology. The Medical and Surgical Cardiac Units at the Massachusetts General Hospital. Boston, Little, Brown, 1980, pp. 110–113.

and supplemented with intravenous theophylline (0.4 mg/kg/hr to obtain plasma levels of 10 to 20 μg/ml).[58] Plasma levels of theophylline should be monitored at least once every 24 hours in the intensive care unit to minimize the chance of toxicity manifested by agitation, arrhythmias, and grand mal seizures.[59] Particularly refractory patients may require a short course of corticosteroids (e.g., methylprednisolone, 0.5 mg/kg every 6 hours for 3 days) to be weaned from the ventilator.[60]

Patients with chronic obstructive pulmonary disease should be weaned from the ventilator slowly. It is helpful to maintain the arterial carbon dioxide tension close to the patient's baseline level to ensure an adequate respiratory drive.[61]

DIAPHRAGMATIC FAILURE. Diaphragmatic dysfunction after cardiac surgical procedures usually occurs as a result of injury to the phrenic nerve(s). An elevated hemidiaphragm may be seen on postoperative roentgenograms in 25 per cent of patients who undergo myocardial preservation, including a topical ice slush and harvesting of an internal mammary artery.[62] Of note, an elevated hemidiaphragm usually is not associated with increased postoperative morbidity or mortality; recovery of the hemidiaphragm to normal position occurs in 80 per cent of patients at 1 year and nearly all patients by 2 years postoperatively. Less than 1 per cent of patients develop clinically important diaphragmatic dysfunction after cardiac surgery because of unilateral or bilateral phrenic nerve injury. Evidence of diaphragmatic failure includes the inability to wean the patient from the ventilator, a vital capacity less than 500 cc, and paradoxical movement of the diaphragm on fluoroscopy or ultrasonography. Because it may take up to 6 weeks for an injured phrenic nerve to recover function, management includes a more prolonged period of mechanical ventilation and, for some patients, transition to a rocking bed.[63] In cases of permanent unilateral phrenic nerve damage, plication of the diaphragm may help to improve respiratory function.[64]

PROLONGED VENTILATORY INSUFFICIENCY. Patients who fail to wean from the ventilator within 48 hours require special medical attention. To maximize the efficiency of mechanical ventilation, such patients should be sedated and consideration given to neuromuscular blockade if the patient is not breathing synchronously with the respirator. Because of the risk of stress-induced gastritis, an H_2-receptor blocker (e.g., ranitidine, 50 mg intravenously every 8 to 12 hours) is administered. To maintain hemodynamic stability, such patients frequently receive large volumes of intravenous fluids; packed red blood cells should be used to maintain an adequate oxygen-carrying capacity. Nutritional support in the form of tube feedings (preferably as a continuous infusion with the patient positioned in the right lateral decubitus position) or parenteral feedings is critical to provide adequate metabolic needs and prevent catabolism of skeletal muscles (e.g., respiratory muscles) (Table 53–3).

If the patient remains intubated beyond 10 to 14 days, the risks of tracheal stenosis, vocal cord damage, retropharyngeal abscess formation, and tracheoesophageal fistula increase. High-compliance, low-pressure cuffs on endotracheal tubes have reduced the risk of such complications, and permit patients to remain intubated continuously for up to 20 or even 30 days, provided the cuff pressures are maintained below 20 mm Hg and meticulous respiratory care technique is used. Placement of a tracheostomy tube is not a trivial decision, since it can be associated with a number of complications that may offset the advantages of improved endotracheal suctioning and reduced risk of upper airway damage, but tracheostomy usually is desirable if it is clear that the patient will remain intubated beyond 3 weeks.

Finally, patients who fail to maintain adequate oxygenation despite adequate sedation, neuromuscular blockade, large tidal volumes, and PEEP, or who develop marked depression of cardiac output, may be candidates for high-frequency jet ventilation.[65] This mode of ventilatory support provides small tidal volumes at high respiratory rates (e.g., 60 breaths per minute) and produces minimal adverse effects on cardiovascular function. In rare cases extracorporeal membrane oxygenators have been used in patients with severe compromise of diffusing capacity caused by ARDS; the mortality remains high in such cases.

HYPERTENSION

Postoperative hypertension has been defined variably in the literature,[66,67] but we consider it to be present if the systolic pressure exceeds 140 mm Hg.[68] The incidence of postoperative hypertension ranges from 40 to 60 per cent of patients.[69] It occurs more commonly in patients with a preoperative history of hypertension, prior maintenance therapy with a beta blocker, and well-preserved left ventricular function.[70] Postoperative hypertension is especially frequent after coronary artery bypass grafting and surgical relief of left ventricular outflow tract obstruction (e.g., aortic valve replacement, correction of coarctation of the aorta).[71]

The mechanisms of postoperative hypertension probably vary from patient to patient, but usually include (1) a "rebound" effect from withdrawal of beta blockade administered preoperatively[26]; (2) excessive sympathetic nervous system activity with elevations of circulating catecholamine levels (especially norepinephrine)[69,70]; (3) pressor reflexes originating in the heart, great vessels, or coronary arteries[72]; and (4) following correction of aortic coarctation, a drop in the aortic pressure proximal to the site of the prior coarctation with resultant stimulation of aortic and carotid baroreceptors by apparent "hypotension." The renin-angiotensin system is stimulated and peripheral resistance is increased. The sudden exposure of vascular beds downstream to the coarctation to "undamped" aortic pressure also has been reported to cause mesenteric arteritis.

The adverse consequences of elevated systemic pressure include an increased risk of postoperative bleeding, suture line disruption, and aortic dissection[73]; elevated left ventricular afterload and consequent reduction of left ventricular output; injury to aortocoronary bypass grafts[74]; and postoperative stroke.

Although a variety of agents may be used for treating acute postoperative hypertension, we prefer those that are rapidly acting and titratable and have a short half-life. Such drugs include sodium nitroprusside (0.5 to 2.0 μg/kg/min),[75] esmolol (50 to 250 μg/kg/min),[76] labetalol (1 to 2 mg/min),[77] and nitroglycerin (25 to 300 μg/min).[66] Many centers are starting to use closed-loop systems designed to titrate the intravenous infusion rate of a drug to a preset pressure level that is constantly being monitored invasively.[78] The need for transition to oral antihypertensive therapy is assessed on an individual basis; chronic treatment usually is required only in the patient with a preoperative history of hypertension.

PERIOPERATIVE MYOCARDIAL INFARCTION

Despite modern intraoperative myocardial protection and improvements in surgical techniques, some degree of ischemia occurs nearly uniformly during coronary artery bypass surgery.[79] Only a minority of patients (5 to 15 per cent of patients undergoing coronary artery bypass graft surgery), however, actually experience a *perioperative myocardial infarction.*[80,81] The potential causes of myocardial ischemia and infarction in the perioperative period include incomplete revascularization; diffuse atherosclerotic disease of the distal coronary arteries; spasm, embolism, or thrombosis of the native coronary vessels or bypass grafts[82–85]; technical problems with graft anastomoses; inadequate myocardial preservation intraoperatively; increased myocardial oxygen needs, as in left ventricular hypertrophy; and hemodynamic derangements in the postoperative period (e.g., hypotension, hypertension, tachycardia). Although initially one might suspect that perioperative myocardial infarction results from occlu-

TABLE 53–8 DIAGNOSIS OF MYOCARDIAL INFARCTION AFTER CARDIAC SURGERY

DIAGNOSTIC FINDING	COMMENT
Symptoms	
Early (<48 hr postop)	Not reliable because of residual effects of anesthesia and postoperative analgesics
Late (>48 hr postop)	Potentially reliable but may be confused with incisional pain and pleuritic pain from chest tubes, pericarditis
Electrocardiogram	
New, persistent Q waves	This is the most reliable diagnostic finding but only if the Q waves persist on serial ECG's over several days.
Evolutionary ST-T changes	Supportive data favoring the diagnosis of MI only if a typical evolutionary pattern is observed. Because of the effects of cardiopulmonary bypass, hypothermia, postoperative pericarditis, mediastinal chest tubes, and medications (e.g., digitalis), a variety of nonspecific ST-Tw abnormalities may be seen and should not be relied on for diagnosing a perioperative MI.
Myocardial specific enzymes	
Total CK	Elevated total CK levels postoperatively may arise from multiple sources, including skeletal muscle in the thorax and calf as well as myocardium.
CK-MB	Myocardial-specific CK may be released from ischemia occurring during cardiopulmonary bypass as well as myocardial and aortic incisions made intraoperatively (e.g., right atrium for cannulation of cavae). Because of the nearly universal release of CK-MB, a diagnosis of MI should not be made unless the CK-MB is significantly elevated (e.g., >30 units/liter).
Echocardiogram	A regional wall motion abnormality is a helpful finding, particularly if it can be shown to be a new finding by comparison with a preoperative study. Paradoxical motion of the high anterior portion of the interventricular septum is a common finding postoperatively in the absence of MI, and should not be taken as the sole evidence of new perioperative myocardial necrosis.
Scintigrams	Abnormal technetium-99m stannous pyrophosphate scintigrams are more sensitive and more specific than the development of new Q waves on the ECG and more specific than the presence of CK-MB in the serum for the diagnosis of perioperative MI. It is important to differentiate between blood pool activity and diffuse left ventricular uptake and to differentiate between rib uptake secondary to operative trauma and localized myocardial uptake.

MI, myocardial infarction; CK, creatine kinase.

sion of bypass grafts placed to diseased coronary arteries, autopsy studies have shown that bypass grafts usually are patent in patients dying of a perioperative myocardial infarction.[86] This observation lends support to the concept that a mismatch between myocardial oxygen supply and demand in the operating room accounts for much of the infarction noted postoperatively.

The diagnosis of a myocardial infarction after cardiac surgery is more difficult than at other times because of the nonspecific ST-T wave abnormalities on the electrocardiogram and nearly universal elevation of creatine-kinase (CK) levels postoperatively. A number of diagnostic findings (Table 53–8) must be carefully interpreted and then integrated along the lines of the algorithm shown in Table 53–9.

A 12-lead electrocardiogram should be obtained immediately on the patient's arrival in the intensive care unit after operation and no less frequently than once every 24 hours for the first 3 postoperative days. Measurements of total CK and CK-MB should be made every 8 hours for the first 24 hours and every 24 hours thereafter for the first 3 postoperative days. If there is clinical suspicion of a perioperative myocardial infarction, the CK measurements are made more frequently (every 8 hours) during the 2nd and 3rd postoperative days and a confirmatory bedside echocardiogram is obtained. It is especially helpful to review new echocardiograms in comparison with the preoperative studies that are almost always available.

The electrocardiogram is the most reliable tool for diagnosing a perioperative myocardial infarction. New and persistent Q waves accompanied by new, persistent, and evolutionary ST-T wave abnormalities are the most helpful criteria. Pathological Q waves owing to perioperative myocardial infarction may appear with an earlier time course (i.e., immediately on arrival from the operating room) than in the nonrevascularized patient; they should be considered diagnostic, however, only if they are seen on serial electrocardiograms once the

TABLE 53–9 ALGORITHM FOR DIAGNOSIS OF PERIOPERATIVE MI AFTER CARDIAC SURGERY

NEW Q's ON ECG	CK-MB >30 IU/LITER	NEW RWMA ON ECHO*	DIAGNOSIS	COMMENT
Yes	Yes	Yes	Definite MI	
Yes	Yes	No	Probable MI	New zone of necrosis not evident on echo. The persistence of new Q waves and abnormally elevated CK-MB suggests that the Q waves are not a "benign" postoperative finding.
Yes	No	Yes	Definite MI	CK-MB peak probably missed because of infrequent sampling.
Yes	No	No	Possible MI	New Q waves may be false-positive finding.
No	Yes	Yes	Probable MI	Non–Q wave MI.
No	Yes	No	MI unlikely	Small non–Q wave MI cannot be entirely excluded.
No	No	Yes	MI unlikely	Removal of "restraining" effect of pericardium may result in new RWMAs, especially in high anterior septal area
No	No	No	No MI	Although small patchy areas of necrosis may be seen histologically, these are not of clinical significance.

* Perioperative echocardiography is not *required* for the diagnosis of a perioperative MI but can provide useful supportive data or aid in the diagnosis in unclear cases, especially if obtained acutely. RWMA, regional wall motion abnormality; MI, myocardial infarction.

early postoperative hypothermia, axis shifts, and any potentially reversible myocardial ischemia have resolved.[87]

Operative variables that have been found to correlate with the development of a perioperative myocardial infarction in patients undergoing coronary bypass grafting include prolonged pump time (>75 minutes) and increased total ischemic time (>50 minutes); although some investigators found that an increased number of grafts also correlated with myocardial infarction, this has not been a uniform finding.[88,89]

Although the unique circumstances of perioperative myocardial infarction (early reperfusion, revascularization of adjacent ischemic zones, potential for early intervention if complications should arise) may lessen the potential adverse impact of myocardial infarction on ventricular function, most patients with a perioperative myocardial infarction have an increased hospital mortality (about 10 per cent) compared with patients undergoing coronary bypass grafting who have not sustained a perioperative myocardial infarction (about 1 per cent).[89,90] Characteristics of patients who are especially at risk of increased short-term mortality after a perioperative myocardial infarction include age over 65 years, unstable angina preoperatively, a myocardial infarction within 1 week before operation, left ventricular aneurysm, intraventricular conduction disturbance (e.g., left bundle branch block), and the need for reoperation for bleeding. About two-thirds of the postoperative mortality is due to pump failure and one-third is due to malignant ventricular tachyarrhythmias.[90] A recent study suggests that perioperative myocardial infarction also affects long-term prognosis, particularly if associated with inadequate revascularization and depressed left ventricular function.[90a]

LOW-OUTPUT SYNDROME AND SHOCK STATES

Sometimes diagnosis of the low-output syndrome and a shock state after cardiac surgery is difficult. Because cold extremities and mottled skin may result from hypothermia postoperatively, these observations lack sufficient specificity. Although reduced systolic pressure is the most striking manifestation of this disorder, a low-output syndrome may be present even if the arterial systolic pressure exceeds 100 mm Hg, since an increased systemic vascular resistance (>1500 dynes-sec-cm^{-5}) may be supporting the peripheral perfusion pressure. It is important to recognize this syndrome, since there is a strong relation between the cardiac index in the early postoperative period and the probability of cardiac death after surgery. Common clinical features of the low-output syndrome and shock states after cardiac surgery include cold extremities, mottled skin, reduced systolic pressure (<90 mm Hg), decreased urine output (<30 ml/hr), low cardiac index (<2.0 liter/min/m^2), low mixed venous oxygen saturation (<50 per cent), and acidosis. One should make careful hemodynamic measurements and integrate them with bedside echocardiographic recordings to confirm the diagnosis of a low-output syndrome and attempt to segregate the findings into one of the patterns (*reduced preload, cardiogenic,* or *septic*) in Table 53–10. Although there is overlap of the hemodynamic findings among these patterns, and coexistence of multiple disorders (e.g., bradycardia and hypovolemia) may blur the distinctions between patterns, they offer a clinically useful approach to the evaluation of the patient with a low-output syndrome. In addition to the specific treatment measures discussed below, a number of general measures are applicable to all patients who are in a shock-like condition after cardiac surgery, including prompt correction of any electrolyte and acid–base disturbances, transfusion to a hematocrit over 30 per cent for improved oxygen-carrying capacity of the blood, and a "low threshold" for mechanical ventilatory support to minimize the work of breathing and thereby reduce total body oxygen needs.

REDUCED PRELOAD

Hypovolemia. Low ventricular filling pressures, a normal systemic vascular resistance, and a reduced cardiac index, coupled with echocardiographic demonstration of small ventricular volumes with preserved systolic function, are indicative of *hypovolemia.* Possible causes of hypovolemia include bleeding, excessive diuresis, the "leaky capillary state" associated with the postpump syndrome, and, less frequently, inadequate vascular volume because of insufficient return of fluids at the conclusion of cardiopulmonary bypass. Rarely, adrenal cortical insufficiency owing to perioperative hemorrhage into the adrenals has been reported as a cause of hypovolemic hypotension after cardiac surgery.

Therapeutic maneuvers include administration of intravenous fluids (normal saline solution, lactated Ringer's solution), transfusion with packed red blood cells if the hemoglobin is less than 10 gm/dl and administration of colloid-type volume expanders. It also is important to discontinue any vasodilators that may have been prescribed during a period when the patient was hypertensive. While waiting for the above measures to take effect, the patient may require a transient infusion of an inotropic pressor agent, usually dopamine (p. 501).

Vasodilatation. Inhibition of sympathetic tone by the effects of anesthetic agents may cause peripheral vasodilatation. In combination with increased venous capacitance that may occur during rewarming, a low-output syndrome may develop owing to a markedly reduced systemic vascular resistance (<1000 dynes-sec-cm^{-5}). This situation is best treated by an infusion of a vasoconstrictor such as epinephrine or norepinephrine in a dose of 1 to 10 μg/min until the systemic vascular resistance returns to a normal level.

CARDIOGENIC SHOCK. When the right ventricular and left ventricular filling pressures are in the normal range and systemic vascular resistance is not reduced, a frequent cause of a cardiac index less than 2 liters/min/m^2 is *bradycardia.* Because cardiac index is the product of stroke volume and heart rate, this abnormality is easily corrected by atrial or atrioventricular pacing at 85 to 100 beats/min.

Left Ventricular Failure. The pattern of predominant *left ventricular failure* is characterized by a disproportionately elevated pulmonary capillary wedge pressure as compared with right atrial pressure, low cardiac index, and normal or elevated systemic vascular resistance. Echocardiography usually reveals a dilated, poorly contractile left ventricle, often exhibiting multiple regional wall motion abnormalities. The differential diagnosis of left ventricular failure after cardiac surgery includes the following conditions (which may coexist in the same patient): preoperative left ventricular dysfunction, inadequate surgical correction of the cardiac lesion (e.g., persistent aortic valve gradient owing to mismatch between the patient's aortic ring and prosthesis, residual left ventricular outflow tract obstruction after repair of idiopathic hypertrophic subaortic stenosis, residual atrial or ventricular septal defect), complication of surgical procedure (e.g., prosthetic valve leak or thrombosis, depression of stroke volume after correction of mitral regurgitation caused by the elevation of afterload), dysrhythmia, depressant effect of pharmacological agent (e.g., antiarrhythmic drug), acid–base or electrolyte disturbance, or myocardial ischemia and/or infarction. Bedside echocardiography usually can help to identify mechanical disorders such as prosthetic valve dysfunction and dysrhythmias, and metabolic abnormalities and toxic drug levels can be readily recognized by electrocardiogram and laboratory measurements.

The objectives of hemodynamic management of patients with *left ventricular failure* postoperatively are to correct hypotension if present, increase forward left ventricular output, and return left and right ventricular filling pressures to the normal range. These parameters are intimately related, and treatment may require careful titration of several intravenous agents for pharmacological support of the failing circulation. Boluses of calcium chloride (0.5 to 1.0 gm) will increase myocardial contractility, but the effect is modest and short-lived. A continuous infusion of dopamine (5 to 10 μg/kg/min) is preferable if the primary goal is to increase systemic arterial

TABLE 53-10 LOW-OUTPUT SYNDROME AND SHOCK STATES AFTER CARDIAC SURGERY

	REDUCED PRELOAD		CARDIOGENIC SHOCK				SEPTIC
Causes	Hypovolemia	Vasodilatation	Bradycardia (Inappropriately slow HR postoperatively)	LV failure	RV failure	Cardiac tamponade	Sepsis
Hemodynamics							
RA	<8	<8	≤10	≥10	>10	≫15	<10
PCW	<15	<15	>15	≫20	≤15*	≫15	<15
CI	<2.0	<2.0	<2.0	<2.0	<2.0	<2.0	≥2.0
SVR	>1200	<1000	>1200	>1000	>1000	≫1000	<1000
Other			HR < 60		PCW > 15 if LV failure is present	RA = PCW = PAd (within 5 mm Hg) unless "asymmetric" tamponade occurs due to pericardial clots	Narrow AV O_2 difference
Echocardiogram	Small ventricular chambers with vigorous systolic contraction unless LV dysfunction was present preoperatively	Small ventricular chambers with normal systolic contraction unless LV dysfunction was present preoperatively	Normal-sized ventricular chambers with vigorous systolic contraction, albeit at a slow rate	Dilated LV with reduced systolic performance; regional wall motion abnormalities may reflect old or new myocardial ischemia and/or infarction.	Dilated RA and RV with reduced RV systolic contraction. TR often present on Doppler study. The contractile performance of LV is variable.	Small cardiac chambers with diastolic collapse of RA and RV. Systolic contraction of RV and LV usually normal unless dysfunction was present preoperatively or coexistent LV or RV failure has occurred postoperatively.	Small ventricular chambers with normal or slightly depressed contractile function (myocardial depressant factor)
Management	IV fluids Transfusion if Hgb <10 Inotropes	Vasopressors	Cardiac pacing	Search for correctible lesion, offending agent, or laboratory abnormality Inotropes Vasopressors and vasodilators Mechanical assistance	Supplemental O_2 Pulmonary vasodilators Inotropes Mechanical assistance	Reexploration Supportive measures: IV fluids, inotropes	IV fluids Antibiotics Vasopressors Inotropes

LV, left ventricular; RV, right ventricular; RA, right atrial; PCW, pulmonary capillary wedge; CI, cardiac index; SVR, systemic vascular resistance; TR, tricuspid regurgitation.

pressure and cardiac output.[91] Dobutamine (2 to 5 μg/kg/min) or amrinone (2 to 5 μg/kg/min) also will both augment cardiac output and should be selected if reduction of ventricular filling pressure is desired; systemic arterial pressure usually will be unchanged or may even drop slightly because of the peripheral vasodilatory effects of these drugs.[92] A commonly used combination is dopamine (2 μg/kg/min) to achieve greater renal perfusion in conjunction with dobutamine (2–5 μg/kg/min) for augmentation of cardiac output. If the arterial pressure is equal to or greater than 90 mm Hg, vasodilator therapy with sodium nitroprusside or nitroglycerin will increase forward cardiac output and lower the pulmonary capillary wedge pressure further. In cases where hypotension is profound (e.g., systolic pressure <70 mm Hg), norepinephrine, 1 to 10 μg/min, may be necessary to prevent coronary hypoperfusion.[93]

We prefer to use an intraaortic balloon pump (Chap. 19) for mechanical support of the circulation along with pharmacotherapy early in the course of management of postoperative left ventricular failure that does not respond to the initial pharmacological maneuvers already discussed. This has the advantages of avoiding a continuous upward titration of the dose of sympathomimetic inotropic agents and vasoconstrictors associated with downregulation of beta adrenoceptors and diminished perfusion of the renal, mesenteric, and coronary vascular beds. Also, intraaortic balloon counterpulsation will not increase myocardial oxygen demand. The intraaortic balloon pump is particularly helpful if significant mitral regurgitation is present, but is contraindicated in the presence of aortic regurgitation and if an abdominal aortic aneurysm is present. If the patient does not improve despite a combination of intraaortic balloon pumping and pharmacotherapy, and cardiac transplantation is decided on, then a left ventricular assist device as a "bridge" to transplantation may be considered until a donor is located (Chap. 19).

Right Ventricular Failure. The pattern of predominant *right ventricular failure* is characterized by a disproportionate elevation of the right atrial pressure in comparison with the pulmonary capillary wedge pressure. In severe cases of postoperative right ventricular failure, the right atrial pressure may exceed 20 mm Hg while the pulmonary capillary wedge pressure remains equal to or less than 15 mm Hg. When left ventricular failure is present simultaneously, the difference between the right atrial and pulmonary capillary wedge pressures lessens and differentiation from cardiac tamponade becomes difficult. Bedside echocardiography is useful for making a proper diagnosis (Table 53–10).

Postoperatively, predominant right ventricular failure may be seen as a result of one or more of the following conditions: elevated pulmonary vascular resistance (persistently elevated from preoperative elevations of pulmonary artery pressure; postoperative hypoxia, pulmonary embolus, or pneumothorax), primary right ventricular ischemia/infarction,[94] or a mechanical lesion (tricuspid regurgitation, residual shunt flow, right ventriculotomy). *Massive pulmonary embolism* is a rare occurrence after cardiac surgery (Chap. 48). The diagnosis should be suspected when sudden deterioration in oxygenation occurs in association with systemic hypotension and elevation of right atrial pressure. Because thrombolytic therapy usually is contraindicated (because of the risk of bleeding postoperatively), management consists of prompt confirmation of the diagnosis with pulmonary arteriography followed by anticoagulation. Pulmonary emboli that cause less hemodynamic compromise (right atrial pressure <15 mm Hg, arterial pressure >90 mm Hg, cardiac index ≥ 2 liters/min/m^2) can be treated with anticoagulation alone. An inferior vena caval filter should be inserted if venography reveals lower-extremity venous thrombosis and recurrences are detected, or if, after the index event, it is felt that the patient could not survive a recurrent embolus. Because a caval filter will not prevent embolization from right atrial or right ventricular thrombi, an echocardiogram should be performed with consideration of surgical removal of any large mobile, nonsessile right heart thrombi.

Hemodynamic management of predominant right ventricular failure should focus on improvement of right ventricular output to allow adequate filling of the left ventricle. Supplemental oxygen is provided to lower the pulmonary artery pressure. Bradycardia (<60 beats/min) is corrected by atrial or atrioventricular pacing. Isoproterenol (1 to 2 μg/min in the average adult) increases right ventricular contractility and also causes pulmonary vasodilatation. Pulmonary hypertension also may be reduced by prostaglandin E_1[95] and intravenous nitroglycerin.[15] Further reduction in right ventricular afterload can be achieved by an infusion of dobutamine to decrease the pulmonary capillary wedge pressure and lower the driving force across the pulmonary vascular circuit. Profound hypotension caused by right ventricular failure that does not respond to the above measures can be treated with an infusion of a pulmonary vasodilator (isoproterenol, phentolamine) directly into the pulmonary artery by way of a Swan-Ganz catheter. Insertion of a counterpulsation balloon catheter directly into the pulmonary artery has been reported, but the survival rate in such cases has been poor.[96] Mechanical support of the failing right ventricle is now being used more frequently (see Chap. 19). Rarely, pulmonary embolectomy may be considered in the presence of refractory failure or shock (p. 1574).

Cardiac Tamponade (see Chap. 45). Postoperative echocardiography has shown that virtually all patients have a pericardial effusion after cardiac surgery.[97] Many such effusions are asymmetrical, with most of the fluid collecting posteriorly; this is probably because the cut anterior surfaces of the pericardium frequently are left unopposed at the conclusion of the operation, and positioning of the patient supine leaves the posterior mediastinum dependent.[98] Even with mediastinal drains in place, it is possible for a patient to develop cardiac tamponade postoperatively; recognition of this condition requires a high index of suspicion and assessment of hemodynamics at the bedside.[99]

Important clinical features of tamponade, such as diminished heart sounds and pulsus paradoxus, may be obscured by mechanical ventilation. Asymmetrical, loculated accumulation of blood and clots in the mediastinum and pericardial space may cause isolated tamponade of one or two cardiac chambers, producing unusual elevations of diastolic pressures (e.g., right atrial tamponade with elevation of central venous pressure without an increase in right ventricular end-diastolic pressure or pulmonary capillary wedge pressure).[100,101] Bedside two-dimensional echocardiography is extremely helpful for diagnosing pericardial effusions and assessing the hemodynamic significance of fluid collections. Diastolic collapse of the right atrium and right ventricle is an indication of a hemodynamically significant external compressive force, and should prompt urgent treatment. Although pericardiocentesis may be helpful in nonsurgical tamponade, it is unlikely to be successful in evacuating the organized pericardial and mediastinal material that develops after cardiac surgery; subxiphoid drainage and/or emergency sternotomy is preferred. Supportive measures that can be attempted in the interim include volume expansion with intravenous fluids (Plasmanate, whole blood), and inotropic agents (dobutamine).

SEPTIC SHOCK. Low ventricular filling pressures, a markedly reduced systemic vascular resistance, and a normal or unexpectedly high cardiac index in the setting of hypotension and a shock-like state should raise the suspicion of the early stages of *sepsis*. With progression of septic shock, a capillary leak syndrome develops (hypovolemia) and myocardial depression may occur, resulting in a somewhat reduced contractile pattern of the ventricles on echocardiography. Combined therapy with intravenous fluids, antibiotics, and inotropic agents is required to interrupt the vicious cycle of hypotension, acidosis, and diminished coronary perfusion. Most patients who are septic during the first 48 hours after cardiac surgery are infected with a skin organism (incision, monitoring lines) or from seeding the bloodstream from a pulmonary or urinary source. Broad antibiotic coverage with one of the following combinations should be instituted: vancomycin plus an aminoglycoside, or ampicillin plus oxacillin and an aminoglycoside. Because the offending organism is likely to be resistant to the prophylactic antibiotic given preoperatively, it is wise not to include it as one of the empiric antibiotics selected to treat sepsis.

ARRHYTHMIAS

EVALUATION AND TREATMENT. There appear to be two peaks in the incidence of arrhythmias perioperatively: the first occurs in the operating room (most commonly during induction of anesthesia, weaning from cardiopulmonary bypass, rewarming) and the second occurs in the intensive care unit between the 2nd and 5th postoperative days. The electrophysiologic mechanisms underlying perioperative arrhythmias are incompletely understood, but they can probably be ascribed to a combination of the effects of circulating catecholamines, alterations in autonomic nervous system tone, transient electrolyte imbalances, myocardial ischemia or infarction, and mechanical irritation of the heart.

The physician caring for the postoperative cardiac surgical patient is frustrated by the lack of clinical data on which to base treatment decisions. Most of the emphasis in the literature is placed on prophylaxis against supraventricular tachyarrhythmias with digoxin (p. 691) and extrapolation of the early (and now outdated) coronary care unit guidelines for treating "warning" ventricular arrhythmias to the postoperative cardiac surgical patient. The availability of newer antiarrhythmic agents (verapamil, esmolol, adenosine) with efficacy against supraventricular arrhythmias coupled with published reports of the successful use of atrial pacing techniques have begun to provide a more rational approach to *supraventricular arrhythmias.* The management of *ventricular arrhythmias* remains controversial, especially in light of data from the nonsurgical ischemic heart disease population that prophylactic and suppressive antiarrhythmic therapy for the asymptomatic or minimally symptomatic patient may be associated with an increased mortality.[31,102] Studies of the prognostic significance of ventricular arrhythmias after cardiac surgery and the impact of antiarrhythmic therapy on postoperative mortality are virtually nonexistent.

In the absence of more definitive data, clinicians can only cautiously apply the information gleaned from arrhythmia-intervention trials in nonsurgical patients and individualize treatment decisions based on the specifics of the patient's medical history and the circumstances present in the intensive care unit. For example, a patient with depressed left ventricular function and a preoperative history of resuscitation from sudden cardiac death who has just undergone coronary revascularization requires an aggressive approach to prevent recurrent ventricular tachycardia or ventricular fibrillation. Alternatively, a young patient with normal left ventricular function who has undergone closure of an atrial septal defect or mitral valve repair for ruptured chordae tendineae probably does not require suppression of ventricular arrhythmias in the absence of sustained ventricular tachycardia causing hemodynamic compromise.

When evaluating rhythm disturbances after open heart surgery, a number of general principles should be kept in mind. Several factors may predispose to the development of arrhythmias, including ventilatory dysfunction, fever, electrolyte imbalance (hypokalemia,[103] hypomagnesemia,[49] hypocalcemia), anemia, myocardial ischemia or infarction, low cardiac output and reflex increase in sympathetic tone, hypertension, pericardial inflammation, and toxic effects of cardioactive medications (e.g., digitalis toxicity, bradycardia induced by diltiazem). *Every effort should be made to look for and eliminate any of the factors that may be provoking the arrhythmia.*

Although antiarrhythmic drug therapy and direct-current cardioversion are traditional methods for treating postoperative arrhythmias, cardiac pacing techniques have a number of advantages. These include a more rapid onset and offset of action, avoidance of potential drug toxicity—especially proarrhythmia—elimination of the need for anesthesia (required for cardioversion), reduced anxiety for the patient, greater safety in patients receiving digitalis, and, perhaps most important, the ability to repeat the pacing protocol if the arrhythmia should recur, a not infrequent event. In addition to terminating arrhythmias, cardiac pacing can be used to suppress arrhythmias in many patients by atrial, atrioventricular sequential, or ventricular stimulation at a critical rate (e.g., 85–100 beats/min).

Surface Electrocardiogram. In an attempt to improve arrhythmia-detection algorithms, many manufacturers have built cardiac monitors that simultaneously record two to four electrocardiograph leads. It usually is unwise, however, to base a treatment decision on monitor lead rhythm strips, especially if one is attempting to analyze a wide-complex tachycardia. The value of a 12-lead electrocardiogram and simultaneously recorded multiple standard electrocardiograph lead rhythm strips cannot be overemphasized in this regard. Unfortunately a number of the criteria for differentiating supraventricular tachycardia with aberrant conduction from ventricular tachycardia (p. 704) may not be applicable to postoperative patients because of previous or newly acquired infarction patterns, transient conduction defects (seen in 5–15 per cent of patients in the early recovery period), and nonspecific repolarization patterns. Although carotid sinus massage and specialized electrocardiograph lead recordings to detect atrial activation may be helpful, it is important to take advantage of the additional recording capabilities provided by the atrial and ventricular epicardial electrodes placed at the conclusion of cardiopulmonary bypass (Fig. 53–3).

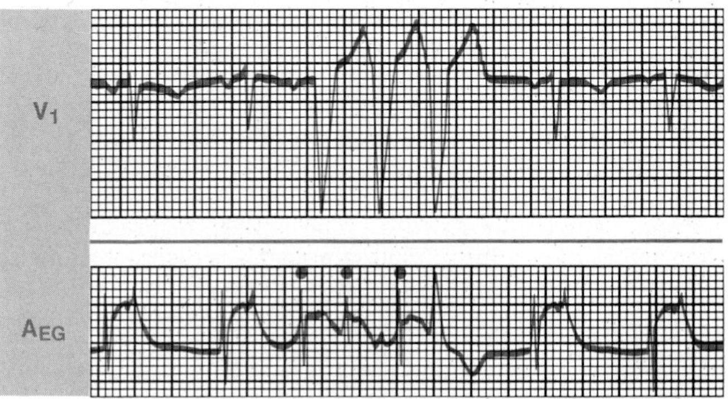

FIGURE 53–3. Simultaneous recordings of electrocardiographic lead V1 and a bipolar atrial electrogram (A_{EG}). The three consecutive beats with wide QRS complexes recorded in the electrocardiogram do not represent ventricular tachycardia, but are due to aberrant ventricular conduction of three premature atrial beats (black dots), as documented in the bipolar atrial electrogram. The appearance of a small ventricular complex after each atrial complex in the bipolar atrial electrogram recording helps to confirm the diagnosis. (From Waldo, A. L., and MacLean, W. A. H.: Diagnosis and Treatment of Cardiac Arrhythmias Following Cardiac Surgery. Mt. Kisco, NY, Futura Publishing Co., 1980.)

Epicardial Electrodes. Although many cardiac surgeons place only single atrial and ventricular pacing wires and a subcutaneous wire for the indifferent electrode, it is preferable that two wires be positioned high on the free wall of the

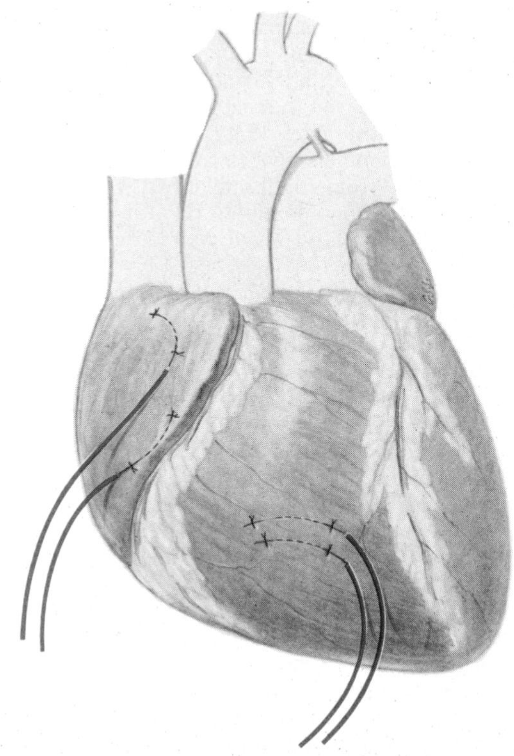

FIGURE 53–4. Placement of atrial and ventricular pacing wires during cardiac surgery. Although two atrial and ventricular electrodes are shown in this diagram (allowing bipolar recording and pacing), some surgeons place only one electrode in each of the sites (restricting recording and pacing to a unipolar configuration). Not shown in this diagram is an indifferent (ground) electrode that is placed in a subcutaneous position. The distal ends of the pacing wires are brought out to the skin through small stab wounds and positioned as shown in Figure 53–2. (From Behrendt, D. M., and Austen, W. G.: Patient Care in Cardiac Surgery. 4th ed. Boston, Little, Brown, 1985.)

Atrial Electrograms

Bipolar

Unipolar

FIGURE 53-5. Simultaneous recording of bipolar and unipolar atrial electrograms utilizing a two-channel electrocardiography machine with the standard right and left arm leads of the electrocardiograph patient cable attached to the two atrial wires and the recording selector set to the standard lead I (bipolar atrial electrogram) and standard lead II (unipolar atrial electrogram) positions. The rhythm disorder is type I (classical) atrial flutter with an atrial rate of 280 beats/min and 2:1 AV conduction. This type of atrial flutter is easily treated with rapid atrial pacing techniques. More rapid forms of atrial flutter (atrial rate 340–430 beats/min) are less responsive to atrial pacing, and have been designated type II flutter. (From Waldo, A. L., and MacLean, W. A. H.: Diagnosis and Treatment of Cardiac Arrhythmias Following Cardiac Surgery. Mt. Kisco, NY, Futura Publishing Co., 1980.)

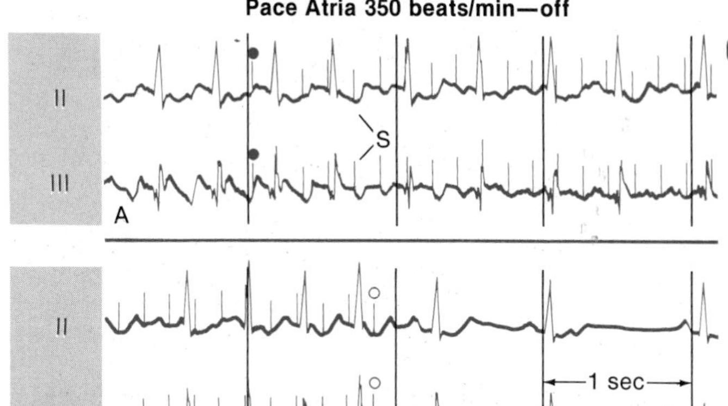

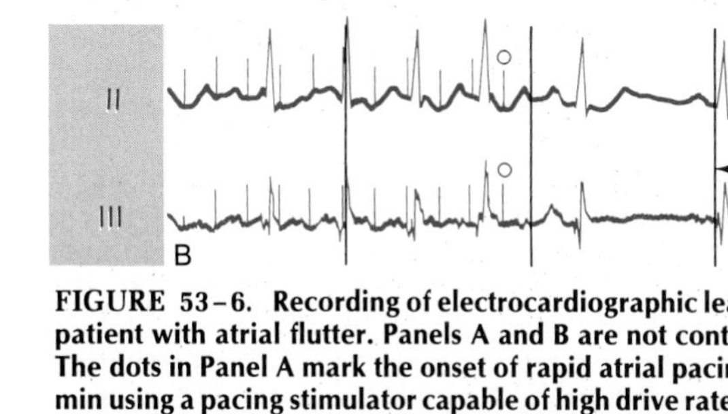

FIGURE 53-6. Recording of electrocardiographic leads II and III in a patient with atrial flutter. Panels A and B are not continuous tracings. The dots in Panel A mark the onset of rapid atrial pacing at 350 beats/min using a pacing stimulator capable of high drive rates. The morphology of the atrial complexes changes dramatically, such that by the end of the trace in Panel A, the atrial complexes are positive in leads II and III. Panel B shows the termination of 30 seconds of atrial pacing at 350 beats/min. The circles represent the last paced atrial beat. With abrupt termination of the rapid atrial pacing, sinus rhythm appears. S = stimulus artifact. Time lines are at 1-second intervals. (From Waldo, A. L., and MacLean, W. A. H.: Diagnosis and Treatment of Cardiac Arrhythmias Following Cardiac Surgery. Mt. Kisco, NY, Futura Publishing Co., 1980.)

right atrium to allow for bipolar atrial recording and pacing. Waldo and MacLean have enumerated the advantages of bipolar pacing, including a smaller stimulus artifact, the ability to record a bipolar atrial electrogram during ventricular pacing, and a reduced likelihood of precipitating undesired atrial arrhythmias if an atrial wire is used as the indifferent electrode during unipolar ventricular pacing.[104] Schematic diagrams showing the suggested intrathoracic positioning of the right atrial wires and recordings of unipolar and bipolar atrial electrocardiograms are shown in Figures 53–4 and 53–5.

SUPRAVENTRICULAR ARRHYTHMIAS

Atrial Premature Depolarizations (see also p. 679). The hemodynamic consequences of atrial premature depolarizations are almost always minor, and one should resist the urge to suppress them with antiarrhythmic drugs. Instead, they should be considered a signal that the patient is possibly hypoxic or that an electrolyte imbalance is present, and a warning that the patient is at risk of developing a more serious arrhythmia, such as atrial fibrillation or atrial flutter. In the absence of such correctable abnormalities, one may want to administer a beta blocker to inhibit the effects of circulating catecholamines and also to slow the ventricular rate if atrial fibrillation should develop. We reserve the practice of "prophylactic" digitalization in response to the emergence of atrial premature depolarizations to those patients with markedly depressed left ventricular function (ejection fraction <30 per cent) in whom atrial fibrillation would cause serious hemodynamic compromise.

Atrial Flutter (see also p. 679). Control of the ventricular rate in atrial flutter is more difficult than atrial fibrillation because of the limited number of ventricular responses to atrial activation (usually 2:1, 4:1, but rarely an odd-numbered multiple). Because atrial flutter may be difficult to terminate with antiarrhythmic agents, electrical procedures such as direct-current cardioversion and rapid atrial pacing often are used clinically. Cardioversion can be expected to terminate atrial flutter in more than 90 per cent of patients, with an energy of 25 to 50 watt-seconds delivered as a single discharge. Atrial flutter can also be terminated by rapid atrial pacing using the temporary epicardial atrial wires placed at the time of operation. The likelihood of success is increased if one uses sufficiently rapid rates of pacing (up to 140 per cent of the spontaneous atrial rate), a sufficient duration of pacing (10 to 30 seconds), and adequate strength (5 to 20 mA). To achieve the high drive rates required, a special stimulator is utilized.[104] A bipolar pacing mode is preferred, although unipolar pacing can be attempted but with a lower chance of success. Difficulty also may be encountered if the spontaneous atrial rate is particularly rapid (i.e., >350 beats/min) and when pacing stimuli are delivered at a distance from the focus initiating the arrhythmia. In the latter instance the pacing protocol may be unable to penetrate and depolarize a portion of the reentrant circuit, allowing the flutter mechanism to persist. Examples of the diagnostic usefulness of atrial electrograms and the successful use of rapid atrial pacing for the termination of atrial flutter are shown in Figures 53–6 and 53–7.

Atrial Fibrillation (see also p. 682). Atrial fibrillation is extremely common after cardiac surgery. Transient symptomatic atrial fibrillation occurs in at least 25 to 30 per cent of patients after coronary artery bypass grafting and 60 per cent of patients after valvular surgery, appearing with greatest incidence on the 2nd or 3rd postoperative day.[105,106] Unless he-

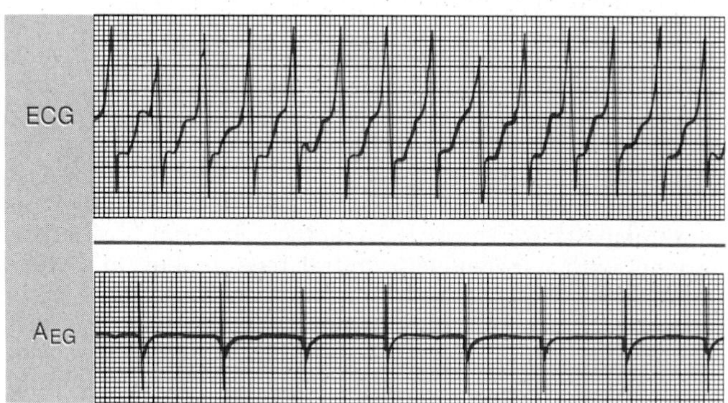

FIGURE 53-7. Monitor electrocardiographic lead recorded simultaneously with bipolar atrial electrogram (A_{EG}) during a wide QRS complex tachycardia at 155 beats/min. The A_{EG} demonstrates the presence of sinus rhythm at 90 beats/min. This observation in conjunction with AV dissociation and fusion beats (second and ninth QRS complexes), establishes that the wide QRS complex tachycardia is ventricular in origin. (From Waldo, A. L., and MacLean, W. A. H.: Diagnosis and Treatment of Cardiac Arrhythmias Following Cardiac Surgery. Mt. Kisco, NY, Futura Publishing Co., 1980.)

modynamic collapse is present—in which case direct-current cardioversion should be performed—the treatment of choice in the postoperative patient is to first slow the ventricular rate. Although many textbooks and manuals of patient care continue to list digitalis glycosides as the drugs of choice, the therapeutic index is especially narrow in the postoperative patient, and the likelihood of achieving a desired level of control of the ventricular rate is reduced in the presence of high circulating catecholamine levels. Provided the patient's ventricular function is adequate, acute intravenous administration of beta blockers (e.g., metoprolol, 5 mg, every 5 minutes for up to three doses) or verapamil (e.g., 5-mg bolus every 5 to 10 minutes for three to four doses) is a more desirable option. Esmolol, an ultrashort-acting cardioselective beta blocker, when administered intravenously in a dose of 50 to 250 μg/kg/min, provides the option of rapid onset of a titratable level of beta blockade with a cardioselective agent; in the event of hemodynamic deterioration, the effects of the drug usually are dissipated within 30 minutes after discontinuation of the infusion. In addition, the probability of conversion to sinus rhythm with esmolol appears to be superior to that with other agents, such as verapamil.[107]

Although direct-current cardioversion with an average energy of 100 watt-seconds is likely to restore sinus rhythm, we prefer to control the ventricular rate by pharmacotherapy, and to postpone the cardioversion procedure until 7 to 10 days postoperatively, when the risk of recurrent atrial fibrillation is decreased because pericardial and mediastinal inflammation have resolved somewhat and the level of sympathetic tone has decreased. In the nonsurgical patient the current recommendation is that anticoagulation be initiated for patients who have been in atrial fibrillation for more than 3 days because of the risk of embolism.[108] We usually do not initiate anticoagulation in the early (<2 weeks) postoperative period before cardioversion if the presence of atrial fibrillation is the only indication for antithrombotic therapy. The advantages of intravenous heparin in reducing the risk of embolism from atrial fibrillation must be weighed against the risk of bleeding as a result of recent surgery. Patients in whom sinus rhythm cannot be successfully restored and who are discharged in chronic atrial fibrillation *should* be considered candidates for anticoagulation.[108]

About 48 hours before cardioversion, antiarrhythmic treatment to possibly restore sinus rhythm pharmacologically (albeit successfully in only 5 to 15 per cent of patients) and to suppress recurrences of atrial fibrillation is started in those patients in whom long-term antiarrhythmic therapy is considered appropriate (e.g., preoperative history of atrial fibrillation, depressed left ventricular function, valvular surgery). Because patients are most likely to relapse into atrial fibrillation during the first 2 months after cardioversion, it is wise to administer suppressive antiarrhythmic therapy for at least this period. Permanent suppressive antiarrhythmic therapy often is still necessary in patients with rheumatic heart disease and a preoperative history of atrial fibrillation despite successful aortic or mitral valve surgery, even if sinus rhythm is present during the early postoperative period. Such patients typically have scarring of enlarged atria that places them at continued risk for intraatrial reentry and atrial fibrillation. Patients with nonrheumatic mitral regurgitation (e.g., ruptured chordae tendineae) who have undergone mitral valve repair or replacement may be observed off antiarrhythmic therapy post cardioversion, despite a preoperative history of atrial fibrillation, since relief of the hemodynamic burden may decrease their propensity to atrial premature depolarizations and atrial fibrillation.

Patients with atrial fibrillation postoperatively are at risk for systemic embolization, but the risk varies with the pattern (chronic > paroxysmal) and underlying cardiovascular pathology (valvular heart disease, dilated or hypertrophic cardiomyopathy, and congestive heart failure > nonvalvular heart disease > lone atrial fibrillator).[108] For patients with persistent atrial fibrillation and mitral valve disease, dilated cardiomyopathy, or a history of systemic embolism, we advocate chronic warfarin therapy designed to achieve a prothrombin time ratio of 1.5 times control.

Paroxysmal Supraventricular Tachycardia (see p. 1715). The reentrant forms of paroxysmal supraventricular tachycardia (PSVT)—atrioventricular nodal reentry tachycardia and atrioventricular reentry tachycardia—occur less frequently in the postoperative patient than atrial fibrillation or atrial flutter, but fortunately retain their responsiveness to vagal maneuvers and pharmacotherapy to inhibit atrioventricular nodal conduction. The antiarrhythmic agent adenosine (p. 650), an endogenous nucleoside, has a number of features making it the drug of choice for treating PSVT in the postoperative patient.[109] A rapid (2 seconds) intravenous bolus of 6 mg will terminate about 60 per cent of episodes of PSVT within 20 seconds; a subsequent bolus of 12 mg administered 1 to 2 minutes later will terminate PSVT in virtually all those cases that failed to respond to the lower dose. Because adenosine is rapidly transported into the cell or degraded enzymatically to inosine, the physiological effects of adenosine are dissipated by 5 minutes. Untoward reactions such as flushing and hypotension are mild and short-lived.

PSVT also may be diagnosed by atrial recordings, and terminated by burst atrial pacing or randomly delivered atrial or ventricular premature depolarizations that invade the reentrant circuit and interrupt the arrhythmia. The automatic form of PSVT (i.e., ectopic automatic atrial tachycardia) is sufficiently unusual postoperatively that its presence should strongly raise the suspicion of digitalis toxicity.

VENTRICULAR ARRHYTHMIAS

Ventricular Premature Depolarizations (see p. 701). Isolated ventricular premature depolarizations (VPDs) commonly occur after cardiac surgery. There may be an increase in the density of VPDs in patients with a preoperative history of VPDs, or they may appear de novo in patients with no history of ventricular arrhythmias. Although there may be a fall in arterial pressure associated with isolated VPDs, this usually is extremely brief and of no significant hemodynamic consequence to the patient unless prolonged periods of bigeminy occur. The emergence of frequent VPDs should trigger a search for any potentially correctable factors. Such a search would include measurement of serum electrolyte levels (potassium, calcium, magnesium), hematocrit, and blood pressure; assessment of the level of oxygenation; estimation of volume status (central venous pressure, pulmonary capillary wedge pressure, urine output); and screening for possible toxic levels of cardioactive agents (digitalis, theophylline).

It is a common, but not uniform practice in most surgical centers to initiate intravenous lidocaine or procainamide to suppress VPDs as prophylaxis against more serious ventricular arrhythmias. These variations in practice reflect the confusion regarding the prognostic significance of VPDs in the postoperative setting. The benefits of prophylactic antiarrhythmic therapy postoperatively have never been adequately addressed in a randomized clinical trial. Because ventricular fibrillation in the early postoperative period is an infrequent event, and probably most often is the result of transitory electrolyte disturbances and/or myocardial ischemia, aggressive correction of electrolyte deficits and antiischemic therapy with intravenous nitroglycerin and beta blockers alone may be effective for preventing ventricular fibrillation without exposing the patient to the potential hazards of antiarrhythmic therapy (myocardial depression, torsades de pointes).

We advocate a conservative approach focusing on prompt detection and correction of provocative factors, liberal use of beta blockers in patients with an ejection fraction greater than 30 per cent, overdrive atrial or atrioventricular sequential pacing between 85 and 100 beats/min, and restriction of suppressive antiarrhythmic therapy to patients with a preoperative history of serious ventricular tachyarrhythmias. If the decision is made to suppress VPDs in patients without a history of symptomatic ventricular arrhythmias, the treatment period should be brief (6 to 24 hours) and the patient should not be automatically converted to an oral antiarrhythmic drug regimen without careful reconsideration of the indications for treatment.

Ventricular Tachycardia (see p. 703). Many of the same arguments cited above for isolated VPDs can be applied for paroxysms of nonsustained ventricular tachycardia (VT). No definitive guidelines are available, but we believe that episodes of VT lasting for 15 to 30 seconds or more in the absence of correctable factors and attempts at overdrive atrial or atrioventricular sequential pacing are an indication for antiarrhythmic therapy, especially if the episodes are associated with hemodynamic compromise. Sustained VT is a serious emergency that should be handled with an orderly approach. If the clinical situation permits, a 12-lead electrocardiogram should be obtained for future reference and confirmation of the diagnosis; simultaneous recording of surface electrocardiographic leads with electrograms from the epicardial wires may be helpful in establishing the mechanism of a wide complex tachycardia (Fig. 53–7). Acute attempts at conversion of the tachycardia include the following maneuvers in the sequence listed: thumpversion, burst ventricular pacing (see p. 705), and boluses of antiarrhythmic agents (lidocaine, 100 mg; procainamide, up to 500 to 1000 mg over 20 minutes; or bretylium, 500 to 1000 mg over 5 to 10 minutes). In urgent circumstances synchronized direct-current cardioversion with a low-energy shock (5 to 50 watt-seconds) may be used. Unsynchronized shocks of 100 to 200 watt-seconds should be used if the tachycardia rate is greater than 160 beats/min and/or has a sinusoidal waveform on the electrocardiogram. After conversion a search for correctable disorders should be undertaken, and if none is found a continuous infusion of lidocaine (2 mg/min), procainamide (2 mg/min), or bretylium (1 to 2 mg/min) is started.

Ventricular Fibrillation (see p. 709). As in the nonsurgical patient, ventricular fibrillation (VF) must be promptly treated with an unsynchronized direct-current shock. Extrapolating from experience in the electrophysiology laboratory, where VF frequently is provoked iatrogenically, it often can be reverted with shocks of 50 to 200 watt-seconds, provided the intervention is performed in less than 1 minute. It should be possible to defibrillate postoperative patients in the intensive care unit expeditiously; therefore, the higher energies (360 to 400 watt-seconds) used in the "field" probably are unnecessary—at least initially. The development of VF should raise the suspicion of a perioperative myocardial infarction. VF may occur in the early postoperative period without any evidence of myocardial necrosis and with electrolyte and drug levels "in the normal range." In such cases reperfusion of previously ischemic zones or transmembrane shifts of electrolytes probably have occurred, and would not be detected by available laboratory measurements. The majority of such patients are not subject to recurrent ventricular tachyarrhythmias, and their prognosis is determined more by overall left ventricular function than by electrical instability.

ATRIOVENTRICULAR JUNCTIONAL RHYTHMS. Nonparoxysmal atrioventricular junctional rhythms (rate >45 beats/min) occur not infrequently after mitral or aortic valve surgery. Trauma and tissue swelling from surgical debridement and suture placement are believed to be the provocative mechanisms. It typically is transient (≤48 hours), and easily treated with atrial or atrioventricular sequential pacing at a rate above that of the intrinsic junctional mechanism.

BRADYARRHYTHMIAS (see pp. 1240–1244) Sinus bradycardia or sinus arrest with emergence of a slow atrioventricular junction escape rhythm may be seen postoperatively when one or more of the following factors are present: advanced age, hypothermia, as a consequence of drug effects (diltiazem, beta blocker, digitalis, procainamide), preoperative sinus node dysfunction, intraoperative trauma to the sinus node, and postoperative elevation of vagal tone. In addition to modifying the dose or discontinuing offending drugs (such as those noted above), atrial pacing at 85 to 100 beats/min should be initiated to maintain an adequate cardiac output and urine flow. Checks of the intrinsic heart rate every 6 hours during the first 24 to 48 hours will indicate when pacing may be discontinued.

Although up to 15 per cent of patients may develop a new conduction defect after cardiac surgery,[110] the majority usually are transient, related to cardioplegia,[111] hypothermia, perioperative electrolyte shifts, or surgical trauma during valve repair or replacement, or closure of septal defects. In the absence of a low cardiac output syndrome related to bradycardia, the development of a new fascicular block or bundle branch alone is not necessarily an indication for initiation of temporary pacing (although it is a common practice in many centers to attach the epicardial wires to an external generator that is either turned off or programmed in the VVI mode with a low escape rate, in the unlikely event that complete heart block occurs). As with nonsurgically related conduction defects, the prognosis of patients with postoperative conduction defects is closely related to the underlying ventricular function. When other factors affecting long-term prognosis (age, left ventricular function, details of graft anatomy) are considered, the presence of a new postoperative bundle branch block or nonspecific intraventricular conduction delay does not clearly have an adverse impact on mortality or cardiovascular-related events over the long term.[111a]

The decision to insert a permanent pacemaker after cardiac surgery should be based on the hemodynamic consequences of bradycardia in the individual patient rather than on a specific heart rate. Most new conduction defects resolve by the 3rd postoperative day, but some persist for as long as 2 weeks. Although we are willing to observe a younger patient (<65 years) with a temporary pacing system for up to 2 weeks postoperatively to see if a conduction defect will resolve, we have a low threshold for implanting a permanent pacemaker if antiarrhythmic therapy or beta blocker treatment is contemplated, since these pharmacologic measures might "stress" a diseased conduction system. We advocate early insertion of a permanent pacemaker in elderly patients with symptomatic bradycardia, since the recuperative process is facilitated, the period of relative immobilization and electrocardiographic monitoring is minimized, and hospital stay is shortened.[112]

CARDIOVERSION (see p. 651). Direct-current cardioversion should be used in the postsurgical patient with the following additional considerations. The recent cardiotomy with resultant pericardial and mediastinal inflammation, presence of chest tubes and/or pleural effusions, and elevated catecholamine levels after surgery may all contribute to higher energy requirements for reversion of arrhythmias such as atrial fibrillation than are commonly required in patients who have not recently undergone cardiac surgery. To achieve the maximum transcardiac spread of current after a median sternotomy, the anterior paddle should be placed to the *right* of the sternum between the third and sixth intercostal spaces, and the other paddle should be positioned in the fourth to sixth intercostal space as far in the left axilla as possible or in a posterior location under the tip of the left scapula. Firm pressure is applied to the paddles to maintain contact with the chest wall as the discharge buttons are depressed.

HEMOSTATIC DISTURBANCES (See Chap. 58)

All patients who undergo cardiopulmonary bypass develop a multifactorial derangement of the hemostatic system. These abnormalities are caused by exposure of the blood to artificial surfaces, hemodilution, and the effects of heparin (Table 53–11). Platelet dysfunction is the most significant hemostatic abnormality that occurs after cardiopulmonary bypass, although diminution of coagulation factor levels may assume greater significance in patients with preoperative deficiencies of hemostasis. Administration of the following drugs before surgery may predispose the patient to excessive bleeding: aspirin, nonsteroidal antiinflammatory agents, thrombolytic agents,[119] certain antibiotics (carbenicillin, ticarcillin, moxalactam, cefamandole, third-generation cephalosporins), dex-

TABLE 53-11 HEMOSTATIC DISTURBANCES AFTER CARDIOPULMONARY BYPASS

ABNORMALITY	CAUSE
Exposure of blood to artificial surfaces	
1. Platelet dysfunction a. Prolonged bleeding time b. Decreased adhesiveness	1. Depletion of platelet α-granules, reduced membrane binding of fibrinogen and α-adrenergic agonists, and increased plasma levels of platelet factor 4 and β-thromboglobulin[113,114]
2. Complement activation	2. C3a and C5a are generated and increase microvascular permeability. C5b-9 complexes are deposited on red cells and platelets, causing hemolysis and platelet activation.[115,116]
Hemodilution	
1. Thrombocytopenia	1. Priming of extracorporeal bypass circuit with crystalloid solutions. Heparin-mediated immune thrombocytopenia may occur in about 5% of patients.[117]
2. Coagulation factor depletion	2. Most coagulation factor levels are reduced by hemodilution by about 50%; factor V is reduced to 20-30% of normal and factor VIII is relatively unaffected. Factor levels usually return to normal within 12 hours after completion of cardiopulmonary bypass. Although plasminogen and fibrinogen levels are decreased by about 50%, fibrin degradation products usually do not appear in the plasma during bypass.[113]
Heparinization*	Thrombus formation is inhibited and excessive bleeding is avoided intraoperatively by maintaining the activated clotting time between 400 and 480 seconds.

* Heparin effects are reversed with protamine sulfate. Vascular collapse has been reported in some patients during protamine treatment.[118]

tran, amrinone, quinidine, cytotoxic agents, gold, phenylbutazone, and fish oils.[120,121] In some institutions, for patients who are undergoing a reoperation or are polycythemic (p. 1749), when the risk of early postoperative bleeding is increased, 2 units of fresh frozen plasma are administered prophylactically after cardiopulmonary bypass.

The most obvious evidence of bleeding in the postoperative cardiac surgical patient is by means of chest tube drainage. "Acceptable" rates of bleeding vary slightly among institutions but usually are less than 100 ml/hr. In our institution, guidelines for returning to the operating room because of excessive bleeding include more than 500 ml/hr for 1 hour, more than 300 ml/hr for 3 hours, and 200 to 300 ml/hr for 5 hours. These guidelines may be tempered by correctable extenuating circumstances, such as uncontrolled hypertension postoperatively, failure to achieve normothermia, or an abnormal coagulation status that is being corrected. Emergency medical maneuvers that can be attempted after sending coagulation studies to the laboratory include the use of PEEP up to 10 cm H_2O for mediastinal tamponade; empirical "correction" of putative platelet dysfunction with desmopressin acetate (DDAVP, a synthetic analog of arginine vasopressin that increases plasma levels of von Willebrand factor), 0.3 μg/kg, infused over 15 to 30 minutes[122,123]; and empirical administration of a small dose of protamine sulfate, 25 to 50 mg, since heparin may be liberated from the patient's fat stores as rewarming occurs.

Once the coagulation profile returns, additional therapy in the form of platelet transfusions for a platelet count less than 100,000/mm^3 and fresh frozen plasma to correct an elevated prothrombin time can be prescribed. When monitoring bleeding from a chest tube, it is important to be alert to a sudden cessation of hemorrhage. This may indicate that the chest tubes have clotted and the fluid is now draining into the mediastinum or the pleural spaces. Serial chest radiographs may be helpful while observing a patient during a bleeding episode. With correct medical management, only about 5 per cent of patients need to return to the operating room for control of bleeding; this should be accomplished within 3 to 4 hours of the original surgery, before hemodynamic destabilization occurs and large volumes of blood products are administered.

ANTITHROMBOTIC THERAPY IN PATIENTS WITH PROSTHETIC HEART VALVES (see p. 1062). Patients who have undergone implantation of a prosthetic heart valve are exposed to a lifelong risk of thromboembolism. The degree of risk varies with the type of valve implanted (mechanical > bioprosthetic), valve location (mitral > aortic), the presence of atrial fibrillation, the size of the left atrium, a history of thromboembolism or the presence of left atrial thrombi at the time of operation, and the adequacy of anticoagulation. For mechanical prosthetic heart valves it is strongly recommended that all patients receive lifelong warfarin therapy designed to prolong the prothrombin time to 1.5 times control (p. 1777).[43,124] Patients with bioprosthetic valves appear to be at greatest risk of thromboembolism in the first 3 months after valve implantation. For patients in sinus rhythm who have a bioprosthetic valve placed in the mitral position, we prescribe warfarin for 3 months, designed to prolong the prothrombin time to 1.3 to 1.5 times control; if atrial fibrillation persists, warfarin is continued permanently. We usually do not anticoagulate patients with bioprosthetic valves inserted in the aortic position, provided the patient is in sinus rhythm.

INFECTION

Despite its nonspecific nature, fever is the most common initial clinical sign of a postoperative infection.[125] It should be emphasized, however, that patients who experience a normal course of convalescence continue to show an elevated temperature for up to 6 days postoperatively (Fig. 53-8).[126] In the absence of infection such early fevers are believed to be caused by alterations in blood components after cardiopulmonary bypass. In addition to infectious causes, fevers that occur beyond 6 days may be due to drug reactions, phlebitis at the site of intravenous lines, atelectasis, pulmonary emboli, or the postpericardiotomy syndrome.

WOUND

Leg. Infections of the leg wound typically present with fever, induration, pain, erythema, local warmth, and drainage from the suture line. The usual infectious agents include staphylococcus, streptococcus, and aerobic gram-negative bacilli. Wound aspiration and Gram's stain should be used to guide antibiotic treatment. More advanced cases require wound debridement and open drainage. Recurrent bacterial cellulitis in the leg used for saphenous vein harvest may be a recalcitrant problem that appears months to years after operation.[127] Antibiotic courses directed against staphylococcus and streptococcus species for each individual occurrence may be insufficient, and a long-term course of antibiotic therapy may be needed. It is important to search for evidence of super-

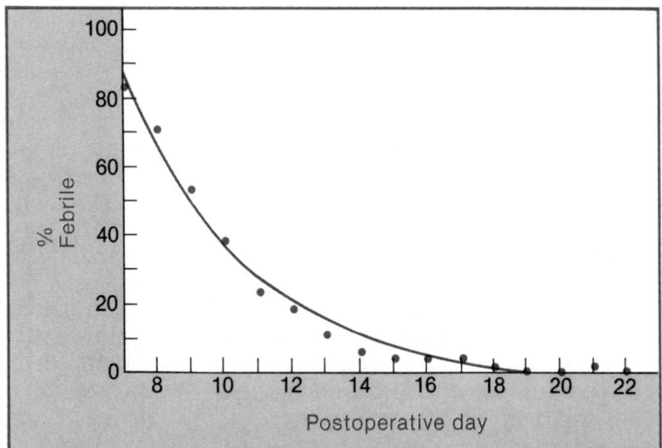

FIGURE 53-8. The decay of fever in a group of 118 retrospectively identified patients with unexplained postoperative fever after postoperative day 6. The percentage of patients that remain febrile is plotted as a function of postoperative day beyond postoperative day 6. A patient is considered febrile if any temperature determination for a given day is equal to or greater than 37.8° C. The percentage of patients febrile on postoperative day 7 is 83 per cent rather than 100 per cent because in 17 per cent of patients fever developed after postoperative day 7. (From Livelli, F. D., Johnson, R. A., McEnany, M. T., et al.: Unexplained in-hospital fever following cardiac surgery. Natural history, relationship to postpericardiotomy syndrome, and a prospective study of therapy with indomethacin versus placebo. Circulation *57*:968, 1978, by permission of the American Heart Association, Inc.)

ficial fungal infections in the affected leg, since persistent tinea pedis infection has been reported to cause recurrent lower-extremity cellulitis.[128] If a fungal infection is identified, treatment with topical miconazole or clotrimazole should be given in addition to antibacterial therapy. Persistent fungal infections (owing to breaks in integrity of the dermal barrier) should be treated with either oral ketoconazole or griseofulvin.

Mediastinitis. Mediastinitis and sternal osteomyelitis are among the most serious complications of a median sternotomy.[129] If one excludes operations that occur after thoracic trauma, it is estimated that mediastinitis occurs in about 2 per cent of patients who undergo median sternotomy.[130]

Most cases present within 2 weeks after sternotomy. Important diagnostic features of patients who develop mediastinitis early after cardiac surgery include persistent fever in excess of 101° F beyond the 4th postoperative day, a systemic toxic condition, leukocytosis, bacteremia, and a purulent discharge from the sternal wound. Wound erythema, abnormal sternal tenderness or instability, and mediastinal widening may all be absent or clinically unapparent early in the development of mediastinitis. Recognition of mediastinitis requires a high index of suspicion and a vigorous, repetitive search for evidence of sternal wound drainage in patients who are persistently febrile late into the 1st week after surgery and in whom there is no other obvious focus of infection, such as pneumonia or urinary tract infection. The diagnosis can be confirmed by needle aspiration from the subxiphoid approach followed by Gram's stain and culture.

In addition to the preoperative risk factors noted in Table 53-4, there are a number of intraoperative and postoperative risk factors for the development of mediastinitis. These include prolonged cardiopulmonary bypass time, excessive postoperative bleeding with reexploration for control of hemorrhage, and diminished cardiac output in the postoperative period. There is an increase in the development of mediastinitis when both internal mammary arteries are mobilized bilaterally for use as bypass conduits.[131] For that reason many surgeons prefer to utilize only the left internal mammary artery, particularly in elderly diabetic patients who may already be predisposed to delayed sternal wound healing. The spectrum of microorganisms that cause mediastinitis includes *Staphylococcus* (*aureus* and *epidermidis*) in about 50 per cent of patients and a variety of gram-negative bacilli in about 40 per cent of cases.[132] Mixed infections and fungal infections are rare. The organism isolated frequently is resistant to the prophylactic antibiotic used preoperatively, especially if the isolate includes a gram-negative bacillus or a β-lactamase-producing *S. aureus*.[133]

Definitive diagnosis of a sternal wound infection requires exploration of the wound and culture of suspicious areas. Specialized radiological techniques such as CT and MRI scanning also have been reported to be helpful in localizing the sites of infection. Although both closed and open methods of treatment of mediastinitis have been reported, most authorities comment on the need for experienced surgical judgment if the closed approach (debridement, reclosure, and antibiotic irrigation) is utilized. The open approach is more frequently used for chronic or extensive infections, and often entails removal of involved bony or cartilaginous structures. Although previously the wound was allowed to heal by secondary intention, current strategy involves formation of a myocutaneous flap over the sternal area. The patient is treated with nutritional (Table 53-3) and respiratory support as needed. With both the closed and open method intravenous antibiotics and sternal antibiotic irrigation are continued for at least 10 to 14 days[134]; 4 to 6 weeks of treatment may be needed in cases of documented sternal osteomyelitis.

The reported mortality associated with mediastinitis varies greatly and appears to be related to the delay in initiation of treatment; patients diagnosed and treated aggressively within 1 month of surgery have a mortality of about 10 per cent, whereas those treated later have a mortality of about 25 per cent.[132,134,135] Surprisingly, the presence of a mediastinal infection does not appear to reduce the likelihood of patency of coronary artery bypass grafts.[136]

INFECTIVE ENDOCARDITIS (see Chap. 35). It has been convincingly shown that perioperative antibiotic prophylaxis is of benefit in patients undergoing cardiac surgery.[137] Although the antibiotic regimen varies, in part related to local differences in microbiological flora and personal preference, it is directed against gram-positive cocci (the most frequent causative pathogen in infections after cardiac surgery) and usually contains a cephalosporin. The regimen utilized in our institution consists of 1 gm of cefazolin intravenously 30 minutes before the skin incision and then repeated at 8-hour intervals for 48 hours after operation.

Cardiac surgery does not appear to increase the risk of endocarditis in patients with abnormal native valves that are not repaired or replaced during the operative procedure, in patients with intracardiac shunts, or in patients with intravascular devices (e.g., permanent pacemaker wires or renal dialysis shunts).[138] Assuming no infection is present preoperatively, such patients need only receive the standard antibiotic prophylaxis regimen in force at the institution in which the surgery is being performed.

Prosthetic Valve Endocarditis (see p. 1081). Prosthetic valve endocarditis is a rare complication of cardiac surgery, estimated to occur in only 2 to 4 per cent of patients; about half of the cases are classified as "early" (<60 days from the date of operation) and half as "late" (>60 days from the date of operation).[139-141] The pooled data from several series indicate that the organism responsible for early prosthetic valve endocarditis includes a *Staphylococcus* species in about 50 per cent of cases.[139,141] The remainder of early cases of prosthetic valve endocarditis are caused by gram-negative bacilli, diphtheroids, and fungi. The microbiological spectrum of late prosthetic valve endocarditis is more characteristic of that seen with native valve endocarditis. Only 30 per cent of cases are due to either *S. epidermidis* or *S. aureus*, and slightly more than one-third are caused by *Streptococcus* species (group *D streptococci* and *Streptococcus pneumoniae*). The nature of the pathology in prosthetic valve endocarditis varies, depending on the type of prosthesis.[141] Mechanical valves typically show a ring abscess or myocardial abscess, whereas porcine heterografts more commonly develop valvar stenosis or regurgitation as a result of the endocarditis.

Features of prosthetic valve endocarditis that have been associated with increased mortality include invasive infection (i.e., extension into the myocardium), congestive heart failure resulting from dysfunction of the prosthesis, and the presence of antibiotic-resistant, virulent microorganisms or a fungal organism.[141] Appropriate antibiotic therapy for prosthetic valve endocarditis is discussed in Chap. 35. The following clinical characteristics indicate the need for early operative intervention[141,142]: (1) moderate to severe congestive heart failure caused by prosthetic valve dysfunction (incompetence or stenosis); (2) signs of extension of the infection into the perivalvular tissue or formation of a myocardial abscess (new electrocardiographic conduction abnormalities, pericarditis, valve dehiscence, persistent unexplained fever beyond 10 days of antibiotic treatment); (3) infection caused by aggressive, invasive organisms or those that are difficult to eradicate (fungi, *S. aureus*, some cases of *S. epidermidis*); (4) persistently positive blood cultures despite appropriate antibiotic therapy; (5) relapse of the clinical syndrome of endocarditis after appropriate antibiotic therapy; and (6) recurrent systemic emboli.

VIRAL. Viral infections that occur after cardiac surgery are almost exclusively the result of infectious complications of transfusion therapy, and usually result in hepatitis. The incidence of viral infections after cardiac operations is decreasing as a result of a reduction in the number of transfusions of blood bank products (e.g., cell-saver techniques and preoperative autologous blood donations) and improved screening techniques in contemporary blood bank practice. The two most common transfusion-related viral infections after cardiac surgery are cytomegalovirus (CMV) infection and non-A, non-B hepatitis (currently referred to as hepatitis C). CMV infection is a febrile syndrome that typically presents 1 month postoperatively. It is characterized by high-spiking fevers, abnormalities of liver function tests, and arthralgias. A self-limited illness, it is best treated with antipyretics and supportive fluid therapy.

Hepatitis C is caused by an RNA virus, and is characterized by a protracted course with fluctuating transaminase levels.[143] About 50 per cent of patients respond to a course of interferon therapy with a reduction in transaminase levels; half of the responders relapse over the long term.[144,145] It is hoped that the incidence of hepatitis C will decrease with improvements in blood bank screening procedures for hepatitis C as are currently in place for hepatitis A and hepatitis B.

FUNGAL. Fungal infections that involve the heart are rare. They typically are seen in cases of fungemia and usually are fatal. Although the problem of fungemia is well described in the immunocompromised host (e.g., heart transplant recipient), in an autopsy study of 60 patients with fungal infections of the heart 25 per cent of cases occurred in association with conventional valvular surgery.[146] About half of fungal infections of the heart are confined to the endocardium, and half involve both the endocardium and the myocardium. Extracardiac involvement is common, with spread of the infection to the lungs, cerebrospinal fluid, urine, and skin. The most commonly encountered organisms, in descending order of frequency, are *Candida*, *Aspergillus*, and *Cryptococcus* species. Patients who appear at particular risk of fungal involvement of the heart are those who have received corticosteroids and long courses of antibiotic treatment postoperatively.

PERIPHERAL VASCULAR COMPLICATIONS

Most adult patients who undergo cardiac surgery—especially coronary revascularization—have atherosclerosis of the peripheral vasculature (e.g., ileofemoral system), and may experience lower-extremity ischemia after surgery because of low flow in the perioperative period with in situ thrombosis, embolism from the heart or aorta, or vascular compromise from an intraaortic balloon pump catheter. Management consists of anticoagulation and removal of indwelling catheters, if clinically feasible. Thrombectomy and even revascularization surgery of the lower extremities (e.g., femorofemoral, femoropopliteal, or axillofemoral bypass) may be required to salvage threatened limbs.

When aggressive preventive measures are not used, asymptomatic deep venous thrombosis of the calf can evolve before hospital discharge in one-third to one-half of patients who receive saphenous vein bypass grafts. Rarely, this causes massive pulmonary embolism. The best strategy is rigorous perioperative prophylaxis against venous thromboembolism in all such patients. The efficacy of "minidose heparin" (5000 units subcutaneously initiated 2 hours preoperatively and continued every 8 to 12 hours postoperatively) has been established. The potential benefit of prevention of deep venous thrombosis with intermittent pneumatic compression devices is under investigation.

OTHER COMPLICATIONS

PERICARDITIS (see Chap. 45). Pericardial friction rubs frequently are audible in the early postoperative period, and probably are the result of mechanical irritation from the mediastinal chest tubes. They usually disappear by the 2nd or 3rd postoperative day and are asymptomatic because of the narcotic analgesics prescribed at that stage of recovery. Although some patients develop pericardial rubs toward the end of the 1st postoperative week, these usually are benign, do not indicate a need for prolongation of hospitalization, and do not require treatment. A separate clinical syndrome that appears late in the 1st postoperative month is the *postpericardiotomy syndrome* (p. 227).[147] The relation between the postpericardiotomy syndrome and chronic constrictive pericarditis is not firmly established, but a number of case reports of patients with *postoperative constrictive pericarditis*[148] include patients with a history of postpericardiotomy syndrome.

RENAL FAILURE (see Chap. 62). All patients who undergo cardiac surgery experience a reduction in renal blood flow and glomerular filtration rate (GFR) as a consequence of both anesthesia and cardiopulmonary bypass. Risk factors for the development of persistent renal failure after cardiac surgery include a preoperative history of renal dysfunction or left ventricular dysfunction, prolonged bypass time (>180 minutes), prolonged aortic cross-clamping (>40 minutes), perioperative hypotension, advanced age (>70 years), and the development postoperatively of medical complications.[149-151] Most cases of acute renal failure after cardiac surgery result from renal ischemia that lowers the GFR directly (prerenal disease) or, if severe or prolonged, can induce acute tubular necrosis. Possible additional contributory factors include sepsis, nephrotoxic drugs, radiocontrast material injections, cholesterol plaque embolization to the renal circulation, increased urine free hemoglobin levels from hemolysis while on cardiopulmonary bypass, and the effects of angiotensin converting enzyme (ACE) inhibitors on glomerular capillary pressure.[150] The detrimental effects of ACE inhibitors are most likely to occur when renal perfusion pressure is low because of renal artery stenosis or systemic hypotension caused by cardiac failure.

Urine output is variable in patients with postoperative acute renal failure. Anuria is uncommon and, if present, should raise the suspicion of urinary tract obstruction (e.g., occluded Foley catheter). More commonly patients are either oliguric (<400 ml/day) or nonoliguric. Oliguric acute renal failure occurs less frequently than nonoliguric renal failure, usually reflects more severe renal injury, and is associated with a greater probability of requiring dialysis during the acute phase.[152,153]

Important diagnostic studies in all patients with acute renal failure include a urinalysis, and estimation of pulmonary capillary wedge pressure and cardiac output by means of pulmonary artery catheterization. Prerenal azotemia should be suspected if the urine sodium level is less than 20 mEq/liter, the fractional excretion of sodium is less than 1 per cent, and the urine osmolality level is greater than 500 mOsm/liter. Acute tubular necrosis should be suspected if the urine sodium level is greater than 40 mEq/liter, the fractional excretion of sodium is greater than 2 per cent, and the urine osmolality level is less than 350 mOsm/liter.

TREATMENT. Essential elements of treatment for both prerenal azotemia and acute tubular necrosis include optimization of intravascular fluid volume and cardiac output. The latter is best accomplished with vasodilators and inotropic agents (p. 1871) rather than with vasopressors, to avoid further reductions in renal blood flow. Experimental studies suggest that several modalities may protect against the development of progressive renal failure in models of acute renal ischemic injury (e.g., renal artery clamping that simulates the effects of suprarenal aortic cross-clamping while on cardiopulmonary bypass). Mannitol (which washes out obstructing casts), a loop diuretic (which decreases energy requirements in the

TABLE 53-12 GASTROINTESTINAL COMPLICATIONS AFTER CARDIAC SURGERY

COMPLICATION	COMMON CAUSES	EVALUATION	TREATMENT	COMMENT
Hyperbilirubinemia				
Early (1–10 days)	"Shock liver" syndrome[162]	Check full chemistry profile	Maximize cardiac output, BP, and oxygenation	Markedly elevated enzyme levels are seen early after onset of shock state
	Hemolysis on cardiopulmonary bypass[163]	↑ Plasma free hemoglobin	Observe	Isolated elevation of direct and indirect bilirubin without enzyme elevation
	Right heart failure[162]	Chest x-ray, hemodynamic monitoring	Digitalis, diuretics, oxygen, consider isoproterenol infusion	Elevated direct bilirubin and alkaline phosphatase but without enzyme elevation
Late (10–90 days)	Infection (cytomegalovirus, hepatitis C)[164]	Viral serology	Observe	Consider interferon for hepatitis C
	Cholecystitis	Ultrasound, biliary isotopic scan (e.g., HIDA, PIPIDA)	General surgical consultation	May require ERCP, cholecystectomy, cholecystotomy
Gastroduodenal disease[160]				
Hemorrhage	Stress gastritis	Nasogastric aspirate (pH and Hematest), CBC	Nasogastric tube, antacids, H_2-receptor antagonists, transfusions	Because of the increased risk of developing this complication, it is important to provide prophylactic treatment (antacids, H_2-receptor antagonists) to patients with COPD and postoperative hypotension, bleeding, or reoperation.[165] Early endoscopy and consideration of surgical intervention are strongly advised if supportive medical care is unsuccessful.
	Peptic ulcer disease	Nasogastric aspirate (pH and Hematest), CBC	Nasogastric tube, antacids, H_2-receptor antagonists, transfusions	Early endoscopy and consideration of surgical intervention are strongly advised if supportive medical care is unsuccessful.
Mesenteric ischemia[166]	Combination of low cardiac output, embolization of atherosclerotic debris or thrombi, and vascular dissection by intraaortic balloon pump	High index of suspicion and early surgical consultation	Early laparotomy with resection of affected bowel and embolectomy when possible	Mortality rate remains high.
Pancreatitis	Hypotension, thromboembolism of vascular supply, splanchnic vasoconstriction	Serum amylase measurements serially, abdominal ultrasonogram	Nasogastric suction and fluid support	Hyperamylasemia is common after cardiac surgery, but clinical pancreatitis is rare.[167] Severe, fulminating acute pancreatitis in postcardiac surgical patients has a poor prognosis despite aggressive surgical treatment.[168]
Miscellaneous				
Intraabdominal bleeding	Trauma (intraop, chest tubes) Preexisting lesion (e.g., hamartoma)	Abdominal lavage	General surgical consultation	
Lower gastrointestinal tract bleed	Colonic pathology (e.g., polyp)	Plain film of abdomen, colonoscopy		
Ileus	Narcotics Adhesions	Plain film of abdomen	Nasogastric suction	

CBC, complete blood count; COPD, chronic obstructive pulmonary disease; ERCP, endoscopic retrograde cholangiopancreatography.

thick ascending limb of the loop of Henle, thereby decreasing ischemic injury), and the combination of dopamine and atrial natriuretic peptide (but neither alone) have all been effective.[154] There are, however, no good clinical trials to confirm the efficacy of these interventions. Several uncontrolled observations suggest that those patients who appear to be protected by a loop diuretic, mannitol, or dopamine were all treated within 12 to 24 hours of the onset of renal dysfunction.[155,156]

It is prudent to undertake a trial of furosemide and mannitol (only if the patient can tolerate the volume load of the latter) within the first 12 to 24 hours after the development of oliguria. The aim of such therapy is to increase urine output. Because of the renal vasodilating effects of dopamine (3 μg/kg/min), patients with both oliguric and nonoliguric renal failure may experience an increase in urine output.[150] There is, however, no evidence that dopamine alone given in this setting is helpful for recruiting salvageable, but nonfunctioning nephrons.[157]

If oliguria persists beyond 12 hours, a number of supportive measures must be activated, including careful attention to electrolyte balance, specifically avoiding hyperkalemia; excessive free water administration that might lead to hyponatremia; correction of acidosis (adding bicarbonate to daily fluids); and adjustment of medication dosages for delayed excretion if the drug is cleared by renal mechanisms.[154] There seems little benefit to instituting dialysis prophylactically for a given level of blood urea nitrogen or creatinine. Rather, dialysis should be carried out for pericarditis, refractory hyperkalemia, uremic encephalopathy, or colitis. Continuous arteriovenous hemofiltration is a simpler modality that can be used to remove excess fluid.

Finally, the patient with chronic renal failure who undergoes surgery is at increased risk of exacerbation of renal dysfunction perioperatively. This may require temporary or even permanent hemodialysis, and these eventualities should be addressed with the patient and the cardiac surgical team preoperatively. Surgery can be safely performed in patients who are already on hemodialysis, but careful coordination of the surgical and dialysis schedules is essential to minimize postoperative problems with fluid and electrolyte management.[158,159] Ultrafiltration can be performed while on cardiopulmonary bypass, to help minimize the intraoperative fluid load received by the patient.

GASTROINTESTINAL COMPLICATIONS (Table 53–12). Serious gastrointestinal complications after cardiac surgery are rare (occurring in about 1 per cent of patients), and usually can be handled by a conservative approach. Only about 0.5 per cent of patients who undergo cardiac surgery require a general surgical operation for a gastrointestinal complication.[160] Patients with circulatory compromise and those who require intraaortic balloon pump support are more likely to develop gastrointestinal complications.[160,161] Despite their relative rarity, gastrointestinal complications are associated with a significant mortality (approaching 40 per cent in some series), highlighting the need for careful monitoring and repeated physical examination in high-risk patients.[160] Most complications occur within 7 days of surgery.

NEUROLOGICAL. Neurologic complications after cardiac surgery are quite common, particularly in the elderly, if one is attentive to the subtle cognitive (short-term memory loss, lack of concentration) and psychological (depression, increased sense of dependency) changes seen early after operation.[169,170] A positive and supportive attitude on the part of the staff and enlistment of the aid of family members help to minimize these problems. Although many patients return to their preoperative state by 4 to 6 weeks after surgery,[171] about 10 per cent will continue to show deterioration of their neuropsychological function over the next 6 months, especially if they are over age 65.[172] More serious neurological complications, such as stroke (Table 53–13), occur in 1 to 5 per cent of patients, but may be seen in as many as 10 per cent of patients over age 65.

Symptomatic visual defects may be seen after cardiac surgery, and result from retinal emboli, occipital lobe infarction, or anterior ischemic optic neuropathy.[176] Risk factors for cerebrovascular accident (CVA) or transient ischemic attack (TIA) after cardiac surgery include preoperative carotid bruit,[177] previous CVA or TIA,[174] postoperative atrial fibrillation,[174] prolonged cardiopulmonary bypass (>2 hours),[177] and preoperative left ventricular mural thrombus.[175] Patients with *symptomatic* carotid bruits should undergo combined carotid endarterectomy along with their cardiac procedure. However, despite the recognition of a carotid stenosis greater than 50 per cent as a risk factor for perioperative CVA, no clinical trial has convincingly shown a benefit of preoperative or simultaneous carotid endarterectomy (which is inherently associated with a 3 to 4 per cent risk of cerebral ischemia) in reducing the incidence of CVA or TIA after cardiac surgical procedures.[178,179]

Neuropathies in the upper extremities have been reported after cardiac operations. The pattern of injury involving predominantly the ulnar nerve and medial antebrachial cutaneous nerve suggests that the lesion involves a brachial plexus compression or traction injury.[180] The average duration of symptoms after such an injury is 2 months, but some patients show a slower time course of improvement extending over 6 to 12 months.

CHYLOTHORAX, CHYLOPERICARDIUM. These are rare postcardiac surgical complications in adults, occurring in less than 0.5 per cent of cases. Treatment of chylothorax consists of prolonged chest tube drainage and dietary support with medium-chain triglycerides. Refractory cases of chylothorax have been successfully treated by the creation of a pleuroperitoneal shunt.[181] Chylopericardium may cause cardiac tamponade (p. 1479), and is treated by creation of a pericardial window into the pleural space and management as above for chylothorax. Persistent chyle leaks may necessitate thoracic duct ligation.

TABLE 53–13 POSSIBLE CAUSES OF STROKE AFTER CARDIAC SURGERY

Embolism
Debridement or replacement of calcified aortic valve
Dislodgment of atherosclerotic plaque during cannulation of aorta
Introduction of air into the arterial circulation intraoperatively[173]
Dislodgment of atherosclerotic plaque from carotid artery stenosis by means of "jet effect" from aortic inflow cannula
Arrhythmia (e.g., atrial fibrillation)[174]
Thrombosis of mechanical prosthetic valve
Dissection of aorta during cannulation
Left ventricular thrombus[175]
Dislodgment of fragment of left atrial myxoma
Endocarditis
Microaggregate formation on cardiopulmonary bypass[173]
Hemorrhage
Anticoagulation perioperatively
Hypertension
Hypotension
Hypoperfusion of cerebral circulation while on cardiopulmonary bypass
Hypoperfusion of cerebral circulation during period of postoperative shock

REHABILITATION AND PREPARATION FOR DISCHARGE

(See Chap. 42)

A coordinated, multidisciplinary cardiac exercise program is essential to overcome the physical deconditioning and psychosocial upheaval associated with cardiac surgery. Emphasis should be placed on early mobilization and progressively more patient self-care, including in the intensive care unit during the first 48 hours postoperatively. After transfer out of the intensive care unit, the patient should be encouraged to engage in low-intensity (2 to 3 METS) isotonic activities such as walking and range-of-motion exercises. The nursing staff should monitor the patient's progress, being alert to any undue acceleration of the heart rate (>120 beats/min) or hemodynamically compromising arrhythmias. Patients also should participate in an education program focusing on instructions regarding postoperative medications and plans for returning to work (by about 6 to 8 weeks). Despite the extensive publicity surrounding coronary bypass surgery and the efforts of many personnel in institutions in which such operations are performed, there is a disappointing rate of return to work reported in several series, even allowing for the advanced age of many patients who undergo coronary artery bypass grafting.[182–184] Innovative strategies are needed to encourage patients to return to work, and society to accept postcardiac surgical patients back into the work force.[185]

REFERENCES

PREOPERATIVE EVALUATION

1. Anderson, E. A.: Preoperative preparation for cardiac surgery facilitates recovery, reduces psychological distress, and reduces the incidence of acute postoperative hypertension. J. Consult. Clin. Psychol. 55:513, 1987.
2. Hanet, C., Marchand, E., and Keyeux, A.: Left internal mammary artery occlusion after mastectomy and radiotherapy. Am. J. Cardiol. *65*:1044, 1990.
3. Kuan, P., Bernstein, S. B., Ellestad, M. H., et al.: Coronary artery bypass surgery morbidity. J. Am. Coll. Cardiol. 3:1391, 1984.
4. Rich, M. W., Kelller, A. J., Schechtman, K. B., et al.: Increased complica-

tions and prolonged hospital stay in elderly cardiac surgical patients with low serum albumin. Am. J. Cardiol. 63:714, 1989.
5. Jeejeebhoy, K. N.: Nutrition in critical illness. *In* Shoemaker, W. C., Ayres, S., Grenovik, A., et al. (eds.): Textbook of Critical Care. Philadelphia, W. B. Saunders, 1989, p. 1093.
6. Gersh, B. J., Kronman, R. A., Frye, R. L., et al.: Coronary arteriography and coronary artery bypass surgery: Morbidity and mortality in patients age 65 years and older. Circulation 67:483, 1983.
7. Naunheim, K. S., Kern, M. J., McBride, L. R., et al.: Coronary artery bypass surgery in patients aged 80 years and older. Am. J. Cardiol. 59:804, 1987.
8. Birnbaum, P. L., Weisel, R. D., Ivanov, J., et al.: The changing pattern of coronary bypass surgery (CABG). Circulation 78(Supp II):II-476, 1988.
9. Loop, F. D., Golding, L. R., MacMillan, J. P., et al.: Coronary artery surgery in women compared with men: Analysis of risks and long term results. J. Am. Coll. Cardiol. 1:383, 1983.
10. Khan, S. S., Nessim, S., Gray R., et al.: Increased mortality of women in coronary artery bypass surgery: Evidence for referral bias. Ann. Intern. Med. 112:561, 1990.
11. Loop, F. D., Lytle, B. W., Cosgrove, D. M., et al.: Sternal wound complications after isolated coronary artery bypass grafting: Early and late mortality, morbidity, and cost of care. Ann. Thorac. Surg. 49:179, 1990.
12. McGrath, L. B., Laub, G. W., Graf, D., and Gonzalez-Lavin, L.: Hospital death on a cardiac surgical service: Negative influence of changing practice patterns. Ann. Thorac. Surg. 49:410, 1990.
13. Weintraub, W. S., Jones, E. L., Craver, J., et al.: Determinants of prolonged length of hospital stay after coronary artery bypass surgery. Circulation 80:276, 1989.
14. Boldt, J., Kling, D., Hempelmann, G.: Right ventricular function and cardiac surgery. Intensive Care Med. 14:496, 1988.
15. Parsons, R. S., Mohandas, K., and Riaz, N.: The effects of an intravenous infusion of isosorbide dinitrate during open heart surgery. Eur. Heart J. 9(Suppl A): 195, 1988.
16. Coriat, P., Daloz, M., Bousseau, D., et al.: Prevention of intraoperative myocardial ischemia during noncardiac surgery with intravenous nitroglycerin. Anesthesiology 61:193, 1984.
17. Hensley, F. A., and Martin, D. E.: The Practice of Cardiac Anesthesia. Boston, Little, Brown, 1990.
18. Knight, P. R., Kroll, D. A., Nahrwald, M. L., et al.: Comparison of cardiovascular responses to anesthesia and operation when intravenous lidocaine or morphine sulfate is used as adjunct to diazepam-nitrous oxide for cardiac surgery. Anesth. Analg. 59:130, 1980.
19. Tyras, D. H., Stothert, J. C. Jr., Kaiser, G. C., et al.: Supraventricular tachyarrhythmias after myocardial revascularization: A randomized trial of prophylactic digitalization. J. Thorac. Cardiovasc. Surg. 77:310, 1979.
20. Csicsko, J. F., Schatzlein, M. H., and King, R. D.: Immediate postoperative digitalization in the prophylaxis of supraventricular arrhythmias following coronary artery bypass. J. Thorac. Cardiovasc. Surg. 81:419, 1981.
21. Johnson, L. W., Dickstein, R. A., Fruehan, C. T., et al.: Prophylactic digitalization for coronary artery bypass surgery. Circulation 53:819, 1976.
22. Chee, T. P., Prakash, N. S., Desser, K. B., and Benchimol, A.: Postoperative supraventricular arrhythmias and the role of prophylactic digoxin in cardiac surgery. Am. Heart J. 104:974, 1982.
23. Ormerod, O. J., McGregor, C. G., Stone, D. L., et al.: Arrhythmias after coronary bypass surgery. Br. Heart J. 51:618, 1984.
24. Selzer, A., Kelly, J. J. Jr., Gerbode, F., et al.: Case against routine use of digitalis in patients undergoing cardiac surgery. J.A.M.A. 195:549, 1966.
25. Lauer, M. S., Eagle, K. A., Buckley, M. J., and DeSanctis, R. W.: Atrial fibrillation following coronary artery bypass surgery. Prog. Cardiovasc. Dis. 31:367, 1989.
26. Oka, Y., Frishman, W., Becker, R. N., et al.: Clinical pharmacology of the new beta adrenergic blocking drugs. 10. Beta adrenoceptor blockade and coronary artery surgery. Am. Heart J. 99:255, 1980.
27. Hammon, J. W. Jr., Wood, A. J., Prager, R. L., et al.: Perioperative beta blockade with propranolol: Reduction in myocardial oxygen demands and incidence of atrial and ventricular arrhythmias. Ann. Thorac. Surg. 38:363, 1984.
28. White, H. D., Antman, E. M., Glynn, M. A., et al.: Efficacy and safety of timolol for prevention of supraventricular tachyarrhythmias after coronary artery bypass surgery. Circulation 70:479, 1984.
28a. Andrews, T. C., Reimold, S. C., Berlin, J. A., and Antman, E. M.: Prevention of supraventricular arrhythmias after coronary artery bypass surgery: A meta-analysis. Circulation 82 (Suppl. III):296, 1990.
29. Davison, R., Hartz, R., Kaplan, K., et al.: Prophylaxis of supraventricular tachyarrhythmia after coronary bypass surgery with oral verapamil: A randomized, double-blind trial. Ann. Thorac. Surg. 39:336, 1985.
30. Gray, R., Conklin, C., Sethna, D., et al.: The role of intravenous verapamil in supraventricular tachyarrhythmias after open-heart surgery. Am. Heart J. 104:799, 1982.
31. Cardiac Arrhythmia Suppression Trial (CAST) Investigators: Preliminary Report: Effect of encainide and flecainide on mortality in a randomized trial of arrhythmia suppression after myocardial infarction. N. Engl. J. Med. 321:406, 1989.
32. Nalos, P. C., Kass, R. M., Gang, E. S., et al.: Life-threatening postoperative pulmonary complications in patients with previous amiodarone pulmonary toxicity undergoing cardiothoracic operations. J. Thorac. Cardiovasc. Surg. 93:904, 1987.
33. Kupferschmid, J. P., Rosengart, T. K., McIntosh, C. L., et al.: Amiodarone-induced complications after cardiac operation for obstructive hypertrophic cardiomyopathy. Ann. Thorac. Surg. 48:359, 1989.
34. Barbieri, E., Conti, F., Zampieri, P., et al.: Amiodarone and desethylamiodarone distribution in the atrium and adipose tissue of patients undergoing short- and long-term treatment with amiodarone. J. Am. Coll. Cardiol. 8:210, 1986.
35. Lamas, G. A., Rebecca, G. S., Braunwald, N. S., and Antman, E. M.: Pacemaker malfunction after nitrous oxide anesthesia. Am. J. Cardiol. 56:995, 1985.
36. Lamas, G. A., Antman, E. M., Gold, J., et al.: Pacemaker back-up mode reversion and injury during cardiac surgery. Ann. Thorac. Surg. 41:155, 1986.
37. Forraris, V., Ferraris, S. P., Lough, F. C., et al.: Preoperative aspirin ingestion increases operative blood loss after coronary artery bypass grafting. Ann. Thorac. Surg. 45:71, 1988.
38. Henderson, W. G., Goldman, S., Copeland, J. G., et al.: Antiplatelet or anticoagulant therapy after coronary artery bypass surgery: A meta-analysis of clinical trials. Ann. Intern. Med. 111:743, 1989.
38a. Buring, J. E., Hennekens, C. H.: Antiplatelet therapy to prevent coronary artery bypass graft occlusion. Circulation 82:1046, 1990.
39. Sethi, G. K., Copeland, J. G., Goldman, S., et al.: Implications of preoperative administration of aspirin in patients undergoing coronary artery bypass grafting. J. Am. Coll. Cardiol. 15:15, 1990.
40. Owings, D. V., Kruskall, M. S., Thurer, R. L., and Donovan, L. M.: Autologous blood donations prior to elective cardiac surgery. Safety and effect on subsequent blood use. J.A.M.A. 262:1963, 1989.
41. Giordano, G. F., Goldman, D. S., Mammana, R. B., et al.: Intraoperative autotransfusion in cardiac operations. Effect on intraoperative and postoperative transfusion requirements. J. Thorac. Cardiovasc. Surg. 96:382, 1988.
42. Dietrich, W., Barankay, A., Dilthey, G., and Richter, J. A.: Autotransfusion and hemoseparation in cardiac surgery. What can be saved in cardiac reoperations and operations of thoracic aortic aneurysms? Thorac. Cardiovasc. Surg. 37:84, 1989.
43. Stein, B., Fuster, V., Halperin, J. L., and Chesebro, J. H.: Antithrombotic therapy in cardiovascular disease. An emerging approach based on pathogenesis and risk. Circulation 80:1501, 1989.
44. Subramanian, V. B., Bowles, M. J., Khurmi, N. S., et al.: Calcium antagonist withdrawal syndrome: Objective demonstration with frequency-modulated ambulatory ST-segment monitoring. Br. Med. J. 286:520, 1983.
45. Gottlieb, S. O., and Gerstenblith, G.: Safety of acute calcium antagonist withdrawal: Studies in patients with unstable angina withdrawn from nifedipine. Am. J. Cardiol. 55:27E, 1985.
46. Mehta, J., and Lopez, L. M.: Calcium-blocker withdrawal phenomenon: Increase in affinity of alpha 2 adrenoceptors for agonist as a potential mechanism. Am. J. Cardiol. 58:242, 1986.

INTRAOPERATIVE EVALUATION

47. Kirklin, J. W., and Barratt-Boyes, B. G.: Cardiac Surgery. New York, John Wiley & Sons, 1986.

POSTOPERATIVE EVALUATION

48. Weber, D. O., and Yarnoz, M. D.: Hyperkalemia complicating cardiopulmonary bypass: Analysis of risk factors. Ann. Thorac. Surg. 34:439, 1982.
49. Keren, A., and Tzivoni, D.: Magnesium therapy in ventricular arrhythmias. Pace 13:937, 1990.
50. Osborn, J. J., Popper, R. M., Kerth, W. J., et al.: Respiratory insufficiency following open heart surgery. Ann. Surg. 156:638, 1962.
51. Chenoweth, D. E., Cooper, S. W., Hugli, T. E., et al.: Complement activation during cardiopulmonary bypass: Evidence for generation of C3a and C5a anaphylatoxins. N. Engl. J. Med. 304:497, 1981.
52. Benumof, J. L., and Wahrenbrock, E. A.: Local effects of anesthetics on regional hypoxic pulmonary vasoconstriction. Anesthesiology 43:525, 1975.
53. Quasha, A. C., Loeber, N., Feeley, T. W., et al.: Postoperative respiratory care: A controlled trial of early and late extubation following coronary artery bypass grafting. Anesthesiology 52:135, 1980.
54. Fountain, S. W., Martin, B. A., and Musclow, C. E.: Pulmonary leukostasis and its relationship to pulmonary dysfunction in sheep and rabbits. Circ. Res. 46:175, 1980.
55. Jorgensen, L., Hoving, T., Rowsell, H. C., et al.: Adenosine diphosphate–involved platelet aggregation and vascular injury in swine and rabbit. Am. J. Pathol. 61:161, 1970.
56. Edmunds, L. H. Jr., and Alexander, J. A.: Effect of cardiopulmonary bypass on the lungs. *In* Fishman, A. (ed.): Pulmonary Disease and Disorders. New York, McGraw-Hill, 1980, p. 1728.
57. Stein, M., and Cassara, E. L.: Preoperative pulmonary evaluation and therapy for surgery patients. J.A.M.A. 211:787, 1970.
58. Aubier, M., and Roussos, S.: Effect of theophylline on respiratory muscle function. Chest 88:915, 1985.
59. Weinberger, M., Hendeles, L., and Ahrens, R.: Pharmacologic management of reversible obstructive airways disease: Symposium on chronic lung obstructrive airways disease. Med. Clin. North Am. 65:579, 1980.
60. Albert, R. K., Martin, T. R., and Lewis, S. W. Controlled clinical trial of methylprednisolone in patients with chronic bronchitis and acute respiratory insufficiency. Ann. Intern. Med. 92:753, 1980.
61. Morgenroth, M. L., Morganroth, J. L., Nett, L. M., et al.: Criteria for wean-

ing from prolonged mechanical ventilation. Arch. Intern. Med. *144*:1012, 1984.

62. Curtis, J. J., Weerachai, N., Walls, J. T., et al.: Elevated hemidiaphragm after cardiac operations: Incidence, prognosis, and relationship to the use of topical ice slush. Ann. Thorac. Surg. *48*:764, 1989.
63. Abd, G. A., Braun, N. M. T., Baskin, M. I., et al.: Diaphragmatic dysfunction after open heart surgery: Treatment with a rocking bed. Ann. Intern. Med. *111*:881, 1989.
64. Graham, D. R., Kaplan, D., Evans, C. C., et al.: Diaphragmatic plication for unilateral diaphragmatic paralysis: A 10-year experience. Ann. Thorac. Surg. *49*:248, 1990.
65. Carlin, G. C., Howland, W. S., Ray, C., et al.: High frequency jet ventilation. A prospective randomized evaluation. Chest *84*:551, 1983.
66. Flaherty, J. T., Magee, P. A., Gardner, T. L., et al.: Comparison of intravenous nitroglycerin and sodium nitroprusside for treatment of acute hypertension developing after coronary artery bypass surgery. Circulation *65*:1072, 1982.
67. Fremes, S. E., Weisel, R. D., Baird, R. J., et al.: Effects of postoperative hypertension and its treatment. J. Thorac. Cardiovasc. Surg. *86*:47, 1983.
68. Gray, R. J., Bateman, T. M., Czer, L. S., et al.: Use of esmolol in hypertension after cardiac surgery. Am. J. Cardiol. *56*:SGF, 1985.
69. Estafanous, F. G., and Tarazi, R. C.: Systemic arterial hypertension associated with cardiac surgery. Am. J. Cardiol. *46*:685, 1980.
70. Cooper, T. J., Clutton Brock, T. H., Jones, S. N., et al.: Factors relating to the development of hypertension after cardiopulmonary bypass. Br. Heart J. *54*:91, 1985.
71. Rocchini, A. P., Rosenthal, A., Barger, A. C., et al.: Pathogenesis of paradoxical hypertension after coarctation resection. Circulation *54*:382, 1976.
72. James, T. N., Hageman, G. R., and Urthaler, F.: Anatomic and physiologic considerations of a cardiogenic hypertensive reflex. Am. J. Cardiol. *44*:852, 1979.
73. Kirklin, J. W., and Barratt-Boyes, B. G.: Postoperative care. *In* Kirklin, J. W., and Barratt-Boyes, B. G. (eds.): Cardiac Surgery. New York, John Wiley & Sons, 1986, p. 139.
74. Brody, W. R., Kosek, J. C., and Angell, W. W.: Changes in vein grafts following aorto-coronary bypass induced by pressure and ischemia. J. Thorac. Cardiovasc. Surg. *64*:847, 1972.
75. Kaplan, J. A., Finlayson, D. C., and Woodward, S.: Vasodilator therapy after cardiac surgery: A review of the efficacy and toxicity of nitroglycerin and nitroprusside. Can. Anaesth. Soc. J. *27*:254, 1980.
76. Gray, R. J., Bateman, T. M., Czer, L. S., et al.: Comparison of esmolol and nitroprusside for acute post-cardiac surgical hypertension. Am. J. Cardiol. *59*:887, 1987.
77. Gabrielson, G., Lingham, R., Dimich, I., et al: Comparative study of labetalol and hydralazine in the treatment of postoperative hypertension. Anesth. Analg. *66*:S63, 1987.
78. Cosgrove, D. M., Petre, J. H., Waller, J. L., et al.: Automated control of postoperative hypertension: A prospective, randomized multicenter study. Ann. Thorac. Surg. *47*:678, 1989.
79. Gray, R. J., Harris, W. S., Shah, P. K., et al.: Coronary sinus blood flow and sampling for detection of unrecognized myocardial ischemia and injury. Circulation 56(Suppl 2):58, 1977.
80. Slogoff, S., and Keats, A. S.: Does perioperative myocardial ischemia lead to postoperative myocardial infarction? Anesthesiology *62*:107, 1985.
81. London, M. J., Hollenberg, M., Wong, M. G., et al.: Intraoperative myocardial ischemia: Localization by continuous 12-lead electrocardiography. Anesthesiology *69*:232, 1988.
82. Lemmer, J. H. Jr., and Krish, M. M.: Coronary artery spasm following coronary artery surgery. Ann. Thorac. Surg. *46*:108, 1988.
83. Lawrence, G. H., McKay, H. A., and Sherensky, R. T.: Effective measures in the prevention of intraoperative aeroembolus. J. Thorac. Cardiovasc. Surg. *62*:731, 1971.
84. Keon, W. J., Heggtveit, H. A., and Leduc, J.: Perioperative myocardial infarction caused by atheroembolism. J. Thorac. Cardiovasc. Surg. *84*:849, 1982.
85. Obarski, T. P., Loop, F. D., Cosgrove, D. M., et al.: Frequency of acute myocardial infarction in valve repairs versus valve replacement for pure mitral regurgitation. Am. J. Cardiol. *65*:887, 1990.
86. Bulkley, B. H., and Hutchins, G. M.: Myocardial consequences of coronary artery bypass graft surgery. The paradox of necrosis in areas of revascularization. Circulation *56*:906, 1977.
87. Albert, D. E., Califf, R. M., LeCocq, D. A., et al.: Comparative rates of resolution of QRS changes after operative and nonoperative acute myocardial infarcts. Am. J. Cardiol. *51*:378, 1983.
88. Gray, R. J., Matloff, J. M., Conklin, C. M., et al.: Perioperative myocardial infarction: Late clinical course after coronary artery bypass surgery. Circulation *66*:1185, 1982.
89. Chaitman, B. R., Alderman, E. L., Sheffield, L. T., et al.: Use of survival analysis to determine the clinical significance of new Q waves after coronary bypass surgery. Circulation *67*:302, 1983.
90. Bateman, T. M., Matloff, J. M., and Gray, R. J.: Myocardial infarction during coronary artery bypass surgery—benign event or prognostic omen? Int. J. Cardiol. *6*:259, 1984.
90a. Force, T., Hibberd, P., Weeks, G., et al.: Perioperative myocardial infarction after coronary artery bypass surgery. Circulation *82*:903, 1990.
91. Salomon, N. W., Plachetka, J. R., and Copeland, J. G.: Comparison of dopamine and dobutamine following coronary artery bypass grafting. Ann. Thorac. Surg. *33*:48, 1982.
92. Makabali, C., Weil, M. H., and Henning, R. J.: Dobutamine and other sympathomimetic drugs for the treatment of low cardiac output failure. Semin. Anesth. *1*:63, 1982.
93. Gray, R., Shah, P. K., Singh, B., et al.: Low cardiac output states after open heart surgery. Chest *80*:16, 1981.
94. Bastien, O., Durand, P. G., George, M., et al.: Evolution of right ventricular performance after CABG. Intensive Care Med. *14*:499, 1988.
95. D'Ambra, M. N., LaRaia, P. J., Philbin, D. M., et al.: Prostaglandin E_1: A new therapy for refractory right heart failure and pulmonary hypertension after mitral valve replacement. J. Thorac. Cardiovasc. Surg. *89*:567, 1985.
96. Miller, D. C., Moreno-Cabral, R. J., Stinson, E. B., et al.: Pulmonary artery balloon counterpulsation for acute right ventricular failure. J. Thorac. Cardiovasc. Surg. *80*:760, 1980.
97. Weitzman, L. B., Tinker, P. W., Kronzon, I., et al.: The incidence and natural history of pericardial effusion after cardiac surgery. Circulation *69*:506, 1984.
98. D'Cruz, I. A., Kensey, K., Campbell, C., et al.: Two-dimensional echocardiography in cardiac tamponade occurring after cardiac surgery. Circulation *5*:1250, 1985.
99. Weeks, K. R., Chatterjee, K., Block, S., et al.: Bedside hemodynamic monitoring—its value in the diagnosis of tamponade complicating cardiac surgery. J. Thorac. Cardiovasc. Surg. *71*:259, 1976.
100. Jones, M. R., Vine, D. L., Attas, M., et al.: Late isolated left ventricular tamponade: Clinical, hemodynamic and echocardiographic manifestations of a previously unreported postoperative complication. J. Thorac. Cardiovasc. Surg. *77*:142, 1979.
101. Bateman, T., Gray, R., Chaux, A., et al.: Right atrial tamponade caused by hematoma complicating coronary artery bypass graft surgery: Clinical hemodynamic and scintigraphic correlates. J. Thorac. Cardiovasc. Surg. *84*:413, 1982.
102. MacMahon, S., Collins, R., Peto, R., et al.: Effects of prophylactic lidocaine in suspected acute myocardial infarction. An overview of results from the randomized, controlled trials. J.A.M.A. *260*:1910, 1988.
103. Rao, G., Ford, W. B., Zikria, E. A., et al.: Prevention of arrhythmias after direct myocardial revascularization surgery. Vasc. Surg. *8*:82, 1974.
104. Waldo, A. L., and MacLean, W. A.: Treatment of cardiac arrhythmias with emphasis on cardiac pacing. *In* Diagnosis and Treatment of Cardiac Arrhythmias Following Open Heart Surgery: Emphasis on the Use of Atrial and Ventricular Epicardial Wire Electrodes. Mount Kisco, Futura, 1980, p. 115.
105. Douglas, P., Hirshfield, J. W., and Edmunds, L. H.: Clinical correlates of postoperative atrial fibrillation. Circulation *70*(Suppl II):165, 1984.
106. Fuller, J. A., Adams, G. G., and Buxton, B.: Atrial fibrillation after coronary artery bypass grafting. Is it a disorder of the elderly? J. Thorac. Cardiovasc. Surg. *97*:821, 1989.
107. Platia, E. V., Fitzpatrick, P., Wallis, D., et al.: Esmolol vs verapamil for the treatment of recent-onset atrial fibrillation/flutter. J. Am. Coll. Cardiol. *11*:170A, 1988.
108. Dunn, M. I., Alexander, J. K., deSilva, R., and Hildner, F.: Antithrombotic therapy in atrial fibrillation. Chest 95(Suppl):119S, 1989.
109. Dimarco, J. P., Miles, W., Akhtar, M., et al.: Adenosine for paroxysmal supraventricular tachycardia: Dose ranging and comparison with verapamil. Assessment in placebo-controlled multicenter trials. Ann. Intern. Med. *113*:104, 1990.
110. Wexelman, W., Lichstein, E., Cunningham, J. N., et al.: Etiology and clinical significance of new fascicular conduction defects following coronary bypass surgery. Am. Heart J. *111*:923, 1986.
111. Gundry, S. R., Sequeira, A., Coughlin, T. R., and McLaughlin, J. S.: Postoperative conduction disturbances: A comparison of blood and crystalloid cardioplegia. Ann. Thorac. Surg. *47*:384, 1989.
111a. Tuzcu, E. M., Emre, A., Goormastic, M., et al.: Incidence and prognostic significance of intraventricular conduction abnormalities after coronary bypass surgery. J. Am. Coll. Cardiol. *16*:607, 1990.
112. Tsai, T., and Matloff, J. M.: Cardiac surgery in the elderly. *In* Gray, R., and Matloff, J. (eds.): Medical Management of the Cardiac Surgical Patient. Baltimore, Williams & Wilkins, 1990, p. 27.
113. Harker, L. A.: Bleeding after cardiopulmonary bypass. N. Engl. J. Med. *314*:1146, 1986.
114. Mammen, E. F., Koets, M. H., Washington, B. C., et al.: Hemostasis changes during cardiopulmonary bypass surgery. Semin. Thromb. Hemost. *11*:281, 1985.
115. Kirklin, J. K., Westaby, S., Blackstone, E. H., et al.: Complement and the damaging effects of cardiopulmonary bypass. J. Thorac. Cardiovasc. Surg. *86*:845, 1983.
116. Salama, A., Hugo, F., Heinrich, D., et al.: Deposition of terminal C5b-9 complement complexes on erythrocytes and leukocytes during cardiopulmonary bypass. N. Engl. J. Med. *318*:408, 1988.
117. Cines, D. B., Tomaski, A., and Tannenbaum, S.: Immune endothelial-cell injury in heparin-associated thrombocytopenia. N. Engl. J. Med. *316*:581, 1987.
118. Horrow, J. C.: Protamine allergy. J. Cardiothorac. Anesth. *2*:225, 1988.
119. Sane, D. C., Califf, R. M., Topol, E. J., et al.: Bleeding during thrombolytic therapy for acute myocardial infarction: Mechanisms and management. Ann. Intern. Med. *111*:1010, 1989.
120. Schrier, S. L.: Disorders of hemostasis and coagulation. *In* Rubenstein, E., and Federman, D. D. (eds.): Scientific American Medicine. New York, Scientific American, 1988 (5 Hematology), p. 1.
121. Sattler, F. R., Weitekamp, M. R., and Ballard, J. O.: Potential for bleeding with the new beta-lactam antibiotics. Ann. Intern. Med. *105*:924, 1986.
122. Czer, L. S., Bateman, T. M., Gray, R. J., et al.: Treatment of severe platelet dysfunction and hemorrhage after cardiopulmonary bypass: Reduction

in blood product usage with desmopressin. J. Am. Coll. Cardiol. *9*:1139, 1987.
123. Salzman, E. W., Weinstein, M. J., Weintraub, R. M., et al.: Treatment with desmopressin acetate to reduce blood loss after cardiac surgery: A double-blind randomized trial. N. Engl. J. Med. *314*:1402, 1986.
124. Saour, J. N., Sieck, J. O., Mamo, L. A. R., and Gallus, A. S.: Trial of different intensities of anticoagulation in patients with prosthetic heart valves. N. Engl. J. Med. *322*:428, 1990.
125. Verkkala, V., Valtonen, V., Jarvinen, A., and Tolppanen, E. M.: Fever, leukocytosis and C-reactive protein after open-heart surgery and their value in the diagnosis of postoperative infections. Thorac. Cardiovasc. Surg. *35*:78, 1987.
126. Livelli, F. D., Johnson, R. A., McEnany, M. T., et al.: Unexplained in-hospital fever following cardiac surgery. Natural history, relationship to postpericardiotomy syndrome, and a prospective study of therapy with indomethacin versus placebo. Circulation *57*:968, 1978.
127. Baddour, L. M., and Bisno, A. L. Recurrent cellulitis after saphenous venectomy for coronary bypass surgery. Ann. Intern. Med. *97*:493, 1982.
128. Greenberg, J., DeSanctis, R. W., and Mills, R. M., Jr.: Vein-donor-leg cellulitis after coronary artery bypass surgery. Ann. Intern. Med. *97*:565, 1982.
129. Spencer, F. C., and Grossi, E. A.: Mediastinitis after cardiac operations. Ann. Thorac. Surg. *49*:506, 1990.
130. Demmy, T. L., Park, S. B., Liebler, G. A., et al.: Recent experience with major sternal wound complications. Ann. Thorac. Surg. *49*:458, 1990.
131. Kouchoukos, N. T., Wareing, T. H., Murphy, S. F., et al.: Risks of bilateral internal mammary artery bypass grafting. Ann. Thorac. Surg. *49*:210, 1990.
132. Bor, D. H., Rose, R. M., Modlin, J. F., et al.: Mediastinitis after cardiovascular surgery. Rev. Infect. Dis. *5*:885, 1983.
133. Kernodle, D. S., Classen, D. C., Burke, J. P., and Kaiser, A. B.: Failure of cephalosporins to prevent *Staphylococcus aureus* surgical wound infections. J.A.M.A. *263*:961, 1990.
134. Culliford, A. T., Cunningham, J. W., Zeaff, R. N., et al.: Sternal and costochondral infections following open heart surgery. J. Thorac. Cardiovasc. Surg. *72*:714, 1976.
135. Engelman, R. M., Williams, C. D., Gouge, T. H., et al.: Mediastinitis following open-heart surgery. Am. J. Surg. *107*:772, 1973.
136. Macmanus, Q., and Okies, J. E.: Mediastinal wound infection and aortocoronary graft patency. Am. J. Surg. *132*:558, 1976.
137. Platt, R., Munoz, A., Stell, J., et al.: Antibiotic prophylaxis for cardiovascular surgery. Efficacy with coronary artery bypass. Ann. Intern. Med. *101*:770, 1984.
138. Keys, T. F.: Antimicrobial prophylaxis for patients with congenital or valvular heart disease. Mayo Clin. Proc. *57*:171, 1982.
139. Wilson, W. R., Danielson, G. K., Giuliani, E. R., and Geraci, J. E.: Prosthetic valve endocarditis. Mayo Clin. Proc. *57*:155, 1982.
140. Ivert, T. S. A., Dismukes, W. E., Cobbs, C. G., et al.: Prosthetic valve endocarditis. Circulation *69*:223, 1984.
141. Cowgill, L. D., Addonizio, V. P., Hopeman, A. G., and Harken, A. H.: A practical approach to prosthetic valve endocarditis. Ann. Thorac. Surg. *43*:450, 1987.
142. Dinubile, M. J.: Surgery in active endocarditis. Ann. Intern. Med. *96*:650, 1982.
143. Alter, H. J., Purcell, R. H., Shih, J. W., et al.: Detection of antibody to hepatitis C virus in prospectively followed transfusion recipients with acute and chronic non-A, non-B hepatitis. N. Engl. J. Med. *321*:1494, 1989.
144. Davis, G. L., Balart, L. A., Schiff, E. R., et al.: Treatment of chronic hepatitis C with recombinant interferon alfa. A multicenter randomized, controlled trial. N. Engl. J. Med. *321*:1501, 1989.
145. DiBisceglie, A. M., Martin, P., Kassiandes, C., et al.: Recombinant interferon ALFA therapy for chronic hepatitis C. N. Engl. J. Med. *321*:1506, 1989.
146. Atkinson, J. B., Connor, D. H., Robinowitz, M., et al.: Cardiac fungal infections: Review of autopsy findings in 60 patients. Human Pathol. *15*:935, 1984.
147. Miller, R. H., Horneffer, P. J., Gardner, T. J., et al.: The epidemiology of the postpericardiotomy syndrome: A common complication of cardiac surgery. Am. Heart J. *116*:1323, 1988.
148. Ng, A. S., Dorosti, K., and Sheldon, W. C.: Constrictive pericarditis following cardiac surgery—Cleveland Clinic experience: Report of 12 cases and review. Cleve. Clin. Q. *51*:39, 1984.
149. Abel, R. M., Buckley, M. J., Austen, W. G., et al.: Etiology, incidence, and prognosis of renal failure following cardiac operations. Results of a prospective analysis of 500 consecutive patients. J. Thorac. Cardiovasc. Surg. *71*:323, 1976.
150. Bhat, J. G., Gluck, M. C., Lowenstein, J., and Baldwin, D. S.: Renal failure after open heart surgery. Ann. Intern. Med. *84*:677, 1976.
151. Alfieri, A., and Kotler, M. N.: Noncardiac complications of open-heart surgery. Am. Heart J. *119*:149, 1990.
152. Gailiunas, P., Chawla, R., Lazarus, J. M., et al.: Acute renal failure following cardiac operations. J. Thorac. Cardiovasc. Surg. *79*:241, 1980.
153. Lange, H. W., Aeppli, D. M., and Brown, D. C.: Survival of patients with acute renal failure requiring dialysis after open-heart surgery: Early prognostic indicators. Am. Heart J. *113*:1138, 1987.
154. Rose, B. D.: Acute renal failure—prerenal disease versus acute tubular necrosis. *In* Rose, B. D. (ed): Pathophysiology of Renal Disease. New York, McGraw-Hill, 1987, p. 63.
155. Luke, R. G., Briggs, J. D., Allison, M. E. M., and Kennedy, A. C.: Factors determining response to mannitol in acute renal failure. Am. J. Med. Sci. *259*:168, 1970.
156. Graziani, G. A., Cantaluppi, S., Casati, A., et al.: Dopamine and furosemide in oliguric acute renal failure. Nephron *37*:39, 1984.
157. Conger, J. D., Falk, S. A., Yuan, B. H., and Schrier, R. W.: Atrial natriuretic peptide and dopamine in a rat model of ischemic acute renal failure. Kidney Int. *35*:1126, 1989.
158. Francis, G. S., Sharma, B., Collins, A. J., et al.: Coronary-artery surgery in patients with end-stage renal disease. Ann. Intern. Med. *92*:499, 1980.
159. Opsahl, J. A., Husebye, D. G., Helseth, H. K., et al.: Coronary artery bypass surgery in patients on maintenance dialysis: Long-term survival. Am. J. Kidney Dis. *12*:271, 1988.
160. Aranha, G. V., Pickleman, J., Pifarre, R., et al.: The reasons for gastrointestinal consultation after cardiac surgery. Am. Surg. *50*:301, 1984.
161. Moneta, G. L., Misbach, G. A., and Ivey, T. D.: Hypoperfusion as a possible factor in the development of gastrointestinal complications after cardiac surgery. Am. J. Surg. *149*:648, 1985.
162. Kumon, K., Kaznihiko, T., Takahiko, H., et al.: Organ failure due to low cardiac output syndrome following open heart surgery. Jpn. Circ. J. *50*:329, 1986.
163. Kleptko, W.: Jaundice after open-heart surgery: A prospective study. Thorax *40*:80, 1985.
164. Tremolada, F., Loreggian, M., Antona, C., et al.: Blood transmitted and clotting factor transmitted non-A, non-B hepatitis. J. Clin. Gastroenterol. *10*:413, 1988.
165. Heikkinen, L., and Alz Kulju, K.: Abdominal complications following cardiopulmonary bypass in open-heart surgery. Scand. J. Thorac. Cardiovasc. Surg. *21*:1, 1987.
166. Wallwork, J.: The acute abdomen following cardiopulmonary bypass surgery. Br. J. Surg. *67*:410, 1980.
167. Svensson, L. G., Decker, G., and Kinsley, R. B.: A prospective study of hyperamylasemia and pancreatitis after cardiopulmonary bypass. Ann. Thorac. Surg. *39*:409, 1985.
168. Rose, D. M., Ranson, J. H., Cunningham, J. N. Jr., and Spencer, F. C.: Patterns of severe pancreatic injury following cardiopulmonary bypass. Ann. Surg. *199*:168, 1984.
169. Heller, S. S., Frank, K. A., Kornfield, D. S., et al.: Psychological outcome following open-heart surgery. Arch. Intern. Med. *134*:908, 1974.
170. Adrian, J., Brankshaw, D. P., Tiller, J. W., et al.: Affective, cognitive and subjective changes in patients undergoing cardiac surgery—a preliminary report. Anaesth. Intensive Care *16*:144, 1988.
171. Fish, K. J., Helms, K. N., Sarnquist, F. H., et al.: A prospective randomized study of the effects of prostacyclin on neuropsychological dysfunction after coronary artery surgery. J. Thorac. Cardiovasc. Surg. *93*:609, 1987.
172. Townes, B. D., Bashein, G., Hornbein, T. F., et al.: Neurobehavioral outcomes in cardiac operations. J. Thorac. Cardiovasc. Surg. *98*:774, 1989.
173. Furian, A. J., and Brener, A. C.: Central nervous system complications of open heart surgery. Stroke *15*:912, 1984.
174. Taylor, G. J., Malik, S. A., Colliver, J. A., et al.: Usefulness of atrial fibrillation as a predictor of stroke after isolated coronary artery bypass grafting. Am. J. Cardiol. *60*:905, 1987.
175. Breuer, A. C., Franco, I., Marzewski, D., et al.: Left ventricular thrombi seen by ventriculography are a significant risk factor for stroke in open heart surgery. Ann. Neurol. *10*:103, 1981.
176. Shahian, D. M., and Speert, P. K.: Symptomatic visual deficits after open heart operations. Ann. Thorac. Surg. *48*:275, 1989.
177. Reed, G. L., Singer, D. E., and Pilard, E. H.: Stroke following coronary artery bypass surgery. A case control estimate of the risk of carotid bruits. N. Engl. J. Med. *319*:1246, 1988.
178. Hertzer, N. R., Loop, F. D., Taylor, P. C., et al.: Staged and combined surgical approach to simultaneous carotid and coronary vascular disease. Surgery *84*:803, 1978.
179. Mehigan, J. T., Buch, W. S., Pipkin, R. D., et al.: A planned approach to co-existent cerebrovascular disease in coronary artery bypass candidates. Ann. Surg. *112*:1403, 1977.
180. Seyfer, A. E., Grammer, N. Y., Bogumill, G. P., et al.: Upper extremity neuropathies after cardiac surgery. J. Hand Surg. [Am.] *10*:16, 1985.
181. Murphy, M. C., Newman, B. M., and Rodgers, B. M.: Pleuroperitoneal shunts in the management of persistent chylothorax. Ann. Thorac. Surg. *48*:195, 1989.
182. Gutmann, M. C., Knapp, D. N., Pollock, M. L., et al.: Coronary artery bypass patients and work status. Circulation *66*:33, 1982.
183. Oberman, A., Wayne, J. B., Kouchoukos, N. T., et al.: Employment status after coronary artery bypass surgery. Circulation *65*:115, 1982.
184. CASS Principal Investigators and Their Associates. Coronary Artery Surgery Study (CASS): A randomized trial of coronary artery bypass surgery. Quality of life in patients randomly assigned to treatment groups. Circulation *68*:951, 1983.
185. Boulay, F. M., David, P. P., and Bourassa, M. G.: Strategies for improving the work status of patients after coronary artery bypass surgery. Circulation *66*:43, 1982.

54

Cost-Effective Strategies in Cardiology

by LEE GOLDMAN, M.D.

The availability of an increasing number of diagnostic and therapeutic technologies, coupled with concerns over the rising costs of health care, has generated increasing interest in determining the costs and effectiveness of cardiologic care. Cost-effectiveness analysis, which initially had been used principally by economists and policymakers, is a potentially useful technique for evaluating how best to diagnose, prevent, and treat medical illnesses. Such analyses highlight the important issues that should guide the physician–decision maker. They can help in identification of gaps in knowledge and establishment of priorities for research to be carried out by clinical investigators. To appreciate the implications of the emerging literature on cost-effectiveness in cardiology, it is important to understand the basic concepts that underlie formal cost-effectiveness analysis.

QUANTITATIVE ANALYSES OF COSTS AND EFFECTIVENESS

Analysts commonly distinguish between *cost-benefit analysis*, in which both costs and benefits are expressed in the same units (such as dollars), and *cost-effectiveness analysis*, in which the costs are commonly expressed in monetary terms while the effectiveness is expressed in terms of the health benefit.[1] The health benefit commonly is measured in units such as the number of lives that are saved, the years of life gained, the quality-adjusted years of life saved,[1-3] the days of disability avoided, or other suitable measurements.

SENSITIVITY ANALYSIS. Cost-effectiveness analyses are critically dependent on the accuracy of the assumptions on which they are based. Therefore, the analysis should include a "sensitivity analysis," in which the calculations are repeated with varying assumptions to determine whether the conclusions are altered.[1,2] It is vital to determine whether the final conclusions are critically dependent on a tenuous estimate by determining whether reasonable variations in important assumptions make major differences in the results of the analysis.

For example, in an analysis of the cost-effectiveness of admitting patients with chest pain and possible uncomplicated acute myocardial infarction in the absence of ST-segment elevation to a full-fledged coronary care unit as opposed to a nonintensive care unit bed with telemetry monitoring, it would be critical to estimate the relative difference, if any, in the rate of successful resuscitation from primary ventricular fibrillation in the two settings. The larger the estimated difference, the more cost-effective the coronary care unit would appear. If the two settings were assumed to be equally effective, the additional cost of the coronary care unit would not yield additional effectiveness for this purpose. Because there are no randomized controlled data to address this issue, any analysis of the relative cost-effectiveness of care of patients with possible myocardial infarction in these two settings depends on the estimates that are made. When a sensitivity analysis was performed, the nonintensive care bed with telemetry monitoring remained the more cost-effective option for patients whose probability of acute myocardial infarction was 10 per cent or less, even if it was assumed that the rate of successful resuscitation from primary ventricular fibrillation in this setting was no better than the success rate among patients seen by trained ambulance personnel within 5 minutes after onset of ventricular fibrillation in the out-of-hospital setting.[4]

THE CLINICAL DECISION TREE. Some cost-effectiveness analyses address difficult clinical problems for which no clear agreement exists, often because available data are not adequate even for the experienced clinician. In such situations, cost-effectiveness analysis may not yield clear answers, usually because the relative differences between competing strategies are small. For example, it may be difficult to decide whether or not to implant a permanent pacemaker in an elderly patient who has symptoms that are suggestive of a pacemaker-responsive arrhythmia but in whom the relation between arrhythmia and symptoms has not been proved. The therapeutic options can be displayed using a decision tree (Fig. 54–1) that explicitly outlines the various possibilities.[5] In this decision analysis, estimates about the relative cost-effectiveness of various therapeutic strategies would depend on the patient's subjective assessment of the quality of life under different scenarios, including persistent symptoms and no pacemaker, persistent symptoms despite a pacemaker, and the pacemaker without symptoms. Because small changes in the assessment of quality of life under these different circumstances would alter the preferred strategy, this particular analysis could not provide a definitive solution for all cases involving this therapeutic dilemma. Nevertheless, this analysis demonstrated that empiric pacing was an attractive option in an elderly patient with unexplained syncope even when there was only about a 25 per cent chance that the syncope was caused by a pacemaker-responsive arrhythmia.

The goal of cost-effectiveness analysis is not to find the greatest possible benefit for the lowest possible cost, because it is not possible to achieve both simultaneously.[2,3,6] Instead, it is necessary either to determine the resources that are available and then find the greatest possible effectiveness that can be purchased for those resources, or to determine the desired effectiveness and then find the lowest cost to achieve it. In either case, it is important to have a preconceived idea of the

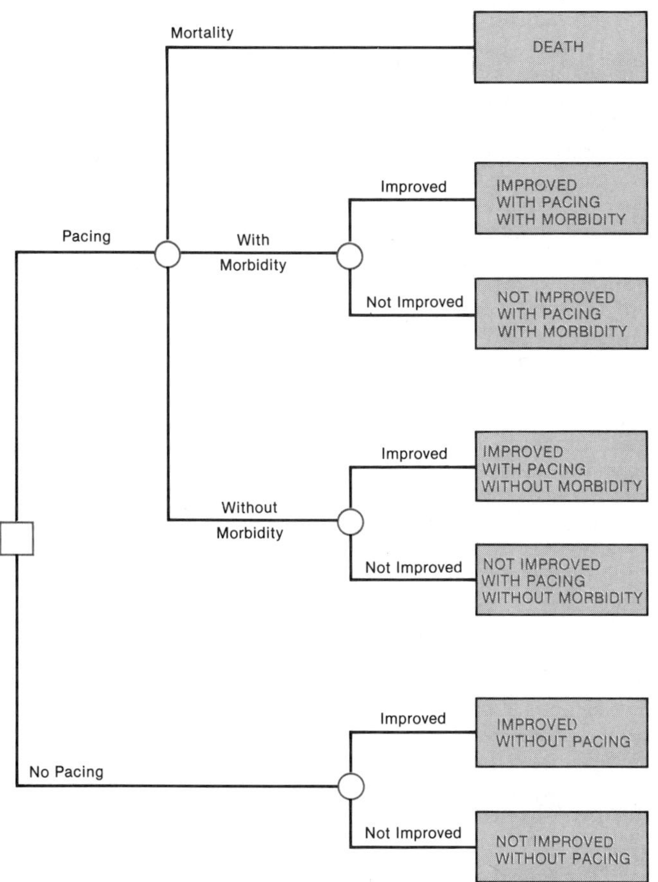

FIGURE 54–1. Decision tree for whether or not to perform empiric pacing in the elderly patient with syncope that may or may not be caused by a pacemaker-responsive arrhythmia. Branches of this decision tree explicitly detail the potential outcomes from the various options. The squares denote the outcomes of decisions that the physician must make, while the circles denote events over which the physician has no control, i.e., occur "by chance." In constructing the decision tree, physicians would use either their own judgment or probabilities derived from the literature to estimate the likelihood of each of the events that can occur at a "chance" node. The sum of the probabilities of these chance events is always 100 per cent. In a cost-effectiveness analysis, each of the potential outcomes, as displayed in the rectangles in the right column, would be assigned a cost and a "utility." The utility would denote how highly the outcome is valued compared to perfect health, which traditionally has a value of 1.0, versus death, which traditionally has a value of 0. Cost-effectiveness calculations would compute the average expected costs and utilities for each of the various options that might be chosen by the physician, in this case the "pacing" and "no pacing" options that emanate from the initial square node. (From Kwoh, C. K., Beck, J R., and Pauker, S. G.: Repeated syncope with negative diagnostic evaluation. Med. Decis. Making *4*:351, 1984.)

desirable or acceptable relative ratio of cost to effectiveness. Although cost-effectiveness analyses determine the ratio of cost to effectiveness, two strategies with the same ratio may have quite different absolute costs and absolute effectiveness. For example, a program that saves 100 lives for $10,000 has the same cost-effectiveness ratio as one that saves 10,000 lives for $1,000,000, but the two programs' absolute costs and absolute effectivenesses vary 100-fold. In cost-effectiveness analyses, any potentially new strategy usually is compared with the current, or baseline, strategy by calculating the *incremental cost : incremental effectiveness* ratio.[1–3,6,7]

CALCULATION OF COSTS

In determining costs, several types must be considered.[7,8] *Operating costs* may include both direct costs such as salaries and indirect costs such as overhead, including utilities and maintenance. Costs also can be categorized as fixed versus variable costs. For example, the first 100 cardiac scans carried out in an imaging center may cost $100,000 for an average cost of $1000 per scan because of the high capital costs of the equipment. If the laboratory were to "increase its output," the incremental cost for the next 100 scans would be much less than the cost for the first 100 scans because the capital costs of the equipment would be nearly the same regardless of whether 100 scans or 200 scans were performed. Thus one could distinguish between the incremental cost of performing the second 100 scans versus the average cost of all 200 scans. In many medical analyses, true costs are not available, and charges are used in the calculation of "cost" effectiveness. Because charges often are the same regardless of volume, they usually do not consider fully the important differences between average and incremental costs.

In calculating net health care costs, a useful approach is shown in Table 54–1. Unfortunately many cost-effectiveness analyses have concentrated only on direct medical costs, without fully taking into account the other terms in the equation.

DISCOUNTING. In virtually all cost analyses, it is important to consider the time frame when costs and effects will be achieved. Because current dollars or benefits are more highly valued than a promise of future dollars or health benefits, a cost or benefit achieved immediately is more highly valued than one that is achieved later.[1] For example, one would be more willing to spend $10,000 today to prevent a death that otherwise would occur tomorrow than to spend $10,000 today to prevent a death that otherwise would occur in 10 years, even if there were no inflation and if there were no interest to be earned on the dollars. There is a preference to achieve an immediate benefit for several reasons. First, other events may intercede so that the projected future death may not occur or might be avoided as a consequence of newly available options that cost less than $10,000. Second, another illness could terminate life during the intervening period. Also, the $10,000 might be spent during the intervening 10 years in ways that are deemed more valuable. Furthermore, there is always a lingering doubt that the money spent now will not actually achieve the desired effect 10 years hence. This principle, by which the promise of future events is less valued than known immediate events, is termed "discounting," and is independent of monetary inflation. It is common practice to "discount" both future costs and future benefits by about 5 per cent per year.

In discussions of cost and effectiveness, several common misconceptions occur.[6] Cost-effective should not be equated with cost-saving because one often must spend to achieve a real benefit. Although a strategy that saves money *and* achieves an equal or better outcome is obviously cost-effective, a program is also cost-effective if it yields an additional benefit that is worth the additional cost. The definition of "worth the cost" may be a somewhat arbitrary value judgment because it is difficult to place a monetary value on years of life and productivity. In many analyses, the approximately

TABLE 54–1 CALCULATION OF NET HEALTH CARE COSTS FOR A PROGRAM

Net costs = direct medical costs*
+ health care costs associated with the adverse effects of treatment
− savings of health care, rehabilitation, and custodial costs owing to prevention or alleviation of disease
+ costs of treating disease that would not have occurred if the patient had not lived longer as a result of the original treatment

* Costs of hospitalization, physician time, medications, laboratory services, and other ancillary services.
See reference 2 for more details.

$30,000 to $35,000 per year cost in 1990 dollars of renal dialysis,[9,10] a program that the United States has decided to support with tax dollars, has been used as the benchmark for the amount of cost that the public appears willing to bear to prolong useful life by 1 year.

Although physicians must be aware of the relative cost-effectiveness of various diagnostic and therapeutic options if they are to make optimal choices for their patients, decisions about the number of dollars that *should* be spent to achieve specific health care benefits will ultimately be determined by society. Physicians have a critical role to play in developing appropriate data on cost-effectiveness issues, but the individual physician's primary responsibility is to the patient, within the confines of the economic limitations that may be imposed on both the physician and the patient by society.

One example of societal constraints on medical care expenditures is the diagnosis-related groups (DRG) system of prospective reimbursement. By defining in advance the number of dollars that a hospital will be reimbursed for the care of certain types of patients, the physician, the hospital, and the patient may all become more concerned with issues of cost-effectiveness. In an analogous manner, capitation systems, in which physicians are prepaid a fixed sum to assume the care of a patient, place an increased emphasis on the determination of cost-effective strategies.

DIAGNOSTIC TESTING

Modern cardiology includes an impressive armamentarium of diagnostic tests. Good clinical judgment requires that the physician choose tests in a cost-effective manner, in which the tests individually or sequentially may lead to improved diagnosis and management. The cost-effective use of diagnostic tests requires the physician to proceed logically through evaluation of the patient, selection of diagnostic tests, integration of the test with clinical data, and formulation of management strategies.[11,12] Each of these steps must be carefully considered for the proper utilization of diagnostic testing.

THE ESTIMATION OF CLINICAL PROBABILITIES. Regardless of the condition in question, the physician must utilize data from the medical history and physical examination to estimate the likelihood of its presence. For example, in evaluating the patient with chest pain, the physician may consider the patient's age and sex, as well as the typicality of the discomfort for angina pectoris.[12-16] The symptom may be categorized as typical angina pectoris, atypical angina pectoris, or nonanginal chest discomfort on the basis of its character, location, provocation, and response to rest or nitroglycerin (p. 1293). Similarly, in estimating the probability of the presence of hemodynamically significant aortic stenosis in an adult with a systolic murmur, one would consider factors such as the intensity, location, and radiation of the murmur, the volume and rate of upstroke of the carotid arterial pulse, and the second heart sound (p. 1038).[17] Although these estimates of clinical probabilities can be based on the judgment of an experienced physician, in some circumstances, the physician can be aided by accumulated data from large series of patients in whom the clinical probability of conditions such as significant coronary artery disease[16] or acute myocardial infarction or unstable angina pectoris[18,19] have been determined.

ORDERING A DIAGNOSTIC TEST. When considering a test that may be ordered, the physician must determine whether the test is efficacious and sufficiently accurate for indications for which it is being considered, that no other test with acceptable efficacy is less hazardous or less expensive, and that this is the most appropriate time for ordering the test.[11,19,20] In one such study carried out in 1977, soon after cardiac nuclear medicine scans became clinically available, 35 per cent were found *not* to have been ordered appropriately.[19] By comparison, the rate of inappropriate ordering for M-mode echocardiograms, which had been routinely available for some time and were presumably well understood by physicians, was only 14 per cent.[20]

Tests may be ordered for such indications as to plan or monitor therapy, to establish a diagnosis, to define the extent of a known disease, to estimate prognosis, or to reassure the physician or the patient.[19-21] Although each of these indications can be a legitimate reason for ordering a diagnostic test, test results that may influence therapeutic action usually are the most valued and are certainly the most cost-effective.

When assessing the accuracy of a test, one must understand terms such as sensitivity, specificity, and positive predictive value (Table 6-2, p. 168).[1,2,11] For some tests, such as a thallium scintiscan, the result is often dichotomized into "normal" versus "abnormal," even though it is understood that the precise distinction between normal and abnormal may be difficult and somewhat arbitrary. Other tests, such as the ejection fraction, commonly are reported on a continuous scale. In some circumstances, such as with the exercise electrocardiogram, a continuous result (e.g., the extent of ST-segment depression) often is dichotomized into normal or abnormal to facilitate the test's interpretation. When a continuous result is dichotomized, an increase in its sensitivity, or the likelihood of a positive test result among patients with the condition, can be obtained only at the expense of decreasing specificity, or the likelihood of a normal test result in patients without the condition.[22] For example, the sensitivity of the exercise electrocardiogram for detecting patients with coronary artery disease can be increased by reducing the depth of ST-segment depression required for a "positive" test result. However, as the definition of a "positive" test result is changed from 2 mm of ST-segment depression to 1 mm of ST-segment depression, the resulting increase in apparent sensitivity will be at the expense of a decreased specificity because patients who have between 1 and 2 mm of ST-segment depression and who do not have coronary artery disease now will be misclassified.

In an era of cost consciousness, the physician often must be asked to decide between two tests that may offer similar types of information. For example, a radionuclide ventriculogram may provide a more accurate assessment of the left ventricular ejection fraction than a two-dimensional echocardiogram, but the latter frequently provides a sufficiently accurate estimate of left ventricular function to obviate the need for the more expensive radionuclide study.

The choice of tests also may depend on the timing of clinical events. For example, a technetium pyrophosphate scan can diagnose a transmural myocardial infarction (p. 315) accurately, but it is unnecessary to order such a test in patients who arrive early enough after the onset of symptoms for enzymes such as creatine kinase isoenzymes to be diagnostic. Technetium pyrophosphate scans can potentially be helpful in patients who arrive long enough after the onset of symptoms so that creatine kinase levels would have returned to normal, but even in such patients, lactic dehydrogenase (LDH) isoenzyme levels appear to be at least as accurate and far less expensive.[23,24]

Thus technetium pyrophosphate scans usually are helpful diagnostically only in patients who arrive long enough after the acute event for creatine kinase isoenzymes to be unhelpful and who have other conditions, such as hemolysis or renal infarction, that make LDH isoenzyme tests unreliable.

INTEGRATING THE TEST RESULT WITH CLINICAL DATA. To use diagnostic tests efficiently, the physician should decide the threshold probability above or below which the future diagnostic or management strategy would be altered.[25,26] For example, consider that a patient has recurrent chest pain, and on the basis of history and physical examination, the physician estimates that there is a 50 per cent probability that it is caused by coronary artery disease. The physician also knows that coronary arteriography would be required to decide whether coronary artery bypass grafting or percutaneous transluminal coronary angioplasty should be carried out if coronary artery disease were present. For cost-effective test ordering, the physician then must estimate how unlikely coronary artery disease would have to be for this

TABLE 54-2 HOW THE POSITIVE AND NEGATIVE PREDICTIVE VALUES OF THE SAME TEST VARY DEPENDING ON THE PRIOR PROBABILITY OF DISEASE

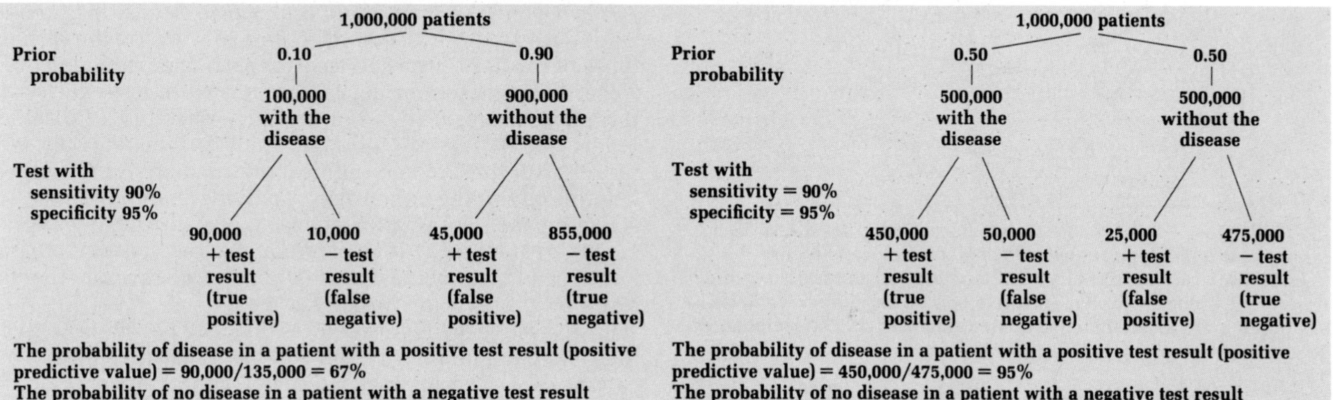

INTERPRETATION OF THE TEST RESULT WHEN 10% OF THE PATIENTS BEING TESTED HAVE THE DISEASE (PRIOR PROBABILITY = 10%)	INTERPRETATION OF THE TEST RESULT WHEN 50% OF THE PATIENTS BEING TESTED HAVE THE DISEASE (PRIOR PROBABILITY = 50%)
1,000,000 patients	1,000,000 patients
Prior probability: 0.10 → 100,000 with the disease; 0.90 → 900,000 without the disease	Prior probability: 0.50 → 500,000 with the disease; 0.50 → 500,000 without the disease
Test with sensitivity 90% specificity 95%	Test with sensitivity = 90% specificity = 95%
90,000 + test result (true positive); 10,000 − test result (false negative); 45,000 + test result (false positive); 855,000 − test result (true negative)	450,000 + test result (true positive); 50,000 − test result (false negative); 25,000 + test result (false positive); 475,000 − test result (true negative)
The probability of disease in a patient with a positive test result (positive predictive value) = 90,000/135,000 = 67%	The probability of disease in a patient with a positive test result (positive predictive value) = 450,000/475,000 = 95%
The probability of no disease in a patient with a negative test result (negative predictive value) = 855,000/865,000 = 99%	The probability of no disease in a patient with a negative test result (negative predictive value) = 475,000/525,000 = 90%

From Goldman, L.: Quantitative aspects of clinical reasoning. *In* Wilson, J. D., et al. (eds.): Harrison's Principles of Internal Medicine 12th ed. New York, McGraw-Hill Book Company, 1991, p. 7.

strategy to be altered. If the physician would proceed with catheterization provided that the probability of coronary artery disease were as low as 10 per cent (or higher), then a test such as an exercise radionuclide ventriculogram, whose negative result might reduce the probability of coronary artery disease to 30 per cent, would not be helpful in decision-making.

Threshold Approach. This concept has been called the "threshold approach" to test utilization and decision-making.[26] In essence, it emphasizes that a test is potentially helpful only if its result would change the pretest probability of disease to a degree that could be sufficient to alter the approach to the patient. If it is highly unlikely that the available diagnostic test could move the probability of disease across such a threshold, the test would not be cost-effective and ordinarily would not be ordered. In some situations, the diagnostic threshold may be redefined because of the special characteristics of the patient at hand. For example, it would be considered important to rule out significant coronary artery disease in an otherwise healthy airline pilot who has atypical chest pain. In this situation, the combination of a normal exercise electrocardiogram and a normal exercise thallium scintiscan would make the presence of coronary disease unlikely. If it were argued that the airline pilot's occupational responsibilities would require even a greater degree of certainty, it would be preferable to proceed directly to the test that usually is considered the benchmark, in this case, coronary arteriography, if it were necessary to be as certain as possible that coronary disease was not present.

BAYES' THEOREM (see also p. 169). One way to understand the concepts of prior probability, thresholds, and the impact of diagnostic tests is through Bayes' theorem.[1,11] When the prior probability (prevalence) of the disease is known in patients who are similar to the patient under consideration, and when the sensitivity and specificity of the test to be ordered are known, the post-test probability that the disease is present can be calculated (Table 54-2). Table 54-2 emphasizes how the physician must consider both the prior (pretest) probability that the patient has a disease and the test result in estimating the post-test probability. For example, if a test has a sensitivity of 90 per cent and a specificity of 95 per cent, a patient whose prior probability of disease was 10 per cent and who has a positive test result would have a 67 per cent probability of disease after the test. By comparison, the same test result in a patient whose prior probability was 50 per cent would yield a post-test probability of 95 per cent.

A test is potentially useful if it changes the probability of disease sufficiently to cross the threshold for decision-making. Unfortunately, available data do not always provide precise guidelines for establishing such appropriate thresholds for diagnostic decision-making. Nevertheless, common clinical judgment is often a sufficient guide. For example, using pooled data from the literature, the effects of exercise electrocardiography and exercise thallium testing can be estimated for a patient with typical angina pectoris (Fig. 54-2), a patient with atypical angina (Fig. 54-3), and a patient with presumably nonanginal chest pain (Fig. 54-4). These estimated probabilities correspond well to the actual probability of disease in patients who have been evaluated.[27]

NONINVASIVE TESTING IN PATIENTS WITH POSSIBLE ANGINA PECTORIS (see also p. 1298). The patient with symptoms typical for angina pectoris already has a high probability of coronary artery disease on the basis of the history alone (80 to 85 per cent); the probability becomes even higher (95 per cent) if the exercise electrocardiogram is positive and becomes overwhelming (99 per cent) after a confirmatory exercise thallium scan. For diagnosing the presence or absence of coronary disease, however, the exercise thallium scan adds little to the results of the exercise test. Although the exercise thallium test may have some additional prognostic value,[28,29] in most situations, the results of the exercise thallium test would be unlikely to add substantial independent

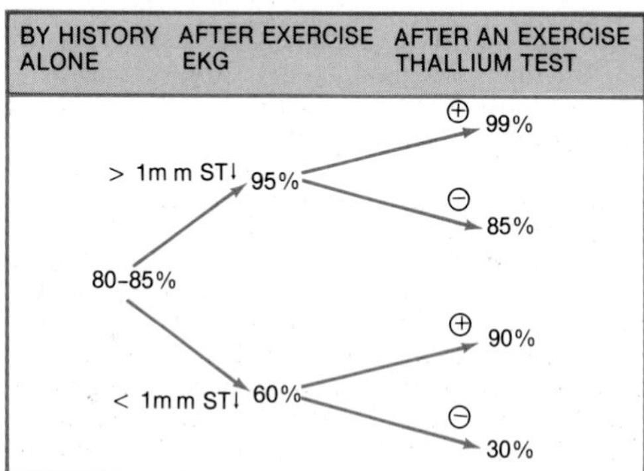

FIGURE 54-2. Approximate probabilities of coronary artery disease in a patient with typical angina pectoris before and after the sequential use of an exercise electrocardiogram and an exercise thallium test. (From Goldman, L.: Non-invasive tests in cardiology. *In* Branch, W., Jr. [ed.]: The Office Practice of Medicine. 2nd ed. Philadelphia, W. B. Saunders Company, 1987.)

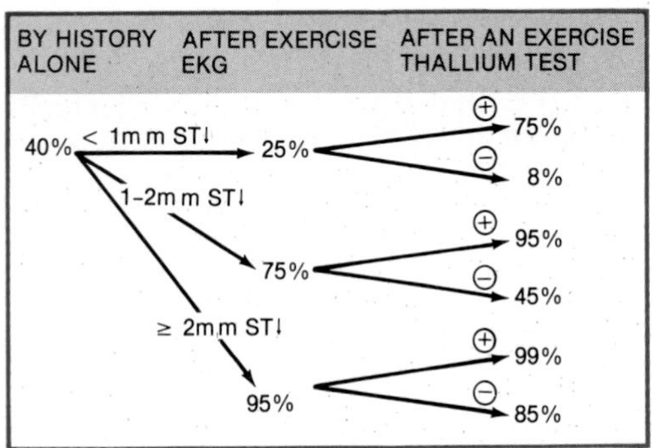

FIGURE 54-3. Approximate probabilities of coronary artery disease in a patient with atypical anginal symptoms before and after the sequential use of an exercise electrocardiogram and an exercise thallium test. (From Goldman, L.: Non-invasive tests in cardiology. *In* Branch, W., Jr. [ed.]: The Office Practice of Medicine. 2nd ed. Philadelphia, W. B. Saunders Company, 1987.)

information regarding the diagnosis of the presence of coronary artery disease. If the exercise electrocardiogram and exercise thallium test give conflicting information, the probability of coronary artery disease in the patient with typical angina pectoris remains similar to what it was before either test was obtained (80 to 90 per cent). If both tests are negative, the patient with typical angina pectoris still has a reasonable probability of having significant coronary artery disease (30 per cent). Thus even two negative tests have not "ruled out" coronary artery disease in a patient with typical angina to an extent to which one could simply reassure the patient, even though they imply a favorable prognosis if coronary artery disease should be present.[28,29] Thus, if one were trying to rule out coronary artery disease in a patient with typical angina pectoris, coronary arteriography still would be required.[12,30]

In the patient with atypical angina (Fig. 54-3), positive results on both exercise electrocardiography and exercise thallium testing would raise the probability of coronary artery disease from 40 to 95 to 99 per cent. Conversely, negative results on both tests would lower the probability of coronary artery disease substantially (to 8 per cent), perhaps to a low enough level that one would not feel compelled to obtain coronary arteriography except in unusual circumstances. If the two tests give conflicting results, the probability of the disease has not been altered appreciably by the two tests.

In asymptomatic healthy people, a resting electrocardiogram appears to have little value as a screening test.[3] Similarly, screening exercise tests have too small a yield to justify their use in healthy people.[32] If, however, an asymptomatic subject who is in the age range in which coronary disease usually occurs has a strongly positive exercise electrocardiogram, the probability of coronary disease is increased substantially (from about 5 to about 50 per cent), and a subsequent negative exercise thallium test is not sufficiently reassuring to eliminate the possibility of coronary disease. Thus one cannot simply use the negative exercise thallium scan to "prove" that the exercise electrocardiogram was a false-positive result.

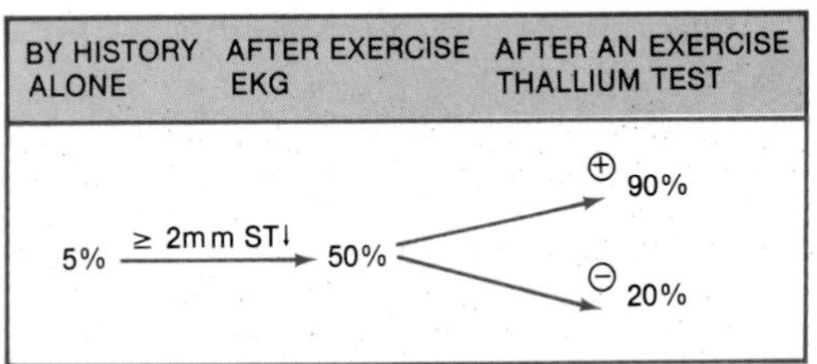

FIGURE 54-4. Approximate probabilities of coronary artery disease in an asymptomatic subject in the coronary artery disease age range before and after the sequential use of an exercise electrocardiogram and an exercise thallium test. (From Goldman, L.: Non-invasive tests in cardiology. *In* Branch, W., Jr. [ed.]: The Office Practice of Medicine. 2nd ed. Philadelphia, W. B. Saunders Company, 1987.)

Coronary arteriography will be required to determine whether the exercise electrocardiogram was a true or false-positive result, and this frequent need to proceed to invasive testing greatly increases the cost of any program that uses screening exercise electrocardiography.

It is beyond the scope of this chapter to discuss the precise guidelines for the most cost-effective use of each of the various types of cardiac diagnostic tests for each possible indication. Nevertheless, test ordering will become more cost-effective if the physician estimates the pretest probability of disease, orders the appropriate test, and properly integrates the test results with the available clinical information. A test will be helpful only to the extent that it provides nonredundant information (i.e., information above and beyond what was previously available).[11,33] It must be emphasized, however, that a test can add incremental information regardless of whether its result is "positive" or "negative."[34]

Cost-effective medicine requires that tests be ordered only if their incremental information will have a positive impact on patient care. The finding that major variations in resource utilization often do not correlate with discernible differences in health outcome suggests that many tests do not meet such criteria.[35] Substantial financial savings can be realized by reducing the utilization of low- or moderate-cost tests as well as by reducing the utilization of expensive procedures.[36-38]

PREVENTION AND TREATMENT

The current and projected future costs of heart disease are substantial. The rate of death from coronary heart disease has been declining in the United States since the late 1960's,[39,40] but the increase in the total population and especially its age portends a rise in the total absolute number of cases of coronary heart disease unless there are major declines in risk factors.[41] Furthermore, the high cost of medical care for prevalent cases of coronary heart disease indicates that coronary disease will remain a major cost for the American public.[41,42]

Among the various preventive and therapeutic modalities in cardiology, some have been studied by means of formal cost-effectiveness analysis, whereas others have been studied in a more qualitative manner. In evaluating the cost-effectiveness of any program, it must be compared with a baseline or standard current approach. In the following sections, selected data on the costs and effectiveness of several modalities for the diagnosis, prevention, and treatment of heart disease are considered.

DETECTION AND TREATMENT OF HYPERLIPIDEMIA

(See also Chap. 37)

Substantial data indicate that the serum cholesterol level is significantly correlated with the risk of coronary artery disease (p. 1116), and after controlling for the cholesterol level, the triglyceride level is not an important independent predictor.[43-45] The high-density lipoprotein cholesterol fraction (p. 1128) appears to be even more important than the low-density lipoprotein fraction for prediction.[44] For primary care settings, the most prudent screening technique is to obtain a total serum cholesterol level. If it is elevated, fasting levels of total cholesterol, high-density lipoprotein cholesterol, and triglycerides can be obtained to define risk more precisely and to determine the hyperlipidemia pattern to guide future dietary and perhaps drug therapy (Chap. 37).[46]

The relation between the intake of dietary fats and the serum cholesterol level is well established.[47,48] There is evidence that increased dietary fat intake is correlated with the progression of coronary atherosclerosis and with long-term coronary mortality,[49,50] whereas reduced intake can retard the progression of atherosclerosis.[51-53] The Lipid Research Clinics Coronary Primary Prevention Trial[54,55] demonstrated that treatment with cholestyramine resulted in a 13.4 per cent reduction in the serum cholesterol level in the group randomized to treatment, whereas cholesterol levels declined by only 4.9 per cent in the randomized control group. The risk of coronary heart disease death was 24 per cent lower and the risk of myocardial infarction was 19 per cent lower in the treated group than in the control group, and the reductions in events were almost exactly what would be predicted on the basis of the reductions in serum cholesterol levels and the known association between cholesterol and event rates.[56]

The Helsinki Heart Study, which used gemifibrozil, demonstrated that the risk of coronary heart disease was lowered because of both a reduction in low-density lipoprotein cholesterol and an increase in high-density lipoprotein cholesterol.[57] In patients treated with niacin in the Coronary Drug Project, a benefit also was found.[58]

Because of the high prevalence of an elevated serum cholesterol level, issues relating to screening and to treatment, with either diet or medications, have major public health implications.[59] One analysis indicated that a 10 mg/dl populationwide reduction in serum cholesterol level in men would yield the same benefit that could be realized by identifying and treating all individual men with serum cholesterol levels above 250 mg/dl and lowering them to 250 mg/dl.[60] This analysis suggested that it would be inadvisable to rely just on a cholesterol reduction program targeted to patients with hypercholesterolemia to reduce national coronary heart disease. Community-based programs in North Karelia, Finland, and in California have achieved about a 3 to 4 per cent net reduction in serum cholesterol levels.[61-66] It is not currently possible to assess the cost-effectiveness of such efforts on a broader regional or national scale.

Although cholesterol-reduction programs targeted to patients with hypercholesterolemia are probably not sufficient for addressing a risk factor such as cholesterol, for which the risk of coronary heart disease is graded and continuous,[43] it is more practical to estimate cost-effectiveness of cholesterol reduction in high-risk groups. Berwick et al.[57] estimated that screening and dietary intervention programs for hypercholesterolemia in the pediatric population would cost about $33,000 (in 1990 dollars) for 10-year-old boys and $29,000 for 10-year-old girls per year of life gained. If the screening was limited to children with a known family history, the cost would be about $21,000 for boys and $24,000 for girls per year of life saved, whereas for children without a family history, the figures would be about $39,000 for boys and $31,000 for girls. Thus, in this example, a "targeted" program, which is limited to children who are at higher risk because of a known family history, would be more cost-effective than a nontargeted program.

In an analysis of the use of screening serum cholesterol levels in asymptomatic adults, it was estimated that screening should be performed about every 5 years in low-risk asymptomatic men and more frequently in high-risk asymptomatic men but was optional in women and in the elderly.[68] Various consensus groups have not currently reached agreement with one another about screening and treatment guidelines in asymptomatic adults.[46,69-73]

Analyses of medication therapy have raised serious questions about the affordability of cholesterol-lowering medications, except in some very high risk groups. As calculated by Weinstein and Stason, the cost per year of life gained for cholestyramine among men aged 45 to 50 years with cholesterol levels above 265 mg/dl would be about $180,000 in 1991 dollars, given a 5 per cent per year discount rate.[73]

Another analysis found that cholestyramine had a cost-effectiveness ratio below about $45,000 per year of life saved only in very selected types of patients, such as those with cholesterol levels of 315 mg/dl or higher in whom treatment was begun between ages 35 and 50 and continued through age 55, or people who smoked, were hypertensive, had diabetes, and in whom new treatment was begun between ages 35 and 49 and continued through age 70.[74] Kinosian and Eisenberg reported that colestipol and cholestyramine, even when used in the less expensive bulk form, cost under $50,000 per year of life saved only when used in relatively high-risk, middle-aged males.[75] Other authors have suggested that cholestyramine is even less cost-effective.[76] In another analysis, in which it was assumed that the relative benefits of cholesterol reduction for secondary prevention in patients who already have coronary heart disease were similar to the benefits of cholesterol reduction for primary prevention,[54,55] secondary prevention was very cost-effective or even cost-saving.[77] Primary prevention with lovastatin was relatively cost-effective only in isolated subgroups, such as people between ages 45 and 74 who had two or more additional risk factors (hypertension, cigarette smoking, or obesity) and whose cholesterol levels were markedly elevated, usually above 300 mg/dl.

In summary, the high prevalence of hypercholesterolemia implies that populationwide interventions, such as dietary changes, will be required if there is to be a major reduction in national coronary heart disease rates. Screening and targeted diet therapy are indicated in high-risk pediatric and adult populations. Medications may be cost-effective in high-risk primary prevention situations and are likely to be very cost-effective and perhaps even cost-saving when used for secondary prevention in people who have existing coronary heart disease, assuming that the benefits to be realized by secondary prevention are truly analogous to those that have been reported for primary prevention.[79-82]

DETECTION AND TREATMENT OF HYPERTENSION

(See also Chaps. 28 and 29)

Most epidemiological data emphasize that the systolic blood pressure is an independent significant predictor of coronary heart disease but that the diastolic blood pressure is not (after controlling for the systolic blood pressure).[56] Nevertheless, it has been common practice to define the threshold for treating hypertension on the basis of the diastolic blood pressure, and virtually all treatment trials use definitions that are based on the diastolic blood pressure level.

About 20 per cent of adults in the United States have diastolic blood pressures above 95 mm Hg, and about another 10 per cent have blood pressures of 90 to 94 mm Hg.[83] There is virtually unanimous agreement that treatment of people whose diastolic blood pressure exceeds about 105 mm Hg will reduce mortality, although the main benefit in the Veterans Administration Trials was to prevent death from conditions other than coronary heart disease.[84-86] Of course, by preventing death from strokes, congestive heart failure, and renal failure, the treatment of hypertension permits more people to survive and potentially to develop coronary heart disease.

Numerous trials have evaluated the benefit of drug treatment for mild hypertension.[87] Many medications that are used to treat hypertension may raise the serum cholesterol and glucose concentrations, thereby theoretically offsetting some of their blood pressure–lowering benefits. Data suggest that the modest elevations in serum cholesterol levels and the occasional precipitation of hyperglycemia are outweighed by the predicted benefit obtained by blood pressure reduction, thus supporting the value of antihypertensive therapy.[87,88] Of course, it would be even more desirable to treat hypertension without raising serum cholesterol or blood sugar.

The Australian National Blood Pressure Study[89] demonstrated that treatment of people with diastolic blood pressure of 95 to 109 mm Hg reduced cardiovascular mortality significantly, and the reduction in incidence of coronary heart disease events was similar to what would be predicted, given the reductions in blood pressure levels using projections from the Framingham equations.[88] The Hypertension Detection and Follow-up Program[90-92a] showed a significant 20 per cent reduction in mortality in the stepped-care group. When data from all the randomized trials of the treatment of mild to moderate hypertension are pooled, there appears to be about a 10 per cent reduction in myocardial infarction in the treated

TABLE 54-3 APPROXIMATE COST PER QUALITY-ADJUSTED YEAR OF LIFE GAINED BY SCREENING AND/OR TREATMENT OF HYPERTENSION (1991 DOLLARS) GIVEN EXPECTED COMPLIANCE

Treat if diastolic blood pressure 105 mm Hg or greater	$20,000
Treat if diastolic blood pressure 95-104 mm Hg	$40,200
Screen for hypertension, treat if blood pressure 95 mm Hg or greater	$41,000

See references 95 and 207.

patients.[87] Treatment is predicted to have the greatest absolute benefit in patients with higher blood pressures[88] and in patients with other risk factors for coronary disease. There is uncertainty as to whether diuretic therapy for hypertensive men with resting electrocardiographic abnormalities would actually increase mortality (p. 852).[93,94]

One recent analysis concluded that screening to detect and treat hypertension was relatively cost-effective for men and women of all ages (Table 54-3).[95] The marginal cost per quality-adjusted year of life gained ranged from about $8000 for men aged 60 to about $29,000 for men aged 20. For women, the cost ranged from about $12,000 at age 60 to about $44,000 at age 20. The results of the analysis were affected relatively little when the authors varied many of the assumptions inherent in their analysis, except that the results were dependent on the cost of medication.

Weinstein and Stason used data from the Framingham Heart Study to calculate the cost-effectiveness of the treatment of mild hypertension.[96] They concluded that the reduction in direct medical care costs for stroke and coronary heart disease would offset about 22 per cent of the cost of treating moderate to severe diastolic hypertension (105 mm Hg and above) and about 15 per cent of the cost for treating mild hypertension (95 to 104 mm Hg), an estimate similar to those made by Stokes and Carmichael.[97] These cost-effectiveness estimates also are similar to those of Littenberg et al.,[95] who found that a program that would screen for hypertension and treat if the diastolic blood pressure was 95 mm Hg or greater would cost about $41,000 per quality-adjusted year of life gained. Treatment programs aimed at people with diastolic blood pressures of 105 mm Hg or greater would be more cost-effective: the cost would be only about $20,000 per year of life gained.

Edelson et al. reported that the cost of primary prevention to treat people 35 to 60 years of age with diastolic blood pressures of 95 mm Hg or greater and no known coronary heart disease was about $11,000 per year of life saved for propranolol and about $16,000 for hydrochlorothiazide.[98] Once again, however, cost-effectiveness was dependent on the cost of the medication and the costs per year of life saved were not estimated to be as favorable for the newer, more expensive medications.

Thus several analyses indicate that screening and treating people with hypertension is reasonably cost-effective and is in the range of the inflation-adjusted annual cost of hemodialysis for chronic renal failure.[9,11] Although hypertension detection and treatment is most cost-effective when it is performed by the patients' own physicians as part of routine medical care,[95,99] worksite programs for the detection and treatment of hypertension can more than pay for themselves by reducing direct medical costs and absenteeism.[100]

CIGARETTE SMOKING

Cigarette smoking is an independently significant correlate of the risk of developing coronary heart disease (p. 1146) and also is a major risk factor for several types of cancer. Many of these risks appear to be reversed after smokers stop smoking. Oster et al. used data from the American Cancer Society and from other sources to estimate the increase in life expectancy that could be realized by smoking cessation (Table 54-4).[101,102]

Although it is not possible to design a trial in which patients are randomized to continue smoking or to guarantee smoking cessation, substantial data confirm that discontinuing smoking improves prognosis. For example, in the Multiple-Risk Factor Intervention Trial,[93] the enrollees who discontinued smoking had a 48 per cent reduction in coronary deaths compared with those who continued smoking, and other data confirm that quitters have lower risks than persistent smokers.[103-107]

There are a variety of interventions to reduce smoking. On average, about 5 per cent of smokers will discontinue the habit for 1 year after receiving a physician's advice, although the rate of quitting will be higher in more highly motivated cohorts.[108-112] Nicotine gum or transdermal patches may increase the 1-year likelihood of smoking cessation by 30 to 100 per cent, suggesting that the cost of a physician's advice plus the availability of nicotine gum per year of life saved will range from about $5700 to $9200 in men aged 35 to 69 and from about $9800 to $13,000 in women aged 35 to 69 in 1990 dollars.[101,113-121] Clonidine has been unsuccessful in the primary care setting.[122]

Group counseling can increase rates of quitting.[121,123] Public programs also are effective, with television advertisements against smoking among the most cost-effective.[124,125] Physicians should not be discouraged by the relatively low rate of quitting that occurs immediately after their advice, since this advice is among the most cost-effective of all the interventions and may be a necessary psychological prelude to the patient's response to subsequent interventions.[126]

OBESITY

In long-term follow-up of the Framingham cohort, obesity emerged as an independently significant risk factor for the development of coronary artery disease (p. 1150). Unfortunately, it is extremely difficult for most adults to lose weight and to maintain the weight loss over the long term. Programs in schools or at the worksite commonly can help to achieve weight losses of 2 to 5 kg at costs that are about $10 to $30 per kilogram lost, which would be highly cost-effective.[128,129] Lay organizations such as Weight Watchers also can aid in producing similar losses at similar costs and are clearly cost-effective despite the high attrition rate.[130] More intensive weight-loss programs for motivated people may still be very cost-effective for those people for whom simpler measures are ineffective.[130] Although physicians may become discouraged over the inability of their patients to lose weight, the usual effects of these other programs are not substantially greater than what may be achieved simply by a physician's advice. Furthermore, it often

TABLE 54-4 INCREASE IN LIFE EXPECTANCY DUE TO SMOKING CESSATION, BY SEX AND AGE AT QUITTING

	UNDISCOUNTED INCREASE IN YEARS OF LIFE EXPECTANCY DUE TO SMOKING CESSATION	
AGE AT QUITTING*	Men	Women
35-39	5.08	3.18
40-44	4.60	2.94
45-49	4.00	2.64
50-54	3.32	2.28
55-59	2.60	1.85
60-64	1.90	1.40
65-69	1.32	0.97

* Median age used for purposes of calculation.

Adapted from Oster, G., Huse, D. M., Delea, T. E., and Colditz, G. A.: Cost effectiveness of nicotine gum as an adjunct to the physician's advice against cigarette smoking. JAMA *256*:131, 1986. Copyright 1986, American Medical Association.

is a physician's advice that influences patients to try other interventions that might not be considered if the physician had not identified overweight as a medical problem.

PHYSICAL ACTIVITY

Substantial data indicate that physical activity reduces coronary heart disease and all-cause mortality, partly because of its beneficial effects on other risk factors but apparently partly independently.[131-137] Unfortunately, it has been reported that less than 10 per cent of physicians recommend exercise for their patients.[138] Many patients, however, both want and expect their physicians to make recommendations regarding physical activity,[138] and in one survey, about 25 per cent of active people ascribed their activity in large part to the advice of a physician.[139]

Worksite exercise programs also are potentially cost-effective independent of their possible effect on the development of clinical coronary artery disease. In one study, employees in the experimental exercise program group missed fewer days of work, were more likely to remain employed, and had fewer hospital days and fewer medical claims, thus resulting in substantial health care savings.[140,141] In fact, some employers have decided to pay their employees directly for participating in exercise programs, such as jogging. Unlike antismoking campaigns, media campaigns advocating exercise seem to encourage people to seek out other programs in the community but not to lead to direct changes in behavior by themselves.[139,142] Thus it appears that a physician's encouragement of increased physical activity, especially if combined with direct guidance on how to implement the suggestion, can lead to major changes in health behavior. Although it is difficult to determine the exact degree of effectiveness to be gained for the cost, there are substantial data linking physical activity to other cardiovascular risk factors and apparently independently to cardiovascular and all-cause mortality.[132-137] These data suggest that efforts to increase physical activity have the potential for being highly cost-effective.

Cardiac rehabilitation in patients who have suffered a myocardial infarction (Chap. 39) appears to lower by about 20 per cent the subsequent rates of reinfarction, cardiovascular mortality, and total mortality.[143] These programs improve the functional and symptomatic status of patients, and the exercise programs themselves are associated with a very small risk of major adverse events.[144-146] Such programs also can help patients return to work earlier after uncomplicated myocardial infarction,[147] and, as a result, can both reduce costs of medical care and increase productivity.[148] Thus the combination of cardiac rehabilitation services and occupational work evaluations appears to be very cost-effective for the post–myocardial infarction patient.

PREVENTION OF INFECTIVE ENDOCARDITIS IN VALVULAR HEART DISEASE

(See also p. 1097)

By extrapolation from cost-effectiveness analyses, penicillin prophylaxis to prevent bacterial endocarditis in patients with rheumatic valvular heart disease appears to have a cost-effectiveness of about $13,000 per year of life gained.[149,150] In patients with prosthetic heart valves, in whom the risk of endocarditis is higher, the cost-effectiveness is likely to be even more favorable. By comparison, two detailed cost-effectiveness analyses indicate that penicillin prophylaxis before dental work to prevent bacterial endocarditis is *not* cost-effective for patients with mitral valve prolapse[149,150] (p. 1035). Using the most likely assumptions, people are as likely to die of penicillin reactions as they are to die of endocarditis, and even given the most optimistic assumptions, it is estimated that routine penicillin prophylaxis for dental procedures in patients with mitral valve prolapse would cost more than a million dollars to save a year of life. In most studies of mitral valve prolapse, the risk of endocarditis is substantially higher in patients with murmurs of mitral regurgitation. Although the cost-effectiveness in this subpopulation of patients with mitral valve prolapse is unclear, the use of prophylactic antibiotics in the presence of a murmur of mitral valve prolapse is often recommended.[151,152]

PREHOSPITAL EMERGENCY SERVICES

(See also Chap. 26)

Prehospital emergency services range from basic life support to advanced life support services. Advanced life support programs, which include interventions such as defibrillation, endotracheal intubation, and intravenous or intramuscular medications, have been instituted throughout much of the United States.[153] Because about 60 per cent of patients whose death certificates list the cause of death as myocardial infarction die outside of the hospital, advances in prehospital emergency services, such as better training in the community or dispatcher-assisted instruction, could have a substantial impact on survival.[154]

Prehospital emergency care appears to be extremely successful in patients who have ventricular fibrillation and who are seen very soon after cardiac arrest (p. 773). For example, in pooled data, about two-thirds of patients who are seen within 5 minutes of a ventricular fibrillation arrest survive to leave the hospital.[155] Unfortunately, many arrests are not caused by ventricular fibrillation, and even the most successful prehospital emergency services often cannot deliver care within 5 minutes. Thus only about 15 to 20 per cent of prehospital cardiac arrest patients commonly survive to leave the hospital in even the best programs.[156,157] These higher rates are achieved principally through advanced life support programs utilizing paramedics, which appear to increase the likelihood of reaching the hospital alive from about 19 to 34 per cent and the likelihood of being discharged alive from the hospital from 7 to 17 per cent.[153] However, the prognosis after hospital discharge of patients who were resuscitated from prehospital arrest is only about 75 per cent as high as age- and sex-matched comparison groups who have survived myocardial infarction without prehospital arrest, and it is only about 60 per cent as high as for age- and sex-adjusted members of the general population.[156]

The cost-effectiveness of prehospital emergency programs is difficult to estimate. One analysis estimated that a mobile coronary care unit has an incremental cost of about $25,000 (in 1991 dollars) per life saved above and beyond the cost of the ambulance system itself.[157] Another analysis estimated that the incremental cost-effectiveness of a mobile coronary care unit was about $100,000 (in 1991 dollars) per life saved and $50,000 (in 1991 dollars) per year of life saved, but this analysis included only the incremental costs of the mobile coronary care unit program and not the costs of the existing emergency medical technician and community training program to which it was added.[158]

Analyses of the cost-effectiveness of prehospital emergency services depend on assumptions about the mean response time and the patients' prognoses, both in terms of life expectancy and in terms of quality of life and neurological impairment. For example, the longer the response time, the more likely it is that survivors of prehospital cardiac arrest will have neurological impairment. If the years of life expectancy that are gained are compromised by such neurological impairment, then the *quality* of those years of life will not be the same as the quality of the years of life that might be gained from preventive measures that delay the onset of disease. Thus, when the calculation of cost-effectiveness is adjusted for the years of life that are gained without major neurological impairment, the apparent benefit of prehospital resuscitation may be reduced. Furthermore, patients whose lives are saved by prehospital emergency services are likely to require careful medical follow-up, sometimes including expensive interventions such as coronary bypass grafting. Most studies have not clearly considered the fact that the survivors of out-of-hospital cardiac arrest will have costs other than those included in the first term of the equation in Table 54–1, such as the costs for rehabilitative and custodial care and the costs for additional diagnosis and therapy of the substantial coronary disease that may have precipitated the arrest. If these costs are taken into account, the relative cost-effectiveness of prehospital emergency services programs would be less appealing than the preceding estimates.

CORONARY CARE UNITS

(See also Chap. 39)

Coronary care units were originally designed to provide the ready availability of resuscitative services to patients with obvious acute myocardial infarction (p. 1223). The mission of these units subsequently has been substantially broadened: patients are now admitted to rule out a myocardial infarction if there is a reasonable suspicion that one may have occurred. The interventions in these units now include prevention of arrhythmias, medical and surgical treatment of acute ischemia, treatment of severe pump failure, and procedures designed to prevent or to limit the size of the acute myocardial infarction. It is difficult, if not impossible, to disentangle each of these potential aspects of coronary care units.

HOME CARE VS. CORONARY CARE. Two trials in Great Britain showed no significant difference in the survival of patients who were admitted to coronary care units compared with randomized controls who were treated at home.[159,160] These studies were too small, however, to detect the expected difference in mortality.[161] Furthermore, patients were eligible for randomization only after prolonged home observation, during which time high-risk patients were excluded and a substantial proportion of patients were actually resuscitated. Thus these studies do not appear to apply to unselected patients coming to American hospitals. In fact, available data suggest that patients who are mistakenly discharged from the emergency room appear to have a significantly higher mortality with their acute myocardial infarctions than patients who are correctly admitted.[162]

REDUCTION OF MORTALITY IN THE CCU. If one assumes that the risk of primary ventricular fibrillation in an acute myocardial infarction is about 4.5 per cent and that the likelihood of successful resuscitation and hospital survival is about 88 per cent in coronary care units, the availability of defibrillation and resuscitation would result in about a 4-percentage-point decline in the in-hospital mortality from acute myocardial infarction compared with the pre–coronary care unit era when defibrillation could not be carried out promptly on a regular nursing unit.[163] Data from the Minnesota area document a positive effect of about this magnitude.[164]

Between the initial development of defibrillation and resuscitation and the subsequent advent of thrombolysis, a variety of intensive care interventions such as intra-aortic balloon counterpulsation, intravenous afterload reduction, and intravenous inotropic agents were used in the care of patients with acute myocardial infarction. Although these interventions certainly saved individual lives, their precise impact on overall mortality rates is less certain.[165,166]

More recently intravenous thrombolysis has been shown to have a statistically significant and clinically important impact on mortality in patients with acute myocardial infarction (p. 1230).[167–172] Depending on the criteria for eligibility for thrombolysis, as few as 15 per cent of patients with acute myocardial infarctions may receive such therapy.[173] The use of prehospital thrombolysis, as well as interventions to speed the access to thrombolysis, could greatly increase the impact of thrombolytic therapy.[174]

Although thrombolytic therapy in the management of acute myocardial infarction has been rapidly adopted,[175] there is still not a broad consensus about which thrombolytic agent is best[176] or about the role of adjunctive aspirin and heparin.[177] The role of subsequent percutaneous transluminal coronary angioplasty also is evolving, with emerging evidence that a conservative strategy of reserving angioplasty for patients with specific clinical indications is as efficacious as routine angioplasty.[178]

Issues related to the choice of thrombolytic agent and the use of angioplasty are critical to the determination of the cost-effectiveness of reperfusion therapy. The cost of thrombolysis per 1-year survivor was estimated to range from about $35,000 for a large myocardial infarction to $200,000 for a moderate-sized myocardial infarction, and $800,000 for a small myocardial infarction when intravenous thrombolysis was followed by catheterization only when the patient was symptomatic or had a positive exercise tolerance test.[179] The cost *per year of life saved* is uncertain, since long-term survival data are still emerging. Another cost-effectiveness analysis also emphasized the importance of the costs of medications and of the additional procedures that are generated in patients who receive thrombolytic therapy.[180]

Another important group to consider are patients who are admitted to the coronary care unit for suspected or "rule-out" myocardial infarction. Coronary care unit admission can be applied selectively only to patients whose probability of myocardial infarction is sufficiently high for it to be cost-effective.[4] Thus, if the probability of myocardial infarction is only 5 per cent, the incremental cost per year of life saved by admission to the coronary care unit compared with an intermediate care unit is about $260,000 (in 1991 dollars); and the cost will fall to about $60,000 (in 1991 dollars) per year of life saved if the potential for acute myocardial infarction is 20 per cent. These estimates suggest that it may be worthwhile for physicians to estimate the probability of acute myocardial infarction from clinical data or from more sophisticated calculations.[17,18] One study indicates that the intermediate-care option, which would be analogous to many "stepdown" units in which electrocardiographic monitoring and resuscitative facilities are available but in which patients do not receive intensive care nursing, is safe for patients who are admitted to rule out a myocardial infarction and in whom this diagnosis is confirmed.[181]

LENGTH OF STAY. The coronary care unit also can be made more cost-effective by limiting the length of stay. Data indicate that, except in patients who have recurrent ischemic pain, 24 hours is nearly always sufficient to determine whether or not a myocardial infarction has occurred.[182] Similar protocols using the electrocardiogram, the history, and serum enzyme levels substantiate that 24 hours is often a sufficient length of stay.[183] If coronary care units were used in this more cost-effective manner, the relative cost-effectiveness for patients with symptoms indicative of but not diagnostic of an acute myocardial infarction would be improved, since the original calculations noted above assumed a longer average length of stay.

When faced with a shortage of coronary care unit beds, physicians can identify correctly which patients are most in need.[184] It is likely that coronary care units can become substantially more cost-effective by limiting admission to patients whose probability of acute myocardial infarction is at about 20 per cent or higher or in whom serious complications are more likely and by shortening the average length of stay for patients who do not have documented myocardial infarctions or complications. Intermediate care (or "stepdown") unit admission appears to be quite cost-effective and safe for patients whose probability of acute myocardial infarction is too high for discharge to be appropriate but not high enough for coronary care unit admission to be worthwhile.

MEDICAL THERAPY OF CORONARY ARTERY DISEASE

(See also Chap. 40)

Although the natural history of patients with medically treated coronary artery disease appears to be improving, it is difficult to measure the impact of specific aspects of the medical treatment. The best-studied intervention is the use of "prophylactic" beta-adrenoceptor antagonists in survivors of a recent myocardial infarction. Numerous studies have shown a substantial benefit from routine use of beta-adrenoceptor antagonists in patients who are ready for discharge after an acute myocardial infarction (p. 1265).[185–189] Several studies indicate that the relative reduction in mortality in years 2 and 3 is similar to the 25 to 30 per cent reduction found in year 1.[185,186,189,191–194] In the fourth, fifth, and sixth years, the benefit appears to be smaller, closer to 8 to 9 per cent.[195] Based on the costs of the medications, and the likely benefits in patients with various risks of short- and long-term complications, cost-effectiveness analysis indicates that the cost of beta-adrenoceptor antagonist therapy to save 1 year of life is about $4700 (in 1991 dollars) in patients at high risk for complications, about $7400 for medium-risk patients, and about $27,000 for low-risk patients. Altering the patients' age from 45 to 65 years had little effect on the analysis. These calculations suggest that beta-adrenoceptor antagonist therapy in the post–myocardial infarction patient is extremely cost-effective in high- and medium-risk patients and is still rather cost-effective even in low-risk patients.[196] It is not possible, as of this writing, to make analogous calculations in patients with angina who have not recently survived a myocardial infarction.

CORONARY ARTERY BYPASS GRAFTING

(See also p. 1320)

Coronary artery bypass grafting prolongs the life of patients with left main coronary artery disease and of patients with three-vessel disease and left ventricular dysfunction.[197–199] Data on patients with less severe degrees of disease are conflicting, with the European trial being the only major randomized study that showed a significant advantage for surgery among patients with two-vessel disease that included the left anterior descending artery.[200,201] The benefit of operation diminishes after about 7 years,[201] presumably because of late graft failure, which appears to be less common with internal mammary grafts than with vein grafts.[202]

In patients with marked symptoms, coronary artery bypass grafting is efficacious in improving symptomatic status. Several studies, however, indicate that coronary artery bypass grafting does not, in general, improve work status[203–205] even though it improves quality of life.[203,206] Weinstein and Stason estimated that the net cost of coronary bypass grafting is about $25,000 to $29,000 (in 1991 dollars).[207] Data also indicate that the initial investment in coronary artery bypass surgery is not offset by lower subsequent treatment costs.[208] The costs vary, depending on postoperative length of stay, which appears to be partly related to predetermined protocol and largely related to postoperative complications.[209,210] Interestingly, professional fees for coronary bypass grafting have not fallen, even as the procedure has become quicker and more routine.[211]

Weinstein and Stason also have performed the most extensive cost-effectiveness analysis of coronary artery bypass grafting in patients with various symptomatic states and extents of disease (Table 54–5).[207] These calculations suggest that in patients with three-vessel disease or left main coronary artery disease, or in patients with two-vessel disease and severe angina, the cost per year of life gained from coronary bypass grafting compares favorably with the cost per year of life gained from renal dialysis in patients with chronic renal failure. It also has been estimated that coronary bypass grafting compares favorably with valve replacement for aortic stenosis and implantation of a pacemaker for heart block in terms of its cost-effectiveness, and that it is more cost-effective than heart transplantation or the treatment of end-stage renal failure and is probably somewhat less cost-effective than hip replacement for disabling arthritis.[212] Of course, patient selection is paramount to maximizing cost-effectiveness, and sometimes a second opinion is helpful in this regard.[213]

TABLE 54–5 ESTIMATED APPROXIMATE COST PER GAIN IN ONE QUALITY-ADJUSTED YEAR OF LIFE FOR CORONARY ARTERY BYPASS GRAFTING (SEE REFERENCE 207; CALCULATIONS ARE UPDATED TO 1991 DOLLARS)

	ONE-VESSEL DISEASE	TWO-VESSEL DISEASE	THREE-VESSEL DISEASE	LEFT MAIN DISEASE
Very mild angina	*	86,000	14,000	6300
Mild angina	850,000	55,000	13,500	6600
Severe angina	55,000	32,000	13,000	7000

* Quality-adjusted life expectancy is reduced.

PERCUTANEOUS TRANSLUMINAL CORONARY ANGIOPLASTY

(See also Chap. 41)

The initial charges for percutaneous transluminal coronary angioplasty (PTCA) have been reported to be about 60 per cent as high as for coronary artery bypass grafting,[214–216] but this estimate included the substantial cost of the availability of standby surgery.[217] The true costs of a treatment strategy, including PTCA, must consider the immediate failure rate, the possible need for urgent coronary artery bypass grafting, and the likelihood of restenosis and its subsequent treatment. If the PTCA can be performed at a time of day when an operating suite and team normally would be "between cases," without causing them to be idle during a period when they would otherwise be in full use, the actual cost of the availability of standby surgery would be minimal and angioplasty becomes more cost-effective.

Even given the full costs of surgical standby, the expenditures for patients undergoing PTCA were significantly lower at 1 year than those of patients treated with coronary artery bypass grafting.[214] Because this study reported a 30 per cent immediate failure rate and a 22 per cent restenosis rate at 1 year, the cost-effectiveness of PTCA is even better now that immediate success rates usually are higher.

SUMMARY

The gratifying reduction in mortality from ischemic heart disease usually is regarded as testimony to the effectiveness of a variety of primary and secondary preventive and therapeutic measures.[218–220] It will be necessary, however, for current and future interventions to be carefully analyzed, so that the benefit of medical care to reduce cardiovascular morbidity and mortality can be maximized within the constraints of the resources that will be available.

Physicians should not view the current emphasis on cost-effective care as contradictory to excellent care. Patients should not be treated as numbers, and optimal medical care cannot be routinely derived from equations. The physician's principal responsibility is to render the best possible medical care to the patient as an individual. An understanding of the principles of cost-effectiveness should allow the physician to improve the choice of diagnostic and therapeutic strategies, and it should assist the physician's ability to determine strategies that are optimal in the aggregate and to adopt or adapt them for the person at hand. In such a context, more cost-effective care implies better care for the individual patient as well as the conservation of resources to improve care for the population as a whole.

REFERENCES

QUANTITATIVE ANALYSES OF COSTS AND EFFECTIVENESS

1. Weinstein, M. C., and Fineberg, H. V.: Clinical Decision Analysis. Philadelphia, W. B. Saunders Company, 1980.
2. Weinstein, M. C., and Stason, W. B.: Foundations of cost-effectiveness analysis for health and medical practices. N. Engl. J. Med. *296*:716, 1977.
3. Sox, H. C., Blatt, M. A., Higgins, M. C., and Marton, K. I.: Cost-effectiveness analysis and cost-benefit analysis. Med. Decis. Making *317*: 1988.
4. Fineberg, H., Scadden, D., and Goldman, L.: Management of patients with a low probability of acute myocardial infarction: Cost-effectiveness of alternatives to coronary care unit admission. N. Engl. J. Med. *310*:1301, 1984.
5. Kwoh, C. K., Beck, J. R., and Pauker, S. G.: Repeated syncope with negative diagnostic evaluation. To pace or not to pace? Med. Decis. Making *4*:351, 1984.
6. Doubilet, P., Weinstein, M. D., and McNeil, B. J.: Use and misuse of the term "cost effective" in medicine (Editorial). N. Engl. J. Med. *314*:253, 1986.
7. Eisenberg, J. M.: Clinical economics: A guide to the economic analysis of clinical practices. JAMA *262*:2879, 1989.
8. Drummond, M., Stoddart, G., LaBelle, R., and Cushman, R.: Health economics: An introduction for clinicians. Ann. Intern. Med. *107*:88, 1987.
9. Roberts, S. D., Maxwell, D. R., and Gross, T. L.: Cost-effective care of end-stage renal disease: A billion-dollar question. Ann. Intern. Med. *92*:243, 1980.
10. Goldman, L. Cost-awareness in medicine. *In* Wilson, J. D., et al. (eds.): Harrison's Principles of Internal Medicine. 12th ed. New York, McGraw-Hill Book Co. 1991, p. 11.

DIAGNOSTIC TESTING

11. Goldman, L.: Quantitative aspects of clinical reasoning. *In* Wilson, J. D., et al. (eds.): Harrison's Principles of Internal Medicine. 12th ed. New York, McGraw-Hill Book Co., 1991, pp. 5–11.
12. Goldman, L.: Noninvasive tests in cardiology. *In* Branch, W., Jr. (ed.): The Office Practice of Medicine. 2nd ed. Philadelphia, W. B. Saunders Company, 1987, p 55.
13. Rifkin, R. D., and Hood, W. B.: Bayesian analysis of electrocardiographic exercise stress testing. N. Engl. J. Med. *297*:681, 1977.
14. Diamond, G. A., Staniloff, H. M., Forrester, J. S., et al.: Computer-assisted diagnosis in the noninvasive evaluation of patients with suspected coronary artery disease. J. Am. Coll. Cardiol. *1*:444, 1983.
15. Goldman, L., Cook, E. F., Mitchell, N., et al.: Incremental value of the exercise test for diagnosing the presence or absence of coronary artery disease. Circulation *66*:945, 1982.
16. Weiner, D. A., Ryan, T. J., McCabe, C. H., et al.: Exercise stress testing: Correlations among history of angina, ST-segment response and prevalence of coronary-artery disease in the coronary artery surgery study (CASS). N. Engl. J. Med. *300*:230, 1979.
17. Hoagland, P. M., Cook, E. F., Wynne, J., and Goldman, L.: Value of noninvasive testing in adults with suspected aortic stenosis. Am. J. Med. *80*:1041, 1986.
18. Goldman, L., Cook, E. F., Brand, D. A., et al.: A computer protocol to predict myocardial infarction in emergency department patients with chest pain. N. Engl. J. Med. *318*:797, 1988.
19. Goldman, L., Feinstein, A. R., Batsford, W. P., et al.: Ordering patterns and clinical impact of cardiovascular nuclear medicine procedures. Circulation *62*:680, 1980.
20. Goldman, L., Cohn, P. F., Mudge, G. H. Jr. et al.: Clinical utility and management impact of M-mode echocadiography. Am. J. Med. *75*:49, 1983.
21. Sox, H. C., Margulies, I., and Sox, C. H.: Psychologically mediated effects of diagnostic tests. Ann. Intern. Med. *95*:680, 1981.
22. McNeil, B. J., Keeler, E., and Adelstein, S. J.: Primer on certain elements of medical decision-making. N. Engl. J. Med. *293*:211, 1975.
23. Lee, T. H., and Goldman, L.: Serum enzyme assays in the diagnosis of acute myocardial infarction. Recommendations based on a quantitative analysis. Ann. Intern. Med. *105*:221, 1986.
24. Vasudevan, G., Mercer, D. W., and Varat, M. A.: Lactic dehydrogenase isoenzyme determination in the diagnosis of acute myocardial infarction. Circulation *57*:1055, 1978.
25. Pauker, S. G., and Kassirer, J. P.: Therapeutic decision-making: A cost-benefit analysis. N. Engl. J. Med. *293*:229, 1975.
26. Pauker, S. G., and Kassirer, J. P.: The threshold approach to clinical decision-making. N. Engl. J. Med. *302*:1109, 1980.
27. Weintraub, W. S., Madeira, S. W., Bodenheimer, M. M., et al.: Critical analysis of the application of Bayes' theorem to sequential testing in the noninvasive diagnosis of coronary artery disease. Am. J. Cardiol. *54*:43, 1984.
28. Pamelia, F. X., Gibson, R. S., Watson, D. D., et al.: Prognosis with chest pain and normal thallium-201 exercise scintigrams. Am. J. Cardiol. *55*:920, 1985.
29. Gordon, D. J., Ekelund, L., Karon, J. M., et al.: Predictive value of the exercise tolerance test for mortality in North American men: The Lipid Research Clinics Mortality Follow-up Study. Circulation *74*:252, 1986.
30. Patterson, R. E., Eng, C., Horowitz, S. F., et al.: Bayesian comparison of cost-effectiveness of different clinical approaches to diagnose coronary artery disease. J. Am Coll. Cardiol. *4*:278, 1984.
31. Sox, H. C., Garber, A. M., and Littenberg, B.: The resting electrocardiogram as a screening test: A clinical analysis. Ann. Intern. Med. *111*:489, 1989.
32. Sox, H. C., Littenberg, B., and Garber, A. M.: The role of exercise testing in screening for coronary artery disease. Ann. Intern. Med. *110*:456, 1989.
33. Harrell, F. E., Califf, R. M., Pryor, D. B., et al.: Evaluating the yield of medical tests. JAMA *247*:2543, 1982.
34. Gorry, G. A., Pauker, S. G., and Schwartz, W. B.: The diagnostic importance of the normal finding. N. Engl. J. Med. *298*:486, 1978.
35. Wennberg, J. E., Freeman, J. L., and Culp, W. J.: Are hospital services rationed in New Haven or over-utilised in Boston? Lancet *1*:1185, 1987.
36. Fineberg, H. V., and Hiatt, H. H.: Evaluation of medical practices. The case for technology assessment. N. Engl. J. Med. *301*:1086, 1979.
37. Moloney, T. W., and Rogers, D. E.: Medical technology—a different view of the contentious debate over costs. N. Engl. J. Med. *301*:1413, 1979.
38. Griner, P. F., and the Medical House Staff, Strong Memorial Hospital, Rochester, New York: Use of laboratory tests in a teaching hospital: Long-term trends. Reductions in use and relative cost. Ann. Intern. Med. *90*:243, 1979.

PREVENTION AND TREATMENT

39. Goldman, L., and Cook, E. F.: The decline in ischemic heart disease mortality rates: An analysis of the comparative effects of medical interventions and changes in lifestyle. Ann. Intern. Med. *101*:825, 1984.
40. Sempos, C., Cooper, R., Kovar, M. G., and McMillen, M.: Divergence of the recent trends in coronary mortality for the four major race-sex groups in the United States. Am. J. Public Health *78*:1422, 1988.
41. Weinstein, M. C., Coxson, P. G., Williams, L. W., et al.: Forecasting coronary heart disease incidence, mortality, and cost: The coronary heart disease policy model. Am. J. Public Health *77*:1417, 1987.
42. Wittels, E. H., Hay, J. W., and Gotto, A. M.: Medical costs of coronary artery disease in the United States. Am. J. Cardiol. *65*:432, 1990.
43. Stamler, J., Wentworth, D., and Neaton, J. D.: Is relationship between serum cholesterol and risk of premature death from coronary heart disease continuous and graded? Findings in 356,222 primary screenees of the Multiple-Risk Factor Intervention Trial (MRFIT). JAMA *256*:2823, 1986.
44. Kannel, W. B., Castelli, W. P., and Gordon, T.: Cholesterol in the prediction of atherosclerotic disease. New perspectives based on the Framingham Study. Ann. Intern. Med. *90*:85, 1979.
45. NIH Consensus Conference: The treatment of hypertriglyceridemia. JAMA *251*:1196, 1984.
46. Expert Panel: Report of the national cholesterol education program. Expert panel on detection, evaluation, and treatment of high blood cholesterol in adults. Arch. Intern. Med. *148*:36, 1988.
47. Keys, A., Anderson, J. T., and Grande, F.: Serum cholesterol response to changes in diet. IV. Particular saturated fatty acids in the diet. Metabolism *14*:776, 1965.
48. Hegsted, D. M., McGandy, R. B., Myers, M. L., and Stare, F. J.: Quantitative effects of dietary fat on serum cholesterol in man. Am. J. Clin. Nutr. *17*:281, 1965.
49. Arntzenius, A. C., Kromhout, D., Barth, J. D., et al.: Diet, lipoproteins, and the progression of coronary atherosclerosis. The Leiden Intervention Trial. N. Engl. J. Med. *312*:805, 1985.
50. Kushi, L. H., Lew, R. A., Stare, F. J., et al.: Diet and 20-year mortality from coronary heart disease. The Ireland-Boston Diet-Heart Study. N. Engl. J. Med. *312*:811, 1985.
51. Blankenhorn, D. H., Alaupovic, P., Wickham, E., et al.: Prediction of angiographic change in native human coronary arteries and aortocoronary bypass grafts: Lipid and non-lipid factors. Circulation *81*:470, 1990.
52. Blankenhorn, D. H., Johnson, R. L., Mack, W. J., et al.: The influence of diet on the appearance of new lesions in human coronary arteries. JAMA *263*:1646, 1990.
53. Blankenhorn, D. H., Nessim, S. A., Johnson, R. L., et al.: Beneficial effects of combined colestipol niacin therapy in coronary atherosclerosis and coronary venous bypass grafts. JAMA *257*:3233, 1987.
54. The Lipid Research Clinics Program: The Lipid Research Clinics Coronary Primary Prevention Trial results. I. Reduction in incidence of coronary heart disease. JAMA *251*:351, 1984.
55. The Lipid Research Clinics Program: The Lipid Research Clinics Coronary Primary Prevention Trial results. II. The relationship of reduction in incidence of coronary heart disease to cholesterol lowering. JAMA *251*:365, 1984.
56. Kannel, W. B., and Gordon, T. (eds.): The Framingham Study: An Epidemiologic Investigation of Cardiovascular Disease. Sections 1–32. Washington, D.C., U.S. Government Printing Office, 1970–1977.
57. Frick, M. H., Elo, O., Haapa, K., et al.: Helsinki Heart Study: Primary-prevention trial with gemfibrozil in middle-aged men with dyslipidemia. N. Engl. J. Med. *317*:1237, 1987.
58. Canner, P. L., Berge, K. G., Wenger, N. K., et al.: Fifteen year mortality in coronary drug project patients; long-term benefits with niacin. J. Am. Coll. Cardiol. *8*:1245, 1986.
59. Sempos, C., Fulwood, R., Haines, C., et al.: The prevalence of high blood cholesterol levels among adults in the United States. JAMA *262*:45, 1989.
60. Goldman, L., Weinstein, M. C., and Williams, L. W.: Relative impact of targeted versus populationwide cholesterol interventions on the incidence of coronary heart disease. Circulation *80*:254, 1989.
61. Pusko, P., Tuomilehto, J., Salonen, J., et al.: Changes in coronary risk

factors during comprehensive five-year community programme to control cardiovascular diseases (North Karelia project). Br. Med. J. *2*:1173, 1979.
62. Puska, P., Salonen, J. T., Nissinen, A., et al.: Change in risk factors for coronary heart disease during 10 years of a community intervention programme (North Karelia project). Br. Med. J. *287*:1840, 1983.
63. Puska, P., Neittaanmaki, L., and Tuomilehto, J.: A survey of local health personnel and decision makers concerning the North Karelia project: A community program for control of cardiovascular diseases. Prev. Med. *10*:564, 1981.
64. Salonen, J. T., Heinonen, O. P., Kottke, T. E., and Puska, P.: Change in health behaviour in relation to estimated coronary heart disease risk during a community-based cardiovascular disease prevention programme. Int. J. Epidemiol. *10*:343, 1981.
65. Salonen, J. T., Puska, P., Kottke, T. E., et al.: Decline in mortality from coronary heart disease in Finland from 1969 to 1979. Br. Med. J. *286*:1857, 1983.
66. Fortmann, S. P., Williams, P. T., Hulley, S. B., et al.: Effect of health education on dietary behavior: The Stanford Three Community Study. Am. J. Clin. Nutr. *34*:2030, 1981.
67. Berwick, D. M., Cretin, S., and Keeler, E.: Cholesterol, Children, and Heart Disease: An Analysis of Alternatives. New York, Oxford University Press, 1980.
68. Garber, A. M., Sox, H. C., and Littenberg, B.: Screening asymptomatic adults for cardiac risk factors: The serum cholesterol level. Ann. Intern. Med. *110*:622, 1989.
69. Basinski, A., Frank, J. W., Naylor, C. D., and Rachlis, M. M.: Detection and Management of Asymptomatic Hypercholesterolemia. A Policy Document by the Toronto Working Group on Cholesterol Policy. Toronto, Ontario Ministry of Health, 1989.
70. The British Cardiac Society Working Group on Coronary Heart Disease Prevention. Lancet *1*:377, 1987.
71. Study Group, European Atherosclerosis Society: Strategies for the prevention of coronary heart disease: A policy statement of the European Atherosclerosis Society. Eur. Heart J. *8*:77, 1987.
72. Assmann, G.: At what levels of total low- or high-density lipoprotein cholesterol should diet/drug therapy be initiated? European guidelines. Am. J. Cardiol. *65*:11F, 1990.
73. Weinstein, M. C., and Stason, W. B.: Cost-effectiveness of interventions to prevent or treat coronary heart disease. Ann. Rev. Public Health *6*:41, 1985.
74. Oster, G., and Epstein, A. M.: Cost-effectiveness of antihyperlipemic therapy in the prevention of coronary heart disease: The case of cholestyramine. JAMA *248*:2381, 1987.
75. Kinosian, B. P., and Eisenberg, J. M.: Cutting into cholesterol: Cost-effective alternatives for treating hypercholesterolemia. JAMA *259*:2249, 1988.
76. Himmelstein, D., and Woolhandler, S.: Free care, cholestyramine, and health policy. N. Engl. J. Med. *311*:1511, 1984.
77. Goldman, L. G., Edelson, J. T., Tosteson, A. A., et al.: Projected cost-effectiveness of lovastatin for cholesterol reduction. Clin. Res. *36*:337A, 1988.
78. Research Committee to the Medical Research Council: Controlled trial of soya-bean oil in myocardial infarction. Lancet *2*:693, 1968.
79. Leren, P.: The Oslo Diet Heart Study: Eleven-year report. Circulation *42*:35, 1970.
80. Group of Physicians of the Newcastle-Upon-Tyne Region: Trial of clofibrate in the treatment of ischaemic heart disease. Br. Med. J. *4*:767, 1971.
81. Coronary Drug Project Group: Clofibrate and niacin in coronary heart disease. JAMA *231*:360, 1975.
82. Research Committee of the Scottish Society of Physicians: Ischaemic heart disease: A secondary prevention trial using clofibrate. Br. Med. J. *4*:775, 1971.
83. National Center for Health Statistics, U.S. Public Health Service: National Health and Nutrition Examination Survey 1976–1980. Public Use Data Tape. Hyattsville, MD, U.S. Department of Health and Human Services, 1982.
84. Veterans Administration Cooperative Study Group on Antihypertensive Agents: Effects of treatment on morbidity in hypertension. Part 1. JAMA *202*:1028, 1967.
85. Veterans Administration Cooperative Study Group on Antihypertensive Agents: Effects of treatment on morbidity in hypertension. Part 2. JAMA *213*:1143, 1970.
86. Veterans Administration Cooperative Study Group on Antihypertensive Agents: Effects of treatment on morbidity in hypertension. Part 3. Circulation *45*:991, 1972.
87. Hebert, P. R., Fiebach, N. H., Eberlein, K. A., et al.: The community based randomized trials of pharmacologic treatment of mild-to-moderate hypertension. Am. J. Epidemiol. *127*:581, 1988.
88. Shea, S., Cook, E. F., Kannel, W. B., and Goldman, L.: Treatment of hypertension and its effect on cardiovascular risk factors: Data from the Framingham Heart Study. Circulation *71*:22, 1985.
89. Australian National Blood Pressure Management Committee: The Australian therapeutic trial in mild hypertension. Lancet *1*:1261, 1980
90. Hypertension Detection and Follow-up Program Cooperative Group: Five-year findings of the Hypertension Detection and Follow-up Program: I. Reduction in mortality of persons with high blood pressure, including mild hypertension. JAMA *242*:2562, 1979.
91. Hypertension Detection and Follow-up Program Cooperative Group: Five-year findings of the Hypertension Detection and Follow-up Program: III. Reduction in stroke incidence among persons with high blood pressure. JAMA *247*:633, 1982.
92. Hypertension Detection and Follow-up Program Cooperative Group: The effect of treatment on mortality in "mild" hypertension: Results of the Hypertension Detection and Follow-up Program. N. Engl. J. Med. *307*:976, 1982.
92a. Hypertension Detection and Follow-up Program Cooperative Group: Effect of stepped care treatment on the incidence of myocardial infarction and angina pectoris: Five-year findings of the Hypertension Detection and Follow-up Program. Hypertension *6* (Suppl I):198, 1984.
93. Multiple-Risk Factor Intervention Trial Research Group: Multiple-Risk Factor Intervention Trial: Risk factor changes and mortality results. JAMA *248*:1465, 1982.
94. The Hypertension Detection and Follow-up Program Cooperative Research Group: The effect of antihypertensive drug treatment on mortality in the presence of resting electrocardiographic abnormalities at baseline: The HDFP experience. Circulation *70*:996, 1984.
95. Littenberg, B., Garber, A. M., and Sox, H. C.: Screening for hypertension. Ann. Intern. Med. *112*:192, 1990.
96. Weinstein, M. C., and Stason, W. B.: Hypertension: A Policy Perspective. Cambridge, Mass., Harvard University Press, 1976.
97. Stokes, J., III, and Carmichael, D. C.: A Cost-Benefit Analysis of Model Hypertension Control. Bethesda, National Heart, Lung and Blood Institute, 1975.
98. Edelson, J. T., Weinstein, M. C., Tosteson, A. N. A., et al.: Long-term cost-effectiveness of various initial monotherapies for mild to moderate hypertension. JAMA *263*:408, 1990.
99. Three-Community Hypertension Control Program. V. Cost-effectiveness of intervention. Mayo Clin. Proc. *56*:11, 1981.
100. Hannan, E. L., and Graham, J. K.: A cost-benefit study of hypertension screening and treatment program at the work setting. Inquiry *15*:345, 1978.
101. Oster, G., Huse, D. M., Delea, T. E., and Colditz, G. A.: Cost effectiveness of nicotine gum as an adjunct to physician's advice against cigarette smoking. JAMA *256*:1315, 1986.
102. Doll, R., and Peto, R.: Mortality in relation to smoking: Twenty years observation of male British doctors. Br. Med. J. *2*:1525, 1976.
103. Friedman, G. D., Petitti, D. B., Bawol, R. D., and Siegelaub, A. B.: Mortality in cigarette smokers and quitters. Effect of base-line differences. N. Engl. J. Med. *304*:1407, 1981.
104. Rosenberg, L., Kaufman, D. W., Helmrich, S. P., and Shapiro, S.: The risk of myocardial infarction after quitting smoking in men under 55 years of age. N. Engl. J. Med. *313*:1511, 1985.
105. Vietstra, R. E., Kronmal, R. A., Oberman, A., et al.: Effect of cigarette smoking on survival of patients with angiographically documented coronary artery disease. JAMA *255*:1023, 1986.
106. Hermanson, B., Omenn, G. S., Kronmal, R. A., and Gersh, B. J.: Beneficial six-year outcome of smoking cessation in older men and women with coronary artery disease. N. Engl. J. Med. *319*:1365, 1988.
107. Rosenberg, L., Palmer, J. R., and Shapiro, S.: Decline in the risk of myocardial infarctions among women who stop smoking. N. Engl. J. Med. *322*:213, 1990.
108. Russell, M. A., Wilson, C., Taylor, C., and Baker, C. D.: Effect of practitioners' advice against smoking. Br. Med. J. *2*:231, 1979.
109. Jamrozik, K., Vessey, M., Fowler, G., et al.: Controlled trial of three different antismoking interventions in general practice. Br. Med. J. *288*:1499, 1984.
110. Stewart, P. J., and Rosser, W. W.: The impact of routine advice on smoking cessation from family physicians. Can. Med. Assoc. J. *126*:1051, 1982.
111. Cohen, S. J., Stookey, G. K., Katz, B. P., et al.: Encouraging primary care physicians to help smokers quit. Ann. Intern. Med. *110*:648, 1989.
112. Cummings, S. T., Coates, T. J., Richard, R. J., et al.: Training physicians in counseling and smoking cessation: A randomized trial of the "Quit for Life" program. Ann. Intern. Med. *110*:640, 1989.
113. Hjalmarson, A. L.: Effect of nicotine chewing gum in smoking cessation. A randomized, placebo-controlled, double-blind study. JAMA *252*: 2835, 1984.
114. Jarvik, M. E., and Schneider, N. G.: Degree of addiction and effectiveness of nicotine gum therapy for smoking. Am. J. Psychiatry *141*:790, 1984.
115. Schneider, N. G., Jarvik, M. E., Forsythe, A. B., et al.: Nicotine gum in smoking cessation: A placebo-controlled, double-blind trial. Addict. Behav. *8*:253, 1983.
116. British Thoracic Society: Comparison of four methods of smoking withdrawal in patients with smoking-related diseases. Br. Med. J. *286*:595, 1983.
117. Hughes, J. R., Gust, S. W., Keenan, R. M., et al.: Nicotine vs placebo gum in general medical practice. JAMA *261*:1300, 1989.
118. Hajek, P., Jackson, P., and Belcher, M.: Long-term use of nicotine chewing gum: Occurrence, determinants, and effect on weight gain. JAMA *260*:1593, 1988.
119. Fortmann, S. P., Killen, J. D., Telch, M. J., and Newman, B.: Minimal contact treatment for smoking cessation. A placebo controlled trial of nicotine polacrilex and self-directed relapse prevention: Initial results of the Stanford Stop Smoking Project. JAMA *260*:1575, 1988.
120. Abelin, T., Muller, P., Buehler, A., et al.: Controlled trial of transdermal nicotine patch in tobacco withdrawal. Lancet *1*:7, 1989.
121. Tonnesen, P., Fryd, V., Hansen, M., et al.: Effect of nicotine chewing gum in combination with group counseling on the cessation of smoking. N. Engl. J. Med. *318*:15, 1988.
122. Franks, P., Harp, J., and Bell, B.: Randomized, controlled trial of clonidine for smoking cessation in a primary care setting. JAMA *262*:3011, 1989.

123. Lando, H. A., McGovern, P. G., Barrios, F. X., and Etringer, B. D.: Comparative evaluation of American Cancer Society and American Lung Association smoking cessation clinics. Am. J. Public Health *80*:554, 1990.
124. Danaher, B. G., Berkanovic, E., and Gerger, B.: Mass media–based health behavior change: Televised smoking cessation program. Addict. Behav. *9*:245, 1984.
125. Pierce, J. P., Macaskill, P., and Hill, D.: Long-term effectiveness of mass media led antismoking campaigns in Australia. Am. J. Public Health *80*:565, 1990.
126. Health and Public Policy Committee, American College of Physicians: Methods for stopping cigarette smoking. Ann. Intern. Med. *105*:281, 1986.
127. Hubert, H. B., Feinleib, M., McNamara, P. M., and Castelli, W. P.: Obesity as an independent risk factor for cardiovascular disease: A 26-year follow-up of participants in the Framingham Heart Study. Circulation *67*:968, 1983.
128. Brownell, K. D., and Kaye, F. S.: A school-based behavior modification, nutrition, education, and physical activity program for obese children. Am. J. Clin. Nutr. *35*:277, 1982.
129. Brownell, K. D., Stunkard, A. J., and McKeon, P. E.: Weight reduction at the worksite: A promise partially fulfilled. Am. J. Psychiatry *142*:47, 1985.
130. Stunkard, A. J.: The current status of treatment for obesity in adults. *In* Stunkard, A. J., and Stellar, E. (eds.): Eating and Its Disorders. New York, Raven Press, 1984.
131. Gibbons, L. W., Blair, S. N., Cooper, K. H., and Smith, M.: Association between coronary heart disease risk factors and physical fitness in healthy adult women. Circulation *67*:977, 1983.
132. Brand, R. J., Paffenbarger, R. S. Jr., Sholtz, R. I., and Kampert, J. B.: Work activity and fatal heart attacks studied by multiple logistic risk analysis. Am. J. Epidemiol. *110*:52, 1979.
133. Paffenbarger, R. S., Hyde, R. T., Wing, A. L., and Hsieh, C. C.: Physical activity, all-cause mortality, and longevity of college alumni. N. Engl. J. Med. *314*:605, 1986.
134. Blair, S. N., Kohl, H. W., Paffenbarger, R. S., et al.: Physical fitness and all-cause mortality: A prospective study of healthy men and women. JAMA *262*:2395, 1989.
135. Leon, A. S., Connett, J., Jacobs, D. R., and Rauramaa, R.: Leisure-time physical activity levels and risk of coronary heart disease and death. The multiple risk factor intervention trial. JAMA *258*:2388, 1987.
136. Slattery, M. L., Jacobs, D. R., and Nichaman, M. Z.: Leisure time physical activity and coronary heart disease death. The US Railroad Study. Circulation *79*:304, 1989.
137. Ekelund, L. G., Haskell, W. L., Johnson, J. L., et al.: Physical fitness as a predictor of cardiovascular mortality in asymptomatic North American men. N. Engl. J. Med. *310*:1379, 1988.
138. Iverson, D. C., Fielding, J. E., Crow, R. S., and Christenson, G. M.: The promotion of physical activity in the United States population: The status of programs in medical, worksite, community, and school settings. Public Health Reports *100*:212, 1985.
139. Gilmore, A.: Canada fitness survey finds fitness means health. Can. Med. Assoc. J. *129*:181, 1983.
140. Cox, M., Shepard, R. J., and Corey, P.: Influence of an employee fitness programme upon fitness, productivity, and absenteeism. Ergonomics *24*:795, 1981.
141. Shepard, R. J., Corey, P., Renzland, P., and Cox, M.: The influence of an employee fitness and lifestyle modification upon medical care costs. Can. J. Public Health *73*:259, 1982.
142. Oldridge, N. B.: Adherence to adult exercise fitness programs. *In* Matarazzo, J. D., Miller, N. E., Herd, J. A., and Weiss, S. M. (eds.): Behavioral Health: A Handbook of Health Enhancement and Disease Prevention. New York, John Wiley and Sons, 1984, pp. 467–487.
143. O'Connor, G. T., Buring, J. E., Yusuf, S., et al.: An overview of randomized trials of rehabilitation with exercise after myocardial infarction. Circulation *80*:234, 1989.
144. AMA-Council on Scientific Affairs. Physician-supervised exercise programs in rehabilitation of patients with coronary heart disease. JAMA *245*:1463, 1981.
145. Greenland, P., and Chu, J. S.: Efficacy of cardiac rehabilitation services. With emphasis on patients after myocardial infarction. Ann. Intern. Med. *109*:650, 1988.
146. U.S. Department of Health and Human Services: Health Technology Assessment Reports, 1987. Cardiac Rehabilitation Services DHHS Publication No. (PHS) 88-3427. Rockville, Md.: National Center for Health Services Research and Health Care Technology Assessment.
147. Dennis, C. A., Houston-Miller, N., Schwartz, R. G., et al.: Early return to work after uncomplicated myocardial infarction: Results of a randomized trial. JAMA *260*:214, 1988.
148. Picard, M. H., Dennis, C., Schwartz, R. G., et al.: Cost-benefit analysis of early return to work after uncomplicated acute myocardial infarction. Am. J. Cardiol. *63*:1308, 1989.
149. Bor, D. H., and Himmelstein, D. U.: Endocarditis prophylaxis for patients with mitral valve prolapse. A quantitative analysis. Am. J. Med. *76*:711, 1984.
150. Clemens, J. D., and Ransohoff, D. F.: A quantitative assessment of predental antibiotic prophylaxis for patients with mitral valve prolapse. J. Chron. Dis. *37*:531, 1984.
151. Clemens, J. D., Horwitz, R. I., Jaffe, C. C., et al.: A controlled evaluation of the risk of bacterial endocarditis in persons with mitral valve prolapse. N. Engl. J. Med. *307*:776, 1982.
152. Mills, P., Rose, J., Hollingsworth, J., et al.: Long-term prognosis of mitral valve prolapse. N. Engl. J. Med. *297*:13, 1977.
153. Eisenberg, M. S., Bergner, L., and Hallstrom, A.: Out-of-hospital cardiac arrest: Improved survival with paramedic services. Lancet *1*:812, 1980.
154. Kellerman, A. L., Hackman, H. B., and Somes, G.: Dispatcher-assisted cardiopulmonary resuscitation—validation of efficacy. Circulation *80*:1231, 1989.
155. Crampton, R. S., Aldrich, R. F., Gascho, J. A., et al.: Reduction of prehospital, ambulance, and community coronary death rates by the community-wide emergency cardiac care system. Am. J. Med. *58*:151, 1975.
156. Eisenberg, M. S., Hallstrom, A., and Bergner, L.: Long-term survival after out-of-hospital arrest. N. Engl. J. Med. *306*:1340, 1982.
157. Cummins, R. O., and Eisenberg, M. S.: Prehospital cardiopulmonary resuscitation: Is it effective? JAMA *253*:2408, 1985.
158. Urban, N., Bergner, L., and Eisenberg, M. S.: The costs of a suburban paramedic program in reducing deaths due to cardiac arrest. Med. Care *19*:379, 1981.
159. Hill, J. D., Hampton, J. R., and Mitchell, J. R. A.: A randomized trial of home-versus-hospital management for patients with suspected myocardial infarction. Lancet *1*:837, 1978.
160. Mather, H. G., Morgan, D. C., Pearson, N. G., et al.: Myocardial infarction: A comparison between home and hospital care for patients. Br. Med. J. *1*:925, 1976.
161. Goldman, L.: Coronary care units: A perspective on their epidemiologic impact. Int. J. Cardiol. *2*:284, 1982.
162. Lee, T. H., Rouan, G., Weisberg, M. C., et al: Clinical characteristics and natural history of patients with acute myocardial infarction sent home from the emergency room. Am. J. Cardiol. *60*:219, 1987.
163. Goldman, L., and Batsford, W. P.: Risk-benefit stratification as a guide to lidocaine prophylaxis of primary ventricular fibrillation in acute myocardial infarction: An analytic review. Yale J. Biol. Med. *52*:455, 1979.
164. Gillum, R. F., Folsom, A., Leupker, R. V., et al.: Sudden death and acute myocardial infarction in a metropolitan area, 1970-1980: The Minnesota Heart Survey. N. Engl. J. Med. *309*:1353, 1983.
165. Goldman, L., Cook, F., Hashimoto, B., et al.: Evidence that hospital care for acute myocardial infarction has not contributed to the decline in coronary mortality between 1973–1974 and 1978–1979. Circulation *65*:936, 1982.
166. Pell, S., and Fayerweather, M. P. H.: Trends in the incidence of myocardial infarction and in associated mortality and morbidity in a large employed population, 1957–1983. N. Engl. J. Med. *312*:1005, 1985.
167. Kennedy, J. W., Martin, G. V., Davis, K. B., et al.: The Western Washington intravenous streptokinase in acute myocardial infarction randomized trial. Circulation *77*:345, 1988.
168. ISIS-2 (Second International Study of Infarct Survival) Collaborative Group: Randomised trial of intravenous streptokinase, oral aspirin, both, or neither among 17,187 cases of suspected acute myocardial infarction: ISIS-2. Lancet *2*:349, 1988.
169. AIMS Trial Study Group: Long-term effects of intravenous anistreplase in acute myocardial infarction: Final report of the AIMS study. Lancet *1*:427, 1990.
170. Mauri, F., Gasparini, M., Barbonaglia, L., et al.: Prognostic significance of the extent of myocardial injury in acute myocardial infarction treated by streptokinase (the GISSI Trial). Am. J. Cardiol. *63*:1291, 1989.
171. Dalen, J. E., Gore, J. M., Braunwald, E., et al.: Six- and twelve-month follow-up of the phase I thrombolysis in myocardial infarction (TIMI) trial. Am. J. Cardiol. *62*:179, 1988.
172. White, H. D., Rivers, J. T., Maslowski, A. H., et al.: Effect of intravenous streptokinase as compared with that of tissue plasminogen activator on left ventricular function after first myocardial infarction. N. Engl. J. Med. *320*:817, 1989.
173. Lee, T. H., Weisberg, M. C., Brand, D. A., et al.: Candidates for thrombolysis among emergency room patients with acute chest pain. Ann. Intern. Med. *110*:957, 1989.
174. Maynard, C., Althouse, R., Olsufka, M., et al.: Early versus late hospital arrival for acute myocardial infarction in the western Washington thrombolytic therapy trials. Am. J. Cardiol. *63*:1296, 1989.
175. Hlatky, M. A., Cotugno, H., O'Connor, C., et al.: Adoption of thrombolytic therapy in the management of acute myocardial infarction. Am. J. Cardiol. *61*:510, 1988.
176. Collen, D.: Coronary thrombolysis: Streptokinase or recombinant tissue-type plasminogen activator? Ann. Intern. Med. *112*:529, 1990.
177. Braunwald, E.: Thrombolytic reperfusion of acute myocardial infarction: Resolved and unresolved issues. J. Am. Coll. Cardiol. *12*:85A, 1988.
178. The TIMI Study Group: Comparison of invasive and conservative strategies after treatment with intravenous tissue plasminogen activator in acute myocardial infarction: Results of the Thrombolysis in Myocardial Infarction (TIMI) Phase II Trial. N. Engl. J. Med. *320*:618, 1989.
179. Laffel, G. L., Fineberg, H. V., and Braunwald, E.: A cost-effectiveness model for coronary thrombolysis/reperfusion therapy. J. Am. Coll. Cardiol. *10*:79B, 1987.
180. Steinberg, E. P., Topol, E. J., Sakin, J. W., et al.: Cost and procedure implications of thrombolytic therapy for acute myocardial infarction. J. Am. Coll. Cardiol. *23*:58A, 1988.
181. Feibach, N. H., Cook, E. F., Lee, T. H., et al.: Outcomes in patients with myocardial infarction who are initially admitted to stepdown units: Data from the Multicenter Chest Pain Study. Am. J. Med. *89*:15, 1990.
182. Lee, T. H., Rouan, G. W., Weisberg, M. C., et al.: Sensitivity of routine clinical criteria for diagnosing myocardial infarction within 24 hours of hospitalization. Ann. Intern. Med. *106*:181, 1987.

183. Mulley, A. G., Thibault, G. E., Hughes, R. A., et al.: The course of patients with suspected myocardial infarction: The identification of low-risk patients for early transfer from intensive care. N. Engl. J. Med. *302*:943, 1980.
184. Singer, D. E., Carr, P. L., Mulley, A. G., and Thibault, G. E.: Rationing intensive care—physician responses to a resource shortage. N. Engl. J. Med. *309*:1155, 1983.
185. Beta-Blocker Heart Attack Trial Research Group: A randomized trial of propranolol in patients with acute myocardial infarction. I. Mortality results. J.A.M.A. *247*:1707, 1982.
186. Norwegian Multicenter Study Group: Timolol-induced reduction in mortality and reinfarction in patients surviving acute myocardial infarction. N. Engl. J. Med. *304*:801, 1981.
187. Hansteen, V., Moinichen, E., Lorensten, E., et al.: One year's treatment with propranolol after myocardial infarction: Preliminary report of Norwegian Multicentre Trial. Br. Med. J. *284*:155, 1982.
188. Multicentre International Study: Improvement in prognosis of myocardial infarction by long-term beta-adrenoreceptor blockade using practolol. Br. Med. J. *3*:735, 1975.
189. Multicentre International Study: Reduction in mortality after myocardial infarction with long-term beta-adrenoceptor blockade. Br. Med. J. *2*:419, 1977.
190. Yusuf, S., Peto, R., Lewis, J., et al.: Beta blockade during and after myocardial infarction: An overview of the randomized trials. Prog. Cardiovasc. Dis. *27*:335, 1985.
191. Alhmark, G., and Saetre, H.: Long-term treatment with beta blockers after myocardial infarction. Eur. J. Clin. Pharmacol. *10*:77, 1976.
192. Australian and Swedish Pindolol Study Group: The effect of pindolol on the two years mortality after complicated myocardial infarction. Eur. Heart J. *4*:367, 1983.
193. Rehnqvist, N., and Olsson, G.: Influence on ventricular arrhythmias by chronic postinfarction treatment with metoprolol. Circulation *68*:III-369, 1983.
194. Wilhelmsson, C., Vedin, J. A., Wilhelmsen, L., et al.: Reduction of sudden deaths after myocardial infarction by treatment with alprenolol. Preliminary results. Lancet *2*:1157, 1974.
195. Pedersen, T. R., and the Norwegian Multicenter Study Group: Six-year follow-up of the Norwegian Multicenter Study on timolol after acute myocardial infarction. N. Engl. J. Med. *313*:1055, 1985.
196. Goldman, L., Sia, S.T.B., Cook, E. F., et al.: Cost-effectiveness of routine long-term beta-adrenergic antagonist therapy following acute myocardial infarction. N. Engl. J. Med. *319*:152, 1988.
197. Takaro, T., Hultgren, H. N., Lipton, M. J., et al.: The VA cooperative randomized study of surgery for coronary arterial occlusive disease. II. Subgroup with significant left main lesions. Circulation *54*(Suppl. III):107, 1976.
198. The Veterans Administration Coronary Artery Bypass Surgery Cooperative Study Group: Eleven-year survival in the Veterans Administration randomized trial of coronary artery bypass surgery for stable angina. N. Engl. J. Med. *311*:1333, 1984.
199. Passamani, E., Davis, K. B., Gillispie, M. J., et al.: A randomized trial of coronary artery bypass surgery. Survival of patients with a low ejection fraction. N. Engl. J. Med. *312*:1665, 1985.
200. European Coronary Surgery Study Group: Prospective randomized study of coronary artery bypass surgery in stable angina pectoris: A progress report on survival. Circulation *65*(Suppl. II):67, 1982.
201. Varnauskas, E., and the European Coronary Surgery Study Group: Twelve-year follow-up of survival in the randomized European coronary surgery study. N. Engl. J. Med. *319*:332, 1988.
202. Cameron, A., Kemp, H. G., and Green, G. E.: Bypass surgery with the internal mammary artery graft: 15 year follow-up. Circulation *74*(Suppl. III):30, 1986.
203. CASS Principal Investigators and their Associates: A randomized trial of coronary artery bypass surgery: Quality of life in patients randomly assigned to treatment groups. Circulation *68*:951, 1983.
204. Charles, E. C., Wayne, J. B., Oberman, A., et al.: Costs and benefits associated with treatment for coronary artery disease. Circulation *66*(Suppl. III):87, 1982.
205. Varnauskas, E., and the European Coronary Surgery Study Group: Survival, myocardial infarction, and employment status in a prospective randomized study of coronary bypass surgery. Circulation *72*(Suppl. V):90, 1985.
206. Kornfeld, D. S., Heller, S. S., Frank, K. A., et al.: Psychological and behavioral responses after coronary artery bypass surgery. Circulation *66*(Suppl. III):24, 1982.
207. Weinstein, M. C., and Stason, W. B.: Cost-effectiveness of coronary artery bypass surgery. Circulation *66*(Suppl. III):56, 1982.
208. Hemenway, D., Sherman, H., Mudge, G. H. Jr., et al.: Comparative costs versus symptomatic and employment benefits of medical versus surgical treatment of stable angina pectoris. Med. Care *23*:133, 1985.
209. Weintraub, W. S., Jones, E. L., Craver, J., et al.: Determinants of prolonged length of hospital stay after coronary bypass surgery. Circulation *80*:276, 1989.
210. Taylor, G. J., Mikell, F. L., Moses, H. W., et al.: Determinants of hospital charges for coronary artery bypass surgery: The economic consequences of postoperative complications. Am. J. Cardiol. *65*:309, 1990.
211. Cromwell, J., Mitchell, J. B., and Stason, W. B.: Learning by doing in CABG surgery. Med. Care *28*:6, 1990.
212. Williams, A.: Economics of coronary artery bypass grafting. Br. Med. J. *291*:326, 1985.
213. Graboys, T. B., Headley, A., Lown, B., et al.: Results of a second opinion program for coronary artery bypass graft surgery. JAMA *258*:1611, 1987.
214. Reeder, G. S., Krishan, I., Nobrega, F. T., et al.: Is percutaneous coronary angioplasty less expensive than bypass surgery? N. Engl. J. Med. *311*:1157, 1984.
215. Jang, G. C., Block, P. C., Cowley, M. J., et al.: Relative cost of coronary angioplasty and bypass surgery in a one-vessel disease model. Am. J. Cardiol. *53*:52C, 1984.
216. Kelly, M. E., Taylor, G. J., Moses, H. W., et al.: Comparative cost of myocardial revascularization: Percutaneous transluminal angioplasty and coronary artery bypass surgery. J. Am. Coll. Cardiol. *5*:16, 1985.
217. Wilson, J. M., Dunn, E. J., Wright, C. B., et al.: The cost of simultaneous surgical standby for percutaneous transluminal coronary angioplasty. J. Thorac. Cardiovasc. Surg. *91*:362, 1986.
218. Goldman, L., and Cook, E. F.: The decline in ischemic heart disease mortality rates. An analysis of the comparative effects of medical interventions and changes in lifestyle. Ann. Intern. Med. *101*:825, 1984.
219. Sytkowski, P. A., Kannel, W. B., and D'Agostino, R. B.: Changes in risk factors and the decline in mortality from cardiovascular disease: The Framingham Heart Study. N. Engl. J. Med. *322*:1635, 1990.
220. Cohn, B. A., Kaplan, G. A., and Cohen, R. D.: Did early detection and treatment contribute to the decline in ischemic heart disease mortality? Prospective evidence from the Alameda County Study. Am. J. Epidemiol. *127*:1143, 1988.
221. Kaplan, G. A., Cohen, B. A., Cohen, R. D., and Guralnik, J.: The decline in ischemic heart disease mortality: Prospective evidence from the Alameda County Study. Am. J. Epidemiol. *127*:1131, 1988.

PART V

HEART DISEASE AND DISORDERS OF OTHER ORGAN SYSTEMS

55

General Anesthesia and Noncardiac Surgery in Patients With Heart Disease

by LEE GOLDMAN, M.D., and EUGENE BRAUNWALD, M.D.

The cardiovascular system of patients undergoing general anesthesia and noncardiac surgical procedures is subject to multiple stresses owing to depression of myocardial contractility and respiration as well as fluctuations in temperature, arterial pressure, ventricular filling pressures, blood volume, and activity of the autonomic nervous system. Complications of anesthesia and operation, such as hemorrhage, infection, fever, pulmonary embolism, and myocardial infarction, impose additional burdens on the cardiovascular system. The patient with cardiac disease who is compensated preoperatively may be unable to meet these increased demands during the perioperative period, in which case arrhythmias, myocardial ischemia, and/or heart failure may develop.[1,2] As a consequence, a substantial proportion of all deaths in most series of noncardiac operations results from cardiovascular complications.

Because both the frequency and the seriousness of cardiovascular complications of general anesthesia and operation are considerably increased in the patient with known cardiovascular disease, the magnitude of these risks must be appreciated to decide on the advisability of noncardiac surgery in the cardiac patient. In addition, both the life expectancy and the quality of life of the patient must be taken into account. For instance, a noncardiac surgical procedure with a high risk, directed to correct a disorder which is not life threatening, may be difficult to justify if the patient's cardiac condition precludes a survival period sufficient to allow the patient to reap the benefits of the operation. Obviously the dangers and disability of the disease for which an operation is being proposed must also be balanced against the risk of the operation itself.

ANESTHESIA

Changes in cardiovascular function during general anesthesia are due to many factors, including direct effects of the anesthetic agent(s) and indirect effects mediated primarily through the autonomic nervous system. In addition, if respiration is inadequately maintained, the resulting hypoxemia, hypercarbia, and acidosis may further depress myocardial contractility and increase cardiac irritability. The interplay of these several variables may produce changes in arterial and central venous pressures, cardiac output, and rate and rhythm. To minimize the risk of operation in the patient with a compromised cardiovascular system, it is essential to minimize these changes.[3]

The choice of the anesthetic approach and the specific anesthetic agents to be used should be made by a qualified anesthesiologist, commonly after careful evaluation of the patient's medical and cardiac condition and often after consultation with the surgeon and the internist or cardiologist. Different anesthesiologists may have preferences for different anesthetic techniques, and the anesthesiological literature clearly indicates that there is little, if any, correlation between the anesthetic route or agents and the likelihood of major clinical complications. Thus, it is the skill and experience of the anesthesiologist, including the ability to monitor hemodynamics and respond quickly, that are far more important than the specific agent that is used. While the cardiological consultant should not expect to dictate the anesthetic approach, the quality of the consultation will be improved if the consultant appreciates the clinical pharmacology of the anesthetic agents and the effects of intubation and extubation.

GENERAL ANESTHESIA

The induction of anesthesia is usually accomplished with intravenous anesthetics. With the exception of ketamine, the agents used for the induction of anesthesia commonly lower systemic arterial pressure by about 20 to 30 per cent in healthy patients, but sometimes by a greater amount in hypertensive patients.[4] During laryngoscopy and tracheal intubation, blood pressure commonly increases by 20 to 30 mm Hg, but it may increase even more in the hypertensive patient,[4] in whom these changes in blood pressure may be associated with electrocardiographic evidence of myocardial ischemia.[5,6] Much of this hypertensive response can be avoided by adequate topical anesthesia of the upper airways, larynx, and trachea, or by blind nasal intubation because the hypertension appears to be caused by the laryngoscopy rather than by the passage of a tube into the trachea.

INHALATION AGENTS. These agents enter the bloodstream by way of the alveoli and are excreted across the alveoli essentially unchanged. In most major operations a combination of inhalation agents and/or intravenous anesthetics is used.[3,7]

Nitrous oxide usually causes a modest decrease of about 15 per cent in cardiac output but usually does not cause substantial hypotension because of reflex vasoconstriction (Table 55–1). Unfortunately, in many patients it is impossible to achieve full anesthesia with concentrations of nitrous oxide that also permit adequate oxygenation.

Halothane and related agents also cause a reduction in myocardial contractility,[8] but unlike nitrous oxide, they are not associated with substantial reflex vasoconstriction. Thus, when halothane is added to nitrous oxide, there are often further reductions in arterial pressure because of reductions in cardiac output without concomitant vasoconstriction.[5] Halothane also appears to sensitize the myocardium to catecholamines, sometimes resulting in arrhythmias. *Enflurane* has properties similar to halothane but appears to result in less sensitization to catecholamines. *Isoflurane* appears to have less of a negative inotropic effect than halothane or enflurane, but it can be associated with marked decreases in systemic vascular resistance, and hence a fall in systemic blood pressure.

INTRAVENOUS ANESTHETICS. Among the narcotic analgesics, *morphine* is generally well tolerated, although it does cause venodilation, thereby decreasing preload and cardiac output. *Fentanyl* is less likely to cause as much hypotension or vasodilation as morphine, and it has a shorter duration of action. Like morphine, it tends not to have major effects on myocardial contractility, but it is more likely than morphine to cause bradycardia. *Sufentanil* and *alfentanil* have cardiovascular effects that are generally similar to those of fentanyl.

Short-acting barbiturates, especially *thiopental*, often cause a fall in blood pressure because of depressive actions on myocardial contractility and sympathetic tone. In patients who have severe hypovolemia or severe cardiac dysfunction, serious reductions in cardiac output can occasionally occur after a small dose of thiopental.

Benzodiazepines can achieve adequate sedation with only mild cardiovascular depression. However, occasionally patients may become apneic or hypotensive after small doses. *Droperidol* causes vasodilation because of its alpha-adrenergic blocking action and its effect on the central nervous system.

Ketamine is unlike other commonly used intravenous anesthetics in that it does not cause cardiovascular depression. Although it may cause minimal direct myocardial depressant activity, this is commonly counterbalanced by an increase in circulating catecholamines.

MUSCLE RELAXANTS. Drugs used for muscle relaxation also may have cardiovascular effects. *Succinylcholine* can cause bradycardia, which can be reversed or prevented by the administration of atropine. In patients anesthetized with halothane, *pancuronium* and *gallamine* cause an increase in heart rate, arterial pressure, and cardiac output, while *tubocurarine* and *metocurine* result in a fall in mean arterial pressure with mild elevations in heart rate and little, if any, change in cardiac output. *Vecuronium* has essentially no cardiovascular side effects.

SPINAL AND EPIDURAL ANESTHESIA

Spinal and epidural anesthesia cause sympathetic denervation, which produces peripheral arteriodilation and venodilation. Systemic vascular resistance may be reduced by 10 to 15 per cent. Venodilation may cause a marked reduction in right ventricular preload as a consequence of sympathetic denervation. Under these circumstances, right ventricular preload depends critically on the effects of gravity on the patient's position, and on the total blood volume (Fig. 13–35, p. 378).

REGIONAL AND LOCAL ANESTHESIA. Regional and local anesthesia cause cardiovascular effects only to the extent that the agents are absorbed into the bloodstream or where there is sympathetic blockade accompanying the local sensory block. A major concern with local or regional anesthesia is whether the technique is adequate for the planned procedure; the cardiological consultant should not underestimate the cardiovascular consequences of inadequate anesthesia.

TABLE 55–1 CARDIOVASCULAR CHANGES WITH NITROUS OXIDE AND AFTER ITS ADDITION TO PREEXISTING GENERAL ANESTHETICS

	EFFECT			
MEASUREMENT	NITROUS OXIDE	NITROUS OXIDE–HALOTHANE	NITROUS OXIDE–ENFLURANE	NITROUS OXIDE–MORPHINE
Blood pressure	None	Increased	None	None
Heart rate	Decreased	None	Decreased	Decreased
Cardiac output	Decreased	None	Increased	Decreased
Systemic vascular resistance	Increased	Increased	None	Increased
Central venous pressure	Increased	Increased	None	Increased

From Tarhan, S. (ed.): Cardiovascular Anesthesia and Postoperative Care. Chicago, Year Book Medical Publishers, 1982.

One study of 53 patients suggested that epidural anesthesia and postoperative analgesia were preferable to standard general anesthesia for high-risk surgical patients.[9] At the present time, however, the potential benefit of regional anesthesia compared to general anesthesia is uncertain,[10–12] in part because the decline in systemic blood pressure from regional anesthesia can cause transient myocardial ischemia.[13] Postoperative epidural analgesia can attenuate sympathetic nervous system hyperactivity, reduce the need for parenteral analgesia, and may be of benefit for patients with coronary artery disease.[14,15]

INTRAOPERATIVE HEMODYNAMICS AND ARRHYTHMIAS

During the operative procedure, it is not uncommon for systolic blood pressure to fall into the range of 95 to 105 mm Hg. Such blood pressure reductions are often brief and may respond to a lightening of the anesthesia or, in 20 to 30 per cent of patients, either to a brisk fluid challenge or the use of intravenous sympathomimetic agents. Any severe reduction in arterial pressure in patients with ischemic heart disease can reduce coronary flow and precipitate myocardial ischemia. In general, such reductions in blood pressure are not associated with major cardiac complications, such as myocardial infarction, unless they are marked and sustained. For example, increased complication rates have been reported for reductions in systolic arterial pressures that exceed approximately 33 per cent of the preoperative blood pressure and that persist for 10 or more minutes, or are more than 50 per cent below the preoperative blood pressure, or for mean arterial pressure reductions of 20 mm Hg or greater for 60 or more minutes, or for 20-mm Hg increases in mean arterial pressure sustained for 15 or more minutes.[16–19] Fluids that are administered to maintain intraoperative blood pressure can potentially cause postoperative fluid overload.

The risk of unplanned intraoperative hypotension is at least as great with spinal or epidural anesthesia as with general anesthesia.[20] However, because spinal and epidural anesthesia are not direct myocardial depressants, they may be advantageous in patients with severe myocardial dysfunction; but even in those circumstances, well-balanced general anesthesia, sometimes including ketamine, has been used successfully.

Transient bradycardias, such as sinus bradycardia and junctional rhythm, may occur during periods of vagal stimulation. These bradyarrhythmias commonly respond to a lightening of the anesthesia or to the administration of atropine or $beta_1$-adrenoceptor agonists such as isoproterenol or epinephrine. Tachyarrhythmias may result from hypovolemia or vasodilation as well as from sensitization of the myocardium to catecholamines that are circulating and/or released by sympathetic nerve endings in the heart. Tachycardia is poorly tolerated by patients with mitral stenosis (p. 1007) and may cause myocardial ischemia in patients with coronary artery disease. Therapy with specific antiarrhythmic medications is usually indicated only when the arrhythmia causes circulatory compromise and does not respond to changes in the depth of anesthesia or to attention to problems such as hypoxemia, hypovolemia, hypotension, or the potentially precipitating surgical manipulation.

Positive-pressure ventilation during general anesthesia reduces the return of blood to the right side of the heart and tends to reduce ventricular preload. Fluid that is administered during positive-pressure ventilation will not increase preload to the extent that it would in the patient who is ventilating spontaneously. When the positive-pressure ventilation of general anesthesia ceases, ventricular preload increases, often abruptly, and hypertension or pulmonary congestion may result. Analogous physiological changes can occur with the cessation of spinal or epidural anesthesia because the venodilation caused by these agents also reduces right ventricular preload.

MONITORING. In patients with severe underlying heart disease undergoing noncardiac surgery, it is mandatory to monitor cardiac function during anesthesia,[21] including cardiac rate and rhythm and directly recorded arterial blood pressure. A radial artery line permits not only monitoring of intraarterial pressure but also frequent sampling for determination of blood gases. In the presence of peripheral vasoconstriction, indirect (cuff) blood pressure measurements may greatly underestimate true arterial pressure. Monitoring of the pulmonary artery (or, preferably, pulmonary artery wedge) pressure and cardiac output is often desirable in patients who are critically ill, who have marginal cardiovascular reserve, who are to undergo prolonged operative procedures in which major blood losses might occur, and in whom hypotensive anesthesia is to be used. Both pulmonary artery wedge pressure and cardiac output can be measured with the aid of a multiple-lumen balloon flotation catheter (Swan-Ganz) and the thermodilution method (Chap. 7). For detection of intraoperative myocardial ischemia, transesophageal echocardiography is about as accurate as 12-lead electrocardiography, and both are preferable to the monitoring of only one or two electrocardiographic leads.[22] Pulmonary capillary wedge pressure is a poor marker of ischemia, but the pulmonary capillary wedge pressure remains the best index of fluid balance.[23] In seriously ill patients, urine output should be monitored with a Foley catheter.

THE OPERATION

Just as consultant cardiologists must understand the pharmacological effects of anesthesia, they must also recognize the physiological effects of surgery, including the direct consequences of the operation and the expected responses to postoperative recuperation.

NATURE OF THE OPERATION. Although ophthalmological surgery[24] and transurethral prostatic resection[25] are almost always safe, even in patients with a history of serious cardiac disease, general surgical mortality is often 25 to 50 per cent higher in patients with underlying cardiovascular conditions than in patients with normal cardiac function.[17,20,26–29] Among noncardiac surgical procedures, the highest cardiovascular complication rates are commonly associated with abdominal aortic aneurysm surgery,[26,30] which causes substantial myocardial stress because of aortic cross-clamping and major shifts in fluid and electrolytes. The risk of cardiac complications is also higher in other major abdominal and thoracic procedures than in procedures on the extremities, in large part because of the more difficult postoperative course. Patients who undergo operation for aortic aneurysm, carotid arterial disease, or peripheral vascular disease often have substantial coronary artery disease as well, and the extent of the latter may be underestimated because of the limitations caused by the peripheral arterial disease.

DURATION. The risk of cardiovascular mortality and morbidity is generally correlated with the duration of anesthesia, but this is principally because the longest operations are more often on the aorta or in the abdomen or chest than on the extremities. In most series[20,28,29] the risk of major cardiovascular complications did not correlate with the duration of surgery after controlling for the type of surgery. However, if the operation is prolonged because of intraoperative complications, it would be expected that the risk of postoperative cardiovascular complications might increase, especially among patients with a prior myocardial infarction[17] or in situations in which the operation takes longer than 5 hours.[20]

EMERGENCY OPERATION. When an operation is carried out under emergency conditions, it is associated with greatly increased mortality in patients with cardiovascular disease. The risk of postoperative cardiac complications, including postoperative myocardial infarction or cardiac death, is increased anywhere from 2.5- to 4-fold in emergency compared with elective surgery.[20,26,28,29] Part of this increased risk is because patients undergoing emergency operations may often have poorly controlled or unappreciated general medical problems, such as fluid and electrolyte imbalance or hepatic dysfunction.[26,28] However, emergency surgery appears to be an important correlate of postoperative complications, even after controlling for the underlying medical disease.[26,28,31]

The application of invasive hemodynamic monitoring to noncardiac surgical procedures in patients with underlying heart disease may reduce the risk of intraoperative and postoperative cardiovascular complications. Thus the risk of a new infarction was reduced from 7.7 to 1.9 per cent when patients with a history of infarction were aggressively monitored during the period from 1977 to 1982 compared with when minimal invasive monitoring was used in the period from 1973 to 1976.[32] Although this nonrandomized study did not control for other secular changes in medical care, it should not be surprising that the application of cardiovascular anesthesiological techniques to noncardiac surgery would have a beneficial effect. Thus, in patients who have suffered a myocardial infarction within the past 3 months, who have angina that is more severe than Canadian Class II (p. 11, 12), who have severe heart failure, or who are at high risk based on indices such as the multifactorial index of cardiac risk in noncardiac surgery[26,28,33–35] (p. 1717), available data support the use of intraarterial and pulmonary artery catheters for careful hemodynamic monitoring. In general, arterial and pulmonary artery pressure should not be allowed to fluctuate by more than 20 per cent of the preinduction values for longer than 5 minutes. For patients with a recent myocardial infarction or severe angina, careful monitoring should usually extend into the postoperative period, usually for at least 24 hours.[32]

INFLUENCE OF UNDERLYING CARDIOVASCULAR DISEASE

ISCHEMIC HEART DISEASE

ASSESSMENT OF RISK

Clinical. Ischemic heart disease is a major determinant of perioperative morbidity and mortality. The incidence of perioperative myocardial infarction is increased 10- to 50-fold in patients who have previously suffered infarcts compared with patients who do not have a clinical history of coronary disease.

During the 1970's, several studies reported about a 30 per cent risk of reinfarction or cardiac death when patients were operated on within 3 months of the previous myocardial infarction, about a 15 per cent risk when the operation was performed 3 to 6 months after a prior infarction, and about a 5 per cent risk when the operation was performed more than 6 months after the infarction.[9,20] However, recent data suggest that the application of invasive hemodynamic monitoring and careful regulation of oxygenation, electrolytes, volume status, and the hematocrit have markedly reduced the complication rate. For example, Wells and Kaplan[36] reported no reinfarctions in 48 patients who were operated on within 3 months after a myocardial infarction, while Rao et al.[32] reported only a 6 per cent reinfarction rate within 3 months after preoperative myocardial infarction and only a 2 per cent reinfarction rate between 3 and 6 months after a myocardial infarction.

Obviously, truly life-saving procedures must be performed almost regardless of the cardiac risk, and purely elective surgery should commonly be delayed for 6 months after infarction, when the cardiovascular risks will have returned to a stable, long-term baseline risk. The more difficult issue is in patients in whom the operation is not truly emergent but is also not purely elective, for example, a patient with severe symptomatic peripheral vascular disease or a patient with a potentially resectable malignant tumor. In such situations one would like to delay operation sufficiently long for cardiac risk to be reduced but not wait a full 6 months. Because full healing of a myocardial infarction usually takes about 4 to 6 weeks, one rational approach is to evaluate the patient with postmyocardial infarction prognostic studies, such as a submaximal exercise tolerance test,[37] and to use the patient's clinical and cardiological conditions as the guide for surgery sometime between 4 weeks and 3 months after the infarction.

A recent preoperative myocardial infarction will increase a patient's relative risk of reinfarction with operation, but the absolute risk depends on a variety of factors in addition to the timing of the infarction. In general, one should be influenced less by whether or not a preoperative myocardial infarction was associated with the development of new Q waves than by the state of left ventricular function and the severity of preoperative angina. Thus, patients who have good exercise tolerance and left ventricular function after infarction and who can resume normal activity levels within 4 to 6 weeks after infarction should be able to undergo operation with relatively small absolute risks, even if their relative risk might be slightly lower if one could wait the full 6 months. By comparison, risks are likely to be substantially higher in patients who have postinfarction angina, large reversible defects on thallium scintigraphy, reduced left ventricular function, marked ST-segment depression with exercise, or other evidence of easily provokable ischemia (p. 1270).

When the patient with angina pectoris is evaluated, the patient's current (preoperative) exercise tolerance should be ascertained and an assessment made as to whether the anginal pattern is stable or unstable (p. 1293). Patients who are Class II by the criteria of the Canadian Cardiovascular Society[38] or the Specific Activity Scale[39,40] can carry objects such as two grocery bags or a young child up a flight of stairs without stopping and without appreciable symptoms. In such patients most surgical procedures are generally well tolerated. Physicians should avoid relying on the *frequency* of angina because patients who voluntarily reduce their activity level may also greatly reduce their symptoms.[40] This phenomenon is especially true in patients whose surgical conditions, such as orthopedic disorders or peripheral vascular disease, limit ambulation.

Laboratory. *Exercise treadmill testing* is an objective means for assessing exercise tolerance and is especially beneficial if the history is unreliable. Unfortunately, the limited sensitivity and specificity of standard electrocardiographic exercise tolerance testing limit the use of this test for diagnosing coronary artery disease (see Chap. 6). In two studies of vascular surgery patients,[41,42] postoperative cardiac complications were significantly less in patients who exercised to higher heart rates and cardiac workloads. The prognostic value of limited exercise tolerance has also been reported in persons over age 65[43,44] in whom the inability to perform 2 minutes of bicycle exercise in a supine position and to raise the heart rate above 99 beats per minute was an independent important predictor of cardiac complications in noncardiac surgery. Of note was that poor exercise capacity was an independent predictor of cardiac complications, but electrocardiographic changes with exercise were not. Although some investigators have used radionuclide ventriculography to predict risk,[45] in other studies data from resting and exercise radionuclide ventriculography did not add important independent information for predicting perioperative cardiac risk.[43,46–48]

In patients who are unable to exercise because of noncardiac disability (e.g., intermittent claudication or orthopedic abnormalities), ambulatory ischemia monitoring and dipyridamole thallium imaging can be used to assess perioperative risk. In one study of vascular surgery patients with normal resting electrocardiograms, the presence of ischemia on ambulatory electrocardiographic monitoring identified more than 90 per cent of patients who had major postoperative cardiac ischemic events.[49] More than one-third of the patients with preoperative ambulatory ischemia had major events. In this study[49] and another report,[50] ambulatory ischemia was a statistically significant independent correlate of major postoperative ischemic events, but asymptomatic postoperative ischemia appears to be an even better predictor of clinical postoperative ischemic events.[50a–c]

Dipyridamole thallium imaging has also been successful in identifying high-risk patients among selected subgroups undergoing vascular surgery, and it is especially appealing for patients who have abnormal resting electrocardiograms or are taking medications such as digoxin that make electrocardiographic monitoring unreliable for the detection of ischemia.[51-55] In one study,[51] all eight postoperative ischemic events, including three myocardial infarctions, occurred in patients who had transient thallium defects precipitated by dipyridamole; there were no such events in 32 patients who had no fixed defects. Among the 16 patients with dipryidamole thallium defects, there were three myocardial infarctions and five additional patients who developed episodes of angina with ST-segment depression postoperatively. In one series, however, dipyridamole thallium imaging was not correlated with the risk of postoperative ischemic events.[56]

The utility of both ambulatory ischemia monitoring and dypyridamole thallium imaging can be improved when these techniques are used in appropriate patient subsets. For example, in patients who do not have Q waves on their electrocardiograms, are less than 70 years of age, and who do not have a history of angina, ventricular ectopic activity requiring treatment, or diabetes mellitus requiring treatment the risk of major postoperative events appears to be sufficiently low that neither technique should be used as a screening test.[49,53]

Patients who have undergone successful coronary revascularization can undergo major noncardiac surgical procedures with a low mortality rate,[21,57] except perhaps in the first 30 days postoperatively. In some circumstances both the coronary artery bypass operation and the noncardiac operation can be performed during the course of the same procedure. It must be remembered, however, that the operative mortality rate for major noncardiac surgery in patients with stable angina and good exercise tolerance is relatively low, usually in the range of 2 per cent. No randomized controlled trials are available to assess the value of coronary artery bypass grafting preoperatively in patients with stable angina pectoris who are about to undergo noncardiac surgery. An analysis of patients in the Coronary Artery Surgery Study registry[57] showed that total operative mortality was 2.4 per cent in 458 patients who had significant coronary artery disease and underwent noncardiac operations without prior coronary artery bypass grafting. By comparison, operative mortality was 0.9 per cent among 399 patients who had had a coronary artery bypass grafting procedure performed before noncardiac surgery. The mortality was higher in patients who had more severe left ventricular dysfunction or dyspnea on exertion and in patients who used nitrates, were older, and had diabetes. The risk of myocardial infarction, however, was not significantly different between the patients with and without preoperative coronary artery bypass grafting. Furthermore, if one considers the mortality associated with coronary artery bypass grafting, which was 1.4 per cent in the Coronary Artery Surgery Study, the overall mortality from combined coronary artery bypass grafting and noncardiac surgery (2.3 per cent) would be as high as for the noncardiac surgery done in the non-bypassed group (2.4 per cent). Thus the data do not argue in favor of prophylactic coronary artery bypass grafting for patients whose symptoms would not otherwise warrant revascularization, who have stable angina with good exercise tolerance, and who do not have other factors that define a high-risk status (see below).

A practical approach to the patient with known or suspected ischemic heart disease should utilize information from the history as well as diagnostic tests.[58-60] If the patient's history indicates reliably that Class I or Class II activities[38,40,61] can be performed, the patient will commonly be raising the double product (the heart rate multiplied by the systolic blood pressure) above the range to be expected with general anesthesia and surgery, and hence should be able to withstand the stress of the procedure. If the history is unreliable, exercise testing to assess physical function[41-44] will aid in risk assessment. If the patient is unable to exercise because of noncardiac conditions, ambulatory ischemia monitoring (in a patient with a normal resting electrocardiogram who is not receiving medication such as digoxin) or dypyridamole thallium imaging should be used unless the patient has no historical risk factors.[49,53]

Patients who can exercise to Class I or II levels, or who have normal ambulatory ischemia monitoring or normal dipyridamole thallium imaging, can undergo most operations with acceptable risk. Patients who cannot perform Class I or II activities or who have positive ambulatory ischemia monitoring or dypyridamole thallium images should have their medical regimens intensified, if possible, and then have repeat testing. If tests remain positive or physical functioning remains limited after optimization of medical management, coronary arteriography will usually be indicated prior to elective surgery to determine whether coronary revascularization, with either percutaneous transluminal coronary angioplasty or coronary bypass surgery, would be feasible. The decision to proceed with revascularization depends more on the functional limitations that result from the coronary lesions than on their anatomical severity. Although the latter is important for long-term prognosis, the former is probably the most relevant correlate of perioperative risk.

COMBINED CAROTID AND CORONARY ARTERY SURGERY. There is some controversy as to the indications for combined coronary revascularization and carotid endarterectomy in patients with coexisting coronary and carotid stenoses. It has been shown experimentally that carotid perfusion is maintained or increased during cardiopulmonary bypass,[62] thus suggesting that nonpulsatile cardiopulmonary bypass per se is unlikely to cause a stroke due to hypoperfusion. Most strokes that occur during coronary revascularization appear to be embolic in origin.[63] Combined coronary and carotid surgery can be performed at an acceptable risk,[64,65] but we recommend combined surgery only when there is severe bilateral or currently symptomatic carotid disease associated with unstable angina, left main coronary disease, or very symptomatic three-vessel coronary disease. If the coronary disease is stable and relatively mild but the carotid disease is symptomatic, the carotid surgery should be performed first and the coronary revascularization at a later date. If the carotid disease is and has always been asymptomatic and is not bilateral and severe, coronary revascularization can be performed without a proven need for prophylactic carotid surgery.[63,64]

USE OF BETA BLOCKERS AND CALCIUM ANTAGONISTS. Although some concern has been expressed about the use of general anesthesia in patients receiving beta-adrenoceptor blocking agents and calcium antagonists, there are no clinical data to indicate that such medications should routinely be discontinued preoperatively. For beta-adrenoceptor blocking agents, early concerns[66] about the safety of propranolol have been contradicted by substantial subsequent data demonstrating the safety of their use[67] and the dangers of discontinuing beta-adrenoceptor blocking agents preoperatively.[68] Propranolol appears to reduce the risk of severe hypertensive episodes and ischemic electrocardiographic responses to the stresses of intubation, anesthesia, and surgery.[69,70] In patients who rely on beta-adrenoceptor blocking agents for the control of severe angina, the medication should be continued up to and including the morning of operation with a small sip of water.[68] Postoperatively, the medication can be resumed orally or sometimes given through a nasogastric tube. However, intravenous propranolol, metoprolol, or esmolol should be used in patients with a prior history of severe angina that required beta-adrenoceptor blocking agents for its control or in patients who have evidence of postoperative myocardial ischemia or otherwise unexplained hypertension or tachycardia.

Propranolol can be given as a 1-mg intravenous bolus, which is repeated up to a total loading dose of 10 mg and followed by 1 mg intravenously every 20 to 60 minutes. The second option is a 5- to 10-mg loading dose given slowly over 60 minutes, followed by a continuous intravenous infusion of

0.01 to 0.05 mg/min.[71,72] Esmolol, an ultra-short-acting beta-adrenoceptor blocker, can be used in doses ranging from 100 to 300 μg/kg/min after a 500 μg/kg/min loading dose.[73] If the patient suffers side effects attributable to administration of a beta-adrenoceptor blocker, treatment should be instituted with isoproterenol or dobutamine, or with glucagon, if the others are not effective.

Nifedipine can be given sublingually, and nitrates can be given sublingually, topically, or intravenously, to aid in the management of the early postoperative patient with angina, but neither of these agents substitutes for beta-adrenoceptor blockers in patients who have relied on the latter for the control of their ischemic heart disease.

HYPERTENSION

Several studies have documented that patients with hypertension have higher risks of suffering major cardiac complications during or shortly after noncardiac operation than do patients who have always been normotensive. However, most, if not all, of this increased risk is because of the ischemic heart disease, left ventricular dysfunction, renal failure, or other abnormalities that often occur in patients with hypertension. Thus, in patients with mild to moderate hypertension, diastolic pressures below 100 mm Hg, and no evidence of serious end-organ damage, general anesthesia and major noncardiac surgery are generally well tolerated.[18] Halothane anesthesia may be more likely than other anesthetic agents to induce intraoperative hypotension in patients with a history of hypertension,[18] and hypertensive patients are at higher risk for labile blood pressures and for hypertensive episodes during surgery and especially just after extubation.

Although uncontrolled early studies suggested that the continuation of any hypertensive agents might increase the risk of perioperative hypotension, substantial subsequent data from more careful studies indicate that patients whose hypertension is well controlled will do at least as well, if not better, if their medications are, in fact, continued up to the time of operation.[5,18,74] Thus, although it is not mandatory to delay noncardiac operation for the weeks or months that may be required to achieve ideal blood pressure control in the stable patient with mild to moderate hypertension who has no complications of the hypertension, there is also no apparent benefit, and some potential harm, from discontinuing successful antihypertensive therapy before surgery.

Thiazide and other diuretics cause some degree of chronic volume depletion,[75] and patients receiving these drugs may require more fluid administration early during the operative procedure. Guanethidine causes depletion of norepinephrine at adrenergic nerve endings, and when hypotension develops in patients receiving these drugs and they require adrenergic agonists, direct-acting agents such as norepinephrine, methoxamine, or phenylephrine should be used rather than indirect-acting agents such as ephedrine. If severe perioperative hypertension develops in a patient who has previously been receiving clonidine, and if the clonidine cannot be given orally, it can be administered intramuscularly in doses about one-half as large as the patient's usual daily dose or it can be administered topically,[76] or the patient can be treated with sublingual captopril, with methyldopa, or with a beta blocker. Although it may be desirable to use propranolol, metoprolol, or esmolol intravenously in patients who rely on beta-adrenoceptor blockers for the control of ischemic heart disease, it is less often necessary to use such agents intravenously in patients who take these medications for their antihypertensive effects. Commonly, intravenous labetolol[77] or nitroprusside can be used for acute episodes of hypertension and methyldopa for nonacute situations.

VALVULAR HEART DISEASE

Patients with valvular heart disease undergoing anesthesia and noncardiac operation are subject to many potential hazards: heart failure, infection, tachycardia, and embolization. As might be expected, patients with no or only mild limitation of activity (i.e., those in Class I or II[38–40]) tolerate operation well[78] and probably require little more than careful perioperative care and prophylaxis for infective endocarditis (p. 1097). Those with more serious impairment of cardiac reserve (i.e., those in Class III or IV) tolerate major noncardiac operations poorly, and their prognosis for surviving major surgery is distinctly worse,[20,29] although as is the case for patients with rheumatic heart disease who face the stress of pregnancy (p. 1796), the risk of operation depends on the functional state of the heart. Patients with symptomatic critical aortic[28] or mitral stenosis are especially prone to sudden death or acute pulmonary edema during the perioperative period; this may occur if demands on cardiac output are suddenly increased or if atrial fibrillation and a rapid ventricular rate are precipitated by anesthesia or operation. Every effort should be made to treat heart failure preoperatively. Patients with severe stenotic or regurgitant valve disease should undergo corrective valvular surgery before an elective operation, while those who require an emergency noncardiac operation may benefit from intraoperative hemodynamic monitoring, afterload reduction, and preload augmentation.[79] In some patients with mitral or aortic stenosis, balloon valvuloplasty (p. 1376) may offer relief of severe obstruction at a low risk when it might not be desirable to carry out valve replacement.[80]

HYPERTROPHIC CARDIOMYOPATHY. Patients with hypertrophic cardiomyopathy are intolerant of hypovolemia, which may lead to both a reduction in the elevated preload necessary to maintain cardiac output and an increase in the obstruction to left ventricular outflow (p. 1404). With careful perioperative, intraoperative, and postoperative care, however, the risk of major cardiac complications in such patients is small. In one series of 56 operations in patients with hypertrophic cardiomyopathy, there were no deaths and the only major complication was a myocardial infarction with congestive heart failure in a patient who also had underlying coronary artery disease. Intraoperative or postoperative hypotension requiring vasoconstrictors occurred in less than 10 per cent of patients.[81] It has been suggested that spinal anesthesia may be relatively contraindicated in patients with hypertrophic obstructive cardiomyopathy because of its tendency to reduce systemic vascular resistance and increase venous pooling and thereby increase the severity of obstruction to outflow.[81] Hemodynamic monitoring is not routinely required but may be helpful when these patients undergo major aortic, abdominal, or thoracic procedures.

PROSTHETIC HEART VALVES. Most patients with mechanical prosthetic heart valves receive anticoagulants on a long-term basis to prevent thromboembolic complications (p. 1062). If these medications are continued through the period of noncardiac operation, hemostasis, hematoma formation, and persistent postoperative bleeding may ensue. Anticoagulants can be temporarily discontinued during the perioperative period with minimal risk of thrombosis. In one study,[82] no thromboembolic complications occurred in 159 patients with prosthetic valves undergoing 180 noncardiac operations when warfarin was discontinued an average of 2.9 days preoperatively and resumed 2.7 days postoperatively.[82] Using a similar approach, Katholi et al. did not observe thromboembolic complications in 25 noncardiac operations on patients with prosthetic aortic valves[83]; however, two such complications occurred in the 10 patients with mitral valve prostheses when anticoagulants were discontinued for noncardiac operations, although these patients had Kay-Shiley caged-disc valves, which are associated with a somewhat higher risk of thromboembolic complications. Because there is a distinct risk of hemorrhagic complications in patients whose anticoagulants have been discontinued for only 2 or 3 days,[82] prothrombin time should be restored to within 20 per cent of normal before one proceeds with the noncardiac surgery.[84] Low molecular weight dextran can be used in the postoperative period to minimize thrombotic complications during the 2 to 3 days when the risk of hemorrhagic complications from resuming anticoagulation is relatively higher. In patients with prostheses that are at high risk for thrombosis, such as caged-disc valves, we recommend discontinuing warfarin, allowing the prothrombin time to come to within about 2 to 3 seconds of normal, using intravenous heparin until about 6 hours before the operation, restarting the heparin about 36 to 48 hours after surgery, and switching to warfarin about 2 to 5 days later. Recent analyses indicate that these various anticoagulation regimens are cost-effective provided that they do not result in lengthening the hospitalization.[85] Even one day of additional hospitalization is relatively costly, and the daily risk of thromboembolic complications is low. Thus, perioperative anticoagulation management should focus on regimens that provide reasonable protection from thromboembolic disease but that permit the patient to be discharged when the surgical condition itself permits.[85]

ENDOCARDITIS PROPHYLAXIS. Patients with valvular heart disease and those with prosthetic heart valves should receive prophylactic antibiotics for surgical procedures likely to be complicated by bacteremias.[86,87] These include incision and drainage of an infected site; oral, lower gastrointestinal, and gallbladder surgery; and genitourinary procedures. Penicillin can be used before operation involving the upper respiratory tract, with erythromycin or vancomycin an acceptable alternative for patients with a penicillin allergy. For gastrointestinal and genitourinary surgery, which can be complicated by either enterococci or gram-negative bacteremia, gentamicin or streptomycin is required in addition to penicillin. (Suggested doses are given on p. 1099).

The value of antibiotic prophylaxis before noncardiac operation in patients with *mitral valve prolapse* is controversial (p. 1035). Most studies indicate that patients with this condition who have murmurs of mitral regurgitation are at substantially higher risk than patients who do not have murmurs,[88] and cost-effectiveness analyses argue *against* routine antibiotic prophylaxis in patients without a murmur.[89,90] At the present time a reasonable compromise is to use antibiotic prophylaxis before surgery in patients with mitral valve prolapse who have clinical evidence of mitral regurgitation.

CONGENITAL HEART DISEASE

Depending on the nature of the malformation, the patient with congenital heart disease may be subject to one or more potentially serious complications, such as infection, bleeding, hypoxemia, and paradoxical embolization during general anesthesia and operation. As is the case for patients with valvular heart disease, patients with congenital heart disease who are to undergo a surgical procedure require prophylaxis to prevent infective endocarditis (p. 1098). Patients with cyanotic congenital heart disease and secondary polycythemia are at increased risk of intraoperative and postoperative hemorrhage as a consequence of coagulation defects and thrombocytopenia (p. 894); this risk can be reduced with careful preoperative phlebotomy, usually to a hematocrit of 50 to 55 per cent.[91]

Patients with cyanotic congenital heart disease tolerate systemic hypotension poorly, since this increases the right-to-left shunt and the severity of hypoxemia. In one large series, induction was commonly accomplished using ketamine or fentanyl to avoid hypotension, and anesthesia was maintained with morphine and nitrous oxide or with large doses of fentanyl with or without nitrous oxide. Halothane in very low concentrations can be used in patients with less severe degrees of cyanosis.[92] With use of careful anesthetic techniques, the risk of major anesthetic complications is extremely low even in very ill and cyanotic patients. However, spinal anesthesia, which causes peripheral arterial vasodilatation and reduces venous return, can have deleterious hemodynamic effects in patients with cyanotic congenital heart disease. Occasionally, infusion of a vasoconstrictor such as phenylephrine may be required to raise systemic vascular resistance and thereby decrease the magnitude of the right-to-left shunt. Because patients with right-to-left shunts are subject to the risk of paradoxical emboli, including air emboli, meticulous techniques with regard to intravenous solutions and injections are mandatory to prevent such complications.

CONGESTIVE HEART FAILURE

Congestive heart failure is a major determinant of perioperative risk, irrespective of the nature of the underlying cardiac disorder. Mortality with noncardiac surgery increases with worsening cardiac class[20,29] and with the presence of pulmonary congestion,[20] especially when a third heart sound is noted.[28] Because the perioperative mortality rate appears to depend more on the patient's condition at the time of operation than on the most severe depression of cardiovascular status the patient has ever experienced, it is clearly advisable to treat the congestive heart failure before the contemplated major elective noncardiac surgery. However, because such a therapeutic regimen almost always includes a diuretic, both hypovolemia and hypokalemia are potential problems for patients treated just before operation. It is therefore desirable, if possible, to stabilize the patient's condition by treating heart failure for approximately 1 week rather than for only 1 or 2 days before the contemplated operation. Also, great care should be taken to avoid dehydration because hypovolemic patients may be especially likely to experience marked hypotension during the early phases of anesthesia. Perioperative cardiogenic pulmonary edema will develop in about 2 per cent of patients over age 40 undergoing major noncardiac surgery without prior congestive heart failure, in about 6 per cent of patients whose heart failure is well controlled, and in about 16 per cent of patients whose heart failure persists on physical examination or chest radiograph before surgery.[20]

Although digitalis can counteract the myocardial depressant actions of many general anesthetic agents,[93] the value of digitalis in patients with congestive heart failure appears to be limited to certain subsets of patients, especially those who have a third heart sound.[94] Digitalis is one of the most common causes of iatrogenic complications in hospitalized patients, and it may be associated with a higher risk of intraoperative bradyarrhythmias.[20] Therefore, preoperative digitalization is *not* recommended except in patients whose congestive heart failure is sufficiently severe that they would normally meet the criteria for long-term digitalization (p. 479).

ARRHYTHMIAS

Arrhythmias may be a manifestation of underlying heart disease, and hence are frequently markers for the likelihood of perioperative cardiac complications. For example, the frequency of ventricular premature contractions correlates with left ventricular dysfunction and the severity of coronary artery disease,[95,96] and thus frequent ventricular premature contractions in patients with coronary artery disease represent a risk factor for the development of cardiac complications.[28] Because patients who have ventricular premature contractions but no evidence of underlying heart disease on detailed examination have an apparently normal cardiac prognosis,[97] ventricular premature contractions in the *absence* of underlying heart disease should not be considered a risk factor for cardiac complications with noncardiac surgery. Atrial arrhythmias are often a manifestation of atrial enlargement, and a supraventricular rhythm other than sinus appears to be a risk factor for the development of perioperative complications.[28]

Although it would be ideal for arrhythmias to be well controlled preoperatively, the risks associated with arrhythmias appear to be related more to the underlying cardiac disease than to the arrhythmias per se. Therefore, there currently is no evidence that asymptomatic ventricular premature contractions require aggressive preoperative control or prophylactic intraoperative suppression. Similarly, in the patient with well-controlled atrial fibrillation, cardioversion need not be carried out specifically because of planned noncardiac surgery if such a management option would not otherwise be appropriate.

Patients who are most at risk for the development of postoperative supraventricular tachyarrhythmias include elderly patients undergoing pulmonary surgery, patients with subcritical valvular stenoses, and patients with prior histories of supraventricular tachyarrhythmias. Although data are less than decisive, there is a suggestion that digitalis may reduce the risk of the development of postoperative supraventricular tachycardia in such patients,[98] and that the rate of the supraventricular tachycardia will be slower in the digitalized patient.[20] Thus, we generally recommend prophylactic preoperative digitalization in elderly patients undergoing major pulmonary surgery, patients with subcritical valvular stenoses, and patients with a prior history of symptomatic supraventricular tachycardias, except if the latter are already taking other medications for the control of such arrhythmias. Verapamil may also be useful in these settings, but its negative inotropic effects make it theoretically less appealing than digitalis for many patients.

CONDUCTION DEFECTS. The patient with *complete heart block* (p. 710) must respond to the demands for an increased cardiac output by augmenting stroke volume, but this compensatory response is prevented in many patients by a concurrent impairment of cardiac contractility. In addition, most anesthetic agents depress myocardial contractility and/or produce peripheral vasodilatation. Furthermore, anesthesia may cause further depression of the automaticity, and therefore the ventricular rate, of the patient with heart block. Thus patients with untreated complete heart block may be unable to meet the increased demands placed on the cardiovascular system by anesthesia and operation, and a permanent or temporary pacemaker should be inserted before general anesthesia, even in asymptomatic patients (Chap. 26).

Another problem is presented by the patient with *chronic bifascicular block* (p. 131).[20,99] A significant fraction of patients developing this abnormality in the course of an acute myocardial infarction progress to complete heart block, often accompanied by sudden severe hemodynamic compromise (p. 1241). In several series, progression from bifascicular to complete heart block has not been documented during the perioperative period in patients without a previous history of third-degree heart block. Therefore, we do *not* recommend prophylactic pacemaker placement for such patients or for patients with first-degree atrioventricular (AV) block or type I second-degree AV block (Wenckebach), although a pacemaker should always be available in the operating room for emergency placement. However, in patients who have bifascicular block, and either type II second-degree AV block or a history of unexplained syncope or transient third-degree AV block, the risk of development of complete heart block is much higher, and a temporary pacemaker should be inserted preoperatively.

THE PATIENT WITH A PERMANENT PACEMAKER. When a patient with a permanent pacemaker in situ is about to undergo operation, the device should be carefully evaluated to insure that it is functioning properly preoperatively (Chap. 26). Demand pacemakers are sensitive to electromagnetic interference, such as that produced by the electrocautery, which may result in failure to pace. The danger of this potentially hazardous interaction can be reduced by placing the indifferent plate of the cautery unit as far as possible from the lead and pulse generator, and the electrocautery should be used in brief bursts rather than continuously. Also, a magnet should be available in the operating room to convert the pacemaker from the demand to the fixed-rate mode. Because the cautery may also interfere with the electrocardiographic monitor and render it temporarily uninterpretable, arterial pressure should be monitored directly when the cautery is being used on patients with permanent pacemakers.

In general, a prophylactic *temporary pacemaker* should be inserted before noncardiac operations only if the patient meets the indications for permanent pacemaker insertion[100] (see also p. 728) and the operation should not be delayed for the time required for a permanent pacemaker insertion, or if the operative course is likely to be complicated by transient bacteremia. In such situations a temporary pacemaker should be placed initially, and the permanent pacemaker can be inserted after the operation. The occasional exception is the patient who has a severe bradycardiac response to vagal stimuli and who might be difficult to manage during a major operation without a pacemaker.

GENERAL MEDICAL PROBLEMS

Patients with heart disease whose general medical status is complicated by renal insufficiency, hepatic abnormalities, hypoxemia, or electrolyte abnormalities have a higher risk of cardiac complications, presumably because these nonmedical conditions exacerbate the stress placed on the heart by the operation.[20,26,28] Morbidity is also higher in markedly obese patients[101] because obesity is often associated with abnormal cardiorespiratory function, metabolic function, and hemostasis. Every effort should be made to correct any of these noncardiac problems before operations, and the potential long-term benefits of surgery must also be interpreted in light of the patient's general prognosis.

POSTOPERATIVE COMPLICATIONS

MYOCARDIAL INFARCTION. Transient intraoperative ischemia does not appear to be a major correlate of postoperative ischemic events in patients undergoing noncardiac surgery,[102] but most clinical postoperative ischemic events are preceded by asymptomatic episodes of postoperative ischemia that can be detected by ambulatory ischemic monitoring.[102,103] Although series from before 1980 showed a peak in the risk of myocardial infarction on about the third postoperative day,[104] more recent series show that a combination of frequent electrocardiograms and cardiac enzymes detects many non-Q-wave infarctions in the first 24 hours postoperatively.[49,105,106] Although care must be taken in interpreting cardiac enzymes in the perioperative period,[107] it may be that supply-demand imbalances cause an early peak in non-Q-wave postoperative infarctions, while the hypercoagulable postoperative state leads to a later (3 to 5 days postoperatively) peak in Q-wave infarctions. For both types of infarction, postoperative stresses include general surgical complications, hypoxia and other pulmonary complications, fluid and electrolyte abnormalities, and the stresses of modern postoperative ambulation protocols. Substantial data indicate that prophylactic anticoagulation with low-dose heparin will reduce the risk of postoperative thromboembolic complications,[108] and such therapy is routinely indicated in most cardiac patients who undergo noncardiac operations. In fact, such anticoagulation regimens may permit a more gradual postoperative ambulation protocol in cardiac patients, and hence possibly lower the incidence of postoperative myocardial infarction.

Myocardial infarction occurring in the perioperative period is often painless. Obviously, then, the incidence of perioperative infarction will be underestimated if electrocardiograms and serial estimations of serum creatine kinase isoenzyme

(MB fraction) are not obtained routinely during the postoperative period in high-risk patients.[105]

HYPERTENSION. Postoperative hypertension is most likely to occur soon after the cessation of positive-pressure ventilation or in the recovery room, and it is more common after carotid endarterectomy and major abdominal vascular procedures.[18]

Common precipitants include fluid overload after cessation of positive-pressure ventilation, hypoxemia, anxiety, and pain.[109] The principal therapeutic approaches should therefore concentrate on assuring adequate oxygenation, pain control, and fluid control. In general, supplemental oxygen, morphine, and diuretics are the mainstays of the treatment of postoperative hypertension. Nitroprusside (p. 869) and labetalol[77] (p. 866) are the preferred medications for more severe hypertension. Intravenous hydralazine in small doses is effective for treating postoperative hypertension, but it has the potential of precipitating supraventricular tachyarrhythmias. Methyldopa will not be helpful in the emergency situation, but it may be an important part of the overall regimen because it will have its onset of effect about 4 hours after administration, at a time when one would like to be able to discontinue more vigorous intravenous antihypertensive regimens.

CONGESTIVE HEART FAILURE. Although postoperative heart failure may be precipitated by myocardial infarction or ischemia, a substantial proportion of the cases are directly caused by excess fluid administration. Heart failure tends to occur soon after cessation of positive-pressure ventilation and again at about 24 to 48 hours after operation, when the fluid that was given in the perioperative period is mobilized from the extravascular sites. Diuretics, often given intravenously, and rarely supplemented by digitalis glycosides, are usually sufficient therapy for postoperative congestive heart failure.

POSTOPERATIVE ARRHYTHMIAS. Arrhythmias are common after operation and are often a manifestation of a noncardiac complication, such as bleeding, infection, or an acid-base or electrolyte imbalance occurring in a patient with heart disease. Management of such arrhythmias often requires recognition and correction of extracardiac factors.

In one study of 916 patients with sinus rhythm throughout the course of major noncardiac surgery, 35 patients (4 per cent) developed new supraventricular tachyarrhythmias postoperatively.[110] Of these 35 patients, 46 per cent had acute cardiac conditions, 31 per cent had major infections, 29 per cent had preexisting hypotension, 26 per cent had anemia, 23 per cent had metabolic derangements, 23 per cent had received new parenteral drugs that could be implicated, and 20 per cent were hypoxic. Forty per cent of the patients required no new therapy with cardiac medications, and only two patients required electrical cardioversion; the arrhythmias of all treated patients reverted to sinus rhythm. No deaths were related to the supraventricular tachyarrhythmias per se, but a substantial proportion of the patients in whom these arrhythmias occurred died as a result of the concurrent medical problems. Thus, a new postoperative supraventricular tachyarrhythmia should prompt a search for remediable medical problems. Direct antiarrhythmic therapy is often unnecessary and is usually secondary in importance to correction of the underlying cause of the arrhythmia.

Sinus tachycardia is the most common rhythm disturbance in the postoperative patient. Multiple noncardiac etiologic factors have been identified, including pain, hypovolemia, hypervolemia, fever, anemia, hypoxemia, pulmonary emboli, anxiety, infection, hypotension, and electrolyte abnormalities (especially hypokalemia). These noncardiac factors are much more common causes of sinus tachycardia in the postoperative cardiac patient than is either myocardial infarction or heart failure. Sinus tachycardia not caused by congestive heart failure will not slow with cardiac glycosides. The therapeutic:toxic ratio of these drugs is actually reduced by most of the above-mentioned noncardiac causes of sinus tachycardia, and therefore digitalis glycosides are not considered appropriate for postoperative patients unless the sinus tachycardia is caused by impaired cardiac function.

Atrial fibrillation is also a common postoperative arrhythmia. Atrial dilatation, which lowers the threshold for development of this arrhythmia, may result from heart failure, mitral valve disease, and/or hypervolemia. Noncardiac precipitants include pneumonia, atelectasis, and pulmonary emboli. Initially, the postoperative patient with atrial fibrillation should be treated with a digitalis glycoside or verapamil; in addition, a beta-adrenoceptor blocker can be used to help gain rapid control of the ventricular rate. Cardioversion is usually delayed until the precipitating factors have been eliminated, since in the patient who has cardioversion before clearing of the atelectasis or pneumonia there is frequently reversion to atrial fibrillation, while in the patient whose pulmonary problem or congestive heart failure is adequately treated there is often spontaneous reversion to sinus rhythm.

Atrial flutter is often poorly tolerated because of the rapid ventricular rate and the difficult pharmacological management. Cardioversion is usually the treatment of choice, along with quinidine or procainamide administered to prevent recurrence (p. 681).

IMPLICATIONS OF POSTOPERATIVE COMPLICATIONS FOR LONG-TERM MANAGEMENT. When a patient develops a perioperative myocardial infarction, the evaluation and the recuperative process generally should be analogous to when a myocardial infarction occurs in other patients (see Chap. 39). Because postoperative congestive heart failure is commonly precipitated by iatrogenic fluid overload, the patient commonly will not need long-term therapy for congestive heart failure. Similarly, perioperative arrhythmias are often precipitated by specific stimuli, and the patient with a postoperative arrhythmia should not automatically be consigned to long-term antiarrhythmic therapy. In patients who develop either postoperative congestive heart failure or arrhythmias, it is often appropriate to discontinue new cardiac therapies several days before discharge and observe the patient to see whether long-term therapy is indicated.

THE ROLE OF THE MEDICAL CONSULTANT

The physician called on to evaluate the status of a patient with suspected or overt cardiac disease before elective or emergency noncardiac surgery must first determine whether cardiovascular disease is present and, if it is, must identify those factors that may increase the risk of operation. It may be necessary to invest considerable time and effort to prepare the patient for operation. In addition, the patient must be followed carefully after operation to detect and manage the cardiac problems that frequently complicate the postoperative period.

ESTIMATION OF RISK

A few patients have such compelling reasons for operation (e.g., rupturing aortic aneurysm, perforated or necrotic bowel, life-threatening hemorrhage, or some forms of intestinal obstruction) that estimation of operative risk is an academic exercise, since failure to operate almost certainly will result in the patient's death. Often, however, the timing or even the performance of an operation is elective, and under these circumstances estimation of risk is an important aspect of the medical consultant's role. Certain cardiovascular problems, such as recent myocardial infarction (less than 1 month), inadequately treated congestive heart failure, and severe mitral or aortic stenosis, are *absolute contraindications* to *elective* surgery. *Relative contraindictions*, which commonly require further clinical or laboratory evaluation or treatment before elective surgery, include more remote myocardial infarction (1 month to 6 months previously), angina pectoris, mild heart failure, cyanotic congenital heart disease with severe polycythemia, and a coagulation abnormality. Several other problems should be recognized and treated before operation: ane-

TABLE 55-2 COMPUTATION OF THE CARDIAC RISK INDEX

CRITERIA	POINTS
1 History	
(a) Age > 70 yr	5
(b) MI in previous 6 mo	10
2 Physical examination	
(a) S_3 gallop or JVD	11
(b) Important VAS	3
3 Electrocardiogram	
(a) Rhythm other than sinus or PACs on last preoperative ECG	7
(b) > 5 PVCs/min documented at any time before operation	7
4 General status	
$Po_2 < 60$ or $Pco_2 > 50$ mm Hg, $K < 3.0$ or $HCO_3 < 20$ mEq/liter, BUN > 50 or Cr > 3.0 mg/dl, abnormal SGOT, signs of chronic liver disease, or patient bedridden from noncardiac causes	3
5 Operation	
(a) Intraperitoneal, intrathoracic, or aortic operation	3
(b) Emergency operation	4
Total possible	53 points

To calculate a patient's score, the number of points from all factors he or she possesses are summed. MI, myocardial infarction; JVD, jugular vein distention; VAS, valvular aortic stenosis; PACs, premature atrial contractions; ECG, electrocardiogram; PVCs, premature ventricular contractions; Po_2, partial pressure of oxygen; Pco_2, partial pressure of carbon dioxide; K, potassium; HCO_3, bicarbonate; BUN, blood urea nitrogen; Cr, creatinine; and SGOT, serum glutamic oxalacetic transaminase.

Reprinted by permission from Goldman, L., et al.: Multifactorial index of cardiac risk in noncardiac surgical procedures. N. Engl. J. Med. *297*:845, 1977.

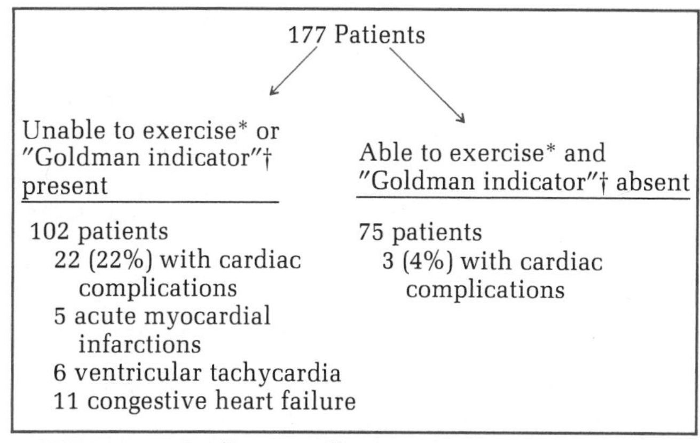

FIGURE 55-1. Cardiac complications in patients over age 65 having intraperitoneal or intrathoracic surgery.[43,44] *Ability to exercise = ability to pedal a supine bicycle for at least 2 minutes to a heart rate of ≥100; †Goldman indicator = factor on cardiac risk index[28] other than age or type of operation. (Data from Gerson, M.C., et al.: Prediction of cardiac and pulmonary complications related to elective abdominal and noncardiac thoracic surgery in geriatric patients. Am. J. Med. *88*:101, 1990.)

mia, hypovolemia, polycythemia, pulmonary disease causing hypoxemia, adrenal hyporesponsiveness secondary to long-term administration of adrenal steroids, hypertension, electrolyte abnormalities, as well as the entire gamut of cardiac arrhythmias. Considerable judgment must be exercised when one or more of the above-mentioned problems are present and when a patient requires prompt surgical treatment but the situation is not a true emergency, as for neoplastic disease.

To identify those preoperative factors associated with the development of cardiac complications after major noncardiac operation in patients over 40 years of age, one analysis[20] identified nine independently significant correlates of life-threatening and fatal cardiac complications. When these factors were weighted based on their relative significance as predictors of cardiac outcome, a multifactorial index was developed for predicting perioperative risk (Table 55-2). Notably, *unimportant* factors included smoking, glucose intolerance, hyperlipidemia, hypertension, peripheral atherosclerotic vascular disease, stable Class I or II angina, and remote myocardial infarction.

The value of the information in this index has been confirmed in two large prospective series of general surgical patients[33,34] (Table 55-3) and in several other studies.[21,43,105,111-113] In one series,[34] risk stratification was equally good when several minor modifications were made in point assignment and when a prior history of Class III or IV angina, unstable angina, and pulmonary edema was included in the index.

However, because the index was derived from unselected general surgical patients above age 40, it appears to underestimate risk by about 40 per cent in patients who undergo resection of an abdominal aortic aneurysm,[30] and it also underestimates risk in patients who are selected on the basis of any high-risk status. One way to take into account the fact that some patients have higher baseline risks is to know the baseline probability of cardiac complications for specific types of patients or types of surgery and then to modify these "pretest" probabilities on the basis of the patient's cardiac condition.[34,113-115] As shown in Table 55-4, this can be a useful approach to estimating the risk of major cardiac complications. Even at its best, however, any index for predicting cardiac complications should be viewed as an aid and not as a crutch; it should supplement, not substitute for, clinical judgment.

TABLE 55-3 MAJOR COMPLICATION* RATES IN FOUR STUDIES THAT HAVE ANALYZED THE MULTIFACTORIAL CARDIAC RISK INDEX[18]

	GOLDMAN ET AL[28]	ZELDIN[33]	DETSKY ET AL.[34]†	JEFFREY ET AL[30]‡		
TYPE OF PATIENTS	UNSELECTED NONCARDIAC SURGERY ≥ 40 y.o.	UNSELECTED NONCARDIAC SURGERY ≥ 40 y.o.	PREOPERATIVE MEDICAL CONSULTATIONS	ABDOMINAL AORTIC ANEURYSM SURGERY	POOLED	POOLED LIKELIHOOD RATIO (Sensitivity/ 1-specificity)
Overall complication rate	58/1001 (6%)	35/1140 (3%)	27/268 (10%)	11/99 (11%)	131/2508 (5.2%)	
Complication rate by class						
Class I (0-5 points)†	5/537 (1%)	4/590 (1%)	8/134 (6%)	4/56 (7%)	21/1317 (1.6%)	.29
Class II (6-12 points)	21/316 (7%)	13/453 (3%)	6/85 (7%)	4/35 (11%)	44/889 (5%)	.94
Class III (13-25 points)	18/130 (14%)	11/74 (15%)	9/45 (20%)	3/8 (38%)	41/257 (16%)	3.4
Class IV (≥ 26 points)	14/18 (78%)	7/23 (30%)	4/4 (100%)	0	25/45 (56%)	22.7

* Documented myocardial infarction, cardiogenic pulmonary edema, ventricular tachycardia, or cardiac death.
† Actual unpublished numbers provided by Dr. Detsky.
‡ See Table 55-2 for calculation of point total.
From Goldman, L.: Multifactorial index of cardiac risk in noncardiac surgery: Ten-year status report. J. Cardiothorac. Anesth. *1*:237, 1987.

TABLE 55-4 ESTIMATION OF PROBABILITY OF CARDIAC COMPLICATIONS

TYPE OF PATIENT	APPROXIMATE BASELINE RISK (%)	APPROXIMATE RISK AS ADJUSTED USING MULTIFACTORIAL INDEX (%)[18]*			
		CLASS I	CLASS II	CLASS III	CLASS IV
Minor surgery	1	0.3	1	3	19
Unselected consecutive patients over age 40 who have major noncardiac surgery	4	1.2	4	12	48
Patients who have abdominal aortic aneurysm surgery or who are over age 40 and have medical consultations before major noncardiac surgery	10	3	10	30	75

*Calculated by multiplying the prior odds of complications by the likelihood ratio for each class; see Table 55-3.

From Goldman, L.: Multifactorial index of cardiac risk in noncardiac surgery: Ten-year status report. J. Cardiothorac. Anesth. *1*:237, 1987.

PREPARATION OF THE PATIENT FOR ANESTHESIA AND OPERATION

Careful preparation of the cardiac patient for operation may diminish the frequency and seriousness of intraoperative and postoperative complications. The medical consultant should, after appropriate discussion with the surgeon, be prepared to urge postponement or cancellation of an elective operation or to insist on sufficient time to institute any measures that are necessary to minimize risk. The consultant should attempt to be brief and to the point, and to provide a limited number of explicit, relevant suggestions.[116-118] The cardiological consultant should work closely with the anesthesiologist and the surgeon so that their talents may be combined to maximize the likelihood of a favorable outcome.

REFERENCES

ANESTHESIA

1. Breslow, M. J., Miller, C. F., and Rogers, M. (eds.): Perioperative Management. St. Louis, C. V. Mosby Co., 1990.
2. Mangano, D. T. (ed.): Perioperative Cardiac Assessment. Philadelphia, J. B. Lippincott Co., 1990.
3. Kaplan J. A. (ed.): Cardiac Anesthesia. Ed. 2. Orlando, Grune & Stratton, 1987.
4. Prys-Roberts, C., and Meloche, R.: Management of anesthesia in patients with hypertension or ischemic heart disease. Int. Anesthesiol. Clin. *18*:181, 1980.
5. Prys-Roberts, C., Meloche, R., and Foex, P.: Studies of anesthesia in relation to hypertension: I. Cardiovascular responses of treated and untreated patients. Br. J. Anaesth. *43*:1112, 1971.
6. Prys-Roberts, C., Foex, P., Greene, L. T., and Waterhouse, T. D.: Studies of anesthesia in relation to hypertension: IV. The effects of artificial ventilation on the circulation and pulmonary gas exchanges. Br. J. Anaesth. *44*:335, 1972.
7. Tarhan, S. (ed.): Cardiovascular Anesthesia and Postoperative Care. Chicago, Year Book Medical Publishers, 1982.
8. Rusy, B. F., and Komai, H.: Anesthetic depression of myocardial contractility: A review of possible mechanisms. Anesthesiology *67*:745, 1987.
9. Yeager, M. P., Glass, D. D., Neff, R. K., and Brinck-Johnsen, T.: Epidural anesthesia and analgesia in high-risk surgical patients. Anesthesiology *66*:729, 1987.
10. Scott, N. B., and Kehlet, H.: Regional anaesthesia and surgical morbidity. Br. J. Surg. *75*:299, 1988.
11. Yeager, M. P.: Regional anesthesia for the patient with heart disease. Pro: Regional anesthesia is preferable to general anesthesia for the patient with heart disease. J. Cardiothorac. Anesth. *3*:793, 1989.
12. Beattie, C.: Con: Regional anesthesia is not preferable to general anesthesia for the patient with heart disease. J. Cardiothorac. Anesth. *3*:797, 1989.
13. Saada, M., Duval, A. M., Bonnet, F., et al.: Abnormalities in myocardial segmental wall motion during lumbar epidural anesthesia. Anesthesiology *71*:26, 1989.
14. Breslow, M. J., Jordan, D. A., Christopherson, R., et al.: Epidural morphine decreases postoperative hypertension by attenuating sympathetic nervous system hyperactivity. JAMA *261*:3577, 1989.
15. Diebel, L. N., Lange, P. M., Schenider, F., et al.: Cardiopulmonary complications after major surgery: A role for epidural analgesia? Surgery *102*:660, 1987.
16. Mauney, R. M., Jr., Ebert, P. A., and Sabiston, D. C., Jr.: Postoperative myocardial infarction: A study of predisposing factors, diagnosis and mortality in a high risk group of surgical patients. Ann. Surg. *172*:497, 1970.
17. Steen, P.A., Tinker, J. H., and Tarhan, S.: Myocardial reinfarction after anesthesia and surgery. JAMA *239*:2566, 1978.
18. Goldman, L., and Caldera, D. L.: Risks of general anesthesia and elective surgery in the hypertensive patient. Anesthesiology *50*:285, 1979.
19. Charlson, M. E., MacKenzie, C. R., Gold, J. P., et al.: The preoperative and intraoperative hemodynamic predictors of postoperative myocardial infarction or ischemia in patients undergoing noncardiac surgery. Ann. Surg. *210*:637, 1989.
20. Goldman L., Caldera, D. L., Southwick, F. S., et al.: Cardiac risk factors and complications in non-cardiac surgery. Medicine *57*:357, 1978.
21. Kaplan J. A., and Dunbar, R. W.: Anesthesia for noncardiac surgery in patients with cardiac disease. *In* Kaplan, J. A. (ed.): Cardiac Anesthesia. Orlando, Grune & Stratton, 1979, p. 377.
22. Smith, J. S., Cahalan, M. K., Benefiel, D. J., et al.: Intraoperative detection of myocardial ischemia in high risk patients: Electrocardiography versus two-dimensional echocardiography. Circulation *72*:1015, 1985.
23. Van Daele, M. E. R. M., Sutherland, G. R., Mitchell, M. M., et al.: Do changes in pulmonary capillary wedge pressure adequately reflect myocardial ischemia during anesthesia? Circulation *81*:865, 1990.

THE OPERATION

24. Backer, C. L., Tinker, J. H., Robertson, D. M., and Vliestra, R. E.: Myocardial reinfarction following local anesthesia for ophthalmic surgery. Anest. Analg. *59*:257, 1980.
25. Erlik, D., Valero, A., Birkhan, J., and Gersh, I.: Prostatic surgery and the cardiovascular patient. Br. J. Urol. *40*:53, 1968.
26. Larsen, S. F., Olesen, K. H., Jacobsen, E., et al.: Prediction of cardiac risk in non-cardiac surgery. Eur. Heart J. *8*:179, 1987.
27. Knorring, J.: Postoperative myocardial infarction: A prospective study in a high-risk group of surgical patients. Surgery *90*:55, 1981.
28. Goldman, L., Caldera, D. L., Nussbaum, R. R., et al.: Multifactorial index of cardiac risk in noncardiac surgical procedures. N. Engl. J. Med. *297*:845, 1977.
29. Skinner, J. R., and Pearce, M. L.: Surgical risk in the cardiac patient. J. Chronic Dis. *17*:57, 1964.
30. Jeffrey, C. C., Kunsman, J., Cullen, D. J., and Brewster, D. C.: A prospective evaluation of cardiac risk index. Anesthesiology *58*:462, 1983.
31. Lewin, I., Lerner, A. G., Green, S. H., et al.: Physical class and physiological status in the prediction of operative mortality in the aged sick. Ann. Surg. *174*:217, 1971.
32. Rao, T. L. K., Jacobs, K. H., and El-Etr, A. A.: Reinfarction following anesthesia in patients with myocardial infarction. Anesthesiology *59*:499, 1983.

INFLUENCE OF UNDERLYING CARDIOVASCULAR DISEASE

33. Zeldin, R. A.: Assessing cardiac risk in patients who undergo noncardiac surgical procedures. Can. J. Surg. *27*:402, 1984.
34. Detsky, A. S., Abrams, H. B., McLaughlin, J. R., et al.: Predicting cardiac complications in patients undergoing non-cardiac surgery. J. Gen. Intern. Med. *1*:211, 1986.
35. Shah, K., Kleinman, B., Rao, T., et al.: Reduction in mortality from cardiac causes in Goldman class IV patients. J. Cardiothorac. Anesth. *2*:789, 1988.
36. Wells, P. H., and Kaplan, J. A.: Optimal management of patients with ischemic heart disease for noncardiac surgery by complementary anesthesiologist and cardiologist interaction. Am. Heart J. *102*:1029, 1981.
37. DeBusk, R. F., Blomqvist, C. G., Kouchoukos, N. T., et al.: Identification and treatment of low-risk patients after acute myocardial infarction and coronary-artery bypass graft surgery. N. Engl. J. Med. *314*:161, 1983.
38. Campeau, L.: Grading of angina pectoris. Circulation *54*:522, 1975.
39. Goldman, L., Hashimoto, B., Cook, E. F., and Loscalzo, A.: Comparative reproducibility and validity of systems for assessing cardiovascular functional class: Advantages of a new Specific Activity Scale. Circulation *64*:1227, 1981.
40. Goldman, L., Cook, E. F., Mitchell, N., et al.: Pitfalls in the serial assessment of cardiac functional status. J. Chronic Dis. *35*:763, 1982.
41. McPhail, N., Calvin, J. E., Shariatmadar, A., et al.: The use of preoperative exercise testing to predict cardiac complications after arterial reconstruction. J. Vasc. Surg. *7*:60, 1988.

42. Cutler, B. S., Wheeler, H. B., Paraskos, J. A., and Cardullo, P. A.: Applicability and interpretation of electrocardiographic stress testing in patients with peripheral vascular disease. Am. J. Surg. *141*:501, 1981.
43. Gerson, M. C., Hurst, J. M., Hertzberg, V. S., et al.: Cardiac prognosis in noncardiac geriatric surgery. Ann. Intern. Med. *103*:832, 1985.
44. Gerson, M. C., Hurst, J. M., Hertzberg, V. S., et al.: Prediction of cardiac and pulmonary complications related to elective abdominal and noncardiac thoracic surgery in geriatric patients. Am. J. Med. *88*:101, 1990.
45. Pasternack, P. F., Imparato, A. M., Riles, T. S., et al.: The value of the radionuclide angiogram in the prediction of perioperative myocardial infarction in patients undergoing lower extremity revascularization procedures. Circulation 72 (Suppl. 2):13, 1985.
46. Franco, C. D., Goldsmith, J., Veith, F. J., et al.: Resting gated pool ejection fraction: A poor predictor of perioperative myocardial infarction in patients undergoing vascular surgery for infrainguinal bypass grafting. J. Vasc. Surg. *10*:656, 1989.
47. McCann, R. L., and Wolfe, W. G.: Resection of abdominal aortic aneurysm in patients with low ejection fractions. J. Vasc. Surg. *10*:240, 1989.
48. Kazmers, A., Cerqueira, M. D., and Zierler, R. E.: The role of preoperative radionuclide ejection fraction in direct abdominal aortic aneurysm repair. J. Vasc. Surg. *8*:128, 1988.
49. Raby, K. E., Goldman, L., Creager, M. A., et al.: Correlation between preoperative ischemia and major cardiac events after peripheral vascular surgery. N. Engl. J. Med. *321*:1296, 1989.
50. Pasternack, P. F., Grossi, E. A., Baumann, F. G., et al.: The value of silent myocardial ischemia monitoring in the prediction of perioperative myocardial infarction in patients undergoing peripheral vascular surgery. J. Vasc. Surg. *10*:617, 1989.
50a. Mangano, D. T., Browner, W. S., Hollenberg, M., et al.: Association of perioperative myocardial ischemia with cardiac morbidity and mortality in men undergoing noncardiac surgery. N. Engl. J. Med. *323*:1781, 1990.
50b. Mangano, D. T., Hollenberg, M., Fegert, G., et al.: Perioperative myocardial ischemia in patients undergoing noncardiac surgery—I. Incidence and severity during the 4 day perioperative period. J. Am. Coll. Cardiol. *17*:843, 1991.
50c. Mangano, D. T., Wong, M. G., London, M. J., et al.: Perioperative myocardial ischemia in patients undergoing noncardiac surgery—II. Incidence and severity during the first week after surgery. J. Am. Coll. Cardiol. *17*:851, 1991.
51. Boucher, C. A., Brewster, D. C., Darling, R. C., et al.: Determination of cardiac risk by dipyridamole-thallium imaging before peripheral vascular surgery. N. Engl. J. Med. *312*:389, 1985.
52. Leppo, J., Plaja, J., Gionet, M., et al.: Noninvasive evaluation of cardiac risk before elective vascular surgery. J. Am. Coll. Cardiol. *9*:269, 1987.
53. Eagle, K. A., Coley, C. M., Newell, J. B., et al.: Combining clinical and thallium data optimizes preoperative assessment of cardiac risk before major vascular surgery. Ann. Intern. Med. *110*:859, 1989.
54. Lette, J., Waters, D., Lapointe, J. et al.: Usefulness of the severity and extent of reversible perfusion defects during thallium-dipyridamole imaging for cardiac risk assessment before noncardiac surgery. Am. J. Cardiol. *64*:276, 1989.
55. McPhail, N. V., Ruddy, T. D., Calvin, J. E., et al.: A comparison of dipyridamole-thallium imaging and exercise testing in the prediction of postoperative cardiac complications in patients requiring arterial reconstruction. J. Vasc. Surg. *10*:51, 1989.
56. Marwick, T. H., and Underwood, D. A.: Dipyridamole thallium imaging may not be a reliable screening test for coronary artery disease in patients undergoing vascular surgery. Clin. Cardiol. *13*:14, 1990.
57. Foster, E. D., Davis, K. B., Carpenter, J. A., et al.: Risk of noncardiac operation in patients with defined coronary disease: The Coronary Artery Surgery Study (CASS) registry experience. Ann. Thorac. Surg. *41*:42, 1986.
58. Weitz, H. H., and Goldman, L.: Noncardiac surgery in the patient with heart disease. Med. Clin. North Am. *71*:413, 1987.
59. Freeman, W. K., Gibbons, R. J., and Shub, C.: Preoperative assessment of cardiac patients undergoing noncardiac surgical procedures. Mayo Clin. Proc. *64*:1105, 1989.
60. Deron, S. J., and Kotler, M. N.: Noncardiac surgery in the cardiac patient. Am. Heart J. *116*:831, 1988.
61. McPhail, N., Menkis, A., Shariatmader, A., et al.: Statistical prediction of cardiac risk in patients who undergo vascular surgery. Can. J. Surg. *28*:404, 1985.
62. Lunder, T., Lindegaard, K. F., Froysaker, T., et al.: Cerebral perfusion during nonpulsatile cardiopulmonary bypass. Ann. Thorac. Surg. *40*:144, 1985.
63. Jones, E. L., Craver, J. M., Michalik, R. A., et al.: Combined carotid and coronary operations: When are they necessary? J. Thorac. Cardiovasc. Surg. *87*:7, 1984.
64. Hertzer, N. R., Loop, F. D., Beven, E. G., et al.: Surgical staging for simultaneous coronary and carotid disease: A study including prospective randomization. J. Vasc. Surg. *9*:455, 1989.
65. Matar, A. F.: Concomitant coronary and cerebral revascularization under cardiopulmonary bypass. Ann. Thorac. Surg. *41*:431, 1986.
66. Viljoen, J. F., Estafanous, G., and Kellner, G. A.: Propranolol and cardiac surgery. J. Thorac. Cardiovasc. Surg. *64*:826, 1972.
67. Should propranolol be stopped before surgery? Med. Lett. *18*:41, 1976.
68. Goldman, L.: Noncardiac surgery in patients receiving propranolol. Case reports and a recommended approach. Arch. Intern. Med. *141*:193, 1981.
69. Prys-Roberts, C., Foex, P., and Roberts, J. G.: Studies of anaesthesia in relation to hypertension. Br. J. Anaesth. *45*:671, 1973.
70. Prys-Roberts, C.: Hemodynamic effects of anesthesia and surgery in renal hypertensive patients receiving large does of beta-receptor antagonists. Anesthesiology *51* (Suppl.):122, 1979.
71. Woolsey, R. L., and Shand, D. G.: Pharmacokinetics of antiarrhythmic drugs. Am. J. Cardiol. *41*:986, 1978.
72. Smulyan, H., Weinberg, S. E., and Howanitz, P. J.: Continuous propranolol infusion following abdominal surgery. JAMA *247*:2539, 1982.
73. Reves, J. G., and Flezzani, P.: Perioperative use of esmolol. Am. J. Cardiol. *56*:57F, 1985.
74. Prys-Roberts, C.: Hypertension and anesthesia—fifty years on. Anesthesiology *50*:281, 1979.
75. Tarazi, R. C., Dustan, H. P., and Frohlich, E. D.: Long-term thiazide therapy in essential hypertension. Evidence for persistent alteration in plasma volume and renin activity. Circulation *41*:709, 1970.
76. Bruce, D. L., Croley, T. F., and Lee, J. S.: Preoperative clonidine withdrawal syndrome. Anesthesiology *51*:90, 1979.
77. Orlowski, J. P., Vidt, D. G., Walker, S., and Haluska, J. F.: The hemodynamic effects of intravenous labetalol for postoperative hypertension. Cleve. Clin. J. Med. *56*:29, 1989.
78. O'Keefe, J. H., Shub, C., and Rettke, S. R.: Risk of noncardiac surgical procedures in patients with aortic stenosis. Mayo Clin. Proc. *64*:400, 1989.
79. Stone, J. G., Hoar, P. F., Calabro, J. R., et al.: Afterload reduction and preload augmentation improve the anesthetic management of patients with cardiac failure and valvular regurgitation. Anesth. Analg. *59*:737, 1980.
80. Hayes, S. N., Holmes, D. R., Jr., Nishimura, R. A., and Reeder, G. S.: Palliative percutaneous aortic balloon valvuloplasty before noncardiac operations and invasive diagnostic procedures. Mayo Clin. Proc. *64*:753, 1989.
81. Thompson, R. C., Liberthson, R. R., and Lowenstein, E.: Perioperative anesthetic risk of noncardiac surgery in hypertrophic obstructive cardiomyopathy. JAMA *254*:2419, 1985.
82. Tinker, J. H., and Tarhan, S.: Discontinuing anticoagulant therapy in surgical patients with cardiac valve prostheses. JAMA *239*:738, 1978.
83. Katholi, R. E., Nolan, S. P., and McGuire, L. B.: Living with prosthetic heart valve. Subsequent noncardiac operations and the risk of thromboembolism or hemorrhage. Am. Heart J. *92*:162, 1976.
84. Tinker, J. H., Noback, C. R., Vliestra, R. E., and Frye, R. L.: Management of patients with heart disease for noncardiac surgery. JAMA *246*:1348, 1981.
85. Eckman, M. H., Beshansky, J. R., Durand-Zaleski, I., et al.: Anticoagulation for noncardiac procedures in patients with prosthetic heart valves. JAMA *263*:1513, 1990.
86. Simmons, N. A.: Antibiotic prophylaxis of infective endocarditis. Lancet *335*:88, 1990.
87. Millard, H. D., Sanders, W. E., Schwartz, R. H., and Watanakunakorn, C.: Prevention of bacterial endocarditis. A statement for health professionals by the Committee on Rheumatic Fever and Infective Endocarditis of the Council on Cardiovascular Disease in the Young. Circulation *70*:1123A, 1984.
88. Clemens, J. D., Horwitz, R. I., Jaffe, C. C., et al.: A controlled evaluation of the risk of bacterial endocarditis in persons with mitral-valve prolapse. N. Engl. J. Med. *307*:776, 1982.
89. Bor, D. H., and Himmelstein, D. U.: Endocarditis prophylaxis for patients with mitral valve prolapse. Am. J. Med. *76*:711, 1984.
90. Clemens, J. D., and Ransohoff, D. F.: A quantitative assessment of predental antibiotic prophylaxis for patients with mitral valve prolapse. J. Chronic Dis. *37*:531, 1984.
91. Sommerville, J., McDonald, L., and Edgill, M.: Postoperative haemorrhage and related abnormalities of blood coagulation in cyanotic congenital heart disease. Br. Heart J. *27*:440, 1965.
92. Hickey, P.R., Hansen, D. D., Norwood, W. I., and Castaneda, A. R.: Anesthetic complications in surgery for congenital heart disease. Anesth. Analg. *63*:657, 1984.
93. Goldberg, A. H., Maling, H. M., and Gaffney, T. E.: The value of prophylactic digitalization in halothane anesthesia. Anesthesiology *23*:207, 1962.
94. Lee, D. C., Johnson, R. A., Bingham, J. B., et al.: Heart failure in outpatients. A randomized trial of digoxin versus placebo. N. Engl. J. Med. *306*:699, 1982.
95. Schulze, R. A., Jr., Rouleau, J., Rigo, P., et al.: Ventricular arrhythmias in the late hospital phase of acute myocardial infarction: Relation to left ventricular function detected by gated cardiac blood pool scanning. Circulation *52*:1006, 1975.
96. Schulze, R. A., Jr., Strauss, H. W., and Pitt, B.: Sudden death in the year following myocardial infarction: Relation to ventricular premature contractions in the late hospital phase and left ventricular ejection fraction. Am. J. Med. *62*:192, 1977.
97. Kennedy, H. L., Whitlock, J. A., Sprague, M. K., et al.: Long-term follow-up of asymptomatic healthy subjects with frequent and complex ventricular ectopy. N. Engl. J. Med. *312*:193, 1985.
98. Bergh, N. P., Dottori, O., and Malmberg, R.: Prophylactic digitalis in thoracic surgery. Scand. J. Resp. Dis. *48*:197, 1967.
99. Pastore, J. O., Yurchak, P. M., Janis, K. M., et al.: The risk of advanced heart block in surgical patients with right bundle branch block and left axis deviation. Circulation *57*:677, 1978.
100. Frye, R. L., Collins, J. J., DeSanctis, R. W., et al.: Guidelines for permanent cardiac pacemaker implantation, May 1984. A report of the Joint Amer-

ican College of Cardiology/American Heart Association Task Force on Assessment of Cardiovascular Procedures (Subcommittee on Pacemaker Implantation). J. Am. Coll. Cardiol. *4*:434, 1984.

101. Pasulka, P. S., Bistrian, B. R., Benotti, P. N., and Blackburn, G. L.: The risks of surgery in obese patients. Ann. Intern. Med. *104*:540, 1986.

POSTOPERATIVE COMPLICATIONS

102. Raby, K. E., Goldman, L., Creager, M. E., and Selwyn, A. P.: Detection of intraoperative and postoperative myocardial ischemia in peripheral vascular surgery (abstract). Circulation *78*:(Suppl. 2):333, 1988.

103. Ouyang, P., Gerstenblith, G., Furman, W. R., et al.: Frequency and significance of early postoperative silent myocardial ischemia in patients having peripheral vascular surgery. Am. J. Cardiol. *64*:1113, 1989.

104. Salem, D. N., Homans, D. C., and Isner, J. M.: Management of cardiac disease in the general surgical patient. *In* Harvey, W. P. (ed.): Current Problems in Cardiology. Vol. 5. Chicago, Year Book Medical Publishers, 1980.

105. Charlson, M. E., MacKenzie, C. R., Ales, K. L., et al.: Surveillance for postoperative myocardial infarction after noncardiac operations. Surg. Gynecol. Obstet. *167*:407, 1988.

106. Charlson, M. E., MacKenzie, C. R., Ales, K. L., et al.: The post-operative electrocardiogram and creatine kinase: Implications for diagnosis of myocardial infarction after non-cardiac surgery. J. Clin. Epidemiol. *42*:25, 1989.

107. Lee, T. H., and Goldman, L.: Serum enzyme assays in the diagnosis of acute myocardial infarction. Recommendations based on a quantitative analysis. Ann. Intern. Med. *105*:221, 1986.

108. Oster, G., Tuden, R. L., and Colditz, G. A.: Prevention of venous thromboembolism after general surgery. Cost-effectiveness analysis of alternative approaches to prophylaxis. Am. J. Med. *82*:889, 1987.

109. Goldman, L.: Anesthesia and surgery in the hypertensive patient. *In* Amery, A. (ed.): Hypertensive Cardiovascular Disease: Pathophysiology and Treatment. The Hague, Martinus Nijhoff Publishing, 1982, p. 916.

110. Goldman, L.: Supraventricular tachyarrhythmias in hospitalized adults after surgery. Chest *73*:450, 1978.

THE ROLE OF THE MEDICAL CONSULTATION

111. Weathers, L. W., and Paine R.: The risk of surgery in cardiac patients. Intern. Med. *2*:57, 1981.

112. Perry, M. O., and Calcagno, D.: Abdominal aortic aneurysm surgery: The basic evaluation of cardiac risk. Ann. Surg. *208*:738, 1988.

113. Rivers, S. P., Scher, L. A., Gupta,S. K., and Veith, F. J.: Safety of peripheral vascular surgery after recent acute myocardial infarction. J. Vasc. Surg. *11*:70, 1990.

114. Detsky, A. S., Abrams, H. B., Forbath, N., et al.: Cardiac assessment for patients undergoing noncardiac surgery. A multifactorial clinical risk index. Arch. Intern. Med. *146*:2131, 1986.

115. Goldman, L.: Multifactorial index of cardiac risk in noncardiac surgery: Ten-year status report. J. Cardiothorac. Anesth. *1*:237, 1987.

116. Lee, T., Pappius, E. M., and Goldman, L.: Impact of inter-physician communication on the effectiveness of medical consultations. Am. J. Med. *74*:106, 1983.

117. Horwitz, R. I., Henes, C. G., and Horwitz, S. M.: Strategies for improving the diagnostic and management efficacy of medical consultations. J. Chronic Dis. *36*:213, 1983.

118. Lee, T. H., and Goldman, L.: Role of consultant. *In* Breslow, M. J., Mullen, C. F., and Rogers, M. (eds.): Perioperative Management. St. Louis, C. V. Mosby Co., 1990.

Rheumatic Fever and Other Rheumatic Diseases of the Heart

by GENE H. STOLLERMAN, M.D.

Two groups of diseases that affect connective tissues are the so-called rheumatic diseases and the heritable disorders of connective tissues. The *rheumatic diseases* have many clinical features in common and are often classified together because they produce acute or chronic arthritis, or both, associated with a variety of systemic inflammatory manifestations. Pathologically, they are characterized by diffuse vascular lesions with varying degrees of exudation and fibrosis, and some seem to be associated with hyperimmune phenomena. In some of the syndromes the etiology has been established as complications of well-recognized infections; however, several of the rheumatic diseases remain obscure in regard to both etiology and pathogenesis. They all involve the heart differently and to varying degrees, as would be expected considering the variety of connective tissue structures that make up the heart's "skeleton"—its valve rings, valves, septa, and pericardial sac and the myocardial interstitium, through which courses its rich blood supply.

The *heritable disorders of connective tissue* are rare, genetically determined biochemical lesions of collagen, elastic tissue, or the mucopolysaccharides. In all, structural lesions are produced when cardiac action stresses the defective cardiac skeleton. These conditions are presented in Chapter 51.

Rheumatic Fever

Rheumatic fever (RF) is frequently classified as a connective tissue disease because its anatomical hallmark is damage to collagen fibrils and to the ground substance of connective tissue (especially in the heart). Of major clinical importance is the presence of potentially lethal myocarditis during the acute attack or, more commonly, the fibrosis of the heart valves, which leads to the crippling hemodynamics of chronic rheumatic heart disease. Its uniqueness from other rheumatic diseases is that it is specifically a delayed nonsuppurative sequel of pharyngeal infection with group A streptococci.

EPIDEMIOLOGY

The relation between the epidemiology of RF and that of streptococcal infection has been reviewed extensively.[1] The current confusion concerning the epidemiology of RF stems from the dramatic decline in incidence and prevalence of the disease despite the fact that group A streptococcal pharyngitis still appears to be common among populations in which RF has become rare.[2] In recent years, focal outbreaks of RF in military and civilian populations in the United States have been found to correlate with the reappearance of virulent, encapsulated, M protein–rich strains belonging to M-serotypes previously noted to be associated with epidemic rheumatic fever, and thus referred to as "rheumatogenic" group A streptococci.[3]

THE CHANGING PATTERN OF RHEUMATIC FEVER

(Fig. 56–1)

Reasons for the spectacular decline in RF in the 60's, 70's, and early 80's are undoubtedly multiple. Certainly antibiotics for the treatment and prevention of streptococcal infection have been a factor, as demonstrated particularly in military populations.[4,5] However, the incidence and death rate from the disease were decreasing before the introduction of antibiotics. Changes in the virulence and serotypes of group A streptococci have been most noteworthy[3] (see below). Improved social conditions, such as better housing and slum clearance, have contributed to the decline, since crowding because of inadequate housing is probably the chief reason for the magnified risk of streptococcal infection and acute rheumatic fever (ARF) in certain ethnic and disadvantaged populations. Improvement in the delivery of health care in defined populations may also be significant.[6]

Notwithstanding its decline, rheumatic heart disease still

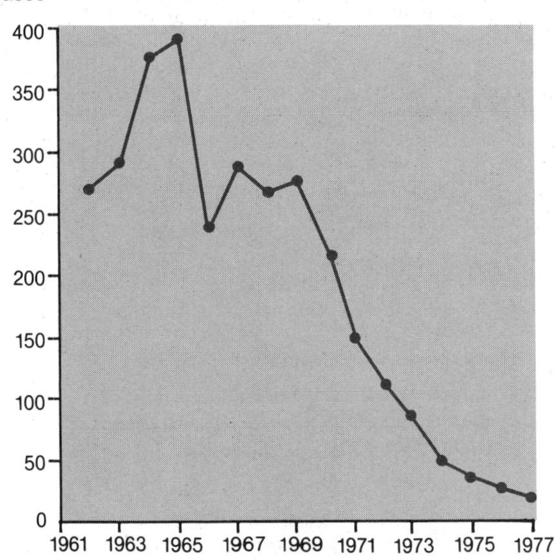

FIGURE 56-1. Acute rheumatic fever attacks reported from 1962 to 1977 to the rheumatic fever registry of the Chicago Department of Health. (From Stollerman, G. H.: Global changes in group A streptococcal diseases and strategies for their prevention. Adv. Intern. Med. 27:373, 1982.)

constitutes the leading cause of death from heart disease in the 5- to 24-year-old age group in many parts of the world and continues to be a serious public health problem, particularly in the slums of the industrializing nations of the Third World.[6-8] The surprising reappearance of outbreaks of RF associated with concomitant reappearance of highly virulent group A streptococcal strains (Fig. 56-2) has made the need for intensified treatment and prevention of streptococcal pharyngeal infection compelling, especially in individuals with rheumatic heart disease (see below, "Prevention").

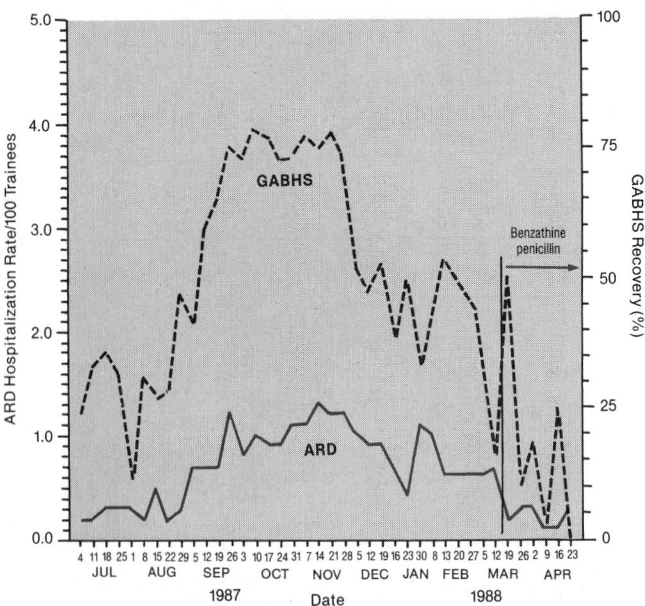

FIGURE 56-2. Hospitalization for acute respiratory disease (ARD, left ordinate) and present recovery of group A streptococci (GABHS, upper curve, right ordinates) among army trainees at Fort Leonard Wood, Missouri, plotted for July 1987 to April 1988. Thirteen cases of ARF were diagnosed between October 1987 and February 1988. No new cases had been reported since the second week of March when benzathine penicillin G was given once to all nonallergic soldiers and thereafter to all new trainees on arrival at the base (From Centers for Disease Control: Acute rheumatic fever among army trainees—Ft Leonard Wood, MO, 1987-1988. MMWR *37*:519, 1988.)

FACTORS IN THE ATTACK RATE OF RHEUMATIC FEVER

QUANTITATIVE FACTORS. One factor is the severity of the antecedent pharyngeal streptococcal infection. The clearest relationship of group A streptococcal infection to RF is found in military populations subject to epidemic streptococcal sore throat. In patients with frank, exudative streptococcal pharyngitis caused by rheumatogenic strains of virulent group A streptococci, RF followed at a fairly predictable attack rate (approximately 3 per cent) regardless of the age, race, or ethnic group studied and regardless of the year or season in which the study was made.[4] The major variables which seem to be related to this attack rate in such studies are the magnitude of the immune response to the antecedent streptococcal infection[9] and the duration of convalescent carriage of the organism.[10] Weak antistreptolysin O (ASO) responses are associated with ARF attack rates considerably less than 1 per cent, whereas strong responses are associated with rates well in excess of 5 per cent. If the infecting organism in the pharynx was not eradicated during convalescence, treatment of streptococcal pharyngitis failed to reduce the attack rate of rheumatic fever.

In contrast to the military studies, reports from civilian medical practice indicate that RF occurs less frequently or not at all following endemic, sporadic streptococcal disease.[3,11-14]

VARIATION IN GROUP A STREPTOCOCCAL INFECTIONS. Variations in the rheumatogenicity of group A streptococcal strains are a factor influencing the attack rate of RF.[3] In several laboratories where regular serotyping of group A streptococci isolated from pharyngeal infections is performed with available antisera prepared against known M-protein serotypes, the frequency of identification of such strains has decreased. Furthermore, the prevalence of several of the virulent M types notorious for causing epidemic RF (e.g., types 5, 14, and 24) has apparently declined, and attention has shifted to the study of "new" M types among both pharyngeal strains and "skin" strains.[2,15] The issue of whether there are "nonrheumatogenic group A streptococci"[16] has been sharpened by the clear demonstration that group A streptococcal pyoderma, with or without complicating acute glomerulonephritis (AGN), does not cause ARF.[17] These skin infections are nonrheumatogenic. Since the pharyngeal route of infection is now an accepted requirement for the pathogenesis of ARF[18] (see below), the question of whether such pyoderma strains can cause RF when they produce pharyngitis is of particular interest. Studies in the southwestern United States have clearly shown seasonal epidemiological separation of ARF and AGN.[19] A study of the streptococcal strains in an island population such as Trinidad shows a clear distinction between the serotypes associated with AGN and those associated with ARF.[20,21] In the past, several studies suggested that RF was associated with infections due to virulent encapsulated ("mucoid") strains capable of causing strong type-specific immune responses to M protein and other streptococcal antigens. Such strains belong to the classic M serotypes known to cause ARF.[22,23] The reappearance of severe epidemic rheumatic fever associated with the reappearance of these virulent strains has greatly strengthened the concept of rheumatogenic strains of group A streptococci.[3] Thus, qualitative and quantitative changes in streptococcal pharyngitis have affected greatly the epidemiology of rheumatic fever in various parts of the world.

GEOGRAPHY AND CLIMATE. The relationship of RF to the intensity and severity of streptococcal disease is the same in the tropics as in the temperate climates.[24] In *prospective* studies in which all patients suspected of having ARF were admitted and recurrent attacks were excluded, the frequency of the clinical manifestations of rheumatic fever is the same as in the studies in the United States.[25,26]

Host Factors

AGE, SEX, AND RACE. Like streptococcal sore throat, ARF occurs most commonly in the young school-age child, median age between 9 and 11 years, and very rarely in early infancy. It is estimated that 40 per cent of streptococcal infections in pediatric populations occur in children 2 to 6 years of age, suggesting that repeated streptococcal infections and early sensitization of the host are prerequisite to the development of RF. No true differences in sex, race, or ethnic group susceptibility have been established. Crowded living conditions account for whatever apparent increased susceptibility has been reported.

ACQUIRED SUSCEPTIBILITY. Because ARF develops in only a relatively small percentage of patients following even the most virulent bouts of streptococcal pharyngitis, the question of host predisposition is often raised. Once RF is acquired, its activation following subsequent streptococcal infection is many times greater in rheumatic subjects than in the general population. The recurrence rate per infection, which is as high as 50 per cent during the first year after the initial attack, decreases sharply until 4 to 5 years after the attack.[27,28] It then levels off at approximately 10 per cent and does not seem to fall much lower.[29] Although the persistently high attack rate in individuals having had RF suggests genetic predisposition (see below), the diminishing recurrence rate per infection also suggests loss of acquired hyperreactivity. An alternative explanation may be acquired sensitization in a genetically predisposed host that persists throughout life.

GENETIC FACTORS. Many investigators have sought genetic markers for rheumatic hosts without more than suggestive results.[30] Only a few adequate studies in identical twins have been made and these have shown a relatively low concordance of RF (less than 20 per cent), actually considerably lower than the concordance found in identical twins with other infectious diseases such as tuberculosis or poliomyelitis.[1,30] No clear correlation of conventional HLA genotypes with rheumatic fever has yet been shown. In contrast, non-HLA B cell alloantigens have been found to be expressed more frequently in rheumatic fever probands than in their unaffected siblings and parents.[31-33] Thus, these B cell alloantigens are not unique to the rheumatic hosts but may be more expressible in them if they are stimulated by putative rheumatogenic antigens of group A streptococci (see below). The uniqueness of the group A streptococcus in initiating a cardiodestructive disease in a limited segment of the human species, regardless of race or ethnic group, continues to make the quest for a unique host response to a specific streptococcal antigen a persisting challenge, particularly for investigators interested in autoimmunity.[34]

ETIOLOGY

The lines of evidence establishing the group A streptococcus as the sole agent causing initial and recurrent attacks of RF (described below) are of necessity indirect, because group A streptococci cannot be recovered from the lesions of RF and no satisfactory experimental model of the disease has been demonstrated.

CLINICAL EVIDENCE. Although the frequency with which septic sore throat preceded ARF has been recognized for over 100 years, inconsistencies in this relationship have been pointed out repeatedly.[1] Almost one-third of patients with ARF deny the occurrence of antecedent sore throat. Throat and blood cultures in such patients show that the former is frequently negative and the latter virtually always sterile at the onset of the rheumatic attack. Recurrences of RF appeared even more mysterious when antecedent streptococcal sore throat was unrecognized and particularly when the chronicity of a rheumatic attack and the hemodynamic complications of rheumatic heart disease made it difficult to distinguish continued versus reactivated rheumatic carditis. On clinical grounds alone, therefore, it is difficult to establish the group A streptococcus as the *sole* etiological agent.

EPIDEMIOLOGICAL EVIDENCE. Such factors as latitude, altitude, crowding, dampness, economic factors, and age all affect the incidence of RF because they are related to the incidence and severity of streptococcal infections in general (see above). Careful epidemiological studies over a period of 20 years show a clear sequential relationship between outbreaks of streptococcal pharyngitis and RF.

IMMUNOLOGICAL EVIDENCE. Initial (primary) or recurrent (secondary) RF does not occur without a streptococcal antibody response.[35] Furthermore, the magnitude of the antibody response is a major variable determining the attack rate (but not the severity or duration) of RF following streptococcal pharyngitis.[9] This is true for both primary and secondary attacks.[27] Indeed, the streptococcal immune response is an important criterion for the diagnosis of RF (see below).

PROPHYLACTIC EVIDENCE. The final and perhaps most convincing evidence is the prevention of both initial and recurrent attacks of RF by, in the former case, penicillin therapy and, in the latter, continuous chemoprophylaxis against streptococcal infections. Completely effective prophylaxis of streptococcal infections in rheumatic subjects allows us to conclude that RF cannot be reactivated by any other infection, illness, or trauma.[27,35]

PATHOGENESIS

Despite the elusiveness of the pathogenesis of RF, there are a few well-established requirements for the development of this postinfectious sequel: (1) the presence of the group A streptococcus, (2) a streptococcal antibody response indicative of actual recent infection, (3) persistence of the organism in the pharynx for a sufficient period, and (4) location of the infection in the throat.

THE ROLE OF TOXINS. Despite the popularity of the concepts of hyperimmunity and autoimmunity in the pathogenesis of RF (see below), none of the antibodies described to date, including those reactive with the heart, has been shown to be cytotoxic. A direct toxic effect, therefore, of some streptococcal product, particularly on the heart, has not yet been ruled out as a pathogenetic mechanism.[1]

IMMUNOLOGICAL THEORIES

The most popular pathogenic theory is that RF results from some type of hyperimmune reaction due either to bacterial allergy or autoimmunity. This view is supported by strong evidence, since RF patients are, in general, the population most intensively hyperimmune to all streptococcal products.

The mean antibody titer to virtually every streptococcal antigen that has been studied is increased in patients during the acute stage of RF.[1] Yet no single humoral mechanism of tissue injury has been defined. Complement levels are increased rather than decreased, and autoantibodies associated with immune complex disease (e.g., rheumatoid factor, anti-DNA, and others) are not present. Although low-grade microscopic hematuria may occur, frank lesions of glomerulonephritis are absent. Careful studies have identified circulating immune complexes, but they are of small size and not high titer and quickly disappear after the acute stage of polyarthritis.[36]

AUTOIMMUNITY. Modern theories of the possible autoimmune pathogenetic mechanisms of RF have been extensively reviewed.[34,37] It has been known for many years that the serum of some patients with ARF contains autoantibodies to heart tissues, and numerous reports using a variety of techniques, mostly immunofluorescence, have confirmed this finding.[38-40] Antiheart antibodies are gamma globulins with specificity for cardiac components reacting primarily with the sarcolemma. Their binding is also associated with deposition of large amounts of complement component C3.

CROSS-REACTIVE ANTIBODIES AND AUTOIMMUNITY. In the early 1960's Kaplan and his associates demonstrated that rabbit antisera against certain group A streptococci react with human heart preparations in the immunofluorescent test.[40,41] Since then, many additional immunological cross reactions have been described between streptococci and human tissues[42-47] (Fig. 56–3). The immunological details of these reactions and their possible relation to the pathogenesis of RF[1,34,37] are summarized below.

Group A streptococci have a number of structural components that are related to mammalian tissues.[1] The hyaluronate capsule of the organism, for example, is identical with human hyaluronate. Antibodies to the group A cell wall polysaccharide cross-react with glycoproteins of heart valves.[43] Membrane antigens of group A streptococci cross-react with sarcolemma and smooth muscle of endocardial and myocardial arteries.[42]

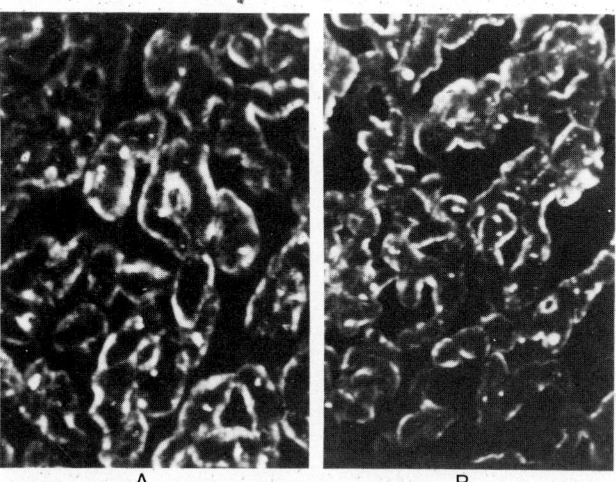

FIGURE 56–3. Immunofluorescent staining patterns of cryostat sections of heart tissue stained with sera containing heart-reactive antibody. *A,* The pattern obtained with a serum sample from a patient with acute rheumatic fever. *B,* The pattern seen with serum from a rabbit immunized with group A streptococcal membranes. (From Zabriskie, J. B.: Rheumatic fever. The interplay between host, genetics, and microbe. Circulation *71*:1077, 1985, by permission of the American Heart Association, Inc.)

Antibodies that are of specific interest for their potential relationship to autoimmune injury of the heart are those absorbable by streptococcal products. A sustained rise in titer of antibodies that cross-react with the cardiac tissue often precedes an attack of RF, but such antibodies do not correlate clearly with the presence or severity of rheumatic carditis, and they have not been shown to be cytotoxic. Antibody to the streptococcal group A polysaccharide has received particular attention because of prolonged persistence of elevated levels in the serum of patients with rheumatic mitral valvular disease in contrast with its more rapid decline in patients with RF without cardiac involvement and in patients with transient mitral insufficiency, including those with mitral valve prolapse.[44,45] Antibodies reactive with cytoplasm of neurons in the subthalamic and caudate nuclei have been found more frequently in rheumatic patients with Sydenham's chorea than in those rheumatic patients without this manifestation.[46] Most recently, delineation of the molecular structure of several streptococcal M proteins has led to the demonstration of epitopes of these serotypes cross-reactive with myosin.[47-50] The tertiary structure of streptococcal M protein has been demonstrated to be that of a helical-coiled coil[50] and to be similar to other coiled proteins in human tissues which include not only myosin but keratin and other connective tissue structures.[47-49] Moreover, the M protein in rheumatogenic strains has been shown to be a very large molecule[51] containing not only the type-specific epitopes that make it capable of producing protective opsonic antibodies but also containing moieties that are powerful blastogens for human T lymphocytes. These moieties are so-called "superantigens" that may stimulate subsets of T cells with specificity for self-antigens (e.g., cardiac tissues) above a threshold of tolerance needed to permit an autoimmune response.[52]

Little doubt remains that streptococcal antigens of various kinds are shared with human myocardium, but it has not yet been shown that they are actually responsible for tissue injury in certain hosts and are thus related to the pathogenesis of rheumatic fever.[33]

PATHOLOGY

There is often considerable disparity between the severity of the clinical manifestations of RF and the extent of the morbid anatomical changes it produces. Sydenham's chorea, cardiac atrioventricular conduction blocks, and erythema marginatum all appear to be related more to functional disturbances than to visible lesions. In contrast, the persistent focal inflammatory lesions of the myocardium, such as the Aschoff nodule, do not always correlate with clinical manifestations of active carditis and have led to differences of opinion between pathologists and clinicians with regard to the definition of rheumatic activity. In general, however, the acute phase of RF is characterized by diffuse exudative and proliferative inflammatory reactions in the heart, joints, and skin. Small blood vessels and arterioles are commonly involved, but unlike the arteritis of some other connective tissue diseases, thrombotic lesions are not seen.

The term *fibrinoid degeneration* describes the basic structural changes

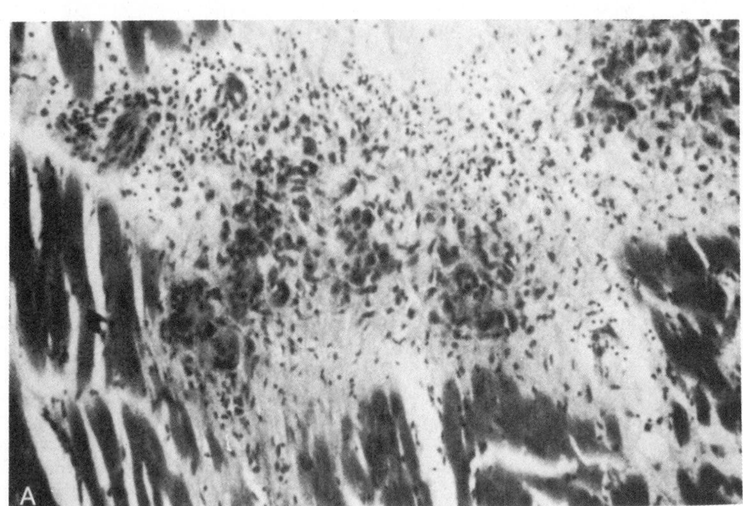

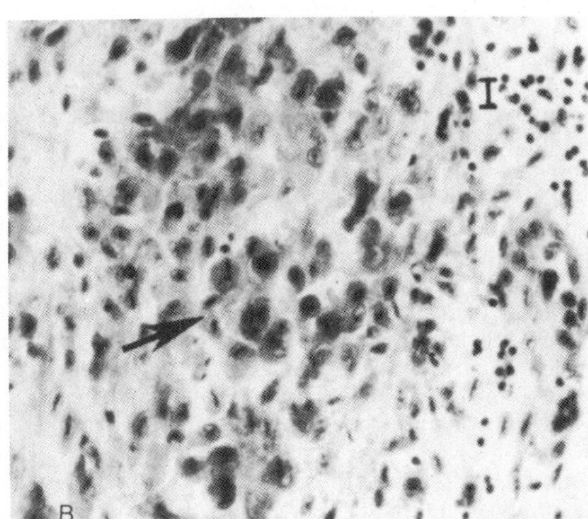

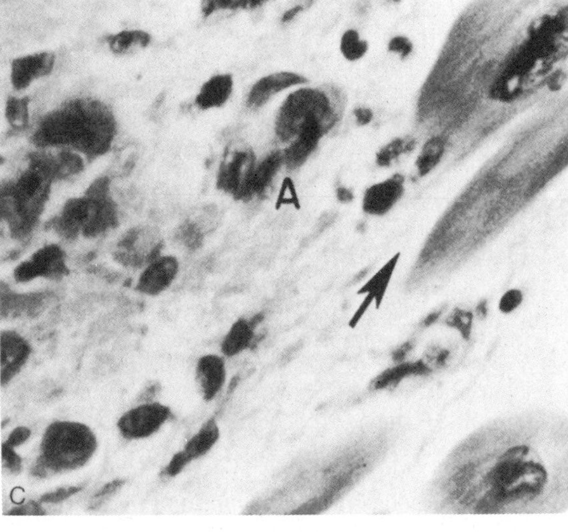

FIGURE 56-4. *A,* Multiple Aschoff lesions in the left ventricle, showing confluence of large monocyte macrophage-appearing cells surrounded by cell infiltrate and dissolution of adjacent myocardial muscle with fibrous tissue replacement. *B,* Higher-power view showing large mononuclear cells *(arrow)* and interstitial lymphocytes (I). *C,* High-power view. (From Husby, G., et al.: Immunofluorescent studies of florid rheumatic Aschoff lesions. Arthritis Rheum. *29*:207, 1986.)

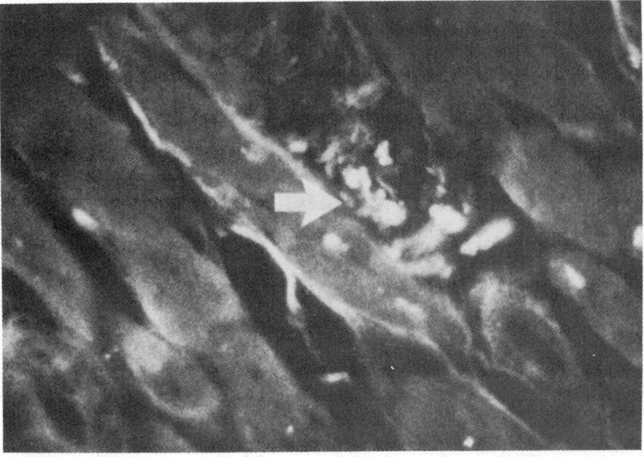

FIGURE 56-5. Postmortem myocardial specimen from a 20-year-old patient with severe rheumatic carditis. Immunofluorescent staining shows many large monocytoid cells that appear to have ingested myosin *(arrow).* (From Husby, G., et al.: Immunofluorescent studies of florid rheumatic Aschoff lesions. Arthritis Rheum. *29*:207, 1986.)

in the collagen of connective tissues. The fibrinoid substance resembles and stains like fibrin and is a feature of the earliest phase of the myocardial lesions. The collagen fibers in these mucoid areas become swollen and eosinophilic, forming a meshwork of rigid, waxlike fibers. This exudative-degenerative phase lasts for 2 to 3 weeks, following which the most characteristic lesion of RF develops—the myocardial *Aschoff nodule.* The proliferative and healing phase then follows and may persist for many months or even years (Figs. 56–4 and 56–5).

Ironically, the only lesion pathognomonic of RF is vague with regard to its origin, functional impact on the heart, and relation to the course and severity of the rheumatic attack.[54] Aschoff nodules do not seem to account for the acute dilatation of the heart in first attacks of severe carditis. The persistence of Aschoff nodules for many years after a rheumatic attack has been well recognized by pathologists. Biopsies of the left atrial appendage obtained during mitral valve surgery for mitral stenosis have shown persistence of Aschoff nodules in patients who no longer have clinical or laboratory evidence of rheumatic activity[55–57] and who have no recent evidence of streptococcal infection.[58] The persistence of Aschoff nodules seems to be correlated, however, with progressive fibrosis and stenosis of the mitral valve. One series[56,57] showed such lesions in 21 per cent of 191 surgically excised left atrial appendages in patients with mitral stenosis. In the same series, of 91 patients with pure mitral regurgitation, Aschoff nodules were present in the left atrial appendage of only one patient.

CARDIAC LESIONS

On gross inspection of the heart, a pancarditis is almost always evident, with fresh exudative pericardial lesions, dilatation of the heart, and verrucous endocardial lesions on the valves.[59]

PERICARDITIS (see also p. 1501). Both layers of the pericardium are thickened and covered with a fibrinous exudate, and serosanguineous pericardial fluid may be present. With healing, fibrosis and adhesions develop which partially or completely obliterate the pericardial sac, but constrictive pericarditis does *not* occur.

MYOCARDITIS. In addition to the Aschoff bodies, a diffuse cellular infiltrate is present in interstitial tissues. The cells are usually lymphocytes, but polymorphonuclear leukocytes, histiocytes, and eosinophils may also be present. Exudate may be associated with damaged muscle. This interstitial myocarditis may be more important than the nodular Aschoff bodies in producing heart failure. Myocardial fibers are also damaged, and the greatest damage occurs in the vicinity of Aschoff nodules and around blood vessels.[60,61] Macrophages containing cardiac myosin have been identified in Aschoff nodules by immunofluorescent studies of florid acute myocarditis (Fig. 56–5).[61]

THE CONDUCTION SYSTEM. Despite the high frequency of prolonged atrial ventricular conduction in ARF, visible changes in the bundle of His are seen in the minority of autopsy cases of ARF. The evanescence of heart block and its easy reversibility in most cases by the administration of atropine fit the concept that a pathophysiological defect rather than an anatomical lesion is responsible for this conduction defect.

ENDOCARDITIS. The verrucous lesions at the valve edge appear as a mass of eosinophilic material staining as fibrin. At the base and edges of the valve, the cells line up in palisades at right angles to the base and often have elongated Aschoff-like nuclei. As the lesions progress, granulation tissue develops and vascularization and progressive fibrosis take place. The changes involve the annulus as well as the cusps and chordae tendineae, which, as a result of scarring, thicken and shorten.

RHEUMATIC VALVULAR DEFORMITIES

(See also Chap. 34)

MITRAL REGURGITATION. Incompetence or regurgitation may result from shortening of one or both cusps, from shortening and fusing of chordae and papillary muscles, or from dilatation of the valve ring. By far, the most common clinically apparent lesion of rheumatic heart disease is mitral regurgitation, and such lesions often occur subclinically when extracardiac symptoms of ARF are absent. Dilatation of the valve ring occurs in active carditis more frequently as a result of acute dilatation of the left ventricle. Marked mitral regurgitation also occurs, however, without acute left ventricular dilatation when the valve cusps and the musculotendinous structures are severely swollen and disorganized by the rheumatic process without coexisting severe myocarditis.

MITRAL STENOSIS. This lesion occurs with varying degrees of mitral regurgitation. When stenosis is severe, regurgitation may be relatively unimportant, and the main hemodynamic problem is obstruction to blood flow during diastole. The gross changes in the mitral valve are variable. The cusps may fuse, leaving an ovoid opening, but the cusps themselves may remain thin and pliable. In other instances the cusps become thick, rigid, or even calcified. A "funnel-shaped valve" with its opening at the apex may result when fusion of the cusps occurs with shortening and thickening of the chordae tendineae and papillary muscles.

AORTIC VALVE DEFORMITIES. The most common aortic lesion is a combination of stenosis and regurgitation. Pure aortic stenosis is relatively uncommon, but a minimal degree of aortic regurgitation occurs frequently in mild rheumatic involvement. In most cases of symptomatic rheumatic aortic disease, both stenosis and regurgitation occur, but one or the other may be functionally predominant. Deformity of the valve results from fusion of the cusps at the commissures, rigidity and shortening of the cusps alone, or combinations of both processes with calcification superimposed (Fig. 56–6).

TRICUSPID VALVE DEFORMITIES. These almost always exist in association with mitral and aortic lesions and occur in approximately 10 per cent of patients with chronic rheumatic heart disease.[59]

PULMONARY VALVE DEFORMITIES. Pulmonary valve deformities are rarest of all. When they occur, stenosis is more usual than is incompetence. The pathological changes in the pulmonary valve are similar to those in the aortic valve.

PROGRESSIVE PATHOLOGICAL CHANGES IN HEALED RHEUMATIC HEART DISEASE. There are manifestations of progressive changes and continued inflammation that seem unrelated to the original rheumatic process. Disruption of red blood cells ("cardiac hemolytic anemia") can result from valvular defects; platelet turnover and destruction have recently been proved to be excessive in rheumatic heart disease[62]; and resultant thrombosis and fibrosis can occur along with calcification. Recurrent congestive heart failure may cause fatty changes in the myocardium and progressive fibrosis. The endocardium, especially the left atrium in mitral valvular deformity, is prone to develop organized thrombi, to stretch and dilate progressively, and to develop chronic inflammatory changes that are not exudative or clearly due to the rheumatic process at all.

EXTRACARDIAC LESIONS

JOINTS. Swelling and edema of the articular and periarticular structures with serous effusion into the joint space occur without erosion of the joint surface or pannus formation. The synovial membrane is reddened and thickened and covered with fibrinous exudate. Histologically there is marked edema, engorgement and dilation of blood vessels, and diffuse and focal infiltrates of lymphocytes and polymorphonuclear leukocytes, the latter more numerous initially. Later, focal fibrinoid lesions with histiocytic granulomas may appear, but these lesions heal also without residua.

SUBCUTANEOUS NODULES. A central zone of fibrinoid necrotic material is surrounded by histiocytes and fibroblasts, and lymphocytes and polymorphonuclear leukocytes collect around small vessels. The structure resembles Aschoff bodies and may heal very rapidly, leaving no apparent scars.

CHOREA. Considerable confusion exists concerning the pathology of Sydenham's chorea because (1) few patients die of "pure" chorea, (2) those who die of severe carditis may have inflammatory lesions of the central nervous system without chorea,[63] (3) no single site is consistently involved, (4) Aschoff bodies are not found in the brain,[64,65] and (5) it has not been possible to correlate clinical findings with pathological changes. Changes found in the central nervous system include arteritis, cellular degeneration, perivascular round cell infiltration, and occasional petechial hemorrhages, but on the whole these are not impressive and are scattered throughout the cortex, cerebellum, and basal ganglia.[66,67]

RHEUMATIC PNEUMONITIS. Because this finding usually occurs with severe carditis only, there has been argument about whether the pulmonary lesion is a form of the acute respiratory distress syndrome secondary to heart failure or part of the rheumatic process itself. It has been described, however, in the absence of heart failure.[68]

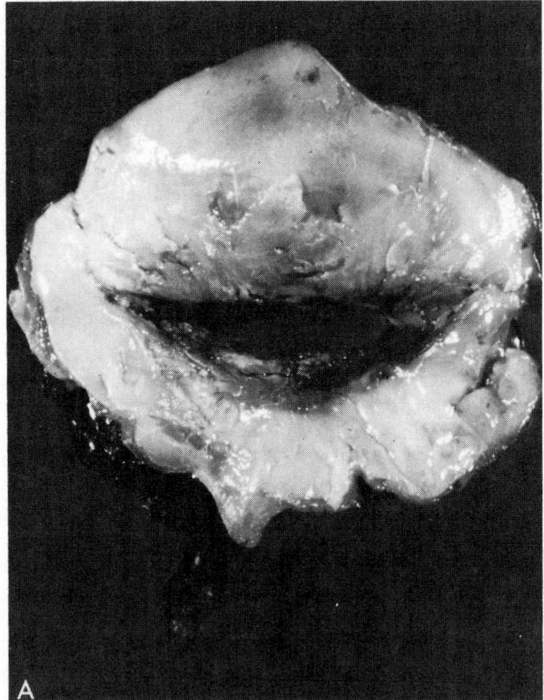

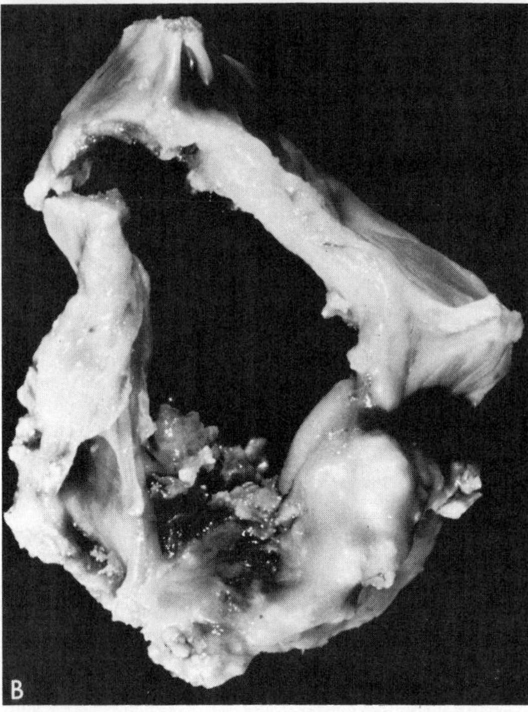

FIGURE 56-6. **Excised rheumatic valve.** ***A,*** **"Fishmouth" mitral valve.** ***B,*** **Aortic valve fixed in open position. (Courtesy of James W. Pate, M.D. From Stollerman, G. H.: Rheumatic Fever and Streptococcal Infection. New York, by permission of Grune and Stratton, 1975.)**

CLINICAL MANIFESTATIONS

The signs and symptoms of ARF vary greatly and are determined by the systems involved, the severity of the lesions and when they appear in the course of the disease, and the stage of the disease when the patient is first observed by the physician. Certain manifestations that follow streptococcal infections (with a frequency far exceeding chance) occur simultaneously, in close succession, or singly. They have been called *major manifestations* and consist of carditis, arthritis, chorea, subcutaneous nodules, and erythema marginatum. The word "major" refers to their importance as diagnostic criteria and not to their importance in the severity of the process or its activity, or to the prognosis.

Minor manifestations of ARF are frequently present and helpful in recognizing the disease. They are too nonspecific, however, to be of major importance in diagnosis. Minor manifestations include such findings as fever, arthralgia, acute phase reactants in the blood, heart block, and a history of previous ARF or rheumatic heart disease.

ANTECEDENT STREPTOCOCCAL INFECTION. Clinical evidence for an antecedent streptococcal infection may not be apparent. As many as one-third of patients do not remember having had any illness in the preceding month (see above). Furthermore, in patients with previous RF who were followed prospectively for recurrences, asymptomatic streptococcal infections accounted for 54[27] to 70 per cent[29] of recurrences of RF. The average interval between onset of symptoms of pharyngitis and the symptoms of RF (the latent period) was 18.6 days in one prospective study,[69] but may be as short as 1 week or as long as 5 weeks. The latent period is no shorter in patients with previous RF than in those without.

ARTHRITIS. The manifestation occurs in about three-fourths of patients during the acute stage of the disease. In general, joint involvement becomes more common with increasing age of the patient, a trend related to the concomitant decrease in the incidence of carditis and chorea.[70,71] The arthritis of RF usually involves the large joints, particularly the knees, ankles, elbows, and wrists. Almost any joint, however, may be affected. In the classic attack, several joints are involved in quick succession, each for a brief time, resulting in the typical picture of migratory polyarthritis. Each joint remains inflamed for usually no more than a week before the inflammation begins to subside, and the inflammation usually abates spontaneously in 2 or 3 weeks.[72-74] Acute polyarthritis rarely occurs more than 35 days after the onset of the streptococcal infection, and *for that reason, it is almost always associated with a rising or peak titer of streptococcal antibodies.* This fact aids in identifying an isolated bout of polyarthritis as rheumatic or in *excluding* RF as a cause for a given bout of polyarthritis when streptococcal antibodies are not increased.

CARDITIS

VARIATIONS IN ONSET AND COURSE. The most important manifestation of ARF is carditis, which, in its most severe form, causes death from acute cardiac failure. Much more commonly, however, carditis is less intense, and the predominant effect is scarring of the heart valves. In contrast to the seriousness of its prognosis, rheumatic carditis most often causes no symptoms of its own and is usually diagnosed in the course of the examination of a patient with arthritis or chorea, which directs the physician's attention to the heart, where murmurs are detected. Carditis, therefore, does not come to medical attention if other symptoms of rheumatic fever are absent or if the carditis is not severe enough to cause heart failure, prolonged or severe fever, or the pain of pericarditis. Patients with undiagnosed carditis may later prove to have rheumatic heart disease and usually give no history of a previous rheumatic attack.

Murmurs indicative of carditis are usually present during the first week of the illness in about three-fourths of all patients in whom carditis is eventually diagnosed.[75] By the second or third week, murmurs become evident in 85 per cent of those in whom they will eventually develop.

Acute heart failure in a young patient who has had rheumatic heart disease previously but who has been well compensated *should always be suspected as a recurrence of acute rheumatic carditis.* Young hearts with rheumatic disease rarely fail abruptly because of hemodynamic handicaps alone except when the latter are severe and protracted. On the other hand, it is often not possible to detect carditis during mild rheumatic recurrences in patients with old rheumatic valvular lesions. Like most episodes of carditis, heart failure or signs of pericarditis will be absent, and the diagnosis of a recurrence will depend on other major and minor criteria in cases in which changing heart murmurs (the most common sign of carditis in first rheumatic attacks) are undetectable.

CLINICAL SIGNS AND CRITERIA. The four major criteria for the clinical diagnosis of rheumatic carditis are (1) an organic heart murmur or murmurs not previously present, (2) enlargement of the heart, (3) congestive heart failure, and (4) pericardial friction rubs or signs of effusion. If any one of these is unequivocal in a patient with active RF, the diagnosis of carditis is justified.

MURMURS OF ACUTE RHEUMATIC CARDITIS. Organic murmurs are almost invariably present. They may not be heard when the heart rate is too rapid, when cardiac output is very low in severe congestive heart failure, when they are obscured by a loud pericardial rub, or, rarely, when there is marked pericardial effusion. Otherwise, the signs of endocarditis are always associated with those of involvement of other layers of the heart, although the latter may not be clinically apparent.

Apical Systolic Murmur. The mitral valve is the most common site of rheumatic inflammation—about three times as frequently involved as the aortic valve. Inflammation ("valvulitis") causing edema, thickening, and verrucae leads to mitral regurgitation early in the course of the disease and often with mild cardiac involvement. The systolic murmur is heard best at the apex, usually grade 3 or more on a scale of 6 in intensity, and, most important, it has a high-pitched blowing quality.

Apical Mid-diastolic Murmur (Carey-Coombs Murmur). This murmur begins directly after the onset of the third heart sound and ends before the first heart sound. The mid-diastolic murmur is often transient, low pitched, and easily missed. The presence of this murmur makes the diagnosis of "mitral valvulitis" more definite, confirms the significance of the apical systolic murmur, and adds to the seriousness of the prognosis for permanent valve injury.

Aortic Diastolic Murmur. This murmur may appear early in the course of the disease as an expression of aortic valvulitis and may occur alone or with mitral valvulitis. The aortic diastolic blow may be audible only intermittently, depending, again, on cardiac output. The murmur is a soft, high-pitched, decrescendo blow heard immediately after the second heart sound. A diastolic cooing or crying "sea gull" murmur is rarely heard, but can be present evanescently in the aortic valvulitis of acute carditis.

CARDIAC ENLARGEMENT AND FAILURE. The most reliable clinical expression of rheumatic myocarditis from the standpoint of diagnosis and prognosis is *dilatation*, particularly of the left atrium and ventricle. In two careful cooperative studies designed to evaluate treatment of rheumatic carditis, cardiomegaly occurred in a little more than half the children who developed carditis.[72,76,77]

Congestive heart failure is the least common but most serious manifestation of rheumatic carditis. It is reported in 5 to 10 per cent of first attacks of rheumatic carditis. It is more common, however, to encounter severe and fatal heart failure as a manifestation of a *rheumatic recurrence* than of a primary attack.

PERICARDITIS. Pericarditis occurs in approximately 5 to 10 per cent of most large series of ARF.[72,75] Occasionally, pericardial reaction and effusion will be more striking and prominent than the degree of myocarditis. In such cases the regression in apparent heart size and the rate of healing of the attack can be rapid. Conversely, the pericarditis may be a relatively minor aspect of a profound case of heart failure due to severe myocarditis. One rarely sees tamponade without severe heart failure as well.

ARRHYTHMIAS. Delayed atrioventricular (AV) conduction, as reflected in prolongation of the P-R interval, occurs with a frequency similar to that of the polyarthritis of ARF, whether or not clear evidence of carditis is present. The prolongation of AV conduction is easily reversed with atropine,[78] suggesting that this feature is usually due to functional effects of the disease on AV conduction rather than to direct inflammation and fibrosis of the conduction system. Prolongation of AV conduction may lead to second-degree and, rarely, even third-degree block.[79] The latter is usually of brief duration and reverts spontaneously. Interference and dissociation phenomena are also characteristic of occasional nodal rhythms.

EXTRACARDIAC MANIFESTATIONS

SUBCUTANEOUS NODULES. These are a major manifestation of ARF.[80] However, they are not pathognomonic of RF, since they occur in rheumatoid arthritis and systemic lupus erythematosus as well. They rarely occur as an isolated manifestation and are associated most often with severe carditis, appearing usually several weeks after its onset.[81]

Nodules are round, firm, painless subcutaneous lesions varying in size from approximately 0.5 to 2.0 cm. The skin over them is freely movable and not inflamed. They are located over bony surfaces or prominences and over tendons, particularly the extensor of the fingers and toes and flexors of the wrists and ankles. They occur in crops and vary in number from one to usually three or four dozen; when numerous, they tend to be symmetrical. Nodules are evanescent, disappearing sometimes within several days but usually lasting a week or two and rarely more than a month. They tend, therefore, to be much smaller and less persistent than rheumatoid nodules.

ERYTHEMA MARGINATUM. This is a less common feature of RF, but is so characteristic that it has taken its rightful place among the five major diagnostic manifestations of the disease. However, it cannot be considered pathognomonic of ARF because it has been reported in sepsis, particularly staphylococcal, in drug reactions, in patients with glomerulonephritis, and in children in whom no etiological factor can be identified.

Erythema marginatum appears as a bright-pink "smoke ring" spreading serpiginously through pale skin. It is nonpruritic, nonpainful, and neither indurated nor raised. It blanches completely on pressure and is evanescent. The individual lesions usually appear on the trunk and the proximal parts of the extremities but not on the face; they rarely extend distally beyond the elbows or knees. Erythema marginatum may recur intermittently for months, uninfluenced by antirheumatic agents, and when all other signs of rheumatic activity are gone, one can allow the patient to begin to ambulate without fear of a relapse.

CHOREA (SYDENHAM'S CHOREA, ST. VITUS' DANCE). This neurological disorder, characterized by involuntary, purposeless, rapid movements, muscular weakness, and emotional lability, may be associated with other manifestations of ARF, but it also may appear as the sole expression of the disease—so-called pure chorea. After puberty it is present exclusively in women, and even in them it declines rapidly after adolescence. Chorea has decreased strikingly in frequency compared with arthritis and carditis. In a recent outbreak of rheumatic fever in children in Utah, however, the frequency of chorea in the acute attack was as high as that described in the United States several decades ago—approximately 25 per cent of cases.[82]

The movements of chorea are abrupt and erratic, not rhythmic or repetitive. In even the most violent attacks, all choreiform movements disappear during sleep and are less violent during rest and sedation.[1]

Chorea may last from 1 week to more than 2 years, but usually about 8 to 15 weeks, with a mean of 13.7. Chorea is never seen simultaneously with arthritis, but often coexists with carditis. When chorea appears alone, however, the other minor clinical and laboratory signs of ARF may be entirely absent. The erythrocyte sedimentation rate and C-reactive protein may be normal. Even more confusing, in such cases the ASO and other streptococcal antibody titers may not be increased because chorea appears only after a relatively long latent period (as long as 1 to 6 months) following the antecedent streptococcal infection, and after the longest latent period, both the acute phase reactants and the streptococcal antibody titers may have returned to normal.[83,84]

FEVER. Some degree of fever accompanies almost all rheumatic attacks at their onset. Temperature usually ranges from 101° to 104°F (38.4° to 40°C), is rarely higher, and has no characteristic pattern. In the usual attack, fever decreases in approximately a week without antipyretic treatment and may become low grade for another week or two. It rarely lasts for more than several weeks. When antirheumatic agents are used, however, a "rebound" of fever may occur after 4 to 6 weeks of treatment, but it usually subsides spontaneously within a few days except in unusually persistent attacks.

ABDOMINAL PAIN. The abdominal pain of RF, which occurs in fewer than 5 per cent of patients with ARF, resembles that seen in other conditions in which acute microvascular mesenteric disease occurs, such as sickle cell crises, sepsis, endotoxin or anaphylactic shock, transfusion reactions, and anaphylactoid purpura.

EPISTAXIS. In the past, the incidence of epistaxis was reported from as high as 48 per cent in the early 1930's to a low of 4 to 9 per cent in the late 1950's,[70] and perhaps it is even less frequent now.

LABORATORY FINDINGS

Although there are no pathognomonic tests for RF, laboratory findings are helpful in two major ways: (1) in establishing the antecedent streptococcal infection and (2) in documenting the presence or persistence of an inflammatory process.

ANTECEDENT STREPTOCOCCAL INFECTION. The diagnosis of recent streptococcal infection can be made only tentatively by throat culture but definitely by antibody determinations. Throat cultures are usually negative by the time RF appears. When they are positive, one still cannot be certain whether the organism isolated represents convalescent carriage of the antecedent infection or an intercurrent acquisition of a different strain. Streptococcal antibodies are therefore more useful because they reach a peak titer shortly after the onset of ARF and indicate true infection rather than transient carriage.

ANTIBODIES. The specific antibodies used to diagnose streptococcal infections are primarily antistreptolysin O and anti-DNAase B. Antistreptolysin O has been the most extensively used test and is generally available in hospitals in the United States.

ASO titers vary with age, geographical area, and other factors influencing the frequency of streptococcal infection. Titers of 200 to 300 units/ml are common in healthy children 6 to 14 years of age who live in crowded cities in the temperate zone of the United States.

The chance of detecting a significant antibody response is greatest 2 to 3 weeks after the onset of ARF, which is usually 4 to 5 weeks after the antecedent streptococcal infection. Thereafter, antibody titers fall off rapidly in the next few months, and after 6 months the decline levels off slowly. For this reason, evidence of increased streptococcal antibodies should be present in all patients at the onset of the rheumatic attack if such onset is well defined. Acute polyarthritis always occurs within a latent period of no more than 4 to 5 weeks after the antecedent streptococcal infection and therefore at or near the peak of the antibody response.

Anti-DNAase B, together with the ASO, has become most generally recommended for diagnosis, with antihyaluronidase a third choice.[85]

ACUTE PHASE REACTANTS. Acute phase reactants include leukocyte counts, erythrocyte sedimentation rate (ESR), C-reactive protein (CRP),[86] serum mucoprotein, serum hexosamine, serum protein electrophoresis, and several others. The two tests that have gained widest use are the CRP and the ESR. These tests are, of course, not specific for RF, but they are almost always abnormal during the active rheumatic process if it is not suppressed by antirheumatic drugs.

ANEMIA. The anemia of RF is the normocytic normochromic anemia of chronic inflammation and is of mild to moderate degree. Suppression of inflammation usually corrects the anemia partially or completely, and corticosteroids are particularly potent in this regard. Anemia is a good index of the severity and chronicity of RF.

ELECTROCARDIOGRAPHIC FINDINGS. The electrocardiogram in RF has no characteristic pattern, and the diagnosis of rheumatic carditis should never be made on the basis of ECG changes alone. Too often the diagnosis of carditis has been made incorrectly when a doubtful systolic murmur has been associated with a prolonged P-R interval or nonspecific ST-T changes. Neither the course of the acute rheumatic attack nor the subsequent development of valvular or myocardial damage can be predicted from the electrocardiographic changes.[74,87] Patients with ECG changes but with no other signs of carditis recover completely without the stigmata of rheumatic heart disease.[88]

DIAGNOSIS

JONES CRITERIA. When T. Duckett Jones formulated his criteria for the diagnosis of ARF in 1944,[89] there was immediate recognition of their value and considerable agreement about their use. These criteria were adopted in modified form in 1955 by the American Heart Association's Council on Rheumatic Fever and Congenital Heart Disease and were further revised by the same Council's committee in 1965.[90] The current criteria (Table 56–1) emphasize the importance of establishing the presence of the antecedent streptococcal infection by demonstration of increased streptococcal antibodies. If supported by such evidence, two major (or one major and two minor) manifestations indicate a high probability of ARF. However, because virtually all patients with Sydenham's chorea are rheumatic subjects, the diagnosis can be made even when chorea is the sole manifestation. Because of the numerous causes of polyarthritis, the diagnosis of RF is weakest when this manifestation appears alone, and particularly in the adolescent or adult population in which other arthritides are common.

CARDITIS

Functional ("Innocent") Murmurs. When functional or organic murmurs are typical, there is little problem for the experienced physician. At times, however, a nondescript murmur, especially in an obese or heavy-chested person, may defy sharp distinctions, and repeated examinations and other studies may be required. Such murmurs are often classified as "doubtful" or "questionable" when no other decision can be made.

Myocarditis. In its severe and chronic form, myocarditis due to other diseases may be impossible to distinguish from chronic rheumatic carditis if the heart is dilated and mitral regurgitation is prominent. This situation occurs when patients with ARF have heart failure with no associated extracardiac manifestations to provide clues. In rheumatic carditis, as the patient recovers cardiac compensation, the valvular lesions persist, and the murmurs become, if anything, louder.

Pericarditis. Rheumatic carditis does not produce an isolated pericarditis. At the onset of RF, however, pericarditis may appear before valvulitis and myocarditis are evident. Although many causes of pericarditis can be listed (Chap. 45), primary viral pericarditis most often enters the differential diagnosis in children.

COURSE AND PROGNOSIS

The clinical course of RF can be quite variable, but in general there is a characteristic sequence of the major manifestations and usually a predictable duration. The latent period between streptococcal infection and the onset of ARF is shortest in arthritis and erythema marginatum and longest in chorea, with that of carditis and subcutaneous nodules in be-

TABLE 56–1 JONES CRITERIA (REVISED)

MAJOR MANIFESTATIONS	MINOR MANIFESTATIONS
Carditis	Fever
Polyarthritis	Arthralgia
Chorea	Previous rheumatic fever or rheumatic heart disease
Erythema marginatum	
Subcutaneous nodules	Elevated ESR or positive CRP
	Prolonged P-R interval
Plus supporting evidence of preceding streptococcal infection: history of recent scarlet fever; positive throat culture for group A streptococcus; increased ASO titer or other streptococcal antibodies.	

From Jones Criteria (revised) for guidance in the diagnosis of rheumatic fever. Circulation *32*:664, 1965, by permission of the American Heart Association, Inc.

tween. The usual duration of a rheumatic attack is rarely longer than 3 months. When severe carditis is present, clinical rheumatic activity may continue for 6 months or more. In fewer than 5 per cent of patients, ARF may remain active for more than 6 months.[91] These cases are classified as "chronic" rheumatic fever.

CARDITIS. Of the patients in whom carditis develops, murmurs occur during the first week of illness in 76 per cent. In 93 per cent of patients there is evidence of carditis in the first 3 months. Age of onset and severity of carditis influence its chronicity. Before the age of 3 years, 92 per cent of patients in one study[92] and 90 per cent in another[93] had carditis. The incidence of carditis decreased to 50 per cent in the 3- to 6-year age group and to 32 per cent in the 14- to 17-year age group[70] in first attacks. Carditis occurs occasionally after the age of 25 in what are apparently first attacks of ARF. When carditis is mild or evidence for it is borderline, it usually disappears rapidly. Severe carditis prolongs the attack. When severe carditis subsides, low-grade fever and tachycardia often continue, cardiac enlargement usually persists, and new murmurs may appear. Congestive heart failure may occur at any time while carditis is still active.

PROGNOSIS. RF does not recur when streptococcal disease is prevented. The prognosis is excellent for the rheumatic subject who escapes carditis during an initial attack of RF. In one 5-year follow-up, rheumatic heart disease did not develop when the acute attack was not accompanied by the appearance of organic heart murmurs.[87] In the United Kingdom–United States Cooperative Study on the treatment of RF,[73,74] similar patients without carditis (defined as the absence of organic murmurs) during the acute attack showed virtually no evidence of late or insidious development of rheumatic heart disease. The percentage of this group of patients with "no carditis" who subsequently had normal hearts was 96 at 5 years and 94 at 10 years. The prognoses become poorer with the increasing severity of initial carditis, so that the percentage of those with congestive heart failure during the acute attack showing complete healing was 30 at 5 years and 40 at 10 years. It is apparent that the healing rate of rheumatic carditis is remarkably high if recurrences are prevented.

Prospective cooperative studies[74] have shown, at 5 years, that the frequency of mitral stenosis was equally distributed between the sexes and was related to the severity of the initial attack of carditis. In fact, a large percentage of the deaths within 5 years was due to such severe mitral valvular deformity. The analysis at 10 years, however, showed the emergence of another group—those whose initial mitral lesion had been relatively mild and who showed slow, progressive obstruction without evidence of recurrent RF or streptococcal disease. This group consisted of predominantly female subjects. It is apparent, therefore, that host factors, as yet undefined, influence the course of valvular sclerosis once mitral deformity has occurred and that progression of rheumatic heart disease may be related to more than the rheumatic inflammation itself. In addition, the tendency of stenotic mitral valves that have been fractured or incised surgically to restenose without evidence of recurrent or active RF is quite apparent in several long-term follow-up studies.[94]

Recurrences. First attacks of RF in the general population following epidemic streptococcal pharyngitis due to rheumatogenic strains average 3 per cent, whereas such infections in patients with a history of recent RF may produce a secondary attack rate as high as 65 per cent.[27] In the Irvington House study,[95] rheumatic attack rate per infection (R/I) in children decreased from 23 to 11 per cent between the first and fifth year after a rheumatic attack.[28] In adults with rheumatic heart disease, this rate was 4.8 per cent 10 or more years after the last attack.[29] Recurrence rates decline, therefore, with the length of time elapsed since the last attack.

A second factor that clearly increases the chance that a streptococcal infection will be followed by a rheumatic attack is the presence of residual rheumatic heart disease. In the Irvington House studies, the recurrence rate in children with rheumatic heart disease and cardiomegaly was 43 per cent; in patients with rheumatic heart disease and no cardiomegaly, 27 per cent; and in patients without apparent residual heart disease, 10 per cent.[28]

A third factor influencing the R/I is the magnitude of the immune response to the antecedent streptococcal disease as reflected in the increase of ASO titer. The decline in first attacks of ARF is also associated with a decline in rheumatic recurrences, and both may be due to the disappearance of rheumatogenic strains of group A streptococci.[3] In the absence of such strains in a rheumatic population, even those subjects with rheumatic heart disease who develop intercurrent streptococcal infections associated with a rise in antistreptococcal antibodies do not have reactivated rheumatic fever.[96]

THE CHANGING NATURAL HISTORY OF RHEUMATIC HEART DISEASE. The current longevity of patients in the United States with inactive rheumatic heart disease can be projected from a subgroup of such patients followed prospectively for more than 30 years as part of the Framingham Study.[97] As expected, compared with a cohort control group, there was a relatively sharp decline in survival during the first half of the study, reflecting, no doubt, hemodynamic changes in the more severely involved hearts, because rheumatic recurrences were extremely rare. Nonetheless, a large proportion of patients with rheumatic heart disease survived. After 36 years of follow-up, in males the percentage surviving in the rheumatic heart disease group was only slightly below 40, compared with somewhat more than 40 per cent in their cohorts without rheumatic heart disease. Among the women the discrepancy in survival between the patients with rheumatic heart disease and their cohorts was greater.[96] The reservoir of relatively benign rheumatic valvular disease in the elderly population has been well recognized by clinicians for many years, but because of the sharp decline in new cases of rheumatic fever, rheumatic heart disease in the United States is becoming a "geriatric" disease. This phenomenon also contributes to the increasing mean age of patients with infective endocarditis.

TREATMENT

GENERAL MANAGEMENT. In any given case of RF, general management depends upon the manifestations and severity of the attack. Patients should remain in bed for the duration of the acute and febrile portion of the illness until clinical and laboratory evidence of inflammation abates.

The administration of antiinflammatory or suppressive therapy should ordinarily be delayed until the disease process is clearly expressed in order to establish the diagnosis. Aspirin or corticosteroids administered prematurely to a patient with arthralgia or early monoarticular arthritis and fever may mask the disease process and cause diagnostic confusion. Furthermore, in isolated polyarthritis a trial of penicillin therapy is often essential to eliminate the diagnosis of septic arthritis, especially gonococcemia, and the therapeutic response to the antibiotic must be carefully evaluated.

Once the diagnosis is established, treatment can begin, usually with a *course of penicillin* adequate to eradicate residual group A streptococci. Massive penicillin treatment has been used by some investigators in an attempt to alter the frequency of cardiac damage, but without success.[98] The usual course of penicillin consists of a single injection of 1.2 million units of benzathine penicillin intramuscularly, or 600,000 units of procaine penicillin intramuscularly, daily for 10 days. This is followed by continuous (secondary) prophylaxis (see below).

ANTIRHEUMATIC THERAPY. The selection of an antirheumatic agent is not critical to the outcome of most attacks of RF.[72–77] Corticosteroids and salicylates can be regarded as valuable symptomatic and supportive therapy, but they are not curative and may actually prolong the course of the disease. However, both steroids and salicylates control the toxic manifestations of the disease; contribute to the comfort of the

focal degenerative changes of elastic and muscle fibers of the aortic media; and patchy inflammatory lesions in all layers of the aorta, predominantly in the region adjacent to the aortic valve ring[117-119] (Fig. 56-7). The lesions resemble those of syphilis except that in ankylosing spondylitis they remain close to the valve ring and do not affect the rest of the aorta. In addition, the basal rather than distal portion of the aortic cusps is thickened in ankylosing spondylitis and the dense adventitial scarring extends into the endocardium in the immediate subaortic region. This extension may involve the base of the anterior mitral leaflet and the upper portion of the ventricular septum. In view of the enthesopathical lesions that characterize the pathology of this condition, patients may present with insertional tendinitis at any site, and the heart valve lesions may reflect this connective tissue localization.

Aortic regurgitation results from thickening and shortening of the cusps and from their displacement caudally by the mass of fibrous tissue behind the commissures, the subaortic ridge or bump, and by dilatation of the aortic valve root consequent to the destruction of elastic tissue (Figs. 56-7 and 56-8). Mitral regurgitation is infrequent and usually insignificant but can result from dilatation of the left ventricle from mitral valve prolapse, an extension of the subaortic bump[120] and from fibrous thickening of the basal portion of the anterior mitral leaflet. The frequent heart block and conduction defects of ankylosing spondylitis are due to the extension of fibrosis into the muscular septum and destruction of the bundle of His and proximal bundle branches.[122-124]

The lesions of the myocardium are rather nonspecific, consisting of fibrosis, perivascular lymphocytic infiltration, and increased mucinous ground substance. Cardiac enlargement without any apparent cause and hypertrophy and dilatation of the left ventricle are often described.[125]

Chronic fibrous obliteration of the pericardial cavity has been found at autopsy, but pericarditis is not a prominent clinical feature of the disease. Pericardial rubs and chest pain have been described, however, during more severe, acute, toxic episodes when there is active peripheral polyarthritis and in association with presumably early phases of the disease, especially in association with early Reiter's syndrome or dysentery with polyarthritis.

CLINICAL CARDIAC FEATURES. In many patients there is evidence of active carditis before aortic regurgitation appears. Precordial pain, pericardial friction rubs, marked tachycardia, cardiac enlargement not explained by hypertension, or other recognizable forms of heart disease and varying P-R intervals greater than 0.24 sec are frequently described, usually when patients have active peripheral arthritis and/or spondylitis with fever and increased erythrocyte sedimentation rates. Remarkably few critical studies have been made of myocardial function in patients with ankylosing spondylitis before evidence of aortic regurgitation draws attention to cardiac involvement, but it is clear that cardiomyopathy may precede valvular involvement.[125] Indeed, the high cardiovascular morbidity and mortality in these diseases may be due to myocardial abnormalities in the absence of valve disease.[125] The usual cardiac features of ankylosing spondylitis are the gradual evolution of aortic regurgitation and varying degrees of AV block. The prevalence of the valve lesion is related to the duration of spondylitis and peripheral joint involvement, reaching an incidence in one series of 10 per cent in those with spondylitis for 30 years or more and of 18 per cent if peripheral joint involvement was also present. The incidence of AV block in each of the above groups was 8.5 and 15.5 per cent, respectively.[117]

In one long follow-up of 97 patients with ankylosing spondylitis, of whom 14 had cardiovascular lesions, aortic regurgitation occurred in 10 patients. Mitral regurgitation and AV block appeared as isolated findings in 1 and 3 patients, respectively. Nine of the 14 patients had peripheral arthritis, and 3 had iritis.[118] Anterior uveitis and extraspinal disease may also precede the articular lesions of ankylosing spondylitis by months or years. Hence the discovery of isolated aortic regurgitation in young or middle-aged men requires that ankylosing spondylitis be considered in the differential diagnosis. In addition, the aortic regurgitation of ankylosing spondylitis is now well documented to occur in so-called secondary forms of the disease such as spondylitis associated with psoriasis, regional enteritis,[118] ulcerative colitis,[126] and Reiter's disease.[127]

Aortic valve replacement (p. 1052) has been performed successfully in several centers, and patients with ankylosing spondylitis may be suitable candidates when such a procedure is indicated. Cardiac pacemakers have been implanted for AV block.

REITER'S DISEASE

Cardiac involvement in the acute stages of Reiter's disease has been described frequently and consists most commonly of acute pericarditis, apical systolic murmurs, gallops, and cardiac conduction abnormalities, particularly AV block. These changes disappear rapidly, and long-term follow-up of large series reveals only an occasional case of cardiac failure or third-degree AV block.[128] This acute form of Reiter's disease usually features nonspecific urethritis, nonsuppurative migratory polyarthritis, conjunctivitis, circinate balanitis, and keratoderma blenorrhagica. Initial attacks usually subside spontaneously, but second attacks occur in about 15 per cent of cases, and chronic manifestations (almost always in B27-positive individuals[114]) may then ensue, with recurrent anterior uveitis, painful mutilating deformities of the feet, sacroiliitis, spondylitis, AV block, and an aortic valve lesion leading to aortic and occasionally to mitral regurgitation.

Postmortem studies of the aortic valves have shown the cusps to be thickened, with rolled edges, and the aorta to incur changes similar if not identical to the lesions described in AS.[129,130]

The development of Reiter's disease in patients with *Yersinia arthritis* or associated with various other dysentery-producing bacteria has emphasized the role of the B27 antigen in the frequency of expression of various clinical features of the syndrome, including its cardiac manifestations.[131-133] Of 19 patients with Reiter's syndrome observed at one institution, all 5 who had conduction abnormalities were B27-positive.[134]

RELAPSING POLYCHONDRITIS

This relatively poorly known condition is a rheumatic vasculitis characterized by recurrent inflammation of cartilage and most commonly auricular and nasal and seronegative arthritis. Both mitral and aortic regurgitation, sometimes severe enough to require valve replalcement, have been reported,[135-137] as have aneurysms of the aorta and its major branches.

RHEUMATOID ARTHRITIS

PATHOLOGY. The heart is frequently involved in the inflammatory process of rheumatoid arthritis (RA), yet its function is seldom compromised by the lesions produced.[135,136] The exudative type of rheumatoid inflammation affects the pericardial surfaces, producing a fibrinous pericarditis that is usually low grade and subclinical. Pericardial inflammation becomes symptomatic and clinically significant in its more florid form and may even be the presenting complaint.

The most characteristic pathological lesion of RA, the nodular granuloma, involves the myocardium, endocardium, and valves of the heart.[140,141] The extent of this kind of involvement is generally proportionate to the severity of the disease and is almost always associated with diffusely distributed rheumatoid nodules, subcutaneously and elsewhere. These granulomas rarely compromise the function of the myocardium, however, nor do they often affect the function of the heart valves unless they become large and numerous enough to distort them (Fig. 56-8).

Diffuse arteritis, when present, affects small vessels, causing round cell infiltration, edema, fibrosis, and proliferation of the intima. Such involvement of the pericardial vessels may be extensive when it reflects an intense systemic form of RA, and the disease may begin in the pericardium before the joints become involved. Coronary arteritis is often observed at necropsy in severe RA, but it very rarely results in clinically apparent myocardial ischemia.

Clinical Features

PERICARDITIS (see also p. 1501). The frequency of rheumatoid pericarditis in necropsy studies ranges from 11 to 50 per cent, with an overall estimate of about 30 per cent.[142] Clinically, the diagnosis of pericarditis is made in about 2 per cent of cases in the adult form and in about 6 per cent in the juvenile form of RA. In careful studies of the more severe forms of the disease which require hospital admission, approximately 10 per cent of patients with rheumatoid arthritis have clinical

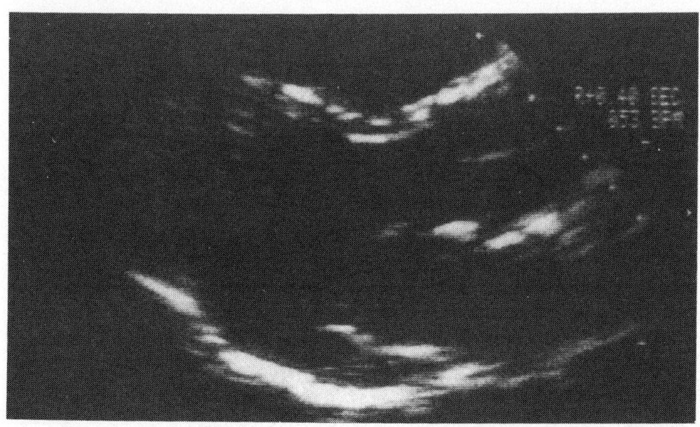

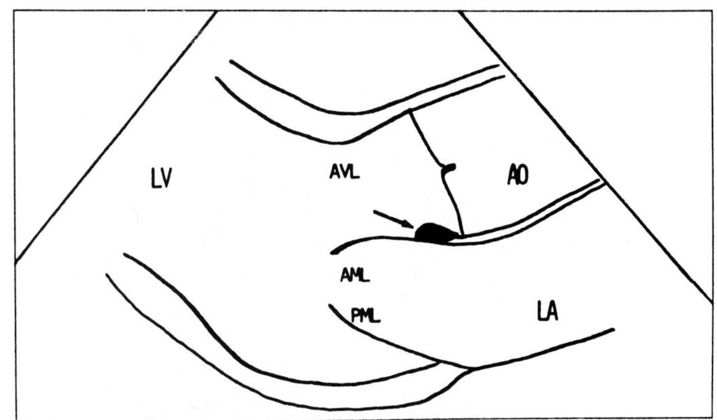

FIGURE 56-8. Long-axis view in a patient with ankylosing spondylitis. Subaortic thickening (*arrow*) is present, and there is an increase in aortic diameter and thickening of the aortic walls and aortic root echodensity. AML = anterior mitral leaflet; AO = aortic root; AVL = aortic valve leaflets; LA = left atrium; LV = left ventricle; PML = posterior mitral leaflet. (From Labresh, K. A., et al.: Two-dimensional echocardiographic detection of preclinical aortic root abnormalities in rheumatoid variant diseases. Am. J. Med. *78*:908, 1985.)

evidence of rheumatoid pericarditis during the lifetime course of their disease. Part of the disparity between clinical and autopsy findings is due to the fact that the chest pain may be overshadowed by arthritic pains and may be masked by antirheumatic agents or mistaken for arthritic pain in neighboring joints.

The pathophysiology of the acute fibrinous pericarditis of RA is not clear, but in severe cases the pericardial fluid, like synovial fluid, shows decreased hemolytic complement (CH_{50}) and C3 levels. Immunofluorescence staining of the pericardium shows plasma cell infiltration and deposits of IgG, IgM, IgA, or C3 in the pericardial vessels.[143] Moreover, the polymorphonuclear leukocytes in the pericardial fluid may show cytoplasmic inclusions which stain for IgM, indicative of ingested immune complexes such as are also seen in the polymorphonuclear cells of synovial fluid in the same patients. These findings are associated with extremely low levels of glucose, indicative of active phagocytosis, as observed in pleural and synovial rheumatoid fluids. About half the patients with overt rheumatoid pericarditis also have rheumatoid pleural and lung lesions.

In reports of patients with rheumatoid arthritis studied by echocardiography, pericardial effusion was demonstrated in 30 per cent of all patients studied and in 50 per cent of those with subcutaneous nodules.[135,144] This incidence is as high as the reported frequency of postmortem findings of rheumatoid pericarditis.

Pericarditis may appear without relation to the duration of rheumatoid arthritis[145] and sometimes may even be the harbinger of the onset of a severe form of the disease. It occurs most often in middle-aged men in whom arthritis was of acute onset. Most often, the clinical course is benign, and symptoms and signs will respond to moderate amounts of prednisone. Occasionally, however, the disease may be more protracted and severe, leading to hemopericardium,[146] cardiac tamponade,[147] and constrictive pericarditis.[145,148]

In its florid form the disease has the usual symptoms and signs of pericarditis, and when persistent, it imitates closely tuberculous pericarditis, from which it must be carefully differentiated. Although some fatal cases have been described in which a true pancarditis was present,[149] such cases are exceptional, and even severe rheumatoid pericarditis usually spares myocardial and endocardial function.

Treatment of rheumatoid pericarditis is the same as that for the arthritic disease. Although corticosteroids tend to be used more liberally in pericarditis to suppress inflammation, there is no evidence that such suppression will prevent adhesive or constrictive pericarditis.

RHEUMATOID MYOCARDITIS. Except for rare cases of myocarditis with diffuse granulomas or amyloid infiltration of the myocardium associated with very severe rheumatoid arthritis, myocarditis is mostly nonspecific and subclinical in the great majority of patients. The histological lesions may be focal or generalized infiltrations of lymphocytes, plasma cells, palisading histiocytes, and fibroblasts.[140] The incidence of myocarditis in autopsies of rheumatoid arthritis patients is reported as 19 per cent. Most of such cases are associated with severe arthritis, vasculitis, and endocarditis or pericarditis.

Although left ventricular function may be compromised by a variety of pathological processes in severe rheumatoid arthritis, the typical case is remarkable for its characteristic sparing of the myocardial musculature despite extensive involvement of the fibrous structures of the heart. Nevertheless, when there are unusually severe systemic manifestations of rheumatoid arthritis, rheumatoid pancarditis with congestive heart failure has been well described and confirmed by necropsy. Such patients exhibit the whole spectrum of rheumatoid inflammation of the heart.[149]

CORONARY ARTERY DISEASE. Clinicopathological correlation suggests that the nature of the coronary artery disease analyzed in some studies of patients with rheumatoid arthritis is probably rheumatoid rather than arteriosclerotic. Coronary arteritis is observed in about 20 per cent of patients with rheumatoid arthritis at autopsy. This arteritis is probably a manifestation of generalized vasculitis often seen in rheumatoid arthritis. Inflammation with edema of the intima of the artery may lead to severe narrowing or occlusion of its lumen, to necrosis, and to angina or infarction.[150] Nevertheless, myocardial necrosis secondary to this form of arteritis is rare.

Rheumatoid vasculitis of the pulmonary arteries causing severe pulmonary hypertension and right heart failure has been reported.[151]

VALVULAR AND ENDOCARDIAL LESIONS. As in myocarditis, the histological picture of the valves and adjacent endocardial areas of patients with rheumatoid arthritis shows nonspecific inflammation with fibrotic and sclerotic changes and infiltrations of histiocytes, plasma cells, lymphocytes, and occasional eosinophils.[140] The most characteristic lesions, however, are granulomas resembling rheumatoid nodules. Usually these do not interfere with valvular function unless they reach large enough proportions to produce frank valvular regurgitation by destroying the base of the valve and its cusps. Such regurgitation may be of sufficient magnitude and rapidity of onset to cause severe cardiac decompensation and death unless valve replacement is undertaken in a timely manner[152] (Chap. 34).

All valves may be involved, but the descending order of frequency is similar to that in rheumatic fever, i.e., mitral, aortic, tricuspid, and pulmonary. Echocardiographic studies have shown a significant slowing of mitral valve movement in patients with rheumatoid arthritis correlating with the duration of the disease and the extent of the formation of subcutaneous nodules.[144] In a few well-described cases, however, mitral and aortic valvular deformity with marked regurgitation due to rheumatoid nodules was the characteristic pathological picture.[149]

ELECTROCARDIOGRAPHIC ABNORMALITIES. Studies of the electrocardiogram in patients with rheumatoid arthritis and in matched controls show that first degree AV block is the most significant finding in rheumatoid arthritis. Complete heart block causing Adams-Stokes syndrome has been described,[152] and other abnormalities include left bundle branch block, atrial fibrillation, and atrial and ventricular ectopic beats.

JUVENILE RHEUMATOID ARTHRITIS (STILL's DISEASE)

This syndrome, one of the more common chronic illnesses of childhood, may also have its onset in adults and is particularly noteworthy for involvement of the serosal surfaces, producing pleuritis and pericarditis as well as arthritis, and is featured by a characteristic rash.[154] Pericarditis can be diagnosed clinically in approximately 7 per cent of children with juvenile rheumatoid arthritis. As in rheumatoid arthritis, postmortem examinations show a much higher incidence of pericarditis, and echocardiography is needed to reveal its clinical frequency.[155] Pericardial tamponade has been reported in both children and adults with this syndrome, but it is very rare. Myocarditis is less common than pericarditis, but may produce cardiac enlargement and heart failure, especially in adult Still's disease.[156-158] Valvular heart disease is rare, but severe aortic regurgitation requiring valve replacement has been described in a young adult.[147]

SYSTEMIC LUPUS ERYTHEMATOSUS

PATHOLOGICAL FEATURES. The hallmark of this disease is the presence of a number of antibodies to nuclear components, the antinuclear antibodies (ANA), as well as antibodies against phospholipids that may participate in the pathogenesis of SLE by forming antigen-antibody-complement complexes that are found in many of the lesions. These and other hyperimmune phenomena explain many of the protean clinical manifestations of SLE. Although anti-heart antibodies have been described in the sera of patients with SLE, they bear no clear relationship to the frequency and severity of cardiac lesions and may be a result rather than a cause of cardiac inflammation, presumably owing to release of myocardial antigens into the circulation.[160]Other etiological ad pathogenetic processes associated with autoimmunity have been extensively reviewed.

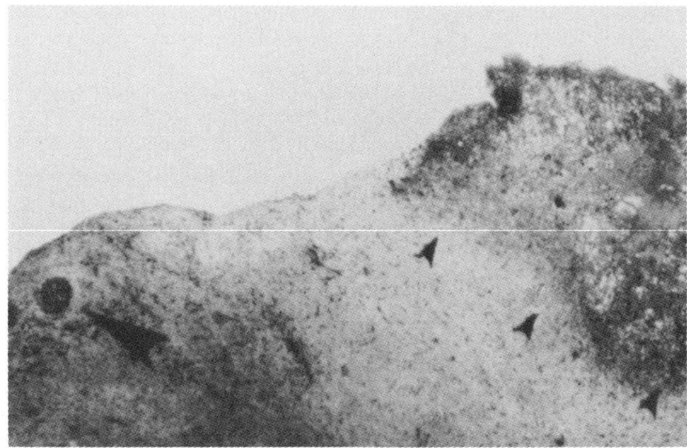

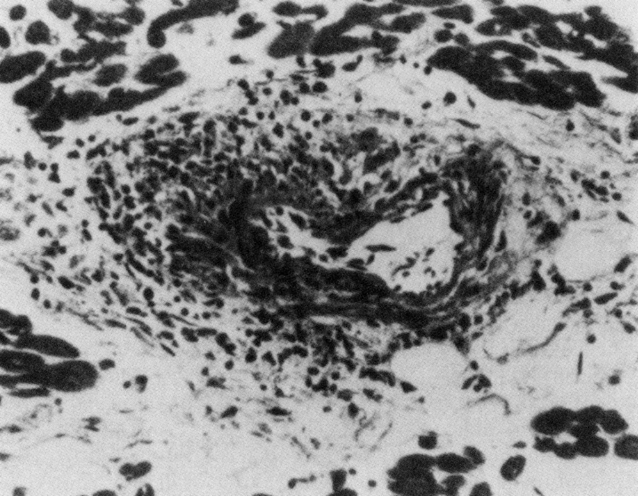

FIGURE 56-9. *Top,* Vasculopathy (large arrow) and necrosis (small arrows) of mitral valve in SLE (original magnification 40×). *Bottom,* Vasculitis of sinus node artery in SLE (original magnification 100×). (From Straaton, K. V., Chatham, W. W., Reveille, J. D., et al.: Clinically significant valvular heart disease in systemic lupus erythematosus. Am. J. Med. *85*:645, 1988.)

Cardiac Abnormalities

Because the basic anatomical lesion of SLE is a diffuse microvasculitis (Fig. 56-9)[161,162] the heart is almost always found to be involved at autopsy.[163] The clinical manifestations, however, are usually overshadowed by the symptoms and signs related to involvement of other organs, and attention is drawn to the heart only when the lesions of pericarditis, myocarditis, or endocarditis are florid. Clinical evidence of cardiac abnormalities has been observed, however, in as many as 50 to 60 per cent of cases in two large series.[164,165] As diagnostic methods become more sophisticated, detection of cardiac involvement during life begins to approach that found at necropsy (see below).

PERICARDITIS. This is found in approximately two-thirds to three-fourths of autopsies and is the most common cardiac lesion of SLE (p. 1501). The acute pericardial inflammation may extend into the sinoatrial and AV nodes, with destruction of conducting fibers.[166,167] Pericardial fluid may be clear or sanguineous and has a high protein content. Effusions may be voluminous and occasionally cause tamponade.[168] Histologically, the pericardium shows fibrinoid degeneration, edema, and necrosis of connective tissue when the process is acute, and various stages of fibrosis with the formation of adhesions are found during the healing or chronic phase. Constrictive pericarditis occurs only rarely;[169] however, pericardial tamponade and constrictive pericarditis both have been reported in cases of procainamide-induced lupus erythematosus.[170,171] Pericarditis, which is frequently detected in lupus patients by echocardiography,[172,173] like arthritis, tends to be episodic and to heal well in remissions rather than to become chronic and sclerosing.

MYOCARDITIS. Subclinical myocarditis manifested as left ventricular dysfunction on echocardiography is common.[172-174] Its severity is proportionate to the severity of the systemic disease process. The lesions observed at autopsy and endomyocardial biopsy[175] consist of fibrinoid necrosis involving interstitial tissues and blood vessels, and only rarely are the cardiac myofibrils destroyed. Small vessel changes include an arteriopathy of vessels 0.1 to 1.0 mm in diameter. The abnormal vessels are located in the conduction system of patients selected for study because of the presence of arrhythmias. Segmental arteritis and periarteritis with some occlusions of the arterial lumen and small areas of fibrosis distal to the obstruction are found. Involvement of the AV as well as the sinoatrial node in the inflammatory process of SLE has been shown at autopsy. Rare cases of myocardial infarction, presumably due to arteritis of larger coronary vessels, have been reported.[178]

ENDOCARDITIS. This is the most characteristic cardiac lesion of SLE.[166,179] The Libman-Sacks verrucous valvular lesions are wartlike, varying from pinhead size to 3 to 4 mm. The lesions may be discrete or in clumps and are composed of degenerating valve tissue apparently extruded beyond the endothelium and accompanied by some fibrosis of the underlying leaflet. The lesions usually contain granular, basophilic masses of cellular debris, the characteristic so-called hematoxylin bodies composed of basophilic fragments in the cytoplasm of cells. They may be found anywhere on the endocardial surface of the heart, but are most common in the angles of the AV valves and on the underside of the base of the mitral valve. They may also extend onto the chordae tendineae or papillary muscles. Generalized involvement of the entire thickness of the heart valves with inflammatory and fibrous changes may also occur. Aortic valve involvement is rare, but has been well described.[180] Despite the frequency and extent of the endocardial lesions of SLE , they profoundly affect the function of the valves in only a minority of cases and, unlike rheumatic fever, do not produce serious regurgitation during the acute phase of the disease. Only rarely do they lead to marked scarring and deformity during healing, requiring valve replacement. The subclinical nature of the valvular lesions has been demonstrated by prospective clinical and echocardiographic studies (Fig. 56–10).[172,173]

Clinical Features

Although autopsy shows that at least two-thirds of patients have pericarditis at some time during the course of SLE, only one-third have recognizable symptoms and signs during life.[164,165] Typical pericardial pain may occur, but often the friction rubs, characteristic electrocardiographic changes, or enlargement of the cardiac silhouette on chest x-ray due to pericardial effusion may be found in the absence of symptoms, and therefore evidence of pericarditis should always be suspected and sought by clinical means and at intervals by echocardiography in *all* patients with SLE, even in those without clinical manifestations. Cardiac tamponade is rare but can occur,[168] requiring repeated aspirations of fluid. Systolic and diastolic murmurs at the mitral area, and less often at the aortic area, seem to come and go during the course of acute exacerbations of the disease and are presumably due to Libman-Sacks endocarditis. However, at autopsy the presence of these lesions is not always confirmed, and other factors such as anemia, tachycardia, fever, myocarditis, transient papillary muscle dysfunction, and the adventitious sounds of pleuropericarditis must be considered. Hemodynamically significant and permanent valvular regurgitation from lupus carditis is rare, but such cases have been reported and have even required valve replacement.[181–183]

Although myocardial dysfunction may be present, overt congestive heart failure due primarily to SLE is uncommon[184] except when associated with hypertension secondary to renal disease. Heart failure may be mistakenly diagnosed in the presence of edema due to renal disease or pericardial effusion

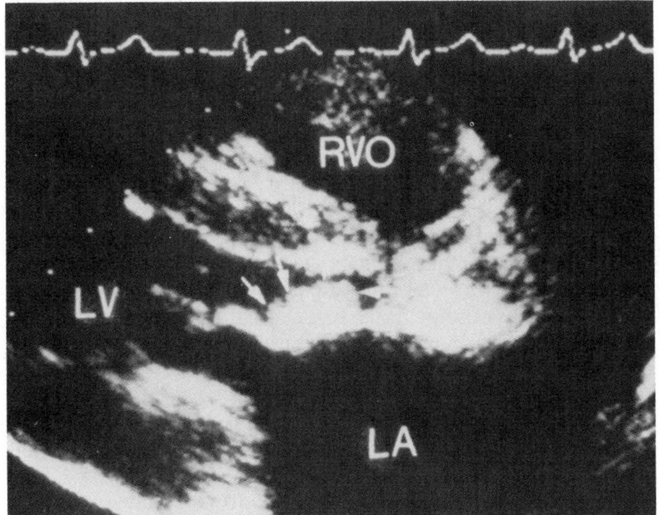

FIGURE 56–10. Parasternal long-axis view of the heart from a patient with systemic lupus erythematosus and high levels of anticardiolipin antibodies. A massive vegetation on ventricular surface of the anterior mitral leaflet (*arrows*) not interfering with the valve mobility, is clearly visualized. LA = left atrium, LV = left ventricle, RVO = right ventricular outflow. (From Nihoyannopoulos, N., et al.: Cardiac abnormalities in systemic lupus erythematosus: Association with raised anticardiolipin antibodies. Circulation *82*:369, 1990, by permission of the American Heart Association.)

or both. Clinically apparent myocarditis, like that of rheumatic fever, producing tachycardia, gallop rhythm, and cardiac dilatation, is usually a feature of very toxic cases of SLE when high fever and other multisystem manifestations of acute vasculitis are present. Arrhythmias are also relatively uncommon and consist of atrial flutter and fibrillation with varying degrees of AV block.[184] The latter may be associated with myocarditis and circulating antibodies to nuclear ribonucleoprotein.[185] Attention has been called to the development of congenital complete heart block, a lupus-like syndrome, and pericarditis in infants born to mothers with active SLE.[188,189] The observation suggests that transplacental transfer of abnormal antibodies may be of pathogenetic importance in these cases. During examination of a pregnant woman with SLE, fetal bradycardia should be recognized as a possible complication of lupus rather than fetal distress from other causes. The maternal antibodies that damage the fetal conduction system appear to be approximately 50 kD and to the SSA/Ro-55b/La system.[186]

Echocardiography may be useful in SLE for demonstrating pericardial involvement and for evaluating valve function in the presence of various murmurs.[176] Extensive hemodynamic studies carried out on patients who had had SLE for 2½ to 7 years prior to heart catheterization and who had no obvious clinical findings of cardiac involvement nonetheless showed considerable evidence of impairment of myocardial function.[190] Myocardial involvement has also been detected by magnetic resonance imaging.[191] More sophisticated studies will be necessary to sort out the complex factors that may compromise myocardial function in a disease that can affect all layers of the heart and the coronary vascular bed as well.[192]

TREATMENT. To the extent that their antiinflammatory effect can control active myocarditis, corticosteroids may be necessary to manage severe cardiac involvement in SLE. Control of hypertension is also helpful in the treatment and prevention of congestive heart failure. There is no evidence that corticosteroid treatment can prevent the rare cases of constrictive pericarditis or valvular deformity. Although the inflammatory reaction may be dramatically suppressed, the basic disease process and tissue injury are not altered by corticosteroid therapy, which is at most supportive and sometimes causes problems (hypertension and fluid retention). Immunosuppressive therapy is usually reserved for the most severe, corticosteroid-resistant forms of the disease and especially for renal involvement. Death from the cardiac disease of SLE compared with other causes of fatality in this disease is rare, so that cardiac manifestations usually do not determine the choice of antiinflammatory therapy.

Among the antibodies found in high concentrations in patients with SLE are a variety of antiphospholipid antibodies, which include the lupus "anticoagulant," the antibodies responsible for a positive VDRL, and more specific anti-phospholipid antibodies such as the anticardiolipin antibody. Elevated levels of these antiphospholipid antibodies are associated with a syndrome consisting of recurrent venous and/or arterial thromboses, placental thrombosis leading to abortion, thrombocytopenia, and cutaneous vascular abnormalities such as livedo reticularis.[193,194] Occasionally, this clinical complex occurs in patients without lupus.[196] High levels of anticardiolipin antibodies have been found in patients with SLE to be highly associated with cardiac abnormalities, especially valvular heart disease.[196–198]

POLYARTERITIS NODOSA

As noted above, necrotizing inflammation of blood vessels is a common finding in immune complex diseases of known and unknown etiology; however, because the origin and nature of the offending agent are unknown in most instances the vasculitides continue to be classified on the basis of their histological and clinical features. These depend largely upon the size of the involved blood vessels, their anatomical sites, the stage of the inflammation, and the characteristics of the lesions.

The clinical features of most cases fit into one of the following five major categories: polyarteritis nodosa (PAN; also termed periarteritis nodosa), allergic granulomatosis, Wegener's granulomatosis, hypersensitivity vasculitis, and giant cell arteritis.

PATHOLOGICAL FEATURES. The muscular arteries, adjacent veins, and occasionally arterioles and venules (but not the capillaries) are involved in a necrotizing inflammation. Segments of vessels, at times only part of the circumference being affected, are involved in the lesions, especially at the bifurcation of arteries. Small aneurysms may form and rupture. In the acute stage of inflammation the lesions contain predominantly polymorphonuclear leukocytes whereas in chronic lesions mononuclear cell infiltration and partial healing are apparent. However, both phases may be present at once, suggesting repeated or continuous insults.

The lesions are commonly found in the coronary arteries as well as kidneys, muscles, and vasa nervorum, but the lungs are usually spared. *Myocardial infarction* is therefore relatively common, and this leads to patchy myocardial fibrosis and left ventricular enlargement. The latter is also secondary to hypertension, frequently present owing to renal involvement. Hemorrhage into the pericardial sac with tamponade and death, inflammatory pericarditis, and uremic pericarditis are causes of pericardial involvement. Endocardial or valvular lesions do not occur unless the papillary muscle is injured by ischemia.

CLINICAL FEATURES. PAN may occur at any age, produces fever and multisystem involvement, and may persist for months or years. Pericarditis may be clinically evident, frequently associated with pleuritis, but is not a prominent feature of the disease. Chest pain due to true angina pectoris is also relatively rare[199] despite the occurrence of myocardial infarction. In one series of 41 cases of PAN and myocardial infarction, only three were diagnosed clinically.[200] The most common form of heart involvement is congestive failure and hypertension due to renal disease, which causes most deaths. Cardiac arrhythmias, most often atrial flutter and fibrillation, can occur. Death from ruptured aneurysms, particularly gastrointestinal bleeding, is not uncommon.

COURSE AND TREATMENT. The prognosis of PAN is grave; one-half to two-thirds of patients died within a year when series comprised hospitalized cases. Treatment with corticosteroids is frequently followed by temporary improvement with doses of 40 to 60 mg of prednisone or prednisolone per day. Five-year survival of untreated patients is estimated at 13 per cent. Studies with immunosuppressive drugs have been encouraging in apparently prolonging the course in some cases, but adequate controlled studies have not been made.[202]

Other Forms of Diffuse Vasculitis

ALLERGIC GRANULOMATOSIS (CHURG-STRAUSS VASCULITIS, HYPEREOSINOPHILIC SYNDROME)

This disease involves the vessels of the heart in the same way as PAN, but eosinophils tend to be more abundant in the lesions, and granulomatous collections of epithelioid and giant cells are formed, accounting for the name of the condition.[202] Pulmonary involvement, especially asthma, dominates the clinical picture, and patients tend to have a history of respiratory infection and fever, often with a striking peripheral eosinophilia. The heart, however, may be a primary target organ. Pericarditis, occasionally constrictive, myocarditis with acute heart failure, and myocardial infarction have been reported, as well as endomyocardial fibrosis in some variants of the syndrome.[203]

WEGENER'S GRANULOMATOSIS

This syndrome is distinguished by necrotizing granulomas of the upper respiratory tract, especially the destructive lesions of the nasopharynx and paranasal sinuses, middle ear, and bronchial tree. Necrotizing inflammation extends into the smaller pulmonary vessels of the lungs and other organs, particularly the kidneys. Pericardial and myocardial involvement is not uncommon, but the clinical picture is dominated by respiratory and renal involvement, without which the diagnosis cannot be made. The special feature of treatment is the encouraging response of this particular syndrome to cyclophosphamide therapy, resulting in dramatic remissions, often complete, and in prolonged survival.[202,204] Although cardiac complications are considered unusual in Wegener's granulomatosis, they have been found in 12 per cent of some recent series[204] and in sporadic case reports that include constrictive pericarditis, high-grade AV block, supraventricular tachycardia, as well as complications secondary to involvement of the coronary arteries.[205,206]

HYPERSENSITIVITY VASCULITIS (LEUKOCYTOBLASTIC VASCULITIS)

Hypersensitivity vasculitis is also called small-vessel vasculitis or angiitis and is characterized by involvement of arterioles, venules, and capillaries only. Antigen-antibody complexes present in the lesions all tend to be of the same age. It is difficult to tell at the inception of the disease whether it is part of a larger syndrome, such as SLE, subacute infective endocarditis, mixed cryoglobulinemia, Henoch-Schönlein purpura, or a drug reaction except by the course and distinguishing features of the other syndromes. Hypersensitivity vasculitis is the most common form of immune complex disease. Muscular and large arteries are spared, so that the tissue lesions are due to microinfarcts and hemorrhagic and exudative reactions at the capillary level rather than to thrombosis of large vessels with resulting ischemia and necrosis. The most common cardiac finding is pericarditis, but such involvement occurs along with that of many other organs, skin, mucous membranes, joints, and so on.

GIANT CELL ARTERITIS[202-208]

Giant cell arteritis, also called cranial or temporal arteritis, affects predominantly older individuals. Large or medium-sized arteries, including the superficial temporal artery, are involved without small-vessel or capillary lesions. The lesions are usually cellular and granulomatous and contain multinucleated giant cells. Involvement of the arteries is spotty and segmented and tends to produce thrombosis at the site of involvement. The aorta is often involved and aneurysms and dissection can result (p. 1547). External and internal carotids and vertebral arteries can be affected, and thrombosis of the ophthalmic or central retinal artery leads to blindness. Thrombosis of the coronary, iliac, femoral, or mesenteric arteries produces ischemia and infarctions. Aortic regurgitation is a rare but well-documented complication.[209]

BEHÇET'S SYNDROME

This diffuse vasculitis causes recurrent genital and oral ulcerations and uveitis.[210] Cardiac manifestations occur in about 5 per cent of patients and include pericarditis, aortic and mitral regurgitation, and endomyocardial fibrosis involving the right side of the heart.[211]

PROGRESSIVE SYSTEMIC SCLEROSIS (DIFFUSE SCLERODERMA)

Progressive systemic sclerosis (PSS) is an insidious, chronic, fibrosing condition that presents as progressive tightening and thickening of the skin (scleroderma), developing over a period of many years. Raynaud's phenomenon occurs at some time in almost all patients. Visceral involvement may occur at any time during the course of the disease, affecting the gastrointestinal tract, lungs, heart or kidney. Much attention has been given to the classification of various subgroups of this syndrome that include patients with diffuse scleroderma, those without diffuse skin changes but with other shared features, such as calcinosis, Raynaud's phenomenon, esophageal dysfunction, sclerodactyly, and telangiectasia (the CREST syndrome), and those with features overlapping polymyositis or systemic lupus erythematosus or both.[212-214]

Pathological Features and Pathogenesis

In contrast to the acute exudative forms of vasculitis associated with the necrotizing lesions described above, PSS seems to be a disease at the opposite end of the inflammatory scale, in which very slow scarring and fibrosis result from gradual obliteration of small vessels. It is difficult to classify PSS pathophysiologically because the cause of the extensive fibrosis is not known, but the importance of small artery spasm and the possibility of its reversal by arterial vasodilators has received considerable attention.[215-225] Pulmonary hypertension has been at least temporarily reduced with such vasodilators as captopril,[221] nifedipine,[223] and verapamil,[224] as have attacks of Raynaud's phenomenon. Left ventricular regional wall motion abnormalities have been demonstrated during cold exposure in 9 of 16 patients with Raynaud's phenomenon and PSS or the CREST syndrome, and in most of these cases treatment with nifedipine blunted the severity of the abnormal ventricular response.[225] Short-term improvement in myocardial perfusion with nifedipine, demonstrated by thallium-201 single-photon-emission computed tomography, was observed in a study of 29 patients with diffuse scleroderma and Raynaud's phenomenon.[217]

Hereditary factors have not been identified. Qualitative abnormalities of collagen are not documented. The disease apparently results from injury or spasm at the level of very small arteries, 150 to 500 μm in diameter, and capillaries are gradually obliterated.[215] Early in the course of lesions, mononuclear cell infiltrates occur around small arteries and in the interstitium. The basement membrane of the capillaries appears thickened. Fibroblastic proliferation and overproduction of collagen result from the low-grade inflammatory process. Narrowing and obliteration of small arteries result in decreased vascularization of the skin, skeletal muscles, lung, and heart, followed by fibrosis. The interlobular arteries of the kidney are involved by intensive intimal proliferation, which causes rapid renal failure, often with severe hypertension.

CARDIAC LESIONS. The importance of primary cardiac involvement in the natural history of the disease has been repeatedly emphasized,[213-221] but only with the advent of noninvasive cardiac evaluation methods of thallium-201 scintigraphy, rest and exercise radionuclide ventriculography, continuous 24-hour Holter ECG monitoring, two-dimensional echocardiography, and pulmonary-function testing has the full picture of the frequency and extent of cardiac dysfunction become apparent.[215-221] Thallium scintigraphy may show fixed defects, but even more common are cold-induced reversible defects[226] compatible with severe coronary vasospasm. Defective perfusion of organs by spastic small arteries may account for the general observation that functional disability of the myocardium and lungs exceeds anatomical changes.[216-225] Heart involvement is a frequent cause of death and second only to involvement of the kidneys as a factor shortening the surival of patients with this disease. Confusion concerning the question of primary involvement of the heart by the sclerosing process has been caused by the frequency of cor pulmonale resulting from pulmonary involvement of PSS and severe hypertension and hypertensive heart disease resulting from the renal involvement. In one study of patients with systemic sclerosis, ambulatory electrocardiography revealed ventricular ectopy in 67 per cent of patients, with more serious ventricular arrhythmias in 25 per cent.[227] These arrhythmias tend to be more severe in patients with other evidence of cardiac disease and are an independent risk factor for death.

"Scleroderma heart" is primarily a myocardial disease, and the heart's small vessels are all vulnerable to the sclerosing process. Atherosclerosis of the major coronary arteries occurs to the same degree in patients with PSS as in age- and sex-matched controls. PSS patients, however, have much more intimal sclerosis of the small coronary arteries than do controls, and such involvement may lead to ischemia, small infarctions, and fibrosis. The combination of vascular insufficiency and fibrosis produces a cardiomyopathy with congestive heart failure and conduction system abnormalities.[215-221] Acute and chronic pericarditis, even in the absence of uremia, is common but usually asymptomatic. At times the resulting effusion can be large enough to cause tamponade,[228] although this degree of effusion is rare. Pericardial fluid, when obtainable, has the features of an exudate but lacks evidence of autoantibodies, immune complexes, or complement depletion, such as that seen in rheumatoid arthritis or SLE.[229] Endocardial involvement is rare, and the deformities of mitral and aortic valves that have been reported probably have little hemodynamic significance.

Clinical Features

The primary clinical manifestations of scleroderma heart disease are those of pericarditis (see also p. 1502) and congestive heart failure. In one series, pericarditis patients had a 7-year cumulative survival rate of 33 per cent, whereas none of the PSS patients with heart failure survived for 7 years.[230] Men have significantly worse survival rates than women, as do blacks and older patients. Although cardiac symptoms may appear months or even years before the skin is involved, as a rule overt heart disease is not a prominent part of the clinical picture of PSS until late in its course, when myocardial involvement and resultant heart failure indicate a grim prognosis. The relative risk of death for a PSS patient with an S_3 gallop indicative of myocardial disease was reported to be many times that for a patient without an S_3 gallop.[231] Pericarditis, however, may be intermittently symptomatic for long periods.

When dyspnea with exertion or at rest occurs in the patient with PSS, primary myocardial failure must be distinguished from myocardial failure secondary to hypertension from renal disease and pulmonary insufficiency from pulmonary fibrosis due to PSS. Cardiac murmurs are not usually due to valvular deformity but to cardiac dilatation and to anemia or to papillary weakness. Chest pain simulating ischemic heart disease as well as typical pericardial pain may occur.

The *roentgenogram of the chest* may reveal cardiac enlargement from pericardial effusion, cardiomyopathy, or hypertension. The electrocardiographic findings are also nonspecific and may, indeed, be normal when the heart is seriously involved. All degrees of AV conduction blocks, right and left ventricular hypertrophy, and all varieties of arrhythmias have been described,[227] but conduction defects are found most often in patients with the primary cardiomyopathy of PSS.[218-221]

Echocardiographic studies reveal patterns consistent with a congestive cardiomyopathy or a restrictive cardiomyopathy, and pericardial effusion can be demonstrated often when not suspected clinically.

TREATMENT. The value of corticosteroids is limited to improvement of the early edematous phase of the disease, but this effect on the heart has not been systematically evaluated and probably will not influence the eventual course of the disease.

As noted above, the most interesting and encouraging recent therapeutic development is the demonstration of improved perfusion of the heart, lungs, and, in the case of Raynaud's phenomenon, the hands, of patients with PSS or the CREST syndrome by the administration of calcium channel blockers such as nifedipine[217,223] and verapamil[225] and other vasodilators such as captopril.[222,232] The possible benefits of long-term therapy with these agents remain to be defined.

POLYMYOSITIS AND DERMATOMYOSITIS

Polymyositis is a diffuse inflammatory disease of unknown cause affecting primarily proximal striated muscles and various connective tissues of the body, especially skin and joints.[233] When the disease also involves the skin, it is called *dermatomyositis*. Polymyositis may be due to a pathological process common to several etiologies because it is seen in association with a variety of syndromes. It is grouped with the connective tissue or rheumatic diseases because of its overlapping clinical and laboratory features, especially when it is associated with rheumatoid arthritis and PSS but also with SLE or polyarteritis. Involvement of the heart in polymyositis has just begun to be fully appreciated in the past decade and was mentioned in earlier publications only as a rare finding, if at all.

Pathological Features

Polymyositis is either increasing in incidence and/or is being more frequently diagnosed, and it is now well recognized as one of the most common myopathies. The principal changes in muscle tissue consist of widespread destruction of muscle fibers with phagocytosis of destroyed cells. There may be focal infiltrates of inflammatory cells, such as lymphocytes, mononuclear leukocytes, plasma cells, and, only rarely, neutrophilic leukocytes. Regeneration of destroyed muscle in the form of proliferating sarcolemmal nuclei, basophilic sarcoplasm, and new myofibrils is a prominent feature. Residual muscle fibers may be small. In any given biopsy specimen, either degeneration of muscle fibers or infiltrations of inflammatory cells may predominate. In electron microscopic studies, the most significant changes, in addition to those in muscle fibers, are found in the endothelium and basement

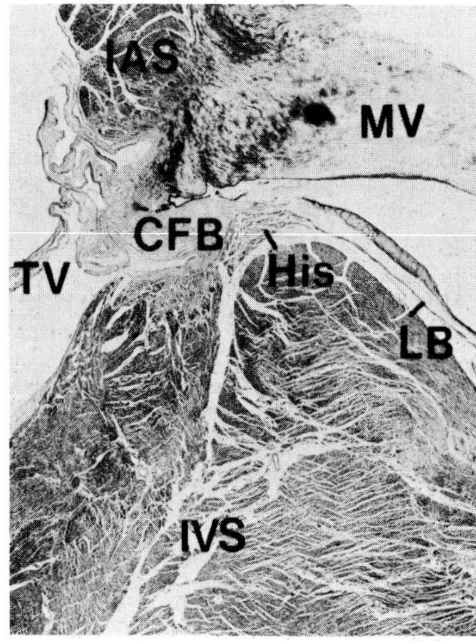

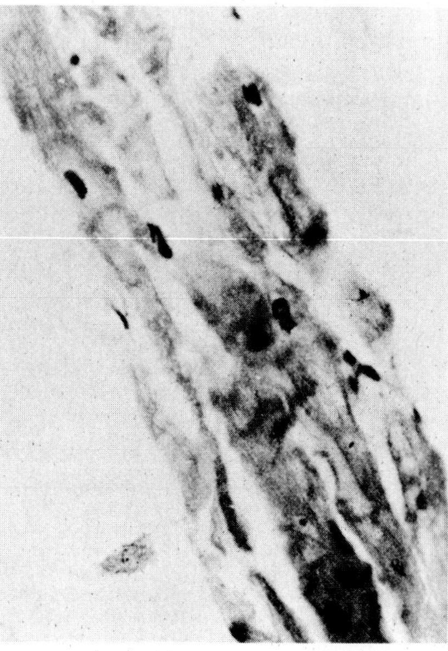

FIGURE 56–11. Cardiac conduction system in a 53-year-old woman with polymyositis-dermatomyositis left bundle branch block. *Left,* the left bundle (LB) and distal portion of the His bundle (His). The interatrial septum (IAS) is at the top and the interventricular septum (IVS) below. The mitral (MV) and tricuspid (TV) valves are attached to the central fibrous body (CFB). *Right,* contraction band necrosis of the left bundle. The myocytes of the bundle show irregular coarse transverse condensations of sarcoplasm and their nuclei are pyknotic. (From Haupt, H. M., and Hutchins, G. M.: The heart and conduction system in polymyositis-dermatomyositis: A clinicopathologic study of 16 autopsied patients. Am. J. Cardiol. *50*:998, 1982.)

membrane of capillaries and small arterioles, much like those described in scleroderma and SLE. Inclusions in the cytoplasm of endothelial cells that are identical to those found in SLE and scleroderma have been described.[234]

CARDIAC PATHOLOGY.[235–239] The cardiac lesions involve the conducting system predominantly but also can produce an extensive cardiomyopathy and pericarditis. The latter may appear far more often than would be suspected on clinical grounds. The cardiac valves and coronary arteries are spared except in overlap syndromes. The sinoatrial node shows conspicuous fibrosis, swelling and degeneration of collagen, and focal or complete replacement. The fibrosis extends into the adjacent myocardium of the right atrium. The AV node, bundle of His, and both bundle branches all may be involved in the degenerative and fibrotic processes (Fig. 56–11). Cardiac muscle fibers in the atria and ventricles are replaced in scattered areas by fibrosis, and, in some cases, the pattern of focal myocardial necrosis and inflammation is the same as that seen in skeletal muscle. Pericarditis is described more often clinically than pathologically.

CLINICAL FEATURES. Almost all authors comment on the rarity of cardiovascular manifestations in polymyositis, and, indeed, the best reported studies of survivorship do not relate death to cardiac causes but rather to pneumonitis, which is relatively common from aspiration secondary to respiratory muscle weakness and dysphagia. However, more careful studies of the heart for subtle signs of involvement in polymyositis patients without cardiac symptoms and signs[238,239] and careful review of autopsied patients with polymyositis-dermatomyositis syndromes[237] show a much higher frequency of cardiac involvement in polymyositis than was previously appreciated. When standard 12-lead electrocardiograms are analyzed systematically, arrhythmias may be quite frequent.[239] These usually consist of supraventricular tachycardia, but ventricular tachycardia and advanced heart block associated with syncope or cardiac arrest have also been observed. Deaths have been attributed directly to myocardial failure or arrhythmias or both in some cases, and cardiac muscle histology has been found to be abnormal on autopsy. Sudden death is not unusual, especially in patients with documented heart block.[239] Constrictive pericarditis has been reported.[235]

TREATMENT. Corticosteroids and immunosuppressive drugs may be of benefit in the treatment of polyositis-dermatomyositis, but only a controlled prospective study can settle this issue. The course of the disease, including myocardial involvement, may not be truly modified by corticosteroids, but the complications of muscle weakness, especially of the respiratory and deglutitional muscles, which lead to pulmonary disease and death, might be diminished by the frequent improvement of muscle strength observed after this treatment.

In the absence of malignancy, survival statistics are favorable for all groups (87 to 91 per cent) in several studies. The leading causes of death, which in one series were metastatic malignant disease (24 per cent), sepsis (19 per cent), profound muscular weakness (9.5 per cent), and cardiovascular and cerebrovascular disorders (unspecified percentage), suggest that at least some of these may be modified by supportive therapy and management to improve the prognosis.

MIXED CONNECTIVE TISSUE DISEASE

As its name implies, this condition is characterized by overlapping features and combinations of rheumatoid arthritis, progressive systemic stenosis, polymyositis, and systemic lupus erythematosus. Patients have high titers of circulating antibodies to nuclear ribonucleoprotein.[240] Cardiac involvement includes pericardial effusion and thickening as well as valvular, usually mitral, regurgitation.[241]

REFERENCES

REUMATIC FEVER

1. Stollerman, G. H.: Rheumatic Fever and Streptococcal Infection. New York, Grune and Stratton, 1975.
2. Bisno, A. L.: The rise and fall of rheumatic fever. J.A.M.A. *254*:538, 1985.
3. Stollerman G. H.: Rheumatogenic group A streptococci and the return of rheumatic fever. Adv. Intern. Med. *35*:1, 1990.
4. Ramelkamp, C. H., Denny, F. W., and Wannamaker, L. W.: Studies on the epidemiology of rheumatic fever in the armed services. *In* Thomas, L. (ed.): Rheumatic Fever. Minneapolis, University of Minnesota Press, 1952, pp. 72–89.
5. Frank, P. F., Stollerman, G. H., and Miller, L. F.: Protection of a military population from rheumatic fever. J.A.M.A. *193*:775, 1965.
6. Gordis, L.: The virtual disappearance of rheumatic fever in the United States; lessons in the rise and fall of disease. Circulation *72*:1155, 1985.
7. Markowitz, M.: The decline of rheumatic fever, role of medical intervention. J. Pediatr. *106*:545, 1985.
8. Argarwal, B. L.: Rheumatic heart disease unabated in developing countries. Lancet *2*:910, 1981.
9. Stetson, C. A.: The relation of antibody response to rheumatic fever. *In* McCarty, M. (ed.): Streptococcal Infections. New York, Columbia University Press, 1954, pp. 208–218.
10. Rammelkamp, C. H., Jr.: The Lewis A. Conner Memorial Lecture. Rheumatic heart disease—A challenge. Circulation *17*:842, 1958.
11. Siegel, A. C., Johnson, E. E., and Stollerman, G. H.: Controlled studies of streptococcal pharyngitis in a pediatric population: I. Factors related to the attack rate of rheumatic fever. N. Engl. J. Med. *265*:559, 1961.
12. Stollerman, G. H.: Factors determining the attack rate of rheumatic fever. J.A.M.A. *177*:823, 1961.
13. Stollerman, G. H., Siegel, A. C., and Johnson, E. E.: Variable epidemiology of streptococcal disease and the changing patterns of rheumatic fever. Mod. Concepts Cardiovasc. Dis. *34*:45, 1965.
14. Kaplan, E. L., Top, F. H., Dudding, B. A., and Wannamaker, L. W.: Diagnosis of streptococcal pharyngitis: Differentiation of active infection from the carrier state in the symptomatic child. J. Infect. Dis. *123*:490, 1971.
15. Top, F. H., Wannamaker, L. W., Maxted, W. R., and Anthony, G. V.: M antigens among group A streptococci isolated from skin lesions. J. Exp. Med. *126*:667, 1967.
16. Stollerman, G. H.: Nephritogenic and rheumatogenic group A streptococci. J. Infect. Dis. *120*:258, 1969.
17. Wannamaker, L. W.: Medical progress. Differences between streptococcal infections of the throat and of the skin. N. Engl. J. Med. *282*:23 and 78, 1970.
18. Wannamaker, L. W.: The chain that links the heart to the throat. Circulation *48*:9, 1973.
19. Bisno, A. L., Pearce, I. A., Wall, H. P., et al.: Contrasting epidemiology of acute rheumatic fever and acute glomerulonephritis. Nature of the antecedent streptococcal infection. N. Engl. J. Med. *283*:561, 1970.
20. Poon-King, T., Mohammed, I., Cox, R., et al.: Recurrent epidemic nephritis in South Trinidad. N. Engl. J. Med. *277*:728, 1967.
21. Potter, E. V., Svartman, M., Poon-King, T., and Earle, D. P.: The families of patients with acute rheumatic fever or glomerulonephritis in Trinidad. Am. J. Epidemiol. *106*:130, 1977.
22. Widdowson, J. P., Maxted, W. R., Notley, C. M., and Pinney, A. M.: The antibody responses in man to infection with different serotypes of group A streptococci. J. Med. Microbiol. *7*:483, 1974.

23. Bisno, A. L.: The concept of rheumatogenic and nonrheumatogenic group A streptococci. *In* McCarty, M., and Zabriskie, J. B. (eds.): Streptococcal Diseases and the Immune Response. New York, Academic Press, 1980, p. 789.
24. Stollerman, G. H.: The streptococcus, rheumatic fever and rheumatic heart disease. *In* Shaper, A. G., Hutt, M. S. R., and Fejfar, Z. (eds.): Cardiovascular Disease in the Tropics. London, British Medical Associates, 1974.
25. Sanyal, S. K., Berry, A. M., Duggal, S., et al.: Sequelae of the initial attack of rheumatic fever in children from North India. Circulation *65*:375, 1982.
26. Sanyal, S. K., Thapar, M. K., Ahmed, S. H., et al.: The initial attack of acute rheumatic fever during childhood in North India. A prospective study of the clinical profile. Circulation *49*:7, 1974.
27. Taranta, A.: Rheumatic fever in children and adolescents. A long-term epidemiologic study of subsequent prophylaxis, streptococcal infections, and clinical sequelae: IV. Relation of the rheumatic fever recurrence rate per streptococcal infection to the titers of streptococcal antibodies. Ann. Intern. Med. *60*(Suppl. 5):47, 1964.
28. Taranta, A., Kleinberg, E., Feinstein, A. R., et al.: Rheumatic fever in children and adolescents. A long-term epidemiologic study of subsequent prophylaxis, streptococcal infections, and clinical sequelae: V. Relation of the rheumatic fever recurrence rate per streptococcal infection to pre-existing clinical features of the patients. Ann. Intern. Med. *60*(Suppl. 5):58, 1964.
29. Johnson, E. E., Stollerman, G. H., and Grossman, B. J.: Rheumatic recurrences in patients not receiving continuous prophylaxis. J.A.M.A. *190*:74, 1964.
30. Taranta, A.: Rheumatic fever made difficult. A critical review of pathogenetic theories. Paediatrician 5:74, 1976.
31. Pattarroyo, M. E., Winchester, R., Vejerano, A., et al.: Association of B-cell alloantigen with susceptibility to rheumatic fever. Nature *278*:173, 1979.
32. Zabriskie, J. B., Lavenchy, D., Williams, R. C., Jr., et al.: Rheumatic fever associated B cell alloantigen as identified by monoclonal antibodies. Arthritis Rheum. *28*:1047, 1985.
33. Khanna, A. K., Buskirk, D. R., Williams, R. C., Jr., et al.: Presence of a non-HLA B cell antigen in rheumatic fever patients and their families as defined by a monoclonal antibody. J. Clin. Invest. *83*:1710, 1989.
34. Stollerman, G. H.: Streptococci and Rheumatic Heart Disease. *In* De Vries, RRP, Cohen, I. R., and van Rood, J. J. (eds.): The Role of Microorganisms in noninfectious diseases. London, Springer-Verlag, 1990, pp. 9–20.
35. Stollerman, G. H.: The epidemiology of primary and secondary rheumatic fever. *In* Uhr, J. W. (ed): The Streptococcus, Rheumatic Fever and Glomerulonephritis. Baltimore, Williams and Wilkins, 1964, pp. 331–337.
36. Yoshimoya, S., and Pope, R. M.: Detection of immune complexes in acute rheumatic fever and their relationship to HLA-B5. J. Clin. Invest. *65*:136, 1980.
37. Stollerman, G. H.: Autoimmunity and rheumatic fever. *In* Cohen, I. R. (ed.): Perspectives in Autoimmunity. Boca Raton, Fl., CRC Press, 1986.
38. Kaplan, M. H., Meyeserian, M., and Kishner, I.: Immunologic studies of heart tissue: IV. Serologic reactions with human heart tissue as revealed by immunofluorescent methods. Isoimmune, Wassermann, and auto-immune reactions. J. Exp. Med. *113*:17, 1961.
39. Hess, E. V., Fink, C. W., Taranta, A., and Ziff, M.: Heart muscle antibodies in rheumatic fever and other diseases. J. Clin. Invest. *43*:886, 1964.
40. Kaplan, M. H.: Immunologic relation of streptococcal and tissue antigens. I. Properties of an antigen in certain strains of group A streptococci exhibiting an immunologic cross-reaction with human heart tissue. J. Immunol. *90*:595, 1963.
41. Kaplan, M. H., and Suchy, M. L.: Immunologic relation of streptococcal and tissue antigens. II. Cross reactions of antisera to mammalian heart tissue with a cell wall constituent of certain strains of group A streptococci. J. Exp. Med. *119*:643, 1964.
42. Zabriskie, J. B., and Freimer, E. H.: An immunological relationship between the group A streptococcus and mammalian muscle. J. Exp. Med. *124*:661, 1966.
43. Goldstein, I., Halpern, B., and Robert, L.: Immunological relationship between streptococcus A polysaccharide and the structural glycoproteins of heart valves. Nature *213*:44, 1967.
44. Dudding, B. A., and Ayoub, E. M.: Persistence of streptococcal group A antibody in patients with rheumatic valvular disease. J. Exp. Med. *129*:1081, 1968.
45. Appleton, R. S., Victoria, B. C., Tamer, D., and Ayoub, E. M.: Specificity of persistence of antibody to the streptococcal group A carbohydrate in rheumatic valvular heart disease. J. Lab. Clin. Med. *105*:114, 1985.
46. Husby, G., van de Rijn, I., Zabriskie, J. B., et al.: Antibodies reacting with cytoplasm of subthalamic and caudate nuclei neurons in chorea and acute rheumatic fever. J. Exp. Med. *144*:1094, 1976.
47. Dale, J. B., and Beachey, E. H.: Epitopes of streptococcal M proteins shared with cardiac myosin. J. Exp. Med. *162*:583, 1985.
48. Cunningham, M. W., and Swerlick, R. A.: Polyspecificity of antistreptococcal murine monoclonal antibodies and their implications in autoimmunity. J. Exp. Med. *164*:998, 1987.
49. Bronze, M. S., Beachey, E. H., and Dale, J. B.: Protective and heart cross-reactive epitopes within the NH2 terminus of type 19 streptococcal M protein. J. Exp. Med. *167*:1849, 1988.
50. Manjula, B. N., Trus, B. L., and Fischetti, V. A.: Presence of two distinct regions in the coiled-coil structure of the streptococcal pep M5 protein: relationship to mammalian coiled-coil proteins and implications to its biological properties. Proc. Natl. Acad. Sci. *82*:1064, 1985.
51. Bessen, D., Jones, K. F., and Fischetti, V. A.: Evidence for two distinct classes of streptococcal M protein and their relationship to rheumatic fever. J. Exp. Med. *169*:269, 1989.
52. Tomai, M., Kotb, M., Majundar, G., and Beachey E. H.: Superantigenicity of streptococcal M protein. J. Exp. Med. *172*:359, 1990.
53. Murphy, G. E.: Nature of rheumatic heart disease with special reference to myocardial disease and heart failure. Medicine *39*:289, 1960.
54. Aschoff, L.: The rheumatic nodules in the heart. Ann. Rheum. Dis. *1*:161, 1939.
55. Kuschner, M., Ferrer, M. I., Harvey, R. M., and Wylie, R. H.: Rheumatic carditis in surgically removed appendages. Am. Heart J. *43*:286, 1952.
56. Virmani, R., and Roberts, W. C.: Aschoff bodies in operatively excised atrial appendages and in papillary muscles. Frequency and clinical significance. Circulation *55*:559, 1977.
57. Roberts, W. C., and Virmani, R.: Aschoff bodies at necropsy in valvular heart disease. Evidence from an analysis of 543 patients over 14 years of age that rheumatic heart disease, at least anatomically, is a disease of the mitral valve. Circulation *57*:803, 1978.
58. Stollerman, G. H., Lynch, W. F., Dolman, M. A., et al.: Immunologic evidence of streptococcal infection in patients undergoing mitral commissurotomy. Circulation *15*:267, 1957.
59. Lanningan, R.: Cardiac Pathology. London, Butterworth and Co., 1966.
60. Becker, C. G., and Murphy, G. E.: On the pathology of rheumatic heart disease. *In* Read, S. E., and Zabriskie, J. B. (eds.): Streptococcal Diseases and the Immune Response, New York, Academic Press, 1980, p. 23.
61. Husby, G. H., Arora, R., Williams, R. C., et al.: Immunofluorescent studies of florid rheumatic Aschoff lesions. Arthritis Rheum. *29*:207, 1986.
62. Steele, P. P., Weily, H. S., Davies, H., and Genton, E.: Platelet survival in patients with rheumatic heart disease. N. Engl. J. Med. *290*:537, 1974.
63. Winkelman, N. W., and Eckel, J. L.: The brain in acute rheumatic fever. Nonsuppurative meningoencephalitis rheumatica. Arch. Neurol. Psychiatr. *28*:844, 1932.
64. Neubuerger, K. T.: The brain in rheumatic fever. Dis. Nerv. System *8*:259, 1947.
65. Costero, I.: Cerebral lesions responsible for death of patients with active rheumatic fever. Arch. Neurol. Psychiatr. *62*:48, 1949.
66. Buchanan, D. N.: Pathologic changes in chorea. Am. J. Dis. Child. *62*:443, 1941.
67. Kernohan, J. W., Woltman, H. W., and Barnes, A. R.: Involvement of the nervous system associated with endocarditis. Neuropsychiatric and neuropathologic observations in 42 cases of fatal outcome. Arch. Neurol. Psychiatr. *42*:789, 1939.
68. Raz, I., Fisher, J., Israel, A., et al.: An unusual case of rheumatic pneumonia. Arch. Intern. Med. *145*:1130, 1985.
69. Rammelkamp, C. H., Jr., and Stolzer, B. L.: The latent period before the onset of acute rheumatic fever. Yale J. Biol. Med. *34*:386, 1961.
70. Feinstein, A. R., and Spagnuolo, M.: The clinical patterns of acute rheumatic fever: A reappraisal. Medicine *41*:279, 1962.
71. Ben-Dov, I., and Berry, E.: Acute rheumatic fever in adults over the age of 45 years: An analysis of 23 patients together with a review of the literature. Semin. Arthritis Rheum. *10*:10, 1980.
72. United Kingdom and United States Joint Report on Rheumatic Fever: The treatment of acute rheumatic fever in children. A cooperative clinical trial of ACTH, cortisone and aspirin. Circulation *11*:343, 1955.
73. United Kingdom and United States Joint Report on Rheumatic Heart Disease: The evolution of rheumatic heart disease in children. Five-year report of a cooperative clinical trial of ACTH, cortisone and aspirin. Circulation *22*:503, 1960.
74. United Kingdom and United States Joint Report on Rheumatic Heart Disease: The natural history of rheumatic fever and rheumatic heart disease. Ten-year report of a cooperative clinical trial of ACTH, cortisone and aspirin. Circulation *32*:457, 1965.
75. Massell, B. V., Fyler, D. C., and Roy, S. B.: The clinical picture of rheumatic fever. Diagnosis, immediate prognosis, course and therapeutic implications. Am. J. Cardiol. *1*:436, 1958.
76. Combined Rheumatic Fever Study Group, 1960: A comparison of the effect of prednisone and acetylsalicylic acid on the incidence of residual rheumatic heart disease. N. Engl. J. Med. *262*:895, 1960.
77. Combined Rheumatic Fever Study Group, 1965: A comparison of the short-term, intensive prednisone and acetylsalicylic acid therapy in the treatment of acute rheumatic fever. N. Engl. J. Med. *272*:63, 1965.
78. Robinson, R. W.: Effect of atropine upon the prolongation of the P-R interval found in acute rheumatic fever and certain vagotonic persons. Am. Heart J. *29*:378, 1945.
79. Lenox, C. C., Zuberbuhler, J. R., Park, S. C., et al.: Arrhythmias and Stokes-Adams attacks in acute rheumatic fever. Pediatrics *61*:599, 1979.
80. Meynet, P.: Rheumatisme articulaire subaigu avec production de tumeurs multiples dans les tissus fibreux periarticulaires et sur le périoste d'un grand numbre d'os. Lyons Med. *19*:495, 1875.
81. Baldwin, J. S., Kerr, J. M., Kuttner, A. G., and Loyle, E. F.: Observations on rheumatic nodules over a 30-year period. J. Pediatr. *56*:465, 1960.
82. Veasy, L. G., Wiedmeier, S. E., Garth, S. O., et al.: Resurgence of acute rheumatic fever in the intermountain area of the United States. N. Engl. J. Med. *316*:421, 1987.
83. Taranta, A., and Stollerman, G. H.: The relationship of Sydenham's chorea to infection with group A streptococci Am. J. Med. *20*:170, 1956.
84. Bland, E. F.: Chorea as a manifestation of rheumatic fever. A long-term perspective. Trans Am. Clin. Climatol. Assoc. *73*:209, 1961.
85. Whitnack, E., and Stollerman, G. H.: Antistreptococcal antibodies in the diagnosis of rheumatic fever: *In* Cohen, A. S., (ed.): Laboratory Diagnostic Procedures in Rheumatic Diseases, 3rd Ed. Boston, Little, Brown and Co., 1985, pp. 273–292.
86. Gewurz, H., Mold, C., Siegel, J., and Fiedel, B.: C-reactive protein and the acute phase response. Adv. Intern. Med. *27*:345, 1982.
87. Feinstein, A. R., and DiMassa, R.: Prognostic significance of valvular involvement in acute rheumatic fever. N. Engl. J. Med. *260*:1001, 1959.
88. Feinstein, A. R., Wood, H. F., Spagnuolo, M., et al.: Rheumatic fever in children and adolescents: VII. Cardiac changes and sequelae. Ann. Intern. Med. *60*(Suppl. 5):87, 1964.
89. Jones, T. D.: The diagnosis of rheumatic fever. J.A.M.A. *126*:481, 1944.
90. Jones Criteria (revised) for guidance in the diagnosis of rheumatic fever. Circulation *32*:664, 1965.
91. Taranta, A., Spagnuolo, M., and Feinstein, A. R.: "Chronic" rheumatic fever. Ann. Intern. Med. *56*:367, 1962.
92. McIntosch, R., and Wood, C. L.: Rheumatic infections occurring in the first three years of life. Am. J. Dis. Child. *49*:835, 1935.
93. Rosenthal, A., Czoniczer, G., and Massell, B. F.: Rheumatic fever under three years of age. A report of ten cases. Pediatrics *41*:612, 1968.
94. Ellis, L. B.: Recurrent mitral stenosis. Mod. Concepts Cardiovasc. Dis. *33*:851, 1964.
95. Wood, H. F., Simpson, R., Feinstein, A. R., et al.: Rheumatic fever in children and adolescents. I. Description of the investigative techniques and of the population studied. Ann. Intern. Med. *60*(Suppl. 5):6, 1964.
96. Bisno, A. L., Pearce, I. A., and Stollerman, G. H.: Streptococcal infections that fail to cause recurrences of rheumatic fever. J. Infect. Dis. *136*:278, 1977.
97. Goetzler, R., Stokes, J., III, and Anderson, K.: Prognosis of subjects in the Framingham Study with rheumatic heart disease. J. Am. Geriatr. Soc. *33*:693, 1985.
98. Vaisman, S., Guasch, J., Vignau, A., et al.: The failure of penicillin to alter acute rheumatic valvulitis. J.A.M.A. *194*:1284, 1965.
99. Lockman, L. A.: Movement disorders. *In* Swaiman, K., and Wright, F. (eds.): Practice of Pediatric Neurology. St. Louis, C. V. Mosby Co., 1975.
100. Centers for Disease Control: Acute rheumatic fever—Utah. M.M.W.R. *36*:108, 1987.
101. Centers for Disease Control: Acute rheumatic fever in a Navy training center—San Diego, California. M.M.W.R. *37*:101, 1988.
102. Centers for Disease Control: Acute rheumatic fever among Army trainees —Ft. Leonard Wood, MO 1987–1988. M.M.W.R. *37*:519, 1988.
103. Kaplan, E. L., Johnson, D. R., and Cleary, P. P.: Group A streptococcal serotypes isolated from patients and sibling contacts during the resurgence of rheumatic fever in the United States in the mid-1980's. J. Infect. Dis. *159*:101, 1989.
104. Stollerman, G. H., Rusoff, J. H., and Hirschfeld, I.: Prophylaxis against group A streptococci in rheumatic fever. The use of single monthly injections of benzathine penicillin G. N. Engl. J. Med. *252*:787, 1955.
105. Albam, B., Epstein, J. A., Feinstein, A. R., et al.: Rheumatic fever in children and adolescents. A long-term epidemiologic study of subsequent prophylaxis, streptococcal infections, and clinical sequelae. Ann. Intern. Med. *60*(Suppl. 5): No. 2, Part II, 1964.
106. American Heart Association, Committee on Rheumatic Fever and Bacterial Endocarditis: Prevention of rheumatic fever. Circulation *78*:1082, 1988.
107. Wannamaker, L. W., Rammelkamp, C. H., Jr., Denny, F. W., et al.: Prophylaxis of acute rheumatic fever by treatment of the preceding streptococcal infection with various amounts of depot penicillin. Am. J. Med. *10*:673, 1951.
108. Wannamaker, L. W., Denny, F. W., Perry, W. D., et al.: The effect of penicillin prophy-

laxis on streptococcal disease rates and the carrier state. N. Engl. J. Med. *249*:1, 1953.
109. Dale, J. B., and Beachey, E. H.:Localization of protective epitopes of the amino terminus of type 5 streptococcal M protein. J. Exp. Med. *163*:1191, 1986.
110. Beachey, E. H., Stollerman, G. H., Johnson, R. H., et al.: Human immune response to immunization with a structurally defined polypeptide fragment of streptococcal M protein. J. Exp. Med. *150*:862, 1979.
111. Beachey, E. H., Grus-Masse, H., Tarter, A., et al.:Opsonic antibodies evoked by hybrid peptide copies of types 5 and 24 streptococcal M proteins synthesized in tandem. J. Exp. Med. *163*:1451, 1986.
112. Bluestone, R., and Pearson, C. M.: Ankylosing spondylitis and Reiter's syndrome: The interrelationships and association with HLA B27. Adv. Intern. Med. *22*:1, 1977.
113. Khan, M. A., and Khan, M. K.: Diagnostic value of HLA-B27 testing in ankylosing spondylitis and Reiter's syndrome. Ann. Intern. Med.*96*:70, 1982.
114. Calin, A. (ed.): Spondyloarthropathies. Orlando, Fl., Grune and Stratton, 1984.
115. Laitinen, O., Leirisalo, M., and Skylv, G.: Relation between HLA-B27 and clinical features in patients with Yersinia arthritis. Athritis Rheum. *20*:1121, 1977.
116. Schachter, J.: Can chlamydial infections cause rheumatic disease? *In* Dumonde, D. C. (ed.): Infection and Immunology in Rheumatic Diseases. Oxford, Blackwell Scientific Publications, 1976, pp. 151–157.

ANKYLOSING SPONDYLITIS

117. Alves, M. G., Espirito-Santo, J., Queiroz, M. V., et al.: Cardiac alterations in ankylosing spondylitis. Angiology *39*:567, 1988.
118. Thomas, D., Hill, W., Geddes, R., et al.: Early detection of aortic dilatation in ankylosing spondylitis using echocardiography. Aust. N.Z. J. Med. *12*:10, 1982.
119. LaBresh, K. A., Lally, E. V., Sharma, S. C., and Ho, G.: Two-dimensional echocardiographic detection of preclinical aortic root abnormalities in rheumatoid variant diseases. Am. J. Med. *78*:908, 1985.
120. Shah, A.: Echocardiographic features of mitral regurgitation due to ankylosing spondylitis. Am. J. Med. *82*:353, 1987.
121. Roberts, W. C., Hollingsworth, J. F., Bulkley, B. H., et al.: Combined mitral and aortic regurgitation in ankylosing spondylitis. Angiographic and anatomic features. Am. J. Med. *56*:237, 1974.
122. Nitter-Hauge, S., and Otterstad, J. E.: Characteristics of atrioventricular conduction disturbances in ankylosing spondylitis. Acta Med. Scand. *210*:197, 200, 1981.
123. Bergfeld, E. L.: HLA-B27-associated rheumatic diseases with severe cardiac bradyarrhythmias. Clinical features in 223 men with permanent pacemakers. Am. J. Med. *75*:210, 1983.
124. Bulkley, B. H., and Roberts, W. C.: Ankylosing spondylitis and aortic regurgitation. Description of the characteristic cardiovascular lesion from study of eight necropsy patients. Circulation *48*:1014, 1973.
125. Ribiero, P., Morley, L. M., Shapiro, R. A., et al.: Left ventricular function in patients with ankylosing spondylitis and Reiter's disease. Eur. Heart J. *5*:419, 1984.
126. Cowan, G. O.: Aortic incompetence associated with ulcerative colitis and ankylosing spondylitis. Proc. Roy. Soc. Med. *63*:4, 1970.

REITER'S DISEASE

127. Good, A. E.: Reiter's disease: A review with special attention to cardiovascular and neurologic sequelae. Semin. Arthr. Rheum. *3*:253, 1974.
128. Sairanen, E., Paronen, I., and Mahonen, H.: Reiter's syndrome: A follow-up study. Acta Med. Scand. *185*:57, 1969.
129. Paulus, H. E., Pearson, C. M., and Pitts, W., Jr.: Aortic insufficiency in five patients with Reiter's syndrome: A detailed clinical pathological study. Am. J. Med. *53*:464, 1972.
130. Collins, P.: Aortic incompetence and active myocarditis in Reiter's disease. Br. J. Vener. Dis. *48*:300, 1972.
131. Ahvonen, P., Hiisi-Brummer, L., and Aho, K.: Electrocardiographic abnormalities and arthritis in patients with *Yersinia enterocolitica* infection. Ann. Clin. Res. *3*:69, 1971.
132. Aho, K., Ahvonen, P., and Lassus, A.: HLA B27 in reactive arthritis. A study of Yersinia arthritis and Reiter's disease. Arthritis Rheum. *17*:521, 1974.
133. Hakansson, U., Eitrem, R., Löw, B., and Winblad, S. W.: HLA-antigen B27 in cases with joint affects in an outbreak in salmonellosis. Scand. J. Infect. Dis. *8*:245, 1976.
134. Ruppert, G. B., Lindsay, J., and Barth, W. F.: Cardiac conduction abnormalities in Reiter's syndrome. Am. J. Med. *73*:335, 1982.
135. Mody, G. M., Stevens, J. E., and Meyers, O. L.: The heart in rheumatoid arthritis—a clinical and echocardiographic study. Q. J. Med. *65*:921, 1987.
136. Esdaile, J., Hawkins, D., Gold, P., et al.: Vascular involvement in relapsing polychondritis. CMA J. *116*:1019, 1977.
137. Balsa-Criado, A., Garcia-Fernandez, F., and Roldan, I.: Cardiac involvement in relapsing polychondritis. Int. J. Cardiol. *14*:381, 1987.
138. Mutru, O., Laakso, M., Isomaki, H., and Koota, K.: Cardiovascular mortality in patients with rheumatoid arthritis. Cardiology *76*:71, 1989.
139. VanDecker, W., and Panidis, I. P.: Relapsing polychondritis and cardiac valvular involvement. Ann. Intern. Med. *109*:340, 1988.

RHEUMATOID ARTHRITIS

140. Lanningan, R.: Cardiac Pathology. London, Butterworth and Co., 1966.
141. Bonfiglio, T., and Ativater, E. C.: Heart disease in patients with seropositive rheumatoid arthritis. A controlled autopsy study and review. Arch. Intern. Med. *124*:714, 1969.
142. Khan, A. H., and Spodick, D. H.: Rheumatoid heart disease. Semin. Arthritis Rheum. *1*:327, 1972.
143. Butman, S., Espinoza, L. R., Del Carpio, J., and Osterland, C. K.: Rheumatoid pericarditis. Rapid deterioration with evidence of local vasculitis. J.A.M.A. *238*:2394, 1977.
144. MacDonald, W. J., Jr., Crawford, M. H., Klippel, J. H., et al.: Echocardiographic assessment of cardiac structure and function in patients with rheumatoid arthritis. Am. J. Med. *63*:890. 1977.
145. Kelly, C. A., Bourke, J. P., Malcolm, A., and Griffiths, I. D.: Chronic pericardial disease in patients with rheumatoid arthritis: A longitudinal study. Q. J. Med. *75*:461, 1990.
146. Stables, R. H., Campbell, S., and Ormerod, O.J.M.: Haemopericardium in rheumatoid arthritis. Int. J. Cardiol. *23*:268, 1989.
147. Breut, C., Drouelle, S., Lognone, T., et al.: Complications des pericardites rhumatoides: Constriction et tamponnade. Presse Med. *18*:1151, 1989.
148. Thould, A. K.: Constrictive pericarditis in rheumatoid arthritis. Ann. Rheum. Dis. *45*:89, 1986.
149. Roberts, W. C., Kehoe, J. A., and Carpenter, D. F.: Cardiac valvular lesions in rheumatoid arthritis. Arch. Intern. Med. *122*:141, 1968.
150. Morris, P. B., Imber, M. J., Heinsimer, J. A., et al.: Rheumatoid arthritis and coronary arteritis. Am. J. Cardiol. *57*:689, 1986.
151. Young, I. D., Ford, S. E., and Ford, P. M.: The association of pulmonary hypertension with rheumatoid arthritis. J. Rheumatol. *16*:1266, 1989.
152. Linch, D. C., GIllmer, D. J., Whimster, W. F., and Keates, J.R.W.: Rheumatoid aortic valve prolapse requiring emergency valve replacement. Br. Heart J. *43*:237, 1980.
153. Ahern, M., Lever, J. W., and Cash, J.: Complete heart block in rheumatoid arthritis. Ann. Rheum. Dis. *42*:389, 1983.
154. Cassidy, J. T.: Juvenile rheumatoid arthritis. *In Kelly*, W. N., Harris, E. D., Ruddy, S., and Sledge, C. B. (eds.): Textbook of Rheumatology, 2nd ed. Philadelphia, W. B. Saunders Company, 1985.
155. Bernstein, B.: Pericarditis in juvenile rheumatoid arthritis. Arthritis Rheum. *20*:241, 1977.
156. Bank, L., Marboe, C. C., Redberg, R. F., and Jacob, J.: Myocarditis in adult Still's disease. Arthritis Rheum. *28*:452, 1985.
157. Bank, I., Marboe, C. C., Redberg, R. F., and Jacobs, J.: Myocarditis in adult Still's disease. Arthritis Rheum. *28*:452, 1985.
158. Sachs, R. N., Talvard, O., and Lanfranchi, J.: Myocarditis in adult Still's disease. Int. J. Cardiol. *27*:377, 1990.
159. Kramer, P. H., Imboden, J. B., Waldman, F. M., et al.: Severe aortic insufficiency in juvenile chronic arthritis. Am. J. Med. *74*:1088, 1983.
160. Hah, B. H.: Systemic lupus erythematosus. *In* Wilson, J. D., et al. (eds.): Harrison's Principles of Internal Medicine. 12th ed. New York, McGraw-Hill, 1991, pp. 1432–1437.
161. Klemperer, P., Pollack, A., and Baehr, G.: Pathology of disseminated lupus erythematosus. Arch. Pathol. *32*:569, 1941.
162. Liberthson, R. R., Homcy, C., Fallon, J. T., et al.: Systemic lupus erythematosus and heart disease. Primary Cardiol. *9*:77, 1983.
163. Gross, L.: Cardiac lesions in Libman-Sacks disease with consideration of its relationship to acute diffuse lupus erythematosus. Am. J. Pathol. *16*:375, 1940.
164. Harvey, A. M., Shulman, L. E., Tumulty, P. A., et al.: Systemic lupus erythematosus: A review of the literature and clinical analyses of 138 cases. Medicine *33*:291, 1954.
165. Hejtmancik, M. R., Wright, J. C., Quint, R., and Jennings, F.: The cardiovascular manifestations of systemic lupus erythematosus. Am. Heart J. *68*:119, 1964.
166. Bulkley, B. H., and Roberts, W. C.: The heart in systemic lupus erythematosus and the changes induced in it by corticosteroid therapy: A study of 36 necropsy patients. Am. J. Med. *58*:243, 1975.
167. Bharati, S., de la Fuente, D. J., Kallen, R. J., et al.: Conduction system in lupus erythematosus with atrioventricular block. Am. J. Cardiol. *35*:299, 1975.
168. Porcel, J. M., Selva, A., Tornos, M. P., et al.: Resolution of cardiac tamponade in systemic lupus erythematosus with indomethacin. Chest *96*:1193, 1989.
169. Wolf, R. E., King, J. W., and Brown, T. A.: Antimyosin antibodies and constrictive pericarditis in lupus erythematosus. J. Rheumatol. *15*:1284, 1988.
170. Sunder, S. K., and Shah, A.: Constrictive pericarditis in procainamide-induced lupus erythematosus syndrome. Am. J. Cardiol. *36*:960, 1975.
171. Ghose, M. K.: Pericardial tamponade. A presenting manifestation of procainamide-induced lupus erythematosus. Am. J. Med. *58*:581, 1975.
172. Enomoto, K., Kaji, Y., Mayumi, T., et al.: Frequency of valvular regurgitation by color Doppler echocardiography in systemic lupus erythematosus. Am. J. Cardiol. *67*:209, 1991.
173. Leung, W-H., Wong, K-L., Lau, C-P., et al.: Cardiac abnormalities in systemic lupus erythematosus: A prospective M-mode, cross-sectional and Doppler echocardiographic study. Int. J. Cardiol. *27*:367, 1990.
174. Murai, K., Oku, H., Takeuchi, K., et al.: Alterations in myocardial systolic and diastolic function in patients with active systemic lupus erythematosus. Am. Heart J. *113*:966, 1987.
175. Salomone, E., Tamburino, C., Bruno, G., et al.: The role of endomyocardial biopsy in the diagnosis of cardiac involvement in systemic lupus erythematosus. Heart Vessels *5*:52, 1989.
176. Elkayam, U., Weiss, S., and Laniado, S.: Pericardial effusion and mitral valve involvement in systemic lupus erythematosus: Echocardiographic study. Ann. Rheum. Dis. *36*:349, 1977.
177. Doherty, N. E., and Siegel, R. J.: Cardiovascular manifestations of systemic lupus erythematosus. Am. Heart J. *110*:1257, 1985.
178. Takatsu, Y., Hattori, R., Sakuguchi, K., et al.: Acute myocardial infarction associated with systemic lupus erythematosus. Chest *88*:147, 1985.
179. Libman, E., and Sacks, B.: A hitherto undescribed form of valvular and mitral endocarditis. Arch. Intern. Med. *33*:701, 1924.
180. Rawsthorne, L., Ptacin, M. J., Choi, H., et al.: Lupus valvulitis necessitating double valve replacement. Arthritis Rheum. *24*:561, 1981.
181. Dajee, H., Hurley, E. J., and Szarnicki, R. J.: Cardiac valve replacement in systemic lupus erythematosus. A review. J. Thorac. Cardiovasc. Surg. *85*:718, 1983
182. Straaton, K. V., Chatham, W. W., Reveille, J. D., et al.: Clinically significant valvular heart disease in systemic lupus erythematosus. Am. J. Med. *85*:645, 1988.
183. Galve, E., Candell-Riera, J., Pigrau, C., et al.: Prevalence, morphologic types, and evolution of cardiac valvular disease in systemic lupus erythematosus. N. Engl. J. Med. *319*:817, 1988.
184. Maier, W. P., Ramirez, H. E., and Miller, S. B.: Complete heart block as the initial manifestation of systemic lupus erythematosus. Arch. Intern. Med. *147*:170, 1987.
185. Gur, H., Keren, G., Averbuch, M., and Levo, Y.: Severe lupus congestive cardiomyopathy complicated by an intracavitary thrombus: A clinical and echocardiographic followup. J. Rheumatol. *15*:1278, 1988.
186. Bilazarian, S. D., Taylor, A. J., Brezinski, D., et al.: High-grade atrioventricular heart block in an adult with systemic lupus erythematosus: The association of nuclear RNP (U1 RNP) antibodies, a case report, and review of the literature. Arthritis Rheum. *32*:1170, 1989.
187. Buyon, J. P., Ben-Chetrit, E., Karp, S., et al.: Acquired congenital heart block: Pattern of maternal antibody response to biochemically defined antigens of the SSA/Ro-SSB/La system in neonatal lupus. J. Clin. Invest. *84*:627, 1989.
188. Scott, J. S., Maddison, P. J., Taylor, P. V., et al.: Connective-tissue disease, antibodies to ribonucleoprotein and congenital heart block. N. Engl. J. Med. *309*:209, 1983.
189. Litsey, S. E., Noonan, J. A., Connor, W. N., et al.: Maternal connective tissue disease and congenital heart block. N. Engl. J. Med. *312*:98, 1985.
190. Strauer, B. E., Brune, I., Schenk, H., et al.: Lupus cardiomyopathy: Cardiac mechanics, hemodynamics, and coronary blood flow in uncomplicated systemic lupus erythematosus. Am. Heart J. *92*:715, 1976.
191. Been, M., Thomson, B. J., Smith, M. A., et al.: Myocardial involvement in systemic lupus erythematosus detected by magnetic resonance imaging. Eur. Heart J. *9*:1250, 1988.
192. Homcy, C. J., Liberthson, R. R., Fallon, J. T., et al.: Ischemic heart disease in systemic lupus erythematosus in the young patient: Report of six cases. Am. J. Cardiol. *49*:478, 1982.
193. Hughes, G.R.V., Harris, N. N., and Gharavi, A. E.: The anticardiolipin syndrome. J. Rheum. *13*:486, 1986.
194. Sontheimer, R. D.: The anticardiolipin syndrome: A new way to slice an old pie, or a new pie to slice? Arch. Dermatol. *123*:590, 1987.
195. O'Rourke, R. A.: Antiphospholipid antibodies: A marker of lupus carditis? Circulation *82*:636, 1990.

196. Nihoyannopoulos, P., Gomez, P. M., Joshi, J., et al.: Cardiac abnormalities in systemic lupus erythematosus. Circulation *82*:369, 1990.
197. Khamashta, M. A., Cervera, R., Asherson, R. A., et al.: Association of antibodies against phospholipids with heart valve disease in systemic lupus erythematosus. Lancet *335*:1541, 1990.
198. Chartash, E. K., Lans, D. M., Paget, S. A., et al.: Aortic insufficiency and mitral regurgitation in patients with systemic lupus erythematosus and the antiphospholipid syndrome. Am. J. Med. *86*:407, 1989.

POLYARTERITIS NODOSA

199. Zeek, P. M.: Periarteritis nodosa and other forms of necrotizing angiitis. N. Engl. J. Med. *148*:764, 1953.
200. Schrader, M. L., Hockman, J. S., and Bulkley, B. H.: The heart in polyarteritis nodosa: A clinicopathologic study. Am. Heart J. *109*:1353, 1985.
201. Frayha, R. A.: Trichinosis-related polyarteritis nodosa. Am. J. Med. *71*:307, 1981.
202. Cupps, T. R., and Fauci, A. S.: The vasculitis syndromes. Adv. Intern. Med. *27*:315, 1982.
203. Lonham, J. G., Elkon, K. B., Pusey, C. D., and Hughes, G.R.V.: Systemic vasculitis with asthma and eosinophilia: A clinical approach to the Churg-Strauss syndrome. Medicine *63*:65, 1984.
204. Fauci, A. S., Haynes, B. F., Katz, P., and Wolff, S. M.: Wegener's granulomatosis: Prospective clinical and therapeutic experience with 85 patients for 21 years. Ann. Intern. Med. *98*:76, 1983.
205. Forstot, J. Z., Overlie, P. A., Neufeld, G. K., et al.: Cardiac complications of Wegener granulomatosis: A case report of complete heart block and review of the literature. Semin. Arthritis Rheum. *10*:148, 1980.
206. Schiavone, W. A., Ahmad, M., and Ockner, S. A.: Unusual cardiac manifestations of Wegener's granulomatosis. Chest *88*:5, 1985.
207. Sams, W. M., Jr., Claman, H. N., and Kohler, P. F.: Human necrotizing vasculitis: Immunoglobulins and complement in vessel walls of cutaneous lesions and normal skin. J. Invest. Derm. *64*:441, 1975.
208. Huston, K. A., and Hunder, G. G.: Giant cell (cranial) arteritis: A clinical review. Am. Heart J. *100*:99, 1980.
209. Klinkhoff, A. V., Reid, G. D., and Moscovich, M.: Aortic regurgitation in giant cell arteritis. Arthritis Rheum. *28*:582, 1985.
210. Moutsopoulos, H. M.: Behçet's syndrome. *In* Wilson, J. D., et al. (eds.): Harrison's Principles of Internal Medicine. 12th ed. New York, McGraw-Hill, 1991, pp. 1455–56.
211. Bletry, O., Monhattane, A., Wechsler, B., et al.: Atteinte cardiaque de la maladie de Behçet: Douze observations. Presse Med. *17*:2388, 1988.

PROGRESSIVE SYSTEMIC SCLEROSIS

212. Masi, A. T., and Rodnan, G. P.: Preliminary criteria for the classification of systemic sclerosis (scleroderma). Bull. Rheum. Dis. *31*:1, 1981.
213. Botstein, G. R., and LeRoy, E. C.: Primary heart disease in systemic sclerosis (scleroderma): Advances in clinical and pathologic features, pathogenesis, and new therapeutic approaches. Am. Heart J. *102*:913, 1981.
214. Weiss, S., Stead, E., Warren, J., and Bailey, O.: Scleroderma heart disease. Arch. Intern. Med. *71*:749, 1943.
215. LeRoy, E. C.: The heart in systemic sclerosis. N. Engl. J. Med. *310*:188, 1984.
216. Follansbee, W. P., Curtiss, E. I., Medsger, T. A., Jr., et al.: Physiologic abnormalities of cardiac function in progressive systemic sclerosis with diffuse scleroderma. N. Engl. J. Med. *310*:142, 1984.
217. Kahan, A., Devaux, J. Y., Amor, B., et al.: Nifedipine and thallium-201 myocardial perfusion in progressive systemic sclerosis. N. Engl. J. Med. *314*:1397, 1986.
218. Roberts, N. K., Cabeen, W. R., Jr., Moss, J., et al.: The prevalence of conduction defects and cardiac arrhythmias in progressive systemic sclerosis. Ann. Intern. Med. *94*:38, 1981.
219. Ferri, C., Bernini, L., Gongiorni, M. G., et al.: Noninvasive evaluation of cardiac dysrhythmias and their relationship with multisystemic symptoms in progressive systemic sclerosis patients. Arthritis Rheum. *28*:1259, 1985.
220. Follansbee, W. P., Curtiss, E. I., Rahko, P.S., et al.: The electrocardiogram in systemic sclerosis (scleroderma). Am. J. Med. *79*:183, 1985.
221. Kahan, A., Nitenberg, A., Foult, J. M., et al.: Decreased coronary reserve in primary scleroderma myocardial disease. Arthritis Rheum. *28*:637, 1985.
222. Niarchose, A. P., Whitman, H. H., Goldstein, J. E., and Laragh, J. H.: Hemodynamic effects of captopril in pulmonary hypertension of collagen vascular disease. Am. Heart J. *104*:834, 1982.
223. Ocken, S., Reinitz, E., and Strom, J.: Nifedipine treatment for pulmonary hypertension in a patient with systemic sclerosis. Arthritis Rheum. *26*:794, 1983.
223a. Morgan, J.M., Griffiths, M., duBois, R. M., and Evans, T. W.: Hypoxic pulmonary vasoconstriction in systemic sclerosis and primary pulmonary hypertension. Chest *99*:551, 1991.
224. O'Brien, J. T., Hill, J. A., and Pepine, C. J.: Sustained benefit of verapamil in pulmonary hypertension with progressive systemic sclerosis. Am. Heart J. *109*:380, 1985.
225. Ellis, W. W., Baer, A. N., Robertson, R. M., et al.: Left ventricular dysfunction induced by cold exposure in patients with systemic sclerosis. Am. J. Med. *80*:385, 1986.
226. Gustafsson, R., Mannting, F., Kazzam, E., et al.: Cold-induced reversible myocardial ischaemia in systemic sclerosis. Lancet August 26, 1989, pp. 475–479.
227. Kostis, J. B., Seibold, J. R., Turkevich, D., et al.: Prognostic importance of cardiac arrhythmias in systemic sclerosis. Am. J. Med. *84*:1007, 1988.
228. McWhorter, J. E., and LeRoy, E. C.: Pericardial disease in scleroderma (systemic sclerosis). Am. J. Med. *57*:566, 1974.
229. Gladman, D. D., Gordon, D. A., Urowitz, M. B., and Levy, H. L.: Pericardial fluid analysis in scleroderma (systemic sclerosis). Am. J. Med. *60*:1064, 1976.
230. Medsger, T. A., Jr., and Masi, A. T.: Survival with scleroderma. II. A life-table analysis of clinical and demographic factors in 358 male U.S. veteran patients. J. Chron. Dis. *26*:647, 1973.
231. Wynn, J., Fineberg, N., Matzer, L., et al.: Prediction of survival in progressive systemic sclerosis by multivariate analysis of clinical features. Am. Heart J. *110*:123, 1985.
232. Whitman, H. H., Case, D. B., Laragh, J. H., et al.: Variable response to oral angiotensin-converting enzyme blockade in hypertensive scleroderma patients. Arthritis Rheum. *25*:241, 1982.
233. Bohan, A., Peter, J. B., Bowman, R. L., and Pearson, C. M.: A computer assisted analysis of 153 patients with polymyositis and dermatomyositis. Medicine *56*:255, 1977.
234. Norton, W. L., Velayos, E., and Robison, L.: Endothelial inclusions in dermatomyositis. Ann. Rheum. Dis. *29*:67, 1970.
235. Tamir, R., Pick, A. J., and Theodor, E.: Constrictive pericarditis complicating dermatomyositis. Ann. Rheum. Dis. *47*:961, 1988.
236. Oka, M., and Raasakka, T.: Cardiac involvement in polymyositis. Scand. J. Rheumatol. *7*:203, 1978.
237. Haupt, H. M., and Hutchins, G. M.: The heart and conduction system in polymyositis-dermatomyositis: A clinicopathologic study of 16 autopsied patients. Am. J. Cardiol. *50*:998, 1982.
238. Raju, N.V.R., Hart, N., Maloney, J., et al.: Cardiac involvement in polymyositis: A case report and review of the literature. Cleve. Clin. Q. *51*:89, 1984.
239. Stern, R., Godbold, J. H., Chess, Q., and Kogan, L. J.: ECG abnormalities in polymyositis. Arch. Intern. Med. *144*:2185, 1984.
240. Sharp, G. C.: Mixed connective tissue diseases. *In* Wilson, J. D., et al. (eds.): Harrison's Principles of Internal Medicine. 12th ed. New York, McGraw-Hill, 1991, pp. 1448–1449.
241. Leung, W-H., Wong, K-L., Lau, C-P., et al.: Echocardiographic identification of mitral valvular abnormalities in patients with mixed connective tissue disease. J. Rheumatol. *17*:485, 1990.

57

Hematological-Oncological Disorders and Heart Disease

by DAVID S. ROSENTHAL, M.D., and EUGENE BRAUNWALD, M.D.

The increased frequency of cardiovascular abnormalities in patients with hematological and neoplastic disorders and, conversely, of blood disorders in patients being treated for a variety of cardiovascular diseases has led to greater interaction between cardiologists and hematologist-oncologists. Blood dyscrasias often complicate the use of cardiac medications and prosthetic heart valves and cardiovascular surgery. Hematologist-oncologists must often consult cardiologists regarding clinical problems that range from interpreting abnormal physical findings and electrocardiographic and echocardiographic changes in their patients to obtaining advice about how to treat heart failure, pericardial effusion, or other cardiac complications common among patients with anemia and hematological malignant diseases.

Anemia and Cardiovascular Disorders

(See also p. 458)

Anemia is one of the most common causes of increased cardiac output and when extremely severe sometimes results in heart failure due to a high-output state in the absence of heart disease. As discussed in Chapter 16, tissue hypoxia combined with reduced blood viscosity leads to a reduction in systemic vascular resistance, which is associated with an increase in cardiac output.[1-3] Acutely induced anemia lowers coronary vascular resistance, whereas chronic anemia enhances formation of intercoronary collaterals and causes increases in preload and reduction of afterload.[4] When the normal hemoglobin concentration is restored, all signs and symptoms of cardiovascular disease usually disappear. The gradual development of severe anemia may lead to cardiac hypertrophy, by causing vasodilation, which increases venous return (and thereby preload) and reduces peripheral resistance (and thereby afterload). Left ventricular end-diastolic volume is increased in patients with chronic anemia, and afterload reduction, as reflected in left ventricular end-systolic stress, has been demonstrated. Such changes may favor maintaining a sufficiently high stroke volume.[5] Another mechanism of enhanced left ventricular function in chronic anemia has been attributed to increased levels of catecholamine and noncatecholamine inotropic factors in plasma.[6,7] For example, papillary muscles placed in serum obtained from patients with chronic anemia exhibit increased contractility.[7]

CARDIAC SYMPTOMS OF ANEMIA. The severity of reduction of cardiac reserve, of fatigue, exertional dyspnea, and edema depend on the severity of the anemia and the presence of an underlying cardiovascular disorder such as myocardial, coronary arterial, or valvular heart disease. Severely anemic patients without heart disease have few if any cardiac symptoms. When hemoglobin values decline below 9 gm/dl, resting cardiac output increases[1,8-10] Symptoms also depend on the rapidity with which the anemia develops, as well as the physical activity of the patient. For example, if the anemia develops gradually in a normal person, patients with hemoglobin levels as low as 7 gm/dl may be able to carry out all but the most strenuous activities, whereas in the presence of coronary artery disease, anemia lowers the threshold for development of angina pectoris, so that patients with mild anemia may develop intensified angina.

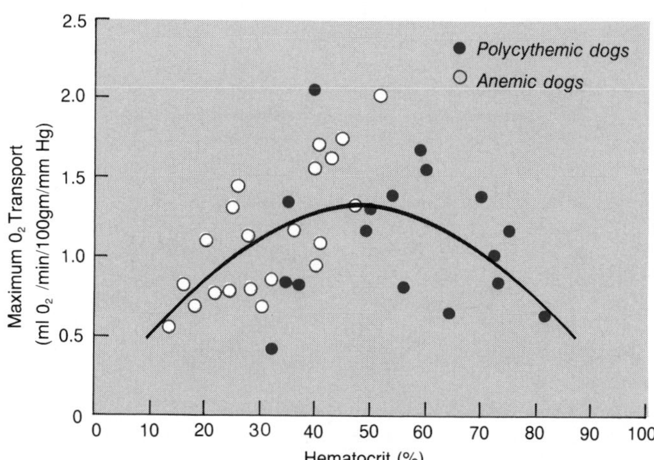

FIGURE 57-1. Maximum oxygen transport adjusted per unit perfusion pressure is shown as a function of hematocrit in anemic and polycythemic dogs. (From Baer, R. W., et al.: Maximum myocardial oxygen transport during anemia and polycythemia in dogs. Am. J. Physiol. *252*:H1086, 1987.)

Although uncommon, congestive heart failure with pulmonary edema can occur solely on the basis of very severe anemia (Hb < 4 gm/dl) even in the absence of underlying heart disease. It may be difficult to distinguish congestive heart failure secondary to chronic anemia from that related to myocardial iron infiltration secondary to transfusion-related hemosiderosis (p. 1747). However, the symptoms of reduced cardiac reserve secondary to anemia alone are usually relieved when the anemia is corrected and a normal red cell mass has been restored.

Electrocardiographic findings are not uncommon as the anemia progresses. With hemoglobin levels below 7 gm/dl, T-wave depression and inversion may be found, simulating myocardial disease. With transfusions, these findings usually return to normal.

Studies in anesthetized dogs have shown that maximal myocardial oxygen delivery far exceeds the supply at all levels of hematocrit. When one is plotting maximum oxygen transport against hematocrit, an "inverted U-shaped" relationship results (Fig. 57–1.)[11] In otherwise normal subjects, the gradual occurrence of severe anemia rarely if ever results in myocardial hypoxia, because of several compensatory mechanisms, including oxygen dissociation, 2,3-diphosphoglycerate (2,3-DPG) levels in red cells, and its effect on the hemoglobin-oxygen dissociation curve, as described below.

OXYGEN DISSOCIATION AND LEVELS OF 2,3-DIPHOSPHOGLYCERATE IN RED CELLS

To account for the circulatory adaptation that occurs in chronic anemia, it is important to appreciate that factors other than hemoglobin concentration and blood flow play a role in the quantity of oxygen delivered to tissues. These factors include tissue oxygen tension and the position of the hemoglobin-oxygen (Hb-O_2) dissociation curve. Normally, 1 gm of hemoglobin binds 1.34 ml of O_2. With a hemoglobin concentration of 15 gm/dl, 100 ml of arterial blood contains 20 ml of O_2. As can be calculated from the Hb-O_2 dissociation curve (Fig. 57–2), 100 ml of mixed venous blood having a PO_2 of 40 mm Hg will contain 15.5 ml of O_2. The difference (i.e., 4.5 ml of O_2 per 100 ml of arterial blood) would be available for delivery to tissues.

SHIFTS OF THE HEMOGLOBIN-OXYGEN DISSOCIATION CURVE. In most patients with anemia, the Hb-O_2 dissociation curve shifts to the right, and more oxygen is released from hemoglobin as the PO_2 declines. The red cell concentrations of 2,3-diphosphoglycerate (2,3-DPG), which are known to vary in a number of disease states,[10] profoundly affect the binding and release of O_2 by hemoglobin. Deoxygenated hemoglobin, which is more alkaline than oxyhemoglobin, stimulates the production of 2,3-DPG, a byproduct of glycolysis. As a consequence, the intraerythrocytic ratio of deoxyhemoglobin to oxyhemoglobin serves as a critical regulator of 2,3-DPG concentration. For example, the decreased oxygen affinity present in chronic anemia can be accounted for by this increase in red cell 2,3-DPG. At a normal arterial PO_2, arterial oxygen saturation remains high despite the reduction in oxygen affinity. However, at the lower PO_2 in the venous blood, elevated 2,3-DPG displaces the Hb-O_2 dissociation curve to the right, enabling greater release of oxygen from the cells at any level of PO_2. Oski et al. have calculated that decreased oxygen affinity mediated by increased red cell 2,3-DPG may compensate for up to half the oxygen deficit in anemia.[12] High levels of 2,3-DPG have also been found in subjects exposed to altitude[13] and in patients with pulmonary disease.[14]

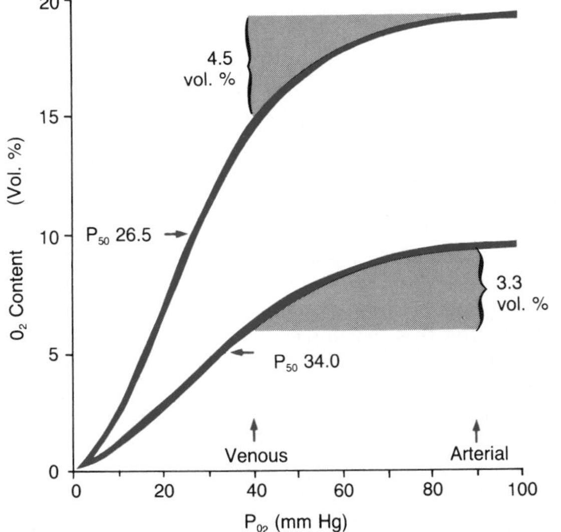

FIGURE 57–2. Enhancement of oxygen unloading by decreased red cell oxygen affinity in anemia with an increase in P_{50} from 26.5 to 34.0. (From Klocke, R. A.: Oxygen transport and 2,3-diphosphoglycerate. Chest *62*:7951, 1972.)

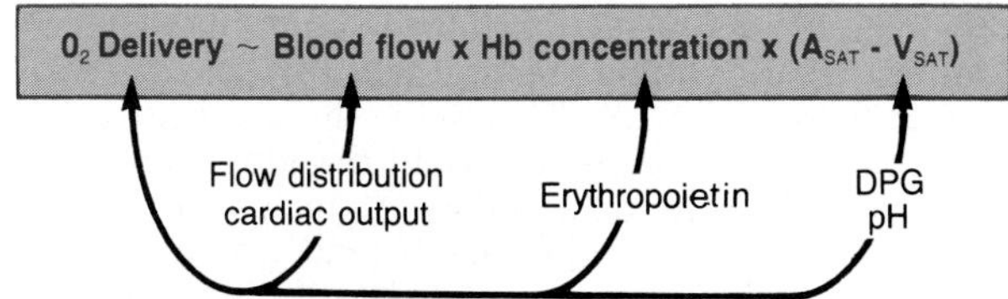

FIGURE 57–3. Oxygen delivered to an organ or tissue is directly proportional to blood flow, hemoglobin concentration, and the difference in oxygen saturation between arterial and venous blood. Patients with various types of hypoxia may compensate in the following ways: (1) Blood flow distribution may be altered to maintain oxygenation of vital organs, with an increase in total cardiac output when hypoxia is severe. (2) Increased erythropoietin production may stimulate erythropoiesis. (3) Oxygen unloading may be enhanced by a shift to the right in the oxygen dissociation curve, mediated by an increase in red cell 2,3-DPG. (From Bunn, H. F.: Pathophysiology of the anemias. *In* Wilson, J. E. et al. (eds.): Harrison's Principles of Internal Medicine. 12th ed. New York, McGraw-Hill Book Co., 1990, p.1517.)

The position of the Hb-O_2 dissociation curve can be expressed by the value of P_{50}, i.e., the partial pressure of O_2 at which hemoglobin is 50 per cent saturated. A reduction of the oxygen affinity of hemoglobin, i.e., a shift of the dissociation curve to the right, is reflected in an elevation of P_{50}. With a P_{50} of 34 mm Hg (instead of the normal P_{50} of 26.5 mm Hg), 3.3 ml of O_2 is unloaded per 100 ml of blood. As a consequence, an anemic individual with a 50 per cent reduction in red cell mass would suffer only a 27 per cent reduction in oxygen unloading (Fig. 57–2).

RESPONSE TO HYPOXIA. Figure 57–3 summarizes the factors responsible for oxygenation in response to hypoxia. O_2 delivery to the metabolizing tissues depends directly on three principal factors: (1) blood flow; (2) hemoglobin concentration (i.e., the O_2-carrying capacity of the blood), and (3) the O_2 unloaded per unit of blood, as represented by the difference between arterial and venous blood oxygen saturations. Each of these three factors varies independently. Blood flow to any tissue is a function of total cardiac output and its fractional distribution. The red cell mass is regulated by erythropoietin in response to tissue oxygenation. The position of the Hb-O_2 dissociation curve is determined primarily by red cell 2,3-DPG levels and blood pH. Chronic anemia is usually well tolerated when these compensatory mechanisms operate effectively, i.e., with an increased cardiac output, redistribution of blood flow, and decreased O_2 affinity.

CARDIAC EXAMINATION. The cardiac enlargement that develops with severe, chronic anemia usually results from dilatation and eccentric hypertrophy with a normal ratio of wall thickness to cavity diameter, as occurs in other forms of volume overload (see Fig. 14–8, p. 400). The precordium is usually hyperactive, not unlike that in mitral regurgitation (Fig. 2–16, p. 27). Third and fourth heart sounds are frequently present, and a midsystolic murmur, maximal at the left sternal border, is usually audible.[15,16] The murmur is probably secondary to the combined effects of increased velocity of blood flow across the pulmonic and aortic valve orifices and reduced blood viscosity. Less frequently, an early, midsystolic rumbling murmur may be heard at the apex or along the left sternal border. This diastolic murmur is probably related to the increase in blood flow across the mitral or tricuspid valves and may be difficult to distinguish from the murmurs of mitral or tricuspid stenosis, although the murmur follows a third heart sound rather than an opening snap. Accurate diagnosis may require echocardiography as well as reexamination after correction of the anemia.

In patients with chronic anemia whose hearts are compensated at a reduced concentration of hemoglobin, blood volume expansion achieved by the transfusion of whole blood may be poorly tolerated. Expanding the blood volume and augmenting left ventricular filling pressure will risk precipitating or aggravating heart failure. Therefore, the slow infusion of packed red blood cells accompanied by the administration of a diuretic would be more useful. Intravenous nitroglycerin therapy may also produce a favorable redistribution of circulating blood volume and antagonize the hemodynamic changes caused by transfusion.[17]

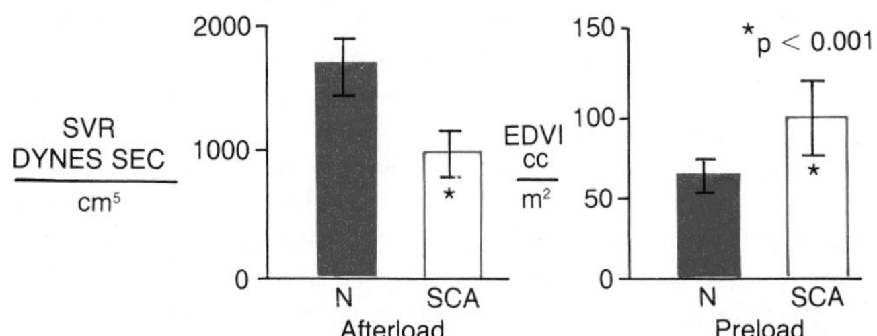

FIGURE 57–4. **Loading conditions in 11 patients with sickle cell anemia (SCA) and 11 normal subjects (N).** ***Left,*** **Afterload, as indicated by systemic vascular resistance (SVR), was significantly decreased in patients with SCA.** ***Right,*** **Preload, as indicated by end-diastolic volume index (EDVI), was significantly increased in patients with SCA. (From Dennenberg, B. S., et al.: Cardiac function in sickle cell anemia. Am. J. Cardiol. *57*:1675, 1983.)**

CARDIAC DISORDERS ASSOCIATED WITH HEMOLYTIC ANEMIA

Cardiomegaly, congestive heart failure, and sudden death have been reported frequently in patients with chronic hemolytic anemias such as sickle cell disease and thalassemia. In addition, hemolysis secondary to cardiac disease may cause acute symptoms. Hemolytic anemias are usually characterized by marked reticulocytosis and erythroid hyperplasia of the bone marrow. Indirect hyperbilirubinemia, increased serum lactic dehydrogenase, and reduced haptoglobin are also common findings. If lysis of red cells occurs within the circulation (intravascular hemolytic anemia), hemoglobinemia and hemoglobinuria may occur and will reflect the severity of hemolysis. Specific laboratory investigations will identify the type of hemolytic anemia, examples being a positive antiglobulin (or Coombs) test in immunohemolytic anemia, increased red cell osmotic fragility in hereditary spherocytosis, and abnormal hemoglobin electrophoresis in sickle cell anemia and the thalassemic syndromes. Acquired hemolytic anemias may occur precipitously, and the resulting symptoms may resemble those of acute blood loss with peripheral vasoconstriction, hypotension, tachycardia, fatigue, lightheadedness, and dyspnea on exertion.

HEMOGLOBINOPATHIES

Sickle Cell Disease

Sickle hemoglobin results from a mutation in the codon for the sixth amino acid of the beta globin chain from glutamic acid to valine (alpha-2, beta-$2^{6glu \rightarrow val}$). Eight to 10 per cent of black Americans are heterozygous for this trait. In certain regions of central Africa, the gene frequency is as high as 20 per cent, and it is likely that the high frequency of hemoglobin S in these areas is associated with resistance to or protection against falciparum malaria. With decreased oxygen tension, red cells containing hemoglobin S acquire an elongated crescent (sickle) shape. Electron microscopy demonstrates bundles of fibers running parallel to the long axis of the cells.[18] If sickle cells are reoxygenated within a short time, their normal red shape can be restored. However, as red cells remain sickled in vivo, their membranes become damaged and rigid, resulting eventually in irreversibly sickled cells that have a shortened survival and may block small blood vessels. The continuous formation and destruction of irreversibly sickled cells contribute to the symptoms of sickle cell disease. Factors that decrease oxygen affinity, such as acidosis and increased red cell 2,3-DPG levels, lead to the deoxygenation of hemoglobin and promote the formation of sickled cells.

Persons who are heterozygous for sickle cell disease are not anemic and rarely have symptoms except at high altitudes or as a result of marked hypoxia. In contrast, the signs and symptoms in patients homozygous for sickle cell anemia (SS) begin at about 6 months of age, when the conversion from fetal to adult hemoglobin production is completed.

The cardiopulmonary system is frequently involved in sickle cell anemia.[19–27] As in other chronic anemias, both cardiac output and oxygen extraction by tissues are increased, and the reduced oxygen content of these red cells leads to further sickling. In addition, for any given value of hematocrit, the elevation of cardiac output and the auscultatory findings associated with anemia are greater in sickle cell anemia[24] compared with other anemias. A normal left ventricle is able to tolerate the volume overload of chronic, moderately severe anemia for indefinite periods with no deterioration in functional capacity.[25] The increased preload and decreased afterload characteristic of chronic anemia (Fig. 57–4) compensate for any left ventricular dysfunction and maintain a normal ejection fraction and high cardiac output in sickle cell anemia.[26] When cardiac decompensation occurs in patients with sickle cell anemia, it is usually the result of other coexisting complications of the SS disease or the presence of underlying cardiovascular abnormalities. Deaths secondary to congestive heart failure occurring in children and young adults with sickle cell anemia are usually precipitated by chronic renal failure, pulmonary thrombosis, or infections.[27,28]

Acute myocardial infarction is a rare complication of sickle cell disease and has been confirmed at postmortem examination in a few patients without significant coronary atherosclerosis.[29–31] More O_2 is extracted by the myocardium than by any other tissue, and transmural infarction due to in situ thrombosis by sickled cells is rare. However, infarction of the papillary muscles of the heart does occur. This should not be surprising, since the papillary muscles are at the terminal portion of the coronary circulation, where collateral vessels are scant and hypoxia is marked.

Pulmonary infarction, a common complication of sickle cell anemia, is probably due to thrombosis in situ rather than to embolization.[32] Although infrequent, fat and bone marrow emboli to the lungs have been reported, the latter resulting from necrosis caused by sickling within the marrow sinusoids. Patients with sickle cell anemia are unusually susceptible to infection. In addition, damage to the lung caused by repeated vascular insults creates a suitable milieu for bacterial growth; as a consequence, pneumonia is a frequent and serious complication. Mortality and morbidity are high in the setting of pneumonia and hypoxia, so that treatment of these complications must be immediate and vigorous. However, it may be difficult to differentiate pulmonary infection from infarction in patients with sickle cell anemia. Although impaired pulmonary function in sickle cell anemia is common, pulmonary hypertension and cor pulmonale are rarely encountered.[24]

In almost all patients with sickle cell anemia the heart ultimately becomes enlarged, and at autopsy strikingly high heart weights are noted in a majority of patients despite the absence of other causes of cardiomegaly such as hypertension, atherosclerosis, or coronary artery disease.[33] In patients who have received multiple blood transfusions, myocardial iron deposition (hemosiderosis) may contribute both to the cardiac enlargement and to the associated impairment of cardiac function. However, this complication occurs much less frequently in sickle cell anemia than in homozygous thalassemia (see below). Histological studies have suggested that the increase in heart weight is secondary to fibrosis, presumably caused by the combination of anemia and papillary muscle infarction. With time, children with sickle cell disease exhibit progressive cardiac chamber enlargement with a progressive increase in left ventricular mass.[34]

There are no specific electrocardiographic changes in sickle cell anemia. However, almost 80 per cent of patients with sickle cell anemia have an abnormal electrocardiogram. These abnormalities include left ventricular hypertrophy and first-degree atrioventricular (AV) block as well as nonspecific ST-segment and T-wave changes and abnormal septal Q waves; this last finding is believed to be secondary to excessive septal thickness.[20,35,36] Arrhythmias rarely occur with sickle cell anemia, although continuous electrocardiographic monitoring during painful crises has revealed both atrial and ventricular arrhythmias in the majority of patients.[36] Echocardiographic measurements in patients with cardiac symptoms are useful in documenting both cardiac hyperactivity and depressed left ventricular performance.[20] Radiological studies may be entirely normal. With exercise, cardiac dysfunction may be manifested by an abnormal ejection fraction response, abnormalities of wall motion, and slowed left ventricular filling.[37-40] M-mode echocardiographic studies demonstrated an incidence of mitral valve prolapse in 25 per cent of SS patients,[21,41] far in excess of that expected. More recent two-dimensional echo and Doppler ultrasonography performed in adult patients with SS disease demonstrated a 22 per cent incidence of diastolic murmurs but no instances of myxomatous valvular degeneration or mitral valve prolapse.[21]

Thalassemic Syndromes

The thalassemias are a group of inherited disorders caused by an imbalance in the synthesis of hemoglobin chains rather than by a single amino acid substitution, as in sickle cell disease. The two principal types are referred to as α-thalassemia, in which α-chain synthesis is absent or reduced (a condition found mainly in Asians), and β-thalassemia, in which β-chain synthesis is absent or reduced. The homozygous form of β-thalassemia is also referred to as Cooley's or Mediterranean anemia and is common in persons of Greek and Italian descent. Heterozygous α- and β-thalassemias are also common in American blacks, particularly in association with sickle cell trait. These inherited autosomal dominant defects have been linked to molecular lesions that interfere with the synthesis of globin subunits. The net result in both types of thalassemia is decreased production of hemoglobin A (Hb A) and therefore hemoglobin-deficient red cells that are both microcytic and hypochromic. In addition, the red cells are target shaped and demonstrate basophillic stippling.

The diagnosis of β-thalassemia is confirmed by quantitative hemoglobin electrophoresis in which levels of Hb A are decreased or absent and levels of Hb A_2 and fetal hemoglobin (Hb F) are increased. The anemia in homozygous β-thalassemia results from a combination of hemolysis and ineffective erythropoiesis. Children have a characteristic "chipmunk" appearance owing to marked hyperplasia of the marrow in the facial bones and massive hepatosplenomegaly owing to extramedullary hematopoiesis. Occasionally, the expanding marrow extrudes from the ribs, sternum, and vertebrae, forming a mass resembling a lymphoma on chest roentgenogram.

CARDIAC ABNORMALITIES IN THALASSEMIA. Cardiac complications are the major cause of death in patients with thalassemia.[42] As with sickle cell disease, these events may be due in part to chronic anemia. In addition, cardiac siderosis is a frequent problem in thalassemia, unlike the situation in sickle cell anemia or many other chronic anemias.[43,44] Iron overload results from a combination of extravascular hemolysis, frequent transfusions, and an inappropriate increase in intestinal iron absorption. Consequently, heart failure and arrhythmias are the common causes of death in children with this condition.[43] Although anemia per se undoubtedly contributes to cardiomegaly, iron overload of the heart is the most likely cause of myocardial damage.[45-47]

Prior to the era of hypertransfusion and chelation therapy, patients with transfusion-dependent, chronic, severe refractory thalassemia regularly manifested serious cardiac involvement, usually by the second decade of life. Although most died within months of the development of congestive heart failure, occasional patients died suddenly, presumably secondary to an arrhythmia. Intensive treatment of heart failure and antiarrhythmic therapy do not appear to change the natural history. At postmortem examination, widespread iron deposition characteristic of hemochromatosis is found in all viscera, including the heart, which is hypertrophied and sometimes twice its normal weight; it is often a deep brown, with large quantities of iron in myocardial cells, demonstrated by staining with Prussian blue dye. The sinoatrial node is usually spared, but the AV node is frequently involved. Apparently cardiac dysfunction depends on the quantity of iron deposited in the ventricles, and it has been suggested that myocardial damage results from iron-induced release of acid hydrolases from lysosomes.[14]

Pericarditis occurs in about half of all patients with thalassemia and is often recurrent and associated with fever, precordial pain, and electrocardiographic changes characteristic of acute pericarditis (p. 1469). Pericardial effusion is common; in rare cases, creation of a pericardial window is necessary to relieve tamponade or a recurrent effusion.

The *electrocardiogram* often shows left ventricular hypertrophy, nonspecific ST-segment and T-wave abnormalities, supraventricular or ventricular premature contractions, and first- or second-degree AV block. The His bundle electrogram may show prolongation of the P-R interval, signifying abnormal conduction through the AV node. The chest roentgenogram may show slight to moderate cardiac enlargement, and *echocardiographic* assessment may disclose increased left ventricular end-diastolic, left atrial, and aortic root dimensions as well as a thickened left ventricular wall[44] and diastolic abnormalities.[44a] At cardiac catheterization, the usual findings comprise a normal or elevated cardiac index with moderate elevations in left ventricular end-diastolic pressure and volume and end-systolic volume with a reduced ejection fraction.

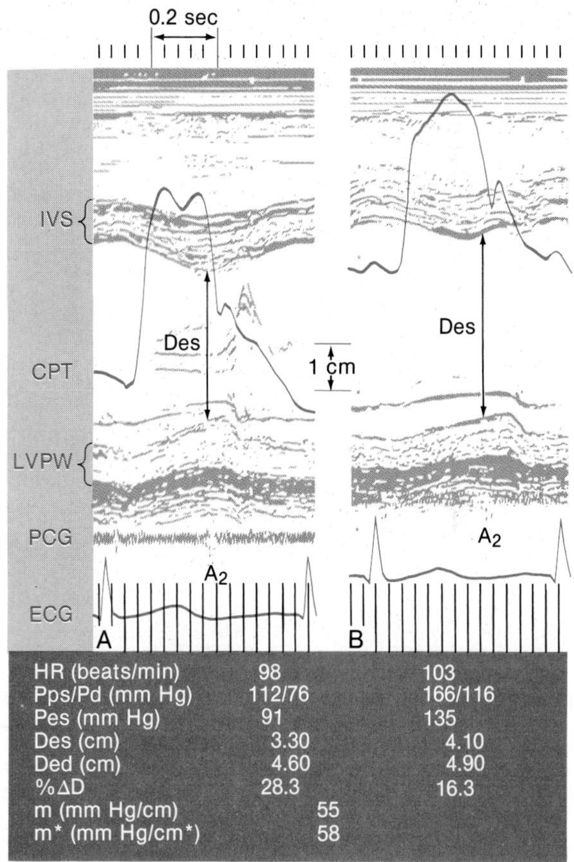

FIGURE 57–5. **Recordings from a 16-year-old patient with thalassemia major during baseline conditions (*A*) and at peak methoxamine effect (*B*). Both the actual and corrected slope values (m and m*) were abnormal despite normal resting fractional shortening (%ΔD). The 44-mm Hg increase in end-systolic pressure (Pes) resulted in a 0.80-cm increase in end-systolic dimension (Des). For the control population, a comparable change in Pes resulted in a 0.40 ± 0.05-cm increase in Des. IVS = interventricular septum; LVPW = left ventricular posterior wall; A_2 = aortic component of the second heart sound; HR = heart rate; Pps = peak systolic pressure; Pd = aortic diastolic pressure; %ΔD = per cent fractional shortening; m = slope; m* = corrected slope. (From Borow, K. M., et al.: The left ventricular end-systolic pressure-dimensions relation in patients with thalassemia major. A new noninvasive method for assessing contractile state. Circulation 66:980, 1982, by permission of the American Heart Association, Inc.)**

There has been considerable interest in defining abnormalities of cardiac performance noninvasively in asymptomatic patients. Valdes-Cruz et al. have reported that in asymptomatic children with thalassemia major[48] the left ventricular posterior wall thinned more slowly than normal during diastole. Utilizing the relationship between ventricular fractional shortening and end-systolic pressure (p. 431), Borow et al. identified preclinical left ventricular dysfunction (Fig. 57–5),[49] an approach that may be useful in the serial assessment of left ventricular contractility in response to chelation therapy.

Management. Supportive therapy consisting primarily of an adequate transfusion program (and even hypertransfusions), splenectomy, and early treatment of infections has prolonged the life of many patients with thalassemia.[51] Roentgenographic evidence of cardiomegaly in children often regresses when hemoglobin is maintained above 10 gm/dl. Indeed, in one study, in four of seven patients with significant cardiomegaly, heart size returned to normal 1 week after multiple transfusions restored hemoglobin to near-normal levels. The use of chelating agents for both treatment and prevention of iron overload and left ventricular systolic function is necessary and is discussed on page 1749).

HEMOLYTIC ANEMIA IN PATIENTS WITH VALVULAR HEART DISEASE

In 1964, Dameshek described an interesting patient with aortic, mitral, and tricuspid stenosis and mitral regurgitation who had hemolytic anemia with distorted and fragmented red cells, including helmet cells, burr cells, and schistocytes.[52] At autopsy, numerous calcified excrescences were present on the mitral valve and the free margins of the aortic valve. The presence of excess iron deposits in the kidney suggested intravascular hemolysis, but it could not be established whether the cardiac abnormalities were the cause. Subsequently, shortened red cell survival was demonstrated in other patients with aortic valve disease, some of whom had anemia.[53] In patients with rheumatic aortic valve disease with mild hemolytic anemia, red cell survival may be significantly reduced during periods of exercise.[54] Although this form of hemolytic anemia is probably uncommon, it should be considered in patients with valvular heart disease and unexplained anemia.

HEMOLYTIC ANEMIA DURING CARDIAC SURGERY. In the past, hemolysis frequently occurred as a consequence of extracorporeal circulation. When the blood of many donors must be transfused or is mixed in a pump-oxygenator, as may occasionally be the case in patients undergoing cardiac surgery, the question arises whether the samples should be crossmatched with each other as well as with the patient. The plasma of one donor may contain a potent antibody that might interact with cells from a donor who has the antigen specific for that antibody. Although infrequent, this phenomenon may explain some cases of mild-to-moderate hemolysis and hemoglobinemia seen after cardiopulmonary bypass.

With the use of earlier heart-lung machines, red cells became damaged as they passed through the pump-oxygenator, presumably as a result of shear forces, leading to slight hemolysis and causing hemoglobinemia and hemoglobinuria. This problem has been largely avoided with newer machines, which also require little if any blood for priming. As a consequence, hemolytic complications have become far less frequent. In addition, the use of autologous blood and aspirated blood filtered for reuse during the operation has been helpful in this regard.

HEMOLYTIC ANEMIA AFTER CARDIAC SURGERY. In 1954, following surgical implantation of Hufnagel valves in the descending aorta for the treatment of aortic regurgitation, a significant number of patients developed anemia,[55] presumably on a hemolytic basis. The potentially serious nature of the hemolytic anemia associated with an intracardiac prosthesis was not really appreciated until chronic and severe hemolytic anemia characterized by microangiopathic red cell changes (consisting of fragmented red cells, burr cells, and schistocytes) was noted after a Teflon patch repair of an ostium primum atrial septal defect (Fig. 57–6).[56] Chromium-51 red cell survival studies confirmed that the half-life of not only autologous red cells but also of donor cells was shortened, indicating a defect extrinsic to the red cell. In keeping with intravascular hemolysis, high concentrations of hemoglobin in the plasma and urine were noted along with hemosiderinuria. At reoperation a jet of blood was found regurgitating through a cleft in the mitral valve that had been impinging on the prosthetic interatrial Teflon patch. Part of the septum had become denuded of endothelium and had formed a small cul-de-sac in contact with the jet of blood. With repair of the cul-de-sac and reendothelialization of the area, hemolysis ceased. Torn cusps of porcine mitral valve or dehiscence of an implanted mitral ring can also cause the sudden onset of a hemolytic anemia.[57,58]

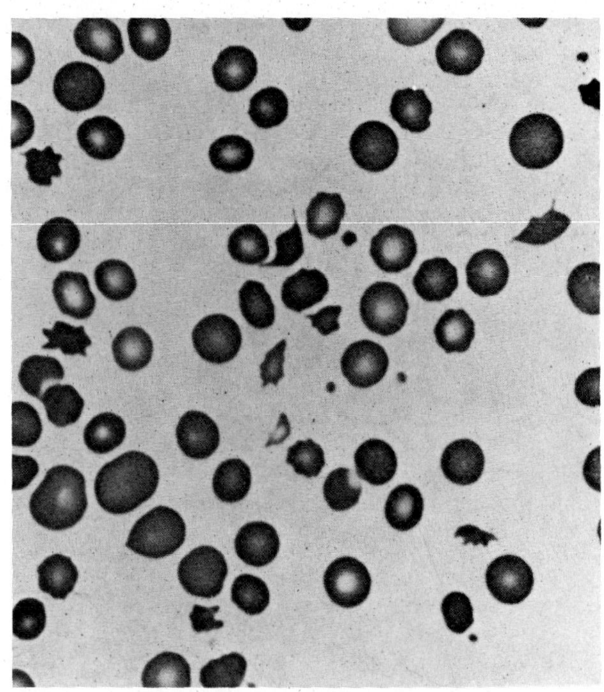

FIGURE 57–6. **Peripheral blood smear from patient with microangiopathic hemolytic anemia secondary to abnormal prosthetic heart valve (×1000).**

Microangiopathic Hemolytic Anemia

This condition has now been reported in association with many cardiac defects (Table 57–1). Its incidence after valve surgery depends on many variables, including the specific operation, the surgical technique, and the tests used to determine hemolysis, and varies widely.[59] In many instances, diurnal variations occur, with greater intravascular hemolysis during physical activity.[60]

CLINICAL PRESENTATION. With newer surgical techniques and prosthetic valves, the incidence of microangiopathic hemolytic anemia appears to be declining.[61] Symptoms and signs may develop suddenly or gradually, usually with no associated splenomegaly. Rarely, a vicious circle develops in a

TABLE 57–1 CAUSES OF MACROVASCULAR HEMOLYTIC ANEMIA

I. Abnormalities of heart and large vessels
- **A. Without surgery**
  - **1. Aortic stenosis**
  - **2. Ruptured sinus of Valsalva**
  - **3. Ruptured chordae tendineae**
  - **4. Coarctation of aorta**
  - **5. Aortic aneurysm**
- **B. Following surgery**
  - **1. "Patching" operations**
    - **a. Ostium primum repair, especially if mitral regurgitation present**
    - **b. Aortic aneurysm repair (aortofemoral bypass)**
    - **c. Hemodialysis shunt**
  - **2. Valvular replacement**
    - **a. Uncomplicated**
      - **(1) Outflow too small**
      - **(2) Large area of exposed plastic**
      - **(3) Cloth-covered struts**
      - **(4) Two or more valves replaced**
      - **(5) Xenograft**
    - **b. Complicated**
      - **(1) Ball variance**
      - **(2) Regurgitation around seating of valve**
      - **(3) Rupture of cloth-covered strut**

From Ersley, A. J.: Traumatic cardiac hemolytic anemia. *In* Williams, W. J. et al. (eds.): Hematology. 4th ed. New York, McGraw-Hill Book Co., 1990, p. 656.

patient with a perivalvular leak: the resultant shear stress produces hemolytic anemia, increasing stroke volume and shear stress, and in turn intensifying the anemia. While it is agreed that direct mechanical trauma to the red cells is the cause of hemolysis, the relative contributions of valve closure, denuded endothelium, turbulence, and the development of antierythrocyte autoantibodies are still not clear and probably vary among patients. In some instances, the hemolytic anemia observed in the early postoperative period is probably due simply to multiple intraoperative transfusions or to the lymphocyte-splenomegaly syndrome (post–pump-oxygenator syndrome) associated with cytomegaloviral infection.

CAUSE. Excessive blood turbulence is the most common feature of all hemolytic anemias due to valvular disease and cardiac surgery. For example, after insertion of a prosthetic valve, perivalvular regurgitation will increase the stroke volume and therefore the turbulence of flow through the narrowed orifice. Experiments in vitro have demonstrated that shearing stresses in excess of 3000 dynes/cm^2 can easily cause hemolysis and that such degrees of stress may readily develop with perivalvular leaks, causing regurgitation from the aorta to the left ventricle,[62] as well as in situations in which the lumen of the aortic valve prosthesis is small relative to the stroke volume or when the ball is large relative to the diameter of the aorta. Although much less common, similar phenomena can occur with prosthetic mitral valves.[57,58] Rarely, chronic intravascular hemolytic anemia may occur in the presence of hypertrophic cardiomyopathy, probably secondary to abnormal turbulence due to the primary underlying cardiac disease.[63] This rare condition may be managed by reducing the outflow gradient by beta-adrenoceptor blocker or calcium antagonist therapy, or by operation (p. 1412).

Definitive treatment of the hemolytic syndrome secondary to turbulence consists of surgical repair of the cardiac abnormality, i.e., either replacement or correction of the prosthesis or correction of the perivalvular leak. If a patient is not readily operable, rest should alleviate the condition, and iron and folate replacement may be helpful.

Hemochromatosis and Hemosiderosis

(See also p. 1419)

A number of disease states are characterized by excessive iron stores in the body (Table 57–2). The deposition of a significant amount of iron in the myocardium, liver, and pancreas may lead to varying degrees of dysfunction of these organs.[64] Insofar as the heart is concerned, myocardial deposits of iron may lead to congestive heart failure, conduction disturbances, and arrhythmias. Significant siderosis is most often encountered in patients with idiopathic hemochromatosis or in anemic patients with large and longstanding transfusion requirements.

IDIOPATHIC HEMOCHROMATOSIS. In this condition, inappropriately large quantities of iron are absorbed from the gastrointestinal tract. This inherited disorder, with a variable clinical expression, develops slowly and depends in part upon environmental factors, such as the magnitude of dietary iron intake, alcohol intake, and the severity of any underlying liver disease. HLA subtyping associated with HLA-A3, HLA-B14, and HLA-B7 antigens has suggested a recessive mode of transmission, has linked the disease to chromosome 6, and has helped to distinguish idiopathic hemochromatosis from iron overload secondary to liver disease.[65]

Clinical manifestations of hemochromatosis occur more frequently in men than in women, and the disease rarely becomes manifest before age 20 years, reaching its peak in the fifth decade. Diabetes is the most common initial manifestation, occurring in half of the patients. The classic clinical presentation includes increased pigmentation of the skin, hepatomegaly, and cardiac dysfunction. Loss of libido and other endocrinopathies, such as hypopituitarism, may also become apparent. Cellular damage results from iron-induced release of lysosomal acid hydrolases.[66]

The incidence of cardiac symptoms increases with time.[66,67] Dyspnea, edema, and ascites are noted early in the course in 15 to 20 per cent of the patients, but eventually about one-third develop symptoms referable to the heart, and approximately the same fraction of patients eventually die of cardiac failure.[67] Arrhythmias are common and include paroxysmal atrial tachycardia and flutter, chronic atrial fibrillation, and frequent premature ventricular contractions; varying degrees of AV block have also been noted. Of all men with second and third degree heart block requiring pacemaker insertion, idiopathic hemochromatosis[68] is retrospectively diagnosed in a significant percentage. Heart block and arrhythmias are often associated with iron deposits in the AV node[69] and supraventricular arrhythmias with deposits in the atria. Low-voltage and nonspecific T-wave changes are also frequently present.

Radiographic studies in symptomatic patients usually reveal a globular heart with biventricular enlargement and weak pulsations. Some patients may have elevated right ventricular and right atrial pressures[70] consequent to the restrictive cardiomyopathy secondary to iron deposition in the myocardium as well as involvement of the pericardium itself.[71]

TRANSFUSIONAL HEMOSIDEROSIS. Iron overload may become a clinical problem in patients with severe chronic anemia who survive long enough to accumulate toxic quantities of iron from transfused blood. For example, patients with thalassemia, other serious chronic refractory anemias, myeloid metaplasia, pure red cell aplasia, and aplastic anemia may accumulate 50 gm of iron from transfusions, resulting in a variety of clinical problems similar to those encountered in idiopathic hemochromatosis. Indeed, children with β-thalassemia major maintained on hypertransfusion programs, while spared the cardiac consequences of severe anemia, generally die of heart failure in the second decade as a consequence of myocardial siderosis.[43] In adults with chronic anemias, cardiac iron deposition secondary to transfusional hemosiderosis may contribute to cardiovascular disability, which is often inappropriately attributed solely to high-output heart failure. Undoubtedly, the combination of impaired cardiac function

TABLE 57–2 CAUSES OF IRON OVERLOAD

GENETIC
Hereditary hemochromatosis
Thalassemia major
Hereditary sideroblastic anemia
Certain hereditary hemolytic anemias
Pyruvate kinase deficiency
Glucose-6-phosphate dehydrogenase deficiency
Congenital dyserythropoietic anemia
Neonatal hemochromatosis
Congenital atransferrinemia
ACQUIRED
Chronic ingestion of medicinal iron
Transfusional iron overload
Acquired sideroblastic anemia
Porphyria cutanea tarda
African nutritional hemochromatosis
Shunt siderosis

From Fairbanks, V. F., and Baldus, W. P.: Production of erythrocytes. *In* Williams, W. J. et al. (eds.): Hematology. 4th ed. New York, McGraw-Hill Book Co., 1990, p. 752.

secondary to iron deposition and the increased burden on the heart imposed by the persistent, incompletely treated anemia is responsible.

Pathological Findings. In a review of 135 hearts studied at autopsy, including four from patients with hemochromatosis and 131 from patients with chronic anemia requiring repeated transfusions, 19 were found to have iron deposits.[72] Grossly visible iron deposits in the heart were always associated with a prior history of cardiac dysfunction and usually of chronic heart failure. Deposits were usually most extensive in idiopathic hemochromatosis and in patients who received more than 100 units of blood without evidence of blood loss. In patients with cardiac hemosiderosis, histological examination revealed that the ventricular free wall and septum contained heavier deposits than did the atrial wall (Fig. 57–7). The quantity of iron in the various layers of the ventricular myocardium is variable, with the epicardium and papillary muscles containing the most iron, the subendocardium containing intermediate amounts, and the midmyocardium and conduction tissue containing the least.

Diagnosis. It is often difficult to determine whether myocardial dysfunction results from the chronic anemia or hemosiderosis. Two techniques are useful: with the use of atomic absorption spectrophotometry, the exact concentrations of iron can be determined in various body organs or tissues. Iron-stained endomyocardial biopsy specimens can confirm hemochromatosis as a cause of cardiac dysfunction.[73] Rarely is iron deposition limited to the heart in these conditions. Since the liver is easily accessible by biopsy and its iron concentration is closely related to that in the myocardium, liver biopsy is a convenient way of confirming a diagnosis of myocardial siderosis. In some patients, echocardiography may detect early left ventricular dysfunction prior to the development of symptoms.[44,74,75] In a group of patients with severe β-thalassemia or transfusion-dependent anemias without clinical cardiac symptoms, left ventricular dysfunction measured by radionuclide angiography was demonstrated during exercise but not at rest.[74] Noninvasive assessment of the left ventricular end-systolic pressure-dimension relation (using a methoxamine challenge) can identify preclinical left ventricular dysfunction not evident on resting or dynamic exercise studies and not due to chronic anemia per se. This technique is a sensitive means of monitoring therapeutic response or iron overload diseases to prevent cardiac complications.[76,77]

Management. Since the majority of patients with myocardial siderosis ultimately die of irreversible cardiac failure and arrhythmias, reversal of the iron overload should be attempted. In patients with idiopathic hemochromatosis, it is possible to mobilize iron stores by repeated phlebotomies, which is the preferred mode of therapy.[75,77–79] Decreases in hepatic iron stores and fibrosis, improvement of liver function, amelioration of diabetes, and reversal of cardiomyopathy have all occurred with such treatment. Since the average patient with idiopathic hemochromatosis has 20 to 40 gm of stored iron, weekly to bimonthly phlebotomies usually have to be continued for 2 to 3 years. Initially the hematocrit will drop but will then return toward normal despite repeated phlebotomies. Removal of excess body iron by phlebotomy has been possible in patients with hematocrits as low as 30 per cent.

The distribution of iron in the tissues differs somewhat between individuals with idiopathic hemochromatosis and those with transfusion siderosis, who have relatively more iron stored in the reticuloendothelial cells. However, repeated

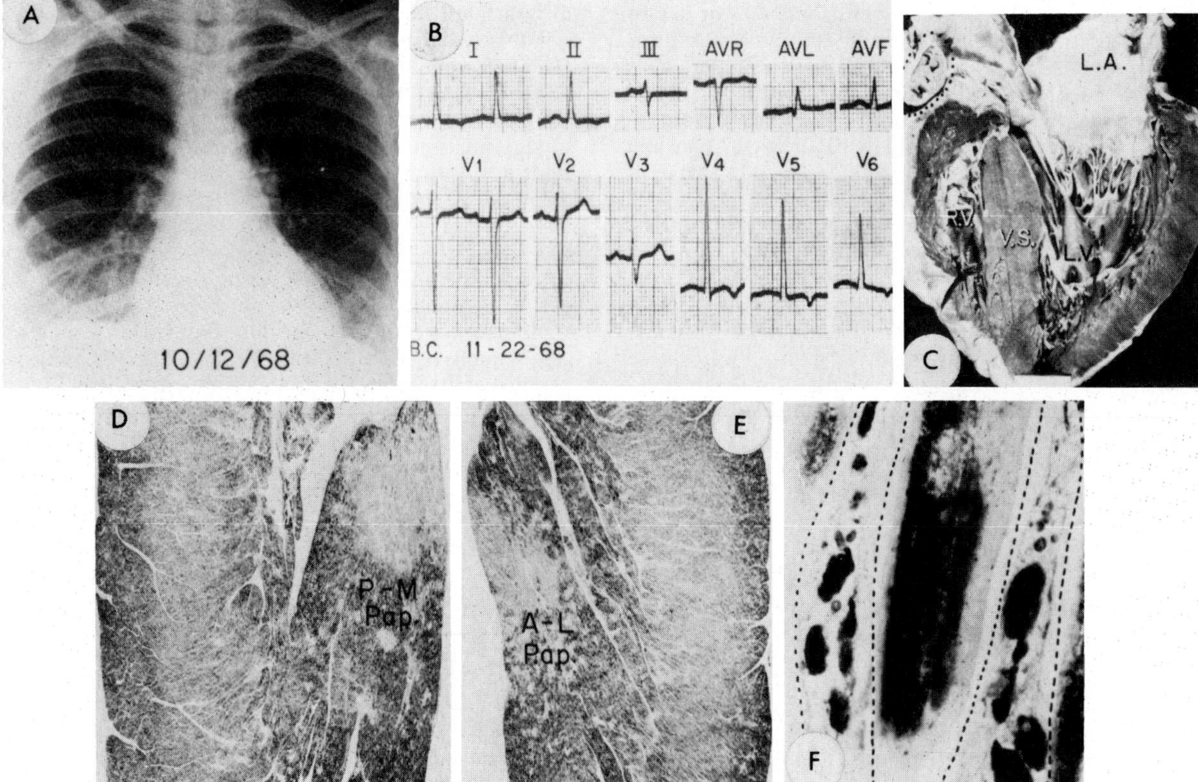

FIGURE 57–7. Observations in a 42-year-old woman with sickle cell anemia who developed congestive heart failure after cumulative transfusions of 260 units of blood. By the time of death, she had received a total of 359 units of blood (90 gm iron). *A,* Chest roentgenogram 2 weeks prior to death, showing cardiomegaly. *B,* Ischemic ST-segment and T-wave changes can be seen on the electrocardiogram. *C,* At autopsy the walls of the right (R.V.) and left (L.V.) ventricles and left atrium (L.A.) and the atrial and ventricular (V.S.) septa were rusty brown, owing to extensive iron deposits. The right atrial wall (partially enclosed by dotted line), in contrast, was tan; only minute particles of iron were present on microscopic examination. *D* and *E,* Large areas of replacement fibrosis (pale areas) were present in both left ventricular papillary muscles. *F,* Severely degenerated myocardial fibers (enclosed by dotted lines) that also contained iron deposits were often found adjacent to viable myocardial fibers. (Prussian blue stains.) (From Buja, L. M., and Roberts, W. C.: Iron in the heart. Am. J. Med. *51*:209, 1971.)

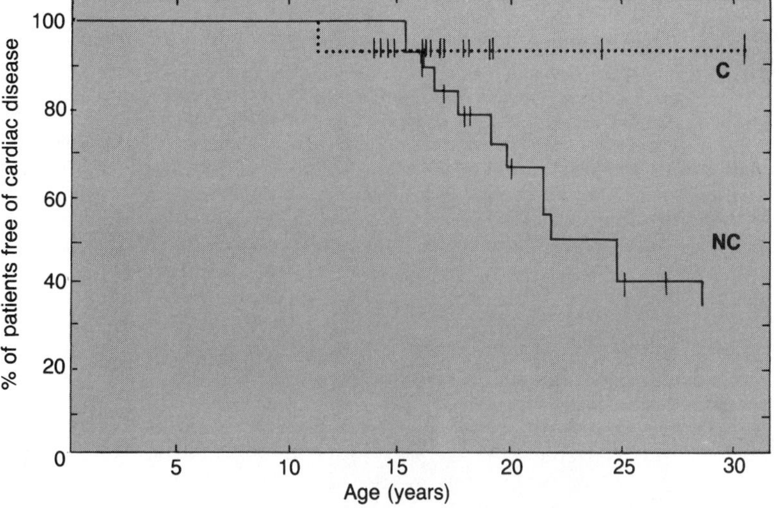

FIGURE 57–8. Life-table depiction of survival free of cardiac disease in patients with thalassemia major treated with desferrioxamine. Dotted line represents the compliant group (C) and solid line represents the current ages of patients still free of cardiac disease. (Reprinted by permission from Wolfe, L., et al.: Prevention of cardiac disease by subcutaneous desferrioxamine in patients with thalassemia major. N. Engl. J. Med. *312*:1600, 1985.)

transfusions in the latter result in a pattern of organ dysfunction similar to that in idiopathic hemochromatosis.[80] Phlebotomy is, of course, not a therapeutic alternative in the management of iron overload due to chronic blood transfusion therapy for anemia or in some patients with idiopathic hemochromatosis and chronic anemia. Rather, chelation therapy is the only approach available for removing iron in these anemic patients.[67–69,81–88]

Deferoxamine is the most widely studied iron chelator. This hydroxamic acid compound has a very high affinity for trivalent iron. It must be administered parenterally, and most of the chelated iron will be excreted in the urine within 4 hours of the injection. Initial studies with intramuscular deferoxamine were unsuccessful in achieving sustained negative iron balance. The addition of oral ascorbic acid doubles iron excretion[81]; when ascorbic acid loading was combined with the continuous, subcutaneous administration of deferoxamine, a negative iron balance was achieved in children with thalassemia.[89] However, ascorbate supplementation in patients with iron overload may be hazardous. Clinical cardiotoxicity manifested by fatal congestive heart failure and arrhythmias has been reported in patients treated simultaneously with deferoxamine and ascorbic acid. Not only does ascorbate make more cellular iron available for chelation, but it also liberates free intracellular iron, which can generate membrane-damaging free oxygen radicals.[90] The adverse effect of ascorbate may be prevented by using this agent *after* the patient has been started on chelation therapy.[91]

Long-term deferoxamine iron chelation therapy is effective not only in delaying but in reversing organ damage caused by transfusional iron overload.[84,86,87] Early and regular treatment with iron chelation appears to protect children with thalassemia major from developing cardiac disease induced by iron overload[85] (Fig. 57–8). An orally active chelator of iron may be just as effective and more easily administered.[91a]

Disorders Associated with Increased Blood Viscosity

As discussed on p. 1743, delivery of oxygen to an organ or tissue is directly proportional to blood flow, hemoglobin concentration, and the difference in oxygen saturation between arterial and venous blood (Fig. 57–3). In anemic patients, an increase in blood flow, due in part to reduced blood viscosity, and enhanced oxygen delivery through elevated levels of red cell 2,3-DPG compensate for the reduced hemoglobin levels. In contrast, conditions associated with increased viscosity cause an increase in resistance to flow and a reduction in blood flow. Disorders with increased viscosity and abnormal blood rheology include the erythrocytoses, such as polycythemia vera, and disease states associated with hypergammaglobulinemia, such as multiple myeloma and cryoglobulinemia.

POLYCYTHEMIA

Polycythemia is characterized by an increase in red cells, as determined by hematocrit, hemoglobin, and/or red blood cell count.[92] However, the terms *polycythemia* and its synonym *erythrocytosis* do not refer to a specific disease entity but to a variety of conditions. *Absolute* polycythemias refer to conditions in which there is an absolute increase in red cell mass (as measured by ^{51}Cr labeling or other dilution techniques). The absolute erythrocytoses are subclassified as primary or secondary, depending whether the elevation in red cell mass is autonomous (primary) or under hormonal (erythropoietin) control. *Primary* polycythemia, i.e., polycythemia vera, is part of the spectrum of myeloproliferative disorders. *Secondary* polycythemia is further classified into those disorders which cause an appropriate increase in erythropoietin secretion (e.g., disorders associated with hypoxemia, such as cyanotic forms of congenital heart disease and pulmonary disease) and those which cause an inappropriate increase in erythropoietin production, as occurs with tumors and a variety of renal diseases. In the *relative* polycythemias, red cell mass is normal but plasma volume is decreased, causing hematocrit, hemoglobin, and red cell values to be elevated.

Although the symptoms of secondary polycythemia depend on the underlying disease state, they are also usually a consequence of increased blood volume and viscosity; the latter increases exponentially with increased hematocrit.[93] When flow rate through a capillary tube is determined at various levels of hematocrit, flow decreases as an essentially linear function of hematocrit (Fig. 57–9). The product of flow rate and arterial oxygen content provides a relative measure of the rate of oxygen transport through a single blood vessel; optimal hematocrit is just below 40 per cent. Delivery of oxygen to the body depends on the product of total blood flow and the oxygen content of arterial blood, which tends to be high in polycythemia vera, in which blood volume, cardiac output, and arterial blood oxygen content are all increased, despite the increase in viscosity (Fig. 57–10). Although the increases in oxygen content, blood volume, and cardiac output in polycythemia vera are not required for adequate tissue oxygenation, in the polycythemias secondary to hypoxemia the increases in blood oxygen content and cardiac output represent an attempt to improve oxygen delivery.

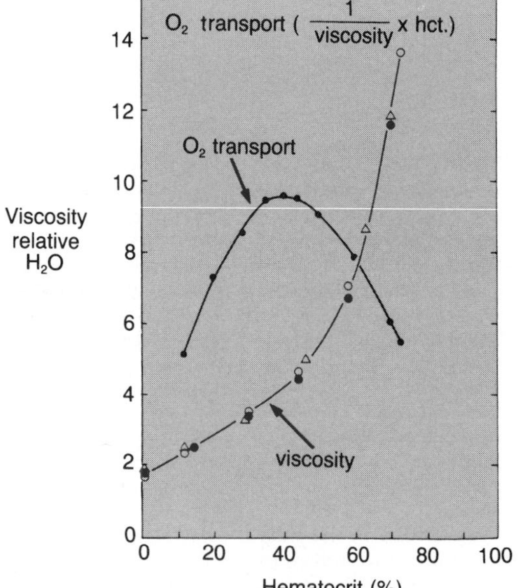

FIGURE 57–9. Viscosity of heparinized normal blood related to hematocrit. Viscosity was measured with an Ostwald viscosimeter at 37° C and expressed in relation to viscosity of water. Oxygen transport was calculated from the product of hematocrit and 1/viscosity and is recorded in arbitrary units. (From Williams, W. J. [ed.]: Hematology, 2nd ed. New York, McGraw-Hill Book Co., 1977, p. 256.)

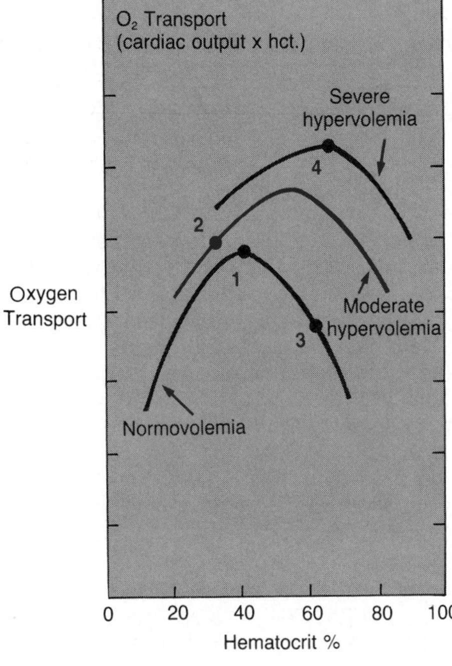

FIGURE 57–10. Oxygen transport at various hematocrit levels in normovolemic, mildly hypervolemic, and severely hypervolemic individuals. The oxygen transport is estimated by multiplying hematocrit by cardiac output. As can be seen in 1, the optimal oxygen transport for the normovolemic subjects is at a hematocrit of about 45 percent with a progressive rise in the optimal hematocrit as the blood volume increases. A suboptimal hematocrit in a hypervolemic person (anemia of pregnancy), as in 2, may be associated with a higher oxygen transport than that of a normovolemic person with normal hematocrit. However, a high hematocrit without increase in blood volume (3) may be associated with an absolute reduction in oxygen transport and tissue hypoxia. Only high hematocrit coupled with high blood volume (4) enhances oxygen transport to the tissues. (From Erslev, A. J.: Clinical manifestations and classification of erythrocyte disorders. *In* Williams, W. J., et al. (eds.): Hematology. 4th ed. New York, McGraw-Hill Book Co., 1990, p. 428.)

POLYCYTHEMIA VERA

Although the pathogenesis of polycythemia vera is not understood, this condition has been classified as a myeloproliferative disorder.[94] All hematopoietic cells are monoclonal based on assays of glucose-6-phosphate dehydrogenase (G-6-PD) isoenzymes,[95] an enzymatic marker that has been used as evidence of the clonal origin of tumors. In black patients heterozygous for G-6-PD, normal tissues possess both isoenzymes A (phenotype: Gd-A) and B (phenotype: Gd-B); if only one isoenzyme is present in the neoplastic cells of such a patient, a clonal origin of the neoplasm or, in this case, the disease polycythemia vera is likely. Thus, erythropoietin is not the stimulus for increased red cell production; indeed, erythropoietin concentrations may be low in this condition.

If erythrocytosis is accompanied by an increased red cell mass, arterial oxygen saturation more than 92 per cent, and splenomegaly, the diagnosis of polycythemia vera is confirmed. In the absence of splenomegaly, any two of the following laboratory findings will satisfy the diagnostic criteria: thrombocytosis, leukocytosis (in the absence of infection), elevated leukocyte alkaline phosphatase activity, or a combination of elevated serum vitamin B_{12} concentration and unsaturated B_{12}-binding capacity.[96]

CLINICAL MANIFESTATIONS. Symptoms are divided into those secondary to the increased red cell mass and increased blood volume, including headache, plethora, pruritus, dyspnea, and bleeding; those due to increased blood viscosity, including paresthesias and thrombosis; and those due to hypermetabolism, including weight loss despite a good appetite and night sweats. Angina pectoris, intermittent claudication, and arterial hypertension occur frequently.

It seems paradoxical that both bleeding and thrombosis can be complications of this disease; however, each occurs in 33 to 50 per cent of patients, and they are the major causes of morbidity and mortality. Bleeding is caused by the distention of veins and capillaries due to the increased blood volume, defective platelet function, or both. Thrombosis has been thought to be related to increased blood viscosity, thrombocytosis, and abnormally increased aggregation of platelets. Thrombotic sites include coronary and cerebral arteries as well as those in the extremities. Less frequently, thrombosis may involve the mesenteric and portal veins. Surgical morbidity is high in patients with polycythemia vera who are inadequately treated, and anesthesia and the stress of operation increase further the risk of hemorrhagic and thrombotic events during the immediate postoperative period.

TREATMENT. Therapy is aimed primarily at decreasing the potential for both hemorrhage and thrombosis. Ideally, this consists of phlebotomy alone. If control of thrombocytosis is necessary, hydroxyurea appears to be the most efficacious agent.[96]

MECHANISMS OF SYMPTOMS. The clinical severity of polycythemia is usually related to the degree of hypervolemia and increased viscosity.[93,94] Myocardial oxygen transport is not impaired with high hematocrit values.[11] In older patients with underlying atherosclerotic vascular disease, cardiac output tends not to be elevated, and as a consequence of the increased viscosity without increased flow, the incidence of ischemic episodes may be higher. In vitro studies suggest that white blood cells can contribute significantly to blood viscosity[97]; since leukocytosis is characteristic of polycythemia vera, white cells undoubtedly play a role in the increased viscosity seen in this disease.

Cerebral blood flow is significantly reduced and is associated with cerebral symptoms in about half the patients with hematocrit values averaging 53.6 per cent, confirming the relationship between cerebrovascular insufficiency and blood viscosity.[98] When hematocrit is lowered to approximately 45 per cent, viscosity declines by 30 per cent and cerebral blood flow increases substantially. With hematocrit values ranging from 46 to 52 per cent, cerebral blood flow is still less than normal, suggesting that even slight increases in red cell mass may interfere with cerebral perfusion. These results imply that patients with polycythemia vera should undergo phlebotomy until hematocrit levels reach the low 40's rather than the previously recommended level of about 47 per cent.

SECONDARY POLYCYTHEMIAS

The secondary polycythemias may be divided into two subgroups: (1) those in which the increased red cell mass compensates for a reduction in oxygen transport with appropriate stimulation by erythropoietin and (2) those in which erythrocytosis is associated with an inappropriate increase in erythropoietin production. It has been suggested that any hypoxic stimulus will cause production of the enzyme erythrogenin in the kidney, which generates erythropoietin by acting enzymatically on a proposed plasma protein substrate, possibly of hepatic origin (Fig. 57–11). If an individual living at sea level is transported to a high altitude, hemoglobin concentrations will rise[99] accompanied by an increase in erythropoietin. Similarly, with severe degrees of chronic hypoxemia in chronic obstructive pulmonary disease, an arterial PO_2 less than 60 mm Hg usually leads to an increase in red cell mass. Although in some instances hemoglobin has been reported to be as high as 24 gm/dl and the hematocrit as high as 75 per cent, in most patients with chronic pulmonary disease these values do not exceed 17 gm/dl and 57 per cent, respectively.[100] In cyanotic congenital heart disease, red cell mass increases as resting arterial oxygen saturation falls (p. 895). Hematocrits as high as 86 per cent may be seen with red blood cell masses almost three times normal.[101] Although plasma volume may be diminished, total blood volume remains significantly elevated because of the striking increase in red cell mass. The most common congenital malformations producing these elevations include tetralogy of Fallot, transposition of the great arteries, and persistent truncus arteriosus (see Chap. 31).

CLINICAL MANIFESTATIONS. Signs and symptoms of hyperviscosity generally occur as hematocrit exceeds 60 per cent; cardiac function may be compromised because of the combination of hypervolemia and the constant volume load and augmented vascular resistance secondary to the increased viscosity of the blood. Ruddy cyanosis, headache, dizziness, roaring in the ears, thrombotic episodes, and bleeding are the major clinical findings and may be treated with phlebotomy.[102] Careful monitoring of arterial pressure, heart rate, and general condition is necessary during phlebotomy, and the acute reduction in blood volume may have to be avoided by the simultaneous administration of plasma expanders.[103] After isovolemic phlebotomy to reduce the hematocrit from the 70's to the 60's, cardiac output rises, and despite the fall in arterial oxygen content, systemic oxygen transport usually increases. These favorable changes are attributed to the reduced blood viscosity and vascular resistance. Although the erythrocytosis is a homeostatic mechanism compensating for the chronic arterial hypoxemia, greatly increased hematocrits are generally undesirable. Studies by Erslev and Caro suggest that secondary polycythemia is not necessarily a boon but could be a burden, and that secondary erythrocytosis cannot always be considered optimal for overall oxygen transport.[104] Secondary polycythemia due to cyanotic congenital heart disease has been reported to cause myocardial infarction without manifestations of coronary atherosclerosis.[105,106]

MANAGEMENT. Phlebotomy, or preferably erythropheresis, in secondary polycythemia reduces blood viscosity, increases systemic oxygen transport without lowering peripheral oxygen consumption, and simultaneously increases effective renal plasma flow.[107,108] The optimal hematocrit for patients with cyanotic congenital heart disease and other chronically hypoxemic states is poorly defined and presents an interesting and perplexing dilemma. The clinical presentation of the patient must be carefully considered. Cerebral blood flow is reduced in secondary erythrocytosis as well as in polycythemia vera and improves with phlebotomy.[109,110] As might be expected from the decreased oxygen transport associated with right-to-left shunts, P_{50} and red cell 2,3-DPG are increased, but the relationship between decreased arterial PO_2 and the rise in P_{50} and red cell 2,3-DPG varies greatly.[111] Successful surgical correction of the cardiac defect will result in normal saturation and obviate the adaptive mechanism, and hematocrit and blood volume will return to normal.

HEMOGLOBIN VARIANTS WITH INCREASED AFFINITY FOR OXYGEN. In 1966, it was first recognized that a hemoglobin variant with *increased* oxygen affinity could be associated with erythrocytosis.[112] These variants, which generally have amino acid substitutions at structural sites crucial to hemoglobin function and individually are quite rare, now number over 40. They are transmitted in an autosomal dominant fashion and cause a shift in the oxygen dissociation curve to the left with reduced levels of P_{50}. The shift to the left of the Hb-O_2 dissociation curve results in a marked reduction in oxygen extraction by the tissues. Increased hemoglobin concentration and blood flow are available compensatory mechanisms to maintain oxygen delivery (Fig. 57–3). However, the primary response appears to be erythrocytosis mediated by increases in erythropoietin.[113–115] The cardiac output is usually normal. Polycythemia constitutes the primary adjustment for oxygen delivery in patients with these hemoglobin variants, who have no increased incidence of myocardial ischemia or other forms of organ hypoxia.

OTHER CAUSES. True erythrocytosis without demonstrable cause, other than excessive cigar and cigarette smoking, has also been noted in a significant number of individuals.[116] All had elevated levels of carboxyhemoglobin with shifts of the Hb-O_2 dissociation curve to the left, stimulating erythropoiesis. In most cases of polycythemia secondary to inappropriate erythropoietin production, such as tumors, renal cysts, and hydronephrosis, the red cell mass, although increased, does not generally cause symptoms of hyperviscosity.

RELATIVE POLYCYTHEMIA. This is a distinct and commonly encountered entity that is also referred to as spurious polycythemia, *Gaisböck syndrome,* and *stress erythrocytosis.* It is not a primary disease process and may be merely a physiological state in which the plasma volume is slightly reduced and the red cell mass is slightly increased. Hematocrit rarely exceeds 60 per cent, and other blood constituents are normal. This disorder can be distinguished from polycythemia vera by measuring the red cell mass, which by definition is normal in relative polycythemia and increased in polycythemia vera. Patients are often hypertensive, prone to thromboembolic complications,[117] and obese; however, these complications appear to be unrelated to the hematological changes, so that reducing the red cell mass by phlebotomy, radiation therapy, or chemotherapy is not appropriate. When present, hypertension and thromboembolic complications should be treated in the usual manner.

THROMBOCYTOSIS

Occasionally thrombocytosis value may be seen alone as a manifestation of a myeloproliferative disorder without an increased hematocrit.[118–123] Essential thrombocytosis has been associated in several instances of sudden catastrophic events such as massive arterial thrombosis in the cerebral and coronary arteries, occurring even in young adults without underlying atherosclerosis.[118–122] Such complications rarely occur in the thrombocytosis secondary to nonmyeloproliferative states such as iron deficiency or postsplenectomy states unless coexistent with severe anemia.[123] Rheological changes in the blood have been found to be associated with myocardial infarction, but it is not clear whether these changes are secondary to infarction or whether they play an initiating role.[124–126] Changes in blood viscosity, plasma viscosity, and red cell filterability occur in patients with myocardial infarction or unstable angina and may play an important role in its pathogenesis. Although these changes may not contribute to disease in many other parts of the body, they may be significant in the coronary microcirculation.

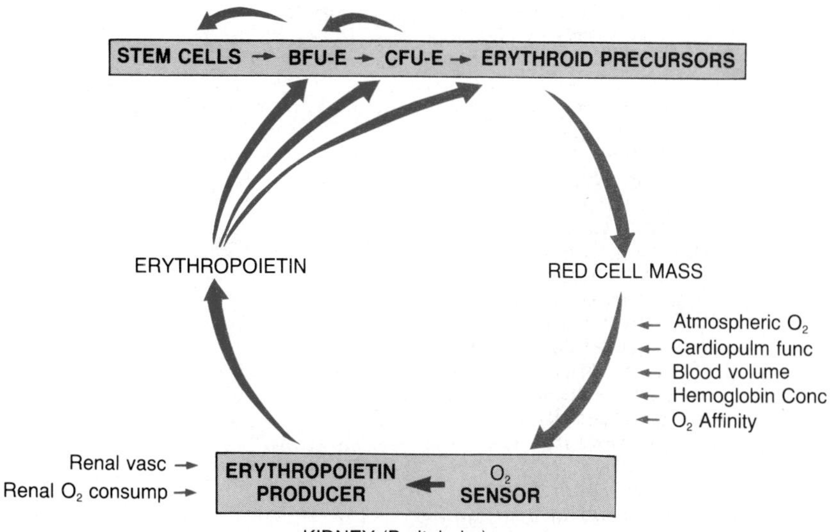

FIGURE 57–11. Feedback circuit linking an oxygen sensor in the kidney with erythroid progenitor cells in the bone marrow. The circuit is moved in one direction by red cells containing oxygen and in the opposite direction by erythropoietin. Oxygen sensing and erythropoietin production may also take place in the liver and in some macrophages. The target for erythropoietin is primarily the erythropoietin-dependent progenitor cells (CFU-E), with milder actions on the burst-forming progenitor cells (BFU-E) and the precursor cells. (From Erslev, A. J.: Production of erythrocytes. *In* Williams, W. J., et al. (eds.): Hematology. 4th ed, New York, McGraw-Hill Book Co., 1990, p. 395.)

INCIDENCE. Primary tumors of the heart which are discussed in Chap. 44, are rare, occurring in less than 0.1 per cent of autopsies. Here we deal with tumors metastatic to the pericardium or heart, which are far more common, ranging from 1.5 to 20.6 per cent (average 6 per cent) of autopsies on patients with malignant diseases, and actually appear to be increasing in incidence.[127] Prolonged survival of cancer patients may be the reason for this higher incidence. Usually the metastases involve the pericardium and myocardium, with the valves or endocardium rarely affected, and the right side of the heart appears to be affected more frequently than the left.[128] Solitary metastases to the heart are rare. Although metastatic nodules in the heart are generally multiple (Fig. 57–12), they may become diffuse and lead to the manifestations of restrictive cardiomyopathy (p. 1415). The mode of spread to the heart may be by direct extension, as occurs in lung cancer; via the hematogenous route, as in malignant melanoma; or through lymphatic channels, as in lymphoma.

The most common primary tumor producing cardiac metastases is carcinoma of the bronchus (Fig. 57–12), with carcinoma of the breast, malignant melanoma, lymphomas, and leukemias next in order of frequency (Table 57–3).[128,129] At autopsy, 15 to 35 per cent of patients dying with primary lung cancer show cardiac involvement, while over 60 per cent of patients with melanoma have cardiac metastases.[130] Hematological malignant tumors, especially lymphomas, have been reported to account for 15 per cent of all cardiac and pericardial metastases,[131] and about 15 per cent of patients dying of malignant lymphomas show metastases to the heart. Metastatic cardiac lesions secondary to mesothelioma and sarcoma, as well as melanoma and breast cancer, are all increasing in number.

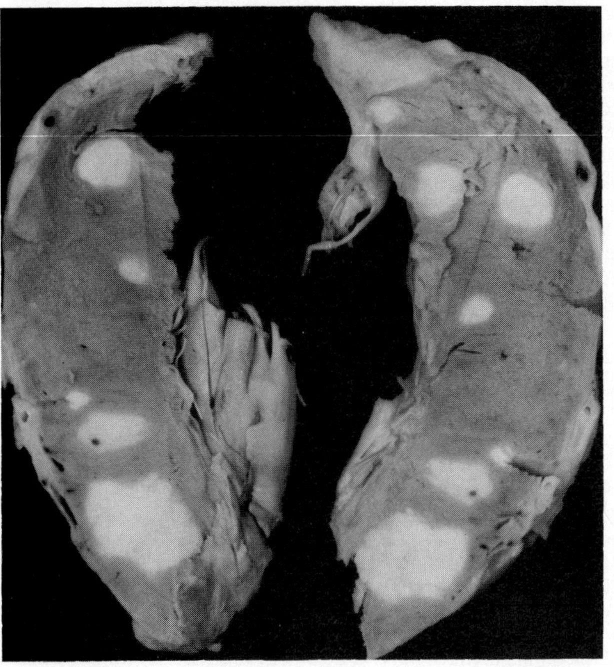

FIGURE 57–12. **Sections of left ventricle showing metastatic nodules in the myocardium. Primary tumor was in a bronchus. (From Edwards, J. E.: Effects of malignant noncardiac tumors upon the cardiovascular system. *In* Brest, A. N. [ed.]: Cardiovascular Clinics, Vol. 4. Philadelphia, F. A. Davis, 1972, p. 282.)**

CLINICAL MANIFESTATIONS

Many metastatic cardiac lesions are clinically silent and are found only at necropsy. For example, despite massive heart involvement with melanoma ("charcoal heart"), sometimes there is surprisingly little evidence of cardiac dysfunction.[132] Specific clinical manifestations of cardiac involvement by cancer may be divided into those due to pericardial, myocardial, or endocardial involvement; cardiac compression by extracardiac tumors[133]; indirect consequences of tumor complications of circulating mediators; embolization in patients in a hypercoagulable state; or the effects of specific tumor therapy, such as chemotherapy and radiation therapy (Table 57–4).[128,129] The most common clinical manifestations result from pericardial effusion with tamponade, tachyarrhythmias, AV block,[134] or congestive heart failure.[133] Metastatic cardiac disease is rarely the presenting symptom of a tumor. The mode of spread may be by direct extension via the hematogenous route or through lymphatic channels. Routine chest radiographs, computed chest tomography, magnetic resonance imaging, echocardiography, and/or radionuclide imaging with gallium or thallium are often helpful in diagnosis.[135–138] Osteogenic sarcoma, which may metastasize to the heart, is unique because the metastases contain bone and may be radiographically visible.[139]

TABLE 57–3 METASTATIC CARDIAC DISEASE

TUMOR TYPE	TOTAL NO.	METASTASES Heart	Pericardial	Both
Bronchogenic carcinoma	402	43 (10.2)	66 (15.7)	23 (5.4)
Breast carcinoma	289	24 (8.3)	34 (11.8)	3 (1.4)
Malignant melanoma	59	20 (34.0)	14 (23.7)	12 (20.4)
Colonic carcinoma	214	2 (0.9)	6 (2.8)	0
Esophageal carcinoma	65	5 (7.7)	5 (7.7)	2 (3.6)
Hypernephroma	95	5 (5.3)	0	0
Ovarian carcinoma	115	6 (5.7)	8 (7.0)	3 (2.6)
Prostatic carcinoma	186	5 (2.7)	2 (1.0)	0
Gastric carcinoma	308	11 (3.6)	10 (3.2)	3 (0.9)
Sarcoma*	207	19 (9.2)	19 (9.2)	8 (3.9)
Hodgkin's disease	75	—	11 (14.6)	—
Acute leukemia	420	227 (53.9)	95 (22.4)	—
Total	2,435	367 (15.1)	270 (11.1)	54 (2.2)

* Reticulum cell sarcoma and lymphosarcoma.
Note: Numbers in parentheses represent percentages.
From Applefeld, M. M., and Pollock, S. H.: Cardiac disease in patients who have malignancies. Curr. Probl. Cardiol. 4(6):5, 1980.

PERICARDIAL INVOLVEMENT (see also p. 1415). Ten to 25 per cent of all patients with cancer have pericardial involvement at autopsy, with slightly more than half being due to tumor, the rest due to therapy or other causes.[140] Signs and symptoms of pericarditis with pericardial effusion and cardiac tamponade are particularly common in patients with carcinoma of the lung and breast as well as in Hodgkin's disease, non-Hodgkin's lymphoma,[141] and the leukemias,[142] particularly acute myelogenous, lymphoblastic leukemia and the blast crisis of chronic myelogenous leukemia. Pericardial involvement is usually diagnosed ante mortem because of the resultant symptomatology and radiographic and echocardiographic evidence. Clinically, this takes the form of either cardiac tamponade or adhesive pericarditis, associated with extensive nodular tumor infiltration of the pericardium.[143–147] The finding of chylous pericardial effusion is usually characteristic of lymphoma.[148] Echocardiography is a key tool in the diagnosis of neoplastic involvement of the pericardium[119,120,136,149] (Fig. 57–13) (see also Fig. 4–102, p. 103 and Fig. 45–27, p. 1506). Pericardiocentesis may be necessary to differentiate tumor from radiation effects.[150] Computed tomography and magnetic resonance imaging are also helpful in detecting pericardial tumors.

TABLE 57-4 CLINICAL MANIFESTATIONS OF CARDIAC INVOLVEMENT IN MALIGNANT DISEASE

Pericardial involvement
Pericarditis
Cardiac tamponade
Superior vena caval syndrome
Arrhythmias
Supraventricular tachycardia
Carotid sinus syncope
Atrioventricular block
Cardiomegaly and congestive heart failure
Unexplained heart murmur
Unexplained hypotension
Noninfective (marantic) endocarditis

Pericardial tumor or fibrosis secondary to radiation therapy may mimic chronic constrictive pericarditis or chronic effusive pericardial disease and cause problems in differential diagnosis (p. 1499). In patients with carcinoma of the lung, Hodgkin's disease, and non-Hodgkin's lymphoma, who commonly undergo irradiation of the thorax, radiation-induced pericarditis is common, and it was believed that this condition could be differentiated from tumor involvement because it occurred usually within a year of such therapy. However, it has become clear that radiation-induced pericarditis may occur as late as 8 years after therapy.[151]

MYOCARDIAL METASTASES. Direct myocardial or endocardial involvement by tumor such as lung cancer, lymphoma, or melanoma may result in arrhythmias, congestive heart failure, ventricular outflow tract obstruction, and peripheral emboli.[131,152] Cardiac metastases can be detected on two-dimensional echocardiography (Figs. 57-12 and 57-14),[136] computed tomography, and magnetic resonance imaging (Fig. 11-36, p. 330).[136,153,154]

VENA CAVAL OBSTRUCTION. The superior vena caval syndrome, resulting from obstruction of this vessel by tumor, is also a recognized complication in patients with carcinoma of the lung and malignant lymphoma.[155] Enlarged mediastinal nodes or the primary tumor itself may impinge upon or even occlude the superior vena cava, causing dyspnea, distention of the neck veins, edema of the face and arms, proptosis, headache, and syncope. Because of the potential life-threatening nature of these problems, local irradiation may have to be initiated prior to any diagnostic procedure. Similar enlargement of nodes or tumor may cause obstruction of the inferior vena cava, with massive leg edema, congestive hepatomegaly, and hypotension.[156]

CARDIAC AMYLOIDOSIS (see also p. 1416). The heart is involved in the majority of cases of primary amyloidosis and also in many instances of amyloidosis secondary to multiple myeloma. Symptoms often include congestive heart failure, hypotension, arrhythmias, and conduction disturbances.[157,158] Echocardiographic examination, contrast tomography, and endomyocardial biopsy have made it easier to confirm this

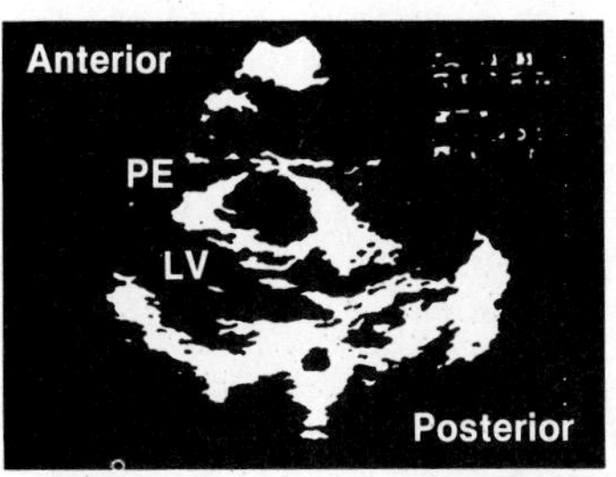

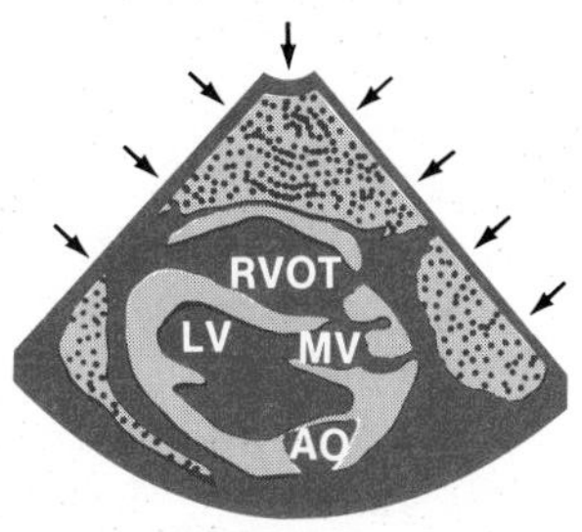

FIGURE 57-13. Two-dimensional, parasternal, long-axis view *(left)* with schematic diagram *(right)* in lymphoblastic lymphoma involving the pericardium. Note a small amount of pericardial effusion (PE) and extensive thickening of the pericardium encasing the heart (arrowheads in right panel). AO = aorta; LV = left ventricle; MV = mitral valve; RVOT = right ventricular outflow tract. (From Kutalek, S. P., et al.: Metastatic tumors of the heart detected by two-dimensional echocardiography. Am. Heart J. *109*:343, 1985.)

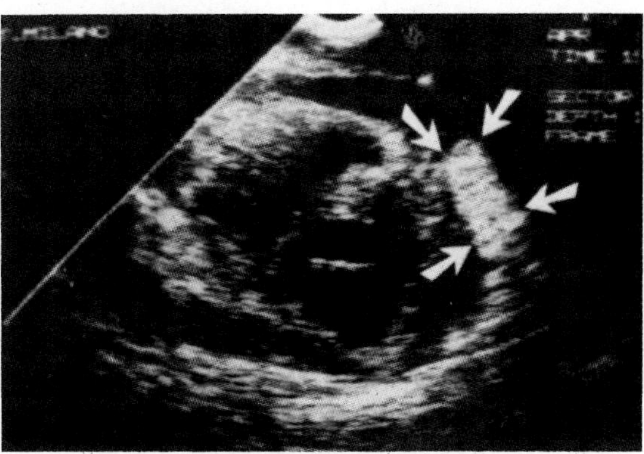

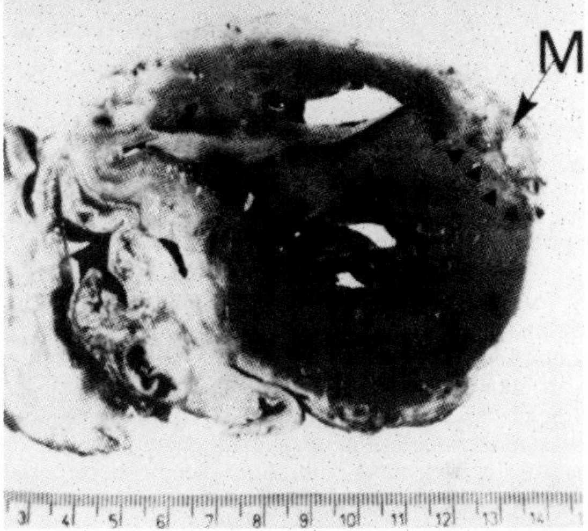

FIGURE 57-14. *Top,* Echocardiogram in parasternal short-axis view. A large echogenic mass (arrows) infiltrates the left lateral ventricular wall and the septum. *Bottom,* Postmortem specimen (cross section). The neoplastic mass (M) infiltrates the epicardium and the subepicardial myocardium (arrowheads). (From Lestuzzi, C., et al.: Secondary neoplastic infiltration of the myocardium diagnosed by two-dimensional echocardiography in seven cases with anatomic confirmation. J. Am. Coll. Cardiol. 9:439, 1987.)

diagnosis. A low myocardial density on contrast-aided tomography, diffuse myocardial thickening, and diffuse hypokinetic wall motion may be the result of cardiac amyloidosis and may simulate hypertrophic cardiomyopathy. Endomyocardial biopsy may be necessary to confirm the diagnosis.[159-161]

ELECTROCARDIOGRAPHIC AND ROENTGENOGRAPHIC FINDINGS. Arrhythmias and a wide variety of electrocardiographic changes are common in patients with metastatic disease. Although they may certainly be caused by tumor involvement of the heart, they are more often due to concomitant factors, such as altered electrolyte concentrations, anemia, and hypoxia. Nonspecific ST-segment and T-wave changes, low voltage, and sinus tachycardia are frequent electrocardiographic abnormalities and cannot be considered diagnostic.[162] Clinically it may be difficult to determine whether any such abnormality is attributable to cardiac metastases or is due to an associated cardiac problem, irradiation, or the cardiotoxic effects of drugs. Atrial arrhythmias, such as fibrillation and flutter, may occur secondary to either neoplastic involvement of autonomic fibers supplying the atria or tumor invasion of the coronary arteries perfusing the atria, with resulting atrial infarction, or to neoplastic infiltration of the atrial myocardium or sinus node. Similarly, electrocardiographic changes of acute myocardial infarction can be produced by tumor infiltration or hemorrhage into the ventricle or occlusion of one of the coronary arteries. Occasionally, the exact area of tumor involvement may be pinpointed based on the acute electrocardiographic changes.[163] Involvement of the

AV node is a rare cause of complete heart block but may be the presenting symptom of the tumor.[164] In addition, tumor involvement of cervical lymph nodes without mediastinal involvement has been associated with carotid sinus syncope.[165]

Roentgenographic evidence of cardiac enlargement and the development of congestive heart failure may be the only clinical signs of malignant involvement of the heart. New systolic murmurs may occur with intraluminal invasion or external compression of the carotid or pulmonary arteries by the tumor. In addition to coincidental atherosclerosis, coronary artery disease in cancer patients can be caused by tumor emboli, extrinsic compression of the coronary arteries or ostia, or thromboemboli brought about by tumor-associated coagulation disorders.

If myocardial metastases are suspected from clinical or electrocardiographic data, a two-dimensional echocardiogram is often helpful diagnostically.

MYOCARDIAL INFARCTION. In a necropsy study of 816 patients with solid tumors, 33 (4 per cent) died of myocardial infarction.[166] Patients with carcinoma of the lung, malignant lymphoma, and leukemia are most commonly afflicted; less frequently affected were patients with cancer of the breast and gastrointestinal tract and malignant melanoma.[167] In general, the etiology of coronary artery disease in patients with cancer is most likely coincidental spontaneous atherosclerosis.[168] The most common cause of tumor-related myocardial infarction is extrinsic compression of a coronary artery, occurring in 60 per cent of cases, whereas tumor emboli are responsible for about 35 per cent.[167,169] Widespread thromboses, including coronary artery thromboses due to disseminated intravascular coagulation, occasionally occur in patients with metastatic tumors, most commonly mucin-secreting adenocarcinomas. Approximately half of all patients with acute myocardial infarction secondary to malignant disease had a history of typical chest pain prior to death. An acute myocardial infarction in a patient with advanced malignant disease is a particularly poor prognostic sign, since more than two-thirds of such patients die within 3 weeks of the event.

VALVULAR EFFECTS: NONBACTERIAL THROMBOTIC ENDOCARDITIS (NBTE). Metastatic tumors may affect cardiac valves in a variety of ways, including direct invasion of valves, interference with valvular function by compression, valvular dysfunction secondary to malignant carcinoid (p. 1424), but most commonly by NBTE.[170-172] Although the pathogenesis is unclear, this condition is associated with adenocarcinomas—especially of the pancreas and lung—as well as hematological malignant disease and lymphomas.[173] It has been suggested that immune complexes elicited by the underlying malignant process play a role in the formation of thrombi.[174] Other causes of NBTE include disseminated intravascular coagulation and nonneoplastic causes of debilitation and cachexia.[173] The fibrin matrix is attached to, but does not destroy, valve leaflets that may be normal or show degenerative changes.[171,172] NBTE involves principally the aortic and mitral valves equally. (The pulmonic valve may be involved in patients with catheters in place for long periods in the right heart and pulmonary artery.[175])

Patients may have clinical evidence of arterial embolization and microembolic events resembling those of infective endocarditis (p. 1083), and changing murmurs, often without fever or leukocytosis (unless an unrelated infection is present). The most serious complications are cerebral emboli with neurological sequelae. Rarely coronary embolization may occur, causing myocardial infarction.

The diagnosis is aided immensely by two-dimensional echocardiography. Antiplatelet therapy with aspirin or anticoagulants has been employed to prevent recurrent embolization, but its effectiveness has yet to be demonstrated.

ENDOCARDIAL INVOLVEMENT. There is a high correlation between eosinophilia in the bone marrow and peripheral blood and the occurrence of endomyocardial fibrosis,[176] which may cause restrictive cardiomyopathy (p. 1415). Ever since Loeffler described the entity "endocarditis parietalis fibroplastica" with eosinophilia, this association has been of interest but remains unexplained. In some patients, the cardiac manifestations predominate, most commonly cardiomegaly, congestive heart failure, arrhythmias, and heart murmurs, whereas in others, all or most of the clinical manifestations are secondary to the *eosinophilic leukemia*. Pathologically, these syndromes are characterized by local or widespread eosinophilic infiltrates with fibrous scarring and thickening of the endocardium, including the atrioventricular valves. In many patients, the course is chronic and insidious, but death is usually the direct result of cardiac involvement.

CARDIAC EFFECTS OF RADIATION THERAPY AND CHEMOTHERAPY

With the advent of intensive radiation therapy and aggressive chemotherapy, cardiac toxicity of antitumor treatment has increased greatly. Formerly, the heart was considered one of the most radioresistant organs and seemed to be spared most of the side effects of chemotherapy. However, radiation can cause myocardial damage.[177] The incidence of cardiovascular complications has risen sharply with the use of curative forms of radiation therapy for Hodgkin's disease and non-Hodgkin's lymphoma involving the mediastinum and the addition of one of the most potent classes of chemotherapeutic agents, the anthracyclines. The addition of growth factors and cytokines such as interferon and interleukin-2 to the armamentarium of the therapist has also brought on unexpected cardiac complications.

RADIATION THERAPY

Therapeutic radiation can cause heart damage by injuring various structures either acutely or chronically (Table 57–5). Most commonly affected is the pericardium, with less damage to the myocardium, endocardium, and papillary muscles, and the least damage to the heart valves and coronary arteries

TABLE 57–5 EFFECT OF RADIATION ON THE HEART

EARLY CHANGES
Cytoplasmic damage
Capillary injury
DNA damage
Local chemical reactions
von Willebrand factor release
Platelet and fibrin deposition
Acute inflammatory reaction
Increased vascular permeability
Protein damage
Transient pericardial effusion
INTERMEDIATE CHANGES
Cellular immune response
Vascular compromise
Attempts at repair
Organized fibrin formation
Endothelial proliferation
Collagen deposition
LATE CHANGES
Compromised vascular supply
Cell death
Fibroblastic proliferation
Altered cell morphology
Enhanced atherosclerosis
Thickening of pericardium
Loss of adventitial tissue
Pericardial effusion
Endocardial thickening
Valvular heart disease
Arrhythmias

From Niemtzow, R. C., and Reynolds, R. D.: Radiation therapy and the heart. In Kapoor, A. S. (ed.): Cancer and the Heart. New York, Springer-Verlag, 1986, p. 240.

TABLE 57-6 CLASSIFICATION OF RADIATION-RELATED CARDIAC DISEASE

1. Acute pericarditis (caused by necrosis of tumor adjacent to the heart)
2. Delayed pericarditis
   a. Acute radiation-induced pericarditis, without effusion
   b. Acute radiation-induced pericarditis, with effusion, with/without cardiac tamponade
   c. Chronic effusive pericarditis
   d. Effusive constrictive pericarditis
   e. Chronic pericardial constriction
   f. Occult constrictive pericarditis
3. Myocardial fibrosis
4. Occlusive coronary artery disease
5. Conduction abnormalities
6. Valvular regurgitation or stenosis

(Table 57-6).[178,178a] Severe pericardial damage with pericarditis,[179-181] acute myocardial infarction,[151,182-186] valvular disease,[187-190] cardiomyopathy,[191] and arrhythmias[192] are the most frequently observed complications.

PERICARDIAL EFFECTS (see also p. 1499). Radiation-induced pericardial abnormalities can be divided into early, intermediate, and late changes (Table 57-5).[178,193,194] The most common acute cardiovascular complication of radiation therapy is pericarditis.[180] Acute pericarditis occurs in 10 to 15 per cent of patients with Hodgkin's disease who receive over 4000 rads to the mediastinum.[181] These episodes are characterized by fever, pleuritic pain, pericardial friction rub, and electrocardiographic and echocardiographic changes typical of this condition (p. 1500). The time from completion of radiotherapy to the clinical onset of pericarditis ranges from 0 to 85 months, with the peak incidence occurring between 5 and 9 months. Echocardiography demonstrates a pericardial effusion in almost all patients with clinical evidence of pericarditis.[195] With long follow-up of patients cured of their underlying neoplastic disease, the clinical manifestations of pericarditis may not develop for 8 to 10 years.[151,193,194] The incidence of pericarditis appears to be a function of the fractional and total dose of radiation to the pericardium and the quantity of the heart irradiated. When the entire dose of radiation is delivered through an anterior port, the incidence of pericarditis is increased. However, when chest irradiation is delivered in divided doses to anterior and posterior ports and with a subcarinal shield, the incidence of pericarditis has decreased to 2.5 per cent, without increasing the risk of relapse of Hodgkin's disease.[196] If the entire heart receives therapeutic doses of radiation, up to 50 per cent of patients may develop pericardial complications.[197] As a consequence whole-heart irradiation has been replaced with chemotherapy for many patients with large mediastinal masses.

It has been suggested that routine follow-up during the first year after radiation of the mediastinum should consist of frequent echocardiography and chest roentgenography. If any evidence of increased cardiac diameter is noted, or if clinical manifestations suggestive of pericarditis or pericardial effusion develop and there is no reason to suspect another cause of pericarditis, patients may be treated symptomatically but occasionally may require pericardiocentesis and/or pericardiectomy.[150,151]

MYOCARDIAL AND ENDOCARDIAL EFFECTS. Echocardiographic studies carried out before and within 6 months after conventional irradiation therapy in women with breast cancer revealed an asymptomatic decrease of the fractional systolic shortening of the left ventricular minor-axis diameter and of the systolic blood pressure/end-systolic diameter ratio. These changes, which reflect slight transient depression of left ventricular function, occurred within the first 6 months after postoperative radiation and disappeared by 6 months.[198]

Radiation-induced endocardial fibrosis may cause manifestations of restrictive cardiomyopathy[191,199] (p. 1415) and a variety of nonspecific electrocardiographic changes[200] as well as varying degrees of AV block.[192] Mitral regurgitation may develop secondary to radiation-induced papillary muscle dysfunction and aortic regurgitation as a consequence of endocardial valvular thickening.[187,189] The onset of new murmurs occurring after radiation therapy should alert the physician to these possibilities. In an autopsy study of the cardiac effects of radiation exposure, three-fourths of the patients exposed to more than 3500 rads, with a field resulting in a large exposure of the anterior thorax, developed interstitial myocardial fibrosis, with more extensive involvement of the right than the left ventricle. Functional abnormalities demonstrated on echocardiography and radionuclide angiocardiography may occur 5 to 15 years after radiation but, as with pericarditis, should become less frequent with new techniques of radiotherapy.[179]

CORONARY AND CAROTID ARTERIAL EFFECTS. Since the report in 1967 of a 15-year-old boy suffering a fatal myocardial infarction 16 months after receiving 4000 rads to the heart for Hodgkin's disease, a number of similar occurrences have been reported.[151,182-186,201-203] Supportive evidence for radiation-induced coronary artery disease includes (1) its occurrence in subjects who are very young with no predisposing factors and disease limited to coronary vessels within the path of the radiation beam, (2) the lack of atherosclerosis in arteries not exposed to irradiation, (3) reports of occlusive lesions in other arteries such as the carotid artery after irradiation,[204] (4) the presence of distinctive pathological changes, and (5) the production of similar lesions in experimental models.

Occlusive coronary and carotid artery disease following irradiation generally occurs 6 to 12 years after exposure. In rabbits, 2500 rads has produced coronary atherosclerosis similar to that in humans.[205] However, rabbits do not develop radiation-induced atherosclerosis unless they also receive a diet high in lipids and cholesterol, which by itself is insufficient to produce the atherosclerotic lesion. Coronary artery lesions presumably induced by radiotherapy in patients appear to be distinct pathologically and to contain severe medial and adventitial fibrosis in continuity with overlying epicardial fibrous tissue and a marked paucity of lipid in the intimal lesions.[206] In affected young patients examined at autopsy, the proximal portions of the arteries are significantly more narrowed than the distal portions. In addition, there is significant loss of smooth muscle cells from the media.[206]

Radiation-induced coronary artery or carotid artery obstruction or occlusion may require surgical treatment. Because of the relatively low incidence of this complication and the concern that lowering the dose of radiation might preclude effective treatment of the neoplastic process, no systematic attempts have been made to try to prevent this complication other than considering chemotherapeutic alternatives if whole-heart irradiation is otherwise deemed necessary for curative purposes. It is anticipated that with changes in radiotherapeutic techniques and available curative chemotherapy, the incidence of all forms of radiation-induced heart disease will continue to decline.

CHEMOTHERAPY

Since the late 1960's there have been major advances in the management of a variety of neoplastic disorders using combination chemotherapy. Therapies have become more aggressive and new agents have been introduced, resulting in significant responses and longer survival. Unfortunately, concomitant with this increased response rate has been an increase in toxicity. Although most complications due to drugs are limited to rapidly proliferating tissues such as the bone marrow and gastrointestinal tract, cardiotoxicity, both early and late, has been recognized with increasing frequency (Table 57-7).[207-210]

TABLE 57–7 MAJOR CARDIOVASCULAR COMPLICATIONS OF CHEMOTHERAPEUTIC AGENTS

AGENT	CARDIAC TOXICITY
Amsacrine	Arrhythmia, cardiomyopathy
Busulfan	Pulmonary fibrosis Pulmonary hypertension Endocardial fibrosis
Cisplatin	ECG changes, vaso-occlusion
Cyclophosphamide	Cardiac necrosis, cardiomyopathy
Cytosine arabinoside	Congestive heart failure Pericarditis
Diethylstilbestrol	Cardiovascular deaths
Doxorubicin	ECG changes, cardiomyopathy
Etoposide	Myocardial infarction
5-Fluorouracil	Vaso-occlusion, myocarditis
Methotrexate	ECG changes
Mitomycin	Myocardial damage
Mitoxantrone	Cardiomyopathy
Vincristine	Hypotension

For many years, the only notable cardiopulmonary complications of chemotherapy for neoplastic disease were orthostatic hypotension and the rare myocardial infarctions that occurred in the course of therapy with vincristine, a periwinkle alkaloid, and the interstitial lung disease and mild pulmonary hypertension secondary to pulmonary fibrosis created by bleomycin or busulfan.[211] However, with the use of higher doses of conventional therapy for curative intent and the addition of the anthracycline group of drugs (doxorubicin, daunorubicin), the incidence of cardiac toxicity as a consequence of chemotherapy for neoplastic disease has increased greatly.

ANTHRACYCLINE CARDIOTOXICITY. Doxorubicin is a glycoside antibiotic (Fig. 57–15). Its potent antitumor effect is attributed to its ability to inhibit nucleic acid synthesis by binding to both strands of the DNA helix, intercalating between base pairs, and thereby inhibiting the normal function of DNA and RNA polymerases. Doxorubicin has received more attention than the related compound daunorubicin because of its wider spectrum of antitumor activity in solid tumors and hematological malignant disease.[212] Complete remissions in 30 to 40 per cent of patients with Hodgkin's disease and non-Hodgkin's lymphoma and all types of acute leukemia have been reported with doxorubicin treatment alone. However, its effectiveness is enhanced when it is combined with other chemotherapeutic agents. Remission rates of 60 to 80 per cent have been attained in adults with acute leukemia when doxorubicin was used in combination with cytosine arabinoside and in patients with lymphomas when it was combined with bleomycin, cyclophosphamide, vincristine, and corticosteroids.[212] Although the majority of toxic manifestations produced by these drugs, including alopecia, gastrointestinal distress, myelosuppression, and mucositis, had been predicted on the basis of animal studies, the occurrence of cardiac toxicity and the interactions with radiation therapy were unexpected. Anthracycline cardiotoxicity can be divided into early and late (Table 57–8).

TABLE 57–8 DOXORUBICIN CARDIAC TOXICITY

EARLY OR ACUTE
Arrhythmias
ECG changes
Left ventricular dysfunction
Pericarditis-myocarditis syndrome
Myocardial infarction
Sudden death
LATE OR CHRONIC
Cardiomyopathy
Sinus tachycardia
Pericardial effusion
Left ventricular dysfunction
Low-output heart failure

Modified from Kapoor, A. S.: Doxorubicin toxicity. *In* Kapoor, A. S. (ed.): Cancer and the Heart. New York, Springer-Verlag, 1986, p. 228.

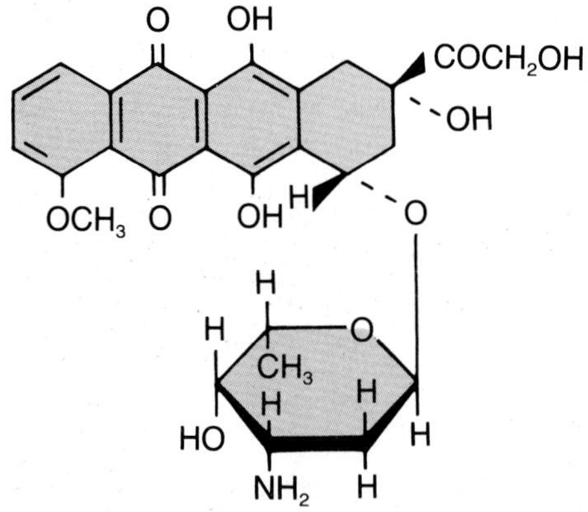

FIGURE 57–15. Structure of doxorubicin.

Early or Acute Cardiotoxicity. This includes arrhythmias, electrocardiographic abnormalities, left ventricular dysfunction, a pericarditis-myocarditis syndrome, and rarely sudden death and myocardial infarction. Arrhythmias, which include supraventricular tachyarrhythmias and premature atrial and ventricular contractions, and abnormalities of conduction such as left axis deviation, decreased QRS voltage, and a variety of nonspecific ST-segment and T-wave abnormalities occur in approximately 11 per cent of patients (range 0 to 41.2 per cent).[213,214] These electrocardiographic changes are usually transient, may occur even at low doses of the anthracycline, and are usually seen within several days after administration of the drug.

The pericarditis-myocarditis syndrome and acute left ventricular dysfunction are rare events. The latter may occur in patients with marginal cardiac reserve, while the acute pericarditis-myocarditis syndrome has been seen in patients with no previous cardiac history.[215] Sudden death may occur as a result of an arrhythmia, myocardial infarction, or acute left ventricular dysfunction.[216]

Late or Chronic Cardiotoxicity. This is primarily due to the development of a dose-dependent degenerative cardiomyopathy.[217] The clinical manifestations consist of sinus tachycardia, tachypnea, cardiomegaly, peripheral and pulmonary edema, hepatomegaly, venous congestion, and pleural effusion. Cardiomyopathy is usually secondary to a cumulative effect of the drug, occurring with increasing frequency at higher doses. Most commonly, congestive heart failure occurs from 9 to 192 days, with a median of 34 days, after the administration of the last dose. It is usually refractory to therapy; when it is severe, as in patients with marked dyspnea and with evidence of heart failure within 4 weeks of the last dose of doxorubicin, survival is short, usually less than 2 weeks.[217,218] The majority of patients with less severe symptoms may be treatable with digitalis and diuretics, but the incidence of cardiac death is high (Fig. 57–16).[217] With long-term follow-up of cancer survivors, there are many reports of congestive heart failure developing 6 to 10 years after doxorubicin therapy. Although in some cases the occurrence may be associated with other risk factors for heart failure, the development of symptoms in childhood survivors suggests a direct relationship with previous anthracycline therapy.[219–221]

Pathological Examination. In chronic anthracycline toxicity, the heart is enlarged, pale, and flabby, with dilated ventricles. Mural thrombi are occasionally found, but the coronary arteries and cardiac valves appear normal. Light microscopy reveals a severe cardiomyopathy with fewer myocardial cells, which show degenerative changes. Electron microscopy shows extensive depletion of myofibrillar bundles, myofibrillar lysis, and distortion and disruption of the Z lines; the mitochondria are swollen with disrupted cristae and inclusion bodies[214,218] (Fig. 57–17). There may be almost complete loss of contractile elements.[222] Routine autopsy studies on patients who had received anthracycline chemotherapy have revealed that clinical evidence of toxicity may be

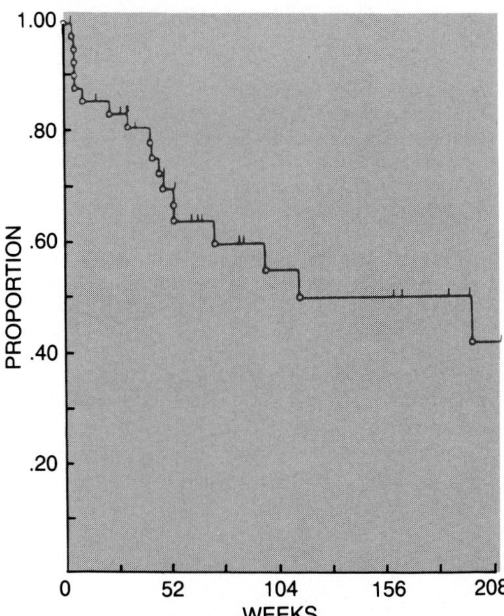

FIGURE 57–16. Actuarial survival plotted for all patients with doxorubicin-induced congestive heart failure. Eighteen patients died of congestive heart failure, 1 died from tumor, and 25 were alive. (From Haq, M. M., et al.: Doxorubicin-induced congestive heart failure in adults. Cancer *56*:1361, 1985.)

present without histological signs; conversely, histological signs of drug toxicity may be seen in the absence of a history of clinical manifestations.[223]

Incidence. The incidence of cardiomyopathy with doxorubicin is 1.7 per cent and with daunorubicin 4.4 per cent. It is fatal in over half the cases.[213] With anthracycline, there is a clear dose-related incidence of cardiomyopathy. None of 764 patients who received a cumulative dose of less than 500 mg/m^2 showed cardiomyopathy, but a progressive increase in the frequency of this complication was noted with higher doses (Table 57–9).[218] It is therefore recommended that cumulative doses of doxorubicin be held to less than 450 to 500 mg/m^2 and 500 to 600 mg/m^2 for daunorubicin. However, cardiomyopathy is being reported with increasing frequency with doxorubicin doses below 450 mg/m^2.[214,218,224] It has been suggested that use of these agents in combination with other modalities of therapy, such as radiation or cyclophosphamide, may be synergistic in the pathogenesis of the cardiomyopathy in some patients, since both radiation and cyclophosphamide alone have been described as potentially cardiotoxic.[206,244–227]

Mechanism. No mechanism for doxorubicin cardiotoxicity has been established, although numerous proposals have been put forward.[228,228a,229] For example, lipid peroxidation may be caused by the binding of DNA by the drug, specifically bound to spectrin, actin, or cardiolipin.[230] Doxorubicin inhibits ATP production, interferes with the sarcolemmal sodium-potassium pump, inhibits oxidative phosphorylation, may provoke an autoimmune response, binds to DNA precursors, interferes with mitochondrial respiration by inhibiting coenzyme Q, and causes myocardial necrosis by allowing the buildup of myocardial calcium.[231–234] A rat myocardial cell culture model has been adapted to study the toxic mechanism.[235,236] Tumor cells and myocardial cells cultured in media containing anthracycline are similarly damaged.[237] Drug-exposed cells have decreased alpha-actin synthesis, which morphologically correlates with the disruption of the thin filaments and the Z lines and relates to poor contractility.[235]

TABLE 57–9 CORRELATION OF CARDIOMYOPATHY (CMY) AND THE TOTAL DOSE OF DOXORUBICIN IN ADULTS

TOTAL DOSE (mg/m^2)	PATIENTS AT RISK	PATIENTS WITH CMY	FREQUENCY (%)
<450	738	0	0
451 to 500	26	0	0
501 to 550	32	3	9
551 to 600	15	3	20
>600	37	15	41
1 Total >550	52	18	35
Total <550	796	3	0.4

Early Detection. Because of the importance of these drugs in cancer chemotherapy and the high incidence of serious cardiac toxicity, several approaches have been suggested for early detection of this complication and for predicting susceptibility.[238–241] Noninvasive studies include serial follow-up of systolic time intervals, in particular the pre-ejection period/left ventricular ejection time (PEP/LVET) ratio, and radionuclide angiogram (p. 297). The PEP/LVET ratio was at first thought to be a sensitive parameter for monitoring toxicity; however, this has not been confirmed on further study and, in fact, has been criticized, since false-positive changes may have been responsible for the inappropriate withholding of potentially life-saving doxorubicin therapy.[242] Radionuclide angiography appears to provide a sensitive and reproducible measurement of left ventricular dysfunction due to

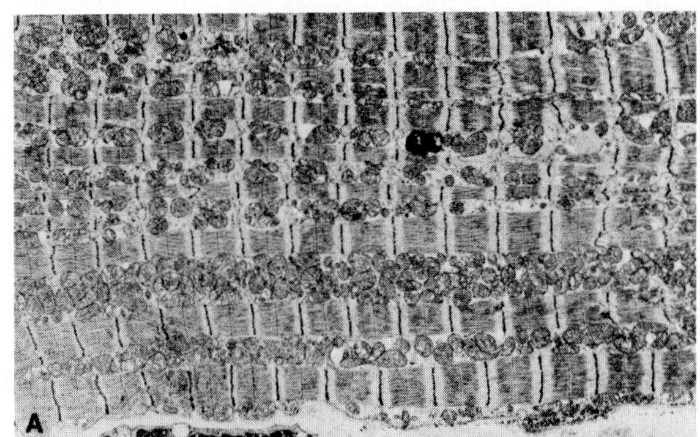

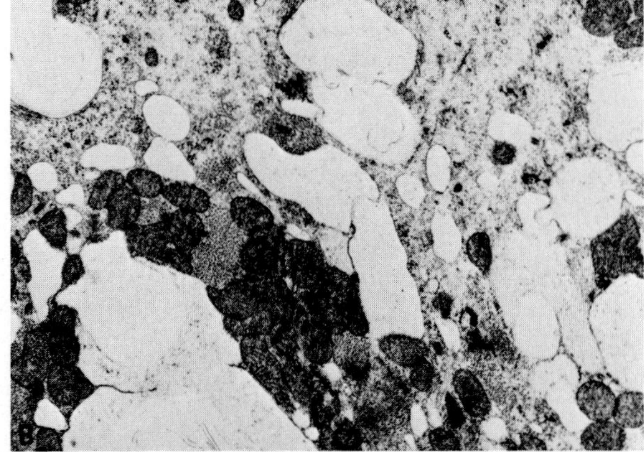

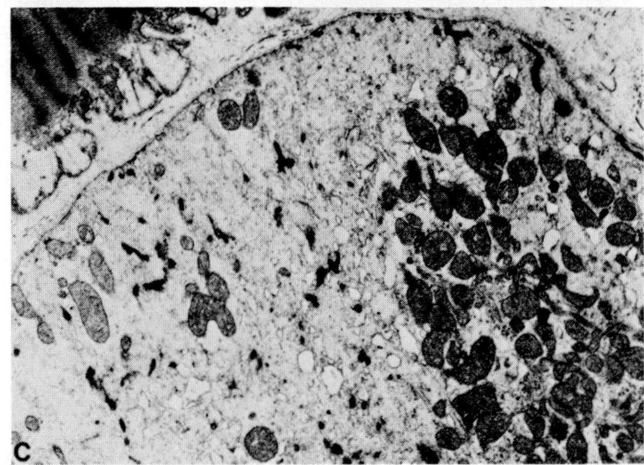

FIGURE 57–17. Electron microscopic images of cardiac biopsy specimens. *A,* Normal cardiac muscle fiber (grade O). *B,* Vacuolation. *C,* Myofibrillar dropout (×3,575). (From Ali, M. D., and Ewer, M. S.: Cancer and the Cardiopulmonary System. New York, Raven Press, 1984, pp. 62 and 63.)

doxorubicin cardiotoxicity.[240,241,243] Sequential studies demonstrate the frequent presence of subclinical left ventricular abnormalities. However, the increased incidence of abnormal results may not be clinically significant if the studies are performed after exercise. Since left ventricular diastolic function can occur before systolic dysfunction, both measurements may be necessary.[241,243,244]

Endomyocardial biopsy appears to be more diagnostic of toxicity than are any of the noninvasive evaluations. In the hands of trained personnel, this technique may be considered a safe procedure[245] (p. 199). Administration of doxorubicin was associated with a dose-related increase in the degree of myocyte damage; drug-associated degenerative changes were identified in 27 of 129 patients at doses greater than or equal to 240 mg/m². Simultaneous studies using endomyocardial biopsy and radionuclide angiography demonstrate good correlation; while the noninvasive studies reveal an accelerating decrease in myocardial function with drug levels exceeding 400 mg/m², biopsy studies show a fairly constant progression of myocardial damage as a function of cumulative dose.[246] These findings suggest that compensatory mechanisms are available to maintain myocardial function despite pathological damage.

It is helpful to grade the hemodynamic abnormalities that occur in patients undergoing doxorubicin chemotherapy[247,248] (Table 57–10). Cardiac monitoring has demonstrated a reduction in the severity and mortality of doxorubicin-associated cardiac failure. Unfortunately, endomyocardial biopsy is invasive and moderately expensive. It has been suggested that different strategies be devised for patients at high risk for cardiotoxicity. Risk factors for the development of drug cardiotoxicity are shown in Table 57–11.[222,224,249–252]

TABLE 57–10 HEMODYNAMIC GRADING OF PATIENTS UNDERGOING DOXORUBICIN CHEMOTHERAPY

GRADE	HEMODYNAMIC FINDINGS
0 Normal	Mean RA <7 mm Hg RVEDP <8 mm Hg LVEDP/Mean PAW <12 mm Hg Cardiac index >2.5 L/min/m² Exercise factor >5.0
1 Mildly abnormal	Any of the following: Mean RA = 7 to 10 mm Hg RVEDP = 8 to 12 mm Hg at rest with increase on exercise = 5 to 9 mm Hg LVEDP/Mean PAW = 12 to 15 mm Hg at rest with increase on exercise = 5 to 11 mm Hg Cardiac index = 2.2 to 2.5 L/min/m² Exercise factor = 4.0 to 5.0
2 Moderately abnormal	Any of the following: Two or more grade 1 features Mean RA = 10 to 15 mm Hg RVEDP = 12 to 17 mm Hg at rest with increase on exercise ≥9 mm Hg Cardiac index = 1.8 to 2.2 L/min/m² Exercise factor <4.0
3 Severely abnormal	Any of the following: Two or more grade 2 features Mean RA ≥16 mm Hg RVEDP ≥19 mm Hg LVEDP/Mean PAW ≥20 mm Hg Cardiac index <1.8 L/min/m²

RA = right atrium; RVEDP and LVEDP = right and left end-diastolic pressure, respectively; PAW = pulmonary artery wedge pressure. Abnormal cardiac index is accompanied by elevated AV oxygen content difference (>5 vol%). Exercise factor = increase in cardiac output (ml/min)/increase in total body oxygen consumption.

From Bristow, M. R., et al.: Efficacy and the cost of cardiac monitoring in patients receiving doxorubicin. Cancer *50*:32, 1982.

TABLE 57–11 RISK FACTORS FOR DEVELOPMENT OF DOXORUBICIN CARDIOTOXICITY

Cumulative dose (>550 mg/m²)
Age extremes
Prior history of cardiac disease
Hypertension
Coronary artery disease
Valvular disorders
Metastatic pericardial or myocardial disease
Prior mediastinal irradiation
Coexistent chemotherapy with alkylating agents
Hypoxic

On the basis of large retrospective analyses of high-risk and normal-risk individuals treated with anthracyclines, guidelines have been recommended as to when to discontinue the drug without any acute or late consequences. Guidelines include radionuclide angiocardiography alone[253] (Table 57–12) or radionuclide studies plus the histopathological findings of an endomyocardial biopsy[222] (Table 57–13).

Prevention. The best management of anthracycline cardiac toxicity is prevention by limiting dosage. However, several possibilities for preventing doxorubicin-induced cardiotoxicity have been suggested. The use of free-radical scavengers (vitamin E),[231] ICRF-187 (a bispiperazine[232–234]), sulfhydryl compounds,[254] coenzyme Q10 (a mitochondrial quinone),[255] cardiac glycosides,[256] calcium-channel antagonists,[257] doxorubicin bound to liposomes,[258,259] and histaminergic and adrenergic blockade have all been reported to lessen cardiac toxicity; prospective studies to determine the efficacy of these interventions are now in progress. Lowering the peak blood levels of the drug appears to offer the best means of reducing cardiac toxicity. In a controlled study monitoring cardiac toxicity by both noninvasive techniques and endomyocardial biopsy, drug-related damage was significantly reduced but not eliminated when the drug was administered by prolonged continuous intravenous infusion rather than by bolus injection; the reduction in toxicity clearly appears to be related to reduced peak plasma levels.[260–262] Similarly, lower dosages given more frequently reduce peak plasma levels and seem to lower the incidence of cardiac toxicity.[263] Antitumor activity does not appear to be compromised by altering the technique of administration in these ways.[260]

Another approach to this problem has been the develop-

TABLE 57–12 GUIDELINES FOR MONITORING PATIENTS RECEIVING DOXORUBICIN

Perform baseline radionuclide angiocardiography at rest for calculation of left ventricular ejection fraction (LVEF) prior to administration of 100 mg/m² doxorubicin. Subsequent studies are performed at least 3 wk. after the indicated total cumulative doses have been given, before consideration of the next dose

PATIENTS WITH NORMAL BASELINE LVEF (≥50%)

Perform the second study after 250 to 300 mg/m².

Repeat study after 400 mg/m² in patients with known heart disease, radiation exposure, abnormal ECG results, or cyclophosphamide therapy, or after 450 mg/m² in the absence of any of these risk factors.

Perform sequential studies thereafter prior to each dose.

Discontinue doxorubicin therapy once functional criteria for cardiotoxicity develop, i.e., absolute decrease in LVEF ≥10% (EF units) associated with a decline to a level ≤50% (EF units).

PATIENTS WITH ABNORMAL BASELINE LVEF (<50%)

Doxorubicin therapy should not be initiated with baseline LVEF ≤30%.

In patients with LVEF >30% and <50%, sequential studies should be obtained prior to each dose.

Discontinue doxorubicin with cardiotoxicity: absolute decrease in LVEF ≥10% (EF units) and/or final LVEF ≤30%.

TABLE 57-13 SEMIQUANTITATIVE SCALE OF BIOPSY-DETERMINED ANTHRACYCLINE MYOCARDIAL DAMAGE

BIOPSY GRADE	HISTOPATHOLOGICAL FEATURES
0	No detectable change from normal
1	Scant number of cells (≤5%) showing distended sarcoplasmic reticulum and/or early myofibrillar loss
1.5	Small numbers of cells (5 to 15%), some showing definite cytoplasmic vacuolization and/or myofibrillar loss
2	Groups of cells (16 to 25%), some showing definite cytoplasmic vacuolization and/or myofibrillar loss Biopsy grades up to 2 carry <10% risk of heart failure with 100 mg/m² incremental dose of doxorubicin
2.5	Groups of cells (26 to 35%), some showing definite cytoplasmic vacuolization and/or marked myofibrillar loss Biopsy grade of 2.5 carries a 10 to 25% risk of heart failure with 100 mg/m² incremental dose of doxorubicin
3	Diffuse cell injury (>35%) showing advanced loss of organelles, total loss of myofibrils, and mitochondrial and nuclear degeneration Biopsy grade 3 is associated with >25% risk of heart failure if more doxorubicin is given

From Fowles, R. E.: Cardiac catheterization and endomyocardial biopsy. *In* Kapoor, A. S. (ed.): Cancer and the Heart. New York, Springer-Verlag, 1986, p. 48.

ment of anthracycline analogs that retain their antitumor effect but do not cause cardiac toxicity. However, most agents that have been studied, such as epirubicin, 4-demethyl-6-demethyl-doxorubicin, rubidazone, and aclacinomycin, continue to show toxicity, either clinically or in animal models.[264,264a] To date, more than 16 such analogs have been described. The 4′-substituted derivatives, i.e., 4′-epi-adriamycin (epirubicin), 4′-deoxydoxorubicin, 4′-deoxy-u′-iodo-doxorubicin (idarubicin), and other analogs have been associated with decreased histological abnormalities in animal models but turn out to have decreased antitumor effect.[265-270]

CHEMOTHERAPY AND VASO-OCCLUSION. Vaso-occlusive complications, including acute myocardial infarction, often occur in patients with malignant tumors. There is increasing suspicion that chemotherapeutic agents such as 5-fluorouracil[271-274] may be the sole precipitating factor in a small but significant percentage of cases. Ischemic coronary complications have also been reported after treatment with cisplatinum,[275,276] bleomycin,[277] and vinca alkaloids,[278-280] such as vincristine, vinblastine, and VP-16-213 (etoposide). Acute endothelial injury, vasospasm and/or autonomic dysfunction, hypomagnesemia, autoimmune response, increases in platelet aggregability and a synergistic effect of irradiation to the heart are all possible mechanisms.

CYCLOPHOSPHAMIDE. As noted in Table 57-7, cardiomyopathies have been reported secondary to high doses of intravenous cyclophosphamide.[227,267-269] In contrast to doxorubicin, the cardiotoxicity of cyclophosphamide is acute and not due to cumulative doses. It causes reductions in ECG voltage and systolic function and an increase in myocardial mass, presumably secondary to edema. Cyclophosphamide may also cause acute pericarditis. A prior history of heart failure and a pretreatment ejection fraction less than 50 per cent correlate with clinical cardiotoxicity. Although mortality is appreciable, survivors exhibit no residual cardiac abnormalities.[281] Ifosfamide, an active compound related to cyclophosphamide, may also cause cardiac side effects in the form of supraventricular arrhythmias and ST-T wave changes.[282]

OTHER ANTINEOPLASTIC AGENTS. *Amsacrine* (AMSA) has been associated with acute cardiac arrhythmias and cardiomyopathy. Although AMSA-related cardiac events are frequent, they are less common than those due to doxorubicin. Manifestations of toxicity include ECG abnormalities, sudden death, and congestive heart failure. Hypokalemia appears to be a risk factor for the development of severe arrhythmias with this agent.[250,283-285] The anthraquinones, mitoxantrone and nonvantrone, are a new group of antineoplastic agents with significant clinical activity.[286] They have been shown to produce favorable results in leukemias as well as in advanced breast cancer. Deterioration in ejection fraction and congestive heart failure have been reported.[287-289] The anthraquinones are being compared in a randomized fashion with the anthracyclines in terms of both therapeutic efficacy and incidence of cardiac toxicity.[290]

5-Fluorouracil has been reported to cause angina pectoris and other manifestations of myocardial ischemia, presumably secondary to coronary vasospasm.[291,291a] Supportive therapy given to cancer patients may also be cardiotoxic when combined with chemotherapeutic agents. Lithium, which is occasionally used to increase the white blood cell count so that more therapy can be given, has been associated with sudden death in patients who are simultaneously receiving combination chemotherapy that includes an anthracycline agent.[250] In addition, antiemetic drugs such as domperidone have been associated with cardiac arrhythmias and cardiac arrest in several patients receiving antineoplastic agents.[292,293] As new antineoplastic agents are brought to trial, lessons learned in the evaluation of cardiac toxicity with doxorubicin are likely to prove helpful.

Bone marrow transplantation, either allogeneic or autolo-

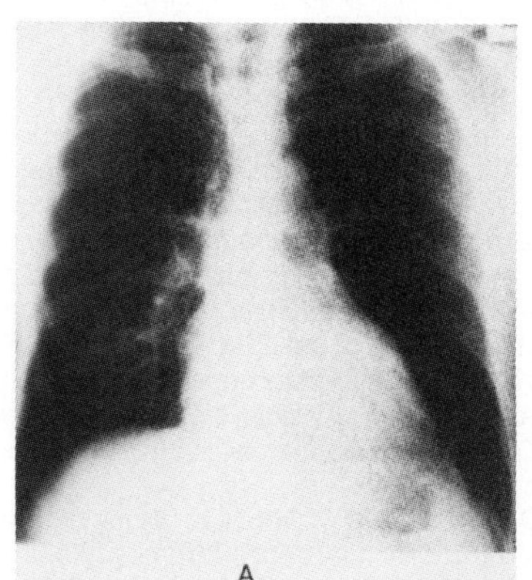
A

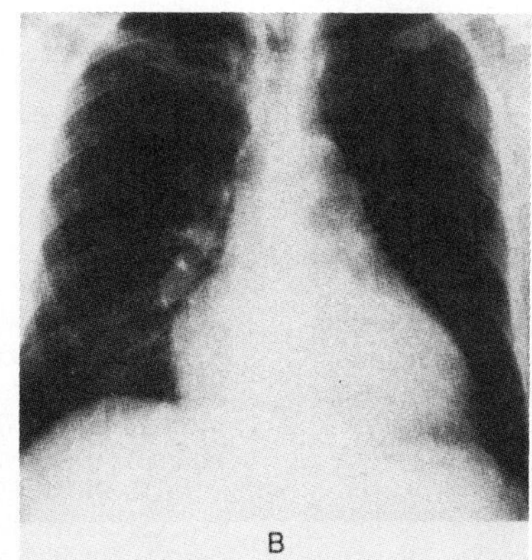
B

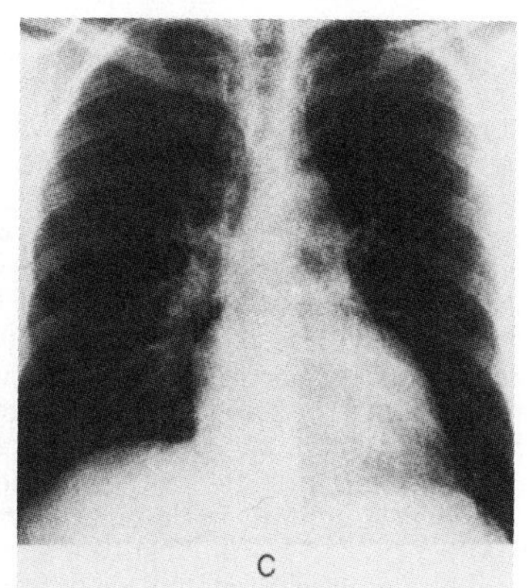
C

FIGURE 57-18. ***A*** **shows a base-line chest radiograph before treatment,** ***B*** **the development of congestive cardiomyopathy during interferon alpha therapy, and** ***C*** **its subsequent resolution after the drug was discontinued. The increased cardiac silhouette was shown on echocardiography to be due to left ventricular enlargement and a moderate pericardial effusion.**

gous, involves the combination of large doses of whole-body irradiation therapy with high-dose chemotherapy. Cardiac complications are frequent during these transplant procedures and may be an important factor in limiting the success rate.[294] Fatal cardiomyopathies, pericarditis, and significant arrhythmias are not infrequent. High-dose cyclophosphamide and cytosine arabinoside are commonly associated with cardiotoxicity. In addition, the effect of whole-heart irradiation in conjunction with anthracycline drugs and cyclophosphamide appears to be additive.

Hematopoietic growth factors and cytokines are leukocyte /lymphocyte-derived glycoproteins that are antiviral, immunomodulating, and antiproliferative as well as cell-specific stimulative. The glycoproteins of the interferon and interleukin family have become potential agents in treating many refractory cancers. Interferon alpha is effective against hairy cell leukemia, chronic myelogenous leukemia, and condyloma acuminatum and also is approved for use in treating Kaposi's sarcoma. In high doses, interferon can cause a severe congestive cardiomyopathy with severe myocardial dysfunction, usually reversible with discontinuation of the agents (Fig. 57-18).[295,296]

Recombinant interleukin-2 (rIl-2) used in association with lymphokine-activated killer (LAK) cells can cause significant tumor destruction in renal cell cancer and malignant melanoma. Eight to thirty per cent of the patients experience myocardial ischemia during or immediately after this infusional therapy. Most affected patients had no or minimal cardiac risk factors, and several cardiac deaths have been directly related to the therapy.[297-301] Despite vasopressor support during the therapy, there has been evidence of reduced left ventricular stroke work and decreased cardiac contractility.[300] Although radionuclide ventriculography and echocardiography may suggest a localized wall motion disorder, no coronary arterial abnormalities have been reported, raising the question of toxic myocarditis or a peripheral vascular effect and not endovascular injury.[301,302] Patients need to be closely monitored while receiving these experimental therapies and the infusions immediately discontinued when any clinical cardiac or electrocardiographic abnormality occurs.

Hematological Abnormalities Related to Cardiac Drugs

Blood dyscrasias are frequent complications of drugs used to treat cardiac disorders. The development of unexplained anemia, leukopenia or thrombocytopenia in a patient receiving a diuretic, antihypertensive, or antiarrhythmic agent should immediately raise the suspicion that a drug used in the treatment of cardiac disease might be responsible.

Many different types of blood dyscrasias occur secondary to drug ingestion. The anemias may be of the aplastic, hemolytic, megaloblastic, or sideroblastic type; other disorders may include granulocytopenia and agranulocytosis, thrombocytopenia, thrombocytosis, defects of platelet function, and a variety of miscellaneous disorders (Table 57-14). Underlying mechanisms include suppression of one or more of the three cellular elements in the bone marrow as well as a variety of immune phenomena with increased peripheral destruction of the formed elements. The drug effect may be dose related or idiosyncratic.

APLASTIC ANEMIA. Many chemical agents are capable of suppressing marrow function and producing hypoplasia or aplasia. Chloramphenicol, benzene, cytostatic agents used in the treatment of malignant disease, and phenylbutazone are the drugs most commonly implicated. Less frequently involved, and perhaps less well documented, are antibiotics such as sulfonamides, hypoglycemic agents, and insecticides. Among drugs used to treat cardiovascular disease, the antiarrhythmic agent phenytoin (p. 641), the diuretic agent acetazolamide, and the angiotensin-converting enzyme inhibitor captopril[303] (p. 867) have been reported, on rare occasion, to lead to such reactions. The onset of aplastic anemia is usually insidious, and the symptoms are directly related to the degree of pancytopenia. If the causative agent is immediately discontinued upon detection of the blood dyscrasia, the latter can often be reversed.

MEGALOBLASTIC ANEMIA. A pancytopenia characterized by macrocytic red cells due to impairment of DNA synthesis may be caused by vitamin B_{12} or folate deficiency or by purine and pyrimidine inhibitors. Most commonly, drugs cause megaloblastic anemia by impairing the absorption of folic acid or acting as folate antagonists. Phenytoin (p. 632), oral contraceptives, and a variety of other drugs can impair folate absorption by interfering with the liver conjugases needed to break down the polyglutamate structure of naturally occurring folates to the monoglutamate form appropriate for absorption by the gastrointestinal tract. Triamterene, a potassium-sparing diuretic (p. 474), is a pteridine analog that exhibits antifolate activity, similar to aminopterin, in vitro. Its propensity to produce a megaloblastic anemia appears to be dose related.

IMMUNOHEMOLYTIC ANEMIAS. There are four different causes for the development of a positive direct Coombs or antiglobulin test, two of which involve cardiac medications: the first mechanism, which is uncommon, involves some drugs that bind to plasma protein and thereby become antigenic, including quinidine and the sulfonamides. The resultant antigen-antibody complex may deposit on the red cell surface and cause agglutinability by anticomplement sera. Hemolysis may be severe, but rapid improvement follows withdrawal of the drug.

The second type of reaction that results in a positive Coombs' test involves the antihypertensive drug alpha-methyldopa[304] (p. 863). The mechanism of antibody formation is unknown, but presumably antibody induced by alpha-methyldopa has an affinity for the Rh locus of the red cell, similar to that of IgG antibodies in idiopathic immunohemolytic anemia. The frequency of positive results on Coombs' test varies from 11 per cent for patients who are receiving 0.75 gm per day for over 3 months to 40 per cent for those receiving 2 gm per day for the same time. Fortunately, the affinity of the alpha-methyldopa antibody for red cells is low, and fewer than 1 per cent of patients whose antiglobulin test is positive will manifest significant hemolytic anemia. Nonetheless, alpha-methyldopa surpasses all other drugs in causing immunohemolytic anemia. On withdrawal of the drug, hemolysis improves within 1 or 2 weeks, with full recovery in 1 month, although the positive Coombs' test may persist for 6 to 24 months. A positive Coombs' test without hemolysis is not an indication to discontinue alpha-methyldopa if its administration is otherwise indicated in the treatment of hypertension.

The other two mechanisms of drug-related positive antiglobulin reactions do not involve cardiovascular drugs. The third is represented by penicillin, in which the drug binds to the red cell membranes, creating a cell-drug complex and antigenic stimulation of an IgG antibody. The fourth mechanism involves cephalothin, which is bound to the red cell membrane; normal serum proteins adhere nonspecifically to red cell membranes.

GRANULOCYTOPENIA AND AGRANULOCYTOSIS. A reduction in circulating neutrophils is the most toxic hematological effect of drugs. It may be secondary to depression of the marrow, or it may be an immune mechanism causing peripheral destruction. When there is immune suppression, examination of the marrow reveals active myeloid precursors, whereas the absence of myeloid elements suggests suppression of synthesis. The marrow-depressive effect is dose related.[305] Anticoagulants such as phenindione, antiarrhythmics such as procainamide and tocainide,[306-308] antihypertensives such as captopril, and diuretics such as the thiazides have all been reported to produce granulocytopenia. Procainamide is the most dangerous and most frequently implicated cardiac drug in granulocytopenia.[309] Presenting symptoms may include a sore throat, ulcerations of mucous membranes, fever, malaise, fatigue, and weakness. Discontinuation of the drug may be followed by a rebound in the white blood cell count and occasionally a leukemoid picture. Because laboratory tests are not conclusive for white cell antibodies, an accurate definition of the immune mechanism responsible for white cell destruction remains unclear.

DRUG-INDUCED THROMBOCYTOPENIA. Many of the drugs used to treat cardiovascular disorders may cause thrombocytopenia, either by a direct effect on the bone marrow or by inducing formation of drug-specific antibody.[310] For example, the thiazide diuretics (p. 860) directly suppress megakaryocyte production. Thiazide-induced thrombocytopenia is usually mild, with the platelet count rarely falling below 50,000/μl. This condition is unique, since it persists for 6 to 8 weeks after drug withdrawal.

TABLE 57–14 BLOOD DYSCRASIAS ASSOCIATED WITH CARDIAC MEDICATIONS

	ANEMIA					
	Aplastic	Megaloblastic	Hemolytic	NEUTROPENIA	THROMBOCYTOPENIA	OTHER
Antiarrhythmics						
Digitoxin	−	−	−	−	+	L
Phenytoin	+	+	−	+	+	L,P
Procainamide	−	−	−	+(A)	−	−
Propranolol	−	−	−	+	−	−
Quinidine	−	−	+	+	+	−
Tocainide	+	−	−	+(A)	−	−
Moricizine	−	−	−	−	+	−
Propafenone	−	−	−	+(A)	−	−
Anticoagulants						
Heparin	+*	−	−	−	+	−
Phenindione	−	−	−	+	−	−
Antihypertensives						
Captopril	+	−	−	+	+	−
Glutethimide	+*	−	−	−	−	P
Hydralazine	−	−	−	−	+	L
Methyldopa	−	−	+	+	+	P
Reserpine	−	−	−	−	+	−
Diuretics						
Acetazolamide	+	−	−	+	+	−
Chlorothiazide	−	−	−	−	+	−
Chlorthalidone	−	−	−	+	+	−
Diazoxide	−	−	−	−	+	−
Ethacrynic acid	−	−	−	+	−	−
Hydrochlorothiazide	−	−	−	+	−	−
Mercurials	−	−	−	+	+	−
Spironolactone	−	−	−	−	+	−
Triamterene	−	+	−	−	−	−
Coronary dilators						
Amyl nitrite	−	−	−	−	−	M
Nitroglycerin	−	−	−	−	−	M
Other						
Amrinone	−	−	−	−	+	−

* Pure red cell aplasia.
L = lupus-like syndrome; P = porphyria; A = agranulocytosis; M = methemoglobinemia.

Thrombocytopenia caused by amrinone, a positive inotropic agent with vasodilator properties (p. 503), is less well studied but is clearly related to the total dose of drug administered and to peripheral destruction of platelets.[311] Other common agents like alcohol and some estrogen preparations may cause thrombocytopenia by a direct depressant effect on the bone marrow. Shortened platelet survival secondary to antibody or complement binding to platelets can cause severe thrombocytopenia and life-threatening hemorrhage. The onset is abrupt and is not related to the dose of medication or the duration of its use. In most cases of immunological thrombocytopenia, the offending agent induces a specific antibody. The resulting drug-antibody complex then binds to the platelet, thereby shortening its survival. Quinidine, one of the first cardiac drugs to produce this response, has been well studied as a cause of thrombocytopenia. The defect can be transferred to a normal individual by administering serum from a patient with quinidine-induced thrombocytopenia, followed by a quinidine challenge to the normal subject.[312] A similar defect can be caused by antibodies to quinine, including the small quantities present in tonic drinks. Acetaminophen (a common analgesic given to cardiac patients), acetazolamide, digitoxin, phenytoin, ethacrynic acid, alpha-methyldopa, and spironolactone have all been implicated in various cases of suspected drug-induced thrombocytopenia, although the mechanism has not always been well defined.

Although in vitro laboratory tests for drug-dependent platelet antibody are available, the results do not always correlate with clinical events. The best proof of drug-induced thrombocytopenia is prompt recovery of the platelet count after drug withdrawal followed by a second episode of thrombocytopenia upon readministration of the suspected drug. (Because of this potential hazard, the drug challenge is not advised.) If serious hemorrhage persists after the drug is withdrawn, treatment with 1 mg/kg prednisone or its equivalent may be necessary. Corticosteroids may hasten the return of a normal platelet count and may also protect capillaries and small vessels even without altering the platelet count. Platelet transfusions are not usually helpful but can be tried in desparate situations in which hemorrhage is life threatening. They are most useful if thrombocytopenia persists well after the drug-antibody complex has been cleared. In this situation, a gratifying elevation in platelet count sometimes occurs.

Heparin. Treatment with this drug is one of the most important causes of thrombocytopenia in cardiac patients (p. 1780). The incidence varies from 5 to 25 per cent among patients receiving heparin; it is more common in those given heparin derived from beef lung and has been associated with all modes and doses of heparin administration.[313] Heparin has a direct platelet-aggregating effect that may contribute to thrombocytopenia. This property is most marked in those fractions with the highest molecular weight and the lowest affinity for antithrombin. There is an increase in platelet-associated immunoglobulin in many of the cases, suggesting an immune etiology. However, the nature of the offending antigen in heparin and its relationship to the biologically active heparin fractions remain unclear. In addition, some patients with heparin-induced thrombocytopenia develop paradoxical thrombosis and disseminated intravascular coagulation. The development of thromboembolism in association with thrombocytopenia is unique to heparin.

OTHER HEMATOLOGICAL ABNORMALITIES CAUSED BY CARDIAC DRUGS. Amyl nitrite, sodium nitrite, and nitroglycerin can oxidize hemoglobin to methemoglobin, which cannot effectively carry oxygen. The patient with methemoglobinemia appears cyanotic but has a normal arterial PO_2, and oxygen therapy will not improve the pallor. Although symptomatic methemoglobinemia may occur in adults, most cases are seen in children who accidentally ingest medications prescribed for adults. Occasionally, adults with mild congenital methemoglobinemia will become markedly symptomatic when exposed to small doses of these same medications. With the increasing use of intravenous nitroglycerin, this complication may become more frequent.[314] If venous blood is chocolate brown and this color persists after the blood is shaken in air, the diagnosis of methemoglobinemia is almost certain. The diagnosis is confirmed by the addition of a few drops of 10 per cent potassium cyanide, which results in the rapid production of the bright red cyanmethemoglobin. Symptoms are nonspecific and consist of dyspnea, headache, fatigue, and dizziness. They are usually self-limited if the responsible drugs are discontinued, since normal red cells can enzymatically reduce the methemoglobin. In severe cases or in patients with enzyme defects, methylene blue may be administered to stimulate reduction of the methemoglobin.

Other medications may interfere with oxygen delivery to tissues. For example, sodium nitroprusside used to treat hypertensive emergencies and to reduce afterload in the management of heart failure may cause fatigue, nausea, abnormal behavior, and muscle spasm as the agent reacts with oxyhemoglobin, producing cyanmethemoglobin and free cyanide ions.[315]

Hydralazine (p. 1051), procainamide (p. 630), and rarely phenytoin (p. 641) can cause a lupus erythematosus-like syndrome, with urticaria, erythema multiforme, photosensitivity, delirium, and immune-mediated blood cell destruction.[316] Although patients with drug-induced lupus have positive antinuclear antibody tests and many of the clinical manifestations of the systemic form, renal function is not usually impaired, and all these manifestations usually remit within several months if the drugs are discontinued. The syndrome is of particular importance in cardiac patients, since the onset of chest pain, pleurisy, or pericardial effusion in the patient with heart disease could lead to an erroneous diagnosis unless drug-induced lupus is suspected.

REFERENCES

ANEMIA AND CARDIOVASCULAR DISORDERS

1. Graettinger, J. S., Parsons, R. L., and Campbell, J. A.: A correlation of clinical and hemodynamic studies in patients with mild and severe anemia with and without congestive heart failure. Ann. Intern. Med. *58*:617, 1963.
2. Ali, M. K., and Ewer, M. S.: Cancer and the cardiopulmonary system. New York, Raven Press, 1984, p. 242.
3. Datta, B. N., and Silver, M. D.: Cardiomegaly in chronic anemia in rats; an experimental study including ultrastructural, histometric and stereological observations. Lab. Invest. *2*:503, 1975.
4. Eckstein, R. W.: Development of interarterial coronary anastomoses by chronic anemia. Disappearance following correction of anemia. Circ. Res. *3*:306, 1955.
5. Reichek, N., Wilson, J., Sutton, M. S., et al.: Noninvasive determination of left ventricular end systolic stress: Validation of the method and initial application. Circulation *65*:99, 1982.
6. Rossi, M. A., Carillo, S. V., and Oliveria, J.S.M.: The effect of iron deficiency anemia in the rat on catecholamine levels and heart morphology. Cardiovasc. Res. *15*:313, 1981.
7. Florenzano, F., Diaz, G., Regonesi, C., and Escobar, E.: Left ventricular function in chronic anemia: Evidence of noncatecholamine positive inotropic factor in the serum. Am. J. Cardiol. *54*:638, 1984.
8. Duke, M., and Abelmann, W. H.: The hemodynamic response to chronic anemia. Circulation *39*:503, 1969.
9. Varat, M. A., Adolph, R. J., and Fowler, N. O.: Cardiovascular effects of anemia. Am. Heart J. *83*:415, 1972.
10. Torrance, J. D., Jacobs, P., Restrepo, A., et al.: Intraerythrocyte adaptation to anemia. N. Engl. J. Med. *283*:165, 1970.
11. Baer, R. W., Vlahakes, G. J., Uhlig, P. N., and Hoffman, I. E.: Maximum myocardial oxygen transport during anemia and polycythemia in dogs. Am. J. Physiol. *252*:H1086, 1987.
12. Oski, F. A., Marshall, B. D., Cohen, P. J., et al.: Exercise with anemia. The role of the left or right shifted oxygen-hemoglobin equilibrium curve. Ann. Intern. Med. *74*:44, 1971.
13. Lenfant, C., Torrance, J., English, E., et al.: Effect of altitude on the oxygen binding by hemoglobin and on organic phosphate levels. J. Clin. Invest. *47*:2652, 1968.
14. Oski, F. A., Gottlieb, A. J., Delivoria-Papadopoulos, M., and Miller, W. W.: Red-cell 2,3-diphosphoglycerate levels in subjects with chronic hypoxemia. N. Engl. J. Med. *280*:1165, 1969.
15. Hunter, A.: The heart in anemia. Q. J. Med. *15*:107, 1946.
16. Harris, T. N., Friedman, S., Tuncali, M. T., and Hallidie-Smith, K. A.: Comparison of innocent murmur of childhood with cardiac murmurs in high output states. Pediatrics *33*:341, 1964.
17. Varriale, P., Kwa, R. P., and Vyas, P.: Intravenous nitroglycerin in transfusion therapy for severe anemia. Association with congestive heart failure. Arch. Intern. Med. *144*:401, 1984.
18. Bunn, H. F.: Disorders of hemoglobin. *In* Wilson, J., and Braunwald E. et al. (eds.): Harrison's Principles of Internal Medicine, 12th ed. New York, McGraw-Hill, 1991, pp. 1543–1552.
19. Denenberg, B. S., Criner, G., Jones, R., and Spann, J. F.: Cardiac function in sickle cell anemia. Am. J. Cardiol. *51*:1674, 1983.
20. Falk, R. H., and Hood, W. B.: The heart in sickle cell anemia. Arch. Intern. Med. *142*:1680, 1982.
21. Simmons, B. E., Santhanam, V., Castaner, A., et al.: Sickle cell heart disease. Two dimensional echo and doppler ultrasonographic findings in the hearts of adult patients with sickle cell anemia. Arch. Intern. Med. *148*:1526, 1988.
22. Miller, G. J., Serjeant, G. R., Sivapragasam, S., and Petch, M.: Cardiopulmonary responses and gas exchange during exercise in adults with homozygous sickle cell disease. Clin. Sci. *44*:113, 1973.
23. Sharache, S., Scott, J. C., and Sharache, P.: "Acute chest syndrome" in adults with sickle cell disease: Microbiology, treatment and prevention. Arch. Intern. Med. *139*:67, 1979.
24. Shubin, H., Kaufmann, R., Shapiro, M., and Levinson, D. C.: Cardiovascular findings in children with sickle cell anemia. Am. J. Cardiol. *6*:875, 1960.
25. Gaffney, J. W., Bierman, F. Z., Donnelly, C. M., et al.: Cardiovascular adaptation to transfusion/chelation therapy of homozygote sickle cell anemia. Am. J. Cardiol. *62*:121, 1988.
26. Estrade, G., Pointrineau, D., Bernasconi, F., et al.: Left ventricular function and sickle-cell anemia. Echocardiographic Study. Arch. Mal. Coeur *82*:1975, 1989.
27. Perrine, R. P., Pembrey, M. E., John, P., et al.: Natural history of sickle cell anemia in Saudi Arabs: A study of 270 subjects. Ann. Intern. Med. *88*:1, 1978.
28. Gerry, J. L., Bulkley, B. H., and Hutchins, G. M.: Clinicopathologic analysis of cardiac dysfunction in 52 patients with sickle cell anemia. Am. J. Cardiol. *42*:211, 1978.
29. Barrett, O., Saunders, D. E., McFarlend, D. E., and Humphries, J. O.: Myocardial infarction in sickle cell anemia. Am. J. Hematol. *16*:139, 1984.
30. Martin, C. R., Cobb, C., Tatter, D., et al.: Acute myocardial infarction in sickle cell anemia. Arch. Intern. Med. *143*:830, 1983.
31. McCormick, W. F.: Massive nonatherosclerotic myocardial infarction in sickle cell anemia. Am. J. Forensic Med. Pathol. *9*:151, 1988.
32. Rubler, S., and Fleischer, R. A.: Sickle cell states and cardiomyopathy. Sudden death due to pulmonary thrombosis and infarction. Am. J. Cardiol. *19*:867, 1967.
33. Burnheimer, J., and Haywood, L. J.: Prevalence of hemoglobinopathies in patients with ischemic heart disease. J. Natl. Med. Assoc. *68*:312, 1976.
34. Balfour, I. C., Covitz, W., Davis, H., et al.: Cardiac size and function in children with sickle cell anemia. Am. Heart J. *108*:345, 1984.
35. Lippman, S. M., Niemann, J. T., Thigpen, T., et al.: Abnormal septal Q waves in sickle cell disease. Prevalence and causative factors. Chest *88*:543, 1985.
36. Maisel, A., Friedman, H., Flint, L., et al.: Continuous electrocardiographic monitoring in patients with sickle cell anemia during pain crisis. Clin. Cardiol. *6*:339, 1983.
37. Covitz, W., Eubig, C., Balfour, I. C., et al.: Exercise-induced cardiac dysfunction in sickle cell anemia. Radionuclide study. Am. J. Cardiol. *51*:570, 1983.
38. Manno, B. V., Burka, E. R., Hakki, A., et al.: Biventricular function in sickle cell anemia: Radionuclide angiographic and thallium-201 scintigraphic evaluation. Am. J. Cardiol. *52*:584, 1983.
39. Willens, H. J., Lawrence, C., Frishman, W. H., and Strom, J. A.: A noninvasive comparison of left ventricular performance in sickle cell anemia and chronic aortic regurgitation. Clin. Cardiol. *6*:542, 1983.
40. Alpert, B. S., Dover, E. V., Strong, W. B., and Covits, W.: Longitudinal exercise hemodynamics in children with sickle cell anemia. Am. J. Dis. Child. *138*:1021, 1984.
41. Lippman, S. M., Ginzton, L. E., Thigpen, T., et al.: Mitral valve prolapse in sickle cell disease: Presumptive evidence for a linked connective tissue disorder. Arch. Intern. Med. *145*:435, 1985.
42. Sanakul, D., Thakerngpol, K., and Pacharee, P.: Cardiac pathology in 76 thalessemic patients. Birth Defects *23*:177, 1988.
43. Ohene-Frempong, K., and Schwartz, E.: Clinical features of thalassemia. Pediatr. Clin. North Am. *27*:403, 1980.
44. Ehlers L. H., Levin, A. R., Klein, A. A., et al.: The cardiac manifestations of thalassemia major: Natural history, noninvasive cardiac diagnostic studies, and results of cardiac catheterization. *In* Engle, M. A. (ed.): Pediatric Cardiovascular Disease. Cardiovascular Clinics II. Philadelphia, F. A. Davis Co., 1981, pp. 171–186.

44a. Spirito, P., Lupi, G., Melevendi, C., and Vecchio, C.: Restrictive diastolic abnormalities identified by Doppler echocardiography in patients with thalassemia major. Circulation *82*:88, 1990.

45. Sapoznikov, D., Lewis, N., Rachmilewitz, E. A., et al.: Left ventricular filling and emptying patterns in anemia due to beta-thalassemia. A computer-assisted echocardiographic study. Cardiology *69*:276, 1982.
46. Sapoznikov, D., Lewis, N., Degan, I., et al.: Studies of left ventricular function in anemia due to beta-thalassemia. Isr. J. Med. Sci. *18*:928, 1982.
47. Lau, K. C., Li, A.M.C., Hui, P. W., and Yeung, C. Y.: Left ventricular function in β thalassemia major. Arch. Dis. Child. *64*:1046, 1989.
48. Valdes-Cruz, L. M., Reinecke, C., Rutkowski, M., et al.:Preclinical abnormal segmental cardiac manifestations of thalassemia major in children on transfusion-chelation therapy: Echographic alterations of left ventricular posterior wall contractions and relaxation patterns. Am. Heart J. *103*:505, 1982.
49. Borow, K. M., Propper, R., Bierman, F. Z., et al.: The left ventricular end-systolic pressure-dimensions relation in patients with thalassemia major. A new noninvasive method for assessing contractile state. Circulation *66*:980, 1982.
50. Canale, C., Terrachini, V., Vallebena, A., et al.: Thalassemic cardiomyopathy: Echocardiographic difference between major and intermediate thalassemia at rest and during isometric effort: Yearly follow-up. Clin. Cardiol. *11*:563, 1988.
51. Yee, H., Mra, R., and Nyunt, K. M.: Cardiac abnormalities in the thalassemia syndromes. Southeast Asian J. Trop. Med. Public Health *15*:414, 1984.
52. Dameshek, W., and Roth, S. I.: Case Records of the Massachusetts General Hospital—Weekly Clinicopathological exercises. Case 52. N. Engl. J. Med. *271*:898, 1964.
53. Westring, D. W.: Aortic valve disease and hemolytic anemia. Ann. Intern. Med. *65*:203, 1966.

54. Miller, D. S., Mengel, C. E., Kremer, W. B., et al.: Intravascular hemolysis in a patient with valvular heart disease. Ann. Intern. Med. *65*:210, 1966.
55. Rose, J. C., Hufnagel, C. A., Freis, C. D., et al.: The hemodynamic alterations produced by a plastic valvular prosthesis for severe aortic insufficiency in man. J. Lab. Clin. Med. *33*:891, 1954.
56. Sayed, H. M., Dacie, J. V., Handley, D. A., et al.: Hemolytic anemia of mechanical origin after open-heart surgery. Thorax *16*:356, 1961.
57. Sonaer, D. H., Cheng, T. O., and Aaron, B. L.: Hemolytic anemia and acute mitral regurgitation caused by a torn cusp of a porcine mitral prosthetic valve 7 years after its implantation. Am. Heart J. *113*:404, 1987.
58. Mok, P., Lieberman, E. H., Lilly, L. S., et al. Severe hemolytic anemia following mitral valve repair. Am. Heart J. *117*:1171, 1989.
59. Dacie, J. V.: The Hemolytic Anemias. Part III. 2nd ed. New York, Grune and Stratton, 1967, p. 957.
60. Sears, A. D., and Crosby, W. H.: Intravascular hemolysis due to intracardiac prosthetic devices. Diurnal variations related to activity. Am. J. Med. *39*:341, 1965.
61. DiSosa, V. J., Collins, J. J., Jr., and Cohn, C. H.: Hematological complications with the St. Jude valve and reduced-dose coumadin. Ann. Thorac. Surg. *48*:280, 1989.
62. Nevaril, C. G., Lynch, E. C., Alfrey, C. P., Jr., and Hellums, J.: Erythrocyte damage and destruction induced by shearing stress. J. Lab. Clin. Med. *71*:784, 1986.
63. Zezulka, A., Schapiro, L., and Sind, S.: Chronic haemolytic anemia in hypertrophic cardiomyopathy. Br. Heart J. *52*:474, 1984.

HEMOCHROMATOSIS AND HEMOSIDEROSIS

64. Schafer, A. I.: Iron overload. *In* Fairbanks, V. F. (ed.): Current Hematology. New York, John Wiley and Sons, 1981, pp. 191–218.
65. Edwards, C. Q., Dadone, M. M., Skolnick, M. H., and Kushner, J. P.: Hereditary hemochromatosis. Clin. Hematol. *11*:411, 1982.
66. Swan, W.G.A., and Dewar, H. A.: The heart in hemochromatosis. Br. Heart J. *14*:117, 1952.
67. Finch, S. C., and Finch, C. A.: Idiopathic hemochromatosis, an iron storage disease. Medicine *34*:381, 1955.
68. Rosenqvist, M., and Hultcrantz R.: Prevalence of haemochromatosis among men with clinically significant bradyarrhythmias. Eur. Heart J. *10*:473, 1989.
69. James, T. N.: Pathology of the cardiac conduction system in hemochromatosis. N. Engl. J. Med. *271*:92, 1964.
70. Wasserman, A. J., Richardson, D. W., Baird, C. L., and Wyso, E. M.: Cardiac hemochromatosis simulating constrictive pericarditis. Am. J. Med. *32*:316, 1962.
71. Cutler, H. J., Isner, J. M., Bracey, A. W., et al.: Hemochromatosis heart disease: An unemphasized cause of potentially reversible restrictive cardiomyopathy. Am. Heart J. *69*:923, 1980.
72. Buja, L. M., and Roberts, W. C.: Iron in the heart. Etiology and clinical significance. Am. J. Med. *51*:209, 1971.
73. Olson, L. J., Edwards, W. D., Holmes, D. R., et al.: Endomyocardial biopsy in hemochromatosis: Clinicopathologic correlates in six cases. J. Am. Coll. Cardiol. *13*:116, 1989.
74. Leon, M. D., Borer, J. S., Bacharach, S. L., et al.: Detection of early cardiac dysfunction in patients with severe beta-thalassemia and chronic iron overload. N. Engl. J. Med. *301*:1143, 1979.
75. Candell-Riera, J., Permanger-Miralda, G., and Soler-Soler, J.: Cardiac hemochromatosis. Primary Cardiol. *12* (October):123, 1986.
76. Grisaru, D., Goldfarb, A. W., Gotsman, M. S., et al.: Deferoxamine improves left ventricular function in β-thalassemia. Arch. Intern. Med. *146*:2344, 1986.
77. Rivers, J., Garrahy, P., Robinson, W., and Murphy, A.: Reversible cardiac dysfunction in hemochromatosis. Am. Heart J. *113*:216, 1987.
78. Easley, R. M., Schreiner, B. F., and Yu, P. N.: Reversible cardiomyopathy associated with hemochromatosis. N. Engl. J. Med. *287*:866, 1972.
79. Skinner, C., and Kenmore, C. F.: Haemochromatosis presenting as congestive cardiomyopathy and responding to venesection. Br. Heart J. *35*:466, 1973.
80. Schafer, A. I., Cheron, R. G., Dluhy, R., et al.: Clinical consequences of acquired tranfusional iron overload in adults. N. Engl. J. Med. *304*:319, 1981.
81. Schafer, A. I.: Treatment of iron overload with parenteral deferoxamines. *In* Isselbacher, K. J. et al. (eds.): Update III to Harrison's Principles of Internal Medicine. New York, McGraw-Hill Book Co., 1982, pp. 157–166.
82. Wolfe, L., Olivieri, N., Sallan, D., et al.: Prevention of cardiac disease by subcutaneous deferoxamine in patients with thalassemia major. N. Engl. J. Med. *312*:1600, 1985.
83. Schafer, A. I., Rabinowe, S., LeBoff, M. S., et al.: Long term efficacy of deferoxamine iron chelation therapy in adults with acquired transfusional overload. Arch. Intern. Med. *145*:1217, 1985.
84. Rahko, P. S., Salerni, R., and Uretsky, B. F.: Successful reversal by chelation therapy of congestive cardiomyopathy due to iron overload. J. Am. Coll. Cardiol. *8*:436, 1986.
85. Maurer, H. S., Lloyd-Still, J. D., Ingrisano, C., et al.: A prospective evaluation of iron chelation therapy in children with severe beta-thalassemia. A six year study. Am. J. Dis. Child. *142*:287, 1988.
86. Freeman, A. P., Giles, R. W., Berdoukas, V. A., et al.: Sustained normalization of cardiac function by chelation therapy in thalassemia major. Clin. Lab. Haematol. *11*:299, 1989.
87. Cohen, A. R., Mizanin, J., and Schwartz, E.: Rapid removal of excessive iron with daily, high-dose intravenous chelation therapy. J. Pediatr. *115*:151, 1989.
88. Freeman, A. P., Giles, R. W., Berdoukas, V. A., et al.: Sustained normalization of cardiac function by chelation therapy in thalassaemia major. Clin. Lab. Haematol. *11*:299, 1989.
89. Cohen, A., and Schwartz, E.: Iron chelation therapy with deferoxamine in Cooley anemia. J. Pediatr. *92*:643, 1978.
90. Nienhuis, A. W.: Vitamin C and iron. N. Engl. J. Med. *304*:170, 1981.
91. Bridges, K. R., and Hoffman, K. E.: The effects of ascorbic acid on the intracellular metabolism of iron and ferritin. J. Biol. Chem. *261*:14273, 1986.
91a. Kontoghiorges, G. T., Aldouri, M. A., Sheppard, L., and Hoffbrand, A. V.: 1, 2-Dimethyl-3-hydroxypyrid-4-one, an orally active chelator for treatment of iron overload. Lancet *1*:1294, 1987.

DISORDERS ASSOCIATED WITH ABNORMAL BLOOD FLOW DISTRIBUTION OR INCREASED VISCOSITY

92. Braunwald, E.: Cyanosis, hypoxia, and polycythemia. *In* Braunwald, E., et al. (eds.): Harrison's Principles of Internal Medicine, 11th ed. New York, McGraw-Hill Book Co., 1987, pp. 145–149.
93. Castle, W. B., and Jandl, J. H.: Blood viscosity and blood volume: Opposing influences upon oxygen transport in polycythemia. Semin. Hematol. *3*:193, 1966.
94. Adamson, J. W.: The myeloproliferative disease. *In* Braunwald, E., et al. (eds.): Harrison's Principles of Internal Medicine, 11th ed. New York, McGraw-Hill, 1987, pp. 1527–1533.
95. Adamson, J. W., and Fialkow, P. J.: Polycythemia vera: Stem cell and probable clinical origin of the disease. N. Engl. J. Med. *245*:913, 1976.
96. Berlin, N. I. (ed.). Polycythemia vera: An update. Semin. Hematol. *23*:131, 1986.
97. Dintenfass, L.: Viscosity of the packed red and white blood cells. Exp. Molec. Pathol. *4*:597, 1965.
98. Thomas, D. J., Marshall, J., Russell, R. W., et al.: Effect of hematocrit on cerebral blood flow in man. Lancet *2*:941, 1977.
99. Torrance, J. D., Lenfant, C., and Cruz, J.: Oxygen transport mechanisms in residents at high altitude. Respir. Physiol. *11*:1, 1970.
100. Balcerzak, S. P., and Bromberg, P. A.: Secondary polycythemia. Semin. Hematol. *12*:353, 1976.
101. Rosenthal, A., Button, L. N., and Nathan, D. G.: Blood volume changes in cyanotic congenital heart disease. Am. J. Cardiol. *29*:162, 1971.
102. Golde, D. W., Hocking, W. G., Koeffler, H. P., and Adamson, J. W.: Polycythemia: Mechanism and management. Ann. Intern. Med. *95*:71, 1981.
103. Rosenthal, A., Nathan, D. G., Marty, A. T., et al.: Acute hemodynamic effects of red cell production in polycythemia of cyanotic congenital heart disease. Circulation *42*:197, 1970.
104. Erslev, A. J., and Caro, J.: Secondary polycythemia: A boon or a burden? Blood Cells *10*:177, 1984.
105. Yeager, S. B., and Freed, M. D.: Myocardial infarction as a manifestation of polycythemia in cyanotic heart disease. Am. J. Cardiol. *53*:952, 1984.
106. Grant, P., Patel, P., and Singh, S.: Acute myocardial infarction secondary to polycythemia in a case of cyanotic congenital heart disease. Int. J. Cardiol. *9*:108, 1985.
107. Wallis, P. J., Skehan, J. D., Newland, A. C., et al.: Effects of erythropheresis on pulmonary hemodynamics and oxygen transport in patients with secondary polycythemia and cor pulmonale. Clin. Sci. *70*:91, 1986.
108. Wallis, P. J., Cunningham, J., Few, J. D., et al.: Effects of packed cell volume reduction on renal hemodynamics and the renin angiotensin aldosterone system in patients with secondary polycythemia and hypoxic cor pulmonale. Clin. Sci. *70*:81, 1986.
109. Willison, J. R., Thomas, D. J., and duBoulay, G. H., et al.: Effect of high hematocrit on alertness. Lancet *1*:846, 1980.
110. York, E. L., Junes, R. L., Menon, D., and Sproule, B. J.: Effects of secondary polycythemia on cerebral blood flow in chronic obstructive pulmonary disease. Am. Rev. Respir. Dis. *121*:813, 1980.
111. Rosenthal, A., Mentzer, W. C., and Eisenstein, E. B.: The role of red blood cell organic phosphates in adaptation to congenital heart disease. Pediatrics *47*:537, 1971.
112. Charache, S., Weatherall, D. J., and Clegg, J. B.: Polycythemia associated with hemoglobinopathy. J. Clin. Invest. *45*:813, 1966.
113. Adamson, J. W., and Finch, C. A.: Erythropoietin and the polycythemias. Ann. N. Y. Acad. Sci. *149*:560, 1968.
114. Bromberg, P. A., Padilla, F., Boy, J. T., and Balcerzak, S. P.: Effect of a new hemoglobin (Hb Little Rock) on the physiology of oxygen delivery. J. Lab. Clin. Med. *78*:837, 1971.
115. Charache, S., Achuff, S., Winslow, R., et al.: Variability of the homeostatic response to P50. Blood *52*:1156, 1978.
116. Smith, J., and Landow, S. A.: Smoker's polycythemia. N. Engl. J. Med. *298*:6, 1978.
117. Weinreb, N. J., and Shih, C. F.: Spurious polycythemia. Semin. Hematol. *12*:397, 1975.
118. Saffitz, J. E., Phillips, E. R., Temesy-Armos, P. N., and Roberts, W. C.: Thrombocytosis and fetal coronary heart disease. Am. J. Cardiol. *52*:651, 1983.
119. Pick, R. A., Glover, M. U., Nanfro, J. J., et al.: Acute myocardial infarction with essential thrombocythemia in a young man. Am. Heart. J. *106*:406, 1983.
120. Hanger, K. H., Kilgore, J., and James, E.: Essential thrombocythemia and coronary artery disease. Chest. *86*:933, 1984.

121. Virmani, R., Popuvsky, M. A., and Roberts, W. C.: Thrombolysis, coronary thrombosis and acute myocardial infarction. Am. J. Med. *67*:498, 1979.
122. Mitus, A. J., Barbui, R., Shulman, L. N., et al.: Hemostatic complications in young patients with essential thrombocythemia. Am. J. Med. *88*:371, 1990.
123. Knizley, H., Jr., and Noyes, W. D.: Iron deficiency anemia, papilledema, thrombocytosis and transient hemiparesis. Arch. Intern. Med. *129*:480, 1972.
124. Karwinski, B., and Svendsen, E.: Trends in cardiac metastasis. Acta Pathol Microbiol Immunol Scand *97*:1018, 1989.
124a. Fuchs, J., Weinberger, I., Rotenberg, Z., et al.: Plasma viscosity in ischemic heart disease. Am. Heart J. *108*:435, 1984.
125. Zannad, F., Stoltz, J. F., Laprevote-Heully, M. C., et al.: Hemorrhagic disorders in the threatened myocardial infarct syndrome. Arch. Mal. Coeur. *78*:1237, 1985.
126. Strano, A., Avellone, G., Novo, S., et al.: Evaluation of blood viscosity and erythrocyte filterability in chronic ischemic heart disease. Ric. Clin. Lab. *1*:179, 1985.

CARDIAC MANIFESTATIONS OF NEOPLASTIC DISEASE

127. Israeli, A., Rein, A.J.J.T., Kriski, M., et al.: Right ventricular outflow tract obstruction due to extracardiac tumors: A report of three cases diagnosed and followed up by echocardiographic studies. *149*:2105, 1989.
128. Kapoor, A. S.: Clinical manifestations of neoplasia of the heart. *In* Kapoor, A. S. (ed.): Cancer and the Heart. New York, Springer-Verlag, 1986, pp. 21–25.
129. Schoen, F. J., Berger, B. M., and Guerina, N. G.: Cardiac effects of noncardiac neoplasms. Cardiol. Clin. *2*:657, 1984.
130. Roberts, W. C., Glancy, D. L., and DeVita, V. T.: Heart in malignant lymphoma. A study of 196 autopsy cases. Am. J. Cardiol. *22*:85, 1968.
131. Petersen, C. D., Robinson, Q. A., and Kurnich, J. E.: Involvement of the heart and pericardium in the malignant lymphomas. Am. J. Med. Sci. *272*:161, 1976.
132. Waller, B. F., Gottdiener, J. S., Virmni, R., and Roberts, W. C.: Structure-function correlations in cardiovascular and pulmonary diseases. The charcoal heart. Chest *77*:671, 1980.
133. McBride, W., Jackman, J. D., Gammon, R. S., and Willerson, J. T.: High output cardiac failure in patients with multiple myeloma. N. Engl. J. Med. *319*:1651, 1988.
134. Almange, C., Lebrestec, T., Louvet, M., et al.: Bloc auriculo-ventriculaire complet par metastase cardiaque: A propos dune observation. Sem. Hop. Paris *54*:1419, 1978.
135. McDonnell, P. J., Becker, L. C., and Bulkley, B. H.: Thallium imaging in cardiac lymphoma. Am. Heart J. *101*:809, 1981.
136. Kutalek, S. P., Panidis, I. P., Kotler, M., et al.: Metastatic tumors of the heart detected by two-dimensional echocardiography. Am. Heart J. *109*:343, 1985.
137. Moncada, R., and Posnik, H.: Computed tomograph of neoplastic disease in the pericardium. *In* Kapoor, A. S.: Cancer and the Heart. New York, Springer-Verlag. 1986, pp. 26–41.
138. Goldman, A. P., Kotler, M. N., and Perry, W. R.: Arterial tumors. *In* Kapoor, A. S. (ed.): Cancer and the Heart. New York, Springer-Verlag, 1986, pp. 82–109.
139. Seibert, K. A., Rettenmier, C. W., Waller, B. F., et al.: Osteogenic sarcoma metastatic to the heart. Am. J. Med. *73*:136, 1982.
140. Kralstein, J., and Frishman, W.: Malignant pericardial disease: Diagnosis and treatment. Am. Heart J. *113*:785, 1987.
141. Lloyd, E. A., and Curcio, C. A.: Lymphoma of the heart as an unusual cause of pericardial effusion. S. Afr. Med. J. *58*:937, 1980.
142. Haedersdal, C., Hasselbach, H., Devantier, A., and Saunamak, K.: Pericardial hematopoiesis with tamponade in myelofibrosus. Scand. J. Haematol. *34*:270, 1985.
143. Hancock, E. W.: Pericardial disease in patients with neoplasm. *In* Reddy, R. S., Leon, D. F., and Shaver, J. A. (eds.): Pericardial Disease. New York, Raven Press, 1981, p. 327.
144. Ramarkrishnan, S., Marshall, A. J., Richard, J. G., and Tyrell, C. J.: Pericardiocentesis and systemic cytotoxic chemotherapy in the management of cardiac tamponade secondary to disseminated breast carcinoma. Br. Heart J. *60*:162, 1988.
145. Leung, W., Tai, Y., Lau, C., et al.: Cardiac tamponade complicating leukaemia: Immediate chemotherapy or pericardiocentesis? Postgrad. Med. J. *65*:773, 1989.
146. Press, O. W., and Livingston, R.: Management of malignant pericardial effusion and tamponade. JAMA *256*:2301, 1987.
147. Rudoff, J., Perey, R., Benrubi, G., and Ostrewski, M. L.: Recurrent squamous cell carcinoma of the cervix presenting as cardiac tamponade. Case report and subject review. Gynecol. Oncol. *34*:226, 1989.
148. Barton, J. C., and Durant, J. R.: Isolated chylopericardium associated with lymphoma. South. Med. J. *73*:1551, 1980.
149. Buck, M., Ingle, J. N., Giuliani, E. R., et al.: Pericardial effusion in women with breast cancer. Cancer *60*:263, 1987.
150. Posner, M. R., Cohen, G. I., and Skarin, A. T.: Pericardial disease in patients with cancer. The differentiation of malignant from idiopathic and radiation-induced pericarditis. Am. J. Med. *71*:407, 1981.
151. Applefeld, M. M., Spicer, K. M., Slawson, R. G., et al.: The long-term cardiac effects of radiotherapy in patients treated for Hodgkin's disease. Cancer Treat. Rep. *66*:1003, 1982.
152. Gouldesbrough, D. R., and Carder, P. J.: Rapidly progressive cardiac failure due to lymphomatous infiltration of the myocardium. Postgrad. Med. J. *65*:668, 1989.
153. Lestuzzi, C., Biasi, S., Nicolosi, G. L., et al.: Secondary neoplastic infiltration of the myocardium diagnosed by two-dimensional echocardiography in seven cases with anatomic confirmation. J. Am. Coll. Cardiol. *9*:439, 1987.
154. Wig, I. L., Mehva, S., Azueta, V., and Rosner, F.: Cardiac metastasis from adenocarcinoma of the lung. Echocardiographic pathologic correlation. Am. J. Med. *80*:108, 1986.
155. Perez, C. A., Presant, C. A., and Amburg, A. L.: Management of superior vena caval syndrome. Semin. Oncol. *5*:123, 1978.
156. Lopez, M. I., and Vincent, R. J.: Malignant superior vena cava syndrome. *In* Kapoor, A. S. (ed.): Cancer and the Heart. New York, Springer-Verlag, 1986, p. 206.
157. Wahlin, A., Olofsson, B., Eriksson, A., and Backman, C.: Myeloma-associated cardiac amyloidosis. Acta Med. Scand. *215*:189, 1984.
158. Alpert, M. A.: Cardiac amyloidosis. *In* Kapoor, A. S. (ed.): Cancer and the Heart. New York, Springer-Verlag, 1986, p. 162.
159. Sedlis, S. P., Saffitz, J. E., Schwob, V. S., and Jaffe, A. S.: Cardiac amyloidosis simulating hypertrophic cardiomyopathy. Am. J. Cardiol. *53*:969, 1984.
160. Laurent, M., Taulet, R., Ramee, M. P., et al.: Light-chain disease with terminal myocardiopathy. Arch. Mal. Coeur *78*:943, 1985.
161. Ursell, P. C., and Fenogolio, J. J.: Spectrum of cardiac disease diagnosed by endomyocardial biopsy. Pathol. Annu. *19*:197, 1984.
162. Koiwaya, Y., Nakamura, M., and Yamamoto, K.: Progressive ECG alterations in metastatic cardiac mural tumor. Am. Heart J. *105*:339, 1983.
163. Hartman, R. B., Clark, P. I., and Schulman, P.: Pronounced and prolonged ST segment elevation. A pathognomonic sign of tumor invasion of the heart. Arch. Intern. Med. *142*:1917, 1982.
164. Cole, T. O., Attah, E. B., and Onyemelukwe, G. C.: Burkitt's lymphoma presenting with heart block. Br. Heart J. *37*:94, 1975.
165. Ballentyne, F., VanderArk, C. R., and Holick, M.: Carotid sinus syncope and cervical lymphoma. Wis. Med. J. *74*:91, 1975.
166. Inagaki, R., Rodriguez, V., and Brody, G. P.: Causes of death in cancer patients. Cancer *33*:568, 1974.
167. Kopelson, G., and Herwig, K. J.: The etiologies of coronary artery disease in cancer patients. Int. J. Radiat. Oncol. Biol. Phys. *4*:895, 1978.
168. Stewart, J. R., and Fajardo, L. F.: Cancer and coronary artery disease. Int. J. Radiat. Oncol. Biol. Phys. *4*:915, 1978.
169. Ackerman, D. M., Hyma, B. A., and Edwards, W. D.: Malignant neoplastic emboli to the coronary arteries. Report of two cases and review of the literature. Hum. Pathol. *18*:955, 1987.
170. Parker, B. M.: Valvular involvement in cancer. *In* Kapoor, A. S. (ed.): Cancer and the Heart. New York, Springer-Verlag, 1986, p. 64.
171. MacDonald, R. A., Robbins, S. L.:The significance of nonbacterial thrombotic endocarditis: An autopsy and clinical study of 78 cases. Ann. Intern. Med. *46*:255, 1957.
172. Chino, F., Kodama, A., Otake, M., and Dock, D. S.: Nonbacterial thrombotic endocarditis in a Japanese autopsy sample. A review of eighty cases. Am. Heart J. *90*:190, 1975.
173. Gonzalez Quintela, A., Candela, M. J., Vidal, C., et al.: Nonbacterial thrombotic endocarditis in cancer patients. Acta Cardiologica *XLVI*:1, 1991.
174. Lehto, V. P., Stenman, S., and Somer, T.: Immunohistological studies on valvular vegetations in nonbacterial thrombotic endocarditis. Arch. Pathol. Microbiol. Scand. *90*:207, 1982.
175. Lange, H. W., Galliani, C. A., and Edwards, J. E.: Local complications associated with indwelling Swan-Ganz catheters: Autopsy study of 36 cases. Am. J. Cardiol. *52*:1108, 1983.
176. Yam, L. T., Li, C. Y., Necheles, T. F., and Katayama, I.: Pseudoeosinophilic, eosinophilic endocarditis and eosinophilic leukemia. Am. J. Med. *53*:193, 1972.
177. Cilliers, G. D., Harper, I. S., and Lochner, A.: Radiation-induced changes in the ultrastructure and mechanical function of the rat heart. Radiotherapy Oncol. *16*:311, 1989.
178. Niemtzow, R. C., and Reynolds, R. D.: Radiation therapy and the heart. *In* Kapoor, A. S. (ed.): Cancer and the Heart. New York, Springer-Verlag, 1986, pp. 232–237.
178a. Geist, B. J., Lauk, S., Bornhausen, M., and Trott, K-R.: Physiologic consequences of local heart irradiation in rats. Int. J. Radiat. Oncol. Biol. Phys. *18*:1107, 1990.
179. Gottdeiner, J. S., Katin, M. J., Borer, J. S., et al.: Late cardiac effects of therapeutic mediastinal irradiation: Assessment by echocardiography and radionuclide angiography. N. Engl. J. Med. *308*:569, 1983.
180. Applefeld, M. M., and Wiernik, P. H.: Cardiac disease after radiation therapy for Hodgkin's disease. Analysis of 48 patients. Am. J. Cardiol. *51*:1679, 1983.
181. Taymor-Luria, H., Kohn, K., and Pasternak, R. C.: Radiation heart disease. J. Cardiovasc. Med. *8*:113, 1983.
182. Iqbal, S. M. Hanson, E. L., and Gensini, G. G.: Bypass graft for coronary arterial stenosis following radiation therapy. Chest *71*:664, 1977.
183. Miller, D. D., Waters, D. D., Dangoisse, V., and David, P. R.: Symptomatic coronary artery spasm following radiotherapy for Hodgkin's disease. Chest *83*:284, 1983.
184. Stegaru-Hellring, B., Keller, H., Bode, H. et al.: Ostium stenosis of both coronary arteries and latent hypothyroidism as sequelae of radiotherapy in Hodgkin's disease. Z. Kardiol. *74*:485, 1985.
185. Simon, E. B., Ling, J., Mendizabal, R. C., and Midawell, J.: Radiation-induced coronary artery disease. Am. Heart J. *108*:1031, 1984.

186. Tracy, G. P., Brown, D. E., Johnson, L. W., and Gottlieb, A. J.: Radiation-induced coronary artery disease. JAMA *228*:1660, 1974.
187. Shashaty, G. G.: Aortic insufficiency following mediastinal radiation for Hodgkin's disease. Am. J. Med. Sci. *287*:46, 1984.
188. Warda, M., Kahn, A., Massumi, A., et al.: Radiation-induced valvular dysfunction. J. Am. Coll. Cardiol. *2*:180, 1983.
189. Detrano, R. C., Yiannikas, J., and Salcedo, E. E.: Two-dimensional echocardiographic assessment of radiation-induced valvular heart disease. Am. Heart J. *107*:584, 1984.
190. Rummeny, E., Hausen, W., Lorbacher, P., and Willems, D.: Acquired infundibular pulmonary stenosis. Possible late complication following radiotherapy of Hodgkin's disease. Z. Kardiol. *73*:641, 1984.
191. Gomez, G. A., Park, J. J., Panahoh, A. M., et al.: Heart size and function after radiation therapy to the mediastinum in patients with Hodgkin's disease. Cancer Treat. Rep. *67*:1099, 1983.
192. Cohen, I. S., Bharati, S., Glass, J., and Lev, M.: Radiotherapy as a cause of complete atrioventricular block in Hodgkin's disease. Arch. Intern. Med. *141*:676, 1981.
193. Loeffler, J. S., Mauch, P., and Hellman, S.: Late effects of radiation therapy in the treatment of Hodgkin's disease. *In* Lacher, M. J., and Redman, J. R. (eds.): Hodgkin's Disease: The Consequences of Survival. Philadelphia, Lea and Febiger, 1990, pp. 27–46.
194. Gerling, G., Gottdiener, J., and Burer, J. S.: Cardiovascular complications of the treatment of Hodgkin's disease. *In* Lacher, M. J., and Redman, J. R. (eds.): Hodgkin's Disease: The Consequences of Survival. Philadelphia, Lea and Febiger, 1990, pp. 267–295.
195. Akaike, A., Cogure, R., Oyama, K., and Oda, M.: Damage to the heart from tumor irradiation in the thorax: An echocardiographic study. Radiology *25*:430, 1985.
196. Green, D., Gingell, R. L., Pearce, J., et al.: The effect of mediastinal irradiation on cardiac function of patients treated during childhood and adolescence for heart disease. J. Clin. Oncol. *5*:239, 1987.
197. Carmel, R. J., and Kaplan, H. S.: Mantle irradiation in Hodgkin's disease. Cancer *37*:2813, 1976.
198. Ikaheimo, M. J., Niemela, K. O., Linnaluoto, M. M., et al.: Early cardiac changes related to radiation therapy. Am. J. Cardiol. *56*:943, 1985.
199. O'Donnell, L. O., O'Neill, T., Toner, M., et al.: Myocardial hypertrophy, fibrosis and infarction following exposure of the heart to radiation for Hodgkin's disease. Postgrad. Med. J. *62*:1055, 1986.
200. Strender, L. E., Lindhal, J., and Larsson, L. E.: Incidence of heart disease and functional significance of changes in the electrocardiogram 10 years after radiotherapy for breast cancer. Cancer *57*:929, 1986.
201. Lederman, G. S., Sheldon, T. A., Chaffey, J. T., et al.: Cardiac disease after mediastinal irradiation for seminoma. Cancer *60*:772, 1987.
202. Radwanen, B. A., Geringer, R., Goldmann, A. M., et al.: Left main coronary artery stenosis following mediastinal irradiation. Am. J. Med. *82*:1017, 1987.
203. Joesuu, H.: Acute myocardial infarction after heart irradiation in young patients with Hodgkin's disease. Chest *95*:388, 1989.
204. Silverberg, G. O., Britt, R. H., and Goffinet, D. R.: Radiation induced carotid artery disease. Cancer *41*:130, 1978.
205. Amromin, G. G., Gildenhorn, H. C., and Solomon, R. D.: The synergism of x-irradiation and cholesterol-fat feeding on the development of coronary artery lesions. J. Atheroscler. Res. *4*:325, 1975.
206. Brosius, F. C., Waller, B. F., and Roberts, W. C.: Radiation heart disease: Analysis of 16 young (aged 15 to 33 years) necropsy patients who received over 3500 rads to the heart. Am. J. Med. *7*:519, 1981.
207. Kantrowitz, N. E., and Bristow, M. R.: Cardiotoxicity of antitumor agents. Prog. Cardiovasc. Dis. *27*:195, 1984.
208. Sunnenberg, D., and Kramer, B.: Long-term effects of cancer chemotherapy. Compr. Ther. *11*:58, 1985.
209. Perry, M. C.: Effects of chemotherapy on the heart. *In* Kapoor, A. S. (ed.): Cancer and the Heart. New York, Springer-Verlag, 1986, p. 223.
210. Lancaster, L. D., and Ewy, G. A.: Cardiac consequences of malignancy and their treatment. Adv. Intern. Med. *30*:275, 1984.
211. Schoenberger, C. I., and Crystal R.: Drug-induced lung disease. *In* Isselbacher, K. J. (ed.): Update IV to Harrison's Principles of Internal Medicine. New York, McGraw-Hill Book Co., 1982, pp. 49–74.
212. Young, R. C., Oxols, R. F., and Myers, C. E.: The anthracycline antineoplastic drugs. N. Engl. J. Med. *305*:139, 1981.
213. Lena, L., and Page, J. A.: Cardiotoxicity of Adriamycin and related anthracyclines. Cancer Treat. Rev. *3*:111, 1976.
214. Ali, M. K., Soto, P. A., Maroongroge, D., et al.: Electrocardiographic changes after Adriamycin chemotherapy. Cancer *43*:465, 1979.
215. Bristow, M. R., Billingham, M. E., Mason, J. W., and Daniels, J. R.: Clinical spectrum of anthracycline antibiotic cardiotoxicity. Cancer Treat. rep. *62*:873, 1978.
216. Wortman, J. E., Lucas, V. S., Jr., Schuster, E., et al.: Sudden death during doxorubicin administration. Cancer *44*:1588, 1979.
217. Lipshultz, S. E., Colan, S. D., Gelber, R. D., et al.: Late cardiac effects of doxorubicin therapy for acute lymphoblastic leukemia in childhood. N. Engl. J. Med. *324*:808, 1991.
218. Greene, H. L., Reich, S. D., and Dalen, J. E.: How to minimize doxorubicin toxicity. J. Cardiovasc. Med. *7*:306, 1982.
219. Freter, C. E., Leet, C., Billingham, M. E., et al.: Doxorubicin cardiac toxicity manifesting seven years after treatment. Am. J. Med. *80*:483, 1986.
220. Steinherz, L. J., and Steinherz, P.: Cardiac failure more than six years post anthrcyclines. Am. J. Cardiol. *62*:505, 1988.
221. Goorin, A. M., Chauvenet, A. R., Perez-, Perez-Atayde, A. R. *Gruz J*, et al.: Initial congestive heart failure, six to ten years after doxorubicin chemotherapy for childhood cancer. J. Pediatr. *116*:144, 1990.
222. Porembka, D. T., Lowder, J. N., Orlowski, J. P., et al.: Etiology and management of doxorubicin cardiotoxicity. Crit. Care Med. *17*:569, 1989.
223. Isner, J. M., Ferrans, V. J., Cohen, S. R., et al.: Clinical and morphological cardiac findings after anthracycline chemotherapy. Analysis of 64 patients studied at necroscopy. Am. J. Cardiol. *51*:1167, 1983.
224. Merrill, J., Greco, F. A., Zimbler, H., et al.: Adriamycin and radiation: Synergistic cardiotoxicity. Ann. Intern. Med. *82*:122, 1975.
225. Fajardo, L. R., and Stewart, J. F.: Pathogenesis or radiation-induced myocardial fibrosis. Lab. Invest. *29*:244, 1973.
226. O'Connell, T. X., and Berenbaum, M. D.: Cardiac and pulmonary effects of high doses of cyclophosphamide and isophosphamide. Cancer Res. *34*:1586, 1974.
227. Mills, B. A., and Roberts, R. W.: Cyclophosphamide-induced cardiomyopathy. A report of two cases and a review of the English literature. Cancer *43*:2223, 1979.
228. Severs, N. J., Twist, V. W., and Powell, T.: Acute effects of Adriamycin on the macromolecular organization of the cardiac muscle cell plasma membrane. Cardioscience *2*:35, 1991.
228a. Lewis, W., and Gonzalez, B.: Actin isoform mRNA alterations induced by doxorubicin in cultured heart cells. Lab. Invest. *62*:69, 1990.
229. Papoian, T., and Lewis, W.: Adriamycin cardiotoxicity in vivo. Am. J. Pathol. *136*:1201, 1990.
230. Lewis, W., Kleinerman, J., and Poszkin, S.: Interaction of Adriamycin in vitro with cardiac myofibrillar proteins. Circ. Res. *50*:547, 1982.
231. Milei, J., Bovevis, A., Llesoy, S., et al.: Amelioration of Adriamycin-induced cardiotoxicity in rabbits by prenylamine and vitamin A + E. Am. Heart J. *111*:95, 1986
232. Speyer, M., et al.: Protective effect of ICRF against doxorubicin-induced cardiotoxicity in advanced breast cancer. N. Engl. J. Med. *319*:745, 1988.
233. Villani, F., Galimberti, M., Monti, E., et al.: Effect of ICRF-187 pretreatment against doxorubicin-induced delayed cardiotoxicity in the rat. Toxicol. Appl. Pharmacol. *102*:292, 1990.
234. Kajagopalan, S., Puliti, P. M., Sinha, B. K., et al.: Adriamycin-induced free radical formation in the perfused rat heart: Implications of cardiotoxicity. Cancer Res. *48*:4766, 1988.
235. Lewis, W., Perillo, N. L., and Gonzales, B.: α-Actin synthesis changes in cultural cardiac myocytes: Relationship to anthracycline structure. J. Lab. Clin. Med. *112*:43, 1988.
236. Dorr, R. T., Bozak, K. A., Shipp, N. G., et al.: In vitro rat, myocyte cardiotoxicity model for antitumor antibiotics using adenosine triphosphate/protein ratios. Cancer Res. *48*:5222, 1988.
237. Singh, Y., Ulrich, L., Katz, D., et al.: Structural requirements for anthracycline-induced cardiotoxicity and antitumor effects. Toxicol. Appl. Pharmacol. *100*:9, 1989.
238. Binacaniello, T., Myer, R. A., Wong, K. Y., et al.: Doxorubicin cardiotoxicity in children. J. Pediatr. *97*:45, 1980.
239. Danesi, R., Del Tacca, M., Bernardini, N., et al.: Evaluation of the JT and corrected JT intervals as a new ECG method for monitoring doxorubicin cardiotoxicity in the dog. J. Pharmacol Meth. *21*:317, 1989.
240. Boujon, B., Lechat, P., Mantz, J., et al.: Echocardiographic detection of adriamycin cardiotoxicity. Study of the relationship between the shortening fraction-constraint and the systolic shortening fraction-diameter of the left ventricle. Arch. Mal. Coeur *82*:167, 1989.
241. Merchandise, B., Schroeder, E., Bosly, A., et al.: Early detection of doxorubicin cardiotoxicity: Interest of Doppler echocardiographic analysis of left ventricular filling dynamics. Am. Heart J. *118*:92, 1989.
242. Applefeld, M. M., and Pollock, S. H.: Cardiac disease in patients who have malignancies. Curr. Probl. Cardiol. *4*:1, 1980.
243. Hausdorf, G., Morf, G., Beron, G., et al.: Long-term doxorubicin cardiotoxicity in childhood: Noninvasive evaluation of the contractile state and diastolic filling. Br. Heart J. *60*:309, 1988.
244. Lee, B. H., Goodenday, L. S., Muswick, G. J., et al.: Alterations in left ventricular diastolic function with doxorubicin therapy. J. Am. Coll. Cardiol. *9*:184, 1987.
245. Bristow, M. R., Mason, J. W., Billingham, M. E., and Daniels, J. R.: Doxorubicin cardiomyopathy. Evaluation by phonocardiography, endomyocardial biopsy, and cardiac catheterization. Ann. Intern. Med. *88*:168, 1978.
246. Bristow, M. R., Mason, J. W., Billingham, M. E., and Daniels, J. R.: Dose effect and structure-function relationships in doxorubicin cardiomyopathy. Am. Heart J. *102*:709, 1981.
247. Fowles, R. E.: Cardiac catheterization and endomyocardial biopsy. *In* Kapoor, A. S. (ed.): Cancer and the Heart. Springer-Verlag, New York, 1986, pp. 42–50.
248. Bristow, M. R., Lopez, M. R., Mason, J. W., et al.: Efficacy and the cost of cardiac monitoring in patients receiving doxorubicin. Cancer *50*:32, 1982.
249. Von Hoff, D. D., Layard, M. W., Basa, P., et al.: Risk factors for doxorubicin-induced congestive heart failure. Ann. Intern. Med. *91*:710, 1979.
250. Weiss, R. B., Grillo-Lopez, A. J., Marsoni, S., et al.: Amsacrine associated cardiotoxicity: An analysis of 82 cases. J. Clin. Oncol. *4*:918, 1986.
251. Lyman, G. H., Williams, C. C., Dinwoodie, W. R., and Schocken, D. D.: Sudden death in cancer patients receiving lithium. J. Clin. Oncol. *2*:1270, 1984.
252. Bradamante, S., Monti, E., Paracchini, L., and Perletti, G.: Hypoxia as a risk factor for doxorubicin-induced cardiotoxicity: A NMR evaluation. Biochem. Biophys. Res. Commun. *163*:682, 1989.
253. Schwartz, R. G., McKenzie, W. B., Alexander, J., et al.: Congestive heart failure and left ventricular dysfunction complicating doxorubicin therapy. Seven-year experience using serial radionuclide angiocardiography. Am. J. Med. *82*:1109, 1987.

254. Doroshow, H. J., Locker, G. Y., Ifrim, I., and Myers, C. E.: Prevention of doxorubicin cardiac toxicity in the mouse by N-acetylcysteine. J. Clin. Invest. *68*:1053, 1981.
255. Cortes, E. P., Gupta, M., Chew, C., et al.: Adriamycin cardiotoxicity: Early detection by systolic time interval and possible prevention by coenzyme Q. Cancer Treat. Rep. *62*:887, 1978.
256. Somberg, J., Cagin, N., Levitt, L. B., et al.: Blockade of tissue uptake of the antineoplastic agent doxorubicin. J. Pharmacol. Exp. Ther. *204*:226, 1978.
257. Milei, J., Marantz, A., Ale, J., et al.: Prevention of adriamycin-induced cardiotoxicity by prenylamine: A pitot double blind study. Cancer Drug Delivery *4*:129, 1987.
258. Bellelli, A., Giomini, M., Giuliani, A. M., et al.: Antitumor effect and cardiotoxicity of a doxorubicin-lecithin association. Anti Cancer Res. *8*:177, 1988.
259. Storm, G., Hoesel, Q. G., deGroot, G., et al.: A comparative study on the antitumor effect, cardiotoxicity and nephrotoxicity of doxorubicin given as a bolus continuous infusion or entrapped in liposomes in the Lou/M WSI rat. Cancer Chemother. Pharmacol. *24*:341, 1989.
260. Legla, S. S., Benjamin, R. S., MacKay, B., et al.: Reduction of doxorubicin cardiotoxicity by prolonged continuous intravenous infusion. Ann. Intern. Med. *96*:133, 1982.
261. Anders, R. J., Shanes, J. G., and Zeller, F. P.: Lower incidence of doxorubicin cardiomyopathy by one-a-week low-dose administration. Am. Heart J. *111*:755, 1986.
262. Shapira, J., Gotfried, M., Lishner, M., et al.: Reduced cardiotoxicity of doxorubicin by a 6-hour infusion infusion regimen. A prospective randomized evaluation. Cancer *65*:870, 1990.
263. Valdirieso, M., Burgess, M. A., Awer, M. S., et al.: Increased therapeutic index of weekly doxorubicin in the therapy of non small cell lung cancer: A prospective randomized study. J. Clin. Oncol. *2*:207, 1984.
264. Taylor, A. L., Applefeld, M. N., Wiernik, P. H., et al.: Acute anthracycline cardiotoxicity. Comparative morphologic study of three analogues. Cancer *53*:1660, 1984.
264a. Nielsen, D., Jensen, J. B., Dombernowsky, P., et al.: Epirubicin cardiotoxicity: A study of 135 patients with advanced breast cancer. J. Clin. Oncol. *8*:1806, 1990.
265. Leitner, S. P., Casper, E. S., Hakes, T. B., et al.: A phase II trial of 4′-deoxydoxorubicin in patients with advanced breast cancer. Cancer Treat. Rep. *69*:1319, 1985.
266. Bramhilla, C., Rossi, A., Bonfonta, B., et al.: Phase II study of doxorubicin versus epirubicin in advanced breast cancer. Cancer Treat. Rep. *70*:261, 1986.
267. Baello, E. B., Ensberg, M. E., Fergoson, D. W., et al.: Effect of high dose cyclophosphamide and total-body irradiation on left ventricular function in adult patients with leukemia undergoing allogeneic bone marrow transplantation. Cancer Treat. Rep. *70*:1187, 1986.
268. Goldberg, M. A., Antin, J. H., Guinan, E. C., and Rappeport, J. M.: Cyclophosphamide cardiotoxicity. An analysis of dosing as a risk factor. Blood *68*:1114, 1986.
269. Braverman, A. C., Antin, J. H., Plappert, M. T., et al.: Cyclophosphamide cardiotoxicity: A prospective evaluation of new dosing regimens. (Submitted for publication.)
270. Lopez, M., Contegiacomp, A., Vici, P., et al.: A prospective, randomized trial of doxorubicin versus idarubicin in the treatment of advanced breast cancer. Cancer *64*:2431, 1989.
271. Baker, W. P., Dainer, P., Lester, W. M., et al.: Ischemic chest pain after 5-fluorouracil therapy for cancer. Am. J. Cardiol. *57*:497, 1986.
272. Freeman, N. J., and Costanza, M. E.: 5-Fluorouracil-associated cardiotoxicity. Cancer *61*:36, 1988.
273. Cristofini, P., Desnos, M., Guenot, O., et al.: Cardiotoxicity of 5-fluorouracil: Coronary spasm? Apropos of two cases with normal coronarography. Ann. Med. Interne *140*:9, 1989.
274. Ensley, J. F., Patel, B., Kloner, R., et al.: The clinical syndrome of 5-fluorouracil cardiotoxicity. Invest. New Drugs *7*:101, 1989.
275. Doll, D. C., List, A. F., Greco, A., et al.: Acute ventricular ischemic events after cisplatin-based combination chemotherapy for germ-cell tumors of the testis. Ann. Intern. Med. *105*:48, 1986.
276. Anjo, A., Dantchev, D., and Mathe, G.: Notes on the cardiotoxicity of platinum complexes in ultrastructural study. Biomed. Pharmacother. *43*:265, 1989.
277. Burkhardt, A., Haltje, W. J., and Gebbens, J. O.: Vascular lesions following perfusion with bleumycin: Electron-microscopic observations. Virchows Arch. Pathol. Anat. *372*:227, 1976.
278. Mandel, E. M., Lewinski, U., and Djaldetti, M.: Vincristine-induced myocardial infarction. Cancer *30*:1979, 1975.
279. Lejonc, J. L., Vernant, J. P., Macquin, J., and Castaigne, A.: Successful removal of aluminum from patient with dialysis encephalopathy. Lancet *2*:692, 1980.
280. Aisner, J., VanEcho, D. A., Whitacre, M., and Wiernik, P. H.: A phase-I trial of continuous infusion VP-16-213 *(etoposide)*. Cancer Chemother. Pharmacol. *7*:157, 1982.
281. Gottdiener, J. S., Applebaum, F. R., Ferrans, V. J., et al.: Cardiotoxicity associated with high dose cyclophosphamide therapy. Arch. Intern. Med. *141*:758, 1981.
282. Kandylis, K., Vassilomanolakis, M., Tsoussis, S., and Efremidis, A. P.: *Ifosfamide* cardiotoxicity in humans. Cancer Chemother. Pharmacol. *24*:395, 1989.
283. Steinherz, L. J., Steinherz, P. G., Mangiacasale, D., et al.: Cardiac abnormalities after AMSA administration. Cancer Treat. Rep. *66*:483, 1982.
284. Lindpainter, K., Lindpainter, L. S., Wentworth, M., and Burns, C. P.: Acute myocardial necrosis during administration of amsacrine. Cancer *57*:1284, 1986.
285. Weiss, R. B., Grillo-Lopez, A. J., Marsoni, S., et al.: Amsacrine-associated cardiotoxicity: An analysis of 82 cases. J. Clin. Oncol. *4*:919, 928, 1986.
286. Shenkenberg, T. D., and VonHoff, D. D.: Mitoxantrone: A new anticancer drug with significant clinical activity. Ann. Intern. Med. *105*:67, 1986.
287. Colman, R. E., Maisey, M. N., Knight, R. K., and Rubens, R. D.: Mitoxantrone in advanced breast cancer: A phase II study with special attention to cardiotoxicity. Eur. J. Cancer Clin. Oncol. *20*:771, 1984.
288. Pratt, C. G., Vietti, T. J., Etcubanas, E., et al.: Nonvantrone for childhood malignant solid tumors. A pediatric oncology group phase II study. Invest. New Drugs *4*:43, 1986.
289. Landys, K., Bergstom, S., Andersson, T., and Noppa, H.: Mitoxantrone as a first line treatment of advanced breast cancer. Invest. New Drugs *3*:133, 1985.
290. Allegra, J. C., Woodcock, T., Woolf, S., et al.: A randomized trial comparing mitoxantrone with doxorubicin in patients with stage IV breast cancer. Invest. New Drugs *3*:153, 1985.
291. Baker, W. P., Dainer, P., Lester, W. M., et al.: Ischemic chest pain after 5-fluorouracil therapy for cancer. Am. J. Cardiol. *57*:497, 1986.
291a. May, D., Wandl, U., Becher, R., et al.: Kardiale nebenwirkungen von 5-fluorouracil. Dtsch. Med. Wochenschr. *115*:618, 1990.
292. Cameron, H. A., Reyntjens, A. J., and Lake-Bakaar, G.: Cardiac arrest after treatment with intravenous domperidone. Br. Med. J. (Clin. Res.) *290*:160, 1985.
293. Osborne, A. J., Slevin, N. L., Hunter, L. W., and Hamer, J.: Cardiac arrhythmias during cytotoxic chemotherapy: Role of domperidone. Hum. Toxicol. *4*:617, 1985.
294. Cazin, V., Gorin, C., Laport, J. P., et al.: Cardiac complications after bone marrow transplantation. A report on a series of 63 consecutive transplantations. Cancer *57*:2061, 1986.
295. Cohen, M. C., Huberman, M. S., and Nesto, R. W.: Recombinant alpha-2 interferon-related cardiomyopathy. Am. J. Med. *85*:549, 1988.
296. Deyton, L. R., Walker, R. E., Kovacs, J. A., et al.: Reversible cardiac dysfunction associated with interferon alpha therapy in AIDS patients with Kaposi's sarcoma. N. Engl. J. Med. *321*:1246, 1989.
297. Nora, R., Abrams, J., and Silverman, H. J.: Infarction in patients receiving high dose recombinant interleukin-2 (rIl-2). Proc. Am. Soc. Clin. Cardiol. *6*:245, 1987.
298. Margolin, K., Jaffe, H. S., Hawkins, M., et al.: Toxicity of interleukin-2 and lymphokine-activated killer cell therapy. Proc. Am. Soc. Clin. Oncol. *6*:251, 1987.
299. Rosenberg, S. A., Lotze, M. T., Muul, L. M., et al.: A progress report on the treatment of 157 patients with advanced cancer using lymphokine-activated hilar cells and interleukin-2 or high dose interleukin-2 alone. N. Engl. J. Med. *316*:889, 1987.
300. Nora, R., Abrams, J. S., Tait, N. S., et al.: Myocardial toxic effects during recombinant interleukin-2 therapy. J. Natl. Cancer Inst. *81*:59, 1989.
301. Osanto, S., Cluitman, F. H. M., Franks, C. R., et al.: Myocardial injury after interleukin-2 therapy. Lancet *2*:48, 1988.
302. Dorr, R. T., and Shipp, N. G.: Effect of interferon, interleukin-2, and tumor necrosis factor in myocardial cell viability and doxorubicin cardiotoxicity in vitro. Immunpharmacology *18*:31, 1989.

HEMATOLOGICAL ABNORMALITIES RELATED TO CARDIAC DRUGS

303. Gavras, F., Graff, L. G., Rose, B. D., et al.: Fatal pancytopenia associated with the use of captopril. Ann. Intern. Med. *94*:58, 1981.
304. Lundh, B., and Hasselgren, K. H.: Hematological side effects from antihypertensive drugs. Acta Med. Scand. (Suppl.) *628*:73, 1979.
305. Erslev, A. J. Aplastic anemia. *In* Williams, W. J. (ed.): Hematology, 3rd. ed. New York, McGraw-Hill Book Co., 1983, pp. 155–158.
306. Volosin, K., Greenberg, R. M., and Grenspon, A. J.: Tocainide-associated agranulocytosis. Am. Heart J. *109*:1392, 1985.
307. Soff, G. A., and Kadin, M. E.: Tocainide-induced reversible agranulocytosis and anemia. Arch. Intern. Med. *147*:598, 1987.
308. Morrill, G. B., and Gibson, S. M.: Tocainide-induced aplastic anemia (letter). Drug Intell. Clin. Pharm. *23*:90, 1989.
309. Finch, S. C.: Neutropenia. *In* Williams, W. J. (ed.): Hematology. New York, McGraw-Hill, 1983, pp. 777–786.
310. Hackett, T., Kelton, J. G., and Powers, P.: Drug-induced platelet destruction. Semin. Thromb. Hemostas. *8*:116, 1982.
311. Ansell, J., McCue, J., Tiarks, C., et al.: Amrinone-induced thrombocytopenia. Blood *58*(Suppl. 1):187a, 1981.
312. Packman, C. H., and Leddy, J. P.: Drug-related immunologic injury of erythrocytes. *In* Williams, W. J. (ed.): Hematology. New York, McGraw-Hill Book Co., 1983, pp. 647–650.
313. Bell, W. R., and Royall, R. M.: Heparin-associated thrombocytopenia: A comparison of three heparin preparations. N. Engl. J. Med. *303*:902, 1980.
314. Gibson, G. R., Hunter, J. B., Raabe, D. S., et al.: Methemoalbuminemia produced by high-dose intravenous nitroglycerin. Ann. Intern. Med. *96*:615, 1982.
315. Vesey, C. J., and Cole, P. V.: Blood cyanide and thiocyanate concentrations produced by long-term therapy with sodium nitroprusside. Br. J. Anaesth. *57*:148, 1985.
316. Weisbart, R. H., Yee, W. S., Colburn, K. K., et al.: Antiguanosine antibodies: A new marker for procainamide-induced systemic lupus erythematosus. Ann. Intern. Med. *104*:310, 1986.

Hemostasis, Thrombosis, Fibrinolysis, and Cardiovascular Disease

by ROBERT I. HANDIN, M.D., and JOSEPH LOSCALZO, M.D., Ph.D.

Thrombosis and embolism either contribute to the pathogenesis of many cardiovascular disorders or complicate their clinical course. After some initial skepticism, several decades of laboratory and clinical research have established a role for platelets and coagulation proteins in the pathogenesis of atherosclerosis (see Chap. 36). The coagulation system plays a role in the clinically silent evolution and progression of atheroma, and in the events that follow plaque rupture and activation which produce clinical symptoms. This close pathogenic relation has led some authors to refer to the overall process as "atherothrombosis."[1] Not only do many acute cardiovascular events, such as myocardial infarction and stroke, arise from thrombotic occlusion of atherosclerotic arteries, but also patients with preexisting chronic disorders such as congestive heart failure, cardiomyopathy, and valvular or congenital heart disease are at increased risk of venous or arterial thromboembolism. As a result of these clinical and experimental observations, anticoagulant, antiplatelet, and, most recently, fibrinolytic agents have become increasingly important therapeutic tools for the cardiologist.

In this chapter the pathophysiology of normal hemostasis is reviewed, and those disorders are described that cause failure of hemostasis with hemorrhage as well as those that increase the risk of thrombosis. The inherited prethrombotic or hypercoagulable states, including fibrinolytic disorders, are used to illustrate more general mechanisms of venous and arterial thromboembolism in patients with cardiovascular disorders. Finally, methods for preventing and treating thromboembolism associated with cardiovascular diseases are discussed, including new options for clot dissolution—an area in which rapid and impressive strides have been made over the past few years.

HEMOSTASIS

Unactivated *platelets* circulate as individual, smooth-surfaced discs that do not interact with other cells in the blood or with the endothelial cells that line the blood vessels. Platelets will adhere, however, to subendothelium that has been exposed as a result of vascular injury or to any foreign or prosthetic material in contact with blood. Adherent, activated platelets generate potent mediators that cause vasoconstriction and leukocyte chemotaxis. The platelets then degranulate, releasing materials that attract platelets, forming a multicellular aggregate or hemostatic plug on the adherent monolayer. These events, collectively referred to as *primary hemostasis*, are the first line of defense against hemorrhage after vascular injury. They are particularly important in capillaries and small arterioles where shear forces are high and the formation of a platelet plug is critical for effective hemostasis.

The *plasma coagulation system*, or secondary hemostatic system, is simultaneously activated in response to vascular injury and, within several minutes, generates insoluble fibrin strands that interdigitate with and strengthen the primary platelet plug. Fibrin is produced by the action of thrombin on fibrinogen. Thrombin is generated by a series of linked proteolytic reactions that take place on phospholipid-rich cell surfaces and are regulated by plasma cofactors and calcium, which accelerate coagulation, and by a series of naturally occurring inhibitors, or anticoagulants. Although platelet activation and fibrin production are described as separate processes, they actually are closely linked and interdependent. For example, the surface of the activated platelet provides the optimal locus for several critical coagulation reactions and accelerates them several hundredfold. Conversely, thrombin generated during plasma coagulation also is a potent agonist, and stimulates platelet secretion and aggregation. The endothelial cells that line the blood vessels also bind coagulation proteins, accelerate their interactions, and secrete both inhibitory and procoagulant molecules.

Although the hemostatic system has evolved to minimize blood loss from injured vessels, there is little difference between the physiological process of normal hemostasis and the pathological events that lead to thrombosis and embolism. Because of this similarity, thrombosis has been described as hemostasis occurring in the wrong place or at the wrong time. Although both inherited and acquired disorders may predispose a patient to thrombosis, in many cases the triggering event is simply the interaction of normal blood components with an abnormal surface such as a diseased or atherosclerotic vessel, a prosthetic cardiac valve, or a vascular graft. Furthermore, bleeding caused by failure of a component in the hemostatic system is similar to the purposeful or therapeutic failure of hemostasis induced by anticoagulant agents used to prevent recurrent thromboembolism. Most of the available anticoagulant drugs are not selective and have a relatively poor therapeutic index. Thus, the dose of drug needed to produce the desired antithrombotic effect also may cause undesirable hemorrhage. Finally, because pathological thrombi may coexist with physiological and vital hemostatic plugs, even the more selective drugs, such as the relatively fibrin-specific plasminogen activators, cannot discriminate between fibrin within pathological thrombi and that within physiological hemostatic plugs.

PLATELETS IN COAGULATION

PLATELET ADHESION TO THE VESSEL WALL. Platelet adhesion, the initial event in both normal hemostasis and thrombosis, is a complex process that involves constituents of the vascular subendothelium, receptor sites on the platelet membrane, and plasma glycoproteins (Fig. 58–1). In normal hemostasis, platelets adhere to exposed subendothelial collagen after the traumatic removal of endothelial cells that normally line the blood vessel. In addition, thrombus formation may be initiated by the adhesion of platelets to damaged endothelial cells or denuded atherosclerotic plaques. Although several candidates have been proposed as the platelet collagen receptor, the collagen-binding site is probably located on the platelet glycoprotein Ia/IIa complex.[2,3] The initial bond between the platelet and the vessel wall is strengthened by the interaction of several adhesive glycoproteins.

Fibronectin. This 440,000-dalton dimeric protein binds to collagen and to platelets through receptor sites on the platelet glycoprotein IIb/IIIa (GpIIb/IIIa) complex.[4,5] Fibronectin binding facilitates both initial platelet attachment to the vessel wall and subsequent spreading over the subendothelial surface.[6]

von Willebrand's Factor (vWF). This protein circulates as a heterogeneous series of high molecular weight multimers and also binds to collagen[7] and to two separate platelet receptor sites. The best defined receptor site for vWF is on the platelet glycoprotein Ib/IV complex.[8] Binding to this site is critically important for normal platelet adhesion. vWF binding to a second platelet receptor site on glycoproteins IIb/IIIa may facilitate both adhesion and platelet-platelet cohesion or aggregate formation.[9] This factor plays a critical role in hemostasis, since it stabilizes the attachment of platelets to the vessel wall under conditions of high shear stress.[10,11] Neither the initial collagen-GpIa/IIa interaction nor the secondary interposition of fibronectin between platelets and collagen is sufficient to sustain platelet adhesion in the face of the high shear stresses encountered with normal blood flow. This unique property of vWF is clinically important, since bleeding and abnormal platelet function are found in patients with a mild or moderate deficiency in vWF despite normal interactions between the platelet membrane and subendothelial collagen and normal binding of fibronectin to the platelet and vessel wall.

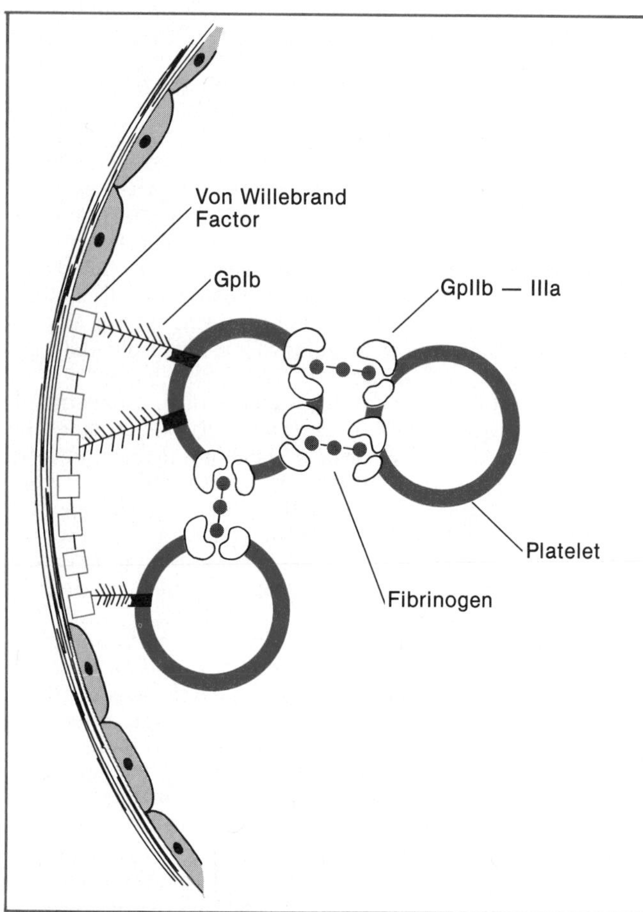

FIGURE 58–1. Molecular mechanisms of platelet attachment to vascular subendothelium (platelet adhesion) and of platelet-platelet interactions (platelet aggregation) in a cross-sectional view of a blood vessel. von Willebrand's multimers attach to exposed vascular subendothelial collagen and to a platelet membrane receptor site on glycoprotein Ib (GpIb). This is the initial interaction in hemostasis and stabilizes platelets so that they remain attached despite the high shear forces generated by flowing blood. Receptor sites on platelet membrane glycoproteins IIb and IIIa (GpIIb–IIIa) then become available to bind fibrinogen. The fibrinogen molecule links platelets together to form the hemostatic plug.

PLATELET ACTIVATION AND SECRETION

Platelet activation follows the adhesion of platelets to vascular subendothelium, or the binding of soluble agonists to platelet membrane receptors, and culminates in granule release and the formation of a platelet aggregate or hemostatic plug. Platelets have specific binding sites for adenosine diphosphate (ADP), thrombin, serotonin, and alpha$_2$-adrenergic agonists.[12] As shown in Figure 58–2, occupancy of these receptors by the appropriate agonists activates two intracellular enzymes, protein kinase A [the cyclic adenosine monophosphate (AMP)–dependent protein kinase] and protein kinase C, which then catalyze the phosphorylation of critical regulatory proteins within the platelet. Protein kinase A activity is regulated by the level of intracellular cyclic AMP and protein kinase C by diacylglycerol (DAG), a product of phospholipid hydrolysis. Inhibition of platelet adenylate cyclase activity activates protein kinase A, which then phosphorylates myosin light chain and enhances the contractile activity of platelet actomyosin. In contrast, the major substrate for protein kinase C is a 47,000-dalton protein that may serve as a feedback inhibitor of platelet activation, as described below. Although the specific target proteins may differ slightly, the sequence of reactions resembles that seen after the activation of beta-adrenoceptors in heart muscle (p. 363).

MECHANISMS OF ACTIVATION. Although there are two separate signal transduction pathways, mediated by protein kinases A and C within the platelet, their relative contributions to platelet activation are still being debated. Agonists like epinephrine clearly inhibit adenylate cyclase activity in platelet membrane fractions; however, incubating intact platelets with epinephrine does not reduce intraplatelet cyclic AMP to below basal levels, suggesting that cyclic AMP levels do not regulate platelet signal transduction and activation.[13] Alternatively, because cyclic AMP is compartmentalized within the platelet, regulation of cyclic AMP content within a specific compartment may be an important mechanism for signal transduction by certain agonists. The bulk of recent evidence suggests that the adenylate cyclase–cyclic AMP system provides a mechanism to *inhibit* platelet activation. In fact, many agents that stimulate platelet adenylate cyclase activity and raise intraplatelet cyclic AMP levels, such as prostaglandins E_1, D_2, and I_2, are potent platelet inhibitors.[14,15]

Transduction of the signal initiated by platelet agonist binding to membrane receptors is more likely to be mediated by the intracellular enzyme phospholipase C, which hydrolyzes a trace membrane phospholipid, phosphatidylinositol 4,5-bisphosphate (PIP_2), yielding inositol 1,4,5,-trisphosphate (IP_3) and DAG.[16,17] Although the role of cyclic AMP in platelet activation may be unclear, the two products of PIP_2 hydrolysis are clearly important mediators of platelet signal transduction. IP_3 acts as a calcium ionophore, transiently raising intraplatelet calcium levels, while DAG activates protein kinase C, which then phosphorylates several intracellular proteins.[18,19] One prominent substrate is a 47,000-dalton protein present in platelets and leukocytes called *plekstrin*.[20] The function of this phosphoprotein is unknown. There also is pharmacological evidence that IP_3 and DAG themselves mediate signal transduction directly. The ability of a calcium ionophore to initiate platelet signal transduction has been well established. Furthermore, incubation of platelets with DAG analogs like oleylacylglycerol, which cross the platelet membrane, can mimic the effect of endogenous DAG.[21] Likewise, incubation of platelets with phorbolmyristate acetate, an agent that directly activates protein kinase C, eliminates the requirement for phospholipid hydrolysis and DAG generation for platelet activation.[22]

ROLE OF ARACHIDONIC ACID AND PROSTAGLANDINS

Arachidonic acid (5,8,11,14-eicosatetraenoic acid), a 20-carbon polyunsaturated fatty acid derived from dietary linoleic acid, is the precursor of the prostaglandins, leukotrienes, and thromboxane—eicosanoid mediators generated by activated platelets, leukocytes, and endothelial cells.[23,24] Arachidonate is taken up by the platelet from plasma and is esterified into platelet phospholipids. As outlined in Figures 58–2 and 58–3, the combined action of phospholipase C and diglyceride lipase on phosphatidylinositol rapidly releases arachidonic acid early in platelet acti-

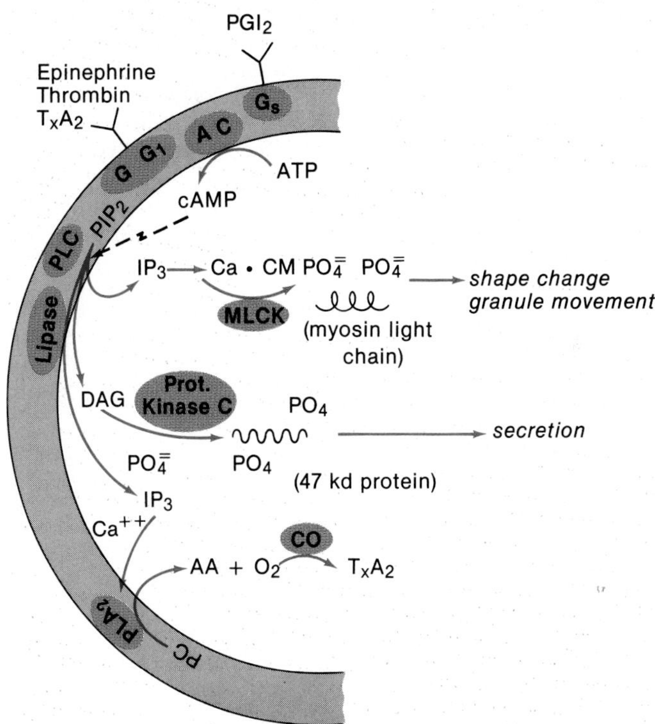

FIGURE 58-2. Biochemical pathways for stimulus-response coupling in the platelet. Platelets contain receptors that bind various agonists, including epinephrine, thrombin, and thromboxane A_2 (TxA_2) and the antagonist prostaglandin I_2 (PGI_2). Receptors for agonists and antagonists are coupled to two enzymes, adenylate cyclase (AC) and phospholipase C (PLC), by means of guanine nucleotide binding (G) proteins. Coupling to AC occurs by way of separate G_i (inhibitory) and G_s (stimulatory) proteins. It is not yet known whether coupling of receptors to PLC is by the same or a different set of G proteins. Activation of AC by PGI_2 raises intracellular cyclic AMP (cAMP) and inhibits platelet function, whereas inhibition of AC facilitates platelet activation by an incompletely worked-out set of reactions. PLC hydrolyzes the membrane phospholipid phosphatidylinositol bisphosphate (PIP_2) to yield diacylglycerol (DAG) and inositol triphosphate (IP_3). IP_3 functions as a calcium ionophore and transiently increases intracellular ionized calcium (Ca), which facilitates several important intraplatelet reactions. In one, Ca bound to calmodulin (CM) activates myosin light chain kinase (MLCK), which then phosphorylates the light chain of platelet myosin. The phosphorylated light chain participates in contractile force generation within the platelet, which causes shape change and granule movement. DAG activates protein kinase C, which, in turn, phosphorylates several other intracellular proteins that regulate secretion. Two mechanisms hydrolyze arachidonic acid (AA) from membrane phospholipids. First, DAG generated by PLC is the substrate for an intramembrane diglyceride lipase. Second, the IP_3-induced calcium flux activates a second enzyme, phospholipase A_2 (PLA_2), which hydrolyzes AA from phosphatidylcholine (PC). AA is then oxygenated by the enzyme cyclo-oxygenase (CO) and subsequently converted to TxA_2, a potent platelet agonist and vasoconstrictor. TxA_2 then stimulates additional platelet activation by way of the previously described pathways. Aspirin and nonsteroidal antiinflammatory agents act as antiplatelet agents by irreversibly acetylating CO and preventing TxA_2 generation.

vation.[25] Additional arachidonate subsequently is liberated from phosphatidylcholine by a phospholipase A_2 enzyme.[26] Released arachidonate is rapidly oxygenated by cyclo-oxygenase or lipoxygenase enzymes in platelets, leukocytes, and endothelial cells to yield various prostanoid and eicosanoid mediators.

THROMBOXANE A_2 (TxA_2). This potent vasoconstrictor and platelet agonist is the most important platelet eicosanoid mediator.[24] The generation of TxA_2 by activated platelets may explain the vasoconstriction and vessel retraction that accompany vascular injury and may contribute to the vasospasm observed in partially occluded atherosclerotic coronary and cerebral vessels. Inhibition of TxA_2 synthesis by agents like aspirin may explain their beneficial antithrombotic effect.[23] The principal platelet lipoxygenase product, 12-hydroxyeicosatetraenoic acid (12-HETE), has no direct role in hemostasis but may serve as a chemotactic agent for neutrophils and contribute to the inflammatory response.[27]

PROSTACYCLIN (PGI_2). The endothelial cell converts arachidonic acid into PGI_2, a labile cyclic prostaglandin.[28] In contrast to TxA_2, PGI_2 is a potent vasodilator that inhibits platelet aggregation and secretion by activating platelet adenylate cyclase and elevating intraplatelet cyclic AMP. Thrombin, calcium ionophore, bradykinin, serotonin, platelet-derived growth factor, and mechanical injury can all induce the synthesis of PGI_2 by endothelial cells. Although it is tempting to postulate that a balance between TxA_2 and PGI_2 synthesis by their respective cells regulates platelet vessel wall interactions and vessel tone, it is difficult to test this hypothesis, since both eicosanoids have very short half-lives, are produced in small quantities, and function locally within the microcirculation. Whole-body turnover studies that assess the excretion of thromboxane and prostacyclin metabolites in urine by gas chromatography and mass spectrometry demonstrate that the production of both eicosanoids is increased in thrombotic states and vascular disease.[29,30]

THE LEUKOTRIENES AND LIPOXINS. A relatively new class of eicosanoid mediators, the leukotrienes, play an important role in inflammation (Fig. 58-3).[31] The major derivative of arachidonic acid in polymorphonuclear leukocytes is 5-hydroxyeicosatetraenoic acid (5-HETE), which is converted to leukotriene A_4 (LTA_4). LTA_4 is then converted to LTB_4 by the addition of a 12-OH group. LTA_4 also is converted to leukotrienes C_4, D_4, and E_4 by the addition and subsequent metabolism of glutathione. The mediator responsible for acute anaphylaxis, formerly called the slow reacting substance of anaphylaxis, or SRS-A, is actually a mixture of the peptidolipid leukotrienes C_4, D_4, and E_4, which are potent bronchoconstrictors and vasoconstrictors. These leukotrienes also may be important in hemostasis, since they constrict the microvasculature and coronary arteries. The lipoxins are conjugated tetraene derivatives of arachidonic acid.[32] They tend to oppose the actions of leukotrienes. Because leukotrienes and lipoxins are products of lipoxygenase reactions, their biosynthesis is not inhibited by cyclo-oxygenase inhibitors such as aspirin.

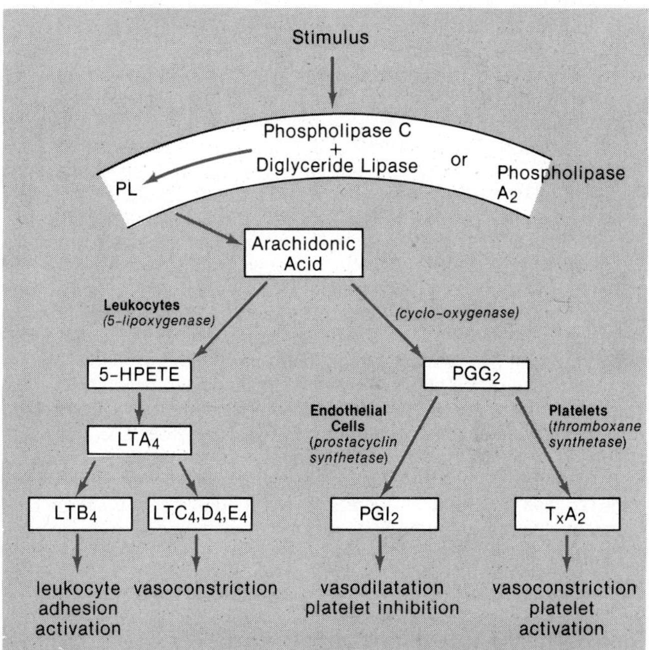

FIGURE 58-3. Liberation of arachidonic acid from membrane phospholipids and its subsequent conversion into biologically active mediators in leukocytes, platelets, and endothelial cells. Arachidonic acid is liberated from membrane phospholipids after cellular activation by the combined effects of the enzymes phospholipase C and diglyceride lipase or by the action of a phospholipase A_2 enzyme. In leukocytes, arachidonic acid is converted to an unstable intermediate, 5-hydroperoxyeicosatetraenoic acid (5-HPETE), by a 5-lipoxygenase enzyme. 5-HPETE is then converted into the leukotrienes (LT). Leukotriene B_4 (LTB_4) stimulates leukocyte adhesion to endothelial cells; leukotrienes C_4, D_4, and E_4 are potent vasoconstrictors. In platelets and endothelial cells the principal pathway for arachidonic acid metabolism is by way of cyclo-oxygenase, which forms the unstable intermediate prostaglandin G_2 (PGG_2). It is then converted to prostaglandin I_2 (PGI_2, or prostacyclin) by means of prostacyclin synthetase within endothelial cells. Prostacyclin, a labile compound, is a potent vasodilator that inhibits platelet activation. Within the platelet, PGG_2 is converted to thromboxane A_2 (TxA_2), another labile compound that is a potent vasoconstrictor and platelet agonist. Aspirin and other nonsteroidal antiinflammatory agents interfere with hemostasis by inhibiting the enzyme cyclooxygenase. They have no effect on leukotriene biosynthesis.

There also is active transcellular metabolism of eicosanoids. For example, two of the prostaglandin endoperoxide precursors, PGG_2 and PGH_2, can leave the platelet and enter the endothelial cell to be converted to PGI_2. Thus, a byproduct of platelet activation is transformed into a platelet inhibitor and acts as a feedback regulator, a phenomenon referred to as the "endoperoxide steal."[33,34] There also is evidence that unmetabolized arachidonic acid derived from aspirin-treated platelets may be converted into the vasoactive leukotrienes by polymorphonuclear leukocytes.

GRANULE SECRETION OR RELEASE

Platelets contain two classes of secretory granules, which are most readily classified by their density on electron micrographs. The most electron-dense (delta) granules contain adenine nucleotides (ADP and ATP), calcium, and serotonin, whereas the least electron-dense alpha granules contain enzymes, adhesive and coagulation proteins, and growth factors.[35] After platelet activation, both granule classes release their contents into the vicinity of the platelet plug, where they diffuse into plasma and into the vessel wall.[36] Platelet-derived growth factor and transforming growth factor beta (TGF-beta), which are both released by activated platelets, stimulate smooth muscle cell and fibroblast migration and proliferation.[37] This may be of importance both in wound healing and in the pathogenesis of atherosclerosis. TGF-beta also may inhibit the migration and proliferation of endothelial cells. Other secreted molecules enhance vascular permeability, bind glycosaminoglycans, and induce the chemotaxis of leukocytes to sites of vascular injury.[38]

PLATELET AGGREGATION

Fibrinogen is an essential cofactor for platelet aggregation. Although platelets circulate in a milieu rich in fibrinogen, they do not bind to it but remain as single, disc-shaped particles. Contact with ADP, derived from damaged tissue and red cells as well as from platelet secretory granules, initiates both platelet aggregate formation and fibrinogen binding. The binding of ADP to a platelet receptor induces platelets to become spherical and to extend large pseudopods. A protein, aggregin, has been proposed as the ADP receptor.[39] In addition, the conformation of the platelet membrane glycoprotein IIb/IIIa (GpIIb/IIIa) complex changes, so that it binds plasma fibrinogen (Fig. 58–1).[40] A unique dodecapeptide sequence on the gamma chain of fibrinogen as well as a second tripeptide sequence (Arg-Gly-Asp-RGD in the single letter amino acid code) on the alpha chain each binds to the platelet.[41,42] The RGD sequence is also present in 8 other adhesive glycoproteins and may represent a universal adhesive protein recognition sequence. Because the fibrinogen molecule contains pairs of alpha and gamma chain binding sites, it can link platelets together into aggregates. Patients with the rare platelet defect *thrombasthenia* have reduced or absent GpIIb/IIIa, reduced fibrinogen binding, markedly diminished or absent platelet aggregation, and severe bleeding, underscoring the importance of the platelet-fibrinogen interaction in hemostasis. The infusion of monoclonal antibodies directed against GpIIb/IIIa, which prevent aggregation and fibrinogen binding in vivo, protects laboratory animals from thrombus formation.[43] Synthetic peptides that block fibrinogen binding to platelet receptors may have a similar antithrombotic effect.[44] These studies document the importance of fibrinogen binding in thrombus formation and provide prototypes for new platelet-modifying drugs with potential antithrombotic activity.

Endothelial Inhibition of Platelet Aggregation

Under normal circumstances, the vascular endothelium presents an antithrombotic surface which inhibits platelet activation. Factors produced by the endothelial cell that are inhibitory include prostacyclin, endothelium-derived relaxing factor (EDRF), tissue-type plasminogen activator (t-PA), and an endothelial surface ADPase. Prostacyclin activates adenylate cyclase and increases intraplatelet cyclic AMP, and EDRF, one form of which is nitric oxide or an S-nitrosothiol derivative, activates platelet guanylate cyclase,[45,46] raising intraplatelet levels of cyclic GMP. Both antagonists inhibit platelet activation, prevent intraplatelet calcium flux, and reduce surface fibrinogen binding.[47] t-PA released from the endothelial cell binds to the platelet surface and activates platelet-bound plasminogen.[48–50] Finally, an endothelial surface ADPase may hydrolyze ADP released from damaged tissue or other platelets. These four independent endothelial-dependent reactions can be synergistic and effectively inhibit platelet plug formation and maintain blood fluidity,[51] and endothelial removal, injury, or dysfunction can enhance platelet plug formation.

Summary of the Role of Platelets

The sequence of reactions just described and summarized in Figure 58–4 represents primary hemostasis and provides the first line of defense against blood loss after injury to a blood vessel. Hemostasis usually is initiated when injury is sufficient to remove the endothelial lining and expose the vascular subendothelium to flowing blood. Platelets then adhere to collagen fibrils in the vessel wall, become activated, and degranulate, thereby releasing granule constituents and mediators into plasma and the vessel wall. Some of these materials, principally ADP and TxA_2, diffuse into plasma and activate circulating platelets, which become linked to the adherent platelet monolayer. The layers of platelets eventually fill the lumen of the vessel, forming a platelet aggregate or hemostatic plug.

The processes of adhesion and aggregation are mediated by the interaction of specific platelet membrane receptors with components of the vessel wall or with plasma proteins like fibronectin, vWF, and fibrinogen, which link platelets to the vessel wall and to one another. Signal transduction pathways in the platelet are complex, and regulated by specific agonists that bind to platelet receptors and activate the hydrolysis of phosphatidylinositol. These products of hydrolysis can then induce transient increases in intracellular calcium and activate an intracellular protein kinase that phosphorylates intraplatelet regulatory proteins. Finally, the eicosanoids derived from arachidonic acid in platelets, leukocytes, and endothelial cells provide short-acting biological mediators that can optimize the degree of platelet activation and vasoconstriction during local hemostasis. The plasma coagulation, or secondary hemostatic, system then generates fibrin strands that are interposed into the platelet plug to provide a stronger and more permanent hemostatic plug.

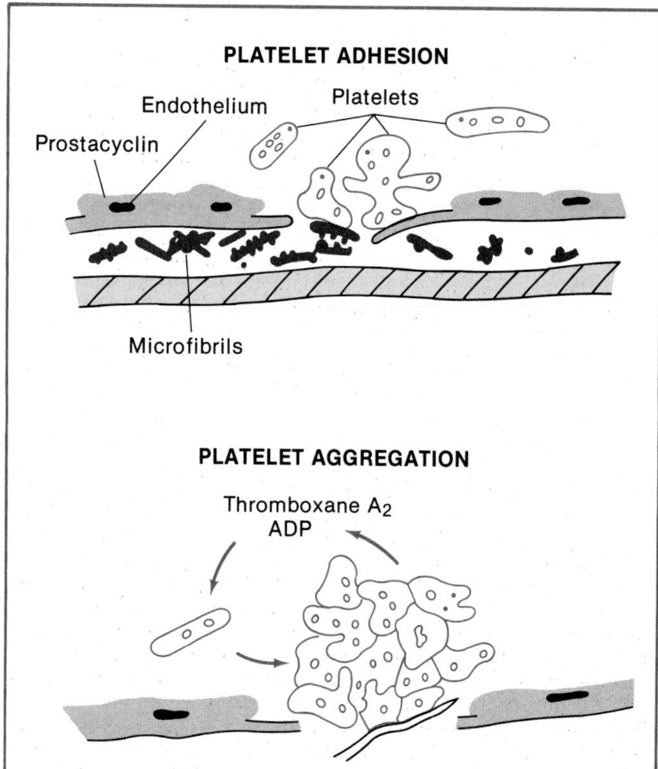

FIGURE 58–4. Overview of primary hemostasis. The initial event is adhesion of platelets to areas of the vessel wall in which the subendothelium has been exposed by endothelial cell disruption or injury. After adhesion, platelets become activated and, under the influence of mediators like ADP and thromboxane A_2, recruit additional circulating platelets to bind to the adherent monolayer and form a platelet aggregate.

FIBRIN GENERATION AND CLOT FORMATION

Blood coagulation is initiated by the interaction of flowing blood with vascular subendothelium or tissue thromboplastin (tissue factor) exposed on cell surfaces after cellular injury. Although the blood coagulation reactions often are referred to as the "fluid phase" of hemostasis, the reactions actually occur on vascular subendothelium or negatively charged, phospholipid-rich surfaces, such as the plasma membrane of suitably activated platelets or endothelial cells. The adsorption of coagulation proteins onto these surfaces increases their concentration, effectively increasing reaction rates and localizing their activity. As shown in Figure 58–5, the interactions among the procoagulants can be conveniently grouped into a series of surface-bound enzyme–cofactor complexes. Several of the coagulation proteins, including factors II, VII, IX, and X, are bound to surfaces by means of bridges formed between calcium, the negatively charged cell surface, and digamma-carboxyglutamic acid (Gla) residues on the proteins.[52] Other proteins are bound by electrostatic or hydrophobic interactions. After adsorption and complex formation, precursor proteins, or zymogens, are converted to active enzymes by limited proteolysis. Reaction rates are controlled by high molecular weight protein cofactors like factors V and VIII that markedly accelerate proteolysis. In each case, the cleavage of one or more relatively small peptides from the parent molecule converts it to an active protease, which then acts on another zymogen in the coagulation cascade.

INTRINSIC COAGULATION PATHWAY. The intrinsic, or contact activation, pathway of coagulation is initiated by the formation of a complex among three plasma proteins—Hageman factor (factor XII), high molecular weight kininogen (HMWK), and prekallikrein (PK) (Fig. 58–6*A*). HMWK and PK circulate in plasma as a noncovalent complex. This complex, when adsorbed onto a suitable surface, binds factor XII and slowly converts some of it to an active enzymatic form called factor XIIa (Fig. 58–6*B*). Factor XIIa then converts a second component of the complex, PK, to kallikrein (Fig. 58–6*C*). The resulting protease, kallikrein, both liberates the vasoactive peptide bradykinin from the third member of the complex, HMWK, and accelerates the conversion of factor XII to XIIa (Fig. 58–6*D*). In a subsequent reaction, factor XI is attached to this trimolecular complex and converted to its active form, XIa, by the proteolytic action of surface-bound XIIa.

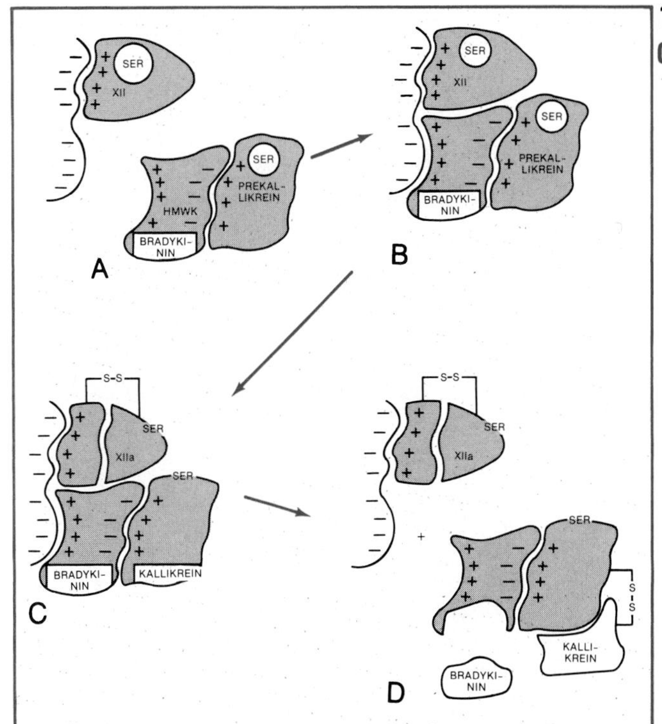

FIGURE 58–6. Reactions comprising the contact activation or intrinsic pathway of coagulation. *A* and *B*, High molecular weight kininogen (HMWK) and prekallikrein (PK), which circulate as a noncovalent complex, attach to a surface such as the vascular subendothelium along with Hageman factor (factor XII). *C, D*, This converts PK to the active serine protease kallikrein, which then converts factor XII to its active form, XIIa, and also liberates bradykinin from HMWK. The subsequent reaction (not shown in the figure) is between surface-bound XIIa and factor XI, which initiates coagulation. (From Verstraete, M., and Vermylen, J.: Thrombosis. Oxford, Pergamon Press, 1984, p. 27.)

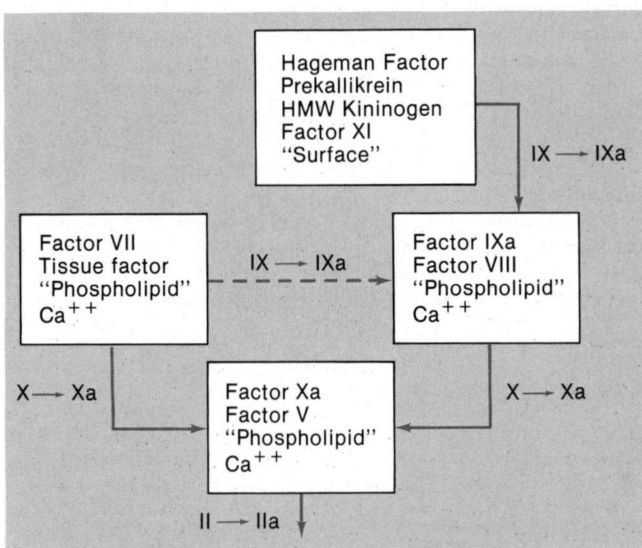

FIGURE 58–5. Major enzyme complexes of the coagulation cascade. The intrinsic, or contact activation, pathway is represented by the box at the top containing Hageman factor, prekallikrein, high molecular weight (HMW) kininogen, and factor XI and the initiating stimulus contact of blood with a "surface." The result of these interactions is formation of an enzyme, factor XIa, that converts factor IX to IXa. In the second reaction, factor IXa along with factor VIII, a source of phospholipid, and calcium assemble to convert factor X to Xa. In the extrinsic, or tissue factor–dependent, pathway, tissue factor and factor VII along with phospholipid and calcium can either directly activate factor X to Xa or activate IX. In the final reaction, factor Xa and factor V along with phospholipid and calcium convert factor II (prothrombin) to IIa (thrombin). Because both initiating pathways can activate factors IX and X, there is no need to make a distinction between intrinsic and extrinsic activation of the coagulation system. (From Mann, K. G., and Fass, D. N.: The molecular biology of blood coagulation. *In* Fairbanks, V. F. [ed.]: Current Hematology. Vol 2. New York, John Wiley & Sons, 1983, p. 347.)

EXTRINSIC COAGULATION PATHWAY. Tissue factor, a ubiquitous cellular lipoprotein, initiates the extrinsic coagulation pathway by forming a calcium-dependent complex with another protein, factor VII, a member of a group of Gla-containing coagulation proteins synthesized in the liver. After complex formation, factor VII develops proteolytic activity (VIIa), which converts factor X to its active form, Xa. The term extrinsic coagulation pathway was derived from an earlier observation that vesicles rich in tissue factor may be released into the blood from damaged tissues or cells. It is now known that endothelial cells still attached to subendothelium, along with circulating leukocytes, may express tissue factor activity and accelerate coagulation reactions after activation by agents like interleukin-1 or bacterial endotoxin.

COMMON PATHWAY. Factor X is activated by products generated by the contact activation or Hageman factor–dependent pathway as well as by the tissue factor–VII complex (Fig. 58–7). Factor XIa first converts factor IX to IXa. Factor X is then activated by IXa, in conjunction with factor VIII, by the formation of a calcium- and lipid-dependent macromolecular complex. Factor VIII has little biological activity until it is converted to VIIIa by traces of thrombin. Formation

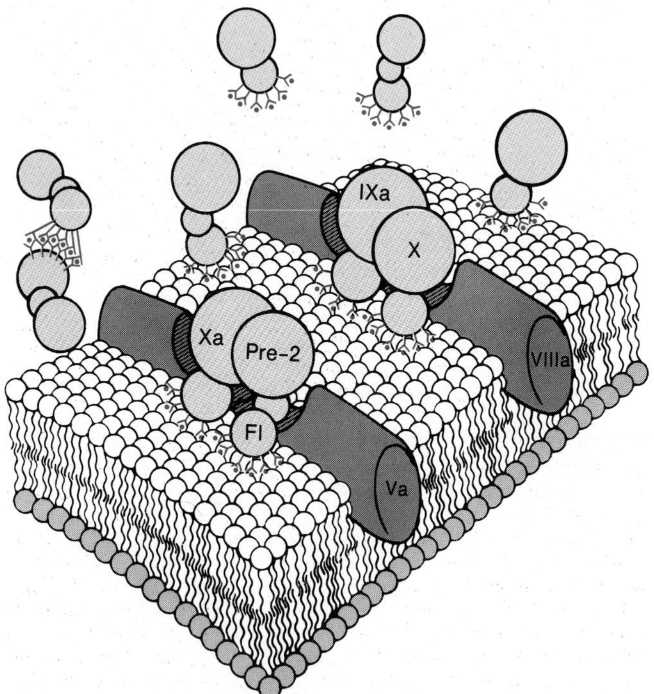

FIGURE 58-7. Hypothetical model of the prothrombinase complex and the complex responsible for factor X activation. Factors Va and VIIIa attach to a model cell membrane by hydrophobic interactions and also develop binding sites for specific coagulation factors. Factors IXa and X bind to factor VIIIa and to the membrane. Binding is partially mediated by gammacarboxyglutamic acid (Gla) residues and calcium. After its activation, factor Xa becomes part of a second adjacent complex with factor Va and prothrombin (depicted here as Pre-2). Again, Xa and prothrombin interact with the cell membrane by means of Gla residues and calcium. Thrombin is then liberated from the surface to participate in additional coagulation reactions. (From Mann, K. G., et al.: The role of factor V in the assembly of the prothrombinase complex. *In* Walz, D. A., and McCoy L. E. [eds.]: Annals of the New York Academy of Sciences. New York, 1981, p. 378.)

of the IXa–X–VIIIa complex occurs on a cell surface, probably on activated endothelial cells or platelets. In addition to activating factor X, the tissue factor–VIIa complex also may activate factor IX. This alternative pathway provides a link between the contact activation and tissue factor–dependent pathways of coagulation, and its existence may help to explain why patients with severe factor VIII or IX deficiency who have a normal tissue factor–dependent mechanism still have defective hemostasis.

Factor Xa then converts prothrombin to thrombin in conjunction with factor Va, calcium, and phospholipid (Fig. 58–7). Prothrombin conversion, which also takes place on activated platelet or endothelial surfaces, requires the assembly of a macromolecular complex among factor Va, Xa, and prothrombin. Thrombin, the product of this reaction, is a potent and versatile protease that has multiple actions in hemostasis, which include activating factors V, VIII, and XIII and binding to and activating platelets and endothelial cells. A most important function is the cleavage of peptides from the A and B chains of fibrinogen to form fibrin of thrombin monomers that subsequently polymerize into large fibrillar polymers (Fig. 58–8). Fibrin polymerization, the basis for the familiar clotting reaction, markedly changes plasma viscosity and converts blood from a sol to a gel. Polymers are initially held together by weak noncovalent bonds that are readily dissociated. They subsequently are cross-linked by a plasma transglutaminase, factor XIIIa, providing optimal mechanical stability.

LIMITING REACTIONS—THE NATURAL ANTICOAGULANTS

During normal hemostasis, only a small quantity of the coagulation protein in plasma is converted into an active protease or cofactor. The rate and extent of serine protease generation are carefully regulated by a group of inhibitor proteins that function as natural anticoagulants (Fig. 58–8). Such tight regulation is critical, since there is enough prothrombin in a single milliliter of blood, if converted to thrombin, to clot the entire volume of blood within 15 seconds. The natural anticoagulants permit coagulation to proceed locally, in response to injury, and prevent it from becoming a systemic and potentially dangerous process. The three most important natural anticoagulants are antithrombin III, protein C, and protein S. Their importance is underscored by the observation that patients with deficiency or dysfunction of any of the three proteins have a prethrombotic or hypercoagulable disorder characterized by recurrent episodes of venous and, rarely, arterial thrombosis and embolism.

ANTITHROMBIN III. This 60,000-dalton protein, which is a member of the serpin or serine protease inhibitor family of proteins, is synthesized in the liver and binds to and inactivates serine proteases within the coagulation cascade. Al-

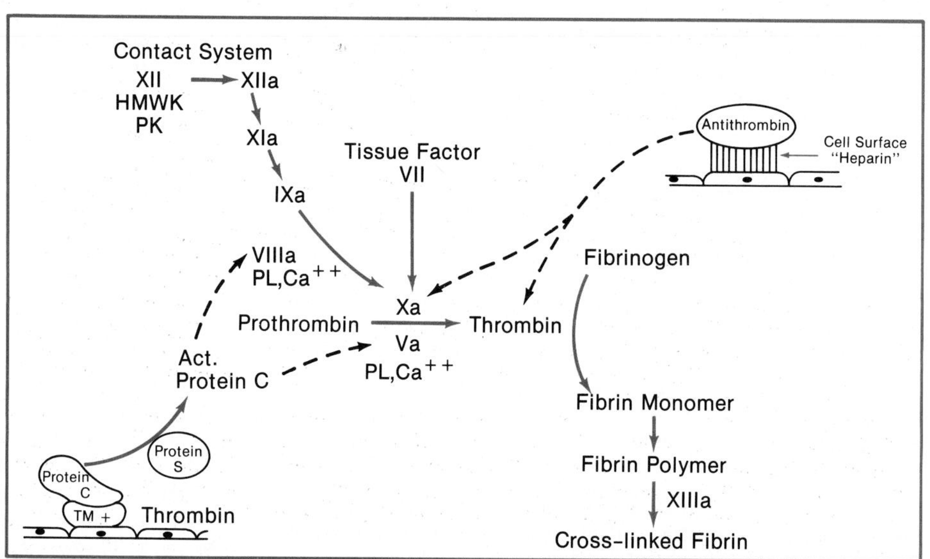

FIGURE 58-8. Overview of the entire coagulation cascade, including the limiting reactions of the natural anticoagulants. There are two major activation pathways: the intrinsic pathway, which involves factors XII, IX, and VIII, and the extrinsic, or tissue factor, system, which involves tissue factor and factor VII. Both pathways result in the conversion of inactive factor X to its active form, Xa. In the third, or common, pathway Xa converts prothrombin to thrombin in a reaction that is accelerated by factor Va. Thrombin then converts fibrinogen to fibrin monomers, which polymerize and are cross-linked by factor XIIIa, a plasma transglutaminase. The interaction of factors VIIIa, IXa, and X; the interaction of the tissue factor–VII complex with factor X; and the conversion of prothrombin to thrombin are all reactions that require phospholipid (PL) and calcium. Two major anticoagulant systems limit coagulation reactions. Antithrombin binds to thrombin, factor Xa, and other coagulation serine proteases except factor VII in a reaction that is accelerated by exogenous heparin or heparin-like molecules on endothelial cells. Protein C is activated by thrombin after it is bound to the endothelial cell protein thrombomodulin. Activated protein C and protein S inactivate the two coagulation cofactors VIIIa and Va, which also limits thrombin generation. (From Handin, R. I.: Bleeding and thrombosis. *In* Wilson, J., et al. [eds.]: Harrison's Principles of Internal Medicine. 12th ed. New York, McGraw-Hill Book Co., 1991, p. 350.)

though named for its interaction with thrombin, it also inactivates factors XIIa, XIa, Xa, and IXa by binding to a serine residue at the active site of these proteases.[53] The kinetics of the interaction vary for the different proteases but, in each case, can be accelerated many times by the addition of heparin. Heparin binds to a site on antithrombin III that is separate from the region that binds proteases, and acts as an "allosteric" regulator. After the formation of a protease–antithrombin complex, heparin is released and can bind to additional antithrombin molecules. In this way its function is analogous to that of an enzyme or catalyst. The "catalytic" acceleration of antithrombin activity by heparin, referred to as its heparin cofactor activity, accounts for the entire anticoagulant action of heparin in plasma. During normal hemostasis, antithrombin is activated by binding to heparin-like glycosaminoglycans (heparans) present on the surface of endothelial cells.

PROTEINS C AND S. The second regulatory system involves protein C, protein S, and an endothelial membrane protein, *thrombomodulin*.[54–56] When bound to thrombomodulin, protein C is converted to an active serine protease by thrombin. Activated protein C then inhibits coagulation by inactivating factors Va and VIIIa. Protein S increases the rate of proteolysis of factors Va and VIIIa by activated protein C. Activated protein C can be inhibited by another serpin plasminogen activator inhibitor 1 (PAI-1). This interaction limits access of activated protein C to Va and VIIIa.[57,58]

RHEOLOGY AND THROMBOSIS

Any discussion of hemostasis should include the effects of blood flow and vascular geometry on thrombus formation.[59] Stress, in rheological terms, is the force per unit area generated during blood flow. When this force is applied at right angles to a surface, it is referred to as "normal" stress, and when applied parallel to a surface, as tangential stress or "shear." Figure 58–9 shows a longitudinal cross section of a blood vessel, with *h* representing wall thickness and *r* the inner radius. The parabola represents the range of velocities, *V*, at which laminar "plates" of blood travel along the longitudinal axis of the vessel at varying distances (*y*) from its center. Normal or circumferential stress (S_c) can be defined mathematically as

$$S_c = Px\eta/h, \qquad (1)$$

where *P* is the distending luminal pressure. In this idealized system of laminar, nonturbulent flow through a vessel of uniform diameter, the shear or tangential stress is

$$S_t = n\eta/Y = P\ Y/2, \qquad (2)$$

where η is blood viscosity and *P* the pressure gradient per unit length of vessel. Finally, the velocity of any laminar plate can be related to the radius of the vessel, the pressure generated, blood viscosity, and vessel length, *L*, as follows:

$$\eta \times \pi Pr^4/8\ \eta L \qquad (3)$$

From Equation 3 one can determine that velocity is maximal at the center of the vessel as it is proportional to the fourth power of the radius and falls off to nearly zero at the vessel wall. In addition, this equation predicts that the greater the viscosity of the blood, the lower its velocity. In addition, from Equation 2, it is clear that an increase in viscosity (η) will increase shear stress. These concepts have some practical applications. First, because plasma proteins, erythrocytes, and platelets require some minimal time to interact with one another and with subendothelial surfaces, conditions of high viscosity and low velocity favor platelet adhesion and thrombus formation. In fact, in the venous circulation, where velocity is low, relatively minor variations in flow, when coupled with minor degrees of injury to venous endothelium, may induce thrombus formation. Venous clots also take on their typical red appearance because of the large numbers of trapped red cells and amount of fibrin that accumulate under conditions of low flow. In the more rapid arterial circulation, platelet-platelet interactions predominate, there is insufficient time for fibrin formation and red cell trapping, and thrombi appear white. Adequate quantities of vWF multimers also are critical to stabilize adhesion of platelets to the vessel wall under conditions of high flow and shear stress. A modest reduction in this protein may lead to impaired hemostasis and clinical bleeding.

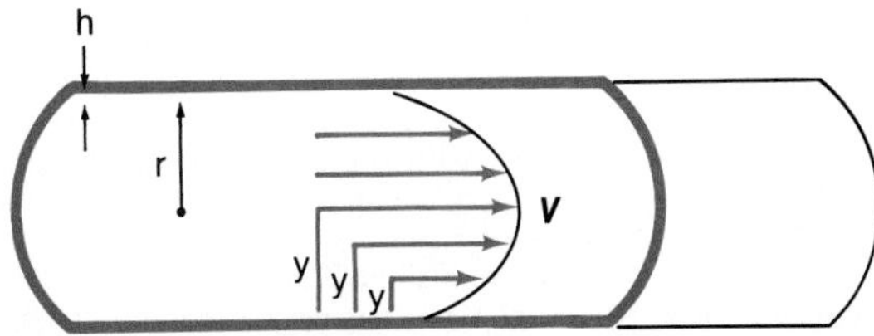

FIGURE 58–9. **Biophysical variables that affect blood shear and rheology in a model cross section of a blood vessel. h = thickness of the vessel wall; r = radius of the vessel. Blood travels at different velocities (*V*), depending on its distance (*Y*) from the vessel wall. These parameters along with measurements of blood viscosity and blood pressure can be used to calculate shear stress on the vessel wall and blood flow.**

Rheology also influences the location of vascular disease, which occurs more frequently at bifurcations. Velocity is reduced as the "plates" of flowing blood are divided. This prolongs the residence time of platelets at the vessel surface and may enhance their deposition onto subendothelium when the bifurcation site is injured. Turbulence, which may occur in a stenotic vessel, adds another variable to the analysis by producing non-Newtonian flow. This also increases the residence time of proteins and platelets, reduces velocity, enhances local viscosity, and promotes platelet and fibrin deposition near flow vortices.

Finally, rheological principles have been applied to the design of therapeutic agents. Improving blood flow and reducing blood viscosity should reduce thrombus formation. There is evidence that cerebral blood flow can be dramatically increased by a slight reduction in the hematocrit.[60] Volume expanders like dextran, which have minimal effects on coagulation reactions, may act as antithrombotic agents by improving flow and reducing viscosity.[61] It also has been suggested that defibrination with agents like *ancrod* or the defibrination that accompanies systemic fibrinolytic therapy may be beneficial, in part, because it markedly reduces blood viscosity and improves blood flow.

CLOT DISSOLUTION—THE FIBRINOLYTIC SYSTEM

The fibrinolytic system, which dissolves fibrin-thrombi and restores blood flow within obstructed blood vessels, is a critically important component of the normal hemostatic system. Orderly, localized clot lysis is achieved by the concerted actions of a complex system that includes proteolytic enzymes, specific activators, and inhibitors of both the proteases and their activators. Although there are several enzymes like leukocyte elastase, which can digest fibrin, the major protease of the fibrinolytic system is *plasmin.* Three principal activators convert the precursor zymogen plasminogen to its active form, plasmin; these are activated Hageman factor fragments, urokinase-type plasminogen activators (UKs), and t-PA. Both the rate and the extent of fibrinolysis are regulated by a circulating inhibitor of plasmin, the alpha$_2$-plasmin inhibitor, a serpin, and endothelial cell–derived inhibitors of the principal activators, the plasminogen activator inhibitors types 1 and 2 (PAI-1 and PAI-2). The fibrinolytic process usually is localized to fibrin clots because plasminogen is selectively incorporated into fibrin thrombi at the time of thrombus formation. In addition, the two endogenous activators UK and t-PA are derived from stimulated endothelial cells at the site of thrombus formation and diffuse into the adjacent thrombus.

PLASMINOGEN

This 92,000-dalton plasma glycoprotein contains 790 amino acids, including 48 cysteines that form 24 intramolecular disulfide bonds, leaving no free sulfhydryl groups. Although the tissue of origin is still debated, plasminogen synthesis has been described in both liver and kidney, and plasminogen is present in eosinophilic leukocytes. The plasma concentration is approximately 21 mg/dl and does not vary greatly during normal blood coagulation. As shown in Figure 58–10, the parent molecule (Glu-plasminogen) has a glutamic acid at its amino terminus. Variable amounts of Glu-plasminogen are converted to Lys-plasminogen by the cleavage of an 8000-dalton polypeptide. Both Glu- and Lys-plasminogen are converted to plasmin by the scission of a single Arg-Val bond,

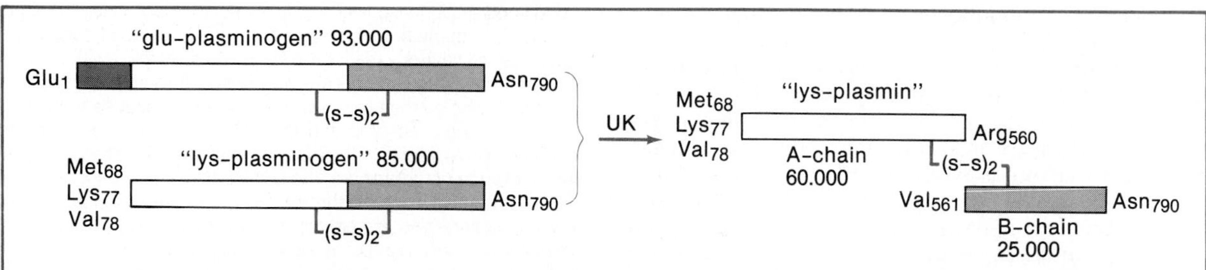

FIGURE 58–10. Molecular forms of plasminogen in plasma. The native molecule has 790 amino acids and a molecular weight of 93,000 daltons, with a glutamic acid as the initial or amino terminal amino acid residue (Glu-plasminogen). In plasma an 8000-dalton preactivation peptide is cleaved from Glu-plasminogen to produce a somewhat smaller form of plasminogen, with lysine as the amino terminal amino acid (Lys-plasminogen). Both Glu- and Lys-plasminogen circulate in plasma and can be converted to plasmin.

This requires two steps for Glu-plasminogen, cleavage of the 8000-dalton peptide, and scission of an internal peptide bond. Lys-plasminogen is activated by the internal bond scission alone. Plasmin is a two-chain molecule linked by disulfide bonds that has proteolytic activity against fibrinogen and fibrin as well as a number of other blood and cellular substrates. (Modified from Verstraete, M., and Vermylen, J.: Thrombosis. London, Pergamon Press, 1984, p. 46.)

through which the single-chain precursor is converted into a disulfide-linked, two-chain protease. Plasmin is a potent protease with broad reactivity. In addition to fibrin, it can digest fibrinogen, coagulation factors V and VIII, and platelet membrane glycoprotein Ib.

The complete covalent structure of plasminogen has been determined by direct protein sequencing and has been deduced from sequencing of plasminogen cDNA. As summarized in Figure 58–11, there are important structural similarities between plasminogen and the various plasminogen activators. Within the plasminogen molecule are five repeated regions of sequence homology that begin at the amino terminus of the molecule. These homologous repeats form looped structures held together by disulfide bonds and referred to as "kringles." (Kringles are a Danish breakfast pastry with a similar twisted, pretzel-like shape.) Plasminogen binds to fibrin through lysine binding sites located on the five nodular "kringle" domains, shown in Figure 58–11 as K_1 through K_5. These noncovalent interactions permit plasminogen to become concentrated within fibrin-rich thrombi for more effective and localized fibrinolysis.[62]

ENDOGENOUS PLASMINOGEN ACTIVATORS

(See also p. 1785)

As already mentioned, three endogenous plasminogen activators have now been identified.[63] They can be distinguished by their mechanism of plasminogen activation and the ability of fibrin to enhance their activity. Hageman factor (factor XII) fragments, generated during the early phase of coagulation, are relatively weak plasminogen activators (Fig. 58–6). Their activity is not enhanced by the adsorption of plasminogen to fibrin.

Tissue-type Plasminogen Activator

The major physiological activator is t-PA, a 70,000-dalton protein synthesized predominantly in endothelial cells. Be-

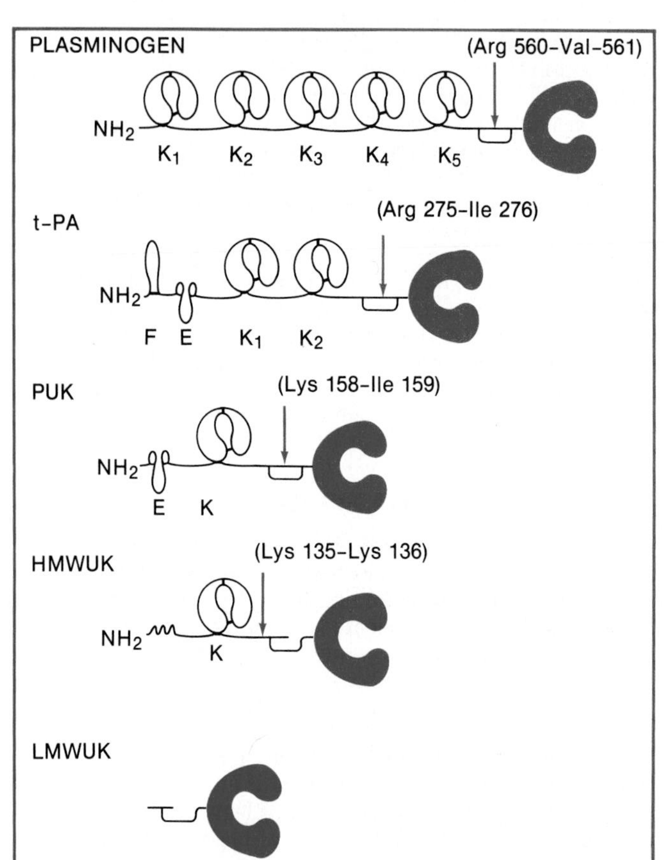

FIGURE 58–11. Structural homologies between plasminogen and the major activators of the fibrinolytic system. Plasminogen, tissue plasminogen activator (t-PA), pro-urokinase (PUK), and the high molecular weight form of urokinase (HMWUK) all contain "pretzel-like" kringle domains which are held together by disulfide bonds. In addition, t-PA contains a finger-like projection (F) at its amino (NH_2) terminus, also held together by disulfide bonds, which is homologous to a finger structure first recognized in the adhesive glycoprotein fibronectin. t-PA and PUK also contain a second slightly differently shaped projection (E) first noted in another molecule, the epidermal growth factor, and now recognized in many other proteins. The large "C"-shaped region on the right-hand end of each molecule represents the proteolytically active region. The K domains numbered 1 through 5 on various molecules and the F domains are the sites on each molecule which interact with fibrin and confer fibrin "specificity." The varying numbers of K domains, in combination with the F domains, confer differing affinities for fibrin. The arrows indicate sites in each of the proteins that are cleaved by proteolytic enzymes. Plasminogen is a single-chain zymogen or precursor which has no proteolytic activity. The scission of the peptide bond between arginine 560 and valine 561 converts it to a two-chain molecule, plasmin, which can proteolyze fibrinogen, fibrin, and various other substrates. As shown in Figure 58–10, a second peptide bond is cleared from Glu-plasminogen to produce Lys-plasminogen. Both forms are converted to plasmin. t-PA is synthesized as a single-chain form which has proteolytic activity and can activate plasminogen. It is quickly converted to a two-chain form with somewhat enhanced proteolytic activity, by the scission of a single bond between arginine 275 and isoleucine 276. PUK, unlike t-PA, has no proteolytic activity until the bond between lysine 158 and isoleucine 158 is clipped, converting it to a two-chain protease. Both HMWUK and LMWUK circulate as two-chain active proteases. Scission of a bond between lysines 135 and 136 removes the single K domain but does not appreciably alter the specificity or biological activity of UK, which has no fibrin specificity.

cause there are only trace quantities of this protein in normal plasma, it had been difficult to purify and characterize t-PA until the cDNA-encoding t-PA was cloned and the recombinant molecule expressed in heterologous cells (Fig. 58–12).[64] As shown in Figures 58–11 and 58–12, t-PA is synthesized as a single-chain molecule, which is readily converted to a two-chain form by the proteolytic cleavage of a single plasmin-sensitive site. Unlike most other serine proteases, both the single-chain and the two-chain forms have proteolytic activity. t-PA is a relatively selective or fibrin-specific activator, since it converts plasminogen to plasmin two to three orders of magnitude more efficiently in vitro in the presence of fibrin than in plasma free of fibrin. Based on preliminary clinical studies, a similar degree of specificity may not be achieved in vivo. As shown in Figure 58–11, the A chain of t-PA, which is derived from the NH_2 terminal portion of single-chain t-PA, has a molecular weight of 40,000 daltons and contains two "kringle" domains (K_1 and K_2 in Fig. 58–11), a fibronectin-like "finger" domain, and an epidermal growth factor domain (EGF). The fibronectin-like finger domain is indicated in Figure 58–11 as F and the EGF homolog as E. The K_2 and F domains of t-PA both interact with fibrin. The smaller (30,000-dalton) B chain of t-PA contains the proteolytic site that converts plasminogen to plasmin. The B chain is homologous to the active site of other serine proteases like elastase, urokinase, trypsin, and plasmin.

Urokinase-type Plasminogen Activators

Endothelial and renal tubular epithelial cells synthesize urokinase-type plasminogen activators (u-PAs) in addition to t-PA. The u-PAs are immunologically distinct from t-PA,[54] but convert plasminogen to plasmin by hydrolyzing the same Arg-Val bond as t-PA. They are derived from a parent single-chain molecule, single-chain u-PA, or scu-PA (also called pro-urokinase or PUK). scu-PA has a molecular weight of 54,000 daltons and only minimal proteolytic activity in the absence of fibrin. scu-PA is quantitatively converted to the high molecular weight two-chain form (HMW-tc-UK), which has full proteolytic activity.[65,66] The ability to activate plasminogen is somewhat enhanced by the presence of fibrin. HMW-tc-UK is converted to a lower molecular weight species of 33,000 daltons (LMW-tc-UK) that is not fibrin-specific, but is proteolytically active. scu-PA and HMW-tc-UK have a single kringle domain (K), like t-PA, although its role in conferring fibrin specificity has not been established. Fibrin selectivity may be conferred by an increased affinity for plasminogen bound to internal lysine sites on fibrin that are exposed by partial clot lysis.[55] Because scu-PA has only minimal proteolytic activity, the mechanism by which it activates plasminogen in a relatively fibrin-specific manner is not fully understood. One possible explanation is that t-PA secreted from endothelial cells in the vicinity of a thrombus generates small quantities of plasmin which, in turn, rapidly converts scu-PA to HMW-tc-UK, and thereby activates additional plasminogen.

Endogenous Inhibitors of Fibrinolysis

PLASMINOGEN ACTIVATOR INHIBITORS. Activity of the endogenous fibrinolytic system is carefully regulated. Endothelial cells and platelets both secrete a plasminogen activator inhibitor (PAI-1) that irreversibly inactivates t-PA and UK[67] monocytes, and placental cells also secrete a second species, PAI-2, that is a more selective inhibitor of u-PA than of

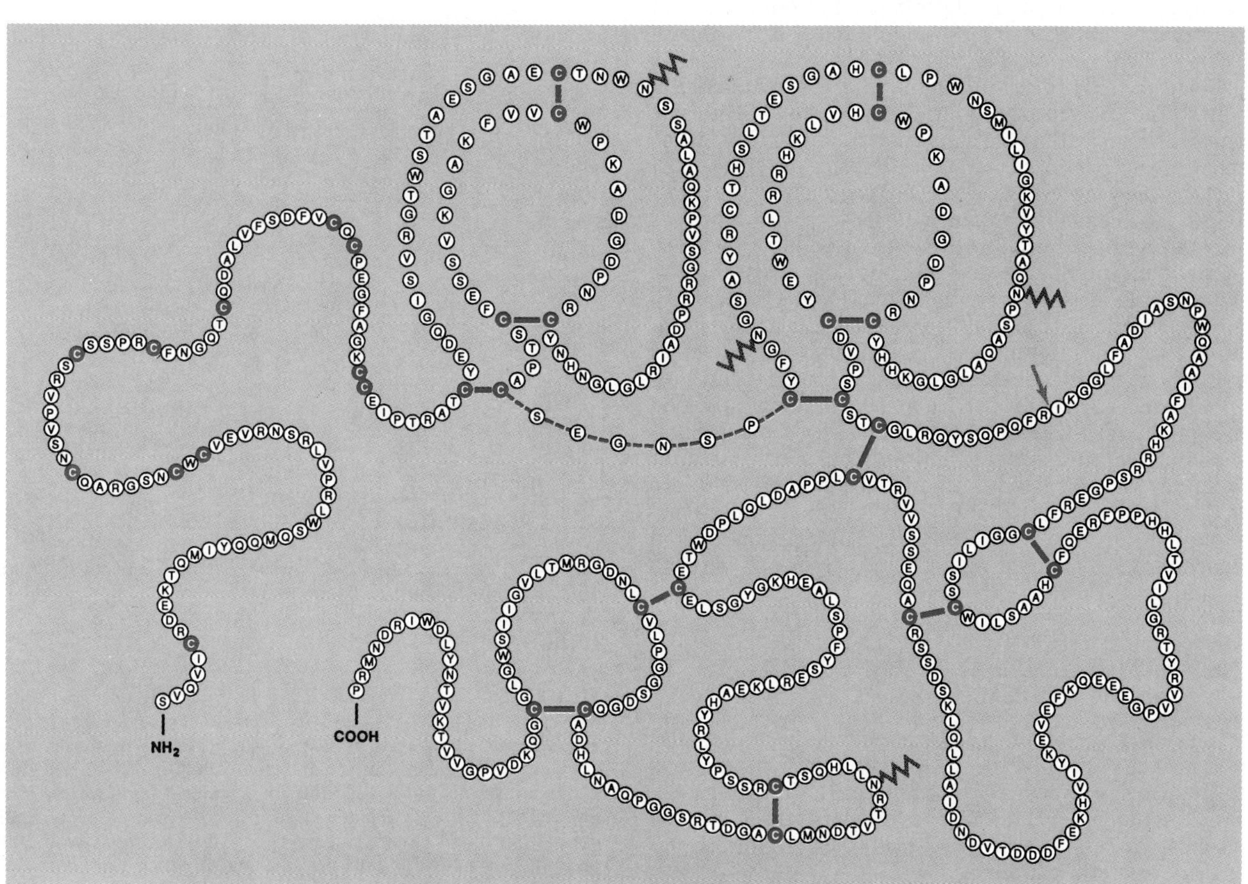

FIGURE 58–12. Structure of tissue plasminogen activator deduced from cDNA cloning and sequencing. The one-letter abbreviations for amino acid residues are used. Solid bars mark sites for potential disulfide bonds between cysteine residues, and zigzag lines mark attachment sites for *N*-linked carbohydrate. The arrow marks the position of the bond scission, which converts one-chain t-PA to the two-chain form. Finally, the broken line indicates the short stretch of six amino acids that connects the two kringle domains. (From Pennica, D., et al.: Cloning and expression of human tissue-type plasminogen activator cDNA in *E. coli.* Nature *301*:214, 1983.)

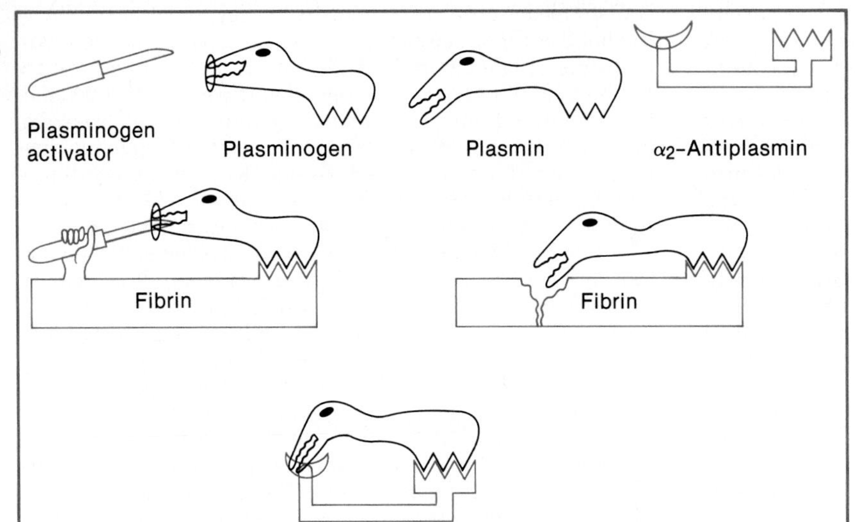

FIGURE 58–13. Schematic view of the interactions among a plasminogen activator (such as tissue plasminogen activator, which binds to fibrin), a fibrin clot, and the alpha$_2$-plasmin inhibitor. The plasminogen activator both binds to fibrin and converts fibrin-bound plasminogen to the active protease plasmin. Plasmin then digests the fibrin clot. Alpha$_2$-plasmin inhibitor binds to and inhibits free plasmin but cannot neutralize plasmin when it is bound to the fibrin clot, since it must bind to both the protease active site and the fibrin-binding site. This mechanism helps to limit fibrinolysis to areas of fibrin clot formation and prevents plasmin from entering the circulation. (From Verstraete, M., and Vermylen, J.: Thrombosis. London, Pergamon Press, 1984, p. 43.)

t-PA. The PAIs are structurally homologous to other serpins such as alpha$_1$-antitrypsin and antithrombin III.

ALPHA$_2$-PLASMIN INHIBITOR. As shown in Figure 58–13, another molecule circulating in plasma, alpha$_2$-plasmin inhibitor (α_2PI), rapidly neutralizes free plasmin.[68] However, the lysine-binding "kringle" domains as well as the active-site serine of plasmin must be available for binding and neutralization by α_2PI. Thus, when it is bound to fibrin, plasmin is protected from the neutralizing effect of α_2PI. This helps to sustain the fibrinolytic activity of plasmin within a thrombus and minimizes systemic fibrinolysis, since α_2PI rapidly neutralizes any release of "free" plasmin. α_2PI also may inhibit fibrinolysis by competing for lysine-binding sites on fibrinogen.

The fibrin clot plays a key role in the regulation of fibrinolysis. Fibrin binds plasminogen, enriching this key fibrinolytic enzyme precursor within the clot. The presence of fibrin also enhances the activity of t-PA and inhibits the activity of α_2PI and PAI-1. Finally, products generated during fibrin clot formation, such as thrombin, enhance the local release of t-PA as well as its principal inhibitor PAI-1 from endothelial cells. The surface of endothelial and mononuclear cells and the platelet also provide sites for enhanced or more efficient conversion of plasminogen to plasmin. These cells express specific surface receptors for plasminogen and for t-PA, as well as u-PA. Binding to these receptors enhances plasminogen activation. This cell surface property may help to maintain blood fluidity, facilitate production of inflammatory mediators on the mononuclear cell surface, and enhance clot lysis after tissue injury. Unregulated systemic fibrinolysis is a rare event, and occurs only in patients with disseminated intravascular coagulation, those with advanced liver disease, and those receiving systemic infusions of fibrinolytic activators to lyse pathological thrombi.

SUMMARY OF COAGULATION AND FIBRINOLYTIC REACTIONS

The plasma coagulation and fibrinolytic systems are complicated because they involve the closely linked interactions of multiple serine proteases. In addition, the reactions are carefully regulated by plasma and cell surface activators, plasma cofactors, and a series of naturally occurring anticoagulants or fibrinolytic inhibitors.

The major coagulation reactions are summarized in Figure 58–8 and the fibrinolytic pathway in Figure 58–14. Two major stimuli initiate coagulation — contact of blood with vascular subendothelium and liberation of tissue thromboplastin or tissue factor. The net result of activation of these two pathways is the generation of thrombin, a potent protease that converts fibrinogen to fibrin. Fibrin then polymerizes and is cross-linked to form a stable clot. There are two critical plasma cofactors — factors Va and VIIIa — that regulate the rates of factor Xa generation by the contact or intrinsic pathway and the rate of thrombin generation from Xa produced by either the extrinsic or the intrinsic pathway. The most impor-

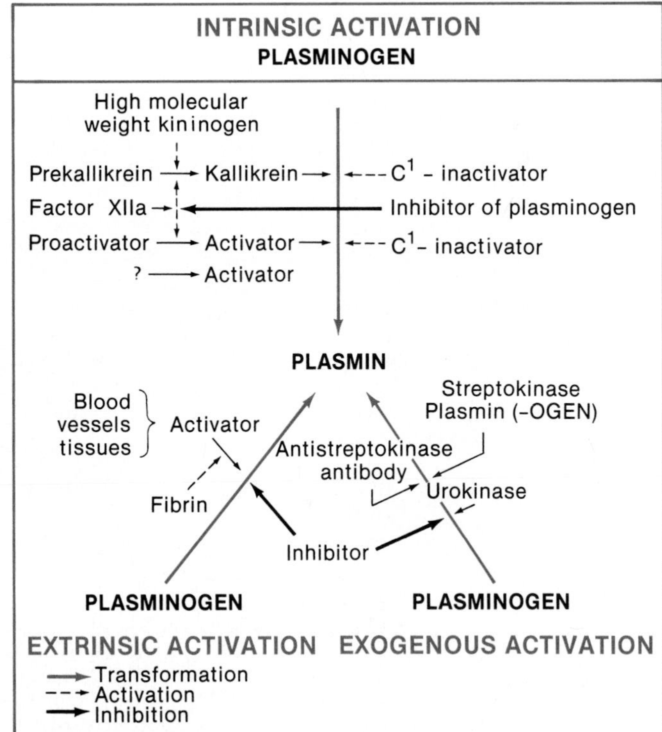

FIGURE 58–14. Overview of the fibrinolytic pathways. There are three principal pathways for the conversion of plasminogen to plasmin. The intrinsic pathway is activated during the early phases of blood coagulation by Hageman factor fragments. This is a relatively weak activation system of questionable physiological significance. The most important physiological mechanism is the extrinsic pathway. Endothelial cells in blood vessels release two fibrin-specific activators, tissue plasminogen activator and pro-urokinase, which rapidly and effectively convert plasminogen to plasmin. Finally, several potential exogenous activators are used in fibrinolytic therapy. The bacterial protein streptokinase and the urinary product urokinase are two standard nonspecific activators. In addition, the two physiological and fibrin-specific activators, tissue plasminogen activator and prourokinase, are now available and being used in clinical trials. (From Verstraete, M., and Vermylen, J.: Thrombosis. London, Pergamon Press, 1984, p. 41.)

tant naturally occurring anticoagulants are antithrombin III, which is activated by cell surface heparin-like molecules (heparans) and rapidly neutralizes coagulation proteases, and protein C, which is activated by thrombin and cell surface thrombomodulin. Along with protein S, activated protein C inactivates factors Va and VIIIa.

The fibrinolytic system may be activated by two endogenous substances: t-PA and the u-PAs. In each case activation is accomplished by converting plasminogen to plasmin directly. Plasmin then digests fibrin thrombi. The rate of plasminogen activation by t-PA, scu-PA, or HMW-tc-UK is enhanced by the presence of fibrin and permits the activation process to be localized to areas that contain fibrin thrombi. t-PA and scu-PA are secreted from endothelial cells after the generation of thrombin. Fibrinolytic activity is regulated at two levels. First, there is endothelial PAI (PAI-1), which may bind to any free plasminogen activator. In addition, there is another serpin, α_2PI, which binds to any free plasmin and rapidly neutralizes its proteolytic activity. In normal hemostasis, fibrinolysis is activated shortly after thrombus formation to restore vessel patency and reestablish normal blood flow rapidly.

EVALUATION OF HEMOSTASIS IN CARDIOVASCULAR PATIENTS

Many patients with cardiovascular disorders require corrective surgery or invasive diagnostic and therapeutic procedures such as cardiac catheterization, coronary angiography, or transluminal angioplasty. Although special precautions usually are not necessary, a specific evaluation of the hemostatic system may be necessary in three clinical situations. First, some patients may have a suspected or poorly documented hemorrhagic disorder that may have produced only minimal symptoms but might cause excess bleeding after an invasive diagnostic or surgical procedure. For example, many patients with mild von Willebrand's disease have little or no spontaneous bleeding but may bleed profusely after an operation. Second, the antiplatelet or anticoagulant medications administered to cardiac patients increase their risk of hemorrhage. This problem is especially serious when patients are to undergo invasive cardiovascular or surgical procedures, since they may have few bleeding symptoms before surgery. Finally, although most cardiovascular disorders do not increase the risk of hemorrhage, certain types of cardiac disease perturb hemostasis and cause bleeding.

Although it may be tempting to order a battery of screening laboratory tests on all cardiac patients with a suspected hemorrhagic disorder, the most useful part of the evaluation is still a careful history. For example, a past history of excessive bleeding after dental extractions or tonsillectomy, bleeding after minor trauma, recurrent epistaxis, abnormal menses, or recurrent joint or muscle bleeding without antecedent trauma all suggest an inherited coagulation disorder. Many, but not all, patients also have a family history of bleeding. Finally, a careful drug history is essential, since many commonly used drugs, including aspirin and other nonsteroidal antiinflammatory agents, may cause platelet dysfunction and clinical bleeding.

Patients with deficits in platelet number or function usually bleed into the skin and mucous membranes and may present with epistaxis, gastrointestinal bleeding, or abnormal menses. Bleeding develops immediately after surgery or trauma and may respond to local pressure or packing. The most common platelet disorders are (1) thrombocytopenia, (2) platelet dysfunction secondary to ingestion of medications such as aspirin, and (3) von Willebrand's disease. Platelet function is readily evaluated by a platelet count and bleeding time. Current techniques for measuring bleeding time are reproducible and sensitive and can detect even mild platelet dysfunction. In most laboratories, the average bleeding time is 5 ± 2 (S.D.) min, so that a value greater than 10 min probably indicates impaired primary hemostasis.

In contrast, in patients with plasma coagulation defects, musculoskeletal and soft tissue bleeding occurs hours or days after surgery or trauma, and usually requires specific replacement therapy. The most common inherited abnormalities are the hemophilias—specifically, deficiencies in the activity of factors VIII and IX, which are sex-linked recessive disorders that cause recurrent hemorrhage and joint deformity. The most common acquired defects are those associated with (1) vitamin K deficiency, (2) liver disease, and (3) disseminated intravascular coagulation (DIC).

The integrity of the plasma coagulation system is readily assessed with a group of simple laboratory tests—the partial thromboplastin time (PTT), prothrombin time (PT), and, in some cases, thrombin time (TT) or fibrinogen level. In rare cases additional assays of clot solubility and fibrin cross-linking may be useful. The PTT exclusively measures the activity of coagulation factors in the intrinsic or contact activation pathway, which include Hageman factor (factor XII), high molecular weight kininogen, prekallikrein, and factors XI, IX, and VIII (Fig. 58–8). The PT, which is used to assay the extrinsic or tissue factor–dependent pathway of coagulation, exclusively measures factor VII. The PT and PTT both assess the integrity of factors in the common pathway, which include factors X and V, prothrombin, and fibrinogen. When a patient has an isolated increase in either the PT or the PTT, the group of factors that are potentially defective can be readily pinpointed. When both PT and PTT are prolonged, fibrinogen level or function also should be assessed, since either reduced or dysfunctional fibrinogen or a common pathway defect involving factor X or V or prothrombin will prolong both tests. Defective fibrin cross-linking and abnormal clot solubility are extremely rare and should be suspected only when a patient has a severe bleeding disorder with a normal PT and PTT.

THROMBOCYTOPENIA

The platelet count normally ranges between 150,000 and 450,000/μl. Low counts may be due to decreased marrow production, accelerated peripheral destruction, or platelet sequestration in an enlarged spleen. The most common causes of decreased production are exposure to marrow toxins, including chemotherapeutic agents, binge consumption of alcohol, and thiazide diuretics. Accelerated destruction can occur from platelet interaction with a prosthetic valve, Dacron vascular grafts or intracardiac patches, or activation of the coagulation system and platelet entrapment in fibrin thrombi. This is particularly prominent in patients with DIC but also occurs in disorders like thrombotic thrombocytopenic purpura and the hemolytic uremic syndrome. Finally, destruction may result from the interaction of antibodies or immune complexes with the platelet surface. Antibodies may arise in response to viral infections or the administration of drugs like quinidine, procainamide, or heparin.

PLATELET DYSFUNCTION

The most common cause of platelet dysfunction is the ingestion of aspirin and related nonsteroidal antiinflammatory agents. Patients usually have a mildly prolonged bleeding time, although in some susceptible individuals bleeding time may be as long as 20 to 30 minutes. This is accompanied by reduced platelet aggregation in response to agents like collagen, ADP, or epinephrine. Aspirin and the nonsteroidal antiinflammatory drugs inhibit platelet synthesis of TxA_2 and other eicosanoids by inhibiting platelet cyclo-oxygenase. Aspirin irreversibly acetylates cyclo-oxygenase; because the platelets cannot synthesize new enzyme, hemostasis is impaired for 5 to 7 days after a single dose of aspirin. The other common nonsteroidal compounds like indomethacin and ibuprofen are competitive inhibitors of cyclo-oxygenase, and induce transient and dose-dependent inhibition of the enzyme. Administration of other drugs, including large doses of penicillin G or semisynthetic penicillins, also may impair platelet function. In addition, certain metabolic disturbances, including uremia, may impair platelet adhesion, release, and aggregation.

VON WILLEBRAND'S DISEASE

The most common inherited defect of primary hemostasis is von Willebrand's disease, which affects as many as 1 in 800 to 1000 persons in the general population.[69] Patients almost always have a prolonged bleeding time; normal platelet aggregation with ADP, epinephrine, and collagen;

and variable defects in vWF concentration and function. In the most common form, type I, vWF content is modestly reduced to less than 50 per cent of normal. There is a parallel reduction in biological activity, as measured by ristocetin-dependent platelet agglutination, and in factor VIII activity, since vWF serves as the intravascular carrier for this factor. Less commonly, patients have variant syndromes (type II) characterized by a severe reduction in vWF activity despite a normal quantity of circulating protein. Patients with von Willebrand variants have a selective loss of the largest and most hemostatically effective multimers.[70] In type IIa disease, this is due to the rapid proteolysis and catabolism of genetically altered forms of vWF after normal synthesis. In type IIb disease, the large multimers spontaneously bind to circulating platelets, causing intravascular aggregation and mild thrombocytopenia. Rarely, patients will present with type III disease, in which there is an almost total absence of antigen or activity. These patients probably have homozygous or doubly heterozygous forms of von Willebrand's disease. No patient with von Willebrand's disease should receive antiplatelet agents, and all patients require treatment before surgery or cardiac catheterization with either cryoprecipitate, which replaces vWF, or 1-deamino-8-D-arginine vasopressin (DDAVP), which can transiently raise vWF levels and improve hemostasis in type I patients.[71]

HEMOPHILIA AND RELATED COAGULATION DEFECTS

Deficiencies in factors VIII and IX are the two most common inherited coagulation disorders. They are both X-linked recessive traits and cause recurrent musculoskeletal bleeding and hemarthroses in male patients. There is a close relation between factor level and clinical severity. Patients with levels of less than 1 per cent have severe disease and bleed frequently, even after minimal trauma; those with 1 to 5 per cent have more moderate disease; and those with greater than 5 per cent activity have mild disease with infrequent bleeding. Patients with factor VIII or IX levels above 15 to 20 per cent may be especially difficult to diagnose, since bleeding may occur only after major trauma or surgery. The third most common disorder is factor XI deficiency, an autosomal recessive trait frequently found among Ashkenazi Jews. Hemarthroses are uncommon, and many patients present with postoperative bleeding. There is little correlation between factor XI activity or antigenic level and clinical severity. All these disorders cause an increase in PTT with no change in PT. It is of interest that in patients with deficiencies in factors XII, HMWK, and PK, PTT is markedly prolonged but bleeding does not occur. Patients with true hemorrhagic disorders are treated with plasma fractions (VIII and IX deficiency) or fresh frozen plasma (XI deficiency), whereas those with laboratory abnormalities of no clinical significance (XII, HMWK, and PK deficiency) do not require therapy.

VITAMIN K DEFICIENCY AND LIVER DISEASE

Patients with biliary obstruction, liver disease, or inadequate food intake and those receiving broad-spectrum antibiotics may rapidly become deficient in vitamin K. The earliest manifestation of vitamin K deficiency is prolongation of the PT due to a fall in the factor VII level. Later, as the other prothrombin complex proteins with a longer half-life decline, the PTT also becomes prolonged. Patients should rapidly be treated with parenteral vitamin K, which can reverse the hemostatic defect in 8 to 10 hours. More rapid correction can be achieved with infusion of fresh frozen plasma. In contrast, patients with liver disease have a more complex coagulation defect, with a combination of vitamin K deficiency, impaired production of multiple coagulation factors, including fibrinogen, production of abnormal clotting proteins, systemic fibrinolysis, intravascular coagulation, and thrombocytopenia secondary to splenomegaly and platelet sequestration. These patients do not tolerate therapy with prothrombin complex concentrates, many of which contain trace quantities of activated coagulation factors, since they cannot clear activated coagulation proteins effectively. Inadvertent infusion has caused fatal thromboembolism. The best therapy for these patients is a combination of vitamin K, platelet concentrates, and fresh frozen plasma.

DISSEMINATED INTRAVASCULAR COAGULATION (DIC)

DIC begins as a thrombotic disorder with the rapid generation of thrombin, extensive fibrin deposition in the microvasculature, and intense secondary fibrinolysis. In some patients this leads to thrombosis of peripheral vessels and tissue damage. If untreated, there is progressive depletion of coagulation proteins and platelets, and diffuse hemorrhage. Various pathological events trigger DIC, including tissue damage from extreme heat, cold, or trauma; malignant tumors; bacterial or viral infections; extensive vascular malformations (Kasabach-Merritt syndrome); and obstetrical mishaps such as abruptio placentae. Treatment of DIC should focus on identifying and removing the triggering mechanism. Plasma and platelet transfusions are indicated to stop diffuse bleeding, and heparin is used to treat patients with microvascular thrombosis. Occasionally heparin also is administered to patients with intractable bleeding despite adequate plasma and platelet replacement.

CARDIAC DISORDERS WITH HEMOSTATIC DEFECTS

As previously mentioned, certain cardiovascular disorders may impair hemostasis. For example, patients with chronic right-sided heart failure may develop liver dysfunction and cardiac cirrhosis. This results in impaired vitamin K absorption, impaired production of the prothrombin complex proteins, and thrombocytopenia from splenomegaly and platelet sequestration. Patients with severe cyanotic congenital heart disease, who have a markedly expanded red cell volume and increased whole blood viscosity, may develop a DIC-like syndrome characterized by thrombocytopenia, shortened platelet survival, and increased consumption of fibrinogen and other coagulation proteins. The factors which trigger DIC in this setting are unknown, although reduced blood flow and increased viscosity because of the marked increase in red cell mass are implicated. The coagulation abnormalities are corrected by red cell removal and plasma replacement.[72] Patients with acute bacterial endocarditis may develop subclinical DIC, which may be exacerbated by insertion of a prosthetic valve. Patients undergoing cardiopulmonary bypass may develop a complex platelet disorder that can cause postoperative bleeding. Platelet dysfunction is due to platelet activation and secretion during bypass and plasmin-mediated proteolysis of glycoproteins Ib/IX and IIb/IIIa.[73]

EVALUATION OF THROMBOTIC AND PRETHROMBOTIC PATIENTS

Although the clinical and laboratory evaluation of hemorrhagic disorders has become straightforward, there are, as yet, no clinically useful laboratory tests that detect either subclinical thrombosis or the prethrombotic state. Several tests have been devised to measure platelet activation in patients with thrombosis and vascular disease. First, intravascular platelet survival, as measured by the infusion of autologous radiolabeled platelets, is shortened in patients with arterial vascular disease as well as in patients with vascular grafts, arteriovenous shunts, and prosthetic cardiac valves.[74] There also is evidence that this shortened survival may be corrected by the administration of antiplatelet agents.[75] The plasma content of platelet alpha granule proteins such as platelet factor 4 (PF-4) and β-thromboglobulin (β-TG) is increased in patients with thrombosis or embolism but usually is not elevated in patients with prethrombotic disorder.[76,77] These radioimmunoassays are difficult to standardize, since their interpretation depends on the ability to totally suppress the secretion of platelet proteins during blood collection. In addition, extraneous metabolic factors that do not affect platelet activation and release may affect plasma measurements. PF-4 has a very short intravascular half-life, since it has a high affinity for glycosaminoglycans and binds to heparans on the surface of endothelial cells. The administration of heparin is accompanied by a transient rise in plasma PF-4 as the endothelial cell surface pool of PF-4 binds to intravascular heparin.[78] In contrast, β-TG, which does not bind to the endothelial cell, is cleared exclusively by a renal mechanism. Thus, the plasma β-TG level is inversely related to creatinine clearance and increases with serum creatinine independent of platelet activation.[79] Measuring β-TG levels to monitor platelet activation may therefore prove inaccurate in patients with renal insufficiency.[80]

Laboratory tests that detect coagulation system activation rather than platelet activation, although equally cumbersome, may be more useful. The pioneering studies of Nossel and colleagues demonstrated an increase in fibrinopeptide A (FPA), one of the peptides cleaved from fibrinogen by thrombin, in patients with deep venous thrombosis and pulmonary embolism.[81] The elevated FPA level returns to normal after the administration of heparin. More recent studies have used radioimmunoassays for a prothrombin activation fragment and for circulating thrombin–antithrombin complexes.[82] Both products are elevated in patients with thromboembolism. The ambient levels of prothrombin fragment and thrombin–antithrombin complex also are elevated in elderly patients with vascular disease and in patients with inherited prethrombotic disorders like antithrombin III or protein C deficiency. The protein elevations in these patients can be suppressed by the administration of warfarin-type anticoagulants. These studies provide the first definitive evidence for activation of the coagulation system in patients with inherited or acquired prethrombotic disorders as well as in patients with asymptomatic vascular disease. However, despite these promising results, neither of the tests is yet available in routine clinical laboratories, since they require specialized reagents and meticulous venipuncture technique.

PRETHROMBOTIC OR HYPERCOAGULABLE DISORDERS

There are no clearly identified disorders in which well-documented abnormalities in platelet function can be linked to arterial or venous thrombosis. Certain patients with myeloproliferative disorders and patients with Types I and II diabetes mellitus are said to have "hyperactive" platelets based on standard platelet aggregation assays.[83] In addition, there is evidence that lipid abnormalities such as those seen in familial hypercholesterolemia may increase platelet membrane cholesterol content, decrease membrane fluidity, and enhance platelet reactivity to agonists in vitro.[84] Patients with homozygous homocystinuria clearly have an increased incidence of cerebrovascular thrombosis and develop premature atherosclerosis.[85] In some studies intravascular platelet survival also was shown to be reduced in patients with homocystinuria.[86] These patients are readily recognized because they may have a "marfanoid" body habitus (resembling the Marfan syndrome), ectopia lentis, and mild mental retardation. In laboratory animals, infusion of homocysteine induces similar arterial lesions, which are accompanied by patchy desquamation of endothelial cells. Platelets then adhere to exposed subendothelium and induce smooth muscle cell proliferation and vascular lesions. There also is evidence that environmental changes can enhance platelet reactivity. One group has reported that the circadian variation in incidence of myocardial infarction is accompanied by a diurnal variation in platelet aggregation in vitro.[87]

DEFICIENCY OR DYSFUNCTION OF THE NATURAL ANTICOAGULANTS

The most thoroughly characterized of the prethrombotic or hypercoagulable disorders are those caused by inherited deficiency or dysfunction of one of three natural anticoagulants: antithrombin III, protein C, or protein S.[88–90] The true incidence of these disorders in the general population is not clear, although preliminary surveys of antithrombin III levels have suggested an incidence of antithrombin III deficiency as high as 1 in 2000 persons. When the clinical experience of large centers that treat venous thromboembolism is reviewed, the congenital disorders identified to date account for no more than 20 per cent of patients with recurrent venous thromboembolism and fewer than 5 per cent of all patients with deep venous thrombosis.

CLINICAL MANIFESTATIONS. Patients with a congenital deficiency of any one of the natural anticoagulants present with remarkably similar histories of familial, recurrent venous thrombosis and pulmonary embolism. Rarely, these patients also have arterial thrombosis. Thromboembolic events are uncommon in infancy and childhood. The incidence of venous thrombosis and pulmonary embolism increases during each ensuing decade, and 90 per cent of patients will have had a thromboembolic episode by the third decade of life. Each of the three abnormalities usually is inherited as an autosomal dominant trait, although a few patients with homozygous protein C deficiency have now been identified. These rare patients become symptomatic shortly after birth and develop neonatal purpura fulminans and DIC.[91] Patients with the heterozygous or autosomal dominant forms of antithrombin III, protein C, or protein S deficiency have only a modestly decreased level of circulating protein. In fact, in many cases, values are just below the normal range. This is quite different from the majority of the X-linked or autosomal recessive coagulation protein disorders, in which patients are not symptomatic until levels are well below normal. Thus, it is important to pay attention to modest deficiencies in the natural anticoagulants.

To date, most patients with antithrombin III deficiency have had a modest reduction in antithrombin level, and no cases of homozygous antithrombin deficiency have been reported. However, families have been identified who have dysfunctional antithrombin molecules. In these cases, the plasma antithrombin level is normal based on immunoassay even though the dysfunctional molecule may not neutralize thrombin effectively or may not bind or become activated by heparin.[92] Effective screening of patients with suspected antithrombin deficiency must include both an immunoassay for total content of the protein and functional assays that measure both the thrombin-neutralizing and heparin cofactor activities of the protein. Families with protein C and S deficiency have shown either a reduction in protein or dysfunctional molecules. Accurate immunoassays for protein C and S are readily available. Functional assay of proteins is complicated by the partitioning of protein S into two compartments—free (active) and bound to C4 binding protein (inactive).

MANAGEMENT. Any patients with symptomatic thromboembolism should be treated acutely with heparin and then placed on an oral anticoagulant. To prevent recurrent thromboembolism, which may be fatal, patients should remain on anticoagulants for life. The only group who may not respond to acute heparin therapy are those rare patients with antithrombin variants that are not activated by heparin. In these cases, patients also should receive infusions of plasma or antithrombin concentrates to provide a source of normal antithrombin. Treatment of protein C and S deficiencies poses a special problem, since administration of warfarin to these patients may further depress protein C and S levels and increase the risk of thrombosis. This is thought to be the mechanism underlying hemorrhagic skin necrosis, a rare complication of warfarin therapy.[93] In several retrospective surveys, all identified cases have had protein C deficiency. Patients with either abnormality who require anticoagulant therapy should receive plasma infusions to raise the protein C or S level or should continue anticoagulation with heparin during the first week of warfarin administration.

It is important to carry out thorough family studies and identify all the affected members of a kindred who are deficient in the natural anticoagulants. Asymptomatic family members, particularly those under the age of 30, need not be placed on oral anticoagulants; however, they should receive prophylactic plasma or antithrombin concentrate replacement and perhaps heparin therapy during any period of prolonged immobility owing to a fracture, trauma, or surgery.

OTHER CAUSES OF VENOUS AND ARTERIAL THROMBOSIS

The inherited prethrombotic disorders account for a small but important fraction of patients with thromboembolism. They also provide interesting model systems in which the relation betweeen a discrete molecular defect and thrombosis can be accurately correlated. In the majority of patients, however, the etiology or pathophysiology remains unclear. Nonetheless, certain acquired disorders or physiological states predispose patients to the development of venous thrombosis. Immobilization, especially when coupled with trauma or surgery, may precipitate deep venous thrombosis. In most patients, the thrombi are small and limited to the calf veins. Proximal extension to the femoral system greatly increases the risk of pulmonary embolism.[94] Calf vein thrombi can be detected by venography as well as by Doppler flow and impedance plethysmographic measurements. Patients with certain primary or metastatic malignancies, particularly those with cancer arising in the pancreas, stomach, and kidney, as well as patients with chronic congestive heart failure or women who take oral contraceptives, are at increased risk for venous thrombosis and embolism. The association of malignancy and thromboembolism has been referred to as *Trousseau's syndrome,* and occasionally the thromboembolic complications may present well before the tumor can be diagnosed. In most of these cases, the pathological mechanism is unclear. A combination of tissue factor generation from tumor or damaged tissue and venous stasis may explain many cases of thrombosis in surgical and cancer patients. Oral contraceptive use also lowers antithrombin III levels and may place some patients in the symptomatic range.[95]

Arterial thrombosis seldom occurs de novo in a normal, uninjured vessel, and usually develops in a stenotic or atherosclerotic artery. One of the best clinical examples of arterial thromboembolism is the transient ischemic attack (TIA) syndrome. In this condition, platelet thrombi form on ulcerated atherosclerotic carotid vessel plaques. After the thrombus reaches a critical size, fragments break off and embolize to the distal cerebral or retinal circulation. In most patients, the distal emboli will break up, so that blood flow is restored to normal and visual impairment or neurological symptoms disappear. Occasionally, emboli can cause permanent neurological dysfunction and produce a completed stroke or cerebrovascular accident (CVA). Patients may have repeated TIAs without suffering a CVA and can be effectively treated with antiplatelet agents that prevent or reduce platelet plug formation on the ulcerated carotid plaque.

Firm evidence has emerged supporting a similar mechanism underlying transient or permanent obstruction of coronary arteries.[96] In fact, it is now clear that the majority of transmural myocardial infarcts are due to coronary thrombosis after the fracture or disruption of an atherosclerotic coronary arterial plaque, producing a surface which activates coagulation reactions. In addition, many patients with unstable angina (p. 1334), like those with TIAs, may have repeated bouts of thrombosis and embolism causing their cardiac instability and chest pain. In addition, their symptoms may abate with antiplatelet therapy, which also may reduce the risk of subsequent myocardial infarction (p. 1340). In addition to forming thrombi in diseased coronary arteries, cardiac patients may develop intracavitary or intracardiac thrombi. For example, patients who have had a transmural myocardial infarction may have residual endocardial scarring or hypokinesis. The damaged endocardium may provide a site for development of a mural thrombus, which may then break up and produce systemic emboli. Similarly, in patients with mitral stenosis, left atrial enlargement, and atrial fibrillation, thrombi often develop in the left atrium or on the mitral valve and can embolize into the systemic circulation. Patients with prosthetic cardiac valves also are at risk for systemic embolization. Although these intracavitary cardiac thrombi are "arterial," they form in areas of low blood flow and are rich in fibrin. In this respect, they more closely resemble the fibrin and red cell–rich thrombi that form in the venous circulation. Thus, effective treatment of intracavitary thrombi requires anticoagulants such as heparin or warfarin or a combination of anticoagulants and antiplatelet drugs.

DISORDERS OF FIBRINOLYSIS

Until recently, the study of potential disorders of the fibrinolytic system and their relation to thromboembolism has been been hampered by a lack of precise assays for components of the system. Now, with the molecular cloning of t-PA, scu-PA, and the fibrinolytic inhibitors PAI-1 and -2, it is possible to analyze fibrinolysis with more precision. In fact, several congenital or acquired abnormalities of the fibrinolytic system have been described that may increase the risk of thrombosis. Both a decreased concentration of plasminogen and abnormal plasminogen molecules have been associated with recurrent thrombosis.[97] Production of abnormal fibrinogen molecules (dysfibrinogenemias) usually causes bleeding; however, in certain dysfibrinogenemias, fibrin thrombi are formed that are unusually resistant to the action of plasmin and can predispose patients to thrombosis.[98] In addition, reduced fibrinolytic activity has been described in patients with CVAs,[99] recurrent venous thrombosis,[100] and mesenteric venous thrombosis.[101] In one case, defective release of t-PA from endothelial cells has been postulated as the cause of the fibrinolytic defect and recurrent venous thrombosis.[102] In a provocative report, elevated levels of PAI-1 have been noted in the plasma of young patients who survive myocardial infarction.[103] This raises the interesting possibility that coronary thrombosis might be due to a failure to lyse intracoronary thrombi owing to rapid neutralization of t-PA.

LIPOPROTEIN (a) (see also Fig. 37–3, p. 1129). A unique lipoprotein particle, lipoprotein (a), also impairs fibrin enhancement of plasminogen activation by t-PA and impairs the binding of t-PA to endothelial cells.[104] This lipoprotein is composed of low-density lipoprotein linked by a disulfide bridge(s) to a unique apolipoprotein, apo(a).[105] Apo(a) is 80 to 90 per cent homologous to plasminogen and contains a serine protease active site, a single kringle 5–like domain, and 37 copies of a kringle 4–like domain. Because of a crucial substitution of serine for arginine at the active site in the homolog, protease activity cannot be generated. The molecule is of particular interest, since elevated levels are highly predictive of atherosclerotic coronary disease. In addition, the lipoprotein colocalizes with fibrin in atheroma, where it may impair fibrinolysis. Thus, lipoprotein (a) may provide a link between the pathological processes of thrombosis and atherosclerosis.

Finally, there is one fibrinolytic abnormality that can cause bleeding rather than thrombosis. Absence of α_2PI, the principal plasmin inhibitor, permits excessively rapid fibrinolysis of hemostatic plugs and recurrent hemorrhage.[106] In *summary,* it is now clear that inherited molecular defects in the fibrinolytic system, like the inherited defects in the natural anticoagulants, may be added to the growing list of disorders that predispose patients to both arterial and venous thromboembolism.

ANTICOAGULANT THERAPY FOR CARDIOVASCULAR DISORDERS

HEPARIN

Heparin is clearly the most effective anticoagulant agent available for the treatment of thromboembolic disorders. Since the pioneering studies by Barrett and Jordan that demonstrated the efficacy of parenteral heparin in patients with pulmonary embolism, it has become the standard therapy for acute venous and arterial thrombosis and embolism.[107] Heparin activity resides in a heterogeneous series of sulfated glycosaminoglycans that function as anticoagulants by binding to and activating antithrombin III.[108] For pharmaceutical applications, heparin is extracted from porcine intestinal mucosa. There is now abundant evidence that heparin-like molecules also are present on endothelial cells throughout the vascular tree, where they regulate the rate of normal coagulation reactions and help to maintain blood fluidity.[109] Commercial heparin preparations are heterogeneous with respect to both the molecular size and the biological activity of the glycosaminoglycans. In fact, only a small fraction of the molecules in commercial heparin (usually about 20 per cent) have anticoagulant activity.

MECHANISM OF ACTION. Heparin can be conveniently fractionated on the basis of its molecular size and antithrombin affinity. Those heparin species with a low affinity for antithrombin—and therefore little or no anticoagulant activity—may have other biological properties of potential importance. For example, such species inhibit the proliferation of vascular smooth muscle cells in culture and prevent smooth muscle cell migration and proliferation within the arterial wall after experimental injury.[110] In the future, this antiproliferative property of heparin could be exploited to produce agents that inhibit atherogenesis. These low-affinity, high molecular weight forms of heparin also bind to and agglutinate platelets and may be the cause of heparin-induced thrombocytopenia. Heparin size also affects the kinetics of substrate neutralization by antithrombin III. For example, high and low molecular weight species neutralize factor Xa equally well. However, the high molecular weight species are more effective in facilitating the neutralization of thrombin by antithrombin III. This difference could be of importance as various heparin fractions are utilized clinically as antithrombotic agents.

Heparin is administered continuously by intravenous pump, by intermittent intravenous infusion, or subcutaneously. It is metabolized within the liver by the enzyme heparinase and excreted unchanged by the kidney. This explains the increased sensitivity and erratic metabolism of heparin by some patients with renal or hepatic disease. The dose and route of administration vary with the clinical situation and the therapeutic goal. As shown in Figure 58–15, varying methods of heparin administration have a marked effect on plasma heparin level and on the magnitude and duration of impaired hemostasis. Administration of a bolus of heparin followed by a continuous infusion of the drug will maintain heparin levels within the "therapeutic" range with minimal oscillation. Intermittent bolus infusion causes a more dramatic increase and subsequent fall in heparin level. After subcutaneous heparin, levels are not as high but are more sustained. The standard heparin regimens are summarized in Table 58–1.

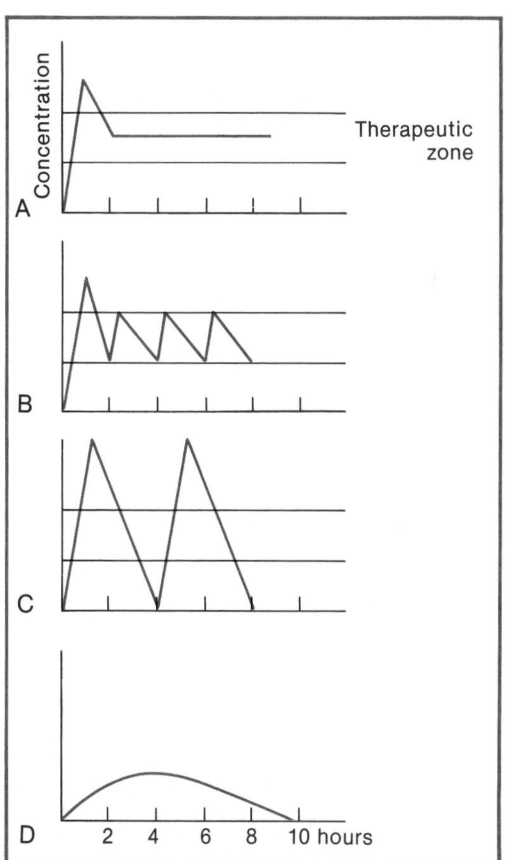

FIGURE 58–15. Concentration of heparin in blood after various routes of administration. *A*, Effect of a heparin bolus followed by a continuous intravenous infusion, the most common method of heparin administration for patients with acute thromboembolism. *B* and *C*, Effects of intermittent intravenous infusions. With this route, heparin levels oscillate widely and frequently are outside the broadly defined "therapeutic zone." This may increase the risk of bleeding and increase the rate of rethrombosis. *D*, Effects of subcutaneous injection, the route used for prophylactic "low-dose" heparin, in which there is a low but sustained level of heparin in the blood. (From Verstraete, M., and Vermylen, J.: Thrombosis. London, Pergamon Press, Copyright 1984, p. 85.)

TABLE 58–1 CLINICAL USE OF HEPARIN

INDICATION	DOSE (USP UNITS)	FREQUENCY	ROUTE
Prophylaxis in elective general surgery	5000	q12h	SC
Prophylaxis in congestive heart failure, cardiomyopathy, myocardial infarction	10,000	q12h	SC
Venous thromboembolism	5000 (bolus)	1000/hr	IV
Massive pulmonary embolism*	20,000 (bolus)	2000/hr	IV

* Reported to be effective in small studies; no randomized trials. Fibrinolytic therapy is a better alternative. SC = subcutaneous; IV = intravenous.

INDICATIONS. The most frequent indications for heparin in cardiac patients are (1) to prevent proximal extension of deep venous thrombosis or the recurrence of pulmonary embolism (p. 1568); (2) to prevent the recurrence of cerebral or other systemic embolism from intracardiac sources in the left atrium, left ventricle, or mitral valve; (3) to preclude development of deep venous thrombosis or pulmonary embolism in high-risk patients, such as those who are immobilized or have congestive heart failure, acute myocardial infarction, or cardiomyopathy or those who are undergoing abdominal surgery; and (4) as long-term therapy for the occasional patient who has recurrent thrombosis or embolism on warfarin or who cannot receive warfarin therapy.

METHOD OF ADMINISTRATION. When full-dose heparin is required, the usual procedure is to administer 5000 USP units of heparin rapidly intravenously followed by a continuous infusion of approximately 1000 USP units per hour. The dose of heparin is adjusted to prolong the PTT to 1.5 times the patient's PTT before instituting heparin therapy. Alternatively, patients may be given an intermittent intravenous infusion of 5000 units four to six times daily. There is good evidence that the risk of bleeding is less with continuous infusion and careful monitoring of the PTT. A less desirable third alternative is to administer 5000 units every 4 to 6 hours by subcutaneous injection. The administration of full-dose heparin is continued for 5 to 7 days, with close monitoring of the PTT and hematocrit along with examination of the stool for occult blood and periodic urinalysis for hematuria. Even with careful control, 10 to 20 per cent of patients experience some bleeding and 1 to 5 per cent have a major hemorrhage. Patients usually are begun on an oral anticoagulant such as warfarin within the first 3 to 5 days of heparinization, although heparin is continued while the dose of warfarin is adjusted.

Low-Dose Heparin. The rationale for low-dose heparin to prevent initial thrombus formation has evolved from extensive clinical studies conducted by Kakkar and colleagues.[111] Their studies demonstrated a clear reduction in both the incidence of and mortality from pulmonary embolism in a large cohort of middle-aged men undergoing major abdominal surgery. Because the incidence of fatal pulmonary embolism also was low in the control group, a multicenter study that enrolled more than 4000 patients was required to prove efficacy. The recommended regimen is 5000 USP units of heparin subcutaneously every 8 to 12 hours beginning 2 hours before surgery. This regimen reduced the rate of deep venous thrombosis by 60 per cent and the risk of fatal pulmonary embolus by 71 per cent in the Kakkar studies. A recent study has shown that the efficacy of low-dose heparin can be improved by monitoring the PTT for minor but reproducible prolongations.[112]

Theoretically, a low-dose heparin regimen should be successful in other surgical and medical settings in which the risk of venous thrombosis and embolism is high. Patients with acute myocardial infarction as well as hospitalized patients with chronic congestive heart failure and low output states, including those with cardiomyopathy, might benefit from prophylactic heparin administration. The regimen does not prevent venous thrombosis and embolism in gynecological patients undergoing pelvic surgery or in orthopedic patients undergoing open reduction and nailing of hip fractures. In addition, in patients who require ophthalmological or neurosurgical procedures, the risk of bleeding, even with low-dose heparin, is prohibitive, and the medication should not be given. Thus, despite careful clinical trials, the use of prophylactic heparin has not become widespread. The trend toward early mobilization of patients after major surgery may have lowered the incidence of venous thrombosis and embolism in the absence of heparin and may limit physician enthusiasm for this regimen.

COMPLICATIONS. The major complication of heparin therapy is hemorrhage caused by interruption of normal hemostasis. Patients may bleed from surgical wounds or catheterization sites or around indwelling vascular catheters and tubes. Patients also may develop gastrointestinal, genitourinary, or retroperitoneal bleeding. Age of the patient, dose and route of administration, presence of pathological lesions in the gastrointestinal or genitourinary tract, and concomitant administration of medications that impair platelet function all affect the incidence and severity of bleeding. Heparin also causes thrombocytopenia in as many as 20 per cent of recipients.[113] More rarely, heparin may provoke intravascular platelet agglutination and paradoxical thrombosis.[114] The antiplatelet effect of heparin is more pronounced with beef lung heparin preparations and, as previously described, is largely caused by the heparin species having low antithrombin affinity and high molecular weight. Because of this adverse effect, beef lung heparin is no longer manufactured. Heparin administration also may induce osteoporosis, although substantial bone loss is not apparent until the 6th to 8th week of therapy.[115] Fortunately, this exceeds the usual duration of heparin therapy for acute thrombosis, but it can become a problem in the occasional patient who requires prolonged intravenous heparin for recurrent thromboembolism.

To reduce complications and improve efficacy, heparin species of low molecular weight and high antithrombin affinity have been prepared by the fractionation of commercial heparin and currently are being tested clinically and in experimental models.[108] Although low molecular weight heparin fractions are effective antithrombotic agents, they are more expensive to produce than standard heparin. Because they are less likely to cause thrombocytopenia, they are the agents of choice in patients with a history of heparin-associated thrombocytopenia who require heparin therapy.

CHRONIC ORAL ANTICOAGULATION

The oral anticoagulants, which are all derivatives of the parent compound warfarin, are the agents of choice for preventing the recurrence of thrombosis and embolism after an initial course of therapy with heparin. The most frequent *indications* for therapy are patients with (1) established deep venous thrombosis and pulmonary embolism, (2) cerebral embolism, (3) atrial fibrillation[116] or mitral stenosis with a history of embolism, (4) prosthetic cardiac valves, and (5) an inherited prethrombotic disorder. The duration of therapy varies. Most patients with a single episode of thromboembolism receive treatment for 3 to 6 months. There is evidence that 90 per cent of patients with deep venous thrombosis will relapse if they do not receive oral anticoagulant therapy and that the risk decreases markedly by 3 months and plateaus by the 6th month. Patients with a noncorrectable cardiac disorder or an inherited prethrombotic state may require prolonged or even lifelong oral anticoagulation. Prophylactic anticoagulation has been proposed for patients (1) with atrial fibrillation who are to undergo cardioversion, (2) with chronic congestive heart failure or low output states such as cardiomyopathy, and (3) who have undergone hip surgery to prevent perioperative thrombosis.

Warfarin-Type Drugs

These are vitamin K antagonists, which prevent the reduction of vitamin K to its active epoxide form by blocking an intrahepatic epoxide reductase. This, in turn, prevents the formation of Gla residues on prothrombin and factors VII, IX, and X as well as on the proteins C and S. The net effect of warfarin administration is to reduce coagulation factor activity and prolong the PT and PTT. The reduction in coagulation factor activity is directly related to the half-life of each plasma factor. Factor VII, which has the shortest half-life, decreases first, followed by proteins C and S, factors IX and X, and prothrombin. Although therapy with warfarin derivatives usually is evaluated by the degree to which the PT is prolonged, prevention of thrombosis requires a reduction in factors IX and X, which are not measured by the PT. Paradoxically, a profound reduction in factor VII, which prolongs the PT, may not protect a patient from recurrent thrombosis but may increase the risk of bleeding. Although warfarin therapy decreases the activity of both procoagulant and anticoagulant molecules, the net effect is to impair coagulation and reduce the rate of thrombus formation. In patients with congenital protein C or S deficiency, who already have low levels of these proteins, the net balance may shift toward thrombus formation, since protein C and S may have fallen to dangerously low levels while the procoagulant proteins are still elevated. This may predispose patients to a rare thrombotic event, hemorrhagic skin necrosis.

PHARMACOKINETICS. The warfarin derivatives are readily absorbed in the stomach and jejunum and, after absorption, are bound to albumin and become distributed in the intravascular and interstitial spaces. Free drug is then taken up by hepatocytes, where it blocks vitamin K metabolism. Warfarin, like many other drugs, is inactivated by hepatic microsomal enzymes, and the resulting metabolites are either excreted into the bowel by way of the enterohepatic circulation or filtered and excreted by the kidneys. The plasma half-life of the different warfarin derivatives varies considerably. In addition, each of the derivatives is optically active and is produced as a racemic mixture of D and L isomers. The D isomers have a longer half-life, so that varying the ratio of D to L isomers also could influence intravascular half-life. The most frequently used derivative, sodium warfarin, has a half-life of 42 hours.

METHOD OF ADMINISTRATION. Oral anticoagulant therapy with an agent like warfarin is initiated by administering 10 to 15 mg/day of the drug for 3 days to the average-sized adult. The daily dose is then adjusted to maintain the PT at 1.5 to 2.0 times the control value. It is important to recognize that laboratory reagents used to measure the PT are not standardized, so that the patient's PT before therapy should be used as a guideline. Ideally, all measurements should be made in the same laboratory with the same reagents, since the correlation between prolongation of the PT and reduction in activity of the prothrombin complex proteins II, VII, IX, and X varies among PT reagents. One approach, used in Great Britain, has been to supply a reference thromboplastin to each clinical laboratory. Each laboratory can then calibrate its local thromboplastin reagent against the British National thromboplastin standard. Another approach has been to introduce new assays that measure the prothrombin complex proteins but do not rely on the PT reagent. In one study, a conformation-specific antibody that recognized the biologically inactive Gla-deficient prothrombin molecules produced by warfarin therapy was used to assess therapeutic efficacy and was slightly superior to the conventional PT-based test.[117]

DRUG INTERACTIONS. The pharmacology of warfarin is complex. It is well recognized that the anticoagulant effect of warfarin derivatives is dramatically affected by the simultaneous administration of other drugs that may enhance or reduce their activity.[118] The biological effect of a given dose also depends on the rapidity of its uptake by the liver, the integrity and vitamin K stores of the hepatocyte, and the activity of hepatic microsomal degrading enzymes. As shown in Table 58–2, some drugs commonly prescribed for patients with heart disease such as quinidine, cimetidine, and clofibrate may enhance warfarin activity. These drugs compete for albumin-binding sites, displace warfarin from the blood, and increase its rate of delivery to the liver. Conversely, drugs such as glutethimide and other common sedatives reduce the potency of a given warfarin dose by increasing liver microsomal enzyme activity and enhancing drug catabolism. In addition, some drugs like antacids and cholestyramine may impair intestinal absorption of the drug and reduce the activity of a given dose.

In addition to these well-documented drug interactions, metabolic abnormalities that alter hepatic or renal function or that lower albumin levels or vitamin K stores can make patients more sensitive to a given dose of warfarin. Conversely, ingestion of foods rich in vitamin K or the presence of a hypometabolic state such as hypothyroidism may require administration of a larger than usual dose of warfarin. In patients with fever, sepsis, or hyperthyroidism, catabolism of the vitamin K–dependent coagulation factors may have increased, so they require less warfarin for an equivalent anticoagulant effect. In addition to these effects on drug absorption and metabolism, the concomitant administration of drugs that impair platelet function, like aspirin, may cause hemorrhage without altering the PT or warfarin level.

COMPLICATIONS. Hemorrhagic complications occur in 7 to 10 per cent of patients who are anticoagulated for more than 4 months.[119] Death from hemorrhage occurs in approximately 1 per cent of patients who receive warfarin for a similar duration. The frequency of bleeding increases with anticoagulant dose and the degree to which the PT is prolonged, but it also is affected by the patient's age and associated medical conditions. For example, in one large study, bleeding occurred during 7 of 1000 days of warfarin treatment when the residual PT activity was between 10 and 29 per cent of normal. This is equivalent to a PT of 18 to 20 seconds. The rate of hemorrhage increased to 85 per 1000 days of treatment when residual PT activity was less than 10 per cent (PT above 20 seconds).[120]

TABLE 58–2 FACTORS INFLUENCING THE DOSE OF COUMARIN NEEDED FOR A CONSTANT ANTICOAGULANT EFFECT

METABOLIC AND DIETARY FACTORS	
Decrease dose:	*Increase dose:*
Decreased oral intake and vitamin K stores (surgery, antibiotics)	**Increased vitamin K intake (liver, cauliflower, green vegetables like broccoli, spinach, green beans)**
Liver disease	**Hypometabolism (hypothyroidism)**
Renal disease leading to hypoalbuminemia	**Hereditary resistance**
Malignancy, sepsis	
Diarrhea, malabsorption syndromes	
Hypermetabolism (hyperthyroidism, fever)	
DRUG INTERACTIONS	
Decrease dose:	*Increase dose:*
Antibiotics	**Vitamin K**
Cimetidine	**Antacids**
Anabolic steroids	**Cholestyramine**
D-Thyroxine	**Barbiturates**
Clofibrate	**Griseofulvin**
Sulfinpyrazone	**Rifampin**
Phenylbutazone	**Antihistamines**
Quinidine	
Alpha-methyldopa	

Modified from Chesebro, J., et al.: Antithrombotic therapy in valvular heart disease. By permission of The American College of Cardiology. J. Am. Coll. Cardiol. 8:52B, 1986.

Because of this unacceptably high rate of hemorrhage, modified regimens have been introduced that use less intense anticoagulation.[121] In these regimens, the warfarin dose is adjusted so that the PT is prolonged to no more than 1.5 times the control value. In one study of "low-dose" warfarin, the frequency of bleeding was markedly reduced when compared with standard therapy (4 vs. 22 per cent), whereas the frequency of recurrent venous thromboembolism remained at 2 per cent in both groups.[122]

RECOMMENDATIONS. It is hard to develop a general set of recommendations regarding the duration and intensity of anticoagulation with warfarin-type drugs. Based on the available evidence, however, the authors recommend that patients who receive prophylactic anticoagulation, such as those with prosthetic cardiac valves, chronic atrial fibrillation or mitral stenosis, cardiomyopathy, or chronic congestive heart failure, or those undergoing hip surgery, receive sufficient warfarin to prolong the PT to 1.5 times the control value. Patients given warfarin after an episode of deep venous thrombosis or pulmonary embolism, who are at high risk for recurrent thromboembolism, or patients with a mechanical cardiac valve, should probably receive a slightly higher dose of warfarin to keep the PT prolonged to 1.5 to 2.0 times the control value. Additional clinical studies coupled with the introduction of more reliable assays to monitor biological effects should make warfarin therapy safer and more effective and will allow the dose to be adjusted to the needs of the individual patient.

ANTIPLATELET DRUG THERAPY IN CARDIOVASCULAR DISEASE

Agents that modify platelet function have now been administered to patients with a wide range of cardiovascular disorders. These drugs have been given to patients with unstable angina, at high risk for arrhythmia and sudden death, with prosthetic cardiac valves or saphenous vein bypass grafts, or undergoing percutaneous transluminal angioplasty as well as to those with a history of acute myocardial infarction, stroke, or transient ischemic attacks. In each of these clinical situations there is evidence for platelet participation in the pathophysiology of the clinical disorder and there are some reports of clinical efficacy.[123,124]

Four fundamental problems have made evaluation of antiplatelet therapy difficult: (1) a lack of firm guidelines regarding disorders or clinical events that might potentially benefit from such therapy; (2) the variable quality of clinical trials on which therapeutic decisions must be based; (3) a lack of correlation between in vitro inhibition of platelet function and a clinical antithrombotic effect; and (4) the inability of available drugs to inhibit platelet participation in thrombus formation completely. The ideal antiplatelet drug, which is not yet available, should substantially reduce arterial thrombosis and embolism without causing undue bleeding or other undesirable side effects. This last limitation of antiplatelet therapy may be most important, since an ideal procedure for patient selection and a perfectly organized clinical trial are of limited value if the agent to be tested has minimal or no efficacy.

PHARMACOLOGY OF ANTIPLATELET DRUGS

CYCLO-OXYGENASE INHIBITORS. The most widely studied antiplatelet agents interfere with platelet signal transduction and stimulus-response coupling. One group of drugs, which includes aspirin and other nonsteroidal antiinflammatory agents such as indomethacin, sulfinpyrazone, and ibuprofen, inhibits platelet cyclo-oxygenase. Aspirin is unique in that it is the only drug that irreversibly inhibits cyclo-oxygenase. Because the platelet cannot synthesize any new enzyme, the antiplatelet effect of a single dose of aspirin can persist for 5 to 7 days. In contrast, other tissues rapidly recover from aspirin inhibition by synthesizing new cyclo-oxygenase. Thus endothelial cells regain their capacity to synthesize prostacyclin within a few hours of aspirin administration.[125] The concept of using low doses of aspirin to selectively inhibit platelet function has gained considerable popularity. In fact, it is possible to inhibit platelet thromboxane production effectively with as little as 20 to 100 mg aspirin per day.[126] There is, as yet, no convincing clinical evidence that low-dose aspirin is more effective than the conventional daily doses of 625 to 1250 mg or that these higher doses are harmful. The antiplatelet effect of the competitive inhibitors is much less dramatic than that of aspirin when measured by in vitro laboratory tests as well as by clinical studies assessing thrombus formation in vivo, and they are not frequently used in clinical trials.

DIPYRIDAMOLE. This agent (Persantine) inhibits platelet phosphodiesterase activity and raises platelet cyclic AMP levels in vitro, although the usual doses do not alter in vitro tests of platelet function or prolong the bleeding time in patients. Like aspirin, dipyridamole has undergone extensive clinical testing[127] but has limited clinical efficacy.[128]

OTHER ANTIPLATELET AGENTS. In addition to aspirin and dipyridamole, a number of new antiplatelet agents have been introduced that have more selective effects on arachidonic acid metabolism or affect other steps in the platelet activation process. Several *thromboxane synthetase inhibitors* have been designed to circumvent the fact that aspirin inhibits both thromboxane and prostacyclin synthesis. Unfortunately drugs in this class, such as *dazoxiben,* increase the concentration of the prostaglandin endoperoxide precursors of TxA_2 to levels that can activate the platelets.[129] Several *thromboxane receptor antagonists* that are active in vitro may soon become available for clinical testing, possibly in conjunction with the thromboxane synthetase inhibitors.[130] *Inhibitory prostaglandins* (e.g., PGD_2) or stable synthetic analogs of prostacyclin, prostaglandin-like BW 245C, or carbacyclin have been administered to normal volunteers and to a small number of patients with occlusive vascular disease or fulminant thrombotic thrombocytopenic purpura.[131,132] Although some beneficial effects were noted, the potent hypotensive effects of these compounds may limit their utility for in vivo studies. Inhibitory prostaglandins have been used to prevent the interaction of platelets with artificial surfaces during ex vivo perfusion and may be of value during hemodialysis and cardiopulmonary bypass.[133]

Ticlopidine is a novel platelet inhibitor with a poorly defined mechanism of action. It has the unique property of having little effect on platelets after direct addition in vitro, although it markedly prolongs the bleeding time and platelet response to aggregating agents after administration to patients. It is thought to alter membrane reactivity to multiple agonists and currently is under study in several multicenter trials.[134] Other agents currently under study are inhibitors of platelet-activating factor (1-alkyl-2-acetyl-sn-glycero-3-phosphorylcholine), a lipid mediator generated from leukocytes during allergic and immunological reactions, that aggregates platelets.[135] In addition, peptides that inhibit fibrinogen binding to platelets and monoclonal antibodies to platelet surface glycoproteins may block platelet aggregation and are being tested in laboratory animals as well as in clinical trials.[136] Several well-known cardiovascular drugs such as nitroglycerin[137] and the calcium channel antagonists[138] may have antiplatelet effects, although their possible utility as antithrombotic agents has only recently been the subject of clinical investigation.

ANTIPLATELET AGENTS IN TREATMENT OF MYOCARDIAL ISCHEMIA AND INFARCTION

It is now well accepted that a majority of acute transmural myocardial infarctions are caused by thrombotic occlusion of a diseased coronary artery.[139] The occluding thrombus, which forms on an ulcerated or ruptured atherosclerotic plaque, can be demonstrated in 90 per cent of patients by means of prompt angiography. Although platelets may initiate thrombus formation, fibrin deposition occurs secondarily. These fibrin-rich thrombi are effectively removed by the administration of fibrinolytic agents that restore vascular patency. Platelets also are implicated in the pathogenesis of coronary arterial vasospasm, which may cause transient ischemia and angina pectoris or, less frequently, myocardial infarction. Activated platelets produce TxA_2, a potent vasoconstrictor that may produce or enhance vasospasm. The concentration of the stable metabolite TxB_2 is elevated in coronary sinus blood obtained during pacing or exercise-induced angina and in blood obtained soon after spontaneous anginal episodes.[140] It also is elevated in patients with variant anginal syndromes who have pain at rest and ST-segment elevation, as well as in those with the clinical syndrome of unstable angina.

UNSTABLE ANGINA (see also p. 1340). Three large randomized placebo-controlled double-blind trials of aspirin in patients with unstable angina have yielded impressive positive results.[141-143] In the first study, the Veterans Administration Cooperative Trial, 1266 men with unstable angina were given 324 mg of aspirin daily, with a 51 per cent decrease in the number of subsequent infarctions and an identical reduction in mortality. A second, Canadian cooperative trial confirmed these results, reporting a 55 per cent reduction in myocardial infarction and a 43 per cent reduction in mortality. In the Theroux study,[143] the number of patients given aspirin who progressed to infarction was reduced by 75 per cent compared with those given placebo. In contrast, there is no evidence that aspirin or any other antiplatelet agents affect the frequency of, duration of, or precipitating events that cause spontaneous or exercise-induced angina pectoris, despite clear evidence for platelet activation in these patients. This striking difference in aspirin's efficacy in various forms of myocardial ischemia as well as the marginal results in most other patients with stable coronary artery disease highlights the problems facing investigators who design clinical trials as well as physicians who must recommend appropriate treatment for their patients. Aspirin currently can be unequivocally recommended only for patients with unstable angina. The differing efficacy may relate to differences in the pathophysiology of unstable angina as compared with chronic angina.

MYOCARDIAL INFARCTION (see also p. 1266). Over the past 12 years there have been several randomized double-blind trials of antiplatelet therapy for the secondary prevention of myocardial infarction.[123] The results are summarized in Table 58–3. Five trials utilized aspirin alone, two had a combination of aspirin and dipyridamole (Persantine), and two used sulfinpyrazone (Anturane). The doses of aspirin varied from 160 to 1500 mg/day, and the studies enrolled 600 to 17,000 patients, predominantly men, who had a well-documented myocardial infarct. Although aspirin therapy was reported to reduce mortality from subsequent infarcts by from 17 to 30 per cent in various studies, none of these trends reached statistical significance. In the second International Study of Infarct Survival, one finds the strongest evidence for the use of aspirin. More than 17,000 patients were randomized to receive either aspirin or streptokinase, both drugs, or placebo. Mortality 5 weeks post infarct was reduced 23 per cent with aspirin, 25 per cent with streptokinase, and 42 per cent with both drugs—all statistically significant reductions.[144]

The first sulfinpyrazone trial reported a striking reduction in sudden death and mortality during the first 6 months of therapy, and the second trial reported a reduction in reinfarction rate. These studies have been criticized, however, on technical grounds relating to the method of patient exclusion and the time of enrollment of subjects.

One investigator has suggested that the lack of statistical significance in many of the aspirin studies may be an insurmountable problem, given the relatively small numbers of patients enrolled in each of these secondary prevention trials. However, when data from all the aspirin trials are pooled to increase the number of evaluable patients, a statistically significant reduction in mortality can be demonstrated. The use of this statistical technique, meta analysis, is subject to the criticism that the study populations may be dissimilar.

The benefits of antiplatelet agents in the primary prevention of cardiovascular disease have been documented in the U.S. Physicians' Health Study.[145] In this study 22,071 male physicians, half of whom received 325 mg of aspirin every other day, were followed for 4.8 years. Aspirin use reduced the incidence of myocardial infarction by 44 per cent, from 0.4 to 0.25 per cent per year, but did not reduce cardiovascular mortality. In the British primary prevention trial, 5139 male physicians, 66 per cent of whom received 500 mg aspirin daily,

TABLE 58-3 ANTIPLATELET THERAPY IN SECONDARY PREVENTION OF MYOCARDIAL INFARCTION

STUDY	DRUGS (DOSAGE)	PATIENTS (DURATION)	OUTCOME*
Elwood et al., 1974	ASA (300 mg/day)	1239 (30 mo)	Mortality ↓ 25%
CDP, 1976	ASA (1 gm/day)	1529 (24 mo)	Mortality ↓ 30%
Breddin et al., 1977	ASA (1.5 gm/day)	946 (24 mo)	No change
Elwood and Sweetman, 1979	ASA (900 mg/day)	1682 (12 mo)	Mortality ↓ 17%
AMIS, 1980	ASA (1 gm/day)	4524 (36 mo)	No change
ART, 1980	Sulfinpyrazone (800 mg/day)	1558 (16 mo)	Reinfarction ↓ 57%
ARIS, 1982	Sulfinpyrazone (800 mg/day)	727 (9 mo)	Reinfarction ↓ 56%
PARIS I, 1980	ASA (1 gm/day) Dipyridamole (225 mg/day)	2206 (36 mo)	Reinfarction ↓ 50%
PARIS II, 1986	Same as PARIS I	3128 (24 mo)	30% ↓ reinf. at 1 yr; 24% ↓ reinf. at 2 yr

All studies cited in Harker, L.A.: Circulation *23*:206, 1986 except PARIS II, which is in Klimt, C.R., et al.: J. Am. Coll. Cardiol. *7*:251, 1986.

* The reduction in reinfarctions in PARIS II was statistically significant at one and two years. Although trends are given, reductions in mortality were not statistically significant.

Abbreviations: CDP = Coronary Drug Project; AMIS = Acute Myocardial Infarction Study; ART = Anturane Reinfarction Trial; ARIS = Anturane Reinfarction Study; PARIS = Persantine-Aspirin Reinfarction Study; ASA = aspirin.

were followed for 6 years.[146] In contrast to the much larger U.S. trial, no significant difference in myocardial infarction or cardiovascular death was noted in the two groups. In both studies, a slight increase in the incidence of severe or disabling stroke was observed in the men who received aspirin.

ANTIPLATELET THERAPY AFTER CORONARY BYPASS GRAFTING OR PROSTHETIC VALVE INSERTION. The efficacy of antiplatelet therapy for patients who undergo coronary bypass grafting has been extensively studied.[147,148] (Although the majority of the studies have demonstrated a beneficial effect of platelet-modifying drugs, differences in dosage regimens, timing of the onset of therapy, and surgical technique, which may affect the incidence of graft occlusion in placebo groups, complicate interpretation of the data.) Although several early studies utilizing aspirin were begun shortly after surgery improved graft patency, the most dramatic results are those of Chesebro et al., who used a combination of ASA and dipyridamole.[148a] Dipyridamole was begun before surgery and continued by gastric lavage throughout the perioperative period. In addition, they began patients on aspirin within 24 hours of surgery. Their results, which are summarized in Figure 58-16, show a marked improvement in graft patency both 1 month and 1 year after surgery in patients who received the prescribed antiplatelet therapy. To date, all studies support the use of antiplatelet therapy for at least the first year after coronary bypass grafting. Although perioperative regimens that involve aspirin improve graft patency, the incidence of postoperative bleeding and the need for reoperation also increase. A prospective trial currently is under way to address this important issue.

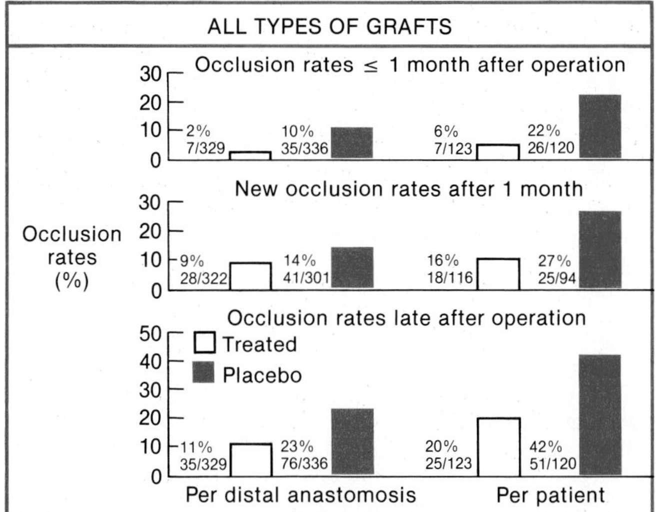

FIGURE 58-16. Occlusion rates of saphenous vein grafts to the coronary artery after treatment with a combination of aspirin (625 mg/day) and dipyridamole (500 mg t.i.d.) beginning at the time of surgery. Rates are expressed per distal anastomosis and per patient. Occlusion is shown 1 month after surgery and as new events beyond 1 month. Data include only patients who underwent angiography 1 month and 1 year after surgery. Below each percentage of occlusion is the total number of anastomoses or patients. (Reprinted by permission from Chesebro, J. H., et al.: Effect of dipyridamole and aspirin on late vein-graft patency after coronary bypass operations. N. Engl. J. Med. *310*:211, 1984.)

Some of the earliest studies of antiplatelet drug efficacy involved patients with prosthetic cardiac valves who had cerebral embolic episodes while receiving warfarin.[149] At least six separate studies have demonstrated a beneficial effect of antiplatelet drugs when used with conventional warfarin-type anticoagulants. The regimens have used aspirin alone, aspirin and dipyridamole, and dipyridamole alone. Although all three regimens have been effective, the combination of aspirin and warfarin causes gastrointestinal bleeding. The type of valve and its position in the heart also affected study outcome. The highest incidence of thromboembolism is seen with older types of prostheses in the mitral position. The increasing use of less thrombogenic porcine homograft or "bioprosthetic" valves has lowered the incidence of thromboembolism. Current recommendations are to use warfarin and, if embolism should occur, 400 mg/day of dipyridamole in patients who receive prosthetic valves. Patients who receive bioprosthetic valves should be treated with anticoagulants for 3 months after valve replacement and then should require no further anticoagulant therapy unless they continue to have atrial fibrillation or their valve is placed in the mitral position.

THROMBOLYTIC THERAPY

(See also pp. 1176, 1190, and 1230)

As discussed earlier, there are two general classes of plasminogen activators: the endogenous agents that are derived from human sources—t-PA and the u-PAs—and the exogenous agents that are derived from nonhuman sources—streptokinase (SK) and its anisoylated derivative complexed to plasminogen (APSAC). These agents differ in their mechanism of action, pharmacokinetics, degree of fibrin selectivity, and side effects.

STREPTOKINASE AND ANISOYLATED PLASMINOGEN-STREPTOKINASE COMPLEX

SK, a 47,000-dalton single-chain protein produced by β-hemolytic streptococci, is the oldest available plasminogen activator. It does not enzymatically activate plasminogen but forms a stoichiometric complex with the proenzyme, thereby leading to a conformational change that confers plasmin-like activity on the bimolecular species.[150] This complex then converts uncomplexed plasminogen molecules to plasmin, which initiates fibrinolysis. APSAC is an inactive derivative produced by acylation of the plasminogen active site. This molecular complex does not interact with plasminogen until spontaneous deacylation occurs in plasma.[151] APSAC is not inhibited by α_2PI.

SK and APSAC have been used in a number of clinical settings and can effectively lyse thrombi. They do, however, produce a number of side effects, including febrile reactions, urticarial skin lesions, angioedema, bronchospasm, and hypotension. Serum sickness–like reactions have been reported 7 days after the completion of therapy owing to the formation of immune complexes. In addition, the presence of neutralizing antibodies can make dosage calculations unpredictable. Antibodies induce platelet aggregates in as many as 15 per cent of patients who receive the drug.[152] Clots in these patients, paradoxically, may propagate rather than lyse. Given the allergic potential of SK and APSAC, some investigators believe that patients should be pretreated with diphenhydramine and hydrocortisone, although this approach is infrequently taken in practice.

SK has a plasma half-life of 30 minutes, whereas APSAC has a longer half-life of 70 minutes. For the therapy of acute myocardial infarction, a dose of 1.5 million units of SK is infused over 1 hour, whereas APSAC is administered as an intravenous bolus (30 units over 5 minutes). Therapeutic regimens for deep venous thrombosis and pulmonary embolism commonly call for prolonged infusions of SK over 24 to 72 hours. These lengthy infusions increase the incidence of hemorrhagic complications.

UROKINASE-TYPE PLASMINOGEN ACTIVATORS

As discussed earlier (p. 1775), the u-PAs are synthesized by endothelial cells and renal tubular epithelial cells as a single-chain species (scu-PA or PUK) with minimal endogenous plasminogen activator activity.[153] This proenzyme is converted to a fully active high molecular weight two-chain form and to a smaller form, the conventional UK species used clinically in North America. Low molecular weight two-chain UK (LMW-tc-UK) has a plasma half-life of 10 minutes, whereas scu-PA has an initial plasma half-life of 5 minutes and a terminal half-life of 6 to 7 hours in rabbits and dogs.[154] LMW-tc-UK has been used to treat deep venous thrombosis and also is approved for intracoronary administration in acute myocardial infarction. Because they are of human origin, allergic reactions are rare with this group of activators.

TISSUE-TYPE PLASMINOGEN ACTIVATOR

t-PA also is secreted by the endothelial cell as a single-chain polypeptide with significant plasminogen activator activity.[155] It is converted to a two-chain species which predominates in plasma. t-PA is a relatively unique plasminogen activator, as it is more than 300-fold more efficient at activating plasminogen in the presence of fibrin. Two-chain t-PA is somewhat less fibrin-selective.[156] Fibrin-binding site requires the second kringle domain of t-PA, a triple-looped structure containing lysine residues present in a number of coagulation proteins, and the fibronectin finger-like domain.[157]

Traditionally, a continuous infusion of 100 mg of t-PA is administered over 3 hours to patients with acute myocardial infarction. Newer regimens which use t-PA administered as a bolus may be even more efficacious[158] and may become the preferred treatment mode. t-PA also has been approved for the treatment of pulmonary embolism (p. 1571). Although not yet approved for use in these disorders, in clinical trials t-PA also is effective in the treatment of deep venous thrombosis and peripheral arterial occlusion as well as thrombotic cerebrovascular occlusion.[159–162] Single-chain t-PA has an initial plasma half-life of 4 minutes and a terminal half-life of approximately 46 minutes.[163] Two weeks after treatment with t-PA one group of investigators failed to detect antibodies in patient plasma.[164]

Indications and Contraindications for Thrombolytic Therapy

There is a general consensus that this form of therapy is indicated in patients with acute myocardial infarction, extensive deep venous thrombosis, major pulmonary embolism with hypotension and/or severe hypoxia, and acute peripheral arterial occlusion. Thrombolytic therapy also has been effective in restoring the patency of indwelling vascular catheters and arteriovenous shunts, as well as in treating patients with axillary vein thrombosis, a condition that is not effectively treated with conventional anticoagulants. General *contraindications* for use of these agents include a history of abnormal bleeding (particularly from the gastrointestinal or genitourinary tract), uncontrolled hypertension, central nervous system disease, conditions such as peptic ulcer or gastrointestinal neoplasm that potentially can be associated with bleeding, and recent major surgery or organ biopsy.

Limitations of Thrombolytic Therapy

Although thrombolytic therapy usually can restore vessel patency and may be of considerable benefit to selected patients, it is sometimes difficult to demonstrate that pharmacological clot lysis improves clinical outcome. For example, studies of thrombolytic therapy in patients with deep venous thrombosis have not demonstrated any significant reduction in the incidence of postphlebitic complications in treated patients. The often-cited urokinase in pulmonary embolism trial clearly demonstrated superior resolution and lung perfusion in patients treated with urokinase.[165] Until recently,[166] however, this benefit had been shown to correlate with improved long-term outcome.

The appropriate approach to patients with acute coronary thrombosis (see also p. 1230) presents a particularly vexing problem, and highlights the three major shortcomings of thrombolytic therapy for arterial disorders. First, it is clear that treating patients with acute myocardial infarction opens occluded vessels in a timely manner in most patients (70 to 80 per cent), improves mortality rates (at 5 weeks), and leads to improved ventricular function, regardless of the agent chosen. All agents and regimens, however, are plagued by (1) delay in time to patency or, in some cases, resistance to lysis; (2) reocclusion rates of 10 to 20 per cent; and (3) hemorrhagic complications that cannot be predicted in a given patient and that do not correlate with the degree of systemic lysis.

Delays in lysis have been explained on the basis of the relative platelet content of the clot, its degree of organization and age, and a cell surface or plasma plasminogen "steal" of systemically administered activator which might decrease the availability of activator for the thrombus itself. Newer approaches to the administration of the activators as well as the design of mutants with longer half-lives or different surface-binding properties may overcome these problems.

The problem of reocclusion is intimately related to the problem of hemorrhage, since agents that intensify the systemic lytic state reduce reocclusion. The use of antiplatelet drugs to temper the transient increase in platelet activity that occurs after the initiation of lytic therapy may reduce the magnitude of this problem. The simultaneous administration of agents that reverse the bleeding tendency caused by plasminogen activators, like recombinant PAI-1 or DDAVP, may attenuate the hemorrhagic complications.[167]

Management of Patients Receiving Thrombolytic Agents

All candidates for thrombolytic therapy should have screening tests of hemostasis, including a platelet count, PT, and PTT, as well as a bleeding time. The bleeding time correlates fairly well with the likelihood of a hemorrhagic complication. During fibrinolytic therapy, surgical and invasive cardiovascular procedures should be avoided whenever possible. Intramuscular injections also should be avoided. In patients undergoing coronary thrombolysis it is common practice to administer aspirin before infusion of the thrombolytic. Approximately 2 to 4 hours after the completion of treatment, heparin is initiated, and continued for 24 to 72 hours. There is no need to routinely measure fibrinogen, fibrin degradation products, plasminogen consumption, or α_2PI consumption, since changes in these parameters predict neither efficacy nor complications arising from therapy.

Bleeding that develops during thrombolytic therapy is best managed by applying direct pressure whenever possible, discontinuing the thrombolytic agent, reversing heparin with protamine, and transfusing the patient with fresh frozen plasma and packed erythrocytes. In extreme cases ϵ-aminocaproic acid (Amicar) may be administered.

REFERENCES

HEMOSTASIS

1. Loscalzo, J.: Lipoprotein a—a unique risk factor for atherothrombotic disease. Arteriosclerosis *10*:672, 1990.
2. Nieuwenhuis, H. K., Akkerman, J.W.M., Houdjik, W.P.M., and Sixma, J. J.: Human blood platelets showing no response to collagen fail to express glycoprotein Ia. Nature *318*:470, 1985.
3. Santoro, S. A.: Identification of a 160,000-dalton platelet membrane protein that mediates the initial divalent cation-dependent adhesion of platelets to collagen. Cell *46*:913, 1986.
4. Yamada, K. M., and Olden, K.: Fibronectins—adhesive glycoproteins of cell surface and blood. Nature *275*:179, 1978.
5. Plow, E. F., and Ginsberg, M. H.: Specific and saturable binding of plasma fibronectin to thrombin-stimulated human platelets. J. Biol. Chem. *256*:9477, 1981.
6. Haverstick, D. M., Coawa, J. F., Yamada, K. M., and Santoro, S. A.: Inhibition of platelet adhesion to fibronectin, fibrinogen, and von Willebrand factor substrates by a synthetic tetrapeptide derived from the cell binding domain of fibronectin. Blood *66*:946, 1985.
7. Bockenstedt, P., McDonagh, J., and Handin, R. I.: The binding and covalent crosslinking of purified von Willebrand's factor to native monomeric collagen. J. Clin. Invest. *77*:743, 1986.
8. Michelson, A. D., Loscalzo, J., Melnick, B., et al.: Partial characterization of a binding site for von Willebrand factor on glycocalicin. Blood *67*:19, 1986.
9. Ruggeri, Z. M., DeMarco, L., Gatti, L., et al.: Platelets have more than one binding site for von Willebrand factor. J. Clin. Invest. *72*:1, 1983.
10. Baumgartner, H. R., Tschopp, T. B., and Weiss, H. J.: Platelet interaction with collagen fibrils in flowing blood. II. Impaired adhesion and aggregation in bleeding disorders. Thromb. Haemost. *37*:17, 1977.
11. Houdjik, W.P.M., Sakariassen, K. S., Nievelstein, P.F.E.M., and Sixma, J. J.: Role of factor VIII–von Willebrand factor and fibronectin in the interaction of platelets in flowing blood with monomeric and fibrillar human collagen types I and III. J. Clin. Invest. *75*:531, 1985.
12. Shattil, S. J.: Platelets and their membranes in hemostasis: Physiology and pathophysiology. Ann. Intern. Med. *94*:108, 1981.
13. Cooper, B., Handin, R. I., Young, L. H., and Alexander, R. W.: Agonist regulation of the human platelet alpha-adrenergic receptor. Nature *274*:703, 1978.
14. Schafer, A. I., Cooper, B., O'Hara, D., and Handin, R. I.: Identification of platelet receptors for prostaglandins I_2 and D_2. J. Biol. Chem. *254*:2914, 1979.
15. Moncada, S., and Vane, J. R.: Arachidonic acid metabolites and the interactions between platelets and blood vessel walls. N. Engl. J. Med. *300*:1142, 1979.
16. Berridge, M. J.: Inositol triphosphate and diacylglycerol as second messengers. Biochem. J. *220*:345, 1984.
17. Majerus, P. W., Connolly, T. M., Deckman, H. et al.: The metabolism of phosphoinositide-derived messenger molecules. Science *234*:1519, 1986.
18. Berridge, M. J., and Irvine, R. F.: Inositol triphosphate: A novel second messenger in cellular signal transduction. Nature 312:315, 1984.
19. Nishizuka, Y.: The role of protein kinase C in cell surface signal transduction and tumour promotion. Nature *308*:693, 1984.
20. Tyers, M., Rachubirski, R. A., Stewart, M. I., et al.: Molecular cloning and expression of the major protein kinase L substrate of platelets. Nature *2*:470, 1988.
21. Chaffoy de Courcelles, D., Roevens, P., and Van Belle, H.: 1-Oleoyl-2-acetyl-glycerol (OAG) stimulates the formation of phosphatidylinositol-4-phosphate in intact human platelets. Biochem. Biophys. Res. Commun. *123*:589, 1984.
22. Halenda, S. P., Zavoico, G. B., and Feinstein, M. B.: Phorbol esters and oleoyl acetoyl glycerol enhance release of arachidonic acid in platelets stimulated by Ca^{2+} ionophore A23187. J. Biol. Chem. *260*:12484, 1985.
23. Majerus, P. W.: Arachidonate metabolism in vascular disorders. J. Clin. Invest. *72*:1521, 1986.
24. Hamberg, M., Svensson, J., and Samuelsson, B.: Thromboxanes: A new group of biologically active compounds derived from prostaglandin endoperoxides. Proc. Natl. Acad. Sci. U.S.A. *72*:2994, 1975.
25. Rittenhouse, S. E.: Activation of phospholipase C in human platelets. *In* Hayaishi, O. (ed.): Advances in Thromboxane and Prostaglandin Research. Vol. 15. New York, Raven Press, 1985, pp. 113–114.
26. Rittenhouse-Simmons, S., and Deykin, D.: The mobilization of arachidonic acid in platelets exposed to thrombin or ionophore A23187. J. Clin. Invest. *60*:495, 1977.
27. Turner, J. R., and Tainer, J. A.: Biogenesis of chemotactic molecules by the arachidonate lipoxygenase system of platelets. Nature *257*:680, 1975.
28. Gerrard, J. M., and White, J. G.: Prostaglandins and thromboxanes: "Middlemen" modulating platelet function in hemostasis and thrombosis. *In* Spaet, T. H. (ed.): Progress in Hemostasis and Thrombosis. Vol. 4. New York, Grune and Stratton, 1982, pp. 87–126.
29. Fitzgerald, G. A., Oates, J. A., Hawiger, J., et al.: Endogenous synthesis of prostacyclin and thromboxane and platelet function during aspirin administration in man. J. Clin. Invest. *71*:767, 1983.
30. Fitzgerald, G. A., Smith, G. K., Pedersen, A. K., and Brash, A. R.: Increased prostacyclin biosynthesis in patients with severe atherosclerosis and platelet activation. N. Engl. J. Med. *310*:1065, 1984.
31. Samuelsson, B.: Leukotrienes: Mediators of immediate hypersensitivity and inflammation. Science *220*:568, 1983.
32. Samuelsson, B., Dahlen, S-E., Lindgren, J. A., et al.: Leukotrienes and lipoxins: Structures, biosynthesis and biological effects. Science *237*:1171, 1987.
33. Marcus, A. J., Weksler, B. B., Jaffe, E. A., and Broekman, M. J.: Synthesis of prostacyclin from platelet-derived endoperoxides by cultured human endothelial cells. J. Clin. Invest. *66*:979, 1980.
34. Schafer, A. I., Crawford, D. D., and Gimbrone, M. A.: Unidirectional transfer of prostaglandin endoperoxides between platelets and endothelial cells. J. Clin. Invest. *73*:1105, 1984.
35. White, J. G.: Electron microscopic studies of platelet secretion. *In* Spaet, T. H. (ed.): Progress in Hemostasis and Thrombosis. Vol. 2. New York, Grune and Stratton, 1974, pp. 49–98.
36. Goldberg, I. D., Stemerman, M. B., and Handin, R. I.: Vascular permeation of platelet factor four following endothelial injury. Science *209*:611, 1980.
37. Sporn, M. B., Roberts, A. B., Wakefield, L. M., and Assoian, R. K.: Transforming growth factor-beta: Biological function and chemical structure. Science *233*:532, 1986.
38. Deuel, T. F., and Huang, J. S.: Platelet-derived growth factor. Structure, function, and roles in normal and transformed cells. J. Clin. Invest. *74*:664, 1984.
39. Colman, R. W.: Aggregin—a platelet ADP receptor that mediates activation. FASEB J. *4*:1425, 1990.
40. Bennett, J. S., Vilaire, G., and Cines, D. B.: Identification of the fibrinogen receptor on human platelets by photoaffinity labeling. J. Biol. Chem. *257*:8049, 1982.
41. Kloczewiak, M., Timmons, S., Lukas, T. J., and Hawiger, J.: Platelet receptor recognition site on human fibrinogen: Synthesis and structure-function relationship of peptides corresponding to the carboxy terminal segment of the gamma chain. Biochemistry *23*:1767, 1984.
42. Plow, E. F., Srouji, A. H., Meyer, D., et al.: Evidence that three adhesive proteins interact with a common recognition site on activated platelets. J. Biol. Chem. *259*:5388, 1984.
43. Coller, B. S., Folts, J. D., Scudder, L. E., and Smith, S. R.: Antithrombotic effect of a monoclonal antibody to the platelet glycoprotein IIb/IIIa receptor in an experimental animal model. Blood *68*:783, 1986.
44. Ruggeri, Z. M., Houghten, R. A., Russel, S. R., and Zimmerman, T. S.: Inhibition of platelet function with synthetic peptides designed to be high affinity antagonists of fibrinogen binding to platelets. Proc. Natl. Acad. Sci. U.S.A. *83*:5708, 1986.
45. Azuma, H., Ishikawa, M., and Sezizaki, S.: Endothelium-dependent inhibition of platelet aggregation. Br. J. Pharmacol. *88*:411, 1986.
46. Stamler, J., Mendelsohn, M. E., Amarante, P., et al.: N-acetylcysteine potentiates platelet inhibition by endothelium-drived relaxing factor. Circ. Res. *65*:789, 1989.
47. Mendelsohn, M. E., and Loscalzo, J.: The effect of S-nitrosothiols on fibrinogen binding to human platelets. Blood *74*:4030, 1989.
48. Vaughan, D. E., Mendelsohn, M. E., Dallerck, P. J., et al.: Characterization of the binding of human tissue-type plasminogen activator to platelets. J. Biol. Chem. *264*:15869, 1989.
49. Loscalzo, J., and Vaughan, D. E.: Human tissue-type plasminogen activator facilitates platelet disaggregation. J. Clin. Invest. *79*:12749, 1987.
50. Stamler, J. S., Vaughan, D. E., and Loscalzo, J.: Synergistic disaggregation of platelets by tissue-type plasminogen activator, prostaglandin E_1 and nitroglycerin. Circ. Res. *65*:756, 1989.
51. Marcus, A. J.: Thrombosis and inflammation as multicellular processes. Blood *76*:1903, 1990.
52. Mann, K. G., Nesheim, M. E., Church, W. R., et al.: Surface-dependent reactions of the vitamin K–dependent enzyme complexes. Blood *76*:1, 1990.
53. Rosenberg, R. D., and Rosenberg, J. S.: Natural anticoagulant mechanisms. J. Clin. Invest. *74*:1, 1984.
54. Clouse, L. H., and Comp, P.: The regulation of hemostasis: The protein C system. N. Engl. J. Med. *314*:1298, 1986.

55. Esmon, N. L., Owen, W. G., and Esmon, C. T.: Isolation of a membrane-bound cofactor for thrombin-catalyzed activation of protein C. J. Biol. Chem. *257*:859, 1982.
56. Walker, F. J.: Regulation of activated protein C by a new protein: A possible function for protein S. J. Biol. Chem. *255*:5521, 1980.
57. De Fouw, N. J., von Hirsbergh, V.W.M., de Jong, W. F., et al.: The interaction of activated protein C and thrombin with the plasminogen activator inhibitor release from human endothelial cells. Thromb. Haemost. *57*:176, 1987.
58. Fay, W. P., and Owen, W. G.: Platelet plasminogen activator inhibitor: Purification and characterization of interaction with plasminogen activators and activated protein C. Biochemistry *28*:5773, 1989.
59. Chien, S.: Transport across arterial endothelium. *In* Spaet, T. H. (ed.): Progress in Hemostasis and Thrombosis. Vol. 4. New York, Grune and Stratton, 1978, pp. 1–36.
60. Thomas, D. J.: The influence of blood viscosity on cerebral blood flow and symptoms. *In* Greenhalsh, R. M., and Rose, F. L. (eds.): Progress in Stroke Research. Kent, England, Pitman Medical Publishing Company, 1979, pp. 47–55.
61. Segal, A.: The Clinical Use of Dextran Solutions. New York, Grune and Stratton, 1964.

CLOT DISSOLUTION—THE FIBRINOLYTIC SYSTEM

62. Adams, L. M., Fretto, L. J., and McKee, P. A.: The binding of human plasminogen to fibrin and fibrinogen J. Biol. Chem. *258*:4249, 1983.
63. Collen, D., and Lijnen, H. R.: The fibrinolytic system in man: An overview. *In* Collen, D., Lijnen, H. R., and Verstraete, M. (eds.): Thrombolysis: Biological and Therapeutic Properties of New Thrombolytic Agents. New York, Churchill Livingstone, 1985, pp. 1–14.
64. Pennica, D., Holmes, W. E., Kohr, W. J., et al.: Cloning and expression of human tissue-type plasminogen activator. Nature *301*:214, 1983.
65. Steffens, G. J., Günzler, W. A., Otting, F., et al.: The complete amino acid sequence of low molecular mass urokinase from human urine. Physiol. Chem. *363*:1043, 1982.
66. Pannell, R., Block, J., and Gurewich, V.: Complementary modes of action of tissue-type plasminogen activator and pro-urokinase by which their synergistic effects on clot lysis may be explained. J. Clin. Invest. *81*:853, 1988.
67. Ginsburg, D., Zeheb, R., Yang, A. Y., et al.: cDNA cloning of human plasminogen activator-inhibitor from endothelial cells. J. Clin. Invest. *78*:1673, 1986.
68. Moroi, M., and Aoki, N.: Isolation and characterization of alpha$_2$-plasmin inhibitor from human plasma. A novel proteinase inhibitor which inhibits activator-induced lysis. J. Biol. Chem. *251*:5956, 1976.

EVALUATION OF HEMOSTASIS IN CARDIOVASCULAR PATIENTS

69. Meyer, D., and Zimmerman, T. S.: von Willebrand's disease. *In* Colman, R. W., Hirsh, J., Marder, V. J., and Salzman, E. W. (eds.): Hemostasis and Thrombosis. Philadelphia, J. B. Lippincott, 1982, pp. 64–74.
70. Ruggeri, Z. M., and Zimmerman, T. S.: Variant von Willebrand's disease. Characterization of two subtypes by analysis of multimeric composition of factor VIII/von Willebrand factor in plasma and platelets. J. Clin. Invest. *63*:1318, 1980.
71. Mannucci, P. M., Canciani, M. T., Rota, L., and Donovan, B. S.: Response of factor VIII/von Willebrand factor to DDAVP in healthy volunteers and in patients with von Willebrand's disease. Br. J. Haematol. *47*:283, 1981.
72. Milan, J. D., Austin, S. F., Nihill, M. R., et al.: Use of sufficient hemodilution to prevent coagulopathies following surgical correction of cyanotic heart disease. J. Thorac. Cardiovasc. Surg. 89:623, 1985.
73. Michelson, A.: Pathomechanism of defective hemostasis during and after extracorporeal circulation: The role of platelets. *In* Hetzer, R. (ed.): Blood Use in Cardiac Surgery. Darmstadt, Steinkopff (*in press*).
74. Abrahamsen, A. F.: Platelet survival studies in man with special reference to thrombosis and atherosclerosis. Scand. J. Haematol. *3*(Suppl.):1, 1968.
75. Harker, L. A., and Slichter, S. J.: Studies of platelet and fibrinogen kinetics in patients with prosthetic heart valves. N. Engl. J. Med. *283*:1302, 1970.
76. Handin, R. I., McDonough, M., and Lesch, M.: Elevation of platelet factor 4 in acute myocardial infarction: Measurement by radioimmunoassay. J. Lab. Clin. Med. *91*:340, 1978.
77. Kaplan, K. L., Nossel, H. L., Drillings, M., and Lasznik, G.: Radioimmunoassay of platelet factor 4 and B-thromboglobulin: Development and application to studies of platelet release in relation to fibrinopeptide A generation. Br. J. Haematol. *39*:129, 1978.
78. Dawes, J., Smith, R. C., and Pepper, D. S.: The release, distribution and clearance of human B-thromboglobulin and platelet factor 4. Thromb. Haemost. *37*:73, 1977.
79. Guzzo, J., Niewiarowski, S., Musial, J., et al.: Secreted platelet proteins with antiheparin and mitogenic activities in chronic renal failure. J. Lab. Clin. Med. *96*:102, 1980.
80. Ludlam, C. A., and Cash, J. D.: Studies on the liberation of B-thromboglobulin from human platelets in vitro. Br. J. Haematol. *33*:2339, 1976.
81. Yudelman, I., Nossel, H. L., and Kaplan, K. L.: Fibrinopeptide A levels in symptomatic thromboembolism. Blood *51*:1189, 1978.
82. Bauer, K. A., Goodman, T. L., Kass, B. L., and Rosenberg, R. D.: Elevated factor Xa activity in the blood of asymptomatic patients with congenital antithrombin deficiency. J. Clin. Invest. *76*:826, 1985.
83. Halushka, P. V., Lurie, D., and Colwell, J. A.: Increased synthesis of prostaglandin E–like material by platelets from patients with diabetes mellitus. N. Engl. J. Med. *297*:1306, 1977.
84. Carvalho, A., Colman, R. W., and Lees, R. S.: Platelet function in hyperbetalipoproteinemia. N. Engl. J. Med. *290*:434, 1974.
85. Gerritsen, T., and Waisman, H. A.: Homocystinuria. Cystathionine synthase deficiency. *In* Stanbury, J. B., et al. (eds.): The Metabolic Basis of Inherited Disease. 3rd ed. New York, McGraw-Hill Book Co., 1972, pp. 404–412.
86. Harker, L. A., Slichter, S. J., and Scott, C. R.: Homocystinemia. Vascular injury and arterial thrombosis. N. Engl. J. Med. *291*:537, 1974.
87. Tofler, G. H., Brezinski, D., Schafer, A. I., et al.: Concurrent morning increase in platelet aggregability and the risk of myocardial infarction and sudden cardiac death. N. Engl. J. Med. *316*:1514, 1987.
88. Winter, J. H., Fenech, A., Ridley, W., et al.: Familial antithrombin III deficiency. Q. J. Med. *51*:373, 1982.
89. Broekmans, A. W., Veltkamp, J. J., and Bertina, R. M.: Congenital protein C deficiency and venous thromboembolism: A study of three Dutch families. N. Engl. J. Med. *309*:340, 1983.
90. Comp, P. C., Nixon, R. R., Cooper, M. R., and Esmon, C. T.: Familial protein S deficiency is associated with recurrent thrombosis. J. Clin. Invest. *74*:2082, 1984.
91. Seligson, U., Berger, A., Abend, M., et al.: Homozygous protein C deficiency manifested by massive venous thrombosis in the newborn. N. Engl. J. Med. *310*:559, 1984.
92. Bauer, K. A., Ashenhurst, J. B., Chediak, J., and Rosenberg, R. D.: Antithrombin "Chicago": A functionally abnormal molecule with increased heparin affinity causing thrombophilia. Blood *62*:1242, 1983.
93. McGehee, W. G., Klotz, T. A., Epstein, D. J., and Rapaport, S. I.: Coumarin necrosis associated with hereditary protein C deficiency. Ann. Intern. Med. *101*:59, 1984.
94. Moser, K. M., and LeMoine, J. R.: Is embolic risk conditioned by location of deep venous thrombosis? Ann. Intern. Med. *94*:855, 1981.
95. Sagar, S., Thomas, D. P., Stamatakis, J. D., and Kakkar, V. V.: Oral contraceptives, antithrombin-III activity, and post-operative deep-vein thrombosis. Lancet *1*:509, 1976.
96. Rentrop, P., Blanke, H., Karsch, K. R., et al.: Selective intracoronary thrombolysis in acute myocardial infarction and unstable angina pectoris. Circulation *63*:307, 1981.
97. Aoki, N., Moroi, M., Sakata, Y., and Yoshida, N.: Abnormal plasminogen. A hereditary molecular abnormality found in a patient with recurrent thrombosis. J. Clin. Invest. *61*:1186, 1978.
98. Carrell, N., Gabriel, D. A., Blatt, P. M., et al.: Hereditary dysfibrinogenemia in a patient with thrombotic disease. Blood *62*:439, 1983.
99. Mettinger, K. L., Nyman, D., Kjellin, K. G., et al.: Factor VIII related antigen, antithrombin III, spontaneous platelet aggregation, and plasminogen activator in ischemic cerebrovascular disease. J. Neurosci. *41*:31, 1979.
100. Isacson, S., and Nilsson, I. M.: Defective fibrinolysis in blood and vein walls in recurrent "idiopathic" venous thrombosis. Chir. Scand. *138*:313, 1972.
101. Boyko, O. B., and Pizzo, S. V.: Mesenteric vein thrombosis and vascular plasminogen activator. Arch. Pathol. Lab. Med. *107*:541, 1983.
102. Latham, B., Kafoy, G. A., Barrett, O., Jr., et al.: Deficient tissue plasminogen activator release with recurrent deep vein thrombosis. Am. J. Med. *88*:199, 1990.
103. Hamsten, A., Wiman, B., deFaire, U., and Blomback, M.: Increased plasma levels of a rapid inhibitor of tissue plasminogen activator in young survivors of myocardial infarction. N. Engl. J. Med. *313*:1551, 1985.
104. Loscalzo, J., Weinfeld, M., Fless, G., and Scanu, A. M.: Lipoprotein (a), fibrin binding and plasminogen activation. Arteriosclerosis 10:240, 1990.
105. Scanu, A. M., and Fless, G. M.: Lipoprotein (a). Heterogeneity and biological relevance. J. Clin. Invest. *85*:1709, 1990.
106. Aoki, N., Saito, H., Kamya, T., et al.: Congenital deficiency of alpha$_2$ plasmin inhibitor associated with severe hemorrhagic tendency. J. Clin. Invest. *63*:877, 1979.

ANTICOAGULANT THERAPY FOR CARDIOVASCULAR DISORDERS

107. Barrett, D. W., and Jordan, S. C.: Anticoagulant drugs in the treatment of pulmonary embolism. A controlled clinical trial. Lancet *1*:1309, 1960.
108. Rosenberg, R. D.: The heparin-antithrombin system. *In* Colman, R. W., Hirsh, J., Marder, V. J., and Salzman, E. W. (eds.): Hemostasis and Thrombosis: Basic Principles and Clinical Practice. Philadelphia, J. B. Lippincott, 1982, p. 962.
109. Marcum, J. A., McKenney, J. R., and Rosenberg, R. D.: Acceleration of thrombin-antithrombin complex formation in rat hindquarters via heparin-like molecules bound to the endothelium. J. Clin. Invest. *74*:341, 1984.
110. Castellot, J. J., Beeler, D. L., Rosenberg, R. D., and Karnovsky, M. J.: Structural determinants of the capacity of heparin to inhibit the proliferation of vascular smooth muscle cells. J. Cell. Physiol. *120*:315, 1984.
111. Kakkar, V. V., Corrigan, T., and Spindler, J.: Efficacy of low doses of heparin in prevention of deep-vein thrombosis after major surgery: A double blind, randomized trial. Lancet *2*:101, 1972.
112. Turpie, A. G., Robinson, J. G., Doyle, D. J., et al.: Comparison of high-dose with low-dose subcutaneous heparin to prevent left ventricular mural thrombosis in patients with acute transmural anterior myocardial infarction. N. Engl. J. Med. *320*:352, 1989.

113. Bell, W. R., and Royall, R. M.: Heparin-induced thrombocytopenia. A comparison of three heparin preparations. N. Engl. J. Med. *303*:902, 1980.
114. Ansell, J., and Deykin, D.: Heparin-induced thrombocytopenia and recurrent thromboembolism. Am. J. Haematol. *8*:235, 1980.
115. Jaffe, M. D., and Willis, P. W.: Multiple fractures associated with heparin therapy. J.A.M.A. *193*:158, 1965.
116. Petersen, P., Roysen, G., Godtfredsen, J., et al.: Placebo-controlled randomized trial of warfarin and aspirin for prevention of thromboembolic complications in chronic atrial fibrillation. Lancet *1*:175, 1989.
117. Furie, B., Liebman, H. A., Blanchard, R. A., et al.: Comparison of native prothrombin antigen and the prothrombin time for monitoring oral anticoagulant therapy. Blood *64*:445, 1984.
118. O'Reilly, R. A.: Vitamin K antagonists. *In* Colman, R. W., Hirsh, J., Marder, V. J., and Salzman, E. W. (eds.): Hemostasis and Thrombosis: Basic Principles and Clinical Practice. Philadelphia, J. B. Lippincott, 1982, p. 955.
119. Deykin, D.: Warfarin therapy. N. Engl. J. Med. *283*:691–694 and 801–803, 1970.
120. Husted, S., and Andreasen, F.: Problems encountered in long-term treatment with anticoagulants. Acta Med. Scand. *200*:379, 1976.
121. Hull, R., Delmore, T., Carter, C., et al.: Adjusted subcutaneous heparin versus warfarin sodium in the treatment of venous thrombosis. N. Engl. J. Med. *306*:189, 1982.
122. Hirsh, J., Deykin, D., and Poller, L.: "Therapeutic range" for oral anticoagulant therapy. Chest *82*(Suppl. 2):11S, 1986.

ANTIPLATELET DRUG THERAPY IN CARDIOVASCULAR DISEASE

123. Stein, B., Fuster, V., Israel, D. H., et al.: Platelet inhibitor agents in cardiovascular disease—an update. J. Am. Coll. Cardiol. *14*:813, 1986.
124. Antiplatelet Trialists' Collaboration: Secondary prevention of vascular disease by prolonged antiplatelet treatment. Br. Med. J. *296*:320, 1988.
125. Jaffe, E. A., and Weksler, B. B.: Recovery of endothelial cell prostacyclin production after inhibition by low doses of aspirin. J. Clin. Invest. *63*:532, 1979.
126. FitzGerald, G. A., Brash, A. R., Oates, J. A., and Pedersen, A. K.: Endogenous prostacyclin biosynthesis and platelet function during selective inhibition of thromboxane synthase in man. J. Clin. Invest. *71*:1336, 1983.
127. Hanson, S. R., Harker, L. A., and Bjornsson, T. D.: Effects of platelet-modifying drugs on arterial thromboembolism in baboons: Aspirin potentiates the antithrombotic actions of dipyridamole and sulfinpyrazone by mechanism(s) independent of platelet cyclooxygenase inhibition. J. Clin. Invest. *75*:1591, 1985.
128. FitzGerald, G. A.: Dipyridamole. N. Engl. J. Med. *316*:1247, 1987.
129. Lewis, P., and Taylor, H. M.: Dazoxiben—Clinical prospects for a thromboxane synthase inhibitor. Br. J. Clin. Pharmacol. *15*:1S, 1983.
130. Brittain, R. T., Boutal, L., Carter, M. C., et al.: AH23848: A thromboxane receptor blocking drug that can clarify the pathophysiologic role of thromboxane A_2. Circulation *72*:1208, 1985.
131. Kelton, J. G., and Blajchman, M. A.: Prostaglandin I_2 (prostacyclin). Can. Med. Assoc. J. *122*:175, 1980.
132. FitzGerald, G. A., Maas, R. L., Stein, R., et al.: Intravenous prostacyclin in thrombotic thrombocytopenic purpura. Ann. Intern. Med. *95*:319, 1981.
133. Zussman, R., Rubin, R. H., Cato, A. E., et al.: Hemodialysis using prostacyclin instead of heparin as the sole antithrombotic agent. N. Engl. J. Med. *304*:934, 1981.
134. Haes, W. K., and Kamm, B.: The North American Ticlopidine Aspirin Stroke Study: Structure, stratification, variables and patient characteristics. Ticlopidine: quo vadis? Agents Actions *15*(Suppl.):273, 1984.
135. Voelkel, N. F., Chang, S. W., Pfeffer, K. D., et al.: PAF antagonists: Different effects on platelets, neutrophils, guinea pig ileum and PAF-induced vasodilation in isolated rat lung. Prostaglandins *32*:359, 1986.
136. Gold, H. K., Coller, B. S., Yasuda, T., et al: Rapid and sustained coronary artery recanalization with combined bolus injection of recombinant tissue-type plasminogen activator and monoclonal antiplatelet GpIIb/IIIa antibody in a canine preparation. Circulation *77*:670, 1988.
137. Schror, K., Ahland, B., Darius, H., and Weiss, P.: Stimulation of vascular PGI_2 by organic nitrates and its significance for the antianginal effect. Scand. J. Lab. Clin. Invest. *173*(Suppl.):33, 1984.
138. Pumphrey, C. W., Fuster, V., Dewarjee, M. K., et al.: Comparison of the antithrombotic action of calcium antagonist drugs with dipyridamole in dogs. Am. J. Cardiol. *51*:591, 1983.
139. DeWood, M. A., Stifter, W. F., Simpson, C. S., et al.: Coronary arteriographic findings soon after non-Q-wave myocardial infarction. N. Engl. J. Med. *315*:417, 1986.
140. Mehta, J., Mehta, P., Feldman, R. J., and Horalek, C.: Thromboxane release in coronary artery disease: Spontaneous angina versus pacing-induced angina. Am. Heart J. *107*:286, 1984.
141. Lewis, H. D., David, J. W., Archibald, D. G., et al.: Protective effects of aspirin against acute myocardial infarction and death in men with unstable angina. N. Engl. J. Med. *309*:396, 1983.
142. Cairns, J., Gent, M., Singer, J., et al.: Aspirin, sulfinpyrazone or both in unstable angina. Results of a Canadian multicenter trial. N. Engl. J. Med. *313*:1369, 1985.
143. Theroux, P., Ouimet, H., McCano, J., et al.: Aspirin, Heparin or both to treat acute unstable angina. N. Engl. J. Med. *319*:1105, 1988.
144. ISIS-2 Collaborative Group: Randomized trial of intravenous streptokinase and aspirin both or neither among 17, 187 cases of suspected acute myocardial infarction. Lancet *2*:348, 1988.
145. The Steering Committee of the Physicians' Health Study Research Group: Final report of the aspirin component of the ongoing physicians' health study. N. Engl. J. Med. *321*:129, 1989.
146. Peto, R., Gray, R., Collins, R., et al.: A randomized trial of the effects of prophylactic daily aspirin among male British doctors. Br. Med. J. *296*:313, 1988.
147. Sethi, G., Copeland, J. G., Goldman,. S., et al.: Implications of preoperative administration of aspirin to patients undergoing coronary bypass grafting. J. Am. Coll. Cardiol. *15*:15, 1990.
148. Goldman, S., Copeland, J., Moritz, T., et al.: Improvement in early saphenous vein graft patency after coronary artery bypass surgery with antiplatelet therapy: Results of a Veterans Administration Cooperative Study. Circulation *77*:1324, 1988.
148a. Chesebro, J. H., Fuster, V., Elveback, L. R., et al.: Effect of dipyridamole and aspirin on late vein-graft patency after coronary bypass operations. N. Engl. J. Med. *310*:209, 1984.
149. Goldman, S., Copeland, J., Moeritz, T., et al.: Saphenous vein graft patency one year after coronary artery bypass surgery and effects of antiplatelet therapy: Results of a Veterans Administration Cooperative Study. Circulation *80*:1190, 1989.

THROMBOLYTIC THERAPY

150. Reddy, K.N.N.: Mechanism of activation of human plasminogen by streptokinase. *In* Kline, D. L., and Reddy, K. N. (eds.): Fibrinolysis. Boca Raton, CRC Press, 1980, p. 71.
151. Anderson, J. L.: Development and evaluation of anisoylated plasminogen-streptokinase activator complex (APSAC) as a second generation thrombolytic agent. J. Am. Coll. Cardiol. *10*:228, 1987.
152. Vaughan, D. E., Kirshenbaum, J., and Loscalzo, J.: Streptokinase-induced, antibody-mediated platelet aggregation: A potential cause of clot propagation in vitro. J. Am. Coll. Cardiol. *11*:1343, 1988.
153. Hussain, S. S., Gurewich, V., and Lipinski, B.: Purification and partial characterization of a single chain high molecular weight form of urokinase from human urine. Arch. Biochem. Biophys. *220*:31, 1983.
154. Gurewich, V., Pannell, R., Louie, S., et al.: Effective and fibrin-specific clot lysis by a zymogen precursor form of urokinase (pro-urokinase). J. Clin. Invest. *73*:1731, 1984.
155. Rijken, D. C., and Collen, D. C.: Purification and characterization of the plasminogen activator secreted by human melanoma cells in culture. J. Biol. Chem. *257*:7035, 1981.
156. Loscalzo, J.: A structural and kinetic comparison of recombinant human single-chain and two-chain tissue plasminogen activator. J. Clin. Invest. *82*:1391, 1988.
157. vanZonnenveld, A. J., Veerman, H., and Pannekoek, H.: Autonomous functions of structural domains on human tissue-type plasminogen activator. Proc. Natl. Acad Sci. U.S.A. *83*:4670, 1986.
158. Neuhaus, K. L., Feuerer, W., Jeep-Tebbe, S., et al.: Improved thrombolysis with a modified dose regimen of recombinant tissue-type plasminogen activator. J. Am. Coll. Cardiol. *14*:1566, 1989.
159. Goldhaber, S. Z., Vaughan, D. E., Markis, J. E., et al.: Acute pulmonary embolism treated with tissue plasminogen activator. Lancet *2*:886, 1986.
160. Goldhaber, S. Z., Meyerowitz, M. F., Green, D., et al.: Randomized controlled trial of tissue plasminogen activator in proximal deep venous thrombosis. Am. J. Med. *88*:235, 1990.
161. Graor, R. A., Risius, B., Young, J. R., et al.: Peripheral artery and bypass graft thrombolysis with recombinant tissue-type plasminogen activator. J. Vasc. Surg. *3*:115, 1986.
162. DelZoppo, G. J.: Investigational use of t-PA in acute stroke. Ann. Emerg. Med. *17*:1196, 1988.
163. Garabedian, H. D., Gold, H. K., Leinbach, R. C., et al.: Comparative properties of two clinical preparations of recombinant human tissue-type plasminogen activator in patients with acute myocardial infarction. J. Am. Coll. Cardiol. *9*:599, 1987.
164. Jang, I. K., van Haecke, J., and de Geest, H.: Coronary thrombolysis with recombinant tissue-type plasminogen activator: Patency rate and regional wall motion after three months. J. Am. Coll. Cardiol. *8*:15, 1986.
165. The Urokinase Pulmonary Embolism Trial: A national cooperative study. Circulation *47*:II-1, 1973.
166. Sharma, G.V.R.K., and Sasahara, A. A.: Long-term benefits of treatment of pulmonary embolism with thrombolytic therapy. J. Am. Coll. Cardiol. (in press).
167. Loscalzo, J.: Shortcomings of thrombolytic therapy. J. Myocard. Isch. *2*:48, 1990.

59

Pregnancy and Cardiovascular Disease

by URI ELKAYAM, M.D.

CARDIOVASCULAR PHYSIOLOGY DURING PREGNANCY AND THE PUERPERIUM

Pregnancy and the peripartum period are associated with substantial cardiocirculatory changes. In the woman with heart disease, these changes can lead to rapid clinical deterioration and result in greater morbidity and possibly death.[1] Therefore, the management of these disorders in the pregnant patient requires an understanding of cardiovascular physiology during gestation, labor, delivery, and the puerperium. Hemodynamic changes occurring during pregnancy are summarized in Table 59–1.

BLOOD VOLUME. Blood volume increases substantially during pregnancy, starting as early as the sixth week of gestation and rising rapidly until midpregnancy, when the volume continues to rise, but at a much slower rate.[1a] Although the degree of volume expansion varies considerably in the individual patient (20 to 100 per cent), the augmentation averages 50 per cent of the volume in the nonpregnant state.[2] This increase is reported to correlate with fetal weight, placental mass, weight of the products of conception, neonatal weight, and maternal weight. A higher increment in blood volume is reported in multigravidas and in women with multiple pregnancies.[1]

Because the increase in blood volume is more rapid than the increase in red blood cell mass (Fig. 59–1), hemoglobin concentration falls during pregnancy, causing the "physiological anemia of pregnancy."[3] Hematocrit and hemoglobin levels are frequently as low as 33 to 38 per cent and 11 to 12 gm/100 ml, respectively.[1] Changes in blood volume during pregnancy may be attributable to estrogen-mediated stimulation of renin,[4] which then promotes aldosterone secretion and hypervolemia as a result of sodium and water retention.[3,5] (Fig. 59–2). Chorionic somatomammotropin, a hormone-like substance in the placenta, may also be a factor.[3]

CARDIAC OUTPUT, STROKE VOLUME, AND HEART RATE. Augmentation of blood volume alters stroke volume and cardiac output (Table 59–1). Cardiac output during pregnancy is estimated to exceed the output during the nonpregnant state by 30 to 50 per cent.[1,3,6] It begins to rise around the fifth week and peaks between the middle of the second and the third trimesters. After that time, cardiac output seems to be maintained at the same level. Changes in body position can induce substantial changes in cardiac output with levels rising in the lateral position and declining in the supine position, owing to caval compression by the gravid uterus and thus decreased venous return to the heart. The increase in cardiac output early in pregnancy can be attributed predominantly to the augmentation in stroke volume; during the third trimester, the increase is largely due to an accelerated heart rate, while stroke volume declines toward prepregnancy values as a result of caval compression.

Heart rate also increases, peaking during the third trimester. The average rise in heart rate is 10 to 20 beats per minute.[6] Although the rate may on occasion be markedly faster, it may decrease slightly in the lateral position compared with the supine position.[7]

BLOOD PRESSURE AND SYSTEMIC VASCULAR RESISTANCE. Systemic arterial pressure begins to fall during the first trimester, reaches a nadir in midpregnancy, and returns toward pregestational levels before term.[1] Since the fall in diastolic blood pressure is substantially greater than the fall in systolic pressure, the pulse pressure widens.[1,8] The reduction in blood pressure results from a decline in systemic vascular resistance due to vasodilation, probably mediated by gestational hormonal activity,[9] increased levels of circulating prostaglandins,[10] increased heat production by the developing fetus, and the creation of low-resistance circulation in the pregnant uterus.[11] A phenomenon unique to pregnancy and described as the supine hypotensive syndrome of pregnancy or the uterocaval syndrome presents with significant decreases in heart rate and blood pressure and occurs in up to 11 per cent of pregnant women.[1-7] These hemodynamic changes are associated with weakness, lightheadedness, nausea, dizziness, and even syncope and are explained by acute occlusion of the inferior vena cava by the enlarged uterus. When the

TABLE 59–1 HEMODYNAMIC CHANGES DURING NORMAL PREGNANCY

PARAMETER	1ST TRIMESTER	2ND TRIMESTER	3RD TRIMESTER
Blood volume	↑	↑↑	↑↑↑
Cardiac output	↑	↑↑ to ↑↑↑	↑↑↑ to ↑↑
Stroke volume	↑	↑↑↑	↑, ↔, or ↓
Heart rate	↑	↑↑	↑↑↑
Systolic blood pressure	↔	↓	↔
Diastolic blood pressure	↓	↓↓	↓
Pulse pressure	↑	↑↑	↔
Systemic vascular resistance	↓	↓↓↓	↓↓

↔ = no change compared to nonpregnant level; ↑ = small increase; ↑↑ = moderate increase; ↑↑↑ = large increase; ↓ = small decrease; ↓↓ = moderate decrease; ↓↓↓ = large decrease

Modified from Elkayam, U., and Gleicher, N.: Hemodynamics and cardiac function during normal pregnancy and the puerperium. *In* Elkayam, U., and Gleicher, N. (eds.): Cardiac Problems in Pregnancy: Diagnosis and Management of Maternal and Fetal Disease. 2nd ed. New York, Alan R. Liss, Inc., 1990, p. 5.

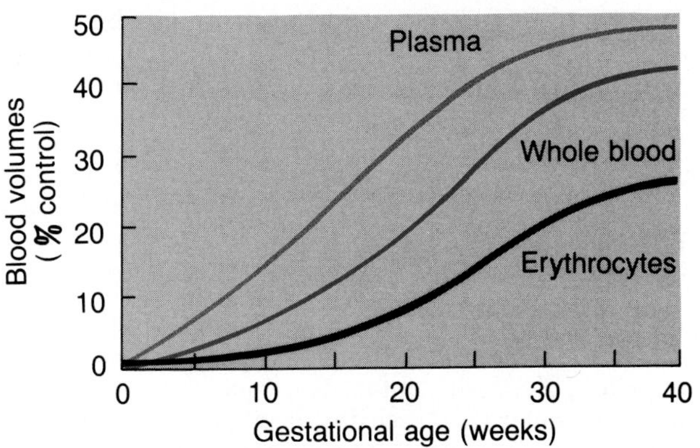

FIGURE 59-1. **Alterations in plasma volume, blood volume, and erythrocyte mass during pregnancy. Predominance of increase in plasma volume results in the "physiological anemia of pregnancy." (From Longo, L. O.: Maternal blood volume and cardiac output during pregnancy: A hypothesis of endocrinologic control. Am. J. Physiol. *245*:R720, 1983.)**

supine position is abandoned, these hemodynamic effects and symptoms usually are promptly relieved.

HEMODYNAMIC CHANGES DURING LABOR AND DELIVERY. Anxiety, pain, and uterine contractions all alter hemodynamics substantially during labor and delivery. Cardiac output increases by up to 50 per cent during contractions, mainly owing to changes in stroke volume,[12] and total cardiac output is higher in the lateral position than in the supine position.[13] The effect of uterine contractions on the heart rate varies[12] and may be influenced by the woman's position during labor and the form of sedation used. Both systolic and diastolic blood pressures increase markedly during contractions, with greater augmentation during the second stage.[1,12]

Hemodynamic changes during labor are associated with a threefold increase in oxygen consumption and are greatly influenced by the form of anesthesia or analgesia used.[1,14,15] In general, reducing the pain and apprehension associated with local and caudal anesthesia will limit the rise in cardiac output; however, these forms of anesthesia will not prevent the increase in cardiac output related to uterine contractions.

HEMODYNAMIC EFFECTS OF CESAREAN SECTION. To avoid the hemodynamic changes associated with vaginal delivery, cesarean section is frequently recommended for women with cardiovascular disease. However, this form of delivery can also be associated with considerable hemodynamic fluctuation related largely to intubation, the form of anesthesia, the anesthetic and analgesic agent(s), the extent of blood loss during the procedure, abdominal surgery, the relief of caval compression, extubation, and postoperative awakening.[14,15]

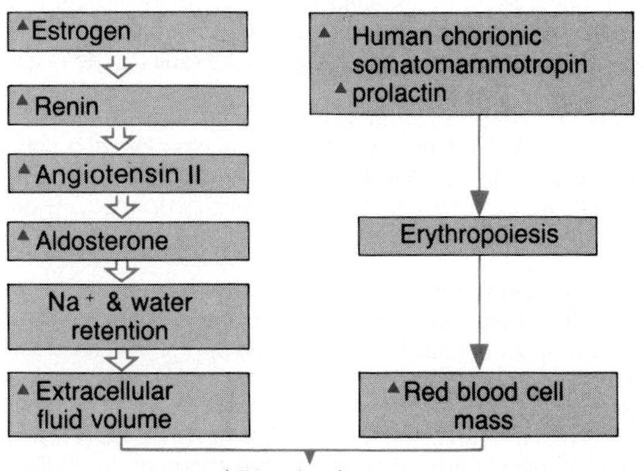

FIGURE 59-2. **Potential mechanisms of hypervolemia of pregnancy. (From Elkayam, U., and Gleicher, N.: Hemodynamics and cardiac function during normal pregnancy and the puerperium. *In* Elkayam, U., and Gleicher, N. [eds.]: Cardiac Problems in Pregnancy: Diagnosis and Management of Maternal and Fetal Disease. 2nd ed. New York, Alan R. Liss, Inc., 1990, p. 5.)**

HEMODYNAMIC CHANGES POST PARTUM. Clinical status often deteriorates in the immediate postpartum period when venous return increases after the fetus is removed and caval compression has been relieved.[1] In addition, blood shifting from the contracting, emptied uterus into the systemic circulation (autotransfusion) increases the preload. This change in effective blood volume occurs despite blood loss associated with delivery and leads to a substantial rise in stroke volume and cardiac output immediately after delivery. Within the first hour, however, the reduction in heart rate decreases cardiac output, which falls to prepregnancy levels 24 hours post partum as stroke volume normalizes.[12]

HEMODYNAMIC RESPONSE TO EXERCISE. Exercise-mediated increases in cardiac output are limited during gestation; in the third trimester output during exercise may be more than 20 per cent lower than it is in nonpregnant women.[16] This attenuated rise in cardiac output is due to the lower responses of heart rate and stroke volume; the latter is probably the result of a reduction in venous return during pregnancy.[17] In normal women during the third trimester, uterine blood flow is reduced 25 per cent during mild exercise.[18] Such reductions may be associated with fetal hypoxia, manifested by brief episodes of fetal bradycardia.[18,19] Strenuous physical activity may be associated with fetal compromise and is therefore not recommended during pregnancy.[18]

CARDIAC EVALUATION DURING PREGNANCY

The evaluation of cardiac disease in pregnancy may be complicated by the normal anatomical and functional changes of the cardiovascular system during gestation. Such changes may result in signs and symptoms that can either simulate or obscure heart disease.[20] In addition, the diagnostic approach to cardiac disease in pregnancy is influenced by the potential risk to the fetus posed by certain diagnostic methods.

HISTORY AND PHYSICAL EXAMINATION

(Table 59-2)

Normal pregnancy is often accompanied by symptoms of fatigue, decreased exercise capacity, dyspnea, lightheadedness, and, rarely, syncope.[20] Respirations are often shallow and rapid and may be erroneously interpreted as dyspnea. In addition, distention of the jugular veins due to increased blood volume and the leg edema often observed in late pregnancy could lead to an inappropriate diagnosis of heart failure or overestimation of its severity. Systemic arterial pulses are full and collapsing and are similar to those palpated in patients with aortic regurgitation or hyperthyroidism. A left ventricular impulse is easily detected in most women in late pregnancy; usually it is hyperactive, brisk, and unsustained and may be displaced to the left. The quality of the impulse may simulate a volume overload state such as that seen in aortic or mitral valve regurgitation. The pulmonary trunk, right ventricle, and pulmonic valve closure are often palpable, and this group of findings may lead to the misdiagnosis of pulmonary hypertension.

CARDIAC AUSCULTATION. Especially after the first trimester, auscultation often reveals an increased first heart sound (S_1) with exaggerated splitting[21] that may be misinterpreted as S_4 or as a systolic click. The physiological increase in the amplitude of the second element of S_1 during inspiration should help differentiate it from an abnormal auscultatory event. S_2 is often increased in late pregnancy and may exhibit expiratory splitting when the patient is examined in the lateral position. These changes in S_2 may be interpreted as signs of pulmonary hypertension (loud S_2) or atrial septal defect (fixed splitting of S_2). Although S_3 and S_4 have been reported to be extremely frequent during gestation,[21] in the author's experience, auscultation of these sounds is actually uncommon in normal pregnancy, and their presence warrants further investigation to detect possible underlying disease.

TABLE 59-2 CARDIAC SYMPTOMS AND FINDINGS DURING NORMAL PREGNANCY

SYMPTOMS
- Decreased exercise capacity
- Tiredness
- Dyspnea
- Orthopnea
- Lightheadedness
- Syncope

PHYSICAL FINDINGS
- Inspection
  - Hyperventilation
  - Peripheral edema
  - Distended neck veins with prominent A and V waves and brisk *x* and *y* descents
  - Capillary pulsation
- Precordial palpation
  - Brisk, diffuse, and displaced left ventricular impulse
  - Palpable right ventricular impulse
  - Palpable pulmonary trunk impulse
- Auscultation
  - Pulmonary basilar rales
  - Increased S_1 with exaggerated splitting
  - Persistent splitting of S_2
  - Early and midsystolic ejection-type murmurs at the lower left sternal edge and/or over the pulmonary area
  - Continuous murmurs (cervical venous hum, mammary souffle)
  - Diastolic murmurs

ELECTROCARDIOGRAM
- QRS-axis deviation
- ST-segment and T-wave changes
- Small Q wave and inverted P wave in lead III (abolished by inspiration)
- Increased R-wave amplitude in lead V_2
- Frequent sinus tachycardia
- Increased incidence of arrhythmias

CHEST X-RAY
- Straightening of the left upper cardiac border
- Horizontal position of the heart
- Increased lung marking
- Small pleural effusion early post partum

ECHO-DOPPLER
- Increased left and right ventricular dimensions
- Unchanged or slightly improved left ventricular systolic function
- Enlargement of the ventricular dimensions
- Mild increase in left and right atrial size
- Small pericardial effusion
- Increased diameter of tricuspid annulus
- Functional tricuspid and pulmonary insufficiency

Modified from Elkayam, U., and Gleicher, N.: Changes in cardiac findings during normal pregnancy. *In* Elkayam, U., and Gleicher, N. (eds.): Cardiac Problems in Pregnancy: Diagnosis and Management of Maternal and Fetal Disease. 2nd ed. New York, Alan R. Liss, Inc., 1990, p. 31.

Innocent Systolic Murmurs. These can be heard in most pregnant women[20,21] and are the result of the hyperkinetic circulation of pregnancy. They are heard best at the lower left sternal edge and over the pulmonic area radiating to the suprasternal notch and to the left and, at times, also to the right side of the neck. The murmurs often sound like those associated with atrial septal defect or stenosis of one of the semilunar valves. Two benign continuous murmurs that can be heard frequently during gestation are the cervical venous hum and the mammary souffle. The *venous hum* is usually heard maximally over the right supraclavicular fossa but can radiate to the contralateral area and sometimes to the area below the clavicle.[22] The *mammary souffle*, which is heard mostly over the breast late in gestation or in the lactating woman post partum, is caused by increased flow in the mammary vessels and can be either systolic or continuous. Characteristically, the murmur decreases or vanishes when pressure is applied to the stethoscope or when the patient moves into the upright position.[23] The continuous murmurs may be incorrectly attributed to patent ductus arteriosus or arteriovenous fistulas. In addition, these murmurs can be misinterpreted as systolic and/or diastolic murmurs, leading to erroneous diagnosis.

A soft, medium- to high-pitched diastolic murmur has been reported in normal pregnant women.[21] However, in the author's experience, such a finding is infrequent in the healthy pregnant woman and therefore requires a careful diagnostic work-up to rule out organic disease.

Increases in blood volume and flow across the various cardiac valves may augment systolic murmurs of aortic or pulmonic stenosis and the diastolic murmur of mitral stenosis. In contrast, the murmurs associated with mitral or aortic regurgitation may decrease in intensity secondary to a reduction in systemic vascular resistance during pregnancy.[24] The physiological increase in blood volume with gestation may also affect auscultatory findings in other volume-dependent abnormalities, such as mitral valve prolapse and obstructive hypertrophic cardiomyopathy; the change in volume may abolish the systolic click and murmur commonly heard in patients with mitral valve prolapse[25] and may decrease the systolic murmur typical of hypertrophic cardiomyopathy.[26,27]

FUNCTIONAL CLASSIFICATION

Functional classification, as recommended by the New York Heart Association, attempts to define a cardiac patient's status according to symptoms at different levels of activity.[28] Traditionally, this classification has also been used to assess the severity of cardiac disease and prognosis during pregnancy.[29] In general, pregnancy is considered safe for cardiac patients in Classes I and II (prior to pregnancy). For Class III patients, special attention during pregnancy and early admission before delivery are recommended. Pregnancy is generally contraindicated for patients in Class IV. Although the functional classification has been widely accepted, it is important to note that this method (which relies on signs and subjective symptoms) may be inaccurate and misleading owing to the major anatomical and functional changes in the cardiovascular system that take place during pregnancy. It is therefore imperative to use additional diagnostic tools to obtain objective and reliable information about cardiac status.

LABORATORY EXAMINATIONS

ELECTROCARDIOGRAPHY (Table 59-2). In normal pregnancy, the QRS axis shifts to either the left or the right.[20] Transient ST-segment depressions and T-wave changes are common. A small Q wave and an inverted P wave in lead III that vary with respiration[20] as well as a greater R-wave amplitude in lead V_2 are often present.[30] The pregnant woman's increased susceptibility to arrhythmias[31] can also be apparent in the frequent finding of sinus tachycardia and atrial and/or ventricular premature beats. Arrhythmias with a high incidence during labor and delivery include atrial and ventricular premature beats, sinus arrhythmia, sinus tachycardia, sinus bradycardia, wandering atrial pacemaker, sinus arrest with nodal escape rhythm, and supraventricular tachycardia.[32]

CHEST X-RAY (Table 59-2). Although the radiation dose associated with a routine chest x-ray is minimal (the average dose to the skin in the primary beam is 70 to 150 mrad, while the estimated dose to the uterus is 0.2 to 43.0 mrad),[33,34] this diagnostic test is best avoided during pregnancy because of the potential for adverse biological effects from *any* amount of radiation. When chest radiography is performed, the pelvic area should be shielded by a protective lead material from accidental direct exposure.

Since changes seen on chest x-rays in normal pregnancy may simulate cardiac disease, they should be interpreted with caution.[20,35] Straightening of the left upper cardiac border because of prominence of the pulmonary conus is often seen and may mimic the left atrial enlargement commonly associated with rheumatic mitral valve disease. The heart seems enlarged on radiography in many pregnant women because of its horizontal positioning secondary to the elevated diaphragm. In addition, an increase in lung markings may simulate the flow redistribution seen with increased pulmonary venous pressure due to left ventricular failure or mitral valve disease. Pleural effusion early post partum has been a frequent finding[36,37]; the effusion is usually small and resorbs 1 to 2 weeks after delivery.

DOPPLER ECHOCARDIOGRAPHY (Table 59-2). Despite concern regarding the use of ultrasound during pregnancy, no hazard has been

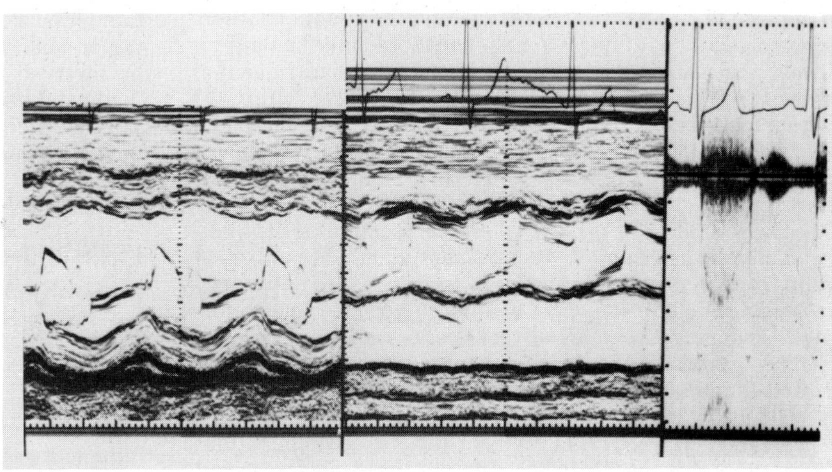

FIGURE 59–3. M-mode echocardiogram at the level of the mitral valve *(left panel)* and the aortic valve *(middle panel)* and Doppler aortic blood flow study *(right panel)* in a 27-year-old woman with congenital bicuspid valve and aortic stenosis at 32 weeks' gestation. The patient had symptoms of fatigue and shortness of breath. Peak instantaneous pressure gradient across the aortic valve by the Doppler technique was 81 mm Hg. The patient had successful pregnancy, labor, and delivery of a normal baby. Small pericardial effusion seen on the left is a common benign finding in pregnancy.

identified in humans, so that both maternal and fetal echocardiography may be considered safe.[38] Normal gestational changes in the cardiovascular system are reflected echocardiographically and should be taken into consideration. When the patient is examined in the left lateral position, an increase in left and right ventricular end-diastolic dimensions is to be expected as a result of volume overload.[39,40] These changes progress with the pregnancy but return to baseline dimensions post partum. Left ventricular systolic dimension and function are either unchanged or increased during pregnancy, and the left and right atria may increase slightly in size.

Pericardial effusion, usually minimal, has been noted in 40 per cent of normal pregnant women late in pregnancy (Fig. 59–3).[41,42] Recent studies have demonstrated mild tricuspid and pulmonary regurgitation, mainly near term,[40,43] that seem related to right-sided chamber enlargement and dilatation of the valve annulus. These findings do not appear to be important clinically but need to be considered when one is interpreting Doppler echocardiograms obtained during pregnancy.

STRESS TESTING. An exercise test using bicycle ergometry or a treadmill may be carried out during pregnancy to help establish the diagnosis of ischemic heart disease and to assess functional capacity and cardiac reserve. The safety of such testing in pregnancy has not been fully established. Since fetal bradycardia has been reported with maximal but not with submaximal exercise,[44] a low-level exercise protocol with fetal monitoring is recommended when stress testing is indicated.[45]

PULMONARY ARTERY FLOTATION CATHETERIZATION. Hemodynamic monitoring with the aid of a pulmonary artery catheter can be of great help in managing patients at high risk during pregnancy, labor, delivery, and the postpartum period. The ability to insert and position the flotation catheter under pressure monitoring without the need for fluoroscopy makes it particularly attractive for use during pregnancy.[46] Hemodynamic monitoring can provide useful diagnostic and prognostic information and should be used without hesitation at any time during pregnancy if a noninvasive cardiac work-up does not provide conclusive information.

Hemodynamic monitoring is recommended throughout labor and delivery for any patient with symptomatic cardiac disease during pregnancy or with the potential for deterioration due to valvular, vascular, myocardial, or ischemic heart disease. Since significant circulatory changes that may lead to hemodynamic deterioration occur in the early postpartum period,[1] hemodynamic monitoring should be continued for 24 hours after delivery to assure stability.

CARDIAC CATHETERIZATION. When cardiac decompensation occurs during pregnancy, particularly if cardiac surgery or balloon valvuloplasty is being considered, cardiac catheterization may be required. Although this technique provides high-quality images, it is associated with a relatively high dose of radiation. The median dose to the skin is 47 rads per examination with 10 to 15 per cent exposure to an unshielded abdomen and approximately 500 mrad estimated dose to the conceptus, even with an appropriate pelvic shield.[33,34]

The potentially deleterious effect of ionizing radiation is linearly proportional to the absorbed dose and is present at all times after fertilization. The type and likelihood of this effect vary with the stage of fetal development and the dose of radiation. An increase in the incidence of fetal malformation appears to be highly unlikely with doses below 5 rads, even when these are delivered at a time when the induction of any specific type of maldevelopment is critical.[47] In general, radiation exposure during the first week of pregnancy may result in absorption or resorption of the preimplanted blastocyst, whereas the risk of teratogenic effects predominates during the second to sixth weeks of gestation. Developing brain cells can be affected by radiation during the seventh to fifteenth weeks, which may lead to alterations in neurological function or behavior. In addition, irradiation at any time during the entire pregnancy may increase the risk for childhood cancer[48]; this risk seems to be higher with exposure during the first trimester.

Therefore, because of its risk to the fetus, cardiac catheterization during gestation should be performed only if information cannot be obtained by alternative noninvasive methods. The procedure should involve the brachial rather than the femoral approach to minimize radiation to the pelvic and abdominal areas, which should be appropriately shielded, and x-ray exposure should be kept to a minimum. To minimize the use of ionizing radiation, techniques such as contrast[49] and Doppler echocardiography with cardiac catheterization should be combined for a complete evaluation.

RADIONUCLIDE IMAGING. A potential limitation of these techniques during pregnancy is radiation exposure to the fetus. The dose estimated to reach the fetus with the radiopharmaceuticals generally used for cardiac imaging is equal to or less than 800 mrad.[50] However, calculations of the dose to the conceptus are only approximations and can vary from person to person owing to differences in the uptake of radionuclides by maternal organs, metabolism, and placental uptake and transfer. Because of these uncertainties and the potential risk, *use of radionuclide imaging should be avoided if possible during gestation and in particular during the first trimester.* In addition, such imaging should be performed only when the information desired cannot be obtained by other, noninvasive techniques, such as two-dimensional and Doppler echocardiography.

Cardiovascular Diseases and Pregnancy

CONGENITAL HEART DISEASE (CHD)

(See also Chap. 32)

PRECONCEPTION COUNSELING. The management of patients with CHD should begin before conception. An accurate diagnostic and functional evaluation is supplemented by counseling of both the patient and her family regarding potential maternal and fetal risks of pregnancy, expected maternal morbidity, and, when appropriate, long-term survival as well as the risk that the offspring will inherit CHD. In addition, guidance concerning anticoagulation and prophylactic antibiotics, if needed, should be provided.[51]

MATERNAL AND FETAL OUTCOME. Maternal outcome is determined by the nature of the disease, surgical repair, the presence of cyanosis, and functional capacity.[52,53] Whittemore et al.[53,54] reported no maternal deaths in 237 women with CHD involving 488 pregnancies. Congestive heart failure, arrhythmias, and hypertension are commonly seen in patients with impaired functional status and with cyanosis.[52,53] Other reported complications in patients with CHD during pregnancy include angina and infective endocarditis.

Maternal functional capacity and the presence of cyanosis also determine fetal outcome. Fetal wastage was reported in 45 per cent of cyanotic mothers, compared with 20 per cent of acyanotic mothers with CHD.[53] Low birth weight for gestational age and prematurity are common in cyanotic mothers and correlate with maternal hemoglobin and hematocrit levels.[54] Risk of substantial cardiac and noncardiac congenital defects is increased for the offspring of mothers with CHD with a reported incidence of CHD of about 10 per cent (3.4 to 16.1 per cent).[53-55] In addition, there are a greater number of noncardiac abnormalities as well as mental and physical impairments in children born to mothers with CHD.[53]

LABOR AND DELIVERY. Cesarean section is not indicated in most patients with CHD[53-55] and should be performed primarily for obstetrical reasons or in response to deteriorating maternal status. Oxygen should be given to hypoxemic mothers during labor and delivery, and hemodynamic as well as blood gas monitoring is recommended in patients with impaired functional capacity, cardiac dysfunction, pulmonary hypertension, and cyanotic malformations.[46]

ANTIBIOTIC PROPHYLAXIS. Official recommendations for antibiotic prophylaxis proposed by the American Heart Association (p. 1806) do not include patients with CHD who are undergoing uncomplicated vaginal delivery unless they have a prosthetic heart valve or a surgically constructed systemic-to-pulmonary shunt.[56] Despite these recommendations, the use of antibiotic prophylaxis is not uncommon in many hospitals for patients with CHD, with the exception of those with an isolated secundum type of atrial septal defect and those who underwent ligation and division of a patent ductus arteriosus more than 6 months earlier. The risk for endocarditis may be increased after manual removal of the placenta, so that antibiotic prophylaxis is recommended for this procedure in patients with CHD.[55]

Atrial Septal Defect (ASD) (see also p. 977)

This common type of maternal CHD is frequently discovered during pregnancy when the murmur is first elicited. This condition is usually well tolerated in pregnancy, even among patients with large left-to-right shunts. Pulmonary hypertension rarely occurs until the fourth decade of life, and the same is true for atrial arrhythmias, which are uncommon before age 40. Because endocarditis is rare, antibiotic prophylaxis is not indicated in patients with secundum-type ASD. Recommendations concerning pregnancy in such patients should be made on an individual basis, account being taken of the functional status and the level of pulmonary artery pressure.

Ventricular Septal Defect (VSD) (see also p. 971)

Women with isolated VSD usually tolerate pregnancy well, although congestive heart failure and arrhythmias have been reported in patients with uncorrected lesions.[46] The risk posed by pregnancy after closure of an uncomplicated VSD should not differ from that in patients without heart disease. The incidence of CHD was found to be as high as 22 per cent among live-born offspring in one report, with a recurrence of VSD in 50 per cent of this group.[53] Marked reduction in blood pressure during or after delivery as a result of blood loss or anesthesia may lead to shunt reversal in patients with pulmonary hypertension. The use of vasopressors and volume replacement to stabilize blood pressure promptly should prevent further complications.

Patent Ductus Arteriosus (PDA) (see also p. 977)

This common congenital defect occurs predominantly in women (2 : 1 female/male ratio). With early diagnosis and surgical correction in early childhood, a patent ductus has become a rare finding in pregnancy.[57] Although maternal outcome in patients with PDA is usually favorable,[58] some patients deteriorate clinically because of congestive heart failure.[55] Although early reports cited a maternal mortality rate of approximately 5 per cent, more recent experience has revealed no maternal deaths among a large number of patients with PDA.[52,53,57] The occasional patient with heart failure should be treated with bed rest, diuretics, and digitalis. Although surgical intervention or catheter-induced closure during pregnancy may be successful,[58] these procedures should be reserved for patients with heart failure unresponsive to medical therapy. In the early postpartum period, shunt reversal may occur in women with pulmonary hypertension who develop systemic hypotension, so that any decrease in systemic blood pressure should be immediately corrected by means of volume replacement or vasopressor agents.

Congenital Aortic Valve Disease (see also p. 978)

A bicuspid aortic valve is the most common type of CHD, occurring in 1 per cent to 2 per cent of the population. This defect may lead to significant aortic stenosis in women of childbearing age. Obstruction of left ventricular outflow can also result from unicuspid or tricuspid valves or supravalvular and subvalvular obstruction. Aortic stenosis, especially if mild, can easily be missed on physical examination, since its murmur may be attributed to the flow-related systolic murmur commonly heard in the normal pregnant woman. The presence of a sustained left ventricular impulse, aortic ejection sound, and S_4 should raise the level of suspicion.

Although data concerning pregnancy in women with surgically uncorrected aortic stenosis are limited, they indicate the potential for clinical deterioration, due to the development of heart failure, hypertension, and angina, and even for death during pregnancy and the peripartum period.[52,53,59] Whittemore et al.[53] reported a high incidence (20 per cent) of cardiac defects in live-born infants of mothers with left heart obstruction.

The author's experience with several patients with moderate to severe aortic stenosis indicates that with early diagnosis and appropriate care, including hemodynamic monitoring during labor and delivery and appropriate anesthesia, the outcome will be favorable in most cases (Fig. 59–3).[55] Patients with severe aortic stenosis (aortic valve area $< 1.0\ cm^2$) should be advised against pregnancy or should agree to an early abortion so that the valve can be corrected surgically. When clinical deterioration after the 22nd week of gestation does not respond to medical therapy, surgical intervention is indicated.

Percutaneous balloon valvuloplasty (p. 1377) has been performed successfully in pregnant women with aortic stenosis.[60] Although this procedure obviates the general anesthesia and cardiopulmonary bypass required for surgery, it is associated with significant and often unpredictable radiation exposure and hemodynamic fluctuations that may lead to immediate and late fetal complications.[33,34,37] In addition, significant restenosis may occur within 6 months of the procedure. For all of these reasons, percutaneous balloon valvuloplasty should be considered only in patients with severe symptoms not manageable with drug therapy and should be performed as late as possible during gestation.

Coarctation of the Aorta (see also p. 967)

Uncorrected coarctation of the aorta is found less commonly during pregnancy, since surgical correction is usually performed prior to the childbearing age.[57] In uncomplicated coarctation, pregnancy is usually safe for the mother; however, fetal development may be impaired since uteroplacental blood flow is decreased owing to the aortic obstruction. In a review of reports published since 1958, Metcalfe et al.[58] found 13 cases of maternal death among 230 women with aortic coarctation involving 565 pregnancies. Whittemore et al.[53] found no deaths, but reported complications such as hypertension, congestive heart failure, and angina. Aortic dissection and rupture have also been associated with coarctation of the aorta during pregnancy.[61] In addition, a higher incidence of CHD has been shown in infants of mothers with surgically uncorrected coarctation compared with mothers whose coarctation had been corrected.[53] For all of these reasons, it seems advisable to correct aortic coarctation *prior* to pregnancy.

Treatment to reduce the incidence of aortic rupture and

cerebral aneurysms during pregnancy consists of limiting physical activity and controlling blood pressure. Excessive reduction of blood pressure, however, may compromise uteroplacental blood flow and should be avoided. Surgical correction of coarctation has been performed successfully during pregnancy[62] and may be indicated in patients with uncontrollable, severely elevated systolic blood pressure or severe heart failure refractory to medical therapy. Contrary to earlier opinion, most pregnancy-related aortic ruptures and dissections in patients with coarctation of the aorta occur prior to labor and delivery.[62]

Pulmonic Stenosis (see also p. 1059)

Over 175 pregnancies in women with pulmonic stenosis have been reported since 1960.[55,57] Although complications such as congestive heart failure have been described, recent reports suggest that the incidence of heart failure is low, and most pregnant women seem to tolerate the additional hemodynamic load.[51,63] In the rare instance of persistent heart failure despite appropriate drug therapy, surgical valvotomy should be considered. Percutaneous balloon valvuloplasty of the pulmonic valve during pregnancy has not been reported. Although this procedure may be attractive since it obviates surgery, it is not free of side effects and may be associated with considerable radiation exposure and acute hemodynamic changes, possibly harming the fetus.

Tetralogy of Fallot (see also p. 971)

Tetralogy of Fallot is the most common type of cyanotic CHD in adults. As a result of palliative or definitive surgical repair in most children with this defect, more patients are reaching childbearing age.[64]

Hemodynamic changes associated with pregnancy may become severe and cause clinical deterioration in women with tetralogy of Fallot. Increases in blood volume and venous return to the right atrium raise right ventricular pressure, and the fall in peripheral vascular resistance can cause or exacerbate a right-to-left shunt and cyanosis.

Maternal hematocrit above 60 per cent, arterial oxygen saturation below 80 per cent, right ventricular hypertension, and syncopal episodes are poor prognostic signs. Close monitoring of hemodynamic parameters and blood gases during labor and delivery is recommended for cyanotic or symptomatic patients. Palliative or corrective surgery will reduce the risks posed by pregnancy. Although reports of pregnancies in 37 women with corrected tetralogy of Fallot described no maternal deaths,[53] worsening of the clinical condition necessitating interruption of the pregnancy is not uncommon. Cardiac defects were reported by Whittemore in 15 and 17 per cent of infants born, respectively, to cyanotic and acyanotic mothers with tetralogy of Fallot.[53] In contrast, an incidence of only 3 per cent has been reported by other authors.[58]

Since maternal and fetal outcomes seem to be markedly improved in women whose defects have been surgically repaired, this procedure should be performed prior to conception. Patients who have undergone only palliative procedures or who have significant residual defects after repair are still at higher risk during pregnancy. Although mortality associated with complete repair is slightly increased in older patients who have previously undergone a palliative procedure,[64,65] surgical repair is recommended *prior* to pregnancy in patients in the absence of contraindications. Since revision of an incompletely repaired defect is recommended in patients with residual VSD when the pulmonary/systemic flow ratio is greater than 1.5:1, in those with right ventricular outflow obstruction (right ventricular systolic pressure > 60 mm Hg), and in those with right ventricular failure due to pulmonic regurgitation,[64] such revision should be performed prior to conception in a woman who plans to conceive.

Inhalation analgesia and paracervical or pudendal block have been recommended for labor and vaginal delivery.[66] Epidural block could result in systemic hypotension and shunt reversal and should therefore be used with great care. To minimize potential hemodynamic problems, a segmental epidural block for the first stage of labor with pudendal or caudal block for the second stage has been recommended along with opiates to decrease the concentration of anesthetics injected epidurally.

EBSTEIN'S ANOMALY (see also p. 970). Most patients with Ebstein's anomaly survive to childbearing age. Long-term prognosis depends on the severity of tricuspid regurgitation, the presence of right ventricular failure, cyanosis due to shunting from right to left through a patent foramen ovale, and the performance and adequacy of surgical intervention. Several successful pregnancies have been reported in patients with Ebstein's anomaly.[55] At the same time, pregnancy may be complicated by right ventricular failure, infective endocarditis, and paradoxical embolism. The incidence of maternal and fetal complications is increased among cyanotic patients.[53,54] The approach to labor and delivery in symptomatic or cyanotic patients with Ebstein's anomaly includes antibiotic prophylaxis, hemodynamic monitoring, oxygen administration, and efforts to prevent a drop in systemic blood pressure in response to peripheral vasodilation or blood loss.

COMPLEX CYANOTIC CHD. The more widespread use of palliative and corrective surgical procedures for complex cyanotic congenital cardiac anomalies has allowed more of these women to reach childbearing age.[55] Although successful pregnancies have been reported in patients with tricuspid atresia,[67] corrected and uncorrected transposition of the great vessels,[68,69] truncus arteriosus,[55] and a single ventricle,[68,70] pregnancy is risky in these patients and cannot be recommended. A high incidence of hemodynamic and functional deterioration with increased maternal morbidity and even mortality may occur.[52,53,71,72] In addition, a high incidence of fetal wastage, premature deliveries, and both cardiac and noncardiac congenital malformations should be anticipated, as well as small-for-gestational-age newborns.[52,53,70,72]

Patients should be informed prior to conception about expected maternal and fetal complications. When the potential mother is believed to be at risk, pregnancy should be discouraged prior to conception or should be interrupted early if it has already begun. If the patient wishes to continue the pregnancy, the hemodynamic load should be reduced by restricting physical activity, and the patient should be closely observed for early detection and management of heart failure and/or arrhythmias. Antibiotic prophylaxis and oxygen therapy are recommended for delivery, and hemodynamic and blood gas monitoring are essential to assure stability. Although vaginal delivery appears to be tolerated by most women, attempts should be made to shorten the second stage by the use of forceps or vacuum extraction.

In providing anesthesia or analgesia for labor and vaginal delivery, the physician should try to avoid increasing the right-to-left shunt. For that reason, regional anesthetic techniques should be avoided; systemic medication, inhalation analgesia, nerve blocks, and intrathecal morphine have been recommended.[66,73]

EISENMENGER'S SYNDROME (see also p. 971). In an extensive review of the literature published in 1979, Gleicher et al.[74] described the outcome of 70 pregnancies among 44 patients with documented Eisenmenger's syndrome and reported a maternal mortality rate of 52 per cent. A more recent review of 24 women with this syndrome revealed a mortality rate of 38 per cent.[55] Recently, more emphasis has been placed on reporting successful rather than unsuccessful pregnancy outcomes in patients with Eisenmenger's syndrome.

Eisenmenger's syndrome is also associated with a poor fetal outcome. Only 26 per cent of all pregnancies reported by Gleicher et al. reached term.[74] In addition, more than 55 per cent of the live-born infants were premature, 30 per cent had intrauterine growth retardation, and perinatal death occurred in 28 per cent.

Because of the high maternal mortality associated with Eisenmenger's syndrome, patients should be advised against pregnancy, and early abortion should be recommended for patients who are already pregnant. Management of a pregnant patient with Eisenmenger's syndrome who decides to proceed to term must include both close medical follow-up to detect deterioration early and restriction of physical activity to minimize the hemodynamic burden. Because of the increased incidence of thromboembolic events—which are often the cause of death in such patients—anticoagulant therapy seems indicated for at least the last 8 to 10 weeks of gestation and for 4 weeks post partum. Since premature delivery is common, these women should be hospitalized if there is any sign of premature uterine activity. For this reason and to assure restriction of activity and close follow-up, early elective hospitalization is recommended. Spontaneous labor is preferred to induction and should lower the chance of prematurity or the need for cesarean section. Hemodynamic, electrocardiographic, and blood gas monitoring are essential during labor and delivery to ensure the early detection and correction of problems; high concentrations of oxygen may be helpful.[75] Most patients in stable condition will tolerate vaginal delivery; however, an attempt should be made to shorten the second stage of labor by the use of forceps or vacuum extraction.

Since epidural anesthesia may lead to peripheral vasodilation and increased shunting from right to left, local anesthetics should be titrated carefully to achieve the epidural block.[66] Delivery has been successful with lumbar epidural block for the first stage of labor and caudal block for delivery; other authors have preferred the use of systemic medication, inhalation analgesia, and paracervical or pudendal block.[66,76] For cesarean section, general anesthesia with a drug having a minimal negative inotropic effect is recommended.[66,76] In addition, segmental epidural anesthesia has been used successfully for cesarean section in patients with Eisenmenger's syndrome.[66,77]

RHEUMATIC HEART DISEASE

Although the incidence of rheumatic heart disease is declining in the United States,[78] it continues to be prevalent in many parts of the world[79] and still frequently complicates pregnancy.[57]

ACUTE RHEUMATIC FEVER

(See also Chap. 56)

This disease occurs most commonly in children, before puberty, and may recur during pregnancy. Acute rheumatic fever associated with carditis and congestive heart failure may be fatal in the pregnant woman.[80] The incidence of Sydenham's chorea, like acute rheumatic fever itself, has been reported to be increased in pregnancy (chorea gravidarum). Chorea gravidarum has been reported to cause preterm labor and fetal and maternal death. Because of the problems faced by women with recurrent rheumatic fever during pregnancy, it is prudent to continue antibiotic prophylaxis against streptococcal infection in the pregnant patient with a history of this condition.[56] The recommended antibiotic regimen is discussed in detail on p. 1729.

CHRONIC RHEUMATIC VALVULAR DISEASE

(See also Chap. 34)

Significant valve deformities due to rheumatic valvular disease may increase morbidity and even mortality during gestation and the peripartum period. Although patients with chronic rheumatic valvular disease should be managed individually according to the location and severity of the lesion, certain general guidelines apply to the care of all patients. These include rheumatic fever prophylaxis, restriction of physical activity, antibiotic prophylaxis for bacterial endocarditis, and hemodynamic monitoring during labor and delivery.

To reduce the cardiovascular load and prevent hemodynamic and symptomatic worsening, physical activity should be restricted for symptomatic patients. All those with chronic rheumatic heart disease should be treated prophylactically with antibiotics to prevent streptococcal infection and recurrence. Although antibiotic prophylaxis during labor and delivery has not been uniformly recommended,[56] it is commonly used for vaginal and abdominal deliveries.[80]

Hemodynamic monitoring is strongly recommended from the onset of labor to 24 hours post partum in any patient who experiences symptoms of heart failure during pregnancy and for those with severe valvular disease, left ventricular dysfunction, or pulmonary hypertension.[46]

Mitral Valve Disease

MITRAL STENOSIS (see also p. 1007). This condition is The most common rheumatic valvular lesion in pregnancy.[57] The status of patients with mitral stenosis may deteriorate significantly during gestation. Although mitral stenosis is often accompanied by some degree of mitral regurgitation, hemodynamic problems are related predominantly to flow obstruction. The pressure gradient across the narrowed mitral valve may increase greatly as left ventricular diastolic filling time decreases secondary to the physiological increase in heart rate and the increased cardiac output of pregnancy.[1] Increased left atrial pressure and the arrhythmogenic effect of pregnancy[31] may result in atrial flutter or fibrillation, substantially accelerating the ventricular rate and further elevating left atrial pressure. In addition to the decreased serum colloid osmotic pressure—often a result of peripartum intravenous fluid administration—these changes predispose to pulmonary edema during the peripartum period.

The therapeutic approach to patients with significant mitral stenosis is designed to reduce the heart rate and decrease blood volume. Both heart rate and symptoms can be controlled effectively by restricting physical activity and administering beta-adrenergic receptor blockers. In patients with atrial fibrillation, digoxin may control further the ventricular rate. Blood volume can be decreased through the restriction of salt intake and the use of oral diuretics; the aggressive use of diuretic agents should be avoided to prevent hypovolemia, which may reduce uteroplacental perfusion (p. 1014).

Vaginal delivery can be allowed in most patients with mitral stenosis. In symptomatic patients or those with moderate or severe stenosis (mitral valve area < 1.5 cm²), hemodynamic monitoring is recommended during labor, delivery, and the puerperium. By inserting a pulmonary artery catheter at the start of labor, one can optimize hemodynamic status by means of intravenous diuretics, digoxin (in case of atrial fibrillation), beta blockers, or nitroglycerin and prevent a rise in left atrial pressure during labor and delivery.[81] With delivery and thus relief of venocaval obstruction due to the gravid uterus, there is an immediate increase in venous return, and one sees a substantial increase in pulmonary artery wedge pressure (Fig. 59–4).[82] For this reason, hemodynamic monitoring should be continued for at least 24 hours post partum.[46]

Epidural anesthesia is the most appropriate form of analgesia in patients with mitral stenosis[66,81,83] and is often associated with a significant fall in pulmonary arterial and left atrial pressures due to systemic vasodilation. By the same mechanism, systemic hypotension may occur and can be prevented by fluid replacement. With this approach, the great majority of patients with mitral stenosis, even if it is severe, can be delivered with few complications.

Mitral Valvuloplasty. Surgical (p. 1016) or percutaneous balloon mitral valvuloplasty (p. 1376) or mitral valve replacement (p. 1027) has been performed in severely symptomatic patients with mitral stenosis during pregnancy.[57,84–86] Becker[86] described 101 cases of closed surgical mitral commissurotomy during pregnancy in which there were no maternal deaths and the fetus survived in 98 of the cases. The same author reported similar favorable results in 23 cases of open

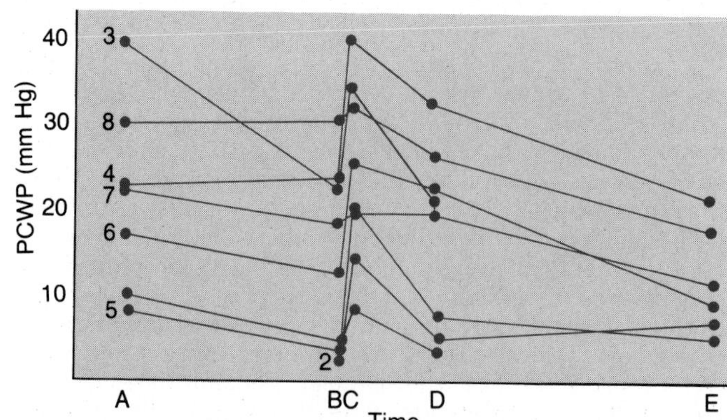

FIGURE 59–4. Intrapartum alterations in pulmonary capillary wedge pressure (PCWP) in eight patients with mitral stenosis. *A*, First-stage labor; *B*, Second-stage labor 15 to 30 minutes before delivery; *C*, 5 to 15 minutes post partum; *D*, 4 to 6 hours post partum; *E*, 18 to 24 hours post partum. (From Clark, S. C., et al.: Labor and delivery in the presence of mitral stenosis: Central hemodynamic observations. Am. J. Obstet. Gynecol. *152*:984, 1985.)

mitral commissurotomy. Mitral valve replacement in 19 cases resulted in a single maternal death due to hepatitis, occurring 7 weeks after surgery; fetal death in four cases; and cerebral palsy in one infant, thought to be due to heparin management. Recently, successful percutaneous mitral balloon valvuloplasty has been reported in two cases during pregnancy and has been recommended for palliation of symptoms.[85,87] Although repair or replacement of the valve may be indicated in some patients with severe mitral stenosis, these procedures are not free of risk and can result in fetal loss (surgery) and irradiation (balloon valvuloplasty). For this reason, they should be recommended only for women who fail to respond to adequate medical therapy.

The author's experience with patients with critical mitral stenosis (mitral valve area < 1.0 cm^2) indicates that careful medical therapy, with particular emphasis on lowering the heart rate, should allow successful completion of pregnancy in the great majority without the need for valve correction or replacement. When a surgical procedure seems indicated, closed mitral valvotomy will avoid the fetal complications that may be associated with the use of extracorporeal circulation and is therefore preferable to the open technique.[86,88] However, this procedure should be recommended only in centers where it is performed routinely. Although percutaneous balloon valvuloplasty is an attractive alternative to surgery, it is limited by the high radiation exposure and hemodynamic fluctuations attending this procedure. When valve replacement is indicated, selection of the type of prosthesis should be based on its hemodynamic profile and durability and the need for anticoagulation (p. 1015).

MITRAL REGURGITATION. This lesion is usually well tolerated in pregnancy,[46] presumably because of the unloading resulting from the physiological fall in systemic vascular resistance. In symptomatic patients, drug therapy with diuretics is indicated, and digoxin may be useful in those with impaired left ventricular systolic function. Since hydralazine has been shown to be safe for use during pregnancy,[89] its use should be considered as a means of reducing left ventricular afterload and mitral regurgitation and preventing the hemodynamic worsening associated with isometric exercise during labor.[90]

Aortic Valve Disease

Aortic valve involvement occurs in conjunction with mitral valve disease in approximately 10 per cent of pregnant patients with rheumatic valvular disease.[91]

AORTIC STENOSIS (see also p. 1035). Rheumatic aortic valve stenosis is uncommon in pregnancy. However, a severe form of this deformity presents significant risk to the mother. Reported clinical experience with aortic stenosis is limited, with information based mostly on anecdotal reports. A survey of the literature by Arias and Pineda[59] revealed a maternal mortality rate of 17 per cent and high rates of therapeutic abortion and fetal mortality among 23 patients with aortic stenosis. These data illustrate the potential hazard posed by this lesion in pregnancy. Nevertheless, recent improvements in diagnostic capabilities, hemodynamic monitoring, and fetal monitoring have increased maternal and fetal safety for pregnant women with aortic stenosis.[46] Management of patients with rheumatic aortic stenosis is similar to that for congenital aortic stenosis (p. 1035).

AORTIC REGURGITATION (see also p. 1043). This lesion is more common during pregnancy than is aortic stenosis.[57,80,91] Similar to mitral regurgitation, aortic regurgitation is also tolerated well during pregnancy, probably because systemic vascular resistance is reduced and heart rate and thus diastolic time are increased. In symptomatic patients, diuretics, digoxin, and hydralazine for afterload reduction can be safely used during pregnancy. Since hydralazine has been shown to prevent an increase in pulmonary artery wedge pressure during isometric exercise,[92] it can be administered intravenously in increments of 2.5 to 5.0 mg during labor with the aid of hemodynamic monitoring to prevent the hemodynamic changes associated with the Valsalva maneuver during labor.

MITRAL VALVE PROLAPSE (MVP) (see also p. 1029). As diagnosed by M-mode echocardiography, MVP has been reported in approximately 15 per cent of women of childbearing age.[93] However, when the diagnosis was based on two-dimensional echocardiographic criteria, the incidence was reported to be only about 2 per cent.[94] In a review of heart disease in pregnancy, MVP was found in only two of 145 pregnant women, and Rayburn et al. reported that MVP was clinically suspected in 1.2 per cent of women examined in prenatal clinics.[95] A combined experience involving 128 pregnant women showed that MVP has no effect on maternal or fetal outcome.[86,97]

Pregnancy has been reported to reduce the incidence of prolapse-related auscultatory and echocardiographic changes that result from an increase in left ventricular end-diastolic volume.[25,95] For the few patients with chest pain or cardiac arrhythmias, the emphasis should be on reassurance and attempts to avoid the use of medications. Beta-adrenergic blocking agents are recommended if symptomatic arrhythmias or chest pain persists, with periodic reassessment of the need to continue drug therapy. Patients with MVP, especially those with a thickened mitral valve and regurgitation, are at increased risk for infective endocarditis. Although antibiotic prophylaxis for uncomplicated vaginal delivery has not been uniformly recommended,[56] the development of bacteremia during vaginal delivery and cesarean section cannot always be predicted,[80] so that some authors have recommended prophylaxis for labor and delivery in patients with MVP accompanied by valve thickening and/or regurgitation.[96]

THE MARFAN SYNDROME

(See also p. 1641)

A review of the literature revealed a high incidence of aortic dissection and death (mostly occurring during the peripartum period) among 32 pregnant patients with the Marfan syndrome. Most of these women had preexisting cardiovascular problems, including aortic dilatation, aortic regurgitation, aortic coarctation, hypertension, cardiomegaly, and patent ductus arteriosus.[98] In addition, the incidence of spontaneous abortion was increased, suggesting their susceptibility to recurrent abortions. In contrast, a retrospective analysis of 105 unselected pregnancies among 26 women with this syndrome revealed only one death from endocarditis in a patient with severe mitral regurgitation.[99] Similarly, no cardiovascular complications were reported among 10 women with this condition and an aortic diameter of less than 45 mm involving 12 term pregnancies.[100] These findings suggest that anecdotal reports in the literature represent a selected group of patients at high risk in which pregnancy-related complications in women with the Marfan syndrome are overrepresented.

The management of pregnant women with the Marfan syndrome should include preconception counseling to discuss potential maternal and fetal risks, including the 50 per cent chance that this syndrome will be inherited.[99] Based on available information, women with significant cardiac involvement, including asymptomatic dilatation of the aorta, should be advised against conception or, if they are already pregnant, to agree to early abortion. In contrast, the risk is significantly lower in patients with no cardiac complications and a normal aortic diameter. Still, a favorable outcome is not guaranteed, and aortic dissection can occur, albeit infrequently, in patients without aortic dilatation.[100] During pregnancy, physical activity should be limited. Beta blockers, which have been shown to reduce the rate of aortic dilatation and the risk of complications in patients with the Marfan syndrome, should be administered.[101]

In women with aortic dilatation or other cardiac complications, abdominal delivery by cesarean section may be preferred to prevent the potential deleterious effect of bearing down.

HYPERTROPHIC CARDIOMYOPATHY

(See also p. 1404)

A review of 82 pregnancies among 35 patients with hypertrophic cardiomyopathy (HC) revealed a favorable outcome in most cases; however, the development or worsening of cardiac symptoms was common.[26] Congestive heart failure was first diagnosed or became worse in 21 per cent of patients, and a few patients experienced chest pain, palpitations, dizzy spells, and syncope. Two patients had ventricular arrhythmias, which proved fatal in one.[102] Fetal outcome does not seem to be affected by maternal HC; however, the risk of inheriting this condition may be as high as 50 per cent in familial cases and less in sporadic cases.[26]

Diagnosis of HC may be missed during pregnancy, since the systolic murmurs associated with obstructive HC may be attributed to the innocent heart murmurs frequently heard in pregnancy. The presence of left ventricular hypertrophy, an S_4, a systolic thrill along the lower left sternal border and apex, and a more intense murmur in the upright position or during the strain phase of the Valsalva maneuver warrants further evaluation using echocardiography, the key definitive diagnostic test for HC.[103]

The therapeutic approach to the pregnant patient with HC depends on the presence of symptoms and left ventricular outflow obstruction. No treatment is indicated in the asymptomatic patient without resting or provocable left ventricular obstruction. In the symptomatic patient with obstructive HC, blood loss during delivery, vasodilation, and sympathetic stimulation during anesthesia must be avoided. Indications for drug therapy include symptoms and the presence of arrhythmias. Symptoms associated with elevated left ventricular filling pressures should be treated with beta-adrenergic blocking agents, with diuretics added if beta blockers alone are not sufficient. While calcium antagonists appear to be useful in nonpregnant patients,[104] the fetal effect of administration of these drugs has not been established.[105]

Although pregnancy per se does not seem to increase the risk for sudden death in patients with HC, such events are most commonly seen during the childbearing years.[106] The presence of ventricular arrhythmias—an important prognostic sign—should be sought on Holter monitoring, and complex ventricular arrhythmias should be treated with drugs that will not harm the fetus, such as quinidine, procainamide, and beta blockers (if effective). The safety of amiodarone during pregnancy, shown to prevent sudden death in nonpregnant patients with HC, has not been established.[105] Amiodarone should therefore be used only in patients with life-threatening arrhythmias that do not respond to other drugs.[107] Supraventricular arrhythmias, especially atrial fibrillation, should be treated with Class 1A antiarrhythmic drugs (p. 634) during pregnancy. Electrical cardioversion can be used when patients with symptomatic atrial fibrillation do not respond to medical therapy.[108] Since digoxin may have unfavorable hemodynamic effects in obstructive HC and the long-term safety of calcium antagonists is unknown, beta blockers are the drugs of choice for controlling heart rate in patients with resistant atrial fibrillation.

Vaginal delivery has been shown to be safe in women with HC. In those with symptoms or outflow obstruction, the second stage of labor may be shortened by the use of forceps.[26,104] The use of prostaglandins to effect uterine contractions may be unfavorable owing to their vasodilatory effect, whereas oxytocin seems to be tolerated well.[102] Since beta-sympathomimetic tocolytic agents may aggravate left ventricular outflow tract obstruction, magnesium sulfate is preferred.[102] Similarly, spinal and epidural anesthetics should be avoided in obstructive HC because of their vasodilatory effect,[109] and excessive blood loss should be avoided or replaced promptly with intravenous fluid or blood.[26]

Because the risk for infective endocarditis is increased in HC, especially the obstructive form, antibiotic prophylaxis should be considered for labor and delivery.

PERIPARTUM CARDIOMYOPATHY

(See also p. 1398)

This form of dilated cardiomyopathy has signs and symptoms of heart failure due to left ventricular systolic dysfunction that become manifest for the first time in the peripartum period. Rarely for the most part, symptoms occur during the last month of gestation or immediately post partum, although occasional cases may appear at any time during the last 3 months of pregnancy or the first 6 months post partum (Fig. 59–5).[110] Any other causes of left ventricular dilatation and systolic dysfunction must be excluded to establish the diagnosis of peripartum cardiomyopathy (PPCM).[111] The reported incidence of the disease in the United States varies from one in 1300 to one in 15,000, with a higher incidence (one in 100) in certain parts of Africa.[112]

Patients usually have symptoms of congestive heart failure, chest pain, palpitations, and occasionally peripheral or pulmonary embolization.[110-113,113a] Physical examination often reveals an enlarged heart and an S_3, and murmurs of mitral and tricuspid regurgitation are not uncommon.[110,112,114] The electrocardiogram may show left ventricular hypertrophy, ST-T changes, conduction abnormalities, and arrhythmias. Chest x-ray may reveal cardiomegaly, pulmonary venous congestion with interstitial or alveolar edema, and occasionally pleural effusion. On Doppler echocardiography, all four chambers are enlarged, with marked reduction in left ventricular systolic function. Small-to-moderate pericardial effusion may be found; mitral, tricuspid, and pulmonic regurgitation may be evident. Hemodynamic changes are indistinguishable from those other forms of dilated cardiomyopathy.[114] A few patients with high-output heart failure have been reported.[113a]

The incidence of PPCM is greater in women with twin pregnancies and in women who are multiparous, over 30 years of age, and black.[110-112] Although the etiology of PPCM is still unknown, the unique nature of this syndrome is suggested by its occurrence at a relatively young age compared with other forms of dilated cardiomyopathy, the recovery of cardiac size and function in a large number of patients, and its relation to pregnancy. It has been postulated that PPCM may be due to myocarditis, nutritional deficiency, small-vessel coronary artery abnormalities, hormonal effects, toxemia, or the maternal immunological response to fetal antigen.[110,112,114] Recently, the use of endomyocardial biopsy in patients with PPCM has revealed a greater incidence of myocarditis[115] compared with other forms of dilated cardiomyopathy. Although biopsy results were normal for myocarditis in some investigations,[116,117] the incidence of this condition in other reports ranged from 29 per cent to 100 per cent.[110,114,115] These findings may suggest an etiological role for myocarditis in patients with PPCM.

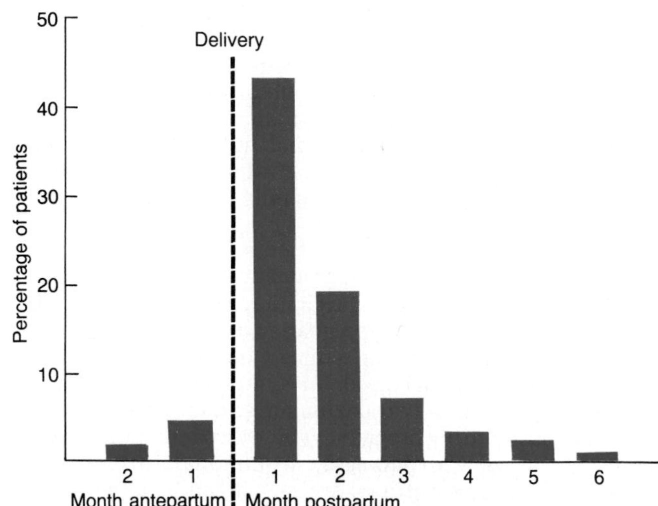

FIGURE 59–5. Onset of peripartum cardiomyopathy in relation to time of delivery in 347 patients. (From Homans, D. C.: Peripartum cardiomyopathy. N. Engl. J. Med. *312*:1432, 1985.)

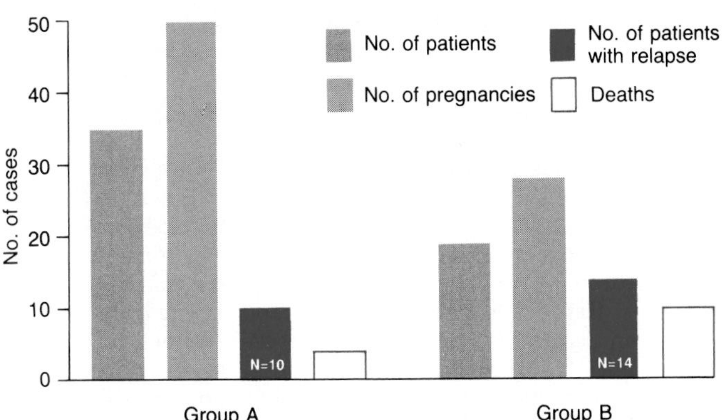

FIGURE 59-6. **Incidence of relapse and death in subsequent pregnancies in patients with peripartum cardiomyopathy (PPCM). Group A, patients with PPCM demonstrating clinical improvement with normalization of heart size on chest X-ray or left ventricular size and function by echocardiography. Group B, patients with PPCM with persistent cardiomyopathy and/or left ventricular dysfunction. N, number. Data are derived from previous reports of 54 patients (references 111, 125–132).**

The clinical course of PPCM varies. Approximately 50 per cent of patients show complete or near-complete recovery of cardiac function and clinical status within the first 6 months post partum; the other 50 per cent demonstrate either continuous clinical deterioration, leading to early death, or persistent left ventricular dysfunction and chronic heart failure, with high morbidity and mortality.[110–112, 117]

Acute heart failure should be treated vigorously with oxygen, diuretics, inotropic support with digitalis, and vasodilator agents. The use of hydralazine as an afterload-reducing agent is safe during pregnancy.[90] Experience with organic nitrates is limited, although hypotension secondary to an excessive dose has been associated with fetal bradycardia.[118] Nitroprusside has been used successfully during pregnancy, but experiments in animals have shown the potential for fetal toxicity.[105] Angiotensin-converting enzyme inhibitors have had deleterious effects on blood pressure control and renal function in the fetus[119] and are therefore *not* recommended for antepartum therapy. Because of the increased incidence of thromboembolic events in PPCM, anticoagulant therapy is recommended. Since the disease may be reversible, the temporary use of an intraaortic balloon pump may help stabilize the patient's condition pending improvement.[120]

Recent data have provided circumstantial evidence of the potential benefits of immunosuppression in patients with PPCM.[115,121] Midei et al.[115] recently reported both objective and subjective improvement in nine of ten patients with PPCM who had biopsy evidence of myocarditis. However, significant clinical improvement as well as the rapid improvement of left ventricular function was also reported in patients with PPCM given supportive therapy alone.[116,117] Since information about the effect of immunosuppressive therapy in PPCM is insufficient,[122] no recommendation can be made at the present time. However, such treatment seems reasonable in patients with acute clinical deterioration who do not respond to conventional therapy. Because of the high mortality and morbidity among patients who do not recover early, such patients should also be considered for cardiac transplantation.[117,123,124]

Subsequent pregnancies in women with PPCM are often associated with relapses and a high risk for maternal mortality. Although the likelihood of such relapse is greater in patients with persistently abnormal heart size and/or function, it has also been reported in women in whom left ventricular function is restored after the first episode[111,125–132] (Fig. 59–6). For these reasons, subsequent pregnancies should be discouraged in patients with PPCM who have persistent cardiac dysfunction; women in whom cardiac function is recovered after one episode of PPCM should be informed about the increased risk that attends later pregnancies.

CORONARY ARTERY DISEASE

(See also Chaps. 39 and 40)

PATHOGENESIS. Coronary artery disease (CAD) is rare among women of childbearing age, and the incidence of peripartum acute myocardial infarction (AMI) is estimated to be less than one in 10,000 pregnancies.[133]

Risk factors for CAD in women under age 50 include high levels of total plasma cholesterol, low levels of high-density lipoproteins, cigarette smoking, diabetes mellitus, hypertension, a family history of CAD, toxemia of pregnancy, and the use of oral contraceptives.[134,135] The combination of heavy smoking and concurrent use of oral contraceptives has been shown to be a powerful predictor of AMI.[136] In addition, an increased risk has been related to the age of the mother at the time of delivery of the first child (below the age of 20)[137] and to a lifelong irregular pattern of menstruation.[138]

Several mechanisms have been proposed to explain the relationship between oral contraceptives and AMI (see also p. 1153). For example, these drugs may trigger clot formation and embolization, as suggested by the increased incidence of venous thrombosis, pulmonary embolism, and cerebral thromboembolism.[133] In addition, oral contraceptives may raise serum levels of triglycerides, total cholesterol, and low-density lipoprotein; lower the level of high-density lipoprotein; increase the incidence of hypertension; and precipitate the ulceration of atherosclerotic plaques.[133] To reduce the risk for AMI, oral contraceptives should be avoided or formulations with lower effective doses of estrogen should be used in women over age 35, cigarette smokers, and those who develop hypertension while using this form of birth control.

Peripartum AMI is often associated with normal coronary angiographic findings[138]; this suggests a decrease in coronary perfusion, possibly due to spasm or in situ thrombosis, as a relatively common etiological factor in this patient population.[133,139,140] Although the cause of spasm is not clear, it has often been associated with pregnancy-induced hypertension and in some instances with the use of ergot derivatives to suppress lactation.[139] Coronary arterial dissection that occurs immediately post partum is another relatively common cause of peripartum AMI.[141,142] Advanced maternal age and parity may predispose to the development of coronary arterial dissection, and nearly all reported cases have involved the left anterior descending coronary artery.[141] Another potential cause of AMI during pregnancy has been collagen vascular disease.[143]

DIAGNOSIS. The diagnostic approach to ischemic myocardial disease in pregnancy is influenced to some extent by whether a diagnostic procedure could harm the fetus. No information is available regarding the safety of exercise testing during pregnancy. Because fetal bradycardia has been reported during maximal exercise in normal women,[44] a submaximal exercise protocol with fetal monitoring is recommended to evaluate ischemic myocardial disease during pregnancy.[45] Radionuclide myocardial perfusion scans and radionuclide ventriculography expose the fetus to radiation and should be used only when the potential benefits seem to outweigh fetal risk.[45] For similar reasons, cardiac catheterization involving fluoroscopy and cineangiography should be used only when relevant information cannot be obtained by other, noninvasive methods.[45]

MANAGEMENT. Fetal safety should also influence the therapeutic approach to ischemic heart disease during pregnancy. Since the safety of long-term therapy with organic nitrates and calcium antagonists in pregnancy has not been established, beta blockers appear to be the most appropriate choice for the treatment of ischemia during gestation. Coronary reperfusion by means of percutaneous transluminal coronary angioplasty or coronary artery bypass graft surgery has been reported to be successful during pregnancy,[144,145] although experience is still limited. Such procedures should be avoided during the first trimester, if possible, owing to the potential deleterious effects on the fetus of both ionizing radiation and cardiopulmonary bypass.[133]

Myocardial infarction is associated with high maternal mortality, especially when it occurs during the third trimester and labor,[146] and is probably related to a delay in diagnosis due to a low level of suspicion as well as the normal increase in cardiovascular work and myocardial oxygen consumption during gestation. Intrapartum management should focus on reducing cardiovascular stress during pregnancy and the peripartum period. Pulmonary artery catheterization with monitoring of pressure and cardiac output can help in the early detection and correction of hemodynamic abnormalities during labor and delivery. During labor, adequate analgesia and supplemental oxygen should be given, and if desired, cardiac output can be increased by placing the patient in the left lateral decubitus position. Labor in the supine position may decrease venous return and thus reduce right and left ventricular filling pressures. Low forceps can be used to shorten the second stage of labor. Although elective cesarean section is not indicated in every case, it should be used in patients with active ischemia or hemodynamic instability despite adequate medical therapy. Epidural anesthesia can reduce hemodynamic fluctuations during labor and is associated with left ventricular unloading due to vasodilation. If general anesthesia is indicated, *halothane should be avoided* in patients with depressed left ventricular systolic function.[66] In addition, atropine and ketamine should be used with caution to prevent tachycardia. Continued hemodynamic monitoring is advisable for 24 hours post partum to prevent hemodynamic worsening associated with the postpartum hemodynamic changes described earlier.[1]

CARDIAC ARRHYTHMIAS

Although the exact prevalence of arrhythmia during pregnancy is not known, anecdotal reports and clinical experience suggest a gestational arrhythmogenic effect, in women both with and without organic heart disease.[31] Palpitations, dizziness, and syncope are relatively common symptoms during pregnancy. Recently, 24-hour Holter monitoring was employed in 86 women referred for such symptoms and found multiple ventricular premature beats, atrial premature beats, or both in 18 per cent of the patients; no supraventricular or ventricular tachycardia was noted.[147] The presence of multiple premature beats was not associated with any adverse maternal or fetal effect, and there was marked reduction in the number of premature beats post partum.

Early studies reported an incidence of supraventricular tachycardia (SVT) during pregnancy of 1.5 per cent to 3.0 per cent in women with heart disease. However, since continuous electrocardiographic monitoring was not performed, these studies probably underestimated the incidence of SVT in such patients. Reports of paroxysmal SVT occurring only during gestation support the arrhythmogenic effect of pregnancy.[31,148,149] Atrial flutter and fibrillation are rare during normal pregnancy and are usually associated with rheumatic mitral valve disease. Ventricular tachycardia or fibrillation is also rare in pregnancy and is usually associated with structural heart disease,[150] although sustained symptomatic ventricular tachycardia in otherwise healthy pregnant women has been described in a few cases.[151]

Among pregnant women who were otherwise healthy, Copeland and Stern[152] reported type I (Wenckebach) second degree atrioventricular (AV) block on six of 26,000 electrocardiograms. However, similar findings were noted for nonpregnant women.[153] Complete heart block has been described during pregnancy; although usually congenital, it can be acquired[154] as a result of myocarditis, congenital heart disease, acute myocardial infarction, or infective endocarditis. Symptomatic patients have been treated with pacemakers, and numerous pregnancies have been reported in patients after a pacemaker has been implanted.[155] A rate-adaptive pacemaker (p. 742) seems to be indicated in women of childbearing age. Reports of skin irritation and ulceration at the implant site due to enlargement of the breast and abdomen during pregnancy have led to placement of the battery under the breast in such women.[108]

Figure 59–7 shows an approach to management of patients with arrhythmias. A complete evaluation is indicated to rule out a cardiac cause as well as electrolyte imbalance, thyroid disease, and arrhythmogenic effects due to drugs, alcohol, caffeine, and cigarette smoking. The identified cause should be treated and antiarrhythmic drug therapy initiated only if the

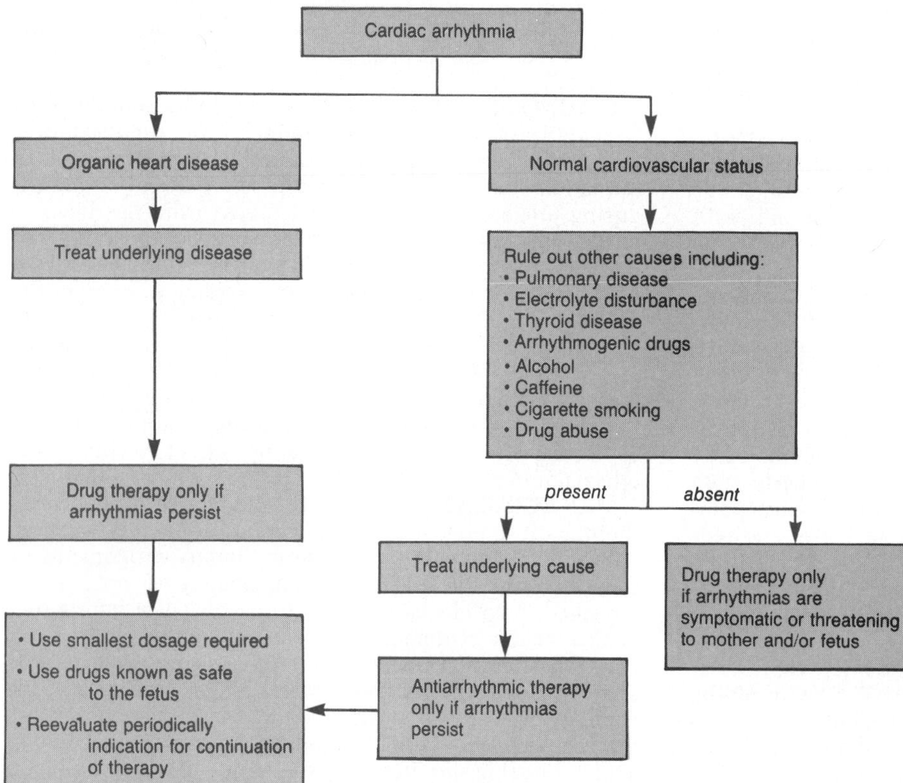

FIGURE 59–7. Management of cardiac arrhythmias during pregnancy. (From Rotmensch, H. H., et al.: Management of cardiac arrhythmias during pregnancy: Current concepts. Drugs *33*:623, 1987.)

arrhythmia persists and is symptomatic or threatens the mother and/or fetus. When drug therapy seems necessary, drugs known to be safe for the fetus (p. 1803) should be used at the smallest dose required to achieve effect and/or therapeutic blood levels, and the indication(s) for continuous drug therapy should be reevaluated periodically.[107]

OTHER CARDIOVASCULAR DISEASES

Aortic Dissection (see also p. 1535)

Although aortic dissection occurs two to three times more frequently in males than in females, a predisposition to this condition during gestation has been suggested.[141,156] Over the last 50 years, approximately 200 cases of aortic dissection in association with pregnancy have been reported.[141] The incidence is increased among women over age 30, multiparous women, and patients with coarctation of the aorta and Marfan syndrome (see p. 1641).[157] Pregnancy-related aortic dissection seems to occur most often during the third trimester and peripartum period.[141]

The diagnostic approach to the pregnant patient suspected of having aortic dissection is similar to that for the nonpregnant patient. Since contrast aortography is often required to establish the diagnosis, an attempt should be made to minimize the radiation dose, and the fetus should be appropriately shielded. The use of transesophageal echocardiography has provided a powerful tool for diagnosing aortic dissection in pregnancy (p. 1538).[158] This method is preferable to computed tomography (CT), which involves radiation exposure, and to magnetic resonance imaging, the safety of which during gestation has not yet been established.

The combination of nitroprusside and propranolol is currently recommended to control hypertension in patients with aortic dissection. Since nitroprusside may result in fetal toxicity (see p. 1804) it should be used only in patients refractory to other drugs. Hydralazine, either intravenously or orally, is the drug of choice for blood pressure reduction in pregnant women with aortic dissection. To avoid the pressure elevation associated with labor and vaginal delivery in women with aortic dissection, abdominal delivery by cesarean section under epidural anesthesia is recommended.[141]

Takayasu's Arteritis (see also p. 1544)

A review of the literature revealed 116 pregnancies in 89 women with Takayasu's disease.[141,159–162] Cerebral hemorrhage, heart failure, and even death have been reported in pregnant patients with Takayasu's arteritis.[159,162] In addition, systolic blood pressure was markedly elevated during uterine contractions in some patients.[159] Low birth weights were noted when the disease was complicated by retinopathy, hypertension, aortic regurgitation, or arterial aneurysms. The management of pregnant patients with Takayasu's arteritis includes treatment of hypertension to prevent complications such as congestive heart failure and cerebral hemorrhage. However, to avoid compromising uteroplacental blood flow, blood pressure should not be reduced excessively in patients with aortic narrowing. Adrenal glucocorticoids have been used in some cases of Takayasu's arteritis during pregnancy[159,161]; however, since pregnancy does not seem to change the inflammatory activity of this disorder, glucocorticoids should be reserved for patients who become pregnant during the acute phase of the disease. Prophylactic antibiotics may be given for labor and delivery in patients with aortic regurgitation and vascular stenoses.

Vaginal delivery is likely to be tolerated in the majority of patients with Takayasu's arteritis. Abdominal delivery may be considered for those with severe systemic hypertension and heart failure that does not respond to medical therapy. Vacuum extraction or forceps can be used to shorten the second stage of labor in patients with a marked increase in blood pressure during uterine contractions. In patients with substantial aortic narrowing, epidural anesthesia may markedly reduce blood pressure distal to the narrowing and compromise placental perfusion.

The use of oral contraceptives may accelerate the progression of Takayasu's arteritis[163] and should therefore be avoided in patients with this condition.

Primary Pulmonary Hypertension (PPH) (see also p. 806)

PPH is one of the few cardiovascular conditions in which pregnancy may be associated with a high maternal mortality rate. A review of the literature as well as of our own experience has revealed that 15 of 37 patients with PPH (41 per cent) died during pregnancy or in the early postpartum period.[164,165] Clinical deterioration or death during pregnancy cannot always be predicted on the basis of the patient's preconception clinical status. Symptomatic deterioration usually occurs in the second trimester and is manifested by fatigue, dyspnea, syncope, chest pain, and right ventricular failure. Death occurs most often during late gestation or in the early postpartum period. Since hemodynamic or electrocardiographic information has not been available, the exact cause of death in patients with PPH is not clear. However, right ventricular ischemia and failure due to an increased hemodynamic load that leads to cardiac arrhythmias and pulmonary embolism are likely mechanisms. In addition to high maternal risk, the incidence of spontaneous abortions and of neonatal deaths due to congenital heart disease is high.[164]

Because of the potentially deleterious effect of pregnancy on both mothers with PPH and their fetuses, pregnancy seems contraindicated in these patients. Since an etiological link between pulmonary hypertension and oral contraceptives has been suggested,[166] this form of birth control is not recommended for women with PPH. Tubal ligation should provide maximum protection against the undesired risks of pregnancy; however, this procedure should be carried out under local or epidural anesthesia and in conjunction with hemodynamic as well as electrocardiographic monitoring. Early abortion is indicated in patients who become pregnant. If the patient elects to continue the pregnancy, physical exertion should be restricted to reduce the circulatory load. In addition, elective early hospitalization is recommended to ensure limited activity and close follow-up. The incidence of premature deliveries is increased in patients with PPH and should be anticipated.

Because of the beneficial effect of anticoagulation in patients with PPH[167] and the increased incidence of thromboembolism during pregnancy, such therapy is recommended throughout gestation and at least during the early postpartum phase. Hemodynamic monitoring and blood gas measurements should be performed regularly during labor and delivery. Oxygen should be provided to prevent hypoxemia, and every effort should be made to prevent or immediately replace blood lost during delivery.[164]

Segmental epidural anesthesia and intrathecal morphine have been successful in relieving pain in these patients.[168,169] Because right ventricular dysfunction is likely, anesthetics having a negative inotropic effect should be avoided in patients with PPH. Most patients can tolerate vaginal delivery, and spontaneous labor is preferable to induction. Continued hemodynamic monitoring for 24 to 48 hours after delivery and a hospital stay of 10 to 14 days are recommended to prevent the complications commonly seen post partum.

CARDIAC SURGERY DURING PREGNANCY

Since heart disease that requires surgery is usually diagnosed and treated prior to pregnancy, cardiac surgery during gestation is uncommon. In general, cardiac surgery in the pregnant woman is not associated with increased maternal risk but may lead to fetal wastage.[86,170] Although many cardiac operations during gestation have been reported in the last 40 years, little information is available regarding the effects of anesthesia and the procedure, especially cardiopulmonary bypass, on the uteroplacental circulation and fetal outcome.[170] Therefore, surgery should be recommended only for patients who do not respond to medical therapy, and procedures not requiring cardiopulmonary bypass are preferred.[88,171] To minimize the risk of teratogenicity, surgery should be avoided during the first trimester.[170] Since heart surgery is indicated when medical therapy has not led to satisfactory improvement, many of these patients will be hemodynamically unstable and will require hemodynamic monitoring for stabilization and careful anesthetic technique. Anesthetic agents should be selected on the basis of their hemodynamic effects and fetal safety.[66] When the patient is at or near term, abdominal delivery by cesarean section can be performed at the same time as cardiac surgery, once fetal maturity has been confirmed.[172] Fetal monitoring is essential for early detection of the fetal bradycardia commonly seen in surgery involving cardiopulmonary bypass. This finding most likely indicates fetal distress due to a decrease in placental blood flow, so that bradycardiac episodes can frequently be managed by increasing the flow rate.[173,174]

PREGNANCY IN PATIENTS WITH VALVE PROSTHESES

(See also p. 1061)

The risk of pregnancy in women with a valve prosthesis is multifactorial and should be assessed and discussed with the patient and her family before conception. Potential problems may be related to an increased hemodynamic load, the hypercoagulable state of pregnancy with the increased likelihood of thromboembolic events, and risk to the fetus due to anticoagulants (p. 1805) and other cardiovascular drugs. In addition, the expected limitation in maternal functional capacity as well as postpartum morbidity and mortality should be taken into consideration. Most patients with an adequately functioning mechanical prosthesis, including those with two and three prosthetic valves, can tolerate the hemodynamic load of pregnancy. This fact was well demonstrated by Salazar et al.,[175] who reported favorable outcomes in 223 pregnancies in women with prosthetic heart valves. Although functional classification was not reported, 60 per cent of these patients required digitalis and diuretics, and 30 per cent were in atrial fibrillation, indicating advanced disease in many cases. In questionable cases, exercise testing prior to conception may be used to predict whether a patient with a prosthetic heart valve can tolerate the increased hemodynamic load of pregnancy.[29]

Significant changes in the levels of coagulation factors increase the risk for thrombosis during gestation.[176] Although thrombosis of prosthetic valves during pregnancy has been reported in isolated cases despite anticoagulation,[177-180] the anticoagulant regimen used was inadequate in most of these cases. In the combined experience of Salazar et al.[175,177] involving women with mechanical valves treated with anticoagulation during pregnancy, thromboembolic events occurred in 6 of 165 patients with mitral prostheses (3.6 per cent) and in none of 37 patients with aortic prostheses.[181] Considering the fact that a fixed dose of heparin (5000 units every 12 hours) rather than adjusted dose was used in some of these patients, the incidence of thromboembolic events in patients with prosthetic heart valves who are adequately treated with anticoagulants during pregnancy is probably comparable to that in the nongravid population.[182] (The approach to and hazards of anticoagulation therapy during pregnancy are described on p. 1805.)

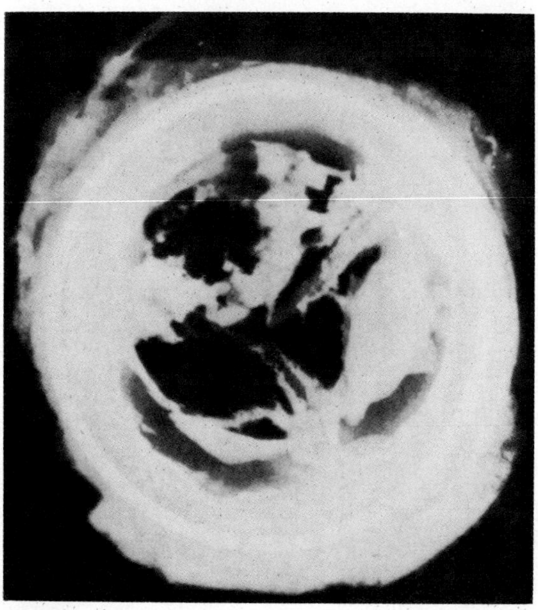

FIGURE 59–8. X-ray examination of a calcified mitral porcine bioprosthesis. This valve was recovered at reoperation, performed shortly after delivery, for severe prosthetic stenosis. (From Bortolotti, U., et al.: Pregnancy in patients with porcine valve bioprostheses. Am. J. Cardiol. *50*:1051, 1982.)

The selection of a prosthetic valve for pregnant patients or women of childbearing age should be individualized (p. 1065). Since it is desirable to avoid anticoagulation during pregnancy, the use of tissue valves is often recommended.[175,183,184] However, the long-term durability of these valves is limited, and frequently reoperation is required, with its related morbidity and mortality. In addition, tissue valves deteriorate more rapidly in young patients, and the incidence of calcification appears to be increased during pregnancy (Fig. 59–8).[185] A mechanical valve is recommended for patients who are willing to follow a strict regimen of anticoagulation and for those who require anticoagulation therapy for other conditions such as thrombophlebitis, atrial fibrillation, rheumatic mitral valve disease with an enlarged left atrial diameter, intracardiac thrombus, or a history of pulmonary embolism.

A review of the literature has suggested that fetal complications significantly increase with anticoagulation.[186] However, more recent prospective studies have demonstrated a normal fetal outcome when an adjusted dose of heparin is given throughout pregnancy, or at least during the first trimester.[175,177,187] Similar results have been reported with the use of oral Coumadin during pregnancy.[188]

In summary, the cumulative experience involving over 450 pregnancies reported by numerous groups from different parts of the world has demonstrated that asymptomatic or mildly symptomatic women with prosthetic heart valves can tolerate the hemodynamic load of pregnancy without difficulties. The incidence of thromboembolic events during pregnancy in women treated with anticoagulation is comparable to that in the nonpregnant population[181,182] and can be further reduced by the careful adjustment and monitoring of therapy during gestation.[187] Thus, pregnancy is not absolutely contraindicated in women with prosthetic heart valves, including mechanical prostheses.[175]

Cardiovascular Drugs in Pregnancy

(Table 59–3)

Because of their potentially unfavorable effects on the developing fetus, all drugs should be avoided, if possible, during pregnancy. When drugs are needed, however, risk/benefit ratio must be evaluated carefully, and the smallest effective dose should be used. Another source of concern is the transfer of drugs into breast milk and subsequently to the neonates during lactation. Generally, only 1 per cent to 2 per cent of the maternal dose appears in breast milk.[189] Most data regarding drug excretion in human milk are anecdotal, and except for some drugs that are clearly contraindicated, there is not enough information to allow or prohibit breast-feeding in mothers receiving medications. Because the mechanisms involved in drug excretion into breast milk are complex, the various models and formulas used to estimate plasma/milk ratios are of limited clinical value. Therefore, close monitoring of the infant's ingested dose and plasma levels, as well as close observation for adverse effects or toxicity, is necessary to ensure safety.

Cardiac Glycosides (see also p. 479)

Recommendations for the gestational use of cardiac glycosides are based on their extensive use in maternal congestive heart failure and supraventricular arrhythmias.[190] During the past decade, digoxin alone or combined with a second drug, such as verapamil[191] or quinidine,[192] has been employed with increasing frequency to treat fetal supraventricular tachycardia and congestive heart failure.[191–193] Digoxin's volume of distribution is markedly increased during pregnancy. Since the drug is only 20 per cent to 25 per cent bound to proteins, its concentration is not greatly affected by the decrease in albumin levels during gestation. Transplacental passage of digoxin has been extensively documented, and the fetomaternal serum digoxin concentration ratio has been shown to range from 0.5 to 1.0.[190]

Pregnancy, especially when complicated by hypertension, is associated with increased levels of digoxin-like substances.[194,195] This phenomenon can interfere with digoxin radioimmunoassay and may cause errors of up to 2 μg/ml.[190,194,195]

To date, few adverse effects have been observed in fetuses of mothers who have undergone long-term treatment with digoxin. Low birth weight has been reported and has been postulated to be secondary to the effect of digoxin on amino acid transport through the placenta, with consequent growth retardation.[105] However, since the duration of pregnancy has been noted to be shorter in mothers with long-term digoxin therapy, it is possible that the reported low birth weight has been due to prematurity rather than intrauterine growth retardation.[105]

Despite these concerns, the gestational use of digoxin is considered safe, and to date there are no reports of teratogenesis in humans.[105,190] Caution is advised in digitalis administration, however, since overdose can be detrimental to the mother and may be lethal to the fetus.[105]

EFFECTS ON THE FETUS. Digoxin is excreted in breast milk and the milk/plasma ratio ranged from 0.59 to 0.90.[189] The total amount of digoxin ingested daily by the infant has been estimated to be approximately 1/100 of the pediatric recommended dose. No apparent clinical effects have been demonstrated in newborns, so that digoxin therapy of the mother should not affect breast-feeding decisions.[189]

Antiarrhythmics (see also Chap. 23)

QUINIDINE (see also p. 633). There is substantial clinical experience with the use of quinidine for the treatment of maternal arrhythmias.[105,108] One report has demonstrated successful treatment of fetal supraventricular tachycardia with quinidine and digoxin.[192] Since the drug is 60 per cent to 80 per cent bound to protein, the unbound fraction may increase owing to the hypoalbuminemia of pregnancy. Transplacental passage of quinidine has been demonstrated with a fetomaternal serum concentration ratio ranging from 0.25 to 0.8.[105]

Effects on the Fetus. Fetal thrombocytopenia has been associated with quinidine treatment, and minimal oxytocic activity has been reported mostly during development of spontaneous uterine contractions. Toxic doses of quinidine, however, may cause premature labor, abortion, or damage to the fetal eighth cranial nerve.[105,108] Although these side effects are of concern, they are rare, and the drug is considered safe for the treatment of both maternal and fetal arrhythmias. Quinidine is secreted in breast milk, with a milk/plasma ratio of 0.71.[189] The calculated total dose of quinidine likely to be ingested by the infant is far below the recommended therapeutic daily pediatric dose.

PROCAINAMIDE (see also p. 636). Information regarding the use of procainamide in pregnancy is limited. Transplacental transfer of procainamide is well documented by its use in the treatment of fetal supraventricular tachycardia.[196] Fetomaternal drug level ratios have been found to be 0.28 and 1.32 in two different patients.[105] At present, no information is available concerning procainamide pharmacokinetics in the maternofetal unit. No teratogenic effects have been reported; however, because of the limited experience with procainamide, quinidine should be used as the drug of choice during pregnancy.

Translactal passage of procainamide was reported, with a milk/plasma ratio of 4.3 ± 2.4 for procainamide and 3.8 ± 1.8 for *N*-acetylprocainamide (NAPA).[197] Although the high ratio may indicate accumulation in the milk, the amount of both procainamide and NAPA ingested daily by the infant is not expected to produce significant plasma levels.[189]

DISOPYRAMIDE (see also p. 638). Reports regarding disopyramide treatment in pregnancy are limited to only a few patients treated for ventricular and supraventricular arrhythmias.[105,108,198] No teratogenic effects have been reported; however, the use of disopyramide for refractory supraventricular tachycardia in a pregnant patient with mitral valve prolapse triggered uterine contractions that abated upon withdrawal of the drug.[105]

Disopyramide is secreted in breast milk in concentrations similar to those in plasma. The estimated dose likely to be ingested by the infant is less than 2 mg/kg/day.[189] Although no adverse effects were noted in such infants,[199] until further investigation provides sufficient information re-

TABLE 59–3 SAFETY AND ADVERSE EFFECTS OF CARDIOVASCULAR DRUGS DURING PREGNANCY

DRUG	POTENTIAL FETAL ADVERSE EFFECTS	SAFETY
Digoxin	Low birth weight	Safe
Quinidine	Toxic dose may induce premature labor and damage to the fetal eighth cranial nerve.	Safe
Procainamide	None reported	*
Disopyramide	May initiate uterine contractions	*
Lidocaine	In high blood levels and fetal acidosis may cause central nervous system depression	Safe
Mexiletine	None reported	*
Admiodarone	Fetal hypothyroidism	*
Calcium antagonists	None reported	*
Beta-adrenergic blocking agents	Intrauterine growth retardation, apnea at birth, bradycardia, hypoglycemia, hyperbilirubinemia. $Beta_2$ blockade may initiate uterine contractions.	Safe
Sodium nitroprusside	Potential thiocyanate toxicity with high dose, fetal mortality in animal studies	Potentially unsafe
Organic nitrates	Fetal heart rate deceleration and bradycardia	*
ACE inhibitors (captopril and enalapril)	Skull ossification defect, premature deliveries, low birth weight, oligohydramnios, neonatal anuria, and renal failure	Unsafe
Diuretic agents	Impairment of uterine blood flow, thrombocytopenia, jaundice, hyponatremia, bradycardia	Potentially unsafe

* To date, only limited information is available and safety during pregnancy cannot be established.

garding its safety, use of disopyramide should be limited to patients with arrhythmias refractory to treatment with more established drugs.

LIDOCAINE (see also p. 639). This drug has been used during pregnancy mainly for epidural or local anesthesia; occasional reports describe its use as an antiarrhythmic agent.[105,108,200] Lidocaine crosses the placenta and can be detected rapidly in the umbilical cord after maternal administration. The fetomaternal plasma concentration ratio is 0.5 to 0.7.[105,189] Elevated lidocaine levels have been associated with infant central nervous system depression and apnea, hypotonia, dilated pupils, and seizures. Bradycardia has also been described. These side effects were reversible with appropriate treatment. As a weak base, lidocaine may be trapped by an acidic environment. For this reason, fetal acidosis may be associated with increased blood levels of the drug and the likelihood of toxicity. Lidocaine use during pregnancy has *not* been associated with teratogenic effects.

In *summary*, the available data indicate that lidocaine is safe for use during pregnancy as long as blood levels are closely monitored. Caution should be exercised in cases with fetal distress when fetal acidosis is likely. To prevent toxicity, maternal lidocaine levels should be maintained below 4 μg/ml.[105]

MEXILETINE (see also p. 640). A limited number of pregnant women have been reported to have been treated for cardiac arrhythmias with mexiletine at doses between 600 and 800 mg/day.[105,201,202] This drug appears to cross the placenta freely, and the fetomaternal ratio ranges from 0.7 to 1.0. Fetal bradycardia, infants small for gestational age, low Apgar score, and neonatal hypoglycemia have all been reported in cases of maternal treatment with mexiletine.[105] Despite these concerns, no teratogenic or long-term adverse effects have been reported. Mexiletine is secreted in breast milk and was found in higher concentrations in breast milk than in maternal plasma (the milk/plasma ratio varied between 0.8 and 1.9)[105,189]; however, the calculated daily quantity ingested by the infant appears to be below the therapeutic range, and drug levels were undetectable in infants' blood. Owing to very limited information and reported untoward effects, mexiletine cannot be recommended for use during gestation until its safety is further investigated.

AMIODARONE (see also p. 646). The use of amiodarone during pregnancy for the treatment of maternal and fetal arrhythmias has been reported in several cases.[105,189,203-205] Transplacental transfer of amiodarone and its metabolite desethylamiodarone has been reported to be 10 to 25 per cent.[105]

Although fetal outcome has been favorable in most cases, side effects, including congenital hypothyroidism with goiter, premature birth, hypotonia, bradycardia, and large anterior and posterior fontanelles, have been reported,[105,204-206] casting doubts on amiodarone's safety during pregnancy. Pending further studies, amiodarone should be used only in refractory cases of maternal or fetal tachyarrhythmias. Close monitoring of maternal and neonatal thyroid size and function is important for early detection of abnormalities.

Amiodarone is secreted in breast milk in quantities significant enough to be detected in the infant's blood.[105,189] The effect of long-term amiodarone exposure in infants is unknown; however, because of the well-known potential side effects of this drug, breast-feeding is *not* recommended in women being treated with amiodarone.[105]

Calcium Channel Antagonists (see also p. 867)

VERAPAMIL (see also p. 648). This drug has been used in pregnancy for various indications, including maternal and fetal supraventricular arrhythmias, premature labor, severe preeclampsia, and severe gestational proteinuric hypertension.[105,207,208]

Transplacental passage of verapamil forms the basis for in utero treatment of fetal tachycardias, which is often successful with this drug alone or combined with digoxin.[191,208] Although dysfunctional labor or postpartum hemorrhage attributable to verapamil has not been reported, discontinuation of the drug at the onset of labor has been recommended. More data are required to establish the safety of long-term therapy during pregnancy. Verapamil is excreted in breast milk[105,209]; its concentration ranges from 23 to 94 per cent of maternal blood level. The estimated total amount of verapamil secreted in milk is less than 0.01 to 0.04 per cent of the administered dose, and no pharmacological effects have been observed in neonates.

NIFEDIPINE (see also p. 867). Limited use of nifedipine in pregnancy as a tocolytic agent[210] and for the acute treatment of hypertensive emergencies[211] and chronic essential hypertension has also been reported.[212] The drug was reported to lower blood pressure without any apparent reduction in uteroplacental blood flow.[213] Constantine et al.[212] combined nifedipine with beta blockers for long-term treatment of hypertensive patients who were pregnant and found a high rate of cesarean section, abnormal antenatal cardiotocograph, premature delivery, and small-for-date infants. For these reasons and until further information is available regarding the safety of nifedipine in pregnancy, long-term use of this agent during gestation cannot be recommended.

Beta-Adrenoceptor Blocking Agents (see also p. 644)

PROPRANOLOL (see also p. 644). This drug has been used in pregnancy for the treatment of cardiac arrhythmias, hypertrophic cardiomyopathy, and hyperthyroidism.[105,108] Propranolol readily crosses the placenta; at delivery, fetal serum concentrations are equal to or lower than maternal concentrations. Because of decreased hepatic metabolism and altered protein binding, serum concentration and half-life may be increased in the neonate during the first 10 days of life. Several adverse effects on the fetus and neonate have been reported, including intrauterine growth retardation, delayed onset of respiration in the newborn, bradycardia, hypoglycemia, and hyperbilirubinemia.[105] Although increasing experience with the use of propranolol in pregnancy has demonstrated the rarity of these side effects, they should be anticipated by the clinician. Since blockade of myometrial beta$_2$-adrenergic receptors with propranolol may stimulate uterine contractions, selective beta$_1$-receptor blockers may be preferable for use during gestation.

Propranolol is excreted in breast milk, with a milk/plasma ratio of approximately 0.5 to 1.0.[105,189] No adverse effects were observed in infants breast-fed by mothers treated with propranolol. However, careful observation of such infants is recommended, since propranolol may accumulate owing to the immature hepatic microsomal enzyme system of the neonate.

METOPROLOL. This drug has been used alone or in combination with hydralazine to treat hypertensive pregnant patients without causing teratogenic or major side effects.[214] Metoprolol is secreted in breast milk[189]; however, the daily quantity ingested by the neonate is very small. Unless hepatic function in the newborn is markedly impaired, breast-feeding is probably safe.

ATENOLOL. Several studies have reported the use of atenolol in the treatment of hypertension during gestation.[105] Transplacental transfer of atenolol has been well documented with a fetomaternal ratio of 1.0.[105,189] Although available data indicate that the safety of atenolol is similar to that of other beta blockers, low birth weight has been reported in association with its use during pregnancy.[105] Atenolol is secreted in breast milk. No adverse effects have been noted in babies exposed to breast milk of women treated with atenolol, so that breast-feeding need not be discontinued.

LABETALOL (see also p. 866). This drug is an antihypertensive agent with selective alpha$_1$ nonselective beta-adrenergic blocking activity and low beta-agonist activity. Labetalol crosses the placenta, and the fetomaternal ratio is 0.5.[189,215] Its clearance and volume of distribution are not altered during pregnancy. A number of favorable reports have described the efficacy and safety of labetalol in the treatment of hypertensive pregnancies.[105,215,216] Despite significant reduction in blood pressure, uterine blood flow has not been affected.[216] Labetalol is secreted in breast milk, and no adverse effects have been noted in neonates.[217]

Sodium Nitroprusside

During pregnancy, nitroprusside (NP) has been used to control blood pressure and heart failure in patients with intracranial aneurysm, surgery, or severe gestational hypertension.[105,218,219] Data concerning the effect of NP on uterine blood flow are conflicting. The drug has been demonstrated to cross the placenta, both in animals and in humans. In pregnant ewes, maternal and fetal levels achieved equilibrium within 20 minutes. A large dose of NP in animals resulted in significant accumulation of maternal and fetal cyanide and fetal death.[218] In the limited number of patients treated with NP during pregnancy, no unfavorable drug-related effect on the fetus was noticed.[105,218] Therefore, NP is a very effective but potentially toxic drug. It has been employed in pregnancy mostly in gravely ill patients, and the data available are small. Until further studies clarify its pharmacodynamics, kinetics, and safety during pregnancy, caution is recommended.

Organic Nitrates

Intravenous nitroglycerin has been used effectively and safely to control severe pregnancy-induced hypertension.[89,118] In one report, however, the reduction of blood pressure with nitroglycerin was associated with fetal heart rate deceleration and bradycardia in a few patients and attenuation of spontaneous beat-to-beat variability, probably owing to loss of cerebral autoregulation and increased intracranial pressure. It appears, therefore, that treatment with nitrates may not be free from side effects. Further studies are needed to clarify the effects of these drugs on uterine blood flow and fetal safety before they can be recommended for use during pregnancy.

Angiotensin-Converting Enzyme (ACE) Inhibitors (see also p. 867)

Both captopril and enalapril have been used in the treatment of hypertension in pregnancy.[220,221] Passage of captopril from the mother to the fetus has been reported in two patients with maternal/fetal plasma concentration quotients of 3.4 and 1.0.[220] In animals, exposure to ACE inhibitors during pregnancy has been reported to produce prolonged fetal hypotension and death.[221] Although there are no reports of direct teratogenicity, two cases have been reported of a rare skull ossification defect in fetuses born to mothers treated with ACE inhibitors.[222] In addition, increased risk of early delivery, low birth weight, severe oligohydramnios, and/or neonatal anuria and renal failure that may be fatal has been reported.[218,222] Despite the limited and anecdotal nature of the available information, the published data indicate a potential risk and suggest that, for the time being, ACE inhibitors should not be used during gestation.[89]

Diuretic Agents

Diuretics have been used in pregnancy for the management of hypertension, heart failure, fluid retention, and prophylactically to prevent preeclampsia.[89,218] Because of the benign nature of dependent edema in pregnancy and the potential impairment of uterine blood flow and placental perfusion due to decreased blood volume, diuretics are not recommended for dependent edema. The prophylactic use of diuretics has not been proved effective in patients with preeclampsia; moreover, further volume restriction with these drugs may be deleterious.[89] Although diuretic therapy during pregnancy in patients with chronic hypertension is controversial, the continuation of diuretic therapy initiated prior to conception does not seem unfavorable. However, because of the potential for a decrease in placental perfusion, initiating diuretics during pregnancy is not recommended. Recent data have shown, however, that thiazide diuretics are safe and effective when used in combination with methyldopa.[223] Placental transfer of both hydrochlorothiazide and furosemide[224,225] has been documented, with similar maternal and fetal serum levels. Although no teratogenic effects have been described, case reports of neonatal thrombocytopenia, jaundice, hyponatremia, and bradycardia have been reported with the use of thiazides.[218]

In *summary*, because of the potential fetal adverse effects, the use of diuretics in pregnancy should be limited to the treatment of heart failure and selected cases of hypertension. The *routine* use of these drugs for the treatment of hypertension or dependent edema is *not* recommended.

Anticoagulant Therapy

Anticoagulants may be necessary to prevent or control the following cardiovascular conditions during pregnancy: venous thrombophlebitis, pulmonary embolism, rheumatic mitral valve disease, prosthetic heart valves, peripartum cardiomyopathy, primary pulmonary hypertension, and Eisenmenger's syndrome.[176]

Because of its large molecular size, heparin does not cross the placenta and is the drug of choice during pregnancy. In a review of anticoagulation during pregnancy, Hall et al.[186] reported a high incidence of maternal and fetal complications associated with heparin; however, other prospective studies have demonstrated a favorable outcome with heparin therapy.[175,177,187]

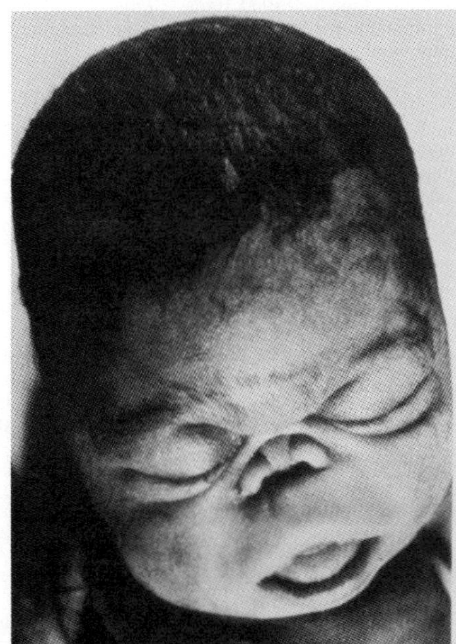

FIGURE 59-9. Severe nasal deformity in a newborn from a mother with aortic valve prosthesis taking Coumadin throughout pregnancy. (From Becker, M. H., et al.: Chondrodysplasia punctata. Is maternal warfarin therapy a factor? Am. J. Dis. Child. *129*:356, 1975.)

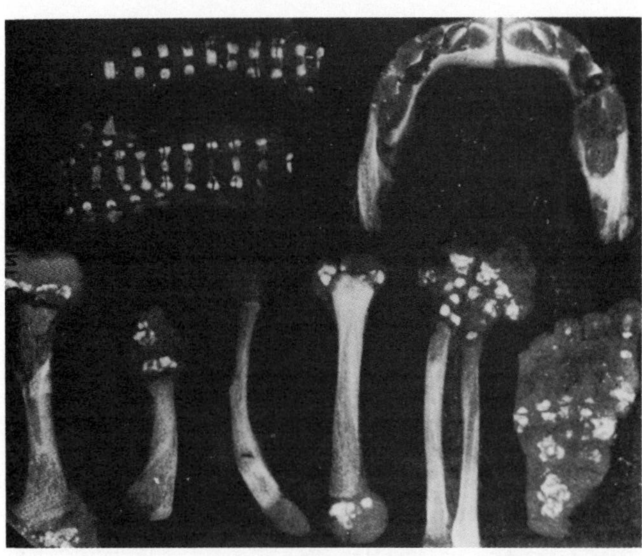

FIGURE 59-10. Roentgenograph of dissected skeleton showing stippling in cartilaginous portions of skeleton. Same case as Figure 59-9. (From Becker, M. H., et al.: Chondrodysplasia punctata. Is maternal warfarin therapy a factor? Am. J. Dis. Child. *129*:356, 1975.)

The use of Coumadin during pregnancy is associated with substantial teratogenic risk, including a high incidence of fetal wastage due to spontaneous abortion and stillbirths[176,179,226]; central nervous system disease such as optic nerve atrophy and blindness, mental retardation, microcephaly, and spasticity; and even death secondary to intracranial hemorrhage.[176,226] Use of this drug during the first trimester has been associated with "coumarin embryopathy" in 5 to 30 per cent of newborns.[176,177,226] This syndrome includes nasal bone hypoplasia (Fig. 59-9) and epiphyseal stippling (chondrodysplasia punctata[227]; Fig. 59-10). Labor and delivery while the patient is taking Coumadin places both the mother and fetus at risk of hemorrhage. Because the drug(s)' half-life is longer in the fetus, the effect of Coumadin may persist for 7 to 10 days after its administration has been discontinued. Our recommended strategy for peripartum anticoagulation therapy is shown in Figure 59-11.

Patients of childbearing age who are taking anticoagulants on a long-term basis should be advised prior to conception regarding the maternal and fetal risks of these agents. If pregnancy is planned, oral anticoagulants should be discontinued and subcutaneous heparin started. To avoid prolonged treatment with heparin prior to conception, the fertility of both parents should be investigated before heparin administration is begun. In cases of conception during Coumadin therapy, heparin should be substituted. A brief period of hospitalization is advisable to establish the required heparin dose and assure continuity of effective anticoagulation.

Self-injection of an adjusted dose of heparin subcutaneously is the recommended approach for the duration of pregnancy. Because of interpatient dose variability and changes in the dose requirement as pregnancy progresses,[176,187] a fixed dose of heparin may not prevent thromboembolic events and cannot be recommended.[228,229] Heparin is administered into the lower abdominal subcutaneous tissue at 12-hour intervals, with dose adjustment to prolong the activated partial thromboplastin time to 1.5 to 2.0 times normal. To reduce pain, concentrated heparin (20,000 units/ml) should be used.[176]

Complications related to long-term heparin therapy may occur and include sterile abscesses and hematomas in the abdominal wall, thrombocytopenia, and osteoporosis.[176,230,231] To reduce the risk of bleeding at delivery, subcutaneous heparin should be replaced in the hospital with intravenous heparin at 38 weeks' gestation. If heparin is needed, it can be substituted with oral Coumadin, adjusted to increase protime 1.5 to 2.0 times normal value, at the end of the first trimester.[177] Heparin and Coumadin should be given concomitantly for 4 days before heparin is stopped.[232]

Heparin should be discontinued at the onset of labor to allow clotting time to normalize prior to delivery. It has been recommended that heparin be continued into early labor when longer labor is anticipated, such as for primigravidas.[233] Since anticoagulation is reinstituted soon after delivery in patients who require this form of therapy, epidural anesthesia may increase the risk of bleeding into the epidural and subarachnoid space.[233] Pudendal anesthesia may also be associated with increased risk of bleeding complications in patients who have had anticoagulative therapy, since pudendal blood vessels are commonly punctured. Hemostatic stitches should be used to avoid bleeding in patients undergoing episiotomy, and uterine contraction should be stimulated by massage and Pitocin or ergot derivatives. Intravenous heparin can be resumed after delivery once he-

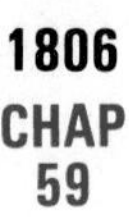

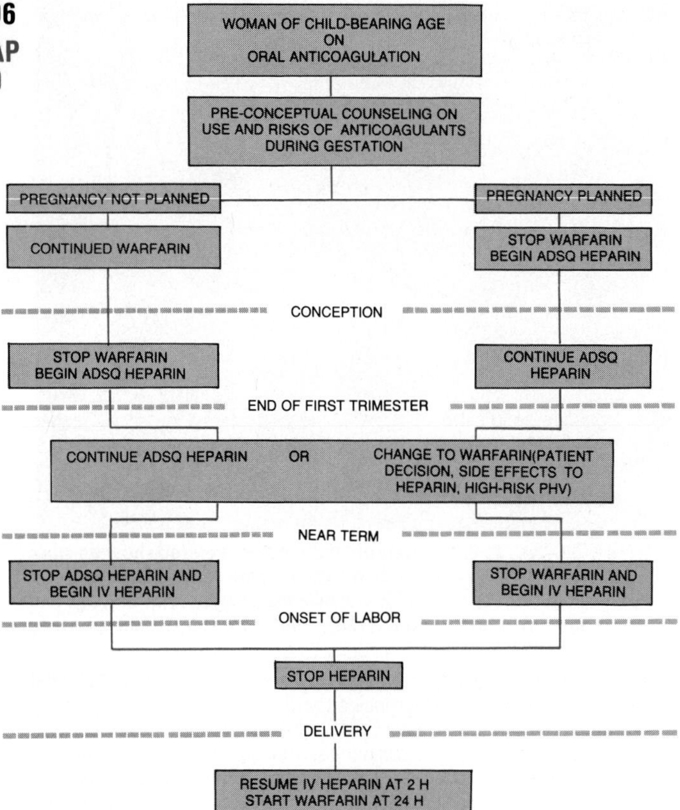

FIGURE 59-11. Recommended strategy for peripartum anticoagulation therapy. ADSQ, adjusted dose subcutaneous; H, hours; IV, intravenous; PHV = prosthetic heart valve. (From McGehee, W.: Anticoagulation in pregnancy. *In* Elkayam, U., and Gleicher, N. [eds.]: Cardiac Problems in Pregnancy: Diagnosis and Management of Maternal and Fetal Disease. 2nd ed. New York, Alan R. Liss, Inc., 1990, p. 397.)

mostasis is deemed adequate, and oral anticoagulation can be started 24 hours post partum after bleeding and hemorrhage have been ruled out.[176,233] Oral anticoagulation can be safely used after delivery, even in lactating women.[176]

Prophylactic Antibiotics

Antibiotic prophylaxis is indicated to prevent recurrent acute rheumatic fever in patients with a history of this disease and to prevent bacterial endocarditis in patients with certain types of underlying heart disease.

The recommended regimen for the prevention of rheumatic fever is the same as in the nongravid state (p. 1729) and includes 1.2 million units of benzathine penicillin G intramuscularly every 4 weeks, 250,000 units of oral penicillin V twice a day, or 1 gm/day of sulfadiazine.[234] Because of predisposition to kernicterus with the use of sulfadiazine, these drugs are not recommended during the third trimester of pregnancy and in women with a previous history of children with neonatal jaundice or blood-group incompatibility.[235]

Similar to the nongravid state, antibiotic prophylaxis for infective endocarditis is indicated during gestation in patients with prosthetic heart valves, congenital heart disease, rheumatic valvular disease, obstructive hypertrophic cardiomyopathy, and mitral valve prolapse with thickened mitral valve and mitral insufficiency who are undergoing procedures likely to result in bacteremia.[56] Since the incidence of bacteremia associated with uncomplicated vaginal delivery has been reported to be low (0 to 5 per cent),[236] the indication for antibiotic prophylaxis is questionable.[234]

The Committee on Bacterial Endocarditis, formed by the American Heart Association, has recommended routine prophylaxis for anticipated normal delivery only in patients with prosthetic heart valves.[56] Despite these recommendations, and since complications and bacteremia are not always predictable, we routinely administer prophylactic antibiotics to all patients susceptible to bacterial endocarditis. The antibiotic regimen recommended for delivery is 2 gm of ampicillin intramuscularly or intravenously, plus 1.5 mg/kg of gentamicin (maximum of 80 mg) intramuscularly or intravenously 30 minutes to 1 hour before the procedure. A second dose may be given 8 hours later. In patients allergic to penicillin, 1 gm of vancomycin is given intravenously, slowly over 1 hour, plus 1.5 mg/kg of gentamicin (to a maximum of 80 mg) intramuscularly or intravenously 1 hour before the procedure. This may be repeated 8 to 12 hours later.[56,234]

REFERENCES

CARDIOVASCULAR PHYSIOLOGY DURING PREGNANCY AND THE PUERPERIUM

1. Oakley, C. M.: Cardiovascular disease in pregnancy. Can. J. Cardiol. *6*:(Suppl B):33B, 1990.
1a. Elkayam, U., and Gleicher, N.: Hemodynamics and cardiac function during normal pregnancy and the puerperium. *In* Elkayam, U., and Gleicher, N. (eds.): Cardiac Problems in Pregnancy: Diagnosis and Management of Maternal and Fetal Disease, 2nd ed. New York, Alan R. Liss Inc., 1990, p. 5.
2. Ueland, K.: Maternal cardiovascular dynamics: VII. Intrapartum blood volume changes. Am. J Obstet. Gynecol. *126*:671, 1976.
3. Longo, L. D.: Maternal blood volume and cardiac output during pregnancy: A hypothesis of endocrinologic control. Am. J. Physiol. *245*:R720, 1983.
4. Hsueh, W. A., Luetscher, J. A., Carlson, E. J., et al.: Changes in active and inactive renin throughout pregnancy. J. Clin. Endocrinol. Metab. *54*:1010, 1982.
5. Cheek, D. B., Petrucco, O. M., Gillespie, A., et al.: Muscle cell growth and the distribution of water and electrolyte in human pregnancy. Early Hum. Dev. *11*:293, 1985.
6. Robson, S. C., Hunter, S., Boys, R. J., et al.: Serial study of factors influencing changes in cardiac output during human pregnancy. Am. J. Physiol. *256*:H1060, 1989.
7. Kjeldsen, J.: Hemodynamic investigations during labor and delivery. Acta Obstet. Gynecol. Scand. *89*(Suppl.):20, 1979.
8. Katz, R., Karliner, J. S., and Resnik., K. R.: Effects of a natural volume overload state (pregnancy) on left ventricular performance in normal human subjects. Circulation *58*:434, 1978.
9. Bryant, E. E., Douglas, B. H., and Ashburn, A. D.: Circulatory changes following prolactin administration. Am. J. Obstet. Gynecol. *115*:53, 1973.
10. Gerber, J. G., Payne, N. A., Murphy, R. R., et al.: Prostacyclin produced by the pregnant uterus in the dog may act as a circulating vasodepressor substance. J. Clin. Invest. *67*:632, 1981.
11. Metcalfe, J., and Ueland, K.: Maternal cardiovascular adjustment to pregnancy. Prog. Cardiovasc. Dis. *16*:363, 1974.
12. Robson, S. C., Dunlop, W., Boys, R. J., et al.: Cardiac output during labour. Br. Med. J. *295*:1169, 1987.
13. Ueland, K., and Hansen, J. M.: Maternal cardiovascular dynamics: II. Posture and uterine contractions. Am. J. Obstet. Gynecol. *103*:1, 1969.
14. Ueland, K.: Cardiovascular physiology of the normal pregnancy. *In* Gleicher, U., Elkayam, U., Galbraith, R. M., et al. (eds.): Principles of Medical Therapy in Pregnancy. New York, Plenum, 1985, p. 643.
15. Ueland, K., and Hansen, J. M.: Maternal cardiovascular dynamic: III. Labor and delivery under local and caudal analgesia. Am. J. Obstet. Gynecol. *103*:8, 1969.
16. Artal, R., Khodiguian, N., Rutherford, S., et al.: Cardiopulmonary and metabolic responses to bicycle ergometry in pregnancy. *In* Proceedings of the Society for Gynecologic Investigation, 1987, p. 48.
17. Morton, M. J., and Metcalfe, J.: Changes in maternal hemodynamics during pregnancy. *In* Artal, R., and Wiswell, R. (eds.): Exercise in Pregnancy. Baltimore, Williams and Wilkins, 1986.
18. Artal, R.: Cardiopulmonary responses to exercise in pregnancy. *In* Elkayam, U., and Gleicher, N. (eds.): Cardiac Problems in Pregnancy: Diagnosis and Management of Maternal and Fetal Disease, 2nd ed. New York, Alan R. Liss, Inc., 1990, p. 25.
19. Artal, R., Romem, Y., Paul, R. H., et al.: Fetal bradycardia induced by maternal exercise. Lancet *2*:258, 1984.

CARDIAC EVALUATION DURING PREGNANCY

20. Elkayam, U., and Gleicher, N.: Changes in cardiac findings during normal pregnancy: Cardiovascular physiology of pregnancy: *In* Elkayam, U., and Gleicher, N. (eds.): Cardiac Problems in Pregnancy: Diagnosis and Management of Maternal and Fetal Disease. 2nd ed. New York, Alan R. Liss, Inc., 1990, p. 31.
21. Cutforth, R., and MacDonald, C. B.: Heart sounds and murmurs in pregnancy. Am. Heart J. *71*:741, 1966.
22. Perloff, J. K.: Normal or innocent murmurs. *In* Perloff, J. K. (ed.): The Clinical Recognition of Congenital Heart Disease. 3rd ed. Philadelphia, W. B. Saunders Company, 1987, p. 8.
23. Tabaznik, B., Randall, T. W., and Hersch, C.: The mammary souffle of pregnancy and lactation. Circulation *22*:1069, 1960.
24. Marcus, F. L., Ewy, G. A., O'Rourke, R. A., et al.: The effect of pregnancy on the murmurs of mitral and aortic regurgitation. Circulation *41*:795, 1970.
25. Haas, J. M.: The effect of pregnancy on the midsystolic click and murmur of the prolapsing posterior leaflet of the mitral valve. Am. Heart J. *92*:407, 1976.
26. Kumar, A., and Elkayam, U.: Hypertrophic cardiomyopathy in pregnancy: *In* Elkayam, U., and Gleicher, N. (eds.): Cardiac Problems in Pregnancy: Diagnosis and Management of Maternal and Fetal Disease. 2nd ed. New York, Alan R. Liss, Inc., 1990, p. 129.
27. Perloff, J. K.: Pregnancy and cardiovascular disease. *In* Braunwald, E. (ed.): Heart Disease. 2nd ed. Philadelphia, W. B. Saunders Company, 1984, p. 1763.
28. Criteria Committee of the New York Heart Association: Nomenclature and Criteria for Diagnosis of Diseases of the Heart and Great Vessels. 6th ed. Boston, Little, Brown and Co., 1964, p. 1.
29. Elkayam, U., and Gleicher, N.: Cardiac problems in pregnancy: I. Mater-

nal aspects: The approach to the pregnant patient with heart disease. JAMA *251*:2838, 1984.
30. Elkayam, U.: Unpublished data.
31. Hong, R. A., and Bhandari, A. K.: Cardiac arrhythmias and pregnancy. *In* Elkayam, U., and Gleicher, N. (eds.): Cardiac Problems in Pregnancy: Diagnosis and Management of Maternal and Fetal Disease. 2nd ed. New York, Alan R. Liss, Inc., 1990, p. 167.
32. Upshaw, C. B., Jr.: A study of maternal electrocardiograms recorded during labor and delivery. Am. J. Obstet. Gynecol. *107*:17, 1970.
33. Department of Health Services: Syllabus on Diagnostic X-ray Radiation Protection for Certified X-ray Supervisors and Operators. Sacramento, Calif., Department of Health Services, 1982, p. 71.
34. Wagner, C. K., Lester, R. G., and Saldana L. R.: Exposure of the pregnant patient to diagnostic radiation. A Guide to Medical Management. Philadelphia, J. B. Lippincott Co., 1985, p. 52.
35. Turner, A. F.: The chest radiograph in pregnancy. Clin. Obstet. Gynecol. *183*:65, 1975.
36. Hughson, W. G., Friedman, P. J., Feigin, D. S., et al.: Postpartum pleural effusion: A common radiologic finding. Ann. Intern. Med. *97*:856, 1982.
37. Austin, J.H.M.: Postpartum pleural effusions. Ann. Intern. Med. *98*:555, 1983.
38. Bioeffects Committee of the American Institute of Ultrasound in Medicine. J. Ultrasound Med. Biol. *2*:R14, 1983.
39. Katz, R., Karliner, J. S., and Resnik, R.: Effects of a natural volume overload state (pregnancy) on left ventricular performance in normal human subjects. Circulation *58*:434, 1978.
40. Limacher, M. C., Ware, J. A., O'Meara, M. E., et al.: Tricuspid regurgitation during pregnancy. Am. J. Cardiol. *55*:1059, 1985.
41. Haiat, R., and Halphen, C.: Silent pericardial effusion in late pregnancy: A new entity. Cardiovasc. Intervent. Radiol. *7*:267, 1984.
42. Enein, M., Aziz, A., Zima, A., et al.: Echocardiography of the pericardium in pregnancy. Obstet. Gynecol. *69*:851, 1987.
43. Campos, O., Martinez, E., Andrade, J. L., et al.: Detection of right-sided valve regurgitation during normal pregnancy by Doppler echocardiography. J. Am. Coll. Cardiol. *15*:139A, 1990.
44. Carpenter, M. W., Sady, S. P., Hoegsberg, B., et al.: Fetal heart rate response to maternal exertion. JAMA *259*:3006, 1988.
45. Elkayam, U., and Gleicher, N.: Diagnostic approaches to maternal heart disease. *In* Elkayam, U., and Gleicher, N. (eds.): Cardiac Problems in Pregnancy. 2nd ed. New York, Alan R. Liss, Inc., 1990, p. 41.
46. Lee, W., Shah, P. K., Amin, D. K., et al.: Hemodynamic monitoring of cardiac patients during pregnancy. *In* Elkayam, U., and Gleicher, N. (eds.): Cardiac Problems in Pregnancy: Diagnosis and Management of Maternal and Fetal Disease. 2nd ed. New York, Alan R. Liss, Inc., 1990, p. 47.
47. Medical Radiation Exposure of Pregnant and Potentially Pregnant Women: Recommendations of the National Council on Radiation Protection and Measurements. Washington, National Council on Radiation Protection and Measurements, 1977, p. 13.
48. Bithell, J. F., and Stewart, A. M.: Pre-natal irradiation and childhood malignancy: A review of British data from the Oxford survey. Br. J. Cancer *31*:271, 1975.
49. Elkayam, U., Kawanishi, D., Reid, C. L., et al.: Contrast echocardiography to reduce ionizing radiation associated with cardiac catheterization during pregnancy. Am. J. Cardiol. *52*:213, 1983.
50. Kereiakes, J. J., and Rosenstein, M.: Handbook of Radiation Doses of Nuclear Medicine and Diagnostic X-ray. Boca Raton, Fl, CR Press, 1980, p. 170.

CARDIOVASCULAR DISEASES AND PREGNANCY

51. Canobbio, M. M.: Counseling the adult with congenital heart disease. *In* Roberts W. C. (ed.): Adult Congenital Heart Disease. Philadelphia, F. A. Davis Co., 1987, p. 733.
52. Shime, J., Mocarski, E.J.M., Hastings, D., Webb, G. D., and McLaughlin, P. R.: Congenital heart disease in pregnancy: Short- and long-term implications. Am. J. Obstet. Gynecol. *156*:313, 1987.
53. Whittemore, R., Hobbins, J. C., and Engle, M. A.: Pregnancy and its outcome in women with and without surgical treatment of congenital heart disease. Am. J. Cardiol. *50*:641, 1982.
54. Whittemore, R.: Congenital heart disease: Its impact on pregnancy. Hosp. Pract. *18*:65, 1983.
55. Elkayam, U., Cobb, T., and Gleicher, N.: Congenital heart disease and pregnancy. In Elkayam, U., and Gleicher, N. (eds.): Cardiac Problems in Pregnancy. 2nd ed. New York, Alan R. Liss, Inc., 1990, p. 73.
56. Shulman, S. T., Amren, D. P., Bisno, A. L., et al.: Prevention of bacterial endocarditis. Circulation *70*:1123A, 1984.
57. McFaul, P. B., Dorman, J. C., Lamki, H., et al.: Pregnancy complicated by maternal heart disease. A review of 519 women. Br. J. Obstet. Gynecol. *95*:861, 1988.
58. Metcalfe, J., McAnulty, J. H., and Ueland, K.: Heart Disease and Pregnancy, Physiology and Management. Boston, Little, Brown and Co., 1986, p. 223.
59. Arias, F., and Pineda, J.: Aortic stenosis and pregnancy. J. Reprod. Med. *4*:229, 1978.
60. Angel, J. L., Chapman, C., Knappel, R. A., et al.: Percutaneous balloon aortic valvuloplasty in pregnancy. Obstet. Gynecol. *72*:438, 1988.
61. Wachtel, H. L., and Czarnecki, S. W.: Coarctation of the aorta and pregnancy. Am. Heart J. *72*:251, 1966.
62. Barash, P. G., Hobbins, J. C., Hook, R., et al.: Management of coarctation of the aorta during pregnancy. J. Thorac. Cardiovasc. Surg. *69*:781, 1975.
63. Togo, T., Sugishita, Y., Tamura, T., et al.: Uneventful pregnancy and delivery in a case of multiple peripheral pulmonary stenosis. Acta Cardiol. *18*:143, 1983.
64. Garson, H., McNamara, D. G., and Cooley, D. A.: Tetralogy of Fallot in adults. *In* Roberts, W. C. (ed.): Congenital Heart Disease in Adults. Philadelphia, F. A. Davis Co., 1987, p. 493.
65. Zitnik, R. S., Bradenburg, R. O., Sheldon, R., et al.: Pregnancy and open heart surgery. Circulation *39*(Suppl. I):257, 1969.
66. Geller, E., Rudick, V., and Niv, D.: Analgesia and anesthesia during pregnancy. *In* Elkayam, E., and Gleicher, N. (eds.): Cardiac Problems in Pregnancy: Diagnosis and Management of Maternal and Fetal Disease. 2nd ed. New York, Alan R. Liss, Inc., 1990, p. 283.
67. Hatjis, C. G., Gibson, M., Capeless, E. L., et al.: Pregnancy in a patient with tricuspid atresia. Am. J. Obstet. Gynecol. *145*:114, 1983.
68. Baumann, H., Schneider, H., Drack, G., et al.: Pregnancy and delivery by cesarean section in a patient with transposition of the great arteries and single ventricle. Case report. Br. J. Obstet. Gynaecol. *94*:704, 1987.
69. Neukermans, K., Sullivan, T. J., Pitlick, P. T.: Successful pregnancy after the Mustard operation for transposition of the great arteries. Am. J. Cardiol. *62*:838, 1988.
70. Ahmed, S., Hawes, D., Dooley, S., et al.: Intrathecal morphine in a patient with a single ventricle. Anesthesiology *54*:515, 1981.
71. Simon, D. L., and Lustberg, A.: A case of truncus arteriosus communis compatible with full-term pregnancy. Am. Heart J. *42*:617, 1951.
72. Mandel, A., and Hirsch, V.: Cor triloculare biatriatum: Report of a case with survival to the age of 29 years. Am. Heart J. *66*:104, 1963.
73. Copel, J. A., Harrison, D., Whittemore, R., et al.: Intrathecal morphine analgesia for vaginal delivery in a woman with a single ventricle. A case report. J. Reprod. Med. *31*:274, 1986.
74. Gleicher, N., Midwall, J., Hochberger, D., et al.: Eisenmenger's syndrome and pregnancy. Obstet. Gynecol. Surv. *34*:721, 1979.
75. Midwall, J., Jaffin, H., Herman, M. V., et al.: Shunt flow and pulmonary hemodynamics during labor and delivery in the Eisenmenger's syndrome. Am. J. Cardiol. *42*:299, 1978.
76. Mangano, D. T.: Anesthesia for the pregnant cardiac patient. *In* Shnider, S. M., and Levinson, G. (eds.): Anesthesia for Obstetrics. Baltimore, Williams and Wilkins, 1986, p. 345.
77. Rosenberg, B., Simon, K., Peretz, B. A., et al.: Eisenmenger's syndrome in pregnancy. Controlled segmental epidural block for cesarean section. Reg. Anaesth. *7*:131, 1984.
78. Gordis, L.: The virtual disappearance of rheumatic fever in the United States: Lessons in the rise and fall of disease. Circulation *72*:1155, 1985.
79. Argarwal, B. L.: Rheumatic heart disease unabated in developing countries. Lancet *2*:910, 1981.
80. Ueland, K.: Rheumatic heart disease and pregnancy. *In* Elkayam, U., and Gleicher, N. (eds.): Cardiac Problems in Pregnancy. 2nd ed. New York, Alan R. Liss, Inc., 1990, p. 99.
81. Jacobi, P., Adler, Z., Zimmer, E. Z., et al.: Effect of uterine contractions on left atrial pressure in pregnant woman with mitral stenosis. Br. J. Med. *298*:27, 1989.
82. Clark, S. L., Phelan, J. P., Greenspoon, J., et al.: Labor and delivery in the presence of mitral stenosis: Central hemodynamic observations. Am. J. Obstet. Gynecol. *152*:984, 1985.
83. Hemmings, G. T., Whalley, D. G., O'Connor, P. H., et al.: Invasive monitoring and anesthetic management of a patient with mitral stenosis. Can. Anaesth. Soc. J. *34*:182, 1987.
84. Bernal, J. M., and Miralles, P. J.: Cardiac surgery with cardiopulmonary bypass during pregnancy. Obstet. Gynecol. Surv. *41*:1, 1986.
85. Palacios, I. F., Block, P. C., Wilkins, G. T., et al.: Percutaneous mitral balloon valvotomy during pregnancy in a patient with severe mitral stenosis. Cathet. Cardiovasc. Diagn. *15*:109, 1988.
86. Becker, R. M.: Intracardiac surgery in pregnant women. Ann. Thorac. Surg. *36*:453, 1983.
87. Safian, R. D., Berman, A. D., Sachs, B., et al.: Percutaneous balloon mitral valvuloplasty in a pregnant woman with mitral stenosis. Cathet. Cardiovasc. Diagn. *15*:103, 1988.
88. Goon, M. S., Raman, S., and Sinnathuray, T. A.: Closed mitral valvotomy in pregnancy—A Malaysian experience. Aust. N. Z. J. Obstet. Gynaecol. *27*:173, 1987.
89. Myers, S. A.: Antihypertensive drug use during pregnancy. *In* Elkayam, U., and Gleicher, N. (eds.): Cardiac Problems in Pregnancy: Diagnosis and Management of Maternal and Fetal Disease. 2nd ed. New York, Alan R. Liss, Inc., 1990, p. 381.
90. Roth, A., Rahimtoola, S., and Elkayam, U.: Enhancement of hemodynamic effects of hydralazine with nitroglycerin in patients with chronic mitral regurgitation. Circulation *76*(Suppl. IV):89, 1987.
91. Panja, M., Nutra, K., Kar, A. K., et al.: A clinical profile of heart disease in pregnancy. Indian Heart J. *38*:392, 1986.
92. Elkayam, U., McKay, C. R., Weber, L., et al.: Favorable effects of hydralazine on the hemodynamic response to isometric exercise in chronic severe aortic regurgitation. Am. J. Cardiol. *53*:1604, 1984.
93. Savage, D. D., Garrison, R. J., Devereux, R. B., et al.: Mitral valve prolapse in the general population: I. Epidemiology features: The Framingham Study. Am. Heart J. *106*:571, 1983.
94. Wann, L. S., Grove, J. R., Hess, T. R., et al.: Prevalence of mitral prolapse by two-dimensional echocardiography in healthy young women. Br. Heart J. *49*:334, 1983.

95. Rayburn, W. F., LeMire, M. S., Bird, J. L., et al.: Mitral valve prolapse: Echocardiographic changes during pregnancy. J. Reprod. Med. *32*:185, 1987.
96. Rayburn, W. F.: Mitral valve prolapse and pregnancy. *In* Elkayam, U., and Gleicher, N. (eds.): Cardiac Problems in Pregnancy. 2nd ed. New York, Alan R. Liss, Inc., 1990, p. 181.
97. Tank, L.C.H., Chan, S.Y.W., Wong, V.C.W., et al.: Pregnancy in patients with mitral valve prolapse. Int. J. Gynaecol. Obstet. *23*:217, 1985.
98. Pyeritz, R. E.: Maternal and fetal complications of pregnancy in the Marfan syndrome. Am. J. Med. *71*:784, 1981.
99. Pyeritz, R. E.: The Marfan syndrome. Am. Fam. Physician *34*:83, 1986.
100. Rosenblum, N. G., Grossman, A. R., Mennuti, M. T., et al.: Failure of serial echocardiographic studies to predict aortic dissection in pregnant patient with Marfan's syndrome. Am. J. Obstet. Gynecol. *146*:470, 1983.
101. Pyeritz, R. E.: Propranolol retards aortic root dilatation in the Marfan syndrome. Circulation *68*(Suppl. III):365, 1983.
102. Shah, D. M., and Sunderji, S. G.: Hypertrophic cardiomyopathy and pregnancy: Report of the maternal mortality and review of the literature. Obstet. Gynecol. Surv. *40*:444, 1985.
103. Maron, B. J., Bonow, R. D., Cannon, R. O., et al.: Hypertrophic cardiomyopathy. Interrelations of clinical manifestations, pathophysiology and therapy. N. Engl. J. Med. *316*:844, 1987.
104. Rosing, D. R., Idanpaan-Heikkila, U., Maron, B. J., et al.: Use of calcium-channel blocking drugs in hypertrophic cardiomyopathy. Am. J. Cardiol. *55*:185B, 1985.
105. Widerhorn, J., Rubin, J. N., Frishman, W. H., et al.: Cardiovascular drugs in pregnancy. Cardiol. Clin. *5*:651, 1987.
106. McKenna, W. J., Deanfield, J. F., Faruqui, A. M., et al.: Prognosis in hypertrophic cardiomyopathy: Role of age and clinical, electrocardiographic, and hemodynamic features. Am. J. Cardiol. *47*:532, 1981.
107. Rotmensch, H. H., Rotmensch, S., and Elkayam, U.: Management of cardiac arrhythmia during pregnancy; Current concepts. Drugs *33*:623, 1987.
108. Rotmensch, H. H., Pines, A., and Donchin, Y.: Antiarrhythmic drugs in pregnancy. *In* Elkayam, U., and Gleicher, N. (eds.): Cardiac Problems in Pregnancy. 2nd ed. New York, Alan R. Liss, Inc., 1990, p. 361.
109. Boccio, R. V., Chung, J. H., and Harrison, D. M.: Anesthetic management of cesarean section in a patient with idiopathic hypertrophic subaortic-stenosis. Anesthesiology *65*:663, 1986.
110. Homans, D. C.: Peripartum cardiomyopathy. N. Engl. J. Med. *312*:1432, 1985.
111. Demakis, J. G., Rahimtoola, S. H., Sutton, E. C., et al.: Natural course of peripartum cardiomyopathy. Circulation *44*:1053, 1971.
112. Ribner, H. S., and Silverman, R. I.: Peripartal cardiomyopathy. *In* Elkayam, U., and Gleicher, N. (eds.): Cardiac Problems in Pregnancy: Diagnosis and Management of Maternal and Fetal Disease. 2nd ed. New York, Alan R. Liss, Inc., 1990, p. 115.
113. McAdams, S. A., and Maguire, F. E.: Unusual manifestations of peripartal cardiac disease. Crit. Care Med. *14*:910, 1986.
113a. Marin-Neto, J. A., Maciel, B. C., Teran Urbanetz, L. L., et al: High output failure in patients with peripartum cardiomyopathy: A comparative study with dilated cardiomyopathy. Am. Heart J. *121*:134, 1990.
114. O'Connell, J. B., Rosa Costanzo-Nordin, M., Subramanian, R., et al.: Peripartum cardiomyopathy: Clinical, hemodynamic, histologic and prognostic characteristics. J. Am. Coll. Cardiol. *8*:52, 1986.
115. Midei, M. C., DeMent, S. H., Feldman, A. M., et al.: Peripartum myocarditis and cardiomyopathy. Circulation *81*:922, 1990.
116. Cole, P., Cook, F., Plappert, T., et al.: Longitudinal changes in left ventricular architecture and function in peripartum cardiomyopathy. Am. J. Cardiol. *60*:871, 1987.
117. Carvalho, A., Brandao, A., Martinez, E. E., et al.: Prognosis in peripartum cardiomyopathy. Am. J. Cardiol. *64*:540, 1989.
118. Cotton, D. B., Longmire, S., Jones, M. M., et al.: Cardiovascular alterations in severe pregnancy-induced hypertension: Effects of intravenous nitroglycerin coupled with blood volume expansion. Am. J. Obstet. Gynecol. *154*:1053, 1986.
119. Rosa, F. W., Bosco, L. A., Graham, C. F., et al.: Neonatal anuria with maternal angiotensin-converting enzyme inhibitors. Obstet. Gynecol. *74*:371, 1989.
120. Brantigan, C. O., Grow, J. B., and Schoonmaker, F. W.: Extended use of intra-aortic balloon pumping in peripartum cardiomyopathy. Ann. Surg. *183*:1, 1976.
121. Melvin, R. R., Richardson, P. J., Olesen, E.G.J., et al.: Peripartum cardiomyopathy due to myocarditis. N. Engl. J. Med. *307*:731, 1982.
122. Mason, J. W., and O'Connell, J. B.: A model of myocarditis in humans. Circulation *81*:1154, 1990.
123. Hovsepian, P. G., Ganzel, B., Sohi, G. S., et al.: Peripartum cardiomyopathy treated with a left ventricular assist device as a bridge to cardiac transplantation. South. Med. J. *82*:527, 1989.
124. Aravot, J. J., Banner, N. R., Dhalla, N., et al.: Heart transplantation for peripartum cardiomyopathy. Lancet *2*:1024, 1987.
125. Meadows, W. R.: Idiopathic myocardial failure in the last trimester of pregnancy and the puerperium. Circulation *15*:903, 1957.
126. Seffel, H., and Susser, M.: Maternal and myocardial failure in African women. Br. Heart J. *23*:43, 1961.
127. Willmer, G.: Postpartal heart disease. South. Med. J. *56*:803, 1963.
128. Walsh, J., and Burch, G.: Idiopathic cardiomyopathy of the puerperium (postpartal heart disease). Circulation *32*:19, 1965.
129. Stuart, K. L.: Cardiomyopathy of pregnancy and the puerperium. Q. J. Med. *37*:463, 1968.
130. Brockington, I. F.: Postpartum hypertensive heart failure. Am. J. Cardiol. *27*:650, 1971.
131. Lee, W., and Cotton, D. B.: Peripartum cardiomyopathy: Current concepts and clinical management. Clin. Obstet. Gynecol. *32*:54, 1989.
132. St. John Sutton, M., Cole, P., Saltzman, D., et al.: Risks of cardiac dysfunction in peripartum cardiomyopathy (PPCM) with subsequent pregnancy. Circulation *80*:II-320, 1989.
133. Goldman, M. E., and Meller, J.: Coronary artery disease in pregnancy. *In* Elkayam, U., and Gleicher, N. (eds.): Cardiac Problems in Pregnancy. 2nd ed. New York, Alan R. Liss, Inc., 1990, p. 153.
134. Sullivan, J. M., and Ramanathan, K. B.: Management of medical problems in the pregnancy—severe cardiac disease. N. Engl. J. Med. *313*:304, 1985.
135. La Vecchia, C., Franceschi, S., Decarli, A., et al.: Risk factors for myocardial infarction in young women. Am. J. Epidemiol. *125*:832, 1987.
136. Croft, P., and Hannaford, P. C.: Risk factors for acute myocardial infarction in women: Evidence from the Royal College of General Practitioners' Oral Contraception Study. Br. Med. J. *298*:165, 1989.
137. La Vecchia, C., Decarli, A., Franceschi, S., et al.: Menstrual and reproductive factors and the risk of myocardial infarction in women under fifty-five years of age. Am. J. Obstet. Gynecol. *157*:1108, 1987.
138. Raymond, R., Lynch, J., Underwood, D., et al.: Myocardial infarction and normal coronary arteriography: A 10-year clinical and risk analysis of 74 infants. J. Am. Coll. Cardiol. *11*:471, 1988.
139. Ruch, A., and Duhring, J. L.: Postpartum myocardial infarction in a patient receiving bromocriptine. Obstet. Gynecol. *74*:448, 1989.
140. Sonel, A., Erol, C., Oral, D., et al.: Acute myocardial infarction and normal coronary arteries in a pregnant woman. Cardiology *75*:218, 1988.
141. Elkayam, U., Rose, J., and Jamison, M.: Vascular aneurysms and dissections during pregnancy: *In* Elkayam, U., and Gleicher, N. (eds.): Cardiac Problems in Pregnancy. 2nd ed. New York, Alan R. Liss, Inc., 1990, p. 215.
142. Movsesian, M. A., and Wray, R. B.: Postpartum myocardial infarction. Br. Heart J. *62*:154, 1989.
143. Rallings, P., Exner, T., and Abraham, R.: Coronary artery vasculitis and myocardial infarction associated with antiphospholipid antibodies in a pregnant woman. Aust. N. Z. J. Med. *19*:347, 1989.
144. Madjan, J. F., Walinsky, P., Cowchuck, J. F., et al.: Coronary bypass surgery during pregnancy. Am. J. Cardiol. *52*:1145, 1983.
145. Cowan, N. C., de Belder, M. A., and Rothman, M. T.: Coronary angioplasty in pregnancy. Br. Heart J. *59*:588, 1988.
146. Hankins, G.D.V., Wendel, G. D., Jr., Leveno, K. J., et al.: Myocardial infarction during pregnancy: A review. Obstet. Gynecol. *65*:139, 1985.
147. Elkayam U: Unpublished data.
148. Szekely, P., and Snaith, L.: Paroxysmal tachycardia in pregnancy. Br. Heart J. *15*:195, 1953.
149. Gleicher, N., Meller, J., Sandler, R. Z., et al.: Wolff-Parkinson-White syndrome in pregnancy. Obstet. Gynecol. *58*:748, 1981.
150. O'Donnell, M., Meecham, J., Tosson, S. R., et al.: Ventricular fibrillation and reinfarction in pregnancy. Postgrad. Med. J. *63*:1095, 1987.
151. Brodsky, M. A., Sato, D. A., Oster, P. D., et al.: Paroxysmal ventricular tachycardia with syncope during pregnancy. Am. J. Cardiol. *58*:563, 1986.
152. Copeland, G. D., and Stern, T. N.: Wenckebach periods in pregnancy and puerperium. Am. Heart J. *56*:291, 1958.
153. Sobotka, P. A., Mayer, J. H., Bauernfeind, R. A., et al.: Arrhythmias documented by 24-hr continuous ambulatory electrocardiographic monitoring in young women without apparent heart disease. Am. Heart J. *101*:753, 1981.
154. Schonbaum, M., Rowland, W., and Quiroz, A. C.: Complete heart block in pregnancy. Successful use of an intravenous pacemaker in 2 patients during labor. Obstet. Gynecol. *27*:243, 1966.
155. Jaffe, R., Gruber, A., Fejgin, M., et al.: Pregnancy with an artificial pacemaker. Obstet. Gynecol. Surv. *42*:137, 1987.
156. Barrett, J. M., Van Hooydonk, J. E., and Boehm, F. H.: Pregnancy related rupture of arterial aneurysms. Obstet. Gynecol. Surv. *37*:557, 1982.
157. Konishi, Y., Tatsuta, N., Kumada, K., et al.: Dissecting aneurysms during pregnancy and the puerperium. Jpn. Circ. J. *44*:726, 1980.
158. Chandrasekaran, K., and Currie, P. J.: Transesophageal echocardiography in aortic dissection. J. Invasive Cardiol. *1*:328, 1989.
159. Ishikawa, K., and Matsuura, S.: Occlusive thromboaortopathy (Takayasu's disease) and pregnancy: Clinical course and management of 33 pregnancies and deliveries. Am. J. Cardiol. *50*:1293, 1982.
160. Wong, V.C.W., Wang, R.Y.E., and Tse, T. F.: Pregnancy and Takayasu's arteritis. Am. J. Med. *75*:597, 1983.
161. Sise, M. J., Couniham, C. M., Shackford, S. R., et al.: The clinical spectrum of Takayasu's arteritis. Surgery *104*:905, 1988.
162. Winn, H. N., Setaro, J. F., Mazor, M., et al.: Severe Takayasu's arteritis in pregnancy: The role of central hemodynamic monitoring. Am. J. Obstet. Gynecol. *159*:1135, 1988.
163. Ask-Upmark, E.: Case of Takayasu's syndrome accelerated (initiated?) by oral contraceptives. Acta Med. Scand. *185*:119, 1969.
164. Elkayam, U., and Gleicher, N.: Primary pulmonary hypertension and pregnancy. *In* Elkayam, U., and Gleicher, N., (eds.): Cardiac Problems in Pregnancy. 2nd ed. New York, Alan R. Liss, Inc., p. 189, 1990.
165. Takenchi, T., Nishii, O., Okamura, T., et al.: Primary pulmonary hypertension in pregnancy. Int. J. Gynaecol. Obstet. *26*:145, 1988.
166. Rich, S., Dantzker, D. R., Ayres, S. M., et al.: Primary pulmonary hypertension: A national prospective study. Ann. Intern. Med. *107*:216, 1987.
167. Fuster, V., Steele, P. M., Edwards, W. D., et al.: Primary pulmonary hypertension: Natural history and the importance of thrombosis. Circulation *70*:580, 1984.
168. Nelson, D. M., Main, E., Crafford, W., et al.: Peripartum heart failure due to primary pulmonary hypertension. Obstet. Gynecol. *62*:59S, 1983.

169. Abboud, T. K., Raya, J., Noueihed, R., et al.: Intrathecal morphine for relief of labor pain in a parturient with severe pulmonary hypertension. Anesthesiology 59:477, 1983.
170. Gazzaniga, A.: Cardiac surgery during pregnancy. *In* Elkayam, U., and Gleicher, N. (eds.): Cardiac Problems in Pregnancy. 2nd ed. New York, Alan R. Liss, Inc., 1990, p. 259.
171. El-Maraghy, M., Abon Senna, I., El-Tehewy, F., et al.: Mitral valvotomy in pregnancy. Am. J. Obstet. Gynecol. *145*:708, 1983.
172. Martin, M. C., Pernall, M. L., Borhszak, A. N., et al.: Cesarean section while on cardiac bypass. Report of a case. Obstet. Gynecol. *6*:41S, 1981.
173. Levy, D. L., Warriner, R. A., Burgess, G. E.: Fetal response to cardiopulmonary bypass. Obstet. Gynecol. *56*:112, 1980.
174. Eilen, B., Kaiser, I., Becker, R., et al.: Aortic valve replacement in the third trimester of pregnancy. Obstet. Gynecol. *57*:119, 1981.
175. Salazar, E., Zajarias, A., Gutierrez, N., et al.: The problem of cardiac valve prosthesis, anticoagulants and pregnancy. Circulation *70*(Suppl. 1):169, 1984.
176. McGehee, W.: Anticoagulation in pregnancy. *In* Elkayam, U., and Gleicher, N. (eds.): Cardiac Problems in Pregnancy. 2nd ed. New York, Alan R. Liss, Inc., 1990, p. 397.
177. Iturbe-Alessio, I., Del Carmen Fonseca, M., Mutchinik O., et al.: Risks of anticoagulant therapy in pregnant women with artificial heart valve. N. Engl. J. Med. *315*:1390, 1986.
178. Donzeau, G. P., Nguyen, A., Touchot, B., et al.: Acute thrombosis of a St. Jude medical aortic prosthesis in a pregnant woman. Thorac. Cardiovasc. Surg. *33*:248, 1985.
179. Shemin, R. J., Phillippe, M., and Dzau, V.: Acute thrombosis of a composite ascending aortic conduit containing a Björk-Shiley valve during pregnancy. Successful emergency cesarean section and operative repair. Clin. Cardiol. *9*:299, 1986.
180. Gonzaelz-Santos, M. L., Horno, R., and Garcia-Dorado, D.: Thrombosis of a mechanical valve prosthesis late in pregnancy. Thorac. Cardiovasc. Surg. *34*:335, 1986.
181. Elkayam, U., and Gleicher, N.: Anticoagulation in pregnant women with artificial heart valves. N. Engl. J. Med. *316*:1663, 1987.
182. Norris, D. C.: Management of patients with prosthetic heart valves. Curr. Probl. Cardiol. *7*:1, 1982.
183. Guidozzi, F.: Pregnancy in patients with prosthetic cardiac valves. S. Afr. Med. J. *64*:961, 1984.
184. Cohn, L. H.: Anticoagulation in pregnant women with artificial heart valves. N. Engl. J. Med. *316*:1662, 1987.
185. Deviri, E., Yechezkel, M., Levinsky, C., et al.: Calcification of a porcine valve xenograft during pregnancy: A case report and review of the literature. Thorac. Cardiovasc. Surg. *32*:266, 1984.
186. Hall, J., Pauli, R. M., and Wilson, K. M.: Maternal and fetal sequelae of anticoagulation during pregnancy. Am. J. Med. *68*:122, 1980.
187. Lee, P. K., Wang, R.Y.C., Chow, J.S.F., et al.: Combined use of warfarin and adjusted subcutaneous heparin during pregnancy in patients with an artificial heart valve. J. Am. Coll. Cardiol. *8*:221, 1986.
188. Oakley, C.: Valve prosthesis and pregnancy. Br. Heart J. *58*:303, 1987.

CARDIOVASCULAR DRUGS IN PREGNANCY

189. Mitani, G. M., Steinberg, I., Lien, E., et al.: The pharmacokinetics of antiarrhythmic agents in pregnancy and lactation. Clin. Pharmacokinet. *12*:253, 1987.
190. Mitani, G. M., Harrison, E. C., Steinberg, I., et al.: Digitalis glycosides in pregnancy. *In* Elkayam, U., and Gleicher, N. (eds.): Cardiac Problems in Pregnancy. 2nd ed. New York, Alan R. Liss, Inc., 1990, p. 417.
191. Lilja, H., Karlsson, K., Lindecranz, K., et al.: Treatment of intrauterine supraventricular tachycardia with digoxin and verapamil. J. Perinat. Med. *12*:151, 1984.
192. Spinnato, J. A., Shaver, D. C., Flinn, G. S., et al.: Fetal supraventricular tachycardia: In utero therapy with digoxin and quinidine. Obstet. Gynecol. *64*:730, 1984.
193. Gleicher, N., and Elkayam, U.: Intrauterine therapy of rhythm and rate disorders and heart failure. *In* Elkayam, U., and Gleicher, N. (eds.): Cardiac Problems in Pregnancy. 2nd ed. New York, Alan R. Liss, Inc., 1990, p. 749.
194. Valdes, R., Jr.: Endogenous digoxin-like immunoreactive factors: Impact on digoxin measurements and potential physiologic implications. Clin. Chem. *31*:1525, 1985.
195. Fievet, P., Gregoire, I., Fournier, A., et al.: Ouabain-like natriuretic factor and atrial natriuretic factor in pregnancy. Kidney Int. *34*(Suppl. 25):A-89, 1988.
196. Given, B. D., Phillippe, M., Sanders, S. P., et al.: Procainamide cardioversion of fetal supraventricular tachyarrhythmia. Am. J. Cardiol. *53*:1460, 1984.
197. Pittard, W. B., II, and Glazier, H.: Procainamide excretion in human milk. J. Pediatr. *102*:631, 1984.
198. Ellsworth, A. J., Horn, J. R., Raisys, V. A., et al.: Disopyramide and N-monodesalkyl disopyramide in serum and breast milk. Drug Intell. Clin. Pharmacy *23*:56, 1989.
199. Hopper, K., Neuvonen, P. J., and Korte, T.: Disopyramide and breast feeding. Br. J. Clin. Pharmacol. *21*:553, 1986.
200. Juneja, M. M., Ackerman, W. E., Kaczorowski, D. M., et al.: Continuous epidural lidocaine infusion in the parturient with paroxysmal ventricular tachycardia. Anesthesiology *71*:305, 1989.
201. Lownes, H. E., and Ives, T. J.: Mexiletine use in pregnancy and lactation. Am. J. Obstet. Gynecol. *157*:446, 1987.
202. Gregg, A. R., and Tomich, P. G.: Mexiletine use in pregnancy. J. Perinat. *8*:33, 1988.
203. Foster, C. J., and Love, H. G.: Amiodarone in pregnancy: Case report and review of literature. Int. J. Cardiol. *20*:307, 1988.
204. DeWolf, D., De Schlepper, H., Verhaaren, H., et al.: Congenital hypothyroid goiter and amiodarone. Acta Paediatr. Scand. *77*:616, 1988.
205. Arnoux, P., Seyral, P., Llurens, M., et al.: Amiodarone and digoxin for refractory fetal tachycardia. Am. J. Cardiol. *59*:166, 1987.
206. Laurent, M., Betremieux, P., Biron, Y., et al.: Neonatal hypothyroidism after treatment by amiodarone during pregnancy. Am. J. Cardiol. *60*:142, 1987.
207. Belfort, M. A., and Moore, P. J.: Verapamil in the treatment of severe postpartum hypertension. S. Afr. Med. J. *74*:265, 1988.
208. Maxwell, D. J., Crawford, D. C., Curry, P.V.M., et al.: Obstetric importance: Diagnosis and management of fetal tachycardia. Br. Heart J. *297*:107, 1988.
209. Miller, M. R., Withers, R., Bhamra, R., et al.: Verapamil and breast feeding. Eur. J. Pharmacol. *301*:125, 1986.
210. Read, M. D., and Wellby, D. E.: The use of calcium antagonist (nifedipine) to suppress preterm labor. Br. J. Obstet. Gynecol. *93*:933, 1986.
211. Seabe, S. J., Moodley, J., and Becker, P.: Nifedipine in acute hypertensive emergencies in pregnancy. S. Aft. Med. J. *76*:248, 1989.
212. Constantine, G., Beevers, D. G., Reynolds, A. L., et al.: Nifedipine as a second line antihypertensive drug in pregnancy. Br. J. Obstet. Gynecol. *94*:1136, 1987.
213. Lindow, S. W., Davey, N., Davy, D. A., et al.: The effect of sublingual nifedipine on uteroplacental blood flow in hypertensive pregnancy. Br. J. Obstet. Gynecol. *95*:1276, 1988.
214. Högstedt, S., Lindebey, S., Axelsson, O., et al.: A prospective controlled trial of metroprolol-hydralazine treatment in hypertension during pregnancy. Acta Obstet. Gynecol. Scand. *64*:505, 1985.
215. Plokin, P. F., Breart, G., Maillard, F., et al.: Comparison of antihypertensive efficacy and prenatal safety of labetalol and methyldopa in the treatment of hypertension in pregnancy: A randomized controlled trial. Br. J. Obstet. Gynaecol. *95*:868, 1988.
216. Jouppilla, P., Kirkinen, P., Koivula, A., et al.: Labetalol does not alter the placental and fetal blood flow or maternal prostanoids in pre-eclampsia. Br. J. Obstet. Gynaecol. *93*:543, 1986.
217. Lunrel, N. O., Kulas, J., Rane, A.: Transfer of labetalol into amniotic fluid and breast milk in lactating women. Eur. J. Clin. Pharmacol. *28*:597, 1985.
218. Dicke, J. M.: Cardiovascular drugs in pregnancy. *In* Gleicher, N., Elkayam, U., Galbraith, R. M., et al. (eds.): Principles of Medical Therapy in Pregnancy. New York, Plenum, 1985, p. 646.
219. Shoemaker, C. T., and Meyers, M.: Sodium nitroprusside for control of severe hypertensive disease of pregnancy: A case report and discussion of potential toxicity. Am. J. Obstet. Gynecol. *149*:171, 1984.
220. Boutroy, M. J.: Fetal effects of maternally administered clonidine and angiotensin-converting enzyme inhibitors. Dev. Pharmacol. Ther. *13*:199, 1989.
221. Rosa, F. W., Bosco, L. A., Graham, C. F., et al.: Neonatal anuria with maternal angiotensin converting enzyme inhibition. Obstet. Gynecol. *74*:371, 1989.
222. Are ACE inhibitors safe in pregnancy? Lancet *2*:482, 1989.
223. Ferris, T. F.: Toxemia and hypertension. *In* Burrow, G. N., and Ferris, T. F. (eds.): Medical Complications During Pregnancy. Philadelphia, W. B. Saunders Company, 1982, p. 1.
224. Garnet, J. D.: Placental transfer of chlorothiazide. Obstet. Gynecol. *21*:123, 1963.
225. Riva, E., Farina, P., Tognoni, G., et al.: Pharmacokinetics of furosemide in gestosis of pregnancy. Eur. J. Clin. Pharmacol. *14*:361, 1978.
226. Sareli, P., England, M. J., Berk, H. R., et al.: Maternal and fetal sequelae of anticoagulation during pregnancy in patients with mechanical heart valve prosthesis. Am. J. Cardiol. *63*:1462, 1989.
227. Becker, M. H., Genieser, N. B., Finegold, M., et al.: Chondrodysplasia punctata: Is maternal warfarin therapy a factor? Am. J. Dis. Child. *129*:356, 1975.
228. Matorras, R., Reque, J. A., Usandizaga, J. A., et al.: Prosthetic heart valve and pregnancy. A study of 59 cases. Gynecol. Obstet. Invest. *19*:21, 1985.
229. Wang, R.Y.C., Lee, P. K., Chow, J.S.F., et al.: Efficacy of low dose subcutaneously administered heparin in the treatment of pregnant women with artificial heart valves. Med. J. Aust. *2*:126, 1983.
230. Hatjis, C. G.: Heparin-induced thrombocytopenia in pregnancy. A case report. J. Reprod. Med. *29*:337, 1984.
231. DeSwiet, M., Dorrington, W., Fidler, J., et al.: Prolonged heparin therapy in pregnancy causes bone demineralization. Br. J. Obstet. Gynaecol. *90*:1129, 1983.
232. Hirsh, J.: Mechanism of action and monitoring of anticoagulants. Semin. Thromb. Hemostas. *12*:1, 1986.
233. Noller, K. L.: Cardiac surgery and pregnancy. *In* Gleicher, N., Elkayam, U., and Galbraith, R. M. (eds.): Principles of Medical Therapy in Pregnancy. New York, Plenum, 1985, p. 713.
234. Cesario, T. C.: Antibiotic therapy in pregnancy. *In* Elkayam, U., Gleicher, N. (eds.): Cardiac Problems in Pregnancy. 2nd ed. New York, Alan R. Liss, Inc., 1990, p. 437.
235. McCans, J., and Wenger, N.: Problems in management of the pregnant patient with rheumatic heart disease and valve prosthesis. South. Med. J. *69*:1007, 1976.
236. Sugrue, D., Blake, S., Troy, P., et al.: Antibiotic prophylaxis against infective endocarditis after normal delivery. Is it necessary? Br. Heart J. *5*:44, 1980.

60

Neurological Disorders and Heart Disease

by JOSEPH K. PERLOFF, M.D.

Cardiovascular disorders occur as consequences of diseases of the nervous system, and disorders of the nervous system occur secondary to diseases of the heart and circulation. This chapter deals with the varied and complex interplay between cardiology and neurology and focuses on six general topics: (1) major heredofamilial neuromyopathic disorders in which cardiac disease is an inherent part; (2) less common neuromyopathic disorders that are sometimes associated with diseases of the heart; (3) acute cerebral disorders accompanied by cardiovascular abnormalities; (4) cardiac complications of drugs used in treating neuromuscular diseases; (5) neurological complications of therapy for cardiovascular diseases; and (6) cardiac denervation. Cardiac causes of syncope are discussed in Chapter 30. Neurological complications associated with congenital and acquired heart disease are discussed in the chapters dealing specifically with those disorders.

MAJOR HEREDOFAMILIAL NEUROMYOPATHIC DISORDERS

Cardiac involvement is an inherent part of three major categories of heredofamilial neuromyopathic disorders: the progressive muscular dystrophies, myotonic muscular dystrophy, and Friedreich's ataxia.[1-4] The majority of nonmyotonic progressive muscular dystrophies are classified as:

1. X-linked progressive muscular dystrophies
   a. Early-onset, rapidly progressive (classic Duchenne dystrophy)
   b. Late-onset, slowly progressive (Becker muscular dystrophy)
2. Limb-girdle dystrophy of Erb
3. Facioscapulohumeral dystrophy of Landouzy-Dejerine

PROGRESSIVE MUSCULAR DYSTROPHIES

Early-Onset, Rapidly Progressive X-Linked (Duchenne) Dystrophy

Classic Duchenne muscular dystrophy is a sex-linked recessive disorder, transmitted by the mother to one-half of her sons as overt disease and to one-half of her daughters as a carrier state.[5,6] The average incidence of Duchenne dystrophy in the general population is around 1 in 5000 male births, but it is believed that the true incidence is as high as 1 in 3000 male births.[7] Assuming that the mutation rate is equal in the two sexes, one-third of cases represent new mutations in either the patient or his mother.[8] Duchenne muscular dystrophy is caused by a defective gene located on the X chromosome. *Dystrophin,* the high-molecular-weight protein product of the gene, is localized to the sarcolemmal membrane of normal skeletal muscle but is absent from skeletal muscle of patients with Duchenne dystrophy.[9] The rare but well-documented cases of clinical Duchenne dystrophy in females have been attributed to X translocation of a single mutant gene at band Xp21 of the X-chromosome short arm.[7,10] The normal X is inactivated, so the mutant X-linked recessive gene expresses itself. Creatine kinase has had important but limited use in the detection of carrier females, but quantification of dystrophin on skeletal muscle biopsies has been a major step forward in carrier identification.[9]

Overt clinical manifestations usually begin in the second year of life, although there is histological and enzymatic evidence that the disease exists from birth.[5] The clumsy, waddling gait and frequent falls often go unnoticed in a child just learning to walk, and the boy's difficulty in rising from the floor by "climbing up" himself (Gowers' sign) tends to be initially ignored by parents and physicians. Because of the seemingly good muscle development and early pseudohypertrophy of the calves (Fig. 60–1), reduced strength is not ascribed to an abnormality of skeletal muscle. Lumbar lordosis, hyperextension of the knees, and shortening of the Achilles tendons contribute to a precarious balance on the toes (Fig. 60–1). Kyphoscoliosis becomes marked, and in terminal stages of the disease the boy sits in a wheelchair, twisted like a pretzel, with his head lolling unsupported because of inadequate neck muscles. Dystrophy of thoracic muscles and diaphragm together with kyphoscoliosis compromises coughing and breathing. Patients are likely to succumb to pulmonary infection in the second decade, although cardiac disease is an important and sometimes dramatic cause of death. Rapidly progressive preterminal heart failure may follow years of circulatory stability during which the chief, if not only, suspicion of cardiac involvement is an abnormal electrocardiogram (Fig. 60–2). Pulmonary emboli have been reported in patients with end-stage Duchenne dystrophy, and systemic emboli can originate in the left ventricle.[11,12]

Physical and radiological examinations of the heart disclose thoracic deformities and the high diaphragm of diaphragmatic dystrophy. A reduction in anteroposterior chest dimension is often striking and is commonly responsible for a systolic im-

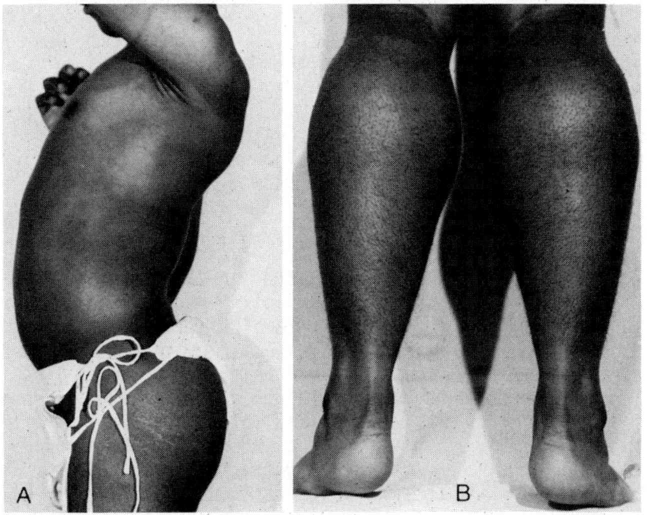

FIGURE 60-1. Classic X-linked Duchenne muscular dystrophy. *A,* Exaggerated lumbar lordosis. *B,* Calf pseudohypertrophy and shortening of the Achilles tendons.

pulse at the left sternal edge, a grade 1-3/6 short impure midsystolic murmur in the second left interspace, and a loud pulmonic component of the second heart sound. These signs should *not* be taken as evidence of pulmonary hypertension, which if present at all, occurs in the terminal stage of the disease with respiratory failure.[13] An increase in transverse heart size on x-ray examination is more often than not caused by the narrow anteroposterior chest dimension and high diaphragm rather than by ventricular dilatation.[1] The murmur of mitral regurgitation has a relatively firm anatomical basis, namely, dystrophic involvement of the posterior papillary muscle and contiguous posterobasal left ventricular wall.[14,15]

ELECTROCARDIOGRAPHY. Twenty-four-hour electrocardiographic recordings show that the most common rhythm disturbance is inappropriate sinus tachycardia,[16,17] which may be labile and gradual or abrupt in onset. The cause(s) of the rate acceleration or of relatively frequent sinus arrhythmias is(are) unknown but may involve abnormal autonomic regulation.[16,18] Alternatively, "dystrophic" disease of the sinoatrial node may prove to be the substrate not only for abnormal sinus node automaticity but also for sinus node reentry and labile sinus tachycardia, especially the abrupt-onset type.[16] Intraatrial or interatrial conduction abnormalities are not uncommon. An abnormal P-terminal force in lead V_1 in the presence of normal left atrial size on the echocardiogram implies an intrinsic disorder of left atrial or interatrial conduction.[17] It is unclear whether the conduction disorder sets the stage for unstable atrial rhythms (see below).

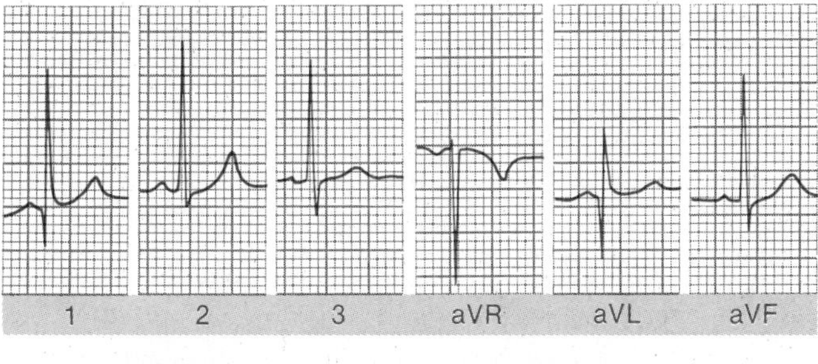

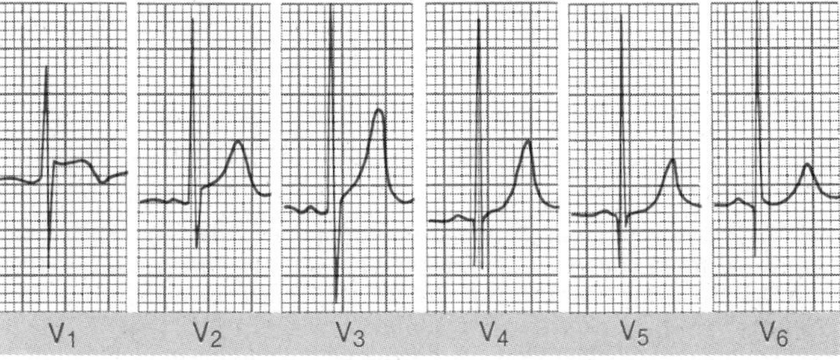

FIGURE 60-2. Electrocardiogram from a 10-year-old boy with classic Duchenne muscular dystrophy. The P-R interval is short (100 msec in lead 2). The QRS complex is typical of Duchenne dystrophy, showing an anterior shift in the right precordial leads and deep but narrow Q waves in leads I, aVl, and V_{4-6}. (From Perloff, J. K.: Cardiac rhythm and conduction in Duchenne's muscular dystrophy. Reprinted by permission of the American College of Cardiology. J. Am. Coll. Cardiol. *3:*1263, 1984.)

In approximately 50 per cent of patients, atrioventricular (AV) conduction, as judged by the P-R interval, is either definitely or marginally accelerated without delta waves (Fig. 60-2).[16] Short P-R intervals may represent atriofascicular bypass tracts or accelerated conduction within the AV node (p. 696).[16] Paroxysmal rapid heart action via bypass tracts is, however, unknown in Duchenne dystrophy, and atrial flutter, a common preterminal arrhythmia, has not been reported with 1:1 AV conduction.[16,19,20] Proximal infranodal conduction abnormalities sometimes take the form of a rightward QRS axis that implies left posterior fascicular block.[16] Significant electrical ventricular instability seldom occurs despite regional left ventricular dystrophy. Multiform ventricular premature complexes, couplets, and episodes of ventricular tachycardia are uncommon but not unknown, especially as the disease advances.[16] Death is occasionally sudden.

Disorders of atrial rhythm are more common than are disturbances of ventricular rhythm, even though involvement of atrial myocardium is relatively scant.[14,15,20,21] These observations suggest that ectopic atrial rhythms are prompted by abnormalities of specialized conduction tissues. A similar speculation applies to the observed or reported disorders of infranodal conduction.[16]

The standard scalar electrocardiogram is the simplest and most reliable tool for detecting cardiac involvement in Duchenne dystrophy (Fig. 60-2).[1,15,22,23] Abnormal electrocardiograms are present even in early childhood.[23,24] Tall right precordial R waves and increased R/S amplitude ratios together with deep Q waves in leads 1, aV_l, and $V_{5,6}$ are characteristic of the classic rapidly progressive pseudohypertrophic X-linked dystrophy of Duchenne (Fig. 60-2).[15,17,20,25] A reduction in or a loss of electromotive force caused by myocardial dystrophy in the posterobasal left ventricular wall (anterior shift of the QRS) and contiguous lateral wall (deep Q waves in leads 1, aV_l, and $V_{5,6}$) is believed to be responsible for the characteristic electrocardiogram.[1,15,17] Necropsy studies have disclosed that these regions are the initial and most extensive sites of myocardial fibrosis (Fig. 60-3),[15,17,20] which is preceded by ultrastructural (subcellular) abnormalities.[17] Electron microscopic examination of right ventricular endomyocardial biopsy specimens has identified abnormalities of mitochondria, C bands, sarcoplasmic reticulum, and nuclei.[26] Primary posterobasal involvement spreads to the epicardial third of the contiguous lateral left ventricular free wall, with progressive transmural fibrous replacement.[17,21] There is relative sparing of the ventricular septum and comparatively little involvement of right ventricular and atrial myocardia.[15,17,21] Based on these observations, Duchenne dystrophy emerges as a unique form of heart disease characterized by a genetically determined predilection for specific regions of the heart—the posterobasal and lateral left ventricular walls.[1,15,17,25] Interestingly, relatively specific electrocardiographic and histopathological abnormalities have been reported in dystrophic hamsters with cardiomyopathy.[27]

HISTOLOGICAL FINDINGS. Light microscopy has disclosed fatty infiltration and mild fibrosis in the sinus and AV nodes, although there is little or no evidence of degeneration of the conduction fibers themselves in either of these nodes or in the His bundle.[28] However, the peripheral conduction system (Purkinje fibers) shows significant degeneration (eosinophilic, necrotic, and vascular changes with fibrosis).[28] In two light microscopic studies, fibers in the sinus node, His bundle, and proximal bundle branch were normal.[15,29] Ultrastructural data on specialized cardiac tissues are scanty and inconclusive.[17] The small intramural coronary arteries are sometimes

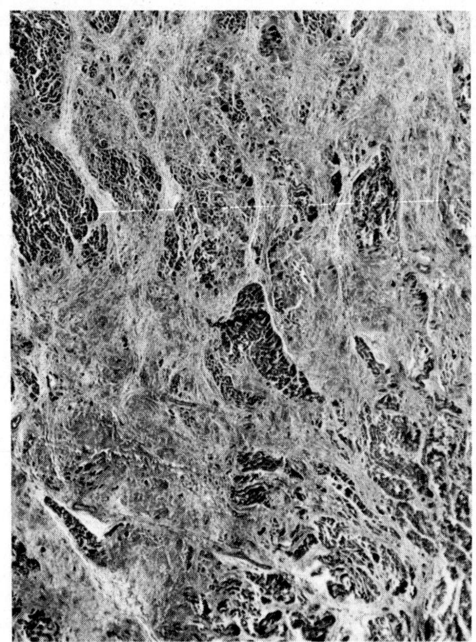

FIGURE 60–3. **Photomicrograph from an 18-year-old boy who died of classic Duchenne progressive muscular dystrophy. The posterobasal left ventricular wall is extensively scarred (hematoxylin and eosin stains). (From Perloff, J. K., et al.: The distinctive electrocardiogram of Duchenne's muscular dystrophy. Am. J. Med. *42:*179, 1967.)**

thick walled, with varying degrees of luminal narrowing.[15,21,29] The arteriopathy occasionally involves sinus nodal and AV nodal arteries,[15,20,29] but an association between the small-vessel coronary arteriopathy and abnormalities of rhythm and conduction remains speculative.

Mitral regurgitation may occur in Duchenne dystrophy. The cause is papillary muscle dysfunction (dystrophic involvement of the posterolateral papillary muscle and contiguous left ventricular wall) rather than an abnormality of leaflets, chordae tendineae, and annulus.[14]

Malignant hyperthermia and cardiac arrest have occurred during anesthesia in a number of children with Duchenne muscular dystrophy after use of halothane, suxamethonium, isoflurane, and succinylcholine.[30,31]

POSITRON EMISSION TOMOGRAPHY (see also p. 302)

Investigators have sought to ascertain whether regional metabolic, perfusion, or wall-motion abnormalities were present during life in patients with Duchenne dystrophy.[2,32] To determine whether segmental abnormalities of the left ventricular wall were present in living subjects, noninvasive methods, including positron-emission tomography (see p. 304) using radioactive tracers for metabolism, supplemented by thallium-201 perfusion scans, gated equilibrium radionuclide angiography, and two-dimensional echocardiography, were employed.[2,32] Accelerated exogenous glucose (^{18}F fluorodeoxyglucose) utilization in the posterobasal and contiguous lateral left ventricular walls (Fig. 60–4) provided evidence of a regional myocardial metabolic abnormality[2] (p. 536). $^{13}NH_3$ activity was reduced in segments in which uptake of exogenous glucose was accelerated (Fig. 60–4). These sites corresponded to those of primary dystrophic replacement found at necropsy.[15,17,20]

The observed regional increases in ^{18}F fluorodeoxyglucose concentrations are believed to indicate a segmental alteration in membrane permeability, an increase in the rate of phosphorylation due to the abnormality in adenyl cyclase identified in skeletal muscle,[33,34] or a compensatory increase in glycolysis in response to a decline in fatty acid oxidation.[2] Regional decreases in $^{13}NH_3$ activity in Duchenne dystrophy (Fig. 60–4) are believed to reflect a metabolic abnormality, a regional decrease in flow, or both of these causes.[2]

EARLY FINDINGS. Early in the natural history (i.e., in very young patients), segmental reductions in $^{13}NH_3$ probably reflect altered regional myocardial metabolic uptake and trapping of the isotope.[2] If these alterations in the myocardium are analogous to those in skeletal muscle in Duchenne dystrophy, a longer diffusion distance of an altered ionic milieu could decrease the extraction fractions of $^{13}NH_3$.[2] Regional depletion of the pool of glutamic acid, which binds the tracer in tissue, might also contribute to a segmental reduction in $^{13}NH_3$.[2]

LATE FINDINGS. Regional perfusion defects sometimes occur in older patients with Duchenne dystrophy, as demonstrated by thallium scintigraphy. In these late stages of the disease, decreased perfusion might contribute to segmental reductions in $^{13}NH_3$ activity.[2] It is likely that the mechanism(s) governing a regional reduction in myocardial blood flow relate(s) to a decrease in the number of myofibers per unit mass (fibrous replacement) and/or to an increase in the number of intrinsically injured but viable posterobasal and lateral left ventricular myocardial cells that require less oxygen and, accordingly, less flow.[2] Necropsy studies (light microscopy) identified no luminal narrowing of extramural or intramural coronary arteries in the involved segments.[15]

MECHANISM OF ABNORMAL POSITRON-EMISSION TOMOGRAPHY FINDINGS. It has been hypothesized that the regional myocardial abnormalities of ^{18}F fluorodeoxyglucose and $^{13}NH_3$ activity represent secondary metabolic alterations initiated by the basic defect in cardiac plasma cell membrane[2] represented in skeletal muscle by absence from the sarcolemmal membrane of dystrophin, the protein product of the Duchenne muscular dystrophy gene (see earlier).[9] Current evidence—both ultrastructural and biochemical—supports the proposition that the fundamental structural and biochemical abnormalities in Duchenne dystrophy reside in plasma cell membranes, not only in those of striated (skeletal and cardiac) muscle fibers but also in those of red blood cells and probably also of fibroblasts.[35–38]

If a reduction in or loss of posterolateral left ventricular electrical forces is the cause of the distinctive electrocardiogram in Duchenne dystrophy,[1,15,17] this loss of forces does not require transmural replacement of

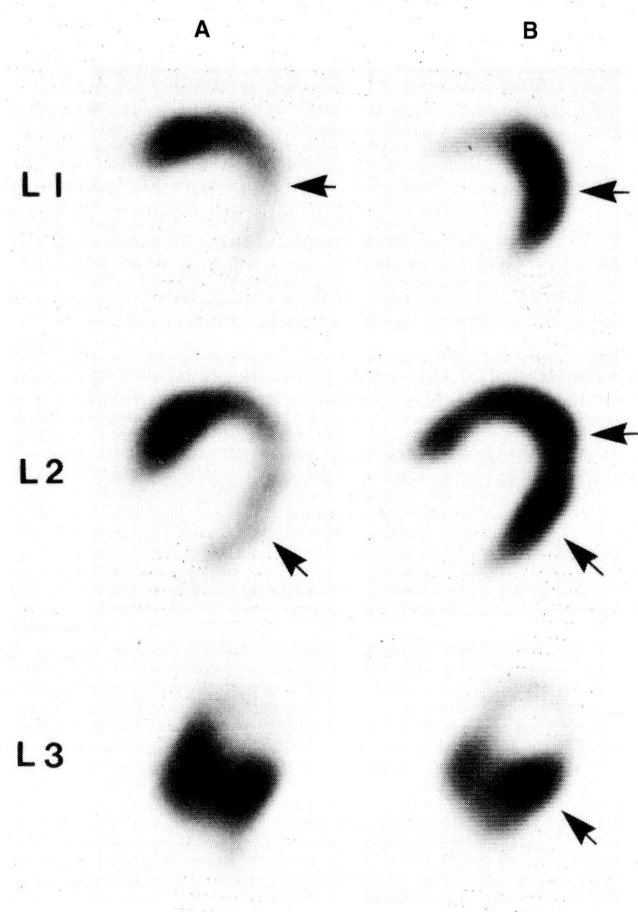

FIGURE 60–4. **Regional myocardial uptake of $^{13}NH_3$ (*A*) and ^{18}F fluorodeoxyglucose (*B*) visualized in three contiguous positron CT images of left ventricular myocardium in a 24-year-old man with classic Duchenne dystrophy. There is a segmental decrease in $^{13}NH_3$ activity in the posterolateral wall (arrows) with a discordant increase in ^{18}F fluorodeoxyglucose concentration in the same region (arrows). This patient had a moderate posterolateral thallium-201 defect, posterolateral akinesis on technetium-99m radionuclide imaging, and a left ventricular ejection fraction of 46 per cent. (From Perloff, J. K., et al.: Alterations in regional myocardial metabolism, perfusion and wall motion in Duchenne muscular dystrophy studied by radionuclide imaging. Circulation 69:33, 1984, by permission of The American Heart Association, Inc.)**

myocardium by inert connective tissue. Increased ^{18}F fluorodeoxyglucose concentrations in these areas together with normal regional wall motion are consistent with the presence of abnormal but viable (metabolically active) contracting myofibers or the preservation of a sufficient population of normal myofibers.[2]

RELEASE OF MUSCLE ENZYMES

Skeletal muscle enzymes are copiously released into the plasma in Duchenne dystrophy. It was hoped that distinctive profiles of an isozyme, such as MB creatine phosphokinase (CPK), might be used to identify active myocardial dystrophy, but the isozyme originates in dystrophic skeletal muscle and not in cardiac muscle, thus compromising the specificity of the determination.[39,40] CPK quantification is a useful but limited means of identifying carrier females in families with Duchenne dystrophy.[41,42] However, dystrophin quantification in skeletal muscle biopsies has been the major step forward in diagnosing carrier females[9] who sometimes manifest occult or overt muscle weakness and mild calf pseudohypertrophy[41,43] in addition to electrocardiographic evidence of cardiac involvement.[41,42,44–46] Electrocardiograms in carrier females differ significantly from those of normal adult women, with R/S ratios larger in leads V_{1-2} in the carrier group.[42,44] Cardiac involvement in female carriers is occasionally expressed overtly as dilated cardiomyopathy.[44,46]

Late-Onset, Slowly Progressive X-Linked (Becker) Dystrophy

A type of X-linked recessive muscular dystrophy that resembles Duchenne dystrophy was first described by Becker.[5,6,47–49] Becker dystrophy can now be distinguished from Duchenne dystrophy by dystrophin assays of skeletal muscle biopsies. In Becker dystrophy, the protein product of the gene is present but abnormal in molecular weight, while in Duchenne dystrophy the protein product is absent or scanty but of normal molecular weight.[9] The Becker and Duchenne muscular dystrophy genes are on separate but close regions of the short arm of the X chromosome.

Becker dystrophy is later in onset and slower in progression than Duchenne dystrophy, with most patients remaining ambulant into adulthood[5] (Fig. 60–5). Becker dystrophy has been called benign sex-linked muscular dystrophy,[48] a designation more appropriate for the skeletal muscle disease than for the heart disease.[1,50] Skeletal muscle impairment is sometimes relatively mild and slowly progressive, while the cardiomyopathy is severe and rapidly progressive.[51–53]

Because the diagnosis of Becker dystrophy was less than secure before the advent of dystrophin assays, some reports of the incidence and type of associated heart disease are open to question. There is evidence, however, that the frequency of cardiac involvement increases after adolescence, and patients who reach adulthood not only have cardiomyopathy but may succumb to it[51,54] (Fig. 60–6). The type of cardiac disease differs substantially from that of Duchenne dystrophy.[51–53,55] All four chambers are involved, with dilatation and failure of the ventricles (Fig. 60–6) in addition to abnormalities of the His bundle and of infranodal conduction that express themselves as fascicular block and complete heart block (Fig. 60–6).

LIMB-GIRDLE DYSTROPHY OF ERB

The heterogeneous collection of conditions designated limb-girdle dystrophy is perhaps the most poorly defined group within the major muscular dystrophies.[5] There is variation in the mode of inheritance, the age of onset, and progression of the illness, as well as in the distribution of muscle weakness. If there is a dominant theme, it is represented by the combination of onset in late childhood or adolescence with difficulty walking; the pelvic girdle is chiefly affected, the upper limbs and shoulder girdle less so, and the face spared. Because of disproportionate pelvic involvement, the patient is often confined to a wheelchair even though skeletal deformities are infrequent.[5] Calf pseudohypertrophy occurs but is relatively late in onset and mild to moderate in degree. Because limb-girdle dystrophy has been poorly defined, conclusions regarding the type and prevalence of heart disease cannot be drawn with confidence. Disorders of cardiac muscle (cardiomyopathy) and of the cardiac conduction system have been reported.[56,57]

FACIOSCAPULOHUMERAL DYSTROPHY (LANDOUZY-DEJERINE)

Facioscapulohumeral dystrophy is inherited as an autosomal dominant with strong penetrance and an incidence estimated at three to ten cases per million population.[5] The disease typically becomes overt at the end of the first decade or the beginning of the second. Facial weakness may be signaled initially by no more than inability to whistle or drink through a straw. More distinctive and troublesome is inability to close the eyes, even during sleep. The face ultimately becomes smooth and the forehead unlined; loss of the normal upward curvature of the lower lip creates a pouting appearance, and the only marks on an otherwise expressionless face are the dimples on either side of the angles of the mouth (Fig. 60–7). Concurrently, the muscles of the arms and shoulders (scapulohumeral) are involved, and winging of the scapulae becomes apparent (Fig. 60–7). Infrequently, the disease expresses itself in infancy and runs a rapid course that leads to death in adolescence.[58] Asymptomatic or minimally affected parents may have severely affected offspring with the infantile form of the disease.[58]

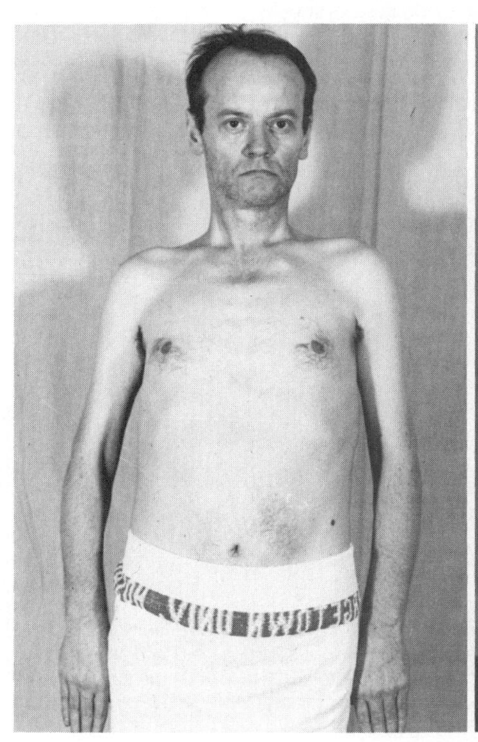

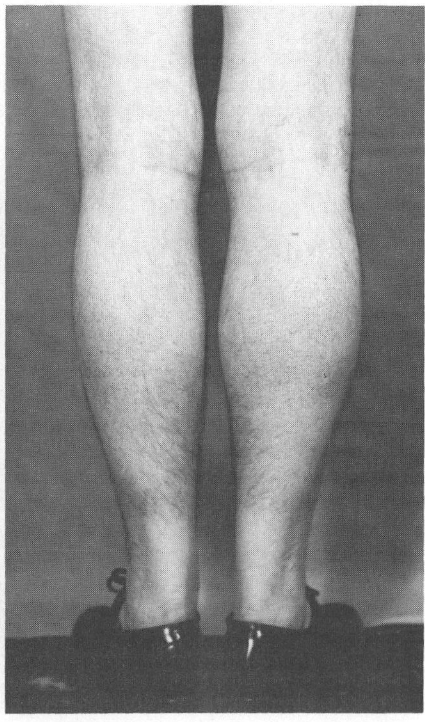

FIGURE 60–5. A 40-year-old man believed to have late-onset, slowly progressive Becker dystrophy. He died because of cardiomyopathy and complete heart block. Dystrophy of shoulder girdle, arms, pelvic girdle, and proximal leg muscle is seen, with mild asymmetrical pseudohypertrophy of the calves. (From Perloff, J. K., et al.: The cardiomyopathy of progressive muscular dystrophy. Circulation *33:*625, 1966, by permission of The American Heart Association, Inc.)

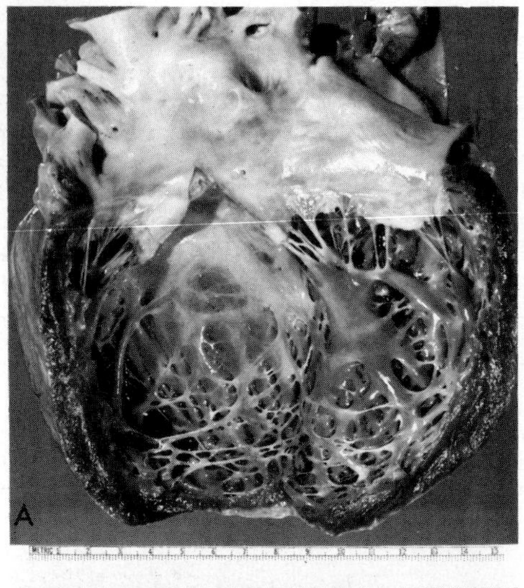

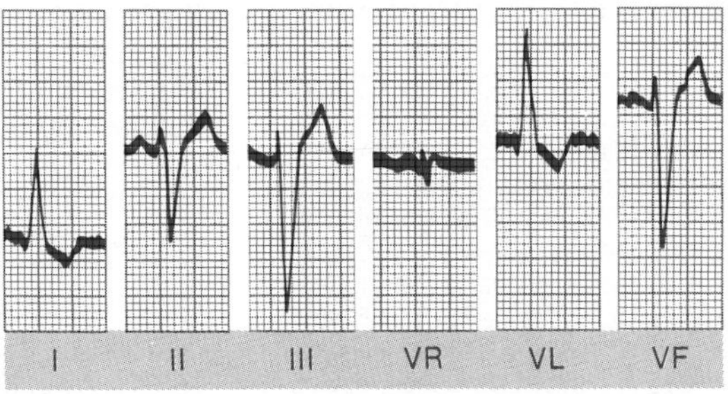

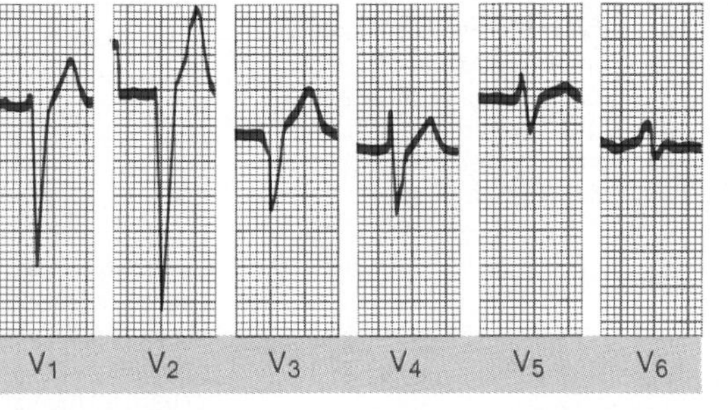

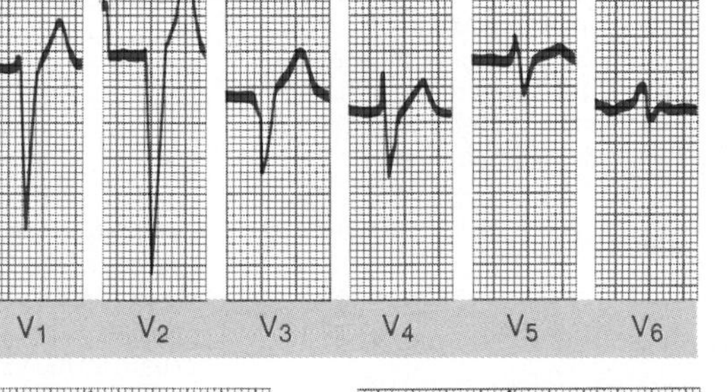

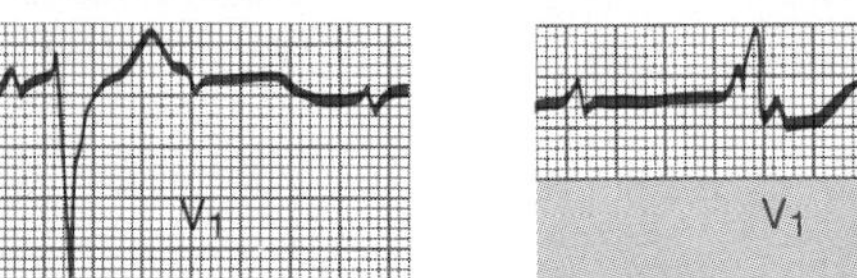

FIGURE 60–6. Gross and microscopic cardiac pathological specimens and the electrocardiogram from a 45-year-old man with late-onset, slowly progressive Becker muscular dystrophy. *A,* Dilated, flabby left ventricle with focal endocardial thickening. The left atrium is also dilated. *B,* Microscopic section from the left ventricle shows marked confluent scarring with variations in fiber size; there was no significant coronary artery disease. *C,* Electrocardiogram recorded at age 40 years. The 12-lead tracing shows left-axis deviation, a QRS of 0.14 sec, small Q waves in leads I and aVl and loss of R-wave amplitude in leads V_2 and V_3. The lower tracings, taken 4 years later (a year before death), show complete heart block with a variable QRS configuration. (From Perloff, J. K., et al.: The cardiomyopathy of progressive muscular dystrophy. Circulation *33:*625, 1966, by permission of The American Heart Association, Inc.)

CARDIAC FINDINGS. The type of cardiac abnormality previously ascribed to facioscapulohumeral dystrophy (adult form) was a unique variety of heart disease — permanent atrial paralysis. However, the cases reported as facioscapulohumeral dystrophy[59–61] are now believed to have been phenotypically similar to Emery-Dreifuss dystrophy (see below).[62] The first secure evidence of cardiac involvement in facioscapulohumeral dystrophy was reported only recently in a prospective investigation of the electrophysiological properties of the atria and AV node and infranodal conduction in 30 rigorously documented cases.[62] The involvement was not represented by atrial paralysis but by a relatively high susceptibility to induced atrial flutter or fibrillation during electrophysiological study, together with less frequent evidence of abnormal sinus node function and abnormal AV nodal or infranodal conduction.[62] It was hypothesized that the genetic marker for facioscapulohumeral dystrophy resulted in a form of cardiac involvement analogous to but much more benign than that in phenotypically similar but genetically distinct Emery-Dreifuss dystrophy and its variants.[62]

EMERY-DREIFUSS MUSCULAR DYSTROPHY

Emery-Dreifuss dystrophy has been separated from facioscapulohumeral dystrophy, which it superficially resembles.[63–65] Scapulohumeral and scapuloperoneal muscular dystrophy are believed to be genetic variants of the Emery-Dreifuss form.[66–69] Emery-Dreifuss dystrophy is an X-linked disorder characterized by slowly progressive muscle wasting and weakness with a humeral-peroneal distribution and early contractures of the elbows, Achilles tendons, and postcervical muscles. Permanent paralysis of the atria (atrial standstill) is the unusual if not unique form of electrophysiological heart disease that occurs in Emery-Dreifuss dystrophy; partial or permanent atrial standstill has also been reported as an isolated disorder in adults, rarely in children, and occasionally in families.[70–74] Criteria for the diagnosis of atrial paralysis include absence of P waves on scalar, esophageal, and intracardiac electrocardiograms; lack of response to direct (intracardiac) electrical or mechanical stimulation of the atria; absence of *a* waves in the jugular venous and right atrial pressure pulses; a supraventricular QRS; and immobility of the atria on fluoroscopy or on two-dimensional echocardiography.[72] The entire atrial myocardium ultimately becomes inexcitable, but prior to this stage, atrial standstill appears to be regional, with certain focal areas that are inert while others are subject to enhanced atrial electrical activity (atrial tachycardia or flutter).[71,73,74] Permanent atrial paralysis, atrial fibrillation, and atrial flutter are features of Emery-Dreifuss dystrophy, but the greatest threats are abnormalities of infranodal conduction with slow junctional

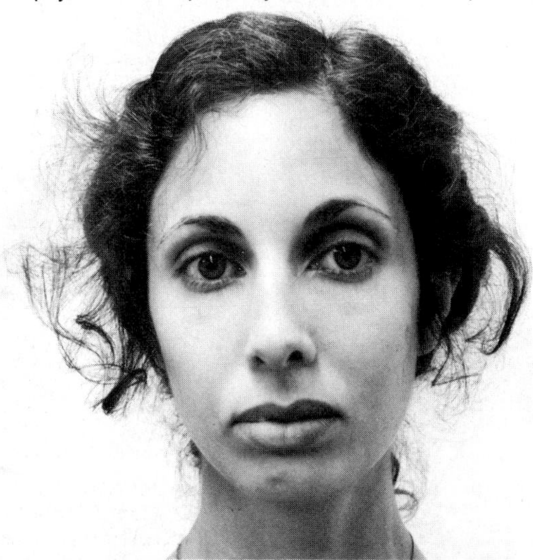

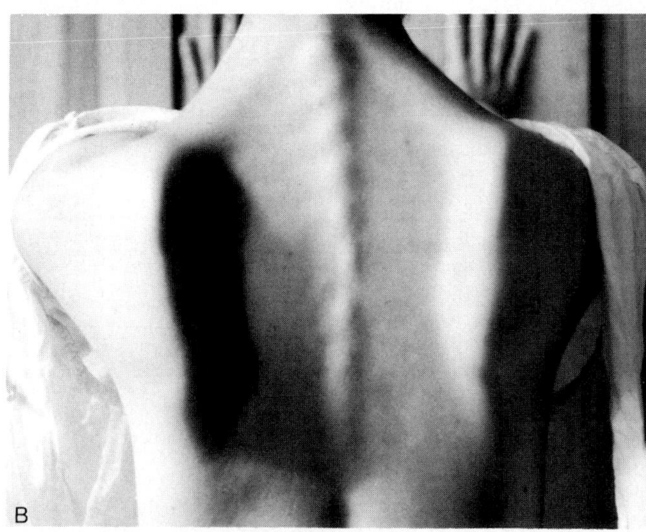

FIGURE 60–7. Facioscapulohumeral muscular dystrophy in 32-year-old woman. *A,* The face is in repose (myopathic). *B,* Typical winging of the scapulae.

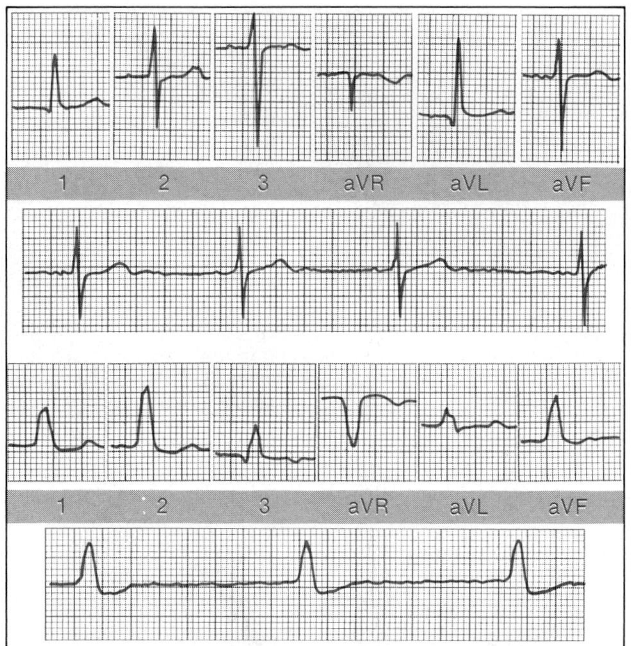

FIGURE 60-8. Limb leads and rhythm strips from two patients, a 16-year-old son (*upper*) and his 38-year-old father (*lower*) with Emery-Dreifuss muscular dystrophy. The son's tracing shows left anterior fascicular block. The P waves are low voltage and bifid, and the rate is bradycardiac. The father's tracing shows complete left bundle branch block. There is fine atrial fibrillation with a slow ventricular response. A pacemaker was inserted a month later.

rhythms or complete AV block[64,67,75,76,79-82] (Fig. 60-8). A permanent pacemaker is often required. It is the cardiac involvement, not the systemic neuromuscular disease, that places the patient at risk. In addition to the defects in rhythm and conduction in Emery-Dreifuss dystrophy and its genetic variants, myocardial fibrosis has been described at necropsy[78] and on myocardial biopsy.[67]

MYOTONIC MUSCULAR DYSTROPHY

Myotonic muscular dystrophy (Steinert's disease) is a multisystem disorder inherited as an autosomal dominant (locus on chromosome 19) with an estimated incidence between three and five per 100,000 population, making it a relatively common neuromuscular disease.[83,84] A consistent and early feature is weakness of the flexor muscles of the neck; atrophy of the sternocleidomastoid muscles often progresses to virtual disappearance. The phenotype of the adult with myotonic dystrophy is characteristic.[5,83] The presence of myotonia (delayed relaxation after contraction) is provoked by voluntary, mechanical, or electrical stimulation of muscles of the hands, forearms, tongue, and jaw. Myotonic responses are best elicited by tapping the thenar eminence (percussion myotonia), especially after patients rapidly open and close their fists. Myotonic dystrophy is a systemic disease with important non-myotonic/nonmyopathic features, including cataracts, testicular atrophy, premature baldness, mental deterioration, and involvement of smooth muscle (esophagus, colon, uterus).[83]

Clinically important cardiac manifestations generally reside in specialized tissues rather than in myocardium.[3,85-87] Involvement is relatively specific, primarily assigned to the His-Purkinje system. At necropsy the most frequent histopathological lesions of the cardiac conduction system are fibrosis, fatty infiltration, and atrophy involving the sinus node, AV node, His bundle, and bundle branches.[88] Involvement of cardiac muscle, generally occult, takes the form of dystrophy rather than myotonia and is not selective, appearing with approximately equal distribution in all four chambers.[3] Myocardial dystrophy may be responsible for atrial and ventricular arrhythmias, including sinus bradycardia, premature atrial beats, atrial flutter (Fig. 60-9), atrial fibrillation, premature ventricular beats, and ventricular tachycardia.[89-91] Preferential selection of the His-Purkinje system (80 per cent of patients) is reflected in intraventricular conduction defects, prolongation of the H-V interval and of the effective refractory period of the right bundle branch, the development of right bundle branch block, or some other abnormal response to atrial pacing or extrastimuli.[3] The most common electrocardiographic abnormalities—prolongation of the P-R interval, left anterior fascicular block, increased QRS duration—reflect the His-Purkinje disease that can progress rapidly, although neither the scalar electrocardiogram nor a single H-V interval predicts the rate of progression.[92] His-Purkinje disease can culminate in fatal Stokes-Adams episodes unless anticipated and treated by pacemaker insertion[90,93,94] (Fig. 60-9). Although sudden death caused by AV block is relatively rare, it is the most grave cardiac threat in myotonic dystrophy. Ventricular tachycardia has also been held responsible for sudden death.[87,91]

The myocardium is seldom involved extensively enough to cause clinically overt signs or symptoms.[3] Fewer than 10 per cent of patients have clinical evidence of heart failure.[88] The electrocardiogram is a sensitive determinant of involvement of specialized cardiac tissues but not of myocardium. Nevertheless, abnormal Q waves with normal coronary arteries indicate regional myocardial dystrophy (Fig. 60-10). Findings on light microscopic examination of the myocardium vary from few or no changes to focal or diffuse fatty infiltration and fibrosis in all four cardiac chambers.[90,95-97] Apart from abnor-

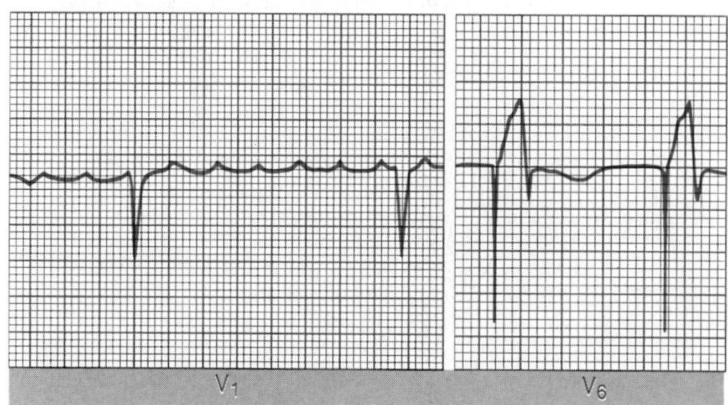

FIGURE 60-9. Rhythm strip from a 34-year-old man with myotonic muscular dystrophy. Lead V_1 shows atrial flutter, with high degree heart block. A syncopal episode prompted insertion of a right ventricular pacemaker (lead V_6).

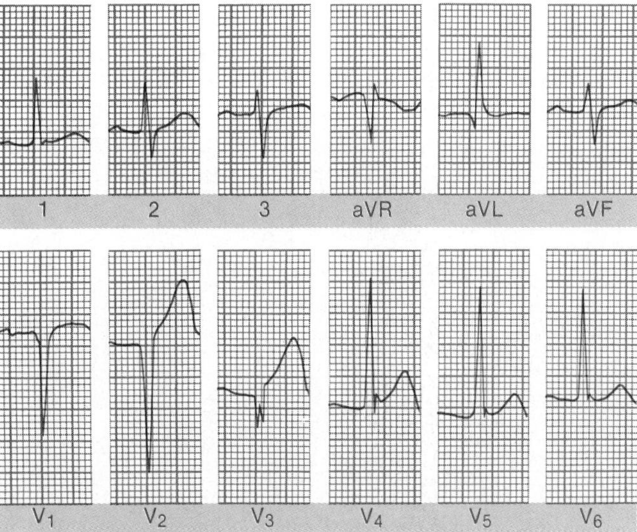

FIGURE 60-10. Electrocardiogram from a 38-year-old man with myotonic muscular dystrophy. Prominent QS deformities are present in leads V_{1-3}. The P-R interval is 0.21 sec and the frontal plane QRS axis is horizontal. (From Perloff, J. K., et al.: Cardiac involvement in myotonic muscular dystrophy [Steinert's disease]: A prospective study of 25 patients. Am. J. Cardiol. *54:*1074, 1984.)

malities of initial forces in the electrocardiogram, occult clinical involvement of the myocardium can be assessed by radionuclide angiography during exercise.[3,98]

Myotonia in skeletal muscle reflects the inability of the muscle cell membrane to reestablish its resting membrane potential quickly after contraction. Whether significant myotonia occurs in cardiac muscle is unproven. Should that be the case, the physiological derangement would, in all probability, be a relatively mild abnormality of diastolic relaxation. There is recent evidence that this, in fact, may be so.[99]

Myotonic dystrophy is genetically transmitted, with complete expression of the gene toward striated muscle tissue, whether skeletal or cardiac.[3] Because specialized cardiac tissues and myocardium have close embryological origins, it is not surprising that the genetic marker affects both. Cardiac involvement is therefore an integral part of myotonic dystrophy with the genetic marker targeting the infranodal conduction system, the sinus node to a lesser extent, and still less specifically the myocardium.[3,100]

An important variation from the above pattern is seen in the offspring of mothers with myotonic dystrophy.[83] The disorder in infants expresses itself as hypotonia and facial paralysis with no evidence of myotonia, at least initially. Respiratory distress is largely responsible for neonatal death from congenital myotonic dystrophy.[83] Affected children have characteristic facies with the upper lip forming a cupid's bow. Studies on cardiac involvement are limited but have reportedly disclosed atrioventricular and intraventricular conduction defects, less commonly reduced left ventricular systolic function.[101] Apart from genetic transmission from the mother (cytoplasmic inheritance), pregnancy is hazardous to the gravida with myotonic dystrophy.[83]

Myotonia congenita (Thomsen's disease) and *paramyotonia congenita* must be distinguished from myotonic muscular dystrophy.[83] Thomsen's disease is characterized by myotonia but not dystrophy. In fact, the skeletal muscles are well developed, even hypertrophied.[5,83] Because the natural history of Thomsen's disease is benign, longevity permits secure conclusions regarding cardiac involvement, which is conspicuously absent. In a single case, cardiac conduction abnormalities similar to those found in myotonic dystrophy were reported.[102] *Paramyotonia* congenita is an uncommon to rare autosomal dominant disorder characterized by prolonged myotonic reaction to cold.[5,103,104] Dystrophy of skeletal muscle is absent, and cardiac involvement is unknown.

FRIEDREICH'S ATAXIA

The hereditary ataxias are divided into (1) the hereditary spinocerebellar ataxia of Friedreich, (2) hereditary ataxia with muscular atrophy (Roussy-Lévy syndrome), (3) hereditary spinocerebellar ataxia, and (4) olivopontocerebellar atrophy.[105] Despite a century of lively interest, Friedreich's ataxia has resisted precise clinical and biochemical definition, and there is still disagreement about where this spinocerebellar degenerative disease fits into the complex framework of the hereditary ataxias.[105-107] It is important to underscore, however, that the disorder is essentially neurological rather than myopathic.[105-107] Friedreich's ataxia is inherited as an autosomal recessive trait and is characterized by ataxia of the limbs and trunk, absence of tendon reflexes, extensor plantar responses, and loss of proprioceptive sensations in the limbs.[107] There are no remissions; instead, ataxia of gait and muscle weakness progress relentlessly, affecting first the lower limbs and then all four extremities. Pes cavus (Friedreich's foot) (Fig. 60-11) and kyphoscoliosis develop within a few years of onset.

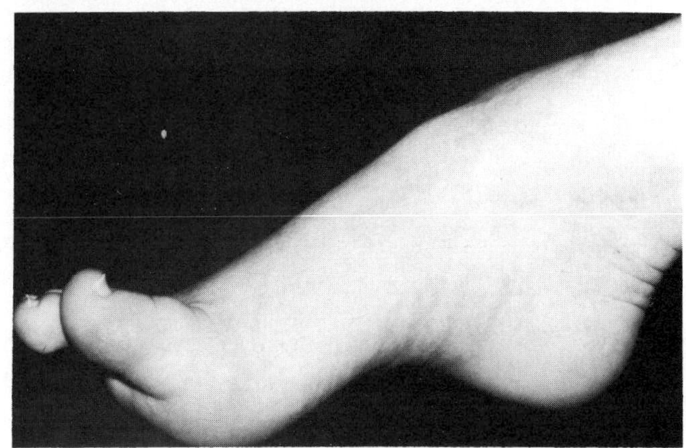

FIGURE 60-11. Pes cavus with hammer toe (Friedreich's foot).

When strict neurological and genetic criteria were used to identify a clinically homogeneous group of patients with Friedreich's ataxia, the incidence of cardiac involvement exceeded 90 per cent.[4,108-114] Severe ataxia occurs long before overt heart disease, and there is no relationship between the degrees of neurological and cardiac involvement.[4] Nevertheless, cardiac disease is often the cause of death.[4,115] There is reason to believe that phenotypically identical Friedreich patients are not genetically homogeneous, so the cardiac expressions might be expected to vary. This, in fact, proved to be the case in a prospective study of 75 patients.[4] Cardiac involvement, usually occult and asymptomatic, is the rule.[115,116] Scalar electrocardiography and echocardiography detected one or more abnormalities in 95 per cent of study patients.[4]

HYPERTROPHIC CARDIOMYOPATHY. The most com-

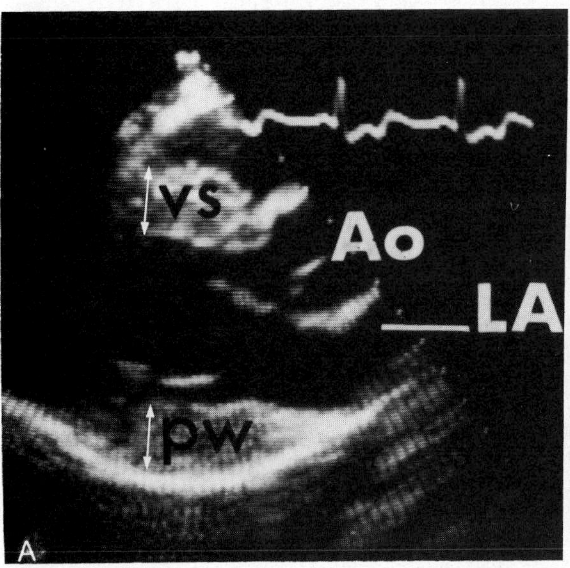

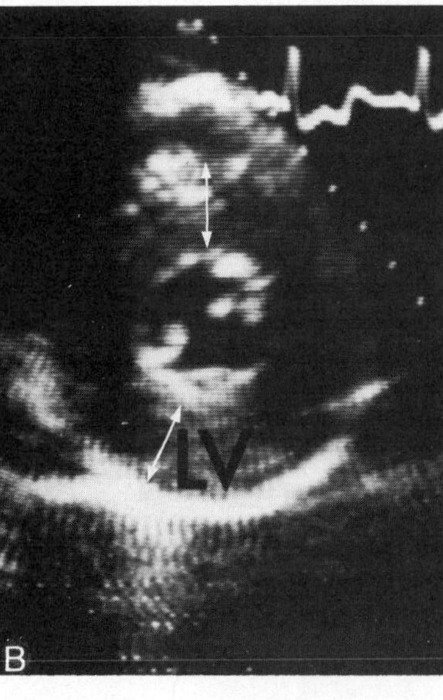

FIGURE 60-12. Two-dimensional echocardiographic parasternal long-axis view (*A*) and short-axis view (*B*) in a 16-year-old boy with Friedreich's ataxia and concentric left ventricular hypertrophy. When he was 13 years of age, the echocardiogram was normal. Ao = aorta; LA = left atrium; LV = left ventricle; PW = posterior wall; VS = ventricular septum. (From Child, J. S., et al.: Cardiac involvement in Friedreich's ataxia. Reprinted by permission of the American College of Cardiology. J. Am. Coll. Cardiol. *7*:1370, 1986.)

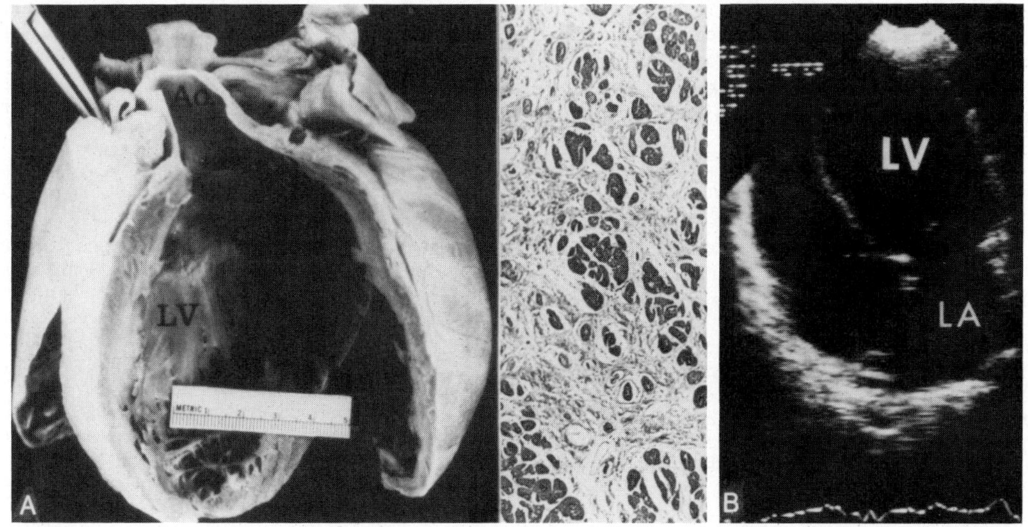

FIGURE 60–13. *A,* Gross and histological specimens from a 17-year-old boy with Friedreich's ataxia whose echocardiogram progressed from normal at age 13 years to a minimally dilated, hypocontractile left ventricle 3 to 4 years later. The gross specimen shows a mildly dilated left ventricle with normal wall thickness; the walls were flabby. The microscopic section from the left ventricular free wall shows marked connective tissue replacement. Although specifically sought, small-vessel coronary artery disease was not identified. *B,* Two-dimensional echocardiogram (apical window) showing the mildly dilated, thin-walled left ventricle (LV). LA = left atrium. (From Child, J. S., et al.: Cardiac involvement in Friedreich's ataxia. Reprinted by permission of the American College of Cardiology. J. Am. Coll. Cardiol. *7:*1370, 1986.)

mon echocardiographic finding has been concentric (symmetrical) left ventricular hypertrophy (Fig. 60–12); asymmetrical septal thickening occurs, but less frequently.[110,112,117–119] Left ventricular outflow gradients have been reported in some cases with disproportionate septal thickness[112] but not in others.[110] Importantly, septal cellular disarray—the histological hallmark of genetic hypertrophic cardiomyopathy (p. 1636)—has been absent or only focal in necropsy studies of Friedreich's ataxia.[108,111,120,121] This observation may, in part, explain why the potentially malignant ventricular arrhythmias common in genetic hypertrophic cardiomyopathy are essentially unknown in Friedreich's ataxia.[122] In the hypertrophic cardiomyopathy of Friedreich's ataxia, systolic ventricular function is normal, not supernormal, and diastolic function is not deranged as in genetic hypertrophic cardiomyopathy.[123,124]

DILATED CARDIOMYOPATHY. A second and much less common form of cardiac involvement in Friedreich's ataxia is dilated cardiomyopathy that may initially express itself as global hypokinesis with normal left ventricular internal dimensions (Fig. 60–13).[4,119] There is one report of dilated cardiomyopathy, chiefly involving the right ventricle, with ventricular tachyarrhythmias.[125] In contrast to the favorable prognosis of Friedreich's ataxia with hypertrophic cardiomyopathy, the outlook is poor in dilated cardiomyopathy patients who experience relentless, progressive cardiac deterioration.[4,119] There is convincing evidence that the dilated form of cardiomyopathy in Friedreich's ataxia is distinct from the hypertrophic form (i.e., not a transition) and represents a fundamentally different type of cardiac involvement designated dystrophic.[4] This view is supported by the flabby myocardium with normal wall thickness in necropsy cases that exhibited premortem progression on echocardiography from normal to dilated globally hypofunctional left ventricles with normal wall thickness (Fig. 60–13).[4] The initial force deformities on electrocardiograms and vectorcardiograms (Fig. 60–14)[4,113] are believed to represent areas of regional ventricular myocardial dystrophy which, if sufficiently widespread, might result in depressed systolic function.[4] Atrial arrhythmias (flutter, fibrillation) and ventricular arrhythmias are features of the dilated cardiomyopathy of Friedreich's ataxia.[4,125] Disease of the coronary arteries, especially small intramural coronary arteries, has been reported in Friedreich's ataxia,[121] but a relationship between the coronary arteriopathy and regional wall abnormalities is doubtful.

In summary, there appear to be two distinct types of cardiac involvement in Friedreich's ataxia: (1) hypertrophic cardiomyopathy, represented by symmetrical (less commonly asymmetrical) left ventricular hypertrophy with normal cavity size and ventricular function, and (2) relatively uncommon dilated cardiomyopathy, represented by depressed systolic function with normal or increased ventricular cavity size. Whether the frequently observed initial force abnormalities on the scalar electrocardiogram represent regional "dystrophic" disease that anticipates dilated cardiomyopathy remains to be proven.

Why a nonmyopathic spinocerebellar corticospinal disorder is accompanied by two widely disparate types of cardiac disease is unknown. An important implication is that phenotypically indistinguishable patients are genetically different.[126,127] The relationship between the spinocerebellar-corticospinal disorder and an increase in ventricular

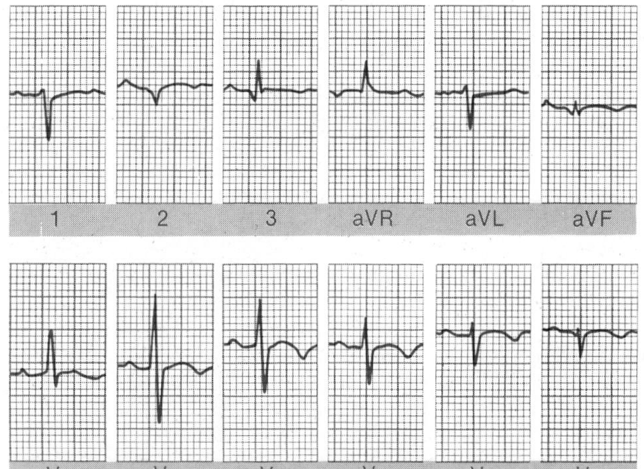

FIGURE 60–14. Electrocardiogram in a 28-year-old man with Friedreich's ataxia. The QRS shows marked right-axis deviation. There are 40-msec Q waves in leads 2, 3, and aVl. A prominent 60-msec R wave appears in lead V_1. A vectorcardiogram and echocardiogram showed no evidence of right ventricular hypertrophy. The ECG pattern reflects loss of inferior and posterior electrical forces without a corresponding regional wall motion abnormality on echocardiography. (From Child, J. S., et al.: Cardiac involvement in Friedreich's ataxia. Reprinted by permission of the American College of Cardiology. J. Am. Coll. Cardiol. *7:*1370, 1986.)

mass—hypertrophic cardiomyopathy—is also an enigma. A unifying thread may be the "catecholamine hypothesis," which has been a focus of interest in the pathogenesis of genetic hypertrophic cardiomyopathy.[128] Plasma catecholamine levels are reportedly increased in patients with Friedreich's ataxia.[129,130]

LESS COMMON NEUROMYOPATHIC DISEASES SOMETIMES ASSOCIATED WITH HEART DISEASE

PERONEAL MUSCULAR ATROPHY (CHARCOT-MARIE-TOOTH SYNDROME). Peroneal muscular atrophy includes several genetic disorders (the hereditary motor and sensory neuromyopathies) characterized by distal weakness of the legs with predilection for muscles innervated by the peroneal nerves, particularly the everters of the foot and occasionally intrinsic muscles of the hands.[131] Peroneal muscular atrophy is an autosomal dominant disorder; one form begins during the first 20 years of life, while the other form begins later, with initial symptoms appearing in early life or not until middle age. Cardiac involvement is not a feature of peroneal muscular atrophy.[114,132,133] Arrhythmias, conduction abnormalities, and dilated heart failure have been sporadically reported in patients with peroneal muscular atrophy,[134-138] but are believed to be chance associations.[133]

MYOTUBULAR MYOPATHY (CENTRONUCLEAR MYOPATHY). Centronuclear myopathy typically exhibits internal nuclei, i.e., structures resembling fetal myotubes (rows of nuclei separated by spaces).[139-140] The disorder is characterized clinically by slow but progressive wasting and weakness of skeletal muscle beginning at birth. Ptosis is the rule, and patients are hyporeflexic or areflexic. Few examples are available for study, but presumptive evidence indicates that myotubular myopathy can be associated with extensive myocardial fibrosis, cardiac dilatation, and early death.[139] In an illustration in one report on skeletal muscle in "idiopathic cardiomyopathy," numerous internal nuclei could be seen.[141] Centronuclear myopathy had apparently presented as cardiomyopathy before the neuromuscular disease was identified.

KEARNS-SAYRE SYNDROME (PROGRESSIVE EXTERNAL OPHTHALMOPLEGIA WITH PIGMENTARY RETINOPATHY). Kearns-Sayre syndrome is a mitochondrial myopathy characterized by progressive external ophthalmoplegia (Fig. 60–15), pigmentary retinopathy, and *heart block*.[142-144] Morphological alterations in skeletal muscle are identified in the trichrome stain as ragged red fibers.[142] Cardiac involvement primarily afflicts the specialized conduction pathways.[145,146] Clinically overt myocardial disease is the exception, despite the fact that ultrastructural abnormalities, especially of mitochondria, are well established.[147-149] Occasional patients exhibit dilated cardiomyopathy with progressive heart failure.[147-149] Patients are chiefly at risk because of the abnormalities of the specialized conduction pathways. Two derangements in cardiac conduction coexist: (1) gradually progressive impairment of infranodal conduction (left anterior hemiblock, right bundle branch block, complete heart block) (Fig. 60–16*A*) and (2) concomitant enhancement of AV nodal conduction.[145,150] The morphological basis for impaired infranodal conduction lies in the extensive changes in distal portions of the bundle of His extending to the origins of the bundle branches.[150] Evidence of enhanced AV nodal conduction has been identified by His bundle electrocardiography[145] (Fig. 60–16*B*). A short or relatively short P-R interval should not be used to weigh against the risk inherent in trifascicular disease in patients with Kearns-Sayre syndrome, right bundle branch block, and left anterior hemiblock.[145] Pacemaker implantation is often necessary.

GUILLAIN-BARRÉ SYNDROME. This syndrome is the most common of the acquired demyelinative neuropathies.[151] The incidence gradually increases with age, but the disease may occur at any age, and both sexes are equally affected. The syndrome often appears days to weeks after a viral respiratory or gastrointestinal infection, with neurological symptoms comprising symmetrical weakness of the limbs often accompanied by paresthesias. The incidence of the acute polyneuropathy is higher in patients with Hodgkin's disease, and the disorder may be precipitated by pregnancy, general surgery, or vaccinations. Myocardial infarction was believed to be the precipitating cause in two cases.[152] Important and characteristic features of the syndrome are flaccid motor paralysis with a distinctive tendency to ascend (Landry's ascending paralysis) and elevation of the cerebrospinal protein concentration without an increase in the number of white blood cells. Involvement of thoracic muscles often requires assisted ventilation. Despite respiratory support, the Guillain-Barré syndrome is fatal in approximately 20 per cent of children with significant involvement of trunk muscles and associated pulmonary insufficiency.[153]

Cardiac Findings. When sudden death occurs, postmortem studies have shed little or no light on the cause. There is substantial evidence, however, that deaths are often if not invariably related to cardiac arrhythmias.[153-155] Bradyarrhythmias (sinus arrest, complete heart block) and tachyarrhythmias (supraventricular and ventricular) as well as premature atrial and ventricular beats are relatively frequent occurrences and may be increased by the use of a respirator.[154] Occasionally, patients exhibit autonomic dysfunction, especially sympathetic hyperactivity, reflected in orthostatic hypotension, transient hypertension, wide fluctuations in blood pressure and in heart rate, and variations in the R-R interval.[156-158] Pacemaker support has been required because of recurrent asystole.[154] In one patient, tracheal aspiration produced an idioventricular rhythm of 40 beats per minute that reverted to sinus rhythm when aspiration ceased.[153] Cardiac monitoring is advisable, especially when the Guillain-Barré syndrome is sufficiently severe to warrant assisted ventilation.[153] ECG occasionally shows widespread deep T-wave inversions.[158]

NEMALINE MYOPATHY. This condition is characterized by myriads of small, rodlike particles in striated muscle.[159-160,160a] Inheritance is either autosomal dominant or recessive, with occasional sporadic cases. The most common clinical manifestation is hypotonia with diffuse weakness of limbs and trunk beginning at an early age. Children are often dysmorphic with an elongated, narrow face, high arched palate, and slender musculature.[5] Alternatively, symptoms begin in adolescence or adult life and are characterized by scapuloperoneal weakness and footdrop.[161] Nemaline myopathy is only rarely associated with cardiac involvement, but nemaline rods in the myocardium and in the cardiac conduction tissues have been held responsible for cardiac dilatation and conduction defects.[162,163]

MYASTHENIA GRAVIS. This is a "neuroimmunological" disease caused by a disorder of neuromuscular transmission due to antibodies to

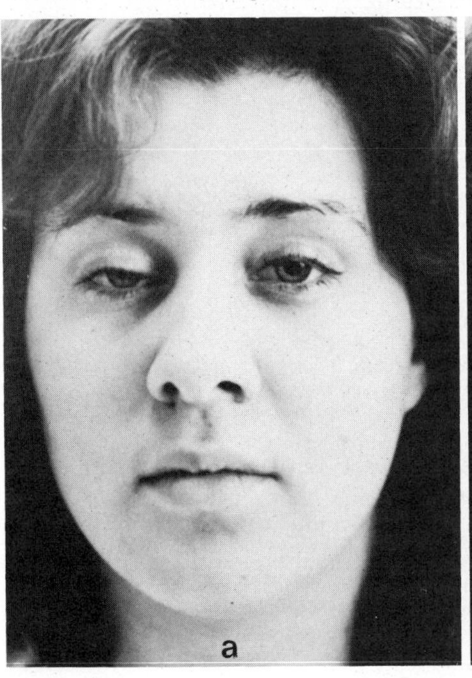

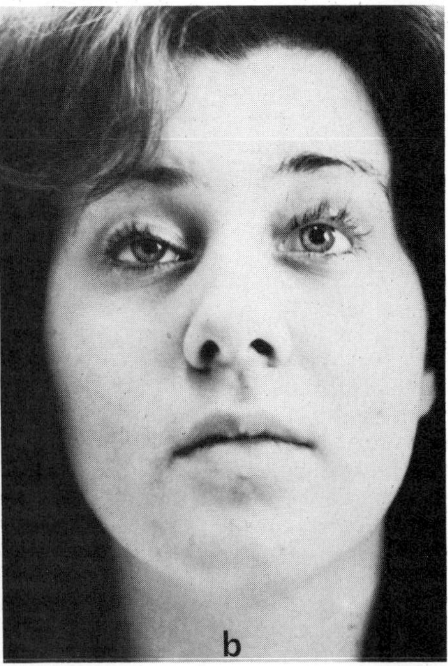

FIGURE 60–15. An 18-year-old girl with Kearns-Sayre syndrome and bilateral asymmetrical ptosis. Within 24 months, her electrocardiogram changed from normal to bifascicular block (complete right bundle branch block and left anterior fascicular block). *A,* The asymmetrical ptosis when the patient looks straight ahead. *B,* Ptosis of the right lid persists when the patient looks up. She also had atypical pigmentary retinopathy.

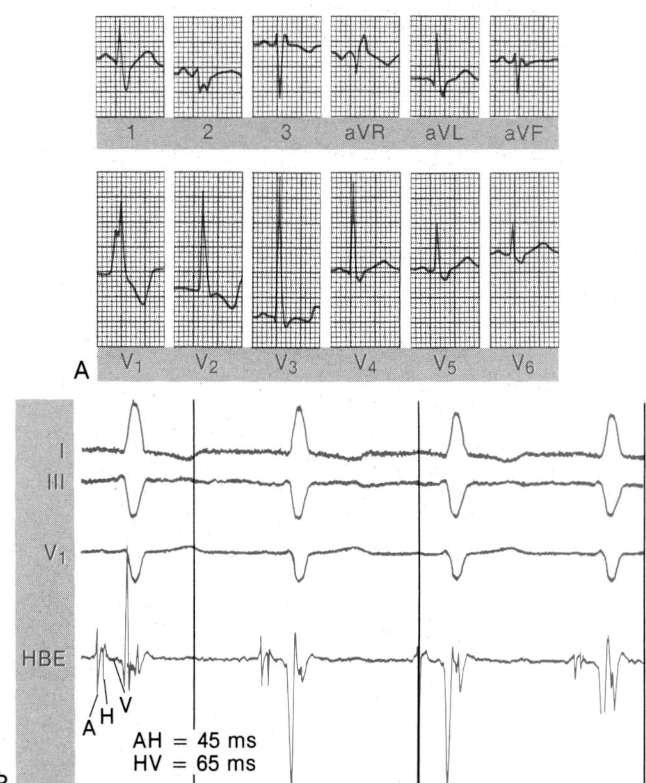

FIGURE 60-16. *A,* **Electrocardiogram from a 13-year-old boy with Kearns-Sayre syndrome. There is a short P-R interval (110 msec), left anterior hemiblock, and complete right bundle branch block.** ***B,*** **Leads I, III, and V_1 with His bundle electrogram (HBE) in a 21-year-old woman with Kearns-Sayre syndrome. Time lines are at 1-sec intervals. The A-H interval is 45 msec (short) and the H-V interval is 65 msec (prolonged). (From Roberts, N. K., et al.: Cardiac conduction in Kearns-Sayre syndrome. Am. J. Cardiol.** ***44:*****1396, 1979.)**

acetylcholine receptors.[164,165] The abnormality may become manifest at any age but is most common in the second to fourth decades. Overt pathological evidence of myasthenia gravis is primarily in the thymus, which shows lymphoid hyperplasia and numerous lymphoid follicles with germinal centers in the medulla. Ocular muscles are affected first, and weakness characteristically fluctuates during the course of a single day, sometimes within minutes. The association of myocardial disease with thymoma, especially malignant thymoma, is generally accepted, whereas the association of myasthenia gravis with heart disease is less clear despite a considerable body of suggestive evidence.[166] Specific cardiac involvement is unproven even though clinical, electrocardiographic, and vectorcardiographic data implicate the myocardium.[166]

Early in this century quinine was used as a provocative diagnostic test for myasthenia gravis. Quinidine and procainamide, like quinine, have anticholinergic properties that depress neuromuscular conduction.[167] These antiarrhythmic agents can unmask previously unsuspected myasthenia gravis and can exacerbate symptoms in previously well controlled patients.[167,168] Accordingly, quinidine and procainamide should be avoided in this disorder.

McARDLE SYNDROME. This metabolic myopathy (muscle phosphorylase deficiency) results in inadequate skeletal muscle glycolysis.[169] The disease is characterized by exercise-induced muscle cramps. The electrocardiogram occasionally reveals sinus bradycardia, increased QRS voltage, and prolongation of the P-R interval, but the most common feature is a rapid acceleration of heart rate and respiratory rate with the beginning of exercise.[5,169] McArdle syndrome differs from the metabolic mitochondrial myopathy of skeletal and cardiac muscle with exercise-induced lactic acidemia and storage of glycogen and lipid.[170]

KUGELBERG-WELANDER SYNDROME. Proximal spinal muscular atrophies are autosomal recessive.[171] The childhood form is subdivided into three groups: the acute Werdnig-Hoffmann, the intermediate Werdnig-Hoffmann, and the Kugelberg-Welander.[171] The last variety of spinal muscular atrophy is characterized by onset in childhood or adolescence, atrophy and weakness principally of proximal limb muscles, slowly progressive clinical course, development of fasciculations, and evidence of neurogenic changes in the electromyogram and on muscle biopsy. There have been a few reports of cardiac involvement in the Kugelberg-Welander syndrome, including atrial fibrillation, atrial standstill, conduction defects (H-V prolongation, complete AV block), and dilated heart failure.[172]

POLIOMYELITIS. Cardiac involvement is believed to occur only rarely in childhood poliomyelitis but may simply be clinically occult.[173,174] In adults, the infrequency of symptomatic involvement of the heart contrasts with a relatively high incidence of electrocardiographic abnormalities, especially of rhythm and conduction.[173,174] Disturbances of rhythm take the form of premature beats (atrial and ventricular) and atrial fibrillation or flutter; disturbances in conduction are manifested by impaired AV conduction (first, second, and third degree heart block) and abnormalities of infranodal conduction (left-axis deviation and bundle branch block).[173,174] Respiratory failure can provoke hypoxemia-induced pulmonary hypertension[175] and multifocal atrial tachycardia.

At necropsy, the sinoatrial node, distal His bundle, and left and right bundle branches show infiltration, degeneration, and fibrous replacement that wholly or in part account for the conduction defects.[173,174] Pathological changes in the myocardium tend to be similar to those in skeletal muscle, including diffuse mononuclear cell infiltration and myofibril degeneration, regeneration, and fibrosis.

PERIODIC PARALYSIS. Periodic paralysis is characterized by recurrences of flaccid weakness accompanied by either abnormally high or abnormally low levels of serum potassium.[176,177] *Hypokalemic attacks* typically begin in late childhood or adolescence, usually occur at night, tend to be severe, and last a day or longer.[177] *Hyperkalemic attacks* have their onset at a younger age. Episodes occur more frequently than with hypokalemia but tend to be milder and shorter in duration (minutes or hours). Many features are common to both varieties of periodic paralysis, including familial recurrence (autosomal dominant inheritance), heightened susceptibility immediately after cessation of strenuous exercise, termination of incipient attacks by *mild* exercise, onset of weakness in the lower extremities with progression to the arms but not to the respiratory muscles, intensification by cold, and persistent weakness between attacks even though potassium levels may be normal.[176,178] During hyperkalemia, the electrocardiogram exhibits peaked T waves, and during hypokalemia there are low-voltage T waves and digitalis sensitivity.

More important are the cardiac arrhythmias that accompany periodic paralysis, including ventricular ectopic beats, ventricular bigeminy, and fusion beats producing multiform complexes.[177-179] Of particular interest is bidirectional tachycardia that is believed to originate in the left ventricle, that is refractory to antiarrhythmic therapy, that occurs independent of attacks of muscle weakness, that exhibits no correlation with serum electrolyte concentrations, and that is regularly converted to sinus rhythm with mild exercise.[180,181] Hypokalemic episodes are best treated with oral potassium chloride, and hyperkalemic episodes, with glucose and insulin, but it should be pointed out that administration of potassium does not necessarily suppress the ventricular electrical instability during hypokalemic attacks.[179]

ALCOHOLIC CARDIOMYOPATHY (see also p. 1819). Dilated cardiomyopathy associated with long-term ingestion of large amounts of ethyl alcohol may be accompanied by clinically occult skeletal myopathy.[182-184] The teratogenic potential of alcohol, exemplified by the fetal alcohol syndrome, afflicts the central nervous system but not the fetal myocardium, although congenital malformations of the heart are not uncommon in the offspring of alcoholic mothers.[185]

ACUTE CEREBRAL DISORDERS ACCOMPANIED BY CARDIOVASCULAR ABNORMALITIES

Acute cerebral injury can provoke cardiovascular abnormalities, and abnormalities of the heart can set the stage for acute cerebral injury. A connection between certain acute cerebral events—subarachnoid hemorrhage, intracranial hemorrhage, space-occupying lesions—and overt cardiovascular abnormalities has been recognized for nearly a century, and a relationship between head trauma and cardiac abnormalities was proposed 50 years ago.[186] The cardiac abnormalities that were emphasized in these settings were disturbances in rhythm and conduction and abnormalities of repolarization. *Neurogenic pulmonary edema* (p. 559) has been reported with a variety of disorders of the central nervous system[187,188] and with brain stem hemorrhage.[189] A rise in systemic blood pressure in response to cerebral injury[190] was known to Harvey Cushing at the turn of the century (the *Cushing pressor response*),[191] and experimentally induced intense cerebral compression in rats evokes a marked increase in systemic vascular resistance, a profound decrease in cardiac output, pulmonary venous congestion, and hemorrhagic pulmonary edema.[187] Interest has also focused on the importance of damage to the myocardium in response to cerebral injury, especially severe brain injury caused by craniocerebral trauma.[192–197]

ARRHYTHMIAS, CONDUCTION DEFECTS, AND REPOLARIZATION ABNORMALITIES. Approximately 90 per cent of patients with *acute cerebral accidents*—most notably spontaneous cerebral or subarachnoid hemorrhage or acute cerebral trauma—exhibit electrocardiographic abnormalities that consist chiefly of disturbances of cardiac rhythm and repolarization.[189,195,196,198–207] Disturbances in cardiac rhythm include sinus bradycardia (sometimes profound), sinus tachycardia, atrial arrhythmias (ectopic beats, fibrillation, flutter, or supraventricular tachycardia), junctional rhythms, and ventricular arrhythmias (ectopic beats, ventricular tachycardia, or fibrillation).[199,208,209] Conduction disturbances include first, second, or third degree AV block.[196] Repolarization abnormalities closely resemble those of ischemic heart disease and consist mainly of abnormal ST segments and T waves in addition to prominent U waves, and a prolonged Q-T interval.[189,202,210] ST segments may be dramatically elevated and T waves dramatically inverted (Fig. 60–17).

MYOCARDIAL INJURY. There is substantial evidence that the "catecholamine storm"—copious release of norepinephrine at cardiac beta$_1$-receptor sites—is responsible for myocardial damage, reflected in an increase in serum cardiac enzymes (CK MB), in left ventricular wall motion abnormalities,[197] in evidence of myofibrillar degeneration on light microscopy, and in subendocardial injury.[190,194,205] Potentially additive effects of glucocorticoids combined with catecholamines have been emphasized in the genesis of stress myocardial injury.[199] The myocardial damage associated with acute cerebral injury puts patients at additional risk (see above). It is important to emphasize that the major sources of donor hearts for cardiac and for heart and lung transplantation are motor vehicle accident or gunshot wound victims who have suffered massive cerebral injury and, in all probability, have varying degrees of catecholamine- and stress-induced myocardial and lung injury.[195,209]

NEUROGENIC PULMONARY EDEMA AND CARDIOPULMONARY ARREST. Cerebrogenic hemorrhagic pulmonary edema has been experimentally induced by cranial compression in rats,[187] and neurogenic pulmonary edema sometimes accompanies acute cerebral injury in patients[187–189] (p. 559). Myocardial damage may aggravate the pulmonary edema but is not necessary for its genesis. Respiratory arrest without circulatory collapse is more common than cardiac arrest in patients with acute cerebral injury.[211] Cardiac arrest per se is likely to be triggered by disturbances in ventricular rhythm (see above). Cerebrogenic cardiac arrhythmias and neurogenic pulmonary edema have been reported following generalized tonic-clonic epileptic seizures without acute cerebral injury.[212,213] Acute injury to the cervical spinal cord without cerebral damage is frequently accompanied by disturbances in cardiac rhythm and conduction and occasionally by sudden death.[214] Bradyarrhythmias are most prevalent, but supraventricular and ventricular tachyarrhythmias and AV block also occur, in addition to marked hypotension. The cardiac abnormalities are believed to arise from acute autonomic imbalance imposed on the heart by the cervical cord injury.[214]

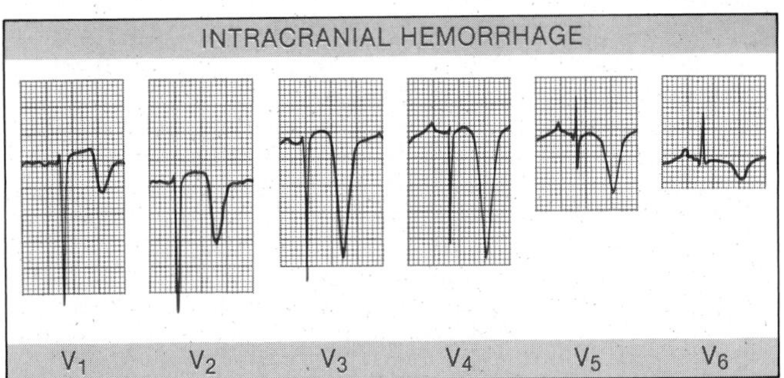

FIGURE 60–17. Deep, symmetrical T-wave inversions in precordial leads of a patient with a cerebral hemorrhage. (Courtesy of John H. Phillips, M.D., Tulane Medical Center, New Orleans, Louisiana.)

Coexistence of Cerebrovascular Disease and Coronary Heart Disease

The preceding section pointed out that acute cerebrovascular accidents in patients with normal hearts (i.e., without coronary artery disease) often result in electrocardiographic abnormalities resembling those of myocardial ischemia or infarction with release of CK MB; however, in older patients, these electrocardiographic abnormalities and isoenzyme elevations may in fact represent an accompanying acute myocardial ischemic event caused by coexisting atherosclerotic coronary artery disease.[215,216] Because ST-segment elevations, deep T-wave inversions, and an increase in CK MB occur in patients with cerebrovascular accidents *without* ischemic heart disease, one cannot rely on these criteria to diagnose ischemic injury due to coronary artery obstruction. Accordingly, earlier estimates of the incidence of acute myocardial infarction in such patients[217] must be reevaluated.[218] Differential diagnosis is important, because mortality is relatively high in patients with coexisting acute cerebrovascular accident and acute myocardial infarction.[210]

DIAGNOSIS. Patients with clinically overt atherosclerotic coronary artery disease should be examined for occult carotid artery disease, and those with overt carotid artery disease should be assessed for occult atherosclerotic coronary artery disease. Cervical arterial murmurs were found in 4.4 to 12.6 per cent of persons 45 years of age and older with no history of stroke, transient cerebral ischemia, or overt ischemic heart disease.[219–221] The prevalence of these asymptomatic murmurs increased with age and was higher among women and among patients with systemic hypertension. In a prospective study of 735 unselected patients over age 55 years who were scheduled for elective surgery, 14 per cent had cervical arterial murmurs.[222] Pooled data on 2205 patients undergoing elective surgery disclosed cervical arterial murmurs in 15 per cent but no difference in stroke distribution between patients with and without carotid murmurs.[222] It was concluded that strokes in patients undergoing operations other than coronary artery bypass are so rare that further evaluation seems unnecessary. Still, it is important to distinguish between hemodynamically mild carotid stenosis with an exceedingly low risk of stroke and hemodynamically significant lesions in which the risk of even nonfatal cerebral infarction is appreciable.[221,223,224]

The need to identify hemodynamically significant carotid artery obstruction—either symptomatic or asymptomatic—was underscored in the Framingham Study, in which attention was called to the relative frequency of cerebral infarction in vascular territories different from that predicted based on an asymptomatic carotid artery murmur.[225] Ruptured aneurysm, embolism from the heart, and lacunar infarction were the mechanisms of stroke in nearly half the cases (see later).

The *physical examination* serves to detect carotid artery murmurs but does not accurately determine the severity of carotid obstruction. Of the currently available noninvasive neurovascular tests that reliably assess carotid artery disease, the first choice is ultrasonic duplex scanning that combines B-mode imaging to visualize specific arterial segments with the pulsed Doppler technique to determine the physiological significance of the obstruction.[226,227]

MANAGEMENT. Expert opinion regarding carotid endarterectomy for prevention of stroke has varied widely.[224] Given relatively secure information regarding the carotid and coronary circulations, however, judgments concerning management before coronary revascularization can be based on the following suppositions[221,224,228–230]: (1) in patients with symptomatic carotid artery murmurs (prior stroke or transient ischemic attacks) and hemodynamically significant carotid artery obstruction (especially bilateral) in whom myocardial revascularization *cannot* safely be deferred (left main coronary obstruction, unstable angina pectoris, severe multivessel disease), *combined* carotid endartectomy and coronary bypass grafting are recommended: (2) in patients with symptomatic carotid artery murmurs and hemodynamically significant carotid obstruction in whom myocardial revascularization *can* safely be deferred, carotid endarterectomy should be carried out first, followed at a later date by coronary revascularization: (3) in patients with asymptomatic carotid artery murmurs and obstruction that is considered hemodynamically insignificant, myocardial revascularization alone can proceed as clinically indicated; (4) less clear is the management of patients with asymptomatic carotid artery murmurs and hemodynamically significant carotid obstruction.[221,224] It has been argued that elective myocardial revascularization can be performed either alone or, if clinically urgent (as already defined), combined with carotid endarterectomy.[228]

An important corollary to these observations is the incidence of neurological complications unassociated with carotid artery obstruction in patients undergoing coronary artery bypass grafting.[228,230–233] These complications are in addition to and distinct from those accompanying open-heart surgery per se.[234,325] Major central nervous system events are associated with coronary bypass operations in 1 to 2 per cent of cases.[230,232,233] The majority of cerebral events complicating coronary bypass grafting are believed to be related to embolization of atheromatous material from the ascending aorta or embolization from a postinfarction left ventricular mural thrombus.[230,233]

Cardiogenic Brain Embolism

Aggregate clinical data on cardiac sources of embolic stroke (the Cerebral Embolism Task Force) emphasize "nonvalvular" atrial fibrillation, ischemic heart disease (acute myocardial infarction, ventricular aneurysm), rheumatic heart disease (mitral stenosis), and prosthetic cardiac valves.[236] Important but less common sources include nonischemic dilated cardiomyopathy, infective endocarditis, nonbacterial thrombotic endocarditis, mitral valve prolapse, mitral annular calcification, calcific aortic stenosis, left atrial myxoma, atrial septal aneurysm, and paradoxical embolization especially but not necessarily with congenital heart disease.[236] Nonvalvular atrial fibrillation encompasses a wide spectrum, from "lone atrial fibrillation" without other clinical evidence of heart disease to ventricular dilatation with congestive heart failure. Nonvalvular atrial fibrillation is the most common cardiac disorder believed to be associated with cerebral embolic events, accounting for almost one-half of cardiogenic embolic strokes.[236] Although some studies report a low stroke incidence in patients with lone atrial fibrillation,[237] other studies conclude that atrial fibrillation unassociated with structural heart disease predisposes to cerebral embolism.[238] Preliminary results indicate that aspirin or Coumadin (given separately) is effective in preventing systemic embolism and ischemic stroke and is comparatively safe in patients with nonvalvular atrial fibrillation. The absolute reduction in risk according to the Stroke Prevention in Atrial Fibrillation Study Group[238] was 6.8 per cent per year, exceeding the incremental risk of clinically important hemorrhage (<1 per cent per year). When that report was compiled, it was not possible to establish an advantage of either warfarin or aspirin over the other.

Focal neurological signs are occasionally seen in patients with *mitral valve prolapse* (p. 1029) and are believed to be embolic (platelet fibrin aggregates).[239–240] *Left atrial myxomas* (p. 1452) result in peripheral emboli in about 45 per cent of cases, and the brain is affected in one-half of these. Occasionally, patients with left atrial myxoma are initially seen by neurologists because of predominantly or exclusively neurological manifestations.[241] *Left ventricular mural thrombi* set the stage for cerebral emboli, most commonly in patients with myocardial infarction because of the prevalence of ischemic heart disease, but left ventricular mural thrombi in patients with dilated cardiomyopathy are much more likely to give rise to cerebral emboli than are mural thrombi associated with myocardial infarction.[182] Infants with endocardial fibroelastosis of the dilated type also suffer strokes caused by emboli from left ventricular endocardial thrombi.[242] *Infective endocarditis* (p. 1078) on native or prosthetic cardiac valves gives rise to neurological complications, including stroke, toxic confusion, and meningitis. Rupture of a mycotic aneurysm is a catastrophic event associated with 80 per cent mortality.[243–245] Septic cerebral emboli may give rise to acute intracranial hemorrhage or cerebral abscess after a misleading interval of quiescence.

Bland emboli from *marantic endocarditis* (p. 1551), especially on the aortic valve, are believed to be more common than clinically recognized.[246] The use of anticoagulants coupled with improved rigid prostheses has decreased the incidence of cerebral emboli after *left cardiac valve replacement.* Drug abuse not only causes infective endocarditis but, depending on the drug and vehicle (embolism of foreign matter), may be associated with intracranial or subarachnoid hemorrhage, cerebral emboli, and ischemic stroke.[247]

Paradoxical emboli reach the brain when peripheral venous blood enters the systemic arterial circulation via right-to-left shunts of cyanotic congenital heart disease.[242,248] An important variation on this theme is what are believed to be paradoxical emboli in acyanotic patients with interatrial communications (ostium secundum atrial septal defect or patent foramen ovale).[248–250] Especially vulnerable are pregnant women with an ostium secundum atrial septal defect; inferior caval to left atrial streaming provides a pathway into the left atrium.[251] Recent interest has focused on younger adults with embolic stroke ascribed to paradoxical emboli through a patent foramen ovale[249] (Fig. 60–18). Evidence in this regard has been considered sufficient to warrant sealing the patent foramen using interventional catheterization techniques. Atrial septal aneurysm, an uncommon localized malformation of the interatrial septum, protrudes into the right or left atrium and is a potential occult source of cerebral embolism[252] (Fig. 60–19).

Focal discrete neurological deficits are well-known sequelae of cerebral emboli; less well known are the diffuse cerebral symptoms believed to result from recurrences of multiple small corticoemboli that cause agitated confusion, dulled sensorium, and seizures.[253]

CYANOTIC CONGENITAL HEART DISEASE WITH NEUROLOGICAL MANIFESTATIONS

Brain damage, mental retardation, venous sinus thromboses, paradoxical cerebroembolism (see earlier), and brain abscess constitute a formidable list of central nervous system complications in cyanotic congenital heart disease.[242,254] Cyanotic spells of tetralogy of Fallot may culminate in syncope, seizures, and rarely in hemiplegia[255] (p. 935). The erythrocytosis of cyanotic congenital heart disease is a risk of stroke chiefly in infants under 2 years of age with iron deficiency, but the risk of stroke is low in cyanotic adults, whether the erythrocytosis is compensated (normochromic) or decompensated (hypochromic) and irrespective of hematocrit level.[254]

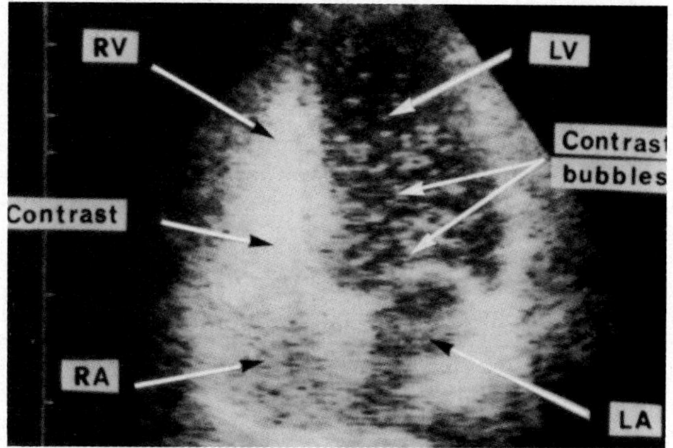

FIGURE 60–18. Two-dimensional contrast echocardiograms (apical four-chamber view) in a patient with a patent foramen ovale. Isotonic saline containing microbubbles was injected into a peripheral vein. Contrast material fills the right atrium (RA) and right ventricle (RV) and appears in the left atrium (LA) and left ventricle (LV) through a patent foramen ovale. (From Lechat, P., et al.: Prevalence of patent foramen ovale in patients with stroke. N. Engl. J. Med. *318:*1148, 1988.) Relabeled for clarity.

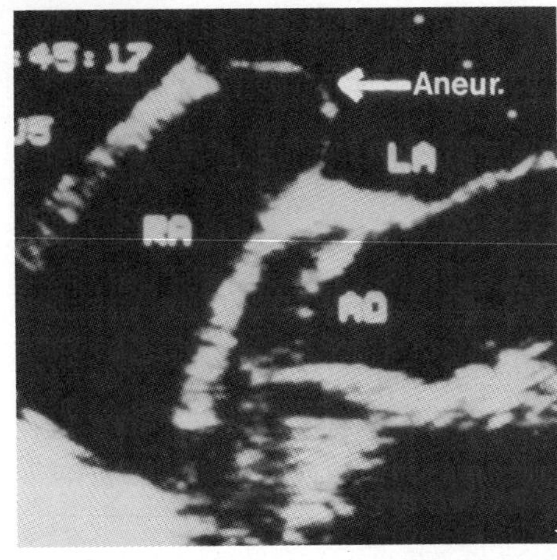

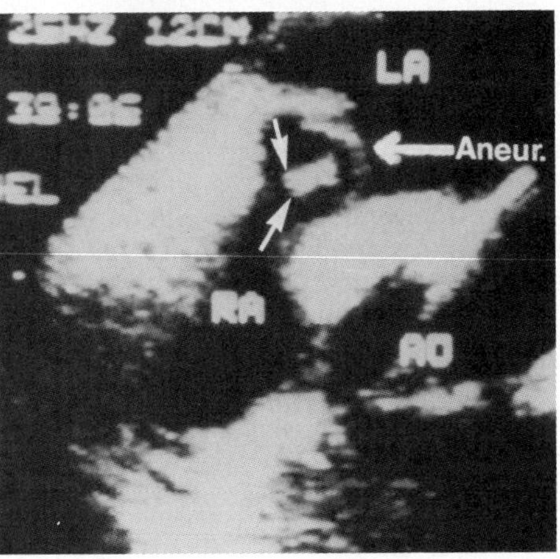

FIGURE 60-19. *Left panel,* Early systolic frame of a thin atrial septal aneurysm (Aneur.) on transesophageal echocardiogram. LA = left atrium; Ao = aorta. *Right panel,* A mobile thrombus (paired arrows) on the right atrial side of an atrial septal aneurysm. (From Schneider, B., Hannath, P., Vogel, P., and Meinertz, T.: Improved morphologic characterization of atrial septal aneurysm by transesophageal echocardiography: Relation to cerebrovascular events. Reprinted by permission of the American College of Cardiology. J. Am. Coll. Cardiol. *16:*1000, 1990.) Relabeled for clarity.

NEUROLOGICAL COMPLICATIONS AFTER CARDIAC ARREST

Broadly speaking, neurological outcomes cover a broad spectrum, ranging from complete recovery to the vegetative state.[256-258] A reversible "metabolic encephalopathy" occurs in patients with brief episodes of systemic circulatory arrest and mild degrees of cerebral hypoxia. Recovery is rapid and complete. In contrast, patients with severe cerebral hypoxia suffer structural damage to specific areas of the brain, as if they had had a stroke, and on awakening manifest permanent focal or multifocal motor, sensory, and intellectual deficits.[256-258] Still other patients with more widespread brain injury remain hospitalized in a state of wakefulness without awareness (vegetative state) or die a neurological death (brain death). Of patients discharged from a hospital, serious neurological deficits are seen in only about 10 per cent because severe postarrest neurological complications frequently lead to death.[257] Preexisting neurological deficits bode ill in survivors of cardiopulmonary resuscitation. Early return to consciousness, and return of cranial nerve function and electroencephalographic function imply a better cerebral prognosis, but do not guarantee a good overall outcome.[257] Delayed electroencephalographic return signifies a poor neurological prognosis.

CARDIAC COMPLICATIONS OF DRUGS USED IN TREATING NEUROMUSCULAR DISEASE

Neuromuscular and cardiovascular diseases may be related to cardiac complications of certain drugs used by the neurologist.

Methysergide prescribed for migraine headache is occasionally accompanied by inflammatory retroperitoneal fibrosis and by a similar fibrotic disease of pleura, systemic arteries, cardiac valves, endocardium, and pericardium.[259-261] Methysergide-induced lesions do little or no damage to underlying cardiac structures, but instead a layer of fresh collagen is deposited on the surfaces of otherwise unharmed cardiac tissue.[260] The aortic valve lesion induced by methysergide causes both stenosis and regurgitation, while the mitral lesion generally causes regurgitation. If the drug is continued, the valvular abnormalities generally progress; however, in some patients, regression or complete disappearance (at least of the cardiac murmurs) has followed discontinuation of methysergide.[260]

In *Parkinson's disease,* neurons are selectively destroyed and cannot release the neurotransmitter dopamine.[262] Accordingly, levodopa (L-dopa), the precursor of dopamine, is used in treatment. A relatively large dose is required for a therapeutic response because only a small percentage of oral L-dopa penetrates the blood-brain barrier. Such doses are seldom tolerated without side effects. L-dopa provokes hypotension (supine and postural) as well as ventricular ectopic beats.[262] The drug must therefore be used cautiously in patients with cerebral ischemia, angina pectoris, recent myocardial infarction, or cardiac arrhythmias, even though after weeks (sometimes months) of use, tolerance improves and side effects diminish. The cardiovascular effects are mediated by the action of L-dopa on the central and peripheral nervous systems.

Bromocriptine, an ergot derivative, stimulates dopamine-sensitive receptors and is also useful in parkinsonism.[262] In high doses, the drug may cause a significant postural fall in blood pressure, and the hypotensive effect may persist for as long as 6 weeks. Rarely, severe hypotension, both supine and erect, occurs after the initial dose of bromocriptine.

Cyclosporine neurotoxicity is only one of the neuropathological concerns accompanying cardiac transplantation.[263] Cyclosporine may produce a wide range of neurological disorders, including coma, encephalopathy, cortical blindness, tremor, ataxia, peripheral neuropathy, and paraparesis.[263] There is no necessary correlation between blood levels and neurotoxic effects of the drug. However, while withdrawal of cyclosporine or reduction in dose generally results in resolution of the signs and symptoms, cases of fatal convulsions and coma have been reported.[263] Perioperative neurological complications of cardiac transplantation (first 2 weeks) include cerebrovascular disorders, encephalopathy, acute psychosis, and mononeuropathy.[264,265] Late neurological complications are related primarily to the use of chronic immunosuppressive therapy (see above), with cerebrovascular disorders becoming less frequent.[264,265]

NEUROLOGICAL COMPLICATIONS OF THERAPY FOR CARDIOVASCULAR DISEASE

Certain therapies for cardiovascular disease can result in serious neurological sequelae, such as those that are sequelae of cardiac arrest and resuscitation (see above). Systemic emboli related to cardioversion for chronic atrial fibrillation occur either at the time of reversion to sinus rhythm or on recurrence of atrial fibrillation. If an anticoagulant is administered for prophylaxis, it must not only precede cardioversion but must be maintained until stable sinus rhythm seems assured.[266]

Several commonly used cardiac drugs have important, although relatively rare, central or peripheral nervous system effects. The adverse responses to quinidine and procainamide in patients with myasthenia gravis were mentioned already (p. 1819). *Lidocaine neurotoxicity* (p. 640) includes drowsiness, dizziness, dysarthria, blurred vision, muscular fasciculations, and occasionally convulsions.[267] Beta-adrenoceptor blockers (p. 1309), in addition to causing drowsiness and lightheadedness, sometimes result in mental depression. Even digitalis glycosides are not exempt from neurotoxic effects[268] (p. 490). William Withering reported that, "The Foxglove when given in very large and quickly repeated doses occasions giddiness, confused vision, objects appearing green or yellow . . . cold sweats, convulsions, syncope, death." [269]

CARDIAC DENERVATION

The most common cause of cardiac denervation is transplantation of the heart (Chap. 18). Less well known is the remarkable denervation of the heart's intrinsic nervous system that occurs in Chagas heart disease (p. 1432).[270,271] Chagasic dysautonomia is associated with pathological changes in the cardiovascular, digestive, and autonomic nervous systems.[271] The cardioneuropathy is characterized by bradycardia, absence of postural reflexes, arterial hypotension, and an abnormal hyperventilation response.[271] The increased capacity of the coronary arteries (judged at necropsy by the volume of barium sulfate–gelatin mass taken up by the coronary arterial bed relative to heart weight) has been attributed to relative sympathetic overdrive in this disease.[270]

REFERENCES

MAJOR HEREDOFAMILIAL NEUROMYOPATHIC DISORDERS

1. Perloff, J. K., deLeon, A. C., and O'Doherty, D.: The cardiomyopathy of progressive muscular dystrophy. Circulation *33*:625, 1966.
2. Perloff, J. K., Henze, E., and Schelbert, H. R.: Alterations in regional myocardial metabolism, perfusion and wall motion in Duchenne muscular dystrophy studied by radionuclide imaging. Circulation *69*:33, 1984.
3. Perloff, J. K., Stevenson, W. G., Roberts, N. K., et al.: Cardiac involvement in myotonic muscular dystrophy (Steinert's disease): A prospective study of 25 patients. Am. J. Cardiol. *54*:1074, 1984.
4. Child, J. S., Perloff, J. K., Bach, P. M., et al.: Cardiac involvement in Friedreich's ataxia. J. Am. Coll. Cardiol. *7*:1370, 1986.
5. Brooke, M. H.: A Clinician's View of Neuromuscular Disease. 2nd ed. Baltimore, Williams and Wilkins Co., 1986.
6. Kunkel, L. M.: Analysis of deletions in DNA from patients with Becker and Duchenne muscular dystrophy. Nature *322*:73, 1986.
7. Boyd, Y., Buckle, V., Holt, S., et al.: Muscular dystrophy in girls with X; autosome translocations. J. Med. Genet. *23*:484, 1986.
8. Roses, A. D.: Progressive muscular dystrophies. *In* Rowland, L. P. (ed.): Merritt's Textbook of Neurology. 7th ed. Philadelphia, Lea & Febiger, 1984.
9. Ervasti, J. M., Ohlendieck, K., Kahl, S. D., et al.: Deficiency of a glycoprotein component of the dystrophin complex in dystrophic muscle. Nature *345*:315, 1990.
10. Boyd, Y., and Buckle, V. J.: Cytogenetic heterogeneity of translocations associated with Duchenne muscular dystrophy. Clin. Genet. *29*:108, 1986.
11. Riggs, T.: Cardiomyopathy and pulmonary emboli in terminal Duchenne's muscular dystrophy. Am. Heart J. *119*:690, 1990.
12. Gaffney, J. F., Kingston, W. J., Metlay, L. A., and Gramiak, R.: Left ventricular thrombus and systemic emboli complicating the cardiomyopathy of Duchenne's muscular dystrophy. Arch. Neurol. *46*:1249, 1989.
13. Yotsukura, M., Miyagawa, M., Tsuya, T., et al.: Pulmonary hypertension in progressive muscular dystrophy of the Duchenne type. Jpn. Circ. J. *52*:321, 1988.
14. Sanyal, S. K., Johnson, W. W., Dische, M. R., et al.: Dystrophic degeneration of papillary muscle and ventricular myocardium. A basis for mitral valve prolapse in Duchenne's muscular dystrophy. Circulation *62*:430, 1980.
15. Perloff, J. K., Roberts, W. C., deLeon, A. C., and O'Doherty, D.: The distinctive electrocardiogram of Duchenne's progressive muscular dystrophy. Am. J. Med. *42*:179, 1967.
16. Perloff, J. K.: Cardiac rhythm and conduction in Duchenne's muscular dystrophy. J. Am. Coll. Cardiol. *3*:1263, 1984.
17. Sanyal, S. K., Johnson, W. W., Thapar, M. K., and Pitner, S. E.: An ultrastructural basis for the electrocardiographic alterations associated with Duchenne's progressive muscular dystrophy. Circulation *57*:1122, 1978.
18. Miller, G., D'Orsogna, L., and O'Shea, J. P.: Autonomic function and the sinus tachycardia of Duchenne muscular dystrophy. Brain Dev. *11*:247, 1989.
19. Zalman, F., Perloff, J. K., Durant, N. N., and Campion, D. S.: Acute respiratory failure following intravenous verapamil in Duchenne's muscular dystrophy. Am. Heart J. *105*:510, 1983.
20. Rubler, S., Perloff, J. K., and Roberts, W. C.: Clinical Pathological Conference—Duchenne's muscular dystrophy. Am. Heart J. *94*:776, 1977.
21. Frankel, K. A., and Rosser, R. J.: The pathology of the heart in progressive muscular dystrophy. Hum. Pathol. *7*:375, 1976.
22. Skyring, A., and McKusick, V. A.: Clinical, genetic and electrocardiographic studies in childhood muscular dystrophy. Am. J. Med. Sci. *242*:54, 1961.
23. Slucka, C.: The electrocardiogram in Duchenne's progressive muscular dystrophy. Circulation *38*:933, 1968.
24. Fitch, C. W., and Ainger, L. E.: The Frank vectorcardiogram and the electrocardiogram in Duchenne muscular dystrophy. Circulation *35*:1124, 1967.
25. Ronan, J. A., Perloff, J. K., Bowen, P. J., and Mann, O.: The vectorcardiogram in Duchenne's progressive muscular dystrophy. Am. Heart J. *84*:588, 1972.
26. Wakai, S., Minami, R., Kameda, K., et al.: Electron microscopic study of the biopsied cardiac muscle in Duchenne muscular dystrophy. J. Neurol. Sci. *84*:167, 1988.
27. Bhattacharya, S. K., Crawford, A. J., and Pate, J. W.: Electrocardiographic, biochemical, and morphologic abnormalities in dystrophic hamsters with cardiomyopathy. Muscle Nerve *10*:168, 1987.
28. Nomura, H., and Hizawa, K.: Histopathological study of the conduction system of the heart in Duchenne progressive muscular dystrophy. Acta Pathol. *32*:1027, 1982.
29. James, T. N.: Observations on the cardiovascular involvement, including the cardiac conduction system, in progressive muscular dystrophy. Am. Heart J. *63*:48, 1962.
30. Chalkiadis, G. A., and Branch, K. G.: Cardiac arrest after isoflurane anaesthesia in a patient with Duchenne's muscular dystrophy. Anaesthesia *45*:22, 1990.
31. Sethna, N. F., and Rockoff, M. A.: Cardiac arrest following inhalation induction of anaesthesia in a child with Duchenne's muscular dystrophy. Can. Anaesthes. Soc. J. *33*:799, 1986.
32. Schelbert, H. R., Benson, L., Schwaiger, M., and Perloff, J. K.: Positron emission tomography. *In* Friedman, W. F., and Higgins, C. B. (eds.): Pediatric Cardiac Imaging, Cardiology Clinics. Philadelphia, W. B. Saunders Company, 1983.
33. Mawatari, S., Miranda, A., and Rowland, L. P.: Adenyl cyclase abnormality in Duchenne muscular dystrophy: Muscle cells in culture. Neurology *67*:1016, 1976.
34. Wilner, J. H., Cerri, C., and Wood, D. S.: Adenyl cyclase in human genetic myopathies. *In* Schotland, D. L. (ed.): Disorders of the Motor Unit. New York, John Wiley and Sons, 1982, p. 431.
35. Carpenter, S., and Karpati, G.: Duchenne muscular dystrophy. Plasma membrane loss initiates muscle cell necrosis unless it is repaired. Brain *102*:147, 1979.
36. Mokri, B., and Engel, A. G.: Duchenne dystrophy: Electronmicroscopic findings pointing to a basic or early abnormality in the plasma membrane of the muscle fiber. Neurology *25*:1111, 1975.
37. Bonilla, E., Schotland, D. L., and Yakayama, Y.: Duchenne dystrophy: Focal alterations in the distribution of concanavalin A binding sites at the muscle cell surface. Ann. Neurol. *4*:117, 1978.
38. Roses, A. D., Harwig, G. B., Mabry, M., et al.: Red blood cell and fibroblast membranes in Duchenne and myotonic muscular dystrophy. Muscle Nerve *3*:36, 1980.
39. Pennington, R.J.T.: Serum enzymes. *In* Rowland, L. P. (ed.): Pathogenesis of Human Muscular Dystrophies. Amsterdam-Oxford, Excerpta Medica, 1977, p. 341.
40. Sutton, T. M., O'Brien, J. F., Kleinberg, F., et al.: Serum levels of creatine phosphokinase and its isoenzymes in normal and stressed neonates. Mayo Clin. Proc. *56*:150, 1981.
41. Yoshioka, M.: Clinically manifesting carriers in Duchenne muscular dystrophy. Clin. Genet. *20*:6, 1981.
42. Lane, R.J.M., Gardner-Medwin, D., and Roses, A. D.: Electrocardiographic abnormalities in carriers of Duchenne muscular dystrophy. Neurology *30*:497, 1980.
43. Fowler, W. M., Gardner, G. W., Taylor, R. G., et al.: Quantitative measurements in female siblings and mothers of boys with Duchenne dystrophy. Arch. Phys. Med. Rehab. *50*:301, 1969.
44. Mann, O., deLeon, A. C., Perloff, J. K., et al.: Duchenne's muscular dystrophy: The electrocardiogram in female relatives. Am. J. Med. Sci. *255*:376, 1968.
45. Paillonry, M., Citron, B., Hersch, B., et al.: Electrocardiograms of women carriers of Duchenne-type muscular dystrophy. Ann. Cardiol. Angiol. *31*:47, 1982.
46. Wiegand, V., Rahlf, G., Meinck, M., and Kreuzer, H.: Cardiomyopathy in female carriers of the Duchenne gene. Z. Kardiol. *73*:188, 1984.
47. Becker, P. E.: Two new families of benign sex-linked recessive muscular dystrophy. Rev. Can. Biol. *21*:551, 1962.
48. Markand, O. N., North, R. R., D'Agostino, A. N., and Daly, D. D.: Benign sex-linked muscular dystrophy. Neurology *19*:617, 1969.
49. Borgeat, A., Goy, J. J., and Sigwart, U.: Acute pulmonary edema as the inaugural symptom of Becker's muscular dystrophy in a 19-year-old patient. Clin. Cardiol *10*:127, 1987.
50. Vrints, C., Mercelis, R., Vanagt, E., et al.: Cardiac manifestations of Becker-type muscular dystrophy. Acta Cardiol. *38*:479, 1983.
51. Yazawa, M., Ikeda, S., Owa, M., et al.: A family of Becker's progressive muscular dystrophy with severe cardiomyopathy. Eur. Neurol. *27*:13, 1987.
52. Lazzeroni, E., Favaro, L., and Botti, G.: Dilated cardiomyopathy with regional myocardial hypoperfusion in Becker's muscular dystrophy. Int. J Cardiol. *22*:126, 1989.
53. Casazza, F., Brambilla, G., Salvato, A., et al.: Cardiac transplantation in Becker muscular dystrophy. J. Neurol. *235*:496, 1988.
54. Nigro, G., Comi, L. I., Limonselli, F. M., et al.: Prospective study of X-linked progressive muscular dystrophy in Campania. Muscle Nerve *6*:253, 1983.
55. Levin, R. N., and Narahara, K. A.: Right axis deviation and anterior wall thallium-201 defect in Becker's muscular dystrophy. Am. J. Cardiol. *56*:203, 1985.
56. Kawashima, S., Ulno, M., Kondo, T., et al.: Marked cardiac involvement in limb girdle muscular dystrophy. Am. J. Med. Sci. *299*:411, 1990.
57. Hoshio, A., Kotake, H., Saitoh, M., et al.: Cardiac involvement in a patient with limb-girdle muscular dystrophy. Heart and Lung *16*:439, 1987.
58. Bailey, R. O., Marzulo, D. C., and Hans, M. B.: Infantile facioscapulohumeral muscular dystrophy: new observations. Acta Neurol. Scand. *74*:51, 1986.
59. Bloomfield, D. A., and Sinclair-Smith, B. C.: Persistent atrial standstill. Am. J. Med. *39*:335, 1965.
60. Caponnetto, S., Patorini, C., and Tirelli, G.: Persistent atrial standstill in a patient affected with facioscapulohumeral dystrophy. Cardiologia *53*:341, 1968.
61. Baldwin, A. J., Talley, R. C., Johnson, C., and Nutter, O.: Permanent paral-

ysis of the atrium in a patient with facioscapulohumeral muscular dystrophy. Am. J. Cardiol. *31*:649, 1973.
62. Stevenson, W. G., Perloff, J. K., Weiss, J. N., and Anderson, T. L.: Facioscapulohumeral muscular dystrophy: Evidence for selective, genetic electrophysiologic cardiac involvement. J. Am. Coll. Cardiol. *15*:292, 1990.
63. Emery, A.E.H., and Dreifuss, F. E.: Unusual type of benign X-linked muscular dystrophy. J. Neurol. Neurosurg. Psychiatry *29*:338, 1966.
64. Emery, A.E.H.: X-linked muscular dystrophy with early contractures and cardiomyopathy (Emery-Dreifuss type). Clin. Genet. *32*:360, 1987.
65. Hopkins, L. C., Jackson, J. A., and Elsas, L. J.: Emery-Dreifuss humeroperoneal muscular dystrophy: An X-linked myopathy with unusual contractures and bradycardia. Ann. Neurol. *10*:230, 1981.
66. Fenichel, G. M., Sul, Y. C., Kilroy, A. W., and Blouin, R.: An autosomal-dominant dystrophy with humeropelvic distribution and cardiomyopathy. Neurology *32*:1399, 1982.
67. Takamoto, K., Hirose, K., and Nonaka, I.: A genetic variant of Emery-Dreifuss disease. Arch. Neurol. *41*:1292, 1984.
68. Tanaka, K., Yoshimura, T., Muratani, H., et al.: Familial myopathy with scapulohumeral distribution, rigid spine, cardiomyopathy and mitochondrial abnormality. J. Neurol. *236*:52, 1989.
69. Bergia, B., Sybers, H. D., and Butler, I. J.: Familial lethal cardiomyopathy with mental retardation and scapuloperoneal muscular dystrophy. J. Neurol. *49*:1423, 1986.
70. Woolliscroft, J., and Tuna, N.: Permanent atrial standstill: The clinical spectrum. Am. J. Med. *49*:2037, 1982.
71. Ward, D. E., Ho, S. Y., and Shinebourne, E. A.: Familial atrial standstill and inexcitability in childhood. Am. J. Cardiol. *53*:965, 1984.
72. Disertori, M., Guarnerio, M., Vergara, G., et al.: Familial endemic persistent atrial standstill in a small mountain community. Eur. Heart J. *4*:354, 1983.
73. Levy, S., Pouget, B., Bemurat, M., et al.: Partial atrial electrical standstill: Report of three cases and review of clinical and electrophysiological features. Eur. Heart J. *1*:107, 1980.
74. Effendy, F. N., Bolognesi, R., Bianchi, G., and Visioli, O.: Alternation of partial and total atrial standstill. J. Electrocardiol. *12*:121, 1979.
75. Miller, R. G., Layzer, R. B., Mellenthin, M. A., et al.: Emery-Dreifuss muscular dystrophy with autosomal dominant transmission. Neurology *35*:1230, 1985.
76. Rowland, L. P., Fetell, M., Alarte, M., et al.: Emery-Dreifuss muscular dystrophy. Ann. Neurol. *5*:111, 1979.
77. Fenichel, G. M., Sul, Y. C., Kilroy, A. W., and Blouin, R.: An autosomal dominant dystrophy with humeropelvic distribution and cardiomyopathy. Neurology *32*:1399, 1982.
78. Hopkins, L. C., Jackson, J. H., and Elsas, L. J.: Emery-Dreifuss humeroperoneal muscular dystrophy: An X-linked myopathy with unusual contractures and bradycardia. Ann. Neurol. *10*:230, 1981.
79. Dickey, P. P., Ziter, F. A., and Smith, R. A.: Emery-Dreifuss muscular dystrophy. J. Pediatr. *104*:555, 1984.
80. Oswald, A. H., Goldblatt, J., Horak, A. R., and Beighton, P.: Lethal cardiac conduction defects in Emery-Dreifuss muscular dystrophy. S. Afr. Med. J. *72*:567, 1987.
81. Wyse, D. G., Nath, F. C., and Brownell, A.K.W.: Benign X-linked (Emery-Dreifuss) muscular dystrophy is not benign. PACE *10*:533, 1987.
82. Yoshioka, M., Saida, K., Itagaki, Y., and Kamiya, T.: Follow up study of cardiac involvement in Emery-Dreifuss muscular dystrophy. Arch. Dis. Child. *64*:713, 1989.
83. Harper, P. S.: Myotonic Dystrophy. 2nd ed. Philadelphia, W. B. Saunders Company, 1989.
84. Wieringa, B., Brunner, H., Hulsebos, T., et al.: Genetic and physical demarcation of the locus for dystrophia myotonica. Adv. Neurol. *48*:47, 1988.
85. Bharati, S., Bump, F. T., Bauernfeind, R., and Lev, M.: Dystrophica myotonia. Correlative electrocardiographic, electrophysiologic and conduction system study. Chest *86*:444, 1984.
86. Moorman, J. R., Coleman, R. E., Packer, D. L., et al.: Cardiac involvement in myotonic muscular dystrophy. Medicine *64*:371, 1985.
87. Hiromasa, S., Ikeda, T., Kubota, K., et al.: Ventricular tachycardia and sudden death in myotonic dystrophy. Am. Heart J. *115*:914, 1988.
88. Nguyen, H. H., Wolfe, J. T., III, Holmes, D. R., Jr., and Edwards, W. D.: Pathology of the cardiac conduction system in myotonic dystrophy: A study of 12 cases. J. Am. Coll. Cardiol. *11*:662, 1988.
89. Hiromasa, S., Ikeda, T., Kubota, K., et al.: A family with myotonic dystrophy associated with diffuse cardiac conduction disturbances as demonstrated by His bundle electrocardiography. Am. Heart J. *111*:85, 1986.
90. Olofsson, B., Forsberg, H., Andersson, S., et al.: Electrocardiographic findings in myotonic dystrophy. Br. Heart J. *59*:47, 1988.
91. Grigg, L. E., Chan, W., Mond, H. G., et al.: Ventricular tachycardia and sudden death in myotonic dystrophy: Clinical, electrophysiologic and pathologic features. Am. J. Cardiol. *6*:254, 1985.
92. Prystowsky, E. N., Pritchett, E.L.C., Roses, A. D., and Gallagher, J. J.: The natural history of conduction system disease in myotonic muscular dystrophy as determined by serial electrophysiologic studies. Circulation *60*:1360, 1979.
93. Uemura, N., Tanaka, H., Niimura, T., et al.: Electrophysiological and histological abnormalities of the heart in myotonic dystrophy. Am. Heart J. *86*:616, 1973.
94. Petkovich, N. J., Dunn, M., and Reed, W.: Myotonia dystrophica with AV dissociation and Stokes-Adams attacks. Am. Heart J. *68*:391, 1964.
95. Motta, J., Guilleminault, C., Bilingham, M., et al.: Cardiac abnormalities in myotonic dystrophy: Electrophysiologic and histopathologic studies. Am. J. Med. *67*:467, 1979.
96. Ludatscher, R. M., Kerner, H., Amikam, S., and Gellei, B.: Myotonia dystrophica with heart involvement: An electron microscopic study of skeletal, cardiac, and smooth muscle. J. Clin. Pathol. *31*:1057, 1978.
97. Tanaka, N., Tanaka, H., Takeda, M., et al.: Cardiomyopathy in myotonic dystrophy: A light and electron microscopic study of the myocardium. Jpn. Heart J. *14*:202, 1973.
98. Hartwig, G. R., Ran, K. R., Radoff, F. M., et al.: Radionuclide angiocardiographic analysis of myocardial function in myotonic muscular dystrophy. Neurology *33*:657, 1983.
99. Child, J. S., and Perloff, J. K.: Diastolic properties of the left ventricle in myotonic muscular dystrophy (Steinert's disease). To be published.
100. Hiromasa, S., Ikeda, T., Kubota, K., et al.: A family with myotonic dystrophy associated with diffuse cardiac conduction disturbances as demonstrated by His bundle electrocardiography. Am. Heart J. *111*:85, 1986.
101. Forsberg, H., Olofsson, B., Eriksson, A., and Andersson, S.: Cardiac involvement in congenital myotonic dystrophy. Br. Heart J. *63*:119, 1990.
102. Anderson, M.: Probable Thomsen's disease with cardiac involvement. J. Neurol. *214*:301, 1977.
103. Subramony, S. H., Malhotra, C.P., and Mishra, S. K.: Distinguishing paramyotonia congenita and myotonia congenita by electromyography. Muscle Nerve *6*:374, 1983.
104. Streib, F. W., Sun, S. F., and Hanson, M.: Paramyotonia congenita: Clinical and electrophysiologic studies. Electromyogr. Clin. Neurophysiol. *23*:315, 1983.
105. Rosenberg, R. N.: Hereditary ataxias. *In* Rowland, L. P. (ed.): Merritt's Textbook of Neurology. Philadelphia, Lea & Febiger, 1984, p. 499.
106. Barbeau, H.: Friedreich's ataxia 1980. Our overview of the pathophysiology. J. Can. Sci. Neurol. *7*:455, 1980.
107. Harding, A. E.: Friedreich's ataxia: A clinical and genetic study of 90 families with an analysis of early diagnostic criteria and intrafamilial clustering of clinical features. Brain *104*:589, 1981.
108. Brumback, R. A., Panner, B. J., and Kingston, W. J.: The heart in Friedreich's ataxia. Arch. Neurol. *43*:189, 1986.
109. Grenadier, E., Goldberg, S. J., Stern, L. Z., and Feldman, J.: M-mode and two-dimensional echocardiographic examination of patients with Friedreich's ataxia. J. Cardiovasc. Ultrasonog. *3*:5, 1984.
110. Gottdiener, J. S., Hawley, R. J., Maron, B. J., et al.: Characteristics of the cardiac hypertrophy in Friedreich's ataxia. Am. Heart J. *103*:525, 1982.
111. Barbeau, A.: Pathophysiology of Friedreich's ataxia. *In* Matthews, W. B., and Glaser, G. H. (eds.): Recent Advances in Clinical Neurology, No. 3. Edinburgh, Churchill Livingstone, 1982, p. 129.
112. Pasternac, A., Drol, R., Petitclerc, R., et al.: Hypertrophic cardiomyopathy in Friedreich's ataxia: Symmetric or asymmetric? J. Can. Sci. Neurol. *7*:379, 1980.
113. Harding, A. E., and Hewer, R. L.: The heart disease of Friedreich's ataxia: A clinical and electrocardiographic study of 115 patients, with an analysis of serial electrocardiographic changes in 30 cases. Q. J. Med. *28*:489, 1983.
114. Zimmermann, M., Gabathuler, J., Adamec, R., and Pinget, L.: Unusual manifestations of heart involvement in Friedreich's ataxia. Am. Heart J. *111*:184, 1986.
115. Hawley, R. J., and Gottdiener, J. S.: Five-year follow-up of Friedreich's ataxia cardiomyopathy. Arch. Intern. Med. *146*:483, 1986.
116. Unverferth, D. V., Schmidt, W. R., Baker, P. B., and Wooley, C. F.: Morphologic and functional characteristics of the heart in Friedreich's ataxia. Am. J. Med. *82*:5, 1987.
117. Pentland, B., and Fox, K.A.A.: The heart in Friedreich's ataxia. J. Neurol. Neurosurg. Psychiatry *46*:1138, 1983.
118. Hawley, R. J., and Gottdiener, J. S.: Five-year follow-up of Friedreich's ataxia cardiomyopathy. Arch. Intern. Med. *146*:483, 1986.
119. Alboliras, E. T., Shub, C., Gomez, M. R., et al.: Spectrum of cardiac involvement in Friedreich's ataxia: Clinical, electrocardiographic and echocardiographic observations. Am. J. Cardiol. *58*:518, 1986.
120. Pentland, B., and Fox, K.A.A.: The heart in Friedreich's ataxia. J. Neurol. Neurosurg. Psychiatry *46*:1138, 1983.
121. James, T. N., Cobbs, B. W., Coghlan, H. C., et al.: Coronary disease, cardioneuropathy, and conduction system abnormalities in the cardiomyopathy of Friedreich's ataxia. Br. Heart J. *57*:446, 1987.
122. Spach, N. S., and Kootsey, J. M.: The nature of electrical propagation in cardiac muscle. Am. J. Physiol. *244*:H3, 1983.
123. Palagi, B., Picozzi, R., Casazza, F., et al.: Biventricular function in Friedreich's ataxia: A radionuclide angiographic study. Br. Heart J. *59*:692, 1988.
124. Giunta, A., Maione, S., Biagini, R., et al.: Noninvasive assessment of systolic and diastolic function in 50 patients with Friedreich's ataxia. Cardiology *75*:321, 1988.
125. Zimmermann, M., Gabathuler, J., Adamec, R., and Pinget, L.: Unusual manifestations of heart involvement in Friedreich's ataxia. Am. Heart J. *111*:184, 1986.
126. Rowland, L. P.: Molecular genetics, pseudogenetics and clinical neurology. Neurology *33*:179, 1983.
127. Rosenberg, R. N.: Biochemical genetics of neurologic disease. N. Engl. J. Med. *305*:1181, 1981.
128. Perloff, J. K.: Pathogenesis of hypertrophic cardiomyopathy. *In* Goodwin, J. F. (ed.): Heart Muscle DIsease. Lancaster, MTP Press Ltd., 1985.
129. Pasternac, A., Wagniart, P., Olivenstein, R., et al.: Increased plasma catecholamines in patients with Friedreich's ataxia. J. Can. Sci. Neurol. *9*:195, 1982.
130. Merkel, A. D., and Barbeau, A.: Plasma catecholamines in Friedreich's ataxia assayed using high performance liquid chromatography with electrochemical detection. J. Can. Sci. Neurol. *9*:205, 1982.

LESS COMMON NEUROMYOPATHIC DISEASES SOMETIMES ASSOCIATED WITH HEART DISEASE

131. Pleasure, D. E., and Schotland, D. L.: Hereditary neuropathies. *In* Rowland, L. P. (ed.): Merritt's Textbook of Neurology. Philadelphia, Lea & Febiger, 1984.
132. Isner, J. M., Hawley, R. J., Weintraub, A. B., and Engel, W. K.: Cardiac findings in Charcot-Marie-Tooth disease. Arch. Intern. Med. *139*:1161, 1979.
133. Dyck, P. J., Swanson, C. J., Nishimura, R. A., et al.: Cardiomyopathy in patients with hereditary motor and sensory neuropathy. Mayo Clin. Proc. *62*:672, 1987.
134. Leak, D.: Paroxysmal atrial flutter in peroneal muscular atrophy. Br. Heart J. *23*:326, 1961.
135. Littler, W. A.: Heart block and peroneal muscular atrophy. Q. J. Med. *39*:431, 1970.
136. Kaj, J. M., Littler, W. A., and Meade, J. B.: Ultrastructure of the myocardium in familial heart block and peroneal muscular atrophy. Br. Heart J. *34*:1081, 1972.
137. Lowry, P. I., and Littler, W. A.: Peroneal muscular atrophy associated with cardiac conduction tissue disease. Postgrad. Med. J. *59*:530, 1983.
138. Martin-Du Pan, R. C., Juse, C., and Perrenoud, J. J.: Congestive cardiomyopathy and pyruvate elevation in a case of Charcot-Marie-Tooth disease. Schweiz. med. Wochenschr. *5*:114, 1984.
139. Spiro, A. J., Shy, G. M., and Gonatas, N. K.: Myotubular myopathy. Arch. Neurol. *14*:1, 1966.
140. Verhiest, W., Brucher, J. M., Goddeeris, P., et al.: Familial centronuclear myopathy associated with cardiomyopathy. Br. Heart J. *38*:504, 1976.
141. Shafiq, S. A., Sande, M. A., Carruthers, R. R., et al.: Skeletal muscle in idiopathic cardiomyopathy. J. Neurol. Sci. *15*:303, 1972.
142. Berenberg, R. A., Pellock, J. M., DiMauro, S., et al.: Lumping or splitting? "Ophthalmoplegia-plus" or Kearns-Sayre syndrome? Ann. Neurol. *1*:37, 1977.
143. Lowes, M.: Chronic progressive external ophthalmoplegia, pigmentary retinopathy and heart block (Kearns-Sayre syndrome). Acta Ophthalmol. *53*:610, 1975.
144. Charles, R., Holt, S., Kay, J. M., et al.: Myocardial ultrastructure and the development of atrioventricular block in Kearns-Sayre syndrome. Circulation *63*:214, 1981.
145. Roberts, N. K., Perloff, J. K., and Kark, P.: Cardiac conduction in Kearns-Sayre syndrome. Am. J. Cardiol. *44*:1396, 1979.
146. Schwartzkopff, B., Frenzel, H., Losse, B., et al.: Heart involvement in progressive external ophthalmoplegia (Kearns-Sayre syndrome): Electrophysiologic, hemodynamic and morphologic findings. Z. Kardiol. *75*:161, 1986.
147. Schwartzkopff, B., Frenzel, H., Breithardt, G., et al.: Ultrastructural findings in endomyocardial biopsy of patients with Kearns-Sayre syndrome. J. Am. Coll. Cardiol. *12*:1522, 1988.
148. Channer, K. S., Channer, J. L., Campbell, M. J., and Rees, J. R.: Cardiomyopathy in the Kearns-Sayre syndrome. Br. Heart J. *59*:486, 1988.
149. Kenny, D., and Wetherbee, J.: Kearns-Sayre syndrome in the elderly: Mitochondrial myopathy with advanced heart block. Am. Heart J. *120*:440, 1990.
150. Clark, D. S., Myerburg, R. J., Morales, R. R., et al.: Heart block and Kearns-Sayre: Electrophysiologic-pathologic correlation. Chest *68*:727, 1975.
151. Pleasure, D. E., and Schotland, D. L.: Acquired neuropathies. *In* Rowland, L. P. (ed.): Merritt's Textbook of Neurology. 7th ed. Philadelphia, Lea & Febiger, 1984.
152. McDonagh, A.J.G., and Dawson, J.: Guillain-Barré syndrome after myocardial infarction. Br. Med. J. *294*:613, 1987.
153. Emmons, P. R., Blume, W. T., and DuShane, J. W.: Cardiac monitoring and demand pacemaker in Guillain-Barré syndrome. Arch. Neurol. *32*:59, 1975.
154. Greenland, P., and Griggs, R. C.: Arrhythmic complications in the Guillain-Barré syndrome. Arch. Intern. Med. *140*:1053, 1980.
155. Narayam, D., Huang, M. T., and Matthew, P. K.: Bradycardia and asystole requiring pacemaker in Guillain-Barré syndrome. Am. Heart J. *108*:426, 1984.
156. Fagius, J., and Wallin, B. G.: Microneurographic evidence of excessive sympathetic outflow in the Guillain-Barré syndrome. Brain *106*:589, 1983.
157. Persson, A., and Solders, G.: R-R variations in Guillain-Barré syndrome: A test of autonomic dysfunction. Acta Neurol. Scand. *67*:294, 1983.
158. Palferman, T. G., Wright, I., Doyle, D. V., and Amiel, S.: Electrocardiographic abnormalities and autonomic dysfunction in Guillain-Barré syndrome. Br. Med. J. *284*:1231, 1982.
159. Shy, G. M., Engel, W. K., Somers, J. E., and Wanko, T.: Nemaline myopathy; a new congenital myopathy. Brain *86*:793, 1963.
160. Conen, P. E., Murphy, G. E., and Donohue, W. L.: Light and electron microscopic studies of "myogranules" in a child with hypotonia and muscle weakness. Can. Med. Assoc. J. *89*:983, 1963.
160a. Ishibashi-Veda, H., Imakita, M., Yutani, C., et al.: Congenital nemaline myopathy with dilated cardiomyopathy: An autopsy study. Hum. Pathol. *21*:77, 1990.
161. Kinoshita, M., and Satoyoshi, E.: Type I fiber atrophy and nemaline bodies. Arch. Neurol. *31*:423, 1974.
162. Meier, C., Gertsch, M., Zimmerman, A., et al.: Nemaline myopathy presenting as cardiomyopathy. N. Engl. J. Med. *308*:1536, 1983.
163. Meier, C., Voellmy, W., Gertsch, M., et al.: Nemaline myopathy appearing in adults as cardiomyopathy: A clinicopathologic study. Arch. Neurol. *41*:443, 1984.
164. Penn, A. S., and Rowland, L. P.: Neuromuscular junction. *In* Rowland, L. P. (ed.): Merritt's Textbook of Neurology. 7th ed. Philadelphia, Lea & Febiger, 1984, p. 561.
165. Barnes, D. M.: Nervous and immune system disorders linked in a variety of diseases. Science *232*:160, 1985.
166. Gibson, T. C.: The heart in myasthenia gravis. Am. Heart J. *90*:389, 1975.
167. Kornfeld, P., Horowitz, S. H., Genkins, G., and Papatestas, A.: Myasthenia gravis unmasked by antiarrhythmic agents. Mt. Sinai J. Med. *43*:10, 1976.
168. Niakan, E., Bertorini, T. E., Acchiardo, S. R., and Werner, M. F.: Procainamide-induced myasthenia-like weakness in a patient with peripheral neuropathy. Arch. Neurol. *38*:378, 1981.
169. Ratinov, G., Baker, W. P., and Swaiman, K. F.: McArdle's syndrome with previously unreported electrocardiographic and serum enzyme abnormalities. Ann. Intern. Med. *62*:328, 1965.
170. Sengers, R.C.A., ter Haar, B.G.A., Trijhels, J.M.F., et al.: Congenital cataract and mitochondrial myopathy of skeletal and heart muscle associated with lactic acidosis after exercise. J. Pediatr. *86*:873, 1975.
171. Melki, J., Abdelhak, S., Sheth, P., et al.: Gene for chronic proximal spinal muscular atrophies maps to chromosome 5q. Nature *344*:767, 1990.
172. Kimura, S., Yokota, H., Tateda, K., et al.: A case of the Kugelberg-Welander syndrome complicated with cardiac lesions. Jpn. Heart J. *21*:417, 1980.
173. Gottdiener, J. S., Sherber, H. S., Hawley, R. J., and Engel, W. K.: Cardiac manifestations in polymyositis. Am. J. Cardiol. *41*:1141, 1978.
174. Singsen, B., Goldreyer, B., Stanton, R., and Hanson, V.: Childhood polymyositis with cardiac conduction defects. Am. J. Dis. Child. *131*:72, 1976.
175. Farber, H. W., and Make, B.: Physiologic closure of a symptomatic patent foramen ovale with oxygen therapy. Am. Rev. Resp. Dis. *131*:181, 1985.
176. Lisak, R. P., Lebeau, J., Tucker, S. H., and Rowland, L. P.: Hyperkalemic periodic paralysis and cardiac arrhythmias. Neurology *22*:810, 1972.
177. Buruma, O. J., Schipperheyn, J. J., and Bots, G. T.: Heart muscle disease in familial hypokalemic periodic paralysis. Circulation *64*:12, 1981.
178. Klein, R., Ganelin, R., Marks, J. F., et al.: Periodic paralysis with cardiac arrhythmia. J. Pediatr. *62*:371, 1963.
179. Kastor, J. A., and Goldreyer, B. N.: Ventricular origin of bidirectional tachycardia. Circulation *48*:897, 1973.
180. Karpawich, P. P., Hart, Z. H., Perry, B. L., et al.: Childhood periodic paralysis with dysrhythmias: Electrophysiologic and histopathologic evaluation. Am. Heart J. *114*:186, 1987.
181. Fukuda, K., Ogawa, S., Yokozuka, H., et al.: Long-standing bidirectional tachycardia in a patient with hypokalemic periodic paralysis. J. Electrocardiol. *21*:71, 1988.
182. Perloff, J. K. (ed.): The Cardiomyopathies. Philadelphia, W. B. Saunders Company, 1988.
183. Meyer, J. G., and Urban, K.: Electrolyte changes and acid-base balance after alcohol withdrawal. With special reference to rum fits and magnesium depletion. J. Neurol. *215*:135, 1977.
184. Rubin, E.: Alcoholic myopathy in heart and skeletal muscle. N. Engl. J. Med. *301*:28, 1979.
185. Clarren, S. K., and Smith, D. W.: The fetal alcohol syndrome. N. Engl. J. Med. *298*:1063, 1978.

ACUTE CEREBRAL DISORDERS ACCOMPANIED BY CARDIOVASCULAR ABNORMALITIES

186. Bramwell, C.: Can head injury cause auricular fibrillation? Lancet *1*:8, 1934.
187. Chen, H. I., Liao, J. F., and Ho, S. T.: Centrogenic pulmonary hemorrhagic edema induced by cerebral compression in rats. Circ. Res. *47*:366, 1980.
188. Schell, A. R., Shenoy, M. M., Friedman, S. A., and Patel, A. R.: Pulmonary edema associated with subarachnoid hemorrhage. Arch. Intern. Med. *147*:591, 1987.
189. Yamour, B. J., Sridharan, M. R., Rice, J. F., and Flowers, N. C.: Electrocardiographic changes in cerebrovascular hemorrhage. Am. Heart J. *99*:294, 1980.
190. Robertson, C. S., Clifton, G. L., Taylor, A. A., and Grossman, R. G.: Treatment of hypertension associated with head injury. J. Neurosurg. *59*:455, 1983.
191. Cushing, H.: Concerning a definite regulatory mechanism of the vasomotor center which controls blood pressure during cerebral compression. Bull. Johns Hopkins Hosp. *12*:390, 1901.
192. Sciarra, D.: Head injury. *In* Rowland, L. P. (ed.): Merritt's Textbook of Neurology. 7th ed. Philadelphia, Lea & Febiger, 1984, p. 277.
193. Hackenberry, L. E., Miner, M. E., Rea, G. L., et al.: Biochemical evidence of myocardial injury after severe head trauma. Crit. Care Med. *10*:641, 1982.
194. Clifton, G. L., Robertson, C. S., Kyper, K., et al.: Cerebrovascular response to severe head injury. J. Neurosurg. *59*:447, 1983.
195. McLeod, A. A., Neil-Dwyer, G., Meyer, C.H.A., et al.: Cardiac sequelae of acute head injury. Br. Heart J. *47*:221, 1982.
196. Tobias, S. L., Bookatz, B. J., and Diamond, T. H.: Myocardial damage and electrocardiographic changes in acute cerebrovascular hemorrhage: A report of three cases and review. Heart Lung *16*:521, 1987.
197. Pollick, C., Cujec, B., Parker, S., and Tator, C.: Left ventricular wall motion abnormalities in subarachnoid hemorrhage: An echocardiographic study. J. Am. Coll. Cardiol. *12*:600, 1988.
198. Baur, H. R., Gobel, F. L., and Pierach, C. A.: Electrocardiographic changes after cervical laminectomy. Int. J. Cardiol. *1*:37, 1981.
199. Samuels, M. A.: Electrocardiographic manifestations of neurologic disease. Semin. Neurol. *4*:453, 1984.

200. Carruth, J. E., and Silverman, M. E.: *Torsades de pointes* atypical ventricular tachycardia complicating subarachnoid hemorrhage. Chest *78*:886, 1980.
201. Mikolich, J. R., Jacobs, W. C., and Fletcher, G. F.: Cardiac arrhythmias in patients with acute cerebrovascular accidents. J.A.M.A. *246*:1314, 1981.
202. Goldberger, A. L.: Recognition of ECG pseudoinfarct patterns. Mod. Concepts Cardiovasc. Dis. *49*:13, 1980.
203. Taylor, A. L., and Fozzard, H. A.: Ventricular arrhythmias associated with CNS disease. Arch. Intern. Med. *142*:232, 1982.
204. Gould, L., Reddy, R. C., Kollali, M., et al.: Electrocardiographic normalization after cerebral vascular accident. J. Electrocardiol. *14*:191, 1981.
205. Myers, M. G., Norris, J. W., Hachinski, V. C., et al.: Cardiac sequelae of acute stroke. Stroke *13*:838, 1982.
206. Stober, T., Anstätt, T., Sen, S., et al.: Cardiac arrhythmias in subarachnoid haemorrhage. Acta Neurochir. *93*:37, 1988.
207. Rudehill, A., Olsson, G. L., Sundqvist, K., and Gordon, E.: ECG abnormalities in patients with subarachnoid haemorrhage and intracranial tumours. J. Neurol. Neurosurg. Psychiatry *50*:1375, 1987.
208. Melin, J., and Fogelhohm, R.: Electrocardiographic findings in subarachnoid hemorrhage. Acta Med. Scand. *213*:5, 1983.
209. Brunninkhuis, L.G.H.: Electrocardiographic abnormalities suggesting myocardial infarction in a patient with severe cranial trauma. PACE *6*:1336, 1983.
210. Gascon, P., Ley, T. J., Toltzis, R. J., and Bonow, R. O.: Spontaneous subarachnoid hemorrhage simulating acute transmural myocardial infarction. Am. Heart J. *105*:511, 1983.
211. Tabbaa, M. A., Ramirez-Lassepas, M., and Snyder, B. D.: Aneurysmal subarachnoid hemorrhage presenting as cardiorespiratory arrest. Arch. Intern. Med. *147*:1661, 1987.
212. Fredberg, U., Bøtker, H. E., and Rømer, F. K.: Acute neurogenic pulmonary oedema following generalized tonic clonic seizure. A case report and a review of the literature. Eur. Heart J. *9*:933, 1988.
213. Oppenheimer, S. M., Cechetto, D. F., and Hachinski, V. C.: Cerebrogenic cardiac arrhythmias. Arch. Neurol. *47*:513, 1990.
214. Lehmann, K. G., Lane, J. G., Piepmeier, J. M., and Batsford, W. P.: Cardiovascular abnormalities accompanying acute spinal cord injury in humans: Incidence, time course and severity. J. Am. Coll. Cardiol. *10*:46, 1987.
215. Miah, K., von Arbin, M., Britton, M., et al.: Prognosis in acute stroke with special reference to some cardiac factors. J. Chronic Dis. *36*:279, 1983.
216. Komrad, M. S., Coffey, C. E., Coffey, K. S., et al.: Myocardial infarction and stroke. Neurology *34*:1403, 1984.
217. Chin, P. L., Kaminski, J., and Rout, N.: Myocardial infarction coincident with cerebrovascular accidents in the elderly. Age Ageing *6*:29, 1977.
218. Gillum, R. F., Fortmann, S. P., Prineas, R. J., and Kottke, T. E.: International diagnostic criteria for acute myocardial infarction and acute stroke. Am. Heart J. *108*:150, 1984.
219. Sandok, B. A., Whisnant, J. P., Furlan, A. J., and Mickell, J. L.: Carotid arterial bruits. Mayo Clin. Proc. *57*:227, 1982.
220. Heyman, A., Wilkinson, W. E., Heyden, S., et al.: Risk of stroke in asymptomatic persons with cervical arterial bruits. N. Engl. J. Med. *302*:838, 1980.
221. Sundt, T. M., Jr., Whisnant, J. P., Houser, O. W., and Fode, N. C.: Prospective study of the effectiveness and durability of carotid endarterectomy. Mayo Clin. Proc. *65*:625, 1990.
222. Roper, A. H., Wechsler, L. R., and Wilson, L. S.: Carotid bruit and the risk of stroke in elective surgery. N. Engl. J. Med. *307*:1388, 1982.
223. Busuttil, R. W., Baker, J. D., Davidson, R. K., and Machleder, H. I.: Carotid arterial stenosis: Hemodynamic significance and clinical course. J.A.M.A. *245*:1438, 1981.
224. Matchar, D. B.: Decision making in the face of uncertainty: The case of carotid endarterectomy. Mayo Clin. Proc. *65*:756, 1990.
225. Wolf, P. A., Kannel, W. B., Sorlie, P., and McNamara, P.: Asymptomatic carotid bruit and risk of stroke. J.A.M.A. *245*:1442, 1981.
226. Langlois, Y., Roederer, G. O., Chan, A., et al.: Evaluating carotid arterial disease. Ultrasound Med. Biol. *9*:51, 1983.
227. Cebul, R. D., and Ginsberg, M. D.: Noninvasive neurovascular tests for carotid artery disease. Ann. Intern. Med. *97*:867, 1982.
228. Jones, E. L., Craver, J. M., Michalik, R. A., et al.: Combined carotid and coronary operations: When are they necessary? J. Thorac. Cardiovasc. Surg. *87*:7, 1984.
229. Rice, P. L., Pifarre, R., Sullivan, H. J., et al.: Experience with simultaneous myocardial revascularization and carotid endarterectomy. J. Thorac. Cardiovasc. Surg. *79*:922, 1980.
230. Breslau, P. J., Fell, G., Ivey, T. D., et al.: Carotid arterial disease in patients undergoing coronary artery bypass operations. J. Thorac. Cardiovasc. Surg. *82*:765, 1981.
231. Breuer, A. C., Hanson, M. R., Furlan, A. J., et al.: Central nervous system complications of myocardial revascularization. A prospective analysis of 400 patients. Stroke *11*:136, 1980.
232. Gonzalez-Scarano, F., and Hurtig, H. I.: Neurologic complications of coronary artery bypass grafting: Case-control study. Neurology *31*:1032, 1981.
233. Bojar, R. M., Najafi, H., De Laria, G. A., et al.: Neurological complications of coronary revascularization. Ann. Thorac. Surg. *36*:427, 1983.
234. Sotaniemi, K. A.: Brain damage and neurological outcome after open heart surgery. J. Neurol. Neurosurg. Psychiatry *43*:127, 1980.
235. Ferry, P. C.: Neurologic sequelae of cardiac surgery in children. Am. J. Dis. Child. *141*:309, 1987.
236. Cerebral Embolism Task Force: Cardiogenic brain embolism. Arch. Neurol. *43*:71, 1986.
237. Kopecky, S. L., Gersh, B. J., McGoon, M. D., et al.: The natural history of lone atrial fibrillation. N. Engl. J. Med. *317*:669, 1987.
238. Stroke Prevention in Atrial Fibrillation Study Group Investigators: Preliminary report of the stroke prevention in atrial fibrillation study. N. Engl. J. Med. *322*:863, 1990.
239. Perloff, J. K., and Child, J. S.: Clinical and epidemiological issues in mitral valve prolapse. Am. Heart J. *113*:1324, 1987.
240. Wolf, P. A., and Sila, C. A.: Cerebral ischemia with mitral valve prolapse. Am. Heart J. *113*:1308, 1987.
241. Yufe, R., Karpati, G., and Carpenter, S.: Cardiac myxoma: A diagnostic challenge for the neurologist. Neurology *26*:1060, 1976.
242. Perloff, J. K.: The Clinical Recognition of Congenital Heart Disease. 3rd ed. Philadelphia, W. B. Saunders Company, 1987.
243. Salgado, A. V., Furlan, A. J., and Keys, T. F.: Mycotic aneurysm, subarachnoid hemorrhage, and indications for cerebral angiography in infective endocarditis. Stroke *18*:1057, 1987.
244. Salgado, A. V., Furlan, A. J., Keys, T. F., et al.: Neurologic complications of endocarditis: A 12-year experience. Neurology *39*:173, 1989.
245. Grandsden, W. R., Eykyn, S. J., and Leach, R. M.: Neurological presentations of native valve endocarditis. Q. J. Med. *73*:1135, 1989.
246. Baron, K. D., Siqueira, E., and Hirano, A.: Cerebral embolism caused by nonbacterial thrombotic endocarditis. Neurology *10*:391, 1960.
247. Caplan, L. R., Hier, D. B., and Banks, G.: Stroke and drug abuse. Curr. Concepts Cerebrovasc. Dis. *17*:9, 1982.
248. Biller, J., Johnson, M. R., Adams, H. P., Jr., et al.: Further observations on cerebral or retinal ischemia in patients with right-left intracardiac shunts. Arch. Neurol. *44*:740, 1987.
249. Lechat, P., Mas, J. L., Lascault, G., et al.: Prevalence of patent foramen ovale in patients with stroke. N. Engl. J. Med. *318*:1148, 1988.
250. Harvey, J. R., Teague, S. M., Anderson, J. L., et al.: Clinically silent atrial septal defects with evidence for cerebral embolization. Ann. Intern. Med. *105*:695, 1986.
251. Pitkin, R. M., Perloff, J. K., Koos, B. J., and Beall, M. H.: Pregnancy and congenital heart disease. Ann. Intern. Med. *112*:445, 1990.
252. Schneider, B., Hanrath, P., Vogel, P., and Meinertz, T.: Improved morphologic characterization of atrial septal aneurysm by transesophageal echocardiography: Relation to cerebrovascular events. J. Am. Coll. Cardiol. *16*:1000, 1990.
253. Dodge, R. P., Richardson, E. P., and Victor, M.: Recurrent convulsive seizures as a sequel to cerebral infarction. Brain *77*:610, 1959.
254. Perloff, J. K., Rosove, M. H., Child, J. S., and Wright, G. B.: Adults with cyanotic congenital heart disease: Hematologic management. Ann. Intern. Med. *109*:406, 1988.
255. Daniels, S. R., Bates, S. R., and Kaplan, S.: EEG monitoring during paroxysmal hyperpnea of tetralogy of Fallot: An epileptic or hypoxic phenomenon? J. Child Neurol. *2*:98, 1987.
256. Longstreth, W. T., Inui, T. S., Cobb, L. A., and Copass, M. K.: Neurologic recovery after out-of-hospital cardiac arrest. Ann. Intern. Med. *98*:588, 1983.
257. Bircher, N. G.: Neurologic management following cardiac arrest. Neurol. Crit. Care *5*:773, 1989.

CARDIAC COMPLICATIONS OF DRUGS USED IN TREATING NEUROMUSCULAR DISEASE

258. Bircher, N. G.: Brain resuscitation. Resuscitation *18*:S1, 1989.
259. Orlando, R. C., Moyer, P., and Barnett, T. B.: Methysergide therapy and constrictive pericarditis. Ann. Intern. Med. *88*:213, 1978.
260. Bana, D. S., MacNeal, P. S., LeCompte, P. M., et al.: Cardiac murmurs and endocardial fibrosis associated with methysergide therapy. Am. Heart J. *88*:640, 1974.
261. Dorne, H. L., and Satin, R.: Methysergide-induced lower extremity arterial insufficiency. J. Can. Assoc. Radiol. *37*:210, 1986.
262. Yahr, M. D.: Parkinsonism. *In* Rowland, L. P. (ed.): Merritt's Textbook of Neurology. 7th ed. Philadelphia, Lea & Febiger, 1984, p. 526.
263. Lane, R.J.M., Roche, S. W., Leung, A.A.W., et al.: Cyclosporin neurotoxicity in cardiac transplant recipients. J. Neurol. Neurosurg. Psychiatry *51*:1434, 1988.
264. Hotson, J. R., and Enzmann, D. R.: Neurologic complications of cardiac transplantation. Neurol. Clin. *6*:349, 1988.
265. Ang, L. C., Gillett, J. M., and Kaufmann, J.C.E.: Neuropathology of heart transplantation. Can. J. Neurol. Sci. *16*:291, 1989.
266. Francis, D. A., Heron, J. R., and Clarke, M.: Ambulatory electrocardiographic monitoring in patients with transient focal cerebral ischaemia. J. Neurol. Neurosurg. Psychiatry *47*:256, 1984.
267. Benorvitz, N. L.: Clinical applications of the pharmacokinetics of lidocaine. Cardiovasc. Clin. *6*:77, 1974.
268. Weidler, D. J., Jallad, N. S., Keener, D. B., et al.: The effects of acute focal cerebral ischemia on digoxin toxicity and pharmacokinetics. Pharmacology *20*:188, 1980.
269. Withering, W.: An account of the Foxglove. *In* Willius, F. A., and Keys, T. E.: Classics of Cardiology. Vol. 1. Malabar, Fla., Robert E. Krieger Publishing Co., 1983, p. 244.
270. Oliveira, J.S.M., dos Santos, J.C.M., Muccillo, G., and Ferreira, A. L.: Increased capacity of the coronary arteries in chronic Chagas' heart disease: Further support for the neurogenic pathogenetic concept. Am. Heart J. *109*:304, 1985.
271. Iosa, D., DeQuattro, V., Lee, D. D., et al.: Plasma norepinephrine in Chagas' cardioneuromyopathy: A marker of progressive dysautonomia. Am. Heart J. *117*:882, 1989.

Endocrine and Nutritional Disorders and Heart Disease

by GORDON H. WILLIAMS, M.D., and EUGENE BRAUNWALD, M.D.

In 1835, Robert Graves described "three cases of violent and long-continued palpitation in females" with thyrotoxicosis.[1] Twenty years later, Thomas Addison reported that patients with disease of the "suprarenal capsules" had a "pulse, small and feeble . . . excessively soft and compressible." As the disease progressed, "the body wastes . . . the pulse becomes smaller and weaker, and . . . the patient at length gradually sinks and expires."[2] Thus, since the mid-19th century, it has been known that deranged hormonal secretion can significantly alter cardiovascular function. The purpose of this chapter is to summarize the more important cardiovascular manifestations of endocrine and nutritional diseases.

ACROMEGALY

The anterior pituitary gland secretes at least seven polypeptide hormones. Four (ACTH and related peptides, FSH, LH, and TSH) primarily produce their biological effect indirectly by altering hormonal secretion from a specific target gland (adrenal cortex, gonad, or thyroid). Thus, the pathophysiological manifestations of a derangement in their secretion are the same as those of their target organs and will be discussed later. There are no cardiovascular manifestations of altered prolactin secretion or growth hormone deficiency; however, acromegaly (growth hormone excess) is associated with a number of clinical signs and symptoms related to the cardiovascular system.

ACTIONS OF GROWTH HORMONE. Growth hormone is only one of a family of peptides whose overall function is to regulate growth of the organism.[3,4] Two hormones secreted by the hypothalamus (somatotropin-releasing hormone and somatostatin) regulate the release of growth hormone from the anterior pituitary.[5,6] After growth hormone is released into the circulation, it stimulates the production of insulin-like growth factors (IGF-I and IGF-II).[7] These growth factors are primarily made under the influence of growth hormone in the liver. They are homologs of the proinsulin molecule and therefore have biological effects that are qualitatively similar to those of insulin. It is uncertain whether either or both can be produced in the absence of growth hormone, although presently available data suggest that at least IGF-II, the weaker growth-promoting hormone, may not require growth hormone for synthesis. Thus, it is likely that IGF-I (somatomedin C) may be the major final mediator of growth hormone's biological effects.[3,4] It feeds back on the pituitary, modifying mRNA levels in the pituitary and growth hormone secretion.[8] In this chapter, by convention the term *growth hormone effects* is used, although most of these effects are probably mediated by the insulin-like growth factors, particularly somatomedin C.

Growth hormone effects influence many metabolic processes, but the net effect is anabolic. Thus, when growth hormone is administered to a growth hormone–deficient individual, positive nitrogen balance, with retention of calcium, sodium, potassium, magnesium, and chloride, is manifest within days.[3,4] While many facets of nitrogen metabolism following administration of growth hormone have been studied, its primary effect has not been assessed definitively. Growth hormone increases the synthesis of both transfer and messenger RNA.[9] It reduces the breakdown of amino acids to urea and increases the transport of amino acids into skeletal and cardiac muscle, thus augmenting the substrate available for protein synthesis.[10] However, direct measurement of intracellular amino acid content has not documented the increase expected if these actions were the only ones responsible for the increased protein synthesis.

Growth hormone also induces changes in both fat and carbohydrate metabolism.[3] When administered for a short time, it increases the uptake and utilization of glucose by fat cells, thus increasing lipogenesis. However, when administered over a long period, it promotes lipolysis, thus increasing plasma free fatty acid levels and their oxidation and promoting ketogenesis, particularly in diabetic patients or animals. Growth hormone reduces glucose uptake by fat and muscle cells, increases gluconeogenesis, and increases peripheral resistance to insulin; as a consequence, plasma glucose levels rise. Because of this reduced tissue uptake of glucose and the increased blood levels of free fatty acids and ketones, those tissues, like the myocardium, that are able to use these latter compounds as energy substrates do so. Growth hormone also increases the synthesis and/or accumulation of sulfated mucopolysaccharides in connective tissue.

EFFECT OF GROWTH HORMONE AND SOMATOSTATIN ON THE HEART. Short-term administration of growth hormone to normal subjects, which produces changes in growth hormone levels similar to those observed in patients with mild acromegaly, increases heart rate and myocardial contractility, the latter reflected in fractional shortening of the left ventricle and mean circumferential shortening of velocity, determined by echocardiography.[11] There is no effect on mean arterial blood pressure. *Somatostatin* has an effect on the heart beyond that induced by its effect on growth hormone secretion. Infusion of somatostatin causes bradycardia and a fall in cardiac output. Furthermore, in some cases of supraventricular arrhythmias somatostatin administration restores sinus rhythm.[12] Finally, cardiac nerves have been shown to contain somatostatin, suggesting that this hormone may be an important physiological regulator of cardiac conduction.[13]

CLINICAL AND BIOCHEMICAL MANIFESTATIONS. Acromegaly is almost invariably the result of a growth hormone–producing chromophobic or eosinophilic pituitary adenoma, although rarely it may be secondary to ectopic production of growth hormone or somatotropin-releasing hormone.[14] Characteristically, the disease is a slowly progressive one with signs and symptoms often predating diagnosis by more than 10 years. The striking physical findings (broad, spadelike hands and feet) are the result of growth hormone's effect on bone, muscle, and connective tissue. Osteoarthritis is common, as are organomegaly, hypertrichosis, hyperhidrosis, and modest weight gain.[15]

A derangement in carbohydrate metabolism is the most common metabolic consequence of chronic overproduction of growth hormone. Impaired glucose tolerance is found in half the patients, and hyperinsulinism is present in nearly all; thus a state of insulin resistance exists. However, clinical diabetes mellitus is present in only 10 per cent of patients, which suggests that only those who are predisposed and have limited insulin reserve actually develop overt disease.[16] The insulin-resistant state also may contribute to other features of the disease, e.g., the hypertension. While it might be anticipated that hyperlipidemia would be common in acromegaly, it is in fact infrequently observed except in patients with clinical diabetes mellitus.[3,4,16] Even in these patients, it is probably secondary to the decreased secretion of insulin rather than to the increased secretion of growth hormone.

CARDIOVASCULAR MANIFESTATIONS

The cardiac manifestations of acromegaly include cardiac enlargement that is greater than would be anticipated for the generalized organomegaly. In addition, the frequency of a number of other cardiovascular disorders is increased in acromegaly: hypertension, premature coronary artery disease, congestive heart failure, and cardic arrhythmias, particularly frequent ventricular premature beats and intraventricular conduction defects.[17,18] Indeed, because of the frequent occurrence of congestive heart failure and cardic arrhythmias in patients who otherwise have no predisposing factors (e.g., no hypertension or arteriosclerosis), it has been suggested that a specific acromegalic cardiomyopathy exists[19] (see below).

CARDIOMEGALY. Nearly all patients with acromegaly have cardiomegaly (Fig. 61–1), particularly after the fifth decade.[20,21] Echocardiographic assessment suggests that frequently there is an increase in cardiac mass, particularly asymmetrical septal hypertrophy, and in a sizable minority left ventricular dilatation and a reduced ejection fraction.[21] Although the cardiomegaly may be related to the generalized effect of growth hormone on protein synthesis, some data suggest that other factors may also be important. For example, enlargement of the heart is often greater than that of other organs. Furthermore, there is no direct relationship between the degree of cardiomegaly and the level of circulating growth hormone.[17] While there is a correlation between the duration of acromegaly and the severity of cardiac hypertrophy,[19] other factors which may be important in the genesis of cardiomegaly include hypertension and atherosclerosis, both of which occur with increased frequency in acromegaly. Focal cardiac interstitial fibrosis and a myocarditis with lymphocytic infiltrate also have been reported in the majority of cases.[19,22] The former is probably due to the effect of growth hormone on collagen synthesis. Additionally, small-vessel disease of the myocardium occasionally may be present.[19] The resultant dysfunction in cardiac contraction secondary to any of these pathological changes could also contribute to the cardiac hypertrophy. Finally, the cardiomyopathy characteristic of acromegaly may also contribute to the cardiomegaly.

HYPERTENSION. This is the most common cardiovascular manifestation of acromegaly, occurring in 15 to 50 per cent of patients if individuals with hypopituitarism are excluded. Hypertensive acromegalic patients tend to be older and to have had their acromegaly longer than nonhypertensive acromegalic patients. The underlying pathophysiology is uncertain. However, the hypertension usually is mild, uncomplicated, and readily responsive to drugs.[17] Most investigators either have searched for factors other than growth hormone that could cause hypertension or have attempted to determine how growth hormone itself may produce hypertension. In many respects, in patients with acromegaly there appears to be volume expansion; the presence of an increase in glomerular filtration rate, renal plasma flow, extracellular fluid volume and sodium space, and reduction in plasma renin activity all support this hypothesis.[4,23] Indeed, there is a striking increase in total exchangeable sodium in active acromegaly that is reduced following treatment. Thus, several studies have assessed the secretion of aldosterone in acromegaly; while increased secretion has been reported, this is an uncommon finding.[23] What does appear to occur frequently in acromegalics, however, is a change in tissue responsiveness to angiotensin II. Thus, with a sodium-restricted intake the response of aldosterone production to angiotensin II is decreased, but the vasoconstrictor response is increased when compared to normal subjects. This abnormality is present in both hypertensive and normotensive acromegalics.[24] Whether this is related to the pathogenesis of the elevated arterial pressure or is simply a reflection of an expanded extracellular fluid volume is unclear.

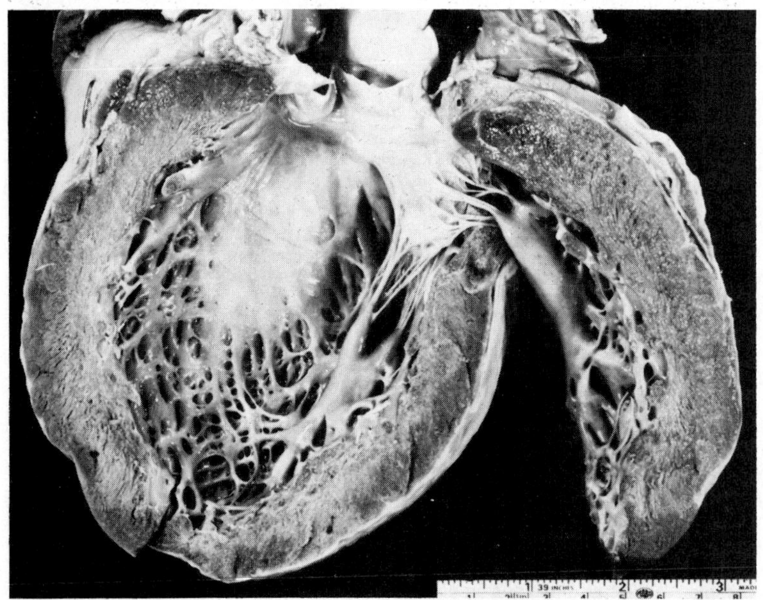

FIGURE 61–1. Opened left ventricle of the heart, showing the marked dilatation and hypertrophy, with fibrosis in the left septal endocardium. (From Rossi, L., et al.: Dysrhythmias and sudden death in acromegalic heart disease. A clinicopathologic study. Chest *72*:496, 1977.)

A number of studies have suggested that growth hormone itself may be responsible for the hypertension. Thus, pituitary irradiation or hypophysectomy significantly reduces arterial pressure in hypertensive acromegalic patients, even when full glucocorticoid replacement is carried out, unless growth hormone levels are not normalized.[18,24] Indeed, the apparent volume expansion may be directly related to the elevated growth hormone levels, since administration of growth hormone can produce retention of sodium, expansion of extracellular fluid volume, and abnormalities in white blood cell sodium transport.[25,26] It has been proposed that the pathophysiology of the hypertension in acromegaly may be similar to that in essential hypertension. In both conditions, there may be initial elevation of cardiac output secondary to expansion of extracellular fluid volume (Chap. 28). This could elevate arterial pressure and lead ultimately to changes in the peripheral vasculature producing fixed hypertension.

ATHEROSCLEROSIS. In view of the alterations in carbohydrate and lipid metabolism caused by growth hormone (see above) as well as the high incidence of hypertension, it is not surprising that premature atherosclerosis occurs in patients with acromegaly. What is uncertain is its frequency.[19] Coronary atherosclerosis could also contribute to the cardiomegaly observed in these patients.

ACROMEGALIC CARDIOMYOPATHY. Some patients with acromegaly without evidence of hypertension or atherosclerosis have significant cardiac dysfunction.[19] They primarily have cardiomegaly, congestive heart failure, and/or cardiac dysrhythmias[22]; the congestive heart failure is particularly resistant to conventional therapy. It has been suggested that these are manifestations of an acromegalic cardiomyopathy which is related to the higher collagen content per gram of heart than in normal myocardium.[19] Histological observations show cellular hypertrophy, patchy fibrosis, and myofibrillar degeneration (Fig. 61–2). Sudden death has been associated with inflammatory and degenerative damage to the sinoatrial perinodal nerve plexus and degeneration of the AV node.[22]

It is not clear whether acromegalic cardiomyopathy is a specific entity. The evidence favoring this view, though indirect, comes from five types of observations: (1) Nearly 50 per cent of acromegalic patients have electrocardiographic abnormalities.[27] The most common findings are ST-segment depression with or without T-wave abnormalities, patterns consistent with left ventricular hypertrophy, intraventricular conduction disturbances—specifically, bundle branch block—and, infrequently, supraventricular or ventricular ectopic rhythms. While hypertension or signs of atherosclerosis are present in many, 10 to 20 per cent of patients with acromegaly and electrocardiographic changes have no evidence of these conditions. (2) Ten to twenty per cent of acromegalics have overt congestive heart failure. In perhaps a fourth of these there is no known predisposing cause. (3) The majority of patients with acromegaly but without hypertension or atherosclerosis have subclinical evidence for cardiac, particularly diastolic, dysfunction.[28,29] (4) Approximately half of all patients with acromegaly, including patients without hypertension, have echocardiographic evidence of left ventricular hypertrophy.[30,31] These patients have growth hormone levels that are significantly higher than those of patients without left ventricular hypertrophy. Half of the patients with left ventricular hypertrophy exhibit asymmetrical septal hypertrophy, and these patients have a significantly greater percentage of internal dimensional shortening during systole than either the patients with concentric hypertrophy or those without left ventricular hypertrophy. (5) In one series of 256 acromegalic patients, 10 had cardiac abnormalities that could not be explained by diabetes, valvular disease, thyroid disease, angina, or myocardial ischemia. In six of these 10 patients, biochemical cure was achieved with surgery, but cardiac function did not improve appreciably. In one of these, who died, there was histological evidence of myocarditis. Of those patients in whom acromegaly remained active, three died; in one, postmortem examination revealed interstitial cardiac fibrosis.

DIAGNOSIS AND TREATMENT

The *diagnosis* of acromegaly is established by documenting the nonsuppressibility of serum growth hormone levels following glucose loading.[4] In most laboratories, growth hormone concentrations in normal subjects are less than 2 ng/ml 120 minutes after the oral administration of 100 gm of glucose. It is also important to evaluate the integrity of the other pituitary hormones, and, in hypertensive patients, to rule out an associated pheochromocytoma or aldosteronoma. The presence of sinus tachycardia or atrial fibrillation in a patient with acromegaly warrants a careful search for coexisting hyperthyroidism.

Surgery and irradiation remain the mainstays of treatment. The surgical approach is more often transsphenoidal rather than transfrontal; heavy particle (proton beam) instead of conventional irradiation is often used.[32] Because of the delayed reduction in growth hormone levels with the latter method, progression of cardiovascular disease in acromegalics continues even though growth hormone levels are falling. In a 10-year follow-up of 11 acromegalic patients, myocardial infarction, dysrhythmias, hypertension,

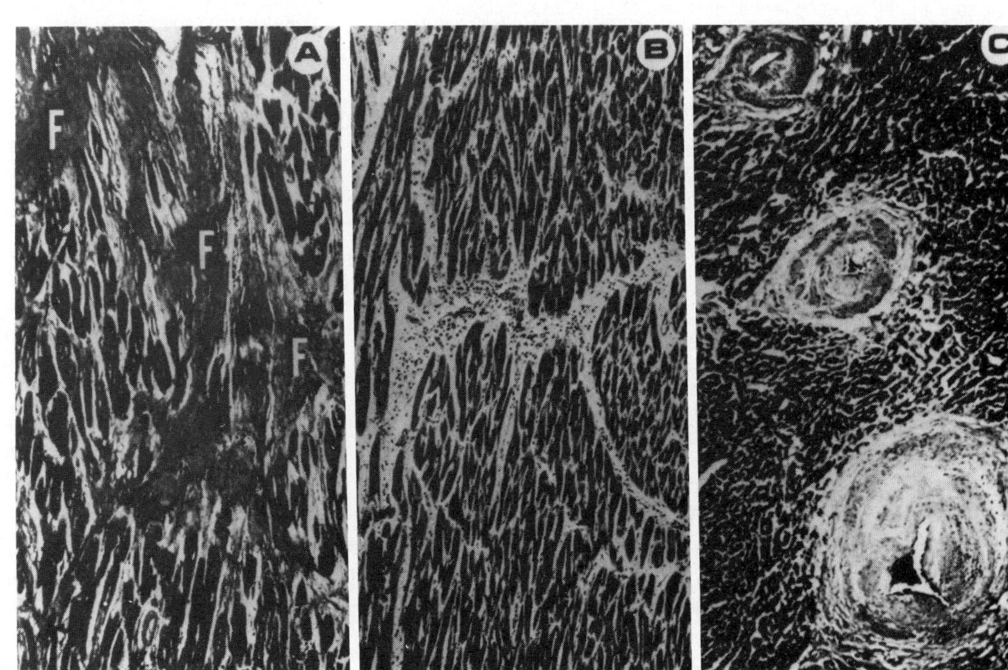

FIGURE 61–2. Histopathological features of acromegalic heart disease. *A,* Nonspecific myocardial hypertrophy and interstitial fibrosis (F). *B,* Myocarditis with predominantly lymphomononuclear cell infiltrate. *C,* Small-vessel disease (proliferative fibrous wall thickening) or intramural coronary artery branches. (Reproduced with permission from Lie, J. T.: Acromegaly and heart disease. Primary Cardiol. *7*:53, 1981. Copyright PW Communications, Inc.)

major artery disease, and heart failure all increased significantly even though the growth hormone levels were falling.[18] The secretion of growth hormone can be suppressed in some acromegalics with the dopamine agonist bromocriptine, and somatostatin.[33,34] Whether these agents have any effect on tumor growth, however, is unclear.

Acromegalic patients with cardiovascular abnormalities usually respond to conventional therapeutic measures for hypertension, heart failure, and arrhythmias. Two caveats: (1) those with hypertension appear to be particularly responsive to volume-depleting maneuvers, i.e., diuretics and sodium restriction, perhaps even more so than patients with essential hypertension; (2) on the other hand, some patients with congestive heart failure, primarily those *without* underlying hypertensive heart disease (i.e., those who are considered to have acromegalic cardiomyopathy), appear to be particularly resistant to therapy.

THYROID DISEASE

Thyroid hormone has a profound effect on a number of metabolic processes in virtually all tissues, with the heart being particularly sensitive to its effects. Therefore, it is not surprising that thyroid dysfunction can produce dramatic cardiovascular effects, often mimicking primary cardiac disease.

ACTION OF THYROID HORMONE. Two biologically active hormones are secreted by the thyroid: thyroxine (T4) and triiodothyronine (T3). Most studies support the hypothesis that T3 is the final mediator and that T4 is a prohormone, primarily because of the universal presence of T3 but not T4 nuclear receptors in tissues responsive to thyroid hormone, specifically the heart.[35-39]

Even though the mechanism of action of thyroid hormone has been intensively investigated over the past three decades, uncertainty still exists about its principal effects. The preponderance of evidence now suggests that the major site of initiation of action of thyroid hormone is on the cell nucleus.[36] It has been observed that thyroid hormone is specifically bound to a chromatin-bound nonhistone nucleoprotein in the nucleus. As a result of this binding, alterations occur in protein synthesis, leading to many of the biochemical and metabolic effects observed with T4 administration.[37,38] According to this hypothesis, the increased oxygen consumption results not from a direct interaction between thyroid hormone and mitochondria, an older hypothesis, but rather indirectly via an increase in mitochondrial protein synthesis secondary to the effect of the thyroid hormone on the nucleus. Support for this hypothesis comes from several sources: (1) specific binding of T3 and, much less strongly, of T4 to nuclear receptor sites has been documented[39]; (2) those tissues sensitive to thyroid hormone have nuclear binding sites[36]; (3) the addition of thyroid hormone in vitro produces an increase in O_2 consumption only after a significant time lag; (4) an early metabolic effect of T4 is an increased rate of incorporation of a labeled precursor into nuclear RNA[40]; (5) inhibitors of protein synthesis prevent many, if not most, of thyroid hormone's effects[41]; and (6) treatment of hypothyroid animals with T3 causes increases in in vivo synthesis of specific messenger RNA's in several tissues, including the heart.[42]

Effect on Na^+, K^+-ATPase. Guernsey and Edelman have extended this hypothesis one step further.[43] They postulated that not only does thyroid hormone enhance protein synthesis, but it specifically increases the activity of Na^+, K^+-ATPase. Thus, the augmented hydrolysis of ATP at the site of the sodium pump in the sarcolemma stimulates cellular (mitochondrial) oxygen consumption. Support for this hypothesis includes the observations that (1) hypothyroid rats treated with T3 exhibit a reduction in active sodium transport in crude homogenates and membrane-rich fractions and a decrease in intracellular Na^+/K^+ ratio in liver, diaphragm, and kidney, and (2) the number of renal Na^+ pump sites and the incorporation of radiolabeled methionine into renal cortical Na^+, K^+-ATPase are both increased, suggesting an increase in protein synthesis as the primary event. Some reports, however, have suggested that the effect of thyroid hormone on cellular respiration cannot be entirely secondary to a change in the activity of this enzyme[44,45] and that thyroid hormone also affects other cellular processes, e.g., the transport of glucose and calcium, particularly in the heart.[46-48]

RELATION BETWEEN THE THYROID AND THE SYMPATHETIC NERVOUS SYSTEM

While the effects of thyroid hormone on the heart are varied and complex, it has been proposed that some of them are indirect, being secondary to changes in the activity of the sympathetic nervous system (Table 61-1). For example, many of the cardiovascular effects of hyperthyroidism, i.e., tachycardia, systolic hypertension, increased cardiac output, and myocardial contractility, can be abolished or reduced by blocking the activity of the sympathetic nervous system.[49] It has been proposed that thyroid hormone may alter the relationship between the sympathetic nervous and cardiovascular systems, either by increasing the activity of the sympathoadrenal system or by enhancing the response of cardiac tissue to normal sympathetic stimulation.[50] Also, it has been suggested that sympathetic stimuli merely exert a direct additive effect on cardiovascular function above that produced by thyroid hormone. On the other hand, there is also evidence that hyperthyroidism reduces the sensitivity of cardiac tissue to sympathetic stimuli.[51]

Thus the results of experiments on the relationship between the sympathoadrenal system and hyperthyroidism have evoked considerable controversy. The plasma and urine levels of norepinephrine, epinephrine, dopamine, and beta-hydroxylase are either low or normal in hyperthyroidism and either normal or elevated in hypothyroidism.[52] These data suggest that the sympathomimetic features of hyperthyroidism cannot be due simply to an overall increase in adrenergic activity but rather are due to a change in the affinity of catecholamines for their receptors or to a modification of a postreceptor mechanism. Previously such changes were difficult to document, primarily because thyroid hormone appears to have different effects on adrenoceptors in different tissues. For example, the effect of thyroid hormone in the rat liver is different from that in the rat heart. Thyroid hormones reduce beta-adrenoceptor number in the rat liver, and hypothyroid animals show an increase in these receptors.[53,54] In contrast, in the rat heart, which has been the organ most extensively studied, administration of thyroid hormone causes both an increase in the number of receptors and their affinity for their ligand, while hypothyroidism induces the opposite effect.[50,55,56]

These changes in receptor number and affinity lead to appropriate changes in sensitivity of the myocardium to beta-adrenoceptor agonists. For example, stimulation of adenylate cyclase activity by isoproterenol is increased in hyperthyroidism and reduced in hypothyroidism. Finally, there are also changes in the force of contraction with increased sensitivity of the ventricular muscle to isoproterenol-induced contraction in hyperthyroidism and reduction in hypothyroidism.[50] That this effect is specific is shown by an unaltered change in calcium-stimulated contractility in hypo-

TABLE 61-1 CLINICAL FEATURES OF HYPERTHYROIDISM

DIRECT THYROID HORMONE EFFECT†	BETA-ADRENERGIC-LIKE EFFECT†
Resting heart rate >90/min (90%)	Resting heart rate >90/min (90%)
Palpitations (85%)	Palpitations (85%)
Atrial fibrillation (10%)	Exertional dyspnea (80%)
Pedal edema (30%)	Increased pulse pressure (systolic hypertension)
Increased oxygen consumption (basal metabolism)	Active apical impulse
Weight loss	Loud first heart sound and pulmonic component of second heart sound
Skeletal muscle myopathy	Midsystolic murmur, usually basal
Increased bone turnover (occasional osteoporosis or hypercalcemia)	Third heart sound (occasional)
Fair skin	Means-Lerman scratch (rate)‡
Fine brittle hair	Tremor
Brittle nails	Brisk reflexes
Oligomenorrhea or amenorrhea	Increased perspiration
Increased bowel frequency	Heat intolerance
	Insomnia
	Anxiety
	Stare, lid lag§

The numbers in parentheses are approximate prevalences of the findings, compiled from several large series. Goiter is almost always present, though in elderly patients the thyroid enlargement may be minimal or absent.

† Both types of effects contribute to the tachycardia and palpitations.

‡ A systolic scratch or click in the second left intercostal space that is probably generated by the pleura and pericardium rubbing together.

§ These reflect upper-lid retraction. Infiltrative ophthalmyopathy with exophthalmos is found only when Graves' disease is the cause of the hyperthyroidism and is not related to the hyperthyroid state per se.

Reproduced with permission from Kaplan, M. M.: The thyroid and the heart: How do they interact? J. Cardiovasc. Med. 7:893, 1982.

thyroid animals.[55] These effects were also observed in vivo in dogs in which propranolol-induced reductions of heart rate and myocardial contractility were greater in hyperthyroid than in euthyroid animals.[57]

Further support comes from the study by Guarnieri et al., who showed that hyperthyroid rats have enhanced activation of protein kinase and contractile response following administration of a threshold dose of the beta-adrenoceptor agonist isoproterenol.[58] In the aforementioned study in conscious hyperthyroid dogs,[57] however, we found no alteration in the sensitivity of the inotropic response to isoproterenol and norepinephrine.

Circulating blood elements have also provided additional evidence in support of the concept that thyroid hormone "up-regulates" beta-adrenoceptors. When patients are used as their own control, both the number of beta-adrenoceptors and the sensitivity of adenylate cyclase to isoproterenol stimulation in mononuclear cells are increased by thyroid hormone.[59] Additionally, in circulating reticulocytes of hypothyroid animals, the number of receptors is decreased.[60]

While there is compelling evidence for changes in the receptor number and affinity induced by thyroid hormone, it is unclear whether thyroid hormone also has additional effects by which it could alter sensitivity to adrenergic stimuli. There are no data regarding the effect of thyroid hormone on cardiac nucleotide regulatory (G) protein (Fig. 13–12, p. 380), although the presence of hypothyroidism does reduce the concentration of N protein in erythrocyte membranes.[60] On the other hand, no change in N-protein concentration has been observed in adipose tissue.[61] Yet in adipose tissue, hypothyroidism does reduce the lipolytic response to catecholamines.[62] Thus, in this tissue, in which there is no alteration in the number of beta-adrenoceptors, the mechanism underlying the hypothyroid-induced alteration in tissue effect is unclear, but probably occurs downstream from the interaction of the agonist with its receptor.

EFFECT OF THYROID HORMONE ON THE HEART

There is abundant evidence that thyroid hormone may alter cardiac function directly. Thus the addition of thyroid to fragments of chick embryonic heart increases the frequency of beating of the cells.[63] Additionally, the increased heart rate and myocardial contractility observed in experimental hyperthyroidism are not completely reversed by either sympathetic or parasympathetic blockade.[51,57] Finally, T4 enhances the rate of contraction of cardiac muscle even in the presence of adrenergic blockade.[64] Right ventricular papillary muscles isolated from cats rendered hyperthyroid exhibited augmented myocardial contractility, as reflected in an upward shift of the myocardial force-velocity curve,[51] with a greatly increased velocity of myocardial fiber shortening, a reduced time to peak tension during isometric contraction, and an augmented peak tension development (Fig. 61–3). Single ventricular myocytes isolated from hyperthyroid rats exhibited a marked augmentation of twitch velocity and abbreviated both the time required for contraction and relaxation.[64a] Prior catecholamine depletion by pretreatment of the hyperthyroid cats with reserpine did not alter this inotropic effect of hyperthyroidism, providing further evidence for a direct cardiac effect.[51] This hypothesis has been assessed in the intact conscious calf. The results suggest that the major actions of T4 on the left ventricle are (1) a direct positive inotropic effect and (2) an increase in the size of the ventricular cavity without a change in the end-diastolic pressure or length of the sarcomere in diastole, although hypothyroidism does not necessarily impair pump function.[65,66]

The available data suggest that the direct effect of thyroid hormone on the heart is mediated via a change in protein synthesis.[67,68] Thyroid hormone increases the activity of the sodium pump in myocardial cells as it does in other tissues. Philipson and Edelman have documented that the activity of both the Na^+, K^+-ATPase and K^+-dependent *p*-nitrophenyl phosphatase in the heart is increased by more than 50 per cent when T3 is administered to hypothyroid rats.[69] The hearts of euthyroid rabbits rendered hyperthyroid exhibited a doubling of myofibrillar ATPase activity.[70] Reverse T3 (a biologically inactive analog) has no effect. Curfman et al. have suggested that this increased activity is the result of an increase in the number of functional enzyme complexes.[71] There is evidence that thyroid hormone both increases the synthesis of myosin and alters its structure, increasing its con-

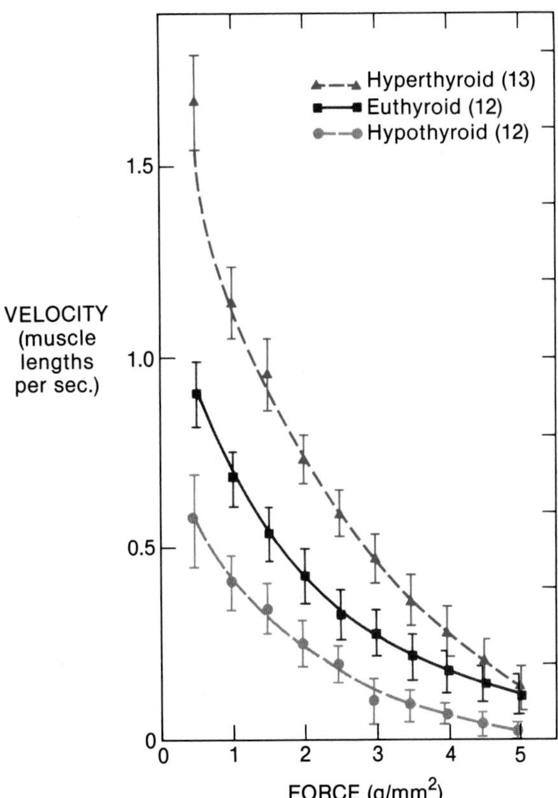

FIGURE 61–3. The average force-velocity relationship for papillary muscles from hyperthyroid, euthyroid, and hypothyroid cats. Initial velocity of shortening is normalized in terms of muscle lengths per second; load, corrected for cross-sectional area of individual muscles, is expressed in gm/mm². Brackets represent ± SEM. (From Buccino, R. A., et al.: Influence of the thyroid state on the intrinsic contractile properties and the energy stores of the myocardium. J. Clin. Invest. *46*:1669, 1967.)

tractile properties, particularly by increasing the more mobile myosin isoenzyme (V_1) as determined by polyacrylamide gel electrophoresis, which is composed of two alpha myosin heavy chains (alpha MHC).[68,72] The mRNA for alpha MHC is substantially increased when hypothyroid rats are given T3, while the beta MHC mRNA, which primarily forms the slower V_3 myosin isoform, is substantially reduced.[68] Thus, the heart appears to respond to thyrotoxicosis by enhancing synthesis of a myosin isoenzyme with a fast ATPase activity.[68,70–73] In addition, α-actin mRNA is increased transiently in hyperthyroidism.[68] The augmented myosin ATPase activity of the hyperthyroid heart appears to contribute to the enhanced contractile response of the hyperthyroid heart, since the activity level of this enzyme is thought to regulate the rate of turnover of actin-myosin cross-bridge links in cardiac muscle. Hypothyroidism induces the opposite effects.[73,74] Goto et al. demonstrated in the hyperthyroid rabbit heart that the increase in myosin isoform V_1/V_3 is associated with decreased contractile efficiency and increased energy costs of excitation-contraction coupling.[75]

Thyroid hormone's effect on cardiac contractility also appears to be mediated in part by changes in intracellular calcium handling. Thyroid hormone increases the number of slow calcium channels, which augments transsarcolemmal calcium influx in cultured ventricular cells.[47] In ferret ventricular muscle, hypothyroidism reduces peak tension and prolongs the duration of contraction in association with changes in cytosolic calcium that are decreased and prolonged in relation to ventricular muscle obtained from euthyroid animals (Fig. 61–4). Hyperthyroidism produces the opposite changes. Thus, alteration in intracellular calcium handling, specifically related to recycling of calcium by the sarcoplasmic reticulum, may account for the thyroid-induced changes in myocardial contractile function.[48,76] Finally, the effect of

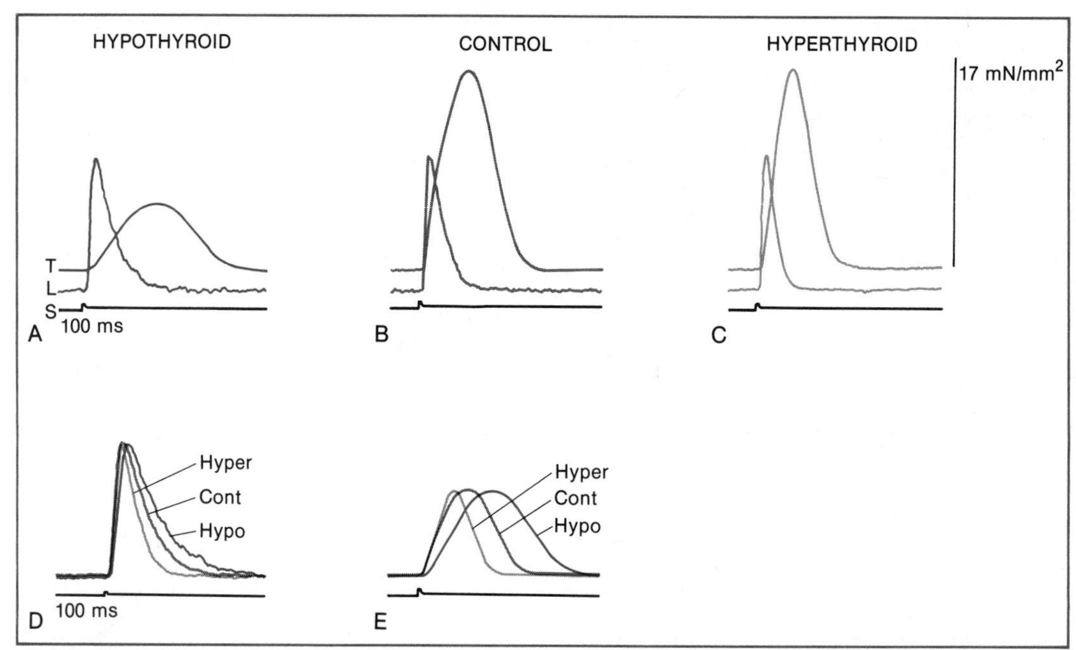

FIGURE 61-4. The thyroid state influences the time course of the isometric contraction and the Ca^{++} transient. The isometric tension (T) and the aequorin light signal, reflecting intracytoplasmic $[Ca]^{++}$ (see p. 357) (L), were recorded from myocardium obtained from a hypothyroid (*A*), euthyroid (*B*), and hyperthyroid (*C*) ferret at 30°C; 0.33 Hz stimulation. I is expressed in milliNewtons/m² muscle cross-sectional area. The Ca^{++} transients (aqueorin signals) are scaled to equal amplitudes and superimposed in *D*. In *E*, the tensions have been scaled to equal amplitudes and superimposed. The time from the beginning of the stimulus sweep (S) to the stimulus represents 100 msecs. (From MacKinnon, R., et al.: Modulation by the thyroid state of intracellular calcium and contractility in ferret ventricular muscle. Circ. Res. *63*:1084, 1988. Used with permission from the American Heart Association.)

thyroxine on myosin isoenzyme appears to be localized primarily to the ventricles with atrial isoenzymes relatively unaltered by changes in thyroid hormone.[72] Klein and Hong, using heterotopic cardiac isografts, have suggested that thyroid's effect on protein synthesis in the heart is, for the most part, secondary to changes in cardiac work rather than a direct effect of thyroid hormone. Indeed, they suggested that even the changes in myosin isoenzyme may in part be secondary to changes in workload, although it is clear that thyroid hormone can induce a separate direct effect.[77,78]

The tachycardia observed in hyperthyroidism appears to be due to a combination of an increased rate of diastolic depolarization and a decreased duration of the action potential in the sinoatrial node cells.[79] The propensity for the development of atrial fibrillation may be due to the shortened refractory period of atrial cells.[80]

HYPERTHYROIDISM

Hyperthyroidism is the clinical state resulting from the excess production of T3, thyroxine (T4), or both. The most common cause is a diffuse toxic goiter (Graves' disease). Although the etiology of this condition is still unknown, the hyperproduction of T4 and T3 is thought to result from circulating IgG autoantibodies that bind to the thyrotropin receptor on the thyroid gland. The second most common form of hyperthyroidism is nodular toxic goiter, a condition in which localized areas of the gland function excessively and autonomously. Less common causes include a single toxic adenoma, ingestion of excessive amounts of thyroid hormone, and subacute thyroiditis, in which there may be a self-limit phase of hyperthyroidism. Rarely, hyperthyroidism may also occur as a result of the production of thyroid hormone by a thyroid carcinoma or production of a thyrotropic substance (probably HCG) by a hydatidiform mole or choriocarcinoma.[81]

Hyperthyroidism is a relatively common disease, occurring four to eight times more commonly in women than in men, with a peak incidence in the third and fourth decades. The commonly associated signs and symptoms (Table 61-1) include fatigue, hyperactivity, insomnia, heat intolerance, palpitations, dyspnea, increased appetite with weight loss, nocturia, diarrhea, oligomenorrhea, muscle weakness, tremor, emotional lability, increased heart rate, systolic hypertension, hyperthermia, warm moist skin, lid lag, stare, and brisk reflexes. In the vast majority of cases a goiter can be palpated. Hyperthyroidism in childhood occurs most frequently just before or during adolescence. It is usually associated with a diffuse goiter. The most common early manifestations in juvenile hyperthyroid patients are excessive movements and emotional lability.

T3 levels are invariably elevated, and serum T4 levels are usually increased as well. In addition to the signs and symptoms directly related to increased production of thyroid hormone, patients with Graves' disease often have exophthalmos and occasionally circumscribed areas of thickening of the skin, particularly of the lower extremities; presumably these are related to the immunological aspects of the disease.

Particularly in older patients, the typical clinical picture is occasionally absent. In these individuals with so-called *apathetic hyperthyroidism*, few clinical manifestations are apparent except for cardiovascular dysfunction. Thus, cardiac arrhythmias and heart failure resistant to conventional forms of therapy are common.

CARDIOVASCULAR MANIFESTATIONS. The heart is among the most responsive organs in thyroid disease, and cardiovascular signs and symptoms are therefore important clinical features of hyperthyroidism.[81,82] Palpitations, dyspnea, tachycardia, and systolic hypertension are common findings. Diastolic hypertension can also occur. Typically, there is a hyperactive precordium with a loud first heart sound, an accentuated pulmonic component of the second heart sound, and a third heart sound; occasionally, a systolic ejection click is heard. Midsystolic murmurs along the left sternal border are common, and a systolic scratch, the so-called Means-Lerman scratch, is occasionally heard in the second left intercostal space during expiration. It is presumed to be secondary to the rubbing together of normal pleural and pericardial surfaces by the hyperdynamic heart.

As would be anticipated, and as described on page 458, cardiac and stroke volume index, mean systolic ejection rate, velocity and extent of wall shortening (Fig. 61-5), and coronary blood flow[83] are all increased, the systolic ejection period and preejection period are abbreviated, the pulse pressure is widened, and systemic vascular resistance is reduced in hyperthyroidism.[84] The changes in left ventricular performance

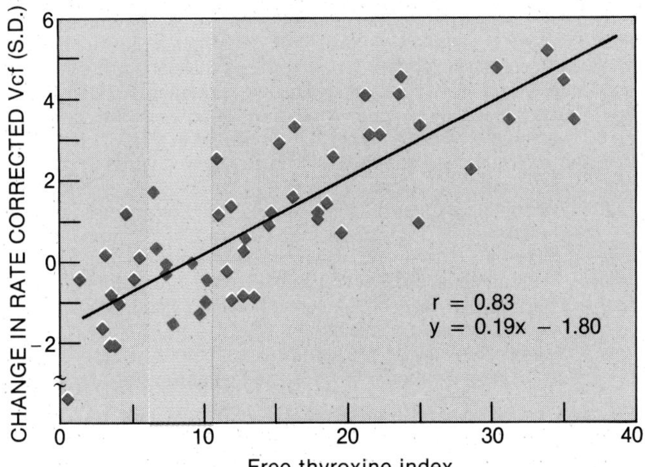

FIGURE 61-5. Rate-corrected velocity of shortening (V_{cf}) in SD units from the normal mean regression line obtained from 11 patients at varying levels of the free thyroxine index. There is a strong positive correlation between the level of thyroid hormone and the change in contractile state. The shaded area represents the normal range for serum free thyroxine index. (From Feldman, T., et al.: Myocardial mechanics in hyperthyroidism: Importance of left ventricular loading conditions, heart rate and contractile state. By permission of the American College of Cardiology. J. Am. Coll. Cardiol. *7*:972, 1986.)

induced by thyroid hormone appear to be secondary to augmented contractility rather than to reduction in afterload or change in heart rate.[85] If the hyperthyroidism is relatively mild, many of the indices of left ventricular function are normal, with exercise needed to bring out abnormalities.[86,87] It has been suggested that many of the changes in cardiac function are secondary to the increased metabolic demands of peripheral tissue. However, the increase in cardiac output is greater than would be predicted on the basis of the increased total body oxygen consumption, supporting the view that thyroid hormone exerts a direct cardiac stimulant action independent of its effect on general tissue metabolism. Furthermore, normalization of myocardial contractile response to exercise may not occur until several months after normalization of thyroid function.[88]

Roentgenographic and electrocardiographic changes are common but are nonspecific in hyperthyroidism.[81] Thus the left ventricle, the aorta, and the pulmonary artery are prominent, and, in some cases, there is generalized cardiac enlargement, which may be accompanied by signs and symptoms of heart failure. In patients with sinus rhythm, the magnitude of the tachycardia, in general, parallels the severity of the disease. Sinus tachycardia, i.e., a rate exceeding 100 beats/min, is present in 40 per cent of patients with hyperthyroidism, occurring most frequently in the younger age groups, and often at night.[89] Fifteen to twenty-five per cent of patients with hyperthyroidism have persistent atrial fibrillation, which is often heralded by one or more transient episodes of this arrhythmia.[90,91] There is shortening of the A-V conduction time and functional refractory period, resulting in an increased frequency at which the A-V conduction system transmits rapid atrial impulses.[91] Intraatrial conduction disturbances, manifested by prolongation or notching of the P wave and prolongation of the P-R interval in the absence of treatment with digitalis, occur in 15 per cent and 5 per cent of patients with hyperthyroidism, respectively. Occasionally, second- or third-degree heart block may result.[82] The cause of the A-V conduction disturbance is not clear, since animal experiments have shown that the functional refractory period of the A-V conduction system and the conduction time were shortened in dogs with hyperthyroidism and prolonged in dogs with hypothyroidism.[92] Intraventricular conduction disturbances, most commonly right bundle branch block, occur in about 15 per cent of patients with hyperthyroidism without associated heart disease of other etiology.[82] Paroxysmal supraventricular tachycardia and flutter are rare in hyperthyroidism. Finally, occult thyrotoxicosis may underlie either chronic or paroxysmal isolated atrial fibrillation. Ciaccheri et al. reported a frequency of thyrotoxicosis of 12.5 per cent in 40 consecutive patients with isolated atrial fibrillation.[91]

Both angina pectoris and congestive heart failure occur in patients with hyperthyroidism, and for many years it was assumed that these were seen only in the presence of underlying cardiovascular disease. Support for this position came primarily from the absence of these symptoms in young persons with significant hyperthyroidism. More recently, however, four lines of evidence have suggested otherwise: (1) Congestive heart failure has been produced in experimental animals by simply administering T4. (2) Children with thyrotoxicosis without underlying cardiac disease may develop congestive heart failure.[93] (3) Angina has been reported in a patient with normal coronary arteries, presumably secondary to thyroid-induced coronary artery spasm.[94] (4) Abnormal left ventricular function observed during exercise in hyperthyroid subjects is not reversed by beta blockade but is reversed by treating the hyperthyroidism.[95] Thus, when it is severe enough, thyrotoxicosis can overtax even the normal heart, although, in most instances, the development of clinical manifestations of heart failure and myocardial ischemia in patients with hyperthyroidism signifies the presence of underlying cardiac or coronary vascular disease. There is also increased frequency of hyperthyroidism in patients with familial hypertrophic cardiomyopathy. In one kindred, 3 of 17 members with hypertrophic cardiomyopathy also had hyperthyroidism.[96] Finally, hyperthyroidism has been associated with mitral valve prolapse in more than a third of cases.[97,98]

TREATMENT OF CARDIOVASCULAR DISEASE IN HYPERTHYROIDISM. Hyperthyroid patients with cardiovascular disease are particularly resistant to therapy. For example, it has been well documented that both congestive heart failure and cardiac arrhythmias are resistant to conventional doses of the cardiac glycosides. While the specific mechanisms underlying these altered responses remain obscure, they may be related to both systemic and local effects.[81,99] First, serum levels of cardiac glycosides are diminished in hyperthyroidism, not because there is an augmentation of its metabolism but because there is an increase in its volume of distribution. Second, experimental hyperthyroidism reduces the enhancement of the myocardial contractile force and the prolongation of the atrioventricular nodal refractory period produced by these agents.[99] Because of this decreased sensitivity to cardiac glycosides, toxicity may develop at a dose that has relatively little therapeutic effect.

DIAGNOSIS AND THERAPY OF HYPERTHYROIDISM

The diagnosis is made on the basis of elevated levels of thyroid hormone in the blood. Because only serum T3 is increased in some individuals, it is important to obtain serum levels of *both* T3 and T4 and an index of the thyroid-binding capacity of the patient's serum (resin thyroxine uptake). In most laboratories hyperthyroidism is confirmed when the levels of serum T4 are greater than 10.5 μg/dl or T3 levels are greater than 180 ng/dl with normal resin thyroxine uptakes. Occasionally, patients will have hyperthyroidism with both T3 and T4 within the normal range. If suspected, confirmation may be obtained by measuring the TSH (thyroid-stimulating hormone) basally (if a supersensitive assay is used) or in response to TRH (thyrotropin-releasing hormone), which should be blunted in hyperthyroidism. However, caution needs to be exercised in using the TRH test, since false-positive results are common.[81]

The definitive treatment of hyperthyroidism is surgical removal of the gland or irradiation using radioactive iodide. In severely ill patients, particularly those with thyroid storm or significant cardiovascular symptoms or both, neither of these therapies is appropriate. Thus, medical therapy is directed at reducing both the production and biological effect of thyroid hormone. Since many of the cardiovascular symptoms of thyrotoxicosis are related to increased beta-adrenoceptor activity, treatment with beta-adrenoceptor blocking agents has been useful.[100] Tachycardia, palpitations, tremor, restlessness, muscle weakness, and heat intolerance are reversed by these agents, which offer the additional benefit of inhibiting the conversion of T4 to the biologically active T3 in peripheral tissues.

Treatment of Cardiovascular Manifestations of Hyperthyroidism

Prompt treatment of the hyperthyroid state can significantly reduce, if not eliminate, the associated cardiovascular symptoms. About half of patients with concurrent onset of hyperthyroidism and angina pectoris experience complete remission of symptoms after treatment of hyperthyroidism.[101] Furthermore, in 62 per cent of 163 thyrotoxic patients with atrial fibrillation sustained for 1 week or longer, spontaneous reversion to sinus rhythm was found when they became euthyroid.[102] Arterial embolization is not common in patients with thyrotoxicosis and atrial fibrillation, but it does occur. In one series, 8 per cent of 262 patients with both conditions had embolization.[103] Thus it is important to determine quickly whether hyperthyroidism is present in patients with cardiovascular disease, since treatment often results in dramatic improvement. In elderly patients with apathetic hyperthyroidism, cardiovascular manifestations, specifically atrial fibrillation and/or congestive heart failure, predominate, and therefore evaluation of thyroid function in such patients is particularly important. However, it should be noted that these individuals are particularly resistant to cardiac glycosides.

Beta blockers (p. 505) can be administered orally or intravenously, but since these drugs interfere with the effects of sympathetic stimulation on the heart, they must be used with caution in patients with congestive heart failure. However, if the heart failure is in part related to the tachycardia, beta blockade may be beneficial. These agents can be administered in small doses while the patient is under close observation and being treated with digitalis and diuretics and reduction in physical activity. Beta-blocking drugs and cardiac glycosides act synergistically to slow ventricular rate in atrial fibrillation by increasing the refractoriness of the A-V conduction system. Thus, the combination may produce benefit that would require toxic doses of either agent used alone. Beta-adrenoceptor blockade improves many peripheral manifestations of thyrotoxicosis.[81]

While beta-adrenoceptor blockade can produce significant improvement of the cardiovascular status in patients with hyperthyroidism, correction of the basic metabolic defect requires specific therapy directed at reducing the production of thyroid hormone.[81] The most useful agents are the thionamides, such as propylthiouracil. These drugs should be administered concurrently with a beta-blocking agent to reduce the total production of thyroid hormone, as well as to block its effect. The usual starting dosage of propylthiouracil is 300 to 800 mg in divided doses daily; it not only reduces thyroid hormone production but also has the advantage of reducing the peripheral conversion of T4 into T3. Usual maintenance doses range from 50 to 300 mg. The thionamides are not without risk, since between 1 and 5 per cent of patients have significant side effects—usually gastrointestinal disturbances or a suppression of the bone marrow; infrequently, a generalized vasculitis has been reported.

Iodine, most commonly administered in the form of 2 drops of saturated solution of potassium iodide three times daily, inhibits the release of thyroid hormones from the thyrotoxic gland, and its beneficial effects occur rapidly, indeed, more rapidly than those of agents that inhibit the synthesis of the hormone. It is therefore useful in the rapid amelioration of the hyperthyroid state in patients with thyroid heart disease. It may also be utilized along with antithyroid agents to control thyrotoxicosis following ^{131}I treatment until the radioactive iodide has had time to take effect. Most hyperthyroid patients, however, escape from the effects of iodide after 10 to 14 days.

Ipodate, an agent for oral cholecystography, has been reported to be beneficial in the treatment of early hyperthyroidism, particularly in the early treatment of cardiac manifestations of thyrotoxicosis.[104]

HYPOTHYROIDISM

Hypothyroidism results from reduced secretion of both T4 and T3, occurring in most cases as a consequence of destruction of the thyroid gland itself, usually by an inflammatory process. In some cases, it is secondary to decreased secretion of TSH, due to either pituitary or hypothalamic disease. In secondary hypothyroidism, the signs and symptoms associated with deficiency of other pituitary hormones are also usually present. The incidence of hypothyroidism peaks between the ages of 30 and 60 years and is twice as common in women as in men. The following signs and symptoms are common: cold intolerance, dryness of the skin, weakness, impairment of memory, personality changes, shortness of breath, constipation, hoarseness, menorrhagia and other forms of menstrual dysfunction, and, occasionally, heart failure. In addition, in the more severe forms of the disease, there is facial puffiness, particularly around the eyes, a characteristic nonpitting form of edema (myxedema) of the lower extremities, slow speech, decreased hearing, and a yellow hue to the skin due to decreased conversion of carotene into vitamin A. These signs and symptoms may be present for years before treatment is initiated, particularly in patients in whom the disease has developed gradually.

EFFECTS OF AMIODARONE ON THYROID FUNCTION. The antiarrhythmic agent amiodarone (p. 646) has three effects on thyroid function. Its first effect is to antagonize thyroid hormone action on pituitary cells by binding to the intranuclear thyroid hormone receptor, and it thereby inhibits T3-induced changes in mRNA levels and TSH response to TRH.[105,106] Its second effect is to inhibit peripheral conversion of T4 to T3. Thus, in nearly all patients who receive long-term treatment with this drug, there is reduction in serum T3 levels and a transient rise in TSH. Within a few days to weeks this causes an increase in serum T4 levels and a return of serum TSH to normal. Clinically and metabolically, these patients are euthyroid even though their T4 levels are elevated.[107] Amiodarone's third effect is due to its high iodide content (35 per cent by weight). Thus, when it is metabolized there is a massive increase in the available inorganic iodide, resulting in acute inhibition of thyroid organification (Fig. 61–6). Depending upon the state of iodine intake before its administration, patients may develop either hypothyroidism (common in the United States) or thyrotoxicosis (more common in Europe).[107–109] As would be anticipated, amiodarone administration in experimental animals produces changes in serum lipids and lipoprotein lipase levels similar to those found in hypothyroidism.[110]

In addition to the more direct effects of amiodarone on thyroid function, in susceptible individuals this agent can also induce a marked increase in Ia-positive T cells (an abnormality found in patients with spontaneous Graves' disease). These T-cell abnormalities disappear after discontinuation of the amiodarone. Thus, amiodarone may induce T-cell abnormalities leading to an autoimmune state.[111] Because of amiodarone's long half-life, the biochemical and clinical abnormalities can persist for months after it is stopped.

CARDIOVASCULAR MANIFESTATIONS. The heart in overt myxedema is often pale, flabby, and grossly dilated. Histological examination discloses myofibrillar swelling, loss of striations, and interstitial fibrosis. With the development of methods that reliably and easily measure the circulating levels of thyroid hormone, the diagnosis of hypothyroidism is being made with increasing frequency at an earlier stage of the disease. Treatment is therefore also initiated earlier, resulting in a reduction in the incidence of cardiovascular signs and symptoms. Thus, the classic findings of cardiac enlargement, cardiac dilatation, significant bradycardia, weak arterial pulses, hypotension, distant heart sounds, low electrocardiographic voltages, nonpitting facial and peripheral edema, and evidence of congestive heart failure, such as ascites, orthopnea, and paroxysmal dyspnea, are now seen only infrequently. However, exertional dyspnea and easy fatigability continue to be common complaints.

Myxedema is associated with increased capillary permeability and subsequent leakage of protein into the interstitial space, resulting in pericardial effusion, a common clinical finding in overt myxedema, occurring in about one-third of all patients (p. 1505). Rarely, it or the presenting symptom is complicated by cardiac tamponade.[112] Cardiomegaly on chest radiograph and low voltage in the electrocardiogram are not reliable indicators of pericardial effusion; echocardiography is

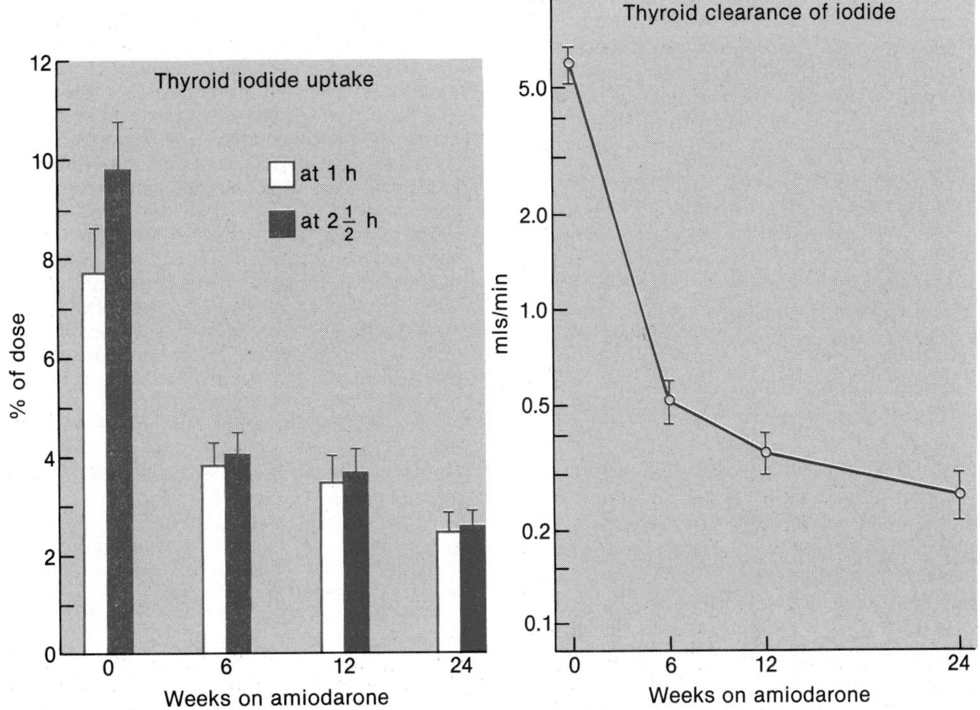

FIGURE 61–6. Effect of amiodarone on mean (±SEM) thyroid iodide uptake (*left*) and thyroid iodide clearance (*right*) in 15 euthyroid patients. (Note that the ordinate of the right panel is plotted on a log scale.) (From Rao, R. H., McCready, V. R., and Spathis, G. S.: Iodine kinetic studies during amiodarone treatment. J. Clin. Endocrinol. Metab. *62*:563, 1986) © by The Endocrine Society, 1986.

the most useful method of establishing the diagnosis (p. 102). The effusions disappear with thyroid replacement therapy.[113]

The electrocardiographic changes observed in patients with hypothyroidism other than sinus bradycardia include prolongation of the Q-T interval, but since the T-wave amplitude is low, precise measurement of this interval is often impossible.[27] The P-wave amplitude is usually very low, and in some cases this wave is not even discernible. Sinus tachycardia is very rare, whereas bradycardia is common. It is possible that hypothermia may contribute to reentrant ventricular arrhythmias by slowing the heart rate and increasing the duration of the QRS and the Q-T intervals, which can rarely lead to severe ventricular tachyarrhthmias.[27,114] The incidence of atrioventricular and intraventricular conduction disturbances is about three times greater in patients with myxedema than in the general population.[25] Other electrocardiographic changes are those associated with pericardial effusion.[113] Thus, flattening or inversion of the T waves and low P-, QRS-, and T-wave amplitudes are commonly observed in patients with pericardial effusion. In most cases these revert to normal with the removal of the fluid. In some cases, however, the electrocardiographic changes persist even though the pericardial fluid is removed, which suggests that the lack of thyroid hormone may produce a primary myocardial abnormality suggestive of a cardiomyopathy.[115] Incomplete or complete right bundle branch block has been observed, but other forms of arrhythmias are uncommon.

There is increased frequency of hypertension in patients with hypothyroidism, although not in severe myxedema.[116] In one study of 477 patients, 15 per cent of hypothyroid subjects had a blood pressure greater than 160/95, compared to 5.5 per cent in age-matched euthyroid subjects. Replacement of thyroid hormone resulted in substantial reduction in blood pressure in the hypertensive patients.[117] In a study of 688 consecutive hypertensive patients, hypothyroidism was found in 25 (3.5 per cent). In nearly one-third of this subgroup, treatment of the hypothyroidism lowered the blood pressure to within the normal range.[116] Thus, individuals with mild to moderate hypothyroidism have an increased possibility of developing hypertension, particularly diastolic hypertension, while individuals with severe hypothyroidism are more likely to have normal or slightly low blood pressures.[116,117]

Cardiovascular manifestations of congenital hypothyroidism are similar except for the rarity of pericardial effusion. Thus the size of the left ventricle, its capacity, and the posterior wall thickness are all less in the hypothyroid infant. Since heart rate is also lower, cardiac output is reduced. There is also a prolongation of the preejection period of the left ventricle.[118]

MYOCARDIAL EFFECTS. Hypothyroid patients have reduced cardiac output, stroke volume, and blood and plasma volumes.[119,120] Circulation time is prolonged, but right and left heart filling pressures are usually within normal limits unless they are elevated by the pericardial effusion. There is a redistribution of blood flow with mild reductions in cerebral and renal flow and significant reductions in cutaneous flow. A delay in the relaxation of skeletal muscle is a well-known finding in hypothyroidism; measurements of isovolumetric relaxation time, by a combination of apex cardiography and phonocardiography, have revealed a prolongation of this interval with an abbreviation to normal during T4 replacement.[121] In addition, there is lengthening of the preejection period and an increased ratio of the preejection period to the left ventricular ejection time (PEP/LVET); these changes are the opposite of those observed in hyperthyroidism.[122]

Cardiac muscle isolated from cats with experimentally produced hypothyroidism exhibited reduced contractility, characterized by a depression of the myocardial force-velocity curve, a reduction of the rate of tension development, and a prolongation of the contractile response (Figs. 61–3 and 61–4).

There is little evidence from either experimental or clinical studies that congestive heart failure is common in myxedema or that it occurs in the absence of other cardiac disease.[123] Presumably the depressed myocardial contractility is sufficient to sustain the reduced workload placed on the heart in hypothyroidism. However, it may be difficult to distinguish between the heart in myxedema and heart failure. Dyspnea, edema, effusions, cardiomegaly, and T-wave changes occur in both conditions. In left heart failure, pulmonary arterial pressure is usually elevated during exercise, cardiac output fails to rise normally, and the Valsalva response is normal, while the opposite occurs in myxedema.[123] The hemodynamic changes in myxedema respond to thyroid hormone administration.

Cardiac catecholamine levels are not reduced in hypothyroidism. Neither the sensitivity of the mechanical performance of the heart to sympathetic nerve stimulation nor the response of the cardiac adenylate cyclase to norepinephrine is altered in hypothyroidism. However, there is a reduction in the total number of myocardial beta receptors.[55] In addition to the effects of hypothyroidism on the beta receptor there also is evidence that the lack of thyroid hormone may modify the contractile process itself. Thus, both isoproterenol-stimulated contractility and the accumulation of cyclic AMP are reduced in hearts obtained from hypothyroid rats.[124] In experimental hypothyroidism, calcium in isolated myocardial sarcoplasmic reticulum particles is reduced, which may explain the altered contractile state.[75] As already noted, thyroid hormone can affect the quantity and function of myosin ATPase activity through a change in protein synthesis. The activity of cardiac myosin ATPase and the rate of calcium uptake and the calcium-dependent ATP hydrolysis by isolated myocardial sarcoplasmic reticulum in the excitation-contraction-relaxation process[74] are reduced in hypothyroidism.

ATHEROSCLEROSIS. It has been suggested that patients with hypothyroidism are at increased risk of developing atherosclerosis, since this disease is accompanied by significant changes in lipid metabolism. Thus, hypercholesterolemia and hypertriglyceridemia, which are associated with the development of premature coronary artery disease, are found in patients with hypothyroidism. Support for this hypothesis has come from several sources, including the documentation that coronary atherosclerosis occurs with twice the frequency in patients with myxedema than in age- and sex-matched controls and that the development of atherosclerosis in cholesterol-fed animals is enhanced by the presence of hypothyroidism and reduced when thyroid hormone is administered.[125] Additionally, hypothyroidism has a deleterious effect on dogs in which a myocardial infarction has been induced. Infarct size was increased, dysrhythmias were more severe, and abnormalities in the microvasculature were present.[126] Yet myocardial infarction and angina pectoris are relatively uncommon occurrences in patients with hypothyroidism. The latter was present in only 7 per cent of a group of patients with hypothyroidism.[127] This low frequency of cardiac complications from atherosclerosis may simply reflect the decreased metabolic demand on the myocardium in hypothyroidism. A definitive study which examines the frequency of atherosclerosis in euthyroid individuals and persons who are now euthyroid but had once been myxedematous has not been reported. However, in one series of treated hypothyroid patients, angina pectoris improved more frequently than it became worse,[127] suggesting that the development of lipid abnormalities may not have the same implications in hypothyroid as in euthyroid individuals.

Other Metabolic Changes in Hypothyroidism

The evaluation of patients with myxedema and chest pain is complicated by the known effects of hypothyroidism on serum enzyme concentrations commonly used to assess myocardial damage. Thus, creatine kinase (CK), lactic dehydrogenase (LDH), and serum glutamic-oxaloacetic transaminase (SGOT) may be moderately or significantly increased in hypothyroidism.[128] The mechanism for the increase in enzymes is uncertain, but it may be related to mild cardiac or skeletal muscle damage with release of enzymes or decreased clearance of normal enzyme concentrations.

DIAGNOSIS AND TREATMENT OF HYPOTHYROIDISM

Caution must be exercised in treating hypothyroid patients who are elderly and who may have underlying heart disease, to avoid precipitating myocardial infarction or severe congestive heart failure; a slow replacement program is indicated in these individuals.

Some have suggested using T3 rather than T4 to treat patients with myxedema; since it has a shorter half-life, if toxic effects develop they will be dissipated more quickly. However, because it has a quicker onset of action, T3 also induces complications more rapidly. Thus, it appears to us more desirable to treat myxedema with T4, usually beginning with a dose as small as 0.0125 mg daily and doubling this every 14 days until a dosage of 0.1 to 0.125 mg is reached. During this process the patient's cardiovascular status is monitored frequently, and, if untoward events occur, the dose is reduced or maintained constant. The measurement of serum TSH levels provides a useful biochemical marker of adequacy of the replacement therapy.

The treatment of congestive heart failure is particularly difficult in patients with myxedema, both because of the effect of thyroid hormone on the heart and because the heart's response to cardiac glycosides is altered.[99] Patients with severe angina pectoris and untreated myxedema pose a difficult clinical dilemma because angina may be exacerbated by thyroid hormone replacement, and the usual medical management of angina with propranolol may induce severe bradycardia. Coronary arteriography often shows severe coronary artery disease in these patients, and an excellent surgical team can perform successful coronary revascularization with minimal thyroid replacement. Full thyroid replacement can then be safely achieved during the postoperative period, without the recurrence of angina.[129]

An increasingly common problem in ill patients is the so-called euthyroid sick syndrome.[130] This occurs in acutely or chronically ill patients who have low serum T4 and T3 levels yet do not have hypothyroidism. The low T3 levels are secondary to decreased extrathyroidal conversion of T4 to T3. The low T4's are often due to a decrease in the concentration of thyroxine-binding globulin, resulting in a decrease in total but only minimal changes in the free hormone levels. In very severe illness, there can be central (CNS) suppression of TSH release and an induced secondary hypothyroid state. Prolonged dopamine infusions can produce this situation also, by direct suppression of TSH secretion. In the euthyroid sick syndrome the serum TSH usually will be normal, whereas in hypothyroidism TSH will be increased, thus providing a biochemical mechanism for distinguishing them.[130,131] T4 therapy is not of benefit in these patients.[132]

DISEASES OF THE ADRENAL CORTEX

Since Addison's description in 1849 of adrenal insufficiency,[2] it has been appreciated that steroids secreted by the adrenal cortex exert a significant effect on the cardiovascular system, primarily by altering blood pressure. Adrenal insufficiency is characterized by significant hypotension, while excessive production of adrenal steroids is often accompanied by hypertension.

Three classes of steroids are secreted by the adrenal cortex: glucocorticoids, e.g., cortisol; mineralocorticoids, e.g., aldosterone; and androgens, e.g., dehydroepiandrosterone. In this section, the physiology and pathophysiology of glucocorticoid and mineralocorticoid secretion will be addressed.

HORMONE ACTIONS

CORTISOL. The primary glucocorticoid, cortisol, is synthesized from cholesterol in the inner layers of the adrenal cortex by a series of enzymatic transformations. After release into the circulation, it is bound to a high-affinity, low-capacity globulin, transcortin. Thus, most of the circulating cortisol is biologically inactive. The daily secretion rate of cortisol ranges from 15 to 30 mg with a pronounced diurnal cycle. Its average plasma concentration is 15 μg/dl in the morning, falling to 5 μg/dl by early evening.[133] The fundamental mechanism of action of the glucocorticoids is similar to that of other steroid hormones. They enter a target tissue by diffusion and combine with a specific high-affinity cytoplasmic receptor protein. The receptor-cortisol complex is then transferred to specific acceptor sites on nuclear chromatin tissue (promoter region) where it produces an increase in RNA and later protein synthesis.

The division of adrenal steroids into glucocorticoids and mineralocorticoids is somewhat arbitrary in that most glucocorticoids have some mineralocorticoid-like properties and vice versa. The major action of glucocorticoids is to promote gluconeogenesis, and, in that respect, they are both catabolic and antiinsulin. They mobilize amino acid precursors from peripheral supporting structures, such as bone, skin, muscle, and connective tissue, and inhibit protein synthesis and amino acid uptake in these same tissues. Gluconeogenesis is also indirectly enhanced by an increase in glucagon secretion secondary to the glucocorticoid-induced hyperaminoacidemia.

Glucocorticoids also have antiinflammatory properties related to their effects on both the microvasculature and the lymphatic system. They maintain normal vascular responsiveness to circulating vasoconstrictors, such as norepinephrine, and have a major effect on both the distribution and excretion of body water. For example, patients with Addison's disease cannot effectively excrete a water load. Finally, glucocorticoids can alter calcium absorption from the gastrointestinal tract by interfering with the activation of vitamin D in the liver and/or blocking its effect on the gastrointestinal tract.[133]

CONTROL OF CORTISOL SECRETION. This is primarily under the control of a negative feedback loop involving the adrenal cortex and the pituitary gland. Thus, as cortisol concentrations fall, ACTH secretion from the pituitary increases, stimulating the adrenal cortex to produce more cortisol and vice versa. The hypothalamus also interacts with this system by releasing corticotropin-releasing hormone, thus modifying ACTH release and the response of the pituitary to the inhibitory effect of cortisol. In addition to this primary negative feedback loop, there is an intrinsic diurnal rhythm in the release of both ACTH and cortisol, probably mediated by changes in the release of corticotropin-releasing hormone from the hypothalamus.

ALDOSTERONE. The major mineralocorticoid produced by the human adrenal gland is aldosterone. It is also synthesized from cholesterol but almost exclusively in the outer layer (glomerulosa) of the adrenal cortex. Aldosterone has two important functions: (1) it is a major regulator of extracellular fluid volume by its effect on sodium retention, and (2) it is a major determinant of potassium metabolism. Aldosterone acts predominantly on the distal convoluted tubule and/or collecting duct of the kidney where it promotes the reabsorption of sodium. Potassium then diffuses into the lumen of the tubules because of the change in electrochemical gradient produced by the active reabsorption of the positively charged sodium ion. Hydrogen ion may also be more freely excreted because of this change in the electrochemical gradient. While aldosterone also acts on salivary and sweat glands and on the endothelial cells of the gastrointestinal tract, these have little impact on total body sodium and potassium homeostasis.

There are three well-defined control mechanisms for aldosterone release.[133,134]

1. The renin-angiotensin system is the major system for the control of extracellular fluid volume by regulating aldosterone secretion. Aldosterone is linked in a negative feedback loop with the renin-angiotensin system. Thus, during periods registered as volume deficiency there is increased release of the enzyme renin from the juxtaglomerular cells of the kidney. Renin then increases the production of angiotensin I from its substrate. Angiotensin I is rapidly converted into the biologically active angiotensin II, which increases aldosterone secretion. Angiotensin II also produces vasoconstriction, thereby raising blood pressure and reducing blood flow to a variety of tissues, especially the kidney.

2. Potassium ion also regulates aldosterone secretion independent of the renin-angiotensin system; elevation of potassium concentration increases aldosterone secretion and vice versa. The adrenal cortex is very sensitive to changes in potassium concentration with as little as a 0.1 mEq/liter increment producing significant changes in the plasma aldosterone levels.

3. ACTH also has been documented to affect aldosterone secretion profoundly. However, because the control of aldosterone release is not appreciably altered in patients who have been on a long-term regimen of steroid therapy, ACTH probably has a smaller role than the other two factors in maintaining normal aldosterone secretion.

In addition to these major stimuli controlling aldosterone secretion, salt-losing hormones such as atrial natriuretic peptide (p. 1858) and dopamine inhibit aldosterone secretion, particularly in response to angiotensin II.[134] Finally, the prior dietary intake of both sodium and potassium alters the magnitude of the aldosterone response to acute stimulation, sodium restriction, and potassium loading, both enhancing the response of the adrenal, perhaps by modifying the local (adrenal) renin-angiotensin system.[133,134]

Diseases of the adrenal cortex, therefore, primarily affect the cardiovascular system via changes in blood pressure or volume homeostasis. Three specific conditions will be discussed next: glucocorticoid excess (Cushing's syndrome), mineralocorticoid excess (primary aldosteronism), and adrenal insufficiency (Addison's disease).

CUSHING'S SYNDROME

(see also p. 839)

In 1932 Harvey Cushing reported a syndrome characterized by truncal obesity, hypertension, fatigue, weakness, amenorrhea, hirsutism, purple abdominal striae, glucosuria, edema, and osteoporosis.[135] Since his original description, a number of specific causes for this syndrome have been described. However, the majority are secondary to bilateral adrenal hyperplasia, with the predominant feature being excess production of glucocorticoids and androgens.[136] Some cases are due to ACTH-producing tumors, of either the pituitary gland (Cushing's disease) or nonendocrine tissue (ectopic ACTH production). Fifteen to twenty per cent of the cases are due to primary adrenal neoplasia, either adenoma or carcinoma. Three times as many women as men are afflicted, and the onset is usually in the third or fourth decade of life. Most patients have the typical body habitus: central obesity and slender extremities with proximal muscle weakness. Hypertension is present in 80 to 90 per cent of patients, and diabetes occurs in 20 per cent, probably in those individuals with a predisposition.[133,136] Evidence of androgen excess may also be present, including hirsutism, amenorrhea, clitoromegaly, and, in some cases, deepening of the voice. The majority of patients also have significant emotional changes ranging from lability of mood to severe depression, confusion, or even frank psychosis.

Laboratory tests disclose evidence of excess production of both glucocorticoids and androgens in the majority of cases. Thus, urinary metabolites of these steroids, 17-ketosteroids and 17-hydroxysteroids, are characteristically increased. Most patients show some evidence of glycosuria or hyperglycemia. There is usually generalized osteoporosis, most marked in the spine and pelvis; polycythemia is frequently encountered. In severe cases, hypokalemia, a mineralocorticoid manifestation, may also occur.

CARDIOVASCULAR MANIFESTATIONS. Prior to the development of effective treatment for Cushing's syndrome, accelerated atherosclerosis was a common finding. Early death usually occurred from myocardial infarction, congestive heart failure, or stroke. While the pathophysiology of the accelerated atherosclerosis is not clear, the hypertensive process probably contributes. However, it is unlikely to be the sole reason, since the hypertension of patients with primary aldosteronism may be as significant, and yet atherosclerosis is unusual. Some of the atherosclerotic changes may be mediated by the lipid-mobilizing effect of cortisol. Chronic excess production of cortisol leads to hyperlipidemia and hypercholesterolemia, both of which may promote the development of atherosclerosis.[137]

The pathophysiology of the hypertension in Cushing's syndrome has been much debated. Early studies suggested that it was secondary to volume expansion due to cortisol's mineralocorticoid properties. However, recent studies have not supported this hypothesis. Alternative hypotheses include glucocorticoid potentiation of response of vascular smooth muscle to vasoconstrictive agents and ACTH- or cortisol-induced increases in renin substrate.[137] The latter thesis suggests that the increased blood pressure is secondary to increased generation of angiotensin II. Thus, the pathophysiology of the hypertension may be multifactorial, being related to volume expansion, increased production of vasoactive agents, e.g., angiotensin II, and increased sensitivity of vascular smooth muscle to vasoactive agents.

The hemodynamic, electrocardiographic, and roentgenographic studies of patients with Cushing's syndrome have revealed no specific abnormalities except those that are, in general, associated with either hypertension or hypokalemia. The P-R intervals tend to be shorter than normal.

Over the past several years, a new familial syndrome has been described: Cushing's syndrome and cardiac myxoma occurring in the same individual (p. 1454). In addition to having these two conditions, 80 per cent of the patients have a cutaneous abnormality. In most it is a pigmented lesion; in some it is a subcutaneous myxoma. Histologically the adrenal glands show nodular hyperplasia.[138]

DIAGNOSIS AND TREATMENT. The diagnosis of Cushing's syndrome is established by the lack of appropriate suppression of cortisol secretion by dexamethasone. The best screening test is the administration of 1 mg of dexamethasone at bedtime with measurement of plasma cortisol between 7 and 10 the next morning.[133] In normal subjects cortisol levels will be less than 5 μg/dl. Some patients, particularly the obese, may have false-positive responses, but false-negative responses occur only rarely. The definitive diagnosis of Cushing's syndrome is made by administration of 0.5 mg of dexamethasone every 6 hours for 2 days with measurement either of plasma cortisol levels at the end of the second day (normal <5 μg/dl) or of the 24-hour 17-OH excretory rate on the second day of dexamethasone suppression (normal <3 mg/24 hours).[137,139]

Therapy of Cushing's syndrome is usually directed at the

specific cause. Thus, patients with adrenal carcinoma or adenoma or an ACTH-producing pituitary tumor are treated surgically. In some cases, patients with adrenal carcinoma have nonresectable lesions, and therefore surgery is combined with chemotherapy. The treatment of patients with bilateral hyperplasia without an evident ACTH-producing tumor is controversial, since the cause is often unknown. In some centers, bilateral adrenalectomy is the treatment of choice, while in others, therapy directed at the pituitary (either surgery or irradiation) is used.[140,141]

The treatment of the *cardiovascular abnormalities* associated with Cushing's syndrome is directed at lowering blood pressure and correcting the hypokalemia if present. Caution should be exercised in treating the hypertension with potassium-losing diuretics because of the tendency for these patients to develop hypokalemia. Thus, potassium-sparing diuretics or potassium supplements are often required. Hypertension in patients with Cushing's syndrome should be treated with agents that block the action or production of renin, such as beta blockers or converting-enzyme inhibitors. As in all clinical conditions in which hypokalemia may be present, cardiac glycosides should be used with caution in patients with Cushing's syndrome.

HYPERALDOSTERONISM

(See also p. 838)

CLINICAL AND BIOCHEMICAL MANIFESTATIONS. Aldosteronism is a syndrome associated with hypersecretion of aldosterone. Primary aldosteronism signifies that the stimulus for the excess aldosterone production resides within the adrenal. In secondary aldosteronism, the stimulus is of extraadrenal origin. These two conditions have similar effects on potassium metabolism.

In patients with primary aldosteronism, which most commonly is due to an aldosterone-producing adrenal adenoma, hypertension, hypokalemia, and metabolic alkalosis are common.[133,142] Polyuria may exist because of the hypokalemia, and glucose intolerance is increased in frequency. Muscle cramps due to the hypokalemia may be present, but little else distinguishes this from other forms of hypertension. Laboratory studies confirm the presence of hypokalemic alkalosis with a low specific gravity of urine and normal levels of adrenal glucocorticoids. The incidence of primary aldosteronism is between 0.5 and 2 per cent of the hypertensive population and it occurs twice as frequently in females as in males, with an initial presentation usually between the ages of 30 and 50 years.[133]

CARDIOVASCULAR MANIFESTATIONS. Many of the cardiovascular effects of aldosteronism are nonspecific, being related to aldosterone's effect on atrial pressure and potassium balance. Thus, T-wave flattening or U-wave prominence on the electrocardiogram (p. 150) and the presence of premature ventricular contractions and other arrhythmias due to hypokalemia are observed.[27] Evidence of left ventricular hypertrophy, either on the electrocardiogram or on the chest roentgenogram, may also be present in patients with longstanding hypertension and hyperaldosteronism. Malignant hypertension and changes in renal function secondary to severe hypertensive angiopathy are infrequent.

DIAGNOSIS AND TREATMENT. The diagnosis of primary aldosteronism is made by the presence of diastolic hypertension without edema, hypersecretion of aldosterone that fails to suppress appropriately during volume expansion, hyposecretion of renin, and hypokalemia with inappropriate urinary potassium loss during salt loading. The state of the renin-angiotensin system is often used to distinguish primary aldosteronism from other conditions that produce hypertension and hypokalemia. For example, hypertension and hypokalemia may be part of the clinical picture of secondary aldosteronism that accompanies malignant or accelerated hypertension or is associated with renal artery stenosis. Secondary aldosteronism can be readily distinguished from primary aldosteronism by the plasma renin activity, which is increased in the former and reduced in the latter. However, the combination of hypertension and a low plasma renin activity does not necessarily mean primary aldosteronism. Between 15 and 30 per cent of patients with essential hypertension have low renin levels, so-called low-renin essential hypertension.[142] The possibility of excess mineralocorticoid secretion has been extensively evaluated in these patients; however, no definitive evidence for such exists (Chap. 28).

The principal treatment for primary aldosteronism is surgical removal of the aldosterone-producing adenoma. In some cases, this is not possible because of the excessive risk imposed by the general physical status of the patient; then, spironolactone, which pharmacologically blocks the effects of aldosterone, is used long term. This form of therapy may be of limited benefit in males, since compliance is reduced by the undesirable side effects of gynecomastia and impotency, particularly when doses greater than 200 mg per day are required.[143]

Although congestive heart failure occurs infrequently in patients with primary aldosteronism, treatment of patients with this condition with cardiac glycosides must be cautious because of the hypokalemia.

In some patients, primary aldosteronism is due not to a solitary adenoma but to bilateral hyperplasia.[142] While the clinical characteristics of these two conditions are similar, their responses to surgery are different. In both cases hypokalemia is corrected, but patients with bilateral hyperplasia often do not exhibit reduction in arterial pressure. Patients with bilateral hyperplasia are best treated with spironolactone and other antihypertensive agents. Thus, preoperative distinction between bilateral hyperplasia and an adrenal adenoma, using adrenal venography or adrenal scanning, is important.

ADRENAL INSUFFICIENCY

Hypofunction of the adrenal cortex includes all conditions in which the level of secretion of adrenal steroids is less than the needs of the body. There are two major categories: those associated with primary damage to the adrenal cortex and those associated with secondary failure due to the lack of a stimulator such as ACTH. Clinically, patients with adrenal insufficiency can be divided into four types:[133] (1) the most common, primary insufficiency (Addison's disease); (2) secondary insufficiency due to a lack of ACTH; (3) selective hypoaldosteronism; and (4) enzyme deficiency (congenital adrenal hyperplasia).

CLINICAL AND BIOCHEMICAL MANIFESTATIONS. Addison's disease may occur at any age and affects both sexes equally. It is commonly due to a destructive process involving both adrenal glands; this process is sometimes infectious, but most often it is autoimmune.[144] Nearly all patients with primary adrenal insufficiency have weakness, increased skin pigmentation, significant weight loss, anorexia, nausea, vomiting, and hypotension, particularly postural. A significant minority also complain of abdominal pain, salt craving, and diarrhea or constipation. In mild forms, baseline laboratory studies are usually within normal limits. However, as the disease progresses, there is a gradual reduction in serum levels of sodium, chloride, and bicarbonate and an increase in potassium levels. The hyponatremia is due to extravascular loss of sodium, both into the urine (because of aldosterone deficiency) and into the intracellular compartment. The hyperkalemia is due both to the deficiency of aldosterone and to the impaired glomerular filtration rate and acidosis present in these patients. Other nonspecific findings include a reduction in basal metabolic rate with normal thyroid function and a normocytic anemia with relative lymphocytosis. While Addison's disease is often thought of as a common cause of significant eosinophilia, this is observed only occasionally.

CARDIOVASCULAR MANIFESTATIONS. The most common cardiovascular finding in adrenal insufficiency is arterial hypotension. In severe cases the pressure may be in the range of 80/50 mm Hg, with postural accentuation. Indeed, syncope occurs in a significant percentage of patients. In severe cases, heart size and peripheral pulses decrease. The electrocardiogram is abnormal in the majority of patients with Addison's disease.[27] The most common abnormalities are low or inverted T waves, sinus bradycardia, prolonged $Q\text{-}T_c$ interval, and low voltage. Conduction defects also occur, with first-degree block present in 20 per cent of patients. Changes secondary to the hyperkalemia are not common even though the serum potassium levels may be elevated. It is of interest that the electrocardiographic abnormalities, other than those secondary to hyperkalemia, do not respond to mineralocorticoids but require glucocorticoid replacement. Cardiac failure in prolonged adrenocortical insufficiency has also been reported rarely, secondary to a high-output state.[145,146]

DIAGNOSIS AND TREATMENT. Decreased response of the adrenal cortex to ACTH establishes the diagnosis of Addison's disease. The best screening test is the administration of synthetic ACTH (cosyntropin), 0.25 mg intramuscularly or intravenously, with measurement of plasma cortisol levels 30 to 60 minutes later. Cortisol levels double or increase by 10 μg/dl in normal subjects. Definitive evaluation is by prolonged (usually 24-hour) infusion of ACTH with assessment of either plasma cortisol or excretion of cortisol or both.[133]

It is possible to differentiate primary adrenal insufficiency from secondary adrenal insufficiency, isolated hypoaldosteronism, or congenital adrenal hyperplasia because one of the adrenal hormonal functions is normal in each of the latter three conditions. Thus in secondary adrenal insufficiency due to ACTH deficiency, aldosterone secretion is normal and the biochemical effects of mineralocorticoid deficiency, i.e., hyperkalemia, are not present. In isolated hypoaldosteronism, glucocorticoid function is normal. Female patients with congenital adrenal hyperplasia have evidence of androgen excess, such as virilization and hirsutism, and hypertension may also be present with a deficiency of 11-hydroxylase[147] (p. 841).

An increasingly common form of hypoaldosteronism is that associated with *hyporeninism.* Most commonly this syndrome is observed in older diabetic patients with a mild degree of renal impairment and hypertension; acidosis is also common. Usually these patients present with unexplained hyperkalemia. The cause is unknown, but may be secondary to damage to the juxtaglomerular apparatus and/or reduced conversion of a renin precursor into the active enzyme.[148] This clinical syndrome is particularly important in terms of cardiovascular diseases. Furthermore, commonly used drugs (beta blockers and calcium antagonists) can exacerbate this condition by further compromising aldosterone release.[149]

The treatment of adrenal insufficiency is accomplished by replacement of the deficient steroid. In adults with primary or secondary insufficiency, hydrocortisone, 20 to 30 mg daily, is administered in divided doses, usually two-thirds in the morning and one-third in midafternoon. In those patients with associated aldosterone deficiency, 9-α-fluorohydrocortisone, 0.05 to 0.10 mg daily, is given. During periods of significant stress (surgery, infection, or trauma), the dose of glucocorticoids should be increased. However, caution needs to be exercised in patients with myocardial infarction, as high-dose steroids could promote early infarct expansion.[150] Occasionally, acute adrenal insufficiency in patients who previously had apparently normal adrenal function is precipitated by the stress of cardiac surgery.[151]

PHEOCHROMOCYTOMA

(See also p. 840)

In 1859, Oliver and Shafer demonstrated that adrenal extract raised blood pressure when injected into experimental animals. In 1901, one active ingredient, epinephrine, was isolated and characterized, and in 1922 a syndrome of paroxysmal hypertension associated with an adrenal medullary tumor, pheochromocytoma, was reported.

EFFECTS OF CATECHOLAMINES ON THE CARDIOVASCULAR SYSTEM

The adrenal medulla and sympathetic nervous system are linked morphologically, biochemically, and physiologically and are often referred to as the sympathoadrenal system.[152] The sympathoadrenal system differs from other endocrine systems in several respects, including the fact that plasma levels of the secretory product, catecholamines, are not regulated by a direct feedback mechanism. Instead, catecholamine secretion is the efferent branch of a reflex arc involving centers in the brain stem, the hypothalamus, and perhaps the cerebral cortex as well. The human adrenal medulla contains about 1 mg of catecholamine per gram of tissue, approximately 85 per cent of which is epinephrine. The strategic location of the adrenal medullary cells within the cortex is associated with their capacity to form epinephrine, since high-dose glucocorticoids induce the formation of phenylethanolamine-*N*-methyltransferase, the enzyme needed to convert norepinephrine into epinephrine.[153]

In addition to their important effects on the cardiovascular system, catecholamines also have significant metabolic effects, stimulating glycogenolysis and gluconeogenesis, that is, increasing the production of glucose from glycogen and amino acid precursors and stimulating lipolysis, thereby mobilizing free fatty acids and inhibiting secretion of insulin. The absence of the adrenal medulla does not produce definable disease in humans. However, the presence of a hormonally active adrenal medullary tumor produces a number of significant findings.

CLINICAL AND BIOCHEMICAL MANIFESTATIONS. A pheochromocytoma is a catecholamine-producing tumor derived from chromaffin cells. Those arising from extraadrenal chromaffin cells are called nonadrenal pheochromocytomas or paraganglionomas. Probably less than 0.1 per cent of patients with hypertension have a pheochromocytoma. Despite the fact that it is an uncommon disease, pheochromocytomas generate a great deal of interest, largely because the morbidity and mortality associated with these tumors are significant, with detection often resulting in cure. Pheochromocytomas are highly vascular tumors; less than 10 per cent are malignant as indicated by local invasion or metastasis, but, as with other endocrine tumors, malignancy cannot always be determined by microscopic appearance alone.

While the vast majority of tumors occur sporadically, approximately 5 per cent are inherited as an autosomal trait, by which they are often part of a pluriglandular neoplastic syndrome,[152] which, in addition to pheochromocytoma, may consist of medullary carcinoma of the thyroid, parathyroidadenoma, and retinal or cerebellar hemangioblastomas. Most pheochromocytomas are solitary adrenal tumors, with 10 per cent being bilateral and 10 per cent nonadrenal. However, in the familial form of pheochromocytoma nearly half the patients have bilateral adrenal tumors.

The features that suggest pheochromocytoma in hypertensive patients are (1) paroxysmal attacks of any kind, (2) headaches, (3) excessive sweating, (4) signs of hypermetabolism, (5) orthostatic hypotension, and (6) unusual blood pressure elevations due to trauma or operation.[152] Many of the features are similar to those of hyperthyroidism. While paroxysmal attacks are the hallmark of pheochromocytoma, more than half the patients have fixed hypertension and nearly 10 per cent are normotensive.

CARDIOVASCULAR MANIFESTATIONS. Hypertension is the major cardiovascular manifestation of pheochromocytoma. Its lability sometimes distinguishes it from other forms of hypertension; however, only clinical awareness of the entity and specific laboratory testing permit establishment of the proper diagnosis. The lability of blood pressure in patients with pheochromocytoma has been suggested to be due not only to episodic discharge of catecholamines but also to a reduction in plasma volume, as well as to impaired sympathetic reflexes. A number of observations suggest that chronic volume depletion is present.[154] For example, alpha-adrenoceptor blockade or removal of the tumor produces severe hypotension, which is correctable by volume expansion.[155] Cardiac output has been reported to be normal, whereas heart rate is increased, and orthostatic hypotension is accompanied by decreased stroke volume and inadequate adjustments in peripheral resistance indicative of impaired peripheral vascular reflexes.[154] An occasional patient will have markedly elevated central aortic pressure and severe systemic hypotension due to severe arterial vasoconstriction. Patients with pheochromocytoma may also have acute pulmonary edema.[155a]

The electrocardiogram is abnormal in as many as 75 per cent of patients with pheochromocytoma.[27] The changes consist of T-wave inversion, left ventricular hypertrophy, sinus tachycardia, and, in some cases, other alterations in rhythm, such as frequent supraventricular ectopic beats or paroxysmal supraventricular tachycardia.[156] An occasional patient will have a short P-R interval and a narrow QRS complex, suggesting that catecholamines are modifying the A-V conduction system. When arterial pressure increases markedly, changes suggestive of myocardial damage, including transient ST-segment elevations, marked diffuse T-wave inversions, and depression of ST segments, are present. These changes are usually transient, and the electrocardiographic pattern reverts to normal after removal of the tumor or pharmacological blockade.[152,155,157] Some of the electrocardiographic abnormalities are presumably due to hypertensive heart disease or myocardial ischemia. However, a specific catecholamine-induced myocarditis[158] and/or cardiomyopathy[159–161] has also been suggested.

The echocardiogram often shows left ventricular hypertrophy with normal left ventricular function.[162] During a hypertensive crisis it may show systolic anterior involvement of the anterior mitral leaflet, paradoxical septal motion, and proximal exclusion of the posterior wall.[163]

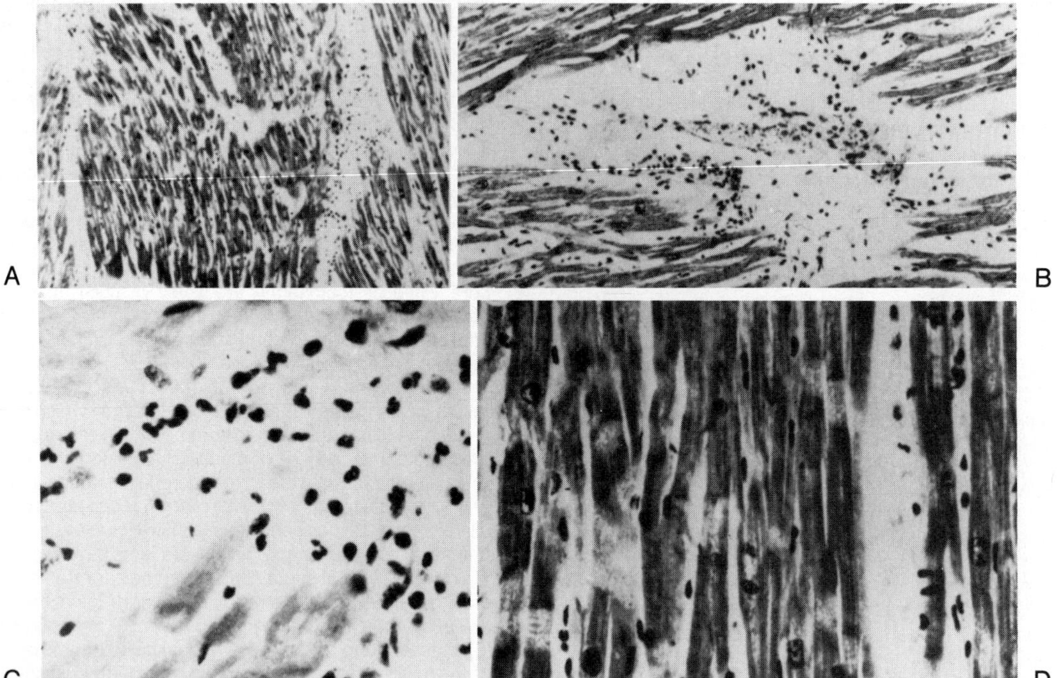

FIGURE 61–7. Left ventricular myocardium with acute myocarditis and contraction band necrosis in a patient with pheochromocytoma dying of catecholamine crisis. *A*, Diffuse infiltration by inflammatory cells through myocardium. *B*, Perivascular inflammation. *C*, Close-up of the inflammatory infiltrate. *D*, Contraction-band necrosis of myocytes. H&E; original magnification ×20 (*A*), ×45 (*B*), ×540 (*C*), ×330 (*D*). (From McManus, B. M., et al.: Fatal catecholamine crisis in pheochromocytoma: Curable cause of cardiac arrest. Am. Heart J. *102*:930, 1981.)

Myocarditis. Pathologically, the myocarditis consists of focal necrosis with infiltration of inflammatory cells, perivascular inflammation, and contraction band necrosis[164] (Fig. 61–7), finally resulting in fibrosis. In some studies, 50 per cent of patients who died from pheochromocytoma had myocarditis,[155] usually accompanied by left ventricular failure and pulmonary edema. Although coronary atherosclerosis is usually present, medial thickening is the most characteristic lesion of the coronary arteries. When norepinephrine is infused into the rabbit, there is sustained coronary vasoconstriction that within 48 hours leads to histologically documented myocardial damage.[165] Occasionally, patients with pheochromocytoma have manifestations of cardiomyopathy which may be reversed when the tumor is removed[159–161] (Fig. 61–8). Finally, the myositis is not necessarily limited to the myocardium, as it also may occur in skeletal muscle.[166]

DIAGNOSIS AND TREATMENT. The diagnosis of pheochromocytoma is established by documenting increased urinary or plasma levels of catecholamines or one of their metabolites.[152,155] Three tests are commonly employed: (1) total catecholamines, (2) vanillylmandelic acid (VMA), and (3) metanephrine. The last two are metabolites of catecholamine and were first used to screen for pheochromocytoma because they are present in greater quantities. When reliably performed, these tests are probably equivalent in accuracy. The probability of a pheochromocytoma being present in a hypertensive patient with a single normal urine level is less than 5 per cent. It is most desirable to measure both the catecholamines and one of the two metabolites, preferably metanephrine, in screening for pheochromocytoma. If the blood pressure fluctuates, it is particularly important to collect the urine at a time the pressure is elevated. Specific pharmacological tests to screen for pheochromocytoma are of limited benefit, usually hazardous, and therefore warranted only in unusual circumstances. Clonidine has been proposed as a useful definitive test for pheochromocytoma, although it is necessary only in unusual cases. Catecholamine levels are suppressed in normal subjects via stimulation of central alpha-adrenoceptors; following clonidine administration in patients with pheochromocytoma they are not.[152] Unfortunately, profound and prolonged hypotension has been reported in some patients during the course of this test.

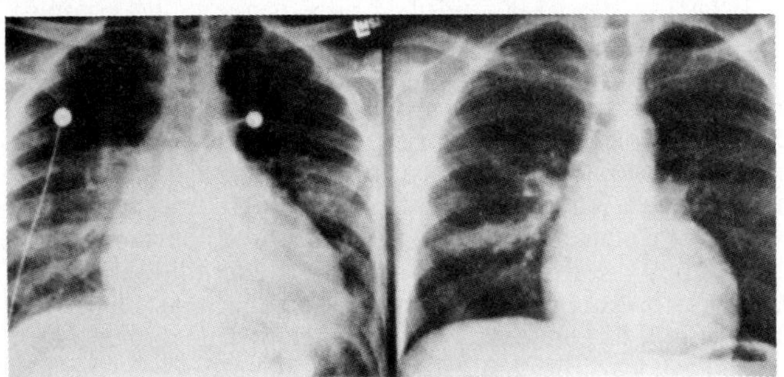

FIGURE 61–8. Pheochromocytoma-induced cardiomyopathy. *Left,* Chest x-ray on admission. Cardiomegaly, right pleural effusion, and signs of congestive heart failure. *Right,* One month after removal of the tumor. No signs of congestion and significant decrease of the heart size. (From Velasquez, G., et al.: Phaeochromocytoma and cardiomyopathy. Br. J. Radiol. *57*:89, 1984.)

Once the diagnosis of pheochromocytoma is established, specific pharmacological blockade should be initiated.[152,155] Administration of phenoxybenzamine hydrochloride should be begun, with the initial dosage 10 mg every 12 hours; the dose is then gradually increased every 2 to 3 days until the arterial pressure is restored to normal. Alternatively, prazosin may be used. However, it should be noted that alpha-adrenoceptor blockade may induce a decline in arterial pressure accompanied by serious postural hypotension, presumably because of the vasodilatation occurring in the presence of hypovolemia. This hypotensive response can be prevented by adequate sodium intake; if the response is very striking, infusion of saline may be required. Adequate control of arterial pressure is essential prior to any arteriographic procedure, before initiating beta-adrenoceptor blockade, and before operation. Serfas and colleagues have suggested that calcium antagonists may be useful both in treating the hypertension associated with pheochromocytoma and in reducing catecholamine production.[167]

Beta-adrenoceptor blockade is useful in patients with pheochromocytoma who have significant tachycardia, palpitations, and catecholamine-induced arrhythmias. However, beta blockade with a drug affecting $beta_2$ receptors must *not* be initiated prior to inadequate alpha blockade, since severe *hypertension* may occur as a result of unopposed alpha-stimulating activity of the circulating catecholamines.

Definitive treatment is surgical removal of the tumor, usually after localization with computed tomography, arteriography, or scanning using a radioactive iodide derivative of guanethidine as the scanning agent.[155] Scanning may be particularly important in localizing extraadrenal, e.g., thoracic, pheochromocytomas. Although rare, of particular importance to the cardiologist is the presence of a cardiac pheochromocytoma (p. 1457). Precise definition of the anatomical boundaries of this tumor is important preoperatively if surgery is to be successful.[168] In those patients with inoperable lesions, long-term use of the combination of alpha- and beta-adrenoceptor blockers has been helpful. Drugs that inhibit the biosynthesis of catecholamines, such as alpha-methyltyrosine, and generalized chemotherapeutic agents have also been used in patients with malignant pheochromocytoma.[155]

PARATHYROID DISEASE

Disordered parathyroid secretion is associated with two cardiovascular disturbances, cardiac arrhythmias and hypertension. Changes in calcium metabolism as well as a direct effect of parathyroid hormone on the cardiovascular system appear to be responsible.

CLINICAL AND BIOCHEMICAL MANIFESTATIONS. Parathyroid hormone (PTH) is a single-chain polypeptide of 84 amino acids. Its major biological effect is to increase mobilization of calcium into the extracellular fluid from a variety of tissues; this action is linked in a negative feedback loop with serum unbound calcium concentration. Thus, an increase in serum calcium concentration reduces PTH release and vice versa.[169] PTH also increases urinary excretion of phosphate, augments bone resorption, and reduces the urinary excretion of calcium. It also indirectly increases the absorption of calcium from the gastrointestinal tract by increasing the rate of conversion of 25-hydroxyl vitamin D into the biologically active 1,25-dihydroxyvitamin D.[169]

Primary hyperparathyroidism, the excess production of PTH, is usually secondary to a solitary parathyroid adenoma. Occasionally, generalized parathyroid hyperplasia exists, and, infrequently, carcinoma of the parathyroid gland is found. In many cases, hyperparathyroidism is asymptomatic; 10 to 20 per cent of cases are first diagnosed as the result of a routine chemical screening test. *Secondary* hyperparathyroidism is at least equal in frequency to primary hyperparathyroidism. It is most commonly associated with renal disease and chronic hypocalcemia.

The signs and symptoms of primary hyperparathyroidism are related to direct effects of PTH on kidney or bone or those associated with the hypercalcemia. Nearly half the patients have signs and symptoms of renal dysfunction, such as polyuria, nocturia, renal stones, and, in severe cases, nephrocalcinosis and renal failure. In many patients, there are also nonspecific joint and back symptoms, and in unusual circumstances spontaneous fractures occur. Hypercalcemia reduces the excitability of the neuromuscular system, which can lead to such diverse effects as significant myocardial dysfunction and decreased auditory acuity.

Cardiac hypertrophy is found with increased frequency in patients with hyperparathyroidism, even in the absence of hypertension. In one study, five of 18 patients with hypertrophic cardiomyopathy had raised serum PTH levels but normal serum calcium levels. In contrast, left ventricular hypertrophy did not occur in six patients with hypercalcemia alone.[170]

Hypocalcemia is the common biochemical abnormality in both hypoparathyroidism and secondary hyperparathyroidism. Gastrointestinal disturbances and tetany secondary to the hypocalcemia may both occur.

CARDIOVASCULAR MANIFESTATIONS OF PARATHYROID DISEASES

(See also p. 841)

CARDIAC EFFECTS. While most of the effects of parathyroid hormone on the heart are probably secondary to a change in extracellular calcium, PTH also has a direct effect on the heart, resulting in an increased beating rate of isolated heart cells and a positive inotropic action.[171,172] These effects are probably mediated by PTH binding to specific receptors, leading to increased entry of calcium into cardiac cells, and by the PTH increasing the release of endogenous myocardial norepinephrine. The direct effect of PTH may be deleterious, since it causes necrosis of rat myocytes and may be directly responsible for the increased accumulation of calcium in dystrophic muscles and for the heart damage found in uremia.[171,173] Whether these effects are clinically relevant is uncertain. Gafter and colleagues reported no change in cardiac performance in seven patients with end-stage renal disease who underwent parathyroidectomy for hyperparathyroidism.[174] On the other hand, hypoparathyroidism may cause a dilated cardiomyopathy, presumably secondary to the hypocalcemia. However, since longstanding hypocalcemia does not necessarily produce left ventricular dysfunction,[175] hypomagnesemia and reduced circulating PTH may also be involved.[176] PTH also has a direct effect on vascular smooth muscle, causing vasodilatation. Presently available data suggest that this vasodilating effect is more closely related to the portion of the PTH molecule responsible for its phosphaturic rather than its hypercalcemic effect.[177]

In addition to any direct action of PTH on the heart, hypercalcemia also has an adverse effect. Chronic hypercalcemia from a variety of causes is associated with increased deposition of calcium in the fibrous skeleton of the heart and valvular cusps as well as in coronary arteries and in myocardial fibers[178] (Fig. 61–9). Chronic hypercalcemia also may be a risk factor for accelerated coronary atherosclerosis.[179,180]

The plateau of the action potential of cardiac fibers is prolonged by low and shortened by high extracellular calcium concentrations (Chap. 22). Lengthening of the plateau prolongs the duration of the action potential, whereas shortening of the plateau has the opposite effect. The changes in duration of action potential are accompanied by corresponding changes in the duration of the refractory period, of the ST segment, and of the Q-T interval.[27] Thus the major electrocardiographic change in hypercalcemia is shortening of the Q-T interval. Less frequently, disorders of intraventricular conduction

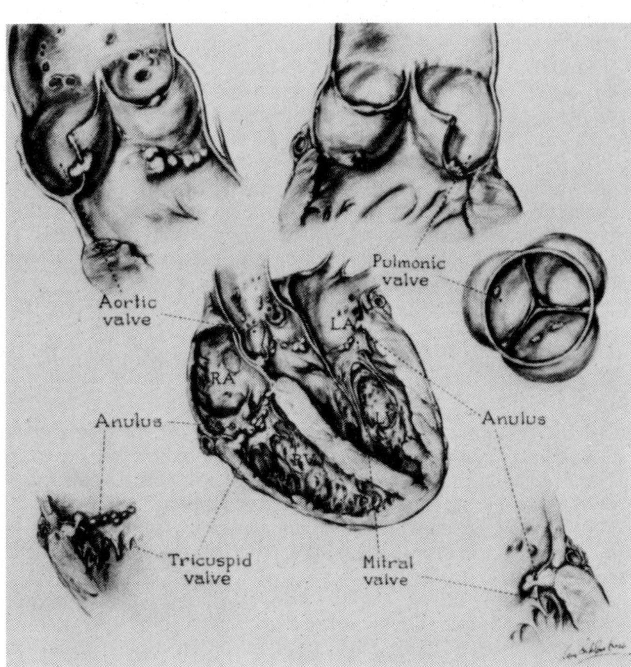

FIGURE 61–9. Heart showing distribution of calcific deposits in the tricuspid and mitral valve annuli and at the bases of both pulmonic and aortic valve cusps in a 43-year-old woman with hypercalcemia secondary to primary hyperparathyroidism. (From Roberts, W. C., and Waller, B. F.: Effect of chronic hypercalcemia on the heart: An analysis of 18 necropsy patients. Am. J. Med. *71*:371, 1981.)

have been reported with shortening of the P-R interval.[27] Complete heart block occurs only rarely.

Hypocalcemia produces the opposite effect on the electrocardiogram with prolongation of the Q-T interval and nonspecific ST- and T-wave changes. Normal contractile function of cardiac muscle requires calcium, and heart failure has been reported in patients with chronic hypocalcemia secondary to hypoparathyroidism.[181]

HYPERTENSION. Hypercalcemic patients detected by routine serum calcium screening techniques have higher arterial pressure than do matched normocalcemic subjects.[182] Yet in patients with hyperparathyroidism, the level of serum calcium is similar in those who are normotensive and those who have hypertension, suggesting that hypercalcemia per se is not the dominant cause for the hypertension. Thus, the pathophysiology of the hypertension is uncertain.[183] For example, hypercalcemia produces nephrocalcinosis, which may lead to renal failure and hypertension. Thus, reversal of hypertension after successful parathyroid surgery is more likely to occur when renal function is normal. Increased serum calcium also increases myocardial contractility, peripheral resistance, and release of or vascular sensitivity to vasoconstrictor agents, such as angiotensin II and norepinephrine. While hypercalcemia can increase cardiac contractility and arterial pressure acutely, it is unlikely that this action produces a significant alteration in cardiac output or performance on a long-term basis in the absence of PTH.[183] Thus an elevation of peripheral resistance is the most likely cause of the hypertension associated with hyperparathyroidism. While the mechanism of hypertension in these patients remains to be elucidated, (1) it may be renin dependent; (2) it is associated with increased circulating PTH, but not necessarily with the level of hypercalcemia; and (3) it is curable surgically in a significant number of patients.[184]

DIAGNOSIS AND TREATMENT

If hypercalcemia is *not* due to primary hyperparathyroidism, circulating concentration of PTH should be suppressed. Thus, an elevated or even a normal concentration of PTH in the presence of hypercalcemia establishes the diagnosis of hyperparathyroidism; many patients with this condition manifest hypercalcemia for the first time after starting thiazide therapy for the associated hypertension. Treatment consists of surgical removal of the parathyroid tumor of hyperplastic glands.

Patients with hypertension should have a determination of serum calcium levels before therapy is begun. If thiazide diuretics are used in treatment, serum calcium levels should be determined every 6 months. If thiazide-induced hypercalcemia occurs, the serum calcium should be determined for 2 to 3 months after discontinuation of the thiazides. Persistence of the hypercalcemia suggests that the patient has primary hyperparathyroidism.[182]

Patients with hypoparathyroidism and hypocalcemia usually are treated with calcium supplementation and vitamin D or one of its metabolites. To minimize the development of nephrolithiasis, serum calcium levels are titrated only to the lower end of the normal range.

DIABETES MELLITUS

Diabetes mellitus is one of the leading public health problems in the industrialized world, and it has a profound effect on the cardiovascular system. Nearly 10 million people are afflicted with this disease in the United States; it is the eighth health-related cause of death. Nearly all the morbidity from diabetes is related to cardiovascular dysfunction—coronary artery disease, hypertension, or renal failure secondary to microvascular disease.

ACTIONS OF INSULIN. Insulin is a double-chain polypeptide derived from proinsulin, which is synthesized in the islet cells of the pancreas. Many stimuli, such as glucose, glucagon, amino acids, catecholamines, and gastrointestinal hormones, can promote insulin secretion, which usually occurs in two phases. The rapid early phase releases preformed insulin stored in granules in the beta cells, while the prolonged late phase results from increased biosynthesis of insulin.[185]

Insulin is an anabolic hormone affecting all metabolic substrates, i.e., carbohydrates, fats, and proteins, as well as nucleic acids. All target tissues for insulin have specific membrane-bound receptors; thus, binding to the receptor is the first step in initiating its metabolic effect. The concept that insulin is the "fed" hormone has been popularized.[185] Thus the ingestion of fuel substrates provokes a rapid rise in the concentration of circulating insulin, which then facilitates the transfer of these substances into their respective depots. According to this theory, in the fasted state insulin levels are low; as a result, there is increased gluconeogenesis by the liver, decreased lipogenesis with lipolysis and fatty acid release from fat tissue, and decreased glucose uptake in cardiac and skeletal muscle. On the other hand, in the fed state insulin levels are high; gluconeogenesis by the liver is reduced; and in cardiac and skeletal muscle glucose and amino acid uptake and protein synthesis are increased. In adipose tissue there is increased glucose and triglyceride uptake, lipogenesis, and absence of release of fatty acids.

In the patient with diabetes, because insulin release is decreased in response to the ingested fuel, there is a delay in the uptake and the disposal of these fuels into their respective depots, which leads to abnormal circulating levels of the substrates. The increased concentrations of lipids in the circulation may be the underlying pathophysiological effect producing a number of the clinical complications of diabetes mellitus.

CLINICAL AND BIOCHEMICAL MANIFESTATIONS. Relatively recently, our understanding of the pathogenesis of diabetes mellitus has been significantly altered. Several lines of evidence suggest that in many instances the insulin-dependent (IDDM) form may be infectious or autoimmune in origin, while in most cases the noninsulin-dependent form (NIDDM) is probably the result of a genetic predisposition.[186]

Most of the signs and symptoms of this disease either are related to the increased levels of blood glucose or are secondary to changes in the cardiovascular system. Thus, the classic presenting symptoms (observed in about 25 per cent of IDDM patients) are polyuria, polydipsia, and polyphagia, all due to the glucosuria. The major pathophysiological consequence of diabetes mellitus is related to changes in the vascular system. The specific target organs include the heart, the eye, the kidney, the autonomic nervous system, and the peripheral vasculature.

CARDIOVASCULAR CHANGES IN DIABETES

PATHOLOGY. The vascular disease associated with diabetes mellitus can be nonspecific (atherosclerosis and arteriosclerosis) or specific (microangiopathic or endothelial proliferative changes of arterioles). The former primarily involves large vessels (especially in the lower extremities), heart, and brain of older patients, while the latter is localized to small vessels and may be seen in patients of all ages. The atherosclerosis tends to be more extensive and more severe than in nondiabetics, resulting in an increased frequency of myocardial infarction and cerebral and peripheral vasculature disease.[187] Indeed, coronary heart disease is the leading cause of death among adult diabetics and accounts for about three times as many deaths among diabetics as among nondiabetics. The incidence of coronary artery disease correlates more closely with the duration of diabetes than with its severity. Of interest is the documentation that diabetics have an increased mortality for noncardiovascular diseases (e.g., cancer) as well.[188] The mechanism(s) responsible for this generalized increased mortality is unclear.

Certainly, diabetes should be considered to be a separate risk factor for coronary heart disease[189-190] (p. 1151). Since each risk factor for vascular disease is thought to add independently (although not equally) to the likelihood for the development of ischemic disease, the diabetic should be considered a high-risk patient in whom all correctable factors should be managed.[191-192] It is logical to approach cigarette smoking and even moderate elevation of blood pressure and plasma lipids more intensively in diabetic than in nondiabetic patients. Contraceptive drugs that suppress ovulation probably should be avoided, since they may contribute to the metabolic abnormalities that underlie their increased risk for vascular disease. The obese diabetic patient should lose weight; this is often accompanied by gratifying improvement of hypertension, hyperglycemia, hyperinsulinemia, and hypertriglyceridemia.

The microangiopathy produces a characteristic thickening of the basement membrane of the capillaries in the retina, conjunctiva, glomerulus, brain, pancreas, and myocardium.[193] In some cases there is also proliferation of the epithelial cells, leading to occlusion of small arterioles similar to that observed in immune arteritis.

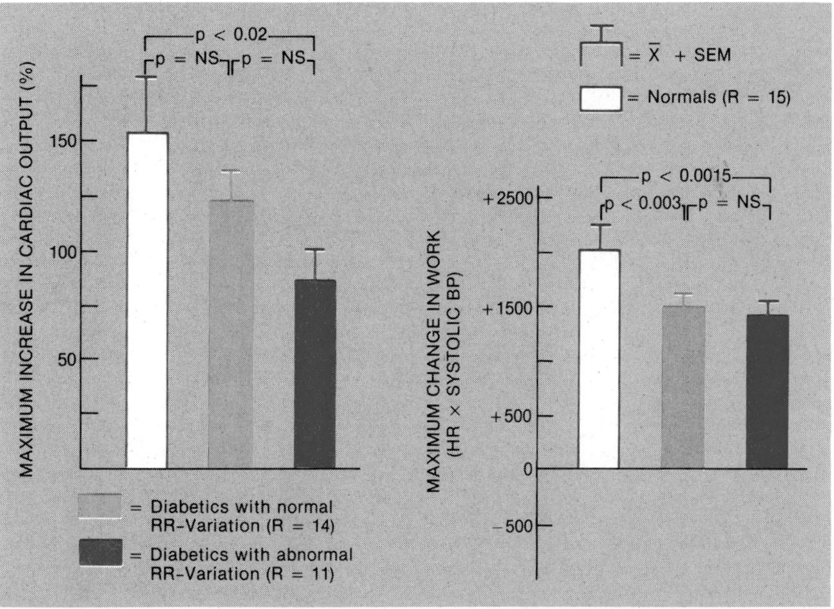

FIGURE 61-10. Per cent maximum increase in cardiac output and heart rate × blood pressure product in response to exercise achieved in 15 normal subjects and 14 diabetics with normal and 11 with abnormal RR variation. The decreased cardiac output response suggests an abnormality in cardiac parasympathetic nervous system activity in patients with abnormal RR variation. (From Roy, T. M., et al.: Autonomic influence on cardiovascular performance in diabetic subjects. Am. J. Med. *87*:385, 1989.)

CARDIAC INVOLVEMENT. Not only is the frequency of acute myocardial infarction increased in diabetic patients,[190,191] but also the treatment of the infarct is more complicated than in the nondiabetic patient. Patients with acute myocardial infarction, regardless of the control of their diabetes before hospital admission, exhibit significantly higher mortality and morbidity than do nondiabetics.[189,191,192] Several factors contribute to the increased mortality of diabetic patients with acute myocardial infarction. The size of the infarct tends to be greater in the diabetic than in the nondiabetic; diabetic patients have a greater frequency of both congestive heart failure and shock than do nondiabetics; and the patient is often in a precarious metabolic status compounded by the difficulty of adjusting insulin therapy to prevent ketoacidosis while not precipitating hypoglycemia.[189,192,194]

The occurrence of myocardial infarction has a distinctly adverse effect on carbohydrate and fat metabolism and often leads to stimulation of the sympathetic nervous system and increased catecholamine concentration[195] (p. 1212). Subsequent increases in circulating free fatty acid levels and reductions in glucose tolerance appear to be related to a number of physiological functions—adipose tissue lipolysis, hepatic and muscle glycogenolysis, catecholamine-induced suppression of insulin release, and increased circulating concentrations of growth hormone and cortisol. The net result is that carbohydrate intolerance is common after myocardial infarction, even in nondiabetics. Also, the high concentrations of free fatty acid in the acute phases of myocardial infarction may lead to ventricular arrhythmias.[196] The suppression of insulin release as a consequence of increased catecholamine activity may decrease glucose utilization by a myocardium that may require this fuel for glycolytic activity.[197]

Diabetic patients with acute myocardial infarction differ from nondiabetics in that their pain patterns are more variable, and infarction may actually occur without pain.[198] Also, survival after infarction is more limited than in the nondiabetics, with fatality rates being as high as 25 per cent during the first year after infarction.[189,191,192] Recurrent infarction, heart failure, and dysrhythmias all contribute to this higher death rate.[189-192,194] Administration of beta blockers to diabetics appears to reduce the overall mortality, at least in the immediate postmyocardial infarction period, similar to what has been reported in nondiabetics.[199]

Peripheral somatic neuropathy is a common complication of diabetes mellitus; also, diabetic autonomic neuropathy leading to diarrhea, vomiting, and other gastrointestinal disturbances is well known in this disease. *Cardiac autonomic dysfunction* also exists in many diabetic patients,[200,201] and the anginal threshold is increased, presumably as a consequence of autonomic and sensory neuropathies.[202a] In two large series it was present in more than a third of the patients and accompanied by depression of left ventricular function. The severity of cardiac dysfunction was directly related to the severity of the cardiac autonomic neuropathy[202,203] (Fig. 61-10). Occasionally it may be present before clinical symptoms of generalized autonomic neuropathy are demonstrable. Furthermore, the neuropathy may involve the sympathetic nervous system and/or the parasympathetic nervous system. Indeed, it may become so severe as to lead to total cardiac denervation. These changes in adrenergic nervous system function result in tachycardia and a fixed, rapid heart rate that barely responds to physiological stimuli, such as the Valsalva maneuver, carotid sinus pressure, or tilting,[204a] or to drugs, such as phenylephrine, atropine, or propranolol. Rarely, these denervated hearts develop arrhythmias.

CONGESTIVE HEART FAILURE. IDDM appears to increase the likelihood of the development of congestive heart failure from all causes. The role of diabetes in congestive heart failure in the Framingham study was analyzed,[192] and the risk of developing heart failure was found to be increased substantially. Even when patients with prior coronary or rheumatic heart disease were excluded, diabetic subjects had a four- to fivefold increased risk of congestive heart failure. Furthermore, this increased risk persisted after age, blood pressure, weight, and cholesterol values, as well as coronary heart disease, were taken into account. On the basis of these findings it appeared that the excessive risk of heart failure in diabetic patients is caused by factors other than accelerated atherogenesis and coronary heart disease. One suggested possibility is a diabetes-induced cardiomyopathy.

Diabetic Cardiomyopathy. There is a substantial increase in the coincidence of diabetes mellitis and cardiomyopathy. The cardiomyopathy occurs in patients who have no evidence of large-vessel disease or abnormalities in myocardial capillary basal lamina documented by endomyocardial biopsies.[205,206] The most common histological abnormalities are interstitial fibrosis (Fig. 61-11) and arteriolar hyalinization (Fig. 61-12). Evidence supporting the presence of cardiomyopathy even in children with diabetes mellitus has been reported. Both systolic and diastolic dysfunction have been observed. The severity of this dysfunction is related to the degree of metabolic control, and there is no clinical evidence of cardiovascular or microvascular disease.[207] Taken together, these studies strongly suggest that in some diabetic patients there is a nonischemic cardiomyopathic process.

ABNORMALITIES OF VENTRICULAR FUNCTION. Several abnormalities of ventricular function, using echocardiographic techniques, have been reported in diabetics. In young

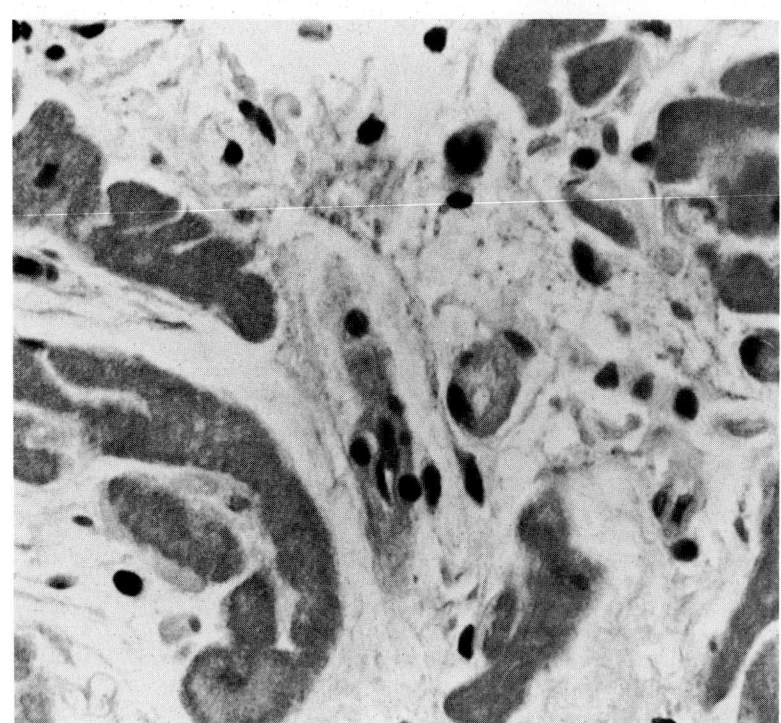

FIGURE 61-11. Myocardium of diabetic patient showing atrophied myocytes on right side (compare with more normal fibers on left), increased interstitial fibrous tissue, and thickening of small arteriolar walls. H & E × 300. (From Sutherland, C. G. G., et al.: Endomyocardial biopsy pathology in insulin-dependent diabetic patients with abnormal ventricular function. Histopathology *14*:596, 1989.)

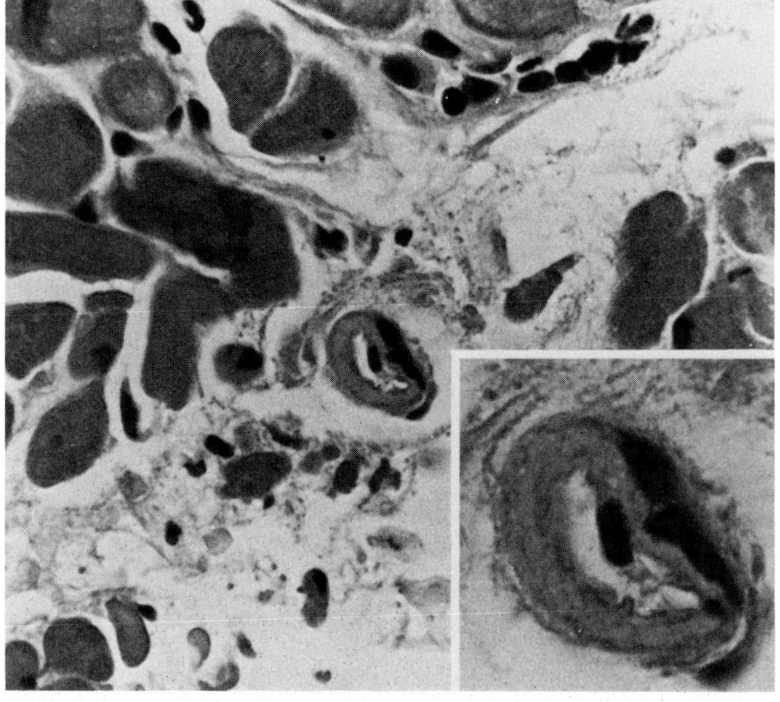

FIGURE 61-12. Hyalinization without luminal narrowing of small arteriole in myocardium of diabetic patient. H & E, ×300. Inset, Same arteriole. (H & E, ×750.) (From Sutherland, C.G.G. et al.: Endomyocardial biopsy pathology in insulin-dependent diabetic patients with abnormal ventricular function. Histopathology *14*:597, 1989.)

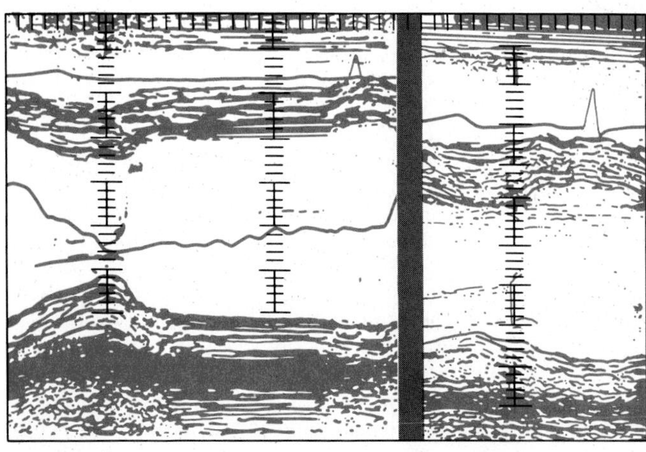

FIGURE 61-13. M-mode echocardiograms from a healthy woman (*left*) and a diabetic woman (*right*). The rate of ventricular filling is much slower in the latter. (From Airaksinen, J., et al.: Impaired left ventricular filling in young female diabetics. An echocardiographic study. Acta Med. Scand. *216*:509, 1984.)

asymptomatic patients, the ratio of early to peak filling velocity is significantly decreased while atrial filling velocity is significantly increased (Fig. 61–13). There is no relationship between the left ventricular diastolic filling abnormalities and evidence of severity of the diabetes, i.e., retinopathy, nephropathy, or peripheral neuropathy.[208] Other reported abnormalities in diabetic subjects include left ventricular asynergy on two-dimensional echocardiograms[208,209]; reduction in the peak diastolic filling rate[210]; an abnormal left ventricular ejection fraction in response to exercise[211,212]; and evidence of diastolic dysfunction, even in normotensive diabetic patients.[213,213a]

Several factors have been reported to contribute to the abnormalities in left ventricular function in diabetics: (1) The role of hypertension with a concomitant increase in left ventricular mass.[214] (2) The potential role of growth hormone. Patients with difficult-to-control diabetes often have increased growth hormone levels. Several investigators have reported that this metabolic abnormality could account for the increased collagen levels present in the left ventricular wall of diabetic humans and animals[215] (Fig. 61–11). Regan et al., however, have reported that in experimental diabetes induced in dogs the collagen accumulation in the myocardium is not related to or dependent on an increase in plasma growth hormone levels.[216] (3) The increased cardiac sorbitol level.[217] (4) The impairment in Ca^{++} handling with hypersensitivity of the myocardium to Ca^{++} secondary to increased sarcolemmal Ca^{++} ATPase activity[218,219] (Fig. 61–14). In a rat model of non-insulin–dependent diabetes mellitus, the abnormalities in myocardial Ca^{++} ATPase activity have also been demonstrated.[220] Further support for this hypothesis comes from the beneficial effect of a calcium antagonist (verapamil), which prevented diabetes-induced myocardial changes in experimental diabetes.[221] (5) Finally, Okumura et al. have suggested that increased 1,2-diacylglycerol levels with resultant activation of protein kinase C may underlie the cardiomyopathy, at least in experimentally induced diabetes.[222] Despite these observations in experimental models, it should be noted that when insulin is administered, the cardiac abnormality is not necessarily corrected. Thus, the relationship between the hyperglycemic state and the abnormalities in myocardial function and metabolism present in experimental diabetes is still unclear.

Pathological Changes. In postmortem studies of 11 diabetic patients, 9 of whom were without significant obstructive disease of the proximal coronary arteries and had died of cardiac failure, all exhibited positive periodic acid–Schiff (PAS) staining material in the interstitium, but none had luminal narrowing of the intramural vessels. Collagen accumulation was present in perivascular loci, between the myofibers, or as replacement fibrosis. Multiple samples of left ventricle and septum revealed abnormally increased deposits of triglyceride and cholesterol.[223] Thus these observations, taken in toto, suggest that a diffuse abnormality, either extravascular or involving the microvasculature, may be the basis for the cardiomyopathic features of diabetes. However, a recent morphological study casts some doubt on small-vessel disease as the producer of cardiac myopathy, because similar findings have been reported in NIDDM subjects. Unsitupa et al., studying 133 patients with NIDDM (Type 2), found a high incidence of impaired left ventricular function already present at the time of initial diagnosis.[224] Hypertension appears to accelerate this process, both in humans and animals, as severe interstitial fibrosis, focal scars, and myocytolytic activity were significantly more frequent in hypertensive diabetics with chronic heart failure examined post mortem than in normotensive diabetics.[225]

Other (nondiabetic) cardiomyopathies may exhibit similar hemodynamic abnormalities; an abnormal rise of ventricular filling pressure without a stroke volume increase in response to afterload increments has also been observed in the preclinical phase of alcoholic cardiomyopathy, in which the interstitium is also altered.[225] More severely altered interstitial changes may be the predominant lesion in the incipient stages of amyloid heart disease.[226]

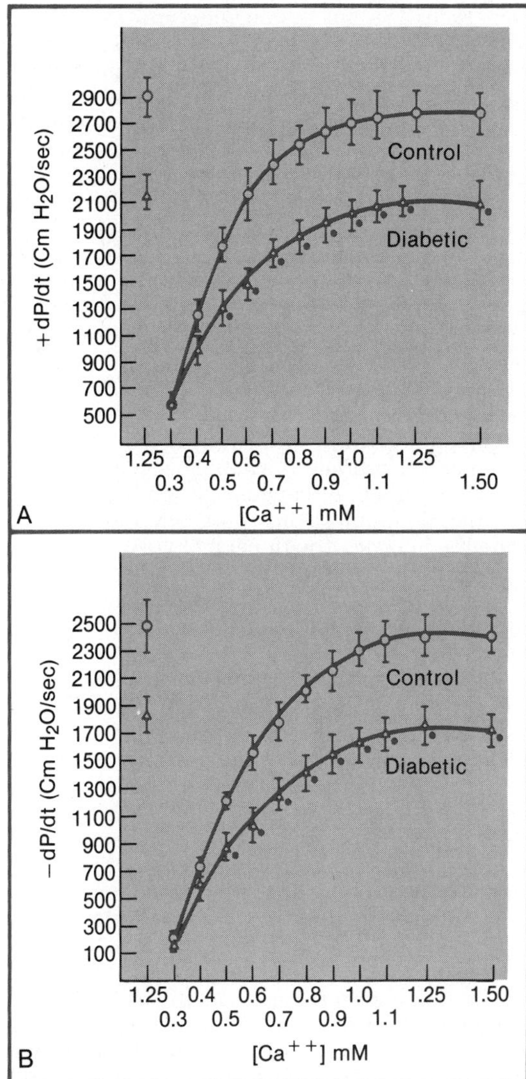

FIGURE 61–14. **Effect of non-insulin–dependent diabetes mellitus on myocardial contractility (+dp/dt, *top*) and relaxation (−dp/dt, *bottom*). Hearts from 12-month-old diabetic rats (triangles) and the age-matched controls (circles) were perfused during the initial 20–minute stabilization period with Krebs-Henseleit buffer containing 11 mM glucose and a calcium concentration of 1.25 mM. At each calcium concentration, +dP/dt (first derivative of left ventricular function, an index of contractility) (*A*) and −dP/dt (an index of relaxation) (*B*) were measured. Each data point represents mean ± SE of five to seven hearts. *Significant difference from control ($P < 0.05$). (From Schaffer, S. W., et al.: Basis for myocardial mechanical defects associated with noninsulin-dependent diabetes. Am. J. Physiol. *256*:E27, 1989.)**

Diabetes mellitus is associated with another form of cardiomyopathy. Approximately half the infants of diabetic mothers have either radiographic cardiomegaly or clinical features suggesting congestive heart failure[227] (p. 995). The cardiomyopathy in these infants may be transient and secondary to hematological, respiratory, and metabolic problems or a more protracted form of nonobstructive or obstructive hypertrophic cardiomyopathy, which appears to be secondary to maternal hormonal influences and to be reversible.

Electrocardiographic changes are commonly observed in patients with diabetes.[27] While many of the changes are predictable on the basis of the associated hypertension or coronary artery disease, in some there is an unexplained diffuse T-wave abnormality that may be related to the cardiomyopathy.

VASCULAR DISEASE. Peripheral vascular disease is a frequent and significant manifestation of diabetes mellitus, sometimes leading to gangrene and requiring amputation. The smaller arteries below the knee are more likely to be involved in patients with diabetes, in contrast to iliac or femoral artery disease in nondiabetic patients. Cerebral vascular disease is also more frequent, with a greater incidence of cerebral infarction though not cerebral hemorrhage. The increased atherosclerosis of the cerebral vessels and the proliferative changes in the cerebral arterioles both contribute to this increased rate of infarction. In addition to the effect of diabetes on cardiac function, insulin itself can cause salt and water retention by mechanisms still obscure. In most cases this fluid retention is self-limiting. However, in individuals who have underlying cardiovascular disease it may lead to overt cardiac failure.[228]

The renal vasculature is affected in a number of ways: atherosclerosis is common in the larger vessels, with proliferative endothelial changes occurring in small vessels. Capillary basement membrane thickening is common, particularly in the glomerular tuft where a pathognomonic change—nodular glomerulosclerosis—is often found. These vascular changes, in concert with parenchymal changes secondary to pyelonephritis and altered renal hemodynamics (increased glomerular pressure),[229,230] lead to a variety of renal disorders, including the nephrotic syndrome, hypertension, and renal failure.

The mechanism underlying the development of atherosclerosis in diabetes is multifactorial (p. 1151). Hyperinsulinemia itself has been shown to enhance lipid synthesis in arterial walls and may be a major factor contributing to the macroangiopathy.[231] Most studies have reported an increased incidence of hypertension in diabetes. Indeed, more than one-third of diabetic patients have hypertension, an incidence that is higher than that of the general population.[232] The hypertension is in part related to the increased frequency of renal disease. Volume overload may be an additional factor.

Recently the association of hypertension with diabetes and obesity has led some investigators to propose that there is a causal link between these conditions: the link being insulin resistance. Resistance to the metabolic actions of insulin is a prominent feature of NIDDM. It has been suggested that the increased frequency of hypertension in this condition is secondary to selective insulin resistance—the autonomic nervous system and/or the kidney is not insulin-resistant. Elevated levels of insulin acting on the kidney will induce volume retention, while an increased insulin effect on the adrenergic nervous system will increase sympathetic outflow. Either of these can then lead to elevation of blood pressure.[233,234] In the past, the hypertension was assumed to be treated best by diuretics and sodium restriction. This therapy has two substantial drawbacks: (1) diuretics impair glucose homeostasis and (2) they probably accelerate renal deterioration. Because converting-enzyme inhibitors have theoretical advantages both in terms of glucose control and in retarding the deterioration of renal function, they may be the treatment of choice for hypertension in diabetics.[229,235,236]

DIAGNOSIS AND TREATMENT OF DIABETES MELLITUS

It is generally agreed that therapy directed at the control of excessive fatty acid mobilization and oxidation and protein catabolism is essential in diabetes mellitus. On the other hand, disagreement still exists regarding the usefulness of treating asymptomatic hyperglycemia. It has been documented that the synthesis of polyols and basement membrane glycoproteins is increased by hyperglycemia.[193,237] Thus, "tight control" of blood glucose may be important if the long-term complications of diabetes mellitus are to be reduced.

Diet, insulin, and oral hypoglycemic agents have been the mainstays of treatment. However, a controversy has arisen concerning the efficacy of oral hypoglycemic agents, such as the sulfonylureas.[238] While hyperglycemia is better controlled with these agents than it is with diet alone, an increased frequency of myocardial infarction has been reported. Although the interpretation and implications of these findings are controversial, there is some experimental evidence suggesting that sulfonylureas may have an adverse effect on the myocardium. Wu and colleagues have reported increased "stiffness" of the myocardium secondary to interstitial accumulation of PAS-staining material that reduced left ventricular function in dogs treated with tolbutamide.[239]

On the basis of available information, in our judgment patients with diabetes who should use oral hypoglycemic agents, preferably one of the second-generation agents (glyburide or glipizide),[240] are those who are not ketosis prone and whose hyperglycemia cannot be controlled with diet alone. It should also be recognized that beta-adrenoceptor blockers reduce the hyperglycemic reaction to stress, and it is possible that beta-adrenoceptor blocker therapy may require a downward adjustment of insulin dosage, since patients receiving beta blockers may be more susceptible to hypoglycemia, particularly in the elderly.[240] Since many of the symptoms of which the hypoglycemic patient is aware are due to the effects of the epinephrine which is released, both physician and patient must be alert to the possibility that hypoglycemia occurring in the beta blocker–treated diabetic may be relatively asymptomatic. Since certain diuretics, such as the thiazides and furosemide, may result in hypokalemia, and because hypokalemia can inhibit insulin release, these drugs may intensify the glucose intolerance of diabetic patients.

In patients with diabetes mellitus and impairment of left ventricular function, a sudden change in the glucose concentration of extracellular fluid, as occurs with the development of insulin deficiency, may result in the movement of fluid from the intracellular to the extracellular space and the intensification of heart failure. The hyperosmolar state has been shown experimentally to reduce cardiac contractility.[241] This hyperosmolar state responds to the lowering of blood glucose by insulin.[242]

OBESITY

There are two types of obesity: adult onset and lifelong. Adult-onset obesity is extremely common, probably occurring to a varying extent in nearly all individuals in developed countries. Its clinical course consists of normal weight patterns during childhood and adolescence, with a gradual increase in weight beginning between 20 and 40 years of age; it reflects an imbalance between caloric intake and utilization.[243] Much less common is lifelong obesity, characterized by the development of obesity early in childhood, with significant increase in weight during adolescence and, in women, during and after pregnancy. These individuals are usually grossly obese, weighing more than 150 per cent of their ideal weight as adults. The underlying cause of obesity in either condition is unclear.

Hirsch has documented an increase both in the size and the number of adipose cells in individuals with lifelong obesity, while in adult-onset obesity only an increase in cell size occurs.[244] With weight reduction the size of the adipose cells decreases in both conditions; however, the number does not change in either. Whether the increased number of adipose cells in lifelong obesity is determined by genetic or environmental factors is uncertain. However, it has been documented that there is no significant change in the number of adipose cells when obesity develops after late childhood in both experimental animals and humans. On the other hand, some evidence suggests that early infant feeding habits may significantly alter their number.[244] The metabolic consequences of obesity include decreased sensitivity to insulin, with resultant hyperinsulinemia, glucose intolerance, hypercholesterolemia, hypertriglyceridemia, and hyperaminoacidemia.

CARDIOVASCULAR CONSEQUENCES OF SEVERE OBESITY

During the past decade the health risk of obesity has been intensively studied. A conference analyzing data from two national health and nutrition surveys and the Framingham 30-year follow-up study concluded that a significant excess in mortality is evident in individuals with an obesity mass index greater than 27. A value greater than this is present in 34 million adult United States citizens. There is a direct correlation between the levels of blood pressure and cholesterol and the degree of obesity.[245] *Hypertension* is common in the grossly obese,[246] although it must be recognized that indirect measurement of blood pressure frequently leads to overestimation of the arterial pressure by the standard cuff method (p. 20). Nonetheless, direct measurement of arterial pressure frequently shows moderate elevations that can usually be promptly restored to normal by means of weight reduction and salt restriction.

Evidence of circulatory dysfunction in the massively obese, associated with cardiac enlargement during life and at autopsy, was first described by Smith and Willius in 1933.[247] It is now widely appreciated that massive obesity is accompanied by a marked increase in blood volume and cardiac output, which are proportional to the excess of body weight and the duration of obesity[248–250]; the hematocrit is often slightly elevated as well. The increased cardiac output is secondary to increased end-diastolic left ventricular volume[249–250] and stroke volume, since heart rate is normal; the cardiac output rises normally during exercise. Left ventricular filling pressures are at or close to the upper limits of normal in the supine position in the basal state, but increase with passive leg raising, and reach strikingly elevated levels during exercise. These increases in ventricular filling pressure are associated with a high resting central blood volume, which also increases significantly with exertion. A tendency to leftward deviation of the electrical axis correlates significantly with increasing obesity independent of age and blood pressure. However, this association is usually confined to the normal QRS-axis range. Thus, abnormal left-axis deviation is not necessarily a reflection of obesity.[251] The maximum velocity of myocardial fiber shortening and the ratio of stroke work index to left ventricular end-diastolic pressure were reduced, even in relatively young obese persons, without any other evidence of heart disease[248] (Fig. 61–15). Massive edema may occur as a consequence of the elevated ventricular filling pressure, despite elevation of the cardiac output.

Examination of the gross and microscopic anatomy of the heart in patients with marked chronic obesity showed heart weight to be considerably greater than predicted for ideal body weight, with left ventricular dilatation and eccentric hypertrophy and, in a few instances, right ventricular hypertrophy as well[252–253] (Fig. 61–16). Left atrial abnormalities (increased size and reduced emptying index) also have been reported.[254] This increase in cardiac weight is not due to excess epicardial fat and fatty infiltration of the myocardium, which were previously considered to be the principal features of the obese heart. However, in at least one study the frequency of atherosclerosis was not increased in persons who were morbidly obese. Obesity-induced cardiac hypertrophy is different from that induced by hypertension. Instead of the concentric left ventricular hypertrophy associated with hypertension, the hypertrophy is eccentric, with chamber dilatation and some wall thickening, as seen in other conditions in which cardiac output is chronically increased (Fig. 61–17). Also, in contrast to the increased afterload associated with systemic hypertension, obesity produces an elevated preload. When hypertension accompanies severe obesity, a combination of concentric and eccentric hypertrophy is present. Obese patients with clinically evident ventricular hypertrophy have an increased propensity to ectopy, in comparison with obese persons without left ventricular hypertrophy or with lean persons.[254] In part, this increased ectopy may be secondary to cardiac autonomic dysfunction.[255] Thus, when these clinical, hemodynamic, and pathological observations are taken together, it appears that manifestations of myocardial dysfunction occur in very obese subjects without evidence of other heart disease and that, in the absence of the obesity hypoventilation syndrome (p. 1593), cor pulmonale is not a presenting feature.

Heart failure in the markedly obese is usually chronic. The pulmonary and systemic congestion with symptoms of dyspnea and edema are, at first, simply related to the reductions in ventricular compliance and elevations of filling pressures. Later, these symptoms are related also to increases in ventricular end-diastolic volume and the reduction of myocardial

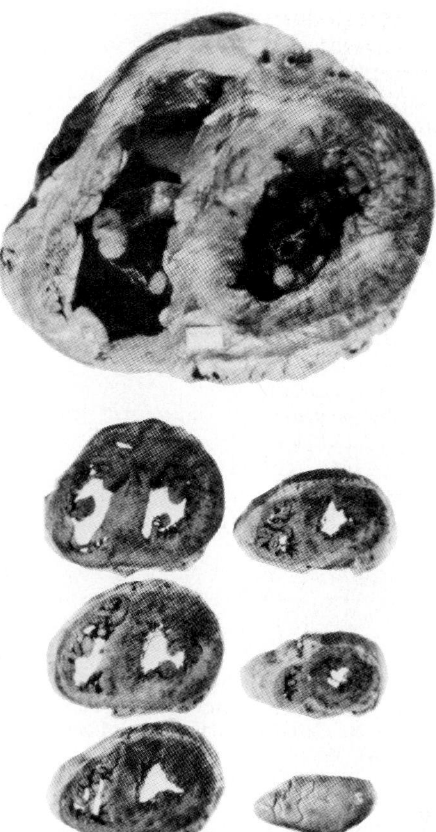

FIGURE 61–16. Cross section of the heart of a 34-year-old man who weighed more than 500 lb. Both ventricular walls are hypertrophied and both cavities are dilated. The heart weight (825 gm) was greatly increased. (From Warnes, C. A., and Roberts, W. C.: The heart in massive [more than 300 pounds or 136 kilograms] obesity: Analysis of 12 patients studied at necropsy. Am. J. Cardiol. *54*:1090, 1984.)

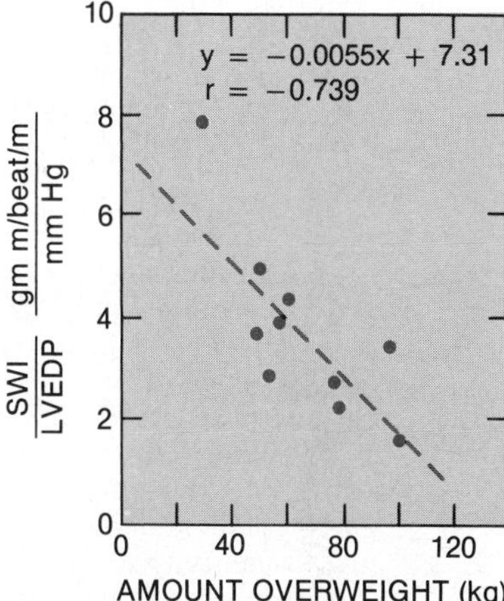

FIGURE 61–15. The significant negative correlation between the ratio of the stroke work index (SWI) to the left ventricular end-diastolic pressure (LVEDP) and the amounts of overweight shows that the higher the degree of obesity, the greater the impairment of left ventricular function. (From Divitiis, O., et al.: Obesity and cardiac function. Circulation 64:477, 1981, by permission of the American Heart Association, Inc.)

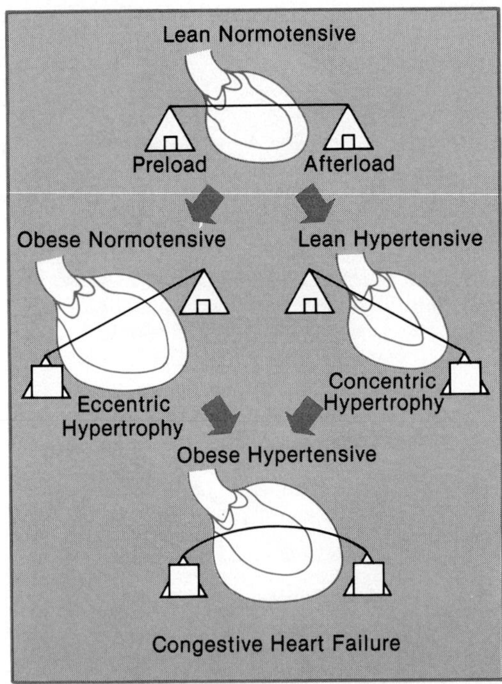

FIGURE 61–17. Adaptation of the heart to obesity and hypertension. (From Masserli, F. H.: Cardiovascular effects of obesity and hypertension. Lancet *1*:1165, 1982.)

contractility. Thus, the marked chronic increase in cardiac work, i.e., in cardiac output and arterial pressure, ultimately leads to heart failure.

Fortunately, weight reduction is beneficial in the majority of patients, even those with heart failure. It usually improves the exercise capacity of patients with chronic exogenous obesity and decreases total body oxygen uptake, the cardiothoracic ratio on chest roentgenogram, systemic arterial pressure, blood volume, cardiac output, arteriovenous oxygen difference, and left ventricular filling pressure at rest.[256] MacMahon et al. have documented that weight loss of as little as 8 kg is associated with a significant decrease in left ventricular mass, particularly the thickness of the posterior and central walls.[257] Alpert and colleagues, studying cardiac function in grossly obese individuals, noted a substantial reduction in left ventricular chamber enlargement and an improvement in systemic function with an average weight loss of 55 kg.[258] However, they were unable to show a change in septal or posterior wall thickness, suggesting that some of the beneficial effects of weight loss on cardiac function may occur only if the obesity is mild or of short duration. Supporting this conclusion is the persistence of elevated left ventricular filling pressure with exercise in obese patients following weight reduction.[259]

Treatment of heart failure in these patients consists of maintenance of the reduced body weight, dietary sodium restriction, cardiac glycosides, and diuretics. Often, patients with massive obesity have associated arteriosclerotic coronary artery disease and the salutary results of weight reduction may be particularly striking in them.

TREATMENT

Most cases of adult-onset obesity are the result of imbalance between intake and output. Thus, reduction of intake is the most significant factor in treating this disease. While abnormalities in endocrine function, particularly of the thyroid or adrenal, have often been implicated in the pathophysiology of obesity, this thesis is rarely substantiated by detailed evaluation. The amount and rate of weight loss with a given level of caloric restrictions depend on the degree of energy expenditure. Energy expenditure depends on both the physical activity and mass of the individual. Thus, with a fixed level of intake and activity, the rate of weight loss decreases as the total weight decreases. There is no evidence that a specific type of diet has any intrinsic benefit except as it is related to its caloric regimen. Thus the claim that high-protein diets are more efficacious is related not to their caloric content but rather to the accompanying ketosis that suppresses appetite.

CARDIAC COMPLICATIONS OF WEIGHT LOSS. Rapid weight loss has been associated with cardiac arrhythmias and sudden death.[260] In some cases, this is probably secondary to inadequate electrolyte supplementation. In others, it may be related to a reduction in myocardial protein and cardiac atrophy, similar to what has been reported in severe malnutrition[261] (Fig. 61–18) (see below). While initially associated with a liquid protein diet, sudden death may occur under any circumstance in which there is rapid weight loss.[262] In nearly all cases, prolongation in the Q-T interval as well as ventricular arrhythmias has been reported, providing strong support for the need for an ECG in any patient undergoing significant rapid weight loss.

MALNUTRITION

Malnutrition, particularly protein-calorie deficiency, is prevalent in many underdeveloped areas of the world. However, in recent years, it has also become a concern in developed countries in those individuals who have chronic diseases, in whom it exists as a result of both anorexia and hypermetabolism. The clinical picture is similar to that of adult kwashiorkor reported from underdeveloped countries, described below.

Protein-calorie malnutrition of childhood refers to syndromes of nutritional deficiency, which range from marasmus to kwashiorkor and which result from a stress like a serious infection superimposed upon an inadequate diet.[263] *Marasmus* is a state of malnutrition in an infant who has been weaned early and fed a diet grossly deficient in calories, protein, and other essential nutrients. *Kwashiorkor* usually occurs in children 1 to 4 years of age and is due to deficiency of protein relative to calories.

CARDIAC CHANGES IN MALNUTRITION. The circulatory status of patients with severe nutritional depletion and electrolyte imbalance is precarious; the cardiac output, systolic pressure, and pulse pressure are abnormally low, and there may be massive, generalized edema; the P-R interval may be shortened (Table 61–2). There is loss of subcutaneous fat and general wasting and atrophy of most organs, including the heart, which is thin-walled, pale, and flabby on gross examination. Histological study reveals atrophy of the muscle fibers, sometimes with interstitial edema. In experimental chronic protein-calorie undernutrition, not only is the heart atrophic, but also left ventricular function may be normal. In the dog there are reductions in left ventricular compliance and contractility, the latter secondary to loss of cardiac tissue, not altered function,[264] whereas in the rat this apparently does not occur, although there is striking atrophy of the heart.[265] The treatment of the dehydrated or severely anemic patient with protein-calorie malnutrition involves correction of hematological, fluid, and electrolyte imbalance and the treat-

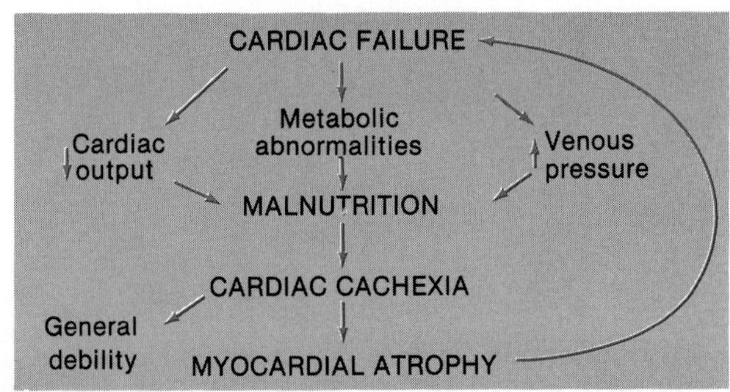

FIGURE 61–18. Possible pathogenesis of cardiac cachexia: Cardiac failure leads to poor nutrition and relative myocardial atrophy. (From Webb, J. G., et al.: Malnutrition and the heart. Can. Med. Assoc. J. *135*:755, 1986.)

TABLE 61-2 SPECTRUM OF CARDIAC EFFECTS DUE TO STARVATION AND ANOREXIA NERVOSA

Cellular
- Diminished protein synthesis
- Activation of calcium-dependent proteinase
- Mitochondrial swelling
- Decreased glycogen content
- Interstitial edema
- Myofibrillar atrophy and destruction

Physiological
- Decreased contractile force
- Decreased cardiac output
- Diminished diastolic compliance

Clinical
- Bradycardia
- Relative hypertension
- Nonspecific electrocardiographic changes
- Ectopic rhythms
- Mitral valve prolapse
- Diminished exercise capacity
- Heart failure, worsened or precipitated by refeeding

Adapted from Schocken, D. D., Holloway, J. D., and Powers, P. S.: Weight loss and the heart. Effects of anorexia nervosa and starvation. Arch. Intern. Med. *149*:878, 1989.

ment of infection. Congestive failure can be avoided if care is taken to avoid overloading with sodium, water, or blood. Digitalis must be given cautiously when these patients are in heart failure because of their sensitivity to glycosides.

In parts of the world where pediatric kwashiorkor is common, there are also cases of adults with similar clinical features. These features include loss of subcutaneous fat and muscle with edema, weakness, depression, anorexia, diarrhea, abdominal distention, hair loss, and thinning of the skin. Classically, plasma albumin and amino acid levels are low, as are serum concentrations of sodium, magnesium, and phosphorus. Urinary excretion of nitrogen is reduced, as is total body potassium. On the other hand, total body and extracellular water and plasma volume are usually increased. The primary pathophysiological event is protein malnutrition. All the clinical signs and symptoms are related to this basic defect.

Anorexia nervosa, a condition more frequently observed in developed countries, produces symptoms similar to those observed in kwashiorkor. Hypomagnesemia with hypocalcemia and hypokalemia frequently occurs in this condition, resulting in heart failure and sometimes sudden death. Cardiac output is low and regional myocardial contraction may be impaired in anorexia nervosa, contributing to the abnormalities in both systolic and diastolic ventricular dysfunction. Congestive heart failure may occur, particularly in the early refeeding phases, probably secondary to an exacerbation of the hypophosphatemia when hyperalimentation and/or oral intake is rich in glucose. Finally, heart rate and blood pressure response to exercise are substantially reduced.[266-269]

MALNUTRITION IN CARDIAC DISEASE

Assessment of protein-calorie nutritional status in cardiac patients has not been extensively evaluated. However, during the last several decades there has been increasing awareness that some patients with cardiovascular disease have clinical features similar to those described above. In these cases, instead of involuntary protein deprivation, anorexia plays a significant role. For example, chronic congestive heart failure leads to cellular hypoxia as well as hypermetabolism. Gastrointestinal hypoxia produces anorexia, which then initiates a vicious cycle. Decreased protein intake produces cardiac atrophy, increased right atrial pressure, tricuspid regurgitation, and increasing congestive heart failure, which produces more cellular hypoxia, greater anorexia, and finally death.[270]

A similar condition has been described in some patients undergoing open-heart surgery for correction of rheumatic valvular disease. In some malnourished patients the mortality reaches 20 per cent, significantly greater than the 1 to 2 per cent in normally nourished patients undergoing the same procedure. The underlying pathophysiology is uncertain but probably includes (1) decreased cardiac mass, (2) reduction of biosynthetic activity of liver, (3) poor healing due to reduced levels of substrate, and (4) impairment of cell-mediated immunity.[271] As a result, wound healing is retarded, skin ulcers occur, and requirements for artificial ventilation are prolonged. Abel and colleagues have suggested that hyperalimentation in the immediate postoperative period does not significantly alter the increased morbidity.[272] This has led Blackburn et al. to suggest that both preoperative and concurrent nutritional support are necessary.[271] However, definitive studies to distinguish between nutritional status and severity of the cardiovascular disease as the cause for the increased morbidity have not been reported.

Cardiovascular Manifestations of Vitamin Deficiency

(see p. 461)

OTHER VITAMIN DEFICIENCIES. Deficiencies of other vitamins have not led to specifically definable cardiovascular abnormalities, except for the hypocalcemia-accompanied vitamin D deficiency. However, vitamin deficiencies, particularly of the B group and folic acid, have been diagnosed with increasing frequency in patients with cardiovascular disease. For example, nearly a third of infants and children with congenital heart disease have been reported to be deficient in a number of the B vitamins.[273] Folic acid deficiency has been documented in a significant number of patients with congestive heart failure. While the deficient state may simply be related to decreased intake, abnormal intestinal absorption or increased rates of excretion may also contribute.

ALTERATIONS IN GONADAL HORMONE SECRETION

There are no specific cardiovascular abnormalities associated with altered gonadal function except for occasional cardiac structural abnormalities in Kallman's syndrome,[274] a genetic form of hypogonadotropic hypogonadism, and a rare form of cardiomyopathy associated with primary hypogonadism.[275] However, gonadectomy in rats is associated with an impairment of left ventricular filling and left ventricular function, and androgen receptors have been found in the heart.

GONADAL FUNCTION AND CARDIOVASCULAR DISEASE

Middle-aged men are at a higher risk for developing cardiovascular disease than are age-matched women. Because the discrepancy between male and female mortality disappears in older, postmenopausal women, some investigators have suggested that estrogen reduces the rate of development of coronary atherosclerosis (p. 1153). Support for this thesis includes the observation that total cholesterol is lower and HDL cholesterol is higher in postmenopausal women who are taking estrogens than in those who are not.[276] Additionally, the risk ratio of coronary artery disease death varies from 0.3 to 0.7 in postmenopausal estrogen users compared to nonusers.[277-279] Several studies, however, have disputed this thesis. First, it has been documented that the development of coronary artery disease in oophorectomized women is no different from that in age-matched nonoophorectomized women,[280] although the study of Colditz et al. has substantially dampened this objection. The latter reported in 121,700 women that bilateral oophorectomy *increases* the risk of coronary heart disease, which can be prevented by estrogen replacement therapy.[281] Second, widespread use of oral contraceptives, most of which contain estrogen, has proved that estrogen administration is not without cardiovascular risk, since it can increase total cholesterol and beta-lipoprotein (LDL) cholesterol and decrease alpha-lipoprotein (HDL) cholesterol in premenopausal women,[282] although low-dose estrogen therapy, even if combined with a progestational agent, appears to have a beneficial effect on lipid profiles in postmenopausal women.[283,284] Additionally, estrogen administration has been shown to increase the degree of abnormality in postexercise electrocardiograms in those individuals who had abnormal tests prior to estrogen therapy.[285] In summary, in addition to the usual variables (age and smoking), the beneficial effect of estrogen therapy in postmenopausal women is, in part, dependent on (1) whether menopause is induced surgically or is natural; (2) whether low- or normal-dose estrogen is used; and (3) what type of progestational agent, if any, is used. The preponderance of evidence suggests that low-dose estrogen therapy will reduce the risk of cardiovascular disease in the postmenopausal woman.

Hyperestrogenemia in men has been reported to be associated with an increased risk of myocardial infarction.[286] In support of this hypothesis, Wilson and colleagues, using information from the Framingham study, reported an increased risk of cardiovascular morbidity in postmenopausal women taking estrogen.[287] Yet other workers have found no association between estrogen levels and heart disease in men, but have observed an increased frequency of coronary artery disease in patients with lower testosterone levels.[288] Thus, whether estradiol levels are an actual risk factor or an associated finding is unclear.[289] Since, in general, higher levels of estrogen are usually associated with lower levels of testosterone in men, separating effects due to androgens from those due to estrogens is difficult. On the basis of these studies, however, some investigators have suggested that it is not an increased estrogen level but a *decreased* testosterone level that is protective in premenopausal *women.* They base this suggestion on the documented reduction in serum cholesterol levels and the incidence of atherosclerosis in castrated men and the negative correlation between plasma testosterone and HDL cholesterol levels.[290,291] However, the similar frequency of coronary artery disease in postmenopausal women and men of similar age with significantly different testosterone levels is unexplained by this suggestion.

CARDIOVASCULAR EFFECTS OF ORAL CONTRACEPTIVES

Several studies have documented that the use of oral contraceptives may be accompanied by an increased risk of cardiovascular morbidity and mortality in premenopausal females.[282,285,292] Specifically there is increased frequency of diabetes mellitus, hypertension, and thromboembolic disease. While the increased risk is small, caution in the use of oral contraceptive agents by individuals who may be predisposed to the development of these diseases is nevertheless warranted. Fortunately, prior use does not increase risk of subsequent cardiovascular disease.[293]

HYPERTENSION (see also p. 832). The hypertension associated with estrogen administration is probably related to its effect in increasing the production of renin substrate by the liver.[294] It has been clearly documented that oral contraceptives increase the concentration of renin substrate and blood angiotensin II.[295] However, most individuals do not develop clinical hypertension, which suggests that a counterregulatory mechanism(s) is activated, reducing the vascular effect of angiotensin II. Alternatively, blood pressure may increase in all patients, but only the predisposed will develop hypertension. Thus, individuals who have a personal or family history of renal disease are more likely to develop hypertension with estrogen administration.

THROMBOEMBOLIC DISEASE. At least two clearly defined alterations in the clotting system are produced by oral contraceptive agents; either or both could be responsible for the increased frequency of thromboembolic disease.[292] (1) Estrogen enhances the biosynthesis by the liver of a number of the clotting factors. (2) Oral contraceptives increase both the blood viscosity and platelet adhesiveness.

REFERENCES

1. Graves, R. J.: Clinical lectures. London Med. Surg. J. (Part II):*7*, 516, 1835.
2. Addison, T.: On the Constitutional and Local Effects of Disease of the Suprarenal Capsules. London, Highley, 1855.

ACROMEGALY

3. Frohman, L. A.: Diseases of the anterior pituitary. *In* Felig, P., et al. (eds.): Endocrinology and Metabolism. 2nd ed. New York, McGraw-Hill Book Co., 1987, p. 247.
4. Faglia, G., Arosio, M., Ambrosi, B.: Recent advances in diagnosis and treatment of acromegaly. *In* Imura, H. (ed.): The Pituitary Gland. New York, Raven Press, 1985, p. 363.
5. Gomez-Pan, A., and Rodriguez-Arnao, M. D.: Somatostatin and growth hormone releasing factor: Synthesis, location, metabolism and function. J. Clin. Endocrinol. Metab. *12*:469, 1983.
6. Frohman, L. A., and Jansson, J.: Growth hormone releasing hormone. Endocr. Rev. *7*:223, 1986.
7. Clemmons, D. R., and Van Wyk, J. J.: Somatomedin: Physiological control and effects on cell proliferation. *In* Baserga, R. (ed.): Handbook of Experimental Pharmacology. Berlin, Springer-Verlag, 1981, p. 161.
8. Yamashita, S., Weiss, M., and Melmed, S.: Insulin-like growth factor I regulates growth hormone secretion and messenger ribonucleic acid levels in human pituitary cells. J. Clin. Endocrinol. Metab. *62*:730, 1986.
9. Moore, D. D., Walker, M. D., Diamond, D. J., et al.: Structure, expression, and evolution of growth hormone genes. Recent Prog. Hormone Res. *38*:197, 1982.
10. Frelin, C.: The regulation of protein turnover in newborn rat heart cell cultures. J. Biol. Chem. *255*:11149, 1980.
11. Thuesen L., Christiansen J. S., Sorensen, J. O. L. et al.: Increased myocardial contractility following growth hormone administration in normal man. Dan. Med. Bull. *35*:193, 1988.
12. Greco, A. V., Ghirlanda, G., Barone, C., et al.: Somatostatin in paroxysmal supraventricular and junctional tachycardia. Br. Med. J. *288*:28, 1984.
13. Day, S. M., Gu, J., Polak, J. M., and Bloom, S. R.: Somatostatin in the human heart and comparison with guinea pig and rat heart. Br. Heart J. *53*:153, 1985.
14. Thorner, M. O., Perryman, R. L., Cronin, M. J., et al.: Somatotroph hyperplasia: Successful treatment of acromegaly by removal of a pancreatic islet tumor secreting a growth hormone-releasing factor. J. Clin. Invest. *70*:965, 1982.
15. Melmed, S., Braunstein, G., Chang, R. J., and Becker, D.: Pituitary tumors secreting growth hormone and prolactin. Ann. Intern. Med. *105*:238, 1986.
16. Aloia, J. F., Roginsky, M. D., and Field, R. A.: Absence of hyperlipidemia in acromegaly. J. Clin. Endocrinol. *35*:921, 1972.
17. McGuffin, W. L., Sherman, B. M., Roth, J. et al.: Acromegaly and cardiovascular disorders. Ann. Intern. Med. *81*:11, 1974.
18. Baldwin, A., Cundy, T., Butler, J., and Timmis, A. D.: Progression of cardiovascular disease in acromegalic patients treated by external pituitary irradiation. Acta Endocrinol. *108*:26, 1985.
19. Lie, J. T., and Grossman, S. J.: Pathology of the heart in acromegaly: Anatomic findings in 27 autopsied patients. Am. Heart J. *100*:41, 1980.
20. Mather, H. M., Boyd, M. J., and Jenkins, J. S.: Heart size and function in acromegaly. Br. Heart J. *41*:697, 1979.
21. Csanady, M., Gaspar, L., Hogye, M., et al.: The heart in acromegaly: An echocardiographic study. Int. J. Cardiol. *2*:349, 1983.
22. Rossi, L., Thiene, G., Caregaro, L., et al.: Dysrhythmias and sudden death in acromegalic heart disease. A clinicopathologic study. Chest *72*:495, 1977.
23. Cain, J. P., Williams, G. H., and Dluhy, R. G.: Plasma renin activity and aldosterone secretion in patients with acromegaly. J. Clin. Endocrinol. *34*:73, 1972.
24. Moore, T. J., Thein-Wai, W., Dluhy, R. G., et al.: Abnormal adrenal and vascular responses to angiotensin II and an angiotensin antagonist in acromegaly. J. Clin. Endocrinol. Metab. *51*:215, 1980.
25. Souadjian, J. V., and Schirger, A.: Hypertension in acromegaly. Am. J. Med. Sci. *254*:629, 1967.
26. Ng, L. L., and Evans, D. J.: Leukocyte sodium transport in acromegaly. Clin. Endocrinol. *26*:471, 1987.
27. Surawicz, B., and Mangiardi, M. L.: Electrocardiogram in endocrine and metabolic disorders. *In* Rios, J. C. (ed.): Clinical Electrocardiographic Correlations. Philadelphia, F. A. Davis Co., 1977, p. 243.
28. Jonas, E. A., Aloia, J. F., and Lane, F. J.: Evidence of subclinical heart muscle dysfunction in acromegaly. Chest *67*:190, 1975.
29. Hayward, R. P., Emanuel, R. W., and Navarro, J. D. N.: Acromegalic heart disease: Influence of treatment of the acromegaly on the heart. Q. J. Med. *62*:41, 1987.
30. Smallridge, R. C., Rajfer, S., Davis, J., and Schaaf, M.: Acromegaly and the heart. Am. J. Med. *66*:22, 1979.
31. Rodrigues, E. A., Caruana, M. P., Lahiri, A., et al.: Subclinical cardiac dysfunction in acromegaly: Evidence for a specific disease of heart muscle. Br. Heart J. *62*:185, 1989.
32. Molitch, M. E.: Acromegaly. *In* Collu, R., Brown, G. M., and Vanloon, G. R. (eds.): Clinical Neuroendocrinology. Boston, Blackwell Scientific Publications, Inc., 1988, p. 189.

33. Vance, M. L., Evans, W. S., and Thorner, M. O.: Bromocriptine. Ann. Intern. Med. *100*:78, 1984.
34. Barkan, A. L., Kelch, R. P., Hopwood, N. J., et al.: Treatment of acromegaly with the long-acting somatostatin analogue SMS 201-995. J. Clin. Endocrinol. Metab. *66*:16, 1988.

THYROID DISEASE

35. Kaplan, M. M.: The thyroid and the heart; how do they interact? J. Cardiovasc. Med. *7*:893, 1982.
36. Oppenheimer, J. H.: The nuclear receptor–triiodothyronine complex: Relationship to thyroid hormone distributions, metabolism, and biological action. *In* Oppenheimer, J. H., and Samuels, H. H. (eds.): Molecular Basis of Thyroid Hormone Action. New York, Academic Press, 1983, p. 1.
37. Ladenson, P. W., Kieffer, J. D., Farwell, A. P., and Ridgway, E. C.: Modulation of myocardial L-triiodothyronine receptors in normal, hypothyroid, and hyperthyroid rats. Metabolism *35*:5, 1986.
38. Jump, D. B., and Oppenheimer, J. H.: Association of thyroid hormone receptors with chromatin. Mol. Cell. Biochem. *55*:159, 1983.
39. Apriletti, J. W., David-Inouye, Y., Baxter, J. D., and Eberhardt, N. L.: Physiochemical characterization of the intranuclear receptor. *In* Oppenheimer, J. H., and Samuels, H. H. (eds.): Molecular Basis of Thyroid Hormone Action. New York, Academic Press, 1983, p. 67.
40. Narayan, P., Liaw, C. W., and Towle, H. C.: Rapid induction of a specific nuclear precursor by thyroid hormone. Proc. Natl. Acad. Sci. USA *81*:4687, 1984.
41. Seelig, S. A., Jump, D. B., Towle, H. C., et al.: Parodoxical effects of cycloheximide on the ultra-rapid induction of two hepatic mRNA sequences by triiodothyronine (T3). Endocrinology *110*:671, 1982.
42. Seelig, S., Liaw, C., Towle, H. C., and Oppenheimer, J. H.: Thyroid hormone attenuates and augments hepatic gene expression at a pretranslational level. Proc. Natl. Acad. Sci. USA *78*:4733, 1981.
43. Guernsey, D. L., and Edelman, I. S.: Regulation of thermogenesis by thyroid hormones. *In* Oppenheimer, J. H., and Samuels, H. H. (eds.): Molecular Basis of Thyroid Hormone Action. New York, Academic Press, 1983, p. 298.
44. Fain, J. N., and Rosenthal, J. W.: Calorigenic action of triiodothyronine on white cells: Effects of ouabain, oligomycin, and cathecholamines. Endocrinology *89*:1205, 1971.
45. Primack, M. P., and Buchanan, J. L.: Control of oxygen consumption in liver slices from normal and T4-treated rats. Endocrinology *95*:619, 1974.
46. Gordon, A., Schwartz, H., and Gross, J.: The stimulation of sugar transport in heart cells grown in a serum-free medium by picomolar concentrations of thyroid hormones: The effects of insulin and hydrocortisone. Endocrinology *118*:52, 1986.
47. Kim, D., Smith, T. W., and Marsh, J. D.: Effect of thyroid hormone on slow calcium channel function in cultured chick ventricular cells. J. Clin. Invest. *80*:88, 1987.
48. MacKinnon, R., Gwathmey, J. K., Allen, P. D., et al.: Modulation by the thyroid state of intracellular calcium and contractility in ferret ventricular muscle. Circ. Res. *63*:1080, 1988.
49. Knight, R. A.: The use of spinal anesthesia to control sympathetic overactivity in hyperthyroidism. Anesthesiology *6*:225, 1945.
50. Hammond, H. K., White, F. C., Buxton, I. L. O., et al.: Increased myocardial beta-receptors and adrenergic responses in hyperthyroid pigs. Am. J. Physiol. *252*:H283, 1987.
51. Buccino, R. A., Spann, J. F., Pool, P. E., and Braunwald, E.: Influence of the thyroid state on the intrinsic contractile properties and the energy stores of the myocardium. J. Clin. Invest. *46*:1669, 1967.
52. Nishizawa, Y., Hamada, N., Fujii, S., et al.: Serum dopamine-beta-hydroxylase activity in thyroid disorders. J. Clin. Endocrinol. Metab. *39*:599, 1974.
53. Malbon, C. C., and Greenberg, M. L.; 3,3′,5′-Triiodothyronine administration in vivo modulates the hormone sensitive adenylate cyclase system of rat hepatocytes. J. Clin. Invest. *69*:414, 1982.
54. Malbon, C. C.: Liver cell adenylate cyclase and β-adrenergic receptors. J. Biol. Chem. *255*:8692, 1980.
55. Brodde, O. E., Schumann, H. J., and Wagner, J.: Decreased responsiveness of the adenylate cyclase system in left atria from hypothyroid rats. Mol. Pharmacol. *17*:180, 1980.
56. Whitsett, J. A., Pollinger, J., and Matz, S.: β-Adrenergic receptors and catecholamine-sensitive adenylate cyclase in developing rat ventricular myocardium: Effect of thyroid status. Pediatr. Res. *16*:463, 1982.
57. Rutherford, J. P., Vatner, S. F., and Braunwald, E.: Adrenergic control of myocardial contractility in conscious hyperthyroid dogs. Am. J. Physiol. *237*:590, 1980.
58. Guarnieri, T., Filburn, C. R., Beard, E. S., and Lakatta, E. G.: Enhanced contractile response and protein kinase activation to threshold levels of β-adrenergic stimulation in hyperthyroid rat heart. J. Clin. Invest. *65*:861, 1980.
59. Andersson, R. G. G., Nilsson, O. R., and Kuo, J. F.: β-Adrenoceptor adenosine 3′,5′-monophosphate system in human leukocytes before and after treatment for hyperthyroidism. J. Clin. Endocrinol. Metab. *56*:42, 1983.
60. Stiles, G. L., Stadel, J. M., De Lean, A., and Lefkowitz, R. J.: Hypothyroidism modulates beta-adrenergic receptor-adenylate cyclase interactions in rat reticulocytes. J. Clin. Invest. *68*:1450, 1981.
61. Malbon, C. C.: The effects of thyroid status on the modulation of fat cell β-adrenergic receptor agonist affinity by guanine nucleotides. Mol. Pharmacol. *18*:193, 1980.
62. Ling, E., O'Brien, P. J., Salerno, T., et al.: Effects of different thyroid treatments on the biochemical characteristics of rabbit myocardium. Can. J. Cardiol. *4*:301, 1988.
63. Markowitz, C., and Yater, W. M.: Response of explanted cardiac muscle to thyroxine. Am. J. Physiol. *100*:162, 1932.
64. Murayama, M., and Goodkind, M. J.: Effect of thyroid hormone on the frequency-force relationship of atrial myocardium from the guinea pig. Circ. Res. *23*:743, 1968.
64a. Josephson, R. A., Spurgeon, H. A., and Lakatta, E. G.: The hyperthyroid heart: An analysis of systolic and diastolic properties in single rat ventricular myocytes. Circ. Res. *66*:773, 1990.
65. Goldman, S., Olajos, M., Friedman, H., et al.: Left ventricular performance in conscious thyrotoxic calves. Am. J. Physiol. *242*:H113, 1982.
66. McDonough, K. H., Chen, V., and Spitzer, J.: Effect of altered thyroid status on in vitro cardiac performance in rats. Am. J. Physiol. *252*:H788, 1987.
67. Crie, J. S., Wakeland, J. R., Mayhew, B. A., and Wildenthal, K.: Direct anabolic effects of thyroid hormone on isolated mouse heart. Am. J. Physiol. *245*:C328, 1983.
68. Gustafson, T. A., Markham, B. E., and Morkin, E.: Effects of thyroid hormone on alpha-actin and myosin heavy chain gene expression in cardiac and skeletal muscles of the rat: Measurement of mRNA content using synthetic oligonucleotide probes. Circ. Res. *59*:194, 1986.
69. Philipson, K. D., and Edelman, I. S.: Thyroid hormone control of Na^+,K^+ATPase and K^+-dependent phosphatase in rat heart. Am. J. Physiol. *232*:C196, 1977.
70. Litten, R. Z., Martin, B. J., Howe, E. R., et al.: Phosphorylation and adenosine triphosphate activity of myofibrils from thyrotoxic rabbit ears. Circ. Res. *48*:498, 1981.
71. Curfman, G. D., Crowley, T. J., and Smith, T. W.: Thyroid-induced alterations in myocardial sodium- and potassium-activated adenosine triphosphatase, monovalent cation active transport and cardiac glycoside binding. J. Clin. Invest. *59*:586, 1977.
72. Samuel, J. L., Rappaport, L., Syrovy, I., et al.: Differential effect of thyroxine on atrial and ventricular isomyosins in rats. Am. J. Physiol. *250*:H333, 1986.
73. Litten, R. Z., III, Martin, B. J., Low, R. B., and Alpert, N. R.: Altered myosin isozyme patterns from pressure overloaded and thyrotoxic hypertrophied rabbit hearts. Circ. Res. *50*:856, 1982.
74. Holubarsch, C., Goulette, R. P., Litten, R. Z., et al.: The economy of isometric force development, myosin isoenzyme pattern and myofibrillar ATPase activity in normal and hypothyroid rat myocardium. Circ. Res. *56*:78, 1985.
75. Goto, Y., Slinker, B. K., and LeWinter, M. M.: Decreased contractile efficiency and increased nonmechanical energy cost in hyperthyroid rabbit heart: Relation between O_2 consumption and systolic pressure-volume area or force-time integral. Circ. Res. *66*:999, 1990.
76. Poggesi, C., Everets, M., Polla, B., et al.: Influence of thyroid state on mechanical restitution of rat myocardium. Circ. Res. *60*:142, 1987.
77. Klein, I., and Hong, C.: Effects of thyroid hormone on cardiac size and myosin content of the heterotopically transplanted rat heart. J. Clin. Invest. *77*:1694, 1986.
78. Korecky, B., Zak, R., Schwartz, K., et al.: Role of thyroid hormone in regulation of isomyosin composition, contractility, and size of heterotopically isotransplanted rat heart. Circ. Res. *60*:824, 1987.
79. Johnson, P. N., Freedberg, A. S., and Marshall, J. M.: Action of thyroid hormone on the transmembrane potentials from sinoatrial cells and atrial muscle cells in isolated atria of rabbits. Cardiology *58*:273, 1973.
80. Arnsdorf, M. D., and Childers, R. W.: Atrial electrophysiology in experimental hyperthyroidism in rabbits. Circ. Res. *26*:575, 1970.
81. Utiger, R. D.: The thyroid: Physiology, hyperthyroidism, hypothyroidism, and the painful thyroid. *In* Felig, P., et al. (eds.): Endocrinology and Metabolism. 2nd ed. New York, McGraw-Hill Book Co., 1987, p. 389.
82. Skelton, C. L.: The heart and hyperthyroidism. N. Engl. J. Med. *307*:1206, 1982.
83. Talafih, K., Briden, K. L., and Weiss, H. R.: Thyroxine-induced hypertrophy of the rabbit heart. Effect on regional oxygen extraction, flow, and oxygen consumption. Circ. Res. *52*:272, 1983.
84. Friedman, M. J., Okada, R. D., Ewy, G. A., and Hellman, D. J.: Left ventricular systolic and diastolic function in hyperthyroidism. Am. Heart J. *104*:1303, 1982.
85. Feldman, T., Borow, K. M., Sarne, D. H., et al.: Myocardial mechanics in hyperthyroidism: Importance of left ventricular loading conditions, heart rate and contractile state. J. Am. Coll. Cardiol. *7*:967, 1986.
86. Iskandrian, A. S., Rose, L., Hakki, A. H., et al.: Cardiac performance in thyrotoxicosis: Analysis of 10 untreated patients. Am. J. Cardiol. *51*:349, 1983.
87. Maciel, B. C., Gallo, L., Marin-Neto, J., et al.: Autonomic control of heart rate during dynamic exercise in human hyperthyroidism. Clin. Sci. *75*:209, 1988.
88. Forfar, J. C., Matthews, D. M., and Toft, A. D.: Delayed recovery of left ventricular function after antithyroid treatment: Further evidence for reversible abnormalities of contractility in hyperthyroidism. Br. Heart J. *52*:215, 1984.
89. Olshausen, K., Bischoff, S., Kahaly, G., et al.: Cardiac arrhythmias and heart rate in hyperthyroidism. Am. J. Cardiol. *63*:930, 1989.
90. Agner, T., Almdal, T., Thorsteinsson, B., and Agner, E.: A reevaluation of atrial fibrillation in thyrotoxicosis. Dan. Med. Bull. *31*:157, 1984.

91. Ciaccheri, M., Cecchi, F., Arcangeli, C., et al.: Occult thyrotoxicosis in patients with chronic and paroxysmal isolated atrial fibrillation. Clin. Cardiol. 7:413, 1984.
92. Goel, B. G., Hanson, C. S., and Han, J.: A-V conduction in hyper- and hypothyroid dogs. Am. Heart J. 83:504, 1972.
93. Cavallo, A., Joseph, C. J., and Casta, A.: Cardiac complications in juvenile hyperthyroidism. Am. J. Dis. Child. 138:479, 1984.
94. Featherstone, H. J., and Stewart, D. K.: Angina in thyrotoxicosis: Thyroid-related coronary artery spasm. Arch. Intern. Med. 143:554, 1983.
95. Forfar, J. C., Muir, A. L., Sawers, S. A., and Toft, A. D.: Abnormal left ventricular function in hyperthyroidism: Evidence for a possible reversible cardiomyopathy. N. Engl. J. Med. 307:1165, 1982.
96. Wilson, R., Gibson, T. C., Terrien, C. M., and Levy, A. M.: Hyperthyroidism and familial hypertrophic cardiomyopathy. Arch. Intern. Med. 143:378, 1983.
97. Brauman, A., Algom, M., Gilboa, Y., et al.: Mitral valve prolapse in hyperthyroidism of two different origins. Br. Heart J. 53:374, 1985.
98. Noah, M. S., Sulimani, R. A., Famuyiwa, F. O., et al.: Prolapse of the mitral valve in hyperthyroid patients in Saudi Arabia. Int. J. Cardiol. 19:217, 1988.
99. Morrow, D. H., Gaffney, T. E., and Braunwald, E.: Studies on digitalis: VIII. Effect of autonomic innervation and of myocardial catecholamine stores upon the cardiac action of ouabain. J. Pharmacol. Exp. Ther. 140:236, 1963.
100. Ingbar, S. H.: The role of antiadrenergic agents in the management of thyrotoxicosis. Cardiovasc. Rev. Rep. 2:683, 1981.
101. Sandler, G., and Wilson, G. M.: The nature and prognosis of heart disease in thyrotoxicosis. A review of 150 patients treated with ^{131}I. Q. J. Med. 28:347, 1959.
102. Nakazawa, H. K., Sakurai, K., Hamada, N., et al.: Management of atrial fibrillation in the postthyrotoxic state. Am. J. Med. 72:903, 1982.
103. Staffurth, J. S., Gibberd, M. C., and Fui, S. T.: Arterial embolism in thyrotoxicosis with atrial fibrillation. Br. Med. J. 2:688, 1977.
104. Chopra, I. J., Huang, T.-S., Hurd, R. E., and Solomon, D. H.: A study of cardiac effects of thyroid hormones: Evidence for amelioration of the effects of thyroxine by sodium ipodate. Endocrinology 114:2039, 1984.
105. Norman, M. F., and Lavin, T. N.: Antagonism of thyroid hormone action by amiodarone in rat pituitary tumor cells. J. Clin. Invest. 83:306, 1989.
106. Lambert, M., Burger, A. G., DeNayer, P., et al.: Decreased TSH response to TRH induced by amiodarone. Acta Endocrinol. 118:449, 1988.
107. Gammage, M. D., and Franklyn, J. A.: Amiodarone and the thyroid. Q. J. Med. 62:83, 1987.
108. Bambini, G., Aghini-Lombardi, F., Rosner, W., et al.: Serum sex hormone–binding globulin in amiodarone-treated patients. Arch. Intern. Med. 147:1781, 1987.
109. Martino, E., Bartalena, L., Mariotti, S., et al.: Radioactive iodine thyroid uptake in patients with amiodarone iodine–induced thyroid dysfunction. Acta Endocrinol. 119:167, 1988.
110. Kasim, S. E., Bagchi, N., Brown, T. R., et al.: Effect of amiodarone on serum lipids, lipoprotein lipase, and hepatic triglyceride lipase. Endocrinology 120:1991, 1987.
111. Rabinowe, S. L., Larsen, P. R., Antman, E. M., et al.: Amiodarone therapy and autoimmune thyroid disease. Am. J. Med. 81:53, 1986.
112. Zimmerman, J., Yahalom, J., and Bar-On, H.: Clinical spectrum of pericardial effusion as the presenting feature of hypothyroidism. Am. Heart J. 106:770, 1983.
113. Khaleeli, A. A., and Memon, N.: Factors affecting resolution of pericardial effusions in primary hypothyroidism: A clinical, biochemical and echocardiographic study. Postgrad. Med. J. 58:1073, 1982.
114. Kumar, A., Bhandari, A. K., and Rahimtoola, S. H.: Torsade de pointes and marked QT prolongation in association with hypothyroidism. Ann. Intern. Med. 106:712, 1987.
115. Shenoy, M. M., and Goldman, J. M.: Hypothyroid cardiomyopathy: Echocardiographic documentation of reversibility. Am. J. Med. Sci. 294:1, 1987.
116. Streeten, D. H. P., Andersen, G. H., Howland, T., et al.: Effects of thyroid function on blood pressure: Recognition of hypothyroid hypertension. Hypertension 11:78, 1988.
117. Saito, I., Kunihiko, I., and Saruta, T.: Hypothyroidism as a cause of hypertension. Hypertension 5:112, 1983.
118. Fouron, J. C., Bourgin, J. H., Letarte, J., et al.: Cardiac dimensions and myocardial function of infants with congenital hypothyroidism: An echocardiographic study. Br. Heart J. 47:584, 1982.
119. Graettinger, J. S., Muenster, J. J., and Checchia, C.: A correlation of clinical and hemodynamic studies in patients with hypothyroidism. J. Clin. Invest. 37:502, 1958.
120. Wieshammer, S., Keck, F. S., Waitzinger, J., et al.: Left ventricular function at rest and during exercise in acute hypothyroidism. Br. Heart J. 60:204, 1988.
121. Vora, J., O'Malley, B. P., Petersen, S., et al.: Reversible abnormalities of myocardial relaxation in hypothyroidism. J. Clin. Endocrinol. Metab. 61:269, 1985.
122. Hillis, W. S., Bremner, W. F., Lawrie, T. D. V., and Thomson, J. A.: Systolic time intervals in thyroid disease. Clin. Endocrinol. 4:617, 1975.
123. McBrion, D. J., and Hindle, W.: Myxoedema and heart failure. Lancet 1:1065, 1963.
124. Levey, G. S., Skelton, C. L., and Epstein, S. E.: Decreased myocardial adenyl cyclase activity in hypothyroidism. J. Clin. Invest. 48:2244, 1969.
125. Steinberg, A. D.: Myxedema and coronary artery disease—a comparative autopsy study. Ann. Intern. Med. 68:338, 1968.
126. Karlsberg, R. P., Friscia, D. A., Aronow, W. S., and Sekhon, S. S.: Deleterious influence of hypothyroidism on evolving myocardial infarction in conscious dogs. J. Clin. Invest. 67:1024, 1981.
127. Keating, F. R., Parkin, T. W., Selby, J. B., and Dickinson, L. S.: Treatment of heart disease associated with myxedema. Progr. Cardiovasc. Dis. 3:364, 1960.
128. Griffiths, P. D.: Serum enzymes in diseases of the thyroid gland. J. Clin. Pathol. 18:660, 1965.
129. Drucker, D. J., and Burrow, G. N.: Cardiovascular surgery in the hypothyroid patient. Arch. Intern. Med. 145:1585, 1985.
130. Wehmann, R. E., Gregerman, R. I., Burns, W. H., et al.: Suppression of thyrotropin in the low-thyroxine state of severe nonthyroidal illness. N. Engl. J. Med. 312:546, 1985.
131. Hamblin, P. S., Dyer, S. A., Mohr, V. S., et al.: Relationship between thyrotropin and thyroxine changes during recovery from severe hypothyroxinemia of critical illness. J. Clin. Endocrinol. Metab. 62:717, 1986.
132. Brent, G. A., and Hershman, J. M.: Thyroxine therapy in patients with severe nonthyroidal illnesses and low serum thyroxine concentration. J. Clin. Endocrinol. Metab. 63:1, 1986.

DISEASES OF THE ADRENAL CORTEX

133. Williams, G. H., and Dluhy, R. G.: Diseases of the adrenal cortex. *In* Wilson, J., et al. (eds.): Harrison's Principles of Internal Medicine. 12th ed. New York, McGraw-Hill Book Co., 1991, p. 1713.
134. Quinn, S. J., and Williams, G. H.: Regulation of aldosterone secretion. Annu. Rev. Physiol. 50:409, 1988.
135. Cushing, H.: The basophil adenomas of the pituitary body and their clinical manifestations (pituitary basophilism). Bull. Johns Hopkins Hosp. 50:137, 1932.
136. Liddle, G. W.: Pathogenesis of glucocorticoid disorders. Am. J. Med. 53:638, 1972.
137. Krieger, D. T.: Physiopathology of Cushing's disease. Endocr. Rev. 4:22, 1983.
138. Carney, J. A., Gordon, H., Carpenter, P. C., et al.: The complex of myxomas, spotty pigmentation, and endocrine overactivity. Medicine 64:270, 1985.
139. Sindler, B. H., Griffing, G. T., and Melby, J. C.: The superiority of the metyrapone test vs. the high dose dexamethasone test in the differential diagnosis of Cushing's syndrome. Am. J. Med. 74:657, 1983.
140. Boggan, J. E., Tyrrell, J. B., and Wilson, C. B.: Transsphenoidal microsurgical management of Cushing's disease: Report of 100 cases. J. Neurosurg. 59:195, 1983.
141. Nolan, P. M., Sheeler, L. R., Hahn, J. F., and Hardy, R. W., Jr.: Therapeutic problems with transsphenoidal pituitary surgery for Cushing's disease. Cleve. Clin. Q. 49:199, 1982.
142. Weinberger, M. H.: Primary aldosteronism: Diagnosis and differentiation of subtypes. Ann. Intern. Med. 100:300, 1984.
143. Rose, L. I., Underwood, R. H., Newmark, S. R., et al.: Pathophysiology of spironolactone-induced gynecomastia. Ann. Intern. Med. 87:398, 1977.
144. Rabinowe, S. L., Jackson, R. A., Dluhy, R. G., and Williams, G. H.: Ia-positive T lymphocytes in recently diagnosed idiopathic Addison's disease. Am. J. Med. 77:597, 1984.
145. Knowlton, A. I., and Baer, L.: Cardiac failure in Addison's disease. Am. J. Med. 74:829, 1983.
146. Dorin, R. I., and Kearns, P. J.: High output circulatory failure in acute adrenal insufficiency. Crit. Care Med. 16:296, 1988.
147. New, M. I., and Levine, L. S.: Recent advances in 21-hydroxylase deficiency. Ann. Rev. Med. 35:649, 1984.
148. Schambelan, M., Sebastian, A., and Biglieri, E. G.: Prevalence, pathogenesis and functional significance of aldosterone deficiency in hyperkalemic patients with chronic renal insufficiency. Kidney Int. 17:89, 1980.
149. Lee, T. H., Salomon, D. R., Rayment, C. M., and Antman, E. M.: Hypotension and sinus arrest with exercise-induced hyperkalemia and combined verapamil/propranolol therapy. Am. J. Med. 80:1203, 1986.
150. Mannisi, J. A., Weisman, H. F., Bush, D. E., et al.: Steroid administration after myocardial infarction promotes early infarct expansion. J. Clin. Invest. 79:1431, 1987.
151. Alford, W. C., Meador, C. K., Mihalevich, J., et al.: Acute adrenal insufficiency following cardiac surgical procedures. J. Thorac. Cardiovasc. Surg. 78:489, 1979.

PHEOCHROMOCYTOMA

152. Bravo, E. L., and Gifford, R. W.: Pheochromocytoma: Diagnosis, localization, and management. N. Engl. J. Med. 311:1298, 1984.
153. Wurtman, R. J., and Axelrod, J.: Control of enzymatic synthesis of adrenaline in the adrenal medulla by adrenal cortical steroids. J. Biol. Chem. 241:2301, 1966.
154. Levenson, J. A., Safar, M. E., London, G. M., and Simon, A. C.: Haemodynamics in patients with phaeochromocytoma. Clin. Sci. 58:349, 1980.
155. Landsberg, L., and Young, J. B.: Catecholamines and adrenal medulla. *In* Wilson, J. D., and Foster, D. W. (eds.): Williams' Textbook of Endocrinology. 7th ed. Philadelphia, W. B. Saunders Company, 1985, p. 891.
155a. Sardesai, S. H., Mourant, A. J., Sivathandon, Y., et al.: Phaeochromocytoma and catecholamine induced cardiomyopathy presenting as heart failure. Br. Heart J. 63:234, 1990.
156. Strenstrom, G., and Swedberg, K.: QRS amplitudes, QT_c intervals and ECG

abnormalities in pheochromocytoma patients before, during and after treatment. Acta Med. Scand. *224*:231, 1988.
157. Haas, G. J., Tzagournis, M., and Boudoulas, H.: Pheochromocytoma: Catecholamine-mediated electrocardiographic changes mimicking ischemia. Am. Heart J. *116*:1363, 1988.
158. Van Vliet, P. D., Burchell, H. B., and Titus, J. L.: Myocarditis associated with pheochromocytoma. N. Engl. J. Med. *274*:1102, 1966.
159. Imperato-McGinley, J., Gautier, T., Ehlers, K., et al.: Reversibility of catecholamine-induced dilated cardiomyopathy in a child with a pheochromocytoma. N. Engl. J. Med. *316*:793, 1987.
160. Scott, I., Parkes, R., and Cameron, D. P.: Pheochromocytoma and cardiomyopathy. Med. J. Aust. *148*:94, 1988.
161. Behrana, A. J., Haselton, P., Leen, C. L. S., et al.: Multiple extra-adrenal paragangliomas associated with catecholamine cardiomyopathy. Eur. Heart J. *10*:182, 1989.
162. Shub, C., Cueto-Garcia, L., Sheps, S. G., et al.: Echocardiographic findings in pheochromocytoma. Am. J. Cardiol. *57*:971, 1986.
163. Cueto, L., Arriaga, J., and Zinser, J.: Echocardiographic changes in pheochromocytoma. Chest *76*:600, 1979.
164. McManus, B. M., Fleury, T. A., and Roberts, W. C.: Fatal catecholamine crisis in pheochromocytoma: Curable form of cardiac arrest. Am. Heart J. *102*:930, 1981.
165. Simons, M., and Downing, S. E.: Coronary vasoconstriction and catecholamine cardiomyopathy. Am. Heart J. *109*:297, 1985.
166. Bhatnagar, D., Carey, P., and Pollard, A.: Focal myositis and elevated creatine kinase levels in a patient with phaeochromocytoma. Postgrad. Med. J. *62*:197, 1986.
167. Serfas, D., Shoback, D. M., and Lorell, B. H.: Phaeochromocytoma and hypertrophic cardiomyopathy: Apparent suppression of symptoms and noradrenaline secretion by calcium-channel blockade. Lancet *2*:711, 1983.
168. David, T. E., Lenkei, S. C., Marquez-Julio, A., et al.: Pheochromocytoma of the heart. Ann. Thorac. Surg. *41*:98, 1986.

PARATHYROID DISEASE

169. Brown, E. M.: Physiology of calcium metabolism. *In* Becker K. L. (eds.): Principles and Practice of Endocrinology and Metabolism. Philadelphia, J. B. Lippincott. Co., 1990, p. 423.
170. Symons, C., Fortune, F., Greenbaum, R. A., and Dandona, P.: Cardiac hypertrophy, hypertrophic cardiomyopathy, and hyperparathyroidism—an association. Br. Heart J. *54*:539, 1985.
171. Bogin, E., Massry, S. G., and Harary, I.: Effect of parathyroid hormone on rat heart cells. J. Clin. Invest. *67*:1215, 1981.
172. Katoh, Y., Klein, K. L., Kaplan, R. A., et al.: Parathyroid hormone has a positive inotropic action in the rat. Endocrinology *109*:2252, 1981.
173. Palmieri, G. M., Nutting, D. F., Bhattacharya, S. K., et al.: Parathyroid ablation in dystrophic hamsters: Effects of Ca content and histology of heart, diaphragm, and rectus femoris. J. Clin. Invest. *68*:646, 1981.
174. Gafter, U., Battler, A., Eldar, M., et al.: Effect of hyperparathyroidism on cardiac function in patients with end-stage renal disease. Nephron *41*:30, 1985.
175. Vered I., Vered, Z., Perez, J. E., et al.: Normal left ventricular performance documented by Doppler echocardiography in patients with long-standing hypocalcemia. Am. J. Med. *86*:413, 1989.
176. Giles, T. D., Iteld, B. J., and Rires, K. L.: The cardiomyopathy of hypoparathyroidism. Chest *79*:225, 1981.
177. Ellison, D. H., and McCarron, D. A.: Structural prerequisites for the hypotensive action of parathyroid hormone. Am. J. Physiol. *246*:F551, 1984.
178. Roberts, W. C., and Waller, B. F.: Effect of chronic hypercalcemia on the heart: An analysis of 18 necropsy patients. Am. J. Med. *71*:371, 1981.
179. Roberts, W. C., and Waller, B. F.: Chronic hypercalcemia as a risk factor for coronary atherosclerosis. Cardiovasc. Rev. Rep. *4*:1275, 1983.
180. Slavich, G. A., Antonucci, F., and Sponza, E.: Primary hyperparathyroidism and angina pectoris. Int. J. Cardiol. *19*:266, 1988.
181. Csanady, M., Forster, T., and Julesz, J.: Reversible impairment of myocardial function in hypoparathyroidism causing hypocalcaemia. Br. Heart J. *63*:58, 1990.
182. Kleerekoper, M., Rao, D. S., and Frame, B.: Hypercalcemia, hyperparathyroidism and hypertension. Cardiovasc. Med. *3*:1283, 1978.
183. Daniels, J., and Goodman, A. D.: Hypertension and hyperparathyroidism: Inverse relation of sodium phosphate level and blood pressure. Am. J. Med. *75*:17, 1983.
184. Resnick, L. M.: Calcium, parathyroid disease, and hypertension. Cardiovasc. Rev. Rep. *3*:1341, 1982.

DIABETES MELLITUS

185. Halban, P. A., and Weir, G. C.: Islet cell hormones: Production and degradation. *In* Becker, K. L. (ed.): Principles and Practice of Endocrinology and Metabolism. Philadelphia, J. B. Lippincott Co., 1990, p. 1068.
186. Eisenbarth, G. S., and Kahn, C. R.: Etiology and pathogenesis of diabetes mellitus. *In* Becker, K. L. (ed.): Principles and Practice of Endocrinology and Metabolism. Philadelphia, J. B. Lippincott Co., 1990, p. 1074.
187. Waller, B. F., Palumbo, P. J., Lie, J. T., and Roberts, W. C.: Status of the coronary arteries at necropsy in diabetes mellitus with onset after age 30 years: Analysis of 229 diabetic patients with and without clinical evidence of coronary heart disease and comparison of 183 control subjects. Am. J. Med. *69*:498, 1980.
188. Yano, K., Kagan, A., McGee, D., and Rhoads, G. G.: Glucose intolerance and nine-year mortality in Japanese men in Hawaii. Am. J. Med. *72*:71, 1982.
189. Stone, P. H., Muller, J. E., Hartwell, T., et al.: The effect of diabetes mellitus on prognosis and serial left ventricular function after acute myocardial infarction: Contribution of both coronary disease and diastolic left ventricular dysfunction to the adverse prognosis. J. Am. Coll. Cardiol. *14*:49, 1989.
190. Woods, K. L., Samanta, A., and Burden, A. C.: Diabetes mellitus as a risk factor for acute myocardial infarction in Asians and Europeans. Br. Heart J. *62*:118, 1989.
191. Herlitz, J., Malmberg, K., Karlson, B. W., et al.: Mortality and morbidity during a five-year follow-up of diabetics with myocardial infarction. Acta Med. Scand. *224*:31, 1988.
192. Abbott, R. D., Donahue, R. P., Kannel, W. B., et al.: The impact of diabetes on survival following myocardial infarction in men vs women. The Framingham Study. JAMA *260*:3456, 1988.
193. Factor, S. M., Okun, E. M., and Minase, T.: Capillary microaneurysms in the human heart. N. Engl. J. Med. *302*:384, 1980.
194. Savage, M. P., Krolewski, A. S., Kenien, G. G., et al.: Acute myocardial infarction in diabetes mellitus and significance of congestive heart failure as a prognostic factor. Am. J. Cardiol. *62*:665, 1988.
195. Ceremuzynski, L.: Hormonal and metabolic reactions evoked by acute myocardial infarction. Circ. Res. *48*:767, 1981.
196. Flink, E. B., Brick, J. E., and Shane, S. R.: Alterations of long-chain free fatty acid and magnesium concentrations in acute myocardial infarction. Arch. Intern. Med. *141*:441, 1981.
197. Opie, L. H., Tansey, M. J., and Kennelly, B. M.: The heart in diabetes mellitus: II. Acute myocardial infarction and diabetes. S. Afr. Med. J. *56*:256, 1979.
198. Nesto, R. W., Phillips, R. T., Kett, K. G., et al.: Angina and exertional myocardial ischemia in diabetic and nondiabetic patients: Assessment by exercise thallium scintigraphy. Ann. Intern. Med. *108*:170, 1988.
199. Gunderson, T., and Kjekshus, J.: Timolol treatment after myocardial infarction in diabetic patients. Diabetes Care *6*:285, 1983.
200. Roy, T. M., Peterson, H. R., Snider, H. L., et al.: Autonomic influence on cardiovascular performance in diabetic subjects. Am. J. Med. *87*:382, 1989.
201. Sato, N., Hashimoto, H., Takiguchi, Y., et al.: Altered responsiveness to sympathetic nerve stimulation and agonist of isolated left atria of diabetic rats: No evidence for involvement of hypothyroidism. J. Pharmacol. Exp. Ther. *248*:367, 1989.
202. Fernandez-Castaner, M., Figuerola, D., Sorribas, A., et al.: Evaluation des epreuves cardiovasculaires dans le diagnostic des neuropathies diabetiques autonomes. Diabetes Metab. *9*:264, 1983.
202a. Ambepityia, G., Kopelman, P. G., Ingram, D.: Exertional myocardial ischemia in diabetes: A quantitative analysis of anginal perceptual threshold and the influence of autonomic function. J. Am. Coll. Cardiol. *15*:72, 1990.
203. Zola, B., Kahn, J. K., Juni, J. E., and Vinik, A. I.: Abnormal cardiac function in diabetic patients with autonomic neuropathy in the absence of ischemic heart disease. J. Clin. Endocrinol. Metab. *63*:208, 1986.
204. Pfeifer, M. A., Cook, D., Brodsky, J., et al.: Quantitative evaluation of cardiac parasympathetic activity in normal and diabetic man. Diabetes *31*:339, 1982.
204a. Weise, F., Heydenreich, F., Gehrig, W., and Runge, U.: Heart rate variability in diabetic patients during orthostatic load—a spectral analytic approach. Klin. Wochenschr. *68*:26, 1990.
205. Zoneraich, S.: Diabetes and the Heart. Springfield, Ill., Charles C Thomas, Publisher, 1978, p. 303.
206. Sutherland, C. G. G., Fisher, B. M., Frier, B. M., et al.: Endomyocardial biopsy pathology in insulin-dependent diabetic patients with abnormal ventricular function. Histopathology *14*:593, 1989.
207. Hausdorf, G., Rieger, U., and Koepp, P.: Cardiomyopathy in childhood diabetes mellitus: Incidence, time of onset, and relation to metabolic control. Int. J. Cardiol. *19*:225, 1988.
208. Zarich, S. W., Arbuckle, B. E., Cohen, L. R., et al.: Diastolic abnormalities in young asymptomatic diabetic patients assessed by pulsed Doppler echocardiography. J. Am. Coll. Cardiol. *12*:114, 1988.
209. Takenakam K., Sakamoto, T., Amano, K., et al.: Left ventricular filling determined by Doppler echocardiography in diabetes mellitus. Am. J. Cardiol. *61*:1139, 1988.
210. Ruddy, T. D., Shumak, S. L., Liu, P. P., et al.: The relationship of cardiac diastolic dysfunction to concurrent hormonal and metabolic status in Type I diabetes mellitus. J. Clin. Endocrinol. Metab. *66*:113, 1988.
211. Mustonen, J. N., Uusitupa, M. I. J., Tahvanainen, K., et al.: Impaired left ventricular systolic function during exercise in middle-aged insulin-dependent and noninsulin-dependent diabetic subjects without clinically evident cardiovascular disease. Am. J. Cardiol. *62*:1273, 1988.
212. Danielsen, R., Nordrehaug, J. E., and Vik-Mo, H.: Left ventricular function in young long-term Type I (insulin-dependent) diabetic men during exercise assessed by digitized echocardiography. Eur. Heart J. *9*:395, 1988.
213. Bouchard, A., Sanz, N., Botvinick, E. H., et al.: Noninvasive assessment of cardiomyopathy in normotensive diabetic patients between 20 and 50 years old. Am. J. Med. *87*:160, 1989.
213a. Paillole, C., Dahan, M., Paycha, F., et al.: Prevalence and significance of left ventricular filling abnormalities determined by Doppler echocardiography in young Type I (insulin-dependent) diabetic patients. Am. J. Cardiol. *64*:1010, 1989.
214. Danielsen, R.: Factors contributing to left ventricular diastolic dysfunc-

tion in long-term Type I diabetic subjects. Acta Med. Scand. *224*:249, 1988.

215. Ramandaham, S., Rodrigues, B., and McNeill, J. H.: Growth hormone and diabetes-induced cardiomyopathy. J. Lab. Clin. Med. *110*:257, 1987.
216. Regan, T. J., Altszuler, N., Eaddy, C., et al.: Relation of growth hormone and myocardial collagen accumulation in experimental diabetes. J. Lab. Clin. Med. *110*:274, 1987.
217. Nakada, T., and Kwee, I. L.: Sorbitol accumulation in heart: Implication for diabetic cardiomyopathy. Life Sci. *45*:2491, 1989.
218. Schaffer, S. W., Mozaffari, M. S., Artman, M., et al.: Basis for myocardial mechanical defects associated with noninsulin-dependent diabetes. Am. J. Physiol. *256*:E25, 1989.
219. Borda, E., Pascual, J., Wald, M., et al.: Hypersensitivity to calcium associated with an increased sarcolemmal Ca^{++}-ATPase activity in diabetic rat heart. Can. J. Cardiol. *4*:97, 1988.
220. Pierce, G. N., Lockwood, K., and Eckhert, C. D.: Cardiac contractile protein ATPase activity in a diet induced model of noninsulin dependent diabetes mellitus. Can. J. Cardiol. *5*:117, 1989.
221. Afzal, N., Ganguly, P. K., Dhalla, K. S., et al.: Beneficial effects of verapamil in diabetic cardiomyopathy. Diabetes *37*:936, 1988.
222. Okumura, K., Akiyama, N., Hashimoto, H., et al.: Alteration of 1,2-diacylglycerol content in myocardium from diabetic rats. Diabetes *37*:1168, 1988.
223. Sunni, S., Bishop, S. P., Kent, S. P., and Geer, J. C.: Diabetic cardiomyopathy. Arch. Pathol. Lab. Med. *110*:375, 1986.
224. Uusitupa, M., Siitonen, O., Pyorala, K., and Lansimies, E.: Left ventricular function in newly diagnosed noninsulin-dependent (Type 2) diabetes evaluated by systolic time intervals and echocardiography. Acta Med. Scand. *217*:379, 1985.
225. Fein, F. S., Capasso, J. M., Aronson, R. S., et al.: Combined renovascular hypertension and diabetes in rats: A new preparation of congestive cardiomyopathy. Circulation *70*:318, 1984.
226. Regan, T. J., Wu, C. F., Weisse, A. B., et al.: Acute myocardial infarction in toxic cardiomyopathy without coronary obstruction. Circulation *51*:453, 1975.
227. Deorari, A. K., Saxena, A., Singh, M., et al.: Echocardiographic assessment of infants born to diabetic mothers. Arch. Dis. Child. *64*:721, 1989.
228. Sheehan, J. P., Sisam, D. A., and Schumacher, O. P.: Insulin-induced cardiac failure. Am. J. Med. *79*:147, 1985.
229. Zatz, R., Dunn, B. R., Meyer, T. W., et al.: Prevention of diabetic glomerulopathy by pharmacological amelioration of glomerular capillary hypertension. J. Clin. Invest. *77*:1925, 1986.
230. Marre, M., Leblanc, H., Suarez, L., et al.: Converting enzyme inhibition and kidney function in normotensive diabetic patients with persistent microalbuminuria. Br. Med. J. *294*:1448, 1987.
231. Falholt, K., Cutfield, R., Alejandro, R., et al.: The effects of hyperinsulinemia on arterial wall and peripheral muscle metabolism in dogs. Metabolism *34*:1146, 1985.
232. The Working Group on Hypertension in Diabetes: Statement on hypertension in diabetes mellitus. Final report. Arch. Intern. Med. *147*:830, 1987.
233. Ferrannini, E., and DeFronzo, R. A.: The association of hypertension, diabetes, and obesity: A review. J. Nephrol. *1*:3, 1989.
234. Reaven, G. M., and Hoffman, B. B.: Hypertension as a disease of carbohydrate and lipoprotein metabolism. Am. J. Med. *87*:2S, 1989.
235. Williams, G. H.: Converting enzyme inhibitors in the treatment of hypertension. N. Engl. J. Med. *319*:1517, 1988.
236. Houston, M. C.: Treatment of hypertension in diabetes mellitus. Am. Heart J. *118*:819, 1989.
237. Beyer, T. A., and Hutson, N. J.: Introduction: Evidence for the role of the polyol pathway in the pathophysiology of diabetic complications. Metabolism *35*:1, 1986.
238. University Group Diabetes Program: A study of the effects of hypoglycemic agents on vascular complications in patients with adult-onset diabetes: V. Evaluation of phenformin therapy. Diabetes *24* (Suppl. I):65, 1975.
239. Wu, C. F., Haider, B., Ahmed, S. S., et al.: The effects of tolbutamide on the myocardium in experimental diabetes. Circulation *55*:200, 1977.
240. Regan, T. J.: Cardiac disease in the older diabetic: Management considerations. Geriatrics *44*:91, 1989.
241. Bielefeld, D. R., Pace, C. S., and Boshell, B. R.: Hyperosmolarity and cardiac function in chronic diabetic rat heart. Am. J. Physiol. *245*:E568, 1983.
242. Axelrod, L.: Response of congestive heart failure to correction of hyperglycemia in the presence of diabetic nephropathy. N. Engl. J. Med. *293*:1243, 1975.

OBESITY

243. Salan, S.: The obesities. *In* Felig, P., et al. (eds.): Endocrinology and Metabolism. 2nd ed. New York, McGraw-Hill Book Co., 1987, p. 1203.
244. Hirsch, J.: The adipose cell hypothesis. N. Engl. J. Med. *294*:389, 1976.
245. Foster, W. R., and Burton, B. T. (eds.): Health implications of obesity: NIH consensus development conference. Ann. Intern. Med. *103*:979, 1985.
246. Messerli, F. H., Sundgaard-Riise, K., Reisin, E., et al.: Disparate cardiovascular effects of obesity and arterial hypertension. Am. J. Med. *74*:808, 1983.
247. Smith, H. L., and Willius, R. A.: Adiposity of the heart. A clinical and pathological study of one hundred and thirty-six obese patients. Ann. Intern. Med. *52*:911, 1933.
248. De Divitiis, O., Fazio, S., Petitto, M., et al.: Obesity and cardiac function. Circulation *64*:477, 1981.
249. Egan, B., Fitzpatrick, M. A., Juni, J., et al.: Importance of overweight in studies of left ventricular hypertrophy and diastolic function in mild systemic hypertension. Am. J. Cardiol. *64*:752, 1989.
250. Nakajima, T., Fujioka, S., Tokunaga, K., et al.: Correlation of intraabdominal fat accumulation and left ventricular performance in obesity. Am. J. Cardiol. *64*:369, 1989.
251. Zack, P. M., Wiens, R. D., and Kennedy, H. L.: Left-axis deviation and adiposity: The United States health and nutrition examination survey. Am. J. Cardiol. *53*:1129, 1984.
252. Ventura, H. O., Messerli, F. H., Dunn, F. G., and Frohlich, E. D.: Left ventricular hypertrophy in obesity: Discrepancy between echo and electrocardiogram. J. Am. Coll. Cardiol. *1*:682, 1983.
253. Warnes, C. A., and Roberts, W. C.: The heart in massive (more than 300 pounds or 136 kilograms) obesity: Analysis of 12 patients studied at necropsy. Am. J. Cardiol. *54*:1087, 1984.
254. Lavie, C. J., Amodeo, C., Ventura, H. O., et al.: Left atrial abnormalities indicating diastolic ventricular dysfunction in cardiopathy of obesity. Chest *92*:1042, 1987.
255. Rossi, M., Marti, G., Ricordi, L., et al.: Cardiac autonomic dysfunction in obese subjects. Clin. Sci. *76*:567, 1989.
256. Reisin, E., Frohlich, E. D., Messerli, F. H., et al.: Cardiovascular changes after weight reduction in obesity hypertension. Ann. Intern. Med. *98*:315, 1983.
257. MacMahon, S. W., Wilcken, D. E. L., and Macdonald, G. J.: The effect of weight reduction on left ventricular mass: A randomized controlled trial in young, overweight hypertensive patients. N. Engl. J. Med. *314*:334, 1986.
258. Alpert, M. A., Terry, B. E., and Kelly, D. L.: Effect of weight loss on cardiac chamber size, wall thickness and left ventricular function in morbid obesity. Am. J. Cardiol. *55*:783, 1985.
259. Backman, L., Freyschuss, U., Hallberg, D., and Melcher, A.: Reversibility of cardiovascular changes in extreme obesity: Effects of weight reduction through jejunoileostomy. Acta Med. Scand. *205*:367, 1979.

MALNUTRITION

260. Frank, A., Graham, C., and Frank, S.: Fatalities on the liquid protein diet: An analysis of possible causes. Int. J. Obes. *5*:243, 1981.
261. Webb, J. G., Kiess, M. C., and Chan-Yan, C. C.: Malnutrition and the heart. Can. Med. Assoc. J. *135*:753, 1986.
262. Pringle, T. H., Scobie, I. N., Murray, R. G., et al.: Prolongation of the QT interval during therapeutic starvation: A substrate for malignant arrhythmias. Int. J. Obes. *7*:253, 1983.
263. Bergman, J. W., Human, D. G., DeMoor, M. M. A., et al.: Effect of kwashiorkor on the cardiovascular system. Arch. Dis. Child. *63*:1359, 1988.
264. Alden, P. B., Madoff, R. D., Stahl, T. J., et al.: Left ventricular function in malnutrition. Am. J. Physiol. *253*:H380, 1987.
265. Nutter, D. O., Murray, T. G., Heymsfield, S. T., and Fuller, E. O.: The effect of chronic protein-calorie undernutrition in the rat on myocardial function and cardiac function. Circ. Res. *45*:144, 1979.
266. Isner, J. M., Roberts, W. C., Heymsfield, S. B., and Yager, J.: Anorexia nervosa and sudden death. Ann. Intern. Med. *102*:49, 1985.
267. Fonseca, V., Havard, C.W.H.: Electrolyte disturbances and cardiac failure with hypomagnesaemia in anorexia nervosa. Br. Med. J. *291*:1680, 1985.
268. Goldberg, S. J., Comerci, G. D., and Feldman, L.: Cardiac output and regional myocardial contraction in anorexia nervosa. J. Adolesc. Health Care *9*:15, 1988.
269. Schocken, D. D., Holloway, J. D., and Powers, P. S.: Weight loss and the heart. Arch. Intern. Med. *149*:877, 1989.
270. Carr, J. G., Stevenson, L. W., Walden, J. A., et al.: Prevalence and hemodynamic correlates of malnutrition in severe congestive heart failure secondary to ischemic or idiopathic dilated cardiomyopathy. Am. J. Cardiol. *63*:709, 1989.
271. Blackburn, G. L., Gibbons, G. W., Bothe, A., et al.: Nutritional support in cardiac cachexia. J. Thorac. Cardiovasc. Surg. *73*:489, 1977.
272. Abel, R. M., Fischer, J. E., Buckley, M. J., et al.: Malnutrition in cardiac surgical patients. Arch. Surg. *111*:45, 1976.
273. Steier, M., Lopez, R., and Cooperman, J. M.: Riboflavin deficiency in infants and children with heart disease. Am. Heart J. *92*:139, 1976.

ALTERATIONS IN GONADAL HORMONE SECRETION

274. Dimitrovski, C., Plaseski, A., Bogoev, M., and Sadikario, S.: Kallmann's syndrome associated with atrial septal defect. J.A.M.A. *248*:1358, 1982.
275. Warren, S. E., Schnitt, S. J., Bauman, A. J., et al.: Late onset dilated cardiomyopathy in a unique familial syndrome of hypogonadism and metabolic abnormalities. Am. Heart J. *114*:1520, 1987.
276. Wallace, R. B., Hoover, J., Barrett-Conner, E., et al.: Altered plasma lipid and lipoprotein levels associated with oral contraceptive and estrogen use. Lancet *2*:112, 1979.
277. Stampfer, M. J., Willett, W. C., Colditz, G. A., et al.: A prospective study of postmenopausal estrogen therapy and coronary heart disease. N. Engl. J. Med. *313*:1044, 1985.
278. Petitti, D. B., Perlman, J. A., and Sidney, S.: Postmenopausal estrogen use and heart disease. N. Engl. J. Med. *315*:131, 1986.
279. Hillner, B. E., Hollenberg, J. P., and Pauker, S. G.: Postmenopausal estro-

gens in prevention of osteoporosis: Benefit virtually without risk if cardiovascular effects are considered. Am. J. Med. *80*:1115, 1986.

280. Ritterband, A. B., Jaffee, I. A., and Densen, P. M.: Gonadal function and the development of coronary heart disease. Circulation *27*:237, 1963.

281. Colditz, G. A., Willett, W. C., Stamper, M. J., et al.: Menopause and the risk of coronary heart disease in women. N. Engl. J. Med. *316*:1105, 1987.

282. Webber, L. S., Hunter, S. M., Baugh, J. G., et al.: The interaction of cigarette smoking, oral contraceptive use, and cardiovascular risk factor variables in children: The Bogalusa Heart Study. Am. J. Publ. Health *72*:266, 1982.

283. Fletcher, C. D., Farish, E., Dagen, M. M., et al.: The effects of conjugated equine estrogens plus cyclical dydrogesterone on serum lipoproteins and apoproteins in postmenopausal women. Acta Endocrinol. *117*:339, 1988.

284. Wolfe, B. M., and Huff, M. W.: Effects of estrogen and progestin administration on plasma lipoprotein metabolism in postmenopausal women. J. Clin. Invest. *83*:40, 1989.

285. Jaffe, M. D.: Effect of oestrogens on postexercise electrocardiogram. Br. Heart J. *38*:1299, 1976.

286. Luria, M. H.: Estrogen and coronary arterial disease in men. Int. J. Cardiol. *25*:159, 1989.

287. Wilson, P. W. F., Garrison, R. J., and Castelli, W. P.: Postmenopausal estrogen use, cigarette smoking, and cardiovascular morbidity in women over 50: The Framingham Study. N. Engl. J. Med. *313*:1038, 1985.

288. Chute, C. G., Baron, J. A., Plymate, S. R., et al.: Sex hormones and coronary artery disease. Am. J. Med. *83*:853, 1987.

289. Gutin, B., Alejandro, D., Duni, T., et al.: Levels of serum sex hormones and risk factors for coronary heart disease in exercise-trained men. Am. J. Med. *79*:79, 1985.

290. Gutai, J., LaPorte, R., Kuller, L., et al.: Plasma testosterone, high density lipoprotein cholesterol and other lipoprotein fractions. Am. J. Cardiol. *48*:897, 1981.

291. Kiel, D. P., Baron, J. A., Plymate, S. R., et al.: Sex hormones and lipoproteins in men. Am. J. Med. *87*:35, 1989.

292. Merians, D. R., Haskell, W. L., Vranizan, K. M., et al.: Relationship of exercise, oral contraceptive use, and body fat to concentrations of plasma lipids and lipoprotein cholesterol in young women. Am. J. Med. *78*:913, 1985.

293. Stampfer, M. J., Willett, W. C., Colditz, G. A., et al.: A prospective study of past use of oral contraceptive agents and risk of cardiovascular diseases. N. Engl. J. Med. *319*:1313, 1988.

294. Boyd, W. N., Burden, R. P., and Aber, G. M.: Intrarenal vascular changes in patients receiving estrogen-containing compounds—A clinical, histological and angiographic study. Q. J. Med. *44*:415, 1975.

295. Hollenberg, N. K., Williams, G. H., Burger, B., et al.: Renal blood flow and its response to A II: An interaction between oral contraceptive agents, sodium intake and the renin-angiotensin system in healthy young women. Circ. Res. *38*:35, 1976.

62

Renal Disorders and Heart Disease

by STEPHEN O. PASTAN, M.D., and EUGENE BRAUNWALD, M.D.

Disorders of the heart and of the kidneys are intimately related. On the one hand, some of the principal clinical manifestations of impairment of the heart's performance as a pump are due to renal retention of sodium and water; a number of diseases of the heart, such as infective endocarditis and cardiogenic shock, may result in serious renal disease or dysfunction. On the other hand, renal failure frequently results in hypertension and lipid abnormalities, which often lead to accelerated atherosclerosis, so that coronary artery disease is a common cause of death in patients being treated for chronic renal insufficiency. Also, uremia often causes pericarditis and thereby may lead to cardiac tamponade or constrictive pericarditis; renal failure also can cause secondary hyperparathyroidism, which can produce cardiac calcification and lead to various disturbances of cardiac function.

EFFECTS OF CARDIAC DISEASE ON RENAL FUNCTION

HEART FAILURE

J. P. Peters at Yale is credited with developing the concept that the kidney in heart failure is physiologically similar to the kidney in hypovolemia: because of inadequate cardiac output in both states, salt and water are retained in an attempt to restore the effective arterial blood volume—an as yet poorly defined parameter of filling of the arterial tree that is somehow related to the ratio of arterial blood volume to the capacity of the vascular bed.

Total body sodium is uniformly elevated in edematous patients with congestive heart failure.[1] Modulation of the tubular transport of sodium provides the most important mechanism for regulating sodium excretion. The proximal tubule is the primary site of sodium reabsorption in the nephron, with approximately 60 per cent of filtered sodium being reabsorbed isotonically at this site. Current conceptions of the forces governing proximal tubular reabsorption of sodium in the normal state and in heart failure are shown in Figure 62–1. As cardiac output falls, several stimuli—including augmented alpha-adrenergic neural activity, circulating catecholamines, and increased circulating and locally produced angiotensin II—cause renal vasoconstriction, particularly of the efferent arterioles (Figs. 62–2 and 62–3). As a consequence, the glomerular filtration rate declines, but there is a proportionately greater fall in renal blood flow and, therefore, a rise in the filtration fraction (i.e., the ratio of glomerular filtration rate to renal blood flow). This results in an elevated protein concentration in the peritubular capillaries and a decline in the postglomerular capillary hydrostatic pressure; thus, the transcapillary hydraulic pressure gradient falls.[2]

SODIUM RETENTION IN HEART FAILURE. The combination of these events, i.e., the reduction of peritubular capillary hydrostatic pressure and an elevation of peritubular on-

Editor's note: The pathophysiology of congestive heart failure is described in Chaps. 14 and 16; the use of diuretics in treating heart failure is discussed in Chap. 17; and the alterations in renal function in congestive heart failure are reviewed here.

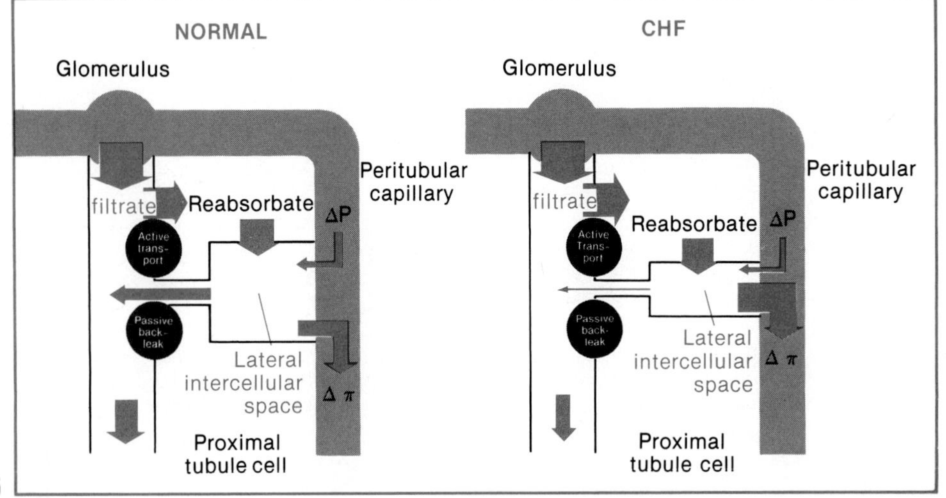

FIGURE 62–1. Peritubular control of proximal tubule fluid reabsorption. Current concept of the role of peritubular capillary physical forces in the regulation of proximal tubule fluid reabsorption in the normal state *(left)* and in congestive heart failure (CHF) *(right)*. ΔP and $\Delta\pi$ are, respectively, the transcapillary hydraulic and oncotic pressure differences operating across the peritubular capillary. The increase in filtration fraction causes $\Delta\pi$ to rise in CHF. The increase in renovascular resistance in CHF is thought to reduce ΔP. Both the increase in $\Delta\pi$ and the fall in ΔP enhance peritubular capillary uptake of proximal reabsorbate and thus increase absolute sodium reabsorption by the proximal tubule. (From Humes, H. D., et al.: The kidney in congestive heart failure. *In* Brenner, B. M., and Stein, J. H. [eds.]: Contemporary Issues in Nephrology. Vol. 1. New York, Churchill Livingstone, 1978, p. 51.)

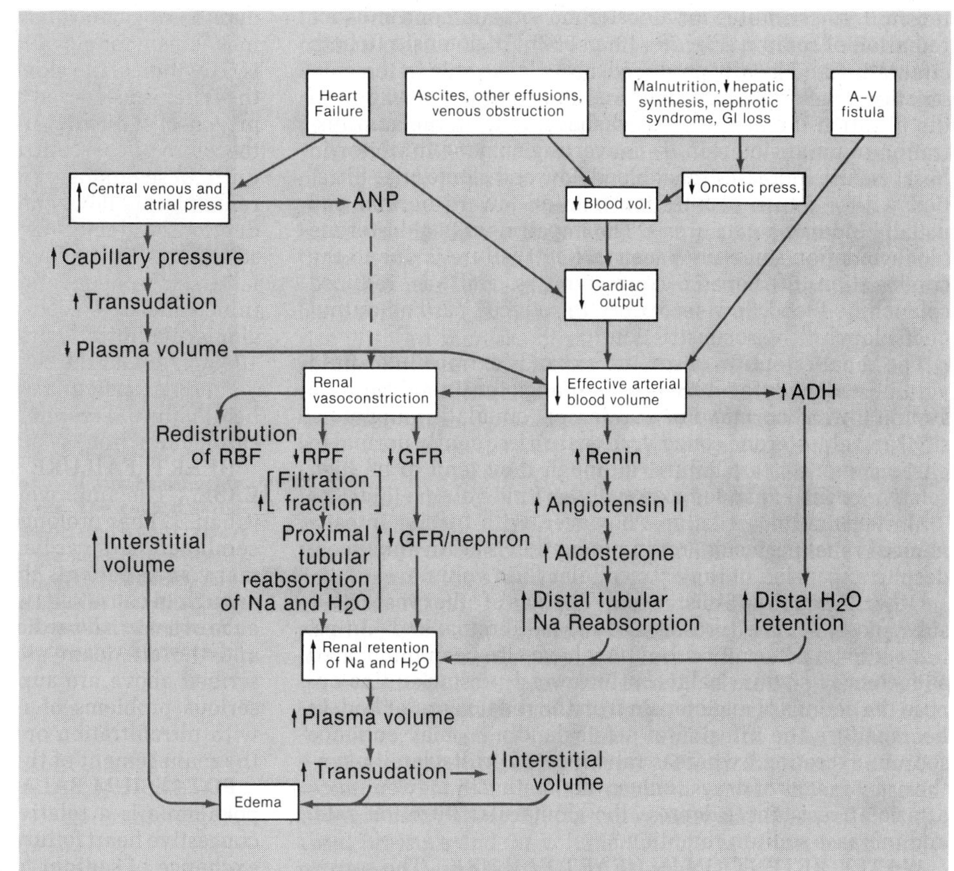

FIGURE 62–2. Major pathophysiological mechanisms leading to salt and water retention and the development of edema. The contribution of heart failure is shown, as well as other major causes. ANP = atrial natriuretic peptide; dotted line indicates inhibition of renal vasoconstriction. (From Braunwald, E.: Edema. *In* Harrison's Principles of Internal Medicine. New York, McGraw-Hill Book Co., 1991, p. 220.)

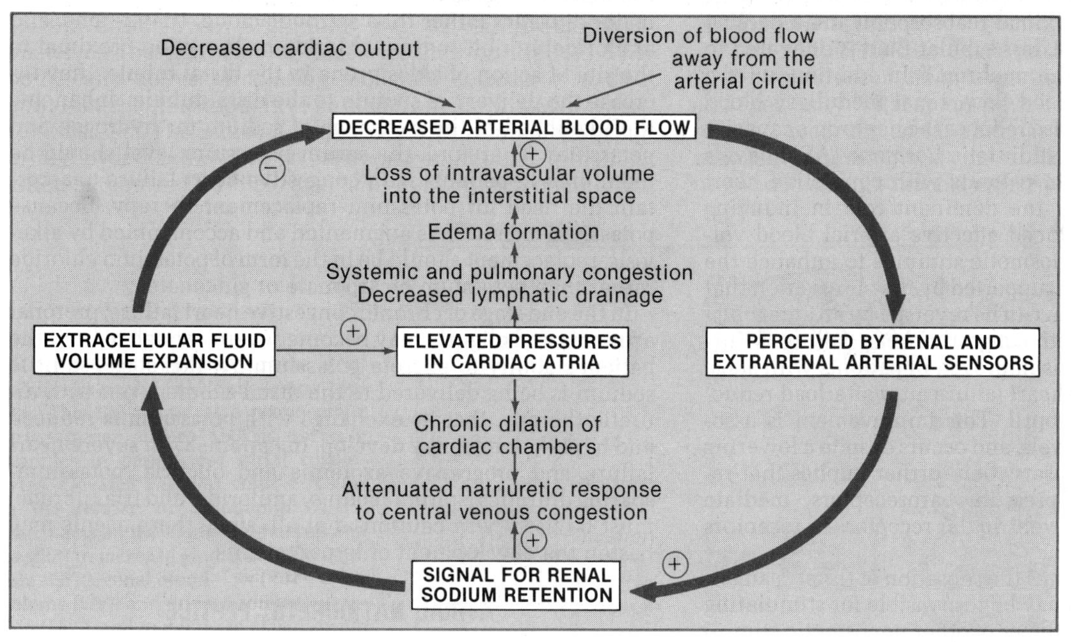

FIGURE 62–3. Sensing mechanisms that initiate and maintain renal sodium retention in congestive heart failure. (Reproduced with permission from Skorecki, K. L., and Brenner, B. M.: Body fluid homeostasis in congestive heart failure and cirrhosis with ascites. Am. J. Med. *72*:323, 1982.)

cotic pressure, enhances the peritubular capillary uptake of proximal tubular fluid, and thereby increases the absolute quantity of sodium reabsorbed by the proximal tubule.[3,4] An additional proposed mechanism for sodium retention in heart failure is the redistribution of blood flow from cortical to juxtamedullary nephrons that contain longer loops of Henle and are therefore capable of greater sodium reabsorption.

In addition to the more avid sodium reabsorption in the proximal convoluted tubule, sodium reabsorption also increases in distal nephron sites, including the collecting duct segments. This results from the operation of Starling forces, i.e., a lowering of capillary hydrostatic pressure and an elevation of oncotic pressure, such as those described for the proximal tubule.

The Renin-Angiotensin-Aldosterone System (see also p. 829). In addition, aldosterone, the sodium resorbing activity of which is limited to the terminal segment of the nephron, distal tubule, and collecting duct system, has been recognized as an important factor in sodium retention associated with congestive heart failure. The absolute concentration of circulating aldosterone is increased in some patients with congestive heart failure owing to both the enhanced production of aldosterone stimulated by the renin-angiotensin axis and its diminished metabolism. In acute heart failure, decreased renal perfusion (whether caused by a reduction in total cardiac output or by a decrease in the renal fraction of the cardiac output) activates the juxtaglomerular apparatus to enhance renin release; this in turn augments the generation of angio-

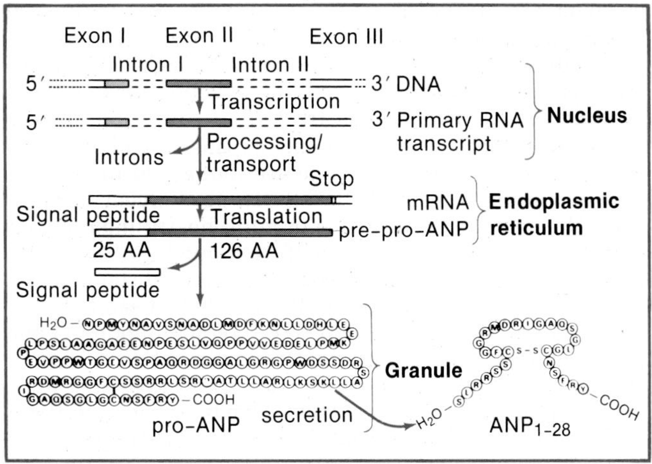

FIGURE 62–6. The biosynthetic pathway, and the sequences of the human pre-pro-ANP gene, pro-ANP, and ANP_{1-28}. ANP_{1-28} is numbered from amino- to carboxyterminus. Specific amino acids in the pro-ANP and ANP sequences are given by single-letter code: alanine = A, arginine = R, asparagine = N, aspartic acid = D, cysteine = C, glutamine = Q, glutamic acid = E, glycine = G, histidine = H, isoleucine = I, leucine = L, lysine = K, methionine = M, phenylalanine = F, proline = P, serine = S, threonine = T, tryptophan = W, tyrosine = Y, valine = V. The pre-pro-ANP gene is present in a single copy on the short arm of chromosome 1. The DNA is transcribed into RNA, and the exon segments are spliced together to form messenger RNA. This is translated to form the initial pro-ANP precursor (pre-pro-ANP). The signal peptide is removed and pro-ANP is stored in atrial myocyte granules. When the peptide is released, the active 28–amino acid fragment is cleaved off and enters the circulation. (From Ballermann, B. J., and Brenner, B. M.: Role of atrial peptides in body fluid homeostasis. Circ. Res. *58:*619, 1986, by permission of the American Heart Association, Inc.)

clear circulating ANP, resulting in its short half-life of about 3 minutes.[46] The biologically active receptor itself is unique, as it both binds ANP *and* catalyzes the formation of cyclic guanosine monophosphate, which serves as a second messenger for ANP action.[47]

PHYSIOLOGICAL EFFECTS OF ANP. The major direct renal effects of ANP occur in the glomerulus, which has an abundance of receptors,[48] and the inner medullary collecting duct, where sodium uptake is decreased by the inhibition of a membrane sodium channel.[49] Intravenous infusion of ANP in animals and humans results in a brisk natriuresis and diuresis (Fig. 62–7*A*). An increase in excretion of chloride, potassium, calcium, magnesium, and phosphorus also has been noted.[50,51] Two consistent and dramatic findings have been increases in both glomerular filtration rate and filtration fraction, despite a drop in blood pressure (Fig. 62–7*B*). In the rat this is associated with constriction of the efferent glomerular arterioles, dilation of afferent arterioles, and an increase in glomerular pressure.[52] Other glomerular effects include an increase in the glomerular capillary ultrafiltration coefficient[52] and inhibition of tubuloglomerular feedback.[53] ANP inhibits renal vasoconstriction, but differing effects of ANP on total renal blood flow have been described, depending on the species studied and on experimental conditions.[50,54] Although changes in the glomerular filtration rate account for the preponderance of the natriuresis in response to ANP, inhibition of distal nephron sodium transport probably contributes as well.[55]

More prolonged effects of ANP on salt balance and hemodynamics may be mediated through changes in the renin-angiotensin-aldosterone system. Renal renin secretion is known to be suppressed by ANP.[56] Aldosterone secretion also is blocked by ANP in vitro and in vivo,[57] as is angiotensin-induced vascular constriction[58] and angiotensin-stimulated aldosterone release. Thus, ANP may play a special role in antagonizing each aspect of the renin-angiotensin-aldosterone axis (Fig. 62–8).

ANP is known to relax smooth muscle, including that found in the renal, coronary, and other vascular beds.[59,59a] However, infusions of ANP into intact animals may increase or decrease vascular resistance, depending on experimental conditions.[50] Thus the fall in blood pressure seen after ANP infusion seems to result mostly from a reduction in cardiac output, which is associated with a decrease in venous return.[60] This hypotensive effect may be augmented by a direct effect of ANP on vascular permeability, resulting in a reversible extravascular fluid shift, and is associated with a rise in hematocrit and total plasma proteins out of proportion to the degree of natriuresis and diuresis.[51]

Other actions of ANP include a suggested role in maintaining sodium balance in chronic renal failure[61] and in mediating the "escape" phenomenon seen with chronic mineralocorticoid administration.[62] Finally, immunoreactive ANP has been found in the central nervous system and may relate to cardiovascular regulatory functions.[63,64]

Despite the multiplicity of actions of ANP in a variety of tissues, the differences between its physiological and pharmacological effects are not clearly delineated. Although it is certain that ANP will take its place as an important regulatory hormone, further studies are needed to define its role in both normal and pathophysiological conditions, as well as a therapeutic agent.

RENAL MANIFESTATIONS OF CARDIAC DISORDERS

INFECTIVE ENDOCARDITIS (see also Chap. 35). The association between glomerulonephritis and bacterial endocarditis has been appreciated for many years. In 1920, before the availability of antibiotics and when infective endocarditis was uniformly fatal, 11 per cent of patients with this infection ultimately died of renal failure.[65] It was initially thought that the glomerular lesion was secondary to septic embolization to the kidney from infected valvular vegetations, but little firm evidence supports this theory. Instead, the pathogenesis of the renal lesions appears to be more in keeping with the generally accepted pathogenesis of most types of glomerulonephritis.[66] Soluble antigenic components of the infecting organism and antibody directed against these antigens have been demonstrated in the glomeruli. As indicated in Chapter 35, many organisms have been responsible for the infective endocarditis that may be associated with glomerulonephritis. By immunofluorescence, the presence of immune complexes and the third component of complement (C3) can be demonstrated in the glomeruli of patients with endocarditis and glomerulonephritis[66]; early in the course there is a decline in the serum level of C3 and of another component of the complement system, Clq. It now appears that the glomerular lesion of endocarditis results from the deposition of immune complexes along the glomerular basement membrane and in the mesangium.[67]

The most commonly observed abnormality by light microscopy is a focal, proliferative glomerulonephritis, often with focal fibrinoid necrosis. Less commonly, the lesions may be more diffuse, and in some instances extracapillary epithelial proliferation (crescents), such as that seen in rapidly progressive glomerulonephritis, has been observed.[66] Clinically, patients have the typical manifestations of acute or rapidly progressive renal failure, often with hypertension, hematuria, and red cell casts, usually without marked proteinuria and edema. The retention of sodium and water is due to reductions in the glomerular filtration rate and the fractional excretion of sodium. Azotemia usually is progressive, unless rapid bacteriological cure occurs.

Other causes of impaired renal function in patients with infective endocarditis include hypovolemia, congestive heart failure, antibiotic-induced

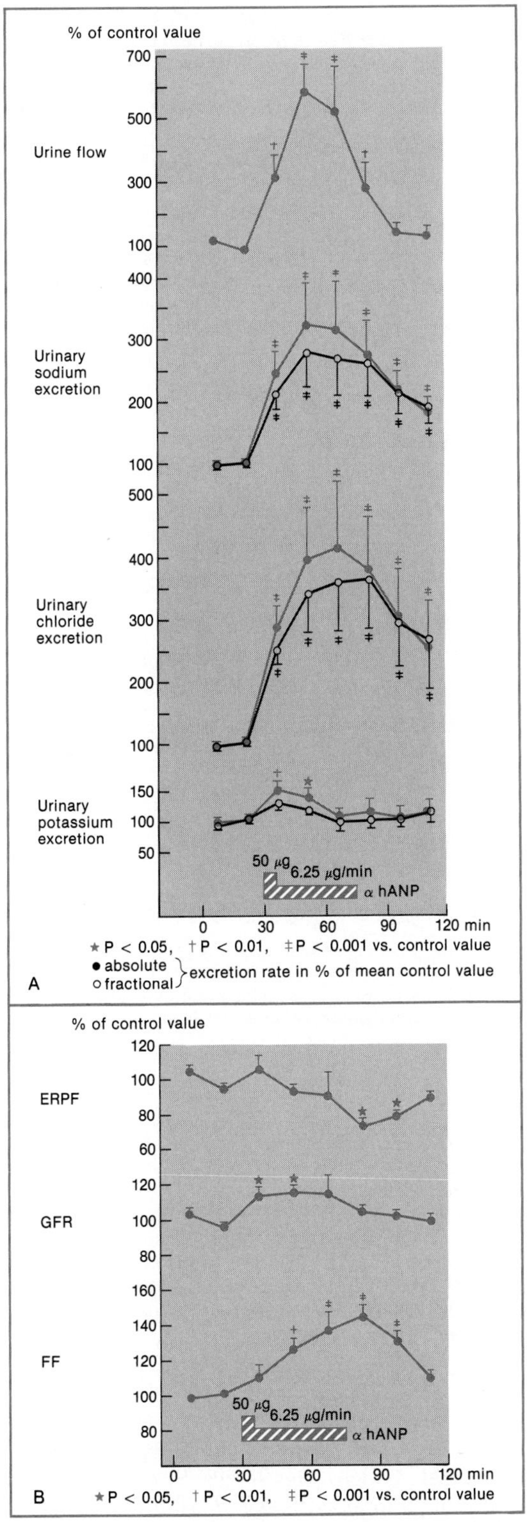

FIGURE 62-7. *A*, Effect of ANP (50 = μg bolus followed by maintenance infusion of 6.25 μ/min) on urine flow and sodium, chloride, and potassium excretion rates in 10 normal subjects (mean ± S.E.M.). The mean of the two control values is taken as 100 per cent. Closed circles are the absolute excretion rates. Open circles are calculated fractional excretion rates (urine/plasma Na, Cl, or K divided by urine/plasma creatinine). *B*, Effect of ANP on ERPF = estimated renal plasma flow; GFR = glomerular filtration rate; FF = filtration fraction. (Reproduced from Weidmann, P., et al.: Blood levels and renal effects of atrial natriuretic peptide in normal man. J. Clin. Invest. *77*:734, 1986, by copyright permission of the American Society for Clinical Investigation.)

nephrotoxicity, and acute allergic interstitial nephritis secondary to antibiotic therapy.

ANTIBIOTIC TREATMENT IN RENAL FAILURE. Many of the antibiotics used in the treatment of infective endocarditis are excreted by the kidney. These include vancomycin, the penicillins, cephalosporins, and aminoglycosides. It is therefore important to modify the dosage and/or the interval of administration of antibiotics with respect to the degree of renal dysfunction. Because many antibiotics are removed by hemodialysis or peritoneal dialysis, supplementary doses may need to be administered in patients receiving these therapies. Guidelines for antibiotic therapy are presented in Table 62–1. Aminoglycoside and vancomycin levels should be monitored to insure adequate therapeutic dosage and to avoid toxic levels that may contribute to further renal impairment or to ototoxicity. Serum bactericidal titers also may be monitored to assess the adequacy of antibiotic therapy.

The most common cause of endocarditis in dialysis patients is *Staphylococcus aureus*,[68] with *Streptococcus viridans*, enterococci, *Staphylococcus epidermidis*, and gram-negative rods accounting for most of the other cases. Therefore, initial antibiotic therapy should include a penicillinase-resistant penicillin, or vancomycin, and an aminoglycoside, until culture results are available.

ACUTE RENAL FAILURE SECONDARY TO CARDIOGENIC SHOCK (see also p. 574). Prerenal azotemia and, less commonly, acute renal failure (acute tubular necrosis) may occur in association with massive acute myocardial infarction. The mechanism of prerenal azotemia has been discussed above. Acute renal failure occurs when there is a marked, sudden reduction of renal perfusion. The myoglobinuria accompanying excessive myocardial necrosis may play a contributory role. It is critically important to distinguish between prerenal azotemia and acute renal failure, since the former usually responds to measures that improve cardiac output, whereas acute renal failure, once established, is a more serious problem that usually does not respond to extrarenal manipulation. Brief periods of modest hypotension (usually lasting less than an hour) often elicit reversible derange-

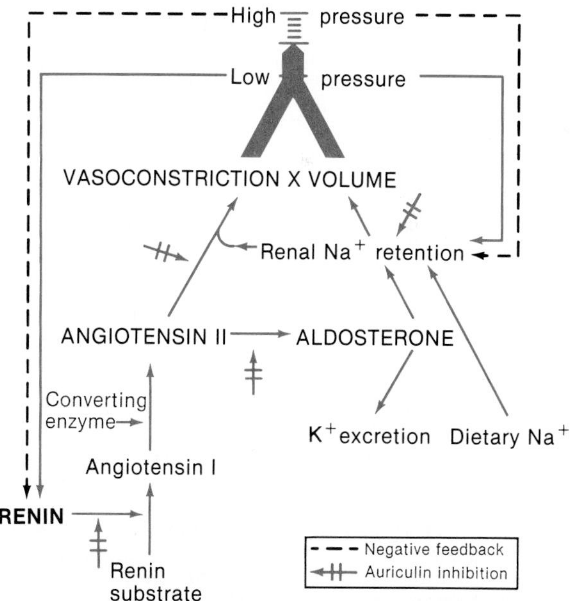

FIGURE 62-8. Atrial natriuretic peptide and the renin-angiotensin-aldosterone system. Renin, secreted in response to reduced renal arterial pressure or a reduction in the sodium supply in the distal tubule, acts to release angiotensin II. Angiotensin II raises blood pressure and stimulates aldosterone secretion, which leads to retention of sodium and water and to improved flow. These pressure and volume effects turn off the renin release. Auriculin opposes the renin system at four points. Within the kidney its natriuretic action opposes aldosterone's action and stops renin secretion. The atrial hormone also opposes the vasoconstrictor action of angiotensin on blood vessels and, at the adrenal cortex, blocks angiotensin's stimulation of aldosterone release. Broken lines = negative feedback; crossed arrows = auriculin inhibition. (Reprinted with permission from Laragh, J. H.: Atrial natriuretic hormone, the renin-aldosterone axis, and blood pressure-electrolyte homeostasis. N. Engl. J. Med. *313*:1330, 1985.)

TABLE 62-1 ANTIBIOTIC THERAPY IN RENAL FAILURE

	PHARMACOKINETIC PARAMETERS					ADJUSTMENT FOR RENAL FAILURE				
		Half-life					GFR (ml/min)			
DRUG	Elimination and Metabolism	*Normal (hr)*	*ESRD (hr)*	Plasma Protein Binding (%)	Volume of Distribution (liters/kg)	Method	*>50*	*10–50*	*<10*	Removed by Dialysis
Aminoglycosides[a]										
Amikacin	Renal	2–3	30	<5	0.22–0.29	D	60–90	30–70	20–30	Yes (H, P)
						I	12	12–18	24	
Gentamicin	Renal	2	24–48	<5	0.23–0.26	D	60–90	30–70	20–30	Yes (H, P)[b]
						I	8–12	12	24	
Streptomycin	Renal	2.5	100	35	0.26	I	24	24–72	72–96	Yes (H)
Tobramycin	Renal	2.5	56	<5	0.22–0.25	D	60–90	30–70	20–30	Yes (H, P)
						I	8–12	12	24	
Cephalosporins										
Cefazolin	Renal	1.4–2.2	18–36	80	0.13	I	8	12	24–48	Yes (H), No (P)
Cephalothin	Renal (hepatic)	0.5–0.9	3–18	65	0.26	I	6	6	8–12	Yes (H, P)
Penicillins										
Ampicillin	Renal (hepatic)	0.8–1.5	7–20	8–20	0.17–0.31	I	6	6–12	12–16	Yes (H), No (P)
Azlocillin	Renal (hepatic)	0.8–1.5	5–6	25–30	0.18–0.23	I	4–6	6–8	8	Yes (H), No (P)
Carbenicillin	Renal (hepatic)	1.5	10–20	30–50	0.12–0.20	I	8–12	12–24	24–48	Yes (H), No (P)
Methicillin	Renal (hepatic)	0.5–1.0	4	35–60	0.31	I	4	4–8	8–12	No (H, P)
Nafcillin	Hepatic (renal)	0.5	1.2	80–90	0.31–0.38	D	U	U	U	No (H)
Oxacillin	Renal (hepatic)	0.4	1	85–95	0.12–0.4	D	U	U	U	No (H, P)
Penicillin G[c]	Renal (hepatic)	0.5	6–20	40–60	0.3–0.42	D	U	75	25–50	Yes (H),
						I	6–8	8–12	12–16	No (P)
Piperacillin	Renal (hepatic)	0.8–1.5	3.3–5.1	16–22	0.18–0.30	I	4–6	6–8	8	Yes (H)
Ticarcillin	Renal	1.0–1.5	16	45	0.14–0.21	I	8–12	12–24	24–48	Yes (H, P)
Aztreonam	Renal	1.7–2.9	6–8	50–60	0–20	D	U	50–75	25	Yes (H), No (P)
Imipenem	Renal (hepatic)	1	3.5–4.0	20	0.24–0.27	I	6	8	12	Yes (H)
						D	100	75	50	
Rifampin	Hepatic	2–5	2–5	60–90	0.9	I	U	U	U	No (H)
Vancomycin[d]	Renal	6–8	200–250	10	0.47–0.84	I	24–72	72–240	240	No (H, P)

From Bennett, W. M.: Drug therapy in renal disease. *In* Rubenstein, E., and Federman, D. D. (eds.): Scientific American Medicine. New York, Scientific American, Inc. 1990.

[a] Need usual loading dose in renal failure. [b] Poor clearance from blood to peritoneum in CAPD. [c] Upper limit of 4 to 6 million units/day in severe renal failure. [d] Elimination is variable in renal failure; best guide to therapy is serum level before next dose.

$T_{1/2}$ = biological half-life; ESRD = end-stage renal disease; GFR = glomerular filtration rate; I = interval extension method of dosage adjustment in hours between maintenance doses; D = dose reduction method of dosage adjustment in percentage of usual maintenance dose; H = hemodialysis; P = peritoneal dialysis; U = unchanged.

ments, but more prolonged or profound hypotension lasting for 1 hour or longer usually leads to acute tubular necrosis.

DIFFERENTIAL DIAGNOSIS. The distinction between prerenal azotemia and acute tubular necrosis in the oliguric patient (i.e., urine output less than 400 ml/24 hr) usually can be made by measurements of serum urea nitrogen and creatinine levels and the sodium, urea, and creatinine concentrations and osmolality of a concurrent sample of urine. In the absence of recent diuretic therapy, patients with prerenal azotemia retain their ability to conserve sodium; therefore, urine sodium concentration is low, usually less than 20 mEq/liter. Tubular function is well preserved, as reflected in urine osmolality exceeding 500 mOsm, and the urine : plasma ratios for urea and creatinine exceed 8 and 40, respectively. The BUN level is more than 10 times the serum creatinine concentration.

In acute tubular necrosis, tubular function is impaired and the urine sodium concentration usually exceeds 40 mEq/liter; the impairment of tubular function also is reflected in a urine osmolality less than 350 mOsm; the urine : plasma values for urea and creatinine are below 2 and 20, respectively; and the BUN level exceeds the serum creatinine level by a ratio of less than 10 to 1. The urinary sediment also may be helpful in the differential diagnosis; patients with prerenal azotemia usually have a relatively clear sediment with a few granular or hyaline casts, whereas those with acute tubular necrosis have many tubular cells and casts in the urine.

MANAGEMENT. As in patients with other causes of acute renal failure, the treatment of acute renal failure secondary to myocardial infarction and pump failure consists of controlling fluid intake to levels in accord with urine output and insensible losses, as well as modifying the dosages of medications that are excreted by the kidneys, observing the patient closely for hyperkalemia, and intervening with dialysis for severe hyperkalemia or azotemia. Dialytic therapy, either hemodialysis or peritoneal dialysis, is initiated when serum creatinine levels reach 8 to 10 mg/dl and no reversible component for the renal failure is apparent. In addition, efforts must be made to maintain left ventricular filling pressure at levels that will optimize cardiac output and therefore renal perfusion (18 to 22 mm Hg). Given sufficient time and with no other associated problems, the prognosis for acute renal failure, when appropriately treated, is excellent. When failure of the cardiac pump is severe enough to lead to acute renal failure, myocardial insufficiency rather than the renal failure is the determinant of the patient's poor prognosis.

ATHEROEMBOLIC DISEASE (see also p. 1552). Atheromatous embolization to the kidneys, which results in chronic, fibrotic interstitial disease, is relatively uncommon.[69] It may occur spontaneously but more commonly follows operation on the aorta and renal arteries and catheter manipulation and aortography in patients with severe atheromatous disease of the aorta. Patchy areas of necrosis develop, followed by fibrosis with cholesterol clefts, as well as a foreign body response containing multinucleated giant cells. The disorder may be suspected if there has been some manipulation of the atheromatous aorta preceding the onset of progressive renal insufficiency. Examination of the urine is seldom helpful in confirming the diagnosis; when it is allowed to sediment, fat may be found floating at the top. Careful ophthalmological examination may reveal cholesterol emboli in the retinal arteries. Treatment consists of avoiding further arterial and aortic manipulation, but progressive destruction of renal tissue occurs with subsequent renal insufficiency; the prognosis for improvement of renal function is guarded.

EFFECTS OF RENAL DISEASE ON THE CARDIOVASCULAR SYSTEM

The successful treatment of end-stage renal disease by dialysis and transplantation is widely considered to be one of the major advances of modern medicine. Cardiovascular disease is the principal cause of mortality in dialysis patients, accounting for 30 to 50 per cent of deaths[70] compared with less than 15 per cent of deaths in an age-corrected control population. Heart failure accounts for about 15 per cent of this dialysis-associated mortality, myocardial infarction for about 10 per cent, and pericarditis for about 3 per cent.

CORONARY ATHEROSCLEROSIS

Numerous risk factors for atherosclerosis have been identified in patients with end-stage renal disease.[71] Of these, hypertension is the most important.[72] Uremia itself has been proposed as an independent risk factor,[73] but recently this suggestion has been questioned. It is unclear whether coronary atherosclerosis is unusually prevalent or accelerated in uremic patients when compared with nonuremic patients of comparable age and with similar risk factors.[70,74] The National Cooperative Dialysis Study demonstrated a clear increase in cardiovascular morbid events in patients who received shorter dialysis treatments or who had elevated (time-averaged) BUN concentrations.[75] These observations imply that the adequacy of a dialysis regimen has a significant impact on cardiovascular morbidity.

Coronary bypass surgery has been carried out successfully in patients with renal failure and angina pectoris that is refractory to medical therapy,[76] although postoperative morbidity is increased compared with that of patients without renal disease. Although the short-term results of coronary angioplasty are satisfactory in patients on chronic dialysis, these patients have a high incidence of restenosis, so that coronary bypass surgery is the preferred therapy.[76a] In addition, angina unassociated with coronary atherosclerosis is being increasingly recognized in chronic renal failure, presumably related to the combination of severe hypertension, left ventricular hypertrophy, and anemia.[70] It also has been suggested that reduced coronary artery compliance owing to calcification may restrict coronary vasodilation and limit myocardial oxygen delivery.[74]

HYPERTENSION

(See also p. 833)

Most patients with chronic renal failure that requires dialysis also have hypertension, which is probably the most important risk factor in the development of atherosclerotic cardiovascular disease. Hemodynamic studies in patients with end-stage renal disease have shown an elevated cardiac index and mean arterial pressure but a normal systemic vascular resistance.[70] The elevated cardiac index and normal systemic vascular resistance are related to the anemia; when the anemia is corrected, the cardiac index falls, and both arterial pressure and systemic vascular resistance rise.[77] Many patients with end-stage renal disease who are treated with erythropoietin experience an elevation of blood pressure, related to an increase in peripheral vascular resistance and an increased blood viscosity, when hematocrit rises to more normal levels.[78] This blood pressure elevation may be associated with seizures, and requires initiation of or an increase in blood pressure medication in approximately 25 per cent of patients. Most patients with end-stage renal failure who develop hypertension have so-called *volume-dependent hypertension* (p. 834). Many studies in patients with end-stage renal failure have shown that arterial pressure is exquisitely dependent on blood volume[79] and that blood pressure control may be achieved by ultrafiltration during dialysis and control of salt and water intake in the interdialytic interval. A minority of patients with chronic renal failure have hypertension that is not volume-related but rather secondary to elevation of plasma renin activity; the hypertension is uncontrollable by lowering blood volume but does respond to bilateral nephrectomy with a consequent reduction in plasma renin activity. Dustan and Page demonstrated the volume-dependent nature of hypertension but also showed that arterial pressure was higher for any given volume when the kidneys were present than after they had been removed.[80] Subsequently a significant correlation between *plasma renin* levels and arterial pressure was demonstrated.[81] The importance of plasma renin also is reflected in observations on patients with renal failure, hypertension, and expanded blood volume who exhibited renin values which, although normal, were higher than expected for the expanded state of their extracellular volume and which therefore may have contributed to the maintenance of hypertension.[82] There also is evidence that local production and action of angiotensin II plays an important part in the hypertension of chronic renal failure.[83]

A third mechanism, which operates in patients whose blood pressure cannot be controlled by either volume reduction or bilateral nephrectomy or explained by elevations in plasma renin activity, may be related to *sympathetically mediated vasoconstriction*. Reduced baroreceptor activity has been demonstrated in patients with chronic renal failure by their response to the inhalation of amyl nitrite and the Valsalva maneuver.[84] Inhalation of amyl nitrite causes peripheral vasodilation, and therefore a fall in blood pressure, which normally results in reflex vasoconstriction and tachycardia. A blunted response in heart rate elevation is taken as evidence of reduced baroreceptor function. Autonomic insufficiency, as evidenced by an inadequate response to the Valsalva maneuver, is said to be present if both bradycardia and arterial pressure overshoot are absent after release of forced expiration against a standard pressure (40 mm Hg) for a set time (12 sec). Many patients with renal insufficiency whose hypertension is caused by sympathetically mediated vasoconstriction exhibit an exaggerated response to the cold pressor test and elevated plasma levels of dopamine beta-hydroxylase as indices of increased adrenergic function but become hypotensive during dialysis.

A fourth mechanism that has been proposed is the *absence of vasodepressor substances* of renal origin, such as the prostaglandins, which may play a role in the genesis of essential hypertension and of renoprival hypertension.[85]

MANAGEMENT. Because volume-dependent hypertension is the most common mechanism in chronic renal disease, the reduction of plasma volume should be the central theme in the management of hypertension in these patients. Before renal function has deteriorated to the point at which dialysis is required, an attempt should be made to reduce plasma volume, but not to the point at which glomerular filtration will decline further; dietary sodium intake should be restricted to the lowest level consistent with a normal sodium balance. Because many patients may have difficulty with this degree of sodium restriction on a long-term basis, and because they may be unable to excrete even this low quantity of sodium, it is often necessary to add diuretics. For most patients with creatinine clearances that exceed 40 ml/min, thiazide diuretics are effective. When the glomerular filtration rate falls below this level, furosemide is required, sometimes in very high doses.

If the arterial pressure remains elevated despite sodium restriction and potent diuretics such as furosemide, antihypertensive agents are required and usually effective. These include calcium channel antagonists, angiotensin converting enzyme (ACE) inhibitors, beta blockers, clonidine, prazosin, hydralazine, and alpha-methyldopa. For the patient whose condition is refractory to these agents, minoxidil may be required. Sympatholytic agents such as guanethidine are not advisable, since they may be associated with particularly profound postural changes in blood pressure in patients with renal failure.

The problem of the control of hypertension is simpler in patients with chronic renal failure who are maintained on intermittent hemodialysis. In addition to dietary restriction of sodium intake, lowering of blood volume by ultrafiltration during hemodialysis may be used. In patients in whom volume reduction does not control blood pressure, pharmacological treatment is indicated, as described above.

Bilateral nephrectomy is seldom used except in those patients who do not respond to antihypertensive drugs, cannot comply with antihypertensive regimens, or experience intolerable side effects with this medication. Although aggressive therapy of hypertension for the patient with renin-mediated malignant hypertension may transiently compromise renal function to the point at which dialysis is required, the increased survival associated with control of the hypertension[86] outweighs the risks attending maintenance hemodialysis.

Hypertension After Renal Transplantation

Hypertension occurs in 30 to 80 per cent of patients during the posttransplant period.[87] Multiple factors have been implicated in its etiology, including acute and chronic rejection, recurrent disease in the transplanted kidney, stenosis of the transplanted renal artery[88], large doses of steroids, and cyclosporin A (CSA).[89] During acute rejection episodes the levels of renin and angiotensin are markedly elevated. In addition, the renin-angiotensin-aldosterone system appears to be of pathogenic importance in the hypertension associated with stenosis of the artery to the transplanted kidney, a complication that occurs in up to 30 per cent of transplant patients who undergo arteriography for refractory hypertension as well as in some patients in whom the diseased native kidneys release renin. CSA-related hypertension is associated with renal vasoconstriction as manifest by decreased renal blood flow, increased renovascular resistance, and decreased glomerular filtration rate, but in humans it is not associated with elevations of renin levels.[89]

MANAGEMENT. To treat hypertension in the posttransplant period the underlying mechanisms of the disorder must be elucidated. Because of activation of the renin-angiotensin-aldosterone system, ACE inhibitors have been found to be effective antihypertensive agents in this setting. Furthermore, ACE inhibitor–induced reversible acute renal insufficiency has been described in patients with functionally significant transplant renal artery stenosis, and its occurrence may serve as a diagnostic test for this entity.[90] In patients with severe refractory hypertension that cannot be ascribed to rejection, angiography and determination of renin activity in venous blood from both the native and the transplanted kidneys are indicated. Surgical revision or angioplasty of a stenosed renal artery or nephrectomy of the native kidney may be in order. Calcium antagonists have been found to counteract some of the adverse effects of CSA on the kidney, and are probably the most effective agents for posttransplant hypertension related to CSA.[91] Also, in some patients, switching from CSA to azathioprine has resulted in noticeable lowering of the blood pressure.[92]

Whereas hypertriglyceridemia is the predominant lipid abnormality in patients with chronic renal failure (see below), hypercholesterolemia Types IIA and B tend to predominate after renal allotransplantation, although in some transplanted patients hypertriglyceridemia persists.[93] The cause of these lipid abnormalities in the posttransplant period is unclear, but they may be related in part to the large doses of glucocorticoids administered to these patients. Furthermore, CSA has been associated with an increased incidence of hypercholesterolemia.[94] In view of the combination of hypertension and lipid abnormalities in a substantial fraction of patients after transplantation, it is not surprising that cardiovascular disease is the most common cause of death greater than 10 years post transplant.[95]

LIPID ABNORMALITIES (see also Chap. 37)

Hypertriglyceridemia with elevations of very low density lipoproteins (VLDL), i.e., Type IV hyperlipoproteinemia (p. 1135), is common in patients with chronic renal failure.[96,96a] There appears to be no relation between the duration of dialysis or the cause of the renal disease and the severity of the hyperlipidemia. A second abnormality in lipid metabolism, *reduced concentration of high-density lipoprotein (HDL) cholesterol,* has also been documented in chronic renal failure,[96,97] a finding of potential importance in view of the strong negative correlation between HDL concentration and the risk of the development of ischemic heart disease. An inverse correlation has been noted between plasma triglyceride and HDL cholesterol levels in both uremic and nonuremic subjects.

MECHANISMS. Several suggestions have been made to explain the elevation of plasma triglycerides in chronic renal failure. The first is that there is increased hepatic synthesis of triglycerides, presumably secondary to increased basal insulin, growth hormone, and glucagon. However, measurements in uremic animals and patients have suggested that the contribution of increased hepatic synthesis is small.[98] A second, more likely possibility[99,100] centers on deficiencies in lipoprotein lipase and hepatic triglyceride lipase known to be necessary for the removal of triglycerides from plasma and their ultimate catabolism; this deficiency also may result from elevated insulin levels, from direct inhibition of these lipases by a nondialyzable factor in uremic serum,[100] or from a deficiency of apoprotein CII in both HDL and VLDL. The reduction of lipoprotein lipase, which is believed to be more important in the generation of hypertriglyceridemia than hepatic lipase, causes a defect in the catabolism of triglyceride-rich lipoproteins, which in turn leads to the accumulation of VLDL[101] and enrichment of intermediate-density lipoproteins and low-density lipoproteins with triglyceride; it also is associated with the appearance of apoprotein B48, an increased concentration of apoprotein AIV, and the presence in LDL of apoproteins C and E (proteins not normally found in LDL). It has been suggested that these abnormal substances may be atherogenic.[100]

Because HDL turnover is diminished in patients with chronic renal failure compared with controls, a decrease in HDL synthesis probably accounts for low HDL levels.[97] In one study HDL cholesterol was significantly reduced in patients with renal failure on chronic hemodialysis (average = 26 mg/dl) compared with normal people (average = 52 mg/dl).[99] This reduction of HDL was due to a reduced protein content in all its subfractions. Apoprotein electrophoresis showed an increase in "arginine-rich" peptide in the VLDL and the HDL fraction and, as noted, a reduction of apoprotein CII, which is transferred to VLDL from HDL and which functions as an activator of the enzyme lipoprotein lipase.[102]

TREATMENT. The standard dietary therapy of patients with type IV hyperlipoproteinemia in the absence of renal failure consists of weight reduction, limitation of alcohol intake, and a reduction in carbohydrate consumption (p. 1140). In patients with chronic renal failure the lipid abnormality usually is not associated with excessive body weight or alcohol consumption, and a reduction in carbohydrate intake is somewhat difficult to achieve, owing to the limitations imposed on the patient's diet by virtue of the reduced protein intake. A reasonable therapeutic approach is to provide caloric replacement through increases in polyunsaturated fat in the diet.[103] With this diet, a significant reduction in plasma triglyceride levels has been observed, both in conservatively treated patients with chronic renal failure and in patients on dialysis.[104]

If conservative measures are unsuccessful, drug therapy may be necessary. *Clofibrate* normally is metabolized by the kidney, and active metabolites can accumulate in patients with severely compromised renal function[105]; patients with renal failure may develop severe myositis in association with the ingestion of the usual doses of this drug.[106] A reduction in total dosage of clofibrate to 1.5 gm per week may lead to a lowering of plasma triglyceride concentration without producing myositis. However, even with this reduced dosage, an increase in serum creatine kinase levels has been reported, presumably as a consequence of damage to skeletal muscle. The metabolism of *gemfibrozil,* another fibric acid derivative, is not dependent on renal function. Modification of the usual dosage of 600 mg twice daily is *not* necessary in patients with renal failure.[106] Although it may be an effective lipid-lowering agent, experience with gemfibrozil in patients with renal dynsfunction is small. Neither clofibrate nor gemfibrozil is effectively removed by hemodialysis or peritoneal dialysis. The efficacy and safety of *lovastatin,* an HMG-CoA reductase inhibitor, in patients with chronic renal failure is still being evaluated but appears to be promising. Because less than 10 per cent of the drug is excreted into the urine, it is not necessary to adjust the dosage, which should start at 10 mg twice daily and be slowly increased as needed over a period of months up to a dose of 40 mg twice daily.[106] *Nicotinic acid* also may be used in uremic patients but should be introduced slowly to avoid side effects, starting with a low dose of 100 mg three times daily.

HEART FAILURE

Chronic renal failure can impair cardiac performance by a variety of mechanisms (Table 62–2). It has been found that left ventricular stroke work index, end-diastolic pressure, and size are increased in many patients with end-stage renal disease.[107] Left ventricular hypertrophy also is a frequent finding. In addition, an increase in pulmonary capillary permeability tending to lead to pulmonary edema, even in the absence of elevation of pulmonary capillary wedge pressure, has been reported in renal insufficiency.[108] Impairment of cardiac performance also occurs secondary to ischemic heart disease (see above). The possibility must be considered that dialysis results in the depletion of essential substances; water-soluble vitamins are dialyzable, and it has been suggested that their loss can lead to beriberi heart disease.[109] Therefore, it seems desirable to provide appropriate vitamin supplements for patients on maintenance hemodialysis. Long-term dialysis may deplete other, as yet unidentified, substances necessary for normal cardiac performance, but this has not been established.

The possibility that the uremic state depresses myocardial function is intriguing. As early as 1944, Raab suggested that specific myocardial toxins might be present in uremia.[110] Depression of cardiac function in isolated rat heart preparations perfused with urea, creatinine, guanidinosuccinic acid, and methyl-guanidine—singly and in combination—has been reported.[111] Uremia produces serious disturbances in monovalent cation transport. Red blood cells, leukocytes, lung, and bone from patients with renal insufficiency have an elevated sodium content and a reduction in ouabain-sensitive Na-K–activated adenosinetriphosphatase activity.[112] It is possible that the same fundamental abnormality is responsible for the observed reduction in human skeletal muscle transmembrane potential, which returns toward normal with vigorous hemodialysis.

The observation that cardiac function in patients with renal failure improves after parathyroidectomy has led to the suggestion that parathyroid hormone (PTH) may depress myocardial function.[113] PTH itself stimulates myocardial cell cyclic adenosine monophosphate production, which has been shown to impair energy metabolism, increase cell calcium content, and result in myocardial cell death.[114] Furthermore, abnormally increased myocardial calcium content has been found to correlate with depression of left ventricular ejection fraction in dialysis patients.[115] Thus, PTH-enhanced myocardial calcium uptake may result in myocardial dysfunction. However, data on the cardiosuppressive effects of PTH have been conflicting.[116]

IMPAIRMENT OF VENTRICULAR FUNCTION IN UREMIA. Although the presence of *cardiomyopathy* in uremic patients has been suggested, its existence as a specific entity has been difficult to document in view of the many other possible causes of cardiac dysfunction in such patients.[117] One study involving patients not on dialysis has documented abnormal left ventricular function with exercise early in renal disease that was unrelated to the degree of anemia or the presence of an arteriovenous fistula or of hypertension.[118] This suggests that cardiac performance can become abnormal relatively early in renal failure. Other studies have failed to show an abnormal left ventricular response to exercise in end-stage renal disease patients compared with controls.[118a]

In a study of dialysis patients carefully selected for the absence of coronary disease, valvular abnormalities, diabetes, or hypertension, left ventricular dilatation and hypertrophy were both present.[118b] Furthermore, the ratio of left ventricular radius to left ventricular wall thickness was higher in dialysis patients compared with controls. This observation implies an impaired ability of the uremic myocardium to hypertrophy, resulting in a ventricular mass inadequately adapted to chamber size and pressure.

There is suggestive evidence that uremia-induced myocardial dysfunction may be reversible. Hemodialysis has been found to raise the left ventricular ejection fraction, both acutely and chronically,[119,120] the greatest improvement occurring in patients with dilated hearts. Reductions in ventricular dilatation and hypertrophy also have been noted with hemodialysis. Some investigators have concluded that an increase in contractile state accounts for the beneficial effects of hemodialysis on cardiac performance.[119,121] In one study comparing different isovolemic dialysis regimens, an increase in ionized plasma calcium was identified as a key factor in this increased contractility.[119] Others suggest that changes in preload and afterload constitute the dominant mechanism.[110,120] It is likely that a combination of these factors is important, depending on the clinical status of the patient and the type of dialysis procedure performed.[121] Left ventricular function also has been found to improve with peritoneal dialysis.[122]

Chronic anemia is another important factor leading to myocardial dysfunction in dialysis patients. Increases in both left ventricular mass index[123] and left ventricular end-diastolic diameter[124] have been found to correlate with the severity of the anemia. Recent studies with recombinant human erythropoietin in hemodialysis patients have shown decreases in

TABLE 62–2 POSSIBLE CAUSES OF HEART FAILURE IN RENAL INSUFFICIENCY

Cause	Effect
Hypertension	Increased ventricular afterload
Hypervolemia	Increased ventricular preload
Anemia	Increased cardiac work (high-output state)
Lipid abnormalities	Increased atherogenesis
Pericarditis	Restriction of ventricular filling
Ionic alterations Hyperkalemia Hypocalcemia Hypermagnesemia Metabolic acidosis	Negative inotropic effect
Disordered calcium and vitamin D metabolism	(A) Metastatic calcification (cardiac and vascular) (B) ? Vitamin D deficiency cardiomyopathy
Arteriovenous shunt for hemodialysis	Increased cardiac work (high-output state)
Thiamine depletion by dialysis Beriberi (?)	Increased cardiac work (high-output state)
Uremic toxins (?)	Depressed contractility; ? cardiomyopathy

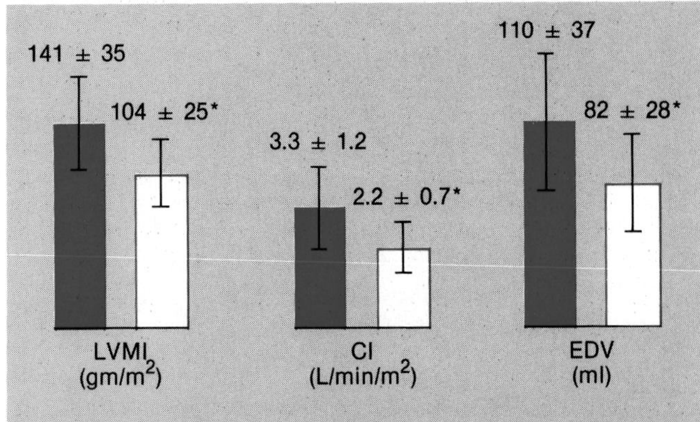

FIGURE 62–9. Echocardiographic changes after kidney transplantation. In 41 patients there were significant decreases in left ventricular mass index (LVMI), cardiac index (CI), and end-diastolic volume (EDV), as measured by echocardiography. Shaded bars = before transplantation; open bars = after transplantation (*p < .05). (From Himmelman, R. B., Landzberg, J. S., Simonson, J. S. et al.: Cardiac consequences of renal transplantation: Changes in left ventricular morphology and function. J. Am. Coll. Cardiol. *12*:915, 1988, by permission of the American College of Cardiology.)

venticular diameters and improved contractility as hematocrit increases.[125,125a] However, no change in ventricular wall thickness was noted in this short-term study; long-term studies need to be performed to assess the full impact of this hormone on the heart.

After kidney transplantation, serial echocardiograms have documented regression of left ventricular hypertrophy.[126,127] Posttransplant decreases in cardiac index and left ventricular end-diastolic volume also have been found, indicating an improvement over the pretransplant hyperdynamic state (Fig. 62–9). In addition to improvements in lipid profile and blood pressure, these hemodynamic changes may contribute to a decreased cardiac mortality in renal transplant patients.[128] Of interest, no improvement in indices of diastolic function has been noted, which may reflect irreversible myocardial calcification or fibrosis in end-stage renal disease. Finally, dialysis patients with dilated nonischemic cardiomyopathy and class III or IV heart failure have shown symptomatic improvement, as well as increases in ejection fraction, after kidney transplantation.[129] Therefore, patients should not necessarily be denied kidney transplantation, if they are otherwise good transplant candidates.

CARDIOVASCULAR COMPLICATIONS OF HEMODIALYSIS

TECHNICAL CONSIDERATIONS

Hemodialysis is designed to accomplish three objectives. It may (1) remove solutes, (2) alter the electrolyte concentration of the extracellular fluid, and (3) remove as much as 1 liter of extracellular fluid per hour. These three processes should be viewed as being essentially independent of one another, and in the course of a single dialysis it often is desirable to carry out only one or two of these three functions.

HYPOTENSION. A significant fall in blood pressure is a common problem in patients undergoing hemodialysis, occurring in 25 to 50 per cent of dialysis procedures. Many interacting factors appear to be responsible (Fig. 62–10). Ultrafiltration of fluid leads to hypovolemia with a concomitant reduction of venous return and cardiac output. Plasma osmolarity, which falls during dialysis, favors water movement out of the extracellular and into the intracellular space.[130] Autonomic dysfunction, which occurs in up to 50 per cent of dialysis patients,[84] prevents normal compensatory cardioacceleration and an increase in vascular tone. The most common defect seems to reside in the afferent limb of the baroreceptor reflex arc.[84,130] High extracorporeal blood volume, a high blood flow rate, and an underestimation of "dry weight" after dialysis also predispose to hypotension. Drugs that lower blood pressure, such as antihypertensives, some antiarrhythmics, narcotic analgesics, and anxiolytic medications, are commonly prescribed to dialysis patients.

Cardiac disorders that may cause or contribute to hypotension during dialysis include arrhythmias, pericardial effusion with tamponade, cardiomyopathy, and myocardial ischemia. Hypoxemia also should be considered (see below). Finally, acetate, a common dialysate base, has been implicated as a vasodilator and myocardial depressant.[131] Because acetate is metabolized to bicarbonate primarily in muscle cells, it appears to be most poorly tolerated by patients with low muscle mass, typically elderly women. Patients with autonomic insufficiency also may be particularly intolerant of acetate.[132]

The incidence of hypotensive episodes can be reduced by identifying and treating the conditions discussed. Simple measures such as decreasing the size of the dialyzer, removing less fluid during the treatment, or withholding antihypertensive medications before dialysis may be effective. A change in dialysate solution also may be useful. A dialysate sodium concentration that exceeds 135 mEq/liter will reduce the fall in plasma osmolarity and has been shown to improve hemodynamic stability.[133,134] Substituting bicarbonate for acetate as the dialysate base also may be helpful.[131] Finally, sequential ultrafiltration followed by isovolemic dialysis can ameliorate the occurrence of hypotension.[135]

ELECTROLYTE SHIFTS. In adjusting electrolyte concentrations, it is important to appreciate that most dialysates contain 1.5 to 3.0 mEq/liter of potassium and 3.0 to 3.5 mEq/liter of calcium (6 to 7 mg/dl of ionized Ca^{++}). Because most patients commence dialysis with somewhat high serum potassium levels, serum potassium may fall precipitously when dialysis begins, whereas the concentration of ionized calcium rises, setting the stage for digitalis intoxication in digitalized patients (p. 490). This complication is even more likely in cases of digoxin excess, which might come about if the dosage has not been adjusted downward to take into consideration the markedly prolonged half-life of this drug in patients with renal failure (p. 489). A close correlation between the rise in ionized serum calcium and improved myocardial performance has been noted (see above).[119]

ARTERIOVENOUS FISTULAS. To achieve vascular access for dialysis, an arteriovenous fistula must be created. These shunts have a flow rate of 250 to 750 ml/minute, and thereby add to the cardiac workload. As discussed on page 459, in association with the anemia characteristic of chronic renal failure, this may contribute to the development of high-output heart failure.[136] This form of heart failure can be readily controlled if any excess fluid accumulation is prevented by ultrafiltration during dialysis and if the anemia is partially treated by transfusion. It is desirable to use only a single vascular access site at any one time and to limit the size of the anastomosis to the smallest required for successful dialysis. The contribution of the fistula to the heart failure state can be determined by studying the effect of occlusion of the fistula on left ventricular function, as assessed by echocardiography or radionuclide ventriculography.

Infection is a major complication of arteriovenous shunts and may become metastatic. Septic pulmonary emboli and infective endocarditis, most often staphylococcal, have been reported.[68] Because patients on hemodialysis often have functional systolic and occasionally even diastolic murmurs, which may change with the patient's altered hemodynamic

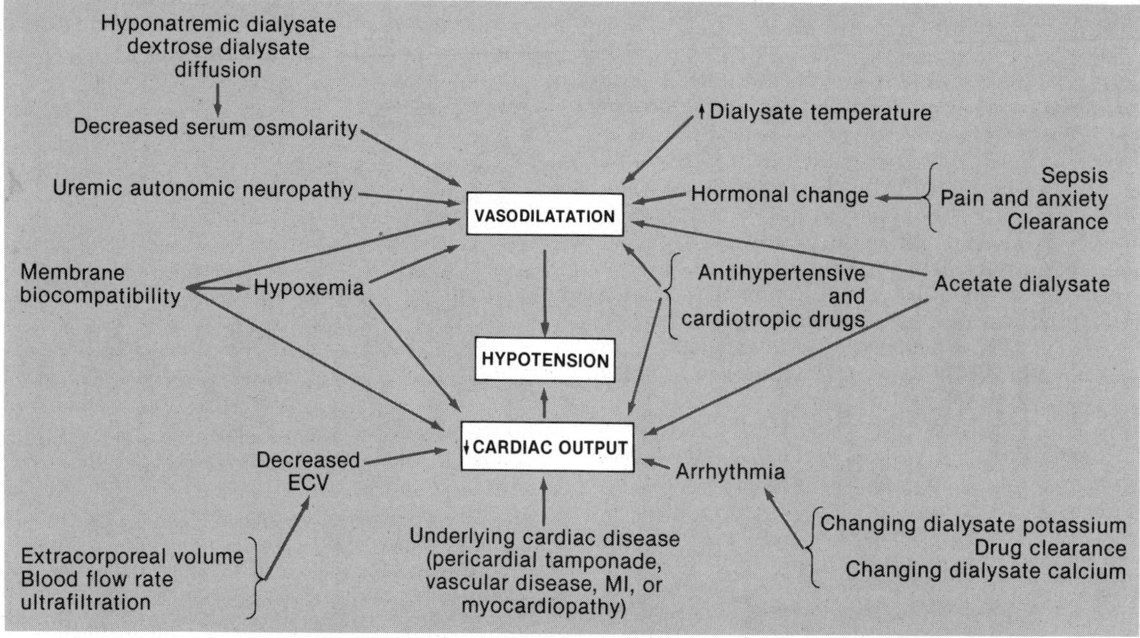

FIGURE 62–10. Major factors leading to dialysis-induced hypotension. (From Hakim, R. M., and Lazarus, J. M.: Medical aspects of hemodialysis. *In* Brenner, B. M., and Rector, F. C. [eds.]: The Kidney. Philadelphia, W. B. Saunders Company, 1986. p. 1820.)

status, the diagnosis of endocarditis may be missed. Therefore, the *early* diagnosis of endocarditis in patients with infected vascular access sites depends on a high index of clinical suspicion and immediate blood cultures. The diagnosis of infective endocarditis may be difficult, since an infected vascular access site without infection of the endocardium can also give rise to positive blood cultures.

HYPOXEMIA. A fall in arterial oxygen tension of 10 to 15 mm Hg frequently occurs within the first 30 minutes of hemodialysis and persists throughout the procedure.[137] This event is undesirable in patients with heart or lung disease, and may lead to serious hypoxemia in patients with even mild arterial desaturation at the commencement of the hemodialysis. Together with the electrolyte changes during hemodialysis referred to above, it may lower the threshold for the development of arrhythmias. Also, the PEP : LVET ratio may increase significantly during dialysis,[138] an increase that correlates significantly with the fall in arterial oxygen tension, suggesting that the latter actually impairs left ventricular function.

The mechanism responsible for the decline in arterial PO_2 during dialysis is in some dispute and is probably multifactorial. It has been reported that activation of complement leads to aggregation of neutrophils in the lungs, which interferes with normal oxygenation.[139] This is particularly observed with cuprophane membranes and not with more biocompatible membranes such as polyacrylonitryl.[140] An additional explanation is that physiological hypoventilation occurs secondary to diffusion of carbon dioxide across the dialyzer. Changing from an acetate- to a bicarbonate-buffered dialysate may prevent this loss of carbon dioxide and lessen the decrease in arterial PO_2.[139]

Of interest, mechanically ventilated patients show a decrease in arterial oxygen tension during dialysis; this indicates that hypoventilation alone cannot account for the observed hypoxemia.[141] Whatever the mechanism, patients with impaired pulmonary function and severe heart disease should be monitored for arterial hypoxemia during the early phase of dialysis and may require inhalation of oxygen during the procedure.

POTASSIUM BALANCE

Life-threatening hyperkalemia may occur in acute oliguric renal failure, in end-stage chronic renal failure, and, rarely, in terminal heart failure (p. 455). The principal detrimental effect of hyperkalemia is in its electrical effect on the heart. The progressive electrocardiographic abnormalities associated with hyperkalemia are shown in Figure 5–51, p. 150. The earliest electrocardiographic sign of hyperkalemia usually is peaking of the T waves, followed progressively by an increase in T-wave amplitude, a widening of the QRS complex, and loss of atrial activity. Finally, with extreme hyperkalemia, a sine wave pattern is noted on the electrocardiogram, followed by cardiac arrest. Unfortunately only a rough correlation exists between the level of serum potassium and the electrocardiographic changes, although in any given patient directional changes in the serum potassium level can be estimated from the electrocardiogram. Even severe hyperkalemia per se produces few, if any, symptoms; occasionally weakness of skeletal muscles or dyspnea presumably secondary to paralysis of respiratory muscles may be noted.

TREATMENT. Severe hyperkalemia is a medical emergency, and its treatment usually can be divided into acute and chronic phases. The most rapid means of counteracting the toxic cardiac effects of potassium is with the administration of intravenous calcium, given in the form of 10 to 20 ml of 10 per cent *calcium chloride* with electrocardiographic monitoring to assure that the signs of hyperkalemia have been reversed. Although administration of calcium chloride is an effective emergency measure, it does not lower the elevated serum potassium concentration.

The second aspect of therapy relies on lowering the serum potassium level. In patients with hyperkalemia and acidosis, *sodium bicarbonate* will reduce the level of serum potassium; the usual dose is 1 to 2 ampules (44 to 88 mEq) administered intravenously. The reduction in $[K^+]$ is caused in part by an exchange of hydrogen and potassium ions across cell membranes as well as enhanced secretion of potassium in the distal tubule. Bicarbonate administration lowers serum $[K^+]$ in hyperkalemic patients even if the serum pH is not affected, implying a specific effect of the bicarbonate anion itself.[142] The administration of 10 units of regular insulin will result in the redistribution of $[K^+]$ from the extracellular to the intracellular space. This should be followed by 50 ml of 50 per cent *glucose* to prevent hypoglycemia. The effects of bicarbonate or glucose and insulin administration can be observed within 15 to 30 minutes and may last for several hours. Although these forms of therapy are useful for rapidly lowering the serum $[K^+]$ concentration, they do *not* lower total body potassium stores.

Further treatment of hyperkalemia involves removal of potassium from the body, which can be accomplished by the administration of *cation exchange resins* by enema or orally. The resin most commonly used is sodium polystyrene sulfonate (Kayexalate), 1 gm of which administered orally exchanges approximately 1 mEq of sodium for potassium. The usual dose is 50 gm two or three times daily. When administered orally, it is desirable to accompany it with an osmotic cathartic to prevent intestinal obstruction as a consequence of inspissation of the resin in the gut.

The most effective means of reducing the body's potassium stores is by means of *dialysis*, either hemodialysis or peritoneal dialysis. However, when using these modalities, one must exercise care not to lower the serum potassium too precipitously, especially in those patients who are receiving cardiac glycosides. This can be accomplished by beginning with a dialysis solution having a potassium concentration of approximately 4 mEq/liter and then progressively lowering it as serum potassium declines.

SECONDARY HYPERPARATHYROIDISM (see also p. 1841)

Ectopic calcification in a variety of tissues, including the heart and arterial bed, is a common manifestation of secondary hyperparathyroidism. This frequent complication of chronic renal failure may involve the sinoatrial and atrioventricular nodes, the intima and media of epicardial coronary arteries, the interventricular septum, the ventricular myocardium, and the valvular annuli and cusps, particularly the mitral annulus and the aortic valve, as shown in Figure 62–11.[143–146] One prospective echocardiographic study identified aortic valve calcification in 28 per cent, and mitral valve calcification in 36 per cent, of 87 maintenance hemodialysis patients.[147] Furthermore, clinically significant valvular stenosis of a tricuspid aortic valve, and less frequently of the mitral valve, may occur. Other clinical and electrocardiographic changes resulting from tissue calcification include varying degrees of atrioventricular block, sinus node dysfunction, supraventricular arrhythmias, infective endocarditis, embolism, mitral regurgitation, and left ventricular failure (see above).[148]

As many as half the patients on maintenance hemodialysis have been reported to have radiological evidence of arterial calcification[149]; calcium deposition usually is in the media, leading to Mönckeberg's sclerosis.[150] Calcium deposition may be associated with almost complete obliteration of the vascu-

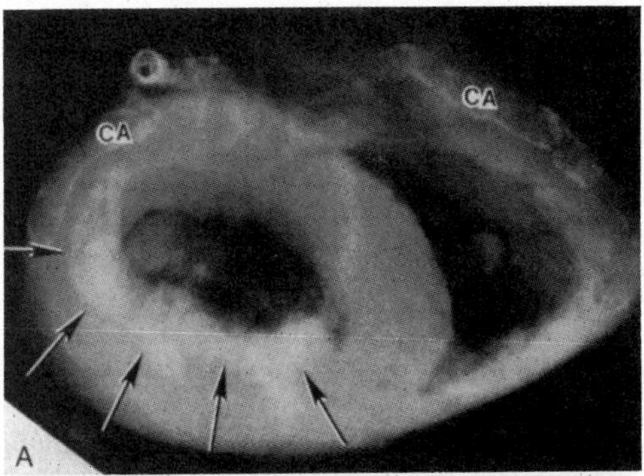

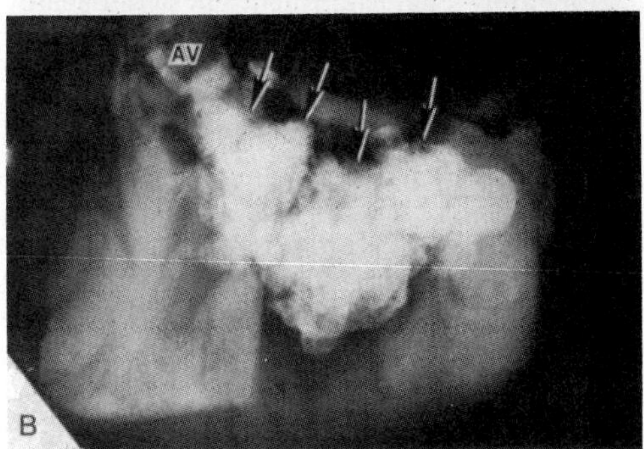

FIGURE 62–11. Postmortem roentgenograms showing severe mitral annular calcification in two patients on hemodialysis. *A*, Superior view of heart showing extensive posterior mitral annular *(arrows)* and coronary arterial (CA) calcification in a patient on dialysis for 14.5 years. *B*, Posteroanterior view of heart revealing extensive calcific deposits in mitral valve apparatus (arrows) and mild calcific deposits in the aortic valve (AV) in a patient on hemodialysis for 7 years. (From Forman, M. B., et al.: Mitral annular calcification in chronic renal failure. Chest *85*:367, 1984.)

lar lumen, and may result in ischemia and, ultimately, gangrene of tissue distal to the involved vessels.[149,150] Case-control studies have shown mitral annular calcification in those dialysis patients with higher ionized calcium, phosphorus, and calcium–phosphorus product levels. These findings suggest that vigorous attempts to normalize calcium–phosphorus metabolism may decrease the incidence of this complication in patients with chronic renal failure.[143,144]

The most effective *treatment* of secondary hyperparathyroidism consists of kidney transplantation or subtotal parathyroidectomy. For patients maintained on dialysis, dietary phospate restriction, calcium supplementation, nonabsorbable aluminum-containing antacids, and oral dihydrotachysterol (a synthentic analog of vitamin D) given in doses of 0.125 to 1.0 mg daily, or 1,25-dihydroxycholecalciferol (1,25$(OH)_2D_3$) in a dose of 0.25 to 1.0 μg daily also are useful measures.[151,152] Intravenous doses of up to 4.0 μg of 1,25$(OH)_2D_3$ after hemodialysis have been shown to markedly suppress PTH levels.[153] Whether this "medical parathyroidectomy" will control secondary hyperparathyroidism over the long term is unknown.

UREMIC PERICARDITIS (see also p. 1496)

Pericarditis is a common complication of both acute and chronic renal failure. Before the era of dialysis the appearance of pericarditis in the uremic patient usually was taken as a sign of terminal renal failure.[154] The incidence of clinically significant pericarditis appears to be declining with the increasing use of early dialysis before progression to advanced uremia. Echocardiography has revealed pericardial effusions in 32 to 56 per cent of patients at the initiation of dialysis, most of which are asymptomatic.[155] The mechanism by which pericarditis and pericardial effusions develop is not clear, but is probably related to the accumulation of uremic toxins, which are responsible for an inflammatory serositis. Volume overload also has been implicated as an important causative factor.[155] The serositis most commonly involves the pericardium but also can involve the pleura.[156] Fibrinous pleuritis, pleural friction rubs,[157] hemorrhagic pleural effusion, and pneumonitis[156] also have been reported to occur in uremia.

A review of published studies reveals that approximately 15 per cent of end-stage renal disease patients develop pericarditis at some time. In renal failure patients, pericarditis carries an average mortality rate of nearly 13 per cent, and in total accounts for about 2.8 per cent of deaths of dialysis patients.[158] Pericarditis that occurs in patients on stable chronic dialysis may be related to inadequate dialysis or to an intercurrent illness, such as a viral infection. In patients with renal failure, pericarditis may be preceded by an otherwise benign respiratory tract infection. Bacterial infection, cytomegalovirus infection, and other conditions such as systemic lupus erythematosus, polyarteritis nodosa, and acute myocardial infarction also have been implicated as causes.[159] In most stable chronic dialysis patients the cause of pericarditis is not certain; the incidence appears to be less in patients on peritoneal dialysis than in those on hemodialysis.

CLINICAL MANIFESTATIONS. The clinical features of uremic pericarditis are summarized in Table 62–3. The diagnosis is made by the same clinical criteria used for other forms of pericarditis, i.e., chest pain usually ameliorated by sitting up and leaning forward, typical echocardiographic changes, increases in heart size on chest roentgenogram, and, with severe pericarditis, evidence of circulatory embarrassment. With echocardiography, small asymptomatic pericardial effusions can be found in approximately one-third of patients on chronic maintenance hemodialysis.[159–161] On electrocardiogram atrial arrhythmias are the most common abnormality, occurring in about 15 per cent of cases. The development of hypotension during dialysis that cannot be readily attributed to changes in intravascular volume is a useful clue to the presence of significant pericardial effusion. A pericardial friction rub is present in almost every patient at some time during the course of pericarditis, and should be diligently looked for. However, the diagnosis of pericarditis may be made in error. Many uremic patients develop a systolic ejection murmur, probably related to the high-output state secondary to chronic anemia. Some patients with chronic renal failure and hypertension develop diastolic blowing murmurs resembling those caused by aortic regurgitation, and the combination of these two murmurs may be mistaken for a to-and-fro pericardial friction rub.

TABLE 62–3 CLINICAL FEATURES OF UREMIC PERICARDITIS

FEATURE	FREQUENCY (%)
Pain	66
Pericardial friction rub	93
Fever	84
Leukocytosis	56
Arrhythmias	23
Hypotension	56
Hepatomegaly	60
Elevated venous pressure	71
Abnormal electrocardiogram	90
Enlarged cardiac silhouette	96

For sources of above data, see Chap. 45.

Cardiac tamponade, described on page 1473, complicates uremic pericarditis in about 20 per cent of patients[162,163]; it is the major serious complication of pericarditis, and can be lethal. Pericardial fluid usually is exudative and bloody; the heparinization required for hemodialysis may cause serious bleeding into the pericardial cavity in patients with pericarditis. Therefore, it is important to limit the degree of heparinization during hemodialysis as much as possible in the presence of active pericarditis and large effusions. However, systemic heparinization can be used safely in patients with small pericardial effusions without associated physical signs and symptoms of active pericarditis. Chronic constrictive pericarditis is an unusual complication of uremic pericarditis, and has been reported to develop in less than 5 per cent of patients.[162]

TREATMENT. A distinction should be made between "uremic pericarditis" in patients who have not previously been dialyzed, or have initiated dialysis within a few weeks of the episode of pericarditis, and "dialysis pericarditis" in patients on a stable peritoneal or hemodialysis regimen. In a literature review, 50 of 65 reported patients with uremic pericarditis responded to dialysis therapy alone, whereas only 8 of 64 patients with dialysis pericarditis responded to dialysis alone.[158] This difference indicates that uremic toxins are more likely to be responsible for pericardial inflammation in previously undialyzed patients.

Dialysis patients with moderate or large effusions are unlikely to improve with dialysis.[159,163] Elective pericardiocentesis has previously been advocated to drain the pericardial space in such patients, and may be accompanied with the instillation of nonabsorbable corticosteroids into the pericardial cavity.[164] In most centers elective pericardiocentesis is associated with an unacceptable mortality rate approaching 10 per cent,[165] and it is successful in only about 25 per cent of cases.[158] In contrast, surgical drainage is a safe and effective method of draining the pericardial space. Placement of a pericardial window of at least 4 × 4 cm, using the subxiphoid approach, appears to be the safest surgical drainage procedure.[166] The choice of operation should depend on the local experience of the thoracic surgeon, and may include thoracotomy with pericardial window or total pericardiectomy, subxiphoid tube drainage, or pericardiectomy by way of median sternotomy.[167] Oral indomethacin has been suggested as an adjunct to the therapy of pericarditis, but a controlled study has failed to show an effect of this drug on the duration of chest pain, pericardial friction rub, the amount of effusion, or the need for surgery.[163]

It is our practice to treat pericarditis in end-stage renal disease patients with vigorous dialysis if the patient is hemodynamically stable. The size of the effusion should be followed by serial two-dimensional echocardiography. If hemodynamic instability develops, the effusion does not decrease in size, or the effusion enlarges over a period of 1 to 2 weeks, then a subxiphoid pericardial window is placed. In patients already on a stable dialysis regimen who have a moderate or large effusion, immediate elective surgical drainage is strongly considered, as the likelihood of responding to intensive dialysis is small. Emergency pericardiocentesis is reserved for patients with cardiac tamponade, and is closely followed by surgical decompression. Pericardial stripping is the treatment of choice in the rare patient with subacute or chronic constrictive pericarditis.[168]

MANAGEMENT OF PATIENTS WITH CARDIAC DISEASE AND RENAL FAILURE

With the greater availability of dialysis facilities and broader criteria for acceptance of patients into treatment programs for end-stage renal disease, this patient population now encompasses people in whom other diseases may be present, including cardiac disease that may require surgical treatment. Because of the high frequency of coronary artery disease among patients with chronic renal failure and the occasional presence of coexisting valvular heart disease, cardiopulmonary bypass often is a consideration. Patients on maintenance hemodialysis can undergo major operations without excess mortality or morbidity, and several series have been published documenting the ability of patients with renal failure to tolerate open heart surgery, both coronary revascularization and valve replacement.[169] Among patients with end-stage renal disease, cardiac operations may be performed with equal success regardless of whether the renal failure has been treated by dialysis or transplantation.

The major problems associated with operation in patients with chronic renal failure include the development of hyperkalemia, fluid overload, and arrhythmias. With the appropriate use of hemodialysis both before and after operation and careful monitoring of the patient's hemodynamic and electrolyte status, the excess risks have been contained. Although many observers think that patients who have severely impaired renal failure but who do not yet require hemodialysis may undergo cardiac surgery without hemodialysis, others dialyze patients who have a glomerular filtration rate less than 20 per cent of normal on several occasions in the days before and after such operations.

The management of patients with hypertrophic obstructive cardiomyopathy (p. 1404) and chronic renal failure presents a unique problem. It is well established that these patients are particularly sensitive to acute changes in blood volume and to tachyarrhythmias. During hemodialysis, blood volume ordinarily is reduced. Although most patients tolerate this volume depletion without difficulty, many of those with hypertrophic cardiomyopathy develop an acute increase in obstruction to left ventricular outflow. This complication can be avoided by using a dialysis apparatus that requires a low extracorporeal volume and allows precise control of ultrafiltration. In addition, these patients are treated with beta-adrenergic receptor blockers or calcium antagonists and are treated with erythropoietin to maintain a hematocrit in the range of 30 per cent.

MODIFICATION OF COMMON CARDIAC MEDICATIONS IN PATIENTS WITH RENAL FAILURE

Because many drugs (and/or their active metabolites) used in the treatment of heart disease are excreted by the kidney, renal failure affects the pharmacokinetics of many agents, including those commonly used to treat heart disease. Information on the pharmacokinetics of important cardiac medications and dosage adjustments in renal failure are listed in Table 62–4.

CARDIAC GLYCOSIDES (see also p. 479). *Digoxin* is filtered by the glomeruli, and its renal excretion is directly proportional to the glomerular filtration rate. It is not altered by the rate of urine flow and therefore by the administration of diuretics[170]; only very small quantities of digoxin may be secreted by the distal convoluted tubule.[171] The ratio of the clearance of digoxin to endogenous creatinine is 0.8, and the percentage of the body's total stores of digoxin lost per day can be calculated as 14 + 0.2 × creatinine clearance in milliliters per minute. Thus 85 per cent of administered digoxin normally is excreted in the urine, most in unchanged form, and only 10 to 15 per cent is eliminated in the stool through biliary excretion. Normally, 38 per cent of the body's stores of digoxin are either metabolized or excreted per day,[172] whereas in anephric patients only 14 per cent of total body digoxin stores are eliminated per day by way of the biliary tree. Therefore, in the patient with impaired renal function, digoxin elimination is reduced to approximately 37 per cent of normal, and digoxin dosage should be modified accordingly.

In patients with end-stage renal disease who require treatment with digoxin, a loading dose of 0.25 mg and maintenance doses of 0.125 mg every other day are recommended. Digoxin levels are determined 1 week later, and depending on the clinical response, the dose is modified, usually upward, to 0.125 mg orally daily. However, in the emergency setting, when rapid digitalization is required, the *loading* dose of digoxin does not need to be reduced. In contrast to digoxin, the half-life of *digitoxin* is not greatly affected by impaired renal function,[173] and therefore dosage does not need to be altered in patients with renal failure. Because of high tissue and protein binding of both digoxin and digitoxin, little removal occurs with either hemodialysis or peritoneal dialysis.[174] Therefore, these methods are ineffective in the treatment of digitalis overdose in which Fab fragments are the treatment of choice in life-threatening cases.[175]

ANTIARRHYTHMIC DRUGS (see also Chap. 23). The dose of *procainamide* (p. 636) must be modified in patients with end-stage renal disease because this drug normally is eliminated by both renal excretion and hepatic metabolism. Procainamide is readily dialyzable.[176]

Quinidine (p. 634) is metabolized by a variety of tissues, including the liver, mostly to hydroxy derivatives; no specific modification of the dose is necessary in patients with impaired renal function. Quinidine prolongs the half-life of digoxin in patients with renal failure. Therefore, a decrease in digoxin dosage may be required when both drugs are administered.[177] Because quinidine is about 80 per cent protein-bound and is widely distributed in tissue, clearance by dialysis would be expected to be quite poor; indeed, clearance by peritoneal dialysis has been found to be less than 10 ml/min.[178]

The half-life of *lidocaine* (p. 639) is about an hour, and its deactivation largely depends on hepatic metabolism; no dosage modification is necessary in patients with renal failure.[179] It is not removed by hemodialysis.

The liver also is the principal site of inactivation of *phenytoin* (p. 641).[180] Because of the diminished protein-binding of the drug in patients with renal failure, the ranges of therapeutic and toxic levels of total drug are lower than those in patients with normal renal function. Alternatively, free levels of the drug can be measured. No alteration in dosage is necessary in chronic renal failure. As is the case for most antiarrhythmic agents, phenytoin is poorly dialyzed.

Propranolol (p. 644) is used extensively in patients with renal failure for its effects on arterial pressure, angina pectoris, and, less commonly, cardiac arrhythmias. Because it is metabolized primarily by the liver, its half-life is not altered by renal failure.[181] It is largely protein-bound (90 per cent) and has a large volume of distribution[182]; therefore, it is not surprising that it is poorly dialyzed. The long-acting beta blockers *atenolol* and *nadolol* are cleared by the kidney, so that toxic levels may accumulate in patients with renal failure if dosage is not adjusted. They may both be removed by hemodialysis.[183]

Mexiletine (p. 640) is an antiarrhythmic agent which is he-

TABLE 62–4 CARDIOVASCULAR DRUG THERAPY IN RENAL DISEASE

	PHARMACOKINETIC PARAMETERS					ADJUSTMENT FOR RENAL FAILURE				
		Half-life					GFR (ml/min)			
DRUG	Elimination and Metabolism	*Normal (hr)*	*ESRD (hr)*	Plasma Protein Binding (%)	Volume of Distribution (liters/kg)	Method	*>50*	*10–50*	*<10*	Removed by Dialysis
Adrenergic modulators and blockers										
Clonidine	Renal	6–23	39–42	20–40	3–6	D	U	U	50–75	No (H)
Guanethidine	Renal (nonrenal)	Biphasic: 48–72 and 96–196[a]	?	0	?	I	24	24	24–36	?
Methyldopa[b]	Renal (hepatic 18%–48%)	Biphasic: 1.4 and 5.8[a]	3–6 and 7–16[a]	<15	0.51	I	6	9–18	12–24	Yes (H, P)
Prazosin	Hepatic (renal)	2–3[c]	?	97	1.2–1.7	D	U	U	U	No (H, P)
Reserpine	Hepatic (GI)	Biphasic: 4.5 and 50–170[a]	87–320	40	?	D	U	U	Avoid	No (H, P)
Angiotensin-converting enzyme inhibitors										
Captopril	Renal (hepatic)	1.9	21–32	25–30	0.7	D	U	U	50	Yes (H)
						I	8–24	24–72	72–108	
Enalapril	Hepatic	24–36	40–60	50–60	?	D	100	75–100	50	Yes (H)
Lisinopril	Renal	12–36	36–48	0–10	1.2–1.4	D	100	75	25–50	Yes (H)
Antiarrhythmic agents[d]										
N-Acetylprocainamide	Renal	6–8	42–70	10	1.5–1.7	I[e]	U	6	12	Yes (H)
						D[e]	U	50	25	
Amiodarone	Hepatic	3–100 Days	U	96	Variable: 1–148	D	U	U	U	No (H)
Bretylium	Renal (non-renal 20%)	6 (PO) 13.6 (IV)	16–32	6	8	D	U	25–50[f]	Avoid[f]	?
Disopyramide	Renal and hepatic	5–8	10–18	5–80	0.8–2.6	I	U	12–24	24–40	No (H)
Encainide	Hepatic	1–3	1–3	71–78	2.7	D	U	50	25	?
Flecainide	Hepatic (renal)	14–20	19–26	50	8–9.5	D	U	U	50–75	No (H)
Lidocaine	Hepatic (renal <20%)	1.2–2.2	1.3–3.0	60–66	1.3–2.2	D	U	U	U	No (H)
Lorcainide	Hepatic	7–13	?	80–85	6–17	D	U	U	U	?
Mexiletine	Hepatic (renal)	8–13	16	75	5.5–6.6	D	U	U	50–75	Yes (H), No (P)
Phenytoin	Hepatic (renal)	24	8	90	0.64	D	U	U	U	No (H)
Procainamide	Renal (hepatic 7%–24%)	2.5–4.9	5.3–5.9	14–23	1.4–2.5	I	4	6–12	8–24	Yes (H)[g]
Quinidine	Hepatic (renal 10%–50%)	5.0–7.2	4–14	70–95	2.0–3.5	I	U	U	U	Yes (H, P)[h]
Tocainide	Hepatic (renal)	11–19	22	10–20	1.6–3.2	D	U	U	50	Yes (H)
Beta blockers										
Acebutolol	Renal (hepatic)	8–9	7	25	1.2	D	U	50[i]	30–50[i]	No (H)
Atenolol	Renal	6–9	15–35	<5	0.7	D	U	50	25[i]	Yes (H),
						I	24	48	96[i]	No (P)
Labetalol	Hepatic	3–8	3–8	50	3–10	D	U	U	U	No (H)
Metoprolol	Hepatic	2.5–4.5	2.5–4.5	12	5–6	D	U	U	U	Yes (H)
Nadolol	Renal	14–24	45	25–30	2	D	U	50	25[i]	Yes (H)
Pindolol	Hepatic (renal)	3–4	3–4	40–57	2	D	U	U	U	?
Propranolol	Hepatic	3.5–6.0	2.3	90–96	3–4	D	U	U	U	No (H)
Sotalol	Renal	5–8	40–50	54	0.7	D	U	30	15–30	Yes (H)
Timolol	Hepatic	3–4	4	10	2–4	D	U	U	U	No (H)
Calcium-channel blockers										
Diltiazem	Hepatic	2–8	2–8	80–86	3–5	D	U	U	U	No (H)
Isradipine	Hepatic	2–5	8.5–14.0	?	1–2	D	U	U	75	?
Nicardipine	Hepatic	1	1	95–98	0.7–0.9	D	U	U	U	No (H)
Nifedipine	Hepatic	4.0–5.5	?	92–98	?	D	U	U	U	No (H)
Nimodipine	Hepatic	1.0–2.8	22	98	0.9–2.3	D	U	U	U	No (H)
Nitrendipine	Hepatic	12	12	98	3–6	D	U	U	U	No (H)
Verapamil	Hepatic	3–7	2.4–4	83–93	3–6	D	U	U	50–75	No (H)
Cardiac glycosides										
Digitoxin	Hepatic (renal)	144–200	210	94	0.6	D	U	U	50–75	No (H, P)
Digoxin	Renal (nonrenal 15%–40%)	36–44	80–120[i]	20–30	5–8	D	U	25–75	10–25	No (H, P)
						I	24	36	48	

TABLE 62-4 CARDIOVASCULAR DRUG THERAPY IN RENAL DISEASE *Continued*

	PHARMACOKINETIC PARAMETERS					ADJUSTMENT FOR RENAL FAILURE				
		Half-life					GFR (ml/min)			
DRUG	**Elimination and Metabolism**	***Normal (hr)***	***ESRD (hr)***	**Plasma Protein Binding (%)**	**Volume of Distribution (liters/kg)**	**Method**	***>50***	***10–50***	***<10***	**Removed by Dialysis**
Vasodilators										
Diazoxide	Renal (hepatic)	17–31	>30	>90	0.2–0.3	D	U	U	U	Yes (H, P)
Hydralazine	Hepatic (nonrenal)	2.0–4.5	7–16	87	0.5–0.9	I	8	8	8–16 (fast) 12–24 (slow)	No (H, P)
Minoxidil	Hepatic	2.8–4.2	U	0	2–3	D	U	U	U	Yes (H)
Sodium nitroprusside	Nonrenal	<10 min	<10 min	0	0.20	D	U	U	U[k]	Yes (H)[k]
Agents used for hyperlipoproteinemia										
Cholestyramine	Not absorbed	—	—	—	—	D	U	U	U	—
Clofibrate	Hepatic (renal)	17	46–110	96	0.14	I[l]	6–12	12–18	24–48	No (H)
Colestipol	Not absorbed	—	—	—	—	D	U	U	U	—
Gemfibrozil	Renal (fecal)	1.5	?	Low	?	D	U	50	25	?
Lovastatin	Hepatic	6–8	?	95	?	D	U	U	U	?
Nicotinic acid	Hepatic (renal)	0.5–1.0	?	?	?	GD	U	50	25	?

From Bennett, W. M.: Drug therapy in renal disease. *In* Rubenstein, E., and Federman, D. D. (eds.): Scientific American Medicine. New York, Scientific American, Inc. 1990.

[a] Biexponential pharmacokinetics. [b] Prolonged hypotension due to retention of active metabolites in severe renal failure. [c] $T_{1/2}$ increased to 6–7 hr in congestive heart failure. $T_{1/2}$ may be prolonged in heart disease, or with reduced hepatic blood flow, or both. [c] In practice, a combination of dose and interval adjustment may be necessary. [d] $T_{1/2}$ may be prolonged in heart disease, or with reduced hepatic blood flow, or both. [e] In practice, a combination of dose and interval adjustment may be necessary. [f] No specific data in ESRD. [g] May be able to treat poisoning with hemodialysis. [h] Hemodialysis with low potassium bath may be effective for poisoning. [i] Drug or active metabolite with long $T_{1/2}$ accumulates in ESRD. [j] Volume of distribution and total body clearance decreased in ESRD. [k] Need to monitor thiocyanate levels to keep <10 mg/dL; $t_{1/2}$ for thiocyanate is 1 wk; thiocyanate dialyzable. [l] Daily dose should not exceed 0.5 gm for each gram/dl of serum albumin.

$T_{1/2}$ = biological half-life; ESRD = end-stage renal disease; GFR = glomerular filtration rate; I = Interval extension method of dosage adjustment in hours between maintenance doses; D = dose reduction method of dosage adjustment in per cent of usual maintenance dose; H = hemodialysis; P = peritoneal dialysis; U = unchanged.

patically excreted and does not need dose adjustment with renal failure.[184] It is not removed by peritoneal dialysis, but studies of its removal by hemodialysis have been conflicting. Metabolites of *encainide* (p. 642) are more active than encainide itself and are renally excreted.[185] Thus marked dose reductions of this drug are required and 7 days allowed to pass before steady-state levels are achieved in renal failure patients.[186] *Amiodarone* (p. 646) does not require dosage adjustments in patients with renal disease and is not removed by hemodialysis.[184]

OTHER CARDIOVASCULAR DRUGS. The nitrates and the calcium channel antagonists diltiazem, nifedipine, and verapamil are metabolized by the liver, so that no specific dosage reduction is required in end-stage renal disease.[183]

Acknowledgment

The assistance of Dr. T. Dwight McKinney in the preparation of this chapter is gratefully acknowledged.

REFERENCES

EFFECTS OF CARDIAC DISEASE ON RENAL FUNCTION

1. Birkenfeld, L. W., Liebman, J., O'Meara, M. P., and Edelman, I. S.: Total exchangeable sodium, total exchangeable potassium, and total body water in edematous patients with cirrhosis of the liver and congestive heart failure. J. Clin. Invest. *37:*687, 1958.
2. Ichikawa, I., Pfeffer, J. M., Pfeffer, J. A., et al.: Role of angiotensin II in the altered renal function in congestive heart failure. Circ. Res. *55:*669, 1984.
3. Skorecki, K. L., and Brenner, B. M.: Body fluid homeostasis in congestive heart failure and cirrhosis with ascites. Am. J. Med. *72:*323, 1982.
4. Hostetter, T. H., Pfeffer, J. M., Pfeffer, M. A., Braunwald, E., and Brenner, B. M.: Cardiorenal hemodynamics and sodium excretion in rats with myocardial infarction. Am. J. Physiol. *245:*H98, 1983.
5. Francis, G. S.: Neurohumoral mechanisms involved in congestive heart failure. Am. J. Cardiol. *55:*15A, 1985.
6. Higgins, C. B., Vatner, S. F., Franklin, D., and Braunwald, E.: Effects of experimentally produced heart failure on the peripheral vascular response to severe exercise in conscious dogs. Circ. Res. *31:*186, 1972.
7. Cannon, P. J.: Prostaglandins in congestive heart failure and the effects of nonsteroidal anti-inflammatory drugs. Am. J. Med. *81*(Suppl. 2B):123, 1986.
8. DiPerri, T., Forconi, S., Puccetti, F., et al.: Effects of prostaglandin A_1 on renal handling of salt and water in congestive heart failure. J. Cardiovasc. Pharmacol. *2:*215, 1980.
9. Raymond, K. H., and Lifschitz, M. D.: Effects of prostaglandins on renal salt and water excretion. Am. J. Med. *80*(Suppl. 1A):22, 1986.
10. Berliner, R. W., and Davidson, P. G.: Production of hypertonic urine in the absence of pituitary antidiuretic hormone. J. Clin. Invest. *36:*1416, 1957.
11. Schrier, R. W.: Pathogenesis of sodium and water retention in high-output and low-output cardiac failure, nephrotic syndrome, cirrhosis, and pregnancy. N. Engl. J. Med. *319:*1065, 1988.
12. Ishikawa, S., Saito, T., Okada, K., et al.: Effect of vasopressin antagonist on water excretion in inferior vena cava constriction. Kidney Int. *30:*49, 1986.
13. Bichet, D. G., Korta, S. C., Mettauer, B., et al.: Modulation of plasma and platelet vasopressin by cardiac function in patients with heart failure. Kidney Int. *29:*1188, 1986.
14. Hakumeki, M. O., Wang, B. C., Sundet, W. D., et al.: Aortic baroreceptor discharge during nonhypotensive hemorrhage in anesthetized dogs. Am. J. Physiol. *249:*H393, 1985.
15. Fitzsimmons, J. T.: Thirst, Physiol. Rev. *52:*468, 1972.
16. Badr, K. F., and Ichikawa, I. I.: Pre-renal failure: A deleterious shift from renal compensation to decompensation. N. Engl. J. Med. *319:*623, 1988.
17. Cogan, M. G.: Atrial natriuretic peptide. Kidney Int. *37:*1148, 1990.
18. Smith, H. W.: Salt and water volume receptors: An exercise in physiologic apologetics. Am. J. Med. *23:*623, 1957.
19. Fried, T.: Atrial natriuretic factor: A historic perspective. Am. J. Med. Sci. *294:*134, 1987.
20. Jamieson, J. D., and Palade, G. E.: Specific granules in atrial muscle. J. Cell. Biol. *23:*151, 1964.
21. DeBold, A. J.: Heart atria granularity: Effects of changes in water-electrolyte balance. Proc. Soc. Exp. Biol. Med. *161:*508, 1979.
22. DeBold, A. J., Borenstein, H. B., Veress, A. T., and Sonnenberg, H.: A rapid and potent natriuretic response to intravenous injection of atrial myocardial extract in rats. Life Sci. *28:*89, 1981.
23. Genest, J., and Cantin, M.: Atrial natriuretic factor. Circulation *75*(Suppl. I):118, 1987.
24. Oikawa, S., Imai, M., Ueno, A., et al.: Cloning and sequence analysis of cDNA encoding a precursor for human atrial natriuretic polypeptide. Nature *309:*724, 1984.

25. Baxter, J. D., Lewieki, J. A., and Gardner, D. G.: Atrial natriuretic peptide. Bio/technology *6*:529, 1988.
26. Saito, Y., Nakao, R. K., Arai, H., et al.: Augmented expression of atrial natriuretic polypeptide gene in ventricle of failing human heart. J. Clin. Invest. *83*:298, 1989.
27. Greenwald, J. E., Apkon, M., Hruska, K. A., et al.: Stretch-induced atriopeptin secretion in the isolated rat myocyte and its negative modulation by calcium. J. Clin. Invest. *83*:1061, 1989.
28. Dietz, J. R.: Release of natriuretic factor from rat heart-lung preparations by atrial distention. Am. J. Physiol. *247*:R1093, 1984.
29. Goetz, K. L., Wang, B. C., Geer, P. G., et al.: Atrial stretch increases sodium excretion independently of release of atrial peptides. Am. J. Physiol. *250*:R946, 1986.
30. Shenker, Y., Sider, R. S., Ostafin, E. A., and Grekin, R. J.: Plasma levels of immunoreactive atrial natriuretic factor in healthy subjects and in patients with edema. J. Clin. Invest. *76*:1684, 1984.
31. Yamaji, T., Ishibashi, M., and Takaku, F.: Atrial natriuretic factor in human blood. J. Clin. Invest. *76*:1705, 1985.
32. Brenner, B. M., Ballerman, B. J., Gunning, M. E., and Zeidel, M. L.: Diverse biological actions of atrial natriuretic peptide. Physiol. Rev. *70*:655, 1990.
33. Kimura, T., Abe, K., Ota, K., et al.: Effects of acute water load, hypertonic saline infusion, and furosemide administration on atrial natriuretic peptide and vasopressin release in humans. J. Clin. Endocrinol. Metab. *62*:1003, 1986.
34. Tikkanen, I., Fyhrquist, F., Metsarinne, K., and Leidenius, R.: Plasma atrial natriuretic peptide in cardiac disease and during infusion in healthy volunteers. Lancet *2*:66, 1985.
35. Raine, A.E.G., Enre, P., Burgisser, E., et al.: Atrial natriuretic peptide and atrial pressure in patients with congestive heart failure. N. Engl. J. Med. *315*:533, 1986.
36. Nicholls, M. G., and Richards, A. M.: Human studies with atrial natriuretic factor. Endocrinol. Metab. Clin. North Am. *16*:199, 1987.
37. Genest, J., Larochelle, P., Cusson, J. R., et al.: The atrial natriuretic factor in hypertension. Hypertension *11*(Suppl. I):13, 1988.
38. Yamaji, T., Ismibasi, M., Nakaoka, H., et al.: Possible role for atrial natriuretic peptide in polyuria associated with paroxysmal atrial arrhythmias. Lancet *1*:1211, 1985.
39. Espiner, E. A., Crozier, I. G., Nicholls, M. G., et al.: Cardiac secretion of atrial natriuretic peptide. Lancet *2*:398, 1985.
40. Hu, J. R., Bethinger, U. G., and Lang, R. E.: Endothelin stimulates atrial natriuretic peptide (ANP) release from rat atria. Eur. J. Pharmacol. *158*:177, 1988.
41. Manning, P. T., Schwartz, D., Katsube, N. C., et al.: Vasopressin-stimulated release of atriopeptin: Endocrine antagonists in fluid homeostasis. Science *229*:395, 1985.
42. Napier, M. A., Vandlen, R. L., Albers-Schonberg, G., et al.: Specific membrane receptors for atrial natriuretic factor in renal and vascular tissue. Proc. Natl. Acad. Sci. USA *81*:5946, 1984.
43. Hirata, Y., Tomita, M., Yoshimi, H., and Ikeda, M.: Specific receptors for atrial natriuretic factor (ANF) in cultured vascular smooth muscle cells of rat aorta. Biochem. Biophys. Res. Commun. *125*:562, 1984.
44. DeLean, A., Gutkowska, J., NcNicoll, N., et al.: Characterization of specific receptors for atrial natriuretic factor in bovine adrenal zona glomerulosa. Life Sci *35*:2311, 1984.
45. Quirion, R., Dalpe, M., DeLean, A., et al.: Atrial natriuretic factor (ANF) binding sites in brain and related structures. Peptides *5*:1167, 1984.
46. Fuller, F., Porter, J. G., Arfsien, A. E., et al.: Atrial natriuretic clearance receptor: Complete sequence and functional expression of cDNA clones. J. Biol. Chem. *236H*:9395, 1988.
47. Schulz, S., Chinkers, M., and Garbers, D. L.: The guanylate cyclase/receptor family of proteins. FASEB J. *3*:2026, 1989.
48. Cogan, M. G.: Renal effects of atrial natriuretic factor. Annu. Rev. Physiol. *52*:699, 1990.
49. Light, D. B., Schwiebert, E. M., Karlson, K. H., et al.: Atrial natriuretic peptide inhibits a cation channel in renal inner medullary collecting duct cells. Science *243*:383, 1989.
50. Ballermann, B. J., and Brenner, B. M.: Role of atrial peptides in body fluid homeostasis. Circ. Res. *58*:619, 1986.
51. Weidmann, P., Hasler, L., Gnadinger, M. P., et al.: Blood levels and renal effects of atrial natriuretic peptides in normal man. J. Clin. Invest. *77*:734, 1986.
52. Dunn, B. R., Ichikawa, I., Pfeffer, J. M., et al.: Renal and systemic hemodynamic effects of synthetic atrial natriuretic peptide in the anesthetized rat. Circ. Res. *59*:237, 1986.
53. Huang, C. L., and Cogan, M. G.: Atrial natriuretic factor inhibits maximal tubuloglomerular feedback response. Am. J. Physiol. *252*:F825, 1987.
54. Pollock, D. M., and Arendshorst, W. J.: Effect of atrial natriuretic factor on renal hemodynamics in the rat. Am. J. Physiol. *251*:F795, 1986.
55. Seymore, A. A., Smith, S. G. III, and Mazack, E. K.: Effects of renal perfusion pressure on natriuresis induced by atrial natriuretic factor. Am. J. Physiol. *253*:F234, 1987.
56. Henrich, W. L., McAllister, E. A., Smith, P. B., et al.: Guanosine 3′,5′ cyclic monophosphate as a mediator of inhibition of renin release. Am. J. Physiol. *255*:F474, 1988.
57. Laragh, J. H.: Atrial natriuretic hormone, the renin-aldosterone axis, and blood pressure-electrolyte homeostasis. N. Engl. J. Med. *313*:1330, 1985.
58. Kleinert, H. D., Maack, T., Atlas, S. A., et al.: Atrial natriuretic factor inhibits angiotensin-, norepinephrine-, and potassium-induced vascular contractility. Hypertension *6*(Suppl. 1):1143, 1984.
59. Bolli, P., Muller, F. B., Linder, L., et al.: The vasodilator potency of atrial natriuretic peptide in man. Circulation *75*:221, 1987.
59a. Chu, A., Morris, K. G., Kuehl, W. D., et al.: Effects of atrial natriuretic peptide on the coronary arterial vasculature in humans. Circulation *80*:1627, 1989.
60. Lappe, R. W., Smits, J.F.M., Todt, J. A., et al.: Failure of atriopeptin II to cause arterial vasodilation in the conscious rat. Circ. Res. *56*:606, 1985.
61. Smith, S., Anderson, S., Ballermann, B. J., and Brenner, B. M.: Role of atrial natriuretic peptide in the adaption of sodium excretion with reduced renal mass. J. Clin. Invest. *77*:1395, 1986.
62. Ballermann, B. J., Bloch, K. D., Seidman, J. G., and Brenner, B. M.: Atrial natriuretic peptide transcription, secretion, and glomerular receptor activity during mineralocorticoid escape in the rat. J. Clin. Invest. *78*:840, 1986.
63. Saper, C. B., Standaert, D. B., Currie, M. G., et al.: Atriopeptin-immunoreactive neurons in the brain: Presence in cardiovascular regulatory areas. Science *227*:1047, 1985.
64. Jacobowitz, D. M., Skofitsch, G., Keiser, H. R., et al.: Evidence for the existence of atrial natriuretic factor-containing neurons in the rat brain. Neuroendocrinology *40*:92, 1985.
65. Baehr, G., and Laude, H.: Glomerulonephritis as a complication of subacute streptococcus endocarditis. JAMA *75*:789, 1920.
66. Neugarten, J., and Baldwin, D. S.: Glomerulonephritis in bacterial endocarditis. Am. J. Med. *77*:297, 1984.
67. Bayer, A. S., Theofilopoulos, A. N., Tillman, D. B., et al.: Use of circulating immune complex levels in the serodifferentiation of endocarditis and nonendocarditic septicemias. Am. J. Med. *66*:58, 1979.
68. Keane, W. F., and Maddy, M. F.: Host defenses and infectious complications in maintenance hemodialysis patients. *In* Maher, J. F. (ed.): Replacement of Renal Function by Dialysis. 3rd ed. Dordrect, Kluwer, 1989.
69. Colt, H. G., Begg, R. J., Saporito, J. J., et al.: Cholesterol emboli after cardiac catheterization. Medicine (Baltimore) *67*:389, 1988.

EFFECTS OF RENAL DISEASE ON THE CARDIOVASCULAR SYSTEM

70. Rostand, S. G., and Rutsky, E. A.: Ischemic heart disease in chronic renal failure: Management considerations. Semin. Dialysis *2*:98, 1989.
71. Hahn, R., Oette, K., Mondorf, H., et al.: Analysis of cardiovascular risk factors in chronic hemodialysis patients with special attention to the hyperlipoproteinemias. Atherosclerosis *48*:279, 1983.
72. Vincenti, F., Amand, W. J., Abele, J., et al.: The role of hypertension in hemodialysis-associated atherosclerosis. Am. J. Med. *68*:363, 1980.
73. Hopkins, P. N., and Williams, R. R.: A survey of 246 suggested coronary risk factors. Atherosclerosis *40*:1, 1981.
74. Rostand, S. G., Kirk, K. A., and Rutsky, E. A.: Dialysis-associated ischemic heart disease: Insights from coronary angiography. Kidney Int. *25*:653, 1984.
75. Sreepada Rao, T. K., Roxe, D. M., Laird, N. M., and Santiago, G. C.: Hemodynamic and cardiac correlates of different hemodialysis regimens: The National Cooperative Dialysis Study. Kidney Int. *23*(Suppl. 13):S-89, 1983.
76. Deutsch, E., Bernstein, R. C., Addonizion, V. P., et al.: Coronary artery bypass surgery in patients on chronic hemodialysis, a case-control study. Ann. Intern. Med. *110*:369, 1989.
76a. Kahn, J. K., Rutherford, B. D., McConahay, D. R., et al.: Short- and long-term outcome of percutaneous transluminal coronary angioplasty in chronic dialysis patients. Am. Heart J. *119*:484, 1990.
77. Nonast-Daniel, B., Creutzig, A., Kuhn, K., et al.: Effect of treatment with recombinant erythropoietin on peripheral hemodynamics and oxygenation. Contrib. Nephrol. *66*:185, 1988.
78. Eschbach, J. W., Haley, N. R., and Adamson, J. W.: New insights into the treatment of anemia of chronic renal failure with erythropoietin. Semin. Dialysis *3*:112, 1990.
79. Heyka, R. J., and Vidt, D. G.: Control of hypertension in patients with chronic renal failure. Cleve. Clin. J. Med. *56*:65, 1989.
80. Dustan, H. P., and Page, I. H.: Some factors in renal and renoprival hypertension. J. Lab. Clin. Med. *64*:948, 1964.
81. Wilkinson, R., Scott, D. F., Uldall, P. R., et al.: Plasma renin and exchangeable sodium in the hypertension of chronic renal failure. The effect of bilateral nephrectomy. Q. J. Med. *39*:377, 1970.
82. Cangiano, J. L., Ramirez-Muxo, O., Ramirez-Gonzalez, R., et al.: Normal renin uremic hypertension. Arch. Intern. Med. *136*:17, 1976.
83. Dzau, V.: Significance of the vascular renin-angiotensin pathway. Hypertension *8*:553, 1986.
84. Nakashima, Y., Fouad, F. M., Nakamoto, S., et al.: Localization of autonomic nervous system dysfunction in dialysis patients. Am. J. Nephrol. *7*:375, 1987.
85. Cinotti, G. A., Mene, P., and Pugliese, F.: Prostaglandins in experimental hypertension. Contrib. Nephrol. *54*:9, 1987.
86. Isles, C. G., McLay, A., and Jones, J. M.: Recovery in malignant hypertension presenting as acute renal failure. Q. J. Med. *53*:439, 1984.
87. Huysmans, F. T., Hoitsma, A. J., and Koene, R. A.: Factors determining the prevalence of hypertension after renal transplantation. Nephrol. Dial. Transplant. *2*:34, 1987.
88. Tilney, N. L., Rocha, A., Strom, T. B., and Kirkman, R. L.: Renal artery stenosis in transplant patients. Ann. Surg. *199*:454, 1984.
89. Curtis, J. J., Luke, R. G., Jones, P., et al.: Hypertension in cyclosporine-treated renal transplant recipients is sodium dependent. Am. J. Med. *85*:134, 1988.
90. Curtis, J. J., Luke, R. G., Whelchel, J. D., et al.: Inhibition of angiotensin-converting enzyme in renal-transplant recipients with hypertension. N. Engl. J. Med. *308*:377, 1983.

91. Steinmuller, D. R.: Refractory hypertension post renal transplantation. Cleve. Clin. J. Med. 56:377, 1989.
92. Chapman, J. R., Marcen, R., Arias, M., et al.: Hypertension after renal transplantation: A comparison of cyclosporine and conventional immunosuppression. Transplantation 43:860, 1987.
93. Kasiske, B. L., and Uman, A. J.: Persistent hyperlipidemia in renal transplant patients. Medicine (Baltimore) 66:309, 1987.
94. Markel, M. S., and Friedman, E. A.: Hyperlipidemia after organ transplantation. Am. J. Med. 87(Suppl. 5N):5N, 1989.
95. Markell, S. S., Brown, C. D., Butt, K.M.H., et al.: Prospective evaluation of changes in lipid profiles in cyclosporine-treated renal transplant patients. Transplant. Proc. 21:1497, 1989.
96. Maschio, G., Oldrizzi, L., Rugiu, C., et al.: Serum lipids in patients with chronic renal failure on long-term, protein-restricted diets. Am. J. Med. 87(Suppl. 5N):5, 1989.
96a. Appel, G. Lipid abnormalities in renal disease. Kidney Int. 39:169, 1991.
97. Fuh, M.M.T., Lee, C-M., Jeng, C-Y., et al.: Effect of chronic renal failure on high-density lipoprotein kinetics. Kidney Int. 37:1295, 1990.
98. Chan, M. K., Varghese, Z., Persaud, J. W., et al.: Hyperlipidemia in patients on maintenance hemo- and peritoneal dialysis: The relative pathogenetic roles of triglyceride production and triglyceride removal. Clin. Nephrol. 17:183, 1982.
99. Rapoport, J., Aviram, M., Chaimovitz, C., and Brook, J. G.: Defective high density lipoprotein composition in patients on chronic hemodialysis. N. Engl. J. Med. 299:1326, 1978.
100. Nestel, P. J., Fidge, N. H., and Tan, M. H.: Increased lipoprotein-remnant formation in chronic renal failure. N. Engl. J. Med. 307:329, 1982.
101. Drueke, T., Lacour, B., Roullet, J. B., and Funcke-Brentano, J. L.: Recent advances in factors that alter lipid metabolism in chronic renal failure. Kidney Int. 24(Suppl. 16):S-134, 1983.
102. Grutzmacher, P., Marz, W., Peschke, B., et al.: Lipoproteins and apolipoproteins during progression of chronic renal disease. Nephron 50:103,1988.
103. Uraemia, lipoproteins and atherosclerosis. Lancet 2:1151, 1981.
104. Sanfelippo, M. L., Swensen, R. S., and Reaven, G. M.: Reduction of plasma triglycerides by diet in subjects with chronic renal failure. Kidney Int. 11:54, 1977.
105. Merk, W., Graben, N., Hartmann, H., et al.: Serum levels of free nonprotein bound clofibrinic acid after single dosing to patients with impaired renal function of various degrees—a multicenter study. Int. J. Clin. Pharmacol. Ther. Toxicol. 25:59, 1987.
106. Guba, E. A., Abel, S. R., and Golper, T. A.: Practical guidelines for drug therapy in dialysis: Lipid lowering agents. Semin. Dialysis 2:186, 1989.
107. Lai, K. N., Barnden, L., and Mathew, T. H.: Effect of renal transplantation on left ventricular function in hemodialysis patients. Clin. Nephrol. 18:74, 1982.
108. Crosbie, W. A., Snowden, S., and Parsons, V.: Changes in lung capillary permeability in renal failure. Br. Med. J. 4:388, 1972.
109. Gotloib, L., and Servadio, C.: A possible case of beriberi heart failure in a chronic hemodialysis patient. Nephron 14:293, 1975.
110. Raab, W.: Cardiotoxic substances in the blood and heart muscle in uremia. J. Lab. Clin. Med. 29:715, 1944.
111. Scheuer, J., and Stezoski, S. W.: The effects of uremic components on cardiac function and metabolism. J. Mol. Cell. Cardiol. 5:287, 1973.
112. Patrick, J., and Jones, N. F.: Cell sodium, potassium and water in uremia and the effects of regular dialysis as studies in the leukocyte. Clin. Sci. Mol. Med. 46:583, 1974.
113. Drüeke, T., Fleury, J., Toure, Y., et al.: Effect of parathyroidectomy on left ventricular function in haemodialysis patients. Lancet 1:112, 1980.
114. Baczynski, R. F., Massry, S. G., Kohan, R., et al.: Effect of parathyroid hormone on myocardial energy metabolism in the rat. Kidney Int. 27:718, 1985.
115. Rostand, S. G. Sanders, C., Kirk, K. A., et al.: Myocardial calcification and cardiac dysfunction in chronic renal failure. Am. J. Med. 85:651, 1988.
116. Gafter, U., Battler, A., Eldar, M., et al.: Effect of hyperparathyroidism on cardiac function in patients with end stage renal disease. Nephron 41:30, 1985.
117. London, G. M., Guerin, A. P., Marchais, S. J., et al.: Cardiomyopathy in end-stage renal disease. Semin. Dialysis 2:102, 1989.
118. Pehrsson, S. K., Jonasson, R., and Lins, L. E.: Cardiac performance in various stages of renal failure. Br. Heart J. 52:667, 1984.
118a. Blake, J. W., Solangi, K. B., Herman, M. V., et al.: Left ventricular response to exercise and autonomic control mechanisms in end-stage renal disease. Arch. Intern. Med. 149:433, 1989.
118b. London, G. M., Fabiani, F., Marchais, S. J., et al.: Uremic cardiomyopathy: An inadequate left ventricular hypertrophy. Kidney Int. 31:973, 1987.
119. Henrich, W. L., Hunt, J. M., and Nixon, J. V.: Increased ionized calcium and left ventricular contractility during hemodialysis. N. Engl. J. Med. 310:19, 1984.
120. Blaustein, A. S., Schmitt, G., Foster, M. C., et al.: Serial effects on left ventricular load and contractility during hemodialysis in patients with concentric hypertrophy. Am. Heart J. 111:340, 1986.
121. Nixon, J. V., Mitchell, J. H., McPhaul, J. J., Jr., and Henrich, W. L.: Effect of hemodialysis on left ventricular function. Dissociation of changes in filling volume and in contractile state. J. Clin. Invest. 71:377, 1983.
122. Leenen, F. H., Smith, D. L., Khanna, R., and Oreopoulos, D. G.: Changes in left ventricular hypertrophy and function in hypertensive patients started on continuous ambulatory peritoneal dialysis. Am. Heart J. 110:102, 1985.
123. Silverberg, J. S., Tahal, D. P., Patton, R., et al.: Role of anemia in the pathogenesis of left ventricular hypertrophy in end-stage renal disease. Am. J. Cardiol. 64:222, 1989.
124. London, G., de Vernejoul, M., Fabiani, F., et al.: Secondary hyperparathyroidism and cardiac hypertrophy in haemodialysis patients. Kidney Int. 32:900, 1987.
125. Low, I., Grutzmacher, P., Bergmann, M., et al.: Echocardiographic findings in patients on maintenance hemodialysis substituted with recombinant human erythropoietin. Clin. Nephrol. 31:26, 1989.
125a. Cannella, G., La Canna, G., Sandrini, M., et al.: Renormalization of cardiac output and of left ventricular size following long-term recombinant human erythropoietin treatment of anemic dialyzed uremic patients. Clin. Nephrol. 34:272, 1990.
126. Himmelman, R. B., Landzberg, J. S., and Simonson, J. S., et al.: Cardiac consequences of renal transplantation: Changes in left ventricular morphology and function. J. Am. Coll. Cardiol. 12:915, 1988.
127. Cueto-Garcia, L., Herrera, J., Arriaga, J., et al.: Echocardiographic changes after successful renal transplantation in young nondiabetic patients. Chest 83:56, 1983.
128. Washer, G. F., Schroter, G.P.J., Starzl, T. E., et al.: Causes of death after kidney transplantation. JAMA 250:49, 1983.
129. Burt, R. K., Gupta-Burt, S., Wadi, W. N., et al.: Reversal of left ventricular dysfunction after renal transplantation. Ann. Intern. Med. 111:635, 1989.
130. Henrich, W. L.: Hemodynamic instability during hemodialysis. Kidney Int. 30:605, 1986.
131. Diamond, S. M., and Henrich, W. L.: Acetate dialysate versus bicarbonate dialysate: A continuing controversy. Am. J. Kidney Dis. 9:3, 1987.
132. Velez, R. L., Woodward, T. D., and Heinrich, W. L.: Acetate and bicarbonate hemodialysis in patients with and without autonomic dysfunction. Kidney Int. 26:59, 1984.
133. Van Stone, J. C., Bauer, J., and Carey, J.: The effects of dialysate sodium concentration on body fluid distribution during hemodialysis. Trans. Am. Soc. Artif. Intern. Organs 26:383, 1980.
134. Henrich, W. L., Woodard, T. D., and McPhaul, J. J., Jr.: The chronic efficacy and safety of high sodium dialysate: Double-blind, crossover study. Am. J. Kidney Dis. 2:349, 1982.
135. Rouby, J. J., Rottembourg, J., Durande, J. P., et al.: Hemodynamic changes induced by regular hemodialysis and sequential ultrafiltration hemodialysis: A comparative study. Kidney Int. 17:801, 1980.
136. Arduson, C. B., Codd, J. R., Graff, R. A., et al.: Cardiac failure in upper extremity arteriovenous dialysis fistulae. Arch. Intern. Med. 136:292, 1976.
137. Aurigemma, N. M., Feldman, N. T., Gottlieb, M. N., et al.: Arterial oxygenation during hemodialysis. N. Engl. J. Med. 297:871, 1977.
138. Thayssen, P., Anderson, K. H., and Pindborg, T.: Noninvasive monitoring of cardiac function during haemodialysis. Scand. J. Urol. Nephrol. 15:313, 1981.
139. Cardoso, M., Vinay, P., Vinet, B., et al.: Hypoxemia during hemodialysis: A critical review of the facts. Am. J. Kidney Dis. 11:281, 1988.
140. Wiegmann, T. B., MacDougall, M. L., and Diederich, D. A.: Dialysis leukopenia, hypoxemia, and anaphylatoxin formation: Effect of membrane, bath, and citrate anticoagulation. Am. J. Kidney Dis. 11:418, 1988.
141. Jones, R. H., Broadfield, J. B., and Parsons, V.: Arterial hypoxemia during hemodialysis for acute renal failure in mechanically ventilated patients: Observations and mechanisms. Clin. Nephrol. 14:18, 1980.
142. Fraley, D. S., and Adler, S.: Correction of hyperkalemia by bicarbonate despite constant blood pH. Kidney Int. 12:354, 1977.
143. D'Cruz, I. A., Jain, M., Fishman, S., et al.: Calcification of the mitral region in patients with chronic renal failure: 2-D echocardiographic, hormonal and autopsy correlation. J. Am. Coll. Cardiol. 1:625, 1983.
144. Nestico, P. F., DePace, N. L., Kotler, M. N., et al.: Calcium and phosphorus metabolism in dialysis patients with and without mitral anular calcium. Analysis of 30 patients. Am. J. Cardiol. 51:497, 1983.
145. Ferman, M. B., Virmani, R., Robertson, R. M., and Stone, W. J.: Mitral annular calcification in chronic renal failure. Chest 85:367, 1984.
146. Depace, N. L., Rohrer, A. H., Kotler, M. N., et al.: Rapidly progressing, massive mitral annular calcification. Arch. Intern. Med. 141:1663, 1981.
147. Maher, E. R., Yound, G., Smyth-Walsh, B., et al.: Aortic and mitral valve calcification in patients with end-stage renal disease. Lancet 2:875, 1987.
148. Osterberger, L. E., Goldstein, S., Khaja, F., and Lakier, J. B.: Functional mitral stenosis in patients with massive mitral annular calcification. Circulation 64:472, 1981.
149. Rosen, H., Friedman, S. A., Raizner, A. E., and Gerstmann, K.: Azotemic arteriopathy. Am. Heart J. 84:250, 1972.
150. Ejerblad, S., Ericsson, J.L.E., and Eriksson, I.: Arterial lesions of the radial artery in uraemic patients. Acta Chir. Scand. 145:415, 1979.
151. Verberckmoes, R., Bouillon, R., and Krempien, B.: Disappearance of vascular calcifications during treatment of renal osteodystrophy. Ann. Intern. Med. 82:529, 1975.
152. Landsberg, K. F., and Landsberg, D. N.: Vitamin D preparations and their role in renal osteodystrophy. Can. J. Hosp. Pharm. 38:10, 1985.
153. Slatapolsky, E., Weerts, C., Thielan, K., et al.: Marked suppression of secondary hyperparathyroidism by intravenous administration of 1,25-dihydroxycholecalciferal in uremic patients. J. Clin. Invest. 74:2136, 1984.
154. Wacker, W., and Merrill, J. P.: Uremic pericarditis in acute and chronic renal failure. JAMA 156:764, 1954.
155. Frommer, J. P., Young, J. P., and Ayus, J. C.: Asymptomatic pericardial effusion in uremic patients: Effect of long-term dialysis. Nephron 39:296, 1985.